Harrison's

Principles of Internal Medicine

EDITORS OF PREVIOUS EDITIONS

T. R. Harrison, Editor-in-Chief, Editions 1, 2, 3, 4, 5

W. R. Resnik, Editor, Editions 1, 2, 3, 4, 5

M. W. Wintrobe, Editor, Editions 1, 2, 3, 4, 5
Editor-in Chief, Edition 6

G. W. Thorn, Editor, Editions 1, 2, 3, 4, 5, 6

R. D. Adams, Editor, Editions 2, 3, 4, 5, 6

P. B. Beeson, Editor, Editions 1, 2

I. L. Bennett, Jr., Editor, Editions 3, 4, 5, 6

E. Braunwald, Editor, Edition 6

K. J. Isselbacher, Editor, Edition 6

R. G. Petersdorf, Editor, Edition 6

Harrison's

Principles of Internal Medicine

Seventh Edition

EDITORS

MAXWELL M. WINTROBE *B.A., M.D., B.Sc. (Med.), Ph.D., D.Sc. (Hon., Manit.), D.Sc. (Hon. Utah), M.A.C.P., Distinguished Professor of Internal Medicine, University of Utah College of Medicine, Salt Lake City.*

GEORGE W. THORN *M.D., M.A. (Hon.), LL.D. (Hon.), D.SC. (Hon.), M.D. (Hon.), F.R.C.P. Hersey Professor of the Theory and Practice of Physic, Emeritus, Harvard Medical School; Samuel A. Levine Professor of Medicine, Emeritus, Harvard Medical School; Physician-in-Chief, Emeritus, Peter Bent Brigham Hospital, Boston.*

RAYMOND D. ADAMS *B.A., M.A., M.D., M.A. (Hon.), D.Sc. (Hon.), M.D. (Hon.) Bullard Professor of Neuropathology, Harvard Medical School; Chief of Neurology Service and Neuropathologist, Massachusetts General Hospital, Boston.*

EUGENE BRAUNWALD *A.B., M.D., M.A. (Hon.) Hersey Professor of the Theory and Practice of Physic (Medicine), Harvard Medical School; Physician-in-Chief, Peter Bent Brigham Hospital, Boston.*

KURT J. ISSELBACHER *A.B., M.D. Mallinckrodt Professor of Medicine, Harvard Medical School; Physician and Chief, Gastrointestinal Unit, Massachusetts General Hospital, Boston.*

ROBERT G. PETERSDORF *A.B., M.D. Professor and Chairman, Department of Medicine, University of Washington School of Medicine; Physician-in-Chief, University of Washington Hospital, Seattle.*

McGraw-Hill Book Company *New York St. Louis San Francisco Düsseldorf Johannesburg Kuala Lumpur London Mexico Montreal New Delhi Panama Paris São Paulo Singapore Sydney Tokyo Toronto*

A BLAKISTON PUBLICATION

Library of Congress Cataloging in Publication Data
Harrison, Tinsley Randolph, date ed.
Harrison's principles of internal medicine.
"A Blakiston publication."
Includes bibliographies.
1. Internal medicine. I. Wintrobe, Maxwell Myer, date ed. II. Title. [DNLM: 1. Internal medicine. WB100 H322p 1974a]
[RC46.H32 1974b] 616'.026 73-18223 (2 vol. ed.)
ISBN 0-07-071134-8 (2 vol. edition) 73-18001
ISBN 0-07-071133-X

Harrison's

Principles of Internal Medicine

1 2 3 4 5 6 7 8 9 0 D O D O 7 9 8 7 6 5 4

Foreign Editions
FRENCH (Sixth Edition)—Flammarion, © 1972
ITALIAN (Seventh Edition)—Casa Editrice Dr. Francesco Vallardi, © 1974
POLISH (Fifth Edition)—Panstwowy Zakland Wydawnictw Lekarskich, © 1971
PORTUGUESE (Sixth Edition)—Editora Guanabara Koogan, S.A., © 1974
SPANISH (Sixth Edition)—La Prensa Medica Mexicana, © 1973
TURKISH (Sixth Edition)—Mentes, © 1974 (est.)
JAPANESE (Sixth Edition)—Hirokawa, © 1972

This book was set in Times Roman by Black Dot, Inc.
The editors were Joseph J. Brehm and Stuart D. Boynton;
the designer was Barbara Ellwood; and the production supervisor was Sally Ellyson.
The drawings were done by John Cordes, J & R Technical Services, Inc.
R. R. Donnelley & Sons Company was printer and binder.

To all those who have taught us,
and especially to our younger colleagues
who continue to teach and inspire us

NOTICE

Medicine is an ever-changing science. As new research and clinical experience broaden our knowledge, changes in treatment and drug therapy are required. The editors and the publisher of this work have made every effort to ensure that the drug dosage schedules herein are accurate and in accord with the standards accepted at the time of publication. The reader is advised, however, to check the product information sheet included in the package of each drug he plans to administer to be certain that changes have not been made in the recommended dose or in the contraindications for administration. This recommendation is of particular importance in regard to new or infrequently used drugs.

Contents

PART SIX DISORDERS DUE TO CHEMICAL AND PHYSICAL AGENTS

Section 1 Chemical intoxications

Section 2 Disorders caused by venoms, bites, and stings

Section 3 Physical agents

PART SEVEN DISORDERS CAUSED BY BIOLOGIC AGENTS

Section 1 Basic considerations

Section 2 Infections of specific tissues and anatomic sites

Section 3 Diseases caused by gram-positive cocci

Section 4 Diseases caused by gram-negative cocci

Section 5 Diseases caused by enteric gram-negative bacilli

Section 6 Diseases caused by other gram-negative bacilli

Section 4 Disorders of the kidneys and urinary tract

Section 5 Disorders of the alimentary tract

Section 6 Disorders of the hepatobiliary system

Section 11 Psychiatric disorders

Section 12 Diseases of striated muscle

Section 13 Disorders of bone and bone mineral metabolism

Section 14 Disorders of the joints and connective tissues

Section 15 Genetic disorders of supporting tissues

Section 16 Skin cancer and cutaneous manifestations of malignancy

List of contributors

AMERICO ABBRUZZESE, M.D.
Assistant Professor of Medicine, Harvard Medical School; Associate in Medicine, Peter Bent Brigham Hospital, Boston.

RAYMOND D. ADAMS, B.A., M.A., M.D., M.A. (HON.), D.Sc. (HON.), M.D. (HON.)
Bullard Professor of Neuropathology, Harvard Medical School; Chief of Neurology Service and Neuropathologist, Massachusetts General Hospital, Boston.

DAVID H. ALPERS, M.D.
Professor of Medicine, Washington University School of Medicine; Associate Physician, Barnes Hospital, St. Louis.

ELLIOT ALPERT, M.D.
Assistant Professor of Medicine, Harvard Medical School; Assistant in Medicine, Massachusetts General Hospital, Boston.

ARTHUR K. ASBURY, M.D.
Professor and Vice Chairman, Department of Neurology, School of Medicine, University of California, San Francisco; Chief of Neurological Service, San Francisco Veterans Administration Hospital.

KARL-ERIK ASTROM, M.D.
Associate Professor of Neuropathology, Harvard Medical School; Associate Neuropathologist, Massachusetts General Hospital, Boston.

K. FRANK AUSTEN, M.D.
Theodore Bevier Bayles Professor of Medicine, Harvard Medical School; Physician-in-Chief, Robert B. Brigham Hospital, Boston.

ROBERT AUSTRIAN, M.D.
John Herr Musser Professor of Research Medicine, University of Pennsylvania School of Medicine, Philadelphia.

ROSS J. BALDESSARINI, M.D.
Associate Professor of Psychiatry, Harvard Medical School; Associate Psychiatrist and Chief, Neuropharmacology Laboratory, Massachusetts General Hospital, Boston.

HARRY N. BEATY, M.D.
Associate Professor of Medicine, University of Washington School of Medicine; Medical Director, Providence Hospital, Seattle.

ALBERT R. BEHNKE, B.A., M.D., M.S. (Hon.)
Consultant, Clinical Investigation Center, U.S. Naval Hospital, Oakland, California.

IVAN L. BENNETT, JR., M.D.
Vice President for Health Affairs for New York University; Provost of New York University Medical Center; Dean, New York University School of Medicine, New York.

THOMAS C. BITHELL, M.D.
Associate Professor of Internal Medicine and Clinical Pathology, University of Virginia, Charlottesville.

GERALD P. BODEY, M.D.
Associate Internist and Associate Professor of Medicine, The University of Texas M.D. Anderson Hospital and Tumor Institute at Houston, Houston.

DANE R. BOGGS, M.D.
Professor of Medicine; Chief, Hematology Section, Department of Medicine, University of Pittsburgh, Pittsburgh.

STUART BONDURANT, M.D.
Professor and Chairman, Department of Medicine, Albany Medical College; Physician-in-Chief, Albany Medical Center, Albany, New York.

AREND BOUHUYS, M.D.
Professor of Medicine and Epidemiology; Director, Yale University Lung Research Center, Yale University School of Medicine, New Haven.

ABRAHAM I. BRAUDE, M.D.
Professor of Medicine; Head, Division of Infectious Diseases, University of California at San Diego School of Medicine, La Jolla.

EUGENE BRAUNWALD, A.B., M.D., M.A. (Hon.)
Hersey Professor of the Theory and Practice of Physic (Medicine), Harvard Medical School; Physician-in-Chief, Peter Bent Brigham Hospital, Boston.

STANLEY A. BRILLER, M.D.
Associate Professor of Medicine, Department of Medicine, School of Medicine, University of Pennsylvania; Director of Electrocardiology, Hospital of the University of Pennsylvania, Philadelphia.

ROGER BULGER, M.D.
Executive Officer, Institute of Medicine, National Academy of Sciences, Washington, D.C.

GEORGE F. CAHILL, JR., M.D., M.A. (Hon.)
Professor of Medicine, Harvard Medical School; Director, Elliott P. Joslin Research Laboratories; Physician, Peter Bent Brigham Hospital, Boston.

JACQUES R. CALDWELL, M.D.
Assistant Professor of Medicine, Division of Infectious Diseases, Department of Medicine, University of Florida, Gainesville.

EVAN CALKINS, A.B., M.D.
Professor and Chairman, Department of Medicine, School of Medicine, State University of New York, Buffalo; Head, Department of Medicine, Edward J. Meyer Memorial Hospital, Buffalo.

E. J. MORAN CAMPBELL, M.D., Ph.D., F.R.C.P.(L), F.R.C.P.(C)
The R. Samuel McLaughlin Professor and Chairman, Department of Medicine, McMaster University, Hamilton, Ontario.

CHARLES B. CARPENTER, M.D.
Associate Professor of Medicine, Harvard Medical School; Senior Associate in Medicine, Peter Bent Brigham Hospital, Boston.

CHARLES C. J. CARPENTER, M.D.
Professor and Chairman, Department of Medicine, Case-Western Reserve School of Medicine; Physician-in-Chief, University Hospitals, Cleveland.

GEORGE E. CARTWRIGHT, B.A., M.D.
Professor and Chairman, Department of Medicine, University of Utah College of Medicine, Salt Lake City; Chief of Medicine, University Hospital, Salt Lake City, Utah.

LEIGHTON E. CLUFF, M.D.
Professor and Chairman, Department of Medicine, University of Florida, Gainesville.

JOHN F. CRIGLER, JR., M.D.
Associate Professor of Pediatrics at The Children's Hospital, Harvard Medical School; Chief, Division of Endocrinology, Department of Medicine, The Children's Hospital Medical Center, Boston.

EUGENE P. CRONKITE, M.D., D.SC. (Hon.)
Chairman, Medical Department, Brookhaven National Laboratory; Professor of Medicine, State University of New York, Stony Brook; President of the Staff and Attending Physician, Hospital of the Medical Research Center, Brookhaven National Laboratory, Upton, New York.

CHANDLER R. DAWSON, M.D.
Associate Professor in Residence, F.I. Proctor Foundation, University of California Medical Center; Director, WHO International Reference Center for Trachoma, San Francisco.

ROBERT DELONG, M.D.
Assistant Professor of Neurology at Massachusetts General Hospital, Harvard Medical School; Assistant Neurologist, Massachusetts General Hospital, Boston.

JAMES J. DINEEN, M.D.
Instructor in Medicine, Harvard Medical School; Assistant Physician, Massachusetts General Hospital, Boston.

JOSEPH F. DINGMAN, M.D.
Lecturer in Medicine, Harvard Medical School; Senior Associate in Medicine, Peter Bent Brigham Hospital, Boston.

FRANK J. DIXON, M.D.
Professor and Chairman, Department of Experimental Pathology, Scripps Clinic and Research Foundation, La Jolla.

ROBERT G. DLUHY, M.D.
Assistant Professor of Medicine, Harvard Medical School; Senior Associate in Medicine, Peter Bent Brigham Hospital, Boston.

KENDALL EMERSON, JR., M.D.
Clinical Professor of Medicine at the Peter Bent Brigham Hospital, Harvard Medical School; Physician, Peter Bent Brigham Hospital; Physician-in-Chief, Boston Lying-in Hospital, Boston.

KARL ENGELMAN, M.D.
Associate Professor of Medicine and Pharmacology, Chief, Hypertension and Clinical Pharmacology Section; Director, Clinical Research Center, University of Pennsylvania School of Medicine, Philadelphia.

EDWIN ENGLERT, JR., M.D.
Professor of Medicine, University of Utah College of Medicine; Chief, Gastrointestinal Section, Veterans Administration Hospital, Salt Lake City.

FRANKLIN H. EPSTEIN, M.D.
Herrman L. Blumgart Professor of Medicine and Director, Thorndike Memorial Laboratory, Harvard Medical School; Physician-in-Chief, Beth Israel Hospital, Boston.

STEFAN S. FAJANS, M.D. B.S.
Professor of Internal Medicine, University of Michigan Medical School, Ann Arbor.

ALVAN R. FEINSTEIN, M.D.
Professor of Medicine and Epidemiology, Yale University School of Medicine; Chief, West Haven Veterans Administration Cooperative Studies Program Support Center, West Haven, Connecticut.

HARRY A. FELDMAN, M.D.
Professor and Chairman, Department of Preventive Medicine, State University of New York Upstate Medical Center, Syracuse.

RICHARD A. FIELD, A.B., M.D.
Associate Clinical Professor of Medicine, Harvard Medical School; Senior Scientist, Retina Foundation, Associate Physician, Beth Israel Hospital, Clinical Associate in Medicine, Massachusetts General Hospital, Boston.

C. MILLER FISHER, M.D.
Professor of Neurology, Harvard Medical School; Neurologist, Massachusetts General Hospital, Boston.

RUSSELL S. FISHER, B.S., M.D.
Professor of Forensic Pathology, University of Maryland Medical School; Lecturer in Forensic Pathology, Johns Hopkins University School of Medicine; Associate in Forensic Pathology, Johns Hopkins University School of Hygiene and Public Health, Baltimore.

ALFRED P. FISHMAN, M.D.
William Maul Measey Professor of Medicine, University of Pennsylvania; Attending Physician, Hospital of the University of Pennsylvania, Philadelphia.

THOMAS B. FITZPATRICK, M.D., Ph.D.
Edward Wigglesworth Professor of Dermatology, and Head, Department of Dermatology, Harvard Medical School; Chief of the Dermatology Service, Massachusetts General Hospital, Boston.

JOHN FOERSTER, M.D.
Assistant Professor, Department of Medicine, The University of Manitoba, Winnipeg.

EDWARD C. FRANKLIN, M.D.
Professor of Medicine and Head, Division of Rheumatology, New York University Medical Center, School of Medicine, New York.

DONALD S. FREDRICKSON, M.D.
Chief, Molecular Disease Branch and Director, Division of

Intramural Research, National Heart and Lung Institute, National Institutes of Health, Bethesda.

LAWRENCE R. FREEDMAN, M.D.
Professor and Chairman, Department of Internal Medicine, University of Lausanne; Chief of Medicine, Hôpital Cantonal Universitaire, Lausanne, Switzerland.

EMIL FREI, III, M.D.
Professor of Medicine, Harvard Medical School; Physician-in-Chief, The Children's Cancer Research Foundation, Boston.

WILLIAM F. FRIEDMAN, M.D.
Professor of Pediatrics and Medicine, School of Medicine, University of California, San Diego; Chief of Pediatric Cardiology, University Hospital, San Diego.

ALVIN E. FRIEDMAN-KIEN, M.D.
Associate Professor of Dermatology and Microbiology, School of Medicine, New York University Medical Center, New York.

HARRY W. FRITTS, JR., M.D.
Professor and Chairman, Department of Medicine, State University of New York, Stony Brook, New York.

J. BERNARD L. GEE, M.D.
Associate Professor of Medicine, Yale University School of Medicine and Attending Physician, Yale-New Haven Hospital, New Haven.

BRUCE C. GILLILAND, M.D.
Associate Professor of Laboratory Medicine and Medicine; Head, Division of Immunology, Department of Laboratory Medicine, University of Washington, Seattle.

GERALD GLICK, A.B., M.D.
Director, Cardiovascular Institute, Department of Medicine, Michael Reese Hospital and Medical Center, Chicago.

ROBERT M. GLICKMAN, M.D.
Assistant Professor of Medicine, Harvard Medical School; Assistant in Medicine, Massachusetts General Hospital, Boston.

STEPHEN E. GOLDFINGER, M.D.
Associate Professor of Medicine, and Associate Dean for Continuing Education, Harvard Medical School; Associate Physician, Massachusetts General Hospital, Boston.

PAUL GOLDHABER, D.D.S., A.M. (Hon.)
Professor of Periodontology; Dean, Harvard School of Dental Medicine, Boston.

J. THOMAS GRAYSTON, M.D.
Vice President for Health Affairs, Health Sciences Center; Professor, Department of Epidemiology and International Health, University of Washington, Seattle.

NORTON J. GREENBERGER, M.D.
Professor and Chairman, Department of Medicine, University of Kansas School of Medicine, Kansas City, Kansas.

JOHN F. GRIFFITH, M.D.
Associate Professor, Department of Pediatrics, Duke University; Chief, Division of Pediatric Neurology, Duke University Hospital, Durham.

THOMAS P. HACKETT, M.D.
Associate Professor of Psychiatry, Harvard Medical School; Chief, Psychiatric Consultation Service, Massachusetts General Hospital, Boston.

JAMES P. HARNISCH, M.D.
Instructor, Department of Medicine, University of Washington, Seattle

DONALD H. HARTER, M.D.
Professor of Neurology, College of Physicians and Surgeons, Columbia University; Associate Attending Neurologist, Columbia–Presbyterian Medical Center, New York.

HARLEY A. HÁYNES, M.D.
Assistant Professor of Dermatology, Harvard Medical School; Chief, Dermatology Clinic, Massachusetts General Hospital, Boston.

ARTHUR HAUT, A.B., M.D.
Professor of Medicine and Head, Section on Hematology, University of Arkansas School of Medicine, Little Rock.

THOMAS R. HENDRIX, M.D.
Professor of Medicine; Chief, Gastroenterology Division, Johns Hopkins University School of Medicine, Baltimore.

ROGER B. HICKLER, M.D.
Professor and Chairman, Department of Medicine, University of Massachusetts Medical School; Chief of Medicine, The Memorial Hospital, Worcester.

PAUL D. HOEPRICH, M.D.
Professor of Medicine and Pathology; Chief, Section of Infectious and Immunologic Diseases, Department of Internal Medicine, School of Medicine, University of California—Davis.

KING K. HOLMES, M.D., PH.D.
Assistant Professor of Medicine, University of Washington School of Medicine; Chief, Division of Infectious Diseases, U.S. Public Health Service Hospital, Seattle.

EDWARD W. HOOK, M.D.
Professor and Chairman, Department of Medicine, University of Virginia School of Medicine; Physician-in-Chief, University of Virginia Hospital, Charlottesville.

SIDNEY H. INGBAR, M.D.
Professor of Medicine, School of Medicine, University of California, San Francisco; Chief, Endocrinology Section, San Francisco Veterans Administration Hospital; Senior Medical Investigator, Veterans Administration Hospital, San Francisco.

KURT J. ISSELBACHER, M.D.
Mallinckrodt Professor of Medicine, Harvard Medical School; Physician and Chief, Gastrointestinal Unit, Massachusetts General Hospital, Boston.

PAUL I. JAGGER, M.D.
Associate Professor of Medicine, School of Medicine, University of California—San Diego

LEONARD W. JARCHO, A.B., M.A., M.D.
Professor and Head, Department of Neurology; Associate Professor of Medicine, University of Utah College of Medicine, Salt Lake City.

MICHEL JÉQUIER, M.D.
Professor de Neurologie, Faculté de Medecine, Université de Lausanne, Lausanne.

CAROL J. JOHNS, M.D.
Associate Professor of Medicine, Director Medical Clinics, The Johns Hopkins Medical Institutions, Baltimore.

JOSEPH E. JOHNSON, III, M.D.
Professor and Chairman, Department of Medicine, Bowman-Gray School of Medicine, Winston-Salem, North Carolina.

NORMAN L. JONES, M.D. F.R.C.P., C.R.C.P. (C)
Associate Professor of Medicine and Coordinator, Regional Respiratory Program, McMaster University Medical Centre, Hamilton, Ontario.

RICHARD L. KAHLER, M.D.
Head, Division of Cardiopulmonary Diseases, Scripps Clinic and Research Foundation, La Jolla; Adjunct Associate Professor of Medicine, University of California, San Diego, School of Medicine.

BYRON A. KAKULAS, M.D.
Professor of Neuropathology, University of Western Australia, Perth; Senior Neuropathologist, Royal Perth Hospital.

MARTIN J. KELLY, M.D.
Assistant Professor of Psychiatry at the Peter Bent Brigham Hospital, Harvard Medical School; Senior Associate in Medicine, Peter Bent Brigham Hospital, Boston.

WILLIAM M. M. KIRBY, M.D.
Professor of Medicine, Department of Medicine, University of Washington, School of Medicine, and Head, Division of Infectious Disease, University of Washington Hospital, Seattle.

VERNON KNIGHT, M.D.
Professor and Chairman, Department of Microbiology, Professor of Medicine, Baylor College of Medicine; Senior Attending Physician, The Methodist Hospital, Houston.

JAN KOCH-WESER, M.D.
Associate Professor of Pharmacology, Harvard Medical School; Associate Physician and Chief, Hypertension and Clinical Pharmacology Unit, Massachusetts General Hospital, Boston.

M. GLEN KOENIG, M.D. (Deceased)
Formerly Professor of Medicine, Vanderbilt University School of Medicine, Nashville.

RAYMOND S. KOFF, M.D.
Assistant Professor of Medicine, Boston University School of Medicine; Chief, Hepatology Section, Veterans Administration Hospital, Boston.

STEPHEN M. KRANE, M.D., A.M. (Hon.), A.B.
Professor of Medicine, Harvard Medical School; Physician and Chief, Arthritis Unit, Massachusetts General Hospital, Boston.

J. THOMAS LA MONT, M.D.
Instructor in Medicine, Harvard Medical School; Assistant in Medicine, Massachusetts General Hospital, Boston.

G. RICHARD LEE, M.D.
Professor of Medicine, Department of Medicine, University of Utah College of Medicine, Salt Lake City.

A. MARTIN LERNER, M.D.
Professor of Medicine and Head, Division of Infectious Diseases, Department of Medicine, Wayne State University School of Medicine; Chief, Hutzel Hospital Medical Unit, Detroit.

BERNARD LOWN, M.D.
Associate Professor in Medicine, Harvard School of Public Health and Physician and Director, S. A. Levine Cardiac Center, Peter Bent Brigham Hospital, Boston.

BERNARD LYTTON, M.B., F.R.C.S.
Professor of Urology, Chief of Urology, Yale-New Haven Medical Center, New Haven.

GEORGE V. MANN, Sc. D., M.D.
Associate Professor, Biochemistry and Medicine, Vanderbilt University Hospital, Nashville.

MART MANNIK, M.D.
Professor of Medicine and Adjunct Professor of Microbiology, Head Division of Rheumatology, Department of Medicine, University of Washington, Seattle.

JANET W. McARTHUR, M.S., M.D.
Professor of Obstetrics and Gynecology, Harvard Medical School; Associate Physician, Massachusetts General Hospital, Boston.

VICTOR A. McKUSICK, M.D.
Chief, Division of Medical Genetics and Professor, Department of Medicine, Johns Hopkins University School of Medicine; Physician-in-Chief, Johns Hopkins Hospital, Baltimore.

ALBERT I. MENDELOFF, M.D.
Professor of Medicine, Johns Hopkins University School of Medicine; Physician-in-Chief, Sinai Hospital, Baltimore.

JOHN P. MERRILL, M.D., D.Sci. (Hon.)
Professor of Medicine, Harvard Medical School; Director, Cardiorenal Section, Peter Bent Brigham Hospital, Boston.

JAY P. MOHR, M.D.
Assistant Professor of Neurology at Massachusetts General Hospital, Harvard Medical School; Assistant Neurologist, Massachusetts General Hospital, Boston.

HUGO MOSER, M.D.
Professor of Neurology at Massachusetts General Hospital, Harvard Medical School; Neurologist, Massachusetts General Hospital, Boston.

KENNETH M. MOSER, M.D.
Professor of Medicine and Director, Pulmonary Division, Department of Medicine, School of Medicine, University of California, San Diego.

JOHN F. MURRAY, M.D.
Professor of Medicine, School of Medicine, University of California, San Francisco.

DON H. NELSON, M.D.
Professor of Medicine, University of Utah College of Medicine; Chief of Medicine, Latter-day Saints Hospital, Salt Lake City.

JAMES C. NIEDERMAN, M.D.
Associate Clinical Professor of Epidemiology and Medicine, Yale University School of Medicine, New Haven.

PHILIP S. NORMAN, M.D.
Associate Professor of Medicine, Department of Medicine; Chief, Clinical Immunology Division, The Johns Hopkins University School of Medicine, Baltimore.

JOHN A. OATES, M.D., B.S.
Professor of Medicine and Pharmacology, Attending Physician, Vanderbilt University Hospital, Nashville, Tennessee.

ROBERT A. O'ROURKE, M.D.
Associate Professor of Medicine, Director, Clinical Cardiology Section, School of Medicine, University of California, San Diego.

JACK H. PETAJAN, M.D., PH.D.
Professor of Neurology, University of Utah College of Medicine, Salt Lake City.

ROBERT G. PETERSDORF, A.B., M.D.
Professor and Chairman, Department of Medicine, University of Washington School of Medicine; Physician-in-Chief, University of Washington Hospital, Seattle.

JAMES J. PLORDE, M.D.
Associate Professor of Medicine, University of Washington School of Medicine, Seattle.

PETER E. POOL, M.D., F.A.C.C.
Associate Clinical Professor of Medicine, Cardiovascular Division, University of California, San Diego, School of Medicine, La Jolla; Director of Cardiology, Encinitas Hospital, Encinitas, California.

DAVID C. POSKANZER, M.D., M.P.H.
Associate Professor in Neurology, Harvard Medical School; Associate Neurologist, Massachusetts General Hospital, Boston.

JOHN T. POTTS, JR., M.D.
Associate Professor of Medicine, Harvard Medical School; Associate Physician, Massachusetts General Hospital, Boston.

CHARLES H. RAMMELKAMP, JR., M.D., D. Sc. (Hon.)
Professor of Medicine and Preventive Medicine, Case–Western Reserve University School of Medicine; Director, Department of Medicine, Cleveland Metropolitan General Hospital, Cleveland.

JEAN J. REBEIZ, M.D.
Assistant Professor of Neurology and Neuropathology, American University of Beirut; Active member of the American Association of Neuropathologists.

PETER REICH, M.D.
Associate Professor of Psychiatry at the Peter Bent Brigham Hospital, Harvard Medical School; Physician, Peter Bent Brigham Hospital, Boston.

WILLIAM H. RESNIK, M.D.
Clinical Professor of Medicine Emeritus, Yale University; Consultant Physician, Yale-New Haven Hospital and Stamford Hospital.

JOHN C. RIBBLE, M.D.
Associate Professor of Pediatrics, New York Hospital–Cornell Medical Center; Associate Attending Pediatrician, New York Hospital, New York.

E. PIERSON RICHARDSON, JR., M.D.
Professor of Neuropathology at Massachusetts General Hospital, Harvard Medical School; Neurologist, Massachusetts General Hospital, Boston.

ELI ROBINS, M.D.
Wallace Renard Professor and Head of the Department of Psychiatry; Psychiatrist-in-Chief, Barnes and Allied Hospitals, St. Louis.

DAVID E. ROGERS, M.D.
President, Robert Wood Johnson Foundation, Princeton, New Jersey.

LESLIE I. ROSE, M.D.
Assistant Professor of Medicine, Harvard Medical School; Associate Director, Endocrine-Metabolic Unit, Peter Bent Brigham Hospital, Boston.

EUGENIA ROSEMBERG, M.D.
Research Director, Medical Research Institute of Worcester, Inc.; Research Professor, University of Massachusetts Medical School, Worcester.

JOHN ROSS, JR., M.D.
Professor of Medicine, Director, Cardiovascular Division, School of Medicine, University of California, San Diego.

RICHARD S. ROSS, M.D.
Professor of Medicine and Clayton Professor of Cardiovascular Disease, Director of Cardiovascular Division, Johns Hopkins University School of Medicine; Physician, Johns Hopkins Hospital, Baltimore.

ROBERT H. RUBIN, M.D.
Clinical and Research Fellow, Infectious Disease Unit, Massachusetts General Hospital, Research Fellow in Medicine, Harvard Medical School, Boston.

DAVID C. SABISTON, JR., M.D.
James B. Duke Professor of Surgery and Chairman of the Department, Duke University Medical Center, Durham, North Carolina.

FUAD SABRA, M.D., F.A.C.P.
Professor of Neurology and Head of Division of Neurology, The Medical School of the American University of Beirut.

MARIA Z. SALAM, M.D.
Assistant Professor of Neurology (Pediatrics) at Massachusetts General Hospital, Harvard Medical School; Research Associate in Neurology, Massachusetts General Hospital, Boston.

HAROLD H. SANDSTEAD, M.D.
Director, USDA Human Nutrition Laboratory; Research Professor of Biochemistry and Medicine, University of North Dakota School of Medicine; Associate Physician, the United Hospital, Grand Forks, North Dakota.

JAY P. SANFORD, M.D.
Professor of Internal Medicine; Head, Division of Infectious Diseases, University of Texas–Southwestern School of Medicine, Dallas.

ARNOLD M. SELIGMAN, M.D.
Professor of Surgery, Johns Hopkins University School of Medicine; Chief, Department of Research Oncology and Cell

Biology, Sinai Hospital, Baltimore; American Cancer Society Research Professor.

WALTER H. SHELDON, M.D.
Professor of Pathology, Johns Hopkins University School of Medicine, Baltimore.

CHARLES C. SHEPARD, M.D.
Chief, Leprosy and Rickettsial Diseases Unit, Virology Section, Center for Disease Control, Health Services and Mental Health Administration, Public Health Service, U.S. Department of Health, Education, and Welfare, Atlanta.

JAY B. SHUMAKER, M.D.
Instructor in Medicine, Tufts University School of Medicine; Chief of Gastroenterology, Newton–Wellesley Hospital, Newton, Massachusetts.

WILLIAM SILEN, M.D.
Professor of Surgery, Harvard Medical School; Surgeon-in-Chief, Beth Israel Hospital, Boston.

LLOYD H. SMITH, JR., M.D., D. SC. (Hon.)
Professor and Chairman, Department of Medicine, University of California, San Francisco; Chief of the Medical Service, Moffitt Hospital, San Francisco.

PHILIP J. SNODGRASS, M.D.
Professor of Medicine, Indiana University School of Medicine; Chief, Medical Service, Veterans Administration Hospital, Indianapolis.

BURTON E. SOBEL, M.D.
Associate Professor of Medicine, Washington University and Director, Cardiovascular Division, Barnes Hospital, St. Louis, Missouri.

J. STUART SOELDNER, B.S., M.D.
Associate Professor of Medicine, Harvard Medical School, and Associate Director, Elliott P. Joslin Research Laboratory, Boston.

EDMUND H. SONNENBLICK, M.D.
Associate Professor of Medicine, Harvard Medical School, Director, Cardiovascular Research, Peter Bent Brigham Hospital, Boston.

WESLEY W. SPINK, M.D., D. Sc. (Hon.)
Professor of Medicine, Emeritus, University of Minnesota Medical School, Minneapolis.

WILLIAM W. STEAD, M.D.
Professor of Medicine, University of Arkansas School of Medicine; Chief, Pulmonary Disease Service, Veterans Administration Hospital, Little Rock.

JURGEN STEINKE, M.D. (Deceased)
Formerly Chief of Endocrinology and Metabolism, Rancho Los Amigos Hospital; Associate Professor of Medicine, School of Medicine, University of Southern California, Los Angeles.

D. EUGENE STRANDNESS, JR., M.D.
Professor of Surgery, Department of Surgery, University of Washington School of Medicine, Seattle.

MELVIN L. TAYMOR, M.D.
Associate Professor of Gynecology, Harvard Medical School; Surgeon (Gynecology), Peter Bent Brigham Hospital; Assistant Obstetrician-Gynecologist, Boston Hospital for Women, Boston.

HENRY M. THOMAS, III, M.D.
Assistant Professor of Medicine, College of Physicians & Surgeons, Columbia University; Assistant Attending Physician, Columbia–Presbyterian Hospital, New York.

GEORGE W. THORN, M.D., M.A. (Hon.), LL.D. (Hon.), D.SC. (Hon.), M.D. (Hon.), F.R.C.P.
Hersey Professor of the Theory and Practice of Physic, Emeritus, Harvard Medical School; Samuel A. Levine Professor of Medicine, Emeritus, Harvard Medical School; Physician-in-Chief, Emeritus, Peter Bent Brigham Hospital, Boston.

WILLIAM A. TISDALE, M.D.
Professor and Chairman, Department of Medicine, University of Vermont College of Medicine; Chief of Medical Service, Medical Center Hospital of Vermont, Burlington.

GENNARO M. TISI, M.D.
Associate Professor of Medicine, School of Medicine, University of California, San Diego.

MARVIN TURCK, M.D.
Professor of Medicine, University of Washington School of Medicine; Chief of Medicine, Harborview Medical Center, Seattle.

FRANK H. TYLER, M.D.
Acting Dean, University of Utah College of Medicine, Salt Lake City.

HENRI VANDER EECKEN, H.M., M.D.
Professor of Neurology, Faculty of Medicine, University of Ghent; Head of the Department of Neurology, Akademisch Ziekenhuis, Ghent.

THEODORE B. VAN ITALLIE, M.D.
Professor of Medicine, College of Physicians & Surgeons, Columbia University; Director of Medicine, St. Luke's Hospital Center, New York.

MAURICE VICTOR, M.D.
Professor of Neurology, Case–Western Reserve University, School of Medicine; Director, Neurology Service, Cleveland Metropolitan General Hospital, Cleveland.

JOSEPH W. WALIKE, M.D.
Clinical Associate Professor of Otolaryngology, University of Washington School of Medicine, Seattle.

JAMES F. WALLACE, M.D.
Associate Professor of Medicine, Department of Medicine, University of Washington School of Medicine, Seattle.

HENRY deF. WEBSTER, M.D.
Head, Section on Cellular Neuropathology, National Institute of Neurological Disease and Stroke, National Institutes of Health, Bethesda.

LOUIS WEINSTEIN, M.S., PH.D., M.D.
Professor of Medicine, Tufts University School of Medicine; Chief, Infectious Disease Service, New England Medical Center Hospital, Boston.

LOUIS G. WELT, A.B., M.D.
Professor of Medicine and Chairman, Department of Internal

Medicine, Yale University School of Medicine; Chief, Medical Service, Yale-New Haven Hospital, New Haven.

JOHN B. WEST, M.D., PH.D.
Professor of Medicine, School of Medicine, University of California, San Diego; Physician, University of San Diego, San Diego.

GORDON H. WILLIAMS, M.D.
Associate Professor of Medicine, Harvard Medical School; Director, Endocrine-Metabolic Unit, Peter Bent Brigham Hospital, Boston.

MAXWELL M. WINTROBE, B.A., M.D., B.Sc. (Med.), PH.D., D.Sc. (Hon., Manit.), D.Sc. (Hon. Utah), M.A.C.P.
Distinguished Professor of Internal Medicine, University of Utah College of Medicine, Salt Lake City.

KENNETH A. WOEBER, M.D.
Professor of Medicine and Chief, Division of Endocrinology, University of Texas Health Science Center, San Antonio.

SHELDON M. WOLFF, M.D.
Clinical Director, National Institute of Allergy and Infectious Diseases; Chief, Laboratory of Clinical Investigation, National Institute of Allergy and Infectious Diseases, National Institutes of Health, Bethesda.

THEODORE E. WOODWARD, M.D.
Professor of Medicine and Head, Department of Medicine, University of Maryland School of Medicine, Baltimore.

RICHARD J. WURTMAN, M.D.
Professor of Endocrinology and Metabolism, Department of Nutrition and Food Science, Massachusetts Institute of Technology; Clinical Assistant in Medicine, Massachusetts General Hospital; Lecturer in Medicine, Harvard Medical School, Boston.

JAMES B. WYNGAARDEN, M.D., F.A.C.P.
Frederic M. Hanes Professor and Chairman, Department of Medicine, Duke University School of Medicine; Chief of Medical Services, Duke University Medical Center, Durham, North Carolina.

ROBERT R. YOUNG, M.D.
Associate Professor of Neurology, Harvard Medical School; Associate Neurologist and Chief, Clinical Neurophysiology, Massachusetts General Hospital, Boston.

Preface

It often is asked why prefaces are written and whether they are ever read. In his famous preface to *Cromwell*, Victor Hugo pointed out that one seldom inspects the cellar of a house after visiting its salons nor examines the roots of a tree after eating its fruit. Admittedly, the readers of this book will judge it by the substance of its contents and its style, not by the pretexts offered by its editors. It could be added that if the guest has returned several times, then surely he knows that the cellar is well stocked. Why then a preface to a seventh edition?

This preface is intended to indicate the ways in which the present edition maintains or diverges from, as the case may be, the original objectives of this book. By doing this, it will be possible to present the objectives of this textbook of medicine to readers unfamiliar with earlier editions.

When the first group of editors met together almost thirty years ago, they decided to write a textbook of medicine which would conform to the *clinical method* which they had found most useful both as students and as teachers. It was thought that such a book should recapitulate the steps in the process of thinking by which a physician reaches a diagnosis, these being the recording of the patient's symptoms and signs, the consideration of the various disorders that can give rise to them, and the effective utilization of measures which will support and confirm or alter the first impressions and lead ultimately to a firm diagnosis.

The logical first step consistent with this clinical approach is the consideration of the cardinal manifestations of disease. Patients present themselves with symptoms, not diagnoses. Consequently it is basic to good clinical medicine to appreciate the different causes of various manifestations of disease and to understand how they may be produced. This requires an understanding of physiology and of the ways in which deviations from the normal lead to disorders of one kind or another. For this reason material of fundamental biologic importance was incorporated in the first edition of this book and has been regarded as an essential component ever since.

The revolutionary changes in the curricula of many American medical schools, particularly the abbreviation of the standard courses in the sciences basic to clinical medicine and the substitution of shorter "core" courses, has imposed, we believe, additional responsibilities on the modern teacher of clinical medicine and on the modern textbook of medicine. The student who embarks on his clinical training now, although far more sophisticated in many ways than his predecessor of even one generation ago, may not possess as much understanding of the mechanisms of symptoms and disease processes as is required to deal intelligently with clinical problems. This book recognizes the challenge to education posed by such curricula. Clinical biochemistry and pathophysiology form an integral part of this book but, insofar as possible, are considered within the clinical setting.

The interpretation of symptoms usually is most effectively achieved by proceeding from the general to the particular. Symptoms often can be grouped as syndromes. Syndromes are the consequence of a variety of etiologic factors or disease mechanisms and, if these can be recognized and understood, measures to restore the normal physiologic state can be designed and carried out in a logical, systematic fashion. Furthermore, the method of approaching a diagnosis which is based on an analysis of the symptoms, recognition of the syndrome, and consideration of the various disease mechanisms which may have produced it, ensures consideration of the many possible interpretations of the clinical picture which the patient presents. By pursuing such an approach, it is less likely that a disorder which should be considered will be overlooked. The problem-oriented record, which is discussed in a special chapter in this edition (Chap. 4) facilitates such a logical approach to the consideration of the patient's complaints.

The plan of this book is consistent with this approach. Following a discussion of the editors' general philosophy regarding the approach to the patient (Part One), the Cardinal Manifestations of Disease are considered (Part Two). The mechanisms whereby various symptoms are produced are discussed and an approach to the recognition of the diseases of which they may be manifestations is outlined. Laboratory findings are discussed in relation to the clinical manifestations. Part Three provides a discussion of the basic concepts involved in our understanding of the inheritance of human disease.

Recognition of the importance of altered immune responses as fundamental mechanisms in the pathogenesis of disease led to the introduction in the sixth edition of this textbook of Part Four, Disorders Due to Hypersensitivity and Altered Immune Response. This very active area of scientific investigation has been expanded and brought up to date in the seventh edition.

The remainder of the book is concerned with more specific disorders and disease entities. In all these sections, the syndromic approach is emphasized insofar as possible. The reader will find at the beginning of most of the sections, either in the Introduction and/or in the first chapter, a discussion of the approach to the patient whose clinical manifestations suggest the type of disease considered in that section.

Treatment is discussed in relation to specific disorders or categories of disease (e.g., Chapter 125, Chemotherapy of Infection; Chapter 235, Principles of Pharmacologic Treatment of Cardiovascular Disorders) and is described in terms which are as specific as practical.

A deliberate attempt has been made to avoid long bibliographies. The references at the end of the chapters are limited, for the most part, to reviews and monographs which contain comprehensive bibliographies, as well as to a few of the most significant recent articles.

With the sixth edition, two of the original editors, Doctors T. H. Harrison and William H. Resnik, retired, and their places were taken by Doctors Eugene Braunwald and Kurt J. Isselbacher. The influence of Doctors Harrison and Resnik is still evident in the seventh edition and can confidently be predicted to outlast the lives of all the present editors. Their role in the planning of this textbook was profound, and the present editors are deeply indebted to them. But time, like the science of medicine, moves on. In this edition Dr. Robert G. Petersdorf replaces Dr. Ivan L. Bennett whose valuable role in previous editions is gratefully acknowledged.

Once again the editors take pleasure in expressing appreciation to our many colleagues who have so generously responded to editorial suggestions. We continue to be indebted to numerous friends and colleagues for valuable criticisms. Among these are: Doctors David Baylink, John Butler, Alexander Fefer, Clement Finch, Joseph Goodner, William Green, Laurence Harker, William Hazzard, Robert Hillman, Victor Lavis, Mart Mannik, Daniel Porte, Peter Simkin, and Paul Strandjord of Seattle, Washington; Leroy Fass of Long Beach, California; Virginia Beamer, Eugene L. Bliss, H. Allan Bloomer, James W. Freston, Burton Janis, Leonard W. Jarcho, Hiroshi Kuida, John G. Moore, Attilio Renzetti, Gerasim Tikoff, T. J. Tsagaris, Frank H. Tyler, and Donald

West of Salt Lake City; Thomas P. Hackett and Peter Reich of Boston; Eliot Slater of London, Eli Robins of St. Louis, David A. Hamburg of Palo Alto, and Paul R. McHugh of Portland, Ore.

Of immeasurable help have been our secretarial coworkers. We are especially indebted to Mrs. Nancy Ehret, Ms. Clo Flahive, Ms. Freda Foster, Mrs. Beatrice A. Fraser, Mrs. Trudy Geissler, Mrs. Mary Jackson, Miss Kathy Nielson, Mrs. Kathy Rees, Mrs. Cynthia Reid, Miss Betty Sanders, Ms. Caryn Sandrew, Mrs. Georgette B. Simchowitz, Mrs. Jana Spellman, and Miss Doris Williams.

Maxwell M. Wintrobe
George W. Thorn
Raymond D. Adams
Eugene Braunwald
Kurt J. Isselbacher
Robert G. Petersdorf

Harrison's

Principles of Internal Medicine

PART ONE | THE PHYSICIAN AND THE PATIENT

1
APPROACH TO THE PATIENT

THE EDITORS

No greater opportunity, responsibility, or obligation is given to an individual than that of serving as a physician. In treating the suffering he needs technical skill, scientific knowledge, and human understanding. He who uses these with courage, with humility, and with wisdom will provide a unique service for his fellowman, and will build an enduring edifice of character within himself. The physician should ask of his destiny no more than this; he should be content with no less.

THE ART OF MEDICINE In the practice of medicine the physician employs a discipline which seeks to utilize scientific methods and principles in the solution of its problems, but it is one in which, in the end, both science and art are wedded. The crucial importance of understanding the scientific base of modern medicine is well known; the significance of the art of medicine is not as well appreciated. Thus, to extract the telltale clue from a maze of confusing symptoms, to determine from a mass of conflicting physical signs and laboratory data the ones that are of crucial significance, to know in a borderline case when to initiate and when to refrain from a line of investigation or treatment involves judgments based on "assimilated" experience. Skill in accomplishing these necessities of medical art is not usually the outcome of laboratory study alone.

Intuition and maturing wisdom are called upon in developing the more personal relations with the patient and the understanding and capacity to peer beyond surface motivations into his behavior. The astute physician will recognize when the casual mention of an apparently trivial complaint is a device for seeking reassurance regarding a feared disorder such as cancer or heart disease. He will at once know when to probe the more intimate aspects of the patient's life, and when to leave them undiscussed; when to express a bright and reassuring prognosis, and when and how to utter doubt and caution.

Medicine is an art also in the sense that the physician can never be content with the sole aim of endeavoring to clarify the laws of nature; he cannot proceed in his labors with the cool detachment of the scientist whose aim is the winning of the truth, and who, in doing so, conducts a "controlled experiment." It is essential that he maintain objectivity in the study and care of his patient, for this is in the patient's interest; nevertheless, he must use wise judgment and must never forget that his primary and traditional objectives are utilitarian—the prevention and cure of disease and the relief of suffering, whether of body or of mind.

THE PATIENT AS A PERSON The same type of illness presents in a variety of ways depending on the age, personality, and social situation of the patient. This is one of the basic principles in psychologic medicine. Relevant here is the progressive change in social relationships, from a state of complete dependence on parent, family, and teacher, who must supply much of the historical details of an illness, to one of relative independence. At the same time, there are variable degrees of maturation which involve the partial suppression of egocentric drives. These trends and their modification during life experience are the basis of personality; and deviations in these natural developments prevent satisfactory social adjustment and result in neuroticism. The latter may be the sole reason for seeking medical help, but more often it complicates other illness.

Another aspect of illness that influences the physician-patient relationship is the real or implied significance of disease in the mind of the patient. Any departure from good health carries a potential threat of physical disintegration or crippling disability, and even the most intelligent and best-informed patient should not be considered immune to forebodings just because he refrains from mentioning them. In fact, most patients are more concerned with the possibility of being rendered dependent by illness than with the disease itself. It is especially important that these fears be borne in mind when dealing with the elderly patient, who is rarely unmindful that "the trap is laid" and death is always near.

The attitude of the patient approaching the doctor must always be tinged, for the most part unconsciously, with distaste and dread; his deepest desire will tend to be comfort and relief rather than cure, and his faith and expectation will be directed towards some magical exhibition of these boons. Do not let yourselves believe that however smoothly concealed by education, by reason, and by confidential frankness these strong elements may be, they are ever in any circumstances altogether absent. (Wilfred Trotter)

Illness also constitutes a threat to the individual's status in his social group. Prolonged invalidism during childhood tends inevitably to leave behind an excessive egocentricity, which may become the basis of a lifelong neurosis. In the adult, illness often enforces a return to a posture of dependency, a change usually accompanied by feelings of apprehension and discouragement, sometimes leading to frank anxiety and depression. This explains a number of common psychologic defenses which the patient exercises against illness. He may refuse medical aid; or, if he summons the courage to consult a physician, he may minimize or even fail to mention the very symptom about which he is most deeply concerned. Then, too, there are persons whose emotional stability has been tenuous and uncertain, so that the position of dependency imposed by illness comes as a welcome relief from adult responsibility. They appear to enjoy illness and to resent anything that menaces their state of invalidism. Lesser degrees of this tendency are to be noted among those who consult the physician at the appearance of every new symptom and who are continuously preoccupied with their past illnesses and operations.

Especially when examining a draped patient in the relatively neutral domain of the hospital ward or even in the private examining room, a patient's emotional life seems relatively unimportant. Organic lesions have a way of compelling attention to themselves, and further, it may be less exhausting to limit one's focus to the sphere of physical disease. More time, energy, and experience frequently are necessary to view the patient as an active participant in an enormous moving pageant which includes the personal eccentricities of his forebears, his own fears and patterns of reaction, the roles of poverty, insecurity, and perhaps poor vocational and domestic relations. Yet every experienced physician knows that to explain many of the manifestations of illness, it is necessary to view the patient comprehensively as an organism with a vast repository of past experiences, many of which are vaguely remembered, yet have become the foundation of his current system of meeting daily problems.

THE PHYSICIAN'S RESPONSIBILITIES The physician seeks to respond to and alleviate the patient's complaints, to search out signs of ill health not yet apparent to the patient or of abnormalities which may lead to ill health, and to maintain the patient in a state of well-being. To achieve these goals requires a broad orientation. Illness is never limited to one system, nor necessarily to a single disease, and whether the physician is a general practitioner, an internist who provides "primary care," or a specialist, the patient must be viewed not as an organ system but as a person.

EXAMINATION OF THE WELL PERSON The intelligent practice of preventive medicine is often considered undramatic; yet few areas of medicine are of greater importance to a single individual or to an entire population. In this aspect of medical practice, the physician and his aides deal with individuals or groups who are not overtly ill or whose complaints may be unrelated to the disease process which he wishes to prevent. The use of the periodic physical examination by large companies, unions, various other groups, and single individuals and the ready availability of multiphasic screening tests allow the physician to detect and to intervene in disease processes earlier in their course, often before the first symptom becomes manifest. Disease now becomes a biologic phenomenon occurring in a population, not merely an illness reported to a physician.

The physician who examines well individuals is not "wasting his training" when he is not constantly dealing with serious organic disease. More skill is required to recognize the early signs of ill health than to deal with what is obvious to the patient or his family. The discovery and cure of potentially serious disease represent a far greater service to one's patient than ministrations in the course of an incurable condition.

The finding of an elevated arterial blood pressure or an elevated blood sugar, serum uric acid, or cholesterol level in an asymptomatic person or the discussion of milder degrees of nervousness or depression provides an unparalleled opportunity to prevent or retard events of serious consequence. It is not always easy to persuade an asymptomatic person to face a situation he has hoped to avoid or to alter his habits or diet in order to follow a therapeutic program throughout the rest of his life. Nevertheless the compensation for these efforts, in terms of a patient's increased longevity and well-being, is so great that it fully justifies the effort and attention of every physician.

CHANGING PATIENT-PHYSICIAN RELATIONSHIPS The one-to-one patient-physician relationship which traditionally has been the goal of all physicians is changing, primarily because of the changing setting in which medicine is increasingly being practiced. In many cases the management of the individual patient requires the active participation of a variety of trained professional personnel—not only physicians and psychiatrists, but also nurses, physicians' assistants, dietitians, biochemists, psychologists, and other paramedical personnel. The patient can benefit greatly from such collaboration, but it is the duty of his physician to guide him through his illness. In order to carry out this increasingly difficult task the physician must have some familiarity with the techniques, skills, and objectives of his colleagues in the fields allied to medicine. He must also be able to interpret their findings not as isolated phenomena but rather in terms of the total clinical picture. In giving his patient an opportunity to receive the full benefits resulting from the important advances of science, the physician must retain responsibility for the crucial decisions concerning diagnosis and treatment.

An increasing number of patients is being cared for by groups of physicians, by clinics, and by hospitals rather than by a single, independent practitioner. There are many potential advantages in the use of such organized medical groups, but there also are hazards, both to the patient and the physician. The identity of the physician who is primarily and continuously responsible for each particular patient must be clearly defined. It is this physician who must have an overview of a patient's illnesses and who must maintain familiarity with his patient's reaction to illness, to drugs, and to the problems of daily living. In addition, since a number of physicians may, at any one time, contribute to the care of a particular patient, and since patients as well as physicians are becoming increasingly mobile, accurate and detailed record keeping assumes progressively greater importance. It is imperative that the physician promptly commit all pertinent data obtained from the clinical and laboratory examinations to his patient's permanent medical record. Only in this way can continuity and high quality in the care of the patient be provided.

THE PHYSICIAN HIMSELF The examining physician is himself a human instrument, subject to reactions arising from events in his own biography. The problem of understanding and responding appropriately to the patient is strongly influenced by this fact. The student receives much expert coaching in the methods of physical and laboratory diagnosis, and it is in these areas that he will most easily develop the skills which permit him to be comfortable with the patient. Mastery of the more intangible psychologic aspects of medicine is not so easily acquired. The young physician may feel himself inadequate in his dealings with the patient, for not only does he experience an inevitable sense of insecurity with respect to the patient's problems, but he may feel equally uneasy about his newly acquired role of authority and responsibility. Moreover, he may find it difficult to control his own reactions: disinterest because the patient presents no fascinating problems of organic disease, irritation at the patient's verbosity or lack of clarity and consistency in reciting his history, or even disappointment because the patient's illness fails to respond to treatment in the expected manner. The same factors can affect even the kindest and most conscientious physician.

To perceive and understand the problems of the patient depends not simply on instruction but on the emotional maturity of the physician and his interest in and concern for other human beings. By sensitive self-cultivation the physician must learn to be at ease and to establish rapport with persons of every walk of life, realizing that everyone is born with manifold potentialities determined by his genes and has a personality and character shaped by the emotional climate in which he grows and develops. The physician must relate as much to the person who is ill as to the illness for which he seeks relief.

The physician has a special function in society and should be skilled as a psychologist in human behavior as well as a biologist in human disease. He brings highly technical knowledge and skills to bear upon the patient's physiologic functioning. He should also bring to the suffering patient a feeling of humaneness, a sense of confidence and security based upon the conviction that all will be done that can be done. Such an atmosphere will develop a wholesome personal relationship. The patient must be made to realize that his unique individuality is recognized and that his life's problems are appreciated. These facts are important to patients with well-defined organic disease as well as to those suffering primarily from psychologic and emotional problems. If one can accept the principle of causality in human behavior, one can, with patience and diligence, learn to fathom some of the patient's motivations even though many of the details often will remain obscure.

To the physician nothing human is strange or repulsive. The misanthrope may become a clever diagnostician of organic disease, but he can scarcely hope to succeed as a physician. The true physician has a Shakespearean breadth of interest in the wise and the foolish, the proud and the humble, the stoic hero and the whining rogue. He cares for people.

2
APPROACH TO DISEASE

THE EDITORS

HISTORY The written history of an illness should embody all the fact of medical significance in the life of the patient up to the time that he consults the physician; but, of course, his most recent diseases attract the most attention, for these, obviously, are the reason that he seeks medical advice. Ideally the narration of symptoms should be in the patient's own words, the principal events being presented in the temporal order in which they occurred. However, few patients possess the necessary powers of observation and talent for lucid, coherent description. Usually the help of the physician is needed. He must guide them by questions but at the same time must avoid influencing them by inserting his own ideas.

Often a symptom which has concerned a patient possesses little significance, whereas a seemingly minor complaint may be of importance. Therefore the mind of the physician must be constantly alert to the possibility that any event related by the patient, any symptom however trivial or apparently remote, may be the key to the solution of the medical problem. As data are gained from the physical and laboratory examinations, the problems which are presented should be clearly identified.

An informative history is more than an orderly listing of symptoms. Something always is gained by listening to the patient and noting the way in which he talks about his symptoms. Inflection of voice, facial expression, and attitude may betray important clues as to the meaning of the symptoms to the patient. Thus, listening to this recitation, one discovers not only something about the disease but also something about the patient.

With experience one learns the pitfalls of history taking. What patients relate for the most part consists of subjective phenomena filtered through minds that vary in their background of past experience. Patients obviously differ widely in their responses to the same stimuli. Their remarks are variably colored by fear of disease, disability, and death, and by concern over the consequences of illness to their families. Additional difficulties are created by language barriers, by failing intellectual powers which deprive the subject of accurate recall, or by a disorder of consciousness that makes him unaware of his illness. It is not surprising, then, that even the most careful physician may at times despair of collecting factual data; and often he is forced to proceed with evidence that represents little more than an approximation of the truth.

Viewed in another way, the symptom marks, in the patient's mind, a departure from normal health; in the physician's mind, it initiates a process of inductive and deductive reasoning that culminates in diagnosis. In pondering the various possible explanations of a given symptom or clinical state the physician begins a search for other data, elicited by further questioning of the patient and his family, by physical examination, or by special laboratory tests. The symptoms alone sometimes will provide the most certain clue, as in angina pectoris or epilepsy, where physical findings and laboratory data collected between attacks may give no evidence of the existence of heart or brain disease even when it is manifestly present. In most illnesses, however, the history will not be so decisive, though it may still narrow the number of diagnostic possibilities and guide the subsequent investigation.

It is in the taking of the history that the physician's skill, knowledge, and experience are most clearly in evidence. He has learned from experience how to weigh each given symptom, depending on its nature and the context in which it occurs. He knows when to be incredulous and turn to more reliable sources of information, but he never lets his skepticism blind him to an unusual symptom, a manifestation of some new condition that has previously been beyond the reach of medical knowledge. Moreover, he knows when to press an interrogation more deeply in a search for further details and when to cast about more broadly, realizing that "disease often tells its secrets in a casual parenthesis." And, finally, he knows how to take advantage of the interview in which the history is gathered to obtain the confidence of his patient and to allay apprehension and fear, the first steps in therapy.

The family history, all too often obtained in a routine, cursory fashion, is a leading tool of clinical genetics and can provide important evidence regarding the nature of the patient's complaints. The use of the family history will be discussed further in Chap. 62, but here it may be pointed out that information regarding symptoms like those of the patient which have occurred in blood relatives, or "run in the family," and knowledge of the ethnic origin of the parents and of consanguinity may be exceedingly helpful. The information must be obtained with tact, however, for patients may be embarrassed by such inquiries. Finally it should be emphasized that the best family history is that which is supported by actual examination of other members of the family. Frequently it is found that some physical deviation from the normal, too subtle to be recognized by a lay person, is quite apparent to the trained observer and that a minor deviation in laboratory data assumes significance when evaluated against a family constellation.

PHYSICAL EXAMINATION Little need be said about the importance of the physical examination, for early in his training the physician learns that physical signs are the objective and verifiable marks of disease. The physical sign represents a solid, indisputable fact. However, its significance is enhanced when it confirms a functional or structural change already evidenced by the patient's history. At other times, the physical sign may stand as the only evidence of disease, especially in those instances in which the history has been inconsistent and confused or is completely lacking.

If full advantage is to be derived from the physical examination, it must be performed methodically and thoroughly. Although attention has usually been directed by the history to the offending organ or part of the body, the examination must extend to all parts of the body. The patient literally must be scrutinized from top to bottom in an objective search for abnormalities that may yield information concerning present and possible future illnesses. Unless the examination procedure is systematic, important parts of it may be forgotten, an error against which even the most skilled clinician must guard. The results of the examination, like the details of the history, should be recorded at the time they are elicited, not hours later when they are subject to the distortions of memory. Many inaccuracies stem from the careless practice of writing or dictating notes long after the examination has terminated. As problems are presented they should be identified.

Skill in physical diagnosis is acquired with experience, but it is not merely technique that determines success in eliciting signs. The detection of a few scattered petechiae or a faint diastolic murmur or a small mass in the abdomen is not a question of keener eyes and ears or more sensitive fingers, but of a mind directed to be alert to these findings. Skill in physical diagnosis reflects a way of thinking more than a way of doing.

All investigations of the body should be regarded as part of the physical examination. The use of various instruments, such as the ophthalmoscope, sphygmomanometer, galvanometer, microscope, or roentgen tube, are mere extensions of the examination to less accessible structures. Proficiency in their use is part of internal medicine.

LABORATORY EXAMINATIONS The marked increase in the number and availability of laboratory diagnostic procedures has inevitably augmented reliance on the knowledge gained from these special means of study in the solution of clinical problems. It is essential that one bear in mind the limitations of such procedures, which by virtue of their impersonal quality and the complexity of the technique involved often gain an aura of authority regardless of the fallibility of the persons carrying out the technical procedures or interpreting the data. One must not be misled by the "magic of numbers!"

Accumulation of laboratory data cannot release the physician from the necessity of careful observation and study of his patient. The wise physician understands the merits and limitations of each source of information, whether it be history, physical examination, or laboratory investigation. The physician also must weigh carefully the hazards and the expense involved in every laboratory procedure.

It is not unusual for a specific disease process to present initially with nonspecific symptoms; an example is the generalized weakness and increased fatigability associated with hypercalcemia. In such situations the classical approach to diagnosis and treatment does not always suggest the appropriate laboratory tests, and the underlying disorder may remain undetected for a long period. It is in this setting that a selected group of biochemical screening tests may provide an early clue to the correct diagnosis and exclude a number of other possibilities. With present-day instrumentation, it is possible to determine on a single specimen of blood the concentration of sodium, potassium, calcium, magnesium, chloride, inorganic phosphate, and carbon dioxide–combining power.

The ability to compare values for several electrolytes is especially useful. For example, an elevated serum sodium value with a corresponding increase in serum chloride and potassium suggests the presence of dehydration, whereas an elevated serum sodium value with low serum chloride and potassium levels suggests a hypochloremic, hypokalemic alkalosis such as occurs in primary hyperaldosteronism (Conn's syndrome). Low serum sodium and chloride levels with a normal blood urea nitrogen level suggest excessive hydration (e.g., inappropriate antidiuretic hormone syndrome). Low serum sodium, chloride, and potassium levels with *elevated serum uric acid* level suggest excessive diuretic therapy, whereas low serum sodium and chloride levels with *elevated* potassium and blood urea levels suggest renal salt-losing syndrome or adrenal insufficiency. An elevation of serum calcium level in the presence of low serum inorganic phosphorus level suggests primary hyperparathyroidism, whereas elevated serum calcium with normal serum phosphorus levels is consistent with metastatic tumor, multiple myeloma, or sarcoid. Tetany or convulsive seizures require determination of blood sugar, serum calcium, and magnesium levels and carbon dioxide–combining power for differential diagnosis.

Release of certain enzymes into the circulation follows injury of any type. In mild or early organic disease, elevated blood enzyme levels may be the sole indicators of underlying disease. The extent to which blood enzyme levels reflect the pathologic process depends upon the nature and degree of tissue injury and the capacity of cells to produce the enzyme examined. For example, a large increase in plasma alkaline phosphatase level may be observed in the presence of relatively mild intrahepatic cholestasis (chlorpromazine, methyltestosterone), whereas the late stage of acute yellow atrophy with widespread total destruction of hepatic parenchymal cells may be accompanied by relatively low levels of alkaline phosphatase, lactic dehydrogenase, and serum glutamic oxalacetic transaminase, the enzymes having already been poured into the body fluids prior to the time the examinations were made.

The thoughtful use of screening tests is not to be confused with indiscriminate laboratory testing; it is based on the fact that a group of laboratory determinations which are known to be frequent harbingers of disease can now be carried out on a single specimen of blood at relatively low cost. The biochemical measurements discussed above, together with simple laboratory examinations such as blood count, urinalysis, and sedimentation rate, often provide the clue to the presence of a pathologic process. This is particularly helpful in identifying organic disease in a patient with evident psychologic or emotional problems.

Discrimination in the ordering of laboratory procedures and judgment in appraising their risk and expense as against the value of the information to be derived from them are important indicators of the effectiveness with which the art and science of medicine have been fused by the individual physician.

THE COMPUTER IN MEDICINE Very properly, there is an increasing interest among those responsible for the nation's health in identifying occult disease and in preventing ill health. The shortage of physicians compels the recruitment of assistance from "paramedical personnel" and the full exploitation of the potential contributions of improved technology. Though the basis of good medical practice is, and undoubtedly always will be, a careful history and physical examination, the searching out of disease in a community need no longer depend on these measures alone. The automation of quantitative biochemical determinations and the "read-out" potential of computerized data will permit broad-scale screening of large segments of our population.

There are some who hold that computer science will facilitate and, in some cases, largely supplement the intellectual functions of the physician. No doubt such a development will, if successful, prove beneficial. The study of patients may be made more comprehensive and more precise. Advantage must be taken of such opportunities. But reliance on the computer will inevitably create psychologic, organizational, legal, economic, and technical problems. It should not and, in fact, cannot replace the interpersonal relationship between physician and patient which is the essence of effective medical care.

THE CLINICAL METHOD AND THE SYNDROMIC APPROACH TO DISEASE The clinical method has as its object the collection of accurate data concerning all the diseases to which human beings are subject, namely, all conditions that "limit life in its powers, enjoyment, and duration." But much more is required in making a diagnosis. Each datum must be interpreted in the light of the known facts of anatomy, physiology, and chemistry. The synthesis of these interpretations yields information concerning the affected organ or body system. Further, from the vantage point afforded by such an anatomic diagnosis the physician may then turn to other data, such as the mode of onset and clinical course of the illness, and to the results of laboratory tests, in order to ascertain the cause of the disease and degree of physiologic impairment.

The clinical method always proceeds in a series of logical steps. The perceptive student will note certain similarities between the clinical method and the scientific method. Each begins with observational data which suggest a series of hypotheses. The latter are tested in the light of further observations, some clinical, others contrived laboratory procedures. Finally, a conclusion is reached, which in science is called a *theory* and in medicine a *working diagnosis.* The modus operandi of the clinical method, like that of the scientific method, cannot be reduced to a single principle or a type of inductive or deductive reasoning. It involves both analysis and synthesis, the essential parts of cartesian logic. The physician does not start with an open mind any more than does the scientist, but with one prejudiced from knowledge of recent cases; and the patient's first statement directs his thinking in certain channels. He must struggle constantly to avoid the bias occasioned by his own attitude, mood, and interest.

It is particularly in the study of more difficult patients that one observes most clearly the logical order of the clinical method. Here in particular the physician must carefully list each problem indicated by the patient's complaints and physical and laboratory findings and seek answers to each. Anatomic diagnosis regularly precedes etiologic diagnosis. One seldom succeeds in determining the cause and mechanism of a disease before ascertaining which organ has been involved. An intermediate step is syndromic diagnosis. Most physicians attempt consciously or unconsciously to fit a given problem into one of a series of syndromes. The syndrome, in essence, is a group of symptoms and signs of disordered somatic function, related to one another by means of some anatomic, physiologic, or biochemical peculiarity of the organism. It embodies a hypothesis concerning the deranged function of an organ, organ system, or tissue. Congestive heart failure, Cushing's disease, and dementia are examples. In congestive heart failure dyspnea, orthopnea, cyanosis, dependent edema, engorged neck veins, pleural fluid, pulmonary rales, and enlarged liver are known to be connected by a single pathophysiologic mechanism—failure of the heart, leading to salt and water retention and high venous pressure. In Cushing's disease the moon facies, hypertension, diabetes, and osteoporosis are the recognized effects of excess corticosteroids acting on many target organs. In dementia deterioration of memory, incoherent thinking, faulty judgment, etc., are related through a neuroanatomic and a neurophysiologic principle, i.e., all these disordered intellectual functions are related to slow impairment of the function and destruction of the association areas of the cerebrum.

A syndromic diagnosis usually does not necessarily identify the precise cause of an illness, but it greatly narrows the number of possibilities and, thus, suggests whatever further clinical and laboratory studies are required. The derangements of each organ system in human beings are reducible to a relatively small number of syndromes. Diagnosis is greatly simplified if a given clinical problem conforms neatly to a well-defined syndrome. Then one need only turn to a book for a list of the various diseases that may cause it. The search for the cause of an illness that does not conform to a syndrome is much more difficult, for a seemingly infinite number of diseases may then have to be considered. Nevertheless, the principle remains: the clinical method is an orderly intellectual activity which proceeds almost invariably from symptom to sign, to syndrome, to disease.

3
CARE OF THE PATIENT

THE EDITORS

The care of the patient begins with the development of an interpersonal relationship between the patient and his physician, as discussed in Chap. 1. In the absence of a sense of trust and confidence on the part of the patient, the effectiveness of therapeutic measures is diminished. In many instances, when there is confidence in the physician, reassurance alone suffices and is all that is needed. In those cases which for the time being are insusceptible of solution or for which no effective remedy is available, a feeling on the part of the patient that his physician is doing all that is possible is one of the most important therapeutic measures that his doctor can provide.

When little was known about the pathogenesis of a disorder and when, with rare exceptions, practically all the drugs in the huge pharmacopoeias were virtually worthless, the medical decisions of the physician were seldom of crucial importance. The thoughtful physician of the time was led to an attitude of therapeutic nihilism. Being aware that most of the drugs available to him were of no real value, he could best display his skill by not tampering with the natural recuperative powers of the body.

O. W. Holmes phrased the status of pharmacotherapy in 1860 when he remarked:

Throw out the opium, which the Creator himself seems to prescribe, for we often see the scarlet poppy growing in the cornfields as if it were foreseen that wherever there is hunger to be fed there must also be pain to be soothed; throw out a few specifics which our art did not discover and is hardly needed to apply; throw out wine which is a food and the vapors of which produce the miracle of anesthesia, and I firmly believe that if the whole materia medica, as now used, could be sunk to the bottom of the sea it would be all the better for mankind,—and all the worse for the fishes.

The discovery during the past several decades of therapeutic agents capable of exerting decisive influence on the course of disease has made it essential that the physician have some understanding not only of the disturbed functions induced by disease, but also of the manner of treatment most likely to exert a beneficial effect, and of the risks involved in the proposed therapeutic plan.

Ideally, treatment should strive for the complete restoration of the patient's physical and mental health. When this goal is not attainable, remedies may still be available which will postpone the progress of incurable disease and delay its evil consequences; or, when they can no longer be postponed, they can be rendered tolerable.

IATROGENIC DISORDERS It is the responsibility of the doctor to use the new and powerful therapeutic measures wisely, with due regard for their action, cost, and potential dangers. Every medical procedure, whether diagnostic or therapeutic, contains within it the potentiality of harm, but it would be impossible to afford the patient all the benefits of modern scientific medicine if reasonable steps in diagnosis and therapy were withheld because of possible risks. "Reasonable" here implies that the physician has weighed the pros and cons of a procedure and has concluded on rational grounds that the step is advisable or essential for the relief of discomfort or the cure or amelioration of disease. When the deleterious effects of the physician's action exceed the advantages that could have been anticipated, one is justified in designating these undesirable effects as iatrogenic. It is necessary only to recall the dangerous or fatal reactions that occasionally follow the use of antibiotics given for trivial respiratory infections, the gastric hemorrhage or perforation caused by cortisone administered for a mild arthritis, or the fatal homologous serum hepatitis that followed needless transfusions of blood or plasma.

But the harm that a physician can do to a patient is not

limited to the imprudent use of medication. Equally important are ill-considered or unjustified remarks. Since the patient, no matter how apparently placid, approaches the physician with apprehension, his anxiety may be enhanced by a too-serious demeanor, a flippant remark, or an unexplained conference concerning his illness. Many persons have been led to a cardiac neurosis because the physician expressed a grave prognosis on the basis of a misinterpreted electrocardiogram. The good physician appreciates that he is always in a position to cause injury by his treatment, by his words, and by his behavior.

The physician must never become so much absorbed in the disease that he forgets the patient who is its victim. This exhortation cannot be repeated too often. As the science of medicine advances, it is all too easy to become so much fascinated by the manifestations of a malady that one disregards the ailing person; his fears, his concerns about his job and the future of his family, the cost of medical care, and the specter of economic insecurity. Treatment of a patient consists of more than the dispassionate confrontation of a disease. It embodies also the exercise of warmth, compassion, and understanding. In the now famous words of Peabody, "One of the essential qualities of the clinician is interest in humanity, for the secret of the care of the patient is in caring for the patient."

INCURABILITY AND DEATH No problem is more distressing than that presented by the patient with incurable disease, particularly when death is imminent and inevitable. What should the patient and his family be told, what measures should be taken to maintain the patient's life, and how is death to be defined?

There is no ironclad rule that the patient must be told "everything," even if he is an adult and the head of his family. How much the patient is told will depend upon his own desires and character, the wishes of his family, the state of his affairs, and perhaps his religious convictions. First of all, the patient must be given an opportunity to speak to his physician and to ask questions. Patients may find it easier to share their feelings about death with their physician because they realize that he is likely to be more objective and less emotional than their own family members.

One thing is certain: it is not for you to don the black cap and, assuming the judicial function, take hope away from any patient . . . hope that comes to us all. (William Osler)

Even when the patient directly inquires, "Doctor, am I dying?" the physician must be circumspect and must attempt to determine whether this is a request for information, a demand for reassurance, or even an expression of hostility. Only further exchanges between the patient and his physician can resolve these questions and guide the doctor in what he should say and how he should say it.

The physician should provide or arrange for emotional, physical, and spiritual support. He must be compassionate, unhurried, and open. Pain should be adequately controlled, human dignity maintained, and isolation from family avoided. The last two, in particular, tend to be overlooked in hospitals, where the intrusion of life-sustaining apparatus can so easily detract from attention to the whole person and instead concentrate on the life-threatening disorder.

The physician must also be prepared to deal with sentiments in the family commonly experienced at a time of impending death. He must deal wisely with the expiatory attitude of the family when a member becomes gravely or hopelessly ill. The meager resources that may represent the savings of a lifetime may be dissipated in weeks in payment for needlessly expensive rooms, nursing services, and futile therapeutic measures. It is difficult for the physician to oppose these gestures too strenuously. He must be mindful that they serve more to bring consolation to the family than to assuage the distress of the patient, but they need not be encouraged.

He also must be prepared to deal with the feelings of guilt that almost invariably afflict the members of a family when parent or child or spouse has died. He must tender what assurance is possible that no fault or stigma of neglect need be attached to the living.

Apart from the anguish of facing the terminal phases of disease, to which patient and family react in highly individualistic ways according to temperament, personal philosophy, and religion, important biologic and medical problems arise as death approaches. One must at each stage in an illness ascertain whether a fatal outcome is inevitable and also whether the patient, should he survive, will suffer a degree of disability that would make life unbearable for him and his family. New concepts of death must also be considered.

Traditionally, in every society, arrest of heart action has been taken as the only valid medical criterion of death. Law books cite this as the only certain proof that human life has ended. But, as every modern physician knows, the heart may sometimes be miraculously restored to action minutes after it has stopped. On the other hand, other vital organs such as the brain may be destroyed, leaving the individual essentially dead as far as his psychic life and personality are concerned, while heart action and circulation are maintained.

Biologically speaking, life, when viewed at a cellular level, is an intricate process of growth and decay in varying proportions at different ages. When decay exceeds growth in organs composed of postmitotic cells such as the musculature and nervous system, where each cell must endure for the lifetime of the individual, death proceeds gradually. This might be termed *cellular death,* and in its most advanced forms organ function may be impaired to a point incompatible with useful life. Of all the organs of man it is the central nervous system, more specifically the brain, that imparts meaningful qualities to life. Without a functioning cerebrum man has none of the attributes that distinguish him from another individual of his own species or from beasts. All awareness of self is permanently effaced; no longer can he think, respond to his physical or social environment, speak, or move. Most thoughtful physicians and many lay people concede that such a state is equivalent to death even though the heart still beats.

Criteria, clinical and electrographic, are at hand which permit the reliable diagnosis of cerebral death. According to the report of the staff of the Massachusetts General Hospital and the Harvard Committee on Brain Death, one may assume that death has occurred when, as a consequence usually of hypoxia and hypotension, all signs of receptivity and responsivity are in abeyance, including all brainstem and spinal reflexes (pupillary reactions, ocular movement, blinking, swallowing, breathing, tendon and other spinal reflexes), and the electroencephalogram is isoelectric. Occasionally, intoxications and metabolic disorders may simulate this state; hence the diagnosis requires expert medical evaluation. Under the aforementioned circumstances, to continue with heroic, highly costly, supportive measures merely for the purpose of preserving cardiac function is in actuality against the best interests of patient, family, and society.

Here the physician, on contemplating the broad implications of his actions, must either involve himself in fruitless supportive care or may have to make the difficult decision to abandon his traditional role of making every effort to preserve life at any cost. If the medical profession, in accord with social sanction, can be brought to redefine life as a state in which cerebral action subserves awareness of environment and the possibility of expressing intellect, emotion, personality, and character, and can equate the opposite of this with death, the dilemma could be avoided.

A practice which has been adopted and which has proved most acceptable is as follows:

1 The diagnosis of brain death, based on the above criteria, should be corroborated by another physician, and the clinical examination and EEG should be repeated one or more times over a period of 24 hr.
2 The family and nurses should be informed of the irreversibility of brain function but should not be asked or permitted to make the decision as to the continuation of medical treatment.
3 The physician may withdraw supportive medical measures, assuming that nothing more can be offered and that extraordinary measures to maintain heart function need not be employed (in agreement with recommendations of Pope Pius XII and others of the clergy).
4 The possibility that such patients may become sources of organs for grafting should not enter into such decisions, although prior to the cessation of heart action the family may be approached by surgeons and asked whether this would be their wish, or the family may suggest that organs be used for this purpose.

4 PROBLEM-ORIENTED MEDICAL RECORD

STEPHEN E. GOLDFINGER
JAMES J. DINEEN

Whatever can be said, can be said clearly.
Whereof one cannot speak, thereof one ought remain silent.
Ludwig Wittgenstein

Medical records, as kept for years, have often failed the purposes of lucid communication, education, and rapid retrieval of stored information. Poorly supported diagnoses, incomplete progress notes, chaotically entered laboratory results, and inadequately expressed plans of management are embarrassingly common findings in records existing at some of the most sophisticated medical institutions. In response to this, the Problem-Oriented Medical Record (POMR) has been devised with the object of providing a means whereby the medical record will better reflect the health problems of patients and the professional responses to them on the part of physicians, nurses, and other major participants in care.

Central to its formulation is the view that the patient's record must be designed so that it expresses specifically what physicians deal with most frequently—the *problems* of patients. While the ultimate goal of clinical taxonomy is directed toward identification of etiology, pathology, and pathologic physiology, in view of their importance as guides in therapy, it would be both unrealistic and dangerous to require a specific diagnosis for a severely dyspneic patient in the absence of reasonably convincing information concerning the reason for his dyspnea. Until the cause can be established, all diagnostic modalities and therapeutic interventions are oriented to the real and immediate problem—*dyspnea.* The same is true of a great variety of symptoms, signs, and laboratory findings which are derived in the process of patient care. A high serum calcium reported in an SMA screening study, a suspicious pigmented skin lesion, or a sudden unexplained deterioration of intellect are examples of worrisome findings that are most appropriately expressed, initially, as problems. In each instance, a more refined diagnosis in the absence of further data can only represent guesswork; hence, it may be wrong. As data pertaining to each problem become available, the problem may then be expressed at a higher level of understanding, i.e., hyperparathyroidism, malignant melanoma, or subdural hematoma. By offering the physician a system of record keeping compatible with his most frequent focus of attention in the practice of medicine—the problem—an opportunity is provided to reduce distortion and error.

The second and more fundamental aspect of problem orientation is the systematized display of patient care embodied in records. This is best described by considering the elements of medical care and their dynamic interrelationship, as proposed by Weed (Fig. 4-1).

THE DATA BASE All clinical care must start with a data base. A careful and complete history and a physical examination are of fundamental value to the physician. The POMR stresses the importance of this traditional approach to data collection. However, there may be

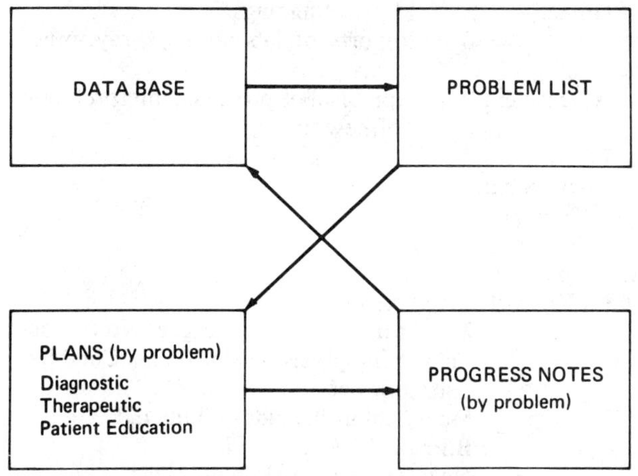

FIGURE 4-1

instances when full information is unobtainable as, for example, in the case of an unidentified unconscious patient brought into the emergency room. His management is, nevertheless, contingent on data, even though incomplete—primarily the initial physical examination, lumbar puncture, and laboratory results. At the other extreme, one might safely argue that no data base can be absolutely complete on any patient, for a lifetime of psychic and biological events can never be fully recalled, much less transcribed. The POMR brings into focus a defined data base, highlights its deficiencies, and serves as the nucleus for its expansion whenever possible. Elements of the data base include:

1 Identifying information (i.e., name, age, sex, race, religion, insurance information, etc.)
2 Patient profile (i.e., occupation, education, marital status, children, hobbies, worries, moods, sleep patterns, habits, etc.)
3 Medical history
  a Chief complaints
  b History of present illnesses
  c Past medical history
  d Review of systems
  e Family history
  f Medications
4 Physical examination
5 Laboratory data and physiologic tests (i.e., complete blood count, electrocardiogram, chest x-ray, creatinine, urinalysis, vital capacity, tonometry, etc.)

It is evident that these components do not constitute anything new to the conscientious physician. In using the POMR, he is asked to *define* the data base and to highlight the abnormalities revealed by it as *problems* with which he must deal. Admittedly, an *ideal* data base has not yet been conceived. Such a construct would depend in part on the population served, the resources at hand, and, most importantly, on the relative cost-benefit of various screening studies in regard to prevention of morbidity. Studies of the value of such tests in these terms may lead to the development of a series of risk-related data bases, each applicable to different groups of individuals. Material obtained for each part of the data base is often organized in the record by standardized formats for display. Although some rather sophisticated examples of such data sheets have been designed, it must be emphasized that the ultimate value of a data base depends on the validity of the information that is entered. An inaccurate history, careless examination of the heart, or a faulty piece of laboratory equipment will yield inaccurate data no matter how efficiently the results are recorded. Moreover, it should be recognized that the data base must constantly be supplemented by later entries into the record.

THE PROBLEM LIST From the data at hand, a Master Problem List is formulated. It should include those features in the patient's psychobiological makeup that require continuing attention by the physician and other members of the health team. Thus, the Problem List may contain entries relating to social history (e.g., marital discord), risk factors (e.g., familial polyposis of the colon), symptoms (e.g., hemoptysis), physical findings (e.g., splenomegaly), laboratory tests (e.g., anemia), etc. All problems are expressed at a level of highest understanding. For example, if the cause of gastrointestinal bleeding is known to be a duodenal ulcer, the latter becomes the appropriate entry, unless severe bleeding in itself constitutes a major health hazard.

The Problem List is a *dynamic* entity which is altered as new information and events dictate. All entries are dated, and a separate column permits the recording of resolved and inactive problems (Fig. 4-2).

When kept in this manner, a Problem List featured at the beginning of a patient record provides a succinct summary of all important health matters and, moreover, serves as a table of contents for entries within the record

FIGURE 4-2

PROBLEM LIST

No.	Active	Date	Inactive	Date
1	Hypertension	1953		
2	Recurrent bronchitis	1958		
3	Penicillin allergy	1958		
4			S/P pyelonephritis	1960
5	Gallstones	Oct 1972	resolved → Cholecystectomy	Mar 1973
6	Arthralgias	Mar 1973	resolved → #9	June 1973
7	Pleurisy	Mar 1973	resolved → #9	June 1973
8	Proteinuria	Apr 1973	resolved → #9	June 1973
9	SLE	June 1973		
10	Unemployment	Nov 1973		

which are properly labeled according to problem (see below). Satisfactory problem listing clearly requires periodic revision of this inventory. Also necessary is a sense of proportion, so that a variety of minor, self-limited problems (e.g., colds, sprains, minor gastrointestinal upsets) are excluded from the Master Problem List, which might otherwise be unduly cluttered with trivial illnesses. When a number of clearly psychosomatic complaints predominate, they may be grouped together as a single entry, e.g., "Functional Symptoms."

PROBLEM-RELATED PLANS Problems regarded as "active" generally require planning for their proper management. The display of these plans, separately listed for each problem, is of critical importance as a reflection of the physician's response to the problems that have been identified. Plans are recorded under three categories:

1 Diagnostic: i.e., laboratory tests, radiological studies, consultations, continued observation, etc.
2 Therapeutic: i.e., medications, diet, physiotherapy, corrective surgery, etc.
3 Patient Education: i.e., instruction of the patient in various aspects of self-care, education regarding the goal of therapy, the prognosis that has been given to him, etc.

It is not necessary that all three sections be completed for each problem, inasmuch as planning may at times be concerned with only one or two of them. For example:

1 Diarrhea
- *Dx* Stool for occult blood, culture, ova, and parasites, microscopic fat; and muscle fibers
  Sigmoidoscopy
  Barium enema if persistent
- *Rx* Avoid foods that exacerbate
  Propantheline 30 mg 3 i.d.
- *Pt.Ed.* Informed that more information is needed to make a diagnosis, will aim for symptomatic therapy for now.

2 Pyuria
- *Dx* BUN
  Repeat urinalysis
  Urine culture

3 Obesity
- *Rx* 1500 kcal diet
  Weight Watchers
- *Pt.Ed.* Dangers of obesity cited. *Goal:* 170 lb

PROGRESS NOTES Progress notes are structured on the basis of those problems which have received attention during the office or hospital visit. (Thus, all problems on the list need not be entered.) In a sense, these notes update the course and management of the problem, following the same general schema already described. They are sturctured in the following manner:

 # Problem
- Subjective(S): Interval history
  Adherence to program
- Objective(O): Physical findings
  Reports of laboratory, x-ray, other tests
- Assessment(A): Appraisal of progress, interpretation of new findings, etc.
- Plan(P):
  Diagnostic:
  Therapeutic:
  Patient Education:

Example:
#3 RHD with mitral stenosis
- *S:* 2 flight dyspnea, mild fatigue. No orthopnea, hemoptysis, ankle edema. Child has strep throat.
  Meds: chlorothiazide 500 mg q.d.
- *O:* B.P. 120/70 P. 78 regular.
  Neck veins normal, lungs clear.
  Grade iii diastolic rumble, wide opening snap. P_2 slightly ↑.
  EKG: Early P mitrale, otherwise normal.
- *A:* Stable. Catheterization still not indicated. Risk of strep throat present.
- *P:*
  - *Dx:* Cardiac fluoroscopy
  - *Rx:* Continue chlorothiazide and penicillin V 250 mg b.i.d.—2 weeks
  - *Pt.Ed:* Reinstructed about antibiotic coverage for tooth extractions, scheduled for next month. (Will contact oral surgeon.)

DATA FLOW SHEETS At times, the course and management of a particular problem may be succinctly recorded by using data flow sheets. Many physicians are familiar with this method of making brief-interval record entries on patients with diabetic ketoacidosis or acute gastrointestinal hemorrhage. A number of other conditions—both acute and chronic—lend themselves to this manner of sequential description. Data flow sheets for such problems as hypertension, renal failure, and respiratory insufficiency serve as excellent adjuncts to effective patient care within the POMR.

CLINICAL JUDGMENT This intangible element of patient care is so crucial that it is cited to emphasize that the style of recording in itself is no guarantee of excellence. The *content* of the record—the problems selected from the data base, the nature of the plans evolved, the choice of therapeutic programs—reflects the true quality of the care provided. In this respect, the initials "C.J." might appropriately be placed alongside every arrow in Fig. 1 to represent the absolute need for clinical judgment in effectively catalyzing the process of sound medical care.

POTENTIAL BENEFITS OF THE PROBLEM-ORIENTED MEDICAL RECORD Allied health personnel Several aspects of the POMR facilitate the team approach to patient care. First, the requirement that all members of the health team systematically display their thoughts and actions improves communications and potentiates supervision. Second, the existence of a list of the patient's problems that the health team must manage reduces errors of omission and treatment out of context. Furthermore, the establishment of a plan for each problem leads to clearer assignment of specific tasks to each of its members. Most importantly, the dissection of the health care process into gathering a data base, formulating problems, and designing a plan for the management of each problem provides a useful road map for the intelligent expansion of the role of various allied health personnel. This breakdown helps the physician as team leader to rethink his role in the health care process and concentrate on the more difficult aspects such as identifying problems from the data base and organizing approaches to these problems, while assigning more routine tasks to other members of the team. Practical experiences in clinical settings as varied as large hospital clinics and rural offices have shown the value of the POMR in the team approach to patient care.

Education and audit In addition to facilitating patient care, a good medical record should educate its readers and also be subject to audit in its own right. By clearly outlining the physician's logic, the POMR reveals the process of patient care in a manner which can be evaluated. This, in itself, is an educational process. It deemphasizes rote memory and substitutes a record of the logical steps which are being taken to recognize the patient's problems and the physician's capacity to act as a guide in attempting to solve them. Such an endeavor, if begun early, can set the stage for a life-long educational process of self and peer evaluation through effective record audit.

Clinical research Any record system that clarifies the details of patient-physician interaction can be a powerful tool in clinical research. A clear data base, an organized system for record entries, and the use of data flow sheets serve to facilitate rapid extraction and analysis of clinical information. Efforts to computerize the POMR, if successful, will amass a spectrum of clinical and epidemiologic data that may prove extremely valuable in our understanding of illness and the process of health care.

THE ROLE OF THE POMR IN PATIENT CARE The POMR is a system of record keeping which greatly facilitates data retrieval and at the same time highlights the decision-making role of the physician as he responds to the problems of patients. It should be evident, nevertheless, that it can only serve the goal of improved health care when it is used with a sound intellectual appreciation of disease, based on a full understanding of pathophysiology and a scientific approach to therapy. The tendency for the POMR to compartmentalize problems must not preclude creative, synthetic thinking. At some institutions an Initial Assessment entry is placed before the Problem List to provide an opportunity for the physician to express an overall perspective and to distinguish the major problems from others which are less important. Finally, as emphasized in the preceding chapters, compassion is an element of medical care that can never be adequately displayed by any record system. A possible danger of the POMR is that the emotional needs of patients may receive even less attention by the busy doctor who is intent on writing excellent notes. The patient and not the record must remain as the primary focus of physician care.

REFERENCES

Bjorn JC, Cross HD: *Problem Oriented Practice,* Chicago: Modern Hospital Press, McGraw-Hill Publications Company, 1970

Goldfinger SE: The problem-oriented record: A critique from a believer. N Engl J Med 288:606, 1973

Hurst W, Walker HK: *The Problem Oriented System.* New York: Medcom Press, 1972

Weed LL: *Medical Records, Medical Education and Patient Care.* Cleveland: Case University Press, 1969

PART TWO | CARDINAL MANIFESTATIONS AND APPROACH TO DISEASE

section 1 | Pain

5
GENERAL CONSIDERATIONS

RAYMOND D. ADAMS
WILLIAM M. RESNIK

Pain, it has been said, is one of "Nature's earliest signs of morbidity." Few will deny that it stands preeminent among all the sensory experiences by which man judges the existence of disease within himself. There are relatively few maladies that do not have their painful phases, and in many of them pain is a characteristic without which diagnosis must always be in doubt. It seems appropriate, therefore, to begin a section on the cardinal manifestations of disease with a discussion of the more general aspects of pain.

The painful experiences of the sick pose manifold problems for the practioner of medicine, and the student should know something of these problems in order to prepare himself properly for the task ahead. He must be ready to diagnose disease in patients who have felt only the first rumblings of discomfort, before other symptoms and signs of disease have appeared. To cope effectively with problems of this type requires a sound knowledge of the sensory supply of the viscera and a familiarity with the typical symptoms of many diseases. He will be consulted by some patients who seek treatment for pains that appear to have no obvious structural basis, and further inquiry will disclose that worry, fear, and other troubled emotional states may have aggrandized relatively minor aches and pains. To understand problems of this type requires insight into the psychologic factors which influence behavior and a knowledge of psychiatric disease. Next, he must manage the "difficult pain cases," in which no amount of investigation will bring to light either medical disease or psychiatric illness, and it is here that he will sense the need of a sound and assured clinical approach to the pain problem. Finally, he must care for the patients with intractable pain, often from an established and incurable disease, who demand relief either by drug or by the "less moderate means of surgery." Assessing the possibilities of the latter requires a comprehension of the anatomic pathways of pain.

END ORGANS, AFFERENT TRACTS, AND NUCLEI OF TERMINATION OF PAIN PATHWAYS Pain is a sensation which has its own sensory apparatus. The receptors in the skin and deep structures are fine, freely branching nerve endings which form an intricate network throughout the body. A single primary pain neuron with its cell body in the posterior root ganglion subdivides into many small peripheral branches to supply an area of skin of several square millimeters. The cutaneous area of each neuron overlaps with those of other neurons, so that every spot of skin lies within the domain of two to four neurons. These freely branching nerve endings are also found in many of the other specialized sensory receptors in the skin, such as the Krause end bulbs, the Ruffinian plumes, the Pacinian corpuscles, which may explain why the extremes of hot, cold, and pressure sensation become painful. Free nerve endings may also serve as receptors for other types of sensation. They are the only end organ in the cornea, where touch and temperature as well as pain are felt.

The sensory nerve fibers for pain, as they course through somatic and visceral nerves, are mixed with other sensory and motor fibers. All sensory fibers enter the spinal cord through the posterior roots and enter the brainstem through certain of the cranial nerves. The pain fibers are of two sizes, one very small (2 to 4 μm in diameter), called "C fibers," with a slow conducting velocity, the other somewhat larger (6 to 8 μm), called "A-delta fibers," with more rapid transmission rates. As the posterior root enters the spinal cord it separates into two divisions, medial and lateral. The medial division, heavily myelinated, synapses either with large secondary sensory neurons in the posterior horn or with anterior horn cells (serving segmental reflexes), or it passes upward in the posterior columns to the medulla. The lateral division, of thinly myelinated and nonmyelinated fibers, enters the substantia gelatinosa, where it synapses with

(1) many small neurons whose axons pass into the posterior and anterior horns of the same and adjacent segments of the spinal cord, also effecting reflex connections, of (2) large secondary sensory neurons which will form the lateral spinothalamic tract. The fibers of the lateral division of the root thus give rise to two secondary pathways for pain from the spinal cord to the brain. One is the lateral spinothalamic tract, the cell bodies of which lie in the posterior horns, with axons crossing through the anterior commissure of the spinal cord within one to two segments of the level of entry. The other is a less well-defined, multineuronal chain which extends upward along the reticular part of the gray matter. The lateral spinothalamic tract, joined in the brainstem by the trigeminothalamic tract, courses through the lateral part of the medulla, pons, and midbrain, giving off many collaterals before terminating in the nucleus ventralis posterolateralis and probably in other thalamic nuclei as well (Fig. 5-1). The reticular chain of neurons extends cephalad and finally makes connections through the interlaminar nuclei of the thalamus with the limbic portions of the cerebrum.

The secondary spinothalamic and trigeminothalamic tracts synapse with the tertiary sensory neurons of the thalamus, whose axons extend to the cortex of the parietal lobe. Physiologists are not agreed as to the cortical terminus for the pain fibers, for electrical stimulation of the cortex in the conscious human being seldom produces a painful sensation, and parietal lobe lesions seldom cause central pain. Most of the pain fibers from the periphery cross to the opposite side of the brain; only a small contingent remains ipsilateral.

As a means of quick orientation to the anatomy of the peripheral pain pathways, it should be remembered that the facial structures and anterior cranium lie in the field of the trigeminal nerves; the back of the head, second cervical; the neck, third cervical; epaulet area, fourth cervical; deltoid area, fifth cervical; radial forearm and thumbs, sixth cervical; index finger, seventh cervical; middle finger, eighth cervical; little finger and inner forearm, first thoracic; nipple segment, fifth thoracic; umbilical, tenth thoracic; groin, first lumbar; medial side of knee, third lumbar; great toe, fifth lumbar; little toe, first sacral; back of thigh, second sacral; genitosacral areas, third, fourth, and fifth sacral. The first to fourth thoracic nerve roots are the important sensory pathways for the intrathoracic viscera; the sixth to eighth thoracic, for the upper abdominal organs (Figs. 21-1 and 21-2).

PHYSIOLOGY AND PSYCHOLOGY OF PAIN The stimuli that arouse pain vary for each tissue. Generally the adequate stimuli for skin are those which injure tissue, i.e., pricking, cutting, crushing, burning, and freezing. Interestingly, these same forms of stimulation have little effect when applied to the stomach and intestine. Pain in the gastrointestinal tract is produced instead by local trauma of an engorged or inflamed mucosa, distention or spasm of smooth muscle, and traction on the mesenteric attachment. Pain is induced in skeletal muscles by ischemia (the basis for the condition known as intermittent claudication), as well as by tears of connective tissue sheaths, necrosis, hemorrhage, or the injection of irritating solutions. Prolonged contraction of muscles evokes an aching type of pain. Ischemia, the only proved source of pain in the heart muscle, is responsible for angina pectoris and for the pain of myocardial infarction. Joints are insensitive to pricking, cutting, and cautery, but pain is induced in the synovial membrane by hypertonic saline solution and inflammation. Arteries give rise to pain when pierced with a needle, when induced to pulsate excessively (as in migraine), and in certain diseases of their walls such as exemplified by atherosclerotic thrombosis and arteritis of cranial arteries. Traction and displacement of intracranial vessels and the meningeal structures by which they are supported may cause headache.

In these painful lesions which damage tissues, irritating substances are believed to be liberated and to stimulate nerve endings. Acetylcholine, 5-hydroxytryptamine, histamine, bradykinin, and other similar polypeptides

FIGURE 5-1
Radiation and sites of reference of cardiac pain (upper), *gallbladder pain* (lower).

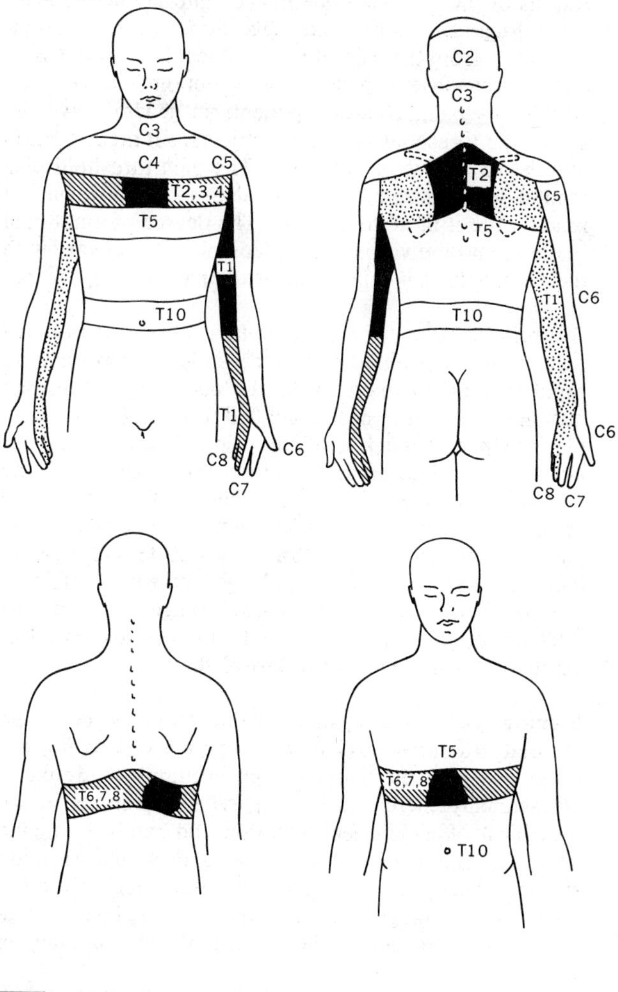

released by tissue injury have been found to elicit pain when injected intraarterially or applied to the base of a blister. Such substances are viewed as the "mediators" for pain.

The sensory experiences resulting from these several modes of stimulation in the skin and in deep skeletomuscular and visceral structures differ in quality. Integumentary stimuli, at the lowest levels of intensity, evoke sensations of touch, pressure, warmth, cold, or tickle. When increased to the point approaching tissue destruction, pain is added, and the resulting experience is thereafter a mixed one. The painful experience itself is one of pricking or burning. The threshold for burning pain from a thermal stimulus is approximately 2,000 times the threshold for warmth. This relationship of pain to tissue destruction is the basis of a biologic principle—that pain has a protective, or self-preserving, value to the organism.

The threshold for the perception of pain, i.e., the lowest intensity of stimulus recognized as pain, is approximately the same in all persons. It is lowered by inflammation and raised by local anesthetics (e.g., procaine), lesions of the nervous system, and centrally acting analgesic drugs. Distraction and suggestion, by turning attention away from the painful part, reduce the awareness of and the response to pain. Strong emotion (fear or rage) suppresses pain. Neurotic patients in general have the same pain threshold as normal subjects, but their reaction may be excessive or abnormal. The pain threshold of a frontal lobotomized subject is also unchanged, but he reacts little if at all to his pain. The degree of emotional reaction and the verbalization (complaint) also vary with the personality and character of the patient.

Superficial pain Sensory impulses subserving pricking pain, being transmitted by larger pain fibers, have a more rapid rate of conductivity to the nervous system than burning pain. A hot needle applied to the toe, for example, produces a quick, pricking pain and, only 1 to 2 sec later, a burning pain. Together they constitute the "double response" of Lewis. Ischemia of nerve, by the application of a tourniquet to a limb, abolishes pricking pain before burning pain. Both types of dermal pain are localized with precision ("local sign"), made possible by the overlap of sensory neurons. Analgesia means the interruption of all pain neurons to an area, and hypalgesia, the interruption of only part of them.

Visceral pain Deep pain (including that of visceral and skeletal structures) has basically the quality of aching, but if intense may be sharp and penetrating ("knifelike"). Occasionally there is a burning type of pain, as in the heartburn of esophageal irritation and rarely in angina pectoris. The pain is felt as being deep to the body surface. The double response is absent, localization is poor, and the margins of the pain are not well delineated, presumably because of the paucity of nerve endings in viscera.

Actually, the pain originating in deep skeletomuscular and visceral structures cannot be localized closer than two to three sensory segments. For example, pain from myocardial disease is felt to arise within the first to fourth or possibly fifth thoracic segments (see Fig. 5-1, showing theoretic distribution of heart pain). Unfortunately, from the standpoint of diagnosis, these spinal segments also receive sensory fibers from other structures—the esophagus, mediastinal contents, osseous structures, muscular structures, etc.; and diseases of these structures may cause pain that is difficult to distinguish from cardiac pain.

Deep musculoskeletal pain Since deep skeletal pain and visceral pain are mediated through a common deep sensory system, it is not surprising that their characteristics (type, localization, and referral) should be similar. Kellgren has mapped the topography of muscle and tendinous pain by injecting a few milliliters of normal saline solution into the various muscles and noting the location of induced pain. The ache is usually segmental and may spread one to two segments above (less often below) the site injected. A tear or injury in a lumbar muscle may give rise to a pain which, in quality and localization, including radiation into the groin and scrotum, is indistinguishable from the pain of renal colic. A hemorrhage into the right upper rectus muscle mimics the pain of gallbladder colic; and a lesion in a muscle or ligament deep in the chest wall causes pain referred to the left arm, like that of angina. The differentiation of these pains must be made on grounds other than location and reference.

Referred pain Deep visceral and somatic pains tend always to be referred superficially to those structures within a given spinal segment that have the most extensive nerve ramifications and therefore the widest cerebral representation (e.g., there are more sensory nerves in the integument than in the viscera, hence the pain in the latter is projected to the body surface). In the case of myocardial pain, sensory impulses entering the first to fourth thoracic nerves activate a pool of sensory neurons, the largest number of which also receive afferents from the skin of the inner side of the arm ($T_{1\text{-}2}$) and the anterior precordium ($T_{3\text{-}4}$). More of the sensory neurons from the heart enter the left side of the spinal cord than the right. These anatomic and physiologic data explain why cardiac pain is referred predominantly to the substernal, left precordial, and inner brachial zones.

Aberrant reference of pain occurs not infrequently and is explained in terms of the physiologic status of the spinal pool of sensory neurons. As was stated, a single sensory neuron entering one spinal root presynaptically depolarizes to a varying degree a pool of spinal neurons over four or five spinal segments. Pain then should spread to segments adjacent to the painful lesion, where it also causes cutaneous hyperesthesia and, by activating motor neurons, involuntary muscle contraction. If some preexistent disease in *adjacent* somatic segments has already partially depolarized the spinal pool of sensory neurons, a new painful disease which will further depolarize them causes the pain to spread to them. For example, if gallbladder disease, which activates sensory fibers entering at the sixth to eighth thoracic nerve, or cervical arthritis (at the second to eighth cervical nerve was present before a myocardial infarct, the cardiac pain may then be referred to the upper part of the abdomen or neck. Generally these aberrant referrals occur in segments that are cephalad to the normal segmental distribution of pain because their inhibitory connections are more abundant than those of caudal ones.

Hyperesthesia, hyperalgesia, hyperpathia, and involuntary spasms It has been customary to use the first two of these terms to designate a lowering of the threshold to touch and pain stimuli and the third for a state of pain with a normal or raised threshold but overreaction. The latter may even occur with anesthesia, as in *anesthesia dolorosa.* Any real distinction between these states is ephemeral. Probably only with inflammation of the skin is the pain threshold consistently lowered. What is most characteristic of all chronically painful states, and these frequently implicate nerves or central nervous structures, is that the part is unusually sensitive to all stimuli, even those which normally do not evoke pain; and the elicited pain is unnatural, radiant, outlasts the initiating stimulus, and is unusually modifiable by fatigue, emotion, etc. One sees listed here many of the characteristics of causalgia, spinal cord pain, phantom pain, zoster neuralgia, thalamic pain, etc. The explanation currently offered for these states is that at the peripheral as well as the central level the system of pain fibers is no longer in equilibrium with other sensory fibers. A kind of inhibition is exerted on the pain system at all times by the small neurons in the substantia gelatinosa, under the control of other afferent as well as descending pathways. Since the largest afferent peripheral nerve fibers suppress the secondary spinal neurons receiving pain impulses, nerve injury, which tends often to destroy some of the larger fibers, then permits their overresponse. According to Melzack and Wall, the small neurons of the substantia gelatinosa constitute a kind of "gate control system," which modulates input. The activation of large afferent fibers in a peripheral nerve most effectively inhibits the gateway cells. But the latter are also under the influence of descending pathways from the cerebrum and from other spinal segments. One might suppose that the activation of some of the sensory fibers controlling "gateway neurons" could be the basis of the effectiveness of *acupuncture.* The associated muscle contractions are reflexive, and their biologic function is to splint the diseased area and thereby to facilitate healing. The protective reflexes are usually of flexor type. The cutaneous tenderness of corresponding segments can be easily demonstrated by scraping skin with the head of a pin or by picking up a fold of skin.

As pain sensation may be induced by stimulation of the receptors or by irritation of peripheral nerves or roots, it may be abolished by diseases which affect the peripheral or central nervous system, or by a surgical procedure which accomplishes the same result. Pain in a circumscribed region may be terminated by section of the nerve which supplies that region (neurotomy) or by section of the spinal roots (posterior rhizotomy); pain in a limb or one side of the trunk may be abolished by section of the anterolateral spinothalamic tract (lateral spinal tractotomy in the spinal cord or tractotomy in the lateral medulla or mesencephalon).

Perception of pain The arrival of pain impulses at the thalamocortical level of the nervous system is attended by conscious awareness of the pain stimulus. Clinical study has not informed us of the exact localization of the nervous apparatus for this mental process. It is not entirely abolished by a total hemispherectomy, including the thalamus on one side. It is often said that impulses reaching the thalamus create awareness of the attributes of sensation and that the parietal cortex is necessary for the appreciation of the intensity and localization of the sensation. This seems to be an oversimplification. Probably a close and harmonious relationship between thalamus and cortex must exist in order for a sensory experience to be complete. The traditional separation of sensation (in this instance awareness of pain) and perception (awareness of the nature of the painful stimulus) has been abandoned in favor of the view that sensation, perception, and the various conscious and unconscious responses to a pain stimulus comprise an indivisible process.

Although similar to other sensory or perceptive phenomena in certain respects, such as predictable response to given intensity of stimulus, pain differs in other ways. One of its most remarkable characteristics is the strong feeling tone, or affect, with which it is endowed, nearly always one of unpleasantness. Furthermore, pain does not appear to be subject to negative adaptation. Most stimuli, if applied continuously, soon cease to be effective, whereas pain may persist as long as the stimulus is operative; and, by establishing a central excitatory state, may even outlast the stimulus.

Stereotaxic surgery on the thalamus in cases of intractable pain permits dissection of the anatomy of the pain experience. Lesions in the terminus of the lateral spinothalamic tract in the posterolateral nucleus are said to abolish pain and temperature sensation in the contralateral side of the body while leaving the patient with all his misery or affect of pain. Lesions in the centrum medianum relieve the painful state without altering pain and temperature sensation. Thus, at this level there must also be a balance of inhibitory and facilitatory sensory systems, for one cannot explain intractable pain simply in terms of continuous stimulation of chains of neurons.

Psychologic aspects of pain A discussion of this problem could hardly be complete without some reference to the influence of emotional states or to the importance of racial, cultural, and religious factors on the pain response, especially its overt expressions. It is common knowledge that some individuals, by virtue of training, habit, or phlegmatic character, are relatively stoical and that others are excessively responsive to pain. And there are rare individuals who are totally incapable of experiencing pain throughout their lifetime, either from a lack of sensory endings or peripheral sensory apparatus, or from some peculiarity of central reception.

Lastly, it is important to keep in mind the devastating effects of chronic pain. As Ambroise Paré remarked, "There is nothing that abateth so much the strength as paine." Continuous pain can be observed to have an adverse effect on the entire nervous system. There are increased irritability, fatigue, troubled sleep, poor appetite, and loss of emotional stability. Courageous men are reduced to a whimpering, pitiable state that may arouse only the scorn of a healthy person. They are irrational about illness and may make unreasonable demands on family and physician. This condition, which may be termed *pain shock*, once established, requires delicate but firm management. Depression (reactive?) is common. Of course, demand for and dependency on narcotic drugs often complicates the picture.

CLINICAL APPROACH TO THE PATIENT WITH PAIN AS THE PREDOMINANT SYMPTOM One of the first points to keep in mind is that not all pain is the consequence of serious disease. Otherwise healthy individuals have thousands of pains which are part of their daily sensory experience. To mention but a few, there is the momentary, hard pain over an eye, in the temporal region, or in the ear or jaw, which strikes with alarming suddenness; the more persistent ache which arises in some fleshy part, such as the shoulder, neck, thigh, or calf, the darting pain in an arm or leg, the fleeting precordial discomfort that arouses momentarily the thought of heart disease, the breath-taking catch in the side, the cluster of abdominal pains with their associated intestinal rumblings, and the brief discomfort upon movement of a joint. These *normal pains*, as they should be called, occur at all ages, tend to be brief, and depart as obscurely as they come. They acquire medical significance only when elicited by an inquiring physician, or when presented as a complaint by a worried patient; and, of course, they must always be distinguished from the *abnormal pains* of disease.

When pain, by its intensity, duration, and the circumstance of its occurrence, appears to be abnormal or constitutes one of the principal symptoms of disease, an attempt should be made to reach a tentative decision as to its cause and the mechanism of its production. This can usually be accomplished by a thorough interrogation of the patient, in which he is encouraged to relate as accurately as possible the main characteristics of the pain and the circumstances under which it occurs. The physical examination is directed towards a search for evidences of suspected disease and the reproduction of the pain.

Location of pain When the pain is caused by a superficial lesion, the cause and effect are usually so obvious that no problem is posed. It is the deep lesion, whether involving somatic or visceral structures, that causes trouble, and here exact localization becomes especially important. We have already seen that the pain originating from such tissues is no longer sensed as coming from them, but is instead only roughly segmental, i.e., within the territory of the cord segments innervating the structure. The identification of the segments involved is of value, for it sets the limit on the diagnostic possibilities that must be considered, i.e., they are limited to those structures having a corresponding innervation. Thus an epigastric or subxiphoid pain, or one in the opposite region in the back, obliges one to search for its cause in all those structures innervated by the sixth through eighth thoracic cord segments, i.e., the esophagus, stomach, duodenum, pancreas, biliary tract, the upper retroperitoneal structures, as well as the deep somatic tissues in this region. Also, one must consider the possibility that a lesion in a viscus innervated by spinal segments above or below the sixth through eighth thoracic cord segments may at times be the source of pain that has spread outside its normal boundaries and involved the epigastrium (Fig. 5-1).

Provoking and relieving factors These factors are of greater value than quality of pain in providing important data concerning its mechanism. Pain related to breathing, swallowing, and defecation focuses attention on the respiratory apparatus, the esophagus, and the lower part of the intestinal tract, respectively. A pain coming on a few minutes after the beginning of general bodily movement and relieved almost at once by rest indicates ischemia or a neural mechanism as the probable cause (see Chaps. 9 and 10). Pain occurring several hours after meals and relieved by food or alkali suggests the irritative effect of acid on the raw lining of the stomach or duodenum. Pain that is brought on or relieved by certain movements or postures of parts of the body is usually due to diseased skeletal structures (bones, muscles, ligaments). Pain that is enhanced by cough, sneeze, and strain is usually radicular in origin or arises in ligamentous structures. Pain that is increased or altered by cutaneous stimuli is due to disease in sensory tracts in the peripheral or central nervous system.

Quality and time-intensity characteristics of the pain Much reliance is put on the patient's choice of words and his account of the intensity of pain. Unfortunately this will depend, in part at least, on his intelligence, his vocabulary, and on what he imagines is taking place. "Crushing" and "squeezing" are commonly employed to describe an anginal pain, and this implication of pressure has some significance, since the pain may depend on an associated involuntary contraction of the pectoral muscles. Another patient with the same disease, however, may describe the pain as "exploding" or "burning." Far more important than the adjective used for pain is the information that it is steady and does not fluctuate. Similarly, the pain of peptic ulcer is frequently designated as "gnawing," but again, the deep, steady quality is more important than the word used to denote it. Gallbladder colic and renal colic are misnomers, if by colic is meant a "paroxysmal abdominal pain due to spasm, obstruction, or distention of any of the hollow viscera." *In both these disorders, the pain tends to be steady.* The aching quality of all deep pains is usually characteristic, but there are also several other informative attributes. A true colicky pain, one that is rhythmic and cramping, suggests an obstructive lesion in a hollow viscus. If the patient is a woman and has had children, it is a good idea to ask whether her "cramp" resembles the pains she had during childbirth. A pain that is steady and varies little or not at all from moment to moment means that the stimulus to pain is steady and unwavering, as in angina pectoris and peptic ulcer. Thus, a pain in the anterior midsternal region whose intensity fluctuates appreciably within the space of a minute or two is not due to angina, even though the history may appear to suggest a relation to exertion. Similarly, a high epigastric pain appearing several hours after a meal and even apparently relieved by food is not caused by an ulcer if the pain fluctuates perceptibly within seconds or a few minutes. The stimulus to ulcer pain does not quickly vary in intensity. A throbbing pain indicates that an arterial pulsation is giving rise to painful stimuli. Sharp, recurrent stabs of pain are caused by disease of nerve roots or sensory ganglions, as exemplified by tic douloureux or tabes, or a single episode may be due to a tear of a muscle or ligament. Once started, in each instance there may be a background of dull, aching pain. Particularly noteworthy here is the abrupt intensification of the dull ache of root pain by cough, sneeze, or strain which momentarily stretches or alters the position of the root.

Mode of onset of the pain This factor is also important. A pain reaching its full intensity almost immediately after its appearance suggests a rupture of tissue. The pain of a dissecting aortic aneurysm often develops in this manner. In fact, the suddenness and the severity of the pain, reaching a peak of intensity within seconds or minutes, sometimes provides the first clue in differentiating this type of chest pain from that caused by myocardial infarction. A similarly rapid accession of pain may occur with the rupture of a peptic ulcer.

Duration of pain This is another useful diagnostic attribute. Anginal pain, for example, rarely lasts less than 2 or 3 min. or more than 10 to 15 min. Ulcer pain may continue for an hour or more, unless terminated by the ingestion of food or alkali or a tumbler of water.

Severity of pain In any given disease, the severity of pain is subject to wide variation, and also patients differ in their tolerance to it. Therefore, one cannot judge the gravity of an illness solely by the patient's report of the intensity of pain. As a rule, pains that completely interrupt work or pleasurable activity, require opiates for relief, enforce bed rest, or awaken the patient from sound sleep are to be taken more seriously than those which have the opposite characteristics.

Time of occurrence An accurate determination must be made of the temporal aspects of the pain. The relationship of ulcer pain to the preceding meal has already been mentioned. Postural aches come after prolonged activity and disappear with rest; arthritic pains are usually most severe during the first movements after prolonged inactivity. The mechanisms for this latter phenomenon are not known, nor do we understand why painful lesions of the bone, such as those caused by metastatic cancer, are likely to be most disturbing during the night. It is possible that the occurrence or aggravation of the latter types of pain is due to enhanced awareness of painful stimuli at a time when the mind is not distracted by other stimuli; or it may be that the pains are now more easily evoked by unconscious movements made during sleep when protective reflexes are in abeyance.

It should be obvious from these remarks that the full significance of a pain is usually not revealed by any one single characteristic. It is only by combining all these data that one can determine its anatomic site and its mechanism. In general, *the most important and revealing clues are obtained from the answers to the questions: What brings on the pain? What relieves it?* Pain is a subjective manifestation, not a state to be observed or measured. The accuracy of our data depends on the skill with which we frame our questions and on the powers of observation and memory of the person answering them.

Finally, the diagnostic value of measures which *reproduce* and *relieve the pain* should be stressed. Not only are they important for diagnosis, but they convince the patient that the physician understands and can control his pain and the illness behind it. Climbing several flights of stairs under the physician's supervision may settle the question of the presence or absence of angina pectoris. An injection of procaine into the tender area in the chest wall or some other skeletal structure, with complete disappearance of the pain, may establish its skeletal origin and exclude the possibility of visceral disease. Reproducing the distress sometimes caused by aerophagia merely by distending the esophagus or stomach with air, or reproducing the vague but sometimes alarming sensation of pressure in the chest caused by unconscious hyperventilation by having the patient deliberately hyperventilate are other examples of how the principle of the reproduction of pain may be usefully employed.

A systematic interrogation of the patient will not lead to accurate diagnosis in every instance, but the habit of searching for the identifying characteristics of pain will enable the physician to increase his skill in this difficult field. Furthermore, after becoming familiar with the customary responses to these questions, he becomes more alert to the anxious, the hysterical, or the depressed patient who, while complaining of pain, seems incapable of describing any of its details, or is unwilling to do so. Instead, there is preoccupation with theories of what is wrong or with the treatments or mistreatments already given.

Finally, there will always be cases that defy solution, when the physician can proceed only by repeatedly reexamining the patient, explaining the need for continued observation, and enlisting his aid and forbearance during this trying period. Asking the patient to tolerate a certain amount of pain without the use of powerful analgesics is usually effective, particularly when the possibility of drug addiction is explained to him.

INTRACTABLE PAINS In the relatively rare circumstances when all manner of investigation has failed to throw light on the cause and mechanism of the pain, demands for pain-relieving surgery may become increasingly insistent. The physician may, in desperation, turn to measures which are more dangerous than the disease. Here the commonest source of error is to operate unnecessarily on the hysterical patient (see Chap. 339), only to discover too late that each operative procedure is followed by a new pain often at a higher level than the first. Depressive psychosis may masquerade as a painful state, and electric shock therapy may dramatically terminate the illness. Sometimes a half dozen or more operations are unsuccessfully performed on a single patient. The safest rule to follow in these cases is not to use opiates continuously or to recommend operation for the relief of pain unless a reasonable diagnosis has been made. For the pains of metastatic cancer, the thalamic pain of vascular disease of the brain, and other incurable diseases, the relative advantages of the controlled use of opiates versus lateral spinothalamic tractomy or frontal lobotomy must be carefully weighed in each patient. The age of the patient, other diseases, life expectancy, and mental state are all of importance in selecting the treatment procedure. Too often an operation on the spinal cord or brain is chosen in preference to narcotics and the controlled use of drugs. Forgotten is the fact that many patients with cancer were formerly kept relatively comfortable and active by the judicious use of morphine and its analogues and were never subjected to costly operations or deprived of any of those qualities of mind and character which are so treasured by their families.

TREATMENT Superficial pain arising in integumentary structures rarely presents a problem in therapy. Acetylsalicylic acid, 0.30 to 0.60 g orally every 4 hr, usually suffices. Acetophenetidin may be added. These two drugs are a particularly effective combination when one element of pain is integumentary. Commercial proprietary preparations of these drugs containing caffeine or amphetamines such as ASA compound, Empirin compound, aspirin, or Edrisal are available in most pharmacies. The caffeine or amphetamine is particularly useful if there is central nervous system depression, and often there is advantage to adding a sedative drug. When this type of pain is not effectively controlled by nonnarcotic analgesics, codeine should be given. Usually the addition of small amounts (8 to 30 mg) of codeine phosphate to the standard dose of acetylsalicylic acid and acetophenetidin is effective. A preparation containing codeine phosphate 8 to 30 mg, acetylsalicylic acid 0.23 g, acetophenetidin 0.16 g, and caffeine 0.032 g is commercially available (Empirin compound with codeine phosphate). Codeine, 20 to 45 mg every 3 hr, gives fairly effective analgesia with minimal side effects. Adequate rest and relief of muscle tension should also be encouraged. The application of moist heat is usually beneficial. Occasionally cold applications are preferred, but with the exception of cooling packs applied to an inflamed, burning skin or to a causalgia, cold is more likely to aggravate than to soothe the painful condition.

Occasionally integumental and deep pains of skeletal structures are of such severity as to require more powerful narcotic analgesics, such as meperidine hydrochloride (Demerol) in doses of 50 to 100 mg orally or intramuscularly, methadone hydrochloride, 5 to 10 mg orally or subcutaneously, or dihydromorphine hydrochloride (Dilaudid), 1 to 2 mg orally and subcutaneously. These drugs are most useful when sedation is not required. When pain is unusually severe and some degree of euphoria is desired, one of the new drugs such as pentazocine hydrochloride (Talwin) should be given in doses of 50 mg orally or subcutaneously every 3 to 4 hr. Morphine, although still a valuable drug in doses of 8 to 15 mg, is not used much because of its habit-forming tendency and the frequently associated nausea and vomiting. Since all these narcotic analgesics are, for the most part, detoxified by the liver, they either should not be used or should be given in only half the usual dosage in cases of liver disease, myxedema, adrenal insufficiency, and other states in which the metabolic rate is reduced. Morphine and related narcotic analgesics tend to cause pruritus and, therefore, should be used with care in patients with skin irritability. The possibility of initiating addiction in susceptible persons must be carefully evaluated in every instance (cf. Chap. 112).

If the patient exhibits mental tension, insomnia, and restlessness, a sedative drug such as phenobarbital or Sodium Amytal may be given with the analgesic agents. Sedative medication, especially the quick-acting barbiturates, should not be used alone for the control of pain, because they sometimes cause excitement and confusion under these circumstances.

Visceral pain originating in the stomach, gallbladder, intestines, or heart is usually very poorly controlled by the nonnarcotic analgesics. The narcotic analgesics are the agents of choice, but of course, they should never be given until the physician is certain that the relief of the pain will not mask the state of his patient. If sedation is not desirable and if constipation is a troublesome problem, the newer synthetic analgesics, meperidine in doses of 50 to 100 mg orally or intramuscularly or methadone 5 to 10 mg by mouth or subcutaneously every 4 to 6 hr, are recommended. Like morphine, these drugs are habit-forming but less so because they induce milder analgesia, sedation, and euphoria. Patients with severe visceral pain who are also anxious or fearful and unable to relax or sleep should be given morphine sulfate in doses of 8 to 15 mg subcutaneously. The well-known spasmogenic effects of morphine are partially counteracted by atropine sulfate, 0.3 to 0.4 mg. Aminophylline, 0.5 g intravenously, also overcomes much of this undesirable spastic action; a rectal suppository of 0.5 g, although less effective, may be substituted. When pain is due to benign, chronic diseases, every effort should be made to avoid opiate addiction. Here the judicious use of propoxyphene (Darvon), 65 mg q. 4 to 6 hr; oxycodone hydrochloride (Percodan), 4.5 mg q. 6 hr, or pentazocine hydrochloride, 50 mg q. 3 to 4 hr, may prove to be adequate.

Intractable pain due to incurable diseases, such as metastatic carcinoma, is one of the most difficult therapeutic problems. As a rule, one resorts to narcotic drugs because of their strong analgesic action, and habituation is accepted as the lesser of two evils. An alternative is "pain-relieving surgery." Section of peripheral nerves, the lateral spinothalamic tracts in the spinal cord (cordotomy) or the lateral part of the medulla, stereotaxic thalamotomy, and lobotomy are relatively safe procedures which have advantages over the continuous use of opiates in selected cases.

REFERENCES

Feindel WH et al: Pain sensibility in deep somatic structures. J Neurol Neurosurg Psychiatry 11:113, 1948

Hardy JD et al: *Pain Sensations and Reactions,* Baltimore: Williams & Wilkins, 1952

Lewis T: *Pain,* New York: Macmillan, 1942

Melzack R, Wall PD: Interaction of fast and slow conducting fiber systems involved in pain and analgesia, in *Pharmacology of Pain,* eds RKS Lim et al, London: Pergamon, 1968

Ryle JA: *The Natural History of Disease,* London: Oxford University Press, 1936

White JC, Sweet WH: *Pain and the Neurosurgeon—A Forty Years Experience*, Springfield, Ill.: Charles C Thomas, 1969

6 HEADACHE

JOHN F. GRIFFITH
RAYMOND D. ADAMS

The term *headache* should encompass all aches and pains located in the head, but in common language its application is restricted to unpleasant sensations in the region of the cranial vault. Facial, pharyngeal, and cervical pain are put aside as something different and are discussed in Chaps. 9 and 324.

Headache, along with fatigue, hunger, and thirst, represent man's most frequent discomforts. Medically speaking, its significance is often abstruse, for it may stand as a symptomatic expression of disease or of some minor tension or fatigue, incident to the affairs of the day. Fortunately, in most instances it reflects the latter, and only exceptionally does it warn of serious disease seated in intracranial structures. But it is this dual significance, benign and potentially malignant, that keeps the physician on the alert. Systematic approach to the headache problem necessitates a broad knowledge of the medical and surgical diseases of which it is a symptom and a clinical methodology which leaves none of the common and treatable causes unexplored.

GENERAL CONSIDERATIONS In the introductory chapter on pain reference was made to the necessity, when dealing with any painful state, of determining its quality, location, duration and time course, and conditions which produce, exacerbate, or relieve it. When headache is considered in these terms, a certain amount of useful information is obtained by careful history, but perhaps less than one might expect. Unfortunately, physical examination of the head itself is seldom useful.

As to quality of cephalic pain, the patient is rarely helpful in his description. In fact persistent questioning on that point occasions surprise, for the patient usually assumes that the word *headache* should have conveyed enough information to the examiner about the nature of the discomfort. Most headaches are dull, deeply located, and of aching character, a pain recognizable as of the type that usually arises from structures deep to the skin. Seldom is there reported the superficial burning, smarting, or stinging type of pain localized to the skin. When asked to analogize the sensation to another sensory experience, the patient may make some allusion to tightness, pressure, or bursting feeling, terms which then give clue to a muscular tension or psychologic state.

Queries about the intensity of the pain are seldom of much value since they reflect more the patient's attitude toward the condition and his customary way of reporting things that happen to him than the true severity. As usual, the bluff, hearty person tends to minimize his discomfort, whereas the neurotic dramatizes it. Degree of incapacity is a better index. A severe migraine attack seldom allows performance of the day's work. The pain which awakens the patient from sleep at night, or prevents sleep, is also more likely to have a demonstrable organic basis. As a rule, the most intense cranial pains are those which accompany subarachnoid hemorrhage and meningitis, which have grave implications, or migraine and paroxysmal nocturnal orbitotemporal ("cluster") headaches, which are benign.

Data regarding *location* of the headache are apt to be more informative. If the source is in deep structures (extracranial, subdermal, or intracranial), as is usually the case, the correspondence with the site of the pain is fairly precise. Inflammation of an extracranial artery causes pain well localized to the site of the vessel. Lesions of paranasal sinuses, teeth, eyes, and upper cervical vertebras induce less sharply localized pain but one that is still referred in a regional distribution that is fairly constant. Intracranial lesions in the posterior fossa cause pain in the occipital-nuchal region, homolateral if the lesion is one-sided. Supratentorial lesions induce frontotemporal pains, again homolateral to the lesion if it is on one side. But localization can also be very uninformative or misleading. Ear pain, for example, although it may mean disease in the ear, more often is referred from other regions, and eye pain may be referred from parts as remote as the occiput or cervical spine.

Duration and *time-intensity curve* of headaches in both the attack itself and the life profile are most useful. Of course, the headache of bacterial meningitis or subarachnoid hemorrhage occurs usually in single attacks over a period of days. Single, brief, momentary (1 to 2 sec) pains in the cranium are presently uninterpretable and are significant only because they indicate no serious underlying disease. Migraine of the classic type has its onset in the early morning hours or daytime, reaches its peak of severity in a half hour or so, and lasts, unless treated, for several hours up to 1 to 2 days, often terminated by sleep. In the life history a frequency of more than a single attack every few weeks is exceptional. A migraine patient having several attacks per week usually proves to have a combination of migraine and tension headaches. In contrast to this is the nightly occurrence (2 to 3 hr after onset of sleep) over a period of several weeks to months of the rapidly peaking, nonthrobbing orbital or supraorbital pain of cluster headache, which tends to dissipate within an hour. The headache of intracranial tumor characteristically can occur at any time of day or night, interrupt sleep, vary in intensity, and last a few minutes to hours, only to recur later in the day. The life profile is one of increasing frequency and intensity over a period of months. Tension headache, once commenced, may persist continuously for weeks or months, though waxing and waning from hour to hour.

Headache that bears a more or less constant relationship to certain biologic events and also to physical environmental changes may prove to be informative. Premenstrual headaches most typically relate to premenstrual tension during the period of oliguria and edema formation; they usually vanish after the first day of vaginal bleeding. The headaches of cervical arthritis are most typically intense after a period of inactivity, and the first stiff movements are both difficult and painful. Hypertensive headaches, like those of cerebral tumor, tend to occur on waking in the morning, but, as with all vascular headaches, excitement and tension may provoke them. Headache from infection of nasal sinuses may appear, with clocklike regularity, upon awakening and in midmorning, and is characteristically worsened by stooping. Eye-strain headaches naturally follow prolonged use of the eyes, as in reading, peering for a long time against glaring headlights in traffic, or watching cinema. Atmospheric cold may evoke pain in the so-called "fibrositic" or "nodular" headache or when the underlying condition is arthritic or neuralgic. Anger, excitement, or irritation may initiate common migraine in certain disposed persons; this is more typical of common migraine than of the classic type.

PAIN-SENSITIVE STRUCTURES AND MECHANISMS OF HEADACHE Understanding of headache has been greatly augmented by the observations of surgeons during operations on man. They inform us that the following cranial structures are sensitive to mechanical stimulation: (1) skin, subcutaneous tissue, muscles, arteries, and periosteum of skull; (2) delicate structures of eye, ear, and nasal cavity; (3) intracranial venous sinuses and their tributary veins; (4) parts of the dura at the base of the brain and the arteries within the dura mater and piarachnoid; (5) the trigeminal, glossopharyngeal, vagus, and first three cervical nerves. The bony skull, much of the piarachnoid and dura, and the parenchyma of the brain lack sensitivity. Interestingly, pain is practically the only sensation produced by stimulation of the listed structures.

The pathways whereby sensory stimuli, whatever their source, are conveyed to the central nervous system are the trigeminal nerves for structures above the tentorium in the anterior and middle fossae of the skull, and the first three cervical nerves for those in the posterior fossa and infradural structures. The ninth and tenth cranial nerves supply part of the posterior fossa and refer the pain to the ear and throat. The tentorium is the border zone between the trigeminal and cervical innervation. The central connections through spinal cord and brainstem to thalamus have already been described and depicted in Chap. 5.

The pain of intracranial disease is referred, by a mechanism already discussed, to some part of the cranium lying within the areas supplied by the aforementioned nerves (the fifth, ninth, and tenth cranial nerves and the first three cervicals). There may be an associated local tenderness of the scalp at the site of reference. Dental or jaw pain may also have cranial reference. The pain of disease in other parts of the body is not referred to the head, although it may initiate headache by other means.

By analysis of several types of headache, Wolff and his colleagues have demonstrated that most "spontaneous" cranial pains can be traced to the operation of one or more of the following mechanisms:

1 Distention, traction, and dilatation of the intracranial or extracranial arteries
2 Traction or displacement of large intracranial veins or the dural envelope in which they lie
3 Compression, traction, or inflammation of sensory cranial and spinal nerves
4 Voluntary or involuntary spasm and possibly interstitial inflammation of cranial and cervical muscles

More specifically, the intracranial mass lesions only cause headache if in a position to deform, displace, or exert traction on vessels and dural structures at the base of the brain, and this may happen long before intracranial pressure rises. In fact the artificial induction of high intraspinal and intracranial pressure by the subarachnoid or intraventricular injection of sterile saline solution does not result in headache. Some have interpreted this to mean raised intracranial pressure does not cause headache, a conclusion which is called into question by the demonstrable relief of headache by lumbar puncture and lowering the cerebrospinal fluid (CSF) pressure in some patients. Actually, most patients with high intracranial pressure complain of recurrent bioccipital and bifrontal headache, probably due to traction on vessels or dura. As to localization, the pains follow the patterns mentioned above; those deflecting the falx or pressing on superior longitudinal or straight sinuses induce pain behind or above the eye; if the lateral part of the lateral sinus is involved, the pain is felt in the ear. Displacement of tentorium elicits pain felt in the supraorbital region.

Dilatation of the temporal arteries with stretching of surrounding sensitive structures is believed to be the mechanism of most of the pain of migraine. Extracranial, temporal, and occipital arteries, when involved in giant-cell arteritis (cranial or "temporal" arteritis), a disease which usually afflicts individuals over fifty years of age, give rise to headache of dull aching and throbbing type, at first localized and then more diffuse. Characteristically it is severe and persistent over a period of weeks or months. The offending artery, strangely, is not always tender to pressure, yet section of it, as in biopsy, may relieve the pain (Chap. 326). Evolving atherosclerotic thrombosis of internal carotid, anterior, and middle cerebral arteries is sometimes accompanied by pain in the forehead or temple; with vertebral artery thrombosis, the pain is postauricular, and basilar artery thrombosis causes pain to be projected to the occiput and sometimes the forehead.

In *infection* or *blockage* of *paranasal sinuses,* accompanied usually by pain over the antrum or in the forehead (from the ethmoid and sphenoid sinuses the pain localizes around the eyes on one or both sides or in the vertex or other part of the cranium, especially in disease of the sphenoid sinuses), the mechanism involves changes in pressure and irritation of pain-sensitive sinus walls. Usually it is associated with tenderness of the skin in the same distribution. The pain may have two remarkable properties: (1) When throbbing, it may be abolished by compressing the carotid artery on the same side. (2) It tends to recur and subside at the same hours, i.e., on awakening, with gradual disappearance when the person is upright, and coming again in the late morning hours. The time relations are believed to yield information concerning the mechanism; morning pain is ascribed to the sinuses filling at night, and its relief on arising, from emptying after the erect posture has been assumed.

Stooping intensifies the pain by pressure change, as does blowing the nose, sometimes; and inhalant sympathomimetic drugs such as Neo-synephrine, which reduce swelling and congestion, tend to relieve the pain. Some believe that the highly sensitive orifice of the sinus is the source, but more probably, the pain arises in the sensitive mucous membrane of the sinus. However, it may persist after all purulent secretions have disappeared, probably because of mechanism of blockage of the orifice by boggy membranes and a vacuum or suction effect on the sinus wall (*vacuum sinus headaches*). The condition is relieved when aeration is restored. During air flights both earache and sinus headache tend to occur on descent, when the relative pressure in the blocked viscus falls.

Headache of ocular origin, located as a rule in the orbit, forehead, or temple, is of steady, aching type and tends to follow prolonged use of the eyes in close work. Ocular muscle imbalance is believed to be the mechanism. The main faults are hypermetropia and astigmatism (not myopia), which result in sustained contraction of extraocular as well as frontal, temporal, and even occipital muscles. Correction of the refractive error abolishes the headache. Traction on the extraocular muscles during eye surgery and on the iris will evoke pain. Another mechanism is involved in the raised intraocular pressure seen in acute glaucoma or iridocyclitis, which causes steady, aching pain in the region of the eye. When intense, it may radiate throughout the distribution of the ophthalmic division of the trigeminal nerve. As for ocular pain in general, it is important that the eyes should always be refracted, but eyestrain is probably not as frequent as one would expect from the wholesale dispensing of spectacles.

The mechanism of *headaches accompanying disease of ligaments, muscles, and apophyseal joints* in the upper part of the spine, which are referred to occiput and nape of neck on the same side, can be in part reproduced by the injection of hypertonic saline solution into these structures. Such pains are especially frequent in late life in rheumatoid and hypertrophic arthritis and tend also to occur after whiplash injuries to the neck. If the pain is arthritic in origin, the first movements after being still for some hours are both stiff and painful. In fact, evocation of pain by active and passive motion of the spine should indicate traumatic or other disease to movable parts. The pain of myofibrositis, evidenced by tender nodules near the cranial insertion of cervical and other muscles, is more obscure. There are no pathologic data as to the nature of these vaguely palpable lesions, and it is uncertain whether the pain actually arises in them. They may represent only the deep tenderness felt in the region of referred pain or the involuntary secondary protective spasm of muscles. Characteristically, the pain is steady (nonthrobbing) and spreads from one to both sides of the head. Exposure to cold or draft may precipitate it. Though severe at times, it seldom prevents sleep. Massage of muscles and heat have unpredictable effects but relieve the pain in some cases.

The *headache of meningeal irritation* (infection or hemorrhage), which is of acute onset, severe, generalized, deep-seated, constant, and especially intense at the base of the skull and associated with stiffness of neck on bending forward, has been ascribed by some authorities to increased intracranial pressure. Indeed the withdrawal of cerebrospinal fluid may afford some relief. But dilatation and congestion of inflamed meningeal vessels must also be a factor. It seems more probable, therefore, that the pain is due to the chemical irritation of nerve endings in the meninges.

Lumbar puncture headache, which is characterized by a steady occipital-nuchal pain but also by frontal pain coming on a few minutes after arising from a recumbent position and relieved within a few minutes by lying down, has as its cause a persistent leakage of CSF into the lumbar tissues through the needle site. The CSF pressure is low (often 0 in the lateral decubitus position), and the injection of sterile isotonic saline solution intrathecally relieves it. The headache is usually increased by compression of the jugular veins and is unaffected by digital obliteration of one carotid artery. It seems probable that in the upright position a low intraspinal and negative intracranial pressure exerts traction on dural attachments and dural sinuses by caudal displacement of the brain. Understandably, then, headache following cisternal puncture is rare. As soon as the leakage of CSF stops and CSF pressure is gradually restored (usually from a few days up to a week or so), the headache disappears. "Spontaneous" low-pressure headache may follow a sneeze or strain, presumably because of rupture of the spinal arachnoid along a nerve root.

The mechanism of the throbbing or steady headache which accompanies febrile illnesses, located in frontal or occipital regions or generalized, is probably vascular. It is much like histamine headache in being relieved on one side by carotid artery compression and on both sides by jugular vein compression or the subarachnoid injection of saline solution. It is increased by shaking the head. It seems probable that the meningeal vessels pulsate unduly and stretch pain-sensitive structures around the base of the brain. In certain cases, however, the pain may be lessened by compression of temporal arteries, and in these cases a component of the headache seems to be derived from the walls of extracranial arteries, as in migraine.

PRINCIPAL VARIETIES OF HEADACHE Usually there is no difficulty in diagnosing the headache of glaucoma, purulent sinusitis, bacterial meningitis, and brain tumor, and a fuller account of these special headaches will be found where these diseases are described in later sections of the book. It is when headache is chronic, recurrent, and unattended by other important signs of disease that the physician faces one of his most difficult medical problems.

The following types of headache should then be considered:

Migraine There are two identifiable, closely related syndromes, *classic* and *common.* In classic migraine there are a positive family history in 80 percent of cases, onset in childhood or adolescence, early neurologic symptoms (such as homonymous hemianopia, paresthesias, aphasia, and hemiparesis) which precede the unilateral throbbing pain, sensitivity to light and sound, nausea and sometimes vomiting, and relief by ergotamine. When all are present diagnosis is easy, but with only one or two there may be uncertainty. In common migraine the family history is less often positive, there are no initial neurologic symptoms, the age of onset may be later, frequency of attacks may be greater, and response to ergot less definite. Also, if the headache is more clearly provoked by psychologically stressful situations, the possibility of psychiatric illness is introduced. Special difficulties are also raised by unusual neurologic manifestations (see Chap. 336).

Cluster headache This headache is also called *paroxysmal nocturnal cephalalgia, migrainous neuralgia,* and *histamine headache* (Horton's syndrome). It is characterized by male predominance, constant, unilateral orbital localization, and onset within 2 or 3 hr after falling asleep (it is infrequent during the waking hours). The pain is usually intense, with lacrimation, blocked nostril, then rhinorrhea, and sometimes flush, miosis, ptosis, and edema of cheek, all lasting approximately an hour. It tends to recur nightly for several weeks or a few months (hence the term *cluster*), followed by complete freedom for years. The pain of a given attack may leave as rapidly as it began. Clusters may recur over the years, being possibly more likely in times of stress, prolonged strain, overwork, and with upsetting emotional experiences. Rarely, the condition may continue for 6, 7, or 8 years. The picture is so characteristic that it cannot be confused with any other disease, though to those unfamiliar with it the possibility of a carotid aneurysm, hemangioma, brain tumor, or sinusitis may be suggested. Appropriate roentgenograms and carotid arteriography will always exclude such conditions but usually are unnecessary. In the differential diagnosis orbital (nasociliary, supraorbital, Sluder's sphenopalatine) neuralgias must also be considered (see Chap. 324).

In the life history profile the clusters of headache may last for weeks. The clusters may be single or recur two, three or more times, with years of freedom in between, during which such precipitating factors as alcohol are no longer effective. Often the pain involves the same orbit in each cluster.

The relationship of the cluster headache to migraine remains conjectural. A portion of the cases have a background of migraine, which led to the earlier postulation of migrainous neuralgia, but the majority do not.

Tension headache and various other cranial pains with psychiatric disease The headache is usually bilateral, often with diffuse extension over the top of the cranium. Occipital-nuchal localization is also common. Although the sensation may be described as pain, close questioning may uncover other sensations, viz., fullness, tightness, pressure (as if the head is surrounded by a band or in a vise), on which waves of aching pain are engrafted. The onset of a given attack is more gradual than in migraine and not infrequently is added intermittently to a pressure ache which lasts unremittingly for weeks or months. In fact, this is the only type of headache that exhibits the peculiarity of being absolutely continuous day and night for long periods of time. Although sleep may be possible, whenever the patient awakens, the headache is present; and the common analgesic remedies have no beneficial effect unless the pain is intense and of aching type.

As to mechanism, the ascription of it to sustained muscle activity, shown by the electromyogram, is only a partial explanation. The continuous pressing quality of milder cephalic sensations at times when the patient is relaxed hardly seems to be attributable to physiologic stimulation and suggests instead that the condition is maintained by focused attention on the head (occasioned sometimes by worry and fear of intracranial disease). Moreover, it must be remembered that all types of headache in their late stages may give rise to muscle tension and that this is of an aching rather than a pressure type. In contrast to migraine, in which pain is periodic and lifelong, with tendency to lessen in late adult years, tension headache occurs more often in middle age and usually coincides with anxiety and depression in the trying times of life. Many premenstrual headaches are of this type, and there is an increased incidence of this type of tension headache at menopause.

Psychologic studies of groups of patients with tension headaches have revealed prominent symptoms of anxiety, hypochondriasis, and, to a lesser extent, depression. When psychiatric syndromes are searched for in headache patients, it is evident that the majority of those with anxiety neurosis, hysteria, obsessive-compulsive neurosis, and schizophrenia, in which anxiety is a prominent symptom, exhibit this type of headache. With endogenous and reactive depressions it is less frequent, though the incidence is increased in the late-life involutional and hypochondriacal states (see Chap. 341). Migraine and traumatic headaches may be complicated by tension headache.

Other odd cephalic pains, e.g., boring pains, "clavus hystericus," may occur in hysteria and raise perplexing problems in diagnosis. Their bizarre character, persistence in the face of every known therapy, absence of other signs of disease, and the presence of the stigmata of the hysterical personality provide the basis for correct diagnosis (see Chap. 339).

Headache of angioma and aneurysm The temporal profile of any given attack shows the onset to be sudden or very acute, with the pain reaching a peak within minutes. Neurologic disturbances such as unilateral numbness, weakness, or aphasia tend to occur after the onset of headache and to outlast it. Should hemorrhage occur, the headache is often extremely severe and localizes more towards the occiput and neck, lasting many days in association with stiff neck. A cranial or cervical bruit and, of course, blood in the cerebrospinal fluid establish the diagnosis, but it may require verification by arteriography. The claim that vascular malformations may give rise to migraine is probably untenable. Statistical data show migraine to be no more frequent in this group of patients than in the general population. Of course, vascular lesions may exist for long periods of time without headache, or the latter may develop many years after other manifestations, such as epilepsy and hemiplegia (see Chap. 326).

TRAUMATIC HEADACHE Severe, chronic, continuous or intermittent headaches appear as the cardinal symptom of two posttraumatic syndromes, separable in each instance from the headache that immediately follows head injury (i.e., that of scalp laceration and contusion with sanguineous cerebrospinal fluid and increased intracranial pressure). The latter lasts several days or a week or two.

The headache of chronic subdural hematoma

Headache and dizziness of fluctuating severity, followed by drowsiness, stupor, coma, and hemiparesis, are the usual manifestations of chronic subdural hematoma. The head injury may have been minor and forgotten by patient and family. The headaches are deep-seated, steady, unilateral or generalized, and respond to the usual analgesic drugs. The typical attack profile of the headache and other symptoms is one of increasing frequency and severity over several weeks or months. Diagnosis is now established by arteriography (see Chap. 327).

Headache of posttraumatic nervous instability

Here, headache is a prominent feature of a complex syndrome comprised of giddiness, fatigability, insomnia, nervousness, trembling, irritability, inability to concentrate, and tearfulness. The pain undergoes many variations from one day to another and also a highly individualized pattern of localization. Often it centers on the site of injury, where there is also tenderness. Reference to throbbing pain as well as pressure is obtained. Particular importance is attached to its persistence, intensification by mental and physical effort, stooping, noise, bright light, and confusion. The patient looks and acts much like a person in an agitated depression, and indeed, many neurologists believe such a state to be a posttraumatic neurosis or depression. The severity and duration of the headache bear no relation to the magnitude of the injury; some of the worst cases have had minor injuries without loss of consciousness, and major injuries may leave no headache in their wake. Unsettled litigation surely prolongs the discomfort and disability. The observation that histamine may reproduce some of the more severe headaches has suggested to some a vascular origin. Cephalic tenderness and aching pain sharply localized to the scar of the scalp laceration represent in all probability a different problem, raising the question of a traumatic neuralgia. With whiplash injuries to the neck, unilateral retroauricular or occipital pain suggests trauma of the corresponding nerves (see Chaps. 9 and 327).

Headaches of brain tumor Headache is the outstanding symptom of cerebral tumor. Unfortunately, the quality of the pain has no specific feature. It tends to be deep-seated, nonthrobbing (or throbbing), and aching or bursting. Attacks last a few minutes to an hour or more and occur once or many times during the day. Activity and frequent change in the position of the head may provoke pain, while rest in bed diminishes its frequency. Nocturnal awakening because of pain, although typical, is by no means diagnostic. Unexpected forceful (projectile) vomiting may punctuate the illness in its later stages. As the tumor grows the pain becomes more frequent and severe; it sometimes is nearly continuous terminally. But there are exceptions, some headaches being mild and tolerable, others as agonizing as that of the headache of bacterial meningitis and subarachnoid hemorrhage. If unilateral, the headache is homolateral to the tumor in 9 out of 10 patients. Supratentorial tumors are felt anterior to the interauricular circumference of the skull; posterior fossa tumors behind this line. Bifrontal and bioccipital headache, coming on after unilateral headaches, signifies the development of increased intracranial pressure.

APPROACH TO THE PATIENT WITH HEADACHE

Obviously very different possibilities are raised by a patient who presents himself for the first time in his life with severe headache and another one who has had recurrent headache over a period of years. The chances of uncovering the cause in the first instance are much greater than in the latter, and some of the underlying conditions (meningitis, subarachnoid hemorrhage, epidural hematoma, glaucoma, and purulent sinusitis) are more serious.

In searching for the cause of recurrent headache one should investigate the status of cardiovascular and renal systems by blood pressure and urine examination, eyes (fundoscopic, intraocular pressure, and refraction), the sinuses by transillumination and x-rays, the cranial arteries by palpation (and biopsy?), the cervical spine by effect of passive movement and x-rays, the nervous system by neurologic examination, and psychic function by mental status.

Hypertension is, of course, frequent in the general population and is always difficult to prove as a cause of recurrent headaches. Minor elevations of blood pressure may be a result rather than the cause of nervous tension. No doubt severe hypertension with diastolic blood pressures of over 100 mm Hg is regularly associated with headache, and measures which reduce blood pressure can be shown to relieve the headache. But it is the moderate hypertensive when subject to numerous and severe headaches who gives concern. If headache is severe and frequent, there is usually an underlying anxiety or tension state or a common migraine syndrome that is exacerbated by blood vessel disease. The mechanism of the puzzling hypertensive phenomenon of occipital pain, present on awakening in the morning and wearing off during the day, is uncertain.

The adolescent with daily frontal headaches represents a special type of problem. Often their relationship to eyestrain is unclear, and refraction of the eyes and new eyeglasses do not relieve the condition. Anxiety or tension is probably a factor in such cases, but it is difficult to be certain of a causal relationship. Some of the most persistent and inexplicable headaches, which have led to a survey by a battery of diagnostic procedures for tumor, have proved in the end to be caused by depression.

Equally puzzling is the somber, tense adult whose primary complaint is headache, or the migrainous person who in late life or at menopause begins to have daily headaches. Here it becomes important to assess mental status along the lines suggested in Chaps. 14, 26, and 338, looking for evidences of anxiety, depression, and hypochondriasis. The quality and persistence of the headache are suggestive of the possibility of psychiatric illness. Sometimes, a direct question as to the patient's idea of what is the matter may elicit suspicion and fear of brain tumor.

The most worrisome type of patient is the one who has only headache of increasing frequency and severity over a period of months or a year or so. Usually it becomes necessary to resort to a complete neurologic survey, including careful inspection of optic disk and roentgenograms of skull, electroencephalogram, lumbar puncture, and radioactive-isotope scanning to rule out brain tumor, abscess, or subdural hematoma.

Every elderly person with severe headache of some few days, or weeks, duration should be considered as possibly having cranial arteritis. Increased sedimentation rate, fever, and anemia may be conjoined, but only in a minority of cases, unfortunately. The finding of a thickened temporal artery is important, and arterial biopsy and response to corticosteroids establish the diagnosis; treatment with corticosteroids often relieves the pain.

TREATMENT The most important steps in the treatment of headache are those measures which uncover and remove the underlying disease or functional disturbance.

For the common everyday headache due to fatigue, stuffy atmosphere, or excessive use of alcohol and tobacco, it is simple enough to advise avoidance of the offending activity or agent, and symptomatic therapy in the form of acetylsalicylic acid, 0.6 g (in the form of aspirin or Anacin) will suffice. Some patients who invariably have headache when constipated and hypochondriacs who not infrequently suffer incapacitating headache, fatigue, and depression whenever bowel elimination does not meet their expectation, are not easily helped. Certainly, simple explanation, an anticonstipation regimen, and drugs which counteract depression (see Chap. 341) are preferable to the continuous use of analgesics. Premenstrual headache, if troublesome, can usually be helped by the use of a diuretic compound for the week preceding the menstrual period and a mixture of mild analgesic and tranquilizing medications (acetylsalicylic acid, 0.6 g, and phenobarbital, 30 mg). If the headaches are severe and incapacitating, they should be treated as common migraine (see Chap. 336).

Hypertensive headaches respond to agents which lower blood pressure and relieve muscle tension. Chlorothiazide (Diuril), 250 to 500 mg twice a day, and methyldopa (Aldomet), 250 to 500 mg per day, when combined with a small amount of phenobarbital, 15 mg t.i.d., have given the best results. Meprobamate, 200 mg t.i.d., or chlordiazepoxide HCl (Librium), 5 mg t.i.d., may be administered in place of phenobarbital. For the morning occipital ache a capsule containing sodium nitrite, 30 mg, caffeine sodium benzoate, 0.5 g, and acetophenetidin, 0.6 g, has been useful. A simplified method of treating this kind of headache is to supply the caffeine in a cup of strong black coffee and to give with it acetylsalicylic acid. Blocks under the head of the bed may be helpful.

The muscle tension headaches respond best to massage, relaxation, and a combination of drugs which relieve anxiety (phenobarbital, amobarbital, meprobamate, and chlordiazepoxide HCl) and pain [acetylsalicylic acid, propoxyphene HCl (Darvon), or oxycodone (Percodan)]. Stronger analgesic medication may be needed (codeine or meperidine HCl). Psychotherapy is usually not beneficial in this group of patients.

Recurrent vascular headaches (common migraine) and classic migraine should be treated according to the plan outlined in Chap. 336.

The headache of the syndrome of posttraumatic nervous instability requires supportive psychotherapy in the form of reassurance and frequent explanation of its benign and transient nature, a program of increasing physical activity, and drugs which allay anxiety and depression. Tender scars from scalp laceration may be novocainized repeatedly (subcutaneous injection of 5 ml of 1% procaine) with some degree of success. Settlement of litigation as soon as possible works to the patient's advantage.

Heat, massage, salicylates, and indomethacin (Indocin) or phenylbutazone (Butazolidine) usually effect some improvement in those arthritic diseases of the cervical spine which are associated with cervicocranial pain (see Chap. 9).

Corticosteroid therapy is indicated in cranial arteritis to prevent disastrous blindness by occlusion of the ophthalmic arteries. The headaches of cranial tumor often respond surprisingly well to large doses of methylprednisolone acetate and like compounds.

In conclusion, it is well to mention the importance of general hygienic measures. Young physicians in particular are apt to seek a specific therapy for each headache syndrome and give little thought to the general health of the patient. We have observed that most of the recurrent and chronic headaches are likely to be more severe and disabling whenever the patient becomes nervous, sick, and tired. A well-rounded diet, adequate rest, a reasonable amount of physical exercise, and a balanced view of the sources of daily anxieties and how to cope with them should be the goal of all therapeutic programs.

REFERENCES

FRIEDMAN AP: *Research and Clinical Studies in Headache,* Baltimore: Williams & Wilkins, 1967

LANCE JW: *The Mechanism and Management of Headache,* London: Butterworth, 1969

VINKEN PJ, BRUYN GW: *Handbook of Clinical Neurology,* vol. 5, *Headache and Cranial Neuralgias,* Amsterdam: North-Holland Publishing Company, 1968

WOLFF HG: *Headache and Other Pain,* Fair Lawn, N.J.: Oxford University Press, 1947

7 PAIN IN THE CHEST

EUGENE BRAUNWALD
T. R. HARRISON

There is little parallelism between the severity of chest pain and the gravity of its cause. Therefore, a frequent problem in patients who complain of chest pain involves the distinction of disorders of trivial significance from coronary artery disease and other serious disorders. An incorrect positive diagnosis of a hazardous condition such as angina pectoris is likely to have harmful psychologic and economic consequences, while failure to recognize a serious disorder, such as coronary artery disease or mediastinal tumor, may result in the dangerous delay of much-needed treatment.

The apparently bizarre radiation of pain arising in the thoracic viscera can usually be explained in terms of the known facts concerning nerve supply (Chap. 5). One occasionally sees a patient with extension of pain to a location which cannot be logically explained. In most instances, such a person will be found to have more than one disorder capable of causing pain in the chest. The presence of one condition may affect the radiation of the pain produced by the other disorder. For example, when the pain of angina pectoris extends to the back or abdomen, the patient may be found to have also a significant degree of spinal arthritis or an upper abdominal disorder, such as hiatus hernia, disease of the gallbladder, pancreatitis, or peptic ulcer. The common tendency to assume that the presence of an objective abnormality, such as a hiatus hernia or an electrocardiographic abnormality, necessarily means that an atypical chest pain arises in the stomach or the heart is to be strongly condemned. Such an assumption is justified only if a careful history indicates that the behavior of the pain is entirely compatible with the site of origin suggested by the objective finding.

THE LEFT-ARM MYTH There is a long tradition, widely accepted by physicians and laymen, that pain in the left arm, especially when appearing in conjunction with chest pain, has a unique and ominous significance as being almost certain evidence of the presence of ischemic heart disease. This is a myth that has neither theoretic nor clinical foundation. From a theoretic standpoint, any disorder involving the deep afferent fibers of the left upper thoracic region should be capable of causing pain in the chest, the left arm, or both areas. Hence a pain of trivial significance arising in skeletal tissues innervated by upper (first to fourth) thoracic nerves may produce left-arm-area pain; almost any condition capable of causing pain in the chest may induce radiation to the left arm. Such localization is common not only in patients with coronary disease but also in those with numerous other types of chest pain. Although pain due to myocardial ischemia most frequently is substernal, radiates down the ulnar aspect of the left arm (Chap. 240), and is pressing and constricting in nature, the location, radiation, and quality of pain are of less diagnostic significance than the behavior of the pain, in terms of the conditions which induce it and relieve it.

Most persons also believe that cardiac pain is situated in the region of the left breast, and therefore left inframammary pain is one of the common symptoms that bring the patient to seek medical advice. It differs radically from the pain due to myocardial hypoxia, i.e., angina pectoris, in that it is usually a long-lasting, dull ache, occasionally accentuated by sharp stabs. Such pain, is frequently observed in patients who are tense, easily fatigued, unusually anxious, or psychoneurotic, or who have neurocirculatory asthenia. In contrast to angina pectoris, such precordial pain has no relationship to exertion and may be accompanied by tenderness over the precordium.

Only the more important or common conditions causing chest pain will be considered in this chapter.

PAIN DUE TO OXYGEN DEFICIENCY OF THE MYOCARDIUM

PHYSIOLOGIC CONSIDERATIONS OF THE CORONARY CIRCULATION Pain due to myocardial ischemia occurs when the oxygen supply to the heart is deficient in relation to the oxygen need. The oxygen consumption of this organ is closely related to the physiologic effort made during contraction. It is dependent primarily on three factors: (1) the tension developed by the myocardium, (2) the contractile (inotropic) state of the myocardium, and (3) the heart rate. When these three factors remain constant, or almost so, an elevation of stroke volume produces an efficient type of response because it leads to an increase in the external work of the heart (i.e., in the product of cardiac output and arterial pressure) with little accompanying augmentation of myocardial oxygen requirements. Thus, a rise in flow load causes less increment in myocardial oxygen consumption than does a comparable increase in cardiac work per minute brought about by elevation either of pressure or of heart rate. However, the net effects of these hemodynamic variables depend not on oxygen need alone, but rather on the balance between the demand and the supply of oxygen. The heart is always active, and the coronary venous blood is normally much more desaturated than that from other areas of the body. Thus the removal of more oxygen from each unit of blood, which is one of the adjustments commonly utilized by exercising skeletal muscle, is already employed in the heart, even in the basal state. Therefore, the heart must rely on an increase in the coronary blood flow for obtaining additional oxygen.

It follows, from hydrodynamic considerations, that the flow of blood through the coronary arteries is directly proportional to the pressure gradient between the aorta and the ventricular myocardium during systole and the ventricular cavity during diastole, but is proportional to the fourth power of the radius of the coronary arteries. Thus a relatively slight alteration in coronary diameter will produce a large change in coronary flow, provided that other factors remain constant. In the normal heart, coronary blood flow occurs primarily during diastole, when it is unopposed by myocardial constriction of the coronary vessels. Coronary flow is regulated primarily by myocardial oxygen needs, probably through the release of vasodilator metabolites. Although changes in coronary blood flow occur with activation of autonomic nerves to the coronary vessels, these alterations result primarily from the effects of these nervous stimuli on myocardial contraction and therefore on the heart's oxygen consumption.

The coronary dilatation which normally occurs during exercise and emotion results from the increased myocardial metabolism during these conditions and is impaired in patients with fixed coronary narrowing due to coronary arteriosclerosis. Thus, any condition in which increased heart rate, arterial pressure, or myocardial contractility occurs tends to precipitate anginal attacks by increasing myocardial oxygen needs in the face of impaired oxygen delivery. Bradycardia usually has the opposite effects, and this apparently explains the rarity of angina in patients with complete heart block, even when this disorder is associated with coronary disease.

CAUSES OF MYOCARDIAL HYPOXIA By far the most frequently underlying cause is organic narrowing of the coronary arteries secondary to coronary atherosclerosis. Less frequently, narrowing of the coronary orifices due to syphilitic aortitis or to distortion by a dissecting aneurysm may be responsible. There is no evidence that systemic arterial constriction or increased cardiac contractile activity (rise in heart rate or blood pressure, or increase in contractility due to liberation of catecholamines or adrenergic activity) due to emotion can precipitate angina unless there is also structural narrowing of the coronary vessels.

Aside from conditions which narrow the lumen of the coronary arteries, the only other frequent causes of myocardial hypoxia are disorders, such as aortic stenosis and/or regurgitation (Chap. 239), which cause a marked disproportion between the perfusion pressure and the ventricular work. Under such conditions the rise in left ventricular systolic pressure is not, as in hypertensive states, balanced by a corresponding elevation of aortic perfusion pressure. Therefore, an increase in heart rate is especially harmful in patients with aortic stenosis, because it shortens diastole more than systole and thereby decreases the total available perfusion time per minute.

Patients with marked *right ventricular hypertension* may have exertional pain which is, in most respects, identical with that of the common type of angina. It is likely that this discomfort results from relative ischemia of the right ventricle brought about by the increased oxygen needs and by the elevated intramural resistance, with sharp reduction of the normally large systolic pressure gradient which perfuses this chamber. Angina is common in patients with *syphilitic aortitis*, and the relative roles of aortic regurgitation and of coronary ostial narrowing are difficult to assess. The importance of tachycardia, decline in arterial pressure, thyrotoxicosis, or diminution in arterial oxygen content (such as occurs in anemia or arterial hypoxemia) in the production of myocardial hypoxia will be apparent from the above discussion. However, these are precipitating and aggravating factors rather than the underlying cause of angina; as already noted, the latter is, in almost all instances, coronary atherosclerosis.

EFFECTS OF MYOCARDIAL HYPOXIA The most common of these is anginal pain, which is considered in some detail in Chap. 240. It is usually described as a heavy pressure or squeezing, a sensation of strangling or constriction of the chest, or difficulty in breathing, and it occurs particularly on walking, especially after meals, on cold days against a wind or uphill. It is not a stabbing pain. It occurs with anger, excitement, and other emotional states; it is not precipitated by coughing or respiratory movements. When anginal pain is induced by walking, it forces the patient to stop or to reduce his speed; it is characteristically relieved by rest and nitroglycerin. The exact mechanism of the pain stimulus is still unknown, but it is probably related to an accumulation of metabolites within the heart muscle. The more severe the attack, the greater the radiation from the substernal areas to the left arm, especially its ulnar aspect. There is considerable variability in the amount of effort required to bring on anginal pain.

As a rule, myocardial infarction is associated with a pain similar in quality and distribution to that of angina but of great intensity and longer duration. The pain of myocardial infarction is not relieved by rest or by coronary dilator drugs and may require large doses of narcotics. It may be accompanied by diaphoresis, nausea, and hypotension.

In addition to chest pain, a second effect of myocardial ischemia consists of electrocardiographic changes (Chaps. 229 and 240). Many patients with angina have normal tracings between attacks, and the record may even remain normal during the episode of pain. However, often depression of the S–T segments appears in leads I, II, AVL, or in those from the left precordium during exertion. The finding of S–T segment depressions of a deep, ischemic type during an attack of pain, with a return to normal after the pain subsides, strongly suggests that the pain is anginal in origin. There is strong experimental evidence that such depressions, as well as the elevations which are usually seen in patients with infarction and are observed in a few patients during anginal attacks, are related to alterations in cellular ionic balance (Chap. 229). The value and limitation of electrocardiographic changes occurring after exercise in the diagnosis of angina pectoris are discussed in Chap. 240.

A third effect of myocardial hypoxia is an alteration in myocardial contraction. It has been shown that the left ventricular end-diastolic and pulmonary vascular pressures may rise during anginal attacks, particularly if they are prolonged. This indicates transient depression of left ventricular function, which is presumably induced by the decreased contractility of the ischemic areas. On auscultation a fourth heart sound is also frequently heard during the anginal episode; paradoxic pulsations may be evident on palpation of the precordium and can be recorded by apex cardiography.

Another characteristic effect of myocardial hypoxia is liability to sudden death (Chap. 34). This may never occur, despite thousands of anginal episodes. However, it may supervene early in the disease and even in the first attack. The usual mechanism is probably ventricular fibrillation, but occasionally in patients with impaired atrioventricular conduction sudden death may be due to ventricular standstill.

PAIN DUE TO IRRITATION OF SEROUS MEMBRANES OR JOINTS

PERICARDITIS The visceral surface of the pericardium is ordinarily insensitive to pain, as is the parietal surface, except in its lower portion, which has a relatively small number of pain fibers which are carried in the phrenic nerves. The pain associated with pericarditis is believed to be due to inflammation of the adjacent parietal pleura. These observations explain why noninfectious pericarditis (that associated with uremia and with myocardial infarction) and cardiac tamponade with relatively mild inflammation are usually painless or accompanied by mild pain, whereas infectious pericarditis, being nearly always more intense and spreading to the neighboring pleura, is usually associated with pain having some pleuritic features i.e., it is aggravated by breathing, coughing, etc. Since the central part of the diaphragm receives its sensory supply from the phrenic nerve (which arises from the third to fifth cervical segments of the spinal cord), pain arising from the lower parietal pericardium and central tendon of the diaphragm is felt characteristically at the tip of the shoulder, the adjoining trapezius ridge, and the neck. Involvement of the more lateral part of the diaphragmatic pleura, supplied by branches from the sixth to ninth intercostal nerves, causes pain not only in the anterior part of the chest but also in the upper part of the abdomen or corresponding region of the back, thus sometimes simulating the pain of acute cholecystitis or pancreatitis.

Pericarditis causes three distinct types of pain. (1) By far the commonest is the pleuritic pain, related to respiratory movements and aggravated by cough or deep inspiration, sometimes brought on by swallowing, because the esophagus lies just beyond the posterior portion of the heart, sometimes by change of bodily position. It is sharper, more left-sided, is frequently referred to the neck or flank, and lasts longer than the pain of angina pectoris. This type of pain is due to the pleuritic component of the pleuropericarditis so commonly present in the infectious forms. (2) The next commonest pericardial pain is the steady, crushing substernal pain which mimics that of acute myocardial infarction. The mechanism of this steady substernal pain is not certain, but the pain may arise from marked inflammation of the relatively insensitive inner parietal surface of the pericardium, or from irritated afferent cardiac nerve fibers lying in the periadventitial layers of the superficial coronary arteries. (3) The third type of pain, which is quite uncommon, is synchronous with the heartbeat and is felt at the left border of the heart and left shoulder. Occasionally two and rarely all three types of pain may be present simultaneously.

The painful syndromes which may follow trauma to or operations on the heart (i.e., the postcardiotomy syndrome) or myocardial infarction, are discussed in later chapters (Chaps. 240 and 241). Such pains often but not always arise in the pericardium.

Pleural pain is very common; it generally results from stretching of inflamed parietal pleura and may be identical with that of pericarditis. It occurs in fibrinous pleurisy, as well as when pneumonic processes reach the periphery of the lung. Pneumothorax and tumors involving the pleural space may also irritate the parietal pleura and cause pleural pain; the latter is sharp, knifelike, superficial in quality, and its aggravation by each breath and by coughing readily distinguishes it from the deep dull steady unwavering pain of myocardial ischemia.

The pain resulting from pulmonary embolism may resemble that of acute myocardial infarction, and in massive embolism it is located substernally. In patients with smaller emboli the pain is located more laterally and is pleuritic in nature. The pain of mediastinal emphysema (Chap. 261) may be intense and sharp and may radiate from the substernal region to the shoulders; often a distinct crepitus is heard. The pain associated with mediastinitis and mediastinal tumors usually resembles that of pleuritis but is more likely to be maximal in the substernal region, and the associated feeling of constriction or oppression may cause confusion with myocardial infarction. The pain due to *acute dissection of the aorta* or to an expanding aortic aneurysm results from stimulation of the adventitia; it is usually extremely severe, is localized to the center of the chest, lasts for hours, and requires unusually large amounts of analgesics for relief. It often radiates into the back but is not aggravated by changes in position or respiration.

The *costochondral and chondrosternal articulations* are the commonest sites of anterior chest pain. Objective signs in the form of swelling (Tietze's syndrome), redness, and heat are rare, but sharply localized tenderness is common. The pain may be "neuritic," i.e., darting and lasting for only a few seconds, or a dull ache enduring for hours or days. An associated feeling of tightness due to muscle spasm (see below) is frequent. When the discomfort endures for a few days only, a story of minor trauma or of some unaccustomed physical effort can often be obtained. The variety of this discomfort is common in persons with arthritis of the spine and also in patients with ischemic heart disease, but in many instances no associated disorder is found. It should be emphasized that *pressure on the chondrosternal and costochondral junctions is an essential part of the examination of every patient with chest pain.* A large percentage of patients with costochondral pain, especially those who also have minor and innocent T-wave alterations (Chap. 229), are erroneously labeled as having coronary disease. The dire consequences of such a mistake have already been emphasized.

Pain secondary to *subacromial bursitis* and *arthritis of the shoulder and spine* may be precipitated by exercise of the local area but not by general exertion. It may be brought about by passive movement of the involved area as well as by coughing.

PAIN DUE TO TISSUE DISRUPTION

Rupture or tear of a structure may give rise to pain that sets in abruptly and reaches its peak of intensity almost instantly. Such a story should arouse the suspicion of dissecting aortic aneurysm, pneumothorax, mediastinal emphysema, a cervical disk syndrome, or rupture of the esophagus. However, the patient may be too ill to recall the precise circumstances, or the pain may be atypical and increase gradually in severity. Likewise, other and more benign conditions, such as a slipped costal cartilage or an intercostal muscle cramp, may also produce pain with an abrupt onset.

PAIN DUE TO INCREASED MUSCLE TENSION

This is of two varieties, depending on whether the discomfort arises in skeletal or smooth muscle. Pain arising from skeletal muscle is very frequent, and the usual causes are discussed later in some detail. A very rare type is *intercostal cramp,* which, except for the location, is identical with the common night cramp in the calves. Here again, the coexistence of minor variations in the electrocardiogram may lead to a false positive diagnosis of ischemic heart disease.

It is likely that increased tension in visceral musculature is responsible for the chest pain associated with some esophageal disorders, the splenic flexure syndrome, aerophagia, and diverticulum of the stomach. There is uncertainty whether the same mechanism or pinching of nerve fibers causes the discomfort of hiatal hernia, a disorder that can mimic the pain of myocardial ischemia exactly as regards location, quality, and intensity but not as regards precipitating and alleviating factors.

CLINICAL ASPECTS OF THE COMMONER CAUSES OF CHEST PAIN

Some of the features of pericarditis have already been described, and those of the more serious causes of chest pain such as myocardial ischemia (angina pectoris and infarction), dissecting aneurysm, and disorders of the pleura, esophagus, stomach, duodenum, and pancreas are considered in the appropriate chapters dealing with these problems. Here, we are concerned with the discussion of those causes which are not considered in more detail elsewhere.

PAIN ARISING IN THE CHEST WALL OR UPPER EXTREMITY This may develop as a result of muscle or ligament strains brought on by unaccustomed exercise and felt in the costochondral or chondrosternal junctions or in the chest wall muscles. We mention the upper extremities and especially the left because of the deeply ingrained legend that pain in the left arm has a specific significance in indicting the heart. Other causes are *osteoarthritis* of the dorsal or thoracic spine and *ruptured cervical disks.* Pain in the left upper extremity and precordium may be due to compression of portions of the brachial plexus by a cervical rib or by spasm and shortening of the scalenus anticus muscle secondary to high fixation of the ribs and sternum. Finally, pains in the upper extremity (shoulder-hand syndrome) and in the pectoral muscles may, through unknown mechanisms, occur in patients with ischemic heart disease.

Skeletal pains in the chest wall or shoulder girdles or arms are usually recognized quite easily. Localized tenderness of the affected area is usually present, and the pain is sometimes clearly related to movements involving the painful locus. Thus deep breathing, turning or twisting of the chest, and movements of the shoulder girdle and arm will elicit and duplicate the pain of which the patient complains. The pain may be very brief, lasting only a few seconds, or full and aching and enduring for hours. The duration is, therefore, likely to be either longer or shorter than untreated anginal pain, which usually lasts for only a few minutes.

These skeletal pains often have a sharp or sticking quality. In addition, there is frequently a feeling of tightness, which is probably due to associated spasm of intercostal or pectoral muscles. This may produce the "morning stiffness" seen in so many skeletal disorders. The discomfort is unaffected by nitroglycerin but often is abolished by infiltration of the painful areas with procaine (Novocain). When chest wall pain is of recent origin and follows trauma, strain, or some unusual activity involving the pectoral muscles, it presents no problem in diagnosis. However, *long-standing skeletal pain is frequent in persons who also have angina pectoris.* Since both disorders are very common, this association may be coincidental. In other instances, the coronary disease appears to be responsible for the chest wall pain; the exact mechanism is uncertain but probably is similar to that responsible for the well-known shoulder-hand syndrome. This coexistence of the two different types of chest pain in the same patient is a frequent cause of a confusing history, because in the patient's mind the anginal needle may be hidden in the skeletal haystack. Thus every middle-aged or elderly patient who has long-standing anterior chest wall pain merits careful study for the presence of ischemic heart disease.

Detailed questioning may reveal that what was originally thought by the patient to be a single type of discomfort actually comprises two different pains, which, though similar in quality and area, differ as regards duration and initiating factors. When the history is inconclusive, the exercise electrocardiogram may furnish useful information concerning the existence of myocardial ischemia. It may be necessary also to learn by direct observation whether exercise alone or postprandial exertion, or even postprandial effort undertaken holding an ice cube, is capable of producing it. Repeated tests may be required, the effects of preceding placebos, as compared to nitroglycerin, on the amount of exertion required to induce the pain being compared. *The confusion created by the presence of innocent skeletal pain impairs the reliability of the history and is probably the commonest cause of errors—both positive and negative—in the diagnosis of angina pectoris.*

ESOPHAGEAL PAIN This usually presents as deep thoracic pain; it results from chemical (acid) irritation of the esophageal mucosa or from spasm of the esophageal muscle in the presence of an intraluminal obstruction, and characteristically follows deglutition. Accompanying dysphagia, regurgitation of undigested food, and weight loss direct attention to the esophagus (see Chaps. 37 and 281).

EMOTIONAL DISORDERS These are also common causes of chest wall pain. Usually, the discomfort is experienced as a sense of "tightness," sometimes called "aching," and occasionally it may be sufficiently severe as to be designated a pain of considerable magnitude. Since the discomfort has almost always the additional quality of tightness or constriction, and, furthermore, since it is often localized across the sternum, although it may be felt in other areas of the anterior part of the chest, it is not surprising that this type of pain is frequently confused with that of myocardial ischemia. Ordinarily, it lasts for a half hour or more and may persist for a day or less with slow fluctuation of intensity. The association with fatigue or emotional strain is usually clear, although this may not be recognized by the patient until called to his attention. The pain probably develops through unconscious and prolonged increase of muscle tone (as in frowning in the face, or as can be quickly produced in the hand by rigidly clenching the fist), often enhanced by an accompanying hyperventilation (by causing a contraction of the chest wall muscles similar to the painful tetany of the extremities). When the hyperventilation and/or the associated adrenergic effect due to anxiety also causes innocent changes in the T waves and S–T segments, the confusion with coronary disease is strengthened. However, the long duration of the pain, the lack of any relation to exertion but association rather with fatigue or tension, and the usually periodic occurrence on successive days without any limitation of capacity for exercise usually make the differentiation from ischemic pain quite clear.

As compared with these two causes (the chest wall muscle and ligament strains and the contraction of the pectoral muscles due to reflex influences, fatigue, or tension), the various other conditions that may cause skeletal discomfort are uncommon and readily recognized after appropriate observation: spinal arthritis, herpes zoster, anterior scalene and hyperabduction syndromes, malignant disease of the ribs, etc.

OTHER CAUSES OF CHEST PAIN The several *abdominal disorders* which may at times mimic anginal pain may usually be suspected from the history, which, as in esophageal pain, ordinarily indicates some relationship to swallowing, eating, belching, etc. Pain resulting from gastric or duodenal ulcer (Chap. 282) is epigastric or substernal, commences about 1 to 1½ hr after meals, and is usually promptly relieved by antacids or milk. The gastrointestinal roentgenogram will be of crucial significance, and roentgenographic examination is also often helpful in differentiating biliary, gastrointestinal, aortic, pulmonary, and skeletal disease pain from angina pectoris. It should be emphasized again that the demonstration of the presence of a coexistent abdominal disorder such as a hiatus hernia does not constitute proof that the chest pain of which the patient complains is due to this. Such disorders are frequently asymptomatic and are not at all uncommon in patients who also have angina pectoris.

Substernal discomfort also frequently occurs in the presence of *tracheobronchitis;* it is described as a burning sensation accentuated by coughing. A variety of *disorders involving the breast,* including inflammatory breast disease, benign and malignant tumors, as well as mastodynia, are common causes of thoracic pain. The localization and superficial swelling and tenderness are of diagnostic importance.

APPROACH TO THE PATIENT WITH PAIN IN THE CHEST

Most persons with this complaint will fall into one of two general groups. The first consists of persons with prolonged and often severe pain without obvious initiating factors. Such persons will frequently be gravely ill. The problem is that of differentiating such serious conditions as myocardial infarction, dissecting aneurysm, and pulmonary embolism from each other and from less grave causes. In some such instances, the careful history will provide significant clues, while objective evidence of crucial importance will appear within the subsequent 2 or 3 days. Thus, when the initial examinations are not decisive, a watch-and-wait policy, with repeated electrocardiograms coupled with measurements of serum enzymes, lung scans, and chest roentgenograms, will commonly provide the correct answer.

The second group of patients comprises those who have brief episodes of pain and are otherwise in apparently excellent health. Here, the resting electrocardiogram will rarely supply decisive information, but records taken during or immediately after exercise will often reveal characteristic changes (Chap. 240). However, in many instances it is the study of the subjective phenomenon, i.e., of the pain itself, that will lead to the diagnosis. Of the several methods of investigation which are available for such patients, three are of cardinal importance.

A detailed and *meticulous history* of the behavior of the pain is the most important method. The location, radiation, quality, intensity, and, especially, duration of the episodes are important. Even more so is the story of the aggravating and alleviating factors. Thus a history of sharp aggravation by breathing, coughing, or other respiratory movements will usually point toward the pericardium (because of the associated pleuropericarditis) or mediastinum as the site, although chest wall pain is likewise affected by respiratory motions. Similarly, a pain which regularly appears on rapid walking and vanishes within a few minutes upon standing still suggests the diagnosis of angina pectoris, although here, once again, a similar story will rarely be obtained from patients with skeletal disorders.

When the history is inconclusive, the *study of the patient at the time of the spontaneous episode* will often supply crucial information. Thus the electrocardiogram, which may be normal both at rest and after exercise in the absence of pain, will occasionally demonstrate striking changes when recorded during an anginal episode. Similarly, radiographic study of the esophagus or of the stomach may show no evidence of cardiospasm or of hiatal hernia except when the observation is made during the pain.

The third method of study represents the *attempt to produce and alleviate the pain at will.* This procedure is necessary only when doubt exists following the history or when needed for psychotherapeutic purposes. Thus the demonstration that a localized pain, which can be reproduced by pressure on the chest, is completely relieved by local infiltration with procaine will often be of conclusive importance in convincing the patient that the heart is not the site. The discomfort due to distention of the stomach or of the splenic flexure with air is frequently mistaken by the patient, and occasionally by the physician, for pain of cardiac origin. The simple demonstration that the pain can be reproduced exactly by passing a tube in the appropriate area and inflating it with air may be not only of diagnostic but also of psychotherapeutic value. However, the demonstration that such procedures will reproduce the patient's pain may be misleading in persons who have angina in addition to another disorder. It may, therefore, be necessary to study also the effect of exercise on the pain and on the electrocardiogram.

When, as is not rarely the case, the history is atypical, the correct diagnosis of angina pectoris will often depend in large measure on the response to nitroglycerin. Here, a number of pitfalls should be avoided. If the patient has previously had the drug, careful questioning may be necessary to avoid errors. Thus, relief of pain after its sublingual administration does not necessarily prove that there is a cause-and-effect relationship. It is necessary to be certain that the pain vanishes more rapidly (usually within 5 min) and more completely when the drug is used than when it is not employed. A false negative impression concerning the effect of nitroglycerin may be the result of the use of a deteriorated preparation which has been exposed to light. In doubtful instances, repeated exercise tests, with and without preceding administration of nitroglycerin, are necessary. The demonstration that the time required for a given exercise to produce pain is consistently and considerably longer when it is undertaken within a few minutes after a sublingual nitroglycerin pill than after a placebo may, in some instances, represent the sole method for accurate recognition of angina pectoris. A completely negative response to such repeated tests constitutes almost conclusive evidence against angina.

In patients in whom the question of whether there is coronary disease cannot be resolved despite the aforementioned clinical and laboratory tests, including exercise electrocardiography (Chap. 240), cardiac catheterization and coronary arteriography may be required. A useful stress test that can be carried out at the time of catheterization is to elevate cardiac frequency in stepwise fashion; the development of S–T segment depressions on the electrocardiogram and the reproduction of the pain support the diagnosis of myocardial ischemia. Coronary arteriography will show severe (more than 60 percent) reduction of the lumen in patients with obstructive coronary artery disease (see Chaps. 231 and 240).

REFERENCES

BRAUNWALD E: The determinants of myocardial oxygen consumption. Physiologist 12:65, 1969

BURCH GE et al: Cardiac causalgia. Am Heart J 76:725, 1968

DRESSLER W: Angina pectoris, chap. IV in *Clinical Aids in Cardiac Diagnosis,* New York: Grune & Stratton, 1970

HURST JW, LOGUE RB: Symptoms due to heart disease, chap. II in *The Heart,* 2d ed., New York: McGraw-Hill, 1970

KEELE KD: Pain complaint threshold in relation to pain of cardiac infarction. Br Med J 1:670, 1968

Pain and its clinical management. Med Clin North Am 52:1, 1968

SMITH JR, PAINE R: Thoracic pain, chap. 8 in *Signs and Symptoms,* 5th ed., eds CM Mac Bryde, RS Blacklow, Philadelphia: Lippincott, 1970

WEHRMACHER WH: *Pain in the Chest,* Springfield, Ill.: Charles C Thomas, 1964, p. 403

WOOD P: The chief symptoms of heart disease, chap. 1 in *Diseases of the Heart and Circulation,* 3d ed., Philadelphia: Lippincott, 1968

8 ABDOMINAL PAIN

WILLIAM SILEN

The correct interpretation of acute abdominal pain is one of the most challenging demands made of any physician. Since proper therapy often requires urgent action, the luxury of the leisurely approach suitable for the study of other conditions is frequently denied. Few other clinical situations demand greater experience and judgment, because the most catastrophic of events may be forecast by the subtlest of symptoms and signs. Nowhere in medicine is a meticulously executed detailed history and physical examination of greater importance. The etiologic classification in Table 8-1, although not complete, forms a useful frame of reference for the evaluation of patients with abdominal pain.

The diagnosis of "acute or surgical abdomen" so often heard in emergency wards is not an acceptable one because of its often misleading and erroneous connotation. The most obvious of "acute abdomens" may not require operative intervention, and the mildest of abdominal pains may herald the onset of an urgently correctible lesion. Any patient with abdominal pain of recent onset requires early and thorough evaluation with specific attempts at accurate diagnosis.

SOME MECHANISMS OF PAIN ORIGINATING IN THE ABDOMEN

Inflammation of the parietal peritoneum The pain of parietal peritoneal inflammation is steady and aching in character and is located directly over the inflamed area, its exact reference being possible because it is transmitted by overlapping somatic nerves supplying the parietal peritoneum. The intensity of the pain is dependent upon the type and amount of foreign substance to which the peritoneal surfaces are exposed in a given period of time. For example, the sudden release into the peritoneal cavity of a small quantity of *sterile* acid gastric juice causes much more pain than the same amount of grossly contaminated neutral fecal material. Enzymatically active pancreatic juice incites more pain and inflammation than does the same amount of sterile bile containing no potent enzymes. Blood and urine are often so bland as to go undetected if exposure of the peritoneum has not been sudden and massive. In the case of bacterial contamination, such as in pelvic inflammatory disease, the pain is frequently of low intensity early in the illness until bacterial multiplication has caused the elaboration of irritating substances.

So important is the rate at which the irritating material is applied to the peritoneum that cases of perforated peptic ulcer may be associated with entirely different

TABLE 8-1
Some important causes of abdominal pain

- *I* Pain originating in the abdomen
  - *A* Parietal peritoneal inflammation
    - *1* Bacterial contamination, e.g., perforated appendix, pelvic inflammatory disease
    - *2* Chemical irritation, e.g., perforated ulcer, pancreatitis, mittelschmerz
  - *B* Mechanical obstruction of hollow viscera
    - *1* Obstruction of the small or large intestine
    - *2* Obstruction of the biliary tree
    - *3* Obstruction of the ureter
  - *C* Vascular disturbances
    - *1* Embolism or thrombosis
    - *2* Vascular rupture
    - *3* Pressure or torsional occlusion
    - *4* Sickle-cell anemia
  - *D* Abdominal wall
    - *1* Distortion or traction of mesentery
    - *2* Trauma or infection of muscles
    - *3* Distention of visceral surfaces, e.g., hepatic or renal capsules
- *II* Pain referred from extraabdominal sources
  - *A* Thorax—e.g., pneumonia, referred pain from coronary occlusion
  - *B* Spine—e.g., radiculitis from arthritis
  - *C* Genitalia—e.g., torsion of the testicle
- *III* Metabolic causes
  - *A* Exogenous
    - *1* Black widow spider bite
    - *2* Lead poisoning and others
  - *B* Endogenous
    - *1* Uremia
    - *2* Diabetic coma
    - *3* Porphyria
    - *4* Allergic factors (C′1 esterase deficiency)
- *IV* Neurogenic causes
  - *A* Organic
    - *1* Tabes dorsalis
    - *2* Herpes zoster
    - *3* Causalgia and others
  - *B* Functional

clinical pictures dependent only upon the rapidity with which the gastric juice enters the peritoneal cavity.

The pain of peritoneal inflammation is invariably accenturated by pressure or changes in tension of the peritoneum, whether produced by palpation or by movement, as in coughing or sneezing. Consequently, the patient with peritonitis lies quietly in bed, preferring to avoid motion, in contrast to the patient with colic, who may writhe incessantly.

Another of the characteristic features of peritoneal irritation is tonic reflex spasm of the abdominal musculature, localized to the involved body segment. The intensity of the tonic muscle spasm accompanying peritoneal inflammation is dependent upon the location of the inflammatory process, the rate at which it develops, and the integrity of the nervous system. Spasm over a perforated retrocecal appendix or perforated ulcer into the lesser peritoneal sac may be minimal or absent because of the protective effect of overlying viscera. As in pain of peritoneal inflammation, a slowly developing process often greatly attenuates the degree of muscle spasm. Catastrophic abdominal emergencies such as a perforated ulcer have been repeatedly associated with minimal or occasionally no detectable pain or muscle spasm in obtunded, seriously ill, debilitated elderly patients or in psychotic patients.

Obstruction of hollow viscera The pain of obstruction of hollow abdominal viscera is classically described as intermittent, or colicky. Yet the lack of a truly cramping character should not be misleading, because distention of a hollow viscus may produce steady pain with only very occasional exacerbations. Although not nearly as well localized as the pain of parietal peritoneal inflammation, some useful generalities can be made concerning its distribution.

The colicky pain of obstruction of small intestine is usually periumbilical or supraumbilical and is poorly localized. As the intestine becomes progressively dilated with loss of muscular tone, the colicky nature of the pain may become less apparent. With superimposed strangulating obstruction, pain may spread in the lower lumbar region if there is traction on the root of the mesentery. Pain arising in the colon is usually perceived in the region involved by the pathologic process.

Sudden distention of the biliary tree produces a steady rather than colicky type of pain; hence the term "biliary colic" is misleading. Acute distention of the gallbladder usually causes pain in the right upper quadrant with radiation to the right posterior region of the thorax or to the tip of the right scapula, and distention of the common bile duct is often associated with pain in the epigastrium radiating to the upper part of the lumbar region. Considerable variation is common, however, so that differentiation between these may be impossible. The typical subscapular pain or lumbar radiation is frequently absent. Gradual dilatation of the biliary tree as in carcinoma of the head of the pancreas may cause no pain or only a mild aching sensation in the epigastrium or right upper quadrant. The pain of distention of the pancreatic ducts is similar to that described for distention of the common bile duct but in addition is very frequently accentuated by recumbency and relieved by the upright position.

Obstruction of the urinary bladder results in dull suprapubic pain, usually low in intensity. Restlessness without specific complaint of pain may be the only sign of a distended bladder in an obtunded patient. In contrast, acute obstruction of the intravesicular portion of the ureter is characterized by severe suprapubic and flank pain which radiates to the penis, scrotum, or inner aspect of the upper region of the thigh. Obstruction of the ureteropelvic junction is felt as pain in the costovertebral angle, whereas obstruction of the remainder of the ureter is associated with flank pain, which often extends into the corresponding side of the abdomen.

Vascular disturbances A frequent misconception, despite abundant experience to the contrary, is that pain associated with intraabdominal vascular disturbances is sudden and catastrophic in nature. The pain of embolism or thrombosis of the superior mesenteric artery or that of impending rupture of an abdominal aortic aneurysm certainly may be severe and diffuse. Yet just as frequently, the patient with occlusion of the superior mesenteric artery has only mild continuous diffuse pain for 2 or 3 days before vascular collapse or findings of peritoneal inflammation appear. The early, seemingly insignificant discomfort is caused by hyperperistalsis rather than peritoneal inflammation. Indeed, absence of tenderness and rigidity in the presence of continuous diffuse pain in a patient likely to have vascular disease is quite characteristic of occlusion of the superior mesenteric artery. Abdominal pain with radiation to the sacral region, flank, or genitalia should always signal the possible presence of a rupturing abdominal aortic aneurysm. This pain may persist over a period of several days before rupture and collapse occur.

Abdominal wall Pain arising from the abdominal wall is usually constant and aching. Movement and pressure accentuate the discomfort and muscle spasm. In the case of hematoma of the rectus sheath, now most frequently encountered in association with anticoagulant therapy, a mass may be present in the lower quadrants of the abdomen. Simultaneous involvement of muscles in other parts of the body usually serves to differentiate myositis of the abdominal wall from an intraabdominal process which might cause pain in the same region.

REFERRED PAIN IN ABDOMINAL DISEASES Pain referred to the abdomen from the thorax, spine, or genitalia may prove a vexing problem in differential diagnosis, because diseases of the upper part of the abdominal cavity such as acute cholecystitis, perforated ulcer, or subphrenic abscesses are frequently associated with intrathoracic complications. A most important, yet often forgotten, dictum is that the possibility of intrathoracic disease must be considered in every patient with abdominal pain, especially if the pain is in the upper part of the abdomen. Systematic questioning and examination directed towards detecting the presence or absence of myocardial or pulmonary infarction, pneumonia, pericarditis, or esophageal disease (the intrathoracic diseases which most often masquerade as abdominal emergencies) will often provide sufficient clues to establish the proper diagnosis. Diaphragmatic pleuritis resulting from pneumonia or pulmonary infarction may cause pain in the right upper quadrant and pain in the supraclavicular area, the latter radiation to be sharply distinguished from the referred subscapular pain caused by acute distention of the extrahepatic biliary tree. The ultimate decision as to the origin of abdominal pain may require deliberate and planned observation over a period of several hours, during which time repeated questioning and examination will provide the proper explanation.

Referred pain of thoracic origin is often accompanied by splinting of the involved hemithorax with respiratory lag and decrease in excursion more marked than that seen in the presence of intraabdominal disease. In addition, apparent abdominal muscle spasm caused by referred pain will diminish during the inspiratory phase of respiration, whereas it is persistent throughout both respiratory phases if it is of abdominal origin. Palpation over the area of referred pain in the abdomen also does not usually accentuate the pain and in many instances actually seems to relieve it. The frequent coexistence of thoracic and abdominal disease may be misleading and confusing, so that differentiation might be difficult or impossible. For example, the patient with known biliary tract disease often has epigastric pain during myocardial infarction, or biliary colic may be referred to the precordium or left shoulder in a patient who has suffered previously from angina pectoris. For the explanation of the radiation of pain to a previously diseased area see Chap. 5.

Referred pain from the spine, which usually involves compression or irritation of nerve roots, is characteristically intensified by certain motions such as cough, sneeze, or strain and is associated with hyperesthesia over the involved dermatomes. Pain referred to the abdomen from the testicles or seminal vesicles is generally accentuated by the slightest pressure on either of these organs. The abdominal discomfort is of dull aching character and is poorly localized.

METABOLIC ABDOMINAL CRISES Pain of metabolic origin may simulate almost any other type of intraabdominal disease. Here several mechanisms may be at work. In certain instances, such as hyperparathyroidism, the metabolic disease itself may produce an intraabdominal process such as pancreatitis. Primary hyperlipemia may also be accompanied by severe pancreatitis, which can lead to unnecessary laparotomy unless recognized. C′1 esterase deficiency associated with angioneurotic edema is also often associated with episodes of severe abdominal pain. Whenever the cause of abdominal pain is obscure, a metabolic origin must always be considered. Abdominal pain is also the hallmark of familial Mediterranean fever (Chap. 225).

The problem of differential diagnosis is often not readily resolved. The pain of porphyria and of lead colic usually is difficult to distinguish from that of intestinal obstruction, because severe hyperperistalsis is a prominent feature of both. The pain of uremia or diabetes is nonspecific, and the pain and tenderness frequently shift in location and intensity. Diabetic acidosis may be precipitated by acute appendicitis or intestinal obstruction, so that if prompt resolution of the abdominal pain does not result from correction of the metabolic abnormalities, an underlying organic problem should be suspected. Black widow spider bites produce intense pain and rigidity of the abdominal muscles and of the back, an area infrequently involved in disease of intraabdominal origin.

NEUROGENIC CAUSES Causalgic pain may occur in diseases which injure nerves of sensory type. It has a burning character and is usually limited to the distribution of a given peripheral nerve. Normal stimuli such as touch or change in temperature may be transformed into this type of pain, which is also frequently present in a patient at rest. A helpful finding is the demonstration that cutaneous pain spots are now irregularly spaced, and this may be the only indication of an old nerve lesion underlying causalgic pain. Even though the pain may be precipitated by gentle palpation, rigidity of the abdominal muscles is absent, and the respirations are not disturbed. Distention of the abdomen is uncommon, and the pain has no relationship to the intake of food.

Pain arising from spinal nerves or roots comes and goes suddenly and is of a lancinating type (see p. 35). It may be caused by herpes zoster, impingement by arthritis, tumors, herniated nucleus pulposus, diabetes, or syphilis. Again it is not associated with food intake, abdominal distention, or changes in respiration. Severe muscle spasm, as in the gastric crises of tabes dorsalis, is common but is either relieved or is not accentuated by abdominal palpation. The pain is made worse by movement of the spine and is usually confined to a few dermatome segments. Hyperesthesia is very common.

Psychogenic pain conforms to none of the aforementioned patterns of disease. Here the mechanism is hard to define. The most common problem is the hysterical adolescent or young woman who develops abdominal pain; she frequently loses an appendix and other organs because of it. Ovulation or some other natural event that causes brief mild abdominal discomfort may be maximized as an abdominal catastrophe.

Psychogenic pain varies enormously in type and location but usually has no relation to meals. It is often at its onset markedly accentuated during the night. Nausea and vomiting are rarely observed, although occasionally the patient reports these symptoms. Spasm is seldom induced in the abdominal musculature and if present does not persist, especially if the attention of the patient can be distracted. Persistent localized tenderness is rare, and, if found, the muscle spasm in the area is inconsistent and often absent. Restriction of the depth of respiration is the most common respiratory abnormality, but this is in the nature of a smothering or choking sensation and is part of an anxiety state (see Chap. 14). It occurs in the absence of thoracic splinting or change in the respiratory rate.

APPROACH TO THE PATIENT WITH ABDOMINAL PAIN There are few abdominal conditions which require such urgent operative intervention that an orderly approach need be abandoned, no matter how ill the patient. Only those patients with exsanguinating hemorrhage must be rushed to the operating room immediately, but in such instances only a few minutes are required to assess the critical nature of the problem. Under these circumstances, all obstacles must be swept aside, adequate access for intravenous fluid replacement obtained, and the operation begun. Many patients of this type have died in the radiology department or the emergency room while awaiting such unnecessary examinations as electrocardiograms or films of the abdomen. *There are no contraindications to operation when massive hemorrhage is present.* Although exceedingly important, this situation fortunately is relatively rare.

Nothing will supplant an orderly painstakingly *detailed history*, which is far more valuable than any laboratory or roentgenologic examination. This kind of history is laborious and time-consuming, making it not especially popular even though a reasonably accurate diagnosis can be made on the basis of the history alone in the majority of cases. The *chronological sequence of events* in the patient's history is often more important than emphasis on the location of pain. If the examiner is sufficiently open-minded and unhurried, asks the proper questions, and listens, the patient will often himself provide the diagnosis. Careful attention should be paid to the extraabdominal regions which may be responsible for abdominal pain. An accurate menstrual history in a female patient is essential. Narcotics or analgesics should be withheld until a definitive diagnosis or a definitive plan has been formulated, because these agents often make it more difficult to secure and to interpret the history and physical findings.

In the examination, simple critical inspection of the patient, e.g., of his facies, position in bed, and respiratory activity, may provide valuable clues. The amount of information to be gleaned is directly proportional to the *gentleness* and thoroughness of the examiner. Once a patient with peritoneal inflammation has been examined in a brusque manner, accurate assessment by the next examiner becomes almost impossible. For example, eliciting rebound tenderness by sudden release of a deeply palpating hand in a patient with suspected peritonitis is cruel and unnecessary. The same information can be obtained by gentle percussion of the abdomen (rebound tenderness on a miniature scale), a maneuver which can be far more precise and localizing. Asking the patient to cough will elicit true rebound tenderness without the need for placing a hand on the abdomen. Furthermore, the brusque demonstration of rebound tenderness will startle and induce protective spasm in a nervous or worried patient in whom true rebound tenderness is not present. A palpable gallbladder will be missed if palpation is so brusque that voluntary muscle spasm becomes superimposed upon involuntary muscular rigidity.

As in history taking, there is no substitute for sufficient time spent in the examination. It is important to remember that abdominal signs may be minimal but nevertheless, if accompanied by consistent symptoms, may be exceptionally meaningful when carefully assessed. Signs may be virtually or actually totally absent in cases of pelvic peritonitis, so that careful *pelvic and rectal examinations are mandatory in every patient with abdominal pain.* The presence of tenderness on pelvic or rectal examination in the absence of other abdominal signs must not lead the examiner to exclude such important operative indications as perforated appendicitis, diverticulitis, twisted ovarian cyst, and many others.

Much attention has been paid to the presence or absence of peristaltic sounds, their quality, and their frequency. Auscultation of the abdomen is probably one of the least rewarding aspects of the physical examination of a patient with abdominal pain. Severe catastrophes, such as strangulating small-intestinal obstruction or perforated appendicitis, may occur in the presence of normal peristalsis. Conversely, when the proximal part of the intestine above an obstruction becomes markedly distended and edematous, peristaltic sounds may lose the characteristics of borborygmi and become weak or absent even when peritonitis is not present. It is usually the severe chemical peritonitis of sudden onset which is associated with the truly silent abdomen. Assessment of the patient's state of hydration is important. The hematocrit and urinalysis permit an accurate estimate of the severity of dehydration, so that adequate replacement can be carried out.

Laboratory examinations may be of enormous value in the assessment of the patient with abdominal pain, yet with but a few exceptions they rarely establish a diagnosis. Leukocytosis should never be the single deciding factor as to whether or not operation is indicated. A white blood cell count greater than 20,000 may be observed with perforation of a viscus, but pancreatitis, acute cholecystitis, pelvic inflammatory disease, and intestinal infarction may be associated with marked leukocytosis. A normal white blood cell count is by no means rare in cases of perforation of abdominal viscera. The diagnosis of anemia may be more helpful than the white blood cell count, especially when combined with the history.

The urinalysis is also of great value in indicating to some degree the state of hydration or to rule out severe renal disease, diabetes, or porphyria. Determination of the blood urea nitrogen, blood sugar, and serum bilirubin levels may also be helpful. The serum amylase determination is overrated, since in carefully controlled series of patients with proved pancreatitis where the determination has been done within the first 72 hr, the amylase was less than 200 Somogyi units in one-third of the cases, between 200 and 500 in another one-third, and greater than 500 in one-third. Since many diseases other than pancreatitis, e.g., perforated ulcer, strangulating intestinal obstruction, and acute cholecystitis, may be associated with very marked increase in the serum amylase, great care must be exercised in denying an operation to a patient solely on the basis of an elevated serum amylase level. The determination of the output of urinary amylase is probably more accurate than the estimation of the serum amylase in the diagnosis of pancreatitis.

Abdominal paracentesis has proved to be a safe and effective diagnostic maneuver in patients with acute abdominal pain. It is of special value in patients with blunt trauma to the abdomen where evaluation of the abdomen may be difficult because of other multiple injuries to the spine, pelvis, or ribs and where blood in the peritoneal cavity produces only a very mild peritoneal reaction. The gallbladder is the only organ which may continue to seep fluid following accidental perforation, so that the region of this organ must be assiduously avoided. Determination of the pH of the aspirated fluid to ascertain the site of a perforation is misleading, because even highly acid gastric juice is rapidly buffered by peritoneal exudate.

Plain and upright or lateral decubitus roentgenograms of the abdomen may be of the greatest value. They are usually unnecessary in patients with acute appendicitis or strangulated external hernias. However, in intestinal obstruction, perforated ulcer, and a variety of other conditions, films may be diagnostic. During a search for free air, the patient should be kept in the decubitus or upright position for at least 10 min before the appropriate film is taken lest a small pneumoperitoneum be missed. In rare instances, barium or water-soluble medium examination of the upper part of the gastrointestinal tract may demonstrate partial intestinal obstruction which may elude diagnosis by other means. If there is any question of obstruction of the colon, oral administration of barium sulfate should be avoided. On the other hand, barium enema is of inestimable value in cases of colonic obstruction and should be used with greater frequency where the possibility of perforation does not exist.

Sometimes, even under the best of circumstances with all available auxiliary aids and with the greatest of clinical skill, a definitive diagnosis cannot be established at the time of the initial examination. Nevertheless, despite lack of a clear anatomic diagnosis it may be abundantly clear to an experienced and thoughtful physician and surgeon on clinical grounds alone that operation is indicated. Should that decision be questionable, watchful waiting with repeated questioning and examination will often elucidate the true nature of the illness and indicate the proper course of action.

REFERENCES

COPE Z: *The Early Diagnosis of the Acute Abdomen,* 13th ed., Fair Lawn, N.J.: Oxford University Press, 1968

FITZ RH: Perforating inflammation of the vermiform appendix: With special reference to its early diagnosis and treatment. Trans Assoc Am Physicians 1:107, 1886

SILEN W et al: Strangulation obstruction of the small intestine. Arch Surg 85:121, 1962

STANILAND JR et al: Clinical presentation of acute abdomen: Study of 600 patients. Br Med J 2:393, 1972

9 PAIN IN THE BACK AND NECK

MICHEL JÉQUIER
RAYMOND D. ADAMS

The following remarks concern mainly the lower part of the back, since it is most frequently the site of disabling pain. The lower portions of the spine and pelvis, with their many muscular and tendinous attachments, are relatively inaccessible to palpation and also to inspection, even through the medium of x-ray. For want of reliable physical signs and laboratory tests, it is often necessary to depend on the patient's description of his pain, which may not be altogether accurate, and his behavior during the execution of certain maneuvers. Seasoned clinicians, for these reasons, come to appreciate the need of a systematic clinical approach, the description of which will be one of the main purposes of this chapter.

ANATOMY AND PHYSIOLOGY OF THE LOWER PART OF THE BACK The spine is roughly divisible into two parts: an anterior column of articulated vertebral bodies and intervertebral disks held together by the anterior and posterior longitudinal ligaments and annulus fibrosus which together constitute the supporting pillar of the body; and a posterior segment, consisting of pedicles and laminas, fused to form the walls of the spinal canal, which provides protection for the spinal cord, and for the attachment of muscles.

The stability of the spine depends on two types of

supporting structures, the ligamentous (passive) and muscular (active). Active muscular support and movement are contributed by the sacrospinalis, abdominal, glutei maximi, psoas, and hamstring muscles.

The vertebral and paravertebral structures derive their innervation from the recurrent branches of the spinal nerves. Pain endings and fibers have been demonstrated in the ligaments, muscles, periosteum of bone, outer layers of annulus fibrosus, and synovium of the articular facets. The sensory fibers from these structures and the sacroiliac and lumbosacral joints join to form the sinovertebral nerves which pass via the recurrent branches of the spinal nerves of the first sacral and the fifth to first lumbar vertebras into the gray matter of the corresponding segments of the spinal cord. Efferent fibers emerge from these segments and extend to the muscles through the same nerves. The sympathetic nerves contribute only to the innervation of blood vessels and appear to play no part in voluntary and reflex movement, though they do contain sensory fibers.

The parts of the back that possess the greatest freedom of movement and hence are most frequently subject to injury, are the lumbar and cervical. The majority of their movements are reflex and are the basis of posture.

GENERAL CLINICAL CONSIDERATIONS

Types of low back pain Of the several symptoms of disease of the spine (pain, stiffness or limitation of movement, and deformity), pain is of foremost importance by virtue of its frequency and its disabling effects. Four types of pain may be differentiated: local, referred, radicular, and that arising from secondary (protective) muscular spasm. One must identify these several types of pain by the patient's description, and here reliance is placed mainly on the character, location, and the conditions which modify them. The mechanism of the several types of pain has already been described in Chap. 5.

Local pain is caused by any pathologic process which impinges upon or irritates sensory endings. Involvement of structures which contain no sensory endings is painless. The substance of the vertebral body may be destroyed by tumor, for example, without evocation of pain, whereas lesions of periosteum, synovial membranes, muscles, annulus fibrosus, and ligaments are often exquisitely painful. Although painful states are often accompanied by swelling of the affected tissues, this is not apparent if a deep structure of the back is the site of disease. Local pain is steady, sometimes intermittent, of the aching type, and rather diffuse but is always felt in or near the affected part of the spine. Often there is involuntary splinting of the spine segments by paravertebral muscles, and certain movements or postures which alter the position of the injured tissues aggravate or relieve the pain. Firm pressure upon superficial structures in the region of the involved structure usually evokes tenderness which is of aid in identifying the site of the abnormality.

Referred pain is of two types, that projected from the spine into regions lying within the area of the lumbar and upper sacral dermatomes and that projected from the pelvic and abdominal viscera to the spine. Pain due to diseases of the upper part of the lumbar spine is usually referred to the anterior aspects of the thighs and legs; and that from the lower part of the lumbar spine is referred to the gluteal regions, posterior thighs, and calves. Pain of this type, although of deep, aching quality and rather diffuse, tends at times to be superficially projected. In general the referred pain parallels in intensity the local pain in the back. In other words, maneuvers which alter local pain have a similar effect on referred pain, though not with such precision and immediacy as in "root pain." Pain from visceral disease usually is felt within the abdomen or flanks and may be modified by the state of activity of the viscera. Its character and temporal relationships are those of the particular visceral structure involved, and posture and movement of the back have relatively little effect, either on the local pain or on that referred to the back.

Radicular, or "root," *pain* has some of the characteristics of referred pain but differs in its greater intensity, distal radiation, circumscription to the territory of a root, and the factors which excite it. The mechanism is distortion, stretching, irritation, or compression of a spinal root, most often central to the intervertebral foramen. The pain is sharp and often quite intense; it nearly always radiates from a central position near the spine to some part of the lower extremity. It is usually superimposed on the dull ache of referred pain. Cough, sneeze, and strain characteristically evoke this sharp radiating pain, though these maneuvers may also jar or move the spine and enhance local pain. Any motion which stretches the nerve, e.g., forward bending with the knees extended or "straight-leg raising" in disease of the lower part of the lumbar spine, excites radicular pain; and jugular vein compression, which raises intraspinal pressure and may cause a shift in the position of the root, may have a similar effect. The fourth and fifth lumbar and first sacral roots, which form the sciatic nerve, cause pain which extends mainly down the posterior aspects of thigh, the postero- and anterolateral aspects of the leg, and into the foot, in the distribution of this nerve—so-called "sciatica." Tingling, paresthesias, and numbness or sensory impairment of the skin, soreness of the skin, and tenderness along the nerve usually accompany radicular pain. Also reflex loss, weakness, atrophy, fascicular twitching, and often stasis edema may occur if motor fibers are involved in the anterior roots.

Pain resulting from muscular spasm is usually mentioned in relation to local pain. Muscle spasm is associated with most conditions which result in local pain. Muscles in a state of persistent tension give rise to a dull ache, called "secondary pain." One can feel the tautness of the sacrospinalis and gluteal muscles and demonstrate by palpation that the pain is localized to them.

Other pains often of undetermined origin are sometimes described by patients with chronic disease of the lower part of the back. In the legs drawing, pulling, cramping sensations (without involuntary muscle spasm), tearing, throbbing, or jabbing pains, feelings of burning or coldness are difficult to interpret and, like paresthesias and numbness, should always suggest the possibility of nerve or root disease.

Since it is often difficult to obtain physical or laboratory confirmation of painful disease of the lower region of the spine, the importance of an accurate history and description of symptoms cannot be overemphasized. Frequently the most important lead comes from the knowledge of the mode of onset and circumstances which initiated the pain. Inasmuch as many painful affections of the back are the result of injury incurred during work or in an accident, the possibility of exaggeration or prolongation of pain for personal reasons, or even hysteria or malingering, must always be kept in mind.

Examination of the lower part of the back *Inspection* of the spine, buttocks, and legs when standing erect, walking, stooping, and squatting is of value. The patient's resting posture should be noted because faulty posture predisposes to pain in the lumbosacral and sacroiliac regions. With sciatica the lumbar region of the spine is often scoliotic, with the convexity toward the normal side, though the converse may occur. Also, a slight flexion or flattening of the lumbar lordosis is common with acute painful states. The presence of a definite kyphosis usually signifies deformity of one of the vertebral bodies, e.g., fracture. Spasm of paravertebral muscles on one or both sides is often obvious during inspection. One may also notice a hypotonia of the gluteus maximus on the affected side with drooping of the gluteal fold.

The next step in the examination is observation of the spine, hips, and legs during certain motions. During the procedure it is well to remember that no advantage accrues from trying to find out how much the patient can be hurt. Instead, it is much more important to determine when and under what conditions the pain commences. One looks for limitation of the natural motions of the patient as he disrobes and while he is standing, sitting, and reclining. When standing, the motion of forward bending normally produces flattening and reversal of the lumbar lordotic curve and exaggeration of the dorsal curve. With lesions of the lumbosacral region which involve the posterior ligaments, articular facets, or sacrospinalis muscle and with ruptured lumbar disks protective reflexes prevent stretching of these structures. As a consequence, the sacrospinalis muscles remain taut and prevent motion in the lumbar part of the spine. Forward bending then occurs at the hips and at the lumbar-thoracic junction. With disease of the lumbosacral joints and spinal roots, the patient bends in such a way as to avoid tensing the hamstring muscles and putting undue leverage upon the pelvis. In unilateral "sciatica," with its increased curvature toward the side of the lesion, lumbar and lumbosacral motions are splinted and bending is mainly at the hips; at a certain point the knee on the affected side is flexed to relieve hamstring spasm and tilting of the pelvis, and to slacken the lumbosacral roots and sciatic nerve.

Lateral bending is usually less instructive than forward bending. However, in unilateral ligamentous or muscular strain, bending to the opposite side aggravates the pain by stretching the damaged tissues. Moreover, in lateral disk lesions, bending of the spine toward the side from which the trunk lists is restricted.

In diseases of the lower part of the spine, flexion while sitting can normally be performed easily, even to the point of bringing the knees in contact with the chest. The reason for this is that knee flexion relaxes the hamstring muscles and relieves stretch of the sciatic nerve.

The study of motions in the reclining position yields the same information as study of motions in the standing and sitting positions, with the difference that there is less pressure on the disks. With lumbosacral lesions and sciatica, passive lumbar flexion causes little pain and is not limited as long as the hamstrings are relaxed and there is no stretching of the sciatic nerve. With lumbosacral and lumbar spine disease (e.g., arthritis), passive flexion of the hips is free, whereas flexion of the lumbar spine is impeded and painful. Passive straight-leg raising (possibly up to 90° except in those who are congenitally stiff), like forward bending in the standing posture with the legs straight, places the sciatic nerve and its roots, also the hamstrings, under tension, thereby producing pain. It also rotates the pelvis, thus causing lumbar joint pain. Consequently, in diseases of the lumbosacral joints and of the lumbosacral roots, this movement is limited on the affected side and, to a lesser extent, the opposite side. Lasègue's sign (pain and limitation of movement during elevation of the leg when the knee is extended) is a useful test of this condition. Straight-leg flexion of the opposite leg may also cause some degree of contralateral pain. That is to say, the evoked pain is always referred to the diseased side, no matter which leg is flexed. In disease of the lumbosacral joints there may also be slight limitation of straight-leg raising.

The motion of hyperextension is best performed with the patient standing or lying prone. If the condition causing back pain is acute, it may be difficult to extend the spine in the standing position. A patient with lumbosacral strain can usually extend or hyperextend the spine without aggravation of pain. If there is an active inflammatory or other acute process, vertical pressure upon these joints will increase the pain. If there is ligamentous strain, no enhancement of pain will occur because the posterior segments of the spine are relaxed during extension. The converse is true if there is strain of extensor muscles, for hyperextension places the muscular attachments to the periosteum under tension. Although disease of articular facets may limit extension, little or no pain is produced. In lumbar disk disease (except in the acute phase of the illness), extension of the spine is usually tolerated well, though in some patients with a displaced disk fragment situated posterolaterally, pain is evoked by extension rather than flexion. A reversed Lasègue's sign suggests spinal nerve involvement at the midlumbar level or a lesion of the lumbosacral joint.

Palpation and percussion of the spine are the last steps in the examination. The approach must always be gentle since rough percussion of the designated area of pain only confuses the physician and antagonizes the patient. It is preferable to palpate first those regions which are the least likely to evoke pain. At all times the examiner should know what structures are being palpated (see Fig. 9-1). Localized tenderness is seldom pronounced in disease of the spine because the involved structures are so deep that they rarely give rise to surface tenderness. Mild superficial and poorly localized tenderness signifies only a disease process within the affected segment of the body, i.e., dermatome.

Tenderness over the costovertebral angle often indicates genitourinary disease, adrenal disease (Rogoff's

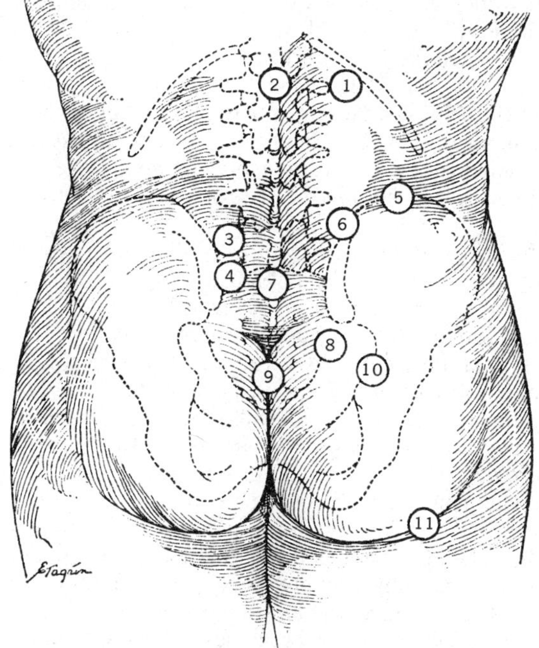

FIGURE 9-1
(1) Costovertebral angle. (2) Spinous process and interspinous ligament. (3) Region of articular fifth lumbar to first sacral facet. (4) Dorsum of sacrum. (5) Region of iliac crest. (6) Iliolumbar angle. (7) Spinous processes of fifth lumbar to first sacral vertebras (tenderness = faulty posture or occasionally spina bifida occulta). (8) Region between posterior superior and posterior inferior spines. Sacroiliac ligaments (tenderness = sacroiliac sprain, often tender with fifth lumbar to first sacral disk). (9) Sacrococcygeal junction (tenderness = sacrococcygeal injury, i.e., sprain or fracture). (10) Region of sacrosciatic notch (tenderness = fourth to fifth lumbar disk rupture and sacroiliac sprain). (11) Sciatic nerve trunk (tenderness = ruptured lumbar disk or sciatic nerve lesion).

sign), or an injury to the transverse processes of the first or second lumbar vertebra [Fig. 9-1 (1)]. Hypersensitivity on palpation of the transverse processes of the other lumbar vertebras as well as the overlying sacrospinalis muscles may signify fracture of the transverse process or a strain of muscle attachments.

Upon palpation of the spinous processes and interspinous ligaments any deviation in the anteroposterior or lateral plane must be particularly noted. Such a deviation usually indicates spondylolisthesis. Tenderness of the interspinous ligaments is indicative of disk lesions [Fig. 9-1 (2)].

Tenderness in the region of the articular facets between the fifth lumbar and first sacral vertebras is consistent with a lumbosacral disk disease [Fig. 9-1 (3)]. It is also not infrequent in rheumatoid arthritis.

Rectal and pelvic examinations to exclude inflammatory and neoplastic diseases of these parts, constitute an essential part of the diagnostic study of all cases of low back pain and sciatica.

Upon completion of the examination of the back a search for motor, reflex, and sensory changes (see Protrusion of Lumbar Intervertebral Disks, ahead), particularly in the lower extremities, should be made.

Special laboratory procedures Laboratory tests often aid in diagnosis. Depending on the circumstances, these may include measurement of the serum proteins, phosphatases (alkaline and acid), calcium, phosphorus, uric acid, serum electrophoresis (myeloma proteins), tuberculin, agglutination for *Brucella,* sedimentation rate, and rheumatoid factor. Roentgenograms should be taken in every case of low back pain and sciatica, preferably with the patient standing, in the anterior-posterior, lateral, and oblique planes of the lumbar part of the spine. Stereoscopic or laminographic films may provide further information in certain cases. Examination of the spinal canal with a contrast medium (myelogram) is necessary. This study can be combined with tests of dynamics of the cerebrospinal fluid, and a sample of the fluid should always be removed for cytologic and chemical examination prior to the installation of the contrast medium (Pantopaque, Myodil, air, or some of the newer contrast media which are resorbed). Injection and removal of Pantopaque require special skill and should not be attempted without previous experience with the procedure. If done properly, the procedure is harmless. Recently a new absorbable substance, Dimer X, has been introduced. It is nonirritating, gives excellent visualization, and makes the entire procedure easier. Injection of contrast medium directly into the intervertebral disk (diskograms) has recently become popular but is still controversial. The technique of this procedure is more complicated than that of myelographic examination, and the risk of damage to nerve roots or the introduction of infection is not inconsiderable. In the authors' opinion, the results do not warrant the risk involved.

PRINCIPAL CONDITIONS WHICH GIVE RISE TO DISABLING PAIN IN THE LOWER PART OF THE BACK

CONGENITAL ANOMALIES OF THE LUMBAR SPINE Anatomic variations of the spine are not at all infrequent, and although not of themselves the source of pain and functional derangement, they may dispose to strain by permitting excessive mobility or the adoption of abnormal postures.

There may be a lack of fusion of the laminas of the neural arch—a spina bifida—of one or several of the lumbar vertebras, or of the sacrum. Hypertrichosis or hyperpigmentation in the sacral area may betray the condition, but it may remain entirely occult until disclosed by x-ray. The anomaly when accompanied by malformation of vertebral joints induces pain only when aggravated by injury. The significance of all congenital abnormalities of the spine in the genesis of back pain is highly controversial.

Spondylolysis consists of a bony defect in the pars interarticularis, which is replaced by cartilage, permitting a forward displacement of the vertebral body, pedicles, and superior articular processes, leaving the laminas, inferior articular processes and spinous processes behind (spondylolisthesis). Although of congenital origin, the first symptoms of disordered function (low back pain radiating to the thighs, tightness of back muscles, and signs of involvement of spinal roots—paresthesias and sensory loss, muscle weakness, and reflex impairment) may not appear until later in life and are often precipitated by an injury.

Articular facets of the vertebras may be set in an unusual plane, either oblique or frontal, rather than the sagittal one as in the normal lumbar spine; there may also be an abnormality in the number of mobile lumbar vertebras (either six or four). The lowest vertebra may be asymmetric in its relation to the sacrum. Although these abnormalities have been blamed for chronic low back pain, large surveys suggest that they bear no relationship to it.

TRAUMATIC AFFLICTIONS OF THE LOWER PART OF THE BACK Trauma constitutes the most frequent cause of low back pain.

In severe acute injuries, the examining physician must be careful to avoid further damage. In tests of motility, all movements must be kept to a minimum until an approximate diagnosis has been made and adequate measures have been instituted for the proper care of the patient. If the patient complains of pain in his back and cannot move his legs, his spine may have been fractured. His neck should not be flexed, nor should he be allowed to sit up. (See Chap. 325 for further discussion of spinal cord injury.)

Sprains and strains The terms *strain* and *sprain* are used loosely by most physicians. It is probably impossible to differentiate between them. Here we shall use only the word strain. Strain should designate a minor injury which does not produce gross structural damage. The abnormal mechanical force may be acute, as in heavy lifting, or mild and persistent, owing to maintenance of an abnormal posture. The latter is often occupational. Rest and relaxation promptly alleviate the discomfort, attesting to the lack of major structural change. What formerly was regarded as sacroiliac strain or sprain is now known to be due to disk disease in most instances. This is caused by lifting heavy objects with the spine in a position of imperfect mechanical balance, as when lifting and turning at the same time. Sudden unexpected motion is particularly likely to cause this injury.

The diagnosis of lumbosacral and sacroiliac strains with injury of the various structures of the lower part of the back depends upon the description of the injury, the localization of the pain by the patient, the finding of localized tenderness, and the augmentation of pain when tension is exerted on the involved structures by the appropriate maneuvers. The prompt alleviation of the pain by rest and relaxation indicates the existence of a strain. The rate of recovery depends on the degree of damage, preexisting disk disease, etc. Pain may, however, be relieved by local infiltration of an anesthetic agent, a finding which is also helpful in diagnosis.

Sacroiliac strain, once so popular as an explanation of unilateral back pain, is now highly controversial. Because of their irregular surfaces, the sacroiliac bones are interlocked; joint movement is minimal and is further restricted by strong sacroiliac ligaments. Only violent injury could derange this well-protected and stable joint. Multiple pregnancies close together may be another cause. When the joint is injured, the principal symptom is a localized ache which is made worse by compression of the pelvis. It must be remembered that involvement of a spinal nerve root (fifth lumbar or first sacral) associated with injury to the disk is the more common cause of pain and local tenderness in the area of the sacroiliac joint.

Vertebral fractures Fractures of the lumbar vertebral body are usually the result of flexion injuries. This is most likely to occur in falls from a height; often the calcaneus is also fractured. Nearly always there is localized tenderness over the fractured vertebra. Spasm of the lower lumbar muscles, limitation of movements of the lumbar section of the spine, and the roentgenographic appearance of the damaged lumbar portion (with or without neurologic abnormalities) are the basis of clinical diagnosis. The pain is usually immediate, though occasionally it may be delayed for days. Some patients are found to have had crushed fractures of the vertebral body without being able to recall any traumatic episode; usually it will be found that they had had an osteoporosis of the spine.

Fractured transverse processes, which are almost always associated with tearing of the paravertebral muscles, are diagnosed by the finding of deep tenderness at the site of the injury, local muscle spasm on one side, and limitation of all movements which stretch the lumbar muscles. Radiologic evidence provides the final confirmation.

Protrusion of lumbar intervertebral disks This condition is now recognized as the major cause of severe and chronic or recurrent low back and leg pain. It is most likely to occur between the fifth lumbar and first sacral vertebras and, with lessening frequency, between the fourth to fifth lumbar, the third to fourth lumbar, the second to third lumbar, and the first to second lumbar vertebras. Rare in the thoracic portion of the spine, it is next most frequent at the sixth to seventh and fifth to sixth cervical vertebras. The cause is usually a flexion injury, but in a considerable proportion of cases no trauma is recalled. Degeneration of the posterior longitudinal ligaments and the annulus fibrosus, which occurs in most adults of middle and advanced years, may have taken place silently or have been manifested by mild, recurrent lumbar ache. A sneeze, lurch, or other trivial movement may then cause the nucleus pulposus to extrude through the frayed ligament.

The fully developed syndrome of ruptured intervertebral disk consists of backache, abnormal posture, and limitation of motion of the spine (particularly flexion). Nerve root involvement is indicated by radicular pain, sensory disturbances (paresthesias, hyper- and hyposensitivity in dermatome pattern), coarse twitching and fasciculation, muscle spasms, and impairment of a tendon reflex. Motor abnormalities (weakness and muscle atrophy) may also occur but are usually less prominent than the pain and sensory disorder. Since herniation of the intervertebral lumbar disks most often occurs between the fourth and fifth lumbar vertebras and the fifth lumbar and first sacral vertebras with irritation and compression of the fifth lumbar and first sacral roots, respectively, it is important to recognize the clinical characteristics of lesions of these two roots. *Lesions of the fifth lumbar root* produce pain in the region of the hip, groin, posterolateral thigh, lateral calf to the external malleolus, dorsal surface of the foot, and the first or second and third toes. Paresthesias may be in the entire territory or only in the distal parts of these territories. The tenderness is in the lateral gluteal region and near the head of the fibula. Weakness, if present, involves the extensors of the big toe and of the foot. The knee and ankle reflex seldom are definitely diminished; they are usually unchanged. Walking on the heels may be more difficult, because of weakness of dorsiflexion, and more uncomfortable than walking on the toes. In *lesions of the first sacral root* the pain is felt in the midgluteal region, posterior part of the thigh, posterior region of the calf to the heel, and the plantar surface of the foot and fourth and fifth toes. Tenderness is most pronounced over the midgluteal region (sacroiliac joint), posterior thigh area, and calf. Paresthesias and sensory loss are mainly in the lower leg and outer toes, and weakness, if present, involves the flexor muscles of the foot and toes, abductors of the toes, and hamstring muscles. The ankle reflex is diminished to absent in the majority of cases. Walking on the toes is more difficult, because of weakness of plantar flexors, and more uncomfortable than walking on the heel. With lesions of either root there may be limitation of straight-leg raising during the acute, painful stages.

Low back pain may also be caused by degeneration of the intervertebral disk, without frank extrusion of a fragment of disk tissue. Or the herniation may occur into the adjacent vertebral body, giving rise to a Schmorl's nodule. In such cases there are no signs of nerve root involvement though the back pain may be referred to the thigh and leg.

The rarer *lesions of the fourth and third lumbar roots* give rise to pain in the anterior part of the thigh and knee, with corresponding sensory loss. The knee-jerk is diminished or abolished. An inverted Lasègue sign is positive when the third lumbar root is affected.

The lumbar disk syndromes are usually unilateral. Only with massive derangements of the disk do bilateral symptoms and signs occur, and these may then be associated with paralysis of the sphincters. The pain may be mild or severe. All or part of the above syndrome may be present. There may be back pain with little or no leg pain; rarely only leg pain may be experienced. The rupture of multiple lumbar or lumbar and cervical disks is not infrequent, attesting to a basic disorder of the entire disk including the annulus fibrosus.

When all components of the syndrome are present, the diagnosis is easy; when only one part is present, particularly backache, it may be difficult, especially if there has been no accident. Since similar symptoms may occur without demonstrable disk rupture, other diagnostic procedures are required. Plain roentgenograms usually show no abnormality or at most a narrowing of the intervertebral space, sometimes more on the side of the rupture, or traction spurs, which are indicative of disk degeneration; hence one must resort to Pantopaque or air myelography. This will reveal in most cases an indentation of the lumbar subarachnoid space or deformity of the root sleeve. Unfortunately, a small ruptured disk may not show, especially at the fifth lumbar to first sacral level. Some clinics use diskograms (opaque material is injected into the disk, to reveal any evidence of extrusion), but the procedure is risky and the results are difficult to interpret. The electromyogram is helpful in showing denervation of leg muscles (see Chap. 353). The protein level of the cerebrospinal fluid is elevated in some instances.

Tumor of the spinal canal, epidural or intradural, may produce a syndrome similar to that of ruptured disk (see Chap. 325).

ARTHRITIS Arthritis of the spine is a major cause of backache, cervical pain, and occipital headache.

Osteoarthritis This, the more frequent type of arthritis (see Chap. 359), occurs usually in later life and may involve all or any part of the spine, which of course determines the localization of the symptoms. The pain is centered in the spine and is associated almost invariably with stiffness and limitation of motion. There is a notable absence of systemic symptoms such as fatigue, malaise, and fever. The severity of the symptoms bears little relation to the radiologic findings; pain may be present when there is little to be seen by x-ray, and often osteophytic overgrowth with spur formation, ridging, and breaking of vertebras is seen in middle and late life without pain. The latter changes in the cervical spine are probably of traumatic origin and are incorrectly called arthritic. When pronounced, however, they may compress cervical roots or spinal cord, giving rise to the spondylitic form of myelopathy (see Chap. 325).

Rheumatoid arthritis Rheumatoid arthritis of the spine may take two forms: (1) affection of some part of the spine is associated with active inflammation of other joints; (2) affection is limited to the spine and sacroiliac joints. The former may be localized to the cervical apophyseal joints and atlantoaxial articulation; the pain, stiffness, and limitation of motion are then in the neck and back of the head. In advanced stages of the disease the upper vertebras may be displaced anteriorly; or a synovitis of the atlantoaxial joint may damage the transverse ligament of the atlas, resulting in posterior displacement of the odontoid process. In either instance serious and even life-threatening compression of the spinal cord may occur gradually or suddenly (see Chap. 325). Lateral roentgenograms in flexion and extension, performed cautiously, are useful in visualizing atlantoaxial dislocation. In the second form of ankylosing spondylitis (also called Marie-Strümpell arthritis) the pain is usually centered in the low region of the back and is recurrent. Often it radiates to the back of the thighs and groins. At first the symptoms are vague (tired back, "catches" in the back, sore back). As with all types of arthritis there are characteristic limitation of movement and worsening of pain and stiffness after a period of inactivity, which may provide clues as to the nature of the disease, many years before radiologic changes are manifest. Signs of systemic infection are variable; they may be absent. Ultimately the entire spine is immobilized and the pain subsides (see Chap. 354). Spondylitis pain may also accompany Reiter's syndrome, psoriasis, and inflammatory diseases of the intestine.

OTHER DESTRUCTIVE DISEASES **Infectious, neoplastic, and metabolic diseases** Metastatic carcinoma (breast, bronchus, prostate, thyroid, hypernephroma, stomach, uterus), multiple myeloma, and reticulum-cell sarcoma are the common tumors which involve the spine; tuberculosis and pyogenic osteomyelitis are the most frequent infections, though brucellosis, typhoid fever, actinomycosis, and blastomycosis are known to occur.

Special mention should be made of the spinal *epidural abscess* (usually staphylococcal), which necessitates urgent surgical treatment. The symptoms are a localized pain, occurring spontaneously and with percussion and palpation, often with radicular radiation, and a rapidly developing flaccid paraplegia appearing in a febrile patient.

Destructive lesions of any type may develop silently, i.e., without any pain, as long as they are limited to the osseous tissue. Upon spreading to the periosteum or to the adjacent spinous structures, however, they become the source of much pain of both local and referred type, and often one or more spinal roots are implicated as well, with the typical radicular type being added to the clinical picture. A "spontaneous" fracture may initiate pain. Pain caused by neoplasms of the spine tends to be of aching character and more or less steady, though occasionally waxing and waning. It is especially severe at night, seeming to be only slightly benefited by rest; yet activity during the day also worsens the pain. As the disease progresses, the pain increases in duration and severity. It may then be of a throbbing character. The most important physical finding, which should lead one to suspect a destructive lesion, is an intensification of the pain by jarring the spine, by percussing the spinous processes gently with the fist or a reflex hammer, or by exerting a steady pressure upon these parts. Axial compression (downward pressure exerted on the head or dropping on the heels from the toe position) may also serve to intensify the pain. Nocturnal pain, spinal ache, and percussion sensitivity are also characteristic of tuberculous spondylitis (Pott's disease) and osteomyelitis. The establishment of the cause of the pain is often delayed because the first roentgenograms may not disclose the lesion. (Nearly a cubic centimeter of bone must be destroyed in a vertebral body before the destruction is visible in a plain roentgenogram, although tomography may reveal the defect). The roentgenograms should be repeated after an interval of a few weeks. Other laboratory data, such as white blood cell count and smear, sedimentation rate, and electrophoresis of serum proteins and acid and alkaline phosphatase in the serum are helpful.

In so-called "metabolic bone diseases" (osteoporosis of either the postmenopausal or senile type or osteomalacia) a considerable degree of loss of bone substance may occur without any symptoms whatsoever. Many patients with such conditions do, however, complain of aching in the lumbar or thoracic area. This is most likely to occur following an injury, sometimes of trivial degree, which leads to collapse or wedging of a vertebra. Certain movements greatly enhance the pain, and certain positions relieve it. One or more spinal roots may then be involved. Paget's disease of the spine is nearly always painless. It may lead to compression of the spinal cord. The recognition of these bone disorders is discussed in some detail elsewhere (Chaps. 325 and 351).

REFERRED PAIN FROM VISCERAL DISEASE The pain of disease of the pelvic, abdominal, or thoracic viscera is often felt in the region of the spine; i.e., it is referred to the more posterior parts of the spinal segment which innervates the diseased organ. Occasionally back pain may be the first and only sign. The general rule is that pelvic diseases are referred to the sacral region, lower abdominal diseases to the lumbar region (centering around the second to fourth lumbar vertebras), and upper abdominal diseases to the lower thoracic spine (eighth thoracic to the first and second lumbar vertebras). Characteristically there are no local signs, no stiffness of the back, and motion is of full range without augmentation of the pain. However, some positions, e.g., flexion of the lumbar area of the spine in the lateral recumbent position, may be more comfortable than others.

Low thoracic and upper lumbar pain in abdominal disease Peptic ulceration or tumor of the wall of the stomach and of the duodenum most typically induces pain in the epigastrium (see Chaps. 7, 8, and 282); but if the posterior wall is involved, and particularly if there is retroperitoneal extension, the pain may be felt in the region of the spine. The pain is central in location or more intense on one side, or it may be felt in both locations. If very intense, it may seem to encircle the body. It tends to retain the characteristics of pain from the affected organ; e.g., if due to peptic ulceration, it appears about 2 hr after a meal and is relieved by food and soda.

Diseases of the pancreas (peptic ulceration with extension to the pancreas, cholecystitis with pancreatitis, tumor) are apt to cause pain in the back, being more to the right of the spine if the head of the pancreas is involved and to the left if the body and tail are implicated.

Diseases of retroperitoneal structures, e.g., lymphomas, sarcomas, and carcinomas, may evoke pain in this part of the spine with some tendency toward radiation to the lower part of the abdomen, groins, and anterior thighs. A secondary tumor of the iliopsoas region on one side often produces a unilateral lumbar ache with radiation toward the groin and labia or testicle; there may also be signs of involvement of the upper lumbar spinal roots. An aneurysm of the abdominal aorta may induce a pain which is localized to this region of the spine but may be felt higher or lower, depending on the location of the lesion.

The sudden appearance of obscure lumbar pain in a patient receiving anticoagulants should arouse the suspicion of retroperitoneal bleeding.

Lumbar pain with lower abdominal diseases Inflammatory diseases of segments of the colon (colitis, diverticulitis) or tumor of the colon cause pain which may be felt in the lower part of the abdomen between the umbilicus and pubis, or in the midlumbar region, or in both places. If very intense, the pain may have a beltlike distribution around the body. A lesion in the tranverse colon or first part of the descending colon may be central or left-sided, and its level of reference to the back is to the second to third lumbar vertebras. If the sigmoid colon is implicated, the pain is lower, in the upper sacral region and anteriorly in the midline suprapubic region or left lower quadrant of the abdomen.

Sacral pain in pelvic (urologic and gynecologic) diseases Although gynecologic disorders may manifest themselves by back pain, the pelvis is seldom the site of a disease which causes obscure low back pain. For the most part the diagnosis of painful pelvic lesions is not difficult, for a thorough palpation of structures by abdominal, vaginal, and rectal examination may be supplemented by methods (sigmoidoscopy, barium enema, pyelography, and culdoscopy) which permit adequate visualization of all these parts.

Menstrual pain itself may be felt in the sacral region. It is rather poorly localized, tends to radiate down the legs, and is of a crampy nature. The most important source of chronic back pain from the pelvic organs, however, is the uterosacral ligaments. Endometriosis or carcinoma of the uterus (body or cervix) may invade these structures, while malposition of the uterus may pull on them. The pain is localized centrally in the sacrum below the lumbosacral joint but may be more on one side. In endometriosis the pain begins during the premenstrual phase and often continues until it merges with menstrual pain. Malposition of the uterus (retroversion, descensus, and prolapse) characteristically leads to sacral pain, especially after the patient has been standing for several hours. Postural adjustments may also evoke pain here when a fibroma of the uterus pulls on the uterosacral ligaments. Carcinomatous pain due to implication of nerve plexuses is continuous and becomes progressively more severe; it tends to be more intense at night. The primary lesion may be inconspicuous, being overlooked upon pelvic examination. Papanicolaou smears and a pyelogram are the most useful diagnostic procedures. X-ray therapy of these tumors may produce sacral pain consequent to swelling and necrosis of tissue, the so-called "radiation phlegmon of the pelvis." Low back pain with radiation into one or both thighs is a common phenomenon during the last weeks of pregnancy.

Chronic prostatitis, evidenced by prostatic discharge, burning and frequency of urination, and slight reduction in sexual potency, may be attended by a nagging sacral ache; it may be mainly on one side, with radiation into one leg if the seminal vesicle is involved on that side. Carcinoma of the prostate with metastases to the lower part of the spine is another more common cause of sacral or lumbar pain. It may be present without urinary frequency or burning. Spinal nerves may be infiltrated by tumor cells, or the spinal cord itself may be compressed if the epidural space is invaded. The diagnosis is established by rectal examination, roentgenograms of the spine, and measurement of acid phosphatase (particularly the prostatic phosphatase fraction). Lesions of the bladder and testes are usually not accompanied by back pain. When the kidney is the site of disease, the pain is ipsilateral, being felt in the flank or lumbar region.

Visceral derangements of whatever type may intensify the pain of arthritis, and the presence of arthritis may alter the distribution of visceral pain. With disease of the spine in the lumbosacral region, for example, distention of the ampulla of the sigmoid by feces or a bout of colitis may aggravate the arthritic pain. In patients with arthritis of the cervical or thoracic spine, the pain of myocardial ischemia may radiate to the back.

OBSCURE TYPES OF LOW BACK PAIN AND THE QUESTION OF PSYCHIATRIC DISEASE The practitioner is consulted by many persons who complain of low back pain of obscure origin. A safe rule is to assume that all of them have some type of primary or secondary disease of the spine and its supporting structures or of the abdominal or pelvic viscera. If the pain is of acute onset and short duration, it may be due to only a minor trauma, a so-called "fibrositis," or some form of articular disease. If it is recurrent, the possibility of a ruptured disk causing an instability of the spine must be considered. If it is severe and progressive, neoplasia, a tuberculous infection, and rheumatoid spondylitis should be kept in mind.

Adolescent girls and boys are subject to an obscure form of epiphyseal disease of the spine (Scheuermann's disease) which may cause low back pain upon exercise over a period of 2 to 3 years.

Postural back pain Many slender asthenic individuals and some fat middle-aged individuals have discomfort in the back. Their backs ache much of the time, and the pain interferes with effective work. The physical examination is negative except for slack musculature and poor posture. The pain is diffuse in the mid or low region of the back and characteristically is relieved by bed rest and induced by the maintenance of a particular posture over a period of time. Pain in the neck and between the shoulder blades is a common complaint among thin, tense, active women and seems to be related to taut trapezius muscles.

Psychiatric illness Low back pain may be encountered in compensation hysteria and malingering, in anxiety or neurocirculatory asthenia (formerly called neurasthenia), in depression and hypochondriasis, and in many nervous persons whose symptoms and complaints do not fall within any category of psychiatric illness.

Again it is probably correct to assume that pain in the back in such patients usually signifies disease of the spine and adjacent structures, and this should always be carefully looked for. However, the pain may be exaggerated, prolonged, or woven into a pattern of invalidism or disability because of coexistent or secondary psychologic factors. This is especially true when there is the possibility of personal gain (notably compensation). Patients seeking compensation for protracted low back pain without obvious structural disease tend, after a time, to become suspicious, hostile toward the medical profession or anyone who might question the authenticity of their illness, and uncooperative. One notes in them a tendency to describe their pain poorly and to prefer, instead, to discuss the degree of their disability and their mistreatment in the hands of the medical profession. These features and a negative examination of the back should lead one to suspect a psychologic factor. A few patients, usually frank malingerers, adopt the most bizarre attitudes, such as being unable to straighten up or walking with the trunk flexed at almost a right angle (camptocormia) (see Chap. 339).

The depressed and hypochondriac patient represents a troublesome problem, and a common error is to minimize the importance of anxiety and depression or to ascribe them to worry over the illness and its social effects. The more common and minor back ailments, e.g., those due to osteoarthritis and postural ache, are enhanced and rendered intolerable by the irritable moodiness and self-concern. Such patients are often subjected to surgical procedures, which prove ineffective. The disability seems excessive for the degree of spinal malfunction, and misery and despair are the prevailing features of the syndrome. One of the most reliable diagnostic measures is the response to drugs which alleviate the depression (see Chap. 341).

PAIN IN THE NECK AND SHOULDER This topic has been discussed to some extent in Chap. 7, Pain in the Chest, and further references will be found in Chap. 10, Pain in the Extremities.

It is useful to distinguish here three major categories of painful disease—that of the spine, cervical plexus, and shoulder. Although the pains in these three regions of the body may overlap, the patient himself usually can indicate their site of origin. Pain arising from the cervical part of the spine is felt in the neck and back of the head (though it may be projected to the shoulder and arm), is evoked or enhanced by certain movements or positions of the neck, and is accompanied by tenderness and limitation of motions of the neck. Similarly, pain of brachial plexus origin is experienced in and around the shoulder, in the supraclavicular region, or between the shoulders, is induced by the performance of certain tasks with the arm and by certain positions, and is associated with tenderness of structures above the clavicle. There may be a palpable abnormality above the clavicle (aneurysms of the subclavian artery, tumor, cervical rib). The combination of circulatory symptoms and signs referable to the lower part of the brachial plexus, manifested in the hand by obliteration of pulse when the patient takes and holds a full breath with the head tilted back or turned (Adson's test), unilateral Raynaud's phenomenon, trophic changes in the fingers, and sensory loss over the ulnar side of the hand with or without interosseous atrophy, complete the clinical picture. Roentgenograms showing a cervical rib or deformed thoracic outlet or superior sulcus tumor of the lung (Pancoast's syndrome) offer confirmation of the diagnosis. Pain, localized to the shoulder region, influenced by motion, and associated with tenderness and limitation of motions (extension, abduction, external and internal rotation), points to a tear of one of the rotator cuffs of those muscles surrounding the shoulder joint or a tendinitis with calcium deposition. Often the term *bursitis* has been used loosely to designate this tendinitis, capsulitis, or muscular tear. Spine, plexus, and shoulder pain all may radiate into the arm or hand, but sensory, motor, and reflex changes which always indicate disease of nerve roots, plexus, or nerves are absent.

Osteoarthritis of the cervical part of the spine may cause pains which radiate into the back of the head, shoulders, and arms on one or both sides of the thorax. Coincident involvement of nerve roots is manifested by paresthesias, sensory loss, weakness, or tendon reflex change. Should bony ridges form in the spinal canal (spondylosis), the spinal cord may be compressed, with resulting weakness and atrophy and sometimes sensory disturbances in the arms and spastic weakness and ataxia with loss of vibratory and position sense in the legs. A Pantopaque or air cervical myelogram reveals the degree of encroachment on the spinal canal (narrowing of the canal to 14 mm in the anteroposterior diameter) and the level at which the spinal cord is affected. The authors have experienced the greatest difficulty in distinguishing spondylosis with or without disk rupture and spinal cord compression from primary neurologic diseases (syringomyelia, amyotrophic lateral sclerosis, or tumor) with an unrelated osteoarthritis of the cervical portion of the spine, particularly at the fifth to sixth and sixth to seventh cervical vertebras, where the disk spaces are often narrowed in the adult (see Chap. 325 for differential diagnosis). A combination of nervous tension with osteoarthritis of the cervical part of the spine or a painful injury to ligaments and muscles after an accident in which the neck is forcibly extended and flexed (e.g., whiplash injury to spine) raises extremely vexatious clinical syndromes. If the pain is persistent and limited to the neck, the problem will sometimes prove to have been due to disruption of a disk, but it is often complicated by psychologic factors.

Ruptured cervical disks One of the commonest causes of neck, shoulder, and arm pain is disk herniation in the lower cervical region. As with rupture of the lumbar disks, the syndrome includes the disorder of spinal function and evidence of neural involvement. It develops after a trauma which may be major or minor (sudden hyperextension of the neck, diving, forceful manipulations, chiropractic treatment, etc.). Virtually every patient exhibits an abnormality in full motion of the neck (limitation and pain). Hyperextension is the movement that most consistently aggravates the pain. With laterally situated disk lesions between the fifth to sixth cervical vertebras, the symptoms and signs are referred to the sixth cervical roots, i.e., pain felt at the trapezius ridge, tip of the shoulder, anterior upper part of the arm, radial forearm, and often in the thumb; paresthesias and sensory impairment or hypersensitivity in the same regions; tenderness in the area above the spine of the scapula and in the supraclavicular and biceps regions; weakness in flexion of the forearm; diminished to absent biceps and supinator reflexes (triceps retained or exaggerated). With sixth to seventh cervical disk disease and involvement of the seventh cervical root, the pain is in the region of the shoulder blade, pectoral region and medial axilla, posterolateral upper arm, dorsal forearm and elbow, index and middle fingers, or all the fingers; tenderness is most pronounced over the medial aspect of the shoulder blade opposite the third to fourth thoracic spinous processes, in the supraclavicular area and triceps region; paresthesias and sensory loss are most pronounced in the second and third fingers or tips of all the fingers; weakness is seen in extension of the forearm (occasionally wristdrop is present) and in the hand grip; the triceps reflex is diminished to absent, and the biceps and supinator reflexes are preserved. Cough, sneeze, and downward pressure on the head in the hyperextension position exacerbate pain, and traction (even manual) tends to relieve it.

Unlike lumbar disks, the cervical ones, if large and centrally situated, may result in compression of the spinal cord (central disk, all of the cord; paracentral disk, part of the cord). The central disk is often nearly painless, and the cord syndrome may simulate a degenerative disease (amyotrophic lateral sclerosis, combined system disease). A common error is to fail to think of a ruptured disk in the cervical region in patients with obscure symptoms in the legs. The diagnosis of ruptured cervical disk should be confirmed by the same laboratory procedures that were mentioned under lumbar disk.

OTHER CONDITIONS Metastases in the cervical spine may be very painful, but the problem is not different from that of secondary deposits of tumor in other parts of the spine.

Shoulder injuries (rotator cuff), subacromial or subdeltoid bursitis, the frozen shoulder (periarthritis or capsulitis), tendinitis, and arthritis may develop in patients who are otherwise well, but these conditions are also frequent in hemiplegics or in individuals suffering from coronary heart disease. The pain is often severe and extends toward the neck and down the arm into the hand. The dorsum of the latter may tingle without other signs of nerve involvement. Vasomotor changes also may occur in the hand (shoulder-hand syndrome), and after a time, osteoporosis and atrophy of cutaneous and subcutaneous structures occur (Sudeck's atrophy or Sudeck-Leriche syndrome). These conditions fall more within the province of orthopedics than of medicine and will not be discussed in detail. The physician, however, must know that they can be prevented by proper exercises.

The carpal tunnel syndrome, with paresthesias and numbness in palmar distribution of the median nerve and aching pain which extends up into the forearm, may be mistaken for disease of the shoulder or neck.

MANAGEMENT OF BACK PAIN A muscular strain is always benign in character, and one may expect full recovery in 2 to 4 weeks. Ligamentous strains, if severe, may last longer, from 6 to 12 weeks. The underlying principle of therapy in both is immobilization in a recumbent position that relaxes and removes pressure from the injured structure. Usually lying on the side with knees and hips flexed is the favored position. If the sacrospinalis muscles are strained, the optimal position is hyperextension; the same is true of strains of the posterior and sacroiliac ligaments. This position is best maintained by having the patient lie with a small pillow or blanket under the lumbar portion of the spine or lie face down. During the acute phase of any injury of this type, application of cold, in the form of an ice bag or cold water bottle (ethyl chloride spray of the skin is said to give dramatic relief at times), is indicated. It reduces the circulation and consequently the swelling. If a lumbar puncture is to be performed, the intrathecal injection of 10 to 20 mg depo-prednisone (Ultracortenol) often reduces the pain of acute radicular disease. After the third or fourth day, heat is desirable to improve the circulation and to relax protective muscle spasm. Analgesic medication should be given liberally during the first few days [codeine, 30 mg, and aspirin, 0.6 g, pentazocine (Talwin), 50 mg, propoxyphene (Darvon), 65 mg, meperidine (Demerol) 50 mg]. When ready for ambulation, after some days in bed, the patient may need protection of the injured part, preferably adhesive strapping, in cases of muscle strain, or a belt or brace. Plaster casts should be avoided. Ambulatory treatment is supplemented by corrective exercises designed to strengthen trunk muscles, especially the abdominal, overcome faulty position, and to increase the mobility of the spinal joints. Only if these measures prove inadequate and the patient is partially disabled over long periods of time by an unstable, painful lower back (recurrent lumbosacral backache) should operative intervention be considered.

In the treatment of an acute rupture of a lumbar or cervical disk, complete bed rest is essential and strong analgesic medication is required. Traction is of little value in lumbar disk disease, and it is best to permit the patient to find the most comfortable position. Later, traction, if of any value, keeps the patient confined to bed. In contrast, traction is of great help in rupture of cervical disks. Often the pain subsides after 2 to 3 weeks in bed, and the patient may remain free of pain upon resuming normal activities. He may suffer some minor recurrence of the pain but be able to carry on his usual activities, and eventually he will recover. There is always danger of relapse. To prevent this, mild muscle-strengthening exercises of the spine after the pain has subsided and avoidance of activities which favor spine injury are recommended. If the pain does not subside after a trial of prolonged bed rest (several weeks) and the myelogram demonstrates a large disk, an operative removal, without spine fusion (which is rarely successful), should be undertaken. The final decision as to the time and necessity of surgery depends on the duration and gravity of the pain and the neurologic disorder.

For the many patients with back pain whose condition does not fall in any one of the above categories, simple measures are beneficial. For the adolescent with a suspicion of epiphyseal disease, restricted activity (avoidance of vigorous sports) for a few months or years and a supporting garment help. Muscle-strengthening exercises and a physical conditioning program are indicated for postural backache. The value of spine fusion remains debatable.

Spondylosis of the cervical part of the spine, if painful, is helped by bed rest and traction; if signs of spinal cord involvement are present, a collar to limit movement may halt the progression and even lead to improvement. Decompressive laminectomy with sectioning of denticulate ligaments is reserved for severe instances of the disease with advancing neurologic symptoms. The shoulder-hand syndrome may benefit from stellate ganglion blocks or ganglionectomy, but the basic treatment is physiotherapy, with or without prednisone, and surgical procedures are used only as measures of last resort.

10
PAIN IN THE EXTREMITIES

D. EUGENE STRANDNESS, JR.

INTRODUCTION Pain in the extremities occurs from a wide variety of diseases of the skin and of the musculoskeletal, vascular, and nervous systems. The commoner ones seen in clinical practice will be the subject of this chapter.

In the diagnosis of pain of the limbs it is important to classify the pain and localize the site of involvement. Pain may be classified as superficial, deep, and referred. *Superficial pain* arising from either the skin or spreading from adjacent structures such as joints is well localized and is associated with tenderness and hyperalgesia. Often there are accompanying paresthesias, itching, tingling, and in some cases even hypalgesia. *Deep pain* arising from fascia, vessels, periosteum, joints, and supporting structures is often poorly localized and dull, and may be associated with muscular rigidity and deep tenderness. *Referred pain* is usually well localized and similar to pain arising from deep structures (Chap. 5). In persons with acute ischemia of the limbs, with threatened loss of viability, both superficial and deep pain are present.

A thorough examination of the limbs must include inspection for evidence of cutaneous manifestations, palpation for masses and tenderness, and auscultation for arterial bruits. Examination of the peripheral pulses at their accessible sites must always be done. A careful neurologic examination looking for changes in reflexes and sensation is also essential.

In most instances an accurate diagnosis can be made or strongly suspected by history and physical examination. Special tests such as arteriography, myelography, and nerve conduction studies are often helpful but are primarily reserved for accurate localization of the disease and determination of the extent of involvement.

PAINFUL SKIN DISEASE The common bacterial and fungous infections may occasionally produce pain, and it can occur in or remote to the involved areas. This is especially true when bacteria have entered the dermis and subcutaneous tissues via the base of the nails or interdigital areas. Depending upon the infecting agent, cellulitis with or without lymphangitis may rapidly ensue and produce local swelling, pain, erythema, and systemic signs of toxicity. If the infection develops in areas such as the pulp of the digits or in plantar or palmar spaces, the pain is severe, throbbing and may secondarily extend to tendons and joints.

Fungous infections, particularly those of the interdigital areas of the feet, may also become secondarily infected by bacteria, resulting in a spreading cellulitis and lymphangitis. There are also nonbacterial forms of cellulitis. The lymphangitis is diagnosed by the presence of the "red lines" in the involved areas. Pain may also occur in the region of the lymph nodes which drain the infected area and may be the first sign of secondary infection.

Cellulitis, particularly of the lower extremities, may be confused with thrombophlebitis. Differentiating features supporting the diagnosis of cellulitis include: (1) rapidity of onset, (2) prominent cutaneous hyperemia and tenderness, (3) presence of a portal of entry for the infective agent, and (4) the nature of the systemic response (fever, leukocytosis), which is usually much more severe than with thrombophlebitis.

Erythema nodosum (Chap. 57) should be suspected when tender erythematous nodules appear in or under the skin and are associated with fever and joint pains. The articular manifestations often precede the appearance of the nodules. These lesions can be associated with a wide variety of diseases, some of which include tuberculosis, sarcoidosis, coccidioidomycosis, streptococcal infections, and ulcerative colitis. However, in the majority of cases, no underlying disease is found.

MUSCULOSKELETAL PAIN **Bursitis and tendonitis** *Inflammation* of one or more of the bursae may occur as a result of trauma, rheumatoid arthritis, gout, connective tissue disorders, and bacterial infection. The commonly involved bursae are the subdeltoid, olecranon, trochanteric, calcaneal, and prepatellar. When the process is acute it is characterized by severe local pain and tenderness with marked limitation of activity and mobility. In long-standing cases the symptoms and physical findings are less pronounced. Calcific deposits within the involved bursa develop in some patients and may be seen in an x-ray.

Tenosynovitis of the tendon sheaths of hands or wrists produces pain in restricted regions. Tenosynovitis may arise in association with infection, rheumatoid arthritis, osteoarthritis, or trauma, or occur without explanation. When the sheath of the thumb's abductor longus and extensor brevis tendons at the radial styloid are affected, the condition is called *de Quervain's disease.* The flexor tendons in the palm and finger and the extensor sheaths on the dorsum of the wrist may also be the site of the inflammation. Typically, the pain and tenderness occur in the region of the tendon, and the pain is aggravated by stretching the involved tendons as their muscles contract.

An important variant of tenosynovitis is the *carpal tunnel syndrome,* the symptoms of which may be confused with the thoracic outlet syndrome, cervical disk disease, and local vascular insufficiency. Thickening or swelling of the tendons as they pass through the flexor compartment at the wrist, amyloid deposit with multiple myeloma, or bone enlargement (acromegaly) can exert pressure on the median nerve, causing nocturnal paresthesias and pain in the fingers, wrist, and forearm. As the condition worsens atrophy of the thenar eminence develops, as well as weakness and sensory loss in the territory of the median nerve. There may be tenderness on pressure over the carpal ligament and electrical tingling in the fingers when the wrist is tapped (Tinel's sign). Nerve conduction may be delayed at the wrist, confirming the diagnosis.

Calcific and *noncalcific tendonitis* is common in the bicipital and supraspinatus tendons, and in the common tendon of origin for the forearm extensors and flexors at the lateral and medial epicondyle of the humerus, respectively (tennis elbow). The diagnosis is suspected by the location of the pain and the hurtful limitation of motion involved by movement of these tendons.

Painful synovial cysts Cysts of the popliteal space (so-called Baker's cysts) can be an obscure source of pain in the leg. The lesion consists of a cyst in the popliteal fossa, which frequently communicates with the knee joint. While the cause is unknown, such cysts are frequently associated with rheumatoid or osteoarthritis. Trauma may be an inciting factor. Unruptured cysts produce only mild aching in the popliteal space with associated stiffness of the joint. If the cyst ruptures there is an acute, extensive inflammation of the lower leg with swelling and pain which may be severe. The clinical picture is commonly confused with thrombophlebitis. The diagnosis can easily be made by instilling radiopaque material into the knee joint.

Painful arthritis of extremities Most causes of arthritis can be classified into one of five major groups: (1) infectious, (2) degenerative, (3) posttraumatic, (4) metabolic, and (5) unknown etiology. The synovial membranes and periarticular structures are primarily involved in rheumatoid disease, infectious arthritis, and gout whereas the cartilage and bone are mainly affected in osteoarthritis and rarer varieties. With acute pyogenic arthritis, gout, and rheumatic fever, the pain is severe even at rest and greatly intensified by even the slightest motion. The local findings of swelling, redness, and heat may be pronounced.

The principal symptom of *osteoarthritis* is pain which is brought on by use and is relieved by rest. Stiffness after sitting and immediately upon rising in the morning is common but seldom persists for more than a few minutes. Some of the more common locations are the terminal phalanges, knees, hips, and spine.

Rheumatoid arthritis most commonly involves the proximal interphalangeal and metacarpophalangeal joints, toes, wrists, ankle, knee, elbow, hip, and shoulder. The onset is often insidious with general fatigue, paresthesias in the extremities, joint pain, and stiffness. The most common symptoms include joint pain at rest which is aggravated by motion. Thickening of the periarticular structures may be marked and accompanied by atrophy of adjacent muscles. Subcutaneous nodules are often found over pressure points. Many of the patients are also subject to cold sensitivity of Raynaud's type. (See Chaps. 356 and 360.)

Gout, a disease usually of men over thirty years of age, manifests itself often in acute episodes. Most frequently the metatarsophalangeal joint is involved; the affected joint is extremely painful and swells markedly within a few hours, becoming hot and dusky red. The process particularly in the acute form may be difficult to distinguish from acute rheumatic fever, gonococcal arthritis, atypical rheumatoid arthritis, traumatic arthritis, cellulitis, suppurative arthritis and Reiter's syndrome. The presence of tophi and an elevated uric acid clarify the diagnosis. Finding the rod-like crystals of sodium urate in a tophus or synovial fluid establishes the diagnosis with certainty. (See Chap. 100.)

Pyogenic arthritis localizes usually in large joints (hip, knee, and shoulder). Such infections are usually metastatic in origin and remain monoarticular. The cardinal signs of infection, pain, and swelling, and a local increase in temperature with cutaneous hyperemia and fever, usually leave little doubt as to the nature of the condition. In suspected cases the joint must be aspirated to identify the organism by Gram's stain and culture.

Hypertrophic osteoarthropathy, with its characteristic clubbing, periostitis at the ends of long bones, arthritis, and autonomic disorder, causes pain which varies from mild to severe. It is deep and aching pain and along with tenderness is localized to the involved joints and adjacent long bones. This syndrome usually appears in relation to malignancies or suppurative conditions of the lungs, mediastinum, or pleura.

Osteomyelitis Osteomyelitis may occur following open fractures, open surgical reduction of fractures, or from a distant infective focus. Usually the symptoms commence abruptly with severe pain (aggravated by motion), local swelling, exquisite tenderness, chills, and fever. There is nearly always a neutrophilic leukocytosis and elevated sedimentation rate, and blood cultures may be positive. X-ray changes may not be evident until the second week or later. The differential diagnosis includes acute pyogenic arthritis, hemarthrosis (particularly in children), cellulitis, and erysipelas.

Painful disorders of muscle Disorders of muscles are common causes of severe pain in the limbs. Localized tenderness and pain with motion is most commonly seen after trauma or severe exercise. An acute suppurative myositis is nearly always associated with injury and direct innoculation with bacteria. Clostridial myositis (Chap. 154) must be considered in every case of a deep infection occurring secondary to a puncture wound.

A condition frequently confused with ischemic rest pain is the *nocturnal muscle cramp.* This process of unknown cause occurs in both sexes at all ages but is most often a source of complaints in pregnant women, the middle aged, and the elderly. Unusually strenuous activity in the daytime increases the liability to cramp at night especially when the feet are cold. The onset is sudden, usually in one of the muscles of the foot or leg, and it may awaken the patient. The pain subsides with vigorous massage and stretching (Chap. 348) of the part. If frequent and troublesome, 50 mg benadryl taken at bedtime will usually prevent the cramps.

When there is generalized muscle tenderness, weakness, increasing fatigability, and other systemic symptoms, the possibility of polymyositis and dermatomyositis must be considered.

ACUTE ARTERIAL OCCLUSION The clinical picture that results from acute arterial occlusion regardless of its cause is dependent upon the location and extent of the obstruction. If critical areas of the vasculature are involved a sequence of events unfolds the first part of which is pain in the most distal portion of the limb. Coldness, paresthesias, numbness, and finally paralysis follow in rapid succession. Irreversible tissue damage, leading to gangrene, will result within 4 to 6 hr if the occlusion is complete. Examination of the limb reveals loss of pulses distal to the obstruction, decreased skin temperature, and pallor. It is not possible on clinical grounds alone to distinguish arterial thrombosis from embolism, although a cardiac source of emboli, mitral stenosis, atrial fibrillation, and myocardial infarction tend to favor the latter.

If the collateral circulation is adequate to maintain viability of the tissues, the symptoms are often mild. Under these circumstances there may be no more than a subjective sensation of numbness and coldness of the limb.

Cholesterol emboli arising from ulcerating plaques in the aorta can result in a confusing clinical picture. The emboli are small and may pass to the kidney, gut, and lower extremities, giving rise to hematuria and abdominal pain. In the legs they occlude the digital arteries, manifested as ischemic rest pain which is often bilateral and symmetrical. The skin of the foot may exhibit a curious mottling (livedo reticularis). Cutaneous infarction (gangrene) of the toes may result. Similar changes in the digits may be caused by intravascular clotting (cold agglutinins, platelet thrombosis, etc.).

Certain parts of the leg are especially vulnerable to circulatory insufficiency. For example the pretibial compartment containing the extensor muscles of toes and foot are enveloped by tight sheaths. If overexerted to the point of injury with attendant pain and swelling the muscles become infarcted and permanently weakened, and even fatal myoglobinuria has been known to occur.

CHRONIC ARTERIAL OCCLUSION **Arteriosclerosis obliterans** Atherosclerosis of large- and medium-sized arteries, the most common vascular disease of man, often leads to symptoms which are induced by exercise (intermittent claudication) but may occur also at rest (ischemic rest pain). The diabetic patient is especially susceptible. The muscle pain which is brought on by exercise and promptly relieved by rest most frequently involves the calf and thigh muscles. If the atherosclerotic narrowing or occlusion involves the aortic and iliac arteries it may also cause hip and buttock claudication and impotence in the male (Leriche syndrome). Ischemic rest pain, and sometimes attendant ulceration and gangrene, is usually localized to the foot and toes and is usually the consequence of multiple sites of vascular occlusion. Pain at rest is characteristically worse at night and totally or partially relieved by dependency.

The examination of such patients will reveal a loss of one or more peripheral pulses, trophic changes in skin and nails (in advanced cases), and the presence of bruits or thrills over or distal to sites of narrowing. A search should always be made in such patients for an abdominal aortic aneurysm since it is prone to rupture and can be corrected by operation. Arteriography is necessary only for confirmation of the location and extent of the occlusive involvement in planning surgical therapy. The upper extremities distal to the origin of the subclavian artery are rarely involved. Aneurysms of the peripheral arteries do not usually produce pain unless they compress adjacent nerves. Aneurysms of peripheral arteries are of importance primarily because they become the source of distal arterial embolization or undergo thrombosis.

Thromboangiitis obliterans This is a disease of young and middle-aged male cigarette smokers which involves the more distal small and medium arteries of the arms and legs. A spectrum of symptoms occur which is useful in establishing the diagnosis. These symptoms include (1) instep claudication, (2) migratory thrombophlebitis, (3) cold sensitivity, and (4) hand and forearm claudication. The disease is usually bilateral and should be suspected on physical examination by the location of the pulse deficit. The pedal and wrist pulses are often absent. There is marked rubor of the feet even in the supine position. Ischemic rest pain and ulcers when present are usually very severe, leading to early amputation of the involved part. Some clinicians doubt the existence of this entity, pointing out that most such patients on investigation prove to have an unusually severe form of atherosclerosis (Chaps. 344 and 326).

PAINFUL VASOSPASTIC DISORDERS In evaluating patients with cold sensitivity it is important to distinguish *Raynaud's disease* from *Raynaud's phenomenon. Raynaud's disease* is a benign, symmetrical disorder of unknown cause which usually has its onset in the late teens or early twenties. Females are most commonly afflicted and cold and emotional stimuli are the factors which trigger the response in the digits. The fingers become white, then blue, and finally red (the triphasic color response). Pain and paresthesias are common during the ischemic phase. Ulcerations are rarely observed.

Raynaud's phenomenon is always secondary to some underlying problem. The onset may occur at any period of life and may be asymmetrical. Excessive use of hands (e.g., sculling, working with a pneumatic drill) may give rise to it, and often it is associated with one of the connective tissue diseases. When severe it is accompanied by tender, painful fingertip ulcers. It may be the first symptom of the underlying disease. The common disorders associated with this problem are collagen vacular disease, rheumatoid arthritis, thromboangiitis obliterans, dysproteinemias, occupational trauma, and the thoracic outlet syndromes.

ERYTHROMELALGIA This rare disorder of the microvasculature produces a burning pain usually in the toes and forefoot associated with changes in ambient temperature. Each patient has a temperature threshold above which symptoms appear and the feet become bright red and warm. Those afflicted rarely wear stockings or regular shoes since these tend to bring out the symptoms. Patients characteristically relieve the pain by walking on a cold surface or soaking their feet in ice water. On physical examination, the peripheral pulses are intact. The foot and toes have a bright red appearance during the attacks. The disease is usually of unknown cause but has been associated in rare cases with myeloproliferative disorders. In some instances it is the manifestation of a painful neuropathy (Chap. 323).

VENOUS THROMBOSIS The common varieties of inflammation and thrombosis (thrombophlebitis) of the superficial and deep veins during severe illness, prolonged bed rest, trauma, and malignancy may produce pain in the extremities. When the superficial veins are involved the afflicted areas are tender and firm, with associated edema and erythema of the overlying skin. Leg swelling is not then prominent.

Deep venous thrombosis is often more subtle and difficult to diagnose. Classically there is a dull, diffuse pain associated with muscle tenderness and leg edema. Calf pain with dorsiflexion of the foot may be present. The first symptom of this disorder is often pulmonary embolism, which can be life-threatening or fatal. The physical findings are nonspecific and the only certain way of establishing the diagnosis is venography. The method of scanning the leg for radioactive fibrinogen (^{125}I) is becoming increasingly important.

Venous thrombosis destroys the valves of veins. This is the principal cause of the *postphlebitic syndrome.* In the upright position the contraction of leg muscles forces blood not only toward the heart but also in the direction of the foot and through the perforating veins. The consequence of the latter is edema, subcutaneous hemorrhage (usually in the region of the medial malleolus), deposition of hemosiderin pigment, cutaneous fibrosis, and ulceration. Dull diffuse pain that is prolonged by dependency and relieved by elevation of the legs is the usual manifestation. Congenital arteriovenous fistulas can also produce venous hypertension, incompetence of the venous valves, and a clinical picture indistinguishable from the postphlebitic syndrome.

LYMPHEDEMA Obstruction of the lymphatics, either congenital or acquired, leads to the development of brawny edema which may also be associated with a dull, deep pain. The pain is similar to that seen in venous disorders. The edema is firm and does not pit readily. The pattern and location of the swelling provide clues as to its nature. In the legs, involvement of the dorsum of the foot is diagnostic. The swelling does not rapidly disappear with bed rest.

THORACIC OUTLET SYNDROMES Compression of the neurovascular bundle as it leaves the thorax can produce symptoms of numbness, tingling, and pain in the hand or portions of it. The pain and tingling occur only in certain positions depending upon the anatomic defect present. They immediately disappear when the compression is removed. The diagnosis is suspected by reproducing the symptoms and confirming disappearance of the radial pulse with the arm in the position associated with the problem. It is important to x-ray the neck and shoulder girdle looking for cervical ribs. Exact classification of the anatomic defect depends upon establishing the site of compression and the position in which symptoms appear. The common causes include not only cervical ribs but also scalenus anterior, costoclavicular, and Wright's syndromes (Chap. 9).

NEUROGENIC LIMB PAIN Many diseases may affect the peripheral nerves and cause pain in the limbs. These include beri-beri, rheumatoid arthritis, collagen vascular diseases, and diabetes mellitus. Clues to diagnosis are areflexia, which is usually most prominent in the lower limbs and distal or other sensory impairment. The pain tends to be of a persistent, burning, and tearing nature and is often associated with tenderness of deep tissues.

Diabetic neuritis may be difficult to diagnose. The diabetic patient often exhibits a loss of deep pain sensation and develops painless, nonhealing ulcers over weight-bearing or pressure-supporting areas. Motor involvement is less common. The ankle and knee jerks are usually absent. There is often a loss of sympathetic tone and as a result the feet are warm and dry. The problem in such patients is to determine whether the pain is neuropathic, vascular, arthritic, or diskogenic (see Chaps. 9, 323, and 355 for differential diagnosis).

Nerve root compression syndromes A herniated nucleus pulposus is a common disorder which results in nerve root compression with pain radiating into the limbs. The pain is deep and poorly localized to the level of the spine where the disk rupture has occurred and is accompanied by involuntary spasm of paravertebral muscles. If the adjacent nerve roots are compressed, the pain radiates along the corresponding nerve distribution and there are also numbness and paresthesias. The neurological findings are discussed in Chap. 9. Degenerative disk disease and osteoarthritis can also bring symptoms similar to those observed with a herniated disk. Plain films of the vertebral column and in some cases myelography may be required to establish the diagnosis.

It has been recognized that degenerative joint disease of the spine or hip, spinal cord neoplasm, and a herniated disk can all cause symptoms in the limbs which gradually develop with activity and are promptly relieved by rest. Since it mimics intermittent claudication this sequence has been called the *pseudoclaudication syndrome.* Findings which help distinguish this entity from true claudication include the following (1) extreme variation in the walk-pain-rest cycle; with ischemic claudication the walking distance is usually constant, with prompt pain relief upon cessation of exercise. (2) The pain most often occurs in the thigh and buttock without calf pain; this variation is not usually seen in chronic arterial occlusion. (3) There is an attendant low back pain or discomfort. (4) Sensory, motor, and reflex changes are present. (5) There are no pulse deficits or associated bruits.

Reflex sympathetic dystrophies *Causalgia* is a syndrome characterized by a constant, spontaneous, severe burning pain which follows partial or more rarely, complete, injury to a peripheral nerve trunk. It is frequently associated with hyperalgesia, hyperesthesia, and vasomotor and sudomotor disturbances. In far advanced cases, there may be associated trophic changes. The diagnosis is not difficult if the clinical picture can be related to evidence of a previous injury.

While causalgia is considered a reflex sympathetic dystrophy, it is often classified separately because of its numerous entities which can lead to similar complaints and it is better to classify them more broadly as minor reflex sympathetic dystrophies. The causes include trauma, surgery, occupational use, myocardial infarction, neurological disorders (central and peripheral), infections, and vascular disorders. The shoulder-hand syndrome which may follow myocardial infarction is considered to be a reflex dystrophy.

A useful diagnostic test for patients suspected of having a reflex sympathetic dystrophy is to carry out a sympathetic block. The pain is usually completely relieved, with concomittant modification of the physical findings.

Glomus tumor This neoplasm is a benign tumor which develops at the level of the neuromyoarterial glomus. The lesion is small (a few millimeters in diameter) and most frequently located beneath the nails. These small tumors are exquisitely tender to palpation, which distinguishes them from fibromas, neurofibromas, nevi, angiomas, and subungual melanomas.

Interdigital neuroma When pain occurs in the plantar aspect of the foot and is related to walking or local pressure, an interdigital neuroma should be suspected. Essentially this is a compression neuropathy of a plantar nerve, sometimes called "Morton's toe." The lesion usually develops near the ball of the foot and during weight bearing there is a numbness of two or three toes (usually 3–4). Applied pressure will reproduce the symptoms described by the patient. Occasionally the small nodule may be palpable. Excision of the affected nerve relieves the pain (Chap. 336).

REFERENCES

BRAIN L, WALTON JN: *Brain's Diseases of the Nervous System,* 7th ed., London: Oxford University Press, 1969

FAIRBAIRN JF II et al: *Peripheral Vascular Diseases,* 4th ed., Philadelphia: Saunders, 1972

HOLLANDER JL (ed): *Arthritis and Allied Conditions,* 7th ed., Philadelphia: Lea and Febiger, 1966

section 2 | Alterations in body temperature

11 DISTURBANCES OF HEAT REGULATION

ROBERT G. PETERSDORF

CONTROL OF BODY TEMPERATURE

INTRODUCTION In health, the body temperature of man is maintained within a narrow range despite extremes in environmental conditions and physical activity. This is also true for most birds and mammals, and such animals are termed *homeothermic,* or warm-blooded. An almost invariable accompaniment of systemic illness is a disturbance in temperature regulation, usually an abnormal elevation, or *fever.* In fact, fever is such a sensitive and reliable indicator of the presence of disease that thermometry is probably the commonest clinical procedure in use. Even in the absence of a frank febrile response, interference with heat regulation by disease is evident. This may take the form of flushing, pallor, sweating, shivering, and abnormal sensations of cold or warmth, or it may consist of erratic fluctuations of body temperature within normal limits when a patient is at bed rest.

HEAT PRODUCTION The principal source of body heat is the combustion of foods. The greatest amount of heat is generated in the liver and the voluntary muscles. Heat production by muscle is of particular importance because the quantity can be varied according to the need. In most circumstances this variation consists of small increases and decreases in the number of nerve impulses to the muscles, causing inapparent tensing or relaxing. When, however, there is a strong stimulus for heat production, muscle activity may increase to the point of shivering, or even to a generalized rigor.

HEAT LOSS Heat is lost from the body in several ways. Small amounts are used in warming food or drink and in the evaporation of moisture from the respiratory tract. Most heat is lost from the surface of the body, by *convection,* i.e., the transfer of heat to a fluid medium. Heat loss by convection depends on the existence of a temperature gradient between the body surface and the ambient air. A second mechanism for heat loss is *radiation,* which may be defined as an exchange of electromagnetic energy between the body and the radiant environment. *Evaporation* is the third major mechanism for dissipating heat and is particularly important when the ambient temperature exceeds that of the body.

The principal method of regulating heat loss is by varying the volume of blood flowing to the surface of the body. A rich circulation in the skin and subcutaneous tissues carries heat to the surface, where it can escape. In addition, sweating increases heat loss by providing water to be vaporized. The sweat, or eccrine, glands are under the control of the sympathetic nerves which, in this instance, mediate cholinergic stimuli. Heat loss by sweating may be tremendous and as much as 1 liter per hr of sweat may be elaborated. The amount of heat loss through sweating is also dependent upon the humidity in the air. The greater the humidity, the less the ability to lose heat through sweat.

When there is need for conservation of heat, adrenergic autonomic stimuli cause a sharp reduction in the blood flow to the surface. This causes vasoconstriction and transforms the skin and subcutaneous tissue into layers of insulation.

HEAT TRANSFER WITHIN THE BODY This depends upon *conduction,* i.e., the transfer of heat between adjacent organs, and by *circulatory convection,* which is governed by bulk movement of body fluids and which is responsible for the transfer of heat between the cells and the bloodstream. It is useful, although oversimplified, to visualize the body as a central core at uniform temperatures surrounded by an insulating shell. The role of the shell as a mediator for heat conservation and heat loss is determined in part by its blood supply and on vasoconstriction or vasodilatation. The importance of insulation is underscored by the susceptibility of the digits to cold; despite intense vasoconstriction these organs are protected by little insulation and hence may be severely cooled. Insulation may be enhanced by the addition of clothing.

NEURAL CONTROL OF TEMPERATURE The control of body temperature, integrating the various physical and chemical processes for heat production or loss, is a function of cerebral centers located in the hypothalamus. A high-decerebrate animal displays a normal temperature if the hypothalamus is left intact. On the other hand, an animal whose brainstem has been sectioned loses ability to control body temperature, which consequently tends to vary with the environment, a condition referred to as *poikilothermia.* Although the centers in the anterior hypothalamus were generally thought to be responsible for heat loss and those in the posterior hypothalamus to control heat conservation, this separation may be an oversimplification. In fact, an area anterior to the hypothalamus may have important integrating functions in temperature control. The spinal cord is also involved in the integration of temperature-regulating responses, particularly vasomotor and sudomotor activity.

Factors affecting neural control of temperature The temperature-regulating system is a negative feedback control system, and possesses three elements essential to such a system: (1) receptors which sense the existing central temperatures; (2) effector mechanisms, consisting of the vasomotor, sudomotor, and metabolic effectors, and (3) integrative structures which determine whether the existing temperature is too high or too low and which activate the appropriate motor response. It is a negative feedback system because a rise in central temperature initiates mechanisms for losing heat while a fall in central temperature activates mechanisms for heat production and heat conservation. The activation of these mechanisms depends on a central reference temperature, which may be compared to a thermostat and which responds to a variety of stimuli, such as the sensory impulses engendered in flushing or sweating, behavioral impulses, exercise, endocrine influences, and probably the temperature of the blood circulating through the hypothalamic centers. In a sense all of these stimuli reset the thermostat.

A classical example of the endocrine influence on temperature is the effect of menstruation. The mean body temperature of women is higher during the second half of the menstrual cycle than it is between the onset of menstruation and the time of ovulation. The sensations of intense heat followed by diaphoresis that characterize the vasomotor instability experienced by some women at the menopause are undoubtedly the result of endocrine imbalance. The activation of the adrenal medulla in response to cold is another example of the relationship between the endocrine system and the thermoregulatory apparatus.

NORMAL BODY TEMPERATURE It is not practical to designate an exact upper level of normal body temperature because there are small differences among normal persons. There are rare individuals whose temperatures are always elevated slightly above accepted "normal" levels, and there is considerable variation in temperature in a given individual. In general, however, it is safe to regard an oral temperature above 99°F (37.2°C) in a person who has been lying in bed as an indication of disease, this oral temperature in a person who has been engaged in moderate activity has the same significance. The temperature may be as low as 96.5°F (35.8°C) in healthy persons. Rectal temperature is usually 0.5 to 1.0 F° higher than oral temperature. In very hot weather the body temperature may be elevated by 0.5 or even 1.0 F°.

There is a distinct diurnal variation in body temperature in healthy man. Oral readings of 97°F (36.1°C) are relatively common on arising in the morning. Body temperature rises steadily through the day, reaches a peak of 99°F (37.2°C) or greater between 6 P.M. and 10 P.M., and then drops slowly to reach a minimum at 2 A.M. to 4 A.M. Although it has been postulated that this diurnal variation is dependent upon increasing activity during the day and rest at night, the pattern is not reversed in individuals who work at night and sleep during the day for long periods of time. The febrile patterns of most human diseases also tend to follow this normal diurnal pattern. Fevers tend to be higher, to "spike," in the evening, and many patients with febrile disease have relatively normal temperatures in the early morning hours.

Severe or prolonged exercise or very hot baths can produce a transient elevation in body temperature, which is quickly compensated for by increased dissipation of heat from the skin and lungs. Such elevations are not properly classified as fevers. Body temperature is more labile in young children, and transient elevations after relatively slight exertion in warm weather are frequently observed in them.

DISORDERED THERMOREGULATION In fever, the temperature-regulating mechanism does not break down. The system behaves normally, except that, as in exercise, the thermostat is reset. At the beginning of fever, the body temperature as sensed by the thermoreceptors is low and the individual responds physiologically as if he were cold. *Heat production* is increased by shivering and *heat loss* is decreased by vasoconstriction. These events explain the sensation of cold or the chills that characterize the beginning of fever. Conversely, when the cause of fever is removed, the reference temperature (thermostat) returns to normal, and the individual responds as if he were warm. Cutaneous vasodilatation, sweating, and inhibition of shivering are the compensatory responses.

Deviations of 5 F° (approx. 3.5 C°) from the normal

body temperature do not interfere appreciably with most bodily functions. Convulsions are common at temperatures higher than 106°F (41.1°C), and irreversible brain damage, presumably due to protein denaturation (impairment of normal enzymic functions), is common when temperatures of 108°F (42.2°C) are reached. Fortunately, when hyperthermia reaches dangerous levels, the mechanisms for heat loss are suddenly activated; consequently, oral temperatures above 106°F (41.1°C) are rare in man. Conversely, when temperatures are lowered to 91°F (32.8°C), loss of consciousness occurs; at 86°F (30°C) poikilothermia sets in, and between 83 and 84°F (28.5°C) slow atrial fibrillation supervenes. Ventricular fibrillation during hypothermia is comparatively rare.

The systemic symptoms accompanying deviations in temperature are poorly understood. For example at temperatures of 102°F (39°C) many patients have malaise, drowsiness, weakness, and generalized aches and pains. Many others, however, feel entirely well. Why some individuals are able to tolerate fever so well while others become markedly ill remains an enigma. Perhaps the inciting stimulus rather than fever per se is the major determinant of systemic complaints.

Diseases of the nervous system Disease of the regulatory centers in the hypothalamus may affect body temperature. Cases have been observed in which there was destruction of the centers controlling heat-conserving mechanisms, with resulting hypothermia. More commonly, cerebral lesions are manifested by hyperthermia; this may occur with tumors, infections, degenerative diseases, or vascular accidents. It is not uncommon in cerebral apoplexy for the temperature to rise to 105 to 107°F (42 to 43°C) during the last few hours before death. Central fever is accompanied by lack of a diurnal variation, absence of sweating, resistance to antipyretic drugs, excessive response to external cooling and loss of consciousness.

Heat stroke ("sunstroke") (see below), is an interesting example of fever due to interference with the controlling mechanism. Here the central mechanisms for cooling seem suddenly to fail and the patient ceases to sweat, despite the fact that his temperature is rising. Some of the highest temperatures ever observed in human beings (112 to 113°F) (44.4°C) have been in cases of heat stroke. A temperature higher than 114°F (45.5°C) is not compatible with life.

Increased heat production Patients with thyrotoxicosis frequently have an elevation in temperature 1 to 2 F° above the normal range. This is ascribable to the increased amount of heat produced by an increase in the activity and rate of the metabolic processes. Dinitrophenol, a drug which was formerly used for weight reduction in obese persons, causes elevation of temperature; this too seems to be caused by increased metabolic activity.

Impairment of heat loss Patients with *congestive heart failure* often have an elevation of body temperature between 0.5 and 1.5 F°. Perhaps this elevation is caused by impairment of heat dissipation as a result of diminished cardiac output, decline in cutaneous blood flow (with increasing insulation of the central temperature core), the insulating effect of edema, and the increased heat production incident to the muscular activity of dyspnea. On the other hand, patients with congestive heart failure are likely to have other causes of fever, such as venous thrombosis, pulmonary embolism and infarction, myocardial infarction, rheumatic fever, and urinary tract infection. However, since slight fever is so regularly present even in the absence of such complications, the circulatory disturbance may be responsible.

Patients with skin disorders such as *ichthyosis* or *congenital absence of sweat glands* may have fever in a warm environment because of inability to lose heat from the surface of the body. Similarly, individuals taking *drugs which impair sweating,* such as atropine or propantheline (Pro-Banthine), may have fever in warm weather.

DISEASES ASSOCIATED WITH HIGH TEMPERATURES (HEAT SYNDROMES)

Three clinical syndromes are associated with high environmental temperature: *heat cramps, heat exhaustion,* and *heat pyrexia.* Although each entity may be identified clinically, there is considerable overlapping in the changes produced by a high environmental temperature. These alterations are especially prevalent during the first days of a heat wave before effective acclimatization can occur. Prophylaxis by augmenting sodium chloride intake prior to exposure, or by restoring a physiologic balance prior to the onset of overt morbidity, can help prevent the full-blown syndrome, especially heat pyrexia. Children and elderly individuals are particularly susceptible to heat stress. Strenuous physical activity or the presence of an acute or chronic disease may hasten the development of one of the heat syndromes.

ACCLIMATIZATION The basic mechanism by which man accommodates to excessive temperatures in unknown. Acclimatization does not increase the threshold for sweating. However, sweating is the most effective natural means of combating heat stress, and can occur with little or no change in the core temperature of the body. As long as sweating continues, man can withstand remarkably high temperatures, provided water and sodium chloride, the most important physiologic constituents of sweat, are replaced. The concentration of sodium chloride varies between that of interstitial fluid and very low concentrations, and the ability to secrete sweat of low NaCl content is a major mechanism for the conservation of salt in hot weather. Dilatation of the peripheral blood vessels in an attempt to dissipate heat is another well-known phenomenon in hot temperatures. Other alterations include a decrease in total circulating blood volume, a decrease in renal blood flow, an increase of the antidiuretic hormone (ADH) as well as aldosterone. Hyperaldosteronism may result in severe potassium loss, which may be aggravated by replacement of sodium without concomitant repletion of potassium. Initially there is an increase in cardiac output but as heat stress persists, venous return diminishes and heart failure may occur. If environmental temperatures in excess of the body's temperature persist, heat is retained and hyperpyrexia develops.

HEAT CRAMPS Heat cramps, called "miner's cramps" and "stoker's cramps," is the most benign heat syndrome. Cramps are characterized by painful spasms of the voluntary muscles and usually follow strenuous exercise. In general, only individuals in good physical condition develop this syndrome. External temperatures need not exceed the body temperature, and direct exposure to the sun is not necessary. The body temperature is usually not elevated. Muscle cramps usually occur after excessive sweating and may even be precipitated by strenuous exercise in cold environments in untrained persons heavily clothed. Muscles of the extremities bear the brunt of physical activity and hence show the highest incidence of cramps. Physical examination of the patient is normal between the paroxysms. Examination of the blood reveals a concentration of the formed elements and a decreased sodium and chloride concentration. Excretion of these ions in the urine is characteristically low. Treatment consists of sodium chloride; cessation of cramps with replacement of sodium chloride and water is striking and supports the hypothesis that the cause of heat cramps is depletion of these essential electrolytes. Occasionally cramps involve the abdominal musculature, mimicking an intraabdominal emergency. Such patients have had mistaken exploratory surgery performed, often with disastrous results. Replacement of saline prior to surgery would have obviated such operations.

HEAT EXHAUSTION Heat prostration, or heat collapse, is probably the most common heat syndrome. Weakness, vertigo, headache, nausea, anorexia, and faintness may precede collapse. Heat collapse occurs in both physically active and sedentary individuals. The onset is usually sudden and the duration of collapse brief. During the acute stage, the patient looks ashen-gray. The skin is cold and clammy. The pupils are dilated. The blood pressure may be low and the pulse pressure elevated. Since prostration develops before exposure to heat is prolonged, body temperature is subnormal or normal. The duration of exposure and the extent to which sweat is lost determine the degree of hemoconcentration. Treatment consists of removal of the patient to a cool area, and spontaneous recovery then usually takes place. Intravenous administration of saline solution or whole blood is necessary only rarely. The pathogenetic mechanism of heat prostration is not primarily a depletion of water and salt, but it is likely that maintenance of these electrolytes will prevent heat prostration in individuals exposed to high temperatures.

HEAT PYREXIA Heat hyperpyrexia, heat stroke, or sunstroke is most common in individuals with preexisting chronic disease. Among these are arteriosclerosis, diabetes mellitus, alcoholism and disorders in which it may be difficult to lose heat such as ectodermal dysplasia, congenital absence of the sweat glands, or severe scleroderma. Direct exposure to the sun is not a necessary prerequisite. Heat pyrexia may develop during any period of hot weather, but the incidence in temperate climates increases during prolonged heat waves. High humidity is a prerequisite to heat stroke, and patients usually stop sweating before onset of acute symptoms. The cessation of sweating is due to an intrinsic breakdown of the heat regulatory mechanism for reasons not known. There may be few premonitory symptoms of heat stroke, and loss of consciousness may be the first sign. Other patients may complain of headache, vertigo, faintness, abdominal distress, or confusion. Delirium may develop in more severe cases.

Pyrexia and prostration are the significant findings on physical examination. A rectal temperature greater than 106°F (41.1°C) is common and is a grave prognostic sign. Internal body temperatures as high as 110°F (43.3°C) have been recorded. The skin is hot and dry, and sweating is absent. The pulse rate is increased, and respirations are rapid and weak. The systolic blood pressure may be elevated. The muscles are flaccid, and tendon reflexes may be diminished. Shock is common in fatal cases. Examination of the blood and urine may show few abnormalities. Leukocytosis is characteristic as are proteinuria, cylinduria, and an elevation in BUN. At the onset electrolytes are normal, although the potassium may be diminished. The electrocardiogram may show, in addition to tachycardia and sinus arrhythmia, flattening and subsequent inversion of the T wave and depression of the S-T segment. Diffuse myocardial necrosis with ECG evidence of myocardial infarction has been reported. Other major laboratory abnormalities include thrombocytopenia; prolonged bleeding, clotting, and prothrombin times; afibrinogenemia and fibrinolysis; and consumptive coagulopathy. All of these may be responsible for diffuse bleeding. Liver damage is common; it appears 24 to 36 hr after admission and is characterized by clinically apparent jaundice and, often, by abnormalities in hepatocellular enzymes. Renal failure is a common complication of heat stroke.

Patients with heat stroke may die within a few hours after being discovered, or may die of complications such as acute renal failure. However, a number of patients will die several weeks after the acute episode, usually of myocardial infarction, heart failure, renal failure, bronchopneumonia or complicating bacteremia. In them autopsy may show extensive parenchymal damage to various organs, either from hyperpyrexia per se or from petechial hemorrhages in the brain, heart, kidneys, or liver.

Treatment Heat stroke requires heroic emergency measures. Time is most important. The patient should be placed in a cool place with adequate circulation of fresh air and with most of the clothing removed. Because the pathogenesis of heat stroke involves failure of the heat-regulating mechanism with cessation of sweating, external means of heat dissipation must be employed. The most effective measure is to immerse the patient in an ice-water bath, and there is no effective substitute for this seemingly drastic treatment. An ice-water bath does not induce shock or stimulate significant cutaneous vasoconstriction. The bath should be given with a minimum of delay. The patient should be watched constantly by a nurse or physician and the rectal temperature monitored. The bath may be discontinued when the core temperature falls below 103°F (39.5°C), but treatment should be resumed if there is a febrile rebound. Compared to immersion in ice water, other forms of therapy are ineffective.

Following the bath the patient should be placed in a cool, well-ventilated room. Massage of the skin aids the acceleration of heat loss and stimulates return of the cool peripheral blood to the overheated brain and viscera. Stimulants such as epinephrine and narcotics are contraindicated. Intravenous fluids should be given but only with monitoring of the central venous pressure and in the absence of cardiac failure. Fresh blood and fibrinogen solutions should be given (without waiting for laboratory confirmation) in case of bleeding and afibrinogenemia.

DISEASES ASSOCIATED WITH LOW TEMPERATURES

COLD ACCLIMATIZATION Cold acclimatization represents a state of increased resistance to cold injury and is the result of exposure to a cold but tolerable environment. Adaptive responses consist of circulatory adjustments protecting the temperatures of exposed portions of the body; metabolic adaptation results in greater heat production to compensate for increased heat loss; and behavioral and neural adaptations minimize either the actual cold stress or the discomfort resulting from physiologically tolerable hypothermia. In contrast with heat acclimatization, it is not possible to delineate adaptive physiologic changes to cold. Nevertheless, primitive people live at zero temperatures wearing little or no clothing; pain perception is less in persons, such as fishermen, who work periodically with their hands in ice water; and military personnel shiver less during cold exposure after training in the Arctic. Adaptation may take place either by shivering, with production of excess heat, or, as is the case in Australian aborigines, by a drop of internal temperature with only minimal shivering.

HYPOTHERMIA Hypothermia is far less common than is elevation in temperature but is of considerable importance because it represents a medical emergency which lends itself to treatment.

Accidental hypothermia This is a well-known complication of exposure, and has often been reported in Great Britain during the winter months. It has also been reported in the United States. It usually occurs in elderly individuals after prolonged exposure, not necessarily to excessively low external temperatures. It is attributed not only to exogenous factors such as a low external environment but also to unknown endogenous factors. The diagnosis of hypothermia has proved elusive largely because *clinical thermometers do not record temperatures below 95°F (35°C), and whenever a patient presents with a temperature in this range the true temperature should be determined with an incubator thermometer or a thermocouple.* Accidental hypothermia has been found in association with myxedema, pituitary insufficiency, Addison's disease, hypoglycemia, cerebrovascular disease, myocardial infarction, terminal cirrhosis, pancreatitis, and ingestion of drugs or alcohol. For example, it is not uncommon to find a derelict in a railroad yard or under a bridge following an alcoholic debauche with a temperature between 85 and 90°F (28.5–32.3°C) or lower. These patients usually appear cold and pale and, when the temperatures are very low, give the appearance of having rigor mortis, so stiff is their musculature. Patients with temperatures less than 80°F (26.7°C) are usually unconscious. The pupils are usually miotic, respirations tend to be shallow and slow, there is bradycardia, and most patients are hypotensive. There is often generalized edema. Laboratory data tend to show hemoconcentration, mild azotemia, and metabolic acidosis. Some patients have hypoglycemia while others show evidence of diabetes mellitus. Thyroid function tests give results typical of myxedema in a number of these patients. Some patients have elevations in serum amylase and a few show pancreatitis at autopsy. The electrocardiogram is distorted by muscular tremors, and may show bradycardia or slow atrial fibrillation, and a characteristic J wave (occurring at the junction of the QRS complex and S-T segment).

TREATMENT Therapy should be instituted at once and consists of maintenance of the airway and intravenous administration of glucose and saline and low molecular weight dextran, both to expand blood volume and to prevent the infarctions which have been a hallmark in fatal cases. *External rewarming is contraindicated* because, while it tends to dilate the constricted peripheral blood vessels, it diverts blood from the visceral organs; most patients who have been rewarmed externally have died. On the other hand, restoration of the core temperature by hemodialysis during which the blood is warmed externally or by peritoneal dialysis during which the dialysate is warmed to 98.6°F is helpful. Corticosteroids, vasopressors, and prophylactic antibiotics have not proved valuable. Large volumes of fluid, supplemented by dialysis, is the treatment of choice. The prognosis in accidental hypothermia remains poor, primarily because many of these patients are old and have associated debilitating disease. One young patient was saved even after her temperature dropped to 69°F (20.6°C).

Immersion hypothermia Responses to cold water immersion may be classified as (1) stimulatory, with deep body temperature normal to 35°C (95°F); (2) depressant, with deep body temperature 35 to 30°C (95–86°F); and critical, with deep body temperature 30 to 25°C (86 to 77°F).

The long-distance swimmer is able to maintain a normal body temperature for periods of 15 to 25 hr or more in water that may plunge skin temperature to 15°C (59°F) or lower, which is some 28°F below deep body temperature, lending support to the concept of a body core insulated by a body shell. The vasoconstriction operative in cold water greatly reduces heat loss. However, there is great individual variability in heat loss in cold water. The relatively obese swimmer may maintain a normal rectal temperature for 2 hr without shivering in 16°C (61°F) water. A lean man under the same conditions, despite violent shivering, may experience a fall in rectal temperature of several degrees and become incapacitated from the rigor. In hypersensitive persons, immersion in cold water may be followed by vascular spasm, vomiting, and syncope.

Other compensatory responses include bradycardia, a slight rise in blood pressure, and an early rise in rectal temperature followed by a fall. At 86°F (30°C), atrial fibrillation is common.

TREATMENT Although rewarming in hot water has been recommended in the treatment of immersion hypothermia, the same objections to sudden diversion of cardiac output to peripheral tissues described above apply. Individuals with this problem should be covered with a light blanket and placed in a room with a moderate ambient temperature. Hemodialysis or peritoneal dialysis should be considered.

LOCAL COLD INJURIES Mechanisms of freezing injury These can be divided into phenomena which affect cells and extracellular fluids (direct effects) and those which disrupt the function of organized tissues and the integrity of the circulation (indirect effects).

DIRECT EFFECTS When tissue freezes, ice crystals form and, concomitantly, solutes in the residual liquid become concentrated. The physical dislocation during slow freezing is extreme. Ice crystals many times the size of individual cells form but only in the extracellular spaces. Large ice crystals can develop between cells in soft tissue without producing irreversible injury as long as the percentage of water frozen does not exceed a critical amount. A major source of damage to living cells during freezing and thawing appears to be the strong salt solutions which develop during formation and dissolution of ice; changes in the proportions of lipids and phospholipids in the cell membrane are also of great importance. The discovery of the protective value of such substances as glycerol and dimethylsulfoxide, which enter cells and prevent freezing injury during comparatively slow cooling to low temperatures and rewarming from them, represents a significant advance. This method has been used extensively in banking spermatozoa for subsequent artificial insemination. It has not been possible, however, to protect organs in this manner since the protective substance must be delivered to all cells.

INDIRECT EFFECTS The fulminating vascular reaction and stasis which supervene are associated with production of histamine-like substances which increase the permeability of the capillary bed. Within blood vessels, cellular elements aggregate. Irreversible occlusion of small blood vessels by cell masses has been demonstrated in thawed tissue following freezing injury. The damaged frozen tissue simulates tissue damage produced by burns.

Manifestations Local cold injury may be divided into freezing (frostbite) and nonfreezing (immersion-foot) injuries. The two types may be observed in the same extremity or in different extremities in the same individual, e.g., trench foot and freezing of the hands but not the feet of shipwreck survivors. The diagnosis of freezing versus nonfreezing injury generally can be made on the basis of history and clinical manifestations.

IMMERSION FOOT This entity is observed in shipwreck survivors or in soldiers (trench foot) whose feet have been wet but not freezing cold for prolonged periods. There is primarily injury to nerve and muscle tissue, but no gross or irreparable pathologic changes occur in blood vessels and skin. The clinical picture reflects primary hypoxic trauma giving rise to three clearly recognizable conditions: (1) *ischemia,* denoted by a pale pulseless extremity; (2) *hyperemia,* characterized by a bounding pulsatile circulation in red swollen painful feet; and (3) the *posthyperemic* or recovery period. The initial cold-induced vasoconstriction, increased blood viscosity, and impaired oxygen transport in the ischemic state are aggravated by such factors as malnutrition, general hypothermia, dehydration, and trauma from relatively fixed, pendant extremities. The problem of rewarming is critical in these patients during the stage of ischemia, when overheating of tissue may lead to gangrene. In the state of hyperemia, the red swollen feet require judicious cooling. Severe cases may show muscular weakness, atrophy, ulceration, and gangrene of superficial areas. Sensitivity to cold and pain on weight bearing, which may cause discomfort for many years, are sequelae even of milder injuries.

FROSTBITE In contrast with immersion foot, in frostbite the blood vessels may be severely and irreparably injured, the circulation of blood ceases, and the vascular bed of the frozen tissue is occluded by agglutinated cell aggregates and thrombi. The cutaneous injury consists in part of separation of the epidermal-dermal interface. Early, the intravascular clumping is reversible. However, with the passage of time, clumped red cells within vessels in injured tissue lose their morphologic identity and take on the appearance of a homogenous, hyalinaceous plug. It has been shown in some, but not all, experimental studies that much of the intravascular aggregation following freezing injury can be reversed and microcirculatory perfusion improved if low molecular weight dextran is given intravenously shortly after injury. Frostbitten tissues unfortunately are often neglected and with thawing become macerated; if this is the situation the method of rewarming is not important. The method of rewarming has been a matter of controversy. It seems most rational to warm the core of the body before treating the local area of frostbite. Following restoration of the core temperature to normal, warming of a frostbitten limb should begin in water at 10 to 15°C, which is then increased 5 C° every 5 min to a maximum of 40°C.

Most cold injuries do not require warming and treatment should be conservative and consists of bed rest, elevation of the injured part, tetanus antitoxin, and antibiotics, when indicated; early drainage of blebs and bullae; daily washes with pHisoHex; and early institution of physiotherapy. Surgical amputation and reconstruction is usually not necessary. Regional sympathectomy performed 24 to 48 hr after thawing is followed by rapid resolution of edema, earlier demarcation of destroyed tissue, and faster healing. The effect of regional sympathectomy is probably due to ablation of persistent vasospasm and to restoration of cold perception.

Some patients with frostbite have residua consisting of excessive sweating, pain, cold feet, numbness, abnormal color, and pain in the joints. The symptoms are generally worse in the winter and following exposure to cold. These patients also often show abnormal nails, discoloration and pigmentation, hyperhydrosis, and by x-ray, osteosporsis and cystic defects near the joints. These abnormalities tend to be milder in patients who have had sympathectomies. Most cold injuries are preventable by graded exposure to cold, as well as appropriate clothing in freezing temperatures.

CLINICAL USES OF LOW TEMPERATURES

Localized application Low temperature has been used extensively in recent years. Two outstanding examples are selective destruction by freezing in cryosurgery and preservation of biologic material. Practical advantages of cryogenic surgery are safety and hemostasis; the results in therapeutic management of tumors have been encouraging. The preservation of red blood cells, spermatozoa, and other viable material by low temperature has become possible through use of glycerol to protect cells against freezing. Hypothermia combined with hyperbaric oxygenation has been employed with notable success in preserving organs, chiefly kidneys, for transplantation.

Use of hypothermia in surgery Periods of ischemia sufficient to permit surgical intervention can be tolerated by organs such as the brain and heart, provided that tissue temperature has been lowered to reduce metabolism before blood supply is interrupted. Hypothermia can be induced with light anesthesia and surface cooling or, more effectively, by means of a pump-oxygenator to provide extracorporeal circulation. Prior to the introduction of this technique, surgical hypothermia was limited to temperatures of about 28°C and temperatures below 25°C were dangerous. At present, extracorporeal circulation has extended the application of hypothermia to temperatures of 10°C or lower. The principal medical problem arises from disturbances in acid-base balance, including large fluctuations in dissolved CO_2 in relation to temperature change, the oxygen debt incurred by some tissues, and an excess in lactic acid production. The oxygen debt is present not only during induction of hypothermia but also during the period of recovery when cardiac function is less than optimal. The body's buffer mechanisms are often inadequate to cope with the shifts in pH and to regulate pH. Therefore intravenous amine type buffers (Tris or THAM) may need to be used. The addition of hyperbaric oxygen has also improved pH control and has enhanced the period during which ischemia may be maintained safely.

REFERENCES

Brengelman G: Temperature regulation, in *Physiology and Biophysics,* eds TC Ruch and HD Patton, Philadelphia: Saunders, 1973

Clinicopathologic Conference: A sixty-five-year-old woman with heat stroke. Am J Med 43:113, 1967

David DM et al: Accidental hypothermia treated by extracorporeal blood-warming. Lancet 1:1036, 1967

Duguid H, Simpson RG: Accidental hypothermia. Lancet 2:1213, 1961

Golding MR et al: The role of sympathectomy in frostbite, with a review of 68 cases. Surgery 57:774, 1965

Knochel JP et al: The renal, cardiovascular, hematologic and serum electrolyte abnormalities of heat stroke. Am J Med 30:299, 1961

Lash RF et al: Accidental profound hypothermia and barbiturate intoxication: A report of rapid "core" rewarming by peritoneal dialysis. JAMA 201:123, 1967

O'Donnel TF, Jr, Clowes GHA, Jr: The circulatory abnormalities of heat stroke. New Engl J Med 287:734, 1972

Penn I, Schwartz SI: Evaluation of low molecular weight dextran in the treatment of frostbite. J Trauma 4:784, 1964

Shibolet S et al: Fibrinolysis and hemorrhages in fatal heatstroke. New Engl J Med 266:169, 1962

Tolman KG, Cohen A: Accidental hypothermia. Can Med Assoc J 103:1357, 1970

12 CHILLS AND FEVER

ROBERT G. PETERSDORF

In view of the extensive knowledge of physiologic mechanisms controlling body temperature mentioned in Chap. 11, it is surprising that so little is known about the ways in which disease upsets thermoregulation.

Some bacteria, particularly gram-negative species, produce endotoxins which are pyrogenic, and a few viruses also cause fever when injected into man or animals. Many microorganisms, however, possess no demonstrable pyrogenic toxin and, of course, fever accompanies diseases which do not involve invasion of the body by any known parasite. Omitting disorders which may involve cerebral thermoregulatory centers directly, such as brain tumors, intracranial hemorrhage or thrombosis, or heat stroke, the following disease states may be accompanied by fever: (1) All *infections,* whether caused by bacteria, rickettsias, viruses, or more complex parasites, cause fever. (2) *Mechanical trauma,* e.g., a crushing injury, frequently gives rise to fever lasting 1 or 2 days. Not infrequently, however, complicating infection sets in. (3) Many *neoplastic diseases* are associated with fever. In most patients, fever in patients with cancer is related to obstruction or infection produced by the tumor. In some solid tumors, however, fever may be due to the tumor per se, particularly following metastasis to the liver. Tumors which are associated with fever include hypernephroma, carcinoma of the pancreas, lung, or bone, and hepatoma. In tumors of the reticuloendothelial system, including Hodgkin's disease, lymphosarcoma, reticulum cell sarcoma, and acute leukemias, fever may be one of the prominent early manifestations. (4) *Hematopoietic disorders,* e.g., acute hemolytic episodes, may be characterized by pyrexia. (5) *Vascular accidents* of any magnitude e.g., myocardial, pulmonary, and cerebral infarctions, nearly always cause fever. (6) *Diseases due to immune mechanisms* are almost always febrile. These include the collagen diseases, drug fevers, and serum sickness. (7) Certain *acute metabolic disorders,* such as gout, porphyria, and Addisonian or thyroid crises, sometimes are associated with fever.

PATHOGENESIS OF FEVER Several hypotheses have been offered to explain disturbed temperature regulation in disease. One attributes fever to shifts in body water which interfere with heat production and heat loss. It is true that newborn infants may become febrile when fluid intake is inadequate and that the temperature elevation subsides promptly when fluid is administered. In adults, there are occasional instances of fever associated with extracellular fluid deficit when the ambient temperature is above 90°F. On the other hand, "dehydration" is not ordinarily associated with fever in adults, and the clinical practice of attributing fever to this cause has little basis in fact.

There is little evidence to implicate abnormal thyroid and adrenal function in the pathogenesis of fever. Temperature regulation is normal in Addison's disease and in Cushing's syndrome. Body temperature is slightly above normal in thyrotoxicosis and a little low in myxedema, but these differences are entirely in keeping with the metabolic rate and there is no real evidence of impaired thermoregulation in either disease.

There was a renewal of interest in a role of the endocrines in the pathogenesis of fever with the finding that abnormalities of etiocholanolone metabolism exist in some patients with "periodic fever" (Chap. 225). Although administration of progesterone and some of its congeners, and of etiocholanolone, results in fever in man, there is no evidence that specific steroid fevers (notably etiocholanolone fever) exist.

Tissue injury Because fever is associated with so many diverse disease processes, it seems reasonable that it is determined by some common mechanism, and the common factor in febrile diseases, whether or not they are infectious in origin, is *tissue injury.* The hypothesis which best fits clinical and experimental observations is that fever results from disturbance of cerebral thermoregulation brought about by a product or products of tissue injury. It has been shown experimentally that inflammatory exudates cause fever when injected intravenously into normal animals, and similar results have been obtained in human subjects. Probably the major source of pyrogenic material is the polymorphonuclear leukocyte, although other cells, notably mononuclear cells, also may release fever-producing substances.

The elements of the febrile response can be illustrated by the sequence of events that follow intravenous injection of killed bacteria or of purified bacterial endotoxin. Following administration of a small amount of typhoid vaccine intravenously in man, the body temperature does not begin to rise until about an hour after the injection. During this interval, the patient notes no discomfort and his appearance is unchanged. Then, rather suddenly, there is malaise, he complains of cold, and within minutes he is burrowing down into the bedclothes, asking for more blankets. He begins to shiver and is soon having a shaking chill which lasts 10 to 20 min. During this time, the skin is pale and cold but the rectal temperature rises steeply. After subsidence of the rigor, the patient gradually feels warmer, the skin circulation increases, and within 2 hr he is flushed and complains of feeling feverish. After another hour, profuse sweating begins and the body temperature begins to return toward normal.

Endogenous pyrogen The pathophysiologic counterpart of these clinical events has been worked out to a large extent in experimental animals. Following its injection, endotoxin is removed rapidly from the bloodstream by the fixed phagocytes of the reticuloendothelial system. At the same time there is, in most species, a profound leukopenia, and the leukocytes are marginated along blood vessel walls. During this period, they appear to be activated, probably by the endotoxin, to release a fever-producing substance into the circulation. This humoral factor, which has been called *endogenous pyrogen,* is presumably the substance which acts on the thermoregulatory centers to produce fever. Endogenous pyrogen has been found in the bloodstream of animals given endotoxin, antigens (in previously sensitized animals), antigenantibody complexes, and those with experimental pneumococcal, streptococcal, staphylococcal, and viral infections. Biologically, endogenous pyrogen found in serum is similar to leukocytic pyrogen derived from sterile inflammatory exudates. Leukocytic pyrogen has undergone partial but not complete purification and has been found to be a low molecular weight basic protein which is heat-labile and which may be closely related to lysozomal enzymes. Its biochemical structure has not been worked out, but evidence suggests that it exists in cells in an inactive precursor form. Whether endogenous pyrogen is the sole mediator of fever or whether some of the agents which incite its release—such as endotoxin—can activate the thermoregulatory centers directly is unknown.

ACCOMPANIMENTS OF FEVER

Systemic symptoms The perception of fever by patients varies enormously. Some persons can tell with considerable accuracy whether their body temperatures are elevated; others, notably patients with tuberculosis, may be wholly unaware of body temperatures as high as 103°F. Often, also, patients may pay no attention to fever because of other unpleasant symptoms such as headache and pleuritic pain. Pain in the back, generalized myalgias, and arthralgia without arthritis are common in fever. Whether these symptoms reflect the presence of an infectious agent or are merely a nonspecific accompaniment of pyrexia is not clear.

Chills Abrupt onset of fever with a *chill* or *rigor* is characteristic of some diseases and, in the absence of antipyretic drugs, rare in others. Although repeated rigors are typical of pyogenic infection with bacteremia, a similar pattern of fever may occur in noninfectious diseases such as lymphoma. It is important to differentiate a true chill, which is accompanied by teeth chattering and bed shaking, from the chilly sensation which occurs in almost all fevers, particularly those in viral infections. In some instances, however, a true rigor occurs in viremia. Chills may be evoked or perpetuated by the intermittent administration of aspirin or other antipyretics. These agents may cause a sharp depression in temperature, which is followed by compensatory involuntary muscular contractions, i.e., a chill. This unpleasant side effect of antipyretic drugs can be averted by administering these agents frequently and in low doses.

Herpes labialis, so-called fever blister, results from activation of the herpes simplex virus by elevation in temperature and occurs frequently in patients undergoing artificial fever therapy. For reasons which are obscure, fever blisters are common in pneumococcal infections, streptococcosis, malaria, meningococcemia, and rickettsoises but are rare in mycoplasma pneumonia, tuberculosis, brucellosis, smallpox, and typhoid.

Delirium may result from elevation of body temperature and is particularly common in patients with alcoholism or cerebral arteriosclerosis.

Convulsions are not infrequent in febrile children, especially those with a family history of epilepsy, although febrile convulsions do not, in general, reflect serious cerebral disease.

CLINICAL IMPORTANCE OF FEVER The temperature is a simple, objective, and accurate indicator of a physiologic state and is much less subject to external and psychogenic stimuli than the other vital signs, i.e., the pulse, respiratory rate, and blood pressure. For these reasons, determination of the body temperature assists in estimating the severity of an illness, its course and duration, and the effect of therapy, or even in deciding whether a person has an organic illness.

Benefit of fever There are few infections of man in which pyrexia appears definitely to be beneficial to the host, examples being neurosyphilis and perhaps chronic brucellosis. Certain other diseases, such as uveitis and rheumatoid arthritis, sometimes improve after fever therapy. In experimental animals some pneumococcal and cryptococcal infections have been influenced in favor of the host animal by raising the body temperature. Aged and debilitated patients with infection may have little or no fever, and this is generally interpreted as a bad prognostic sign. In the great majority of infectious diseases, however, there is no reason to believe that pyrexia accelerates phagocytosis, antibody formation, or other defense mechanisms.

Detrimental aspects of fever Fever accelerates all metabolic processes and accentuates weight loss and nitrogen wastage. The work and the rate of the heart are increased. Sweating aggravates loss of salt and water. There may be discomfort due to headache, photophobia, general malaise, or unpleasant sensation of warmth. The rigors and profuse sweats of hectic fevers are particularly unpleasant for the patient. In elderly individuals with overt or potential cardiac or cerebral vascular disease, fever may be particularly deleterious.

MANAGEMENT OF FEVER Since fever ordinarily does little harm and imposes no great discomfort, antipyretic drugs are rarely necessary and may obfuscate the effect of a specific therapeutic agent or of the natural course of the disease. There are situations, however, in which lowering of the body temperature is of vital importance; e.g., heat stroke, postoperative hyperthermia, delirium due to hyperpyrexia, or shock associated with fever and heart failure. Under these circumstances lowering the temperature is indicated. Cooling blankets which can be set at hypothermic temperatures are a highly effective means for external cooling. Alternatively, sponging the body surface with cool saline solution or the application of cool compresses to the skin and forehead may be employed. There is no advantage in sponging with alcohol, which, because of its pungent odor, makes some patients ill. When high internal temperature is combined with cutaneous vasoconstriction, as in heat stroke or postoperative hyperthermia, the cooling measures should be combined with massage of the skin in order to bring blood to the surface, where it may be cooled. Immediate immersion in a tub of ice water should be considered a lifesaving emergency procedure in patients with heat stroke if the internal body temperature is in excess of 108°F. If cooling blankets are available, they are preferable to immersion into ice in most instances.

If antipyretic drugs, such as aspirin (0.3 to 0.6 g), are employed to bring about a fall in temperature, the ill effects of the unpleasant diaphoresis, sometimes associated with an alarming fall in blood pressure and the subsequent return of fever, occasionally accompanied by a chill, can be mitigated by enforcing a liberal fluid intake and by administering the drug regularly and frequently at 2- to 3-hr intervals. Although adrenal steroids are also potent antipyretics, they must be used with caution because of their tendency to precipitate abrupt falls in temperature accompanied by hypotension. The capacity of these drugs to mask other manifestations of infection also constitutes a relative contraindication to their use.

The discomfort of a rigor can be alleviated in many patients by the intravenous injection of calcium gluconate. This procedure will stop the shivering and chilliness but has no influence on the ultimate height of the fever. Severe disruptive rigors sometimes need to be abolished with morphine sulfate (10 to 15 mg subcutaneously).

DIAGNOSTIC CONSIDERATIONS IN FEVER

In many illnesses fever is the most prominent and often the only manifestation of disease. It is not an indication of any particular type of disease; rather it should be considered a reaction to injury comparable to an elevated leukocyte count or a rapid erythrocyte sedimentation rate.

TYPES OF FEVER Fever is classically described as intermittent, remittent, sustained, and relapsing.

An intermittent fever is one in which the temperature falls to normal each day. When the variation between the peak and the nadir is very large the fever is called *hectic* or *septic*. Intermittent fevers are characteristic in pyogenic infections (notably those in the right upper quadrant), lymphomas, and miliary tuberculosis.

In remittent fever the temperature falls each day but does not return to normal. Most fevers are remittent, and this type of febrile report is in no way characteristic.

A sustained fever is characterized by persistent elevation without significant diurnal variation. It is exemplified by the fever of untreated typhoid or typhus.

A relapsing fever is one in which short febrile periods occur between one or several days of normal temperature. Examples of relapsing fever are seen in the following conditions:

Malaria (Chap. 210) had vanished from the United States almost completely, but Vietnam war veterans constitute an important and sizable reservoir of this infection, as do other persons recently arrived from foreign countries. It is most unusual, however, for malaria to recur after a symptom-free interval of 1 year or more. Seizures recur at 2- or 3-day intervals, or more irregularly in falciparum infections, depending on the maturation cycle of the parasite. The diagnosis depends on demonstration of the parasites in the blood.

Relapsing fever (Chap. 162) occurs in the Southwest part of the United States, as far east as Texas, and in many other parts of the world. The recurrences are related to the cyclic development of parasites. Diagnosis is by demonstration of the spirochetal organisms in stained films of the blood.

Rat-bite fever is brought about by two agents—*Spirillum minus* (Chap. 163) and *Streptobacillus moniliformis* (Chap. 145), both transmitted by the bite of a rat. Both may cause an illness characterized by periodic exacerbations of fever. The clue to the diagnosis depends on obtaining a history of rat bite 1 to 10 weeks previous to the onset of symptoms. The cause can be established by appropriate laboratory procedures.

Localized *pyogenic infections* in rare instances, give rise to periodic bouts of fever separated by afebrile and relatively symptom-free intervals. The so-called "Charcot's intermittent biliary fever," i.e., cholangitis with biliary obstruction due to stones, is an example. *Urinary tract infection,* with episodes of ureteral obstruction due to small stones or inspissated puss, can also cause recurrent fever.

In *Hodgkin's disease,* perhaps 5 to 10 percent of cases, there is at sometime the so-called "Pel-Ebstein fever"—bouts of fever lasting 3 to 10 days, separated by afebrile and asymptomatic periods of 3 to 10 days. These cycles may be repeated regularly over a period of several months. In rare instances this periodicity of the fever has been sufficiently striking to suggest the correct diagnosis before lymphadenopathy or splenomegaly became evident. However, Pel-Ebstein fever may be caused by other diseases, not related to Hodgkin's disease.

EPIDEMIOLOGY OF FEVER The diagnosis of febrile illnesses must take into consideration the context of the epidemiologic setting. For example, an acute 6-day febrile illness in a soldier in Vietnam is probably due to dengue or Chikungunya fevers (Chap. 208), malaria (Chap. 210), scrub typhus (Chap. 181), or leptospirosis (Chap. 161); in a college student in the United States it may represent infectious mononucleosis or some other viral infection; and in an octogenarian following prostatectomy it is probably an indication of urinary tract infection, wound infection, pulmonary infarction, or aspiration pneumonia. Likewise, travelers returning from short trips to foreign countries are much more likely to have febrile illnesses indigenous to their home than to the foreign country they have visited.

RARE VERSUS COMMON DISEASES Most of the time fever is a manifestation of a common disease, and fever associated with a pulmonary infiltrate is much more likely to be due to pneumococcal than to pneumocystis pneumonia. Failure to appreciate this cardinal principle has led to many prolonged and futile diagnostic work-ups.

FEBRILE ILLNESSES OF SHORT DURATION Acute febrile illnesses of less than 2 weeks' duration are a common occurrence in medical practice. In many instances they run their course, progressing to complete recovery, and a precise diagnosis is not made. In most instances, however, it is safe to assume that the illness is of infectious origin. Although short febrile illnesses may be noninfectious (e.g., allergic fevers due to drugs or serums, thromboembolic disease, hemolytic crises, or gout), they are decidedly in the minority.

Most undiagnosed acute febrile infectious diseases are probably viral and remain undiagnosed because diagnostic methods are unavailable or cumbersome. It is not practical to carry out tests needed to identify all the known viruses, and, furthermore, there must be a considerable number of still unidentified viruses pathogenic for man. In bacterial infections, on the other hand, laboratory diagnosis is simpler, and these infections are often rapidly controlled with chemotherapy.

The following characteristics, though not restricted solely to acute infections, are highly suggestive that infection is present:

1 Abrupt onset
2 High fever, i.e., 102 to 105°F, with or without chills
3 Respiratory symptoms—sore throat, coryza, cough
4 Severe malaise, with muscle or joint pain, photophobia, pain on movement of the eyes, headache
5 Nausea, vomiting, or diarrhea
6 Acute enlargement of lymph nodes or spleen
7 Meningeal signs, with or without spinal fluid pleocytosis
8 Leukocyte count above 12,000 or below 5,000 per mm^3

None of the symptoms or signs listed is encountered only in infection. Many of these features could be seen in acute leukemia or disseminated lupus erythematosus. Nevertheless, in a given instance of acute febrile illness with some or all of the manifestations listed, the probabilities strongly favor infection, and the patient may be given reasonable reassurance that he will probably recover in a week or two, regardless of a precise diagnosis.

It is desirable, of course, to establish an accurate diagnosis, and whatever steps are practicable in the circumstances to establish the cause should be taken. Cultures of the throat, blood, urine, or feces should be obtained before institution of antibacterial chemotherapy. Skin and/or serologic tests should be carried out when indicated.

PROLONGED FEBRILE ILLNESSES Some of the knottiest problems in the field of internal medicine are found in cases of prolonged fever in which the diagnosis remains obscure for weeks or even months. Eventually, however, the true nature of the illness usually reveals itself, since a disease which causes injury sufficient to evoke temperature elevations to 101°F or higher for several weeks does not often subside without leaving some clue as to its nature. The elucidation of problems of this sort calls for skillful application of all diagnostic methods—careful history, thorough physical examination, and the carefully considered use of laboratory examinations and roentgenograms.

Fever of unknown origin (FUO) In some patients fever becomes the dominant sign or symptom in a patient's illness, and when its cause escapes detection it is defined as fever of unknown origin (FUO). It is appropriate to use this term only in patients who have elevations in temperature (>101°F) for a prolonged period (at least 2 to 3 weeks) and in whom the diagnosis cannot be made during at least 1 week of intensive studies. These rigid criteria eliminate from this diagnostic category patients with common bacterial or viral infections, those in whom the diagnosis is obvious, and those whose fever is due to a sequential occurrence of etiologically unrelated diseases, e.g., one who is febrile following a myocardial infarction, who then develops thrombophlebitis that is associated with fever, and in whom this is followed by multiple pulmonary emboli, also a febrile disease. Much of the confusion in the literature concerning causes of FUO is due to failure to define the criteria employed in classifying patients who have had fever of unknown origin.

DISEASES CAUSING PROLONGED FEVERS

Table 12-1 lists some of the diseases which are responsible for prolonged fever. Some of these disorders must initially be considered to be FUO; in others the diagnosis comes to mind readily.

TABLE 12-1
Common disease entities causing prolonged fever in the United States

I Infections
- *A* Granulomatous infections
  - *1* Tuberculosis
  - *2* Deep-seated fungus infections
- *B* Pyogenic infections
  - *1* Upper abdominal infections
    - *a* Cholecystitis (stone), empyema of gallbladder
    - *b* Cholangitis
    - *c* Liver abscess
    - *d* Subhepatic abscess
    - *e* Subphrenic abscess
    - *f* Lesser sac abscess
  - *2* Lower abdominal infections
    - *a* Diverticulitis
    - *b* Appendicitis
  - *3* Pelvic inflammatory disease
  - *4* Renal infections
    - *a* Pyelonephritis (rare)
    - *b* Intrarenal abscess
    - *c* Perinephric abscess
    - *d* Ureteral obstruction
  - *5* Retroperitoneal infections: Infected aortic aneurysm
- *C* Bacterial endocarditis (acute and subacute)
- *D* Bacteremias with overt primary focus
  - *1* Meningococcemia
  - *2* Gonococcemia
  - *3* Vibriosis
  - *4* Listeriosis
  - *5* Brucellosis
- *E* Viral, rickettsial, and viral-like illness
  - *1* Infectious mononucleosis
  - *2* Cytomegalovirus
  - *3* Coxsackie B virus diseases
  - *4* Q fever (including endocarditis)
  - *5* Psittacosis
- *F* Parasitic diseases
  - *1* Amebiasis
  - *2* Malaria
  - *3* Trichinosis
- *G* Spirochetal infections: Leptospirosis

II Neoplasms
- *A* Solid (localized)
  - *1* Kidney
  - *2* Lung
  - *3* Pancreas
  - *4* Liver
  - *5* Atrial myxoma
- *B* Metastatic
  - *1* From gastrointestinal tract
  - *2* From lung, kidneys, bone
  - *3* Melanoma
- *C* Tumors of the reticuloendothelial system
  - *1* Lymphoma, Hodgkin's disease
  - *2* Leukemias
  - *3* Reticulum cell sarcoma, multiple myeloma (rare)
- *D* Unclassified: Diffuse sarcoma of bone

III Connective tissue disease
- *A* Rheumatic fever
- *B* Systemic lupus erythematosus
- *C* Rheumatoid arthritis (including Still's disease)
- *D* Temporal arteritis (polymyalgia rheumatica)

IV Miscellaneous
- *A* Drug fever
- *B* Multiple pulmonary emboli
- *C* Sarcoidosis
- *D* Thyroiditis
- *E* Hemolytic states
- *F* Cryptic trauma with bleeding into enclosed space
- *G* Regional enteritis and Whipple's disease
- *H* Granulomatous hepatitis

V Pseudogenic fevers
- *A* Habitual hyperthermia
- *B* Factitious fever

VI Periodic fevers
- *A* Familial Mediterranean fever
- *B* Etiocholanolone fever (?)

VII Undiagnosed

Infection

Infections occupy a less prominent position among causes of prolonged fever now than formerly because of the common practice of administering antibiotics to any patient in whom fever persists for more than a few days. Consequently, many infections are at present being eradicated by more or less "blind" therapy without accurate determination of their nature or location. Nevertheless, patients with infections comprise the greatest percentage of any group with FUO.

TUBERCULOSIS (Chap. 156) Tuberculosis remains the most prominent cause of FUO. The diagnosis should be considered strongly in young dark-skinned persons. Most of these patients do not have pulmonary tuberculosis but extrapulmonary or miliary disease involving the bones, lymph nodes, genital or urinary organs, peritoneum, or liver. Extrapulmonary or miliary tuberculosis may not be detectable by x-ray until late in the course of the disease. Skin test is an important diagnostic tool because, except in severely debilitated patients with overwhelming disease, a negative result, if the test has been properly executed, rules out the possibility of tuberculosis. A positive skin reaction, on the other hand, does not prove that tuberculosis is causing the illness but requires that the diagnosis be kept in mind until another cause for the fever is found.

PYOGENIC INFECTIONS Upper abdominal infections These commonly occur in the right upper quadrant and are related to the gallbladder or liver. Patients with such conditions tend to have mild jaundice, abnormality of liver function, high spiking fevers, and leukocytosis. Bacteremia, often due to enteric pathogens or *Salmonella,* is common. In these patients, exploratory laparotomy is usually necessary for diagnosis and may achieve cure as well.

Lower abdominal infections Appendicitis with perforation and abscess formation is a remarkably common cause of prolonged fever, particularly in elderly patients. Persistent right lower quadrant physical signs along with x-ray abnormalities require surgical exploration.

Renal infections Ordinary pyelonephritis is rarely accompanied by prolonged fever; if pyrexia occurs in these patients, intrarenal or perinephric abscess should be considered. Ureteral obstruction by either a mass of leukocytes or renal epithelium, as in papillary necrosis, may be accompanied by prolonged fever.

Retroperitoneal infection Aneurysms that have become filled with organizing clot and debris may become infected. Enteric pathogens (including *Escherichia coli,* bacteroides, and *Salmonella*), have been isolated frequently from patients with such infections. Surgery is mandatory for both diagnosis and therapy.

BACTERIAL ENDOCARDITIS In the classical subacute form of the disease, a heart murmur is nearly always present; therefore, absence of murmur largely eliminates this disease from consideration. The correct diagnosis is likely to be missed in middle-aged or elderly patients, in whom a heart murmur may not be given much weight. For example, an elderly patient with subacute bacterial endocarditis may first come to the physician's attention following the occurrence of a cerebral embolus and may be regarded as having had a hemorrhage or thrombosis because of arteriosclerosis. The best clinical practice is to culture the blood of *every* patient who has fever and a heart murmur. Bacterial endocarditis without cardiac murmurs is seen most frequently in intravenous drug users who develop infection on the tricuspid valve; every such person with fever should be assumed to have endocarditis until proved not to have. In addition, antibiotics mask subacute bacterial endocarditis (SBE) because they often render the blood culture negative until they have been excreted or metabolized. For this reason, patients suspected of having SBE and who have received antimicrobials should have blood cultures taken for several days after administration of the drugs is discontinued.

BACTEREMIA Neisseria Chronic meningococcemia (Chap. 131), although rare, is a well-known cause of prolonged fever. The arthralgia and rash of this disease are sufficiently evanescent to be missed. When this syndrome appears in a young woman, gonococcemia is much more likely (Chap. 132).

Salmonella (Chap. 136) Typhoid fever is not often a cause of prolonged fever of obscure origin because cultures of feces and blood will be positive and specific antibodies will be found in the serum. Other *Salmonella* organisms may, however, cause prolonged febrile illness and may present greater diagnostic difficulties. Repeated culture of the blood or bone marrow may yield the cause of this organism. Eventually, the infection may localize in a joint, pleural cavity, or some other metastatic focus.

BRUCELLOSIS (Chap. 140) This infection should be considered primarily in farmers, veterinarians, or slaughterhouse workers. Arthralgia and myalgia are common, but arthritis is rare. These patients tend to have normal or depressed leukocyte counts, and their sedimentation rate is often normal. In active febrile disease the blood and bone marrow cultures are frequently positive and specific agglutinins are nearly always present in the serum.

VIRAL INFECTIONS These are rarely the cause of prolonged fevers, but occasionally patients with viral infections may have febrile illnesses, which are often characterized by spontaneous remissions and exacerbations. Psittacosis may look much like typhoid fever, and Q-fever endocarditis has been a particularly puzzling illness.

PARASITIC DISEASES Amebiasis presents as an FUO, primarily in the form of liver abscess. The diagnosis of malaria demands a history of recent exposure.

Neoplasms

CARCINOMAS AND SARCOMAS Certain malignant processes are especially likely to cause fever. Notable are sarcomas involving bone or lymphoid tissue, hypernephroma, carcinoma of the pancreas or stomach, and primary or metastatic cancer of the liver. Occasionally, the clinical picture is strongly suggestive of pyogenic infection, with hectic fever, chills, sweats, and marked leukocytosis; and patients have been subjected to laparotomy with preoperative diagnoses such as empyema of the gallbladder, localized peritonitis, or liver abscess. An elevated alkaline phosphatase level and abnormal retention of BSP (Bromsulphalein) are important clues to intrahepatic malignancy.

HODGKIN'S DISEASE AND LYMPHOMAS Fever may be the principal symptom and only objective finding early in the course of Hodgkin's disease, especially when the principal involvement is in the abdominal viscera or the retroperitoneal regions. Pel-Ebstein fever is seen in a minority of cases of Hodgkin's disease. The diagnosis of this disorder is usually made by biopsy.

LEUKEMIAS It is not uncommon for acute leukemia to be mistaken for acute infection at the onset. The acute leukemias are nearly always accompanied by fever, sometimes as high as 105°F. The correct diagnosis is suggested by rapid development of anemia and characteristic changes in peripheral blood and bone marrow. Chronic lymphatic or granulocytic leukemia may be characterized by fever, but such fever is usually due to concomitant infection; because of the typical changes in circulating leukocytes, fever does not often cause a diagnostic problem. Before it is assumed that fever in a patient with leukemia is due to the blood dyscrasia, infection must be ruled out by appropriate tests and cultures, and sometimes attempts to treat the "most likely" pathogen must be made.

ATRIAL MYXOMA Patients with changing heart murmurs, peripheral embolic phenomena, and joint pains are usually suspected of having bacterial endocarditis, rheumatic fever, or occasionally some other connective tissue disease such as lupus erythematosus. In the face of persistence of these symptoms and signs without a positive diagnosis, angiography should be performed with the possibility that an atrial myxoma may be responsible.

Connective tissue diseases

RHEUMATIC FEVER Though rheumatic fever is generally easy to detect in children, the diagnosis in adults may be difficult. Attention to unexplained heart murmurs, arrhythmias, pleural and pericardial rubs, arthralgias, and skin rashes should call the diagnosis to mind. These findings, along with an elevated antistreptolysin titer, C-reactive protein, and other acute phase reactants, contribute to the diagnosis. A prompt response to large doses of aspirin is characteristic of rheumatic fever and provides another diagnostic clue.

SYSTEMIC LUPUS ERYTHEMATOSUS Fever is a common accompaniment of this disease. Of course, in the presence of arthritis, pleuritis, pericarditis, the classical malar rash, and renal failure, the diagnosis is easy. However, often these findings are absent and fever is the major manifestation. Biopsy of many organs, including the kidney, is generally not helpful; the diagnosis must be made by finding LE cells in the blood or bone marrow or by detecting a high titer of antinuclear antibody.

RHEUMATOID ARTHRITIS In its classical form, this disease is not difficult to recognize, but in certain patients who initially have FUO arthritis is absent early in the course of the illness; these patients have primarily fever, hepatosplenomegaly, lymphadenopathy, anemia, and leukocytosis. Joint changes do not appear until late in the disease. The diagnosis is made usually only after prolonged observation, in part because serologic tests for rheumatoid disease are characteristically negative.

TEMPORAL ARTERITIS (POLYMYALGIA RHEUMATICA) This is a disease of elderly persons who complain of fever, headache, and pain in the muscles and joints. Overt arthritis is unusual. The sedimentation rate tends to be very rapid, and there may be anemia, leukocytosis, or eosinophilia. Occasionally, the temporal or occipital arteries are inflamed and tender; when this is the case, the diagnosis is easily made by temporal artery biopsy. There may be accompanying visual defects or blindness because of the involvement of the retinal artery. This disease responds extremely well to steroids, which may be used as a therapeutic trial.

Miscellaneous causes of fever

SARCOIDOSIS Ordinarily fever is not characteristic of sarcoidosis, but it is prominent in a minority of cases, especially those characterized by arthralgia, hilar lymphadenopathy, and cutaneous lesions resembling erythema nodosum, or in those with extensive hepatic lesions. Diagnosis is suggested by lymphoid enlargement, ocular lesions, and hyperglobulinemia and is clinched by biopsy of skin, lymph nodes, muscle, and liver.

REGIONAL ENTERITIS Inflammatory lesions of the large and small intestine rarely present as FUO, but an occasional patient who has only fever, abdominal pain, and subtle changes in bowel habits will be found to have regional enteritis. Likewise, Whipple's disease may make itself known by fever, without arthritis or malabsorption.

DRUG FEVER This is an important cause of cryptic fever; a careful history of drug intake should be taken in every patient with unexplained fever. Fever due to allergy to one of the antibiotics may become superimposed on the fever of the infection for which the drug was given, resulting in a very confused picture. Often fever is due to common drugs, including sulfonamides, arsenicals, iodides, thiouracils, barbiturates, and laxatives, especially those containing phenolphthalein. Any questions of drug fever can be resolved rapidly by discontinuing all medications. The diagnosis can be further substantiated by giving a test dose of the drug after fever has subsided, but this may result in a very unpleasant or even dangerous reaction.

MULTIPLE PULMONARY EMBOLI Symptomless thrombosis of deep calf or pelvic veins may cause prolonged febrile illness as a result of repeated small pulmonary emboli. These emboli may not be manifested by pleuritic pain or hemoptysis, but cough, dyspnea, or vague thoracic discomfort is likely to be present. Careful examination of the legs and repeated examination of the lungs should reveal the diagnosis. Sometimes these patients come to the physician's attention with a nephrotic syndrome due to renal vein thrombosis.

HEMOLYTIC EPISODES Most hemolytic diseases are characterized by bouts of fever, and acute hemolytic crises may give rise to shaking chills and marked elevations of temperature. The difficulty sometimes encountered in differentiating sickle-cell disease from acute rheumatic fever is well known. The presence of these hemolytic disorders is suggested by the more rapid development of anemia than occurs in other febrile illnesses and by the usual accompaniment of reticulocytosis and jaundice. Fever is not characteristic of severe anemia due to external blood loss or of the anemia of uremia.

CRYPTIC TRAUMA Perisplenic and perivesical hematomas, with or without superimposed infection, are among the sites in which accumulated old blood and pus have resulted in prolonged fever.

GRANULOMATOUS HEPATITIS This disease of unknown etiology is not an uncommon cause of FUO. It is probably a manifestation of hypersensitivity. Liver biopsy shows only nonspecific granulomas. The fever generally subsides spontaneously over a period of weeks or months. Sometimes defervescence can be achieved with steroids, but because the diagnosis of tuberculosis can never be ruled out completely, patients in whom steroid therapy is given should also be given antituberculous medication.

HABITUAL HYPERTHERMIA Not infrequently, a patient while not appearing acutely ill has been subject to elevation of body temperature above the "normal" range level, i.e., his temperature has been in the range of 99.0 to 100.5°F. Prolonged low-grade fever may be a manifestation of serious illness, or it may be a matter of no real consequence. Possibly there are some persons whose "normal" temperatures are in this range. However, there is no certain way of identifying such individuals. The possibilities to be considered in such cases vary considerably according to the age groups concerned. A special problem termed *habitual hyperthermia,* is encountered in young females. The patient may have temperatures of 99.0 to 100.5°F regularly or intermittently for years and also usually has a variety of complaints characteristic of psychoneurosis, such as fatigability, insomnia, bowel distress, vague aches, and headache. Prolonged careful study and observation fail to reveal evidence of organic disease. Unfortunately, many of these people go from doctor to doctor and are subjected to a variety of unpleasant, expensive, and even harmful tests, treatments, and operations. The diagnosis of this syndrome can be made with reasonable certainty after a suitable period of observation and study, and if the patient can be convinced of its validity, a real service will have been rendered.

In a patient past middle age, even low-grade fever should always be regarded as a probable indication of organic disease. The possibilities to be considered in this age group are the same as those discussed earlier under Prolonged Febrile Illness.

FACTITIOUS FEVER Rarely, a patient will produce purposeful elevations in temperature. Many methods have been employed to cause the thermometer to register higher than the true temperature. If malingering is suspected, all that is necessary to prove it is to repeat the temperature determination immediately after a high reading has been obtained, with someone remaining at the bedside while the thermometer is in place. Other clues to false elevations in the temperature are a dissociation between pulse and temperature, absence of the normal diurnal variation in temperature, and excessively high fevers (greater than 106°F in adults) in the absence of chills, sweats, or tachycardia. Malingerers who elevate their temperature falsely usually have severe character disorders and are notoriously refractory to psychotherapy.

Periodic fevers
(See Chap. 225)

DIAGNOSTIC PROCEDURES IN FEVER

With so large a number of possibilities, it is obvious that no single plan can be outlined for the systematic study of every problem in unexplained fever. In any given patient, the history, physical examination, and, most importantly, the epidemiologic setting must determine the diagnostic approach. If the features suggest infectious disease, the main dependence will be upon bacteriologic and immunologic methods, whereas when a person in the "cancer age group" has an obscure febrile disorder the best chance of early diagnosis may lie in x-ray studies and biopsy.

HISTORY Careful elicitation of the patient's past history and the chronologic development of his symptoms may provide important leads. Places of recent residence, contact with domestic or wild animals and birds, preceding acute infectious diseases such as diarrheal illness or boils, or contact with persons with tuberculosis may provide clues to infection. Localizing symptoms may provide a lead to an organ system affected by neoplasm or infection.

PHYSICAL EXAMINATION Careful search is made for skin lesions and for petechial hemorrhages in the ocular fundi, conjunctivas, nail beds, and skin. The lymph nodes are carefully palpated, with special attention to the retrocalvicular, axillary, and epitrochlear areas. The finding of a heart murmur may be important. Detection of an abdominal mass may be the first lead to diagnosis of neoplastic disease. Palpable enlargement of the spleen suggests infection, leukemia, or lymphoma and points away from a diagnosis of solid tumors. Enlargement of the liver and spleen suggests lymphoma, leukemia, chronic infection, or cirrhosis. A large liver without palpable spleen points to liver abscess or metastatic cancer. The rectum and the female pelvic organs may reveal masses or abscesses; the testicles may reveal teratoma or tuberculosis.

LABORATORY TESTS Useful examinations include:

1 Cultures of blood, bone marrow (*Brucella* or *Salmonella*), or other body fluids
2 Serum enzymes, particularly *alkaline phosphatase* and enzymes that measure hepatocellular function
3 Blood smears for abnormal morphology, parasites, LE cells
4 Bone marrow examinations for tumor cells, granulomas, LE cells, and abnormal red or white cells
5 Immunologic tests, i.e., ASLO titers and other acute-phase reactants, antinuclear antibodies, latex fixation tests, and a variety of febrile agglutinins.

ROENTGENOGRAMS The following should be considered:

1 Chest films, which need to be repeated at intervals.
2 Bone x-rays are useful for detecting foci of osteomyelitis or primary or metastatic bone tumors.
3 Intravenous urograms are helpful in finding tumors of the kidney or perinephric or intrarenal abscesses. However, if a renal tumor is suspect on clinical grounds a negative IVP does not rule out the diagnosis, and an aortogram should be performed.
4 Abdominal aortography is useful for diagnosing tumors of the kidney, retroperitoneal mass lesions, and, if selective arterial catheterization is performed, tumors of the liver, pancreas, and gut.
5 Intravenous cholangiograms may be helpful in delineating right upper quadrant pathologic change if the patient is not jaundiced.
6 Cardiac angiograms should reveal atrial myxoma.
7 Lymphangiograms are helpful in the diagnosis of abdominal or retroperitoneal lymphomas but may be misleading.
8 Upper gastrointestinal x-rays are rarely useful; films of the small intestine may provide clues to Whipple's disease or regional enteritis, and a barium enema may show diverticulitis or tumor.

RADIOACTIVE SCANS *The liver scan is the single most useful test in the diagnosis of disease in the right upper quadrant.* Lung scans may reveal pulmonary emboli, and simultaneous liver and lung scans are useful in delineating subphrenic abscess. Bone scans are said to detect osseous metastases more readily than x-rays.

BIOPSIES Biopsy often is the best means of definitive diagnosis.

1 Bone marrow biopsy may be helpful not only in clarifying the histologic nature of the marrow but also for occasional demonstration of other disease processes such as metastatic carcinoma or granulomas, and for culture.
2 Needle biopsy of the liver is a very useful procedure and can be done with reasonable safety. It may be helpful not only in primary or metastatic disease of the liver, but also because the liver may reveal existence of other diseases such as histoplasmosis, schistosomiasis, brucellosis, tuberculosis, sarcoidosis, or lymphoma.
3 Lymph node biopsy is helpful in diagnosis of many diseases, including the lymphomas, metastatic cancer, tuberculosis, and mycotic infections. However, inguinal nodes are notoriously unsatisfactory for biopsy and are too frequently chosen because of their easy accessibility. Axillary, cervical, and supraclavicular nodes are much more likely to yield helpful information, and the node excised need not necessarily be large.
4 Muscle biopsy may be of assistance in the recognition of dermatomyositis, periarteritis nodosa, sarcoidosis, and trichinosis.
5 Lung biopsy may be performed with a needle under direct fluoroscopy. It is of value only in solitary mass lesions; diffuse pulmonary disease is rarely diagnosed by needle biopsy; instead, open lung biopsy should be performed.
6 Renal biopsy is rarely helpful, even in connective tissue disease.
7 Pleural and pericardial biopsy with the hook needle technique should be attempted in the presence of effusion.
8 Biopsy of the temporal artery (see above).
9 Biopsy of other accessible masses should not be neglected.

EXPLORATORY LAPAROTOMY Exploratory laparotomy has been advocated as the most definitive diagnostic maneuver in connection with FUO, but is valuable only when other investigations including history, physical examination, x-rays, and laboratory data point to the abdomen as a likely source of disease. Blind exploration of the abdomen simply because the diagnosis is obscure is to be deprecated. Moreover, often the tissue that is obtained at laparotomy could just as easily have been sampled by external biopsy techniques.

THERAPEUTIC TRIALS It is common practice to give a trial of antibiotic therapy to patients with unidentified febrile disorders. Occasionally, this kind of marksmanship is effective, but in general, "blind" therapy does more harm than good. Undesirable features include drug toxicity, superinfection due to resistant pathogenic bacteria, and interference with accurate diagnosis by cultural methods. Furthermore, a coincidental fall in temperature not due to therapy is likely to be interpreted as response to treatment, with the conclusion that an infectious disease is present. If therapeutic trials are instituted, they should be as specific as possible. Examples are *isoniazid and streptomycin or PAS or ethambutol* for tuberculosis; *aspirin* for rheumatic fever; *chloroquine and/or emetine* for hepatic amebiasis; *penicillin and streptomycin* for enterococcal endocarditis; and *chloramphenicol* for *Salmonella* bacteremia. Shotgun broad-spectrum therapy is contraindicated, because it is unlikely to yield useful information and is more likely to be toxic. Similarly, cortisone or ACTH is nonspecific. These drugs do have an antipyretic effect and produce euphoria in many persons, but the apparent improvement induced by them tells little about the nature of the underlying disease. Temporal arteritis is an exception to this statement.

PROGNOSIS IN FUO The intelligent application of the diagnostic maneuvers should provide the answer in approximately 90 to 95 percent of patients with prolonged obscure febrile illness. Fortunately, the remainder recover spontaneously. Because many of the procedures involved in the diagnosis of FUO are painful, time-consuming, and expensive, it is essential that they be chosen with thoughtfulness and care.

REFERENCES

ATKINS E: Fever, in *Signs and Symptoms,* 5th ed., eds McBryde and Blacklow, Philadelphia: Lippincott, 1972

BAKER RR, TUMULTY PA et al: The value of exploratory laparotomy in fever of undetermined etiology. Johns Hopkins Med J 125:159, 1969

DELLER JJ, RUSSELL PK: An analysis of fevers of unknown origin in American soldiers in Vietnam. Ann Intern Med 66:1129, 1967

PETERSDORF RG, BEESON PB: Fever of unexplained origin: Report of 100 cases. Medicine 40:1, 1961

——, BENNETT IL, JR: Factitious fever. Ann Intern Med 46:1039, 1957

——, WALLACE JF: Fever of unknown origin, in *Diagnostic Approaches to Presenting Syndromes,* ed JA Barondess, Baltimore: Williams & Wilkins, 1971, pp. 301–332

WOLSTENHOLME AND BIRCH (eds): *Pyrogens and Fever,* Edinburgh and London: Churchill, Livingstone, 1971

section 3 | Alterations in nervous function

13
GENERAL CONSIDERATIONS

RAYMOND D. ADAMS

The symptoms and signs of nervous disease are probably the most frequent and complex in all of medicine. Of course they are of prime concern to neurologists and psychiatrists but are so often observed in patients who do not have classifiable diseases of the nervous system that they necessarily become of interest to every physician.

A lucid exposition of all the diverse manifestations of nervous diseases is difficult, in part because the more complex phenomena may be viewed from either a neurologic or psychologic standpoint. Naturally our bias, as physicians, is toward the neurologic for it draws on all the accepted principles of medicine and biologic science. The aim, therefore, throughout this section will be to describe as accurately as possible all the more common expressions of disordered nervous function and to offer the most generally accepted explanations in terms of anatomy, biochemistry, and physiology. However, in discussion of the most complex cerebral derangements, a particular effort will be made to present both the neurologic and psychologic conceptions, for the latter have received much attention in medical circles in recent years.

NEUROLOGIC AND PSYCHOLOGIC VIEWPOINTS OF DISORDERED NERVOUS FUNCTION An understanding of what is embodied in these two concepts of derangements of the nervous system is necessary to appreciate some of the theoretic problems in neuropsychiatry. The terms *neurologic* and *psychologic* designate two different methodologies and clinical approaches; they do not denote the respective activities of neurologists and psychiatrists. The neurologic methodology, which embraces all the principles of medicine applied to diseases of the brain, spinal cord, and nerves, is used by physicians, neurologists, and the majority of modern psychiatrists. The psychologic methodology comprises another set of ideas of value in medicine but falling more strictly within the province of psychiatry and psychology.

To be more explicit, the *neurologic conception* starts with the assumption that a disease exists, the manifestations of which relate to the type and locations of a pathologic process within the nervous system. This process may be obvious, e.g., a cerebral infarct or tumor; or it may be impossible to see with a light or even an electron microscope, e.g., the encepholopathy of delirium tremens, status epilepticus, or schizophrenia. In these latter states the inference as to the existence of disease depends not on a demonstrable lesion but on a combination of factors such as genetic background, circumstances and mode of development, stereotypy of clinical syndrome, clinical course, and associated laboratory data. In all instances the symptoms and signs are the result of some physical or chemical change which usually induces a variety of parenchymal derangements, of which the visible lesion represents only the most advanced and often irreversible stage. The symptoms and signs of the disease express the deficit occasioned by the impaired functioning of certain parts of the diseased nervous system and also the excessive activity of intact but disinhibited systems of neurons (the negative and positive symptoms, respectively). These clinical manifestations vary widely in type and include, on the one hand, the relatively simple, easily elicited, stereotyped objective symptoms and signs, such as motor paralysis or spasticity, and, on the other, the most complex, difficult to evoke, highly individualized subjective signs, such as an hallucination, paraphasic utterance, or mood disturbance.

This is perhaps the most difficult idea for the student to grasp—that in the neurologic conception no real distinction is drawn between what are commonly called the "physical" and "mental," or the "organic" and "functional" symptoms. Another unique feature of nervous disorders is that all have their objective (behavioral) as well as their subjective (conscious) aspects. All except the most complex nervous disorders (in which insight is lost) are known to the patient through introspection and to the physician through extrospection. Of course the intelligence and personality of the patient, which are products of his inheritance and early life experiences, influence the manner of perceiving and of reporting and analyzing the nervous disorder, as well as his feelings and emotional reaction to it, but these latter are secondary phenomena in that they do not figure directly in pathogenesis.

The neurologic examination, upon which so much depends in this branch of medicine, is the means by which the physician assesses systematically the activities of the altered nervous system during one or several brief periods of time. Special physiologic and psychologic tests serve only to refine and quantify the clinical defects.

The goals of the neurologic method, or of neuropathology (the scientific study of disease), are to define the essential pathologic processes underlying the disease, and to ascertain their cause and mechanism, thereby providing a rational basis for prevention and treatment. A complete medical theory of a disease of the nervous system must embrace all aspects of it, the anatomic, pathologic, biochemical, and physiologic as well as the psychologic.

The *psychologic conception* assumes that disordered nervous functioning may, like the content of the mind, be traced to past life experiences. Since certain features of personality, the degree of emotional maturity, the capacity to adjust to social situations are regarded as learned patterns of reaction, abnormalities in these spheres are also thought to be the product of unfavorable past experiences and inadequate training and education leading to immature and unstable reactions. This is not to deny that intelligence and certain qualities of character are to some extent genetic and may be of themselves sources of difficulty, but only to point out that some of the most modifiable, pathologic aspects are traceable to environmental influences.

Some of the most critical of life experiences in personality development as well as social adjustment are easily remembered, i.e., "conscious"; others have been forgotten, i.e., they are "unconscious," or can be recalled with difficulty and sometimes only through the free-association method of psychoanalysis. But in either case the principal step in the methodology involves an exhaustive review of the patient's autobiography and a search for patterns of behavior and social interaction that may reveal connections between present symptoms and past experiences. In the sense that the symptoms may relate to psychic conflicts in the patient's life, often occasioned by certain unfortunate incidents, they are psychogenic. By repeated interviews and frank discussions the psychiatrist endeavors to expose these relationships to the patient and to assist him in making new adaptations to them (psychotherapy). The aim of the psychologic approach is to discover the origins of abnormal mental processes. Their scientific study, i.e., psychopathology, has led to the identification of a number of basic psychologic mechanisms such as conflict, projection, repression, patterning, and conditioning.

It is held, chiefly by psychoanalysts, that all psychologic theories must be couched in psychologic terms and that reference to anatomy, biochemistry, physiology, and pathology of the brain has no place in such formulations. Of course this is true in a strictly logical system, but it overlooks another use of the term "psychologic" in psychiatry and medicine—that which designates many of the more complex cognitive and affective disorders of cerebral function such as perception, thinking, learning, volition, and emotion which can be deranged by diseases of the nervous system.

The authors would suggest that both the neurologic and psychologic concepts of a nervous disorder have their place in medicine. Most modern neurologists and psychiatrists believe that the two methodologies are applicable to different types of nervous abnormalities—the neurologic to disease, the psychologic to social maladjustments; further, that they operate at different levels in medical work and are not mutually exclusive. In *diagnostic neuropsychiatry* where one begins always with the accurate elicitation of symptoms and signs, the methodology is strictly that of neurologic medicine. Yet even at this stage one takes advantage of psychologic techniques and knowledge in calming and reassuring the patient, in skillfully directing his thinking, in history taking, in obtaining cooperation; and one immediately attempts to size up the personality, character, and intelligence. But a search for psychologic explanations of the symptoms not only is too time-consuming but commits one prematurely to a formula that may be irrelevant to the disease. In the interpretation of symptoms and signs one utilizes the factual data of anatomy and physiology of the nervous system to ascertain which parts of the nervous system have been damaged. Admittedly, the precise form and content of certain complex symptoms, such as a hallucination, may be divulged only by a thorough exploration of the psychology of the patient, i.e., his premorbid and morbid personality and past experiences, but these are of secondary importance in diagnosis. In the *therapy and management* of many diseases, including those for which there is no known treatment, detailed information as to the patient's personality, intelligence, and general reactions is quite indispensable. As in all branches of medicine, success depends on the physician's rapport and his ability to understand and deal with the patient as a troubled human being. The approach involves a kind of practical skill in human psychology; the neurologic methodology has little to offer. In *theorizing* about diseases of the nervous system the neurologic method offers the only rational approach, for it embraces data from all the sciences. A psychologic theory can never provide a complete explanation of a disease of the nervous system.

Thus we are confronted with one of the central issues in neuropsychiatry—that of defining a disease of the nervous system. The authors propose to designate by this term any disorder of nervous function in which there is actual or presumptive evidence of a lesion in the nervous system. Diseases in this sense should be distinguished from an abnormal psychologic reaction, which is defined as a disorder in psychic life and behavior, occasioned usually by a maladjustment in social relations. Worry over the loss of a job or the ill health of one's child, protracted grief, or fear of dying, with all their potential visceral reverberations, would obviously not be classified as diseases. These and countless other daily problems are best looked upon as natural psychologic and physiologic reactions to environmental circumstances and dealt with either by changing the situation or helping the patient to adjust to them psychologically. The classification of a persistent anxiety state without obvious cause in a previously healthy person is much more difficult. Most psychiatrists consider it a reaction to some threat or fear in the unconscious mind, whereas neurologists tend to think of it as an unexplained biochemical disorder, perhaps evoked by a social situation, but still as mysterious as was hyperthyroidism a century ago. Mania and depression, and schizophrenia, which constitute two of the major problems in psychiatry, also have, unfortunately, a controversial status. Despite the absence of a visible lesion, most psychiatrists and virtually all neurologists now agree that they are genetically determined diseases of the nervous system, rather than deviate ways of living or abnormal psychologic reactions. They differ from other nervous diseases in their lifelong duration, their fluctuating course, and the importance of social stimuli in their evocation.

NEUROLOGY, PSYCHIATRY, AND PSYCHOSOMATIC MEDICINE The fields of neurologic and psychiatric medicine are broad and touch every medical and surgical specialty. Common to both is a concern about diseases which disturb emotional control, learning, memory, perception, and thinking. In addition, neurology includes in its subject matter many diseases that do not alter the mind, and psychiatry is occupied to a large extent with countless problems of adjustment which cause unhappiness and disability, yet have not been defined as nervous diseases.

In the following chapters, which cover the whole subject matter of both neurology and psychiatry, no attempt is made to subdivide their cardinal manifestations. This is in the best tradition of eclecticism. Emphasis will assuredly be placed on the conditions most likely to be encountered by general practitioners and internists. A comprehensive account of the major neuroses and psychoses and of the major types of nervous diseases will be presented in the second half of the book.

There is still another area of neuropsychiatry, not heretofore mentioned, and one that has received much attention in recent years—that of *psychosomatic medicine.* Included here are such conditions as peptic ulcer, mucous colitis, ulcerative colitis, bronchial asthma, atopic dermatitis, urticaria and angioneurotic edema, hay fever, Raynaud's disease, hypertension, hyperthyroidism, amenorrhea and other disturbances of menstruation, enuresis, dysuria, paroxysmal tachycardia, rheumatoid arthritis, and migraine. These psychosomatic diseases are set apart by three lines of evidence. (1) A large series of observations made by Cannon, H. Wolff, Mittelman, S. Wolf, Cobb, Finesinger, Jones, and others, which have revealed that the function of the offending organ is excited and possibly deranged by strong emotions and restored toward normalcy by tranquility and feelings of security. (2) A careful analysis of the biographies of such patients which has shown what is believed to be an inordinately high incidence of resentment, hostility, dependence, suppressed emotionality, and inability to communicate to others about matters of emotional concern (cf. studies by Lindemann, Dunbar, French, Alexander). (3) A demonstrable relationship between onset and exacerbation of symptoms and the occurrence of disturbing and frustrating incidents in the patient's life and the demonstration that medical therapy which neglects these emotional factors is often unsuccessful.

The psychosomatic diseases differ from the psychoneuroses in that they have different symptoms, last longer, have a known or demonstrable pathologic basis, and often a known cause (e.g., allergy in asthma, atopic dermatitis, and hay fever). Treatment has been most effective when simply directed toward the relief of symptoms. Finally, the incidence of frank neuroses in this group of patients is no greater than in the population at large, and neurotic individuals are not more liable than normal ones to psychosomatic disorders.

Despite more than 30 years of intensive investigation by psychiatrists published in a voluminous literature, no complete proof of psychogenesis has been established for a single one of the psychosomatic diseases. Moreover, the concepts that have emerged about them, although educationally useful, have not been of much theoretic value. The therapeutic results obtained by a thoughtful, understanding physician, unsophisticated in psychologic theory, are no less successful than those of the most experienced psychiatrist. Lastly, advances in medical science have uncovered in one after another of these diseases new nonpsychologic mechanisms (e.g., milk sensitivity in mucous colitis, a defect of an α_2-globulin inhibitor in certain forms of urticaria); and surely, others will be found. For these many reasons we have made no effort to group the psychosomatic diseases or to discuss them further in the neurology and psychiatry sections of our book.

Finally, a few words of caution must be given lest the reader be misled into thinking that expert clinicians believe all neurologic and psychiatric problems are reducible to a clear-cut disease or a straightforward situational reaction. Medicine is never that simple. Most patients have several diseases and exhibit a multitude of reactions and defenses that are difficult to classify. Never does a given disease look the same in two patients. Experience makes one appreciate the wisdom of Claude Bernard's, Walter Cannon's, and Adolph Meyer's view of man as "an infinitely complex psychobiologic unit functioning in relationship to his physical and uniquely social environment." In the broadest sense disease represents a faulty or inadequate adaptation of the organism to its environment. Sometimes the maladaptation can be traced to a single agent in the environment, such as the tubercle bacillus, without which the disease tuberculosis could not develop, but even here previous exposure, general health, nutrition, the individual's family, and even racial resistance play a part. The natural compounding of all the variables relating not to one but to a multitude of diseases and reactions makes it understandable why every sick patient stands as a unique combination of problems to be resolved medically, not by referring back to earlier cases of the same type, but by the application of certain general medical principles derived from all branches of medicine. Confusion is maximum in neurology and psychiatry, where the diseases of man's nervous system, which number into the hundreds, many not even known or catalogued, are combined with a great diversity of behavioral states that may be either primary or secondary.

One hears it said that more than half of all medical ailments are "psychologic" or "psychosomatic," but this is a gross misstatement. What is meant is that many patients present problems too vague and complex to be understood in terms of medicine and psychology. Fortunately many of these illnesses are benign and trivial and disappear in the course of time, so that no more than kindly reassurance and simple explanation are necessary. The student and physician must acquire a sensitivity to psychologic problems without becoming so mindful of them that every illness is cast in a naive psychologic formula. Above all an open mind should be maintained, one that will permit a critical, periodic reevaluation of all new hypotheses in this field and acceptance only of those based on the valid data of controlled, clinical observation and scientific experiment.

14 NERVOUSNESS, ANXIETY, AND DEPRESSION

RAYMOND D. ADAMS

The majority of patients who enter a physician's office or hospital will admit to being nervous, anxious, or depressed. The stress of contemporary society or the prospect of real or imaginary illness is thought to induce these reactions. If they stand in clear relationship to a stressful event or situation, such as worry over economic reverses or grief over the death of a loved one, such states can be accepted as normal. Only when excessively intense and uncontrollable or when accompanied by derangements of visceral function do they become the basis for medical consultation.

The problems become more abstruse when similar symptoms occur in persons who are not being subjected to immediately stressful or unhappy experiences, and knowledge of such threatening situations, if it exists at all, lies buried in the subconscious mind of the patient. One may assume that it has either been suppressed from consciousness or is part of an elaborate subjective interpretation. The relationship between social stimulus and prevailing anxiety or nervousness can then be discovered only by gentle probings by the psychologically sophisticated physician. But once the connection is established and the problem dealt with realistically, the symptoms become understandable and disappear. One recognizes here all the elements of a *psychoneurotic reaction.* The line of separation between the latter and normal emotional reactions is admittedly ambiguous.

There is still another category of nervousness, anxiety, and depression wherein the emotional states are intense and prolonged but without obvious explanation. Such states may overwhelm the individual and derange him in all his activities. Delving into his unconscious mind or studying his lifelong reaction pattern fails to reveal a plausible psychogenesis. One recognizes here all the elements of a more complete, pervasive *psychotic reaction.* In many such instances a genetic factor appears to operate and the features of the illness are so stereotyped as to indicate a disease of the parts of the nervous system which control the affective, emotional life. Yet consistent biochemical change in the blood or brain tissue has not been found, and no lesion has been discerned. Therefore treatment must proceed along nonpsychologic lines.

The problem confronting every physician is to recognize all these nuances of reaction and disease which obviously shade into one another, and to determine to what extent they dominate the medical condition of his patient. Some type of therapeutic maneuver must then be initiated, varying from simple reassurance and realistic management of existing personal difficulties, to suppression of symptoms by drugs. Often referral to a psychiatrist is necessary for more expert management, including electrotherapy.

In this chapter the cardinal features of these states will be described, together with currently accepted views of their origins. The major diseases of which they may be a part are discussed in Chaps. 339 and 341.

NERVOUSNESS By this vague term the lay person usually refers to a state of restlessness, tension, uneasy apprehension, irritability, or hyperexcitability. But it may connote other states, such as thoughts of suicide, fear of killing one's child or spouse, a distressing hallucination, a paranoid idea, or a frankly hysterical outburst. Careful inquiry as to what the patient means when he complains of nervousness is always a necessary first step.

In its most common signification, a period of nervousness may represent no more than a psychic and behavioral state in which an organism is maximally challenged by difficult personal problems, and there are periods in normal life when this is more likely to happen. For example, adolescence rarely passes without its period of turmoil as the person attempts to emancipate himself from parental dominance or to adjust to scholastic demands or to the opposite sex. The menses are regularly accompanied by increased tension and moodiness, and, of course, the menopause is another critical period. Some persons, because of early patterning or character formation, claim to have been nervous in all their social relationships throughout life; one should then suspect a psychoneurosis or depressive character formation even though performance within the family unit, at school, and at work were adequate. Others complain of a recent development of nervousness, and one must consider such conditions as an upheaval in personal affairs, the first attack or exacerbation of a psychoneurosis, an endogenous depression, an endocrine disease (hyperthyroidism, adrenal corticism, or corticosteroid therapy), or withdrawal from a sedative drug (alcohol, barbiturate). Some patients complain of a nervousness that attends the onset of a medical or neurologic disease; it would then appear to be secondary, occasioned by fear of disability, dependency, or death.

Nervousness, even in its simplest form, is reflected in many important activities of the human organism. There are often a mild somberness of mood, an increased tendency to tears and anger (irritability). Fatigue that bears no proper relationship to activity and rest is frequent, and sleep is often disturbed, as are eating and drinking habits. Headaches may increase in number and intensity. There is a tendency to sweat, tremble, be aware of heart action, feel a bit "queer in the head" or giddy, have an upset stomach, and urinate more often, though these recognized autonomic accompaniments of anxiety are seldom as conspicuous as in anxiety neurosis. Thus, it would appear that nervousness and anxiety constitute a graded series of reactions, the latter in many instances being only a more intense and protracted form of nervousness (see Chap. 339).

THE ANXIETY STATE Anxiety is "the fundamental phenomenon and central problem of the neurosis . . . a nodal point, linking up all kinds of most important questions, a riddle of which the solution must cast a flood of light upon our whole mental life" (Freud). From the viewpoint of the social historian, anxiety is said to be "the most prominent mental characteristic of Occidental civilization" (Willoughby). These comments should inform the reader of the broad implications of this reaction.

The more strictly medical meaning of the term *anxiety*, and the one used in this chapter, is a state characterized by a subjective feeling of fear and uneasy anticipation (apprehension), usually with a definite topical content and associated with the physiologic accompaniments of strong emotion, i.e., breathlessness, choking sensation, palpitation, restlessness, increased muscular tension, tightness in the chest, giddiness, trembling, sweating, and flushing. By topical content is meant the idea, person, or object about which the person is anxious. The several vasomotor and visceral alterations that underlie the symptoms are mediated through the autonomic nervous system, particularly the sympathetic part of it, and involve also the thyroid and adrenal glands.

Forms of anxiety Anxiety is manifested in acute episodes, each lasting a few minutes, or as a protracted state that may last for weeks, months, or years. In the acute *attacks*, or *panics* as they are called, the patient is plunged into an inexplicable mental state in which he fears he will die, lose his reason or self-control, become insane, or commit some horrible crime. He is breathless, has a racing heart, chokes, sweats, trembles, and feels gastric distress and anorexia. As a persistent protracted state he experiences fluctuating degrees of nervousness, restlessness, irritability, fatigue, insomnia, intolerance of physical exertion, and pressure or tension headaches. Discrete anxiety attacks and chronic states of anxiety merge into one another.

Episodic anxiety without disorder of mood (i.e., depression) is usually classified as *anxiety neurosis*. The chronic form with prominent exercise intolerance is called *neurocirculatory asthenia*. Anxiety may, however, be combined with other somatic symptoms in hysteria and may be the restraining factor in *phobic neurosis*. Persistent anxiety with insomnia, lassitude, and fatigue, regardless of mood, should always raise suspicion of a *depressive psychosis*. Panic attacks may also occur at the beginning of a schizophrenic illness. Both anxiety and depression are prominent features of the syndrome of posttraumatic nervous instability (see Chaps. 327, 341, 342).

Thus, the differential diagnosis of an anxiety state requires that the physician consider all the major syndromes in psychiatry. Often it is but one component of a far more serious condition, one which may result in suicide or some other antisocial act. Also, without the psychic counterparts of fear and apprehension, the visceral symptoms alone should arouse suspicion of thyrotoxicosis, autonomic epilepsy, corticosteroid overdosage, pheochromocytoma, hypoglycemia, and menopause.

Physiologic and psychologic basis The cause, mechanism, and biologic meaning of anxiety have been the subjects of much speculation, and completely satisfactory explanations are not possible. The psychologist regards anxiety as anticipatory behavior, i.e., a state of uneasiness about something which may happen in the future. William McDougall spoke of it as "an emotional state arising when a continuing strong desire seems likely to miss its goal." The primary emotion, somewhat muted perhaps, is that of fear, and its arousal under conditions not overtly threatening may be explained by conditioning to some recondite component of a formerly threatening stimulus.

The only well-systematized theory is that put forth by the school of psychoanalysis, which looks upon anxiety as a response to a situation that in some manner undermines the security of the individual. The topical content or cause of potential danger lies in the unconscious mind. The postulated danger is internal rather than external; a primitive drive has been aroused that is not compatible with current social practices, and it can be satisfied only at risk of harm to the person.

Physicians have searched for evidence of impairments of visceral function without success. The neurocirculatory asthenic is in poor physical condition, has an elevated blood lactate level after exercise, and will not tolerate the work or exercise needed to build up his stamina. The urinary excretion of epinephrine has been found elevated in some patients; in others, there is an increased urinary excretion of norepinephrine. Aldosterone excretion is raised to two or three times the normal level during intense anxiety. Medical students experiencing fear and anxiety while preparing for an examination also excrete increased amounts of aldosterone. The interpretation of these data (whether primary or secondary) is not certain, but it is becoming increasingly evident that prolonged and diffuse anxiety is a pattern of behavior related to certain biochemical abnormalities of blood, and probably of the brain.

DEPRESSION There are few persons who do not experience periods of discouragement and despair, and these periods become manifestly more frequent in modern society where individual freedom is constrained and one's impulses must be inhibited. As with nervousness and anxiety, depression of mood that is appropriate to a given situation in life is a natural, healthy reaction and seldom is the basis of medical complaint. The patient tends to seek help only when he cannot control his grief or unhappiness. But there are numerous instances in which the patient is miserable, unhappy, and hopeless for reasons that are not apparent. Many of his symptoms are interpreted as ill health, being so similar to those of many disease states as to bring him first to the internist. Sometimes another disease is found (such as chronic hepatitis, brucellosis, postinfluenzal asthenia infections), in which a chronic fatigue is confused with depression; but often an endogenous depression is itself the essential problem. Since the risk of suicide is not inconsiderable if the illness is mistaken for another or overlooked as a complication, an error in diagnosis may be life-threatening.

Information about depressions, like that of all psychiatric syndromes, is gained from three sources: the history obtained from the patient, the history obtained from the family or close friend, and the findings on examination.

From the patient and his family it is learned that he has been "feeling unwell," "low in spirits," "blue," "glum," "unhappy," or "morbid." There has been a change in emotional reactions of which the patient may not be fully aware. Activities that were formerly pleasant are no longer so. Often, however, change in mood is less conspicuous than reduction in psychic and physical energy. Fatigue is almost invariable; not uncommonly, it is worse in the morning after a night of restless sleep. The words "loss of pep," "weak," "tired," "no energy to work," "my job seems more trying and difficult" appear in the conversation. The outlook is pessimistic. The patient is preoccupied with uncontrollable worry over trivialities. With excessive worry the ability to think with accustomed efficiency is reduced; there is complaint that the mind does not function properly, of being forgetful and unable to concentrate. If the patient is naturally of suspicious nature, paranoid tendencies may assert themselves.

Particularly troublesome in medical diagnosis is the patient's tendency to become hypochondriacal about associated diseases. Indeed, most cases formerly diagnosed as hypochondriasis are now regarded as depression. Pain from whatever cause—a stiff joint, a toothache, fleeting abdominal pains, or other troubles such as constipation, frequency of urination, insomnia, pruritus, burning tongue, weight loss—may become an obsessive focus of complaint. The patient passes from doctor to doctor seeking relief from symptoms that would not trouble the average person, and no amount of reassurance relieves the state of mind. The nervousness and anxiety felt by many of these persons may be obscured by their preoccupation with visceral functions.

When examined, the patient's facial expression is often plaintive, troubled, pained, or anguished. His attitude and manner betray his prevailing mood of depression, discouragement, and despondency. In other words, the affective response, which is the outward expression of feeling, is consistent with the depressed mood. During the interview the patient's eyes may be tearful, or he may cry openly. In some there is a kind of immobility of the face that mimics parkinsonism, though others are restless and agitated (pacing, wringing their hands, etc). Occasionally the patient will smile, but the smile impresses one as more of a social gesture than an expression of feeling.

The stream of speech, from which the ideational content is determined, is slow. At times the patient is mute and speaks neither spontaneously nor in response to questions. Again there may be a long pause between questions and answers. The latter are brief and may be monosyllabic. There is a paucity of ideas. The retardation extends to all topics of conversation and affects movement of limbs as well. The most extreme forms of decreased motor activity, rarely seen in the medical clinic, border on stupor.

Content of speech is found to be abnormal if examined carefully. Conversation is replete with pessimistic thoughts, fears, expressions of unworthiness, inadequacy, inferiority, and sometimes guilt. In severe depressions bizarre ideas, delusions about the body ("blood drying up," "bowels are blocked with cement," "I am half dead") may be expressed.

Etiology of mechanism Three theories have emerged concerning the cause of the pathologic depressive state: (1) the endogenous form is hereditary; (2) a biochemical abnormality results in a periodic depletion in the brain of serotonin and norepinephrine; (3) a basic fault in character development exists. These theories, which are not mutually exclusive, will be elaborated upon in Chap. 339.

It is the writer's belief that depression is one of the most commonly overlooked diagnoses in clinical medicine. Part of the trouble is with the word itself, which implies being unhappy about something. The persistent or recurrent endogenous depression or involutional depression should be suspected in all chronic states of ill health, hypochondriasis, disability that exceeds manifest signs of a medical disease, neurasthenia, and suicide attempts. Inasmuch as recovery is the rule, the suicide is a tragedy for which the medical profession must often share responsibility.

REFERENCES

Freedman AM, Kaplan HI: *Comprehensive Textbook of Psychiatry*, chaps. 17, 23, Baltimore: Williams & Wilkins, 1967

15
LASSITUDE AND ASTHENIA

RAYMOND D. ADAMS

The term *weakness* is used by patients to describe a variety of subjective complaints which vary in their import and prognostic significance. The different meanings can usually be fitted into the following classification:

1 Lassitude, fatigue, lack of energy, listlessness, and languor. (These terms, though not synonymous, shade into one another; all refer to a weariness and a loss of that sense of well-being typically found in persons healthy of body and mind.)

2 Weakness, loss of strength, paresis, paralysis. These may be persistent or episodic.

a Persistent weakness: This may be (1) restricted to certain muscles or groups of muscles (see Chap. 17) or (2) more or less generalized, i.e., involving the entire masculature (see Chaps. 17 and 343).

b Episodic, often recurrent: Attacks of weakness may occur in the periodic paralyses. [Many patients confuse "attacks of weakness" with a diminished sense of alertness, lightheadedness, feeling of faintness. These usually turn out to be episodes of partial or threatening syncope, attacks of anxiety or vertigo, or seizures (see Chaps. 16, 19, 337).]

LASSITUDE AND FATIGUE Of all the symptoms in this group these are among the most frequent and abstruse. More than half of all patients entering a general hospital register direct complaint of fatigability or admit to it when questioned. During the Second World War fatigue was so prominent as to be given a separate place in medical nosology, viz., "combat fatigue," which referred to all acute psychiatric illnesses that happened on the battlefield. The common clinical antecedents and accompaniments of fatigue, its significance, and its physiologic and psychologic bases should, therefore, be matters of common medical knowledge.

Patients who complain of weariness and tiredness have a more or less characteristic way of describing their condition. They say that they "are all in," "have lost pep," "have no ambition" or "no interest," are "turned off" or "fed up." They manifest their condition by showing an indifference to the tasks at hand, by talking much about how hard they are working; they are inclined to sit around or lie down, occupying themselves with trivial tasks. On closer analysis one finds a difficulty in initiating activity and also in sustaining it.

This condition is the familiar aftermath of prolonged labor or great physical exertion, and under such circumstances it is accepted as a normal, physiologic reaction. When, however, the same symptoms or similar ones appear in no relation to such antecedents, they are suspected as being the manifestations of disease.

The physician's task begins, then, with an attempt to determine whether his patient is merely suffering from the physical and mental effects of overwork without realizing it. Overworked, overwrought people are everywhere observable in our society. Their actions are both instructive and pathetic. They seem to be impelled by notions of duty and refuse to think of themselves. Or, as is often the case, some personal inadequacy seems to prevent them from deriving pleasure from any activity except their work, in which they indulge themselves as a kind of defense mechanism. Such persons show their fatigue by other symptoms, such as irritability, restlessness, and sleeplessness. Their symptoms and behavior are best understood by referring to psychologic studies of the effect of fatigue on the normal individual.

Effects of fatigue on the normal person According to several authoritative sources, fatigue has both explicit and implicit effects, grouped under: (1) a series of biochemical and physiologic changes in many organs of the body, (2) an overt disorder in behavior, a reduced output of work, known as *work decrement,* and (3) an expressed dissatisfaction and a subjective feeling of tiredness.

As to the biochemical and physiologic changes, continuous muscular work leads to depletion of muscle glycogen and an accumulation of lactic acid and other metabolites, which in themselves reduce the power of contraction and delay recovery. Extreme degrees of muscle work, in which activity exceeds provision of substrate, results in necrosis of fibers and rise in serum levels of creatine phosphokinase and aldolase even in normal persons. The muscles are slightly swollen and sore for several days. It is said that the injection of blood from a fatigued animal into a rested one will produce overt manifestations of fatigue in the latter. During repeated contractions of muscle its action is observed to become tremulous, movements are less adept, and the coordination of agonist, antagonist, and synergic muscles is less perfect. The rate of breathing increases, the pulse quickens, the blood pressure rises and pulse pressure widens, and the white blood cell count and metabolic rate are increased. These alterations bear out the hypothesis that fatigue is in part a manifestation of altered metabolism.

The decreased capacity for work or productivity which is a direct consequence of fatigue has been investigated by industrial psychologists. Their findings show clearly the importance of the motivational factor on work output, whether it be in manual or clerical tasks. Individual differences in energy potential appear to be important, as are differences in physique, intelligence, and temperament.

The subjective feelings of fatigue have been carefully recorded. Aside from feeling weary the tired person is unable to deal effectively with complex problems and tends to be unreasonable, often about trivialities. The number and quality of his associations in psychologic tests are reduced. The ability to deliberate and to reach judgments is impaired; decisions made late at night may appear unsound the next day. The worker after a long, hard day is unable to perform adequately his duties as head of a household; the example of the tired businessman who becomes the proverbial tyrant of the family circle is well known. A disinclination to try and the appearance of ideas of inferiority are other characteristics of the fatigued mind.

Instances of fatigue and lassitude resulting from overwork are not difficult to recognize. A description of the patient's daily routine and a talk with his associates and family will usually suffice. Moreover if he can be persuaded to live at a more reasonable pace and allow time for outside pleasurable activities, his symptoms will promptly subside. A common error in diagnosis, however, is the ascription of fatigue to overwork when actually it is a manifestation of a psychoneurosis or depression.

Fatigue as a manifestation of psychiatric disorder The great majority of patients who enter a hospital because of unexplained chronic fatigue and lassitude have been found to have some type of psychiatric illness. Formerly this state was called *neurasthenia;* but since fatigue rarely exists as an isolated phenomenon, the current practice is to label such cases according to the total clinical picture. The usual associated symptoms are nervousness, irritability, anxiety, depression, insomnia, headaches, difficulty in concentrating, sexual disorders, and loss of bodily appetites. In one series in a general hospital 75 percent of persons admitted because of chronic fatigue and nervousness were diagnosed, finally, as having *anxiety neurosis* and *tension states.* Depression accounted for another 10 percent, and the remainder of the patients had a miscellany of medical and psychiatric illnesses.

Several features are common to the psychiatric group. The fatigue may be worse in the morning. There is an inclination to lie down and rest, but sleep does not come. The fatigue relates more to some activities than to others. Inquiry as to what was happening when the fatigue was first experienced may reveal an unpleasant event, a grief reaction, a surgical operation, or a medical illness. The feeling of fatigue interferes with mental as well as physical activities. As to the psychic aspects, it is difficult to concentrate during the solution of a problem, or in carrying on a conversation.

Depressing emotion, as was already remarked in the previous chapter, has its characteristic effect on impulse life and energy. Also, sleep is poor, with a tendency to early-morning waking, so that such persons are at their worst in the morning, both in spirit and in energy output. Their tendency is to improve as the day wears on, and they even feel fairly normal by evening. It is difficult to decide whether the fatigue is a primary manifestation of disease or is secondary to a lack of interest.

Many physicians question whether all chronically fatigued individuals deviate enough from normal to justify the diagnosis psychoneurosis or depression. Many people in society, because of circumstances beyond their control, have no purpose in life and much idle time. They are bored with the monotony of their routine. Such circumstances are conducive to fatigue, just as the opposite is also true—that a new enterprise that excites optimism and enthusiasm will dispel their fatigue. Other individuals seem normal until some adversity is encountered, arousing worry or fear, and then it becomes apparent that their adjustment was unstable. Such reactions are understandable to anyone who has ever had stage fright or "buck fever" and who remembers the sense of physical weakness, the utter incapacity to act, the intellectual chaos that overwhelms the previously well-ordered mind, and the exhaustion which follows.

Psychologic theories The enervating effect of a strong emotion such as anxiety is well known, and it might be supposed that the simple prolongation of the emotional experience would provide a rational explanation for a chronic fatigue of anxiety. Even if true, however, this explanation does not account for the occurrence of emotion at a time when there is no reason for it.

The dynamic schools of psychiatry, particularly the psychoanalytic, have postulated that chronic fatigue, in the broadest sense, is like the anxiety from which it derives; it is a danger signal that something is wrong—that some attitude or activity has been too intense or too persistent. The fatigue is self-preservative, serving not merely as a protection against physical injury but also as a protection of the individual's self-esteem and his confidence in himself. As to mechanism, it is claimed that the fatigue is the result of exhaustion of the store of psychic energy required to maintain repression of unacceptable ideas. Others, however, claim to have evidence that fatigue is not a negative symptom, a lack of or depletion of energy, but an unconscious desire for inactivity. A reciprocal relationship is said to exist between fatigue and anxiety. Both are protective, but anxiety is the more imperative. It calls for the individual to take some positive action to extricate himself from a predicament, whereas fatigue calls for inactivity. Both operate blindly, however, for the person cannot perceive what it is that must be done or stopped. All this happens at the unconscious level.

Some persons are low in impulse and energy throughout life, being more so at times of stress; some psychiatrists believe that they have a constitutional inadequacy. Kahn classifies such individuals as "psychopaths weak in impulse," and points out in his description their inability throughout life to play games vigorously, to compete successfully, to work hard without exhaustion, to withstand or recover quickly from illness, or to assume a dominant role in a social group.

It is obvious that these several psychologic hypotheses could not all be correct, nor could they be applicable to all situations in which chronic fatigue is the complaint. Undoubtedly there are persons who are underactive and weak because of genetic factors or early life experiences. It is equally clear that psychic and physical energy are closely linked to mood. The more chronic varieties of acquired fatigue, without a basis in medical disease, have in nearly all instances a psychologic basis.

Lassitude and fatigue in chronic infection and in endocrine and other medical diseases Infection is another cause of chronic fatigue, though a much less frequent one. Everyone has at some time or other sensed the abrupt onset of extreme exhaustion, the tired ache in the muscles, an inexplicable listlessness, only to discover later that he is "coming down with the flu." In chronic infections such as hepatitis, tuberculosis, brucellosis, infectious mononucleosis, the infection may not be at once evident. But it should always be suspected when the fatigue is out of proportion to other symptoms such as mood change, nervousness, and anxiety. Often this syndrome will begin with an obvious infection but will persist for several weeks after it should have terminated, and it may then be difficult to decide whether there is still a lingering infection or the infection has been complicated by psychiatric illness during convalescence. In many diseases such as infectious hepatitis and brucellosis, infectious mononucleosis, and a host of other systemic viral infections, long-standing neurotic symptoms appear to have been uncovered. Nevertheless it is difficult to dismiss an obscure secondary metabolic disorder consequent to the infection. (See Chap. 341.)

Metabolic and endocrine diseases (see Chaps. 83 and 85) of various types may cause inordinate degrees of lassitude and fatigue. Sometimes there is in addition a true muscular weakness (see Chaps. 16 and 347). In Addison's disease and Simmonds' disease fatigue may dominate the clinical picture. Aldosterone deficiency is another established cause of fatigue (see Chap. 86). In persons with hypothyroidism, with or without frank myxedema, lassitude and sluggishness are frequent complaints. These same symptoms may also be present in patients with hyperthyroidism but are usually less troublesome than nervousness. Uncontrolled diabetes mellitus may be accompanied by excessive fatigability, as are hyperparathyroidism, hypogonadism, and Cushing's disease.

Anemia, when moderate or severe, should be considered as a possible cause of unexplained lassitude. Mild grades of anemia are usually asymptomatic; lassitude is far too often ascribed to it.

Any type of nutritional deficiency may, when severe, cause lassitude, and in its earlier stages this may be the chief complaint. Weight loss and the history of dietary inadequacy may provide the only other clues to the nature of the illness. Many patients feel weak and tired after a myocardial infarct, but usually there is an accompanying depression.

Among neurologic diseases in which fatigability is a prominent symptom should be mentioned the posttraumatic nervous instability syndrome, Parkinson's disease, and multiple sclerosis. The fatigue of Parkinson's disease may precede the recognition of neurologic signs by months or even years. It is probably a reaction to the increasing disability occasioned by subjective awareness of the akinesia. The majority of patients who recover from a stroke complain of being weak and tired. Hot temperatures worsen the symptoms of the multiple sclerotic patient.

Differential diagnosis If one looks critically at the patients who enter a university hospital because of lassitude and fatigability (sometimes incorrectly called weakness), it is clear that the most common overlooked diagnoses are psychoneurosis and depression. The correct conclusion can usually be reached by keeping these illnesses in mind as one elicits the principal symptoms of these psychiatric illnesses from patient and family. Difficulty arises when such symptoms are so inconspicuous as not to be appreciated; one comes then to suspect the psychiatric diagnosis only by having eliminated the common medical causes. Observations in the hospital may bear out the existence of a tension state or gloomy mood, as the patient resists attempts to be mobilized. Strong reassurance in combination with a therapeutic trial of 5 to 10 mg dextro-amphetamine morning and noon and 100 to 200 mg sodium amobarbital three times a day may suppress symptoms of which the patient was barely aware and may clarify diagnosis. The danger of mistaking a depression for a neurosis has already been mentioned above. Of course the asthenic psychopath is recognized by his actions as revealed in his biography.

Obscure infections such as pulmonary tuberculosis, brucellosis, subclinical hepatitis, subacute bacterial endocarditis, malaria, hookworm, and parasitic infections should be sought by the characteristic symptoms and signs described elsewhere in the book. An endocrine survey is in order in all obscure cases. There should also be a search for occult tumors. The use of a simple "water excretion test" may prove very helpful in identifying an organic component in a patient's fatigue syndrome, since a wide variety of systemic disorders is associated with a delayed diuresis following the ingestion of water. It is thought that the "sick-cell" with impaired permeability of cell membrane "traps" water and then releases it slowly. The test consists in the administration of 500 ml water at 8 A.M., 8:15 A.M., and 8:30 A.M. for a total intake of 1,500 ml with the patient fasting and lying in a horizontal position. Smoking is not permitted. The water should be room temperature, *not cold.* Urine volume is measured hourly for 3 to 4 hr. A normal response will usually include a diuresis of 400 to 600 ml in the first, second, and third hours, with a total volume of at least 80 percent in 3 to 4 hr (1,200 ml). An impaired response in the horizontal position suggests *organic disease.* The test is inexpensive and simple to administer! It should be remembered that chronic intoxications with barbiturates, alcohol, or bromides, some of which are given to suppress nervousness, may contribute to fatigability.

Finally, when onset of fatigue is rapid and recent, the cause is likely to be an infection, a disturbance in fluid balance, or rapidly developing circulatory failure of either peripheral or cardiac origin.

GENERALIZED WEAKNESS AND ASTHENIA As can be judged from the foregoing remarks, weakness must be distinguished from lassitude and fatigue. The demonstration of reduced muscular power sets the case analysis along rather different lines, for it raises consideration more particularly of diseases of the nervous system or of the musculature.

True neural or myopathic weakness is probably never due to psychologic factors, though the hysteric or malingering patient may claim weakness. Usually this can be detected by the criteria outlined in Chap. 343. In anemia, chronic infection, malignancy, and nutritional depletion (except when polyneuropathy is present), the thin muscles are always stronger during tests of peak contraction than one would expect, though of course strength falls short of that of a healthy individual (see Chap. 343 for description of tests of peak, power, and endurance of muscles).

The proper ascertainment of muscular weakness depends on two lines of inquiry: (1) a history of reduced efficiency; and (2) demonstrable failure in ability to contract the muscles forcefully one or more times. If one proceeds to test each of the major groups of muscles from head to foot, comparing the patient's performance with one's idea of normalcy for man and woman, one may ascertain whether all or certain groups fall below standard. Quantitative and qualitative changes (myasthenia, inverse myasthenia, myotonia, paramyotonia, pathologic cramping) may also be detected by the methods to be outlined in Chap. 343. The topography of weakness and associated neurologic findings permit distinction between the various types of spinal, peripheral nerve, and myopathic pareses. Rare diseases, difficult to diagnose, that cause inexplicable muscle weakness are masked hyperthyroidism, hyperparathyroidism, ossifying hemangiomas with hypophosphatemia, some of the kalemic periodic paralyses, and hyperinsulinism.

REFERENCES

ADAMS RD: *Principles of Clinical Myology,* Thayer Lectures, Johns Hopkins Medical Journal, 131:24, 1972

MAYER-GROSS W et al: *Clinical Psychiatry,* 3d ed., Baltimore: Williams & Wilkins, 1969

WALTON JN (ed): *Disease of Voluntary Muscle,* 2d ed., Boston: Little, Brown, 1969

16
FAINTNESS, SYNCOPE, AND EPISODIC WEAKNESS

RAYMOND D. ADAMS
EUGENE BRAUNWALD

Episodic faintness, lightheadedness or giddiness, and reduced alertness are frequently difficult to distinguish, tending to shade into one another. And the difference between faintness and frank syncope is only quantitative. Since syncope, though less common, is more definite, it will be considered in greater detail. Types of episodic weakness, such as myasthenia gravis and familial periodic paralysis, which cause striking reduction of muscular strength but no impairment of consciousness, should be set apart (see Chaps. 15 and 347); epilepsy, which is also associated with episodic unconsciousness, differs from syncope in most other respects and is discussed in Chap. 24.

CARDINAL FEATURES

The term *syncope* literally means "cutting short," "cessation," or "pause," and it is synonymous with *faint.* Syncope comprises a generalized weakness of muscles, with inability to stand upright, and an impairment of consciousness. The term *faintness,* in contrast, refers to lack of strength, with sensation of impending loss of consciousness.

The syncopal attack usually develops rapidly, but it is doubtful whether consciousness is ever terminated with the absolute suddenness of an epileptic seizure. At the beginning of the attack the patient is nearly always in the upright position, either sitting or standing [the Stokes-Adams attack (cf. Chap. 234) is exceptional in this respect]. Usually the patient is warned of the impending faint by a sense of "feeling badly." He is assailed by giddiness, the floor seems to move, and surrounding objects begin to sway. His senses become confused, he yawns or gapes, there are spots before his eyes, his vision may dim, and his ears may ring. Nausea and sometimes vomiting accompany these symptoms. There is a striking pallor or ashen-gray color of the face, and very often the face and body are bathed in cold perspiration. The deliberate onset may enable the patient to protect himself as he slumps; a hurtful fall is exceptional. If the patient can lie down promptly, the attack may be averted without complete loss of consciousness.

The depth and duration of unconsciousness vary. Sometimes the patient is not completely oblivious of his surroundings, or there may be complete lack of awareness and of capacity to respond. The patient may remain in this state for seconds to minutes or even as long as half an hour. Usually he lies motionless with skeletal muscles relaxed, but a few clonic jerks of the limbs and face may occur in exceptional cases, shortly after the beginning of the unconsciousness. Generalized tonic-clonic convulsions are never a part of syncope. Sphincter control is usually maintained. The pulse is feeble or cannot be felt; the blood pressure is low, and breathing is almost imperceptible. The reduction in vital functions and pallor simulate death. Once the patient is in a horizontal position, perhaps from having fallen, gravitation no longer hinders the flow of blood to the brain. The strength of the pulse then improves, color begins to return to the face, breathing becomes quicker and deeper, and consciousness is quickly regained. There is from this moment onward a correct perception of the environment. The patient is, nevertheless, keenly aware of physical weakness, and if he rises too soon, another faint may be precipitated. Headache and drowsiness, which, with mental confusion, are the usual sequelae of a convulsion, do not follow a syncopal attack.

CLASSIFICATION OF CAUSES OF RECURRENT WEAKNESS, FAINTNESS, AND DISTURBANCES OF CONSCIOUSNESS

The following list is based on established or assumed physiologic mechanisms.

I Circulatory (deficient quantity of blood to the brain)
- *A* Inadequate vasoconstrictor mechanisms
  - *1* Vasovagal (vasodepressor)
  - *2* Postural hypotension
  - *3* Primary autonomic insufficiency
  - *4* Sympathectomy (pharmacologic or surgical)
  - *5* Diseases of central and peripheral nervous systems (Chap. 323)
  - *6* Carotid sinus syncope (see also Bradyarrhythmias, below)
- *B* Hypovolemia
- C Mechanical reduction of venous return
  - *1* Valsalva's maneuver
  - *2* Cough
  - *3* Micturition
  - *4* Atrial myxoma, ball valve thrombus
- *D* Reduced cardiac output
  - *1* Obstruction to left ventricular outflow: aortic stenosis, hypertrophic subaortic stenosis
  - *2* Obstruction to pulmonary flow: pulmonic stenosis, primary pulmonary hypertension, pulmonary embolism
  - *3* Myocardial: massive myocardial infarction with pump failure
  - *4* Pericardial: cardiac tamponade
- *E* Arrhythmias (Chap. 234)
  - *1* Bradyarrhythmias

a Atrioventricular (AV) block (11° and 111°), with Stokes-Adams attacks
b Ventricular asystole
c Sinus bradycardia, sinoatrial block, sinus arrest
d Carotid sinus syncope (see also Inadequate Vasoconstrictor Mechanisms, above)
e Glossopharyngeal neuralgia (and other painful states)

2 Tachyarrhythmias
a Episodic ventricular fibrillation with or without associated bradyarrhythmias
b Ventricular tachycardia
c Supraventricular tachycardia without AV block

II Other causes of weakness and episodic disturbances of consciousness
A Altered state of blood to the brain
1 Hypoxia – ex: acute hemorrhage
2 Anemia
3 Diminished CO_2 due to hyperventilation (faintness common, syncope seldom occurs)
4 Hypoglycemia (episodic weakness common, faintness occasional, syncope rare)

B Cerebral
1 Cerebrovascular disturbances (cerebral ischemic attacks, see Chap. 326)
a Extracranial vascular insufficiency (basilar-vertebral, carotid)
b Diffuse spasm of cerebral arterioles (hypertensive encephalopathy)

2 Emotional disturbances, anxiety attacks, and hysterical seizures (see Chaps. 14 and 339)

The list of conditions which cause weakness and faintness and disturbances of consciousness is deceptively long and involved. Close study, however, reveals that the commoner types of faint are reducible to a few simple mechanisms. Syncope results essentially from a sudden impairment of brain metabolism usually brought about by a hypotensive reduction of cerebral blood flow.

Nature has provided man with several mechanisms by which his circulation adjusts to the upright posture. Approximately three-fourths of the systemic blood volume is contained in the venous bed, and any interference with venous return may lead to a reduction in cardiac output. Cerebral blood flow may still be maintained, as long as systemic arterial vasoconstriction occurs; but when this adjustment fails, serious hypotension with resultant cerebral underperfusion to less than half of normal results in syncope. Normally, the pooling of blood in the lower parts of the body is prevented by (1) pressor reflexes which induce constriction of peripheral arteries and arterioles; (2) reflex acceleration of the heart by means of aortic and carotid reflexes; (3) improvement of venous return to the heart by activity of the muscles of the limbs and by increased rate of respiration. Placing a normal person on a tilt table to relax his muscles and tilting him upright slightly diminishes cardiac output, and blood accumulates in the legs to a slight degree. This may then be followed by a slight transitory fall in systolic arterial pressure, and thus may be a means of reproducing faints in patients with defective vasomotor reflexes.

TYPES OF SYNCOPE

VASOVAGAL (VASODEPRESSOR) SYNCOPE This is the common faint that may be experienced by normal persons; it is frequently recurrent, and tends to take place during emotional stress (especially in a warm, crowded room), after an injurious, shocking accident, and during pain. Mild blood loss, poor physical condition, and fasting are other factors which increase the possibility of fainting in susceptible individuals. A short premonitory phase is characterized by nausea, perspiration, yawning, epigastric distress, hyperpnea, tachypnea, weakness, confusion, and pupillary dilation. Clonic convulsive movements may occur 15 to 20 sec after loss of consciousness. Physiologically, there is first a marked fall in arterial pressure and systemic resistance. Cardiac output declines when vagal activity leads to marked bradycardia, resulting in further lowering of arterial pressure and reducing cerebral perfusion. Assumption of the supine posture with elevation of the legs and removal of the offending stimulus will rapidly restore consciousness.

POSTURAL HYPOTENSION WITH SYNCOPE This type of syncope affects persons who have a chronic defect in or variable instability of vasomotor reflexes. Though the character of the syncopal attack differs little from that of the vasovagal or vasodepressor type, the effect of posture is its cardinal feature; sudden arising from a recumbent position or standing still are the circumstances under which it is most likely to happen.

Postural syncope tends to occur under the following conditions: (1) in otherwise normal persons who for some unknown reason have defective postural reflexes; (2) rarely, as part of a syndrome named *primary autonomic insufficiency,* which includes chronic orthostatic hypotension, as well as symptoms of peripheral preganglionic autonomic and extrapyramidial disorder; (3) after physical deconditioning, e.g., after prolonged illness with recumbency, especially in elderly individuals with flabby muscles; (4) after a sympathectomy that has abolished vasopressor reflexes; (5) in diabetic and other neuropathies, tabes dorsalis, and diseases of the nervous system which cause muscular atrophy and paralysis of vasopressor reflexes; (6) in persons with varicose veins, because of pooling of blood in the abnormally enlarged venous channels; (7) in patients receiving antihypertensive and certain sedative and antidepressive drugs.

In the otherwise normal individuals who faint if tilted on a table, it has been found that at first the blood pressure diminishes slightly and then stabilizes at a lower level. Shortly thereafter the compensatory reflexes suddenly fail, and the arterial pressure falls precipitously. This reaction also may be observed in some of the conditions listed above. In others, e.g., after surgical sympathectomy, in diseases of the sympathetic nervous system, and in the unusual condition known as chronic orthostatic hypotension, the arterial pressure never stabilizes after tilting but falls steadily to a level at which cerebral circulation cannot be maintained.

CHRONIC ORTHOSTATIC HYPOTENSION In this condition, occurring as a consequence of *primary autonomic insufficiency,* there is a degeneration of preganglionic and probably postganglionic autonomic neurons, with anhydrosis and other symptoms of sympathetic and parasympathetic paralysis (sphincteric disturbances, impotence, lack of tears, lack of saliva, pupillary paralysis). Extrapyramidal disorders (tremor, ataxia, rigidity) appear in the more advanced stages of the disease. As remarked above, the hypotension differs from that already described in that the systolic and diastolic pressures fall rapidly as soon as the patient assumes an upright position, but there are no compensatory tachycardia, pallor, sweating, nausea, or other symptoms. The loss of consciousness is usually abrupt. Recumbency restores the circulation of the brain, with a prompt return to consciousness. The pooling of blood in the abdomen and legs fails to excite a normal degree of vasoconstriction of systemic arterioles, presumably because of the abnormality in the autonomic nervous system. There is also evidence that patients with this type of postural hypotension are deficient in release of norepinephrine and epinephrine. Repeated attacks may result in mental confusion, slurred speech, and other neurologic signs, though the extrapyramidal disorder appears to be due to the same degenerative process that affects autonomic motor neurons. The combination is called the Shy-Drager syndrome.

Micturition syncope, a condition usually seen in the elderly when they arise from bed at night to urinate, is probably a special type of postural syncope. It has been suggested that vasomotor reflexes from the bladder itself play a contributory part and that vagally mediated bradycardia forms a significant component.

SYNCOPE OF CARDIAC ORIGIN (CARDIAC SYNCOPE) Cardiac syncope results from a sudden reduction in cardiac output, resulting most commonly from a cardiac arrhythmia. In normal individuals slow ventricular rates, between 35 and 40 beats per min and fast ones of 120 to 175 beats per min do not reduce cerebral blood flow, especially if the person is in the supine position, but changes in pulse rate outside these limits impair cerebral circulation and functions. The upright posture, cerebrovascular disease, anemia, and coronary, myocardial or valvular disease all reduce the tolerance to alterations in rate.

Complete atrioventricular block is the commonest arrhythmia that leads to fainting, and syncopal episodes associated with this arrhythmia are known as the Stokes-Adams-Morgagni syndrome. The etiology of disturbances in atrioventricular conduction is considered elsewhere (Chap. 234), but in patients with these attacks the block may be persistent or intermittent; it is often preceded by disturbed conduction in one or two of the three fascicles through which the ventricles are normally activated or by second degree atrioventricular block (Mobitz type II). When the block is complete and the pacemaker below the block fails to function, syncope occurs. Less commonly a brief bout of ventricular tachycardia or fibrillation is responsible for the syncopal episode. Familial instances of recurrent syncope due to ventricular fibrillation, characterized by a prolonged Q-T interval (sometimes associated with congenital deafness), have been reported.

Stokes-Adams attacks occur usually without more than a momentary sense of weakness, the patient suddenly losing consciousness. This may occur at any time of the day or night, regardless of the position of the body. When the patient is upright, the unconsciousness will develop after a more brief period of asystole than with the recumbent position. After cardiac standstill of more than several seconds, the patient turns pale, falls unconscious, and, as in other types of fainting, may exhibit a few clonic jerks. With longer periods of asystole, up to 5 min, the ashen-gray pallor gives way to cyanosis, stertorous breathing, fixed pupils, incontinence, and bilateral Babinski signs. Prolonged confusion and neurologic signs due to the relative ischemia of parts of the brain supplied by narrowed, arteriosclerotic arteries may persist in some patients, and permanent impairment of mental function may also occur. With the resumption of the heartbeat, the face and neck become flushed. Cardiac faints of this type may recur several times a day. Occasionally the heart block is transitory, and the electrocardiogram taken later shows only evidence of myocardial disease.

Less commonly, a decreased rate of discharge of the sinoatrial node, resulting from sinoatrial block or from sinus pauses, leads to syncope. The sinoatrial function may be impaired by inflammatory disease, by acute myocardial infarction, by augmented vagal activity, by cardiodepressant drugs such as quinidine, and immediately following cessation of tachycardia. Recurrent attacks of tachyarrhythmias—including atrial flutter and paroxysmal atrial and ventricular tachycardia with normal AV conduction—may also suddenly reduce cardiac output, to a degree sufficient to cause syncope.

In another form of cardiac syncope the heart block is reflexive and is due to irritation of the vagus nerves. Examples of this phenomenon have been observed with esophageal diverticula, mediastinal tumors, gallbladder disease, carotid sinus disease, glossopharyngeal neuralgia, and pleural and pulmonary irritation. However, in these conditions reflex bradycardia is more commonly of the sinoatrial than the atrioventricular type.

Cardiac syncope may also result from *acute massive myocardial infarction,* particularly when associated with cardiogenic shock; fright, severe pain, or arrhythmias may also be involved. *Aortic stenosis* often sets the stage for exertional syncope, most commonly by limiting cardiac output, with resultant myocardial and cerebral ischemia and arrhythmias. *Idiopathic hypertrophic subaortic stenosis* may also lead to exertional syncope, because of intensified obstruction and/or ventricular arrhythmias. In *primary pulmonary hypertension* a relatively fixed cardiac output and bouts of acute right ventricular failure may be associated with syncope (Chap. 259). However, vagal reflexes may be involved in this condition as well as with the syncope that occurs with *pulmonary embolism.* Ball valve thrombus in the left atrium, left atrial myxoma, or thrombosis or malfunction of a prosthetic valve may produce sudden mechanical obstruction of the circulation and syncope. Cardiac tamponade and dissecting aneurysm of the thoracic aorta are occasionally responsible. *Tetralogy of Fallot* is the congenital malformation most commonly responsible for syncope. In this condition systemic vasodilatation, perhaps associated with infundibular spasm, greatly increases the right-to-left shunt and produces arterial hypoxia, which leads to syncope.

CAROTID SINUS SYNCOPE The carotid sinus is normally sensitive to stretch and gives rise to sensory impulses carried via the nerve of Hering, a branch of the glossopharyngeal nerve, to the medulla oblongata. Massage of one or both of the carotid sinuses, particularly in elderly persons, causes (1) a reflex cardiac slowing (sinus bradycardia, sinus arrest, or even atrioventricular block), the so-called vagal type of response, (2) a fall of arterial pressure without cardiac slowing, the so-called depressor type of response, and (3) an interference with the circulation of the ipsilateral cerebral hemisphere, the so-called central type. Two or three types of carotid sinus response may coexist.

Syncope due to carotid sinus sensitivity may be initiated by turning of the heart to one side, by a tight collar, or, as in a few reported cases, by shaving over the region of the sinus. But the absence of such stimuli is of no aid in diagnosis, since spontaneous attacks may occur. The attack nearly always begins when the patient is in an upright position, usually when he is standing. The onset is sudden, often with falling. Clonic convulsive movements occur quite frequently in the vagal and depressor types of carotid sinus but not in the cerebral type of syncope. Unilateral paresthesias or motor deficits characterize the latter. The period of unconsciousness seldom lasts longer than a few minutes. The sensorium is immediately clear when consciousness is regained. The majority of the reported cases have been in males.

In a patient displaying faintness on compression of one carotid sinus, it is important to distinguish between the benign disorder (hypersensitivity of one carotid sinus) and a much more serious condition—atheromatous narrowing of the opposite carotid or of the basilar artery (see Chap. 326).

Other forms of vasovagal syncope have been described. Exceptionally intense pain of visceral origin may inhibit cardiac action through vagal stimulation, e.g., cardiac standstill during an attack of gallbladder colic, a lesion of esophagus or mediastinum, bronchoscopy, needling of body cavities, etc.

VAGAL AND GLOSSOPHARYNGEAL NEURALGIA This is known occasionally to induce a reflex type of fainting. Again the sequence is always pain, then syncope; in this instance the pain is localized to the base of the tongue, pharynx or larynx, tonsillar area, and ear. It may be triggered by pressure at these sites. Section of the appropriate branches of the ninth or tenth cranial nerve relieves the condition. It has been suggested that the cardiovascular effects are attributable to excitation of the dorsal motor nucleus of the vagus via collateral fibers from the nucleus of the tractus solitarius. The rare vertiginous faint which accompanies intense vertigo from labyrinthine or vestibular disease, as well as the syncope following prostatic massage or pleural or peritoneal taps, may be other examples of reflex vagal stimulation.

TUSSIVE SYNCOPE ("LARYNGEAL VERTIGO") This is a rare condition that results from a paroxysm of coughing. Patients with this type of syncope are usually males with chronic bronchitis. After hard coughing the patient suddenly becomes weak and loses consciousness momentarily. The unconsciousness that results from breath holding in infants is probably similar. The intrathoracic pressure becomes elevated and interferes with the venous return to the heart. The Valsalva maneuver of trying to exhale against a closed glottis is believed to produce an identical effect. Episodes of faintness and lightheadedness are not infrequent in pertussis and chronic laryngitis. Exceptionally, other kinds of strenuous activity such as laughing, straining at stool, running upstairs, or lifting may produce a similar syndrome.

SYNCOPE ASSOCIATED WITH CEREBROVASCULAR DISEASE This is infrequent and has usually been caused by partial or complete occlusion of the large arteries in the neck. The best examples are found in the "aortic arch syndrome" (pulseless disease), in which the brachiocephalic and common carotid and vertebral arteries have become narrowed. Physical activity may then critically reduce blood flow to the upper part of the brainstem, causing abrupt loss of consciousness (cf. Chap. 326). Stenosis or occlusion of vertebral arteries and the "vertebral steal syndrome" are other examples. Fainting is said also to occur occasionally in patients with congenital anomalies of the upper cervical part of the spine (Klippel-Feil syndrome) or cervical spondylitis, in which the vertebral circulation is compromised. Head turning may then cause neck pain, nausea, vomiting, vertigo, visual scotomas, and finally unconsciousness. If one carotid artery is occluded, heavy massage or pressure on the other may cause loss of consciousness, a kind of carotid syncope.

PATHOPHYSIOLOGY OF SYNCOPE

In the final analysis the loss of consciousness in these different types of syncope must be caused by a change in the nervous elements in those parts of the brain which subserve consciousness. Syncope resembles epilepsy in this respect; yet there is an important difference. In epilepsy, whether major or minor, the arrest in mental function is almost instantaneous, and, as revealed by the electroencephalogram, it is accompanied by a paroxysm of activity in certain groups of cerebral neurons. Syncope, on the other hand, is not so sudden. The difference relates to the essential pathophysiology—a sudden spread of an electric discharge in epilepsy, and the more gradual failure of the cerebral circulation in syncope.

During syncopal attacks, there are demonstrable reductions in cerebral blood flow, cerebral oxygen utilization, and cerebral vascular resistance. The electroencephalogram reveals high-voltage slow waves, two to five per second, coincident with the loss of consciousness. If the ischemia lasts only a few minutes, there are no lasting effects on the brain. If it persists for a longer time, it may result in necrosis of the border zones between the major cerebral and cerebellar arteries.

in a person who exhibits the general personality and behavioral characteristics of hysteria.

DIFFERENTIAL DIAGNOSIS

OF CONDITIONS OFTEN ASSOCIATED WITH EPISODIC WEAKNESS AND FAINTNESS BUT NOT WITH SYNCOPE

Anxiety attacks and the hyperventilation syndrome These are discussed in detail in Chaps. 14, 19, and 339. The giddiness of anxiety is frequently interpreted as a feeling of faintness without actual loss of consciousness. Such symptoms are not accompanied by facial pallor and are not relieved by recumbency. The diagnosis is made on the basis of the associated symptons, and part of the attack can be reproduced by hyperventilation. Two of the mechanisms known to be involved in the attacks are reduction in carbon dioxide as the result of hyperventilation and the release of epinephrine. Hyperventilation results in hypocapnia, alkalosis, increased cerebrovascular resistance, and decreased cerebral blood flow.

Hypoglycemia Another frequent cause of obscure episodic weakness is hypoglycemia. When severe, hypoglycemia is usually traceable to a serious disease, such as a tumor of the islets of Langerhans or advanced adrenal, pituitary, or hepatic disease. The clinical picture is one of confusion or even a loss of consciousness. When mild, as is usually the case, hypoglycemia is of the reactive type (Chap. 90), occurring 2 to 5 hr after eating, and is not usually associated with a disturbance of consciousness. The diagnosis depends largely upon the history, the documentation of reduced blood sugar during an attack, and the reproduction by an injection of insulin or an oral dose of tolbutamide of a symptom complex exactly similar to that occurring in the spontaneous attacks.

Acute hemorrhage Acute blood loss, usually within the gastrointestinal tract, is an occasional cause of syncope. Peptic ulcer is the commonest source of the hemorrhage. In the absence of pain and hematenesis the cause of the weakness, faintness, or even unconsciousness may remain obscure until the passage of a black stool.

Cerebral ischemic attacks These occur in some patients with arteriosclerotic narrowings or occlusion of the major arteries of the brain. The main symptoms vary from patient to patient and include dim vision, hemiparesis, numbness of one side of the body, dizziness, and thick speech, and to these may be added an impairment of consciousness. In any one patient all attacks are of identical type and indicate a temporary deficit of the function in a certain region of the brain due to inadequate circulation. The mechanism of the deficit has not been fully elucidated; recurrent embolism is the probable explanation (see Chap. 326).

Hysterical fainting Hysterical fainting is rather frequent and usually occurs under dramatic circumstances (Chap. 339). The attack is unattended by any outward display of anxiety. The evident lack of change in pulse and blood pressure or color of the skin and mucous membranes distinguishes it from the vasodepressor faint. The diagnosis is based on the bizarre nature of the attack in a person who exhibits the general personality and behavioral characteristics of hysteria.

OF SEIZURE AND SYNCOPE

More typical varieties of syncope must be distinguished from other disturbances of cerebral function, the most frequent of which is akinetic or some other form of epilepsy (see Chap. 24). The epileptic attack may occur day or night, regardless of the position of the patient; syncope rarely appears when the patient is recumbent, the only common exception being the Stokes-Adams attack. The patient's color does not usually change in epilepsy; pallor is an early and invariable finding in all types of syncope, except chronic orthostatic hypotension and hysteria, and it precedes unconsciousness. Epilepsy is more sudden in onset, and if an aura is present, it rarely lasts longer than a few seconds before consciousness is abolished. The onset of syncope is usually more deliberate and without aura. Injury from falling is frequent in epilepsy and rare in syncope, for the reason that only in epilepsy are protective reflexes instantaneously abolished. Tonic-convulsive movements with upturning eyes are a feature of epilepsy and not of syncope. The period of unconsciousness tends to be longer in epilepsy than in syncope. Urinary incontinence is frequent in epilepsy and rare in syncope, but since it may be observed occasionally in syncope, it cannot be used as a means of excluding epilepsy. The return of consciousness is prompt in syncope, slow in epilepsy. Mental confusion, headache, and drowsiness are common sequelae in epilepsy; physical weakness with clear sensorium characterizes the postsyncopal state. Repeated spells of unconsciousness in a young person at a rate of several per day or month are much more suggestive of epilepsy than of syncope. No one of these points will absolutely differentiate epilepsy from syncope, but taken as a group and supplemented by electroencephalograms, they provide a means of distinguishing the two conditions.

Of different types of syncope Differentiation of the several conditions that diminish cerebral blood flow is discussed in some detail in Chap. 33, and only a few points need to be repeated here.

When faintness is related to reduced cerebral blood flow resulting directly from a disorder of cardiac function, there is likely to be a combination of pallor and cyanosis, with pronounced dyspnea, and often the jugular veins are distended. When, on the other hand, the peripheral circulation is at fault, pallor is usually striking but is not accompanied by cyanosis or respiratory disturbances, and the veins are collapsed. When the primary disturbance lies in the cerebral circulation, the face is likely to be florid and the breathing slow and stertorous. During the attack a heart rate faster than 150 beats per minute indicates an ectopic cardiac rhythm, while a striking bradycardia (rate of less than 40) suggests complete heart block. In a patient with faintness or syncope attended by bradycardia, one has to distinguish between the neurogenic reflex and the cardiogenic (Stokes-Adams) types. The electrocardiogram is decisive, but even without it, the Stokes-Adams seizures can be recognized clinically by their longer duration, by the greater constancy of the slow heart rate, by the presence of audible sounds synchronous with atrial contraction, and by marked variation in intensity of the first sound, despite the regular rhythm (Chap. 234). The clinical diagnosis may at times be difficult or impossible.

The color of the skin, the character of the breathing, the appearance of the veins, and the rate of the heart are therefore valuable data in diagnosis if the patient is seen during the attack. Unfortunately, the physician does not have the opportunity to see most patients during their "spells" of weakness, hence he must obtain the proper clues from the patient's story. It is therefore of primary importance that the physician be familiar with the circumstances and the precipitating and alleviating factors in a given episode of weakness or fainting. The following points are also helpful in the differential diagnosis of syncope:

Type of onset When the attack begins with relative suddenness, i.e., over the period of a few seconds, carotid sinus syncope, postural hypotension, or sudden atrioventricular block is likely. When the symptoms develop gradually during a period of several minutes, hyperventilation or hypoglycemia should be considered. Onset of syncope during or immediately after exertion suggests aortic stenosis and, in elderly subjects, postural hypotension. Exertional syncope is seen occasionally in persons with aortic insufficiency and with severe occlusive disease of cerebral arteries.

Position at onset of attack Attacks due to hypoglycemia, hyperventilation, hypertensive encephalopathy, or heart block are likely to be independent of posture. Faintness associated with a decline in blood pressure (including carotid sinus attacks) and with ectopic tachycardia usually occurs only in the sitting or standing position, whereas faintness resulting from orthostatic hypotension or orthostatic tachycardia is apt to set in shortly after change from the recumbent to the standing position.

Associated symptoms The associated symptoms during an attack are important; palpitation is likely to be present when the attack is due to anxiety or hyperventilation, to ectopic tachycardia, or to hypoglycemia. Numbness and tingling in the hands and face are frequent accompaniments of hyperventilation. Irregular jerking movements and generalized spasms without loss of consciousness or change in the electroencephalogram are typical of the hysterical faint. Genuine convulsions during the attack, although characteristic of epilepsy, may occasionally occur with heart block and with hypertensive encephalopathy.

Duration of attack When the duration is very brief, i.e., a few seconds to a few minutes, carotid sinus syncope or one of the several forms of postural hypotension is most likely. A duration of more than a few minutes but less than an hour suggests hypoglycemia or hyperventilation.

SPECIAL METHODS OF EXAMINATION

In many patients who complain of recurrent weakness or syncope but do not have a spontaneous attack while under observation of the physician, an attempt to reproduce attacks is of great assistance in diagnosis.

When hyperventilation is accompanied by faintness, the pattern of symptoms can be reproduced readily by having the subject breathe rapidly and deeply for 2 to 3 min. This test is often of therapeutic value also, because the underlying anxiety tends to be lessened when the patient learns that he can produce and alleviate the symptoms at will simply by controlling his breathing.

Among other conditions in which the diagnosis is commonly clarified by reproducing the attacks are carotid sinus hypersensitivity (massage of one or the other carotid sinus), orthostatic hypotension and orthostatic tachycardia (observations of pulse rate, blood pressure, and symptoms in the recumbent and standing positions), and tussive syncope (by inducing the Valsalva maneuver). In all these instances the crucial point is not whether symptoms are produced (the procedures mentioned frequently induce symptoms in healthy persons) but whether the exact pattern of symptoms that occurs in the spontaneous attacks is reproduced in all of the artificial ones. Careful continuous monitoring of the electrocardiogram in the hospital or the recording of the electrocardiogram over several hours using a portable lightweight tape recorder in an ambulatory patient may be extremely useful in identifying an arrhythmia responsible for the syncopal episode. Monitoring is most helpful if it shows that the syncopal episode is characterized by a bout of cardiac standstill, extreme bradycardia, or severe tachyarrhythmia.

The electroencephalogram may be helpful in differentiating syncope from epilepsy. In the interval between epileptic seizures it may show some degree of abnormality in 40 to 80 percent of cases. In the interval between syncopal attacks it should be normal.

TREATMENT

Fainting in most instances is relatively benign. In dealing with patients who have fainted the physician should think first of those causes of fainting that constitute a therapeutic emergency. Among them are massive internal hemorrhage and myocardial infarction, which may be painless, and cardiac arrhythmias. In an elderly person a sudden faint, without obvious cause, should arouse the suspicion of complete heart block, even though all findings are negative when the physician sees the patient.

If the patient is seen during the preliminary stages of fainting or after he has lost consciousness, he should be placed in a position which permits maximal cerebral blood flow, i.e., with head lowered between the knees, if sitting, or in the supine position. All tight clothing and other constrictions should be loosened and the head turned so that the tongue does not fall back into the throat, blocking the airway. Peripheral irritation, such as sprinkling or dashing cold water on the face and neck or the application of cold towels, is helpful. If the temperature is subnormal, the body should be covered with a warm blanket. If available, aromatic spirit of ammonia may be given cautiously by inhalation. Since emesis is frequent, one should be prepared for a possible aspiration of vomiting. Nothing should be given by mouth until the patient has regained consciousness. Then one-half a teaspoon of aromatic spirit of ammonia in one-half a glass of cold water, or a sip of brandy or whiskey, may be given. The patient should not be permitted to rise until his sense of physical weakness has passed, and he should be watched carefully for a few minutes after rising.

As a rule, the physician sees the patient after he has recovered from the faint, and he is asked to explain why it happened and how it can be prevented in the future. The prevention of fainting depends on the mechanisms involved. In the usual vasovagal faint of adolescents, which tends to occur in periods of emotional excitement, fatigue, hunger, etc., it is enough to advise the patient to avoid such circumstances. In postural hypotension the patient should be cautioned against arising suddenly from bed. Instead, he should first exercise his legs for a few seconds, then sit on the edge of the bed and make sure he is not lightheaded or dizzy before he starts to walk. He should sleep with the headposts of the bed elevated on wooden blocks 8 to 12 in. high. A snug elastic abdominal binder and elastic stockings are often helpful. Drugs of the ephedrine group (ephedrine sulfate, 40 to 50 mg) may be useful if they do not cause insomnia. If there are no contraindications, a high intake of sodium chloride, which expands the extracellular fluid volume, may be beneficial.

In the syndrome of chronic orthostatic hypotension, special corticosteroid preparations (Florinef acetate tablets, 1 to 2 mg per day in divided doses) have given relief in some cases. Binding of the legs (G suit) and sleeping with head and shoulders elevated are helpful.

The treatment of carotid sinus syncope involves first of all instructing the patient in measures that minimize the hazards of a fall (see below). Loose collars should be worn, and the patient should learn to turn the whole body, rather than the head alone, when looking to one side. Atropine or the ephedrine group of drugs should be used, respectively, in patients with pronounced bradycardia or hypotension during attacks. If atropine is not successful, a demand pacemaker should be inserted into the right ventricle. Radiation or surgical denervation of the carotid sinus has apparently yielded favorable results in some patients, but it is rarely necessary. Once it has been concluded that the attacks are due to a narrowing of major cerebral arteries, some of the surgical measures discussed in Chap. 326 must be considered.

The treatment of the various cardiac arrhythmias which may induce syncope is discussed in Chap. 234. The treatment of hypoglycemia will be found in Chap. 90 and of the hyperventilation syndrome and hysterical fainting in Chaps. 14 and 339, respectively.

The chief hazard of a faint in most elderly persons is not the underlying disease but rather fracture or other trauma due to the fall. Therefore, patients subject to recurrent syncope should cover the bathroom floor and bathtub with rubber mats and should have as much of their home carpeted as is feasible. Especially important is the floor space between the bed and the bathroom, because faints are common in elderly persons when walking from bed to toilet. Outdoor walking should be on soft ground rather than hard surfaces, and the patient should avoid standing still, which is more likely to induce an attack than walking.

REFERENCES

FRIEDBERG CK: Syncope: pathological physiology: differential diagnosis and treatment. Mod Concepts Cardiovasc Dis 40:55–60, 1971

LEE JE et al: Episodic unconsciousness, in *Diagnostic Approaches to Presenting Syndromes,* ed JA Barondess, Baltimore: Williams & Wilkins, 1971, pp. 133–167

WRIGHT KE JR, MCINTOSH MD: Syncope: review of pathophysiological mechanisms. Prog Cardiovasc Dis 13:580–594, 1971

17 MOTOR PARALYSIS

RAYMOND D. ADAMS

The motor system may undergo dissolution in several ways during the course of nervous disease. In diffuse progressive disorders of the cerebrum there may be disintegration first of the highest, most complex nervous organizations, including learned patterns of volitional movement. Thus, concepts or memories of specialized, learned movement patterns may be lost while less complicated semivolitional or automatic movements are retained. As cerebral decortication proceeds there may be a paralysis of all voluntary movements without change in or even with exaggeration of reflex movements. In lesions of basal ganglions and cerebellum, volitional movements and normal postures are altered or hampered by the presence of abnormal movements (tremor, chorea, athetosis), abnormal postures (dystonia), or incoordination (ataxia). In lesions of the brainstem, all volitional movements are abolished on one or both sides of the body, often with release of certain obligatory postural states (decerebrate) but with spinal reflex activities left either normal or enhanced. In lesions of the spinal cord, paralysis of voluntary movement may occur with either increase or abolition of reflex activity. In complete lesions of peripheral nerves and skeletal muscles, all movements—learned, instinctual, automatic, postural, and reflex—are lost, since these are the final common motor pathway and the apparatus of movement, respectively.

These and other impairments of motor function may be somewhat arbitrarily subdivided into (1) paralysis due to affection of lower motor neurons, (2) paralysis due to disorder of upper motor (corticospinal and cortico-brainstem) neurons, (3) abnormalities of coordination (ataxia) due to lesions in the cerebellum, (4) abnormalities of movement and posture due to disease of the extrapyramidal motor system, (5) apraxic or nonparalytic disturbances of purposive movement due to involvement of the cerebrum. The first two types of motor disorder and the cerebral disorders of movement will be discussed briefly in the following pages; cerebellar ataxia and extrapyramidal motor abnormalities will be considered in Chap. 18.

DEFINITIONS The term *paralysis* is derived from two Greek words, *para,* beside, and *lysis,* a loosening. In medicine it has come to refer to an abolition of function, either sensory or motor. When applied to voluntary muscles, paralysis means loss of contraction due to interruption of one of the motor pathways from the cerebrum to the muscle fiber. Lesser degrees of paralysis are sometimes spoken of as *paresis,* but in everyday medical parlance motor paralysis usually stands for either partial or complete loss of function. The word *plegia* comes from the Greek word meaning stroke; and the word *palsy,* from an old French word, has the same meaning as paralysis. All these words are used interchangeably in medical practice, though it is preferable to use paresis for slight and paralysis or plegia for severe loss of motor function.

PARALYSIS DUE TO DISEASE OF THE LOWER MOTOR NEURONS Some of the essential facts concerning the anatomy and physiology of this system of motor nerve cells are well known. A few of them deserve brief comment because they explain important clinical phenomena.

Each motor nerve cell, through the extensive arborization of the terminal part of its fiber, comes into contact with 100 to 200 or more muscle fibers; altogether they constitute "the motor unit." All the variations in force, range, and type of movement are determined by differences in the number and size of motor units called into activity and the frequency of their action. Feeble movements involve only a few small motor units; powerful movements recruit many more units of increasing size. Motor units involved in slow, tonic contractions (type I) have muscle fibers rich in oxidative enzymes and more mitochondria, and those involved in fast, phasic contractions (type II), more phosphorylase, histochemical methods show. When a motor neuron becomes diseased, as in progressive muscular atrophy, it may manifest increased irritability, and all the muscle fibers that it controls may discharge sporadically, in isolation from other units. The result of the contraction of one or several such units is a visible twitch, or *fasciculation,* which can be seen and recorded in the electromyogram as a large diphasic or multiphasic action potential. If the motor neuron is destroyed, all the muscle fibers to which it is attached undergo a profound atrophy, namely, denervation atrophy. For some unknown reason the individual denervated muscle fibers now begin to be hypersensitive and to contract spontaneously, though they can no longer do so in response to a nerve impulse as a part of a motor unit. This isolated activity of individual muscle fibers is called *fibrillation* and is so fine that it cannot be seen through the intact skin but can be recorded only as a repetitive short-duration spike potential in the electromyogram (Chap. 344).

The motor nerve fibers of each ventral root intermingle as the roots join to form plexuses, and although the innervation of the muscles is roughly metameric, or according to segments of the spinal cord, each large muscle comes to be supplied by two or more roots. In contrast a single peripheral nerve usually provides the complete motor innervation of a muscle or group of muscles. For this reason the distribution of paralysis due to disease of the anterior horn cells or anterior roots differs from that which follows a lesion of a peripheral nerve.

All motor activity, even of the most elementary reflex type, requires the cooperation of several muscles. The analysis of a relatively simple movement, such as clenching the fist, affords some idea of the complexity of the underlying neural arrangements. In this act the primary movement is a contraction of the flexor muscles of the fingers, the flexor digitorum sublimis and profundus, the flexor pollicis longus and brevis, and the abductor pollicis brevis. In the terminology of Beevor, these muscles act as *agonists,* or *prime movers,* in this act. In order that flexion may be smooth and forceful the extensor muscles (antagonists) must provide a diminishing contraction, i.e., relax, at the same rate as the flexors contract. The muscles which flex the fingers also flex the wrist; and since it is desired that only the fingers flex, the muscles which extend the wrist must be brought into play to prevent its flexion. The action of the wrist extensors is *synergic,* and these muscles are called synergists in this particular act. Lastly the wrist, elbow, and shoulder must be stabilized by appropriate flexor and extensor muscles, which serve as *fixators.* The coordination of agonists, antagonists, synergists, and fixators involves reciprocal innervation and is managed entirely by segmental spinal reflexes under the guidance of proprioceptive sensory stimuli. Only the agonist movement in a voluntary act is believed to be initiated at a cortical level.

In addition there are many basic motor activities, such as the maintenance of certain postures, stepping movements and others, which do not involve reciprocal innervation. Agonists and antagonists contract simultaneously. The alternating movements of spinal stepping represent an even more basic type of coordination. In the support of the body in an upright posture, when the limb must be as rigid as a pillar, and in shivering the agonists and antagonists must act together. In general, the more delicate the movement, the more precise the coordination between agonist and antagonist muscles.

If all or practically all peripheral motor nerves supplying a muscle are destroyed, all voluntary, postural, and reflex movements are abolished. The muscle becomes soft and yields excessively to passive stretching, a condition known as *flaccidity.* Muscle tone—the slight resistance that normal relaxed muscle offers to passive movement—is reduced (hypotonia or atonia). The denervated muscles undergo extreme atrophy, usually being reduced to 20 or 30 percent of their original bulk within 3 months. The reaction of the muscle to sudden stretch, as by tapping its tendon, is lost. And, finally, it may be demonstrated that the muscle will no longer respond to electric stimuli of short duration, i.e., faradic stimuli, but still responds to currents of long duration, i.e., to galvanic stimuli. This alteration of electric response is known as *Erb's reaction of degeneration.* If only a part of the motor units in the muscles is affected, partial paralysis or paresis will ensue. The atrophy will be less, the tendon reflexes will be weakened instead of lost, and the reaction of degeneration may not be obtained. Quantitative testing by determination of strength-duration curves is a means of showing partial denervation, and electromyographic evidence of fibrillations and fasciculations may also be obtained.

The tonus of muscle and the tendon reflexes are known to depend on the muscle spindles and the afferent fibers to which they give origin and on the small anterior horn cells whose axons terminate on the small muscle fibers within the spindles. These small spinal motor neurons are called *gamma neurons*, in contrast to the large *alpha neurons*. Two different gamma neurons are now recognized, one, connected with nuclear bag spindle muscle fibers for phasic actions; the other, with nuclear chain spindle fibers for tonic actions. A tap on a tendon, by stretching the spindle muscle fibers, activates afferent neurons which transmit impulses to alpha motor neurons. The result is the familiar brief muscle contraction or tendon reflex. The spindle muscle fibers are then relaxed (unloaded), which terminates the reflex. Thus the setting of the spindle fibers and the state of excitability of the gamma neurons (normally inhibited by the corticospinal fibers and other supranuclear neurons) determine the level of activity of the tendon reflexes and the responsiveness of muscle to stretch. Other mechanisms of an inhibitory nature, involving Golgi tendon organs, are brought into play in more powerful stretching of muscle.

Lower motor neuron paralysis is the direct result of physiologic arrest or destruction of anterior horn cells or their axons in anterior roots and nerves. The signs and symptoms vary according to the location of the lesion. Probably the most important question for clinical purposes is whether sensory changes coexist. The combination of flaccid, areflexic paralysis and sensory changes usually indicates involvement of mixed motor and sensory nerves or affection of both anterior and posterior roots. If sensory changes are absent, the lesion must be situated in the gray matter of the spinal cord, in the anterior roots, in a purely motor branch of a peripheral nerve, or in motor axons alone. The distinction between nuclear (spinal) and anterior root (radicular) lesions may at times be impossible to make. Spasticity in muscles weakened by a spinal lesion points to the integrity of the segments below the level of the lesion.

PARALYSIS DUE TO DISEASE OF THE CORTICOSPINAL AND CORTICO-BRAINSTEM NEURONS

Several anatomic and physiologic facts concerning the upper motor neurons are worthy of note. It was formerly believed that the corticospinal tract originated from the large motor cell of Betz in the fifth layer of the precentral convolution. However, there are only about 25,000 to 30,000 Betz cells, whereas the corticospinal tract at the level of the medulla contains approximately 1 million axons. This tract must, therefore, contain many fibers that arise not from the giant Betz cells of the motor cortex (area 4 of Brodmann) but rather from the smaller Betz cells of area 4, the cells of the adjacent precentral cortex (area 6), as well as those of the secondary motor cortex in the superior frontal convolution and postcentral cortex (areas 1, 2, 3, 5, 7). The most critical degeneration studies of van Crevel, however, have shown that when areas 4, 6, 1, 2, 3, 5, and 7 are removed in the cat, if one waits several months, all will be found degenerated and none can be traced to other parts of the cerebral cortex. The corticospinal tract is the only long-fiber connection between the cerebrum and the spinal cord. At the level of the internal capsule these corticospinal fibers are intermingled with many others destined to end in the globus pallidus, substantia, nigra, red nucleus, and reticular substance and with others ascending from the thalamus. The fibers to the cranial nerve nuclei become separated at about the level of the midbrain and cross the midline to the contralateral cranial nerve nuclei (Fig. 17-1). These fibers form the corticomesencephalic, corticopontine, and corticobulbar tracts and, since they have functions similar to those of the corticospinal tract, may be included in the pyramidal system of motor neurons. The decussation of the corticospinal tract at the lower end of the medulla is variable in different persons. A small number of fibers, 10 to 20 percent, do not cross but descend ipsilaterally as the uncrossed corticospinal tract. Exceptionally, all of them cross; rarely, none. The termination of the corticospinal tract is in relation to nerve cells in the intermediate zone of gray matter, and not more than 10 to 15 percent establish direct synaptic connection with anterior horn cells. These facts, derived from degeneration studies, must of necessity modify current views of the anatomy of the corticospinal tract and suggest new interpretations.

The motor area of the cerebral cortex is difficult to define. It includes that part of the precentral convolution which contains Betz cells (area 4), but, as already mentioned, it probably extends anteriorly into area 6 and the

FIGURE 17-1
Diagram of the corticospinal and corticobulbar tracts. Lesion at A *produces ipsilateral oculomotor palsy and contralateral paralysis involving face, arm, and leg. Lesion at* B *causes ipsilateral facial paralysis of peripheral type and contralateral paralysis of arm and leg. Lesion at* b *results in ipsilateral facial weakness of upper motor neuron of central type and contralateral paralysis of arm and leg. (Courtesy of Bergmann and Staeheln:* Krankheiten des Nervensystems. *Berlin: Springer-Verlag, 1939.)*

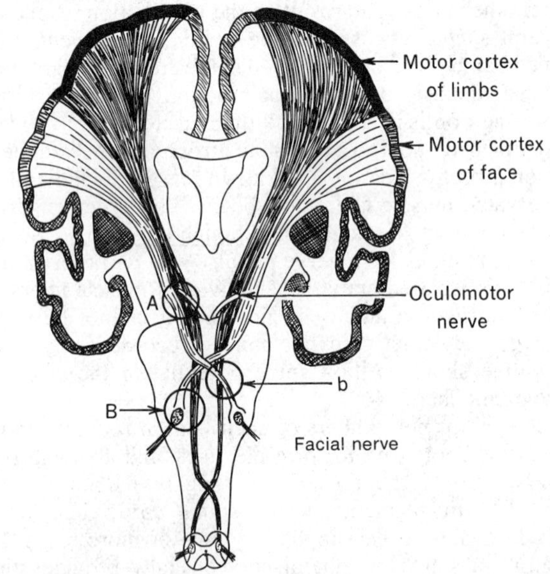

secondary motor area of the superior frontal convolution and posteriorly into the anterior parietal lobe, where it overlaps the sensory areas. Physiologically it is defined as the region of electrically excitable cortex from which isolated movements can be evoked by stimuli of minimal intensity. The muscle groups of the contralateral face, arm, trunk, and leg are represented in the motor cortex, those of the face being at the lower end of the precentral convolution and those of the leg in the paracentral lobule on the medial surface of the cerebral hemisphere. These motor points are not fixed but vary somewhat with the conditions of previous stimulation. The parts of the body capable of the most delicate movements have, in general, the largest cortical representation. Area 6, the premotor area, and the secondary motor area are also electrically excitable but require more intense stimuli to evoke movements, and the movements produced are more complex than those evoked from area 4. Very strong stimuli elicit movements from a wide area of premotor frontal and parietal cortex, and the same movements may be obtained from several points. From this it may be assumed that one of the functions of the motor cortex is to synthesize simple movements into an infinite variety of finely graded, highly differentiated patterns.

Corticospinal motor neuron paralysis may be due to lesions in the cerebral cortex, subcortical white matter, internal capsule, brainstem, or spinal cord. Usually much more is involved than the corticospinal, or pyramidal, tract; hence the term pyramidal paralysis is a misnomer. The distribution of the paralysis varies with the locale of the lesion, but there are also other typical features. Paralysis due to a lesion of these supranuclear motor neurons always involves a group of muscles, never individual muscles, and if any movement is possible, the proper relationships between antagonists, synergists, and fixators, are always preserved. The paralysis never involves all the muscles on one side of the body, even in the hemiplegia resulting from a complete lesion of the internal capsule. Movements that are invariably bilateral, such as those of the eyes, jaw, pharynx, larynx, neck, thorax, and abdomen, are little if at all affected. The hand and arm muscles suffer most severely, the leg muscles next, and of the cranial musculature only the muscles of the lower part of the face and tongue are involved to any significant degree. Broadbent was the first to call attention to this distribution of paralysis, and this predilection of certain muscles to paralysis with pyramidal disease is referred to as *Broadbent's law.* Corticospinal motor paralysis is rarely complete for any long period of time; in this respect it differs from the total and absolute paralysis due to a complete destruction or interruption of anterior horn cells and their axons. The paralyzed arm may suddenly move during yawning and stretching, and various spinal reflexes can be elicited at all times.

Acute disorders of the corticospinal motor system, at lower levels such as the cervical cord, may not only cause a paralysis of voluntary movement but may also abolish temporarily the spinal reflexes subserved by segments below the lesion. This condition is known as *spinal shock.* After a few days to weeks it disappears and gives way to a phenomenon known as *spasticity.* The latter is a feature of all acute and chronic lesions of the pyramidal system at cerebral, capsular, midbrain, and pontine levels. In cerebral and brainstem levels it does not usually appear immediately, and in exceptional cases the paralyzed limbs remain flaccid but with reflexes. Spasticity is related to the excessive activity of the released or disinhibited spinal motor neurons. The tendon reflexes are hyperactive, and clonus may appear. The posture of the arm and leg inform us that certain spinal neurons are more active than others. The arm, for example, is maintained in a pronated, flexed position and the leg in an adducted, extended position. Any attempts to extend the arm or flex the leg passively will encounter, after a brief free interval, a resistance which quickly yields (clasp-knife phenomenon). When the limb is left in the new position, the resistance reappears (lengthening and shortening reactions). The nocifensive spinal flexion reflexes, of which Babinski's sign is a part, are also released and the cutaneomuscular abdominal and cremasteric reflexes abolished. The flexion reflexes are not an essential component of spasticity. In the hemiplegic patient they are less prominent than in the spinal paraplegic or quadriplegic patient. With cerebral lesions exaggerated stretch and cutaneous cranial reflexes can also be elicited in cranial as well as limb and trunk muscles, and when the corticospinal disorder is bilateral there is pseudobulbar (dysarthria, dysphonia, and dysphagia and bifacial paralysis). Flexor and extensor spasms may occur with lesions of the spinal cord but not the cerebrum.

Spasticity may be present when the limbs are not paralyzed but only paretic, and it then produces interesting effects on voluntary movements. Attempts by the patient to move the hemiplegic limbs voluntarily may result in a variety of associated movements. Flexion of the arms results in involuntary pronation; flexion of the leg

TABLE 17-1
Differences between paralysis of corticospinal and lower motor neurons

Upper, corticospinal motor paralysis	*Lower, spinomuscular, or nuclear-infranuclear paralysis*
Muscle groups affected diffusely, never individual muscles	Individual muscles may be affected
Atrophy slight and due to disuse	Atrophy pronounced, 70 to 80 percent of total bulk
Spasticity with hyperactivity of the tendon reflexes	Flaccidity and hypotonia of affected muscles with loss of tendon reflexes
Extensor plantar reflex, Babinski's sign	Plantar reflex, if present, is of normal flexor type
Fascicular twitches not produced	Fascicular twitches may be present
Normal reactions to galvanic and faradic current	Loss of faradic reaction, retention of galvanic action (reaction of degeneration)

causes the foot to dorsiflex and evert automatically (Strümpell's tibialis sign). When asked to rotate one arm, the quadriparetic patient makes the same movement in the other (mirror movement). Flexion of one leg is associated with involuntary extension of the other.

Table 17-1 shows the main difference between corticospinal and lower motor neuron syndromes.

APRAXIC OR NONPARALYTIC DISORDERS OF MOTOR FUNCTION Aside from upper and lower motor neuron paralysis with cerebral lesions, there may be loss of purposive movement without paralysis. This is called *apraxia* and may be explained as follows. Many simple actions are acquired by learning or practice. These depend on the formation of movement patterns, particularly those which involve manufacture, i.e., the use of tools and instruments as well as gestures. Once established, they are remembered and may be reproduced under the proper circumstances. Any purposive act may be conceived as occurring in several stages. First, the idea of an act must be aroused in the mind of the subject by an appropriate stimulus situation, perhaps by a spoken command to do something. This idea, or concept, is then translated into action by excitation of patterns of premotor or motor cortical neurons in proper sequence, which are transmitted to lower centers by the corticospinal tracts. These initiate particular movements of individual muscle groups but also modify or suppress the subcortical mechanisms that control the basic attitudes and postures of the body. In right-handed and most left-handed persons the neural mechanisms for the formulation of an idea of an act (motor schema or image) in response to a spoken command or a verbal stimulus and its reproduction are believed to be centered in the posterior and inferior parts of the left parietal lobe; these areas, near the language mechanism, are connected with the left premotor regions for the control of the right hand and thence with the motor areas of the right cerebral hemisphere through the corpus callosum for the control of the left side.

A failure to execute certain acts in the correct context while retaining the ability to carry out the individual movements upon which such acts depend is the main feature of *apraxia.* The most adequate clinical test of motor deficits of this type is to observe a series of self-initiated actions such as using a comb, a razor, a toothbrush, or a common tool, or gesturing, e.g., waving goodbye, saluting, shaking the fist as though angry, or blowing a kiss. These actions may be called forth by a command or a request to imitate the examiner. Of course, failure to follow a spoken or written request may be due to an aphasia that prevents understanding of what is asked, or an agnosia may prevent recognition of the tool or object to be used. But when these difficulties are excluded, there remains a peculiar motor deficit in which the patient appears to understand but has lost his memory of how to perform a given act, especially if it is called for in an unnatural setting. He may have the idea of what he wants to do or what others command him to do, but he cannot translate the idea of the sequence of movements into a precise well-executed act. This is sometimes called *ideomotor apraxia.* The failure is evident both after spoken command and in requests to imitate the gestures of the examiner. Sometimes these two conditions may be dissociated; the patient, while not aphasic, cannot execute a spoken command but can still imitate the act if it is called forth by gesture. Also if merely given the tool he may use it properly in an automatic fashion.

Apraxia may be limited to one group of muscles, such as tongue or lips, as in Broca's aphasia (Chap. 25), or the loss of commanded actions of the left arm and leg (sympathetic apraxia).

If this motor deficit can be singled out, it reflects a specific loss of certain learned patterns of movement (a "specific amnesia," so to speak, analogous to the amnesia of words in aphasia). The added element of mental confusion tends often to obscure the disorder.

A kind of ideational apraxia, hard to demonstrate, is most often manifest in diffuse or bilateral cerebral lesions; whereas ideomotor apraxis means major hemisphere parietal disease, and the effect is bilateral; left-sided ideomotor apraxia with right hemiplegia indicates a lesion in the corpus callosum and adjacent white matter of one or other hemisphere; motor (kinetic) apraxia signifies a lesion in the premotor cortex opposite the affected hand (see Chap. 27 for further discussion of disconnection syndromes).

DIFFERENTIAL DIAGNOSIS OF PARALYSIS The diagnostic consideration of paralysis may be simplified by the following subdivisions, which relate to the location and distribution of weakness.

1 *Monoplegia* refers to weakness or paralysis of all the muscles in one limb, whether leg or arm. It should not be applied to paralysis of isolated muscles or groups of muscles supplied by a single nerve or motor root.
2 *Hemiplegia* is the commonest distribution of paralysis —loss of strength in arm, leg, and sometimes face on one side of the body.
3 *Paraplegia* indicates weakness or paralysis of both legs. It is most commonly found in spinal cord disease.
4 *Quadriplegia* indicates weakness of all four extremities. It may result from lesions involving peripheral nerves, gray matter of the spinal cord, or corticospinal tracts bilaterally in the cervical cord, upper brainstem, or cerebrum. *Diplegia* is a special form of quadriplegia in which the legs are affected more than the arms.
5 *Isolated paralyses* refer to weakness localized to one or more muscle groups

Monoplegia The physical examination of patients who complain of weakness of one extremity often discloses an unnoticed weakness in another limb, and the condition is actually hemiplegia or paraplegia. Or instead of weakness of all the muscles in a limb, only isolated groups are found to be affected. Ataxia, sensory disturbances, or pain in an extremity will often be interpreted by the patient as weakness, as will the mechanical limitation resulting from arthritis or the rigidity of parkinsonism.

In general, the presence or absence of atrophy of muscles in a monoplegic limb can be of diagnostic help.

PARALYSIS WITHOUT MUSCULAR ATROPHY Long-continued disuse of a limb may lead to atrophy, but this is usually not so marked as in diseases that denervate muscles; the tendon reflexes are normal, and the response of the muscles to electric stimulation and the electromyogram are unaltered.

The most frequent cause of monoplegia without muscular wasting is a lesion of the cerebral cortex. Only occasionally does it occur in diseases which interrupt the cortiocospinal tract at the level of the internal capsule, brainstem, or spinal cord. A vascular lesion (thrombosis or embolus) is the commonest, and of course, a tumor or abscess may have the same effect. Multiple sclerosis and spinal cord tumor, early in their course, may cause weakness of one extremity, usually the leg. Weakness due to damage to the corticospinal system is usually accompanied by spasticity, increased reflexes, and an extensor plantar reflex (Babinski's sign), and the electric reactions and electromyogram are normal. However, acute diseases that destroy the motor tracts in the spinal cord may at first (for several days) reduce the tendon reflexes and cause hypotonia (*spinal shock*). This does not occur in partial or slowly evolving lesions and occurs only to minimal degree in lesions of brainstem and cerebrum. In acute diseases affecting the lower motor neurons the tendon reflexes are always reduced or abolished, but atrophy may not appear for several weeks. Hence one must take into account the mode of onset and the duration of the disease in evaluating the tendon reflexes, muscle tone, and degree of atrophy before reaching an anatomic diagnosis.

PARALYSIS WITH MUSCULAR ATROPHY This is more frequent than paralysis without muscular atrophy. In addition to the paralysis and reduced or abolished tendon reflexes, there may be visible fasciculations. If completely paralyzed, the muscles exhibit an electric reaction of degeneration, and the electromyogram shows reduced numbers of motor units (often of large size), fasciculations at rest, and fibrillations. The lesion may be in the spinal cord, spinal roots, or peripheral nerves. Its location can usually be decided by the distribution of the palsied muscles (whether the pattern is one of nerve, spinal root, or spinal cord involvement), by the associated neurologic symptoms and signs, and by special tests (cerebrospinal fluid examination, roentgenogram of spine, and myelogram).

Brachial atrophic monoplegia is relatively rare, and when present, it should suggest in an infant a brachial plexus trauma, in a child poliomyelitis, in an adult poliomyelitis, syringomyelia, amyotrophic lateral sclerosis, or brachial plexus lesions. Crural monoplegia is more frequent and may be caused by any lesion of thoracic or lumbar cord, i.e., trauma, tumor, myelitis, multiple sclerosis, etc. Multiple sclerosis almost never causes atrophy, and ruptured intervertebral disk and the many varieties of neuritis rarely paralyze all or most of the muscles of a limb. Muscle dystrophy may begin in one limb, but by the time the patient is seen the typical more or less symmetric pattern of proximal limb and trunk involvement is evident. A unilateral retroperitoneal tumor may paralyze the leg by implicating the lumbosacral plexus.

Hemiplegia This is the most frequent distribution of paralysis in man. With rare exceptions (a few unusual cases of poliomyelitis or motor system disease) this pattern of paralysis is due to involvement of the corticospinal tract.

LOCATION OF LESION PRODUCING HEMIPLEGIA The site or level of the lesion, i.e., cerebral, capsular, brainstem, or spinal cord, can usually be deduced from the associated neurologic findings. Diseases localized in the cerebral cortex, cerebral white matter (corona radiata), and internal capsule usually evoke weakness or paralysis of the face, arm, and leg on the opposite side. The occurrence of convulsive seizures or the presence of a defect in speech (aphasia), a cortical type of sensory loss (astereognosis, loss of two-point discrimination, etc.), anosognosia, or defects in the visual fields suggest a cortical or subcortical location.

Damage to the corticospinal and cortico-brainstem tracts in the upper portion of the brainstem (see Fig. 17-1) may cause paralysis of the face, arm, and leg on the opposite side. The lesion in such cases is localized by the presence of a paralysis of the muscles supplied by the oculomotor nerve on the same side as the lesion (Weber's syndrome) or other neurologic findings. With low pontine lesions a unilateral abducens or facial palsy is combined with a contralateral weakness or paralysis of the arm and leg (Millard-Gubler syndrome). Lesions of the lowermost part of the brainstem, i.e., in the medulla, affect the tongue and sometimes the pharynx and larynx on one side and arm and leg on the other side. These "crossed paralyses," so common in brainstem diseases, are described in Chap. 324.

Rarely, a homolateral hemiplegia may be caused by a lesion in the lateral column of the cervical spinal cord. At this level, however, the pathologic process often induces bilateral signs, with resulting quadriparesis or quadriplegia. Homolateral paralysis if combined with a loss of vibratory and position sense on the same side and a contralateral loss of pain and temperature (Brown-Séquard syndrome) signifies disease of the spinal cord on one side.

Muscle atrophy of minor degree often follows lesions of the corticospinal system but never reaches the proportions seen in diseases of the lower motor neurons. The atrophy is due to disuse. When the motor cortex and adjacent parts of the parietal lobe are damaged in infancy or childhood, the normal development of the muscles and the skeletal system in the affected limbs is retarded. The palsied limbs and even the trunk on one side are small. This does not occur if the paralysis begins after the greater part of skeletal growth is attained (after puberty). In the hemiplegia due to spinal cord injury muscles at the level of the lesion atrophy as a result of damage to anterior horn cells or ventral roots.

CAUSES OF HEMIPLEGIA In this condition vascular diseases of the cerebrum and brainstem exceed all others in frequency. Trauma (brain contusion, epidural and subdural hemorrhage) ranks second, and other diseases such as brain tumor, brain abscess and encephalitis, demyelinative diseases, complications of meningitis, tuberculosis, and syphilis are of decreasing order of importance.

Most of these diseases can be diagnosed by the mode of evolution and the conjoined clinical and laboratory data presented in the chapters on neurologic diseases. For further discussion see Chap. 326.

Paraplegia Paralysis of both lower extremities may occur in diseases of the spinal cord and the spinal roots or of the peripheral nerves. If onset is acute, it may be difficult to distinguish spinal from neural paralysis, for in any acute myelopathy spinal shock may result in abolition of reflexes and flaccidity. As a rule in acute spinal cord diseases with involvement of corticospinal tracts, the paralysis affects all muscles below a given level; and often, if the white matter is extensively damaged, sensory loss below a particular level (loss of pain and temperature sense with lateral spinothalamic tracts and loss of vibratory and position sense with posterior columns) is conjoined. Also, in bilateral disease of the spinal cord, the bladder and bowel sphincters are paralyzed. Alterations of cerebrospinal fluid (dynamic block, increase in protein or cells) are frequent. In peripheral nerve diseases both sensory and motor loss tend to involve the distal muscles of the legs more than the proximal ones (an exception is acute idiopathic polyneuritis), and the sphincters are often spared or only briefly deranged in function. Sensory loss, if present, is more likely to consist in distal impairment of touch, vibration, and position sense, with pain and temperature sense spared in many instances. The cerebrospinal fluid protein level may be normal or elevated.

For clinical purposes it is helpful to consider separately the acute and the chronic paraplegias and to divide the chronic ones into two groups, those which occur in infancy and those which begin in adult life.

Acute paraplegia, beginning at any age, is relatively infrequent. Fracture dislocation of the spine with traumatic necrosis of the spinal cord, spontaneous hematomyelia with bleeding from a vascular malformation (angioma, telangiectasis), thrombosis of a spinal artery with infarction (myelomalacia), and dissecting aortic aneurysm or atherosclerotic occlusion of nutrient spinal arteries arising from the aorta with resulting infarction (myelomalacia) are the commonest varieties of sudden paraplegia (or quadriplegia, if the cervical cord is involved). Postinfectious or postvaccinal myelitis, acute demyelinative myelitis (Devic's disease if the optic nerves are affected), necrotizing myelitis, and epidural abscess or tumor with spinal cord compression tend to develop somewhat more slowly, over a period of hours or days, or they may have a subacute onset. Poliomyelitis and acute idiopathic polyneuritis, the former a purely motor disorder with meningitis, the latter predominantly motor but often with minimal sensory disturbances (paresthesias or objectively demonstrated impairment), must be distinguished from the other acute myelopathies and from each other.

In pediatric practice, delay in starting to walk and difficulty in walking are common problems. These conditions may be associated with a systemic disease such as rickets or may indicate mental deficiency or, more commonly, some muscular or neurologic disease. Congenital cerebral disease accounts for a majority of cases of infantile diplegia (weakness predominant in the legs, with the arms minimally affected). Present at birth or manifest in the first months of life, it may appear to progress; but actually it is stationary and only becomes apparent as the motor system develops. Later there may seem to be slow improvement as a result of the normal maturation processes of childhood. Congenital malformation of the spinal cord or birth injury of the spinal cord are other possibilities. Friedreich's ataxia and familial paraplegia, progressive muscular dystrophy, and the chronic varieties of polyneuritis tend to appear later during childhood and adolescence and are slowly progressive.

In adult life multiple sclerosis, subacute combined degeneration, spinal cord tumor, ruptured cervical disk and cervical spondylosis, syphilitic meningomyelitis, chronic epidural infections (fungous and other granulomatous diseases), Erb's spastic paraplegia and motor system disease, and syringomyelia represent the most frequently encountered forms of spinal paraplegia. (See Chap. 325 for discussion of these spinal cord diseases.) The several varieties of polyneuritis and polymyositis must be considered in their differential diagnosis, for they, too, may cause paraparesis.

Quadriplegia All that has been written about the common causes of paraplegia applies to quadriplegia. The lesion is usually in the cervical rather than the thoracic or lumbar segments of the spinal cord. If it is situated in the low cervical segments and involves the anterior half of the spinal cord, as in occlusion of the anterior spinal artery, the arm paralysis may be flaccid and areflexic and the leg paralysis spastic (anterior spinal syndrome). There are only a few points of difference between the common paraplegic and quadriplegic syndromes. In infants, aside from developmental abnormalities and anoxia of birth, an inherited cerebral disease (Schilder's disease, metachromatic leukoencephalopathy, lipid storage disease) may be responsible for a quadriparesis or quadriplegia. Congenital forms of muscular dystrophy may be recognized soon after birth and also infantile muscular atrophy (Hoffmann-Werdnig disease).

In adults repeated cerebral vascular accidents may lead to bilateral hemiplegia, usually accompanied by pseudobulbar palsy.

Isolated paralysis Paralysis of isolated muscle groups usually indicates a lesion of one or more peripheral nerves. The diagnosis of a lesion of an individual peripheral nerve is made on the presence of weakness or paralysis of the muscle or group of muscles and impairment or loss of sensation in the distribution of the nerve in question. Complete transection or severe injury to a peripheral nerve is usually followed by atrophy of the muscles it innervates and by loss of their tendon reflexes. Trophic changes in the skin, nails, and subcutaneous tissue may also occur.

Knowledge of the muscular and sensory function of each individual nerve is needed for a satisfactory diagnosis. Since lesions of the peripheral nerves are relatively uncommon in civil life, it is not practical for the general physician to keep all these facts in his memory, and a textbook of anatomy or Chap. 323 of this text should be consulted. It is, however, of considerable importance to decide whether the lesion is a temporary one of conduction only (neuropraxia) or whether there has been a pathologic dissolution of continuity, requiring nerve regeneration for recovery. Electromyography may be of value here.

EXAMINATION SCHEME FOR MOTOR PARALYSIS AND APRAXIA The first step is to inspect the paralyzed limb, taking note first of its posture and of the presence or absence of muscle atrophy, hypertrophy, and fascicular twitchings. The patient is then called upon to move each muscle group, and the power and facility of movement are graded and recorded. The range of passive movement is then determined by moving all the joints. This provides information concerning alterations of muscle tone, i.e., hypotonia, spasticity, and rigidity. Dislocations, disease joints, and ankyloses may also be revealed by these same maneuvers. Muscle bulk is then inspected. Slight atrophy may be due to disuse from any cause, i.e., pain, fixation as the result of a cast, or any type of paralysis. Pronounced atrophy usually occurs only with denervation of several weeks' or months' standing.

The tendon reflexes are then tested. The usual routine is to try to elicit the jaw jerk (increased in pseudobulbar palsy) and the supinator, biceps, triceps, quadriceps, and Achilles tendon reflexes. Two cutaneous reflexes are then tested, the abdominal and plantar reflexes.

If there is no evidence of upper or lower motor neuron disease, but certain acts are nonetheless imperfectly performed, one should look for a disorder of postural sensibility or of cerebellar coordination or rigidity with abnormality of posture and movement due to disease of the basal ganglions (Chap. 18). In the absence of these disorders, the possibility of an apraxic disorder may be investigated by watching the patient's own movements and those called forth by specific command and gesture.

Hysterical paralysis may pose problems. Usually it is easily distinguished from chronic lower motor neuron disease by absence of areflexia and severe atrophy. Diagnostic difficulty arises only in certain acute cases of upper motor neuron disease that lack all the usual changes in reflexes and muscle tone. In hysterical paralysis one arm or one leg or all one side of the body may be affected. The hysterical gait is sometimes diagnostic (Chap. 19). Often there is loss of sensation in the paralyzed parts and sometimes loss of sight in the eye, of hearing in the ear, and of smell in the nostril on the paralyzed side, a group of sensory changes that is never seen in organic brain disease. The patient should be asked to move the affected limbs; as he does so, the movement is seen to be slow and jerky, often with contraction of both agonist and antagonist muscles simultaneously or intermittently. Hoover's sign and Babinski's combined leg flexion test are helpful in distinguishing hysterical from organic hemiplegia. To elicit Hoover's sign, the patient, lying on his back, is asked to raise one leg from the bed against resistance; in a normal individual the back of the heel of the contralateral leg is pressed firmly down, and the same is true when the patient with organic hemiplegia attempts to lift the paralyzed leg. The hysteric exerts little force with the good leg or will contract it more strongly under these circumstances than as a primary willed action. To carry out Babinski's combined leg flexion test, a patient with an organic hemiplegia is asked to sit up without using his arms; when he does so, the paralyzed or weak leg flexes at the hip, and the heel is lifted from the bed while the heel of the sound leg is pressed into the bed. This sign is absent in hysterical hemiplegia.

MUSCULAR PARALYSIS AND SPASM UNATTENDED BY VISIBLE CHANGE IN NERVE OR MUSCLE A discussion of motor paralysis would not be complete without some reference to a group of diseases that appear to have no basis in visible structural change in motor nerve cells, nerve fibers, motor end-plates, and muscular fibers. This group is comprised of myasthenia gravis, myotonia congenita (Thomsen's disease), familial periodic paralysis, disorders of potassium, sodium, calcium, and magnesium metabolism, tetany, tetanus, botulinus poisoning, black widow spider bite, and the thyroid myopathies. In these diseases, each of which possesses a fairly distinctive clinical picture, the abnormality is purely biochemical, and even if the patient survives for a long time, no visible microscopic changes develop. An understanding of these diseases requires knowledge of the processes involved in nerve and muscle excitation and in the contraction of muscle. They will be discussed in Chaps. 347 and 348.

REFERENCE

BRODAL A: *Neurological Anatomy in Relation to Clinical Medicine,* New York: Oxford, 1969

18
TREMOR, CHOREA, ATHETOSIS, ATAXIA, AND OTHER ABNORMALITIES OF MOVEMENT AND POSTURE

RAYMOND D. ADAMS

In this chapter are discussed the automatic, static, and less modifiable postural activities of the human nervous system. These are believed, on good evidence, to be an expression of the function of the *older motor system,* meaning, according to S. A. K. Wilson, who introduced this term, the motor structures in the basal ganglions and brainstem.

In health, the activities of the motor systems of basal ganglions and cerebellum are blended and modulate the corticospinal and cortico-brainstem-spinal systems. The static postural activities of the former are indispensable to the voluntary or willed movements of the latter.

This close association of the corticospinal (formerly pyramidal) and extrapyramidal systems is shown by human disease. Lesions of the corticospinal tracts result not only in paralysis of volitional movements of the contralateral half of the body but in the appearance of a fixed posture or attitude in which the arm is maintained in flexion and the leg in extension (predilection type of Wernicke-Mann or hemiplegic dystonia of Denny-Brown). Similarly, decerebration from a lesion in the upper pons or midbrain releases another posture in which all four extremities are extended and the cervical and thoracolumbar spine dorsiflexed. In these released action patterns one has evidence of extrapyramidal postural and righting reflexes which are mediated through bulbospinal and other brainstem-spinal systems.

The student may be dismayed to read in current articles trenchant criticism of the validity of the concept of the corticospinal tract and the division of the motor system into corticospinal and extrapyramidal. Extremists claim the corticospinal tract may be severed in animals and even in man without lasting motor deficits. But it must be remembered that this tract is so puny in most mammals, even in small monkeys, that it can hardly be compared to that of man, and there has yet to be a pathologically proved example in man of complete interruption of this tract with preserved voluntary motor function.

If an oversimplification may be permitted for clarity of exposition, the extrapyramidal motor system may be subdivided into two parts: (1) the striatopallidonigral and (2) the cerebellar. Disease in either of these parts will result in disturbances of movement and posture without significant paralysis. These two major systems and the symptoms that result when they are diseased are reviewed on the following pages.

THE BASAL GANGLIONS: PHARMACOLOGY AND PATHOLOGIC ANATOMY

As an anatomic entity the basal ganglions have no precise definition. The list of basal structures originally thought to have some part in motor function, such as the caudate and lenticular nuclei, has been greatly expanded by physiologists to include the field of Forel and zona incerta, subthalamic nucleus of Luys, substantia nigra, red nucleus, dentate nucleus of cerebellum, and the reticular formation of the brainstem. The anatomic connections between these structures and other parts of the brain, such as the cerebral cortex and afferent sensory systems, are too intricate to present in a textbook of medicine (cf. Brodal's monograph on neurologic anatomy).

The principal new anatomic datum to emerge in recent years is the central physiologic role of the ventrolateral (and anterior) nucleus of the thalamus. It is a vital link in an ascending fiber system from the lenticular nucleus and cerebellum to the motor cortex. Indeed it would seem that most of the basal ganglionic and cerebellar influence on the motor system is funneled through the ventral plane of thalamic nuclei, thus effecting a number of corticocortical circuits. Descending pathways to the spinal cord are disputed; probably there are polysynaptic descending fibers through the reticular formation of the pons and medulla to the motor neurons of the spinal cord. It is noteworthy that these ascending thalamocortical fibers pass through the internal capsule and cerebral white matter; hence lesions in these parts may simultaneously affect both corticospinal and extrapyramidal systems.

Another exciting development has been the discovery that certain drugs such as the phenothiazines produce extrapyramidal syndromes (Parkinson's disease, athetosis, dystonia, etc.); this has led to a major advance in the chemistry of central neurotransmitters. In man it has been found that the substantia nigra, putamen, and caudatum are rich in dopamine, serotonin, and norepinephrine. Of these substances dopamine has excited the greatest attention; the following steps in the metabolic pathway have been revealed:

L-Tyrosine

↓ *tyrosine hydroxylase + pteridine (cofactor)*

L-Dopa (3,4-hydroxyphenylalanine → → dopaquinone indolquinone → melanin)

↓ *decarboxylase + vitamin B_6 (cofactor)*

L-Dopamine → homoprotocatechuric acid → homovanillic acid

↓ *dopamine beta-hydroxylase + vitamin C (cofactor)*

Norepinephrine

↓ *methyl transferase*

L-Epinephrine

Dopa is seen to be a step in the metabolism not only of norepinephrine but also of melanin. Norepinephrine is an important intercellular transmitter substance in the hypothalamus and peripheral autonomic system; melanin is contained in certain of the neurons of the substantia nigra and other pigmented nuclei of the brainstem. Dopamine has physiologic properties of its own; probably it, too, is a transmitter substance in the parts of the brain where it is concentrated.

The metabolic pathway of serotonin, or 5-hydroxytryptamine, is rather like that of the aforementioned catecholamines. It starts with L-tryptophan, which is converted into 5-hydroxytryptophan by tryptophan hydrolase (+ pteridine cofactor). The latter enzymatic step is rate-limiting in the formation of 5-hydroxytryptamine (serotonin). The latter reaction is catalyzed by the same decarboxylase which converts dopa to dopamine.

In Parkinson's disease the lenticular nuclei and globus pallidus have a reduced content of dopamine, serotonin, and norepinephrine, and the content of the major metabolite, homovanillic acid, is decreased in these parts and in the cerebrospinal fluid (CSF). A number of the tranquilizing medications, such as reserpine and chlorpromazine, deplete the basal ganglions of these substances. The quantity of L-dopa in the striatum and substantia nigra is also decreased, and the administration of this substance orally or intravenously replenishes the stores in the basal ganglions, with concomitant improvement in extrapyramidal symptoms. Further information concerning the biochemistry of catecholamine, serotonin, and norepinephrine may be found in the U.S. Department of Health, Education and Welfare monograph on Parkinson's disease (1968).

Some of the most significant facts about clinicopathologic relationships in man are to be found in the writings of a number of famous neurologists. In 1912 S. A. K. Wilson delineated the syndrome of familial lenticular degeneration, and at about the same time Van Woerkem observed a disturbance of basal ganglionic and cerebral function in acquired forms of liver disease. The putamen and globus pallidus were thought to be the main anatomic sites of both types of hepatocerebral degeneration. In 1920 Oskar and Cecile Vogt described a number of other motor disturbances associated with lesions limited to the striatum (putamen and caudatum). Lewy was one of the first to describe the pathology of paralysis agitans, and with the work of Tretiakoff (in postencephalitic forms) and Hassler (in paralysis agitans) at least some of the lesions were localized in the substantia nigra. The thorough studies of Huntington's chorea by Bielschowsky in 1919 related the choreoathetosis to lesions in the caudate nucleus and putamen. A long series of observations, the most recent ones being those of J. Purdon Martin, have related hemiballismus to lesions in the subthalamic nucleus of Luys.

Unfortunately, many of the classic cases leave much to be desired. In some instances the disease process was diffuse, and many other parts of the brain were affected, as in Wilson's hepatolenticular degeneration. Also, lack of quantitative neuropathologic methods hampered progress in the field. Even now the topography of the pathologic findings in several of these diseases (e.g., dystonia musculorum deformans) has not been fully determined.

Table 18-1 presents clinicopathologic correlations accepted by many neurologists; however, there is still much uncertainty as to finer details.

TABLE 18-1
Clinicopathologic correlations

Symptoms	*Principal location of morbid anatomy*
Unilateral plastic rigidity with static tremor (Parkinson's syndrome)	Contralateral substantia nigra plus (?) other structures
Unilateral hemiballismus and hemichorea	Contralateral subthalamic nucleus of Luys, prerubral area, and Forel's fields
Chronic chorea of Huntington's type	Caudate nucleus, putamen
Athetosis and dystonia	Contralateral putamen
Cerebellar ataxia, i.e., intention tremor; slowness in starting and stopping alternating voluntary movements; hypotonia; rebound phenomenon	Homolateral cerebellar hemisphere or middle and inferior cerebellar peduncles, superior brachium conjunctivum (ipsilateral if below the decussation, contralateral if above)
Decerebrate rigidity, i.e., opisthotonos, extension of arms and legs	Lesion usually bilateral in tegmentum, involving upper brainstem, particularly red nucleus or structures between red nucleus and vestibular nuclei
Palatal and facial myoclonus (rhythmic)	Lesion in the central tegmental tract, inferior olivary nucleus, and olivodentate connections
Diffuse myoclonus	Cerebellar cortex (?), thalami (?)

The symptoms that lend themselves best to clinical analysis are akinesia, rigidity, chorea, athetosis, dystonia, myoclonus, and tremor.

AKINESIA

When extrapyramidal disease is analyzed along classic neurologic lines into primary functional deficits and secondary release effects, akinesia stands as the principal negative or deficit symptom. By the term *akinesia* one refers to the disinclination of the patient to use an affected part of the body, to engage it freely in all the natural actions of the body. In contrast to paralysis, the negative symptom of corticospinal lesions, strength is undiminished in the part and it can be used effectively in the desired movement. In this respect, too, it is unlike apraxia, where movements are lost because of a lesion which erases the memory of the motor schema that forms a sequence of movements for intended action. The parkinsonian patient exhibits the phenomenon of akinesia most clearly in his extreme underactivity. He sits motionless for long times. In looking to the side he moves his eyes, not his head. In arising from a chair he fails to make all the little adjustments needed (putting feet back, putting hands on arms of chair, etc.). He neglects his affected arm. Yet he is not weak (paretic) or apraxic. Formerly, akinesia was attributed to rigidity, which could reasonably hamper all movements, but now that stereotaxic surgery has been shown to abolish both tremor and rigidity, it becomes clear that the motor deficit, or akinesia, is still there. Strictly interpreted it would appear that, apart from their contribution to the maintenance of postures, the basal ganglions must provide something essential to the performance of the large variety of semiautomatic actions that make up the full repertoire of natural human motility.

A point of interest is whether akinesia is an invariable manifestation of all extrapyramidal diseases, without which there could be no secondary release effects such as flexion dystonia, athetosis, chorea, and rigidity. The question has no clear answer. Though akinesia always seems to be present in Huntington's and Sydenham's chorea, double athetosis, and Parkinson's disease, one cannot be sure of the existence of either akinesia or paralysis in hemiballismus.

ALTERATIONS OF MUSCLE TONE (SPASTICITY, RIGIDITY, HYPOTONIA)

It has been pointed out that muscle tone (the small resistance to muscle stretch offered by healthy muscle) is enhanced in the many conditions that cause a paralysis of voluntary movement by interrupting the corticospinal tract. The special distribution of the increased tone (i.e., greater in antigravity muscles—leg extensors and arm flexors in man), the sudden augmentation of tone with gradual yielding upon quick movement (the lengthening reaction or clasp-knife phenomenon), the absence of resistance upon slow movement and its disappearance in relaxed muscle with "electromyographic silence," and exaggerated tendon reflexes are the identifying characteristics of spasticity. This type of hypertonus is believed to be due in some instances to hyperactivity of the small gamma motor neurons, resulting in increase in the sensitivity of the spindle muscle fibers to stretch; in other instances it seems clearly related to excessive activity (or disinhibition) of the larger alpha motor neurons. The "gamma spasticity" is abolished by procaine injection of the motor nerve, which paralyzes the small gamma motor and sensory fibers, leaving the larger ones intact, without weakening the willed contractions of the muscle; the "alpha spasticity" is not affected.

In the state known as *rigidity* the muscles are continuously or intermittently firm, tense, and prominent; and the resistance to passive movement is intense and even, like that noted in bending a lead pipe or in stretching a strand of toffee. Although rigidity is present in all muscle groups, both flexor and extensor, on the whole it tends to be more prominent in those which maintain a flexed posture, i.e., the flexor muscles of trunk and limbs. It appears to be somewhat greater in the large muscle groups, but this may be merely a question of muscle mass. Certainly the smaller muscles of the face and tongue and even those of the larynx are often affected. The tendon reflexes are not enhanced. Nevertheless, like "gamma spasticity," this rigidity is said to be abolished by procaine, and Foerster earlier demonstrated that it is eradicated by posterior root section. In the electromyographic tracing, motor unit activity is more continuous than in spasticity, persisting even after relaxation.

A special type of rigidity, first noted by Negro in 1901, is the *cogwheel phenomenon.* When the hypertonic muscle is passively stretched, the resistance may be rhythmically jerky, as though the resistance of the limb were controlled by a ratchet. A number of different explanations of this phenomenon have been suggested. Wilson postulated that it might be due to a minor form of the lenthening-shortening reaction, but a more likely explanation is an associated static tremor that is masked by rigidity during an attitude of repose but emerges faintly during manipulation.

Rigidity is prominent in extrapyramidal diseases such as paralysis agitans, postencephalitic Parkinson's syndrome, and dystonia musculorum deformans.

The *tension hypertonus of athetosis* differs from both spasticity and rigidity. Strictly speaking, it takes two forms, one which occurs during the involuntary athetotic movement, and another which appears in the absence of any involuntary motion. Clinically these forms of hypertonus are variable from one moment to the next and are paradoxic in that they sometimes disappear during a rapid passive movement or when the limb is passively shaken. The tendon reflexes may be normal or brisk. The lengthening and shortening reactions are absent. This form of variable hypertonus is found in double athetosis and choreoathetosis and in some cases of dystonia musculorum deformans. Usually in Sydenham's and Huntington's chorea a state of hypotonia prevails, sometimes as strikingly as in sensory polyneuropathies and lower motor neuron paralyses.

CHOREA Derived from the Greek word meaning "dance," chorea refers to widespread arrhythmic movements of a forcible, rapid, jerky type. These movements are involuntary and are noted for their irregularity, variability, relative speed, and brief duration. They may be simple or quite elaborate and of variable distribution. In some respects they resemble a voluntary movement in their complexity, yet they are never combined into a coordinated act. The patient may, however, incorporate them into a deliberate movement, as if to make them less noticeable. When superimposed on voluntary movements, they may take on a grotesque and exaggerated character. Grimacing and peculiar respiratory sounds may be other expressions of the movement disorder. Usually the movements are discrete, but if very numerous, they may flow into one another; the resultant picture then resembles athetosis. They may be limited to a limb or an arm and leg on one side (hemichorea), or they may involve all parts of the body. Normal volitional movements are, of course, possible, for there is no paralysis, but they too may be excessively quick and poorly sustained. The limbs are often unusually slack, or hypotonic. A choreic movement may be superimposed on a tendon reflex, giving rise to the "hung-up reflex." The tendon reflexes tend to be pendular because of the associated hypotonia; when the knee jerk is elicited with the patient sitting, the leg swings back and forth four or five times, like a pendulum, rather than one or two times as in a normal person.

Chorea appears in typical form in Sydenham's chorea and was noted also in the acute stages of epidemic encephalitis lethargica. It is a feature also of Huntington's chorea (chronic chorea), where the movements tend more typically to be choreoathetotic. Vascular lesions in the subthalamus, particularly those in and near the subthalamic nucleus of Luys, may result in wild flinging movements of the opposite arm and leg (hemiballismus). As these subside, they become almost indistinguishable from chorea. Phenothiazine drugs and, rarely, hyperthyroidism may cause chorea.

ATHETOSIS This term is from a Greek word meaning "unfixed" or "changeable." The condition is characterized by an inability to sustain the fingers and toes, tongue, or any other group of muscles in one position. The maintained posture is interrupted by continuous, slow, sinuous, purposeless movements. These are most pronounced in the digits and the hands but often involve the tongue, throat, and face. One can detect as basic patterns of movement an extension and pronation and flexion and supination of the arm, and alternating flexion and extension of the fingers. They may be unilateral, especially in children who have suffered a hemiplegia at some previous date (posthemiplegic athetosis). The movements are slower than those of chorea, but in many cases gradations between the two (choreoathetosis) are seen. Most athetotic patients exhibit variable degrees of motor deficit due in some instances to associated corticospinal tract disease. Discrete individual movements of the tongue, lips, and hand are often impossible, and attempts to perform such voluntary movements result in a contraction of all the muscles in the limb (an *intention spasm*). Variable degrees of rigidity are generally associated, and these may account for the slower quality of athetosis, in contrast to chorea. It must be admitted, however, that in some cases it is almost impossible to distinguish between chorea and athetosis.

Athetosis or choreoathetosis of all four limbs is a cardinal feature of a curious state known as *double athetosis*, which begins in childhood. Athetosis appearing in the first months of life usually represents a congenital or postnatal condition such as hypoxia, kernicterus, or birth injury. Postmortem examination in some of the cases has disclosed a peculiar pathologic change of probable hypoxic etiology, a status marmoratus in the striatum; in others there has been a loss of medullated fibers, a status dysmyelinisatus, in the same regions. In adults athetosis may occur as an episodic illness or persistently in acquired hepatocerebral degeneration, in postphenothiazine dyskinesias, and in certain degenerative diseases (see Chap. 18).

TORSION SPASM OR DYSTONIA Torsion spasm is closely allied to athetosis, differing only in that the larger axial muscles (those of the trunk and girdle) rather than appendicular muscles are involved. It results in bizarre, grotesque movements and positions of the body. The word *dystonia* has been given to these movements but, unfortunately, is also applied to any fixed posture which may be the end result of a disease of the motor system. Thus Denny-Brown speaks of hemiplegic dystonia, the flexion dystonia of parkinsonism, and extensor dystonia with retraction of the head and arching or twisting of the back. If the latter meaning is given, it would be better to speak of athetosis of the trunk as torsion spasms or phasic dystonia, in contrast to fixed dystonia. The former, like athetosis, may show remarkable fluctuations; sometimes the whole musculature of the body may be thrown into spasm by an effort to move an arm or to speak. If mild, the torsion spasm may be limited to the lumbar or cervical muscles or those of one limb and may cease when the body is at rest.

Torsion spasm may be seen in the condition of double athetosis after hypoxic damage to the brain, in kernicterus, and, rarely, in Wilson's hepatolenticular degeneration. It is most characteristic of the syndrome designated *dystonia musculorum deformans* but also occurs in other conditions such as the postphenothiazine dyskinesias and Hallevorden-Spatz disease (Chap. 333).

Chorea, athetosis, and torsion spasm are all closely related. The movements are elaborate and depend for their expression on cortical mechanisms. Paralytic lesions involving the corticospinal tract abolish the involuntary movements. The hypotonia in chorea and some cases of athetosis, the pendular reflexes, and some degree of interference with the natural movements are also reminiscent of the syndrome that follows disease of the cerebellum. Lacking, however, are intention tremor and true incoordination or ataxia.

MYOCLONUS This term refers to several different motor disorders, some localized, others diffuse. As in chorea, the myoclonic movement is involuntary and arrhythmic, but it is much faster than chorea, being concluded in a few hundred milliseconds. Variations in degree are noteworthy; it may consist of no more than a flick of a single muscle or part of a muscle, but the larger movements always betray its nature, involving as they do a group of muscles. Thus myoclonus may be distinguished from fasciculation. Sensory relationships are another prominent attribute. Flickering light, a series of loud sounds, or abrupt contact with some part of the body may regularly initiate a jerk, sometimes as a direct sensorimotor effect, again through the mechanism of startle. One special variety is evoked by willed movement, presumably through a proprioceptive mechanism. Hence, one may speak of action or intention myoclonus, auditory or visual myoclonus. A series of intense stimuli may recruit a series of myoclonic jerks into a full-blown seizure, as happens often in the familial myoclonic epilepsy syndrome of Unverricht-Lundborg. The pathologic disturbance in the latter is usually a lipid storage disease or an amyloid nerve cell inclusion (Chap. 333).

Familial types of myoclonus may persist in almost pure form or in association with mild ataxia over a period of many years. In the child and adult, herpes simplex encephalitis may present as a confusional state and dementia with myoclonus. In the elderly adult diffuse myoclonus and a rapidly evolving dementia are prominent symptoms in Creutzfeldt-Jakob disease. Intention myoclonus is often a sequela to anoxic encephalopathy. Postsomnolescent myoclonus jerks of arms for 20 to 30 min after a night's sleep are reported by some patients with idiopathic epilepsy. In all these diseases the pathologic changes are so widespread that anatomic localization is impossible. The least degrees of lesion causing myoclonus are seemingly located in the thalamus and cerebellum. Indeed cerebellar incoordination and intention tremor are combined with diffuse myoclonus of the action or intention type in several of the aforementioned diseases, i.e., lipidoses and the Lafora body type of myoclonus.

The term *myoclonus* unfortunately has also been assigned to a rather different motor phenomenon—that of repetitious, rhythmic clonus of some part of the "branchial cleft" or craniocervical musculature. An example is "nystagmus of the palate" (rhythmic contractions at the rate of 10 to 50 or more per minute of the soft palate, pharyngeal muscles, vocal cords, facial muscles, and diaphragm). The lesions producing this state, which we would prefer to designate as a form of continuous *bulbar, facial*, or *diaphragmatic clonus*, have been situated in all instances in the central tegmental tract, inferior olivary nucleus, or olivocerebellar tract. The causative lesions have been infarcts, tumors, and encephalitic processes.

The main fault with our concept of myoclonus is that it covers too many motor disorders. When movements are grouped according to their brevity or involuntary nature, one must include the normal dormescent start or jerk of a limb as one falls asleep, and the motor components of a natural startle reaction. The obligatory Moro response also falls within the group, as well as the form of epilepsy known as infantile or salaam spasms and the falling spells of the petit mal triad. Metrazol injections cause myoclonus of the limbs, which has been shown to depend on a lower brainstem (medullary reticular) mechanism. Another problem arises on the clinical side in distinguishing diffuse myoclonus from other abrupt involuntary movements such as tremors, chorea, and restricted forms of epilepsy (epilepsia partialis continua). Speed of movement, lack of rhythmicity, and relationships to sensory stimulation prove to be the most reliable identifying features of the larger group of myoclonic disorders. There is an advantage in trying to separate the arrhythmic diffuse from the rhythmic restricted form in that each stands as a diagnostic attribute of a whole category of nervous diseases.

TREMOR This consists of a more or less regular rhythmic oscillation of a part of the body around a fixed point. The rate varies from three to eight oscillations per second; in one person the rate is fairly constant in all affected parts, regardless of the size of the muscle or of the part of the body. Tremors usually involve the distal part of the limbs, the head, tongue, or jaw, and rarely the trunk.

There are many different types of tremor, and only a few are recognized as bearing any meaningful relationship to disease of the extrapyramidal motor system; but since tremors have not been discussed elsewhere, all the different types will be considered here.

Tremors may be classified in several ways. They may be subdivided according to their distribution, amplitude, regularity, and relationship to volitional movement. The tremors described in the following paragraphs should be familiar to every physician.

Static (parkinsonian) tremor. This is a coarse, rhythmic tremor, with an average rate of four to five beats per second, most often localized in one or both hands, and occasionally, in the jaw or tongue. Its most characteristic feature is that it occurs when the limb is in an attitude of repose, and willed movement at least temporarily suppresses it. If the tremulous limb is completely relaxed, the tremor usually disappears, but the average patient rarely achieves this state. In some cases the tremor is constant; in others it varies from time to time and with the progress of the disease extends from one group of muscles to another. In paralysis agitans the tremor tends to be rather gentle and more or less limited to the distal muscles, whereas in postencephalitic parkinsonism and hepatolenticular degeneration it often has a wider range and involves proximal muscles. In many cases there is a variable degree of rigidity of a plastic type. The tremor interferes with voluntary movements surprisingly little; it is not uncommon to see a patient who has been trembling violently raise a full glass of water to his lips and drain the contents without spilling a drop. The handwriting of these patients is often small and cramped (micrographia). The gait may be of a festinating type. It is the combination of static tremor, slowness of movement, rigidity, and flexed postures without true paralysis that constitutes Parkinson's syndrome (also called amyostatic syndrome).

The exact pathologic anatomy of static tremor is unknown. In paralysis agitans and postencephalitic Parkinson's syndrome, the visible lesions are predominantly in the substantia nigra. In hepatocerebral degeneration, where this syndrome is mixed with cerebellar ataxia, the lesions are more diffuse. A similar tremor, without rigidity, slowness of movement, flexed postures, or masked facies, is seen in senile persons. Unlike Parkinson's disease, it does not progress.

Action tremor This term refers to a tremor present when the limbs are actively maintained in a certain position, as when outstretched, and throughout voluntary movement. It may increase slightly as the action of the limbs becomes more precise, but it never approaches the degree of augmentation in fine movement seen in intention tremor. It is easily made to disappear when the limbs are relaxed. Probably some of the *action tremors* are but an exaggeration of normal or physiologic tremor, which ranges from six to eight per second, being slower in childhood and old age. More particularly, in adults the tremor is of small excursion, has a frequency of seven to eight per second, and is somewhat irregular. The tremor involves the outstretched hand, head, and, less often, the lips and tongue, and it interferes little with voluntary movements such as handwriting and speech. This type of tremor is seen in numerous medical, neurologic, and psychiatric diseases and is therefore more difficult to interpret than static tremor. When occurring as the only neurologic abnormality in several members of a family, it is known as *familial* or *hereditary tremor.* Familial tremor may begin in childhood, but usually comes on later and persists throughout adult life. Being worse when the patient is under observation, it becomes a source of embarrassment because it suggests to the onlooker that the patient is nervous. A curious fact about familial tremors is that one or two drinks of an alcoholic beverage may abolish them, and they may become worse after the effects of the alcohol have worn off. Similar tremors are seen in delirious states, such as delirium tremens, in chronic alcoholism as an isolated symptom ("the morning shakes"), and in general paresis. An action tremor, usually more rapid than the above, is also characteristic of hyperthyroidism and other toxic states, and a similar tremor is frequently observed in patients suffering intense anxiety. In fact it can be reproduced by injections of epinephrine. Severe action tremor may also accompany certain diseases of the basal ganglions, including parkinsonism. The fast-frequency action tremors are suppressed by beta-adrenergic blocking agents (propanolol, 40 mg t.i.d.).

Intention tremor The word *intention* is ambiguous in this context because the tremor itself is not intentional. The term means, instead, that the tremor requires for its full expression the performance of an exacting, precise, willed movement. The term *ataxic tremor* has been suggested because it is always combined with and adds to cerebellar ataxia. The tremor is absent when the limbs are inactive and during the first part of a voluntary movement, but as the action continues and greater precision of movement is demanded (e.g., in touching a target such as the patient's nose or the examiner's finger), a jerky, more or less rhythmic interruption of forward progression, with side-to-side oscillation, appears. It continues for a fraction of a second or so after the act is completed. The tremor may seriously interfere with the patient's performance of skilled acts. Sometimes the head is involved (titubation). This type of tremor invariably indicates disease of the cerebellum and of its connections. When the disease is very severe, every movement, even the lifting of a limb, results in a wide-ranging tremor of such violence as to throw the patient off balance. This latter state is occasionally seen in multiple sclerosis, Wilson's disease, and vascular and other lesions of the midbrain and subthalamus.

Hysterical tremor Hysterical tremors may simulate any of the aforementioned varieties and are difficult to diagnose. One notable feature is that they usually do not correspond to any of the better-known types of organic tremor. Most often they are restricted to a limb, and they are seldom as regular as the static tremors of paralysis agitans. If the affected limb is restrained by the examiner, the tremor may move to another part of the body. It persists during movement and at rest and is less subject to the modifying influences of posture and willed movement than organic tremors are. This manifestation of hysteria is exceedingly rare.

OTHER INVOLUNTARY MOVEMENTS There are other abnormalities of movement, about which only a few words can be said. They vary from simple irritative phenomena to complex psychologically related phenomena, such as compulsions.

Spasmodic torticollis This is an intermittent or continuous spasm of sternomastoid, trapezius, and other neck muscles, usually more pronounced on one side, with turning or tipping of the head. It is involuntary and cannot be inhibited and thereby differs from habit spasm or tic. This condition should be considered a form of dystonia. It is worse when the patient sits, stands, or walks, and usually contactual stimulation of the chin or of the back of the head partially alleviates the muscle imbalance. Psychiatric treatment is ineffectual. In severe cases muscle sectioning, neurectomy, or section of the anterior cervical roots has given favorable results.

Other craniocervical spasms Blepharoclonus (inability to keep the eyes open), lingual spasms, "spastic" dysphonia, facial spasms, and cervicothoracic spasms are all special varieties of involuntary movement, appearing usually in late middle life and the senium. Facial, cervical, and thoracic spasms have occurred with striking frequency during phenothiazine medication. Transiency, or nonprogressivity, unresponsiveness to psychotherapy, and uncertain amelioration by all pharmacologic agents characterize most of them. Exceptionally, these disorders are induced by drugs of the phenothiazine class (see Chap. 18) and persist after their discontinuance (tardive or postphenothiazine dyskinesias).

Tics and habit spasms Many persons throughout life are given to habitual movements, such as sniffing, clearing the throat, protruding the chin, or blinking, whenever they become tense. The patient admits that the movements are voluntary and that he feels compelled to make them in order to relieve tension; they can be inhibited for a time by an effort of will but reappear when attention is diverted. In certain cases they become so ingrained that the person is unaware of them and unable to control them. Children between five and ten years of age are especially likely to have habit spasms. The movements are often purposive coordinated acts which normally serve the organism; it is only their incessant repetition when uncalled for that constitutes a habit. Stereotypy is their main identifying feature. Multiple convulsive tics (*Gilles de la Tourette's disease*) constitute a more severe form of the same condition. In children it is best to ignore the habit spasm and at the same time to arrange for more rest and a calmer environment. In adults relief of nervous tension by tranquilizing drugs and psychotherapy is helpful, but the disposition to tic formation persists. Mentally backward children and adults often display, when idle, a wide variety of rhythmic body-rocking, head-bobbing, arm-and-finger movements. These are of the nature of mannerisms and have no known basal ganglion anatomy.

Writer's cramp and other so-called "occupational spasms" should be mentioned here if only to indicate their unclassifiable status. Usually a middle-aged man or woman begins to observe upon attempting to write that all the muscles of thumb and fingers either go into a spasm or are in some way inhibited. Usually it is the spasm that interferes, and it may be painful and spread into the forearm or even the shoulder. Sometimes the spasm fragments into a tremor which interferes with the execution of fluid, cursive movements. Although limited to writing, exceptionally it may involve other equally demanding motor acts. At all other times and in the execution of grosser movements the hand is normal. Psychogenesis has been claimed, but careful clinical analysis will disprove it. Many patients learn to write in new ways or to use the other hand though that, too, may be involved. Hypnosis is usually without effect. Liversedge has stated that about half the patients can be helped by a deconditioning procedure that delivers an electric shock whenever the spasm occurs. His results have not been verified by others. Aside from the spasm there is no other neurologic abnormality.

EXTRAPYRAMIDAL MOTOR DISTURBANCES DUE PRIMARILY TO DISEASES OF THE CEREBELLUM

Isolated lesions in the midline flocculonodular lobe result in grave disturbances of equilibrium. Often the symptoms are exhibited only when the patient attempts to stand and walk. He sways, staggers, titubates, and reels (see below under Disturbance of Movement and Posture). There may be no disturbance in coordination and no intention tremor of the limbs. A midline tumor of the cerebellum, hemorrhage, or other lesion such as medulloblastoma usually produces this syndrome.

Extensive lesions of one cerebellar hemisphere, especially the anterior lobe, cause disturbances of coordination in volitional movements of the ipsilateral arm and leg. This is known as *ataxia*. The movements are characterized by an inappropriate range, rate, and strength of each of the various components of the motor act and by an improper combination of those components. Electromyographic analysis has shown that ataxia is manifested as a decomposition of movement consisting of abnormal duration and timing of bursts of contraction and relaxation of agonists and antagonists of a joint, usually a large one (Carrera and Mettler). This incoordination is also called *asynergia.* The defects are particularly noticeable in acts that require rapid alternation of movements. Slowness in acceleration and deceleration, which is almost invariably present, impedes the performance (dysdiadochokinesis). The direction of projected (purposive) movement is frequently inaccurate. Owing to delay in arresting a movement, the patient may overshoot his mark. The antagonist muscles do not come into play at the proper time, possibly because of the hypotonia that is almost always present. This may be demonstrated by having the patient flex his arm against a resistance that is suddenly released. The patient with cerebellar disease will sometimes strike his face because he fails to check the flexion movement (Holmes's rebound phenomenon). In movements requiring accurate direction, as the limb approaches its destination it may stop short and then advance by a more or less rhythmic series of jerks and oscillations (intention tremor). In addition to hypotonia, there may be, in acute cerebellar lesions, some slight weakness.

A similar ataxia, asynergia, and dysmetria, usually with hypotonia and only a little intention tremor, may accompany lesions of the lateral and inferior parts of the cerebellar hemisphere. Bilateral lesions of the cerebellar hemispheres and midline flocculonodular lobe lead to such a severe disturbance in all movements that the patient may be unable to stand or walk or use his limbs effectively. In addition, there are ocular and speech disturbances, namely, nystagmus, dysmetria, and skew deviation of the eyes, and dysarthria. Lesions of the cerebellar penduncles have the same effect as extensive hemispheral lesions. This syndrome, due to involvement of one cerebellar hemisphere, may be observed in a tumor or abscess or in vascular lesions of the brainstem and cerebellar penduncles. The ataxia tends to be bilateral and symmetric in primary atrophy or degeneration of the cerebellum. There have been numerous attempts to explain in physiologic terms the hypotonia, mild degrees of weakness and fatigability, and abnormalities in the rate and regularity of projected movement that accompany cerebellar lesions in man. It has been found that depression of fusimotor (spindle) efferent activity in the spinal cord leads to decreased spindle afferent discharge and lessened tonic facilitation of alpha motor neuron activity. The cerebellar facilitation that is lost with acute lesions is normally mediated through two systems of fibers—the fastigioreticulospinal and the dentatorubrothalamocortical. The latter, acting specifically on cortical areas 4 and 6, is the more important in man. Although the corticospinal tract is probably essential for the expression of cerebellar deficits in man, in the primate any pathway subserving specifically projected movements into environment may support tremor and other parts of the syndrome. Tremor ataxia and hypotonia seem to be separable, independent entities, but all are believed related to the disturbed fusimotor activity.

A kind of pseudoataxia, especially of gait, may be caused by the improper timing of the components of complex actions, e.g., with defects in postural sense (sensory ataxia and with slow relaxation of muscles in hypothyroidism (myxedema with ataxia).

SOME GENERAL FEATURES OF ALL EXTRAPYRAMIDAL MOTOR DISTURBANCES

From the above discussion of many special types of motor disorder the reader must not think that they always appear in pure form. Various combinations occur in diseases. For example, Wilson's disease usually presents with a Parkinson-like picture of tremor, rigidity, slowness of movement, and flexion dystonia of trunk, but exceptionally there is athetosis, tonic innervation (inability to relax a voluntary movement), phasic dystonia, and action myoclonus. Hallevorden-Spatz disease may take the form of universal rigidity and flexion dystonia or choreoathetosis. Occasionally the degeneration of Huntington's chorea leads to rigidity rather than choreoathetosis. Corticospinal and various of these extrapyramidal disorders may be associated in patients with cerebral diplegia. Nonetheless certain combinations tend to occur with greater or lesser frequency in certain diseases, as will be pointed out in Chaps. 330, 332, and 333. The benign restricted or localized spasms and twitches are the most obscure disorders with reference to both their pathologic anatomy and physiology.

In broad terms all the extrapyramidal disorders should be viewed in terms of the primary deficit (negative symptom) and the new phenomena (movements, abnormal postures, tremors, etc.) which have appeared. These latter (positive symptoms) are presently ascribed to release from or disequilibrium of undamaged motor parts of the nervous system. The clearest negative effect is usually evidenced as an akinesia, or disinclination to use the affected muscles. The difficulty in rapid alternating sequences of movement stands as another negative effect in diseases of both the basal ganglions and the cerebellum. In fact this latter symptom, presenting as a clumsiness, may be the only fault manifest in certain maladroit children. Stress and nervous tension characteristically worsen both the motor deficiency and the abnormal movements in all these extrapyramidal syndromes, just as relaxation helps the motor performance. All the movement disorders are abolished in sleep.

One of the most remarkable discoveries of recent years, to be credited largely to the pioneering efforts of neurosurgeons (Meyer, Cooper), has been the abolition of tremors, rigidity, and involuntary movements of the limbs by a surgical lesion in the medial segment of the globus pallidus or the ventrolateral nucleus of the thalamus. The effects are contralateral. Usually the lesion has been made first by the injection of procaine (Novocain) and then by use of alcohol, cooling and freezing (Cooper), or electrocoagulation (White and Sweet and Leksell). The operation has been successful in temporarily alleviating tremor or rigidity (or both) on one side. The procedure is successful in approximately 80 percent of cases of paralysis agitans, and the postural abnormality in dystonia musculorum deformans and double athetosis has responded somewhat less consistently. The operations have been perfected to the point at which the mortality rate is less than 1 percent, and the risk of hemiplegia or some other sequel is less than 10 percent. Of course, as the disease progresses, the beneficial effects are lost. The therapeutic procedure indicates that the pallidum and ventrolateral nucleus, probably through their connections with the cerebral cortex (motor cortex and its corticospinal pathway), are essential for the expression of these extrapyramidal syndromes. The indications for these surgical procedures are discussed in Chap. 333.

DISTURBANCE OF MOVEMENT AND POSTURE: EXAMINATION AND DIFFERENTIAL DIAGNOSIS

In Chap. 17 the methods of examining the motor system were described at some length, so only a few additional remarks concerning extrapyramidal disorders need be made there. These abnormalities are best demonstrated by seeing the patient in action. If he complains of a limp after walking a distance or of difficulty in climbing stairs, he should be observed under these conditions. Tests of rate, regularity, and coordination of voluntary movement must be sufficiently varied and demanding of the patient's motor coordination to bring out the defect. The physician must cultivate the habit of accurately observing and describing abnormalities of movement and must not be content merely to give the condition a name or to force it into some category such as chorea or tic or myoclonus. The main postures of the body in all common acts should be noted. Aside from the assessment of muscle power and of gait, the usual test applied to the upper limb is to ask the patient to touch the examiner's fingertip and then the tip of his own nose repeatedly (*finger-to-nose test*). In testing the leg the patient is asked to place his heel on one knee and then to run it down his shin and back to the knee (*heel-to-knee-to-shin test*). Finer movements of the hand may be tested by having the patient successively touch each finger to his thumb, pat his thigh rapidly, or use tools or handle objects. Rapidly alternating movements such as repeatedly touching the index finger with the thumb, pronation and supination, or opening and closing the hands are valuable tests.

The fully developed extrapyramidal motor syndromes can be recognized without difficulty once the physician has become familiar with the typical pictures. The mental picture of Parkinson's syndrome, with its slowness of movement, poverty of facial expression, and static tremor and rigidity, should be fixed in mind. Similarly, the gross distortions and postural abnormalities of dystonia, whether widespread in trunk muscles or involving only neck muscles, as in spasmodic torticollis, once seen should thereafter be familiar. Athetosis, with its instability of postures and ceaseless movements of fingers and hands; intention spasm; chorea, with its more rapid and complicated movements; and the abrupt movements of myoclonus that flit over the body are other standard syndromes. Characteristic of all is a mild defect in the voluntary use of the affected parts.

The clinical differences between corticospinal and extrapyramidal disorders are summarized in Table 18-2.

TABLE 18-2
Clinical differences between corticospinal and extrapyramidal syndromes

	Corticospinal	*Extrapyramidal*
Character of rigidity	Clasp-knife effect	Plastic, equal throughout passive movement or intermittent cogwheel rigidity)
Distribution of rigidity	Flexors of arms, extensors of legs	Flexors of all four limbs and trunk
Shortening and lengthening reaction	Present	Absent
Involuntary movements	Absent	Presence of tremors, chorea, athetosis, dystonia
Tendon reflexes	Increased	Normal or slightly increased
Babinski's sign	Present	Absent
Paralysis of voluntary movement	Present	Absent or slight

Early or mild forms of these conditions, like all medical diseases, may offer special difficulties in diagnosis. Cases of paralysis agitans, seen before the appearance of tremor, are often overlooked. The patient may complain of being nervous and restless or may have experienced an indescribable stiffness and aching in certain parts of the body. Because of the absence of weakness or of reflex changes, the case may be considered psychogenic or rheumatic. It is well to remember that Parkinson's syndrome often begins in a hemiplegic distribution, and for this reason the illness may be misdiagnosed as cerebral thrombosis. A slight masking of the face, a suggestion of a limp, blepharoclonus (uninhibited blinking of eyes when the bridge of the nose is tapped), a mild rigidity, failure of an arm to swing naturally in walking, or loss of certain movements of cooperation will help in diagnosis at this time. Every case presenting the syndrome of Parkinson or other abnormality of movement and posture in adolescence or early adult life should be surveyed for hepatolenticular degeneration by tests of liver function and split-lamp examination for corneal pigmentation (Kayser-Fleischer ring); if facilities are available, urinary amino-nitrogen excretion and copper excretion should be determined.

Mild or early chorea is often mistaken for simple nervousness. If one sits for a time and watches the patient, the diagnosis will often become evident. There are cases, nonetheless, in which it is impossible to distinguish simple nervousness from early Sydenham's chorea, especially in children, and there is no laboratory test upon which one can depend. The first postural manifestation of dystonia may suggest hysteria, and it is only later, when the fixity of the postural abnormality, the lack of the usual psychologic picture of hysteria, and the relentlessly progressive character of the illness become evident, that accurate diagnosis is reached. Another common error is to assume that a bedfast patient who has complained of dizziness, staggering, and headaches and exhibits no other neurologic abnormality is suffering from hysteria. The flocculonodular cerebellar syndrome is demonstrable only when the patient attempts to stand and walk.

The uncertainty of balance and short-stepped gait (marche-a-petits-pas) in the elderly is often incorrectly attributed to loss of confidence and fear of falling.

REFERENCES

BRODAL A: *Neurological Anatomy in Relation to Clinical Medicine,* New York: Oxford, 1969

COOPER IS: *Involuntary Movement Disorders,* New York: Hoeber, 1969

CUMINGS JN: Biochemistry of the basal ganglia, chap. 4 in *Handbook of Clinical Neurology,* vol. 6, eds PJ Vinken and GW Bruyn, Amsterdam: North Holland Publishing Company, 1968, p. 116

DENNY-BROWN, D: Clinical symptomatology of disease of the basal ganglia, in *Handbook of Clinical Neurology,* vol. 6, eds PJ Vinken and GW Bruyn, Amsterdam: North Holland Publishing Company, 1968, p. 133

19 DIZZINESS, VERTIGO, AND DISORDERS OF GAIT

MAURICE VICTOR
RAYMOND D. ADAMS

Dizziness and other sensations of unbalance occur in a wide variety of diseases. In many instances the clue to an important medical disorder is afforded by the correct analysis of the complaint.

In everyday language the term dizziness covers a number of different sensory experiences—true vertigo, which refers to a feeling of whirling or rotation, as well as nonrotatory swaying, weakness, faintness, and lightheadedness. Blurring of vision, feelings of unreality, syncope, and even petit mal may be incorrectly called dizzy spells; hence a close questioning as to how the patient is using the term becomes a necessary first step in clinical study. A distinction is sometimes drawn between subjective vertigo, meaning a sense of turning one's body, and objective vertigo, an illusion of movement of objects in the environment, but its validity is doubtful.

In this chapter the term *vertigo* will be used to refer to all subjective and objective illusions of rotation. *Giddiness* will refer to a swaying type of dizziness. *Equilibrium,* the state of equipoise whereby the posture of the body is maintained against the forces of gravity, is deranged in vertigo but is also affected by other disorders as well, e.g., loss of joint or muscle sense (sensory ataxia), cerebellar disease (cerebellar ataxia), and motor abnormalities (spasticity and rigidity, myotonia, and the pseudomyotonia of hypothyroidism). Although these latter conditions are described in Chaps. 17, 18, and 348, their effects on stance and gait are appropriately reviewed in this context.

ANATOMIC, PHYSIOLOGIC, AND PSYCHOLOGIC CONSIDERATIONS Several mechanisms maintain balanced posture and awareness of the body's positions in relation to its surroundings. The most important of these are:

1 Impulses from the retinas of the two eyes which are coordinated by ocular motor mechanisms to supply information about the position and movement of the body and its surroundings.
2 Impulses from the labyrinths of the inner ears—specialized spatial proprioceptors whose primary function is to register changes in the direction of motion (either acceleration or deceleration) and position of the body. [N.B. The semicircular canals respond to movement and angular momentum, whereas the otoliths (sense organs of the utricle and saccule) are mainly concerned with orienting the organism with reference to gravitational force.]
3 Impulses from the proprioceptors of joints and muscles—essential to all reflex, postural, and volitional movements. Those of the neck are of special importance in relating the position of the head to that of the rest of the body.

The cerebellum and certain ganglionic centers in the brainstem (particularly the vestibular nuclei, oculomotor nucleus, and red nucleus) and in the basal ganglions are the important coordinators of these sensory data and provide for postural adjustment, upright stance, and locomotion.

Important psychophysiologic mechanisms are also involved in the maintenance of equilibrium and the proper relationship of our bodies to the external world. Early in life we come to coordinate the parts of our body in relation to one another and to perceive that portion of space occupied by our bodies. The construct of these integrated sensory data has been designated by Russell Brain as the *body schema.* The space around our body is said to be represented by another set of data, the *environmental schema.* These two schemata are dynamic and interdependent, since both are simultaneously changed in every activity. For example, we learn to see objects as being stationary when we are moving. Thus, the motion of ourselves and of objects in space is always relative. At times, when sensory information is incomplete, we mistake movement of our surroundings for those of our own body, as in the illusion caused by motion of a neighboring train. A disturbance in the awareness of one's own body schema is postulated by some psychiatrists as the basis of neurotic disorientation and feelings of unreality.

CLINICAL CHARACTERISTICS OF VERTIGO AND GIDDINESS The clinical recognition of *vertigo* proves to be relatively easy when the patient states that objects in the environment turned or moved in one direction or that his head and body whirled. Often, however, he is not so explicit. The feeling may be described as oscillation, or of veering, of being pulled to one side or to the ground, as though drawn by a magnet. Again, the floor or walls may seem to tilt or to sink or rise up. The feeling of impulsion is particularly characteristic. If the patient is ambiguous he should be asked to compare his feelings with those he has experienced when coming to a halt after rapid rotation.

All but the mildest forms of vertigo are accompanied

by perspiration, pallor, nausea, and vomiting. The nystagmus which is invariably present, causes objects in the field of vision to move rhythmically in one direction. As a rule the patient can walk only with difficulty, or not at all should the vertigo be intense. A sudden attack may even catapult him to the ground, and only when down does he experience vertigo. Forced to lie down he realizes that one position, usually on one side with eyes closed, reduces the vertigo and nausea, and that the slightest motion of the head aggravates them. One form of vertigo, the benign positional vertigo of Bárány occurs only for a few seconds after lying down and sitting up. If the vertigo is less severe the patient can walk unsteadily but may veer to one side. The ataxia of gait with vertigo (vertiginous ataxia) is recognized always as being a "dizziness in the head," not a trouble in the control of the legs and trunk. It is noteworthy that in these circumstances the coordination of the individual movements of the limbs is not impaired—a point of difference from cerebellar disease. There may be headache, especially in the region of the offending ear. Loss of consciousness as part of a vertiginous attack nearly always signifies another type of disorder (seizure or faint).

Giddiness and other types of pseudovertigo are usually described as feelings of swaying, lightheadedness, a swimming sensation, and, more rarely, as though walking on air, "queer in the head," uncertain, about to fall or "pass out." These sensory experiences are particularly common in psychoneurotic and other psychiatric illnesses featured by anxiety attacks. They may be reproduced by hyperventilation, and then it is appreciated that panic and apprehensiveness, palpitation, breathlessness, trembling, and sweating are concurrent.

Other pseudovertiginous symptoms are less definite. In severe anemic states weakness and languor may be attended by a lightheadedness related to postural change and exertion, the basis of which must be a mild hypoxia. In the emphysematous patient physical effort may be associated with weakness and peculiar cephalic sensations, and coughing may lead to giddiness and even fainting (tussive syncope) because of impaired return of venous blood to the heart. The dizziness that so often accompanies hypertension is more difficult to evaluate. Sometimes it is an expression of anxiety, or it may be due to an unstable adjustment of cerebral blood flow. *Postural dizziness* is another example of unstable vasomotor reflexes preventing a constancy of cerebral circulation and is notably frequent in persons recently bedfast, in the weak and ill, and the elderly. Abrupt arising from a recumbent or sitting position is followed immediately by a swaying type of dizziness, dimming of vision, and spots before the eyes which last a few seconds. The patient is forced to stand still and steady himself by holding onto a nearby object. A syncopal attack may occur at this time (see Chap. 16).

In practice it is not difficult to separate these types of pseudovertigo from true vertigo for there is none of the feeling of rotation or impulsion so characteristic of the latter. Lacking also are the other ancillary symptoms of true vertigo, namely, nausea, vomiting, tinnitus and deafness, and staggering.

THE NEUROLOGIC AND OTOLOGIC CAUSES OF VERTIGO Vertigo may constitute the aura of an epileptic seizure, but this event is rare. The lesion is then on the posterolateral aspects of the temporal lobe near the Sylvian fissure. A sensation of movement, either of the body away from the side of the lesion or of the environment in the opposite direction, lasts for a few seconds before being submerged in other seizure activity. Vertiginous sensations may rarely serve as a stimulus for *reflex epilepsy* (see page 337), and the test for this form of vertigo provokes the seizure.

Oculomotor disorders are a source of a spatial disorientation simulating dizziness. This is maximal when the patient looks in the direction of action of the paralyzed muscle; it is attributable to the receipt of two conflicting visual images. In fact some normal people even experience dizziness for a time when adjusting to bifocal glasses or when looking down from a height.

Whether lesions of the cerebellum can produce vertigo seems to depend on the part of it involved. Large destructive processes in the cerebellar hemispheres and vermis cause no vertigo, unless they extend to central vestibulocerebellar connections.

The observations of DeJong document a kind of vertigo induced by disturbances of upper cervical roots and the structures which they innervate (so-called cervical vertigo), but its existence, or at least this interpretation of it, is still open to question.

Labryinthine (aural) lesions are the usual causes of paroxysmal vertigo. In the classical variety, that of Ménière's disease, the onset is abrupt, the vertigo is clearly of the rotary type, and it lasts a few minutes to hours. Concomitant tinnitus, fullness in the ear, high-tone deafness with auditory recruitment (see Chap. 20), nystagmus, nausea, vomiting, and staggering comprise the full syndrome. The patient preferentially lies with the faulty ear uppermost and is disinclined to look toward the normal side because of exaggeration of the nystagmus and dizziness. The nystagmus is fine, rotatory, and most pronounced when the eyes are turned away from the offending ear. Vertiginous attacks of this type may recur and give rise to mild, chronic states of disequilibrium which may persist for days. Seldom does it last, however, for central mechanisms compensate for permanent deficits of one labyrinth. Chronic vertigo may be complicated by the giddiness of a secondary anxiety state. *Vestibular neuronitis* is a term that refers to severe vertigo, often of several days' duration, without tinnitus or deafness. Its pathologic basis is uncertain. It occurs in Bárány's benign positional vertigo and the more malignant positional vertigo of posterior fossa tumors and other lesions, and lasts only a few seconds.

Vertigo of acoustic nerve origin, the commonest cause of which is an acoustic neuroma, tends usually to be mild and intermittent (lasting weeks or months). Seldom does it come in discrete attacks separated by free intervals. Vertigo has rarely been observed as the initial symptom with eighth nerve tumors, but the usual sequence is deafness of high-frequency type (without recruitment), followed some years later by chronic vertigo and impaired caloric responses, then cranial nerve palsies (involving the eighth, fifth, and tenth nerves), ipsilateral ataxia of limbs, and headache, the other common signs of a cerebellopontine angle tumor.

Vertigo of brainstem origin implicates vestibular nuclei and their connections. In these cases auditory function is nearly always spared, since the vestibular and cochlear fibers separate upon entering the medulla and pons. The nystagmus which accompanies such central lesions tends to be coarse and protracted; it is more marked on lateral gaze to one side than the other. There may also be a nonrotatory vertical component. The central localization is evidenced further by the attendant signs of involvement of other structures within the brainstem (cranial nerves, sensory and motor tracts, etc.). Mode of onset, duration, and other features of the clinical picture depend upon the nature of the causative disease, usually vascular, neoplastic, or demyelinative.

DIFFERENTIAL DIAGNOSIS As already stated, a careful history and physical examination of the dizzy patient usually afford a basis for separating true vertigo from the swaying dizziness of the hyperventilating, anxious patient and from the other types of pseudovertigo. If it is discovered that the patient is unobservant or imprecise in his descriptions, a helpful tactic is to provoke a number of dissimilar sensations by rotating the patient, irrigating his ears with warm or cold water, by asking him to stoop for a minute and straighten up, and to hyperventilate for 3 min. Should the patient be unable to distinguish among these several types of induced dizziness or to ascertain the similarity of one of the types to his own condition, his history is probably too inaccurate for purposes of diagnosis.

When vertigo is mild or poorly described, small items of the patient's history, such as disinclination to walk during an attack, tendency to list to one side, aggravation by riding in a vehicle, preference for one position, are helpful.

In some patients an attack of vertigo is so abrupt and violent that they are virtually flung to the ground, sometimes with a serious injury. These attacks have been called by the quaint term "otolithic crises of Tumarken," but without proof of involvement of the utricle or saccule. The diagnosis is usually substantiated by the presence of vertigo, nausea, and vomiting while on the ground, distinguishing it from a seizure or faint. Probably it differs from other forms of labyrinthine vertigo only in its severity.

In the differentiation of types of labyrinthine and vestibular nerve disease, inspection of eardrums, x-rays of mastoids, middle ears, and inner ears, and auditory and caloric tests are useful, especially in excluding labyrinthitis. In caloric testing, the patient's head is tilted forward 30° from the horizontal (bringing the horizontal semicircular canal into a vertical plane), which is the position of maximal sensitivity to thermal stimuli. The external auditory meatus are irrigated in turn for 40 sec with water at 30°C and 44°C (7° below and above body temperature). Cold water induces nystagmus to the opposite side (direction of the fast phase), and warm water to the same side. The nystagmus begins in 20 sec and should persist 90 to 120°. Comparison of the two ears reveals which one is paretic or hypersensitive. Special rotational chairs and electronystagmography are other more refined means of assessing disordered labyrinthine function. The diagnosis of benign positional vertigo is settled at the bedside by reproducing a brief vertigo and nystagmus (lasting up to a minute) by moving the patient from the sitting position to recumbency with head to one side in one trial and to the other in the second. Going from a recumbent to a sitting position reverses the direction of vertigo and nystagmus. This specific pattern and its reversibility are not observed in the more malignant positional vertigo of posterior fossa tumors and other lesions.

The association of vertigo with auditory signs and symptoms signifies always a disease process of end organ or eighth nerve. Labyrinthine and auditory tests and neurologic signs of structures adjacent to the eighth cranial nerve separate these two groups of diseases.

Pure vertigo as a manifestation of disease of the brainstem is rare, and the rule we have found trustworthy is that unless other symptoms and signs appear within 1 to 2 weeks, one can nearly always postulate an aural origin and exclude vascular disease of the brainstem. This is true of multiple sclerosis, which may be the explanation of a persistent vertigo in some adolescents or young adults.

DISTURBANCES OF EQUILIBRIUM AND OF GAIT

All that has been said above refers in large measure to the patient's awareness of a disorientation in space; but there are forms of neurologic abnormality with a prominent disequilibrium of the body but no dizziness whatsoever. Since these are manifested most clearly as an impairment of upright stance and locomotion, their evaluation depends on a knowledge of the nervous mechanisms underlying these peculiarly human functions. Analysis of gaits is a particularly rewarding medical exercise. With some experience a neurologic diagnosis may be reached merely by noting the manner in which the patient stands and walks.

The normal gait seldom attracts attention, but it should be observed with care. The body is erect, the head straight, and the arms hang loosely and gracefully at the sides, each moving rhythmically forward with the opposite leg. The feet are slightly everted, and the steps are of moderate length and approximately equal, the internal malleoli of the tibias almost touching one another. With each step there is coordinated flexion of hip and knee, dorsiflexion of foot, and a barely perceptible elevation of the hip so that the foot clears the ground. The heel strikes the ground first, and inspection of shoes will show that this part is most subject to wear. In the erect posture, the muscles of greatest importance in maintaining equilibrium are the erector spinae and the extensors of the hips and knees.

When analyzed in greater detail, the requirements for locomotion in an upright, bipedal position may be reduced to the following elements: (1) antigravity support of the body; (2) stepping; (3) an adequate degree of equilibrium; and (4) a means of propulsion. The support of the body is provided by the antigravity reflexes which maintain firm extension of knees, hips, and back muscles, but modifiable by position of the head and neck. These reflexes depend on the integrity of the spinal cord and lower parts of the brainstem (pontine transection leads to exaggeration of these antigravity reflexes—decerebrate rigidity). Stepping, the second element, is a basic movement pattern, present at birth, and integrated at the midbrain level. Its appropriate stimulus is contact of the sole with a flat surface and inclination of the body forward and alternately from side-to-side. Equilibrium involves the maintenance of balance at right angles to the direction of movement. The center of gravity during the continuously unstable equilibrium which prevails in walking must shift from side to side within narrow limits as the weight is borne first on one foot then the other. Propulsion is provided by leaning forward and slightly to one side and permitting the body to fall a certain distance before being checked by the support of the leg. Here both forward and alternating lateral movements must occur. But in running, where at one moment both feet are off the ground, a forward drive or thrust by the hind leg is also needed. Locomotion may fail in the course of neurologic diseases when one or more of these mechanical principles is prevented from operating, as we shall see.

There are many individual variations of gait, and it is a commonplace observation that the sound of an individual's footsteps, notably his pace and heaviness of tread, may identify him. The manner of walking and the carriage of the body may even provide clues to character, personality, and occupation. Furthermore, the gaits of men and women differ, the steps of women being quicker and shorter and the movement of their trunk and hips more graceful and delicate. Certain female characteristics of gait, if observed in the male, immediately impart an impression of femininity; or male characteristics in the female, one of masculinity.

Since normal body posture and locomotion require visual information (we see where we are going and pick our steps), labyrinthine function, and proprioception, it is of interest to note the effect of deficits in these senses on normal function. A blind man or a normal one who is blindfolded may walk very well. He moves cautiously, to avoid collision with objects, and on smooth pavement shortens his step slightly; with the shortening there is less rocking of the body and he seems unnaturally stiff. A man without labyrinthine function (as may happen after prolonged administration of streptomycin) shows a slight unsteadiness in walking and an inability to descend stairs without holding onto a banister. Running is also difficult. Characteristically, he has great difficulty in focusing on a stationary object when he is moving, so that he cannot drive a car. Proof that he is dependent on visual cues comes from his performance blindfolded, when his unsteadiness and staggering increase to some extent, but usually not to the point of falling. A loss of proprioception, as in a complete lesion in the posterior columns of the spinal cord in the high cervical region, abolishes for a long time the capacity for independent locomotion. After years of training the patient will still have difficulty in starting to walk and in propelling himself forward. As Purdon Martin has illustrated, he holds his hands in front of his body, bends body and head forward, walks with a wide base with irregular uneven steps but does rock his body. If he loses his balance, he shows no reactions to his posture. If he falls, he cannot arise without help, and he cannot get up from a chair. He is unable to crawl or to get into an "all-fours" posture. When standing, if blindfolded, he immediately falls. Thus the postural reactions are demonstrably more dependent on proprioceptive than on visual or labyrinthine information.

When confronted with a disorder of gait, the examiner must observe the patient's natural stance and the attitude and dominant positions of the legs, trunk, and arms. It is good practice to watch the patient as he walks into the examining room, because he is apt to walk more naturally then than during special tests. He should be asked to stand with his feet together, head erect, with eyes first open and then closed. Swaying due to nervousness may be overcome by asking him to touch the tip of his nose with the finger of first one hand and then the other. Next the patient should be asked to walk forward and backward, with his eyes first open and then closed. Any tendency to reel to one side, as in cerebellar disease, can be checked by having him walk around a chair. When the affected side is toward the chair, the patient tends to walk into it; and when it is away from the chair, he veers outward in ever-widening circles. More delicate tests of gait are walking a straight line heel to toe or having the patient arise quickly from a chair, walk briskly, and then stop or turn suddenly. If all these tests are successfully executed, it may be assumed that any difficulty in locomotion is not due to disease of the proprioceptive mechanisms or cerebellum. Detailed neurologic examination is then necessary in order to determine which of the many other possible diseases is responsible for the patient's disorder of gait.

The following abnormal gaits are so distinctive that with a little practice they can be recognized at a glance.

Cerebellar gait The main features of this gait are *wide base* (separation of legs), *unsteadiness, irregularity,* and *lateral reeling.* Steps are uncertain, some are shorter and others longer than intended, and the patient may lurch to one side or the other. The unsteadiness is more prominent on quickly arising from a chair and walking, on stopping suddenly while walking, or on turning abruptly. If the ataxia is severe, the patient cannot stand without assistance. If it is lesser in degree, standing with feet together and head erect, with eyes either open or closed, may be difficult. In its mildest form the ataxia is best demonstrated by having the patient walk a line heel to toe. After two or three steps he loses his balance and must place one foot to the side to avoid falling. Romberg's sign, i.e., marked swaying or falling with the eyes closed but not with the eyes open, is not a feature of cerebellar disease. Compensation may be effected by shortening the step and shuffling, i.e., keeping both feet simultaneously on the ground. The defect in the cerebellar gait is not in antigravity support, steppage, or propulsion but in the coordination of proprioceptive, labyrinthine, and visual information in reflex coordination of movements. The abnormality of gait may or may not be accompanied by other signs of cerebellar incoordination and intention tremor of the arms and legs. The presence of the latter signs depends on involvement of the superior midline structures as distinct from cerebellar hemispheres; if the lesion is unilateral, the signs are always on the same side.

Cerebellar gait is most commonly seen in multiple

sclerosis, cerebellar tumors, particularly medulloblastoma of the cerebellar vermis, and the cerebellar degenerations. In certain forms of cerebellar degeneration (e.g., the type associated with chronic alcoholism) the disease process reaches a plateau and then remains stable for many years, and the gait disorder, in these circumstances, becomes altered to some extent. The base is wide and the steps are still short, but more regular; the trunk is inclined slightly forward, the arms are held away from the sides, and the gait assumes a somewhat rhythmic quality. In this way the patient can walk for long distances, but he lacks the capacity to make the necessary postural adjustments in response to sudden changes in his position. In this respect, among others, ataxia of cerebellar disease differs from that due to drunkenness (see below).

A slowness in muscle relaxation as myxedema may also lead to a kind of gait disorder that simulates a cerebellar defect.

Gait of sensory ataxia This gait is due to an impairment of proprioception resulting from interruption of afferent nerve fibers in the peripheral nerves, posterior roots, posterior columns of the spinal cords, or medial lemnisci; it may also be produced occasionally by a lesion of both parietal lobes. Whatever the location of the lesion, the patient is deprived of knowledge of the position of his limbs. The principal features of the resulting gait disorder are *uncertainty, irregularity,* and the *stamp* of the feet. Hunt characterized this type of gait very well when he said that the ataxic patient is recognized by "his stamp and stick." This form of ataxia is characterized by varying degrees of difficulty in standing and walking, and in advanced cases there is a complete failure of locomotion, although muscular power is retained. The legs are kept far apart to correct the instability, and the patient carefully watches the ground and his legs. As he steps out, the legs are flung abruptly forward and outward, often lifted higher than necessary. The steps are of variable length, and many are attended by an audible stamp as the foot is banged down on the floor. The body is held in a slightly flexed position, and the weight may be supported on the cane that the severely ataxic patient often carries. The incoordination is greatly exaggerated when the patient is deprived of visual cues, as in walking in the dark. Most patients, when asked to stand with feet together and eyes closed, show greatly increased swaying or actual falling (Romberg's sign). It has been said that a lame man whose shoes are not worn in any one place is probably suffering from sensory ataxia. There is invariably a loss of vibratory and position sense in the feet and legs. A disordered gait of this type is observed in tabes dorsalis, Friedreich's ataxia, subacute combined degeneration, syphilitic meningomyelitis, chronic polyneuritis, and those cases of multiple sclerosis in which posterior column disease predominates.

Hemiplegic and paraplegic (spastic) gait In hemiplegia the leg is held stiffly and does not flex freely and gracefully at the knee and hip. It tends to rotate outward and describes a semicircle, first away from and then toward the trunk (circumduction). The foot scrapes along the floor, and the toe and outer side of the sole of the shoe are worn. One can diagnose the hemiplegic gait by hearing the slow rhythmic scuff of the foot along the floor. The other muscles of the body on the affected side are weak and stiff to a variable degree, particularly the arm, which is carried in a flexed position and does not swing naturally. This type of gait disorder is most frequently associated with vascular disease of the brain.

The spastic paraplegic gait is entirely different from the gait of sensory ataxia, though the two may be combined. Each leg is advanced slowly and stiffly with restricted motion at the knee and hip. The patient looks as though he were wading in water. The legs are extended or slightly bent at the knees and may be strongly adducted at the hips, tending almost to cross ("scissors" gait). The steps are regular and short. Movements of the legs are slow, and the patient may be able to advance only with great effort. An easy way to remember the main features of the hemiplegic and paraplegic gait is by the letter S, which begins each of its descriptive adjectives—spastic, slow, scuffing. The defect is in the stepping mechanism and in propulsion, not in support or equilibrium. Cerebral spastic diplegia, multiple sclerosis, syringomyelia, spinal syphilis, combined system disease, spinal cord compression, and familial spinal spastic ataxia are the common causes of spastic paraparesis.

Festinating gait The term *festinating* comes from the Latin *festinare,* to hasten, and appropriately describes the involuntary increase or hastening of the gait that characterizes both paralysis agitans and postencephalitic Parkinson's syndrome. *Rigidity* and *shuffling,* in addition to *festination,* are the cardinal features of this gait. When they are joined to the typical tremors, rigidity, and slowness of movement, there can be little doubt as to the diagnosis.

The general attitude of the patient is one of flexion; rigidity and immobility of the body are other conspicuous features. There is a paucity of the automatic movements made in sitting, standing, and walking; the head does not turn in looking to one side, the arms are seldom folded, and the legs are rarely crossed. The arms are held stiffly as though in preparation for writing, and the facial expression is unblinking and masklike.

In walking, the trunk is bent forward and the arms are carried ahead of the body and do not swing. The legs are stiff and bent at the knees and hips. The steps are short, and the feet barely clear the ground as the patient shuffles along. Once forward or backward locomotion is started, the upper part of the body advances ahead of the lower part, as though the patient were chasing his center of gravity. His steps become more and more rapid, and he may fall if not assisted. This is the festination, and it may occur when the patient is walking forward or backward, taking the form of either propulsion or retropulsion. The defect is in rocking the body from side to side so as to clear the floor and in moving the legs quickly enough to catch the center of gravity in forward propulsion. Other unusual gaits are sometimes observed in the postencephalitic patient. For example, he may be unable to take his first step forward because he cannot lift one foot, or he may be unable to step forward until he hops or takes one step backward; walking may be initiated by a series of short steps that give way to a more normal gait;

occasionally such a patient may run better than he walks or walk backwards better than forward.

Athetotic, dystonic, and choreic gaits Diseases that are characterized by involuntary movements and abnormal postures seriously affect gait. In fact, a disturbance of gait may be the initial and dominant manifestation of these diseases, and the testing of gait often serves to provoke abnormalities of movement and posture that are otherwise not conspicuous. The *athetotic* patient often assumes the most grotesque postures. One arm may be held aloft and the other one behind the body with wrist and fingers alternately undergoing slow flexion, extension, and rotation. The head may be inclined in one direction, the lips alternately retract and then purse, and the tongue intermittently protrudes from the mouth. The legs advance slowly and awkwardly, the result of superimposed involuntary movements and postures. Sometimes the foot is plantar-flexed at the ankle, and the weight is carried on the toes; or it may be dorsiflexed or inverted. This type of gait is typical of congenital athetosis and Huntington's chorea.

In *dystonia musculorum deformans* the first symptom may be a limp due to inversion or plantar flexion of the foot or a distortion of the pelvis. The patient stands with one leg rigidly extended or one shoulder elevated. The trunk may be in a position of exaggerated lordosis, and the hips are partly flexed, with a tilting forward of the pelvis. Because of the muscle spasms that deform the body in this manner, the patient may have to walk with knees flexed. The gait may seem normal as the first steps are taken, but as the patient walks, one or both legs become flexed, giving rise to the "dromedary gait." In the more advanced stages walking becomes impossible, owing to torsion of the trunk or the continuous flexion of one leg.

In *Sydenham's chorea* the gait is often bizarre. As the patient stands or walks there is a continuous play of irregular "choreic" movements affecting the face, neck, hands, and, in the advanced stages, the large proximal joints and trunk. The positions of the trunk and upper parts of the body vary with each step. There are jerks of the head, grimacing, squirming, twisting movements of the trunk and limbs, and peculiar respiratory noises. The general features of these conditions are described more fully in Chap. 333.

Drop-foot, steppage, or equine gait This is caused by paralysis of the pretibial and peroneal muscles. The legs must be lifted abnormally high in order for the feet to clear the ground. There is a slapping noise as the foot strokes the floor. The anterior and lateral borders of the sole of the shoe become worn. The steps are regular and even; otherwise, walking is not remarkable. Foot drop may be unilateral or bilateral and occurs in diseases that affect the peripheral nerves of the legs or motor neurons in the spinal cord, such as poliomyelitis, progressive muscular atrophy, and Charcot-Marie-Tooth disease (peroneal muscular atrophy). It may also be observed in patients with peripheral types of muscular dystrophy. The most common cause of unilateral foot drop is compression of the anterior tibial nerve, where it crosses the head of the fibula.

Waddling gait This gait is characteristic of progressive muscular dystrophy. The attitude of the body may be straight, but more often the lumbar lordosis is accentuated. The steps are regular but a little uncertain. With each step there is an exaggerated elevation of one hip and depression of the other; once the weight is on the hip it yields to an abnormal degree, so that the upper trunk then inclines to that side. This alternation of lateral trunk movements results in the rolling gait, or *waddle,* a term suggested by Oppenheim. The gluteal musculature is weak and inefficient, although leg muscles may appear well developed. Muscular contractures leading to an equinovarus position of the foot may complicate childhood cases, so that the waddle is combined with circumduction of the legs and "walking on the toes."

Staggering or drunken gait This is characteristic of alcoholic and barbiturate intoxication. The drunken patient totters, reels, tips forward and then backward, threatening each moment to lose his balance and fall. Control over trunk and legs is greatly impaired. The steps are irregular and uncertain. The patient appears stupefied and indifferent to the quality of his performance, but under certain circumstances he can momentarily correct his defect.

The frequently used adjectives *drunken* and *reeling* do not describe aptly the gait of cerebellar disease, except, perhaps, the most acute and severe cases. The intoxicated patient reels in many different directions, unlike the patient with cerebellar disease, and no effort is made to correct the staggering by watching the legs or the ground, as in cerebellar or sensory ataxia. In the drunken patient, despite a wide diversity of excursions of all parts of the body, balance may be exquisitely maintained. In contrast, the patient with cerebellar disease has great difficulty in maintaining his balance if he sways or lurches too far to one side.

Hysterical gait This may take any one of several forms—monoplegic, paraplegic, or hemiplegic. The monoplegic or hemiplegic patient does not lift the foot from the floor while walking; instead, he drags it as a useless member or pushes it ahead of him as though it were a skate. The characteristic circumduction is absent in hysterical hemiplegia, and the typical hemiplegic posture, hyperactive tendon reflexes, and Babinski sign are missing. The hysterical paraplegic cannot very well drag both legs and usually he depends on a crutch or remains helpless in bed; the muscles may be rigid with contractures or flaccid. The gait may be quite dramatic. Some patients look as though they were walking on stilts, and others lurch wildly in all directions, actually demonstrating by their gyrations a remarkable ability to make rapid postural adjustments.

Astasia-abasia, in which the patient, though unable to either stand or walk, retains normal use of his legs while in bed, is nearly always hysterical. When such a patient is placed on his feet, he takes a few normal steps and then becomes unable to advance his feet; he lurches wildly and crumples to the floor if not assisted.

Frontal lobe ataxia Equilibrium and the capacity to stand and walk may be severely disturbed by diseases that affect the frontal lobes, particularly their medial parts. Although this disorder of gait is sometimes spoken of as an ataxia or as an *apraxia,* since the difficulty in walking cannot be accounted for by weakness or loss of sensation, it is probably neither. It most likely represents a loss of integration at the cortical and basal ganglionic level of the essential elements of stance and locomotion which were acquired in infancy and are often lost in senility.

The patient assumes a posture of slight flexion, with the feet placed farther apart then normal. He advances slowly, with small, shuffling, hesitant steps. At times the patient halts, unable to advance without great effort, although he does much better with a little assistance. Turning is accomplished by a series of tiny, uncertain steps which are made with one foot, the other being planted on the floor as a pivot. The initiation of walking becomes progressively more difficult, and in advanced cases the patient may be unable to take a step, as though his feet were glued to the floor. Finally he becomes unable to stand or even to sit, and without support he falls backward or to one side.

Some patients are able to make complex movements with their legs, such as drawing imaginary figures, at a time when their gait is seriously impaired. Eventually, however, all movements of the legs become slow and awkward, and the limbs, when passively moved, offer variable resistance (Gegenhalten). An inability to turn in bed is highly characteristic, and may eventually become complete. These motor disabilities are usually associated with dementia, but there need be no parallelism in their evolution. Grasping, groping, hyperactive tendon reflexes, and Babinski signs may or may not be present. The end result in many cases is a "cerebral paraplegia in flexion" (Yakovlev), in which the patient lies curled up in bed, immobile and mute, his limbs fixed by contractures in an attitude of flexion.

Senile gait Elderly persons often complain of difficulty in walking, and examination may disclose no abnormality other than the slightly flexed posture of the senile and short uncertain steps, *marche-a-petits-pas.* Speed, balance, and all the graceful, adaptive movements are lost. The exact nature of this gait disorder is not understood. Probably it is the frontal lobe gait disorder. It should be noted, however, that a short-stepped, cautious gait lacks specificity, being a general defensive reaction to all forms of defective locomotion.

REFERENCES

ALTMANN F: Diagnostic significance of vertigo, in *The Vestibular System and Its Diseases,* ed RJ Wolfson, Philadelphia: University of Pennsylvania Press, 1966, p. 353

BIEMOND A, DEJONG JMBV: On cervical nystagmus and related disorders. Brain 92:437, 1969

DIX MR: Modern tests of vestibular function, with special reference to their value in clinical practice. Br Med J 3:317, 1969

FISHER CM: Vertigo in cerebrovascular disease. Arch Otolaryngol 85:529, 1967

SPECTOR M: *Dizziness and Vertigo,* New York: Grune & Stratton, 1967

WEISS AD: Neurological aspects of the differential diagnosis of vertigo. Ann Otol Rhinol Laryngol 77:216, 1968

20 COMMON DISTURBANCES OF VISION, OCULAR MOVEMENT, AND HEARING

MAURICE VICTOR
RAYMOND D. ADAMS

Diseases of the eyes and ears, by virtue of their frequency, unusual nature, and serious consequences, comprise separate medical specialties and, therefore, fall outside the field of internal medicine. Yet disturbances of visual and auditory function may be the initial or leading manifestations of many systemic diseases. Of more general interest is the fact that these two senses represent the most finely developed parts of the entire afferent apparatus of the nervous system; hence the study of their disorders may yield important information about neurologic diseases.

THE EYE AND DISORDERS OF VISION The diverse composition of the eye, with its epithelial, vascular, collagenous, neural, and pigmentary tissue, explains why it is a medical microcosm susceptible to manifold diseases. Moreover its transparency makes it accessible to direct inspection by means of an instrument found in the consulting room of every physician and affords an opportunity to inspect directly during life many of the specific lesions of medical diseases.

Since the eye is the organ of vision, it is obvious that degrees of impairment of visual acuity to the point of blindness should stand as the most frequent symptom of eye disease. Strabismus and diplopia, ocular pain, irritation, redness and photophobia, inability to read or recognize objects and people, and drooping or closure of the eyelids are of less importance. The impairment of eyesight may be unilateral or bilateral, sudden or gradual, episodic or enduring. The common causes vary with age. In late childhood and adolescence increasing difficulty in focusing the eyes and in seeing clearly usually can be traced to *myopia,* though an optic nerve or suprasellar tumor must be excluded. In middle age *presbyopia* is almost invariable and requires eye refraction and spectacles. Still later in life *cataracts, glaucoma, retinal hemorrhages,* and *detachments* are the most frequent causes of visual disturbance. Episodic blindness in early life is usually due to migraine; later, amaurosis fugax is caused by stenosis of the carotid artery or cranial arteritis. Cerebrovascular disease deranges vision with increasing frequency in late life.

Thus failing eyesight may be due to an abnormality of the refractive media of the eye or to a lesion of the retina or optic nerve or the parts of the brain with which they are connected. In approaching this problem one begins always by inquiring as to precisely what the patient means when he says he cannot see properly, for he may be referring to symptoms as varied as excessive tearing, diplopia, partial syncope, or even giddiness or dizziness. Fortunately his statements can be checked by the measurement of visual activity, a technique which is the single most important part of the ocular examination. If visual acuity is less than 20/20 and cannot be improved by refraction and if the media of the eye are transparent, there is some sensory defect, the nature of which must be ascertained.

In the measurement of visual acuity the *Snellen Chart,* which contains rows of letters of diminishing size (those of each row subtending 5 min of an arc when held at various distances from the eye), is utilized. The letters at the top of the chart subtend 5 min of an arc at a distance of 200 ft; those at the bottom subtend an arc of 5 min at 20 ft. Thus if the patient can see only the top letters at 20 ft, rather than 200 ft, his vision is 20/200; if he sees those at the bottom at this distance, the acuity is 20/20. The patient with a corrected refractive error should wear his eyeglasses for the test; if the visual acuity is then less than 20/20, either his refractive error has not been properly corrected or there is some other reason for it. The former possibility can be ruled out if the patient sees clearly while looking through a pinhole of 2 to 3 mm in a cardboard with his glasses still on. The pinhole permits a narrow shaft of light to fall on the fovea without being refracted.

Light entering the eye is focused on the outer layer of the retina (the rods and cones). Consequently the media (tissue and fluids) through which the light passes must be transparent. These media are the cornea, the aqueous humor of the anterior chamber, the lens, the vitreous humor of the vitreous cavity, and the retina itself. The clarity of these media can be determined ophthalmoscopically, but this examination requires that the pupil be dilated to at least 6 mm in diameter. This is best accomplished by instilling a few drops of 10% phenylephrine (Neo-Synephrine) in each eye after the visual acuity is measured, the pupillary response recorded, and the intraocular pressure estimated. *An attack of angle-closure glaucoma may be precipitated by pupillary dilatation, but this happens rarely and can be controlled by 4% pilocarpine.* The cycloplegic action of phenylephrine lasts only an hour or two. Looking through a +6 ophthalmoscopic lens from a distance of 15 to 20 cm permits the visualization of any opacity in refractive media against the diffuse bright red of reflexed light from the retina. By adjusting the lens of the ophthalmoscope from high + to 0 or − one can "depth-focus" from the cornea to the retina. Clarity of all media means that reduced vision uncorrected by glasses must be due to a lesion in the macula, optic nerve, or structures further back in the visual system.

More specifically the alterations in the refractile media that affect vision have certain medical implications, as follows.

Corneas In hypercalcemia [secondary to sarcoid (Chap. 223)], hyperparathyroidism (Chap. 350), and vitamin D intoxication (Chap. 349), calcium phosphates and

carbonates precipitate within the cornea, primarily beneath the epithelium—so-called *band keratopathy;* cystine crystals are deposited in cystinosis (Chap. 97), cholesterol esters in hypercholesterolemia (*arcus senilis*) (Chap. 106), chloroquine crystals in treatment of discoid lupus by this drug, and copper in hepatolenticular degeneration [Kayser-Fleischer ring (Chap. 103)]. Opacification (keratitis) of the cornea may also occur after herpes simplex and herpes zoster infections (Chaps. 200 and 202); or it may be combined with uveitis and iritis in Behcet's disease (Chap. 202), Reuter's disease (Chap. 201), Stevens-Johnson disease (Chap. 71), and idiopathic infections. Keratitis may be a manifestation also of congenital syphilis (Chap. 159) and of more innocent states such as drying and injury of eyes during coma.

Aqueous humor The common problem is one of high pressure due to impediment of the outflow of the aqueous fluid. This is termed *glaucoma.* In 90 percent of cases (of the wide-angle type) the cause is unknown; in 5 percent the angle between pupil and lateral cornea is narrow and blocked when the pupil is dilated; and in the remaining 5 percent the condition is secondary to some disease process that blocks outflow channels (inflammatory debris of uveitis, or red blood cells from hemorrhage in the anterior chamber, i.e., hyphema). Glaucoma occurs in 2 percent of all patients over the age of forty; it may be asymptomatic and go unrecognized for years before it progresses to rapid loss of vision. Therefore, the intraocular pressure should be measured routinely, using a Schiotz tonometer. This is a simple procedure which should be practiced by every physician. With the patient supine, a drop of local anesthetic is put into each eye and the tonometer is then placed on the cornea so that the instrument is perfectly vertical. When the tonometer is pressed against the eye, the scale is read and the units are converted into millimeters of mercury from the chart in the tonometer case. The normal pressure is about 15 mm Hg. Pressures of 20 to 30 may damage the optic nerve, leading first to a nasal quadrant defect and finally to blindness. With the ophthalmoscope one can see also that the optic disk is excavated.

The lens Opacities form in diabetes mellitus (Chap. 88) and galactosemia ("sugar cataracts," from sustained high levels of blood glucose and galactose, which are changed to sorbitol or dulcitol, the accumulation of which leads to a high osmotic gradient within the lens fibers); in hypoparathyroidism (Chap. 350), which by lowering the concentration of Ca in the aqueous opacifies newly forming lens fibers; after prolonged high doses of chlorpromazine, triparanol, and corticosteroid therapy, which are believed to result in lenticular opacities; and in myotonic dystrophy (Chap. 346), which is associated with a special type of cataract. Weakening of zonular ligaments of lens allows a dislocation (iridodonesis) in both Marfan's syndrome (Chap. 364) and homocystinuria (Chap. 96).

Vitreous humor Hemorrhage may occur from rupture

of a retinal vessel, causing a shower of black or red dots. It is also seen in diabetes mellitus, where it may occur following rupture of newly formed retinal vessels, in *retinitis proliferans,* or after a retinal tear which may progress to retinal detachment. The vitreous humor may also be affected by deposition of calcium soaps (seen as glistening objects with the ophthalmoscope)—so-called *asteroid hyalosis* of diabetes mellitus.

The search for neurologic explanations of reduced vision begins with an examination of the retina with an ophthalmoscope. This thin (0.4-mm) sheet of transparent tissue and the optic nerve head into which the visual information is channeled are the only parts of the central nervous system that can be inspected during life.

Light entering the eye passes through the full thickness of the retina to reach the receptor layer of rods and cones and underlying pigment epithelium, which contains the visual pigment (rhodopsin). Impulses arising in these photoreceptors are transmitted via secondary neurons, the bipolar cells, to the innermost ganglion cell layer, the axons of which in turn travel through the optic nerve head, optic nerve, chiasm, and optic tracts to the lateral geniculate bodies. These retinal neurons normally acquire a myelin sheath only after piercing the lamina cribrosa. The macular region (two disk diameters or 3 mm lateral to the optic disk) is the most sensitive part of the retina. The vascular supply comes from the ophthalmic branch of the internal carotid artery, which in turn gives origin to the central retinal artery. The latter, upon issuing from the optic disk, divides into four arterioles, which supply the four quadrants of the retina. The ganglion cells and bipolar cells receive their blood supply from these arterioles and their capillaries, whereas photoreceptor elements receive nourishment from the underlying choroidal vascular bed.

These small vessels react in disease like those of corresponding size in the brain. Since the walls of the retinal arterioles are transparent with the ophthalmoscope, what is seen is a column of blood. In arteriosclerosis (usually coexistent with hypertension), the lumens of the vessels are narrowed because of fibrous tissue replacement of the media and thickening of the basement membrane. The light reflection from the vessel then has a different refractive index than the adjacent retinal tissue. Tortuosity of vessels, arteriole-venous compressions, and narrowed segments are other signs of hypertension and arteriolosclerosis. In malignant hypertension there are, in addition, cotton-wool exudates, splinter hemorrhages, and papilledema, and they correlate with similar changes in the intracranial arterioles. Atheromatous deposits, which form in larger arteries, are seldom observed in the retina because of the small size of the vessels, although occasionally atheromatous and other emboli from the carotid and aorta may reach them. Capillary-venular aneurysms may develop, most often in diabetes mellitus. Since the central retinal vein and artery share a common adventitial sheath, atheromatous plaques in the artery may result in thrombosis of the vein. Round, punctate hemorrhages always lie in the bipolar layer, and flame-shaped ones in the outer ganglion cell layer. Rupture of arterioles on the inner surface of the retina, as occurs with ruptured intracranial saccular aneurysms, hemangiomas, and other conditions causing sudden high elevations of intracranial pressure, permits blood to cover the retina and extend beneath the vitreous humor (subhyaloid hemorrhage).

Aside from visible vascular lesions, other more specific alterations of the retina may impair vision. The most important of these are tears and separations and detachments and degenerations.

1 *Degeneration of the outer receptor layer and subjacent pigment epithelium* occurs as a hereditary trait in retinitis pigmentosa and also in Laurence-Moon-Biedl syndrome, progressive ophthalmoplegia, Bassen-Kornzweig disease (Chap. 106), Refsum's disease (Chap. 323), Batten-Mayou juvenile lipid storage disease, and idiopathic senile macular degeneration (Chaps. 106 and 333).
2 *Degeneration in Bruch's membrane* (which supports the layer of pigment epithelium next to the rods and cones) and its repair by fibrosis give rise to angioid-streaks typical of pseudoxanthoma elasticum (Chap. 364), Paget's disease (Chap. 351), hyperphosphatemia, and acromegaly.
3 *Deposits of phenothiazine conjugate with the melanin* of the pigment layer with resulting degeneration of the outer retinal layers. When these drugs are used, the doses should be kept low and the central visual fields tested with small color-test objects.

Sarcoidosis, toxoplasmosis, and *histoplasmosis* involve both the retina and the choroid. The latter is the site of noninfective inflammatory reactions, often in association with iridocyclitis.

The optic nerves, chiasm, and tracts which constitute the third visual neuron can be inspected only in part, from the foveal or macular region to the optic disk. The latter reflects raised intracranial pressure (papilledema or choked disk), papillitis, (a demyelinative disease of the optic nerve), optic nerve atrophy, and glaucoma.

Central visual disturbances (caused by defects in the retina, optic nerves and tracts, lateral geniculate bodies, geniculocalcarine path, and striate cortex of occipital lobes) are evidenced by changes in the visual fields. In good light, using a cotton pledget on a stick and covering first one eye, then the other, the periphery of the patient's visual field can be compared with that of the examiner. The types of visual field defect resulting from lesions in different parts of the visual pathways are shown in Fig. 20-1. A prechiasmal lesion causes either a scotoma (an island of impaired vision within the visual field) or a cut in the peripheral part of the visual field. A small scotoma in the macular part of the visual field may seriously impair visual acuity. Demyelinative, toxic (methyl alcohol, quinine, and certain of the phenothiazine tranquilizing drugs), nutritional (so-called "tobacco-alcohol" amblyopia), and vascular diseases are the usual causes of scotomas. The toxic states are characterized by symmetric bilateral scotomas, and the nutritional disorders by more or less symmetric central scotomas (involving the fixation point) or centrocecal ones (involving both the fixation point and the blind spot). These latter scotomas are predominantly in the distribution of the papillomacular bundle, but does not establish whether the primary effect is on the nerve fibers or the ganglion cells. Demyelinative diseases are characterized by unilateral or asym-

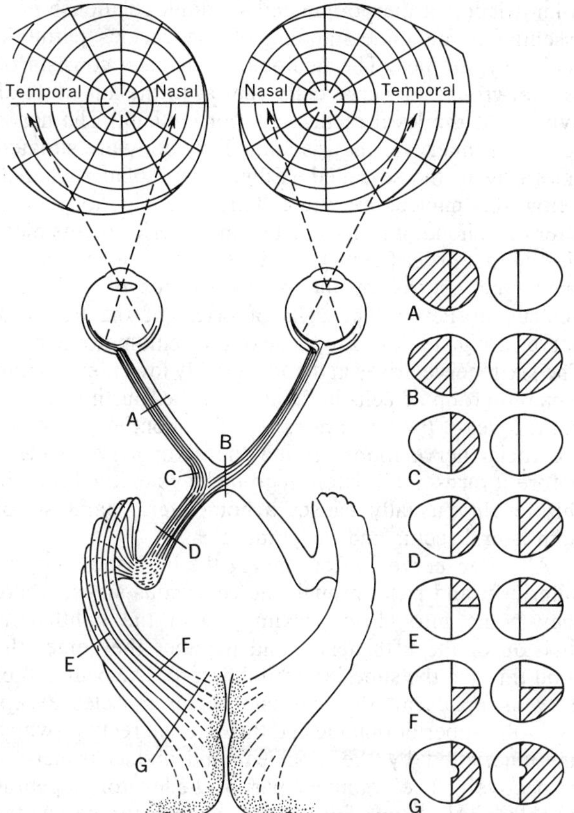

FIGURE 20-1
Diagram showing the effects on the fields of vision produced by lesions at various points along the optic pathway. A *Complete blindness in left eye;* B *bitemporal hemianopsia;* C *nasal hemianopsia of left eye;* D *right homonymous hemianopsia;* E *and* F *right upper and lower quadrant hemianopsias;* G *right homonymous hemianopsia with preservation of central vision. (From Homans,* A Textbook of Surgery, *Springfield, Ill.: Charles C Thomas, 1945)*

metric bilateral scotomas. If the lesion is near the optic disk, there may be swelling of the optic nerve head, i.e., papillitis, which can usually be distinguished from papilledema by the marked impairment of vision it produces. Vascular lesions as a rule give rise to unilateral scotomas. The lesions take the form of retinal hemorrhages or hard exudates or occluded vessels which cause infarction of the retina or, rarely, of the optic nerve. The common "cotton-wool patches" are in reality small retinal infarcts. Large zones of retinal infarction may follow occlusion of a branch of the central retinal artery.

Another common defect encountered on visual field examination is concentric constriction. This may be due to papilledema, in which case it is usually accompanied by an enlargement of the blind spot. A concentric constriction of the visual field, at first unilateral and later bilateral, and pallor of the optic disks (optic atrophy) should suggest chronic syphilitic optic neuritis. Glaucoma is another cause of this type of field defect. Tubular vision, i.e., constriction of the visual field to the same degree regardless of the distance of the visual test stimulus from the eye, is a sign of hysteria. In organic disease, e.g., chorioretinitis, the area of the constricted visual field naturally enlarges as the distance between the patient and the stimulus increases.

With most diseases of the optic nerve the optic disk will eventually become pale (optic atrophy). This may require several weeks or months to occur, as illustrated by the delay between the sudden blindness of a traumatic severance of one optic nerve and the pallor. If the optic nerve degenerates [e.g., in multiple sclerosis, Leber's hereditary optic atrophy (Chap. 333), or syphilitic optic atrophy], the disk becomes chalk-white, with sharp, clean margins. If the atrophy is secondary to papillitis or papilledema, the margins are obscure and irregular, with pigment deposits in the adjacent retina.

Hemianopsia means blindness in one-half the visual field. *Bitemporal hemianopsia* indicates a lesion of the decussating fibers of the optic chiasm and is due usually to tumor of the pituitary gland or of the infundibulum or third ventricle, to meningioma of the diaphragm of the sella, or occasionally to a large suprasellar aneurysm of the circle of Willis. *Homonymous hemianopsia* (a loss of vision in corresponding halves of the visual fields) signifies a lesion of the visual pathway behind the chiasm and, if *complete,* gives no more information than that. *Incomplete homonymous hemianopsia* has more localizing value: if the field defects in the two eyes are identical (*congruous*), the lesion is likely to be in the calcarine cortex; if *incongruous,* the visual fibers in the parietal or temporal lobe are more likely to be implicated. Since the fibers from the peripheral lower quadrants of the retina extend for a variable distance into the temporal lobe, lesions of this lobe may be accompanied by a homonymous upper quadrantic field defect. Parietal lobe lesions may affect the lower quadrants more than the upper.

If the entire optic tract or calcarine cortex on one side is destroyed, there is complete homonymous hemianopsia, including that part of the field supplied by the macula. Incomplete lesions of the optic tract and radiation usually spare central (macular) vision. Apparent macular sparing is frequently due to imperfect fixation of gaze. A lesion of the tip of one occipital lobe produces central homonymous hemianopsia because half the macular fibers of both eyes terminate there. Lesions of both occipital poles (as in embolization of the posterior cerebral arteries) result in bilateral central scotomas; and if all the calcarine cortex on both sides is completely destroyed, there is "cortical" blindness. Altitudinal or horizontal hemianopsias are more often due to lesions of the occipital lobes below or above the calcarine sulcus than to lesions of the optic chiasm.

In addition to blindness, i.e., "visual anesthesia," there is another category of visual impairment, which consists of a defect of visual perception, i.e., *visual agnosia.* The patient can see but cannot recognize objects unless he hears, smells, tastes, or palpates them. The failure of visual recognition of words alone is called *alexia.* The ability to recognize visually presented objects and words depends upon the integrity not only of the visual pathways and primary visual areas of the cerebral cortex (area 17 of Brodmann) but also of those cortical areas which lie just anterior to them (areas 18 and 19 of the occipital lobe) and the angular gyrus of the dominant hemisphere. Visual-object agnosia and alexia result from lesions of these latter areas or from a lesion of the left calcarine cortex combined with one which interrupts the fibers crossing from the right occipital lobe. These subjects are discussed further in Chaps. 21 and 27.

Other disturbances of vision include various types of distortion in which the perceived objects appear too small (micropsia), too large (macropsia), or askew. If this disturbance is in only one eye, a local retinal lesion should be suspected. When bilateral, such phenomena suggest disease of the temporal lobes; the latter may be accompanied by attacks with complex visual hallucinations which actually represent a sensory seizure (Chap. 24).

The optic nerves also contain the afferent fibers for the pupillary reflexes. These fibers leave the optic tract and terminate in the superior colliculi. A lesion of the optic nerve or tracts may abolish the pupillary light reflex; the pupil is dilated and unreactive. Cerebral lesions, on the other hand, leave the pupillary light reflex unaltered. The lack of direct reflex in the blind eye and of consensual reflex in the sound one means that the afferent limb of the reflex arc (optic nerve) is the site of the lesion. A lack of direct light reflex with retention of the consensual reflex places the lesion in the efferent limb of the reflex (the homolateral oculomotor nucleus or nerve). Loss of light reflex without visual impairment or ocular palsy (Argyll Robertson pupillary phenomenon) is thought to be due to a lesion in the superior colliculi or periaqueductal region (see below).

Amaurosis refers to blindness from any cause. *Amblyopia* refers to an impairment or loss of vision which is not due to an error of refraction or to other disease of the eye. Nyctalopia means poor twilight or night vision and is associated with vitamin A deficiency and pigmentary degeneration of the retina.

DIPLOPIA, STRABISMUS, AND DISORDERS OF THE THIRD, FOURTH, AND SIXTH NERVES *Strabismus* (squint) refers to a muscle imbalance that results in improper alignment of the two eyes. It may be due to paralysis of an eye muscle, the ocular deviation resulting from the unrestrained activity of the opposing muscle; or it may be due to inequality of tone in the muscles that yoke the two eyes together in a central position. The former is called *paralytic strabismus* and is primarily a neurologic problem; the latter is *nonparalytic strabismus* (referred to as concomitant strabismus if the squinting eye has a full range of movement) and is an ophthalmologic problem. Once binocular fusion is established, any type of ocular imbalance causes diplopia, for the reason that images then fall on disparate or noncorresponding parts of the two retinas. After a time, however, the patient learns to suppress the image of one eye. This almost invariably happens early in concomitant strabismus of congenital nature, and the person grows up with a diminished visual acuity in that eye (*amblyopia exanopsia*). The vision may remain normal in both eyes when the eyes are used alternately for fixation; this is *alternating strabismus.*

The oculomotor, trochlear, and abducens nerves innervate the extrinsic and intrinsic musculature of the eye. A knowledge of their origin and anatomic relationships is essential to an understanding of the various paralytic ocular syndromes. The oculomotor nucleus consists of several groups of nerve cells ventral to the aqueduct of Sylvius, at the level of the superior colliculi. The nerve cells that innervate the iris and ciliary body are situated anteriorly in the so-called "Edinger-Westphal nucleus." Below this nucleus are the cells for the superior rectus, inferior oblique, internal rectus, and inferior rectus muscles, in that order from above downward. Convergence is under the control of the medial groups of cells, the nucleus of Perlia. The cells of origin of the trochlear nerves are just inferior to those of the oculomotor nerves. The sixth nerve arises at a considerably lower level, from a paired group of cells in the floor of the fourth ventricle at the level of the lower pons. The intrapontine portion of the facial nerve loops around the sixth nerve nucleus before it turns anterolaterally to make its exit; a lesion in this locality usually causes a homolateral paralysis of both lateral rectus and facial muscles.

All three nerves, after leaving the brainstem, course anteriorly and pass through the cavernous sinus, where they come into close proximity with the ophthalmic division of the fifth nerve, and together they enter the orbit through the superior orbital fissure. The oculomotor nerve supplies all the extrinsic ocular muscles except two—the superior oblique and the external rectus—which are innervated by the trochlear and abducens nerves, respectively. The voluntary part of the levator palpebrae muscle is also supplied by the oculomotor nerve, the involuntary part being under the control of autonomic fibers. Other autonomic fibers supply the sphincter pupillae and the ciliary muscles (muscles of accommodation).

Although all the extraocular muscles probably participate in every movement of the eyes, particular muscles move the eyes in certain fields. The lateral rectus rotates the eye outward; the medial rectus, inward. The function of the vertical recti and the oblique muscles varies according to the position of the eye. When the eye is turned outward, the elevators and depressors of the eye are the superior and inferior recti; when the eye is turned inward, they are the inferior and superior oblique muscles, respectively. In contrast, torsion of the eyeball is effected by the oblique muscles when the eye is turned outward, and by the recti when it is turned inward.

Accurate binocular vision is achieved by the associated action of the ocular muscles, which allows a visual stimulus to fall on exactly corresponding parts of the two retinas. Conjugate movement of the eyes is controlled by centers in the cerebral cortex and brainstem. Area 8 in the frontal lobe is the center for voluntary conjugate movements of the eyes to the opposite side. In addition, there is a center in the occipital lobe concerned with contralateral following movements. Fibers from these centers pass to the opposite sides of the brainstem, where they connect with lower centers for conjugate movements: those for the right lateral gaze are thought to be in the proximity of the right abducens nucleus; those for the left lateral gaze are near the left abducens. Simultaneous innervation of one internal rectus and the other external rectus during lateral gaze is a function of the medial longitudinal fasciculus. The arrangements of nerve cells and fibers for vertical gaze and convergence are situated in the pretectal areas and paramedian zones of the midbrain tegmentum.

OCULAR MUSCLE AND GAZE PALSIES There are three types of paralysis of extraocular muscles: (1) paralysis of isolated ocular muscles, (2) paralysis of conjugate movements (gaze), and (3) syndromes of mixed gaze and ocular muscle paralysis.

Characteristic clinical disturbances result from single lesions of the third, fourth, or sixth cranial nerves. A complete third nerve lesion causes ptosis (since the levator palpebrae is supplied mainly by the third nerve), an inability to rotate the eye upward, downward, or inward; a divergent strabismus due to unopposed action of the lateral rectus muscle; a dilated nonreactive pupil (iridoplegia); and paralysis of accommodation (cycloplegia). When only the muscles of the iris and ciliary body are paralyzed, the condition is termed *internal ophthalmoplegia.* Fourth nerve lesions result in an extorsion of the eye and a weakness of downward gaze most marked when the eye is turned inwards, so that patients commonly complain of special difficulty in going downstairs. Head tilting, to the opposite shoulder, is especially characteristic of fourth nerve lesions. This maneuver causes a compensatory intorsion of the lower part of the eye, enabling the patient to obtain binocular vision. Lesions of the sixth nerve result in paralysis of abduction and a convergent strabismus, owing to the unopposed action of the internal rectus muscles. With incomplete sixth nerve palsies, turning the head toward the side of the paretic muscle may overcome diplopia. (The foregoing signs may occur with various degrees of completeness, depending on the severity and site of the lesion or lesions.)

Ocular palsies may be central, i.e., due to a lesion of the nucleus or the intramedullary portion of the cranial nerve, or peripheral. Ophthalmoplegia due to a lesion in the brainstem is usually accompanied by involvement of other cranial nerves or long tracts. Peripheral lesions, which may or may not be solitary, have a great variety of causes; the most common are *aneurysm of the circle of Willis,* tumors of the base of the brain, carcinomatosis of the meninges, herpes zoster, *syphilitic* and other chronic forms of *meningitis.* The third nerve palsy that occurs with diabetes is most often due to infarction of the third nerve, and the prognosis for recovery in such cases, as with other nonprogressive diseases of the peripheral nerve, is usually excellent. The points of difference between lesions within and outside the brainstem are tabulated in Table 20-1, and the various intramedullary and extramedullary cranial nerve syndromes are described in Tables 325-1 and 325-2. See also the diagrams in Chap. 326.

When the ocular palsy is slight, there may be no obvious squint or defect in ocular movement; yet the patient experiences diplopia. Study of the relative positions of the images of the two eyes then becomes the most accurate way of determining which muscle is involved. The image seen by the affected eye is usually less distinct, but the most reliable way of distinguishing the two images is by the red glass test. *A red glass is placed in front of the patient's right eye.* He is then asked to look at the flashlight, held at a distance of a meter, to turn his eyes in various segments of his visual fields, and to state the position of the red and white images. The relative

TABLE 20-1
Comparison of lesions within and outside the brainstem

Effect	*Lesions within the brainstem*	*Lesions external to the brainstem*
Involvement of multiple contiguous nerves	±	+
Involvement of sensorimotor tracts	+, often "alternating" or crossed sensory or motor palsies	±
Disturbance of consciousness	+	0 (+ late)
Evidence of other segmental disturbances of the brainstem such as decerebrate rigidity, tonic neck reflexes, pseudobulbar palsy	+	0 (+ late)
X-ray evidence of erosion of cranial bones or enlargement of foramens	0	+

positions of the two images are plotted as indicated in Fig. 20-2.

Three rules aid in the analysis of ocular movements by the red glass test. (1) The direction in which the distance between the images is at a maximum is the direction of action of the paretic muscle. For example, if the greatest separation is in looking to the right, either the right abductor or the left abductor muscle is weak. (2) The image projected farther to the side belongs to the paretic eye. If the patient looks to the right and the red image is farther to the right, then the right abducens muscle is weak. If the white image is to the right of the red, then the left internal rectus muscle is weak. (3) In testing vertical movements, again the image of the eye with the paretic muscle is the one projected most peripherally in the direction of eye movement. One ignores lateral separation at this time. It must be remembered that there are two elevator and two depressor muscles. The responsible muscle may be either one of the obliques or of the vertical recti muscles. For example, if the maximum separation of images occurs on looking downward and to the left, and the white image is projected farther down than the red, the paretic muscle is the left inferior rectus. If the maximum separation occurs on looking down and to the right, and the white image is lower than the red, the paretic muscle is the left superior oblique. Separation of images on looking up and to the right or left will similarly distinguish paresis of the inferior oblique and superior rectus muscles.

Monocular diplopia or polyopia may occur and is related to diseases of the lens and refractive media of the eye. The acute onset of convergence paralysis, due to lesions of the upper midbrain in the midline, may give rise to diplopia and blurred vision at a near point.

Paralysis of conjugate movement (gaze) The term *conjugate gaze,* or *conjugate movement,* refers to the

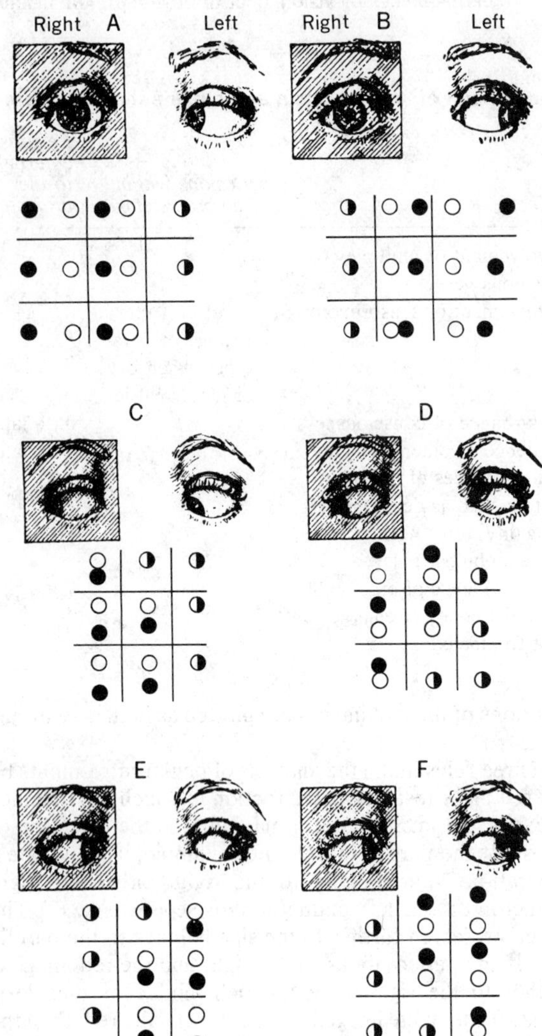

FIGURE 20-2
Diplopia fields with individual muscle paralysis. The dark glass is in front of the right eye, and the fields are projected as the patient sees the images. A *Paralysis of right external rectus. Characteristic: right eye does not move to the right. Field: horizontal homonymous diplopia increasing on looking to the right.* B *Paralysis of right internal rectus. Characteristic: right eye does not move to the left. Field: horizontal crossed diplopia increasing on looking to the left.* C *Paralysis of right inferior rectus. Characteristic: right eye does not move downward when eyes are turned to the right. Field: vertical diplopia (image of right eye lowermost) increasing on looking to the right and down.* D *Paralysis of right superior rectus. Characteristic: right eye does not move upward when eyes are turned to the right. Field: vertical diplopia (image of right eye uppermost) increasing on looking to the right and up.* E *Paralysis of right superior oblique. Characteristic: right eye does not move downward when eyes are turned to the left. Field: vertical diplopia (image of right eye lowermost) increasing on looking to left and down.* F *Paralysis of right inferior oblique. Characteristic: right eye does not move upward when eyes are turned to the left. Field: vertical diplopia (image of right eye uppermost) increasing on looking to left and up. (From Cogan,* Neurology of the Ocular Muscles, *2d ed., Springfield, Ill.: Charles C Thomas, 1956)*

simultaneous movement of the two eyes in the same direction. An acute lesion, such as an infarct, in one frontal lobe may cause paralysis of contralateral gaze, and the eyes will turn toward the side of the lesion. The ocular disorder in this circumstance is temporary (several days' duration). In bilateral frontal lesions the patient may be unable to turn his eyes voluntarily in any direction—up, down, or to the side—but retains fixation and following movements, which are believed to be occipital lobe functions. Gaze paralysis of cerebral origin is not attended by strabismus or diplopia. The usual causes are vascular occlusion with infarction, hemorrhage, and abscess or tumor of the frontal lobe. With certain extrapyramidal disorders, e.g., postencephalitic parkinsonism, Huntington's chorea, and Steele-Richardson disease, ocular movements may be limited in all directions, especially upward. Lesions of the superior colliculi and tegmentum, near the posterior commissure, interfere with voluntary upward gaze, and often movements of convergence as well as the pupillary light reflexes are abolished (Parinaud's syndrome). There also exists a pontine center for conjugate lateral gaze, probably in the vicinity of the abducens nuclei. A lesion here causes ipsilateral gaze palsy, with the eyes turning to the opposite side. Vertical and lateral gaze palsies are combined in the supranuclear ophthalmoplegia syndrome of Steele-Richardson. The palsy tends to last longer than with cerebral lesions and is frequently accompanied by other signs of pontine disease. Fully developed forms of gaze paralysis are readily discerned, but lesser degrees may be overlooked unless one pays special attention to the predominant position of the eyes and tests the ability to sustain conjugate movement.

In skew deviation, a poorly understood disorder of gaze, the eyes diverge, one looking down, the other up. The deviation is constant in all fields of gaze. It may occur with any lesion of the posterior fossa but particularly with one in the brainstem. The lesion is on the side of the lower eye.

Mixed gaze and ocular paralyses These are always a sign of intrapontine or mesencephalic disease. A lesion of the lower pons in or near the sixth nerve nucleus causes a homolateral paralysis of the lateral rectus muscle and a failure of adduction of the opposite eye, i.e., a combined paralysis of the sixth nerve and of conjugate lateral gaze. Lesions of the medial longitudinal fasciculi interfere with lateral conjugate gaze in another way. When the patient looks to the right, the left eye fails to adduct; when he looks to the left, the right eye fails to adduct. The abducting eye shows nystagmus. This condition is referred to as *internuclear ophthalmoplegia* and should always be suspected when only adduction of the eyes is affected. If the lesion is in the higher (midbrain) part of the medial longitudinal fasciculus, convergence may be lost, along with paralysis of the medial recti on attempted lateral gaze (anterior internuclear ophthalmoplegia); if the lesion is in the lower (pontine) part, convergence is normal but there may be some degree of associated limitation of conjugate lateral gaze or sixth nerve palsy (posterior internuclear ophthalmoplegia).

NYSTAGMUS This refers to involuntary rhythmic movements of the eyes; it is of two types, oscillating (pendular) and rhythmic (jerk). In jerk nystagmus, the movements are distinctly faster in one direction than the other; in pendular nystagmus, the oscillations are roughly equal in rate for the two directions, although on conjugate lateral gaze, the pendular type may resemble the jerk type, with the fast component to the side of the gaze.

In testing for nystagmus, the eyes should first be examined in the central position and then during upward, downward, and lateral movements. If nystagmus is monocular (as described below), each eye should be tested separately, with the other one covered. Labyrinthine nystagmus is most obvious when visual fixation is prevented by shielding the eyes or using Frenzel's spectacles, which also magnify the eyes and aid nystagmus detection; brainstem nystagmus and cerebellar nystagmus are brought out best by having the patient fixate on a finger. Labyrinthine nystagmus may vary with the position of the head; hence, these various tests should be performed with the head in several different positions. In particular, the postural nystagmus of Barany is evoked by hyperextension of the neck, with the patient in the supine position. Optokinetic nystagmus should be tested by asking the patient to look at a rotating cylinder on which several stripes have been painted or at a striped cloth moved across the field of vision.

A few irregular jerks are observed in many normal individuals when the eyes are turned far to the side. These so-called "nystagmoid movements" are probably similar to the tremulousness of a muscle that is contracted maximally. Occasionally a fine rhythmic nystagmus may be found in extreme lateral gaze, but if it is bilateral and disappears as the eyes move a few degrees toward the midline, it usually has no clinical significance.

Pendular nystagmus is found in a variety of conditions in which central vision is lost early in life, such as albinism and in various other diseases of the retina and refractive mediums. Occasionally it is observed in patients with multiple sclerosis and as a congenital abnormality, even without poor vision. The syndrome of miners' nystagmus, formerly a common cause of industrial disability, occurs after many years of work in comparative darkness. The oscillations of the eyes are very rapid, increase on upward gaze, and are often associated with vertigo, head tremor, and intolerance of light. *Spasmus nutans* is a specific type of pendular nystagmus of infancy and is accompanied by head nodding and occasionally by wry positions of the neck. The prognosis is good; most infants recover within a few months.

Jerk nystagmus is the commoner type. It may be lateral or vertical, particularly on ocular movement in these planes, or it may be rotary. By custom, the direction of the nystagmus is named according to the direction of the fast component. There are several varieties of jerk nystagmus. When one is watching a moving object—e.g., the passing landscape from a train window or a rotating drum with vertical stripes—a rhythmic jerk nystagmus, *optokinetic nystagmus,* normally appears. The slow phase is a result of visual fixation; the quick phase is compensatory. With unilateral cerebral lesions, particularly in the parietooccipital region, optokinetic nystagmus is lost when the moving stimulus, e.g., the drum, moves toward the side of the lesion.

Aside from optokinetic nystagmus, lateral and vertical nystagmus are most frequently due to barbiturate intoxication. Jerk nystagmus may signify disease of the labyrinthine-vestibular apparatus. Labyrinthine stimulation or irritation produces a nystagmus with the fast phase to the opposite side. The slow component reflects the effect of impulses derived from the semicircular canals, and the fast component is a corrective movement. Vestibular-labyrinthine nystagmus may be horizontal, vertical, or, most characteristically, rotary. Vertigo, nausea, vomiting, and staggering are the usual accompaniments (see Chap. 19). Brainstem lesions often cause a coarse unidirectional nystagmus, which may be horizontal or vertical; the latter is brought out usually on upward gaze and rarely on downward gaze. The presence of vertical nystagmus is pathognomonic of disease in the tegmentum of the brainstem. Vertigo is inconstant, and signs of disease of other nuclear structures and tracts in the brainstem are frequent. Upward jerk nystagmus of this type is frequent in demyelinative or vascular disease, in tumors, and in Wernicke's disease and syringobulbia. Vertical downward nystagmus is most often associated with the Arnold-Chiari malformation. Cerebellopontine angle tumors cause a coarse bilateral horizontal nystagmus, coarser to the side of the lesion. Nystagmus probably does not occur with cerebellar disease unless the fastigial nuclei and their connections with the vestibular nuclei are involved. The nystagmus that occurs only in the abducting eye and is said to be a pathognomonic sign of multiple sclerosis probably represents an incompletely developed form of internuclear ophthalmoplegia. The movement of the adducting eye (which does not show nystagmus) is impaired.

Convergence nystagmus is a rhythmic oscillation in which a slow abduction of the eyes in respect to each other is followed by a quick movement of adduction. It is usually accompanied by other types of nystagmus and by one or more features of Parinaud's syndrome. Occasionally there is also a jerky retraction movement of the eyes (*nystagmus retractorius*) or eyelids, or a maintained spasm of convergence, best brought out on attempted elevation of the eyes to command. These unusual phenomena all point to a lesion of the upper midbrain tegmentum and are usually manifestations of vascular disease or of pinealoma. *Seesaw nystagmus*—one eye moving up, the other down—is occasionally observed in conjunction with bitemporal hemianopia. Its mechanism is unknown.

Oscillopsia refers to illusory movement of the environment, in which objects seem to move back and forth, to jerk or to wiggle. It may or may not occur with turning of the eyes and consequent displacement of the image on the retina. *Opsoclonus* is the term applied to sustained, irregular, conjugate "dancing" movements of the eyes in a horizontal, rotatory, and vertical direction. The neurologic basis for these movements is not clear, but in most cases they are associated with other signs of cerebellar disease.

Ocular dysmetria consists of an overshoot of the eyes on attempted fixation, followed by several cycles of oscillations of diminishing amplitude until precise fixation is attained. The overshoot may occur on eccentric fixation or on refixation in the primary position of gaze. This sign occurs in disease of the cerebellum or its pathways and is analogous to cerebellar dysmetria of the limbs.

ALTERATIONS OF PUPILS Pupil size is determined by the balance of innervation between the dilator and constrictor fibers. The pupillodilator fibers arise in the posterior part of the hypothalamus and descend in the lateral tegmentum of the midbrain, pons, medulla, and cervical spinal cord to the eighth cervical and first thoracic segments, where they synapse with the lateral horn cells. These give rise to preganglionic fibers that synapse in the superior cervical ganglion; the postganglionic fibers course along the internal carotid artery and traverse the cavernous sinus to join the first division of the trigeminal nerve, finally reaching the eyes as the long ciliary nerves. The pupilloconstrictor fibers arise in the nucleus of Edinger-Westphal, join the oculomotor nerve, and synapse in the ciliary ganglion with the postganglionic neurons that innervate the iris and ciliary body.

The pupils are usually equal in size, though if the eyes are turned to one side, the pupil of the abducting eye dilates slightly. Pupil size varies with light intensity; as one pupil constricts under a bright light (direct reflex), the other unexposed pupil does likewise (consensual reflex). Pupillary constriction is also part of the act of convergence and accommodation for near objects.

Interruption of the sympathetic fibers either centrally, between the hypothalamus and their point of exit from the spinal cord (first thoracic segment), or peripherally, (superior cervical ganglion in the neck or along the carotid artery), results in miosis and ptosis (because of paralysis of the levator palpebrae), with loss of sweating of the face, and occasionally enophthalmos (Bernard-Horner syndrome). Stimulation or irritation of the pupillodilator fibers has the opposite effect, i.e., lid retraction, slight proptosis, and dilatation of the pupil. The ciliospinal pupillary reflex, evoked by pinching the neck, is effected through these efferent sympathetic fibers. Abnormal dilatation of the pupils (mydriasis), often with loss of pupillary light reflexes, may result from midbrain lesions and is a frequent finding in cases of deep coma. Extreme constriction of the pupils (miosis) is commonly observed with pontine lesions, presumably because of bilateral interruption of the pupillodilator fibers.

The functional integrity of the sympathetic and parasympathetic nerve endings in the iris may be determined by the use of certain drugs. Atropine and homatropine dilate the pupils by paralyzing the parasympathetic nerve endings; physostigmine and pilocarpine constrict them, the former by inhibiting cholinesterase activity at the neuromuscular junction, and the latter by direct stimulation of the sphincter muscle of the iris. Cocaine dilates the pupils by stimulating the sympathetic nerve endings. Morphine acts centrally to constrict the pupils.

In chronic syphilitic meningitis and other forms of late syphilis, particularly tabes dorsalis, the pupils are usually small, irregular, and unequal; they do not dilate properly in response to mydriatic drugs and fail to react to light, although they do constrict on accommodation. In some cases there is an associated atrophy of the iris. This is known as the *Argyll Robertson pupil*. The exact locality of the lesion is not certain; it is generally believed to be in the tectum of the midbrain proximal to the oculomotor nuclei, where the descending pupillodilator fibers are in close proximity to the light-reflex fibers. The possibility of a partial third nerve lesion or a lesion of the ciliary ganglion has not been excluded. A dissociation of the light reflex from the accommodation-convergence reaction is sometimes observed with other midbrain lesions, e.g., pinealoma, multiple sclerosis, and diabetes mellitus; in these diseases miosis, irregularity of pupils, and failure to respond to a mydriatic are not constantly present. Another interesting pupillary abnormality is the myotonic reaction, sometimes referred to as *Adie's pupil*. The patient may complain of blurring of vision or may have suddenly noticed that one pupil is larger than the other. The reaction to light and convergence are absent if tested in the customary manner, although the size of the pupil will change slowly on prolonged stimulation. Once contracted or dilated, the pupils remain in that state for some minutes. The affected pupil reacts promptly to the usual mydriatic and miotic drugs but is usually sensitive to a 2.5% solution of Mecholyl, a strength that will not affect a normal pupil. The myotonic pupil usually appears during the third or fourth decade of life; it may be associated with absence of knee or ankle jerks and hence be mistaken for tabes dorsalis.

Ocular movement, pupillary contraction, and visual acuity may be affected by diseases which alter the contents of the orbit. Usually this is accompanied by bilateral exophthalmos, as in thyroid or pituitary disease (see Chap. 85), or unilateral exophthalmos with orbital tumors (dermoids, adenoma of lacrimal gland, optic nerve glioma, neurofibroma, metastatic carcinoma, meningioma) or granuloma, or cavernous sinus thrombosis (see Chap. 329). Progressive paralysis of the eyelids, which may obstruct vision, occurs separately or as part of an external paralysis, as in the ocular dystrophy of Kiloh and Nevin or in oculopharyngeal dystrophy.

DISTURBANCES OF HEARING *Tinnitus* and *deafness* are frequent symptoms and always indicate disease of the ear or of the auditory nerve and its central connections.

Tinnitus, or ringing in the ears, is a purely subjective phenomenon and may also be reported as a buzzing, whistling, hissing, or roaring sound. It is a very common symptom in adults and may be of no significance, as, for example, when a hissing sound is due to wax in the external auditory canal or a blocked eustachian tube. On the other hand, it is regularly associated with disease of the eighth nerve, inner ear, or ossicles. Severe and prolonged tinnitus in the presence of normal hearing is very rare. If tinnitus is localized to one ear and is described as having a tonal character, such as ringing or a bell-like tone, and particularly if there is reduced hearing with the recuitment phenomenon (see below), it is probably cochlear in origin. Noises described as rushing water or escaping steam point more to disease of the nerve or even the brainstem. Clicking sounds are caused by intermittent contraction of the tensor tympani. A pulsating tinnitus synchronous with the pulse may be related to an intracranial vascular malformation; however, this symptom must be carefully judged, since introspective persons often report hearing their pulse when lying with one ear on a pillow. Certain drugs such as salicylates and quinine produce tinnitus and transient deafness. Nervous persons are less tolerant of tinnitus than more stable ones; depressed or anxious patients may demand relief from tinnitus that has existed for years.

Examination of hearing should always begin with inspection of the external auditory canal and the tympanic membrane. A ticking watch or whispered words are suitable means of testing hearing at the bedside, the opposite ear being closed by the finger. If there is any suspicion of deafness or a complaint of tinnitus or vertigo, or if the patient is a child with a speech defect, then hearing must be tested further. This can be done with the use of tuning forks of different frequencies, but the most accurate results are obtained by the use of an electric audiometer and the construction of an audiogram which reveals the entire range of hearing at a glance.

Deafness is frequent. In the United States it is estimated that there are more than 6 million persons with hearing loss; in one-third to one-half these persons the loss is hereditary. The deafness is of two types: (1) nerve deafness (also called sensorineural), due to cochlear disease or interruption of nerve fibers, and (2) conduction deafness, due to disease of the middle ear, such as otosclerosis or chronic otitis, or to occlusion of the external auditory canal or eustachian tube. In differentiating these two types, the tuning fork tests are of value. When a vibrating fork of 256 DV frequency is held several inches from the ear (the test for air conduction), sound waves can be appreciated only as they are transmitted through the middle ear and will be reduced with disease in this location. When the fork is applied to the skull (test for bone conduction), the sound waves are conveyed directly to the cochlea, without the intervention of the middle ear apparatus, and will therefore not be reduced or lost. Normally air conduction is better than bone conduction. These principles form the basis for several tests of auditory function.

In *Weber's test,* the vibrating fork is applied to the forehead in the midline. In middle ear deafness the sound is localized in the affected ear; in nerve deafness, in the normal ear. In *Rinné's test* the fork is applied to the mastoid process, the other ear being closed by the observer's finger. At the moment the sound ceases the fork is held at the auditory meatus. In middle ear deafness the sound cannot be heard by air conduction after bone conduction has ceased (abnormal or negative Rinné's test). In nerve deafness the reverse is true (normal or positive Rinné's test), although both air and bone conduction may be quantitatively decreased. In *Schwabach's test,* the patient's bone conduction is compared with that of a normal observer. In general, high-pitched tones are lost in nerve deafness and low-pitched ones in middle ear deafness, but there are frequent exceptions to this rule.

The following audiologic tests, taken together, help distinguish between cochlear and retrocochlear (nerve) lesions: (1) *auditory recruitment:* the difference in hearing between the two ears is estimated, and the loudness of the stimulus delivered to each ear is then increased by regular increments. In nonrecruiting deafness (characteristic of nerve trunk lesion) the original difference in hearing persists in all comparisons of loudness above threshold. In recruiting deafness (as occurs in Ménière's disease) the more defective ear gains in loudness and finally is equal to the better one. (2) *Speech discrimination:* retrocochlear lesions are indicated by scores above 25 percent. (3) Short-increment sensitivity index (SISI), in which the patient responds to a series of twenty 1-decibel (dB) increments in amplitude superimposed on a steady tone of the same frequency presented at a sensation level of 20 dB. The patient's score is the percentage of these 20 increments which he is able to detect at a given frequency. Low SISI scores, below 60 percent, point to an end-organ lesion. (4) Threshold sensitivity recorded via *Békésy audiometry* for both continuous and interrupted tonal stimuli: four types of tracing may be obtained; the type II tracing is obtained in patients with end-organ lesions, and type III or IV, usually the former, characterizes retrocochlear lesions. (5) Threshold tone decay: this test quantifies auditory adaptation and requires only a conventional pure tone audiometer. Retrocochlear lesions yield greater amounts of decay than cochlear ones.

The common causes of middle ear deafness are otitis media, otosclerosis, and rupture of the eardrum. Nerve deafness has many causes. The internal ear may be aplastic from birth (hereditary deaf-mutism), or it may be damaged by rubella in the pregnant mother. Acute purulent meningitis or chronic infection spreading from the middle ear may cause nerve deafness in childhood. The auditory nerve may be involved by tumors of the cerebellopontine angle or by syphilis. Deafness may also result from a demyelinative plaque in the brainstem. A large series of genetically determined syndromes which feature a neural type of deafness, some congenital, others progressive, has recently come to light (see article by Konigsmark). The most interesting of these are dominant progressive nerve deafness, dominant unilateral deafness, dominant low-frequency hearing loss, recessive congenital deafness, sex-linked congenital neural deafness, several types of deafness (neural and conductive) with malformations of external ears, face, and neck (Treacher-Collins disease and Engelmann's diaphyseal dysplasia); hereditary deafness with nephritis (Alport's syndrome); hereditary deafness with goiter (Pendred's disease); hereditary heart disease with deafness; hereditary deafness with renal disease and digital anomalies; hereditary deafness with various combinations of mental retardation, retinitis pigmentosa, and polyneuropathy (as in Hallgren's disease, Alstrom's disease, Refsum's disease); hereditary deafness with skin abnormalities such as albinism, lentigines, piebaldness, white forelock (Waardenburg's disease), onchydystrophy and pegged teeth, atopic dermatitis, anhydrosis.

Of the types of progressive conduction deafness, hereditary otosclerosis is the most frequent (cause of 50 percent of deafness in adulthood). Hysterical deafness may be difficult to distinguish from organic disease. In the case of bilateral deafness, the distinction can be made by observing a blink (cochleoorbicular reflex) or an alteration in skin sweating (psychogalvanic skin reflex) in response to a loud sound. Unilateral hysterical deafness may be detected by an audiometer, with both ears connected, or by whispering into the bell of a stethoscope attached to the patient's ears, closing first one and then the other tube without the patient's knowledge.

In otosclerosis and hereditary sensorineural deafness, vestibular function is usually retained (caloric responses are normal).

REFERENCES

BENDER MB: Neurophthalmology, in *Clinical Neurology*, vol. 1, chap. 4, ed AB Baker, New York: Hoeber-Harper, 1962

COGAN DG: *Neurology of the Ocular Muscles*, 2d ed., Springfield, Ill.: Charles C Thomas, 1956

KONIGSMARK BW: Medical progress. Hereditary deafness in man. N Engl J Med 281:713–720; 774–778; 827–832, 1969

TILLMAN TW: Special hearing tests in otoneurologic diagnosis. Arch Otolaryngol 89:25–30, 1969

21 DISORDERS OF SENSATION

MAURICE VICTOR
RAYMOND D. ADAMS

Loss or perversion of somatic sensation not infrequently is the principal manifestation of disease of the nervous system. The reason for this is clear enough, since the major anatomic pathways of the sensory system are distinct from those of the motor system and may be selectively disturbed by disease. An understanding of these sensory disorders may provide important leads to neurologic diagnosis.

Ideally, one should be familiar with the sensory organs in the skin and deep structures, the distribution of the peripheral nerves and the spinal roots, and the pathways by which the sensory impulses are conveyed through the spinal cord and brainstem to the thalamus and parietal lobe cortex. These topics were introduced in Chap. 5.

GENERAL CONSIDERATIONS Unfortunately, space does not permit here a more detailed review of the anatomy of the sensory system or of its physiology. The interested reader may turn to the references at the end of the chapter. The cutaneous distribution of sensory spinal roots and peripheral nerves may be observed in Figs. 21-1 and 21-2.

Disorders of the somatic sensory apparatus pose special problems for the patient. He is confronted with derangements of sensation which may be unlike anything he has previously experienced, and he has few words in his vocabulary to describe what he feels. He may say that a limb feels "numb" and "dead" when in fact he means it is weak. Observant individuals may occasionally discover a loss of sensation, for example, inability to feel discomfort on touching an object hot enough to blister the skin or unawareness of articles of clothing and other objects in contact with the skin. But more often disease has induced a new and unnatural series of sensory experiences. If nerves, spinal roots, or spinal tracts are only partially interrupted, a touch may arouse tingling or pricking (Novocain feeling), meaning presumably that at least some of the remaining touch and pain fibers are functional but are acting abnormally. Tightness and drawing and pulling sensations, a feeling of a band or girdle around the limb or trunk, are common with partial involvement of pressure fibers. Similarly, burning and pain (causalgia) may represent overactivity of surviving thermal and pain fibers. The responsible lesion may be in the peripheral nerve, the lateral spinothalamic tract in the spinal cord or brainstem, or the thalamus. Also, hyperesthesia and hyperpathia are frequent. These abnormal sensations are called *paresthesias*, or *dysesthesias*, if they are unpleasant; and their character and distribution inform us of the anatomy of the lesion involving the sensory system.

EXAMINATION OF SENSATION The examination of sensation is the most difficult part of the neurologic examination. For one thing, test procedures are relatively crude and inadequate. And, embarrassingly often, no objective sensory loss can be demonstrated despite symptoms that clearly indicate the presence of such a deficit. Also, a response to a sensory stimulus is difficult to evaluate objectively, since the examiner's conclusions depend on the patient's interpretations of sensory experiences. This presupposes a general responsiveness, alert-

FIGURE 21-1
Distribution of the sensory spinal roots on the surface of the body. (From G Holmes, Introduction to Clinical Neurology, *2d ed., Baltimore: Williams & Wilkins, 1952)*

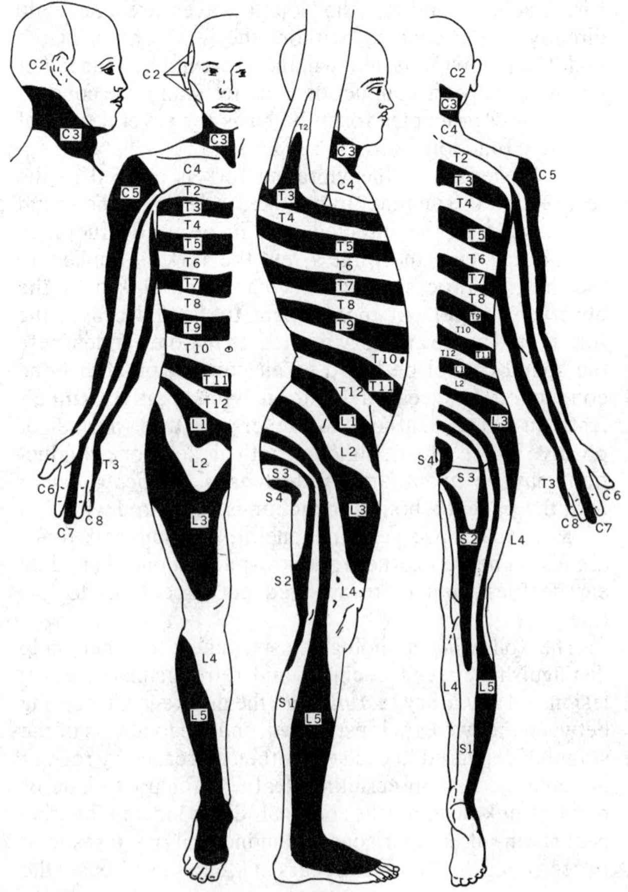

ness, and a desire to cooperate, as well as intelligence and a certain level of education. Hypersuggestibility and fatigue may interfere with the obtaining of accurate test data.

The detail in which sensation is tested will be determined by the clinical situation. If the patient has no sensory complaints, it is sufficient to examine vibration and position sense in the fingers and toes, to test the appreciation of pain over the face, trunk, and extremities, and to determine whether the sensory findings are the same in symmetric parts of the body. A rough survey of this sort may detect sensory defects of which the patient is unaware. On the other hand, more thorough testing is in order if the patient has complaints referable to the sensory system, or if there is localized atrophy or weakness, ataxia, trophic changes of joints, or painless ulcers.

A few other general principles should be mentioned. One should not press the sensory examination in the presence of fatigue, for an inattentive patient is a poor witness. The examiner must also avoid suggesting symptoms to the patient. After having explained in the simplest terms what is required, he should interpose as few questions and remarks as possible. Consequently, the patient must not be asked, "Do you feel that?" each time he is touched; he should simply be told to say "yes" or "sharp" every time he has been touched or feels pain. The patient should not be permitted to see the part under examination. For short tests it is sufficient that he close his eyes; during more detailed testing it is preferable to screen his eyes from the part being examined. Finally, the findings of the sensory examination should be accurately recorded on a chart.

Sensation is frequently classified as *superficial* (cutaneous, exteroceptive) and *deep* (proprioceptive); the former comprises the modalities of light touch, pain, and

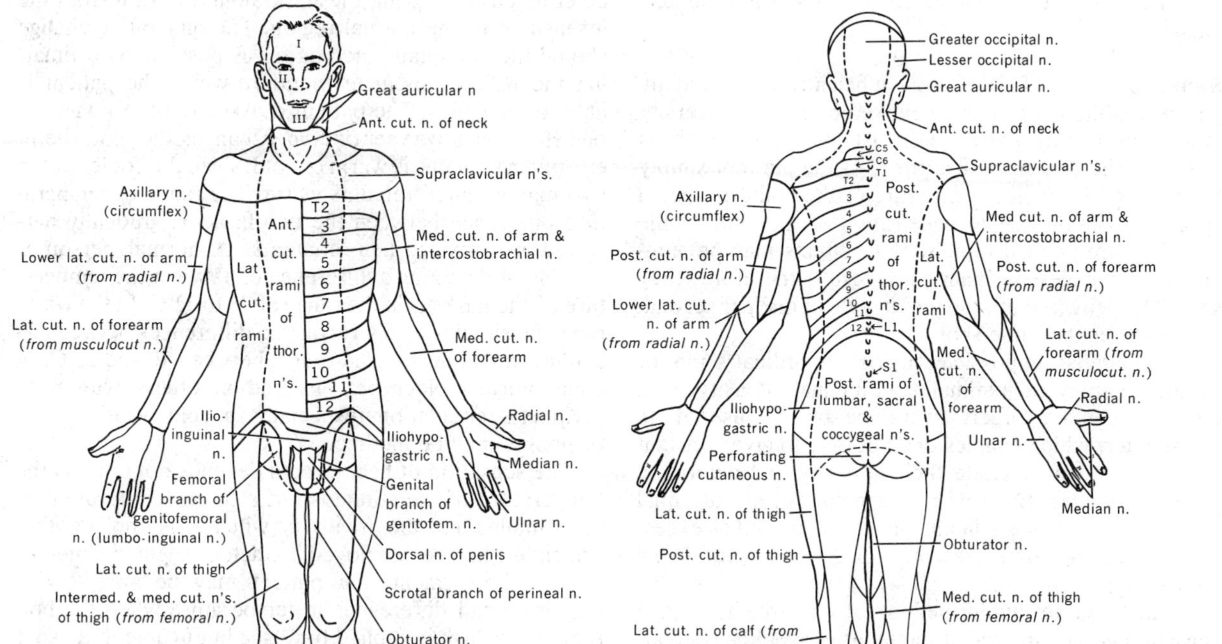

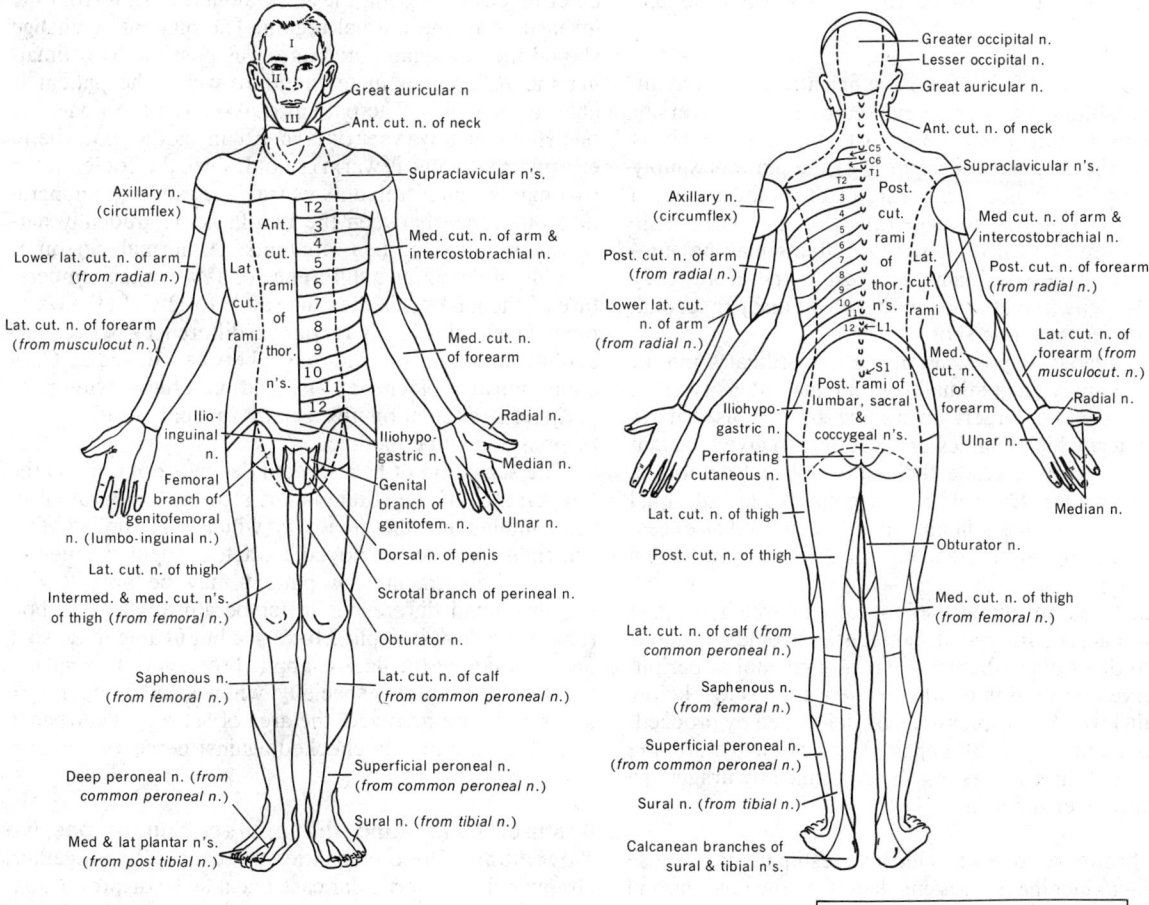

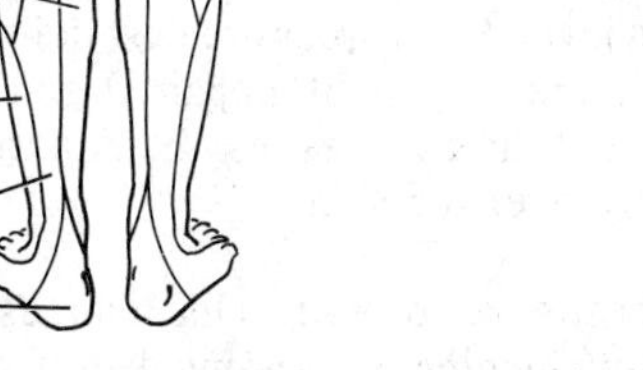

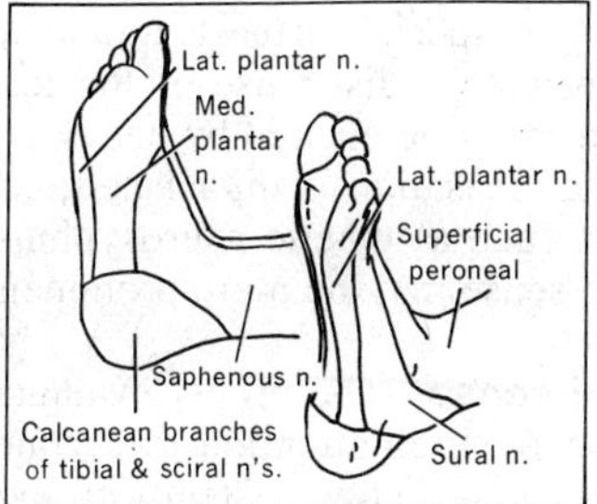

FIGURE 21-2
The cutaneous fields of peripheral nerves. (From Haymaker and Woodhall, Peripheral nerve injuries, in Principles of Diagnosis, *2d ed., Philadelphia: Saunders, 1953)*

temperature; the latter includes the sense of position, passive motion, vibration, and deep pain.

Sense of touch This is usually tested with a wisp of cotton. The patient is first made acquainted with the nature of the stimulus by applying it to a normal part of the body. Then he is asked to say "yes" each time various other parts are touched. A patient simulating sensory loss may say "no" in response to a tactile stimulus. Cornified areas of skin, such as the soles and palms, will require a heavier stimulus than normal, and the hair-clad parts a lighter one because of the numerous nerve endings around the follicle. The patient is more sensitive to a moving contactual stimulus of any kind than a stationary one. The application of the examiner's or preferably the patient's finger tips is a useful method of mapping out an area of tactile loss, as Trotter originally showed.

More precise testing is possible by using a von Frey hair. By this method, a stimulus of constant strength can be applied and the threshold for touch sensation determined.

Sense of pain This is most efficiently estimated by pinprick, although it may be evoked by a great diversity of noxious stimuli. The patient must understand that he is to report the degree of sharpness of the pin, not simply the feeling of contact or pressure of the point or even a special sensation due to penetration of the skin. If the pinpricks are applied rapidly, their effects may be summated and excessive pain may result; therefore, they should be delivered not too rapidly, about one per second, and not over the same spot.

It is almost impossible, using an ordinary pin or needle, to apply each stimulus with equal intensity. This difficulty can be largely overcome by the use of an algesimeter, which enables one not only to give constant stimuli but also to grade their intensity and determine threshold values. Even when the pinpricks are of equal intensity, an isolated stimulus may be reported as excessively sharp, apparently because of direct contact with a pain spot.

If an area of diminished or absent touch or pain sensation is encountered, its boundaries should be demarcated to determine whether it has a segmental or peripheral nerve distribution or whether sensation is lost below a certain level. Such areas are best delineated by proceeding from the region of impaired sensation toward the normal, and the changes may be confirmed by dragging a pin lightly over the skin.

Deep pressure sense One can estimate this sense simply by pinching or pressing deeply on the tendons and muscles; no special virtue is attached to the traditional and somewhat sadistic use of the testicle for this test. Pain can often be elicited by heavy pressure even when superficial sensation is diminished; conversely, in some diseases, such as tabetic neurosyphilis, the loss of deep pressure sense may be more prominent.

Thermal sense The proper evaluation of this form of sensation requires attention to certain details of procedure. One may fail consistently to evoke a sensation of hot or cold, if small test objects are used. The perception of thermal stimuli is relatively delayed, especially if the test objects are applied only lightly and momentarily against the skin. At a temperature below 10°C or above 50°C, sensations of cold or warmth become confused with pain. As the temperature of the test object approaches that of the skin, the patient's response will be modified by the temperature of the skin itself.

The following procedure for testing thermal sensation is therefore suggested. The areas of skin to be tested should be exposed for some time before the examination. The test objects should be large, preferably Erlenmeyer flasks containing hot and cold water. Thermometers, which extend into the water through the flask stoppers, indicate the temperature of the water at the moment of testing. At first, extreme degress of heat and cold (e.g., 10 and 45°C) may be employed to delineate roughly an area of thermal sensory disturbance; the patient will report that the flask feels "less hot" or "less cold" over such an area than over a normal part. If areas of impaired sensation are found, the borders may be accurately determined by moving the flask along the skin from the insensitive to the normal region. The qualitative change should then be quantitated as far as possible by estimating the *differences in temperature* which the patient is able to recognize. The patient is asked to report whether one stimulus is *warmer or colder* than another not whether a given stimulus is warm or cold, since the cooler of the two may be interpreted as warm. The range of temperature difference between the two flasks is gradually narrowed by mixing their contents. A normal person is capable of detecting a difference of 1° when the temperature of the flasks is in the range of 28 to 32°C. In the warm range he should readily recognize differences between 35 and 40°C, and in the cold range, between 10 and 20°C. In many normal older persons and in others with poor peripheral circulation (especially in cold weather), the responses may be modified.

The sensation of heat or cold depends not only on the temperature of the stimulus but also on the duration of the stimulus and the area over which it is applied. This principle may be employed to detect slight degrees of sensory impairment; the patient may be able to distinguish small differences in temperature when the bottom of the flask is applied for 3 sec but unable to do so if only the side of the flask is applied for 1 sec. Throughout the test procedure, especially when small temperature differences are involved, the area of sensory disturbance should be continually checked against perception in normal parts.

Postural sense and the appreciation of passive movement These modalities are usually lost together, although in any particular case one may be disproportionately affected.

Abnormalities of postural sensation may be revealed in several ways. When the patient extends his arms in front of him and closes his eyes, the affected arm will wander from its original position; if the fingers are spread apart, they may undergo a series of slow-changing postures ("piano-playing" movements, or *pseudoathetosis*). In attempting to touch the tip of the nose with his index finger, the patient may miss the target repeatedly.

The lack of position sense in the legs may be demonstrated by displacing the limb from its original position and asking the patient to point to his large toe. If postural sensation is defective in both legs, the patient will be unable to maintain his balance with feet together and eyes closed (Romberg's sign). This sign should be interpreted with caution. Even a normal person in the Romberg position will sway slightly more with his eyes closed than open. A patient with lack of balance due to motor disorders or cerebellar disease will also sway more if his visual cues are removed. Only if there is a marked discrepancy between the state of balance with eyes open and closed can one confidently state that the patient shows Romberg's sign, i.e., loss of proprioceptive sensation. Mild degrees of unsteadiness in nervous or suggestible patients may be overcome by diverting their attention, e.g., by having them alternately touch the index finger of each hand to their nose while standing with their eyes closed.

The appreciation of passive movement is first tested in the fingers and toes, and the defect, when present, is reflected maximally in these parts. It is important to grasp the digit firmly at the sides opposite the plane of movement; otherwise the pressure applied by the examiner in displacing the digit may allow the patient to identify the direction of movement. This applies to the testing of the more proximal segments of the limb as well. The patient should be instructed to report each movement as "up" or "down" in relation to the previous stationary position. It is useful to demonstrate the test with a large and easily identified movement, but once the idea is clear to the patient, the smallest detectable changes in position should be tested. The range of movement normally appreciated in the digits is said to be as little as 1°. Clinically, however, defective appreciation of passive movement is judged by comparison with a normal limb or, if bilaterally defective, on the basis of what the examiner has through experience learned to regard as normal. Slight impairment may be disclosed by a slow response or, if the digit is displaced very slowly, by a relative unawareness that movements have occurred; or after the digit has been displaced in the same direction several times, the patient may misjudge the first movement in the opposite direction; or after the examiner has moved the toe, the patient may make a number of small voluntary movements of the toe, in an apparent attempt to determine its position or the direction of the movement.

The sense of vibration This is a composite sensation comprising touch and rapid alterations of deep pressure sense. Its conduction depends on both cutaneous and deep afferent fibers which ascend in the dorsal columns of the cord. It is therefore rarely affected by lesions of single nerves but will be disturbed in cases of polyneuritis and disease of the dorsal columns, medial lemniscus, and thalamus. For this reason, vibration and position sense are usually lost together, although one of them (usually vibration sense) may be affected disproportionately. With advancing age, vibration sense may be diminished at the toes and ankles.

Vibration sense is tested by placing a tuning fork with a low rate (and long duration) of vibration (128 DV) over the bony prominences. The examiner must make sure that the patient responds to the vibration, not simply to the pressure of the fork. Although there are mechanical devices to quantitate vibration sense, it is sufficient for clinical purposes to compare the point tested with a normal part of the patient or the examiner. Thus, if the fork is allowed to run down until vibration is no longer appreciated but is still felt at an analogous point on the opposite limb, and if this finding is consistent, one can be certain of a significant impairment of vibration sense. In a similar way, the appreciation of vibration at the tibial tuberosity after it has disappeared in the ankle, or at the iliac portion of the spine after it has disappeared at the tibial tuberosity, is an indication of a peripheral nerve lesion. The level of vibration-sense loss due to spinal cord lesions may be estimated by placing the fork over successive vertebral spines.

DISCRIMINATIVE SENSORY FUNCTIONS Damage to the sensory cortex or to the sensory projections from thalamus to cortex results in a special type of disturbance that affects mainly the patient's ability to make sensory discriminations. Lesions in these structures may disturb postural sense but leave the so-called "primary modalities" (touch, pain, temperature, and vibration sense) relatively little affected. In such a situation, or if a cerebral lesion is suspected on other grounds, discriminative function should be tested further by the following tests:

Two-point discrimination The ability to distinguish two points from one is tested by using a compass, the points of which should be blunt and applied simultaneously and painlessly. The distance at which such a stimulus can be recognized as double varies greatly; 1 mm at the tip of the tongue, 2 to 3 mm on the lips, 3 to 5 mm at the fingertips, 8 to 15 mm on the palms, 20 to 30 mm on the dorsa of the hands and feet, and 4 to 7 cm on the body surface. It is characteristic of the patient with a lesion of the sensory cortex to mistake two points for one, although occasionally the opposite occurs.

Cutaneous localization and number writing The ability to localize cutaneous stimuli is tested by touching various parts of the patient's body and asking him to point to the part touched or to the corresponding part on the examiner's limb. Recognition of numbers or letters (these should be larger than 4 cm) or of the direction of lines drawn on the skin also depends on localization of tactile stimuli.

Appreciation of texture, size, and shape Appreciation of texture depends mainly on cutaneous impressions, but the recognition of shape and size of objects is based on impressions from deeper receptors as well. The lack of recognition of shape and form, therefore, though frequently found with cortical lesions, may also be present with lesions of the spinal cord and brainstem because of interruption of tracts transmitting postural and tactile sensation. The latter type of sensory defect, called stereoanesthesia, should be distinguished from astereognosis, which connotes an inability to identify an object by palpation, the primary sense data (touch, pain temperature, and vibration) being intact. In practice, a pure astereognosis is rarely encountered, and the term is employed where the impairment of superficial and vibratory sensation in the hands is of insufficient severity to account for the defect. Defined in this way, astereognosis may be the product of a lesion in *either* hemisphere, in the postcentral gyrus or the thalamoparietal projections. Astereognosis may be confused with *tactile agnosia.* The latter disorder is due to a lesion lying posterior to the postcentral gyrus of the *dominant* parietal lobe, and causes an inability to recognize an object by touch or handling in *both* hands. In contrast to tactile agnosia the patient with astereognosis may appreciate the size, form, consistency, and weight of an object placed in his hand, but he cannot identify it.

Extinction of sensory stimuli and sensory inattention In response to bilateral simultaneous testing of symmetric parts, the patient may acknowledge only the stimulus on the sound side, or he may improperly localize the stimulus on the affected side, whereas stimuli applied to each side separately are properly appreciated. This phenomenon of extinction, or cortical inattention, is characteristic of parietal lobe lesions, the symptoms of which are considered in Chap. 27.

A few other terms require definition, since they may be encountered in reading about sensation. Most of them are pedantic, and it is recommended that the simplest terms possible be used. Anesthesia refers to a loss of all forms of sensation and hypesthesia to a diminution of all sensation. Loss or impairment of specific cutaneous sensations is indicated by an appropriate prefix or suffix, e.g., thermoanesthesia or thermohypesthesia, analgesia (loss of pain) or hypalgesia, tactile anesthesia (loss of sense of touch), and pallanesthesia (loss of vibratory sense). The term hyperesthesia requires special mention; although it implies a heightened receptiveness of the nervous system, careful testing will usually demonstrate an underlying sensory defect, i.e., an elevated threshold to tactile, painful, or thermal stimuli; once the stimulus is perceived, however, it may have a severely painful or unpleasant quality (hyperpathia).

SENSORY SYNDROMES Sensory changes may be due to interruption of a single peripheral nerve. These changes will vary with the composition of the nerve involved, depending on whether it is predominantly muscular, cutaneous, or mixed. In lesions of cutaneous nerves, the area of tactile anesthesia is more extensive than the one for pain, because of greater overlapping of pain fibers. Also, because of overlap from adjacent nerves, the area of sensory loss following division of a cutaneous nerve is always less than its anatomic distribution. If a large area of skin is involved, the sensory defect characteristically consists of a central portion, in which all forms of cutaneous sensation are lost, surrounded by a zone of partial loss, which becomes less marked as one proceeds from the center to the periphery. The sense of deep pressure and passive movement is intact because it is carried by special nerve fibers from subcutaneous structures and joints. Along the margin of the hypesthetic zone the skin becomes excessively sensitive. A light contact may be felt as a smarting, mildly painful sensation. According to Weddell, this is because of collateral regeneration from surrounding healthy nerves into the denervated region (see Chap. 5).

Particular types of lesion differentially affect the fibers in a sensory nerve. Compression paralyzes large touch and pressure fibers more than the small pain, thermal, and autonomic motor fibers; procaine and cocaine have opposite effects.

In lesions involving the brachial and lumbosacral plexuses, the sensory disturbance is no longer confined to the territory of a single nerve and is accompanied by muscle weakness and reflex change.

Sensory changes due to multiple nerve involvement (polyneuropathy) In most instances of polyneuropathy the sensory changes are accompanied by varying degrees of motor and reflex loss. Usually the sensory impairment is symmetric, with notable exceptions in some instances of diabetic and periarteritic neuropathy. Since the longest and largest fibers tend to be the most affected, the sensory loss is most severe over the feet and legs and less severe over the hands. The abdomen, thorax, and face are spared except in the most severe cases. The sensory loss usually involves all the modalities, and although it is manifestly difficult to equate the impairment of pain, touch, temperature, vibration, and position sense, one of these may seemingly be impaired out of proportion to the others (exceptions are discussed in Chap. 323). One cannot accurately predict, from the patient's symptoms, which mode of sensation will be disproportionately affected. The term glove-and-stocking anesthesia is frequently employed to describe the sensory loss of polyneuropathy and draws attention to the predominantly distal pattern of involvement. It is an inaccurate term insofar as the border between normal and impaired sensation is not so sharp; the sensory loss shades off gradually. In hysteria, by contrast, the border between normal and absent sensation is usually sharp.

Sensory changes due to involvement of multiple spinal nerve roots Because of considerable overlap from adjacent roots, division of a single sensory root does not produce complete loss of sensation in any area of skin. Compression of a single sensory cervical or lumbar root (e.g., in herniated intervertebral disks) causes varying degrees of impairment of cutaneous sensation in a segmental pattern, however. When two or more roots have been completely divided, a zone of sensory loss can be found in which reduction of pain perception is greater in extent than touch. Surrounding the area of complete loss is a narrow zone of partial loss, in which a raised threshold accompanied by overreaction (*hyperpathia*) may or may not be demonstrated. The presence of muscle paralysis atrophy and reflex loss indicates involvement of ventral roots as well.

The tabetic syndrome This results from damage to the large proprioceptive and other fibers of the posterior lumbosacral roots. It is usually caused by neurosyphilis, less often by meningeal tumors, diabetes mellitus, etc. Numbness or paresthesias and lightning pains are frequent complaints, and areflexia, atonicity of the bladder, abnormalities of gait (Chap. 19), and hypotonia without muscle weakness are found on examination. The sensory loss may consist only of loss of vibration and position sense in the lower extremities, but in severe cases, loss or impairment of superficial or deep pain sense or of touch may be added. The feet and legs are most affected, much less often the arms and trunk.

Complete spinal sensory syndromes In a complete transverse lesion of the spinal cord, all forms of sensation are abolished below a level that corresponds to the lesion. There may be a narrow zone of "hyperesthesia" at the upper margin of the anesthetic zone. It is important to remember that during the evolution of such a lesion there may be a discrepancy between the level of the lesion and that of the sensory loss, the latter ascending as the lesion progresses. This can be understood if one conceives of a lesion evolving from the periphery to the center of the cord, affecting first the outermost fibers carrying pain and temperature sensation from the legs. Conversely, a lesion advancing from the center of the cord may affect these modalities in the reverse order.

Partial spinal sensory syndromes (hemisection of the spinal cord—Brown-Séquard syndrome) In rare instances disease is confined to one side of the spinal cord; pain and heat sensation are affected on the opposite side, and proprioceptive sensation is affected on the same side as the lesion. The loss of pain and temperature sensation begins two or three segments below the lesion. An associated motor paralysis on the side of the lesion completes the syndrome. Tactile sensation is not involved, since the fibers from one side of the body are distributed in tracts (posterior columns and anterior spinothalamic) on both sides of the cord.

Lesions of the central gray matter (syringomyelic syndrome) Since fibers conducting pain and temperature cross the cord in the anterior commissure, a lesion in this location will characteristically abolish these modalities on one or both sides but will spare tactile sensation. The commonest cause of such a lesion is syringomyelia, less often, tumor and hemorrhage. This type of dissociated sensory loss usually occurs in a segmental distribution, and since the lesion frequently involves other parts of the gray matter, varying degrees of segmental amyotrophy and reflex loss may be added. If the lesion has spread to the white matter, corticospinal, spinothalamic, and posterior column signs will be present as well.

Posterior column syndrome There is loss of vibratory and position sense below the lesion, but the senses of pain, temperature, and touch are affected relatively little or not at all. This condition may be difficult to distinguish from an affection of large fibers in sensory roots (tabetic syndrome). In some diseases vibratory sensation may be involved predominantly, whereas in others position sense is more affected. It should be stressed that an interruption of proprioceptive fibers may interfere with discriminative sensory function, such as two-point discrimination and recognition of size, shape, and weight; and that impairment of this function may occur with posterior column disease alone. Paresthesias in the form of tingling and "pins-and-needles" sensations or girdle sensations are a common complaint with posterior column disease, and pain stimuli may also produce unpleasant sensations.

The anterior spinal artery syndrome With occlusion of the anterior spinal artery or other destructive lesions that predominantly affect the ventral portion of the cord, there is a relative or absolute sparing of proprioceptive sensation and loss of pain and temperature sensation below the level of the lesion. Since the corticospinal tracts and the ventral gray matter also fall within the area of distribution of the anterior spinal artery, paralysis of motor function forms a prominent part of this syndrome.

Disturbances of sensation due to lesions of the brainstem A characteristic feature of lesions of the medulla and lower pons is that in many instances the sensory disturbance is crossed, i.e., there is loss of pain and temperature sensation of one side of the face and of the opposite side of the body. This is accounted for by involvement of the trigeminal tract or nucleus and the lateral spinothalamic tract on one side of the brainstem. This is nearly always due to a lateral medullary infarction (Wallenburg's syndrome). In the upper pons and midbrain, where the spinothalamic tracts and the medial lemniscus become confluent, an appropriately placed lesion may cause a loss of all superficial and deep sensation over the contralateral side of the body. Cranial nerve palsies, cerebellar ataxia, or motor paralysis are often associated, as indicated in Chaps. 324 and 326.

Sensory loss due to a lesion of the thalamus (syndrome of Dejerine-Roussy) Involvement of the nucleus ventralis posterolateralis of the thalamus, usually due to a vascular lesion or tumor, causes loss or diminution of all forms of sensation on the opposite side of the body. Position sense is affected more frequently than any other sensory function, and deep sensory loss is usually, but not always, more profound than cutaneous loss. There may be spontaneous pain or discomfort ("thalamic pain"), sometimes of the most torturing and disabling type, on the affected side of the body; and any form of stimulus may have a diffuse, unpleasant, lingering quality. Emotional disturbance also aggravates the painful state. This overresponse is usually associated with an elevated threshold; i.e., a stronger stimulus than normal is necessary to produce a sensation of pain, in spite of the greater discomfort experienced by the patient once the sensation had been evoked. The thalamic pain syndrome may occasionally accompany lesions of the white matter of the parietal lobe (see Chap. 326).

Sensory loss due to lesions in the parietal lobe There is a disturbance mainly of discriminative sensory functions on the opposite side of the body, particularly the face, arm, and leg. Loss of position sense, impaired ability to localize touch and pain stimuli, elevation of two-point threshold, a general inattentiveness to sensory stimuli on one side of the body, and astereognosis (if the lesion is in the dominant hemisphere) are the most prominent findings. It is generally taught that the primary modalities of sensation (pain and temperature, touch and vibratory sense) are not affected by lesions which are confined to the cerebral cortex, but this statement requires modification. In acute, deep parietal lesions the primary modalities may be abolished, and as was said, they may rarely be followed by the "thalamic pain syndrome," but usually the impairment takes a different form from that due to thalamic lesions. Thus, with cortical lesions, the patient's reports are variable; one examination may disclose no sensory abnormalities, whereas another does. This type of response is often attributed to hysteria. Other features of parietal lobe symptomatology and the differences between dominant and nondominant parietal lobe syndromes will be considered in Chap. 27.

Sensory loss due to suggestion and hysteria The possibility of suggesting sensory loss to a patient has already been mentioned. In fact, hysterical patients almost never complain spontaneously of cutaneous sensory loss, although they may use the term *numbness* to indicate a paralysis of a limb. Complete hemianesthesia, often with reduced hearing, sight, smell, and taste, as well as impaired vibration sense over only half the skull, is a common finding in hysteria. Anesthesia of one entire limb or a sharply defined sensory loss over part of a limb, not conforming to the distribution of root or cutaneous nerve, is also frequently observed. Postural sensation is rarely affected. The diagnosis of hysterical hemianesthesia is best made by eliciting the other relevant symptoms of hysteria or, if this is not possible, by noting the discrepancies between this type of sensory loss and that which occurs as part of the usual sensory syndromes.

REFERENCES

Brodal A: The somatic afferent pathways, chap. 2 in *Neurological Anatomy,* New York: Oxford, 1969

Holmes, Gordon: Chaps. 8 and 9 in *Introduction to Clinical Neurology,* 2d ed., Baltimore: Williams & Wilkins, 1952

Mayo Clinic: *Clinical Examinations in Neurology,* 3d ed., Philadelphia: Saunders, 1972

Melzack R, Wall P: Pain mechanisms: a new theory. Science 150:971, 1965

Mountcastle VB: Central nervous mechanisms in sensation, chaps. 61, 62, and 63, in *Medical Physiology,* 12th ed., ed VB Mountcastle, vol. 2, St. Louis: Mosby, 1968

22
COMA AND RELATED DISTURBANCES OF CONSCIOUSNESS

RAYMOND D. ADAMS

The practitioner of medicine is frequently called upon to treat patients whose principal abnormality is an impairment of consciousness, which varies from inattentiveness and simple confusion to coma. In large municipal hospitals it is estimated that as many as 3 percent of total admissions to the emergency ward are due to diseases that have caused coma; although this figure seems high, it serves to emphasize the importance of this class of neurologic diseases and the necessity for every student of medicine to acquire a theoretic as well as a practical knowledge of them.

The terms *consciousness, confusion, stupor, unconsciousness,* and *coma* have been endowed with so many different meanings that it is almost impossible to avoid ambiguity in their usage. They are not strictly medical terms, but literary, philosophic, and psychologic ones as well. The word *consciousness* is the most difficult of all. William James once remarked that everyone knew what consciousness was until he attempted to define it. To the psychologist consciousness denotes a state of awareness of one's self and one's environment. Knowledge of one's self, of course, includes all "feelings, attitudes and emotions, impulses, volitions, and the active or striving aspects of conduct" (English)—in short, an awareness of all one's own mental functioning, particularly of the cognitive processes. These can be judged only by the patient's verbal account of his introspections and, indirectly, by his actions. Physicians, being practical men for the most part, have learned to place greater confidence in their observations of the patient's general behavior and his reactions to overt stimuli than in what he says. For this reason when they employ the term *consciousness,* they usually do so in its commonest and simplest signification, namely, a state of awareness of the environment. This narrow definition has another advantage in that the word *unconsciousness* is its exact opposite—a state of unawareness of environment or a suspension of those mental activities by which man is made aware of his environment. To add to the ambiguity, psychoanalysts have given the word *unconscious* a still different meaning; for them it stands for a repository of impulses and memories of previous experiences that cannot immediately be recalled to the conscious mind.

DESCRIPTION OF STATES OF NORMAL AND IMPAIRED CONSCIOUSNESS The following definitions, though admittedly unacceptable to most psychologists, are of service to medicine, and they will provide the student with a convenient terminology for describing the mental states of his patients.

Normal consciousness This is the condition of the normal person when fully awake, in which he is responsive to psychologic stimuli and "indicates by his behavior and speech that he has the same awareness of himself and his environment as ourselves." This normal state may fluctuate during the course of the day from keen alertness or deep concentration with a marked constriction of the field of attention to general inattentiveness and drowsiness.

Sleep Sleep is a state of physical and mental inactivity from which the patient may be aroused to normal consciousness. A person in sleep gives little evidence of being aware of himself or his environment, and in this respect he is unconscious. Yet he differs from a comatose patient in that he may still respond to unaccustomed stimuli and at times is capable of some mental activity in the form of dreams, which leave their traces in memory.

And, of course, he can be recalled to a state of normal consciousness when stimulated.

Inattentive, confusional, and cloudy states of consciousness In these conditions the patient does not take into account all elements of his immediate environment. Like delirium, these states always imply an element of sensorial clouding or imperceptiveness and distractibility of attention. The term *confusional* lacks precision, for often it is meant to denote an inability to think with customary speed and coherence. Here the difficulty is in defining thinking, a term which variably refers to problem solving and coherence of ideas about a subject.

An inattentive, severely confused person is usually unable to do more than carry out a few simple commands. Few if any thought processes are in operation. His capacity for speech may be limited to a few words or phrases, or he may be voluble. He is unaware of much that goes on around him and does not grasp his immediate situation. A moderately confused person can carry on a simple conversation for short periods of time, but his thinking is slow and incoherent, and he is unable to stay on one topic. He is distractible and at the mercy of every stimulus. Often he is disoriented in time and place. In mild degrees of confusion the disorder may be so slight that it is overlooked unless the examiner is searching in his analysis of the patient's behavior and conversation. The patient may even be roughly oriented as to time and place and able to speak freely on almost any subject. Only occasional irrelevant remarks betray an incoherence of thinking. Patients with mild or moderately severe confusion may be subjected to psychologic testing. The degree of confusion often varies from one time of day to another and tends to be least pronounced in the early morning. Severe confusion or stupor may resemble semicoma during periods when the patient is drowsy or asleep. Many events that happen to the confused patient leave no trace in his memory; in fact, capacity to recall later the events that transpired in any given period is one of the most delicate tests of mental clarity. However, careful analysis will show the defect to be one of inadequate registration and fixation of items rather than a fault in retentive memory.

Some neurologists regard *delirium* as a state of confusion with excitement and hyperactivity, and in some medical writings the terms *delirium* and *confused-cloudy states* are used interchangeably. It is undoubtedly true that the delirious patient is nearly always confused. However, the vivid hallucinations which characterize delirious states, the relative inaccessibility of the patient to other events than those to which he is reacting at any one moment, his extreme agitation and tremulousness, and the tendency to convulse suggest a cerebral disorder of a somewhat different type. The clearest evidence of the relationship of inattention, confusion, stupor, and coma is that the patient may pass through all these states as he becomes comatose or emerges from coma. The author has not observed any such relationship between coma and delirium. These distinctions are drawn with greater clarity in Chap. 26.

At times a patient with certain types of aphasia, especially jargon aphasia, may create the impression of confusion, but close observation will reveal that the disorder is confined to the sphere of language and that behavior is otherwise natural.

Stupor In stupor mental and physical activity are reduced to a minimum. Although inaccessible to many stimuli, the patient opens his eyes, looks at the examiner, and does not appear to be unconscious. Response to spoken commands is either absent or slow and inadequate. As a rule tendon or plantar reflexes are not altered. On the other hand, tremulousness of movement, coarse twitching of muscles, restless or sterotyped motor activity, and grasping and sucking reflexes are not infrequent, depending on the way in which disease affects the nervous system. In psychiatry the term *stupor* means a state in which impressions of the external world are normally received but activity is suspended or marked by negativism, e.g., catatonic schizophrenia.

Coma The patient who appears to be asleep and is at the same time incapable of sensing or responding adequately to either external stimuli or inner needs is in a state of coma. Coma may vary in degree, and in its deepest stages no reaction of any kind is obtainable. Corneal, pupillary, pharyngeal, tendon, and plantar reflexes are all absent. With lesser degrees of coma pupillary reflexes and ocular movements and other brainstem reflexes are preserved, and there may or may not be extensor rigidity of the limbs and opisthotonos, signs which, as Sherrington showed, indicate decerebration. Respirations are often slow or rapid and may be periodic, i.e., Cheyne-Stokes breathing. In still lighter stages, referred to as *semicoma,* most of the above reflexes can be elicited, and the plantar reflexes may be either flexor or extensor (Babinski's sign). Moreover, pricking or pinching the skin, shaking and shouting at the patient, or an uncomfortable distention of the bladder may cause the patient to stir or moan and his respirations to quicken.

THE ELECTROENCEPHALOGRAM AND DISTURBANCES OF CONSCIOUSNESS One of the most delicate confirmations of the fact that these states of altered consciousness are expressions of neurophysiologic changes is the electroencephalogram. In the normal waking state the electrical potentials of the cortical neurons are integrated into regular waves of two frequency ranges, from 8 to 15 per second (alpha rhythm) and from 16 to 25 per second (beta rhythm). These wave forms are established by adolescence, but certain individual differences in general pattern and dominance of alpha waves are maintained throughout adult life. With sleep these cortical potentials slow down and amplitude (voltage) of the individual waves increases. At one stage in light sleep characteristic bursts of 14 to 16 waves per second appear, the so-called "sleep spindles," and in deep sleep all the waves of normal frequency and amplitude are replaced by slow ones of high voltage ($1^1/_4$ to 3 per second). In rapid eye movement (REM) sleep the brain waves return to normal (see Chap. 23). Similarly, some alteration in brain waves occurs in all disturbances of consciousness except the milder degrees of confusion.

This alteration usually consists of a disorganization of the electroencephalographic pattern, which shows random, slow waves of high voltage in stages of confusion; more regular, slow, two to three per second waves of high voltage in stupor and semicoma; and slow waves or even suppression of all organized electrical activity (isoelectric state) in the deep coma of hypoxia and ischemia, the so-called "brain death syndrome". The electroencephalograms of deep sleep and of light coma resemble each other. However, not all diseases that cause confusion and coma have the same effect on the electroencephalogram. Some, such as barbiturate intoxication, may cause an increase in frequency and amplitude of the brain waves. In epilepsy the disturbance of consciousness is usually attended by paroxysms of "spikes" (fast waves of high amplitude) or by the characteristic alternating slow waves and spikes of petit mal. Other diseases, such as hepatic coma, characteristically cause a slowing in frequency and an increasing amplitude of "brain waves" and special triphasic waves. Whether all metabolic diseases of the brain induce similar changes in the electroencephalogram has not been determined. Probably there are differences among them, some of which may be significant (see Chap. 322).

MORBID ANATOMY AND PHYSIOLOGY OF COMA

In recent times there has been some clarification and amplification of earlier neuropathologic observations that the smallest lesions associated with protracted coma are always to be found in the midbrain and thalamus. The essence of more recent neurophysiologic studies, to be found in the writings of Bremer, of Morison and Dempsey, and of Moruzzi and Magoun, is that an ascending series of destructive lesions of spinal cord, medulla, pons, and cerebellum has no effect on the state of consciousness until the level of midbrain and diencephalon (thalamus) is reached. High brainstem transections invariably induce states of prolonged unresponsiveness, whereas stimulation of the upper brainstem reticular formation causes a drowsy or sleeping animal to become suddenly alert and his EEG to change correspondingly. As anesthetic agents abolish consciousness, they are found to suppress the activity of the upper reticular activating system, without interfering, at least at certain levels, with the transmission of specific sensory impulses.

Anatomic studies show the reticular activating system of the upper brainstem to receive collaterals from the specific sensory pathways and to project, not just to the sensory cortex of the parietal lobe, as do the thalamic relay nuclei for somatic sensation, but to the whole of the cerebral cortex. The latter has corticofugal connections which feed back nerve impulses to the reticular formation. Sensory stimulation, it would seem, then, has the double effect of conveying to the brain information about the outside world but also of providing some of the energy for activating those parts of the nervous system on which consciousness depends.

These new data are in line with the older ideas of Herbert Spencer and Hughlings Jackson—that the diencephalon and cerebral cortex always function together as a unit and represent the highest levels of integrative nervous activity, called by Penfield *centrencephalic.* Though anatomic details have yet to be worked out and the precise physiology of the reticular activating system leaves much to be desired, being more complicated than this simple formulation would suggest, nevertheless, as a working idea it will make some of the following neuropathologic observations more comprehensible.

The study of a large series of human cases in which coma has preceded death by several days will bring to light two major types of lesion. In the first group a macroscopically visible lesion such as a tumor, abscess, intracerebral, subarachnoid, subdural, or epidural hemorrhage, massive infarct, or meningitis is demonstrable; usually the lesion involves a portion only of the cortex and white matter, leaving much of the cerebrum intact. Rarely, it is located in the thalamus or midbrain, which would make the coma understandable. But in the other instances the coma will always be related to a temporal lobe–tentorial herniation with compression, ischemia, and secondary hemorrhage in the midbrain and lower thalamus or with downward displacement of the brainstem. A detailed clinical record will show the coma to have coincided with these secondary displacements and herniations. Exceptionally, widespread bilateral damage to the cortex and subcortical white matter will be found—the result of bilateral infarcts or hemorrhages, viral encephalitis, hypoxia, or ischemia—without thalamic or midbrain lesions. In the second group (and this is larger than the first) no visible lesion is seen by the naked eye, and often no abnormality is divulged by any technique of pathology. The lesion, here caused by a metabolic or toxic state, is subcellular or molecular. In some instances the grossly normal brain will reveal a demonstrable cellular change under the light microscope which may be characteristic, e.g., hepatic coma. Usually the microscopic lesions are too diffuse for clinicoanatomic correlation. Thus, pathologic changes are compatible with physiologic deductions—that the state of prolonged coma correlates with lesions of all parts of the cortical-diencephalic systems of neurons, but it is only in the upper brainstem that they may be small and discrete.

MECHANISMS WHEREBY CONSCIOUSNESS IS DISTURBED IN DISEASE Knowledge of diseases of the nervous system is so limited that it is not possible to identify all the different mechanisms by means of which consciousness is disturbed. Already several ways in which the mesencephalic-diencephalic-cortical systems are deranged have been identified; there are probably many others.

In a number of disease processes there is direct interference with the metabolic activities of the nerve cells in the cerebral cortex and the central cerebral nuclear masses of the brain. Hypoxia, hypoglycemia, hyper- and hypoosmolar states, acidosis, alkalosis, hyper- and hypokalemia, hyperammonemia, and deficiencies of thiamine, nicotinic acid, vitamin B_{12}, pantothenic acid, and pyridoxine are well-known examples (see Chap. 332). The relevant points for our discussion are that cerebral metabolism or blood flow is reduced in all the metabolic disorders leading to coma. Oxygen values of below 2 ml per 100 g of brain tissue are incompatible with an alert state. In hypoglycemia the cerebral blood flow is normal or above normal, whereas the cerebral metabolic rate is diminished, owing to deficiency of substrate. In thiamine and vitamin B_{12} deficiency the cerebral blood flow is normal or slightly diminished, and the cerebral metabolic rate is diminished, presumably because of insufficiency of coenzymes. Extremes of body temperature, either hyperthermia (temperature over 106°F) or hypothermia (temperature below 97°F), probably induce coma by exerting a nonspecific effect on the metabolic activity of neurons.

Diabetic acidosis, uremia, hepatic coma, and the coma of systemic infections are examples of endogenous intoxications. The identity of the toxic agents is not entirely known. In diabetes acetone bodies (acetoacetic acid, β-hydroxybutyric acid, and acetone) are present in high concentration, and in uremia there is probably accumulation of dialyzable toxin, perhaps phenolic derivatives of the aromatic amino acids. In both conditions "dehydration" and serum acidosis may also play an important role. In many cases of hepatic coma, elevation of blood NH_3 to levels five to six times normal has been found. Lactic acidemia and other organic acids may affect the brain by lowering its pH to less than 7.3. The mode of action of bacterial toxins is unknown. In all these conditions the cerebral metabolic rate tends to be reduced, whereas cerebral blood flow remains normal. In water intoxication the membrane excitability of nerve cells is altered by hyponatremia and changes in intracellular K levels.

Drugs such as barbiturates, bromides, Dilantin, alcohol, glutethimide, and phenothiazines induce coma by their direct suppressive effect on the neurons of the cerebrum and diencephalon. Others such as methyl alcohol, ethylene glycol, and paralydehyde result in metabolic acidosis. Many additional pharmacologic agents have no direct action on the nervous system but lead to coma through the mechanism of circulatory collapse and inadequate cerebral blood flow. In toxic and metabolic diseases, although the patient usually approaches coma through a state of drowsiness, confusion, and stupor, and the reverse sequence occurs as he emerges from it, each disease has its special effects, manifesting itself by a characteristic clinical picture. This means that the mechanism and topography of the lesion will be different.

A critical decline in blood pressure, usually to a systolic level below 70 mm Hg, affects neural structures by causing a decrease in cerebral blood flow and, secondarily, a diminution in cerebral metabolic rate. If decline in blood pressure is episodic, the corresponding clinical picture is syncope (see Chap. 16). Here the clinical picture is one of physical weakness usually preceding and following the loss of consciousness, the whole process being acute and promptly reversible.

The sudden, violent, and excessive discharge of *epilepsy* is another mechanism. Usually a Jacksonian convulsion has little effect on consciousness until it spreads from one side of the body to the other. Coma immediately ensues, presumably because the spreading of the seizure discharge to central neuronal structures paralyzes their function. Other types of seizure in which consciousness is interrupted from the very beginning are believed to originate in the diencephalon.

Concussion exemplifies still another special pathophysiologic mechanism. In "blunt" head injury it has been shown that there is an enormous increase in intracranial pressure of the order of 200 to 700 lb per in.^{2}, lasting a few thousandths of a second. Either the vibration set up in the skull and transmitted to the brain or this sudden high intracranial pressure is believed to be the basis of the abrupt paralysis of the nervous system that follows head injury. That the increased pressure itself may be the main factor has been suggested by experiments in which raising the intraventricular pressure to a level approaching diastolic blood pressure has abolished all vital functions.

As was pointed out above, large, destructive, and space-consuming lesions of the brain, such as hemorrhage, tumor, or abscess, interfere with consciousness in two ways. One is by direct destruction of the midbrain and diencephalon; the other, far more frequent, is by producing herniation of the medial part of the temporal lobe through the opening of the tentorium and crushing the upper brain against the opposite free edge of the tentorium. Here the mechanism is again mechanical, and probably circulatory as well.

CLINICAL APPROACH TO THE COMATOSE PATIENT Coma is not an independent disease entity but is always a symptomatic expression of disease. Sometimes the underlying disease is perfectly obvious, as when a healthy individual is struck on the head and rendered unconscious. All too often, however, the patient is brought to the hospital in a state of coma, and little or no information about him is immediately available. The physician must then subject the clinical problem to careful scrutiny from many directions. To do this efficiently, he must have a broad knowledge of disease and a methodical approach to the problem that leaves none of the common and treatable causes of coma unexplored.

It should be pointed out that when the comatose patient is seen for the first time, simple therapeutic measures take precedence over diagnostic procedures. A quick survey should make sure that the comatose patient has a clear airway and is not in shock (circulatory collapse) or, if trauma has occurred, that he is not bleeding from a wound. In patients who have suffered a head injury there may be a fracture of the cervical vertebras, and therefore one must be cautious about moving the head and neck lest the spinal cord be inadvertently crushed. There must be an immediate inquiry as to the previous health of the patient: whether the patient had suffered a head injury or had been seen in a convulsion, and the circumstances in which he was found. The persons who accompany the comatose patient to the hospital should not be permitted to leave until they have been questioned.

Diagnosis The temperature, pulse, respiratory rate, and blood pressure are of aid in diagnosis. Fever suggests a severe systemic infection such as pneumonia, bacterial meningitis, or a brain lesion that has disturbed the temperature-regulating centers. An excessively high body temperature, 107 to 110°F, associated with dry skin should arouse the suspicion of heat stroke. Hypothermia is frequently observed in alcoholic or barbiturate intoxication, extracellular fluid deficit, peripheral circulatory failure, or myxedema. Slow breathing points to morphine, barbiturate intoxication, or hypothyroidism, whereas deep, rapid breathing suggests pneumonia but may occur in diabetes or uremic acidosis (Kussmaul's respiration) or with intracranial diseases, as a central neurogenic hyperpnea. The rapid breathing of pneumonia is often accompanied by an expiratory grunt, cyanosis, and fever. Diseases that elevate the intracranial pressure or damage the brain, especially the brainstem, often cause slow, irregular, or periodic (Cheyne-Stokes) breathing. The pulse rate is less helpful, but if exceptionally slow, it should suggest heart block, or if combined with periodic breathing and hypertension, an increase in intracranial pressure. A tachycardia of 140 heartbeats per minute or above calls attention to the possibility of an ectopic cardiac rhythm with insufficiency of cerebral circulation. Marked hypertension occurs in patients with cerebral hemorrhage and hypertensive encephalopathy and, at times, those with increased intracranial pressure; whereas hypotension is the usual finding in the coma of diabetes, alcohol or barbiturate intoxication, or internal hemorrhage, myocardial infarction, dissecting aortic aneurysm, gram-negative bacillary septicemia, and Addison's disease.

Inspection of the skin may also yield valuable information. Cyanosis of the lips and nail beds means inadequate oxygenation. Cherry-red coloration indicates carbon monoxide poisoning. Multiple bruises, and in particular a bruise or boggy area in the scalp, favor cranial trauma. Bleeding from an ear or nose or orbital hemorrhage also raises the possibility of trauma. Puffiness and hyperemia of face and conjunctivas and telangiectasia are the usual stigmas of alcoholism; marked pallor suggests internal hemorrhage. The presence of a maculohemorrhagic rash indicates the possibility of meningococcal infection, staphylococcus endocarditis, typhus, or Rocky Mountain spotted fever. Pellagra may be diagnosed from the typical skin lesions on face and hands. The face may be myxedematous. In pituitary hypoadrenalism the skin is sallow. Excessive sweating suggests hypoglycemia or shock, and dry skin, diabetic acidosis and uremia. Skin turgor is reduced in dehydration. Hemorrhagic blisters will have formed over pressure points if the patient has been motionless for a time.

The odor of the breath may provide clues to the nature of a disease causing coma. The odor of alcohol is easily recognized (except for vodka, which is odorless). The spoiled-fruit odor of diabetic coma, the uriniferous odor of uremia, and the musty fetor of hepatic coma are distinctive enough to be identified by physicians who possess a keen sense of smell.

The next step in the physical examination should give special attention to the status of the nervous system. Although the examination is limited in many ways, careful observation of the stuporous or comatose patient may yield considerable information concerning the function of different parts of the nervous system. One of the most helpful procedures is to sit at the patient's bedside for 5 to 10 min and observe what he does. The predominant postures of the body, the position of the head and eyes, the rate, depth, and rhythm of respiration, and the pulse should be noted. The state of responsiveness should then be estimated by noting the patient's reaction when his name is called and his capacity to execute a simple command or to respond to painful stimuli. The most effective painful stimuli are supraorbital pressure, sternal pressure, or pinching the side of the neck or inner parts of the upper arms or thighs. By grading these stimuli, one may titrate the response, so to speak, and evaluate both the degree of coma and changes from hour to hour in the course of the disease. Vocalization may persist in stupor and light coma and is the first response to be lost. Deft avoidance movements of parts stimulated, and grimacing are preserved in light coma and substantiate the integrity of corticomedullary and corticospinal tracts.

Usually it is possible to determine whether or not the coma is accompanied by meningeal irritation or focal disease in the cerebrum or brainstem. With meningeal irritation from either bacterial meningitis or subarachnoid hemorrhage, there is resistance to active and passive flexion of the neck but not to extension, turning, or tipping the head. Resistance to movement of the neck in all directions indicates disease of the cervical spine or is part of generalized rigidity. In infants, bulging of the anterior fontanel is at times a more reliable sign of meningeal irritation than stiff neck. A temporal lobe or cerebellar pressure cone or decerebrate rigidity may also limit passive flexion of the neck and may be confused with meningeal irritation.

Evidence of disease of a cerebral hemisphere, diencephalon, midbrain, pons, or medulla can be obtained even though the patient is comatose by noting the residual movement, prevailing postures of the body, respiratory rhythm and frequency, and status of cranial nerves. This is of more than passing importance, because severe and persistent derangements of these functions are frequent with mass lesions of the brain and rare in metabolic disorders (except in terminal stages). A hemiplegia, in most instances, reflects a contralateral hemispheral lesion and is revealed by lack of restless movements, grasp reflex, and avoidance movements. The paralyzed limbs are slack and remain in uncomfortable positions. If lifted from the bed, they "fall flail." The cheek puffs out in expiration on the paralyzed side, and the eyes are often turned away from the paralysis (toward the lesion). Painful stimuli may provoke a moan or grimace on one side and not the other, reflecting a hemianesthesia. A homonymous hemianopsia in a stuporous patient is revealed by attraction of eyes to visual stimuli presented on one side and not the other or lack of blink in reaction to threat on one side.

Of the various tests of brainstem function those which have been most useful are pattern of breathing, pupillary size and reactivity, and ocular movement and oculovestibular reflexes. As to patterns of abnormal breathing in progressive lesions which reduce the state of consciousness from confusion and inattention to stupor and coma, the earliest abnormality with cerebral lesions is the appearance of posthyperventilation apnea (period of apnea after 5 to 10 deep breaths). Its presence indicates bifrontal disease, wherein lies the mechanism, according to Plum, for activating rhythmic breathing when CO_2 is reduced. In coma due to massive cerebral lesions the rate of respiration increases slightly, and as it progresses an irregularity appears which gives way to the waxing-waning Cheyne-Stokes respiration (CSR). This means that the centers in the midbrain now isolated from the cerebrum are rendered more sensitive than usual to CO_2 (hyperventilation drive); and by intermittently reducing plasma CO_2 to low levels a temporary apnea follows. With midbrain—upper pontine lesions a state of *central neurogenic hyperpnea* (CNH), rather like Kussmaul breathing, supervenes. Here respirations are increased in rate (up to 100 per min) and in depth, to the extent that respiratory alkalosis may result. The reflex mechanisms for respiratory control in the lower brainstem have in this instance been released, and the threshold of respiratory activation is low. This respiratory drive continues despite low arterial CO_2 tensions and elevated pH. Oxygen therapy (unlike the hyperventilation of pneumonia, pulmonary congestion, etc.) does not modify the pattern. Low pontine-level lesions sometimes cause *apneustic breathing* (where there is a pause of 2 to 3 sec after full inspiration) or other abnormal patterns, such as short cycle clusters (three to four respirations without a waxing or waning followed by a pause (Biot respirations); or respiration alternans, in which a few breaths are omitted from time to time. With lesions of the medulla the rhythm of breathing is chaotic, being irregularly interrupted, the breath varying in rate and depth. This has been called "ataxia of breathing," not a very appropriate term. The latter progresses to apnea, as may also CSR or CNH; in fact, respiratory arrest is the mode of death of most patients with serious central nervous system disease. As Plum and Fisher both point out, when certain supratentorial brain lesions progress to the point where the temporal lobe and cerebellum herniates, one may observe a succession of respiratory patterns (CSR—CNH—Biot breathing to ataxic breathing), indicating extension of the functional disorder from upper to lower brainstem.

With midbrain lesions the pupils dilate to 4 to 5 mm and become unreactive to light; and with severe destruction of the tissue at this level (anoxic pannecrosis), they will finally dilate widely and not respond. Pontine tegmental lesions cause miotic pupils with only slight reaction to strong light. Thus, the preservation of pupillary light reflexes indicates integrity of the pupillary dilatation and constrictive mechanisms in the midbrain. Ciliospinal pupillary dilatation is also lost in brainstem lesions (see Chap. 20). Unilateral Horner's syndrome (miosis, ptosis, exophthalmos, and reduced sweating) may be observed homolateral to a predominantly one-sided lower brainstem lesion, usually medullary. The pupillary reactions are of great importance, because drug intoxications and metabolic disorders which cause coma leave the pupils unaffected. Exceptions are glutethimde (Doriden) and deep ether anesthesia, which cause the pupils to be of medium size of slightly enlarged and unreactive for several hours; opiates (heroin and morphine), which cause pinpoint pupils with light reflex so small that it can be seen only with a magnifying glass, and atropine poisoning, in which the pupils are widely dilated and fixed.

Ocular movements are altered in a variety of ways. In light coma from metabolic abnormalities the eyes rove from side to side in random fashion like the slow eye movements of light sleep. They disappear as brainstem function becomes depressed. Oculocephalic reflexes (doll's eye movements), elicited by briskly turning or tilting the head, with eyes moving conjugately in the opposite direction, are exaggerated. They are not present in the normal person, and if they are elicitable, evidence is obtained of the integrity of the tegmental structures of the midbrain and pons, which integrate ocular movements, and of the third, fourth, and sixth cranial nerves. Irrigation of each ear with 30 to 100 ml ice water (or just cold water if the patient is not completely comatose) will normally cause nystagmus away from the stimulated side (see Chap. 20). In comatose patients in whom the fast corrective "cortical" phase of nystagmus is lost, the eyes are deflected to the side irrigated with cold water or away from the side irrigated with hot water. The position is held for 2 to 3 min. These oculovestibular reflexes are also lost in brainstem lesions. If only one eye abducts and the other fails to adduct in the lateral conjugate movement, there is indication of interruption of the medial longitudinal fasciculus (on the side of adductor paralysis). Irrigating both ears with ice water with the head extended to 60° will sometimes induce vertical conjugate movements. An abducens palsy (sixth nerve) is reflected by a turning in of the eye because of unopposed action of the internal rectus muscle, and oculomotor palsy results in abduction from the unopposed action of the abducens muscle. The eyes may be held conjugately to one side at all times in a coma—away from the side of the paralysis with large cerebral lesions (looking at the lesion) and toward the side of the paralysis with unilateral pontine lesions (looking away from the lesion). And, during a one-sided seizure the eyes jerk toward the convulsing side of the face, arm, and leg (opposite to the irritative focus). The eyes may be turned down and inward (looking at the nose) in thalamic and upper midbrain lesion (Parinaud's syndrome, see Chap. 20). Retraction and convergence nystagmus and ocular bobbing [brisk downward movements of both eyes with slow elevation to the original position (two to three times a minute)] occur with lesions in the midbrain tegmentum and lower pons respectively. The major brainstem structural lesions, including temporal lobe herniation, abolish most, if not all, conjugate ocular movements when producing coma, whereas metabolic disorders do not. Of the intoxications, barbiturates and diphenylhydantoin (Dilantin) are the only common drugs which affect ocular movements, but they leave pupillary reactions intact.

As to the meaning of the forced postures and movements in the comatose patient, it may be said that restless, grasping, picking movements of one arm or arm and leg or all four extremities signify that the corticospinal tract(s) is intact; variable resistance to passive movement (paratonic rigidity) and strong grasping or complex avoidance movements have the same signification, and if they are bilateral, the coma usually is not deep. Focal seizures require an intact corticospinal motor system and are seldom seen in the paralyzed side with massive destruction of a cerebral hemisphere. Often these elaborate forms of semivoluntary movement are present on the "good side" in patients with extensive disease in one hemisphere and probably represent some type of disequilibrium of cortical and subcortical movement patterns. Definite choreic, athetotic, or even hemiballismic movements indicate disorder of the subthalamic and basal ganglionic structures, just as they do in the alert patient. *Decerebrate rigidity,* with jaw clenched, neck retracted, arms and legs stiffly extended and internally rotated, appears in the condition of diencephalic-midbrain suppression by temporal lobe pressure cone, with hemorrhages and infarction of the upper pons and midbrain and with certain metabolic disorders such as hypoglycemia and hypoxia. Occasionally the mechanism of the decerebrate posture is unclear, as with certain bilateral subacute encephalitic, demyelinative, and infarctive cerebral lesions. In some instances the lesions are clearly in the cerebral white matter or basal ganglions. *Decorticate rigidity,* with arm or arms in flexion and adduction and leg(s) extended, signifies higher lesions in cerebral white matter, internal capsules, and thalamus. *Diagonal postures,* opposite arms and legs flexed and extended, probably mean supratentorial lesions; extended arms and flexed legs are probably fragments of decerebrate postures and point to midpontine lesions. *Abolition of all postures and movements* indicates acute bilateral corticospinal interruption and low pontine-medullary lesions involving reticular facilitatory (extrapyramidal) mechanisms. The coma is usually profound.

Lower brainstem reflexes are seldom helpful in the analysis of coma. Only in the most profound metabolic comas and intoxications and in the hypoxemic pannecrosis of the entire brain (brain-death syndrome) are coughing, swallowing, and spontaneous respirations all abolished. Further, the tendon and plantar reflexes give little indication of what is happening. Tendon reflexes may be preserved until late and may be normal or slightly reduced on the hemiplegic side. The plantar reflexes may be absent or extensor. Only in deep coma or in states of decerebrate rigidity will a cerebral hemiplegia not be detected by flaccidity and motionless arm and leg.

A history of headache before or at the onset of coma, recurrent vomiting, and papilledema affords the best clues to increased intracranial pressure. This can be confirmed by lumbar puncture, which is usually safe unless there is a herniation of the temporal lobe through the tentorium or of the cerebellum through the foramen magnum. In the latter instance the cerebrospinal fluid pressure may not reflect intracranial pressure. Papilledema may develop within 12 to 24 hr in brain trauma and brain hemorrhage but, if pronounced, usually signifies brain tumor or abscess, a lesion of longer duration. Multiple retinal or large subhyaloid hemorrhages are usually associated with ruptured saccular aneurysm or hemorrhage from an angioma. Papilledema, with widespread retinal exudates, hemorrhages, and arteriolar changes, is an almost invariable accompaniment of hypertensive encephalopathy. In patients with evidence of increased intracranial pressure, lumbar puncture, although admittedly dangerous because it may promote further herniation, is nevertheless necessary in some instances. See Chap. 20 for further discussion of retinal changes.

Laboratory procedures Unless the diagnosis is established at once by history and physical examination, it is necessary to carry out a number of laboratory procedures. If poisoning is suspected, the gastric contents must be aspirated and saved for later chemical analysis. A catheter is passed into the urinary bladder, and a specimen of urine is obtained for determination of specific gravity, sugar, acetone, and albumin content. Urine of low specific gravity and high protein content is nearly always found in uremia, but proteinuria may also occur for 2 or 3 days after a subarachnoid hemorrhage or with fever. Urine of high specific gravity, glycosuria, and acetonuria are almost invariable in diabetic coma; but glycosuria and hyperglycemia may result from a massive cerebral lesion. If diphenylhydantoin, bromide, or barbiturate intoxication is suspected, it can be verified by special tests for these substances. A blood count is made, and in malarial districts a blood smear is examined for malarial parasites. Neutrophilic leukocytosis occurs in bacterial infections and also with brain hemorrhage and softening. Venous blood should be examined for glucose, nonprotein nitrogen, CO_2, sodium bicarbonate, pH, NH_3, sodium, potassium, chlorides, and Ca. The cerebrospinal fluid must be drawn, and the pressure, presence of blood, white cell count, and results of Pandy's test should be recorded. Bloody cerebrospinal fluid occurs in cerebral contusion, subarachnoid hemorrhage, brain hemorrhage, and occasionally with hemorrhagic infarcts due to thrombophlebitis or arterial embolism. If there is pleocytosis, a stained smear of the sediment should be searched for bacteria, and a rough quantitative sugar determination should be done. The standard cerebrospinal fluid formula in bacterial meningitis is elevated pressure, high white cell count (5,000/20,000), elevated protein level, and subnormal sugar values. The fluid should be saved for quantitative tests for sugar and protein, and a bacterial culture and Wassermann reaction should be performed. If it is suspected that the pressure is elevated, a No. 22 needle should be used. A very high pressure must be slowly reduced by removal of 10 to 15 ml over a period of 15 to 20 min, and urea, mannitol, or other hypertonic solutions should be given intravenously. Also, a corticosteroid may be given to reduce brain swelling over a longer period of time. Jugular compression tests are obviously contraindicated. X-rays of the skull should be obtained as soon as possible after these procedures, preferably between the emergency ward and the hospital room.

CLASSIFICATION OF COMA AND DIFFERENTIAL DIAGNOSIS The demonstration of focal brain disease or meningeal irritation, with cerebrospinal fluid abnormality, helps in differential diagnosis. The diseases that frequently cause coma may be conveniently divided into three classes, as follows:

I Diseases that cause no focal or lateralizing neurologic signs or alteration of the cellular content of the cerebrospinal fluid
- *A* Intoxications (alcohol, barbiturates, opiates, etc.) (Chaps. 111, 112, and 113)
- *B* Metabolic disturbances (diabetic acidosis, uremia, Addisonian crises, hepatic coma, hypoglycemia, hypoxia (Chap. 332)

C Severe systemic infections (pneumonia, typhoid fever, malaria, Waterhouse-Friderichsen syndrome)
D Circulatory collapse (shock) from any cause, and cardiac decompensation in the aged (Chap. 16)
E Epilepsy (Chaps. 24 and 337)
F Hypertensive encephalopathy and eclampsia (Chap. 326)
G Hyperthermia or hypothermia
H Concussion (Chap. 327)

II Diseases that cause meningeal irritation, with either blood or an excess of white cells in the cerebrospinal fluid, usually without focal or lateralizing signs
A Subarachnoid hemorrhage from ruptured aneurysm, occasionally trauma (Chap. 326)
B Acute bacterial meningitis (Chap. 329)
C Some forms of virus encephalitis (Chap. 330)
D Acute hemorrhagic leukoencephalitis (Chap. 331)

III Diseases that cause focal or lateralizing neurologic signs, with or without changes in the cerebrospinal fluid
A Brain hemorrhage (Chap. 326)
B Brain softening due to thrombosis or embolism (Chap. 326)
C *Brain abscess* (Chap. 329)
D Epidural and subdural hemorrhage and brain contusion (Chap. 327)
E Brain tumor (Chap. 328)
F Miscellaneous, i.e., thrombophlebitis, some forms of virus encephalomyelitis (Chap. 330)

With the clinical tests outlined above clearly in mind one can usually ascertain whether a patient with coma falls in one of the above categories. Concerning the group of comas without focal, lateralizing, or meningeal signs, which includes most of the secondary metabolic diseases of the brain, intoxications (both exogenous and endogenous), concussion, and postseizure states, it should be pointed out that a previous neurologic disease may have left residues which confuse the clinical picture. An earlier hemiparesis from vascular disease or trauma may reveal itself in an alcoholic or hepatic coma, uremia, or hyperglycemic encephalopathy. Also, in hypertensive encephalopathy, transitory focal signs may sometimes be present. And occasionally, for no understandable reason one leg may seem to move less or one plantar reflex be extensor in a metabolic coma. In actuality, the diagnosis of postepileptic coma or concussion depends on observation of the precipitating event or indirect evidence thereof; usually the diagnosis is not too long obscure, for another fit may occur and recovery of consciousness, once the seizures cease, is usually prompt. The final determination of the exact toxic or metabolic disorder requires the synthesis of a variety of clinical and laboratory data, which will be described in other parts of the book.

With respect to the comas of group II, the signs of meningeal irritation (head retraction, stiffness of neck or forward bending, Kernig and Brudzinski leg flexion signs) can usually be elicited in both bacterial meningitis and subarachnoid hemorrhage. However, if the coma becomes deep, stiff neck may disappear or be absent from the beginning. In such cases diagnosis is established by CSF examination. In the coma of bacterial meningitis, unless it is associated with brain swelling and cerebellar herniation, the CSF pressure is not exceptionally high (usually less than 400 mm); if the pressure is high, as death approaches there are signs of compression of the medulla, with fixed, dilated pupils, arrest of respiration, and fall in arterial blood pressure. Patients in coma from ruptured aneurysms also have high CSF pressure and often a massive hemispheral and ventricular extension of the hemorrhage.

In patients with group III type of coma it is the inequality of sensory-motor disturbances in the two arms and legs and the aforementioned changes in respiratory pattern, pupillary and ocular reflexes, and the remaining postural states that provide clues to serious structural lesions in the segmental brainstem apparatus. As the latter become prominent, they may obscure earlier signs of cerebral disease. It is noteworthy that bilateral cerebral infarction or hemorrhage or traumatic necrosis and hemorrhage may resemble the comatose state of metabolic and toxic diseases, since brainstem mechanisms may be preserved; contrariwise, hepatic, hypoglycemic, and hypoxic coma will sometimes look like the coma of brainstem lesion by causing decerebrate postures. Usually, however, the CSF pressure is elevated and the fluid sanguineous in massive cerebral hemorrhage. Unilateral infarction due to anterior, middle, or posterior cerebral artery occlusion seldom produces more than a stupor or light coma; if infarction is bilateral, however, coma may be profound. Evidence of brainstem displacement and temporal lobe herniation is manifested by increased or altered ventilation (CSR, CNH), bilateral Babinski signs, dilated pupil and drooped eyelid on the side of the lesion, decerebrate postures, later dilated pupils, and loss of full ocular movements. The coma itself gives no clue as to the nature of the original mass lesion. The terminal pattern of a descending gradient of diencephalic, mesencephalic, pontomedullary paralysis of nervous paralysis is identical in all. Differential diagnosis must depend on the other data.

An error which must be cautioned against is the diagnosis of irreversible coma (brain-death syndrome) on the basis of complete abolition of all brainstem and cerebral activity and isoelectric (flat) EEG if there is hypothermia or evidence of intoxication. Only with hypoxia and cerebral ischemia can this diagnosis be made securely.

Diagnosis has as its prime purpose the direction of therapy, and it matters little to the patient whether or not we diagnose a disease for which we have no treatment. The treatable forms of coma are drug intoxications, toxemia from systemic infections, epidural and subdural hematoma, brain abscess, bacterial and tuberculous meningitis, diabetic acidosis, and hypoglycemia.

RELATIVE INCIDENCE OF DISEASES THAT CAUSE COMA There have been only a few attempts to determine the relative incidence of diseases that lead to coma. A report from the Boston City Hospital (Solomon and Aring) included the largest series of clinical cases but was heavily skewed by the large local problem of chronic alcoholics, which made up 60 percent of all admissions in coma. Trauma (13 percent), cerebral vascular disease (10 percent), poisonings (3 percent), epilepsy (2.4 percent), diabetes, bacterial meningitis, pneumonia, uremia, and eclampsia followed in that order. In a series of 386 cases of coma of uncertain cause Plum and Posner observed that approximately 40 percent turned out to be metabolic; 25 percent, drug intoxications; and the remainder, neurologic disease of supra- or infratentorial structures.

Of course, figures like these do not provide information concerning coma caused by multiple factors. For example, a patient with a cerebral vascular lesion, old or recent, and diabetes mellitus may lapse into coma during an insulin reaction at a time when there is still sugar in the urine. Only by appreciating the interplay of these several common factors is one likely to reach the correct diagnosis.

The differential diagnosis of diseases that cause focal or lateralizing signs and meningitis will be taken up under the discussions of traumatic, neoplastic, vascular, and infective diseases of the brain.

CARE OF THE COMATOSE PATIENT Impaired states of consciousness, regardless of their cause, are often fatal because they not only represent an advanced stage of many diseases but also add their own characteristic burden to the primary disease. The main objective of therapy is, of course, to find the cause of the coma, according to the procedures already outlined, and to remove it. It often happens, however, that the disease process is one for which there is no specific therapy; or, as in hypoxia or hypoglycemia, the disease process may already have expended itself before the patient comes to the attention of the physician. Again, the problem may be infinitely complex, for the disturbance may be attributable not to a single cause but rather to several possible factors acting in unison, no one of which could account for the total clinical picture. In lieu of direct therapy, supportive measures must be used, and, indeed, it may be said that the patient's chances of surviving the original disease often depend in large measure on their effectiveness.

The physician must give attention to every vital function in the insensate patient. The following is a brief outline of the more important procedures. In order for them to be carried out successfully a well-coordinated team of nurses under constant guidance of a physician is needed.

1 If the patient is in shock, this takes precedence over all other abnormalities. The treatment of shock is discussed in Chap. 32.

2 Shallow and irregular respirations and cyanosis require the establishment of a clear airway and oxygen. The patient should be placed in a lateral position so that secretions and vomitus do not enter the tracheobronchial tree. Pharyngeal reflexes are usually suppressed, and therefore an endotracheal tube can be inserted without difficulty. Stagnant secretions should be removed with a suction apparatus as soon as they accumulate, since they will lead to atelectasis and bronchopneumonia. Oxygen can be administered by mask in a 100 percent concentration for 6 to 12 hr, alternating with 50 percent concentration for 4 hr. The depth of respiration can be increased by the use of 5 to 10 percent carbon dioxide for periods of 3 to 5 min every hour. Atropine should not be given; edema of the lungs and fluid in the tracheobronchial passages are not glandular secretions. Furthermore, atropine thickens this fluid and also may disturb temperaure regulation of the body. Aminophylline is helpful in controlling Cheyne-Stokes breathing. Respiratory paralysis dictates the use of endotracheal intubation and a positive-pressure respirator, but in the author's experience neither has been effective in comatose states in which there is disorganization of respiratory centers.

3 The temperature-regulating mechanisms may be disturbed, and extreme hypothermia, hyperthermia, or an unrecognized poikilothermia may occur. In hyperthermia, removal of blankets and use of alcohol sponges and cooling solutions are indicated.

4 The bladder should not be permitted to become distended. If the patient does not void, a retention catheter should be inserted. If more than 500 ml urine is found in the bladder, decompression must be carried out slowly over a period of hours. Urine excretion should be kept between 500 and 1,000 ml per day. The patient should not be permitted to lie in a wet or soiled bed.

5 Diseases of the central nervous system may upset the control of water, glucose, and salt. The unconscious patient can no longer adjust his intake of food and fluids by hunger and thirst. Salt-losing and salt-retaining syndromes have both been described with brain disease. Water intoxication and severe hyponatremia may of themselves prove fatal. The maintenance of water and electrolytes will be discussed in Chap. 84. If coma is prolonged, the insertion of a stomach tube will ease the problem of feeding the patient and maintaining fluid and electrolyte balance.

6 Aspiration pneumonitis should be avoided by prevention of vomiting (stomach tube), position, and restriction of oral fluids. Should it occur, corticosteroid therapy is beneficial. The legs should be examined each day for signs of phlebothrombosis.

7 If the patient is capable of moving, suitable restraints should be used to prevent a possible fall out of bed.

8 Convulsions should be controlled by measures outlined in Chap. 337.

REFERENCES

FISHER CM: Neurological examination of the comatose patient. Acta Neurol Scand, 1969

PLUM F, POSNER J: *Diagnosis of Stupor and Coma,* Philadelphia: Davis, 1966

23 SLEEP AND ITS ABNORMALITIES

RAYMOND D. ADAMS

Sleep, that familiar but inexplicable condition of repose in which consciousness is in abeyance, is obviously not abnormal, yet there is no absurdity in considering it in connection with abnormal phenomena. Irregularities of sleep which approach serious extremes are the source of much complaint, as are also unnatural forms of waking. Then, too, there are many disorders of the nervous system that affect sleep mechanisms and not a few medical conditions that are modified by sleep. For these several reasons the careful student of medicine is required to keep abreast of such research in this field as may bear on clinical symptoms and to know something of the diseases which alter the sleep-waking cycles.

NORMAL SLEEP Sleep, as everyone knows, is an elementary phenomenon of life and an indispensable phase of man's existence. It represents one of the basic functions of the nervous system, traceable through all mammalian, avian, and reptilian species.

Observations of the human sleep-waking cycle show it to be age-linked. The baby sleeps up to 20 hr a day, the child, 10 to 12 hr, and the adult, approximately 7 hr. But wide individual differences, due apparently to genetic factors, early-life conditioning, and the physical and psychologic state, are to be noted in the amount of required sleep.

The pattern of sleeping, which in terrestrial life is adjusted to the 24-hr day, also varies in the different epochs of life. A nocturnal predominance begins to appear only after the first few weeks of postnatal life; first the morning nap is omitted, then by the fifth year the afternoon nap, and the night's sleep becomes consolidated into a single long period. This biphasic pattern of sleeping and waking persists throughout adolescence and adult years, unless altered by disease, and not until old age does it progressively break down. Night awakenings then increase in frequency, and the daytime waking period becomes interrupted frequently by paroxysmal bursts of sleep lasting 1 to 10 sec (microsleep) and longer naps. Throughout most of life the female needs about an hour more of sleep than the male.

One of the most interesting and valuable discoveries about sleep was made by Loomis and his associates and by Dement and Kleitman through electroencephalographic analysis. Five stages of sleep, representative of two alternating physiologic mechanisms, were defined: Relaxed wakefulness was found to be accompanied by sinusoidal alpha waves of 8 to 12 cycles per second (cps) and low-voltage fast activity of mixed frequency in the EEG; and there are the usual associated blinks, eye and limb movements, and moderate tone in all the skeletal muscles. As a person falls asleep and the muscles relax, the eyelids droop, the eyes begin to roll from side to side, and the EEG pattern changes to one of progressively lower voltage and mixed frequency. This is called Stage I sleep. As sleep deepens into Stage II, bursts of 12 to 14 cps waves (sleep spindles) and high-amplitude sharp slow-wave (K) complexes appear. By now eye movements have ceased, but muscle tone is maintained. The deep sleep of Stages III and IV is featured by an increasing proportion of high-voltage, slow-wave activity in the EEG. In Stage V, rapid eye movements return and muscle tension increases in the jaw, whereas the neck, trunk, and limb muscles, after a few quivering, tremulous or myoclonic movements, become completely slack. The first four stages are called nonrapid eye movement sleep (NREMS); the last stage is variously designated as rapid eye movement sleep (REMS), paradoxic sleep (PS), or activated sleep (AS) (see Fig. 322-1).

In a typical night the normal drowsy adult passes successively through Stages I, II, III, and IV of NREMS. After about 70 min, mostly spent in Stages III and IV, the first REMS period occurs, usually heralded by an increase in body movements and a shift in the EEG pattern from Stage IV to II. This NREMS-REMS cycle (activity-rest cycle of Kleitman) is repeated at about the same interval four to six times during the night, depending on the length of sleep. The first REMS cycle may be brief, and the later cycles include less Stage IV NREMS. The newborn infant has much more REMS than NREMS (though it may not be of the same quality as that of the adult), and with age the sleep cycle lengthens to 70 to 90 min. About 20 to 25 percent of sleep time in young adults is spent in REMS, 5 percent in Stage I, 50 percent in Stage II, and 20 percent in Stages III and IV combined. The cycle is fairly stable from time to time in any one person and is believed to continue to operate during wakefulness in relation to cyclic gastric motility, hunger, degrees of alertness, and capacity for cognitive activity.

The discovery of the activated REMS has encouraged the exploration of its physiologic basis and its relationship to anatomic structures. It was already known that the body temperature falls during sleep; now this fall seems to occur only in NREMS, and the same is true of the heart beat and respiration, both of which become slow and more regular in NREMS. Oxygen consumption diminishes in NREMS and increases markedly in REMS. Urine excretion and osmolarity are elevated in REMS: the opposite happens in NREMS. Levels of plasma 1–corticosteroids rise throughout the night, but more in REMS. Cortical neurons tend to discharge in synchronized bursts during NREMS and randomly in wakeful states; in REMS the activity is intermediate. Most dreaming occurs in REMS and is most consistently recalled if the subject is awakened at this time.

On closer study, REM was found to have two components—one tonic, the other phasic. During the phasic period the eyes move rapidly in all directions, the pupils dilate, the blood pressure, pulse, and respiration increase and become more irregular, and little jerky myoclonic or trembling motions appear in the limbs. This phase is traced to bursts of activity in the medial and spinal vestibular nuclei, and their activities are mediated through the medial longitudinal fasciculi and ocular nuclei, the median raphe nuclei, and the corticospinal tract. In the tonic phase the alpha and gamma spinal neurons are inhibited and both postural and flexor reflexes diminish or are abolished. This tonic phase is traced to ponto-geniculate-occipital systems of neurons and to a descending reticulospinal fiber system.

There is some evidence that these two alternating physiologic sleep mechanisms for NREMS and REMS which lie in the brainstem contain and are influenced by biogenic amines, particularly 5-hydroxytryptamine (serotonin) and norepinephrine. The serotonin neurons are known to be located in the medial tegmentum of the pons and lower midbrain and to project upward to the hypothalamus and thalamus and to the orbital frontal and medial temporal (limbic) cortex. The norepinephrine-rich neurons project downward to the lateral horn cells of the spinal cord and upward to the posterior hypothalamus and limbic zones. These latter are the hypothalamic-limbic zones, which, if stimulated, will alert the animal or, if destroyed, will cause prolonged hypersomnia. Destruction of serotonergic neurons in the medial tegmentum of the pons or their pharmacologic suppression by serotonin antagonists results in insomnia, with disappearance of both NREMS and REMS. Monoamine oxidase inhibitors selectively diminish or abolish REMS. Thus, a serotonergic mechanism appears to subserve NREMS and to trigger the catecholaminergic or adrenergic mechanism of REMS. Unfortunately, the details of this neuropharmacology of sleep are not yet fully ascertained, nor do we know how these structures are normally activated at regular intervals to produce sleep. In some mysterious way, a product (or products) of fatigue or some obscure hypnotoxin activates the neurons subserving NREMS at the same time that afferent stimulation of the upper reticular formation diminishes. Neuronal systems of REMS are suppressed for a time during NREMS but periodically become active and interrupt it. The plasma and cerebrospinal fluid of drowsy or sleeping animals have been shown by Monnier and Pappenheimer to contain a substance with properties that induce somnolence and increase REMS in alert animals. Its origin and specific nature are unknown.

These data are necessary to understand some of the derangements of sleep described below.

THE EFFECTS OF TOTAL AND PARTIAL SLEEP LOSS Of all the conditions that make for human efficiency and sense of well-being, sleep is one of the most important. Deprived of sleep, experimental animals will die within a few days, no matter how well they are fed, watered, and housed, and under similar circumstances human beings suffer a variety of unpleasant symptoms that must be separated from the diseases that cause insomnia.

Despite many studies of the deleterious effects of sleeplessness, we still know all too little about them. Human beings deprived of sleep (NREM and REM) for periods of 60 to 200 hr experience increasing fatigue and irritability and find it difficult to concentrate, to perceive accurately, and to maintain their orientation. Illusions and hallucinations intrude in consciousness, primarily in the visual and tactile sensory fields, becoming more intense as the period of sleeplessness is prolonged. Performance of motor tasks deteriorates. If the tests are of short duration and of slow pace, the subject can keep up; if speed and perseverance are demanded, he cannot. Incentive to work weakens, and sustained action is interrupted by lapses of attention. Neurologic signs to be noted include a mild and fleeting nystagmus, a slight tremor of the hands, ptosis of eyelids, expressionless face, and thickness of speech, with mispronunciation and incorrect choice of words. A decrement of alpha waves appears in the EEG, and closing of the eyes no longer generates alpha activity. The concentration of 17-hydroxycorticosteroids increases in the blood, and catecholamine output rises.

Occasionally, probably only in predisposed persons, loss of sleep provokes psychotic episodes. Rarely, the subject may suddenly go beserk, with screaming, sobbing, and incoherent muttering about seeing things. Fragmentary delusions and paranoid thoughts are more frequent.

Recovery after prolonged sleep deprivation shows that the amount of sleep required is never equal to the amount lost. At first, the subject rapidly falls into Stage IV of NREMS and remains there, at the expense of Stage II sleep; Stage IV is interrupted from time to time by REM sleep which remains in the usual proportion. But by the second night, REMS rebounds and exceeds that of the predeprivation period. Stage IV NREMS seems, then, to be the most valuable in restoring the flagging functions of the nervous system.

The effects of partial and differential deprivation are somewhat different. If prevented night after night from having REMS, subjects show a greater tendency to become hyperactive, emotionally labile, and less able to control their impulses, a state which corresponds to the heightened activity, excessive appetite, and oversexuality of REMS-deprived animals. Differential deprivation of NREMS (Stages III and IV) leads, instead, to hyporesponsiveness.

Of course, since the need for sleep is known to vary from person to person in everyday life, it is difficult to decide what is partial sleep deprivation. Some individuals function perfectly on as little as 3 to 4 hr per night, and others, who sleep long hours, claim not to obtain the maximum benefit from it.

DERANGEMENTS OF SLEEP **Insomnia** This word signifies want of sleep, and is used popularly to indicate any impairment in its duration, depth, or restorative properties. Quantitative precision as to what constitutes insomnia is impossible because of our uncertainty as to the natural requirement of sleep and also its role in the economy of the human body.

Two classes of insomniacs may be defined: one in which there appears to be a primary disturbance of the normal sleep mechanism, the other in which sleep impairment is secondary to another disease or condition. The latter condition is encountered frequently in medical practice and may usually be ascribed to pain or some other annoying sensation or to nervousness, anxiety, and worry.

The term *primary insomnia* should be reserved for those persons who throughout their lives have never enjoyed restful slumber, and in whom none of the usual symptoms of neurosis, depression, or other psychiatric or medical diseases can be elicited. Unlike the rare individuals who seem to thrive on 3 to 4 hr of sleep a night, they suffer the effects of partial sleep deprivation and resort to all manner of drugs and various techniques to induce or maintain sleep. Their life comes so obviously to revolve around sleep that they have been called "sleep pedants" or "sleep hypochondriacs." Although their statements are much to be distrusted, Rechtschaffen confirms that they do indeed sleep poorly. They sleep for shorter periods, awaken more often than normal persons, spend less time in REM sleep and more in Stage II NREMS, move more often, and show a heightened physiologic arousal. Personality inventories have revealed a slightly higher incidence of psychopathy in this group of patients, but whether this is cause or effect is not known.

While there is no doubt that the victims of insomnia, regardless of the cause of their wakefulness, are likely to exaggerate the amount of sleep lost, *primary insomnia* should be recognized as an entity and not passed off as a quirk of the neurotic.

Of the sensory disorders conducive to abnormal wakefulness, pain in the spine with or without nerve root involvement stands out, and also abdominal discomfort from peptic ulcer and carcinoma. Tired, aching, restless legs, an obscure benign state known as the "restless leg syndrome" (anxietas tibialis), may regularly delay the onset of sleep. And excessive fatigue may give rise to many abnormal muscular sensations of similar nature. Acroparesthesias, a peculiar nocturnal tingling, numbness of palms and fingers due to tight carpal ligaments (carpal tunnel syndrome) may awaken the patient at night, as does also cluster or histamine headache, which nearly always occurs 2 to 3 hr after falling asleep.

But severe insomnia is a more frequent complaint of patients suffering from psychiatric disease. Its simplest form is that occurring in a reactive nervous state in which domestic and business worries keep the patient's mind in a turmoil. Also, vigorous mental activity late at night or excitement which leaves the muscles tense counteracts drowsiness and sleep. Under these circumstances there is difficulty in falling asleep and a tendency to sleep late in the morning. Sleeplessness is also commonly recorded in the histories of patients suffering from psychoneuroses and psychoses.

Illnesses in which anxiety and fear are prominent symptoms usually result in difficulty in falling asleep and light, fitful, or intermittent sleep. Also, disturbing dreams are frequent and may awaken the patient; exceptionally, he may even try to stay awake in order to avoid them. The sleep pattern is altered, but quality and quantity are little if at all diminished. In contrast, the depressive illnesses, particularly the manic-depressive or involutional type cause either light sleep in the early part of the night or early-morning waking and inability to return to sleep. Quantity of sleep is reduced, and nocturnal motility is increased. The REMS, although not reduced, comes earlier in the night; this is termed the "increased pressure of REMS." If anxiety is combined with depression, both the above patterns are observed. In states of mania, sleep diminishes and REMS may be abolished. The sleep rhythm may be totally deranged in acute confusional states and delirium, and REMS increases. In the latter the patient may only doze for short periods, both day and night. The total amount and depth of sleep in a 24-hr period are reduced. Frightening hallucinations may prevent sleep. The senile and arteriosclerotic patient tends to catnap during the day and then refuse to go to bed at night. His nocturnal sleep is intermittent; its total amount may be either increased or decreased.

Disturbances in the transitional period of sleep (somnolescent starts, sensory paroxysms, and nocturnal paralysis) As sleep comes on, it would appear that certain nervous centers may be excited to a burst of insubordinate activity. The result is a sudden start that rouses the incipient sleeper. It may involve one or both legs or the trunk, less often, the arms. If the start occurs repeatedly during the process of falling asleep and is a nightly event, it may become a matter of great concern to the patient. These starts are more apt to occur in individuals in whom the sleep process develops slowly, and it has been observed that they are especially frequent in tense, nervous persons. It is probable that some relationship exists between these nocturnal starts and the sudden isolated jerk of a leg, or arm and leg, which may occur in healthy, fully conscious persons. It does not appear to be related to epilepsy, despite certain superficial resemblances. Disturbances of this nature may be the stimulus for night terrors. These somnolescent starts must be distinguished from flexor spasms of the legs, which occur in patients who have suffered disease of the pyramidal tracts and from a rare condition known as nocturnal myoclonus in which the legs are involved in brusque flexion or extension movements of such force as to awaken the patient.

Sensory centers may be disturbed in a similar way, either as an isolated phenomenon or in association with phenomena that induce motion. As the patient drops off to sleep, he may be roused by a sensation that darts through his body. A sudden clang or crashing sound disturbs commencing sleep. Sometimes there is a sudden flash of light or a sensation of being lifted and dashed to earth or of being turned. These latter are probably similar sensory paroxysms involving the labyrinthine mechanism.

Curious paralytic phenomena, so distressing to a patient as to cause him to seek medical advice, may also occur in the transition from the sleeping to the waking state. Sometimes in an otherwise healthy individual a state supervenes in the morning in which, although awake, conscious, and fully oriented, he is unable to innervate a single muscle. He lies as though still asleep with eyes closed and is all the while engaged in a struggle for movement. He has the impression that if he could move a single muscle, the spell would instantly vanish and he would regain full power. It has been reported that the slightest cutaneous stimulus such as the touch of a hand may abolish the paralysis. Such attacks are usually transient and of no special significance. They have also been reported to occur during the development of sleep. They may be related to narcolepsy.

Nightmares and night terrors (pavor nocturnus) Awakening in a state of terror has happened to nearly everyone. Children are especially susceptible. Fevers dispose to it, as may any upsetting condition of the body, such as indigestion. Bad dreams, stimulated directly by the reading of blood-curdling stories or seeing exciting television programs before bedtime, may be followed by a night terror.

Sometimes a distinction is drawn between a terrifying dream which awakens the individual in a state of fear and one which causes him to run about wildly in his sleep as though to avoid a frightening hallucination. But probably the difference is only one of degree. The child usually seeks the security of the parental bed and needs to be calmed; the adult, once awakened, realizes it is all a dream and soon goes back to sleep. Recent studies have shown that all night terrors occur during REMS.

Such phenomena are of little significance as isolated events in childhood. Only if persistent and frequent do they become matters of pressing medical complaint. Then they are often found to be part of a behavioral disturbance or neurosis. Of greater importance is their differentiation from nocturnal epilepsy, which also may have a tendency to occur only during a specific stage of sleep. Interfering with the metabolism of either serotonin or norepinephrine offers a possible pharmacotherapeutic approach to both night terrors and nocturnal epilepsy.

Somnambulism and sleep automatism Examples of sleepwalking come to the attention of the practicing physician not infrequently. This condition likewise occurs more often in children than in adults. After being asleep for a time, the patient arises from his bed and walks about the house. He may turn on a light or perform some other familiar act. There is no outward sign of emotion; the eyes are open, and the sleeper is guided by vision, thus avoiding familiar objects. The sight of an unfamiliar object may awaken him. If spoken to, he makes no response; if told to return to bed, he may do so but more often must be led back to it. Sometimes he will mutter strange phrases or sentences over and over. The following morning he usually has no memory of the episode.

Most psychiatrists hold that these are dissociated mental states similar to the hysterical trance and fugue, except that they begin during sleep. To them sleepwalking is accepted as evidence of a nervous disorder, probably of psychoneurotic variety. Some observations are at variance with this interpretation, for somnambulism was found to arise almost exclusively from Stages III and IV of NREM sleep. And the entire nocturnal sleep pattern of such individuals does not differ from normal. Also, there are examples of this condition in adults who have no other signs of mental illness. It is probably allied to talking in one's sleep, although the two conditions seldom occur together.

Half-waking somnambulism, or sleep automatism, is a state in which an adult patient, half-roused from sleep, goes through a fairly complex routine such as going to a window, opening it, and looking out, but afterward recalls only a part of the episode. The patient may injure himself during sleepwalking.

Nocturnal epilepsy Paroxysmal abnormalities of the brain waves of the type seen in epilepsy tend to occur in epileptic patients during or shortly after the onset of sleep. This characteristic electroencephalographic pattern has been found so frequently in the epileptic patient that the practice of artificially inducing sleep in order to obtain confirmation of epilepsy has been adopted in many laboratories. Of course, it has long been known that epilepsy occurs during sleep, either in Stage IV of NREM sleep or in REM sleep.

The sleeping epileptic patient attracts attention to his condition by a cry, violent motor activity, or labored breathing. As in the diurnal seizure, after the tonic-clonic phase, he becomes quiet and falls into a state resembling sleep but from which he cannot be aroused. His appearance depends on the phase of the seizure he happens to be in when first observed. Seizures of this type may occur at any time during the night, and some patients may have all their seizures at night. If the seizure during the night is unobserved, the only indication of it may be disheveled bedclothes, a few drops of blood on the pillow, wet bed linen from urinary incontinence, a bitten tongue, or sore muscles. In some the occurrence of a seizure is betrayed only by incoherent behavior or a headache, the common aftermath of a convulsive disorder that was unnoticed. Rarely, a patient may die in an epileptic seizure during sleep, presumably from being smothered by bedclothes, aspirating vomitus, or for some more obscure reason.

Other less well-defined types of seizure occur at night. The patient may arise as though in a night terror and perform complex acts. He may be excited and overactive and, if restrained, become combative. After some minutes he is subdued and returns to sleep. The following morning he disclaims all memory of the episode. In most instances, this does not represent a psychomotor seizure but is instead a night terror. An electroencephalographic study may be helpful in such cases.

Nocturnal jerks of the legs, also called *nocturnal myoclonus,* are another troublesome symptom because they interfere with sleep night after night. Only recently has this condition been classified as a myoclonic form of epilepsy. It is unaccompanied by all other epileptic manifestations. Anticonvulsant drugs are said to control it, though in two cases the author has had better success with an occasional dose of Pántopon. It differs from the restless leg syndrome in that involuntary movements occur.

Epilepsy may occur in conjunction with both night terrors and somnambulism, and the question then arises whether the latter is in the nature of postepileptic automatism. Usually, no such relationship is established.

Prolonged states of sleep and reversal of sleep-waking rhythm Encephalitis lethargic, or "epidemic encephalitis," that remarkable illness which appeared on the medical horizon during the great pandemic influenza following the First World War, has provided some of the most dramatic instances of prolonged somnolence. In fact, protracted sleep lasting from days to weeks was such a prominent symptom that the disease was called "sleeping sickness." The patient appeared to be in a state of continuous sleep, or "somnosis," and remained awake only while stimulated. Although the infective agent was never isolated, the pathologic anatomy was fully divulged by many excellent studies, all of which demonstrated a destruction of neurons in the midbrain, subthalamus, and hypothalamus. Patients surviving the acute phases of the illness often had difficulty in reestablishing the normal sleep-waking rhythm. As the somnolence disappeared, some patients exhibited a reversal of sleep rhythm, tending to sleep by day and stay awake at night; they also showed a tendency toward Parkinson's syndrome.

Hypersomnia also occurs in trypanosomiasis, the common cause of sleeping sickness in Africa, and with a variety of diseases localized to the floor and walls of the third ventricle. Small tumors in the posterior hypothalamus and midbrain have been associated with arterial hypotension, diabetes insipidus, and somnolence lasting many weeks. Such patients can be aroused, but if left alone, they immediately fall asleep. Tumors of the brain, in general, show a tendency to cause drowsiness and increased amounts of sleep, but those of the diencephalon more so than any others (e.g., than posterior fossa ones). Traumatic brain lesions and other diseases have been found to produce similar clinical pictures. Myxedema, if severe, may cause hypersomnia.

Pathologic wakefulness This state has been induced in animals by lesions in the tegmentum (median raphe nuclei) of the pons. Comparable states are known to occur in man, but must be rare. The commonest causes of asomnia in the hospital are delirium tremens and drug-withdrawal psychoses. Drug-induced psychoses and hypomania may cause hyposomnia.

Narcolepsy and cataplexy The term *narcolepsy* has been used rather loosely. According to most authorities, it should refer to peculiar brief recurrent attacks of sleep, not to prolonged or continuous sleep. *Cataplexy* is a sudden brief loss of muscular power evoked by strong emotion, usually laughter. Although a few of the reported cases are doubtless examples of hysteria, there is unquestionably a well-defined clinical entity which bears no relationship to neurosis or any other known psychiatric condition. This will be discussed further in Chap. 335.

Sleep palsies and acroparesthesias Curious and at times distressing paresthetic disturbances develop during sleep. Everyone is familiar with the phenomenon of an arm or leg falling asleep. The immobility of the limbs and the maintenance of uncomfortable postures without being aware of them permits pressure to be applied to exposed nerves. The ulnar, radial, and peroneal nerves are quite superficial in places; pressure of the nerve against an underlying bone may interfere with intraneural circulation of the compressed segment. If such pressure is continued for half an hour or longer, a sensory and motor paralysis sometimes referred to as *sleep palsy* may develop. This condition usually lasts only a few hours or days, but if the compression is prolonged, the nerve may be severely damaged so that functional recovery awaits regeneration. Unusually deep sleep, as in alcoholic intoxication, or anesthesia renders the patient especially liable to sleep palsies merely because he does not heed the discomfort of an unnatural posture.

Acroparesthesias are frequent in adult women and are not unknown to men. The patient will say that after being asleep for a few hours she is awakened by an intense numbness, tingling, prickling, a feeling of "pins and needles" in her fingers and hands. There are also aching, burning pains or tightness and other unpleasant sensations. At first there is a suspicion of having slept on the arm, but the usual bilaterality and the occurrence regardless of the position of the arms dispel this notion. Usually the paresthesias are in the distribution of the median nerves. Vigorous rubbing of the hands restores normal sensation, and the paresthesias subside within a few minutes, only to return later on upon first awakening in the morning. The condition never occurs during the daytime unless the patient is lying down or sitting with the arms and hands in one position. When acroparesthesias are frequent, the hands may at all times feel swollen, stiff, clumsy, slightly numb, and sometimes distressingly painful. Careful examination discloses little or no objective sensory loss, though in some cases touch and pain sensation have been slightly altered in parts supplied by the median nerves. Slight atrophy and weakness of the abductor pollicis brevis and opponens pollicis muscles have been noted, and in a few cases it has been marked (carpal tunnel syndrome). The use of the hands for heavy manual work during the day seems to aggravate the condition, and a holiday or a period of hospitalization may relieve it. It often occurs in young housewives with a new baby or in factory workers who perform a routine skill. It has been demonstrated that there is a compression of the median nerves in the carpal tunnel of the wrist by thickened carpal ligaments, tenosynovitis, bony overgrowth (as in acromegaly), or amyloid deposit (multiple myeloma). The injection of 50 mg hydrocortisone beneath the carpal ligament and the use of Diuril or one of its analogues has given immediate relief in a respectable number of cases. The section of the carpal ligament has nearly always cured recalcitrant cases.

OTHER MEDICAL CONDITIONS RELATED TO SLEEP Nocturnal enuresis, or bedwetting (with daytime continence), is a frequent disorder of sleep during childhood but may persist into adult life. Approximately one of five children four to fourteen years of age is affected, boys more frequently than girls. Though the condition was formerly thought to be functional, i.e., psychogenic, the studies of Gastaut have revealed a peculiarity of bladder physiology. Intravesicular pressures periodically rise to much higher levels in enuretic patients than in normal persons, and their arousal time under such conditions is prolonged. Also, the bladders of enuretic patients tend to be smaller. This suggests a maturational failure of certain modulating nervous influences. The urinary incontinence has been found to occur usually during the first third of the night, during Stages III and IV of NREMS. Recall of dreams upon awakening is nearly always absent. Imipramine (Tofranil), which increases Stage II and decreases REMS, improves the condition in 75 to 85 percent of patients. Diseases of the urinary tract, diabetes mellitus and insipidus, epilepsy, and sickle-cell anemia must be differentiated as causes of symptomatic enuresis.

Duodenal ulcer patients secrete more HCl during sleep (peaks coincide with REMS) than normal subjects. Patients with coronary arteriosclerosis show ECG changes during REMS, and nocturnal angina has been recorded at this time. Asthmatic patients are observed to have their attacks at any time of night, not concomitantly with REMS, but they have less Stage IV NREMS. Somnolent myxedema patients have shown a decrease in Stage III and IV and more Stage II NREMS.

The senile dement exhibits reduced amounts of REMS and Stage IV NREMS, as do mongolian idiots, phenylketonurics, and brain-damaged children. A correlation has been demonstrated between the level of intelligence and the amount of REMS in all these conditions, and in normal persons as well. Barbiturates and alcohol, which suppress REMS, permit extraordinary excesses of it to appear during withdrawal periods, which may in part account for the hyperactivity and confusion seen in these states.

TREATMENT In general, there are three varieties of wakefulness. For best management, treatment should be based on the type exhibited by the patient. In younger patients the most infrequently observed type of insomnia is the inability to fall asleep. These individuals have become more and more tense during the day and are unable to relax. This type of insomnia usually lasts from 1 to 3 hr, and then the individual sinks into an exhausted, deep sleep which continues through the night. For these patients a quick-acting, fairly rapidly destroyed hypnotic such as secobarbital (Seconal), 0.1 g given 15 to 20 min before going to bed, is useful.

The second group consists of patients who are able to go to sleep but who awaken in 2 or 3 hr and lose sleep in the middle of the night. They awaken during the period when sleep normally lightens, and some are alternately awake and asleep all the rest of the night. Often these are sick persons with a debilitating or painful illness which generates more pain and restlessness as muscles relax and leave painful areas unsplinted. In others, fever, sweats, dyspnea, or other distressful symptoms develop and demand attention. Frequently, these patients secure relief from pentobarbital (Nembutal), 0.1 g given at bedtime. For cardiac patients who have Cheyne-Stokes respiration or moderate orthopnea, a rectal suppository of aminophylline, 0.5 g given at bedtime, will frequently relieve the respiratory distress and promote sleep. When pain is a factor in insomnia, acetylsalicylic acid, 0.3 to 0.6 g, should be given with the sedative. Occasionally, codeine phosphate, 30 mg, may be required when pain is severe.

The third group of insomnia patients consists of those who go to sleep promptly and sleep well most of the night, only to awaken too early in the morning. Most of these individuals are older persons who turn night into day. They go to bed and get up earlier and earlier so that soon they are sleeping during the day and are alert during the night. Into this category also fall those individuals who are under great tension, worry, or anxiety or are overworked and exhausted. These people sink into bed and sleep through sheer exhaustion, but around 4 or 5 A.M. they awaken with their worries and are unable to get back to sleep. Most of these patients are benefited by barbital, 0.3 g given with fruit juice or milk at bedtime. For debilitated patients the compressed tablets of insoluble material should be crushed to ensure proper absorption, or sodium barbital should be substituted. Chloral hydrate, 1.0 g given with fruit juice at bedtime, is also effective and may be substituted for barbital if desired.

Patients with serious mental agitation, delirium, or excitement who require prompt, easily controlled, relatively safe sedation should receive whiskey, 30 to 60 ml by mouth, or paraldehyde, 15 to 30 ml by mouth in iced fruit juice, or the same dose of the latter by rectum but diluted with 200 ml physiologic saline solution or 120 ml olive oil. For frankly delirious patients 25 to 50 mg chlorpromazine (t.i.d.) has been a most helpful medication. Generally, it is wise to avoid barbiturates with highly agitated patients, since occasionally they may precipitate serious mental confusion, excitement, or even manic tendencies. Chloral hydrate, 1 to 2 g by mouth, is also useful in the management of these individuals and frequently proves more satisfactory than the barbiturates.

A word of caution about oversedation is wise in any discussion of sedative drugs. All too frequently they are abused in that they are given when not needed, the dosage is too great, or the wrong preparation is chosen. These drugs are a common source of constipation, lead to fatigue and lack of energy and strength, and interfere with the patient's recovery from his illness.

When large dosages of quicker-acting barbiturates, 0.4 to 0.6 g daily, are given for more than a few weeks, there is real danger of habituation, which, once developed, is pernicious in character. Withdrawal, unless accomplished skillfully and in graded steps, may cause serious mental disturbance or precipitate convulsions. The chronic insomniac who has no other symptoms should not be permitted to use sedative drugs as a crutch on which to limp through life. The solution of this problem is rarely to be found in medication. One should search out and correct the underlying difficulty, using medication only as a temporary helpful tool. A good book, pleasure in staying awake, and belief that the human organism will always get as much sleep as needed are helpful.

Barbiturate sedatives may be of value in treating night terrors, and if their differentiation from nocturnal epilepsy is impossible, a trial on diphenylhydantoin sodium (Dilantin Sodium) and phenobarbital is indicated. (See Chap. 337 for further information concerning anticonvulsant medication.)

REFERENCES

DEMENT W, KLEITMAN N: Cyclic variations in EEG during sleep and their relation to eye movements, bodily motility and dreaming. Electroencephlog Clin Neurophysiol 9:673, 1957

GASTAUT H, BROUGHTON R: A clinical and polygraphic study of episodic phenomena during sleep. Recent Advances Biol Psychiat 7:197, 1965

LOOMIS AL et al: Cerebral states during sleep as studied by human brain potentials. J Exp Psychol 21:127, 1937

MONNIER M, HOSLI L: Humoral regulation of sleep and wakefulness by hypnogenic and activating dialysable factors, in *Sleep Mechanism,* Prog Brain Res 18:118, 1965

PAPPENHEIMER JR et al: Sleep-promoting effects of cerebrospinal fluid from sleep-deprived goats. Proc Nat Acad Sci USA 58:513, 1967

REICHTSCHAFFEN A, MONROE LJ: Laboratory studies of insomnia, in *Sleep: Physiology and Pathology, A Symposium,* ed A Kales, Philadelphia: Lippincott, 1969, p. 158

24 THE CONVULSIVE STATE

RAYMOND D. ADAMS

The magnitude of the problem of convulsion as a leading manifestation of a medical or neurologic disease can hardly be overstated. The statistics of Lennox show that at least 1 million persons in the United States are subject to recurrent seizures and that at least ten times that number consult a physician or go to a hospital at some time in their lives because of a seizure.

A solitary or brief outburst of convulsions may occur during the course of many medical illnesses; its significance derives from the fact that it indicates involvement of the nervous system and by its very nature, if repeated every few minutes, as in status epilepticus, may threaten life. Practical considerations require of the physician a knowledge of the diseases with prominent convulsive aspects, and of the therapeutic measures most successful in seizure control. Recurrent convulsions over long periods of life, most of the episodes being more or less identical in type, represent a different sort of problem. On the one hand they may be a manifestation of an ongoing primary neurologic disease that demands diagnosis and therapy, as in brain tumor. On the other, they may call attention to an old burnt-out lesion that began some time in the distant past and remains as a glial scar. Not infrequently the original disease was unnoticed; perhaps it occurred *in utero,* at birth, or during childhood in parts of the brain that were too immature to test; or it may have affected a silent area of the brain. Patients with such old lesions, who make up the majority of those with recurrent seizures, are necessarily classified as having "idiopathic epilepsy," because it is impossible to obtain data regarding the original disease. The seizure may be the only sign of the brain abnormality. Inasmuch as idiopathic epilepsy represents one of the most frequent problems in neurologic medicine, it has been assigned a special chapter in our textbook.

The convulsive disorder is the expression of a sudden, excessive, disorderly discharge of neurons in either a structurally normal or diseased cortex. This was the postulation of Hughlings Jackson, the most eminent British neurologist of the nineteenth century, and modern electrophysiology offers no evidence to the contrary. The discharge results in an almost instantaneous disturbance of sensation, loss of consciousness, convulsive movement, or some combination thereof. A terminologic embarrassment arises from the diversity of the clinical manifestations. It seems improper to call a condition a "convulsion" when only an alteration of sensation or of consciousness takes place. The word "seizure" is preferable, as a generic term, and also lends itself to qualification. Motor or convulsive seizure is not, therefore, tautologic, and one may also speak of sensory seizure. The word "epilepsy," which originally meant "falling evil," has many unpleasant connotations, and although a useful term medically, it should be avoided in open discussions until the public becomes more enlightened.

COMMON TYPES OF CONVULSIVE DISORDER

The generalized convulsion ranks as the most frequent type, being both a common expression of a number of ongoing diseases and the lasting mark of some obscure disease in the past. As in petit mal, another special type of brief spell, the location of the causative lesion and its cause are known. Various other patterns of seizure, such as the psychomotor, which is associated with disease of the temporal lobe, usually have a demonstrable cortical focus, either actively progressing or stationary.

When the idiopathic recurrent types of convulsive disorder are analyzed as a group, as in the survey of nearly 2,000 patients by Lennox, it was found that 51 percent had generalized convulsions; 8 percent, petit mal; and the remaining 41 percent, focal and mixed types, of which psychomotor was the most frequent.

Generalized convulsion (other than grand mal) Certain intercurrent medical diseases manifest themselves at one stage by a seizure or a series of seizures beginning as immediate loss of consciousness, with stiffening, then clonic rhythmic jerking of the limbs. The focality of the initiating lesion may be indicated by tonic or clonic spasm of the muscles of only one part of the body or a turning of eyes and head to one side. Consciousness tends to be reinstated soon after the cessation of the motor activity. A single myoclonic jerk or multiple ones may be a prelude to the major seizure or may follow it or be interspersed between seizures. In some instances, especially in metabolic disorders of the brain, the focal motor seizures may appear first on one side of the body, then on the other. Medication may prevent them from becoming generalized.

Generalized convulsion (grand mal) The recurrent generalized seizure of grand mal type is more elaborate and demonstrates more clearly the effect of the epileptic discharge on the physiology of the nervous system. It begins with a sudden loss of consciousness, a cry, a fall to the ground, tonic then clonic movements of muscles of tongue and limbs, sometimes sphincteric incontinence, and other autonomic disorders. The motor activity soon terminates, leaving the patient in a state of coma, which lasts for many minutes or even as long as a half-hour. As the coma recedes, mental confusion, drowsiness, and headache supervene. This type of seizure, which is more fully described in Chap. 337, either may represent the generalized phase of a focal seizure or may constitute the entire attack. Anticonvulsant therapy abbreviates it.

Petit mal (minor epilepsy, l'absence) This type of seizure comes without warning and is notable for its brevity and minimal motor accompaniment. It consists essentially of a brief loss of consciousness, lasting a few seconds. A few three-per-second blinks or jerks of eyelids and sometimes arms may be conjoined. Petit mal may be combined with sudden falling episodes or single, brief generalized myoclonic contractions of limbs (see under Idiopathic Epilepsy, Chap. 337).

COMMON FOCAL SEIZURE PATTERNS Psychomotor epilepsy Certainly this is the most frequent and interesting type of focal seizure pattern. The aura, if it occurs, often takes the form of a complex hallucination or perceptual illusion. There may be an unpleasant smell or taste, or the revival of a complicated visual scene involving people, dwellings, etc., usually taken from past experiences and resembling a dream. Furthermore, the patient's perception of what is seen and heard and his relationship to the outside world are altered. Objects appear to be far away or unreal (*jamais vu*); or strange objects or persons may seem familiar (*déja vu phenomenon*). Hughlings Jackson applied the term *dreamy state* to these psychic disturbances. In the seizure the patient behaves as though he were partially conscious. He may get up and walk about, unbutton or remove his clothes, attempt to speak, or even continue such habitual acts as driving a car. If he is asked a specific question or given a command, it is evident that he is out of contact with the examiner and does not understand. When restrained, he may resist with great energy and at times may be violent. This type of behavior is said to be *automatic,* presumably because the patient behaves like an automaton. Convulsive movements, when present, are likely to consist of chewing, smacking and licking of the lips, and less often, tonic spasms of the limbs or turning of the head and eyes to one side.

In any given case one or several of these phenomena may be observed. In the series studied by Lennox and Lennox, which numbered 414 cases, 43 percent of patients displayed some of these motor or psychomotor phenomena; 32 percent, the automatic state; and 25 percent, the psychic changes. Some psychomotor seizures are very brief, lasting only for seconds, and others continue for hours. This calls to mind that the duration of the seizure is an unsatisfactory criterion for classification.

LOCALIZED MOTOR SEIZURES (CONTRAVERSIVE, FOCAL MOTOR, AND JACKSONIAN SEIZURES) A lesion in one or the other frontal lobe may give rise to a generalized or major convulsive seizure of the type described above, without an introductory aura. In some cases there is a turning movement of the head and eyes to one side, simultaneously with loss of consciousness. It has been postulated that in both types of seizure, the one with and the one without contraversive movements, the discharge from the frontal lobe spreads rapidly into an integrating center such as the thalamus, with immediate loss of consciousness. In patients with head and eye turning, the discharge is believed to reach area 8 (area for contralateral turning of head and eyes), although it has been found that contralateral turning of the head and eyes can be induced in the experimental animal by stimulation of the temporal or occipital region as well as of the premotor cortex.

Do most cases of idiopathic generalized motor seizures (grand mal) that have no focality of onset have a frontal focus? Unfortunately, this question cannot be answered at the moment. Such a focus has been found in only a small number of such cases, and these may not be representative of the whole group.

The *Jacksonian motor seizure* begins usually with a tonic contraction or a clonic rhythmic twitching of the fingers of one hand, the face on one side, or one foot. The twitching may occur in bursts, or paroxysms. The disorder then spreads, or marches, from the part first affected to other muscles on the same side of the body—from the face to the neck, hand, forearm, arm, trunk, and leg; if the first movement is in the foot, the order is reversed. A high incidence of onset in the lips, fingers, and toes probably is related to the greater cortical representation of these parts of the body. The disease process or focus of excitation is usually the Rolandic cortex, area 4 (Fig. 27-1) on the opposite side; in a few cases it has been found in the post-Rolandic convolution. Lesions confined to the premotor cortex (area 6) are said to induce tonic contractions of an arm, face, neck, or all of one side of the body. Perspiration and piloerection, sometimes only of the parts of the body involved in a focal motor seizure, suggest that these autonomic functions have cortical representation in the Rolandic area. Some neurologists distinguish focal motor and Jacksonian motor seizures by the absence of a characteristic march in the former, but both have essentially the same localizing significance.

Another type of focal motor epilepsy, the previously mentioned *epilepsia partialis continua,* consists of rhythmic clonic movements of one group of muscles, usually in the face, arm, or leg. These may continue for a variable period of time, from minutes to weeks or months. The seizure usually does not "march" to other parts of the body. Its localizing value has not been settled. Some patients have a lesion in the opposite sensorimotor areas of the cerebral cortex.

SOMATIC, VISUAL, AND OTHER SENSORY SEIZURES Somatic sensory seizures, either focal or marching to other parts of the body on one side, nearly always indicate a parietal lobe lesion. The usual sensory disorder is described as a numbness, a tingling, or a "pins-and-needles" feeling. Other variations are sensations of crawling (formication), buzzing, electricity, or vibration. Pain and thermal sensations are infrequent. The onset is in the lips, fingers, and toes in the majority of cases, and the spread to adjacent parts of the body follows a pattern determined by sensory arrangements in the postcentral (post-Rolandic) convolution of the parietal lobe. In the series of Kristiansen and Penfield the seizure focus was found in the postcentral convolution in 24 of 55 cases; it was central, either pre- or post-Rolandic, in 18, and precentral in 7 cases. If localized in the cranial muscles, the focus is in the lowest part of the convolution, near the Sylvian fissure; if in the foot or leg, the upper part near the superior sagittal sinus is involved.

Lesions in or near the striate cortex of the occipital lobe usually produce a sensation of lights, of darkness, or of color. The patient may tell of seeing stairs of moving lights in the visual field on the side opposite the lesion. Sometimes they appear to be straight ahead of the patient. Often, if they occur on only one side of the visual field, he believes only one eye to be affected, the one opposite the lesion, probably because the average person is unaware that he has two corresponding visual fields. It is curious that a seizure arising in one occipital lobe may cause momentary blindness in both eyes. It has been noted that seizures arising in the lateral surface of the occipital lobes (Brodmann's areas 18 and 19) are more likely to cause twinkling or pulsating lights. Complex visual hallucinations are usually due to a focus in the posterior part of the temporal lobe, near its junction with the parietal, and they may be associated with auditory hallucinations. Often the visual images, either those of the hallucination or of objects seen, are distorted or seem too small (*micropsia*) or unnaturally arranged.

Auditory hallucinations are rather infrequent as an initial manifestation of a seizure. Occasionally a patient with a focus in the superior temporal convolution on one side will report a buzzing or a roaring in his ears. A human voice sometimes repeating recognizable words has been noted a few times in patients with lesions in the more posterior part of the dominant temporal lobe.

Vertiginous sensations of a type suggesting vestibular stimulation may be the first symptom of a seizure. The lesion is usually localized in the superior posterior temporal region or at the junction between the parietal and temporal lobes. Occasionally, with a temporal focus, vertigo is followed by an auditory sensation.

Olfactory hallucinations are often associated with disease of the inferior and medial parts of the temporal lobe, usually in the region of the hippocampal convolution or the uncus (hence the term *uncinate seizures,* after Jackson). Usually the smell is exteriorized, i.e., projected to someplace in the environment, and is of a disagreeable nature. Gustatory hallucinations have also been recorded in proved cases of temporal lobe disease. Sensations of thirst and salivation may be associated. Stimulation of the upper surface of the temporal lobe in the depths of the Sylvian fissure during neurosurgical operations has produced peculiar sensations of taste.

Visceral sensations arising in the thorax, epigastrium, and abdomen are among the most frequent of the auras. They are described as a vague, indefinable feeling, a sinking sensation in the pit of the stomach, and a weakness in the epigastrium or substernal area that rises to the throat and head. The seizure discharge may be localized to the upper bank of the Sylvian fissure or in the upper intermediate or medial frontal areas near the cingulate gyrus. Palpitation and acceleration of pulse at the beginning of the attack have also been related to a temporal lobe focus.

PSYCHIC PHENOMENA A close relationship between psychic changes and temporal lobe foci has been established. Disease of either temporal lobe may be accompanied by seizures that have many of the characteristics outlined earlier in this chapter under Psychomotor Epilepsy. In addition, complex visual and auditory hallucinations with feelings of unreality, and partial or complete interruption of consciousness may be observed. Compulsive thought or action may recur in a fixed pattern during each seizure. Automatic behavior or even frank psychoses resembling confusional states or even schizophrenia, and lasting for hours or days, may be induced by seizure discharges or electrical stimulation of the temporal lobe.

In addition to these types, the clinicians of the nineteenth century recognized many other special forms of epilepsy, some of which were given descriptive names. The term *myoclonic epilepsy* referred to a syndrome of epilepsy and isolated twitches of a muscle or group of muscles, the latter being the *myoclonus* (see Chap. 18). Random, arrhythmic myoclonus in a sense might be designated as *epilepsia partialis discontinua et disseminata.* It is usually caused by a more or less diffuse disease of the cerebral and cerebellar cortex and possibly of other parts of the nervous system, such as the thalamus. In childhood a number of other forms of epilepsy occur, related presumably to the immaturity of the child's nervous system. The seizures of the newborn (*neonatal epilepsy*) are fragmentary and brief. Infantile or salaam spasms, i.e., brief flexion of neck and limbs, are peculiar to the age period of six months to three to four years. *Febrile seizures* appear only in the age period of eighteen months to six years. *Photic reflex* epilepsy is induced by flickering light in childhood and adolescence (Chap. 334).

The various motor, sensory, or psychic phenomena may be combined in many different sequences. These presumably indicate the spread of a seizure discharge from one cortical area to another. A flash of light followed by tingling of one side of the body suggests that the epileptic discharge began in the occipital lobe and extended to the somatic sensory areas in the parietal lobe. A smell of something burning, followed by chewing and smacking movements, and then loss of speech would be interpreted as a spread of the seizure discharge from the region of the uncus to the upper parts of the temporal and the inferior frontal lobes. A focal motor seizure followed by a tonic contraction of one side of the body and then by turning of the head and eyes contralaterally would indicate a successive involvement of the motor, premotor, and contraversive cortical field for head and eyes. Little is known about the factors that facilitate or inhibit the spread of seizure discharges from one part of the brain to another.

THE EVOCATION OF SEIZURES (REFLEX EPILEPSY) Seizures can sometimes be evoked in susceptible persons by a physiologic or psychologic stimulus. Approximately 1 in every 15 patients will have remarked that their seizures occur under special circumstances, such as being exposed to flickering light, passing from darkness to light or the reverse, being startled by a loud noise, hearing a series of monotonous sounds or music, touching, rubbing, or hurting a particular part of the body, making certain movements (e.g., eating, reading, carrying out some complex mental task), or being subjected to fright or other strong emotion. The evoked seizure may be focal (beginning often in the part of the body that has been stimulated) or generalized. In a few instances this reflex epilepsy, as it is called, has been due to a focal cerebral disease, such as a tumor, but more often its cause cannot be ascertained. A special type of reflex myoclonic epilepsy with a strong tendency to familial incidence can be elicited by photic stimulation (photic epilepsy). Another point of interest in these cases of evoked seizure has been the phenomenon of willfully averting the seizure by undertaking some mental task, e.g., thinking about some distracting subject or counting, or by initiating some physical activity.

The condition of patients of this type informs us that epilepsy is a natural state, a physiologic event resulting from excitation and subsequent inhibition of a damaged part of the cerebrum. The basis of the synchronization and potentiation of the cortical seizure focus has been the subject of much study. Evidently the physiologic event that initiates the seizure is a high-voltage discharge of an assemblage of cortical neurons. There need not be a visible lesion for, under the proper circumstances, it can be initiated in entirely normal cerebral cortex, as when the cortex is activated by a drug or injured by hypoxia. But it is the visible focal lesion that has been the most thoroughly investigated. Some of the electrical properties of the cortical focus suggest that its neurons have been deafferented. Deafferented neurons are known to be hypersensitive; they remain chronically in a state of partial depolarization, and the cytoplasmic membranes have an increased permeability which renders them susceptible to activation by hyperthermia, hypoxia, hypoglycemia, and hyponatremia, as well as by repeated sensory (e.g., photic) stimulation and during certain phases of sleep (where hypersynchrony of neurons is known to occur). Another hypothesis is that the lesion of the cortex has resulted in the removal of a normal diencephalic inhibitory effect.

The biochemical studies of the involved clone of neurons of a seizure focus have not clarified the problem. Epileptic foci are known to be sensitive to acetylcholine and to be slower in binding and removing it than normal cerebral cortex; a deficiency of gamma-aminobutyric acid (GABA), the inhibitory transmitter, a disturbance of cytochrome oxidase with decrease in ATP production, a reduction in the Krebs cycle function with a shift to GABA-succinate shunt, a disturbance in local regulation of extracellular K, Na, Ca, Mg are other hypotheses equally lacking of confirmation.

Once the intensity of the seizure discharge exceeds a certain point, it spreads to adjacent cortical and to thalamic and brainstem nuclei. Then it is that the first clinical manifestation of the convulsion begins. Presumably the excitatory activity is fed back from the thalamus to the original focus and to other parts of the forebrain, giving rise to the characteristic high-frequency discharge in the EEG, and there is propagation downward to spinal neurons via corticospinal and reticulospinal pathways. Shortly thereafter a diencephalocortical inhibition begins and intermittently interrupts the focal and generalized seizure discharge, changing it from the persistent discharge of the tonic phase to the intermittent bursts of the clonic phase. These become less and less frequent and finally cease altogether, leaving in their wake strong inhibition or paralysis of the neurons of the epileptic focus. This latter is the basis of *Todd's postepileptic paralysis* and of the diffuse slow waves in the EEG in all parts of the cerebrum. In petit mal it is thought that the high-voltage spike–slow wave discharge originates in the thalamus, and this may also be true of some cases of grand mal, in both of which consciousness is at once abolished. On the other hand, atypical petit mal and possibly the typical type as well can be induced by a mesial frontal lesion. Temporal lobe seizures are known to arise in foci in the medial temporal lobe amygdaloid nuclei and hippocampus. Electrical stimulation in these areas reproduces loss of conscious contact with environment, feelings of depersonalization, and automatic behavior.

A discovery of no little importance is that a seizure focus, if active for a time, may establish via commissural connections a secondary focus in the corresponding area of cortex in the opposite hemisphere (mirror focus). The nature of this development is not fully understood. This becomes a source of confusion in trying to identify electrographically the side of the primary lesion.

Severe seizures may disturb the chemistry of the brain by causing hypoxia, acidosis with rise in P_{CO_2}, and an accumulation of lactic acid. Some of these effects are secondary to respiratory spasm, blockage of airway, and excessive muscular activity. These biochemical changes give rise to secondary cerebral lesions. These are especially frequent in the temporal lobes and cerebellum and may themselves later become epileptic foci. A violent epileptic discharge of the brain may cause respiratory arrest or cardiac standstill, with death ensuing immediately.

The electroencephalogram provides a delicate proof of Hughlings Jackson's theory of epilepsy—that it is an excessive, disorderly discharge of cortical neurons. At the onset of the focal seizure this is registered in or near the focus as a series of spikes or sharp waves interrupting the normal alpha and beta waves. The clinical spread of the seizure has its electroencephalographic equivalent in the extension of the abnormal electrical waves; and with generalization of the seizure (grand mal), the entire electroencephalographic recording surface of the brain exhibits spikes of high voltage. Petit mal is accompanied by a characteristic three- per-second wave-spike complex occurring simultaneously in all cortical leads and presumably taking origin from a diencephalic focus. At first there was thought to be a characteristic electroencephalographic picture for psychomotor epilepsy, but further studies have not confirmed this. The postseizure state, sometimes called *postconvulsive paralysis of cerebral function,* also has its electroencephalographic correlate in random generalized slow waves. With recovery of normal mentation the electroencephalogram returns to normal. If the electroencephalographic tracing is obtained during the interval between seizures, it is abnormal to some degree in approximately 40 percent of fully conscious and 75 percent of sleeping patients.

The electroencephalographic changes are discussed in Chap. 337.

PATHOLOGY OF THE CONVULSIVE STATE As will be pointed out in Chap. 322, in some cases of idiopathic epilepsy of grand mal and petit mal type the brain has been grossly and microscopically normal, though in all probability in no single case has the brain been subjected to serial sectioning of the entire cerebrum. Certainly the convulsive states attending drug withdrawal, intoxication, etc., must represent derangements at the subcellular level.

Of the innumerable diseases that are epileptogenic (see below) it has not been possible to distinguish the component of lesion that is responsible for the seizures from one that is not. In other words one cannot say from microscopic examination whether or not any given lesion was epileptic. Gliosis, fibrosis, vascularization, meningocerebral cicatrix have all been incriminated, but they occur as well in nonepileptic foci. Partial disconnection of groups of cortical neurons from those of neighboring cortex, of the other cerebral hemisphere, and of the thalamus seems likely to have occurred. Or certain systems of inhibiting neurons may have been destroyed. In the highly epileptic experimental lesions produced by aluminum cream and penicillin one can see that some neurons are surely destroyed, especially in the superficial layers, and the synaptic connections of the remaining ones are reduced in number. Probably a disorganization of these cortical interneural relationships is more important than the nature of the lesion, for diseases as different as, for example, hemorrhage, infarction, and neoplastic invasion are all epileptogenic at times. Once gliotic focus of whatever cause, bordered by groups of discharging neurons, becomes epileptogenic, it may remain so throughout the lifetime of the patient.

DISEASES CAUSING SYMPTOMATIC SEIZURES

Among the medical diseases which may be complicated by a burst of seizures, the following are the most frequent.

Generalized convulsions mixed in some instances with unilateral muscular contractions of clonic type appear prominently during an abstinence or withdrawal period in patients addicted to alcohol or barbiturates. Suspicion of this mechanism is raised by the telltale marks of alcoholic excesses or the history of a prolonged nervousness requiring sedation. Also disturbances of sleep, disorientation, illusions, and visual hallucinations often precede and follow the convulsive phase of the illness. The convulsive period lasts several days and is accompanied and followed for several more by a confusional state.

Bacterial meningitis is another type of illness with a strong convulsive tendency, more pronounced in children than in adults. Fever and stiff neck usually provide the clue, and lumbar puncture yields the salient laboratory data.

Uremia is another condition with a prominent convulsive aspect. Of interest is the sequence of events in complete anuria. This condition is tolerated for 2 to 3 days without neurologic signs, and then there is a rapid onset of twitching, trembling, myoclonic jerks, and generalized motor seizures. Tetany may be added (see Chap. 269). The motor display, one of the most dramatic in medicine, lasts several days until the patient sinks into terminal coma or recovers. When this syndrome accompanies lupus erythematosus, delirium tremens, idiopathic epilepsy, or generalized neoplasia, one can nearly always be sure that it has a basis in renal failure.

Cardiac arrest, suffocation or respiratory failure, NO_2 anesthesia, CO poisoning—the common causes of hypoxic encephalopathy—induce a diffuse myoclonic jerking of all the musculature and generalized seizures as soon as cardiac function is resumed. The convulsive phase of this condition may last only a few days, in association with coma, stupor, or confusion; or it may persist indefinitely as an intention myoclonic-convulsive state.

Other acute illnesses complicated by generalized and multifocal motor seizures are hyponatremia and water intoxication, thyrotoxic storm, hypertensive encephalopathy, porphyria, hypoglycemia, pyridoxine deficiency, argininosuccinic aciduria, and phenylketonuria. Picrotoxin and metrazol are two of the most highly convulsant drugs in use, and lead and arsenic the most frequent convulsive metallic intoxicants.

Generalized seizures with or without twitching may occur in the terminal phases of many other illnesses, such as gram-negative septicemias with shock, liver coma, and intractable congestive heart failure.

There are several primary diseases of the brain which are announced by an acute convulsive state. Myoclonic jerking and seizures appear early in acute inclusion-body encephalitis and other forms of viral, treponemal, and parasitic encephalitis, subacute sclerosing encephalitis, as well as in lipid storage diseases, Jakob-Creutzfeldt disease, and diffuse gliomatosis of the brain.

It seems strange that difficult problems of a convulsive nature seldom occur in patients suffering from cerebrovascular disease. Only exceptionally will a cerebral embolus cause a focal fit, though old cortical infarcts arising therefrom become epileptogenic in 20 percent of cases. The rupture of an aneurysm is occasionally marked by one or two generalized convulsions. Thrombotic occlusions of cerebral arteries are almost never convulsive in the evolving phases of the stroke. Subcortical hemorrhages in malignant hypertension occasionally become sources of recurrent focal epilepsy. The rare thrombophlebitis with cortical ischemia and infarction is probably the most highly convulsive vascular lesion.

The usual causes of focal seizures beginning at any age but especially in adult years are cerebral tumors, trauma, tic scars, suppurative diseases, especially thrombophlebitis, and abscess. Each of these groups of disease will be discussed in Chaps. 327, 328, and 329.

APPROACH TO THE CLINICAL PROBLEM OF RECURRENT SEIZURES

A history of recurrent attacks of loss of consciousness or awareness associated with abnormal movements or confusion is usually sufficient to establish a diagnosis of epilepsy. With such patients a thorough history, a complete physical and neurologic examination, testing of the visual fields, and laboratory studies, including x-ray examination of the skull and an electroencephalogram, should be done. The results of these essential procedures will determine to which of the categories in the above classification the case belongs or whether one must resort to the label of idiopathic epilepsy.

If a patient not known to have been epileptic has an acute illness with frequent generalized or one-sided seizures, a search must be conducted for clinical and laboratory signs of infection, metabolic and endocrine diseases, and intoxications.

If convulsions have occurred in the past, an inquiry as to epilepsy in the family history and occurrence of head trauma or infections in the past must be made; and careful description of the seizure itself, including prodromata, aura, manifestations during the seizure and the postictal period, must be obtained. Seizures in other members of the family favor slightly the diagnosis of idiopathic epilepsy. Signs of pulmonary or ear infection or of congenital heart disease with a right-to-left shunt should suggest, in a patient with recently acquired seizures, the possibility of a brain abscess. The presence of a heart murmur and fever or of atrial fibrillation favors embolism. Head trauma of a serious nature, followed by seizures after an interval of several weeks to 2 years, indicates that an injury may have given rise to convulsions. A regularly recurring aura, especially of a focal nature, may indicate a localized lesion in the brain. Similarly, a focal convulsive movement at the onset of the seizure probably indicates a localized cerebral lesion. A transient monoplegia or hemiplegia (Todd's paralysis) in the postictal period also has considerable significance in localizing a lesion. In fact, its presence may provide the best clue to a focal brain lesion. A history of other neurologic symptoms such as headache, localized paralysis, or mental changes often indicates the need for special diagnostic studies.

A general physical examination may provide clues to the legion of conditions associated with epilepsy. Protuberances over the skull may suggest an underlying pathologic condition. Vascular nevi over the body, especially over the face and in the retina, may be associated with vascular abnormalities within the skull. Small tumors, often pedunculated, distributed over the body surface bring to mind the diagnosis of von Recklinghausen's disease and, when associated with seizures, may indicate an intracranial glioma or neurofibroma. White spots over the trunk and limbs and sebaceous adenomas of the face point to the diagnosis of tuberous sclerosis. Smallness of an arm or leg points to a congenital defect of the brain. Cranial nerve disturbances are also helpful in diagnosis; thus, a sixth-nerve paralysis is often associated with increased intracranial pressure. Localized weakness, differences in reflexes, or the presence of abnormal reflexes, such as Babinski's response, all have localizing value.

The question of what laboratory procedures should be done in cases of epilepsy can be answered only on the basis of the clinical findings. With recent onset of generalized convulsions simple blood chemistry tests are among the first measures to be carried out. The determination of blood glucose helps orient the examiner in instances of hypoglycemia and hyperglycemia; the calcium level provides the main clue to hypocalcemia, the blood urea nitrogen (BUN) to kidney disease, and sodium and potassium levels to multiple metabolic disturbances, including dilutional hyponatremia. X-rays of the skull should be taken in all cases. Significant findings related to increased intracranial pressure include erosion of the clinoid processes and, in infants and children, separation of the sutures. Hyperostoses, erosions of the skull, abnormal vascular markings, and intracranial calcifications are other findings of importance that may appear in skull x-rays. Because of the frequency of cerebral metastases from primary carcinoma of the lung, chest x-rays should be made in all patients suspected of having intracranial neoplasm.

Lumbar puncture can be of considerable value in elucidating the causes of epilepsy. If the history, neurologic examination, or skull x-rays show any abnormality, especially if a focal lesion in the brain is suggested, then a lumbar puncture is mandatory. Of special importance are determination of the pressure, cell count, total protein, and serologic tests. Increased pressure points to an expanding intracranial lesion. An abnormal cell count usually indicates an infectious process. An elevation only of total protein (greater than 100 mg per 100 ml) favors the diagnosis of a tumor. If the pressure is normal but other symptoms or signs point to a recently acquired, localized brain lesion, an arteriogram or pneumoencephalogram may be needed. If, in addition to localizing signs, the patient shows signs of increased intracranial pressure, whether by papilledema or high cerebrospinal fluid pressure, then a ventriculogram may be preferred to a pneumoencephalogram, although arteriography is now used more frequently than air visualization because of its greater safety. The visualization of the cerebral hemisphere by these procedures may be of particular help to the neurosurgeon in localizing the lesion and in planning a surgical approach to it.

The electroencephalogram, although now routinely employed in the definitive diagnosis of cases with epilepsy, is not absolutely conclusive, since it may be normal in some patients, particularly if the seizures are relatively infrequent, or abnormal in diseases that do not cause epilepsy. The test is of particular value in diagnosing petit mal, for here clinical or subclinical attacks are apt to be frequent enough to register during the electroencephalographic test. Abnormal electrical waves may manifest themselves in other types of epilepsy as well, and the electroencephalogram may be abnormal during the interseizure period, demonstrating either focal or generalized abnormalities of cortical activity. Activation of the electroencephalogram by photic stimulation, drug-induced sleep, or Metrazol injection is now standard procedure in many laboratories.

The type of clinical study in any given case is dictated to some extent by the age of the patient. Up until early adulthood the plan should be outlined as below. Most patients in this age group turn out to have idiopathic epilepsy. With increasing age, the incidence of idiopathic epilepsy becomes less and that of symptomatic epilepsy increases. Thus the appearance of convulsions for the first time at a period past middle age should be presumptive evidence of brain tumor until every effort has been made to rule it out.

The most frequent causes of recurrent convulsions in different age groups are presented in Table 24-1.

DIFFERENTIAL DIAGNOSIS The clinical differences between a seizure and a syncopal attack were presented in Chap. 16 and need not be repeated here. It must be emphasized once again that there is no single criterion for distinguishing between them. The author has erred in calling akinetic seizures simple faints and in mistaking cardiac or carotid sinus faints for seizures. Petit mal may be difficult to identify because of the brevity of attacks. One helpful maneuver is to have to the patient count for 5 to 10 min. If he is having petit mal, he will blink or stare, pause in counting, or skip one or two numbers. Psychomotor seizures are the most difficult of all to diagnose. These attacks are so variable in character and so likely to induce minor disturbances in conduct rather than obvious interruptions of consciousness that they may be misdiag-

TABLE 24-1
Causes of recurrent convulsion in different age groups

Age of onset, yr	*Probable cause*
Infancy, 0–2	Congenital maldevelopment, birth injury; metabolic (hypocalcemia, hypoglycemia), vitamin B_6 deficiency, phenylketonuria
Childhood, 2–10	Birth injury, trauma, infections, thrombosis of cerebral arteries or veins, beginning of idiopathic epilepsy
Adolescence, 10–18	Idiopathic epilepsy, trauma, congenital defects
Early adulthood, 18–35	Trauma, neoplasm, idiopathic epilepsy, alcoholism, drug addiction
Middle age, 35–60	Neoplasm, trauma, vascular disease, alcoholism, drug addiction
Late life, over 60	Vascular disease, degeneration, tumor

nosed as temper tantrums, hysteria, psychopathic behavior, or acute psychosis.

A special problem in diagnosis is offered by states of mental dullness and confusion. Epileptic patients as seen in hospital and office practice usually show no mental deterioration, regardless of the type of seizure. Therefore, the appearance of dementia, confusion, or some other derangement of mental function should suggest the possibility of recurrent subclinical seizures not controlled by medication, drug intoxication, postseizure psychosis, or a brain disease that has caused both dementia and seizures. To distinguish these clinical states may require careful observation, along the lines suggested in Chap. 26, and electroencephalography.

TREATMENT Since recurrent seizures with persistent coma in the intervening intervals may prove fatal, some form of anticonvulsant medication should be given immediately to most patients who have had a convulsion. A safe plan of medication is to administer diphenylhydantoin 400 mg and phenobarbital 200 mg per day. Both medications may be given orally or parenterally. The type of disease causing the seizures and its treatment determines the anticonvulsant program thereafter. Antibiotic medications usually arrest the seizure tendency in bacterial meningitis. NaCl in a 3% solution usually terminates the seizures in hyponatremia. $MgSO_4$ and Ca gluconate often help in uremic convulsions. Abstinence seizures terminate naturally within a few days and are rarely severe and frequent during this period. Glucose intravenously stops hypoglycemic convulsions. In all these conditions occasional seizures, if brief, are not of serious consequence, and it is preferable not to give excessive doses of anticonvulsant drugs, which are of themselves dangerous if they add to the coma and obscure the manifestations of the underlying disease.

Status epilepticus or persistent focal seizures with generalization are best treated with diazepam 10 mg intravenously and up to 100 mg given over a 12-hr period. Administration of sodium phenobarbital 200 to 400 mg and then 100 to 200 mg every 4 to 6 hr is another highly effective program. Both drugs may be used with diphenylhydantoinate 100 mg every 6 hr. Paraldehyde intravenously 1 to 3 ml (given slowly) or 5 to 10 mg intramuscularly (avoiding nerves) is useful in recurrent focal seizures. (See Chap. 337 for further data on therapy.)

REFERENCES

JASPER HA et al: *Basic Mechanisms of the Epilepsies,* Boston: Little, Brown, 1969

LENNOX W, LENNOX M: *Epilepsy,* Boston: Little, Brown, 1960

SCHMIDT RP, Wilder BJ: *Epilepsy,* Contemporary Neurology Series, Philadelphia: Davis, 1968

25
AFFECTIONS OF SPEECH

RAYMOND D. ADAMS
JAY P. MOHR

Language or speech functions are of fundamental significance to man in both his social intercourse and his private intellectual life; when they are disordered, as a consequence of developmental anomaly or disease of the brain, the result and physiologic loss exceed in gravity even the results of blindness, deafness, and paralysis. Every sophisticated physician should be informed on this subject.

DEVELOPMENT OF LANGUAGE The acquisition of language by the infant and child has been observed methodically by a number of eminent scientists, and their findings provide a basis for understanding the various derangements of speech.

First, there is the *babbling* and *lalling stage,* during which the infant of a few weeks of age emits a variety of sounds in combinations of vowel and labial or nasoguttural consonants. This predominantly motor speech activity is no doubt stimulated and reinforced by auditory sensations, which become linked to the kinesthetic ones arising from the speech musculature. It is not clear whether the capacity to hear and understand the spoken word precedes or follows the first motor speech. Possibily it varies from one infant to another, but certainly both speaking and auditory perception of words develop very early in life. Soon babbling merges with *echo speech,* in which short sounds are repeated in parrot-like fashion; and then longer syllable groups gradually come to be repeated correctly as the praxic function of the speech apparatus develops. Short sounds and words directly related to seen objects or persons are first to appear. Through experience and correction from parents and siblings the child's vocal behavior is gradually shaped to conform to the system of language of the social group in which he is raised.

To learn the name of an object requires the formation of a link between the visual perceptive (association) region of the occipital lobes and the auditory perceptive region in the left temporal lobe. And in order to learn to say a name it is necessary to form a link between the auditory perceptive region (Wernicke's area) and the center for motor patterns of speech (Broca's area). By the age of eighteen to twenty-four months the average infant can construct a phrase; in the months and years that follow, he learns to speak in full sentences. A six-year-old child has a speaking vocabulary of several thousand words and an even larger understanding vocabulary.

Concurrent exposure to graphic visual symbols encourages association of the auditory and kinesthetic images of words and is the basis of reading. Usually the written word is learned by associating it with the spoken word rather than with the seen object. It is held that the superior plane of the temporal lobe (Wernicke's area) and contiguous parietoocipital areas are essential to the establishment of these cross-modal associations. Writing is learned soon after reading, and the auditory-visual symbols of words now must become linked to cursive movements of the hand. Only those destined to become literate learn to read and write; and to be a complete master of the art of writing is an attainment of only a few select members of our society.

Language development appears to proceed in an orderly manner, but there are individual variations in the actual time at which each successive stage is reached and, to a limited extent, in the order of the different stages. Maturational delays are frequent. The pattern appears to be set by the neurologic equipment of the individual at any given age. Psychologic factors are of minor importance, at least in the beginning. There is, therefore, good reason why educators have found it unprofitable to teach reading and writing before the sixth year.

Anthropologists have suggested that the individual merely recapitulates the language development of his race. It is supposed that gestures and the utterance of simple meaningful sounds first occurred in primitive man as a differentiation of emotional speech. Gradually these movements and sounds became the conventional signs and verbal symbols of concrete objects, then of the abstract qualities of objects. Signs and spoken language were the first means of human communication; graphic records appeared much later. The American Indian, for instance, never attained a written language. Writing began as pictorial representation, and only much later were alphabets devised. The reading and writing of words and propositions have been relatively recent developments.

ANATOMY OF THE LANGUAGE FUNCTIONS The conventional teaching is that there are three language areas, situated, in most persons, in the left cerebral hemisphere (see Fig. 27-1, page 160). Two are receptive and one is executive. The two receptive areas are closely related and embrace what may be referred to as the central language zone. One, subserving auditory language reception, is situated in the posterior part of the first and second temporal convolutions (areas 41 and 42) near the primary auditory receptive area in Heschl's convolutions; the other, subserving visuolexic functions, occupies the angular convolution (area 39) in the inferior parietal lobule anterior to the primary visual receptive areas. The intervening regions of the brain between these auditory and visual language "centers"—the inferior temporal region (area 37) and the supramarginal convolution—are also part of this central language zone and are involved in language formulation. The executive area, situated at the posterior end of the third (inferior) frontal convolution (referred to as Broca's area or area 44), is for motor aspects of speech. Of dubious significance as a unique "writing center" is the premotor area at the foot of the second frontal convolution above Broca's area. These sensory and motor areas are connected by the arcuate bundle of nerve fibers which passes through the isthmus of the temporal lobe, and other connections may traverse the external capsule of the lenticular nucleus (subcortical white matter of the insula). From Broca's area there are fiber connections with the lower Rolandic cortex, which in turn innervates the speech apparatus. These language areas are also connected with the thalamus and to corresponding areas in the minor cerebral hemisphere through the corpus callosum and anterior commissure.

There has been much difference of opinion concerning these cortical areas, and objection has been made to calling them centers, for they do not represent histologically circumscribed structures of constant function and fixed localization. Actually there is relatively little information concerning their anatomy and physiology. A competent neuroanatomist could not distinguish under the microscope some of these cortical speech areas from other parts of the cerebral cortex. Crude electrical stimulation of the parts of the cortex concerned with speech while the patient is alert and talking (during craniotomy under local anesthesia) causes only an arrest of speech. Knowledge of the location of speech functions has come almost exclusively from the study of human beings who have succumbed to focal brain diseases. From the available information it seems almost certain that the whole language mechanism is not divisible into discrete parts, each depending on a certain fixed group of neurons. Instead, speech must be regarded as a complex sensorimotor process, roughly localized in the opercular or peri-Sylvian region of the left cerebral hemisphere; the more complex elaborations of speech probably depend on the entire cerebrum.

Carl Wernicke, more than any other person, must be credited with the anatomic-psychologic scheme upon which contemporary ideas of *aphasia* rest, but earlier Paul Broca, of Paris, had made the fundamental observation that a lesion of the posterior part of the left inferior frontal convolution deprived a man of speech.

Carl Wernicke showed that the primary receptive and executive functions reside in the cerebral cortex of the dominant cerebral hemisphere—in the superior temporal and inferior frontal convolutions, respectively. Lesions that separated the receptive and/or executive areas from each other, or from other regions of the cerebrum, were said to be transcortical. Lesions which interrupted afferent pathways leading to the receptive area and the efferent pathway from the executive or motor area were assumed to be subcortical. This anatomic scheme was the basis of Wernicke's classification, and although it was much criticized by Pierre Marie, Henry Head, von Monakow, Arnold Pick, and Goldstein, the anatomic plans which they offered differed little from that of Wernicke. Careful case analysis has repeatedly documented the cortical receptive type of aphasia (Wernicke's aphasia) in the superior temporal gyrus and Broca's motor aphasia in the inferior frontal convolution and adjacent premotor, motor, and insular regions of the cortex. Subcortical lesions beneath the inferior frontal convolution are known now to cause *pure word muteness;* those of the temporal white matter, *word deafness;* and those beneath the angular gyrus, *pure word blindness.* The existence of a transcortical type of aphasia remains uncertain. The latter concept is especially confusing to modern students of physiology when applied to interruption of pathways between Wernicke's and Broca's zones, because it presupposes a neat separation of compartments for sensory and motor functions, which is not in line with contemporary views of sensorimotor physiology of the rest of the body.

The most that one can say is that human language depends in some way upon the integrity of an anatomic region situated between the primary input zones of the temporal and occipital lobes and the output zones in the inferior frontal lobe of the dominant hemisphere. This places the mechanism in close connection with the cortical sensory association and cross-modal elaboration areas of the superior temporal and inferior parietal lobes, with the corresponding parts of the opposite cerebral hemisphere through the corpus callosum, with the medial parts of the temporal lobes (learning-memory mechanism), and with the diencephalon. The acquisition of language appears to involve, in part, the establishment of specific, item-by-item, cross-modal, verbally mediated associations. But how these regions of the brain are organized, how they can be activated (controlled) by a variety of visual and auditory stimuli, resulting in the complex behavior of which we make casual daily use in interpersonal communication, remains almost totally unknown.

From the available clinical and pathologic data it may be concluded that the locus of the anatomic lesion is more significant than the extent of brain damage. Localization of the lesion is in most instances predictable from the clinical deficit, but there are wide variations in the degree to which a deficit appears following focal brain disease. Inconsistency of anatomic data in certain types of aphasia has been explained in several ways. The most popular explanation has been that the net effect of any lesion depends not only on locus and extent of lesion but also on the degree of cerebral dominance. If cerebral dominance is poorly established, a left-sided lesion has less effect on speech than if dominance is strong. Unfortunately, handedness and cerebral dominance are not recorded in many of the 1,500 cases collected by Henschen from the world's medical literature. Another factor which imparts an element of unpredictability to the anatomy of speech is the poorly understood impression that individuals differ in the way in which they acquire language as children. This is believed to play a role in making available alternate means for accomplishing language tasks when the method initially learned has been impaired through brain disease. The extent to which improvement in language performance represents "recovery" of function or generation of new response methods remains poorly understood at present.

CEREBRAL DOMINANCE AND ITS RELATIONSHIP TO SPEECH AND HANDEDNESS The functional supremacy of one cerebral hemisphere is crucial to language function. There are three ways of determining that the left side of the brain is dominant: (1) the loss of speech when disease occurs in certain parts of the left hemisphere and its preservation in diseases involving corresponding parts of the right hemisphere; (2) the greater facility in the use of the right hand, foot, and eye; (3) the arrest of speech immediately after the injection of amobarbital (Amytal Sodium) or some other drug in the left internal carotid artery. Only (2) and (3) are of use in deciding the cerebral dominance of a living, healthy patient. Unfortunately the Sodium Amytal, or Wada, test does not reproduce the syndrome of major hemisphere inactivation. There is only mutism, followed by a brief period of groping for names. Presumably it gives information about the localization of motor output areas rather than of sensory ones.

Of the general population approximately 90 to 95 percent are right-handed; the remainder prefer the left hand. A person is said to be right-handed if he chooses the right hand for intricate, complex acts and is more skilful with it. The preference is more complete in some persons than in others. Most individuals are neither right-handed nor completely left-handed but favor one hand for more complicated tasks.

The reason for hand preference is still controversial. There is strong evidence of a hereditary factor, but the mode of inheritance is uncertain. Learning is also a factor; many children are shifted at an early age from left to right (shifted sinistrals) because it is a handicap to be left-handed in a right-handed world. Many right-handed persons sight with the right eye, and it has been said that eye preference determines hand preference. Even if true, this still does not account for eye dominance. It is noteworthy that handedness develops simultaneously with language, and the most that can be said at the present is that speech localization and the preference for one eye, one hand, and one foot are all manifestations of some fundamental, inherited tendency not yet defined. Anatomic differences between the dominant and the minor cerebral hemispheres are minor, but the one finding relevant to language laterality is the slightly larger planum temporale, beneath Wernicke's language zone, in the left hemisphere.

Left-handedness may result from disease of the left cerebral hemisphere in early life, and this probably accounts for its higher incidence among the feebleminded and brain-injured. Presumably the neural mechanisms for language then become centered in the right cerebral hemisphere. Handedness and cerebral dominance may fail to develop in some individuals, and this is particularly true in certain families. Developmental defects in speech and reading, stuttering, "mirror writing," and general clumsiness are much more frequent in these families.

Differences in degree of cerebral dominance unquestionably account for some of the inconsistency in the cerebral localization of speech in different persons. In studies of groups of left-handed individuals who suffer cerebral derangements of speech it has been noted that approximately 75 percent of them have had lesions in the left cerebral hemisphere. Further, in those extremely rare cases of aphasia due to right cerebral lesions, the patient is nearly always left-handed, and the speech disorder tends to be less severe and enduring. The latter may take the form of an expressive disturbance rather than inability to read (alexia) or inability to name objects (amnestic aphasia), and visuoconstructive troubles are prominent, as are also faults in calculation and implicit awareness of one's neurologic deficits (anosognosia).

The functional capacities of the minor hemisphere in speech are not fully documented by careful anatomic studies. There is always some uncertainty as to whether any residual function after lesions of the major hemisphere is due to recovery of parts of its language zones or to the activity solely of the minor hemisphere. The following functions are not disturbed in lesions of the left hemisphere: motor responses of mimicry, social anticipation (smiling, handshaking, modesty reactions) and self-care (washing and feeding), avoidance behavior to noxious stimuli, and capability of training in performances of cross-matching visually presented simple words with pictures.

TYPES OF LANGUAGE DISORDERS ENCOUNTERED IN MEDICINE These may be divided into four categories:

1 Disturbances of speech that occur with diseases affecting the higher nervous integrations, namely, delirium and dementia. Speech is seldom lost in these conditions but is instead merely deranged as part of a general impairment of intellectual functions; e.g., in Alzheimer's disease a gradual impairment of all elements of language constitutes an important part of the clinical picture (see Chap. 27). *Palilalia* and *echolalia,* in which the patient repeats, parrot-like, the syllables and words which he hears, are special abnormalities observed only in states of dementia with bilateral cerebral lesions.
2 A cerebral disturbance in which there is a loss more or less exclusively of the production and/or comprehension of spoken and/or written speech. This condition is called *aphasia* or, in milder degrees, *dysphasia.*
3 A defect in articulation with intact mental functions and normal comprehension and memory of words. This is a pure motor disorder of the muscles of articulation and may be due to flaccid or spastic paralysis, rigidity, repetitive spasms (stuttering), or ataxia. The terms *anarthria* and *dysarthria* have been applied to some of these conditions.
4 Loss of voice due to a disease of the larynx or its innervation, with resulting *aphonia* or *dysphonia.* Articulation and internal language are unaffected.

In the practice of medicine the most frequent and troublesome disorders of speech are aphasia, stuttering, dysarthria, and aphonia.

TYPES OF APHASIA Systematic examination will usually enable one to decide whether a patient has a total *aphasia* (with loss of all or nearly all speech functions); a motor aphasia (*Broca's aphasia*), sometimes called verbal or executive aphasia; a central aphasia (*Wernicke's aphasia*), with impairment in all language-dependent behavior; or one of the *dissociative speech syndromes,* such as word deafness (auditory verbal aphasia), word blindness (alexia), amnestic aphasia (dysnomia), and several types of mutism. Impaired ability to communicate by writing (agraphia) is found to some degree in all types of aphasia; rarely is it affected alone.

Total, or global, aphasia This syndrome is due to a lesion that destroys a large part of the speech areas of the major cerebral hemisphere. Usually it is due to occlusion of the left internal carotid or middle cerebral artery, but it may be caused by hemorrhage, tumor, or other lesions, and it may be a postictal effect of grand mal epilepsy. The middle cerebral artery nourishes all the speech areas, and nearly all the aphasic disorders due to vascular occlusion are caused by involvement of this artery or its branches.

Most patients with total aphasia can say at most a few words; they cannot read or write, and they understand only a few words and phrases of the speech of others. Related signs include right hemiplegia, hemianesthesia, and homonymous hemianopia. The state of consciousness may vary from full alertness to semicoma; in the latter condition the lack of verbal response is obviously difficult to interpret, for the very diagnosis of aphasia presupposes a reasonably alert mind and the relative integrity of other cerebral functions. The patient may participate in common gestures of greeting, show modesty and avoidance reactions, and engage in self-help activities. With the passage of time some degree of understanding of spoken speech may be evident and a few words of speech may emerge. Rapid improvement frequently occurs when the main cause is edema, post-convulsive paralysis, or transient metabolic derangements such as infection, hyponatremia, etc., which worsen old dysphasic lesions. Although speech loss from a disintegrating embolus of the left middle artery may be transient, some part of the deficit may persist, being easily demonstrated by presenting the patient with complex words or double negatives in sentences.

Motor speech disorders (Broca's aphasia) Although the nature of Broca's aphasia remains somewhat in doubt, we have chosen to apply the term, as have others, to a primary deficit in motor speech production. In our experience there is a wide range of variation in the motor deficit, from the mildest cortical type of dysarthria, with entirely intact "inner language," to a complete loss of all means of communication through lingual, phonetic, and manual action. Since the muscles that can no longer be used in speech still function in other learned acts, i.e., they are not paralyzed, the term *apraxia* seems applicable to certain elements of the deficit.

In the fully developed syndrome the patient will have lost all power of speaking aloud. No longer can he utter a word spontaneously in conversation, in reading aloud, or in trying to repeat words that he hears. Occasionally, expletives, "yes," or "no" can be spoken, usually in the correct context. One might suspect the lingual and phonetory apparatus of being paralyzed, until the patient is observed to have no difficulty chewing, swallowing, clearing his throat, licking his lips, and even vocalizing without words. Often the lower part of the face is weak on the opposite (right) side, and occasionally the arm and leg on the opposite side are also weak. The tongue may deviate away from the lesion, i.e., to the right. For a time, despite good preservation of auditory comprehension and ability to read, commands to purse the lips, to lick the lips, to blow, smack, and make other purposeful movements are poorly executed, which means that the apraxia has temporarily extended to certain other learned oropharyngeal acts. The coordination of speech and breathing is also deranged. Imitation of the examiner's actions is better performed than execution of acts on command. Self-initiated actions, by contrast, are normal. The patient may repeat his few remaining words over and over again, as if compelled to do so. If he can speak at all, certain sterotyped, automatic expressions, such as "Hi," "Good morning," seem to be the easiest, and the words of well-known songs may be sung. When angered or excited he may explode with an expletive, which makes the point that he is "speechless" but not "wordless." Usually, the patient recognizes his ineptitude and his own mistakes. Repeated failures in speech may cause exasperation or despair.

In the milder form of Broca's aphasia and later in the recovery phase of the severe form, the patient is able to speak aloud to some degree. Then it is noticed that enunciation (articulation) and the melody of his language are at fault. This dysfluency takes the form of improper accent or stress of certain syllables, of incorrect phrasing of words in a series, intonation of sentences, and pacing of the speed of word utterances. All this interferes with communicative effectiveness of the patient's speech.

Most patients with Broca's aphasia have a similar impairment in writing. Should their right hand be paralyzed, they cannot print with their left one; and if manual mobility is spared, they fail as miserably in writing out their replies to questions or requesting their needs as in speaking them. Writing to dictation is impossible, though letters and words can still be copied.

Comprehension of spoken and written language, though normal under many conditions of testing, may break down, especially when novel material is rapidly introduced, since there may be elements of the central aphasia of Wernicke in some of the Broca syndromes. This aspect of the disorder is variable.

Broca's aphasia due to vascular lesions (the common ones) usually regresses in time, but as words begin to emerge, the patient's expressions are noted to be slow, laborious, and slurred, and many of the small words (articles, prepositions, conjunctions) are omitted, giving the speech an agrammatic character (*agrammatism*).

The natural course of Broca's aphasia varies, of course, with the nature of the causative lesion. An embolus in the upper main division (Rolandic) of the middle cerebral artery causes the most abrupt onset and rapid regression (occurring sometimes in hours or days). Because of the distribution of this artery, there are frequently an associated right-sided faciobrachial paresis and a *left*-sided brachial apraxia.

Atherosclerotic thrombosis, tumor, subcortical hypertensive hemorrhage, traumatic hemorrhage, etc., may also declare themselves as a Broca type of aphasia should they involve the premotor cortex, which lies immediately behind the posterior part of the left inferior frontal convolution.

A closely related syndrome, pure word mutism, also causes the patient to be wordless but leaves his inner speech intact. Since this is anatomically more in the nature of a dissociation of the motor cortex for speech from lower centers, it will be described with the dissociative or subcortical syndromes.

Wernicke's aphasia This syndrome is said to have two components: (1) an impairment in the hearing of word elements (phonemic hearing), which reflects involvement of auditory association areas or their separation from the angular gyrus, and the proximity of the lesion to the primary auditory cortex of Heschl's transverse gyri; (2) a general impairment of language-dependent behavior, which reveals the major role the auditory region plays in the regulation of language.

The defect in auditory functions is manifested by impaired ability to repeat spoken words and the inability to match two sequences from a series of identical auditory stimuli or rhythms. The only words that can be repeated are short ones and those of which the component syllables are widely separated in phonemic composition. A few simple commands may still be executed, but there is failure to carry out complex ones.

The patient gestures freely, talks volubly, and appears strangely unaware of his deficit. The words that the patient utters are often inappropriate, in the nature of paraphasia, which means substitution of words similar in sound (literal paraphasia) or similar in meaning to the correct one (verbal paraphasia). Speech elements may appear that are not part of the language (neologisms, or jargon speech). Hesitancy and lack of fluency, which are constant features of motor speech disorders, may also occur in Wernicke's aphasia. Characteristically, however, they tend to occur chiefly in that part of a spoken phrase that contains the central communicative (predicative) item, such as a key noun, verb, or descriptive phrase. The impression is often conveyed that the patient is constantly "searching" for the correct word and that he has difficulty in finding it. When severely disorganized, the speech may be reduced to an incomprehensible gibberish or jargon.

The general impairment of language-dependent behavior may be more or less dissociated from the deficit in the hearing of words. Although all the sensory and motor apparatus required in the activation and expression of language behavior appears to be intact, the patient is unable to function as a social organism because he is deprived of all means of communication, i.e., he has a "central aphasia." As already stated, he cannot understand what is said to him, read aloud or silently with comprehension, tell others what he wants or thinks, or write to them. When trying to refer to an object that he sees or feels, he cannot find the name, even though he may be able to repeat it from dictation; nor can he write from dictation the very words that he can copy from sight or touch. His copying performance is notably slow and laborious and conforms to the exact contours of the model (including the examiner's handwriting style) in a servile fashion. When tested in detail he cannot match words that he hears with those that he sees. Yet he can repeat aloud single words that he hears and can match a single word shown to him with that same word when it is mixed with other words. Performance is also impaired on those tasks which require the recognition, on the basis of past experience, of a relationship between two stimuli which are physically dissimilar but verbally equivalent (e.g., the sound of the word "cat" and the printed letters of the word "cat"). But the patient can still produce a response that is physically identical to that given (e.g., copying from sight the word "cat").

In time there is nearly always improvement, often to the point that the deficits can be detected only by asking the patient to repeat unfamiliar words from dictation, to name unusual objects, to spell difficult words, or to write complex self-generated sentences.

As a rule, the lesion lies in the posterior Sylvian region (temporal and parietal) and is due to an embolic occlusion of the lower division of the left middle cerebral artery. A "slit hemorrhage" in the subcortex of the temporoparietal region or involvement of the temporal isthmus and adjacent white matter by tumor, abscess, or extension of a small putaminal or thalamic hemorrhage may have similar effects.

The posterior Sylvian region, comprising posterior-superior temporal, opercular supramarginal, and posterior insular gyri, appears to encompass a variety of language functions, since seemingly minor changes in size and locale of the lesion are associated with important variations in the elements of Wernicke's aphasia or lead to *conduction aphasia* or to *pure word deafness.* The interesting theoretic problem is whether all the deficits observed are indicative of a unitary language function that resides in the posterior Sylvian region or instead, of a series of separate sensorimotor activities whose anatomic pathways happen to be crowded together in a small region of the brain. In view of the multiple ways in which language deteriorates in disease, the latter hypothesis seems more likely.

DISSOCIATIVE SPEECH SYNDROMES These are characterized by an impairment in the access of nervous impulses to and from the language mechanism, due to an interruption of one of the major afferent or efferent (motor) pathways. Included also, and this is somewhat confusing, are lesions which separate the more strictly receptive parts of language from the purely motor ones, leaving behavior with respect to language-dependent tasks normal (see also p. 163).

Central-type conduction disorder: separation of Wernicke's and Broca's language areas Here the principal abnormality resembles Wernicke's aphasia in certain respects. There is the same paraphasia in self-initiated speech, in repeating what is heard, and in reading aloud. In contrast, no difficulty is shown in comprehending words that are heard or seen. Nor is any element of dysarthria or dysprosody detected. The patient is alert and aware of his deficit. One of the best ways of eliciting the defect is to have the patient repeat nonsense syllables. His mistakes are then manifestly of a type observed in literal paraphasia, i.e., close similarity but detectably different sounds occasioned by improper positioning of the oropharyngeal apparatus. The disorder in repeating from dictation becomes more apparent when the rate of presentation of auditory material is increased and as the uttered words become more polysyllabic. Since nouns are the longest words in the sentence, one may gain an impression that they are specifically affected.

The lesion in autopsied cases is located in the cortex and subcortical white matter in the upper bank of the Sylvian fissure, involving the supramarginal gyrus of the inferior parietal lobule and occasionally the posterior part of the superior temporal region. Presumably fiber systems in the insula are interrupted. The usual cause is an embolus in the ascending parietal or posterior temporal branch of the middle cerebral artery. Deeper, larger lesions in position to interrupt the arcuate fasciculus connecting the temporal and frontal lobes usually involve other pathways as well, giving rise to a more extensive speech deficit (central Wernicke's aphasia, or amnestic aphasia). However, these latter types of aphasia, as they regress, may resolve into conduction aphasia. More anterior insular lesions usually include some degree of Broca's aphasia.

"Pure" word deafness This syndrome is characterized by impaired auditory comprehension and inability to repeat what is said or to write to dictation, being similar in this respect to Wernicke's aphasia. Inner speech, by contrast, is intact, as manifested by correctly phrased self-initiated utterances, correct writing, and reading. The patient may declare that he cannot hear, but shouting does not help him, sometimes to his surprise. By audiometric testing no hearing defect is found. Ordinary sounds can be distinguished. The patient is forced to depend heavily on visual cues in understanding the remarks of others, and frequently he uses these cues well enough to obviate much of his difficulty. But tests which prevent the use of visual cues readily uncover his deficit. If able to describe his auditory experience, the patient says that words sound like a jumble of noises. Often the syndrome is not pure and elements of paraphasia enter, which also help the examiner in distinguishing the condition from true deafness.

In most recorded autopsy studies the lesion has been bilateral in the superior temporal gyrus, in position to damage the primary auditory cortex in the transverse gyrus of Heschl and its relations to the association areas of the superior posterior part of the temporal lobe. The few unilateral lesions are localized in this part of the major (dominant) temporal lobe. Requirements of small size and superficiality of the lesion in the cortex and subcortical white matter are best fulfilled by a small embolic occlusion of a branch of the lower division of the middle cerebral artery.

"Pure" word blindness In this state a literate person loses the ability to read and often to name colors. He can no longer name or point on dictated command to visual letter stimuli or the words of which they are composed. However, understanding spoken language, repetition of what is heard, writing to dictation, and conversation are all intact. Often no complaint about the difficulty is registered; it is discovered almost by accident. In lesser degrees of the affection, reading aloud is possible, but the patient manages only a single letter at a time (this may be seen in otherwise normal patients who have bilateral hemianopia with only central vision remaining); commonly letter or name responses that seem to have little connection with the presented ones are expressed. The response may be corrected and the defect obscured if other visual cues are available, such as the bottle on which the words Coca-Cola appear. The naming of common colors presented singly and of objects is also impaired. When the dominant hemisphere is involved, as it usually is in such cases, there may be a right homonymous hemianopia, an amnestic defect (see Chap. 26), and a hemisensory defect on the right due to involvement of the left occipital lobe, the left fornix and its decussation, and the left thalamus, respectively, a combination which nearly always signifies thrombosis or embolism of the left posterior cerebral artery.

The autopsy of such lesions has usually demonstrated a lesion that destroys the left visual striate cortex (area 17) and visual association areas (18 and 19), as well as the connections of the right visual cortex and association areas with the left angular gyrus. This latter "disconnection" usually occurs in the posterior part (splenium) of the corpus callosum, wherein lie the callosal connections of the visual association areas of the two hemispheres. As the patient is blinded in the right half of each visual field by the left occipital lesion, the only visual information reaching the right occipital lobe must be transferred across the corpus callosum to the angular gyrus of the left (dominant) hemisphere. Less often the lesion is confined to the left occipital lobe and the deep central white matter of the parietal lobe, in a position to sever the connection between both occipital and left parietal lobes. In this case the right homonymous hemianopia may be absent. With purely left cerebral lesions, a primary or secondary tumor or, rarely, multifocal leukoencephalopathy may be the underlying disease. The associated disturbances of color naming are not dependent on a lesion of the corpus callosum. In large lesions of the left parietooccipital region, alexia may be combined with right-left confusion, acalculia, and difficulty in naming of fingers and other parts of the body (Gerstmann's syndrome) (see Chap. 27).

"Pure" word muteness (subcortical motor aphasia) The patient will have lost all capacity to speak, while retaining perfectly the ability to write, to understand spoken words, and to read silently with comprehension. Although usually paretic, the lips, tongue, pharynx, and larynx show none of the apraxic disturbance of Broca's aphasia. With recovery or in milder degrees of the disorder, vocal utterances are dysarthric because of paresis and are extremely slow, with inadequate volume and intonation.

The causative lesion, usually vascular, is located in the premotor cortex, separating it from the motor cortex for face, tongue, and laryngeal movements; or it is located beneath both Broca's convolution and the motor cortex, separating them from subcortical motor centers.

Amnestic-dysnomic aphasia This may be a relatively early or an isolated manifestation of disease of the nervous system. The patient loses only the ability to name objects. There are typical pauses in speech, groping for words, and substitution of another word or phrase that conveys the meaning. When shown a series of common objects, the patient may tell of their use instead of giving their names. The difficulty applies not only to objects seen but to the names of things heard or felt, but this is more difficult to demonstrate. Recall of the names for letters, digits, and other printed verbal material is almost invariably preserved. That the deficit is principally one of naming is shown by the patient's correct use of the object and, usually, by an ability to point to the correct object on hearing or seeing the name. There is a tendency among patients to attribute failure to forgetfulness, or to give some other lame excuse for the disability, suggesting that they are not completely aware of the nature of their difficulty.

The causative lesion is usually deep in the temporal lobe, in position, probably, to interrupt connections of sensory speech areas with the hippocampal-parahippocampal regions concerned with learning and memory. Mass lesions, such as a tumor or an otogenic abscess, are the most frequent, and as they enlarge, an upper contralateral quadrantic visual field defect, or Wernicke's aphasia, is added. Occasionally, dysnomia appears with diseases which occlude the temporal branches of the posterior cerebral artery. Alzheimer's disease and senile dementia may begin with a dysnomic or amnestic type of aphasia. This deficit may also be discovered in testing patients with a confusional state caused by metabolic, infectious, intoxicative, or other acute medical illnesses, but then it has no certain localizing value. By the time the patient's difficulty is fully recognized, other disorders of speech and indifference, apathy, and abulia are conjoined.

Isolation of Broca's and Wernicke's areas In this situation a lesion causes other neurologic manifestations related to destruction of the border zones between anterior, middle, and posterior cerebral arteries. It effectively isolates the auditory and motor speech mechanisms from the rest of the cerebrum. The patient suffers a deficit of auditory and visual word comprehension and is unable to initiate communicative speech. Presumably information from the rest of his cerebrum cannot be transferred to Wernicke's area for conversion into verbal form. What speech there is remains fluent and paraphasic and a dysnomia coexists. There may be a remarkable facility in echoing, parrot-like, word phrases and songs that are heard, unlike the deficit in Wernicke's aphasia. States such as this have followed prolonged hypotension or carbon monoxide poisoning, and at autopsy the cerebral cortex along the upper and lower banks of the Sylvian fissure is preserved. The syndrome is of great theoretic interest and may be more common than is currently appreciated.

DISORDERS IN THE DEVELOPMENT OF LANGUAGE

A close parallelism exists between the symptoms observed in adults who have suffered a loss in language functions as a result of brain injury and those seen during the development of language skills. In the pediatric age period and extending into adult life an interesting series of developmental language disorders has been uncovered. A high percentage of such patients come from families in which similar speech disorders and ambidexterity and left-handedness are frequent. Males predominate; male to female ratios are as high as 10:1.

Developmental disorders of language and congenital deafness are actually far more frequent than aphasia. These include developmental dyslexia (special reading disability), developmental word deafness, developmental speech delay, and developmental apraxia (abnormal clumsiness of the limbs). Here the various stages of language development, described above, are not attained at the usual age and may not even appear by adult life. Disorders of this type are probably due to slowness in the normal processes of maturation rather than to an acquired disease. Visible lesions are probably not to be expected, though it must be admitted that the brains of such individuals have never been studied by a proper method. These conditions are often misunderstood by parents, teachers, and physicians. The unfortunate child or adult is judged to be feebleminded or lazy. Another frequent error is to assume that the condition is due to psychologic factors, since nervousness, depression, poor sleep, and headaches, frequently appear in such persons. Probably they are secondary.

Congenital word deafness If an individual is born deaf, he can learn to talk only after special training; he is "deaf and dumb." As a baby he babbles, but after 6 months or so he becomes relatively silent. Should deafness develop within the first few years of life, after speech has been acquired, the child gradually loses speech but can be retaught by the lip-reading method. But then his speech is harsh, poorly modulated, and unpleasant, and he is apt to make many peculiar throat noises of a snorting or grunting kind. Such patients may be bright and alert and also clever at pantomime and gesturing. They are inattentive to household noises and do not appear to understand what is said to them. The deafness can be demonstrated at an early age by careful observation of the child's responses to sounds, but it cannot be accurately tested before the age of three or four years. The psychogalvanic reflex technique for testing reaction to sounds and tests of the labyrinths, which are frequently unresponsive in deaf-mutes, may be helpful. In contrast, the idiot or moron is stupid in all his actions and talks little because he has nothing to say.

Developmental word deafness may be difficult to distinguish from true deafness. Usually the parents have noted that the word-deaf child responds to loud noises and music, though obviously this does not assure perfect hearing, particularly for high tones. The word-deaf child does not understand what is said, and delay and distortion of speech are evident. In contrast to the deaf child, he is alert, active, and inquisitive and may chatter incessantly. He adopts a language of his own design, and attentive parents come to understand it. This peculiar type of speech is known as *idioglossia* (also observed in the child who has marked difficulty in the articulation of certain consonants). He learns to lip-read very quickly and is clever at acting out his own ideas.

Congenital word blindness (dyslexia) In this unusual condition the patient has good eyesight and is able to see the word but not to grasp its meaning. There is no loss of the ability to recognize the meaning of objects, pictures, and diagrams. Usually with assiduous training, the patient, who is otherwise bright and intelligent, can learn to read individual letters and a few simple words. Spelling is impossible. Often the patient cannot write anything of his own composition but can copy skillfully. Lesser degrees of congenital dyslexia are more common than the severe ones and pose serious problems in the classroom. Some 10 percent of school children have some degree of this disability, and an equal proportion of adults is affected. The problem is complex, for difficulty in learning to read well is unquestionably influenced by the teaching techniques used in the school.

A few of the more severely handicapped children have a right homonymous visual impairment or a right-sided sensory neglect; arithmetic calculation may also be impaired and sometimes recognition of body parts and distinction between right and left, all reminiscent of the Gerstmann syndrome (Chap. 27). The important genetic study of Hallgren shows that dyslexia is inherited as an autosomal dominant trait and is unrelated to psychologic factors; speech delay, articulatory abnormalities, and difficulty in reading digits may be associated. Also, there is a statistically higher incidence of left-handedness among these persons.

Abnormalities of articulation and phonation (lisping, dyslalia) A number of odd varieties of deficient articulation may come to the notice of the physician. One is *lisping,* in which the *s* sound is replaced by *th;* e.g., "thister" for "sister." Another condition, called *lallation* or *dyslalia,* a common speech disorder observed in early childhood, is characterized by multiple substitutions or omissions of consonants. In severe forms, speech may be almost unintelligible. These children are unaware that their speech differs from that of other persons and are distressed at not being understood. Milder degrees consist of the failure to pronounce or distortion of one or two consonants. For example, there may be imperfect enunciation of the sound *r* so that it sounds like *w.* "Running a race" becomes "wunning a wace." The nature of this disorder is not known. It has been suggested that the development of language in some children is so rapid that there is a partial failure of both perceptive and imitative speech. The patient usually recovers spontaneously from this disorder or responds promptly to speech therapy, which is best carried out at about the age of five years. These abnormalities are more frequent among feebleminded than normal children, and mental defect should always be suspected if numerous consonants are mispronounced and the condition persists beyond the age of twelve or thirteen years.

The speech disorder resulting from *cleft palate* is easily recognized. Many of these patients also have a harelip; the two abnormalities together interfere with suckling and later in life with the enunciation of labial and guttural consonants. The voice has an unpleasant nasality, and often, if the defect is severe, there is an audible escape of air through the nose.

Stammering, stuttering, and cluttered speech
Stammering and stuttering are difficult to classify. In some respects they belong to the developmental disorders,

but they differ from them in being largely centered in articulation. They consist of a spasm of the muscles of articulation when an attempt is made to speak. The spasm may be tonic and result in a complete block of speech, sometimes called *stammering,* or repetitive, leading to repeated utterance of the first syllable, i.e., a stutter; or the words may come out in rapid clusters, all poorly enunciated. Certain syllables offer greater difficulty than others. The patient falters on an initial consonant or syllable, which he repeats over and over again before he finally succeeds in enunciating the rest of the word, e.g., p-p-paper, b-b-b-boy. The severity of the stutter is increased by excitement, as in speaking before strangers or a group of people. The spasms may overflow into other muscle groups not directly concerned with speech. Males are affected four times more often than females. The time of onset may be when the child first begins to talk, i.e., at two or three years of age, or between the ages of six and eight years. These latter are the two critical periods of language development. Later onset is not infrequent, however; many of these children also have some degree of reading and writing disability. Slowness in developing hand preference or enforced change from left- to right-handedness is noted in many cases. If stuttering is mild, it tends to develop or to be present only during periods of emotional distress; and it usually disappears spontaneously during adolescent or early adult years. If severe, it persists all through life, regardless of treatment, but tends to improve as the patient grows older.

The essential character of stuttering is difficult to define. There is no detectable paralysis or incoordination of speech musculature, which seems to function normally in other commonplace acts and when the patient is alone and relaxed or singing. Stuttering differs from apraxia in that the muscles, when called upon to perform the specific act, go into voluntary spasm; but since the spasm does not occur during other movements in which these muscles are involved, it differs from the intention (tension) spasm of athetosis. It appears to represent a special category of movement disorder much like writer's cramp, another nonpsychogenic motor disorder of unknown cause.

Everyone who has studied stuttering and stammering has been impressed with the high incidence of similar disabilities in other members of the same family, sometimes going back several generations. This and the preponderance in males suggest a sex-linked characteristic, but the inheritance does not follow a simple pattern.

Many of the patients, probably as a natural result of this impediment to free social intercourse, become increasingly fearful of speaking and have feelings of inferiority after a few years. By the time adolescence and adulthood are reached, emotional factors are so prominent that many physicians have mistaken stuttering for neurosis. Usually there is little or no evidence of any personality deviation before the onset of stuttering, and psychotherapy by competent psychiatrists, though unquestionably helpful in relieving emotional tension and assisting a satisfactory adjustment to the condition, has not significantly modified the underlying defect. Occasionally, stuttering will develop during adult life as a consequence of brain disease.

In recent times, special procedures have been developed using the methods of behavioral science which are helpful in alleviating stuttering.

Aside from these special types of developmental language disorder, there are many other common defects in speech that handicap individuals throughout their life. Wordblocking, multiple substitutions of words, inability to complete spoken sentences, and word clustering are observed in many adults and make their speech inefficient and unpleasant to hear. These abnormalities are often associated with the specific language defects.

DISORDERS OF ARTICULATION AND PHONATION

The third group of speech abnormalities is that of the disorders of articulation. In simple dysarthria there is no abnormality of the cortical centers. The dysarthric patient is able to understand perfectly what he hears, and if literate, he reads and has no difficulty in writing, even though he is unable to utter a single intelligible word. This is the strict meaning of being inarticulate.

The act of speaking is a highly coordinated sequence of contractions of the larynx, pharynx, palate, tongue, lips, and respiratory musculature. These are innervated by the hypoglossal, vagal, facial, and phrenic nerves. The nuclei of these nerves are controlled through the corticobulbar tracts by both motor cortices. As with all movements, there are also extrapyramidal influences from the cerebellum and basal ganglions. A current of air is produced by expiration, and the force of it is finely regulated by the activity of the various muscles engaged in speech. *Phonation,* or the production of vocal sounds, is a function of the larynx. Changes in the size and shape of the glottis and in the length and tension of the vocal cords are controlled by the action of the laryngeal muscles. Vibrations are set up and transmitted to the column of air passing over the vocal cords. Sounds thus formed are modified as they pass through the nasopharynx and mouth, which act as resonators. Articulation consists of contractions of the tongue, lips, pharynx, and palate, which interrupt or alter the vocal sounds. Vowels are of laryngeal origin, as are some consonants; but the latter are formed for the most part during articulation. For instance, the consonants *m, b,* and *p* are labial, *l* and *t* are lingual, and *nk* and *ng* are nasoguttural.

Defective articulation and phonation are recognized at once by listening to the patient during ordinary conversation or while he is reading aloud from a newspaper or a book. Test phrases or attempts at rapid repetition of lingual, labial, and guttural consonants (e.g., la-la-la-la or me-me-me-me) bring out the particular abnormality. Disorders of phonation call for a precise analysis of the voice and its apparatus. The movements of the vocal cords should be inspected with the aid of a hand mirror, or, even better, a laryngoscope, and those of the tongue, palate, and pharynx by direct observation.

Defects in articulation may be subdivided into several types: paretic dysarthria, spastic and rigid dysarthria, and ataxic dysarthria.

Paretic dysarthria This is due to a neural or bulbar (medullary) weakness or paralysis of the articulatory muscles (lower motor neuron paralysis). In the latter condition the shriveled tongue lies inert on the floor of the mouth, and the lips are relaxed and tremulous. Saliva constantly collects in the mouth because of dysphagia, and drooling is troublesome. Speech becomes less and less distinct. There is special difficulty in the correct utterance of vibratives, such as *r;* and as the paralysis becomes more complete, lingual and labial consonants are finally not pronounced at all. Degrees of this abnormality are observed in myasthenia gravis. Bilateral paralysis of the palate may occur with diphtheria, poliomyelitis, and progressive bulbar palsy. Bilateral paralysis of the lips, as in the facial diplegia of idiopathic polyneuritis, interferes with enunciation of labial consonants; *p* and *b* are slurred and sound more like *f* and *v*.

Spastic and rigid dysarthria These are more frequent than the paralytic variety. Diseases that involve the corticobulbar tracts, usually vascular disease or motor system disease, result in the syndrome of pseudobulbar palsy. The patient may have had a minor stroke some time in the past affecting the corticobulbar fibers on one side; but since the bulbar muscles are probably represented in both motor cortices, there is no impairment in speech or swallowing from a unilateral lesion. Should another stroke then occur, involving the other corticobulbar tract and possibly the corticospinal tract at the pontine, midbrain, or capsular level, the patient immediately becomes anarthric or dysarthric and dysphagic. Often the muscles of facial expression on both sides are weakened as well. Unlike bulbar paralysis due to lower motor neuron involvement, this condition entails no atrophy or fasciculation of the paralyzed muscles; the jaw jerk and other facial reflexes soon become exaggerated; the palatal reflexes are retained; emotional control is poor (pathologic laughter and crying); and sometimes breathing becomes periodic (Cheyne-Stokes). When the frontal operculum alone is involved, the speech deficit may be a pure dysarthria but usually without the impairment in emotional control. In the beginning, the patient may be totally anarthric and aphonic, but as he improves, or in mild degrees of the same condition, speech is notably slow, thick, and indistinct, much like that of partial bulbar paralysis.

In paralysis agitans, or postencephalitic Parkinson's syndrome, one observes an extrapyramidal disturbance of articulation. The patient speaks slowly and articulates poorly, slurring over many syllables and trailing off the end of sentences. The voice is low-pitched, monotonous, and lacks inflection. The words are pronounced hastily. In advanced cases speech is almost unintelligible; only whispering is possible. It may happen that the patient finds it impossible to talk while walking but can speak if he sits or lies down.

In chorea and myoclonus, speech may also be affected in a highly characteristic way. Unlike the defect of pseudobulbar palsy or paralysis agitans, chorea and myoclonus entail abrupt interruptions of the words by the abnormal movements. The idea is best conveyed by the phrase "hiccup speech," in that the breaks are as unexpected as in singulitis. Grimacing and other characteristic motor signs must be depended upon for diagnosis.

Pyramidal and extrapyramidal disturbances of speech may be combined in generalized cerebral diseases such as general paresis, in which slurred speech is one of the cardinal signs.

In many cases of capsular hemiplegia or partially recovered Broca's aphasia the patient is left with a dysarthria that may be difficult to distinguish from a pure articulatory defect. Careful testing of other language functions, especially writing, will reveal the aphasic quality.

Ataxic dysarthria This is characteristic of acute and chronic cerebellar lesions. It may be observed in multiple sclerosis, Friedreich's ataxia, cerebellar atrophy, and heat stroke. The principal speech abnormality is slowness; imprecise enunciation, monotony, and unnatural separation of the syllables of words (scanning) are other features. Coordination of speech and respiration are poor. There may not be enough breath to utter certain words, and others may be ejaculated explosively. *Scanning dysarthria* is distinctive, but in some cases, especially if there is a possibility of spastic weakness of the tongue from corticobulbar tract involvement, it is impossible to predict the anatomy of disease from analysis of speech alone. Myoclonic jerks involving the speech musculature may be superimposed on cerebellar ataxia in a number of diseases.

APHONIA AND DYSPHONIA Finally, a few points should be made concerning the fourth group of language disorders, i.e., disturbances of voice. In adolescence and early adult life there may be a persistence of the unstable "change of voice" normally seen in boys soon after puberty. As though by habit, the patient speaks part of the time in a falsetto voice. This condition may persist into adult life. Its basis is unknown. Voice training has been helpful in many patients.

Paresis of the respiratory movements, as in poliomyelitis and acute infectious polyneuritis, may affect voice because insufficient air is provided for phonation and speech. Also, disturbances in the rhythm of respiration may interfere with the fluency of speech. This is particularly noticeable in so-called "extrapyramidal diseases," where one may observe that the patient tries to talk during part of inspiration. In the latter conditions reduced volume of speech due to limited excursion of the breathing muscles is another common feature; the patient is unable to speak above a whisper or to shout. Whispering speech is also a feature of stupor, but strong stimulation may make the voice audible.

Paresis of both vocal cords causes complete aphonia. There is no voice, and the patient can speak only in whispers. Since the vocal cords normally separate during inspiration, their failure to do so when paralyzed may result in an inspiratory stridor. If one vocal cord is paralyzed, the voice becomes hoarse, low-pitched, and rasping. Involvement of one tenth cranial nerve by tumor, for example, may also cause a certain nasality of voice because the posterior nares do not close during phonation. Certain consonants such as *b, p, n,* and *k* are followed by escape of air into the nasal passages. The abnormality is sometimes less pronounced in recumbency and increased when the head is thrown forward. Hoarseness may also be due to structural changes in the vocal cords caused by cigarette smoking, chronic inflammation, polyps, etc.

Another curious condition about which little is known is *spastic dysphonia.* The authors have seen many patients, middle-aged or elderly men and women, otherwise healthy, who gradually lost the ability to speak quietly and fluently. Any effort to speak results in contraction of all the speech musculature so the the patient's voice is strained and phonation is labored. This is apparently a neurologic disorder similar to writer's cramp. The patients are not neurotic, and psychotherapy has been ineffective. This condition differs from the stridor caused by spasm of the laryngeal muscles in tetany. It is nonprogressive but in some instances is combined with other of the restricted extrapyramidal disorders such as blepharospasm and spasmodic torticollis.

CLINICAL APPROACH TO LANGUAGE DISORDERS

Aphasia In investigating a case of aphasia it is first necessary to inquire into the patient's native language, his handedness, and his previous education. Many naturally left-handed children are trained to use their right hand for writing; therefore, in determining this point we must ask which hand is used for throwing a ball, threading a needle, or using a spoon and common tools such as a hammer, saw, or bread knife. It is important before the beginning of the examination to determine whether the patient is alert and can be made to participate reliably in testing, as accurate assessment of language depends on these factors. One should quickly ascertain whether the patient has other signs of a gross cerebral lesion such as hemiplegia, facial weakness, homonymous hemianopia, or cortical sensory loss. When hemiplegia, hemianesthesia, and homonymous hemianopia are present, the aphasic disorder is usually of the total (global) type. Such a constellation of major neurologic signs is seldom associated with the less complete forms of language disorder such as Broca's or Wernicke's aphasia, or one of the dissociative syndromes. Dyspraxia of limbs and speech musculature, in response to spoken commands or to visual mimicry, is generally associated with Broca's aphasia and sometimes with Wernicke's aphasia. Bilateral or unilateral homonymous hemianopia without motor weakness tends often to be linked to "pure" word blindness (alexia or dyslexia) or to amnestic-dysnomic aphasia. Bilateral hemiplegias are associated not infrequently with "pure" word muteness. The special types of aphasia—Broca's, Wernicke's, alexia, or "pure" word deafness—are often associated with evidences of embolism to other parts of the brain or other organs.

Conversational testing permits quick assessment of the motor aspects of speech (praxis and prosody) and apparent language formulation and auditory comprehension.

Disabilities in the purely motor aspects of speech suggest a motor aphasia, and this possibility can be pursued further by tests of repeating from dictation and by special tests of praxis of the oropharyngeal and respiratory apparatus. Disabilities in language formulation in the form of literal paraphasias with impaired comprehension are indicative of Wernicke's aphasia. Impaired comprehension but perfectly normal formulated speech suggest the rare syndrome of pure word deafness. Disorders confined to naming, generally without paraphasias, when other language functions (reading, writing, spelling, etc.) are found adequate, are diagnostic of amnestic dysnomia.

When conversation shows virtually no disabilities, other tests may still be revealing. Reading aloud single letters, words, and text may reveal the dissociative syndrome of pure word blindness, while tests of writing in this syndrome will show little abnormality. Literal and verbal paraphasic errors may appear in milder cases of Wernicke's aphasia as the patient reads aloud from text or from words in the examiner's handwriting. Similar errors appear even more frequently when the patient is asked to explain the text, read aloud, or give his explanation in writing. Should such tests still be unrevealing of deficits, the examiner may find it useful to increase the complexity of the tests. If the patient then succeeds, one may be sure that there is no disorder of adequacy of reception, and adequacy of response channels is next determined, by presenting the patient with tasks that permit a response physically identical with the test stimulus. Copying visual stimuli and repeating aloud from auditory stimuli are examples of this kind of testing. Inadequacy of receptive or response channels will then preclude further analysis of the deficit involving that channel in more complex types of tests, except in the unlikely instance that the more complex test is better performed. If reception and response channels are found adequate in these initial tests, they may then be used in tests requiring all types of language function, such as writing from dictation, vocal naming of visual stimuli, matching physically dissimilar stimuli having a name in common (i.e., the word "cow" and a picture of a cow). By utilizing the same test material used in the earlier tests, direct comparison of performances in spoken naming, written naming, and matching can be compared from visual, auditory, and palpated stimuli. A performance profile can be constructed separately for each type of stimulus material tested (i.e., objects, pictures, words, letters, numbers, colors, etc.). The resultant profile can then be used to determine if the main deficits fall across one or more input or response channels. These data then provide a base line against which later changes may be compared.

Developmental language disorders The general physician is frequently called upon to examine children who show some disorder of speech or delay in language development. From the above remarks it will be seen that these abnormalities fall into several broad categories, of which stuttering, delay in onset of speech, dyslalia, partial or complete deafness, word deafness, cleft palate, lisping, and word blindness are the most frequent. When faced with problems of this type, the physician must ask several questions. "Is the child partially or completely deaf?" "Does he have a more generalized mental or neuromuscular defect—is he feebleminded or suffering from an infantile hemiplegia or spastic diplegia?" "Does he stammer, stutter, or show dyslalia?" In attempting to answer these questions, the physician will find the parents' account of the child's development and his behavior at home most helpful. Failure to respond to noise of any kind suggests deafness. An interest in sounds and music but not in stories or conversation, together with slow development of understanding and use of speech, is indicative of high-tone deafness or word deafness (auditory verbal agnosia). Delayed onset of suckling, head control, sitting or standing, walking, etc., necessitates neurologic examination; one should look particularly for spastic weakness or rigidity of the limbs and poor motor control of the tongue, as well as mental retardation. The latter can be assessed at an early age by intelligence tests, such as the performance part of the Stanford-Binet test. If the child is otherwise normal, recitation of a nursery rhyme will disclose the stammering, stuttering lallation of cleft-palate speech.

Articulatory-phonation disorders Disturbances of articulation point to involvement of a different set of neural structures, such as the motor cortices, the corticobulbar pathways, the seventh, ninth, and tenth nuclei, the brainstem, and extrapyramidal nuclei and tracts. Often it is necessary to use other neurologic findings to decide which of these are implicated in any given case. The important distinction between the pseudobulbar or supranuclear palsies and the bulbar palsies is grasped only with difficulty by the average student. The information obtained by localizing these two major types of dysarthria is extremely helpful in differential diagnosis.

Dysphonia should lead to an investigation of laryngeal disease, either primary or secondary to an abnormality of innervation. Inspection of vocal cords is a necessary step in the clinical study.

TREATMENT The sudden loss of speech would be expected to cause great apprehension, but except for almost pure motor defects, most patients show remarkably little concern. It appears that the very lesion that deprives them of speech also causes at least a partial loss of insight into their own disability. This reaches almost a ludicrous extreme in some cases of Wernicke's aphasia, in which the patient becomes indignant when others cannot understand his jargon. Nonetheless, as improvement occurs, many patients do become discouraged. Reassurance and a positive program of speech rehabilitation are the best ways of helping the patient at this stage.

The contemporary methods of training and reeducation in overcoming an aphasic defect have never been critically evaluated. Most aphasic difficulty is due to vascular disease of the brain, and nearly always this is accompanied by some degree of spontaneous improvement in the days, weeks, and months that follow the stroke. Sometimes recovery is complete within hours or days; at times not more than a few words are regained after a year or two of assiduous speech training. Nevertheless, it is the opinion of many experts in the field that speech training is worthwhile.

One must decide for each patient whether speech training is needed and when it should be started. As a rule, therapy is not advisable in the first few days of an aphasic illness, because one does not know how lasting it will be. Also, if the patient suffers a severe global aphasia and can neither speak nor understand spoken and written words, the speech therapist is helpless. Under such circumstances, one does well to wait a few weeks until some one of the language functions has begun to return. Then the physician may begin to encourage and help the patient to use the function to a maximum degree. In milder aphasic disorders the patient may be sent to the speech therapist as soon as the illness has stabilized.

The methods of speech training are specialized, and it is advisable to call in a person who has been trained in this field. However, inasmuch as the benefit is largely psychologic, an interested member of the family or a schoolteacher can be of help if a speech therapist is not available in the community.

The language problems of children are serious and demand skillful diagnosis and treatment. Often, excellent results are obtained. Most of the well-organized urban school systems have remedial reading teachers who will take over the problem once it has been evaluated medically. The essence of all the training programs is drill by an enthusiastic teacher who can and has time to motivate the patient to work diligently. The emotional problems that often accompany the developmental disturbances of language and of cerebral dominance must be dealt with gently and firmly. Usually once improvement starts they recede in importance as the patient gains in self-confidence.

The physician should, by wise counseling, help the patient understand the nature of this problem and try to avoid some of the secondary and emotional problems that the speech disorder creates. Prolonged psychotherapy helps with the emotional problems but has not, in the authors' experience, corrected the underlying speech defect. Fortunately, the natural course of mild stuttering is toward improvement during adolescence, and many patients recover spontaneously by adult life. The methods of behavioral control are frequently successful in treating symptomatic stuttering, regardless of the age of the patient.

There is no special treatment for the dysarthric disturbance of speech.

REFERENCES

Brain R: Aphasia, apraxia, agnosia, chap. 83 in *Neurology,* 2d ed., eds SAK Wilson, N Bruce, vol. 3, Baltimore: Williams & Wilkins, 1955

Geschwind N: Disconnection syndromes in animals and man. Brain 88:237, 585, 1965

Hallgren B: Specific dyslexia. Acta Psychiat Neurol, suppl 65, 1950

Nielsen JM: *Agnosia, Apraxia, Aphasia: Their Value in Cerebral Localization,* 2d ed., New York: Hafner, 1962

Orton ST: *Reading, Writing and Speech Problems in Children,* New York: Norton, 1937

Sidman M et al: Behavioral studies of aphasia: Methods of investigation and analysis. Neuropsychologia 9:119, 1971

26 DELIRIUM AND OTHER ACUTE CONFUSIONAL STATES

RAYMOND D. ADAMS
MAURICE VICTOR

Every physician sooner or later discovers through clinical experience the need for special competence in assessing the mental faculties of his patients. He must be able to observe with detachment and complete objectivity their character, intelligence, mood, memory, judgment, and other attributes of personality, in much the same fashion as he observes the nutritional state and the color of the mucous membranes. The systematic examination of these affective and cognitive functions permits him to reach certain conclusions regarding mental status, and these are also of value in understanding the patient and his illness. Without the data obtained from the study of the mental status, errors will be made in evaluating the reliability of the patient's history in diagnosing the neurologic or psychiatric disease from which he suffers, and in conducting any proposed therapeutic program.

Perhaps the content of this chapter will be more clearly understood if we repeat a few of the introductory remarks of Chap. 13. The main thesis of the neurologic physician is that mental and physical functions of the nervous system are simply two aspects of the same neural process. Mind and behavior both have their roots in the self-regulating, goal-seeking activities of the organism, the same ones that provide impulse to all forms of mammalian life. The prodigious complexity of man's brain permits, to an extraordinary degree, the solving of difficult problems, the power of reasoning to the logical choice of alternative solutions, a high capacity for the memory of past experiences and the ability to phrase them in a symbolic language that can be written and read, and the imagination of events that have not taken place. Somehow there emerges in the course of these complex cerebral functions a more complete and continuous awareness of one's self and of the operation of one's own psychic processes than is found in any other species. It is this continuous inner consciousness of past experiences and ongoing cognitive activites that is called mind. Any separation of the mental from the observable behavioral aspects of nervous functioning is illusory. Biologists and psychologists have reached the modern monistic view by placing all protoplasmic activities of the nervous system (growth, development, behavior, and mental function) in a continuum and noting the inherent purposiveness and creativity common to all of them. The physician is persuaded of its truth by his daily experiences with disease, in which every known aberration of behavior, intellect, and personality appear as expressions of diseases of the cerebrum.

In this chapter and the next we are concerned with common disturbances of sensorium and intellection which have not been previously discussed and which stand as cardinal manifestations of certain cerebral diseases. The most frequent of these are the acute confusional states, delirium, abnormalities of thinking and reasoning, and disturbances of memory.

DEFINITION OF TERMS

The definition of normal and abnormal states of mind is difficult, because the terms used to describe these states have been given so many different meanings, in both medical and nonmedical writings. Compounding the difficulty is the fact that the pathophysiology of the confusional states, delirium and dementia, is not fully understood, and the definitions depend on their clinical relationships, with all the lack of precision which this entails. The following nomenclature, though tentative, is useful, and will be employed throughout this textbook.

Confusion is a general term denoting an incapacity of the patient to think with customary speed and clarity. This abnormality may depend on one of several factors. In delirium, for example, inattention and the intrusion of illusory and hallucinatory experiences are mainly responsible. At certain stages in the evolution or devolution of stupor and coma, as indicated in Chap. 22, confusion is aligned with a disorder of consciousness, awareness, and perception. In patients with dementia, confusion is related to a derangement of intellectual function, i.e., an inability to learn, remember, calculate, make appropriate deductions from given premises, reason abstractly, etc.

The term *delirium* will be used here to denote a special type of confusional state, acute in onset and transient in nature, and characterized by gross disorientation, alertness and vigilance, disorders of perception in which illusions and vivid hallucinations are prominent, and overactivity of psychomotor and autonomic nervous system functions. Implicit in the definition are certain nonmedical connotations of the term—intense agitation, frenzied excitement, and creations of the imagination. That such a syndrome merits separate classification is not universally acknowledged. Some authors attach no special meaning to the term delirium and make no attempt to distinguish it from any other disorder of behavior or confusional state, such as one that might be associated with stupor and coma or with dementia. However, most stuporous or demented patients, in contrast to those with delirium, show a *reduced* state of alertness and attentiveness, *decreased* psychomotor activity, and a *relatively slight* tendency to hallucinate. For these reasons, and also because of the particular clinical settings in which they occur, it seems worthwhile to set the delirious states apart from those of depressed consciousness on the one hand and of dementia and amnesia on the other. Such a concept is far from new. To a greater or lesser extent, the terms exogenous reaction type, symptomatic psychosis, toxic psychosis, infective-exhaustive psychosis, drug, traumatic or fever delirium all have reference to the syndrome of delirium. All these terms convey the idea of an acute and transient confusional state, occurring in a particular clinical setting and carrying a serious prognosis, by virtue of adding its burden to an already serious medical illness.

The term *amnesia* means loss of the ability to form memories despite an alert state of mind. It presupposes an ability to grasp the problem, to use language normally, and to maintain adequate motivation. The failure is mainly one of retention, recall, and reproduction, and it should be distinguished from states of drowsiness and acute confusion, in which the learned material seems never to have been adequately assimilated.

Dementia, as indicated above, means loss of reason or, more particularly, a deterioration of all intellectual or cognitive functions, without clouding or disturbances of perception. Implied in the word is the idea of a gradual enfeeblement of mental powers in a person who formerly possessed a normal mind. *Amentia,* by contrast, indicates a congenital feeblemindedness.

OBSERVABLE ASPECTS OF BEHAVIOR AND THEIR RELATION TO CONFUSION, DELIRIUM, AMNESIA, AND DEMENTIA

The intellectural, emotional, volitional, and behavioral activities of the human organism are so complex and varied that one may question the possibility of using derangements of them as reliable guides to cerebral disease. Certainly they have not the same reliability and ease of anatomic and physiologic interpretation as sensory and motor paralysis or aphasia. Yet one observes certain of these higher cerebral disturbances recurring with such regularity in certain diseases as to be useful in clinical medicine; and some of them gain in specificity because they are often combined in certain ways to form syndromes, which are essentially what states of confusion, delirium, amnesia, and dementia are.

The components of mentation and behavior that lend themselves to bedside examination are (1) the processes of sensation and perception; (2) the capacity for memorizing; (3) the ability to think, reason, and form logical conclusions; (4) temperament, mood, and emotion; (5) initiative, impulse, and drive; (6) insight. Of these (1), (2), and (3) may be considered cognitive, (4) affective, and (5) conative or volitional. Insight includes essentially all introspective observations made by the patient concerning his own normal or disordered functioning. Each component of behavior and intellection has its objective side, expressed in the manifest effects of certain stimulus conditions on the patient and his behavioral responses, and its subjective side, expressed in what the patient says he thinks and feels.

DISTURBANCES OF PERCEPTION Perception, i.e., the processes involved in acquiring through the senses a knowledge of the "world about" or of one's own body, involves many things aside from the simple sensory process of being aware of the attributes of a stimulus; it includes the selective focusing and maintaining of attention, elimination of all extraneous stimuli, and recognition of the stimulus by knowing its relationship to personal remembered experience. One must appreciate that the perception of an object undergoes predictable types of derangement in disease. Most often one finds a reduction in the number of perceptions in a given unit of time and failure to synthesize them properly and relate them to the ongoing activities of the mind. Or there may be apparent inattentiveness, fluctuations of attention, distractibility (pertinent and irrelevant stimuli now having equal value), inability to persist in an assigned task. Qualitative changes also appear, mainly in the form of sensory distortions and misinterpretation and misidentification of objects and persons (illusions); and these, at least in part, form the basis of hallucinatory experience in which the patient reports and reacts to stimuli not present in his environment. There is an inability to perceive simultaneously all elements of a large complex of stimuli, which is sometimes explained as a "failure of subjective reorganization." These major disturbances in the perceptual sphere, sometimes called "clouding of the sensorium," occur most often in acute confusional states and deliriums, but quantitative deficiency may become evident in the advanced stages of amentia and dementia.

DISTURBANCES OF MEMORY Memory, i.e., the retention of learned experiences, is involved in all mental activities. It may be arbitrarily subdivided into several parts, namely, (1) registration, which includes all that was mentioned under perception; (2) mnemonic integration and retention; (3) recall; and (4) reproduction. As stated above, in disturbances of perception and attention there may be a complete failure of learning and memory for the reason that the material to be learned was never registered and assimilated. In Korsakoff's amnestic syndrome newly presented material appears to be temporarily registered but cannot be retained for more than a few minutes, and there is nearly always an associated defect in the recall and reproduction of memories formed some days, weeks, or months before the onset of the illness (retrograde amnesia). Dislocation of events in time and the fabrication of stories, called *confabulation,* constitutes a third, but not invariable feature of the syndrome. Sound retention with failure of recall is at times a normal state; when it is severe and extends to all events of past life it is usually due to hysteria or malingering. Proof that the processes of registration and retention are intact under these circumstances comes from hypnosis and suggestion, whereby the lost items are fully recalled and reproduced. In Korsakoff's amnestic state the patient fails on all tests of learning and recent memory and his behavior accords with his deficiencies of information. Since memory is involved to some extent in all mental processes, it becomes the most testable component of mentation and behavior.

DISTURBANCES OF THINKING Thinking, which is central to so many important intellectual activities, remains one of the most elusive of all mental operations. If by thinking we mean selective ordering of symbols for problem solving and capacity to reason and form sound judgments (the usual definition), obviously the working units of most complex experiences of this type are words and numbers. The activity of substituting word and number symbols for the objects for which they stand (symbolization) is a fundamental part of the process. These symbols are formed into ideas or concepts, and the arrangement of new and remembered ideas into certain orders or relationships, according to the rules of logic, constitutes another intricate part of thought, presently beyond the scope of analysis. In a general way one may examine thinking for speed and efficiency, ideational content, coherence and logical relationships of ideas, quantity and quality of associations to a given idea, and the propriety of the feeling and behavior engendered by an idea.

Information concerning the thought processes and associative functions is best obtained by analyzing the patient's spontaneous verbal productions and by engaging him in conversation. If he is taciturn or mute, one may then have to depend on his responses to direct questions or upon written material, i.e., letters, etc. One notes the prevailing trends of the patient's thoughts; whether his ideas are reasonable, precise, and coherent or vague, circumstantial, tangential, and irrelevant; and whether his thought processes are shallow and completely fragmented. Disorders of thought are frequent in deliriums and in degenerative and other types of cerebral disease. The organization of thought may be disrupted with fragmentation, repetition, and perseveration. This is spoken of as incoherence and marks many acute confusional and delirious states. The patient may be excessively critical, rationalizing, and hairsplitting; this is a type of thinking often manifest in depressive psychoses. Derangements of thinking may also take the form of a flight of ideas. The patient moves nimbly from one idea to another, and his associations are numerous and loosely linked. This is a common feature in hypomanic or manic states. The opposite condition, poverty of ideas is characteristic both of depression, where it is combined with gloomy thoughts, and of dementing diseases, where it is part of a general reduction in all intellectual activity. Thinking may be distorted in such a way that the patient fails to check his ideas against reality. When a false belief is maintained in spite of normally convincing contradictory evidence, the patient is said to have a delusion. Delusion is common to many illnesses, particularly manic-depressive and schizophrenic states. Ideas may seem to the patient to have been implanted in his mind by some outside agency such as radio, television, or atomic energy. These reflect the passivity feelings characteristic of manic-depressive and schizophrenic psychoses. Other distortions of logical thought, such as gaps or condensations of logical associations, are typical of schizophrenia, of which they constitute a diagnostic feature.

DISTURBANCES OF EMOTION, MOOD, AND AFFECT The emotional life of the patient is expressed in a variety of ways. In the first place, rather marked individual differences in basic temperament are to be observed in the normal population; some persons are throughout their life cheerful, gregarious, optimistic, and free from worry, whereas others are just the opposite. The unusually volatile, cyclothymic person is believed to be liable to manic-depressive psychosis and the suspicious, withdrawn, introverted person to schizophrenia and paranoia. Strong, persistent emotional states such as fear and anxiety may occur as reactions to life situations and may be accompanied by derangements of visceral function. If excessive and disproportionate to the stimulus, they are usually manifestations of an anxiety neurosis or depression. Variations in the degree of responsiveness to emotional stimuli are also frequent and, when excessive and persistent, assume importance. In depression all stimuli tend to enhance the somber mood of unhappiness. Emotional response that is excessively labile, variable from moment to moment, and poorly controlled or uninhibited is a condition common to many diseases of the cerebrum, particularly those involving the corticopontine and corticobulbar pathways. It constitutes a part of the syndrome of pseudobulbar palsy. All emotional expression may be lacking, as in apathetic states or severe depressions, or the patient may be a victim of every trivial problem in daily life; i.e., he cannot control his worries. Finally, the emotional response may be inappropriate to the stimulus, e.g., a depressing or morbid thought may seem amusing and be attended by a smile, as in schizophrenia.

Since there are relatively few overt manifestations of temperament, mood, and other emotional experiences described above, the physician must evaluate these states by the appearance of the patient and by verbalized accounts of his feelings. For these purposes it is convenient to divide emotionality into mood and feeling or affect. By *mood* is meant the prevailing emotional state of the individual without reference to the stimuli immediately impinging upon him. It may be pleasant and cheerful or melancholic. The language, e.g., the adjectives used, and the facial expressions, attitudes, postures, and speed of movement most reliably betray the patient's mood. By contrast, *feelings* (or *affect*) are said to be emotional experiences evoked by environmental stimuli. According to some psychiatrists, feeling is the subjective component and affect, the overt manifestation. Others apply either word to the subjective state. The difference between mood as a prevailing emotional state and feeling and affect as emotional reactions to stimuli may seem rather tenuous, but these distinctions are considered valuable by psychiatrists.

DISTURBANCES IN IMPULSE Impulse, that basic biologic urge, driving force, or purpose, by which every organism is directed to reach its full potentialities, appears to be another extremely important and observable, though somewhat neglected, dimension of behavior. Again, one notes wide normal variations from one person to another in strength of impulse to action and thought, and these individual differences are present throughout life. One of the most conspicuous pathologic deviations is an apparent constitutional weakness in impulse in certain neurotic persons. Moreover, with many types of cerebral disease (particularly those which involve the posterior orbital parts of the frontal lobes) a reduction in impulse is coupled with an indifference or lack of concern about the consequences of actions. In such cases all other measurable aspects of psychic function may be normal. Extreme degrees of lack of impulse, or *abulia*, sometimes take the form of mutism and immobility called *akinetic mutism*. Psychomotor retardation is a lesser degree of the same state and is a feature of cerebral disease or of depression. In the latter instance mood alteration and extreme fatigability are conjoined.

LOSS OF INSIGHT Insight, the state of being fully aware of the nature and degree of one's deficits, becomes manifestly impaired or abolished in relation to all types of cerebral disease that cause complex disorders of behavior. Rarely does the patient with any of the aforementioned states seek advice or help for his illness. Instead, his family usually brings him to the physician. Thus, it appears that the diseases which produce all these abnormalities not only evoke observable changes in behavior but also alter or reduce the capacity of the patient to make accurate introspections concerning his own psychic function. This fact stands as one of the most incontrovertible proofs that the cerebrum is the organ both of behavior and of all inner psychic experiences; that is to say, behavior and mind are but two inseparable aspects of the function of the nervous system.

COMMON SYNDROMES

This entire group of acute confusional and delirious states is characterized principally by clouding of consciousness with prominent disorders of attention and perception that interfere with clarity of thinking and the formation of memories. One syndrome, here called *delirium,* includes overactivity, sleeplessness, tremulousness, and hallucinations. Convulsions often precede the delirium. A second syndrome is a *confusional state* in which there is manifest reduction in alertness and psychomotor activity. A third syndrome consists of a confusional state occurring in a patient with some other cerebral disease. The latter disposes him to the acute psychosis which we have chosen to designate as a *beclouded dementia.* These illnesses tend to develop acutely, to have multiple causes, and to terminate within a relatively short period of time (days to weeks), leaving the patient without residual damage.

Delirium

CLINICAL FEATURES These are most perfectly depicted in the alcoholic patient. The symptoms usually develop over a period of 2 or 3 days. The first indications of the approaching attack are difficulty in concentrating, restless irritability, tremulousness, insomnia, and poor appetite. One or several generalized convulsions are the initial major symptom in 30 percent of the cases. The patient's rest becomes troubled by unpleasant and terrifying dreams. There may be momentary disorientation or an occasional inappropriate remark.

These initial symptoms rapidly give way to a clinical picture that, in severe cases, is one of the most colorful and dramatic in medicine. The state of consciousness becomes altered; it is clouded in that the patient is inattentive and unable to perceive all elements of his situation. He may talk incessantly and incoherently and looks distressed and perplexed; his expression is in keeping with his vague notions of being annoyed or pursued by someone who seeks to injure him. From his manner and from the content of his speech it is evident that he misinterprets the meaning of ordinary objects and sounds around him and has vivid visual, auditory, and tactile hallucinations, often of a most unpleasant type. At first he can be brought momentarily into touch with reality and may in fact answer questions correctly; but almost at once he relapses into his preoccupied, confused state, gives wrong answers, and is unable to think coherently. The clouding of sensorium is revealed by his inability to repeat or reverse series of digits or to do serial additions or subtractions. As a rule he is oriented. Before long he is unable to shake off his hallucinations even for a second and does not recognize his family or his physician. Tremor and restless movements are usually present and may be violent. Sleep is impossible or occurs only in brief naps. The countenance is flushed, the pupils are dilated, and the conjunctivas are injected; the pulse is rapid and soft, and the temperature may be raised. There is much sweating, and the urine is scanty and of high specific gravity. The signs of overactivity of the autonomic nervous system, more than any other, distinguish delirium from all other confusional states.

The symptoms abate, either suddenly or gradually, after 2 or 3 days, although in exceptional cases they may persist for several weeks. The most certain indication of the end of the attack is the occurrence of sound sleep and of lucid intervals of increasing length. Recovery is usually complete.

Delirium is subject to all degrees of variability, not only from patient to patient but in the same patient from day to day and hour to hour. The entire syndrome may be observed in one patient, and only one or two symptoms in another. In its mildest form, as so often occurs in febrile diseases, it consists of an occasional wandering of the mind and incoherence of verbal expression, interrupted by periods of lucidity. This form, lacking motor and autonomic overactivity, is sometimes referred to as a *quiet delirium* (or *hypokinetic delirium*) and is difficult to distinguish from other confusional states. The more severe form of active delirium and tremulousness, best exemplified by delirium tremens, may progress to a "muttering stupor" and in about 10 percent of patients ends fatally.

MORBID ANATOMY AND PATHOPHYSIOLOGY The brains of patients who have died in delirium tremens usually show no pathologic changes of significance. A number of diseases, however, may cause delirium and also give rise to focal lesions in the brain, such as focal embolic encephalitis, viral encephalitis, Wernicke's disease, or trauma. The topography of these lesions is of particular interest. They tend to be localized in the midbrain and subthalamus and in the temporal lobes, where they involve the reticular activating and limbic systems.

Penfield's studies of the human cortex during surgical exploration clearly indicate the importance of the temporal lobe in producing visual, auditory, and olfactory hallucinations. With subthalamic and midbrain lesions, visual hallucinations may occur that are not unpleasant and may be accompanied by good insight (the peduncular hallucinosis of Lhermitte).

The electroencephalogram in delirium shows nonfocal slow activity in the 5- to 7-per-sec range, a state that rapidly returns to normal as the delirium clears. However, in other cases only activity in the fast beta frequency range is seen, and in milder degrees of delirium there is usually no abnormality at all.

An analysis of the several conditions conducive to delirium suggests at least three different physiologic mechanisms. The withdrawal of alcohol, barbiturates, or other sedation drugs, following a period of chronic intoxication is the most common cause of delirium (see Chaps. 111, 113). These drugs are known to have a strong depressant effect on certain areas of the central nervous system; presumably, the release and overactivity of these parts, after withdrawal of the drug, are the basis of delirium. In this respect it is interesting to note that the symptoms of delirium tremens are the antithesis of those of alcoholic intoxication. In the case of bacterial infections and poisoning by certain drugs, such as atropine and scopolamine, the delirious state probably results from the direct action of the toxin or chemical on these same parts of the brain. Thirdly, destructive lesions, such as acute inclusion body encephalitis of the temporal lobes, may cause delirium by disturbing the function of certain areas.

Psychophysiologic mechanisms have also been postulated. It has long been suggested that some persons are much more liable to delirium than others. There is much reason to doubt this hypothesis, for it has been shown that all of a group of randomly selected persons develop delirium if the causative mechanisms are strongly operative. This is not surprising, for any healthy person under certain circumstances may experience phenomena akin to those found in delirium. Thus after repeated auditory and visual stimulation the same impressions may continue to be perceived even though the stimuli are no longer present. Moreover, it has been shown that a healthy person can be induced to hallucinate by being placed for several days in an environment as free as possible of sensory stimulation. A relation between delirium and dream states has been postulated because in both one finds a loss of appreciation of time, a richness of visual imagery, indifference to inconsistencies, and "defective reality testing." Moreover, patients may refer to some of these delirious symptoms as a "bad dream," and normal persons may hallucinate in the so-called hypnagogic period between sleeping and waking. In general, however, formulations in the field of dynamic psychology seem more reasonably to account for the topical content of delirium than to explain its occurrence. Wolff and Curran, having observed the same content in repeated attacks of delirium due to different causes, concluded that the content depends more on age, sex, intellectual endowment, occupation, personality traits, and past experience of the patient than on the cause or mechanism of the delirium.

The main difficulty in understanding delirium arises from the fact that it has not been possible from clinical studies to ascertain which of the many symptoms have physiologic significance. What is the basis of this altered consciousness, this sensorial alteration, the lack of harmony between actual sensory impressions of the present and memory of those in the past? Obviously, something has been removed from the perceptive process, something that leaves the patient at the mercy of certain sensory stimuli and unable to attend to others, yet at the same time incapable of discriminating between sense impression and fantasy. The lack of inhibition of sensory processes may also be the basis of the sleep disturbance (insomnia) and the convulsive tendency.

Acute confusional states associated with reduced mental alertness and responsiveness

CLINICAL FEATURES In the most typical examples, all mental functions are reduced to some degree, but alertness, attentiveness, and the ability to grasp all elements of the immediate situation suffer most. In its mildest form the patient may pass for normal, and only failure to recollect and reproduce happenings of the past few hours or days reveals the inadequacy of mental function. The more obviously confused patient spends much of his time in idleness, but what he does do may be inappropriate and annoying to others. Only the more automatic acts and verbal responses are properly performed, but these may permit the examiner to obtain from the patient a number of relevant and accurate replies to questions about age, occupation, and residence. Reactions are slow and indecisive, and it is difficult for the patient to sustain a conversation. He may doze during the interview and is observed to sleep more hours each day than is natural or the same number at more irregular intervals. Responses tend to be rather abrupt, brief, and mechanical. Perceptual difficulties are frequent, and voices, common objects, and the actions of other persons are frequently misinterpreted. Often one cannot discern whether the patient hears voices and sees things that do not exist, i.e., whether he is hallucinating, or is merely misinterpreting stimuli in the environment. Inadequate perception and forgetfulness result in a constant state of bewilderment. Failing to recognize his surroundings and having lost all sense of time, he repeats the same question and makes the same remarks over and over again. Irritability may or may not be present. Some patients are extremely suspicious; in fact, a paranoid trend may be the most pronounced and troublesome feature of the illness.

As the confusion deepens, conversation becomes more difficult, and at a certain state the patient no longer notices or responds to much of what is going on around him. Replies to questions may be a single word or a short phrase spoken in a soft tremulous voice or whisper. The patient may be mute. In its most advanced stages confusion gives way to stupor and finally to coma. As the patient improves, he may pass again through the stage of stupor and confusion in the reverse order. All this informs us that at least one category of confusion is but a manifestation of the same disease processes that in their severest form cause coma.

In the most typical cases, this type of confusional state is readily distinguished from delirium; in others with more than the usual degree of irritability and restlessness, one cannot fail to notice the resemblance to delirium. Similarly, certain cases of delirium, in which tremor, vivid hallucinations, vigilant excited attitude, insomnia, and the low convulsive threshold are inconspicuous, are difficult to distinguish from other acute confusional states. The same diagnostic difficulty arises when a delirium is complicated by an illness that superimposes stupor (e.g., delirium tremens with pneumonia or meningitis). Difficulty in distinguishing these two states explains why some writers (such as Romano and Engel and Lipowski) insist that there is only one disordered mechanism, the manifestations of which they call *delirium*. The present writers would disagree, for they believe that several pathogenetic mechanisms of different types and involving different parts of the brain are included in this category of acute, reversible cerebral disease.

MORBID ANATOMY AND PATHOPHYSIOLOGY

All that has been said on this subject in Chap 22 is applicable to at least one subgroup of the confusional states. In the others no consistent pathologic change has been found. The electroencephalogram is of interest because it is almost invariably abnormal in more severe forms of this syndrome, in contrast to delirium, where the changes are relatively minor. High-voltage slow waves in the 2- to 3-per-sec (delta) range or the 5- to 7-per-sec (theta) range are the usual finding.

Senile and other dementing brain diseases complicated by medical diseases (beclouded dementia)

Many elderly patients who enter the hospital with medical or surgical illness are mentally confused. Presumably the liability to this state is determined by preexisting brain disease, in this instance senile dementia, which may or may not have been obvious to the family before the onset of the complicating illness. Other cerebral diseases (vascular, neoplastic, demyelinative) may have the same effect of increasing the patient's liability to confusion.

All the clinical features of hypokinetic delirium or of acute confusion may be present. The severity may vary greatly. The confusion may be reflected only in the patient's inability to relate sequentially the history of his illness, or it may be so severe that he is virtually *non compos mentis.*

Although almost any complicating illness may bring out his confusion, it is particularly frequent with infectious disease, especially in those cases which resist the effects of antibiotic medication; with posttraumatic and postoperative states, notably after concussive brain injuries; with the removal of cataracts (in which case the confusion is probably related to being temporarily deprived of vision); and with congestive heart failure, chronic respiratory disease, and severe anemia, especially pernicious anemia. Often it is difficult to determine which of several possible factors is responsible for the confusion in this heterogeneous group of illnesses, and there may be more than one. A cardiac patient with a confusional psychosis may be febrile, have marginally reduced cerebral blood flow, be intoxicated by one or more drugs, or be in electrolyte imbalance. The same is true of a patient in a postoperative confusional state, in which a number of factors such as fever, infection, dehydration, and drug intoxication may be incriminated. Alcoholism may further complicate the problem.

When the patient recovers from the medical or surgical illness, he usually returns to his premorbid state, though his shortcomings, now drawn to the attention of the family and physician, may be more obvious than before.

Coincidental development of acute schizophrenic or manic-depressive psychosis during a medical or surgical illness

A certain proportion of psychoses of the schizophrenic or manic-depressive type first become manifest during an acute medical illness or following an operation or parturition. A causal relationship between the two is usually sought but cannot be established. Usually the psychosis began long before but was not recognized. The diagnostic studies of the psychiatric illness must proceed along the lines suggested in Chaps. 341 and 342. Close observation will usually reveal a clear sensorium and relatively intact memory, which permits differentiation from the acute confusional states.

CLASSIFICATION AND DIAGNOSIS

The syndromes themselves and their main clinical relationships are the only satisfactory basis for classification until such time as the actual cause and pathophysiology are discovered (Table 26-1). The practice of classifying the syndromes according to their most prominent symptom or degree of severity, e.g., "picking delirum," "microptic delirium," "acute delirious mania," 'muttering delirium," has no fundamental value.

The first step in *diagnosis* is to recognize that the patient is confused. This is obvious in most cases, but, as pointed out above, the mildest form of confusion, particularly when some other acute alteration of personality is prominent, may be overlooked. In these mild forms a careful analysis of the patient's thinking as he gives the history of his illness and the details of his personal life will usually reveal an incoherence. Digit span and serial subtraction of 7s from 100 are useful bedside tests of the patient's capacity for sustained mental activity. Memory of recent events is one of the most delicate tests of adequate mental function and may be accomplished by having the patient relate all the details of his entry to the hospital, laboratory tests, etc.

Once it is established that the patient is confused, the differential diagnosis must be made between delirium, acute confusional states associated with psychomotor underactivity and a beclouded dementia. This can be done usually by careful attention to the patient's degree of alertness and wakefulness, his capacity to solve new problems, his memory, accuracy of perception, and hallucinations. The distinction between confusional states and dementia may be difficult at times. It has been said that the patient with the acute confusional psychosis has a clouded sensorium, i.e., he is inattentive and inclined to inaccurate perceptions and hallucinations, whereas the patient with dementia has a clear sensorium. However, some demented patients are as beclouded as those with confusional psychoses, and the two conditions are at times indistinguishable, except for their different time courses. All this suggests that the parts of the nervous system affected may be the same in both conditions. When the physician is faced with this problem, the history of the mode of onset becomes of great value. The confusional psychosis has an acute or subacute onset and is usually reversible, whereas dementia is chronic and more or less irreversible.

Once a case has been classified as delirium or either type of acute confusional state, it is important to determine its clinical associations. A thorough medical and neurologic examination and often a lumbar puncture should be performed. The other medical and neurologic findings are of great value in indicating the underlying disease to be treated, and they also give information concerning prognosis. In the neurologic examination, particular attention should be given to language functions, visual fields and visual-spatial discriminations, cortical sensory functions, and calculations and other test performances that require normal functioning of the temporal, parietal, and occipital lobes. Confusional states are frequent with diseases of these parts of the brain. Moreover, some of the signs of the latter are often mistaken for a confusional psychosis.

Schizophrenia and manic-depressive psychosis can usually be separated from the confusional states by the presence of a clear sensorium and good memory.

CARE OF THE DELIRIOUS AND CONFUSED PATIENT

The physician must be secure in his ability to manage the delirious and confused patient because such illnesses are observed almost daily on the medical and surgical wards of a general hospital. Occurring as they do during an infective fever, in the course of another illness such as cardiac failure, or following an injury, operation, or the excessive use of alcohol, they never fail to create grave problems for the physician, the nursing personnel, and the family. The physician's program of treatment may constantly be threatened by the patient's agitation, sleeplessness, and uncooperative attitude. The nursing personnel are often sorely taxed by the necessity of providing a satisfactory environment for the convalescence of the patient and, at the same time, maintaining a tranquil atmosphere for the other patients on the ward. And the family is appalled by the sudden specter of insanity and all that it entails.

Under such circumstances, it is a great temptation to rid oneself of the clinical problem by transferring the patient to a psychiatric hospital. This is an unwise action, for it may result in the inexpert management of the underlying medical disease and may even jeopardize the patient's life. Furthermore, delirium seldom lasts more

TABLE 26-1
Classification of delirium and acute confusional states

I Delirium
- *A* In a medical or surgical illness (no focal or lateralizing neurologic signs; cerebrospinal fluid usually clear)
  - *1* Typhoid fever
  - *2* Pneumonia
  - *3* Septicemia, particularly erysipelas and other streptococcal infections
  - *4* Rheumatic fever
  - *5* Thyrotoxicosis and ACTH intoxication (rare)
  - *6* Postoperative and posttraumatic states
- *B* In neurologic disease that causes focal or lateralizing signs or changes in the cerebrospinal fluid
  - *1* Vascular, neoplastic, or other diseases, particularly those involving the temporal lobes and upper part of the brainstem
  - *2* Cerebral contusion and laceration (traumatic delirium)
  - *3* Acute purulent and tuberculous meningitis
  - *4* Subarachnoid hemorrhage
  - *5* Encephalitis due to viral causes and to unknown causes, e.g., infectious mononucleosis
- *C* The abstinence states, exogenous intoxications, and postconvulsive states; signs of other medical, surgical, and neurologic illnesses absent or coincidental
  - *1* Withdrawal of alcohol (delirium tremens), barbiturates, and nonbarbiturate sedative drugs, following chronic intoxication (Chaps. 111 and 113)
  - *2* Drug intoxications: camphor, caffeine, ergot, bromides, scopolamine, atropine, amphetamine
  - *3* Postconvulsive delirium

II Acute confusional states associated with psychomotor underactivity
- *A* Associated with a medical or surgical disease (no focal lateralizing neurologic signs; cerebrospinal fluid clear)
  - *1* Metabolic disorders: hepatic stupor, uremia, hypoxia, hypercapnea, hypoglycemia, porphyria
  - *2* Infective fevers, especially typhoid
  - *3* Congestive heart failure
  - *4* Postoperative, posttraumatic, and puerperal psychoses
- *B* Associated with drug intoxication (no focal or lateralizing signs; cerebrospinal fluid clear): opiates, barbiturates, bromides, Artane, etc.
- *C* Associated with diseases of the nervous system (the focal or lateralizing neurologic signs and cerebrospinal fluid changes of these conditions are commoner than in delirium)
  - *1* Cerebral vascular disease, tumor, abscess
  - *2* Subdural hemotoma
  - *3* Meningitis
  - *4* Encephalitis
- *D* Beclouded dementia, i.e., senile or other brain disease in combination with infective fevers, drug reactions, heart failure, or other medical or surgical disease

than a few days, and if the patient can be kept on a medical ward, the social stigma that attaches to incarceration in a mental institution is avoided. Only a few delirious patients are so agitated and noisy as to annoy others, and should this happen, most general hospitals now have facilities for isolating such patients.

The primary therapeutic effort is directed to the control of the underlying medical disease. Other important objectives are to quiet the patient and protect him against injury. A private nurse, an attendant, or a member of the family should be with the patient at all times if this can be arranged. Depending on how active and vigorous he is, a locked room, screened windows that cannot be opened by the patient, and a low bed or mattress on the floor should be arranged. It is often better to let the patient walk about the room than to tie him into bed, which may excite or frighten him so that he struggles to the point of complete exhaustion and collapse. If he is less active, the patient can usually be kept in bed by leather wrist restraints, a restraining sheet, or a net thrown over the bed. Unless it is contraindicated by the primary disease, the patient should be permitted to sit up or walk about the room part of the day.

All drugs that could possibly be responsible for delirium—particularly opiates, barbiturates, bromides, atropine, hyosine, cortisone, adrenocorticortropic hormone (ACTH), and salicylates in large doses—should be discontinued (unless withdrawal effects are believed to underlie the illness). Paraldehyde and chloral hydrate are trustworthy sedatives under these circumstances. Paraldehyde, which is preferred, may be given orally or rectally in doses of 10 to 12 ml. For oral administration, mixing it with fruit juices makes it more palatable, though alcoholic patients will take it in any form and seem to enjoy it. Chlorpromazine, chlordiazepoxide, and diazepam are often extremely effective if given in full doses, and should be continued until natural sleep is restored. One must be cautious in attempting to suppress agitation completely. To accomplish this may require very large doses of drugs, and vital functions may then be dangerously impaired. The purpose of sedation is to assure rest and sleep so that the patient does not exhaust himself. Continuous warm baths or warm packs are also effective in quieting the delirious patient, but very few general hospitals have proper facilities for this valuable method of treatment.

A fluid intake and output chart should be kept, and any fluid and electrolyte deficit should be corrected. The pulse and blood pressure should be recorded at intervals of 2 hr in anticipation of circulatory collapse. Transfusions of whole blood and vasopressor drugs may be lifesaving.

Finally, the physician should be aware of many small therapeutic measures that may allay fear and suspicion and reduce the tendency to hallucinations. The room should be kept dimly lighted at night, and if possible, the patient should not be moved from one room to another. Every procedure should be explained in detail, even such simple ones as the taking of blood pressure or temperature. The presence of a member of the family may enable the patient to maintain contact with reality.

It may be some consolation and also a source of professional satisfaction to remember that most delirious patients tend to recover if they are placed in good hygienic surroundings and competently nursed. The family should be reassured on this point. They must also understand that the abnormal behavior and irrational actions of the patient are not wilful but rather are symptomatic of a brain disease.

See also Chaps. 111 and 113 for specific aspects of management of delirium due to withdrawal of alcohol, barbiturates, and other sedative drugs.

REFERENCES

ENGEL GL: Physiologic and psychologic considerations of delirium. Med Clin North Am 28:629, 1944

LIPOWSKI ZJ: Delirium, clouding of consciousness and confusion. J Nerv Ment Dis 145:227, 1967

WOLFF HG, CURRAN D: Nature of delirium and allied states. Arch Neurol Psychiat 33:1175, 1935

27 DERANGEMENTS OF INTELLECT AND BEHAVIOR DUE TO DIFFUSE AND FOCAL CEREBRAL DISEASE

RAYMOND D. ADAMS
MAURICE VICTOR

Increasingly, as the number of elderly adults in our population rises, the internist is consulted because an otherwise healthy person begins to lose his capacity to function effectively as head of a family or as a worker. This may have several significations—indicating the beginning of a brain tumor, the formation of a chronic subdural hematoma, or the development of a chronic drug intoxication, a chronic meningoencephalitis (syphilis), degenerative cerebral disease, a chronic, low-pressure hydrocephalus, a degenerative brain disease, or a depressive psychosis. In former times when there was little that could be done about any of these clinical states, no great premium was attached to diagnosis. But modern medicine now offers the means of treating several of these conditions and in some instances of restoring the patient to normal health and effectiveness. Early recognition of the underlying pathologic process improves chances of recovery.

THE CLINICAL SYNDROME OF DEMENTIA In current neurologic parlance the term *dementia* usually denotes a clinical state comprised of failing memory and loss of other intellectual functions due to chronic progressive degenerative disease of the brain. It may or may not be associated with signs of disease in one or more of the motor, sensory, or speech areas of the cerebrum. The chronicity of the process is ordinarily emphasized, but the illogic of setting apart any one constellation of cerebral symptoms on the basis of their speed of onset, evolution, or duration is obvious. We would like to propose that the state of dementia be regarded as a generic syndrome of multiple causation and mechanism, and that a diffuse degeneration of neurons is only one of the causes.

The earliest signs of dementia may be so subtle as to escape the notice of even the most discerning physician. Often an observant relative of the patient or an employer is the first to become aware of a certain lack of initiative, irritability, loss of interest, and inability to perform up to the usual standard. Later there is distractibility, inability to think with accustomed clarity, reduced general comprehension, perseveration in speech, action, and thought, and defective memory, especially for recent events. Frequently a change in mood becomes apparent, deviating more often toward depression than elation. The direction of this deviation is said to depend on the previous personality of the patient rather than upon the character of the disease. Excessive lability of mood may also be observed, i.e., easy fluctuation from laughter to tears on slight provocation. Lapses in social graces and conduct occur, and judgment becomes impaired, early in some cases and late in others. Paranoid ideas and delusions may develop. As a rule, the patient has little or no realization of these changes in himself; he lacks insight. As the condition progresses, there is loss of almost all intellectual faculties. Mutism, unresponsiveness, dysarthria, aphasia, and sphincteric incontinence may be added to the clinical picture. In a late stage a secondary physical deterioration also takes place. Food intake, which may be increased in the beginning of the illness, is in the end usually limited, with resulting emaciation. Any febrile illness or metabolic upset induces a marked increase in confusion and even stupor or coma, indicating the precarious state of cerebral compensation. Finally the patient remains in bed most of the time and dies of pneumonia or some other intercurrent infection. This whole process may evolve over a period of months or years, usually the latter.

Many of these alterations of behavior are the direct result of disease of the nervous system; expressed in another way, the symptoms are the primary manifestations of neurologic disease. Others are secondary, i.e., they are reactions to the catastrophe of losing one's mind. For example, the dement is said to seek solitude to hide his affliction and may thus appear asocial or apathetic. Again, excessive orderliness may be an attempt to compensate for failing memory; apprehension, gloom, or irritability may reflect general dissatisfaction with a necessarily restricted life. It would appear that even in a state of fairly advanced deterioration, the patient is still capable of reacting to his illness and to the persons who care for him. Degenerative diseases may progress to virtually complete decortication. The patient is unaware of what is happening but lies with eyes open. He no longer responds to spoken commands or speaks. There is no interest in food or drink though they are swallowed if placed in the mouth. The facial and limb muscles are stiff with increased tendon reflexes and Babinski signs. Grasping and sucking are prominent. The sphincters are incontinent.

Morbid anatomy and pathologic physiology of dementia Attempts to relate failing intellectual function to lesions in certain parts of the brain have been eminently unsuccessful. Two types of difficulty have obstructed progress in this field. (1) There is the problem of defining, analyzing, and determining the significance of the so-called "intellectual" functions. (2) The morbid anatomy of these diseases is often so diffuse and complex that it cannot be fully localized and quantitated. The memory impairment, which is a constant feature, may occur with extensive disease in any part of the cerebrum. Yet it is interesting to note that the function of certain parts of the diencephalon and of the hippocampi may be more fundamental to retentive memory than the rest of the cortex, as will be pointed out below. Failure in tests of verbal function (the most advanced degree of which is aphasia) is closely associated with disease of the dominant cerebral hemisphere, and particularly the speech areas in the frontal, temporal, and parietal lobes and the insula. Loss of capacity for arithmetic, reading, and numerical calculation (acalculia) is related to lesions in the posterior part of the left (dominant) cerebral hemisphere. Impairment in drawing or constructing simple and complex figures with blocks, sticks, picture arrangements, etc., as shown by test of visual construction, is most often observed in right (nondominant) parietal lobe lesions. Thus, the clinical picture resulting from cerebral disease depends in part on the extent of the lesion, i.e., the amount of cerebral tissue destroyed, and on the specific locality of the lesion.

Dementia is related usually to obvious structural disease of the cerebrum and the diencephalon. In some diseases, such as Alzheimer's and Pick's presenile or senile dementia, the main process appears to be a degeneration and loss of nerve cells in the association areas, with secondary changes in the cerebral white matter. In others, such as Huntington's chorea and other cerebro–basal ganglionic degenerations, loss of neurons in the cerebral cortex is accompanied by a similar degeneration of neurons in the putamen and caudate nuclei and cerebellum. Arteriosclerotic vascular disease results in multiple foci of infarction all through the thalami, basal ganglions, brainstem, and cerebrum and, in the latter, in the motor, sensory, or visual projection areas as well as in the association areas. Severe trauma may cause contusions of cerebral convolutions and rarely degeneration of the central white matter (Strich), which result in protracted stupor, coma, or dementia. Most diseases that produce dementia are quite extensive, and the frontal lobes are affected more often than other parts of the cerebrum.

Mechanisms other than the destruction of brain tissue may operate in some cases. Chronic increased intracranial pressure or chronic hydrocephalus (with large ventricles the pressure may not exceed 180 mm), regardless of cause, is often associated with a general impairment of mental function. Compression of cerebral white matter is the main factor. The compression of one or both of the cerebral hemispheres by chronic subdural hematomas may cause a widespread disturbance of cortical function. A diffuse inflammatory process is at least in part the basis for dementia in syphilis and in neurotropic virus infections such as "inclusion body encephalitis"; presumably there are loss of some neurons and also inflammatory derangement of the function of other neurons. Lastly, several of the toxic and metabolic diseases discussed in

Chap. 332 may interfere with nervous function over a period of time and create a clinical picture similar to, if not identical with, that of dementia. One must suppose that the altered biochemical environment has affected the excitability of the neurons.

(Details of all the diseases which cause dementia will be found in Chap. 333.)

Bedside classification of dementing diseases of the brain The conventional classification of dementing diseases of the brain is usually according to etiology, if known, or pathology. Another more practical approach, which follows logically from the method by which the whole subject has been presented in this book, is to subdivide the diseases into three categories on the basis of the associated clinical and laboratory signs of medical disease and the accompanying neurologic signs. Once the physician has determined that the patient suffers a dementing illness, he must then decide, from the medical, neurologic, and laboratory data, into which category the case fits. This classification may at first seem somewhat artificial. However, it is likely to be more useful to the student or physician not conversant with the many diseases that cause dementia than a classification based on pathology.

I Diseases in which dementia is usually associated with clinical and laboratory signs of other medical disease
- *A* Hypothyroidism
- *B* Cushing's disease
- *C* Nutritional deficiency states such as pellagra, the Wernicke-Korsakoff syndrome, and subacute combined degeneration of spinal cord and brain (vitamin B_{12} deficiency)
- *D* Neurosyphilis: general paresis and meningovascular syphilis
- *E* Hepatolenticular degeneration, familial and acquired
- *F* Bromidism

II Diseases in which dementia is associated with other neurologic signs but not with other obvious medical disease
- *A* Invariably associated with other neurologic signs
  - *1* Huntington's chorea (choreoathetosis)
  - *2* Schilder's disease and related demyelinative diseases (spastic weakness, pseudobulbar palsy, blindness, deafness)
  - *3* Amaurotic family idiocy and other lipid-storage diseases (myoclonic seizures, blindness, spasticity, cerebellar ataxia)
  - *4* Myoclonic epilepsy (diffuse myoclonus, generalized seizures, cerebellar ataxia)
  - *5* Jakob-Creutzfeldt disease (diffuse myoclonus)
  - *6* Cerebrocerebellar degeneration (cerebellar ataxia)
  - *7* Cerebral–basal ganglion degenerations (apraxia-rigidity)
  - *8* Dementia with spastic paraplegia (spastic legs)
- *B* Often associated with other neurologic signs
  - *1* Cerebral arteriosclerosis
  - *2* Brain tumor
  - *3* Brain trauma, such as cerebral contusion, mid-brain hemorrhage, chronic subdural hematoma
  - *4* Marchiafava-Bignami disease (often with apraxia and other frontal lobe signs)
  - *5* Low-pressure hydrocephalus (often with ataxia of gait)

III Diseases in which dementia is usually the only evidence of neurologic or medical disease
- *A* Alzheimer's disease and senile dementia
- *B* Pick's disease

Many of these diseases are discussed more fully in other sections of this book. The special features of the dementia that accompanies arteriosclerotic, senile, syphilitic, traumatic, nutritional, and degenerative diseases are discussed in the appropriate chapters.

Differential diagnosis The first task in dealing with this class of patients is to make sure of deterioration of intellect and personality change. It may be necessary to examine the patient several times before one is confident of the clinical findings.

There is always a tendency to assume that mental function is normal if patients complain only of nervousness, fatigue, insomnia, or vague somatic symptoms and to label the patients psychoneurotic. *This will be avoided if one keeps in mind that psychoneuroses rarely begin in middle or late adult life.* A practical rule is to assume that all mental illnesses beginning during this period are due either to structural disease of the brain or to depressive psychosis.

A mild dysphasia must not be mistaken for dementia. The aphasic patient appears uncertain of himself, and his speech may be incoherent. Furthermore, he may be anxious and depressed over his ineptitude. Careful attention to the patient's language performance will lead to the correct diagnosis in most instances. Further observation will disclose that the patient's behavior, except that which is related to the language disorder, is within normal limits.

The depressed patient presents another type of problem. He may remark that his mental function is poor or that he is forgetful and cannot concentrate. Scrutiny of his remarks will show, however, that he actually remembers all the details of his illness and that no qualitative change in mental ability has taken place. His difficulty is either a lack of energy and interest or an anxiety that prevents the focusing of attention on anything except his own problems. Even during mental tests his performance may be impaired by his emotions, in much the same way as that of the worried student during examinations. This condition of emotional blocking is called *experiential confusion.* When the patient is calmed by reassurance, his mental function improves, indicating that intellectual deterioration has not occurred. Thy hypomanic patient fails in tests of intellectual function because of his restlessness and distractibility. It is helpful to remember that the demented patient rarely has sufficient insight to complain of mental deterioration; and if he admits to poor memory, he seldom realizes the degree of his disability. The physician must never rely on the patient's statements as to the efficiency of mental function and must always evaluate a poor performance on tests in the light of the emotional state and motivation at the time the test is given.

The neurologic syndrome associated with metabolic or endocrine disorders, i.e., ACTH therapy, hyperthyroidism, Cushing's disease, Addison's disease, or the postpartum state may be difficult to diagnose because of the wide variety of clinical pictures by which they manifest themselves. Some patients appear to be suffering from a dementia, others from an acute confusional psychosis; or if mood change or negativism predominates, a manic-depressive psychosis or schizophrenia is suggested. In these conditions some degree of clouding of sensorium and impairment of intellectual function can usually be recognized, and these findings alone should be enough to exclude schizophrenia and manic-depressive psychosis. It is well to remember that acute onset of mental symptoms always suggests confusional psychosis or delirium. Inasmuch as many of these conditions are completely reversible, they must be distinguished from dementia (see Chap. 26).

Once it is decided that the patient suffers from a dementing disease, the next step is to determine by careful physical examination whether there are other neurologic signs or indications of a particular medical disease. This enables the physician to place the case in one of the three categories in the bedside classification. X-rays of the skull, electroencephalogram, lumbar puncture, and pneumoencephalogram should be carried out in most cases. Usually these procedures necessitate admission to a hospital. The final step is to determine by the total clinical picture which disease within any one category the patient has.

KORSAKOFF'S PSYCHOSIS (AMNESIC OR AMNESTIC—CONFABULATORY PSYCHOSIS) These terms are used interchangeably to designate a unique but common disorder of cognitive function, in which memory is deranged out of all proportion to all other components of mentation and behavior. It possesses two salient features which may vary in severity but are always conjoined: (1) an impaired ability to recall events and other information that had been well established before the onset of the illness (retrograde amnesia); and (2) an impaired ability to acquire new information, i.e., to learn or to form new memories (anterograde amnesia). Other cognitive functions (particularly the capacity for concentration, spatial organization, visual and verbal abstraction), which depend little or not at all on memory, may also be impaired but to a relatively minor degree. The patient tends to be lacking in initiative and spontaneity. Confabulation, meaning false or fabricated accounts of recent events, is variably present.

The definition of Korsakoff's psychosis demands also that certain aspects of behavior and mental function be intact. The patient should be alert, attentive, responsive, and capable of understanding the written and spoken word, of making appropriate deductions from given premises and solving such problems as can be concluded within his forward memory span. These "negative" features are of particular importance because they help to distinguish Korsakoff's psychosis from a number of other disorders in which the basic defect is not in retentive memory, but in some other psychologic mechanism, e.g., in attention and perception (as in the delirious, confused, or stuporous patient), in recall (as in the hysterical patient), or in volition (as in the patient with frontal lobe disease).

The anatomic structures of particular importance in memory function are the diencephalon (specifically the medial portions of the medial dorsal nuclei of the thalamus) and the hippocampal formations (gyrus dentatus, hippocampus, and parahippocampal gyri). Bilaterally placed lesions in either of these regions derange memory and learning out of all proportion to other cognitive functions, and even unilateral lesions of the dominant hemispheres produce a lesser degree of the same effect. It would appear that these structures are involved in all forms of learning and integration of newly formed memories and that they form a tenuous but vital link between the high-brainstem reticular formation (the integrity of which is necessary to maintain an alert state of mind, a prerequisite for any learning) and the cerebral cortex, which is the locus for special memories such as words, geometric figures, numbers, etc.

The physiologic basis of Korsakoff's psychosis is obscure. An acceptable hypothesis, which is still to be conceived, would have to explain how a single pathologic process, acting over a circumscribed period of time, impairs not only all future learning but also the ability to recall information that has been acquired before the illness began, and why the most recently acquired information is the most vulnerable. Such a hypothesis would also have to explain why the anterograde and retrograde amnesias, in patients who recover, always recover together and why certain types of memory function (immediate recall, long-standing social habits and motor skills, memory for words, etc.) are not damaged at all. Detailed discussions of these subjects will be found in the references at the end of this chapter.

Classification of diseases characterized by an amnesic syndrome The amnesic (Korsakoff's) syndrome, as defined above, may be a manifestation of a number of neurologic diseases that are identified by their mode of onset and clinical course, the associated neurologic signs, and ancillary findings.

I Amnesic syndrome of sudden onset—usually with gradual but incomplete recovery
- *A* Bilateral hippocampal infarction due to atherosclerotic-thrombotic or embolic occlusion of the posterior cerebral arteries or their inferior temporal branches
- *B* Trauma to the diencephalic or inferomedial temporal regions
- *C* Spontaneous subarachnoid hemorrhage
- *D* Carbon monoxide poisoning and other hypoxic states (rare)

II Amnesia of sudden onset and transitory duration
- *A* Temporal lobe seizures
- *B* Postconcussive states
- *C* "Transient global amnesia"

III Amnesic syndrome of subacute onset with varying degrees of recovery, usually leaving permanent residue
  - *A* Wernicke-Korsakoff disease
  - *B* Inclusion body (herpes simplex) encephalitis
  - *C* Tuberculous and other forms of meningitis characterized by a granulomatous exudate at the base of the brain

IV Slowly progressive amnesic states
  - *A* Tumors involving the floor and walls of the third ventricle
  - *B* Alzheimer's disease and other degenerative disorders

SYNDROMES CAUSED BY DISEASES OF SPECIAL PARTS OF THE CEREBRUM Symptoms and signs of disease of one part of the cerebrum may occur by themselves or in combination with dementia; they provide important information about the location of a disease process and at times about its nature. This is an appropriate place, therefore, to review briefly the known effects of disease of various parts of the cerebrum. Agnosia, apraxia, and aphasia will be only mentioned, since they are treated more extensively in Chaps. 21, 25, and 326.

Frontal lobes In Fig. 27-1, it may be seen that the frontal lobes lie anterior to the central, or Rolandic, sulcus and superior to the Sylvian fissure. They consist of several functionally different parts, which are conventionally designated in the neurologic literature by numbers (according to a scheme devised by Brodmann) and by letters (in the scheme of von Economo and Koskinas).

The posterior parts, areas 4 and 6 of Brodmann, are specifically related to motor function. Voluntary movement in man depends on the integrity of these areas, and lesions in them produce spastic paralysis of the contralateral face, arm, and leg. This is discussed in Chap. 17, Motor Paralysis. Lesions limited more or less to the premotor areas (area 6) are accompanied by prominent grasp and sucking reflexes. Lesions in areas 8 and 24 of Brodmann interfere with the mechanism concerned with turning the head and eyes contralaterally. Lesions in areas 44 and 45 of the major hemisphere abolish or reduce verbalization, deglutition, and chewing. Lesions in area 44 of the dominant cerebral hemisphere, usually the left one, have often resulted in loss of verbal expression, the aphasia of Broca. Lesions in the medial limbic or piriform cortex (areas 23 and 24), wherein are bilaterally organized the mechanisms controlling respiration, circulation, and micturition have relatively unclear clinical effects.

The remaining parts of the frontal lobes (areas 9, 10, 11, 12, and 13 of Brodmann), sometimes called the *prefrontal areas*, have less specific and measurable functions. In contrast to the motor areas of the frontal lobes and other areas of the brain, stimulation of the prefrontal areas in man has yielded a paucity of findings. Many patients with gunshot wounds of these areas have shown only mild and inconsistent abnormalities of behavior. Nevertheless, the following groups of symptoms have been observed in patients with large lesions of one or both of the frontal lobes or of the central white matter and the

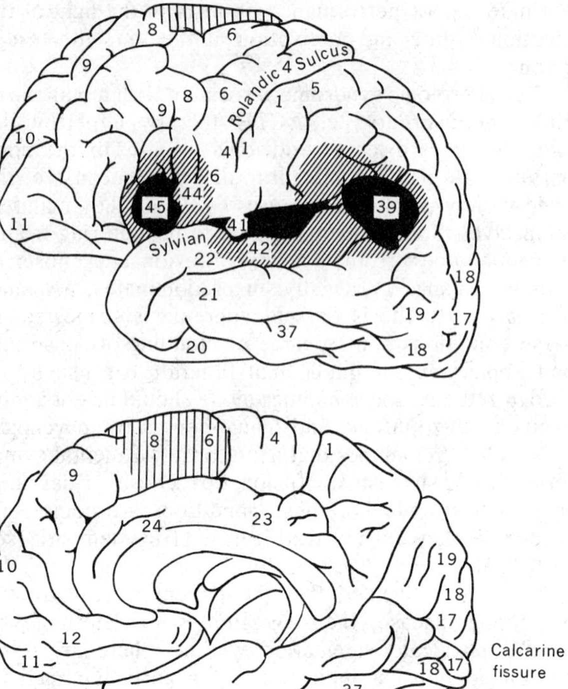

FIGURE 27-1
Diagram to show cortical areas, numbered according to the scheme of Brodmann. The speech areas are in black, the three main ones being 39, 41, and 45. The zone marked by vertical stripes in the superior frontal convolution is the secondary motor area which, like Broca's area 45, if stimulated causes vocal arrest. (Redrawn from Handbuch der Inneren Medizin, *Berlin: Springer-Verlag, 1939)*

anterior part of the corpus callosum by which they are joined.

1 Change of personality, usually expressed as lack of concern over the consequences of any action, which may take the form of a childish excitement (*moria* of Jastrowitz), an inappropriate joking and punning (*witzelsucht* of Oppenheim), or an instability and superficiality of emotion, or irritability

2 Slight impairment of intelligence, usually described as lack of concentration, vacillation of attention, inability to carry out planned activity, difficulty in changing from one activity to another, loss of recent memory, or lack of initiative and spontaneity

3 Motor abnormalities such as decomposition of gait and upright stance, trunk ataxia of Bruns, abnormal postures, reflex grasping or sucking, incontinence of sphincters, and an apathetic-akinetic-abulic state

The most pronounced changes have been observed in cases with bilateral disease of the frontal lobes, and there has been much doubt as to the effect of a lesion involving only one frontal lobe. Nevertheless, the most careful psychologic tests on patients with lesions of either frontal lobe demonstrate a slight elevation of mood, with increased talkativeness and tendency to joke, a lack of tact, inability to adapt to a new situation, and loss of initiative.

Several careful studies of lobotomized patients have now been published. Of course, very few of these patients were normal before the operation, so that base-line measurements of mental ability were not always obtainable. However, some patients of normal intellect have received this treatment for severe neurosis or intractable pain. They are said to have shown little or no loss of ability in their performance on intelligence tests, depending on the extent of the procedure; and if worry, fears, conpulsions, and suffering from pain were incapacitating, the loss of these traits resulted in test scores actually higher than before the operation. However, careful examination of the behavior in everyday tasks usually will disclose a slight lowering of general intelligence, a decrease in drive or energy, a definite change of personality in the form of shallow emotional life, a lack of tact, and inability to direct and sustain activity toward future goals. Also there is a diminution of traits related to neuroticism, such as suggestibility, rigidity of character, self-criticism, and introversion.

Finally it should be emphasized that the function of the frontal lobes or other discrete parts of the brain cannot be determined simply by the study of human beings who have suffered injury or disease of that part. Symptoms from lesions of a part of the nervous system are not identical with the functions of that part. The symptoms of frontal lobe deficit must depend both on a loss of certain parts of the cerebrum and on the functional activity of the remaining portions of the nervous system. To date, a unified concept of frontal lobe function has not emerged. There is no doubt that the human mind is changed by disease of the frontal lobes, but it is difficult to say in what way it is changed. Perhaps at present it is best to regard the frontal lobes as that part of the brain which orients the individual, with all his percepts and concepts formed from past life experiences, toward action that is projected into the future.

Temporal lobes The boundaries of the temporal lobes may be seen in Fig. 27-1. The Sylvian fissure separates the superior surface of each temporal lobe from the frontal and anterior parts of the parietal lobes. There is no definite anatomic boundary between the temporal and occipital lobes or between temporal and parietal lobes. The temporal lobe includes the superior, middle, and inferior temporal, fusiform, and hippocampal convolutions and the transverse convolutions of Heschl, which is the auditory receptive area present on the superior surface within the Sylvian fissure. The hippocampal convolution was once believed to be related indirectly to the olfactory bulb, but now it is known that lesions here do not cause anosmia. The fibers from the homolateral lower quadrant of each retina course through the central white matter en route to the occipital lobes, and lesions that interrupt them characteristically produce a contralateral homonymous upper quadrant defect of visual fields. Hearing and labyrinthine function, also localized in the temporal lobes, are bilaterally represented, which accounts for the fact that unless both temporal lobes are affected, there is no demonstrable loss of hearing. Loss of equilibrium has not been observed with temporal lobe lesions. Extensive disease in the superior and middle convolutions of the left temporal lobe in right-handed individuals results in Wernicke's aphasia. This syndrome, discussed in Chap. 25, Affections of Speech, consists of jargon aphasia and inability to read, to write, or to understand the meaning of spoken words (Wernicke's aphasia).

Between the auditory and olfactory projection areas there is a large expanse of temporal lobe which has no assignable function. This is the temporal association area. Patients with tumors and vascular lesions of this part of the brain have been examined on numerous occasions, but usually the full extent of the disease has not been determined, even by pneumoencephalography, arteriography, or isotopic scanning procedures. Cases of partial or complete temporal lobectomy for tumor have provided more valuable material, but again it has seldom been possible to be certain that other parts of the brain were not involved. Dysnomia has been the most frequent symptom in dominant hemisphere lesions. The most careful psychologic studies have shown a difference between cases involving loss of the dominant and the nondominant temporal lobe. With lesions of the dominant side there is impairment in learning auditorially presented material; with nondominant lesions there is a similar failure in tests with visually presented material. In addition, about 20 percent of both right and left lobectomy patients have shown a syndrome similar to that described for the prefrontal parts of the brain; but more significant is the fact that in the other cases little or no defect in personality was exhibited. The study of cases of uncinate epilepsy, with the characteristic dreamy state, olfactory or gustatory hallucinations, and masticatory movements, suggests that all these functions are organized through the temporal lobes. Similarly, stimulation of the posterior parts of the temporal lobes of fully conscious epileptic patients during surgical procedures has brought to light the interesting fact that complex memories and visual and auditory images, some with strong emotional content, can be aroused. Studies of the effect of stimulation of the amygdaloid nucleus, which is in the anterior and medial part of the temporal lobe, have shed additional light on this subject. Symptoms may be evoked not unlike some of those of schizophrenic patients. Complex emotional experiences that have occurred previously may be revived. There are remarkable autonomic effects. Blood pressure rises, pulse increases, respirations are increased in frequency and depth, and the patient looks frightened. These effects have been discussed in Chap. 24, The Convulsive State. Ablation of these nuclei has eliminated uncontrollable rage reactions in psychotic patients. Hippocampal and adjacent convolutions have been excised bilaterally, with a disastrous loss of ability to learn or to establish new memories (Korsakoff's psychosis). All this indicates an important role of the temporal lobes in auditory and visual perception and imagery, in learning and memory, and in the emotional life of the individual.

Bilateral ablation of temporal lobes, so far studied only in monkeys, produces an animal that displays a curious tendency to react to every visual stimulus without seeming to recognize it (psychic blindness) and to examine every object in its environment by oral and manual contact. Placidity, with lack of the usual emotional response to stimuli, was another prominent feature.

To summarize, in man the temporal lobe syndromes include the following:

I Effects of unilateral disease of the dominant temporal lobe
- *A* Quadrantic homonymous anopia
- *B* Wernicke's aphasia
- *C* Impairment in verbal tests of material presented through the auditory sense
- *D* Dysnomia or anmestic aphasia

II Effects of unilateral disease of nondominant temporal lobe
- *A* Quadrantic homonymous anopia
- *B* Impairment of mental function with inability to judge spatial relationships in some cases
- *C* Impairment in nonverbal tests of visually presented material

III Effects of bilateral disease
- *A* Korsakoff's amnesic defect
- *B* Apathy and placidity
- *C* Loss of sexual capacity
- *D* Loss of other of the unilateral functions

Parietal lobes This part of the human nervous system is the subject of one of the most interesting discussions of cerebral function that has occurred in this century: its role in the formation of the body image or body schema.

It has long been known that the postcentral convolution is the terminus of somatic sensory pathways from the opposite half of the body. It has also been learned that destructive lesions here do not abolish cutaneous sensation but instead cause mainly a defect in sensory discrimination with variable impairment of sensation. In other words, pain, touch, and thermal and vibratory sensation are largely retained, whereas stereognosis, sense of position, distinction between single and double contacts (two-point threshold), and the localization of sensory stimuli are lost. There is also the phenomenon of extinction, i.e., if both sides of the body are touched simultaneously, only the stimulus on the normal side is perceived. This type of sensory disturbance, sometimes called *cortical sensory defect,* is discussed in Chap. 21, Disorders of Sensation. Later it was noted that extensive lesions deep in the white matter of the parietal lobes produce a contralateral homonymous hemianopia, and lesions in the angular gyrus of the dominant hemisphere result in an inability to read.

More recent investigations have centered about the function of the parietal lobes in perception of position in space and of the relationship of the various parts of the body to one another. Since the time of Babinski it has been known that patients with a large lesion of the minor parietal lobe are often unaware of their hemiplegia and hemianesthesia. Babinski called this condition *anosognosia.* Related psychologic disorders are lack of recognition of the left arm and leg, neglect of the left side of the body (as in dressing) and of external space on the left side, and constructional apraxia (an inability to perform the movements of constructing simple figures). All these disorders of parietal lobe function may occur with left-sided lesions as well, but are observed only rarely, being obscured by the commonly associated *aphasia* and *agnosia.*

Another frequent constellation of symptoms, usually referred to as *Gerstmann's syndrome,* occurs only with lesions of the dominant parietal lobe. This consists of inability to write (agraphia), inability to calculate (acalculia), failure to distinguish right from left, and loss of recognition of various parts of the body. This is a true *agnosia,* since it represents a defect in the formulation and use of symbolic concepts, including the significance of numbers and letters and the names of parts of the body. An ideomotor apraxia may or may not be associated. *Agnosia* and *apraxia* are discussed in Chaps. 17 and 21.

The effects of disease of the parietal lobes may be summarized as follows:

I Effect of unilateral disease of the parietal lobe, right or left
- *A* Cortical sensory syndrome and sensory extinction (or total hemianesthesia with large acute lesions of white matter)
- *B* Mild hemiparesis, unilateral muscular atrophy in children
- *C* Homonymous hemianopia or visual inattention, and sometimes anosognosia, neglect of one-half of the body and of extrapersonal space
- *D* Abolition of opticokinetic nystagmus to one side

II Effects of unilateral disease of the dominant parietal lobe (left hemisphere in right-handed patients), additional phenomena
- *A* Disorders of language (especially alexia)
- *B* Gerstmann's syndrome
- *C* Bimanual astereognosis (tactile agnosia)
- *D* Bilateral apraxia of the ideomotor type

In all these lesions, if the disease is sufficiently extensive, there may be a reduction in the capacity to think clearly, inattentiveness, and impaired memory.

It is impossible at this time to present a formula of parietal lobe function in general. It does seem reasonably certain that both the parietal and occipital lobes participate in sensory functions, especially in those which provide consciousness of one's surroundings, of the relationship of objects in the environment to one another, and of the position of the body in space. In this respect, the parietal lobe may be regarded as a suprasensory mechanism for transmodal (intersensory) relationships, particularly tactile and visual, which are the basis of our concepts of space.

Occipital lobes The occipital lobes are the terminus of the geniculocalcarine pathways and are essential for visual sensation and perception. Lesions in one occipital lobe result in homonymous defects in the contralateral visual fields. Most often the defect takes the form of loss of vision in part or all of the homonymous fields. Occasionally patients complain of changes in the form and contour of visually perceived objects (metamorphopsia), illusory displacement of images from one side of the visual field to another (optic alloesthesia), or of abnormal persistence of the visual image after the object has been removed (palinopsia). Bilateral lesions cause "cortical" blindness, a state of blindness without change in optic fundi or pupillary reflexes.

Lesions in Brodmann's areas 18 and 19 of the dominant hemisphere (Fig. 27-1) cause a loss of visual recognition with retention of some degree of visual acuity, a state termed *visual agnosia.* In the classic form of this blindness an individual with intact mental powers is unable to recognize objects, even though by tests of visual acuity and perimetry he appears to see sufficiently well to do so; he is able to recognize objects by tactile or other extravisual sense. In these terms, *alexia,* or inability to read, represents a visual verbal agnosia or "word blindness." The patient can see letters and words but cannot recognize their meaning, although he can still recognize them through tactile or auditory senses.

Several special types of visual agnosia have been described. In the simultanagnosia of Wolpert, the patient, though able to see the individual parts of a picture, is unable to gather the meaning of the whole. Similarly, in prosopagnosia the patient cannot identify the face of a relative or friend, even though he can recognize a face as such and its individual parts. Disturbances of perception of movement may occur in association with simultanagnosia or prosopagnosia. The visual-spatial agnosia with bilateral lesions of the parietooccipital junction is characterized by errors in the localization of objects by sight, not only of objects exposed in the amblyopic fields, but also in total visual space. Associated abnormalities are confusion of right and left and of direction, and a failure to conceive spatial relationships. Such patients may become lost in familiar surroundings; they are truly disoriented in space.

Some authors have questioned whether there is a clinical entity of visual agnosia. Analysis of the reported cases discloses that many patients have had impaired mental function and various degrees of aphasia. Also, in most cases, tests of primary visual sensation or visual acuity have been inadequate. By controlling the time factor in tests of visual perception and the adaptation time, and by testing simultaneous perception of multiple points in the visual field, it is possible to show that the visual function is more often impaired than was first suspected. The division of the visual process into sensation and perception in these cases becomes highly artificial.

CORPUS CALLOSUM AND THE DISCONNECTION SYNDROMES A number of clinical syndromes result from interruption of the connections between the two cerebral hemispheres in the corpus callosum or adjacent white matter (commissural syndromes) or between the several parts of one hemisphere (intrahemispheric dissociation syndromes).

When the entire corpus callosum is missing because of a congenital defect or destroyed by a surgical procedure or anterior cerebral artery occlusion (anterior four-fifths), the speech and perception areas of the left hemisphere are isolated from those of the right hemisphere. The patient, if blindfolded, is unable to match a stimulus object held in one hand with that in the other hand. Further he cannot match an object seen in the right half of his visual fields with one in the left half. If given verbal commands to execute, he performs correctly with the right hand but not with the left. For example, if asked to write from dictation with the left hand he makes only an illegible scrawl. Without vision, objects placed in the right hand are named correctly, but not those in the left. In lesions confined to the posterior fifth of the corpus callosum (splenium), only the visual part of the disconnection syndrome occurs. The occlusion of the left posterior cerebral artery provides the best examples of the latter. Since infarction of the left occipital lobe causes a right homonymous hemianopia, thereafter all visual information needed for activating the speech areas of the left hemisphere must come from the right occipital lobe across the splenium of the corpus callosum. Such a patient cannot read or name colors because the visual information cannot reach the left angular gyrus. There is no difficulty in copying words (though he cannot read what he has written); the visual information for activating the left motor area crosses the corpus callosum more anteriorly. Matching of colors without naming them is done without error.

A disconnection in the anterior third of the corpus callosum, where fiber systems between right and left motor areas pass, results only in failure of the left hand to obey spoken commands, the right one performing perfectly (left-sided motor apraxia). The left one can still imitate the examiner's movements.

Of intrahemispheric disconnections, the following are the most important:

1 Conduction (also called "central") aphasia: the patient has fluent but paraphasic speech and writing with nearly perfect comprehension of spoken or written language. The Wernicke speech area is separated from the Broca motor area by a lesion in the arcuate fasciculus. There is motor apraxia of the left hand.

2 Sympathetic apraxia in Broca's aphasia: a lesion in the subcortical region, by destroying the anterior part of the arcuate fasciculus or the origin of the motor callosal fibers, causes an apraxia of command movements of the left hand. This condition may also result from a left-sided capsular lesion and an anterior corpus callosal lesion.

3 Pure word deafness: Although the patient is able to hear and to identify nonverbal sounds, there is loss of ability to comprehend spoken language. The patient's speech remains normal. The lesion has been a subcortical infarction of the left temporal lobe spanning Wernicke's area. It prevents the left auditory fibers from activating Wernicke's area and also those crossing the corpus callosum from activating the right auditory region. Bilateral temporal lesions have the same effect.

The neglect of these disconnection syndromes in the past shows how fragmentary has been our knowledge of the anatomy of the fiber systems of the brain, and how incomplete have been our methods of examination.

OTHER BEHAVIORAL DISORDERS ASSOCIATED WITH CEREBRAL DISEASE When one attempts to categorize all the patients with relatively acute or subacute disorders of mentation and behavior under the section headings above, there are still a considerable number that remain difficult to classify. They present themselves as an almost infinite variety of syndromes in which the following abnormalities of function may occur: reduced or increased levels of speech, thought, and action; disorientation as to time and place; idleness and lack of interest; loss of spontaneity and sense of humor; muteness and hypokinesia, resistiveness and negativism; hostility, lack of observance of social custom, use of abusive and vulgar language; inexplicable fright, euphoria, and lack of proper concern; complaint of visual distortion, of excess sensitivity to sounds; distortions of smell and taste; inability to find the names of objects, to follow a conversation, to think coherently; sexual indiscretion, lack of modesty, and other signs of disinhibition; seizures; disturbances of sleep. Obviously these many symptoms do not all have the same basic significance and the majority possess only relative localizing value. They may be associated with definite hemiparesis, hemihypesthesia, frank aphasia, or homonymous hemianopia, but even without these lateralizing signs they point to the existence of cerebral disease.

Syndromes comprising these elements may be observed in subacute inclusion body encephalitis, Behcet's meningoencephalitis, adult toxoplasmosis, infectious mononucleosis, acute or subacute demyelinative diseases (acute or subacute recurrent multiple sclerosis), granulomatous and other forms of angiitis, gliomatosis cerebri, carcinomatosis with encephalopathy of multifocal type, multiple tumor metastases, acute and subacute bacterial endocarditis, and thrombopenia with small-vessel thrombosis (Moschcowitz's disease). A fuller account of some of these cerebral symptoms will be found in descriptions of these diseases.

THE APPROACH TO THE CLINICAL PROBLEM OF DEMENTIA The physician presented with a patient suffering from dementia caused by local cerebral disease must adopt an examination technique designed to expose fully the intellectual defect. Abnormalities of posture, movement, sensation, and reflexes cannot be relied upon for the full demonstration of the neurologic deficit, for it must be remembered that the association areas of the brain may be severely damaged without demonstrable neurologic signs of this type.

Three categories of data are required for the recognition and differential diagnosis of dementing brain disease:

1 A reliable history of the illness
2 Findings on mental examination, i.e., so-called "mental status," as well as on the rest of the neurologic examination
3 Special laboratory procedures, lumbar puncture, x-rays of the skull, electroencephalogram, radioactive scanning of the brain, and sometimes pneumoencephalogram

The history should always be supplemented by information obtained from a person other than the patient, because, through lack of insight, the patient is often unaware of his illness; indeed, he may be ignorant even of his chief complaint. Special inquiry should be made about the patient's general behavior, capacity for work, personal habits, and such faculties as memory and judgment.

This performance of an examination of the mental status must be systematic. At a minimum it should include the following:

I Insight (patient's replies to questions about his chief symptoms): What is your difficulty? Are you ill? When did your illness begin?

II Orientation (knowledge of personal identity and present situation): What is your name? What is your occupation? Where do you live? Are you married?
Place: What is the name of the place where you are now? How did you get here? What floor is it on? Where is the bathroom? What are you doing now?
Time: What is the date today? What time of day is it? What meals have you had? When was the last holiday?

III Memory:
Remote: Tell me the names of your children and their birth dates. When were you married? What was your mother's maiden name? What was the name of your first school teacher? What job have you held?
Recent past: Tell me about your recent illness (compare with previous statements). What did you have for breakfast today? What is my name or the nurse's name? When did you see me for the first time? What tests were done yesterday? What were the headlines in the newspaper today? Give the patient a simple story, oral or written, and ask him to retell it after 3 to 5 min.
Immediate recall ("short-term memory"): Repeat these numbers after me (give series of 3,4,5,6,7,8 digits at speed of one per second). Now when I give a series of numbers, repeat them in reverse order.
Visual span: Show the patient a picture of several objects and then ask him to name what he has seen and to note any inaccuracies.

IV General information: Ask about names of presidents, well-known historic dates, the names of large rivers, of large cities, etc.

V Capacity for sustained mental activity:
Calculation: Test ability to add, subtract, multiply, and divide. Subtraction of serial 7s from 100 is a good test of calculation as well as of concentration.
Abstract thinking: See if the patient can detect similarities and differences between classes of objects, or explain a proverb or a fable.

VI General behavior: Attitudes, general bearing, stream of thought, attentiveness, mood, manner of dress, etc.

VII Special tests of localized cerebral functions: grasping, sucking, aphasia battery, praxis with both hands, cortical sensory function, drawing of clock face, map of United States or Europe, floor plan of house, etc.

In order to enlist the patient's full cooperation, the physician must prepare him for questions of this type. Otherwise, the first reaction will be one of embarrassment or anger because of the implication that his mind is not sound. It should be pointed out to the patient that some individuals are rather forgetful and that it is necessary to ask specific questions in order to form some impression about their degree of nervousness when being examined. Reassurance that these are not tests of intelligence or of sanity is helpful.

A more formal and reliable method of examining the mental capacity of adults is the Wechsler-Bellevue test. This can be given by a psychologist or by the physician if he has carefully read the instructions for administering and scoring the test. The *Mental Examiners' Handbook,* by F. L. Wells and J. Ruesch, published by the Psychological Corporation, is helpful to those not familiar with this type of examination. In the Wechsler-Bellevue test the discrepancy between the vocabulary, picture completion information, and object assembly tests as a group (these correlate well with premorbid intelligence and are relatively insensitive to dementing brain disease) and arithmetic, block design, digit span, and digit-symbol tests provide an index of deterioration.

Although the form of confusion or dementia does not indicate a particular disease, certain combinations of symptoms and neurologic signs are more or less characteristic and may aid in diagnosis. The mode of onset, the clinical course, the associated neurologic signs, and the accessory laboratory data constitute the basis of differential diagnosis. It must be admitted, however, that some of the rarer types of "degenerative" brain disease are at present recognized only by pathologic examination. The correct diagnosis of treatable forms of senile (over sixty years of age) or presenile (forty to sixty years) dementias, such as general paresis, subdural hematoma, brain tumor, bromide or other chronic drug intoxication, normal-pressure hydrocephalus, pellagra and other deficiency states, and hypothyroidism, is of greater practical importance than the diagnosis of the untreatable ones.

Management of the demented patient Dementia is a clinical state of the most serious nature, and usually it is worthwhile to admit the patient to the hospital for a period of observation. The physician then has an opportunity to see him several times in a new and fairly constant hospital environment, and certain special procedures such as x-rays of the skull, lumbar puncture, analysis of blood for drugs, basal metabolic rate, an electroencephalogram, and often a pneumoencephalogram can be carried out at this time. The management of the demented patient in the hospital may be relatively simple if he is quiet and cooperative. If the disorder of mental function is severe, a nurse, attendant, or member of the family must stay with him at all times. Provision must be made for adequate food and fluid intake and control of infection, using the same measures outlined for the delirious patient.

Once it is established that the patient has an untreatable dementing brain disease, a responsible member of the family should be apprised of the medical facts. The patient should be told that he has a nervous condition for which he is to be given rest and treatment. Nothing is accomplished by telling him more. The family should be given the prognosis, if the diagnosis is sufficiently certain for this to be done. If the dementia is slight and circumstances are suitable, the patient should remain at home, continuing activities of which he is capable. He should be spared responsibility and guarded against injury that might result from imprudent action. If he is still at work, plans for occupational retirement should be carried out. In more advanced stages of the disease mental and physical enfeeblement become pronounced and institutional care should be advised. Seizures should be treated symptomatically. Nerve tonics, vitamins, and hormones are of no value in checking the course of the illness or in regenerating decayed tissue. They may, however, offer some support to the patient and family. Sometimes stimulants in the form of dextroamphetamine, caffeine, and nicotinic acid cause transitory improvement in mental function. Undesirable restlessness, nocturnal wandering, belligerency, or anxiety may be reduced by some of the tranquilizing drugs (see Chap. 114).

REFERENCES

GASSEL M: Occipital lobe syndromes (excluding hemianopia), in *Handbook of Clinical Neurology,* vol. 2, eds PJ Vinken and GW Bruyn, Amsterdam: North Holland Publishing Company, 1969, p. 640

GESCHWIND N: The clinical syndromes of cortical connections, in *Modern Trends in Neurology,* vol. 5, ed D Williams, London: Butterworth, 1970, p. 29

LURIA AR: Frontal lobe syndromes, in *Handbook of Clinical Neurology,* vol. 2, eds PJ Vinken and GW Bruyn, Amsterdam: North Holland Publishing Company, 1969, p. 725

TALLAND GA: *Deranged Memory,* New York: Academic, 1965

VICTOR M: The amnesic syndrome and its anatomical basis. Can Med Assoc J 100:1115, 1969

section 4 | Alterations in circulatory and respiratory function

28
DYSPNEA

HARRY W. FRITTS, JR.
HENRY M. THOMAS, III

While resting quietly a normal person breathes with effortless ease. Breathing rhythm is leisurely and somewhat irregular; breathing frequency is usually below 16 breaths per minute; for a person of average size, the tidal volume is less than 600 ml. To generate this flow of air a very small amount of energy is expended. Indeed, Otis, Fenn, and Rahn have estimated that the calories needed for 24 hr of quiet breathing are fewer than those contained in a small bar of candy. Translated into more precise terms, this finding indicates that the respiratory muscles of a resting man utilize less than 2 percent of the total energy consumed by the body. It is, therefore, not surprising that quiet breathing is a largely subconscious process.

Even when exercise lifts breathing to the conscious level the normal man does not find the sensation unpleasant. He may complain of breathlessness as he approaches the point of exhaustion, but his discomfort is ameliorated by a feeling of exhilaration or accomplishment. If, however, the motion of his chest is impeded, his awareness of breathing becomes a sensation of distress. Such distress has been characterized by the word *dyspnea,* derived from the Greek roots *dys* (hard) and *pnoe* (breathing). Thus, in broad context *dyspnea* denotes an unpleasant awareness of breathing, ranging in intensity from mild discomfort to agony.

Although *dyspnea* has never been a precise term, its current meaning is ambiguous because the word is used in two different ways. On the one hand physicians remark, "The patient complained of dyspnea," while on the other they say, "The patient appeared dyspneic." In the first instance the physician substitutes the noun *dyspnea* for the words used by the patient to describe his symptoms; in the second the physician employs the adjective *dyspneic* to describe an observed abnormality in the breathing pattern of the patient. Though the choice of definitions is a matter of personal preference, ambiguity can be minimized by using *dyspnea* to denote the overall subject of uncomfortable breathing; by using the words of the patient to describe his symptoms; and by employing precise terms to characterize the breathing pattern, e.g., "a rapid rate with small tidal volumes." This approach has the advantage of separating signs from symptoms, an important distinction because the two are often poorly correlated. Some patients with seemingly normal ventilatory patterns complain bitterly of distress, while others with obviously abnormal frequencies and tidal volumes deny discomfort.

TYPES OF DISCOMFORT The thorax is capable of generating several disagreeable sensations which, to an extent, can be individually identified. There is, for example, the "tight" feeling associated with obstruction to airflow. There is also the sense of "smothering" produced by strapping a belt around the chest. A variant of "smothering" is the "bursting" sensation felt in the lower part of the thorax when one nears the breakpoint of a held breath. A still different sort of distress develops when a person breathes carbon dioxide, thereby raising his blood P_{CO_2}. Here, the discomfort characteristically has a diffuse quality, with typical descriptions being, "I feel awful," or "I have a fullness in my head and chest." A more specific "burning" sensation comes from irritation of the airways or from the cough the irritation produces. In view of these multiple types of discomfort, breathlessness may often represent a mixture of sensations, rather than a single one.

QUANTIFICATION Even though respiratory discomfort cannot be measured directly, a number of indices are available to predict when it will appear. All relate the minute volume of ventilation, *MV*, to the maximum voluntary ventilation, *MVV*, and all provide information about the fraction of the maximal ventilation actually being utilized. For instance, the breathing reserve, calculated as the difference between *MVV* and *MV*, represents the amount of the ventilatory capacity still available. This amount is customarily expressed as a percentage of the *MVV* by the following simple formula:

$$\% = \frac{MVV - MV}{MVV} \times 100$$

Although there is considerable individual variability, most people are asymptomatic when the calculated index is above 70 percent, and most are aware of their breathing when the index is below this level. Accordingly, an average normal man, having an *MVV* of 150 liters per min, would begin to feel discomfort only after his *MV* exceeded 50 liters per min, a rate of air movement adequate for heavy exercise. In contrast, a patient with moderately advanced emphysema, having an MVV of only 50 liters per min, might have distress when his MV reached 15 liters per min, a rate of air movement only slightly greater than that maintained at rest.

CONDITIONS ASSOCIATED WITH RESPIRATORY DISCOMFORT The foregoing considerations suggest that the relation between the actual ventilation and the maximal capacity to move air is one of the determinants of breathlessness. It therefore follows that stimuli which increase ventilation or disorders which reduce capacity will tend to make discomfort appear. Among stimuli known to be associated with increased ventilation are arterial hypoxemia, arterial hypercapnea, arterial acidemia, muscular exercise, fever, hypermetabolism, systemic hypotension, and an elevated pressure in the great veins and chambers of the right side of the heart. Among disorders known to reduce ventilatory capacity are weakened respiratory muscles, an abnormal chest wall, a low total lung volume, and an increased resistance to airflow. While all these factors are obvious sources of respiratory discomfort, other influences are less easily understood. For instance, normal man will experience distress if he breathes into an apparatus which forces him to maintain a small tidal volume; yet he can obtain relief by taking occasional deep breaths. Also, paralyzing the respiratory muscles with curare can lead to discomfort, even though the alveolar ventilation is adequately maintained by a mechanical respirator.

These observations have led to the view that uncomfortable breathing is related not only to the absolute values of ventilation and capacity, but to a variety of other influences. One such influence is any condition which augments the amount of energy required for a particular level of ventilation. Another is any factor which causes the patient to utilize either a frequency or a tidal volume which is not his normal one.

RELATION OF STIMULI TO DISCOMFORT The parts of the respiratory apparatus have been extensively studied, and their sensitivities to various stimuli have been well characterized. The respiratory center, a complex array of cells in the pons and medulla, is particularly sensitive to changes in carbon dioxide tension and hydrogen ion concentration in the blood and cerebrospinal fluid. The carotid and aortic chemoreceptors respond principally to the blood oxygen tension; other receptors in the aortic arch and carotid arteries are sensitive to blood pressure. These peripheral elements transmit impulses centrally through the glossopharyngeal and vagus nerves.

Information about the position and motion of the thorax and lungs travels centrally through several pathways. The intercostal nerves transmit signals from the muscles and joints of the chest wall, while the phrenic nerves subserve the same function for the diaphragm. In addition, vagal fibers carry impulses from airways and parenchymal receptors which sense the state of expansion of the lungs. These latter pathways, constituting the sensory arm of the Hering-Breuer reflex, provide a means of regulating the respiratory cycle, since inflation tends to limit inspiration and to initiate expiration. Though highly developed in animals, this reflex is somewhat weaker in normal man.

Despite this detailed knowledge of the physiology of the respiratory center and peripheral nerves, there is little understanding of the way breathlessness is perceived. Popular theories have suggested that the cortex somehow senses an overloaded respiratory center, fatigue of the respiratory muscles, excessive energy expenditures, or stimulation of stretch or irritant receptors in the upper airways, lower airways, or lungs. Campbell has postulated that sensory elements, particularly muscle spindles, play a central role in comparing the tension in the muscle to the degree of stretch. According to Campbell, respiratory discomfort can arise when the tension is inappropriately large for a particular muscle length. Though the exact role of this mechanism has not been determined, impulses from the respiratory muscles doubtless have importance in some forms of respiratory discomfort.

DIFFERENTIAL DIAGNOSIS The separation of an abnormal breathing pattern from respiratory symptoms is an important first step in the approach to the patient. At times, bizarre patterns may be unassociated with distress. One example is the *Kussmaul breathing* (Chap. 265) seen in diabetic acidosis. The patient's minute ventilation may be greatly increased, yet he will be unaware of this augmentation. Similarly, many patients with *Cheyne-Stokes respiration* (Chap. 233) are oblivious of the change in their breathing pattern. Quite often patients with anemia overventilate, particularly during exercise, but complain chiefly of weakness or tiredness. As a general rule, these diseases produce changes in other organ systems which overshadow the effect on respiration.

Those patients who have breathlessness as a principal symptom usually have one of the following conditions: (1) heart disease, (2) pulmonary emboli, (3) obstructive disease of the lung, (4) interstitial or alveolar disease of the lung, (5) disorder of the chest wall or respiratory muscles, or (6) anxiety neurosis. Fig. 28-1 is a flow chart showing how one might proceed with this differential diagnosis. As may be seen, it cannot always be made on the basis of history alone, or even on history and physical examination. Instead, one combines the information from these sources with data from a number of tests. It is important to emphasize that, arriving at a diagnosis is often a far more complicated procedure than the chart indicates; the latter provides an outline, in skeletal form, as to how the work-up of a patient with dyspnea may be approached. Since each condition listed in the chart is discussed in detail in Part Eight, Sec. Three, the following paragraphs stress only those points in the evaluation of the patient which will help distinguish one of the conditions from the other.

HEART DISEASE (see also Chap. 233) Deciding whether breathlessness originates from disease of the heart or of the lungs may present a problem. Cough, wheezing, rales, or nocturnal attacks of breathlessness may occur in either type of disease. The important clues to a cardiac origin come from associated symptoms and signs of cardiovascular dysfunction, including angina, cardiomegaly, hypertension, abnormal heart sounds, or murmurs signifying aortic or mitral valve disease. Also, electrocardiographic or x-ray evidence of left ventricular or left atrial abnormalities provides additional support for this diagnosis.

In congestive heart failure, tests of pulmonary func-

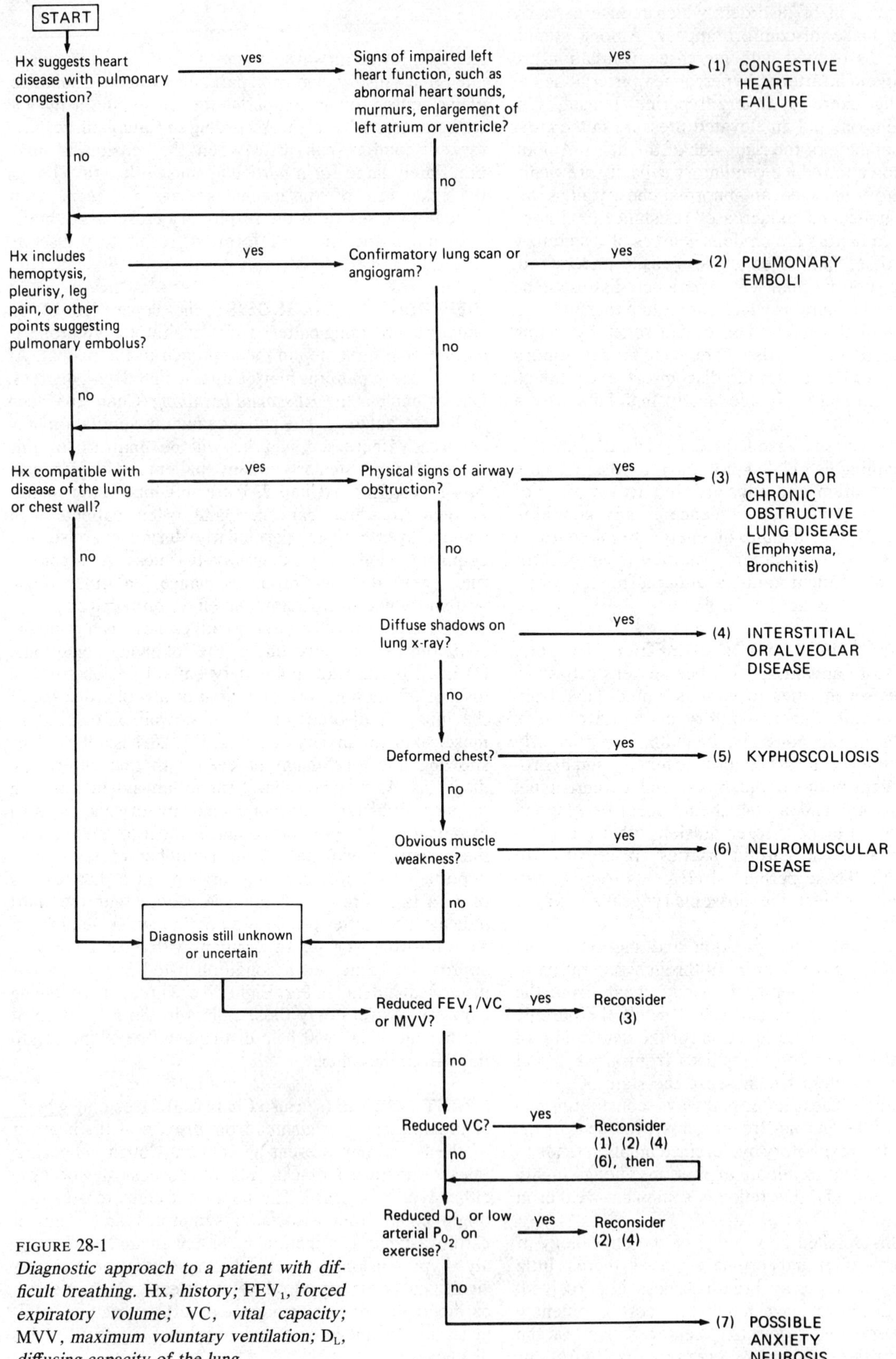

FIGURE 28-1
Diagnostic approach to a patient with difficult breathing. Hx, *history;* FEV$_1$, *forced expiratory volume;* VC, *vital capacity;* MVV, *maximum voluntary ventilation;* D$_L$, *diffusing capacity of the lung.*

tion usually show some reduction in the vital capacity and the ratio of the 1-sec forced expiratory volume to the vital capacity (FEV_1/VC), as well as modest changes in the mechanical properties of the lung. Except in the presence of intracardiac shunts or of obvious pulmonary edema, the arterial saturation in nonpulmonary heart disease is usually above 90 percent, and the carbon dioxide tension is low.

PULMONARY EMBOLI (see also Chap. 256) This is one of the most difficult conditions to recognize. Right-sided heart failure in the absence of signs of intrinsic lung disease should suggest the possibility of multiple emboli, but often the diagnosis is uncertain without angiography or lung scanning. While the arterial tension of oxygen may be subnormal, the carbon dioxide tension is seldom elevated, an important point of distinction between cor pulmonale secondary to emboli and that caused by obstructive pulmonary disease.

OBSTRUCTIVE DISEASE OF THE LUNG (see Chap. 252) Typical diseases causing acute airway obstruction are asthma, bronchiolitis, and croup. In each, a careful history and a detailed physical examination will almost always establish the diagnosis. In contrast, chronic airway obstruction may be more difficult to recognize because in some patients the signs and symptoms are nonspecific or suggest heart disease. Usually, the patient gives a history of having had shortness of breath for many months. At first breathlessness occurs only with heavy exercise; later with moderate activity; and eventually at rest. Frequently, breathlessness is associated with a chronic cough, productive of variable amounts of sputum. Intercurrent respiratory infections augment the cough, the production of sputum, and the breathlessness. The patient may complain of becoming short of breath at night, and he may say that relief comes from bringing up large volumes of secretions. While such an episode can usually be distinguished from the orthopnea or the paroxysmal nocturnal dyspnea that occurs with heart failure, distinction in some instances is impossible. Finally, some patients give a history of wheezing.

The physical examination is especially important. Signs associated with airway obstruction include prolongation of expiration, utilization of the muscles of the neck to lift the anterior part of the upper thorax, retraction of the soft tissues of the thorax during inspiration, and retraction of the lower rib margins as inspiration begins (Hoover's sign). Often better seen than felt, retraction of the ribs usually denotes either a low position of the diaphragm or an abnormally negative intrapleural pressure, both characteristic of obstructive disease. Other signs include expiratory wheezes and, if the disease is advanced, evidence of right-sided heart failure. One of the most useful tests is to have the patient make a forceful expiration while the physician listens with a stethoscope placed over the trachea or upper part of the sternum. Wheezes which were not apparent during quiet breathing may be heard, while expiratory flow continuing beyond 4 or 5 sec will indicate obstruction. Whereas the vital capacity may be low or normal, the FEV_1/VC and MVV are invariably reduced.

Finally, a high hematocrit may reflect chronic arterial hypoxemia, and a high bicarbonate, a chronically elevated tension of carbon dioxide. Whether or not these changes are present, measurement of arterial blood gases will give useful information about gas exchange.

INTERSTITIAL OR ALVEOLAR DISEASE OF THE LUNG (see also Chap. 254) This category embraces a large number of diseases, ranging from acute pneumonia to chronic disorders such as tuberculosis, sarcoid, carcinoma, pneumoconiosis, and idiopathic fibrosis of the lung. The history varies with the cause, and the signs elicited by physicial examination depend on the nature and state of the disease. In almost all these disorders chest roentgenograms will be abnormal. The patients with chronic diseases characteristically have higher than normal ventilations at rest, and even more abnormal values during exercise.

Pulmonary function tests show a reduced vital capacity and an increased stiffness of the lung. Although the oxygen saturation may be low at rest and fall farther with exercise, the carbon dioxide tension is seldom elevated. Indeed, until the late stages of these diseases, the carbon dioxide tension is usually low.

DISEASES OF THE CHEST WALL OR RESPIRATORY MUSCLES (see Chap. 255) Three typical disorders of the bony thorax causing breathlessness are fractured ribs, kyphoscoliosis, and arthritis of the spine. All interfere with the motion of the thorax and consequently impair ventilation. In each instance the history, physical examination, and standard roentgenograms will make the diagnosis.

By way of contrast, evaluating weakness of the respiratory muscles is more difficult unless the weakness is marked. In the latter instance there is usually an obvious diagnosis, such as poliomyelitis or injury to the spinal cord. A reduced vital capacity in a patient whose heart and lungs appear normal may signal neuromuscular disease of milder degree.

ANXIETY NEUROSIS Several clues may suggest that breathlessness has a psychogenic origin. The most important is the patient's tendency to have a larger than normal resting ventilation and periodically to inspire deeply, then expire audibly. He feels as if he were smothering. The breathing pattern is frequently strange, with irregularities in both frequency and tidal volume. At other times the pattern is one of such maintained hyperventilation that the patient complains of tingling in the extremities or even a sensation of faintness. Watching the patient breathe during sleep may give valuable information. If the abnormal breathing pattern disappears, psychogenic causes should be suspected. Similarly, observing the patient when he does not know he is being watched is helpful, because the respiratory pattern may be completely different when he is alone. Having the patient hyperventilate will sometimes reproduce the symptoms. Another clue comes from obvious discrepancies between symptoms, physical signs, and results of pulmonary function tests.

CONCLUSIONS The intimate mechanisms of respiratory distress are poorly understood, even though a large number of conditions associated with breathlessness are well characterized. The history, physical examination, roentgenograms, standard laboratory procedures, and, where indicated, special tests of respiratory and cardiac function will usually lead to the diagnosis. However, there will remain a group of patients with no measurable abnormalities who appear to have genuine distress. The condition of such persons should be carefully followed, with the expectation that if their symptoms have an organic basis, concrete signs will appear.

REFERENCES

CAMPBELL EJM; COMROE J; VON EULER C; SEARS TA: in *Breathlessness,* Oxford: Blackwell, 1966

GAENSLER EA: *Dyspnea: diagnostic and therapeutic implications, DM, May, 1961*

MERTON PA; GODFREY S, CAMPBELL EJM; NOBLE MIM et al; HOWELL JBL; COTES JE et al; DORNHORST AC: in *Breathing: Hering-Breuer Centenary Symposium,* Ciba Foundation ed R Porter, London: Churchill, 1970

RICHARDS DW, JR: The nature of cardiac and pulmonary dyspnea. Circulation 7:15, 1953

WRIGHT GW, BRANSCOMB, BV: The origin of the sensations of dyspnea. Trans Clin Climatol Assoc 66:116, 1954

29 CYANOSIS, HYPOXIA, AND POLYCYTHEMIA

EUGENE BRAUNWALD
RICHARD L. KAHLER
M. M. WINTROBE

CYANOSIS

Cyanosis refers to a bluish color of the skin and mucous membranes resulting from an increased amount of reduced hemoglobin, or of hemoglobin derivatives, in the small blood vessels of those areas. It is usually most marked in the lips, nail beds, ears, and malar eminences. In the last region true cyanosis cannot easily be distinguished from the ruddy color commonly seen in robust elderly subjects. Furthermore, the "red cyanosis" of polycythemia vera (Chap. 311) must be distinguished from the true cyanosis discussed here. A cherry-colored flush, rather than cyanosis, is caused by carboxyhemoglobin (Chap. 109). In *argyria,* the skin is bluish because of the deposition of silver salts, and the discoloration persists despite pressure, unlike cyanotic skin which blanches. The degree of cyanosis is modified by the quality of cutaneous pigment and the color of the blood plasma, as well as by the state of the cutaneous capillaries. The thickness of the skin is particularly important; the thin skin of newborn infants and the mucous membranes of patients of all ages often appear cyanotic. The accurate clinical detection of the presence and degree of cyanosis is difficult, as proved by oximetric studies. Some observers can reliably detect central cyanosis when the arterial saturation has fallen to 85 percent; others may not detect it until the saturation has reached 75 percent.

The increase in the amount of reduced hemoglobin in the cutaneous vessels, which produces cyanosis, may be brought about either by an increase in the quantity of venous blood in the skin as the result of dilatation of the venules and venous ends of the capillaries, or by a decrease in the oxygen saturation in the capillary blood. In general, cyanosis becomes apparent when the mean capillary concentration of reduced hemoglobin exceeds 5 g per 100 ml. It is the absolute rather than the relative amount of reduced hemoglobin which is important in producing cyanosis. Thus, in a patient with severe anemia the relative amount of reduced hemoglobin in the venous blood may be very large when considered in relation to the total amount of hemoglobin. However, since the latter is markedly lowered, the absolute amount of reduced hemoglobin may still be small, and therefore patients with severe anemia and marked arterial desaturation do not display cyanosis. Conversely, the higher the total hemoglobin content, the greater the tendency toward cyanosis; thus, patients with marked polycythemia tend to be cyanotic at higher levels of arterial oxygen saturation than patients with normal hematocrit values. Likewise, local passive congestion, which causes an increase in the total amount of reduced hemoglobin in the vessels in a given area, may cause cyanosis even though the average percentage saturation is not altered. Cyanosis also is observed when nonfunctional hemoglobin is present in the blood; as little as 1.5 g per 100 ml methemoglobin or 0.5 g sulfhemoglobin is sufficient to produce cyanosis (Chap. 312).

True cyanosis may be subdivided into *central* and *peripheral* categories. In the *central* type, there is arterial blood unsaturation or an abnormal hemoglobin derivative, and the mucous membranes and skin are both affected. *Peripheral* cyanosis is due to a slowing of blood flow to an area and abnormally great extraction of oxygen from normally saturated arterial blood. It results from vasoconstriction and diminished peripheral blood flow, such as occurs in cold exposure, shock, congestive failure, and peripheral vascular disease. Often, in these conditions, the mucous membranes of the oral cavity or those beneath the tongue may be spared. Clinical differentiation between central and peripheral cyanosis may not always be simple, and in conditions such as cardiogenic shock with pulmonary edema there may be a mixture of both types.

Differential diagnosis

CENTRAL CYANOSIS Decreased arterial oxygen saturation results from a marked reduction in the oxygen tension in the arterial blood. This may be brought about by a decline in the tension of oxygen in the inspired air without sufficient compensatory alveolar hyperventilation to maintain alveolar oxygen tension. Cyanosis does not occur in a significant degree in an ascent to an altitude of 8,000 ft but is marked in a further ascent to 16,000 ft. The reason for this becomes clear on studying the S shape of the oxygen dissociation curve (Fig. 29-1). At 8,000 ft

TABLE 29-1
Causes of cyanosis

I Central cyanosis
- *A* Decreased arterial oxygen saturation
  - *1* Decreased atmospheric pressure—high altitude
  - *2* Impaired pulmonary function
    - *a* Alveolar hypoventilation
    - *b* Uneven relationships between pulmonary ventilation and perfusion
    - *c* Impaired oxygen diffusion
  - *3* Anatomic shunts
    - *a* Certain types of congenital heart disease
    - *b* Pulmonary arteriovenous fistulas
    - *c* Multiple small intrapulmonary shunts
- *B* Hemoglobin abnormalities
  - *1* Methemoglobinemia—hereditary, acquired
  - *2* Sulfhemoglobinemia—acquired
  - *3* Carboxyhemoglobinemia (not true cyanosis)

II Peripheral cyanosis
- *A* Reduced cardiac output
- *B* Cold exposure
- *C* Redistribution of blood flow from extremities
- *D* Arterial obstruction
- *E* Venous obstruction

the tension of oxygen in the inspired air is about 120 mm Hg, the alveolar tension is approximately 80 mm Hg, and the hemoglobin is nearly completely saturated. However, at 16,000 ft the oxygen tensions in atmospheric air and alveolar air are about 85 and 50 mm Hg, respectively, and the oxygen dissociation curve shows that the arterial blood is only about 75 percent saturated. This leaves 25 percent of the hemoglobin in the reduced form, an amount likely to be associated with cyanosis in the absence of anemia.

Seriously *impaired pulmonary function*, through alveolar hypoventilation, perfusion of unventilated or poorly ventilated areas of the lung, or impaired oxygen diffusion, is a common cause of central cyanosis. This may occur acutely, as in extensive pneumonia or in pulmonary edema, or with chronic pulmonary diseases (e.g., emphysema). In the last situation clubbing of the fingers and polycythemia are generally present. However, in many types of chronic pulmonary disease with fibrosis and obliteration of the capillary vascular bed, cyanosis does not occur because there is relatively little perfusion of underventilated areas.

Another cause of decreased arterial oxygen saturation is shunting of systemic venous blood into the arterial circuit. Certain types of congenital heart disease are associated with cyanosis (Chap 237). Since blood normally flows from a high- to a low-pressure region, in order for a cardiac defect to result in a right-to-left shunt it must ordinarily be combined with an obstructive lesion distal to the defect or with elevated pulmonary vascular resistance. The commonest congenital cardiac lesion associated with cyanosis is the combination of ventricular septal defect and pulmonary outflow tract obstruction (tetralogy of Fallot). The more severe the obstruction, the greater the degree of right-to-left shunting and resultant cyanosis. The mechanisms for the elevated pulmonary vascular resistance which may produce cyanosis in the presence of intra- and extracardiac communications without pulmonic stenosis are discussed elsewhere (Chap. 237). In patients with patent ductus arteriosus, pulmonary hypertension, and right-to-left shunt, differential cyanosis results; i.e., cyanosis occurs in the lower extremities but not in the upper extremities.

Pulmonary arteriovenous fistulas may be congenital or acquired, solitary or multiple, microscopic or massive. The degree of cyanosis produced by these fistulas depends upon their size and number. They occur with some frequency in hereditary hemorrhagic telangiectasia (Chap. 315). Arterial oxygen unsaturation also occurs in some patients with cirrhosis, although it is uncommon in this condition. A number of factors may explain this observation; pulmonary arteriovenous fistulas or portal vein–pulmonary vein anastomoses have been demonstrated in some patients.

In patients with cardiac or pulmonary right-to-left shunts, the presence and severity of cyanosis depend on the size of the shunt relative to the systemic flow as well as on the oxyhemoglobin saturation of the venous blood. In patients with central cyanosis due to arterial oxygen unsaturation, the severity of cyanosis increases with exercise. With increased extraction of oxygen from the blood by the exercising muscles, the venous blood returning to the right side of the heart is more unsaturated than at rest, and shunting of this blood or its passage through lungs incapable of normal oxygenation intensifies the cyanosis. Also, since the systemic vascular resistance normally decreases with exercise, passage of right ventricular blood into the systemic circuit is made easier by exercise in patients with congenital heart disease and communications between the two sides of the heart. Secondary polycythemia occurs frequently in patients with arterial unsaturation and contributes to the cyanosis.

Arterial blood saturation is ascertained by subjecting an arterial blood sample to Van Slyke analysis for determining oxygen content and capacity or by directly determining the hemoglobin saturation by oximetric or spectrophotometric techniques.

Cyanosis is produced by small amounts of circulating methemoglobin and by even smaller amounts of sulfhemoglobin (Chap. 312). Although they are uncommon causes of cyanosis, these abnormal hemoglobin pigments should be sought by spectroscopic analysis when cyanosis is not readily explained by malfunction of the circulatory or respiratory systems. Generally, clubbing does not occur with them.

PERIPHERAL CYANOSIS Probably the most common cause of peripheral cyanosis is generalized vasoconstriction resulting from exposure to cold air or water. This is clearly a normal response to the stimulus and is transient. When the cardiac output is low, as in severe congestive heart failure or shock, cutaneous vasoconstriction occurs as a compensatory mechanism, so that blood is diverted to more vital areas [kidneys, central nervous system, heart (Chap. 233)], and intense cyanosis associated with cool extremities may result. Even though the arterial blood is normally saturated, the reduced volume flow through the skin and the reduced oxygen tension at the venous end of the capillary result in cyanosis.

Acute arterial obstruction to an extremity generally results in pallor and coldness, but there may be associated slight cyanosis. If there is venous obstruction, the extremity is usually congested and markedly cyanotic, and there is true stagnation of blood flow. Venous hypertension, which may be local (as in thrombophlebitis) or generalized (as in tricuspid valve disease or constrictive pericarditis), dilates the subpapillary venous plexuses and intensifies cyanosis. Stasis of a lesser degree resulting from increased blood viscosity probably contributes to the cyanosis in some patients with polycythemia vera, and intensifies the cyanosis in patients with secondary polycythemia. Peripheral cyanosis occurs characteristically in peripheral vascular disease.

Certain features are important in arriving at the proper cause of cyanosis.

1 The history, particularly the duration (cyanosis present since birth is usually due to congenital heart disease); possible exposure to drugs or chemicals which may produce abnormal types of hemoglobin.
2 Clinical differentiation of central as opposed to peripheral cyanosis. Objective evidence by physical or radiographic examination of disorders of the respiratory or cardiovascular systems. Massage or gentle warming of a cyanotic extremity will increase peripheral blood flow and abolish peripheral but not central cyanosis.
3 The presence or absence of clubbing of the fingers. Clubbing without cyanosis is frequent in patients with subacute bacterial endocarditis and in association with ulcerative colitis, it may occasionally occur in healthy persons, and in some instances it may be occupational, e.g., in jack-hammer operators. Slight cyanosis of the lips and cheeks, without clubbing of the fingers, is common in patients with well-compensated mitral stenosis and is probably due to minimal arterial hypoxia resulting from fibrotic changes in the lungs secondary to long-standing congestion combined with reduction of cardiac output. The combination of cyanosis and clubbing is frequent in many patients with certain types of congenital cardiac disease and is seen occasionally in persons with pulmonary disease such as lung abscess or pulmonary arteriovenous shunts. On the other hand, peripheral cyanosis or acutely developing central cyanosis is not associated with clubbed fingers.
4 Determination of arterial blood oxygen tension or oxygen saturation. Spectroscopic and other examinations of the blood for abnormal types of hemoglobin.

HYPOXIA

The fundamental purpose of the cardiorespiratory system is to deliver oxygen (and substrates) to the cells and to remove carbon dioxide (and other metabolic products) from them. Proper maintenance of this function depends on intact cardiovascular and respiratory systems and a supply of inspired gas containing adequate oxygen. Changes in oxygen and in carbon dioxide tension as well as changes in the intraerythrocytic concentration of certain *organic phosphate compounds,* especially, 2,3-diphosphoglyceric acid (2,3-DPG), cause shifts in the oxygen dissociation curve. High concentrations of 2,3-DPG have been found in the red blood cells of most mammals, including man; the levels change in various clinical and environmental conditions. Increased concentrations shift the oxyhemoglobin dissociation curve to the right, thus decreasing the affinity of hemoglobin for oxygen and releasing a greater percentage of oxygen to the tissues. Decreased concentrations of 2,3-DPG lead to a diminished delivery of oxygen because of the greater affinity of hemoglobin for oxygen (Fig. 29-1). Intraerythrocytic concentration of 2,3-DPG increases in chronic anemia, exposure to high altitude, low-output cardiac failure, cyanotic congenital heart disease, and chronic obstructive pulmonary disease; it is one of the important adaptive mechanisms for avoiding tissue hypoxia in these conditions.

When hypoxia occurs as the result of a decline in oxygen tension in the inspired air, respiration is stimulated, alveolar ventilation increases, and the carbon dioxide tension in the alveoli and in the arterial blood falls. This respiratory alkalosis causes a leftward shift in the oxygen dissociation curve, i.e., an increased affinity of hemoglobin for oxygen (Fig. 29-1), and enables a given alveolar oxygen tension to cause a greater degree of oxygen uptake by the hemoglobin (Bohr's effect). Thus, at an alveolar oxygen tension of 55 mm Hg, a rise in pH from 7.44 to 7.64 will cause the arterial saturation to increase from 80 to nearly 90 percent.

However, when hypoxia results from interference with the passage of air into the lungs or from the perfusion of poorly ventilated alveoli, carbon dioxide tension usually remains normal or even rises; and the oxygen dissociation curve tends to remain unchanged or move to the right. Under these conditions the percentage saturation of the hemoglobin in the arterial blood at a given level of alveolar oxygen tension does not rise and may even fall. Thus arterial hypoxia and cyanosis are likely to be more marked in proportion to the degree of depression of alveolar oxygen tension when such depres-

TABLE 29-2
Causes of hypoxia

I Decreased oxygen delivery to the tissues
- *A* Generalized hypoxia
  - *1* Arterial hypoxia
    - *a* Low atmospheric oxygen tension
    - *b* Diminished oxygenation in the lungs
    - *c* Systemic venous-to-arterial shunts
  - *2* Anemic hypoxia
    - *a* Diminished hemoglobin concentration
    - *b* Altered hemoglobin
  - *3* Circulatory hypoxia (ischemia, stagnation)
- *B* Specific organ hypoxia
  - *1* Reflex
  - *2* Organic

II Increased oxygen requirements
- *A* Thyrotoxicosis
- *B* Exercise

III Improper oxygen utilization

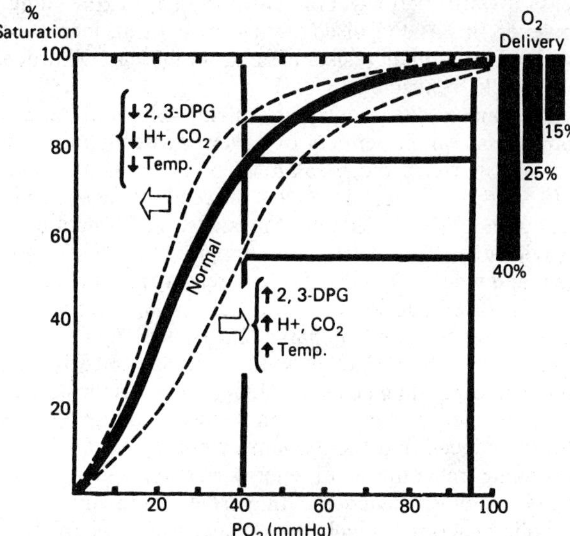

FIGURE 29-1
The oxyhemoglobin dissociation curve and factors which affect it. The percentage saturation of hemoglobin is shown on the ordinate, and the P_{O_2} *in millimeters of mercury is shown on the abscissa. Decreases of 2,3-diphosphoglyceric acid (2,3-DPG) concentration,* P_{CO_2}*, or temperature, or increased pH cause a leftward shift in the curve. Conversely, a rightward shift of the curve results from increased 2,3-DPG concentration, temperature, or* P_{CO_2}*, or a decreased pH. Adjustments in blood pH or body temperature have an immediate effect on the affinity of hemoglobin for oxygen, while shifts mediated through 2,3-DPG changes take several hours to occur. A rightward shift in the curve (decreased affinity of hemoglobin for oxygen) results in the release of a greater percentage of oxygen to the tissues.*

During vigorous muscular effort the blood acidity and temperature increase, and an increase in 2,3-DPG concentration has been demonstrated This causes the dissociation curve to shift rightward and raises the tissue oxygen tension for any given degree of saturation of the hemoglobin, thus making oxygen more available to the exercising muscles. On the other hand, acute exposure to high altitude, with its respiratory alkalosis and rise in pH (opposing the effects of increased 2,3-DPG synthesis), results in a leftward shift of the dissociation curve. (From DR Harkness; by permission of Year Book Medical Publishers)

sion results from pulmonary disease than when the depression occurs as the result of a decline in the partial pressure of oxygen in the inspired air.

The respiratory mechanisms may be considerably impaired without the development of a significant degree of arterial hypoxia. This is because the properties of hemoglobin are such that its dissociation curve is practically flat above 100 mm Hg of oxygen tension, and almost flat to about 80 mm Hg. When the tension of oxygen in the alveoli falls below the point at which the slope of the dissociation curve tends to become more nearly vertical, a rapid decline in the amount of oxygen in the arterial blood occurs.

ANEMIC HYPOXIA This includes various states, one of which is associated with anemia and others in which there is a partial conversion to non-oxygen-carrying derivative pigments (Chap. 312). Any decrease in hemoglobin concentration is attended by a corresponding decline in the oxygen-carrying power. Under such conditions the P_{O_2} in the arterial blood remains normal, but the absolute amount of oxygen transported per unit volume of blood is diminished. As the anemic blood passes through the capillaries, and the usual amount of oxygen is removed from it, the P_{O_2} in the venous blood declines to a greater degree than would normally be the case.

Carbon monoxide intoxication (Chap. 109) This condition is accompanied by the equivalent of anemic hypoxia in that the hemoglobin which is combined with the carbon monoxide (carboxyhemoglobin) is unavailable for oxygen transport. But, in addition to this, the presence of carboxyhemoglobin increases the affinity of normal hemoglobin for oxygen at low levels of P_{O_2} (i.e., shifts the lower portion of the dissociation curve of hemoglobin to the left), so that the oxygen can be unloaded only at lower tensions. By such formation of carboxyhemoglobin a given degree of reduction in oxygen-carrying power produces a far greater degree of tissue hypoxia than the equivalent reduction in hemoglobin due to simple anemia.

CIRCULATORY HYPOXIA As in anemic hypoxia, arterial P_{O_2} is normal but venous and tissue P_{O_2} are reduced as a consequence of reduced tissue perfusion in the face of normal tissue oxygen consumption. For this reason the term *stagnant hypoxia* may be used for this condition. Generalized circulatory hypoxia occurs in heart failure, as discussed in Chap. 233.

SPECIFIC ORGAN HYPOXIA Decreased circulation to a specific organ resulting in localized stagnant hypoxia may be due to organic arterial or venous obstruction or may occur as a reflex phenomenon. The latter may occur when vasoconstriction of, for instance, the limbs results from an attempt to maintain adequate perfusion to more vital organs, as in severe congestive heart failure. When organic arterial obliterative disease develops, ischemic hypoxia results, with accompanying pallor. Localized hypoxia may also result from venous obstruction which results in congestion. Edema, which increases the distance through which oxygen diffuses before it reaches the cells, can also cause localized hypoxia.

INCREASED OXYGEN REQUIREMENTS Even if oxygen diffusion into blood perfusing the pulmonary capillary bed is unhampered and the hemoglobin is qualitatively and quantitatively normal, the P_{O_2} in venous blood (hence, capillary and tissue P_{O_2}) may be reduced if the oxygen consumption of the tissues is elevated without a corresponding increase in volume flow per unit of time. Such a situation may be encountered in febrile states and in thyrotoxicosis. Under such conditions the circulation may be considered deficient relative to the metabolic requirements. Thus, this type of metabolic hypoxia is comparable to circulatory hypoxia, in that in both conditions the volume flow of blood is decreased relative to the needs of the tissues; the difference is that in one case the primary defect is the volume flow of blood and in the other the primary defect is an increased oxygen need by the tissues.

Ordinarily, the clinical picture of patients with hypoxia due to an elevated basal metabolic rate is quite different from that in other types of hypoxia; the skin is warm and flushed, owing to increased cutaneous blood flow which dissipates the excessive heat produced, and cyanosis is absent in these patients.

Exercise is a classic example of increased tissue oxygen requirements. The increased demands are normally met by several mechanisms: (1) by increasing the cardiac output and thus oxygen delivery to the tissues; (2) by preferentially directing the blood to the exercising muscles and away from resting muscles (by changing vascular resistances in various circulatory beds, in some areas by direct effects, in others reflexly); (3) by increasing oxygen extraction from the delivered blood and widening the arteriovenous oxygen differences. If the capacity of these mechanisms is exceeded, then hypoxia, especially of the exercising muscles, will result.

IMPROPER OXYGEN UTILIZATION The administration of cyanide (Chap. 109) and several other similarly acting poisons leads to a paradoxic state in which the tissues are unable to utilize oxygen and as a consequence the venous blood tends to have a high oxygen tension. This condition has been termed *histotoxic hypoxia.* Cyanide produces cellular hypoxia by paralyzing the electron-transfer function of cytochrome oxidase so that it cannot pass electrons to oxygen, whereas diphtheria toxin is believed to inhibit the synthesis of one of the cytochromes and thus interfere with oxygen consumption and energy production by the cells involved.

Effects of hypoxia

When hypoxia is general, all parts of the body may suffer some impairment of function, but those parts which are most sensitive to the effects of hypoxia give rise to symptoms which dominate the clinical picture. The *changes in the central nervous system* are especially important, and here the higher centers are most sensitive. Acute hypoxia, therefore, produces impaired judgment, motor incoordination, and a clinical picture closely resembling that of acute alcoholism. When hypoxia is long-standing, the symptoms consist of fatigue, drowsiness, apathy, inattentiveness, delayed reaction time, severe fatigue, and reduced work capacity. As hypoxia becomes more severe, the centers of the brainstem are affected, and death usually results from respiratory failure. With reduction of arterial oxygen tension, cerebrovascular resistance decreases and cerebral blood flow increases, which tends to minimize the cerebral hypoxia. On the other hand when the reduction of arterial P_{O_2} is accompanied by hyperventilation and diminution of P_{CO_2}, cerebrovascular resistance rises, blood flow falls, and hypoxia is enhanced. Compared with the brain, the phylogenetically older spinal cord and peripheral nerves are relatively insensitive to hypoxia. Hypoxia also causes pulmonary arterial constriction, which serves the useful function of shunting blood away from poorly ventilated areas toward better-ventilated portions of the lung. However, it has the disadvantage of causing increased pulmonary vascular resistance and an increased burden on the right ventricle.

A complex disturbance of cellular functions results from the metabolic effects of severe acute hypoxia. In liver and muscles the breakdown of the primary foodstuff, carbohydrate, normally proceeds anaerobically (i.e., without oxidation) to the stage of formation of pyruvic acid. The breakdown of pyruvate requires oxygen, and when this is deficient, increasing proportions of pyruvate are reduced to lactic acid, which cannot be further broken down (Chap. 72). Hence, there is an increase in the blood lactate, with decrease in bicarbonate and a corresponding acidosis. Under these circumstances the total energy obtained from foodstuff breakdown is greatly reduced and the amount of energy available for continuing resynthesis of energy-rich phosphate compounds becomes inadequate. Impairment of the myriad of anabolic reactions which take place in tissues follows. Since the total energy obtained from foodstuff breakdown is greatly reduced under these circumstances, the amount of energy available for continuing resynthesis of energy-rich phosphate compounds becomes inadequate. As the breakdown of the latter substances is the immediate source of energy driving the myriad of anabolic reactions which take place in tissues, such deficiency of energy-rich phosphate compounds produces a complex disturbance of cellular function.

Most of the useful respiratory response to hypoxia originates in special chemosensitive cells in the carotid and aortic bodies, although the respiratory center is also stimulated directly by oxygen lack. The peripheral chemoreceptors are extremely rugged and continue to function after other tissues have been damaged by hypoxemia. The chemoreceptors are stimulated by a reduction in their oxygen supply below their needs either by lowered arterial P_{O_2} or by lowered blood flow to them. If respiration is stimulated by hypoxia, the resulting increase in ventilation, with loss of carbon dioxide, tends to make the blood more alkaline. On the other hand, the diffusion of additional quantities of lactic acid from the tissues into the blood tends to make the blood more acid. In either case the total amount of bicarbonate, and hence the carbon dioxide–combining power, tends to be diminished. With mild hypoxia there is likely to be respiratory alkalosis; severe hypoxia is attended by metabolic acidosis.

The heart, although relatively sensitive to hypoxia as compared with most of the structures of the body, is less sensitive than the nervous system. Consequently, in the absence of severe coronary artery disease, serious manifestations of cardiac impairment do not commonly occur when there is generalized hypoxia, and the manifestations arising in the nervous system dominate the picture. Diminished oxygen tension in any tissue results in local vasodilatation, and in generalized hypoxia diffuse vasodilatation results in an elevation of total cardiac output. In patients with preexisting heart disease, particularly coronary artery disease, the combination of hypoxia and the requirements of the peripheral tissues for an increase of cardiac output may precipitate congestive heart failure. Prolonged or severe hypoxia may also impair hepatic and renal function.

One of the important mechanisms of compensation for prolonged hypoxia is an increase in the amount of hemoglobin in the blood. This is due not to direct stimulation of the bone marrow but to the effect of an erythropoiesis-stimulating factor (erythropoietin) which originates primarily in the kidneys. Assayable levels of erythropoietin are increased by hypoxia, and its production has been found to be regulated by the balance between tissue oxygen supply and demand.

POLYCYTHEMIA

The term *polycythemia* signifies an increase above the normal in the number of red corpuscles in the circulating blood. This increase is usually, though not always, accompanied by a corresponding increase in the quantity of hemoglobin and in the volume of packed red corpuscles. The increase may or may not be associated with an increase in the total quantity of red blood cells in the body. It is important to distinguish between *absolute* polycythemia (an increase in the total red corpuscle mass) and *relative* polycythemia, which occurs when, through loss of blood plasma, the concentration of the red corpuscles becomes greater than normal in the circulating blood. This may be the consequence of abnormally lowered fluid intake or of marked loss of body fluids, such as occurs in persistent vomiting, severe diarrhea, copious sweating, or acidosis (Chap. 265). Loss of electrolytes from the extracellular compartment, when not accompanied by corresponding loss of water, leads to a decline of osmolar concentration in the extracellular fluid. The resulting shift of water into cells, including red blood cells, may produce relative polycythemia, sometimes of high grade. Loss of plasma into the interstitial fluid may also result in relative polycythemia.

Because the term polycythemia is used loosely to refer to all varieties of increase in the number of red corpuscles, the terms *erythrocytosis* and *erythremia* are preferred in referring to two forms of absolute polycythemia. Erythrocytosis denotes absolute polycythemia which occurs in response to some known stimulus (secondary polycythemia); erythremia (polycythemia rubra vera) refers to the disease of unknown etiology, which is discussed elsewhere (Chap. 311).

Erythrocytosis develops as a consequence of a variety of factors and represents a physiologic response to conditions of hypoxia. Sojourn at high altitudes leads to defective saturation of arterial blood with oxygen and stimulates the production of more red corpuscles. The oxygen saturation, rather than oxygen tension, appears to be the more important determinant of the erythropoietic response to chronic hypoxia (Fig. 29-2). Immediately on ascent to a high altitude, symptoms such as fatigue, dizziness, headache, nausea, vomiting, ringing in the ears, and prostration may appear. In most persons adaptation soon occurs, with the development of polycythemia and other compensatory adjustments. However, a disorder may set in insidiously after several years of continued residence at high altitudes, leading to the development of a condition known as *chronic mountain sickness* or *seroche* (Monge's disease). Two forms have been described, an *emphysematous type,* in which dyspnea is prominent and bronchitis is common; and an *erythremic type,* in which prominent manifestations are a florid color

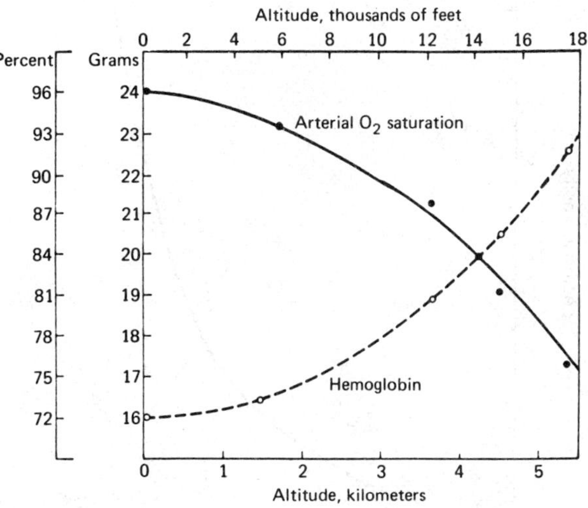

FIGURE 29-2
Relationship between mean arterial oxygen saturation (percent) and the mean hemoglobin content (g per 100 ml) in healthy male residents at various altitudes. (From Hurtado et al, by permission of Archives of Internal Medicine)

which turns to cyanosis on mild exertion, mental torpor, fatigue, and headache. Those affected are usually in the fourth to sixth decades. Return to sea level promptly relieves the symptoms. *Brisket disease of cattle,* a disorder of young calves grazing at high altitudes in Utah and Colorado, which is characterized by pulmonary hypertension and subsequent failure of the right side of the heart, is not a true counterpart of Monge's disease, since it is not associated with sustained oxygen unsaturation or polycythemia.

Any chronic pulmonary disease which alters ventilation-perfusion relationships or seriously impairs gas diffusion may produce chronic hypoxemia and lead to erythrocytosis. *Pulmonary arteriovenous fistulas* or *cavernous hemangioma of the lung* may lead to impaired saturation of arterial blood with oxygen, with the consequent development of erythrocytosis and of a clinical picture resembling closely that of certain types of congenital heart disease. The increased blood viscosity secondary to the polycythemia (Fig. 29-3) elevates pulmonary arterial pressure and, combined with the elevation of pulmonary vascular resistance resulting from hypoxia, further elevates right ventricular pressure, contributing to the development or intensification of cor pulmonale. (Chap. 262).

The *abnormal ventilatory conditions* present in very obese individuals may cause alveolar hypoventilation and result in arterial unsaturation, erythrocytosis, hypercapnea, and somnolence (the Pickwickian syndrome, Chap. 255). This syndrome is observed less commonly in nonobese persons, in whom decreased sensitivity of the respiratory center to CO_2 may play a role.

The partial shunting of blood from the pulmonary circuit, such as occurs in *congenital heart disease,* causes the most striking erythrocytosis resulting from abnormal-

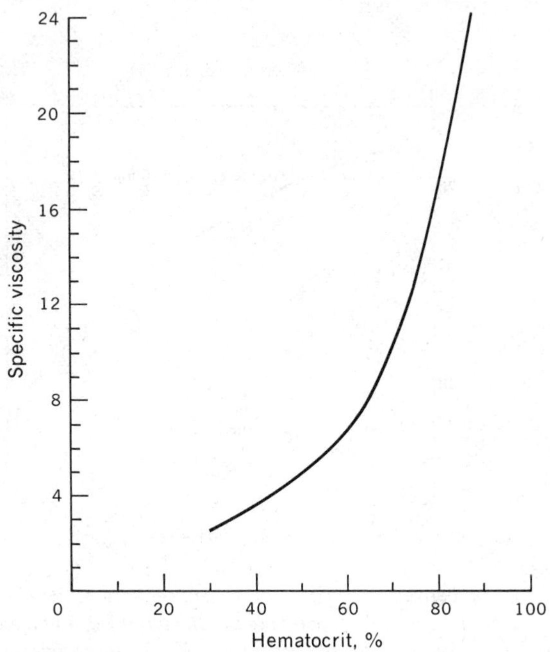

FIGURE 29-3
Correlation of hematocrit value with specific viscosity of the blood. (From Rudolph et al; by permission of Pediatrics*)*

ities in the heart or lungs. Erythrocyte counts as high as 13 million per cubic millimeter, which are possible only when the red corpuscles are smaller than normal, have been observed in such cases, with volumes of packed red blood cells even as high as 86 ml per 100 ml of blood. As the polycythemia develops, there is a progressive rise in blood viscosity (Fig. 29-3), with the sharpest increase beginning when the volume of packed red blood cells reaches 65 to 70 percent. Phlebotomy is sometimes performed in severely symptomatic patients with extremely high hematocrit levels, but it must be carried out slowly and with great caution. It should not be continued if there is no symptomatic improvement. The commonest defect producing such polycythemia is pulmonary stenosis associated with a right-to-left shunt that allows venous blood to enter the systemic arterial tree without traversing the lungs. Other conditions include transposition of the great arteries, tricuspid atresia, persistent truncus arteriosus, and other less-common anomalies, discussed in Chap. 237.

The excessive use of coal-tar derivatives and other forms of chronic poisoning, by producing abnormal hemoglobin pigments such as methemoglobin and sulfhemoglobin (Chap. 312), also may cause erythrocytosis. Carriers of certain abnormal hemoglobins which have a high oxygen affinity, such as hemoglobin Chesapeake (Chap. 307), are slightly polycythemic.

Erythrocytosis is found in *Cushing's syndrome* (Chap. 86) and can be produced by the administration of large amounts of adrenocortical steriods. Especially intriguing are the instances of polycythemia observed in association with various *tumors.* These have been chiefly of two varieties, *infratentorial* and *renal.* The tumors in the posterior fossa of the skull have usually been vascular (hemangioblastomas). The renal tumors have included hypernephroma, adenoma, and sarcoma. Other tumors that have been associated with polycythemia include uterine myoma and hepatic carcinoma. Polycythemia also has been reported in association with polycystic disease of the kidneys and hydronephrosis. However, only a small proportion (0.3 to 2.6 percent) of the various renal disorders mentioned above have been associated with polycythemia. Plasma erythropoietin levels have been found elevated in a number of these patients. Erythropoiesis-stimulating activity has been demonstrated in tumor extracts and in renal cyst fluid, and polycythemia has disappeared after the associated tumor was removed.

The term *stress erythrocytosis* has been applied to the polycythemia seen occasionally in very active, hard-working persons in a state of anxiety, who appear florid but who have none of the characteristic signs of erythremia—no splenomegaly or leukocytosis with immature cells in the blood. In such persons the total red blood cell mass is normal and the plasma volume is below normal.

The differential diagnosis of polycythemia is discussed in the chapter on erythremia (Chap. 311). However, it should be pointed out that in secondary polycythemia with hypoxia, arterial P_{O_2} is reduced, erythropoietin levels are elevated, while levels of leukocyte alkaline phosphatase and serum vitamin B_{12} are normal. In polycythemia vera, erythropoietin levels are normal or decreased and leukocyte alkaline phosphatase and vitamin B_{12} levels are elevated.

REFERENCES

BATES DV et al: *Respiratory Function in Disease,* Philadelphia: Saunders, 1971, p. 584

BAUMAN AW: Polycythemia vera, in *Hematology for Internists,* ed RI Weed, Boston: Little Brown, 1971, p. 325

GUYTON AC: *Textbook of Medical Physiology,* 4th ed., Philadelphia: Saunders, 1971, p. 512

HARKNESS DR: The regulation of hemoglobin oxygenation, in *Advances in Internal Medicine,* ed GH Stollerman, Chicago: Year Book, 1971, p. 189

HURTADO A: Some clinical aspects of life at high altitudes. Ann Intern Med 53:247, 1960

LUKAS DS: Cyanosis, in *Signs and Symptoms,* ed CM Mac Bryde, RS Blacklow, 5th ed., Philadelphia: Lippincott, 1970, p. 358

RUDOLPH AM et al: Hematologic adjustments to cyanotic congenital heart disease. Pediatrics 11:454, 1953.

30 EDEMA

LOUIS G. WELT

Edema is defined as an increase in the extravascular component of the extracellular fluid volume. It may be localized or have a generalized distribution depending on the primary lesion. It is recognized by the clinician in its gross generalized form by puffiness of the face (which is most readily apparent in the periorbital areas) and by the persistence of an indentation of the skin following pressure. This is known as *"pitting" edema.* In its more subtle form it may be detected by the fact that the rim of the bell of the stethoscope leaves an indentation on the skin of the chest that lasts a few minutes. One of the first symptoms a patient may note is the ring on a finger fitting more snugly than in the past. Lastly, it should be cautioned that the volume of the interstitial space may increase by several liters before edema is recognized by the patients from the symptoms or by the physician through physical examination. *Ascites* and *hydrothorax* refer to accumulation of excess fluid in the peritoneal and pleural cavities, respectively. *Anasarca,* or "dropsy," refers to gross generalized edema.

PATHOGENESIS

A more detailed discussion of the volume and distribution of body fluids is presented in Chap. 264. About one-third of the total body water is confined to the extracellular space. This compartment, in turn, is composed of the plasma volume and the interstitial space. Under ordinary circumstances the plasma volume represents about 25 percent of the extracellular space, and the remainder is in the interstitium. The forces that regulate the disposition of fluid between these two components of the extracellular compartment are frequently referred to as the *Starling forces,* owing to the masterful description presented by that noted physiologist.

In general terms, two forces tend to promote a movement of fluid from the vascular to the extravascular space, and these forces are the *hydrostatic pressure within the vascular system* and the *colloid oncotic pressure* in the interstitial fluid. In contrast, the factors which promote a movement of fluid into the vascular compartment are the *colloid oncotic pressure* contributed by the plasma proteins, and the *hydrostatic pressure within the interstitial fluid,* referred to as the *tissue tension.* These forces are balanced so that there is a large movement of water and diffusible solutes from the vascular space at the arteriolar end of the microcirculation and back into the vascular compartment at the venous end.[1] In addition, fluid is returned from the interstitial space into the vascular system by way of the lymphatics, and unless these channels are obstructed, lymph flow tends to increase if there is a tendency toward a net movement of fluid from the vascular compartment to the interstitium. In this fashion, all these forces are usually balanced so that a given steady state exists with respect to the size of the two compartments, and yet a large exchange between them is permitted. However, should any one of these factors be altered significantly, one can see how there may be a net movement of fluid from one component of the extracellular space to the other.

An increase in pressure in the vessels of the microcirculation may readily result from an increase in venous pressure due to local obstructive phenomena in the venous drainage, or to congestive heart failure, or to the simple expansion of the vascular volume by the administration of large volumes of fluid at a rate in excess of the ability of the kidneys to excrete these excesses. The colloid oncotic pressure of the plasma may be reduced owing to any of the factors that may induce hypoalbuminemia, such as malnutrition, liver disease, and loss of protein into the urine or into the gastrointestinal tract, or to a severe catabolic state.

Damage to the capillary endothelium increases the permeability of these vessels, which permits the transfer to the interstitial compartment of a fluid containing more protein than usual. Injury to the capillary walls may be the result of chemical, bacterial, thermal, or mechanical agents. Increased capillary permeability may also be a consequence of a hypersensitivity reaction. Lastly, damage to the capillary endothelium is presumably responsible for inflammatory edema, which is easily recognized by the presence of other signs of inflammation—redness, heat, and tenderness.

In any attempts to formulate a hypothesis concerning the pathophysiology involved in edematous states, it is exceedingly important to discriminate between the primary events, which account for the maldistribution of fluid between the two components of the extracellular space, and the predictable secondary consequences, which include the retention of salt and water. There are instances in which an abnormal retention of salt and water may, in fact, be the *primary* disturbance. In these circumstances the edema is a secondary manifestation of the generalized increase in volume of the extracellular fluid. These special instances are usually related to those conditions characterized by an acute reduction in renal function (such as acute tubular necrosis or acute glomerulonephritis) and other disorders characterized by the primary production of excess mineralocorticoid or inappropriate secretion of the antidiuretic hormone.

These latter circumstances aside, one can create a hypothesis which is admittedly at least incomplete but within which one can begin to understand the concatenation of events in a variety of edematous states and perceive many of the features common in the pathophysiology of each. The basic premise is that the primary disorder concerns one or more alterations in the Starling forces such that there is a net movement of fluid from the vascular system into the interstitium or from the arterial compartment of the vascular space into the chambers of the heart or into the venous circulation itself. In either event, a diminished arterial volume may be anticipated to have certain consequences that lead to retention of salt and water. If retention of an increment of salt and water repairs the volume deficit, the stimuli to retain salt and water should be dissipated and a new steady state achieved. If, on the other hand, retention of salt and water does not repair the volume deficit because the increased volume of fluid cannot be sustained in the appropriate component of the vascular bed, the stimuli are not dissipated and the retention of salt and water continues. The sequence of events can be explored in a variety of circumstances.

OBSTRUCTION OF VENOUS AND LYMPHATIC DRAINAGE TO A LIMB The simplest condition to examine may be the consequences of lymphatic and venous obstruction to a limb. This must increase the

[1] *There is no final resolution of the argument whether the exchange of fluid and solutes occurs between capillary endothelial cells or through the cells themselves. The bulk of the evidence suggests that both routes are employed.*

hydrostatic pressure in the microcirculation so that more fluid is transferred from the circulation than can be reabsorbed at the venous end; furthermore, in this condition the alternate route (i.e., the lymphatic channels) is considered to be obstructed as well. This event must of necessity cause an increased volume of interstitial fluid in the limb at the expense of the plasma volume. The diminished plasma volume has a variety of consequences:

Renal hemodynamic changes The diminished volume of plasma may be expected to reduce the perfusion of the kidney and decrease the glomerular filtration rate. Since one of the most important influences regulating the excretion of salt (and water) may be the filtered load itself, this would promote the excretion of lesser quantities of salt and smaller volumes of water. Other consequences of a hemodynamic nature are presumably conditioned by alterations in plasma volume. For reasons that are as yet unclear, it seems quite well established that an influence of "volume" on the rate of excretion of salt functions independently of its filtered load and independently of mineralocorticoid secretion. The nature of this regulatory mechanism is unknown, but a direct correlation occurs between alterations in volume and alterations in the excretion of salt. The phenomenon may be related to the character and distribution of blood flow to the kidney, but there are other alternatives. In any event, a diminished plasma volume can readily diminish the excretion of salt owing to alterations in renal hemodynamic parameters.

Humoral factors Ample evidence reveals that a diminished volume of plasma in some fashion promotes an increased secretion of aldosterone. This is because of an increase in an aldosterone-stimulating agent, which is dependent on the presence of intact kidneys and may well be angiotensin. This, in turn, may be increased in the plasma owing to some influence on the renal circulation related to alterations in flow or pressure, or to the chemical composition of intraluminal fluid that may stimulate the release of renin from the juxtaglomerular apparatus. In turn, the renin reacts with renin substrate to form angiotensin I, and the latter is converted enzymatically to angiotensin II, which stimulates the secretion of aldosterone. Whatever the precise sequence of events, a diminished plasma volume promotes increased secretion of this mineralocorticoid which implements the renal tubular reabsorption of sodium. (See also Chap. 86.)

The influence of alterations in plasma volume on the excretion of sodium salts was mentioned in relation to possible alterations in renal hemodynamics. Certain data suggest the possibility that the increase in volume of some component(s) of the extracellular space promotes the secretion of a "natriuretic" hormone, also referred to as a *third factor,* or *volume effect.* The unambiguous demonstration of such a hormone, its site(s) of secretion, and its characterization are yet to be presented.

The retention of sodium owing to the hemodynamic and humoral factors alluded to above may, in turn, be accompanied directly by an increased reabsorption of water. If not, then the primary retention of sodium thus dictates some increase in the effective osmolality of body fluids, promotes thirst and the acquisition of water, and promotes the secretion of antidiuretic hormone, which then implements the retention of water.

In the context of the disorder under discussion, the volume of the extracellular fluid (about 140 mmol sodium per liter of water) is increased. This increment tends to accumulate in the interstitium of the limb in which venous and lymphatic drainage are obstructed until the tissue tension is great enough to counterbalance the primary alteration in the Starling forces, at which time no further fluid will accumulate in that limb. At this point the additional accumulation of fluid will repair the deficit in plasma volume, and the stimuli to retain more salt and water are dissipated. The net effect is an increase in the volume of interstitial fluid in a local area, and the secondary responses repair the plasma volume deficit incurred by the primary event.

This same sequence may be translated easily to many other edematous states.

NEPHROTIC SYNDROME (see also Chap. 271) The primary alteration in this disorder is a diminished colloid oncotic pressure due to exorbitant loss of protein into the urine. This should promote a net movement of fluid into the interstitium and initiate the sequence of events described above. However, so long as the hypoalbuminemia is severe, the increment of fluid cannot be restrained within the vascular compartment, and hence the stimuli to retain salt and water are not abated.

CIRRHOSIS (see also Chap. 296) Measurements of blood volume in cirrhosis of the liver are commonly increased when the disorder is accompanied by a fairly large system of dilated venous radicles. Nevertheless, the arterial volume is quite likely diminished in size. If the primary event in the formation of ascites is obstruction of the lymphatic drainage of the liver as well as obstruction of the portal venous system, it is likely that the enlarged venous system has promoted a deficit in the arterial component. Once again, the sequence of events already described will come into play, and salt and water will be retained. So long as the venous bed continues to enlarge and the collection of fluid in the peritoneal cavity increases, the deficit in volume of the arterial side of the circulation is not repaired and the stimuli persist to retain salt and water. In addition, considerable data suggest that there are arteriovenous shunts in this disorder. One consequence of these shunts is a reduced renal blood flow despite an increase in cardiac output. In this fashion the alterations due to renal hemodynamic factors are fortified.

Although the diseased liver admittedly may not inactivate aldosterone and antidiuretic hormone in a competent fashion, it is unlikely that this plays a significant role in salt and water retention.

CONGESTIVE HEART FAILURE In this disorder it is postulated that the defective systolic emptying of the chambers of the heart promotes an accumulation of blood in the heart and venous circulation at the expense of the arterial volume, and the oft-repeated sequence of events is initiated. In many instances of mild heart failure a small increment of volume may be achieved, which may repair the volume deficit and establish a new steady state. This may result because up to a point an increase in the volume of blood within the chambers of the heart appears to promote a more forceful contraction and may thereby increase the volume ejected in systole. However, if the cardiac disorder is more severe, retention of fluid cannot repair the arterial volume deficit. The increment accumulates in the venous circulation, and the increase in hydrostatic pressure therein promotes the formation of edema in the lungs as well as elsewhere. The pulmonary edema impairs gas exchange and may induce hypoxia, which embarasses cardiac function still further. The volume of blood within the chambers of the heart becomes ever larger and reaches a point where this increase affects systolic emptying adversely, thus worsening the heart failure. (See also Chap. 233.)

IDIOPATHIC CYCLIC EDEMA This syndrome, which occurs predominantly, but not exclusively, in women, is characterized by periodic episodes of edema, frequently accompanied by abdominal distention, and is commonly seen in patients with significant psychosocial difficulties. Another feature of the disorder is the observation of fairly large, diurnal alterations in weight, such that the patient may well weigh several pounds more in the evening than in the morning after having been in the upright posture most of the day. Such large diurnal weight changes suggest an increase in capillary permeability which is further enhanced in some fashion episodically. The facts that it occurs most commonly in women and appears to bear a time correlation with the menstrual cycle suggest that there may be some hormonal influence on the permeability of the vessels which permits the loss of plasma volume into the interstitial space and the sequence of events secondary to a contraction in plasma volume.

The treatment of idiopathic cyclic edema includes a reduced salt intake, the employment of appropriate diuretic agents in anticipation of the edematous episode, education in the use of rest in the supine position for several hours each day, the wearing of elastic stockings which are put on prior to arising in the morning, and an attempt to understand the underlying emotional problems.

The general formulation regarding the pathophysiology of edema formation is represented graphically in Fig. 30-1. This picture is certainly incomplete, and the amplification presented in this discussion may well have serious defects of omission and error. Allusion has been made to some of the unknown areas. One more which deserves further comment concerns the precise role of the mineralocorticoid hormone in these problems. Although increased quantities of aldosterone have been demonstrated to be secreted in these various edematous states, it must be emphasized that augmented levels of aldosterone (or other mineralocorticoids) do not always promote the accumulation of edema, as witnessed by the lack of striking fluid retention in most instances of primary aldosteronism. Furthermore, although normal subjects will retain some salt and water under the influence of a potent mineralocorticoid such as deoxycorticosterone

FIGURE 30-1
Sequence of events leading to the formation and retention of salt and water.

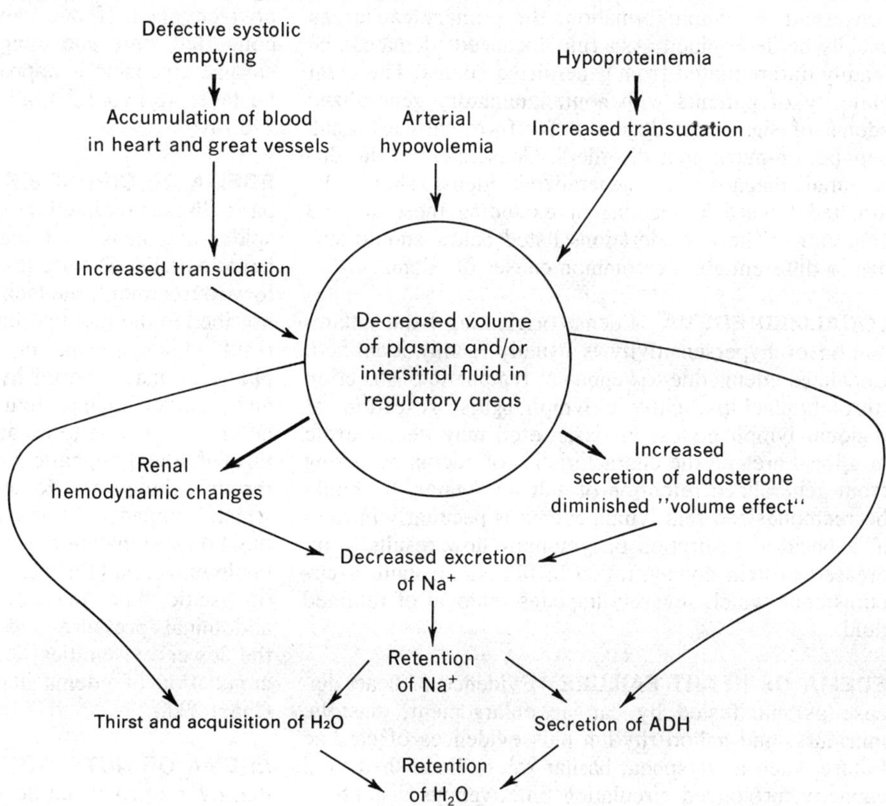

acetate or 9-alpha-fluorohydrocortisone, this accumulation appears to be self-terminative despite continued exposure to the steroid and to salt and water. It is probable that the failure of normal subjects to accumulate fluid indefinitely reflects an increase in glomerular filtration rate, other hemodynamic influences, and the effect of the increase in volume which promotes an increased excretion of salt independent of the filtered load of sodium. The role of aldosterone in the accumulation of fluid in these edematous states discussed above may be more effective because these patients are unable to repair the crucial deficit in volume.

Throughout this discussion it has been assumed that the retention of sodium salts is primary to water retention. This is attested to by (1) the usual failure to accumulate edema if sodium is not available in the diet and (2) the successful use of pharmacologic agents and other measures that promote the excretion of sodium in the urine. In most circumstances the mechanisms responsible for maintaining a normal effective osmolality in the body fluids continue to operate efficiently so that sodium retention promotes thirst and secretion of the antidiuretic hormone, which, in turn, lead to the ingestion and retention of approximately 1 liter of water for each 140 mmol sodium retained. Similarly, measures which promote the loss of sodium into the urine are accompanied by antithetical responses leading to the net loss of an equivalent volume of water from the body.

DIFFERENTIAL DIAGNOSIS

Despite numerous inconsistencies encountered in the explanation for the various factors and mechanisms concerned in edema formation, the primary cause can usually be determined. As a rule, localized edema can be readily differentiated from generalized edema. The great majority of patients with noninflammatory generalized edema of significant degree suffer from cardiac, renal, hepatic, or nutritional disorders. Consequently, the differential diagnosis of generalized edema should be directed toward implicating or excluding these several conditions. The considerations listed below should suffice to differentiate the common causes of edema.

LOCALIZED EDEMA Edema originating from inflammation or hypersensitivity is usually readily identified. Localized edema due to venous or lymphatic obstruction (thrombophlebitis, chronic lymphangitis, resection of regional lymph nodes, filariasis, etc.) may demonstrate in a local area all the characteristics of edema occurring from generalized retention of salt and water. It should be reemphasized that lymph edema is peculiarly intractable because restriction of lymphatic flow results in increased protein concentration in interstitial fluid, a circumstance which severely impedes removal of retained fluid.

EDEMA OF HEART FAILURE Evidence of heart disease as manifested by cardiac enlargement, diastolic murmurs, and gallop rhythm plus evidences of cardiac failure, such as dyspnea, basilar rales, diminished vital capacity, prolonged circulation time, venous distention, increased venous pressure, and hepatomegaly, usually provides abundant evidence of the pathogenesis of edema resulting from heart failure. (See also Chap. 233.)

EDEMA OF THE NEPHROTIC SYNDROME The classic triad—massive proteinuria, hypoproteinemia, and hypercholesterolemia—is usually present. This syndrome may occur during the course of a variety of kidney diseases, which include glomerulonephritis, diabetic glomerulosclerosis, amyloid infiltration, renal vein thrombosis, diffuse connective tissue diseases, and hypersensitivity reactions. A history of previous renal disease may or may not be elicited; more commonly, it is not. (See also Chap. 271.)

EDEMA OF ACUTE GLOMERULONEPHRITIS The edema occurring during the acute phases of glomerulonephritis is characteristically associated with hematuria, proteinuria, and hypertension. Some evidence supports the view that the fluid retention is due to increased capillary permeability; but probably in most instances the edema in this disease results from primary retention of sodium and water by the kidneys owing to acute renal insufficiency and the consequent development of a congested state. However, discrimination between congestive heart failure and a congested state in acute renal insufficiency is often difficult. The congested state differs from congestive heart failure since it is characterized by a normal or increased cardiac output, normal or diminished circulation time, a reduction in the packed cell volume, a normal arteriovenous oxygen difference, and failure to respond to a digitalis preparation. Patients commonly have severe evidence of pulmonary congestion on chest roentgenograms before cardiac enlargement is significant, and these patients frequently lie supine in bed with no tachypnea. If one cannot discriminate between the congested state and congestive heart failure, use of a cardiac glycoside is appropriate, but special care should be taken to avoid digitalis intoxication. (See also Chap. 270.)

EDEMA OF CIRRHOSIS Ascites and evidence of hepatic disease (collateral venous channels, hepatomegaly, spider angiomas, and jaundice) characterize edema of hepatic origin. The ascites is frequently extremely refractory to treatment; the lack of therapeutic response can be ascribed to the fact that intraabdominal fluid collects as a result of a combination of obstruction of hepatic lymphatic drainage, portal hypertension, hypoalbuminemia, and relatively high protein content of the ascitic fluid. The latter may be due to escape of a protein-containing fluid through the lymphatic vessels of the liver capsule or through the portal vessels, the lymphatic drainage of which is impeded. Edema may also occur in other parts of the body in patients with cirrhosis as a result of hypoalbuminemia. Furthermore, the sizable accumulation of ascitic fluid may be expected to increase intraabdominal pressure and impede venous return from the lower extremities; hence, it tends to promote accumulation of edema in these limbs as well. (See also Chap. 296.)

EDEMA OF NUTRITIONAL ORIGIN An inadequate diet over a prolonged period may produce hypoproteinemia and edema. In some instances of extreme malnutrition the degree of transudation appears to be disproportionately great for the degree of serum protein deficit observed. Coexisting beriberi heart disease may augment edema of this origin. In the latter condition, increased cardiac output and blood flow, in addition to those factors usually present in heart failure and capillary dilatation, may further favor edema formation. More striking edema is commonly observed when these famished subjects are provided with an adequate diet. The mechanism is not clear, but the ingestion of more food may increase the quantity of salt taken, which is retained along with water. The edema may be more apparent than under other circumstances, because the subcutaneous tissue is so depleted of fat that modest collections of edema may be more obvious than they would be in an obese subject.

GENERAL DIFFERENTIAL CRITERIA

Aside from the criteria already mentioned, certain other points may help elicit the cause of edema.

The distribution of edema is an important guide to the cause. Thus, edema of one leg or of one or both arms is usually the result of vascular or lymphatic obstruction. Edema resulting from hypoproteinemia characteristically is generalized, but it is especially evident in the eyelids and face and tends to be most pronounced in the morning because of the recumbent posture assumed during the night. Edema associated with heart failure, on the other hand, tends to be more extensive in the legs and to be accentuated in the evening, a feature also determined largely by posture. In the rare types of cardiac disease, such as tricuspid stenosis and constrictive pericarditis, in which orthopnea may be absent and the patient may prefer the recumbent posture, the factor of gravity may be equalized and facial edema observed. Less common causes of facial edema include trichinosis, allergic reactions, and myxedema. Unilateral edema occasionally results from cerebral lesions affecting the vasomotor fibers on one side of the body; paralysis also reduces lymphatic and venous drainage on the affected side.

The color, thickness, and sensitivity of the skin are important. Local tenderness and increase in temperature suggest inflammation. Local cyanosis may signify a venous obstruction. Generalized but usually slight cyanosis commonly indicates congestive heart failure. In individuals who have had repeated episodes of prolonged edema, the skin over the involved area may be thickened, hard, and often red.

The venous pressure is of great importance in evaluating edema. Elevation of this measurement in an isolated part of the body usually reflects venous obstruction. Generalized elevation of venous pressure is almost pathognomonic of congestive heart failure, although it may be present in the congestive state that accompanies acute renal insufficiency. Ordinarily significant increase in venous pressure can be recognized by the level at which cervical veins collapse; in doubtful cases and for accurate recording, the central venous pressure should be measured.

Determination of the concentration of serum proteins, and especially of serum albumin, clearly differentiates those patients in whom edema is due entirely or in part to diminished intravascular colloid osmotic pressure. The presence of proteinuria affords useful clues. The complete absence of protein in the urine is evidence against (but does not exclude) either cardiac or renal disease as a cause of edema. In a patient with edema without proteinuria, the presence of a palpable liver constitutes strong evidence that hepatic disease may be the cause of the edema. Slight to moderate proteinuria is the rule in patients with heart failure, whereas persistent massive proteinuria usually reflects the presence of the nephrotic syndrome. Since the liver may be palpable in subjects with heart failure or hepatic disease, the presence of proteinuria in a patient who does not have a palpable liver suggests the possibility of the nephrotic syndrome. Aside from the points mentioned, which bear directly on the question of the type of edema, much valuable information can be obtained from other features of the examination. Some of these are the presence or absence of heart disease, the character of the urinary sediment, the dietary history, and a history of alcoholism.

It should be emphasized that edema may originate from a variety of abnormal states; it is not, therefore, necessarily a consequence of only one of the disorders enumerated above. For example, in a diabetic patient, edema may be the result of hypoalbuminemia associated with the nephrotic syndrome with intercapillary glomerulosclerosis, increased venous pressure associated with congestive heart failure due to atherosclerotic and hypertensive heart disease, and the anemia consequent to uremia.

SIGNIFICANT QUESTIONS TO ASK WHEN CONFRONTED WITH A PATIENT WITH EDEMA

1 Is the edema localized or general?

2 If localized, concentrate on those phenomena alluded to above that may be responsible. In this context, localized edema may include hydrothorax or ascites or both in the absence of congestive heart failure or hypoalbuminemia. Either of these collections may be a consequence of local venous or lymphatic obstruction, as in inflammatory disease or carcinoma. It is a frequent accompaniment of an inflammatory process which involves the pleura or peritoneum, and the cause of the inflammatory process may vary from bacterial invasion to infarction of underlying parenchyma to a diffuse connective tissue disease with vasculitis, etc. In instances of either hydrothorax or ascites, an examination of the characteristics of the fluid is extremely important. This should include bacterial culture, smear with stains for ordinary and less common infectious agents, determination of protein concentration, cell count, and the presence or absence of blood; the cells should be concentrated by centrifugation and preparation for histologic examination for evidences of malignancy and other characteristics.

3 If the edema is generalized: *(a)* Is there hypoalbuminemia of significant degree, e.g., serum albumin concentration less than 2.5 g per 100 ml? If there is, a history, physical examination, and other laboratory data will help evaluate the question of cirrhosis, malnutrition, protein-losing gastroenteropathy, or the nephrotic syndrome as the underlying disorder. *(b)* Is there evidence of congestive heart failure of a severity to promote generalized edema even in the absence of hypoalbuminemia, or is there evidence of both congestive heart failure and some degree of hypoalbuminemia? The significant factors to be examined are alluded to in the body of this chapter and in other chapters as well. *(c)* Does the patient have an adequate urine output with urine of good quality, or is there significant oliguria or even anuria? Diminished excretion of urine over a period of several days may be accompanied by the ingestion of usual volumes of fluid, leading to a net accumulation of volume, which expresses itself as generalized edema. A variety of renal diseases may be responsible for oliguria or anuria, and these are discussed in Chaps. 268, 269, and 274. The major differential diagnosis in these instances is frequently the discrimination between overload with fluid and a congested state as opposed to congestive heart failure.

REFERENCES

BLYTHE WB et al: Further evidence for a humoral natriuretic factor. Circ Res 28:II-21, 1971

WELT LG: Agents affecting volume and composition of body fluids, chap. 36 in *The Pharmacological Basis of Therapeutics,* eds LS Goodman, A Gilman, New York: Macmillan, 1970

WESTON RE: Pathogenesis and treatment of edema with special reference to use of diuretics, chap. 6 in *Clinical Disorders of Fluid and Electrolyte Metabolism,* 2d ed., eds MH Maxwell, CR Kleeman, New York: McGraw-Hill, 1972

31 PALPITATION

EUGENE BRAUNWALD
WILLIAM H. RESNIK

Palpitation is a common, disagreeable subjective phenomenon which may be defined as an awareness of the beating of the heart. Palpitation is not pathognomonic of any particular group of disorders; indeed, often it signifies not a primary physical disorder but rather a psychic disturbance. Even when it occurs as a more or less prominent complaint, the diagnosis of the underlying disease is made largely on the basis of other associated symptoms and data, rather than from an analysis of the palpitation alone. Nevertheless, palpitation is frequently of considerable importance in the minds of patients. The clear association of the symptom with the function of the heart and the fear that it may represent heart disease account for the patient's apprehension about it. Concern is all the more pronounced in patients who know or who have been told that they may have heart disease; to them palpitation may seem to be an omen of impending disaster. Since the resulting anxiety may be associated with increased activity of the autonomic nervous system, with consequent increases of the cardiac rate and rhythm and the vigor of contraction, the patient's awareness of these changes may then lead to a vicious cycle, which may ultimately be responsible for his total incapacitation.

Palpitation may be described by the patient in various terms, such as "pounding," "fluttering," "flopping," and "skipping," and in most cases it will be obvious that the complaint is of a sensation of disturbed heartbeat. The wide variability in the sensitivity to alterations in cardiac activity among different individuals must be appreciated. Some patients seem to be unaware of the most serious tachycardias; others are seriously troubled by an occasional extrasystole. Patients with anxiety states often exhibit a lowered threshold at which disorders of rate and rhythm result in palpitation. Indeed, it is not unusual for palpitation to be the major manifestation of the emotional disorder. The degree of awareness of the heartbeat also varies at different times in the same individual; it is more common at night, during introspective moments just before falling asleep, but is less marked during activity. Patients with organic heart disease and chronic disorders of cardiac rate, rhythm, or stroke volume tend to accommodate to these abnormalities and are often less sensitive than normal persons to such events. Persistent tachycardia and/or atrial fibrillation may not be accompanied by continual palpitation, in contrast to a sudden, brief alteration in cardiac rate or rhythm which often causes considerable subjective discomfort. Thus, palpitation is particularly prominent when the precipitating cause for increased heart rate or contractility or arrhythmia is recent. Conversely, in emotionally well-adjusted individuals palpitation becomes progressively less disconcerting as the cause (e.g., anemia, frequent extrasystoles, complete atrioventricular block) persists.

PATHOGENESIS OF PALPITATION

Under ordinary circumstances the rhythmic heartbeat is imperceptible to the healthy individual of average or placid temperament. Palpitation may be experienced by normal persons who have engaged in strenuous physical effort or have been aroused emotionally or sexually. This type of palpitation is physiologic and represents the normal awareness of an overactive heart—i.e., a heart that is beating at a rapid rate and with an increased contractility. Since palpitation due to overactivity of the heart may occur also in certain pathologic states, e.g., severe anemia or thyrotoxicosis, it is commonly assumed that it is the overactivity per se that is responsible for the symptom. However, overactivity of the heart is generally associated with several other alterations in cardiac function, including acceleration of heart rate, steeper gradient of development of intraventricular pressure during the period of isometric contraction, increased intensity of the heart sounds, especially of the first sound, a shorter duration of systole, and a greater ejection velocity.

When palpitation is heavy and regular, it is usually caused by an augmented stroke volume, and it should raise the question of a variety of hyperkinetic circulatory states (anemia, arteriovenous fistula, thyrotoxicosis, and the so-called idiopathic hyperkinetic heart syndrome), aortic or mitral regurgitation, and ventricular septal defect. It may also occur immediately following the onset of cardiac slowing, as with the sudden development of heart block, or upon the conversion to sinus rhythm from atrial fibrillation. But unusual movements of the heart within the thorax are also frequently the mechanism of palpitation. Thus, the ectopic beat and/or the compensatory pause may be appreciated, since both are associated with alterations in cardiac motion.

IMPORTANT CAUSES OF PALPITATION

Palpitation due to disorders of the mechanism of the heartbeat

(See also Chap. 234)

EXTRASYSTOLES In most cases the diagnosis will be suggested by the patient's story. The premature contraction and postpremature beat are often described as a "flopping," or the patient may say that he feels as if "the heart turns over." The pause following the premature contraction may be felt as an actual cessation of the heartbeat, in contrast with the complete unawareness of pauses of similar duration when atrial fibrillation with a slow ventricular rate occurs. The patient's apprehensions seem to magnify the duration of the interval and sometimes may make him wonder if the heart will ever resume its beat. The first ventricular contraction succeeding the pause may be felt as an unusually vigorous beat and will be described as "pounding" or "thudding."

Usually the identification of the extrasystole as the cause of palpitation is a simple matter. When extrasystoles are numerous, clinical differentiation from atrial fibrillation can be made by any procedure that will bring about a definite increase in the ventricular rate; at increasingly rapid heart rates, the extrasystoles usually diminish in frequency and then disappear, whereas the irregularity of atrial fibrillation increases. Heart block, with dropped beats, is the only other common arrhythmia with which the premature contraction is likely to be confused; here, simple auscultation will reveal the absence of the premature beat prior to the pause.

ECTOPIC TACHYCARDIAS These conditions, which are considered in some detail in Chap. 234, are common and medically important causes of palpitation. Ventricular tachycardia, one of the most serious arrhythmias, rarely is manifested as palpitation; this may be related to the abnormal sequence, and hence impaired coordination and vigor, of ventricular contraction. If the patient is seen between attacks, the diagnosis of ectopic tachycardia and its type will have to depend on the history, but of course the precise diagnosis can be made only when an electrocardiogram and observations on the effect of carotid sinus pressure are made during the episode. The mode of onset and offset gives the most important lead in distinguishing sinus from one of the various forms of ectopic tachycardias; sinus tachycardia commences and ceases over the course of minutes or seconds, but not instantaneously as is characteristic of the ectopic rhythms. Determining this mode may prove difficult, for in many cases of rapid heart action it is not possible to ascertain with certainty whether there was an actual sudden onset or whether there was a preceding period of anxiety followed by the rapid, but not abrupt, development of sinus tachycardia.

Palpitation dependent on organic or functional disturbance originating outside the circulatory system

THYROTOXICOSIS In its fully developed form, thyrotoxicosis will usually be evident and offers little difficulty in the way of diagnosis except in the elderly, in whom so-called apathetic hyperthyroidism may be present. Thyrotoxicosis is particularly likely to be overlooked in the presence of myocardial failure. The suspicion that thyrotoxicosis is present may be aroused by the detection of any one of its characteristic features, and the diagnosis will be confirmed by the procedures mentioned in Chap. 85.

ANEMIA When mild, anemia may cause palpitation during exertion; when severe, palpitation may be present at rest. In some patients the coloring of the skin may not reveal the cause of the symptoms, but appropriate studies of the blood will clarify the situation.

FEVER Palpitation may be present in acute infections, particularly in the early stages, but here the symptom is merely an insignificant phenomenon in the midst of other obviously more important ones. Palpitation may be a prominent symptom in an individual suffering from one of the chronic and sometimes more obscure febrile illnesses, such as incipient tuberculosis, chronic brucellosis, subacute bacterial endocarditis, or acute rheumatic fever with carditis and relatively few or no joint manifestations. Carditis in acute rheumatic fever and subacute bacterial endocarditis are considered in this group because the presenting symptoms, including palpitation, are often only those of an infection without localizing symptoms that direct suspicion to the heart. The problem is to determine that the cause of the palpitation is an infectious illness and to carry out the usual procedures to reveal the type of infection.

HYPOGLYCEMIA Palpitation is often a prominent feature of this condition and appears to be related to release of epinephrine. The diagnosis is confirmed by appropriate blood sugar estimations, by reproduction of the symptom when insulin is administered, and by prompt relief of all symptoms on the administration of glucose (Chap. 90).

TUMORS OF THE ADRENAL MEDULLA (PHEOCHROMOCYTOMAS) Such tumors may give rise to recurrent attacks, including paroxysms of hypertension and palpitation which are identical to those seen following the injection of epinephrine or norepinephrine. This type of tumor is a rather uncommon cause of palpitation and is mentioned chiefly because cure may be effected by surgical removal (Chap. 87). A similar syndrome may be produced when monoamine oxidase (MAO)–inhibitor drugs are taken concurrently with sympathomimetic drugs, such as ephedrine or amphetamine.

DRUGS The relationship between the development of palpitation and the use of tobacco, coffee, tea, alcohol, epinephrine, ephedrine, aminophylline, atropine, or thyroid extract is obvious.

Palpitation as a manifestation of the anxiety state

Persons who are healthy physically and well adjusted emotionally may have palpitation under certain circumstances. Thus, during or immediately after vigorous physical exertion or during sudden emotional tension, palpitation is common and is usually associated with outspoken tachycardia.

In some patients, palpitation may be one of the outstanding manifestations of a transitory episode of acute anxiety which may never recur, i.e., after this one episode or between infrequent bouts of increased nervous tension, the patient may experience no palpitation. In other persons the palpitation may, with other symptoms, represent prolonged anxiety neurosis or anxious depressions or a lifelong disorder indicative of disturbed autonomic function. The latter condition has been called neurocirculatory asthenia (see Chap. 339). Whether these illnesses are simply an expression of a chronic, deep-seated anxiety state superimposed on a normal autonomic nervous system or whether they depend on instability of the autonomic nervous system is not clear. At any rate, the clinical significance of this differentiation between the transitory and the enduring forms is that the former is often dissipated by firm reassurance from the physician, whereas the latter is usually resistant even to the most thorough and expert psychiatric care. In the latter case, the patient must be treated with most carefully planned psychologic support and tranquilizing medications. This chronic form of palpitation is known by various names, such as *Da Costa's syndrome, soldier's heart, effort syndrome, irritable heart, neurocirculatory asthenia,* and *functional cardiovascular disease.* Aside from palpitation, the chief symptoms are those of an anxiety state.

Physical examination usually reveals the typical findings of the hyperkinetic syndrome. These include a left parasternal lift, a precordial or apical systolic murmur, a wide pulse pressure, a rapidly rising pulse and excessive perspiration. Electrocardiograms may display minor depressions of the S-T junction and inversion of T waves and so occasionally lead to a mistaken diagnosis of coronary disease; this is particularly likely to occur when these findings are associated with complaints by the patients of an aching feeling of substernal tightness, commonly present in emotional stress. The presence of any kind of organic disease is one of the commonest causes of the underlying anxiety which frequently precipitates this functional syndrome.

The diagnosis of this type of anxiety state depends on the presence of the findings mentioned above. Even when a patient presents undoubted objective evidence of structural cardiac disease, a superimposed anxiety state should be considered responsible for the symptoms when the clinical picture is that which has been described. Normal values for vital capacity and for circulation time make it extremely improbable that the dyspnea that accompanies this type of palpitation is due to organic cardiac disease. It is noteworthy that an anxiety state, in contrast to heart disease, causes a sighing type of dyspnea. Also pain localized to the region of the apex, lasting for hours or days, and accompanied by hyperesthesia is due usually to an anxiety state, not to structural cardiac disease. Palpitation associated with organic cardiac disease is nearly always accompanied by arrhythmia or by marked tachycardia, whereas the symptom may exist with regular rhythm and with a heart rate of 80 beats per min or less in patients with the anxiety state. Giddiness due to this syndrome can usually be reproduced by hyperventilation (Chap. 16) or by change from the recumbent to the erect posture.

The treatment of the anxiety cardiac syndrome depends on removal of the cause. In many instances a thorough examination of the heart and a statement that it is normal will suffice. Instructions to take more rather than less physical exercise will reinforce these statements. Frequently, the demonstration that the physician can reproduce not only the palpitation but many other symptoms of the anxiety state merely by the subcutaneous injection of 0.5 to 1.0 ml 1:1,000 epinephrine serves to convince the patient that his symptoms are not the result of some mysterious disorder but are rather the effect of a well-understood physiologic mechanism. This is especially true when the initial anxiety has been mainly the result of fear of heart disease. When the anxiety state is a manifestation of chronic anxiety neurosis or depres-

TABLE 31-1
Items to be covered in history

Does the palpitation occur:	*If so, suspect:*
As isolated "jumps" or "skips"?	Extrasystoles
In attacks, known to be of abrupt beginning, with a heart rate of 120 beats/min or over, of regular or irregular rhythm?	Paroxysmal rapid heart action
Independent of exercise or excitement adequate to account for the symptom?	Atrial fibrillation, atrial flutter, thyrotoxicosis, anemia, febrile states, hypoglycemia, anxiety state
In attacks developing rapidly though not absolutely abruptly, unrelated to exertion or excitement?	Hemorrhage, hypoglycemia, tumor of the adrenal medulla
In conjunction with the taking of drugs?	Tobacco, coffee, tea, alcohol, epinephrine, ephedrine, aminophylline, atropine, thyroid extract, monoamine oxidase inhibitors
On standing?	Postural hypotension
In middle-aged women, in conjunction with flushes and sweats?	Menopausal syndrome
When the rate is known to be normal and the rhythm regular?	Anxiety state

sive psychosis, the symptoms are more likely to persist.

Management of patients with palpitation and the anxiety cardiac syndrome is facilitated by a clear understanding on the physician's part of the mechanisms of the symptoms. The palpitation is probably related to adrenergic stimulation of the heart and to the lower perception threshold. The pain may arise in the intercostal tissues as a result of the pounding of the heart. The hyperventilation with its ensuing train of symptoms (Chap. 16) is analogous to sighing. It is possible that the entire syndrome is related to decline of the normal inhibitory effect of the cerebral cortex on those hypothalamic centers which normally control the sympathetic system. Explanation of these physiologic mechanisms to the patient and reassurance that they are not indicative of serious disease is one of the most important therapeutic steps.

Table 31-1 summarizes the main points of information to be ascertained in the history in elucidating the significance of palpitation. These questions and others formulated according to circumstances of the individual case will serve to suggest the additional lines of inquiry that may be necessary for analysis and appraisal of palpitation. The recording of the electrocardiogram using a portable tape recorder in an ambulatory subject, and the precise temporal correlation of the cardiac rate and rhythm with the presence of palpitation is extremely useful in the identification or exclusion of a rhythmic disturbance. The effectiveness of antiarrhythmia treatment can also be assessed objectively in this manner, without the necessity of relying only on the patient's subjective symptoms.

One point merits special emphasis. *As a rule palpitation produces anxiety and fear out of all proportion to its seriousness.* When the cause has been accurately determined and its significance explained to the patient, his concern is often ameliorated and may disappear entirely.

REFERENCES

DRESSLER W: *Clinical Aids in Cardiac Diagnosis,* New York: Grune & Stratton, 1970, p. 4

MASSIE E: Palpitation and tachycardia, chap. 16 in *Signs and Symptoms,* eds CM MacBryde, RS Blacklow, Philadelphia: Lippincott, 1970

WOOD P: *Diseases of the Heart and Circulation,* 3d ed., Philadelphia: Lippincott, 1968, p. 17

32 HYPOTENSION AND THE SHOCK SYNDROME

KARL ENGELMAN
EUGENE BRAUNWALD

HYPOTENSION The differential diagnosis of hypotensive states and the development of a rational plan of therapy require understanding of the normal regulation of arterial pressure.

Control of arterial pressure Arterial pressure must be maintained at levels sufficient to permit adequate perfusion of the extensive capillary networks in the systemic vascular bed. The level of pressure in the central arterial bed is in a large measure dependent on two factors—the volume of blood ejected by the left ventricle per unit of time, i.e., the cardiac output, and the resistance to blood flow offered by the vessels in the peripheral vascular bed. The resistance of a blood vessel, in turn, varies inversely as the fourth power of its radius, and at any given level of cardiac output arterial pressure is therefore largely dependent upon the degree of constriction of the smooth muscle in the walls of the arterioles. Though resistance to flow also varies with the viscosity of the fluid and the length of the vessels, alterations in these factors are ordinarily of only secondary importance.

Cardiac output is controlled largely by factors which regulate ventricular end-diastolic volume, the level of myocardial contractility, and heart rate (Chap. 232). The autonomic nervous system plays a major role in the maintenance of arterial pressure by its influences on the cardiac output and on the degree of constriction of the resistance (arterioles) and capacitance (venules and veins) vessels. The afferent limbs of the autonomic reflex arcs regulating arterial pressure arise in stretch receptors in the aortic arch and the carotid sinuses. Impulses are transmitted along afferent fibers in the glossopharyngeal and vagus nerves to extensive central autonomic connections in the medulla. Synapses connect not only the sympathetic and parasympathetic nuclei and efferent arcs, but also the cerebral cortex and hypothalamic nuclei which control hormonal secretion via the pituitary gland.

A rapid reduction of arterial pressure diminishes the stimulation of pressoreceptors, which in turn evokes an activation of sympathetic outflow and inhibition of parasympathetic activity. As a result, the vascular smooth muscles in arterioles and veins constrict, while heart rate and myocardial contractility are augmented. In addition, with decreases in arterial pressure, adrenal medullary secretion is increased, as are the output of antidiuretic hormone (ADH), adrenocorticotropic hormone (ACTH), renin, and aldosterone; all these effects act to restore the arterial pressure to control levels. Opposite changes occur if arterial pressure is raised acutely. Thus, the operation of the pressoreceptor and a number of humoral systems normally serve to buffer the body from a variety of influences which would otherwise produce marked alterations in arterial pressure.

Measurement of arterial pressure Arterial pressure is determined clinically with a pneumatic cuff; ordinarily, this indirect method provides slight underestimation of the true arterial pressure. Considerable error may be introduced if proper precautions are not taken in determining blood pressure by this method. The arterial pressure may be significantly underestimated if the air in the cuff is released too rapidly, especially in the presence of bradycardia or an irregular rhythm, or if inadequate inflation of the cuff does not result in complete vascular occlusion. This indirect method is most accurate when, in normal-sized adults, cuffs 12 to 14 cm in width are employed. However, when a cuff of this size is used on children or adults with unusually thin arms, blood pressure may be seriously underestimated, or conversely, it may be overestimated when employed on an arm or thigh greater than 20 cm in girth. Marked vasoconstriction resulting in severely attenuated limb blood flow and/or marked reductions in pulse pressure may also result in serious underestimation of arterial pressure by the auscultatory method. Direct intraarterial recordings may reveal a normal or even an elevated pressure, while the absence of Korotkoff sounds makes the pressure unobtainable by the indirect methods.

The "normal" blood pressure The "normal" blood pressure is difficult to define. Traditional statistical approaches define normality on the basis of values included within two standard deviations of the mean of pressures obtained in a large population of presumably healthy individuals. On this basis 95 percent of the population are defined as being normotensive, with the remaining 5 percent evenly divided between the hypertensive and hypotensive groups. A better definition of abnormality would be based on demonstrated deleterious effects of blood pressure levels exceeding certain limits. Using such criteria chronic hypotension would seem to occur very rarely. However, the incidence of hypertension based on casual blood pressure levels exceeding 160/95 mm Hg (widely accepted as hazardous) is estimated to be approximately 15 percent in the adult population of the United States, with the incidence in the black population exceeding that in the nonblacks by 50 to 100 percent. Even these statistics may understate the prevalence of hypertension if one accepts the validity of actuarial data indicating that longevity is shortened progressively in adults whose blood pressures exceed 100/60 mm Hg. The hazard of hypertension and its major complication, widespread vascular disease, appears to be a function of the level of blood pressure; the hazard rises more steeply with higher levels, especially as they exceed diastolic values of 90 to 95 mm Hg.

ACUTE HYPOTENSION AND SHOCK

Not uncommonly, physicians are called upon to treat patients who acutely develop severe hypotension or shock. These two terms are not synonymous; although shock is usually associated with hypotension, a previously hypertensive patient may be in shock despite an arterial pressure within normal limits, and hypotension may occur in the absence of shock. *Shock* may be defined as a state in which there is widespread, serious reduction of tissue perfusion which, if prolonged, leads to generalized impairment of cellular function.

The most common clinical causes of shock are listed in Table 32-1. Since maintenance of arterial pressure is dependent on cardiac output and peripheral vasomotor tone, marked reductions in either of these variables without a compensatory elevation of the other results in systemic hypotension. Reduction of cardiac output due to hypovolemia or acute myocardial infarction is among the most frequently encountered and easily categorized causes of shock. Failure of neurogenic mechanisms resulting in decreased vasoconstrictor impulses is another

TABLE 32-1
Etiologic factors in shock

I Hypovolemia
- *A* External fluid losses
  - *1* Hemorrhage
  - *2* Gastrointestinal
    - *a* Vomiting (pyloric stenosis, intestinal obstruction)
    - *b* Diarrhea
  - *3* Renal
    - *a* Diabetes mellitus
    - *b* Diabetes insipidis
    - *c* Excessive use of diuretics
  - *4* Cutaneous
    - *a* Burns
    - *b* Exudative lesions
    - *c* Perspiration and insensible water loss without replacement
- *B* Internal sequestration
  - *1* Fractures
  - *2* Ascites (peritonitis, pancreatitis, cirrhosis)
  - *3* Intestinal obstruction
  - *4* Hemothorax
  - *5* Hemoperitoneum

II Cardiogenic
- *A* Myocardial infarction
- *B* Arrhythmia (paroxysmal tachycardia or fibrillation, severe bradycardia)
- *C* Severe congestive heart failure with low cardiac output

III Obstruction to blood flow
- *A* Pulmonary embolus
- *B* Tension pneumothorax
- *C* Cardiac tamponade
- *D* Dissecting aortic aneurysm
- *E* Intracardiac (ball valve thrombus, atrial myxoma)

IV Neuropathic
- *A* Drug induced
  - *1* Anesthesia
  - *2* Ganglion-blocking or other antihypertensive drugs
  - *3* "Ingestion" (barbiturates, glutethimide, phenothiazines)
- *B* Spinal cord injury
- *C* Orthostatic hypotension (primary autonomic insufficiency, peripheral neuropathies)

V Other
- *A* Infection
  - *1* Gram-negative septicemia (endotoxin)
  - *2* Other septicemias
- *B* Anaphylaxis
- *C* Endocrine failure (Addison's disease, myxedema)
- *D* Anoxia

well-defined category; in many patients, particularly in the late stages of shock, multiple factors play a role in the development of circulatory failure.

Hypovolemia has been studied much more extensively than any other cause of shock; the mechanism of development is usually readily evident and well understood, and therapy, i.e., restoration of blood volume, is both simple and effective if applied before irreversible tissue damage occurs. Whether the primary insult is the external loss of blood, plasma, or water and salt or the internal sequestration of these fluids in a hollow viscus or body cavity, the general effect is similar, i.e., reduced venous return and decreased cardiac output. For purposes of a general discussion of shock, hemorrhagic hypovolemia will be used as the model, but the general physiologic consequences of the various etiologies of reduced tissue perfusion are similar.

Depending upon the severity and rate of development of hypovolemia, the shock syndrome may develop abruptly or evolve gradually. If the precipitating factors progress unabated, the endogenous defense mechanisms, while initially competent to maintain adequate circulation, eventually are extended beyond their capacity for compensation. The development of the shock syndrome may be thought to evolve through several stages which merge with one another:

1 The period in which the blood volume deficit is relatively minor and in which the patient may be asymptomatic. In a previously healthy individual compensation for an acute blood loss of as much as 10 percent of the normal blood volume (as with venesection of 500 ml blood from a donor) is achieved acutely by constriction of the arteriolar bed and an augmentation of heart rate. Other responses with more gradual effects include the increased secretion of antidiuretic hormone and aldosterone. Arterial pressure is maintained and cardiac output is normal, or only slightly reduced, primarily as a consequence of selective reductions of blood flow to the skin and muscle beds.

2 With a reduction of blood volume of 15 to 25 percent, cardiac output falls markedly, and despite intense arteriolar constriction in most vascular beds, arterial pressure declines. Generalized venoconstriction occurs, increasing the fraction of the total blood volume in the central circulation and tending to sustain venous return. With this massive reflex adrenergic discharge there are tachycardia, intense cutaneous vasoconstriction, pallor, diaphoresis, piloerection, mesenteric and renal vasoconstriction with oliguria, apprehension, and restlessness.

3 Once the patient has achieved this state of maximal mobilization of compensatory mechanisms, small additional losses of blood result in rapid deterioration of the circulation, with life-threatening reductions of cardiac output, blood pressure, and tissue perfusion. The duration of this shock state, the severity of tissue anoxia, and the age and underlying physical state of the patient are of primary importance in determining the ultimate outcome. If tissue perfusion is restored rapidly, recovery may be expected. However, if shock persists, the severe vasoconstriction may itself become a complicating factor and by reducing tissue perfusion even further may initiate a vicious cycle leading to an irreversible state due to widespread cellular injury. Anoxia, hypercapnia, and acidosis result from hypoperfusion of tissues; these metabolic derangements ultimately result in failure of the energy-requiring active transport systems of cell membranes. The integrity of the cells is compromised, and potassium ions, intracellular lysosomal enzymes, peptides, and other vasoactive compounds are released into the circulation. In profound shock from any cause an additional important factor which may occur to exacerbate stasis of the microcirculation is widespread disseminated intravascular coagulation (DIC) in the bowel, kidney, and other organs. The resultant ischemia produced in the bowel may further complicate the circulatory compensation as a result of breakdown of the mucosal barrier, leading to entry of bacteria and toxic bacterial products into the circulation. Because many of these substances are potent vasodilators, vasoconstrictor mechanisms may be inhibited, with a further decrease in blood pressure despite intense sympathetic activity. Blood flow to the brain, heart, and kidneys is further reduced, and infarction of these vital organs often leads to death.

Just as cardiac output may fall to dangerous or even fatal levels because of actual fluid losses or sequestration with diminished venous return, cardiac failure or intrathoracic obstruction to blood flow may have a similar effect. Furthermore, even in the presence of a normal blood volume and cardiac function, "vasomotor collapse" due to drug-induced or neuropathic failure of sympathetic vasomotor activity can result in shock because of reduction of peripheral resistance and the pooling of blood in the venous bed. Finally, a complex form of shock may result from infection, especially gram-negative bacteremia with endotoxin release, from anaphylaxis, anoxia, and endocrine disorders which affect myocardial function, fluid and electrolyte balance, vasomotor tone, and general tissue metabolic processes.

Treatment of the patient with shock should be directed toward the rapid restoration of cardiac output and tissue perfusion. General supportive measures must be undertaken immediately, sometimes even before the cause of the shock state has been identified. Whether shock results from decreased cardiac output due to a primary reduction in intravascular volume or a reduction of "effective blood volume" with pooling of blood in certain vascular beds, the most effective means of restoring adequate circulation is by the rapid infusion of volume-expanding fluids (whole blood, plasma, plasma substitutes, or isotonic electrolyte solutions). However, when shock is secondary to, or is accompanied by, cardiac failure with increased pulmonary vascular and central venous pressures, the infusion of volume-expanding fluids may result in pulmonary edema. Here attention must be directed toward restoring cardiac function with cardiotonic drugs such as the digitalis glycosides and isoproterenol, and an attempt should be made to support arterial pressure at levels sufficient to maintain the coronary perfusion pressure (Chap. 240). Arrhythmias, which may also contribute to the low cardiac output, should be corrected (Chap. 234).

The appearance of the external jugular veins may be helpful in differentiating between shock with high or low central venous pressure. However, a catheter inserted into the superior vena cava is the best means for continuously monitoring venous pressure and is of considerable value in guiding therapy; such a catheter should be inserted in patients with shock whenever possible. Serial measurements of central venous pressure, urine flow rate, heart rate, and the clinical and mental state of the patient often provide more important indices of the efficacy of therapy than arterial pressure changes. In patients with shock and impaired left ventricular function, e.g., cardiogenic shock due to massive acute myocardial infarction, a balloon (Swan-Ganz) catheter which can be "floated" into the pulmonary artery at the bedside without the aid of fluoroscopy is even more helpful than a central venous pressure catheter in guiding treatment.

There is considerable debate concerning the efficacy of vasoconstrictor drugs in shock. In patients with severe peripheral constriction these agents are often ineffective and may actually reduce the already lowered tissue perfusion. However, these drugs are usually helpful in patients with inadequate vasoconstrictor responses. The use of alpha adrenergic blocking agents or massive doses of adrenal glucocorticoids in shock secondary to gram-negative septicemia with endotoxin release is also a matter of considerable controversy and cannot yet be considered a routine procedure.

CHRONIC HYPOTENSION Although many patients have been treated for chronic "low blood pressure," most of them, with systolic pressures in the range of 90 to 110 mm Hg, are normal and may actually have a greater life expectancy than those with higher pressures. Patients with true chronic hypotension may complain of lethargy, weakness, easy fatigability, and dizziness or faintness, especially if arterial pressure is lowered further when the erect position is assumed. These symptoms are presumably due to a decrease in perfusion of the brain, heart, skeletal muscle, and other organs.

Chronic hypotension occasionally results from severe reductions of the cardiac output. The major endocrine causes of chronic hypotension are associated with deficient gluco- and mineralocorticoid secretion and resultant reductions of the intravascular and interstitial fluid volume. Hypotension is usually more pronounced in patients with primary adrenocortical insufficiency than in those with hypopituitarism because secretion of the salt-retaining adrenocortical hormone, aldosterone, is partially preserved in pituitary insufficiency (Chap. 83).

Malnutrition, cachexia, chronic bed rest, and a variety of neurologic disorders may result in chronic hypotension, especially in the standing position. Interference with the neural pathways anywhere between the vasomotor center and the efferent sympathetic nerve endings on the blood vessels or heart may prevent the vasoconstriction and increase in cardiac output which occur as a normal response to a reduction in arterial pressure. Multiple sclerosis, amyotrophic lateral sclerosis, syringomyelia, syphilitic or diabetic tabes dorsalis, peripheral neuropathies, spinal cord section, diabetic neuropathy, extensive lumbodorsal sympathectomy, and the administration of drugs interfering with nerve transmission in the sympathetic nervous system are all associated with orthostatic hypotension. In addition, *idiopathic orthostatic hypotension* (primary autonomic insufficiency), a rare condition in which there is degeneration of central and/or peripheral autonomic nervous structures, may result in such severe orthostatic hypotension that syncope or seizures occur when the patient arises from recumbency. This condition is progressive and characterized by ascending anhydrosis and loss of hair, decreased BMR, reduced norepinephrine production, deficient secretion of lacrimal and salivary glands, ileus, bladder atony, and absence of tachycardia on standing despite the marked reduction of blood pressure.

Specific therapy is not available for most of the neurologic causes of orthostatic hypotension, and treatment with sympathomimetic drugs has not proved effective over prolonged periods. However, the expansion of extracellular volume, which may be achieved with a high-(10 to 20 g per day) salt diet and/or the potent synthetic salt-retaining steroid, 9α-fluorohydrocortisone (0.1 to 0.5 mg per day) may be helpful. Tight, full-length, elastic supportive hose to reduce orthostatic pooling of blood in the legs may also be helpful in sustaining arterial pressure, and in the most severe cases pressurized aviator suits may be necessary to permit ambulation.

REFERENCES

Christy JH: Pathophysiology of gram-negative shock. Am Heart J 81:694, 1971

Nickerson M: Vascular adjustments during the development of shock. *Can Med Assoc J 103:853, 1971*

Weil MH, Shubin H: *Diagnosis and Treatment of Shock*, Baltimore: Williams & Wilkins, 1967

33
ELEVATION OF ARTERIAL PRESSURE

KARL ENGELMAN
EUGENE BRAUNWALD

Patients with elevations of arterial pressure are usually asymptomatic, and the blood pressure abnormality often arouses attention only incidentally during military, life insurance, or other periodic physical examinations. Because hypertension results in secondary organ damage and a reduced life span, it should be evaluated fully and, when appropriate, treated.

DIAGNOSIS OF HYPERTENSION Often, however, the first question is whether patients with a moderately elevated routine blood pressure recording are truly hypertensive. It is well established that anxiety, discomfort, physical activity, or other stress can acutely and transiently raise arterial pressure. Most persons have a higher pressure when initially examined than after several measurements made in the course of a single visit; in order to establish the diagnosis of hypertension it is necessary to document in the course of several examinations that arterial pressure remains elevated (Chap. 245). Patients with transient or "labile" hypertension may not require immediate treatment but should be reexamined periodically, since over the course of time they often develop sustained hypertension.

Systolic hypertension in the presence of a normal or reduced diastolic pressure is rarely considered to be responsible for organ damage, but usually reflects other pathologic processes. It is most commonly seen in elderly patients with decreased compliance of the aortic wall. In patients with severe bradycardia, thyrotoxicosis, severe anemia, fever, aortic valvular insufficiency, arteriovenous shunts or fistulas, and the hyperkinetic heart syndrome, systolic hypertension is due to an elevated stroke volume, often accompanied by a rapid diastolic runoff.

Patients with true systemic hypertension have an increased mean arterial pressure, with elevations of both systolic and diastolic pressures. Regardless of the primary cause, the hemodynamic abnormality in most of these patients is increased vascular resistance, especially at the level of the smaller muscular arteries and arterioles, though a small number of patients may have an increased cardiac output, particularly in the early stages of the illness. In a small fraction of patients, hypertension is associated with hypervolemia, or increased blood viscosity secondary to polycythemia.

ETIOLOGY OF HYPERTENSION A specific cause for the increase in peripheral resistance which is responsible for the elevated arterial pressure cannot be defined for approximately 90 percent of patients with hypertensive disease. Numerous experimental studies have sought to define the role of a variety of components ultimately responsible for idiopathic, or so-called "essential," hypertension. Evidence for the role played by abnormal psychologic stimuli comes from the finding that chronically stressed animals may become hypertensive, and that sedatives and tranquilizers are helpful in the treatment of many hypertensive patients. Another neurogenic mechanism, the resetting of the sensitivity of the pressoreceptors, occurs in hypertensive dogs so that they appear to recognize elevated arterial pressures as normal. The importance of salt intake is suggested by studies showing that rats can be made hypertensive when given excessive dietary salt, and epidemiologic studies have also suggested this as a factor of possible etiologic significance in man; other studies have indicated that increased water and sodium in the walls of arterioles may result in increased peripheral resistance. In addition, hereditary and racial factors seem to play significant roles in the development of hypertension, since this disease is often found in families and is especially prevalent and virulent among certain ethnic groups, such as the American black population.

It appears that all the above-mentioned factors play some role in patients with essential hypertension, which might be best regarded as a multifactorial disease related to abnormalities of the regulatory mechanisms normally concerned with the homeostatic control of arterial pressure.

TABLE 33-1
Classification of arterial hypertension

- *I* Systolic hypertension with wide pulse pressure
  - *A* Decreased compliance of aorta (arteriosclerosis)
  - *B* Increased stroke volume or cardiac output
    - *1* Arteriovenous fistula
    - *2* Thyrotoxicosis
    - *3* Hyperkinetic heart disease
    - *4* Fever
    - *5* Psychogenic factors
    - *6* Aortic valvular insufficiency
    - *7* Patent ductus arteriosus
- *II* Systolic and diastolic hypertension (increased peripheral vascular resistance)
  - *A* Renal
    - *1* Chronic pyelonephritis
    - *2* Acute and chronic glomerulonephritis
    - *3* Polycystic renal disease
    - *4* Renovascular stenosis or renal infarction
    - *5* Most other severe renal disease (arteriolar nephrosclerosis, diabetic nephropathy, etc.)
  - *B* Endocrine
    - *1* Acromegaly
    - *2* Adrenocortical hyperfunction
      - *a* Cushing's disease and syndrome
      - *b* Primary hyperaldosteronism
      - *c* Congenital or hereditary adrenogenital syndromes (17-α-hydroxylase and 11-β-hydroxylase defects)
    - *3* Pheochromocytoma
    - *4* Myxedema
  - *C* Neurogenic
    - *1* Psychogenic
    - *2* "Diencephalic syndrome"
    - *3* Familial dysautonomia (Riley-Day)
    - *4* Poliomyelitis (bulbar)
    - *5* Polyneuritis (acute porphyria, lead poisoning)
    - *6* Increased intracranial pressure (acute)
    - *7* Spinal cord section
  - *D* Miscellaneous
    - *1* Coarctation of aorta
    - *2* Increased intravascular volume (excessive transfusion)
    - *3* Polyarteritis nodosa
    - *4* Hypercalcemia
  - *E* Unknown etiology
    - *1* Essential hypertension (>90% of all cases of hypertension)
    - *2* Toxemia of pregnancy
    - *3* Acute intermittent porphyria
    - *4* Oral contraceptives

More specific etiologic relationships have been established for a smaller group of patients with systemic hypertension (Table 33-1). Primary renal diseases associated with the development of serious hypertension (as distinguished from renal damage secondary to hypertension) have been recognized for years, although in many cases the exact mechanism of blood pressure elevation is unknown. Hypertension may develop suddenly during the course of acute glomerulonephritis, and it is usually a prominent feature in the late stages of renal damage due to chronic glomerulonephritis (Chap. 270) or pyelonephritis (Chap. 273). Polycystic renal disease, renal infarction, and partial occlusion of the renal artery due to congenital or acquired vascular defects are also implicated as etiologic factors, the latter having been clearly related to activation of the renin-angiotensin-aldosterone pressor system.

The most clearly defined etiologic relationships in the development of hypertension are found among the endocrine disorders. Adrenocortical hormones have also been implicated in the hypertensive syndromes associated with tumors or hyperplasia of the anterior pituitary (Cushing's syndrome, primary hyperaldosteronism, Chap. 86), as well as with various congenital or hereditary enzyme defects (hypertensive adrenogenital syndromes). Secretion of excessive quantities of the pressor catecholamines, norepinephrine and epinephrine, associated with pheochromocytomas i.e., chromaffin cell tumors arising from the adrenal medulla or sympathetic ganglions, is also commonly associated with hypertension (Chap. 87). Up to 50 percent of patients with acromegaly (Chap. 83) may have hypertension, but the mechanism of their blood pressure elevation is less clear. The presence of these endocrinopathies is usually readily recognizable and distinguishable from essential hypertension by their distinctive clinical and biochemical features. The clinical differentiations between primary and the various forms of secondary hypertension are detailed in Chap. 245.

EFFECTS OF HYPERTENSION Following an asymptomatic latent period, clinical manifestations which reflect the underlying pathologic sequelae of the hypertensive state usually become apparent. Cardiac, renal, and central nervous system effects due to accelerated vascular damage are most prominent, and if unaltered by therapy, they often ultimately result in symptomatic illness and death.

Effects on heart Cardiac compensation for the excessive work load imposed by increased systemic pressure is at first sustained by left ventricular hypertrophy. Ultimately, the function of this chamber deteriorates, it dilates, and the symptoms and signs of heart failure appear (Chap. 233). Angina pectoris may also occur because of accelerated coronary arterial disease and/or increased myocardial oxygen requirements as a consequence of the increased myocardial mass, which exceeds the capacity of the coronary circulation. On physical examination the heart is enlarged and has a prominent left ventricular impulse. The sound of aortic closure is accentuated, and there may be a faint murmur of aortic insufficiency. Presystolic (atrial) gallop sounds appear frequently in hypertensive heart disease, and a protodiastolic (ventricular), or summation, gallop rhythm may be present. Electrocardiographic changes of left ventricular hypertrophy are common; evidence of ischemia or infarction may be observed late in the disease. The majority of deaths due to hypertension result from myocardial infarction or congestive heart failure.

Neurologic effects The neurologic effects of longstanding hypertension may be divided into retinal and central nervous system changes. Because the retina is the only tissue in which the arteries and arterioles can be examined directly, repeated ophthalmoscopic examination provides the opportunity to observe the progress of the vascular effects of hypertension. The Keith-Wagener-Barker classification of the retinal changes in hypertension (Table 33-2) has provided a simple and

TABLE 33-2
Classification of hypertensive and arteriolosclerotic retinopathy

	Hypertension					*Arteriolosclerosis*	
	Arterioles						
Degree	*General narrowing A/V ratio**	*Focal spasm†*	*Hemorrhages*	*Exudates*	*Papilledema*	*Arteriolar light reflex*	*AV crossing‡ defects*
Normal	3/4	1/1	0	0	0	Fine yellow line, red blood column	0
Grade I	1/2	1/1	0	0	0	Broadened yellow line, red blood column	Mild depression of vein
Grade II	1/3	2/3	0	0	0	Broad yellow line, "copper wire," blood column not visible	Depression or humping of vein
Grade III	1/4	1/3	+	+	0	Broad white line, "silver wire," blood column not visible	(*a*) Right-angle deviation, tapering, and disappearance of vein under arteriole (*b*) Distal dilatation of vein
Grade IV	Fine, fibrous cords	Obliteration of distal flow	+	+	+	Fibrous cords, blood column not visible	Same as grade III

* This is the ratio of arteriolar/venous diameters.
† This is the ratio of diameters of region of spasm to proximal arteriole.
‡ Arteriolar length and tortuosity increase with severity.

excellent means for serial evaluation of the hypertensive patient. Table 33-2 includes both the criteria for grouping the retinal findings of hypertension and the secondary arteriolosclerotic changes. Increasing severity of hypertension is associated with focal spasm and progressive general narrowing of the arterioles, as well as the appearance of hemorrhages, exudates, and papilledema. These retinal lesions often produce scotomas, blurred vision, and even blindness, especially in the presence of papilledema or hemorrhages of the macular area. Hypertensive lesions may develop acutely, and if therapy results in significant reduction of blood pressure, may show rapid resolution. Rarely, these lesions resolve without therapy. In contrast, retinal arteriolosclerosis results from endothelial and muscular proliferation, and it accurately reflects similar changes in other organs. Sclerotic changes do not develop as rapidly as hypertensive lesions, nor do they regress appreciably with therapy. As a consequence of increased wall thickness and rigidity, sclerotic arterioles distort and compress the veins as they cross within their common fibrous sheath, and the reflected light streak from the arterioles is changed by the increased opacity of the vessel wall.

Central nervous system dysfunction also occurs frequently in patients with hypertension. Occipital headaches, most often in the morning, are among the most prominent early symptoms of hypertension. Dizziness, lightheadedness, vertigo, tinnitus, and dimmed vision or syncope may also be observed, but the more serious manifestations are due to vascular occlusion or hemorrhage. With severe long-standing hypertension, patients develop multiple focal or large vascular infarcts or hemorrhages which result in destruction of brain tissue. The focal changes may be manifested as personality or memory deficits, but the larger lesions which produce major strokes are responsible for up to 10 to 15 percent of deaths occurring secondary to hypertension.

Renal effects Arteriolosclerotic lesions of the afferent and efferent arterioles and the glomerular capillary tufts are the most common renal vascular lesions in hypertension and result in decreased glomerular filtration rate and tubular dysfunction. Proteinuria and microscopic hematuria occur because of glomerular lesions, and approximately 10 percent of the deaths secondary to hypertension result from renal failure. Blood loss in hypertension occurs not only from renal lesions; epistaxis, hemoptysis, and metrorrhagia also occur more frequently in these patients.

Malignant hypertension Although the above-described complications of hypertension are serious and are often eventually fatal after many years of the disease, a small fraction, variously estimated as between 1 and 5 percent, of patients with essential hypertension enter an accelerated phase which usually results in rapid death. This "malignant" phase of hypertension is associated with very high levels of arterial pressure and characteristic rapidly progressive necrosis of the walls of small arteries and arterioles, with concentric collagenous endothelial thickening leading to diminution or occlusion of the vascular lumen. These lesions of arteriolonecrosis result in massive proteinuria, hematuria, and rapidly progressive uremia, grade IV retinopathy with papilledema, and cerebral edema with increased intracranial pressure, mental confusion, and seizures. These manifestations progress rapidly over a period of days to weeks, and if therapy is not effective, death occurs from uremia or an intracranial vascular accident.

TREATMENT As a consequence of the pathologic changes secondary to the elevated arterial pressure, treatment of patients with systemic hypertension is directed toward lowering pressure in an attempt to halt or reverse the progressive organ damage. In certain instances specific therapy or cure of the primary etiologic factor can be achieved by repair of a stenotic renal artery lesion or coarctation of the aorta, or by removal of a tumor which secretes pressor substances. However, because of the unknown cause of the hypertension in the majority of patients, therapy is directed primarily toward the major physiologic abnormality, i.e., it is designed to lower systemic vascular resistance. Because the sympathetic nervous system plays such an important role in the maintenance of peripheral resistance, many effective antihypertensive drugs act by interfering with the vasoconstrictor impulses mediated by this system (Chap. 245). Although arterial pressure can be reduced in the majority of patients, hypertension is a chronic disease, and a therapeutic program must usually be maintained for the duration of the patient's life.

REFERENCES

Combined Staff Conference: Recent advances in hypertension. Am J Med 39:616, 1965

Laragh JH (ed): Symposium on hypertension: mechanisms and management. Am J Med 52:565, 1972

Lund-Johansen P: Hemodynamics in early essential hypertension. Acta Med Scand 181:Suppl. 482, 1967

Page IH, McCubbin JW: The physiology of arterial hypertension, in *Handbook of Physiology*, vol. 3, ed WF Hamilton, Washington: The American Physiological Society, 1965, p. 2163

Scheie HG: Evaluation of ophthalmoscopic changes of hypertension and arteriolar sclerosis. AMA Arch Ophthalmol 49:117, 1953

34 SUDDEN CARDIOVASCULAR COLLAPSE AND DEATH

BURTON E. SOBEL
EUGENE BRAUNWALD

Sudden death claims more than 400,000 lives annually in the United States alone and should be considered a major health problem in the Western world. Despite the liberality of the Joint American Heart Association and International Society of Cardiology Committee definition (death occurring instantaneously or within an estimated 24 hr of the onset of acute symptoms or signs), about half of sudden deaths are virtually instantaneous and unwitnessed, and though most of these deaths are unexpected, approximately one-half the victims have previously known heart disease and an additional quarter have hypertension or diabetes. A brief period of time, usually only several minutes, elapses between sudden cardiovascular collapse (without effective cardiac output) and irreversible ischemic changes in the central nervous system. Therefore, effective therapy must be instituted immediately if sudden cardiovascular collapse is not to terminate in sudden death. However, prolonged survival without functional impairment may be the reward for prompt treatment of certain forms of cardiovascular collapse.

MECHANISMS Sudden cardiovascular collapse may be due to (1) arrhythmias (Chap. 234); (*a*) most commonly, ventricular tachycardia or fibrillation, sometimes following a bradyarrhythmia, or (*b*) less frequently, ventricular asytole or severe bradycardia; (2) a marked, abrupt reduction in cardiac output, such as occurs with mechanical blockade of the circulation; massive pulmonary thromboembolism (Chap. 256) and cardiac tamponade are two examples of this form; (3) sudden ventricular (pump) failure, which may occur in the presence of an acute myocardial infarction (Chap. 240) or critical aortic stenosis (Chap. 239); (4) vasodepressor reflexes, which may contribute to sudden reductions in arterial pressure and heart rate, and which are activated in diverse conditions, including primary pulmonary hypertension (Chap. 259), pulmonary thromboembolism, and the hypersensitive carotid sinus syndrome (Chap. 16).

Sudden death and coronary atherosclerosis Sudden death is primarily a complication of coronary atherosclerosis, more than two-thirds of the cases resulting from this disorder. In the vast majority of such patients sudden death results from precipitous ventricular fibrillation. However, evidence of coronary occlusion and, indeed, of acute myocardial infarction may not be found at autopsy; nonetheless, acute myocardial ischemia appears to be the precipitating event. Only approximately 40 percent of patients dying from coronary artery disease survive long enough to be hospitalized. The remainder (approximately 300,000 patients per year in the United States) die suddenly before they reach the hospital. In fact, in 25 percent of patients with coronary artery disease death is the first indication of the presence of the disorder (Chap. 240). Extrapolating from experience in coronary care units, in which control of electrical activity of the heart has affected mortality favorably, it would appear that the incidence of sudden death in the community might be reduced substantially by prophylactic therapy in populations at particularly high risk, if such therapy could be demonstrated to be effective, of low toxicity, and convenient to the patient.

Other causes of sudden death Sudden cardiovascular collapse may result from a number of disorders other than coronary arteriosclerosis (Table 34-1). Severe aortic stenosis (congenital or acquired) with sudden arrhythmias or pump failure, and myocarditis or cardiomyopathy associated with arrhythmia may be responsible. Massive pulmonary embolism leads to circulatory collapse and death within minutes in approximately 10 percent of patients; some of the remainder succumb gradually with progressive right ventricular failure. Acute circulatory collapse may be presaged by smaller emboli occurring at variable intervals before the lethal attack. Accordingly, implementation of therapy during the premonitory sublethal phase, including anticoagulant administration (Chap. 256), may be lifesaving. Sublethal emboli are common in hospitalized patients and can be recognized in at least 40 percent of postmortem examinations when specialized pulmonary arterial injection techniques are utilized. Their clinical manifestations include unexplained or disproportionate dyspnea or tachypnea, hypoxemia, respiratory alkalosis, and hypocapnia. Sinus tachycardia is common. Atrial flutter, chaotic atrial rhythms, and multiple premature atrial beats are compatible with the diagnosis; thrombophlebitis or conditions predisposing to it are also helpful, suggestive signs.

Sudden death with cardiovascular collapse is a rare but always potential complication of bacterial endocarditis (Chap. 127). In this condition it is usually due to relentless progression of congestive heart failure, but it may also result from ventricular fibrillation, complete atrioventricular block, rupture of a sinus of Valsalva, or a septic embolus to the cerebral or coronary vessels.

Less common causes of sudden death have been recognized increasingly in recent years. Primary degeneration of the atrioventricular conduction system, with or without deposition of calcium or cartilage, may lead to sudden death in the absence of severe coronary atherosclerosis. Trifascicular atrioventricular (AV) block is often seen in these conditions, which account for more than two-thirds of the cases of chronic AV block in adults (Chap. 234). Patients in whom the degree of block is unstable are particularly susceptible to more serious brady- or tachyarrhythmias. Electrocardiographic QT interval prolongation, nerve deafness, and autosomal recessive inheritance seem to be associated with a high

TABLE 34-1
Conditions associated with cardiovascular collapse and sudden deaths in adults

- Ischemic heart disease secondary to coronary atherosclerosis
- Valvular heart disease, especially aortic stenosis
- Bacterial endocarditis
- Myocarditis
- Cardiomyopathies (primary myocardial disease)
- Ruptured or dissecting aortic aneurysm
- Coronary embolism
- Congenital coronary artery disease
- Hereditary QT interval prolongation
- Sinoatrial node disease
- Primary degeneration of the conduction system
- Secondary disease of the conduction system (e.g., amyloid, sarcoid, hemochromatosis, thrombotic thrombocytopenic purpura, myotonia dystrophica)
- Cerebrovascular accident, particularly hemorrhage
- Pulmonary thromboembolism
- Drug toxicity or idiosyncrasy (e.g., digitalis, quinidine)

proportion of cases of ventricular fibrillation. The same electrocardiographic abnormality and electrophysiologic instability without nerve deafness appear to be inherited in an autosomal dominant mode. Electrocardiographic changes in these disorders may be manifest only after exercise, so they may be more important causes of sudden death than has been generally recognized. Sinoatrial arrest or block with depression of lower pacemakers may also lead to asystole. Sudden rupture of a papillary muscle, the ventricular septum, or free wall, usually occurring within the first few days following acute myocardial infarction, occasionally causes sudden death (Chap. 240). Sudden cardiovascular collapse is also a major, frequently the terminal, event in patients with major cerebrovascular accidents (Chap. 326), sudden alterations of intracranial pressure, or lesions affecting the brainstem. It may also occur with asphyxia, and the toxicity of cardioactive drugs such as digitalis and quinidine may result in life-threatening arrhythmias, leading to sudden cardiovascular collapse and, if not treated immediately, to death (Chap. 235).

Electrophysiologic mechanisms underlying sudden death Available data suggest that potentially lethal ventricular arrhythmias in patients with acute myocardial infarction result from (1) enhanced automaticity of His-Purkinje fibers, (2) reentry due to locally impaired conduction of excitability, which is facilitated when temporal dispersion of the refractory periods is present in adjacent regions of myocardium and conduction velocity is depressed; (3) possible focal reexcitation from current flow between adjacent cells repolarized at disparate times. Local myocardial ischemia, electrolyte and pH changes, nonhomogeneous catecholamine release, elevated circulating free fatty acid levels, and digitalis or quinidine toxicity may affect the refractory period and conduction velocity and contribute to electrical instability.

The so-called *vulnerable period,* corresponding to the ascending limb of the T wave (Chap. 236), represents that portion of the cardiac cycle when temporal dispersion of ventricular refractoriness is normally maximum and, accordingly, when reentrant rhythms leading to sustained, repetitive activity can be initiated most readily. In patients with acute myocardial infarction, the vulnerable period is prolonged and the intensity of stimulus required to evoke repetitive tachycardia or ventricular fibrillation is reduced, so that a single ventricular premature contraction may initiate the rhythm. Electrical shocks of low energy or even striking a blow over the precordium ("thumpversion") may terminate ventricular tachycardia, presumably by interrupting a reentrant pathway. Since paroxysms of ventricular ectopic beats progressively increase asynchrony of recovery, such paroxysms frequently augur ventricular fibrillation. In addition, since temporal dispersion of refractoriness may be increased in the presence of a slow heart rate, profound bradycardia due to decreased automaticity of the sinus node or AV block may also be particularly dangerous in patients with acute myocardial infarction. Increased automaticity of subsidiary ectopic pacemakers, driven by myocardial catecholamine release, may contribute further to the development of chaotic ventricular rhythms. Electrophysiologic derangements tend to occur with greatest frequency early following the onset of myocardial infarction. They cause the majority of instantaneous deaths, but they may also occur suddenly and unexpectedly later in the course of an apparently uncomplicated hospitalization.

Asystole is a less common electrophysiologic mechanism underlying sudden death due to coronary atherosclerosis. It may occur when subsidiary pacemakers fail to perform adequately, when impulse formation in the sinus node is deranged, or when AV block precludes supraventricular initiation of the heartbeat.

Factors associated with increased risk of sudden death in nonhospitalized persons When electrocardiograms are recorded for 24 hr during the course of normal activities, supraventricular premature contractions are found to occur in most American men over fifty years of age, ventricular premature contractions and complex ventricular arrhythmias occur in almost two-thirds, and persistent or transient conduction defects in less than 10 percent. Supraventricular arrhythmias do not appear to be associated with increased risk of sudden death. On the other hand, conduction abnormalities and certain types of ventricular premature beats, such as those increased or evoked by exercise or cigarette smoking, those originating from the left ventricle (recognizable by their terminal anterior and rightward vectors), those occurring during the vulnerable period, and those occurring in pairs or salvos do appear to be associated with an increased risk. In general, electrocardiographic findings which may be particularly ominous in the presence of acute ischemia are of less significance in the absence of an acute process. In the asymptomatic patient, ventricular premature contractions should alert the physician to look for more definitive evidence of heart disease, such as other electrocardiographic abnormalities, hypertension, or a history of angina. However, in the absence of such findings, isolated ventricular premature contractions, without the dangerous characteristics described above, probably imply little additional risk.

Overt coronary artery disease, hypertension, or diabetes mellitus is present in more than 75 percent of persons dying suddenly, and, perhaps more significantly, the incidence of sudden death in persons with at least one of the three abnormalities is substantially increased. More than 75 percent of men without known prior coronary artery disease who die suddenly exhibit at least two of the following four risk factors: hypercholesterolemia, hypertension, hyperglycemia, and cigarette smoking. Although cigarette smoking may not augment the atherogenic process, the incidence of sudden death is higher in cigarette smokers than in nonsmokers, perhaps because of the known effects of nicotine on catecholamine and fatty acid metabolism. The proclivity of cigarette smoking to cause sudden death is not cumulative and appears to be entirely reversible when smoking is discontinued. Even though ventricular premature contractions may be increased or made overt by exercise, sudden death generally is not related to unusual exertion. Cardiovascular collapse on exertion occurs occasionally in patients with ischemic heart disease undergoing exercise testing or training, but with appropriate personnel and facilities these episodes respond promptly to electrical defibrillation. Rarely also, acute emotional stress may precipitate acute myocardial infarction and sudden death.

PREVENTION OF SUDDEN DEATH Some patients have prodromata, usually the new development of angina pectoris or an increase in the severity of previously existing angina (Chap. 240), in the weeks or months preceding acute myocardial infarction, and therefore these symptoms also often precede sudden cardiovascular collapse. As already stated, the presence of certain forms of ventricular premature contractions may characterize patients particularly susceptible to sudden death. Although identification of patients at high risk is particularly important, selection of an effective prophylactic regimen remains difficult, and none has clearly demonstrated effectiveness in reducing the risk. For example, although procaine amide is effective in suppressing ventricular arrhythmias in patients in the coronary care unit, drug toxicity militates against its routine prolonged use in a general ambulatory population. Nevertheless, it is reasonable to propose a trial of prophylactic treatment, on an individual basis, of patients with known or suspected coronary artery disease who have recurrent, "hazardous" ventricular contractions and the electrocardiographic characteristics described above. Quinidine gluconate, 330 mg by mouth every 6 hr, is frequently effective in suppressing these arrhythmias. The dose may be increased up to 3 g per day if necessary unless gastrointestinal disturbance or electrocardiographic evidence of toxicity occurs. The long-acting preparation has the obvious advantage of requiring relatively infrequent dose schedules (b.i.d. or t.i.d.). Patients who tolerate quinidine poorly may do well with procaine amide, 500 mg by mouth every 4 hr. However, the incomplete knowledge regarding the pathogenesis of sudden death makes rational prophylactic drug selection and dosage difficult at this time and a stereotyped regimen for all patients impractical.

Delays by the patient, physician, and transportation system and in the emergency room after the occurrence of acute myocardial infarction are the major impediments to prevention of sudden death. The median elapsed time between onset of symptoms and hospitalization averages 5 to 8 hr in most areas of the United States. Indecision by patient and physician and denial by the patient of the seriousness of his condition contribute most to total delay. The availability of special ambulances (mobile coronary care units) equipped and staffed to handle acute cardiac emergencies appears to reduce delay by increasing community and physician awareness of the urgency of prompt medical attention. Such ambulances can also be effective in resuscitating a small fraction of the patients who have undergone cardiovascular collapse. However, the hospital emergency room and its coronary care unit must also be prepared to accept and to handle expeditiously and effectively new patients with potential myocardial infarction.

Therefore, providing instructions to susceptible persons on how to seek medical care on an emergency basis upon the development of symptoms of myocardial infarction is of great importance in the prevention of sudden cardiac death. This strategy includes educating the patient to the fact that prompt entry into an effective emergency care system is not only correct but also what the physician expects of the patient, regardless of whether symptoms suggestive of myocardial infarction (Chap. 240) occur during the day or night; this concept may mean instructing the patient to contact the emergency care system directly if the physician is not immediately available.

APPROACH TO THE PATIENT WITH SUDDEN CARDIOVASCULAR COLLAPSE Sudden death can often be averted even when cardiovascular collapse has occurred. In patients experiencing sudden onset of ventricular fibrillation without prior ventricular failure (primary ventricular fibrillation) while they are under observation in the operating room, the cardiac catheterization laboratory, or the coronary care unit, correction of the arrhythmia is the rule, and the outcome is usually favorable. However, prompt application of definitive therapy for sudden cardiovascular collapse in the community entails formidable, practical obstacles, as outlined above.

The development of transvenous and transthoracic cardiac pacemakers, (Chap. 234), external countershock units (Chap. 236), and the improvement of cardiopulmonary resuscitative maneuvers, including external cardiac massage coupled with artificial respiration, have contributed to effective therapy.

When a patient under close medical observation develops sudden collapse from an arrhythmia, the immediate goal must be restoration of effective cardiac rhythm. Circulatory collapse must be recognized and confirmed immediately. Its cardinal features are (1) impaired cerebration, syncope, and seizures, (2) absent peripheral arterial pulses, and (3) absent heart sounds. When ventilation immediately preceding the collapse has been adequate, cyanosis may be absent or minimal. Since external cardiac massage can provide only limited cardiac output, definitive restoration of effective rhythm should be the immediate goal, and in the absence of evidence to the contrary, abrupt circulatory collapse should be assumed to be due to ventricular fibrillation. If the physician sees the patient within 60 sec of the collapse, time should not be wasted by attempting to achieve oxygenation. An immediate *blow to the precordium* ("thumpversion") may be attempted, since this is occasionally effective and takes only moments. *Electrical defibrillation* (Chap. 236) should be attempted immediately thereafter, without necessarily even pausing first to record an electrocardiogram. Maximum electrical output—usually 400 watt-sec—should be used. If these immediate attempts are unsuccessful, *external cardiac massage* and complete cardiopulmonary resuscitation should be brought into play.

If collapse is due to unequivocal asystole, transthoracic or transvenous *electrical pacing* should be implemented immediately. Intracardiac ephinephrine, 1 ml of 1:1,000 diluted 1:10 with intracavitary blood, may facilitate the heart's response to artificial pacing or be helpful when a slow ventricular focus is present but ineffective. If these initial definitive measures fail despite adequate technical performance, prompt restitution of a favorable metabolic milieu and monitoring are necessary. This is best accomplished by (1) expeditious endotracheal intubation and ventilation; (2) external cardiac massage; (3) correction of acid-base balance, usually requiring intravenous sodium bicarbonate administration (44 mEq intravenously every 5 to 10 min during the arrest period); and (4) assessment and correction of electrolyte imbalance. Definitive efforts to restore an effective cardiac rhythm should be attempted again as soon as possible, certainly within minutes. When effective cardiac rhythm is restored but rapidly degenerates again into ventricular tachycardia or fibrillation, lidocaine should be administered as a bolus, 100 mg intravenously, continued by intravenous infusion at a rate up to 300 mg per hr, and countershock repeated.

Cardiac massage External cardiac massage is designed to lead to the ejection of blood from the heart by manual compression of the ventricles between the sternum and the spine, and cyclic passive ventricular filling. Adherence to several aspects of technique is essential (Fig. 34-1). (1) The patient should be placed supine on a firm surface (a wooden board beneath his back serves well). (2) The frequency of external massage should approximate one per second. (3) The resuscitator's waist must be higher than the patient's chest in order to permit him to administer the necessary force, since approximately a 100-lb force applied with the heel of the hand to the sternum of an adult male is required to depress the anterior chest wall the necessary 5 cm per beat. (4) Depression and release of the chest wall should be smooth, with each occupying 50 percent of the cycle, since sudden compression may elicit a pressure wave palpable at the femoral or carotid artery but may eject little blood. (5) Massage should not be interrupted, even momentarily, since cardiac output increases cumulatively during the first 8 to 10 compressions and even brief interruptions are extended by the time required for cumulation. (6) Ventilations should be continued at a frequency of about 12 per min and monitored by arterial blood gas analyses.

Each external cardiac compression limits venous return, and the optimal anticipated cardiac index during external massage approximates only 40 percent of the lower limit of normal, well below that seen in most patients after spontaneous ventricular contractions have returned or have been induced by ventricular pacing. Therefore, prompt restoration of effective cardiac rhythm is essential. Rarely, organized electrocardiographic activity, unaccompanied by effective cardiac contraction (electromechanical dissociation), may occur and respond to intracardiac epinephrine (1 ml of 1:1,000 solution diluted 1:10 with blood) or calcium gluconate (1 g). Cardiac massage should be terminated as soon as effective cardiac contractions, initiated spontaneously or by ventricular pacing, serve to produce a detectable pulse and systemic arterial blood pressure. Subsequent treatment of arrhythmias and hypotension and adjustment of intravascular volume should be guided by the same general principles underlying their management in circulatory collapse due to cardiogenic shock (Chap. 240).

The therapeutic approach outlined above is based on several considerations: (1) irreversible brain damage often occurs after a few (approximately four) minutes of circulatory collapse; (2) the likelihood of restoring effective cardiac rhythm and successfully resuscitating the patient diminishes rapidly with time; (3) 80 to 90 percent survival can be anticipated in patients developing *primary* ventricular fibrillation, such as those undergoing cardiac catheterization or exercise testing, in whom definitive treatment is prompt; (4) survival rates in the general hospital setting are much lower, approximately 20 percent, depending in part on the coexisting or underlying disease process; (5) survival rates in the community approach zero, probably because of unavoidable delays in initiating definitive therapy and limitations of equipment and available personnel; and (6) external cardiac massage can provide only a limited cardiac output. Thus, *when circulatory collapse is a primary event, therapy must be directed toward prompt restoration of effective cardiac rhythm.*

Complications External cardiac massage is not free from significant complications, including rib fracture, hemothorax, pneumothorax, liver laceration, fat embolus, and ruptured spleen with late, occult blood loss. How-

FIGURE 34-1
External cardiac massage. A *Position of hands during application of external cardiac massage.* B *When pressure is applied, the lower portion of the sternum is displaced posteriorly with the palm of the hand.* C *In order to apply maximal downward pressure the resuscitator leans far forward, so that his arms are at right angles to the sternum.*

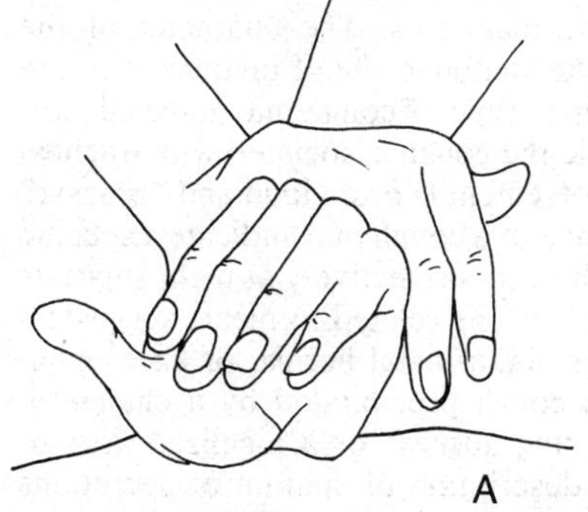

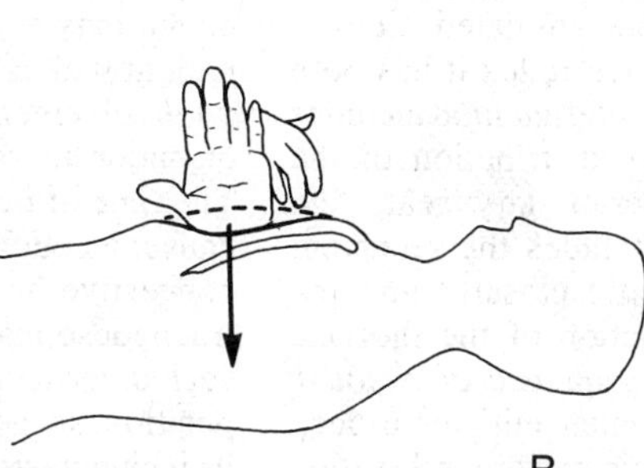

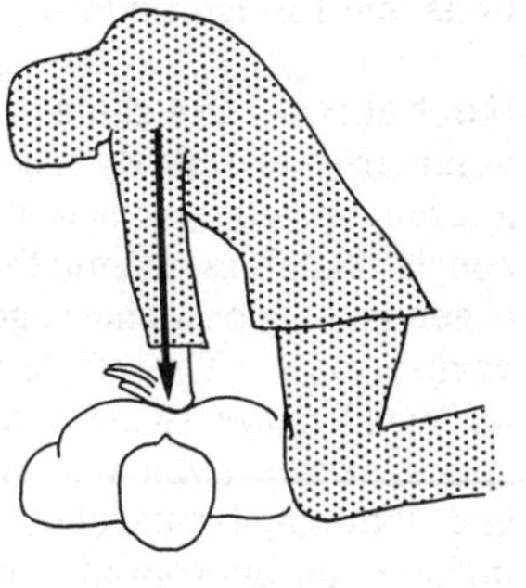

ever, these complications can be minimized by proper technique and if appropriately considered they can be readily recognized and often managed effectively. The decision to terminate unsuccessful cardiopulmonary resuscitation is always difficult. In general, if effective cardiac rhythm has not been restored and if the patient's pupils are fixed and dilated despite 30 min or more of cardiac massage, a successful resuscitation cannot be expected.

An important challenge to the medical system is to provide trained medical or paramedical personnel immediately for patients who develop sudden cardiovascular collapse. The development of appropriately staffed "rescue stations" in large factories, office buildings, and sports arenas is one approach that has been proposed, but its effectiveness is yet to be demonstrated. It is likely that the identification of individuals at high risk and the application of effective preventive measures to this segment of the population will be more satisfactory.

REFERENCES

GORDON T, KANNEL WB: Premature mortality from coronary heart disease. JAMA 215:1617, 1971

HINKLE LE, JR et al: The frequency of asymptomatic disturbances of cardiac rhythm and conduction in middle-aged men. Am J Cardiol 24:629, 1969

JUDE JR: Cardiac arrest, in *Davis-Christopher Textbook of Surgery,* ed DC Sabiston, Jr., Philadelphia: Saunders, 1972, p. 1920

LOVELL RRH, PRINEAS RJ: Mechanisms of sudden death and their implications for prevention and management. Prog Cardiovasc Dis 13:483, 1971

LOWN B, WOLF M: Approaches to sudden death from coronary heart disease. Circulation 44:130, 1971

35 COUGH AND HEMOPTYSIS

GENNARO M. TISI
EUGENE BRAUNWALD

COUGH Cough, one of the most frequent cardiorespiratory symptoms, is an explosive expiration which provides a means of clearing the tracheobronchial tree of secretions and foreign bodies.

Mechanism Coughing may be initiated either voluntarily or reflexly. As a defensive reflex it has both afferent and efferent pathways. The *afferent limb* includes cough receptors within the sensory distribution of the trigeminal, glossopharyngeal, superior laryngeal, and vagus nerves. The *efferent limb* includes the recurrent laryngeal nerve (which causes glottic closure) and the spinal nerves (which cause contraction of the thoracic and abdominal musculature). The *sequence of a cough* includes an appropriate stimulus which initiates a deep inspiration. This is followed by glottic closure, relaxation of the diaphragm, and muscle contraction against a closed glottis so as to produce maximally positive intrathoracic and intraairway pressures. These positive intrathoracic pressures result in a narrowing of the trachea, produced by an infolding of its more compliant posterior membrane. Once the glottis opens, the combination of a large pressure differential between the airways and the atmosphere coupled with this tracheal narrowing produces flow rates through the trachea close to the speed of sound. The shearing forces which are developed aid in the elimination of mucus and foreign materials. A tracheostomy short-circuits glottic closure and therefore decreases the effectiveness of the cough mechanism.

Etiology Cough is produced by inflammatory, mechanical, chemical, and thermal stimulation of the cough receptors. *Inflammatory* stimuli are initiated by edema and hyperemia of the respiratory mucous membranes, and by irritation from exudative processes. Such stimuli may arise either in the airways (as in laryngitis, tracheitis, bronchitis, and bronchiolitis) or in the alveoli (as in pneumonitis and lung abscess). *Mechanical* stimuli are produced by inhalation of particulate matter, such as dust particles, and by compression of the air passages and pressure or tension upon these structures. Lesions associated with airway compression may be either extramural or intramural in type. The former include aortic aneurysms, granulomas, pulmonary neoplasms, and mediastinal tumors; intramural lesions include bronchogenic carcinoma, bronchial adenoma, foreign bodies, granulomatous endobronchial involvement, and contraction of airway smooth muscle (bronchial asthma). Pressure or tension upon the air passages is usually produced by lesions associated with a decrease in pulmonary compliance. Examples of specific causes include acute and chronic interstitial fibrosis (Chap. 254), pulmonary edema, and atelectasis. *Chemical* stimuli may result from inhalation of irritant gases, including cigarette smoke, and of chemical fumes. Finally, *thermal* stimuli may be produced by inhalation of either very hot or cold air.

Diagnostic evaluation When one is considering the above list of causes, answers to the following general questions will significantly narrow the diagnostic possibilities: Is the cough acute or chronic? Is it productive of sputum or nonproductive? Are the findings on physical examination of the chest normal or abnormal? Is the chest roentgenogram normal or abnormal?

Features of the history, physical examination, chest roentgenogram, screening pulmonary function studies (static lung volumes and dynamic flow rates), and sputum examination may indicate a specific cause. The *history* may indicate specific diagnoses. The character of the cough may suggest the anatomic site of involvement: the patient with a "barking" type of cough may have epiglottal involvement, while the cough associated with tracheal or major airway involvement is often loud and "brassy." The time of occurrence of a cough may indicate a specific cause: a cough which occurs selectively at night suggests congestive heart failure; one related to meals suggests a tracheoesophageal fistula, a hiatal hernia, or an esophageal diverticulum; a cough precipitated by a change in position suggests a lung abscess or a localized area of bronchiectasis. The description of sputum or secretions produced in conjunction with the cough may also be helpful: putrid sputum suggests a lung abscess; bloody sputum, bleeding (see Hemoptysis, further on); frothy and pink-tinged sputum, pulmonary edema; mucoid and massive sputum, alveolar cell carcinoma; purulent and/or large amounts of sputum, lung abscess and bronchiectasis. On *physical examination* the character of the auscultatory findings may suggest the site of disease: inspiratory stridor and wheezing may be present in laryngeal disease; inspiratory and expiratory rhonchi favor tracheal and major airway involvement; coarse subcrepitant inspiratory rales may indicate interstitial fibrosis and/or edema; fine crepitant rales may indicate a process such as pneumonitis or pulmonary edema, which fills the alveoli with fluid. The *chest roentgenogram* may show an intrapulmonary mass lesion which may be either central or peripheral, an alveolar filling process which may be pneumonic or nonpneumonic, an area of honeycombing and cyst formation which may indicate an area of localized bronchiectasis, or bilateral hilar adenopathy which may indicate sarcoidosis or a lymphoma. *Screening pulmonary function* studies may also indicate specific diagnoses. Significant expiratory obstruction to airflow (as determined from a forced expiratory flow maneuver), coupled with a history of cough and significant sputum production, indicates that irrespective of other lesions the patient has significant bronchitis. Decreased lung volume (as determined from the static lung volumes) indicates that a restrictive type of lung disease is present—reduction of lung volumes produced by thoracic, pleural, alveolar, or interstitial disease. Finally, a careful *sputum examination* may be more enlightening than a patient's description of the character of his sputum. Examination shows whether the sputum is thin or viscid, purulent or not, foul-smelling or not, blood tinged or not, scant or copious. Gram stain and culture of a deep-cough specimen may reveal a specific bacterial, fungal, or mycoplasmal causation, while sputum cytology may result in a positive diagnosis of a pulmonary neoplasm.

Two features of cough should be highlighted. (1) A cough is often so common in the cigarette smoker as to be ignored or minimized. *Any changes in the nature and character of a chronic cigarette cough should initiate immediate diagnostic evaluation, with particular attention directed to detection of bronchogenic carcinoma.* (2) Female patients are inclined to swallow sputum and not to expectorate as male patients do. This tendency may lead to the incorrect conclusion that a cough in a female patient is irritative and nonproductive.

Complications Three complications may be produced by the coughing mechanism: paroxysms of coughing may precipitate syncope (cough syncope, Chap. 16), and strenuous coughing may produce rupture of an emphysematous bleb and rib fractures. A potential mechanism for cough syncope includes the development of markedly positive intrathoracic and alveolar pressures which decrease venous return, producing a decrease in cardiac output and resultant syncope. Although cough fractures of the ribs may occur in otherwise normal patients, their occurrence should at least raise the possibility of pathologic fractures, which are seen in multiple myeloma, osteoporosis, and osteolytic metastases.

Therapy Specific treatment of cough depends upon the underlying cause. An irritative, nonproductive cough may be suppressed by an antitussive agent, such as codeine or dextromethorphan, 15 mg q.i.d. These drugs are particularly useful in interrupting prolonged, self-perpetuating paroxysms. However, a cough productive of significant quantities of sputum should not be suppressed, since retention of sputum in the tracheobronchial tree may interfere with alveolar aeration and impair the ability of the lung to resist infection. When secretions are tenacious and thick, adequate hydration, expectorants (such as potassium iodide), and humidification of the air with steam are helpful.

HEMOPTYSIS For purposes of definition hemoptysis includes both blood-streaked sputum and gross hemoptysis. It is apparent that any patient with gross hemoptysis should be given appropriate diagnotic tests so that a specific cause may be found. The condition of the patient with blood-streaked sputum should also be studied unless one can be certain that this type of hemoptysis is due to a benign condition. A major pitfall in dealing with hemoptysis is to ascribe recurrent episodes of hemoptysis to a previously established diagnosis, such as chronic bronchiectasis or bronchitis. Such an approach may result in missing a potentially treatable lesion. The safest approach to a recurrent episode of hemoptysis is to treat it as if it were the initial episode and proceed with a complete diagnostic evaluation.

Etiology and incidence Prior to embarking upon an extensive diagnostic workup of hemoptysis, it is essential to determine that the blood is in fact coming from the respiratory tract, not from the nasopharynx or gastrointestinal tract. Once this point is established, the diagnostic tests for hemoptysis may proceed. Although there are numerous single case reports of diseases which have been associated with hemoptysis, Table 35-1 presents the more common disorders.

The incidence of the diagnoses listed in Table 35-1 depends upon the nature of the series reported and whether one includes both gross bleeding and blood streaking of the sputum. If both types of bleeding are included, then the major causes (approximately 60 to 70 percent) are chronic bronchitis and bronchiectasis. If the definition is restricted to gross bleeding (greater than several tablespoons) then the incidence depends upon the type of series reported. Surgical series favor the incidence of mass lesions and operable lesions (carcinoma, 20 percent; bronchiectasis, 30 percent). Those from centers with a large tuberculosis population favor this condition (incidence varying between 2 and 40 percent). Combined medical-surgical series include a wider representation of those lesions which present with hemoptysis (carcinoma, 20 percent; bronchiectasis, 30 percent; bronchitis, 15 percent; other inflammatory lesions including tuberculosis, 10 to 20 percent; other lesions including the vascular, traumatic, and hemorrhagic etiologies listed in Table 35-1, 10 percent). Despite the most extensive of

TABLE 35-1
Causes of hemoptysis

1 Inflammatory
 a Bronchitis
 b Bronchiectasis
 c Lung abscess
 d Pneumonia
 e Tuberculosis
2 Neoplastic
 a Bronchogenic carcinoma
 b Bronchial adenoma
3 Vascular
 a Left ventricular failure
 b Mitral stenosis
 c Pulmonary thromboembolism
 d Primary pulmonary hypertension
 e Arteriovenous malformations
 f Eisenmenger's syndrome
 g Pulmonary vasculitis: Wegener's granulomatosis and Goodpasture's syndrome
4 Traumatic
 a Foreign body
 b Lung contusion
5 Hemorrhagic
 a Hemorrhagic diathesis
 b Anticoagulant therapy

evaluations, 5 to 15 percent of cases entailing gross hemoptysis remain undiagnosed.

Two points should be highlighted with reference to diseases associated with hemoptysis: (1) *hemoptysis is rare in metastatic carcinoma to the lung;* (2) *although hemoptysis may occur at some time during the course of a viral or bacterial pneumonia, it is usually scanty and its occurrence should always raise the question of a more serious underlying process.*

Diagnosis The *history* may suggest specific diagnoses: recurrent, chronic hemoptysis in a young, otherwise asymptomatic female favors the diagnosis of a bronchial adenoma; recurrent hemoptysis with chronic, marked sputum production associated with honeycombing and cyst formation on the roentgenogram suggests a diagnosis of bronchiectasis; putrid sputum production suggests a lung abscess; weight loss and anorexia in a male smoker over the age of forty years raises the possibility of a bronchogenic carcinoma; a recent history of blunt trauma to the chest suggests a lung contusion; and acute pleuritic chest pain raises the possibility of a pulmonary embolism or some other pleurally based lesion (lung abscess, coccidiomycosis cavity, and vasculitis). Several findings on the *physical examination* may also suggest a specific diagnosis: a pleural friction rub suggests those diagnoses just mentioned in connection with pleuritic pain; the findings of pulmonary hypertension raise the diagnostic possibilities of primary pulmonary hypertension, mitral stenosis, recurrent or chronic thromboembolism, and Eisenmenger's syndrome; a localized wheeze over a major lobar airway suggests an intramural lesion such as a bronchogenic carcinoma or a foreign body; systemic arteriovenous communications suggest the diagnosis of Osler-Weber-Rendu disease with pulmonary AV malformation; evidence of significant expiratory obstruction to airflow coupled with sputum production suggests that whatever other lesion may be present, the patient has significant bronchitis. Finally, the *chest roentgenogram* is critical to diagnosis. The presence of honeycombing favors a diagnosis of bronchiectasis; an air-fluid level, the diagnosis of a lung abscess; and a mass lesion, the diagnosis of a central or peripheral pulmonary neoplasm. A mass lesion which may cause hemoptysis should be distinguished from an area of blood pneumonitis caused by aspiration of blood into contiguous areas.

One of the most demanding diagnostic problems is the identification of the side of bleeding in a patient with normal findings on physical examination and a normal roentgenogram of the chest. A patient with hemoptysis tends to keep the bleeding side dependent. If he did not do this, gravitational drainage would cause aspiration into the noninvolved dependent lung. The patient may also be able to give a history of a burning or deep pain which may localize the side of bleeding; bronchoscopy may then be helpful. This procedure generally is most helpful when the bleeding is scant, and of least help when the bleeding is massive, since blood may be aspirated into contiguous airways.

Following the history and physical examination, the diagnostic approach to a patient with hemoptysis includes whatever specialized studies and procedures are required to make a specific diagnosis. The first step is to obtain a roentgenogram. Usually bronchoscopy is the procedure employed next. This endoscopic technique may provide definitive visual, biopsy, or cytologic information. Bronchography is also frequently employed, especially in view of the high incidence of bronchiectasis, but is not useful when there is evidence of active inflammation. It is most helpful when an area of abnormality is identified on the chest roentgenogram. Other frequently employed diagnostic techniques include thoracentesis and pleural biopsy, sputum cytology and bacteriology, tomography, lung scintiphotoscans, and pulmonary angiography. The use of each of these techniques is determined by the clinical presentation.

Therapy Since hemoptysis is such an alarming symptom, there is a tendency to overtreat the patient. Usually hemoptysis is scant and will stop spontaneously without specific therapy. If the hemoptysis is substantial, the mainstays of therapy include keeping the patient calm, instituting complete bed rest, excluding unnecessary diagnostic procedures until the hemoptysis has begun to subside, and suppressing cough if it is present and an aggravating feature of the hemoptysis. Fatal hemoptysis due to exsanguination is very infrequent except in Goodpasture's syndrome, in which it is a common cause of death. The major threat of gross hemoptysis is massive aspiration. Here the objectives of therapy are to stop the bleeding, support the patient's vital signs, and prevent airway obstruction from aspiration. The emergency care of such a patient demands that intubation and suctioning equipment be at the bedside. Management of potentially lethal hemorrhage raises the possibilities of emergency surgical resection. Collapse therapy seems to have little justification today, and surgical resection requires precise identification of the site of bleeding.

REFERENCES

BATES DV et al: *Respiratory Function in Disease,* p. 584 ff, Philadelphia: Saunders, 1971

COMMITTEE ON ETIOLOGY OF CHRONIC BRONCHITIS, MEDICAL RESEARCH COUNCIL: Definition and classification of chronic bronchitis. Lancet 1:775, 1965

COMMITTEE ON THERAPY, AMERICAN THORACIC SOCIETY: The management of hemoptysis. Am Rev Resp Dis 93:471, 1966

LOUDON RG, SHAW GB: Mechanics of cough in normal subjects and in patients with obstructive respiratory disease. Am Rev Resp Dis 96:666, 1967

MAC BRYDE CM, BLACKLOW RS: *Signs and Symptoms,* 5th ed., Philadelphia: Lippincott, 1970, p. 324

section 5 | Alterations in gastrointestinal function

36 ORAL MANIFESTATIONS OF DISEASE

PAUL GOLDHABER

DISTURBANCES OF THE JAWS, TEETH, AND DENTAL TISSUES

DEVELOPMENTAL DISTURBANCES The most serious and common developmental disturbance of the jaws is *cleft palate* (approximately 1 per 1,000 births), which ordinarily presents as a large continuous defect in the midline of the hard and soft palates connecting the nasal and oral cavities and leads to difficulties in eating, drinking, and speech. In mild cases only the soft palate is involved. In more severe cases, the defect may extend anteriorly and follow the line of fusion to the left or right between the premaxilla and the maxilla, producing, in addition, a cleft of the alveolar ridge between the lateral incisor and cuspid, and a cleft lip (*harelip*). Surgery for cleft palate is ordinarily delayed until the patient is about 1½ years old in order to avoid injury to the growth centers in the maxilla. An obturator may be used to close the defect if the cleft is too large. Since tooth structure, unlike bone, does not undergo physiologic remodeling, developmental disturbances severe enough to cause obvious alterations in the morphologic features or integrity of the teeth provide relatively permanent evidence that a systemic disturbance has acted during that particular phase of tooth development.

The most common type of defect is *enamel hypoplasia,* which results from an aberration in enamel formation due to disturbance of those ameloblasts actively secreting enamel matrix. The defects range from deep pits or grooves extending horizontally around the surface of the crown to defective or completely absent incisal edges or occlusal surfaces. The systemic factors thought to be involved are serious gastrointestinal disturbances and deficiencies of calcium, phosphorus, or vitamins A and B.

Mottled enamel is a form of hypoplasia due to excessive fluoride ingestion. It consists of white spotting of the enamel or, in more severe forms, of pitting, brownish staining, and brittleness. It should be noted that these effects occur at levels of fluoride significantly higher than that recommended for the artificial fluoridation of drinking water in order to prevent dental caries.

Amelogenesis imperfecta is a hereditary condition in which enamel is absent or is thin, brown, and easily fractured. *Dentinogenesis imperfecta,* also hereditary and usually associated with *osteogenesis imperfecta,* affects the dentin rather than the enamel, giving the teeth a characteristic translucence. Because the union between the dentin and enamel is defective, the latter chips easily, exposing the underlying dentin, which rapidly wears down or fractures.

Congenital syphilis may give rise to characteristic "screwdriver" upper central incisors with notched incisal edges (Hutchinson's incisors) and first molars with rough, pitted occlusal surfaces (mulberry molars).

Complete or partial *anodontia* may occur in *hereditary ectodermal dysplasia,* a syndrome characterized by partial or complete absence of sweat glands, defective or absent sebaceous glands, hair follicles, and other ectodermal structures. When some teeth are present, they are usually cone-shaped.

Intrinsic *staining* of the teeth may be due to a number of factors. Erythroblastosis fetalis may give rise to green, brown, or blue coloration because of the deposition of blood pigment in the enamel and dentin of the developing teeth. In teeth which develop after birth, when hemolysis has ceased, the stain does not develop. A yellow-brown discoloration may be caused by the administration of *tetracycline* to infants or to women in the last trimester of pregnancy. In *congenital porphyria,* porphyrins are incorporated in the developing teeth, giving rise to a reddish-brown coloration which fluoresces red in ultraviolet light.

ODONTOGENIC TUMORS The odontogenic tumors are neoplasms derived primarily from the tissues involved in odontogenesis. The *ameloblastoma,* an example of an ectodermally derived tumor, is the most aggressive tumor in the group and may occur at any age. Most frequently, it occurs in the molar-ramus area, originating as a central lesion of bone which gradually grows and expands the bone. Although the tumor may recur following resection, the prognosis is favorable, since the tumor is slow-growing and rarely, if ever, metastasizes. The *odontomas* are mixed tumors derived from both ectoderm and mesoderm which usually form a slow-growing mass composed of numerous structures having a morphologic resemblance to miniature teeth.

DENTAL CARIES, PULPAL AND PERIAPICAL INFECTION, AND SEQUELAE Dental caries, the principal cause of tooth loss up to the fourth decade of life, is characterized by a bacteria-induced progressive destruction of the mineral and organic components of the outer enamel and underlying dentin. Numerous long-term studies have clearly shown that the artificial fluoridation of drinking water supplies to a level of 1 part per million leads to a 50 to 75 percent reduction in the occurrence of dental caries in permanent teeth of children, presumably because of an alteration of the developing enamel crystals during tooth formation which makes them more resistant to acid dissolution.

If the carious lesion progresses unchecked, there is eventual infection of the dental pulp, giving rise to an *acute pulpitis.* During the early stages of pulpitis moderately severe pain may result from thermal changes, particularly cold drinks. It is noteworthy that toothache in persons flying at high altitudes (aerondontalgia) occasionally occurs in persons having early pulpal inflammation or recently filled teeth. The cause of this phenomenon is not known. As more of the pulp becomes involved because of advanced caries, heat or reclining may stimulate the onset of even more severe and continuous pain. At this stage, damage to the pulp is irreversible, and treatment consists either of extraction or thorough removal of the remaining contents of the pulp chamber and root canals followed by sterilization and filling with an inert material (root canal therapy).

If the pulpitis is not treated, infection may spread beyond the apex of the tooth into the periodontal ligament, giving rise to pain on chewing or percussion. The most common manifestation of periapical disease is the *periapical granuloma,* a localized mass of chronic granulation tissue which slowly expands at the expense of the surrounding alveolar bone. The *chronic periapical granuloma* may present the above symptoms or may be asymptomatic. If allowed to persist untreated the periapical granuloma may give rise to a *periapical cyst* or a *periapical abscess*—all three lesions appearing as radiolucent areas on roentgenograms. The acute periapical abscess may extend into the surrounding bone marrow, resulting in an *osteomyelitis.* More frequently, the abscess perforates the cortical plate and, following the path of least resistance, spreads through various tissue spaces, giving rise to cellulitis and bacteremia, or discharges into the oral cavity, into the maxillary sinus, or through the skin.

The symptoms produced by cellulitis depend on which tissue space is affected. For example, *Ludwig's angina* originates from an infected mandibular molar, involves the submaxillary space, and subsequently extends into the sublingual and submental spaces. Clinically, this is manifested by swelling of the floor of the mouth, elevation of the tongue, and difficulty in swallowing and breathing. With continued swelling, there may be edema of the glottis, necessitating an emergency tracheotomy. Spread of the infection to the parapharyngeal spaces may lead to cavernous sinus thrombosis.

PERIODONTAL DISEASE

After the third decade chronic destructive periodontal disease (*periodontitis*) is responsible for the loss of more teeth than dental caries. It begins as a marginal inflammation of the gingivae (gingivitis), which slowly spreads to involve the underlying alveolar bone and periodontal ligament. As the disease progresses, the alveolar bone is resorbed, resulting in loss of periodontal ligament fiber attachment from the tooth to the bone. The separation of the soft tissue from the tooth surface results in "pocket" formation, the inner aspect of which bleeds readily on probing or spontaneously during chewing. Frank pus sometimes exudes from under the gingival margin, accounting for the use of the now outmoded term "pyorrhea." With continued loss of alveolar bone the involved teeth become mobile. As the periodontal pockets deepen, the pocket orifice may become occluded, leading to the formation of a *periodontal abscess.* The prognosis for teeth with advanced bone loss, extreme mobility, and recurrent abscess formation is usually poor or hopeless, and the usual treatment is extraction.

The most important local etiologic factors associated with this disease are thought to be *poor oral hygiene,* resulting in the accumulation of grossly visible adherent masses of bacteria (*bacterial plaque*), calculus (mineralized bacterial plaque), and food impaction. The margins of overextended fillings also play a role as local irritating factors. Occlusal trauma, particularly due to grinding and clenching habits, may be involved. Therapy is aimed at elimination of these factors and the development of a local environment which can be maintained in health by good oral hygiene.

Systemic factors are thought to modify the response of the host to the local factors, but their nature is more obscure. In some instances, however, there are characteristic alterations in the gingiva in response to a number of specific systemic conditions. For example, during *pregnancy* the gingiva may become edematous and friable, with a raspberry-like appearance of the interdental papillae. Occasionally, a tumorlike mass may develop in an interdental area; this usually regresses following parturition. The use of the anticonvulsant drug *diphenylhydantoin sodium* (Dilantin) frequently results in fibrous hyperplasia of the gingiva, which may actually cover the teeth, interfere with mastication, and cause a serious esthetic problem. A similar clinical picture, although usually more generalized and extensive, occurs in *idiopathic familial fibromatosis.* The latter condition appears to be hereditary.

A relatively common gingival disease, found predominantly in young adults, is *acute necrotizing ulcerative gingivitis* Vincent's infection; trench mouth). This disease is characterized by tender or painful gingivae, bleeding on pressure, and the pathognomonic sign of papillary or marginal gingival necrosis and ulceration. Clinical evidence suggests that the cause of this disease has a psychosomatic component. Vincent's infection differs from *acute herpetic gingivostomatitis,* with which it is most frequently confused, in that fever or malaise rarely develops, and patients respond rapidly to penicillin or broad-spectrum antibiotics.

It should be noted that both infected periapical lesions and periodontal disease provide potential sources of infection which may spread to other sites. Transient bacteremias have been demonstrated after simple massage of inflamed gingivae, as well as during tooth extraction. The frequent association of tooth extraction with the subsequent occurrence of subacute bacterial endocarditis has led to the prophylactic use of antibiotics in dental patients with a history of rheumatic fever or other evidence of valvular disease.

DISEASES OF THE ORAL MUCOSA AND TONGUE

HEMATOLOGIC DISTURBANCES Oral manifestations are common in both the acute and chronic forms of all types of leukemia, particularly *monocytic leukemia.* They consist of local gingival bleeding, enlargement, and necrosis. Petechiae and ulceration of the oral mucosa may also be evident. Extensive ulcerations of the gingivae, buccal mucosa, lips, soft palate, pharynx, and tonsils may also occur in *agranulocytosis.* In thrombocytopenic states multiple petechiae, ecchymoses, and bleeding gingivae may be observed. The mucous membranes of the oral cavity, including the papillae of the tongue, are atrophic in the *Plummer-Vinson syndrome* (see Chaps. 37, 281). As a result, the tongue is red, smooth, and sore, and there is difficulty in swallowing. Of interest is the finding that the atrophic mucous membranes have a predisposition toward the development of oral carcinoma. The oral symptoms in *pernicious anemia* are similar (see Chap. 305).

VITAMIN DEFICIENCIES *The oral effects of deficiency of the B group of vitamins* involve the soft tissues primarily, giving rise to reddening and ulceration of the oral mucosa and tongue, swelling and burning of the tongue, and fissuring at the corners of the lips (*angular cheilosis*). Severe vitamin C deficiency (*scurvy*) is manifested by petechiae in the oral mucosa; swollen, ulcerated, bleeding gingivae; and loosening of teeth.

PIGMENTATIONS (see Table 36-1) The spread of irregular spots or blotches or brown pigment throughout the oral mucosa, primarily the buccal mucosa, may be the first sign of *Addison's disease.* The pigmentation associated with the *Peutz-Jeghers syndrome* is readily differentiated because of its characteristic distribution around the lips, eyes, and nostrils, as well as its intraoral distribution. Both *lead poisoning* and *bismuth poisoning* may be manifested by a dark line along the gingival

TABLE 36-1
Pigmented lesions of the oral mucosa

Condition	*Usual location*	*Clinical features*	*Course*
Black hairy tongue	Dorsum of tongue	Elongation of filiform papillae of tongue, which take on a brown to black coloration	Long-lasting but may disappear spontaneously
Heavy-metal pigmentation (bismuth, mercury, lead)	Gingival margin	Thin blue-black pigmented line along gingival margin due to prior treatment for syphilis with bismuth or mercury or from accidental absorption of lead	Long-lasting
Amalgam tattoo	Gingiva and mucobuccal fold	Small blue-black pigmented areas associated with embedded amalgam particles in soft tissues; these will show up on radiographs as radiopaque particles	Remains indefinitely
Fordyce's disease	Buccal and labial mucosa	Aggregation of numerous, small yellowish spots just beneath mucosal surface; no subjective symptoms	Remains without apparent change indefinitely
Addison's disease	Any area in mouth but mostly on buccal mucosa	Blotches or spots of bluish-black to dark-brown pigmentation occurring early in the disease accompanied by diffuse pigmentation of skin; other symptoms of adrenal insufficiency	Condition controlled by steroid therapy
Peutz-Jeghers syndrome	Any area in mouth	Dark-brown spots on lips, buccal mucosa, and palate with characteristic distribution of pigment around lips, nose, eyes, and on hands; concomitant intestinal polyposis	Lesions remaining indefinitely
Malignant melanoma	Any area in mouth	May appear as a raised, painless, brown-black lesion or may be amelanotic; may be ulcerated and infected	Early metastasis leading to death

margin, particularly in individuals who have poor oral hygiene. Bismuth poisoning may also demonstrate pigmented patches elsewhere in the oral mucosa.

INFECTIONS See Tables 36-2 and 36-3 and Chap. 126.

DERMATOLOGIC DISEASES See Tables 36-2 and 36-3 and Chap. 363.

TONGUE ALTERATIONS See Table 36-4.

MALODOROUS BREATH A distinctly unpleasant odor of the breath (halitosis) may emanate from any patient with *infections of the upper part of the respiratory tract,* especially in bronchiectasis and lung abscess. Halitosis may occur with oral sepsis as in *stomatitis, gingivitis,* or extensive *caries.* Some persons who smoke excessively may have halitosis. Occasionally otherwise normal persons will have halitosis without obvious cause. A *fishy odor* of the breath is found in patients with hepatic failure, an *ammoniacal or urinary odor* is found in azotemia, and a *sweet, fruity* odor is typical of diabetic acidosis.

TABLE 36-2
Vesicular, bullous, or ulcerative lesions of the oral mucosa

Condition	*Usual location*	*Clinical features*	*Course*
Viral diseases			
Acute herpetic gingivostomatitis (herpes simplex)	Lip and oral mucosa	Labial vesicles which rupture and crust, and intraoral vesicles which quickly ulcerate; extremely painful to pressure; acute gingivitis, fever, malaise, foul odor, and cervical lymphadenopathy; occurs primarily in infants and children	Heals spontaneously in 10–14 days, unless secondarily infected
Recurrent herpes labialis	Mucocutaneous junction of lip	Eruption of groups of vesicles which may coalesce, then rupture and crust; painful to pressure or spicy foods	Lasts about 1 week, but condition may be prolonged if secondary infection occurs
Herpangina (Coxsackie A; also possibly Coxsackie B and echo viruses)	Oral mucosa, pharynx, tongue	Sudden onset of fever, sore throat, and oropharyngeal vesicles usually in children under 4 years, summer months; diffuse pharyngeal injection and vesicles (1–2 mm), grayish white surrounded by red areola; vesicles enlarge and ulcerate	Incubation period 2–9 days; fever for 1–4 days; recovery uneventful
Foot, hand, and mouth disease (Coxsackie A-16)	Oral mucosa, pharynx, palms, and soles	Fever, malaise, headache with oropharyngeal vesicles which become painful, shallow ulcers	Incubation period 2–18 days; lesions heal spontaneously in 2–4 weeks
Bacterial or fungous diseases			
Acute necrotizing ulcerative gingivitis ("trench mouth," Vincent's infection)	Gingiva	Painful, bleeding gingiva characterized by necrosis and ulceration of gingival papillae and margins plus lymphadenopathy and foul odor	Continued destruction of tissue followed by remission, but may recur
Primary syphilis (chancre)	Lesion appears where organism enters body; may occur on lips, tongue, or tonsillar area	Small papule developing rapidly into a large, painless ulcer with indurated border; unilateral lymphadenopathy; chancre and lymph nodes containing spirochetes; serologic tests positive by 3d to 4th weeks	Healing of chancre in 1–2 months, followed by secondary syphilis in 6–8 weeks
Secondary syphilis	Oral mucosa frequently involved with mucous patches, primarily on palate but also at commissures of mouth	Maculopapular lesions of oral mucosa, about 5–10 mm in diameter with central ulceration covered by grayish membrane; eruptions occurring on various mucosal surfaces and skin accompanied by fever, malaise, and sore throat	Lesions may persist from several weeks to a year
Tertiary syphilis	Palate and tongue	Gummatous infiltration of palate or tongue followed by ulceration and fibrosis; atrophy of tongue papillae may produce characteristic bald tongue and glossitis	Gumma may destroy palate, causing complete perforation
Tuberculosis	Tongue, tonsillar area, soft palate	A solitary, irregular ulcer covered by a persistent exudate; ulcer has an undermined, indurated border	Lesion may persist

TABLE 36-2
Vesicular, bullous, or ulcerative lesions of the oral mucosa *(continued)*

Condition	*Usual location*	*Clinical features*	*Course*
Bacterial or fungous diseases (continued)			
Cervicofacial actinomycosis	Swellings in region of face, neck, and floor of mouth	Infection may be associated with an extraction, jaw fracture, or eruption of molar tooth; in acute form resembles an acute pyogenic abscess, but contains yellow "sulfur granules" (gram-positive mycelia and their hyphae)	Acute form may last a few weeks; chronic form lasts months or years. Prognosis excellent. Actinomycetes respond to antibiotics (tetracyclines or penicillin) but not to anti- fungal drugs
Histoplasmosis	Any area in mouth, particularly tongue, gingiva, or palate	Numerous small nodules which may ulcerate; hoarseness and dysphagia may occur because of lesions in larynx, usually associated with fever and malaise	May be fatal
Dermatologic diseases			
Mucous membrane pemphigoid	Primarily mucous membranes of the oral cavity, but may also involve the eyes, urethra, vagina, and rectum	Painful, grayish-white collapsed vesicles or bullae with peripheral erythematous zone; gingival lesions desquamate, leaving ulcerated area	Protracted course with remissions and exacerbations; involvement of different sites occurs slowly; cortico-steroids may control severe cases
Erythema multiforme	Primarily the oral mucosa and skin of hands and feet	Intraoral ruptured bullae surrounded by an inflammatory area; lips may show hemorrhagic crusts; the "iris" or "target" lesion on the skin is pathognomonic; patient may have severe signs of toxicity	Onset very rapid; condition may last 1–2 weeks; may be fatal
Pemphigus vulgaris	Oral mucosa and skin	Ruptured bullae and ulcerated oral areas; mostly in older adults	With repeated recur-rence of bullae, toxicity may lead to cachexia, infection, and death within 2 years
Neoplastic diseases			
Squamous cell carcinoma	Any area in mouth, most commonly on lower lip, tongue, and floor of mouth	Ulcer with elevated, indurated border; failure to heal, pain not prominent; lesions tend to arise in areas of leukoplakia or in smooth or atrophic tongue	Invades and destroys underlying tissues or may metastasize to regional lymph nodes
Acute leukemia	Gingiva	Gingival swelling and superficial ulcerations followed by hyperplasia of gingiva with extensive necrosis and hemorrhage; deep ulcers may occur elsewhere on the mucosa complicated by secondary infection	Fatal
Lymphosarcoma	Gingiva, palate, tongue, and tonsillar area	Elevated, ulcerated area which may pro-liferate rapidly, giving the appearance of a traumatic inflammatory lesion; swelling of regional lymph nodes	Fatal
Other conditions			
Recurrent aphthous stomatitis	Any place on oral mucosa	Single or clusters of painful ulcers with surrounding erythematous border, found anywhere on mucosa; lesions may be 1–15 mm in diameter	Lesions heal in 1–2 weeks but may recur monthly or several times a year
Traumatic ulcers	Any place on oral mucosa; dentures frequently respon-sible for ulcers in vestibule	Localized, discrete ulcerated lesion with red border; produced by accidental biting of mucosa, penetration by a foreign object, or chronic irritation by a denture	Lesion usually heals in 7–10 days when irritant is removed, unless secondarily infected

DISEASES OF THE SALIVARY GLANDS

Conditions affecting the salivary glands include mumps parotitis (Chap. 205), Mikulicz's disease (Chap. 354), and Sjögren's syndrome (Chap. 386). Inflammation of the salivary glands (*sialadenitis*) is usually associated with the presence of a salivary stone (*sialolithiasis*) in the duct of one of the major salivary glands. The classic history of pain and swelling of the gland at mealtimes is due to the partial blockage of salivary flow by the stone. Localization of the stone may be accomplished by palpation or by roentgenograms with or without the use of an intraductal injection of radiopaque material (*sialography*). Acute or recurrent parotitis, with or without a defined microorganism, may occur in children and is marked by sudden onset of swelling of the whole gland or side of the face, accompanied by suppuration from Stenson's duct.

Xerostomia, or dryness of the mouth, is due to salivary gland dysfunction and may be temporary or permanent. Among the factors which cause temporary dryness are emotional factors (such as fear), infection of the glands, and administration of drugs, such as atropine or antihistamines. Radiation to the area may produce a more permanent xerostomia because of atrophy of the glands. A similar dryness may occur in Sjögren's syndrome.

ORAL CANCER

Oral cancer constitutes more than 5 percent of all human cancers. *Squamous cell carcinoma* is the most common malignant oral tumor, accounting for approximately 90 to 95 percent of all oral malignant tumors. Most of these tumors occur on the lips, primarily the lower lip, rather than intraorally. About half the intraoral tumors involve the tongue, primarily the posterior two-thirds and the lateral borders. The major etiologic factor in lip cancer appears to be exposure to intense sunlight. Predisposing factors for intraoral carcinoma include tobacco (usually in the form of cigar or pipe smoking, or snuff placed in the mucobuccal fold), excessive consumption of alcohol, syphilitic glossitis, and the atrophic mucosa of the Plummer-Vinson syndrome. Although numerous instances of carcinoma of the tongue adjacent to a sharp tooth or dental appliance have been reported, animal studies with chronic irritation per se, as well as epidemiologic studies, cast doubt on this apparent relationship. The most common *precancerous lesion* in the oral cavity is *leukoplakia,* a whitish patch on the mucosa that histologically shows hyperkeratosis, acanthosis, and dyskeratosis. *All chronic ulcerative lesions which fail to heal within 1 to 2 weeks should be considered potentially malignant* and must be biopsied in order to make the definitive diagnosis. It is noteworthy that in their early stages intraoral epidermoid carcinomas are rarely painful, in contrast to similar-appearing inflammatory lesions.

The prognosis for patients with carcinoma of the lip is usually good, since these malignant tumors are noted sooner and apparently metastasize later. Patients with carcinoma of the tongue have a poorer prognosis, particularly as the tumor occurs more posteriorly on the tongue. Intraoral carcinomas may spread by direct invasion to the underlying bone. Depending on the site of origin of the intraoral carcinoma, metastases usually spread to the submaxillary or cervical lymph nodes. Death may result

TABLE 36-3
White lesions of oral mucosa

Condition	*Usual location*	*Clinical features*	*Course*
Pachyderma oris	Any area in mouth	Elevated white lesion due to hyperkeratosis and thickening of the oral epithelium secondary to chronic irritation	Removal of irritant leads to healing in 2–3 weeks
Leukoplakia	Any area in mouth	White patch or raised plaque with sharply defined borders; in more severe cases the lesion is indurated and rough, and may be fissured and eroded; pain not present in early lesions	Carcinoma frequently arises in the more severe type of lesion
Lichen planus	Any area in mouth but most often on buccal mucosa	Varied appearance of lesion due to arrangement of grayish-white papules which coalesce to make up the pattern; a reticular network is most common; oral lesions may precede skin lesions	May disappear spontaneously
Moniliasis (thrush)	Any area in mouth	Creamy white curdlike patches which reveal a raw, bleeding surface when scraped; found in sick infants, debilitated elderly patients, or patients receiving high doses or corticosteroids or broad-spectrum antibiotics	Responds favorably to antifungal therapy after correction of predisposing causes
Chemical burns	Any area in mouth	White slough due to necrosis of epithelium and underlying connective tissue caused by contact with agents (e.g., aspirin) applied locally or the use of undiluted sodium perborate or hydrogen peroxide as a mouthwash; removal of slough leaves a raw, painful surface	Lesion heals in several weeks if not secondarily infected

TABLE 36-4
Alterations of the tongue

Type of change	*Clinical features*
Size or morphology changes:	
Macroglossia	Enlarged tongue which may be part of a syndrome found in developmental conditions such as Down's syndrome; may be due to tumor (hemangioma or lymphangioma), metabolic disease (such as primary amyloidosis), or endocrine disturbance (such as acromegaly or cretinism)
Fissured ("scrotal") tongue	Dorsal surface and sides of tongue covered by painless shallow or deep fissures which may collect debris and become irritated
Median rhomboid glossitis	Congenital abnormality of tongue with ovoid, denuded area in the median posterior portion of the tongue
Color Changes:	
"Geographic" tongue ("wandering rash")	Asymptomatic inflammatory condition of the tongue, with rapid loss and regrowth of filiform papillae, leading to appearance of denuded red patches "wandering" across the surface of the tongue
Hairy tongue	Elongation of filiform papillae of the medial dorsal surface area due to failure of keratin layer of the papillae to desquamate normally; brownish-black coloration may be due to staining by tobacco, food, or chromogenic organisms
"Strawberry" and "raspberry" tongue	Appearance of tongue during scarlet fever due to the hypertrophy of fungiform papillae plus changes in the filiform papillae
"Bald" tongue	Complete atrophy of papillae which may occur in pernicious anemia, severe iron-deficiency anemia, pellagra, or syphilis; may be accompanied by painful, burning sensations

from recurrent or uncontrollable disease above the clavicles; metastatic disease beyond the neck; treatment complications; or a second primary cancer, usually in the oral cavity or the upper parts of the gastrointestinal or respiratory tracts.

NEUROLOGIC DISTURBANCES

A number of neurologic disturbances have a direct effect on oral and paraoral structures. *Trigeminal neuralgia* (tic douloureux) is an example of a syndrome involving the trigeminal nerve. It is characterized by extremely severe, unilateral, lancinating pain of the face occurring spontaneously or set off by pressure on a "trigger zone" on the face. Facial palsy is a unilateral disturbance of the motor branch of the facial nerve due to either trauma, surgical sectioning, or tumor involvement. When it is of acute onset and unknown cause, possibly a localized infection in the nerve, it is called *Bell's palsy*. It may be due to cranial herpes zoster in some instances. The condition is manifested by drooping of the corner of the mouth, inability to close the eye on the same side, and difficulty in speech and eating. In mild cases the symptoms may disappear spontaneously within a month. Alteration in taste sensation in the anterior two-thirds of the tongue due to disturbance of the sensory component of the facial nerve occurs in some cases and indicates a more central location of the lesion in the nerve.

The pain associated with the *glossopharyngeal neuralgia syndrome* is similar in type and intensity to that found in trigeminal neuralgia, being set off by a trigger zone in the pharynx and affecting the posterior region of the tongue, pharynx, soft palate, and ear. Disturbance of the hypoglossal nerve leads to dysfunction of the tongue musculature and atrophy. Bilateral nerve involvement prevents protrusion of the tongue; unilateral involvement leads to deviation of the protruded tongue toward the affected side.

DISTURBANCES OF THE TEMPOROMANDIBULAR JOINT

Pain in the area of the temporomandibular joint frequently causes the patient to seek therapy. It may be due to posterior displacement of the condyle in the fossa leading to displacement of the meniscus and chronic trauma. *Dislocation of the condyle anteriorly* beyond the articular eminence due to sudden stretching or tearing of the capsular ligament may result in a locking of the mandible in an open position. In *osteoarthritis* the clinical signs and symptoms may be minimal despite extensive changes in the condyle. Temporomandibular joint involvement occurs less frequently in *rheumatoid arthritis*. When affected the joints are swollen and painful, leading to limitation of movement, particularly on arising in the morning. In children the disease may lead to malocclusion. *Ankylosis* of the joint may occur eventually, necessitating a condylectomy.

The myofascial pain syndrome, the most common disorder of the temporomandibular joint, is characterized by facial pain and mandibular dysfunction. The pain is often localized in the ear or jaw and may extend to the neck and shoulder. The mandibular dysfunction is manifested by limitation of movement, particularly an inability to open the jaw to the fullest extent. It is thought that such patients have increased musculature tension and hyperexcitable reflexes related to emotional tension. The precipitating factor appears to be the stretching of an abnormal focus of pain which initiates a self-sustaining pain-spasm-pain cycle. Treatment of the pain-dysfunction syndrome involves the use of drugs to relieve the pain, lessen cortical excitability, and relax the muscles. Local anesthetics are used intramuscularly in the region of the trigger zone or as superficial sprays in an attempt to break the pain-spasm-pain cycle.

REFERENCES

BHASKAR SN: *Synopsis of Oral Pathology,* St. Louis: Mosby, 1969

GORLIN RJ, PINDBORG JJ: *Syndromes of the Head and Neck,* New York: McGraw-Hill, 1964

LEAKE DL et al: Suppurative parotitis in children. Oral Surg 31:174, 1971

MCCARTHY P, SHKLAR G: *Diseases of the Oral Mucosa,* New York: McGraw-Hill, 1964

MITCHELL DF (ed): *Symposium on Oral Medicine,* Philadelphia: Saunders, 1968

SHAFER WG et al: *A Textbook of Oral Pathology,* Philadelphia: Saunders, 1966

37 DYSPHAGIA

THOMAS R. HENDRIX

Dysphagia, or difficulty in swallowing, is a most reliable symptom and indicates the presence of disease or dysfunction. Dysphagia should never be dismissed as an emotional disturbance or be confused with globus hystericus, a term used to indicate the sensation of a lump or tightness in the throat independent of swallowing.

The most characteristic manifestation of dysphagia is the sensation of food "sticking" somewhere in its passage to the stomach, usually at the level of the obstruction but sometimes referred to the suprasternal notch, even though the obstruction may be at the lower end of the esophagus. Pain may accompany dysphagia, especially if esophageal spasm in induced by the peristaltic waves attempting to force the bolus through the obstruction. If the pain is mild, it tends to be localized to the site of obstruction; if more severe, it radiates more widely, into the base of the neck, angles of the jaw, arms, epigastrium, or back. Sometimes pain, in a sense, may even cause dysphagia, as when the throat is so sore that swallowing is difficult. For further details regarding these symptoms, see Chap. 281.

Normal swallowing is a complex function dependent upon coordination of voluntary muscular structures of the oropharynx, striated muscles protecting the larynx and respiratory passages, as well as relaxation of the esophageal sphincters and the peristaltic wave itself; hence dysphagia may occur as a consequence of derangement or incoordination of any of the elements of the swallowing act as well as narrowing of the lumen by inflammatory stricture or tumor.

For clinical purposes it is useful to consider dysphagia as having either an oropharyngeal or an esophageal origin, because symptoms, etiology, and treatment are usually different for the two types.

OROPHARYNGEAL DYSPHAGIA Symptoms associated with dysphagia caused by disorders of oropharyngeal structures include aspiration with swallowing, regurgitation of fluid into the nose, pharyngeal pain with swallowing, and inability of the tongue to move the bolus into the pharynx. Dilatation and atony of piriform sinuses and pharynx and retention of contrast media in the valleculae are characteristic radiographic findings in patients with pharyngeal dysfunction. In addition, aspiration of contrast medium into the trachea or regurgitation into the nasopharynx and apparent obstruction at the upper esophageal sphincter (cricopharyngeus) may be found.

Neuromuscular disorders are the most common causes of oropharyngeal dysphagia. Examples of these disorders are cerebral vascular accidents which cause pseudobulbar palsy (see Chap. 17) or bulbar palsy, poliomyelitis, motor system disease, diphtheritic polyneuritis, myasthenia gravis, myotonic dystrophies and restricted muscular dystrophies (oculopharyngeal and laryngoesophageal), and dermatomyositis. Ulcerative lesions such as pharyngitis, Vincent's angina, monilia stomatitis, viral infections with herpetic lesions, and retropharyngeal abscess interfere by causing pain and thereby inhibiting the initiation of deglutition. Plummer-Vinson syndrome (Paterson-Kelly syndrome, or sideropenic dysphagia) may also be listed here, since the difficulty in swallowing in this disorder resembles that due to a neuromuscular disorder, although pain may be an additional disturbing feature. Limited pathologic studies have shown both epithelial and muscle atrophy. It is clear that the dysphagia is not due to the characteristic web, or mucosal fold, of the anterior aspect of the cricopharyngeal area, because the web often persists long after the symptoms have been relieved by iron replacement.

Oropharyngeal dysphagia may be caused by narrowing of the lumen of the pharynx or upper esophagus by tumor, granulomatous disease, Zenker's diverticulum, or an enlarged thyroid.

ESOPHAGEAL DYSPHAGIA Symptoms indicating that the cause of dysphagia is to be found in the esophagus range from retrosternal fullness with swallowing to failure of the bolus to pass through the esophagus associated with pain relieved only by regurgitation of the offending bolus. Barium swallows in patients with dysphagia of esophageal origin show segmental narrowing of the esophageal lumen, failure of peristalsis, or both. Abnormalities of peristalsis may be characterized more precisely by intraluminal manometric studies.

Mechanical narrowing of the esophageal lumen is most frequently caused either by carcinoma of the squamous type, arising from the esophagus itself, or by adenocarcinoma of the cardia extending up into the esophagus. Rarely, benign tumors may reach sufficient size to cause dysphagia. Inflammatory strictures most commonly result from reflux esophagitis but are also caused by ingestion of corrosive substances, such as lye, or by trauma from foreign bodies or instrumentation. In addition, a lower esophageal ring may produce dysphagia by obstructing the esophageal lumen. Extrinsic pressure from aneurysms, vascular anomalies, mediastinal tumors, or paraesophageal diaphragmatic hernias may compress the esophageal lumen sufficiently to cause dysphagia. Finally, the motility disturbances associated with diffuse esophageal spasm, cardiospasm, and esophageal reflux may be the basis of dysphagia. Although esophageal peristalsis is absent in the majority of patients with scleroderma, dysphagia does not become a prominent symptom until reflux esophagitis has led to an inflammatory stricture.

DIFFERENTIAL DIAGNOSIS Determination of the basic mechanism responsible for dysphagia is usually a simple matter, but identification of the exact disorder responsible for it may be quite difficult. For example, cancer of the esophagus sometimes presents suddenly rather than gradually, and the roentgenogram may have a smooth, symmetric appearance such as is more commonly seen with benign stricture or cardiospasm; even esophagoscopy may be inconclusive, and biopsy may yield deceptive results if the tissue shows only inflammatory reaction and does not include neoplastic cells. Similarly, neuromuscular disorders and disturbances of esophageal motility interfering with swallowing may be difficult to classify.

Certain symptoms associated with dysphagia, however, have diagnostic value. Hiccups, together with difficulty in swallowing, suggest a lesion at the terminal portion of the esophagus, such as carcinoma, achalasia, or hiatal hernia. Dysphagia followed after an interval of some duration by hoarseness usually means extension of a malignant growth beyond the walls of the esophagus and the involvement of a recurrent laryngeal nerve. When the hoarseness comes first and the dysphagia later, the primary lesion is almost always in the larynx. This combination of laryngeal and pharyngeal symptoms may also occur in polymyositis or dermatomyositis or with any disease causing bilateral involvement of vagus nerves or nuclei (poliomyelitis and polyneuritis). In motor system disease, the most common cause of a mixture of bulbar and pseudobulbar palsy, dysphagia is usually combined with dysphonia and dysarthria; the jaw jerk is hyperactive and the tongue atrophic. Dysphagia and unilateral wheezing virtually always indicate a mediastinal mass involving the esophagus and a main or large bronchus. Coughing with each swallow of food or drink means a fistulous communication between the esophagus and the trachea or a motor disorder in which the larynx is not effectively closed. Coughing occurring some time after swallowing may be due to regurgitation of food, most common in achalasia and Zenker's diverticulum.

DIAGNOSTIC PROCEDURES Examination of the mouth and pharynx should disclose those lesions which impede the transfer of food from the mouth to the esophagus, because of pain or mechanical interference. When lesions of the hypopharynx (e.g., *chronic abscess secondary to tuberculosis of the spine*) or of the larynx (e.g., *tuberculosis* or *carcinoma*) are suspected, examination with a mirror is necessary.

The most important diagnostic technique in the evaluation of dysphagia is a *barium swallow,* which makes it possible to determine whether dysphagia is caused by mechanical obstruction or by esophageal motor abnormality. Absence of esophageal peristalsis can best be demonstrated by barium swallows with the patient in Trendelenburg's position. If there is no peristalsis, barium will remain in the esophagus until the patient is tilted upright. Since the muscular action of the pharynx is so rapid, swallows must be recorded by *cineradiography.* Projection of the film at slow speed permits detection and analysis of abnormalities of pharyngeal function.

If barium swallow shows a lesion within the esophagus or a narrowing of the lumen, *esophagoscopy* is the most direct method for establishing the nature of the lesion. In addition to inspecting the lesion, one should perform biopsies to differentiate inflammatory from neoplastic lesions. A malignant stricture is not ruled out with certainty, however, if the biopsy shows only normal tissue or chronic inflammation, because tumors of the esophagus often spread beneath the mucosa and may be missed by a superificial biopsy. In such circumstances repeated biopsy or exfoliative cytology is necessary. Cytologic studies by experienced personnel are very accurate in the diagnosis of esophageal cancer.

Motor abnormalities of the pharynx and esophagus may be suspected by viewing the movement of a swallowed radiopaque bolus by fluoroscopy, but to characterize these abnormalities definitely the motor response of pharynx and esophagus to swallowing must be studied by recording intraluminal pressure from several points simultaneously. Records are best obtained by use of a train of water-filled, perfused catheters connected to external pressure transducers or strain gages. Examination of manometric records of swallows will demonstrate whether the wave is normally propagated over the length of the esophagus, whether the pressure generated by the peristaltic wave is normal and sufficient to propel the bolus, and, finally, whether sphincter relaxation is complete, of adequate duration, and properly coordinated with the peristaltic wave. Combining manometric with cineradiographic techniques has added greatly to our understanding of pharyngoesophageal function.

REFERENCES

COHEN BR, WOLF BS: Cineradiographic and intraluminal pressure correlations in the pharynx and esophagus, in *Handbook of Physiology,* sec. 6, vol. IV, ed CF Code, Washington: American Physiology Society, 1968, p. 1841

DONNER MW, SILBIGER DL: Cinefluorographic analysis of pharyngeal swallowing in neuromuscular disorders. Am J Med Sci 251:600, 1966

HARRIS LD: The present status of esophageal manometry. Gastroenterology 50:708, 1966

PHILLIPS MM, HENDRIX TR: Dysphagia. Postgrad Med 50:81, 1971

38
INDIGESTION

KURT J. ISSELBACHER
JAY B. SHUMAKER

"Indigestion" is a term frequently used by patients to describe a multitude of symptoms generally appreciated as distress associated with the intake of food. The term is thus nonspecific and may have a different meaning for the patient and the physician. In approaching the patient with indigestion it is important for the physician first to elicit a good description of this complaint. To some patients indigestion refers to a feeling that digestion has not proceeded naturally. They may describe a sense of abdominal fullness, pressure, or actual pain. Others may use the term to describe heartburn, belching, distention, or flatulence. These complaints will be considered in this chapter. Discussed elsewhere are the closely related symptoms of dysphagia, nausea and vomiting, and anorexia (Chaps. 37 and 39).

Indigestion may occur as a result of disease of the gastrointestinal tract or in association with pathologic states in other organ systems. As a result of systematic clinical and laboratory tests, a definable pathophysiologic process often can be shown to be responsible for the symptoms in a given case of indigestion. Frequently, however, clear etiologic explanation for the patient's complaints of indigestion are not established. Such cases are often designated as "functional indigestion," with a strong implication that psychosomatic factors underlie the complaints. Although it is clear that psychic factors may lead to symptoms of indigestion, the designation of "functional indigestion" is rarely if ever a satisfactory explanation, serving only to rephrase the patient's description of his symptoms. A psychogenic cause should not be assumed until organic causes of indigestion have been thoroughly excluded.

After having ascertained the patient's definition of indigestion, it is also important to determine (1) the location and duration of the discomfort, (2) the temporal relation of the symptoms to the ingestion of food, and (3) the possible relation of the symptoms to the ingestion of specific types of food (e.g., fatty foods, milk, and drugs).

PAIN PATTERNS True visceral abdominal pain as seen in indigestion is mediated over visceral afferent nerves which accompany the abdominal sympathetic pathways (see Chap. 8). Visceral pain is generally described as dull and aching in nature (with a diffuse midline localization) or as fullness or pressure. The location of the discomfort corresponds generally to the segmental level of the affected organ. Abdominal visceral pain can be produced experimentally by artificially increasing pressure in a hollow viscus. Usually this type of pain is the result of distention or exaggerated muscular contraction of a viscus. Inflammation generally lowers the threshold to such stimuli.

The visceral pain of indigestion should be distinguished from the sharp, lateralized, and localized pain patterns seen in many acute abdominal processes involving the peritoneum. In contrast to true visceral pain, this pain is mediated over cerebrospinal afferent nerves. Again it is of a dull, aching type, whether from inflammation of the viscera or of peritoneal surfaces.

In view of the diffuse nature of true visceral abdominal pain, the main clue comes from the segmental level of the viscus; in any given segmental region there is no way of determining which of several viscera are the source of it (Table 38-1). The following rules, already given in Chap. 5, are useful: *Substernal pain* of gastrointestinal origin usually arises from disorders in the esophagus or cardia of the stomach. Because pain in this area is frequently of cardiac origin, heart disease must be considered carefully and excluded. *Epigastric pain* is generally of gastric, duodenal, biliary, or pancreatic origin. As the pathologic process in the biliary tract and pancreas becomes more intense, it tends to lateralize and localize, e.g., biliary pain to the right upper quadrant and tip of the right scapula and pancreatic pain to the epigastrium, left upper quadrant, and back. *Periumbilical pain* is generally associated with small-intestinal disease. *Pain below the umbilicus* is often of appendiceal, large-intestinal, or pelvic origin.

TEMPORAL RELATIONSHIPS OF PAIN AND INDIGESTION The unraveling of the temporal relationships of the patient's symptoms often provides the most significant diagnostic information. It is important to ascertain whether the symptoms are *constant* (continually present over extended periods of time), as may occur, for example, with an infiltrating gastric carcinoma, or *intermittent,* as in acute gastritis following an alcoholic binge or in association with the use of certain drugs. The symptoms may have a *diurnal* pattern; e.g., pain occurring

TABLE 38-1
Distribution of visceral pain and examples of disorders frequently involving the specific organ

Organ	*Location of referred pain*	*Frequent disorders*
Esophagus	Substernum, epigastrium	Peptic esophagitis, hiatus hernia stricture, carcinoma
Stomach	Epigastrium	Gastritis, peptic ulcer, carcinoma
Duodenum (first and second portions)	Epigastrium	Peptic ulcer
Duodenum (third portion, jejunum, and ileum)	Periumbilical	Regional enteritis, lymphoma, gastroenteritis (infectious), intestinal obstruction
Gallbladder	Epigastrium, right upper quadrant, right side of back	Cholelithiasis, cholecystitis
Pancreas	Epigastrium, left side of back	Pancreatitis, pancreatic carcinoma
Liver	Right upper quadrant	Passive congestion of liver, hepatitis, cirrhosis
Colon	Below umbilicus	Ulcerative colitis, carcinoma, partial obstruction

nocturnally and with *recumbency* is seen in esophagitis and hiatus hernia. Symptoms are occasionally *seasonal;* this may occur in peptic ulcer disease, in which some patients experience more discomfort in the spring and autumn.

Another important and often diagnostic feature is the relation of pain or indigestion to ingestion of food. This relationship is especially significant or helpful if symptoms occur either during or minutes after the meal or if they occur several hours (four or more) after eating. *Early postprandial symptoms* may reflect esophageal disease, because they may be associated with disordered swallowing function. In such instances, the distress or other symptoms of indigestion often are experienced substernally. Early postprandial complaints occur also in gastric disorders such as acute gastritis or carcinoma. *Late postprandial indigestion,* i.e., that occurring several hours after eating, may reflect failure of the stomach to empty adequately, as in pyloric stenosis or gastric atony. It may also be a symptom of duodenal ulcer, in which case it classically occurs several hours after the meal, when the ulcerated mucosa is exposed to acid secretions of the stomach unbuffered by food. Conversely, the relief of pain following food ingestion is also seen in patients with peptic ulcer and is presumably due to the neutralization of the acid by the ingested food. Late postprandial indigestion also may result from impaired digestive and absorptive processes, as in pancreatic insufficiency.

FOOD INTOLERANCE In a number of situations specific foods or types of foods appear to be related to indigestion. Careful documentation of this relationship is sometimes of great help in arriving at an etiologic diagnosis.

Some foods may be poorly tolerated because of their consistency. Patients with esophageal stricture or carcinoma may tolerate liquids well, but the ingestion of solids may be associated with discomfort, especially substernal distress (see Chap. 281). Certain foods may be tolerated poorly because the intestinal tract cannot assimilate them adequately. This may occur following the ingestion of fatty foods in patients with pancreatic or biliary tract disease. Citrus fruits, with their relatively low pH, often provoke symptoms in patients with peptic ulcer disease.

Individuals may lack a specific enzyme required for assimilation of a certain nutrient. Patients may have a deficiency of the mucosal enzyme lactase, which catalyzes the hydrolysis of lactose. When lactase deficiency exists on a congenital or acquired basis (e.g., in sprue, ulcerative colitis) (Chap. 284), the ingestion of milk (which contains lactose) results in abdominal cramps, distention, flatulence, and diarrhea.

There are a number of other conditions or disorders in which specific foods are poorly tolerated. Foods may be poorly tolerated because they initiate *allergic reactions* or exert a deleterious or *toxic effect* on the intestinal tract of susceptible persons (e.g., gluten in patients with nontropical sprue). Finally certain substances may lead to systemic effects because of biochemical defects in the patient which render them particularly hazardous. An example of the latter is galactose intolerance in galactosemia (Chap. 105).

The above mechanisms do not explain the majority of clinical situations in which indigestion is associated with the eating of specific foods. For example, a history of fatty-food intolerance or an inability to eat cabbage, cucumbers, or spicy foods is commonly obtained from patients with indigestion. However, the mechanisms underlying the production of symptoms in these circumstances is still unclear.

ADDITIONAL SYNDROMES COMMONLY DESCRIBED AS INDIGESTION Gaseousness, flatulence, aerophagia A number of common clinical syndromes which may be described by the patient as "indigestion" appear to be related to increased quantities of gas in the intestinal tract. About 20 to 60 percent of intraluminal gas represents swallowed air. A degree of air swallowing, or *aerophagia,* occurs in normal persons and the swallowed air can be observed by the radiologist at fluoroscopy. Under certain circumstances, such as chronic anxiety, poor eating habits, or actual intestinal disease itself, aerophagia may increase in magnitude and lead to symptoms in its own right.

Early postprandial fullness and pressure, relieved by eructation and accompanied by a large amount of air seen on roentgenogram in the gastric fundus, is often referred to as the *magenblase* (i.e., gastric bubble) *syndrome.* Acute gastric distention by swallowed air can occasionally produce sharp pains which may mimic angina pectoris. This sequence of events may be especially perplexing in older patients with coronary artery disease, because it is well recognized that true angina pectoris may itself be precipitated by the ingestion of a large meal. Fatty meals delay gastric emptying and hence the passage of swallowed air down the intestine. This relationship may explain, in part, the prolonged sense of fullness and eructations experienced by many individuals after a fatty meal.

Swallowed air that is not eructated passes on in the intestinal tract and may either produce diffuse abdominal distention or become trapped in the splenic flexure of the colon. Distention of this segment of the colon produces a sensation of left upper quadrant fullness and pressure with radiation to the left side of the chest. This is known as the *splenic flexure syndrome.* Patients will often describe relief of pain with defecation or with the expulsion of flatus. Diagnosis may be made by demonstrating, on physical examination, a note of increased tympany in the extreme left lateral portion of the upper part of the abdomen or by the visualization of large amounts of air in the splenic flexure of the colon by radiography.

A second major source of intestinal gas is the fermentative action of bacteria on carbohydrates and proteins within the lumen. Increased amounts of intraluminal gas production due to this mechanism have been demonstrated in conditions associated with abnormal bacterial colonization of the small intestine and in patients with carbohydrate malabsorption.

Increased gas production may occur following the ingestion of certain foods (e.g., the legumes) which contain significant quantities of nonabsorbable sugars. As in the case of swallowed air, increased amounts of intraluminally produced gas can produce symptoms by causing distention, pain, increased motility (with diarrhea), or flatulence.

Heartburn Heartburn, or pyrosis, is a sensation of warmth or burning located substernally or high in the epigastrium. Experimental studies in human beings have shown that esophageal distention or increased motor activity is associated in most subjects with a feeling of fullness and burning in this area.

Heartburn may occur with organic disease of the intestinal tract and is usually associated with gastroesophageal reflux. This is frequently the case in hiatus hernia. In this setting, heartburn occurs after a large meal or with stooping or bending. Esophageal reflux of acid contents at these times leads to symptoms by either the production of abnormal motor acitvity or direct mucosal irritation (i.e., esophagitis). Heartburn may arise following the ingestion of certain foods or drugs (e.g., alcohol and aspirin). It may also be seen in the absence of a demonstrable anatomic or motor pathologic condition, in which case it is frequently accompanied by aerophagia and for lack of other explanation is often attributed to psychologic factors.

INDIGESTION DUE TO DISEASE OUTSIDE THE INTESTINAL TRACT A multitude of extraintestinal disease processes may result in indigestion by mechanisms which are poorly understood. Indigestion may be the presenting complaint, for example, in congestive heart failure, uremia, pulmonary tuberculosis, and neoplastic disease. Under these circumstances the symptoms of indigestion may present with no unique features to suggest that they are in fact due to some other systemic disease process. Drugs such as aspirin, corticosteroids, indomethacin, and phenylbutazone affect gastric secretion and are ulcerogenic; thus they may lead to symptoms of indigestion.

DIAGNOSTIC APPROACH TO THE PATIENT WITH INDIGESTION Indigestion represents a challenging and difficult diagnostic problem because of the nonspecific nature of its manifestations. The evaluation of indigestion must include initially a thorough medical work-up, with ultimate confirmation or exclusion of pathophysiologic derangements by the appropriate diagnostic procedures.

A careful history should include an assessment of the patient's general medical health, including the possibility of diseases in extraintestinal organ systems which may produce indigestion. Careful evaluation of psychologic factors is crucial, because they often play an etiologic or contributory role in the patient's problem. Of particular importance are anxiety, depressive reactions, and hysteria (Chaps. 337 and 338). Evaluation of the patient's intestinal problem must include an assessment of his nutritional status, changes in weight, and appetite.

A clear and detailed description of the specific symptoms should be obtained, particularly the patient's definition of the term "indigestion." The nature of the pain, its frequency and time of occurrence, its relationship to meals, and the special circumstances which lead to its exacerbation or relief should be elicited. Associated intestinal symptoms such as nausea and vomiting, abnormal bowel habits, steatorrhea, diarrhea, and melena should also be sought. Physical examination rarely establishes the specific diagnosis, but it may be useful in detecting disease in other organ systems (e.g., congestive heart failure) which can affect intestinal physiology.

X-ray examination of the alimentary tract is crucial to the evaluation of indigestion. This may involve examination of the esophagus, stomach, small intestine, colon, and biliary tract. Esophagoscopy, gastroscopy, colonoscopy, or sigmoidoscopy also may be helpful or necessary. Stools should be examined for appearance, occult blood, fat, and muscle fibers. As stated above, careful attempts must be made to exclude nonintestinal disease, especially cardiac disease.

Unfortunately, even after completion of careful diagnostic studies many cases of indigestion will turn out to have no clear explanation. Some of these are psychogenic and may respond to appropriate psychiatric measures. Others represent physiologic derangements which are undetectable by currently available diagnostic methods. Still others represent actual disease processes in early stages which may be diagnosable by conventional methods at a later date. The ultimate evaluation of indigestion requires, therefore, the utmost in sensitivity, diligence, and patience on the part of the examining physician.

REFERENCES

CALLOWAY DH: Respiratory hydrogen and methane as affected by consumption of gas forming foods. Gastroenterology 51:383, 1966

COGHILL NF: Dyspepsia. Br Med J 4:97, 1967

LEVITT MD, BOND JH JR: Volume, composition and source of intestinal gas. Gastroenterology 59:921, 1970

39
ANOREXIA, NAUSEA, AND VOMITING

KURT J. ISSELBACHER
JAY B. SHUMAKER

ANOREXIA Anorexia, or loss of the desire to eat, is a prominent symptom in a wide variety of intestinal and extraintestinal disorders. It must be clearly differentiated from satiety and from specific food intolerance. Anorexia occurs in many disorders and as a result *by itself is of little specific diagnostic value.* The mechanisms whereby hunger and appetite are modified in various disease states are poorly understood. Normally food intake is regulated by two hypothalamic centers—a lateral "feeding center" and a ventral-medial "satiety center." The latter inhibits the feeding center following a meal leading to the sensation of satiety.

Anorexia is commonly seen in diseases of the gastrointestinal tract and liver. For example, it may precede the appearance of jaundice in hepatitis, or it may be a prominent symptom in gastric carcinoma. In the setting of intestinal disease, anorexia should be clearly differentiated from *sitophobia,* or fear of eating because of subsequent or associated discomfort. In such circumstances, appetite may persist, but the ingestion of food is curtailed nonetheless. Sitophobia may be seen, for example, in regional enteritis (especially with partial obstruction) or in patients with gastric ulcer following partial or total gastrectomy.

Anorexia may also be a prominent feature of severe extraintestinal diseases. For example, anorexia may be profound in severe congestive heart failure and may contribute significantly to the cachexia in these patients. It may be a major symptom in patients with uremia, pulmonary failure, and various endocrinopathies (e.g., hyperparathyroidism, Addison's disease, and panhypopituitarism). Anorexia also often accompanies psychogenic disturbances, such as anxiety or depression.

ANOREXIA NERVOSA Anorexia nervosa is a self-imposed state of cachexia and malnutrition and may at times become life-threatening. It is accompanied by severe psychologic disturbances which lead to an abnormal desire to lose weight. The major clinical feature of anorexia nervosa consists of profound weight loss in the absence of other signs of demonstrable organic illness. Although the name implies loss of appetite, these patients also have abnormal eating patterns, with episodes of anorexia and periods of excessive eating. The severe restriction of dietary intake is often in response to an uncontrollable urge to eat. Once anorexia becomes severe, other peculiar habits may develop which are aimed at limiting weight gain. Patients may surreptitiously dispose of food, induce vomiting, or employ laxatives to produce diarrhea. One of the striking findings in these patients is that in spite of their depleted nutritional state they may show hyperactivity and increased alertness.

Anorexia nervosa is accompanied by other psychologic behavior disorders, including withdrawal, obsessions, depression, and occasionally psychotic delusions. Most often anorexia nervosa is associated with excessive concern about obesity and physical appearance. Commonly patients with anorexia nervosa demonstrate a distorted perception of their physical state, denying the presence of any abnormality, and tend to view their emaciated, wasted appearance as normal. When these manifestations represent the major psychologic disturbance, the disorder is referred to as true or *primary anorexia nervosa.* However profound anorexia may also be a major manifestation of psychiatric disorders. Thus in hysterical patients anorexia may be the prominent symptom. Obsessive-compulsive patients may adhere to ritualistic diets, with resulting malnutrition. With severe depression there may be a loss of interest in eating, while the psychotic patient may avoid eating because of a delusional fear of food. These types of anorexia or malnutrition have been referred to as *secondary anorexia nervosa.*

Physical examination of the patient with anorexia nervosa reveals emaciation, often of extreme degree. There may be multiple vitamin deficiencies. The blood pressure, basal metabolism, and body temperature may be subnormal. The skin is often dry and scaly. Sexual maturity is markedly delayed. In female patients amenorrhea is quite common, and the appearance of axillary and pubic hair may be delayed. In general these patients are alert, outwardly cooperative, and of normal intelligence.

Laboratory tests are of value primarily to exclude systemic diseases such as carcinomatosis, miliary tuberculosis, panhypopituitarism, malabsorption states, regional enteritis, or diabetes mellitus. However, some conditions may be falsely diagnosed as anorexia nervosa either when the underlying organic disease is subtle or when it is in its early stages and the history, physical examination, and laboratory tests are not yet diagnostic. This is especially true in regional enteritis. It is obviously essential to explore fully all possibilities of underlying organic disease before making a diagnosis of anorexia nervosa.

In differentiating anorexia nervosa from panhypopituitarism the most significant findings are the preservation of axillary and pubic hair and breast tissue, as well as thyroid and adrenal function. In addition, physical strength and activity are much greater in patients with anorexia nervosa than in those with panhypopituitarism.

Treatment of this condition is difficult. In extreme cases it may be necessary to nourish the patient with parenteral or nasogastric feedings. Since patients with anorexia nervosa invariably exhibit severe psychologic disturbances, optimal management necessitates resolution of the patient's distorted ideas about eating. In some patients a period of anorexia will terminate spontaneously. Improvement has also been obtained by the use of *operant reinforcement techniques.* With this approach, access to physical activity, recreation, and personal attention is made contingent on weight gain by the patient. More intensive psychotherapeutic measures are frequently employed; yet often the basic conflicts in patients with anorexia nervosa remain unresolved or are likely to recur.

NAUSEA AND VOMITING Nausea and vomiting may occur independently of each other, but generally they are so closely allied that they may conveniently be considered together. *Nausea* denotes the feeling of the imminent desire to vomit, usually referred to the throat or epigastrium. *Vomiting* refers to the forceful oral expulsion of gastric contents; *retching* denotes the labored rhythmic respiratory activity that frequently precedes emesis. Extremely forceful *projectile vomiting* is a special form of vomiting which has significance because it connotes the presence of increased intracranial pressure.

Nausea often precedes or accompanies vomiting. It is usually associated with diminished functional activity of the stomach and alterations of the motility of the duodenum and small intestine. Accompanying severe nausea there is often evidence of altered autonomic (especially parasympathetic) activity: pallor of the skin, increased perspiration, salivation, and the occasional association of hypotension and bradycardia (vasovagal syndrome). Anorexia is also often present.

Following a period of nausea and a brief interval of retching, a sequence of involuntary visceral and somatic motor events occurs, resulting in emesis. The stomach plays a relatively passive role in the vomiting process, the major ejection force being provided by the abdominal musculature. With relaxation of the gastric fundus and gastroesophageal sphincter, a sharp increase in intraabdominal pressure is brought about by forceful contraction of the diaphragm and abdominal wall. This, together with concomitant annular contraction of the gastric pylorus, results in the expulsion of gastric contents into the esophagus. Increased intrathoracic pressure results in the further movement of esophageal contents into the mouth. Reversal of the normal direction of esophageal peristalsis may play a role in this process. Reflex elevation of the soft palate during the vomiting act prevents the entry of the material into the nasopharynx, whereas reflex closure of the glottis and inhibition of respiration help to prevent pulmonary aspiration.

Repeated emesis may have deleterious effects in a number of different ways. The process of vomiting itself may lead to traumatic rupture or tearing in the region of the cardioesophageal junction, resulting in massive hematemesis, the so-called Mallory-Weiss syndrome. Prolonged vomiting may lead to dehydration and the loss of gastric secretions (especially hydrochloric acid) to metabolic alkalosis with hypokalemia. Finally, in states of central nervous system depression (coma, etc.), gastric contents may be aspirated into the lungs, with a resulting aspiration pneumonitis.

Vomiting mechanism The act of vomiting is under the control of two functionally distinct medullary centers: the *vomiting center* and the *chemoreceptor trigger zone*. The vomiting center controls and integrates the actual act of emesis. It receives afferent stimuli from the intestinal tract and other parts of the body, from higher cortical centers, especially the labyrinthine apparatus, and from the chemoreceptor trigger zone. The important efferent pathways in vomiting are the phrenic nerves (to the diaphragm), the spinal nerves (to the abdominal musculature), and visceral efferent nerves (to the stomach and esophagus).

The chemoreceptor trigger zone is also located in the medulla but by itself is incapable of mediating the act of vomiting. Activation of this zone results in efferent impulses to the medullary vomiting center, which in turn initiates the act of emesis. The chemoreceptor trigger zone can be activated by many stimuli, including drugs such as apomorphine, cardiac glycosides, and ergot alkaloids. Certain of the phenothiazine derivatives appear to antagonize the effects of the above-mentioned drugs on the chemoreceptor trigger zone.

Clinical classification Nausea and vomiting are common manifestations of organic and functional disorders. The precise mechanisms triggering vomiting in the various clinical states are poorly understood, making classification of mechanisms difficult. The categories mentioned below serve to illustrate some of the many disorders which may be accompanied by nausea and vomiting.

Acute abdominal emergencies Many of the disorders in this category which lead to the "surgical abdomen" are associated with nausea and vomiting. Notably, vomiting may be seen with inflammation of a viscus as in acute appendicitis or acute cholecystitis, obstruction of the intestine, or acute peritonitis (see Chap. 8).

Chronic indigestion In many of the disorders falling in this category (see Chap. 38) nausea and vomiting may be prominent. Emesis may be either spontaneous or self-induced and may lead to relief of symptoms, as, for example, in uncomplicated peptic ulcer. Nausea and vomiting may accompany the distention and pain seen in the aerophagic syndromes. Often in patients with chronic indigestion, nausea and vomiting may be provoked by specific foods (e.g., fatty foods), for reasons that are poorly understood.

Acute infectious disease Acute systemic infections with fever, especially in young children, are frequently accompanied by vomiting and often by severe diarrhea. The mechanism whereby infections remote from the gastrointestinal tract produce these manifestations is unclear. Viral, bacterial, and parasitic infections of the intestinal tract may be associated with severe nausea and vomiting, often with diarrhea. Severe nausea and vomiting may be prominent in viral hepatitis, even before the appearance of jaundice.

Disorders of the nervous system Central nervous system disorders which lead to increased intracranial pressure may be accompanied by vomiting, often projectile. Brain swelling due to inflammation, anorexia, acute hydrocephalus, neoplasms, etc., may thus be complicated by vomiting. Disorders of the labyrinthine apparatus and its central connections which underlie vertigo may be accompanied by vomiting with nausea and retching. Acute labyrinthitis and Ménière's disease are examples of such disturbances. Migraine headaches, tabetic crises, and acute meningitis are additional examples of disorders of the nervous system which may lead to vomiting. In the reactive phase of hypotension with syncope, there may be nausea and vomiting.

Diseases of the heart Severe nausea and vomiting may be present in acute myocardial infarction, especially of the posterior wall of the heart. Nausea and vomiting may also be seen in congestive heart failure, perhaps in relation to congestion of the liver. The possibility that these symptoms may be due to drugs (e.g., opiates or digitalis) should always be borne in mind in patients with cardiac disease.

Metabolic and endocrine disorders Nausea and vomiting commonly accompany several endocrinologic disorders, including diabetic acidosis and adrenal insufficiency, especially adrenal crises. The morning sickness of early pregnancy is another instance of nausea and vomiting possibly related to hormonal changes.

Drugs and chemicals The side effects of many drugs and chemicals include nausea and vomiting. In some instances this is because of gastric irritation which stimulates the medullary vomiting center.

Psychogenic vomiting This term is applied to the vomiting which may occur as part of any emotional upset on a transitory basis or more persistently as part of a psychic disturbance. Close observation will usually disclose the condition to be one of regurgitation rather than of vomiting, and weight loss may not correspond at all to the patient's description of the frequency and severity of vomiting. As discussed earlier in this chapter, anorexia nervosa is an emotional disturbance which may be associated not only with anorexia but also with vomiting. Often patients with emotional disorders and vomiting maintain a relatively normal state of nutrition, because a relatively small amount of the ingested food is vomited.

Differential diagnosis Vomiting should be distinguished from *regurgitation,* which refers to the expulsion of food in the absence of nausea and without the abdominal diaphragmatic muscular contraction which is a part of vomiting. Regurgitation of esophageal contents may occur with esophageal stricture or diverticula. Regurgitation of gastric contents is generally seen with gastroesophageal sphincter incompetence, especially with hiatus hernia or in association with peptic ulcer, usually when pylorospasm supervenes.

The temporal relationships of vomiting to eating may be of help diagnostically. Vomiting which occurs predominantly in the morning is often seen early in pregnancy and in uremia. Alcoholic gastritis is commonly accompanied by early-morning emesis, the so-called "dry heaves." Vomiting which occurs shortly after eating may suggest pylorospasm or gastritis. On the other hand, vomiting which occurs 4 to 6 hr or longer after eating and involves the elimination of large quantities of undigested food often indicates gastric retention (as in diabetic gastric atony or pyloric obstruction).

The character of the vomitus offers clues to the diagnosis. If the vomitus contains free hydrochloric acid, the obstruction may be due to an ulcer; absence of free hydrochloric acid is more compatible with gastric malignancy. A feculent or putrid odor reflects the results of bacterial action on the intestinal contents. Such vomiting may be seen with low-intestinal obstruction, peritonitis, or gastrocolic fistula. Bile is commonly present in gastric contents whenever vomiting is prolonged. It has no significance unless constantly present in large quantities, when it may signify an obstructive lesion below the ampulla of Vater. The presence of blood in the gastric contents usually denotes bleeding from the esophagus, stomach, or duodenum.

REFERENCES

Blinder BJ et al: Behavior therapy of anorexia nervosa: effectiveness of activity as a reinforcer of weight gain. Am J Psychiatry 126:8, 1970

Bruch H: Changing approaches to anorexia nervosa. Int Psychiatry Clin 7:3, 1970

Crisp AH, Toms DA: Primary anorexia nervosa or weight phobia in the male: report on 13 cases. Br Med J 1:334, 1972

Frazier S: Anorexia nervosa. Dis Nerv Syst 26:155, 1965

Lumsden K, Holden SW: The act of vomiting in man. Gut 10:173, 1969

40 CONSTIPATION, DIARRHEA, AND DISTURBANCES OF ANORECTAL FUNCTION

ALBERT I. MENDELOFF

NORMAL COLONIC FUNCTION

MOTOR AND ABSORPTIVE FUNCTIONS On a normal mixed diet the stomach is nearly empty several hours after food is ingested. By the time the head of the food column reaches the ileocecal valve, most of the carbohydrate, protein, and fat has been broken down into absorbable form and entered the portal venules and the lacteals.

When the intestinal bolus reaches the terminal ileum, it proceeds very sluggishly unless the stomach empties; the so-called "gastroileal reflex" causes the ileum to empty into the cecum by a rapid series of small squirts. The ileocecal valve can probably function as a true sphincter, slowing down the entry of ileal contents into the cecum, but it also serves to prevent reflux, at least of gas, from the cecum into the ileum. The volume reaching the cecum daily is 600 to 800 ml, a slurry churned in the right side of the colon by segmental contractions. Now and then a coordinated wave involving a short length of colon pushes the mass along the colon; eating or walking may initiate an occasional massive contraction; this empties a sizable area of the right and transverse parts of the colon of its contents, which then are packed into the left side of the colon. Defecatory reflexes originate from the rectal walls, which normally are approximated around a small lumen empty of feces; when sigmoid contraction distends the rectal musculature, the defecatory reflex proceeds from sacral cord to brain, resulting in an increase in intraabdominal pressure through descent of the diaphragm, closure of the glottis, contraction of the abdominal wall musculature, and tensing of the pelvic floor. The later descent of the pelvic floor and the inhibition of tone of the external anal sphincter complete the skeletal muscular phase of defecation. Central nervous system impulses simultaneously engage sacral parasympathetic nerves to contract the smooth muscle of the pelvic colon. However, if the external sphincter is voluntarily contracted, the sigmoid colon relaxes, and the fecal mass slips back up into the rectosigmoid.

INNERVATION The colon and rectum are supplied with both sympathetic and parasympathetic nerves carrying both sensory and motor fibers. Sympathetic elements from the lower six thoracic segments travel to the right side of the colon via the superior mesenteric plexus; the left side of the colon receives sympathetic fibers originating in the lumbar segments of the cord gathered into the inferior mesenteric plexus, branches of which follow the inferior mesenteric artery. The rectum receives sympathetic innervation from the hypogastric or presacral nerve. Parasympathetic cholinergic fibers to the right side of the colon are assumed to be part of the vagus, passing through the celiac plexus. The left side of the colon and rectum receive all their parasympathetic innervation via the nervi erigentes, originating in the sacral nerves and joining the sympathetic fibers in the pelvic plexuses, from which some accompany the inferior mesenteric artery. The anus and external anal sphincter are supplied by the inferior hemorrhoidal branch of the internal pudendal nerve and by the perineal branches of the fourth sacral nerves, which nerves also innervate the levatores ani. Sensory nerves from the skin and mucous membrane of the anal canal are plentiful and go to the sacral cord.

The functional significance of the sympathetic supply to the lower part of the intestine is unclear. Careful studies in man following dorsolumbar sympathectomy have failed to reveal any consistent dysfunction of colon or rectum. Attempts to relieve colon pain syndromes by presacral neurectomy have been unavailing. The parasympathetic cholinergic innervation of the colon seems to be of sole importance in the motor and secretory functions of that organ; cholinergic drugs correspondingly activate such functions and result, when large enough dosages are employed, in watery diarrhea, cramps, and pain.

The mechanism of defecation has been previously described, and the important contribution of the abdominal musculature, the levatores ani, and the external anal sphincter noted. The internal anal sphincter, a smooth muscle, relaxes when the rectum is distended and seems to allow gas to escape without full defecatory movements. Sensory innervation of the anal canal permits the brain to discriminate as to whether rectal contents are liquid, gaseous, or solid.

CONTINENCE AND INCONTINENCE

The defecation reflex depends upon the presence of a neuroreceptor system beginning in the smooth muscle of the upper part of the rectum. When its tension reaches a threshold, this musculature contracts, joining and augmenting an entire complex of abdominal wall contraction, internal anal sphincter relaxation, and opening of the external anal sphincter. The reflex is believed to be further augmented by the anal sensation of feces passing though the anal canal, and perhaps also by associated reflexes like that of micturition. The central representation of defecation lies, in experimental animals, in the medulla near the vomiting center, and it may be transiently disturbed by vascular insults to the brain. Voluntary inhibition of defecation, described earlier, is mediated through rapid relaxation of the abdominal musculature and the contraction of the external anal sphincter.

This sequence of events can take place in persons whose sacral cord has been destroyed—i.e., all its elements can function in the absence of an intact peripheral nerve supply—but the strength of such a denervated contraction is weak, and evacuation is generally incomplete unless distention, usually by enema, reinforces the reflex. Cord transection abolishes the cerebral appreciation of the urge to defecate. Thus disease or trauma to the higher region of the spinal cord and the brain can produce in the function of colon and rectum the same range of functional disturbances as occur in the bladder (see Chap. 46). The colon may become hypotonic, the external sphincter ineffective, and the defecatory reflexes dulled; the levatores ani are often weak and the abdominal musculature unable to produce and sustain effective pressure increases.

The inability to appreciate anal sensation, whether due to central disease, peripheral neuritis of sacral nerves, or surgical interruption of anal innervation, as in treatment of hemorrhoids and perirectal abscess, may also weaken the responses and is often particularly troublesome when the stool is semisolid or liquid. The "sensing" of the consistency of rectal contents by anal receptors has been demonstrated only recently; it provides some explanation for the unpleasant fact that many surgical repairs of the anorectal area look anatomically excellent but the patient is incontinent of any fecal material other than a hard dry stool.

Sudden interruption of function of the central nervous system, as by cerebral vascular accident, interferes with this whole defecatory complex at many levels, and usually results in some fecal incontinence. The dysfunction is maximal at the onset of the process, and function generally returns toward normal over a period of weeks. In most forms of neurologic disease resulting in incontinence, the reflex may be satisfactorily activated by rectal distention, most practically produced by a combination of laxatives and enemas, which results in a mass movement in the more proximal part of the intestine, augmenting the reflex evacuation from the rectum. As sensation from the anal area returns, the passage of stool through the anus reinforces the reflex. Since the intestine is filled infrequently, and irrigation techniques are generally effective and not dangerous, fecal incontinence in such patients is usually much less troublesome than is urinary incontinence. Fecal impactions may be prevented by regularly administered enemas, control of diet, use of drugs, and regular exercises for strengthening the voluntary anal muscles.

DISORDERED INTESTINAL FUNCTION

SYMPTOMS Exaggerations of the motor components of normal gastrointestinal activity constitute the most important early symptoms of gastrointestinal diseases. In the small intestine rapid propulsive motility may be associated with dyssynergy, the combination giving rise to cramping contractions. Because of the rather imprecise character of man's system for the detection and recognition of the sources of visceral pain, these cramps are usually projected to the midline—if they originate in the duodenum, to the epigastrium; if from the jejunum, to the umbilicus; if from the lower part of the ileum, to the area just below the umbilicus. In the colon, dyssynergic activity is rarely projected to the midline but usually is lateralized along the general course of the offending organ. Since the colon is large, festooning the abdomen, and full of fluid and partially compressible gas, contractions in one or another area of the intestine may force the contents back toward the cecum; a simultaneous dyssynergic contraction anywhere else in the colonic wall may trap gas in the area intervening, distending a relaxed but otherwise innocent portion of the intestine so that discomfort is referred to the distended site, often in the splenic or hepatic flexure. Gas in the colon is derived partially from swallowed air and partially from bacterial decomposition of sugars not completely hydrolyzed and absorbed by the small intestine. The laxative reputation of beans derives from their content of stachyose and raffinose. The polysaccharides are not broken down by intestinal enzymes, arrive in the right side of the colon, and are metabolized by colonic bacteria, with the production of large amounts of hydrogen and carbon dioxide. Common sugars like lactose, in lactase-deficient populations, also provide colonic bacteria with substrate for gas production. Sharp, unpleasant contractions in the left lower quadrant associated with straining at stool and partially relieved by defecation are called *tenesmus.* A sensation of urgent need to defecate—*rectal urgency*—is an extremely distressing symptom associated with irritability of the rectum. Sharp pain in the anal area is made worse by defecation and is usually associated with an inflammatory response in the skin of the anus—*anal pain.*

After establishing the presence or absence of these deviations, the physician must find out whether or not eating or defecation exacerbates or relieves them, whether the patient tries to mitigate the discomfort by moving about or by lying still, or by holding the abdominal wall immobilized with his hands or against the mattress. Although the general topography of the area of distress may localize findings to the large or small intestine, relief by defecation is a feature of disturbance of the left side of the colon, as exacerbation by eating is usually a feature of malfunction of the small intestine or right side of the colon. Restlessness occurs with colic; peritoneal irritation tends to immobilize the patient. All these disturbances originate as increases in the tone of the intestinal wall, and pressure relationships between adjacent segments of intestine determine not only the tension exerted against the wall but also the speed and character of the flow of the fluid contents along the lumen. As increased tension may compress the vessels nourishing the intestinal wall, so disease or contraction of the nourishing vasculature may deprive the wall of its ability to contract, to absorb, or to secrete. Unabsorbed residue or unduly large volumes of secretions attract more fluid into the lumen, further distending the intestine; if large volumes of swallowed air cannot be passed quickly along the small intestine to the cecum, as is usual, the movements of the air-fluid mixture in the small intestine become loud enough to be noticed by the patient; such *borborygmi* are heard normally in the colon. Sudden changes in volume of the abdomen—*distention*—occur when the intraluminal volume of the small or large intestine increases, because of paralysis of neuromuscular elements, abnormal handling of gas, or mechanical obstruction behind which muscular contractile activity is greatly increased. Bowel sounds may be absent if the wall is paralyzed, faint if the injury is submaximal, or increased if a viable area is forced to raise its intraluminal pressure in order to drive fluid past an obstructed segment. Sudden changes in pain reference occurring during the course of an illness usually indicate that the peritoneal surfaces have become involved, with more accurate cerebral localization of the underlying disturbance, and perhaps with associated development of spasm or guarding of the overlying musculature.

DIARRHEA AND CONSTIPATION *Diarrhea* and *constipation* are terms given to alterations in the normal pattern of human defecation habits. There is no standard definition by which patients or physicians may classify strictly the deviation from normal; the range of variation in bowel habits among apparently healthy persons is extraordinarily wide, so that the deviation must be compared with each patient's previous pattern. Diarrhea may be considered as the frequent passage of unformed stools, and constipation as an undue delay in the evacuation of feces. It is the task of the physician to understand enough of the normal and disturbed physiology of digestion, absorption, and propulsive motility that he may ask pointed questions of the patient which serve to define more precisely the locus, the nature, and the severity of the disturbance.

ACUTE DIARRHEA Acute disturbances of intestinal function are relatively common and usually manifest themselves as diarrhea. The sudden onset of loose stools in a previously healthy person commonly is due to an active infection and much less often to the ingestion of toxins, poisonous chemicals, or drugs. When the patient is first seen, the history will usually point toward the source of the trouble: the eating of a particular meal or food in company with others who have also become similarly ill within 24 hr of eating the suspected food is *prima facie* evidence that a preformed toxin has been ingested; diarrhea developing in a number of patients within 28 to 72 hr after a common meal should make one suspect a salmonella infection. The presence of fever, malaise, muscle aching, and profound epigastric or periumbilical discomfort with severe anorexia suggests inflammatory disease of the small intestine. With acute diarrhea, the stools are characteristically watery, often accompanied by the explosive passage of gas; there is no rectal urgency or tenesmus and little hypogastric cramping. On physical examination one finds a generally tender abdomen without guarding, and one hears "whooshing" peristaltic sounds. The hemogram usually is within normal limits. Commonly, acute diarrhea is produced by infection with a virus, of which a number of species have been identified. Viral gastroenteritis runs an acute course for 2 to 3 days, then gradually subsides. The stool in viral gastroenteritis never contains recognizable exudate—it is singularly free of inflammatory cells, blood, or fibrin. Culture of the stool is usually nonproductive. By contrast, inflammatory diseases of the colon almost always result in leukocytic exudate and fibrin in the feces; stools may give culture positive for organisms of the genus *Salmonella* or *Shigella* or may on microscopic examination show motile forms and/or cysts of various parasites, the most important of which in the United States is *Endamoeba histolytica.* Colonic infections usually are accompanied by hypogastric cramping, tenesmus, and rectal urgency. The patient may not have true anorexia but may be afraid to eat because eating stimulates the urge to defecate. There are usually fever and leukocytosis.

Recently, our understanding of acute diarrhea has advanced with the demonstration that the small intestine can actively *secrete* fluids from the base of the villi while maintaining normal absorption at the villous tips. Relative oversecretion occurs in the presence of the enterotoxins of *Vibrio cholerae* and of *Escherichia coli;* the latter does not seem to bind to the cell and therefore produces a shorter-lived watery diarrhea. The effect of these toxins in stimulating intestinal secretion appears to be mediated by the adenyl cyclase system and by the prostaglandins.

By contrast *Shigella* organisms penetrate the mucosa into the lamina propria, which becomes hyperemic and ulcerated. In addition to this morphologic colitis, the ileum is stimulated to oversecrete its bicarbonate-rich fluid, adding to the total diarrheal stool. *Travelers' diarrhea* cannot yet be considered an etiologic entity, but may result from the activation of any of the above mechanisms by toxins produced by bacteria thought otherwise not to be pathogenic.

Acute diarrhea may be the presenting symptom of any type of systemic infection or of a hitherto-silent chronic gastrointestinal disease, of which the most well-defined are *regional enteritis* and *ulcerative colitis;* the latter may occasionally begin with fulminant dysentery, the former more often presenting as a tender mass in the right lower quadrant with mild diarrhea. Generalized cramping and diarrhea may follow use of a parasympathomimetic drug. Tenesmus, urgency, and left-sided hypogastric tenderness and cramping are classic symptoms of *diverticulitis;* the stool may contain pus, blood, or both, usually with much mucus. A fecal impaction may cause a patient to have rectal urgency but expel only a little watery exudate or nothing. Short-circuiting operations on the intestine and stomach usually result in mild diarrhea for months after the operation.

Differential diagnosis of these varied entities is made by history, physical examination, gross and microscopic appearance of the stools, appropriate bacteriologic studies, and proctoscopy. Since fluid and electrolyte losses in diarrhea may be so great as to be life-threatening, the patient is given supportive care until studies indicate specific treatment. If no definitive etiologic agent can be identified, barium enema and upper gastrointestinal roentgenograms should be carried out. Upper gastrointestinal films may be very misleading when the barium meal is fed within the first few days of an acute enteritis or colitis, and should be reserved for a time when the whole disease has become more quiescent.

CHRONIC DIARRHEA A history of bouts of loose stools extending over a period of months or years, usually intermittent in character, calls for painstaking investigation. One particularly wants to know the circumstances of the first such bout—did it follow an acute infection, an operation, an emotional upset of severe degree? The number of days or weeks lost by the patient from his daily occupation on account of the illness, changes in weight, strength, and appearance give important leads as to the nature and severity of the underlying disease. By the time the patient sees a physician the presenting symptoms may not be diarrhea but rather those of serious malnutrition, since any long-continued illness of this type may interfere with appetite as well as with absorptive and digestive functions. Associated signs and symptoms may reveal that the diarrhea and malnutrition are due to a generalized disorder—hyperthyroidism, tuberculosis, lymphosarcoma, to name a few—which may involve the intestines functionally or structurally.

A long history of intermittent diarrhea unaccompanied by fever, weight loss, blood in the stools, or significant loss of working capacity suggests an *emotional* or *allergic* disorder. A detailed dietary history is important in such cases, in order to establish the adequacy of the nutrient intake and to allow the patient a chance to ventilate his ideas on the relationship of food and eating to his symptoms. In such disordered functional states, the patient usually has a fairly formed stool on arising in the morning but then has one or two loose stools within the next hour. A similar pattern may occur after the evening meal. The stool caliber is usually small, and there may be mild discomfort in the left lower quadrant of the abdomen, relieved by defecation. Such a triad of symptoms makes up the diarrheal component of the "irritable colon" syndrome, an extremely common disorder in anxious, nervous people, in which the symptoms result from exaggeration of normal colonic function.

When diarrheal episodes are characterized by blood in the stools, or by fever, malaise, anorexia, and weight loss, one suspects a chronic inflammatory process involving either the small intestine or the colon or both. *Regional enteritis* may attack any portion of the intestine, producing an encroachment on the lumen and episodes of partial obstruction, mucosal ulcerations, or local abscesses and fistulas of the abdominal or anal skin, of the bladder, or of other loops of intestine. On proctoscopic examination the rectum is often seen to be normal or discretely erythematous. The stools show little microscopic exudate, although they are often positive for occult blood, gross bleeding being infrequently encountered. Tuberculosis and lymposarcoma of the intestine can give similar symptoms and may be impossible to differentiate, although usually the roentgenologic appearances are dissimilar.

The involvement may be primarily colonic, the most important diseases being *ulcerative colitis,* amebic colitis, or Crohn's disease. Here the feces may show pus cells and red blood cells when the disease is active, and proctoscopy is usually diagnostic. Stool cultures and examinations for parasites on numerous occasions are important aspects of the medical investigation.

When the patient presents with diarrhea of more than a few months' duration, with weight loss, weakness, and symptoms of nutritional deficiency disease, but without fever or melena, disorders of the small intestine should be considered. In children celiac disease (gluten-sensitive enteropathy) and cystic fibrosis of the pancreas are the important disorders to be differentiated; in older patients the same distinction between an absorptive defect and a digestive disorder must still be made in order to distinguish gluten-sensitive enteropathy from chronic pancreatitis. In these disorders the stools are light in color, often frothy, and malodorous. See Chap. 284 for differential diagnosis of malabsorption.

A history of progressive disease characterized by arthritis, abdominal pain, diarrhea, and weight loss in middle-aged men suggests the diagnosis of Whipple's disease. Lymphosarcomas may produce malabsorption syndromes by blockage of lymphatic channels from the small intestine. Areas of intestine with relative stasis may become "blind loops" and harbor large numbers of bacteria, which deconjugate bile salts and utilize nutrients needed by the host. The presenting symptoms of such pathologic disturbances may be diarrhea, steatorrhea, and macrocytic anemia. Surgical revisions of the intestine, multiple jejunal diverticulosis, and regional enteritis may result in such conditions. Rarer causes of diarrhea are the enormous hypersecretion of gastric juice due to tumors secreting peptide hormones (as in the Zollinger-Ellison syndrome), and the increased motility due to serotonin in the carcinoid syndrome (see Chap. 99).

Special techniques are often needed to define clearly all these abnormalities. Duodenal intubation and analysis of digestive juices for pancreatic enzymes is of considerable importance in ruling out primary disease of the pancreas. Nevertheless, the aid of the skilled radiologist is probably more useful than any test in interpreting all but the earliest manifestations of these syndromes. Pancreatic calcification, fistulas, distortions of the duodenal loop, diffuse granulomatous diseases of the small intestine, diverticula, polyps, ulcerated areas, stenosis, and obstruction, all can be identified by modern radiologic techniques.

CONSTIPATION Whereas diarrhea may be a dangerous symptom per se, with its accompaniment of dehydration and loss of cations, constipation of itself is not debilitating. The acute onset of severe constipation in an apparently normal person signifies that something has disturbed the neural, cascular, or muscular integrity of the intestine or associated defecatory reflexes and muscles. Such disturbances may result from severe infections, particularly of the central nervous system, from acute mesenteric circulatory catastrophes, renal colic, cerebrovascular accidents, mechanical obstruction of large or small intestine, painful anal lesions, certain drugs, or fecal impaction. Rapid and complete physical examination including a digital examination of the rectum and proctoscopy is called for in all cases of acute constipation. If no other physical signs to explain the sudden constipation are elicited, a low-pressure barium enema should be given to establish the site of obstruction, if present, and appropriate measures taken.

A long history of intermittent bouts of constipation, accompanied by abdominal distress, relieved by defecation and by passage of hard stools of small caliber, with or without mucus, is characteristic of the "irritable colon" syndrome, one of the most common forms of anxiety met by the physician. The abuse of laxatives over many years frequently aggravates the underlying clinical picture. The symptoms are essentially exaggerations of normal physiologic activity of the colon and in mild degrees are usually experienced by most normal individuals. Extensive studies of sigmoid motility in patients with this syndrome have shown that disturbed motor function correlates closely with emotional conflicts. Proctoscopic examination of these patients demonstrates an unremarkable rectum and a rectosigmoid which is often spastic, the lumen smaller than normal, the veins prominent, and the mucus more abundant than usual. The stools are negative for blood, parasites, and pathogenic bacteria; the x-ray examination usually reveals nothing abnormal.

Another common disorder is atonic constipation. Patients with this disorder, whether as the result of childhood training or of a perverted understanding of the necessity for daily bowel movements, have equated general health with "bowel regularity." This leads to a dependence on laxatives or enemas to hasten the "overdue" evacuation, so that over the years they lose the sensitivity of the rectal defecatory reflexes. Consequently, they do not have a regular schedule for moving their bowels, which for most normal people is most easily accomplished after breakfast and, if needed, after the heaviest meal of the day; over the years they no longer demonstrate any rhythmicity in defecation, take laxatives whenever they feel "run down," and have stools which may be alternately voluminous and watery or small and hard. Lax abdominal muscles and a pelvic floor weakened by multiple deliveries may contribute to poor defecatory performance. On physical examination these patients often have a palpable colon filled with feces, and on rectal examination feces fill the ampulla, the patient being unaware of this.

In both the above types of constipation, it is obvious that a thorough analysis of dietary and defecatory habits, use of laxatives, mode of living, and emotional problems must be made before proper therapy can be instituted. At the same time it must be stressed that such patients are not immune to the development of colonic neoplasms, and it is a most difficult task to decide how often complete studies should be carried out on patients with longstanding, apparently static, complaints. The simplest solution is to do repeated stool examinations for occult blood and digital and proctoscopic examinations, remembering that in patients who have difficulty with evacuation, anal diseases—fissures, ulcers, and hemorrhoids—are more common than in the general population.

A lifelong history of obstinate constipation may be associated with the enormous dilatation of the large intestine seen in *idiopathic* or acquired megacolon. In the former condition, the rectosigmoid is contracted and obstructing because of its lack of the ganglionic cells necessary to pass on the propulsive waves of the proximal portion of the colon; in the latter condition, severe contraction of the voluntary anal sphincter produces enormous dilatation of the rectal ampulla and colon. Radiologic studies are usually helpful in differentiating these two conditions.

When constipation is of recent onset and progressive, the investigation should be thorough and extremely comprehensive. General physical and psychiatric examination may reveal a systemic disorder such as hypothyroidism, hyperparathyroidism, tuberculosis, urinary tract disease, or congestive heart failure. A major psychosis, profound depression, parkinsonism, or a recent cerebrovascular accident may be responsible for progressive constipation. A careful history of drug ingestion may reveal that the patient received ganglionic-blocking agents, opiates, or heavy sedation prior to onset of symptoms. A marked change in dietary regimen, particularly in combination with sedative drugs, may produce a marked decrease in frequency of bowel movements.

If the digital and proctoscopic findings fail to explain the constipation, a barium enema and upper gastrointestinal roentgenograms are indicated. Tumors of the gastrointestinal tract comprise nearly half of all cancers, and patients with colonic cancers have a better prognosis for survival after surgical resection than those with gastric and esophageal lesions. A high index of suspicion for a neoplastic origin of changes in bowel habits, repeated tests for occult blood in the stools, and careful proctoscopy and x-ray studies will usually justify in salvaged lives the money and time spent.

PROCTALGIA See Chap. 288.

REFERENCES

DAVENPORT HW: *Physiology of the Digestive Tract,* 3d ed., Chicago: Year Book, 1971

GRADY GF, KEUSCH GT: Pathogenesis of bacterial diarrheas. N Engl J Med 285:831, 891, 1971

PHILLIPS, SF: Diarrhea: A current view of the pathophysiology. Gastroenterology 63:495, 1972

41 HEMATEMESIS AND MELENA

KURT J. ISSELBACHER
RAYMOND S. KOFF

Hematemesis is defined as the vomiting of blood, and *melena* as the passage of black, tarry stools. These dramatic symptoms of gastrointestinal hemorrhage should not only bring the patient to prompt medical attention but, within certain limits, help define the anatomic site of bleeding. Only rarely will exsanguinating gastrointestinal hemorrhage occur without the appearance of altered or gross blood passed by mouth or rectum. The color of vomited blood will vary from red to black depending upon the duration of contact of the blood with gastric acid in the stomach. Thus if vomiting occurs shortly after the onset of bleeding, the vomitus is likely to be red; if there is delay in vomiting, the appearance will be dark-red, black, or of "coffee grounds" appearance. Since blood entering the gastrointestinal tract below the duodenum rarely reenters the stomach, hematemesis usually indicates that the bleeding is proximal to the jejunum.

Melena may occur independently of, or be associated with, hematemesis. Bleeding of sufficient volume to produce hematemesis usually results in melena. The altered color of the blood results from prolonged contact with gastric juice to produce hematin. In contrast to hematemesis, melena may result from hemorrhage into the jejunum or ileum provided that transit through the intestine is slow. At least 50 to 100 ml blood must rapidly enter the upper part of the gastrointestinal tract to produce a single black, tarry stool. Following a single-liter episode of hemorrhage, tarry stools will persist for 1 to 3 days. Subsequently the stools return to normal color, but tests for occult blood may be positive for 3 to 8 days.

The passage of red blood per rectum usually denotes lower intestinal bleeding, i.e., bleeding originating below the duodenum. However, if bleeding is massive and rapid enough, red blood may appear per rectum from an upper intestinal or gastric lesion.

Not all black or red stools are due to blood. Black stools may result from the ingestion of iron, charcoal, or bismuth. Red or purple stools are occasionally seen after ingestion of beets or following intravenous administration of sulfobromophthalein. Gastrointestinal bleeding, even if detected only by positive tests for occult blood in the stool or clear aspirate of the gastric contents, indicates potentially serious disease and must be investigated.

The clinical manifestations of gastrointestinal bleeding are dependent upon the extent of hemorrhage, the rate of bleeding, and associated or coincidental diseases. Unless anemia is present prior to the onset of bleeding, loss of less than 500 ml blood is usually not associated with systemic symptoms. Rapid hemorrhage of greater volume will result in decreased venous return to the heart, decreased cardiac output, reflex vasoconstriction, and increased peripheral resistance. The patient may experience syncope, lightheadedness, nausea, sweating, and thirst. He may appear anxious and restless. When blood loss approaches 40 percent of the blood volume, shock with tachycardia and a thready peripheral pulse are usually present. The skin is cold and clammy, and pallor is prominent. Hematocrits will not reflect the blood loss accurately until several hours after the start of the hemorrhage, when hemodilution has occurred. The platelet count rises, and leukocytosis is found 2 to 5 hr after onset of bleeding. Occasionally blood in the intestinal tract is associated with mild fever (100 to 102°F), and the blood urea nitrogen level becomes variably elevated 24 to 48 hr after bleeding, because of the breakdown of blood proteins to urea by intestinal bacteria.

ETIOLOGY OF UPPER GASTROINTESTINAL BLEEDING Swallowed blood resulting from epistaxis, hemoptysis, dental extractions, and tonsillectomy may be vomited or result in melena. A careful history and physical examination will exclude these sources.

The three most common causes of upper gastrointestinal hemorrhage are (1) variceal bleeding, (2) peptic ulceration, and (3) erosive gastritis. These three entities encompass 90 to 95 percent of all cases of upper gastrointestinal bleeding in which a definite lesion can be found.

Variceal bleeding Bleeding from esophageal or gastric varices is most frequently associated with portal hypertension due to cirrhosis of the liver. Although in the United States alcoholic cirrhosis is by far the most prevalent form of this disease, variceal hemorrhage may occur in other forms of cirrhosis associated with portal hypertension, especially postnecrotic cirrhosis. Portal vein thrombosis may also lead to variceal hemorrhage in the absence of cirrhosis. Bleeding from varices tends to be abrupt and often massive; however, minor bleeding may occur for days from esophageal varices before it is discovered. Upper gastrointestinal bleeding in a patient with cirrhosis suggests a variceal source, but because patients with cirrhosis have a higher incidence of peptic ulceration, bleeding from the latter must be excluded. Furthermore, in the alcoholic patient with cirrhosis who has continued to drink prior to the onset of bleeding, bleeding from gastritis is quite common.

Peptic ulcer Peptic ulcer disease is probably the most common cause of upper gastrointestinal bleeding. The majority of these ulcers are situated in the duodenum. About 20 to 30 percent of patients with peptic ulcer will have at least one episode of significant gastrointestinal bleeding. When a patient with known peptic ulcer has gastrointestinal hemorrhage, the ulcer is the most probable site of bleeding.

Gastritis Gastritis may be associated with recent heavy alcohol ingestion or with a history of ingestion of salicylates or other drugs. Similarly gastric erosions and ulcerations may occur in "stressful" situations and are not infrequently found in patients with intracranial disease, burns, or recent trauma. Erosive gastritis can rarely be diagnosed by radiologic techniques, and gastroscopy is necessary to confirm this diagnosis.

Other lesions Less common sources of upper gastrointestinal bleeding originating in the esophagus include esophagitis (with or without hiatus hernia), carcinoma, and peptic ulcer of the esophagus. Lacerations of the mucosa of the distal end of the esophagus associated with severe vomiting (the Mallory-Weiss syndrome) are suggested by a history of nonbloody vomiting followed by hematemesis. Though sudden severe hemorrhage is seen in a small number of patients with carcinoma of the stomach, particularly in association with mucosal ulceration, chronic blood loss is a more frequent complication of gastric carcinoma. Mesenteric venous or arterial occlusion by embolism or thrombosis may produce either occult or overt blood loss.

Lymphoma, polyps, and other tumors of the stomach and proximal small intestine are relatively uncommon lesions and are therefore unusual sources of hemorrhage. The Peutz-Jeghers syndrome of small-intestinal polyposis and melanin pigmentation of the lips, mucosa, fingers, and toes may be associated with recurrent melena.

Saccular arteriosclerotic aortic aneurysms may rupture into the upper part of the intestine and are almost invariably fatal. Most commonly rupture occurs into the third portion of the duodenum. Sudden intestinal bleeding may occur following abdominal trauma and hepatic laceration. Such bleeding should suggest the entry of blood from a damaged liver into the bile ducts, i.e., hemobilia.

Primary blood dyscrasias, including leukemia, thrombocytopenic states, and the hemophilias, may result in significant gastrointestinal bleeding. Polycythemia vera, although associated with an increased incidence of peptic ulceration, may also result in gastrointestinal bleeding because of mesenteric or portal vein thrombosis. Periarteritis nodosa, Henoch-Schönlein purpura, and other vasculitides may lead to gastrointestinal blood loss.

Gastrointestinal bleeding, usually mild although occasionally persistent, may accompany amyloidosis. , Osler-Rendu-Weber disease, pseudoxanthoma elasticum, Turner's syndrome, single or multiple intestinal hemangiomas, neurofibromatosis, Kaposi's sarcoma, and hemangiectatic hypertrophy. Hematemesis and melena occur in uremia, with occult intestinal bleeding being the most common cause. In central nervous system disorders, especially after trauma or surgery, superficial gastric erosions may develop (Cushing's ulcers) and be a cause of upper intestinal bleeding.

ETIOLOGY OF LOWER GASTROINTESTINAL BLEEDING Anal lesions Small amounts of bright-red blood on the surface of the stool and on toilet tissue are most commonly caused by hemorrhoids. Bleeding from internal or external hemorrhoids is frequently precipitated by straining or passage of hard stools. Anal fissures or fistulas likewise first may come to the attention of the patient as a result of rectal bleeding. An anal pathologic condition does not preclude other causes and sources of bleeding, such as carcinoma, and these must be sought and excluded.

Rectum and colonic disease Carcinoma of the rectum, rectal polyps, and ulcerative proctitis are the most common bleeding lesions of the rectum. Bleeding from carcinoma in any area of the colon may result in the appearance of gross blood, whether on the stool or mixed with the fecal contents. Bloody diarrhea is often the presenting feature of ulcerative colitis but is less common in granulomatous ileocolitis, although occult blood may be present in the stool. Bleeding may also accompany diarrhea due to infectious agents.

Diverticula Intestinal diverticula may occur in every part of the intestinal tract but are most commonly found in the sigmoid colon. Diverticulosis per se may be a cause of massive or mild gastrointestinal bleeding. Mild blood loss is more common when inflammation is present, i.e., in diverticulitis. Meckel's diverticulum, a congenital anomaly occurring in about 2 percent of the population and located in the ileum usually 20 to 100 cm proximal to the ileocecal valve, is often associated with bleeding. Ectopic gastric musoca may be present in about 15 percent of these diverticula and may ulcerate, with profuse or recurrent rectal hemorrhage, particularly in children and young adults.

APPROACH TO THE PATIENT WITH GASTROINTESTINAL BLEEDING The approach to the problem presented by the patient with gross bleeding from the gastrointestinal tract is dependent upon the site, extent, and rate of bleeding. In general the patient with hematemesis is more likely to have bled greater amounts and is more likely to exsanguinate than the patient with melena. There is usually a sense of urgency in the immediate diagnosis and treatment of patients with upper gastrointestinal bleeding. When first seen, the patient may be in shock. Before a complete history and physical examination are undertaken, blood must be obtained for typing and cross matching, and an intravenous infusion of saline solution or other plasma expanders must be started at once.

History A history of epigastric pain relieved by food, milk, or antacids strongly suggests peptic ulcer disease. A history of jaundice and alcoholism suggests chronic liver disease. One must carefully inquire about a recent alcoholic binge or the ingestion of drugs such as aspirin, which may be associated with gastritis or precipitate bleeding from peptic ulcer. Attention must be directed to possible previous episodes of bleeding, vomiting, symptoms of gastrointestinal distress, diarrhea, cramps, weight loss, fever, bleeding from other sites such as the skin and mucous membranes, and a family history of intestinal disease or hemorrhagic diathesis.

Physical examination Physical examination is directed to excluding a nonintestinal source of blood (i.e., ruling out epistaxis, hemoptysis, pharyngeal lesions). Careful assessment of the skin may reveal the characteristic telangiectasia of Osler-Rendu-Weber disease, the diffuse melanin pigmentation of hemochromatosis, the localized pigmentation of Peutz-Jeghers syndrome, the soft-tissue tumors and multiple sebaceous cysts which occur with colonic polyposis in Gardner's syndrome, or the dermal neurofibromas of neurofibromatosis. The peripheral stigmas of chronic liver disease with hepatosplenomegaly, ascites, and edema suggest the likelihood of portal hypertension and the possibility of bleeding from varices, gastritis, or peptic ulceration. One must look for abdominal tenderness or masses, determine the frequency and character of the bowel sounds, and look for evidence of malignancy such as a Virchow's node or rectal shelf.

Laboratory studies Initial studies include the hematocrit, hemoglobin, careful assessment of red blood cell morphologic features (hypochromic, microcytic red blood cells suggest that blood loss is chronic), white blood cell count, and differential blood cell count. There should be a platelet count, or the number of platelets should be estimated from the blood smear. Prothrombin time and coagulation studies may be in order to exclude primary or secondary clotting defects. Though the initial studies are valuable and essential, repeated evaluation of the laboratory data is important as one follows the clinical course of the bleeding.

DIAGNOSTIC APPROACH The diagnostic approach (see also Chaps. 282 and 296 for additional and detailed discussions) to the patient with gastrointestinal hemorrhage must necessarily be individualized. The initial management of gastrointestinal bleeding may be under the direction of the internist, but it is prudent to consult a surgeon early in the course of the illness in the event that the bleeding cannot be controlled by medical means. It must be emphasized that demonstration of a lesion in a patient with gastrointestinal bleeding should also be accompanied by evidence that this lesion is the site of bleeding. In recent years the availability of experienced endoscopists as well as radiologists with facilities for selective arteriography has increased to the extent that in many medical centers it is possible to have emergency endoscopy, barium, and angiographic studies performed within hours of the patient's admission to the hospital. It is to be hoped that this "vigorous diagnostic approach" will serve to decrease the morbidity and mortality associated with upper gastrointestinal bleeding.

When there is a history of melena or hematemesis or the suspicion of bleeding from the upper part of the gastrointestinal tract, the patient should have a tube passed to empty the stomach and to determine whether the bleeding is in the upper part of the gastrointestinal tract and is still active. Provided that blood volume is maintained, the next diagnostic step will depend on whether the bleeding continues. This is generally determined by vital signs, gastric aspiration, the number, frequency, and consistency of stools, and requirements for blood.

If gastric aspiration suggests that bleeding has stopped, medical treatment may be initiated. Upper gastrointestinal barium studies may then be obtained when the patient's general condition has stabilized. If the conventional barium study is nondiagnostic, esophagogastroscopy may be performed 8 to 12 hr later. Some consultants recommend, however, that endoscopy be performed first, with barium studies carried out secondarily.

If upper gastrointestinal bleeding persists, ice water or iced saline lavage may be attempted to slow the bleeding. If bleeding persists, and gastroesophagoscopy and barium studies have not revealed the site of bleeding, the patient should be considered for emergency selective angiography. Angiography may demonstrate the site of active bleeding and, if variceal hemorrhage is suspected, may confirm the presence of varices as well as portal hypertension. Occasionally one may be able to observe the leaking of contrast material from esophageal vessels. Angiography is also valuable in providing information on the patency of the portal, splenic, and left renal veins should surgical decompression of the portal system be contemplated.

When bleeding continues and gastric aspiration fails to reveal fresh bleeding into the stomach, blood loss may be occurring from a lesion beyond the pylorus or ligament of Treitz. In that situation, selective celiac axis and mesenteric artery angiography may be useful to localize the cryptogenic bleeding site. However, extravasation of contrast material into the intestinal lumen can be shown only when bleeding is active and at a rate estimated to be greater than 0.5 ml per min. Arteriography is helpful to reveal the *site of bleeding;* however, the *cause of bleeding* often cannot be determined unless an aneurysm, varix, or vascular malformation is present. A promising approach to the control of persistent bleeding is the continuous administration of vasoconstrictors, such as vasopressin, either by selective superior mesenteric artery infusion (in the case of esophageal varices) or in the case of arterial bleeding by direct infusion of the agent into the vessel leading to the bleeding site (Fig. 41-1).

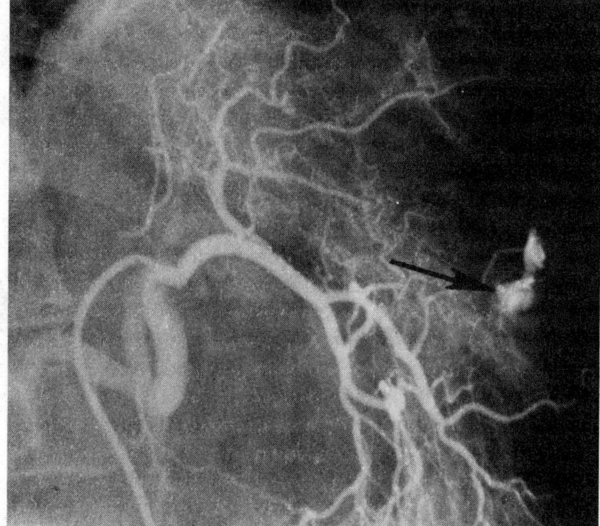

A

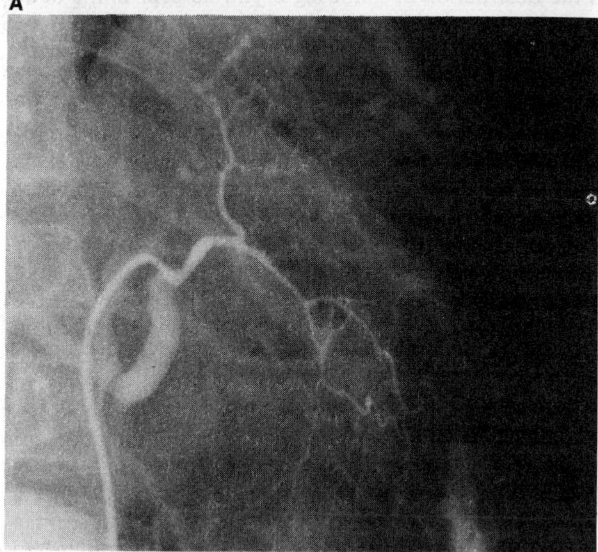

B

FIGURE 41-1
Angiographic findings on a patient with massive upper gastrointestinal bleeding. Angiographic studies revealed the bleeding to be secondary to hemorrhagic gastritis; it was controlled by the selective left gastric arterial infusion of vasopressin. A *Selective left gastric arteriography demonstrates massive extravasation of contrast material (arrow) from a branch of the left gastric artery.* B *Selective left gastric arteriography during the infusion of 0.1 unit of surgical Pituitrin per minute demonstrates a marked decrease in the caliber of the left gastric artery and cessation of hemorrhage.*

If *variceal hemorrhage* is suspected, massive bleeding persists, and angiography is *not* available, the administration of vasopressin into a peripheral vein (10 to 20 units over a 20- to 30-min period and repeated once or twice every 2 to 4 hr) may permit hemostasis by reduction of portal venous pressure. However repeated systemic injections of vasopressin may lead to loss of effectiveness because of tachyphylaxis, and occasionally adverse cardiovascular reactions may occur because of vasoconstrictor effects. It may then be necessary to resort to esophageal tamponade, with a Sengstaken-Blakemore tube. Although tamponade is hazardous because of the occasional occurrence of esophageal erosions or rupture, variceal hemorrhage can frequently be controlled temporarily with this technique. Nevertheless, esophageal tamponade is probably most useful to reduce bleeding and stabilize the patient's condition as a preoperative maneuver.

In the evaluation of *rectal bleeding* (see also Chap. 288) the most important diagnostic procedures are digital examination of the rectum and proctosigmoidoscopy. Biopsy of suggestive lesions may be performed through the sigmoidoscope under direct vision. Barium enema examination and air-contrast studies will aid in localizing lesions above the reach of the sigmoidoscope. Superior and inferior mesenteric angiography is very useful for demonstrating the site of active colonic bleeding, and the local infusion of vasoconstrictors through the angiographic catheter has been successful in controlling hemorrhage. Colonoscopy, by means of a flexible fiber optic instrument capable of permitting visualization of the entire large intestine, is currently being evaluated and may prove useful in determining the site and nature of bleeding lesions proximal to the rectosigmoid area. Bleeding should not be attributed to hemorrhoids or anal fissures unless other lesions have been excluded. When appropriate, stool culture and examination for ova and parasites should be performed.

REFERENCES

Baum S, Nusbaum M: Control of gastrointestinal hemorrhage by selective arterial infusion of vasopressin. Radiology 98:497, 1971

Conn HO, Simpson JA: Excessive mortality associated with balloon tamponade of bleeding varices. JAMA 202:587, 1967

Malt RA: Current concepts: control of massive upper gastrointestinal hemorrhage. N Engl J Med 286:1043, 1972

Palmer ED: The vigorous diagnostic approach to upper-gastrointestinal trace hemorrhage: a 23-year prospective study of 1,400 patients. JAMA 207:1477, 1969

42
JAUNDICE AND HEPATOMEGALY

KURT J. ISSELBACHER

JAUNDICE

Jaundice, or *icterus,* refers to the yellow pigmentation of the skin or scleras by bilirubin. This in turn is a result of elevated levels of bilirubin in the bloodstream. Jaundice may be brought to clinical attention by a darkening of the urine or a yellow discoloration of the skin or sclera; the latter often is the site where clinical icterus may first be detected. Scleral pigmentation is attributed to richness of this tissue in elastin, which has a special affinity for bilirubin. Jaundice must be distinguished from other

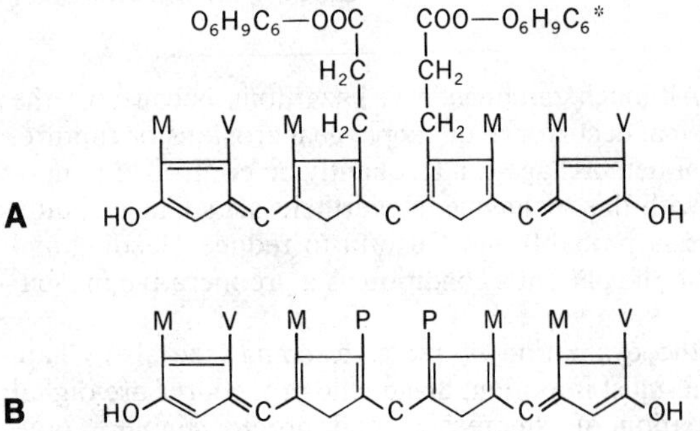

FIGURE 42-1
The chemical structures of conjugated (A) and unconjugated (B) bilirubin. Abbreviations: M = methyl, V = vinyl, P = propionic acid. The asterisk (*) refers to glucuronic acid.

causes of yellow pigmentation such as carotenemia (see Chaps. 55, 80 and 85), which is due to carotenoid pigments in the bloodstream and is associated with a yellowish discoloration of the skin but not of the sclera. Atabrine treatment (see Chap. 211) may produce a yellow color of the skin and urine, but the scleras are usually only minimally discolored, and when pigment is present, it is seen only in the regions of the scleras exposed to light.

Normal serum bilirubin concentrations range from 0.5 to 1.0 mg per 100 ml, and normally most of this is unconjugated (see Fig. 42-1). The precise level at which jaundice becomes clinically evident varies, but usually it can be recognized when the total serum bilirubin exceeds 2 to 2.5 mg per 100 ml. Not infrequently in deep jaundice the skin may take on a greenish hue because of the conversion of bilirubin to biliverdin, an oxidation product of bilirubin. Oxidation occurs more readily with conjugated bilirubin, and hence a greenish hue is seen more frequently in conditions with pronounced conjugated hyperbilirubinemia.

Production and metabolism of bilirubin

NORMAL SOURCES OF BILIRUBIN (Fig. 42-2) The majority of the bilirubin is derived from the catabolism of hemoglobin present in senescent red blood cells. This normally accounts for about 80 to 85 percent of the daily bilirubin production. When a circulating red blood cell reaches the end of its normal life span of approximately 120 days, it is destroyed in the reticuloendothelial system. In the catabolism of hemoglobin, globin is first dissociated from heme, after which the heme moiety is oxidatively cleaved and converted to biliverdin by a microsomal heme oxygenase. This enzyme system requires oxygen and a cofactor, reduced nicotinamide adenine dinucleotide phosphate (NADPH). Bilirubin is then formed from biliverdin by another enzyme, biliverdin reductase.

About 15 to 20 percent of the bilirubin is derived from sources other than senescent erythrocytes. One of these is the *destruction of maturing erythroid cells in the bone marrow,* or so-called "ineffective erythropoiesis" (see Chap. 309). The other is from *nonerythroid components,* especially in the liver, and involves the turnover of heme and heme proteins (such as cytochrome, myoglobin, and heme-containing enzymes). These two sources of bilirubin are collectively referred to as the *early labeled fraction,* a term derived from experiments with labeled glycine and delta-aminolevulinic acid (ALA). Thus when labeled glycine is administered to a normal subject, approximately 15 percent of the label appears in stool stercobilinogen in the first 3 to 5 days; 85 percent of the label appears at about 120 days and reflects the bilirubin produced from the normal destruction of senescent red blood cells.

TRANSPORT OF BILIRUBIN Following liberation of bilirubin into the plasma virtually all the pigment is tightly *bound to albumin.* The maximum binding capacity is 2 moles of bilirubin per mole of albumin. Because in a normal adult this corresponds to plasma unconjugated

FIGURE 42-2
The sources and precursors of plasma bilirubin.

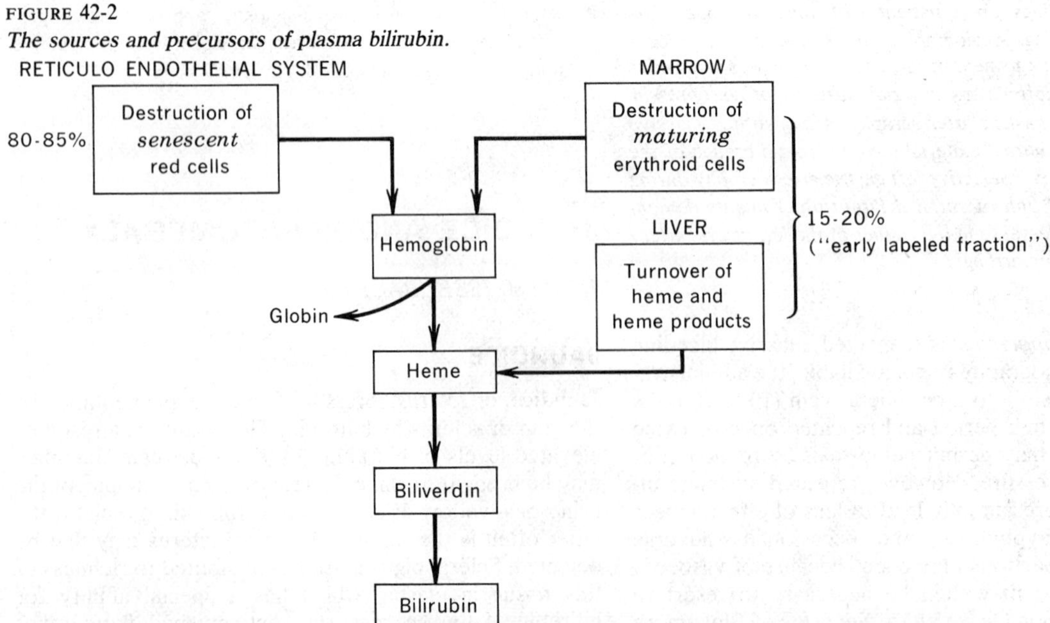

bilirubin concentrations of 60 to 80 mg per ml, saturation of the binding capacity of the plasma almost never occurs. It is clinically relevant that certain organic anions, such as sulfonamides and salicylates, compete with bilirubin for common binding sites on albumin and may displace bilirubin from albumin, permitting it to enter tissues such as the central nervous system. Most of the evidence for albumin binding has been obtained from studies using unconjugated bilirubin. The conjugated pigment also appears to be bound primarily to albumin, although the binding forces may be different. Some conjugated bilirubin in the plasma is ultrafiltrable.

Bilirubin is found in body fluids (cerebrospinal fluid, joint effusions, cysts, etc.) in proportion to the albumin content of the fluids and is absent from true secretions such as tears, saliva, and pancreatic juice. Scar tissue is rarely bilirubin-stained. The appearance of jaundice is also influenced by blood flow and edema. Paralyzed extremities and edematous areas tend to remain uncolored, and "unilateral" jaundice in patients with hemiplegia and edema may be seen if jaundice develops in such patients.

HEPATIC METABOLISM OF BILIRUBIN The liver occupies a central role in the metabolism of the bile pigments. Three distinct phases are recognized: (1) *hepatic uptake,* (2) *conjugation,* and (3) *excretion* into bile. Of these three steps, excretion appears to be the rate-limiting step and the one most susceptible to impairment when the liver cell is damaged.

Uptake Unconjugated bilirubin bound to albumin is presented to the liver cell, and upon entry the pigment and albumin became dissociated. Little is known concerning the uptake phase, but the mechanism is believed to involve the binding of bilirubin to certain cytoplasmic anionic binding proteins referred to as Y and Z proteins or ligandins. Hepatic uptake appears to be reversible.

Conjugation Unconjugated bilirubin is water-insoluble and must be converted to a *water-soluble derivative* in order to be excreted by the liver cell into bile. This is accomplished by the process of conjugation whereby bilirubin is predominantly converted to bilirubin glucuronide (mostly diglucuronide). This reaction occurs in the microsomes or endoplasmic reticulum of the hepatocytes by action of the enzyme glucuronyl transferase. The action catalyzed by glucuronyl transferase is as follows:

Bilirubin + uridine diphosphate glucuronic acid →
bilirubin diglucuronide + uridine diphosphate

As a result of this enzymatic reaction glucuronic acid is attached to the two carboxyl groups of bilirubin (Fig. 42-1). Glucuronyl transferase is also found in kidney and intestine, but the liver is the principal site of conjugated bilirubin formation. The hepatic microsomal glucuronyl transferase system also is involved in the formation of glucuronides of other endogenous and exogenous substances (e.g., conjugates of steroids, antibiotics, and salicylates) (see Chap. 291).

The *major* product of conjugation is *bilirubin diglucuronide.* However, bile also contains various amounts of other derivatives, especially glycosidic conjugates with monosaccharides (e.g., glucose, xylose) and disaccharides (e.g., aldobiuronic acid, hexuronosylhexuronic acid). The role of these other conjugates normally and in disease is unclear.

Excretion or secretion into bile In order for bilirubin to be excreted into bile, *the pigment must be in the conjugated form.* Although the overall process is not well understood, the excretion of conjugated bilirubin into bile appears to be an energy-dependent process and the *rate-limiting* step in the hepatic metabolism of bilirubin. When this step is compromised, two consequences occur: (1) decreased excretion of bilirubin into the bile, and (2) "regurgitation," or reentry of conjugated bilirubin from the liver cells into the bloodstream.

INTESTINAL PHASE OF BILIRUBIN METABOLISM After its appearance in the intestinal lumen, bilirubin glucuronide may be excreted in the stool or metabolized to urobilinogen and related products. Because of its polarity, *conjugated bilirubin is not reabsorbed* by the intestinal mucosa, a mechanism which may serve to rid the body of this pigment.

The formation of urobilinogen from conjugated bilirubin requires the action of bacteria and occurs in the lower part of the small intestine and colon. The bacteria, by stepwise enzymatic reductions, induce the formation of a series of colorless urobilinogens, (Fig. 42-3), which react with Ehrlich's aldehyde reagent to produce red aldehyde complexes. Oxidation of the urobilinogens (i.e., *d*-urobilinogen, mesobilirubinogen, and stercobilinogen) leads to colored products, the urobilins. When urobilin is mixed with Schlesinger's solution (zinc acetate in alcohol), zinc complexes are produced which have an intense green fluorescence. Because these compounds are measured together in most quantitative analyses, they usually are referred to collectively as "urobilinogens."

In contrast to conjugated bilirubin, *urobilinogen is*

FIGURE 42-3
Chemical steps in the reduction of bilirubin to the urobilinogens and urobilins.

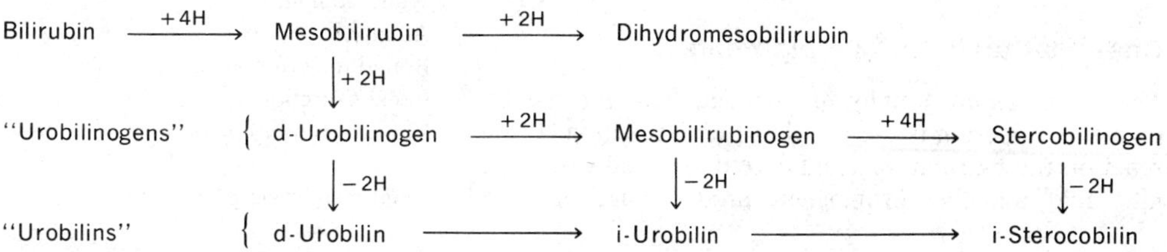

reabsorbed from the small intestine into the portal blood and is thus subject to an enterohepatic circulation. Some urobilinogen is reexcreted by the liver into the bile; the rest is excreted in the urine in an amount usually not exceeding 4 mg daily. When the hepatic excretory mechanism is impaired (e.g., in hepatocellular disease) or the production of bilirubin is greatly increased (e.g., in hemolytic anemia), the urinary urobilinogen may increase significantly.

The normal output of fecal urobilinogen ranges from 50 to 280 mg per day. Under conditions of decreased excretion of conjugated bilirubin into the intestine (e.g., liver disease, bile duct obstruction) or suppression of intestinal flora by antibiotics, fecal output will be diminished. In hemolytic anemia, urinary and fecal urobilinogen excretion is greatly increased.

In a normal person with a blood volume of 5 liters and a hemoglobin concentration of 15 g per 100 ml, the total circulating hemoglobin is 750 g. Because approximately 0.8 percent of the red blood cells are destroyed daily, 6.3 g hemoglobin is released for catabolism. Assuming a quantitative degradation of heme to bilirubin and to urobilinogen, the expected daily output of urobilinogen would be approximately 250 mg plus the additional 15 to 30 mg which would be derived from the other sources described above (i.e., ineffective erythropoiesis, nonhemoglobin heme precursors). Often, however, the amount excreted is considerably less, and it appears likely that there are alternative pathways for hemoglobin degradation not involving bilirubin formation.

RENAL EXCRETION OF BILIRUBIN Normally the urine contains no bilirubin that is detected by the methods usually employed, although traces may be detectable by sensitive spectrophotometric procedures. Unconjugated bilirubin, being tightly bound to albumin, is not filtered by the renal glomerules, and because there is no tubular secretory process for bilirubin, *unconjugated bilirubin is not excreted in urine.* On the other hand, a small fraction of plasma conjugated bilirubin (about 5 percent) is not bound to albumin but is associated with low molecular weight proteins, probably peptides. This non-albumin-bound fraction is dialyzable and is filtered by the renal glomerulus. Thus, in contrast to the unconjugated pigment, a fraction of plasma *conjugated bilirubin appears in the urine.* Bile salts enhance the dialyzability of conjugated bilirubin, and in obstructive jaundice, the elevated level of plasma bile acids may account for an increased renal excretion of conjugated bilirubin. This may also explain why in biliary tract obstruction, serum conjugated bilirubin levels tend to plateau and not to exceed 30 to 40 mg per 100 ml, while with severe hepatocellular injury bilirubin levels higher than this may occur.

Chemical tests for bile pigments

The most widely employed chemical test for the bile pigments in serum is the van den Bergh reaction. In this reaction the bilirubin pigments are diazotized with sulfanilic acid, and the chromogenic products are measured colorimetrically. The van den Bergh reaction can be used to distinguish between unconjugated and conjugated bilirubin because of the different solubility properties of the pigments. When the reaction is carried out in an *aqueous* medium, the water-soluble conjugated bilirubin reacts to give the so-called *direct* van den Bergh reaction. When the reaction is carried out in *methanol,* both conjugated and unconjugated pigments react, giving a measure of the *total* bilirubin level. The total minus the direct-reacting bilirubin give the *indirect* value, which is a measure of the unconjugated bilirubin level.

In the direct van den Bergh reaction, the most accurate measurements are those carried out at 1 min. If the reaction is allowed to proceed longer, a small amount of the unconjugated pigment may begin to react in the aqueous medium. As a result, if the reaction is carried out at 30 min in a patient with unconjugated hyperbilirubinemia, falsely low values for the indirect-reacting bilirubin may be obtained. This serves to emphasize that the direct and indirect van den Bergh reactions represent *approximations* (not absolute measurements) of the conjugated and unconjugated pigments. A summary of the key differences in the properties and reactions of the bilirubin pigments is presented in Table 42-1.

The measurement of bilirubin in the urine may be carried out by the Harrison spot test or with Ictotest[1] tablets. The foam test is also a simple and qualitatively valid procedure. When normal urine is vigorously shaken in a test tube, the foam is absolutely white. In a urine containing bilirubin, the foam will be yellow. This difference may be subtle and may become evident only by comparing a normal urine specimen and one containing bilirubin side by side. Urine urobilinogen may be estimated by the semiquantitative Watson-Schwartz test or the qualitative Diamond test. Fecal measurement must be quantitative to be of value.

Except for concentrated urine, the most common cause of a deep yellow-brown or dark urine is bilirubinuria. However, other mechanisms and diseases associated with a dark urine need to be considered. These include yellow urine due to drugs (e.g., azosulfapyridine); red urine due to porphyria, hemoglobinuria, myoglobinuria, or drugs (e.g., pyridium); and dark-brown or black urine due to homogentisic acid (in ochronosis) or melanin (with melanoma).

[1] *Trademark of Ames Company, Ames, Iowa.*

TABLE 42-1
Comparison of the major differences between conjugated and unconjugated bilirubin

	Bilirubin	
Properties and reactions	*Unconjugated*	*Conjugated*
Water solubility	0	+
Affinity for lipids	+	0
Bound to serum albumin	+++	+
Renal excretion	0	+
Van den Bergh reaction	Indirect (total minus direct)	Direct
Lipid membrane permeability	+	0

APPROACH TO THE PATIENT WITH JAUNDICE

Once jaundice is recognized clinically or chemically, it is important to determine whether it is predominantly due to unconjugated or conjugated hyperbilirubinemia. *A simple clue in this regard is to determine whether bilirubin is present in the urine.* Its absence in the urine suggests unconjugated hyperbilirubinemia (since this pigment is not filtered by the glomerulus); its presence indicates conjugated hyperbilirubinemia. One can then proceed to the direct chemical measurement of the bilirubin pigments in the serum. In predominantly unconjugated hyperbilirubinemia, 80 to 85 percent of the total serum bilirubin is unconjugated (i.e., less than 15 to 20 percent is conjugated). The patient is considered to have predominantly conjugated hyperbilirubinemia when more than 50 percent of the serum bilirubin is of the conjugated type.

An approach to the classification of jaundice based on this important distinction is presented in Table 42-2. Derangements of bilirubin metabolism may occur through any of four mechanisms: (1) overproduction, (2) decreased hepatic uptake, (3) decreased hepatic conjugation, and (4) decreased excretion of bilirubin into bile (due to both intrahepatic and extrahepatic factors). Jaundice may also be described on the basis of the pathogenetic mechanisms or disease processes leading to deranged bilirubin function. Thus, the terms *hemolytic jaundice, hepatocellular jaundice,* and *obstructive* (or cholestatic) *jaundice* are often used.

Though these classifications and terms are helpful, in any one patient more than a single derangement or more than one "type" of jaundice may be present. For example, a patient with cirrhosis may have not only impaired liver cell function (and hence hepatocellular jaundice) but also hemolysis. Furthermore, obstructive jaundice may be due either to *mechanical* obstruction of the biliary radicles or to *functional* factors causing impaired hepatic excretion of bilirubin into bile.

In the present chapter a brief description of the major types of jaundice is given. A more detailed discussion of the individual disease entities is found in Chap. 293.

JAUNDICE WITH PREDOMINANTLY UNCONJUGATED BILIRUBIN IN THE SERUM

Overproduction of bilirubin When an increased amount of hemoglobin is released from red blood cells into either the bloodstream or tissues, increased bilirubin production occurs. Hyperbilirubinemia develops when the capacity of the liver to remove the pigment from the circulation is exceeded. In most cases of hemolysis, the total serum bilirubin concentration ranges from 3 to 5 mg per 100 ml. A slight increase in direct-reacting pigment may also be found, but this usually constitutes less than 15 percent of the total serum bilirubin. This finding is probably analogous to the slight elevations of direct-reacting bilirubin which occur when normal subjects are infused with unconjugated bilirubin. Both instances appear to be a reflection of the fact that the rate-limiting step in hepatic bilirubin metabolism is excretion and that when the excretory capacity of the liver is exceeded, some reentry of conjugated bilirubin into the bloodstream occurs. For a detailed description of the causes of increased bilirubin production, see Chap. 293.

Impaired hepatic uptake of bilirubin As indicated previously, the uptake of bilirubin by the liver cell involves dissociation of the pigment from albumin, and presumably binding to certain cytoplasmic proteins (Y and Z of Arias). In Gilbert's syndrome and some cases of drug-induced jaundice there may be a derangement in this phase of bilirubin metabolism (see Chap. 293).

Impaired glucuronide conjugation Both acquired and genetic derangements in hepatic flucuronyl transferase occur. In the fetus and at birth, glucuronyl transferase activity is low and appears to account in part for the *neonatal jaundice* normally found between the second and the fifth days of life. There is also a rare hereditary disorder, the Crigler-Najjar syndrome, with either an absence (type I) or a deficiency (type II) of glucuronyl

TABLE 42-2
Classification of jaundice based on underlying derangement of bilirubin metabolism

I Predominantly *unconjugated* hyperbilirubinemia
- *A* Overproduction
  - *1* Hemolysis (intra- and extravascular)
  - *2* Ineffective erythropoiesis
- *B* Impaired hepatic uptake
  - *1* Familial (e.g., Gilbert's syndrome)
  - *2* Drugs (e.g., flavaspidic acid)
  - *3* Prolonged fasting
- *C* Impaired bilirubin conjugation (decreased glucuronyl transferase activity)
  - *1* Hereditary absence or deficiency of transferase (type I and type II Crigler-Najjar syndrome)
  - *2* "Immaturity" of transferase (neonatal jaundice)
  - *3* Acquired transferase deficiency
    - *a* Drug inhibition (e.g., pregnanediol, chloramphenicol)
    - *b* Hepatocellular disease (hepatitis, cirrhosis)*

II Predominantly *conjugated* hyperbilirubinemia
- *A* Impaired hepatic excretion (intrahepatic defects)
  - *1* Familial or hereditary disorders
    - *a* Dubin-Johnson syndrome; Rotor syndrome
    - *b* Recurrent (benign) intrahepatic cholestasis
    - *c* Cholestatic jaundice of pregnancy
  - *2* Acquired disorders
    - *a* Hepatocellular disease* (e.g., viral or drug-induced hepatitis)
    - *b* Drug-induced cholestasis (e.g., oral contraceptives, methyltestosterone)
- *B* Extrahepatic biliary obstruction (mechanical obstruction; e.g., stones, stricture, tumor of bile duct)

* *In hepatocellular disease (hepatitis and cirrhosis) there is usually interference in the three major steps of bilirubin metabolism—uptake, conjugation, and excretion. However, excretion is the rate-limiting step and is usually impaired to the greatest extent. As a result, conjugated hyperbilirubinemia predominates.*

transferase leading to pronounced unconjugated hyperbilirubinemia.

Acquired defects in bilirubin glucuronyl transferase activity may be produced by drugs (i.e., enzyme inhibition) or intrinsic liver disease. However, with liver cell damage, the excretory capacity of the liver is impaired to a greater extent than is the conjugating capacity. Therefore in most hepatocellular diseases, the hyperbilirubinemia is predominantly of the conjugated type (see Chap. 293).

JAUNDICE WITH PREDOMINANTLY CONJUGATED BILIRUBIN IN THE SERUM **Impaired excretion of bilirubin by the liver** The impaired excretion of bilirubin into the biliary canaliculi, whether due to functional or mechanical factors, results in predominantly conjugated hyperbilirubinemia and bilirubinuria. The presence of *bilirubin in the urine is evidence of conjugated hyperbilirubinemia* and is a most important point in the differential diagnosis of jaundice. Such findings are identical to those occurring in complete obstruction of the bile duct, emphasizing that *jaundice due to hepatocellular disease can seldom be differentiated from that due to extrahepatic obstruction solely on the basis of changes in bile pigment metabolism.* Indeed there are often instances when the two conditions are not distinguishable by any biochemical criteria and liver biopsy or laparotomy is needed for the definitive diagnosis.

When there is interference in the excretion of conjugated bilirubin into bile, by what mechanism does this pigment enter the systemic circulation? Several postulates have been proposed for this "reentry": (1) rupture of the bile canaliculi secondary to the necrosis of the hepatic cells that constitute their walls; (2) occlusion of the canaliculi by inspissated bile or their compression by swollen hepatic cells; (3) obstruction of the terminal intrahepatic bile ducts (cholangioles) by inflammatory cells; (4) altered hepatic cell permeability; and (5) as a result of impaired excretion, accumulation of conjugated bilirubin in the hepatocytes and secondary diffusion into the plasma. Although some of these postulates are speculative, it is likely that several of these mechanisms occur. For example, occasionally in histologic sections escape of bile through rents in the walls of canaliculi in areas of necrosis is apparent. Also microscopic studies of the liver of rats injected with fluorescent dyes have shown reflux of bile from canaliculi into sinusoids. However, no anatomic damage needs to be invoked, because when unconjugated bilirubin is infused into normal subjects at high rates, conjugated hyperbilirubinemia occurs; this is explained most logically by passive diffusion.

Extrahepatic biliary obstruction Complete obstruction of the extrahepatic bile ducts leads to jaundice with predominantly conjugated hyperbilirubinemia, bilirubinuria, and clay-colored stools. Failure of bile to reach the intestine results in virtual disappearance of urobilinogen from the stool and urine. The concentration of bilirubin rises progressively but then usually plateaus at a level of 30 to 40 mg per 100 ml. To some extent this plateau may be explained by a balance between renal excretion and diversion of bilirubin to other metabolites. In hepatocellular jaundice, such a plateau tends not to occur, and bilirubin levels in excess of 50 mg per 100 ml may be found.

Partial obstruction of the extrahepatic bile ducts can also give rise to jaundice but only if the intrabiliary pressure is increased, because the excretion of bilirubin does not diminish until the intraductile pressure approaches the maximal secretory pressure of approximately 250 mm bile. Jaundice may occur at much lower pressures if the obstruction is complicated by infection of the ducts or hepatocellular injury. Therefore, jaundice, bilirubinuria, and clay-colored stools are inconstant findings in partial biliary obstruction, and the amount of urobilinogen in urine and stool varies with the degree of occlusion.

The functional reserve of the liver is so great that *occlusion of the intrahepatic bile ducts* does not give rise to jaundice unless the drainage of bile from a large segment of the parenchyma is interrupted. Either of the two major hepatic ducts or a large number of secondary radicles may be occluded without production of jaundice. In experimental animals the ducts draining at least 75 percent of the parenchyma must be occluded before jaundice appears.

ADDITIONAL POINTS OF TERMINOLOGY In clinical practice, a patient may be described as having *obstructive,* or *cholestatic,* jaundice. By this is meant that clinically, and especially biochemically, there is little to suggest hepatocellular damage and that the main features point to interference with, or obstruction in, the flow of bile. Typically one would expect such a patient to show (1) predominantly conjugated hyperbilirubinemia, (2) minimal biochemical changes of parenchymal liver damage, and (3) a moderate to a marked increase in the serum alkaline phosphatase level (usually greater than 15 Bodansky units). As emphasized in Chaps. 291 and 292, an *elevated alkaline phosphatase level* in a patient with jaundice or liver disease in the absence of other disorders such as bone disease is most suggestive of interference with bile secretion or an infiltrative process in the liver. However, *laboratory tests alone may not permit differentiation of intrahepatic from extrahepatic cholestasis.*

Some clinicians reserve the term obstructive jaundice for those situations in which anatomic obstruction can be demonstrated and use the term cholestatic jaundice for cases of parenchymal liver disease in which the obstructive phase is on a functional basis. Nevertheless, because these two entities frequently are indistinguishable by clinical and biochemical criteria, the terms obstructive jaundice and cholestatic jaundice are often used interchangeably.

Hepatocellular disorders in which jaundice associated with an obstructive, or cholestatic, phase occurs include (1) occasional cases of viral hepatitis, (2) drug reactions, especially those due to chlorpromazine and methyltestosterone, (3) some cases of alcoholic hepatitis or alcohol-induced fatty liver, (4) jaundice in the last trimester of pregnancy, (5) most cases of Dubin-Johnson or Rotor syndrome, (6) benign recurrent intrahepatic cholestasis, and (7) certain types of postoperative jaundice. These and other conditions are discussed in Chaps. 293 and 294.

In summary, all forms of conjugated hyperbilirubinemia have by definition an impairment in the excretion of bilirubin into bile. In most cases of parenchymal liver disease, a broad derangement is shown by the biochemical tests of liver function. However, when the major detectable alterations of liver function tests include (1) conjugated hyperbilirubinemia and (2) moderate to marked elevation of the serum alkaline phosphatase level, the terms obstructive or cholestatic jaundice may be appropriate. Additional procedures, including operation, are often needed to determine the cause of the cholestasis.

HEPATOMEGALY

In the supine position, the major part of the liver lies beneath the right rib cage. In some normal persons the liver edge may be palpable 1 to 2 cm below the right costal margin, and a palpable liver edge by itself does not necessarily indicate hepatomegaly. In evaluating liver size by physical examination, two factors other than ability to palpate the liver edge need to be considered, namely, (1) the location of the upper border of liver dullness by percussion, and (2) the body habitus.

Normally, the upper edge of liver dullness on the right side in the midclavicular line is at the level of the fifth rib, but in those of asthenic habitus it may be lower. The liver edge normally descends 1 to 3 cm with deep inspiration. In hypersthenic subjects, the liver may extend over to the left side of the abdominal wall, with the lower edge high and not palpable; in hyposthenic subjects with a very acute costal angle, the liver may lie in the right half of the abdomen, the edge being palpable by as much as 6 to 8 cm below the right costal margin lateral to the right rectus abdominis muscle. Thus, palpability does not necessarily imply hepatomegaly.

TABLE 42-3
Causes of a palpable liver and hepatomegaly

I Palpable liver without hepatomegaly
- *A* Right diaphragm displaced downward (e.g., emphysema, asthma)
- *B* Subdiaphragmatic lesion (e.g., abscess)
- *C* Aberrant lobe of liver (Riedel's lobe)
- *D* Extremely thin or relaxed abdominal muscles
- *E* Occasionally present in normal persons

II Hepatomegaly
- *A* Vascular congestion (e.g., congestive heart failure, hepatic vein thrombosis)
- *B* Bile duct obstruction (e.g., lesion in common duct leading to hepatomegaly and subsequently biliary cirrhosis)
- *C* Infiltrative disorders
  - *1* Bone marrow and reticuloendothelial cells
    - *a* Extramedullary hematopoiesis
    - *b* Leukemia
    - *c* Lymphoma
  - *2* Fat
    - *a* Fatty liver (e.g., secondary to alcohol, diabetes, or toxins)
    - *b* Gaucher's disease and some other lipidoses
  - *3* Glycogen (e.g., diabetes, especially after insulin excess)
  - *4* Amyloid
  - *5* Iron (hemochromatosis and hemosiderosis)
  - *6* Granuloma (tuberculosis, sarcoid)
- *D* Inflammatory disorders
  - *1* Hepatitis—due to drugs or infectious agents
  - *2* Cirrhosis—except in late stages when prolonged scarring may lead to a *small,* shrunken liver
- *E* Tumors—primary or metastatic
- *F* Cysts—polycystic disease, congenital hepatic fibrosis

In determining liver enlargement by palpation, one should be certain that the liver is being palpated rather than other right upper quadrant masses such as gallbladder, colonic neoplasm, or fecal material in the colon. Liver enlargement is often confirmed by radiologic studies, including hepatic scintiscans, celiac axis angiography, and splenic venography.

In many cases of generalized liver enlargement, the left lobe will be felt in the epigastrium between the xiphoid and umbilicus. The liver should be carefully palpated during deep inspiration to determine whether the edge is tender, regular or irregular, firm or soft, rounded and thickened or sharp. The edge is tender and often rounded with hepatic inflammation, as in hepatitis, or when the liver is acutely congested, as in cardiac decompensation. Pulsation of the liver may be found with tricuspid valvular incompetence. A carcinomatous liver may be rocklike in hardness; the cirrhotic liver is very firm in consistency. The largest livers are often found with carcinoma (primary or metastatic), marked fatty infiltration, congestive cardiac decompensation, Hodgkin's disease, and amyloidosis. Rapid decrease in liver size may occur with improvement of congestive failure or mobilization of fat from the liver.

In a patient with hepatomegaly, auscultation is sometimes helpful. A friction rub may be audible (and palpable) in the right upper quadrant; it is usually due to a recent biopsy, tumor, or perihepatitis. In portal hypertension a venous hum may be audible between the umbilicus and the xiphoid. An arterial murmur or bruit over the liver may indicate tumor, usually hepatoma.

Some of the causes of a palpable liver and hepatomegaly are given in Table 42-3.

REFERENCES

ARIAS IM: Inheritable and congenital hyperbilirubinemia. N Engl J Med 285:1416, 1971

BILLING BH, JANSEN FH: Enigma of bilirubin conjugation. Gastroenterology 61:258, 1971

CASTELL DO et al: Estimation of liver size by percussion in normal individuals. Ann Intern Med 70:1183, 1969

GARTNER LM, ARIAS IM: Formation, transport and excretion of bilirubin. N Engl J Med 280:1339, 1969

LESTER R, SCHMID R: Bilirubin metabolism. N Engl J Med 270:779, 1964

——, TROXLER RF: Recent advances in bile pigment metabolism. Gastroenterology 56:143, 1969

SCHMID R: Bilirubin metabolism in man. N Engl J Med 287:703, 1972

SHERLOCK S: Jaundice, chap. 10 in *Diseases of the Liver,* 4th ed., Philadelphia: Davis, 1968

WITH TK: *Bile Pigments: Chemical, Biological and Clinical Aspects,* New York: Academic, 1968

43 ABDOMINAL SWELLING AND ASCITES

ROBERT M. GLICKMAN
KURT J. ISSELBACHER

ABDOMINAL SWELLING Abdominal swelling or distention is a common problem in clinical medicine and may be the initial manifestation of a systemic disease or of otherwise unsuspected abdominal disease. *Subjective* abdominal enlargement, often described as a sensation of fullness or bloating, is usually transient and is often related to a functional gastrointestinal disorder when it is not accompanied by objective physical findings of increased abdominal girth or local swelling. *Obesity* and lumbar lordosis, which may be associated with prominence of the abdomen, may usually be distinguished from true increases in the volume of the peritoneal cavity by history and careful physical examination.

Clinical history Abdominal swelling may first be noticed by the patient because of a progressive increase in belt or clothing size, the appearance of abdominal or inguinal hernias, or the development of a localized swelling. Often, considerable abdominal enlargement has gone unnoticed for weeks or months, either because of coexistent obesity or because the ascites formation has been insidious, without pain or localizing symptoms. Progressive abdominal distention may be associated with a sensation of "pulling" or "stretching" of the flanks or groins and vague low back pain. Localized *pain* usually results from involvement of an abdominal organ (e.g., a passively congested liver, large spleen, or colonic tumor). Pain is uncommon in cirrhosis with ascites and when it is present, pancreatitis, hepatoma, or peritonitis should be considered. Tense ascites or abdominal tumors may produce increased intraabdominal pressure, resulting in *indigestion* and *heartburn* due to gastroesophageal reflux or *dyspnea, orthopnea,* and *tachypnea* from elevation of the diaphragm. A coexistent pleural effusion, more commonly on the right, presumably due to leakage of ascitic fluid through lymphatic channels in the diaphragm, may also contribute to respiratory embarrassment. The patient with diffuse abdominal swelling should be questioned about increased alcoholic intake, a prior episode of jaundice or hematuria, a change in bowel habits, or a past history of rheumatic heart disease. Such historic information may provide the clues that will lead one to suspect an occult cirrhosis, a colonic tumor with peritoneal seeding, congestive heart failure, or nephrosis.

Physical examination A carefully executed *general physical examination* can yield valuable clues concerning the etiology of abdominal swelling. Thus palmar erythema and spider angiomas suggest an underlying cirrhosis, while supraclavicular adenopathy (Virchow's node) should raise the question of an underlying gastrointestinal malignancy. *Inspection* of the abdomen is an important but often cursorily performed aspect of the abdominal examination. By noting the abdominal contour one may be able to distinguish localized from generalized swelling. The tensely distended abdomen with tightly stretched skin, bulging flanks, and everted umbilicus is characteristic of ascites. A prominent abdominal venous pattern with the direction of flow away from the umbilicus often is a reflection of portal hypertension; venous collaterals with flow from the lower part of the abdomen toward the umbilicus suggests obstruction of the inferior vena cava; flow downward toward the umbilicus suggests superior vena cava obstruction. "Doming" of the abdomen with visible ridges from underlying intestinal loops is usually due to intestinal obstruction or distention. An epigastric mass, with evident peristalsis proceeding from left to right, usually indicates underlying pyloric obstruction. A liver with metastatic deposits may be visible as a nodular right upper quadrant mass moving with respiration.

Auscultation may reveal the high-pitched, rushing sounds of early intestinal obstruction or a succussion sound due to increased fluid and gas in a dilated hollow viscus. Careful auscultation over an enlarged liver occasionally reveals the harsh bruit of a vascular tumor, especially a hepatoma, or the leathery friction rub of a surface nodule. A venous hum at the umbilicus may signify portal hypertension and an increased collateral blood flow around the liver. A fluid wave and flank dullness which shifts with change in position of the patient are important signs that indicate the presence of peritoneal fluid. In the obese patient, small amounts of fluid may be difficult to demonstrate; on occasion the fluid may be detected by abdominal percussion with the patient on his hands and knees. Doubt about the presence of peritoneal fluid may be resolved by careful paracentesis with a small-gage (No. 19 or 20) needle. Careful percussion should serve to distinguish generalized abdominal enlargement from localized swelling due to an enlarged uterus, ovarian cyst, or distended bladder. Percussion can also outline an abnormally small or large liver. Loss of normal liver dullness may result from massive hepatic necrosis; it may also be a clue to free gas in the peritoneal cavity, as from perforation of a hollow viscus.

Palpation is often difficult with massive ascites, and ballottement of overlying fluid may be the only method of palpating the liver or spleen. A slightly enlarged spleen in association with ascites may be the only evidence of an occult cirrhosis. When there is evidence of portal hypertension, a soft liver suggests that obstruction to portal flow is extrahepatic; a firm liver suggests cirrhosis as the likely cause of the portal hypertension. A very hard or nodular liver is a clue that the liver is infiltrated with tumor, and when accompanied by ascites, it suggests that the latter is due to peritoneal seeding. A pulsatile liver and ascites may be found in tricuspid insufficiency.

An attempt should be made to determine whether a mass is solid or cystic, smooth or irregular, and whether it moves with respiration. The liver, spleen, and gallbladder should descend with respiration unless they are fixed by adhesions or extension of tumor beyond the organ. A fixed mass not descending with respiration may indicate that is is retroperitoneal. Tenderness, especially if localized, may indicate an inflammatory process such as an abscess; it may also be due to stretching of the visceral peritoneum or tumor necrosis. Rectal and pelvic examinations are mandatory; they may reveal otherwise undetected masses due to tumor or infection.

Radiographic and laboratory examinations are essential for confirming or extending the impressions gained on physical examination. Upright and recumbent films of the abdomen may demonstrate the dilated loops of intestine with fluid levels characteristic of intestinal obstruction or the diffuse abdominal haziness and loss of psoas margins suggestive of ascites. A plain film of the abdomen may reveal the distended colon of otherwise unsuspected ulcerative colitis and give valuable information as to the size of the liver and spleen. An irregular and elevated right side of the diaphragm may be a clue to a liver abscess or hepatoma. Studies of the gastrointestinal tract with barium or other contrast media are usually necessary in the search for a primary tumor.

ASCITES In most cases the clinical and laboratory evaluation of the patient with ascites is sufficient to reveal the cause of the fluid accumulation. Often the ascites is a component or complication of cirrhosis, congestive heart failure, nephrosis, or disseminated carcinomatosis. However, even when the cause of ascites seems obvious, it is often important to determine whether another separate or related disease process has supervened. For example, when the patient with compensated cirrhosis and minimal ascites develops progressive ascites that is increasingly difficult to control with sodium restriction or diuretics, the obvious temptation is to attribute the worsening of the clinical picture to progressive liver disease. However, an occult hepatoma, portal vein thrombosis, or even tuberculosis may be responsible for the decompensation. The disappointingly low success of diagnosing tuberculous peritonitis or hepatoma in the patient with cirrhosis and ascites reflects the too-low index of suspicion for the development of such superimposed conditions. Similarly, the patient with congestive heart failure may develop ascites from a disseminated carcinoma with peritoneal seeding. The thorough evaluation of each patient with ascites, even in the presence of an "obvious" cause, will help avoid these errors.

Diagnostic paracentesis (50 to 100 ml) should be part of the routine evaluation of the patient with ascites. The fluid should be examined for its gross appearance, protein content, cell count, and differential cell count, as well as Gram's and acid-fast stains and culture. Cytologic and cell-block examination may disclose an otherwise unsuspected carcinoma. Table 43-1 illustrates some of the features of ascitic fluid typically found in various disease states. In some disorders, such as cirrhosis, the fluid has the characteristics of a transudate (less than 2.5 g protein per 100 ml and a specific gravity less than 1.016); in others, such as peritonitis, the features are those of an exudate. Although there is variability of the ascitic fluid in

TABLE 43-1
Ascitic fluid characteristics in various disease states

				Cell count		
Condition	*Gross appearance*	*Specific gravity*	*Protein, g/100 ml*	*Red blood cells, >10,000/mm^3*	*White blood cells, mm^3*	*Other tests*
Cirrhosis	Straw-colored or bile-stained	<1.016 (95%)*	< 2.5 (95%)*	1%	< 250 (90%)*; predominantly endothelial	
Neoplasm	Straw-colored, hemorrhagic, mucinous, or chylous	Variable, >1.016 (45%)	> 2.5 (75%)	20%	>1,000 (50%); variable cell types	Cytology, cell block, peritoneal biopsy
Tuberculous peritonitis	Clear, turbid, hemorrhagic, chylous	Variable, >1.016 (50%)	>2.5 (50%)	7%	>1,000 (70%); usually >70% lymphocytes	Peritoneal biopsy, stain and culture for acid-fast bacilli
Pyogenic peritonitis	Turbid or purulent	If purulent, >1.016	If purulent, >2.5	Unusual	Predominantly polymorphonuclear leukocytes	+ Gram's stain, culture
Congestive heart failure	Straw-colored	Variable, <1.016 (60%)	Variable 1.5–5.3	10%	<1,000 (90%); usually mesothelial, mononuclear	
Nephrosis	Straw-colored or chylous	<1.016	< 2.5 (100%)	Unusual	< 250; mesothelial, mononuclear	If chylous, ether extraction, Sudan staining
Pancreatitis, pseudocyst	Turbid, hemorrhagic, or chylous	Variable, often >1.016	Variable, often > 2.5	Variable, may be blood stained	Variable	Increased amylase in ascitic fluid and serum

* *Since the conditions of examining fluid and selecting patients were not identical in each series, the percentage figures (in the parentheses) should be taken as an indication of the order of magnitude rather than as the precise incidence of any abnormal finding.*

SOURCE: *The data in this table are a composite of those from several large series (see the first five references).*

any given disease state, some features are sufficiently characteristic to suggest certain diagnositic possibilities. For example, blood-stained fluid with more than 2.5 g protein per 100 ml is unusual in uncomplicated cirrhosis but is consistent with tuberculous peritonitis or neoplasm. Cloudy fluid with a predominance of polymorphonuclear cells, and positive Gram's stain is characteristic of bacterial peritonitis; if the cells are mostly lymphocytes, tuberculosis should be suspected. The complete examination of each fluid is most important, for occasionally only *one* finding may be abnormal. For example, if the fluid is a typical transudate but contains more than 250 white blood cells per cubic millimeter, the finding should be recognized as atypical for cirrhosis, nephrosis, or congestive heart failure and should warrant a search for tumor or infection.

Chylous ascites refers to a turbid, milky, or creamy peritoneal fluid due to the presence of thoracic or intestinal lymph. Such a fluid shows Sudan-staining fat globules microscopically, and an increased triglyceride content by chemical examination. A turbid fluid due to leukocytes or tumor cells may be confused with chylous fluid, and it is often helpful to carry out alkalinization and ether extraction of the specimen. Alkali will tend to dissolve cellular proteins and thereby reduce turbidity; ether extraction will lead to clearing if the turbidity of the fluid is due to lipid. Chylous ascites is most often the result of lymphatic obstruction from trauma, tumor, tuberculosis, filariasis (see Chap. 219), or congenital abnormalities. It may also be seen in the nephrotic syndrome.

Rarely, ascitic fluid may be *mucinous* in character, suggesting either pseudomyxoma peritonei (Chap. 289) or rarely a colloid carcinoma of the stomach or colon with peritoneal implants.

On rare occasions a syndrome may be seen of fever and ascites, without infection, occurring several weeks after abdominal surgery. This seems to result from starch (from surgical gloves) introduced into the peritoneum at the time of surgery, with a subsequent foreign-body reaction and ascites formation. Given the proper index of suspicion, diagnosis can be made by paracentesis and finding double refractile particles (i.e., starch) when polarized light is used.

The etiology of ascites may remain uncertain even after the usual diagnostic procedures have been carried out. Under those circumstances a high proportion of the cases will be due to (1) cirrhosis of the liver, (2) carcinomatosis with peritoneal involvement, (3) tuberculous peritonitis, or (4) hepatoma. In all of these conditions pronounced weight loss, wasting, anorexia, and fever may be found, and hepatomegaly, splenomegaly, and deranged liver function tests may be present. Procedures such as peritoneal biopsy, peritoneoscopy, liver biopsy, splenoportography, or laparotomy may be necessary to provide the diagnosis. Other less common causes of ascites include constrictive pericarditis, hepatic vein obstruction, myxedema and benign tumors of the ovary, particularly fibroma (Meigs' syndrome, with ascites and hydrothorax). The physiologic and metabolic factors involved in the production of ascites are described in Chap. 296.

REFERENCES

BERNER C et al: Diagnostic probabilities in patients with conspicuous ascites. Arch Intern Med 113:687, 1964

BORHANMANESH F et al: Tuberculous peritonitis: Prospective study of 32 cases in Iran. Ann Intern Med 76:567, 1972

CODER DM, OLANDER GA: Granulomatous peritonitis caused by starch glove powder. Arch Surg 105:83, 1972

HYMAN S et al: Mimetic aspects of ascites. JAMA 183:651, 1963

LEVINE H: Needle biopsy of the peritoneum in exudative ascites. Arch Intern Med 120:542, 1967

SHERLOCK S: *Diseases of the Liver and Biliary System,* 4th ed., Philadelphia: Davis, 1968

section 6 | Alterations in body weight

44 LOSS OF WEIGHT (See also Chap. 39)

GEORGE W. THORN

Weight loss, as revealed by history or detected by physical examination, constitutes a cardinal manifestation of disease or disordered bodily function, unless an otherwise normal individual has imposed on himself caloric restriction in an effort to reduce.

Under normal circumstances decreased food intake or total starvation initiates a constellation of metabolic changes designed to reduce energy expenditure and heat loss. Chief among these are reduced basal metabolic rate, lowered body temperature, restricted physical activity, and reduced peripheral blood flow (vasoconstriction). By these means the body attempts to maintain the function of vital organs such as the heart, brain, kidneys, liver, and lungs. These mechanisms are seriously impaired when complications such as fever, vomiting, diarrhea, or dehydration supervene.

Anorexia is a frequent accompaniment of chronic as well as acute disease processes. In the absence of specific abnormalities of gastrointestinal function, loss of appetite may be due to toxic products liberated by microorganisms, by breakdown products of tumor tissue, or by retention of metabolic end products as occurs in late-stage renal and hepatic disease. Hypoosmolality of the body fluid compartment and increased cell water content may give rise to centrally mediated nausea and vomiting through its effect on specific hypothalamic centers. Thus, a patient with malignant hypertension may experience nausea as a consequence of hypertensive cerebrovascular changes in the absence of uremia or, later, as a result of retention of nitrogenous products with progressive renal failure.

In evaluating the implication of weight loss several considerations deserve special attention.

1 Is the patient's history concerning the magnitude and duration of weight loss reliable? Can it be documented by comparison with prior measurements or confirmed by physical examination?
2 Has there been a notable change in appetite or food intake?
3 Has there been evidence of disordered gastrointestinal function with a change in bowel habits?
4 Has there been evidence of polyuria, particularly nocturia?

The determination of the *magnitude of weight loss* is not always easy. Some patients follow changes in weight regularly on bathroom scales or weighing machines, or they have serial physical examinations. Other patients may be vague or uninformed regarding actual changes in weight. Questions regarding a change in waist measurement or collar, suit, dress, or shoe size may provide helpful clues. Physical examination should then confirm this, with its opportunity to detect adipose tissue loss and the presence or absence of edema or dehydration. Special consideration should be given to the valuation of overall weight loss in the presence of edema, as the actual tissue loss in such patients will, of course, greatly exceed the apparent decrease in total body weight.

Weight loss with anorexia and decreased food intake occurs in such a diversified range of acute and chronic diseases as not to be particularly helpful in differential diagnosis. The magnitude of weight loss may reflect either the *seriousness* or the *duration* of the underlying disorder. Thought should be given to the diagnosis of psychologic difficulties such as depression and anorexia nervosa, to generalized endocrine and metabolic disorders such as pituitary-adrenal insufficiency and hyperparathyroidism, and to hepatic and renal disease, as well as to chronic infection, neoplasm, and drug intoxication. Weight loss without a significant change in food consumption would suggest hypermetabolic states, such as thyrotoxicosis and anxiety or gastrointestinal hypermotility.

Of course, particular attention will be given in the history to any abnormality in gastrointestinal function as a cause of weight loss. Here again, one is concerned with *decreased food intake* such as might occur in partial intestinal obstruction; *decreased absorption,* which suggests pancreatic or hepatic disease, spruelike syndromes, regional enteritis, or severe food allergies; or *increased loss of food* and *fluids* through vomiting, diarrhea, or draining fistulas. Disorders of gastrointestinal function accompany systemic disorders so frequently that the physician must always maintain a high index of suspicion that what appears to be primarily a disorder of gastrointestinal function may actually reflect deep-seated infection, tumor, or renal, hepatic, cardiac, or pulmonary disease. On the other hand, *specific gastrointestinal disorders* may complicate systemic disease; thus, the patient with nausea, vomiting, and renal azotemia may have an associated peptic ulcer.

The presence of polyuria, particularly nocturia, in association with anorexia and weight loss suggests diabetes mellitus, diabetes insipidus, chronic renal disease, and disorders giving rise to *hypercalcemia* or *hypokalemia.*

Physicians should encourage patients to weigh regularly and to maintain a lifelong record of changes in body weight, since alterations in weight so frequently mirror abnormalities in bodily function. Loss of weight may be the first indication of serious organic disease or psychologic disorder, the detection and understanding of which may be measurably enhanced by carefully recorded changes in body weight.

TABLE 44-1
Approach to the patient with weight loss

Appetite normal or increased	*Appetite decreased*
1 Increased caloric utilization *a* Hyperthyroidism *b* Anxiety *c* Drugs—thyroid, amphetamines	*1* Predominantly psychologic *a* Depression* *b* Anorexia nervosa
2 Decreased intestinal absorption *a* Hypermotility, carcinoid *b* Sprue, pancreatic deficiency, and enteropathy	*2* Primarily gastrointestinal *a* Decreased absorption *b* Sprue, enteropathy, etc. *c* Obstruction: neoplasm, adhesions *d* Hepatobiliary disease
3 Abnormal loss *a* Diabetes mellitus (glucosuria) *b* Fistulas *c* Intestinal parasites	*3* Systemic disturbances *a* Malignancy *b* Infection *c* Uremia *d* Cardiovascular disease *e* Endocrine-metabolic *(1)* Adrenal insufficiency *(2)* Hypercalcemia *(3)* Hypokalemia *f* Intoxications: lead, alcohol *g* Hematologic disorders *(1)* Myelofibrosis *(2)* Leukemia

* *Depression with reduced food intake occurs frequently in the elderly, with or without concomitant serious organic diseases. Depression is manifested by one or more of the following changes: (1) Sadness, tendency to cry; (2) loss of interest in work; (3) giving up friends; (4) loss of libido; (5) hypochondriasis.*

45 GAIN IN WEIGHT. OBESITY

GEORGE W. THORN
GEORGE F. CAHILL, JR.

GENERAL CONSIDERATIONS In the adult an increase in body weight may reflect an increase in adipose tissue, an accumulation of fluid (edema), or both. Weight gain in excess of 1 kg per day almost invariably implies excess fluid retention. A useful indication of excessive fluid retention can be derived from differences in body weight measured in the morning and again in the evening. Normally the evening weight rarely exceeds the morning weight by more than 1 kg unless the patient is retaining excessive fluid. With a weight gain of 1 kg or less during the day the patient will return to his usual weight the following morning. With a gain of more than 1.5 kg he is likely to demonstrate a gain in weight and, ultimately, edema if the condition persists. The increased fluid retention may reflect increased salt and fluid intake (diet), decreased sodium and water excretion (cardiovascular, renal, or hepatic disease), or both. Excess gain in body weight, as measured by differences in morning and evening weight, often provides subtle or early evidence of organic disease. Dietary indiscretions, licorice, and medications, including steroid hormones, may also be responsible. Obese patients can sequester substantial quantities of excessive fluid without necessarily exhibiting edema. This fact can be readily demonstrated by noting the striking response to a diuretic agent, a method of exploitation often utilized by "lose-weight-fast" schemes.

CYCLIC EDEMA

Idiopathic edema, or *"cyclic edema,"* is a syndrome which occurs predominantly in females and is characterized by periodic swelling in the absence of demonstrable organic disease. For a discussion of this syndrome, see page 179.

OBESITY

Obesity constitutes the single most prevalent metabolic disorder in countries or cultures where food supply is abundant. It occurs when the caloric intake exceeds the energy requirement of the body for physical activity and growth. As a result there is an accumulation of fat, which is stored as adipose tissue (see Chap. 72, page 401). The excessive adipose tissue may be distributed generally over the body, or it may be localized. The factors controlling the location of adipose tissue are not all known, but pituitary, thyroid, adrenal, and sex hormones play an important role. In the female, excessive adipose tissue is distributed predominantly in the lower part of the trunk and extremities; in the male it is frequently more pronounced in the upper part of the trunk, often sparing the extremities.

For the most part, obesity is preventable. Unfortunately, although the prescription for its cure is uniquely simple, the successful application of the treatment for prolonged periods or a lifetime is most difficult. Hence, relapse with return to the obese status is the rule rather than the exception.

For the elderly, a combination of factors, such as a progressive fall in basal metabolic rate, which accompanies the aging process, and a lessened degree of physical activity with sustained enjoyment of food, sets the stage for increased body weight unless caloric intake is appropriately reduced. The association of obesity with serious disorders such as hypertension, diabetes mellitus, cardiovascular disease, and pulmonary insufficiency should stimulate physicians to do everything in their power to acquaint patients with these facts and to be willing to encourage and *supervise* a long-term, rational approach to the problem.

The amount of body fat can be estimated from whole-body specific gravimetric determinations or from measurement of the thickness of subcutaneous fat folds with skin-fold calipers (Montoye et al., 1965). Body fat content can also be determined indirectly from a calculation of lean body mass (radioactive potassium technique). The most practical method, however, uses standard weight-height tables (Table 45-1). The weights recorded in these tables are those associated with the lowest mortality rates as derived from life insurance company data. These data, in which the ideal weight approximates that at age twenty-five, indicate quite clearly that increasing weight during adult life is associated with increased mortality rate. A person is considered overweight if he exceeds the upper range of ideal weight for his body frame. He is considered obese if his weight exceeds by 9 to 10 kg his ideal weight.

ETIOLOGY Hypothalamic relationships It has been shown for years that lesions involving the hypothalamus may lead to obesity. Lesions in the ventromedial nucleus of the hypothalamus induce hyperphagia and obesity, whereas lesions in the lateral hypothalamic area lead to a cessation of eating. On the basis of these findings, a dual mechanism has been postulated for the regulation of food intake: a "satiety" center in the ventromedial nucleus and a "feeding" center in the lateral hypothalamic area. Studies on gold thioglucose–treated mice have demonstrated fiber connections between these two centers. Additional experimental studies suggest that the control of food intake may be mediated by a "glucostat," "lipostat," or "aminostat." It appears that the basic cause of obesity is a derangement of the appetite-controlling mechanisms, permitting the assimilation of more food than is needed.

It has been claimed that certain persons are more efficient than others in their ability to digest, absorb, and utilize food and that they therefore become obese at lower caloric intakes than might be expected. Extensive balance studies on such patients have never substantiated this explanation; at equivalent levels of physical activity and basal metabolism, there seems to be little variation in the required caloric intake. Another consideration concerns the possibility that those patients predisposed to obesity may have been born with more fat cells than the less obese person. Though this possibility cannot be excluded, and may indeed be a factor in a very limited number of individuals, it is apparent that *enlargement of adipose tissue cells* is a uniform accompaniment of obesity.

TABLE 45-1
Desirable weight, in pounds, for adults twenty-five and over (indoor clothing)

Height (in shoes)		*Small frame*	*Medium frame*	*Large frame*
ft.	*in.*			
Men				
5	2	112–120	118–129	126–141
5	3	115–123	121–133	129–144
5	4	118–126	124–136	132–148
5	5	121–129	127–139	135–152
5	6	124–133	130–143	138–156
5	7	128–137	134–147	142–161
5	8	132–141	138–152	147–166
5	9	136–145	142–156	151–170
5	10	140–150	146–160	155–174
5	11	144–154	150–165	159–179
6		148–158	154–170	164–184
6	1	152–162	158–175	168–189
6	2	156–167	162–180	173–194
6	3	160–171	167–185	178–199
6	4	164–175	172–190	182–204
Women				
4	10	92–98	96–107	104–119
4	11	94–101	98–110	106–122
5		96–104	101–113	109–125
5	1	99–107	104–116	112–128
5	2	102–110	107–119	115–131
5	3	105–113	110–122	118–134
5	4	108–116	113–126	121–138
5	5	111–119	116–130	125–142
5	6	114–123	120–135	129–146
5	7	118–127	124–139	133–150
5	8	122–131	128–143	137–154
5	9	126–135	132–147	141–158
5	10	130–140	136–151	145–163
5	11	134–144	140–155	149–168
6		138–148	144–159	153–173

HORMONAL ALTERATIONS **Anterior pituitary deficiency** Anterior pituitary deficiency of a mild degree (Sheehan's syndrome, see Chap. 83) may be accompanied by weight gain. This syndrome, most frequently observed in women after childbirth, is characterized by oligomenorrhea, loss of axillary and pubic hair, secondary hypothyroidism, and adrenal cortical deficiency *without increased pigmentation.*

Hypothyroidism Obesity due to inadequate thyroid hormone may be suspected in a patient who has developed intolerance to cold, whose skin has become dry and coarse, and whose reflexes are prolonged (see Chap. 85). Weight gain associated with a more severe degree of hypothyroidism or myxedema may be due to edema, ascites, and pleural effusion. Gordon and his colleagues believe that some obese patients have a specific block in the utilization of fatty acids by peripheral tissues that can be modified by administration of triiodothyronine, but this observation has not been sustained by other investigators.

Cushing's syndrome Patients exhibit the characteristic "buffalo hump," rounded facies, and truncal obesity with sparing of the extremities (see Chap. 86).

Diabetes mellitus Obesity is both a common accompaniment of and a predisposing factor to the development of diabetes mellitus. As the disease progresses in severity, with glucosuria and ketonuria, weight loss occurs despite an increased appetite. Hypoglycemic manifestations developing 4 to 5 hr after meals are characteristic of the so-called "paradoxic" response (see Chap. 88).

Hyperinsulinism Obesity results from excessive food intake secondary to the hypoglycemia induced by primary excessive insulin secretion. The hypoglycemia occurs under fasting conditions, in contrast to "reactive hyperglycemia," which characteristically develops 1 to 2 hr after a high carbohydrate intake. The latter also may lead to obesity as the symptoms lead to further excessive food intake.

Gonadal deficiency Primary gonadal deficiency appears to predispose to obesity in both males and females. The frequent association of obesity with the menopause and with the eunuchoid state is well documented and suggests a relationship to gonadal deficiency, although psychologic factors may well be an additional factor. It is also well known that the obesity of adolescent children disappears with puberty and that at this time the adult adipose tissue distribution takes place.

FAMILIAL AND CULTURAL EATING HABITS These habits are firmly implanted at an early age. In groups which place great emphasis on food, there is a tendency to overeat. Sometimes the cultural pattern equates success with obesity (witness the common caricature of the obese banker) and encourages the ambitious person to achieve a comfortable corpulence. Moreover, when activity patterns change, eating habits may remain constant, so that the man who has previously been physically active may fail to reduce his caloric intake when he suddenly changes to a sedentary occupation. This tendency may be reinforced by the gradual decline of metabolic rate and of muscular activity which ordinarily accompanies aging.

PSYCHOLOGIC FACTORS Certain persons may have increased appetite for psychologic reasons. Under these circumstances food is used as a substitute for the satisfaction that ordinarily would be derived from other sources. In this respect, these persons resemble the alcoholic, who uses alcohol as a substitute for normal sources of satisfaction, such as friends, family, or success in work. Increased food intake may also be a manifestation of depression or anxiety, and the resulting obesity may aggravate the tendency toward isolation or the ineffectiveness of performance. Reduction of food intake under these circumstances, without recognition and treatment of the underlying emotional disturbance, is usually unsuccessful if not hazardous. Psychologic studies have shown that obese persons eat more as a response to external cues, such as the taste of the food or the environment in which it is served, whereas nonobese individuals eat as a response to as-yet-unidentified "hunger" cues arising from within. Also, obese subjects, once they start eating, continue to do so until either the food is gone or their stomachs are uncomfortably distended. Nonobese subjects more frequently leave food on their plate and stop eating because they have lost their hunger. Again, the analogy with the alcoholic is striking.

THERAPEUTIC CONSIDERATIONS

It is axiomatic that weight reduction, other than that resulting from fluid loss, requires that the caloric intake be less than that utilized. Rapid weight-losing schemes exploit the use of diuretics and dehydration programs which may prove unhealthy as well as illusory. It is essential for patients to appreciate that any program which results in weight loss of more than 0.3 kg per day undoubtedly represents to a considerable extent loss of fluid rather than of tissue. It is also important for a patient to realize that from time to time during the diet program he might gain 0.5 to 1.0 kg as a consequence of cyclic retention of salt and water. This phenomenon may be exaggerated in women at or about the time of ovulation of menstruation. It is also obvious that increased physical activity will assist overall weight loss and that specially designed exercise programs may facilitate the redistribution of adipose tissue.

DIET There is little evidence to support the contention that diets of equivalent caloric value but with differing ratios of carbohydrate, fat, or protein exhibit markedly different weight-reducing potential. Diets relatively high in protein do increase satiety, increase specific dynamic action, and minimize fluctuation in blood glucose level. For long-term weight reduction and maintenance of ideal weight *a diet of modest caloric reduction* has been found more acceptable for most patients. There are patients, however, whose social obligations or temperament require more drastic measures—at least for short periods of time. For such individuals, a "fast" day may be prescribed on a weekly basis. On this day the patient rigidly restricts his diet to 100 to 200 kcal (e.g., clear liquids, tea or coffee without cream or sugar, bouillon, low-calorie carbonated beverages, or skim milk if needed). Or a diet of 800 kcal may be prescribed until sufficient weight reduction has been accomplished, and then the patient may be tested on a diet of 1200, 1500, or 1800 kcal for maintenance (Table 45-2). Prolonged periods of almost total starvation, though providing a very effective means of weight reduction, should be carried out only under strict medical supervision; almost without exception they have proved *ineffective* in the long run in terms of maintaining ideal weight.

Significant reduction in dietary fat will, in many patients, lead to constipation. This will be minimized to some extent by the increased intake of fruit and bulky vegetables, but patients may require supplementary medication such as dioctyl sodium sulfosuccinate (Colace), 100 mg once or twice daily, or liquid petrolatum.

The identification of "chemical diabetes" by means of a glucose tolerance test provides a tremendous incentive for patients to attain their ideal weight. This is also true for patients with cardiovascular disease or those with skeletal disorders which involve the spine, hip, knees, ankles, and feet. Also the value of weight reduction as a means of reducing the level of blood lipids should be emphasized.

Group therapy offers a realistic opportunity for long-term reinforcement of a dietary program. Of the various types of approaches, "behavior modification" appears to have been the most successful. Certainly this approach, which has been publicized by R. B. Stuart in 1967 and by Penick et al. in 1971, yielded results far superior to those in a comparably selected group who received classical supportive psychotherapy. The behavioral type of program involves four general principles:

1 Description of the behavior to be controlled. This is essentially a carefully notated record of when, where, and how food is ingested.
2 Modification and control of the discriminatory stimuli governing eating.

TABLE 45-2
Three suggested diets for weight reduction

600 kcal	*1200 kcal*	*2400 kcal*
Breakfast		
150 kcal	275 kcal	675 kcal
1/2 grapefruit	1/2 grapefruit	1/2 grapefruit
1 slice bread	1 slice bread	2 slices bread
1/2 cup skim milk	1/2 cup skim milk	1/2 cup milk
	1 egg	1 egg
	1 tsp butter	2 tsps butter
		1 1/2 cups dry cereal
		2 tsps sugar
		jelly
Lunch		
215 kcal	350 kcal	800 kcal
1/4 cup cottage cheese	2 oz lean meat	4 in. chicken pie
1 slice bread	2 slices bread	1 slice bread
1 apple	1 apple	1/2 cup salad
	1 tsp mayonnaise	2 tsps butter
		3 oz ice cream
Dinner		
235 kcal	575 kcal	925 kcal
2 oz lean meat	4 oz lean meat	3 in. hamburger
1/2 tomato	1/2 cup peas	1/2 cup beans
1/2 cup spinach	1/2 cup potato	1/2 cup potato
1 orange	1 tsp butter	2 tsps butter
	1 cup skim milk	1 roll
	1 cup salad with diet dressing	1 cup coleslaw
		1 slice pie

3 Development of techniques which control the act of eating.
4 Prompt reinforcement of behavior which delays or controls eating.

It appears that the organization and effective supervision of a program such as this can be carried out by a team with modest psychiatric training.

Patients should understand thoroughly when they undertake a reduction diet that, in all probability, some degree of dietary restriction or discretion will be necessary permanently after ideal weight (Table 45-1) *has been attained.* The desirability of determining body weight each morning should be strongly emphasized and the diet for the day adjusted accordingly. It will be helpful if from time to time the physician or the dietitian reviews the comparative caloric content of foods and alcoholic beverages. Once ideal weight has been attained, a patient should be encouraged to visit his physician every 3 to 6 months. At this time, levels of blood sugar, cholesterol, fatty acids, uric acid, etc., can be checked. Continued interest on the part of the physician is essential for success in this important area of preventive medicine.

EXERCISE (see Chap. 72) Exercise has been endorsed as a method to increase caloric loss. Since body fat has no other way to be eliminated than by oxidation to CO_2, exercise should expedite weight reduction during any hypocaloric regimen. Unfortunately, it is very difficult to induce obese subjects to exercise, particularly for any length of time. Table 45-3 lists the exercise needed to eliminate an extra 200 kcal. It is obvious, therefore, that exercise, although excellent for the circulation and for the psyche, is very minimal in its overall caloric effect when compared to a reduction in caloric intake.

THYROID MEDICATION Obese patients should be examined carefully to rule out endocrine abnormalities. One of the commonest and most treatable of these is hypothyroidism resulting from primary thyroid gland insufficiency (see Chap. 85). The preferable laboratory tests which assist most in evaluating thyroid function are the serum thyroxine (T4D, Murphy-Pattee; normal 4 to 11 μg per 100 ml) and the resin T_3 uptake ratio (RT3, Abbott Laboratories; normal 0.82 to 1.17). The mathematical product of the T4D and the RT3 ratio is the free T4 index (FTI) which correlates well with the patient's metabolic status. Although obesity may accompany hypothyroidism as a complicating disorder, hypothyroidism itself does not cause true adiposity. Thus, correction of hypothyroidism by thyroid therapy does not usually alter the natural course of the associated exogenous obesity. Primary hypothyroidism complicating obesity can be easily corrected by full replacement doses of thyroid. A useful and reliable form of thyroid medication is liotrix (Euthroid, Warner-Chilcott), which contains a physiologic ratio of the two synthetic thyroid hormones, L-thyroxine (levothyroxine, T_4) and L-triiodothyronine (liothyronine, T_3).

A much more controversial situation arises when thyroid replacement therapy is considered as the primary treatment of obesity in the absence of any measurable thyroid abnormality. The rationale for using thyroid in the treatment of obesity may have arisen from a misinterpretation of the basal metabolic rate (BMR) in obese subjects. The BMR may be low normal or slightly reduced in obese patients because of the poor correlation of surface area measurements with true metabolic status. Thus, a low BMR in obesity usually does not represent true hypothyroidism; the diagnosis of thyroid disorder must depend upon more specific thyroid hormone measurements.

Supplemental thyroid therapy does not raise the low BMR of obese patients unless pharmacologic doses are prescribed (viz., greater than liotrix-3 or desiccated thyroid, 180 mg daily). Large doses of thyroid hormone are not recommended in obesity, since they eventually cause thyrotoxicity and may precipitate cardiac arrhythmias or congestive heart failure. This is especially likely to occur from the synergistic actions of thyroid in the presence of hypokalemia which may have been induced by the concomitant use of thiazide diuretics. Even more hazardous to the obese patient is the use of amphetamines in combination with thyroid hormone and thiazide diuretic therapy.

APPETITE DEPRESSANTS Unfortunately, no pharmacologic agent is available at this time which acts primarily by depressing the "appetite center." This type of depression is seen regularly in disease states such as hepatitis and uremia and as a toxic manifestation of drugs such as digitalis.

SUBSTANCES WHICH DEPRESS APPETITE BY INDUCING A SENSE OF WELL-BEING Amphetamine and its derivatives are the prototype of this group of substances. These agents are commonly referred to as "anorexigenic" or "anorectic." There is no evidence to show, however, that their effectiveness results from a depression of the appetite center. Probably as a result of stimulation, or a "lift," the patient's drive toward overeating may be significantly modified, so that as far as he is concerned, the overall effect of the drug is "appetite-depressing." Obviously, drugs which create such a state of euphoria may lead to habituation in certain persons.

At present a large number of derivatives of amphetamine sulfate (Benzedrine) and closely related compounds is available for clinical use; e.g., dextroamphetamine sulfate (Dexedrine), levoamphetamine sulfate and phos-

TABLE 45-3
Some 200 kcal "snacks" and types of exercise required to "burn" 200 kcal

Snacks (200 kcal)	*Exercise equivalent (200 kcal)*
2 apples	Running 12 min
2 Tbsp butter	Swimming 30 min
2 slices bread	Walking 1 hr
53 peanuts	Singing 3 hr
18 marshmallows	Dishwashing 4 hr
24 oz beer	Sitting in front of television 14 hr
1 martini	
3 eggs	

phate, levoamphetamine alginate (Levonor), methamphetamine hydrochloride (Amphedroxyn, Desoxyephedrine, Desoxyn, Desyphed, Dexoval, Desoxyfed, Drinalfa, Efroxine, Methedrine, Norodin, Semoxydrine, Syndrox), phenylpropanolamine (Propadrine), phenmetrazine (Predulin), phenyl-*tert*-butylamine resin (Ionamin), and diethylpropion (Tenuate and Tepanil). The usual dosage of amphetamine sulfate or dextroamphetamine sulfate is 5 mg given 30 to 60 min before meals. It may be necessary in some patients to omit the evening dose because of increased nervousness or sleeplessness. Long-acting preparations which can be given in a single dose of 10 to 15 mg each morning are also useful. These substances may prove helpful for some patients during the early weeks of restricted food intake.

When any one of the drugs related to amphetamine is tested in obese patients under controlled conditions and is given in adequate dosage, it exerts an anorexigenic effect that is clearly beyond that of the placebo. However, after a few weeks (6 to 8 weeks minimum), the weight loss ceases and the patient usually resumes his previous eating and gains weight unless other forms of treatment have been more successful. All the controlled studies utilize a fixed dosage throughout the period of study, since a progressive increase in dosage to overcome whatever process is leading to tolerance would presumably add to the risk of drug misuse or habituation. Periods of treatment with amphetamines for 2 weeks alternating with equal periods without treatment are as effective as continuous treatment.

Although serious reactions are rarely encountered with amphetamine and its congeners, the physician must be alert to the sympathomimetic effect of these agents in causing a rise in blood pressure, increased cardiac rate and work, and the possible development of cardiac arrhythmias. Since tolerance to these drugs develops relatively rapidly, their usefulness is short-lived unless the dosage in increased.

METABOLIC STIMULANTS, INCLUDING HORMONES Repeated efforts have been made to discover a nontoxic agent which would maintain a normal metabolic level in the face of weight loss. Dinitrophenol has had the widest use. The consensus today is that its undesirable toxic side reactions make its use unjustified.

In most instances, substances of this type are being employed by physicians or patients in an attempt to induce *weight loss without caloric restriction.* To do this, it is obviously necessary to raise basal metabolic level *above normal.* There is no known substance which can be used to increase metabolic level above normal for prolonged periods of time without danger of toxicity.

Many laymen think "hormones" the most important cause of obesity and hopefully consider them to be its cure. The well-informed physician recognizes to what a small extent disturbances in hormone secretion are primarily responsible for obesity and how futile most types of hormone therapy are as cures of obesity.

No pituitary preparation now available is useful in weight reduction. Male and female gonadal hormones and adrenal cortical hormones have no place in therapy unless specific deficiency of these hormones exists. One must not underestimate the psychologic reinforcement given to a patient on a reducing program when he reports regularly to his physician for "an injection"!

SURGICAL PROCEDURES

In extreme situations in which the patient's life is threatened by obesity, such as respiratory or cardiac failure, severe hypertension, or marked peripheral edema with ulceration, surgical bypass procedures can be done. A current procedure is anastomosis of the jejunum, about a foot below the ligament of Treitz, to the terminal ileum by an end-to-side procedure. More radical procedures have resulted in iron and vitamin deficiencies, and less radical procedures in little or no weight loss. Nevertheless, a small number of patients still either fail to lose weight or else develop some degree of symptomatic malabsorption necessitating restoration of the original anatomic arrangement.

REFERENCES

Bray GA et al: Obesity: A serious symptom. Ann Intern Med 77:779, 1972

Gordon ES et al: Abnormal energy metabolism in obesity. Trans Assoc Am Physicians 75:118, 1962

Meyers FH et al: CNS stimulants and antidepressants, chap. 28 in *Review of Medical Pharmacology,* 2d ed., Los Altos, Calif.: Lange, 1970

Operations for obesity. Br Med J 4:247, 1971

Penick SB et al: Behavior modification in the treatment of obesity. Psychosom Med 33:49, 1971

Schachter S: Obesity and eating. Science 161:751, 1968

section 7 Alterations in genitourinary function

46 DYSURIA, INCONTINENCE, AND ENURESIS

BERNARD LYTTON
FRANKLIN H. EPSTEIN

NORMAL MICTURITION An appreciation of the anatomic and physiologic mechanisms involved in micturition is necessary for a rational approach to the difficult problems of urinary incontinence, enuresis, and other disorders of bladder function.

The bladder muscle, or detrusor, consists of interlacing bundles of muscle that arch around the internal vesical orifice and continue down into the urethra, where they are interspersed with elastic fibers. The normal tone of these fibers constitutes the internal vesical sphincter. The bladder receives a dual nerve supply from the autonomic system. The sacral parasympathetic nerves, via the pelvic nerves (second, third, and fourth sacral segments), provide the preganglionic fibers to ganglions of the pelvic plexus and bladder wall, and these give off postganglionic fibers to the detrusor and posterior urethra. The sympathetic preganglionic fibers (last two dorsal and first two lumbar segments) pass via the lumbar splanchnic nerves to synapse in the paraaortic and pelvic plexuses. The postganglionic fibers supply mainly the blood vessels in the bladder wall and the muscles around the bladder neck. The sympathetic innervation has little influence on bladder function but is probably concerned with closure of the bladder neck at the time of ejaculation; removal of the first lumbar sympathetic ganglion bilaterally is usually followed by infertility because of retrograde ejaculation.

Afferent fibers subserving the sensations of distention and pain pass mainly via the pelvic nerves to the sacral segments of the spinal cord. Some of these fibers are said to pass via the sympathetic nerves, but it is probable that any residual sensation of bladder filling after section of the sacral nerves results from stretching of the peritoneum overlying the bladder. The internal pudendal nerve supplies motor and sensory fibers, from the second, third, and fourth sacral segments, to the external sphincter muscle, urethra, and perineal muscles. The action of the detrusor and sphincter muscles is, therefore, both reflex and voluntary.

Micturition is normally a voluntary act. As the bladder fills, a fairly constant low pressure is maintained by the detrusor muscle as it accommodates itself to the increasing volume. When it reaches its capacity, 400 to 500 ml in the normal adult, the stretch receptors transmit impulses via the pelvic afferent nerves, the sacral reflex center, and the fasciculus gracilis to the brain. This initiates the desire to void. Impulses from the brain, which arise in the paracentral lobules, are transmitted via descending fibers, just anterior to the corticospinal tracts, to the micturition center in the sacral part of the cord and to the pelvic and pudendal nerves to initiate the act of micturition. An initial relaxation of the perineal muscles is followed by detrusor contraction. At this point there is usually tensing of the abdominal muscles and diaphragm, although the resultant rise in abdominal pressure alone cannot initiate voiding normally and is not essential for evacuation. The intravesical pressure rises rapidly to 18 to 43 cm water, the external sphincter relaxes, the bladder neck opens, and voiding occurs, with a pressure of 50 to 150 cm. The opening of the bladder neck is the result of active detrusor contraction which widens the bladder neck and shortens the urethra, thus lowering the resistance of the bladder outlet. Closure of the bladder neck occurs with relaxation of the detrusor, which assisted by recoil of the elastic fibers, allows a return of the musculature to its normal position. It is apparent that any interference with detrusor activity or the anatomy of the bladder neck will interfere with the opening mechanism and lead to incomplete emptying or some loss of continence.

DYSURIA Dysuria denotes difficulty or pain associated with voiding. It may result from a wide variety of pathologic conditions. Frequency, hesitancy, burning, urgency, and strangury (slow, painful emission of urine) are often referred to under the more general term dysuria.

Urgency occurs as a result of trigonal or posterior urethral irritation by inflammation, stones, or tumor. The urge may be so great and so sudden that a patient voids involuntarily.

Frequency of urination in connection with bladder lesions occurs when there is either a decreased capacity or pain on distention. In acute inflammatory lesions, edema and loss of elasticity of the bladder wall cause pain or an urge to void when only a small quantity of urine is present in the bladder. Chronic inflammatory lesions such as tuberculosis produce a similar effect and may proceed to permanently diminished capacity from scarring. Frequency may be an early presenting symptom of primary malignant disease of the bladder, because of induration of the bladder wall as a result of tumor invasion and reactionary inflammatory changes.

The majority of conditions producing these symptoms arise in the bladder and urethra. Diseases of other organs and systems may, by invading, compressing, or distorting the lower part of the urinary tract, produce dysuria. Diseases of the nervous system, which involve the nerve supply of the bladder either centrally, as in tabes and multiple sclerosis, or peripherally, as in diabetic neuropathy, produce difficulty in voiding and sometimes pain when secondary infection occurs as a result of residual urine.

The *evaluation of the condition of a patient with dysuria* must include a complete history and physical examination as well as a complete urologic examination, together with relevant radiologic or laboratory investigations suggested by abnormalities detected during the clinical examination.

Inflammatory lesions in the bladder, prostate, or urethra are the commonest causes of dysuria and frequency. These include bacterial infections, chronic prostatitis in men, and chronic posterior urethrotrigonitis in women. The latter conditions are characterized by chronic inflammatory changes involving the posterior urethra, the prostatic glands in the male, or their anlage in the female—the paraurethral glands. The cause is obscure, and treatment is directed principally toward drainage by prostatic massage and by urethral sounding with instillation of mild astringents in the female. Meatal revision, internal urethrotomy, and posterior urethral fulguration are also advocated in the more persistent cases of posterior urethritis in women. A great deal may be learned from examination of the external urinary meatus. About 20 percent of children with urinary complaints have a degree of meatal stenosis, which may interfere sufficiently with bladder function to result in recurrent infection. Meatal stenosis may be an important cause in the development and persistence of chronic prostatitis in men and chronic posterior urethritis and trigonitis in women. Unsuspected meatal stenosis of long standing may cause trabeculation of the bladder and other manifestations of obstructive uropathy. Meatotomy results in relief or considerable improvement.

A urethral caruncle may produce symptoms of severe discomfort on voiding. This tumor appears as a small cherry-red polyp which may or may not protrude from the posterior lip of the external meatus and is generally exquisitely tender on palpation. The latter feature helps to distinguish it from the commoner condition of urethral prolapse. Excision and fulguration constitute the treatment of choice.

Benign overgrowth of the *prostate* commonly causes frequency, hesitancy, straining, slowing of the stream, and dribbling in older men. Pain is uncommon unless the condition is complicated by infection or vesical calculi.

Frequency and urgency may follow *radiation injury* to the bladder; this is most frequently seen after treatment for carcinoma of the cervix. In the acute phase this condition may be anemable to treatment with "bladder sedatives" containing antispasmodics and with small doses of steroids to combat the inflammatory reaction. The persistence of symptoms or bleeding may necessitate surgical intervention. Symptoms may not appear until several months or years after radiation treatment. Malignant tumors of the intestine, diverticulitis, regional ileitis, or ulcerative colitis may involve the bladder and cause frequency. Fistula formation may result in severe dysuria and pneumaturia and should be suspected in any patient with a prolonged and persistent urinary infection.

Chronic interstitial cystitis, a nonspecific chronic inflammatory disease of the bladder wall which may be manifested by small, shallow, stellate hemorrhagic mucosal ulcers (Hunner's ulcers), gives rise to a fairly characteristic pattern of dysuria. This condition may be the result of an autoimmune reaction. The patients, generally middle-aged women, complain of persistent frequency and often have severe suprapubic pain, relieved by voiding. There may be associated terminal hematuria. The urine contains a few white cells and red cells but no bacteria. Interstitial cystitis may ultimately lead to fibrosis with permanent contraction of the bladder, which may require cystoplasty or urinary diversion.

Frequency without discomfort on voiding may be associated with a normal bladder capacity and may be due to the polyuria of diabetes, to conditions causing hypercalcemia or hypokalemia, to the nocturia of early congestive heart failure, or to loss of renal parenchyma resulting in the passage of a large volume of poorly concentrated urine. The absence of nocturia in a patient with frequency suggests that it may be of psychogenic origin or may be due to a polyp or irritative lesion in the posterior urethra that is relieved by recumbency. A patient who complains of recent onset of nocturia should be carefully questioned about diuretic medication.

It should always be remembered that frequency may be due to paradoxic incontinence (see below).

Expanding masses in the pelvis that reduce bladder capacity by external compression are exemplified by pregnancy, large ovarian cysts, and uterine fibroids. A retroverted gravid uterus or pelvic tumor which becomes impacted may result in stretching and elongation of the urethra and produce difficulty in voiding and finally complete retention.

INCONTINENCE

Paradoxic incontinence True incontinence must be distinguished from paradoxic incontinence, which accompanies bladder distention caused by mechanical or functional obstruction and is characterized by small, frequent, involuntary "overflow" voidings. Response of the bladder muscle to obstruction may be compared to that seen in striated and heart muscle. With chronic obstruction the detrusor hypertrophies, the bladder becomes trabeculated, and this suffices to increase the force of contraction to overcome the block. As soon as a small quantity of urine is voided, the intravesical pressure drops, leaving a residual urine which gradually increases in amount. Ultimately, the detrusor becomes paralyzed by overdistention and complete retention ensues. Overflow incontinence is seen in flaccid neurogenic bladders, when small involuntary voidings occur, as the pressure of accumulating urine overcomes the resistance at the bladder outlet. With loss of a small amount of urine, pressure falls and a large residual is left. Timed voiding using suprapubic pressure, together with the oral administration of large doses of bethanechol chloride, may be helpful in controlling this type of incontinence. Often both neurologic and obstructive elements contribute, as in elderly arteriosclerotic men with prostatic enlargement or in cases of diabetic neuropathy with secondary bladder neck obstruction. The bladder in these patients is flaccid and painless, which may make it difficult to palpate, and the residual urine predisposes to infection.

Congenital incontinence Congenital incontinence

may be due to malformations such as vesical exstrophy, epispadias, patent urachus, and ectopic ureteral openings in the female, which are frequently associated with duplications of the renal collecting system. Congenital defects in the spinal cord and chorda equina, which occur in association with spina bifida, sacral anomalies, and meningomyelocele, may result in neurogenic vesical dysfunction.

The results of primary reconstructive surgery in cases of exstrophy are cosmetically satisfactory, but sphincter control is rarely achieved. Furthermore, most of these children have persistent vesicoureteral reflux and infection, which may lead to progressive renal damage. The majority, therefore, are still best treated by some form of urinary diversion with excision of the bladder. The results of urethral and bladder neck reconstruction in simple epispadias are better. The management of neurogenic bladder disturbance is principally directed toward establishing timed reflex voiding, decreasing outlet resistance with diminution of residual urine, and controlling infection. The use of electrical stimulators to promote bladder emptying is still in the experimental phase. When there is progressive renal impairment, due to persistent infection and vesicoureteral reflux, urinary diversion is necessary.

Acquired incontinence This may occur as a result of *disease or injury to the spinal cord,* as in tabes, multiple sclerosis, and tumor, or following fractures of the spine. The disruption of the neural mechanism results in complete relaxation of the detrusor and bladder outlet or in ineffective contractions of the detrusor, so there may be overflow incontinence with a flaccid bladder or uncontrollable frequent voidings with a spastic bladder. These contractions are ineffective, so that there is a small amount of residual urine. Wetting can sometimes be controlled by the administration of anticholinergic drugs. Cerebral vascular accidents or senility may produce loss of voluntary control of bladder and bowel function.

Parturition can stretch and disrupt the structures of the pelvic floor and perineum to the point that urethral resistance, though sufficient to maintain continence at rest, gives way under stress of straining or coughing, and incontinence ensues. Such incontinence is probably due to descent of the proximal urethra below the pelvic diaphragm, so that an increase in intraabdominal pressure, which is normally transmitted equally to both bladder and the proximal urethra, is no longer exerted on the proximal urethra. The resultant pressure differential thus exceeds the posterior urethral resistance, and urinary leakage occurs. The descensus is associated with loss of the urethrovesical angle and shortening of the urethra, which may be visualized on cystourethrography. Treatment is directed toward repair of the pelvic floor, with return of the bladder neck above the pelvic diaphragm, restoration of urethral length, and correction of the urethrovesical angle.

Stress incontinence may be aggravated by urgency because of an associated urethrotrigonitis. Relief of the trigonitis will sometimes result in satisfactory control.

Surgical or *radiation injuries* can produce vesicovaginal and ureterovaginal fistulas. Incontinence in ureterovaginal fistula occurs with normal voiding, but in vesicovaginal fistula there is generally no normal evacuation of the bladder. The treatment of these fistulas is always surgical. Temporary urinary diversion will enable spontaneous closure to occur in some instances. Reconstruction of a damaged ureter is the treatment of choice, but mobilization of the bladder to the pelvic brim, anastomosis to the intact ureter, implantation of the ureter into the intestine, or substitution with an ileal segment may be necessary. Nephrectomy is the simplest procedure in the elderly or debilitated patient or when there are serious technical difficulties, provided there is adequate function in the other kidney.

Injury to the sphincter mechanism may occur with pelvic fractures or after prostatic or bladder neck surgery, especially in elderly patients. Gradual improvement may occur for up to a year after injury. Postsurgical incontinence may be controlled with a penile clamp, but this has the disadvantage of producing edema and occasionally ulceration of the penis or a urethral diverticulum. A condom catheter may lead to maceration of the penile skin and is often difficult to apply. An indwelling catheter often leads to problems of chronic infection. A variety of surgical procedures have been devised to improve control by using some mechanical means to increase urethral resistance; they are only partially successful. Urinary diversion may become necessary in certain cases.

ENURESIS Enuresis implies the unintentional voiding of urine, usually at night, when it is synonymously referred to as bedwetting. The term enuresis should be restricted to condition of those children in whom there is no gross urologic abnormality.

Micturition in infancy is governed by a simple spinal reflex. Maturation of the nervous system and development of control over the simple reflexes by the higher centers occur during the second year of life. By the age of thirty months, most children have voluntary control over rectal and urinary sphincters. The child who persistently wets the after the age of three or who, after a period of control, begins to wet the bed again presents a clinical problem. Enuresis then may be a delay in the development or a loss of bladder control. It may be affected by physical and psychologic factors. There appears to be no constant single cause.

It is estimated that 15 percent of boys and 10 percent of girls at the age of five are enuretic, but by the age of nine only 5 percent of all children remain bedwetters. The majority of children with simple enuresis remain dry at night by the time they reach puberty. Bedwetting is more common among children of parents in the lower income groups. This could be because of the later institution of toilet training.

It is important, early in the management of these patients, to distinguish incontinence due to organic urologic disease from enuresis. Diabetes mellitus or insipidus may occasionally present with enuresis. Renal disease due to glomerulo- or pyelonephritis or sickle-cell disease producing papillary necrosis may cause bedwetting as a result of the increased volumes of urine passed by these patients. A careful evaluation at the outset should exclude chronic retention with dribbling incontinence due to either bladder neck obstruction or neurologic disease.

Patients with organic disease of the bladder are usually incontinent during the day as well as at night, although enuretics may also be incontinent during the day. Those with organic disease often have constant dribbling of urine. Occasionally, however, one finds serious degrees of bladder neck obstruction with nocturnal enuresis as the only symptom. A congenital decrease in bladder capacity may be responsible for enuresis; this condition is sometimes familial. The enuresis generally ceases as the child gets older and spends less time asleep. Occasionally a patient with petit mal epilepsy may present the problem of bedwetting. Urinalysis will reveal an unsuspected infection. Enuresis occurring in retarded children or in those with serious psychiatric distrubances requires treatment directed to the management of their primary problem.

Contributory factors such as the child's general health, physical environment, and emotional state should be evaluated, and the parents should be encouraged to adopt an understanding rather than a punitive attitude. Correction of minor urologic abnormalities such as meatal stenosis, balanitis, vulvovaginitis, posterior urethritis, and urethral valves will sometimes lead to relief, but this is perhaps attributable only to dysuria following instrumentation or to the understanding interest shown by the physician. The administration of antiparasympathetic agents to reduce bladder activity, or of amphetamines to lighten sleep, has been advocated, but the results are equivocal. Imipramine (Tofranil), a mood-elevating drug whose effect is reinforced by its anticholinergic and stimulant properties, given at bedtime, has produced a favorable response in over half the children treated, but may require continuation of treatment for some time. The results of psychotherapy are unconvincing. Considerable success has been claimed for alarm systems which attempt to establish a conditioned reflex. The child is awakened when an electrical circuit is completed by wetting; this method seems to be worth a trial in older children who prove resistant to simpler therapy.

REFERENCES

Bors E, Comarr AE: *Neurological Urology*, Baltimore: University Park Press, 1971

Lapides J: Structure and function of internal vesical sphincter. J Urol 80:341, 1958

Poussaint AF , Ditman KS: A controlled study of imipramine (Tofranil) in the treatment of enuresis. J Pediat 67:283, 1965

Werry JS, Cohrssen J: Enuresis: An etiologic and therapeutic study. J Pediat 67:423, 1965

Woodburne RT: Structure and function of the urinary bladder. J Urol 84:79, 1960

47 OLIGURIA, POLYURIA, AND NOCTURIA

LOUIS G. WELT

INTRODUCTION

The kidneys provide the main channel for the excretion of water and solutes, and the urine flow and composition are adjusted so as to maintain the internal environment of the body in a remarkably constant steady state. The volume and solute content of the urine in health may vary widely. They are largely dependent on the magnitude and characteristics of the fluid and food ingested and on the quantity of water lost from other routes such as perspiration and insensible water loss. There are many ways in which urine flow can be varied in both health and disease, and it appears essential to review briefly, and in a general fashion, the manner in which urine is formed so that the vicissitudes of life and the impact of disease on urine volume and osmolality may be better understood.

PHYSIOLOGIC CONSIDERATIONS

The final bladder urine represents the net effect of a host of reactions that begin with the formation of an almost protein-free ultrafiltrate of plasma in the glomeruli. The quantity of fluid filtered at the glomeruli per unit of time is the net effect of the difference in the chemical potential of the water of plasma and that of the ultrafiltrate as well as the surface area available for filtration. These factors apply to the filtrable solutes as well. The volume of water excreted per unit of time is, then, the difference between the volume filtered and the volume reabsorbed. The quantity of solutes excreted per unit of time is the difference between that which is filtered and that which is reabsorbed or secreted by the renal tubules. Many aspects remain obscure about these mechanisms, but there is now a general concept around which a description may be presented and from which implications may be drawn with respect to the influence of a variety of circumstances and disease processes. We are indeed indebted to the brilliant micropuncture studies started by Richards and his group in Philadelphia, and continued more recently by Wirz, by Gottschalk and his colleagues, and now by many others.

The water filtered by the glomeruli is reabsorbed at several areas along the nephron by passive diffusion along osmotic gradients, which, in turn, are established by the active transport of solutes. The osmotic gradient is maximized in the medulla and papilla, owing to the anatomic arrangement of the loops of Henle and their accompanying blood vessels, which permit the establishment of an ever-increasing osmolality as the papilla is approached. This latter mechanism is referred to as the *countercurrent multiplication system.*

The *initial* step in the reabsorption of water, and the step that represents the largest volume, occurs in the proximal convolution of the nephron. The active transport of solutes, which are primarily sodium, chloride, bicarbonate, and glucose, creates an osmotic gradient so that water follows immediately. In this fashion, approximately two-thirds to three-fourths of the filtered solutes and water are reabsorbed by the end of the proximal tubule. The characteristics of this fluid are altered considerably, not only in volume but also in composition. However, it is still isoosmotic with the parent filtrate.

Another phase in the reabsorption of water occurs in the more distal portions of the nephron, which include the loop of Henle, the distal convolution, and, lastly, the collecting ducts. Although the reabsorption at these levels is smaller in volume than that which occurs in the more proximal segment of the nephron, these latter mechanisms are responsible in one circumstance for the formation of a maximally concentrated urine, and in the other circumstances for the formation of a dilute urine. There are, obviously, circumstances wherein the urine osmolality occupies positions intermediate between these polar extremes.

The formation of a *maximally concentrated* urine depends on the presence of antidiuretic hormone, which permits the distal convolution and collecting duct membranes to be completely permeable to water. The micropuncture data reveal that the fluid in the early part of the distal convolution is always hypotonic (whether or not there is maximal antidiuretic hormone activity) to plasma. Furthermore, water is lost between the end of the proximal convolution and the early distal convolution. These two data clearly imply that solutes have been transported in excess of water, and hence some part of the ascending limb is presumably impermeable to water in the presence or absence of the antidiuretic hormone.

In the presence of antidiuretic hormone activity, the fluid within the distal convolution becomes more concentrated. Where one distal convolution meets with another to form a collecting tubule, the fluid is invariably isoosmotic (in the rodent) with the parent filtrate. As the fluid courses through the collecting duct (in the presence of antidiuretic hormone activity) and is exposed to a fluid with an ever-increasing osmolality, a passive movement of water causes the fluid within the collecting ducts to remain in osmotic equilibrium with the fluid in the interstitium; thus, the intraductal fluid increases in concentration until it exits into the pelvis of the kidney and moves down into the bladder for excretion.

Allusion has been made to the mechanism whereby the fluid in the interstitium is rendered continuously more hyperosmotic from outer medulla to papillary tip. It is dependent upon the anatomic arrangement of the loops of Henle and their blood vessels and is achieved by the transport of sodium salts (in excess of water) from the ascending limb of the loop. This renders the fluid in the interstitium hyperosmotic to the fluid entering the descending limb of the loop of Henle. This difference in osmolality promotes a movement of water from the descending limb fluid; and, in addition, there is entry of solutes into this portion of the limb. The net result is an increase in the osmolality of the fluid in the descending limb. This same process is repeated over and over again, and the fluid in the limb and interstitium becomes more concentrated along its course. When the fluid reaches the ascending portion of the limb and solutes are transported out of the luminal fluid, this fluid and the interstitium become ever less concentrated; the fluid becomes hypotonic by the time it reaches the early distal convolution.[1]

In this setting the fluid coursing through the collecting ducts is made more hyperosmotic. Since urea can presumably permeate the collecting ducts largely by passive diffusion, urea moves from the collecting system into the interstitium as water moves along the osmotic gradient. In this fashion, urea contributes significantly to the total solute concentration in the medullary and papillary interstitium and serves to counterbalance the concentration of urea within the collecting ducts.

In man, the maximal concentration of the final urine may be as high as 1,200 to 1,400 mOsm per kg water. This may be considerably higher in rodents, the experimental animals from which the data that permit this formulation have been obtained.

In contrast, in the "complete" absence of antidiuretic hormone, the fluid in the distal convolution is not only hypotonic to plasma in the earliest portions but remains so and is excreted as bladder urine with the same or even lower osmolality. Data reveal that salt is transported from the distal convolutions and from the collecting ducts themselves. In the absence of antidiuretic hormone, this aids and abets formation of minimally concentrated urine.

In this fashion, one can visualize the manner in which a highly concentrated or a minimally concentrated urine can be formed. Varying amounts of antidiuretic hormone between none and maximal provide a graded response.

Furthermore, it must be pointed out that even in the two polar situations of maximal antidiuretic hormone activity, or none, the rate of excretion of solutes determines the volume and osmolality of urine. This is to state that a urine may have an osmolality approaching that of the plasma with no antidiuretic hormone activity in the face of a solute diuresis; in contrast, the urine volume may be large and the osmolality may approach that of plasma despite maximal antidiuretic hormone activity in the presence of a solute diuresis. The manner in which a solute diuresis influences the concentration and the volume of urine is not completely clear.

However, within the context of the discussion presented above, it is apparent that a good deal of the water removed from the initial volume of filtrate depends on the active transport of salt and other solutes from the luminal fluid. Even if a constant *percentage* of filtered salt were reabsorbed in the proximal tubule, an increased filtration *rate* would provide a larger volume of fluid to the descending limb of the loop of Henle. Furthermore, to the extent that limitations are placed on the transport of salt from the proximal tubule (owing to the presence in filtrate of a larger concentration of a poorly reabsorbable solute), less water will be reabsorbed. If less salt is transported out of the loop of Henle, or if the flow of fluid through the loop is hastened, the countercurrent multiplier system will operate less efficiently; hence, the maximal osmolality will not be achieved in the interstitium of the medulla

[1] *The antidiuretic hormone possibly serves to increase the rate of transport of solutes from the ascending limb in addition to its influence on the permeability of the distal tubular and collecting duct permeability.*

and papilla. By the same token, if the reabsorption of solutes is diminished in the distal convolution (e.g., glucose is not reabsorbable at this site), less water will be reabsorbed and a greater volume will reach the collecting duct system. Hence, a large solute excretion will increase the volume and diminish the osmolality of the final urine despite maximal antidiuretic hormone activity.

In contrast, it will be recalled that the efficient transport of solutes prior to, in, and beyond the distal convoluted tubule, coupled with the relative impermeability to water of these latter structures in the absence of antidiuretic hormone, are responsible for the formation of minimally dilute urine. If reabsorption of solutes is less efficient, owing to the filtered load or to the presence of less readily reabsorbable solutes, it is clear that urine osmolality cannot reach minimally dilute levels. As the solute diuresis becomes more intense, urine osmolality will approach that of the plasma.

In summary, a small solute excretion in the absence of antidiuretic hormone would be anticipated to be accompanied by the most dilute urine, and in the presence of antidiuretic hormone, with the most maximally concentrated urine. Varying quantities of antidiuretic hormone will have obvious influences; and the character of the urine anticipated in the presence of maximal antidiuretic hormone activity or none will be modified by the quantity and character of the solute load destined for excretion.

PATHOLOGIC CONSIDERATIONS

OLIGURIA Dehydration There are many causes for oliguria, and the commonest may well be simple dehydration. In the face of a diminished volume of body fluids (especially if the loss has been water in excess of salt to provide an osmotic as well as a volumetric stimulus for the secretion of antidiuretic hormone), one anticipates a diminished filtration rate and a reduced excretion of solutes owing to the influence of a plasma volume deficit on renal hemodynamics. The diminished rate of excretion of solutes accompanied by antidiuretic hormone activity should ensure a small volume of highly concentrated urine.

Congestive heart failure Since the volume of the filtrate plays an important role in the rate of excretion of urine, any circumstance which causes a reduced glomerular filtration rate is likely to be associated with some diminution in the rate of flow of urine. The defective systolic emptying of the heart, which is a characteristic of congestive heart failure, is commonly associated with a reduced flow of blood to the kidney and with a reduced filtration rate. This becomes more and more intense as the failure becomes more profound. Furthermore, in congestive heart failure (see Chap. 30 for more details) the renal excretion of salt is diminished, and the combination is obviously likely to result in a small volume of urine. This may be a striking feature of heart failure.

Cirrhosis of the liver Cirrhosis is frequently accompanied by diminished renal blood flow and filtration rate (despite a coexistent increase in cardiac output) and by a strikingly low urine flow. In cirrhosis of the liver, as in congestive heart failure, the renal tubular reabsorption of salt is presumably more efficient, and this contributes to a diminished urine volume.

Acute renal insufficiency A low urine volume is one of the cardinal manifestations of this condition. In acute glomerulonephritis (or disorders with the same basic pathology) this low volume is presumably almost entirely a consequence of the drastic reduction in filtration rate. In acute tubular necrosis there is almost certainly a reduced filtration rate, but other factors as well may contribute to the striking oliguria. It is quite possible that in this latter disorder, the necrotic epithelium represents a nonfunctioning and simply passive membrane. Under these circumstances the intraluminal fluid would be under the same influences with respect to the Starling forces as is the interstitial fluid of the kidney. It could be anticipated, therefore, that the bulk of the diminished filtrate might be reabsorbed directly into the peritubular vessels, since the tubular walls no longer function as more than a passive diffusion barrier. In other instances the oliguria may be a consequence of nephron obstruction by casts. In many instances, the trivial formation of urine may be a consequence of a combination of these three mechanisms. In renal cortical necrosis, where all elements of the nephron are destroyed, total anuria is common. This may obtain because there is virtually no filtration whatsoever; what little does occur is likely to be subject to the influences suggested above in the context of acute tubular necrosis.

Chronic renal insufficiency The ability to form a maximally concentrated urine is disturbed early in chronic renal insufficiency. This is accredited to at least two factors. One suggestion is that with a reduced population of nephrons and an elevated concentration of urea the filtration rate and the filtered load of urea per nephron are increased, and in this circumstance there is an osmotic diuresis in those nephrons that contribute to the final urine. In the context of the discussion in the section on physiologic considerations, a framework was provided in an attempt to clarify the influence of the rate of excretion of solutes on the urine concentrating mechanism. Furthermore, if the destruction of renal mass occurs primarily in the medulla (as is so common in pyelonephritis) the nephrons with the longest loops of Henle are more likely to be destroyed. Since these longest loops of Henle set up the highest interstitial osmolality, it is apparent why urine concentrating defects are seen early. Hence, although chronic renal insufficiency may be associated with some polyuria, this is usually not striking. In the patient with end-stage kidney disease, striking reductions in urine flow are frequently observed. This is primarily a consequence of the magnitude of the destruction of renal mass.

Obstruction of the urinary tract Obstruction of the lower part of the urinary tract, i.e., from the bladder to the urethral meatus, is common and is due most frequently to stricture, to compression of the prostatic urethra by an enlarged gland, and, less commonly, to congenital malformations with valve formations that make emptying the bladder difficult. These patients may develop fairly striking acute reductions in urine flow, and this should always be a consideration when a patient is seen with oliguria.

Although it is less common to see oliguria as a consequence of obstruction of the upper part of the urinary tract, it does occur. The reason for its rarity is that there are two kidneys and two ureters, and in order to achieve oliguria from obstruction above the bladder, both ureters must be compromised. However, this does occur in a variety of circumstances, which include neoplastic infiltration of the ureters, and bilateral constriction consequent to a retroperitoneal sclerosing inflammatory process. On occasion constrictions may occur at the ureterovesical junctions bilaterally. Hence, although uncommon, bilateral obstruction of the upper part of the urinary tract may cause oliguria. Unilateral ureteral calculus with ureteral spasm on the opposite side is also possible.

Interpretation of oliguria—a summary Oliguria may obtain from the appropriate interplay of normal physiologic responses to a diminished effective plasma volume. It may result from circumstances as diverse as frank dehydration to congestive heart failure or cirrhosis of the liver with edema and ascites. The distinguishing features of each of these circumstances are a diminished glomerular filtration rate, evidence of a large fractional tubular reabsorption of water (i.e., high urine creatinine to plasma creatinine or urine urea to plasma urea ratios), and avid and efficient active renal tubular transport of salt as evidenced by a low urinary concentration of sodium. The latter two phenomena reflect intact tubular structure and function. In contrast, the oliguria that is associated with renal parenchymal destruction is likely to be accompanied by a diminished glomerular filtration rate, as well as by evidence of impaired tubular reabsorption of water and salt. These deficiencies will be reflected by urine to plasma concentration ratios for creatinine and urea which are low, frequently less than 20; and by urinary concentrations of sodium in excess of 20 mM.

POLYURIA Diabetes insipidus This condition results from inability to synthesize and secrete antidiuretic hormone and is the archetype of a disorder accompanied by the excretion of large volumes of dilute urine. In a compilation of several reports, intracranial tumors accounted for 40 percent of the variety of causes for diabetes insipidus, 33 percent were so-called *idiopathic,* and the remainder were scattered among a variety of disorders including trauma. Although not a rare disorder, diabetes insipidus is certainly uncommon. The primary condition from which it must be discriminated is primary polydipsia, which may be due to an intracranial organic lesion but perhaps more often accompanies a basic emotional disorder. These two disorders can be distinguished one from the other in a relatively simple fashion (see Chap. 84).

Nephrogenic diabetes insipidus Inability of the renal tubules to respond to antidiuretic hormone of endogenous or exogenous origin characterizes nephrogenic diabetes insipidus. It is a hereditable disorder, with full expression in males and partial expression in females, which manifests itself quite early in life; these patients are frequently referred to as "water babies." Management of this condition is difficult, since the infants do not respond to any of the available posterior pituitary preparations. However, they do respond to chlorothiazide drugs. The probable manner in which this agent influences the water turnover is by promoting a salt deficit. This, in turn, causes a smaller urine volume. This may be a consequence of a diminished filtration rate but is more likely to be associated with a larger fractional reabsorption of salt, and hence water, in the more proximal portions of the nephron. In this fashion less fluid is delivered to sites where it may escape into the bladder urine.

Acquired renal lesions There are acquired renal lesions associated with inability to concentrate the urine maximally.

Potassium depletion is commonly, if not invariably, associated with inability to concentrate the urine appropriately. The nature of the defect is not clear. Although it is at some risk that one translates data from rodents to human beings, information from rats and hamsters does exclude certain possibilities. Micropuncture data obtained by Gottschalk and his colleagues show that the osmolality of fluid in the distal convolution is the same in potassium-depleted rats as in control animals. Hence, there appears to be no lack of osmotic equilibration at this site. Furthermore, more recent data from the same laboratory utilizing normal and potassium-depleted hamsters reveal that there is no osmotic disequilibrium across the collecting duct epithelium. Other data indicate that the interstitial fluid deep in the papilla is not as hyperosmotic in potassium-depleted as in normal animals. The reasons for this are still unclear. Some published data on rats tend to deny the possibility that this is a consequence of a greater flow of fluid through the loop of Henle, since, if anything, the fractional reabsorption of water in the proximal convolution appears to be greater in a state of potassium depletion. Two obvious influences have not yet been evaluated, namely, the rate of medullary blood flow and the rate of active transport of salt in the ascending limb. An increase in medullary blood flow would tend to diminish the hypertonicity of the medullary and papillary interstitium; and a diminished rate of transport of salt across the ascending limb of the loops of Henle would diminish the efficiency of the countercurrent multiplier mechanism. The defect is reversible with potassium repletion.

Hypercalcemia has been known for some time to be accompanied by diminished ability to concentrate the urine maximally. In this instance as well, the precise mechanism is unknown. At this time the available data are somewhat similar to those discussed with respect to potassium depletion. There is no evidence of an osmotic disequilibrium across the collecting ducts and no evidence of an increased flow of fluid through the loop of Henle. The facets that have not been examined in the state of potassium depletion also raise questions about the hypercalcemic state.

Other examples of acquired renal lesions characterized by inability to concentrate the urine are seen frequently in patients with *chronic renal insufficiency,* as alluded to earlier. In addition, some rather striking examples of extreme polyuria have been seen in patients with multiple myeloma, amyloidosis, and, more commonly, after relief of an obstructive uropathy. Marked diuresis is commonly observed in the recovery phase of acute tubular necrosis from a variety of insults. This is frequently referred to as the "diuretic phase" of acute tubular necrosis and may be due in part to the delivery of accumulated fluid but very likely also due in part to renal tubular abnormalities with reference to the reabsorption of solutes and water.

Solute diuresis Large solute diureses, such as are noted in patients with uncontrolled diabetes mellitus and constant glycosuria, are almost always accompanied by large urine flows and complaint of polyuria. Solute diuresis may also occur in patients suffering a "reaction to injury" who are unable to utilize protein but are given large quantities of this foodstuff. In such instances protein is converted to a very large extent to urea and excreted. This increase in solute excretion promotes a large urine flow, as described earlier.

Polyuria—a summary In the absence of hypokalemia, hypercalcemia, multiple myeloma, amyloidosis, relief of bladder obstruction, solute diuresis, and chronic renal insufficiency, there are three conditions that may be responsible for polyuria: nephrogenic diabetes insipidus, primary polydipsia, and diabetes insipidus. The first of these is an inborn error, is discernible early in life, and is distinguished by an inability to respond to endogenous and exogenous vasopressin. The important discrimination between diabetes insipidus and primary polydipsia is discussed in Chap. 84.

NOCTURIA *The diurnal rhythm* that applies to urine flow is such that a larger volume is excreted in the waking 12 hr than during the 12-hr period spent mostly asleep. The precise mechanisms underlying this particular rhythm are not clear, although the evidence suggests a correlation with filtration rate and solute excretion. This rhythm is lost in several circumstances, and in other instances it may appear to have been lost owing to mechanical problems.

The rhythm characterized by a relatively diminished volume of urine at night is frequently disturbed in patients with *edema.* This may very well be because edema accumulates more during the day owing to activity and the influence of gravity through posture. At night, when the patient is supine, some of the edema may be resorbed into the plasma volume, thereby promoting an alteration in renal hemodynamics that leads to increased excretion of urine.

Nocturia is common in patients with *chronic renal insufficiency,* primarily because they excrete urine at a fairly constant rate, and hence the benefits to sleep of the normal diurnal rhythm are lost. The reason for this may be similar to those relating to a concentrated urine. In this instance it may be due to a constant osmotic diuresis per nephron.

Partial obstruction of the bladder is often accompanied by nocturia simply because the stimulus to void is so frequently present.

For reasons that are certainly unclear, the patient with untreated *adrenal cortical insufficiency* loses the normal diurnal rhythm and hence may complain of nocturia.

Lastly, anything that causes *dysuria* is almost certain to promote nocturia. In this instance, as is the case with obstruction of the bladder, nocturia is characterized by frequent but *small* volumes in contrast to the other cases noted above.

Nocturia—a summary Nocturia may have any of several origins, so that the details of the history are important. It is necessary to know if urination is uncomfortable or painful, whether there is difficulty in starting the stream, whether the urine volumes are small or large. These characteristics will help to discriminate between mechanical disturbances and those that relate to the edematous states, chronic renal insufficiency, and adrenal cortical or anterior pituitary deficiencies.

REFERENCES

GOTTSCHALK CW: Osmotic concentration and dilution of the urine. Am J Med 36:670, 1964

PAPPER S: *Clinical Nephrology,* Boston: Little, Brown, 1971

PITTS RF: *Physiology of the Kidney and Body Fluids,* 2d ed., Chicago: Year Book, 1968

STRAUSS MB, WELT LG: *Diseases of the Kidney,* 2d ed., Boston: Little, Brown, 1971

48 HEMATURIA

BERNARD LYTTON
FRANKLIN H. EPSTEIN

Bleeding from the urinary tract, whether microscopic or gross, is a serious sign. Although a common cause is acute cystitis, it should be regarded with the same gravity as abnormal bleeding from any other body orifice. Women sometimes have difficulty in distinguishing whether bleeding is from the urinary tract, vagina, or rectum. Hematuria is usually classified as initial, terminal, or total. *Total hematuria* indicates that the bleeding occurs throughout the urinary stream and suggests that the bleeding originates from either the kidney or the ureter. *Initial bleeding* is generally associated with lesions in the urethra distal to the bladder neck; terminal bleeding, with lesions in the bladder, usually in the area of the trigone. Severe hermorrhage from the bladder, however, will present as total hematuria. These distinctions as to the type of bleeding are, therefore, only rough indications as to the origin of the bleeding; too much reliance should not be placed on them. About 20 percent of the patients who come to the physician with hematuria have it as the only symptom of their urinary tract disease; it is often difficult to persuade these patients to undergo a complete urologic investigation to establish the origin of the bleeding. Ureteral colic is often associated with renal bleeding and is due to the passage of clots.

The finding of an occasional red blood cell in a

centrifuged specimen of urine is probably of no significance, since Addis showed that up to 500,000 red cells may normally be excreted in the urine in 12 hr. *Vigorous exercise* or even intense excitement may increase the numbers of red cells, epithelial cells, and casts in the urinary sediment of normal subjects. Microscopic hematuria may also be increased during certain *febrile diseases* without implying serious disease of the kidneys. The presence of red blood cell casts is pathologic and further indicates that the source of the bleeding is in the kidneys rather than the lower part of the urinary tract.

Certain *dyes* and *pigments,* such as phenolsulfonphthalein, azo dyes, and the indole alkaloids found in beet roots (Betanin), may produce red discoloration of the urine, which must be distinguished from bleeding. The appearance of the red dye from beet roots occurs only in certain individuals; it is thought to be related to the degree of absorption of the dye from the gastrointestinal tract. Pink or brown discoloration of the urine may occur as a result of hemo- or myoglobinuria. These may be precipitated by cold, exercise, or drug toxicity, especially in susceptible individuals (see Chap. 306).

Diseases of *the renal parenchyma,* such as glomerulonephritis, malignant hypertension, polycystic kidneys, renal infarction, periarteritis, or poisoning with a nephrotoxic agent, will in most instances be detected by a careful history, physical examination, and the usual laboratory tests. Hematuria may result from a disorder of blood clotting, produced by blood dyscrasias, scurvy, or anticoagulant drugs. The increased tendency to bleed in patients on long-term anticoagulant therapy may bring to light another, previously unsuspected, pathologic condition in the urinary tract. Sickle-cell anemia or sickle-cell trait may cause bleeding into the urine from disrupted capillaries and microinfarcts in the renal medulla. The aforementioned conditions account for only a small proportion of all patients with hematuria.

Tumors, urinary tract obstructions, calculi, and *infections* account for the bleeding in about 75 percent of patients with hematuria. Tumors alone account for some 20 percent of all cases. It is therefore mandatory in those patients in whom no other cause is found for the bleeding, to visualize the upper part of the urinary tract by intravenous pyelography supplemented by retrograde pyelography as indicated, and to visualize the bladder and urethra by instrumental examination. Retrograde pyelography may be supplemented by injections of air, rather than opaque dye, when one is trying to delineate suspected small calculi or small tumors in the renal collecting system. Doubtful lesions in the kidney may be further investigated by nephrotomography or aortography (see Chap. 266).

Cystoscopy will readily reveal the presence of acute and chronic cystitis, interstitial cystitis, bladder tumors, and vesical calculi. Bleeding from engorged veins in the prostatic urethra due to benign prostatic hypertrophy is a common source of hematuria. Like prostatitis in men and chronic nonspecific posterior urethritis in women, it should be accepted as the origin of the bleeding only if more serious conditions have been excluded.

Acute cystitis may result in gross hematuria, initially overshadowing all other symptoms. Chronic infections such as tuberculosis of the urinary tract or infection with *Schistosoma haematobium* may also have hematuria as their only presenting symptom. Schistosomiasis causes ulceration of the bladder mucosa at the site of deposition of the ova by the adult flukes which inhabit the venules of the bladder and pelvis. It is probably the commonest cause of hematuria in areas in the Middle East and Africa where it is endemic.

Bleeding associated with the menses should suggest the possibility of endometriosis of the urinary tract, provided contamination from the vagina has been excluded.

Trauma to *the kidney* nearly always manifests itself as hematuria, which is often painless and may persist for several days. The incidence of renal injury is increasing because of the increased number of serious automobile accidents. The majority of these cases may be treated conservatively with bed rest and careful observation. Follow-up intravenous pyelography should be carried out, because occasionally the renal injury may produce an anatomic deformity leading to obstruction, stone

TABLE 48-1
Investigation of hematuria

1 Microscopy of urinary sediment
  a RBCs, WBCs + bacteria (Suggest hemorrhagic cystitis)
  b RBCs, WBCs (Present in calculi, tumors, interstitial cystitis)
  c RBC casts (Indicate parenchymal renal disease)
  d Cytology (May reveal urothelial tumor cells)

2 Hematologic evaluation
  a Complete blood count, platelet count (To rule out leukemias, thrombocytopenia)
  b Bleeding time, prothrombin time, partial thromboplastin time (To exclude clotting disorders, coagulopathy)
  c Hemoglobin electrophoresis (If sickle-cell disease is suspected)
  d Antinuclear factor (Disseminated lupus erythematosus)

3 Radiologic examination
  a Intravenous pyelography (Calculi, tumors, obstruction, renal tumors, polycystic disease, retroperitoneal fibrosis)
  b Retrograde pyelography (Only if inadequate visualization on intravenous pyelography or systemic reactions to contrast)
  c Arteriography (To differentiate tumor from cyst)

4 Cystoscopy (Urethral lesions, prostatic bladder disease, stones, tumors, diverticula, ureteral orifices, site of bleeding)

5 Renal biopsy (To distinguish specific forms of parenchymal disease, especially vascular disease and glomerulonephritis)

formation, or hypertension. A blow on the lower part of the abdomen when the bladder is distended, particularly in children, in whom the bladder is an abdominal organ, may produce a contusion or rupture of the bladder, giving rise to hematuria.

A small group of about 6 to 8 percent of all cases seen have hematuria for which no obvious source can be detected. Further urologic and hematologic investigation 3 to 4 months after the first episode of bleeding will determine the cause in just under half of these. Patients in whom episodes of hematuria persist should have a renal biopsy at a time when they are bleeding. A focal glomerulitis has been found to be responsible for the bleeding in many of these cases. The condition appears to have a good prognosis for normal renal function. A small number of cases, however, still remain undiagnosed and may have persistent hematuria for which no cause is found over a period of many years.

Arteriovenous malformations responsible for intermittent unexplained bleeding may sometimes be detected by renal angiography. These may in some instances be satisfactorily treated by partial nephrectomy.

An outline for the investigation of hematuria is summarized in Table 48-1.

REFERENCE

Leader AJ, Carlton, CE Jr.: Hematuria, in *Urology*, 3d ed., eds MF Campbell, JH Harrison, Philadelphia: Saunders, 1970, p. 202

49 DISTURBANCES OF MENSTRUATION

GEORGE W. THORN

Since normal menstrual cycles depend upon the integrated action of the endocrine and nervous systems, it is to be expected that abnormalities in the menstrual cycle may occur in association with a wide variety of systemic disorders as well as with specific pathologic changes in the reproductive organs. (See Chap. 92 for a discussion of disease of the ovaries and uterus.)

MENARCHE In temperate climates the menstrual cycle usually begins between the ages of twelve to fifteen; in tropical climates it may appear as early as nine or ten. During the first year or two, the menstrual cycles are likely to be irregular, since many are anovulatory.

Uterine bleeding in the newborn may be noted for 3 to 4 days following delivery and is thought to be due to the sudden decrease in circulating estrogen level which had previously induced endometrial growth in the fetus.

Vaginal bleeding in very young girls should suggest injury from a foreign body introduced into the vagina. Very rarely vaginal bleeding will occur in association with precocious development of breasts due to an ovarian or adrenal tumor.

The delayed onset of menses, beyond the age of sixteen years, suggests *abnormalities* in the development *of the reproductive system,* such as imperforate hymen, uterine hypoplasia, and ovarian agenesis; *endocrine dysfunction,* such as anterior pituitary or thyroid deficiency; or *psychologic disturbances,* which mediate their effect through neurohumoral pathways.

MENSES Normally periods occur at intervals of 27 to 32 days, and flow lasts an average of 5 days. Approximately 60 to 250 ml blood is lost, with the greatest quantity lost during the first or second day. The volume of menstrual flow can be estimated by the fact that each well-soaked pad will contain approximately 30 to 50 ml blood.

MENOPAUSE Naturally occurring menopause may be expected by age fifty. Menopause represents the period of change between the years of reproduction and the regression of ovarian function. A gradual reduction in the duration of the menstrual cycle is to be expected at this time. *Irregular bleeding* or *hypermenorrhea* is most often caused by anovulatory cycles, but *neoplasms* should always be suspected. Induced or artificial menopause follows extirpation or irradiation of the ovaries. *Premature menopause* may occur as early as thirty-five without definitive cause; occasionally a familial tendency for this will be noted. However, other causes of amenorrhea such as endocrine abnormalities and emotional factors must be excluded.

ABNORMAL UTERINE BLEEDING During the reproductive cycle abnormal uterine bleeding should always suggest pregnancy and one of its complications, such as threatened abortion, ectopic pregnancy, or hydatid mole. Having excluded the complications of pregnancy by history, physical examination, and a rapid serologic test, one should consider uterine pathologic change, such as polyps, leiomyomas, and carcinoma of the cervix or body of the uterus. To detect these conditions a pelvic examination and diagnostic curettage will be required. Ovarian disease, pelvic inflammation, and hormonal abnormalities such as *hypothyroidism* also can induce abnormal uterine bleeding. Systemic disturbances, particularly those associated with anemia, leukemia, abnormalities in blood clotting, and circulatory disturbances such as hypertension should be excluded. The anemia that follows prolonged menstrual bleeding may predispose a patient to further excessive menstruation. In view of the widespread use of hormones, particularly estrogens, progesterone, and contraceptive pills, one should consider the *administration* or *withdrawal* of sex hormonal preparations as potential causes of abnormal uterine bleeding. Physicians should be alerted to the possibility that vaginal bleeding may be indicative of carcinoma of the vagina in girls whose mothers were treated with diethylstilbestrol during pregnancy. Finally, disturbed emotional states or serious psychologic difficulties may predispose to abnormal uterine bleeding.

Hypermenorrhea, characterized by excessively long or too profuse menstrual bleeding, may result from delay in the repair of the endometrium and, of course, frequently accompanies anovulatory cyclic bleeding.

Polymenorrhea refers to regular menstrual cycles that occur more frequently than every 23 to 24 days. It is the least common of the menstrual irregularities and tends to occur very early or late in menstrual life. It is due to a shortening of the follicular or luteal phase of the menstrual cycle.

Intermenstrual bleeding refers to the occurrence of irregular bleeding between normally spaced periods. Spontaneous bleeding of this type is more likely to be endometrial in origin in contrast to bleeding of the cervix or vagina.

AMENORRHEA AND OLIGOMENORRHEA Physiologic amenorrhea precedes the menarche, follows the menopause, and characterizes pregnancy and lactation. *Primary amenorrhea* indicates that menstruation has never occurred, whereas *secondary amenorrhea* refers to cessation of menstruation.

Uterine abnormalities such as agenesis or hypoplasia give rise to primary amenorrhea, whereas destruction of endometrium by irradiation or excessive curettage or removal of the uterus can induce secondary amenorrhea. *Vaginal abnormalities* include such conditions as imperforate hymen. The continued retention of blood may lead to hematometra, hematosalpinx, and eventually hematoperitoneum.

Ovarian agenesis or dysgenesis (Turner's syndrome) is a cause of primary amenorrhea. The high incidence of genetic defects in girls with primary amenorrhea deserves special emphasis. Polycystic disease of the ovary (Stein-Leventhal syndrome), masculinizing tumors of the ovary or adrenal glands, destruction of ovarian function by irradiation, and hormonal imbalance give rise in most instances to secondary amenorrhea or oligomenorrhea. Hypopituitarism with Simmonds' cachexia, Sheehan's syndrome, or the Chiari-Frommel syndrome will, of course, result in reduced ovarian function and predispose to oligomenorrhea or amenorrhea. With pituitary deficiency, one would expect associated evidence of reduced adrenal and thyroid function (Chap. 83). Diabetes mellitus and hyperthyroidism may induce menstrual abnormalities characterized by oligomenorrhea or hypermenorrhea. Malnutrition, obesity, debilitating disease, intoxication, and severe anemia may be associated with oligomenorrhea or amenorrhea as well as with abnormal uterine bleeding. Fear, anxiety, and grief are frequent causes of temporary amenorrhea, and indeed psychologic factors acting on hypothalamic centers constitute one of the most frequent causes of secondary amenorrhea. Amenorrhea is almost an invariable accompaniment of anorexia nervosa. Postcontraceptive amenorrhea, sometimes associated with lactation, is now commonly encountered in those regions in which the use of oral contraceptives is popular.

DYSMENORRHEA Some form of discomfort normally accompanies ovulatory menstruation, in contrast to anovulation bleeding, which is almost never associated with pain. Dysmenorrhea may reflect itself as lower abdominal cramps, backache, headache, and occasionally nausea and vomiting. Of these symptoms, the commonest is abdominal cramps. Many women suffer some discomfort for a few hours on the first day of menstruation, but in the majority of cases this is not incapacitating. Obviously, the degree of pain and discomfort experienced by any individual will depend upon concurrent involvement of the pelvic organs in disease or anatomic abnormalities. The pain threshold of the patient and the effect of emotional and psychologic problems, particularly those related to ignorance or misconception about the significance of the menstrual cycle, are important factors in evaluating the pathogenesis of dysmenorrhea. In *primary spastic* or *intrinsic dysmenorrhea,* there is no evidence of pelvic disease. It may gradually disappear later in reproductive life, and relief is usually afforded by the birth of a full-term fetus. *Characteristic of secondary dysmenorrhea is the onset of pain after several years of relatively painless periods.* Pain may begin several days before menstrual flow and radiate throughout the entire lower part of the abdomen, into the lower region of the back, and down the legs. It is more constant in nature and not as sharp or cramplike as that noted in the primary type. Secondary dysmenorrhea is usually associated with pelvic disease such as endometriosis, retroversion of the uterus, pelvic neoplasm, or inflammatory disease such as salpingitis or parametritis. In rare instances intense pain at the time of menstruation may accompany the expulsion of a large mass of shaggy, uterine membrane, i.e., membranous dysmenorrhea. Such events are infrequent and isolated and do not occur with successive periods.

PREMENSTRUAL TENSION This term is applied to a constellation of symptoms which increase in intensity for 5 to 10 days before menstruation. The most frequent complaints are a sense of abdominal bloating, breast tenderness, headache, irritability, mental depression, and an increase in weight which may be associated with edema of the legs (see Cyclic Edema, Chap. 30). The abdominal distention and tight feeling may be present without any great increase in weight and often without gaseous distention of the intestines. There is no doubt that the wide fluctuations in female sex hormone levels which occur during the reproductive period, with their important effect on electrolyte and water metabolism as well as upon mood and drive, provide critical "triggering" mechanisms for pathophysiologic changes in peripheral tissues as well as in the central nervous system.

REFERENCES

Charles D (ed): Symposium on menstrual disorders. Clin Obstet Gynecol 12:691, 1969

Philip J et al: Primary amenorrhea: a study of 101 cases. Fertil Steril 16:795, 1965

Rakoff AE: Endocrine mechanisms in psychogenic amenorrhea, chap. 8 in *Endocrinology and Human Behavior,* ed RP Michael, Fair Lawn, N.J.: Oxford University Press, 1968

Shearman RP: A physiological approach to the differential diagnosis and treatment of primary amenorrhea. J Obstet Gynaecol Br Commonw 75:1101, 1968

——, Mayes B: The investigation and treatment of amenorrhea developing after treatment with oral contraceptives. Int J Fertil 13:321, 1968

Teter J: Diagnosis and classification of the syndromes of ovarian deficiency. Med Gynaecol Sociol 4:3, 1969

50 DISTURBANCES OF SEXUAL FUNCTION

GEORGE W. THORN

GENERAL CONSIDERATIONS In men disturbances in sexual function may result from alterations in one or all of three distinct entities.

1 Libido, or the sexual impulse
2 Potentia, or penile erection
3 Ejaculation of semen

In women aberrations of sexual function are more difficult to analyze. Lack or diminution of sexual drive or failure to attain orgasm (frigidity) is much more frequent than in men.

ALTERATIONS IN LIBIDO **Loss of libido** Loss of libido may occur as a result of either psychologic or somatic factors. It may be complete in the presence of serious organic disease or with advanced age. On the other hand, lost or diminished libido may occur only under particular circumstances or in relation to a particular person, indicating the predominance of psychologic factors. In instances such as these, it is not unusual for a patient to experience nocturnal penile erection and emission of semen. Although loss of libido may accompany serious endocrine disorders such as anterior pituitary deficiency, Addison's disease, or diabetic acidosis or ketosis, it is not likely to be a *primary complaint* of the patient under these circumstances since the impairment in general health and activity is so overwhelming. Under these circumstances, it is more likely that the patient's spouse will have noted or called attention to the difficulty. For practical purposes it is important to bear in mind that the primary complaint of lost or decreased libido in male patients, in the absence of *severe* organic disease or *advanced* age, is almost certainly dependent upon *emotional or psychologic disturbances.*

Frigidity Inability on the part of the woman to participate in or to derive a pleasurable experience from the sexual act is a distressing complaint of relatively frequent occurrence. In the past such matters were not brought to the attention of the physician, but fortunately with the changing mores of our society many women now seek medical advice.

In order for the physician to handle frigidity disorders adequately he must have a healthy attitude toward sexual matters and be able to discuss freely even the most intimate of sexual acts. If the physician has difficulty in discussing such matters, cases of frigidity should be referred to a colleague.

The sexual drive of the normal woman is primarily conditioned by psychologic factors, with endocrine functions in a supporting role. The changes in sexual drive produced by alterations in hormonal level are of relatively little importance in contrast to the role of emotional and psychologic factors. In evaluation of patients with frigidity a detailed sexual and social history is a necessity. Frequently, conditioning from birth or early childhood results in a woman's belief that she is frigid. Many experiences in childhood can, later in life, result in incapacity for sexual pleasure. Such experiences develop a climate of fear, insecurity, and dread concerning the whole subject of sex. A common cause of frigidity is a lack of knowledge on the part of either one or both of the partners concerning the basic anatomy and physiology of the male and female genital systems. It is the duty of the physician to teach, by use of detailed diagrams of the genital system, the basic physiology of the sex act. Both partners should be present for the instruction, for rarely is frigidity a unilateral problem. It is important for both of the patients to discuss any problems concerning sex with the physician, either separately or together, in order to achieve any measure of success. Lessening of frigidity is a slow process, but by careful attention to the particular problems of each case, a good result can frequently be achieved. It is important to remember that it is not necessary for a woman to achieve an orgasm but only that she find intercourse a pleasurable experience.

Excessive libido Excessive libido may occur in conjunction with serious neurologic disease such as encephalitis or brain tumor as well as with psychologic and emotional disturbances. *Nymphomania* refers to the abnormal sexual behavior of women with a heightened libido.

ALTERATIONS IN POTENTIA **Impotence** Impotence implies the presence of sexual desires in a patient who cannot obtain or sustain penile erection. Impotence is rarely of endocrine origin. More frequently it accompanies a neurologic or emotional disorder. An important differentiating point is the history of the occurrence of nocturnal or early-morning erections. This implies that the neurologic and circulatory pathways involved in attaining an erection are intact and indicates that more emphasis should be placed on finding a psychologic cause.

In neurologic disorders absence or impairment of parasympathetic nerve activity prevents the development of tumescence of the corpora cavernosa. Impotence is common among patients who suffer disease of the sacral cord segments and their afferent and efferent connections, e.g., cord tumor, tabes, and multiple sclerosis. Approximately one-fourth of male diabetics in the younger age group and about one-half in the fifth decade develop impotence as a consequence of diabetic polyneuritis. Loss of both sexual desire and erection may occur in hypopituitarism, hypothyroidism, and severe eunuchoidism, as well as in association with general debilitating diseases. Patients with trauma to the prostatic urethra and those who have had perineal operations frequently have reduced potentia. Malformation of the genitals such as extreme degrees of epispadias, pseudohermaphroditism, growths and edema of the penis, as well as large hernias, hydroceles, and elephantiasis may interfere with sexual function. In the majority of patients, however, impotence is of psychologic origin and fortunately temporary. Fears and phobias which arise about the sexual act, as well as feelings of guilt, may be responsible.

Priapism True priapism is a state of sustained erection of the penis not accompanied by sexual desire. It is most frequent in the third or fourth decades and is usually accompanied by pain. Two types are recognized: the sustained and the recurrent nocturnal types. Priapism may result from urethral inflammation, from new growth involving the corpora, or from systemic disease such as leukemia or sickle-cell anemia. Diseases of the spinal cord may be accompanied by penile erections, reflexly induced and sustained for long periods of time. The neural apparatus for the control of sexual function is organized through the lower spinal segments, and hence may function effectively even when completely removed from voluntary control by spinal cord lesions. Recurrent nonsustained, painful priapism is of unknown cause, although it is often associated with prostatitis. Since it frequently subsides spontaneously, the efficacy of therapy is difficult to document. The administration of amyl nitrite has been noted to cause relaxation during the early phase of priapism. It has also been suggested that an anticoagulant might be effective in minimizing the venous thrombosis which is likely to occur with prolonged priapism. For this, intravenous administration of heparin is suggested; an initial dose of 100 mg is followed by subsequent doses of 50 mg every 6 hr.

EJACULATION Another type of disturbance consists of *premature ejaculation* of semen, a common complaint in neurotic persons though by no means peculiar to them. After lumbar sympathectomy the semen may be ejected into the bladder because of paralysis of the periurethral muscle at the verumontanum.

DYSPAREUNIA Dyspareunia, or *pain on intercourse,* may be present for a short time at the onset of marriage or sexual intercourse. Pain that continues long after marriage or develops later in life suggests local disease or emotional disturbance. Vaginal and pelvic examination should be made to exclude pelvic inflammatory disease, endometriosis, or tumor. In the absence of demonstrable organic disease, psychologic or emotional factors must be considered. Fear of pregnancy, fear of cancer if contraceptives are used, and tension between husband and wife can prevent enjoyment of intercourse with consequent spasm of vaginal musculature. Explanation of these facts with reassurance by an understanding physician may be followed by appreciable improvement.

STERILITY In the male, sterility may result from lack of or impairment of spermatogenesis due to testicular agenesis, hypogenesis, or cryptorchidism; to castration or exposure to roentgen rays or toxic substances; to injury or inflammation; or to endocrine or nutritional disorders. Obstruction of the seminal vesicles and epididymis and pronounced deformity of the penis interfere with the normal passage of the spermatozoa. Infection of the prostate or seminal vesicles may be injurious to the spermatozoa (Chap. 51).

In the female, sterility may result from impaired oogenesis as a consequence of deficient ovarian tissue (e.g., ovarian agenesis or hypoplasia, polycystic disease of the ovary with thickened capsule), the inability of the ovum to become impregnated due to disease of the fallopian tubes (such as infection and endometriosis), or uterine, cervical, or vaginal abnormalities in structure and function. In addition, debilitating diseases, endocrine abnormalities, and nutritional deficiencies may impair ovulation as well as fertilization and implantation of the ovum.

INFERTILITY The problem of infertility is discussed in Chap. 51.

SEXUAL DEVIATIONS Problems relating to homosexuality, pedophilia, and exhibitionism are discussed in Chap. 340.

REFERENCES

BURNS E, THOMPSON I: Priapism, in *Urology,* 3d ed., eds MF Campbell, JH Harrison, Philadelphia: Saunders, 1970, p. 531

ENGLISH OS: The psychosomatic approach in urology, chap. 52 in *Urology,* 3d ed., eds MF Campbell, JH Harrison, Philadelphia: Saunders, 1970

GRACE DA, WINTER CC: Priapism: An appraisal of management of twenty-three patients. J Urol 99:301, 1968

MASTERS WH, JOHNSON VE: *Human Sexual Inadequacy,* Boston: Little, Brown, 1970

SCHÖFFLING K et al: Disorders of sexual function in male diabetics. Diabetes 12:519, 1963

51 INFERTILITY

MELVIN L. TAYMOR

DEFINITION Infertility may be defined as the inability to conceive during the course of normal sexual activity. It is generally held that a marriage should not be considered infertile until a year of unprotected coitus has been allowed to pass. However, each couple's problems should be judged individually, and diagnosis and treatment instituted at an earlier or later date as indicated.

ETIOLOGY The two fundamental concepts to be kept in mind are (1) the multiplicity of etiologic factors and (2) the equal responsibility of male and female partners. To delineate these possible factors working either singly or in concert, one need only review the pathways of conception in male and female and the disorders of these pathways that may ensue.

Deficiency of sperm production in quantity and quality accounts for the majority of the *male's* contribution to the problem of infertility. Sperm production may be adversely affected by congenital influences such as germinal aplasia or cryptorchidism, by hormonal deficiencies of the pituitary or thyroid glands, by infection such as mumps orchitis, and by environmental factors such as nutritional deficiencies, noxious chemicals and drugs, radiation, excess local heat, and altitude. Often the cause is not ascertainable by diagnostic methods available at present. Sperm transport is affected by congenital malformations, surgical trauma, and infections. Impotency, an important factor in many cases, is commonly on a psychologic basis, although local infection or general systemic disorders may play a contributory role.

Defects in the *female* are related to production of ova and interference with their union with spermatozoa. Vaginal causes are organic or functional. Very often these causes are a combination of organic and psychologic factors. The obstruction may be due to an unruptured hymen, or it may be functional and due to hypertrophy and contraction of the levator ani muscles. Vaginitis itself is not a serious cause of infertility except in its role as a temporary deterrent to coitus. The cervix is one of the most important areas of obstruction to the passage of sperm. During the few days prior to ovulation the endocervical glands secrete a thin, watery mucus that is beneficial to sperm survival and migration. Infection or estrogen deficiency may decrease the quality of the mucus. Too often the offender is an overzealous physician who cauterizes the cervix too deeply and destroys the endocervical glands. Uterine abnormalities are not a common cause of infertility. Infertility can be associated with an anomaly such as bicornate, or double, uterus. Uterine fibroids are more likely to result in repeated abortions rather than the failure to conceive. Tubal occlusion is usually secondary to gonorrheal salpingitis. Bacterial salpingitis, secondary to pelvic peritonitis, appendicitis, abortion, or instrumentation, is more likely to result in partial blockage of the fibrated end of the tube. Nongonorrheal infection is also more likely to result in what is called the peritoneal factor. In this condition adhesions may develop between the tube and ovary, or fixation of the ovary may occur. Under these circumstances the chances of union between the sperm and egg are significantly reduced. In addition to infection, the peritoneal factor may be due to endometriosis. Hormonal or endocrine factors are all-important; these may result in deficient corpus luteum function and absence of ovulation

Immunologic factors may play a significant role in some cases of unexplained infertility.

Finally, emotional factors may play a vital role by interfering with ovulation or initiating tubal spasm or dyspareunia. However, the fact should be stressed that more often than not, the state of infertility with its accompanying diagnostic and therapeutic maneuvers is more likely to produce serious emotional reactions than are primary emotional factors likely to produce infertility.

TREATMENT The treatment of any defects, minor or major, in both the husband or the wife should be carried out concomitantly so that the total fertility potential of the couple will be raised to an optimum level.

In the *male* with azoospermia, in whom spermatogenesis is normal as shown by testicular biopsy, and in whom a block has been demonstrated, epididymovasostomy can result in return of fertility in 10 to 20 percent of cases. When hormonal studies reveal a deficiency of pituitary gonadotropin, an attempt should be made to rule out various causes of pituitary insufficiency, e.g., pituitary tumors. If no tumor is found, then treatment with human chorionic gonadotropin [5,000 units anterior pituitary-like extract (APL) intramuscularly twice weekly for 2 to 6 months] is indicated. However, sperm deficiencies not associated with specific pituitary defects will not respond to pituitary or pituitary-like extract. Azospermia or severe oligospermia will not respond in any significant degree to the administration of hormones, vitamins, thyroid preparations, or diet unless a specific deficiency can be demonstrated. In the present state of knowledge, little can be offered in the vast majority of cases of azoospermia or severe oligospermia.

This degree of pessimism should not be carried over to the infertile male with moderate degree of oligospermia (10 to 30 million sperms per ml) or to the male partner of an infertile couple with only a moderately lowered sperm count (30 to 60 million per ml), particularly if one considers the "couple-as-a-unit" concept of infertility. A modest improvement in the sperm count or motility combined with attention to the factors in the female partner may raise the fertility of the couple above a critical level. Avoidance of excess alcohol and tobacco, sufficient sleep and exercise, an optimum diet, adjustment of local excesses of heat, administration of thyroid preparations in minor degrees of hypofunction—all these singly or together may prove of definite benefit. A varicocele has been shown to be a contributing factor in oligospermia, and high ligation of the varicocele has been shown to improve sperm count and quality in a significant number of cases.

In the *female* specific attention should be directed to the cervical factor by correction of unfavorable coital habits, correction of retroversion of the uterus by a pessary, improvement in quality and quantity of preovulatory mucus by the daily administration of small dosages of estrogen (0.1 mg diethylstilbestrol daily for three or four cycles), by the use of a plastic cervical cap, and by the correction of cervicitis by systemic and local antibiotics or by cervical cauterization. Cauterization must be conservative lest more harm than good be produced by cervical stenosis or obliteration of mucus-secreting glands. When cervical stenosis is found, dilatation under anesthesia is of definite value.

Attempts to overcome tubal occlusion by repeated insufflations, diathermy, and high dosage of estrogen occasionally meet with success. Plastic repair of tubes or cornual implantation is followed by success in only 10 to 20 percent of cases. Surgery for tube-ovarian blockade, due to ovaries fixed by endometriosis, peritubal or periovarian adhesions, but associated with essentially normal tubes, results in a higher percentage of success. Infrequent ovulation accompanied by gross irregularity will respond to thyroid preparations when specifically indicated and to the correction of a specific dietary or vitamin deficiency. Ovulation accompanied by an inadequate luteal phase should be treated with progesterone preparations (Medroxyprogesterone, 2.5 mg daily for 10 days) or injections of human chorionic gonadotropin (HCG, 1,000 units intramuscularly every other day for five doses). Treatment should begin on the fifth or sixth day after the mid-cycle rise in the basal body temperature.

When absence of ovulation is caused by a specific defect in thyroid function, nutrition, adrenal function, or the psyche, correction of these defects often improves the condition. When amenorrhea or anovulation is caused by gonadotropin deficiency, efforts should first be made to diagnose and treat the cause. The amenorrhea itself and associated infertility can be treated effectively by the administration of gonadotropins. The preparation utilized is an extract of gonadotropins, high in FSH (follicle-stimulating hormone) and LH (luteinizing hormone) activity, prepared from the urine of postmenopausal females (HMG). The usual dosage is 150 to 200 FSH units administered intramuscularly daily for 5 to 12 days. When there is evidence of follicular activity, as indicated by increased levels of estrogen in the urine or increasing fern formation in cervical mucus, 8,000 IU of HCG is administered. Each patient responds differently. Overstimulation can result in enlarged cystic ovaries and multiple pregnancies, so the condition of each patient should be followed carefully. Polycystic ovaries are most susceptible to massive enlargement and possible rupture.

Clomiphene citrate, a chemical closely related to stilbestrol, also can stimulate ovulation, and usually should be utilized before gonadotropin therapy is attempted. The mode of action is not completely clarified, but after a 3-to-5-day course of the medication, 100 mg daily, a burst of gonadotropins 3 to 10 days later often stimulates ovulation. It, too, should be used with caution in patients suspected of having polycystic ovaries.

TABLE 51-1
Tests for infertility

I In the male.
- *A* Routine.
  - *1* Semen analysis. The semen is delivered into a clean glass container by withdrawal or masturbation. The following characteristics are considered normal:
    - *a* Volume—3 to 5 ml.
    - *b* Sperm count—above 60 million per ml is unquestionably normal, below 30 million per ml unquestionably indicates reduced fertility. The significance of counts between 30 million and 60 million depends upon the quality of motility and the degree of fertility in the female partner. A highly fertile female would be more susceptible to a count of borderline fertility.
    - *c* Motility—40 percent or more still actively motile 4 to 5 hr after collection.
    - *d* Morphology—at least 60 percent of the spermatozoa should be of normal size and shape.
  - *2* Examination of prostatic smear—excess leukocytes indicate that infection may play a contributory role.
- *B* Special tests—for the male with reduced fertility as indicated by semen analysis.
  - *1* Evaluation of thyroid function by basal metabolic rate, protein-bound iodine, or radioactive iodine uptake.
  - *2* Testicular biopsy—in most cases this will result in a definitive diagnosis. In only a few cases, however, will it demonstrate a remediable defect.
  - *3* Urinary gonadotropins—these may be low in pituitary deficiency. Excretion is high in primary gonadal failure.
  - *4* Sex chromatin determination.

II In the female.
- *A* Routine.
  - *1* Postcoital test—examination of the cervical mucus for its preovulatory qualities of clarity, spinnbarkeit (ability of the mucus to form a thread 5 to 10 cm in length when stretched between slide and cover slip), ferning (ability of the mucus to form fernlike pattern when dried and examined under low power of microscope), and for the number of viable spermatozoa 8 to 12 hr after coitus.
    - *a* Good test—more than 20 active spermatozoa per high-power field.
    - *b* Fair test—5 to 20 spermatozoa per high-power field.
    - *c* Poor test—less than 5 spermatozoa per high-power field. A poor postcoital test in the presence of good preovulatory mucus suggests a semen deficiency, a deficiency of the coital method, or malposition of the cervix. A poor postcoital test combined with poor mucus in the preovulatory phase and a normal semen analysis indicates a hostile cervix either on an inflammatory or an endocrine basis.
  - *2* The evaluation of tubal patency—initially by insufflation with carbon dioxide (Rubin test) and followed at a later date by hysterosalpingography in those cases which show failure of carbon dioxide to pass or who fail to conceive after an interval of time despite a normal Rubin test.
  - *3* Evaluation of ovulation and hormonal factors by:
    - *a* Measurement of basal body temperature, which characteristically shows a sustained rise after ovulation. Studies have shown that actual ovulation may occur as long as 2 days before or 2 days after the beginning of the temperature rise. The value of the temperature chart as an exact indicator of ovulation timing for purposes of timing coitus or insemination treatments can be overestimated.
    - *b* Endometrial biopsy with the demonstration of secretory changes in the endometrium is valid evidence that ovulation has occurred. The presence of endometrium out of phase with the time of biopsy is evidence of a progestational deficiency.
- *B* Special tests should be carried out when indicated.
  - *1* Evaluation of thyroid function.
  - *2* Endocrine assays, such as urinary gonadotropin and 17-ketosteroid determination, in cases of anovulation or inadequate luteal function.
  - *3* Further studies of ovulation timing utilizing vaginal or urinary smears and studies of cervical mucus.
  - *4* Culdoscopy to detect early endometriosis, pelvic adhesions interfering with tube-ovarian function, or polycystic ovaries.

Psychotherapy is of value in improving the coital habits of the couple, in reducing tubal spasm, and in correcting some deficiencies of hormonal nature. Finally, the manner and attitude of the physician play a role in the outcome by preventing undue feelings of guilt and depression from gaining the upper hand, and by instilling sufficient hope and fortitude to allow the couple to carry through with the tedious and sometimes painful diagnostic testing and therapeutic maneuvers.

References

GEMZELL CA: Induction of ovulation with human pituitary gonadotropins. Fertil Steril 13:153, 1962

STONE A, WARD ME: Factors responsible for pregnancy in 500 infertility cases. Fertil Steril 7:1, 1956

TAYMOR ML: The induction of ovulation, in *Davis' Gynecology and Obstetrics,* ed JJ Rovinsky, Hagerstown, Md.: Harper & Row, 1969

——: *Management of Infertility,* Springfield, Ill.: Charles C Thomas, 1969

section 8 | Alterations in the skin

INTRODUCTION AND GENERAL CONSIDERATIONS

T. B. FITZPATRICK
H. A. HAYNES

Dermatologic lesions are indicators of disorders of organ systems other than just the skin. The challenge and the interest of dermatology are that the skin manifests so many visible pathologic changes. If the viscera were as visible to the physician as is the skin, many more diseases would no doubt be listed in the textbooks of medicine and surgery.

Abnormal skin changes are as important signs of multisystem disease as are lymphadenopathy, splenomegaly, or jaundice. A physician concerned about the cause of jaundice should be equally concerned about tender red nodules on the leg, for these may be a presenting sign of carcinoma of the pancreas—a diagnosis confirmable by biopsy of the nodules. The skin is a microcosm of the body tissues, for the epidermis contains epithelial tissue, and the dermis contains the same tissues that are present in much of the rest of the body: blood vessels, lymphatic components, collagen, elastic tissue, ground substance, and nerves. Inflammatory, neoplastic, or metabolic changes occurring in these tissues throughout the body may be clinically apparent only when present in the skin. Such pathologic processes, when they occur in the skin and thereby become readily available for gross and microscope study, provide critical diagnostic clues.

Many of the diseases primarily involving the skin affect the patient only by causing disfigurement or pruritus and thus becloud certain changes in the skin that are important clues to other serious diseases. To recognize these clues and to detect the abnormal changes in the skin, the general physician needs to learn to interpret the skin as well as he is able to interpret a roentgenogram of the chest or a blood smear. He must develop his visual, as well as his aural and tactile, skills. Visual inspection of the patient has been pushed into the background by the increasing number of new and complex diagnostic procedures, but it still is of primary importance in detecting significant clues to internal diseases.

For the general physician, the problem of dermatologic diagnosis is largely related to his inability to recognize specific lesions and aggregates of lesions. The student during medical school usually does not have a chance to become adequately acquainted with the various skin lesions; although he may have been introduced to them, the encounter was too fleeting to permit recognition of even those that are most common. The identification of specific skin lesions requires neither a detailed history nor long contemplation but simply a trained eye. With the increasing number of people seeking medical care, the general physician is confronted more and more with dermatologic problems.

Diseases of the skin impair one's ability to function effectively. For example, dermatitis of the hands may interfere with the performance of skilled tasks in surgery and other activities requiring manual dexterity; pruritus, the paramount symptom of skin disease, causes discomfort and lost sleep to the extent that normal efficiency is impaired. An almost unique feature of dermatologic disease is disfigurement, which leads to social isolation and profound psychologic effects that are often underestimated by the general physician. The patient with a disfigurement realizes that noticeable skin conditions arouse strong feelings in the observer and provoke reactions that range from curiosity to fearfulness or from slight displeasure to open disgust. The patients themselves often assume that the lesions are disgusting or that the skin is "dirty," and have feelings of inadequacy that alter their relation to their social environment. Sometimes, the disfigurement of severe acne produces psychologic changes that persist a lifetime.

Less obvious is the relation of the skin to general body physiology. Yet this is most important. Examples are the systemic disturbances arising after excessive and severe damage by physical burns or those associated with generalized exfoliative dermatitis with its massive loss of epidermal scales. The integumentary system serves critical functions in homeostasis. This system, the stratum corneum, having probably the lowest water permeability of any biologically produced membrane, prevents loss of body fluids, thereby protecting the body against dehydration in a dry atmosphere. The skin, in serving as a barrier membrane, also retards the entrance of potentially toxic agents from the environment, impedes the invasion of most microorganisms, and prevents damage to underlying tissue from many external physical stresses such as ultraviolet radiation, electrical energy, and mechanical forces. The skin is also an essential component of the thermoregulatory mechanisms that maintain the body temperature within narrow limits.

52 INTERPRETATION OF ALTERATIONS IN THE SKIN

T. B. FITZPATRICK
H. A. HAYNES

CLINICAL EXAMINATION OF THE SKIN

The identification of skin lesions, or alterations, is a problem similar to the recognition of cells in a blood smear; the minute details are of the greatest importance. The individual type of skin lesion (e.g., papule, nodule) can be considered as a letter in the alphabet, forming the basic element for the identification of the pathologic change and often leading to the clinical diagnosis. Lesions may be the presenting complaint of the patient or may be incidental findings during the routine physical examination; or they may be incidental to some major presenting complaint such as fever, cough, arthralgia, and the like. The recognition of the important and nonimportant skin lesions commonly encountered during the routine physical examination of the skin is an important part of the physician's task (Plates 1 to 4).

Inasmuch as the identification of skin lesions is the *sine qua non* of dermatologic diagnosis, the examiner's eye is undoubtedly the most important instrument at his disposal. Adequate illumination, preferably with natural light, is necessary. The observation of the skin should begin with an over-all, "low-power" general assessment of the completely disrobed patient. The systematic approach to the examination of skin should be as follows: first the fingernails and then the anterior and posterior aspects of the arm; then, in sequence, the scalp, the face, the trunk, the lower extremities, and the skin between the toes; and then the mucous membranes, including the mouth and anogenital areas. The examiner of dermatologic lesions should consider the following points: (1) the specific *type* of lesion, (2) the *configuration,* or *shape* of the lesion, and (3) the *arrangement* of the groups of lesions, such as linear, arciform, annular, polycyclic, herpetiform, zosteriform, and serpiginous.

Types of skin lesions can be classified by determining the topographic level of the lesions in relation to the normal skin (Table 52-1). For example, it is possible to distinguish lesions that are in or that protrude or are superimposed above or below the level of the normal skin. The lesions that are encompassed within the scope of dermatology are listed in Fig. 52-1 and Table 52-1, and the histologic aspects are illustrated in Figs. 52-2 through 52-13.

The shape of the individual lesion and the arrangement of two or more lesions in relation to each other sometimes constitute important diagnostic clues. A *linear arrangement* of lesions often is indicative of an exogenous cause; also, linear lesions may occur because the pathologic process involves a vein, a lymphatic component, or an arteriole. Linearity can often be seen in various types of cutaneous hamartoma involving epidermal cells or melanocytes or even dermal connective tissue. In contrast, *annular and arciform* lesions and *annular and arciform arrangements* are relatively common and therefore only rarely lead to a specific diagnosis. The *iris* lesion, however, a special and important type of annular lesion, may be an erythematous annular macule or papule, with either a purplish papule or vesicle in the center. Iris lesions are characteristic of the erythema-multiforme syndrome. Annular macules may be observed in drug eruptions, secondary syphilis, and lupus erythematosus. Annular lesions with scale often suggest dermatophytosis or pityriasis rosea or psoriasis. The wheals that occur in creeping eruptions and the nodules that occur in late syphilis are arranged in a *serpiginous* (snakelike) pattern.

Lesions that are close to each other are described as *grouped,* and are of relatively little diagnostic value except in the special pattern, *herpetiform,* which is pathognomonic for herpes simplex or herpes zoster. Similarly, the special arrangement, *zosteriform,* follows a dermatome in a bandlike pattern and is characteristically

TABLE 52-1
Types of skin lesion

Flat lesions (in plane of skin)	*Elevated lesions (above plane of skin)*	*Depressed lesions (below plane of skin)*
Macule	Vesicle and bulla	Atrophy§
Infarct*	Pustule	Sclerosis§†
Sclerosis*†	Abscess‡	Erosion
Telangiectasia†	Cyst‡	Excoriation
	Papule	Scar†
	Wheal	Ulcer
	Plaque	Sinus‡
	Nodule‡	Gangrene§
	Vegetation	
	Keratosis	
	Desquamation (scales)	
	Exudate* (crusts)	
	Lichenification	

* *May also be below the plane of the skin.*
† *May also be above the plane of the skin.*
‡ *May also be in or below the plane of the skin.*
§ *May also be in the plane of the skin.*

SOURCE: *TB Fitzpatrick, DP Johnson: Fundamentals of dermatologic diagnosis, in TB Fitzpatrick et al (eds):* Dermatology in General Medicine, *New York: McGraw-Hill, 1971*

seen in herpes zoster; a zosteriform arrangement of skin nodules is occasionally seen in metastatic carcinoma of the breast. A *reticular* arrangement often results from vascular dilatation and is observed in cutis marmorata and livedo reticularis.

The sites of localization of skin eruptions have been greatly overemphasized, however, in dermatologic diagnosis; of far more importance are the type, shape, and arrangement of the lesions. Eruptions can be classified as *localized* or *generalized;* the term *"total"* (universal) denotes an involvement of all the skin, including the hair and the nails. When the eruption occurs in bilateral and symmetrical distribution, the pathologic stimulus is usually endogenous or is hematogenously disseminated. Bilateral symmetry is characteristic of hypersensitivity and is a common response to a drug. In photosensitivity eruptions, lesions are localized to the parts of the body that are exposed to sunlight. The exposed areas of the face that are usually spared include the fold of skin on the upper eyelids, the skin of the hair-covered scalp, and the skin below the chin.

LABORATORY AND OTHER AIDS IN EXAMINATION OF THE SKIN

There are certain technical, clinical, and laboratory aids and procedures that are indispensable in the clinical examination and interpretation of skin conditions.

Visual aids

MAGNIFICATION Certain diagnostic signs can be revealed only by magnification of the skin lesions; e.g., the follicular plugging indicative of lupus erythematosus, the fine telangiectasia and raised border indicative of basal-cell carcinoma, and, if present, the bluish color indicative

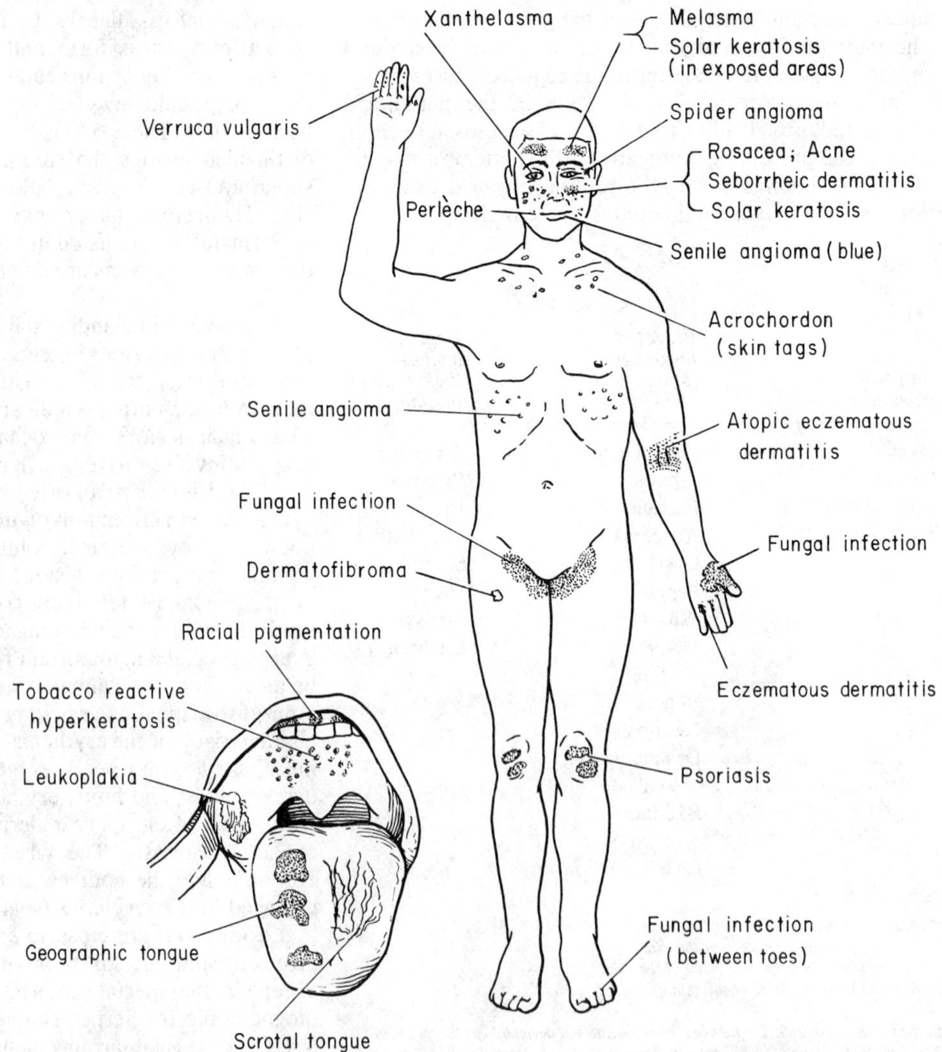

FIGURE 52-1 (THIS PAGE AND OPPOSITE)
Common lesions, shown on anterior and posterior views of the patient, encountered during the physical examination of the skin. See also the Color Atlas, Plates 1 to 4. (Reproduced from TB Fitzpatrick and DP Johnson: "Fundamentals of Dermatologic Diagnosis," in Dermatology in General Medicine, eds TB Fitzpatrick et al, New York: McGraw-Hill, 1971, p. 10)

of early primary malignant melanoma. A pocket magnifier (2 to 7 X) and a binocular microscope (5 to 40 X) are useful.

TRANSILLUMINATION Transillumination, or side-lighting, of skin lesions, which is done in a darkened room, is often required to detect slight degrees of elevation or depression, and is also sometimes useful in estimating the extent of the eruption.

DIASCOPY Diascopy is an indispensable technique for the examination of the skin because it permits the differentiation of purpura from erythematous macules. Diascopy consists of firmly pressing a microscope slide or a piece of clear plastic over the skin lesion; if the lesion is erythematous, the pressure will reveal capillary dilatation rather than an extravasation of blood. Sarcoidosis, lymphoma, and tuberculosis of the skin are suggested if diascopy of the nodules reveals either a characteristic hyaline, yellowish brown or an "apple-jelly" appearance.

LONG-WAVE ULTRAVIOLET LIGHT, OR WOOD'S LAMP Long-wave ultraviolet light (360 nm), or Wood's lamp, is an essential source of illumination for examination of the skin. Wood's lamp consists of a high-pressure mercury arc lamp with a specially compounded glass filter made of nickel oxide and silica (Wood's filter). This filter permits a band of radiation of 360 nm, which, upon impingement, will reveal fluorescence.

This valuable technique can be used for mass screening for the detection of the fluorescence of dermatophytosis *in the hair shaft* in ring worm of the scalp. In internal medicine, however, Wood's lamp is especially important for the detection of the pinkish red fluorescence of the urine of patients with porphyria cutanea tarda; the addition of hydrochloric acid greatly intensifies the fluorescence, owing to the oxidation of porphyrin precursors to porphyrins.

Wood's lamp is also of great help in the estimation of variation in the pigmentation of the skin; it reveals both increased and decreased pigmentation. Inasmuch as melanin is a universal absorber of ultraviolet light, areas of increased melanin will show an increased intensity under Wood's lamp; conversely, areas of decreased melanin will show a decrease in intensity (or an increased reflection) because the ultraviolet light is not absorbed. In this respect, Wood's lamp is the only means of recognizing the sometimes indistinguishable hypomelanotic mac-

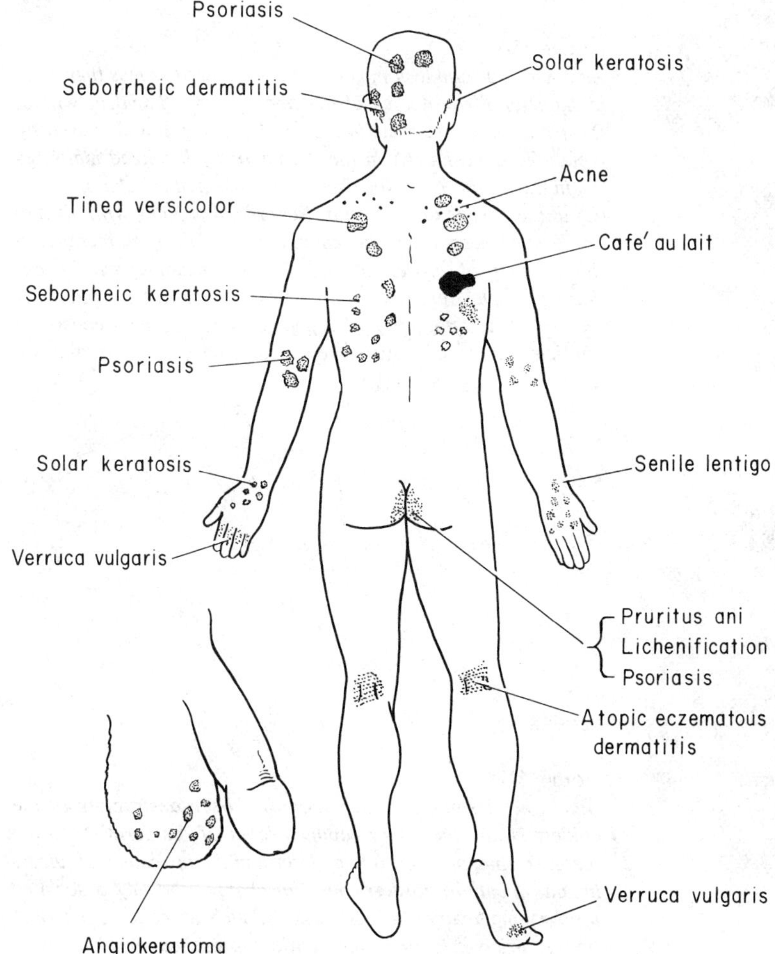

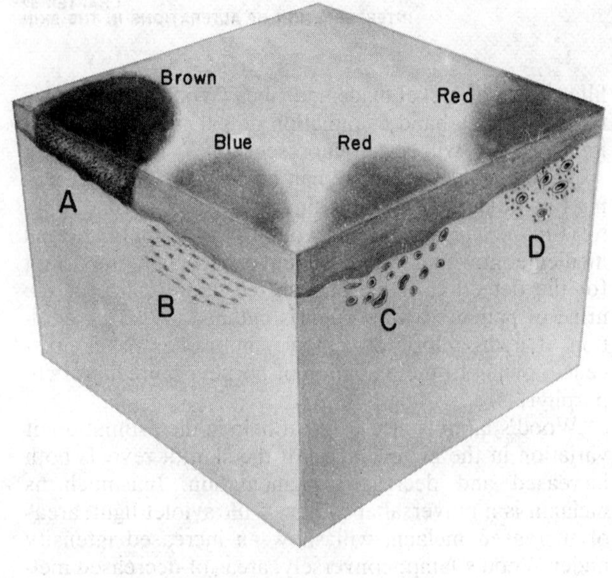

Types of skin lesion

MACULE

FIGURE 52-2
A macule is a circumscribed area of change in normal skin color without elevation or depression of the surface relative to the surrounding skin. The macules may be of any size and are the result of hypopigmentation (e.g., vitiligo) or hyperpigmentation—melanin (A) *or hemosiderin* (D)*—such as café au lait spots and Mongolian spots* (B)*, or permanent vascular abnormalities of the skin, as in a capillary hemangioma or transient capillary dilatation (erythema)* (C)*. Pressure of a glass slide (diascopy) on the border of a red lesion is a simple and reliable method for detecting the extravasation of red blood cells. If the redness remains under the pressure of the slide, the lesion may be purpuric* (D)*; if the redness disappears, the lesion is erythematous and is due to vascular dilatation* (C).

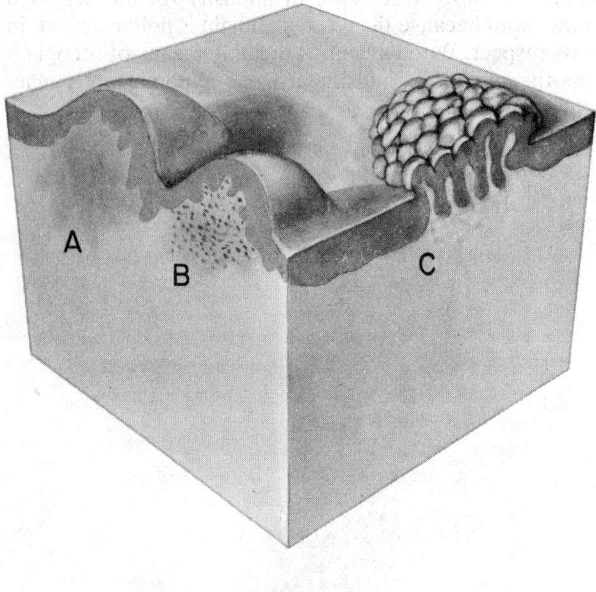

PAPULE

FIGURE 52-3
A papule is a solid lesion, generally considered as less than 1 cm in diameter. Most of it is elevated above, rather than deep within, the plane of the surrounding skin. The elevation is caused by metabolic deposits (A) *in the dermis or by localized infiltrates* (B) *in the dermis or by localized hyperplasia of cellular elements* (C) *in the dermis or epidermis. Superficial papules with distinct borders are seen when the lesion is the result of an increase in the number of epidermal cells* (C) *or melanocytes. Deeper dermal papules resulting from cellular infiltrates have indistinct borders. The topography of a papule or plaque may consist of multiple, small, closely packed, projected elevations that are known as a vegetation* (C).

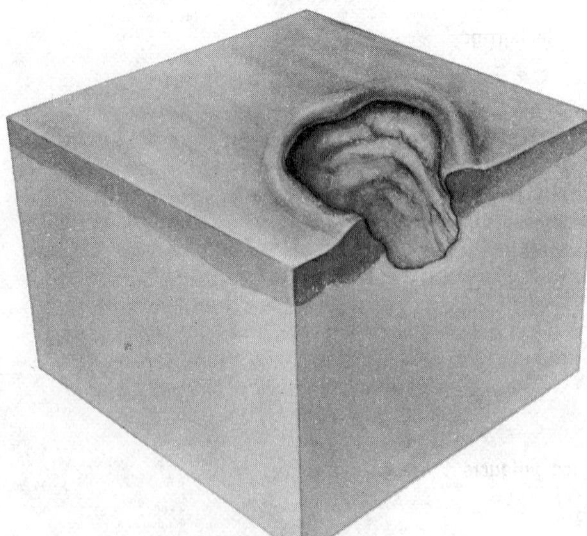

ULCERS

FIGURE 52-4
Ulcers *are lesions in which there has been destruction of the epidermis and the upper papillary layer of the dermis. Certain features that are helpful in determining the cause of ulcers include location, borders, base, discharge, and any associated topographic features of the lesions, such as nodules, excoriations, varicosities, hair distribution, presence or absence of sweating, and adjacent pulses.*

Types of skin lesion (cont.)

NODULE

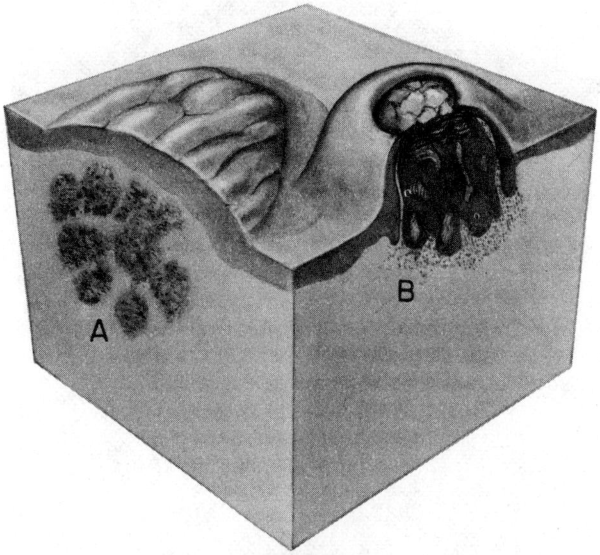

FIGURE 52-5
A nodule *is a palpable solid, round or ellipsoidal lesion deeper than a papule and is in the dermis or subcutaneous tissue* (A) *or in the epidermis* (B). *The depth of involvement rather than the diameter primarily differentiates a nodule from a papule. Nodules result from infiltrates* (A), *neoplasms* (B), *or metabolic deposits in the dermis or subcutaneous tissue and often indicate systemic disease. Late syphilis, tuberculosis, the deep mycoses, lymphoma, and metastatic neoplasms, e.g., can present as cutaneous nodules. Therefore, biopsy should be performed on unidentified persistent nodules, and a portion of excised tissue should be ground in a sterile mortar and cultured for fungi. Nodules can develop as a result of a benign or malignant proliferation of keratinocytes, as in keratoacanthoma* (B), *verruca vulgaris, and squamous-cell and basal-cell carcinoma.*

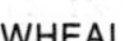

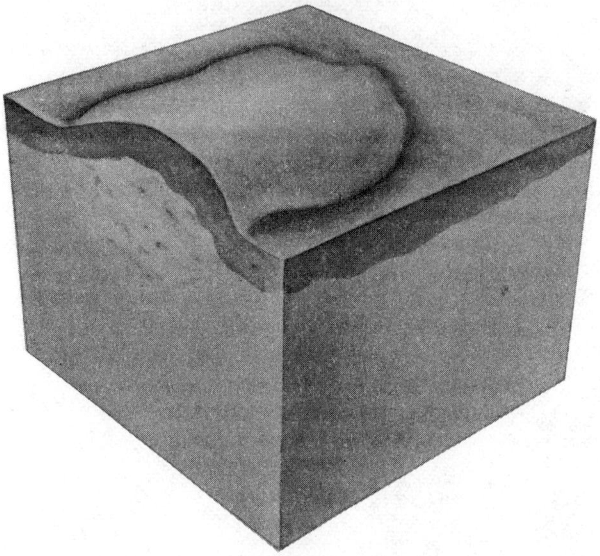

WHEAL

FIGURE 52-6
A wheal *is a rounded or flat-topped, pale-red elevation in the skin that is characteristically evanescent, disappearing within hours. Observation of the borders of wheals that have been traced with a skin-marking pencil reveals that the wheals shift relatively rapidly from the involved to the uninvolved adjacent areas. Wheals are the result of edema in the upper layer of the dermis.*

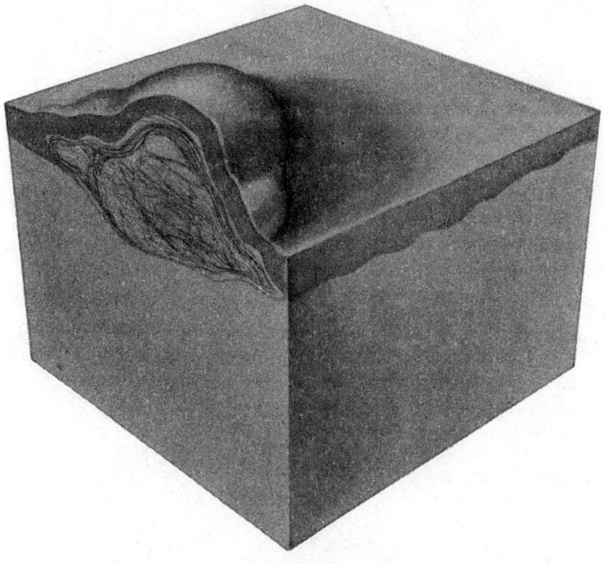

VESICLE

FIGURE 52-7
A vesicle *(less than 0.5 cm) or a* bulla *(more than 0.5 cm) is a circumscribed elevated lesion containing fluid. Often the walls are so thin that they are translucent, and the serum, lymph fluid, blood, or extracellular fluid can be seen. Vesicles and bullae arise from a cleavage at various levels of the skin; the cleavage may be within the epidermis (i.e., intraepidermal vesication), or at the epidermodermal interface (i.e., subepidermal).*

Types of skin lesion (cont.)

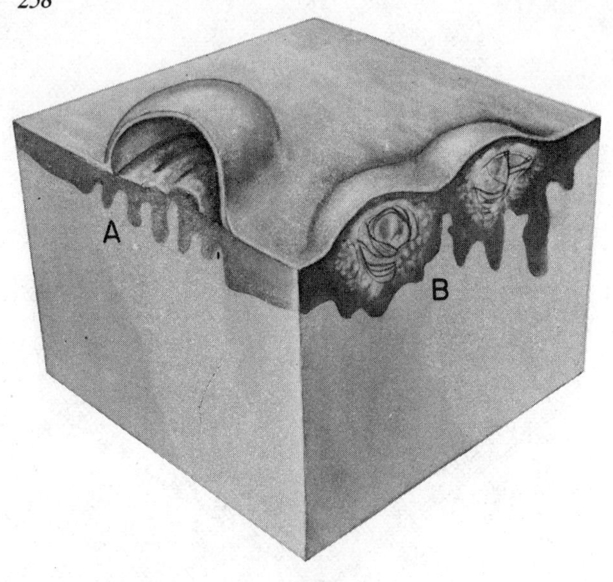

BULLA (A: subcorneal; B: spongiotic)

FIGURE 52.8
When the cleavage is just beneath the stratum corneum, a subcorneal vesicle *or* bulla *results* (A), *as seen in impetigo and subcorneal pustular dermatosis. Intraepidermal vesication may result from intercellular edema, or spongiosis* (B), *as characteristically seen in delayed hypersensitivity reactions of the epidermis (e.g., in contact eczematous dermatitis), and in dyshidrotic eczema* (B). *Spongiotic vesicles may or may not be seen clinically as vesicles.*

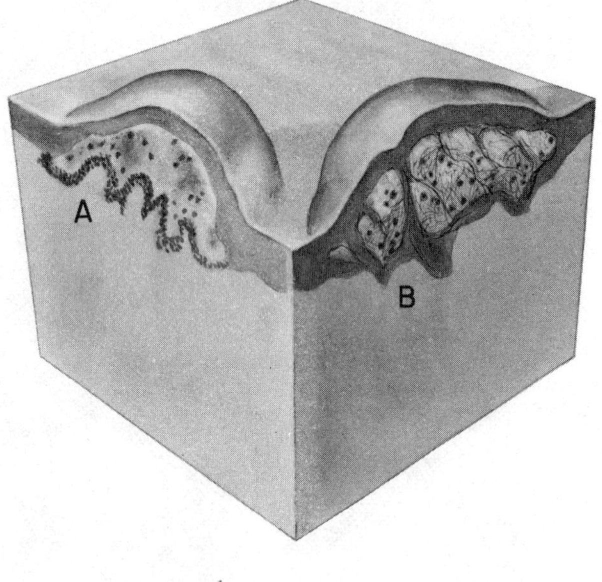

VESICLE (A: acantholytic; B: viral)

FIGURE 52-9
Loss of intercellular bridges, or desmosomes, is known as acantholysis (A), *and this type of intraepidermal vesication is seen in the vesicles or bullae of pemphigus vulgaris; the cleavage is usually just above the basal layer, as in pemphigus vulgaris, but may occur just below the subcorneal layer, as in pemphigus foliaceus. Viruses cause a curious "ballooning degeneration" of epidermal cells* (B), *as in herpes zoster, herpes simplex, variola, and varicella. Viral bullae often have a depressed ("umbilicated") center.*

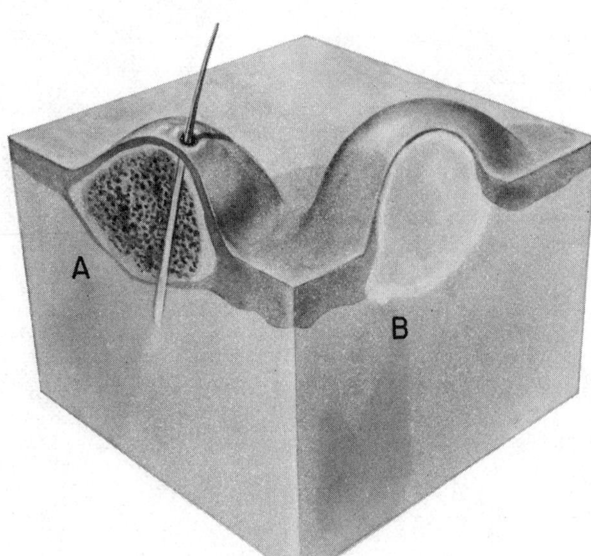

PUSTULE

FIGURE 52-10
A pustule *is a circumscribed elevation of the skin that contains a purulent exudate that may be white, yellow, or greenish yellow. This process may arise in a hair follicle* (A) *or independently* (B). *Pustules may vary in size and shape; follicular pustules, however, are always conical and usually contain a hair in the center. The vesicular lesions of the viral diseases (varicella, variola, vaccinia, herpes simplex, and herpes zoster) may secondarily become pustular. A Gram stain and culture should be done on all pustules.*

Types of skin lesion (cont.)

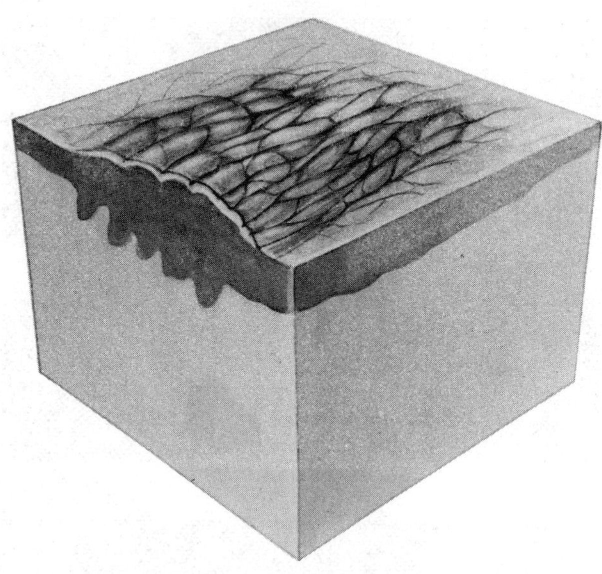

PLAQUE

FIGURE 52-11
A plaque is an elevation above the skin surface that occupies a relatively large surface area in comparison with its height above the skin. Frequently, it is formed by a confluence of papules, as in psoriasis and mycosis fungoides. Lichenification is a proliferation of keratinocytes and stratum corneum forming a plaquelike structure. The skin appears thickened, and the skin markings are accentuated. The process results from repeated rubbing, and frequently develops in persons with atopy. Lichenification occurs in eczematous dermatitis.

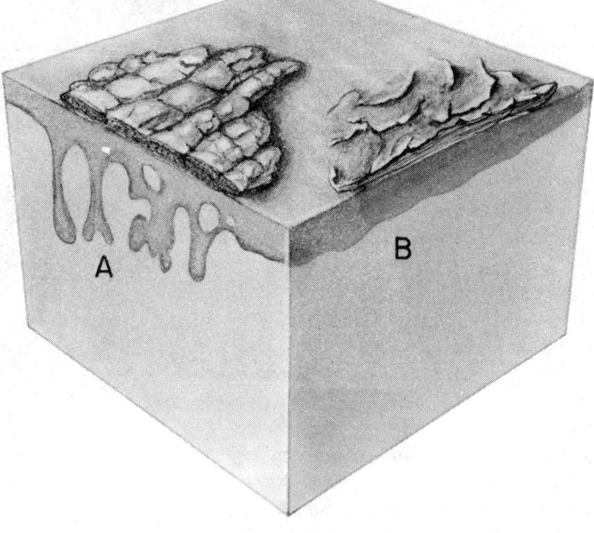

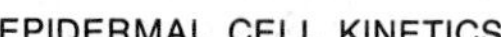

EPIDERMAL CELL KINETICS

FIGURE 52-12
Epidermal cells are completely replaced every 27 days. The end product of this holocrine process is the stratum corneum. This outermost layer of skin, the stratum corneum, normally does not contain nuclei and is imperceptibly lost. With an increased rate of proliferation of epidermal cells, as in psoriasis, the stratum corneum is not formed, and the outermost layer of the skin contains nuclei (parakeratosis) (A) *and remains attached to the Malpighian layer* (A). *These desquamating layers of skin are seen clinically as* scales. *Densely adherent scales that have a gritty feel (like sandpaper) result from a localized increase in the stratum corneum and are typically seen in solar keratosis* (B).

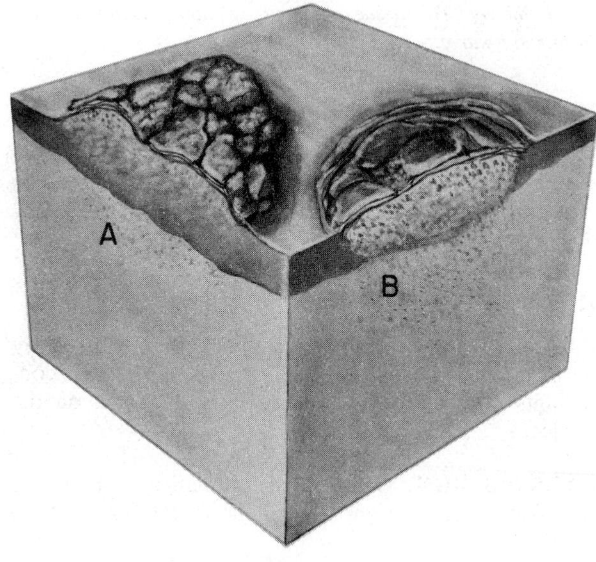

CRUSTS

FIGURE 52-13
Crusts, *resulting when serum, blood, or purulent exudate dries on the skin surface, are the hallmark of pyogenic infection. Crusts may be thin, delicate, and friable* (A) *or thick and adherent* (B). *Crusts are yellow when formed from dried serum, green or yellow-green when formed from purulent exudate, or brown or dark red when formed from blood. Superficial crusts occur as honey-colored, delicate, glistening particulates on the surface* (A) *and are typically seen in impetigo. When the exudate involves the entire epidermis, the crusts may be thick and adherent, and this condition is known as ecthyma* (B).

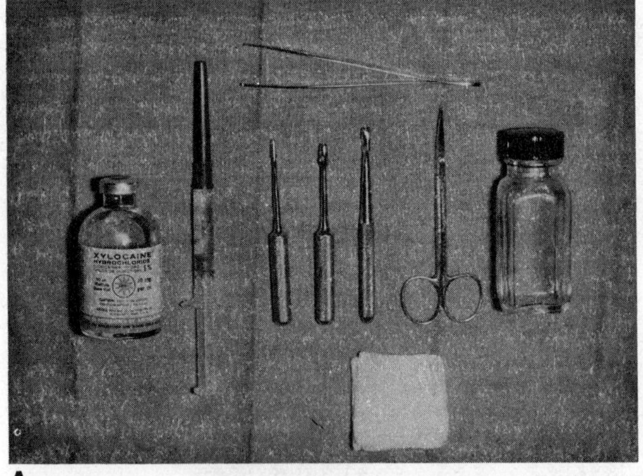

A

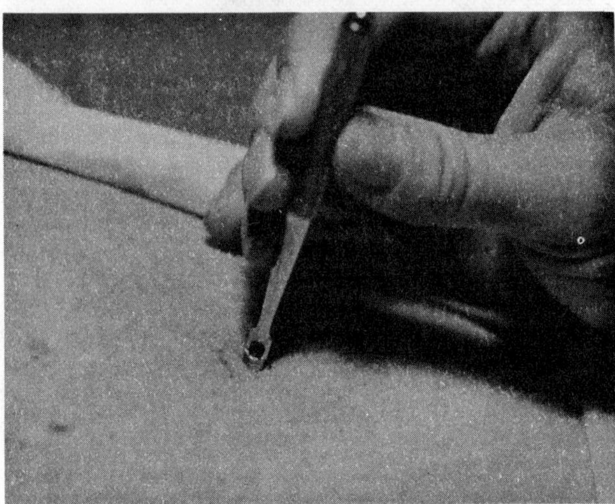

B

FIGURE 52-14

A Biopsy of cutaneous lesions requires the following equipment: a local anesthetic, biopsy punches, forceps, and scissors. Biopsy punches are available in graduated sizes from 2 to 6 mm in diameter. B *Skin sutures are ordinarily not necessary following punch biopsy. The tissue obtained by biopsy is placed in a Formalin fixative.*

ules in tuberous sclerosis, a serious, dominantly inherited, trait associated with mental retardation. The white spots are present at birth and remain throughout life, and therefore represent important markers of this genetic disorder.

Clinical tests

PATCH-TESTING Patch-testing is primarily used by dermatologists to detect contact sensitivity. The contactants are listed in Fisher's 1967 monograph on the subject.

DARIER'S SIGN One very useful clinical response of the skin, Darier's sign, is used as a test for urticaria pigmentosa, and is evoked by the vigorous rubbing of a pigmented macule with the blunt end of an instrument such as a pen. In urticaria pigmentosa (mastocytosis), a palpable wheal occurs in a few minutes after the physical trauma, owing to the release of histamine by the mast cells in the skin.

Laboratory procedures

EXAMINATION FOR BACTERIA IN CRUSTS AND BIOPSY SPECIMENS Gram stains and bacterial cultures of exudates should be performed on all lesions consisting of crusts and purulent exudates. Ulcers and nodules should always be examined by removal of a wedge of tissue consisting of all three layers of skin, that is, tissue extending down to the subcutaneous layer. The biopsy specimen should be minced in a sterile mortar and cultured for bacteria (including typical and atypical mycobacteria) and fungi.

EXAMINATION FOR MYCELIA The presence of mycelia may be ascertained by the application of 10% potassium hydroxide to a single tiny portion of scale, which is then gently heated. For fungi, scales and hair should be cultured on Sabouraud's medium.

TZANCK TEST The Tzanck test, or the microscopic examination of cells from the base of vesicles, is necessary for determination of the presence of giant epithelial cells and multinucleated giant cells (Plate 5-5) that occur in herpes simplex, herpes zoster, and varicella. Material taken from the base of a vesicle by gentle curettage with a scalpel is spread gently on a glass slide and prepared with Giemsa's or Wright's stain for the examination.

DARKFIELD EXAMINATION OF SERUM FOR *TREPONEMA PALLIDUM* Darkfield examination of serum from erosions on the male and female genitalia is essential for the detection of *Treponema pallidum.* Darkfield examination of material obtained from the oral cavity is useless because of the presence of nonpathogenic treponemas that are indistinguishable from *T. pallidum.*

Biopsy

Microscopic examination of tissue is particularly applicable in dermatology because the lesions can be subjected to histologic examination. Although the classic method is an elliptical incision followed by suturing, a satisfactory method for diagnostic purposes is "punch" biopsy. Biopsy of the skin, in contrast to biopsy of the liver, enables correlation of gross and microscope pathology. For punch biopsy, a small tubular blade is rotated between the thumb and index finger to cut through the entire thickness of the abnormal skin; the resulting cylinder of skin is then lifted out with forceps, and the skin is cut off at its base with a pointed scissors (Fig. 52-14). This simple operation can be done under local anesthesia, and the bleeding can be stopped by the use of absorbable foam; suturing is not usually necessary. This technique is as harmless and simple as a venipuncture, and allows enough tissue to permit a definitive histologic diagnosis in most cases.

REFERENCES

FISHER AA: *Contact Dermatitis,* Philadelphia: Lea & Febiger, 1967

FITZPATRICK TB et al (eds): *Dermatology in General Medicine,* New York; McGraw-Hill, 1971

53
SKIN LESIONS OF GENERAL MEDICAL SIGNIFICANCE

T. B. FITZPATRICK
H. A. HAYNES

The skin (Fig. 53-1) is composed of three layers: (1) the *epidermis,* the outermost part, which consists of two main cell types, keratinocytes and melanocytes; (2) the *dermis,* upon which the epidermis rests, composed of a mélange of connective-tissue elements, nerves, blood and lymph vessels, glands, appendages, and a few cells (mast cells, histiocytes); and (3) the *panniculus adiposus* (subcutaneous tissue), which acts as a cushion between the epidermis and dermis and the underlying bone. The specialized cells of the epidermis, the keratinocytes, produce and retain in their cytoplasm the scleroprotein keratin. They are constantly turning over, about 27 days being required to complete differentiation and maturation. Maturation of keratinocytes consists of loss of the nucleus, leaving only the cytoplasm. The latter is made up of a highly ordered, two-phase system of keratin filaments embedded in an amorphous matrix, much like the cellulose-lignin system of wood fiber, which is known to be well adapted to withstand shearing and compression forces. The anucleate outermost portion of the epidermis is the *stratum corneum,* which acts as a tough, keratinous membrane. The stratum corneum functions structurally as a "waterproof" wall between the internal fluid milieu and the environment, and is the major barrier of the skin, protecting the body against loss of fluids and entrance of toxic agents. It also serves as a passive membrane—substances move across the skin by passive diffusion in the direction of the concentration gradient.

The skin has a relatively limited number of pathologic responses. The individual skin lesion (see Table 52-1) represents the letters of the alphabet, and the groups of

TABLE 53-1
Skin alterations and clinical reactions of general medical significance*

I Classification of lesions according to the component of the skin primarily affected
- *A* Affecting the epidermis
  - *1* Scaling macules, papules, or plaques
  - *2* Vesicles and bullae (erosions follow rupture)
  - *3* Pustules
  - *4* Exudative (impetiginized) lesions
  - *5* Eczematous dermatitis
  - *6* Erythroderma syndrome (exfoliative dermatitis)†
  - *7* Atrophy, diffuse† or circumscribed
  - *8* Hypomelanotic macules (discrete or diffuse)
  - *9* Hypermelanotic macules
  - *10* Diffuse brown hypermelanosis syndrome†
- *B* Affecting the dermis
  - *1* Papules and nodules (with and without inflammation)
  - *2* Ulcers
  - *3* Sclerosis, diffuse† or circumscribed
  - *4* Edema†
  - *5* Atrophy, diffuse† or circumscribed
- *C* Affecting the panniculus adiposus
  - *1* Nodules (with and without inflammation)
  - *2* Atrophy, diffuse† or circumscribed
- *D* Affecting the blood vessels
  - *1* Morbilliform and scarlatiniform eruptions
  - *2* Urticaria
  - *3* Erythema multiforme syndrome
  - *4* Erythema nodosum syndrome (including nodular liquefying panniculitis)
  - *5* Purpura (with and without inflammation)
  - *6* Infarcts
  - *7* Telangiectasia

* *Not including benign and malignant primary neoplasms of the skin, or benign hyperplasias.*
† *Pathologic changes affect large areas of skin, and there are no discrete lesions.*

FIGURE 53-1
Anatomy of the skin. (Copyright 1967 CIBA Pharmaceutical Company, division of CIBA-Geigy Corporation. Reproduced, with permission, from the Clinical Symposia, illustrated by Frank H. Netter, M.D. All rights reserved.)

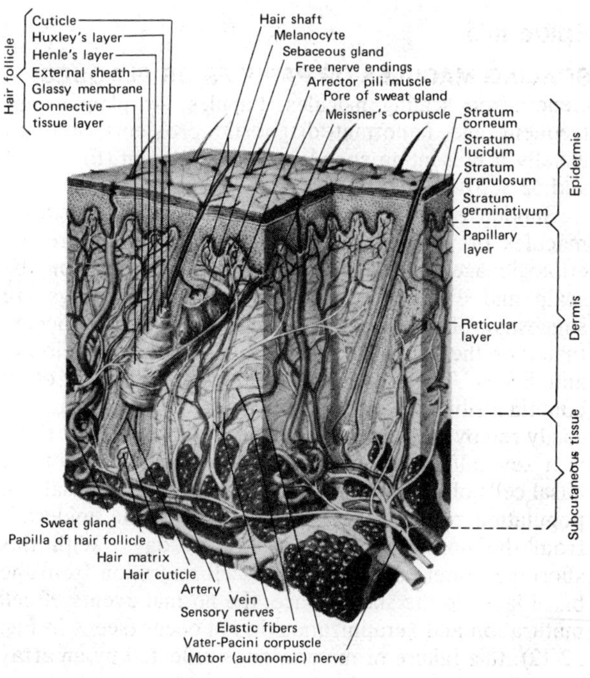

lesions constitute the word or phrase. The lesions in the majority of patients seen by the general physician can be placed in one of the groups of clinical reactions (Table 53-1) or types of skin lesions listed in Table 52-1. These skin lesions or clinical reactions may consist of one type of lesion, such as either a vesicle or a nodule, or may consist of aggregates of various types of lesions, such as papules or vesicles, as in erythema multiforme. Just one lesion or several solitary lesions or one or more groups of lesions may be distributed any place on the body. A pathologic process may involve the skin in the form of isolated lesions, as just mentioned, or the pathologic process may involve all of the skin so that the borders of the lesions may not be defined; this latter type of diffuse involvement occurs in systemic sclerosis and in pigmentation disorders.

In the physician's attempts to identify the specific types of lesions, it is therefore essential that he try to estimate the component of the skin that is *primarily* affected, such as, for example, the epidermis, the dermis, the panniculus adiposus, or the blood vessels. Inasmuch as there is a finite number of disorders that produce pathologic changes in the various individual components, this method of approach will improve the physician's diagnostic acumen. For example, even though erythema multiforme involves the dermis and the epidermis, the *primary component affected* is the blood vessel, and it is this involvement that explains the erythematous macules; the inflammatory process leads subsequently to the development of the cellular infiltrates seen clinically as papules and to destruction of the basement membrane and the development of bullae.

CLASSIFICATION OF LESIONS ACCORDING TO THE COMPONENT OF THE SKIN PRIMARILY AFFECTED

Epidermis

SCALING MACULES OR PAPULES OR PLAQUES

Generalized scaling macules, papules, or plaques are frequent and important diagnostic problems and are usually a presenting complaint of the patient (Figs. 52-2 and 52-3, 52-11).

Sudden onset of symmetrical scaling erythematous macules or papules should suggest that drugs are the etiologic agents. Scaling erythematous papules on the scalp and extensor aspects of the arms and legs are suggestive of *psoriasis;* psoriatic lesions often are accentuated on the sites of repeated trauma, such as the elbows and knees. The papules or plaques of psoriasis often contain a silvery, white, micaceous scale that is relatively easily removed in layers (see Plate 2-6). In psoriasis, there is a severalfold increase in the normal number of the basal cells of the epidermis. This increase in the basal-cell population reduces the turnover time of the epidermis from the normal 27 days to 3 to 4 days. With this shortened interval of epidermal-cell migration from the basal layer to the skin surface, the normal events of cell maturation and keratinization do not occur (see *A* in Fig. 52-12); this failure of maturation is reflected by an array of abnormal morphologic and biochemical changes. In association with the basal-cell hyperplasia, there is enhanced metabolism and accelerated synthesis and degradation of nucleoproteins, resulting in an elevated urinary excretion of nucleic acid metabolites such as uric acid. In addition, there is a proliferation of the subepidermal vasculature that is necessary to support the increased rate of cell division. The large number of cytologic, histologic, histochemical, and biochemical alterations are now known to be the result, rather than the cause, of the disease process. The only main fact known at this time about the fundamental cause of psoriasis is that the predisposition to its development is genetically transmitted.

The treatment of psoriasis still remains in the province of the dermatologist. The most effective treatment in the control of psoriasis, for most patients, is the use of topical corticosteroids with plastic wrap, crude coal tar in combination with artificial ultraviolet light, and, more recently, anthralin incorporated into a zinc oxide paste containing salicylic acid. Corticosteroids can also be injected directly into small resistant plaques. In certain patients who are resistant to topical therapy, it has become necessary to use a variety of systemic chemotherapeutic agents, especially methotrexate, which has the capacity to inhibit cell replication without a proportionate inhibition of cell function, i.e., keratinization. Systemic corticosteroids are not only ineffective in psoriasis but may cause generalization of the process and are absolutely contraindicated. An erosive joint disease, *psoriatic arthritis,* is discussed in Chap. 358.

The general physician does not always appreciate the importance of psoriasis as a major cause of disability and of disfigurement. Psoriasis affects between 2 and 8 million persons in the United States.

Symmetrical scaling macules or papules localized on the palms and soles often are presenting signs of *secondary syphilis;* there is very often generalized lymphadenopathy and there may be mouth lesions occurring as erosions.

A relatively common and often baffling generalized scaling eruption is seen in *pityriasis rosea.* In this condition, the scale at the periphery of the lesion is very thin and forms a collarette; the center of the lesion may or may not be scaly. Pityriasis rosea typically has a "fir-tree" type of distribution, especially evident on the back. Very often, but not always, a preceding, single, isolated, scaling lesion is present for several days before generalization of the lesions.

Rarely, generalized scaling macules and papules are seen in *dermatophytosis* (Plate 2-1) and *candidosis,* and it is therefore necessary that some of the scales be examined for the presence of mycelia.

From the clinician's point of view, *mycotic infections of the skin* may be separated into two major categories, each of which has a different etiology, associated systemic disease, and response to treatment, with only one category responding to the oral antifungal, griseofulvin. The various types of *dermatophytosis* (so-called "ringworm" infections) constitute one category, and they all respond to oral griseofulvin and are confined to the epidermis, hair, toenails, and fingernails. Dermatophytosis is due to three types of fungus: Microsporum, Epidermophyton, and Trichophyton. *Microsporum audouini,* a parasite of humans, is the principal pathogen causing epidemic urban fungous infection of the scalp. *Microsporum canis,* which affects the scalp and also the face, where it causes boggy nodules, is a parasite of animals and originates largely from young (usually) farm animals and pets (kittens, puppies, and calves). *Trichophyton rubrum, Trichophyton mentagrophytes,* and *Epidermophyton floccosum,* which also are parasites of humans, are the agents most usually causing dermatophytosis of the feet, the commonest site of mycotic infection. The type of fungus infecting upper extremities, face, and trunk can be Trichophyton or Microsporum or Epidermophyton.

Inasmuch as Trichophyton, Microsporum, and Epidermophyton are parasites in humans, factors other than just contact might be implicated. Other considerations, such as variation in the host response, based on hereditary factors and mediated, possibly, through increased susceptibility or related to immune factors that have yet to be clearly defined, must be investigated.

The response of these three types of fungus to oral griseofulvin varies. Griseofulvin is highly effective, even in short courses, in fungous infection of the scalp, trunk, and groin, but even prolonged therapy rarely controls infection of the hands, fingernails, or toenails. Topical treatment with any of the antifungals is quite effective in infection of the feet, trunk, and groin, but is without any effect on infection of the fingernails or toenails.

The other major category of mycotic infections is represented by candidiasis (monilial infections). These infections do not respond at all to oral griseofulvin and are caused largely by *Candida albicans,* although occasionally by *C. tropicalis, C. krusei,* and *C. stellatoidea. C. albicans* can exist as a harmless saprophyte in the gastrointestinal tract and in the vagina. It is more common in females, and is most often present in those who are pregnant or who are taking oral contraceptives or broad-spectrum antibiotics. The association with diabetes mellitus, however, is so common that all patients (regardless of sex) with candidiasis should be screened for this disease.

Despite the fact that *C. albicans* is a normal saprophytic fungus in the vagina and gastrointestinal tract, it is rarely isolated from the exposed surface of the normal skin. *C. albicans* can invade the epidermis when the skin is exposed to high humidity and when the skin becomes macerated, and therefore, candidiasis is of common occurrence in the intertriginous areas (under the breasts and in the umbilicus, groin, and axillae), and in the oral, as well as in the vaginal, mucous membranes. Chronic paronychia is usually caused by *C. albicans.* Candidiasis also may involve the lungs, urinary tract, and heart (see Chap. 171).

The treatment of candidiasis of the skin and mucous membranes depends on the site of the infection and the type of lesion. Maceration of the skin should be treated by air-drying of the area. Lotions and dusting powders containing nystatin are also very useful for intertriginous areas. Oral administration of nystatin is not of value in cutaneous moniliasis. Unless the male, as well as the female, sexual partner is treated when candidiasis is present, there will be constant re-transfer of the infection.

Differentiation between dermatophytosis caused by any of the three types of fungus already mentioned and candidiasis may be difficult, if not impossible, without cultures of the fungus (see Laboratory Procedures in Chap. 52). Direct examination of the scales from a scaling eruption in the intertriginous area is not diagnostic because it may reveal mycelia in both dermatophytosis and candidiasis; spores, however, are seen only in candidiasis. Too often, the general physician starts treatment with topical antifungus agents or with griseofulvin without establishing whether the eruption is a type of dermatophytosis or candidiasis. Inasmuch as candidiasis does not respond to systemic griseofulvin or to most of the topical antifungus agents, prescribing these agents for an eruption that is actually candidiasis results in prolonged disability for the patient.

In the past few years, fungous diseases have assumed a new importance in medicine because of the increased number of patients under treatment with chemotherapeutic agents for leukemia and other neoplasms. Almost all of the saprophytic fungi are now known to invade the tissues of patients who are being treated with chemotherapeutic agents or who have had kidney transplants.

VESICLES AND BULLAE Some diseases may occasionally be associated with vesicles or bullae, such as erythema multiforme or porphyria cutanea tarda, but blisters (vesicles and bullae) are the major feature of a number of disorders: certain bacterial and viral infections; allergic contact dermatitis (such as poison ivy); trauma from mechanical, thermal, or chemical agents; and the bullous diseases of unknown cause (such as pemphigus and pemphigoid).

Grouped vesicles occur in herpes zoster and herpes simplex, whereas scattered discrete vesicles occur in varicella. A helpful sign in determining the nature of the vesicles is the Tzanck test (Plate 5-5; see also Laboratory Procedures in Chap. 52). In herpes simplex, herpes zoster, and varicella, there will be clusters of epithelial giant cells, which are absent in vaccinia and variola. Skin biopsy will also establish the nature of the vesicle or bulla, that is, whether it is an intraepidermal (as seen in virus infections and pemphigus) or a subepidermal bulla (as seen in bullous pemphigoid) (Figs. 52-7 to 52-9).

Vesicles arranged in linear streaks are characteristic of poison ivy dermatitis. The most reliable clue to the diagnosis of both allergic and primary-irritant contact dermatitis is the localization of vesicles to the skin areas likely to have been exposed to the agent in question.

Scattered, isolated bullae in adults represent a special and serious problem in diagnosis and treatment. *Bullous pemphigoid* and *pemphigus* are chronic, occurring primarily in adults, and one of them, pemphigus, has serious consequences for the patient. These two disorders need to be distinguished by biopsy of the skin and by the newly available immunofluorescence techniques. It is impossible on the basis of clinical diagnosis alone to distinguish between bullous pemphigoid, which is a chronic and relatively benign disorder and often of limited duration, and *pemphigus vulgaris,* which is a serious disease leading in a relentless course to death, unless treatment with immunosuppressive agents or steroids is instituted. Pemphigus has been divided into four separate entities, but pemphigus vulgaris is the most important for the general physician to recognize. Pemphigus vulgaris may begin in the nasal or oral mucous membrane, and the patient may consult the dentist or otolaryngologist first. The lesions tend to spread in an unpredictable fashion to other parts of the body, but especially seem to localize around the umbilicus and on the scalp and trunk, although there is no specific distribution pattern. Pemphigus vulgaris affects primarily the middle-aged, particularly between the ages of forty and sixty. It rarely occurs before the age of seventeen or after the age of seventy-five years. The clinical lesions appear as flaccid bullae from the beginning; they break easily and rarely become very large. The denuded areas that form at the site of the ruptured bullae increase in size as the epidermis detaches itself. Occasionally, almost the entire surface may be involved by large, denuded areas; this involvement represents a serious problem in the management of secondary infection and in maintenance of fluid balance—more or less the same problems that occur in a severely burned patient. Oral or nasal mucosal lesions occur in nearly all the patients, and more than half have lesions in the mucous membrane of the mouth as the first manifestation of the disease. The disease often starts with only a few lesions in the mouth and may remain limited in extent for several weeks; it then gradually spreads to other parts of the body.

The diagnosis of pemphigus is made on the basis of the light-microscope examination of the biopsy of an early vesicle. The earliest change in pemphigus vulgaris consists of intercellular edema followed by disappearance of intercellular bridges in the lower epidermis (see *A* in Fig. 52-9). This results in loss of cohesion between the epidermal cells (acantholysis) and leads to the formation of clefts and then bullae that are predominantly in the suprabasal locations; in other words, the basal cells, although separated from one another, remain attached to the dermis much like a "row of tombstones."

Immunofluorescence allows detection of antibodies in the serum of patients with pemphigus and bullous pemphigoid and differentiation of these two bullous disorders by the localization of the antibody. The antibodies, which are in the IgG fraction of serum, react with a specific intercellular antigen. The fluorescence is localized to the site of acantholysis in pemphigus; in bullous pemphigoid, however, the antibodies react with the basement membrane, and the fluorescence is localized there.

Treatment of pemphigus with systemic and intradermal corticosteroids, sometimes in combination with methotrexate or azathioprine, is quite successful.

PUSTULES This skin reaction (Fig. 52-10) may result from infections or from sterile inflammation. Pustules may arise from preexisting vesicles of any cause. Infection by pyogenic bacteria, especially staphylococci, as well as by certain fungi and mycobacteria, can produce pustules without a preceding vesicular stage. Noninfectious causes of pustules include acne, pustular psoriasis, and hypersensitivity to drugs, particularly sulfonamides, iodides, or bromides.

EXUDATIVE (IMPETIGINIZED) LESIONS Acute infection with gram-positive cocci can occur as a primary process or may be superimposed on eczematous dermatitis or occasionally on any of the vesicular bullous diseases, and is characterized by the presence of crusts (Fig. 52-13). Such infection on the skin has the same importance as a streptococcal pharyngitis, inasmuch as acute glomerular nephritis develops in a significant percentage of patients with impetiginized dermatitis. Patients with impetiginized dermatitis must therefore be treated with full courses of systemic antibiotics.

ECZEMATOUS DERMATITIS Eczematous dermatitis (Plate 2-2 and 2-3) is not a specific disease entity but a characteristic inflammatory response of the skin due to both endogenous and exogenous agents that cause a delayed hypersensitivity reaction. Eczematous dermatitis therefore requires a qualifying etiologic term, e.g., *atopic eczematous dermatitis*. Eczematous dermatitis is sufficiently serious to account for the highest incidence of skin morbidity, responsible for incalculable losses of time and productivity in industry, with approximately one-third of all patients in the United States seen by dermatologists having one or the other of its forms. In Tables 53-2 and 53-3 some of the types of eczematous dermatitis are summarized (*B* in Fig. 52-8 and 52-11).

ERYTHRODERMA SYNDROME (EXFOLIATIVE DERMATITIS) The erythroderma syndrome is an important dermatologic complication that may occur as the result of an extension of a drug reaction, as a generalized spreading of a preexisting dermatosis, such as psoriasis or atopic dermatitis, or in association with lymphoma and leukemia. This syndrome consists of a generalized erythematous scaling eruption involving all of the skin surface, and has important implications in general medicine because of the systemic effects occasioned by the massive and continuous exfoliation of the skin. The severity of the metabolic response to exfoliation depends on the duration and severity of the process itself. Patients with extensive exfoliative dermatitis may have negative nitrogen balance, edema, hypoalbuminemia, and loss of muscle mass. An important feature also in these patients is the large extrarenal water loss, due to the defective cutaneous barrier that leads to markedly increased transepidermal water loss. Serious metabolic effects of chronic exfoliative dermatitis occur when the rate of scaling reaches 17 g per mm^2 per 24 hr. The etiology of exfoliative dermatitis determines its course: the disease eventually clears in patients with psoriasis or atopic dermatitis, whereas the prognosis is relatively poor in patients with lymphoma and leukemia. Approximately 60 percent of patients with exfoliative dermatitis recover within eight to ten months, 30 percent die, and 10 percent have a persistent problem unresponsive to therapy.

ATROPHY, DIFFUSE OR CIRCUMSCRIBED Epidermal atrophy is manifested by an almost transparent epidermis and is associated with a decrease in the number of epidermal cells. An atrophic epidermis may or may not retain the normal skin markings. Circumscribed epidermal atrophy occurs in discoid lupus erythematosus, in necrobiosis lipoidica diabeticorum, and in striae cutis distensae; diffuse epidermal atrophy occurs with aging and in scleroderma.

The most important atrophic-type disorder is *necrobiosis lipoidica diabeticorum* (NLD) (Plate 5-1). These lesions, which are usually asymptomatic, occur more frequently in women and on areas subject to trauma such as the anterior and lateral surfaces of the lower legs. The lesion begins as a small, reddish, elevated nodule with a sharply circumscribed border, gradually enlarges, and becomes flattened and depressed as the skin becomes atrophic. The brownish yellow color is prominent, and blood vessels are readily seen because of the atrophic

TABLE 53-2
Various types of eczematous dermatitis* of uncertain etiology

Clinical type	*Suspected pathogenesis*	*Diagnostic considerations*
Atopic eczematous dermatitis	Hereditary predisposition plus precipitating factors	Eczematous dermatitis, especially localized to the antecubital and popliteal fossae and to the face
Lichen simplex chronicus	Hereditary predisposition plus repeated local trauma	One or more lichenified plaques (see Fig. 52-11), especially on neck
Prurigo nodularis	Repeated local trauma	One or more nodules, especially on extremities
"Neurodermatitis"	Hereditary predisposition plus repeated scratching	Generalized or localized eczematous eruption at sites of repeated trauma
Stasis dermatitis	Chronic venous insufficiency	Signs of venous insufficiency
Nummular eczematous dermatitis	Various precipitating factors (contact irritants, xerosis, emotional stress, etc.)	Discrete coin-shaped patches, usually on extremities and trunk
"Dyshidrotic" eczematous dermatitis	Emotional stress plus other factors‡	Vesicles and bullae on palms and soles
Seborrheic dermatitis	Constitutional diathesis	Greasy scaling patches on scalp, eyebrows, and nasolabial area
Various patterns of eczematous dermatitis	Association with gastrointestinal malabsorption	Eczematous eruption in patient with steatorrhea and abnormal biopsy specimens of the jejunal mucosa
"Eczematous-like eruptions"† with systemic disease: Wiskott-Aldrich syndrome X-linked agammaglobulinemia Phenylketonuria Ahistidinemia Hurler's syndrome Hartnup disease Acrodermatitis enteropathica	Metabolic and immunologic disorders	Related features of clinical syndrome plus immunologic deficiency or biochemical abnormality

* *This term is used by many clinicians for at least four types of eczematous dermatitis that may be exclusively localized to the hands (atopic eczematous dermatitis, allergic contact eczematous dermatitis, nummular eczematous dermatitis, and "dyshidrotic" eczematous dermatitis). Possibly, contact irritants to which the hands are frequently exposed may precipitate or aggravate one of the above-mentioned basic types of eczematous dermatitis.*

† *These eruptions are reported in the literature as eczematous dermatitis, but clear, careful clinical descriptions with cutaneous biopsy specimens are frequently lacking.*

‡ *Such as constitutional diathesis and contact dermatitis.*

epidermis that is smooth and loses its skin markings entirely. The lesions of NLD are extremely indolent, and shallow ulcerations that are very slow to heal may develop. NLD may occur when diabetes mellitus cannot be detected even by use of the most stringent and provocative tests, such as the cortisone–glucose tolerance test. It is characterized by focal changes in the dermis that present as acellular and intense eosinophilic areas of necrosis bordered by inflammation. The inflammatory cells are granulomatous and include epithelioid cells, histiocytes, and multinucleated giant cells. The blood vessels are always involved with endothelial proliferation and sometimes even occlusion of the arterioles and arteries deep within the dermis; the capillary walls are thickened with focal deposits of PAS-positive material.

HYPOMELANOTIC MACULES See Chap. 55.

HYPERMELANOTIC MACULES See Chap. 55.

DIFFUSE BROWN HYPERMELANOSIS SYNDROME See Chap. 55.

Dermis

PAPULES AND NODULES (WITH AND WITHOUT INFLAMMATION) Papules and nodules without epidermal change (i.e., scaling) may be either skin color or erythematous or even slightly pigmented (yellow or brown). Dermal papules and all nodules require a biopsy for definitive diagnosis because they often represent either processes that have general medical significance, such as sarcoidosis or histiocytosis X, or tuberculosis or lymphoma. Inasmuch as dermal nodules may be present in deep mycotic infections such as coccidioidomycosis, it is necessary to obtain a biopsy, not only to rule out malignancy but to culture a portion of the excised tissue for fungi. Cultures of nodules must be made from minced tissue. The histologic specimen should be carefully studied for the presence of acid-fast bacilli, inasmuch as nodules are the presenting feature of leprosy or tuberculosis; nodules removed from the common areas of localization for leishmaniasis (face and arms) should be carefully examined for the presence of parasites.

Papules and nodules with and without inflammation can occur in disorders of the sebaceous glands. Sebaceous glands are distributed largely on the face and scalp, although they can also occur in the labia minora and on the scrotal skin, trunk, nipples, and eyelids. The sebaceous gland is a holocrine gland in which the entire cell is cast off into the excretory stream. Sebum is a complex lipid mixture of squalene (a major product of the steroid pathway), triglycerides, and wax ester. Sebaceous glands are mostly controlled by direct hormonal stimulation with androgens, derived largely from the gonads in both sexes; in the female, but not in the male, adrenal androgens may be important factors in maintaining sebum production. The major disease of the sebaceous gland in humans is *acne vulgaris* (Plate 1-5), which occurs predominantly

TABLE 53-3
Various types of eczematous dermatitis* of known etiology

Clinical type	*Pathogenesis*	*Diagnostic considerations*
Allergic contact eczematous dermatitis	Chemical allergens (plants, medicaments, cosmetics, metals, fabrics, etc.)	Site and configuration are clues to causal agent; patch tests may confirm diagnosis; avoidance of cause cures eruption
Photoallergic contact eczematous dermatitis	Ultraviolet radiation plus topical chemicals (in soaps, perfumes, citrus fruits, etc.), which then become allergens	Occurs on exposed skin; photopatch tests confirm diagnosis
Polymorphous light-induced eruption—eczematous type	Ultraviolet radiation; sometimes visible light	Occurs on exposed skin; diagnosis implies that all known causes of light-induced eruptions have been eliminated
"Infectious eczematoid dermatitis"	Bacterial products from draining focus (e.g., ear infection)	Occurs near site of infection; responds to treatment of primary infection
Eczematous dermatophytosis	Fungus	Fungi demonstrated in scales or exudate

* *This term is used by many clinicians for at least four types of eczematous dermatitis that may be exclusively localized to the hands (atopic eczematous dermatitis, allergic contact eczematous dermatitis, nummular eczematous dermatitis, and "dyshidrotic" eczematous dermatitis). Possibly, contact irritants to which the hands are frequently exposed may precipitate or aggravate one of the above-mentioned basic types of eczematous dermatitis.*

on the face and, to a lesser degree, on the back, chest, and shoulders. It is characterized by a variety of clinical lesions. These lesions may be either noninflammatory or inflammatory papules and nodules. The noninflammatory papules are called comedones, and these may either be open (blackheads) or closed (whiteheads). The closed comedones are the precursors of large inflammatory nodules and of papules and pustules. In addition, cysts and scars of various sizes may occur, the typical acne scar being a sharply punched-out pit. In the pustular and cystic lesions, despite a large amount of purulent exudate that may be recovered following incision, the lesions are usually sterile but may contain *Corynebacterium acnes.* It is believed that acne develops as a result of a primary inflammation in the follicle wall, and that the follicle partly ruptures, leading to a spilling-out of its components and the development of a perifollicular inflammatory process. The inflammatory infiltrate is lymphocytic but later, as a result of the presence of keratinous material, gram-positive diphtheroids, and sebum, the infiltrate consists essentially of a foreign-body giant-cell reaction.

The initial stimulus to the formation of comedones (both the closed and open type), is not precisely known at this time, but the initial histologic event in comedone formation is excessive keratinization within the follicular canal. It is currently believed that *Corynebacterium acnes* is responsible for lipolysis with a release of fatty acids; it is thought that these fatty acids are capable of producing an inflammatory process in the follicle wall. Acne vulgaris is a serious and important problem, especially common in the adolescent female, and its therapy is complex and prolonged. Moderate to severe acne vulgaris is best treated by a dermatologist utilizing topical agents, incision and drainage of the cystic lesions, ultraviolet-light therapy, and judicious use of systemic antibiotics; x-ray therapy has no place in the treatment of acne vulgaris.

The mechanism of action of antibiotics such as tetracycline is not completely known, but these drugs are known to suppress the number of corynebacteria and cause a reduction of free fatty acids recoverable from the skin. Inasmuch as the organisms have been shown to have lipolytic activity in vitro, it is presumed that the antibiotic causes this reduction of free fatty acids.

Estrogens combined with progestins (oral contraceptives) were initially considered effective in controlling acne; however, they have been of only limited value in the treatment of acne in females and cannot be given to males. There is no evidence suggesting that diet has any effect on the course or severity of acne vulgaris. Acne vulgaris may begin as early as the eighth year or may not appear until the twentieth. It lasts for several years and then subsides spontaneously, usually when the patients are in their early twenties. In some patients, however, acne vulgaris may continue into the third and fourth decades.

Pretibial myxedema (PM) also may cause nodules on the legs and dorsa of the feet (Plate 5-2). The lesions are usually bilateral and consist of elevated, firm, dermal nodules and plaques that are not easily movable. They may be skin-color, pink, or, rarely, brown, and, when diascoped, appear yellow and waxy. The epidermis over the nodules may appear normal or may have a marked verrucous (warty) surface. The pathogenesis of pretibial myxedema is not clear. Pretibial myxedema may occur without hyperthyroidism (Graves' disease) or before or after treatment of hyperthyroidism, and its development does not parallel the ocular changes (if present). The nodules in pretibial myxedema are accumulations of mucopolysaccharides, which can be demonstrated by special staining of the histopathologic material. Long-acting thyroid stimulator (LATS), which is associated in the plasma with immunoglobulin G (7S gamma-globulin), has been implicated in the pathogenesis of pretibial myxedema, exophthalmos, and acropachy; the role of LATS in the pathogenesis of pretibial myxedema has not been established.

ULCERS Ulcers occur as a result of destruction of the epidermis and, at least, the papillary layer of the dermis (Fig. 52-4). All ulcers of the skin that do not heal within a period of a month must be considered to be carcinoma until proved otherwise, and it is essential that a biopsy be obtained to rule out malignancy. Ulcers can be divided into two categories: lesions that occur on the legs and feet, and lesions that occur elsewhere on the body. Ulcers not occurring on the legs are rather uncommon except in primary cancer of the skin or in malignant metastases to the skin. Ulcers arising in nodules with inflammation should be approached in the manner suggested previously for nodules—that is, a biopsy should be obtained, and the tissue examined for bacterial, mycotic, and parasitic diseases. Chancre-like ulcerations and noduloulcerative lesions with regional lymphadenopathy may occur in primary syphilis and primary tuberculosis and in tularemia, anthrax, glanders, and bubonic plague. Isolated noduloulcerative lesions may be seen in sporotrichosis, coccidioidomycosis, leishmaniasis, cryptococcosis, and tertiary syphilis. Except for tertiary syphilis, these disorders can only be detected by biopsy and by culture of minced tissue for the fungi. The organism can be seen in the tissue in leishmaniasis; serologic studies are necessary to detect tertiary syphilis.

The most prominent etiologic factors in ulceration on the legs and feet are disturbances of circulation. Chronic venous insufficiency leads to ulceration, especially on the medial aspect of the ankle or lower leg, and the ulcers develop in areas of skin with brownish hemosiderin pigmentation and occasionally where there is edema or sclerosis of the area. Hypertensive or ischemic ulcerations tend to start on the lateral aspect of the ankle. Ulceration can also occur as a result of tissue infarction in areas supplied by either large or small blood vessels (arteries, arterioles); this infarction may occur as the result of occlusion or constriction due to a variety of etiologic factors, in addition to those already mentioned: emboli, thrombosis, cryoagglutinins, macroglobulinemia, cryoglobulinemia, thrombotic thrombocytopenic purpura, polycythemia, systemic lupus erythematosus, Raynaud's phenomenon, arteriosclerosis obliterans, and thromboangiitis obliterans. Ulceration of the lower extremities also occurs in hemolytic anemia, including sickle-cell anemia, thalassemia, and hereditary spherocytosis.

Some ulcers show extensive necrosis of the edges, such as those in *pyoderma gangrenosum* (Plate 5-3), an indolent ulcer usually on the lower extremities and often associated with ulcerative colitis or regional ileitis. The ulcers in pyoderma gangrenosum have ragged bluish red overhanging edges and a necrotic base. These lesions often start as pustules or tender red nodules at the site of trauma, and then gradually increase in size until liquefaction necrosis occurs and an irregular ulcer develops. The ulcers are often multiple and may cover large areas of the leg. The histopathologic findings are not specific. The healing of the ulcers usually parallels the activity of the ulcerative colitis, and, inasmuch as the ulceration extends into and involves the reticular layer of the dermis and the subcutis, scarring occurs.

The term *"tropical" ulcer,* in addition to cutaneous leishmaniasis, now also includes ulceration due to cutaneous diphtheria, treponemal disorders (syphilis, yaws, and bejel), and phagedenic ulcer, a chronic ulcer of the feet and legs caused by mixed bacteria that occurs in persons suffering from starvation and neglect.

Ulcers can be associated with peripheral neuropathy ("neuropathic" ulcer, or malum perforans) seen in diabetes mellitus, tabes dorsalis, polyneuritis, leprosy, congenital anesthesia, or hereditary sensory radicular neuropathy.

Anal and perianal ulcers are seen in histiocytosis X and in amebiasis. A hanging-drop preparation is necessary to detect *Entamoeba histolytica.*

Ulcers with artificial and bizarre shapes must be suspected of being self-induced by means of destructive agents such as acid and lighted cigarettes. Factitial ulcers are overstudied and, unfortunately, underdiagnosed by most physicians.

Stony-hard, noduloulcerative lesions, especially around joints (elbows, knees, and fingers) are suggestive of calcinosis cutis or gout; roentgenographic examination enables the detection of calcinosis cutis but shows no opaque bodies in gout.

SCLEROSIS, DIFFUSE OR CIRCUMSCRIBED Diffuse sclerosis of the skin is most often seen on the upper extremities, chest, and face in systemic scleroderma (sometimes called progressive systemic sclerosis). Initially, the skin appears yellowish, and shows slight nonpitting edema; later, however, it becomes indurated, bound down, and may be markedly hyperpigmented. Calcinosis cutis and Raynaud's phenomenon occur commonly.

Circumscribed sclerosis occurs in *morphea,* which consists of one or more round or oval firm, reddish plaques up to several centimeters in diameter that become white or yellow centrally, often with a lilac-colored, telangiectatic border. This disorder is not associated with any other organ involvement and is a localized cutaneous form of scleroderma. Another type of localized scleroderma is *linear scleroderma,* in which the morphologic change is the same type that is seen in morphea except that the process occurs in bands extending parallel to the long axis of the extremity or along the paramedian line of the forehead and scalp. This form of scleroderma has no relationship to progressive systemic sclerosis.

EDEMA In addition to the various causes of localized edema and generalized edema there is a type of edema of the lower extremities that is not often recognized by the physician. This is a bilateral pedal edema commonly seen in patients with subacute or chronic dermatitis of the lower extremities. This type of edema is most often seen with chronic eczematous dermatitis but is unrelated to cardiac failure or lymphatic obstruction. It is most probably due to an increased permeability as a result of local capillary damage, which is part of the inflammatory process in the skin. The increased capillary permeability leads to an increased transfer of fluid from the intravascular to the extravascular component of the extracellular-fluid space. This type of edema pits and disappears completely when the dermatitis has resolved.

ATROPHY, DIFFUSE OR CIRCUMSCRIBED Dermal atrophy results from a decrease of the papillary or reticular connective tissue and is manifested in the skin as a depression. Circumscribed dermal atrophy may follow trauma, or may occur in association with epidermal atrophy, as in the striae of pregnancy or in Cushing's disease.

Panniculus adiposus (subcutis)

NODULES (WITH AND WITHOUT INFLAMMATION) Nodules in the subcutis may be recognized by the fact that the skin is usually movable over the nodule; occasionally, however, in inflammatory processes, the nodule may involve both the dermis and panniculus adiposus, and the skin will then not be movable over the nodule. This immobility of the skin occurs especially in *Weber-Christian panniculitis,* in which the subcutaneous nodules, which at first are slightly mobile, become adherent to the overlying skin; then, as the edema subsides in the area of induration, a central depression occurs. Movable nodules occur around joints in rheumatic fever, rheumatoid arthritis, and systemic lupus erythematosus, and in certain metabolic diseases such as xanthoma, gout, and calcinosis. Also, metastatic carcinoma or metastatic malignant melanoma may appear as movable subcutaneous nodules. *Lipomas,* relatively common causes of subcutaneous nodules, are benign tumors composed of adipose tissue and may be single or multiple and are frequently lobulated; they are often rubbery or compressible and occur most often on the trunk and the back of the neck and forearms. Occasionally, subcutaneous lipoma may be painful and associated with marked obesity; this condition, known as Dercum's disease, occurs especially in middle-aged females. Subcutaneous nodules also occur in onchocerciasis and loaiasis. Sarcoidosis may be manifested in the skin solely as subcutaneous nodules on the lower extremities (Fig. 52-5).

ATROPHY, DIFFUSE OR CIRCUMSCRIBED Atrophy of the panniculus adiposus produces depressions in the skin; these depressions are seen in progressive lipodystrophy, in liquefying panniculitis, and in the localized fat atrophy that occurs at the site of injections of insulin. About 25 percent of diabetics who receive insulin have this type of atrophy, and, among them, it is more common in females under the age of twenty. The depressed areas of localized fat atrophy show a complete absence of the panniculus, and there is no inflammation. In lipodystrophy, diffuse atrophy of the skin may involve large portions of the body.

Blood vessels

MORBILLIFORM AND SCARLATINIFORM ERUPTIONS Morbilliform (measles-like) and scarlatiniform eruptions are macular and papular exanthems and can be due to drug hypersensitivities, measles, German measles, erythema infectiosum, viral exanthems, rickettsial diseases including endemic murine typhus and Rocky Mountain spotted fever, scarlet fever, and secondary syphilis. Many of the diseases manifested by macules or papules and occurring in acutely ill patients with a fever are listed in Table 53-4.

URTICARIA Urticaria is characterized by wheals, of which the outstanding feature is their persistence for only a few hours (Fig. 52-6). This short duration differentiates urticarial wheals from the otherwise almost identical papules of erythema multiforme, which persist for more than one or two days rather than for a few hours. An acute onset of urticaria is usually related to ingestion of drugs or certain types of foods (shellfish, fresh berries).

Chronic recurrent urticaria is a special problem, and its causes are not easily established. Most patients with chronic recurrent urticaria require a careful search for cryptic diseases such as lymphoma, systemic lupus erythematosus, primary or metastatic carcinoma, systemic vasculitis, or dermatomyositis. It is especially important, even in chronic urticarias, to carry out a painstaking interrogation of the patient in search of a history of drugs. Aspirin is one of the commonest drugs causing chronic urticaria and can often be missed even in a careful drug history because many patients do not consider aspirin a drug. It is probably true that some patients with chronic urticaria can relate their problem to emotional stress, but this cause should only be considered after excluding all possible organic causes.

ERYTHEMA MULTIFORME SYNDROME Erythema multiforme syndrome is a characteristic response of the skin and mucous membranes that is related to a number of different possible etiologies, including infectious agents (*Herpesvirus hominis, Mycoplasma pneumoniae*), and drugs (especially penicillin, antipyretics, barbiturates, hydantoins, and sulfonamides). The major pathology is an acute inflammatory infiltrate around blood vessels and may include degenerative changes in the endothelial cells of the capillaries.

The lesions occur in a characteristic symmetrical distribution and favor the extensor areas of the distal parts of the limbs, the backs of the hands, and the dorsa of the feet; the palms and soles are often involved, even

TABLE 53-4
Rash and fever in the acutely ill patient: diagnosis according to type of lesion

Diseases manifested by macules or papules	*Diseases manifested by vesicles, bullae, or pustules*	*Diseases manifested by purpuric macules, purpuric papules, or purpuric vesicles*
Drug hypersensitivities	Drug hypersensitivities	Drug hypersensitivities
Scarlet fever	Dermatitis from plants	Bacteremia†:
Erythema infectiosum (fifth disease)	Rickettsial pox	Meningococcemia (acute or chronic)
Measles (rubeola)	Varicella (chicken pox)*	Gonococcemia
German measles (rubella)	Generalized herpes zoster*	Staphylococcemia
Enterovirus infections (echo and Coxsackie)	Disseminated herpes simplex*	Pseudomonas bacteremia
Adenovirus infections	Eczema herpeticum*	Subacute bacterial endocarditis
Typhoid fever	Disseminated vaccinia*	Enterovirus infections (echo and Coxsackie)
Secondary syphilis	Eczema vaccinatum*	Rickettsial diseases:
Typhus, murine (endemic)	Variola*	Rocky Mountain spotted fever
Rocky Mountain spotted fever (early lesions)	Enterovirus infections (echo and Coxsackie), including hand-foot-mouth disease	Typhus, louse-borne (epidemic)
Pityriasis rosea	Toxic epidermal necrolysis	"Allergic" vasculitis
Erythema multiforme	Erythema multiforme bullosum	
Erythema marginatum		
Systemic lupus erythematosus		
Dermatomyositis		
"Serum sickness" (manifested only as wheals)		

* *The characteristic lesion of these exanthems is an* umbilicated *papule or vesicle on an erythematous base.*
† *Often presents as infarcts.*
SOURCE: *Fitzpatrick TB, Fisher M: A color atlas of rashes occurring in the acutely ill febrile patient, in* Dermatology in General Medicine, *eds TB Fitzpatrick et al, New York: McGraw-Hill, 1971*

to the exclusion of the dorsal surfaces. Oral lesions, first as blisters and then erosions, occur on the buccal mucous membrane, gums, and tongue, and there is often swelling and crusting of the lips. The syndrome may also include severe toxemia with prostration, high fever, and cough, and "patchy" inflammation of the lungs. The skin lesions are often characterized by a vivid redness that gradually becomes duller, and they become more indurated, with the development of centers that are pale or may have bullae; these "target" or "iris" lesions, which are characteristic of erythema multiforme but do not invariably occur, are identified by the clear red area at the periphery that surrounds a pale pink zone and a central livid area, which may contain a bulla.

ERYTHEMA NODOSUM SYNDROME (INCLUDING NODULAR LIQUEFYING PANNICULITIS) Acute, tender, red nodules on the leg are characteristically found in two disorders: *erythema nodosum syndrome* and *nodular subcutaneous fat necrosis* associated with pancreatitis.

The erythema nodosum syndrome refers to the occurrence of multiple bilateral tender nodules appearing principally on the anterior aspect of the lower extremities and occasionally on the upper extremities or face. The erythema nodosum syndrome is associated with a number of disorders that are unrelated to each other.

The nodules in erythema nodosum are only slightly elevated, edematous, and sometimes exquisitely tender. Bruising is a characteristic feature of the disease and is due to hemorrhage, leading to the formation of contusions. The lesions never ulcerate or become indurated and very seldom leave any scarring or atrophy. Erythema nodosum is associated with primary tuberculosis and primary coccidioidomycosis, histoplasmosis, beta-hemolytic streptococcal infections, lymphogranuloma venereum, sarcoidosis, ulcerative colitis, regional enteritis, drugs (penicillin, sulfonamides, bromides, iodides), and oral contraceptives containing ethinyl estradiol and norethynodrel.

Tender, red, subcutaneous nodules may also appear on the legs in association with acute pancreatitis and with pancreatic neoplasms, and, when they do, are often erroneously called erythema nodosum. This disorder has been termed *nodular liquefying panniculitis* (NLP). These lesions are distinctive. Their morphologic features are different from those of classic erythema nodosum. The lesions in NLP vary in size from a few millimeters to several centimeters, and, in contrast to the lesions of erythema nodosum, are movable. The lesions of NLP involute in two to three weeks and may leave a hyperpigmented scar that is slightly depressed. The nodules are often associated with abdominal pain and may also be accompanied by fever and arthralgia. Rarely, lesions may be present on other parts of the body besides the legs. Some of the larger nodules may undergo an abscess-like change, becoming fluctuant, and may rupture, exuding a whitish, creamy or oily viscous material; abscess formation with drainage rarely, if ever, occurs in erythema nodosum. The most-common pancreatic neoplasm associated with nodular liquefying panniculitis is an acinous adenocarcinoma of the pancreas.

PURPURA (WITH AND WITHOUT INFLAMMATION) A purpuric eruption demands immediate exploration for its etiology. Purpura arises in the skin of the vascularized dermis and is almost always confined to the dermis. The purpuric macules gradually disappear after days or weeks, depending on their size. Punctate or tiny purpuric spots are termed *petechiae,* larger (>2.0 cm) macules are spoken of as *suggillations,* and extensive purpuric macules are called *ecchymoses* (*D* in Fig. 52-2).

Purpura with inflammation is usually "palpable," i.e., papular, and is seen in systemic vasculitis and in bacteremias such as staphylococcemia, gonococcemia (Plate 5-4), and meningococcemia. In these bacteremias and in vasculitis, the examination of biopsied skin may establish a diagnosis within 8 hr (which is the time required for processing the tissue). Gentle scraping of the purpuric lesions will produce enough material for a Gram stain; intracellular gram-negative diplococci are occasionally found in the lesions in acute, but not in chronic, meningococcemia, and are rarely found in acute gonococcemia. The differential diagnosis of palpable purpuric lesions and infarcts occurring in *systemic vasculitis* as compared with those in chronic meningococcemia is not easy. The skin lesions in systemic vasculitis are usually bilateral, and almost symmetrical, in their distribution. They tend to be concentrated on the lower extremities, especially on the lower portion and around the ankles and the dorsa of the feet. The lesions in chronic meningococcemia are more randomly distributed, with occurrence on the trunk, lower and upper extremities, and face. Nevertheless, in meningococcemia, lesions can occur in a bilateral distribution, which makes the distinction between chronic meningococcemia and systemic vasculitis difficult, if not impossible, at times. The individual lesions in both chronic meningococcemia and systemic vasculitis may be identical, consisting of a mixture of palpable purpura and urticarial-type papules without purpura. Unfortunately, the histologic findings in biopsy specimens of the lesions in both diseases do not permit a distinction. Therefore, a patient with bilaterally distributed palpable purpuric lesions and fever is best treated with antibiotics before the results of blood cultures are available, inasmuch as it is impossible to make a specific diagnosis of either meningococcemia or systemic vasculitis.

Purpura without inflammation is completely macular, and examination of a blood smear can quickly establish the presence of platelets; if platelets are seen in the smear, thrombocytopenic purpura can be safely ruled out as a possibility.

On the lower legs of older people, a great variety of inflammatory skin diseases, including various types of contact dermatitis, may be associated with purpura; under these circumstances, the purpura does not have the same importance as it does when present on the trunk or upper extremities. Perifollicular purpura, however, on the lower extremities (usually accompanied by a follicular hyperkeratosis) is almost pathognomonic of scurvy.

Purpura frequently develops in amyloidosis when the lesions (waxy macules and papules) are pinched. This "pinch" purpura, however, may also occur in the normal skin of patients with thrombocytopenic purpura or in the skin of apparently normal elderly persons. (For a full discussion of the classification and differential diagnosis of purpura, see Chaps. 59 and 313.)

INFARCTS Infarcts in the skin are usually not pale like those that occur in the kidney but have a variegated dusky red, grayish hue. They are irregularly shaped macules, sometimes slightly depressed below the plane of the skin, and often surrounded by a pink zone of hyperemia. Infarcts are usually slightly tender.

Cutaneous infarctions are important and often diagnostic signs of serious multisystem disease, including both acute and chronic meningococcemia, streptococcal and staphylococcal septicemia, gonococcemia, pseudomonas septicemia, systemic vasculitis, purpura fulminans, systemic lupus erythematosus and, rarely, dermatomyositis.

TELANGIECTASIA Redness of the skin is most frequently caused by transient dilatation of blood vessels (erythema). In contrast to the color produced by fixed blood pigments, as in purpura, the erythema will disappear under the pressure of a glass or plastic slide (see Diascopy in Chap. 52). Telangiectasia is the condition in which the redness of the skin is the result of a permanent enlargement in the caliber of the blood vessels (which will be revealed by examination with a hand lens) and an increase in the number of the vessels. Telangiectasia may be composed of fine linear branches of blood vessels appearing distinctly red (i.e., not blue), which are often seen on the nose and face, or of confluent macular areas that appear as a permanent erythema. Telangiectasia is the cause of the erythema in discoid and systemic lupus erythematosus, dermatomyositis, and psoriasis.

Telangiectasia may also occur in a scattered, discrete fashion on the upper trunk or on the extremities and is seen characteristically in progressive systemic sclerosis (systemic scleroderma). Telangiectasia occurring around the nail beds, i.e., periungual telangiectasia, is an important diagnostic sign in lupus erythematosus (both discoid and systemic) and in dermatomyositis; these lesions are seen rarely, if at all, in systemic scleroderma.

Sharply outlined, red macules or papules 1 to 2 mm in diameter, with an area of radiating telangiectasia, are seen in *hereditary hemorrhagic telangiectasia* (Chap. 315). These occur on the lips, nasal mucosa, face, and hands.

Generalized telangiectasia occurring in the form of red macules over most of the body surface may be the presenting sign of mastocytosis or urticaria pigmentosa.

Telangiectasia is a prominent and diagnostic feature of *ataxia telangiectasia,* or Louis-Bar's syndrome. Telangiectasia may be present as early as the second year of life but usually develops by the fifth year; it appears first on the bulbar conjunctiva and subsequently involves the ears, the eyelids, the butterfly area of the face, the upper aspect of the chest, and the extremities.

Telangiectasia may occur in a characteristic form known as the *arterial spider,* or spider nevus, spider angioma, or naevus araneus. The main vessel of the spider is an arteriole, and it is usually faintly pulsating, which will show under the diascope. A less common skin lesion usually found with vascular spiders in liver disorders is the telangiectatic *mat* or net, a small red patch composed of intermeshed fine vessels that blanch on pressure. Spider angiomas, usually three or fewer, occur not infrequently in normal children and adults. Numerous spider angiomas often develop during pregnancy or after the ingestion of progestational agents or in rheumatoid arthritis or thyrotoxicosis. Most patients with numerous and prominent vascular spiders, however, have some form of underlying diffuse liver disease; e.g., in alcoholic cirrhosis. The progression of subacute hepatitis is often paralleled by the appearance of crops of spiders, and, in Laënnec's and postnecrotic cirrhosis, almost half the patients have multiple vascular spiders. The mechanism responsible for the development of spider angiomas in liver disease is not known, nor has it been firmly established that the lesions result from disordered metabolism of estrogens by the liver.

REFERENCES

FARBER EM, COX AJ (eds): Psoriasis, *Proceedings of the International Symposium, Stanford University, 1971,* Stanford, Calif.: Stanford University Press, 1971

FITZPATRICK TB, FISHER M: A color atlas of rashes occurring in the acutely ill febrile patient, in *Dermatology in General Medicine,* eds TB Fitzpatrick et al, New York: McGraw-Hill, 1971

——, JOHNSON DP: Fundamentals of dermatologic diagnosis, in *Dermatology in General Medicine,* eds TB Fitzpatrick et al, New York: McGraw-Hill, 1971

MULLIN GT et al: Arthritis and skin lesions resembling erythema nodosum in pancreatic disease, Ann Intern Med 68:75, 1968

54 GENERALIZED PRURITUS

T. B. FITZPATRICK
H. A. HAYNES

Generalized pruritus is a frequent and important problem in differential diagnosis for the general physician. In many patients, intense generalized pruritus is the only symptom. Unfortunately, there are no good studies that have described in detail the special qualities of pruritus that permit a specific diagnosis; in other words, it is not really known what type of pruritus is seen, for example, in obstructive biliary disease as opposed to lymphoma. In the absence of these data, the clinician must rely on the history, physical examination, and laboratory studies to establish the nature of the pruritus.

The most important cause of pruritus is psychogenic, that is, a reaction to stress and strain. This type of pruritus often affects the skin of the scalp, and may be associated with other sensory complaints such as a bitter taste in the mouth or burning of the tongue. Some patients with psychogenic pruritus are convinced that the itching is caused by some sort of parasite in their skin that cannot be seen by themselves or the physician. The patient scratches his skin until the lesions become excoriated, and then asserts that the itching has disappeared, owing, he believes, to removal of the parasite or "germ" by the bleeding.

Older persons in whom dry skin is a common occurrence may have generalized pruritus unrelated to multisystem disease. Some other older persons, however, usually more than 60 years of age, who do not have obvious dry skin may also have generalized ("senile") pruritus that is intense and does not seem to be caused by emotional stress. This pruritus is usually most severe when the patients disrobe to go to bed, and usually begins in one area, particularly the back, and spreads to involve the entire body. Neither psychogenic nor senile pruritus leads to a loss of sleep.

A subtle and important cause of pruritus without a visible rash may be a reaction to drugs, such as aspirin and, especially, opiates and their derivatives, and quinidine.

The itching that is associated with pediculosis corporis may be so intense that it will interfere with the patient's sleep. This type of eruption is usually relatively easy to diagnose by the linear excoriations that occur along the back, and often the insect can be found in the clothing, particularly along the seams.

For a list of conditions in which generalized pruritus occurs without any evidence of primary skin disease, see Table 54-1.

The pruritus in hepatic disease has no special qualities. Generalized pruritus may frequently be the first sign of biliary cirrhosis and may occur many months before the onset of jaundice. It may be the first sign also of lymphoma, and, rarely, of carcinoma. The pruritus may be of sudden onset and may be very severe from the beginning.

Patients with pruritus associated with obvious skin lesions, such as bullae and papules, should be referred to a dermatologist. Some of the dermatologic disorders in which pruritus is a common symptom include scabies, dermatitis herpetiformis, lichen planus, urticaria, mycosis fungoides, insect bites, and eczematous dermatitis including atopic dermatitis. Many of these disorders require specialized dermatologic approaches, particularly biopsy of the skin, in order to establish the diagnosis.

The treatment of generalized pruritus is unsatisfactory. Not one of the systemic medications has been shown to be effective in generalized pruritus. A topical preparation containing $^{1}/_{2}$% menthol and 1% phenol in Nivea oil is somewhat helpful in relieving pruritus temporarily. The topical anesthetics containing benzocaine should be avoided because of the high risk of allergic sensitization. When the patient with pruritus also has insomnia, a hypnotic or a sedative should be prescribed. Antihistamines are of little value except in pruritus due to urticaria. It is a general clinical impression that aspirin is helpful in pruritus of any origin, but this has not been proved. The development of drugs that control pruritus remains one of the great challenges of medical research, and it is paradoxical that, at this juncture, severe pain can be immediately controlled with a variety of agents but there is not one single agent that can modify or diminish generalized pruritus. The receptors for the itch stimuli reside in the papillary layer of the dermis, but there are no specific end organs for itching. Itching is a sensation carried principally by unmyelinated slowly conducting fibers of the C group to central neuronal pools in the spinal cord. The stimuli are then carried by the posterior roots of the spinal nerves, and, from the anterolateral spinothalamic tracts, enter the thalamus and then proceed to the sensory area of the gyrus postcentralis of the cortex.

TABLE 54-1
Conditions associated with generalized pruritus without primary skin lesions

Psychogenic states	*Metabolic and endocrine disorders*	*Malignant neoplasms*	*Drug reactions*	*Infestations*	*Hematologic disease*	*Miscellaneous conditions*
Periods of emotional stress	Obstructive biliary disease	Lymphoma and leukemia	Sensitivity to opium derivatives	Ancylostomiasis (hookworm)	Polycythemia vera†	Dry skin; pregnancy
Delusions of parasitosis	Primary biliary cirrhosis	Abdominal cancer	Sensitivity (subclinical) to miscellaneous drugs	Onchocerciasis		
	Uremia			Pediculosis corporis		
	Hyperthyroidism					
	Hypothyroidism*					
	Diabetes mellitus*					

* *Not definitely proved as causes.*
† *Especially after a bath.*

55

PIGMENTATION OF THE SKIN AND DISORDERS OF MELANIN METABOLISM

T. B. FITZPATRICK
H. A. HAYNES

THE MELANOCYTE SYSTEM

DEFINITION OF MELANIN Melanin is the principal pigment in the coloration of human skin, hair, and eyes. In humans, it functions primarily as a screen that shields the dermis from the deleterious effects of solar radiation. Inasmuch as the amount and distribution of melanin in skin and hair are changed in a number of diseases, a detailed study of irregularities of pigmentation may provide important diagnostic clues to diseases in other organs.

Melanin, derived from the Greek word *melas* (black), is the name given to a biochrome of high molecular weight formed when tyrosinase oxidizes the phenol tyrosine to dopa. The biochrome is therefore often referred to as tyrosine melanin. Tyrosine melanin is the product of unicellular glands, melanocytes, that secrete melanin particles into epidermal cells. The exact chemical nature of melanin has not been determined because tyrosine melanin (both natural and synthetic) is so extremely insoluble that all attempts to degrade it into identifiable fragments have failed. It is known, however, that all animal melanins contain indoles and are composed basically of indole-5,6-quinone units, in contrast with melanins of plant origin, which contain catechols. From studies with radioactive dopa (dihydroxyphenylalanine) it appears that melanin is a copolymer of dopa-quinone, indole-5,6-quinone, and indole-5,6-quinone-2-carboxylic acid in the ratio of 3:2:1.

BIOSYNTHESIS OF MELANIN Melanocytes are situated at the dermoepidermal interface, in the hair bulb, uveal tract, retinal pigment epithelium, inner ear, and leptomeninges. These scattered groups of cells are known as the melanocyte system, which constitutes a cytologic and biochemical unit, inasmuch as the melanocytes in all these locations (except in the retinal pigment epithelium) are derived from the neural crest (Fig. 55-1) and can hydroxylate tyrosine to dopa and, ultimately, to the pigment tyrosine melanin. The melanocyte system is analogous, but not known to be related, to the chromaffin system. The cells of the chromaffin system also are derived from the neural crest and possess biochemical mechanisms for the hydroxylation of tyrosine to dopa, although by the action of tyrosine hydroxylase, instead of by tyrosinase; unlike melanocytes, they convert dopa to adrenochrome and not to tyrosine melanin. Benign and malignant neoplasms arise in all parts of the melanocyte system except in the retinal pigment epithelium and the hair bulbs.

The melanocytes present at the dermoepidermal interface form a horizontal network that is closely connected to the epidermal cells by means of numerous cytoplasmic processes, or dendrites. This intimate relationship permitting cytocrine transfer of melanin particles (melanosomes) from melanocytes to Malpighian cells has been clearly demonstrated by electron microscopy in a study of the fine structure of cortical cells and hair melanocytes and by tissue culture of human epidermis.

It has been possible to demonstrate by electron microscopy that melanocytes contain specialized organelles with a distinctive internal structure. These organelles, known as melanosomes, contain tyrosinase, the melanin-synthesizing enzyme. Under normal conditions, melanin is progressively formed and deposited on the surface of melanosomes until they become amorphous particles without detectable tyrosinase activity (Fig. 55-2). Melanosomes are believed to originate in the Golgi area, appearing first as unmelanized vesicles that gradually become dark and increasingly dense.

Tyrosinase is one of a large group of copper-containing aerobic oxidases that catalyze the oxidation of both monohydroxy and *o*-dihydroxy phenols to orthoquinones. In man and other mammals, this oxidase catalyzes the hydroxylation of the melanin precursor, tyrosine, to

FIGURE 55-1
Diagram showing the embryonic origin, dispersal, and developmental fate of melanocytes in man. (By permission from JB Stanbury et al, eds: The Metabolic Basis of Inherited Disease, *2d ed., McGraw-Hill 1966)*

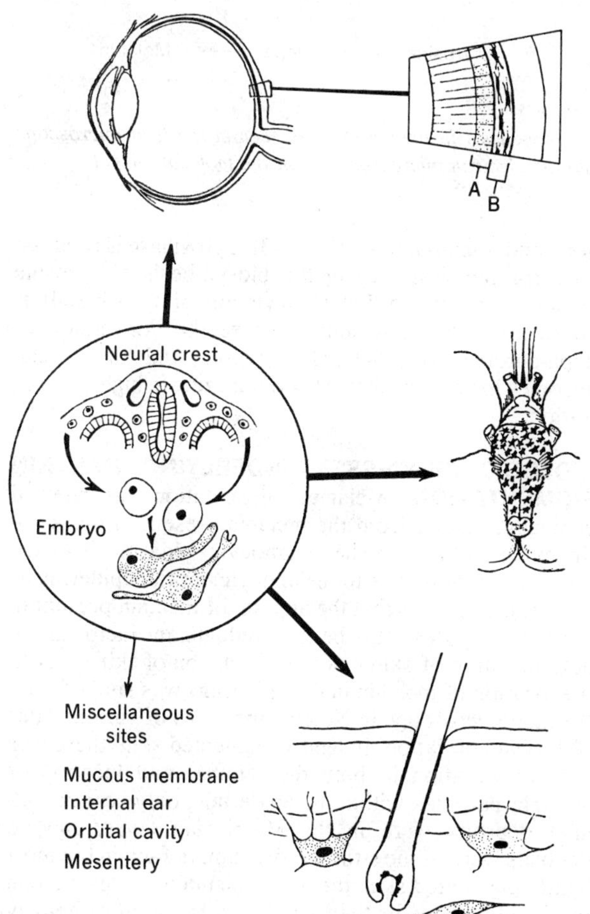

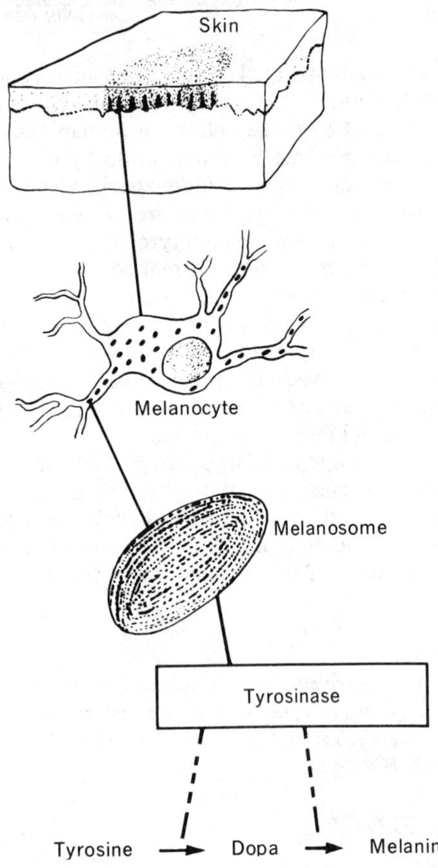

FIGURE 55-2
Melanogenesis in human skin, as seen in the light microscope and the electron microscope and at the molecular level.

dopa and dopa-quinone (Fig. 55-3). Tyrosinase is required only for the first step in the biosynthesis of tyrosine melanin, i.e., the orthohydroxylation of tyrosine. It is noteworthy that zinc ions catalyze the conversion of dopa-chrome to 5,6-dihydroxyindole and that melanosomes have been shown to contain zinc in high concentration.

BIOLOGIC PROCESSES UNDERLYING MELANIN PIGMENTATION Melanin pigmentation, as viewed clinically, results from the melanin present in the keratinocytes and also in the melanocytes. Inasmuch as the ratio of keratinocytes to melanocytes in the epidermis is 36:1, it is apparent that the amount of melanin present in the keratinocytes must be the predominant factor in the determination of skin color. The relation of skin color to the location of melanin in the epidermis was studied with the light microscope in Negro Americans of various hues of brown coloration. In lightly pigmented skin, there was a great variation in both the number and location of melanin particles within the epidermis; only scanty melanin deposits were in the Malpighian layer, and no deposits were in the stratum corneum. In fact, in the most lightly pigmented skin, the only melanin particles were in the keratinocytes of the basal layer. In the most heavily pigmented skin, there were melanin particles in the keratinocytes of the basal layer, throughout the Malpighian cells, and in the stratum corneum.

It is apparent, therefore, from studies of normal skin and of pigmentary disorders, that the intensity of pigmentation, as viewed clinically, depends not only on the rate of melanosome production but also on the number of melanosomes that are transferred to the keratinocytes. Another factor that determines normal and abnormal melanin pigmentation is the degree of melanization of the individual melanosomes. Until recently, three factors—melanosome formation, melanosome melanization, and melanosome secretion—were considered to be the major variables in normal and abnormal melanin pigmentation. In the past few years, however, a fourth variable has been implicated in melanin pigmentation—i.e., the phenomenon of aggregation and degradation of melanosomes that occurs during their transport in the keratinocytes.

Melanosomes are present in melanocytes mainly as nonaggregated (single), membrane-delimited, discrete organelles. In keratinocytes, however, melanosomes occur either as single, or nonaggregated, particles or as aggregates of three or more within a membrane-delimited organelle. These melanosome-containing organelles resemble the melanosome-containing organelles within macrophages that have been identified as lysosomes. In the epidermal keratinocyte, melanosomes appear to undergo a gradual degradation. In heavily pigmented skin, however, intact melanosomes remain in the stratum corneum, indicating that some melanosomes are apparently not degraded within the lysosomes in the epidermis. Numerous studies in recent years have shown that there appears to be a considerable variation in the arrangement of melanosomes in the nonfollicular keratinocytes in different racial groups. In the keratinocytes of the hair follicle in all racial groups, there are, in the growing phase of the hair growth cycle, single, or nonaggregated, melanosomes. In Negroids and Australian aborigines, however, melanosomes are found, in the epidermal keratinocytes, to be nonaggregated (single), whereas in Caucasoids, Mongoloids, and American Indians, melanosomes are found, in the keratinocytes, to be mostly aggregated, and there is often a suggestion of fragmentation of the melanosomes within these lysosome-like organelles. Some recent observations have shown that the size of the melanosome determines whether or not a melanosome becomes aggregated in the keratinocytes. Melanosomes that are smaller than 1 μm can aggregate in the form of a phagosome and undergo degradation—a process that could gradually decrease the intensity of the coloration.

The pigmentation of the skin is related to four biological processes (Fig. 55-4):

1 Formation of melanosomes in melanocytes
2 Melanization of melanosomes in melanocytes
3 Secretion of melanosomes into keratinocytes
4 Transport of melanosomes by keratinocytes with and without degradation in lysosome-like organelles

Inasmuch as these four biological processes are the bases of normal pigmentation and are altered in abnormal melanin pigmentation, a résumé of each is necessary.

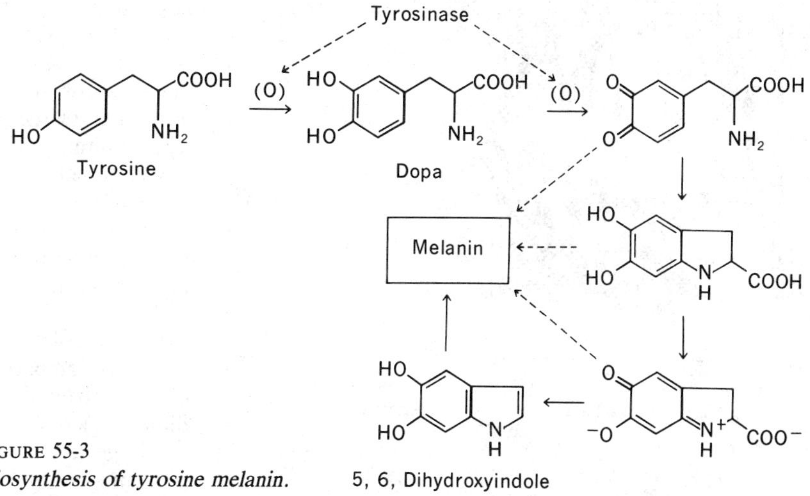

FIGURE 55-3
Biosynthesis of tyrosine melanin.

Aggregation[1] and dispersion of melanosomes probably play no part in the pigmentary anomalies of humans. Such movement has thus far been observed only in specialized effector cells, melanophores, present only in vertebrates below mammals in the phylogenetic scale; this movement of melanosomes is under neural and hormonal control in these animals.

MELANOCYTE-SYSTEM DISTURBANCES AND ETIOLOGIC FACTORS

Disorders of melanin pigmentation are frequent and important signs of disease in other organ systems (Table 55-1). These disorders of the melanocyte system (Table 55-2) may be classed as hypomelanoses and hypermelanoses and can be divided into three main categories: (1) hypomelanosis, in which paucity or absence of pigment renders the skin white or lighter than normal; (2) hypermelanosis (brown), in which excess pigment produces a brown-to-black color; and (3) hypermelanosis (blue), in which excess pigment produces a blue or slate or gray color. Within the three categories, the pigmentary disorders with similar etiology may be grouped together (Table 55-2). Hypomelanosis (decreased pigmentation) may result from loss of melanocytes, as in thermal burns, or from absence or paucity of melanin. Brown hypermelanosis (see Table 55-2) results, in most instances, from an increase in the activity of epidermal melanocytes, i.e., an increase in the number of melanosomes produced, and not from an increase in the number of these cells. Gray or slate or blue hypermelanosis results from the presence of melanin within dermal phagocytes or ectopic dermal melanocytes, and this clinical color change from brown is related to the Tyndall light-scattering phenomenon.

Recognition of hypomelanosis and of gray or slate or blue hypermelanosis is usually not difficult. When the degree of hypomelanosis is very slight, diagnosis may be facilitated by the use of black light (Wood's lamp; see Chap. 52). Differentiation between abnormal diffuse brown hyperpigmentation and normal pigmentation frequently poses a problem because there is such a wide range of coloration in different individuals. It is usually possible, however, to determine whether the patient has been aware of an unusual or progressive or gradual deepening of coloration that has had no obvious cause, such as a summer tan that has not faded. The degree of brown hypermelanosis that develops appears to be related to the basic skin color of the patient. For example, with the onset of primary adrenocortical insufficiency, a patient of Mediterranean extraction (such as Italian, French, or Spanish) may become intensely pigmented, whereas a light-skinned patient will have only a minimal degree of hypermelanosis that may or may not be detectable. Localized pigmentation that develops newly in the mucous membranes and in specific areas, such as the axillas and palmar creases, is usually easier to identify as a pathologic change than is generalized brown hyperpigmentation.

GENETIC FACTORS *Oculocutaneous albinism* is a mendelian autosomal recessive trait and is characterized by paucity or absence of melanin in the eyes and an unpatterned hypomelanosis of the skin and hair; albinism involving the skin only has not been reported. In this disorder, melanocytes and melanosomes are present, but whatever tyrosinase may be synthesized by the melanocytes must be functionally defective and unable to catalyze the oxidation of tyrosine to melanin. The formation of melanosomes is interrupted in the early stages; few or no mature melanosomes are present in albinotic skin or hair. Oculocutaneous albinism is diagnosed and classified on the basis of ocular and cutaneous findings, and is further classified according to the presence or absence of tyrosinase in the plucked hair follicles of the scalp. In some persons with oculocutaneous albinism, the hair follicles darken when incubated in tyrosine, i.e., "*tyro-*

[1] *Aggregation in this sense refers to the clustering of melanosomes around the nucleus of the melanocyte, i.e., the phenomenon that occurs when a frog is placed on a white background; when the frog is placed on a dark background, however, there is movement, or dispersion, of the melanosomes into the dendrites.*

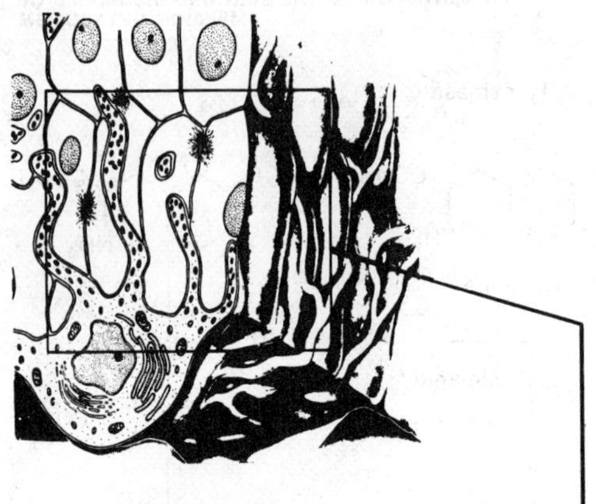

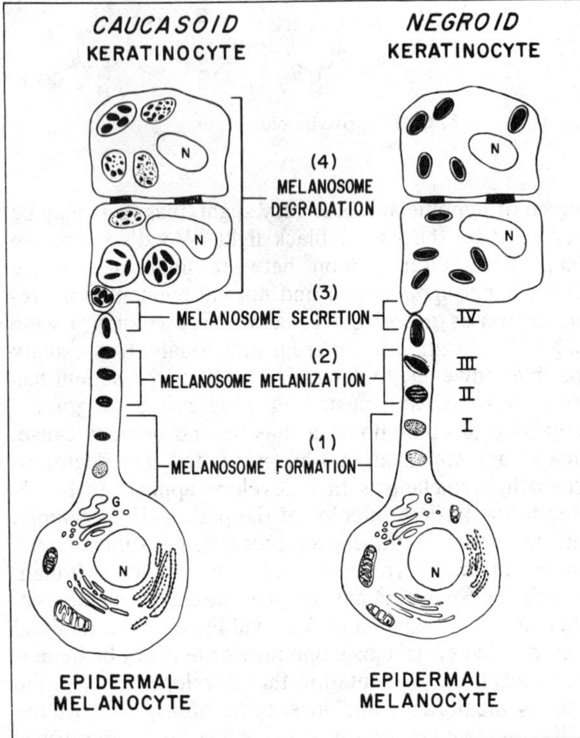

FIGURE 55-4
Four biologic processes underlying melanin pigmentation. (1) Formation of melanosomes in melanocytes; (2) melaninization of melanosomes in melanocytes; (3) secretion of melanosomes into keratinocytes; and (4) transport of melanocytes by keratinocytes, either with degradation of melanosomes within lysosome-like organelles (in Caucasoids) or without apparent degradation of melanosomes (in Negroids).

Note the difference between the melanosomes in the Negroid and Caucasoid keratinocytes. In the Negroid keratinocytes, the melanosomes are nonaggregated. In the Caucasoid keratinocytes, groups of several melanosomes are aggregated within membrane-limited lysosome-like organelles, and the melanosomes often appear fragmented. (G, Golgi apparatus; N, nucleus; I–IV, the four stages in the development of the melanosome.)

The epidermal melanin unit is shown at the top. The melanocyte supplies melanosomes to a group of keratinocytes.

sinase-positive," whereas in others no such darkening occurs, i.e., *"tyrosinase-negative."* These two types are now known to have separate gene loci. The ocular abnormalities in oculocutaneous albinism include hypopigmentation of the fundus oculi, translucence of the irides, and nystagmus. The deficiency of melanin in oculocutaneous albinism has two disturbing consequences for humans: decreased visual acuity and an abnormal degree of intolerance to sunlight. The sensitivity of human albinos to ultraviolet light leads to the development of carcinoma in exposed areas of the skin, especially in albinos living in the tropics.

In *phenylketonuria,* there is a single metabolic block in the conversion of phenylalanine to tyrosine. The condition is associated with subnormal pigmentation of the hair and the iris. The hair of patients with phenylketonuria ranges in color from light blond to dark brown, and it is only by comparison with the hair of siblings that the characteristic dilution of color becomes evident. The diminution of melanin formation results from the fact that the large amounts of phenylalanine and its metabolites present in serum and extracellular fluid act as competitive inhibitors of tyrosinase activity, thus blocking melanin synthesis.

Piebaldism, an autosomal dominant trait, involves the skin and the hair but not the eyes. In piebaldism, in addition to the absence of eye involvement, the hypomelanosis occurs in circumscribed areas on the extremities and anterior surface of the thorax, and there is commonly

TABLE 55-1
Pigmentary disturbances as diagnostic signs in general medicine

Chief complaint or presenting problem	*Pigmentary change*	*Diseases*
"Getting dark"	Generalized diffuse brown hypermelanosis	Addison's disease; hemochromatosis; ACTH-producing tumors; systemic scleroderma
"Abdominal pain"; "brown spots on lips, fingers"	Circumscribed small dark-brown macules	Peutz-Jegher's syndrome
"Brown spots"; hypertension	Circumscribed uniformly brown macules	Neurofibromatosis; Albright's syndrome
"Mole"	Circumscribed polychromic macules and papules (red, white, and blue admixed with brown)	Early primary malignant melanoma
"White spots"	Circumscribed white macules	Leukoderma associated with "vitiligo," Addison's disease, pernicious anemia, thyrotoxicosis
Seizures; mental retardation	Circumscribed leaf-shaped white macules present at birth; poliosis	Tuberous sclerosis
Uveitis; deafness	Circumscribed white macules; poliosis	Vogt-Koyanagi-Harada disease
Deafness	White forelock	Waardenburg's syndrome
"Sun sensitivity"; decreased vision	Generalized diffuse hypomelanosis of skin, hair, and uveal tract	Oculocutaneous albinism

a white forelock. *Waardenburg's syndrome* comprises piebaldism associated with congenital deafness. Electron microscopic studies have revealed that the areas of the skin lacking in pigment lack melanocytes, as in vitiligo (q.v.).

Vitiligo may be localized or generalized. When localized, the hypomelanosis of the skin and hair may be restricted to one region, such as the anogenital area or scalp. When generalized, the pattern of hypomelanosis is quite typical, with lesions particularly on the face, axillas, neck, and extremities, and with loss of pigment in the hair. Idiopathic vitiligo is fairly common, affecting 1 percent of the population. The lesions are completely lacking in pigment, and this snow-whiteness is distinctive and serves to differentiate vitiligo from other hypomelanoses. Vitiligo is believed to be inherited as an autosomal dominant trait with irregular penetrance. In the majority of cases, vitiligo is idiopathic, but typical vitiligo, as just described, is known to occur with a variety of diseases, such as Addison's disease, hyperthyroidism, hypoparathyroidism, pernicious anemia, and alopecia areata; all of these disorders are believed by some investigators to be caused by autoimmunity. In the differential diagnosis of circumscribed hypomelanosis, there are many disorders with vitiligo-type hypomelanosis of the skin and hair that must be considered (see Table 55-3). Electron microscopic studies of idiopathic vitiligo of the skin reveal a marked reduction or, more commonly, a total absence of detectable melanocytes; this phenomenon suggests, presumably, that the hypomelanosis is the result of a structural defect, rather than a metabolic change, in the existing melanocytes.

In about a third of the patients with vitiligo, it is possible to bring about a permanent repigmentation of vitiligo areas by the use of systemically administered psoralens (furocoumarins), which are available in all countries of the world in various forms. The duration of treatment varies from patient to patient and is determined to a considerable extent by the site of the lesions. Hypomelanotic macules on the face show the most rapid response. Usually, repigmentation is not complete in less than a year.

Tuberous sclerosis is an autosomal dominant trait usually causing mental retardation, seizures, and, more rarely, retinal plaques. The most constant visible clinical features of the disease are white macules on the skin, which are present at birth, thus preceding adenoma sebaceum (the typical facial lesion), which does not occur until the second or even the sixth year after birth. Such immediate diagnosis in an infant enables one to advise the parents about a possible genetic defect in any children born to them. The white macules are isolated and irregularly distributed all over the body but are most frequent on the posterior aspect of the trunk, especially on the buttocks. There may be any number from four to more than a hundred. They are not easily detected in fair-skinned infants without the aid of Wood's (ultraviolet) light. The macules occur in two characteristic shapes: (1), lance-ovate lesions in the shape of a leaflet of the mountain-ash tree, usually 3 cm in their longest dimensions (Plate 5-6); and (2) polygonal lesions, like a "thumb print" and approximately 1 cm in diameter. The macules are not pure white as in vitiligo or albino skin but are grayish or "off-white." The macules in tuberous sclerosis are hypomelanotic because the melanosomes in the melanocytes synthesize almost no melanin, in contrast to vitiligo, in which the total absence of melanocytes results in the total lack of pigment.

Neurofibromatosis (*Recklinghausen's disease*) is inherited as a dominant trait. It is characterized by the appearance, usually by the age of three years and primarily on the trunk but also on the extremities, of numerous pale yellowish brown macules (Plate 1-4), or café au lait spots, that vary in diameter from less than 1 to more than 15 cm. Spotty generalized pigmentation may also be present, especially in the axillas. Often, but not always, a few or myriads of soft, rounded, cone-shaped or pendulous cutaneous tumors covered by normal skin are seen; these appear in the second or third decade.

The presence of *six or more café au lait spots* with a diameter greater than 1.5 cm is diagnostic of *neurofibromatosis* even when there is no familial history of the condition. In *polyostotic fibrous dysplasia,* however, there are rarely more than *three or four macules,* unilaterally distributed, usually on the buttocks or cervical area. A single, large, isolated café au lait spot of neurofibromatosis resembles the pigmented macule of polyostotic fibrous dysplasia (*Albright's disease*). It is possible, however, to detect large pigmented globules in whole mounts of epidermis prepared from the café au lait macules of neurofibromatosis; these pigmented globules are not found in the macular pigmented areas present in polyostotic fibrous dysplasia or in the café au lait macules that are observed in 10 percent of the normal population.

METABOLIC FACTORS Generalized brown hypermelanosis of the skin is a characteristic manifestation of *hemochromatosis* and *cutaneous porphyria* (*porphyria cutanea tarda*). The hyperpigmentation observed in hemochromatosis may be grayish brown or brown and be indistinguishable from the hypermelanosis of Addison's disease (see Endocrine Factors). The diagnosis of hemochromatosis is established by the presence of hemosiderin in the sweat glands of the skin. Porphyria may be recognized by the abnormally large amounts of *uroporphyrin* in the urine, stools, and plasma, and by other characteristic clinical features, such as the presence of bullae, atrophic scars, and milia on the exposed surfaces of the face and hands.

NUTRITIONAL FACTORS In *chronic nutritional deficiency* in general, splotches of dirty-brown hyperpigmentation appear, especially on the trunk. In selective deficiencies, such as when the *deficiency* is *of protein,* as in *kwashiorkor,* or when there is *protein loss* as in *chronic nephrosis, ulcerative colitis,* and *malabsorption syndrome,* there is sometimes an associated change in hair color (which is the only pigmentation change), first to reddish brown and eventually to gray. In other selective deficiencies, such as *sprue,* the brown hypermelanosis may be distributed over any area of the body, whereas, in *pellagra,* it is limited to areas of skin that are exposed to light or to irritation, as in the perineum. In *deficiency of vitamin* B_{12}, the hair loses its original color and becomes gray, and there is a general distribution of Addisonian diffuse brown hypermelanosis, which is more prominent around the small joints.

ENDOCRINE FACTORS Diffuse brown hypermelanosis is a striking feature of primary adrenocortical insufficiency (Addison's disease). There is marked accentuation of pigmentation in certain areas, namely, on the pressure points (vertebrae, knuckles, elbows, knees), and in the body folds, palmar creases, and gingival mucous membrane. An identical type of diffuse hyperpigmentation has also been reported to follow adrenalectomy in patients with Cushing's disease. In these patients, there usually are signs and symptoms of pituitary tumors; all

TABLE 55-2
Disturbances of human melanin pigmentation

Causative factors	*Classification*		
	*Hypomelanosis**: *White*	*Hypermelanosis**: *Brown*	*Hypermelanosis**: *Gray, slate, or blue*[m]
Genetic factors	Piebaldism[a] Waardenburg's syndrome[a] Canities, premature[a] Vitiligo[a,b] Albinism, oculocutaneous:[c] tyrosinase-positive tyrosinase-negative Albinism, ocular Cross-McKusick-Breen syndrome[c] Hypomelanotic macules in tuberous sclerosis[a,d] Nevus depigmentosus[a,d] Phenylketonuria[e,f] Fanconi's syndrome[e] Neurofibromatosis[a] Ataxia telangiectasia[a]	Café au lait and frecklelike macules in neurofibromatosis[a] Melanotic macules in polyostotic fibrous dysplasia (Albright's syndrome)[a] Ephelides (freckles)[a] Lentigines[a] Lentigines with cardiac arrhythmias[a] Seborrheic keratosis[a] Melanocytic nevus[a] Neurocutaneous melanosis[a] Xeroderma pigmentosum[a] Acanthosis nigricans, juvenile type[a] Peutz-Jeghers syndrome[a]	Oculodermal melanocytosis (nevus of Ota)[a,m] Dermal melanocytosis (Mongolian spot)[a,m] Blue melanocytic nevus[a,m] Incontinentia pigmenti[a,n] Franceschetti-Jadassohn syndrome[a,n]
Metabolic factors		Hemochromatosis[c] Hepatolenticular disease (Wilson's disease)[c] Porphyria (congenital erythropoietic and porphyria variegata and cutanea tarda)[c] Gaucher's disease[j] Niemann-Pick disease[j]	Hemochromatosis[c]
Endocrine factors	Hypopituitarism[c] Addison's disease[a] Hyperthyroidism[a]	ACTH-producing and MSH-producing pituitary and other tumors[c] ACTH therapy[c] Pregnancy[j] Addison's disease[c] Estrogen therapy[k] Melasma[a,l]	
Nutritional factors	Chronic protein deficiency or loss: [e,g] Kwashiorkor Nephrosis Ulcerative colitis Malabsorption syndrome Vitamin B_{12} deficiency[e]	Kwashiorkor[a] Pellagra[j] Sprue[j] Vitamin B_{12} deficiency[j]	Chronic nutritional insufficiency[a]
Chemical and pharmacologic agents	Monobenzyl ether of hydroquinone[a] Chloroquine and hydroxychloroquine[e] Arsenical intoxication[a]	Arsenical intoxication[c] Busulfan administration[c] Photochemical agents (topical or systemic drugs, tar)[a] Berlock dermatosis[a] Dibromomannitol administration[c]	Fixed (drug) eruption[a,m] Quinacrine toxicity[c] Chlorpromazine administration[j,o]

the tumors recorded have been chromophobe adenomas. A third example of the Addisonian type of melanosis has been reported in patients with tumors of organs (pancreas, lung) other than the adrenal or pituitary glands. The generalized brown hypermelanosis found in all these conditions results from overproduction of melanocyte-stimulating hormone (MSH) and ACTH. Both MSH and ACTH share common amino acid sequences. It appears that an excess of alpha-melanocyte-stimulating hormone plays the dominant role in the pigmentation that occurs in adrenocortical insufficiency. Both MSH and ACTH are increased as a result of the decreased output

TABLE 55-2 *(continued)*
Disturbances of human melanin pigmentation

Causative factors	*Classification*		
	*Hypomelanosis**:	*Hypermelanosis**	
	White	*Brown*	*Gray, slate, or blue*[m]
Physical agents	Burns: thermal, ultraviolet, and ionizing radiation[a,h] Traumatic injury[a,h]	Ultraviolet light (suntanning)[a] Thermal radiation Alpha, beta, and gamma ionizing radiation[a] Chronic rubbing and scratching[a]	
Inflammation and infection	Pinta[a,h] Leprosy[a,d] Fungal infections (tinea versicolor)[a,d] Pityriasis alba[a,d] Eczematous dermatitis[a,d] Psoriasis[a] Lupus erythematosus, discoid[a] Postinflammation hypomelanosis[a,d]	Postinflammation melanosis (exanthems, drug eruptions)[a] Lichen planus[a] Lupus erythematosus, discoid[a] Lichen simplex chronicus[a] Atopic dermatitis[j] Psoriasis[a]	Pinta in exposed areas[a] Erythema dyschromicum perstans[a,n]
Neoplasms	In sites of malignant melanoma after disappearance (therapeutic or spontaneous) of tumor[a] Nevus, "halo"[a]	Malignant melanoma[a] Mastocytosis (urticaria pigmentosa)[a] Adenocarcinoma with acanthosis nigricans[a]	Slate-gray dermal pigmentation with metastatic melanoma and melanogenuria[c]
Miscellaneous factors	Alezzandrini's syndrome[a] Vogt-Koyanagi-Harada syndrome[a] Scleroderma, circumscribed or systemic[a] Canities[e] Alopecia areata[i] Horner's syndrome, congenital and acquired[f] Hypomelanosis, guttate, idiopathic[a]	Scleroderma, systemic[c] Chronic hepatic insufficiency[c] Whipple's syndrome[c] Encephalitis, chronic[a] Lentigo, senile ("liver spots")[a] Catatonic schizophrenia[c]	

* *The listing includes the pigmentation disorder itself or the condition with which it is associated.*
[a] *Pigment change is circumscribed.*
[b] *Total loss of pigment in the skin and hair may occur.*
[c] *Pigment change is diffuse, not circumscribed, and there are no identifiable borders.*
[d] *Loss of pigmentation is usually partial (hypomelanosis); viewed with Wood's lamp, the lesions are not completely devoid of pigment (amelanosis), as in vitiligo.*
[e] *Pigment is decreased in the hair.*
[f] *Pigment is decreased in the iris.*
[g] *Hair is gray or reddish.*
[h] *There is a loss of melanocytes.*
[i] *Regrown hair is white.*
[j] *Pigment change may be diffuse or circumscribed.*
[k] *Nipples are affected.*
[l] *Idiopathic or due to progestational agents.*
[m] *Gray, slate, or blue color results from the presence of* dermal *melanocytes or phagocytized melanin in the dermis.*
[n] *Areas of brown may be admixed with the slate-gray and blue discoloration.*
[o] *Pigment has not been definitely identified as melanin.*
SOURCE: *TB Fitzpatrick, MC Mihm Jr: Abnormalities of the melanin pigmentary system, in* Dermatology in General Medicine, *eds TB Fitzpatrick et al, New York: McGraw-Hill, 1971*

TABLE 55-3
Circumscribed vitiligo-type hypomelanosis of skin

Associated with genetic disorders *Present at birth*	*Delayed onset*
Piebaldism	Vitiligo
Waardenburg's syndrome	
Nevus depigmentosus	
Tuberous sclerosis	
Neurofibromatosis	
Ataxia telangiectasia	
Associated with chemicals (occupational or therapeutic)	
Phenolic germicides ("O-Syl, "Phenocide," etc.)	
Hydroquinone	
Hydroquinone, monobenzyl ether of	
Hydroquinone, monomethyl ether of	
Associated with metabolic or endocrine disorders	
Addison's disease	
Hyperthyroidism	
Pernicious anemia	
Hypoparathyroidism-Addison's disease-candidiasis syndrome	
Associated with neoplasms	
Malignant melanoma (in sites of regression)	
Melanocytic nevi ("halo nevi")	
Associated with infections	
Leprosy	
Pinta	
Tinea versicolor	
Associated with idiopathic conditions	
Vogt-Koyangi-Harada syndrome	
Postinflammation: atopic dermatitis, pityriasis alba, psoriasis	
Morphea (not in the lesion)	

of cortisol by the adrenals. Hypermelanosis of the Addisonian type can be produced in adrenalectomized human subjects by the administration of large amounts of homogeneous ACTH and alpha-MSH.

CHEMICAL FACTORS Chemicals can induce both hypomelanosis and hypermelanosis. Hydroquinone prevents the formation of melanin and is of therapeutic value in treating hypermelanosis. Striking generalized Addisonian hypermelanosis of the skin follows busulfan therapy; the mechanism of action of this drug is not known. Inorganic trivalent arsenicals produce both generalized Addisonian hypermelanosis and scattered macular hypomelanosis, as well as punctate keratoses on the palms and soles. Some phenolic germicides have been shown to cause a vitiligo-like hypomelanosis that may or may not be reversible.

PHYSICAL FACTORS Mechanical trauma, as well as burns caused by heat, ultraviolet light, or alpha, beta, and gamma radiation, can lead to hypomelanosis or hypermelanosis. The effect of these physical agents on pigmentation is determined by the intensity and duration of exposure and is limited to the site of injury. The hypomelanosis results from destruction of melanocytes.

Chronic pruritus (because the skin is constantly scratched and rubbed) such as that associated with chronic biliary tract disease and lymphoma, may lead to generalized brown hypermelanosis.

INFLAMMATORY AND INFECTIOUS FACTORS
Circumscribed hypomelanosis is a characteristic feature of *tuberculoid leprosy.* It occurs in areas of anesthesia, and the degree of pigment loss is only partial; the lesions are lighter in color than the areas of surrounding skin but are not snow-white as in vitiligo. Generalized spotty hyperpigmentation not uncommonly follows *exanthems* and *eruptions due to drugs;* it usually disappears spontaneously within 2 or 3 months.

NEOPLASTIC FACTORS Hypomelanosis is seen in rare instances at the site of a primary or a metastatic *malignant melanoma* that has undergone remission spontaneously or as the result of chemotherapy. During the terminal stages of malignant melanoma, striking generalized blue hypermelanosis of the skin sometimes develops, and large amounts of a conjugated derivative of 5,6-dihydroxyindole are excreted in the urine ("melanogenuria"). This intermediate in the metabolic pathway from tyrosine to melanin can be oxidized to melanin in the absence of tyrosinase, and therefore melanin can be synthesized at almost any site in which oxidation can take place. Consequently, diffuse black pigmentation may develop in the peritoneum, liver, heart, muscle, and dermis of patients during the late stages of malignant melanoma. The brown melanin in the dermal phagocytes appears clinically as blue in the skin because of the Tyndall light-scattering phenomenon.

The multiple, irregular, round or oval, yellowish brown to reddish brown macules and papules characteristic of *urticaria pigmentosa* are related to the presence of melanin in the epidermis that overlies the clusters of mast cells. Urticarial wheals develop when the lesions are stroked vigorously. In rare instances (*systemic mastocytosis*), mast cells infiltrate diffusely into the liver, spleen, gastrointestinal system, and bones, as well as into the skin.

UNKNOWN FACTORS Generalized brown hypermelanosis of the type seen in Addison's disease is not infrequently associated with *systemic scleroderma* and may appear very early in the course of the disorder. Generalized hyperpigmentation occasionally develops in patients with *chronic hepatic insufficiency,* especially that due to portal cirrhosis. The pathogenesis of the pigmentation in both these conditions is unknown.

Melasma (chloasma) (Plate 2-4) occurs in pregnant women and sometimes in women taking oral progestational agents, but it also occurs in nonpregnant women and in men. The lesions consist of large macules with irregular borders on the exposed areas of the face and vary in color from yellow-brown to red-brown and very dark brown.

REFERENCES

Fitzpatrick TB, Quevedo WC Jr: Biologic processes underlying melanin pigmentation and pigmentary disorders, in *Modern Trends in Dermatology,* ed P Borrie, series 4, London: Butterworth, 1971

——: Albinism, in *The Metabolic Basis of Inherited Disease,* ed JB Stanbury et al, New York: McGraw-Hill, 1972

Kawamura T et al (eds): *Biology of Normal and Abnormal Melanocytes,* Tokyo: Tokyo University Press, 1971

Toda K et al: Alteration of racial differences in melanosome distribution in human epidermis after exposure to ultraviolet light. Nature [New Biol] 236:143, 1972

56 PHOTOSENSITIVITY AND OTHER REACTIONS TO LIGHT

T. B. FITZPATRICK
H. A. HAYNES

INTRODUCTION

During the last decade, interest in the reaction of human skin to light has been renewed as a result of (1) the widespread use of certain drugs that produce photosensitivity, such as phenothiazines (tranquilizers) and tetracycline and demethychlortetracycline, which alter the cutaneous responses to sunlight, and a steadily growing awareness among investigators and clinicians that many compounds (e.g., sulfonamides and oral hypoglycemic agents) synthesized for various therapeutic purposes can cause cutaneous photosensitivity as a side effect; (2) the incorporation of certain topical antimicrobial agents (e.g., halogenated salicylanilides) into soaps that produce photosensitivity; (3) the increased recognition of, and better diagnostic and therapeutic approaches to, various skin eruptions (papules, plaques, and eczematous and urticarial reactions) of unknown cause and differing morphologic features (i.e., polymorphic photodermatitis) that follow exposure to ultraviolet and visible light; (4) the general public's obsession with sunbathing, resulting in premature aging of the skin (solar elastosis); (5) the establishment of new demographic data indicating that exposure to sunlight is an important cause of basal-cell and of

TABLE 56-1
Classification of solar radiation

Type of radiation	*Wavelength range*
Middle ultraviolet (sunburn)	290–320 nm
Near ultraviolet (long wave)	320–380 nm
Visible	380–720 nm
Near infrared	720 nm–1.5 μ
Middle infrared	1.5–5.6 μ
Far infrared	5.6–1000 μ

TABLE 56-2
Units of wavelength (equated with 1 cm)

Unit	*Abbreviation*	*Centimeter equivalent*
Nanometer	nm	10^{-7}
Angstrom	A	10^{-8}
Millimicron	mμ	10^{-7}
Millimeter	mm	10^{-1}

squamous-cell carcinoma of the sun-exposed parts of the body; and (6) increased recognition of the fact that sunlight is a major cause of discomfort and photosensitivity reactions in patients with certain types of porphyria, especially erythropoietic protoporphyria.

There are more than 25 human disorders that are either caused by or aggravated by exposure of the skin to sunlight. These range from degenerative and neoplastic changes to disability and discomfort associated with chemically induced photosensitivity reactions.

This discussion will be concerned with: the degenerative and neoplastic conditions associated with solar radiation, such as basal-cell carcinoma, squamous-cell carcinoma, malignant melanoma, solar keratoses (Plate 4-2), and chronic sun-induced degeneration; photosensitivity related to drugs; and photosensitivity related to increased plasma levels of photosensitizing porphyrins in patients with all types of porphyria except acute intermittent porphyria.

To understand the photobiology of man's responses to light, it is essential to know about the solar radiation (Table 56-1) that passes through the atmosphere to the Earth's surface.

Electromagnetic emanations from the sun comprise a wide range of radiation and include electric waves, radio waves, infrared rays, visible light, ultraviolet light, roentgen rays, gamma rays, and secondary cosmic rays. The units of wavelengths in common use are: (1) the nanometer (nm); (2) the angstrom (A); (3) the millimicron (mμ); and (4) the micron (μ) or micrometer (μm). These units are related as shown in Table 56-2. The shortest wavelengths that reach the surface of the Earth through the atmosphere are about 286 to 290 nm. Wavelengths shorter than 290 nm are principally absorbed by ozone in the stratosphere.

The amount and type of solar radiation that reach a given part of the Earth at any given time are determined by a great variety of factors, such as latitude, time of day, season, altitude, local atmospheric conditions (smog, cloudiness, haze, smoke, dust, fog, humidity, aerosol particles), variations in the thickness of the ozone layer, and height of the sun above the horizon.

Approximately 50 percent of the radiant energy emitted by the sun is present in the visible portion of the spectrum (380 to 720 nm), about 40 percent in the infrared region, and about 10 percent in the ultraviolet region. The damage to skin (sunburn, skin cancer) is evoked by 3 percent of the ultraviolet radiation of wavelengths of from 290 to 320 nm.

Protection against this damage to the "normal" skin has long been the subject of much investigation, and there are many commercially available sunscreens that are satisfactory under certain conditions (Table 56-3). For maximum protection, patients should apply, 45 min *before exposure, 5% para*-aminobenzoic acid (PABA) in 50 to 70% ethanol (Table 56-3); PABA-esters in ethanol are less effective. The solution should be re-applied after swimming or after profuse sweating.

SUNBURN AND TANNING

Clinical changes

ERYTHEMA, OR SUNBURN REACTION Erythema is caused principally by radiation of from 290 to 320 nm, with maximum effectiveness at 300 to 307 nm. Light of wavelengths greater than 320 nm (320 to 700 nm) is generally considered to be nonerythemogenic, although prolonged exposure to radiation of 320 to 400 nm (2 hr of midday summer sun in northern latitudes) can produce mild sunburn in normal subjects. Wavelengths of 307 nm are thought to accelerate aging (wrinkling) in the skin and to lead to the development of solar keratoses, carcinoma, and, possibly, some types of malignant melanoma. Wavelengths of the long-wave ultraviolet and visible spectrums are innocuous unless the skin contains either topically applied or ingested photosensitizing agents.

The sunburn reaction is a complex process in which a number of changes occur simultaneously. At present, the nature of the chromophore that absorbs the light energy that initiates the primary photochemical responses is not well established, although the bulk of evidence suggests that nucleic acids (in DNA) are the primary sites for the absorption of radiation of from 290 to 320 nm. Vasodilatation accompanying the sunburn reaction appears to result from the activation and release of one or several chemical mediators (e.g., kinin, serotonin, and also histamine). Ultraviolet radiation appears to have a direct effect on the blood vessels of the upper layer of the dermis (capillaries, venules, and arterioles). The formation of peroxides or peroxy radicals may play an important role in the damage to lysosomal membranes associated with lipid peroxidation.

MELANIN PIGMENTATION, OR TANNING The familiar tanning (increase in melanin pigment) that follows exposure of the skin to solar radiation is known to involve two distinct photobiologic processes. The first, *immediate pigment darkening* (IPD), or darkening of preformed pigment in the epidermis, is elicited by wavelengths of 320 to 700 nm. The second, or *melanogenesis,* is an intricate process that consists of the *erythema response* (*sunburn*) followed in a few days (4 days usually) by formation of new pigment. Immediate pigment darkening probably represents oxidation of melanin through the production of semiquinone-like free radicals in the melanin polymer; redistribution of already existing melanosomes within the keratinocytes also may occur.

Melanogenesis involves: (1) increase in the number of functional melanocytes, resulting from increased proliferation of melanocytes, and activation of dormant melanocytes; (2) increased arborization of melanocytic dendrites; (3) increase in the number of melanosomes in melanocytes; (4) increase in tyrosinase activity; and (5) increase in the transfer of melanosomes.

TABLE 56-3
Topical formulations for protection against ultraviolet and visible light

Wavelength	*Formulation*	*Commercial product*
Short UV: 250–260 nm (germicidal spectrum)	10% 2-hydroxy-4-methoxybenzophenone-5-sulfonic acid	Uval
Middle UV: 290–320 nm (sunburn spectrum)	5% *para*-aminobenzoic acid in 50–70% ethyl alcohol	Pabanol; PreSun
	2.5% ester of *para*-aminobenzoic acid (isoamyl-*p-N,N*-dimethylaminobenzoate)	Block Out; Pabafilm; Spectraban
	10% 2-hydroxy-4-methoxy-benzophenone-5-sulfonic acid	Uval
	3% oxybenzone plus 3% dioxybenzone	Solbar
Long UV: 320–380 nm	10% 2-hydroxy-4-methoxy-benzophenone-5-sulfonic acid	Uval
Visible radiation: 380–700 nm	5–10% opaque and reflecting pigments like zinc oxide, titanium dioxide, calamine	Afil; Rvpaque; Reflecta; Covermark
	3% dihydroxyacetone plus 0.25% 2-hydroxy-1,4-naphthoquinone in isopropanol-water mixture or in cream base	None

Cellular and molecular changes

HYPERPLASIA Within 72 hr after exposure, an increase in the number of epidermal cells is visible in the light microscope and is characterized by a high rate of cell proliferation accompanied by a high rate of mitotic activity. The rate of proliferation of cells decreases after 7 to 10 days, and the thickness of the epidermis gradually returns to normal within the next 30 to 60 days.

DNA AND RNA CHANGES Damage to DNA by sunburn-producing ultraviolet light (230–320 nm) results in cell death. The principal photoproducts formed in the DNA of epidermal cells are pyrimidine dimers, which are of the C_4-cyclobutane type and are formed between adjacent pyrimidine bases. RNA synthesis in the epidermis is inhibited within 1 hr after irradiation. By 24 hr, new synthesis is evident and, by 60 to 70 hr, is maximum.

MITOSIS Inhibition of epidermal mitosis and retardation of basal-cell turnover occurs within 1 hr after irradiation. Inhibition of mitosis can persist for 7 to 24 hr; it is followed by an acceleration of mitotic rate and basal-cell turnover that reaches a peak by 48 to 72 hr and is associated with epidermal hyperplasia. The mitotic cycle appears to be interrupted in the G_2 or in the prophase stage, or in both.

SUN-INDUCED CARCINOMA

The reported epidemiologic evidence clearly implicates solar radiation as a factor in the induction of human skin cancer.

Some studies have established that carcinoma of the skin occurs more frequently on the parts of the body habitually exposed to sunlight; the lesions of the head and hands are concentrated on the nose, central portions of the cheeks, eyelids, and dorsa of the hands. In fair-skinned Caucasoids who easily sunburn, these cancers are limited almost exclusively to the exposed portions of the face, head, neck, arms, and hands. Negroid skin, on the other hand, is remarkably resistant to the development of skin cancer on the exposed surfaces, and a similar resistance is seen among the pigmented Caucasoids (e.g., East Indians), American Indians, and Asiatics. Approximately 80 to 90 percent of basal-cell carcinomas occur on the head and neck, approximately 4 to 8 percent on the trunk, and about 10 to 12 percent on the extremities.

Carcinoma of the exposed skin is more prevalent among persons who are outdoors a great deal (e.g., golfers, farmers, sailors), and is the common cause of cancer in Caucasoids in Australia, South Africa, and the southern parts of the United States.

The reported evidence for a causal relation between sunburn-evoking ultraviolet radiation and the prevalence of human squamous-cell carcinoma and basal-cell carcinoma is overwhelming. The wavelength limit for carcinogenesis by ultraviolet light has been established at about 290 to 320 nm, which is the same as that for sunburn.

It should be emphasized that, of all the radiation emitted by the sun, ranging from x-rays at the short-wave end of the spectrum to radio waves at the long-wave end, only a portion penetrates the Earth's atmosphere; the shortest wavelength of solar radiation recorded at sea level is about 290 nm. This sharp cutoff between the sea level and extraterrestrial distribution in the ultraviolet spectrum is largely, if not exclusively, due to the absorption of harmful radiation by ozone.

Several studies based on the distribution of local populations in the United States, Australia, and Ireland have emphasized that skin cancer develops earlier and more frequently in people who have light skin and freckles, who burn easily and do not tan on exposure to the sun, and who are of mostly Celtic ancestry. Australia, with the highest reported incidence of skin cancer in the world, has a population largely descended from British stock, with about 25 percent claiming Celtic (i.e., Irish, Scottish, and Welsh) extraction. In all three countries surveyed, the persons of Celtic ancestry were found to have a disproportionately high incidence of skin cancer.

All varieties of skin cancer develop in patients with xeroderma pigmentosum, an autosomal recessive trait. This rare defect is representative, in the extreme, of the basic problem of solar radiation and skin cancer. Patients with this disease have a greatly increased susceptibility to malignant tumors of the skin in the light-exposed areas. The characteristic skin manifestations are atrophy, telangiectasia, hyperpigmented macules, keratoses, and ulcerations, all occurring in sun-exposed areas. Within the first few years of life, basal-cell or squamous-cell carcinomas or sarcomas or malignant melanomas develop. An inherited enzyme defect may be responsible, at least in part, for the cancer-forming potential in patients with xeroderma pigmentosum. Cultured fibroblasts from patients with xeroderma pigmentosum are incapable of releasing thymine dimers from DNA and, in consequence, are deficient in their ability to repair their ultraviolet-damaged DNA. It is possible that this enzymatic deficiency results in a high somatic mutation rate of skin cells after sun-exposure and, eventually, in cancer formation.

DEGENERATIVE CHANGES OF THE SKIN

Degenerative changes of the skin (wrinkling, telangiectasia, keratoses) are significantly more frequent in white-skinned people living in areas where the intensity of ultraviolet radiation is great (e.g., southwestern U.S.A., Australia, South Africa). The term "solar degeneration" implies a group of changes in the exposed areas of the skin, including wrinkling, atrophy, hypermelanotic and hypomelanotic macules, telangiectasia, yellow papules and plaques, and keratoses. The furrowed and leathery condition of the skin is seen particularly in persons who have fair skin and poor tanning ability and are constantly exposed to the sun. The most conspicuous and characteristic structural change involves biochemical alterations of connective tissues (elastin, as well as collagen). The sunburn-producing radiation (290–320 nm) and, possibly also, long-wave ultraviolet radiation (320–400 nm) that can penetrate deeply in the dermis are involved in evoking the degenerative changes.

Chronically light-damaged human epidermis shows

shortening or flattening of the rete ridges, thinning of the epidermis (decrease in Malpighian cells), and many abnormal cells in disorderly arrangement. There is a progressive degeneration in the papillary and subpapillary zones of the dermis. Other changes include: (1) the development of vascular ectasia; (2) accumulation of acid mucopolysaccharides; (3) appearance of abnormal fibrocytes; (4) loss of collagen; (5) degeneration of elastic tissue (referred to as "actinic elastosis"), and disorganization of the connective tissue into amorphous masses.

PHOTOTOXICITY AND PHOTOALLERGY

Sensitivity to sunlight is now regarded as a very common clinical problem. Continuous daily exposure to sun alone may be a major factor responsible for irreversible changes in the human skin, e.g., freckles, telangiectasia, wrinkling, keratosis, atrophy, hypermelanotic and hypomelanotic macules, and carcinomas in the sun-exposed regions.

Apart from these chronic changes, human skin can also become hypersensitive to ultraviolet and visible light. The interface between Man and his environment is the skin, and the physical (light) and chemical agents acting directly on it are paramount etiologic or precipitating factors in photosensitivity disorders. Aggravating this situation is the fact that the general public is subjected to an ever-increasing quantity of newer chemicals and is also obsessed with sunbathing.

TO DRUGS AND OTHER CHEMICALS PLUS LIGHT

There is now a growing awareness of the relation between certain chemical agents and light in the causation of certain types of dermatitis. These agents include chemicals and drugs that may not act as contact irritants and are generally innocuous to skin in the absence of exposure to light; when the skin is challenged with proper concentrations of the agent and the appropriate wavelengths of light, however, these agents can induce undesirable reactions in the skin.

Many substances occur in nature that have photosensitizing potential and have for a long time been recognized as potentially "toxic." Large numbers of other substances have been synthesized within the past two decades and are used for clinical and commercial purposes without understanding of their incidental "side-effects" that are usually manifested in skin when it is inadvertently exposed to light. The widespread use of certain chemical agents (e.g., tranquilizers and antibiotics) and the development of antimicrobial agents (e.g., halogenated salicylanilides) that are incorporated into soaps and other topical agents have caused many persons to have adverse reactions to light. Several thousand cases of disabling photosensitivity reactions are recognized each year in the United States and elsewhere in industrial workers, agricultural workers, pharmaceutical and cosmetic manufacturing plants, and users of cosmetic preparations, who, in many instances, cannot avoid contact with the causative agent and exposure to either natural or artificial light.

Cutaneous photosensitivity is a general term used in referring to the abnormal reaction of the human skin to the stimulus of light. Drug photosensitivity reactions may be defined clinically as adverse responses manifested by the skin as a result of combined exposure to certain therapeutic or chemical agents and sunlight. The adverse cutaneous reactions can occur in some individuals who have either ingested certain drugs or have been in contact with certain chemicals (Table 56-4). These reactions may include an abnormal sunburn response: edema, papules, macules, vesicles, bullae, or acute eczematous or urticarial reactions. There may be desquamation and hyperpigmentation or hypopigmentation. These adverse photosensitivity reactions are classified into two broad categories: (1) phototoxic reactions, which are common, and (2) photoallergic reactions, which are uncommon.

Phototoxic reactions are those that can be elicited in almost everyone challenged if enough light energy of the appropriate wave-lengths and appropriate concentration of the agent are either applied topically or given orally. The reaction produced by light and the offending agent is characterized clinically by an exaggerated sunburn reaction with or without painful edema. The reaction occurs within a few hours (5–18 hr) after exposure to the sun.

Hyperpigmentation and desquamation also occur. The reaction is usually confined to the site of exposure. If the applied concentration of the implicated agent is high, there may be bullae or small vesicles.

The phototoxic reactions in general should be regarded as the result of abnormal augmentation, due to an association with drugs and other chemicals, of the sunburn response of the skin. It is believed that a deleterious amount of radiant energy is absorbed by the skin and the photosensitizing agents. The photosensitizers are either in the extracellular fluid of the skin after oral ingestion or in the epidermal cells as a result of passive penetration after topical application. The photosensitizing agent absorbs additional quanta of light not only from the sunburn spectrum (290–320 nm) but also from the long-wave ultraviolet spectrum (320–400 nm) as a result of the formation of a complex between the cellular components (e.g., DNA, RNA, proteins, and lipids) and the sensitizing agent, and thus increases the total amount of absorbed energy. This absorbed energy can directly cause cell damage by creating a covalent linking of the sensitizing molecule to the pyrimidines (e.g., thymine) in the cellular DNA. This linkage, recognized as the formation of cyclobutane photoadducts of the sensitizer and the pyrimidines, can be lethal to the cell. It has been established that potent photosensitizers like 8-methoxypsoralen and 4,5′,8-trimethylpsoralen selectively undergo a photoaddition reaction with epidermal DNA. In addition, the photosensitizing molecule can transfer the absorbed energy and promote formation of free radicals (molecules with unpaired electrons that are highly reactive) and cause damage to the cell membranes and lysosomes. Drug-induced cutaneous phototoxic reactions may, therefore, reasonably be regarded as the undesirable sequelae of augmentation of the primary photochemical reactions that underlie the sunburn response of skin.

Photoallergy to drugs can be considered to represent an acquired and altered capacity of the skin to respond to light energy in the presence of a photosensitizer, and, presumably, is dependent on an antigen-antibody reaction or a delayed hypersensitivity response mediated by mononuclear cells. The absorbed energy of light seems to promote a photochemical reaction between the drug and the proteins of the skin; the drug acting as a haptenic group either combines directly with the protein to form a photoantigen or is altered by the absorbed energy, and this altered haptenic group then reacts with the proteins to form an antigen.

The clinical manifestations in drug-induced photoallergic reactions may range from eczematous or papular lesions, appearing 24 hr or more after an exposure, to acute urticarial lesions developing within a few minutes after exposure. The eruption frequently extends beyond the areas that were exposed. In recurrent cases, flare-ups of distant previously uninvolved sites frequently may also occur. The action spectrum (wavelengths that induce cutaneous reactions) is generally in the long-wave range (320–400 nm), and less energy is required than is necessary for the production of phototoxic reactions. Histologically, the epidermal changes also are characteristic, although not diagnostic of these various responses. A dense perivascular round-cell infiltrate in the dermis is often seen in both the eczematous and papular responses. Spongiosis and vesiculation are prominent in the eczematous lesions, whereas the urticarial or papular lesions show no remarkable epidermal changes. Some edema and vasodilatation are common in most of these eruptions.

The various clinically important therapeutic agents given systemically and their effects on the skin in the presence of light (whether phototoxic or photoallergic reactions) are listed in Table 56-4. The biologic action spectrums are also given, indicating the range of wavelengths that effectively induces either the phototoxic or photoallergic reactions.

TO PLANTS PLUS LIGHT Phytophotodermatitis (phototoxic reactions) can develop as the result of contact with many plants (belonging principally to the families Rutaceae and Umbelliferae) and subsequent exposure of the skin to sunlight. The photodermatitis involves a mild-to-severe erythematous reaction with or without vesicles or bullae. Dense postinflammatory hyperpigmentation is visible within 3 to 5 days. Phytophotodermatitis has also been seen in individuals in contact with carrots, celery, and the oil of Persian limes. Perfumes and colognes containing particular oils are also known to induce hyperpigmentation with or without erythema. The pigmentation in berlock dermatitis occurs in configurations that seem bizarre but actually represent the areas to

TABLE 56-4
Systemic chemicals that induce photosensitivity reactions in humans

Chemical	*Use*	*Clinical findings*	*Action spectrum, nm*
Chlortetracycline; demethylchlortetracycline (Declomycin); oxytetracycline; doxycycline	Antibiotic	Exaggerated sunburn; phototoxicity	290–400
Sulfanilamide; sulfathiazole; sulfapyridine; sulfamethazine; sulfaguanidine; sulfisoxazole; monochlorphenamide	Chemotherapeutic; antibacterial	Phototoxicity; photoallergy	290–320
Carbutamide; tolbutamide (Orinase); chlorpropamide (Diabinase)	Hypoglycemic	Phototoxicity	290–320
Chlorothiazide (Diuril); quinethazone (Hydromox)	Diuretic; antihypertensive	Papules, edema; plaques	290–320
Griseofulvin	Antimycotic	Exaggerated sunburn; phototoxicity; photoallergy	290–400
Nalidixic Acid	Antibacterial	Erythema; bullae	290–400
Chlorpromazine (Thorazine); promethazine (Phenergan); mepazine (Stelazine); trimeprazine (Compazine); promazine (Sparine)	Tranquilizer; antihistamine	Exaggerated sunburn; macules, papules, urticaria; gray-blue hyperpigmentation	320–400
Psoralen; 4,5′, 8-trimethylpsoralen (Trisoralen); 8-methoxypsoralen (Oxsoralen)	Stimulator of melanin synthesis	Erythema; bullae; hyperpigmentation	320–400
Mestranol and norethynodrel; diethylstilbestrol	Oral contraceptive	Melasma; phototoxicity	?
Chlordiazepoxide (Librium)	Tranquilizer	Eczematous dermatitis	290–320
Triacetyldiphenolisatin	Laxative	Eczematous dermatitis	290–320
Calcium cyclamate; sodium cyclohexylsulfamate	Sweetener	Phototoxicity; photoallergy	290–360

which the scent was applied; sometimes the hyperpigmentation may be drop-like or pendant-like, and was therefore named accordingly (*bréloque* or *berlocke*, meaning trinket or pendant). This phytophotodermatitis, as well as that which follows contact with various other plants, is thought to be caused by furocoumarins, particularly 5-methoxypsoralen, 8-methoxypsoralen, and other psoralens that are characteristically present in these plants. The combination of exposure to long-wave ultraviolet radiation (320–400 nm) and furocoumarins greatly enhances the erythema and the pigmentation response.

TO LIGHT ALONE In this category are included several photosensitivity reactions in patients with various types of porphyria. The photosensitivity reactions are related to the overproduction in vivo of proto-, uro- and coproporphyrins and their precursors. In the porphyrias, endogenously synthesized photosensitizing molecules, when exposed to light, cause burning, itching, urticaria, edema, crusting and scarring, vesiculation, atrophy, and many other disabling cutaneous changes. The light-absorbing molecules that are implicated in evoking the cutaneous reactions are undoubtedly the irreversibly oxidized porphyrins that are present in abnormal amounts in red blood cells, plasma, skin, liver, stool, and urine. The photodermatitis is produced by a narrow band of light in the region of 400 to 410 nm, which corresponds to one of the absorption peaks of porphyrins. The most disabling type of photosensitivity reactions are encountered in erythropoietic (congenital) porphyria (Günther's disease) and in erythropoietic protoporphyria (Chap. 102). Symptoms and signs of sensitivity to sunlight occur in early childhood.

The adverse cutaneous responses to sunlight in patients with erythropoietic protoporphyria (EPP) have been found to be ameliorated by oral ingestion of beta-carotene (Chap. 102). Patients who take beta-carotene are able to withstand prolonged exposures to sunlight and experience relief from their usual photosensitivity reactions. In laboratory experiments, beta-carotene was found to be an effective quencher for the "singlet" oxygen generated in certain photosensitivity reactions, and therefore presumably acts in the same manner in vivo. During porphyrin-mediated photosensitivity reactions, peroxides are generated; the peroxy radicals apparently are very damaging to the lipid membranes. It is presumed that beta-carotene is preferentially oxidized and, by quenching the "singlet oxygen," inhibits the lipid peroxide formation.

REFERENCES

Mathews-Roth MM et al: Beta-carotene as a photoprotective agent in erythropoietic protoporphyria. New Engl J Med 282:1231, 1970; Trans Assoc Am Physicians 83:176, 1970

Pathak MA, Epstein JH: Normal and abnormal reactions of man to light, in *Dermatology in General Medicine,* eds TB Fitzpatrick et al, New York: McGraw-Hill, 1971

____ et al: Evaluation of topical agents that prevent sunburn. New Engl J Med 280:1459, 1969

Urbach F (ed): *The Biologic Effects of Ultraviolet Radiation,* Oxford: Pergamon, 1969

57 HIRSUTISM AND ALOPECIA

T. B. FITZPATRICK
H. A. HAYNES

HIRSUTISM Forbes described hirsutism as "more hair than is cosmetically acceptable to a woman living in a certain culture." In other words, whether or not an increased amount of hair is abnormal or normal depends on the ethnic origin of the individual. To determine whether a given degree of hypertrichosis represents hirsutism or a normal quantity of hair for the ethnic group is the major problem for the physician. When hypertrichosis is inherited, it appears at puberty and increases until the early twenties. Forbes suggests that if the menses are regular and the physical examination, including examination of the pelvic organs, does not reveal evidence of a virilizing disorder, then a single assay of urinary 17-ketosteroids and 17-hydroxysteroids should be sufficient to establish whether or not there is a hormonal disorder.

Hirsutism without any evidence of virilism may appear in acromegaly or in disorders with an excess of glucocorticoid hormone, such as Cushing's syndrome. Also, malignant adrenal tumors may cause atypical syndromes, i.e., a combination of Cushing's syndrome and virilism. Hirsutism without virilism can occur in the absence of virilism in porphyria cutanea tarda, in patients receiving androgens or glucocorticoids or diphenylhydantoin sodium (Dilantin).

Hirsutism with virilism may be detected by an assay for testosterone. This assay is particularly indicated in patients with hirsutism and virilism who have urinary 17-ketosteroids that are within the normal range, inasmuch as small amounts of testosterone are capable of causing virilization. Signs of virilism include a low-pitched voice, acne, increased muscularity, and clitoral hypertrophy. Development of male-type recession of the hair line or of general alopecia is a manifestation of virilism and is not a feature of constitutional hirsutism. Hirsutism with virilism may occur as a result of three sources of endogenous androgen: (1) aberrant *testicular* tissue; (2) *ovarian* tumors, such as arrhenoblastoma and hilus-cell tumors; and (3) *adrenal* tumors, especially malignant tumors of the adrenal cortex, as well as congenital adrenal hyperplasia (adrenogenital syndrome).

Constitutional hirsutism with endocrine dysfunction is the commonest type of hirsutism and is often associated with irregular menses and obesity. The hair appears at puberty and increases until the early twenties, making the distinction from ethnic hirsutism difficult. This syndrome of constitutional hirsutism with endocrine dysfunction may or may not be associated with large polycystic ovaries. Virilism is rarely present, and, if present, is very

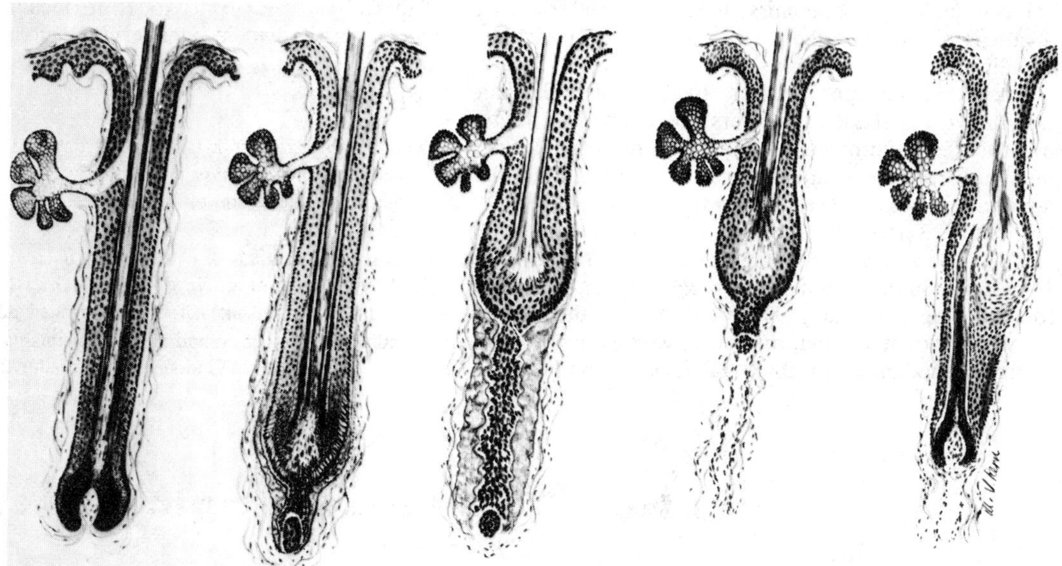

FIGURE 57-1
Stages in hair cycle. Progressive changes from a growing (anagen) hair to a resting club hair (telogen)—second from right. In the normal human scalp, some 10 percent of the hairs are in the resting phase. In various types of alopecia, this percentage rises sharply and may be easily determined by the number of hairs which are easily removed by gentle traction. (DM Pillsbury and WB Shelley)

slight and is represented only by increased serum secretion or acne with no clitoral hypertrophy or male-pattern baldness. The actual etiology of the endocrine dysfunction in constitutional hirsutism is not known at this time.

TABLE 57-1
Alopecia, primarily involving the scalp, without skin changes

Conditions associated with circumscribed alopecia (including male-pattern baldness)	*Conditions associated with diffuse alopecia*	*Cause*
	Hypopituitarism† Hypothyroidism† Hyperthyroidism Hypoparathyroidism Pregnancy Postpartum effects	Endocrine factors
Syphilis, secondary*	Postpyrexia Leprosy†	Infection
Trichotillomania		Psychogenic factors
	Thallium reactions† Anticoagulant administration, prolonged Hypervitaminosis A Methotrexate reaction	Drugs
	Iron deficiency (with and without anemia) Homocystinuria Orotic aciduria, hereditary	Nutritional and metabolic factors
	Lupus erythematosus, systemic Alopecia areata	Idiopathic factors

* *Patchy.*
† *May be limited to lateral one-third of eyebrow.*

There have been reports of increased urinary pregnanetriolone in constitutional hirsutism. Suppression of adrenal function by exogenously administered corticosteroids has possibly brought about some improvement in the menstrual irregularities and in the infertility. That the ovaries may be the source of excess androgen production in constitutional hirsutism is suggested by the effects of ovarian wedge resection, which can be beneficial for the sterility that occurs in such hirsute women. Elevated plasma and urinary testosterone levels have been found in some patients with constitutional hirsutism, but, for the most part, these levels appear to be normal in the majority of patients. There have been some reports of qualitative differences of gonadotropin excretion in constitutional hirsutism, including a relative increase in the luteinizing hormone. The use of estrogens to suppress the production of pituitary gonadotropin is a safe, rational, and effective procedure for the treatment of hirsutism.

The cosmetic approach to the treatment of most types of hypertrichosis is quite unsatisfactory except for the permanent removal of the hair follicles by a competent person using electrolysis.

ALOPECIA Hairs plucked from the scalp can be classified into anagen or telogen by the appearance of the hair bulbs (Fig. 57-1). The anagen, or growing, hair roots usually have a sheath surrounding the hair. If the hair is brown or black, the tips will be dark with melanin; the latter can be more easily seen with transmitted light. Telogen hairs, or resting hairs, are club-shaped, the root sheath is absent, and there is a thin epithelial sac surrounding the club.

The scalp has approximately 100,000 hairs; the hair growth cycle is about 2 to 6 years, and the resting period is 3 months. Approximately 70 hairs are normally lost each day from the scalp; the cycle for beard hair is the same. Eyebrows and eyelashes, however, appear to grow for almost 3 months (10 weeks) and then rest for 9 months. The anagen hairs constitute about 85 percent of the population of scalp hairs. In pregnancy, anagen hairs constitute approximately 90 percent during the second and third trimesters, and, therefore, women in the postpartum period note an abnormal loss of hair about 3 months after delivery. This loss is due to the reestablishment of a normal ratio of telogen to anagen hairs.

Alopecia of the scalp, eyebrows, and eyelashes can occur without any visible associated change in the skin (Table 57-1) or secondary to severe local inflammation or scarring, as in discoid lupus erythematosus.

REFERENCES

BARDIN CW, LIPSETT MB: Testosterone and androstenedione blood production rates in normal women and women with idiopathic hirsutism or polycystic ovaries. J Clin Invest 46:891, 1967

FORBES AP: Hirsutism, in *Dermatology in General Medicine*, eds TB Fitzpatrick et al, New York: McGraw-Hill, 1971

KIRSCHNER MA et al: Effect of estrogen administration on androgen production and plasma luteinizing hormone in hirsute women. J Clin Endocrinol Metab 30:727, 1970

section 9 | Hematologic alterations

58 PALLOR AND ANEMIA

M. M. WINTROBE
G. R. LEE

PALLOR

The color of the skin depends on many factors, including the thickness of the epidermis, the quantity and type of pigment contained therein, and the number and degree of patency of the blood vessels, as well as the quantity and nature of the hemoglobin carried within them. Even the nature and fluid content of the subcutaneous tissue are significant factors. It is obvious, therefore, that pallor does not necessarily indicate that anemia is present.

A sallow complexion is present in certain persons, as it was in their forebears, and may exist in the absence of any true anemia; the flush of excitement, on the other hand, or constant exposure to the sun and wind may produce an appearance which masks an underlying anemia. The number and pattern of distribution of the finer blood vessels vary in different individuals, and in the same person vasoconstriction may produce the appearance of pallor, whereas other factors, such as exercise, may lead to the appearance of a "healthier" color. Certain disorders may affect the skin in such a way that a pallid appearance is produced, even though anemia is absent. These disorders include scleroderma, the various nephrotic states, and myxedema. The last two, however, may be accompanied by actual anemia.

Thus it is evident that the skin itself is an unreliable index of anemia. The mucous membranes, if not inflamed, and the nail beds and palms of the hands, if the hand has not been held in an awkward position and has not been exposed to cold or excessive warmth, are much better. In the palms the color of the creases is especially significant, for they retain their red color even after the intervening skin of the palms has become definitely pale. When the color of the creases is lost, the hemoglobin may be judged as being below 7 g per 100 ml. The color of the conjunctiva may be helpful, but one should not be misled by a coexistent conjunctivitis.

ANEMIA

Definition and detection Anemia might be most accurately defined as a reduction in the circulating red blood cell mass. However, since the size of the red blood cell mass is not easily measured, such a definition is of limited usefulness. Furthermore, from the standpoint of oxygen transport, concentration is probably more important than total amount of red cells or hemoglobin. Certainly, it is more practical to define anemia in terms of concentrations per unit volume of blood. In these terms, anemia is a reduction below normal in the volume of packed red blood cells (VPRC) per 100 ml, the blood hemoglobin (Hb) concentration per 100 ml, and/or the red blood cell (RBC) count per microliter. Under most clinical circumstances, these measurements accurately reflect changes in the red blood cell mass because the total blood volume tends to be kept within relatively narrow limits by a variety of physiologic mechanisms. Nevertheless, in conditions in which blood volume deviates from normal, such as overhydration, dehydration, fluid retention, or significant blood loss, the usual measures of concentration may be misleading. An increase in the plasma volume may give a false impression of anemia. Of greater importance is the fact that an extracellular fluid deficit may mask an underlying anemia.

The VPRC as measured by the standard "macro" method is simple, reproducible, and well suited for routine use in detecting anemia. With little extra effort, the erythrocyte sedimentation rate, volume of packed white blood cells and platelets, and icterus index may be measured at the same time. The macro method requires a venepuncture, since about 1 ml blood is needed, and centrifugation takes 30 min. Micro methods require only a drop of blood and 5 min of centrifugation, and disposable capillary tubes may be used. However, "normal" values obtained with the micro method are 1 to 3 ml per 100 ml lower than with the macro method. Also, when anemia is moderately severe the VPRC measured by a micro method is less reproducible than by the macro method, making it less suitable for use in calculating erythrocyte indexes. "Hematocrit" also may be calculated from the size and number of cells as determined by electronic counters, but such calculated values do not always agree with results of standard centrifugal methods.

Blood hemoglobin concentration, measured by the cyanmethemoglobin method, also provides accurate information, if properly calibrated. The red blood cell count performed by the hemocytometer method lacks accuracy; when it is performed by an electronic counter, reasonable accuracy is possible if the instrument is calibrated and properly maintained.

Normal values for red corpuscles for persons at various ages are presented in the Appendix. These data are for persons living at sea level. At higher altitudes, higher values are found, roughly in proportion to the elevation above sea level. In general, the blood of normal persons tends to approach the mean for the sex. Provided the measurements are accurate, anemia may be defined as a reduction below the mean of more than 10 percent.

Pathologic physiology In normal subjects, erythrocytes are produced by the bone marrow and released to the circulation, where they survive approximately 120 days. They are then removed by the reticuloendothelial system, in which the hemoglobin is broken down to bile pigments, iron, and globin. It is useful to think of the tissues involved in these processes as if they were one organ, the erythron, a concept which is illustrated diagrammatically in Fig. 58-1. It is apparent that the size of the circulating red blood cell mass is related to the rates of production and destruction. In a normal subject, the two rates are equal; therefore, the red blood cell mass remains constant in size, and the subject is said to be in hematologic equilibrium. When destruction exceeds production, the red blood cell mass decreases in size and anemia develops. When production exceeds destruction, the red blood cell mass increases.

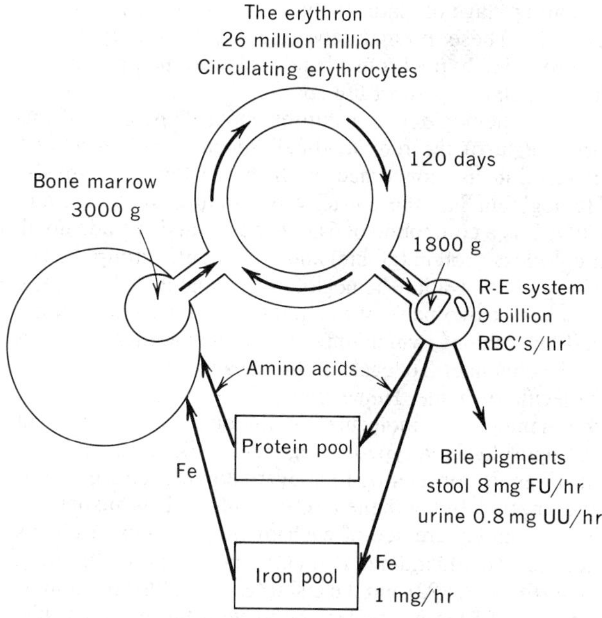

FIGURE 58-1
The amount of blood in circulation represents the balance between production and destruction. In a 70-kg man the circulating red corpuscles carry approximately 770 g hemoglobin. Since the average life span of the red corpuscles normally is 120 days, the turnover rate per day is the total in the circulation divided by 120. In the average man this comes to approximately 2.16×10^{11} red corpuscles per day, or 9 billion per hour, and 6.4 g hemoglobin per day. From this are derived approximately 21 mg iron per day, 250 mg protoporphyrin, and 6.2 g globin. The iron and globin are reutilized. Of the protoporphyrin derived from the destroyed red corpuscles, somewhat less than 250 mg appears as fecal urobilinogen, since there are great variations in completeness of evacuation and also because of variations in the extent to which pigments giving this reaction are produced. Under normal conditions, through increased production and transformation of yellow marrow to red, the bone marrow is capable of approximately a seven- or eightfold increase in production capacity. Consequently, other things being equal, anemia will not develop as the result of increased blood destruction until the life span of the red corpuscles has been reduced to less than about 15 to 17 days.

ERYTHROCYTE PRODUCTION The erythron is maintained within "normal" limits by a well-balanced hormonal mechanism which mediates the response to various normal and abnormal situations. The hormone erythropoietin is a glycoprotein which is thought to be formed by the action of an enzyme produced in the kidney [renal erythropoietic factor (REF) or erythrogenin] that reacts with a plasma substance ("erythropoietinogen") of hepatic origin. The kidney, however, in most species (including man) is not the sole source of erythropoietin; removal of the kidneys does not abolish erythropoiesis or cause the complete disappearance of erythropoietin activity in the plasma.

Erythropoietin induces primitive marrow cells to differentiate into pronormoblasts, thereby bringing about expansion of the erythroid marrow. Fat is replaced by erythroid cells, and formerly inactive or "yellow" marrow becomes active or "red." Under maximum stimulation, the marrow is capable of increasing its production capacity six- to eightfold.

Tissue hypoxia is the ultimate stimulus for erythropoietin production. Tissue oxygen tension depends on the relative rates of oxygen supply and demand which, in turn, depend on blood flow, blood hemoglobin concentration, hemoglobin oxygen saturation, and hemoglobin oxygen affinity, as discussed in Chap. 29.

In addition to inducing hyperplasia of the erythrocyte precursors, erythropoietin secretion causes red blood cell generation time to be shortened, premature denucleation to occur, and reticulocytes to be released to the blood at an earlier stage of maturity than normally ("shift reticulocytes"). These prematurely released erythrocytes are macrocytic, hypochromic, and polychromatophilic and have a relatively short life span.

Since hemoglobin constitutes about 90 percent of the dry weight of the red blood cell, much of red blood cell production is concerned with hemoglobin synthesis. Hemoglobin has the capacity of binding oxygen reversibly. It is a compound of 64,458 mol wt and is made up of a colorless protein (globin) and a prosthetic group, heme. The globin of adult hemoglobin (hemoglobin A) in man consists of two pairs of polypeptide chains, alpha chains and beta chains, which differ from one another in amino acid sequence. To each of the chains is attached one molecule of heme. Heme, which imparts the red color to the hemoglobin molecule, is a complex of iron and protoporphyrin 9, type III (Fig. 58-2). Like other porphyrin rings, it consists of four pyrrole nuclei connected to one another by methene ($=C-$) bridges. It is suspended in a nonpolar crevice of each of the four globin chains between two histidines known respectively as the proximal (F8, α87, β92) and the distal (E7, α58, β63) histidines. The iron forms a covalent bond with the proximal histidine, and oxygen, when bound, is positioned between iron and the distal histidine.

The structure of heme is identical in all mammals, but the properties of hemoglobin, because of differences in the amino acid composition of globin, vary in different species with respect to electrophoretic mobility, solubility, and resistance to denaturation by alkali. In addition, in man a number of different types of hemoglobin, dependent on genetically determined differences in globin structure, have been discovered which in some instances govern the development of hematologic abnormalities and certain clinical manifestations (Chap. 307).

FIGURE 58-2
Chemical structure of heme and its manner of union with globin to form hemoglobin. The carbon atoms derived from the alpha carbon of glycine are represented by ●, those supplied from the methyl carbon of acetate by ▼, and those derived from the carboxyl group of acetate by ×. The unmarked carbons are those derived either from the methyl carbon atom of acetate or from the carboxyl atom.

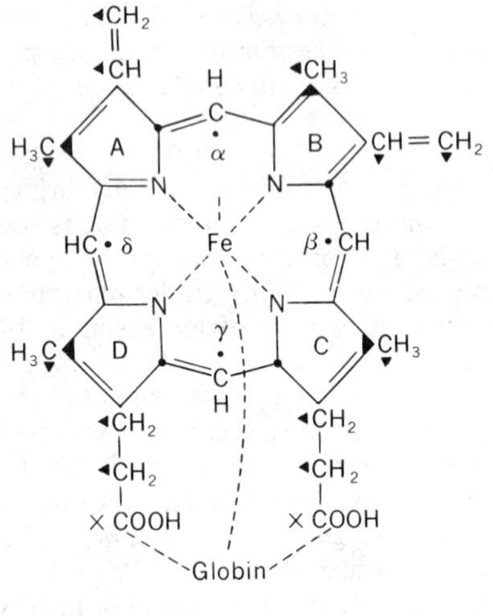

The source materials for the formation of porphyrin are the amino acid glycine and succinyl coenzyme A (CoA), which arises from the tricarboxylic acid cycle. In vitro as well as in vivo studies have clarified the steps in the synthetic process (Fig. 58-3). Acetate is transformed into α-ketoglutarate, and this, in the presence of coenzyme A, gives rise to succinyl CoA. This is the site at which pantothenic acid functions in erythropoiesis, since this vitamin is a component of CoA. Pyridoxine is involved in the next step. The activated form of succinate condenses with a pyridoxal phosphate-glycine-enzyme complex to form delta-aminolevulinic acid (δ-ALA) and carbon dioxide. Two molecules of δ-ALA condense to form a monopyrrole, porphobilinogen. The subsequent steps leading to the formation of protoporphyrin are shown in the diagram. Ultimately protoporphyrin is converted to hemoglobin in the presence of iron, globin, and an enzyme, heme synthetase (ferrochelatase). The first and last two steps in the heme biosynthetic chain occur in mitochondria; the other steps take place in the cytoplasm.

The metabolism of iron is discussed in Chap. 304. Globin is synthesized in the cell by a process common to the synthesis of all proteins (Chap. 62).

RED BLOOD CELL DESTRUCTION The normal red blood cell survives about 120 days. Since it contains no nucleus, all the enzymes necessary to maintain this life span must be in the cell when it enters the circulation. The principal factors essential to normal survival are (1) a source of energy, (2) the ability to maintain a stable fluid and electrolyte content, and (3) a system which protects the cell from endogenous and exogenous oxidants.

About 85 to 90 percent of the energy used by red blood cells is derived from the conversion of glucose to lactate by anaerobic glycolysis (Chap. 72). The high-energy compound synthesized in this pathway is adenosinetriphosphate (ATP), two molecules of which are produced for each molecule of glucose broken down. The remaining 10 to 15 percent of erythrocyte energy is derived from the hexosemonophosphate shunt in which nicotinamide adenine dinucleotide phosphate (NADPH) is formed. Since no mitochondria are found in mature red blood cells, there is no tricarboxylic acid (Krebs) cycle, and energy from this pathway is not available.

The maintenance of the fluid and electrolyte content of the red blood cell is chiefly a function of its membrane. This is made up of structural proteins (40 to 50 percent) and lipids (35 to 45 percent), as well as carbohydrates (7 to 15 percent). The lipids, consisting of free cholesterol, phospholipids, and globosides, exchange freely with plasma lipids. The equilibrium between membrane and plasma is affected by plasma bile salt concentration. Alterations in membrane lipids lead to characteristic distortions of erythrocyte shape; e.g., loss of cholesterol leads to spherocytes, cholesterol gain produces target cells. Thorny cells ("acanthocytes") are characteristic of abetalipoproteinemia (Chap. 106). The structural proteins of the membrane have been only partially characterized. A genetic defect in one of these proteins may lead to the excessive membrane permeability found in hereditary spherocytosis (Chap. 306).

The membrane has the property of selective permeability and is able to facilitate the passage of cations against an ionic gradient. This function is accomplished by a "pump" which exchanges intracellular sodium for extracellular potassium. The pump utilizes ATP, requires an enzyme (ATP-ase), and is inhibited in vitro by cardiac glycosides.

The principal components of the system which protect the red blood cell and its contents from oxidation are glutathione, reduced triphosphopyridine nucleotide (TPNH, NADPH), and the enzymes glucose 6-phosphate dehydrogenase, glutathione reductase, and glutathione peroxidase.

At the end of its life span, the red blood cell is removed by components of the reticuloendothelial sys-

FIGURE 58-3

Chemical steps in the biosynthesis of hemoglobin. The following abbreviations are used: CoA, Coenzyme A, GTP, guanosine triphosphate; GDP, guanosine diphosphate; Pi, inorganic phosphorus; GSH, glutathione; Δ-ALA, delta-aminolevulinic acid; Δ-ALA-DH, delta-aminolevulinate dehydrogenase; PD, porphobilinogen deaminase; UI, uroporphyrinogen isomerase; UD, uroporphyrinogen decarboxylase; COx, coproporphyrinogen oxidase; HS, heme synthetase; Hgb, hemoglobin. (From MM Wintrobe et al, Clinical Hematology, *7th ed., Philadelphia, Lea & Febiger, 1974)*

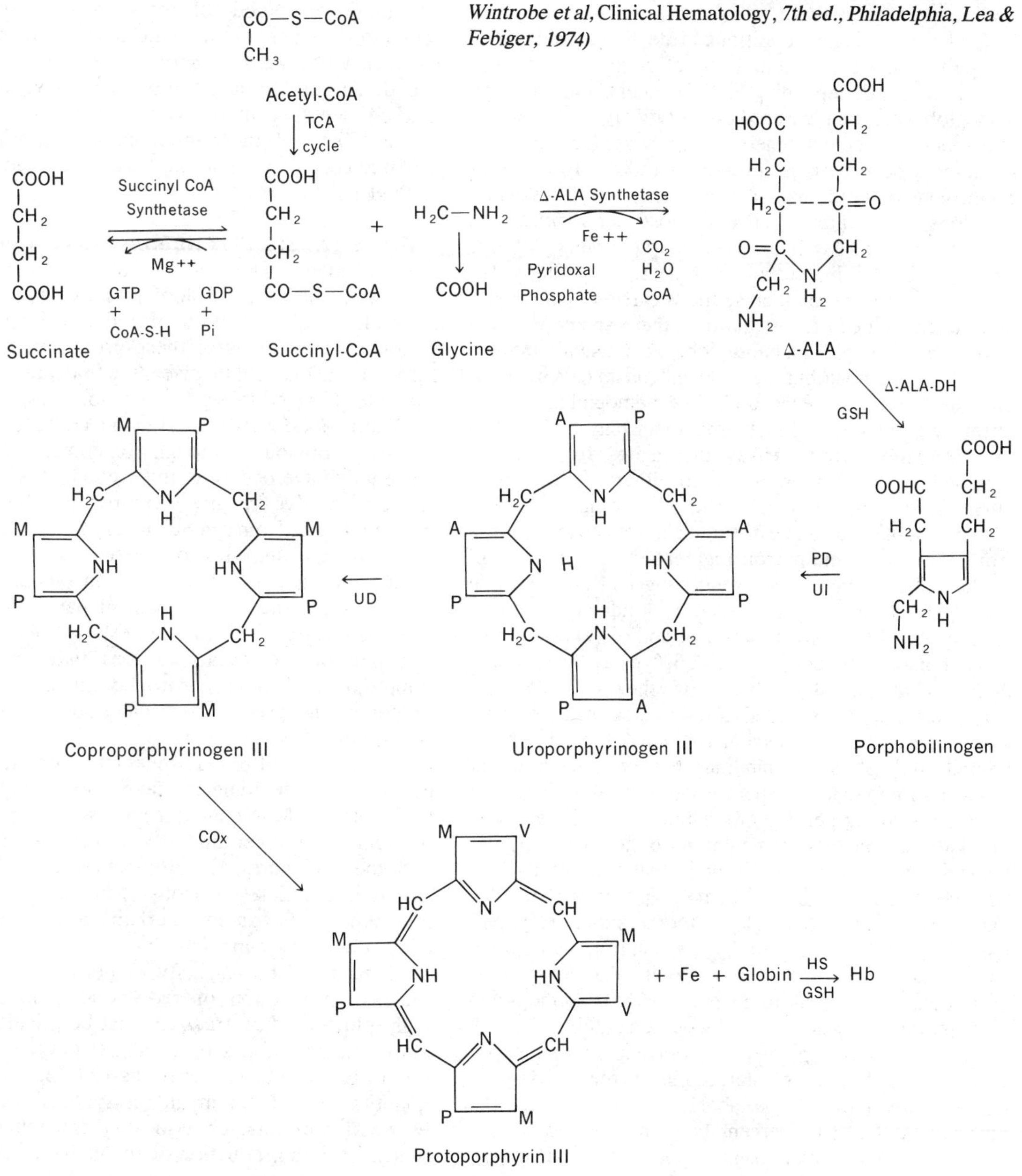

tem, principally the spleen. Within the reticuloendothelial cell, hemoglobin catabolism takes place. Iron and amino acids are extracted and subsequently are reutilized. Most of the liberated iron is transported as "plasma iron" via the transport protein, transferrin, a β_1-globulin, to the bone marrow, where it is used in the synthesis of new hemoglobin. Part of the iron may be retained within the reticuloendothelial cell as ferritin, a ferric iron–protein complex, or as hemosiderin, a more stable and less available form of storage iron. The liberated globin is degraded and is returned to the body pool of amino acids. As outlined in Chap. 42, the porphyrin ring is converted to bile pigments, which are excreted. A byproduct of this reaction is carbon monoxide, and the measurement of this compound can serve as a useful index of the rate of erythrocyte destruction.

Under pathologic conditions, free hemoglobin may escape into the circulation. This colors the plasma faint pink to deep red, depending on the concentration. Plasma hemoglobin can be measured quantitatively by the benzidine reaction. Hemoglobinemia occurs in severe hemolytic states when there is intravascular hemolysis, as in erythroblastosis fetalis, severe hemolytic transfusion reactions, blackwater fever, and *Clostridium welchii* (*C. perfringens*) sepsis (Chap. 154). Liberated hemoglobin is promptly bound by certain globulins with affinity for hemoglobin, the haptoglobins, and is carried to the hepatic parenchymal cell for breakdown there and conversion to bilirubin. The plasma haptoglobins can usually bind 40 to 200 mg hemoglobin per 100 ml plasma. When this binding capacity is exceeded, free hemoglobin, as the tetramer or dimer, and methemoglobin may be found in the circulation. Heme easily dissociates from methemoglobin and becomes bound to either β_1-globulin or albumin, forming methemalbumin. This compound reacts with benzidine and can be distinguished spectroscopically from other heme and pyrrole pigments. Demonstration of methemalbumin in plasma strongly suggests intravascular hemolysis. Protein-bound heme is gradually removed from plasma by the liver over a period of several days.

Hemoglobin dimers (mol wt 32,000) enter the glomerular filtrate, are partially reabsorbed in the proximal tubule, and, if the T_{max} is exceeded, are excreted into the urine. The apparent *renal threshold* for hemoglobin is chiefly related to haptoglobin binding; however, even in the absence of haptoglobins there is a threshold for hemoglobin (about 40 mg per 100 ml). The tubular epithelium of the kidney converts hemoglobin to hemosiderin, and hemosiderin is found regularly in the urine of patients with low concentrations of heme pigments in their plasma. The passage of hemoglobin by the kidney is accompanied and also followed by proteinuria, hemoglobin casts, and precipitates of hemoglobin. The color of the urine ranges from pink to deep red with oxyhemoglobin, from purple to black from reduced hemoglobin.

Not all the bile pigment is derived from senescent erythrocytes. Studies of stercobilin excretion following the administration of ^{15}N-labeled glycine indicate that normally at least 10 percent (and in diseases such as pernicious anemia, thalassemia, and congenital porphyria, the greater proportion) is derived in part from *ineffective erythropoiesis;* i.e., the destruction of newly formed red blood cells within the marrow or very shortly after their release.

In the intestine, as outlined in Chap. 42, bilirubin is converted to urobilinogen. Urobilinogen consists of a series of colorless chromogens, all of which are characterized by a positive Ehrlich's aldehyde reaction, as well as by instability and ease of oxidation to colored pigments, the urobilin group. The transition to urobilins can be hastened by mild oxidizing agents, such as iodine, and this is the basis of Schlesinger's qualitative test (alcoholic zinc acetate) for urobilin.

The amount of urobilinogen excreted in the urine in 24 hr (UU) by the normal adult is 0 to 3.5 mg, most frequently 0.5 to 1.5 mg. The normal range for fecal urobilinogen (FU), as calculated from a 4-day period of collection, is 40 to 280 mg per day, usually 100 to 200 mg. The expected values are related to the size of the circulating red blood cell mass; thus, lower values are found in young children. Mean values have been found to increase with age. An important qualification should be added. The oral administration of tetracyclines causes a marked decrease in the concentration of fecal urobilinogen. The usefulness and limitations of urine and fecal urobilinogen determinations are discussed in a later chapter (Chap. 306).

PATHOGENESIS OF ANEMIA An etiologic classification of anemia is given in Table 58-1. Anemia may develop as the result of blood loss, excessive destruction or inadequate production of red blood cells, or from various combinations of these processes. The different forms of anemia will be discussed in detail in subsequent chapters. Here certain generalizations may be made.

When *blood loss* is acute, the cause of the anemia usually is obvious, although sometimes a large hemorrhage may have occurred under conditions which do not reveal themselves readily. Hemorrhage in the gastrointestinal tract, e.g., from a peptic ulcer, may be dramatic in its symptoms and may be so severe as to cause shock; at other times it may be insidious in character and may occur without the development of pain or of symptoms pointing clearly to the gastrointestinal tract. Hemorrhage into one of the serous cavities may cause puzzling symptoms and signs: profound anemia may develop suddenly, and even icterus may appear as the result of absorption of blood.

Chronic loss of blood occurs most commonly from the pelvic organs in females and from the gastrointestinal tract in the male. A common cause of chronic posthemorrhagic anemia in certain parts of the world is infestation with the hookworm. The ultimate result of chronic blood loss is iron deficiency. Iron-deficiency anemia is a very prevalent form of anemia, perhaps the most common, and is discussed in Chap. 304.

Because of the capacity of normal bone marrow to increase production of red blood cells even six- or eightfold, *blood destruction* must be greatly accelerated above the normal rate for anemia to develop, unless some other abnormality is present as well; e.g., qualitative or quantitative defects in globin synthesis, deficiency of essential nutrients, or associated inflammatory disease which impairs production of red cells. In such instances, red cell survival need not be so greatly shortened before anemia is produced. Hemolytic anemias (Chap. 306) are characterized by evidence of excessive red blood cell breakdown (jaundice, increased serum bilirubin of the unconjugated or "indirect" type, and increased urine and fecal urobilinogen), as well as by signs of accelerated red cell production, such as reticulocytosis, polychromatophilia, and even nucleated red cells in the circulating blood.

The *reticulocyte index* is a crude measure of the degree of accelerated (and effective) erythropoiesis. It is determined by multiplying the value obtained for the reticulocyte percentage by the ratio of the patient's hematocrit to normal hematocrit. This index, however, provides only an approximation of accelerated erythropoiesis. As pointed out earlier, when the bone marrow is greatly stimulated, erythrocytes enter the circulation at an earlier point in maturation than would otherwise be the case and such reticulocytes, shifted from the marrow to the blood, presumably complete their maturation in the blood. Since their stay in the blood as reticulocytes is prolonged, the percentage of reticulocytes is greater than if they had remained in the bone marrow. To allow for this, the value for reticulocyte index is divided by 2. Noteworthy also is the fact that accelerated erythropoiesis *alone* does not indicate increased red blood cell destruction, since reticulocytosis occurs in response to blood loss as well.

As Table 58-1 indicates, there are many different causes of accelerated blood destruction. In some instances the primary fault is failure to produce normal erythrocytes because of deficiency of essential substances. Consequently, these causes are listed also under that heading. Furthermore, the degree to which red blood cell survival is shortened differs in the various forms of hemolytic anemia; as a result, the extent to which the various characteristic features of hemolytic anemia are manifested in the different disorders depends on the degree of accelerated blood destruction.

Inadequate production of mature erythrocytes may occur as the result of deficiency of essential substances or for a variety of other reasons as outlined in Table 58-1. Nutrients which are especially important for normal erythropoiesis are iron, vitamin B_{12}, and folic acid. Iron is an essential component of hemoglobin; the two vitamins are needed in the synthesis of deoxyribonucleic acid (DNA). Deficiencies of any of these three nutrients may lead to severe anemia. The effects of protein deficiency are less striking, but severe deficiency causes moderate anemia in man and in experimental animals. In the latter, anemia associated with protein deficiency has been shown to be due to reduced production of erythropoietin.

The role of ascorbic acid in relation to anemia has not been established clearly; though anemia is seen in scurvy, it has not been shown that it is due directly to lack of vitamin C.

TABLE 58-1
Etiologic classification of anemia

I Blood loss
- *A* Anemia after recent hemorrhage (acute)
- *B* Anemia after persistent hemorrhage (chronic)

II Excessive red cell destruction
- *A* Extracorpuscular factors
  - *1* Antibodies
  - *2* Drugs, chemical and physical agents
  - *3* Physical trauma to erythrocytes
  - *4* Sequestration (especially in the spleen)
  - *5* Increased avidity of the reticuloendothelial system [e.g., certain infections (malaria), inflammatory or neoplastic diseases]
  - *6* Lead poisoning
- *B* Intracorpuscular factors
  - *1* Hereditary
    - *a* Disorders of glycolysis
    - *b* Faulty synthesis or maintenance of reduced glutathione
    - *c* Qualitative or quantitative abnormalities in synthesis of globin
    - *d* Abnormalities of RBC membrane
    - *e* Erythropoietic porphyria
  - *2* Acquired
    - *a* Paroxysmal nocturnal hemoglobinuria
    - *b* Deficiency of iron, vitamin B_{12}, or folate

III Inadequate production of mature erythrocytes
- *A* Deficiency of essential nutrients
  - *1* Iron, folic acid, vitamin B_{12}
  - *2* Protein
  - *3* Possibly ascorbic acid
  - *4* Experimentally: copper, cobalt, pyridoxine, nicotinic acid, riboflavin; possibly pantothenic acid, thiamine
- *B* Deficiency of erythroblasts
  - *1* Atrophy of bone marrow: aplastic anemia
    - *a* Chemical or physical agents
    - *b* Hereditary
    - *c* Idiopathic
  - *2* Isolated erythroblastopenia ("pure red cell aplasia")
    - *a* Thymoma
    - *b* Chemical agents
    - *c* Folic acid antagonists
    - *d* Antibodies
    - *e* Hereditary
- *C* Conditions associated with infiltration of bone marrow
  - *1* Leukemia, lymphoma
  - *2* Multiple myeloma
  - *3* Carcinoma, sarcoma
  - *4* Myelofibrosis
- *D* Sideroblastic anemias
- *E* Endocrine abnormality
  - *1* Myxedema
  - *2* Addisonian adrenal insufficiency
  - *3* Pituitary insufficiency
  - *4* Sometimes, hyperthyroidism
- *F* Chronic renal disease
- *G* Chronic inflammatory diseases
  - *1* Infections
  - *2* Noninfectious diseases, including granulomatous and collagen diseases
- *H* Hepatic disease

Cobalt deficiency has never been demonstrated in man, but a form of copper deficiency associated with hypoproteinemia, iron deficiency, and microcytic hypochromic anemia has been described in infants; this anemia, however, responds to iron in the absence of copper.

The requirement for the B vitamins, other than vitamin B_{12} and folic acid, insofar as erythropoiesis is concerned, has not been definitely established. Experimentally, deficiency of nicotinic acid and riboflavin, and possibly of pantothenic acid and even thiamine, may be associated with the development of some anemia. In man, however, even under the extraordinary circumstances under which he sometimes finds himself, anemia clearly attributable to lack of these vitamins has not been demonstrated.

Anemia due to deficiency of pyridoxine has only once been produced experimentally in the human infant. Otherwise, dietary deficiency of pyridoxine as a cause of anemia has not been clearly demonstrated. However, microcytic hypochromic anemia responding to the administration of pyridoxine in doses far above the physiologic requirement has been reported in a number of patients. Such anemia is more likely to be due to a fault in erythropoiesis related in some fashion to the role of pyridoxine in heme synthesis than to dietary deficiency of this vitamin, as discussed in Chap. 304.

In man, deficiencies which result in anemia often are not due to lack of an essential substance in the diet but are *"conditioned"* by special circumstances. Thus, deficiency of vitamin B_{12} in pernicious anemia results from an inability to absorb this vitamin because of lack of gastric intrinsic factor. Again, in sprue and other malabsorption syndromes (Chap. 284), vitamin B_{12} or folic acid deficiency may develop. Excessive demands in pregnancy and greater needs for growth in childhood and adolescence may "condition" the development of various types of deficiency, and anemia will then ensue (see Table 305-1).

Elsewhere *aplastic anemia* and other conditions associated with aplasia or hypoplasia of the bone marrow, as well as so-called "pure red cell aplasia," will be discussed (Chap. 309). In aplastic anemia granulocytes and platelets as well as red blood cells are reduced in number.

The pathogenesis of the anemia in *leukemia, malignancy with metastases to bone marrow, myelofibrosis,* and other similar conditions is as yet obscure. Such anemia has been classified as myelophthisic. The term implies wasting away of the marrow, but it is usually used to imply encroachment on or replacement of the bone marrow by leukemia or metastases. There is little or no evidence, however, that the erythropoietic tissue is crowded out in these myelophthisic anemias. Measurement of red blood cell production rates has, at times, yielded normal or increased values. A number of studies have shown the life span of the red corpuscles to be reduced, and occasionally frank hemolytic anemia develops. It is possible that no single explanation for the anemia associated with these diseases will be found.

A unique group are the sideroblastic anemias (Chap. 304), which are characterized by the presence of ringed sideroblasts in the bone marrow and by hypochromic stippled red corpuscles in the blood. In these disorders, defective heme synthesis may be the primary fault.

Anemia accompanying *endocrine abnormalities* has not been well studied. It is plausible that the anemias associated with hypothyroidism and hypopituitarism are related to the decreased need for oxygen transport, since when thyroid hormone or growth hormone is lacking, the consumption of oxygen by the tissues is reduced. The anemia of myxedema usually is only moderate in degree, often is normocytic but may be macrocytic, and disappears gradually as thyroid hormone is supplied. This anemia, which is so readily correctible, may be easily overlooked. The pathogenesis of the anemia associated with adrenocortical insufficiency may be similar to that of hypothyroidism.

In the anemia of *renal insufficiency* (Chap. 308), the decrease in red blood cell survival is, in part at least, the consequence of extracorpuscular factors. The nature of these factors has not been completely defined; there is no evidence of an autoimmune mechanism, nor is there a clear relation with any of the products which are retained in renal insufficiency. Mechanical factors resulting in fragmentation or distortion of red blood cells as the effects of injury through contact with diseased vessels, or forced passage between taut strands of fibrin may play an important role ("microangiopathic anemia"). Since the kidney is concerned in erythropoietin production, attention has been directed to a possible defect in synthesis of this hormone as an explanation for the decrease in red blood cell production. Plasma erythropoietin levels have been found to be reduced in comparison to those associated with similar degrees of anemia due to other causes. Furthermore, the radioiron marrow transit time, which becomes shortened as erythropoietin stimulates the marrow, is prolonged in renal disease. Unlike the anemia of other chronic disorders, as described below, the anemia of renal insufficiency is not characterized by hypoferremia as a constant feature.

The anemia accompanying *chronic infection,* cancer, and rheumatoid arthritis (Chap. 308) is unique in that it is associated with a profound disturbance in iron metabolism. This is manifested by a reduced plasma iron concentration, reduced plasma iron-binding capacity, increased iron stores, and decreased marrow sideroblasts. The defect cannot be altered by iron administration, even if iron is given parenterally in large quantities. An increase in free erythrocyte protoporphyrin and in serum copper occurs at the same time. It is probable that the flow of iron to plasma from reticuloendothelial stores is restricted, but the way in which such a restriction is brought about is unknown. This metabolic defect is overcome and anemia is corrected when the underlying disease, e.g., infection, is treated effectively.

Multiple factors are implicated in the pathogenesis of the anemia of *hepatic disease.* Blood loss from esophageal varices may lead to acute or chronic posthemorrhagic anemia. Nutritional folic acid deficiency not uncommonly accompanies cirrhosis in alcoholics. Alcohol itself has been shown to cause reversible depression of red blood cell production. In most cases of liver disease, however, the cause of the anemia is not clearly defined. The red blood cells are normal or increased in size and tend to be thinner than normal, probably because of the effects of serum factors, such as bile salts, and increased amounts of cholesterol and lecithin on the red blood cell membrane. Red blood cell survival tends to be moderately shortened, and red blood cell production is not increased enough to compensate for the reduced survival.

Finally, it must be recognized that in patients with ailments of long standing, more than one factor may play a role in the development of anemia. Thus, nutritional deficiency because of reduced intake of food or faulty absorption from the gastrointestinal tract, blood loss, the negative nitrogen balance associated with long confinement to bed, and impaired iron metabolism such as that associated with chronic inflammatory conditions, all may play a role.

SIGNS AND SYMPTOMS OF ANEMIA Anemia should never be thought of as a diagnosis in itself, but rather as a manifestation of an underlying disease process. Thus, the signs and symptoms found in the anemic patient are a mixture of those due to anemia and those due to the underlying disease. Only those symptoms common to all anemias will be discussed below; symptoms more specifically related to the underlying disease are dealt with in the chapters dealing with those entities.

Cardiorespiratory system Hemoglobin is the vehicle and the cardiovascular system the means of delivery of oxygen to the tissues. When anemia is present, the oxygen-carrying capacity of the blood is reduced. If an equivalent amount of oxygen is to be delivered, blood flow must be increased by means of certain cardiovascular adjustments. These and alterations in oxygen affinity were discussed in Chap. 29. Many of the signs and symptoms of anemia reflect these changes in cardiovascular function.

An increased blood flow is accomplished by increases in cardiac stroke volume and heart rate. The patient may be aware of this increased cardiac activity and complain of palpitation. On examination, tachycardia and an increased pulse pressure may be found, along with increased pulsations over the precordium and major arteries, and even capillary pulsation in the fingertips may be detected. The circulation time may be shortened, and there may be a slight rise in right auricular pressure. Still other signs of the "hyperkinetic syndrome" may be observed (Chap. 233).

The adequacy of the cardiovascular adjustments to anemia depends on the degree of the anemia, the rapidity with which it has developed, and the preexisting status of the cardiovascular system. Symptoms are usually present when the blood hemoglobin concentration is less than 7.5 per 100 ml blood. If anemia has developed so rapidly that there has been little or no time for physiologic adjustment, symptoms are likely to be prominent and to appear comparatively early; on the other hand, if the anemia has been insidious in onset, the adjustment may be so good that the hemoglobin may be as low as 6 per 100 ml, without sufficient functional embarrassment occurring for the patient to be seriously handicapped.

The cardiovascular changes necessarily encroach upon the cardiac reserve; consequently, exercise tolerance is decreased. There may be no symptoms at rest, but signs of oxygen want, such as easy fatigability and dyspnea, develop on exertion. When compensatory adjustments become imperfect or fail, either because of an extreme degree of anemia or because of a previously damaged heart, the clinical picture of cardiac failure ensues. There may be edema, congestion of the neck veins, hepatomegaly, and rales at the base of the lungs.

Severe anemia may produce a systolic murmur, which is usually most marked at the pulmonic area but may be heard elsewhere over the precordium, especially at the apex. Very rarely, diastolic murmurs are heard at the base. Over the vessels of the neck a curious humming sound, the bruit de diable, may be heard.

Neuromuscular system Headache, vertigo, faintness, increased sensitivity to cold, tinnitus or roaring in the ears, black spots before the eyes, muscular weakness, and easy fatigability and irritability are common symptoms associated with anemia. Restlessness is an important symptom of rapidly developing anemia. Drowsiness develops in severe anemia. Headache due to anemia may be very severe. Delirium is seldom seen.

Alimentary system Loss of appetite is not unusual as an accompaniment of anemia. Nausea, flatulence, abdominal discomfort, constipation, diarrhea, vomiting, or abnormal appetite may also be found.

Genitourinary system Menstrual disturbances (most often amenorrhea) in the female, and loss of libido in the male, are frequently encountered in severe anemia. In other instances, excessive menstrual bleeding accompanies anemia. Slight proteinuria and evidence of distinct renal function impairment may be seen in association with anemia.

Epithelial tissues The pallor which accompanies anemia has been discussed. In addition to pallor, loss of normal skin elasticity and tone, thinning of the hair, and purpura and ecchymoses may develop in the chronic forms of anemia.

APPROACH TO THE PATIENT WITH ANEMIA Anemia is not a diagnosis in itself but a manifestation of disease. The challenge to the physician is to diagnose correctly and treat the underlying disease. Failure to appreciate this simple principle may lead to many serious errors in management of the condition. To cite a common example, a patient with anemia secondary to a bleeding cecal carcinoma may be treated with blood transfusions or iron-containing medications or even "hematinic" pills containing a mixture of nutrients and will apparently improve, but the carcinoma will progress to an inoperable stage.

Since literally hundreds of disorders may be associated with anemia, a rational approach to anemia requires that a classification of the causes of anemia be used which forms the basis of a systematic procedure leading to a diagnosis. Classifications of anemia have been based on etiology (as in Table 58-1), and such an approach is effective in many cases. However, the necessary information is often difficult to obtain; accurate evaluation of rates of erythrocyte production and destruction often involves rather elaborate, time-consuming, and expensive procedures that needlessly delay proper management. An example is the determination of red blood cell life span. A more practical approach is based on a morphologic classification of anemia. The advantage is that the information necessary to make the classification is quickly obtained at little cost.

The first step in the morphologic classification of a given anemia is to determine whether it is (1) macrocytic, (2) hypochromic and/or microcytic, or (3) normocytic, normochromic. This is accomplished by the calculation of erythrocyte indexes and the careful examination of the stained blood smear.

There are three erythrocyte indexes, the mean corpuscular volume (MCV), the mean corpuscular hemoglobin concentration (MCHC), and the mean corpuscular hemoglobin (MCH). They are calculated from ratios of the three measures of anemia. Thus,

$$\text{MCV} = \frac{\text{VPRC}}{\text{RBC}}$$

$$\text{MCHC} = \frac{\text{Hb}}{\text{VPRC}}$$

$$\text{MCH} = \frac{\text{Hb}}{\text{RBC}}$$

Normal values for these indexes are given in the Appendix. The major morphologic categories may be defined by deviations from normal in these indexes. Thus, in macrocytic anemia, MCV and MCH are increased and MCHC is normal. In hypochromic, microcytic anemias, MCH and either MCV ("microcytic") or MCHC ("hypochromic"), or both MCV and MCHC, are reduced. The indexes remain within normal limits in the normocytic, normochromic anemias.

Since the above determinations are subject to laboratory error, the erythrocyte indexes should always be confirmed by examination of the blood smear. With experience, an accurate assessment of red blood cell size can be made by observing the average red blood cell diameter under the microscope. Hypochromia is seen as an increase in the area of central pallor. It is always wise to compare the observations made on the patient's blood with those made on a normal blood smear, since the magnification and illumination of microscopes vary. Uncommonly, distortions of red blood cell shape may lead to an erroneous impression from examination of the blood smear, especially when cells are unusually flat (leptocytosis), as they are in liver disease, in thalassemia, and after splenectomy. Such cells appear larger and more hypochromic than the erythrocyte indexes indicate.

The next step in the morphologic approach to anemia varies with the major morphologic category (Table 58-2). Macrocytic anemias are subdivided into two groups, megaloblastic and nonmegaloblastic. The megaloblastic anemias, of which pernicious anemia is the prototype, result from defective synthesis of nucleic acids, usually because of a deficiency of vitamin B_{12} or folic acid. Certain morphologic features are particularly useful in detecting the megaloblastic anemias. The earliest changes are seen in the blood smear and consist of the presence of oval macrocytes and hypersegmented neutrophils. In the bone marrow, characteristic alterations are seen in nucleated red blood cells; they are larger than normal, and the nuclear chromatin is finer and more particulate. These changes are discussed more fully in Chap. 305, along with a more complete subclassification of the megaloblastic anemias.

The nonmegaloblastic macrocytic anemias make up a heterogeneous group. Macrocytosis is found in patients with markedly increased rates of red blood cell production, because young erythrocytes are somewhat larger than mature erythrocytes; in addition, when demands upon the marrow are great, as discussed earlier, the nucleus is prematurely discharged and the red blood cell is released before maturation has progressed fully. Such

TABLE 58-2
Morphologic classification of anemia

I Macrocytic anemias (MCV 94–160 fl; MCH 32–50 pg; MCHC 32–36 g/100 ml)
- *A* Megaloblastic
  - *1* Vitamin B_{12} deficiency (pernicious anemia, etc.)
  - *2* Folate deficiency (malabsorption syndromes, pregnancy, etc.)
  - *3* Inherited abnormalities of DNA synthesis
  - *4* Drug-induced disorders of DNA synthesis
- *B* Nonmegaloblastic
  - *1* Accelerated erythropoiesis
  - *2* Miscellaneous (myxedema, liver disease, hypoplastic anemias)

II Hypochromic microcytic anemias (MCV 50–80 fl; MCH 12–27 pg; MCHC 24–32 g/100 ml)
- *A* Iron deficiency
  - *1* Chronic blood loss (menstrual, gastrointestinal tract, hookworm, etc.)
  - *2* Excessive demands (growth, pregnancy)
  - *3* Dietary deficiency (infancy)
  - *4* Malabsorption (postgastrectomy, sprue, etc.)
- *B* Genetic anomaly: thalassemia alone or with a hemoglobinopathy
- *C* Sideroblastic anemias (pyridoxine-responsive and others)
- D Hypocupremic syndrome of infants
- *E* Chronic disorders (sometimes)

III Normocytic anemias (MCV 82–92 fl; MCH 28–32 pg; MCHC 32–36 g/100 ml)
- *A* Recent loss of blood
- *B* Hemolytic anemias
- *C* Anemias due to bone marrow failure
- *D* Anemia of chronic disorders
- *E* Anemia of renal failure
- *F* Anemia of endocrine disorders
- *G* Myelophthisic anemias
- *H* Overexpansion of plasma volume (not true anemia)

Note: MCV, mean corpuscular volume; MCH, mean corpuscular hemoglobin; MCHC, mean corpuscular hemoglobin concentration; fl, femtoliters (replaces cubic microns).

cells are considerably larger than normal and, since hemoglobin synthesis has not been completed, may be somewhat hypochromic as well. Macrocytosis may also be observed in the anemia accompanying hypothyroidism, liver disease, or aplastic anemia, but the cause of the macrocytosis in these disorders is less clear.

The hypochromic and/or microcytic anemias are disorders in which hemoglobin synthesis is deficient. Normal hemoglobin synthesis requires iron, protoporphyrin, and globin, and an abnormality affecting the availability of any of the three may lead to a hypochromic and/or microcytic anemia. By far, the most common cause of this type of anemia is iron deficiency (see Chap. 304). Hypochromia and microcytosis are also found in most forms of thalassemia and may at times be seen in certain of the hemoglobinopathies (see Chap. 307). The anemia of chronic disorders, such as infection, cancer, and rheumatoid arthritis, is usually normocytic and normochromic, but at times it is hypochromic and occasionally is both hypochromic and microcytic (see Chap. 308). The morphologic changes probably occur because of the disturbance in iron metabolism previously alluded to. Hypochromia and microcytosis are found also in sideroblastic anemias. These are comparatively rare and probably include a variety of entities (Chap. 304). They have in common evidence of excessive iron stores, sometimes producing clinical manifestations of hemochromatosis.

Frequently, a final diagnosis in the hypochromic, microcytic group of anemias can be reached after a careful history and physical examination. Special attention should be given to the dietary history, to evidence of blood loss, and to the possibility of familial transmission. Evaluation of the status of iron metabolism will help to confirm the impression. The principal clinical tools used for evaluating iron metabolism are the serum iron concentration and iron-binding capacity and the quantitation in marrow aspirates stained with Prussian blue of iron stores as well as of iron in nucleated red blood cells (sideroblasts). Results of these procedures are indicated in Table 58-3.

In evaluating the status of a patient with normocytic, normochromic anemia (Table 58-2, III), it is useful to try to draw some preliminary conclusions about the rates of erythrocyte production and destruction. It is rare that measurement of the red blood cell life span with chromium 51 is necessary; simpler methods usually provide the necessary information. The most useful of the simple methods for detecting increased red blood cell production is the reticulocyte count or the reticulocyte supply index (page 1597). Increased red blood cell destruction is detected by evaluating bile pigment metabolism by means of serum bilirubin and urinary and fecal urobilinogen determinations as well as by measurement of CO excretion. The anemia of acute blood loss (Chap. 303) is associated with increased red blood cell production; consequently, the reticulocyte count is usually increased. The hemolytic anemias (Chap. 306) are characterized by evidence of both increased production and destruction. In the anemia of chronic disorders (Chap. 308), a moderate increase in erythrocyte destruction is accompanied by a modest decrease in production; the changes are subtle, so that the reticulocyte count and measures of hemoglobin catabolism remain within normal limits. Alterations in iron metabolism (Table 58-3) may be helpful. The anemias due to bone marrow failure are usually associated with a depressed reticulocyte count; there is no evidence of excessive hemoglobin catabolism, and leukopenia and thrombocytopenia also are present. The myelophthisic anemias are characterized by a bizarre blood smear: marked variations in erythrocyte size and shape, nucleated red blood cells, myeloid immaturity, and enlarged, bizarre platelets.

Examination of bone marrow In some of the above conditions, a final diagnosis is established by study of the bone marrow. This procedure is useful in evaluating not only the condition of the anemic patient but also disorders affecting other formed elements of the blood. There are two basic techniques by which marrow is obtained for study: aspiration from the sternum or iliac crest, and biopsy of the posterior iliac spine with the Westerman-Jensen needle. Thin smears are prepared from bone marrow aspirates; when stained with Wright's stain, such preparations are ideal for the study of cellular morphologic details. These smears may also be stained with the Prussian blue reaction in order to assess the amount of iron in reticuloendothelial cells and sideroblasts. Fixed, thick sections of marrow obtained by biopsy are ideal for evaluating the cellularity of the marrow and for detecting fibrosis or granulomatous disorders.

When the patient's condition has been studied thoroughly in the manner indicated above, the number of

TABLE 58-3
Measures of iron metabolism in the hypochromic-microcytic anemias

Type of anemia	*Serum iron*	*Serum iron-binding capacity*	*Marrow iron stores*	*Marrow sideroblasts*
Iron-deficiency	Decreased	Increased	Absent	Absent
Thalassemia	Normal or increased	Normal	Normal or increased	Normal or increased
Anemia of chronic disorders	Decreased	Decreased	Usually increased	Decreased
Sideroblastic anemias	Increased	Decreased	Markedly increased	Markedly increased

instances in which examination of the bone marrow will be required is small. Table 58-4 lists various types of reaction which may be observed if differential counts on aspirated bone marrow are made. In such preparations, consideration should be given to the following:

1 The myeloid/erythroid (M/E) ratio. By this is meant the proportion of leukocytes of the myeloid series to nucleated red blood cells of all types. The normal values range from 2.5 to 5.0:1. A decrease in the M/E ratio (i.e., a greater-than-normal proportion of nucleated red blood cells) may be the result of a decrease in the number of myeloid cells or of an increase in erythroid cells. In the latter event, one must differentiate between normoblastic and megaloblastic hyperplasia.
2 An increased number of cells other than those of the myeloid or erythroid series. These include lymphocytes, plasma cells, reticulum cells, and other forms (myeloma cells, carcinoma cells, Gaucher's cells, etc.).
3 Megakaryocytes. Since these form so small a proportion of the cells of the bone marrow, specific attention should be given them. It may be necessary to examine several preparations of marrow because of their irregular distribution. One should attempt to determine whether they appear to be increased or greatly decreased in number and whether their structure is normal.
4 The absence of marrow elements. In such cases, biopsy may be necessary.

TABLE 58-4
Conditions in which various types of reaction may be observed, as demonstrated by bone marrow aspiration

M/E ratio increased	*Nonmyeloid cells increased*
Myeloid forms of leukemia	Other forms of leukemia
The majority of infections	Multiple myeloma
Leukemoid reaction	Metastases from carcinoma, etc.
Decrease in nucleated red blood cells	Gaucher's disease, Niemann-Pick disease
	Aplastic anemia (usually relative increase only)
	Infectious mononucleosis

M/E ratio decreased

Decrease in myeloid cells or increase in erythroid cells with

Normoblastic hyperplasia or	*Megaloblastic hyperplasia*
Hemorrhagic anemias	Vitamin B_{12} deficiency:
Iron-deficiency anemia	pernicious anemia, etc.
Hemolytic anemias	Folate deficiency:
Thalassemia	Sprue, idiopathic steatorrhea, resection of small intestine, etc.
Anemia of chronic renal disease	
Cirrhosis of the liver	Nutritional macrocytic anemias (tropical and nontropical)
Sideroblastic anemias	
Polycythemia vera	
	Megaloblastic anemia of infancy
	Megaloblastic anemia of pregnancy
	Inherited and acquired abnormalities of DNA synthesis

Table 58-5 gives normal values for the differential nucleated cell count of bone marrow obtained by aspiration, and representative findings in a number of conditions are presented. These must be regarded only as examples of findings in typical cases; they do not give the range of variation in disease. The latter obviously depends on the stage of the disease and the presence or absence of modifying factors.

Although in all cases the material obtained by sternal puncture is of interest, bone marrow examination is an essential aid in diagnosis only in a limited number of conditions. These include aleukemic leukemia, multiple myeloma, Gaucher's and Niemann-Pick diseases, and certain cases of macrocytic anemia. In the last-mentioned condition the demonstration of megaloblasts is very useful, since it suggests vitamin B_{12} or folate deficiency. In "aleukemic" leukemia, the bone marrow reveals numerous immature forms when they may be absent or scarce in the blood. In addition to these disorders, in disseminated tuberculosis and histoplasmosis, and in parasitic diseases such as kala-azar, the causative organisms may be discovered in the bone marrow when they cannot be found in any other way. Again, the cells of metastatic lesions may be demonstrated by bone marrow examination.

In aplastic anemia the negative character of the aspirated marrow material may be helpful. In cases suspected of being instances of "atypical leukemia," "agnogenic myeloid metaplasia," or "hypersplenism," sternal puncture, followed if necessary by biopsy, may support one of these diagnoses or, instead, may reveal myelosclerosis or myelofibrosis.

MANAGEMENT OF ANEMIA In the sense that by their administration a specific deficiency is corrected, vitamin B_{12}, folic acid, and iron may be considered to be specific agents for the treatment of certain types of anemia. In pernicious anemia and other megaloblastic anemias associated with vitamin B_{12} deficiency, the parenteral administration of vitamin B_{12} corrects the deficiency and the anemia is relieved. In certain other instances of macrocytic megaloblastic anemia, folic acid rather than vitamin B_{12} relieves the anemia. Examples are nutritional megaloblastic anemia, the megaloblastic anemias of infancy and pregnancy, and some cases of the malabsorption syndrome. These agents are valueless in anemias other than those in which the bone marrow is megaloblastic.

Likewise iron therapy is effective in iron-deficiency anemia and is useless in all other types of anemia. Such therapy is almost always effective by mouth; only in the rare instances of severe gastrointestinal intolerance or when blood loss exceeds absorption capacity, and in cases of chronic ulcerative colitis with iron deficiency, is it justifiable to give iron parenterally. Under such circumstances, iron-dextran may be given intramuscularly with reasonable safety.

Whether or not desiccated thyroid and ascorbic acid should be classed as specific therapeutic agents, as they are in Table 58-6, is debatable. It is clear that the anemia accompanying hypothyroidism is relieved only by the administration of thyroid, but whether this is the direct consequence of the relief of a deficiency is less certain. The relationship of ascorbic acid therapy to the anemia of scurvy is even less apparent.

Anemias which are neither due to deficiency of iron nor caused by lack of vitamin B_{12} or folic acid are most difficult to manage. Iron, vitamin B_{12}, folic acid or other vitamins, or combinations of these substances, given orally or parenterally, are useless and wasteful of the patient's funds and the physician's time. These anemias cannot, in the present state of our knowledge, be relieved without modification of the underlying cause. Thus, the anemia of chronic renal disease is difficult to treat unless renal failure can be corrected by transplantation. Likewise, the anemia of chronic infection persists as long as the underlying infection continues. Aplastic anemia in which the bone marrow has been damaged in general carries a very poor prognosis. In some instances the destruction of hematopoietic tissue may not be complete, and in such cases the maintenance of life by transfusion may ultimately be followed by some, or even occasionally by complete, regeneration of bone marrow. High doses of androgens may be useful. The anemia of leukemia is relieved if the leukemic process can be checked by chemotherapy or irradiation. The same is true of the anemia of Hodgkin's disease and other disorders of the lymphoid tissue. In all these conditions the administration of iron, vitamin B_{12}, and folic acid is valueless, and the giving of transfusions is but a temporary measure of limited value. The use of blood transfusions in the treatment of anemia and other hematopoietic disorders is discussed in a separate chapter (Chap. 310).

Adrenocorticosteroids and corticotropin may be very useful in the management of acquired hemolytic anemias, and indirectly, when they affect the leukemic process, they serve to relieve anemia temporarily in acute lymphoblastic leukemia. The corticosteroids and androgens also have some value in other instances of anemia, e.g., certain instances of refractory anemia.

Splenectomy produces permanent relief of the anemia of hereditary spherocytosis and may be valuable in some cases of acquired hemolytic anemia. This is especially true in the more chronic cases and when leukopenia and thrombocytopenia also are present. This operation is also valuable in certain cases characterized by "hypersplenism" (Chap. 317). However, splenectomy should not be

TABLE 58-5
Representative differential counts of bone marrow obtained by puncture

Types of cells	*Normal*[1] *average and range*	*Leukemia, acute*[2,3]	*Leukemia,*[3] *chronic myelocytic*	*Leukemia,*[3] *chronic lymphocytic*	*Multiple myeloma*[4]	*Pernicious anemia*	*Hemolytic anemias*	*Iron deficiency anemia*	*I.T.P.*[7]
Myeloblasts	2.0 (0.3–5.0)	*50–95*[5]	4.0		0.5	0.8	0.8	0.5	
Promyelocytes	5.0 (1.0–8.0)		*10.0*	0.8	1.8	2.7	3.0	2.0	1.5
Myelocytes									
Neutrophilic	12.0 (5.0–19.0)		*26.0*[5]	1.5	1.8	7.7	8.0	9.0	8.0
Eosinophilic	1.5 (0.5–3.0)		2.0	0.7		0.8	2.0	0.8	
Basophilic	0.3 (0.0–0.5)		0.4	0.2		0.3			
Metamyelocytes	22.0 (13.0–32.0)		22.0	8.0	3.3	14.5	18.0	15.0	15.3
Segmented neutrophils	20.0 (7.0–30.0)		29.0	8.5	62.0	14.5	9.0	28.0	31.0
Mature eosinophils	2.0 (0.5–4.0)		0.8	1.0	3.5	0.5	0.6	0.2	0.5
Mature basophils	0.2 (0.0–0.7)		0.4	3.0	1.2	0.2			0.2
Lymphocytes	10.0 (3.0–17.0)		1.4	*60.0*[5]	13.0	9.5	10.0	1.0	2.5
Plasma cells	0.4 (0.0–2.0)				*4.0– 50.0*[4,5]	0.2	0.4	0.7	0.8
Monocytes	2.0 (0.5–5.0)		0.2		0.2	0.3			
Reticulum cells	0.2 (0.1–2.0)		1.2	1.5	1.0	2.0	2.6	0.8	
Mitotic figures	Rare		0.2	0.3		2.7	1.0		
Abnormal cells	0								
Megakaryocytes	0.4 (0.03–3.0)								0.2[6]
Megaloblasts	0					*40.0*[5]			
Pronormoblasts	4.0 (1.0–8.0)			0.2			5.0		4.0
Normoblasts	18.0 (7.0–32.0)		2.4	14.3	9.0	3.0	*43.0*[5]	*40.0*[5]	36.0
M/E ratio	4:1(2.5–5:1)		40:1	1.5:1	8:1	0.7:1.0	*1:1*	1.4:1	1.5:1

[1] *Adapted from MM Wintrobe et al,* Clinical Hematology, *7th ed., Philadelphia: Lea & Febiger, 1974.*

[2] *The immature forms are listed in the table as myeloblasts merely as a matter of convenience. In acute lymphoblastic leukemia the cells are lymphoblasts, not myeloblasts.*

[3] *The bone marrow picture in* aleukemic leukemia *is similar to that of leukemia of the various types, whether or not changes can be demonstrated in the blood.*

[4] *The characteristic cells in multiple myeloma differ somewhat from typical plasma cells in that the nuclear chromatin is relatively fine and the wheel-spoke arrangement of the chromatin is not present; the cytoplasm is basophilic and bright blue, not blue-green as in the plasma cell. A perinuclear clear zone is unusual.*

[5] *The most significant changes are shown in italics.*

[6] *Although the number of megakaryocytes may not appear to be increased, in typical idiopathic thrombocytopenic purpura the majority (64 percent in the case cited) have no platelets about them and most of the remainder (32 percent) have very few.*

[7] *Idiopathic thrombocytopenic purpura.*

TABLE 58-6
Therapeutic agents for anemia

I Specific
  A Vitamin B_{12}
  B Folic acid
  C Iron
  D Desiccated thyroid (?)
  E Ascorbic acid (?)
II Nonspecific
  A Blood transfusions
  B Irradiation and chemotherapy (in leukemia, etc.)
  C Adrenocorticosteroids, androgens
  D Splenectomy

undertaken without a thorough diagnostic study and full knowledge of the risks involved—the operative mortality rate, the possibility of postoperative atelectasis, or other complications, such as postoperative thrombosis. Finally, one must consider the likelihood of failure to achieve the result desired by this operation.

Details of the management of anemia will be discussed in later chapters in connection with the various types of anemia. In dealing with cases of anemia, the value of a diet containing food factors especially useful in blood regeneration, such as animal protein, the B vitamins, ascorbic acid, and iron, should not be overlooked. Such a diet offers much more than can be gained from vitamin capsules. In addition, the physician should ensure a reasonable balance between rest and activity, and attention should be given to the need for reassurance and the necessity of providing the patient with some understanding of his illness. Palliative measures may also be required for various complaints as they arise.

It should be apparent from what has been said already that adequate management of anemia is impossible without a thorough study of the patient and discovery of the nature and cause of the anemia.

59
BLEEDING

T. C. BITHELL
M. M. WINTROBE

Except for that which occurs during menstruation, spontaneous bleeding is abnormal, and blood loss from even large injuries usually is insignificant. This is attributable to the efficiency with which vascular integrity is normally maintained and the rapidity with which it is restored following injury. In general, both these phenomena reflect the function of the hemostatic apparatus. Bleeding may develop spontaneously or following trivial trauma, when any of the components required for normal hemostasis is qualitatively abnormal or quantitatively deficient.

It must be recognized, however, that the adequacy of the hemostatic apparatus is relative. A ruptured esophageal varix will usually result in serious hemorrhage, while the erosion of blood vessels by a gastric tumor will produce less dramatic but continued bleeding, despite the presence of a normal hemostatic mechanism. Thus, bleeding may result from either a failure of the hemostatic apparatus or from localized pathologic processes which produce vascular erosion or malformation. In either case, this symptom is one of the most serious and significant of the cardinal manifestations of disease.

Localized pathologic processes are by far the most common causes of bleeding; such disorders will be discussed here from a general standpoint only. Although less common, bleeding which results from disorders of hemostasis will be covered in more detail.

THE PHYSIOLOGY OF HEMOSTASIS

Hemostasis is the process which stops the flow of blood from injured vessels. Completely efficient hemostasis requires normal blood vessels and extravascular tissue, numerically and functionally normal platelets, and a normal coagulation mechanism. A simplified diagram of the hemostatic process is seen in Fig. 59-1, where for descriptive purposes the process is divided into vascular, platelet, and coagulation "phases."

THE VASCULAR PHASE The active contribution of vessels to hemostasis, as distinguished from the essentially passive maintenance of vascular integrity, still is poorly understood. The most immediate consequence of injury to small vessels is a reduction of blood flow as a result of vasoconstriction and extravasation of blood. Vasoconstriction tends to reduce markedly the blood flow through an injured area. The escape of blood into normal tissue is limited by the extravascular supporting tissue, and the increased tissue pressure ("tamponade") tends to collapse venules and capillaries, which may then rapidly cohere and even become obliterated. The ends of elastic vessels may retract into deeper tissues, and small puncture injuries are immediately sealed because of the elasticity of the skin. These virtually instantaneous phenomena are quickly supplemented by the events of the platelet phase.

THE PLATELET PHASE Within seconds after injury, the platelets begin to adhere to the surface of the injured vessel (*adhesion*). This is the result of a specific biochemical interaction between the platelets and certain subendothelial structures, including collagen fibers, elastin, and the basement membrane. The process of platelet adhesion initiates a complex secretory phenomenon, termed the *release reaction.* This involves the mechanical contraction of the platelet, a marked change in its shape, and the extrusion from storage organelles of numerous biologically active substances, including ATP, ADP, 5-hydroxytryptamine (serotonin), and various enzymes.

Platelets then begin to adhere to one another (*aggregation*), a process which is specifically triggered by ADP. This becomes self-perpetuating as additional ADP is released from aggregated platelets, and rapidly produces a plug or thrombus composed of irreversibly aggregated platelets.

The platelet has been likened to a sponge, since despite its small size, it contains a remarkable variety of

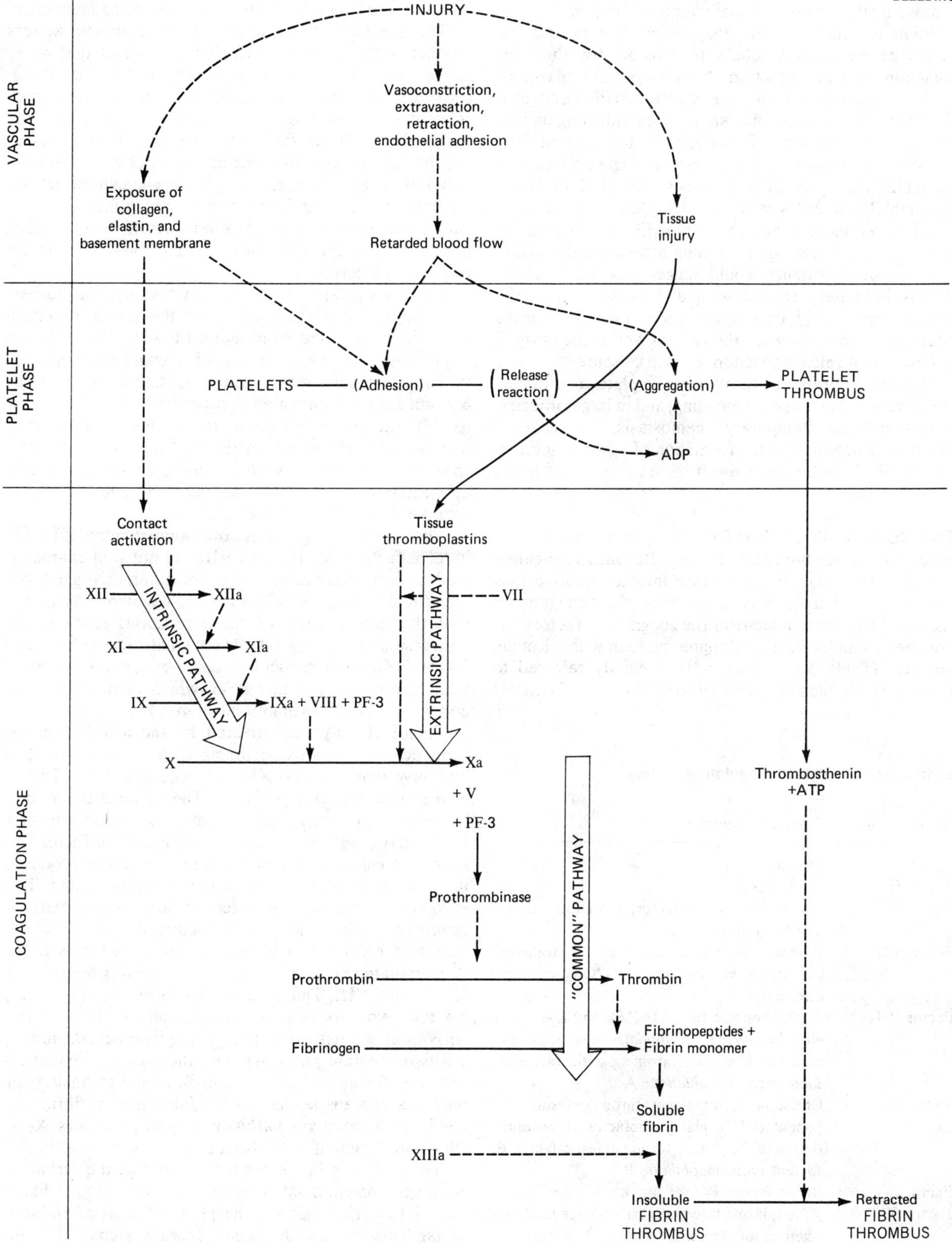

FIGURE 59-1

A simplified diagram of the hemostatic process. Subscript a *denotes the activated forms of the respective factors;* PF-3 *denotes platelet factor 3; solid arrows denote transformation; interrupted arrows denote action. Calcium is required for most processes illustrated but is omitted for the sake of simplicity.*

hemostatically important ingredients. These include, in addition to ADP, various coagulation factors and the substance which is uniquely responsible for the phenomenon of clot retraction. Various platelet phospholipids, generically termed *platelet factor 3 (PF-3)*, are also essential for at least two steps in blood coagulation, namely the activation of factor X by factors IX and VIII, and the formation of prothrombinase (Figure 59-1). It is probable that such PF-3 becomes activated or made "available" on the surface of the platelet membrane, where it serves to bind and orient activated coagulation factors and calcium, thus forming a catalytically active surface. Most evidence would suggest that PF-3 activation is intimately related to and dependent upon the phenomenon of platelet aggregation, but the precise interrelationships between the two, as well as the normally concurrent release reaction, remain obscure.

In small injuries, the formation of a platelet thrombus alone may suffice to arrest bleeding, and in larger injuries, it may provide "temporary" hemostasis. "Permanent" hemostasis depends on the formation of a firm, impermeable fibrin thrombus as a result of the process of blood coagulation.

THE COAGULATION PHASE Blood coagulation is the process by which fluid blood is converted into a coagulum or a clot. This process involves the interaction of various poorly defined trace plasma proteins, the "coagulation factors." The *nomenclature* of the coagulation factors has now been standardized by designating each with a Roman numeral (Table 59-1). Factor III originally referred to tissue thromboplastin, factor IV to calcium, and factor VI to the activated form of factor V. These terms are seldom used. The descriptive terms *fibrinogen* and *prothrombin*, however, are generally preferred to the Roman numerals.

TABLE 59-1
Synonyms for various coagulation factors

International nomenclature	*Common synonyms*
Factor I	Fibrinogen
Factor II	Prothrombin
Factor V	Proaccelerin, labile factor, accelerator globulin (AcG), thrombogen
Factor VII	Proconvertin, stable factor, serum prothrombin conversion accelerator (SPCA), autoprothrombin I
Factor VIII	Antihemophilic factor (AHF), antihemophilic globulin (AHG), thromboplastinogen, platelet cofactor I, plasma thromboplastic factor A, *facteur antihémophilique* A
Factor IX	Christmas factor, plasma thromboplastin component (PTC), platelet cofactor II, autoprothrombin II, plasma thromboplastic factor B, *facteur antihémophilique B*
Factor X	Stuart factor, Prower factor
Factor XI	PTA (plasma thromboplastin antecedent), antihemophilic factor C
Factor XII	Hageman factor
Factor XIII	Fibrin stabilizing factor, Laki-Lorand factor, fibrinase

The mechanism by which the coagulation factors interact is still uncertain. Evidence suggests that many are proenzymes which are normally inert but are transformed into proteolytic enzymes when activated, each sequentially activating the proenzyme next in line (the *"cascade,"* or *"waterfall,"* hypothesis). *Calcium* is essential for most steps in the coagulation process, but remarkably little is known concerning its mechanism of action. Several of the coagulation factors are utilized or consumed during in vitro coagulation (factors V, VIII, XIII, fibrinogen, and prothrombin), whereas the remainder are found in the serum.

Blood coagulation is initiated by two distinct processes, namely, contact activation and the action of certain lipoproteins released from injured tissues (tissue thromboplastins). The phenomenon of *contact activation* involves a molecular rearrangement of factor XII, which as a result acquires enzymatic properties and converts factor XI into its active form. In the test tube, contact activation occurs when shed blood is exposed to electronegative surfaces, such as glass. In vivo, a similar effect may be produced by collagen and other "foreign" extravascular surfaces, e.g., skin.

The reactions which follow contact activation and involve factors XI, IX, and VIII are not well characterized, and there are several plausible alternatives to those illustrated in Fig. 59-1. There is good evidence, however, that the end product of these reactions leads to the conversion of factor X into its enzymatic form. Activated factor X forms a particulate complex (*prothrombinase*) with factor V, Ca^{++}, and PF-3, which then initiates the conversion of prothrombin into thrombin.

Factor X may be activated by the aforementioned sequence of reactions beginning with contact activation and involving factors XII, XI, IX, and VIII. This is termed the *intrinsic pathway*. The production of prothrombinase by means of this pathway is relatively slow but requires neither tissue thromboplastin nor factor VII. A functionally identical prothrombinase can be produced in a matter of seconds by tissue thromboplastins. This involves a sequence of reactions termed the *extrinsic pathway* which, in addition to factors X and V, requires only factor VII. Consequently this pathway bypasses the steps initiated by contact activation involving factors XII, XI, IX, and VIII. Thus, blood coagulation is initiated only by the two processes mentioned above, i.e., contact activation and tissue thromboplastin. It proceeds initially via two separate pathways, i.e., the tissue-activated extrinsic pathway and the contact-activated intrinsic pathway. Later steps leading to the formation of fibrin proceed via a *common pathway*, requiring factors X, V, PF-3, prothrombin, and fibrinogen.

The final step in the coagulation phase, the *thrombin-fibrinogen reaction*, involves the transformation of fibrinogen into fibrin, which is the physical basis of all blood clots. This occurs in three separate steps; viz., the enzymatic proteolysis of fibrinogen by thrombin which removes four peptides (fibrinopeptides), the formation of a visible but unstable fibrin polymer (soluble fibrin), and finally the formation of a stable fibrin polymer (insoluble fibrin) as the result of the action of factor XIII (fibrin-stabilizing factor). Structurally, fibrin resembles the proteins of muscle and skin and provides an extremely strong and stable framework for the "permanent" hemostatic plug.

CLOT RETRACTION This is the result of the mechanical shrinkage of fibrin strands within a clot. The platelets supply both the energy (ATP) and the contractile apparatus required for this process (thrombosthenin, a protein which functions like actomyosin of muscle). Despite the teleologic view that clot retraction may constitute a "physiologic" ligature which pulls the edges of a wound together, the hemostatic significance of the process remains uncertain.

PHYSIOLOGIC INHIBITORS OF COAGULATION AND FIBRINOLYSIS Mechanisms which maintain the normal fluidity of the blood, restrict the processes of hemostasis to the site of injury, and remove the resulting "debris" when its function has been served are homeostatically as important as the processes which lead to hemostasis.

The *physiologic inhibitors of coagulation* are poorly understood substances which neutralize the various enzymes produced during blood coagulation and thus prevent the propagation of a thrombus beyond the wound site. They include plasma inhibitors of most stable enzymes as well as the particulate activators, e.g., antithrombins, antiprothrombinase. These procoagulant substances also are removed from the circulation by cellular mechanisms in the liver and reticuloendothelial system.

Fibrinolysis is usually considered to be the major physiologic means of disposing of fibrin after its hemostatic function has been fulfilled. This process is thus of great importance in wound-healing and in the recanalization of thrombosed vessels. Fibrinolysis (Fig. 59-2) is

accomplished by a proteolytic enzyme (plasmin) which, like the coagulation factors, is formed from an inert precursor in the plasma (plasminogen). Various substances activate plasminogen in vitro, including tissue extracts, certain bacterial enzymes, factor XII*a*, and thrombin. The mechanism of plasminogen activation in vivo is poorly understood. Plasminogen activators are present in vascular endothelium and in the lysosomes of many cells; they are apparently released by a variety of stimuli, including stress, hypoglycemia, anoxia, and even vigorous exercise. Plasminogen is avidly bound to fibrin (Fig. 59-2, step 1) and when activated (step 2), is present both in a bound form and free in the plasma. The antiplasmins in the plasma rapidly destroy free plasmin but are relatively ineffective against bound plasmin, which is thus free to carry out its physiologic function, fibrinolysis (physiologic proteolysis) (step 3). If plasmin is activated in amounts which exceed the capacity of the antiplasmins, however, other proteins in the plasma, including fibrinogen and most of the coagulation factors, may be destroyed. This abnormal process (pathologic proteolysis) (step 4) may lead to a serious coagulation disorder (Chap. 314).

The process of hemostasis is considerably more complicated than the stepwise reactions illustrated in Fig. 59-1 would suggest, and many of the complexities are of fundamental homeostatic importance. For example, although the production of thrombin is a relatively slow process at first, when once formed in even trace amounts,

FIGURE 59-2
A simplified diagram of the fibrinolytic enzyme system. Plasminogen is synonymous with profibrinolysin; plasmin with fibrinolysin. Solid arrows denote transformation; interrupted arrows denote action.

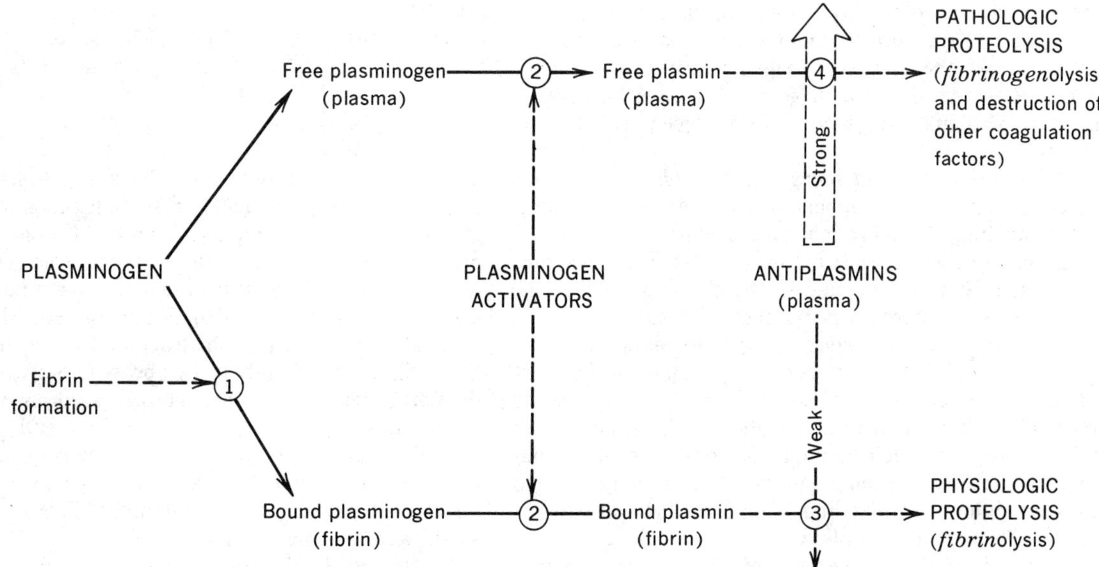

this enzyme acts upon platelets to facilitate the release reaction and further aggregation, and also activates factors V and VIII. As a result of such "autocatalytic" feedback mechanisms, the hemostatic process proceeds at an ever-accelerating rate, and once initiated, fibrin formation is virtually instantaneous. This is of great importance in arresting blood loss from a major injury. In this, and in many other respects, the hemostatic apparatus functions in a remarkably interdependent manner. As a result, hemostatic function compatible with life is maintained even when an essential component is completely lacking, e.g., in hemophilia and severe thrombocytopenia. The physiologic inhibitors of coagulation are also closely integrated with the processes of hemostasis. For example, fibrin, which provides the basis for the permanent thrombus, also restricts the extent of the thrombus by absorbing large amounts of thrombin. Thus, the products of coagulation are themselves potent inhibitors of the process.

TABLE 59-2
The causes of common bleeding manifestations

Location or source of bleeding	*Most common causes*
Gastrointestinal tract (Chap. 41)	Peptic ulcers (Chap. 282), tumors (Chap. 283), gastritis, hiatal hernia, esophageal varices (Chap. 296), colitis, hemorrhoids, hereditary hemorrhagic telangiectasia (Chap. 315)
Respiratory tract (Chap. 35)	Tumors (Chap. 260), pulmonary emboli (Chap. 256), tuberculosis, mitral stenosis (Chap. 239, bronchiectasis (Chap. 253), other infections
Urinary tract (Chap. 48)	Stones (Chap. 275), glomerulonephritis, infections (Chap. 273), cystitis, tumors (Chap. 278), prostatic hypertrophy
Central nervous system (Chap. 22)	Trauma, hypertension, vascular malformations
Vagina (Chap. 49)	Endocrine disorders, tumors, obstetric complications
Nose and paranasal sinuses	Trauma, hypertension, tumors, polyps, inflammation, perforation of nasal septum, hereditary hemorrhagic telangiectasia (Chap. 314)
Ears	Trauma, basal skull fracture
Serous cavities	Trauma, rupture of spleen, ectopic gestation
Nipples	Fissure, breast tumor
Intraocular	Hypertension, nephritis, diabetes, trauma, leukemia
Skin (petechiae and ecchymoses)	Thrombocytopenia or other disorders of blood vessels or platelets (Chap. 313)
Dissecting intramuscular and soft-tissue hematomas	Hemophilia or other coagulation disorders (Chap. 315)
Synovial joints	Hemophilia or other coagulation disorders (Chap. 315)

THE CLINICAL EVALUATION OF BLEEDING

In the evaluation of bleeding, particular attention should be directed to (1) the location or source of the bleeding; (2) the appearance and amount of the blood; (3) the signs and symptoms which result from blood loss; and (4) certain bleeding manifestations which suggest the presence of a disorder of hemostasis.

The most common *locations* and *sources of bleeding*, together with the disorders which are most frequently associated with each, are summarized in Table 59-2. Bleeding into the skin and from the bodily orifices is usually obvious to the patient. An exception is blood loss in the stools, which may be unnoticed but is a common source of significant blood loss.

Hemorrhage into the confined spaces of the central nervous system rapidly produces definite symptoms and neurologic signs. Intracerebral hemorrhage is a common terminating event in hypertension, and spontaneous bleeding into the subarachnoid space from a congenital aneurysm of the circle of Willis may occur in young persons. Subdural hemorrhage must always be kept in mind in patients who have suffered even trivial head trauma.

The *appearance and the amount of blood* should be carefully noted. The appearance of blood originating from the lungs and bronchi varies with the degree of aeration and the presence or absence of mucus, pus, etc. It is usually bright red and frothy in appearance, e.g., hemoptysis in tuberculosis, but if it originates in areas of consolidation or congestion, it appears dark, e.g., the "rusty" sputum of pneumococcal pneumonia. In most infectious processes, the blood is mixed with pus or mucus and is seldom large in amount. An exception is tuberculosis, in which hemoptysis from arteriobronchial fistulas may be alarming. Mitral stenosis may lead to massive pulmonary bleeding when bronchial varicosities rupture (bronchial "apoplexy").

Because of the conversion of red hemoglobin into brown acid hematin by the gastric acid, the appearance of blood from the gastrointestinal tract depends on its site of origin. That originating from the upper gastrointestinal tract (e.g., peptic ulcer, gastritis) resembles coffee grounds if vomited, and if sufficient to discolor the stools, produces a black, tarry appearance (melena). In the presence of achlorhydria or when hematemesis is massive, however, the blood may appear red. Blood which originates in the intestinal tract below the ligament of Treitz imparts a bloody red or brown color to the stools (hematochezia), rather than a tarry appearance. In ulcerative colitis, intussuception, volvulus, and mesenteric thrombosis, a bloody mucoid discharge is usually seen. It must be remembered that blood from the nose, sinuses, or lungs may appear in the stools if swallowed, or may be swallowed and then vomited.

Gastrointestinal bleeding from peptic ulcers, Meckel's diverticula, and esophageal varices may be massive; that which occurs from most polyps, tumors, and infectious processes is seldom so. Esophageal hiatal hernias and hookworm infestation usually produce slow and continued bleeding which is insufficient to change the color of the stools (occult bleeding).

In epistaxis from nasal polyps, various inflammatory processes which produce engorgement of Kiesselbach's plexus, and hypertension, the blood is bright red and bleeding may be rapid. In epistaxis associated with perforation of the cartilagenous nasal septum, e.g., syphilis, small amounts of blood mixed with mucus are usually seen. Profuse and recurrent epistaxis is frequently the initial and often the sole symptom in patients with hereditary hemorrhagic telangiectasia.

Small amounts of blood often impart a smoky color to the urine, e.g., glomerulonephritis, whereas in prostatic hypertrophy, renal stones, etc., the urine may appear grossly bloody, and when bleeding is rapid, clots may be passed per the urethra. With the exception of renal tuberculosis, infections of the urinary tract, e.g., pyelonephritis, are rarely associated with gross bleeding but commonly produce hematuria which is discovered in the examination of the urine sediment (microscopic hematuria).

Abnormal vaginal bleeding is exceedingly common; it may be from an abnormally heavy menstrual period (hypermenorrhea, menorrhagia), e.g., anovulatory cycle bleeding, or may occur between menses (metrorrhagia), e.g., adenocarcinoma of the uterus. Blood originating from the uterus is usually dark and fluid, but may appear bright red and be mixed with clots if bleeding is rapid, e.g., abruptio placentae. Bleeding from disorders of the cervix, e.g., carcinoma or polyps, is usually intermittent and small in amount.

The *signs and symptoms* which result from blood loss per se depend on the amount and the rapidity of the bleeding. Acute and severe blood loss occurring within a matter of a few minutes usually results in syncope, whereas the loss of a comparable amount over a period of hours results in the picture of peripheral circulatory collapse (Chap. 32). In hemorrhage into the serous cavities (e.g., fractures of the pelvis or ribs, rupture of the spleen, ectopic gestation, and hemophilia) large amounts of blood may accumulate in the pleura, peritoneum, or retroperitoneal space, and shock may develop rapidly without external evidence of bleeding. Slow continuous blood loss results in the insidious development of the symptoms of iron-deficiency anemia (Chap.304).

CLINICAL MANIFESTATIONS OF DISORDERED HEMOSTASIS Although any of the varieties of bleeding summarized in Table 59-2 may be encountered, certain *bleeding manifestations* are more or less *characteristic of the disorders of hemostasis.* For example, bleeding into the synovial joints (hemarthrosis) in the absence of obvious trauma, and spontaneous bleeding into the skin are rarely encountered in patients with normal hemostatic function. Moreover, such signs and symptoms fall into two relatively distinct patterns, i.e., those which are most common in disorders of vessels and platelets, and those which are more frequently seen in disorders of coagulation (Table 59-3). *Hemarthrosis* and its sequelae, for example, are almost diagnostic of a severe hereditary coagulation disorder, e.g., hemophilia, and are exceedingly rare in vascular and platelet disorders. Recurrent crops of *petechiae*, on the other hand, are strongly suggestive of an abnormality of the vessels or platelets, e.g., thrombocytopenia, and are rare in the coagulation disorders. Ecchymoses may occur in any disorder of hemostasis, but if they are the result of abnormal blood coagulation, they are usually large and are commonly associated with subcutaneous hematomas which characteristically dissect deeper structures. In hemophilia, such dissecting hematomas may spread to involve an entire limb.

Profuse and often life-threatening hemorrhage following trivial trauma or surgical procedures is a hallmark of the hereditary coagulation disorders, and a history of surgery, major injury, or even multiple tooth extractions without abnormal bleeding is good evidence against the presence of such a disorder. In these conditions, the onset of bleeding is often delayed for several hours. This phenomenon of *delayed bleeding* is rare in disorders of vessels or platelets, where slow but persistent oozing begins immediately following trauma.

The *sex* of the patient, the *age* when abnormal bleeding was first noted, and the *family history* are of particular importance in evaluating the disorders of hemostasis, since most disorders of vessels and platelets are acquired, whereas most serious coagulation disorders are hereditary, and among the latter group, over 90 percent occur only in males. The absence of a family history of bleeding, however, does not exclude the presence of a hereditary coagulation disorder.

THE LABORATORY EVALUATION OF BLEEDING

FINDINGS IN ACUTE BLEEDING The loss of blood stimulates the hematopoietic system (Chap. 303), resulting in leukocytosis with an increase in immature neu-

TABLE 59-3
The clinical distinction between disorders of vessels and platelets and disorders of blood coagulation

Findings	*Disorders of coagulation*	*Disorders of platelets or vessels ("purpuric" disorders)*
Petechiae	Rare	Characteristic
Deep dissecting hematomas	Characteristic	Rare
Superficial ecchymoses	Common; usually large and solitary	Characteristic; usually small and multiple
Hemarthrosis	Characteristic	Rare
Delayed bleeding	Common	Rare
Bleeding from superficial cuts and scratches	Minimal	Profuse
Sex of patient	80–90% of hereditary forms occur only in males	Relatively more common in females
Positive family history	Common	Rare

SOURCE: *Wintrobe et al,* Clinical Hematology, *7th ed., Philadelphia: Lea & Febiger, 1974*

trophils and an elevation of the platelet count (thrombocytosis) and the reticulocyte count (reticulocytosis). Other evidence of accelerated red cell production may be seen in the blood smear (polychromasia and stippling of the erythrocytes), and even nucleated red cells of the normoblastic type may occasionally be found following acute hemorrhage. The erythrocyte sedimentation rate and the indirect-reacting serum bilirubin may be increased as a result of bleeding into the tissues, particularly in the neonate. The laboratory findings in anemia are described elsewhere (Chaps. 58, 303, 304). The various procedures which are valuable in the differential diagnosis of the causes of bleeding, other than those concerned with disorders of hemostasis, are considered in the appropriate chapters, as indicated in Table 59-2.

DIAGNOSIS OF DISORDERS OF HEMOSTASIS No single test is suitable for the laboratory evaluation of the hemostatic process, but numerous methods of varying complexity and utility are now available for testing the vascular, platelet, and coagulation phases of hemostasis.

Tests of the vascular and platelet phases *The enumeration of the platelets* is considerably more difficult than is the case with erythrocytes or leukocytes. This difficulty is due to the tendency of platelets to aggregate in vitro and the difficulty of visualizing these small, highly refractile structures. Among the numerous techniques which have been used, the so-called indirect methods and those hemocytometer methods which employ an ordinary microscope (Rees-Ecker) are very inaccurate and are seldom used. The only satisfactory methods presently available require a phase-contrast microscope (Brecher-Cronkite method) or automated counting equipment, e.g., the Coulter counter. In view of the many variables involved and the relatively large error of even the best methods, the platelet count should always be verified by the examination of a well-prepared peripheral blood smear.

Clot retraction is a specific function of intact platelets. It is usually deficient in thrombocytopenia and in a rare disorder of platelet function (thrombasthenia, Chap. 313). The determination of the presence or absence of clot retraction is not necessary in the diagnosis of thrombocytopenia, however, since the platelets can now be enumerated with reasonable accuracy. Qualitative estimates of the extent of clot retraction can be made by incubating one of the samples obtained for the clotting time, where retraction is normally apparent within 2 hr.

Hemostasis in a small superficial wound, such as that produced in measuring *the bleeding time,* depends on the rate at which a stable platelet thrombus is formed; it thus measures the efficiency of the vascular and platelet phases. Unfortunately, the bleeding time leaves much to be desired in terms of reproducibility, since no two skin areas are exactly the same and it is impossible to produce a truly standard wound. Despite these intrinsic limitations, the bleeding time is valuable when carefully performed. It is prolonged in the majority of patients with von Willebrand's disease and disorders of platelet function. The bleeding time is usually prolonged in thrombocytopenia, but is seldom of diagnostic importance. Contrary to theory, this test is only inconstantly abnormal in the various disorders attributed to dysfunction of the vessels. The bleeding time is occasionally prolonged in severe coagulation disorders.

The *tourniquet test* is an extremely crude index of the efficiency of the vascular and platelet phases. Many normal subjects will develop some petechiae, and many patients with bleeding due to vascular or platelet disorders will not. The tourniquet test correlates poorly with the platelet count, and although it is usually positive in severe thrombocytopenia, petechiae are usually apparent on physical examination of such patients in any case.

The bleeding time, tourniquet test, and platelet count are usually normal in disorders of coagulation.

Tests of the coagulation phase Great care must be used in the collection of blood samples for coagulation studies, and foaming and contamination of the specimen with tissue juice, in particular, must be avoided. A poorly collected blood specimen is a much more common cause of erroneous results than is technical error. Because of the innumerable technical variations which are employed in even the simplest tests, only the normal range for the particular laboratory and technique utilized is meaningful.

In Fig. 59-1, it can be seen that in addition to the coagulation factors normally present in the plasma, the production of fibrin via the intrinsic pathway requires contact activation, factor 3 from platelets or a phospholipid platelet substitute, and calcium. The *partial thromboplastin time (PTT)* is a simple test of this pathway;

FIGURE 59-3
The interpretation of screening tests of blood coagulation.

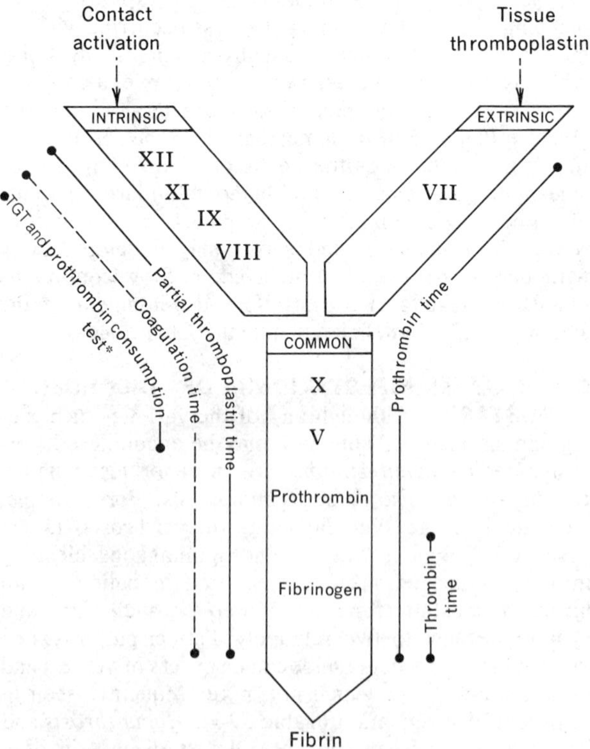

PF-3 is also required for normal prothrombin consumption.

contact activation is provided by a glass tube, and phospholipid is added in the form of a crude cephalin fraction. In the activated PTT, contact activation is further standardized by the addition of various particulate silicates, e.g., kaolin, Celite. When such a mixture is recalcified, fibrin forms at a normal rate only if the factors involved in the intrinsic pathway (i.e., factors XII, XI, IX, and VIII) as well as those required in the common pathway (i.e., factors X, V, prothrombin, and fibrinogen) are present in normal amounts (Fig. 59-3). The platelet substitute provides an excess of phospholipid, and the PTT is thus unaffected by the platelets. Since it bypasses the tissue-activated extrinsic pathway, this test is also unaffected by factor VII. The PTT will be prolonged if the level of any of the required factors is below 15 to 20 percent of normal, and thus detects many patients with mild hereditary coagulation disorders. The test is also prolonged by heparin and by inhibitors of any of the essential factors.

The production of fibrin via the extrinsic pathway (Fig. 59-1) requires only tissue thromboplastin and calcium, in addition to the coagulation factors normally present in the plasma. This pathway is measured by the *plasma prothrombin time,* in which plasma is recalcified in the presence of an excess of tissue thromboplastin. Fibrin forms at a normal rate in such a mixture only if the factors involved in the extrinsic pathway (i.e., factor VII) and the common pathway (i.e., factors X, V, prothrombin, and fibrinogen) are present in normal amounts (Fig. 59-3). This test bypasses the intrinsic pathway and the factors concerned there, i.e., factors XII, XI, IX, and VIII. Since tissue thromboplastin contains phospholipids, the prothrombin time is also insensitive to platelets. Of the five coagulation factors measured in the prothrombin time, three (i.e., factors VII, X, and prothrombin) are depressed by coumarin-like drugs (Chap. 315). As a result, the prothrombin time is the most widely used test for controlling anticoagulant therapy with such drugs. The prothrombin time is relatively more sensitive to deficiencies of factors VII and X than to deficiencies of fibrinogen and prothrombin. It is prolonged by inhibitors of any of the essential factors and by heparin. The expression of the prothrombin time as a "percentage" of normal is not recommended, since the dilution curves used to arrive at this figure may be misleading.

The *clotting time of whole blood* is the most frequently used and most commonly misinterpreted coagulation test. In theory, it would seem that the rate of fibrin formation in whole blood would provide a measurement of the same coagulation factors as the PTT, as well as the platelets, since the coagulation of blood collected without contaminating tissue thromboplastins is initiated by contact with glass, bypasses the extrinsic pathway, and depends on the contained platelets as a source of PF-3 (Fig. 59-3). In fact, the coagulation time measures only the time required to form the first traces of thrombin which suffice to produce a visible clot. Even the small amounts of PF-3 which are available in severe thrombocytopenia are sufficient to produce these requisite traces of thrombin, and consequently, the clotting time is normal even in severe thrombocytopenia. For the same reason, the clotting time is significantly prolonged only in severe deficiencies of coagulation the factors involved in the intrinsic and common pathways (Fig. 59-3) and is usually normal when these factors are present in amounts which exceed 1 percent of normal plasma levels. The clotting time is unaffected by the level of factor VII. It is widely used to monitor heparin therapy.

The *thromboplastin generation test* (TGT) is a valuable method for differentiating between the six factors required for the formation of prothrombinase via the intrinsic pathway, namely, factors XII, XI, IX, VIII, X, and V. Although relatively time-consuming, this technique is helpful in differentiating between the commonest forms of hemophilia—deficiencies of factors VII, IX, and XI (Chap. 315)—since it can be performed without plasma samples from known hemophiliacs. The *prothrombin consumption test* measures the same factors as the TGT but is much less sensitive than the TGT or the PTT. Abnormal results are obtained only when essential factors are below 2 to 3 percent of normal, and the prothrombin consumption test, thus fails, as does the coagulation time, to permit detection of mildly affected patients. The prothrombin consumption test is abnormal in the presence of thrombocytopenia and certain qualitative abnormalities of platelet function.

In the *plasma thrombin time,* preformed thrombin is added to plasma; the time required to form a clot indicates the rate at which the first visible fibrin polymers (soluble fibrin) are formed. The thrombin time is prolonged when the fibrinogen level is low and when the fibrinogen is functionally defective, but is unaffected by the levels of any of the other coagulation factors. It is prolonged by heparin and by abnormal amounts of other antithrombins.

Assays for *plasma fibrinogen concentration* are of increasing clinical importance and have now become widely available. Satisfactory quantitative methods based on gravimetric, nephelometric, and chemical principles have been described, and simple bedside "screening" methods also are available (Fi test—Hyland; Fibrindex—Ortho).

Fibrin-fibrinogen degradation products are protein fragments of various sizes which are produced by the proteolytic degradation of fibrinogen or fibrin by plasmin. These fragments are present in the serum in diffuse intravascular coagulation and abnormal fibrinolysis (Chap. 315), and are thus of considerable diagnostic significance. Assays for fibrinogen degradation products require relatively elaborate techniques, such as hemagglutination inhibition. Unpolymerized fibrin monomers are commonly present in the serum in the same disorders, and may be demonstrated by various *paracoagulation techniques,* e.g., the protamine gelation test.

The *rate of whole blood clot lysis* is a gross measurement of the fibrinolytic enzyme, plasmin. This test requires only the incubation and observation of one of the samples obtained for the clotting time. If fibrinolysis is very rapid, the whole blood clot lysis time may be helpful, but otherwise the time required for lysis, which is normally more than 72 hr, is usually too long to be of diagnostic help. Relatively simple but more definitive tests, such as

TABLE 59-4
The presumptive diagnosis of common bleeding disorders by the "primary" screening tests

	Vascular and platelet phases		*Coagulation phase*			*Common causes*	
Test	*Platelet count*	*Bleeding time*	*Partial thromboplastin time*	*Prothrombin time*	*Presumptive diagnosis*	*Hereditary*	*Acquired*
A	Decreased	Prolonged	Normal	Normal	Thrombocytopenia	Aldrich syndrome, others	ITP, drugs, other secondary forms
B	Normal or elevated	Prolonged	Normal	Normal	Disorder of platelet function	Thrombasthenia, deficient release reaction	Drugs, uremia, dysproteinemias, thrombocythemia
C	Normal	Prolonged	Prolonged	Normal	von Willebrand's disease		
D	Normal	Normal	Prolonged	Normal	Coagulation abnormality in intrinsic pathway	Deficiency of factors VIII, IX, XI, and XII	Inhibitors
E	Normal*	Normal*	Prolonged	Prolonged	Coagulation abnormality in common or multiple pathways	Deficiency of factors V, X, prothrombin and fibrinogen; dysfibrinogenemias	Liver disease, vitamin K deficiency, intravascular coagulation, fibrinogenolysis
F	Normal	Normal	Normal	Prolonged	Coagulation abnormality in extrinsic pathway	Deficiency of factor VII	
G	Normal	Normal	Normal	Normal		Deficiency of factor XIII, telangiectasia	Allergic purpura, scurvy, drugs, autoerythrocyte sensitization

* *May be abnormal in acquired disorders which produce deficiencies of multiple coagulation factors.*
SOURCE: *Wintrobe et al,* Clinical Hematology, *7th ed., Philadelphia: Lea & Febiger, 1974*

the euglobulin lysis time, are available for the study of abnormal fibrinolysis and for monitoring therapy with thrombolytic agents.

Results of all the aforementioned tests of blood coagulation are usually normal in disorders of the vessels or the platelets.

INITIAL LABORATORY STUDY OF THE DISORDERS OF HEMOSTASIS

The definitive diagnosis of the disorders of hemostasis often requires a specially equipped laboratory and relatively elaborate methods. However, the most essential information can usually be obtained from the four simple tests summarized in Table 59-4. The platelet count and the bleeding time together provide the most reliable and reproducible tests of the vascular and platelet phases. The PTT measures all the coagulation factors involved in the intrinsic and common pathways and is generally accepted as the best single screening test for disorders of blood coagulation. This test, and its various modifications, when accurately performed, will be abnormal in over 90 percent of patients with abnormalities of blood coagulation. The plasma prothrombin time provides valuable ancillary information, since it assesses the extrinsic as well as the common pathway.

In view of their availability, simplicity, and low cost, these four tests are admirably suited to serve as primary screening tests. They should be the first laboratory tests obtained, since they direct further laboratory study, and when interpreted in the light of a careful history, a thorough physical examination, and the laws of probability, they categorize the disorder and provide a valuable "presumptive" diagnosis (Table 59-4); i.e., thrombocytopenia, a disorder of the vessels, a qualitative disorder of platelet function, von Willebrand's disease, or a coagulation disorder. Abnormalities of coagulation can usually be localized to one of the three pathways and the factors involved therein if a single abnormality is present, as in most hereditary forms.

Further details concerning the clinical picture, differential diagnosis, and treatment of the various hemorrhagic disorders will be found in subsequent sections concerned with the disorders of blood coagulation (Chap. 315) and disorders of vessels and platelets (Chap. 313).

REFERENCES

BIGGS R, MACFARLANE RG: *Human Blood Coagulation,* 4th ed., Philadelphia: Davis, 1972

BOWIE EJW et al: *Mayo Clinic Laboratory Manual of Hemostasis,* Philadelphia: Saunders, 1971

HIRSHY J, DOERY JCG: Platelet function in health and disease. Prog Hematol 7:185, 1972

RATNOFF OD: *Bleeding Syndromes. A Clinical Manual,* Springfield, Ill.: Charles C Thomas, 1960

WINTROBE MM et al: *Clinical Hematology,* 7th ed., Philadelphia: Lea & Febiger, 1974

60 ENLARGEMENT OF LYMPH NODES AND SPLEEN

M. M. WINTROBE
D. R. BOGGS

LYMPH NODES There are some 500 to 600 *lymph nodes* in the body, varying from less than 1 mm to 1 to 2 cm in size. These structures afford mechanical filtration for the lymph stream, removing cellular debris, foreign particles, and bacteria which may have gained access to the lymph from the various structures drained by the lymph channels. In the normal individual very few lymph nodes are palpable, even on careful physical examination. However, the access of disease-producing bacteria, certain viruses, or other antigens leads to antibody production, with concomitant proliferation in the nodes. Infection of the nodes may also occur, and various types of malignant cells can proliferate there. It has been aptly stated that in the exercise of their function the lymph nodes may sacrifice their own integrity for the welfare of the organism as a whole. One may wonder whether they may not also nourish neoplastic tissue at their own expense.

These structures are also the site of formation of lymphocytes and of antibodies. Furthermore, in certain diseases, lymph nodes may be the site of formation of erythrocytes, neutrophils, and platelets. This is known as myeloid metaplasia and is a reflection of embryonal hematopoietic potentialities. This reaction may be accompanied by lymph node enlargement.

On physical examination the cervical, supraclavicular, axillary, and inguinal nodes are those most often found to be enlarged. Other lymph nodes which may be found to be enlarged on palpation are the epitrochlear, brachial, and very rarely, the popliteal. Enlargement of mediastinal nodes is detected by chest roentgenography. *Lymphangiography* is a technique in which a radiopaque dye is injected into lymphatic channels in the feet. The dye drains into inguinal, iliac, and paraaortic lymph node chains, thereby permitting enlarged nodes to be visualized.

Causes of lymph node enlargement Enlargement of the lymph nodes may be purely local, or it may be widespread. Such enlargement may be accompanied by all the signs of acute inflammation, such as heat, reddening of overlying skin, and tenderness. The nodes may remain discrete, or they may fuse with one another as the result of perilymphangitis. Necrosis may even ensue and may be followed by rupture of the nodes and the formation of a sinus. Rapidly enlarging nodes are likely to be tender, reflecting antibody formation, or there may be actual infection within the node. Inflammation of the skin overlying the tender nodes is usually indicative of an infected node. On the other hand, very great enlargement of the lymph nodes, usually due to infiltration with malignant cells, may take place in the absence of any signs of inflammation.

Enlarged lymph nodes may be discrete or matted together; they may be extremely hard or only moderately so, or they may even be soft or feel cystic. Nontender nodes which feel hard and matted together usually contain metastatic carcinoma or a very aggressive intrinsic neoplasm such as reticulum cell sarcoma. Noninflamed, enlarged lymph nodes usually do not produce serious symptoms unless their enlargement obstructs some vital passageway. Thus, mediastinal lymphadenopathy may be very great and yet produce no symptoms unless the venae cavae or bronchi are obstructed.

The chief causes of lymph node enlargement are listed in Table 60-1.

Infection may cause lymph node enlargement as a result of antibody response or of granulomatous hyperplasia in response to infection within the node; or there may be suppurative infection of the node. Localized infections ordinarily induce lymph node enlargement which is limited to the regional nodes draining the infected area. If infection is systemic, whether it is due to steady "seeding" of the bloodstream with bacteria (as in bacterial endocarditis) or to a systemic virus infection (such as infectious mononucleosis, measles, or chickenpox), generalized lymph node enlargement may be present. This, however, is not of the same degree in all parts of the body. In infectious mononucleosis, for example, generalized lymph node enlargement is characteristic, but cervical glandular enlargement is often more striking than that found elsewhere in the body.

Of the *chronic infections,* syphilis and tuberculosis may produce lymphadenopathy. In syphilis, firm, painless swelling is found in the regional lymph nodes draining the primary lesion; generalized, firm, shotty, nontender nodes accompany the secondary state; and glandular swelling of various degrees may accompany the late stages or the congenital form. Tuberculosis most often involves the cervical, mediastinal, or mesenteric glands. The enlarge-

TABLE 60-1
Chief causes of lymph node enlargement

I Antigenic challenge
- *A* Infection
  - *1* Regional lymph node enlargement in the area draining a localized infection
  - *2* Generalized lymph node enlargement with systemic infection
- *B* Allergic reactions such as serum sickness
- *C* Diseases associated with "autoimmunity" such as systemic lupus erythematosus

II Suppurative infections of lymph nodes [e.g., streptococcus, staphylococcus, *Pasteurella tularensis, Treponema pallidum,* virus of lymphogranuloma venereum, *Pasteurella pestis* (plague)]

III Granuloma formation
- *A* Due to infections such as tuberculosis, syphilis, and histoplasmosis
- *B* Disease of unknown etiology such as sarcoid

IV Primary lymph node diseases: Hodgkin's disease, lymphosarcoma, reticulum cell sarcoma, etc.

V Leukemia

VI Metastases from malignant disease in breast, stomach, etc.

VII Congenital abnormalities (lymphangiomas)

ment usually is slowly progressive and is easily confused with that caused by Hodgkin's disease. However, tuberculous glands frequently are tender and firm and adhere to one another. Sometimes breakdown of the overlying skin occurs, leading to the production of a stubborn draining sinus. Rarely the lymph node enlargement is acute and rapidly developing, and in such cases the glands may remain discrete and freely movable. Other chronic infections in which glandular swelling may be prominent include fungous infections and filariasis.

Serum sickness should not be overlooked as a cause of lymphadenopathy, particularly since it is usually accompanied by fever.

Hodgkin's disease, lymphosarcoma, reticulum cell sarcoma, and giant follicular lymphoma are frequently classed under the single heading of primary lymph node diseases or *"lymphomas"* because, clinically, they are very similar. In these conditions the lymph node enlargement is characteristically localized at first; only as the disease progresses does wider dissemination occur. The node enlargement usually is discrete and firm and ranges greatly indegree. When the adenopathy becomes widespread, nodes may be discovered in locations where the presence of lymphoid tissue may not have been suspected. Such cases of lymph node enlargement are distinguished from those due to leukemia chiefly by the changes in the blood characteristically seen in the latter condition, but also by the asymmetry of the swellings which is often seen in the lymphomas. In leukemia, lymph node enlargement usually is generalized and symmetric, although, especially in acute leukemia, adenopathy may be much more prominent in the neck than elsewhere. Tenderness of lymph nodes suggests infection rather than one of the lymphomas, leukemia, or metastatic involvement. However, some degree of tenderness, as well as pain, may be encountered when the glands have enlarged rapidly, especially in Hodgkin's disease. In the last condition, the presence of connective and fibrous tissue in the nodes may cause them to be harder than usual; occasionally they may have the consistency of cartilage.

In *sarcoidosis* the pre- and postauricular lymph nodes, the submaxillary, submental, epitrochlear, and paratracheal glands are more often affected than in Hodgkin's disease. A history of involvement of the eyes and of the parotid glands (uveoparotid fever) suggests sarcoid, and punched-out areas in the small bones of the hands and feet may be demonstrable by roentgenography (see Chap. 223).

Treatment of convulsive disorders with various *hydantoin or hydantoin-like drugs* may produce a clinical and pathologic syndrome which closely mimics the lymphomas. Lymph node hyperplasia also is encountered in Addison's disease, hyperthyroidism, and hypopituitarism.

Lymph node enlargement due to *metastatic carcinoma,* as a rule, is distinctly localized, and the glandular swelling ordinarily is very hard. Such enlargement may involve nodes which are easily discovered, such as those of the axilla in cases of carcinoma of the breast. Or the lymphadenopathy may be more often heard about than seen, such as Virchow's sentinel node above the clavicle in cases of carcinoma of the stomach or other abdominal organs. When the adenopathy is present in some region of the body inaccessible to physical examination, it is discoverable only by roentgenography or through the indirect effects of pressure produced by enlargement of the nodes.

Of congenital abnormalities which may lead to lymphoid enlargement, simple or capillary lymphangiomas, cavernous lymphangiomas, and the cystic form (cystic hygroma) may be mentioned.

Differential diagnosis of lymph node enlargement

It should be evident from this discussion that the discovery of the cause of lymph node enlargement requires a thorough examination of the patient.

The location of the glandular enlargement may suggest the site of origin of the disease and may sometimes give some clue to its nature. Acute cervical adenitis should direct attention to the mouth and pharynx, mastoid adenitis to scalp infections, axillary adenitis to the upper extremity and the breast, epitrochlear enlargement to involvement of the ulnar side of the hand or forearm, and inguinal swelling to the lower extremities and genitalia. The examination of the patient must be painstaking, for sometimes secondary glandular enlargement may be much more prominent than the primary cause. Thus, for example, cervical metastases from a nasopharyngeal tumor usually overshadow the primary growth, which is characteristically small and easily overlooked unless a careful nasopharyngoscopic examination is made. The study of the patient should include careful palpation of the sternum for tenderness and of the abdomen for hepatic or splenic enlargement, as well as examination of the chest for evidence of mediastinal tumor. Rectal and pelvic examination must not be overlooked.

Important laboratory procedures include the serologic test for syphilis; examination of the blood for agglutination reactions; and blood culture and culture of the throat, sputum, and other possible sources which might reveal infection; as well as examination of the blood and sometimes of the bone marrow for morphologic evidences of disease. Skin tests, such as tuberculin, histoplasmin, and coccidioidin, may also need to be performed.

If a disease known to be associated with lymph node enlargement is uncovered by the above studies, it is reasonable to assume that the enlarged nodes are due to this cause. However, if a definitive diagnosis is not made or if doubt exists, a *lymph node biopsy* should be performed. In addition to microscopic examination of the node, culture for bacteria and fungi may be helpful. As a general rule, if more than one area of lymph node enlargement is present, the cervical and supraclavicular areas are better sites for a lymph node biopsy than are the axillary and inguinal areas. Pathologic interpretation of an inguinal node biopsy often proves difficult, presumably because of the frequency with which this area is called upon to respond to the challenge of chronically traumatized feet and legs of man. The surgeon may have difficulty finding axillary nodes unless they are quite enlarged.

In patients with pulmonary lesions of unknown cause or with a known but apparently localized carcinoma of the lung, mediastinoscopy and biopsy of mediastinal nodes may be required (Chap. 260).

THE SPLEEN A palpable spleen is always a somewhat alarming finding because of the association of splenomegaly with leukemia and lymphoma. If the spleen is palpable, it is presumed to be enlarged. However, a palpable spleen does not necessarily imply the presence of disease. Thus, McIntyre and Ebaugh, as a part of a routine physical examination, were able to palpate the spleen in 3 percent of entering college freshmen. Three years later, 30 percent of these students still had a palpable spleen and had no discernible disease.

Structure and function of the spleen The pulp of the spleen is composed of (1) anastomosing strands of lymphoid tissue (white pulp), (2) a reticular network and branching multipolar cells which are placed about blood sinuses and intermingle with the strands of lymphoid tissue (red pulp), and (3) lymphocytes, granulocytes, and erythrocytes. The spleen is a very vascular organ and is capable of changing substantially in size, depending on its content of blood. It is also contractile; its capsule contains a small amount of elastic tissue. The circulation of the spleen is unique. In the lymphatic sheath, capillaries branch at right angles from arterioles. These capillaries rarely contain blood cells but rather appear to "skim" plasma from the arteriole. They serve as afferent lymphatics terminating within the lymphatic sheath. The sinusoidal structure of the red pulp consists of wide sinuses through which blood flow is rapid. These alternate with much narrower sinuses, termed *cords,* in which only a small amount of blood is normally present. The large sinuses and the cords are separated by a basement membrane containing regularly spaced perforations which provide direct communication between the two types of sinuses. The cords are blind sinuses, and the fenestrations connecting them with the large sinuses provide the only exit for blood cells.

Arterioles terminate in the marginal zone of concentric flattened cells which loosely separates the white and red pulp. Erythrocytes course through the spleen by filtering through these flattened cells and then enter and rapidly traverse the large sinuses. A lesser number of red blood cells circulate slowly through the smaller sinuses (cords). These cells enter the cords from a few arterioles which terminate in the cords or from the marginal zone or the large sinuses through perforations of the basement membrane. Normally, only a small proportion of the blood, perhaps 20 ml, is in the cords.

The spleen, as a lymphoid organ, participates in the cellular events leading to antibody formation. However, splenectomy leads to no detectable defect in antibody production in adults or adolescents. It has been claimed that young children who have been splenectomized are more than normally susceptible to infection.

If the spleen is removed, certain characteristic changes in blood cells are observed. Immediately following splenectomy, normoblasts, target cells, and erythrocytes with Howell-Jolly bodies, diffuse basophilia, basophilic stippling, or siderotic granules appear in the blood. Howell-Jolly bodies and target cells are usually demonstrable indefinitely in such patients, but other erythrocyte abnormalities tend to disappear. Neutrophilia and thrombocytosis are present immediately after splenectomy but disappear in a few weeks in most patients. Changes in the blood following splenectomy have been cited as evidence that the spleen exerts an inhibitory action on the bone marrow. Definitive experimental evidence for any humoral influence by the spleen on the bone marrow has not been forthcoming. Insofar as the red blood cell changes are concerned, there is experimental evidence to support the view that the spleen normally removes the forms which are not usually seen in the blood. The primary site of destruction of senescent erythrocytes is the spleen.

Approximately one-third of the blood platelets are within the splenic circulation, a much higher figure than that for erythrocytes. There is evidence to suggest that the youngest and presumably most viable platelets are preferentially sequestered by the spleen. When the spleen is enlarged, the proportion of the total body pool of platelets which is in the spleen may increase, resulting in thrombocytopenia. Thrombocytopenia due to accelerated rates of platelet destruction by the spleen occurs when platelets are coated with antibody. There is no evidence that the normal spleen sequesters a significant number of neutrophils, and the mechanism of neutropenia which may develop in association with splenomegaly has not been determined.

During embryonic life the spleen plays an important part in blood formation, and the potentialities of this organ for blood formation persist even in adult life. In certain circumstances, foci of extramedullary blood formation can be found in the spleen; thus, when the functional activity of the bone marrow is impaired by processes such as idiopathic myelofibrosis, the hematopoietic potentiality of the spleen may become an important asset.

Enlargement of the spleen This may occur under a great variety of circumstances. The chief ones are listed in Table 60-2.

Of greatest frequency is the enlargement of the spleen which occurs in association with infections. The *"acute splenic tumor"* which accompanies various systemic infections such as typhoid fever and septicemia are examples. It is thought that such splenic enlargement is due to cellular proliferation accompanying antibody formation. Like lymph node enlargement, splenic enlargement is frequently encountered in various contagious diseases and is often seen in infectious mononucleosis. Likewise, various subacute infections, notably bacterial endocarditis, are characteristically accompanied by enlargement of the spleen. *Abscess* of the spleen is rare and is usually secondary to pyemia arising from some other site. Frequently multiple and unrecognized, it is unusual for a splenic abscess to achieve prominence and produce local symptoms such as pain, elevation of the left leaf of the diaphragm, or rupture into the peritoneal cavity.

Malaria is, perhaps, the commonest cause of splenic enlargement when the world population is considered. Infection with other parasites which leads to splenic enlargement includes leishmaniasis, trypanosomiasis, and schistosomiasis. In kala-azar the spleen may be huge.

TABLE 60-2
Chief causes of splenomegaly

I Inflammatory splenomegaly
- *A* "Acute splenic tumor": many acute and subacute infections
  - *1* Bacterial (typhoid, septicemias, subacute bacterial endocarditis, abscess, etc.)
  - *2* Viral and miscellaneous (contagious diseases, infectious mononucleosis)
- *B* Chronic infections (tuberculosis, syphilis, brucellosis, histoplasmosis, malaria, schistosomiasis, leishmaniasis, trypanosomiasis, etc.)
- *C* Miscellaneous diseases (lupus erythematosus, rheumatoid arthritis, sarcoidosis, histiocytosis X, etc.)

II Congestive splenomegaly (Banti's syndrome)
- *A* Cirrhosis of liver
- *B* Thrombosis or stenosis, portal or splenic veins

III Hyperplastic splenomegaly
- *A* Hemolytic anemias, congenital and acquired
- *B* Thalassemia and certain hemoglobinopathies
- *C* Myelofibrosis, myelophthisic anemias
- *D* Polycythemia vera
- *E* Miscellaneous chronic anemias (pernicious anemia, chronic iron deficiency, "pyridoxine-responsive anemia," etc.)
- *F* Thrombocytopenic purpura
- *G* Obscure disorders ("big spleen syndrome," "primary splenic neutropenia," and "panhematopenia")

IV Infiltrative splenomegaly
- *A* Gaucher's disease, Niemann-Pick disease
- *B* Amyloidosis, hemosiderosis

V Neoplasms and cysts
- *A* True cysts (dermoid, echinococcus, etc.)
- *B* False cysts (hemorrhagic, serous, inflammatory, degenerative)
- *C* Benign tumors (lymphangioma, hemangioma, etc.)
- *D* Leukemia, lymphomas
- *E* Malignant tumors (direct invasion or metastatic)

Primary tuberculous splenomegaly is extremely rare, but slight enlargement of the spleen accompanying a widespread tuberculous infection is by no means unusual. Splenomegaly may occur in connection with syphilis, especially congenital syphilis. Enlargement of this organ may also accompany the late stages of syphilis in association with gummas or amyloidosis. Rheumatoid arthritis, brucellosis, and sarcoidosis are other chronic diseases which may be accompanied by splenic enlargement. Splenic enlargement has been observed in about 25 percent of cases of disseminated lupus erythematosus.

The vascularity of the spleen and its location in the portal bed make this organ liable to swelling as the result of increased venous pressure in that region. Such types of enlargement of the spleen may be classed under the general heading of "congestive splenomegaly" and include the syndromes known as *Banti's disease and splenic anemia,* as well as the splenic enlargement which accompanies cirrhosis of the liver and thrombosis of the splenic or portal vein (Chap. 317) and that which may be associated with cardiac failure.

The functions of the spleen in relation to the hematopoietic system result in enlargement of this organ when there is increased blood destruction (acute and chronic hemolytic anemias) or chronic anemia of various types such as pernicious anemia, chronic hypochromic anemia, myelophthisic anemia, thalassemia, hemoglobin-C disease, and other hemoglobinopathies. In polycythemia vera splenomegaly is often encountered, and this finding helps to distinguish the primary disorder from secondary forms of polycythemia, where splenic enlargement is rare. The lymphatic hyperplasia which is associated with hyperthyroidism may be accompanied by splenomegaly. The spleen is also enlarged in myelofibrosis, primary splenic neutropenia, and primary splenic panhematopenia (Chap. 317).

Certain rare diseases such as Gaucher's disease and Niemann-Pick disease are characterized by splenic enlargement. In these conditons the swelling of the organ is probably due to the excessive storage of normal and abnormal metabolic products in the cells of the spleen (see Chap. 317). Deposition of amyloid, whether due to primary or secondary amyloidosis, may produce splenomegaly.

Like other organs, the spleen may be enlarged because of neoplasms of various types. The leukemias, particularly chronic myelocytic and chronic lymphocytic leukemia, regularly produce splenomegaly. Hodgkin's disease, lymphosarcoma, reticulum cell sarcoma, and giant follicular lymphoma are frequent causes of splenomegaly. Other metastatic tumors only rarely cause splenomegaly. Direct extension from carcinoma of the stomach and hematogenous spread from the stomach, lung, pancreas, and breast and from malignant melanoma may occur. Other tumors that may involve the spleen include lymphangioma, hemangioma and endothelial sarcoma (lymphangiosarcoma), fibrosarcoma, leiomyosarcoma, and myoma. A subcapsular cavernous hemangioma may rupture into the peritoneal cavity and produce acute hemorrhagic shock.

Cysts of the spleen may be of parasitic origin or nonparasitic. Of the latter, those containing serous or hemorrhagic fluid and due to trauma are the commonest. They may sometimes be identified roentgenographically because of calcification of the wall. Echinococcus cysts occur more rarely in the spleen than in the liver. "True" cysts are formed from embryonal defects or rests and include dermoids and mesenchymal inclusion cysts.

Differential diagnosis of splenomegaly A thorough physical examination, together with the history and the examination of the blood, will serve to differentiate many of the causes of splenomegaly which have been outlined. Sometimes additional procedures may be required, such as blood culture, marrow aspiration or biopsy, a roentgenogram of the chest, serologic tests including those for syphilis, liver function tests, and spleen or lymph node biopsy. Since certain of the causes of splenomegaly do not induce diagnostic pathologic changes in the spleen, a splenic aspiration or splenic biopsy will not necessarily yield a diagnosis. In most instances the cause of splenomegaly is not determined by studying the spleen itself but by detecting diseases which are known to be associated with splenomegaly.

The absence of fever is more helpful in differential diagnosis here than is its presence, since most of the conditions which have been mentioned may be accompanied by fever. However, at times, as in malaria and undulant fever, the characteristic temperature curve is very helpful in making the diagnosis. In the septicemias the splenic enlargement is, as a rule, obviously only a minor feature of the whole clinical picture. The exanthemas are recognized by the respective characteristic changes in the skin. In their absence the skin should be inspected carefully for evidence of the petechiae which may accompany acute leukemia, thrombocytopenic purpura, or other hematopoietic disorders; the red petechiae occurring in crops together with the larger, slightly nodular and tender Osler nodes so characteristic of subacute bacterial endocarditis; or the spider telangiectases which accompany long-standing liver disease. The plum-red "cyanosis" of polycythemia vera can hardly be overlooked.

Moderate lymph node enlargement accompanying splenomegaly is seen in many infectious diseases as well as in leukemia, but as asymmetric enlargement should arouse suspicion of Hodgkin's disease or lymphosarcoma. Great enlargement of the lymph nodes is seen in the last-named conditions as well as in chronic leukemia, especially in the lymphocytic form. The discovery of icterus suggests hemolytic anemia as a cause or, if there is little or no anemia and the splenic enlargement is only slight, infectious hepatitis. The splenomegaly associated with the Banti syndrome (congestive splenomegaly) is usually substantial in degree, and jaundice may or may not be present under these circumstances.

Lesions in the mucous membranes accompanying splenic enlargement are seen in measles (Koplik's spots), secondary syphilis (mucous patches), infectious mononucleosis (infection of the throat, tonsillar enlargement, sometimes signs of Vincent's angina), and acute leukemia (swollen, thickened gums which may be bleeding or purplish in color). In the leukemias, sternal tenderness may be quite pronounced.

The discovery of very great enlargement of the spleen tends to rule out the acute splenic tumor of various systemic infections, although sometimes the spleen may extend 4 to 6 cm below the costal margin in septicemia and in subacute bacterial endocarditis. Huge spleens are encountered in the chronic leukemias, congestive splenomegaly, kala-azar, schistosomiasis, Gaucher's disease, Hodgkin's disease and lymphosarcoma, and myelofibrosis.

Examination of the blood may indicate at once the nature of the disorder, as in malaria, the frank leukemias, or infectious mononucleosis. The discovery of icterus will lead to examination of the blood smear, a reticulocyte count, examination of the stools and urine for the products of blood destruction, an erythrocyte fragility test, and other studies (see Chap. 306) to rule out the various hemolytic anemias. The discovery of leukopenia should lead to the consideration of malaria, "aleukemic" leukemia, the Banti syndrome, typhoid fever, histoplasmosis, and leishmaniasis. The white blood cell count may sometimes be low also in infectious mononucleosis and in some cases of chronic hemolytic anemia. The demonstration of thrombocytopenia, as well as prolonged bleeding time, poor clot retraction, and positive tourniquet test result, is an important finding, for it suggests acute leukemia. In that condition immature leukocytes will be found in the blood. In the "aleukemic" form, immature cells are absent from the blood or very scarce, but they are readily demonstrated by sternal puncture. In idiopathic thrombocytopenic purpura, the spleen is barely palpable in about 33 percent of cases, but it is never very large. Thrombocytopenia only very rarely accompanies infectious mononucleosis and, though present in other conditions such as pernicious anemia, chronic hypochromic anemia, chronic hemolytic anemias, myelophthisic anemia, the Banti syndrome, Hodgkin's disease, and the related lymph node disorders, it is rarely severe in these diseases.

Sternal puncture may be very helpful if "aleukemic" leukemia, leishmaniasis, or Gaucher's disease is being considered seriously, for the characteristic cells or causative organisms may be demonstrated in this way. Sternal puncture does not often reveal malaria when the parasites have eluded careful study of the blood, but sometimes positive blood cultures for bacteria are obtained by this means when the usual method has failed. Needle biopsy of bone marrow should be done if myelofibrosis or one of the lymphomas is a consideration. Splenic puncture is helpful when parasites, storage cells, signs of myeloid metaplasia, or granulomas are found, but this procedure should not be undertaken when hemorrhagic manifestations are present or in the absence of evidence of distinct splenic enlargement.

Various disorders of the spleen are discussed in a later chapter (Chap. 317).

REFERENCES

Jandl JH, Aster RH: Increased splenic pooling and the pathogenesis of hypersplenism. Am J Med Sci 253:383, 1967

McIntyre OR, Ebaugh FG jr.: Palpable spleens in college freshmen. Ann Intern Med 66:301, 1967

Saltzstein SL, Ackerman LV: Lymphadenopathy induced by anticonvulsant drugs. Cancer 12:164, 1959

Wintrobe MM et al: *Clinical Hematology*, 7th ed., Philadelphia: Lea & Febiger, 1974

61 ALTERATIONS IN LEUKOCYTES

DANE R. BOGGS
M. M. WINTROBE

Unlike the red corpuscles, the leukocytes do not carry out their chief functions in the circulating blood. For them the circulation is mainly a transport system through which they pass from the sites where they are formed to the locations where they are needed. The time that the leukocytes spend in the blood does not reflect their life span, and exact life spans for different types of leukocytes are not known. Their fate, like that of soldiers, probably depends as much on external factors as on the ultimate wearing out of internal metabolic activities.

Little is known about the factors which normally maintain the leukocyte count and the proportion of different types of leukocytes within a rather narrow range of values, nor is much known about the factors which cause these to change. However, it has been possible to infer a great deal about the functions of the leukocytes by observing the alterations associated with various physiologic states and with different disease entities. In many respects the leukocyte and differential counts serve as mirrors which reflect changes taking place in the body, and thereby, these determinations have proved to be of immense value in differential diagnosis.

The only known function of the leukocytic systems is to defend the body from foreign material by means of phagocytosis and antibody formation. These are interrelated functions; phagocytosis is enhanced by antibody specific for the substance being phagocytized, and phagocytosis of antigen may be an initiating step in antibody production. Neutrophils, monocytes, eosinophils, and basophils are phagocytes, while lymphocytes and plasma cells are concerned with antibody production. Each of these six types of leukocytes probably plays a distinct and unique role in body defense mechanisms, although the role of basophils and eosinophils is unclear.

The concentration in blood of each specific type of leukocyte is a much more meaningful value than is total white blood cell count (total leukocyte concentration). The mean and 95 percent confidence limits of various blood leukocytes as found in 291 prisoners from the Utah State Prison are given in Table 61-1. The number of eosinophils and basophils in the blood is so small that the normal range encompasses zero. Thus, eosinopenia and basopenia cannot be determined from results of routine blood examination.

In this chapter current concepts of the physiology of each of the leukocytic systems will be reviewed, and the diagnostic and clinical significance of changes in the concentration of the various blood leukocytes will be considered.

TABLE 61-1
Normal values for concentration* of blood leukocytes

Cell type	*Mean (cells/μl)*	*95% confidence limits (cells/μl)*
Neutrophil	3,650	1,830–7,250
Lymphocyte	2,500	1,500–4,000
Monocyte	430	200–950
Eosinophil	150	0–700
Basophil	30	0–150

* *Total leukocyte counts from venous blood samples were done in a "Coulter counter," and 200 leukocytes were differentiated on Wright's-stained blood smears made on cover glass.*

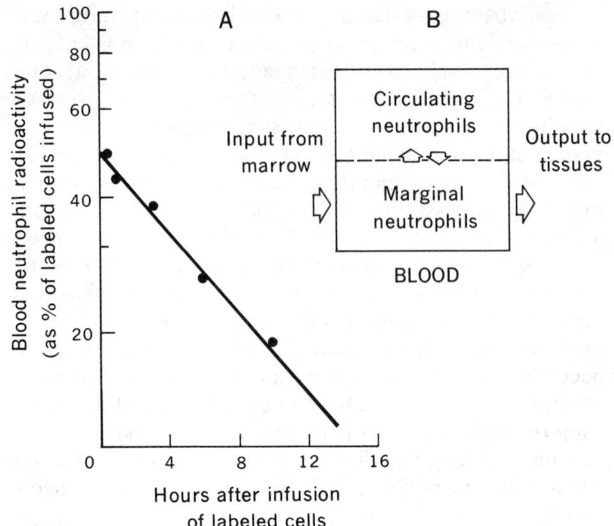

FIGURE 61-1
Disappearance of ^{32}DFP-labeled neutrophils in a normal subject (A) *and a model of blood neutrophil kinetics* (B).

THE PHAGOCYTIC SYSTEM

Neutrophils

NEUTROPHIL PHYSIOLOGY During the first half of the last century a number of investigators noted that leukocytes within the confines of blood vessels often are marginated along venule and capillary walls. Modern techniques have made it possible to show that in man approximately one-half of the intravascular neutrophils are marginated and one-half circulate freely (Fig. 61-1*B*). Blood neutrophil concentration, as determined in venous samples, measures the circulating but not the marginal pool.

Neutrophils enter the blood from a storage reservoir in the bone marrow and leave the blood in random fashion after an average intravascular sojourn of 10 hr (Fig. 61-1*A*). They do not return to the blood after leaving it. There are many more neutrophils and neutrophil precursors in the bone marrow than in the blood. Bone marrow neutrophils comprise two pools of cells, the mitotic production pool and the postmitotic maturation and storage pool (Fig. 61-2). Morphologic subdivisions within these pools necessarily are somewhat arbitrary. The production pool may be considered as consisting of three compartments of increasing maturity: myeloblasts, promyelocytes, and myelocytes. The postmitotic maturation and storage pool consists of metamyelocytes, "bands" or "juveniles," and segmented neutrophils. Under ordinary circumstances, metamyelocytes are not released to the blood. Bands and segmented neutrophils are readily released to the blood, although segmented neutrophils are released in preference to bands. These cells constitute the storage compartment of bone marrow neutrophils. Approximately 60 percent of the postmitotic neutrophil pool of normal marrow consists of bands and segmented neutrophils. Thus the effective storage reservoir is at least fifteen times as large as the blood pool (Fig. 61-2).

From this marrow reserve of neutrophils the rate of cell entry to the blood can be accelerated upon demand before an increase in the rate of cell production occurs. In normal individuals there are enough postmitotic neutrophils to replace those in the blood for approximately 10 days at normal rates of marrow release.

The fate of neutrophils leaving the blood has not been entirely clarified. In a normal subject, neutrophils appear in bronchial secretions, in urine, and in the lumen of the intestine. Whether these sites of egress account for the majority of neutrophils leaving the blood each day or represent but a small proportion of these cells is not known. Following initiation of tissue injury, neutrophils marginate along the walls of the capillaries and venules adjacent to the injured area and by diapedesis traverse the intervening tissue. They enter the area of beginning exudate formation within 1 or 2 hr following the inflammatory stimulus. Diapedesis takes place between endothelial cells of the blood vessels. Neutrophils are delayed for some time at the basement membrane and then move in a seemingly directed fashion through the intervening tissue to enter the exudate. Turnover of neutrophils through an established exudate is almost as rapid as the turnover of neutrophils through the blood.

Neutropenia and neutrophilia may develop by a variety of kinetic mechanisms. Transient changes in blood neutrophil concentration may develop without any change in the rate at which cells enter or leave the blood; rapid shifts of cells between marginal and circulating pools can take place. Since this mechanism does not induce a change in the total number of neutrophils in the confines of the vascular system, it may be designated as producing "pseudoneutrophilia" or "pseudoneutropenia." Strenuous exercise or the administration of epinephrine and perhaps a variety of other stimuli lead to transient demargination of neutrophils with a brief but sometimes striking episode of neutrophilia. Pseudoneutropenia is regularly induced during hemodialysis (page 317).

Persistent neutrophilia is usually accompanied by an accelerated rate of entry of new cells from the bone marrow and is of necessity accompanied by increased production. Conversely, in most instances of persistent neutropenia, the storage pool of the bone marrow is exhausted, and usually production is found to be decreased.

However, changes in egress of neutrophils from the blood can also be the primary cause of changes in blood neutrophil concentration. Administration of pharmacologic doses of hydrocortisone induces neutrophilia, at least in part by reducing the rate of cell loss from the blood. Certain instances of neutropenia, such as those induced by overwhelming infection, by injection of endotoxin, or by administration of antineutrophil antibody, reflect a very marked acceleration in the rate of cell loss from the blood. This acceleration is so great that input from the marrow and increased production cannot keep pace, and neutropenia develops primarily because of accelerated cell loss.

NEUTROPHILIA An increase in blood neutrophil concentration accompanies most *bacterial infections.* With the exception of a few diseases, such as tuberculosis, brucellosis, and typhoid fever, neutrophilia develops during the inception and persists through the acute phases of bacterial infection. Neutrophilia may be present in some fungal infections, such as actinomycosis; a few viral

FIGURE 61-2
Diagrammatic model of neutrophil kinetics. Neutrophils share with platelets and erythrocytes a common precursor (pluripotential stem cell). The marrow mitotic pool is the site of production. The postmitotic pool consists of cells which continue to mature (metamyelocytes and bands) and a marrow reserve of mature neutrophils. From this, cells enter the blood for a brief sojourn on their way to tissues and body cavities. Only the circulating pool is measured in the traditional leukocyte count of the blood. Data for the size of the system and the transit times through various compartments are based upon studies of neutrophils labeled with radioactive diisopropyl fluorophosphate in normal volunteers. Cell ratios, indicated by the numbers posted on each compartment, are based upon 500 cell differential counts of neutrophils and neutrophil precursors in smears of marrow aspirates from 12 normal volunteers.

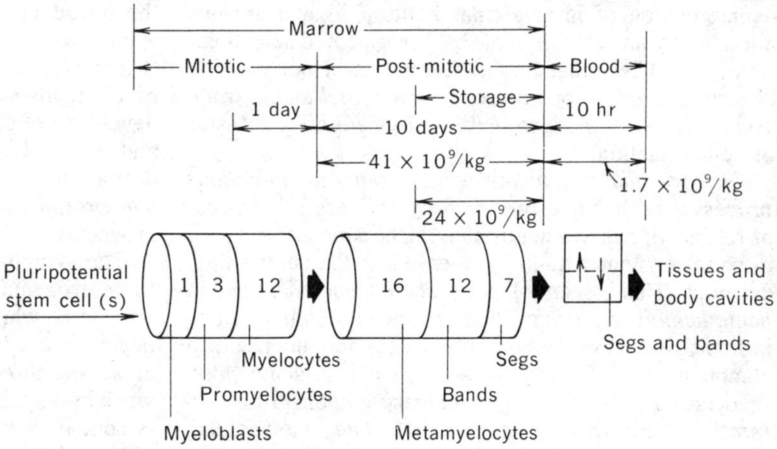

infections, such as rabies and herpes zoster; and a variety of parasitic and rickettsial infestations. The highest neutrophil levels, often exceeding 30,000/μl, commonly are observed in pneumococcal pneumonia or with localized abscesses. Neutrophilia may not persist as infections become chronic. In some chronic infections, such as bacterial endocarditis and pyelonephritis, neutrophil concentration may be normal.

The presence or absence of neutrophilia is a useful diagnostic sign, and serial determination of neutrophil concentration provides prognostic information during the course of infection. The proportion of blood neutrophils which are not segmented ("band"/segmented ratio) is of equal or even greater diagnostic and prognostic significance. In the early stages of infection the rate of release of neutrophils from the marrow storage pool to the blood is accelerated in response to demand for phagocytes at the infected site. As the storage pool is reduced, a greater proportion of bands is released, and band/segmented ratio in the blood increases, leading to a moderate "shift to the left." As the infection is controlled, or as it stabilizes, the demand for neutrophils is reduced or marrow production accelerates to meet continued increased demands. In these circumstances neutrophilia may persist for some time, but as the marrow storage pool is reconstituted, the band/segmented ratio returns toward normal. On the other hand, if the infection is spreading, the demand for neutrophils may steadily increase and may exceed the ability of the marrow to increase production, so that the storage pool either remains small or may actually become exhausted. In such a patient the shift to the left becomes increasingly more pronounced. Thus the characteristic pattern of early infection is neutrophilia with a modest shift to the left; of healing or well-controlled infection, neutrophilia with little or no cell immaturity; and of severe continuing infection, neutrophilia or even neutropenia with an increasing proportion of bands in the blood.

The magnitude of neutrophilia varies with its cause, being greater as a rule in localized in contrast to systemic infections and in highly virulent infections in otherwise healthy patients as compared with debilitated individuals.

The *transient episodes of neutrophilia* induced by injecting *epinephrine* or by *strenuous exercise* are due to demargination of intravascular neutrophils and are not attended by any change in the band/segmented neutrophil ratio. It is likely that the brief episodes of neutrophilia observed in such conditions as *paroxysmal tachycardia, convulsive seizures, and delirium tremens* are the result of demargination.

Neutrophilia accompanying many other noninfectious processes probably is produced by accelerating the rate of release of marrow neutrophils, since a modest increase in band/segmented ratio is observed as the neutrophilia develops. This is seen following *acute hemorrhage* and in *acute hemolytic anemia.* The neutrophilia which develops in many diseases may be attributed to the influence of a combination of factors. In some, such as acute *gout, myocardial infarction, or pulmonary embolism and infarction, burns, and spider and snake bites,* the stimulus for neutrophilia is tissue damage, inflammation, and sterile exudate formation. From what is known about the effects of pharmacologic doses of *hydrocortisone,* described above, it is likely that increased hydrocortisone blood levels, whether resulting from increased production due to stress or decreased degradation, as in hepatic failure, may be, at least in part, responsible for the neutrophilia. Patients with *Cushing's disease* often have mild neutrophilia.

Neutrophilia also is seen in *diabetic acidosis, uremia, eclampsia, Hodgkin's disease,* and sometimes in association with malignant neoplasms. The excessive production of neutrophils, eosinophils, basophils, and platelets, as well as of erythrocytes, so characteristic of *polycythemia vera* may be due to an abnormally functioning pluripotent stem cell compartment.

Unexplained or extreme neutrophilia or the presence of significant numbers of myelocytes and metamyelocytes and other immature cells in the blood suggests leukemia. The diagnosis of leukemia and its differentiation from "leukemoid reactions" is considered in Chap. 316.

NEUTROPENIA Neutropenia may be present when the white blood cell count (total leukocyte concentration) is decreased, normal, or increased. It should be obvious that the precentage of neutrophils in differential leukocyte counts is relatively meaningless unless it is multiplied by the total leukocyte count to obtain neutrophil concentration.

Clinical manifestations Of itself, neutropenia causes no symptoms unless infection supervenes. However, patients with neutropenia of any cause may suffer from frequent and severe bacterial infections. When neutropenia is related to some disease, the clinical manifestations will be those of the underlying disorder.

The decrease in resistance to infection which attends neutropenia is dramatically exemplified by the syndrome of *agranulocytosis or agranulocytic angina,* first recognized in 1922. This disorder is characterized by severe sore throat, marked prostration, and extreme reduction or even complete disappearance of the neutrophils from the blood. Although there may be a prodromal period marked by malaise or moderate fever, the onset is usually acute and fulminating. When first described, agranulocytosis often ended in sepsis and death. It was later recognized that the appearance of this syndrome corresponded with the introduction of certain coal-tar derivatives as therapeutic agents, in particular the antipyretic, aminopyrine (Pyramidon). The course of events was shown to consist of (1) neutropenia; (2) loss of resistance to infection, development of sore throat; and (3) overwhelming sepsis and death. Recognition of the etiologic basis of the syndrome, prohibition of further use of the offending drug, and prompt antibiotic therapy have greatly altered the prognosis.

The symptoms and physical signs directly attributable to neutropenia of any cause are those produced by the infections which attend neutropenia. Infection usually begins in the skin, especially the perineal and axillary areas, the throat, or the lungs, but may be first noted in virtually any area of the body. Initial infections usually are due to common bacteria such as pneumococci, staphylococci, streptococci, and coliform organisms. In patients with recurrent infections, or in patients who receive repetitive courses of antibiotics, more unusual organisms and those resistant to antibiotics, such as *Pseudomonas*, are observed, and infection with fungi, such as *Candida*, becomes more common. With very severe neutropenia infections spread rapidly and bacteremia is common. Patients with a small but significant number of neutrophils in the blood often suffer from chronic, indolent infections which can be contained with proper local and systemic measures but often defy complete cure.

The relationship between the severity of neutropenia and the frequency of infection is far from exact. However, as a general statement, patients with idiopathic neutropenia rarely develop life-threatening infections unless the neutrophil concentration is less than 1,000 per μl. In patients with a count of less than 500, this complication is usually observed.

Absolute numbers of monocytes and eosinophils may be increased, and hypergammaglobulinemia is present in some patients with neutropenia. These changes may be due to a physiologic response of other protective systems in compensation for the decreased resistance to infection secondary to the neutropenia or may merely represent the reaction to repeated or chronic infection. Blood lymphocyte concentration is variable and may be decreased, normal, or increased.

Etiology Neutropenia may exist as an isolated hematologic abnormality or may be associated with anemia and/or thrombocytopenia. All the causes of aplastic anemia (Chap. 309) are also causes of neutropenia. The major causes of neutropenia may be categorized as (1) iatrogenic, (2) secondary to known diseases (or syndromes), (3) familial, (4) antibody-induced, and (5) idiopathic. Examples of each are given in Table 61-2.

Neutropenia induced by *drugs or by physical agents*, such as x-ray, is probably the most common form of neutropenia (Table 61-3). Drugs which induce neutropenia may be divided into two broad classes, those in which neutropenia may be expected if enough of the drug is given and those in which neutropenia is an unpredictable, "hypersensitivity" reaction. Neutropenia is a common side effect of antitumor therapy, since the alkylating agents, antimetabolites, stathmokinetic agents (those which poison the mitotic spindle, thereby leading to cell death in metaphase), and x-ray (Chaps. 316 and 318) all produce neutropenia if given in sufficient dosage. This effect appears to be due to a decrease in neutrophil production, and recovery will usually follow discontinuation of the drug. Certain chemicals, such as benzene, may be added to the above list of agents which produce dose-related neutropenia.

TABLE 61-2
Causes of neutropenia

I Iatrogenic
- *A* Drugs and physical agents (see Table 61-3)
- *B* Hemodialysis

II Diseases
- *A* Infections
  - *1* Bacterial, e.g., overwhelming infections of any type; also certain other, not necessarily overwhelming infections, e.g., typhoid, paratyphoid, brucellosis
  - *2* Viral and rickettsial, e.g., influenza, measles, rubella, hepatitis, Colorado tick fever, psittacosis
- *B* Nutritional deficiency, e.g., selective deficiency of folic acid or vitamin B_{12}
- *C* Hematopoietic diseases, e.g., acute leukemia, chronic lymphocytic leukemia, lymphosarcoma, aplastic anemia, paroxysmal nocturnal hemoglobinuria, thymic alymphoplasia, deficient immunoglobulin production
- *D* Diseases producing splenomegaly, e.g., congestive splenomegaly, Gaucher's disease, Felty's syndrome
- *E* Other diseases, e.g., lupus erythematosus, pancreatic exocrine deficiency

III Familial chronic neutropenia

IV Antibody-induced neutropenia, e.g., autoantibodies and transplacental antibodies

V Idiopathic neutropenic syndromes, e.g., cyclic neutropenia, hypoplastic neutropenia, hyperplastic neutropenia

In addition to those listed in Table 61-3, many other drugs have been suspected as a cause of neutropenia. Neutropenia with certain of the above drugs has been accompanied by virtual absence of neutrophil precursors from the bone marrow, while with others mitotic neutrophil precursors have been abundant in marrow aspirates. Thus it appears that different pathogenetic mechanisms, increased destruction and decreased production, are involved in hypersensitivity reactions.

Certain drugs, notably aminopyrine, appear to destroy mature neutrophils by an immunologic mechanism in sensitized patients. Patients who have recovered from aminopyrine-induced neutropenia become neutropenic again within a few hours following administration of a very small challenging dose of the drug. Blood, withdrawn from such patients 3 hr after a test dose of the drug, induces transient neutropenia when transfused into normal subjects.

Neutropenia associated with sensitivity to such drugs as the phenothiazines apparently is due to interference with neutrophil production in the bone marrow rather than to destruction of mature neutrophils. In such cases few or no neutrophil precursors are demonstrable in the bone marrow. The phenothiazine, chlorpromazine, inhibits in vitro nucleic acid synthesis of suspensions of marrow cells.

Hemodialysis is regularly associated with a profound, although transient, neutropenia. Within minutes of the start of hemodialysis neutrophils practically disappear from the patient's circulating pool. However, within 30 to 60 min the neutropenia disappears and a "rebound" neutrophilia develops despite continuation of dialysis. The neutropenia is due to transient margination of circulating neutrophils, predominantly in the lungs, and thus, is a pseudoneutropenia. Such neutropenia can be produced in normal subjects by infusing autologous blood which has been incubated for 15 min in a dialysis coil.

Many classes of disease are associated with neutropenia (Table 61-2). Mild neutropenia is common in a variety of *viral and protozoal infections* and in infections such as typhoid fever and brucellosis. Neutropenia may also be observed in response to acute, severe, bacterial infections in which neutrophilia is the rule. In the last circumstance neutropenia should be viewed as a very

TABLE 61-3
Drugs and physical agents producing neutropenia

Group I—regularly produce neutropenia if given in sufficient amounts
- Physical agents:
  - Radiation with roentgen rays, gamma rays, beta rays, and neutrons
- Antitumor drugs:
  - Alkylating agents (nitrogen mustard, busulfan, chlorambucil, cyclophosphamide, etc.), antimetabolites (methotrexate, 6-mercaptopurine, etc.), stathmokinetics (vinblastine, etc.), antibiotics (daunomycin, etc.)
- Benzene
- Colchicine

Group II—produce leukopenia in "sensitive" persons only
- Analgesics (aminopyrine, dipyrone, phenylbutazone, etc.)
- Phenothiazines (chlorpromazine, promazine, mepazine, etc.)
- Antithyroid drugs (thiouracil, methimazole, etc.)
- Anticonvulsants (trimethadione, phethenylate, etc.)
- Sulfonamides and derivatives [carbutamide, sulfisoxazole (Gantrisin) etc.]
- Antihistamines (Pyribenzamine, etc.)
- Antimicrobial agents (organic arsenicals, chloramphenicol)
- Tranquilizers (meprobamate, etc.)
- Miscellaneous (dinitrophenol, gold salts, etc.)

poor prognostic sign for recovery from the infection. In experimental studies of induced pneumococcal pneumonia in dogs, neutropenia developed only in those animals in which the infection was so overwhelming that the marrow reserve of neutrophils was exhausted. If an infected patient runs out of phagocytes, a poor prognosis can be expected. Not only are such patients neutropenic, but very few of their remaining neutrophils are fully mature.

Neutropenia often accompanies *diseases of the hematopoietic system* (Table 61-2). Neutropenia was reported to be the first hematologic change in rare instances of copper deficiency in infants, and mild neutropenia occasionally accompanies severe iron-deficiency anemia. Neutropenia may accompany deficient immunoglobulin production (Chap. 64).

A number of children with pancreatic exocrine insufficiency which is not due to cystic fibrosis also have neutropenia. Since neutropenia is not common in cystic fibrosis, the relationship of the pancreatic dysfunction to the neutropenia is unclear.

Removal of the spleen leads to transient neutrophilia, and in certain diseases the presence of neutropenia seems to be correlated with an *enlarged spleen.* Patients with cirrhosis of the liver often have neutrophilia, but when the spleen is congested and enlarged as a result of increased portal pressure in cirrhosis, neutropenia is more common. Congestive splenomegaly of any cause and splenomegaly due to such diseases as Gaucher's disease may be associated with neutropenia. Neutropenia is rarely observed in rheumatoid arthritis unless the spleen is enlarged (Felty's syndrome). In other diseases, such as systemic lupus erythematosus, the presence of neutropenia correlates poorly with the presence of splenomegaly. The role of the spleen in neutrophil kinetics remains to be clarified, but it is likely that in certain of the above circumstances the spleen traps and destroys an abnormally large number of neutrophils.

Familial neutropenia probably exists in at least two forms: severe neutropenia inherited as an autosomal recessive trait, and a milder form inherited as an autosomal dominant.

Antineutrophil antibodies developing in the absence of such drugs as aminopyrine (autoimmune antineutrophil antibodies) may be responsible for many instances of idiopathic neutropenia, but there is no fully satisfactory in vitro test for detecting their presence. The observation that children born of neutropenic mothers may suffer from transient neutropenia suggests the presence of such antibodies.

Transient neonatal neutropenia also has been observed in children born of multiparous mothers without neutropenia. In such cases there is evidence for maternal sensitization to fetal neutrophil antigens, resulting in a situation somewhat analogous to that in erythroblastosis fetalis.

Idiopathic forms of neutropenia are separable into various syndromes, but none of these syndromes is common, and none is very well understood. Neutropenia occurring in regular cycles and sometimes persisting for years has been reported in a number of patients. In some instances the neutropenia has recurred at roughly 3-week intervals. In others the intervals were longer or more irregular. Such cycling of blood levels suggests a disturbance in the regulatory mechanism for neutrophil production. Other examples of chronic idiopathic neutropenia include those with few or no neutrophil precursors *(hypoplastic)* and those with abundant neutrophil precursors in the bone marrow *(hyperplastic neutropenia).* Neutropenia with abundant mature neutrophils in marrow has been described in which defective release of neutrophils from marrow to blood was thought to be the primary problem ("lazy leukocyte" syndrome).

Kinetic mechanism of neutropenia The changes in neutrophil kinetics which can lead to neutropenia are indicated in Fig. 61-3. Blood and/or bone marrow neutrophils can be labeled with radioactive diisopropyl fluorophosphate, and from such in vivo studies the rate of neutrophil production, destruction, blood and marrow transit times, and the sizes of the circulating and marginal pools can be determined. Short-term cultures of bone marrow can be used to study rates of maturation or of proliferation as judged by incorporation of tritiated thymidine into DNA of neutrophil precursors. Colonies of granulocytes also can be grown in vitro from bone marrow cultured on semisolid media. The number of such colonies is believed to reflect the number of stem cells present in bone marrow. Neutrophil migration from the blood into induced inflammatory exudates on the skin can be measured. Administration of epinephrine results in demargination of blood neutrophils, and the resultant increase in neutrophil concentration in venous blood samples provides a rough estimate of the size of the marginal pool. Administration of endotoxin, etiocholanolone, or hydrocortisone "flushes" neutrophils from the marrow storage pool into the blood. If the expected increase in blood neutrophil concentration following administration of these drugs does not take place, it is assumed that the patient's storage pool is exhausted.

Either increased cell loss with compensatory increase in production or decreased production can result in exhaustion of the marrow storage pool. In either case, most of the neutrophils in the blood will be "bands." If the bone marrow is examined in these patients, the ratio of mitotic to postmitotic neutrophil precursors is found to be increased. Assuming that the patient is not anemic, the myeloid/erythroid ratio of the bone marrow should distinguish between an increase or a decrease in the size of the marrow mitotic pool of neutrophils. With neutropenia due to increased cell loss, abundant mitotic neutrophil precursors and metamyelocytes should be observed in the bone marrow, producing a pattern which has been termed *maturation arrest.* This is a misnomer because such a pattern probably signifies the reverse of maturation arrest; except in leukemia, it reflects a marrow in which the storage pool is exhausted and from which bands are released to the blood as soon as they are formed.

Careful examination of the blood smear is very useful in interpreting kinetic changes in patients with neutropenia. If the storage pool is exhausted, band-form neutrophils are released to the blood as soon as they are formed, and very few will have had time to mature into

FIGURE 61-3

Changes in neutrophil kinetics resulting in neutropenia. The bone marrow is represented as two connected tubes which contain the mitotic and postmitotic compartments, as described in Fig. 61-2. The diameters of the tubes reflect the sizes of the pools, and their length represents their morphologic integrity. The normal neutrophil system is shown at the top of the figure, and three types of change in the system which may lead to neutropenia are illustrated diagrammatically below. In pseudoneutropenia there is a change in the ratio of the circulating (CGP)/marginal (MGP) pools, but the bone marrow is normal. Both when there is decreased production or increased cell loss, the storage compartment of the postmitotic pool is drained, leaving only young metamyelocytes. However, the mitotic pools differ greatly in size in these two neutropenic states.

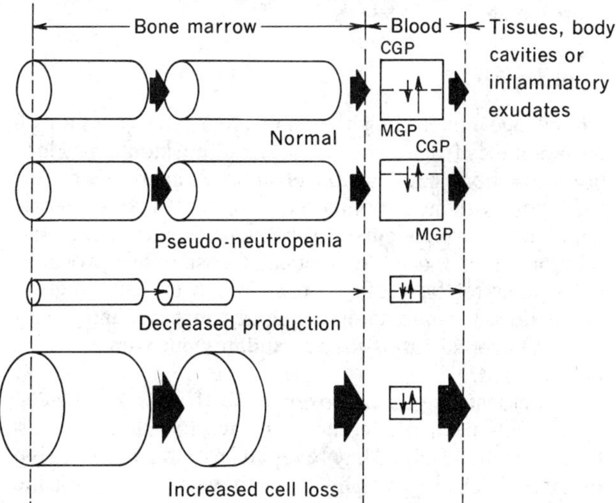

segmented neutrophils. In this circumstance there will be an increase in the band/segmented cell ratio in the blood. In contrast, if pseudoneutropenia resulting from increased margination of neutrophils along vessel walls is present, the band/segmented cell ratio in blood should be normal.

Therapy There is no known method of therapy which will safely and reproducibly accelerate the rate of neutrophil production in a neutropenic patient. Administration of such agents as bacterial endotoxin leads to an accelerated rate of neutrophil production in experimental animals and probably in normal man. However, this acceleration of production appears to be a physiologic response to the acute neutrophil depletion induced by endotoxin. Neutropenic patients would be expected to be under maximal or near-maximal stimulation of neutrophil production through normal physiologic mechanisms. Through the years a number of agents have been reported as efficacious in the therapy of neutropenia, but to date none can be considered of proved benefit.

If the patient is receiving any drugs or has been exposed to any other agents which might possibly be injurious, further exposure to these drugs and agents should be avoided. Drug-induced neutropenia usually responds to discontinuance of the offending agent, although a few patients die of infection before recovery can occur, and a few others develop chronic neutropenia for reasons which are not clear.

Neutropenia secondary to known diseases such as those listed in Table 61-2 improves or is corrected if general improvement in the disease is brought about.

In a limited proportion of cases of neutropenia, improvement has followed splenectomy, particularly in cases with splenomegaly; e.g., in patients with congestive splenomegaly secondary to obstruction in the portal circulation. However, the advisability of the operation must be weighed in the light of the many other problems and complications which may develop. At present there is no means of predicting which patients will respond favorably to splenectomy. Experience with splenectomy in patients who have few neutrophil precursors observable in the bone marrow and who do not have palpable spleens have generally been unfavorable. Only a few of the reported splenectomized patients with idiopathic neutropenia have benefited from the procedure.

Pharmacologic doses of corticosteroids induce neutrophilia in normal human subjects but do so in part by reducing the rate of cell egress from the blood, and such therapy has little or no effect on the rate of neutrophil production. Administration of 40 mg prednisone per day to normal human subjects reduces the number of neutrophils migrating into induced inflammatory exudates to about 10 percent of normal despite doubling of the number of neutrophils in the blood. Even in some patients with neutropenia, blood neutrophils may increase with corticosteroid therapy. However, if the mechanism of increase in these patients is the same as it is in normal subjects, the neutrophil increase in the blood is at the expense of neutrophil outflow to the tissues. In that event, steroid therapy would have to be looked upon as dangerous in neutropenic patients.

ALTERATIONS IN NEUTROPHIL MORPHOLOGY AND FUNCTION

Morphologic abnormalities Microscopically identifiable abnormalities of neutrophils characterize or are associated with a variety of inherited conditions. Most patients, such as those with hereditary hyposegmentation (Pelger-Huët anomaly), hereditary hypersegmentation, or increased, fat-containing azurophilic granulation (Alder's anomaly), do not suffer from frequent infections. It is reasonable to assume that these anomalies do not interfere significantly with neutrophil function. On the other hand, patients who inherit the *Chediak-Higashi syndrome* usually die in childhood of fulminant infection. This anomaly, characterized by the presence of enormous granules (giant lysosomes) in neutrophils and in other leukocytes, is inherited as an autosomal recessive trait and is associated with partial albinism, hepatosplenomegaly, and development of lymphoid neoplasms. The anomalous leukocytes phagocytize bacteria in an apparently normal fashion. However, the giant lysosomes seem to be functionally defective in killing bacteria, thus reducing the resistance of these patients to infection. Also in the *May-Hegglin anomaly* (cytoplasmic crescent- or spindle-shaped inclusions, dominantly inherited) leukocyte dysfunction at inflammatory sites has been described.

Chronic granulomatous disease of childhood Neutrophils of normal morphologic appearance but with decreased ability to kill phagocytized bacteria appear to be responsible for this syndrome. Recurrent infections with bacteria of low virulence develop shortly after birth, and death due to sepsis occurs before adulthood. Chronic lymphadenitis and infected eczematoid dermatitis are usually found in these children. The name of the disease is derived from the granulomas observed in lymph nodes, lungs, liver, spleen, and other viscera. Most patients with the syndrome have been males, and inheritance appears to be sex-linked. However, affected females with normal families have been described; thus more than one form of disease may be responsible for this syndrome. Neutrophils and monocytes from these patients phagocytize bacteria normally, but certain types of bacteria survive for an abnormally long time after being phagocytized. The disorder is thought to be due to defective generation of hydrogen peroxide in the phagosome, and the burst of hexosemonophosphate shunt activity which normally accompanies phagocytosis in missing or blunted. The latter forms the basis for the simplest diagnostic test for the chronic granulomatous disease syndrome; nitrotetrazolium blue is not reduced by the cells during phagocytosis. A similar cellular defect, presumably acquired, has been reported in adults with primary diseases such as cryoglobulinemia. Still other causes of defective bacterial killing, such as familial myeloperoxidase deficiency of neutrophils, have been reported.

Defective phagocytosis may occur but usually reflects the milieu of the cell rather than a defective cell. Inherited defects in poorly defined serum opsonins have been associated with phagocytic defects.

Phagocytosis of bacteria by neutrophils in vitro is inhibited by high concentrations of glucose in the suspending medium. The inhibitory concentrations are within the range of glucose observed in patients with diabetic acidosis. The propensity of such patients for developing bacterial infection possibly is explained by inhibition of phagocytosis.

Defective chemotactic response of neutrophils, whether tested in vitro or in vivo, has been described as a familial defect causing infection.

Monocytes

Monocytes arise in the marrow and share a common stem cell with neutrophils. The blood monocyte is the precursor of the tissue macrophage, and blood transit time for monocytes is brief, approximately 12 hr in experimental animals.

Monocytes migrate into inflammatory exudates at a slower rate and/or in a later phase of inflammation than neutrophils. Monocyte maturation continues in the inflamed tissue, and the monocyte enlarges, synthesizes enzymes, and assumes the morphologic and chemical characteristics of a macrophage. Macrophages are avid phagocytes and probably play a scavenging role, clearing the exudate of dead neutrophils and other debris in addition to engulfing and killing bacteria.

Macrophages may play some role in the initiation of antibody production under certain circumstances, although there is little to suggest that the monocyte itself is capable of antibody production (Chap. 63). Soluble and particulate antigens are pinocytized and phagocytized by macrophages. Small lymphocytes accumulate around the antigen-bearing macrophage, and some form of transfer of antigen or antigen-related material occurs.

Monocytosis is often observed in chronic inflammatory disorders due to infection (tuberculosis, subacute bacterial endocarditis, brucellosis) or other causes, during recovery from infection, in many protozoan (e.g., malaria, trypanosomiasis) and some rickettsial infections (Rocky Mountain spotted fever), and in patients with neutropenia.

Eosinophils

Knowledge concerning the physiology and function of eosinophils is fragmentary. The site of eosinophil production is the bone marrow, and eosinophils share a common stem cell with neutrophils and monocytes. If the eosinophilic cells of rodents are the same type of cell as the eosinophils of man, the kinetics of eosinophils probably are similar to those of neutrophils. Eosinophils migrate into induced inflammatory exudates in man, and eosinophil/neutrophil ratios in the exudate approximate those in the blood.

A modest degree of *eosinophilia* (from 600 to 2,000 eosinophils per μl) is common in overtly allergic conditions such as seasonal hay fever and asthma, in some skin diseases such as pemphigus, in a variety of parasitic infestations, and in such diseases as periarteritis nodosa. It is also seen in Hodgkin's disease and in Addison's disease. Hereditary eosinophilia, unassociated with overt disease, has been described.

Marked eosinophilia, up to and even exceeding 50,000 eosinophils per μl, has been observed in an occasional patient with carcinoma, during acute phases of tissue invasion with parasites such as *Trichina,* and in idiopathic states described as Loeffler's syndrome, tropical eosinophilia, pulmonary infiltration with eosinophilia, and eosinophilic leukemia (Chap. 316).

Eosinophilia usually is present in chronic myelocytic leukemia, myelofibrosis, and polycythemia vera. In these diseases the degree of eosinophilia often parallels the degree of neutrophilia, although in an occasional patient the eosinophilia may be so striking as to overshadow other leukocytic changes. The presence of eosinophilia is useful in distinguishing chronic myelocytic leukemia from leukemoid reactions and polycythemia vera from secondary polycythemia.

During acute bacterial infections eosinophils usually disappear from the blood. Hydrocortisone is known to produce transient eosinopenia.

Basophils

This least common member of the family of normal blood leukocytes is even less well understood than the eosinophil. Whether it is closely related or entirely distinct from tissue mast cells is unclear. However, these two cells are both rich in histamine and may play a role in the allergic response.

Elevated blood basophil concentration is commonly observed in chronic myelocytic leukemia, myelofibrosis, and polycythemia vera. Basophilia is a useful diagnostic sign in distinguishing chronic myelocytic leukemia and polycythemia vera from leukemoid reactions and secondary forms of polycythemia, respectively. A modest increase in basophils may be observed in myxedema, ulceraltive colitis, and other chronic inflammatory diseases.

IMMUNOCYTES

Lymphocytes and plasma cells are concerned with the production of antibody rather than with phagocytosis. The plasma cell develops directly from the lymphoid system as a specialized cell concerned with the production of circulating antibody.

Lymphocytes

LYMPHOCYTE KINETICS Most of the small lymphocytes of the blood, thoracic duct, and lymph nodes constitute a relatively long-lived population. These long-lived lymphocytes are thought to be thymus-derived ("T cells") and are concerned primarily with the process of cellular immunity (see Chap. 63). Lymphocytes in the germinal centers of lymph nodes and in the bone marrow are relatively short-lived. These shorter-lived "B"-type lymphocytes are concerned with humoral immunity and are thought to be influenced by the poorly defined "bursa-equivalent" (see Chap. 63). How long the long-lived population may survive without dividing is indicated by studies in patients who have been irradiated. Chromosome defects of a type which induce cell death upon division can be detected for a number of years following therapeutic irradiation. From such studies an estimate of an average intermitotic time of more than a year has been derived.

Lymphocytes do not remain in the blood for this long a period of time but seem to migrate from blood to lymphoid tissue and back to the blood. Vascular exit is through specialized cells in the postcapillary venules of lymph nodes. In the node, recirculating lymphocytes constitute the majority of cells in the cuff surrounding the germinal centers, and from this cuff they migrate into lymph channels and reenter the blood through the thoracic duct or the right lymphatic duct. The number of lymphocytes entering the blood from the thoracic duct is sufficient to replace the total number in the blood several times each day. Such a recirculatory pattern for cells is indicative of very complex cellular kinetics. Any shift or change in the recirculatory pattern at any point in the circuit can induce a profound change in the concentration of lymphocytes in the blood. However, a change in the rate of lymphocyte production may or may not be reflected by a change in blood lymphocyte concentration, and certainly no conclusions can be drawn concerning lymphocyte production from blood levels. The independence of blood lymphocyte levels in relation to events occurring elsewhere in the lymphocyte system is most dramatically illustrated by the pattern of lymphocyte changes which often accompanies hydrocortisone therapy of chronic lymphocytic leukemia. Therapeutic doses of hydrocortisone and its derivatives usually lead to a reduction of the total number of lymphocytes within the body, but for the first few weeks of therapy blood lymphocyte concentration increases.

Injected antigen is delivered to lymph nodes via lymphatics, when it becomes attached to reticular surfaces in the cortex of the node or may be phagocytized by macrophages in the medulla. A new antigen or the product of antigen cellular interaction stimulates conversion of small "uncommitted" lymphocytes to large cells synthesizing DNA. These large blastlike cells may be capable of antibody production or they or their progeny may mature into plasma cells or lymphocytes specialized for antibody production. Immunoglobulins are synthesized by plasma cells as well as by cells which are morphologically similar to the large lymphocyte. Certain studies suggest that the most 7S immunoglobin is produced by plasma cells while most 19S immunoglobin is produced by large lymphocytes.

From such cellular proliferation in response to an antigenic challenge, a small lymphocyte eventually emerges. This small lymphocyte is not concerned directly with producing antibody, but carries the capacity ("immunologic memory") to produce a specific antibody. Small lymphocytes of this "committed" compartment may remain dormant for years unless once again exposed to the antigen for which they carry antibody-specific "memory." Faced with a second antigenic challenge, these cells hypertrophy and again develop into or produce antibody-producing cells.

The role of the thymus and other organs in the development of the immunocyte system and details concerning the formation of antibody are found in Chap. 63.

The size of the immunocyte system depends, at least in part, upon the degree of antigen exposure. Germ-free animals have fewer lymphocytes than conventional animals but rapidly develop a lymphoid system of normal size when removed from the germ-free environment.

LYMPHOCYTOSIS The diagnostic significance of lymphocytosis depends in part upon whether the increase is due to normal- or abnormal-appearing lymphocytes. Lymphocytosis due to an increase in normal-appearing small lymphocytes may accompany recovery from acute infections and may be present during *chronic infections,* especially in *tuberculosis* and *syphilis.* In *pertussis* and in a rare syndrome of children and young adults termed *infectious lymphocytosis* very striking increases in the concentration of normal-appearing small lymphocytes may occur. Persistent, unexplained lymphocytosis with normal-appearing small lymphocytes in older patients usually proves to be due to *chronic lymphocytic leukemia* (Chap. 316).

Infectious mononucleosis (Chap. 224) is usually accompanied by lymphocytosis as well as by the appearance of abnormal-appearing lymphocytes in the blood. Known viral diseases, such as *measles,* may be accompanied by lymphocyte changes somewhat similar to those seen in infectious mononucleosis. *Acute lymphoblastic leukemia* (Chap. 316) is characterized by very immature lymphoblasts in the blood, and these cells are easily distinguished from those of infectious mononucleosis by their fine, granular chromatin and prominent nucleoli.

LYMPHOPENIA Lymphopenia occurs as a relatively nonspecific response to various forms of *stress,* such as *trauma, acute infection,* or *hemorrhage.* Such lymphopenia usually disappears within a few days. Persistent lymphopenia should raise the suspicion of *Hodgkin's disease.*

Plasma cells

These are but rarely observed in the blood of normal subjects but may appear in small numbers during severe *antigenic challenges,* as in certain *infections* or in *serum sickness.* Large numbers of plasma cells appear in the blood of a few patients with *multiple myeloma* (plasma cell leukemia, Chap. 316). Plasma cells constitute less than 1 percent of the nucleated cells of normal bone marrow, but they are not distributed uniformly throughout the marrow, so that the range of normal is quite wide (up to 5 percent in counts of 500 cells from marrow aspirates of normal nonalcoholic volunteers). An increased percentage of plasma cells on smears of marrow aspirates should raise the suspicion of multiple myeloma or some other protein-secreting tumor, but may also be observed in such conditions as *liver disease,* during antigenic challenge, and in *aplastic anemia. Absence of plasma cells* on smears of marrow aspirates usually is indicative of one of the diseases associated with inadequate production of serum antibody, such as *sex-linked hypogammaglobulinemia* or *chronic lymphocytic leukemia.*

REFERENCES

BOGGS DR: The kinetics of neutrophilic leukocytes in health and in disease. Semin Hemat 4:359, 1967

DOUGLAS SD: Disorders of phagocytic function. Blood 35: 851, 1970

JENSEN DP et al: Hemodialysis-coil-induced transient neutropenia and overshoot neutrophilia in normal man. Blood 41:399, 1973

KAUDER E, MAUER AM: Neutropenias of childhood. J. Pediatr 69:147, 1966

WINTROBE MM et al: *Clinical Hematology,* 7th ed., Philadelphia: Lea & Febiger, 1974

PART THREE | INHERITANCE AND GROWTH

62
GENETICS AND HUMAN DISEASE

VICTOR A. McKUSICK

Increasingly in recent years the importance of genetics to medicine has come to be appreciated. The relative importance of those conditions in which genetic factors play a leading role has increased as some other etiologic categories of disease, e.g., infectious and nutritional, have become better understood and better treated.

The mutant gene should be considered an etiologic agent. The variability, yet predictability, of the clinical picture in a genetic disorder in which the etiologic agent, a gene, operates from within is very similar to that of an infectious disease in which the etiologic agent invades from the environment. In studying progressive muscular dystrophy of the pseudohypertrophic type, one is not searching for its cause. The cause, an X-linked recessive gene, is known. It is the mechanism by which the mutant gene produces the clinical manifestations, as well as methods of interrupting that mechanism or compensating for it, that is sought by research in muscular dystrophy.

In addition to those conditions for which a single mutant gene in single or double dose is quite directly responsible, and in addition to those disorders which result from chromosomal aberrations, there are many disorders, including some of the commonest affections of man (e.g., atherosclerosis, hypertension, and certain malformations) in which genetic factors and environmental factors collaborate in a complex manner. For a majority of the diseases of man, causation must not be viewed in the rigid sense of a single etiologic agent—a pattern of thinking engendered by the bacteriologic era of medicine—but rather as a nexus, a network of multiple interacting factors among which the genetic factor (or factors) is always likely to be important. In coronary artery disease, for example, one cannot say that heredity, high-fat diet, cigarette smoking, particular forms of stress, or any other of many postulated factors is *the* cause. The controversy between genetics and environment, nature and nurture, of an earlier day has now subsided since it is appreciated that both types of factors are important.

The collaboration of heredity and environment is well illustrated by primaquine sensitivity (glucose 6-phosphate dehydrogenase deficiency), in which hemolytic anemia usually occurs only if the genetically predisposed person is exposed to a chemical of a particular type (Chap. 306); and by suxamethonium (succinylcholine) sensitivity (pseudocholinesterase deficiency), in which the genetically predisposed person suffers no obvious ill effects of his defect unless given the agent mentioned as a muscle relaxant in anesthesia.

An important principle of medical genetics is *heterogeneity*. Many genetic disorders which at first were thought to represent single entities have, on close study, been found to consist of two or more fundamentally distinct entities. There are known, for example, to be two types of X-linked hemophilia (Chap. 314), and their genes are at loci rather far apart on the X chromosome. Four or five distinct varieties of hereditary intestinal polyposis can be distinguished on clinical grounds. Several recessively inherited varieties of familial goiter are found to result from separate and distinct biochemical defects. Clarification of genetic heterogeneity in a category of disease is important because the simulating conditions, which by definition involve different basic defects, may have different modes of inheritance and hence will necessitate different genetic counseling.

Many hereditary syndromes are the result of multiple end effects of single mutant genes, a phenomenon called *pleiotropism*. This is also a useful principle in medical genetics, because one or more manifestations of the genes are often external clues valuable in the diagnosis of grave internal effects of the gene. Examples include the long-limbed habitus and ectopia lentis, clues to the nature of aortic disease (in Marfan's syndrome); the Kayser-Fleischer corneal ring, a diagnostic clue in Wilson's disease; characteristic skin changes and angioid streaks of the ocular fundus, which are clues to the "cause" of gastrointestinal hemorrhage in pseudoxanthoma elasticum.

A third important principle of medical genetics is that the clinical manifestations of a mutant gene vary more or less widely depending on the genetic background, i.e., the rest of the genome. Variability in disease caused primarily by a single etiologic factor is not limited to genetic disease. Learning clinical medicine, especially diagnosis, is to a large extent learning how to cope with this variability. As noted later, those conditions which are inherited in the autosomal dominant mode show particularly wide case-to-case variability.

Diseases tend to fall into one or another of three classes as to the role of genetic factors in their causation: (1) Many disorders, most of them individually rare, are determined primarily by mutation at a single genetic locus. This is indicated by the fact that these disorders display simple mendelian pedigree patterns of the autosomal dominant, autosomal recessive, or X-linked type. (2) Many common disorders, such as essential hypertension, and some relatively frequent forms of congenital malformation (e.g., cleft lip/palate) "run in families" but causation is multifactorial. Multiple genetic (polygenic) and multiple exogenous factors collaborate in etiopathogenesis. (3) Since 1959 it has been recognized that many disorders have as their basis an abnormality of chromosome number or structure (see Table 62-2).

DEFINITIONS *Congenital* means "present at birth" and is not synonymous with genetic. Genetic factors may or may not be of importance in the cause of individual congenital malformations. On the other hand, hereditary conditions are not necessarily congenital; at least, clinical manifestations may not appear until much later in life. *Hereditary, genetic,* and *heritable* are roughly synonymous. *Familial* and *heredofamilial* were used previously to designate conditions inherited as recessive traits, i.e., conditions which often occur in multiple siblings with both parents normal. Since a recessive disorder is as genuinely inherited as a dominant one, these terms have little justification. Possibly the only use for the term *familial* is in connection with disorders with a familial aggregation not yet proved to be genetic in basis.

The word *genotype* refers to the genetic constitution of the individual; *phenotype* refers to the outward expression. The phenotype is, of course, what the physician observes, from which he makes deductions about the genotype. The difference is comparable to that between character and reputation—"genotype" and "character" refer to the true nature of the individual, "phenotype" and "reputation" to the apparent nature. *Karyotype* refers to the chromosomal complement of cells. An *ideogram* is a drawing representing the karyotype.

Abiotrophy is a term introduced by Gowers (1902) to describe the behavior of genetic disorders, such as Huntington's chorea and the spinocerebellar ataxias, in which a system functions normally and may be histologically normal up to a stage more or less late in life. The term refers to an inborn defect which leads to premature deterioration of a particular tissue, organ, or system.

The investigation of members of a family with regard to a particular disease trait usually begins from a *proband,* or *propositus (-a).* The proband is the affected person through whom the family is ascertained. The proband is comparable to the *index* case of epidemiologic studies. Often in family studies it is desirable to compare the frequency of a discontinuous trait or the mean level of a biometric trait in the relatives of probands and in the relatives of controls. Data are almost meaningless unless the degree of relationship of the relatives studied is indicated. It means little, for example, to state that 5 percent of the relatives of patients with rheumatoid arthritis have rheumatoid arthritis, but more significance can be attached to the statement that 5 percent of first degree relatives have rheumatoid arthritis. *First degree relatives* are parents, sibs, and offspring; on the average their genetic resemblance to the proband is 0.50. When there is genetic identity (as in monozygotic twins), it is 1.0. *Second degree relatives* are grandparents, aunts and uncles, and grandchildren of the proband; on the average their genetic resemblance to the proband is 0.25.

TABLE 62-1
Correlations of phenotype, sex chromatin, and sex chromosomes

	Sex phenotype	*Barr bodies (maximum number per cell)*	*Sex-chromosome constitution*
Normal male	Male		XY
Testicular feminization syndrome	Female (with testes)		XY
Double Y (or XYY) male	Male		XYY
Turner's syndrome	Female		XO
Normal female	Female		XX
Klinefelter's syndrome	Male		XXY
Klinefelter's syndrome	Male		XXYY
Triple X syndrome	Female		XXX
Triple X-Y syndrome	Male		XXXY
Tetra X syndrome	Female		XXXX
Tetra X-Y syndrome	Male		XXXXY
Penta X syndrome	Female		XXXXX

CYTOGENETICS IN MAN It was not until 1956 that the correct chromosome number in man (46) was known and not until 1959 that a microscopically identifiable chromosomal aberration was reported to be the cause of disease in man. These advances were made possible by the introduction of two modifications of technique: (1) the use of colchicine in cell cultures to cause an accumulation of cells in metaphase of mitosis, the stage most favorable for counting the chromosomes; and (2) the use of hypotonic solutions to produce swelling of the nucleus and separation of the chromosomes. The cells studied have been derived from the bone marrow by the usual aspiration technique or from explants of skin or other tissue. Cells grown from the peripheral blood in short-term culture have been particularly useful for family studies and surveys. Use of the mitosis-stimulating properties of phytohemagglutinin is another technique that has facilitated chromosome study. The chromosomes are studied by light microscopy after appropriate fixing and staining (Figs. 62-1 and 62-2).

Mongolism (mongoloid idiocy, Down's syndrome) was found to be characterized by 47 chromosomes, the extra one being one of the smallest autosomes, or nonsex chromosomes (Fig. 62-2). In *Klinefelter's syndrome* it was found that there are 47 chromosomes and a sex chromosome constitution XXY (Figs. 62-2 and 62-3). In *Turner's syndrome* (gonadal aplasia) it was found that there are 45 chromosomes, there being only one sex chromosome, the so-called XO sex chromosome constitution (Figs. 62-2 and 62-3). In both the latter two cases an abnormality of the sex chromosomes had been suspected because of paradoxic findings on Barr's test of nuclear sex. In Klinefelter's syndrome the subject is ostensibly male but shows the "chromatin-positive" pattern of the normal female; in Turner's syndrome the phenotypic female shows in a majority of cases the "chromatin-negative" pattern of the normal male (Fig. 62-4).

The three conditions above appear to arise through the accident of nondisjunction occurring either during meiosis in one parent (i.e., in spermatogenesis or oogenesis) or in the first mitotic cleavage of the zygote. In meiotic nondisjunction both chromosomes of a given pair pass into one cell product rather than separating. Abnormal cells of two types are produced: one with one chromo-

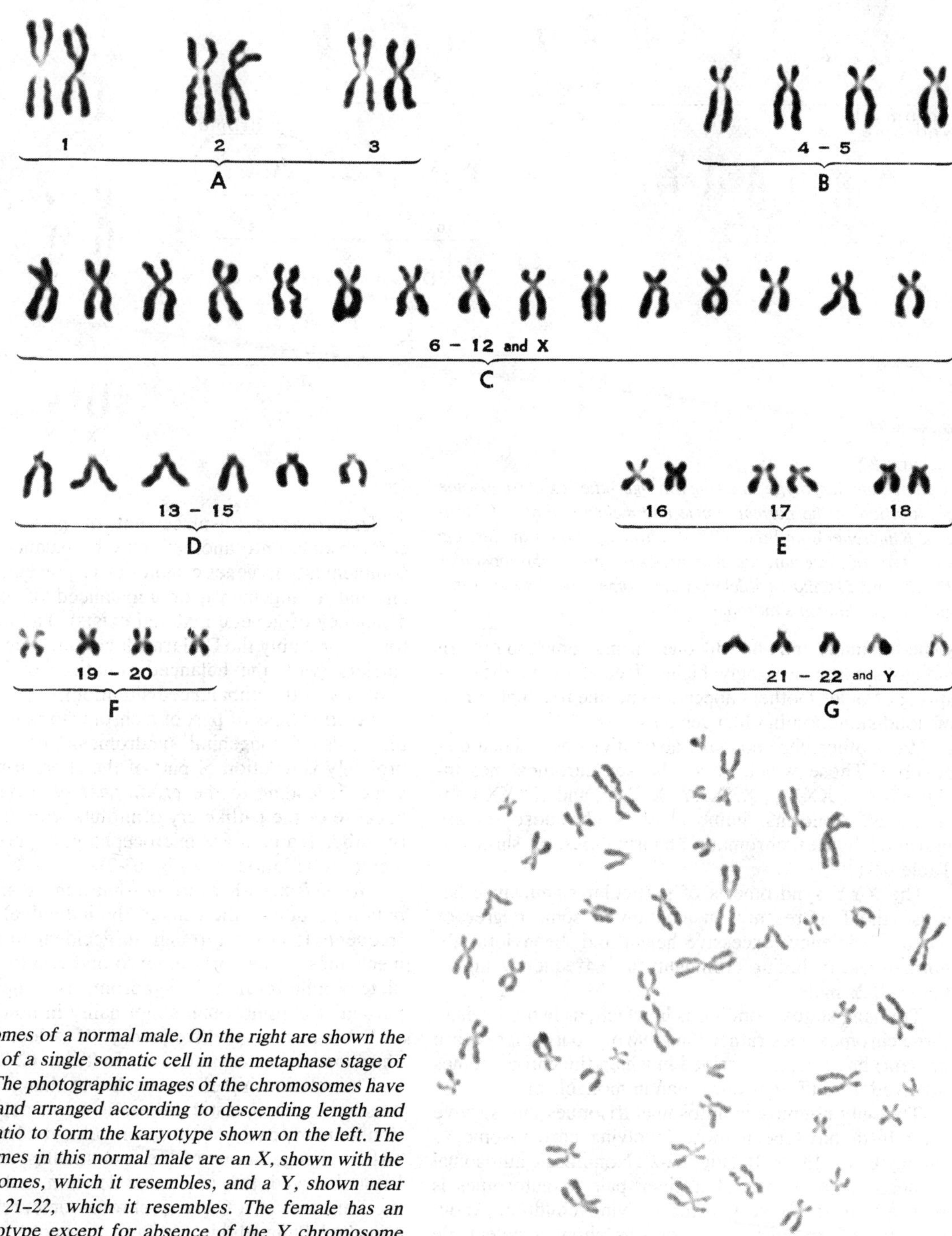

FIGURE 62-1
The chromosomes of a normal male. On the right are shown the chromosomes of a single somatic cell in the metaphase stage of cell division. The photographic images of the chromosomes have been cut out and arranged according to descending length and varying arm ratio to form the karyotype shown on the left. The sex chromosomes in this normal male are an X, shown with the 6–12 chromosomes, which it resembles, and a Y, shown near chromosomes 21–22, which it resembles. The female has an identical karyotype except for absence of the Y chromosome and the presence instead of a second X chromosome in group C.

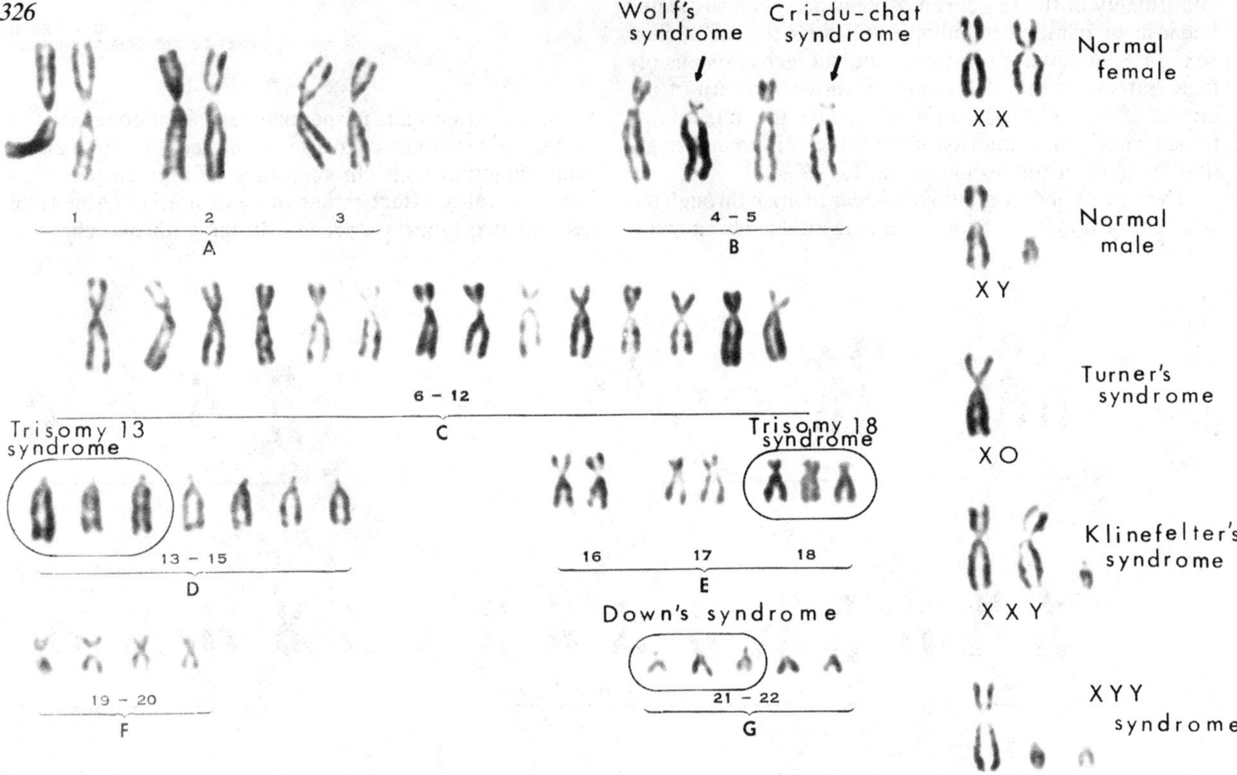

FIGURE 62-2
A composite karyotype, showing (on right) the sex chromosome constitution of the normal female and male and those of Turner's, Klinefelter's and the XYY syndromes; and on the left the karyotype of three autosomal trisomies (involving chromosomes 13, 18, and 21) and two deletion syndromes (Wolf's syndrome and the cri-du-chat syndrome).

some too many and one with one chromosome too few. In mongolism the strikingly higher frequency in the offspring of older mothers appears to be due to a higher risk of nondisjunction in older females.

Many other chromosomal aberrations have been discovered. Those which affect the sex chromosomes include XXX, XXXY, XXXXY, XXYY, and XXXX constitutions. Abnormal numbers of X chromosomes are indicated by sex chromatin abnormalities, as shown in Table 62-1.

The XYY syndrome is of particular significance because the features are, in addition to some degree of mental deficiency, excessive height and behavioral abnormalities, including criminality in a frequency higher than in XY males.

Trisomic states (conditions in which, as in mongolism, three chromosomes rather than two of a particular set are present) have been described in which the chromosomes involved are different ones than in mongolism.

The only nonmosaic autosomal trisomies that survive after birth have been those involving chromosome 21 (mongolism), 13, or 18 (Fig. 62-2). Nonmosaic autosomal monosomy (only one of a given pair of autosomes is present) must be very rare in living children. About one-fifth of spontaneous abortions show a detectable chromosomal abnormality as the probable "cause" of abortion.

Translocation (displacement of part or all of one chromosome onto another) may be balanced (i.e., a full complement of genetic material is present, although in unusual arrangement), or unbalanced (if excess and/or deficiency of genetic material exists). The most frequent form is probably the D-G translocation, which can exist in carriers (with the balanced situation) or in mongoloid idiots (with the unbalanced situation).

Deletion (loss of part of a chromosome) also occurs as the basis of congenital syndromes. The most frequent probably is deletion of part of the short arm of chromosome 5, leading to the *cri-du-chat* syndrome, so called because of the catlike cry of infants with this abnormality; other features are microcephaly, hypertelorism, and mental retardation (see Fig. 62-2).

Mosaicism, with a chromosome abnormality present in only a portion of the cells of the individual, is relatively frequent. It arises through an accident in chromosome mechanics in the early embryo and results in an incomplete or mild form of the syndrome as compared with the particular chromosomal abnormality in nonmosaic form.

Estimates of the frequency of selected congenital chromosomal errors are given in Table 62-2.

The relationship of demonstrable changes in the chromosomes to neoplastic disease is under active investigation. In many cases of chronic myelocytic leukemia a consistent change in one of the four smallest autosomes has been observed. It appears that deletion, or loss, of part of the long arm of a G-group chromosome, resulting in the so-called Philadelphia (or Ph^1) chromosome (Fig. 62-5), may be responsible for most cases of this form of leukemia. Whereas the chromosome aberrations leading to

TABLE 62-2
Frequency of selected chromosomal aberrations

	A *Spontaneous abortions*	*B* *Live-born*
Sex chromosome abnormalities:		
Turner's syndrome (all types)	1/18	1/3,500 "females"
Klinefelter's syndrome (all types)	Probably same as in live-born	1/500 "males"
Extra X chromosomes (females mainly XXX)	Probably same as in live-born	1/1,360 "females"
Autosomal abnormalities:		
Trisomy G	1/40	1/600
Trisomy 18	1/200	1/4,500
Trisomy D	1/33	1/14,500
Trisomy 16	1/33	Almost 0
Triploidy	1/22	Almost 0

abnormalities of sex, soma, and behavior described above are all congenital, the Philadelphia chromosome (which is present only in blood cells) arises in postnatal life through chromosome breakage produced by agents such as radiation and, probably, viruses. New methods of staining the chromosomes, particularly staining with fluorochromes such as quinacrine mustard or with Giemsa stain under special pH and other conditions, give additional information (Fig. 62-6). Among these findings is the fact that the G-group chromosome deleted to form the Philadelphia chromosome is not the same one that is trisomic in Downs's syndrome. Furthermore, fluorescence of the long arm of the Y chromosome when stained with quinacrine produces an *F* body in the nuclei of buccal mucosal cells, so that the male can be identified by buccal smear (Fig. 62-4*C*). The XYY male has two *F* bodies. A complication is that occasional normal males lack the fluorescent segment of the Y chromosome.

A high percentage—at least 20 percent—of spontaneous abortions show a major-grade chromosomal abnormality which was clearly the cause of fetal death. The types of abnormalities found are indicated in Table 62-2. Some other abnormalities, such as trisomy of large chromosomes, are probably lethal at a stage before pregnancy is recognized. The karyotype of Turner's syndrome is found frequently in abortion material, whereas the karyotype of Klinefelter's syndrome is no more frequent than among live-born infants.

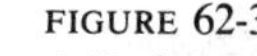

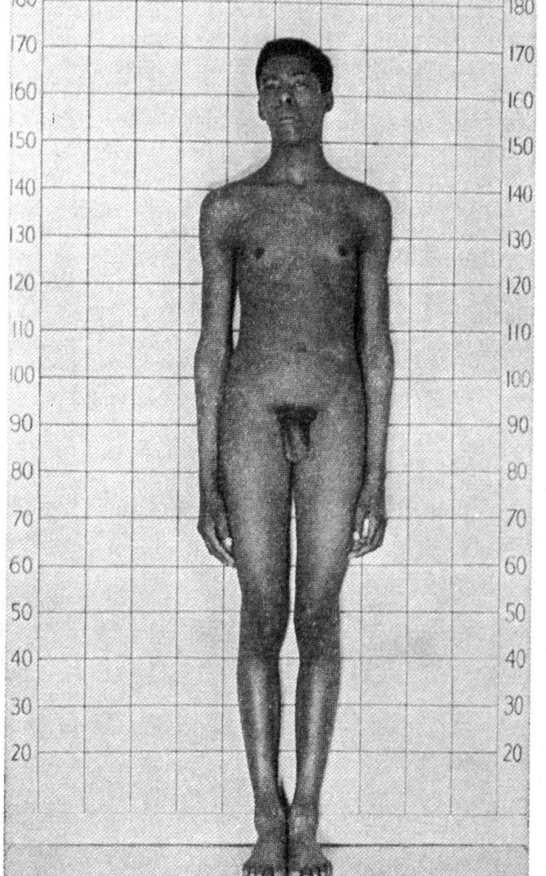

A

FIGURE 62-3
A *Patient with Klinefelter's syndrome. Note the long legs, gynecomastia, and sparse body hair.* B *Patient with Turner's syndrome. Note the short stature, broad shieldlike chest with wide intermammary distance, hypoplastic mandible, low-set ears, and webbed neck. Note the scar of the operation for resection of coarctation of the aorta.*

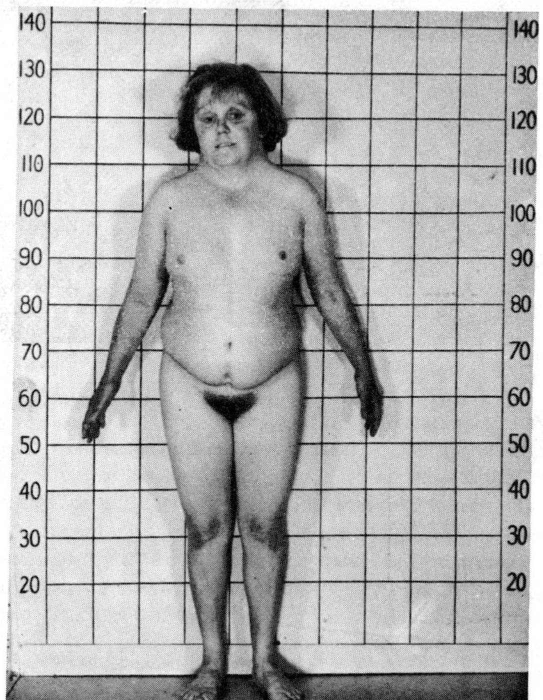

B

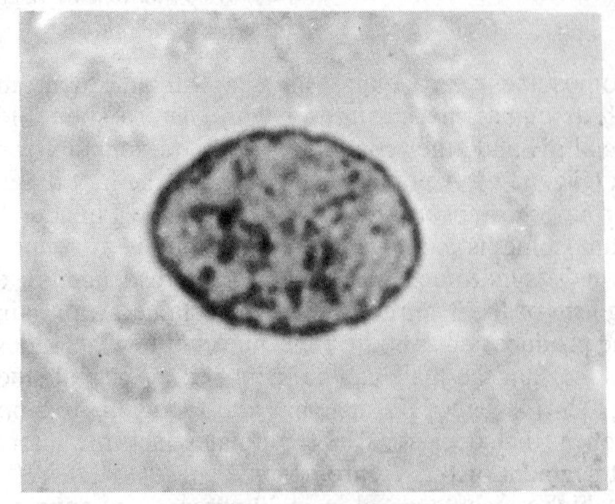

A

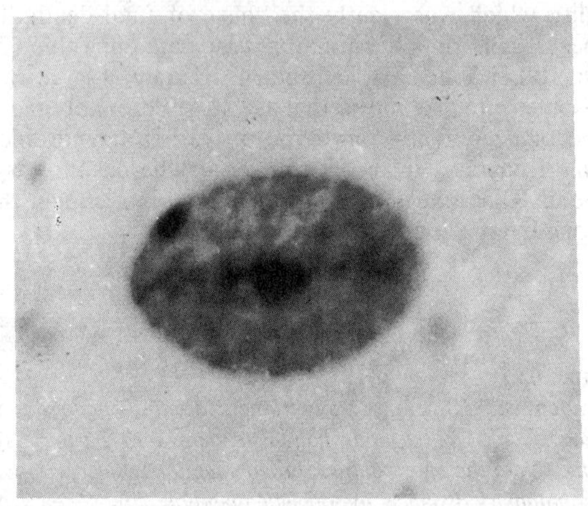

B

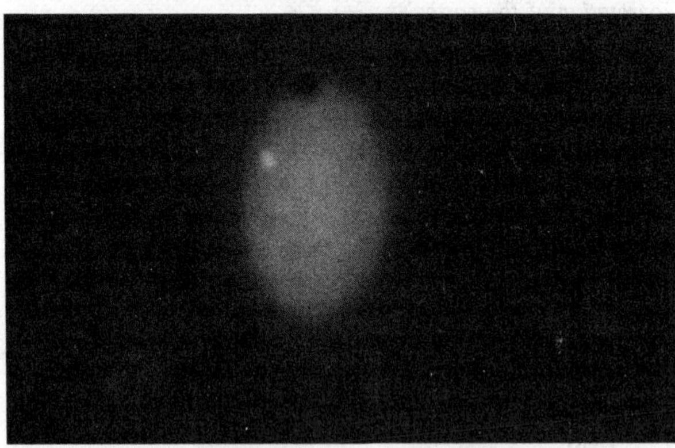

C

FIGURE 62-4
A *Cell in buccal smear from normal male. No sex chromatin mass is seen in this "chromatin-negative" pattern, which is shown also by most patients with Turner's syndrome.* B *Cell in buccal smear from normal female, showing a sex chromatin mass adjacent to the nuclear membrane. This "chromatin-positive" pattern is also shown by patients with Klinefelter's syndrome.* C *Cell in buccal smear of normal male showing fluorescent body representing Y chromosome.*

THE PATTERN OF GENETIC DISEASE IN FAMILIES

In accordance with the laws of Mendel, many diseases in man occur in families in a characteristic pattern. These are, for the most part, rare conditions and result from "point mutation" in the genetic material, as will be discussed later. The specific pedigree pattern depends on whether the responsible mutant gene is located on one of the autosomal chromosomes or on an X chromosome. It also depends on whether the effects of the gene are evident in single dose, i.e., in the heterozygous state, or whether the gene requires double dosage, or the homozygous state, for its expression. According to the type of chromosome bearing the gene in question, a trait is said to be either *autosomal* or *sex-linked* (or, more precisely, *X-linked*). Depending on whether expression of the gene occurs in the heterozygous state or only in the homozygous state, a trait is said to be either *dominant* or *recessive*, respectively.

Figure 62-7 presents an idealized pedigree pattern of an *autosomal dominant trait.* Within the limits of chance, half the sons and half the daughters of an affected person inherit the trait. This follows directly from the fact that the mutant gene is carried by one of a pair of autosomes and that there is a 50 percent chance of the affected parent contributing that chromosome to any given offspring.

As a generalization, dominant traits are less severe than recessive traits. In part an evolutionary or selective reason for this observation can be offered. A dominant mutation which determines a grave disorder that makes reproduction impossible will promptly disappear. On the other hand, even though in the homozygous condition a recessive mutation precludes reproduction, it can gain wide dissemination in heterozygous carriers if it endows these carriers with a selective advantage.

A biochemical explanation is also possible for the greater severity of recessive traits. One might anticipate a greater derangement when both genes specifying a particular protein, let us say an enzyme, are of mutant type than if only one is mutant.

Another characteristic of dominant characters is wide variability in severity. The degree of severity is referred to as the *expressivity*. Sometimes the expressivity is so much reduced that the presence of the gene cannot be recognized at all, at least by the methods at one's disposal. When this is the case, the trait is said to be *nonpenetrant*. Sometimes in pedigrees of families with a dominant trait, so-called "skipped" generations occur. In the skipped individual, expressivity is so low that the presence of the gene is not recognizable, i.e., the trait is nonpenetrant in that person. The variability results from

FIGURE 62-5
The G group chromosomes of bone marrow cell from a female with chronic myelocytic leukemia. One chromosome 21, marked Ph[1] *for Philadelphia chromosome, lacks part of its long arm.*

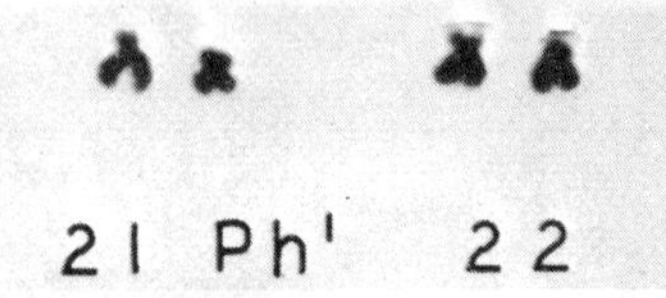

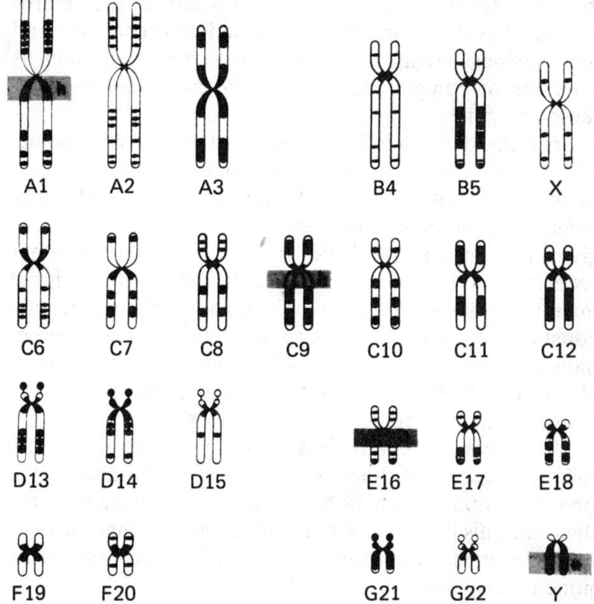

FIGURE 62-6
Idiogram of human chromosomes stained by "banding" techniques (quinacrine, Giemsa stain, etc.). Heterochromatin indicated by special methods is marked "h." The unique and characteristic banding pattern in each chromosome is displayed. (Courtesy of Frederick Hecht and the New England Journal of Medicine.)

differences in the environment and in the rest of the genetic make-up, the *genome.* At least in part the variability of dominant traits may be the result of differences in the "normal" allele which accompanies the mutant allele in the heterozygous affected individual. Evidence of the last is provided when one can demonstrate that sib-sib correlations for behavior of the given disease are stronger than the parent-sibling correlations.

Not every person afflicted with an autosomal dominant disorder has an affected parent because a certain proportion have the abnormal gene as a result of fresh mutation occurring in a germ cell of either the father or the mother. The graver the condition, in terms of average interference with reproduction by affected persons, the larger is the proportion of cases which represent new mutation. This follows from the plausible assumption that the frequency of the particular dominant gene is not changing but that an equilibrium exists between addition of new genes to the gene pool through mutation and the loss of genes from the gene pool through failure of reproduction. For a number of dominant traits, such as achondroplasia and Marfan's syndrome, it has been possible to demonstrate paternal age effect. Fathers of children who are sporadic (new mutation) cases are, on the average, 5 to 7 years older than fathers in general. Maternal age effect in some chromosomal aberrations, notably mongolism, is well known; paternal age effect in point mutation is less well known.

Autosomal recessive traits (Fig. 62-8) likewise occur equally often in males and females, as a rule. The affected individuals usually have normal parents, but both parents are heterozygous carriers of the gene in question. Since related individuals are more likely to be heterozygous for the same mutant gene, consanguineous mating, of first cousins, for example, is more likely to result in offspring affected by a recessive trait. Viewed in another way, a greater proportion of the parental matings in families affected by recessive traits are likely to be consanguineous than is true generally. The rarer the recessive trait, the higher is the proportion of consanguineous parental matings.

On the average, among the offspring of two heterozygous parents one-fourth of males and females are expected to be homozygous affected individuals. One-half will be heterozygous carriers for the trait, and one-fourth will be homozygous for the normal allele.

Affected sibships can usually be ascertained only through the appearance of one or more affected members. Since there is no way to recognize those matings of two appropriately heterozygous parents who are so fortunate as to have no affected children, a collection of sibships containing at least one affected child is a biased sample. More than the expected one-fourth of all children in ascertainable families will be affected. The proportion of affected children among those born after the first affected child in the sibship is indeed 25 percent, but a method for testing the recessive hypothesis based only on sibs born later is inefficient inasmuch as not all the data are used. Efficient methods for correcting for the so-called "bias of ascertainment" are available.

If an individual affected by a recessive trait marries a homozygous normal person, none of the children will be affected, but all will be heterozygous carriers. If an individual affected by a recessive trait marries a heterozygous carrier, one-half of the offspring are likely to be affected. A pedigree pattern superficially resembling that of a dominant trait can result. It was previously thought that two genetic forms of alkaptonuria (Chap. 96) exist—one inherited as an autosomal recessive and one as an autosomal dominant trait. Closer investigation reveals that the apparently dominant form was the same disease as the clearly recessive one. Because of much inbreeding, homozygous affected individuals frequently mated with

FIGURE 62-7
Pedigree pattern of an autosomal dominant trait.

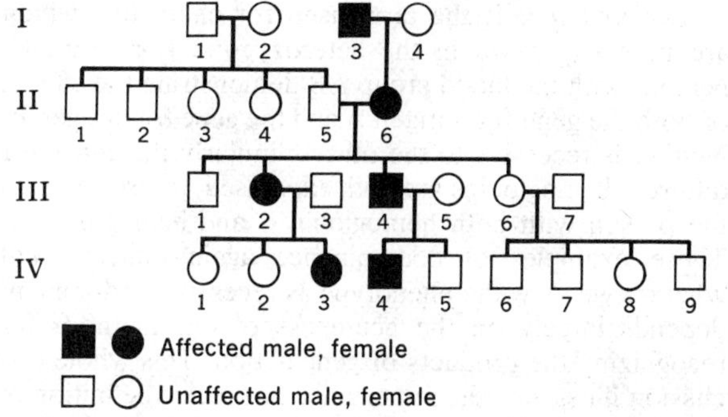

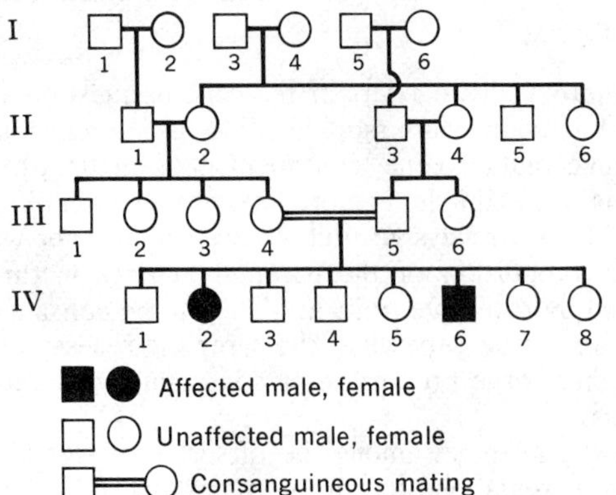

FIGURE 62-8
Pedigree pattern of an autosomal recessive trait.

heterozygous carriers and a quasi-dominant pedigree pattern resulted.

When two individuals affected by the same recessive disease mate, all their offspring are likely to be affected. However, an exception to this generalization occurs if the recessive trait which phenotypically is identical in two parents is in fact determined by genes at different loci. The exception illustrates the genetic axiom: The phenotype is not a necessary indication of the genotype. Different genotypes can result in the same phenotype (so-called "genetic mimics" or "genocopies"). Or an environmental insult can result in a phenotype indistinguishable from that produced by a mutant gene (a so-called "phenocopy").

Dominant and *recessive* are somewhat arbitrary concepts. When our methods are sufficiently acute, the effect of a recessive gene in the heterozygous state can be recognized. Furthermore, a gene which has obvious expression in the heterozygous individual and is therefore considered dominant may have a different effect, quantitatively and even qualitatively, in the homozygous state. The gene for sickle hemoglobin and the states referred to as sickle-cell anemia and sickle-cell trait illustrate the arbitrary nature of the distinction. If sickle-cell anemia is considered as the phenotype, then the condition is recessive, since a homozygous state of the gene is required. The phenotype sickling, however, is dominant since the gene in the heterozygous state is expressed. *Intermediate inheritance* is the term sometimes applied to this type of pedigree pattern (Fig. 62-9).

Codominance is the term used for characters which are both expressed in the heterozygote. For example, persons with the blood group AB demonstrate the effects of both the gene for antigen A and the gene for antigen B. Neither is recessive to the other. Similarly the genes for different hemoglobins are both expressed, for example, in the person with both hemoglobin S and hemoglobin C. These examples of codominance again indicate that whether we view the phenotype as recessive or dominant depends largely on the acuteness of our methods for recognizing the products of gene action. This whole discussion illustrates the importance of precise definition of the phenotype. If the particular phenotype occurs only in the homozygote, it is recessive; if it occurs in the heterozygote, it is dominant. Strictly speaking, dominance and recessiveness are attributes of the phenotype, although as a matter of convenience we may speak of dominant or recessive genes.

In traits determined by genes on the X chromosome, either dominance or recessiveness may be observed, just as in autosomal traits. The female with two X chromosomes may be either heterozygous or homozygous for a given mutant gene, and the trait can demonstrate either recessive or dominant behavior. On the other hand, the male with one X chromosome can have only one genetic constitution, namely, *hemizygous.* Regardless of the behavior of the mutant gene in the female, whether recessive or dominant, the mutant gene, if present in the male, is always expressed.

An important characteristic of sex-linked (X-linked) inheritance, both dominant and recessive, is the absence of male-to-male (i.e., father-to-son) transmission of the disease. This is a necessary result of the fact that the male contributes his X chromosome to all his daughters but to none of his sons.

X-linked recessive inheritance (Fig. 62-10) is illustrated in a classic manner by hemophilia. The pedigree pattern of an autosomal dominant trait is a vertical one, with affected persons in successive generations. The pedigree pattern of an autosomal recessive trait tends to be horizontal, with affected persons confined to a single generation. The pedigree pattern of a X-linked recessive character tends to be oblique because of transmission to the sons of normal carrier sisters of affected males. This pattern has been compared to the knight's move in chess. Tracing X-linked recessive characters through many generations is often difficult because the patronymic of affected persons tends to change with each generation.

To have hemophilia a female must be homozygous for this recessive gene. She must have received a gene for hemophilia from each parent. Such a case can occur, and has been observed, when a hemophilic male marries a carrier female (Fig. 62-10B). As with other recessive traits this homozygous state is more likely to result from consanguineous matings. A hemophilic female may also occur if a carrier mother is impregnated by a mutant sperm from a normal father, or if the phenotypic female has in fact an XO sex chromosome constitution (Turner's syndrome) or an XY constitution (the syndrome of testicular feminization). (In these comments reference is, of course, made to X-linked recessive hemophilia A and B,

FIGURE 62-9
Pedigree pattern of an autosomal intermediate trait as illustrated by sickle state.

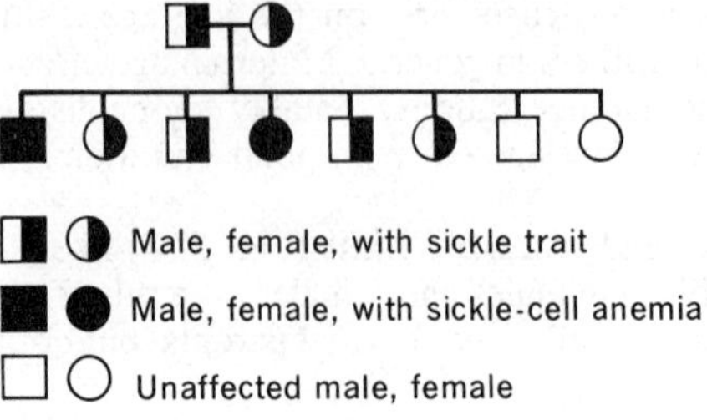

not to other hemophilioid states which occur equally frequently in males and females. Also not considered is the rare possibility that unfortunate lyonization, as described below, in a heterozygous female has resulted in a majority of the cells which produce antihemophilic factor having the mutant-bearing X chromosome as the genetically active one.)

A hemophilic male can have inherited the hemophilia gene *only* from his mother and can transmit it only to his daughters, not to any of his sons. *All* daughters of a hemophilic male are carriers (Fig. 62-10C).

In man one can enumerate more than 60 other diseases inherited as X-linked recessives, including such significant entities as primaquine sensitivity (Chap. 306), the Duchenne type of progressive muscular dystrophy (Chap. 344), and agammaglobulinemia (Chap. 64). In some (e.g., primaquine sensitivity and nephrogenic diabetes insipidus) a partial defect can be demonstrated in the heterozygous female carrier, and one might prefer to call the inheritance X-linked intermediate. In another condition, choroideremia, hemizygous males, but only the males, have severe impairment of vision, and from this point of view the disease is an X-linked recessive trait; but the heterozygous female carriers show striking changes in the fundus oculi on ophthalmoscopy, even though vision is unaffected.

At least one common trait, color blindness, is inherited as an X-linked recessive trait. It is sufficiently frequent (about 8 percent of white males are color blind) that the occurrence of homozygous color blind females is no great rarity.

In X-linked dominant inheritance both females and males are affected and both males and females transmit the disorder to their offspring, just as in autosomal dominant inheritance. Superficially the pedigree patterns in the two types of inheritance are similar, but there is a critical difference (Fig. 62-11). In X-linked dominant inheritance, although the affected female transmits the trait to half her sons and half her daughters, the affected male transmits it to *none* of his sons and to *all* his daughters. Furthermore, in a series of cases females are expected to occur twice as often as males. One of the best studied X-linked dominant traits is vitamin D–resistant rickets, or hypophosphatemic rickets (Chap. 349). In this condition the hemizygous affected male tends to have more severe clinical involvement than does the heterozygous affected female.

One common trait is inherited as an X-linked dominant: the Xg(a+) blood group. In due course, antiserums that directly identify the Xg(a−) blood group will probably be found. These will then be considered codominant traits.

Some rare conditions are thought to be inherited as X-linked dominant traits lethal in the hemizygous male. The characteristics (Fig. 62-12) are (1) occurrence only in females (who are heterozygous for the mutant gene), (2) transmission from affected mother to half her daughters, (3) increased frequency of abortion (male fetus being lost) by affected women. Conditions which appear to have this mode of inheritance include incontinentia pigmenti, focal dermal hypoplasia, and the orofaciodigital (OFD) syndrome. A male with the last condition was found to be no exception to X-linked dominant, male-lethal inheritance, because in fact he was an instance of XXY Klinefelter's syndrome.

Understanding of the behavior of X-linked traits and interpretation of findings in (1) females heterozygous for X-linked genes and (2) persons with an abnormal complement of X chromosomes have been greatly advanced by *Lyon's hypothesis.* There is now good evidence that at an early stage in development one X chromosome of the female becomes relatively inactive genetically (Fig. 62-13). The inactive X chromosome forms the *Barr body.* In each cell it is a random matter whether the X chromosome derived from the mother or that derived from the father is the one that becomes inactive. Once the "decision" is made in a given cell, however, the same X chromosome remains inactive in all descendants of that cell. The adult female is, therefore, a mosaic of two types

FIGURE 62-10

Pedigree patterns of an X-linked recessive trait. A *Note the "oblique" pattern.* B *An affected female can result from the mating of an affected male and a carrier female, as in the consanguineous marriage shown here.* C *An affected male mating with a normal, noncarrier female has all normal sons and all carrier daughters.*

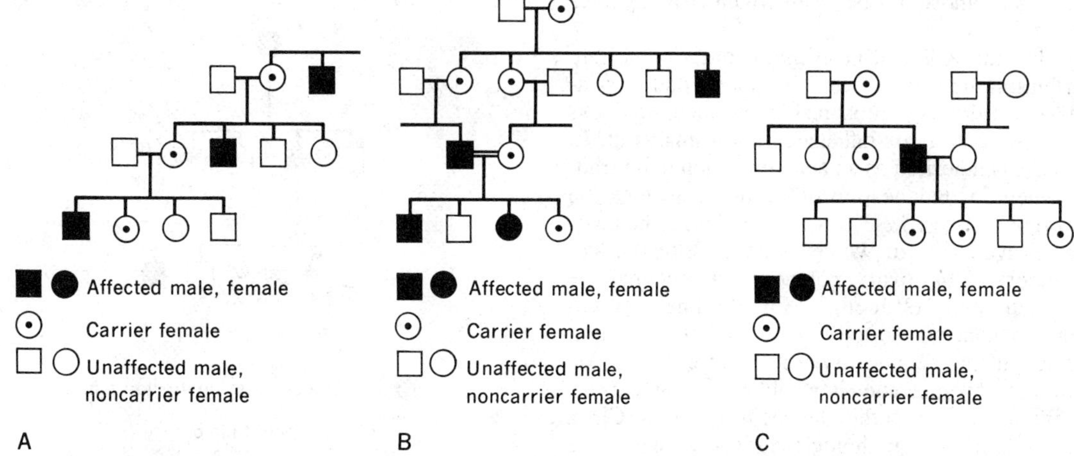

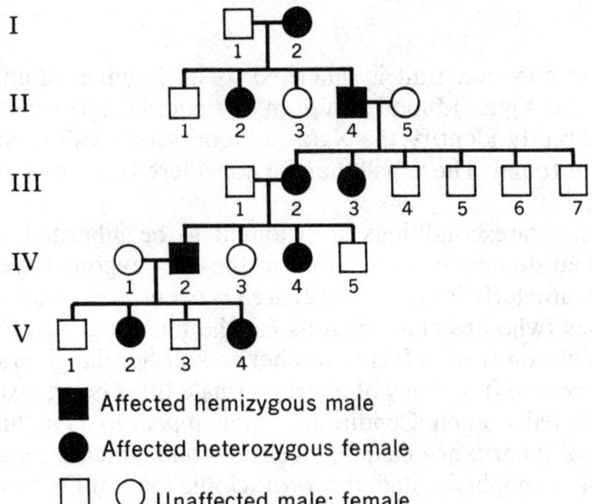

FIGURE 62-11
Pedigree pattern of an X-linked dominant trait.

of cells, those with the mother's X active and those with the father's X active.

Lyon's hypothesis is thought to account for these findings: (1) Heterozygous females tend to vary widely in expression of X-linked recessive genes. As an extreme case, females heterozygous for the hemophilia gene have clinical hemophilia, if most of the pertinent anlage cells destined to produce antihemophilic globulin have the X chromosome with the hemophilia gene active. (2) A mosaic pattern is observed in females heterozygous for conditions such as ocular albinism, an X-linked recessive trait. The fundi in such females show a mosaic of pigmented and unpigmented areas. (3) Persons with multiple X chromosomes, e.g., the XXX female, have two Barr bodies. All X chromosomes in excess of 1 are inactivated. (Table 62-1). These persons have much less drastic abnormalities than would be expected with such excess chromosómal material if relative inactivation did not occur.

Occurrence of the following types of inheritance in man is uncertain: (1) *holandric (all-male) inheritance,* resulting from the possible location of a gene on the Y chromosome, and (2) *partial sex linkage,* resulting from the location of a gene on possibly homologous parts of the X and Y chromosomes between which crossing over might occur.

Before leaving X-linked inheritance, one should note the distribution between such inheritance and sex-influenced (or sex-limited) autosomal inheritance. Baldness appears to be such a sex-influenced autosomal trait. In man baldness is inherited as an autosomal dominant trait, but in women for baldness to occur the gene must be in homozygous state, i.e., in women baldness behaves like a recessive trait. In women who develop masculinizing tumors of the ovary, baldness may occur if the genotype is proper. As another example, one may imagine a mutant gene whose sole effect was that of preventing lactation in the female. Even if it were located on an autosomal chromosome, it would not have expression in the male. Idiopathic hemochromatosis (Chap. 101) results from the pathologic effects of excessive accumulations of iron within the body, probably as a result of a hereditary defect in the intestinal mechanism regulating iron absorption. Although the inheritance seems to be autosomal dominant, females are rather rarely affected because they have a safety valve on excessive iron accumulation—menstruation and pregnancy.

Note the difficulties in distinguishing X-linked recessive inheritance from male-limited autosomal dominant inheritance, if the nature of the disease is such that reproduction of affected males does not occur. The syndrome of testicular feminization (Chap. 91) is an example. The affected individuals are genetic males, but, because of end-organ unresponsiveness to androgens, female external genitalia and all the secondary sex characters of the female develop. The affected male does not reproduce, and normal females are carriers. The pedigree pattern is precisely that of an X-linked recessive trait. However, the inheritance can equally well be X-linked autosomal dominant. In diseases too severe to permit reproduction of affected males—the Pelizaeus-Merzbacher disease (a form of cerebral degeneration), the Duchenne variety of muscular dystrophy (Chap. 344), one variety of gargoylism (Chap. 362)—there is on the basis of pedigree patterns no way to distinguish X-linked and sex-limited inheritance.

Table 62-3 lists some relatively frequent mendelian disorders. McKusick's *Mendelian Inheritance in Man* provides a complete listing which now encompasses over 420 autosomal dominant, 375 autosomal recessive, and 85 X-linked traits, as well as many more in which the particular mode of inheritance has not been firmly established.

Genetic counseling Familiarity with the patterns of disease is useful in diagnosis; if the pedigree pattern is consistent with the mode of inheritance usual for a suspected entity, the diagnosis of that entity is thereby strengthened. Knowing what individuals in a kindred are at risk, one can watch for the earliest signs of hereditary disease.

Furthermore, familiarity with pedigree patterns is essential to genetic counseling. The risk of having an af-

FIGURE 62-12
Pedigree pattern of an X-linked dominant trait lethal in the hemizygous male.

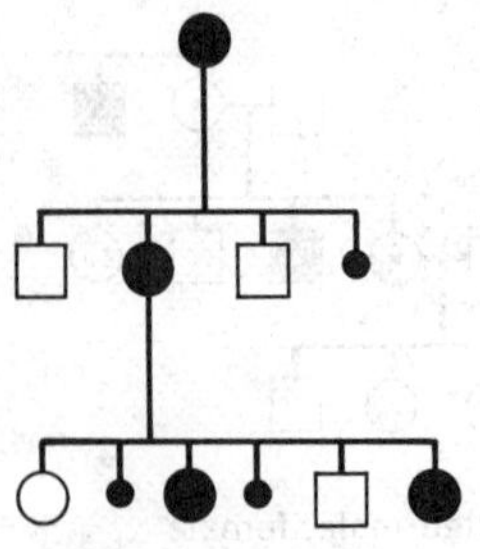

Affected and unaffected female
Unaffected male
Abortion

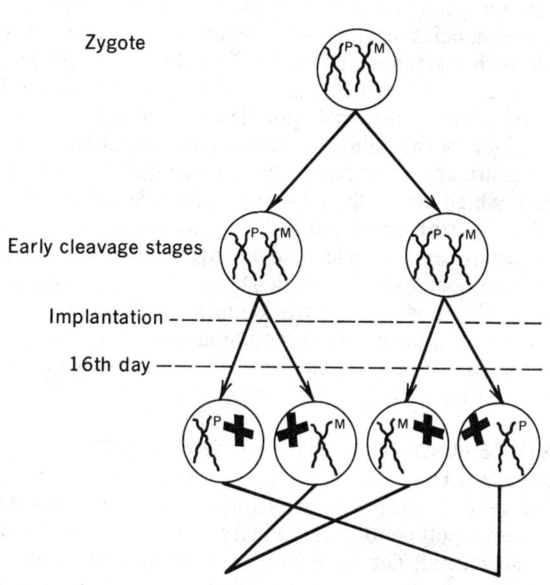

FIGURE 62-13
Schematic representation of the phenomenon underlying Lyon's hypothesis. In the normal female, early in embryogenesis (probably soon after implantation) one X chromosome in each cell becomes inactive. Once it has been "decided" whether the maternal (M) or paternal (P) X chromosome will be the inactive one, all descendants of that cell "abide by the decision."

fected child may be stated as 1 in 2 for a person affected by a dominant trait and as 1 in 4 for a couple which has already had a child affected by a recessive disease. For the sister of a male affected by an X-linked recessive trait the risk of being a carrier is (unless the affected brother represents a new mutation) 1 in 2, of having an affected son one-half that, or 1 in 4, and the risk of having any affected child (considering both sexes) one-half that, or 1 in 8.

In connection with statements of mendelian risk, it should be made clear to the person seeking genetic counseling that the figure is a probability. Parents with one child with cystic fibrosis may take the statement of "1 in 4" to mean that they have had their one affected child and can now have three children who will be normal. The analogy to tossing coins is useful; with each toss of a true coin the chance of "heads" is 50 percent regardless of the result of earlier tosses. "Chance has no memory."

If a given condition is regularly inherited as a dominant trait, and if one can be certain that one parent does not have the condition in *forme fruste,* then the risk to children born later is virtually nil. It can be shown that for a rare X-linked recessive disorder of such a nature that the affected males do not reproduce—Duchenne's muscular dystrophy is such a condition—about one-third of all cases will be the result of fresh mutation in the X chromosome contributed to the affected male offspring by the mother, and in the other two-thirds of cases the mother will be a heterozygous carrier of the mutation which occurred in an earlier generation. If by chance the carrier female has only one affected son and no affected relative, such as a brother, it is impossible to tell from the pedigree whether she is a carrier or not. Special tests for carrier status for various X-linked disorders have been devised. None is completely discriminatory and probably never can be because of the considerations of Lyon's hypothesis. Screening for heterozygous carriers for X-linked recessive traits is much more worthwhile than screening for carriers of autosomal recessive traits. Any X-linked carrier female has a 50 percent chance of having an affected son regardless of the genotype of her husband. An autosomal carrier has a one-fourth chance of having an affected child only if he or she marries another carrier.

TABLE 62-3
Some relatively frequent* mendelian disorders

Autosomal dominant disorders:
- Marfan's syndrome
- Osteogenesis imperfecta tarda
- Hereditary hemorrhagic telangiectasia
- Familial polyposis of colon
- Hereditary spherocytosis
- Cystic kidney disease (adult form)
- Huntington's chorea
- Alzheimer's disease
- Acute intermittent porphyria

Autosomal recessive disorders:
- Congenital deafness (deaf-mutism)†
- Albinism
- Phenylketonuria
- Galactosemia
- Wilson's disease
- Pseudoxanthoma elasticum
- Tay-Sachs disease
- Alkaptonuria
- Sickle-cell anemia
- Cystic fibrosis
- Familial Mediterranean fever

X-linked disorders:
- Hemophilia A
- Hemophilia B
- Lesch-Nyhan syndrome
- Duchenne's muscular dystrophy
- Agammaglobulinemia, Bruton's type
- Glucose 6-phosphate dehydrogenase (G-6-PD) deficiency
- Hypophosphatemic rickets†

* *Good data on frequency are available for few mendelian disorders. Those conditions for which such data are available are mainly recessively inherited inborn errors of metabolism ascertained by screening programs. Recessive disorders tend to show rather wide differences in frequency in different population groups, e.g., sickle-cell anemia and Tay-Sachs disease are frequent among persons of African and Ashkenazic Jewish extraction, respectively, but cystic fibrosis, phenylketonuria, and Wilson's disease, which are relatively frequent disorders in persons of northwestern European extraction, are relatively rare in these groups. For these reasons, no estimates of frequency are given here.*

† *Autosomal dominant and X-linked forms of congenital deafness are known, but autosomal recessive inheritance is the rule. Similarly, autosomal dominant and autosomal recessive forms of hypophosphatemic, or vitamin D–resistant, rickets are known. Genetic heterogeneity is illustrated also by conditions which simulate other disorders listed here.*

Other genetic considerations such as the severity of the disease in question, including its severity in the specific family, must be included in the evaluation. Only the risks should be stated to the persons seeking counsel. The decision as to what action they should follow must be theirs and must take account of factors such as economic status and emotional fortitude. Socially valuable traits partially determined by genetic constitution may be present in the family and outweigh the disadvantage of a mutant gene.

Often the statement of risks is a relief to the persons involved and is not disturbing. For example, a young man with pseudoxanthoma elasticum (Chap. 364), an autosomal recessive trait, was relieved to learn that the likelihood that his children by an unrelated wife would be affected by the severe eye involvement and tendency to hemorrhage is essentially nil. In families affected by a clear-cut, nearly fully penetrant autosomal dominant trait normal persons are sometimes surprised to learn, and considerably relieved, that there is virtually no risk of their offspring being affected.

Genetic counseling has gained a strong ally in prenatal diagnosis by amniocentesis. By 14 weeks of gestation 5 to 10 ml of amniotic fluid can be removed with apparent safety by percutaneous transabdominal puncture. Chromosomal abnormalities (e.g., that of Down's syndrome) and biochemical defects (e.g., that of Tay-Sachs disease) can be detected in amniotic cells grown in culture. If an abnormality is found and if the laws of the state permit, the parents can be offered termination of the pregnancy. The pregnancies in which amniocentesis is considered are those with a significant chance of producing an offspring with a condition which can be diagnosed by available methods. These high-risk families are those in which a previously born child has had a given disorder or the parents are known to have a biochemical or chromosome status which makes them likely to have affected children. In the view of some authorities, any pregnant woman over forty years of age or even over thirty-five should have amniocentesis to exclude Down's syndrome or other serious chromosomal aberration in the offspring.

Genetic counseling in common disorders of multifactor causation presents special problems, which are discussed later.

NATURE AND FUNCTION OF THE GENETIC CODE

The gene is DNA, deoxyribonucleic acid. The function of many genes is to specify the sequence of amino acids that make up a polypeptide chain in a protein, either enzymatic or structural. The code word, or codon, for each amino acid is three-lettered, being spelled in one of four purine or pyrimidine bases: adenine, thymine, guanine, and cytosine (see Table 62-4). The principle of colinearity of the triplet code words in the DNA of the gene and the amino acids in the protein specified by that gene is now well established.

TABLE 62-4
The genetic code

First nucleotide	*Second nucleotide:* **A** or *U*			**G** or *C*			**T** or *A*			**C** or *G*			Third nucleotide
A or *U*	**AAA**	*UUU*	Phe	**AGA**	*UCU*	Ser	**ATA**	*UAU*	Tyr	**ACA**	*UGU*	Cys	**A** or *U*
	AAG	*UUC*		**AGG**	*UCC*		**ATG**	*UAC*		**ACG**	*UGC*		**G** or *C*
	AAT	*UUA*	Leu	**AGT**	*UCA*		**ATT**	*UAA*	Stop	**ACT**	*UGA*	Stop	**T** or *A*
	AAC	*UUG*		**AGC**	*UCG*		**ATC**	*UAG*		**ACC**	*UGG*	Trp	**C** or *G*
G or *C*	**GAA**	*CUU*	Leu	**GGA**	*CCU*	Pro	**GTA**	*CAU*	His	**GCA**	*CGU*	Arg	**A** or *U*
	GAG	*CUC*		**GGG**	*CCC*		**GTG**	*CAC*		**GCG**	*CGC*		**G** or *C*
	GAT	*CUA*		**GGT**	*CCA*		**GTT**	*CAA*	Gln	**GCT**	*CGA*		**T** or *A*
	GAC	*CUG*		**GGC**	*CCG*		**GTC**	*CAG*		**GCC**	*CGG*		**C** or *G*
T or *A*	**TAA**	*AUU*	Ile	**TGA**	*ACU*	Thr	**TTA**	*AAU*	Asn	**TCA**	*AGU*	Ser	**A** or *U*
	TAG	*AUC*		**TGG**	*ACC*		**TTG**	*AAC*		**TCG**	*AGC*		**G** or *C*
	TAT	*AUA*		**TGT**	*ACA*		**TTT**	*AAA*	Lys	**TCT**	*AGA*	Arg	**T** or *A*
	TAC	*AUG*	Met	**TGC**	*ACG*		**TTC**	*AAG*		**TCC**	*AGG*		**C** or *G*
C or *G*	**CAA**	*GUU*	Val	**CGA**	*GCU*	Ala	**CTA**	*GAU*	Asp	**CCA**	*GGU*	Gly	**A** or *U*
	CAG	*GUC*		**CGG**	*GCC*		**CTG**	*GAC*		**CCG**	*GGC*		**G** or *C*
	CAT	*GUA*		**CGT**	*GCA*		**CTT**	*GAA*	Glu	**CCT**	*GGA*		**T** or *A*
	CAC	*GUG*		**CGC**	*GCG*		**CTC**	*GAG*		**CCC**	*GGG*		**C** or *G*

Note: The DNA codons appear in boldface type; the complementary RNA codons are in italics. A = adenine, C = cytosine, G = guanine, T = thymine, U = uridine (replaces thymine in RNA). In RNA, adenine is complementary to thymine of DNA; uridine is complementary to adenine of DNA; cytosine is complementary to guanine, and vice versa. "Stop" = punctuation. The amino acids are abbreviated as follows:

Ala = alanine
Arg = arginine
Asn = asparagine
Asp = aspartic acid
Cys = cysteine
Gln = glutamine
Glu = glutamic acid
Gly = glycine
His = histidine
Ile = isoleucine
Leu = leucine
Lys = lysine
Met = methionine
Phe = phenylalanine
Pro = proline
Ser = serine
Thr = threonine
Trp = tryptophan
Tyr = tyrosine
Val = valine

The triplet code for each of 20 specific amino acids is shown in Table 62-4. Messenger RNA (ribonucleic acid), in which the nucleotides are complementary to those of DNA so that it is a negative copy of the DNA, conveys the blueprint for amino acid sequence from DNA on a chromosome in the nucleus to the site of protein synthesis on the ribosomes in the cytoplasm (Fig. 62-14). The code dictionary summarized in Table 62-4 was deduced from studies of the messenger RNA code, in which uridine substitutes for thymine. In addition to ribosomal RNA and messenger RNA, a third type, transfer or soluble RNA, is involved in the assemblage of amino acids into polypeptide chains. The process by which RNA is copied from DNA is called *transcription;* the process by which the RNA-DNA blueprint determines the amino acid sequence of a protein is called *translation* (Fig. 62-14).

The limits of the gene have become clearer. As a functional unit, called by Seymour Benzer the *cistron,* the gene is that portion of DNA responsible for specification of a single polypeptide, and a *locus* is physically that portion of the linearly arranged genetic material (DNA) occupied by the cistron or gene. The alternative forms of the gene which occur at the same locus are called *alleles.* For example, the genes for A, B, and O blood types are multiple alleles at one locus. Within a locus there are many mutable sites.

The normal process of development occurs by differential gene action; i.e., by activity of some genes but not of others in particular tissues at particular stages. The mechanism controlling differential gene activity, what switches one gene on and another off at a particular stage, is unknown. Dramatic examples of differential gene function are reflected by the shift from synthesis of embryonic hemoglobin to fetal hemoglobin in the first trimester and from fetal hemoglobin to adult hemoglobin in the first months of extrauterine life.

MUTATION This term means change in the genetic material. At least three classes of mutation must be considered. When used without further specification, the term usually refers to "point mutation," i.e., change in a single base with substitution of one for another. As seen in Table 62-4, change in DNA from CTT to CAT causes a substitution of valine for glutamic acid in the product protein. This change is the one which occurs in the beta chain of sickle hemoglobin. Similarly, a change from CTT to TTT causes substitution of lysine for glutamic acid, the situation in hemoglobin C. It was first reported that a variant hemoglobin, called Hb I, had lysine (the sixteenth amino acid in the alpha chain) replaced by aspartic acid. Francis Crick insisted, however, that this is not true because change in a single base cannot result in this amino acid substitution. When the matter was reinvestigated, it was found that, in fact, glutamic acid is substituted for lysine, a change produced by a single base substitution.

A second class of mutation is that which results in the gross chromosomal abnormalities discussed in the next section. This class includes (1) abnormalities of chromosome number, e.g., missing or supernumerary chromosomes as a result of errors in chromosome segregation during cell division; and (2) abnormalities of chromosome structure, i.e., chromosomal deletions, translocations, inversions, and so on, as a result of chromosome breakage.

A third class of mutation results from nonhomologous pairing and unequal crossing over, as shown in Fig. 62-16. During the meiotic process in gametogenesis, homologous chromosomes pair, but if the matching is not precise, unequal crossing over occurs. The result is either duplication (Fig. 62-15*A*) of genetic material or deletion. Gene duplication, like the other forms of mutation, has been demonstrably important in evolution. It is a process by which an organism can experiment with new mutations in one copy of the duplicated gene while retaining an essential function of the original gene. The separate genes that specify the various polypeptide chains of hemoglobin (the beta chain of adult hemoglobin A, the delta chain of

FIGURE 62-14
Schema of the genetic control of protein synthesis. (Courtesy, Dr. Irving M. London.)

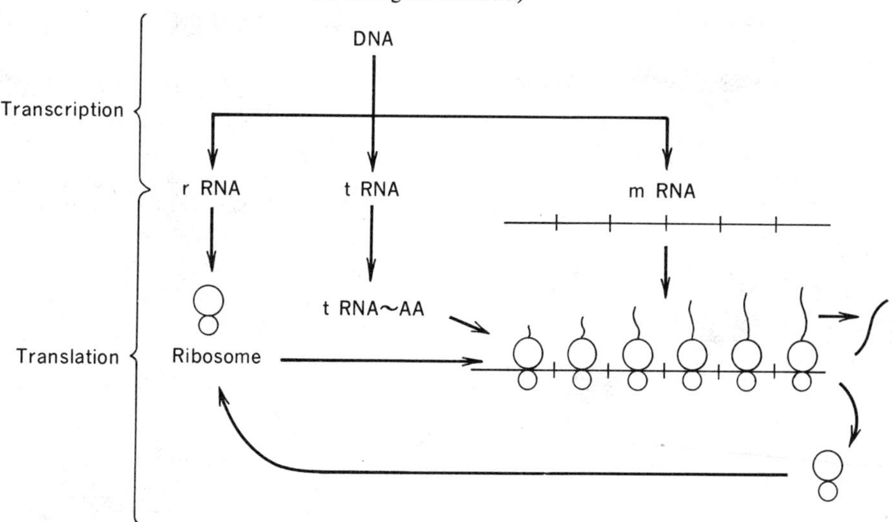

adult hemoglobin A_2, the gamma chain of fetal hemoglobin, the epsilon chain of embryonic hemoglobin, and the alpha chain of all four of these hemoglobins) as well as the gene that specifies the single polypeptide chain of myoglobin appear to have evolved from a primordial common ancestral gene through the process of gene duplication and subsequent independent mutation in the separate genes.

Nonhomologous pairing with unequal crossing over also can cause deletion of part of a gene or of part of two contiguous genes. Study of the amino acid sequence in some abnormal hemoglobins suggests that this was the type of mutation responsible, rather than change in a codon which caused a different amino acid to be specified. For example, in hemoglobin Gun Hill five amino acids are missing from the beta chain (amino acids 93 through 97), so that this hemoglobin is only 141 amino acids long rather than 146. Hemoglobin Lepore is another example of mutation due to unequal crossing over. The gene for the beta chain of hemoglobin A and that for the delta chain of hemoglobin A_2 are probably contiguous. In a person with hemoglobin Lepore, the normal beta and delta chains are replaced by a polypeptide chain that has the structure of the delta chain at one end and of the beta chain at the other. As is diagramed in Fig. 62-15*B*, a fusion gene specifying a hybrid polypeptide chain of this type could have arisen by unequal crossing over. Complementary "ante-Lepore" hemoglobins predicted by the diagram (see question mark above the β-δ fusion product) have been identified—hemoglobin P_{Congo} and hemoglobin Miyada.

FIGURE 62-15

Genetic mutation through nonhomologous pairing and unequal crossing over. A *Gene duplication from crossing over between genes.* B *Creation of a fusion gene through crossing over within a gene, as is thought to have occurred to produce the gene for Lepore hemoglobin.*

BIOCHEMICAL ASPECTS OF GENE ACTION

Biochemical genetics has two parts: One, the chemistry of the genetic material (discussed earlier), had its beginnings with Friedrich Miescher's work on nucleic acid. The second part of biochemical genetics had its origin in the early part of this century, with a physician, Archibald Garrod, and his "inborn errors of metabolism." The disorders he considered were defects in intermediary metabolism resulting from an inherited abnormality of particular enzymes. In its broader implications, biochemical genetics is concerned with the chemical nature of the genetic code and with all the biochemical steps by which that code is translated into an observed characteristic, e.g., an inherited disease.

In accordance with the current views, all properties of a protein are a consequence of its amino acid sequence. Probably the proteins specified by genes not only are enzyme proteins but also may be structural proteins, e.g., collagen, or proteins with other functions and properties, such as hemoglobin. The useful concept of "one gene, one enzyme" requires modification to "one gene, one polypeptide," or (see below) "one cistron, one polypeptide."

In the schema outlined earlier, mutation represents a change in the code, i.e., a change in the base sequence of DNA. Mutations may be of two types. In "mis-sense" mutations a different amino acid is substituted at a given site in the particular protein, e.g., valine for glutamic acid, changing "normal" hemoglobin to sickle hemoglobin. In "non-sense" mutations the change in the base sequence of DNA is such that there is no corresponding amino acid and none of a given protein, e.g., an enzyme, may be found.

The terms borrowed from bacterial genetics, CRM-positive (pronounced "krim-positive") and CRM-negative mutations, correspond to the terms *mis-sense* and *non-sense* mutations, respectively. CRM means cross-reacting material, and in CRM-positive mutations material which reacts in a normal manner in immunologic tests but is functionally (e.g., enzymatically) ineffective is present. In man, a large proportion of enzyme deficiency states are found to show some residual enzyme activity,

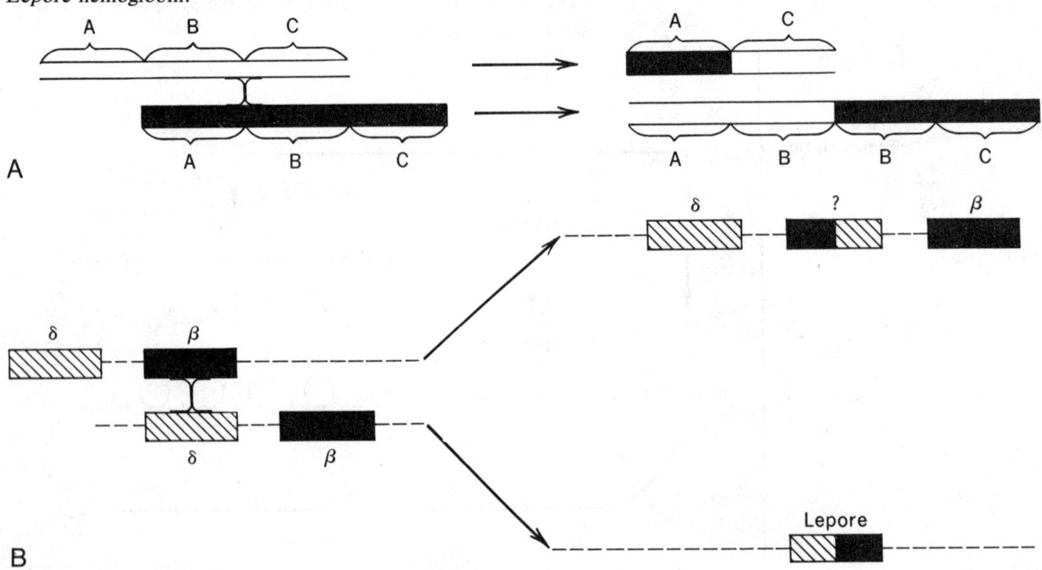

and when the properties of the enzyme are studied it is often found to have either reduced catalytic capacity or increased lability. Sometimes less enzyme is synthesized because of the change in amino acid structure. The fact that some enzyme remains can present problems in detecting deficiency under the conditions of the test tube but at the same time is a more promising result because methods of treating the patient which increase the stability or catalytic capacity of the residual enzyme or increase the amount synthesized become possibilities.

As stated above, the mutant gene can result in the formation of a different protein or of no protein at all of a given type. If the protein in question is an enzyme, none at all may be formed or an enzyme may be formed which is so impaired in its function that the net effect is the same. In intermediary metabolism such a change can have pathogenetic consequences through any of several mechanisms or through some combination of these. We may represent a hypothetical metabolic process as follows:

$$\begin{array}{ccccccc} & \text{Gene}_{AB} & & \text{Gene}_{BC} & & \text{Gene}_{CD} & \\ & \downarrow & & \downarrow & & \downarrow & \\ & \text{Enzyme}_{AB} & & \text{Enzyme}_{BC} & & \text{Enzyme}_{CD} & \\ A & \longrightarrow & B & \longrightarrow & C & \longrightarrow & D \end{array}$$

If a mutant form of gene$_{CD}$ results in no formation of enzyme$_{CD}$ or in the formation of functionally defective enzyme, then the effects may be of several types:

1 The disease characteristic may reflect the deficiency of product D:

$$A \longrightarrow B \longrightarrow C \not\longrightarrow (D)$$

Albinism (Chap. 98) might be cited as an example; melanin is not formed because of a block in tyrosine metabolism. In several forms of genetic cretinism (Chap. 85), thyroid hormone is not formed because of blocks of this type; in the adrenogenital syndrome (Chap. 92), hydrocortisone is not produced.

2 A metabolite just proximal to the block may accumulate in toxic amounts.

$$A \longrightarrow B \longrightarrow \begin{array}{c} C \\ C \\ C \end{array} \not\longrightarrow (D)$$

An example is alkaptonuria. Homogentisic acid is not metabolized normally. It is excreted in the urine in large amounts. Furthermore its increase in the body in some way leads to a form of degenerative arthritis.

3 If the reactions in question are reversible, there may be an accumulation of precursors farther back from the site of the block.

$$\begin{array}{c} A \\ A \\ A \end{array} \rightleftharpoons \begin{array}{c} B \\ B \end{array} \rightleftharpoons C \longrightarrow (D)$$

An example is the accumulation of glycogen in the form of glycogen storage disease (von Gierke's disease) in which the primary defect involves glucose 6-phosphatase (Chap. 104).

Glycogen ⇌ glucose 1-phosphate ⇌ glucose 6-phosphate ⇸ (glucose 6-phosphatase)

4 There may be synthesis of products through an accessory pathway which is normally of minor significance.

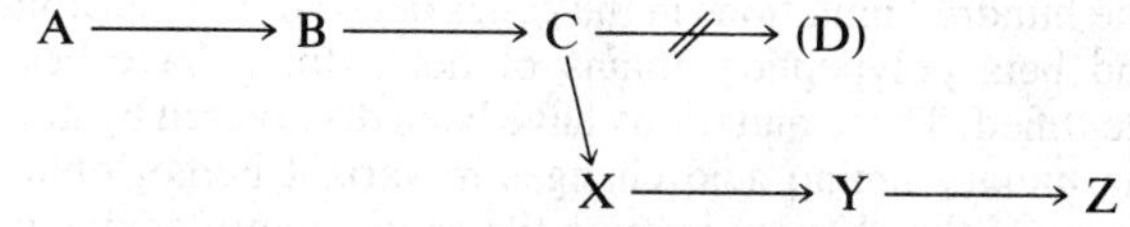

In phenylketonuria, phenylketone products are produced in unusual amounts from phenylalanine, which is not properly metabolized. In hyperoxaluria, an excess production of oxalate may be the result of a defect in the normal metabolism of glyoxylate:

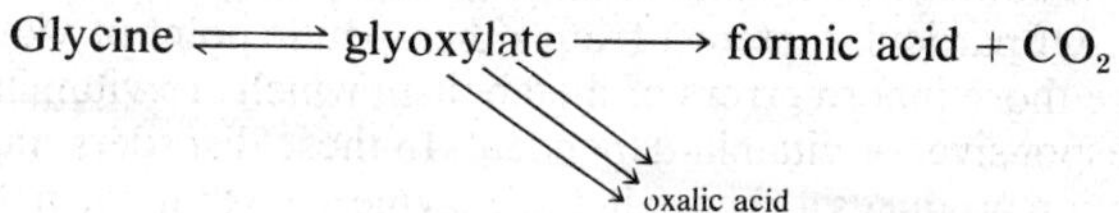

Undoubtedly these do not exhaust the possible mechanisms of a pathogenetic effect from a mutation in a gene controlling an enzyme. For example, interruption of a normal feedback inhibition can result from enzyme deficiency, with the result that more of some substance is formed than is normally the case. In the Lesch-Nyhan syndrome, hyperuricemia results because deficiency of hypoxanthine-guanine phosphoribosyl-transferase (HGPRT) leads to failure of synthesis of guanylic acid, which has an inhibitory effect on the first and rate-limiting step in purine synthesis. In oroticaciduria, not only does orotic acid accumulate as a direct effect of the block, as indicated in diagram 2 above, but an abnormally large amount of the substance (orotic acid) just preceding the enzyme block is synthesized because the inhibitory effect of a later product of the metabolic chain on the first step is removed.

Metabolic processes are in most instances chains, indeed often networks. A mutation in the genes controlling any of several metabolic steps may lead to the same phenotypic result. Thus, the phenotype is not an indication of the specific genotype. Identical diseases may be produced by mutation of different genes; "genetic mimics," they are called.

More than 120 disorders have been traced to a deficiency in the activity of specific enzymes. Almost all behave as recessive traits. Enzyme systems have sufficient margin of safety that the mutant gene must be present in double dose and the deficiency must be complete in order for abnormality to be demonstrable in the phenotype. On the other hand, conditions based on mutation in a gene determining the amino acid sequence of a nonenzymatic protein, e.g., hemoglobin, are likely to be dominant in their inheritance pattern. This is because the physical and functional properties of the product protein may be so altered that abnormality occurs even though only about half the product protein is of mutant type. The above principle concerning dominant and recessive inheritance is nicely demonstrated by the methemoglobinemias (Chap. 312), of which dominant and recessive forms exist. The recessive form is due to deficient activity of an enzyme, methemoglobin reductase, of the red blood cell. The dominant forms have a defect in hemoglobin, these being the several types of hemoglobin M.

The nonenzymatic protein which has been subjected to most extensive study is hemoglobin (Chap. 307). Over one hundred mutations in the genes determining the alpha and beta polypeptide chains of hemoglobin have been identified. These mutations have been discovered by finding unitary amino acid changes in variant hemoglobins. Some of the changes involve the same amino acid; e.g., both hemoglobin S and hemoglobin C have a change in the sixth of the 146 amino acids of the beta polypeptide chain. In other variant hemoglobins the change is present in different amino acids of the chain. Understanding of how the particular amino acid substitution alters the function of hemoglobin is steadily increasing.

Of particular interest from a therapeutic point of view are those inborn errors of metabolism which are vitamin-responsive, or vitamin-dependent. In these disorders mutation produces a change in the enzyme such that when its vitamin cofactor is present in usual amounts it functions inadequately. Pharmacologic doses of the cofactor permit the enzyme to function adequately. Vitamin-dependent disorders cured by the administration of vitamin B_6 and vitamin B_{12} are known. Vitamin B_6-responsive and nonresponsive forms of homocystinuria exist, as well as vitamin B_{12}-responsive and nonresponsive forms of methylmalonicaciduria.

Another type of process, not strictly enzymatic, by which mutations have pathogenetic effects involves changes in membrane transport mechanisms in the kidney and elsewhere. Cystinuria (Chap. 96) is an example. Other active transport systems may be cited, e.g., those involved in the movement of substances such as amino acids across the intestinal mucosa, of substances like bilirubin into and out of the liver cell, and of electrolytes across the muscle cell membrane. All these mechanisms are vulnerable to the effects of mutation in the determinant genes, and diseases for which such mutation is probably responsible may be cited.

Structural genes, i.e., those specifying the amino acid sequence of proteins, have for the most part been discussed to this point. "A pile of bricks is not a house," however. Other genes have a controlling role, ensuring an orderly interplay of the structural genes in development and in the adult organism. Mutation can occur also in these controlling genes, with resultant disease. The evidence is coming mainly from the study of microorganisms; although a number of disorders of man are suspected to result from mutation in controlling genes, critical evidence is not easily assembled.

The complex machinery of protein synthesis, of which the framework is DNA-RNA-ribosomes, has become more clearly understood in recent years. Of potential therapeutic importance is the demonstration that intermediate steps in protein synthesis can be modified by various measures. It is possible, for example, that although a warped and enzymatically weak protein is formed in a given disorder, the amount synthesized can be increased by some means and the disease abolished or ameliorated.

THE GENETICS OF COMMON DISORDERS All disease is in some degree genetic and in some degree environmental in etiology and pathogenesis. As to the relative importance of endogenous and exogenous factors, disease may be thought of as falling on a spectrum (Fig. 62-16). Near the genetic end (G) are simply inherited disorders such as phenylketonuria and galactosemia, but these are not at the extreme end because exogenous factors, diet in these specific examples, can importantly modify the phenotype. Near the environmental end (E) are infectious diseases but again not at the extreme end because twin and other studies indicate a significant role of genotype in susceptibility.

In the analysis of disorders affecting all systems, two classes of disorders, with regard to the role of genetic factors, are evident: (1) rare, simply inherited disorders (near the G end of the spectrum); (2) common disorders in which genetic factors play some role. Examples in the gastrointestinal system are familial polyposis of the colon and peptic ulcer; in the cardiovascular system, hereditary hemorrhagic telangiectasia and coronary artery disease; in the connective tissue system, Marfan's syndrome, lupus erythematosus; in the eye, retinitis pigmentosa and glaucoma.

The common disorders are, for the most part, multifactorial in causation. The etiologic picture is a nexus in which environmental and genetic factors collaborate in a complex way in determining the disease.

Questions asked in connection with common disease are mainly two: How significant are genetic factors in etiology? By what mechanism does the mutant gene contribute to the pathogenesis?

Methods for evaluating the role of genetic factors in common diseases are mainly six:

1 *Family studies.* If genetic factors are important, a familial aggregation for the disorder should be demonstrable. Familial aggregation may have other than a

FIGURE 62-16
Schematic representation of the spectrum of disease in regard to the relative importance of genetics (G) *and exogenous* (E) *factors in etiology and pathogenesis.*

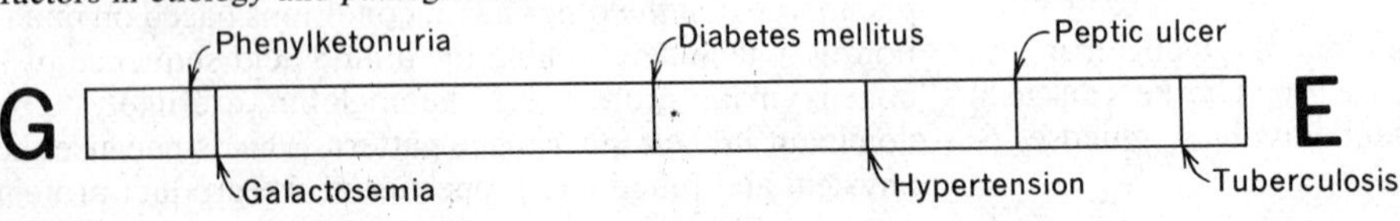

genetic basis; thus, evidence from family studies is per se not critical.

2 *Twin studies.* Monozygotic twins, because of genetic identity, should show a higher concordance rate (i.e., "both affected") than dizygotic twins shown, if genetic factors are significantly involved.

3 *Interracial comparisons.* Races have different frequencies of many genes. If genetic factors are important in etiology, the frequency of common diseases may vary from race to race. A difficulty in interpretation of racial data is the uncertainty of environmental comparability. Races are social as well as biologic entities.

4 *Component analysis.* Whenever a factor is shown to be an important element of the etiologic nexus, its genetics can be studied by family studies, twin studies, racial comparisons, and animal homologies. Lipid metabolism in atherosclerosis is an example.

5 *Blood group and disease association.* A simply inherited trait such as a specific blood group can, in some instances, be shown to occur more frequently with a given common disease than would be expected by chance. Some physiologic peculiarity of the person with that blood group seems to predispose him slightly but definitely to the disorder. The best example is the association between blood group O and peptic ulcer (Chap. 310). Another is the association of non-O blood groups and venous thromboembolic disease. Demonstration of association is evidence of a genetic factor in the disorder. Failure to demonstrate association does not exclude the importance of genetic factors.

6 *Animal homologies.* If one has available in animals a disorder seemingly identical to a common disease of man, then one may be able to do breeding experiments and extensive biochemical and physiologic investigations that will throw light on the two questions stated above.

The collaboration of multiple genes appears to be involved in determining stature; i.e., stature is a polygenic

FIGURE 62-17
Distribution curve for stature in the southeastern part of England. The mean is 68 in., the standard deviation, 2.6 in. (Drawn from data analyzed by Cedric O. Carter)

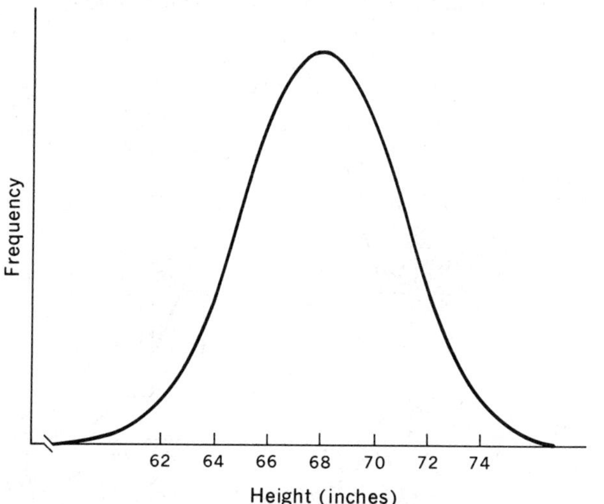

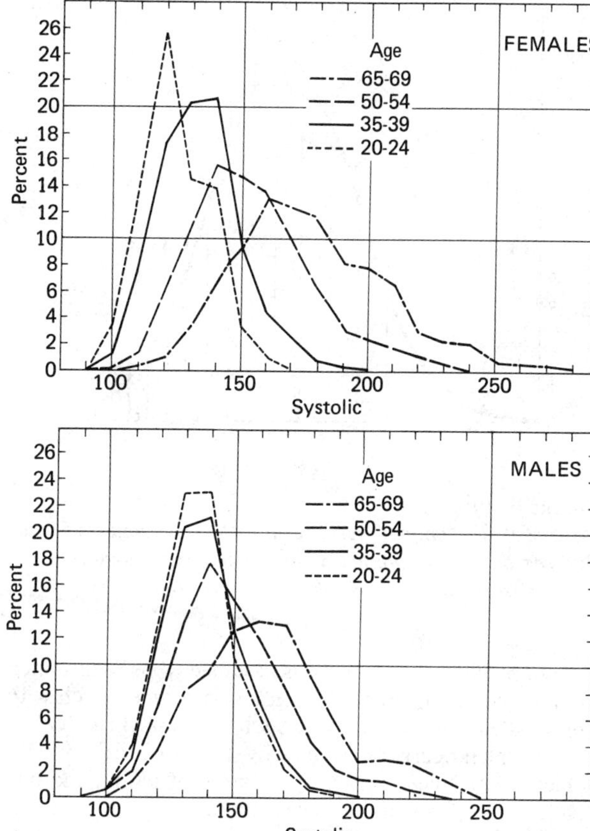

FIGURE 62-18
Distribution curves for blood pressure. Normal blood pressure increases with age and is somewhat different in males and females; hence the separate plots. Note that all show positive skew, i.e., a tail at the end of the curve for higher pressures. [*From Bøe et al, Acta Med Scand 157: (suppl. 321), 1957*]

trait. Environmental factors, such as nutrition and chronic infectious disease, also influence stature; thus, stature is a multifactorial trait, to use the more general term. When the stature of a large group of persons is plotted, the distribution curve is a "normal," bell-shaped gaussian one (Fig. 62-17). This suggests that the multiple genes involved in determining a person's height interact in an additive manner. By way of contrast, the distribution curve for blood pressure is "skewed" (Fig. 62-18), suggesting that the multiple genes determining level of blood pressure interact in a multiplicative manner. This conclusion is supported by the fact that if a logarithmic scale is used for blood pressure, the curve is "normalized" (Fig. 62-19). As a corollary to the view that blood pressure is a polygenic trait, essential hypertension is interpreted as the condition present in those persons whose particular assemblage of genes determines a level of blood pressure at the upper end of the distribution curve. What one calls essential hypertension and what one calls normotension are largely arbitrary decisions.

That a rather small number of genes can produce a continuous distribution is indicated by the example

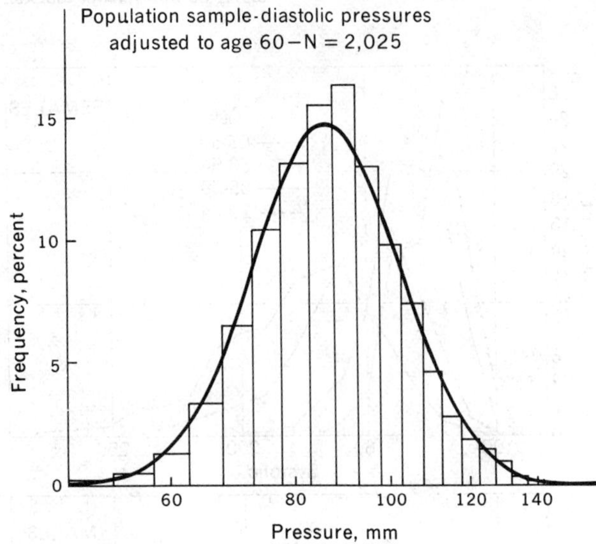

FIGURE 62-19
An essentially "normal" curve results when adjustments for age and sex differences are made and a logarithmic blood pressure scale is used. (Courtesy of J.A. Fraser Roberts)

TABLE 62-6
Proportions of expected types of zygotes

Female gametes	Male gametes: – – 1/16	– 0 1/4	0 0 6/16	0 + 1/4	+ + 1/16
– – 1/16	60 in. 1/256	62 in. 4/256	64 in. 6/256	66 in. 1/64	68 in. 1/256
– 0 1/4	62 in. 4/256	64 in. 1/16	66 in. 6/64	68 in. 1/16	70 in. 1/64
0 0 6/16	64 in. 6/256	66 in. 6/64	68 in. 36/256	70 in. 6/64	72 in. 6/256
0 + 1/4	66 in. 1/64	68 in. 1/16	70 in. 6/64	72 in. 1/16	74 in. 4/256
+ + 1/16	68 in. 1/256	70 in. 1/64	72 in. 6/256	74 in. 4/256	76 in. 1/256

shown in Fig. 62-20. Stature is assumed to be determined by two genetic loci on different chromosomes, each with three alleles in frequencies such that an allele (called "—") which decreases stature by 2 in., one (called "O") which determines the average stature of 68 in., and one (called "+") which increases stature by 2 in. have a relative frequency of 1:2:1. Five classes of gametes produced by each sex have the following frequencies (derived from Table 62-5): ——, 1/16; —0, 1/4; 00, 6/16; +0, 1/4; ++1/16. Zygotes formed from random union of gametes in these proportions have four stature genes (two at each of the two loci), and the possible combinations of +, 0, and – alleles found among the zygotes are nine in number. The relative frequencies of these are derived from Table 62-6 and plotted in Fig. 62-20. A satisfactory approximation to a normal distribution is obtained, particularly when environmental influences blur the separation of groups. This example illustrates that even in conditions, like essential hypertension, which appear to by polygenic, it is worthwhile to search for single-gene–determined biochemical and physiologic mechanisms.

Since blood pressure level is a continuous variable, the analogy to stature serves well to illustrate multifactorial causation. In the case of congenital malformations the multifactorial model requires the additional assumption of a threshold. One can, for instance, represent the distribution of "risk genes" for cleft lip, with or without cleft palate, by a bell-shaped curve (Fig. 62-21). Affected persons have a large number of risk genes, placing them above a postulated threshold. First degree relatives (parents, sibs, and offspring) may be shown to have, on the average, a number of risk genes half way between that of affected probands and that in the general population. Second degree relatives (grandchild, grandparents, aunts,

TABLE 62-5
Proportions of expected types of gametes

Chromosome 2	Chromosome 1: Allele – 1/4	Allele 0 1/8	Allele + 1/4
Allele – 1/4	1/16 – –	1/8 – 0	1/16 – +
Allele 0 1/2	1/8 0 –	1/4 0 0	1/8 0 +
Allele + 1/4	1/16 + –	1/8 + 0	1/16 + +

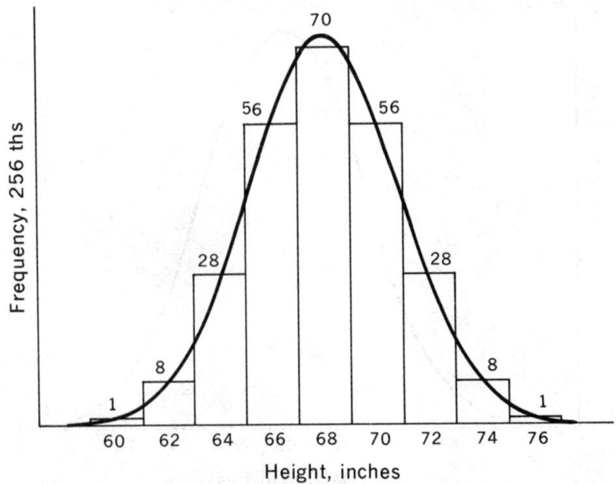

FIGURE 62-20
Distribution curve for stature, assuming that only two loci, each with three alleles, determine this characteristic. A small number of genes combined with environmental influence can result in a continuous distribution. (Example from Cedric O. Carter)

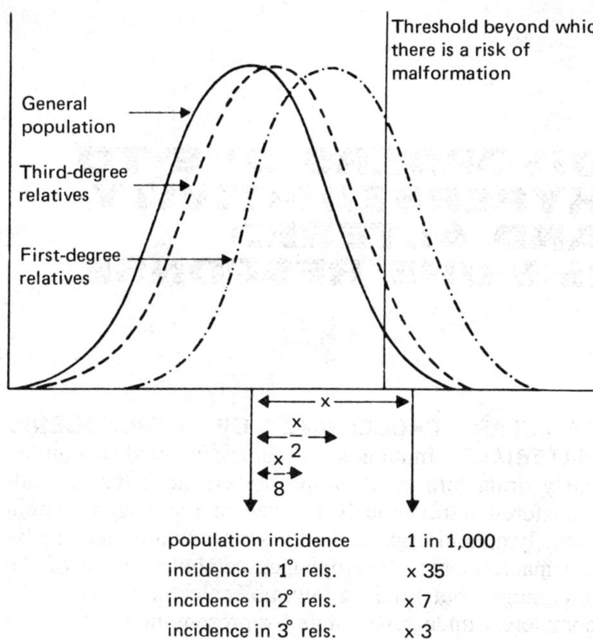

FIGURE 62-21
Model for polygenic inheritance of cleft lip with or without cleft palate. X = deviation of mean of malformed persons from the population mean. (Courtesy of Cedric O. Carter and British Medical Bulletin)

and uncles) have, on the average, a number of risk genes which is one-fourth the difference between the general population number and the number in affected probands; third degree relatives (first cousins) have on the average, a number which is one-eighth the difference. The distribution curves for two of these classes of relatives are presented in Fig. 62-21. The model enables one to predict what proportion of relatives of each class will have the given malformation. Agreement between prediction and observation has been satisfactory for several forms of malformation that have been analyzed from this point of view.

REFERENCES

CARTER CO.: *Human Heredity,* Baltimore: Penguin, 1962

——: Genetics of common disorders. Br Med Bull 25:52, 1972

COURT BROWN WM: *Human Population Cytogenetics,* Amsterdam: North-Holland Publishing Company, 1967

EZDINKI EZ et al: Philadelphia-chromosome-positive and -negative chronic myeloid leukemia. Ann Intern Med 159:175, 1970

HARRIS H: Molecular basis of hereditary disease. Br Med J 1:135, 1968

HECHT F et al: Revolutionary cytogenetics. N Engl J Med 285:1482, 1971

JINK H et al: Venous thromboembolic disease and ABO blood type. Lancet 1:539, 1969

MCKUSICK VA: *Human Genetics,* 2d ed., Englewood Cliffs, N.J.: Prentice-Hall, 1969

——: *Mendelian Inheritence in Man. Catalogs of Autosomal Dominant, Autosomal Recessive and X-linked Phenotypes,* 3d ed., Baltimore: Johns Hopkins, 1971

PERUTZ, MF, LEHMANN G: Molecular pathology of human hemoglobin. Nature 219:902, 1968

ROBERTS JAF: *Introduction to Medical Genetics,* 5th ed., London: Oxford, 1970

ROSENBERG LE: Inherited aminoacidopathies demonstrating vitamin dependency. N Engl J Med 281:145, 1969

ROWLEY JD: Cytogenetics in clinical medicine. JAMA 207:914, 1969

STANBURY JB et al: *The Metabolic Basis of Inherited Disease,* 3d ed., New York: McGraw-Hill, 1972

PART FOUR | DISORDERS DUE TO HYPERSENSITIVITY AND ALTERED IMMUNE RESPONSE

63 INTRODUCTION TO CLINICAL IMMUNOLOGY

K. FRANK AUSTEN

The immunologic response not only constitutes the principal means of man's defense against pathogenic microorganisms, but also is capable of mediating adverse clinical reactions. Whether an immune response is defined clinically as immunity or hypersensitivity is determined by its effect on the host; the distinction does not necessarily imply different mechanisms of elicitation. The components of the immune system may be considered in terms of the sequential manner in which they contribute to the immune response. The principal features include immunogens, capable of initiating the immune response; cellular processing of immunogenic material; products of the immune response; control mechanisms of the response; and consequences, both beneficial and detrimental, of the immune response. Consideration of the immunologic response in terms of these arbitrary divisions affords a basis for a clinical approach to the diagnosis and management of immune deficiency states and hypersensitivity syndromes.

INITIATION OF THE IMMUNE RESPONSE A substance must ordinarily be recognized as foreign in order to elicit an immune response. The ability of a substance to evoke such a response is termed *immunogenicity;* the capacity to react specifically with the antibodies induced is termed *antigenicity*. The distinction is useful because many simple substances of less than 1,000 mol wt are not immunogenic unless coupled covalently or by large numbers of ionic bonds to macromolecules but can react with antibodies of appropriate specificity; such simple substances are termed *haptens.*

Deliberate initiation of the immune response is accomplished most reliably by injection of the immunogen. Feeding is not usually effective because, being proteins, most immunogens are digested in the gastrointestinal tract. The oral route may, however, be utilized under certain circumstances, such as with attenuated poliomyelitis virus. Natural immunization to environmental substances may occur by such diverse routes as inhalation of plant or tree pollens, ingestion of certain foods or drugs, and skin contact with drugs or natural chemicals such as the catechols of poison ivy plants.

CELLULAR PROCESSING OF IMMUNOGENIC MATERIALS Immunogens that are injected subcutaneously drain into local lymph nodes; those that are administered intravenously localize in the spleen. Within these lymphoid organs, the immunogens are taken up by the macrophages. Macrophages catabolize most of the immunogen but retain a few molecules in a partially or completely undegraded state for presentation to the lymphocyte for immune recognition. The macrophages are nonspecific handlers of the immunogen and do not determine the specificity of the immune response. The specificity of the immune response depends on the interaction of the immunogen with lymphocytes which, according to selectional theories, are genetically precommitted to interact with a particular antigen. Two kinds of lymphocytes are present in peripheral lymphoid organs. The so-called *B lymphocytes,* derived from bone marrow stem cells in mammals and cells from the bursa of Fabricius in birds, are situated in the lymphoid follicles and are distinguishable by a large concentration of immunoglobulin molecules on their surface membranes. (Suspensions of B lymphocytes incubated with antibodies to human immunoglobulin conjugated to a fluorescent dye can be shown, when examined under the ultraviolet microscope, to have discrete deposits of immunoglobulin on their surface.) The immunoglobulin on the membrane of the B lymphocyte interacts with antigen, a process which initiates antibody formation. The B lymphocytes, upon this interaction with antigen, differentiate into plasma cells which avidly secrete antibody. The so-called *T lymphocytes,* derived from the thymus, are situated in the areas of recirculation in the lymphoid organs, and do not have demonstrable immunoglobulin molecules on their membranes. Thus the presence or absence of immunoglobulins on lymphocytes can serve to establish whether the cells are T or B in kind. The T lymphocytes also react specifically with antigen and are involved in cell-mediated types of immune reactions. In addition an antibody response to many immunogens requires interaction of both B and T lymphocytes with the macrophage-bound antigen.

Following an immunogenic stimulus the regional lymph nodes (or spleen) become hyperplastic and increase severalfold in weight, and the specific antibody levels in the efferent lymph exceed those in the afferent lymph entering the regional node. Net antibody synthesis by isolated lymph node tissue also has been demonstrated in vitro. The evidence that the plasma cell is particularly active in antibody synthesis includes (1) the prominence of plasma cells as lymphoid tissue becomes hyperplastic in response to an immunogenic stimulus; (2) the approximate relationship between the antibody extractable from such tissue with the plasma cell content; (3) the demonstration by immunofluorescent staining procedures of gamma-globulin in the cytoplasm of plasma cells; and (4) the clinical observations of increased numbers of plasma cells in circumstances of gamma-globulin overproduction and the virtual absence of such cells in heritable disorders of antibody production.

Antibody synthesis by spleen lymphoid cells had also been demonstrated in vitro. A suitable method involves the culture of spleen cell suspensions with foreign red cells; about 4 to 7 days after culture the spleen cells are embedded in a slide or dish with soft agar containing the foreign red cells and complement; if the cell is a plasma cell it will secrete antibody which will lyse the neighboring red cells and form a visible plaque. With this method the actual number of cells making antibody can be readily determined. This in vitro system has confirmed that T and B lymphocytes and macrophages are necessary to produce an in vitro immune response and that the B lymphocyte proliferates after antigenic stimulation and before its conversion into actively secreting plasma cells.

In summary, as shown in Fig. 63-1, the macrophage presents the immunogenic molecules to two types of lymphocytes—B lymphocytes bearing specific immunoglobulin which differentiate into plasma cells and T lymphocytes involved in cell-mediated immunity and serving a helper function in antibody formation.

PRODUCTS OF THE IMMUNE RESPONSE **Structure of gamma-globulins** The gamma-globulins are a group of serum proteins with a distinct electrophoretic mobility and the capacity to behave as antibodies. On the basis of different physicochemical and immunochemical properties, these proteins, termed immunoglobulins, have been divided into a number of major classes. The fundamental molecular unit of all classes of immunoglobulins, as determined by the employment of reducing and denaturing agents, consists of two heavy (H) and two light (L) polypeptide chains linked by interchain disulfide bonds and non-covalent bonds. Each H chain is usually linked to its respective L chain by a single disulfide bond, and two or more disulfide bonds link the heavy chains. IgM macroglobulin consists of five of these subunits joined by disulfide bonds and J chains. IgA can exist either as a monomer or as a polymer held together by J chains. The non-covalent bonds between the polypeptide chains are predominantly hydrophobic bonds. When the enzyme papain is employed, human IgG is split into three fragments; two, termed Fab, are identical and contain the antigen combining sites, and the third, Fc, can be crystallized and is responsible for the unique biologic activities of a class. The Fab fragment consists of an L chain and the N-terminal half of the H chain, termed the Fd fragment, joined by their interchain disulfide bond; the Fc fragment consists of the C terminal portions of the two H chains held by their interchain disulfide bonds. The molecular basis of the specificity of bivalent antibody for antigen resides in the Fab fragments. The combining site is probably constructed predominantly from the Fd fragment of the H chain, while the L chain contributes indirectly by interacting with and stabilizing the neighboring Fd fragment. Differing antibody specificities depend on differing primary amino acid sequences in the region of the combining site; these differences exist in both the H and L chains, which vary in the combining site region but are constant in the C terminal ends of the chains.

For the L chain the constant portion is approximately one-half the chain, whereas in the H chain the invariable portion includes the Fc piece and about one-half the Fd fragment. It is the antigenic differences in the invariable portion of the H chain which permit division of the human immunoglobulins into five major classes (IgG, IgA, IgM, IgD, and IgE). The constant portion of the L chain allows recognition of two types (kappa and lambda), which occur in combination with all five H chains (gamma, alpha, mu, delta, and epsilon). The molecular formulas for the preponderant immunoblogulin class, IgG, would thus be gamma$_2$ lambda$_2$ ($\gamma_2\lambda_2$) and gamma$_2$ kappa$_2$ ($\gamma_2\kappa_2$). IgG is further subdivided into four subclasses, IgG 1 to 4, on the basis of minor intraclass antigenic differences. In addition to the designation of class and subclass by structural differences, there are genetic differences within a class, termed allotypy, expressed by additional discrete structural differences. Genetic control of structural differences in three of the gamma chain subclasses, 1 to 3, has been related to the Gm loci, while allotypic differences in the kappa chain reside in the Inv locus.

Primary immune response The immune response to the first introduction of an immunogen is termed primary. In a primary response, possibly because of the differential sensitivity of the methodology employed, the IgM

FIGURE 63-1
Schematic presentation of the immune response.

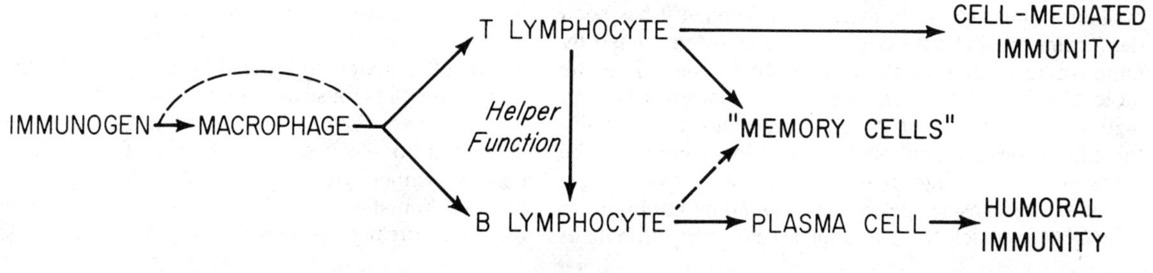

antibodies are recognized somewhat earlier than those of the IgG class. The IgM antibodies are observed within the first week of immunization and decline thereafter as the titer of IgG antibodies increases. This relationship and the finding that formation of IgM antibodies requires appreciable levels of immunogen have been interpreted to indicate that IgG antibodies inhibit synthesis of antibodies of the IgM class. Lymphocytes lodged in the mucosa of the intestine and along the respiratory tract appear to lead to synthesis of antibodies of the IgA and IgE class in response to local deposition of immunogen by ingestion or inhalation. The view that IgM antibodies represent a primitive product of the immune response is supported by the predominant synthesis of this antibody class in the newborn and by phylogenic observations. In addition to sequential changes in immunoglobulin class, heterogeneity of the primary response occurs within the IgG class, expressed as an increasing affinity for the antigen. This may be explicable in terms of continued formation of new antibodies capable of interacting with increasing numbers of diverse antigenic determinants on the macromolecular immunogen.

Secondary immune response When the antibody levels have diminished following initial immunogenic exposure, a subsequent encounter will evoke an enhanced response, termed secondary or anamnestic. The anamnestic response requires a lower threshold dose of immunogen for elicitation and is characterized by a shortened lag phase for appearance of detectable product and a higher and more persistent antibody response. Although the quantity of antibody produced per unit time is usually much greater in the secondary response, the doubling time appears to be about the same as in the primary, which is consistent with the participation of more cells rather than an augmentation in the rate of synthesis per cell. The antibodies formed after the secondary stimulus have a much higher affinity for the corresponding antigenic determinant than those appearing after a comparable time during the primary response. The high-affinity antibodies characteristic of the secondary response are of the IgG class.

Determination of antibody synthesis Studies by immunofluorescent techniques have demonstrated that individual lymph node cells produce only a single class of heavy and light chains at any one time. Preliminary evidence suggests that L chains are made on small polyribosomes and H chains on large ones; and it is held that half the immunoglobulin molecules, consisting of single L and H chains, are assembled through attachment of free L chains to the polyribosomal-bound H chains, and that the product then is released for assembly into a bivalent immunoglobulin molecule. Although it has been demonstrated that antibody specificity is determined by amino acid sequence, there is no real insight into the molecular basis by which a flexibility sufficient to recognize the vast array of potential immunogens is maintained. Theories of antibody production continue to be assessed; they range from instructive (in which the immunogen helps shape the corresponding antibody) to selective (in which the immunogen selectively stimulates a cell or portion of the gene already capable of producing the desired product). This latter theory seems most consistent with the data at hand.

The consequences of the immune response grouped as cellular immunity are of great biologic importance but cannot be presented in physicochemical terms. Accordingly, these cellular phenomena, along with the humoral responses, will be examined in the sections dealing with control mechanisms and the biologic consequences of the immune response.

CONTROL MECHANISMS OF THE IMMUNE RESPONSE Wide variations usually are observed in the amounts of specific antibody formed in different individuals of the same species in response to a similar immunogenic stimulus. Experiments involving inbred strains of mice and guinea pigs have demonstrated genetic control of the immune response to a variety of antigens. The antigens used usually contained few antigenic determinants. While some strains manifested a high immune response to a particular antigen, others responded poorly or not at all. This genetic control follows classical mendelian genetics and in most instances is an autosomal dominant trait. In addition control of this aspect of the immune response is associated with the histocompatibility genes of the strain and resides at the level of thymic cell function. In man there is evidence that the capacity to make antibodies of the IgE class in response to inhaled pollens is associated with an increased incidence of a similar immunoglobulin response to drugs and other environmental antigens.

Role of the thymus The development of the capacity to respond to an immunogen is dependent on a functioning thymus gland as well as on other lymphoepithelial structures arising embryologically as outpouchings of the gut wall and eventually consisting of lymphocyte populations in close proximity to epithelial cells of endodermal origin. Experimental studies have revealed that neonatal thymectomy interferes with the development of the lymphoid system, profoundly impairs the immunologic capabilities termed "cellular immunity" (such as rejection of foreign-tissue grafts and delayed hypersensitivity), and also under certain circumstances diminishes humoral responses. The manner in which the thymus mediates the development of these aspects of immunologic competence is not entirely clear but may include (1) an environment in which "stem" cells, possibly of bone marrow origin, differentiate to become immunologically competent before being distributed peripherally to populate node tissue; (2) elaboration of a humoral factor regulating the maturation of peripheral lymphocytes; and (3) the exertion of "censorship," whereby potentially self-reacting clones are eliminated. It has now been shown principally through experiments in the mouse that some of the cells in the thymus undergo a process of maturation and then enter the recirculating pool of lymphoid cells, mixing with the B type of lymphocytes. The proliferative response of peripheral blood lymphocytes to mitogens like phytohemagglutinin or Concanavalin A is attributed to the presence of these functional thymic derived lymphocytes. The consequences of thymectomy are less dramatic in the adult animal, but there is evidence that the thymus continues to provide a mechanism whereby immunologically uncommitted cells acquire the capacity to respond to specific immunogens.

In birds there is an anatomic separation of the central control of the capacity to develop cellular and humoral immunity; the former is regulated by the thymus and the latter by the bursa of Fabricius. In mammals the precise equivalent of the bursa has not been established, but it is assumed to be some portion of the gut-associated lymphoid tissue. The evidence in man for some division of central control resides in the existence of patients with hereditary lesions expressed predominantly as defects in cellular immunity, humoral immunity, or both.

Tolerance The capacity of an individual's immune response to distinguish between his own and foreign macromolecules was termed "horror autotoxicus" by Ehrlich and "self-tolerance" by Burnet. An operational definition of tolerance sufficient to include a variety of terms developed from special experimental circumstances is "a state of specific immunologic nonreactivity to an immunogenic stimulus which would be followed by a recognizable response in a normal animal." Though moderate doses of an immunogen can initiate the immune response, an excessive dose is followed by a state of tolerance or specific nonreactivity to any subsequent dose of the immunogen, although unrelated immunogens, in appropriate dose, are fully active. The physical state of the antigen is important in inducing or maintaining a state of tolerance; antigens that are soluble and of low molecular weight are highly effective in inducing tolerance, while the same antigen in aggregated forms may trigger an immune response. Tolerance is more easily established in the neonate than in the adult, is maintained by persistence of the immunogen, and can be manifested by impairment of either humoral or cellular immunity. The T lymphocyte is made tolerant with much smaller amounts of antigen than the B lymphocyte, and the tolerance state in the T-cell population is very long-lived in contrast to the short duration of tolerance in the B lymphocytes. Tolerance to an immunogen has been shown experimentally to be associated with the functional absence of the specifically responding cells or clone. It is held that the immunogen destroys the relevant clones as they arise, possibly by bypassing the macrophage and presenting to the small lymphocyte as free immunogen or as an immune complex in the region of great antigen excess.

Autoimmunity The appearance of antibodies in man directed against self represents an autoimmune response. These autoantibodies may reflect a normal response to tissue antigens which are separated anatomically from the immune system during fetal development and appear later as a consequence of tissue breakdown. Autoantibodies also may arise following abrogation of tolerance in a normal immune system by an exogenous antigen cross-reacting with self or because an abnormal immune system has lost the capacity to distinguish self. Autoantibodies do not necessarily indicate an autoimmune disease. This term must be restricted to situations in which the autoimmune response, humoral or cellular, is responsible for tissue injury.

CONSEQUENCES OF THE IMMUNE RESPONSE: HOST RESISTANCE

The consequences of the immune response are termed *immunity* when beneficial to the host and *hypersensitivity*, or *allergy*, when detrimental. This is a clinical judgment and does not imply that the basic pathways leading to immunity or hypersensitivity are different.

The constituents of host defense in normal man are both nonimmunologic and immunologic; those developing as a result of deliberate immunization or overt infection are exclusively immunologic. The nonimmunologic lines of defense include the extrinsic barriers to pathogen penetration, both mechanical and enzymatic, and the intrinsic cellular elements—circulating polymorphonuclear leukocytes and monocytes and fixed mononuclear phagocytic cells. Although these cellular elements are effective in the absence of an immune response, they clearly operate much more effectively in its presence. The so-called *natural antibodies* are present in normal persons who have not been subjected to deliberate immunization or overt infection; these natural antibodies would appear to result from the host's subclinical exposure to the specific pathogen or some cross-reacting pathogen. This makes it possible to consider the role of the immune response in host defense without further reference to a subclinical or overt encounter with the immunogen.

Serum complement The humoral immune response participating in host resistance appears to involve a supporting system, known as serum complement; hence it is relevant to examine this system before evaluating the role of the various immunoglobulin classes in host defense. The complement system (C) consists of distinct serum proteins, numbered 1 through 9, which interact in a well-defined sequence as cytotoxins for target cells and yield a series of by-products representing the essential ingredients of an inflammatory response. When an immune aggregate, or a target cell sensitized by interaction with specific antibody of the IgG1, IgG2, IgG3, or IgM class against some cell-surface antigen, interacts with normal serum, the first component of complement (C1) binds to the complex and is converted from an inactive precursor form to an active enzyme. Complex-bound active C1 ($C\overline{1}$) then acts on its natural substrates, the fourth and second components of complement, yielding a new cell-bound enzymatic activity consisting of major fragments of C4 and C2; the $C\overline{42}$ unit is termed C3 convertase. The action of C3 convertase on C3 results in the binding of the major portion of the molecule, C3b, to the complex, leaving the lesser fragment, C3a or anaphylatoxin, in the fluid phase. The complex bearing C3b can attach to a specific receptor on primate red blood cells or polymorphonuclear leukocytes, a phenemenon known as *immune adherence*, which enhances phagocytosis. The subsequent cleavage of fifth component (C5) yields another fragment with anaphylatoxic properties (C5a), while interaction of the fifth, sixth, and seventh complement components produces a fluid-phase trimolecular complex capable of reacting with unsensitized cells. The target cell, now bearing the products of interaction with the first seven components, interacts with the eighth and ninth components to complete the reaction by osmotic lysis and with alteration of the cell membrane as seen by electron microscopy. The system has biologic meaning because it is lethal for some target cells and results in the elaboration of various by-products capable of mediating an inflammatory response. These include the anaphylatoxins C3a and C5a, which produce a local increase in vascular permeability, bringing more antibody and complement to the site of the lesion; the *chemotactic factors,* C3a, C5a, and $C\overline{567}$, which attract polymorphonuclear leukocytes and monocytes; *complex bound C3b,* which promotes immune adherence and enhanced phagocytosis; and $C\overline{567}$, which prepares unsensitized bystander cells for lysis by C8 and C9. The complement reaction may be beneficial or detrimental to the host, depending entirely on the location of the antigens against which the antibody mediating the reaction is directed.

Several lines of study have recently provided incontrovertible evidence for an alternate pathway to activation of the terminal complement components, C3 through C9. This alternate pathway, formerly recognized in part as the properdin system, is readily activated by complex microbial polysaccharides without a clear requirement for the classical early components, C1, C2, and C4, or specific antibody. The relatively intact phagocytic and bactericidal activity of serums from animal strains or families deficient in the classical early components is attributed to the function of the alternate pathway.

Antibody IgG comprises 70 to 80 percent of the serum antibodies of man and is almost exclusively responsible for the antibodies to viruses, toxins, and gram-positive pyogenic bacteria. It is transported across the placenta, while other maternal immunoglobulins mostly are excluded from the fetal circulation. The interaction of IgG with antigen to activate the complement system leads to the development of anaphylatoxins, a release of chemotactic factors, and the capacity of the complex to undergo immune adherence and enhanced phagocytosis; it may be of great importance in controlling man's pyogenic environment.

Between 5 and 10 percent of the total serum antibody is IgM. Antibodies of this class commonly are directed against lipopolysaccharide antigens typified by the somatic 0 antigens (endotoxins) of gram-negative bacteria. The sensitization of a site on a target cell for subsequent lysis by the nine components of complement can be accomplished either by a single IgM molecule or an IgG doublet.

Antibodies of the IgA class comprise about 10 to 20 percent of serum immunoglobulins and are the predominant immunoglobulin in parotid saliva, tears, colostrum, nasal and bronchial secretions, bile, succus entericus, and urine. Secretory IgA has activity against viruses and bacteria, and a specific immune response to experimental virus infection has been demonstrated in the saliva, nasal secretions, and tears of human volunteers. While serum IgA has a sedimentation coefficient of 7S, secretory IgA is principally 11S protein because of an additional structural unit, the T (transport) piece. The T piece probably is responsible for the movement of the molecules into secretions; and it is presumed that such molecules in the external secretions of the respiratory, gastrointestinal, and genitourinary tract contribute to host resistance. The functions in host resistance of the trace immunoglobulins IgD and IgE are unknown, although there are some studies to implicate IgE in host resistance to parasitic infections.

Specific cellular immunity Specific cellular immunity to intracellular pathogens has been demonstrated experimentally in several models, the most direct of which has involved *Listeria monocytogenes* infection in the mouse. Mice infected with a sublethal dose of this organism developed resistance to a dose 100 times the LD_{50}. Resistance was not associated with the appearance of antibody because agglutination titers were negligible and protection could not be conferred by passive transfer of serum; resistance was, however, correlated in time with the development of delayed-type skin hypersensitivity to listeria culture filtrate. Furthermore, monolayer cultures of normal mouse peritoneal macrophages are destroyed readily by inoculation with listeria, while cultures obtained from resistant animals, previously infected with sublethal challenge, are capable of eliminating the organism. These peritoneal macrophages are demonstrating specific cellular immunity because their activity is not diminished by repeated washing or enhanced by the addition of normal or immune serum to the culture. Furthermore, these macrophages are capable of destroying intracellular pathogens, other than those used to initiate the immune response such as *Brucella abortus* or *Salmonella typhimurium,* indicating that upon specific activation, cellular immunity may be expressed in a nonspecific fashion. On the other hand, the induction of cellular immunity is specific because recall can be initiated only by an organism which has previously been used to initiate a primary response. The association of cellular immunity with the cutaneous reaction of delayed hypersensitivity suggests that the specificity resides in the sensitized lymphocyte, which then "activates" the macrophage to exhibit a nonspecific increased resistance to intracellular pathogens. This is somewhat analogous to humoral immunity, wherein specificity resides with the antibody produced by the plasma cell while the execution involves the nonspecific complement system.

The experimental data considered above imply that a deficiency of IgG would predispose to pyogenic infection, and a defect in cellular immunity to infection with intracellular pathogens. These generalizations are supported by clinical observations in patients illustrating such heritable or acquired defects (Chap. 64).

CONSEQUENCES OF THE IMMUNE RESPONSE: HYPERSENSITIVITY The adverse, or allergic, manifestations of the immune response traditionally have been divided on the basis of their time course following antigen challenge into *immediate, subacute,* and *delayed* hypersensitivity. Clear differences exist in the mechanisms whereby these three broad categories of clinical responses arise; and even differences within a category, such as immediate hypersensitivity, are being appreciated.

Immediate hypersensitivity Immediate hypersensitivity consists of all the allergic responses that begin within minutes of antigen-antibody interaction and may be divided into *cytotoxic* or *anaphylactic* on the basis of the mediation of the clinical response. In a cytotoxic reaction, such as an acute hemolytic transfusion reaction in man, the critical damage is to the primary target cell selected because the responsible complement-fixing antibody is directed against some cell-surface antigen. In an anaphylactic reaction, the interaction of antigen with antibody results in the formation and/or release of chemical mediators which act at secondary sites, namely, smooth muscle and vascular tissue.

Anaphylaxis The chemical mediators of anaphylactic tissue injury known to be specifically formed and/or released from mammalian tissue by antigen-antibody interaction are each under 1,200 in molecular weight and include amines, such as histamine and serotonin; small peptides such as the nonapeptide, bradykinin; an acidic molecule known as slow-reacting substance of anaphylaxis (SRS-A); and the eosinophil chemotactic factor of anaphylaxis (ECF-A). Each mediator except ECF-A has been shown to contract smooth muscles and increase vascular permeability. While the amines, histamine and serotonin, are released from tissue stores, in which they exist in their biologically active form, bradykinin, ECF-A, and SRS-A must be formed as well as released as a result of antigen-antibody interaction. SRS-A and ECF-A are without an established chemical structure but can be recognized because of a unique combination of chemical and pharmacologic characteristics. SRS-A is elaborated in large amounts when lung tissue from individuals with allergic or extrinsic asthma is exposed in vitro to pollen antigen; SRS-A also profoundly constricts the isolated human bronchiole in the presence of specific pharmacologic antagonists of histamine and serotonin.

The anaphylactic reaction may be divided further into *cytotropic* and *aggregate* to indicate whether the critical interaction of antigen with antibody leading to release of chemical mediators requires prior fixation of antibody to a primary target cell, such as a mast cell. The sensitization of human polymorphonuclear leukocytes with antibody of the IgE class for the subsequent antigen-induced release of histamine is an example of a cytotropic reaction. Aggregate anaphylaxis is initiated by antigen-antibody complexes which act directly upon the target cell to release mediators or by complexes which activate the complement system to produce anaphylatoxins which then act on the target cell. The biochemical mechanisms and pharmacologic controls of mediator release from the target cell appear to be similar whether activation is by cytotropic or aggregate anaphylactic pathways.

Because an animal or man can respond to an immunogen by making antibodies of several immunoglobulin classes, the clinical picture termed systemic anaphylaxis, which follows a subsequent challenge with specific antigen by a route or dose sufficient to bring about an immediate reaction, represents a composite response to the interaction of antigen with several different immunoglobulins. It is not surprising, therefore, that man exhibits at least three distinct reaction patterns within the anaphylactic syndrome, perhaps reflecting genetic differences in the immune response or variation in the pattern of exposure to the immunogen. Patients may experience respiratory distress because of edema of the hypopharynx and larynx or as a result of intractable bronchospasm. Hypotension then occurs secondary to the hypoxia. Alternatively, a primary vascular collapse without antecedent respiratory difficulty may ensue. It is possible to speculate on the basis of minimal experimental data in man that the pattern of laryngeal edema is mediated by histamine, the intractable bronchospasm by SRS-A, and primary vascular collapse by bradykinin. However, the critical point is that the anaphylactic syndrome has a variable presentation, probably determined by the relative amounts of the different antibodies involved.

Arthus reaction Subacute hypersensitivity reactions, depending on the deposition of immune complexes, activation of the complement system, and infiltration of polymorphonuclear leukocytes, are termed *Arthus lesions* when produced in the skin and *serum sickness* when they occur systemically. In contrast to the immediate clinical wheal of cutaneous anaphylaxis brought about by the release of chemical mediators, the Arthus lesion is a hemorrhagic reaction which develops over 4 to 10 hr and is associated with a marked polymorphonuclear leukocyte infiltrate of venules with surrounding edema and hemorrhage with or without secondary thrombosis. The reaction is not elicited by precipitating antibodies which do not activate complement and is depressed in experimentally induced C3 deficiencies or in acquired leukopenia. The mechanism of the Arthus lesion appears to be as follows: (1) antigen-antibody aggregates are deposited in vessel walls; (2) the complement system is activated, and the chemotactic principles are elaborated; (3) polymorphonuclear leukocytes enter, resulting in (4) enhanced phagocytosis of the aggregates, which, in turn, (5) leads to release of lysosomal enzymes with secondary focal necrosis of the vessel wall.

Serum sickness Serum sickness (Chap. 69) may be considered a disseminated form of the Arthus lesion, although the polymorphonuclear leukocytic infiltrate is less striking in the arteritis or glomerulitis of serum sickness than in the classical Arthus lesion. When man or an experimental animal receives a foreign or heterologous protein, the disappearance curve is characterized by three phases: (1) distribution throughout the extracellular compartment; (2) metabolic degradation; and (3) immune elimination due to an immune response with the appearance of specific antibody. The manifestations of serum sickness appear just prior to the onset of the immune elimination phase and are attributed to circulating antigen-antibody complexes formed in the region of antigen excess; these complexes apparently escape the usual clearance mechanisms effective against complexes formed at equivalence or in the zone of antibody excess and are trapped at vascular sites. For example, in experimental glomerular lesions, the complexes appearing in association with the complement components are deposited on the epithelial side of the basement membrane. Similarly, immunofluorescent and electronmicrographic techniques have shown deposition of complexes and development of glomerulitis in acute poststreptococcal nephritis and systemic lupus erythematosus in man. However, this is not the only recognized immunologic mechanism of renal disease in man; in Goodpasture's syndrome and certain other instances of nephritis an anti-basement membrane antibody is deposited on the endothelial side of the basement membrane and may produce direct cytotoxic injury.

Delayed hypersensitivity These reactions are exemplified in the skin by the tuberculin skin test or contact sensitivity and are implicated in the classical allograft rejection reaction of the unmodified recipient. The cutaneous response of erythema and induration is evident within 12 hr and reaches a peak in 24 to 48 hr. Granulocytes about small blood vessels are abundant in 12 hr, but by 24 hr a massive accumulation of mononuclear cells predominates. The delayed hypersensitivity response differs from the cutaneous anaphylactic or Arthus lesion because it is not transferred by serum but requires the transfer of viable lymphocytes in experimental animal models. The lymphocyte plays an essential role because (1) transfer of the delayed reaction can be achieved with thoracic duct cells, (2) the reaction can be suppressed in animals or man treated with an antiserum against the lymphocyte, and (3) the capacity to show contact sensitivity or allograft rejection in heritable or acquired lymphocyte deficiency states is absent. In man, the delayed reaction has been transferred with whole cells or an extract of peripheral blood cells termed *transfer factor,* which has a molecular weight of less than 10,000. Elicitation of the delayed skin reaction requires a larger portion of the antigen than does interaction with humoral antibody; this phenomenon, referred to as hapten-carrier specificity, means that the specificity for eliciting a delayed response exceeds that of the reaction requiring humoral antibodies. Although this specificity seems to reside in the sensitized lymphocyte, it is only part of the reaction mechanism. In vitro studies have shown that lymphocytes stimulated by specific antigen or nonspecific mitogens, such as phytohemagglutinin, release soluble mediators whose in vitro effects include chemotaxis, macrophage activation, cytotoxicity, and recruitment of normal lymphocytes into the proliferating lymphocyte pool. Because probably less than 2 percent of the cells at the site of a delayed hypersensitivity reaction are specifically sensitized, it is thought that these mediators, elicited by the stimulation of a relatively small number of sensitive lymphocytes, act as biologic amplifiers of the cellular immune reaction. Consequently, possible causes of anergy in diseases such as sarcoidosis, measles, and Hodgkin's disease include defects in lymphocyte function, in mediator function, and in participation of nonsensitized cells such as macrophages.

CONCLUSION In understanding both heritable and acquired defects in host resistance, it is important to appreciate not only the elements of the immune response contributing specificity, such as the immunoglobulins and the sensitized lymphocytes, but also the role of the nonspecific elements, such as the complement sequence, the polymorphonuclear leukocyte, and the macrophage. These nonspecific elements provide the killing mechanism after a specific immunoglobulin or sensitized lymphocyte has interacted with cell-surface antigens of the pathogen. Defects may occur at any point in the sequential steps in the afferent and efferent arcs of the immune response as well as in the nonspecific humoral and cellular systems which are activated in the final expression of the response. Similarly, in considering hypersensitivity to an exogenous immunogen or an autoantibody, immunochemical and immunopathologic definition of the lesion will assist materially in understanding its mechanism and in arriving at a rational course of therapy, which then may be directed at any point in the afferent and efferent arcs of the immune response or at the nonspecific participants involved in its expression.

REFERENCES

AUSTEN KF, BECKER EL: *Biochemistry of the Acute Allergic Reactions, Second International Symposium,* Oxford: Blackwell Scientific Publications, Ltd., 1971

DAVID JR: Migration inhibitory factor and mediators of cellular hypersensitivity in vitro. Prog Immunol 1:399, 1971

DAVIS BD et al: Immunology, sec. II in *Microbiology,* New York: Hoeber-Harper, 1967

JANEWAY CA et al: *The Gamma Globulins,* Boston: Little, Brown, 1967

MACKANESS GB, BLANDEN RV: Cellular immunity. Prog Allergy 11:89, 1967

MÜLLER-EBERHARD HJ: Chemistry and reaction mechanisms of complement. Adv Immunol 8:1, 1968

RUDDY S et al: The complement system of man. N Engl J Med 287:489, 1972

SCHUR PH: Gamma G subclasses. Prog Clin Immunol 1:71, 1972

UNANUE ER: Regulatory role of macrophages in antigenic stimulation. Adv Immunol 15:64, 1972

WOLSTENHOLME GEW, PORTER R: *Ciba Foundation Symposium on the Thymus,* Boston: Little, Brown, 1966

64 IMMUNOGLOBULINS AND IMMUNOLOGIC DEFICIENCY STATES

EDWARD C. FRANKLIN

IMMUNOGLOBULINS

CLASSIFICATION Antibodies belong to a heterogeneous group of proteins collectively known as the immunoglobulins. Though the bulk of antibody activity resides in the electrophoretically slowly migrating γ-globulin fraction, small amounts of protein related to the immunoglobulins have been identified by serologic techniques in the β- and α_2-globulins. In addition to antibodies, the immunoglobulins comprise a group of structurally related homogeneous proteins which include myeloma proteins and macroglobulins found in several proliferative disorders of plasma cells and lymphocytes. Their structural similarity to classical antibodies has led to their use as models of antibodies, an assumption which has been borne out by the finding of antibody activity in an ever-increasing number of these proteins.

In spite of the fact that antibodies with different specificities differ in their primary structure, all immunoglobulins have certain properties which permit their grouping into at least five major classes and a limited number of subclasses. Their major properties are listed in Table 64-1. There are four subclasses of IgG (IgG1 to 4), which differ in some of their biologic properties; two of IgA (IgA1 and 2); and several less-well-defined subclasses of IgM and IgD. Of all the known characteristics, the antigenic properties of the immunoglobulins have been especially useful in classification and clinical practice, since they have resulted in the development of class- and subclass-specific antiserums which are widely used to quantitate and characterize the immunoglobulin fractions in various body fluids. Antibodies have been identified in each of the four major immunoglobulin fractions; the IgE fraction appears to consist of reaginic (skin-sensitizing) antibodies primarily. Table 64-1 lists the homogeneous proteins corresponding to each of the major immunoglobulin classes. When large series of patients with these proteins are studied, the frequency of each type is closely related to the relative concentration of the corresponding fraction in normal serum. For example, G myeloma proteins occur more frequently than A myeloma proteins, which, in turn, are seen more often than macroglobulins, while D and E myeloma proteins occur only rarely.

The five well-characterized classes of immunoglobulins show striking differences in their distribution in the body and in some of their biologic properties. For example, the IgG fraction is the only one to cross the placental barrier to provide passive immunity to the newborn infant. During intrauterine life and early infancy, both IgM and IgG antibodies are formed by the fetus, while synthesis of IgA globulins does not commence until later. Following an antigenic stimulus later in life, IgM antibodies generally appear rapidly during the primary response and production continues only as long as the antigen persists, while IgG antibodies are formed somewhat later, persist for a longer period, and are largely responsible for "immunologic memory." However, a clear-cut separation between the properties of these two classes of antibodies is not feasible. Although all immunoglobulins exist in the intravascular and, in some instances, the extravascular compartments, the IgA globulins are the major immunoglobulin fraction in external secretions, such as bronchial and intestinal mucus, saliva, colostrum, and lacrimal fluid, where they provide a first line of defense against bacterial and viral antigens. The IgA molecules in these secretions differ from those in the blood since they are covalently linked to an extra structural unit known as a "secretory piece," which is synthesized in the epithelial cells of the exocrine glands, and may play an important role in the secretion of antibodies into these fluids, or possibly in protecting them from proteolysis. The secretory piece has a molecular weight of about 70,000, differs in structure from any of the immunoglobulin subunits, and appears to be under separate genetic control, since it is present in patients with agammaglobulinemia.

STRUCTURAL UNITS The immunoglobulins, like many other complex proteins, are made of two or more types of polypeptide chains, each of which is under separate genetic control. All immunoglobulins consist of a basic subunit composed of four chains held together by disulfide bonds (Fig. 64-1). Two of these, known as light chains, are common to all classes of immunoglobulins and account for their structural and antigenic similarities. There are two major types, each with a molecular weight of about 22,000, known as kappa (κ) and lambda (λ). The other two polypeptide chains have molecular weights between 55,000 and 70,000, and are therefore called heav chains. Because the heavy chains are different in eac class of immunoglobulins, they are identified by th Greek letter corresponding to the class (γ, α, μ, δ, ϵ) fo the IgG, IgA, IgM, IgD, and IgE fractions, respectively. The IgM, or macroglobulin, fraction has a molecular weight of about 850,000, since it is composed of five subunits, each consisting of two heavy and two light chains. The disulfide bonds joining these subunits can be preferentially cleaved by reducing agents, often with a concomitant loss of antibody activity, a property that has been used clinically to identify IgM antibodies, but the method is not infallible. Recent studies suggest that the subunits of IgM and also polymers of IgA are held

TABLE 64-1
Some properties of immunoglobulins

	Immunoglobulin class (Ig)				
Property	*G*	*A*	*M*	*D*	*E*
Molecular weight	145,000	±160,000	900,000	±160,000	200,000
Sedimentation coefficient (Svedberg)	7	7 (9, 11, 13, 15)	19	7	8
Electrophoretic mobility	γ	γ–β	γ–β	γ–β	γ–β
Approx. concentration, mg/100 ml	1,200	200	100	3	0.03
Carbohydrate, %	2.5	10	10	10	10
Valence	2	2	5*	2†(?)	2†(?)
Homogeneous protein	G myeloma	A myeloma	Macroglobulin	D myeloma	E myeloma

* *10 potential.*
† *Not yet measured, but likely.*

together by another polypeptide chain known as the J chain.

The antigen-binding sites reside in the amino terminal half of the molecule, the Fab fragment, and appear to involve both the heavy and light polypeptide chains (Fig. 64-1). The demonstration of several so-called hypervariable segments in the variable regions of both the heavy and light chains suggests that they may be directly involved in the antigen-binding sites and thus be related to the specificity of a given antibody. Many of the other properties of antibodies, for example complement and skin fixation, some of which are class-specific, reside in the carboxy terminal half of the heavy chain known as the Fc fragment. Each Ig^0 molecule, as well as probably all the other 7S immunoglobulins, has two antigen-binding sites. While only five combining sites for protein antigens exist in the intact IgM molecule, it appears likely that 10 binding sites are potentially available to react with antigens.

The elucidation of the amino acid sequence of a number of Bence Jones (light-chain) proteins and parts of many myeloma proteins has clearly demonstrated the existence of several subclasses of variable regions specific for either κ or λ chains, as well as at least four others which are common to all classes of heavy chains.

Studies of the amino acid sequence of the "constant" carboxy-terminal halves of the heavy and light chains, which are similar for all molecules belonging to a particular immunoglobulin class, have demonstrated striking homologies among all the classes and especially the subclasses. These homologies, together with the marked homologies among the variable regions of different species, suggest that the immunoglobulins may have evolved from a common ancestral gene by a series of gene duplications and translocations.

Each of the polypeptide chains is under separate genetic control, and in several instances genetic polymorphisms have been discovered. These have been best studied in the case of the γ chains, where a series of closely linked loci, known as Gm loci, control the synthesis of the four subclasses of γ chains (γ_1 to γ_4); the κ chains, whose constant regions express the effect of the Inv locus; and one of the α chain subclasses. In the case of the Inv factors, molecules having different allotypic specificities differ from one another in a single amino acid residue. It seems likely, also, that in other instances the differences will be more complex but still limited to only a few amino acid residues.

A clear-cut understanding of the genetic control of heavy and light chains has been complicated by the possibility that they may be under the control of more than one gene, since the variable and constant regions of the molecule appear to be under the control of separate genes. Since each polypeptide chain appears to have only a single initiation site, the parts appear to be joined not at the level of the polypeptide chain but possibly at the level of either deoxyribonucleic acid (DNA) or ribonucleic acid (RNA). Though all classes of light and heavy chains exist in any one individual, studies of homogeneous immunoglobulins indicate that individual molecules contain two identical heavy and two identical light chains. Consistent with this finding is the observation that each plasma cell can synthesize only one type of heavy chain and one type of light chain at any one time. Studies of murine and human plasma cell tumors in vitro have shown that the synthesis of heavy and light chains occurs on separate polyribosomes, and that, in general, synthesis of light and heavy chains is almost balanced. The small excess of light chains normally produced may be stored in

FIGURE 64-1

Schematic diagram of γG-globulin. Heavy chains (H) *consist of an Fc fragment, which is the same in all molecules of given sub-classes, and an Fd fragment, part of which is constant and part of which varies in composition in different myeloma proteins. Similarly, light chains L have a constant and a variable half. A light chain and an Fd fragment make up the Fab half. A light chain and an Fd fragment make up the Fab fragment. S—S is a disulfide bond. N and C are N and C terminal ends. Gm and Inv are genetic factors associated with H and L chains respectively. The solid color denotes the constant region while the dashed boxes represent the variable region.*

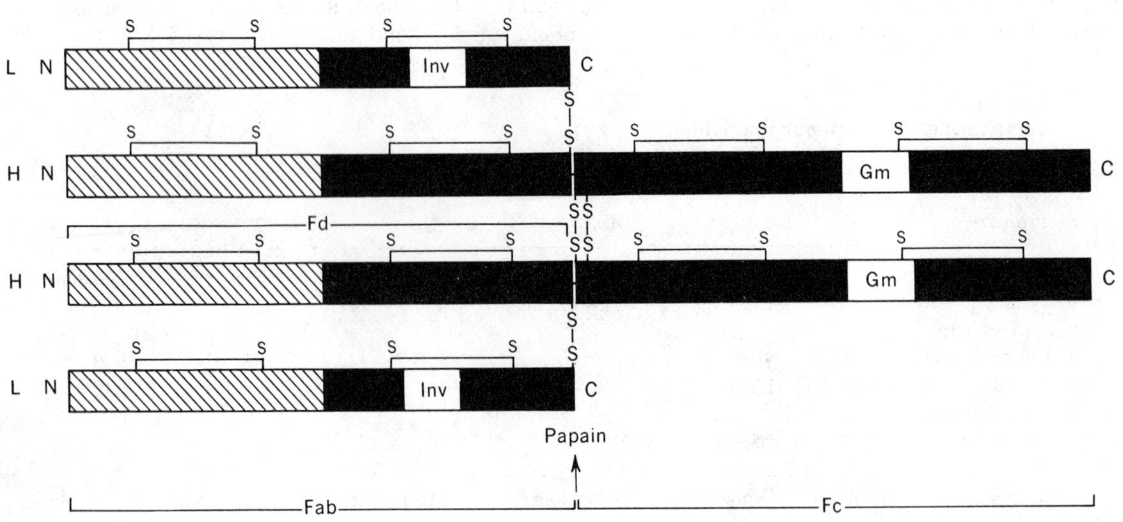

the cell and may play a role in the orderly release of completed antibody molecules.

DISORDERS OF IMMUNOGLOBULINS Several diseases are associated with quantitative alterations in immunoglobulins. A diffuse increase in all or, on occasion, selected immunoglobulins due to an increase in synthesis is of little diagnostic value, since it is a nonspecific manifestation of many chronic diseases, such as infections, liver disease, "connective tissue" diseases, and sarcoidosis (Fig. 64-2). A decrease in one or more of the immunoglobulins (hypogammaglobulinemia) is usually the result of a decrease in synthesis, which may be congenital or on occasion acquired, and is only rarely due to excessive catabolism or loss via the urine or gastrointestinal tract (Chap. 284). Another type of disorder involves the production of antibodies which react with an antigen present in the host. It seems likely that in many instances, these "autoantibodies" are induced initially by foreign antigens and cross-react with tissue or serum constituents of the host. Though autoantibodies may occur in many diseases and be directed against nucleoproteins, autologous or isologous γ-globulin (rheumatoid factors), or against red blood cells, white blood cells, platelets, thyroid antigens, intrinsic factor, etc., their role in the pathogenesis of these disorders remains unclear.

The fourth group of disorders is characterized by the production of immunoglobulin components which appear as homogeneous "spikes" in the electrophoretic pattern of serum or urine (Fig. 64-2*C* and *D*). These diseases include a number of neoplastic processes involving plasma cells and lymphocytes, including multiple myeloma, macroglobulinemia, and "heavy-chain" diseases. The abnormal proteins range in electrophoretic mobility from

FIGURE 64-2
Paper electrophoretic patterns of normal serum (A)*; serum with diffuse hypergammaglobulinemia* (B)*; serum with G myeloma protein ("paraproteinemia")* (C)*; urine with light-chain (Bence Jones) protein* (D)*. Arrow signifies origin.*

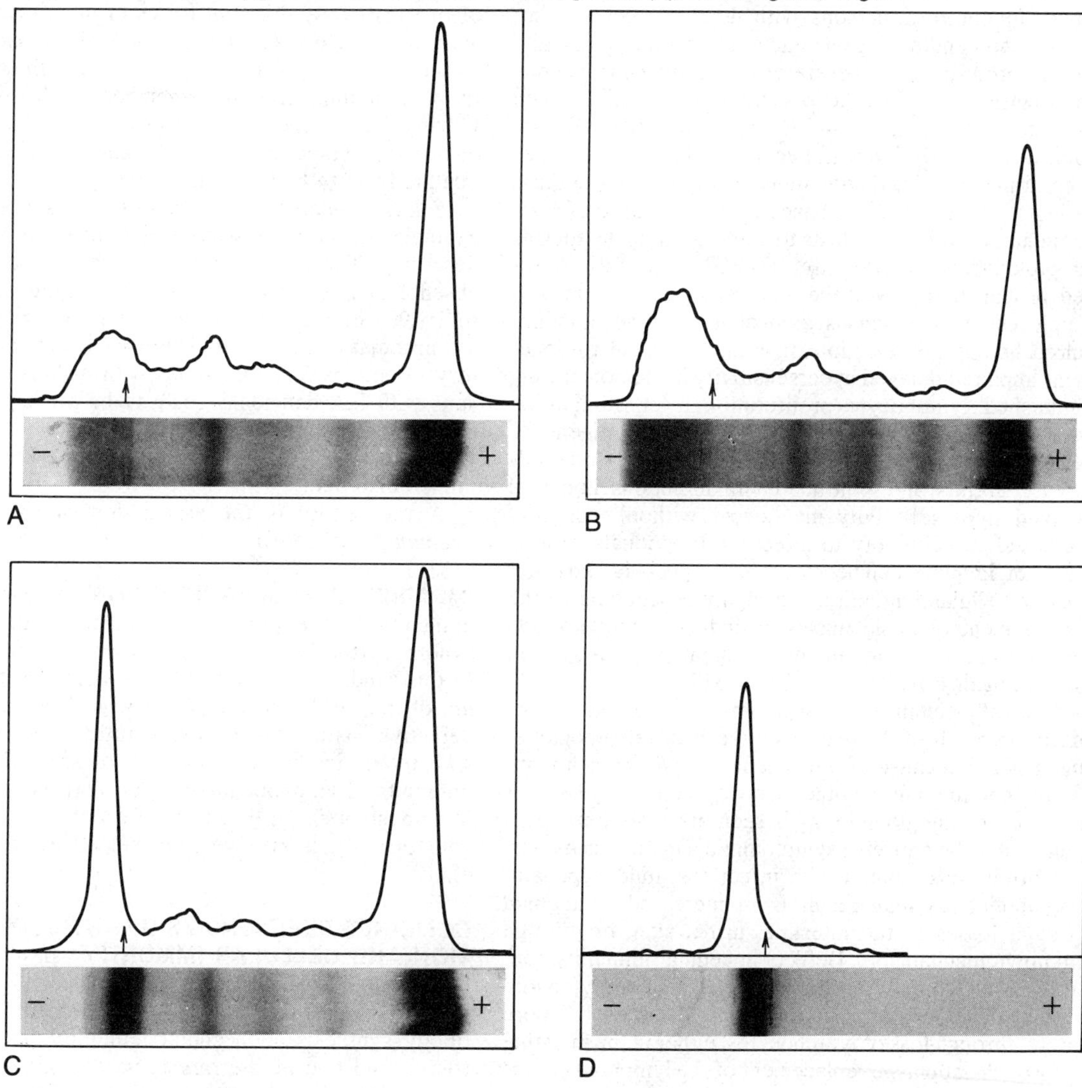

the slow γ-globulin to the fast α_2-globulin fraction. Precise identification is not possible from the appearance or mobility of the spike on paper electrophoresis; it requires immunoelectrophoretic and, in some instances, ultracentrifugal analyses.

IMMUNOLOGIC DEFICIENCY STATES

Immunologic deficiency states are characterized by an increased susceptibility to infection, a feature that may reflect diminished amounts of antibody, a defect in cellular immunity, or a combination of the two. Deficient antibody synthesis results in recurrent bacterial infections in sites which are commonly infected by virulent organisms such as pneumococci, staphylococci, streptococci, and meningococci, while it has no significant effect on resistance to viral infections. The diagnosis is based on the demonstration of low concentrations or absence of one or several of the immunoglobulins, and is supported by the absence of natural antibodies and by a poor immune response following infection or antigenic challenge. In contrast, persons with defective cellular immunity can handle pyogenic bacterial infections normally but are predisposed to severe viral and fungal infections and to infections with otherwise avirulent organisms such as *Pneumocystis carinii* and Enterobacteriaceae. Consequently, immunization with live attenuated viral vaccines is contraindicated and potentially very dangerous in these patients. The diagnosis is based on the presence of lymphopenia; negative skin tests to common antigens such as streptokinase/streptodornase, *Candida,* and PPD (purified protein derivative); the inability to be sensitized to simple chemicals such as dinitrofluorbenzene; and impaired homograft rejection. It is also possible to document impaired delayed hypersensitivity by demonstrating diminished lymphocyte proliferation after stimulation with phytohemagglutinin, allogenic cells, or antigens. In certain disease states, such as sarcoidosis, Hodgkin's disease, uremia, and some acute viral infections, impaired delayed hypersensitivity may occur without markedly increased susceptibility to infection. Individuals with all types of immune deficiency states, especially those involving cellular immunity, are highly susceptible to the development of malignancies, a finding which supports the concept that the immune system plays a role in defense against malignancy (Chap. 319).

Clinically significant hypogammaglobulinemia is most often the result of decreased synthesis of immunoglobulins, usually because of a deficiency of plasma cell number or function. On the other hand, defective synthesis of a single immunoglobulin, as is seen in isolated IgA deficiency, may be entirely asymptomatic. On rare occasions, and often unassociated with infections, mild hypogammaglobulinemia may result from increased catabolism through losses in the intestine, urine, skin, or through unknown mechanisms. Defects in cellular immunity generally result from thymic dysfunction, failure of lymphoid cellular development, certain chronic diseases, or, more rarely, through loss of lymphocytes, either in the intestine or through neoplastic replacement of the lymphoid organs as in malignant lymphomas.

IMPAIRED ANTIBODY PRODUCTION Many defects in antibody production have been described, but only the most important ones will be mentioned:

Transient hypogammaglobulinemia of infancy represents a self-limited exaggeration of the normal hypogammaglobulinemia which results from the catabolism of IgG transmitted to the fetus from the mother before the onset of Ig synthesis by the infant.

Sex-linked familial agammaglobulinemia (*Bruton's*) is the most clear-cut example of severe hypogammaglobulinemia involving all classes of immunoglobulin, with concentrations of immunoglobulins usually less than 50 mg per 100 ml. The basic defect is an almost complete absence of plasma cells and germinal centers. Symptoms appear early in life and can be controlled by the administration of γ-globulin. Ironically, these persons have a high incidence of rheumatoid arthritis and other collagen diseases such as dermatomyositis, scleroderma, and lupus erythematosus.

The common variable form of hypogammaglobulinemia, which includes a series of disorders of immunoglobulin formation differing both in severity and origin, is usually milder and may be idiopathic or the result either of one of several different forms of inheritance or of an accompanying disease such as leukemia, myeloma, etc. It may occur at any age and in either sex. Because of the frequent finding of family members with disorders involving the immune system, such as certain "autoimmune disorders," some investigators also consider the idiopathic form to be familial.

Selective depression of one or two classes of Ig. Many examples of such "dysgammaglobulinemias" have been described. The most important of these is the selective absence of IgA, which is seen with a frequency of 1:500 to 1:1,000 of the general population and may be either asymptomatic or associated with recurrent upper respiratory infections and sometimes with malabsorption. Persons with IgA deficiency seem to be predisposed to the development of rheumatoid arthritis, systemic lupus erythematosus, thyroiditis, and certain other "autoimmune" disorders.

A rare entity is the association of *thymoma with agammaglobulinemia.*

IMPAIRED CELLULAR IMMUNITY Impaired cellular immunity in the pure form is seen in the DiGeorge syndrome (third and fourth pharyngeal pouch syndrome). In this syndrome, failure of development of the epithelium of the third and fourth pharyngeal pouches leads to defective maturation of the parathyroids and thymus, with tetany in the first few days of life and no cellular immunity. Lymphopenia may or may not be present; immunoglobulins are normal. Recently a few children with this condition have been helped by thymus transplants.

COMBINED DEFICIENCIES OF ANTIBODY PRODUCTION AND CELLULAR IMMUNITY In many primary immune deficiency diseases and occasionally in some of the secondary forms, there is a combined defect in antibody synthesis and cellular immunity. The most profound, and one of the rarest, *is reticular dysgenesis,* a rapidly fatal disorder due to failure of development of a primitive stem cell necessary for the development of hematopoietic and immunocompetent cells.

Probably the purest forms of mixed immune deficiency syndromes are the X-linked recessive and autosomal recessive *(Swiss) types of lymphopenic hypogammaglobulinemia* (thymic dysplasia), which are usually fatal in infancy and which are marked by thymic aplasia, lymphopenia, and severe hypo- or agammaglobulinemia (possibly also the result of stem cell dysfunction). These severe forms of immune deficiency syndrome have also been successfully treated in recent years with HLA-matched bone marrow transplants.

Two complex disorders, involving other organ systems as well, are *ataxia telangiectasia* and the *Wiskott Aldrich syndrome*. The former is an autosomal recessive disorder marked by progressive cerebellar ataxia, telangiectasia in many organs, especially skin and conjunctiva, ovarian dysgenesis, and a high frequency of lymphoreticular malignancies. The most commonly observed defect in immunoglobulins is a deficiency in IgA and often also in IgE. This is frequently accompanied by sinopulmonary infections, impaired immune response to certain antigens, significant impairment in cellular immunity, some decrease in tissue and circulating lymphocytes, and a poorly developed thymus.

In the Wiskott Aldrich syndrome there are sex-linked recessive transmission of thrombocytopenia, eczema, increased susceptibility to infection, and impaired delayed hypersensitivity. The major immunoglobulin defect is a depression in IgM, an occasional increase in IgA, and a rather selective failure to form antibodies to polysaccharide antigens. Impaired cellular immunity is manifested by progressive lymphopenia in the blood and lymphoid organs. As in certain other immune deficiency states, lymphoreticular cancers are common. Recent reports have indicated that bone marrow transplants or transfer factor, a soluble substance derived from lymphocytes which can transfer delayed hypersensitivity, may cause temporary remissions in this disorder.

Various degrees of depression of humoral and cellular immunity have been commonly encountered as a result of the use of antilymphocyte serum and cytotoxic agents employed in organ transplantation and in a variety of autoimmune and neoplastic disorders. When contemplating their use, it is important to balance the dangerous side effects of these agents with their potential usefulness. In addition both cellular and humoral immune defects accompanying certain viral infections, especially if they occur in utero, have become apparent. Careful studies of patients with myeloma, Hodgkin's disease, and chronic lymphocytic leukemia have clearly demonstrated significant defects in humoral, cellular, or both types of immunity respectively.

TREATMENT Treatment of these disorders has had limited success. Infections are almost uniformly the presenting problems, and successful management involves accurate microbiologic diagnosis, specific chemotherapeutic or antibiotic treatment, drainage of pus, and general supportive measures. In addition, recognition of the underlying immunologic deficiency state is important. When hypogammaglobulinemia is involved, immediate and chronic replacement therapy with concentrated human γ-globulin is indicated. The half-life of isologous γ-globulin in these patients is generally normal or slightly prolonged. Empirically, resistance to infections in most patients is adequate when the concentration of γ-globulin is about 150 mg per 100 ml. A practical approach is to estimate the amount of γ-globulin which will increase the serum concentration by 100 mg per 100 ml. On the basis of a life of 30 days, monthly administration of 200 mg γ-globulin per kilogram of body weight will maintain this level. Whether therapy is successful should be judged by ensuing resistance to infections, not by the concentration of circulating γ-globulin. Rarely, recurrent infections with the same organism require the use of specific immune γ-globulin. In secondary acquired hypogammaglobulinemia, treatment also is governed by the underlying disease.

Immunologic deficiency states associated with impaired cellular immunity are not amenable to prolonged treatment. Transfer of immunologically competent cells in the form of spleen tissue, bone marrow, or neonatal thymus from normal individuals occasionally will restore cellular immunity. However, these procedures are still in the experimental stage.

REFERENCES

Bergsman D (ed), Good RA (scientific ed): *Immunologic Deficiency Diseases in Man*, vol. IV, no. 1, New York: National Foundation—March of Dimes, 1968 (Birth Defects Original Article Series)

Cohen S, Milstein C: Structural and biological properties of immunoglobulins. Adv Immunol 7:1, 1967

Edelman GM et al: The covalent structure of an entire γG immunoglobulin molecule. Proc Natl Acad Sci USA 63:78, 1969

Franklin EC (ed): Immunoglobulin diseases. Semin Hematol 10, Nos. 1 and 2, p. 1–177, 1973

Johansson SGO, Bennich H: Immunologic studies of an atypical myeloma immunoglobulin. Immunology 13:381, 1967

Kagan BM, Stiehm ER (eds): *Immunologic Incompetence*, Chicago: Year Book, 1971

Metzger H: Structure and function of γM macroglobulins, eds FJ Dixon, KG Kunkel. Adv Immunol 12:57, 1970

——: Myeloma proteins and antibodies. Am J Med 47:837, 1969

Milstein C, Pink JRL: Structure and evolution of immunoglobulins. Prog Biophys Mol Biol 21:209, 1970

Report of a World Health Organization Committee—special article: Primary immunodeficiencies. Pediatrics 47:927, 1971

Rosen FS, Janeway CA: The gamma globulins. III. Antibody deficiency syndromes. N Engl J Med 275:70, 769, 1966

Seligmann M et al: A proposed classification of primary immunologic deficiencies. Am J Med 45:817, 1968

Tomasi T, Bienenstock J: Secretory immunoglobulins. Adv Immunol 9:2, 1968

65 MULTIPLE MYELOMA AND OTHER PLASMA CELL AND LYMPHOCYTE DYSCRASIAS

EDWARD C. FRANKLIN

DEFINITION AND CLASSIFICATION The group of plasma cell dyscrasias consists of several disorders generally characterized by the uncontrolled proliferation of cells normally involved in antibody synthesis. In most instances, this is accompanied by the synthesis of a homogeneous immunoglobulin and/or one of its constituent polypeptide chains. Though precise classification of these disorders based on morphology is difficult, characterization of the proteins produced by the neoplastic cells permits their grouping into three major categories: (1) multiple myeloma—IgG, A, D, and E; (2) macroglobulinemia—IgM; (3) heavy-chain diseases—γ, α, and μ. A closely related variant that is being recognized more frequently as a result of widespread use of serum protein electrophoresis is "benign monoclonal gammopathy," a clinically benign condition in which a serum protein abnormality is noted in the absence of a significant plasma cell abnormality.

ETIOLOGY As is true of most other neoplastic disorders, little is known about etiologic factors. The rare association of chromosomal abnormalities and the occasional familial occurrence do not provide real clues. Viral particles have been demonstrated repeatedly, but in the absence of successful transmission of the disease with cell-free extracts of tissues, it is most likely that these represent superinfections in immunologically debilitated hosts. The available animal models, especially those in mice, have not provided insights into the etiology of the human disease.

MULTIPLE MYELOMA

Multiple myeloma is the most common of the plasma cell dyscrasias. It is characterized by the infiltration of the marrow by neoplastic plasma cells which in most instances produce a myeloma protein and/or one of its constituent polypeptide chains. In the advanced phases of the disease, the proliferating plasma cells result in diffuse osteoporosis, characteristic punched-out bony lesions often involving the skull, with no obvious repair on x-ray films, or pathologic fractures, most frequently of the vertebras and ribs. These lesions may ultimately give rise to hypercalcemia. Though painful fractures and bony lesions have long been considered the hallmark of myeloma, it now appears that the majority of patients with myeloma do not have clinically apparent bony lesions at the time of diagnosis, or even later in the disease, and that such lesions are often a late manifestation of the disease. This is probably in part the result of earlier diagnosis of the disorder in the latent period, which may last from 5 to 20 years and during which the serum electrophoretic pattern is abnormal in the absence of clinical evidence of disease. In spite of the frequent absence of clinically apparent bony lesions, virtually every patient with multiple myeloma (with the possible exception of those rare persons with multiple soft-tissue plasmacytomas) has widespread infiltration of the marrow with malignant plasma cells which can be detected by bone marrow aspiration (see below).

The presence of nonspecific findings such as weakness, anemia, an elevated sedimentation rate, or an unexplained infection, particularly bacterial pneumonia, is grounds for suspecting this disorder and for attempting its diagnosis. Occasionally attention is directed to myeloma through the discovery of a homogeneous protein in the serum or urine or the gradual onset of the nephrotic syndrome. As the disease progresses, the following manifestations may become prominent: (1) Frequent and recurrent infections, most often bacterial pneumonias, which are often the immediate cause of death. They are usually the result of impaired antibody synthesis, but occasionally defects in cellular immunity and a decrease in polymorphonuclear leukocytes, either as a manifestation of the disease or as a result of therapy, are responsible. (2) Chronic renal dysfunction, with several factors contributing to the development of renal failure. Probably the most common is the tubular damage resulting from the reabsorption of large amounts of Bence Jones proteins filtered by the glomeruli, or the occasional development of proteinaceous casts, which can obstruct and destroy entire nephrons. In the initial phases the so-called myeloma kidney is associated with proteinuria, which may progress to the nephrotic syndrome and uremia. Occasionally specific tubular reabsorption defects, including the Fanconi syndrome of adults, are seen. Somewhat rarer are amyloid deposits in the kidney, which may give rise to nephrosis and occasionally to renal failure. Other factors contributing to renal disease are severe hypercalcemia, recurrent pyelonephritis, and hyperuricemia, due either to rapid cellular turnover or to vigorous cytotoxic therapy. Acute renal failure may be precipitated by severe dehydration or by massive uricosuria following a course of chemotherapy. (3) Damage to other organs, such as the nervous system, especially the cord and nerve roots (which may be damaged by a pathologic fracture of a vertebra), the liver and spleen (which may be injured by the deposition of amyloid), and on rare occasions, the lungs and other structures, in which localized plasmacytomas develop. Clinically apparent involvement by myeloma deposits in the liver, spleen, and lymph nodes is very rare and thus distinguishes multiple myeloma from some of the related disorders, such as macroglobulinemia and heavy-chain disease. In about 5 to 10 percent of the patients symptoms are due to the abnormal protein, which can induce symptoms by a variety of mechanisms (see below).

LABORATORY FEATURES A number of nonspecific laboratory abnormalities is noted. A marked elevation of the sedimentation rate is the rule and often provides the first clue to this illness. Anemia, probably the result of many factors (including marrow replacement, hemolysis, infection, renal failure, and effects of therapy) is common, and the blood smear often shows marked rouleau formation. In addition, hyperuricemia (as a result of rapid cell turnover), uremia, and hypercalcemia without an increase in alkaline phosphatase may be seen.

Though multiple myeloma may be suspected on clinical grounds, the diagnosis requires the demonstration of characteristic changes in the marrow and is usually supported by finding a homogeneous spike on serum and urine electrophoresis. Because of the uneven distribution of the lesions and the importance of histologic documentation, a normal marrow aspirate in a patient clinically suspected of having multiple myeloma should be followed by additional aspirates or marrow biopsies from other sites. Characteristically, in the marrow there is an increase in plasma cells, which make up more than 15 percent and often up to 90 percent of myeloid cells, which frequently occur in sheets, which are often binucleate, and which may contain one or two nucleoli. The cytoplasm is usually blue with Wright's stain, because of the abundance of ribonucleic acid but may on occasion be acidophilic; the rough endoplasmic reticulum may contain proteinaceous inclusions known as Russell's bodies. The nuclear chromatin is often finer than that of a normal plasma cell, and the nucleus may show some mitotic figures. In rare instances of plasma cell leukemia, plasma cells can be seen in the peripheral blood. Occasionally, the marrow is infiltrated by lymphocytoid plasma cells rather than by the characteristic plasma cells.

A homogeneous protein component ranging in mobility from the slow γ to the α_2 globulin is seen on serum electrophoresis in about 60 percent of patients, in the urine only in about 20 percent, and in both serum and urine in another 20 percent (Fig. 64-2). Probably fewer than 2 percent of patients, especially those with far-advanced rapidly progressive disease, fail to show a spike; such patients often show a marked depression of all immunoglobulins. The abnormal component is generally first detected on paper or cellulose acetate electrophoresis, and is recognized on the basis of its homogeneity rather than by the absolute concentration. Although in most patients the concentration of γ- or β-globulins is definitely increased, an absolute increase is not required for the diagnosis. Paper electrophoresis alone is incapable of further defining the nature of the protein component; differentiation between the major classes and subclasses of immunoglobulins requires immunoelectrophoretic analyses. Since the frequency of an immunoglobulin class or subclass among myeloma proteins is similar to that of the normal counterpart, IgG myelomas are more common than IgA, IgD myelomas are quite rare, and only five instances of IgE myelomas have been noted. Detection of an abnormal protein in the urine is also best accomplished by electrophoretic and immunoelectrophoretic techniques. In the absence of significant renal disease, only a homogeneous component representing light chains, also known as Bence Jones proteins, is seen. With severe renal damage late in the disease, this component may be obliterated by the presence of most of the serum proteins which pass through the damaged glomeruli. As with normal immunoglobulins, κ light chains are about twice as frequent as λ proteins.

DIAGNOSIS The characteristic clinical features coupled with the results of bone marrow aspirates and serum and urine electrophoresis make definitive documentation relatively easy, although on occasion more than one site has to be aspirated to demonstrate the plasma cellular abnormality. It is important to attempt to differentiate myeloma from "benign monoclonal gammopathy," metastatic tumors to bone, and on occasion hyperparathyroidism. With a proper index of suspicion, multiple myeloma can be documented in many elderly persons with unexplained infections, bone pain, renal disease, and anemia.

PROGNOSIS When this disease is diagnosed in the clinically obvious state, the prognosis is unfavorable; most patients left untreated are dead within a year or two. With the more frequent discovery of the disease during the long latent period between its onset and its clinical perception, more patients now survive for longer periods after diagnosis. In addition, chemotherapy (see below) has significantly improved the prognosis, which is generally not related to the type or amount of myeloma protein but appears to reflect the severity of the disease at the time of diagnosis. In particular, severe renal dysfunction, advanced bony lesions, and marked anemia are poor prognostic signs. Renal failure, recurrent infections, and general debilitation are the most common causes of death.

TREATMENT Proper nutrition, hydration, mobilization, and analgesia are important as supportive measures and help delay the onset of hypercalcemia and some of the renal complications. Allopurinol is of use in preventing hyperuricemia, and steroids aid in the treatment of hypercalcemia. Plasmapheresis is of value when the hyperviscosity syndrome is present (see below). X-ray therapy is used in the treatment of localized lesions, particularly those resulting from the presence of bony lesions, and can be used, together with systemic chemotherapy, under careful supervision.

Chemotherapy with either of two alkylating agents (melphalan or cyclophosphamide) is the treatment of choice and, if properly used, results in clinical improvement and prolongation of survival in more than 50 percent of patients. There are few deleterious side effects. In addition to subjective increase in well-being and a decrease in bone pain, objective signs of improvement include a rise in hematocrit, decrease in the myeloma protein and a concomitant increase in normal immunoglobulin levels, decreased frequency of infections, and lack of progression and sometimes healing of bony lesions. These agents can be given either by continuous therapy (melphalan 2 to 4 mg per day, cyclophosphamide 1 to 4 mg per kg per day), often after an initial loading dose, or by intermittent therapy (melphalan 0.25 mg per kg per day for 4 days every 6 weeks, together with prednisone). Several reports suggest that intermittent therapy may be more effective. Regardless of the regimen employed, the patients must be carefully followed to prevent severe marrow depression. White counts between 2,000 to 4,000 per mm^3 are considered safe; if the levels fall lower, therapy must be discontinued temporarily.

BENIGN MONOCLONAL GAMMOPATHY

A closely related disorder which is often difficult to distinguish from multiple myeloma is the entity known as benign monoclonal gammopathy. This has been recognized through the application of electrophoresis as a routine laboratory procedure. In a large study in Sweden about 1 percent of the population was shown to have a homogeneous serum spike, usually an IgG or IgA globulin. In persons over seventy, the incidence increased to 3 percent. Careful study of these asymptomatic individuals usually reveals only a moderate increase of plasma cells in the marrow and no evidence of anemia, bony lesions, or renal disease. Generally, there is less than 2 g per 100 ml of γ-globulin, and Bence Jones proteins are rarely noted. Long-term follow-up of such cases has not yet been carried out, but up to now few of them have progressed to overt myeloma. Although it seems possible that some of these persons may have multiple myeloma in the latent period and will later develop the clinical manifestations of the disease, it seems likely that many have a benign disorder, possibly a pronounced immune response to some unknown antigen. Homogeneous antibodies in the absence of myeloma have been induced in genetically predisposed mice and rabbits with pneumococcal and streptococcal antigens and may represent the experimental counterpart to this disorder. Regardless of the ultimate nature of this disorder, most investigators now feel that chemotherapy is not warranted.

Closely related to this disease, is the association of a myeloma spike with a variety of neoplasms and certain other diseases. Though it is tempting to speculate that some of these conditions represent an immune response to an underlying disease, there is no evidence to support such a view.

MACROGLOBULINEMIA

Macroglobulinemia includes a spectrum of disorders ranging from a mild, relatively benign, and often slowly progressive lymphocytic infiltration of the marrow and lymphoid organs to malignant and progressive forms of lymphosarcoma or lymphoma, always associated with the presence in the serum of a homogeneous macroglobulin spike. Since this entity is defined by the biochemical abnormality in the serum, it may include the IgM equivalent of the benign monoclonal gammopathies.

Clinically, the disease generally occurs in the elderly and resembles a malignant lymphoma in the advanced stages. Many patients seek medical attention because of weakness, weight loss, and mild anemia, and may continue with mild nonspecific complaints for many years. Later they may develop bleeding from mucous membranes, signs and symptoms of the hyperviscosity syndrome (see below), lymphadenopathy, and hepatosplenomegaly. Not infrequently the disease may become more malignant and assume many of the clinical features of lymphosarcoma or lymphatic leukemia. Bone lesions are rare, and amyloid is occasionally seen as a complication. Not infrequently patients with macroglobulinemia develop the cold agglutinin syndrome (see below). Symptoms related to the abnormal proteins are more common in macroglobulinemia than in multiple myeloma.

LABORATORY FINDINGS As in multiple myeloma, anemia, increased sedimentation rate, and hyperuricemia are common. The diagnosis is suspected on clinical grounds and confirmed by electrophoresis, immunoelectrophoresis, and ultracentrifugation, which reveals a homogeneous IgM protein with a sedimentation coefficient of 19S and smaller amounts of more rapidly sedimenting components. Bence Jones proteins are often seen in the urine. The bone marrow may at times contain plasma cells but generally is infiltrated with lymphocytes or lymphocytoid plasma cells. Many mast cells may be seen. When involved, lymph nodes and spleen have the pathologic features of lymphosarcoma. If indicated, serum viscosity should be measured and cold agglutinins should be looked for.

PROGNOSIS AND TREATMENT Depending on when the diagnosis is made, the disease may be slowly progressive or rapidly fatal. In the early stages, no treatment is needed. Later on, the indications for chemotherapy and the type needed are similar to those in chronic lymphocytic leukemia. Occasionally x-ray therapy is indicated for local lesions. If hyperviscosity is symptomatic, vigorous therapy is indicated (see below).

HEAVY-CHAIN DISEASES

As with macroglobulinemia, this disorder is defined by the demonstration of the characteristic immunoglobulin heavy-chain (H-chain) fragment in serum or urine. Three of the five possible types of heavy-chain disease (γ, α, and μ), each with a characteristic clinical picture, have been recognized since the description of the first patient with γ chain disease in 1963. Though these diseases may be suspected on clinical grounds, a definitive diagnosis is based on finding the appropriate heavy-chain fragment in the serum and/or urine.

GAMMA HEAVY-CHAIN DISEASE Twenty-six patients with γ *heavy-chain disease* have been studied. Most of them were elderly, although one was eighteen years old. Weakness, weight loss, lymphadenopathy (which may wax and wane), hepatosplenomegaly, and recurrent infections are common features. Of particular interest is the frequent involvement of the nodes in Waldeyer's ring, which may give rise to palatal edema and erythema and occasionally to respiratory difficulty. Bony lesions have been noted only once; clinically the disorder resembles a lymphoma more than myeloma.

Anemia, lymphocytosis, eosinophilia, thrombocytopenia, and hyperuricemia are commonly found. Since the marrow and lymph nodes are infiltrated with plasma cells, lymphocytes, or lymphocytoid plasma cells, the diagnosis can not be made on morphologic grounds. It requires the demonstration in the serum and urine of a broad protein peak, usually with a β-globulin mobility, which is reactive with antiserums to γ chains and unreactive with antiserums to light chains. In some patients the protein may be present in trace amounts; in others it is produced in large amounts. The prognosis of this disorder is rather poor; most of the patients have died within 6 months to 4 years after diagnosis, most frequently of overwhelming infections. Chemotherapy has not proved useful. In several instances the disorder has progressed to a less differentiated form of reticulum cell sarcoma with concomitant decrease in heavy-chain production. Amyloidosis has been reported in two of the patients.

ALPHA CHAIN DISEASE This appears to be the most common form of heavy-chain disease. It appears to be the almost invariable accompaniment of a malignant lymphoma of the intestine with severe malabsorption, a disorder that is most often but not exclusively seen in the Mediterranean region. In most instances, the disorder is rapidly progressive, but several spontaneous remissions have been noted. Organs normally involved in the synthesis of IgA are usually affected. Usually, the intestine is infiltrated with plasma cells which have been shown to synthesize the abnormal protein; recently, two patients with involvement of the respiratory tract have been reported. These patients have the same nonspecific laboratory features characteristic of γ heavy-chain disease. The diagnosis is made by the demonstration of a protein in the serum and urine which reacts with antiserums to α chains but not to light chains.

μ CHAIN DISEASE The rarest of these entities is μ chain disease, all three reported cases of which were seen in individuals with long-standing chronic lymphatic leukemia (CLL). Two of these patients also excreted a Bence Jones protein, and one had amyloid. An unusual feature, which should direct attention to the possibility of this entity in patients with CLL, is the finding of plasma cells with large vacuoles in the cytoplasm. This abnormality is only rarely seen in CLL, however, since several surveys of large groups of patients failed to uncover additional instances. The diagnosis is difficult to make, since the protein is present in the serum in amounts too small to give rise to a characteristic spike and is not found in the urine. The abnormality is detected on immunoelectrophoresis by finding a precipitin band reactive with antiserums to μ chains but not to light chains. Although all known patients died shortly after the detection of the protein, no statement can be made about the prognosis, since it is not known how long the disease had been present prior to its discovery.

NATURE OF IMMUNOGLOBULINS

Correlation of the type of protein produced with several clinical syndromes has permitted a more precise classification of these disorders than was possible on morphologic grounds alone. In order to understand the disorders of protein synthesis, two points concerning normal immunoglobulin synthesis should be considered: (1) under normal conditions, synthesis of heavy and light chains is approximately equal, so that only intact immunoglobulins are secreted (a minimal excess of light chains is always noted however); (2) only one type of immunoglobulin is made by a cell at any single point of its existence. Bearing these two assumptions in mind, one may best view the protein components produced in these disorders in the light of the normal immunoglobulins and their structural units (Table 65-1).

Thus if heavy- and light-chain synthesis remains balanced in the markedly expanded cell pool, a patient with myeloma or macroglobulinemia will have a homogeneous myeloma protein or macroglobulin belonging to one of the major classes or subclasses. These proteins resemble normal immunoglobulins, and since many have been shown to possess antibody activity, they represent no more than a normal component produced in excess. In certain instances, asynchronous production of heavy and light chains occurs. If only light chains are produced, a homogeneous protein spike (often with the thermal properties of a Bence Jones protein) appears in the urine and usually no abnormal protein is found in the serum. Since they represent light polypeptide chains and often fail to demonstrate the characteristic thermal properties of precipitating at 56°C and going back in solution at 100°C, it is preferable to refer to them as light-chain proteins and to rely on electrophoretic and immunologic methods for their identification. These cases cannot be classified as belonging to any of the major classes of plasma cell neoplasms and have on occasion been referred to as light-chain disease. If light-chain synthesis exceeds that of heavy chains, both a serum spike, related to one of the major classes of immunoglobulins, and a light-chain component are found in the urine. Occasionally, because of the existence of larger polymers or decreased catabolism, light chains accumulate in the serum and may give rise to a spike. In a small percentage of patients (1 to 2 percent), often late in the course of the disease, synthesis of heavy and light chains ceases so that no homogeneous component is seen. Such patients are often hypogammaglobulinemic, since background immunoglobulin synthesis is depressed.

Structurally altered proteins and polypeptide chains have been noted with increasing frequency. The most striking examples are seen in patients with "heavy-chain disease." To date only γ chain proteins have been studied

TABLE 65-1
Disorders of protein synthesis

*Disorder**	*Serum abnormality*
I Balanced synthesis: H = L	Homogeneous serum protein
II Unbalanced synthesis: L > H	
A Excess L	Homogeneous serum protein + Bence Jones protein
B Only L	Bence Jones protein only
III No synthesis: H + L	Hypogammaglobulinemia
IV Structural mutations:	
A Heavy-chain diseases	Broad serum spike
B Half molecules(?)	Homogeneous serum protein
C Myeloma with deletion	Homogeneous serum protein

* *H = heavy-chain proteins; L = light-chain proteins.*

in sufficient detail to delineate the nature of the defect. At least five instances are known where the proteins represent an incomplete heavy chain having an internal deletion of part of the Fd variable region and all of the Fd constant region, with resumption of synthesis either just before or after the hinge region in the Fc fragment. Although these proteins obviously represent synthetic products, further proteolytic digestion of them seems to have occurred in a few instances.

While the heavy-chain disease proteins represent extreme examples of defective molecules, it has also been demonstrated that apparently intact myeloma proteins have smaller deletions of parts of the heavy or light chain. It seems likely that in these instances, the abnormal protein is the result of a mutation of a structural gene. In patients producing large amounts of intact proteins, normal regulation of protein synthesis persists, although it seems likely that an increased number of cells is no longer subject to feedback regulation. In instances of asynchronous polypeptide chain production it remains to be determined whether two separate clones proliferated or whether possibly there is a defect in a regulatory gene.

EFFECTS OF THE ABNORMAL PROTEINS The clinical manifestations of multiple myeloma and macroglobulinemia generally reflect the existence of a malignant disease and not the presence of the abnormal protein. In some patients, however, the existence of large amounts of the abnormal proteins, the synthesis of proteins with unusual solubility or antibody properties, or occasionally the marked depression of normal γ-globulins may be responsible for certain clinical features outlined below.

Hyperviscosity syndrome The presence in serum in high concentrations of a protein, most often a macroglobulin, may cause a marked rise in viscosity, which in turn may interfere with efficient circulation to the brain, digits, kidneys, or eyes. The fundi may show a characteristic appearance, with extremely dilated venules and many hemorrhages. The hyperviscosity often results in the sudden onset of confusion, which frequently progresses to severe organic central nervous system disturbances. Progressive signs of cardiac and peripheral vascular insufficiency result from the impaired circulation in the small capillaries. The diagnosis may be confirmed by demonstration of increased serum viscosity with an Ostwald viscosimeter. Treatment must be instituted immediately, with repeated plasmaphereses until the viscosity is diminished and symptoms subside, following which a maintenance schedule, in conjunction with appropriate chemotherapy, must be worked out to control the underlying disease. Plasmapheresis is particularly successful in patients with macroglobulinemia, because these high molecular weight proteins are confined largely to the intravascular space. Where indicated chemotherapy should be directed at the primary disorder (myeloma or macroglobulinemia).

Cryoglobulinemia Somewhat similar clinical findings may result from the presence of cryoglobulins, which are proteins that precipitate in the cold and redissolve on warming. Although cryoglobulins are often asymptomatic, they may on occasion cause peripheral vascular insufficiency and even gangrene after exposure to low temperatures. Cryoglobulins are most often associated with multiple myeloma and macroglobulinemia, but they may occur in systemic lupus erythematosus or other "connective tissue" diseases, or even in the absence of any overt illness. About one-third of cryoglobulins are G myeloma proteins, one-third are macroglobulins, and about one-third are mixtures of IgG and IgM molecules. These mixtures are most often found in patients with one of the connective tissue diseases and are associated with purpura and progressive, often fulminant, renal lesions reminiscent of those seen in nephritis caused by antigen-antibody complexes. In more than half these subjects the IgM component is monoclonal, presumably the product of a malignant clone of lymphocytes. The precise mechanism for cryoprecipitation is not known, and in general, there is little correlation between symptoms and the amount of cryoglobulins or the temperature at which precipitation occurs. There is evidence that many cryoglobulins may, in fact, be antibodies to γ-globulins.

Cold agglutinin disease Another disorder directly related to an unusual group of macroglobulins is the hemolytic anemia induced by cold agglutinins. Although antibodies which cause hemolysis after exposure to the cold may be seen transiently in certain infections, such as infectious mononucleosis or atypical pneumonia, they rarely cause severe hemolysis in any disease other than macroglobulinemia or lymphosarcoma. The cold agglutinins are generally directed against the I antigen of the red blood cell and usually possess only κ light chains. Unlike antibodies which interact with red blood cells at body temperature, cold agglutinins usually appear free in the circulation.

Bence Jones proteins Another disorder related to abnormal proteins is the renal disease seen in patients with Bence Jones proteinuria. The filtration of large amounts of these proteins through the glomeruli exposes the tubules to an enormous reabsorptive load, which may cause degeneration of tubular cells, deposition of proteinaceous inclusions in the cells, and the formation of tubular casts. This is often referred to as "myeloma kidney," and may result in renal failure with uremia or in the appearance of the nephrotic syndrome. Severe dehydration preceding certain diagnostic procedures such as intravenous pyelograms may be sufficient to precipitate acute renal failure in these patients. The kidney has been clearly established as the prime site of degradation of small proteins such as light chains. Consequently, the bulk of Bence Jones proteins is catabolized by the normal kidney and only the excess appears in the urine. When renal function becomes impaired, the degradative function is diminished and the amount of Bence Jones protein in the urine often increases markedly.

Amyloid Amyloid is a fibrillar substance often associated with this group of diseases. It is discussed in detail in Chap. 107. It is likely that amyloid associated with plasma cell dyscrasias consists of fragments of light chains and that amyloid-like fibrils can be produced from certain Bence Jones proteins by proteolysis in vitro.

Miscellaneous On rare occasions paraproteins may interact with other substances, such as calcium and some of the clotting factors, or may coat blood platelets and interfere with the normal mechanisms of blood coagulation and hemostasis.

Hypogammaglobulinemias The recurrent infections often seen in patients with hypogammaglobulinemias (Chap. 64) are not directly caused by the presence of abnormal proteins but are probably attributable to the decrease in the immune response which is caused by the diminished production of immunoglobulins.

REFERENCES

ALEXANIAN R et al: Treatment for multiple myeloma. JAMA 208:1680, 1969

FAHEY JL et al: Infection, antibody response and γ-globulin components in multiple myeloma and macroglobulinemia. Am J Med 35:698, 1963

FORTE FA et al: Heavy chain disease of the μ (γM) type: Report of the first case. Blood 37:137, 1970

FRANKLIN EC (ed): Immunoglobulin diseases, eds P Miescher, E Jaffe. Semin Hematol 10, pt. 1, Jan. 1973, pt. 2, April, 1973

——et al: Heavy chain disease—a new disorder of serum gamma globulins. Am J Med 37:332, 1964

HALLEN J: Discrete gammaglobulin (M-) components in serum: Clinical study of 150 subjects without myelomatosis. Acta Med Scand Suppl 462, 1966

MACKENZIE M, FUDENBERG HH: Macroglobulinemia: An analysis of 40 patients. Blood 39:874, 1972

MELTZER M, FRANKLIN EC: Cryoglobulinemia—a study of 29 patients. I. IgG and IgM cryoglobulins and factors affecting cryoprecipitability. Am J Med 40:828, 1966

—— et al: Cryoglobulinemia—a clinical and laboratory study. II. Cryoglobulins with rheumatoid factor activity. Am J Med 40:837, 1966

OSSERMAN K, TAKATSUKI K: Plasma cell myeloma—γ-globulin synthesis and structure: A review of biochemical and clinical data with the description of a newly recognized and related syndrome, $H\gamma_2$ chain (Franklin's) disease. Medicine 42:357, 1963

SELIGMANN M et al: Immunochemical studies in 4 cases of alpha chain disease. J Clin Invest 48:2374, 1969

SOLOMON A, FAHEY JL: Bence Jones proteinemia. Am J Med 37:206, 1964

66 TRANSPLANTATION

JOHN P. MERRILL
CHARLES B. CARPENTER

INTRODUCTION Transplantation of the human kidney is now a justified procedure for the treatment of advanced chronic renal failure. An analysis of more than 8,300 cases performed as of July 1972 shows an 80 percent 2-year survival rate of an adequately functioning graft when the donor-recipient pair were siblings. An additional 6 percent of patients were living on hemodialysis but with a nonfunctioning graft. For a similar period 2-year functional survival for grafts between parent-child are 67 percent, with 83 percent of the patients alive. The data for 2-year survival in transplants between unrelated donor and recipient are 46 percent for graft survival and 65 percent for patient survival. In virtually all the instances the unrelated donor was a cadaver. Where tissue typing demonstrated that very little antigenic difference existed between the tissues of donor and recipient sibling pairs, 2-year survival approaches 95 percent. Though these figures represent important progress since the early days of renal transplantation, it is significant that there has been very little improvement in the past 2 years, suggesting the inadequacy of the methods of immunosuppressive therapy which have been uniformly utilized over the past 4-year period. However, at least for related individuals, the results compare favorably with such accepted procedures as open-heart surgery for acquired valvular heart disease. Human liver, pancreas, bone marrow, heart, and endocrine glands have been transplanted, but with less success. In all, 185 cardiac allografts have been reported. The results of cardiac transplantation in one of the largest and best-studied series in the United States, show 35 transplants in 34 patients, with a 45 percent 1-year survival.

IMMUNOLOGIC CONSIDERATIONS Necessary to the understanding of transplantation immunity are the following terms: *autograft*—the transplantation of tissue from one part of an individual to another part of the same individual; *isograft*—the transplantation of tissues between two individuals of the same inbred strain. Because in these cases the antigens of the donor and recipient are identical, no histocompatibility difference exists and no immune response to the graft occurs. A case in point in man is transplantation between identical twins. In an *allograft*, i.e., a graft of tissues between two individuals of the same species, histocompatibility differences may be strong or weak, depending on the individual and the species. A *xenograft* is a graft between individuals of two different species. The term "heterograft" is still used synonymously with xenograft.

TISSUE TYPING The rejection of an allograft in man is due to an immune response in the recipient against antigens present on the tissues of the donor and absent in the host. Only identical twins share all antigens having relevance to transplantation. Fortunately for clinical transplantation, only two antigen systems appear to play a major role in histocompatibility. First of these is the ABO blood group system, and donor-recipient pairs must be matched for this histocompatibility locus in accordance with the usual rules for blood transfusion. The second system is termed the major histocompatibility (MHC) locus and consists of an unknown number of subloci closely linked on a different chromosome from that which determines ABO antigens. Since chromosomes segregate randomly in each generation, compatibility for ABO does not assure MHC locus compatibility, or vice versa. At present the MHC locus appears to contain two subloci which determine the serologically defined HL-A antigens, more than 30 in number, and another sublocus which determines the proliferative response of recipient lymphocytes to donor cells in a mixed lymphocyte culture (MLC). Current evidence suggests that the gene(s) controlling the MLC response are adjacent to the second sublocus (Fig. 66-1). For several years the MLC response was thought to be determined solely by differences in HL-A antigens, since the MHC locus is inherited intact and HL-A identical siblings generally have negative MLC reactions; however, a small number of exceptions have been noted that are possibly due to gene recombination following chromosomal crossing over in one of the parents.

HL-A antigens are usually detected on lymphocytes by the cytolytic action of human antiserums in the presence of rabbit complement. Agglutination techniques may also be employed. Antiserums are obtained from selected multiparous females, immunized as a normal course of pregnancy, or by deliberate immunization of volunteers. Since one chromosome, or haplotype, is inherited from each parent and contains two subloci, the HL-A antigenic configuration for any individual comprises four HL-A antigens, two derived from each parent. The degree of histocompatibility, or tissue matching, between any two individuals reflects the number of HL-A antigens shared by the two individuals. Thus, if all four antigens are the same in a potential donor-recipient pair, no HL-A incompatibility exists and theoretically tissue could be transplanted from one to the other with minimal stimulation of an immune response, i.e., the tissue would not be rejected. Conversely, if all four HL-A antigens are different, there is marked tissue incompatibility and the likelihood of a strong immune response to transplanted tissue would be expected. It is the antigens present in the donor and lacking in the recipient that are important, since in the case of kidney, at least, only the host mounts an immune response, aimed against antigens not contained in the recipient but present in the donor. For obvious genetic reasons there is a greater probability that siblings carry the same HL-A antigens, while the likelihood that this situation will obtain in an unrelated donor-recipient pair is small; in these cases the MLC sublocus will most likely be mismatched. Various degrees of histocompatibility between the two extremes are possible, depending upon whether three or two antigens are shared. Unfortunately, the number of HL-A mismatches per se does not always correlate with clinical results, emphasizing the role of other loci, and the responsiveness of individuals to various antigens. The different HL-A antigens may vary in their strength, i.e., in the immune response which they elicit when such an antigen is absent in the recipient, but this variation in response seems to be less an inherent feature of certain antigens than a relative state of hyporesponsiveness in certain recipients. Nevertheless, the histocompatibility system and its relation to tissue matching is borne out by the obviously greater clinical success in transplanted kidneys between siblings than in unrelated donor-recipient pairs.

FIGURE 66-1

Current scheme of the human major histocompatibility MHC locus. Shown are the maternal and paternal chromosomes which comprise the diploid genotype of the individual. Phenotypically, the individual has four HL-A antigens; in the example shown, two are from each parent. In addition there are poorly defined determinants at the MLR (mixed lymphocyte response) sublocus, detectable only by a lymphocyte proliferative response in tissue culture. The antigens determined by each parental chromosome are expressed in each generation and are referred to as a haplotype. By definition, therefore, children share one haplotype with each parent. Siblings may share both haplotypes (25 percent), share one haplotype (50 percent), or differ by both haplotypes (25 percent). Occasional examples of apparent crossing over have been noted, resulting in an MLR incompatibility between HL-A identical siblings.

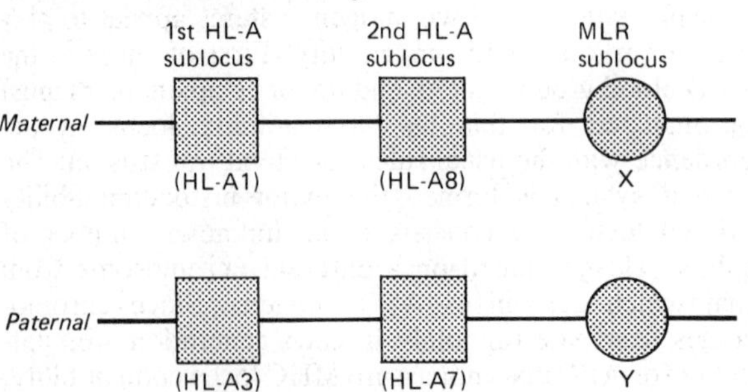

There is renewed interest in techniques for assessing the non-HL-A component of the MHC locus by the mixed lymphocyte reaction. In the usual technique lymphocytes from donor and recipient are incubated together for a period of 6 to 7 days in an MLC. Antigenic disparity will be reflected by stimulation of the lymphocytes with transformation into blasts. The greater the degree of dissimilarity, the greater the number of cells that are transformed. In most cases of organ transplantation the degree to which the recipient responds to donor antigens is most important, and the donor cells are rendered incapable of responding by preincubation with mitomycin prior to mixing. Cell transformation is accompanied by DNA synthesis and thus may be quantitated by the degree to which radioactive tritium-labeled thymidine is incorporated into the transformed recipient cells. In theory, HL-A identical donor-recipient cell mixtures should show no stimulation above control, and marked antigenic disparity should be reflected by marked stimulation. This is not always true, since HL-A identical cells may on occasion show some MLC reaction. The degree of histocompatibility reflects the strength of the immune response expected from the recipient and determines the amount of toxic immunosuppressive therapy which must be used to modify this response. For this reason tissue matching has played an important part in the selection of appropriate donor-recipient pairs when a choice exists. Unfortunately, in the present state of knowledge, the difference between unrelated donor-recipient pairs is only poorly quantitable, and is thus of questionable value except in the rare case in which all four antigens are shared ("full-house" match). Excellent survival has been observed in some recipients of unrelated-donor kidneys when the donor had one or more antigens recognizably foreign to the recipient; however, no real difference was observed in the clinical outcome of patients having between one and four antigen mismatches. Clearly, some recipients, when treated with standard immunosuppressive therapy, do not respond to demonstrable histoincompatibilities.

IMMUNOLOGY OF REJECTION Knowledge of the immunology of tissue transplantation stems largely from animal experimentation. However, enough evidence has accumulated in man, particularly in kidney transplantation, to indicate that the evidence is similar though not identical for the different species. The following observations describe reasonably accurately the events that transpire during the rejection of most human tissue transplants. Spleen and bone marrow grafts differ because in these instances cells capable of reacting against the recipient (graft-versus-host reaction) are transplanted.

From data derived both from animal and human experience, it appears that the rejection of transplanted tissue results from the antigenic stimulus of a two-component lymphoid system (Fig. 66-2). The lymphocytes involved are the offspring of marrow-derived stem cells. As these stem cells mature under the direct or humoral influence of (1) the thymus or (2) a human equivalent to the cells of the avian bursa, they develop antigen receptors so that they can respond in a cooperative manner to make an immune response when stimulated by antigen. The mature lymphocytes comprising the two distinct populations are for convenience abbreviated as (1) thymus-dependent (T) and (2) bone marrow (bursa)-dependent (B). Recent evidence suggests that cooperative interaction between T and B cells, through the mediation of a substance furnished by the T cells after antigenic stimulation, is necessary for initiation of the immune response. This cell interaction may take place upon the dendrites of tissue macrophages. In the case of the renal allograft, donor antigen may stimulate either T or B cells by way of antigen liberated from the kidney and reaching the lymphocytes by the bloodstream or lymphatics; or by contact between the recipient's lymphocytes and donor antigen as the former circulate through the kidney.

Some T cells are long-lived, circulating in the peripheral blood but "homing" in on lymphoid organs. They are responsible for cell-mediated immunity (CMI) such as graft rejection, delayed hypersensitivity (tuberculin skin test), the immune response to intracellular organisms, and possible "surveillance" which protects against growth of spontaneously occurring neoplasia. B cells are short-lived, noncirculating cells, largely responsible for the production of immune globulins, often referred to as "circulating antibody" or "humoral antibody." Both cell types are involved in immunity to transplants. Allografts to recipients previously unexposed to donor antigen are rejected as a "first-set" graft, largely through the T-cell system. Recipients who have previously been immunized to donor allografts by exposure to donor antigens by blood transfusions or by a previous transplant, or who have been the recipients of xenografts, have circulating preformed humoral antibody, and such grafts undergo "humoral rejection" in which the B-cell mechanism predominates. In human renal allografts, specific antigenic determinants (HL-A antigens) exist, over 30 of which have been recognized. These are mostly surface membrane protein moieties, and the immune process directed against them by the recipient is relatively specific for the individual HL-A determinants. It is, however, possible for unrelated individuals to share one or more specific HL-A determinants. Thus, a recipient may become immunized to the tissues of a donor by previous exposure to transfused white cells/or platelets from another individual whose tissues contain the same antigens as the allograft donor. Once a kidney has been in place for several days in a previously unsensitized recipient, humoral immunity may become superimposed upon the cellular rejection; therefore, both types of immune processes may mediate the rejection of an allograft, with one or the other predominating.

The rejection of an allograft by an individual who has not previously been exposed to donor antigens occurs by way of the CMI pathways in which the sensitized lymphocytes predominate. In the case of the kidney, the sensitized lymphocyte first combines with an antigen on vascular endothelium. Very early in the rejection process cells can be seen in contact with the small venules. The precise mechanism of the damage induced by the sensitized "killer" T lymphocytes awaits elucidation, but immunoglobulins and complement are not required. Rather, a cyclic nucleotide (cAMP and cGMP)-dependent secretory process which follows direct cell-to-cell contact has been implicated. Similarly, the interaction of sensitized lymphocytes and antigens at the graft site is likely to release migration inhibitory factor (MIF) which may account for the accumulation of mononuclear (histiocytic) cells at the graft site. Some of these cells migrate through the vessel wall and are seen as perivascular accumulations. Intravascular accumulations result in slowing of flow, stasis, and graft ischemia. B lymphocytes, specifically sensitized, or nonspecifically recruited by the prior formation of immune complexes of antibody and histocompatibility antigens, may also appear in the graft along the endothelial lining of vessels. When significant amounts of circulating immune antibodies, principally IgG and IgM, appear, the complement sequence is initiated. If intense, such activation may release significant amounts of polymorphonuclear (PMN) chemotactic factors, and PMNs are attracted to the graft, where the release of lysosomal enzymes from the leukocytes may result in damage to the vascular wall. In addition, the deposition of platelets is facilitated, with the release of vasoactive kinins and the deposition of fibrinogen and fibrin. This sequence of events is corroborated by histologic observations of rejection demonstrating interstitial infiltration of cells, and damage to vascular endothelium with the deposition of fibrin, complement, and immune globulins. It can be shown also that the earliest evidence of renal allograft rejection is redistribution of blood flow from the cortex to the corticomedullary area, reflecting the primary role of the influence of vascular damage in the rejection process.

When a kidney is transplanted into a heterologous species or an individual previously sensitized to donor antigen, it is immediately perfused by "preformed" humoral antibody directed specifically against graft antigen.

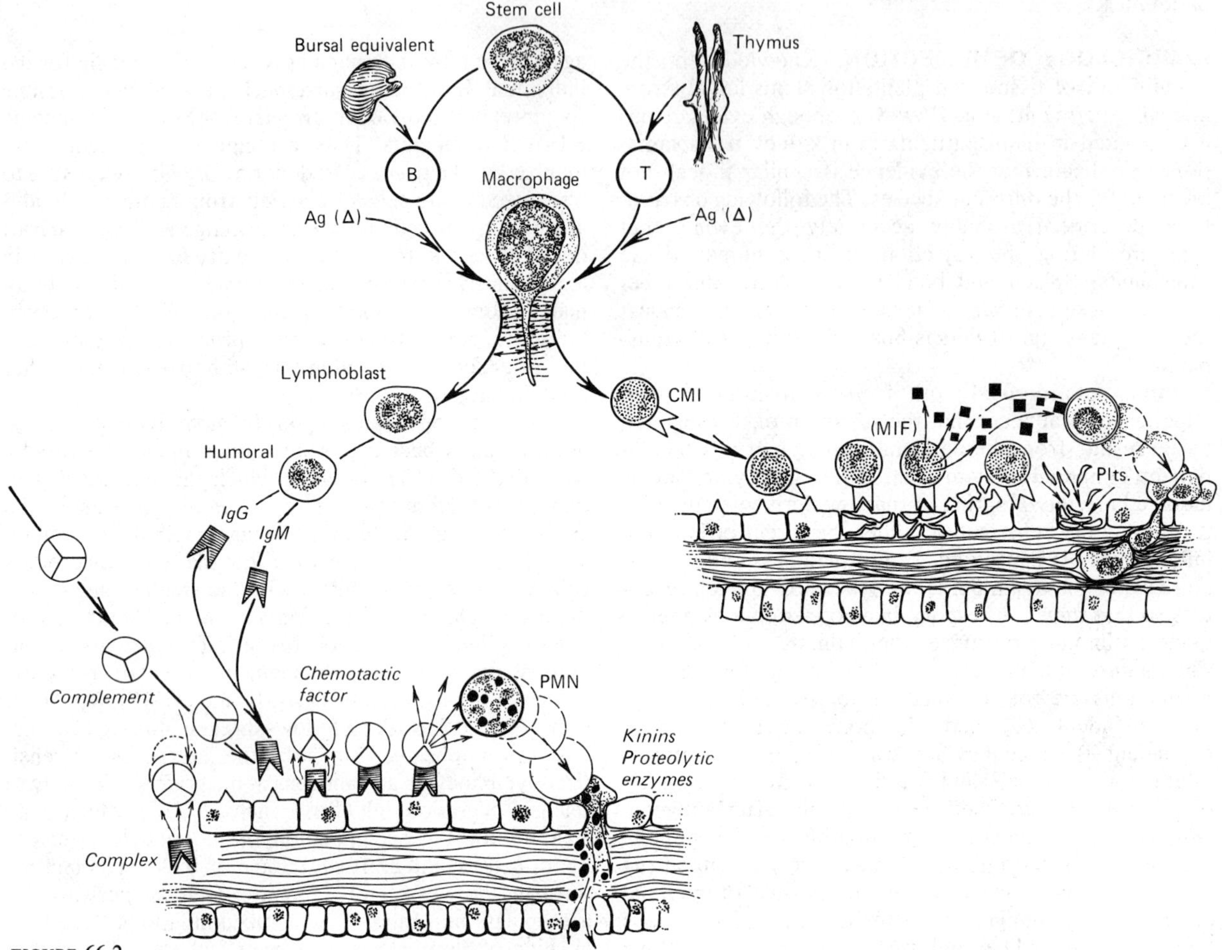

FIGURE 66-2
Overall scheme of the development of effector mechanisms in graft rejection. Bone marrow stem cells differentiate under the influence of the thymus gland into mature thymus-derived (T) lymphocytes, or under the influence of an equivalent to the avian bursa of Fabricius into mature bone-marrow–derived (B) lymphocytes. Exposure to antigen (Δ) results in an interaction between T cells and B cells, and often involves macrophages. The sensitized B cells after mitoses develop into immunoglobulin-secreting cells (e.g., plasma cells), illustrated here by IgG and IgM. Such immunoglobulins may form immune complexes with antigen in the circulation which activate the complement sequence, or they may react directly with antigens on the blood vessel surface. Elaboration of secondary mediators, including the products of complement activation, results in vascular damage as illustrated. Sensitized T lymphocytes are the primary effector cells in cell-mediated immunity (CMI) and may react directly with antigens in the graft to exert a cytotoxic effect. In addition, T cells release factors, such as macrophage migration inhibition factor (MIF) which may accelerate the rate of mononuclear cell infiltration. In addition, it has been shown that unsensitized B lymphocytes can be activated to exert cytotoxic effects by the fixation of IgG to target cells, followed by interaction of the IgG (Fc portion) with a receptor on the B cell (not shown). Finally, platelet aggregation and thrombosis can occur following the endothelial damage induced by any of these mechanisms.

Again, the sequence of events which takes place reflects primarily the vascular site of injury. In such an instance little cellular infiltrate may be seen, but destruction to the vessel wall is violent and immediate, occurring in a matter of minutes in some instances. Platelet thrombi, the deposition of fibrin, and necrosis of vascular endothelium are prominent, and flow through the graft may cease within minutes or hours. Presumably, the same humoral mechanisms discussed above participate, but the sequence of events is accelerated; thus, the term "hyperacute rejection" has been applied.

The failure of transplanted kidneys after 2 or even 3

years of adequate function is due to a form of "chronic rejection." In such kidneys the development of nephrosclerosis, with proliferation of the vascular intima of renal vessels, and intimal fibrosis with marked decrease in the lumen of the vessels take place (Fig. 66-3). The result is renal ischemia, hypertension, widespread tubular atrophy, interstitial fibrosis, and glomerular atrophy with eventual renal failure. Occasionally, lobular or proliferative glomerulonephritis may be the initiating factor and may progress to renal failure. Both long-term vascular lesions and glomerular lesions are probably the result of subclinical episodes of rejection with damage to capillary and vascular epithelium and resultant healing fibrosis and sclerosis.

Finally, there is evidence that humoral antibody, in all probability some fraction of IgG, may actually play a role in promoting the *survival* of the allograft. This enhancing antibody, which is not cytotoxic or complement activating, may block the action of cytotoxic "killer" lymphocytes, thus preventing the disastrous effects of the immune onslaught against the graft.

IMMUNOSUPPRESSIVE TREATMENT When histocompatibility differences exist between donor and recipient, it is necessary to modify or suppress the immune response in order to enable the recipient to accept a graft. Immunosuppressive therapy in general suppresses all immune responses, including those to bacteria, fungi, and even malignant tumors. Agents used in man to suppress the immune response are the following:

Drugs *Azathioprine* (*Imuran*), an analogue of 6-mercaptopurine, is the keystone to immunosuppressive therapy in man. This agent can inhibit synthesis of deoxyribonucleic acid (DNA) or ribonucleic acid (RNA), or both. Because cell division and proliferation result as part of the immune response to antigenic stimulation, suppression may be mediated by the inhibition of mitosis of immunologically competent lymphoid cells interfering with synthesis of DNA. Alternatively, inhibition may be brought about by blocking the synthesis of ribonucleic acid (possibly messenger RNA), which is thought to play an immunologic role in the processing of antigens prior to lymphocyte stimulation. Therapy with azathioprine is generally instituted 2 to 10 days prior to transplantation of the kidney and is continued, at levels of 2 to 3 mg per kg per day, as long as the allograft functions. Because the drug is rapidly metabolized by the liver, its dose need not be varied directly in relation to renal function, even though renal failure results in retention of the metabolites of azathioprine. Some patients are unusually sensitive to this drug, particularly when renal function is compromised, and reduction in dosage is required because of leukopenia and occasionally thrombocytopenia. Excessive amounts of azathioprine may also cause jaundice, anemia, and alopecia. Actinomycin C formerly was employed in the treatment of rejection episodes, but because of its toxicity is now used infrequently.

The *corticosteroids*, usually in the form of prednisone, are important adjuncts to immunosuppressive therapy. Of all the agents employed, prednisone has effects that are easiest to assess, and in large doses it is unquestionably the most effective agent for the reversal of rejection. In general, 150 to 200 mg prednisone is given immediately prior to or at the time of transplantation, and the dosage is reduced to maintenance levels over a period of 2 weeks. The well-known side effects of the corticosteroids, particularly impairment of wound healing and predisposition to infection, make it desirable to taper the dose as rapidly as possible in the immediate postoperative period. Prednisone should be used in large doses (200 to 1,000 mg)

FIGURE 66-3
Biopsy of the renal cadaveric allograft illustrating obliterative endarteritis. Loss of the media is associated with intimal thickening. The elastic tissue shows dissolution of the elastica. The evidence for arteritis with subsequent thrombosis are typically the gaps in the elastica and media. The intimal thickening probably represents organization of a thrombus formed in response to the arteritis. (From GJ Dammin and JP Merrill, Transplantation, tissue rejection and the kidney, Chap. 20 in Structural Basis for Renal Disease, *ed EL Becker, New York: Hoeber-Harper, 1968)*

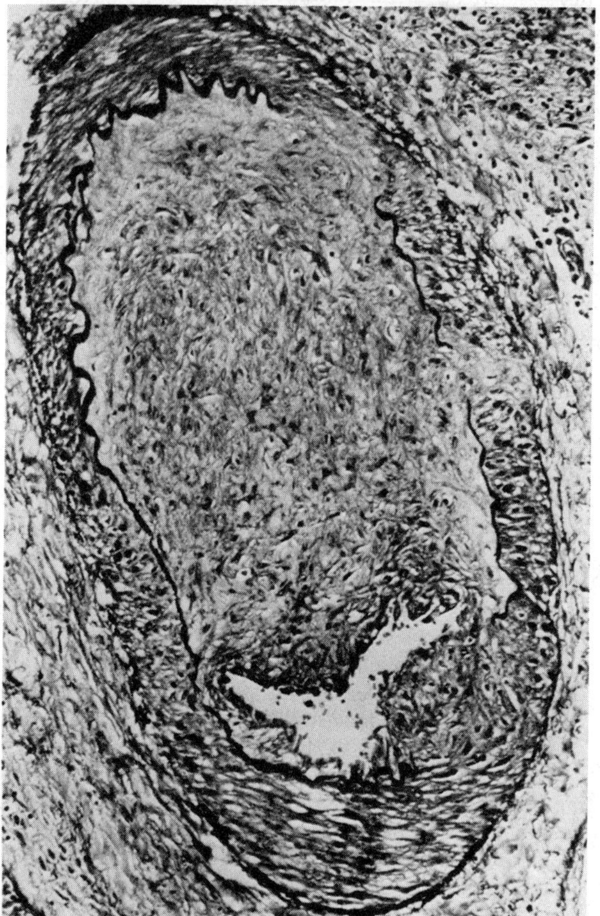

immediately upon detection of beginning rejection. When the drug is effective, the results are usually apparent within 48 to 96 hr, and the dose may subsequently be reduced again. Although most patients whose renal function is stable after 6 months or a year do not require large doses of prednisone, maintenance doses of 20 mg per day are the rule. Many patients tolerate an alternate-day course of steroids better without an increased risk of rejection.

When jaundice or nephritis appears in patients maintained on azathioprine, *cyclophosphamide* may be substituted. It appears to be as effective in the maintenance of renal allografts as Imuran and somewhat more effective in hepatic allografts. Leukopenia, alopecia, cystitis, ovarian fibrosis, and aspermia may result if the dosage is not carefully regulated.

Antilymphocyte globulin (ALG) When serums from animals made immune to host lymphocytes are injected into the recipient, a marked suppression of cellular immunity to the tissue graft results. The action upon CMI is considerably more effective than upon humoral immunity. A globulin fraction of the serum is the agent generally employed. For use in man peripheral human lymphocytes, thymocytes, lymphocytes from cadaver spleens, or those harvested from thoracic duct fistulas have been utilized. More recently, cultured human lymphoblasts, which can be produced in large quantities, offer the advantage of availability. These cells are injected into horses, rabbits, or goats to produce antilymphocyte serum, from which the globulin fraction is then separated. The globulin is injected intramuscularly, or preferably intravenously, 5 days to a week prior to transplantation and continued for 2 to 3 weeks thereafter. A number of shorter and longer treatment protocols have been devised. The exact mechanism of action of ALG remains unclear, but the most likely explanation appears to be its action of the selective depletion of T lymphocytes belonging to the recirculating pool, i.e., those cells primarily responsible for CMI. Once coated with antibody, these cells are either lysed or phagocytized by the reticuloendothelial system in the liver. Pain and swelling may occur at the site of injection, and occasional anaphylaxis has been reported. Two deaths attributable to the use of ALG are known to have occurred in improperly prepared batches of ALG, and fatal anaphylaxis during the course of therapy has been reported. Antiplatelet or anti-red cell antibodies may cause thrombocytopenia and intravascular coagulation or severe anemia. In some batches, horse globulin may be found distributed in a linear pattern upon the glomeruli of the renal allograft; however, this seldom results in glomerulonephritis. Serum sickness reactions, with or without nephritis, have been extremely rare.

Although ALG is unquestionably effective in prolonging grafts in experimental animals, its efficacy in human beings is somewhat less clear, even though an effective preparation of antilymphocyte globulin may result in the disappearance of a previously positive delayed type of hypersensitivity skin reaction. Although ALG should still be used with extreme caution in man, it seems probable that further exploration of this preparation, particularly employing larger doses, may result in development of an effective agent which can be used with relatively little hazard of serum sickness or nephrotoxic nephritis.

Other techniques Of the alternate techniques of immunosuppression, thymectomy and splenectomy have not favorably influenced the course of human kidney transplants. Prolonged drainage of the thoracic duct lymph as a means of lymphocyte depletion, though cumbersome, may have some beneficial effects. In extracorporeal irradiation, arterial blood is circulated around a radioactive cobalt or cesium source where the circulating cells are subjected to gamma radiation. Blood is then returned to the venous end of the shunt. This procedure also is cumbersome, and the results are conflicting. It may, however, have some use in maintaining patients when toxic effects of other immunosuppressive agents necessitate their temporary cessation. Local irradiation to the transplanted kidney in two or three doses of 350 rd each has also been utilized. Current evidence suggests that this technique may result in fewer early rejection episodes in cadaveric transplants than in nonirradiated controls.

COMPLICATIONS OF RENAL TRANSPLANTATION

The complications of human renal transplantation often result from the use of *immunosuppressive therapy*. Wound infection with gram-negative organisms is common, as is breakdown of wounds, particularly the ureteral anastomosis. Pulmonary infections with a variety of unusual organisms, including *Candida* (Chap. 171), *Aspergillus* (Chap. 174), *Nocardia* (Chap. 173), *Pneumocystis* (Chap. 214), and cytomegalovirus (Chap. 206), also occur. Their relationship to a general defect in immunologic integrity is clear. The complications of *corticosteroid* therapy are well known and include gastrointestinal bleeding, hemorrhagic pancreatitis, and impairment of wound healing. Leukopenia, anemia, and jaundice occur as a result of azathioprine administration.

Even identical twins who do not require immunosuppressive therapy develop complications. In 18 sets of identical twins whose original disease was glomerulonephritis, 11 developed a similar histologic lesion in the transplanted kidney. The glomerular lesion is not, however, limited to the isograft, nor is it necessarily a question of "catching" the disease in the transplant because of continuing antiglomerular activity. A number of patients with true allografts treated with immunosuppressive therapy have developed typical glomerular lesions over a period of years. One patient who received a successful allograft from his mother developed a classical nephrotic syndrome with glomerulonephritis $2^1/_2$ years after transplantation. Because the reason for transplantation initially was the accidental removal of a single normal ectopic kidney, the development of glomerulonephritis in the transplant cannot be attributed to "continuing activity."

However, in a few instances glomerular lesions have developed in an allograft, even with immunosuppressive therapy. These lesions so resemble that of the patient's own original disease and there is so little other evidence of rejection, that they must be considered recurrences of the original disease. Finally, in at least one case, glomerulonephritis has developed apparently *de novo* in a patient who had survived 5 years with a normally functioning allograft.

Sensitization of the human recipient to subsequent skin grafts from any donor may occur following the intradermal injection of donor leukocytes, and uremic recipients, particularly when maintained for long periods on hemodialysis, require repeated transfusions and thus have repeated exposure to formed elements in the blood which are capable of sensitizing the recipient to subsequent tissue grafts. Rapid rejection of a first kidney allograft has been documented in a number of patients who presumably have been sensitized by platelets or leukocytes in transfusions administered prior to operation. Antibodies to human leukocytes have been demonstrated in the serum of these patients and are associated in a significant number of instances with a rapid rejection of the renal transplant.

Some patients have not developed cytotoxic antibodies to human tissue in spite of multiple transfusions. This observation has led to the definition of two groups: (1) *responders*, and (2) *nonresponders*. Preliminary evidence suggests that the nonresponders may fare better following allografting. Hyperacute rejection almost invariably follows transplantation of the kidney in the recipient who has been immunized against the specific HL-A antigens of the donor. It is also true that if the recipient carries antibodies against greater than 10 percent of a pool of randomly selected donors (responder), his prognosis following a cadaver allograft will be poorer than that of a nonsensitized individual, even though he appears not to be immunized against the specific donor.

Urinary fistula requiring nephrostomy may be the result of rejection of the ureter, disruption of the ureteral blood supply, infection, or a combination of all three. Wound infection and failure of the wound to heal are not uncommon, particularly when the higher doses of steroids are required.

Tumor cells have been transplanted inadvertently with kidneys taken from cadaver donors dying from bronchogenic carcinoma and other malignancies. The immunosuppressive therapy which allows the kidney to be tolerated in the recipients also apparently permits survival and propagation of the malignant tumor. With cessation of immunosuppressive therapy both the renal allograft and the tumor are destroyed.

The incidence of *tumors arising in patients with immunosuppressive therapy* is approximately twice the incidence in the general population in a comparable age range. Fifty-five percent of the tumors were of epithelial origin, and most of the remainder were mesenchymal tumors. Others included lymphoma of the central nervous system and two reticulum-cell sarcomas which developed at the site of the injection of ALG.

Persistent hyperparathyroidism may necessitate parathyroidectomy as long as 6 months following the resumption of normal renal function by a transplanted kidney. This appears to be due to markedly enlarged parathyroid glands which have developed during the uremic phase and do not spontaneously regress with the resumption of normal renal function. In 11 of 130 patients in one series, *aseptic necrosis of the femoral head* occurred. Similar results have been reported by others. This complication may be due to residual hyperparathyroidism and large doses of prednisone.

SELECTION OF RECIPIENTS FOR KIDNEY TRANSPLANTATION Table 66-1 lists practical considerations in the selection of a recipient for a human renal allograft. Such a procedure should be undertaken only when conservative treatment has failed, when there are no reversible elements in the patient's renal failure, and when he is too sick to be maintained comfortably with the usual methods of treatment. However, the considerable success with kidneys transplanted from blood relatives, reports of success with second or third kidney transplants, and the ability to maintain patients who have had transplant failures on hemodialysis justify consideration of kidney transplantation before the patient is critically ill and possibly even before it is obvious that hemodialysis is the only other course. The recipient should be free of life-threatening extrarenal complications such as cancer, severe coronary artery disease, and cerebrovascular disease. Provided that diffuse vascular involvement is not present, diabetes itself is not a contraindication. Although age may be a limiting factor, the "physiologic" age rather than the chronologic age contraindicates transplantation. A cadaver transplant into an eighty-two-year-old patient is on record, and adult renal allografts have been transplanted into recipients as young as three. Although abnormalities of the bladder and urethra present additional hazards, successful renal allografts have been placed in individuals with these abnormalities by prior construction of an artificial bladder (i.e., ileal conduit) into which the donor ureter is placed. The demonstration of "preformed antibodies" in the potential recipient prior to transplantation is a contraindication when it can be shown that these antibodies react specifically to donor cells.

DONOR SELECTION Donor sources are cadavers or volunteer blood-related living donors. Living volunteer donors should be found completely normal on physical examination and should be of the same major ABO blood group, because there is good evidence that crossing major blood group barriers prejudices survival of the allograft. It is, however, possible to transplant a kidney of a type O donor into an A or B recipient. Selective renal arteri-

TABLE 66-1
Contraindications to human kidney transplantation

1 Absolute contraindications:
- *a* Reversible renal involvement
- *b* Ability of conservative measures to maintain useful life
- *c* Major extrarenal complications (cerebrovascular or coronary disease; neoplasia)
- *d* Active infection
- *e* Active glomerulonephritis
- *f* Previous sensitization to human tissue

2 Relative contraindications:
- *a* Age
- *b* Presence of vesical or urethral abnormalities
- *c* Iliofemoral occlusive disease
- *d* Diabetes mellitus
- *e* Inactive lupus erythematosus
- *f* Psychiatric problems

ography should be performed on volunteer donors to rule out the presence of multiple or abnormal renal arteries, because the surgical procedure is inordinately difficult and the ischemic time of the normal kidney prohibitively long when vascular abnormalities exist. Cadaver donors should be free of malignant neoplastic disease because of possible transmission of cancer to the recipient.

Although tissue typing is not considered mandatory for cadaver donors, direct cross matching for the presence of preformed antibodies against specific donor tissue is. The chances of finding a perfect 4-antigen match between unrelated donor and recipient are calculated to be between 1 in 300 and 1 in 1,000, varying with the incidence of HL-A antigens in the population. This reflects the necessity for a large recipient pool, maintained on hemodialysis. A coordinated regional or national system of computerized information sharing and logistical support for the transportation of cadaver kidneys to the suitable recipient is under development. It is now possible to remove cadaver kidneys and to maintain them for up to 48 hr on cold pulsatile perfusion. This should permit adequate time for various typing, cross matching, transportation, and selection problems to be solved.

CLINICAL COURSE AND MANAGEMENT OF THE RECIPIENT Usually, but not invariably, bilateral nephrectomies are performed prior to transplantation, and the recipient is maintained on intermittent hemodialysis. Removal of the patient's own diseased kidneys obviates one source of infection in the postoperative period and facilitates the diagnosis of rejection of the allograft, since variations in renal function and urine sediment are then related only to changes in the allograft. However, bilateral nephrectomy also potentiates the anemia of the patient maintained on dialysis, and therefore ideally the procedure should be performed as close as is feasible to the projected time of transplantation. It should be ascertained also that the recipient has a normally functioning bladder and lower outflow tract.

Adequate hemodialysis should be performed within 48 hr prior to surgery, and care should be taken that the serum potassium level is not markedly elevated so that intraoperative cardiac arrhythmias can be averted. In patients who have been presensitized to donor tissue, hyperacute rejection may take place on the operating table. Within minutes the kidney will become swollen, tense, and a mottled purple in color, and blood flow may cease soon thereafter. Thrombotic obliterative lesions may be seen by frozen section, and if they are extensive the kidney should be removed. Postoperatively the diuresis that occurs must be carefully monitored; in many instances it may be massive, reflecting the inability of ischemic tubules to regulate sodium and water excretion. Massive potassium losses may occur and occasionally result in cardiac arrhythmias. The chronically uremic patient undoubtedly has some excess of extracellular fluid, and some degree of negative balance should be accomplished provided circulatory hemodynamics remain stable.

Although immunosuppressive regimens vary, a typical program would be the following:

Antilymphocyte globulin is administered daily by the intravenous route for 1 week before and 2 weeks after transplantation of a kidney from a living donor; in recipients of cadaver organs the first dose must be administered on the day of surgery and continued for a 3-week period thereafter. Azathioprine in a dose of 4 mg per kg is given for 2 days preoperatively; on the day of operation it is administered by the intravenous route, and it is continued for about 1 week, depending upon renal function. It is then reduced to 3 mg per kg, and the maintenance dose is $1\frac{1}{2}$ mg per kg by mouth. In recipients of kidneys from living donors the equivalent of 300 to 500 mg cortisone is given on the day of operation; this dose is maintained for 2 days and is decreased gradually to a maintenance dose of 50 to 100 mg cortisone, usually administered as the prednisone equivalent. For rejection episodes, 1 g soluble corticosteroid in the form of methylprednisolone is administered intravenously daily for a 5-day period. This is decreased to 800, 600, and 400 mg over the next 10-day period while oral prednisone dosage is maintained at 25 to 50 mg.

The rejection episode Early diagnosis of rejection is imperative, because prompt institution of vigorous therapy may reverse renal function and prevent irreversible damage due to fibrosis. Clinical evidence of rejection is characterized by fever, swelling, and tenderness over the allograft, and by significant reduction in urine volume. In patients whose renal function is good initially, oliguria may be accompanied by decreased urinary sodium concentration and increased osmolarity. These changes may not be present in the more chronic stages of rejection or when renal function is impaired at the onset of rejection. A transplanted cadaver kidney frequently undergoes a period of anuria which may last as long as 3 weeks without prejudicing the eventual function of the graft. In this instance, the reversible lesion is presumably due to ischemia, and the diagnosis of rejection becomes more difficult. Renal arteriography and radioactive hippuran renograms may be useful in ascertaining changes in the renal vasculature and in renal blood flow, even in the absence of urinary flow. When renal function has been good initially, a rise in the blood urea nitrogen level and a decrease in the creatinine clearance may herald the onset of rejection. The serum creatinine or its clearance is more reliable, because fever and the administration of prednisone may influence the concentration of blood urea nitrogen without necessarily reflecting a decrease in urea clearance. Increase in the 24-hr excretion of urinary lysozyme has been helpful. Increase in proteinuria may reflect rejection, but when it occurs later in the course of the postoperative period, predominant glomerular disease may be present. Hypertension is also a concomitant of rejection. When hypertension responds to prednisone, it is likely that rejection has been responsible for the elevation of blood pressure, because other forms of hypertension usually do not improve with corticosteroid therapy. Treatment of rejection is by the administration of massive doses of corticosteroids, beginning with 1 g methylprednisolone administered intravenously, with the dose gradually reduced after a period of 5 days to maintenance with oral prednisone. If the therapy is effective, improvement in graft function should be seen within a period of 5 days to 1 week.

Modification of the usual clinical manifestations of infection by immunosuppressive therapy is a major problem in the posttransplant period. The signs and symptoms of infection may be masked and distorted, and fever without obvious cause is common. Only after days or weeks will it become apparent that it has a viral or fungal origin. The importance of blood cultures in such patients cannot be overemphasized, because systemic infection without obvious external foci is frequent. Particularly important are rapidly occurring pulmonary lesions, which may result in death within 5 days of onset. When these become apparent, immunosuppressive agents should be discontinued except for maintenance doses of prednisone. In the case of *Pneumocystis carinii*, pentamidine seems to be the treatment of choice; amphotericin B has been used effectively in systemic fungal infections. Involvement of the oropharynx with *Candida* may be treated with local Mycostatin. Small doses (a total of 300 mg) amphotericin given over a period of 2 weeks may be effective in refractory oral candidiasis. The treatment of jaundice in transplant patients should include cessation of Imuran therapy. It is surprising that total cessation of Imuran therapy often does not result in rejection of a graft. In some instances of jaundice, cyclophosphamide may be substituted for Imuran. Antiplatelet agents and anticoagulants, although effective in theory, have not been strikingly successful in the prevention of the chronic vascular lesion.

The condition of patients who have been discharged from the hospital should be closely observed in a specialized outpatient clinic whose physicians are familiar with the problems and complications of the posttransplant patient. When, in spite of repeated efforts to reverse the rejection, renal function progressively fails, the philosophy should be to save the patient, not the graft. Excessive immunosuppressive therapy may lead to fatal infection or bleeding. A biopsy of the graft may establish the irreversibility of the lesion. When such irreversibility is established, the graft should be removed and the patient started again on hemodialysis. Infection and occasionally hemorrhage at the operative sites days and even months following removal of the graft occasionally occur and must be carefully watched. Psychologic complications following transplantation are common. Depression and anxiety may reflect both the difficult, stressful postoperative course and the anxiety and uncertainty of the physician.

TRANSPLANTATION OF OTHER TISSUES Organs other than the kidney which have a potential for clinical transplantation are the liver and heart. Two possible indications for *liver transplantation* are chronic hepatic failure and malignancy which is localized to the liver. Two techniques for liver transplantation have been utilized in man: (1) *Orthotopic*—the recipient's own liver is removed and the transplant is substituted for it in the anatomic position. (2) *Auxiliary*—the recipient's liver is left in place and the allograft is placed in the right paravertebral gutter. The donor's vena cava then is interposed in the recipient terminal inferior vena cava, and the hepatic artery is anastomosed to the right common iliac artery. Finally, the end of the allograft portal vein is anastomosed to the recipient's superior mesenteric vein.

Immunosuppressive regimens are similar to those in kidney transplantation. There is some suggestion that the use of antilymphocyte globulin is more effective in liver allografting. Obviously, the donor source must be a cadaver. Complications of liver transplantation have been strikingly different from those encountered with renal allografts. In many instances an initial hemorrhagic diathesis with fibrinolysis occurs. This is followed by a phase of hypercoagulability in the successfully transplanted recipient, which in one instance resulted in fatal pulmonary emboli. Infections also seem to present a greater problem than with renal allografts. These complications are not insurmountable, however, and there are now a number of liver-transplant recipients who have survived for 2 years or more. Although at this time liver transplantation is not as clinically feasible a procedure as kidney grafting, in a few centers with expertise and experience in this technique liver transplants continue to be performed, it is hoped with steady improvement in the results.

Transplantation of the heart has been accomplished successfully in man in a number of instances. Current results suggest that it is comparable to transplantation of the cadaver kidney and that results certainly will improve. Indications for cardiac transplantation are myocardial insufficiency, usually due to severe coronary artery disease and myocardial fibrosis, and failure to respond to the most rigorous medical measures. The donor must be a cadaver and is usually an individual whose death has resulted from trauma or suicide. The question of the ethics and morals raised by the removal of a heart capable of sustaining life in another individual has been discussed by many medical and lay authors. It seems eminently reasonable that if "death" of the brain has occurred, as evidenced by lack of electrical activity in the electroencephalogram over a period of 24 to 36 hr, dilated pupils, failure of spontaneous respiration, and lack of peripheral reflexes, the ability to maintain respiration or cardiac output by artificial methods is academic. Nevertheless, the decision as to when to discontinue these efforts should be made independently by the physician caring for the prospective donor in consultation with one or two colleagues. The question of whether or not the heart is to be used for transplantation should not affect this decision. Once the decision has been made, the donor can be maintained until the recipient is prepared for operation.

Human *spleen* and *pancreas* have been transplanted with limited success. If it could be shown that normal spleen can produce a useful amount of AHG, transplantation of that organ to some patients with hemophilia would provide a distinct advantage over standard substitution therapy. Transplantation of lymphoid tissue (including spleen) for total agammaglobulinemia has resulted in temporary improvement, but eventually the transplanted lymphoid tissue rejects the host (graft versus host reaction). Temporary success in transplanting pancreas in diabetics also has been reported, but substitution therapy seems more feasible.

Various other *endocrines*, including parathyroid, adrenal, and thyroid, have all been transplanted, with only temporary success. A large percentage of *corneal grafts* survive as allografts in man, primarily because the cornea is not vascularized, which excludes immunologically competent cells. Grafts of bone and blood vessels do not survive as living allografts but act as a "scaffolding" over which host tissue may grow.

Transplantation of allogenic bone marrow in man is of particular interest to patients with leukemia and aplastic anemia and has resulted in a number of attempts to modify these diseases by this means. Similarly, the reconstitution of the genetic defect in congenital or acquired agammaglobulinemia or alymphocytosis has been attempted by grafting into such recipients cells competent to produce cell-mediated immunity or humoral immunity. Some degree of success has been achieved in all these instances when the marrow or spleen cells have been transplanted from identical twin donors or from HL-A matched siblings. However, leukemia has recurred even when the marrow transplant has been successful. In aplastic anemia one series has produced at least one successful survival for more than 1 year. Similar results have been reported in smaller series of patients with agammaglobulinemia or alymphocytosis. Cyclophosphamide or whole-body radiation has been administered to the recipient to prevent rejection of the graft; however, survival of the graft may be accompanied by the appearance of the graft-versus-host reaction, with death of the recipient as a result of anorexia, diarrhea, dermatitis, or, more frequently, opportunistic infection. Some encouraging results in preventing the graft-versus-host reaction have been reported with the use of cyclophosphamide or amethopterin.

Transplantation of a normal allogenic liver to repair the metabolic defect in Wilson's disease has been reported in two instances with some preliminary success, and the transplantation of the kidney not as a functioning excretory organ but as a source of the congenitally absent enzyme has been accomplished with early success in two cases of Fabry's disease.

ORGAN PRESERVATION If it were possible to remove cadaver organs and to store them for a period of weeks or longer under conditions permitting their successful replantation, one of the difficult problems in organ procurement would be solved. Bone marrow is the only organ that can be stored easily for prolonged periods.

XENOGRAFTS Kidneys, lungs, and hearts have been transplanted to human beings from various primates, including chimpanzees and baboons. Although one chimpanzee kidney graft functioned well for more than 7 months, clinical efforts in this area have been abandoned. It seems quite possible, however, that continuing efforts to find other species whose tissues may be more compatible to man's (e.g., the pig) may result eventually in a source of organs which might eliminate many of the present problems. In fact, it might be possible to breed pigs for histocompatibility with man in the same fashion that mice were bred to produce purebred lines with predictable tissue antigenicity.

REFERENCES

Bach ML, Bach FH: The genetics of histocompatibility. Hosp Practice 5:(8)33, 1970

Belzer F et al: Preservation and transplantation of human cadaver kidneys. Transplantation 14:3, 1972

Brent L: Immunological tolerance 1951–1971, in *Immunological Tolerance to Tissue Antigens*, eds NW Nisbet, MW Elves, Oswestry, England: Orthopaedic Hospital, 1971

Briggs WA et al: Aseptic necrosis in the femur after renal transplantation. Ann Surg 175:282, 1972

Lazarus JM, Hampers CL: Renal transplantation. Ann Intern Med 76:(3)504, 1972

Merrill JP: Allograft rejection, chap. 24 in *Immunological Diseases*, 2d ed., ed M Samter, Boston: Little, Brown, 1971

67 ASTHMA, HAY FEVER, AND OTHER MANIFESTATIONS OF ALLERGY

PHILIP S. NORMAN

The most common conditions which arise from immune responses with manifestations of hypersensitivity are the so-called "allergic" diseases—hay fever, asthma, and urticaria. These reactions result from the abnormal production of IgE antibodies to otherwise innocuous antigens (allergens) that are common in the environment.

ALLERGIC RHINITIS (HAY FEVER)

DEFINITION Allergic rhinitis is characterized by sneezing, rhinorrhea, swelling of the nasal mucosa, itching of the eyes, and lacrimation. Hay fever is the common term for allergic rhinitis due to seasonal spread of pollens in the air, but the disease is not necessarily seasonal and may result from exposure to antigens other than pollen. *Vasomotor rhinitis* designates those diseases without allergic or infectious etiology which resemble hay fever.

ETIOLOGY Plants that evolve large amounts of airborne pollen are common sources of antigens responsible for hay fever, whereas flowering plants such as roses or goldenrod, which are pollinated by insects, are not. Ragweed pollen is the principal offender in the central, eastern, and southeastern parts of the United States but is virtually absent west of the Rocky Mountains. Ordinarily ragweed pollinates between early August and late October, the most likely season for hay fever.

In the northern half of the United States, grasses pollinate from May to July; in the South grass may pollinate throughout the year. Although the season when trees pollinate may vary, they ordinarily do so in early spring, and earlier in the South than in the North. Some widespread airborne pollens are nonallergenic; pine pollen, for instance, almost never causes hay fever. Certain molds, found most frequently on decaying vegetation, produce airborne spores, which appear in definite seasons. *Hormodendrum* has a peak incidence in July, and *Alternaria* in October; both may cause seasonal allergic rhinitis.

Most pollens are about 25 to 40 μm in diameter and settle promptly from the air. The settling properties of pollen are used for crude estimations of the "pollen count" in the air by collecting and enumerating particles on a greased glass slide. There is an approximate but regular correlation between the pollen count and the frequency and severity of hay fever in the susceptible population. Pollen particles from plants, grasses, or trees of varying types can be differentiated by microscopic examination, permitting precise definition of the airborne pollens responsible for hay fever.

Pollen particles are relatively large and, when inhaled, will impinge on and be deposited within the nose, whereas few reach the terminal bronchioles. House dust, fungus spores, animal danders, feathers, broken insect parts, facial powders, vegetable dusts, insecticides, and food particles disseminated during cooking also have been incriminated as causes of hay fever; an etiologic relationship between ingested food and respiratory allergy is often suspected but difficult to document.

PATHOGENESIS When pollens and mold spores land on the nasal mucosa, their carbohydrate coat is digested by the lysozyme of respiratory mucus, releasing the contents. Ragweed and grass pollens contain specific proteins, referred to as *allergens,* which account for their sensitizing potential. Allergens are of relatively low molecular weight (10,000 to 40,000) and represent 1 percent or less of the extractable solids of pollen. The biologic potency of these allergens is such that intradermal injection of 1 μμ will cause a wheal and erythema reaction in a sensitive patient. Other pollen, mold, and dander allergens are less well characterized but appear to have similar properties. Presumably, it is the unusual ability of allergic individuals to become sensitized following release of these allergens in the respiratory tract that leads to allergic disease.

The process of sensitization is poorly understood but leads to production of IgE or "reaginic" antibodies in lymphoid tissues lining the respiratory tract. IgE antibodies are cytotrophic for the basophilic leukocytes and tissue mast cells. Although little is known about the life cycle of these cells, they are found in relatively large numbers submucosally in the respiratory and gastrointestinal tracts and in the skin. When an allergen diffuses across the mucous membrane and makes contact with specific IgE antibody fixed to the surface of these cells, they are activated to secrete histamine and probably other mediators such as SRS-A (slow-reacting substance) into the surrounding tissues. This process probably accounts for the major manifestations of respiratory allergies. Drugs which raise intracellular cyclic AMP (adenosine monophosphate) inhibit mediator secretion and are useful agents in the suppression of allergic symptoms.

The sensitivity in hay fever is not confined to the mucous membranes but is general and is exemplified by the ability of the entire skin to react. The IgE antibodies circulate freely until they meet the cells which have a special affinity for them. Nearly everyone can synthesize IgE antibodies; normal persons have serum concentrations of 0.006 to 0.180 mg per 100 ml. They are thought to play a useful role in resistance to intestinal parasites. Furthermore, most people will develop IgE-mediated wheal and erythema skin reactivity to repeated intradermal injections of antigens such as ascaris extract and bovine ribonuclease. Allergic individuals, however, are likely to develop such reactions to antigens instilled into the nose. The nature of the defect responsible for this phenomenon is unknown, but it is probably hereditary, because there is a strong tendency for allergic disease to run in families. The mode of inheritance has not been determined, but when both parents have "atopic" disease, the allergy in the offspring is apt to be unusually severe. In all, from 5 to 15 percent of individuals are atopic—i.e., they are capable of developing allergy to inhaled antigens.

The nasal mucosa of patients with hay fever or allergic rhinitis also appears to be more susceptible to irritants than the normal nasal mucosa. Furthermore, studies in volunteers indicate that persons with allergic rhinitis are more susceptible than normal persons to infection by respiratory viruses. This enhanced reactivity of the nasal mucosa to a variety of stimuli also may explain the effects of emotional disturbances in exaggerating and possibly initiating symptoms of rhinitis in the allergic individual.

MANIFESTATIONS Pruritus about the eyes, nose, throat, and mouth, nasal discharge, sneezing, and lacrimation are the characteristic features of hay fever or allergic rhinitis. Particularly troublesome to the patient is mucosal swelling with occlusion of the airway, making breathing difficult and often causing insomnia. Symptoms vary in severity from day to day.

Occlusion of the nasal passages by swelling of the turbinates and mucous membranes may result in obstruction of the sinus ostiums or the eustachian tube, and infection of the sinuses and middle ear is a relatively common complication of perennial allergic rhinitis but is uncommon in seasonal hay fever. In addition, infection of the sinuses or nose in patients with allergic rhinitis results in formation of nasal polyps. These polyps further obstruct the nasal passages, increase symptoms, and exaggerate infection.

Many persons with hay fever or allergic rhinitis subsequently develop asthma. Retrobulbar neuritis, laryngeal edema with hoarseness, angioedema, urticaria, and other allergic illnesses occasionally accompany allergic rhinitis.

DIAGNOSIS Of great importance in the diagnosis of hay fever is its seasonal occurrence, which coincides with pollination of weeds, grasses, or trees. Allergic rhinitis due to local contamination of the patient's environment is diagnosed by carefully correlating the patient's symptoms with exposure to potential allergens at home, at work, and at play. The continuous character of perennial allergic rhinitis makes an allergic etiology less readily recognizable. The nasal mucosa is typically pale and edematous. The conjunctivas and the skin about the eyes, nose, and occasionally the mouth are reddened. In addition, nasal polyps are characteristic of allergic nasal disease, although often associated with infection in the nose or sinuses. Microscopic examination of nasal secretions shows many eosinophils, and mild blood eosinophilia is common when symptoms are at their maximum. Allergic individuals commonly have serum IgE levels two to six times normal, but this finding is not regular enough to be of great diagnostic usefulness.

The appearance of the mucosa of the nose and eyes is not diagnostic in allergic rhinitis; the same physical signs may occur from exposure to irritants or from upper respiratory infection. Pregnancy may be accompanied by mucosal edema and obstruction of the nose. Certain drugs, notably rauwolfia, may have similar effects. Polycythemia vera and hyperthyroidism may present with nasal and conjunctival hyperemia resembling allergic rhinitis.

Skin tests Approximately 25 percent of the normal population will show wheal and erythema skin reactions following intracutaneous inoculation of strong solutions of common airborne antigens. Not all persons with positive skin reactions, however, have allergic rhinitis. The allergic patient commonly has positive skin reactions to many antigens when from the history only one or two are incriminated as the cause of symptoms. Skin tests with allergenic antigens, therefore, are of more value in detecting an allergic propensity than in detecting the specific antigen responsible for the patient's symptoms. Only careful correlation of the skin reactivity with the environmental circumstances will delineate the responsible antigen.

Tests are performed with crude aqueous extracts of pollen, dust, foods, animal dander, insects, and other substances. These extracts are commercially available, but their potency varies considerably. No method of standardization is very reliable, because the extracts are crude and the measurement of specific antigen has not been possible except in the case of ragweed and a few grasses.

Skin tests are done by applying a drop of antigen to a skin scratch or by intradermal inoculation of 0.01 to 0.02 ml. In the beginning, very dilute extract should be used. The concentration may be increased gradually until there is certainty that the patient has a negative reaction. When a very dilute solution shows a positive reaction, it is more likely that the allergen is significant clinically. The uncertainties in standardization of solutions, however, make this rule of thumb difficult to apply in practice. Ordinarily, it is unwise to test a patient repeatedly on the same day or to test with many extracts at one time. Positive reactions appear within 15 to 20 min and are characterized by wheal and erythema formation and local pruritus. If large doses of extract are given, symptoms of hay fever or even a generalized reaction may be produced. Extracts of foods are available for skin testing, but their use should be limited because it is preferable to diagnose allergy to foods by history and by elimination diets. Identification of bacteria in the respiratory tract which are potentially responsible for infection is more valuable than skin testing with bacterial extracts.

When it is undesirable to perform skin tests in young children or in persons with generalized skin disease, passive transfer of the patient's serum to normal recipients may be performed (Prausnitz-Küstner, or P-K test). Ordinarily, 0.05 to 0.1 ml of the patient's serum is injected intradermally into the recipient, and 24 hr later normal skin and sites injected with serum are tested with the antigenic extracts. In vitro techniques for the detection of specific IgE antibodies may provide a diagnostic tool which measures reagins without the risk of transferring serum hepatitis.

Epinephrine and ephedrine greatly reduce the wheal and erythema response to intradermally injected antigen, as do large doses of antihistamines; these drugs should not be administered before skin testing. Adrenocortical steroids have little effect on these reactions.

THERAPY Specific treatment Elimination of the offending antigen from the patient's environment is the most effective means of controlling allergic disease. This is not always easy, even when the antigen is known. If it is determined that dander from dogs or cats is responsible, then animals should be avoided. When feathers are found to be responsible for allergic symptoms, a feather pillow should be replaced by one of synthetic fiber. Air filtration is often useful in controlling symptoms due to airborne pollens, but occasionally it may be necessary to advise the patient to live in a pollen-free area during the hay fever season. Mechanical obstruction of the nasal airway, which may aggravate the symptoms of rhinitis, should be corrected, and infection should be treated with an antibacterial drug capable of eradicating the specific microorganism. Alleviation of emotional disturbances by the use of drugs, correction of the environment, or psychiatric guidance occasionally will help alleviate the symptoms of allergy.

Immunotherapy (desensitization, hyposensitization) by repeated subcutaneous injections of gradually increasing doses of the allergens specifically responsible for allergic respiratory disease may be helpful. Controlled studies in ragweed and grass hay fever have shown that many patients are partially relieved of their symptoms although there are few cures. Improvement is dose-related, greater doses showing greater evidence of clinical efficacy. Two types of immunologic response are noted: (1) the development of normal circulating IgG antibodies ("blocking" antibodies) which can combine with allergen and block its ability to trigger basophil histamine release, and (2) a blunting of annual seasonal restimulation of specific reagins. There is often also an actual reduction (sometimes complete abolition) of IgE-mediated basophil histamine secretion in the presence of allergen. The reasons for this reduction in cellular reactivity are not clear, because the patient continues to have circulating reagins. The beneficial effects of desensitization persist for some months after treatment is discontinued, but the allergic symptoms tend to recur eventually.

Bacterial vaccines have been employed in desensitizing patients with allergic rhinitis. Because of the lack of evidence for bacterial hypersensitivity as a cause of allergic respiratory disease and the lack of data that such treatment is effective, it cannot be recommended.

Drug treatment Antihistamines, such as tripellenamine, 50 mg; diphenhydramine, 50 mg; chlorpheniramine, 4 mg; and many others, often are effective in controlling hay fever. In moderate to severe cases they are only partially helpful at best and may produce drowsiness and reduce physical and mental dexterity. Orally administered ephedrine, 25 mg, or pseudoephedrine, 60 mg, may also be used to shrink nasal mucous membranes, alone or in combination with antihistamines. Atropine-like drugs may be added to combinations to dry up excessive nasal secretions.

Oral adrenocortical steroids are extraordinarily effective in relieving the symptoms of allergic respiratory disease. Despite the side effects connected with prolonged use, they can safely be used to manage seasonal problems, and in some patients small daily doses will suppress symptoms completely. Hydrocortisone, 25 to 100 mg, prednisone 5 to 20 mg, and methylprednisolone, 4 to 12 mg each day, are usually quite effective. Adrenal steroids can cause a disappearance of nasal polyps when used in patients with perennial rhinitis. The benefit derived from adrenal steroids always must be balanced against the potential side effects of these potent drugs.

Small doses of the water-soluble steroid dexamethasone sprayed into the nose three or four times a day effectively suppress the symptoms of all but the severest hay fever without danger of systemic side effects. The effect of the steroid is local and cannot be duplicated by the same dose given orally. This method offers the best combination of effectiveness with freedom from side effects currently available. Shrinkage of polyps also can be achieved by this treatment. Freon-propelled units delivering properly measured doses of steroid are convenient for this purpose.

ASTHMA

DEFINITION Asthma is characterized by paroxysms of expiratory dyspnea and wheezing, overinflation of the lungs, cough, and rhonchi. It characteristically occurs in attacks of variable duration; between attacks pulmonary function is normal or nearly normal and patients are relatively free of symptoms. Such spasmodic asthma is more frequent at night, and attacks usually last several minutes to several hours. Occasionally spasms last several days, and some asthmatic patients maintain an almost continuous state of airway obstruction nearly every day.

ETIOLOGY Asthma begins before age ten in about one-half of cases and before age thirty in another third, but it may begin *de novo* even in old age. Before age ten, asthma is twice as frequent in boys, but by age thirty the incidence is equal in men and women. Asthma is present in members of the immediate family of about one-third of patients.

In most asthmatics three main factors are thought to interact to a variable degree in producing attacks: (1) allergy to external inhaled allergens; (2) respiratory infections; (3) psychophysiologic reactions to life stress. Although asthma is regarded as an allergic disease, hypersensitivity is found to be the predominant cause in only about one-third of cases and a contributing factor in perhaps another third.

Hay fever and urticaria sometimes precede development of asthma, or occur simultaneously, suggesting that

these infections; presumably the same organisms implicated in respiratory infections in normal individuals are involved.

In about a third of patients, emotional strain and specific stressful life situations appear to be important factors in initiating asthmatic episodes. It would be presumptuous to identify a specific kind of psychologic stress as generating asthma or to describe an "asthmatic personality." Nevertheless, many asthmatic episodes occur when there are no detectable external factors except psychologic stress.

Three variants on the usual asthmatic syndrome are recognized:

1 A syndrome of chronic sinusitis, nasal polyps, poorly remitting asthma, and unusual sensitivity to aspirin has been observed in some adults. These persons have onset of symptoms as adults and may have rapidly developing life-threatening paroxysms of bronchospasm after a single aspirin tablet.
2 *"Tokyo-Yokohama asthma"* or *"New Orleans asthma"* refers to a greatly increased rate of asthmatic attacks which have appeared in well-marked periods of a few weeks in urban areas in individuals not otherwise troubled with asthma. It has been suggested that these "epidemics" result from industrial air pollution, because they occur when conditions of humidity and temperature inversion favor high levels of air pollutants. Air sampling in New Orleans, however, shows that these same conditions also favor increased levels of airborne pollen and mold spores and that these allergens correlate with attack rates as well as or better than inorganic air pollutants. In any event, several surveys in large cities have indicated that emergency room visits for asthma are much more frequent on humid days with temperature inversions.
3 *Allergic bronchopulmonary aspergillosis* (Chap. 174) is a specific infection occurring in asthmatic patients in whom endobronchial growth of *Aspergillus fumigatus* is accompanied by prolonged asthma, expectoration of small brown "plugs" of mycelia, transient pulmonary infiltrates, and eosinophils in the sputum and blood.

The diagnosis may be suspected from the character of the pulmonary infiltrates and the appearance of the sputum and is established by demonstration of mycelia on microscopic examination of the sputum and positive cultures for *A. fumigatus*. These infections have been recognized with increasing frequency in the United States. They respond to the usual measures for asthma but may recur. Treatment with antimycotic agents is not ordinarily indicated.

The etiologic factors which have been incriminated in asthmatic episodes may be acting in individuals with an underlying physiologic defect which predisposes them to bronchospasm. For example, asthmatic patients will react with a greater degree of bronchospasm for a longer period to drugs such as acetylcholine, mecholyl, histamine, serotonin, or cholinesterase inhibitors than normal, and are also unusually sensitive to nonspecific irritants such as dusts, cooking odors, and gaseous air pollutants. They will respond to vigorous exercise with bronchospasm and react more vigorously to the above-mentioned stimuli after treatment with β-adrenergic blocking agents such as propranolol. Therefore, these drugs are contraindicated in asthmatic patients. If there is an acquired or innate physiologic defect in some or all asthmatic patients, its nature is unknown.

In vitro study of specimens of lung from patients with allergic asthma indicate that lung mast cells are sensitized with IgE reagins and will release histamine, serotonin, SRS-A, and possibly other mediators upon exposure to specific allergen. Changes in cellular cyclic AMP appear to operate in this process, and drugs such as catecholamines and xanthines which raise intracellular cyclic AMP tend to inhibit it. If patients are allowed to inhale aerosols of an allergenic extract, an increase in airway resistance and reduction in flow are noted after about 15 to 20 min. This increase is often brief but may be followed in several hours by a more prolonged period (up to 24 hr) of bronchial constriction. It is not clear what mediators are involved in these reactions, but histamine may be less important than it is in allergic rhinitis, and antihistamines are of little use in most asthma. The more prolonged action of SRS-A has given rise to the suggestion that it may be important in asthma. Most asthma is *not* allergic, and the predisposition of allergic individuals to develop the hyperreactivity of airways already noted is not explained.

PATHOLOGY AND PATHOPHYSIOLOGY When asthma is severe, the pathologic changes consist of hypertrophy of bronchial smooth muscle and edema of bronchial walls with extensive infiltration with eosinophils and the presence of thick tenacious secretion. In mild cases there may be no visible anatomic findings. Bronchospasm, mucosal edema, and intraluminal secretion all contribute to the obstruction of airflow, both in smaller and larger airways. At times there may be complete blockage of airflow in some of the small or even medium airways, with resulting areas of atelectasis.

With the constriction of airways there is a tendency to complete closure which can be opposed by an increase in transpulmonary pressure, which in turn increases the intraluminal air pressure distending the bronchi. Asthmatic patients regularly achieve these changes during attacks by breathing at progressively greater lung volume at the end of inspiration thus achieving a markedly negative pleural pressure. The elastic properties of the lung tissue then tend to open the airways. During expiration, which is more passive, pleural pressure rises, intraluminal pressure falls rapidly, the bronchi close, and airflow ceases while the chest is still relatively inflated. The active use of accessory muscles to maintain hyperinflation adds greatly to the work of breathing, oxygen consumption is greatly increased, and the patient rapidly becomes tired.

MANIFESTATIONS The narrowed lumens of the bronchi and increased amounts of tenacious sputum make wheezing a prominent physical sign in *both* inspiration and expiration. Fruitless attempts to raise mucus make cough a prominent symptom. It may become more severe during recovery from an attack, when sputum becomes more liquid and increases in quantity. The sputum is usually mucoid and white and contains no blood or pus. Microscopic examination often shows eosinophils and Charcot-Leyden crystals. As the attack subsides, mucous casts of the smaller bronchi may be seen (Curschmann's spirals). Purulent sputum indicates bronchial or pulmonary infection.

During a mild attack the sensation of obstruction to breathing may cause the patient to hyperventilate and thereby reduce blood CO_2 tension. If airway obstruction becomes more severe, there may be a fall in oxygen tension, with cyanosis and a rise in CO_2 tension due to ventilatory failure. Such rises in P_{CO_2} are often uncompensated and are accompanied by a low plasma bicarbonate concentration. There is also an altered ventilation/perfusion ratio in asthma which arises from regional defects in ventilation due to bronchial plugging. These ventilation defects may reflexly cause transient regional reduction in blood flow, which can be detected during asthmatic attacks by pulmonary scanning techniques.

When an asthmatic episode is prolonged for many hours or days and is resistant to therapy, it is defined as *status asthmaticus*. The chest is greatly distended, the patient works desperately to move air through the obstructed airways, using the accessory muscles of respiration, and breath sounds and wheezes may become very faint because movement of air is poor. Cough is virtually impossible, and the patient is extremely fatigued and often dehydrated. If status does not resolve, the chest becomes almost silent and severe respiratory acidosis ensues. Death from respiratory arrest is possible, and vigorous emergency treatment is necessary.

Asthmatic episodes may be complicated by *atelectasis* due to mucoid plugging of bronchi with subsequent extraction of gases from the unventilated portion of the lung. *Pneumonia* may supervene in poorly ventilated or atelectatic portions of lung. *Spontaneous pneumothorax* and *mediastinal emphysema* are rare complications of an asthmatic attack. Ordinarily, asthma does not affect cardiac function unless the attack is protracted or is accompanied by irreversible emphysema. Under these circumstances, cor pulmonale may develop.

DIAGNOSIS Certain specific causes of local or generalized airway obstruction must be considered when a patient comes initially to the physician with asthma. Generally, wheezing and rhonchi are heard throughout the chest; localized wheezing indicates endobronchial disease, such as foreign body aspiration, neoplasm, or stenosis. The symptoms of airway obstruction in localized endobronchial disease are at times spasmodic and may mimic asthma closely. "Cardiac asthma," or wheezing occurring during cardiac failure, or pulmonary edema usually can be differentiated from paroxysmal asthma by the presence of moist rales, blood-tinged sputum, and other signs of heart failure. Asthma occasionally is a presenting manifestation of polyarteritis nodosa (Chap. 71). Reactions to drugs, particularly aspirin, are an occasional cause of severe asthma. Eosinophilic pneumonia, which is sometimes caused by parasitic infestation of the lungs, is often accompanied by asthma.

Poisoning with cholinergic drugs or insecticides may induce bronchoconstriction and expiratory dyspnea that can be specifically relieved with atropine. Carcinoid tumors which elaborate serotonin may be associated with asthma.

Chemical pneumonias such as silo-filler's disease may be accompanied by difficult breathing resembling asthma. On the other hand, allergic interstitial pneumonitis (Chap. 257), which is a hypersensitivity reaction to inhaled organic dusts, usually is not accompanied by bronchospasm.

LABORATORY FINDINGS Skin tests used for the diagnosis of allergic asthma are no different from those used for the diagnosis of hay fever. There are no specific laboratory tests that prove the etiology to be allergic; indeed, nearly every asthmatic patient, allergic or not, will show an increased number of eosinophils in the sputum at some time during the disease.

Measurements of pulmonary function will demonstrate decreased flow, increased airway resistance, and hyperinflation which are almost completely reversible between attacks. At times, patients are so successful at compensating for bronchoconstriction by hyperinflation of the chest that normal measures of flow or airway resistance are obtained—only an increased thoracic gas volume gives the clue. No pulmonary function test is diagnostic of asthma; demonstration of the spasmodic or reversible nature of the airway disease is required. However, only a few patients have almost continuous airway obstruction; most of them are normal between attacks, and their attacks are so infrequent that abnormal measurements are difficult to document. Occasionally, it may be necessary to demonstrate bronchial hyperirritability by a mecholyl provocation test. Inhalation of mecholyl will produce an abnormal change in serial measurements of the flow or resistance over a period of 15 min.

THERAPY Specific treatment As with hay fever, elimination of the offending allergen from the environment is the most successful means of preventing and treating allergic asthma. When this is not possible, specific immunotherapy or desensitization, employing extracts of the offending allergen in the same manner as already described for allergic rhinitis, may be tried. Although desensitization in allergic asthma has traditionally been considered highly effective, this has not been demonstrated in controlled studies. Much of asthma is not allergic, and immunotherapy with a mixture of common allergens in patients without demonstrable allergy has no rationale.

The frequent occurrence of bronchial infection in adults with nonseasonal or chronic asthma necessitates special consideration. The pneumococcus and *Hemophilus influenzae* are the microorganisms most often isolated from the bronchi and sputum of patients with asthma and chronic bronchitis, and exacerbations of cough and dyspnea may be associated with an increase in the number of these bacteria. These patients may be treated with tetracycline, 1 g per day, erythromycin, or ampicillin in the same dosage continuously during the winter months or at the earliest sign that symptoms are increasing. This approach may lead to a significant decrease in the severity and frequency of exacerbations.

Drug treatment Treatment of acute asthma is most effective when begun soon after onset of the paroxysm. Mild attacks may be readily relieved by inhalation of 50 to 150 μg of nebulized isoproterenol. A variety of commercial products which furnish a measured dose of isoproterenol with inert freon as a propellant are available. The smallest amount consistent with relief should be employed, and administration should not be repeated more often than every 3 hr. With a rapidly developing severe paroxysm, 0.3 to 1.0 ml of 1:1,000 epinephrine should be injected subcutaneously; this dose may be repeated as needed but no more often than every 30 min. Both isoproterenol and epinephrine may become ineffective after repeated use in a prolonged asthmatic attack. There are reports that a single inhalation of isoproterenol may have caused paradoxic bronchospasm (following an initial transient decrease in airway resistance) in a few patients who had used the drug excessively for unremitting asthma over several days. Some asthmatic deaths may be associated with overuse of isoproterenol, as its effectiveness in relieving bronchospasm becomes progressively less.

Early in attacks, a sedative such as amobarbital, 50 or 100 mg, may be desirable to allay agitation and relieve anxiety. As the attack becomes more severe and prolonged, sedatives become less desirable because the patient needs every faculty for the work of breathing. Respiratory arrest has been reported in severely asthmatic patients shortly after injections of sedative or tranquilizing drugs. Drugs which depress respiration such as morphine have been the apparent cause of sudden death and should never be used during asthmatic episodes.

Aminophylline is an active bronchodilator and may be used with, or in preference to, epinephrine. It may be given intravenously or rectally; a dose of 0.5 g is usually required for adequate bronchodilatation. It is ordinarily not possible to give this dose orally without gastric irritation. Intravenous aminophylline must be given slowly, and it is desirable to dilute 0.5 g in 50 ml of 5 percent glucose and to administer it in a drip over a 20-min period. Hydration to prevent inspissation of mucus is important, and it is often convenient to follow intravenous medication with a liter or more of 5 percent glucose.

When epinephrine and aminophylline are ineffective in relieving bronchospasm or there is prompt recurrence, administration of corticosteroids is necessary. Daily doses will range between 15 and 80 mg prednisone, and a favorable response cannot be expected for several hours. Considerable foresight is required to select those patients who will require steroids for adequate control, because the physical signs of asthma are often misleading. Early determination of arterial P_{O_2} and P_{CO_2} will help to recognize those patients who are on the verge of ventilatory failure and who will require prompt and vigorous therapy. Increasing carbon dioxide tension despite treatment is a grave prognostic sign and may mean that tracheostomy and mechanical ventilation will be necessary to prevent death.

When steroids are required, 100 to 300 mg hydrocortisone may be given intravenously, although this route probably is no more effective than the oral route. Once initiated, steroids should be continued to maintain improvement, and then tapered as rapidly as is consistent with continued control of asthma.

Continuous administration of adrenal steroids to patients with chronic asthma or asthmatic bronchitis has been effective and safe in preventing paroxysms. The dose required is usually less than 20 mg prednisone or its equivalent per day. This regimen has been continued for several years in many patients without serious side effects or complications. In fact, patients with severe asthma accompanying infections often have fewer episodes of infection while receiving adrenal steroids continuously. Continuous corticosteroid treatment is contraindicated in children because it interrupts growth.

Prophylactic management of asthmatic patients involves the use of drugs to abort paroxysms. Oral ephedrine, 25 to 50 mg, and phenobarbital, 30 to 60 mg, may be given three or four times a day when the patient is most likely to develop asthma. Recommended doses of oral theophylline or aminophylline preparations contain too little drug to be effective, and effective doses usually cause gastric irritation. Smoking is undesirable in asthmatics, as are obesity, excessive exertion, fatigue, and dietary indiscretion.

Disodium cromoglycate, given by inhaling 20 mg of the dry powder, will prevent allergic bronchospasm if given prophylactically before exposure to an aerosol of an allergen. It appears, therefore, to be useful in allergic asthma, particularly in children, if employed on a regular basis two to four times a day.

ALLERGIC SKIN DISEASE

There are many dermatologic manifestations of allergy, including contact dermatitis, urticaria, angioedema, erythematous rashes, and eczema. These are roughly divisible into those related to "delayed" and "immediate" hypersensitivity. Urticaria and angioedema usually are manifestations of immediate hypersensitivity, while contact dermatitis and many instances of eczematous dermatitis are attributable to delayed hypersensitivity. At times an antigen may induce and elicit both immediate and delayed hypersensitivity reactions, resulting in both urticaria and eczema.

Urticaria, angioedema, contact dermatitis, and erythematous rashes are the principal forms of allergy in which the skin is the major target organ. Many other rashes are attributed to systemic allergic disease, including erythema nodosum, erythema multiforme, exfoliation, bullae, purpura, "fixed" drug eruptions, and photosensitivity. Certain diseases such as systemic lupus erythematosus, dermatomyositis, rheumatic fever, and scleroderma also are characterized by "allergic" skin lesions.

CONTACT DERMATITIS See Chap. 53.

URTICARIA Urticaria (hives) is characterized by white or red evanescent wheals, papules, or macules that are surrounded by erythema and are pruritic. They may be generalized, but commonly appear in areas of skin covered by clothing. Urticaria also may involve mucous membranes such as the stomach and mouth and frequently is accompanied by eosinophilia. It often occurs in serum sickness or in combination with hay fever and allergic asthma. Emotional tension, increased heat, and physical exercise may exaggerate urticaria. Urticaria can be induced by histamine and acetylcholine, and good evidence indicates that liberation of histamine during an allergic reaction is responsible for hives. Urticaria may occur from ingestion, inhalation, injection, or contact with the offending antigen. Foods and drugs frequently are responsible, but hives also have been related to a great variety of inhalants and contactants, such as pollen, dander, dust, feathers, and wool. As in other allergic diseases, the responsible antigen may be detected by careful history, skin test, or elimination diets.

If a specific cause of urticaria is found, it should be corrected or the antigen eliminated from the environment. Acute symptoms usually respond to antihistamines, but adrenal steroids may be needed. Epinephrine, 0.2 to 0.5 ml of 1:1,000 aqueous solution intramuscularly, provides prompt but transient relief. Chronic, idiopathic urticaria is often refractory to treatment, and many of these patients require psychiatric assistance. Prolonged use of adrenal steroids in chronic urticaria is inadvisable.

When first seen, systemic lupus erythematosus occasionally resembles recurrent urticaria.

Angioedema is characterized by edema of the eyelids, lips, external genitalia, and the mucous membranes of the mouth, tongue, or gastrointestinal tract. The swelling may be localized to one area or may be diffuse, and commonly is accompanied by urticaria elsewhere. When the respiratory tract is involved, the patient may have laryngeal edema with hoarseness, stridor, and cyanosis, and rarely death may ensue. Generally, angioedema is attributed to food allergy; shellfish very commonly are incriminated. In addition, the reaction may occur from the many antigens responsible for urticaria. The treatment of angioedema is the same as for urticaria. If respiratory tract obstruction occurs, tracheostomy may prove lifesaving.

A rare form of angioedema is inherited as an autosomal dominant trait and begins in childhood. Nonpruritic angioedematous swellings in the skin characteristically are accompanied by angioedema of the intestine, which may result in abdominal pain and lead to unnecessary laparotomy. The diagnosis is made by demonstrating a specific deficiency of a serum protein that inhibits the first component of complement and the proteolytic enzyme kallikrein. There is no specific treatment.

REFERENCES

Bates DV, Christie RU: *Respiratory Function in Disease*, Philadelphia: Saunders, 1965

Norman PS: Treatment of allergic rhinitis. Johns Hopkins Med J 121:49, 1967

—— et al: Trials of alum-precipitated pollen extracts in the treatment of hay fever. J Allergy 50:31, 1972

Samter M, Alexander HL: *Immunological Diseases*, 2d ed., Boston: Little, Brown, 1971

Williams DA et al: Assessment of the relative importance of the allergic, infective and psychologic factors in asthma. Acta Allergol 12:376, 1958

68
REACTIONS TO DRUGS

LEIGHTON E. CLUFF
JACQUES R. CALDWELL

INTRODUCTION Adverse reactions to drugs are unintended and undesired noxious effects of agents administered for diagnostic, prophylactic, or therapeutic purposes. Illness induced in this manner is a major public health problem. Approximately one million individuals are hospitalized in the United States each year because of diseases caused by medications prescribed by physicians or purchased over the counter (OTC). Patients also experience adverse drug effects during hospitalization, and when these are added, the magnitude of the problem of drug-induced illness becomes exceedingly large.

The importance of adverse drug effects in persons outside the hospital has not been well defined. As reflected by the frequency of hospitalization for drug-induced disease, however, the problem in ambulatory, nonhospitalized persons is probably immense. Although mortality may be low, the morbidity from diseases caused by drugs is considerable. Only during the past decade, however, has there developed a concerted effort to gain understanding of the determinants of adverse reactions to drugs. A few clinical, pharmacological, and immunologic factors responsible for predisposing or leading to drug-induced diseases have been identified. Increased understanding of these factors is essential if adverse drug effects are to be avoided, corrected, or eliminated.

EPIDEMIOLOGY Drug-induced illness has reached epidemic proportions. All drugs may cause adverse reactions, but with varying frequency, severity, and clinical manifestations. The development of adverse reactions depends upon the potential of a drug or drugs for causing illness and is also determined by individual predisposition. Epidemiological studies of adverse drug reactions have been helpful in evaluating the magnitude of the overall problem, in calculating the rate of reactions to individual drugs, and in characterizing some of the determinants of adverse drug effects.

Patients attending medical clinics may have been taking many different drugs in the preceding 30 days, including drugs prescribed by physicians and purchased without a prescription. Patients receive on the average 10 different drugs while hospitalized, and this figure may be as high as 60. The sicker the patient, the more drugs are given, but, as expected, there is a corresponding increase in the likelihood of adverse drug reactions. When fewer than 6 different drugs are given to hospitalized patients, the probability of an adverse reaction is about 5 percent, but if more than 16 drugs are given, the probability is higher than 40 percent. It is likely that the increasing rate of adverse reactions in patients receiving many drugs is attributable in part to untoward drug interactions. In addition to those adverse reactions to drugs occurring during hospitalization, between 3 and 5 percent of medical and pediatric patients are admitted to hospitals because of drug-induced diseases. Retrospective analysis of ambulatory patients has revealed a history of some adverse drug effects in 20 percent of them.

Epidemiologic studies revealing the rates of adverse drug reactions are limited by the unavailability of suitable controls. Some of the minor manifestations and even some major manifestations of presumed drug-induced illness, therefore, are difficult to establish. Despite this deficiency the data convincingly demonstrate an overwhelming problem of drug-induced disease.

Gastrointestinal manifestations, particularly vomiting and diarrhea, account for about one-third; neurological manifestations account for about one-fifth; cardiovascular, metabolic, and cutaneous manifestations each account for about one-tenth; and hematological and other manifestations each account for about 5 percent of adverse drug reactions. Women experience twice as many gastrointestinal manifestations of adverse drug effects as men. The case fatality ratio from drug-induced disease in hospitalized patients varies from 2 to 12 percent.

Most adverse drug effects detected by intensive epidemiologic study are caused by well-established drugs such as digitalis preparations, penicillin, and psychotropic agents, but diuretics, anticoagulants, and antihypertensive drugs are also important causes of drug-induced disease.

Patients admitted to the hospital for a drug-induced illness or with a prior history of an untoward effect are three times more likely than other patients to acquire another adverse drug reaction. This indicates a predisposition to untoward drug effects possibly related to heritable or metabolic factors, causing abnormal degradation, detoxification, or excretion of drugs, associated with renal, hepatic or immunological dysfunction and enzyme defects. Simultaneous administration of different drugs also may inhibit or enhance enzyme production or competition for protein binding, influencing pharmacologic activity and metabolism.

Epidemiologic methods are necessary to determine rates of adverse drug reactions, to characterize patterns of drug utilization, and to identify or evaluate clinical and pharmacological determinants of drug-induced illness. Such studies in relatively small population groups are limited in their ability to detect previously unknown adverse drug effects. Reports by attentive and alert physicians are still the only effective means of recognizing such events. Data derived from vital statistics, retrospective and prospective drug investigation, and animal data also can contribute to elucidation of drug problems.

ETIOLOGY Adverse reactions to drugs may be attributable to pharmacologic or immunologic mechanisms, but in many instances the mechanism is not known. Different descriptive terms have been used to characterize adverse reactions depending upon their manifestations and presumed mechanisms. Pharmacologic effects other than those for which the drug is usually administered have been referred to as *side effects.* Patients showing unusual susceptibility to the pharmacologic actions of a drug are said to have an *idiosyncrasy.* Reactions associated with manifestations often typical of immunologic diseases are often called *allergic. Facilitative* reactions are indirect consequences of drug administration, such as staphylococcal enteritis following administration of oral antibiotics responsible for altering the intestinal microflora. Drugs given to parents and responsible for congenital abnormalities in their infants are called *teratogenic* or *mutagenic. Toxic* reactions due to overdosage may be responsible for serious untoward effects, but can be easily differentiated from other adverse reactions developing in persons given a normal dose of a drug.

For practical purposes it is important only to differentiate adverse reactions to drugs into two classes: those attributable to the drugs' pharmacologic action or those unrelated to it. Reduction in dosage of a drug responsible for a pharmacologic reaction will usually prevent or abort the untoward effect. If the reaction is attributable to immunologic mechanisms, reduction in dose of the drug ordinarily will not terminate the reaction, and in the allergic individual even minute doses may result in catastrophic events. In addition, patients predisposed to an idiosyncratic drug reaction may experience this effect with drug doses significantly lower than that usually given for a therapeutic effect. This predisposition to exaggerated pharmacologic drug action may be related to defective drug metabolism or excretion, to genetic abnormalities, as in patients with glucose-6-phosphate-deficient erythrocytes, or to drug interactions.

Immunologic mechanisms Immunologic mechanisms are responsible for less than 15 percent of all adverse drug reactions. Most pharmacologic agents are poor immunogens, since they are small molecules with molecular weights less than 2,000. Stimulation of antibody synthesis or sensitization of lymphocytes by the drug or one of its metabolites requires in vivo activation and covalent linkage to a protein, peptide, or carbohydrate carrier. Antibodies thus formed may exhibit high specificity for the immunogenic compound or may cross-react with other drugs. Thus, antibodies to penicillin may react with penicillin and its synthetic analogues or may cross-react with related agents such as the cephalosporin antibiotics. Certain drug-induced antibodies may cross-react with antigens present on normal host tissues. For instance, alpha methyldopa administration stimulates the production of antibodies which react with Rh antigens present on host erythrocytes. These antibodies can produce hemolysis if the complement system is activated. Administration of therapeutic agents such as isoniazid, hydralazine, Procainamide, the hydantoin anticonvulsants, and the sulfonamides has been associated with a clinical syndrome resembling systemic lupus erythematosus.

Interaction of drugs with different classes of specific antibodies or with sensitized lymphocytes produces a variety of clinical manifestations. Thus the interaction of a drug dimer or polymer with IgE which is affixed to tissue mast cells can cause release of histamine and produce urticaria, wheezing, and hypotension characteristic of an anaphylactic reaction. Combination of IgG antibodies with drug adsorbed to red blood cells can fix complement and lyse erythrocytes. Circulating complexes of IgG bound to drug can also cause arthralgia, lymphadenopathy, and glomerulonephritis as observed in the serum sickness syndrome. A drug which has interacted with sulfhydryl or amino groups in skin can react with sensitized lymphocytes to produce the rash characteristic of contact dermatitis.

Drug-drug interaction The common practice of treating patients with multiple drugs increases the risk of toxicity from *drug-drug* interaction. Drugs such as phenylbutazone and coumarin may both compete for the same binding site on serum albumin. Since phenylbutazone has higher affinity for the binding site, it can displace coumarin and cause a markedly prolonged prothrombin time and bleeding. Administration of sulfonamides to patients receiving oral tolbutamide can produce hypoglycemia by the same mechanism. Drugs with opposing pharmacologic actions may compete for end organ receptor sites. Thus, an adrenergic stimulating agent such as ephedrine can displace the adrenergic blocker guanethidine from sympathetic receptors and provoke a hypertensive reaction in a patient given both compounds simultaneously. The synergistic action of two drugs given together may result in organ toxicity. Thus, the simultaneous administration of the recommended doses of two drugs with potential ototoxicity, such as ethacrynic acid and gentamicin, can produce marked hearing loss. Alteration of metabolism of one drug by a second drug is another example of drug-drug reaction. For instance, phenobarbital induces microsomal enzymes in the liver which are responsible for metabolizing a variety of compounds such as the coumarin anticoagulants. This increases the hydroxylation of the anticoagulants and thereby necessitates increasing the dose of coumarin required to maintain adequate anticoagulation. The sudden withdrawal of phenobarbital from a patient receiving both compounds without simultaneously altering the coumarin dose may result in marked increase in the prothrombin time and hemorrhage.

Some patients have a peculiar predisposition to allergic and other adverse reactions to therapeutic agents. Persons with atopic illness may have an increased risk of developing drug allergies. The maculopapular rash associated with ampicillin therapy occurs much more frequently in patients with infectious mononucleosis than in individuals with other illnesses. Patients with latent or quiescent acute intermittent porphyria may have an attack precipitated by the administration of barbiturates.

MANIFESTATIONS Adverse effects of drugs attributed to their pharmacologic action are drug-specific. Allergic reactions, however, are often the same irrespective of the incriminated drug. Some presumed allergic reactions, however, are more common with certain drugs than with others.

The commonest manifestations of allergy to drugs are no different from hypersensitivity reactions of other types and include rashes, asthma, and the symptoms of serum sickness. These are easily recognized clinically as allergic in origin. Other features of drug allergy are less easily characterized. The accompanying table of common drug reactions (see Table 68-1) includes some effects that may not be allergic at all.

Skin Morbilliform, urticarial, and maculopapular rashes are probably the most common skin reactions, but many others are observed, including vesicular, bullous, exfoliative, eczematous, and purpuric eruptions. Pruritus is frequent. Although the type of skin lesion usually will not help identify the causative drug, certain skin reactions are relatively specific. Erythema multiforme or nodosum is seen in allergy to Dilantin, bromides, iodides, trimethadione, and sulfonamides. "Fixed" drug eruptions are most frequently due to aminopyrine, phenolphthalein, or Atabrine. Photosensitization during drug therapy occurs characteristically with chlorpromazine, phenothiazine, sulfonamides, and tetracycline derivatives.

Fever Fever may be an isolated manifestation of drug allergy, and most pharmaceuticals in common use can produce a febrile reaction, including most antibiotics and chemotherapeutic agents. However, the tetracycline derivatives are uncommon causes of drug fever, and digitalis has rarely, if ever, been incriminated as the cause of a pyrogenic reaction. Elevation of temperature may appear abruptly after treatment begins, or it may develop in a stepwise fashion during or after the second week of drug administration. Drug fever is often associated with chills and constitutional symptoms and may be accompanied by leukocytosis. Discontinuing therapy usually results in defervescence within a short period, although several days may be required for return of temperature to normal.

Blood Changes in the formed elements of the blood are common during drug allergy. Some drugs have been found to have limited or no effects on the blood, while others produce specific abnormalities. For example, penicillin has not been incriminated as a cause of serious hematologic abnormalities. In therapeutic doses, acetanilid is probably not a cause of anemia, agranulocytosis, thrombocytopenia, or aplastic anemia; in high dosage, however, it may produce leukocytosis, methemoglobinemia, and acute hemolysis. *Methemoglobinemia* also occurs with antipyrine, nitrites, sulfonamides, primaquine, and pamaquine, but this reaction is probably not allergic in origin. Barbiturates, salicylates, and para-aminosalicylic acid rarely, if ever, produce agranulocytosis. *Eosinophilia* may accompany allergic reactions of many types, but it occurs with such frequency as an isolated finding during therapy with streptomycin or nirvanol that it has no significance. *Lymphocytosis* is common in patients receiving Dilantin and Nirvanol, and polymorphonuclear leukocytosis may be found in individuals taking Dilantin or atropine. Studies of the erythrocyte abnormality responsible for the acute hemolytic anemia induced by primaquine, sulfonamides, and nitrofurans in certain individuals indicate that what was thought to be drug allergy is actually a genetically determined enzyme deficiency. Jaundice due to pharmaceutical agents is discussed in Chap. 294.

Nervous system A variety of neurologic manifestations may appear during drug therapy, but in the majority of instances there is little evidence to incriminate allergy as a cause. The commonest reactions consist of psychotic changes or alterations in consciousness and may be seen with digitalis, atropine, thiocyanates, sedatives and steroids. Among other drugs that produce adverse effects on the nervous system (ranging from paresthesia and peripheral neuritis to deafness) are streptomycin, hydralazine, chlorpromazine, Diamox, isoniazid, polymyxin, neomycin, and kanamycin.

Other reactions Nausea, vomiting, and diarrhea are exceedingly common. Abdominal pain in the absence of other symptoms may be produced by quinine, chlorpromazine, and primaquine. Albuminuria and cylindruria occur particularly with heavy metals, bacitracin, polymyxin, colistin, gentamicin, and some of the cephalosporins. Dilantin, chloral hydrate, sulfonamides, trimethadione, Phenurone, colchicine, thiocyanates, gentamicin, kanamycin, cephaloridine, and amphotericin B occasionally produce renal dysfunction, probably because of their direct toxic action. Amphotericin B may produce tubular necrosis and renal calcification, but this is only occasionally associated with significant evidence of renal insufficiency and nitrogen retention. Hypersensitivity to sulfonamides has resulted in acute hemorrhagic nephritis.

Vasculitis Histologic lesions indistinguishable from those of polyarteritis nodosa have been found in the tissues of patients who have experienced allergic reactions to iodides, Dilantin, sulfonamides, and penicillin. Manifestations of systemic lupus erythematosus have appeared during therapy with isoniazid, hydralazine, and a few other drugs but usually have been reversible following discontinuation of the drug (Chap. 70).

Anaphylaxis This may follow the parenteral administration of a variety of drugs, but the agent incriminated most often is penicillin. The risk of any particular patient developing anaphylaxis to penicillin is very small, but because a large number of patients (20 to 30 percent in general hospitals) receive the drug, this reaction may be observed relatively frequently. Radiopaque iodinated dyes, particularly those used for intravenous pyelog-

(Text continues on p. 380.)

TABLE 68-1
Partial list of common adverse drug reactions*

I Gastrointestinal

A GI bleeding

Alkylating agents	Indomethacin
Aminosalicylic acid	Phenindiones
Antimetabolites	Phenylbutazone
Corticosteroids	Rauwolfia
Coumarin derivatives	Salicylates
Heparin	Tolbutamide
Hydralazine	Xanthine derivatives

B Jaundice

Alkylating agents	Methimazole
Aminosalicylic acid	Methyldopa
Anabolic steroids	Methyltestosterone
Antimetabolites	Nitrofurantoin
Benzothiadiazines	Novobiocin
Chloramphenicol (neonates)	Phenindiones
Chlordiazepoxide	Phenothiazines
Chlorpropamide	Phenylbutazone
Erythromycin	Primaquine
Ethynylestradiol	Probenecid
Gold	Propylthiouracil
Hydantoin derivatives	Sulfonamides
Imipramine and amitriptyline	Tetracyclines
Isoniazid	Tolbutamide
MAO inhibitors	Trimethadione

II Cutaneous

A Acneiform eruption

Anabolic steroids	Hydantoin derivatives
Bromides	Iodides
Corticosteroids	Methyltestosterone

B Erythema multiforme

Barbiturates	Phenolphthalein
Bromides	Salicylates
Digitalis	Streptomycin
Gold	Sulfonamides
Hydantoin derivatives	Tolbutamide
Mercurials	Trimethadione
Penicillins	

C Urticaria

(Can occur with almost any drug)

D Purpura (nonthrombocytopenic and thrombocytopenic)

Acetophenetidin	Isoniazid
Antimetabolites	Phenothiazines
Chloral hydrate	Quinidine/quinine
Chloramphenicol	Salicylates
Corticosteroids (ecchymoses)	Sulfonamides
Gold	Tetracyclines
Iodides	Xanthine derivatives

E Fixed eruption

Acetophenetidin	Phenolphthalein
Aminopyrine	Phenothiazines
Barbiturates	Quinidine/quinine
Gold	Salicylates
Iodides	Sulfonamides
Mercurials	

F Photosensitization

Acetazolamide	Chloroquine
Alkylating agents	Coal-tar derivatives
Benzothiadiazines	Ethynylestradiol

Photosensitization (Cont.)

Griseofulvin	Sulfonamides
Phenothiazines	Tetracyclines
Promethamine	Tolbutamide

III Hematologic

A Bone marrow suppression

1 Anemia

Acetazolamide	Gold
Acetophenetidin	Hydantoin derivatives
Alkylating agents	Hydralazine
Amphotericin B	Iodides
Antihistamine	Meprobamate
Antimetabolites	Phenylbutazone
Barbiturates	Streptomycin
Chloramphenicol	Sulfonamides
Chlorpropamide	Tolbutamide
Colchicine	Trimethadione

2 Granulocytopenia

Acetazolamide	Isoniazid
Acetophenetidin	Meprobamate
Alkylating agents	Mercurials
Aminopyrine	Methyldopa
Aminosalicylic acid	Methimazole
Antihistamine	MAO inhibitors
Antimetabolites	Phenindiones
Benzothradianzenes	Phenothiazines
Chloramphenicol	Phenylbutazone
Chlorpropamide	Primaquine
Colchicine	Procainamide
Dimercaprol (BAL)	Propylthiouracil
Gold	Quinidine/quinine
Hydantoin derivatives	Streptomycin
Hydralazine	Sulfonamides
Imipramine and amitriptyline	Tolbutamide
Iodides	Trimethadione

3 Thrombocytopenia

Sedormid (allylisopropyl-acetylurea)	Acetazolamide
Organic arsenicals—	Benzothiadiazines
Mapharsen	Chlorpropamide
Sulfonamides	Colchicine
Quinidine	Diethylstilbesterol
Quinine	Heparin
Ristocetin	Hydantoin derivatives
Chloramphenicol	Hydralazine
Phenylbutazone	Iodides
Gold compounds	Isoniazid
Antimetabolites	Meprobamate
Aminosalicylic acid	Nitrofurantoin
Aminopyrine	Primaquine
Alkylating agents	Salicylates

B Hemolysis

Acetophenetidin	Methyldopa
Aminopyrine	Nitrofurantoin
Aminosalicylic acid	Primaquine
Cephalothin	Probenecid
Chloroquine	Quinidine/quinine
Dimercaprol (BAL)	Salicylates
Hydantoin derivatives	Sulfonamides

C Leukocytosis

Acetophenetidin	Belladonna alkaloids
Aminosalicylic acid	Chlordiazepoxide

* *This list is by no means comprehensive but represents some of the more common complications of drug therapy.*

TABLE 68-1 *(Cont.)*

Partial list of common adverse drug reactions

Leukocytosis (Cont.)

Corticosteroids (also eosinopenia and lymphopenia)
Hydantoin derivatives
Iodides
Iron dextran
Penicillins
Phenindiones
Phenothiazines
Sympathetic amines

D Eosinophilia

Aminosalicylic acid
Chlordiazepoxide
Digitalis (rare)
Hydantoin derivatives
Iodides
Isoniazid
Kanamycin and neomycin
Methimazole
Phenothiazines
Propylthiouracil
Streptomycin
Sulfonamides

E Hypoprothrombinemia

Aminosalicyclic acid
Coumarin derivatives
Phenindiones
Propylthiouracil
Quinidine/quinine
Salicylates

IV Metabolic

A Hypokalemia

Acetazolamide
Benzothiadiazines
Corticosteroids
Ethacrynic acid
Furosemide
Mercurials
Phenolphthalein

B Hyperuricemia

Alkylating agents
Antimetabolites
Benzothiadiazines
Ethacrynic acid
Salicylates

C Hyperglycemia

Benzothiadiazines
Corticosteroids
Sympathetic amines

V Neurologic

A Alterations in consciousness

Barbiturates
Belladonna alkaloids
Bromides
Cocaine (derivatives)
Digitalis
Gold
Griseofulvin
Indomethacin
Isoniazid
MAO inhibitors
Phenothiazines
Primaquine
Procainamide
Quinidine/quinine
Rauwolfia
Spironolactones
Streptomycin
Sulfonamides
Sympathetic amines

B Convulsions

Cocaine (derivatives)
Imipramine and amitriptyline
Insulin
Isoniazid
Methylphenidate
Penicillins (rare)
Phenothiazines
Sympathetic amines
Tolbutamide
Xanthine derivatives

C Peripheral neuropathy

Acetazolamide
Amphotericin B
Chloroquine
Colchicine
Colistin and polymyxin
Digitalis (rare)
Dimercaprol (BAL)
Ergot alkaloids
Gold
Hydantoin derivatives
Hydralazine
Isoniazid
MAO inhibitors
Nitrofurantoin
Phenylbutazone
Streptomycin
Sulfonamides

D Extrapyramidal syndrome

Chlordiazepoxide
Imipramine and amitriptyline
Methyldopa
Phenothiazines

Extrapyramidal syndrome (Cont.)

Rauwolfia

VI Ear and eye

A Auditory nerve damage

Gentamicin
Griseofulvin
Kanamycin and neomycin
Streptomycin
Vancomycin

B Ocular damage

Chloramphenicol
Chloroquine
Corticosteroids
Phenothiazines
Phenylbutazone
Primaquine

VII Allergic

A Anaphylaxis

Aminosalicylic acid
Antihistamines
Cocaine (derivatives)
Colchicine
Heparin
Insulin
Iodides
Meprobamate
Mercurials
Nitrofurantoin
Penicillins
Phenindiones
Phenothiazines
Probenecid
Procainamide
Salicylates
Streptomycin
Sulfonamides

B Fever

(Almost all medications except digitalis and chloramphenicol)

C "Serum sickness"

Aminosalicyclic acid
Antihistamines
Barbiturates
Benzothiadiazines
Heparin
Hydantoin derivatives
Hydralazine
Insulin
Iodides
Mercurials
Penicillins
Phenolphthalein
Phenylbutazone
Probenecid
Procainamide
Propylthiouracil
Quinidine/quinine
Salicylates
Streptomycin
Sulfonamides
Tetracyclines

VIII Cardiorenal

A Arrhythmia

Aminopyrine
Aminosalicyclic acid
Digitalis
Dimercaprol (BAL)
Guanethidine
Heparin
Imipramine and amitriptyline
Methylphenidate
Phenothiazines
Procainamide
Quinidine/quinine
Salicylates
Spironolactones
Sympathetic amines
Xanthine derivatives

B Hypotension

Antihistamines
Chlordiazepoxide
Guanethidine
Hydralazine
Imipramine & amitriptyline
MAO inhibitors
Methylphenidate
Phenothiazines
Procaine inhibitors
Quinidine/quinine
Rauwolfia
Spironolactones
Vancomycin
Xanthine derivatives

C Renal disorders

Acetazolamide
Acetophenetidin
Alkylating agents
Amphotericin B
Benzothiadiazines
Bromides
Chloral hydrate
Colchicine

TABLE 68-1 *(Cont.)*

Partial list of common adverse drug reactions

Renal disorders (Cont.)	
Colistin and polymyxin	Phenylbutazone
Gold	Quinidine/quinine
Griseofulvin	Salicylates
Guanethidine	Sulfonamides
Hydantoin derivatives	Tetracyclines
Kanamycin and neomycin	Tolbutamide
Mercurials	Trimethadione
Methyldopa	Vancomycin
IX Miscellaneous	
A Collagen-vascular syndromes	
Hydantoin derivatives	Procainamide
Hydralazine	Propylthiouracil
Isoniazid	Sulfonamides
Penicillins	Trimethadione
Phenylbutazone	
B Fetal and neonatal effects	
Alkylating agents	Morphine
Anabolic steroids	Novobiocin
Antimetabolites	Phenothiazines
Benzothiadiazines	Progesterone
Chloramphenicol	Propylthiouracil
Corticosteroids	Rauwolfia
Coumarin derivatives	Salicylates
Iodides	Streptomycin
Meperidine	Sulfonamides
Methyltestosterone	Tetracyclines

raphy, and Bromsulphalein are two other common diagnostic agents incriminated in anaphylaxis.

DIAGNOSIS The manifestations of drug-induced diseases, whether attributable to pharmacologic, immunologic, or other mechanisms, resemble those associated with other diseases and may be produced by different and dissimilar drugs. Recognition of the role of a drug or drugs responsible for illness is dependent upon appreciation of the possible implication of adverse reactions to drugs in any disease, identification of a temporal relationship between drug administration and development of illness, and familiarity with the manifestations most often caused by particular drugs. Although reactions have been described with many drugs, there is always a "first," and any drug should be suspected of causing an adverse effect if the clinical setting is appropriate.

Illness induced by a drug's pharmacologic action may be more easily recognized than illness attributable to immunologic or other mechanisms. For example, effects such as development of cardiac arrythmia in a patient receiving digitalis, hypoglycemia in a patient given insulin, or bleeding in a patient receiving anticoagulants are more easily related to the prescribed drug than are symptoms like fever or rash, which may be caused by many drugs or by other factors.

Once an adverse reaction is suspected, discontinuance of the suspected drug followed by disappearance of the reaction is presumptive evidence of a drug-induced illness. Reappearance of the reaction upon readministration of the drug is confirmatory evidence of the relationship. With pharmacologic adverse reactions, lowering the dosage may also be followed by disappearance of the reaction, and increasing the dose may cause it to reappear. When the reaction is thought to be allergic, however, readministration of the drug may be hazardous, since anaphylactic shock may develop. Readministration is unwise under these conditions unless alternate drugs are not available and treatment is mandatory.

If the patient is receiving many different drugs when an adverse reaction is suspected, the drugs most likely to be incriminated can usually be identified. All drugs may be discontinued at once, or they may be discontinued one at a time at intervals of 1 to 2 days. Depending on the excretion or metabolism of the drug and on the nature of the reaction, the manifestation may or may not disappear promptly. If the drug is eliminated slowly, the reaction may persist, but if it is excreted rapidly, the reaction may disappear quickly. Drug fever usually terminates within 24 to 48 hr after administration of a drug is stopped. Rashes and arteritis may persist for a longer period of time.

Blood and urine levels of a drug may be useful in determining whether toxic levels have been reached or whether the drug is eliminated slowly or rapidly. Investigation of potential drug-drug interactions by determining that such interactions have been previously recognized may be useful under some circumstances when more than one drug appears to be involved in the reaction.

Serum antibody has been demonstrated in some persons with drug allergy involving cellular blood elements, as in agranulocytosis, hemolytic anemia, and thrombocytopenia. In other types of drug allergy, precipitation, hemagglutination, or complement fixation tests with drugs or drug degradation products have been clearly related to adverse reactions only rarely. Skin tests with the drug or its degradation products also are often of little value in identifying the allergic individual. This indicates the inadequacy of present methods of testing and is not an argument against an immunologic basis for allergic drug reactions. Demonstration of derivatives (e.g. penicilloyl) responsible for many penicillin allergic reactions have provided tools for testing persons suspected of having penicillin allergy, but even these tests are not completely reliable and many are still experimental.

Eliciting a drug history from patients is important diagnostically. Attention must be directed to nonprescription, or over-the-counter, as well as prescription drugs. Each type can be responsible for adverse drug effects, and recent studies reveal frequent adverse interactions between drugs purchased by patients over the counter and those prescribed by physicians. In addition, it is common for patients to be cared for by several physicians, and duplicative, additive, counteractive, or synergistic drugs may, therefore, be taken by individuals if the physicians are not aware of the patient's drug history. The drugs taken by a patient, at least during the 30 days before he is seen, should be determined by every physician before he prescribes any medications. A previous history of adverse drug effects in patients is common. These patients are predisposed to other drug-induced illnesses, and familiarity with such a history should engender added caution in drug prescribing.

Some patients have a heritable predisposition to reactions to certain drugs, and their predisposition may be recognized by specific biochemical study. For example, erythrocyte G-6-PD deficiency can be identified; patients with the defect are usually black. Such patients may have an acute hemolytic crisis when given sulfonamides, nitrofurantoins, probenecid, tolbutamide, and aminoquinolones. These crises can be avoided by testing for the enzyme defect before administration of these drugs. Similarly, persons with an abnormal serum pseudocholinesterase may have apnea when given succinylcholine.

No drug is completely safe and any drug may cause illness. A high index of suspicion is essential for recognizing adverse drug reactions and for identifying reactions not previously described.

TREATMENT AND PROPHYLAXIS Allergic reactions to drugs usually subside promptly when administration of the agent is discontinued. Occasionally, however, the reaction persists for prolonged periods despite withdrawal of the drug. Recurrent urticaria for many months after a penicillin reaction is a common example. In the event of persistent or severe manifestations of drug allergy, the use of adrenocortical steroids is indicated. Adrenal steroids, antihistamines, and epinephrine are usually ineffective in alleviating pharmacologic reactions due to a drug. Reactions of this type are best managed by withdrawing the offending drug, reducing the dose, and administering appropriate pharmacologic antagonists.

A specific history of hypersensitivity to a given drug contraindicates its readministration unless the clinical situation is serious. When such a situation arises, the procedure of choice is to look for an alternative agent which is just as efficacious. In a number of instances, when it has been judged necessary to prescribe a drug to which a patient is known to be allergic, the concomitant administration of adrenal steroids has completely suppressed the manifestations of hypersensitivity. However, adrenal steroids will not prevent or control anaphylactic shock. Desensitization by administering progressively increasing dosages of a drug such as penicillin should be used only as a last resort. Although desensitization is often successful, there are occasional examples of "desensitized" individuals who experienced a fatal anaphylactic reaction upon receiving a large systemic dose of the drug in question.

The U.S. Food and Drug Administration and the pharmaceutical manufacturers are accumulating information on adverse drug reactions. They solicit the cooperation of all physicians in reporting reactions to them.

REFERENCES

CLUFF LE, JOHNSON JE: Drug fever. Progr Allergy 8:149, 1964

GARDNER P, CLUFF LE: The epidemiology of adverse drug reactions: A review and perspective. Johns Hopkins Med J 126:77, 1970

HANSTEN PD: *Drug Interactions,* Philadelphia: Lea & Febiger, 1971

HOWLING HF: *Medicines for Man,* New York: Knopf, 1970

HURWITZ N: Predisposing factors in adverse reactions to drugs. Br Med J 1:536, 1969

MOSER RH: A study of iatrogenic disease; a contemporary analysis of illness produced by drug and other therapeutic practices, in *Diseases of Medical Progress,* 3d ed., Springfield, Ill.: Charles C Thomas, 1969

STEWART RB, CLUFF LE; Studies on the epidemiology of adverse drug reactions VI: Utilization and interactions of prescription and nonprescription drugs in outpatients. Johns Hopkins Med J 129:319, 1971

VESSELL ES: Drug metabolism in man. Ann NY Acad Sci 179:5, 1971

69 IMMUNE-COMPLEX DISEASES

FRANK J. DIXON

DEFINITION The essential feature of immune-complex diseases is that they are caused by antigen-antibody complexes formed in the circulation or interstitial fluids. These complexes are pathogenic agents and produce disease subsequent to their localization in tissues and interaction with the humoral and cellular mediators of immunologic inflammation.

ETIOLOGY The concept that immunologic injury to specific organs or tissues might occur as a result of antigen-antibody reactions immunologically unrelated to the structures injured was first voiced by von Pirquet more than 60 years ago. In the course of studying serum sickness in human beings, he postulated that the coexistence of foreign serum antigens and homologous antibodies in the circulation resulted in the formation of toxic compounds which were probably the cause of the vascular, renal, cardiac, cutaneous, and joint lesions characteristic of this disease. In the past decade much information has accumulated establishing antigen-antibody complexes as these toxic compounds, which are pathogenic agents capable of inducing a variety of injuries, ranging from acute through chronic inflammation and finally to hyaline degeneration in particular anatomic sites. Apparently, the interaction of antigen with antibody forms a macromolecular complex, which, if soluble, can circulate in the host and, upon further reaction with serum factors and/or cells, can injure any tissue in which it is trapped. Complexes so formed are for the most part taken up and catabolized to harmless end products by reticuloendothelial phagocytes and blood leukocytes, but a small fraction eludes these cells and tends to accumulate throughout the body in filtering structures, such as glomeruli and blood vessels, where they can cause injury. This accumulation is apparently determined by anatomic and physiologic, not immunologic, factors, so that the sites of injury or disease need have no immunologic relationship to the causative antigen or antibody. In this respect immune-complex disease is quite different from the "antitissue-antibody" type of immunologic disease in which the subject makes antibody specifically reactive with an antigenic component of the target or diseased tissue and the distribution of the tissue-fixed antigen determines the location of the disease. Further, immune-complex diseases may involve multiple sites or tissues, depending upon physical and biologic characteristics of the complexes and local permeability factors in the filtering structures.

PATHOGENESIS The pathogenicity of immune complexes is in large part determined by their antigen-antibody ratio; i.e., size and the biologic properties of the antibody. Complexes formed in antibody excess tend to be insoluble and are rapidly phagocytosed, do not circulate, and have little opportunity to accumulate in filtering sites. Complexes formed in extreme antigen excess, i.e., antibody-2 antigen, are usually too small to become trapped in physiologic filters. Further, such antigen-excess complexes do not contain an arrangement of immunoglobulin molecules capable of complement (C) activation, and activation of complement is one of the most important steps in the induction of inflammation by complexes. Also essential in complement activation is the nature of the antibody in the complex, since some antibodies are capable and others are incapable of complement activation. Though the immunochemical character of the antigen does not seem to be an important factor in phlogogenicity, the size of the antigen may play a role, since large protein molecules and even virions themselves acting as antigens would of necessity result in large nonfiltrable antigen-antibody complexes, regardless of antigen-antibody ratio.

Most of the knowledge of the pathogenic mechanisms in immune-complex disease has been derived from the study of experimental and clinical serum sickness. These diseases, resulting from a single large injection of foreign serum protein, are acute phlogogenic, multisystem disorders involving blood vessels, heart, kidneys, lymphoid tissue, skin, and joints, and resembling in part acute glomerulonephritis, rheumatic fever, systemic lupus erythematosus, polyarteritis, and rheumatoid arthritis. Using isotope-labeled bovine serum albumin (BSA) as antigen in rabbits, it was possible to quantitate the various immunologic events involved in this disease. As shown in Fig. 69-1, the immune response to BSA in the rabbit is indicated by the rapid terminal elimination of the circulating antigen, beginning 11 days after injection. The fate of circulating serum protein antigen is characterized by an initial 2-day period during which the antigen equilibrates between intravascular and extravascular spaces, followed by a slower rate of loss lasting a little more than a week, during which the antigen is catabolized nonimmunologically, and finally by a rapid terminal immune elimination. Measurement of circulating antigen-antibody complexes indicates their appearance on day 8, shortly before immune elimination begins, and their increase during the following 2 to 3 days. Coincident with the increase of circulating complexes and the beginning of immune elimination is a fall in the serum complement to levels half normal. Presumably as antibody is formed and complexes increase in size and amount, they are capable of reacting with serum complement, which in turn increases the size of the complexes and makes them more readily phagocytosed, thereby hastening their elimination. The importance of immune-complex size is illustrated by the fact that only rabbits with circulating complexes greater

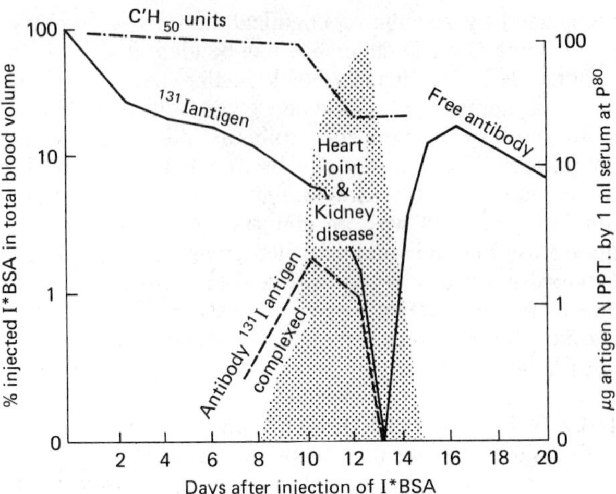

FIGURE 69-1
Immunologic course of experimental serum sickness.

than 19S in size develop significant serum sickness. Once the antigen is eliminated, free antibody appears in the circulation. Simultaneously with the appearance of circulating complexes the clinical and histologic manifestations of serum sickness develop. Following elimination of circulating complexes the serum sickness diminishes. If the immune complexes are truly the etiologic agent of this disease, one would expect to find them in the lesions themselves, and their presence there has been shown, utilizing the fluorescent-antibody technique. BSA, host immunoglobulin, and host complement all have been detected in fine granular deposits along the capillary walls in diseased glomeruli and in arteritic lesions.

These immunologic developments trigger a number of secondary humoral and cellular events capable of mediating an inflammatory response. As the complexes form in the circulation, they act upon basophils, probably via homocytotropic antibodies. The basophils then put out a substance which causes platelets, the major reservoir of histamine and serotonin in the rabbit, to clump and release these substances. This systemic liberation of vasoactive substances is essential for the subsequent localization of complexes in various parts of the vascular bed, presumably by increasing vascular permeability, and this localization can be blocked by antihistamines and antiserotonins. As the complexes begin to localize in glomeruli, arteries, etc., they also activate complement and the complement-derived chemotactic factors attract polymorphonuclear (PMN) leukocytes, which release their proteolytic enzymes and basic proteins, causing local tissue destruction. Complexes also cause endothelial proliferation, a prominent aspect of the glomerular response in acute serum sickness. Since depletion of complement and PMN in animals subjected to serum sickness will not completely suppress the associated glomerulonephritis, it seems that complexes can also cause damage, although less severe, in the sites in which they localize by routes independent of complement and polymorphonuclear leukocytes. The nature of this pathogenic mechanism is not well understood.

A chronic form of serum sickness clinically more similar to the spontaneous human serum sickness-like diseases can be produced by daily injections of relatively small amounts of foreign serum proteins into rabbits. Properly executed, this results in the presence of circulating complexes for at least several hours every day. Such rabbits after several months develop a chronic membranous or necrotizing glomerulonephritis, morphologically distinct from the acute proliferative glomerulonephritis occurring in "one-shot" serum sickness. The complexes accumulate in heavy deposits along the outer aspect of the glomerular capillary basement membranes, apparently interfering with normal glomerular function. The antigen-antibody system and the pathways of mediation of inflammation appear to be similar in both kinds of serum sickness, so the differences in morphologic and functional expressions of disease are presumably related to the quantitative and temporal aspects of exposure to immune complexes, a fact worth remembering when trying to relate particular human disease patterns to certain types of antigen-antibody complexes.

CLINICAL IMMUNE-COMPLEX DISEASES Understanding of the role of immune complexes in serum sickness is reasonably complete because the antigen is known and can be traced via isotope and immunofluorescent techniques, thereby making possible detailed observation of formation and fate of the complexes. In most human diseases suspected of having an immune-complex pathogenesis, the antigen is not known and the search for immune complexes is far from direct, so that suspicions are based on indirect and/or circumstantial evidence. The first suggestion of immune-complex pathogenesis in human disease was based on the clinical and histopathologic similarities of serum sickness on the one hand and glomerulonephritis, rheumatic fever, systemic lupus erythematosus, rheumatoid arthritis, and various vasculitides on the other. The relationship was postulated even before the pathogenesis of serum sickness was well understood. Immunologic and/or physicochemical attempts to demonstrate circulating immune complexes have provided evidence of their presence in some patients with rheumatoid arthritis, systemic lupus erythematosus, hyperglobulinemic purpura, and diseases characterized by the appearance of Australia antigen. Among the more successful techniques employed in the demonstration of circulating immunoglobulin-containing complexes that are possibly antigen-antibody in nature are (1) *analytic ultracentrifugation*—a quantitative but relatively insensitive procedure which gives a measurement of size as well as amount of protein complexes; (2) *cryoprecipitation*—an easily performed, often quite sensitive means of separating complexes with temperature-related solubility; (3) *reaction with the Clq component of complement*—a reaction capable of detecting immunoglobulin-containing complexes, as well as other possible serum substances such as DNA and endotoxin; and (4) *reaction with IgM rheumatoid factors*—selected rheumatoid factors will react with small amounts of immunoglobulin-containing complexes, particularly those found in rheumatoid patients.

The best understood of the various immune-complex diseases is systemic lupus erythematosus. In this disease multiple antibodies are reactive with a variety of cellular antigens of the host. Best known are the diagnostic antinuclear, particularly anti-DNA, antibodies. At times in the course of this disease some of these cellular antigens are detectable in the serum (antigen excess). During shifts from antigen to antibody excess and vice versa, immune complexes would of necessity be present in the serum, a situation very similar to that in serum sickness. These complexes may be evidenced by cryoprecipitation or positive Clq or rheumatoid factor reactions. As would be expected, while immune complexes circulate the manifestations of disease worsen. These complexes are deposited in glomeruli and larger blood vessels associated with the most serious manifestations of this disease, glomerulonephritis and vasculitis. Renal biopsy has been extremely valuable in the study of this kidney disease. Nuclear (DNA) antigens have been found in diseased glomeruli by immunofluorescence, as well as by host immunoglobulin and complement. In addition, antinuclear (DNA) antibodies have been eluted from the kidneys of patients with lupus erythematosus. Thus, all the components of immune complexes have been identified in the diseased organs.

The other disease with a reasonably well-demonstrated immune-complex pathogenesis is glomerulonephritis. About 95 percent of glomerulonephritis appears to be associated with immune-complex deposition in the glomeruli, and 5 percent is caused by antibodies formed against antigenic determinants in the glomerular basement membrane, immune complexes deposited in a characteristic pattern in glomeruli, and with irregular granular to lumpy aggregates along the glomerular basement membranes (Fig. 69-2). Thus, when host immunoglobulin and complement are found in this distribution, it is strong presumptive evidence for immune complexes, even if the nature of the antigen is not known. In immune-complex glomerulonephritis, a number of different antigens have

FIGURE 69-2
Section of glomerulus from patient with chronic membranous glomerulonephritis stained with fluorescein-labeled antihuman immunoglobulin. The immune deposits are present in the glomerular capillary walls in a fine granular form consistent with immune-complex deposition.

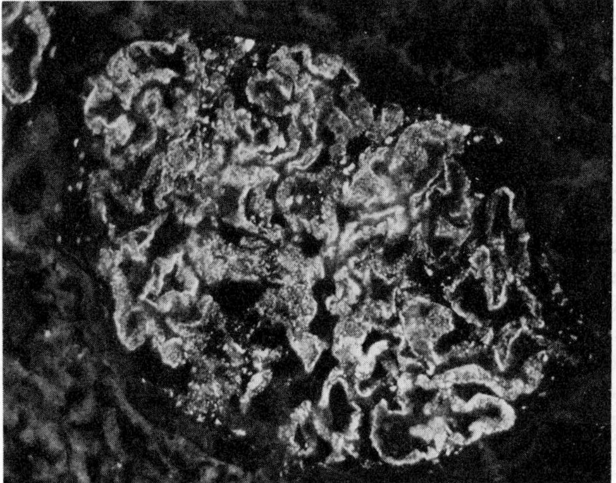

been found capable of forming nephritogenic complexes. In addition to the nuclear antigens in systemic lupus erythematosus, there are streptococcal antigens in acute poststreptococcal glomerulonephritis (Chap. 270); malarial antigens in the nephrosis accompanying quartan malaria (Chap. 211); staphylococcal antigens in the nephritis accompanying infected ventriculoatrial shunts for hydrocephalus; Australia antigen in nephritis and vasculitis accompanying infection with this agent; and thyroglobulin in nephritis associated with autoimmune thyroiditis (Chap. 85). However, taken together, these recognized antigens account for only a small proportion of all immune-complex glomerulonephritis. The great variety of antigens capable of causing this single disease entity, presumably via a single pathogenic mechanism, illustrates the antigenic nonspecificity of immune-complex disease.

In a sense, the study of glomerulonephritis has turned up many more instances of immune-complex disease than there are antigens to account for them, and has prompted a search for other etiologic agents. Examination of spontaneous immune-complex diseases of animals finds many, perhaps most, of them associated with chronic viral infections. In these chronic infections viremia is the rule, and commonly the viruses themselves, and perhaps soluble viral products, serve as antigens to form circulating immune complexes. This situation has been found in chronic infections with the following viruses: lymphochoriomeningitis, lactic dehydrogenase, and Gross, Rauscher, Friend, Aleutian, and equine infectious anemia. Indeed, in the well-studied NZBxW mice with a lupus-like disease, there are not only nuclear antigens involved in immune-complex formation but also antigens derived from the C-type RNA virus which infects them. Thus, in this animal model of human lupus at least two kinds of antigen-antibody systems are simultaneously forming immune complexes, which are then deposited in glomeruli and are causing nephritis. The search for similar viruses which may be involved in human immune-complex disease has just begun; one virus, Australia antigen, has been shown to form circulating complexes with immunoglobulin and to be deposited in glomeruli associated with the development of nephritis.

From this discussion it is apparent that immune complexes are a common means by which immunologic diseases are mediated. The facts that a single kind of antigen-antibody complex may induce disease in a variety of tissues and organs (as in serum sickness); that a large number of different antigens may be able to form complexes, all capable of causing a similar disease (as with the multiple agents involved in immune-complex glomerulonephritis); and that multiple antigen-antibody systems may be found participating simultaneously in immune-complex formation (as in NZBxW mice and patients with systemic lupus erythematosus) indicate the pathogenic complexity of these disorders. However, now that some of the immunologic characteristics of these diseases are recognized, the search for causal agents should yield results, making possible specific immunotherapy and perhaps even immunoprophylaxis.

SERUM SICKNESS IN MAN

MANIFESTATIONS After an incubation period of 4 to 10 days (it may be much shorter in sensitized persons or as long as 21 days in others), there is the onset of *pruritus,* followed shortly by *rash.* The rash may take the form of erythematosus, morbilliform, or petechial eruption, but by far the commonest pattern is urticaria. Often, the skin lesions appear at the local site of injection of the serum several hours before the rash becomes generalized. *Lymphadenopathy,* most prominent in the area draining the injection site, is usual, as is *edema* of the face, lips, eyelids, or, rarely, the glottis. Most patients with serum sickness have fever, which is accompanied often by arthralgia and at times by arthritis, with effusion into one of the large joints. The joint manifestations may be, in fact, the overshadowing feature of serum sickness. Other symptoms include headache, nausea, vomiting, abdominal pain, diarrhea, cardiac arrhythmias, and pericarditis.

The most disabling complications of serum sickness are neurologic disorders, which occur in a minority of cases. Unilateral mononeuritis, which involves the shoulder girdle or arm and is characterized by weakness and sensory deficit, may appear. Isolated facial palsy occurs, and occasionally, there may be extensive polyneuritis or meningoencephalitis.

Apparent relapses or recurrences are not unusual.

LABORATORY FINDINGS There is usually a mild peripheral neutrophilic leukocytosis, and the bone marrow shows an increase in number of plasma cells. Eosinophilia is not a feature of classical serum sickness, but it occasionally accompanies the drug-induced syndrome. The urine may contain protein, casts, and erythrocytes. Electrocardiograms sometimes show transient conduction defects. Slight pleocytosis in the cerebrospinal fluid is frequent, even in the absence of demonstrable neurologic dysfunction.

COURSE Serum sickness is a benign, self-limited disease which subsides within 1 to 3 weeks. In patients with neuropathy, residual weakness may require several weeks to abate, but complete restoration of function is the rule. Rare deaths from edema of the glottis are recorded, but a fatal outcome is more often a result of the intercurrent disease.

TREATMENT Urticaria usually responds to small doses of epinephrine and can be controlled with ephedrine and antihistaminics. Joint pains are usually relieved promptly by aspirin or other salicylates.

For severely ill and uncomfortable patients, adrenal steroids offer prompt relief, and the great efficacy of these compounds has led to their increasing use for symptomatic treatment. They need to be given for only 4 to 7 days in most patients.

Tracheostomy or tracheal intubation is needed at times for sudden respiratory obstruction by edema, and equipment for these procedures should be at hand during the early stages of the disease. Adrenal steroids relieve incipient respiratory obstruction promptly.

In patients who have developed serum sickness as a

result of administration of tetanus or diphtheria horse antiserum, active immunization with toxoid should be initiated before the patient is released from medical care. Once a foreign serum has produced serum sickness it should never be given again.

ANAPHYLAXIS

Occasional patients given an injection of serum, of skin-test antigen, or a drug will become profoundly ill and may collapse and die within minutes. Asthmatic wheezing, cyanosis, and severe pruritus involving the hands often occur at the onset of illness. This reaction is the human counterpart of anaphylactic shock in lower animals. Because it rarely occurs in individuals who give no history of hypersensitivity and because fatalities have followed the injection of tiny amounts of serum for the purpose of determining a patient's state of sensitization, prevention is very difficult. Perhaps the most important step in reducing the incidence of anaphylaxis is to follow the dictum that no serum product or drug should be given to any patient without clear indications. Although most severe reactions occur after parenteral administration of the antigen or drug, fatalities have been reported after oral ingestion.

Treatment consists of the intravenous or intracardiac administration of epinephrine and vigorous support of respiration and circulation. Adrenal steroids may be given parenterally but are of little or no value in treating this acute situation. When the injection site permits, a tourniquet may be applied to slow absorption of the antigen.

REFERENCES

AGNELLO F et al: Clq precipitins in the sera of patients with systemic lupus erythematosus and other hypocomplementemic states: Characterization of high and low molecular weight types. J Exp Med 134:228s, 1971

COCHRANE CG: Mechanisms involved in the disposition of immune complex in tissues. J Exp Med 134:75s, 1971

——, DIXON FJ: Cell and tissue damage through antigen antibody complexes. Calif Med 111:99, 1969

DIXON FJ: The pathogenesis of glomerulonephritis. Am J Med 44:493, 1968

——: *The Harvey Lectures*, vol. 58, New York: Academic, 1962–1963, p. 21

—— et al: Pathogenesis of immune complex glomerulonephritis of New Zealand mice. J Exp Med 134:65s, 1971

—— et al: Experimental glomerulonephritis: The pathogenesis of a laboratory model resembling the spectrum of human glomerulonephritis. J Exp Med 113:899, 1961

KOFFLER D et al: Systemic lupus erythematosus: Prototype of immune complex nephritis in man. J Exp Med 134:169s, 1971

NOWOSLAWSKI AK et al: Tissue localization of Australia antigen immune complexes in acute and chronic hepatitis and liver cirrhosis. Am J Pathol 68:31, 1972

OLDSTONE MBA, DIXON FJ: Immune complex disease in chronic viral infections. J Exp Med 134:32s, 1971

WINCHESTER RJ et al: Occurrence of γ-globulin complexes in serum and joint fluid of rheumatoid arthritis patients: Use of monclonal rheumatoid factors as reagents for their demonstration. J Exp Med 134:286s, 1971

70 SYSTEMIC LUPUS ERYTHEMATOSUS

MART MANNIK
BRUCE C. GILLILAND

INTRODUCTION Systemic lupus erythematosus (subsequently abbreviated SLE) is a disease of unknown cause. However, abundant evidence shows that immunologic mechanisms of tissue injury are important in its pathogenesis. The clinical presentation and the course of SLE are variable. A hallmark of this disease is the presence of a number of antibodies to nuclear components, but other immunologic abnormalities exist as well. Some patients with SLE have spontaneous remissions, others respond favorably to treatment with corticosteroids, and in some patients the course is unresponsive to currently available medications. On the basis of frequent findings of virus-like inclusions in patients with SLE and detailed studies of animal models that resemble SLE, viral infections and genetic predisposition are considered as possible factors in the etiology of SLE.

PATHOGENESIS The serum of patients with SLE contains many antibodies; among them are the antibodies to deoxyribonucleic acid (DNA), nucleoprotein, and other nuclear constituents. These antibodies are collectively termed antinuclear antibodies (ANA) or antinuclear factors (ANF). The antinuclear antibodies alone are harmless; their presence in vivo or in tissue cultures does not harm living cells, since antibodies do not penetrate the membrane of living cells. However, the antinuclear antibodies participate in the pathogenesis of SLE by forming antigen-antibody complexes with their specific antigens. DNA and antibodies to DNA, nucleoprotein and antibodies to nucleoprotein, as well as complement components, have been demonstrated in the renal glomerular basement membrane and in the vascular basement membrane of patients with SLE. These observations resemble the findings in experimental serum sickness (Chap. 69). In acute and chronic experimental serum sicknesses, antigen-antibody complexes circulate transiently. Though the bulk of these materials is removed by the reticuloendothelial system, small amounts of immune complexes are entrapped by vascular and glomerular basement membranes. During the formation of antigen-antibody complexes, complement is consumed and serum concentration of complement is decreased. Similarly, during the active phase of SLE, serum complement and complement components are decreased. Transient presence of circulating DNA has been documented, and some evidence for circulating immune complexes has been marshaled. For these reasons SLE has been classified as an immune-complex disease. Even though DNA and nucleoprotein have been identified in tissue lesions, the source of these antigens has not been clarified. Other antigens may also be involved.

In experimental immune-complex diseases of animals and in human serum sickness, inflammation in joints, pleura, and pericardium occurs because of the presence of antigen and subsequent immune-complex formation. Similar mechanisms may well explain the multitude of clinical manifestations in patients with SLE.

ETIOLOGY The etiology of SLE remains unknown. The reasons for development of the antinuclear and other antibodies are not clear. Furthermore, the origin of the antigens in tissue lesions has not been elucidated—they may be autologous nuclear components, or they may originate from invading microorganisms. The hypothesis that SLE results from a viral infection has been supported by several observations. The endothelial cells of glomerular and peripheral capillaries frequently contain virus-like cytoplasmic inclusions. However, similar inclusions have been encountered in patients with other renal diseases.

A genetic predisposition for SLE has been suggested on the basis of subclinical or clinical abnormalities in relatives of patients with SLE. These abnormalities include the presence of ANA and other "autoantibodies," dysgammaglobulinemia, rheumatoid arthritis, dermatomyositis, etc. These hypotheses find further support from the studies of New Zealand black (NZB) and white (NZW) mice and their F_1 hybrids. The latter, in particular, develop a syndrome analogous to SLE, including renal lesions, decreased complement, and antibodies to DNA as well as other antinuclear antibodies. However, these mice also carry murine leukemia virus concomitantly. Future investigations undoubtedly will clarify the current notions in regard to the etiology of SLE.

PATHOLOGY The pathologic changes in SLE are variable and depend on the stage of the disease. Fibrinoid deposits are commonly seen in blood vessels, among collagen fibers, and on serosal surfaces. Hematoxylin bodies are specific for SLE and are defined as hematoxylin-stained round or oblong masses in areas of inflammation. Hematoxylin bodies are thought to represent degenerated nuclei that have interacted with antinuclear antibodies.

The renal lesions in patients with SLE have been classified into *focal glomerulonephritis, diffuse glomerulonephritis,* and *membranous lupus nephritis.* In focal glomerulonephritis some glomeruli show focal hypercellularity, accumulation of inflammatory cells, and thickening of basement membrane. Immunofluorescent microscopy shows the presence of immunoglobulins and the third component of complement (C3) in involved areas as well as in the mesangium of uninvolved areas. In diffuse glomerulonephritis the same changes are present in all glomeruli, but frequently in an uneven manner. The basement membrane may be considerably thickened. Tubular atrophy and interstitial infiltration with lymphocytes and plasma cells are present. On immunofluorescent microscopy, extensive "lumpy-bumpy" deposits of immunoglobulin and C3 are seen in the basement membrane. On electron microscopy, the basement membrane shows deposits primarily on the endothelial side. In membranous lupus nephritis little hypercellularity is present, but the basement membrane is diffusely thickened. Tubular atrophy and interstitial mononuclear cells are present as well. Immunofluorescent microscopy discloses granular deposits of immunoglobulins and C3. By electron microscopy these deposits are localized on the epithelial side of the basement membrane. The mechanisms for these differences in renal involvement have not been elucidated.

The biopsy of skin lesions in patients with SLE will show atrophy, epidermal hyperkeratosis, and keratotic plugging. The dermis is edematous and infiltrated variably with lymphocytes, plasma cells, and histiocytes. On immunofluorescent staining the epidermal-dermal junction is seen to have IgG and C3 deposits. Similar changes are frequently present in clinically uninvolved skin. The mechanism for such deposits has not been clarified.

Widespread small-vessel vasculitis may be present in many organs. Such lesions exist in the synovium of patients with SLE, showing both mononuclear and polymorphonuclear infiltration. Autopsy studies on SLE patients with central nervous system abnormalities may show necrotizing vasculitis of arterioles and capillaries in many parts of the brain. Microinfarcts of brain tissues may be apparent. The spleen shows marked intimal proliferation of penicillar and central arteries, which gives an "onion skin" appearance to these vessels. The heart valves and chordae tendineae have at times nonbacterial verrucous vegetations (Libman-Sacks endocarditis).

CLINICAL MANIFESTATIONS SLE is predominantly a disease of females (9 females to 1 male) in their second to fifth decades of life, but it spares neither children nor persons of advanced age. The prevalence of SLE is 2 to 3 per 100,000. Most recent estimates indicate that 77 percent of patients with SLE have a 5-year survival and that renal disease and central nervous system involvement decrease this survival. The most frequent causes of death in patients with SLE are uremia, heart failure, hemorrhage, central nervous system disease, or intercurrent bacterial infections.

Patients with SLE may present with a variety of abnormalities, including arthritis and arthralgias, cutaneous manifestations, nephritis, fever, central nervous system manifestations, Raynaud's phenomenon, pleurisy, pericarditis, hemolytic anemia, leukopenia, or thrombocytopenia (Table 70-1).

Arthritis and *arthralgias* are the most frequent presenting complaints, as well as the most common complaints during the course of the illness. The arthralgias are fleeting; they involve the hands or feet and also large joints. Redness, warmth, tenderness, and synovial effusions are frequently present. However, deformities are rare, and the erosions so characteristic of rheumatoid arthritis are unusual. The synovial fluid white cell counts are relatively low (less than 3,000 per mm^3), and mononuclear cells predominate. Aseptic necrosis may occur, in part because of therapy with corticosteroids. Profound muscle weakness and tenderness reflect myositis in some patients.

Fever is frequent during the course of SLE. Fatigue, malaise, anorexia, and weight loss also occur. However,

TABLE 70-1
Clinical manifestations during the course of systemic lupus erythematosus

Manifestation	*Cumulative percentage of patients*
Arthritis and arthralgias	92
Fever	84
Skin eruptions	72
Lymphadenopathy	59
Renal involvement	53
Anorexia, nausea, vomiting	53
Myalgia	48
Pleuritis	45
Central nervous system abnormalities	26

SOURCE: *Modified from EL Dubois, 1966*

systemic complaints may be totally absent in some patients.

Cutaneous manifestations of SLE include a variety of lesions. A facial eruption, with butterfly distribution over the malar areas and bridge of the nose, consists of erythema, atrophy, telangiectasia, and keratotic plugging. This characteristic rash occurs in about 40 percent of patients. Similar eruptions may occur on other parts of the body, particularly in the exposed areas. At times skin eruptions are precipitated or worsened by exposure to ultraviolet rays. Patchy alopecia occurs with similar frequency. Patients with SLE may have short broken hairs above the forehead, the so-called "lupus hairs." Dermal vasculitis can be found in about 20 percent of patients, usually as small infarcts of the digital skin. In some patients only erythema due to excessively large or numerous capillaries around the digits and fingernails is seen. Ulcers may be encountered on nasal and oral mucous membranes. Other cutaneous manifestations include purpura, bullae, hives, and angioneurotic edema. Raynaud's phenomenon is seen in about one-fifth of patients with SLE.

Discoid lupus is a chronic skin ailment with lesions usually confined to face, neck, arms, and scalp. Scaling is prominent, with atrophy, telangiectasia, and keratotic plugging. Deep scars remain when the lesions subside. Only few of these patients go on to develop systemic lupus erythematosus. On the other hand, some patients with SLE also have discoid lesions.

Renal involvement is one of the most serious manifestations in SLE. Clinically detectable evidence of renal involvement is seen in about one-half of all patients with SLE. These abnormalities extend from minimal proteinuria and few red cell casts to massive hematuria, proteinuria, and frank nephrotic syndrome. In some patients renal involvement goes on to total renal failure; in others there is a course of exacerbations and remissions, with eventual renal failure. Some patients respond well to treatment or improve spontaneously, but minimal proteinuria and decreased creatinine clearance may persist as evidence of irreversible damage. In carefully investigated patients electron microscopic or immunofluorescent abnormalities have been observed in the absence of the usual abnormalities of renal function and urinary sediment.

The development of superimposed urinary tract infection should always be kept in mind, since these patients seem liable to such infections.

Cardiopulmonary abnormalities are moderately frequent in patients with SLE. Symptoms and signs of pericarditis or other cardiac abnormalities are encountered in almost 50 percent of them. Pericarditis may be the presenting complaint, with the usual physical and electrocardiographic findings. Tamponade due to SLE pericarditis is unusual. Myocarditis may occur. The nonbacterial verrucous endocarditis is rarely diagnosed clinically but should be suspected when new murmurs develop in the absence of bacterial endocarditis. Pleuritic involvement occurs in nearly half the patients. This may be accompanied by pleuritic pain and effusions, but asymptomatic pleural effusions occur as well. Patchy and transient parenchymal infiltrates have been noted. The cause of these abnormalities is not known, and they are difficult to distinguish from infiltrates caused by infections.

Neurologic manifestations represent another serious aspect of SLE. A variety of central nervous system manifestations has been noted in 20 to 50 percent of patients. Among these are convulsive disorders, followed in frequency by abnormalities in mental functions and cranial nerves. Peripheral neuropathies are infrequent. Occasionally patients present with primarily mental dysfunction, e.g., emotional lability, psychosis, organic brain syndrome, without other significant symptoms. Cerebrospinal fluid of patients with central nervous system involvement may show slight to moderate increase in protein concentration and mild increase in lymphocytes; usually these occur late in the disease. The electroencephalograms are abnormal, with diffuse nonspecific changes.

Lymph node enlargement occurs in many patients with SLE. Such abnormalities may be diffuse or local. Characteristically the nodes are not tender. The enlargement of nodes is thought to occur because of increased activity of the immune system. Splenomegaly occurs in about 10 percent of patients and may be associated with hemolytic anemia. *Hepatomegaly* is found in about 25 percent of patients. The cause for hepatomegaly is not fully known. Lupoid hepatitis is a syndrome of chronic active hepatitis associated with positive tests for LE cells or antinuclear antibodies (Chap. 295).

LABORATORY MANIFESTATIONS A variety of abnormalities in *hematologic* and *immunologic* tests may be encountered in SLE (Table 70-2).

A mild, normochromic, normocytic *anemia* is seen frequently. Most likely this is the hypoproliferative anemia that accompanies many inflammatory processes. Less frequently patients have severe immunohemolytic anemia that requires steroid therapy or splenectomy. Leukopenia is seen in over half the patients. The mechanisms for leukopenia and thrombocytopenia are not fully delineated, but intravascular immune complexes as well as antibodies directed to leukocytes and platelets may contribute to these abnormalities. A potentially serious

TABLE 70-2
Laboratory abnormalities in systemic lupus erythematosus

Abnormality	*Percent of patients*
Hematologic	
Anemia (Hb <11 g/100 ml)	72
Leukopenia (WBC <4,500/mm³)	61
Thrombocytopenia (platelets <100,000/mm³)	15
Positive direct Coombs test	14
Circulating anticoagulants	Rare
Immunologic	
Positive tests for ANA	99
Positive LE cell tests	60–80
Hypocomplementemia	75
Increased γ-globulin (>1.5 g/100 ml)	60–77
Positive tests for rheumatoid factors	20
Biologic false positive tests for syphilis	15

but infrequent problem is the occurrence of *clotting defects* due to antibodies to factor VIII or IX or to the presence of an inhibitor to prothrombin. Prior to a renal biopsy, the integrity of the clotting mechanism must be evaluated.

Urinalysis and renal function studies indicate that over half the patients with SLE have mild to severe damage to the kidneys. With early or focal glomerulonephritis the creatinine clearance may be normal and only mild proteinuria and microscopic hematuria may exist. With more extensive renal involvement proteinuria may become significant (>0.5 g per day) and the urine sediment may contain abundant red cells, white cells, and red cell casts as indicators of glomerular damage.

The serum albumin to globulin ratio becomes reversed because of an increase in immunoglobulins, particularly IgG. Serum electrophoresis reveals that the major elevation is in γ-globulin. In advanced renal involvement with nephrotic syndrome all serum proteins, except α_2 macroglobulin and IgM, become reduced. Small amounts of cryoglobulins, composed of immunoglobulins and complement components, may be present. The erythrocyte sedimentation rate (ESR) tends to be high in patients with active disease.

The most characteristic laboratory abnormalities in SLE are the autoantibodies. The presence of ANA in a patient with active SLE is almost a sine qua non for the diagnosis. These tests are now widely available as a diagnostic aid. The ANA are usually detected by rat kidney or liver sections (other tissues with nucleated cells may also be used); the test serum is applied to the tissue section, antibodies to nuclear antigens interact with the nuclei, other proteins are washed away, and the ANA are detected with an antiserum to human immunoglobulins (these antibodies are coupled with fluorescein isothiocyanate that permits their detection with appropriate microscopy). The ANA include antibodies to a variety of nuclear antigens (antibodies to nucleoprotein, DNA, histones, and other soluble antigens). Patients with SLE also have antibodies to RNA, ribosomes, lysosomes, and other cytoplasmic constituents. The reasons for such a large number of antibodies are not clear. Many of these antibodies persist even when the disease is quiescent, except that the titers of antibodies to DNA tend to be higher during exacerbations of the disease. The lupus erythematosus cell test (LE cell test) is positive less frequently than the test for ANA because more antibodies are required for positivity. A positive test depends on the presence of ANA, particularly on antibodies to nucleoprotein. In this test the buffy coat of the patient's blood is collected and white cells are damaged with glass beads. Thereafter the antibodies to nuclear antigens react with the damaged nuclei, complement is bound, and the resulting material is ingested by living neutrophils. The resulting LE cell contains a large red-purple inclusion body that displaces the segmented nucleus against the cell membrane with virtually no visible cytoplasm.

During flare-ups of SLE the total serum hemolytic complement (expressed in 50 percent hemolytic units —CH_{50}) or individual components of complement are decreased. The most frequently used measurement of complement components is the immunochemically determined C3 level (formerly β_{1c}). The lowering of complement occurs because of activation of complement by immune complexes and thus reflects the primary disease process. Hence these measurements are useful in following the response to therapy or for detecting exacerbations. Occasionally the complement levels remain low in spite of apparent full clinical remission; the reasons for this are not known.

About 20 percent of patients with SLE develop positive tests for rheumatoid factors, but the titers tend to be lower than in rheumatoid arthritis. False positive tests for syphilis are encountered, at times prior to clinical onset of SLE. Antinuclear antibodies occur in many other diseases (rheumatoid arthritis, 20 percent; Sjögren's syndrome, 60 percent; scleroderma, 40 percent) and are induced by several drugs (see below).

DIAGNOSIS The possibility of SLE should be considered in any young or middle-aged female in the presence of three or four of the symptoms or signs listed in Table 70-1 or in the presence of glomerulonephritis, hemolytic anemia, leukopenia, or thrombocytopenia. A positive test for ANA is essential for diagnosis. Other diseases that cause positive tests for ANA must be considered, and they must often be excluded on the basis of clinical observations alone. Major consideration must be given to rheumatoid arthritis, scleroderma, Sjögren's syndrome, and the history of ingestion of drugs that might have induced a positive test for ANA. Pyogenic arthritides should be considered in single severely inflamed joints.

Drug-induced SLE Hydralazine and procainamide clearly induce a syndrome similar to SLE in some patients. This syndrome includes arthralgias, arthritis, myalgias, pleurisy, pericarditis, fever, skin eruptions, lymphadenopathy, positive LE cell preparations, and positive tests for ANA. Renal disease and central nervous system involvement are very unusual in the drug-induced SLE. Prospective studies have shown that almost 70 percent of patients receiving procainamide develop positive tests for ANA within weeks or months. A much smaller proportion become symptomatic. Once the drug is discontinued, the symptoms abate in a few weeks but occasionally may smolder on for months; recovery may be hastened by treatment with corticosteroids. The ANA tests revert to negative in a few months. Isoniazid alone or with para-aminosalicylic acid (PAS), several anticonvulsants (Dilantin, mesantoin), phenothiazine derivatives, alpha-methyldopa, and levodopa have also been associated with positive tests for ANA. In some patients the administration of sulfonamides, penicillin, and oral contraceptives has been associated with exacerbations of SLE.

TREATMENT A cure for SLE is not available. However, abundant experience indicates that appropriate therapy may suppress flare-ups and prolong life. The optimal treatment programs for various manifestations of SLE have not been defined. Adequately designed studies have been difficult to perform because of the variability in the manifestations and course of the disease and the lack of adequate prognostic parameters. Corticosteroids remain the cornerstone of therapy, even though the "immunosuppressive" drugs seem to be helpful in some patients.

Arthralgias, arthritis, myalgias, and fever may respond adequately to rest and salicylates. Antimalarials have been used successfully for the same symptoms, as well as for control of skin eruptions. Chloroquine was used widely in mild SLE, but potential retinal toxicity has decreased its usage. Hydroxychloroquine in small dosages (200 mg per day) seems safe, but the patient should be cautioned about potential toxicity, and careful examination by the ophthalmologist should be conducted at least twice a year. Exposure to ultraviolet light should be avoided, particularly with active and recurrent skin lesions. If skin involvement becomes debilitating and does not respond to conservative therapy, corticosteroids in small to moderate dosages should provide relief.

Central nervous system involvement, pericarditis, myocarditis, pleurisy, severe myositis, severe hemolytic anemia, clotting problems, significant leukopenia, and thrombocytopenia are indications for use of corticosteroids. In desperate situations, particularly in central nervous system involvement with seizures or psychosis, relatively high doses should be used (even up to 2 mg prednisone or prednisolone per kilogram of body weight). Once improvement has occurred, the dose should be tapered and adjusted to maintain control of symptoms. Many of the above manifestations can be controlled with 10 mg prednisone or less per day as a maintenance dose. If a flare-up occurs and is recognized by the patient and the physician, only a moderate (5 to 10 mg) increase of the prednisone dose may provide control of symptoms. Careful follow-up of patients, with judicious use of laboratory tests, is essential in treatment of the above manifestations of SLE. Psychosis or other mental disturbances may be difficult to evaluate in a patient who is receiving steroids for SLE, since such symptoms may be caused by the steroids or by the SLE. With further increase of the steroid dosage the symptoms should decrease if they are due to central nervous system involvement by SLE.

Several approaches to the treatment of SLE nephritis have been advocated, but no currently available program is useful in all patients. Renal biopsy is recommended for establishing the nature of glomerular lesions, since those with focal lupus glomerulonephritis respond to treatment well or improve spontaneously. Perhaps the most useful program is to start with 40 to 60 mg prednisone or prednisolone per day until all clinical symptoms have abated. This may take a few weeks; the urinary sediment should improve, and complement should return toward normal. Thereafter the steroid dose should be reduced gradually to the minimal dose to keep the patient free of symptoms. With severe focal involvement and with diffuse lupus glomerulonephritis or membranous glomerulonephritis, higher doses (up to 150 to 200 mg prednisone or prednisolone) have been tried and found helpful for some patients, with subsequent improvement of renal function. However, the diffuse and membranous lesions do not respond well. For these reasons the use of azathioprine (1 to 2 mg per kg body weight) or cyclophosphamide (100 to 150 mg per day) has been tried and found useful in some patients. These drugs are currently under further evaluation. Their action in SLE is not fully understood, since they are largely immunosuppressive for the primary immune response but also show potent anti-inflammatory activity. Such drugs have serious toxicity in terms of suppression of white cell count, hemorrhagic cystitis, alopecia, sterility, etc., and their long-term risks are not fully known.

Any intercurrent infections must be recognized and treated with appropriate therapy. Patients with SLE, either because of their disease or as a consequence of treatment, are liable to bacterial infections, which are a leading cause of death among them.

Exacerbations of SLE frequently occur during the third trimester of pregnancy or in the immediate post-partum period. Nevertheless, many patients with SLE can be carried to term and successful delivery with appropriate therapy. Therefore, SLE is not an absolute indication for therapeutic abortion, but the procedure is recommended during life-threatening active disease.

REFERENCES

Baldwin DS et al: The clinical course of the proliferative and membranous forms of lupus nephritis. Ann Intern Med 73:929, 1970

Camerford FC, Cohen AS: The nephropathy of systemic lupus erythematosus. Medicine 46:425, 1967

Dubois EL (ed): *Lupus Erythematosus,* New York: McGraw-Hill, 1966

Estes D, Christian CL: The natural history of systemic lupus erythematosus by prospective analysis. Medicine 50:85, 1971

Hurd EF et al: Glomerular cytoplasmic tubular structures in renal biopsies of patients with systemic lupus erythematosus and other diseases. Arthritis Rheum 14:539, 1971

Johnson RT, Richardson EP: The neurological manifestations of systemic lupus erythematosus. Medicine 47:337, 1968

Koffler D et al: Immunological studies concerning the nephritis of systemic lupus erythematosus. J Exp Med 126:607, 1967

Labowitz R, Schumacher HR, Jr: Articular manifestations of systemic lupus erythematosus. Ann Intern Med 74:911, 1971

Rothfield NF et al: Renal disease in systemic lupus erythematosus. N Engl J Med 269:537, 1963

SCHUR PH, SANDSON J: Immunologic factors and clinical activity in systemic lupus erythematosus. N Engl J Med 278:533, 1968

71
VASCULITIS

MART MANNIK
BRUCE C. GILLILAND

Many clinical syndromes of necrotizing inflammation of blood vessels exist. In most of these conditions the etiology is not known, but several descriptive classifications have been offered, depending on the size of the involved blood vessels, the anatomic sites, the stage of the inflammation, and the histologic characteristics of the lesions. In these conditions cellular infiltration, necrosis, and fibrinoid deposits are present in the walls of blood vessels and perivascular areas. These cellular infiltrates are composed of polymorphonuclear leukocytes in acute stages; with progression of the lesion, monocytes, lymphocytes, and plasma cells appear. Giant cells are encountered in some types of vasculitis. Endothelial edema and proliferation, together with hemorrhage, contribute to diminution or occlusion of the vascular lumen and subsequent ischemic symptoms and signs.

Most forms of vasculitis are thought to be caused by immunologic phenomena. Multiple reasons exist for this belief. Necrotizing inflammation of blood vessels is a common finding in experimentally induced immune-complex diseases (Chap. 69). Vasculitis is a known manifestation of human serum sickness (whether due to foreign serum, drugs, or other antigens) and occurs frequently in several known human immune-complex diseases. For example, in systemic lupus erythematosus, DNA, antibodies to DNA, and complement components have been identified in vascular lesions; and in mixed cryoglobulinemia, IgG, antibodies to IgG, and complement components have been seen in involved vessels. Furthermore, in some patients the hepatitis-associated antigen (Australia antigen) has been implicated as the causative agent of polyarteritis with the finding of Au antigen, immunoglobulins, and complement in the lesions. In other types of necrotizing inflammation, immunoglobulins and complement components have been visualized with immunofluorescent microscopy but antigens have not been identified. Not all studies have shown the presence of immunoglobulins in the vascular lesions, perhaps because the immune complexes are ingested and degraded by the inflammatory cells in the lesions. Future work should identify the etiologic factors in many forms of vasculitis. Until then, however, the histologic and clinical features of the vasculitides serve to classify them.

Periarteritis nodosa was delineated by Kussmaul and Maier in the last century. In the early 1950s Zeek's careful descriptive work laid the foundation for most of the classifications of vasculitides. The descriptive classifications of vasculitides have been helpful in predicting the prognosis and response to therapy of individual patients. Upon careful microscopic examination of the lesions, the vasculitides can usually be placed in one of the five categories indicated in Table 71-1. However, at times the clinical problem defies categorization, and even within each of these categories variability from patient to patient is common. The nature of the antigen, the type of antibodies produced, the size of immune complexes formed, and cellular immunity are some of the factors that may

TABLE 71-1
Classification of vasculitis

	Periarteritis nodosa	*Allergic granulomatosis*	*Wegener's granulomatosis*	*Hypersensitivity vasculitis*	*Giant-cell arteritis*
Size of involved blood vessels	Muscular arteries, adjacent veins, occasional arterioles	Muscular arteries, adjacent veins, occasional arterioles	Arteries, arterioles, venules, some capillaries	Arterioles, venules, capillaries	Large and medium arteries
Histology and stage of lesions	Necrotizing inflammation, coexistence of acute and healing lesions, no giant cells	Necrotizing inflammation with granulomas, coexistence of acute and healing lesions, giant cells in granulomas	Necrotizing inflammation with granulomas, coexistence of acute and healing lesions, giant cells in granulomas	Necrotizing inflammation, all lesions in same stage, no giant cells	Inflammation without necrosis, no neutrophils, giant cells present
Anatomic predilections	Widespread, common to branching points of arteries; lungs not involved	Widespread but lungs frequently involved	Upper and lower respiratory tract involved	Widespread but common to skin, serosal surfaces, glomeruli	All large arteries, including aorta, coronary, vertebral, carotid, temporal, mesenteric

play a role in the pleomorphism of the clinical picture in the various vasculitides.

PERIARTERITIS NODOSA Pathology In periarteritis nodosa, the necrotizing inflammation involves muscular arteries, adjacent veins, occasionally arterioles and venules, but not capillaries. The lesions involve segments of vessels, at times affecting only part of the circumference, and there is a predilection for the bifurcation of arteries. These areas may form small aneurysms, which may rupture. During the active disease each patient has acute lesions that show predominantly polymorphonuclear leukocytic infiltration of the vessel walls and perivascular areas, as well as chronic lesions with mononuclear cell infiltration and partial healing. These observations suggest that the disease process is continuous, with repeated insults, and if it is caused by immune mechanisms, then there must be repeated or continuous availability of antigen(s).

The lesions of periarteritis nodosa are widespread throughout the body; they are commonly found in the coronary arteries, mesenteric arteries, kidneys, muscles, vasa nervorum, etc. The extent and location of lesions dictate the severity of clinical symptoms. Central nervous system involvement is unusual. The lungs are usually not involved, but this point has caused controversy and confusion among those contributing to literature in the field. Necrotizing inflammation and granuloma formation in blood vessels accompanied by lung involvement and eosinophilia should be classified as allergic granulomatosis.

Clinical manifestations Periarteritis nodosa is usually a disease of adulthood, but it occurs in childhood and senescence. It affects two to three men for every woman. The onset of the disease is extremely variable. Often an antecedent history of upper respiratory tract infection or reaction to drugs is recorded.

The early complaints of patients with polyarteritis nodosa include fever, weakness, anorexia, weight loss, myalgias, and arthralgias. With the progression of the disease several organs may show involvement. Small, 5- to 10-mm nodules occur along the course of the arteries as a result of aneurysm formation. Vascular occlusion of such vessels leads to ecchymoses, ulceration (often secondarily infected), and gangrene of fingers or toes. Muscle weakness may evolve. Arthralgias are common, but severe and persistent arthritis is uncommon. Mononeuritis multiplex evolves because of involvement of the vasa nervorum. Asymmetric and multiple nerve trunks may be involved. Retinal exudates and hemorrhages may occur.

Pericarditis and pleuritis, with or without effusions are common. Involvement of coronary arteries may lead to myocardial ischemia or infarction, but electrocardiographic abnormalities may be recorded in the absence of symptoms.

Abdominal complaints are frequent (in 60 to 70 percent of patients) and include abdominal pain, nausea, vomiting, diarrhea, and bleeding. All these symptoms are related to the involvement of the mesenteric arteries as they enter the intestinal wall. The mesenteric vasculitis may lead to mucosal ulceration, with hemorrhage, perforation, and infarction. The acute abdominal symptoms early in the disease lead to erroneous diagnoses of intraabdominal catastrophes of other causes, often resulting in unavoidable but unnecessary laparotomy. The liver may be involved, and massive hepatic infarction has been reported. Periarteritis of the gallbladder may cause cholecystitis and perforation.

Renal involvement occurs in over half the patients, and predominantly large vessels are involved. Glomerulosclerosis occurs, with severe involvement. Hypertension may evolve along with renal failure. However, hypertension may occur early in the disease when renal function is normal. The causes of death in polyarteritis nodosa include renal failure, myocardial infarction, infections, congestive heart failure and gastrointestinal bleeding.

Laboratory findings and diagnosis No specific chemical or serologic tests exist for periarteritis nodosa. The leukocyte count is elevated in about 80 percent of patients, principally because of neutrophilia. Anemia may be present because of blood loss and the inflammatory process. The erythrocyte sedimentation rate is often elevated. Other abnormalities depend on the organ involvement, e.g., hematuria, proteinuria, and decreased renal function due to kidney involvement; abnormal electrocardiogram (ECG) due to coronary artery vasculitis, etc.

The diagnosis of periarteritis nodosa often causes difficulties. This diagnosis should be suspected in patients with involvement in several of the systems mentioned above, particularly in adult males. Infections, systemic lupus erythematosus, trichinosis, heart failure, Hodgkin's disease, and most other syndromes can be ruled out. Histologic examination of tissue is essential for proper diagnosis and for distinction from other vasculitides. Clinically involved tissue is best for histologic examinations, and tender subcutaneous nodules, tender muscles, and skin infarcts are suitable. Each tissue should be examined thoroughly because of the segmental nature of the lesions. Blind muscle biopsy has yielded positive information only in one-third of patients shown to have periarteritis later. The frequent finding of vasculitis in testes at autopsy has resulted in the recommendation of testicular biopsy.

Treatment The prognosis of periarteritis nodosa with involvement of many organ systems is grim. Hypertension and renal involvement are thought to predict rapid progression of the disease. In untreated patients one-half to two-thirds have died within a year, but these statistics are heavily biased by postmortem studies and selective inclusion of severely ill patients. Treatment with corticosteroids frequently leads to rapid symptomatic improvement (initial dose 40 to 60 mg prednisone or prednisolone per day, tapered subsequently). In one study 5-year survival in untreated patients was estimated at 13 percent. Controlled studies on the use of cytotoxic (immunosuppressive) drugs have not been recorded, but some experiences suggest that these agents may help when other drugs have failed.

ALLERGIC GRANULOMATOSIS Allergic granulomatosis is separated from periarteritis nodosa because of pathologic and clinical differences, but the etiology is unknown in both.

Pathology The organs and the size of vessels that are segmentally involved are the same in allergic granulomatosis as in periarteritis nodosa. However, in allergic granulomatosis, eosinophils tend to be abundant in lesions, epithelioid cells are numerous, giant cells are present, and a marked accumulation of inflammatory cells occurs, thus leading to the granulomatous appearance. Pulmonary involvement is frequent and striking, with granuloma formation in the vessel walls and perivascular areas.

Manifestations Patients with allergic granulomatosis frequently give a history of an antecedent respiratory infection. Many have asthma that precedes evidence of vasculitis. In contrast to polyarteritis nodosa, fever is common. Fifty-four percent of these patients have peripheral eosinophilia, with eosinophils in excess of 1,500 per mm^3. The radiologic examination is not diagnostic, but parenchymal lung lesions include consolidation in small and large areas. Pleural effusions are not common.

Involvement of other organs is quite similar to that in periarteritis nodosa, and includes the heart, kidneys, intestine, and peripheral nerves.

Treatment This has not been evaluated systematically. Sporadic reports and analogy to other forms of necrotizing vasculitis indicate that corticosteroids, in the same doses used for periarteritis, are the drugs of choice. Cytotoxic (immunosuppressive) drugs might be tried in patients unresponsive to corticosteroids.

WEGENER'S GRANULOMATOSIS Wegener's granulomatosis is separable from other vasculitides by clinical and pathologic criteria, but the etiology is unknown. Usually the disseminated form of the disease progresses to death, but cytotoxic agents have provided dramatic improvement.

Pathology Typical Wegener's granulomatosis is characterized by (1) necrotizing granulomatous lesions in the upper part of the airway, lower part of the respiratory tract, or both; (2) generalized focal necrotizing inflammation of arteries and veins, almost always in the lungs and frequently in other organs; (3) necrotizing glomerulitis. In the nose, paranasal sinuses, nasopharynx, glottis, and middle ear, accumulation of granulation tissue, ulceration, and even destruction of bony tissue may occur. A severe granulomatous reaction, with giant cells, fibrosis, and necrosis, is seen microscopically. Arteries, arterioles, veins, and venules adjacent to and away from granulomas are involved, with severe necrotizing inflammation in variable stages. The trachea, bronchi, and lung parenchyma develop granulomatous masses; those in the lung may cavitate. Massive accumulation of chronic inflammatory cells and giant cells is seen, together with partial necrosis. In addition, necrotizing vasculitis takes place in pulmonary blood vessels. Focal necrotizing glomerulitis and necrotizing vasculitis of small arteries are seen in kidneys. Splenic infarcts are not uncommon. Necrotizing vasculitis with granulomas may occur in every organ.

At times typical lesions of Wegener's granulomatosis may be confined to the lungs or other single organs. These limited forms may go on to rapidly progressive lethal disease.

Clinical manifestations This illness affects males and females equally, usually occurring in middle age. The onset may be insidious, with years of nonbacterial rhinorrhea, sinusitis, or chronic otitis media, at times accompanied by abnormal chest x-ray films. In others, the disease first becomes symptomatic with explosive onset of fever, malaise, and weight loss; abnormalities in the upper and lower parts of the respiratory tract and kidneys develop later. The initial upper respiratory symptoms may last for years, but the generalized disease usually runs a short course with survival for less than 1 year.

The upper respiratory tract involvement manifests itself as rhinorrhea, chronic sinusitis, nasal obstruction, hearing loss, hoarseness, dysphagia, or epistaxis. On examination, accumulation of granulation tissue, ulcerations, and infection may be evident. The disease may extend to the orbit. Cough, hemoptysis, dyspnea, and pleurisy may evolve, but bronchospasm does not occur. Hilar enlargement and multiple or single nodules of varying size may be encountered on x-ray films of the chest. Cavitation, with very thin walls, may be seen. The lesions tend to be bilateral and in the lower lung fields. Abnormal chest films without symptoms have at times led to the diagnosis of "limited" Wegener's granulomatosis. These x-ray patterns are not diagnostic and resemble tumors and other granulomatous processes. Patients may complain of myalgias and arthralgias. Pericardial and myocardial involvement are seen, and the central nervous system and peripheral nerves may be affected. Skin lesions include purpura and nodules that may progress to ulceration. Renal abnormalities tend to progress from microscopic hematuria and proteinuria to renal failure.

No specific serologic or biochemical tests are available for Wegener's granulomatosis. Mild anemia, elevated erythrocyte sedimentation rate, mild leukocytosis without eosinophilia, and urinary abnormalities are common. Tissue examination is essential for proper diagnosis. Infectious granulomas, lethal midline granuloma, sarcoidosis, and other vasculitides should be considered in the differential diagnosis.

Treatment Once patients develop the generalized phase of Wegener's granulomatosis, the clinical course is short, and average survival is 5 to 6 months after the diagnosis is made. Administration of high doses of corticosteroids (prednisone or prednisolone in dosage of 60 mg per day or more) result in some improvement and prolongation of life. Encouraging results have been obtained with the use of cytotoxic (immunosuppressive) drugs such as cyclophosphamide, chlorambucil, and azathioprine. Highly active disease has been suppressed, and patients have survived with mild residual disease. Various dosage schedules of cyclophosphamide have been used, including 75 to 150 mg per day. The cytotoxic drugs have been discontinued in some patients without recurrence, but others have been maintained on low doses. With severe generalized Wegener's granulomatosis use of these drugs seems advisable, but in limited forms of the disease their potential benefits must be weighed against their known hazards.

HYPERSENSITIVITY VASCULITIS (SMALL-VESSEL VASCULITIS) Hypersensitivity vasculitis has been given many names because of its varied clinical picture. The role of immunity in its pathogenesis is inferred by similarity to experimental models, and in some patients with this disorder the involvement of antigen-antibody complexes is documented. Basically, the arterioles, venules, and capillaries of many organs are involved by necrotizing inflammation. In a single patient, all lesions tend to be of the same age. The clinical picture depends on the extent of the disease and on the primary target organ. Systemic lupus erythematosus, rheumatoid arthritis, and mixed cryoglobulinemia are excellent examples of this type of vasculitis in which immune mechanisms have been implicated in the pathogenesis of the blood vessel inflammation. Drugs and microbial infections have also been implicated as the causative agents.

Pathology Hypersensitivity vasculitis (small-vessel vasculitis) is the most frequently encountered vasculitis. The inflammation and necrosis involve arterioles, vessels, and capillaries; muscular and large arteries are spared. As a result, the clinical symptoms do not evolve from large vessel ischemia and infarction but result from hemorrhagic and exudative lesions and microinfarcts. Many organs may be involved, including skin, mucous membranes, brain, lungs, heart, gastrointestinal tract, kidneys, and muscle. Neutrophils have accumulated in small-vessel walls and in perivascular areas. Necrosis, edema, and extravasation of blood are present. Many neutrophils are fragmented; hence some prefer to call this form of vasculitis "leukoclastic angiitis." Healing and hyalinization occur late. Focal or diffuse glomerulonephritis is found. Characteristically all vascular lesions are in the same stage of evolution, in contrast to what occurs in periarteritis nodosa. This observation suggests episodic, rather than continuous, exposure to immune complexes, if indeed this is the mechanism of injury.

Clinical manifestations The clinical manifestations and onset of hypersensitivity vasculitis are variable, and the reasons for this variability are not known. In some patients the skin manifestations are extensive; systemic manifestations and involvement of other organs predominate throughout the course of the illness in others. In some the disease follows a quick course that leads to death, but most patients survive for years and may recover without recurrences.

In youngsters and in some adults hypersensitivity vasculitis may present as the Henoch-Schönlein syndrome, with prodromal headache, anorexia, fever, abdominal pain and bleeding, arthralgias, purpuric eruptions, and evidence of renal involvement. However, in adults the usual criteria for the Henoch-Schönlein syndrome are not frequently fulfilled.

The history of an antecedent respiratory infection may be obtained, drugs may have been ingested (the list is long and includes penicillin, sulfonamides, other antibiotics, salicylates, phenylbutazone, phenacetin, propylthiouracil, busulfan, iodides, vaccines, phenothiazines). Fever is a common systemic symptom. The skin lesions include urticaria, purpura, ecchymoses, papules, nodules, vesicles, and necrotic ulcerations. Lesions may occur anywhere, but they tend to have some symmetry, and the lesions predominate in lower extremities—the legs, ankles, and feet. Patients frequently complain of itching, burning, stinging, and pain in the skin lesions. They may have myalgia, arthralgia, and arthritis. The joints may be warm, red, and painful with acute effusions. However, synovitis of long duration with synovial hypertrophy is unusual, and bony erosions do not develop, unless rheumatoid arthritis is present. Pulmonary infiltrates and pleural effusions may be found on chest roentgenograms. Pericarditis and myocarditis may develop, accompanied by electrocardiographic abnormalities. These patients may have peripheral neuropathy and encephalopathy, manifested by confusion, delirium, and coma. Diffuse electroencephalographic abnormalities may be present. Renal involvement becomes apparent, with microscopic hematuria, proteinuria, and decreasing renal function. Abdominal pain and gastrointestinal bleeding occur.

Similar clinical manifestations accompany the vasculitis associated with systemic lupus erythematosus, rheumatoid arthritis, and mixed cryoglobulinemias. Patients with subacute bacterial endocarditis may have small-vessel vasculitis, as manifested by the Osler's nodes, Roth's spots, arthralgias, and glomerulonephritis.

Laboratory studies Elevation of the erythrocyte sedimentation rate is the most common abnormality. Mild anemia and moderate leukocytosis occur. Complement levels may be reduced, but extensive studies are not available. If vasculitis occurs in systemic lupus erythematosus, antinuclear antibodies will be found, as will rheumatoid factors in patients with rheumatoid arthritis and in mixed cryoglobulinemia. Examination of the urinary sediment and evaluation of proteinuria and renal function are indicated for initial evaluation and follow-up of these patients. Biopsy of lesions is important.

Treatment The mortality figures for this disorder are variable because many series are based on autopsy findings. Spontaneous improvement occurs in some patients; in others the disease lingers. If drugs, toxins, or other environmental factors are suspected, all these exposures should be eliminated. If this disorder is immunologically mediated, then removal of the antigen would be the best treatment. Uncontrolled observations suggest that corticosteroids favorably influence the course of this disorder. The optimal dosages have not been determined; 40 to 60 mg prednisone or prednisolone seems reasonable at the outset, but the dose should be reduced when symptoms, signs, and laboratory tests show improvement. The dose should be increased when flare-ups occur. By analogy to systemic lupus erythematosus and Wegener's granulomatosis, cytostatic (immunosuppressive) drugs might be used in desperate situations. However, the results of controlled clinical trials with this therapy are not yet available.

GIANT-CELL ARTERITIS Giant-cell arteritis (also called temporal or cranial arteritis) is an inflammation of arteries in elderly persons. The cause of the disorder is unknown, and the pathogenesis of arterial inflammation has not been elucidated. Any large or medium-sized arteries may be involved, including the superficial temporal artery. Giant-cell arteritis responds dramatically to treatment with corticosteroids.

Pathology The inflammatory changes of giant-cell arteritis consist of accumulation of lymphocytes, macrophages, and plasma cells, together with giant cells, in the walls of large and medium-sized arteries. The intima shows marked proliferation; the internal elastic lamina and other elastic fibers are fragmented. The lesions are spotty and do not involve long stretches of the vessels. Thrombosis occurs at sites of inflammation. In early lesions only the intima is thought to be involved. Accumulation of neutrophils and fibrinoid necrosis do not occur, and arterioles and capillaries are spared.

The segmental lesions of giant-cell arteritis may involve many arteries, including the superficial temporal artery. The aorta is frequently involved, and aneurysms and dissection have been recorded. The external and internal carotid arteries and the vertebral artery systems are involved. Inflammation and occlusion of the ophthalmic or central retinal artery lead to blindness. Involvement of iliac, femoral, mesenteric, and coronary arteries may cause ischemia and infarction in the respective sites. The distribution and histopathology of the lesions in giant-cell arteritis resemble the pathology of pulseless disease or Takayasu's syndrome.

Clinical and laboratory manifestations Giant-cell arteritis is a disease of the elderly that affects both sexes nearly equally. This illness has rarely been diagnosed before the age of fifty and usually affects those above sixty. The symptomatic involvement of arteries is frequently preceded by systemic symptoms, including fever, sweats, malaise, fatigue, anorexia, and weight loss. The fevers tend to be low grade but may be striking. A fever of unknown origin in an elderly person, accompanied by a very high erythrocyte sedimentation rate, should always raise the diagnostic possibility of giant-cell arteritis.

Patients with giant-cell arteritis often have the *polymyalgia rheumatica* syndrome. This is characterized by an aching pain and stiffness in the neck and shoulders, but it may extend to the upper arms and less frequently to the forearms. The hips and thighs may be similarly involved. Aching is increased with motion. Morning stiffness may be present. The muscles may be tender, and disuse atrophy may ensue. Joint pain in the shoulders, hips, and, less commonly, peripheral joints is reported, but objectively the joints are not inflamed and do not show synovial hypertrophy, even though small effusions may be present. Biopsy of asymptomatic temporal arteries will often make it possible to establish a histologic diagnosis of giant-cell arteritis in patients with polymyalgia rheumatica. The segmental occurrence of the lesions must be kept in mind in interpreting the results of the biopsies. The frequency of positive temporal artery biopsies varies from series to series, but the true prevalence of giant-cell arteritis in polymyalgia rheumatica remains unknown.

Headache is a frequent symptom, particularly in patients who have clinical temporal arteritis, with tender and thickened temporal arteries. The headache has no typical pattern, but marked scalp tenderness is often prominent. Furthermore, these patients may complain of intermittent claudication of the jaws and tongue upon mastication or talking.

Loss of vision is the most serious complication of giant-cell arteritis. Blindness usually develops suddenly without significant warning, but mild visual disturbances may herald total visual loss. Usually for months or weeks these patients will have had other complaints suggestive of giant-cell arteritis or polymyalgia rheumatica. Aortic aneurysms, aortic dissection, mesenteric arteritis, myocardial ischemia, and infarction and claudication of the lower extremities have been attributed to giant-cell arteritis.

Laboratory findings The significant abnormalities in laboratory tests include a very high erythrocyte sedimentation rate (ESR), mild hypoproliferative anemia, and elevation of the α_2-globulins and fibrinogen. The ESR exceeds 50 mm per hr (by Westergren's method) and often reaches values above 100 mm per hr. Important negative findings include normal serum levels of muscle enzymes and normal electromyograms even in the presence of severe polymyalgia. Muscle biopsies disclose no characteristic changes.

In the absence of specific diagnostic tests, the diagnosis of giant-cell arteritis or polymyalgia rheumatica has to rest on clinical findings and a positive biopsy. Polymyalgia rheumatica, or a number of the other symptoms discussed above, in the presence of a high ESR in an elderly person should raise the question of giant-cell arteritis or polymyalgia rheumatica. A temporal artery biopsy should be considered early in the evaluation of such patients. Other causes of a high ESR must, of course, be considered, including occult neoplasms and chronic infections.

Treatment Though patients with the polymyalgia rheumatica syndrome and giant-cell arteritis may obtain some relief from their symptoms with salicylates, indomethacin, and phenylbutazone, the basic process of arteritis does not seem to improve. However, patients with this disorder have a remarkable response to corticosteroid treatment. The clinical symptoms abate in a few days, the ESR and the hypoproliferative anemia return toward normal within 2 weeks, and the reversal of arterial lesions has been documented by arteriography. Several dosage schedules have been recommended. A starting dose of 30 to 40 mg prednisone or prednisolone (or its equivalent) per day has worked well, but the dose should be reduced gradually when symptoms have abated and the ESR has decreased. The maintenance dose is usually less than 10 mg prednisone per day. This drug can be ultimately discontinued altogether in the majority of patients. The hazards of corticosteroids should be considered, and the prolonged use of high doses of corticosteroids should be discouraged.

REFERENCES

CARRINGTON CB, LIEBOW AA: Limited forms of angiitis and granulomatosis of Wegener's type. Am J Med 41:497, 1966

CHURG J, STRAUSS L: Allergic granulomatosis, allergic angiitis and periarteritis nodosa. Am J Pathol 27:277, 1951

DAHL EV et al: Testicular lesions of periarteritis nodosa with special reference to diagnosis. Am J Med 28:222, 1960

FAUCI AS et al: Effect of cyclophosphamide upon the immune response in Wegener's granulomatosis. N Engl J Med 285:1493, 1971

GOCKE DJ et al: Association between polyarteritis and Australia antigen. Lancet 2:1149, 1970

GODMAN GC, CHURG J: Wegener's granulomatosis. Pathology and review of the literature. AMA Arch Pathol 58:533, 1954

HAMILTON CR, JR et al: Giant cell arteritis: including temporal arteritis and polymyalgia rheumatica. Medicine 50:1, 1971

ISRAEL HL, PATCHEFSKY AS: Wegener's granulomatosis of lung: diagnosis and treatment. Ann Intern Med 74:881, 1971

MCCOMBS RP: Systemic "allergic" vasculitis. Clinical and pathological relationships. JAMA 194:1059, 1965

MELTZER M et al: Cryoglobulinemia—a clinical and laboratory study. II. Cryoglobulins with rheumatoid factor activity. Am J Med 40:837, 1966

ROSE GA, SPENCER H: Polyarteritis nodosa. Quart J Med 26:43, 1957

WILSKE KR, HEALEY LA: Polymyalgia rheumatica. A manifestation of systemic giant-cell arteritis. Ann Intern Med 66:77, 1967

WINKELMAN RK, DITTO WB: Cutaneous and visceral syndromes of necrotizing or "allergic" angiitis: a study of 38 cases. Medicine 43:59, 1964

ZEEK PM: Periarteritis nodosa and other forms of necrotizing angiitis. N Engl J Med 248:764, 1953

PART FIVE NUTRITIONAL, HORMONAL, AND METABOLIC DISORDERS

section 1 Basic considerations

72 INTERMEDIARY METABOLISM OF PROTEIN, FAT, AND CARBOHYDRATE

GEORGE F. CAHILL, JR.

Before discussing specific metabolic pathways and their roles in health and disease, a few general biochemical principles should be outlined. The metabolic system, as a whole, is governed by innumerable control mechanisms in cells and tissues whereby a pathway can be activated as needed, or can be inhibited as products accumulate. The net result is a finely integrated summation of an almost infinite number of chemical reactions occurring in all body cells, coordinated by signal systems such as hormones, levels of circulating substrates, and, not infrequently, the nervous system.

ENZYMES AND CONTROL MECHANISMS All biochemical reactions are controlled by specific proteins, the enzymes. Thus, as true catalysts, the enzymes accelerate molecular transformations, and do so by initially binding with the reactant. Thus enzyme (E) plus substrate (S) form a complex (ES) which then dissociates to form enzyme plus the altered molecule (P) or product. Without the enzyme, substrate would yet be converted to product, but much more slowly, frequently years instead of seconds. The concentration of substrate needed to saturate one-half the catalytic sites on the enzyme molecule is referred to as the K_m, or Michaelis constant. Thus the conversion of E to P, in the reaction

$$E + S \rightarrow ES \rightarrow E + P + \text{energy}$$

is a function of the concentration of S, the amount of enzyme E, the concentration of product P, and, most importantly, the release of energy. If there is little or no energy exchanged, the overall reaction is readily reversible. This situation is frequently encountered in most enzymatic sequences not subject to regulatory control. On the other hand, if there is a large energy release, the reaction, although theoretically reversible to a limited degree, is, practically speaking, unidirectional. It is at these "committed" steps where checks and balances are exerted by other regulators in order to control the entire pathway. Frequently involved are other participants in the reaction, which may directly contribute reactants and serve as coenzymes, first binding to the enzyme at a site near where the substrate binds and then transferring a part of their molecule to the substrate to form the product. The enzyme also may be altered by agents which bind to it and do not participate directly in the reaction. These factors, by distorting the three-dimensional structure of the enzyme, can either alter the activity of the enzyme itself or alter the binding affinity of substrate, product, or coenzyme. An enzyme capable of being distorted by such factors is an *allosteric* enzyme and offers a unique mechanism whereby molecules can finely accelerate or decrease the rate of a given enzymatic reaction. The total amount of enzyme available is a function of the genetic code, of its transcription and translation, and of the rate of removal of the enzyme by degradation. Finally, other cofactors, such as metals and inorganic or organic ions, are frequently necessary as part of the enzyme complex and, again, may either inhibit or augment the overall reaction.

Abnormalities resulting in disease have been shown to occur at each of these regulatory sites. The reaction may be altered because of inadequate substrate concentration, or, possibly, similarly structured molecules may competitively displace the substrate from the enzyme. In addition, there can be a lack of necessary coenzymes, or displacement of cofactors by inhibitors, or there may be substances that distort the enzyme (allosteric regulators), thereby increasing or decreasing its activity. Finally, there may be a primary inherited abnormality in the amino acid sequence of the enzyme itself, or in another protein-regulating synthesis of the enzyme. Disease states in man have been demonstrated for each of the possible aberrations described above.

ENERGY Except for organisms capable of using the sun's energy (autotrophs) to drive their metabolic machinery, living matter needs a constant input of fuel not only for growth but for maintenance (homeostasis). The principal storage form of energy in all living matter is the hydrogen-carbon bond. A major part of the metabolic machinery is involved in translating this energy into energy that can be readily used for synthetic reactions, for locomotion, for pumping ions or molecules against concentration gradients, and for many other essential cell processes. The energy requirement for almost all these is provided in the form of the high-energy phosphate bond (Fig. 72-1). The phosphate radical is rich in electrons, and two phosphates adjacent to each other contain much energy, or in biochemical language, a high-energy phosphate bond (~P). Likewise, a phosphate adjacent to other highly negatively charged groups contains much energy (8 to 10 kcal per mole), an example being creatine phosphate. On the other hand, a phosphate in ester linkage to an alcohol contains relatively less energy (2 kcal per mole) and is called a low-energy phosphate bond; it does not participate in energy transfer processes.

The site for most high-energy phosphate formation is in the mitochondria. These intracellular organelles are literally energy transducers which, with the help of enzyme sequences in the cell fluid (the cytosol), prepare and partially degrade the original molecule bearing the hydrogen-carbon bond. The energy from this bond is then converted into an as yet hypothetic high-energy phosphate intermediate (X~P), which, in turn, transfers the ~P to a phosphate on a specific purine (adenine) nucleotide to form adenosine triphosphate (ATP) from adenosine diphosphate (ADP). The ATP is then capable of diffusing from the mitochondria to the site in the cell needing the energy.

In Fig. 72-2 is sketched a single mitochondrion inside a cell. It consists of an aqueous phase containing the enzymes of the tricarboxylic acid cycle (Krebs cycle or citric acid cycle) which receives acetyl CoA and in one turn discharges two molecules of CO_2 and a number of high-energy phosphate bonds (30 ATP). The latter are formed by transfer of the energy of the carbon-hydrogen bond from the original acetyl CoA to specific carriers, nicotinamide-adenine dinucleotide (NAD^+)[1] and flavin adenine dinucleotide (FAD), which enter the solid phase of the mitochondrion, the cristae, where the energy is transformed into high-energy phosphate, and the hydrogen finally meets oxygen to form water. Thus in the presence of oxygen, acetyl CoA, and a need for a high-energy phosphate, the cycle turns, hydrogen is transferred to the sequence of enzymes (the respiratory chain) in the cristae, and water and ~P are produced.

[1] *Formerly called DPN or diphosphopyridine nucleotide.*

FIGURE 72-1
The structure of adenosine triphosphate. Energy is stored in the two terminal high-energy phosphate bonds (denoted in the text as ~P) and is released or transferred to support reactions requiring energy (endergonic).

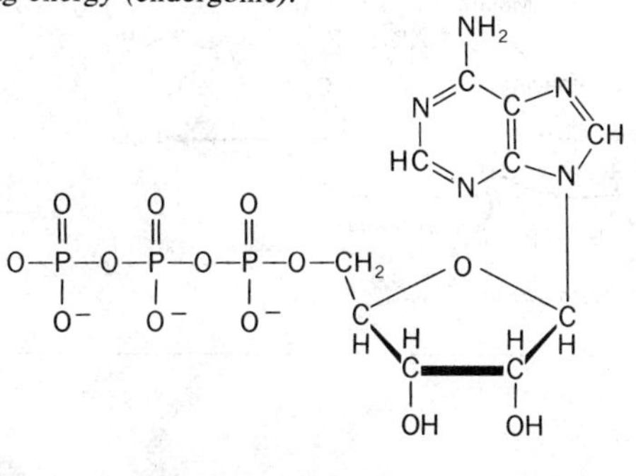

What turns the system on is the need for ~P as signaled by the presence of ADP, and the system runs until the ADP is made into ATP. Thus ADP added to mitochondria initiates oxygen consumption, which continues as long as ADP is available ("respiratory control"). Oxygen consumption, not linked to ~P production, results in heat alone or "uncoupled" oxidative phosphorylation. Normally three ~P molecules are produced for each oxygen molecule in a well-coupled respiratory chain.

Not all the cells' high-energy phosphate is derived from mitochondria; Fig. 72-2 shows two sites where ~P is produced in the metabolism of glucose to pyruvate. Nonmitochondrial generation (anaerobic glycolysis) may occur in the absence of oxygen, and, as discussed below, may be crucial to the cell, or even to the survival of the entire organism.

The acetyl CoA which provides the bulk of mitochondrial fuel can be derived from several sources. It is the final common pathway of the breakdown of all carbohydrates, being formed by pyruvate decarboxylation in the mitochondrion itself with thiamine (vitamin B_1) and lipoic acid as cofactors. Acetyl CoA is also formed from long-chain fatty acids which enter the mitochondria esterified to carnitine where they are again reesterified with coenzyme A (a cofactor containing the vitamin pantothenic acid). The fatty acid coenzyme A molecule then undergoes sequential removal of hydrogen, the hydrogen being transferred to the respiratory chain for energy production as NADH or FADH (cofactors containing the vitamins nicotinamide and riboflavin), and cleavage of two carbons at a time to form acetyl CoA, which in turn enters the tricarboxylic acid cycle. Ketone bodies can also directly contribute acetyl CoA to mitochondrial oxidation, as can certain amino acids after deamination and partial degradation. Thus all three metabolic fuels, carbohydrate, fat, and protein, feed acetyl CoA into mitochondrial metabolism for terminal combustion and generation of high-energy phosphate.

GLUCOSE METABOLISM Mitochondrial generation of ATP, although accounting for more than 90 percent of all energy produced in the cell, is not the only source of utilizable energy. Anaerobic glycolysis in the cytoplasm also produces two ~P molecules per molecule of glucose oxidized, as indicated in Fig. 72-2. The efficiency of energy transformation, the amount of useful energy obtained per molecule of fuel consumed, is much lower in glycolysis than in mitochondrial oxidative phosphorylation; in other words, glycolysis is a very inefficient means of supplying large amounts of energy.

In the utilization of glucose by a cell, it is first phosphorylated to glucose 6-phosphate by the enzyme hexokinase. Adenosine triphosphate is utilized in the process, yielding ADP and glucose 6-phosphate. Thus a high-energy bond is consumed and a low-energy bond generated with loss of heat, which makes the reaction essentially unidirectional and therefore a potential site of metabolic control. Glucose 6-phosphate occupies a strategic position with reference to several biochemical pathways.

Glycolysis This sequence of reactions is the most important route of glucose 6-phosphate metabolism. After the conversion of glucose to glucose 6-phosphate, a step requiring ATP, glucose 6-phosphate is converted to fructose 6-phosphate, to which another high-energy phosphate is added from ATP to form fructose 1,6-diphosphate. This is another step yielding much energy as heat, using a high-energy phosphate, and producing one with low energy, and is therefore essentially unidirectional. It has been suggested that this reaction controls the entire glycolytic pathway. This step is opposed by another enzyme, fructose 1,6-diphosphatase, which converts fructose 1,6-diphosphate back to fructose 6-phosphate. The latter enzyme, as expected, is located in tissues which produce glucose, and therefore is found in liver, where its activity is increased by any one of a group of metabolic stimuli which accelerate gluconeogenesis, e.g., glucocorticoids. Conversely, fructose 1,6-diphosphatase is essentially lacking in tissues such as muscle, adipose tissue, or brain, where the only route of glucose metabolism is via glycolysis to pyruvate and lactate, and then via acetate and the citric acid cycle to CO_2 in the presence of oxygen.

After formation of fructose 1,6-diphosphate, the hexose unit is split into two interconvertible 3-carbon phosphorylated sugars. One of these, glyceraldehyde 3-phosphate, is dehydrogenated and phosphorylated to form NADH and 1,3-diphosphoglyceric acid, which through a series of reactions yields pyruvate and two high-energy phosphate bonds per 3-carbon residue. Thus the overall reaction is:

FIGURE 72-2

A general scheme of energy and molecular transformations in compartments of the cell. Glucose is transported across the cell membrane, phosphorylated through use of high-energy phosphate bond (~P), and then transformed either to store its energy content (upward, glycogenesis) or to release its energy content (downward) via (1) breakdown of glycogen by phosphorylase (A)*; (2) oxidation through the glycolytic cycle to form acetyl CoA; (3) hydrogen transfer* (B) *to enter the mitochondrial apparatus; (4) oxidation through the pentose pathway. Energy is transformed into useful form via the consumption of O_2 in mitochondrial membranes, with concomitant esterification of inorganic phosphate (P_i) to form a (hypothetic) high-energy phosphate intermediate compound (X~P), which can be used to synthesize ATP (see Fig. 75-2); this mitochondrial process is oxidative phosphorylation. The mitochondrial matrix contains enzymes catalyzing the Krebs (tricarboxylic acid) cycle, transforming the energy released from acetyl CoA produced from glucose, amino acids, ketone bodies, or fatty acids. Further details are discussed in the text.*

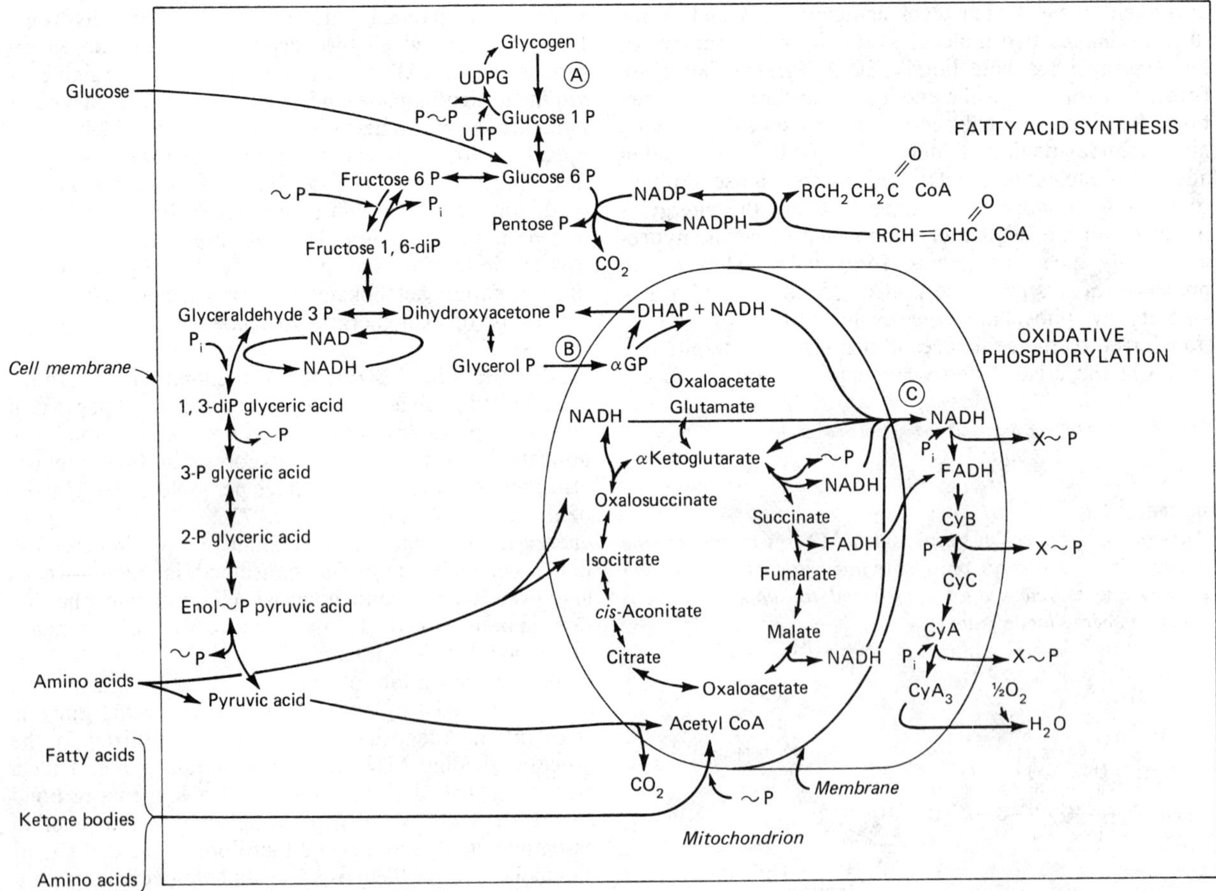

$$\text{Glucose} + 2 \sim P + 2\,P_i + 2\,NAD^+ \rightarrow 2\ \text{pyruvate} + 4 \sim P + 2\,NADH + 2\,H^+$$

where P_i is inorganic phosphate. If oxygen is lacking and the NADH cannot be oxidized to NAD^+, its hydrogen atom can be disposed of in the conversion of pyruvate to lactate, and thereby NAD^+ is replenished for further glycolysis. Thus the overall reaction is:

$$\text{Glucose} + 2 \sim P \rightarrow 2\ \text{lactate} + 4 \sim P$$

or

$$\text{Glucose} \rightarrow 2\ \text{lactate} + 2 \sim P$$

This sequence, termed *anaerobic glycolysis*, since it can occur in the absence of oxygen, can provide a small but, in an emergency, significant and necessary amount of energy. Anaerobic glycolysis is limited, however, by the accumulation of lactic acid which eventually lowers the pH to a degree not compatible with cellular function. Certain tissues, such as the red cell or renal medulla, which are devoid of, or very low in, mitochondria, normally derive their energy by this process, and the lactic acid so produced is released into the circulation to be metabolized by other tissues.

GLYCOGEN Glycogen is a very large, complex polymer of branching chains of glucose units and serves as a storage form of carbohydrate. Although present in all tissues, it plays its most significant role in liver and in muscle, in the former as the reserve for blood glucose maintenance between meals and in the latter as the principal source of fuel during strenuous activity. Glycogen is synthesized from glucose 1-phosphate by an enzyme sequence whose activity, in turn, is regulated by its interconversion into an active form or into an inactive form, each interconversion being controlled itself by a separate enzyme which can exist in an active or inactive form. This highly complex system is increased in overall activity by insulin and glucose and is decreased by physiologic events stimulating glycogen breakdown. For example, in liver, epinephrine or glucagon react with the cell membrane to generate the formation of cyclic AMP (Fig. 72-3) which in turn activates the turning off of the glycogen-synthesizing system.

Glycogen breakdown occurs via a separate pathway, and, as expected, being essentially unidirectional, is a site of metabolic regulation. The same events that turn on the glycogen-synthesizing system turn off the glycogenolytic system, and vice versa. Cyclic AMP therefore activates enzymes which in turn activate other enzymes to activate the enzyme phosphorylase (by its conversion from an inactive phosphorylase) to cleave glucose units off the terminal glycogen chains. The net effect is a mechanism whereby a few molecules of the initial signal, such as epinephrine acting on the muscle or liver cell, or glucagon on the liver cell, can initiate a rapid amplification resulting in an almost instantaneous cessation of glycogen synthesis and a rapid acceleration of glycogen breakdown. In liver, this results in glucose release; in muscle, fuel for aerobic or anaerobic glycolysis.

Not discussed here is the role of the enzymes involved in forming the branch points or in cleaving the branch points; these are discussed in Chap. 104, Disorders of Glycogen Synthesis and Mobilization.

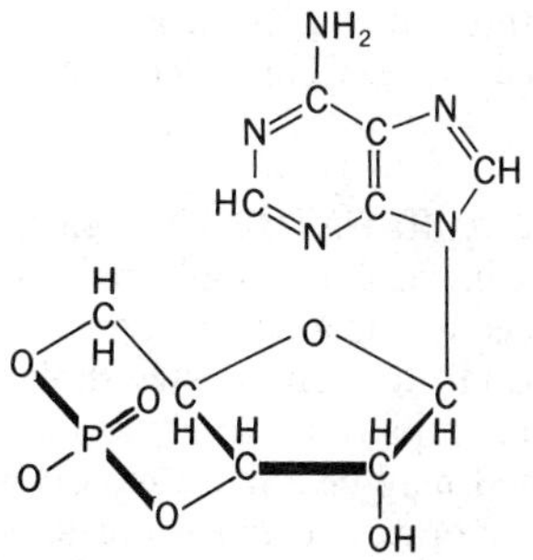

FIGURE 72-3
The structure of cyclic 3′,5′-adenosine monophosphate (cyclic 3′,5′-AMP or cyclic adenylate). It is produced in the cell from adenosine triphosphate.

DIRECT OXIDATIVE PATHWAY In several tissues (adipose, liver, adrenal, mammary) reduced $NADP^+$ (NADPH)[2] is required to provide the hydrogen and electrons for synthesis of lipid. Thus a certain proportion of glucose 6-phosphate is oxidized by glucose 6-phosphate dehydrogenase to 6-phosphogluconic acid and NADPH, and the former then is oxidized to a compound which loses carbon 1 as CO_2 and produces another NADPH and a pentose phosphate, ribulose 5-phosphate. Through a complicated series of reactions, the pentose phosphates return to the main glycolytic sequence as fructose 6-phosphate or triose phosphate. This metabolic route is significant in lipid-synthesizing tissues such as developing brain, in adipose tissue where it is involved in the conversion of dietary glucose into stored fatty acid, and in certain endocrine glands active in synthesizing steroid hormones.

GLUCOSE 6-PHOSPHATASE This enzyme provides yet another pathway of glucose 6-phosphate metabolism and is located only in those tissues capable of producing glucose: liver and kidney, and also placenta. In the liver, it is the final common pathway for glucose production and opposes the action of the glucose phosphorylating system. The activity of glucose 6-phosphatase in liver is increased in states associated with increased glucose production (diabetes, excess adrenal glucocorticoids) and is decreased in those associated with increased insulin or carbohydrate intake. Again there are two "unidirectional" enzymes at an important site of metabolic control, one for the production and the other for the uptake of glucose by liver. The role of the enzyme in kidney is apparently different and may be related to the process of reabsorption of metabolic intermediates which are converted to glucose 6-phosphate and then are released into the bloodstream. It is clearly not related to the renal tubular

[2] *$NADP^+$ is nicotinamide-adenine dinucleotide phosphate and was formerly called TPN^+ or triphosphopyridine nucleotide.*

reabsorption of glucose since this process does not involve phosphorylation or dephosphorylation. In type I glycogenosis, this enzyme is deficient in body tissues, particularly liver (see Chap. 104), resulting in severe hypoglycemia.

GLUCURONIC ACID PATHWAY An alternative route of glucose 6-phosphate metabolism is the oxidation of carbon 6 of glucose, the glucose condensing with uridine triphosphate (UTP) to form uridine diphosphate glucose (UDPG), similar to its route to glycogen. The glucuronic acid thus formed may become a moiety in many of the complex carbohydrates which serve as structural units (glycoproteins) or may be used to conjugate and detoxify endogenous and exogenous compounds prior to their elimination from the body. As part of this pathway, carbon 6 of UDPG can be cleaved to form CO_2 and a 5-carbon sugar which, through a series of reactions, enters the glycolytic pathway. One of the intermediates in this sequence, 1-xylulose, may accumulate and be excreted in the urine in the benign disease, essential pentosuria, which is due to lack of the enzyme that catalyzes the subsequent step in the sequence (Chap. 89).

SORBITOL PATHWAY Another route of glucose metabolism, not involving prior phosphorylation, is one in which glucose is directly reduced at carbon 1 to a polyalcohol, sorbitol. Much attention has been paid to this metabolic route since the enzyme involved has a high K_m for its substrate, and only in hyperglycemia does much sorbitol accumulate in certain tissues such as the lens of the eye or peripheral nerves. This process has been indicted in certain of the complications of diabetes (Chap. 88).

ACETATE AND PYRUVATE METABOLISM Just as glucose 6-phosphate occupies a position at the crossroads of many metabolic reactions, so do acetate and its closely related products. Pyruvate, the terminus of the previously mentioned pathways, to be further metabolized, must be decarboxylated in the presence of NAD^+ and coenzyme A, thiamine, and lipoic acid to form CO_2 and acetyl CoA (see Chap. 78). Free acetate itself is of only minor importance in nonruminants as a metabolic fuel. It is the acetyl CoA, therefore, which can enter the subsequent metabolic routes.

In the process of fatty acid synthesis, the acetyl CoA accepts CO_2 to form malonyl CoA, and through a series of reactions involving condensations and reductions (NADPH derived from glucose oxidation via the direct oxidative pathway) a 16-carbon, saturated, long-chain fatty acid, palmitic acid, is formed; this can then be extended or unsaturated by other enzyme systems. This sequence takes place primarily in adipose tissue but also in liver and to a lesser extent in other tissues. Another route open to acetyl CoA is the formation of ketone bodies, a reaction which occurs exclusively in liver. There is some question as to whether ketones are formed by direct condensation of two acetyl CoAs or via an intermediate comprising three acetyl CoAs, namely, β-hydroxy-β-methylglutaryl CoA. A third route for acetyl CoA metabolism, via β-hydroxy-β-methylglutaryl CoA, is in the formation of the steroid nucleus and the various compounds derived from it by further metabolic changes, such as cholesterol, steroid hormones, and bile salts. The fourth and perhaps most important route is the condensation of acetyl CoA with oxaloacetate to form citrate, the first step in the sequence of intramitochondrial reactions involving the Krebs (or citric or tricarboxylic acid) cycle, as previously described.

Another pathway of pyruvate metabolism is the direct condensation with CO_2 to form oxaloacetate. This sequence is important in liver and is catalyzed by an enzyme, pyruvic carboxylase. In fasting, or in diabetes mellitus in which fat breakdown to acetyl CoA occurs at a rapid rate, the high level of acetyl CoA accelerates this reaction. Normally oxaloacetate would accept the acetyl CoA to form citrate for oxidation via the citric acid cycle, but this reaction is apparently blocked in the fasting state or in diabetes, and under these conditions the oxaloacetate is phosphorylated and decarboxylated to form phosphoenolpyruvate by another enzyme important in liver, phosphoenolpyruvate carboxykinase. By this sequence, pyruvate is converted to phosphoenolpyruvate and then to glucose, a reaction which cannot proceed directly in this direction because of the energy differential.

HYDROGEN SHUTTLES H atoms (reducing equivalents) can be shunted between different metabolic or structural compartments or pathways which eventually generate ATP. Thus, H atoms can be transferred from the low-efficiency mitochondrial apparatus, increasing the generation of ATP. Any metabolite that is reduced in the cytoplasm to a product which is a substrate for an intramitochondrial oxidation can act as an H carrier. One such system is the α-glycerophosphate-dihydroxyacetone shuttle:

$$\alpha\text{-Glycerophosphate} + \text{NAD}^+ \rightleftharpoons \text{dihydroxyacetone phosphate} + \text{NADH} + \text{H}^+$$

A soluble cytoplasmic α-glycerophosphate dehydrogenase uses NAD^+ to oxidize α-glycerophosphate (αGP) to dihydroxyacetone phosphate (DHAP) (both produced by the glycolytic cycle) and NADH. NADH cannot enter mitochondria to act as a carrier of H equivalents from the cytoplasm, but α-glycerophosphate can enter (Fig. 72-3*B*). Then a distinctly different α-glycerophosphate dehydrogenase within mitochondria oxidizes αGP to DHAP, producing intramitochondrial NADH, which in turn generates mitochondrial ATP. The DHAP then diffuses into cytoplasm to reenter the shuttle cycle.

USES OF ATP A detailed listing of specific reactions into which ATP enters is found in standard biochemical texts. A selected few are of illustrative interest. Studies indicate that the mitochondrion, a self-sufficient apparatus in many ways, transforms energy and also has the capacity to maintain high internal electrolyte concentrations when it is functioning in its energy-producing role. Mitochondria can accumulate K^+, Ca^{++}, Mg^{++}, Mn^{++}, and phosphate ions while oxidizing and phosphorylating, but not when phosphorylation is uncoupled. The purpose of the accumulation is as yet obscure, for Ca^{++} ions, for instance, are themselves uncoupling agents. However, demonstrations that parathyroid hormone is capable of affecting phosphate and Ca^{++} exchanges in mitochondria in vitro are of obvious importance in understanding the mechanism of action of the hormone. The contribution of the osmotic work done by mitochondria toward that of the whole cell is not yet clear.

A major role of ATP in the body is to serve as the ultimate energy source for muscle contraction. The details of the molecular events concerned with this physical process are still a matter for investigation, but ATP is necessary for the relaxation phenomenon, whereby the contracted actomyosin fibrils resume their more elongated form, primed for the next contraction. Indeed, so definite is the association between the use of ATP and muscle contraction that the actomyosin molecule is called an *ATPase.* The dependence of muscle contraction on ATP is reflected in the demands of the myocardium, for instance, for a continued supply of utilizable energy derived from oxidation. The myocardium is supplied with large, intricate mitochondria, and interference with the supply of oxygen by a decrease in blood flow produces noncontracting myocardial areas with differences in electrical potential (see Chap. 229). Such changes probably increase cellular permeability so that enzymes (e.g., lactic dehydrogenase and the transaminases from cytoplasm, and intramitochondrial enzymes such as malic dehydrogenase) leak into the circulation to provide biochemical diagnostic criteria of impaired myocardial function. Biochemical lesions of the myocardium that interfere with the generation of ATP occur in anemia, thyrotoxicosis, and beriberi, and result in a myocardial contractile defect which is not susceptible to the beneficial action of digitalis, ordinarily so effective when the contractile mechanism itself operates at a disadvantage but has an adequate energy supply. Defects in energy transformation in skeletal muscle appear to be present in at least two diseases, as demonstrated by functional and structural changes in muscle mitochondria in patients with thyrotoxicosis and in two reported cases of nonthyrotoxic hypermetabolism.

Another significant use of ATP is the generation of heat to maintain body temperature. In the synthesis of ATP by oxidative phosphorylation, for example, only 60 percent of the energy liberated from oxidation of its substrates is transformed by the mitochondrion to phosphate bond energy. An appreciable portion of the liberated energy is evolved as heat, which assists in maintaining body temperature. When the external environment increases the need for heat production, the body responds with an increased rate of oxygen consumption.

The synthesis of the polymeric compounds that store energy in the body requires ATP, e.g., the condensation of glucose 1-phosphate to form glycogen, of acetyl CoA to form fatty acids, of soluble RNA–amino acid complexes to form polypeptides and proteins, and of nucleosides to form nucleotides.

ENERGY TRANSFORMATION To survive, a species must possess mechanisms whereby it can deposit and store fuel during periods of availability and be able to mobilize this fuel at times of increased need; in addition, it must store and mobilize fuel for the necessary chemical reactions required to maintain the integrity of its structure.

The human body contains numerous organic compounds with energy potential: lipids, carbohydrates, proteins, and nucleic acids. The lipids are by far the most quantitatively important form of storage of fuel, in addition to providing other functions such as insulation of the body as a whole or as essential components in the structure of cell walls, myelin, and other membranes. Carbohydrates serve as a lesser form of fuel storage. Protein serves as the structural basis for all enzymes, contracting elements such as muscle, or supporting structures such as collagen, and in addition as a fuel, or precursor for carbohydrate in the process of gluconeogenesis. Nucleic acids form fundamental components in the hereditary and synthetic mechanisms and are usually not available as fuels. The body can be divided into four main metabolic compartments, adipose tissue, nervous tissue, muscle, and liver.

ADIPOSE TISSUE Adipose tissue is composed of between 60 and 90 percent triglyceride and thus contains 6 to 8 kcal per g total wet tissue. A normal 70-kg male may have 12 kg adipose tissue and thereby a potential fuel reserve of approximately 90,000 kcal, which theoretically could support life for well over 2 months. In obesity, 100 kg adipose tissue may be present—an entire year's supply!

Adipose tissue metabolism (Fig. 72-4) is controlled by many factors, which may be grouped into two general classes, anabolic and catabolic. A rise in blood glucose level following ingestion of carbohydrate stimulates insulin production; insulin directly increases glucose uptake into adipose tissue, where, in the process of lipogenesis, it is metabolized via acetyl CoA into fatty acids, which are then esterified with glycerol to form triglycerides. Thus the individual has converted a less efficient fuel on a weight basis (carbohydrate) to a more efficient form of energy storage (lipid). Some of the ingested glucose may also be converted to glycogen in liver, muscle, and adipose tissue. These carbohydrate stores serve two ancillary purposes: (1) as a temporary storage site during ingestion of large amounts of carbohydrate (until the lipogenetic process can store the energy as fat), and (2) as an emergency store of quickly available glucose for anaerobic glycolysis during periods of stress. The economy of storage of energy as lipid far surpasses that as carbohydrate, since triglyceride is deposited in an extra-aqueous phase, whereas glycogen is stored with water and electrolytes; 1 g glycogen-containing tissue yields only 1 to $1\frac{1}{2}$ kcal, and it is therefore one-fourth to one-sixth as efficient for storage of energy as an equivalent unit of lipid-containing tissue (see Chap. 45, Gain in Weight. Obesity).

Insulin appears to exert other effects on adipose tissue. Following a fatty meal, triglycerides enter the bloodstream in the form of lipoproteins—chylomicrons—via the thoracic duct. They may then enter the liver and be chemically modified and released into the circulation, or they may be directly incorporated into adipose tissue where they are hydrolyzed into free fatty acids and reesterified into triglyceride. These many rearrangements of the originally ingested fat may be the animal's mechanism to ensure that the fat which it stores in its adipose tissue contains the correct number and

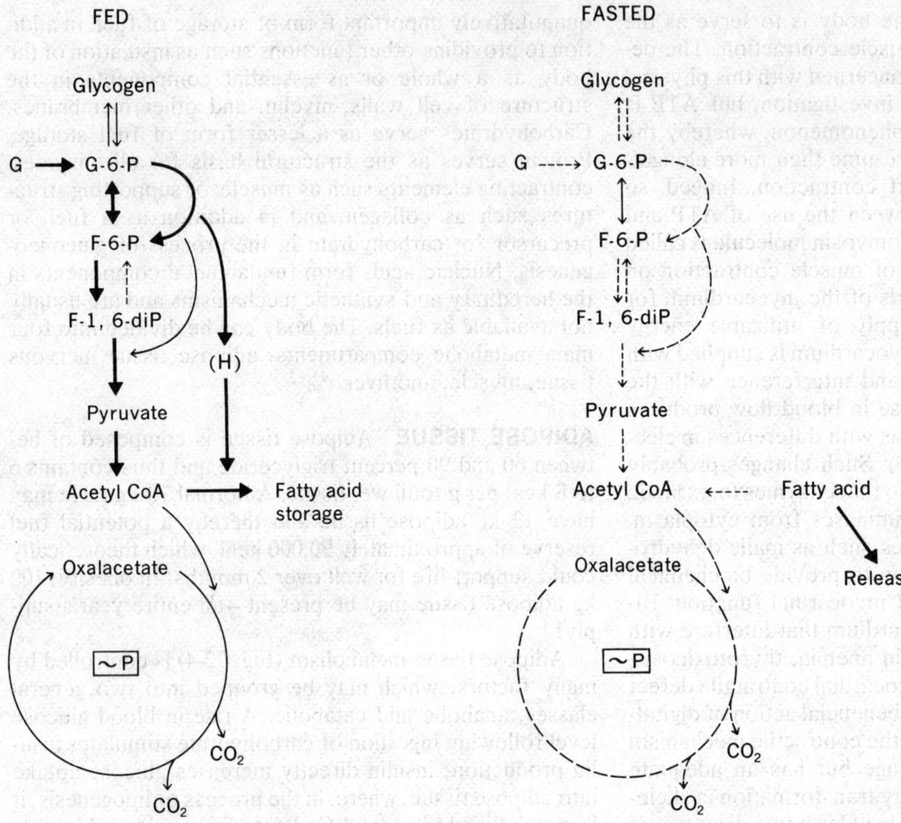

FIGURE 72-4
Comparison of flow of substrate across metabolic pathways in adipose tissue in the fed and fasted state. In the former, glucose (G) is metabolized to acetyl CoA, which is then resynthesized to fat and stored. During fasting, glucose metabolism is limited, and fatty acids are released for fuel for the remainder of the body.

types of fatty acids. Insulin in the fed individual apparently plays an important role in the uptake of circulating triglycerides into adipose tissue, in addition to its role in promoting lipogenesis from glucose.

Fuel stored as adipose tissue triglyceride is released in only one form, free fatty acids. Adipose tissue free fatty acid concentration is in equilibrium with the fatty acid bound to albumin in the circulation; thus, a rise in adipose tissue free fatty acids induces a release of these into the circulation. The level of free acids in adipose tissue is controlled by several factors. Insulin decreases this level by providing increased glucose uptake, which supplies increased glycerol acceptor for esterification of fatty acids in the cell. Insulin also inhibits the breakdown of triglyceride into free fatty acid. Conversely, lack of insulin, as in fasting, increases adipose tissue free fatty acid by a reversal of these processes and thereby augments fatty acid release. Among other substances which increase fatty acid production by adipose tissue are norepinephrine, epinephrine, and growth, thyroid, and adrenal hormones. The action of epinephrine and norepinephrine on free fatty acid mobilization depends on the thyroid status, being increased in hyperthyroidism and decreased or absent in hypothyroidism. The principal physiologic control of free fatty acid release and circulating levels is probably the balance of sympathetic nerve endings producing norepinephrine which causes generation of cyclic AMP (Fig. 72-3) in the adipose cell membrane. Cyclic AMP then activates the intracellular lipolytic system. Insulin, on the other hand, depresses the generation of cyclic AMP and thus inhibits free fatty acid release.

NERVOUS TISSUE Nervous tissues require a continuous supply of glucose (Fig. 72-5). This glucose utilization is independent of insulin, or of glucose concentration (as long as it is adequate), or of the state of nervous activity. Only in severe metabolic derangements producing coma is there a significant decrease in the use of glucose (except for a gradual slight decrease with age probably due to a progressive attrition of neurons). During prolonged starvation, however, and probably in individuals who are consuming a very high fat (ketogenic) diet, the brain may decrease its glucose utilization without loss of function because of its capacity to utilize acetoacetate and β-hydroxybutyrate.

In nervous tissue glucose is totally glycolyzed and then oxidized to CO_2 by the tricarboxylic acid cycle. Thus glucose and oxygen must always be available: if their supply is interrupted, brain function ceases almost immediately. Brain glycogen levels are extremely low and insignificant as an energy source.

MUSCLE Muscle tissue is versatile in that it can utilize several different fuels to support activity (Fig. 72-5). Glucose is readily removed by muscle from the circulating fluids under the stimulus of insulin, although increased muscular activity or anoxia can also increase glucose uptake. The glucose in muscle is readily glycolyzed to lactic acid, and, if there is adequate oxygen, to CO_2 and water. The glucose may also be stored as glycogen to be used as emergency fuel for glycolysis when oxygen is unavailable or relatively inadequate.

Muscle mitochondria also readily utilize fatty acids as fuel. These can come from several sources, from free fatty acids circulating in the blood, having been released from adipose tissue, from fat stored directly in the muscle itself, or possibly from circulating triglyceride derived from the diet or the liver. Whatever the origin, the fatty acid is oxidized completely to CO_2 and water, and it is fat which serves as the major contributor of energy to muscle metabolism.

A third type of fuel for muscle is derived from the liver as a product of the incomplete combustion of fatty acids, namely, acetoacetic and β-hydroxybutyric acids, which, with acetone, form the ketone bodies. These two acids are also completely metabolized to CO_2 and water in muscle and in certain circumstances can provide a major share of muscle fuel.

By mechanisms not yet clarified, muscle selectively metabolizes ketone bodies, then fatty acids, and, as a last resort, glucose. If ketones are unavailable and free fatty acid concentration is low, as after carbohydrate or insulin administration, muscle will then readily metabolize glucose. Conversely, if ketone or fatty acid concentrations are high, glucose metabolism is minimized, even in the presence of insulin, and the glucose which is taken into the tissue is converted to and stored as glycogen.

One major role of muscle is to serve as a storehouse for amino acids. It is now accepted that a primary site of insulin action is in muscle, where insulin stimulates the incorporation of circulating amino acids into muscle protein. This action is biochemically distinct from the effect on glucose. If insulin is lacking, this process is decreased or even reversed, and amino acids are mobilized by proteolysis and release. Adrenocortical hormones oppose the insulin effect. In fasting, amino acids are mobilized from muscle, and during feeding, when insulin increases, amino acids are incorporated into muscle protein. Removal of both insulin and adrenal hormones achieves a new balance, but one without flexibility in either direction.

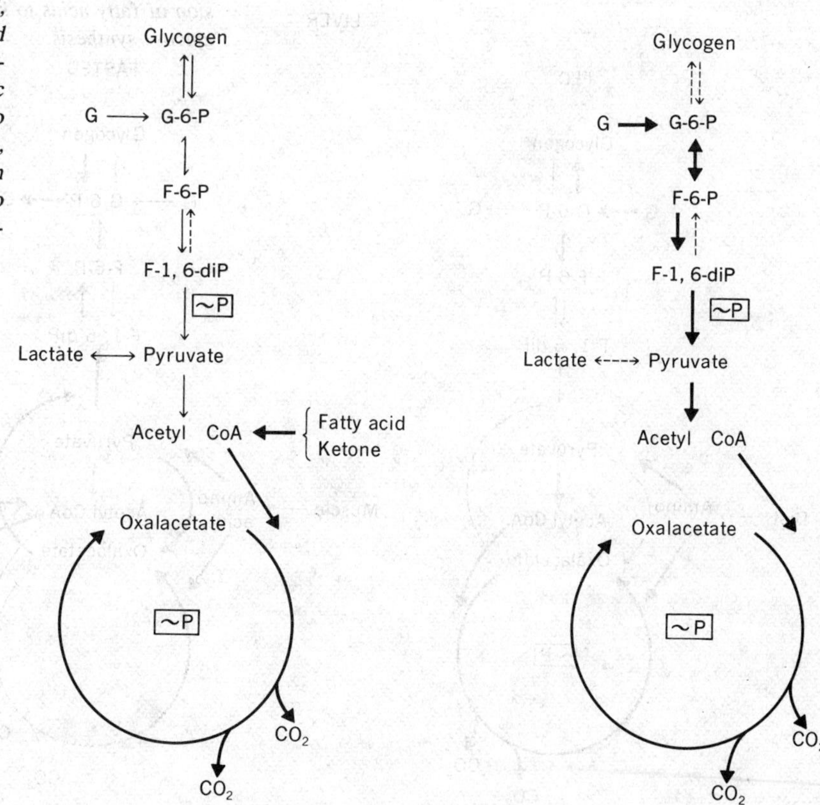

FIGURE 72-5
Muscle tissue utilizes predominantly fatty acid or ketone as a source of fuel, but it is also able to derive limited amounts of energy (~P) from the conversion of glucose to lactate (anaerobic glycolysis). Nervous tissue is able to utilize only glucose as its metabolic fuel, and requires a constant supply of oxygen for total combustion of the glucose to CO_2 in order to derive energy for adequate function.

LIVER Of the four groups of tissues playing a major role in body fuel economy, the liver (Fig. 72-6) serves as the director of traffic and, as such, is metabolically more complicated than adipose, nervous, and muscle tissues. During fasting, it must provide glucose for those tissues requiring glucose for survival (mainly the brain). In contrast, during times of carbohydrate ingestion, it stops producing glucose and, instead, removes and stores glucose as glycogen, transiently if the glycogen reserve is already adequate, or more permanently if the glycogen reserve has been previously depleted by prolonged fasting or other stress.

Unlike peripheral cells, the liver cell is very permeable to glucose, and the concentration of glucose in the blood is approximated by the concentration in the liver cell, being slightly greater if glucose is being produced by the liver and slightly less if glucose is being removed. The net flow of glucose inside the liver cell into and out of the metabolically activated pool of glucose, glucose 6-phosphate, is a function of two enzymes present in liver, glucokinase and glucose 6-phosphatase. The activity of the former is increased by insulin or carbohydrate feeding, and that of the latter by fasting, insulin insufficiency, or adrenal steroids. Thus the activities of these two opposing systems direct the net flow of glucose into and out of the liver, and exercise control over the concentration of glucose in the circulating fluids.

Liver is also unique in possessing other enzymes which are located at metabolic control sites in the sequence of reactions between amino acids and glucose. These enzymes increase in activity during times of increased gluconeogenesis, as in association with early fasting, diabetes, or adrenal steroid administration, and are decreased by carbohydrate feeding or insulin administration.

During fasting, the liver must provide glucose for tissues requiring this fuel, primarily brain, but also spinal cord, peripheral nerve, leukocytes, erythrocytes, renal medulla, and probably others. This it does by synthesizing new glucose (gluconeogenesis) from glycogenic amino acids released into the circulation from muscle, and, to a lesser extent, from lactate or pyruvate returning to the liver from peripheral tissues, as well as from glycerol arising from lipolysis in adipose tissue. Normally liver contains only 80 to 100 g glycogen, about one-half a day's supply of carbohydrate, should gluconeogenesis not be stimulated to provide the glucose needed by the organism. The liver in a briefly fasted normal man produces approximately 180 g glucose daily, of which about 144 g is oxidized by brain to CO_2 and water and 36 g is returned as lactate and pyruvate. The bulk of this glucose is derived from glycogen between meals and during the usual overnight fast. But if man is deprived of food for a more prolonged period, approximately 10 g glycogen is conserved for emergency glycolysis, and blood glucose concentration is then maintained by gluconeogenesis.

FIGURE 72-6
As described in the text, the liver in the fed animal stores glucose as glycogen and derives its own energy from amino acid metabolism. During fasting, its energy (~P) is derived from the conversion of fatty acids to ketone, and amino acids are diverted into glucose synthesis.

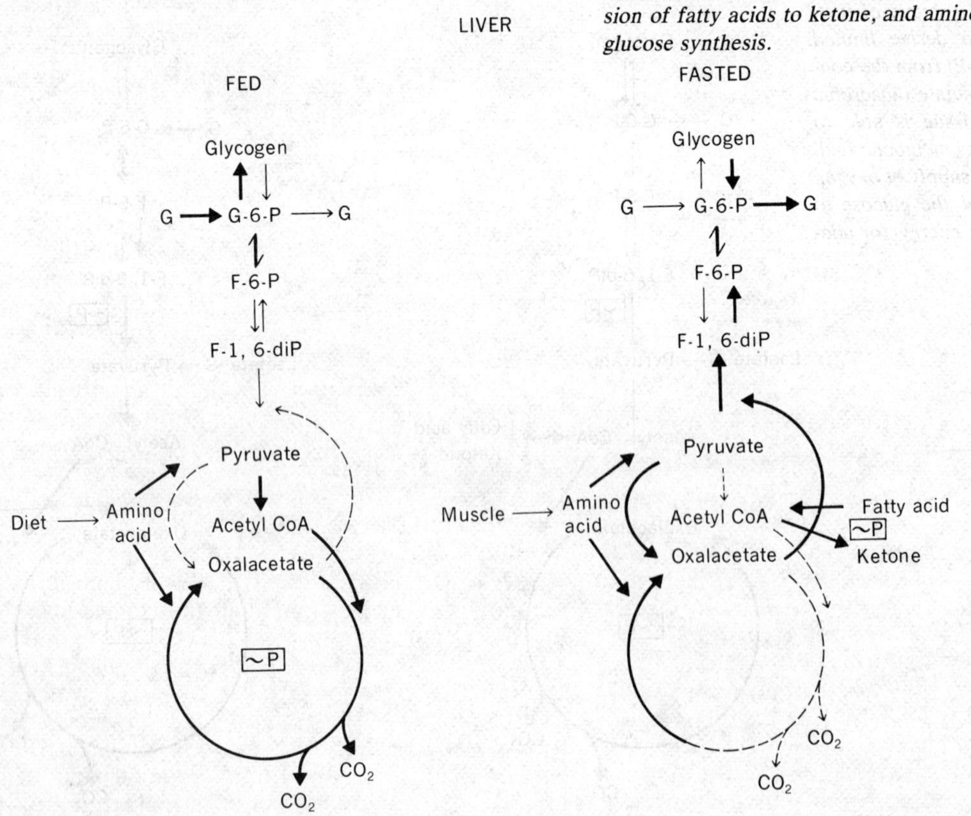

The liver in the normally fed individual mainly uses amino acid as its source of fuel. During fasting, the amino acid which is presented to the liver is diverted, for reasons of economy, into glucose synthesis, and the liver now uses to meet for its own needs the energy derived from the partial oxidation of fatty acids to ketone bodies, from which one-third of the total potential energy of the fatty acid is derived. Thus gluconeogenesis, amino acid metabolism (and therefore urea production), and ketone body production are intimately related.

When the animal is fed, liver metabolism is grossly altered through a number of complicated mechanisms. Gluconeogenesis ceases, those amino acids which enter the liver are metabolized, providing the needed energy for the liver's own metabolic processes, and ketone production ceases. The level of free fatty acids in the circulation falls, since their release from adipose tissue is inhibited by insulin. The liver, however, continues to remove about one-fourth of the total turnover of free fatty acids, but now, since its own energy is adequately provided by amino acid oxidation via its citric acid cycle, the liver esterifies these free fatty acids and returns them as triglyceride to the periphery instead of converting them to ketone bodies. In other words, during fasting, amino acid carbon is diverted into gluconeogenesis, and since the liver's own energy needs are met primarily by ketogenesis, the citric acid cycle of the liver assumes a minor role in the production of energy. During feeding, the citric acid cycle predominates, amino acids are deaminated and their products are oxidized via the cycle, and ketone production essentially ceases.

TOTAL MAN Normal man readily adapts to nutritional and environmental changes by altering hormone levels and responsive metabolic pathways, thereby maintaining a finely regulated "internal environment." Thus homeostasis is closely preserved in the face of diverse nutritional and metabolic alterations such as feeding or fasting, during exercise and acute or chronic stress, whether the stress is physical, as in trauma or infection, or emotional. Several of these states with direct clinical application are discussed below.

THE FASTED STATE In normal postabsorptive man, blood glucose concentration is maintained at approximately 80 mg per 100 ml, with hepatic production equaling utilization, mainly by brain, which oxidizes 100 mg glucose per minute to CO_2 and H_2O. Interruption of brain substrate metabolism by low glucose concentration, by a decrease in circulation, or by a decrease in available oxygen results in dysfunction within minutes of deprivation and in irreversible damage if the deprivation is prolonged. The highest centers usually reflect the metabolic defect first, as evidenced by bizarre behavior, frequently with signs and symptoms of epinephrine discharge (palpitations, cold skin, sweatiness, and piloerection). Unconsciousness follows, and eventually, if the substrate or oxygen availability becomes more restricted, respiratory arrest and death occur (see Chap. 90).

The maintenance of circulating glucose concentration is a most important homeostatic process. Between meals this regulation is achieved mainly by hepatic glycogenolysis. However, since total liver glycogen amounts to 80 to 100 g, hepatic glycogen synthesis and storage begins soon after a meal has been ingested in order to replete the glycogen used between meals. But after more prolonged fasting, as occurs overnight, glucose levels begin to be directly maintained by gluconeogensis as glycogen stores become depleted.

Tissues other than brain, such as red cells, renal medulla, and some smooth muscle, also use glucose as fuel, but, lacking mitochondria for terminal oxidation of glucose to CO_2, derive their energy from glycolysis of the glucose to lactate, returning the latter back into the bloodstream for removal by liver (and kidney) and reincorporation into glucose (the Cori cycle). Thus overall glucose production is slightly greater than that needed by brain, but terminal oxidation of glucose to CO_2 is mainly by this organ.

In the postabsorptive state, glucose is largely excluded from tissues other than brain. Muscle and adipose tissue, which, with brain, are the main glucose consumers in the fed state, markedly diminish their glucose utilization. If the fasting continues for more than a day, glucose is almost totally excluded from these tissues. Instead, muscle uses free fatty acids liberated from adipose tissue, and, should the starvation be of several days duration, uses them both directly and indirectly as ketoacids formed by the partial oxidation and degradation of the fatty acids by liver.

The glucose derived from gluconeogensis is synthesized partly from returning lactate (Cori cycle), partly from glycerol released from the adipose tissue, and mainly from amino acids released from muscle (Fig. 72-7). The overall control appears to be insulin, with glucagon possibly playing a significant secondary role. As glucose levels fall, there is decreased insulin release from the pancreas and, since the half-life of insulin is 10 min, insulin levels fall accordingly. Muscle proteolysis is very sensitive to low levels of insulin, while high levels of insulin slow this process and thereby inhibit amino acid formation and release. As shown in Fig. 72-7, a decrease in insulin as occurs after an overnight fast initiates a release of amino acids from muscle to liver. Liver, in the presence of low levels of insulin and above-normal levels of glucagon, readily converts amino acids into glucose. In fact, early in fasting or simply between meals, it is this bihormonal shift which mobilizes liver glycogen as the first mechanism for the maintenance of blood glucose levels.

STARVATION, MORE PROLONGED Brain in an average-sized individual consumes one-third to one-fourth of the total calories, or about 500 kcal per day. In order to support this rate of glucose consumption by gluconeogenesis from muscle amino acids in prolonged starvation, mobilization of the major share of total body protein over several weeks would be required, an event incompatible with survival. As mentioned above, part of the fatty acids released from adipose tissue are metabolized in liver to keto acids and transported by the blood to muscle. As the level of acetoacetate and β-hydroxybutyrate, the principal keto acids, rise in the blood, brain progressively oxidizes them as fuel and reduces its glucose consumption accordingly. The net effect is a decreased glucose requirement to 20 to 30 mg instead of 100 mg per min. Thus muscle nitrogen is spared and survival is markedly prolonged. The levels of acetoacetate and β-hydroxybutyrate in blood rise to 1.5 and 6 mM respectively, and HCO_3- is reduced accordingly, resulting in a mild but tolerable metabolic acidosis, in marked contrast to the uncontrolled diabetic in whom these organic acids can result in levels of 15 to 20 mM due to overproduction and possibly underutilization as well.

Starvation and protein-calorie malnutrition are further discussed in Chap. 76.

Small carbohydrate intake If one administers 100 mg glucose per min to normal man, the small increase in glucose concentration provokes increased secretion of insulin, and the resulting elevated level, in turn, suppresses muscle proteolysis and amino acid release, liver gluconeogenesis, and keto acid production. Thus, by providing exogenous substrate for brain, liver glucose production is decreased. The net result is a marked sparing of muscle protein; however, some proteolysis and irreversible metabolism of essential amino acids takes place to a small extent. Nevertheless, the amount of muscle protein spared by this carbohydrate administration may be crucial to preservation of effective coughing and clearing of the tracheobronchial tree, in other words, the difference between survival and death. Thus any patient not eating should receive 100 to 150 g glucose daily in order to minimize muscle catabolism until he can again eat.

Large carbohydrate intake Should the influx of carbohydrate surpass that needed by brain, the next priority is the displacement of fatty acid oxidation by glucose, particularly in muscle. This displacement is achieved by the yet higher level of insulin suppressing free fatty acid release from adipose tissue, and circulating levels of free fatty acids decrease accordingly. At the same time glucose forms a greater share of muscle substrate. If the carbohydrate load surpasses the total caloric needs to maintain metabolic processes, the excess glucose has two available metabolic routes. One is to be converted into and stored as glycogen in muscle or liver and the other is to be taken up into adipose tissue, converted into fat, and stored as such. Since normal man usually eats meals rather than nibbling around the clock, lipogenesis and fat storage occurs with each meal, with lipid mobilization occurring between meals. Variations in the concentration of insulin appear to be the message signaling the tissues to either store or mobilize fuel. Inability to achieve a high insulin level postprandially results in delayed uptake of metabolic fuel, i.e., glucose intolerance.

Oral vs. parenteral carbohydrate intake A given amount of carbohydrate, if ingested orally, results in a greater rise in insulin levels when compared with the same amount infused parenterally and, subsequently, in a greater capacity to remove the glucose and other fuels such as amino acid and triglyceride from the circulation. This higher insulin level is probably due to one or more not definitely characterized hormones released from the gut mucosa, which in turn sensitize the beta cells to produce more insulin. Overproduction of these factors may play a role in the postprandial hypoglycemia which

FIGURE 72-7

Quantitative estimation of the flow of metabolic fuels by a normal fasted man for a period of 24 hr, utilizing 1800 kcal.

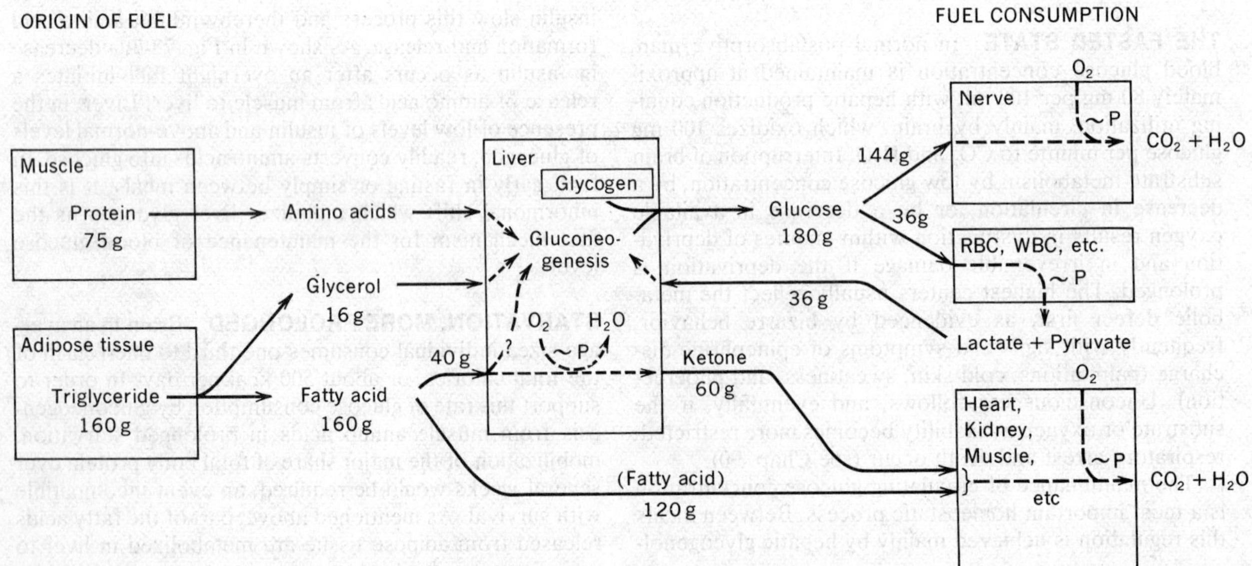

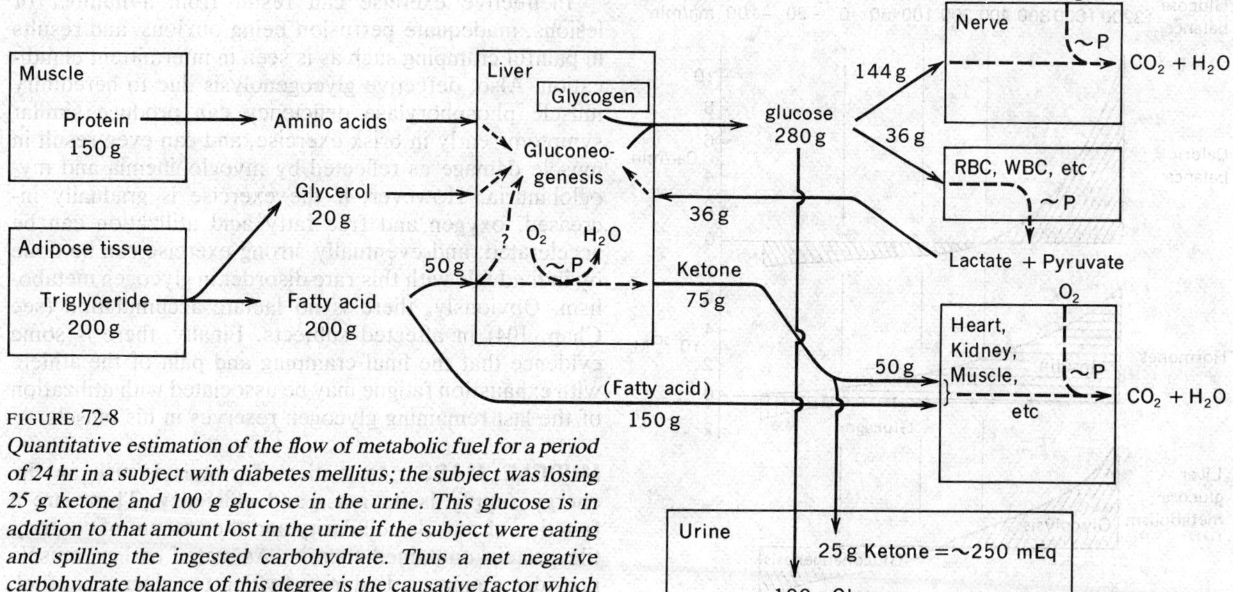

FIGURE 72-8
Quantitative estimation of the flow of metabolic fuel for a period of 24 hr in a subject with diabetes mellitus; the subject was losing 25 g ketone and 100 g glucose in the urine. This glucose is in addition to that amount lost in the urine if the subject were eating and spilling the ingested carbohydrate. Thus a net negative carbohydrate balance of this degree is the causative factor which necessitates increased gluconeogenesis and the resultant ketosis. Net energy loss is 2400 kcal.

may complicate gastric surgery and possibly in other hypoglycemic states (see Chap. 90).

INSULIN DEFICIENCY During fasting, the low insulin level (Fig. 72-7) initiates release of peripheral fuels and augments the capacity for liver gluconeogenesis. The latter is also stimulated by the associated increase in glucagon secretion. Should the insulin be pathologically low, due to defective beta cells, or to resistance to the insulin released, an unopposed release of fuel would occur as well as unopposed gluconeogenesis, hyperglycemia, ketonemia, and all the symptomatology of diabetic ketoacidosis (Fig. 72-8) (Chap. 88). On the other hand, if there is a low but significant amount of insulin, glycogenolysis and inadequate removal of ingested or infused glucose would result in hyperglycemia, glycosuria, and dehydration without a significant degree of ketoacidosis, as demonstrated in the syndrome of nonketotic hyperosmolar coma.

TRAUMA AND INFECTION During stress, be it physical, metabolic, or even emotional, the associated sympathetic activity results in beta cell suppression as well as increased mobilization of fatty acids from adipose tissue and glucose from liver glycogenolysis. Thus a diabetic type of metabolism may occur, resulting in delayed or inadequate removal of circulating fuels and, if severe, in hyperglycemia of sufficient degree to produce hyperosmolar coma. This may be iatrogenically induced in severely ill subjects overenthusiastically given carbohydrate. Another sequela of trauma or severe infection, such as peritonitis or septicemia, is accentuated mobilization of peripheral protein reserves, the "hypercatabolic" state. This process is very resistant to physiologic levels of insulin by an as yet uncharacterized mechanism, and may lead to such severe protein catabolism that the patient dies within several weeks because of ineffective respiratory musculature.

EXERCISE The energy for skeletal muscle during exercise is provided by several metabolic fuels. First there is the expected use of the small intracellular depot of ATP, producing ADP, which is rapidly replenished to ATP by creatine phosphate, until generation of substrate-derived ATP for glycolysis can be initiated. Thus the first few contractions of strong exercise are supported; next there is rapid glycogenolysis due to activation of the phosphorylase system, and ATP and lactic acid are generated from anaerobic glycolysis. Aiding this is augmented glucose uptake from the extracellular fluid which also ends up as lactic acid, later to be made into glucose by liver (Cori cycle) or to be oxidized to CO_2 by other tissues. The brisker the exercise, the more lactate produced and later to be consumed (as part of the "oxygen debt" needed to recharge the entire system back to its prior homeostatic state). In certain animals there are muscles rich in glycogen which can contract rapidly and anaerobically with much force, the so-called white or "twitch" muscles. Chicken breast is an excellent example.

With more sustained exercise, blood flow brings free

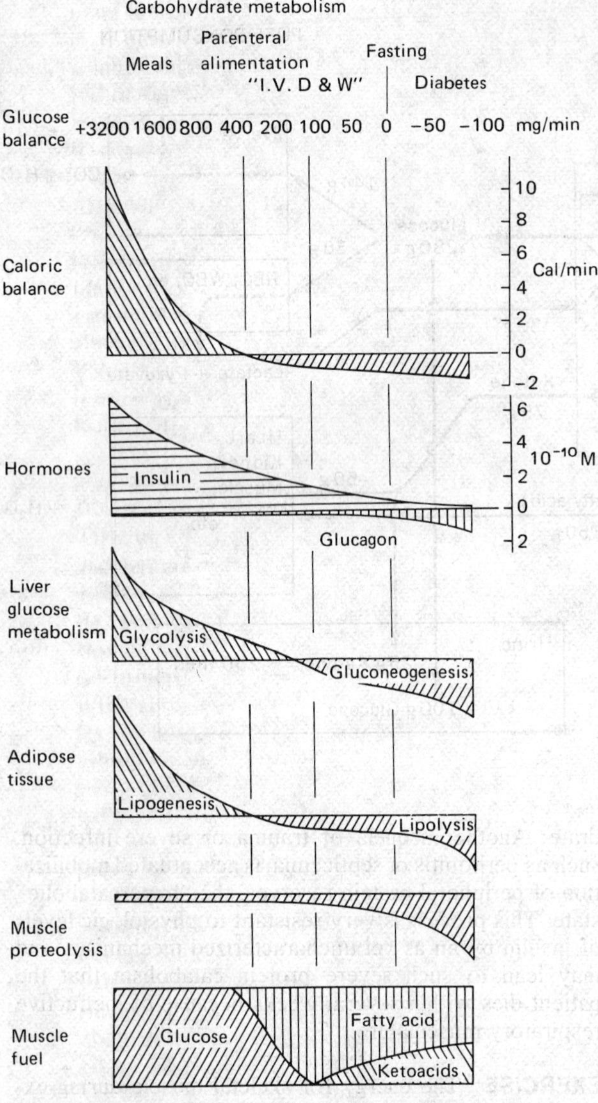

FIGURE 72-9
The spectrum of carbohydrate balance in man, progressing from a large carbohydrate-containing meal to a net negative carbohydrate loss as occurs in uncontrolled diabetes. Also shown are the interrelations and metabolic states of certain tissues as altered by the hormonal and substrate changes. Glucose balance refers to the rate of glucose entering or leaving the body. Thus with large meals, 3,200 mg per min may be absorbed. In fasting, the net balance is 0. In diabetes, there may be a net negative balance due to glucosuria.

fatty acids and oxygen to the muscle for aerobic metabolism, and ATP is produced by mitochondria. Glucose uptake and some glycogenolysis may still ensue, but the bulk of ATP is from fatty acid–derived acetyl CoA metabolized over the citric acid cycle. Again, in certain animals, muscles for long-sustained activity are rich in blood supply, myoglobin, and cytochromes, thanks to the numerous mitochondria, and thus the muscles are "red." In man, muscles are mixtures of these two types of fibers, again leading to a greater physical versatility as compared with lower animals.

With either brief or sustained exercise, the sympathetic nervous system plays an inportant role, initiating free fatty acid release from adipose tissue by augmenting generation of cyclic AMP and, in turn, triglyceride lipolysis. There is also an increase in glucagon which stimulates liver glycogenolysis to provide glucose.

Ineffective exercise can result from a number of lesions, inadequate perfusion being obvious, and results in painful cramping such as is seen in intermittent claudication. Also, defective glycogenolysis due to hereditary muscle phosphorylase deficiency can produce similar symptoms early in brisk exercise, and can even result in muscle damage as reflected by myoglobinemia and myoglobinuria. However, if the exercise is gradually increased, oxygen and free fatty acid utilization can be accelerated, and eventually strong exercise can be done by individuals with this rare disorder in glycogen metabolism. Obviously, there is no lactate accumulation (see Chap. 104) in affected subjects. Finally, there is some evidence that the final cramping and pain of the athlete with exhaustion fatigue may be associated with utilization of the last remaining glycogen reserves in his muscle.

MUSCLE MASS As critical for muscle use as the energy supply is its mass and efficiency. These are a function of muscle cellularity and the amount of contractile protein contained therein. As stated earlier, muscle provides amino acids during fasting for glucogenic fuel, and this process is a function of low insulin levels. During feeding, the higher insulin level promotes resynthesis of the muscle protein catabolized previously. Thus total muscle nitrogen is integrated into the fuel needs of the body as a whole. But for each single muscle, its own content of contractile protein per cell is a function of its use. An unused muscle atrophies in spite of ample insulin and amino acid. This is particularly true of denervated muscle. Conversely, even in the face of overall body catabolism, a given muscle can maintain its mass, or even undergo exercise hypertrophy. The clinical extrapolation is to keep essential muscles, such as the intercostals and diaphragm, active in a debilitated individual by encouraging coughing, even with tracheal suction as a stimulus, and as much other physical exercise as tolerated. Anabolic steroids, as a means of maintaining or augmenting muscle nitrogen, are virtually ineffective as compared with the effect of exercise itself.

The spectrum of carbohydrate balance in man is presented diagrammatically in Fig. 72-9.

REFERENCES

CAHILL GF JR: Physiology of insulin in man. Diabetes 20:799, 1971

HAVEL RJ: Caloric homeostasis and disorders of fuel transport. N Engl J Med 287:1186, 1972

RENOLD AE et al: Diabetes mellitus, in *The Metabolic Basis of Inherited Disease*, 3d ed., eds JB Stanbury et al, New York: McGraw-Hill, 1972, p. 83

73 NUTRITIONAL REQUIREMENTS

THEODORE B. VAN ITALLIE
HAROLD SANDSTEAD
GEORGE V. MANN

Only about 47 of the thousands of substances involved in human metabolism are essential; that is, these materials must be supplied by the diet. All the remaining compounds can be derived through the metabolic processes of the body. Requirements for the essential nutrients vary among and within species, and are influenced by differing physiologic circumstances such as growth, pregnancy, lactation, and level of physical activity. The nature of the diet itself (for example, the relative proportions of fat and carbohydrate) can affect requirements for certain nutrients. Because of these considerations, definitions of nutritional requirements can only be approximations.

The major nutrients, fat, protein, and carbohydrate, were extensively studied during the latter portion of the nineteenth century. Subsequently, certain of the macrominerals indispensable for growth and health were identified. Systematic studies were begun about 1900 by F. G. Hopkins and E. V. McCollum and were extended by H. C. Sherman, H. Steenbock, the Mellanbys, C. Elvejhem, and many others. Laboratory animals or human subjects were fed chemically defined diets; when growth failure or other signs of deficiency appeared, food concentrates or synthetic materials were added to the diet to ascertain which essential nutrient had been lacking. This method made it possible to produce in animals disorders which mimic human disease and to isolate essential organic factors (vitamins). The vitamins were first named alphabetically and then, when they were identified, were given chemical names. One of two or more similar chemical compounds capable of fulfilling a specific vitamin function is known as a *vitamer*.

Since 1943, the Food and Nutrition Board of the National Research Council–National Academy of Sciences has published formulations of daily nutrient intakes that are judged to be adequate for the maintenance of good nutrition in the population of the United States. These formulations have been designated "recommended daily dietary allowances" (RDA) (Table 73-1). With the exception of calories, the RDA allow a margin of safety, often generous, for individual variations. Accordingly, individuals whose diets do not supply the RDA are not necessarily malnourished, nor should diets be judged "poor" simply because they do not precisely meet RDA standards.

The tabulations in the RDA represent value judgments based on the existing knowledge of nutritional science. The physiologic and biochemical bases for the RDA vary for each specific nutrient. In general, the procedure has been to identify the minimum requirement and then provide an additional allowance sufficient to take care of individual variation. In some cases this has entailed adding to the observed mean twice the standard deviation of the distribution of minimal requirement for the subjects measured.

The RDA should not be mistaken for another widely used reference table published, with periodic revisions, since 1941 by the Food and Drug Administration. This is called the "minimum daily requirements" (MDR). It was intended for use in the regulation of food products in commerce. To avoid unnecessary confusion between the RDA and the MDR, the Food and Drug Administration is phasing out MDR in favor of RDA.

TABLE 73-1
Recommended daily dietary allowances of Food and Nutrition Board

						Fat-soluble vitamins			Water-soluble vitamins							Minerals				
	Age,[1] years	Weight, kg	Height, cm	Kcal[2]	Protein, g	A[5], IU	D, IU	E, IU	Ascorbic acid, mg	Folic acid, mg	Niacin,[3] mg Eq.	Riboflavin, mg	Thiamine, mg	B_6, mg	B_{12}, μg	Ca, g	P, g	I_2, μg	Fe, mg	Mg, mg
Infants[4]	0–19	4–9	55–72	kg × 120	kg × 2	1,500	400	5	35	0.05	6	0.4	0.3	0.3	1.5	0.6	0.5	40	10	100
Children	1–10	12–28	81–131	1100–2200	25–40	2,500	400	10	40	0.2	10	1.0	0.7	1.0	4	0.8	0.8	80	10	200
Adolescent																				
Male	10–18	35–59	140–170	2500–3000	45–60	5,000	400	20	50	0.4	18	1.4	1.2	1.8	5	1.4	1.4	135	18	350
Female	10–18	35–54	142–160	2250–2300	50–55	5,000	400	20	50	0.4	15	1.4	0.9	1.8	5	1.3	1.3	115	18	350
Adult[6]																				
Male	18 up	67–70	175 up	2800	60 up	5,000		30	60	0.4	17	1.7	1.0	2.0	5	0.8	0.8	130	10	350
Female	18 up	58 up	163 up	2000	55 up	5,000		25	55	0.4	12	1.7	0.8	2.0	5	0.8	0.8	100	18	300
Pregnant				+200	65	6,000	400	30	60	0.8	15	1.8	1.0	2.5	8	+0.4	+0.4	125	18	450
Lactating				+1000	75	8,000	400	30	60	0.5	20	2.0	1.2	2.5	6	+0.5	+0.5	150	18	450

[1] *Age ranges are more abridged here than in the original table.*
[2] *Calorie adjustment must be made for size and expenditure.*
[3] *Niacin equivalents include preformed niacin and tryptophan, 60 mg being the equivalent of 1 mg niacin.*
[4] *Allowances for calcium, thiamine, riboflavin, and niacin are proportional to calorie requirement.*
[5] *Assuming one-fifth from preformed vitamin A and four-fifths from beta-carotene.*
[6] *These allowances will include a range of individual requirements for persons living in the United States under usual environmental conditions. They can be achieved with a variety of common foods which will also supply other nutrients for which human requirements are uncertain.*
SOURCE: *Adapted from Recommended Dietary Allowances, National Research Council, Food and Nutrition Board, 7th ed., Publication 1694.*

TABLE 73-2
Essential nutrients for human beings*

Elements	Macro	Na, K, Ca, Mg, P, Cl, S, C, H, O, N
	Micro	Fe, Zn, Cu, Mn, Co, I
	Probable	Cr, Ni, V, Sn, Mo, Se, F
Vitamins	Water-soluble	Thiamine, riboflavin, vitamin B_6, niacin, folacin, pantothenic acid, cobalamin, biotin, ascorbic acid
	Fat-soluble	Vitamin A–carotene, vitamins D, E, and K, essential fatty acids (linoleic, arachidonic)
Nitrogenous	Essential amino acids	Lysine, threonine, leucine, isoleucine, methionine, tryptophan, valine, phenylalanine (for children, histidine)
	Nonessential nitrogen	

* *Choline is not considered a vitamin. When optimal amounts of cobalamine, serine, and methionine are available, choline is synthesized from them.*

The essential elements and compounds necessary in the human diet are listed in Table 73-2. The essentiality of a nutrient varies according to species, the stage of growth and development, and metabolic circumstances. Ascorbic acid is necessary for primates and certain rodents and birds because they lack the enzyme necessary for one step in the formation of ascorbic acid from glucose. The essential amino acids illustrate the relativity of the term *essential.* Histidine is essential for growing children but probably not for human adults. Glycine and L-cystine are essential for chickens during periods of feather growth but not at other times.

DIET COMPOSITION The energy for resting metabolism, synthesis of body tissues, physical activity, excretory processes, and for maintenance of thermal balance is supplied by the major foodstuffs, carbohydrate, fat, and protein. In the United States approximately 15 percent of dietary calories is derived from protein, 40 percent from fat, and 45 percent from carbohydrate. A variable portion of dietary protein is used for anabolic purposes, the remainder contributes to the energy pool. The proportion of fat and protein in the American diet has tended to increase since 1900 as the contribution of carbohydrates, especially the polysaccharides from foods such as potatoes and cereal flours, has decreased. Although total carbohydrate intake has decreased by almost 25 percent, the proportion of sugars and syrups within the carbohydrate category has increased by 25 percent.

The human organism has a remarkable versatility in adapting to different food mixtures. Thus, the hunters and pastoralists of the world subsist on meat or milk diets which contain less than 50 g carbohydrate daily, and many agriculturists and vegetarians maintain reasonable health on diets with only 30 to 40 g protein and 25 g or less fat daily. It is important to recognize that dietary adequacy can be obtained with widely different fuel mixtures (Fig. 73-1). By *adequacy* is meant the level of nutrition that permits achievement of the genetic potential of the individual.

CALORIES In the estimation of energy requirements, the RDA uses the concept of the *reference man* and *woman.* The reference man is twenty-two years old and weighs 70 kg; the reference woman also is twenty-two years old and weighs 58 kg. Both are assumed to maintain a "light" activity level (120 to 239 kcal per hr) in an environmental temperature averaging 20°C (68°F). Adjustments must be made when individuals or population averages differ from the reference man or woman in body size, age, or activity. It is known that energy requirements diminish progressively after early adulthood. A proportion of this decline results from the decrease of resting metabolism with age (2 percent per decade); however, the degree of reduction of physical activity associated with aging can only be estimated. The energy cost of physical activity is slightly increased in an ambient temperature below 14°C (57°F) or above 30°C (86°F).

Pregnancy requires an extra allowance of about 40,000 kcal; thus, during pregnancy a daily additional allowance not exceeding 200 kcal is believed adequate. During lactation, an average milk yield of about 850 ml per day is assumed, an amount which requires an additional allowance of about 1000 kcal per day. The major variable affecting energy needs in adults is physical activity. The cost of physical activity covers a wide range. At very high levels of activity, which are necessarily intermittent, energy output may be thirteen times that expended while sitting in a chair. Most of the mild to moderate obesity that develops insidiously with advancing age can be accounted for by the decreases in resting metabolic rate and voluntary energy expenditure that occur without a corresponding reduction in calorie intake. Many obese adolescents and adults are relatively inactive physically. Cultural attitudes and technical developments in the Western world have dramatically decreased the energy expenditure associated with most occupations and have reduced the energy output incident to daily living. Thus, for the average person, an increase in activity level requires a positive effort in a setting which often tends to discourage physical exercise. The consequences of such physical inactivity are obesity and health problems of many kinds, possibly including an increased risk of coronary heart disease.

CARBOHYDRATE With the exception of ascorbic acid, there are no carbohydrates known to be essential in the human diet. However, the body requires carbohydrate as an energy source for the brain and for other specialized purposes. If these needs are not met by carbohydrate from the diet, the body must draw first on its very limited stores of liver glycogen and then use protein from dietary and endogenous sources to maintain glucose homeostasis. Although it is not possible to define a precise minimum requirement for carbohydrate, adults accustomed to normal diets tend to exhibit increasing hyperketonemia and ketonuria as the daily carbohydrate intake is reduced below 75 g per day (see Chap. 72). Nevertheless, adaptation to a diet very low in carbohydrate is possible (Fig. 73-1).

After infancy, a relatively high proportion of nonwhite

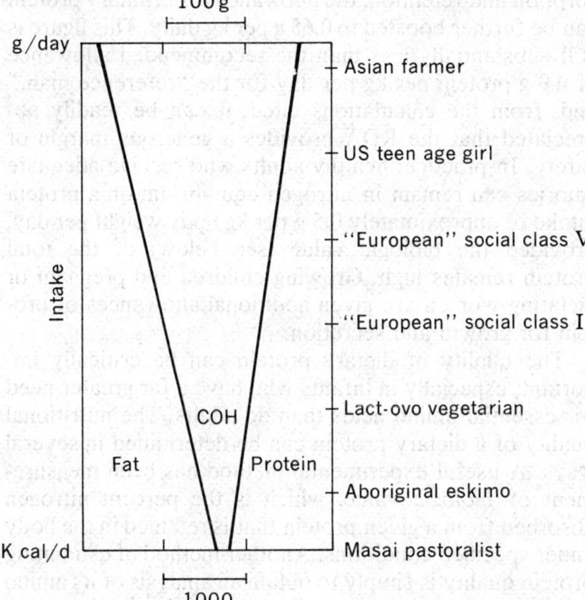

FIGURE 73-1
The range of dietary mixtures compatible with good nutrition encountered in various groups of individuals. Social classes I to V are those designated to the Registrar General of the United Kingdom in accordance with socioeconomic status. Class I refers to professional persons, class V to unskilled laborers.

populations and a considerably smaller proportion of Caucasoids are deficient in the intestinal enzyme lactase and may exhibit a relative intolerance to milk. For the most part, such intolerance is not clinically serious and, in children, may be largely circumvented by taking smaller quantities of milk more frequently. There is evidence that a diet high in sucrose, particularly in the form of candy, may promote dental caries. Moreover, certain individuals with endogenous hypertriglyceridemia (type IV) often exhibit a decrease in plasma triglyceride concentrations when the proportion of carbohydrate in the diet is appreciably reduced. Some investigators believe that simple (refined) carbohydrates are more likely to induce hypertriglyceridemia in susceptible individuals than isocaloric amounts of the more complex polysaccharides of cereals, potatoes, flour, rice, and other vegetables. With these possible exceptions, there are no persuasive reasons to believe that simple carbohydrates in the diet are damaging or predispose to disease.

FAT Dietary fat furnishes 9 kcal per g, while carbohydrate and protein provide 4 kcal per g. Fats add palatability to food, and diets very low in fat tend to be unappetizing and unsatisfying. Along with the gradual rise that has occurred in the total fat content of the diet in the United States there has been a relative decrease of about 10 percent in the proportion derived from animal sources and a corresponding increase in that from vegetable sources. It has been demonstrated repeatedly that manipulation of the fatty acid pattern of the diet can have a pronounced effect on the plasma cholesterol concentration. A diet with a high content of long-chain saturated fatty acids tends to raise the plasma cholesterol level, while one relatively rich in polyunsaturated fatty acids tends to decrease cholesterol. If dietary cholesterol also is rigidly restricted, a further reduction in the plasma cholesterol level may occur. Because approximately two-thirds of men and a smaller proportion of women in the United States maintain plasma concentrations of cholesterol that are thought to be undesirably high in terms of risk of coronary disease (greater than 220 mg per 100 ml), a number of health agencies have recommended that measurement of the plasma lipid "profile" be a routine part of all health maintenance examinations and that, where indicated, dietary modifications designed to lower plasma levels of cholesterol and triglycerides be instituted (see Chap. 244).

Two polyunsaturated fatty acids, arachadonic acid and its precursor, linoleic acid, have been shown to be essential nutrients for laboratory animals and for infants. The prostaglandins appear to derive from arachadonic acid. If the ratio of triene to tetraene fatty acids in serum is used as an index of essential fatty acid deficiency, the minimum requirement of infants appears to be near 2 percent of the caloric intake. The possibility that essential fatty acid (EFA) deficiency can occur in adults would seem remote in view of the extensive stores of linoleate normally present in human adipose tissue. Nevertheless, at least one case of presumed EFA deficiency in an adult has been reported.

Food fat serves as the vehicle for absorption of the fat-soluble vitamins; notably, vitamins A, D, E, and K. Thus, when the diet remains very low in fat or when steatorrhea is chronically present, deficiencies of the fat-soluble nutrients, particularly of vitamin A and carotenes, are much more likely to occur.

In contrast to the long-chain fatty acids that predominate in nature, fatty acids with eight and ten carbons enter the circulation via the portal system and appear to require only minimal amounts of pancreatic lipase and bile salts for their efficient digestion and absorption. Thus, triglycerides composed of these "medium-chain" fatty acids are useful in the nutritional management of patients with chylous fistulas and a variety of forms of intestinal malabsorption.

PROTEIN Amino acids Protein is a dietary essential because of its component amino acids. Food proteins contain various combinations of the 20 natural amino acids, of which at least eight are essential for adult man. Infants also require histidine. More information concerning the amino requirements of man will emerge as further experience is gained with prolonged total parenteral feeding.

After digestion and absorption, the amino acids derived from dietary protein are utilized to meet a variety of needs, depending upon the metabolic circumstances. When sufficient dietary calories are available, amino acids can be used efficiently for anabolic purposes; however, when the caloric intake is insufficient, a large proportion of dietary amino acids may be diverted for the provision of energy. In general, the energy requirements of the body take precedence over its anabolic needs. When dietary carbohydrate is lacking, the glucogenic amino acids are used to provide new glucose as fuel for the central nervous system, intermediates such as oxaloacetate to maintain the machinery of the citric acid cycle, and carbon chains for the nonessential amino acids which the body can synthesize. As described in Chap. 76, there is a spectrum of protein-calorie malnutrition ranging from protein deficiency with sufficient calories to a dietary energy deficiency which is not relieved even by high-quality protein in the diet.

Genetic determinants govern the formation of proteins. Protein in the body can be formed or replaced only with the amino acid mixture appropriate for the protein, and all the constituent amino acids must be present simultaneously in the correct proportions. Lacking one or more of the amino acids, the body cannot make proteins, since it cannot make incomplete ones, and it has a limited ability to conserve an incomplete mixture until the missing amino acids can be obtained. Alpha-keto acids derived from tissue proteins and from carbohydrate intermediates are readily aminated to furnish nonessential amino acids. In addition to the nutritional requirement for each of the essential amino acids there is a need for nitrogen which can be used in the synthesis of both essential and nonessential amino acids from the appropriate carbon skeletons. Knowledge of this biochemical transformation has been applied in the nutritional management of uremia (Chap. 268).

Estimates of amino acid needs of adults are largely based on nitrogen balance studies, while requirements for infants and children are characterized as the least amounts compatible with maximum growth. Balance is a statement of the net economy of a substance, positive during retention, negative during loss. Nitrogen is lost from the body mainly in the urine, the amount being highly dependent upon protein intake. Urea nitrogen tends to predominate in the urine with high protein diets and become negligible on protein-free diets. Fecal nitrogen is relatively constant, averaging about 1 g per day in adults. A small additional quantity of nitrogen is lost through the skin, in the breath, and in various secretions.

Dietary protein requirements Studies of young adults fed protein-free diets have disclosed that obligatory nitrogen losses, including urinary, fecal, cutaneous, and minor routes of nitrogen loss, total about 54 mg nitrogen per kg body weight per day. Because the nitrogen content of protein is about 16 percent, the sum of the excreted nitrogen times 6.25 (derived from 100/16) represents a daily attrition of 0.34 g body protein per kg that has to be replaced by the diet. Since obligatory losses of nitrogen exhibit a coefficient of variation of ±15 percent, it has been calculated that almost all the population represented would fall within the range of ±30 percent. Thus, if the average estimate of protein needs is increased by 30 percent, namely, to 0.45 g per kg body weight, almost all individuals with higher than normal needs will be covered. Finally, if it is reasoned that dietary proteins are only about 70 percent utilized because of limitations of absorption and retention, the allowance for ordinary protein can be further boosted to 0.65 g per kg daily. This figure is still substantially less than the recommended allowance of 0.9 g protein per kg per day for the "reference man," and, from the calculations cited, it can be readily appreciated that the RDA provides a generous margin of safety. In practice, healthy adults who receive adequate calories can remain in nitrogen equilibrium on a protein intake of approximately 0.5 g per kg body weight per day, provided the biologic value (see below) of the total protein remains high. Growing children and pregnant or lactating women are given additional allowances of protein for growth and secretion.

The quality of dietary protein can be critically important, especially in infants who have a far greater need for essential amino acids than do adults. The nutritional quality of a dietary protein can be determined in several ways. A useful experimental method has been measurement of *biologic value*, which is the percent nitrogen absorbed from a given protein that is retained in the body under specified conditions. Another method of estimating protein quality is simply to obtain an analysis of its amino acid composition. The resulting pattern of essential amino acids is then matched with those of several reference proteins, and on the basis of such a comparison a *chemical score* is assigned. Egg protein is generally accepted as having an optimal amino acid composition for the support of growth in the rat and has been assigned a chemical score of 100. Accordingly, this protein, which also has a very high biologic value, is often used as a reference standard. Proteins which are low in biologic value generally are deficient in one or more of the essential amino acids and are designated as having a reduced chemical score. For example, wheat flour, which has a low content of lysine and methionine, has a chemical score of 50. It is possible in animals to produce imbalances of amino acid intake which induce anorexia and growth failure.

Deficiencies of essential amino acids in human beings are not associated with specific signs or symptoms. However, the so-called "pellagragenic" diet may be deficient in available tryptophan (Chap. 77).

Proteins which are low in one or more of the essential amino acids often must be taken in increased amounts in order to furnish a sufficient quantity of the limiting amino acid or acids to permit synthesis of body protein. Two or more proteins, each deficient in different essential amino acids, can complement one another when eaten together. Between them they may furnish a high-grade protein. This is one reason for advising people to eat a variety of foods to ensure a sound diet. It is also the basis for the search for indigenous food proteins in areas of the world where protein malnutrition is prevalent in order to find a combination of native proteins which will yield an adequate mixture of high biologic value. This usually is a more economic and feasible solution than importing a complete protein or introducing entirely new foods.

Generally, the available amino acid pattern of plant proteins is less like that of human tissues than proteins from animal sources. However, since animal proteins require that time, labor, plant proteins, and other foodstuffs be used to feed livestock for their production, a long-term goal has been to find ways in agriculture, food technology, and cookery to make mixtures of complementary plant proteins which will be as nutritious as most animal proteins.

VITAMINS Except for folic acid and vitamin B_{12} which are discussed in Chap. 305, and vitamin D, which is discussed in Chap. 349, the vitamins known to be important to human health are considered in Chaps. 77 to 80.

ESSENTIAL ELEMENTS The essential elements are listed in Table 73-2. They have been classified as macroelements and trace elements on the basis of their concentrations within the body. Carbon, hydrogen, oxygen, nitrogen, and sulfur are components of the organic compounds of which the major foodstuffs are composed. Specific deficiencies of these macroelements therefore do not occur. On the other hand, deficiencies of the other macroelements and of trace elements do occur in man and/or animals. Knowledge of their requirements is therefore of importance to the physician.

Sodium and chloride (see also Chap. 264) The daily consumption of sodium chloride by most people in the United States ranges from 7.5 to 18 g, an amount equivalent to 3 to 7 g sodium. This intake far exceeds the requirement. Though unacclimatized persons may lose as much as 3 g sodium chloride per liter of sweat, following adaptation their losses may decrease to 0.5 g. Because the sodium-conserving mechanisms are extremely efficient, a sodium intake of 50 to 100 mg is adequate for acclimatized normal adults living in an environment of moderate temperature. Thus adaptation and the environment influence the sodium requirement. Needs for sodium and chloride are increased by diseases which increase enteric secretions, or those which adversely affect renal tubular conservation or impair adaptation of the sweat glands.

The possible adverse effect of chronic consumption of sodium in amounts far exceeding the requirement is a subject of current research interest. Studies with rats have shown that high sodium intakes may produce a syndrome which resembles hypertensive cardiovascular disease of man. The genetic attributes of the animals determine their tolerance to excess sodium. Increased dietary potassium has a protective effect on the sodium-sensitive animals. These animal studies and epidemiologic observations on man support the concept that a high consumption of sodium throughout life may have adverse effects on the cardiovascular system of some individuals.

Chloride is associated with sodium in the food chain. Therefore under usual circumstances, its requirement is met when the sodium intake is adequate.

Potassium (see also Chap. 264) Quantitatively, potassium is the principal intracellular cation. Within the cell it is mostly bound to proteins including various enzymes whose reactions it facilitates. It also influences the osmotic equilibrium of the cell and is in part responsible for the transmembrane resting potential. The uptake of glucose and amino acids by cells requires its presence and simultaneous entry. Thus, the requirement for potassium is related to those processes which maintain the intracellular milieu and affect anabolism. The relation of the potassium requirement to these processes is illustrated by the fact that utilization of 1 g dietary nitrogen for anabolic purposes requires the presence of approximately 150 mg (4 mEq) potassium.

Under usual circumstances, the diet provides adequate potassium. Consequently, except for patients with disorders which cause inordinate enteric or renal losses of the cation or who have been given diuretic or cathartic drugs that increase its excretion, the usual mixed diet will provide the potassium requirements. The potassium content of special formula diets or of fluids intended for total intravenous alimentation is of clinical concern. The amount required depends on the patient's previous history and on the quantities of nitrogen, carbohydrate, and fat in the preparation. Previously starved patients or those who have experienced large enteric losses often are severely depleted. When made anabolic by administration of adequate calories and nitrogen, their requirements for potassium are large. Thus it is occasionally necessary to provide 150 to 250 mEq potassium daily to avoid hypokalemia. In contrast, 60 to 120 mEq daily may be sufficient for the previously well-nourished individual. The potassium requirement of patients who are treated clinically with certain diuretic drugs is increased. This can be satisfied by increasing their consumption of potassium-rich foods and/or oral administration of potassium.

Calcium The calcium requirement of man is a subject of controversy. The uncertainty is in part due to incomplete knowledge of the factors which influence its homeostasis. They include the interaction between calcium, phosphorus, magnesium, zinc, and organic ligands present in the diet. In the alkaline intestinal milieu, calcium tends to form insoluble complexes with these minerals and ligands such as phytate or fatty acids. With other organic ligands, calcium may form soluble complexes. Thus the availability of calcium for absorption is influenced by these substances.

The calcium requirement also is related to the physiologic state of the individual. Growth, pregnancy, lactation, physical activity, age, and the ability of the absorptive mechanism to adapt are important determinants.

If one assumes that 30 percent of the dietary calcium can be utilized, a daily intake of 0.50 g to age 20 is sufficient for the accumulation of the 1,000 g present in the average adult. The RDA for calcium substantially exceeds this figure. Observations on populations whose daily intakes are considerably below 0.50 g suggest that the capacity for adaptation is great. It appears that no unequivocal adverse effects can be attributed to the lower intake. Some workers have questioned this interpretation. They believe that osteoporosis may be caused by a prolonged marginal intake of calcium, and that the relatively high phosphate content of man's diet may also be an adverse factor. They have suggested that the calcium intake should be considerably greater than the recommended allowance. There is less debate about the increased need for calcium during lactation and pregnancy. It is recommended that lactating women consume an additional 0.50 g and that pregnant women eat an additional 0.40 g calcium daily.

Phosphorus Little is known about the phosphorus requirements of man. Compared with other mammalian species, man's intake of phosphorus is high relative to his consumption of calcium. Thus, when an ordinary diet adequate in calcium is eaten, the phosphorus needs will be met. Special attention should be given to the phosphorus requirement of persons receiving total parenteral nutrition. In addition to its role in hydroxyapatite formation, phosphate is essential for the anabolic processes. Therefore sufficient phosphate should be added to the parenteral formula to prevent hypophosphatemia.

Magnesium Magnesium is the second most plentiful cation within cells. As a cofactor for many of the ATP-dependent reactions, it plays a critical role in energy metabolism. The usual North American diet contains approximately 120 mg per 1000 kcal, an amount which appears adequate under ordinary conditions. During lactation and pregnancy, an intake of 160 mg per 1000 kcal is recommended. The factors which influence calcium absorption have a similar effect on magnesium. Thus the presence of increased concentrations of free fatty acids in the intestinal milieu increases the amount of dietary magnesium necessary for homeostasis.

The amount of magnesium required by patients receiving total intravenous nutrition depends on their previous nutritional history and the degree of anabolic activity. As much as 240 mg (20 mEq) per day may be required by some adults.

Iron The requirement of normal man for iron, the most abundant transition element in the body (3 to 5 g in adults), is influenced by growth, pregnancy, menstruation, and losses in desquamated cells (intestinal and skin), hair, sweat, and other body secretions. The availability of food iron is a critical factor in the homeostatic equation.

Iron tends to complex with ligands in the intestinal milieu. Some, such as phytate or oxalate, form insoluble complexes with iron, thus decreasing its availability. Others, such as certain amino acids, may form soluble complexes which are readily absorbed. Hence iron in vegetables in general is less available, while iron in meat is more readily absorbed. Under usual circumstances, approximately 10 percent of the dietary iron is absorbed. It is therefore recommended that infants and children consume 10 mg dietary iron daily, while adolescents and adult women eat 18 mg and adult men consume 10 mg (see also Chap. 304).

Zinc Of the transition metals in man, zinc is second in abundance (2.0 to 2.5 g in adults). Assay of North American diets has shown their content to range from 5 to 15 mg daily. Meat and seafood contain the largest amounts of available zinc, while concentrations in vegetables are lower. The factors which affect availability of zinc are similar to those which influence iron absorption.

It is estimated that 20 to 30 percent of dietary zinc is absorbed. On the basis of this figure and recorded values for zinc losses in sweat, urine, and menstrual blood, together with estimates of the amount of zinc needed for tissue growth and repair, the minimum daily dietary requirement of adults for zinc approximates 8 mg. Therefore an allowance of 12 to 15 mg probably provides a reasonable margin of safety. The minimum requirement for pregnant women appears to be 12 mg daily. Thus their recommended allowance is 15 to 20 mg. The minimal daily requirement of infants is approximately 4.3 mg; a reasonable allowance for them is 8 to 12 mg daily. Growing children probably should not receive less than 8 mg daily. An allowance of 12 to 15 mg seems sufficient to meet their needs.

Copper After iron and zinc, copper is third in abundance in the body (75 to 150 mg in adults). It is essential for the action of cytochrome oxidase and a number of other oxidase enzymes and has a critical role in iron metabolism, but the amounts required in the human diet are not established. The usual North American daily diet contains 2 to 5 mg copper. Of this, between 0.6 and 1.6 mg is absorbed. The homeostatic mechanisms controlling copper absorption and excretion appear finely attuned to needs. Thus copper deficiency has not been observed in man except under the most unusual circumstances (Chap. 58), and the dietary content of copper in the North American diet appears adequate.

Iodine (see also Chap. 85) The amount of iodine required is in part dependent on the presence of goitrogenic compounds in the diet or drinking water. Under usual circumstances, a daily intake of 50 to 70 μg is sufficient to meet the requirements for synthesis of thyroid hormone and to prevent goiter. This amount may be insufficient when potent goitrogens are also present. To ensure an adequate intake of iodine by the average individual, salt is iodized in many countries. In the United States, the iodine concentration in iodized salt is 100 ppm, an amount which has proved sufficient to practically eliminate the occurrence of iodine deficiency goiter in the United States.

Fluoride Though fluorine is not essential to man in the same sense as iron or zinc, its beneficial effect on teeth and possibly on bone during the formative years of life has prompted some to classify it as a special type of essential element, i.e., one not necessary for life, but one which improves physiologic performance. When present in drinking water at a concentration of 1 ppm, fluoride strikingly reduces the incidence of later tooth decay. Its apparent beneficial effects on bone are based on epidemiologic observations on the frequency of osteoporosis in certain populations whose drinking water contains 1 to 5 ppm fluorine. Experimental studies suggest that a simultaneously increased consumption of fluorine and calcium results in harder bones, due to the incorporation of fluorine, along with the calcium, into newly formed hydroxyapatite.

Other trace elements The amounts of the other trace elements required by man are unknown. It appears that the usual mixed American diet contains sufficient amounts of them to satisfy requirements. However, experience has shown that this opinion must be considered tentative (see Chap. 81). A requirement for *manganese* is implied from observations in experimental animals. Manganese is concentrated by the mitochondria, and it is essential for the metabolism of cartilage, fat, and pancreatic beta cells. The requirement appears related to the rate of overall metabolism. *Cobalt* requirements are related to its presence in the cobalamine molecule (Chap. 305). It has no other known function. *Chromium* plays a role in glucose metabolism. It is therefore considered essential. Requirements for chromium appear to be very small. In plant and animal tissues, chromium occurs both as a chromium-organic ligand complex and as the inorganic salt. The biologic activity (facilitation of glucose entry into cells in the presence of insulin) of the complex (glucose tolerance factor) is many times greater than that for the inorganic salt. The effect of chromium nutriture on glucose metabolism has stimulated interest in this cation in relation to diabetes mellitus. A need for *selenium* by animals is established. Metabolically at least one of its functions is related to that of vitamin E. Selenium deficiency in rats and swine produces hemorrhagic necrosis of the liver and renal parenchyma. A similar disease has not been recognized in man. The need for *molybdenum* by experimental animals was established with difficulty, requiring the use of antagonistic elements such as tungsten and copper. This element activates xanthine oxidase, and the requirement must be minute. *Nickel* is one of the newest identified essential elements. Experiments with chickens have shown it to have a role in biologic oxidation. Studies in fetal and suckling rats indicate that it is a growth factor which is required in the parts-per-billion range. It seems probable that its requirement by man also is minute and that a mixed diet will provide all that is needed. *Vanadium* has been found to be a growth factor for rats and chicks. It has also been shown to play a role in cholesterol metabolism of experimental animals. Its role in human nutrition and metabolism is undefined. *Tin* also has been shown to be a growth factor for rats. In our society, where the tin can is one of the common containers used for food storage, it seems improbable that man may not receive adequate tin in his diet.

Rapid advances in analytic techniques and improved methods for controlling experimental environments make it likely that in the near future other trace elements will be found essential.

REFERENCES

Evaluation of Protein Quality, Publication 1100, National Academy of Sciences–National Research Council, Washington, 1963

McCollum EV: *A History of Nutrition*, Boston: Houghton Mifflin, 1964

Recommended Dietary Allowances, 7th ed., Publication 1694, National Academy of Sciences, Washington, 1968

Senior JR (ed): *Medium Chain Triglycerides*, Philadelphia: University of Pennsylvania Press, 1968

Underwood EJ: *Trace Elements in Human and Animal Nutrition*, 3d ed., New York: Academic, 1971

section 2 | Nutritional deficiency states

74 MALNUTRITION: CONCEPTS OF PATHOGENESIS AND TREATMENT

THEODORE B. VAN ITALLIE

PATHOGENESIS Human nutritional disease can be divided into two broad etiologic categories, *primary malnutrition* and *secondary*, or *conditioned, malnutrition*. In primary malnutrition, the diet is at fault; in conditioned malnutrition, the diet is potentially adequate but, for a variety of reasons, the affected individual is unable to make use of available foodstuffs properly. Broadly considered, conditioning factors include disorders that affect eating behavior, ingestion, absorption, transport, utilization, and excretion (Table 74-1). When a patient exhibits some form of malnutrition of which the cause is not readily evident, it is helpful to examine both the primary (dietary) and conditioning factors that could be responsible.

Primary malnutrition is prevalent in technically underdeveloped areas where the food supply often is uncertain and the nutritional properties of food are not understood. In such areas and among the poor and underprivileged classes of all countries the problems of too little food and too little choice are compounded by lack of judgment in the selection of food or its preparation. The stress of infection and parasitic infestation often exacerbates the effects of undernutrition in these groups. Human beings cannot select an adequate diet from a variety of foods by instinctive reliance upon taste or the other senses, but require some measure of nutrition education. For the most part, culture determines food behavior, and a child learns early in life how his culture has dealt with food. The most important teacher of nutrition is the mother. Once food habits are established, they are very difficult to change; however, instruction of mothers concerning diet and other matters pertaining to health ("mothercraft") and the teaching of nutrition in elementary schools offer major opportunities to correct or modify poor food habits.

Dietary deficiencies can result from at least two kinds of changes. The food supply may alter; thus, the change

TABLE 74-1
Categories of conditioned malnutrition (with examples)

1 *Altered eating behavior*	4 *Faulty transport*
Anorexia nervosa	Abetalipoproteinemia
Alcoholism	Chyluria
Food "faddism"	Hyperlipoproteinemia
Bulimia	Deficiency of retinol-binding protein (RBP)
2 *Impaired ingestion*	5 *Impaired utilization*
Oropharyngeal disease	Diabetes mellitus
Myasthenia gravis	Insufficient lipoprotein-clearing factor
Esophageal stricture	
3 *Defective absorption*	6 *Excessive excretion*
Intrinsic factor deficiency	Protein-losing enteropathy
Pancreatic insufficiency	Addison's disease
Gluten enteropathy	Primary aldosteronism
Obstructive jaundice	

to polished rice in the Orient led to endemic beriberi. Also, a shift may occur from a wide to a narrow assortment of food choices. For example, nutritional deficiencies may occur when fresh vegetables are replaced by a few canned foods.

Certain principles should be kept in mind in relation to the causes and management of primary malnutrition.

1 *Animals, including man, adapt to the available food.* This adaptation occurs for many nutrients; for example, when the protein supply is low, the adult human organism uses dietary nitrogen with increasing efficiency and eventually can achieve nitrogen equilibrium on as little as 30 g dietary protein per day.
2 *Nutrient deficiencies are often multiple.* An inadequate diet of natural foods rarely will be low in only one essential nutrient. This is important in therapy since treatment with a single nutrient may aggravate coexistent deficiencies of other nutrients.
3 *The nutrient requirements of human beings are known.* There is no foundation for the faddists' argument which advocates unconventional foods for managing ill health because it is contended that "unknown essential nutrients" are supplied by these crude or unprocessed foods.
4 *Frank deficiency disease appearing in a few individuals* often is indicative of subclinical disease in others of the same family or social group.

A type of primary malnutrition can also result from an overabundance of certain dietary constituents. Examples include the dental mottling that results from excess fluoride in the water supply, the hyperlipoproteinemia that may follow a prolonged, excessive intake of foods rich in cholesterol and saturated fats, and the obesity that results from a continuing overgenerous intake of calories.

Despite abundance of food, misguided or misinformed choices can result in dietary imbalance and nutritional deficiency. For example, nutritional surveys have disclosed a surprisingly high incidence of primary malnutrition, clinical and subclinical, among certain population groups in the United States. In a sampling of 10 states during the years 1968 to 1970, the most commonly observed nutrient deficiencies were of iron, vitamin A, vitamin C, and riboflavin. Folic acid deficiency also was found to be relatively common, particularly among pregnant and lactating women. A high prevalence of low hemoglobin and hematocrit values was found throughout all segments of the population that was surveyed. These low levels were associated with low levels of serum iron and serum transferrin saturation and, to a lesser extent, with low levels of serum folic acid. Unexpectedly, many adolescent and adult males had low hemoglobin levels. Apparently, the low levels of hemoglobin in the surveyed population were chiefly due to nutritional iron deficiency. The reported deficiencies of Vitamins A and C and riboflavin were largely based on evidence from biochemical measurements and dietary intake data. In these categories, deficiency states rarely reached the florid, clinical level, but it was judged that the affected individuals were at risk with respect to these nutrients. It must be emphasized that the Ten-State Nutrition Survey was not representative of the country as a whole since it was focused principally on low-income families, although some middle- and upper-income families were included in the survey sample. Prevalence of malnutrition or risk of malnutrition was generally inversely related to income.

The conditioned forms of malnutrition are relatively more prevalent in affluent societies and are the nutritional problems most commonly encountered in hospital practice. In addition to the nutritional deficiencies that are secondary to other diseases, nutritional disorders may result from the use of drugs that induce anorexia or interfere with the absorption, utilization, or excretion of one or more nutrients (Table 74-2). Accordingly, when a drug must be administered for a prolonged period, the physician should be aware of its possible effects on nutritional status.

PRINCIPLES OF THERAPY AND SUPPORTIVE CARE

Treatment of nutritional disease depends in part on whether the malnutrition is primary or conditioned. In primary malnutrition, therapy is a matter of providing the needed nutrients in appropriate amounts. However, some patients with primary malnutrition are gravely ill and must be treated as medical emergencies. In such instances (for example, in patients severely ill with pellagra, beriberi, or vitamin A deficiency), general supportive care is essential, and vitamin therapy may have to be initiated by the parenteral route (Chaps. 77, 78, and 80). When the malnutrition is conditioned, treatment is often much more complicated and prolonged. In order to overcome or circumvent the conditioning effects of the underlying disorder, a program of compensatory nutritional therapy generally is required. The kind of treatment indicated is determined by the nature of the underlying disorder. Compensatory nutritional therapy may involve (1) either increasing or reducing the daily allowance of one or more nutrients; (2) administration of nutrients by upper gastrointestinal tube or parenterally; and (3) feeding of "tailored" nutrients (like medium-chain triglycerides) to circumvent a block in digestion, absorption, or transport. In patients with certain in-born errors of metabolism, e. g., phenylketonuria or galactosemia, diets that rigidly restrict the improperly metabolized nutrient may be required to prevent serious organic damage (Chaps. 96 and 105).

PARENTERAL NUTRITION The commonest form of parenteral nutrition is *short-term intravenous feeding*. This is the conventional procedure used to correct acute deficits of water, electrolytes, vitamins, and other nutrients, or to prevent ketosis and reduce the excessive tissue breakdown that occurs in response to total or semistarvation, or to help maintain patients nutritionally during self-limited acute illnesses and for several days following surgery. This type of parenteral nutrition is relatively safe and simple since the dextrose and saline solutions that are used are not appreciably hypertonic and can be given via peripheral veins.

Unfortunately, sufficient calories to ensure utilization of parenterally given amino acids for anabolic purposes cannot be provided by short-term intravenous feeding unless excessively large volumes of isotonic or mildly hypertonic solutions are administered. Thus, during conventional intravenous alimentation, nitrogen and energy deficits tend to build up and, if a shift to oral feeding is not possible for a protracted period, the patient gradually suffers progressive debility with its attendant complications (Chap. 76).

Hypertonic glucose solutions providing a more adequate supply of calories cannot be given by the peripheral route because of the high risk of local venous thrombosis. Only by the use of fat emulsions suitable for parenteral use is it possible to deliver in isotonic form sufficiently high concentrations of calories. *Total parenteral nutrition* has been employed increasingly in an attempt to meet all the known nutritional needs of certain patients, particularly the need for energy. In the absence of fat emulsions safe for parenteral use, it was found feasible to administer hypertonic glucose solutions via indwelling catheters placed in the vena cava, atrium, or other central vascular sites where the rate of blood flow and intraluminal diameter permit rapid dilution, thereby minimizing the possibility of osmotic damage to the venous endothelium.

Although the use of hypertonic solutions to provide total parenteral nutrition permits administration of an adequate supply of calories in a tolerable volume of fluid, the procedure remains potentially hazardous as well as expensive and time-consuming; accordingly, its use should be reserved for the long-term management of patients who cannot be fed by mouth or by a tube suitably positioned in the upper gastrointestinal tract. The dangers of infection and other potential complications such as hyperosmolar coma, abnormal liver function, osmotic diuresis with dehydration, and hypophosphatemia prohibit the use of the procedure in routine postoperative care or in individuals who are terminal. The complexity

TABLE 74-2
Drug-induced nutrient deficiencies (with examples)

Drug	*Nutrient affected*	*Mechanism*	*Potential clinical result*
Estrogen and progesterone compounds (oral contraceptive agents)	Folic acid	Inhibition of reduction of polyglutamate to active form of folate	Megaloblastic anemia
	Vitamin B_6	Increased requirement for the vitamin	Increased xanthurenic acid excretion after tryptophan loading; "depression, anxiety, hyperirritability"
Isonicotinic hydrazide (INH) (and other hydrazides)	Vitamin B_6	Diversion of vitamin to the inactive INH pyridoxal hydrazone	Peripheral neuritis; hypochromic, microcytic anemia
	Niacin	Interference with niacin synthesis from tryptophan by inactivation of vitamin B_6	Pellagra-like syndrome
Diphenylhydantoin	Folic acid	Inhibition of reduction of folic acid to metabolically active form	Megaloblastic anemia
Phenformin	Vitamin B_{12}	Interference with absorption of the vitamin	Megaloblastic anemia; subacute combined degeneration of the spinal cord
Penicillamine	Vitamin B_6	Binding of vitamin causing inactivation	Peripheral neuritis; convulsions
Cholestyramine	Triglycerides and fat-soluble nutrients	Bile acid binding	Steatorrhea; deficiencies of fat-soluble vitamins

and hazards of the procedure require that total parenteral nutrition be carried out under the close supervision of a properly trained team that includes physicians, nurses, and a pharmacist.

REFERENCES

KALLEN DJ: Nutrition and society. JAMA 215:94, 1971

ROE DA: Drug-induced deficiency of B vitamins. NY State J Med 71:2770, 1971.

SHILS ME: Guidelines for total parenteral nutrition. JAMA 220:1721, 1972

Ten-State Nutrition Survey, 1968–1970. Department of Health, Education, and Welfare Publication no. (HSM) 72:8131, 1972

75
ASSESSMENT OF NUTRITIONAL STATUS

THEODORE B. VAN ITALLIE

Diagnosis of malnutrition requires special attention to the nutritional history (of which the dietary history is part), recognition of physical signs suggestive of nutritional deficiency disease, the use of appropriate laboratory studies, including x-rays, and, on occasion, observation of the patient's response to a therapeutic trial.

NUTRITIONAL HISTORY The nutritional history is not merely concerned with the current and past dietary intake but also takes into consideration the many conditioning factors that may affect nutriture. Examples of such factors are given in Table 74-1.

Although an extensive nutritional history is not routinely required, certain clues in the regular history should alert the physician to the need for further exploration of the patient's nutritional status. In the adult, these include an appreciable change in body weight (5 lb or more), excessive consumption of ethanol, bizarre food practices (e.g., clay eating), "food faddism," use of drugs capable of affecting nutriture (e.g. isoniazid, diuretics), menorrhagia, repeated, closely spaced pregnancies, and chronic anorexia or diarrhea. When appropriate, an attempt should be made to elicit evidence of previous malnutrition, with particular attention to the signs and symptoms of nutrient deficiency states (Table 75-1). It should be kept in mind that the reliability of the dietary history cannot be taken for granted. Some patients, especially alcoholics, are either unwilling or unable to provide accurate information about their dietary intake.

Unless the physician is particularly interested in nutritional problems, the dietary history usually is best obtained from the patient by a trained dietitian or nutritionist; however, the physician should first brief the interviewer concerning the clinical problem to ensure that all pertinent information will be elicited. The most commonly used approaches to the dietary history are the so-called 24-hr dietary recall and the food record. In the former procedure, the interviewer makes a detailed listing of the foods consumed by the patient during the previous 24 hr, obtaining estimates of the quantity of each food item consumed during this period. Usually the nutritionist will also obtain supplementary information such as how often major foods are eaten, food likes and dislikes, and

TABLE 75-1
Deficiency syndromes

Deficiency	*Common suggestive signs*	*Laboratory tests*
Vitamin A	Bitot's spots Conjunctival xerosis Corneal xerosis Keratomalacia Xerosis of skin Follicular hyperkeratosis (without perifollicular hemorrhage)	Plasma vitamin A Plasma carotene: reflects dietary intake of carotenoids Dark adaptation tests, electroretinogram; Electronystagmogram
Thiamine (beriberi)	Calf-muscle tenderness Weakness of legs (squatting test) Loss of ankle and knee jerks Hypesthesia and paresthesia Cardiac enlargement, tachycardia, pulmonary congestion and peripheral edema	Erythrocyte transketolase (ETK) activity and in vitro effect on ETK activity of thiamine pyrophosphate (TPP) Urinary thiamine (μg/g creatinine): reflects dietary intake Blood pyruvate, alpha-ketoglutarate levels: variably useful Erythrocyte thiamine concentration
Riboflavin (ariboflavinosis)	Angular stomatitis (or angular scars) Cheilosis Magenta tongue Atrophic lingual papillae Corneal vascularization Angular palpebritis (angular blepharitis) Dyssebacia Scrotal (or vulvar) dermotosis	Erythrocyte glutathione reductase (EGR) activity and in vitro effect on EGR activity of flavin adenine dinucleotide (FAD) Urinary riboflavin (μg/g creatinine): reflects dietary intake

TABLE 75-1 *(Continued)*
Deficiency syndromes

Deficiency	*Common suggestive signs*	*Laboratory tests*
Niacin (pellagra)	Scarlet and raw tongue Atrophic lingual papillae Tongue fissuring Malar and supraorbital pigmentation Pellagrous dermatosis	Urinary N^1-methylnicotinamide (mg/g creatinine)
Vitamin B_6	Nasolabial seborrhea Glossitis Peripheral neuropathy with symmetric sensory and motor deficits, more likely in the lower extremities Drug-resistant convulsions in infants	Erythrocyte glutamic-oxaloacetic transaminase (EGOT) activity and in vitro effect on EGOT activity of pyridoxal phosphate Tryptophan load test (effect on urinary excretion of xanthurenic and quinolinic acids) Urinary vitamin B_6 excretion (μg/g creatinine): reflects dietary intake
Vitamin C (scurvy)	Spongy and bleeding gums Petechiae Ecchymoses Follicular hyperkeratosis with coiled hairs and perifollicular hemorrhage ("pink halo") Intramuscular or subperiosteal hematoma Painful epiphyseal enlargement	Ascorbic acid concentration in (*1*) plasma, (*2*) whole blood, and (*3*) white blood cells Urinary ascorbic acid Vitamin C load test
Protein-calorie malnutrition (kwashiorkor—marasmus) (young children)	Psychomotor change Dyspigmentation of hair Easy pluckability of hair Thin sparse hair Straight hair Moon face Diffuse depigmentation of skin Flaky-paint dermatosis Edema Muscle wasting Hepatomegaly	Serum albumin concentration Serum amino acid ratio (leucine, isoleucine, valine, methionine, glycine, serine, glutamine, taurine) Urinary excretion of hydroxyproline (hydroxyproline index) Urinary excretion of creatinine per 24 hr Analysis of anagenic hair roots for volume, protein, or DNA
Semistarvation (older children and adults)	Marked loss of subcutaneous fat Muscle wasting Dirty-brown patchy pigmentation of face, especially malar eminences Parotid enlargement Weakness and physical inactivity Bradycardia at rest	Relative weight Measurement of skin-fold thickness Basal metabolic rate Lean body mass (derived from measurement of body density, ^{40}K-counting, or estimation of total body water)
Vitamin D (rickets)	*Active rickets (in young children):* Epiphyseal enlargement (painless) (over six months of age) Beading of ribs Persistently open anterior fontanelle (after eighteen months of age) Craniotabes (under one year of age) Muscular hypotonia *Healed rickets (in older children or adults):* Frontal or parietal bossing Knock knees or bow legs Deformities in thorax (Harrison's sulcus, pigeon chest) *Osteomalacia (in adults)*	Serum alkaline phosphatase concentration Plasma assay for 25-hydroxycholecalciferol (25-HCC)
Iron	Pallor Angular stomatitis Atrophic lingual papillae Thin, brittle nails with spooning (koilonychia)	Plasma iron level Plasma iron-binding capacity Status of marrow iron Hematocrit Blood hemoglobin concentration

TABLE 75-1 *(Continued)*
Deficiency syndromes

Deficiency	*Common suggestive signs*	*Laboratory tests*
Iron *(Cont.)*		Erythrocyte morphology Erythrocyte protoporphyrin concentration
Folic acid	Pallor Glossitis Aphthous stomatitis	Erythrocyte folate concentration Serum folate concentration Urine formiminoglutamic acid (FIGLU) excretion after histidine load Neutrophil and erythrocyte morphology Bone marrow morphology
Vitamin B_{12}	Pallor Mild icterus ("lemon-yellow" color of skin in lightly pigmented subjects) Anorexia, flatulence, diarrhea Paresthesia Ataxia Loss of position and vibratory sense Areflexia with extensor plantar responses Optic neuritis Occasionally dementia, forgetfulness (Each of above can appear as an isolated finding)	Serum vitamin B_{12} concentration Radioactive vitamin B_{12} absorption (Schilling test) Correction of abnormal Schilling test by concomitant administration of intrinsic factor (IF) Urinary methylmalonate excretion Bone marrow morphology Serum bilirubin Tests for circulating IF antibody

SOURCE: *Jelliffe, The Assessment of the Nutritional Status of the Community, World Health Organization, Geneva, 1966*

use of vitamin and mineral supplements. In the latter procedure, the food record, the subject records his own intake for a specified period, in accordance with the instructions of the dietitian. It is of course essential to determine how long a certain type of diet has been consumed, because deficiency states almost always evolve slowly.

Initially, the physician requires only enough information about dietary intake to rule out certain possibilities or to suggest the need for further diagnostic investigation. For example, if the patient is an adolescent girl subsisting principally on a milk diet, primary riboflavin deficiency can be ruled out; however, iron deficiency should be suspected.

The physician will find it useful to obtain a brief history of food taken in a typical day, using as his reference the five major food groups in Table 75-2. In this way he can determine whether there are any apparent problems that require further exploration.

PHYSICAL SIGNS Although very few clinical signs are pathognomonic of specific nutritional deficiency syndromes, many signs strongly suggest nutritional deficiency disease and also provide valuable clues to the nature of the deficiency. When two or more clinical signs characteristic of a deficiency disease are present simultaneously, their diagnostic significance is greatly enhanced. The common suggestive signs associated with a number of deficiency syndromes are listed in Table 75-1 together with pertinent laboratory tests.

Gross obesity and marked emaciation are readily perceived by inspection; however, certain patients appear to be normally nourished until the status of the subcutaneous fat is estimated by measurement of skin-fold thickness, either by means of suitable calipers or by palpation. Such measurements may disclose a marked reduction of subcutaneous fat suggestive of a chronic energy deficit. Or, conversely, an apparently undernourished patient may exhibit adequate fat stores.

TABLE 75-2
A synopsis of U.S. basic food groups and their nutrient contribution*

	Essential nutrient contribution											
Food group	*Calories*	*Protein*	*Ca*	*P*	*Fe*	*Vitamin A and carotene*	*Vitamin D*	*Vitamin C*	*Niacin, thiamine, riboflavin, pyridoxine*	*Folic acid*	B_{12}	*Vitamin E*
Dairy	+	+	+	+	−	+	+	−	+	−	+	−
Meat	+	+	−	+	+	−	−	−	+	−	+	+
Cereal and bread	+	−	−	+	−	−	−	−	+	+	−	+
Vegetables	+	−	+	−	+	+	−	+	+	+	−	−
Fruit	−	−	−	−	−	+	−	+	−	±	−	−

* *Some cereal products are enriched with iron. Liver is rich in vitamin A and folic acid. Fresh orange juice contains significant amounts of folic acid. Most vegetable oils contain abundant amounts of vitamin E.*

TABLE 75-3
Biochemical aids in diagnosing nutritional deficiency (adult values)

Nutrient	*Test**	*Level suggesting deficiency*	*Usual range†*
Protein	Total protein (S), g/100 ml	<6.0	6.5–8.6
	Total albumin (S), g/100 ml	<2.8	3.5–4.2
Vitamin A and carotene	Vitamin A (P), μg/100 ml	<10	20–49
	Carotene (P), μg/100 ml	<20	40–300
Vitamin D	Total calcium (S), mEq/l	<3.5	4.6–5.5
	Phosphorus (S), mEq/l	<0.8	1.5–2.2
	Alkaline phosphatase (S), King-Armstrong units	>20	4–17
	25-Hydroxycholecalciferol (P), ng/ml	<10	20–48
Vitamin E	Tocopherols (P), mg/100 ml	<0.4	0.6–1.5
Vitamin K	Prothrombin activity (P), % of normal	<70	70–100
Vitamin C	Ascorbate, mg/100 ml		
	Buffy coat (leukocytes, platelets)	<10	25–40
	Whole blood	<0.3	0.4–1.0
	Plasma	<0.1	0.20–0.39
	Urinary ascorbate after administration of 100 mg ascorbic acid intravenously, percent of test dose excreted over subsequent 3 hr	<5	>50
Thiamine	Pyruvate (B), mg/100 ml	>1.0	0.3–0.9
	Erythrocyte transketolase (ETK) activity, μg hexose/ml/hr	<800	900–1200
	Thiamine pyrophosphate effect on ETK activity, %	>25	<16
	Urinary thiamine, μg/g creatinine	<27	66–129
Riboflavin	Erythrocyte riboflavin, μg/100 ml RBC	<10	15–19.9
	Urinary riboflavin, μg/g creatinine	<27	80–269
Niacin	Urinary N^1-methylnicotinamide, mg/g creatinine	<0.5	1.6–4.29
Vitamin B_6	Urinary "xanthurenic acid" after 2 g L-tryptophan, μmol/24 hr	>50	<50
Pantothenic acid	Pantothenate (S), ng/ml	<50	100
Folic acid	Folate activity (S), ng/100 ml	<3	6–21
	Folate activity (RBC), ng/100 ml	<140	160–650
	Urinary formiminoglutamic acid (FIGLU) after 15 g L-histidine, mg/24 hr	>35	<17
Vitamin B_{12}	Vitamin B_{12} activity (S), pg/ml *(Euglena gracilis)*	<100	200–960
	Urinary methylmalonate, mg/24 hr	>50	<40
Iron	Iron (S), μg/100 ml	<50	60–160
	Iron-binding capacity (S), percent saturation	<16	20–45
	Erythrocyte protoporphyrin concentration, μg/100 ml RBC	>90	6–40
Copper	Copper (S), μg/100 ml	<75	81–147
Zinc	Zinc (P), μg/100 ml	<70	80–120
Manganese	Manganese (S), μg/100	<0.08	0.08–0.26
Sodium	Sodium (S), mEq/l	<135	136–145
Potassium	Potassium (S), mEq/l	<3.6	3.5–5.0
Magnesium	Magnesium (S), mEq/l	<1.4	1.5–2.5
Iodine	Urinary iodine, μg/g creatinine	<50	>50

* *P, plasma; S, serum; B, whole blood.*
† *Values falling between the* usual range *and the* level suggesting deficiency *may be considered low or marginal in appropriate instances. Values above the* usual range *are not necessarily undesirably high.*

BODY COMPOSITION Techniques for the in vivo measurement of body composition have been developed during the last three decades, starting with studies of body density. A variety of methods has been used to estimate total body fat, "lean body mass," and various fluid "compartments," including total body water, extracellular water, and plasma volume. Isotope dilution procedures have been employed to estimate the pool sizes of certain vitamins and minerals in the human body and their turnover under various conditions. Such methods have provided information about the changes in body composition that are associated with different kinds of malnutrition; however, the more complex measurements are not readily available and are therefore of little practical value in nutritional diagnosis.

ANTHROPOMETRIC MEASUREMENTS Measurement of height and body weight should never be neglected; they are the two most commonly used measures of growth in children and adolescents. In adults, use of the simple concept of *relative weight* is helpful in quantifying percent deviation from the so-called desirable body weight. Desirable weight can be defined as the average weight of individuals of given sex and height at age 22. Relative weight (RW) is calculated by the following formula:

$$RW = 100 \times \text{actual weight/desirable weight}$$

Other anthropometric measurements include determination of skin-fold thickness (mentioned above) to obtain information concerning the amount and distribution of subcutaneous fat and measurements of head, body, and limb circumferences (corrected for subcutaneous fat) at standard sites. The chest/head circumference ratio is useful in detecting protein-calorie malnutrition in early childhood, while poor muscle development or muscle wasting is characteristic of all forms of protein-calorie malnutrition.

BIOCHEMICAL TESTS Biochemical measurements used in assessing nutritional status are listed in Table 75-3. Specimens for analysis should be obtained before the findings are modified by nutritional supplements or by a change in diet.

In addition to the usual measurements of urinary excretion rates of nutrients and their products and of concentrations of nutrients, erythrocytes, and leukocytes in plasma, more sophisticated tests have been devised that are based on the metabolic roles of certain vitamin-dependent cofactors. For example, vitamin B_6 is known to be necessary for the transformation of tryptophan to niacin. In vitamin B_6 deficiency, this pathway is partly interrupted, and hence abnormal quantities of intermediate products, such as kynurenine and quinolinic and xanthurenic acids, are excreted in the urine. This is the basis of the tryptophan load test (Chap. 78). Use of tyrosine loading in ascorbic acid deficiency involves a similar principle (Chap. 79). Employment of biochemical tests in therapeutic trials is discussed below.

THERAPEUTIC TRIALS Therapeutic trials can play an important role in the diagnosis of a deficiency syndrome, particularly if the physical signs and laboratory findings are equivocal. For example, the effect of a given nutrient on the reticulocyte count can be helpful in defining the nutritional etiology of an anemia. Rapid improvement of clinical signs after therapy also may be observed in a variety of nutritional deficiencies, with obvious diagnostic implications. Thus, the clinical response to thiamine administration of patients with beriberi or Wernicke's ophthalmoplegia is often sufficiently prompt and dramatic to confirm the diagnosis. When a therapeutic trial is conducted, however, it is essential that only the test nutrient be administered; the patient should receive an appropriate dose of a single vitamin or mineral rather than the mixtures that are so readily available.

At the biochemical level, measurement of the effect of therapy on excretion of an "abnormal" metabolic product (e.g., the effect of vitamin B_6 on xanthurenic acid excretion) can serve as a useful extension of clinical assessment. Finally, in vitro trials have been devised in which, for example, thiamine pyrophosphate or flavin adenine dinucleotide is added to a system containing an erythrocyte hemolysate. The ability of such vitamin-derived coenzymes to correct a specified biochemical defect in vitro provides a valuable index of the extent of deficiency of the vitamin in question.

REFERENCES

BEHNKE AR: Anthropometric evaluation of body composition throughout life. Ann NY Acad Sci 110:450, 1963

JELLIFFE DB: *The Assessment of the Nutritional Status of the Community*, World Health Organization, Geneva, 1966

Manual for Nutrition Surveys, 2d ed., Bethesda, Md.: Interdepartmental Committee on Nutrition for National Defense. National Institutes of Health, 1963

MOORE FD et al: *The Body Cell Mass and Its Supporting Environment: Body Composition in Health and Disease*, Philadelphia: Saunders, 1963

PEARSON WN: Biochemical appraisal of the vitamin nutritional status in man. JAMA 180:49, 1962

76
STARVATION AND PROTEIN-CALORIE MALNUTRITION

THEODORE B. VAN ITALLIE

STARVATION Although modern technology has greatly reduced the risk of mass starvation in many countries, there still are large areas where famine is endemic and sometimes epidemic. But even if mass hunger were not a problem, the subject of starvation would remain of compelling interest to the physician. This is because "conditioned starvation," namely, the sustained calorie deficiency occurring in association with disease, is one of the important problems he must face. An informed approach requires that the physician be familiar with the clinical and metabolic consequences of starvation. This will also permit him to distinguish the findings directly attributable to the primary disease from those produced by the superimposed calorie deficiency.

Metabolic changes (see also Chap. 72) The most reliable information about the metabolic changes that occur during prolonged human starvation has been obtained from studies of experimentally induced caloric deprivation such as the Carnegie Nutrition Laboratory Experiment (1919) and the Minnesota Experiment (1950). In general, the changes in body composition observed during starvation, whether primary or conditioned, reflect the body's attempt to adapt to undernutrition. Most conspicuously, the fat stores are utilized in order to spare "structural" protein. Thus, body fat diminishes at a considerably more rapid rate than does muscle. Skeletal muscle, thyroid, and pancreas diminish in mass in roughly the same proportion as the body taken as a whole. More extensive losses occur in other soft tissue organs, notably the liver and the intestine. In contrast, the brain and skeleton show minimal gross changes, while the heart, kidneys, and adrenal glands exhibit proportionately less weight loss than that of the total body. In short, the central nervous system and circulation are maintained whatever the cost to less essential parts of the organism.

The body also conserves calories by reducing its output of energy. Basal metabolism decreases substantially as does voluntary physical activity. It is noteworthy that emaciated patients with anorexia nervosa frequently fail to restrict voluntary activity and, indeed, may exhibit marked physical restlessness. This characteristic should help to identify the individual with undiagnosed anorexia nervosa who, in other respects, may be difficult to distinguish from patients suffering from involuntary starvation.

It is difficult to generalize about the metabolic changes that occur in response to starvation since the picture in total caloric deprivation differs markedly from that in semistarvation in a number of respects. For example, hyperketonemia and hyperuricemia are characteristic of total caloric starvation; they are rarely observed in semistarvation. Semistarved individuals are usually ravenously hungry; those undergoing a total fast often report complete absence of hunger.

Insulin secretion diminishes in fasting man while the plasma glucagon concentration remains "normal" or increases slightly. This synergism of low insulin and relative or absolute elevation of glucagon levels has been viewed as a hormonal mechanism controlling the rate of hepatic substrate extraction for gluconeogenesis. With the decrease in plasma insulin concentrations there occurs an increased rate of release of free fatty acids and glycerol from depot fat. Secretion of growth hormone, a lipolytic agent which also may act to conserve protein, is not diminished and, indeed, may increase appreciably during starvation.

As might be expected, adrenocortical function remains normal or is increased during starvation insofar as secretion of cortisol is concerned. Since increased cortisol concentrations stimulate gluconeogenesis and decrease glucose utilization, such an adaptative response would appear to be beneficial for survival.

Fasting glucose tolerance is usually reduced during starvation, and this "intolerance" to glucose appears to reflect resistance at the tissue level that is independent of the insulin supply. Predictably, the enzymes concerned with glucose homeostasis and lipid metabolism exhibit appropriate adaptations to starvation. Thus, the enzymes concerned in fatty acid synthesis decrease, while those involved in lipolysis and fatty acid utilization increase. The enzymes responsible for gluconeogenesis from amino acids increase, and glucose 6-phosphatase, responsible for releasing glucose from the liver, increases. During the early phase of total starvation, when no dietary carbohydrate is available to the body, the human organism is faced with the necessity of supplying the brain with 100 to 145 g glucose per day, a quantity that must be derived largely from glucogenic amino acids. Initially, most of this newly formed glucose is produced by the liver, but later the renal cortex also synthesizes an appreciable quantity of glucose. Evidence is accumulating that, of the amino acids which provide the supply of substrate for hepatic and renal gluconeogenesis, the principal one is alanine. Since alanine makes up less than 10 percent of cell proteins, it is noteworthy that a much higher proportion of this amino acid is released from muscle cells during starvation. Apparently most of the alanine leaving the cells during fasting is synthesized by transamination from pyruvic acid, with the amino groups being supplied by other amino acids liberated during protein catabolism.

The body cannot long tolerate the excessive protein losses (180 to 260 g per day) that would be required to sustain the central nervous system during prolonged fasting; thus, in the absence of dietary carbohydrate, the brain is able to meet most of its energy needs by oxidizing the ketone bodies that are synthesized in quantity by the liver during periods of carbohydrate privation. In this way, the body's supply of protein is further safeguarded, and the fasting fuel economy is maintained almost entirely by substrates derived from stored triglyceride.

Clinical findings The semistarved patient characteristically complains of feeling weak, tired, irritable, and depressed. He may also describe himself as "feeling old," with loss of libido, lack of ambition, and narrowing of interests. Sitting on any hard surface is uncomfortable, and muscle soreness and muscle cramps often are troublesome. He is frequently harassed by polyuria and nocturia. The nails grow slowly and the hair falls out in increasing amounts. The extremities too readily become numb, and cold temperatures are poorly tolerated. The hands and feet feel cold even when the ambient temperature is relatively warm.

On inspection, the semistarved individual looks haggard, pale, and emaciated. Clinical manifestations of specific vitamin deficiencies usually are not evident. The hair is dry, and irregular areas of "dirty-brown" pigmentation are often present, particularly around the mouth, under the eyes, and on the malar eminences. The eyes are dull and the scleras seem to lose their vascularity, looking like unglazed porcelain. At times edema, particularly of the eyelids and cheeks, may mask the degree of emaciation and give the face a swollen appearance. In some cases, the parotid glands may be enlarged.

The neck is thin and looks abnormally long; the clavicles, scapulae, ribs, vertebral column, iliac crests, and other bony protuberances are prominent; the buttocks are thin and sagging. When not edematous, the extremities are sticklike, and the nailbeds and lips may show a slight cyanosis. Goosefleshlike changes are often present in certain skin areas, most commonly on the exterior surfaces of the thighs and upper arms. On palpation, the skin is cold, dry, rough, and inelastic. The skin folds show marked loss of subcutaneous fat. Muscle tone is poor and peripheral edema may be present. The pulse is weak, regular, and very slow at rest. The blood pressure usually is low, with the systolic pressure often 100 mm Hg or less. The heart is small to percussion, but the heart sounds are readily heard owing to the thinness of the chest wall. The abdomen is scaphoid, and the liver and spleen usually are not enlarged. The deep tendon reflexes are diminished or may be absent.

Systemic changes During severe caloric undernutrition marked changes in cardiovascular function take place. Heart size decreases and marked bradycardia (in the range of 34 to 40 beats per min) usually occurs. Electrocardiographic changes are observed, with reduction in amplitude of the P wave and QRS complex. A marked rightward shift of the QRS and T axes also may occur. These parameters return slowly to normal during nutritional rehabilitation. The arterial blood pressure and the pulse pressure tend to diminish as starvation progresses. Venous blood pressure also is reduced, although the plasma and extracellular fluid volumes increase markedly relative to body weight.

Moderate anemia is commonly found in association with semistarvation, and its severity increases gradually with the degree and duration of calorie restriction. In the Minnesota experiment, the mean hemoglobin concentration decreased from 15.1 to 11.7 g per 100 ml after 24 weeks of semistarvation. Leukopenia also occurred with the mean white cell count diminishing from 6,346 to 4,129 per μl. No significant change took place during this time in the relative proportions of polymorphonuclear leukocytes and lymphocytes.

Despite an absolute decrease of 27.5 percent in the "active tissue" compartment (body weight minus the sum of fat plus extracellular water plus bone minerals), plasma protein concentrations in the Minnesota subjects diminished only slightly during semistarvation. Indeed, the small reductions that occurred were more than offset by the average increases in plasma volume. Thus, the changes in circulating hemoglobin reflected more accurately the loss of active tissue (body protein "reserves") during calorie deprivation than did the behavior of the plasma proteins. Moreover, electrophoretic analyses of serum samples from these subjects after 24 weeks of reduced food intake showed only a minimal reduction of the gamma-globulins.

Early in starvation, urea is the chief nitrogenous component of the urine. As the body's adaptive mechanisms permit it to conserve protein more efficiently, urinary urea decreases, being replaced by ammonia. Elaboration of this "basic" ion helps the organism to conserve sodium and potassium. In addition, the decreased solute load reduces the obligate urinary volume and thereby conserves body water.

In contrast to the reduced urinary output during total caloric starvation, polyuria of 2 to 3 liters or more per 24 hr and nocturia are the most commonly described features of renal dysfunction in semistarved patients. Such individuals appear to have a reversible defect in renal concentrating ability.

Populations subjected to prolonged semistarvation often exhibit an increased prevalence of active tuberculosis, and semistarved individuals tend to tolerate infections poorly. Nevertheless, the evidence that semistarvation affects mechanisms of immunity is equivocal. In any case, susceptibility to infection must be distinguished from the increased severity of response to infection.

Starvation edema The edema that occurs in starved persons usually does not result from either hypoalbuminemia or congestive heart failure; indeed, venous pressure during starvation generally is lower than normal. The edema fluid itself is very low in protein. "Famine edema" occurs gradually, usually after the first month of semistarvation, and at first is transient, occurring late in the day. Initially, the crural areas and the eyes are likely to be involved. As undernutrition continues, the edema becomes more constant and more massive. Keys et al. suggested that in ordinary cases of famine the edema is not due to accumulation of new tissue fluid only but to retention in relative excess of the prestarvation level of extracellular fluid. Loss of elasticity and other changes in tissue structure also are thought to play an important role in the pathogenesis of famine edema.

If the body's adaptative mechanisms fail to protect the semistarved individual from still further loss of weight, particularly lean body mass, a preterminal stage of starvation is entered. In this final phase, often accompanied by persistent diarrhea, marked weakness and apathy reduce further the limited intake of liquids and food. Edema yields to progressive dehydration, followed by coma and death.

Psychologic effects Even a loss of about 10 percent of body weight can be accompanied by increased irritability and reduced libido in previously lean individuals. As semistarvation progresses and still more weight is lost, the depleted individual tends to become moody, depressed, and, if the starvation is primary, excessively preoccupied with food. Personal appearance and social behavior deterioriate, and the semistarved individual may be apathetic, lose ability to concentrate, and have difficulty in thinking. Nevertheless, in adults, intellectual performance is affected only minimally by semistarvation.

Medical management With rare exceptions, individuals suffering from starvation uncomplicated by other serious disease respond well to small quantities of ordinary food taken by mouth at frequent intervals. Use of "predigested" products has little if any advantage; indeed, simple foods such as skim milk powder appear to be preferable. Intravenous feeding is beneficial only in the occasional subject who cannot tolerate food by mouth; furthermore, parenteral fluids must be administered with extreme caution in order to avoid precipitating heart failure.

During early rehabilitation from semistarvation, if a large increase in food intake is permitted, there is rapid weight gain and a sharp rise in the resting metabolic rate. Concurrently, the plasma and extracellular fluid volumes remain high, while the cardiac output and cardiac index are still reduced. The venous pressure and pulse rate may rise well above normal, cardiac enlargement and peripheral edema may occur, and borderline or even overt heart failure may develop.

An appropriate rehabilitation diet for patients recovering from starvation uncomplicated by other serious illness is approximately 110 percent of the recommended daily allowances (RDA) for that individual, calculated on the basis of his "desirable" weight. Initially, feedings should be small, however, and offered frequently until the tolerance of the patient to food is established. Vitamin and protein supplementation are of value only in cases complicated by specific deficiency states. The sodium content of the diet should be limited so as to prevent or minimize edema.

Recovery from starvation moves at a frustratingly slow pace. Weakness, easy fatigability, and muscular aches, as well as irritability and depression, may persist for many weeks or even months after the start of rehabilitation. Polyuria also may continue for several months. Recovery of strength and working capacity is slow and seems to parallel the sluggish rate of return to normal of the lean (active) tissue compartment and the blood hemoglobin concentration. The electrocardiogram may require several months to revert to normal. The habit of conserving energy tends to become ingrained, and during rehabilitation the formerly starved patient often must be hectored to return to a more normal level of physical activity.

During rehabilitation, body fat tends to increase to a point well beyond the prestarvation level, and this extra fat deposition may persist for a year or longer after the end of starvation. Thus, the formerly starved person may take on a paradoxically obese appearance during part of his prolonged convalescence.

PROTEIN-CALORIE MALNUTRITION *Protein-calorie malnutrition of early childhood* is an inclusive designation that has been used to embody a spectrum of nutritional disorders of varying severity which range from the protein deficiency syndrome known as *kwashiorkor* at one extreme to *nutritional marasmus* at the other. Protein-calorie malnutrition is by far the major cause of infant and childhood mortality and morbidity in the world because of its very high prevalence in many underdeveloped countries.

The West African term *kwashiorkor* was introduced by Williams in 1933 to describe a syndrome most commonly observed in children between the ages of one and three years. However, the disorder can occur later in childhood and occasionally in adults. The word *kwashiorkor* is said to denote illness in a child displaced from its mother by a subsequent pregnancy. A number of conditioning factors such as parasitism, infectious diarrhea, and childhood exanthems contribute to precipitation of the florid stage of the disease; however, the principal cause is a high carbohydrate diet that provides insufficient protein. A similar syndrome can be induced in pigs and monkeys by feeding a low-protein diet in which the calories are derived principally from carbohydrate. The clinical features of the syndrome are variable, depending on the extent of the dietary imbalance, the age of onset, the duration of the deficiency state, and the severity of the conditioning factors. Characteristically, the child with kwashiorkor is wretched, emotionally unresponsive, and anorexic. He exhibits weakness and retardation of growth and motor development. It is difficult to judge true weight in the child with kwashiorkor because of edema. Although muscle wasting is invariably present, some subcutaneous fat may be retained and, on occasion, as in the case of the frequently cited Jamaican "sugar baby," the child actually may be obese. The status of the subcutaneous fat reflects the child's caloric intake. A "moon-face" appearance is frequently present in kwashiorkor, particularly in obese individuals.

Edema is the principal sign of kwashiorkor and is closely associated with hypoalbuminemia. The edema is of the dependent type, and the presence of pretibial pitting can be readily ascertained. When present, the skin lesions are characteristic; they consist of dyspigmentation, manifested as sharp-edged erythematous patches in white-skinned infants and diffuse depigmentation in darker-skinned groups. Desquamation leading to the virtually pathognomonic flaky-paint dermatosis also may be present. Skin changes are most often confined to the perineum in infants and to exposed surfaces in older

FIGURE 76-1
A child with kwashiorkor. (Courtesy of Nevin S. Scrimshaw)

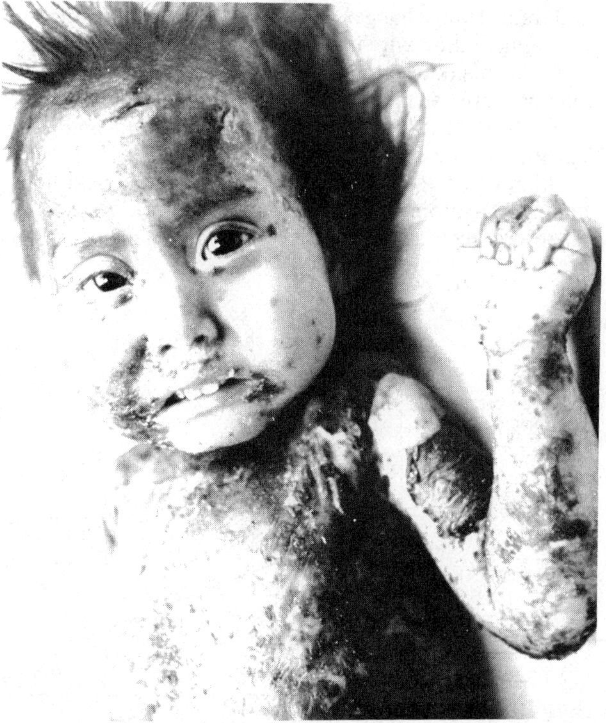

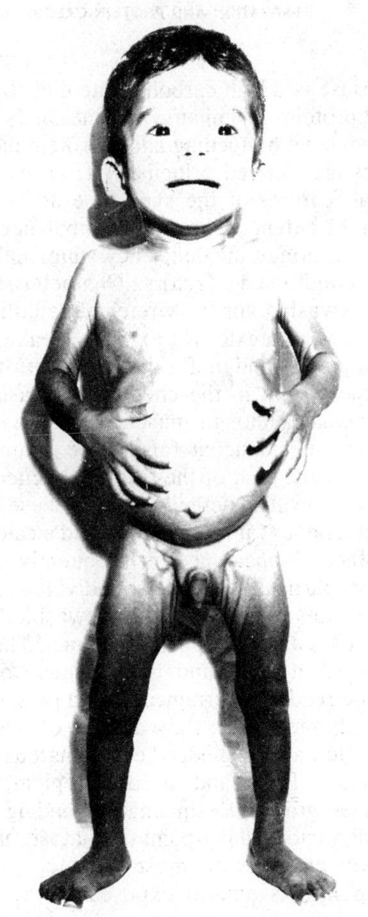

FIGURE 76-2
A child with marasmus. (Courtesy of Nevin S. Scrimshaw)

children. Hair changes are variable and may include dyspigmentation with lightening of color, straightening of curly hair, silkiness of texture, and "easy pluckability." One or more "stripes" of lightened hair color ("flag sign") may attest to alternating intervals of good and poor nutrition in the past (Fig. 76-1).

Although fatty liver is an almost invariable pathologic finding, hepatomegaly occurs inconstantly. Associated disorders include anemia and vitamin deficiency, especially deficiencies of vitamin A and folic acid, as well as a variety of infections and infestations.

Nutritional marasmus is comparable with severe semistarvation in adults, resulting from a very low intake of all nutrients, including protein. This disorder most commonly affects infants during the first year of life, and its most conspicuous features are marked wasting of muscle and fat and retardation of growth. Infants with nutritional marasmus are tiny and have a typically wizened facies which makes them appear prematurely old. The edema and apathy that characterize kwashiorkor are not present; however, minor dyspigmentation of the hair may occur, and associated vitamin deficiencies have been observed (Fig. 76-2). Between the extremes of advanced kwashiorkor and marked marasmus lies a continuum of intermediate syndromes which, in turn, range from "latent" and marginal to forms of marked severity (Fig. 76-3).

Laboratory findings in protein-calorie malnutrition are highly variable, depending in part on the patient's location in the kwashiorkor–nutritional marasmus spectrum and the severity of the disorder. The plasma protein concentration, notably albumin, is greatly reduced in kwashiorkor. However, hypoalbuminemia is a relatively late complication, and measurement of this parameter is of debatable value in the detection of marginal cases. "Plasma aminograms" show a reduction in most of the essential amino acids and normal or higher values for most of the nonessential group. This observation is not surprising in light of the fact that the need of infants for essential amino acids (in milligrams per kilogram of body weight) is approximately eight times that of adults. A shortened form of the plasma aminogram entails measurement by paper chromatography of four essential amino acids (leucine, isoleucine, valine, methionine) and four that are nonessential (glycine, serine, glutamine, taurine). In kwashiorkor the ratio of dispensable to indispensable amino acids is high (5–10:1) as compared with normally fed controls (2:1).

The hydroxyproline index (hydroxyproline/creatinine per g body weight) also offers promise as a means of disclosing marginal malnutrition in children. Abnormal values (0.5 to 1.5) are found in children with varying grades of nutritional marasmus, while marginally malnourished children exhibit values ranging between 1.0 and 2.0 (normal being 2.0 to 5.0). Additional tests of adequacy of protein nutriture include measurement of the urinary

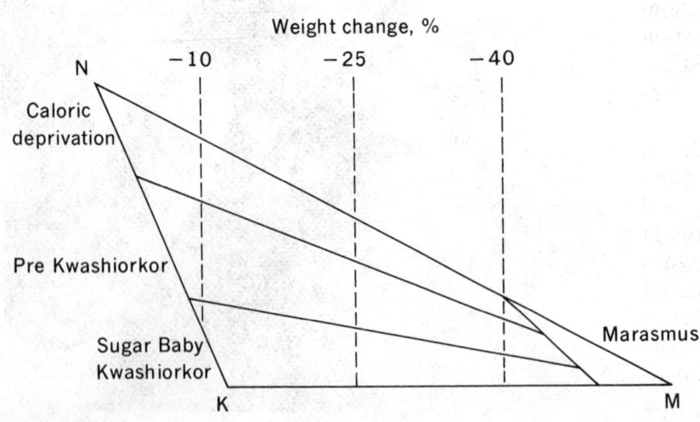

FIGURE 76-3
Relation of marasmus (M) and kwashiorkor (K). The energy depletion is indicated along the abscissa, the extent of protein depletion along the ordinate. The classic example of kwashiorkor, the "sugar baby" fed a pablum of starch, will show but little weight loss because his energy stores are preserved. The child with marasmus is greatly underweight and protein-depleted. Infection may move a child rapidly toward K and M. (Adapted from NS Scrimshaw and M Behar: Malnutrition in underdeveloped countries. N Engl J Med 272:137, 1965)

urea nitrogen/creatinine nitrogen ratio and urinary excretion of creatinine during a 3-hr period or longer.

REFERENCES

BENEDICT FG et al: *Human Vitality and Efficiency under Prolonged Restricted Diet*, Washington: Carnegie Institution, Publication no. 280, 1919

Calorie Deficiencies and Protein Deficiencies: Proceedings of a Colloquium, London: J. & A. Churchill, Ltd., 1968

JELLIFFE DB: Protein-calorie malnutrition in tropical preschool children: A review of recent knowledge. J Pediatr 54:227, 1959

KEYS A et al: *The Biology of Human Starvation*, Minneapolis: University of Minnesota Press, 1950

OWEN OE et al: Brain metabolism during fasting. J Clin Invest 46:1589, 1967

ZIFF M et al: Excretion of hydroxyproline in patients with rheumatic and non-rheumatic diseases. J Clin Invest 35:579, 1956

77 PELLAGRA

RICHARD H. FOLLIS, JR.
THEODORE B. VAN ITALLIE

HISTORY During the eighteenth century, a new disease began to appear with increasing frequency in northern Spain and Italy. First called *mal de la rosa* by Casal (from the erythematous skin lesions), the malady soon came to be known as *pelle agro* (skin, rough), from which the present-day name, pellagra, is derived. Casal described the prominent features: "a horrible crust" involving the skin, particularly of the hands and neck; "painful burning of the mouth"; "perpetual shaking of the body"; and "mania." He also noted the prominence of maize (corn) in the diet of the people whom he had studied.

Pellagra began to appear in epidemic proportions in the southern United States in the early 1900s. Joseph Goldberger, of the U.S. Public Health Service, soon showed in classic studies that diet alone could cure, prevent, or cause the disease. He demonstrated the importance of protein in the diet, and for a time he favored the idea that lack of specific amino acids was the cause. His interest then shifted to the curative effects of yeast and to the identification of an antipellagra vitamin. In 1937, Elvehjem and his coworkers showed that niacin (nicotinic acid) would cure black tongue, a pellagra-like disease, in dogs. Shortly thereafter niacin proved effective in the therapy of clinical pellagra. When it was found that the essential amino acid, tryptophan, is a precursor of niacin, it became clear that pellagra results from a deficiency of dietary tryptophan and/or niacin. Studies of the efficiency of tryptophan conversion to niacin indicate that an average of 60 mg dietary tryptophan is equivalent to 1 mg niacin. Deficiency of other nutrients, such as riboflavin, thiamine, folic acid, and vitamin B_{12}, may complicate the disease. The persistent relation of dietary corn to the development of pellagra has been a subject of recurrent investigative interest. Pellagra is rare in certain populations consuming other grains with an even lower content of niacin and tryptophan than corn. Since most of the niacin in corn is in the "bound" form and may be biologically unavailable, this fact has been invoked to explain the association of corn diets with pellagra. However, other cereals also contain a high proportion of bound niacin; thus, the role of niacin binding in pellagragenic diets awaits clarification.

PREVALENCE After 1940, the prevalence of endemic pellagra diminished greatly in the United States, presumably because of some combination of economic improvement, changed food habits, and enrichment of flour with niacin. The disease is still important in Yugoslavia, Rumania, Egypt, India, and South Africa. Individuals of different age groups are not equally affected by the disease, owing in part to differences in the type of food consumed. The greatest prevalence is in females, aged twenty to forty-five years, i.e., the childbearing, lactating group. In Goldberger's studies the next most commonly affected were children aged nine to fifteen years, but these observations were made at a time when child labor was common and diets in the southern United States were very restricted.

Primary pellagra is extremely rare in the United States today. "Secondary" or "conditioned" pellagra may develop in persons who have some other disease. Chronic alcoholism is the most common cause, although it is more usual for the chronic alcoholic to develop symptoms of thiamine deficiency. Polyneuritis, as well as skin changes and other signs characteristic of pellagra, may be observed in the same individual. Disturbances of the large and small intestine, particularly those that lead to chronic diarrhea, have been known to cause pellagra.

CLINICAL FINDINGS Classically, pellagra was considered to be characterized by the four D's: diarrhea, dermatitis, dementia, and death. However, before pellagra becomes clinically manifest and the patient seeks the help of a physician, certain prodromal symptoms may be present. These include loss of appetite leading to weight loss, indigestion, diarrhea or constipation, generalized weakness, lassitude, burning sensations in the mouth, headache, and insomnia. These symptoms are usually followed after varying periods of time by the manifestations of full-blown pellagra, which affect the skin, alimentary tract, nervous system, and to a lesser extent the blood. Pellagra is a seasonal disease with acute exacerbations in the spring and early summer, when a combination of the winter's impairment of diet and a new exposure to sun and heavier work seem to precipitate the acute episodes.

The skin lesions may begin as an erythema that looks very much like sunburn. Burning or itching may be intense. The initial changes may be followed by the formation of vesicles or by peeling. The erythematous skin may assume a dirty-brown color and then becomes rough and scaly. This stage, which may not necessarily be

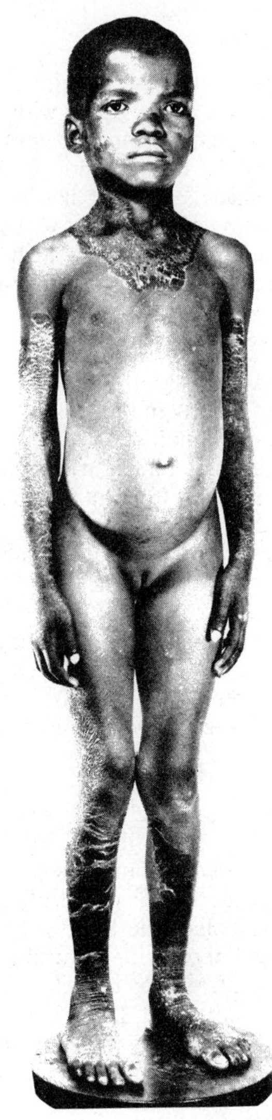

FIGURE 77-1
Pellagra in a young girl. (Courtesy of JG Prinsloo and the American Journal of Clinical Nutrition*)*

preceded by erythema, may remain for prolonged periods. Characteristically, the skin lesions are symmetric and tend to be localized over exposed areas: the backs of the hands, the face, neck, elbows, and knees, and the most exposed areas of the feet. In addition, the scrotum, vulva, and perianal region may be involved. Unilateral dermatitis usually is associated with local pressure, trauma, heat, or sunlight. The evolution of the lesions may differ; erythema of the hands may appear while hyperkeratosis of the legs is already present. Seborrhea about the nose with comedo formation (sometimes attributed to riboflavin deficiency) may be conspicuous (Fig. 77-1).

Sore mouth is a common complaint. Changes in the tongue are conspicuous; in fact, glossitis is thought by some to be a more sensitive gage of the disease than skin lesions. The tip and margins of the tongue become hyperemic, a change that may spread to involve the entire surface so that the structure acquires a beet-red appearance. Small ulcers sometimes appear. Inflammatory lesions may be found in the mucous membranes of the mouth. Secondary infection is common, particularly with fusospirochetal organisms. In advanced stages of the disease, the tongue may be pale with complete atrophy of the papillae. Angular lesions, i.e., gray macerated or ulcerated areas at the corners of the mouth, are frequently present. Pain on swallowing is common. Anorexia, accompanied by epigastric discomfort, is a frequent complaint. Diarrhea has always been a prominent part of the pellagra syndrome. Stools are small, frequent, and watery, and thus quite different from those in sprue. The liver usually is not enlarged.

Neurologic signs and symptoms rarely appear at the beginning of the disease but are common when skin or alimentary manifestations are prominent. Thiamine deficiency may be responsible for a variable proportion of the neurologic findings. Subjectively, the patient may complain of vertigo, weakness, headache, paresthesia, anesthesia, and general aches. Severe pain of the hands and feet may be present. Objectively, tendon reflexes are abnormal, usually diminished. Coarse tremors of the tongue, head, or extremities may be noted on examination. Muscular spasms are sometimes prominent. Mental disturbances are a feature of endemic pellagra; they include general "nervousness," confusion, depression, insomnia, apathy, and delirium.

LABORATORY FINDINGS Chemical examinations of the blood are of little diagnostic help in pellagra. Gastric analysis reveals achlorhydria in about one-half the cases. The two principal metabolites of niacin found in the urine are N^1-methylnicotinamide and its pyridone. In pellagra the combined excretion of these two metabolites in the urine is usually less than 2 mg in 24 hr. In mild deficiency, slightly larger quantities are excreted. Normal subjects receiving adequate diets excrete 12 to 18 mg of the two metabolites per day.

Anemia is present in approximately one-half the cases of pellagra, but in only about one-quarter is it of any consequence. The anemia is not particularly specific; however, a deficiency of folic acid or vitamin B_{12} with macrocytic anemia may develop in some cases.

PATHOLOGY The earliest skin lesions show dilatation of the superficial blood vessels and proliferation of their endothelial cells. The superficial connective tissue elements of the corium assume a spongy appearance. The epidermis, which may already show hyperkeratosis, separates from the corium with the formation of a vesicle. There may be increased pigmentation of the superficial hyperkeratotic layer with decrease in pigment cells in the basal region. Chronic lesions merely show hyperkeratosis. The epithelium of the tongue is atrophic, with loss of papillae; a subacute inflammatory reaction may be present. The esophagus is commonly the site of acute inflammation with loss of epithelium. Alterations in the remainder of the intestinal tract are not particularly noteworthy, except in the colon. Small ulcers may be present in the colon with abscess formation in the submucosa; cystic dilatations of the mucous glands are prominent. The liver may contain excessive fat, which is usually periportal in distribution. The lining of the vagina frequently is acutely inflamed with superficial ulceration.

The neurologic changes are variable and consist of atrophy of cerebral neurons, degeneration of peripheral nerves, nerve roots, and tracts in the spinal cord. The bone marrow may show erythroblastic or, rarely, megaloblastic hyperplasia.

PATHOGENESIS When man subsists on a diet of which the main staple is corn and in which there is little other protein, pellagra is likely to ensue. Corn is nutritionally inferior to other foods in a number of ways, particularly when modern milling procedures are employed. Its protein is low in quantity and, more important, in quality because it is low in two essential amino acids, tryptophan and lysine. Although corn contains appreciable quantities of niacin when assayed chemically, much of this vitamin is present in "bound" form and appears to be biologically available only if it is hydrolyzed. Niacin is found in high concentrations in liver, yeast, red muscle meats, fish, and wheat germ. Vegetables and cereals contain much less. Coffee is a significant source of niacin.

In India, in contrast to many other countries, the use of sorghum and millet (jowar) in the diet, rather than corn, has been associated with the development of pellagra. Since Indian millet contains appreciable amounts of niacin and is not deficient in tryptophan, another conditioning factor, as for example leucine-isoleucine imbalance, may be responsible for its pellagragenic properties.

Meat protein, dairy products, and eggs generally are limited or entirely lacking in the pellagrin's diet. Furthermore, diets that have been associated with pellagra have been deficient not only in protein, but also in available niacin, riboflavin, thiamine, and vitamin B_{12}.

The multiple nutrient deficiency aspects of pellagra have been recognized for some time, and they cause one to ask: What is the definition of pellagra? Some workers would be restrictive and define the disease as pure tryptophan–niacin deficiency. The argument is that since the cardinal symptoms respond to niacin, pellagra should be regarded as a deficiency of this vitamin. Since, however, some of the classic symptoms and signs are alleviated not by niacin therapy but by other nutrients, it may be preferable to define pellagra as a multiple deficiency syndrome produced principally by deficiency of tryptophan–niacin, but usually associated with deficiencies of folic acid, riboflavin, thiamine, and, occasionally, vitamin B_{12}.

It is generally agreed that exposure of the skin to ultraviolet radiation may precipitate the appearance of dermal lesions or may increase the severity of those already present. In addition, the exposure of pellagrous subjects to sunlight may lead to effects in other areas than the skin; for instance, glossitis may be induced, nausea and vomiting may occur, or diarrhea may appear. The effect of sunlight helps to explain the seasonal variations in the prevalence of pellagra in the north temperate zones.

DIAGNOSIS Physical signs in endemic pellagra often are diagnostic. The dietary history is especially important. The diagnosis of incipient pellagra or the recognition of cases without skin manifestations ("pellagra sine pellagra") is more difficult. Here it may be necessary to evaluate the response to therapy with niacin and other nutrients. Measurement of N^1-methylnicotinamide and its pyridone in a 24 hr urine sample may be of help. Fasting plasma concentrations of free tryptophan have been reported to be low in untreated adult pellagrins. The possibility of overt or subclinical pellagra should be considered in every person with a compatible diet history who suffers from gastrointestinal disease, particularly those conditions in which malabsorption occurs (Chap. 284). So, too, with any chronic alcoholic, the question of adequate nutrition with respect to niacin and other vitamins must always be considered.

Three forms of disorder with pellagra-like skin lesions, though uncommon, are worthy of mention. The first is a rare hereditary affliction called *Hartnup disease* (Chap. 98). This syndrome consists of a pellagra-like skin rash following exposure to sunlight, intermittent cerebellar ataxia, renal aminoaciduria, and the excretion of large amounts of indole-3-acetic acid and indican in the urine. Increased quantities of protoporphyrin are found in the stool. Other manifestations of pellagra, such as glossitis, stomatitis, or gastrointestinal symptoms, are not present. The skin lesions respond to niacin therapy.

A second form of pellagra-like disease has been reported in patients receiving isoniazid, the tuberculostatic drug which is also a pyridoxine (vitamin B_6) antagonist. Pyridoxine is needed for the conversion of tryptophan to niacin, and in severe deficiency this conversion may be reduced. In such patients peripheral neuritis and pellagra-like skin lesions appear and may not regress even when the drug is discontinued. Treatment with niacin often is efficacious in curing the skin lesions. Pyridoxine preparations will usually relieve the neurologic manifestations.

The third condition in which pellagra-like skin lesions have been observed is malignant carcinoid tumors (*malignant argentaffinomas*). These tumors produce such large amounts of 5-hydroxytryptamine (serotonin) from tryptophan that a conditioned form of tryptophan deficiency results. In addition to skin lesions, the patients may exhibit other symptoms characteristic of pellagra: mental confusion, diarrhea, and glossitis.

TREATMENT Severely ill pellagrins, particularly those with diarrhea and dementia, should be treated as emergencies. Water and electrolyte deficits must be corrected immediately. Oral administration of niacinamide in doses of 200 mg two or three times a day is recommended until the acute symptoms have subsided and the patient is able to eat properly. Niacinamide is free from the unpleasant vasomotor effects of nicotinic acid. Occasionally it may be necessary to give niacinamide intravenously, but the oral route is preferable and adequate for most patients with pellagra. Riboflavin and thiamine also should be given in therapeutic amounts, since deficiencies of these nutrients are commonly associated with pellagra. A daily maintenance dose of the other vitamins should be a part of the therapeutic regimen, and a high-calorie, high-protein diet is desirable. Frequent small feedings are advocated at first. Stomatitis, diarrhea, or constipation, and oozing of ulcerated lesions of the skin will necessitate symptomatic care.

PROGNOSIS Until the advent of vitamin therapy, the prognosis of pellagra was grave, but now it is excellent. The glossitis begins to decrease in 24 hr; the papillae of the tongue begin to regenerate by the end of the first week. Lesions of the lips begin to heal in 2 to 3 days. Gastrointestinal symptoms improve in 24 to 48 hr, and diarrhea usually ceases by the end of the first week. Demented patients usually become rational after 3 or 4 days, unless irreversible brain damage has occurred. Polyneuritis, if present, may require some time to improve.

REFERENCES

BEAN WB et al: Secondary pellagra. Medicine 23:1, 1944

FOOD AND AGRICULTURE ORGANIZATION: *Maize and Maize Diets*, FOA Nutritional Studies no. 9, Rome, 1953

GILLMAN J, GILLMAN T: *Perspectives in Human Malnutrition: A Contribution to the Biology of Disease from a Clinical and Pathological Study of Chronic Malnutrition and Pellagra in the African.* New York: Grune & Stratton, 1951

GOLDSMITH GA: Niacin: Antipellagra factor, hypocholesterolemic agent. Model of nutrition research yesterday and today. JAMA 194:167, 1965

SYDENSTRICKER VP: The history of pellagra, its recognition as a disorder of nutrition and its conquest. Am J Clin Nutr 6:409, 1958

TRUSWELL AS et al: Plasma tryptophan and other amino acids in pellagra. Am J Clin Nutr 21:1314, 1968

78
THIAMINE DEFICIENCY, ARIBOFLAVINOSIS, AND VITAMIN B_6 DEFICIENCY

THEODORE B. VAN ITALLIE
RICHARD H. FOLLIS, JR.

BERIBERI History During the seventeenth, eighteenth, and nineteenth centuries, as a result of the increasing contacts of European physicians with the Far East, a disease peculiar to that area became known to Western physicians. The principal characteristics of this disease, oriental beriberi, as described by a nineteenth-century physician, were "a feeling of numbness, sense of weight and weakness in the legs, edema of the feet, unsteady and tottering walk with almost total palsy, rigidity and various affections of the nerves, oppression and weight in the precordium, and, occasionally, sudden death." The disease was endemic throughout South China, Southeast Asia, the Philippines, the East Indies, and parts of India.

Studies soon revealed the close relation of rice in the diet to the disease. Beriberi was eradicated from the Japanese Navy by Takaki, who added meat, vegetables, and condensed milk to the rice diet of the common sailor. In Batavia (now Djakarta), Eijkman observed a beriberi-like disease in fowl fed polished rice; the birds could be cured with unpolished grain. By 1912, the therapeutic effectiveness of rice polishings had been demonstrated, particularly in patients with the acute cardiac manifestations of beriberi. This led E. B. Vedder, a U.S. Army physician, to recommend to R. R. Williams, a chemist working in Manila, that the protective substance be isolated. In 1936, Williams and his coworkers announced the chemical structure and synthesis of the active principle, thiamine.

Prevalence Today the prevalence of clinical beriberi in the Far East is much reduced. However, cases are still encountered, particularly in infants and pregnant or lactating women. Thiamine deficiency in the United States is most often seen in alcoholics. The presence of thiamine in enriched flour and white bread has diminished the prevalence of this disorder. Fortification of alcoholic beverages with thiamine has been suggested as well as the provision by public health authorities of thiamine-impregnated snacks on bar counters. The cost of such measures would appear to be less than the present high cost involved in the institutional care of patients suffering from Wernicke-Korsakoff disease.

Clinical findings Three main types of beriberi have been recognized in the Orient: a chronic form in which neurologic involvement is prominent (*dry beriberi*), an acute form with heart failure, and a less acute state in which edema is the most characteristic manifestation (*wet beriberi*). The onset of the chronic neurologic form is insidious. Over the course of days or weeks, the patient comes to be easily fatigued and experiences heavy feelings in the legs, together with stiffness and aching in the muscles. In time the muscles become weaker, acutely painful, and then atrophic. The extensors of the foot usually are first affected, then the muscles of the calf and thigh. Pain followed by atrophy soon occurs in the muscles of the arms; the muscles of the trunk may be affected later. Associated with these signs and symptoms are foot drop and wrist drop, together with loss of ankle and knee reflexes. Paresthesias and anesthesias may be demonstrated, particularly over the lower extremities. Circumoral anesthesia may be present. Aphonia is sometimes a symptom. Walking becomes difficult, and the patient can only shuffle about with a cane or is forced to hold on to objects about him to keep from falling. Evidence of neurologic involvement may fluctuate. In time, however, the patient becomes completely bedridden.

Progressive weight loss occurs, together with persistent anorexia. Diarrhea may further complicate the nutritional picture. Cardiac changes may accompany these neurologic disturbances or may appear suddenly in the absence of any evidence of involvement of the nervous system. The cardiac manifestations consist of palpitation, precordial pain, and dyspnea, which may come on in paroxysms without warning. The heart is found to be enlarged and tachycardia is present. Prominent venous pulsations are noted in the neck. Edema of the lower extremities usually is present. The blood pressure is not elevated, but the pulse pressure is increased and venous pressure is elevated. Death may occur suddenly.

In infants beriberi continues to be a health problem in the Far East. In babies the manifestations may be aphonic, in which the child loses his voice; cardiologic, a sudden episode of labored breathing, cyanosis, and, if not promptly treated, cardiac arrest leading to death; and pseudomeningitic. These babies are typically born of mothers with low dietary intakes of thiamine and consequently low levels in their milk. The infant seems to flourish until quite suddenly it is stricken, usually at three to six months of age. The disorder is prevented by giving the mother thiamine and treated by the administration of thiamine to the infant. This will often bring a dramatic cure in a matter of hours.

In the mid-1930s, observers in large urban clinics in the Occident began to recognize instances of cardiac and neurologic disease occurring predominantly in alcoholics. In some areas the prevalence of these forms of Occidental beriberi, as these entities came to be called, was high. The clinical aspects of this form of heart disease are described in Chap. 233.

The symptoms and signs relative to neurologic involvement in alcoholics have the characteristics of a progressive polyneuritis with sensory and motor defects (Chaps. 111, 332, and 333). Almost invariably there is a history of excessive consumption of alcohol and poor dietary intake. In addition, such patients frequently exhibit manifestations of delirium tremens or Wernicke's disease. To such examples of neurologic involvement in poorly nourished, chronic alcoholics have been added other syndromes in recent years, such as alcoholic amblyopia, central pontine myelinolysis, and corticocerebellar degeneration. None of these changes, including Wernicke's disease, has been described in beriberi occurring in Asian peoples.

Thiamine is involved in a number of key reactions in the glycolytic and pentose phosphate pathways of glucose metabolism. Consequently, disturbances of lactate and pyruvate oxidation and of pentose phosphate shunt reactions would be expected to reflect alterations of these functions.

Pathology Postmortem examinations performed on patients dying with neurologic manifestations of beriberi at the turn of the century in the Orient revealed myelin degeneration of the peripheral nerves, with loss of axoplasm. Lesions in the brain and spinal cord have not been reported from the Orient. Among the sporadic cases designated as neurologic beriberi encountered in the Occident, usually among alcoholics, lesions of peripheral nerves also have been described. More prominent, however, are changes in the brain. Alterations characteristic of Wernicke's disease—bilateral hemorrhagic necrotic foci in the mammillary bodies, the hypothalamic nuclei, and midline structures—are found. Damage to the optic nerve and lesions in the spinal cord have been reported.

The heart is likely to be enlarged, but this increase in size usually is due to dilatation, although hypertrophy of the right ventricle has sometimes been noted. The myocardial fibers do not exhibit necrosis, although swelling and vacuolization may be prominent. No cellular infiltration is present.

Pathogenesis Rice is the principal foodstuff of one-half or more of the inhabitants of the world. The introduction of power milling machinery at the end of the nineteenth century led to a great increase in beriberi in the Far East. When rice is highly milled, most of its vitamin content, such as thiamine, riboflavin, niacin, pantothenic acid, and pyridoxine, is removed. Lipids and minerals, such as calcium, iron, and iodine, which are present in the outer portions of the grain, are lost as well.

Although the rice eater's diet is deficient in a number of nutrients, the principal manifestations of beriberi—the derangements in cardiac and neurologic function—appear to be related to thiamine deficiency. The therapeutic response of the patient with cardiovascular beriberi, whether infant or adult, to thiamine is good evidence for this relation. The development of anatomic lesions in the hearts of experimental animals deprived of thiamine is further proof for the relation of this vitamin to the integrity of the myocardium.

The precise relation of thiamine to maintenance of the integrity of the peripheral nervous system is uncertain. The predilection of the nervous system for injury in thiamine deficiency suggests that the vitamin is especially crucial for those tissues which depend upon carbohydrate metabolism exclusively for their energy sources. Moreover, the pentose phosphate pathway is needed for lipid synthesis. This is one of the ways in which thiamine deficiency could lead to demyelinization. The clinical response of neurologic defects to thiamine usually is not rapid, but this can be explained if the damage has been severe enough to have caused structural loss. Hence, regeneration is necessary if function is to be restored.

In contrast, the ophthalmoplegia of Wernicke's disease may improve within a few hours after thiamine administration, and lesions similar to those observed in Wernicke's disease have been demonstrated in the brains of thiamine-deficient animals. The enigma of the rarity of Wernicke's disease in the Orient (except among Western prisoners of war) remains.

Diagnosis Patients with neuritic (dry) beriberi exhibit tenderness of the calf muscles and have difficulty in rising from a squatting position. Patellar and Achilles tendon reflexes are usually hypoactive or absent. Paresthesias are common, but loss of vibratory and position sense is less common.

Cardiovascular (wet) beriberi is characterized by edema of the lower extremities and varying grades of congestive heart failure. Cardiomegaly and pulmonary congestion are common, together with evidence of high-output failure, including a relatively shortened circulation time. Electrocardiographic changes in cardiovascular beriberi are nonspecific and may include prolongation of the Q-T interval, low voltage, and flat or inverted T waves.

Urinary thiamine levels are valuable in population surveys but of far less use in the diagnosis of individual cases. Although a urinary thiamine excretion rate of less than 65 μg per g creatinine is considered indicative of a low or deficient thiamine status, many apparently healthy individuals have been found to fall within this "deficient" range. Measurement of erythrocyte transketolase (ETK) activity, an enzyme which functions in the pentose phosphate pathway and requires thiamine as a cofactor, and the in vitro response of ETK activity to added thiamine pyrophosphate (TPP) are more helpful. One to two hours after the patient has been treated with thiamine, the ETK activity increases to a level equivalent to or higher than that observed when the initial blood sample was incubated with TPP. An in vitro TPP effect greater than 16 percent strongly suggests thiamine deficiency. Measurement of blood thiamine concentrations and, because of their sensitivity to other factors, the study of blood lactate and pyruvate changes after exercise or glucose loading are of limited diagnostic value.

Beriberi usually is readily identified if it is included in the differential diagnosis. In the Occident, beriberi may be overlooked because of a "low index of suspicion" and failure to obtain an adequate dietary history, particularly in patients suspected of alcoholism. All too frequently, cardiovascular beriberi is considered only after the patient in congestive failure fails to respond appropriately to conventional treatment with digitalis and diuretics. When suitable biochemical tests are not available, the best criterion for the diagnosis of beriberi is the response of the patient to thiamine administration. In cardiovascular beriberi, improvement after administration of thiamine may be dramatic; marked diuresis, decrease in heart rate and size, and clearing of pulmonary congestion may occur with 12 to 48 hr.

In patients with the Wernicke-Korsakoff syndrome irreversible brain damage occurs rapidly; hence early recognition and treatment are vital.

Treatment When there is cardiac involvement, beriberi becomes a medical emergency. Prompt administration of thiamine is essential. Initially, 60 mg thiamine should be given intramuscularly, followed by 25 mg per day in divided doses orally for 1 to 2 weeks. Thereafter, 2.5 mg per day should be sufficient. Ordinarily, increments above individual oral doses of 2.5 mg per day are largely unabsorbed. Since patients with beriberi often exhibit multiple deficiencies, they should also receive the other water-soluble vitamins in therapeutic quantities.

Prognosis The response to thiamine of infants and adults with cardiovascular beriberi in the Orient is one of the most dramatic in medicine. In the Occident, such dramatic responses are seen less often. Although the eye signs of Wernicke's disease improve promptly upon thiamine administration, the loss of memory for the immediate past and the confabulation (Korsakoff's psychosis) respond only if the disease is treated early.

RIBOFLAVIN DEFICIENCY Ariboflavinosis still is a common nutritional deficiency in many developing countries. In the United States, there appears to be a positive correlation between family income and riboflavin intake. Riboflavin deficiency is found sporadically among the poor and in alcoholics, but its prevalence is not known precisely. Deficiency of riboflavin almost always occurs in association with deficiencies of other B vitamins. Riboflavin requirement is related to "metabolic body size," represented as body weight in kilograms taken to the 0.75 power; riboflavin allowances for adults are approximately 1 to 2 mg per day. Milk, eggs, fish, meat (especially liver), and certain vegetables are good sources of riboflavin; when dietary protein intake is adequate in adults, a deficiency of riboflavin usually does not occur. Exposure of milk to direct sunlight destroys a considerable amount of the vitamin content; riboflavin in food also is destroyed by treatment with alkali.

Riboflavin is the precursor of two flavoprotein coenzymes, flavin mononucleotide (FMN) and flavin adenine dinucleotide (FAD) and thereby plays a central role in many important metabolic processes. In the tissues very little of the vitamin is stored as riboflavin; nearly all is in the form of FMN and FAD. Thyroid hormone regulates the conversion of riboflavin to FMN and FAD by increasing the activity of the enzyme flavokinase, which catalyzes the transformation of riboflavin to FMN. Thyroid hormore causes smaller increases in the acitivities of FAD pyrophosphorylase, which converts FMN to FAD, and of FMN phosphatase, which degrades FMN to riboflavin. In hypothyroidism, flavokinase activity decreases, and tissue level of FMN and FAD also are diminished.

Riboflavin is absorbed from the upper intestinal tract, and apparently is phosphorylated to FMN in the intestinal mucosa. The presence of food increases the rate of intestinal absorption. Riboflavin and FMN circulate in plasma both free and bound to plasma proteins. Riboflavin is excreted predominantly in urine.

Lack of riboflavin in young rats results in cessation of growth and extensive skin changes. In adult animals riboflavin deficiency produces enlarged livers with a high content of triglyceride and glycogen. Electron microscopy in mice discloses giant mitochondria within hepatic cells. Deficient rats exhibit abnormalities of tryptophan metabolism and excrete excessive quantities of anthranilic and xanthurenic acids. Apparently riboflavin is required for the formation of pyridoxal phosphate from pyridoxine phosphate. The former coenzyme, in turn, is needed for normal metabolism of tryptophan.

In riboflavin-deficient patients, angular stomatitis, cheilosis, and sore throat are early findings. Subsequently, seborrheic dermatitis of the face and scrotum, glossitis, and a generalized dermatitis involving trunk and extremities may occur. The eyes itch and burn, and the patient may complain of photophobia and visual impairment; corneal vascularization may occur. Late findings include neuropathy and mild anemia. Human riboflavin deficiency has been induced experimentally by means of a riboflavin antagonist, galactoflavin. In such individuals clinical symptoms occur more rapidly and are more marked than in patients with dietary restriction of the vitamin alone.

The anemia of experimentally induced riboflavin deficiency in primates is normochromic and normocytic and is associated with red cell hypoplasia and reduced reticulocytosis. The anemia responds promptly to riboflavin administration, an increase in the reticulocyte count occuring within a few days after initiation of treatment. Apparently, normal utilization of folic acid is dependent upon the integrity of certain flavoprotein enzymes; hence, the anemia of riboflavin deficiency may be related in part to an associated disturbance of folic acid metabolism.

Clinical diagnosis of riboflavin deficiency is often difficult because ariboflavinosis usually occurs in conjunction with other vitamin deficiency states. Moreover, the stomatitis, glossitis, and dermatitis are not specific to riboflavin deficiency. Corneal vascularization, if present, is a useful (but not a pathognomic) sign. A careful dietary history is helpful in suggesting the diagnosis. When suitable laboratory tests are not available, a therapeutic trial is indicated.

In the past, the laboratory diagnosis of riboflavin deficiency has depended on measurement of blood levels of riboflavin and its derivatives. Measurements performed on erythrocytes appear to yield more reliable information about riboflavin nutrition than plasma concentrations. The urinary excretion of riboflavin also has been suggested as providing useful diagnostic information.

An in vitro enzyme assay for glutathione reductase and the increase in its activity induced by FAD (analogous to the TPP-effect for thiamine gives promise of a specific diagnostic test of riboflavin deficiency in man. This test is based on the observation that the magnitude of increase in erythrocyte glutathione reductase activity after ingestion of riboflavin and correlates well with the level of dietary intake of this vitamin. In normal subjects fed a riboflavin-free diet for only 1 week, significant changes in erythrocyte glutathione reductase activity occur when FAD is added to the reaction mixture. The suitability of this determination for large-scale nutritional surveys remains to be established.

The recommended therapeutic dose of riboflavin is about 10 mg orally; treatment at this level should be continued until the manifestations of the deficient state have regressed. Larger doses of riboflavin may be administered safely without untoward effects.

VITAMIN B_6 DEFICIENCY Vitamin B_6 is a collective term for three naturally occuring pyridines: pyridoxine, pyridoxal, and pyridoxamine. Pyridoxal and pyridoxamine are found mainly in animal products, and pyridoxine occurs in plant foods. Of these three vitamers, pyridoxine is the main source of vitamin B_6 activity in the average diet.

Pyridoxal phosphate is known to serve as a coenzyme for the decarboxylases, deaminases, transaminases, and a number of other enzymes. It also appears to be incorporated into the glycogen phosphorylase of muscle. In rats, a deficiency of vitamin B_6 causes cachexia, and anemia; in young pigs, scaling of the skin, and a profound microcytic, hypochromic anemia, epileptiform convulsions, and sensory neuron degeneration develop. Convulsive seizures have occurred in babies fed formulas deficient in vitamin B_6. Nasolabial seborrhea, cheilosis, and angular lesions may reflect a deficiency of vitamin B_6; however, these signs are nonspecific and frequently are not nutritionally related. Rarely, a red, painful tongue with denudation of the epithelum with or without fissures may be associated.

Vitamin B_6 is involved in each sequence of the reactions by which tryptophan is converted to nicotinic acid. Thus, when this vitamin is deficient, increased quantities of intermediate products and their derivatives are formed and excreted in the urine. Of these, xanthurenic acid appears to reflect most reliably the state of vitamin B_6 nutriture. The quantity of xanthurenic acid excreted following a tryptophan load provides a sensitive index of vitamin B_6 deficiency. Use of a 2-g L-tryptophan dose seems least likely to distort the metabolic state through over-loading and has been reported to afford the greatest reproducibility of the quantities of tryptophan metabolic intermediates excreted in the urine. By means of tryptophan loading it has been possible to demonstrate disturbances of tryptophan metabolism, presumably reflecting B_6 deficiency, early in pregnancy and in women using oral contraceptives. Large does of pyridoxine (25 mg per day) were needed to correct the altered vitamin B_6-tryptophan metabolism resulting from oral contraceptive use.

Vitamin B_6 is excreted in the urine together with a number of metabolic products, including 4-pyridoxic acid. The latter disappears from the urine at an early stage of deprivation; hence its continued presence in the urine would appear to rule out vitamin B_6 deficiency. It also has been suggested that in vitro stimulation of erythrocyte glutamic-oxaloacetic transaminase (EGOT) activity by pyridoxal phosphate can serve as a useful measurement in the evaluation of vitamin B_6 nutritional status.

A number of drugs interfere with vitamin B_6 utilization. Isoniazid and hydralazine form inactive derivatives and increase B_6 requirements. Penicillamine and cycloserine act as antimetabolites of vitamin B_6. Polyneuritis may appear as a complication of therapy with these agents and can be relieved by supplying large amounts of pyridoxine hydrochloride.

Certain microcytic anemias have been found to be partially responsive to pyridoxine therapy (Chap. 304). In infants receiving normal diets convulsive seizures have been described which could be relieved by administration of pyridoxine. Such observations have led to the concept of pyridoxine dependency due to a genetically determined requirement for unusually large amounts of pyridoxine.

REFERENCES

Brin M: Erythrocyte transketolase in early thiamine deficiency. Ann NY Acad Sci 98:528, 1962

Lane M et al: The rapid induction of human riboflavin deficiency with galactoflavin. J Clin Invest 43:357, 1964

Luhby AL et al: Vitamin B_6 metabolism in users of oral contraceptive agents: 1. Abnormal urinary xanthurenic acid excretion and its correction by pyridoxine. Am J Clin Nutr 24:684, 1971

Rivlin RS: Riboflavin metabolism. N Engl J Med 283:463, 1970

Sauberlich EH et al: Thiamin requirements of the adult human. Am J Clin Nutr 23:671, 1970

Williams RR: *Toward the Conquest of Beriberi,* Cambridge, Mass.: Harvard, 1961

79 SCURVY

RICHARD H. FOLLIS, JR.
THEODORE B. VAN ITALLIE

HISTORY Although accounts of a disease which might be construed as scurvy are found in ancient writings, the first clear-cut descriptions appear in records of the Crusades. When the long sea voyages of discovery began toward the end of the fifteenth century, scurvy became commonplace and soon ranked first among causes of disability and mortality in sailors. Scurvy on land appeared among military and civilian population groups as a result of the many European wars which led to troop movements and civilian displacement. In 1747 James Lind, a British naval surgeon, in a model experiment, studied the effects of several types of treatment, such as one composed of "two oranges and one lemon given every day." The sailors, who were described as having "putrid gums, the spots and lassitude, with weakness of their knees," responded dramatically, and thus British sailors came to be known as "limeys." Infantile scurvy began to receive attention after 1883, when Barlow described the syndrome as it is recognized today. With increasing use of breast milk substitutes, scurvy became common in the urban areas of Europe and the United States at the turn of the century.

A disease of the growing bones of guinea pigs, quite like that seen in children, was produced by dietary means in 1907. Twenty-five years later, C. G. King and his associates isolated from lemon juice a biologically active, crystalline material. This compound was later synthesized and shown to be ascorbic acid.

PREVALENCE In previous times scurvy in adults tended to occur in epidemic form. Scurvy now is seen only in occasional individuals in the United States, usually in men living alone whose diet is grossly unbalanced and is devoid of sources of ascorbic acid ("bachelor" scurvy). Each year in urban clinics in the United States and Europe such examples of adult scurvy are encountered. Occasional cases of scurvy continue to appear in pediatric clinics, usually as a result of maternal error or neglect.

CLINICAL FINDINGS The principal manifestations of scurvy in the adult include follicular hyperkeratosis with perifollicular hemorrhage, swollen, bleeding gums, petechiae, aching muscles, fatigue, and emotional changes. These changes appear after 2 or more months of depletion. Subsequently, arthralgias involving the large joints occur, and these may be followed by joint effusion. Fatigue and psychologic disturbances may be early symptoms.

Oral lesions occur almost exclusively in individuals who have retained their own teeth and are most severe in those with preexisting gingivitis. Reddening and swelling of the interdental papillae occur first, soon followed by hemorrhage. Less well-known features of scurvy include the appearance of minute hemorrhages and small aneurysms in the bulbar conjunctivas. The development of Sjögren-like (sicca) syndrome also has been noted.

The clinical picture in children is very different from that in adults. The peak age incidence is 8 months; few cases are seen after the first year. The most prominent sign on physical examination is tenderness of the lower extremities, which are also usually somewhat swollen. The legs are characteristically partially flexed and guarded. Involvement of the upper extremities is less common. The extremities are obviously painful, and the child may scream when approached. The costochondral junctions may be enlarged and crepitus of the epiphyseal areas of the ankles and wrists may be felt. The gums are swollen and hemorrhagic when teeth are present, but show little change before teeth erupt. Subcutaneous hemorrhages may be observed; these tend to be in the form of ecchymoses, not the pinpoint hemorrhages seen about the follicles in the adult. Follicular lesions are uncommon in children. Hemorrhages may occur elsewhere: suborbital with proptosis, epistaxis, hematuria, or signs of subdural bleeding.

LABORATORY FINDINGS The concentration of ascorbic acid may be determined in samples of serum (or plasma), whole blood, or in the buffy coat layer. The ascorbate concentration in the buffy coat most faithfully reflects the body pool of L-ascorbic acid (about 1,500 mg in normally nourished adults) and is the preferred measurement; however, this procedure is technically difficult.

Diagnostically, the more conveniently measured serum and plasma concentrations are equivalent to that in whole blood, except when the ascorbate level is low. Thus, when serum levels are in the vicinity of 0.2 mg per 100 ml (a concentration often associated with deficiency), whole blood, because it contains a fraction of the buffy coat, is a somewhat more reliable indicator of vitamin C status. Clinically manifest scurvy is to be expected when the whole blood concentration falls below 0.3 mg per 100 ml.

Saturation or load tests may be of some help in evaluating ascorbic acid nutriture. When adequate amounts of the vitamin are being ingested, the urinary output will be about 25 to 75 mg per 100 ml. Urinary output will be virtually zero when the body stores are depleted. If 200 mg ascorbic acid is administered each day and urinary excretion of the vitamin is small during the first 3 or 4 days, the stores probably were reduced.

PATHOLOGY In adults, the most conspicuous finding at autopsy is the presence of generalized hemorrhage. The perifollicular lesions and ecchymoses noted clinically are conspicuous. In addition, extravasations of blood are found in the pericardial or pleural cavities, the walls of the intestinal tract, bladder, and renal pelves. In young adults separation of the epiphyses or costochondral junctions may be present, as well as subperiosteal hemorrhage.

In children the most characteristic changes at autopsy are in the skeleton. The periosteum is found to be separated or may be easily stripped from the shaft of a bone and the costal or epiphyseal cartilages are separated from the shaft of the rib or a long bone. Microscopic examination at the cartilage-shaft junction shows a dense "lattice" of spicules of calcified cartilaginous matrix, many of which have fractured. Little bone has formed on this lattice which, furthermore, has not been destroyed. In less advanced cases, fractures occur only at the edges or corners of the bone. Hemorrhage may be observed in the marrow or beneath the periosteum. As a result of decreased osteoid formation, the cortex and trabeculae of the shaft are reduced in thickness. Aside from hemorrhages elsewhere—subdural, subpleural, and subcutaneous—little else is found that is specific for scurvy. Rickets frequently coexists in such children.

PATHOGENESIS Scurvy represents the reaction of particular hosts, such as man, other primates, certain birds and fish, and the guinea pig, to a lack of ascorbic acid in the diet. Most other mammalian species can synthesize the vitamin from D-glucose or D-galactose. Ascorbic acid is found in high concentrations in citrus and other fruits, leafy vegetables, tomatoes, tubers, most grasses, and sprouting plants. The vitamin content of human milk varies, since the mother is dependent on dietary sources. Milk from a well-nourished woman contains 5 to 7 mg per 100 ml. Fresh cow's milk contains 1.0 to 2.6 mg per 100 ml; however, storage and sterilized infant formulas prepared from cow's milk or proprietary foods may be expected to produce scurvy in infants if the product has not been fortified or the diet is not supplemented with a source of ascorbic acid.

Scurvy, broadly speaking, is a genetic disease in that the tissues of the susceptible species have lost their ability to synthesize ascorbic acid. The chemical steps in the formation of the vitamin are well known:

$$\text{D-Glucuronate} + \text{NADPH} + H^+ \rightarrow \text{L-gulonate} + \text{NADP}^+$$

$$\text{L-Gulonate} + \text{NAD}^+ \rightarrow \text{L-gulonolactone} + \text{NAD}^+ + H^+$$

$$\text{L-Gulonolactone} \rightarrow \text{L-ascorbate} + H_2O$$

Liver and kidney tissues of all mammalian species so far studied can carry out the first two reactions above. Animals subject to scurvy do not have an enzyme system which permits the third reaction.

In ascorbic acid–deficient organisms, the connective tissue cells can proliferate. However, their microscopic appearance reveals their functional impotency; their cytoplasm is scanty, and virtually no stainable RNA is present. The basic structural disturbance in scurvy is the failure of various types or connective tissue cells to form their respective collagenous matrices. Fibroblasts are unable to elaborate collagen; osteoblasts and adontoblasts do not synthesize osteoid and dentine. The lack of formation of these matrices explains the failure of wounds to heal, the changes in the growing bone of infants and children, and the alterations in the teeth of experimental animals.

Collagen is characterized chemically by large amounts of glycine, proline, hydroxyproline, and hydroxylysine. The presence of hydroxyamino acids makes collagen unique, since these amino acids are not found in other proteins. Hydroxyproline is not synthesized in the absence of ascorbic acid, which appears to be needed for synthesis of an essential protein enzyme. Since exogenous hydroxyproline is not incorporated into collagen, all the hydroxyproline in the collagen molecule must be derived from the hydroxylation of proline in vivo. The point in collagen synthesis at which hydroxylation of proline takes place has been shown to be following the formation of an initial polypeptide of proline, lysine, and glycine called *protocollagen* or *procollagen.* In this reaction an enzyme called *collagen proline hydroxylase* serves as a catalyst.

The role of ascorbic acid in maintaining the integrity of blood vessels is not clear, but since the integrity of collagen is affected as a result of ascorbic acid deficiency, it is probable that the blood vessels lose the support provided by these fibers and, hence, become more liable to the effects of minor trauma.

Certain other metabolic defects may be observed as a result of ascorbic acid deficiency. One of the most interesting aspects of ascorbic acid function is its nonspecific relation to metabolism of the aromatic amino acids, phenylalanine and tyrosine. Premature infants deficient in ascorbic acid excrete relatively large amounts of homogentisic, parahydroxyphenyllactic, and parahydroxyphenylpyruvic acids in the urine when excess phenylalanine and tyrosine are administered. The defect appears to be an inability to metabolize the tyrosine. Ascorbic acid is implicated in the section of the aqueous humor. The vitamin also plays a role in the metabolism of folic acid, i.e., in the transformation of this material to folacin (citrovorum factor). Occasionally, scurvy is associated with a macrocytic anemia which responds to vitamin C and folic acid. Ingestion of ascorbic acid in food also aids in the absorption of dietary iron.

DIAGNOSIS The clinical features of full-blown scurvy in adults or infants are characteristic. Also helpful is the feeding history in infants. If an infant four to six months or older has been bottle-fed with boiled milk or milk substitutes from birth or shortly after and has received no supplemental ascorbic acid, the possibility of scurvy should be considered. The dietary history of adults is likewise important because the disease often is observed in individuals subsisting on diets obviously low in ascorbic acid content.

X-ray examination in the adult is of no particular help in diagnosis, except that one may see alterations in the lamina dura of the jaws. In infants, x-ray examination of the skeleton may be helpful. At the junction between the epiphyseal cartilage and shaft of the long bones, there may be a zone of increased density, which represents the area of excess spicules of calcified cartilaginous matrix, some of which may have fractured (Fig. 79-1). There may also be defects, i.e., areas of rarefaction, at the "corners" of the bones, and these result from fractures at the periphery of the junction between cartilage and shaft. The formation of spurs or projections of the periosteum about the margins of the cartilage also is characteristic. In addition, the bone film will show a "ground-glass" appearance, which reflects the decrease in density due to diminished width of the cortices and size of the medullary trabeculae.

TREATMENT Infants should be given fresh orange

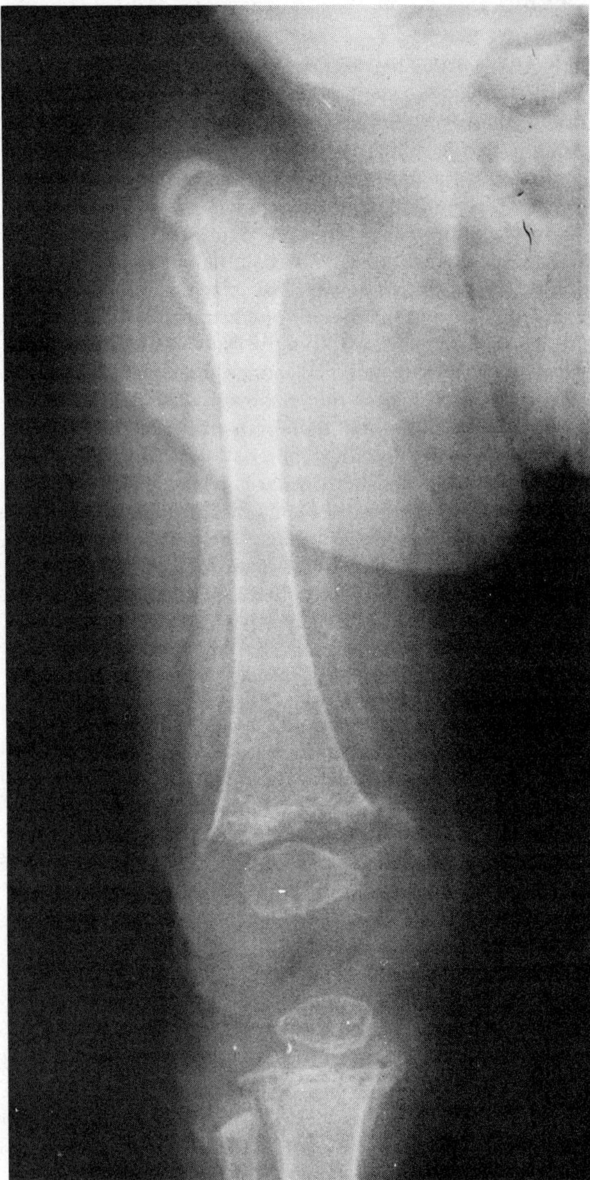

FIGURE 79-1
Four characteristic changes of scurvy. Large subperiosteal hemorrhages are being calcified. The epiphyseal margin shows a translucent line medially, the "corner sign" of Park. The epiphyseal plates are dense, and the bone shaft shows a "ground glass" appearance with lack of trabecular detail. (Courtesy of David Baker, Columbia University)

juice in single or multiple doses each day. This may be sweetened. If orange juice is refused, synthetic ascorbic acid may be employed orally, 100 to 300 mg per day. There is little need for parenteral therapy. In view of the skeletal changes, children in whom the disease is in the stage of healing should be handled as little and as gently as possible. It is not necessary to manipulate any bony deformities, nor should splints or casts be applied.

In adults treatment involves administration of orange juice or ascorbic acid in divided doses up to 500 mg per day. Citrus juices generally contain about 40 to 50 mg ascorbate per 100 ml. A diet rich in vitamin C should be initiated and continued in both children and adults.

About 10 percent of ingested ascorbic acid may be excreted in the urine as oxalate. Acidification of the urine by ingestion of large amounts of ascorbic acid can cause the precipitation of urate, oxalate, or cystine stones in the urinary tract. Large doses of vitamin C also can interfere with the accuracy of clinical tests for glycosuria. In the absence of firm evidence for the usefulness of large doses of ascorbic acid in treatment or prevention of colds or other infections, the use of large amounts of vitamin C for such purposes cannot be recommended, and the potential dangers should be appreciated.

PROGNOSIS Under therapy gum lesions, if present in infants and in adults, begin to regress in 2 to 3 days. Periosteal shadows, resulting from new bone formation, begin to appear in the long bones of infants after approximately a week. Hemorrhages in the skin usually disappear in 2 to 3 weeks.

REFERENCES

BAKER EM et al: Metabolism of ^{14}C-and ^{3}H-labeled L-ascorbic acid in human scurvy. Am J Clin Nutr 23:444, 1971

BARLOW T: On cases described as "acute rickets" which are probably a combination of scurvy and rickets, the scurvy being an essential and the rickets a variable element. Med Chir Trans 66:159, 1883

BURNS JJ: Biosynthesis of L-ascorbic acid: Basic defect in scurvy. Am J Med 26:740, 1959

GOULD BS: *Collagen Biosynthesis*, London: Academic, 1970, p. 139

HESS AF: *Scurvy, Past and Present*, Philadelphia: Lippincott, 1920

HODGES RE et al: Clinical manifestations of ascorbic acid deficiency in man. Am J Clin Nutr 24:432, 1971

80 DEFICIENCIES OF VITAMINS A, E, AND K. HYPERVITAMINOSIS A

THEODORE B. VAN ITALLIE
RICHARD H. FOLLIS, JR.

VITAMIN A History One of the first symptoms of vitamin A deficiency is inability to see in subdued light (night blindness). Treatment of the condition has been known empirically for millennia; Hippocrates recommended the use of ox liver. Over a century ago, Bitot called attention to the simultaneous occurrence of night blindness and lesions of the conjunctiva. At the turn of the century, Mori suggested that ocular lesions seen in Japanese children might be related to a lack of fat in the diet. Early in the twentieth century, two groups of investigators in the United States recognized that a fat-soluble factor was essential for growth, survival, and the prevention of xerophthalmia in rats. In 1924, Bloch reported that xerophthalmia in Danish children could be prevented by feeding them butterfat or cod-liver oil. Somewhat later, the provitamin A status of β-carotene and certain other carotenoids was established. The chemical structures of β-carotene and vitamin A were described in 1930 and 1931, respectively.

The internationally adopted nomenclature for compounds with vitamin A activity is used in this chapter, as follows: *Retinol* denotes vitamin A alcohol; *retinyl ester* is vitamin A ester; *retinal* is vitamin A aldehyde, and *retinoic acid* signifies vitamin A acid.

Prevalence Today, the areas of greatest prevalence of endemic vitamin A deficiency are found in Indonesia, India, Indochina, Central America, the Middle East, and the Philippines. Vitamin A deficiency is the principal cause of blindness in the world, and yet this occurs mostly in tropical areas where the carotenoids that would prevent it are plentiful. Clinically significant vitamin A deficiency is most likely to develop in young children, and the blindness in adults attributed to vitamin A deficiency usually has its origin in childhood. The real need is to educate mothers to change feeding practices which limit intake by children of foods containing vitamin A activity.

Pathogenesis At least two forms of vitamin A alcohol are known (A_1 or retinol and A_2 or 3-dehydroretinol), together with the acid and aldehyde derivatives, retinoic acid and retinal. The vitamins A are intimately related to provitamins, the carotenes, and certain other pigmented compounds. Of these, only dietary β-carotene is of any real significance as a provitamin A. A part of ingested carotene is absorbed by the cells of the intestinal mucosa and transformed into vitamin A. Bile is important in this process. Vitamin A is usually present as retinyl ester in foods; it is hydrolyzed in the intestinal tract and absorbed as retinol. Within the cells of the intestinal mucosa, retinol is esterfied, usually by palmitic acid, and carried in chylomicrons via the thoracic duct to the liver, where it is stored. As needed, retinyl ester is hydrolyzed to the alcohol and transported to the tissues attached to retinol binding protein, an alpha$_1$-globulin which, in turn, is bound to prealbumin. Retinal is found in the retina and is important in the visual process. The interrelations between alcohol, acid, and ester forms of vitamin A have been greatly clarified. Undoubtedly, there is more than one "active form" of vitamin A. In the eye it is 11-*cis*-retinal, but in support of growth, tissue differentiation, and glycopeptide synthesis, retinoic acid is effective. Since retinoic acid does not substitute for retinal in the eye and biologically cannot be reduced to either the alcohol or the acid, there must be at least two "active forms." Moreover, retinoic acid does not substitute for retinal or retinol in the reproductive system.

The greatest concentration of vitamin A in man is found in the liver. Appreciable concentrations are also present in the kidneys, adrenals, lungs, and the retina. Fat depots contain a small amount of the vitamin.

Vitamin A deficiency may result from dietary insufficiency of this vitamin or its precursors or because of some process which interferes with its absorption from the intestinal tract, transport, or storage in the liver. Obstruction of the biliary tract or pancreatic ducts in children or adults may lead to diminished absorption of vitamin A. Diarrhea and the various types of malabsorption syndromes are accompanied by vitamin A deficiency. Of particular importance is the interrelation of vitamin A and protein nutrition, since retinol is transported by a specific protein (retinol binding protein, RBP) which appears to be synthesized in the liver. RBP-retinol complex is further bound to prealbumin which also is thought to be synthesized in the liver. Therefore, protein deficiency may decrease synthesis of these two transport proteins and may possibly alter the activity of the hydrolyzing enzymes necessary for release of retinol from its ester form prior to binding by transport proteins. Small amounts of retinyl ester and carotenoids are present and travel with beta-lipoproteins.

The intricate reactions whereby vitamin A enters into the visual process are summarized in Fig. 80-1. Retinal is the prosthetic group of photosensitive pigment in both rods (*rhodopsin*) and cones (*iodopsin*). All-*trans*-retinol is oxidized to all-*trans*-retinal; this compound isomerizes in the dark to the 11-*cis* form which, combined with *opsin*, forms *rhodopsin*. After absorbing light, the 11-*cis* isomer of retinal is converted back to the corresponding all-*trans* form. Energy to operate this reaction is supplied by light, and the energy exchange stimulates impulses which travel via the optic nerve to the brain.

Pathology The tissues chiefly affected are epithelial in nature, principally those which ordinarily are not keratinized. These include the lining epithelium of the upper and lower respiratory passages, genitourinary tract, eye and paraocular glands, salivary glands, accessory glands of the tongue and buccal cavity, and pancreas. The fundamental change is thought to be metaplasia of the normal nonkeratinized lining cells into a keratinizing type of epithelium. Altered glycoprotein synthesis is associated with the loss of mucous cells. The cornea becomes dry, wrinkled, and hazy owing to intrinsic changes as well as to lack of tears as a result of obstruction of the ducts.

FIGURE 80-1
The reactions whereby vitamin A enters into the visual process.

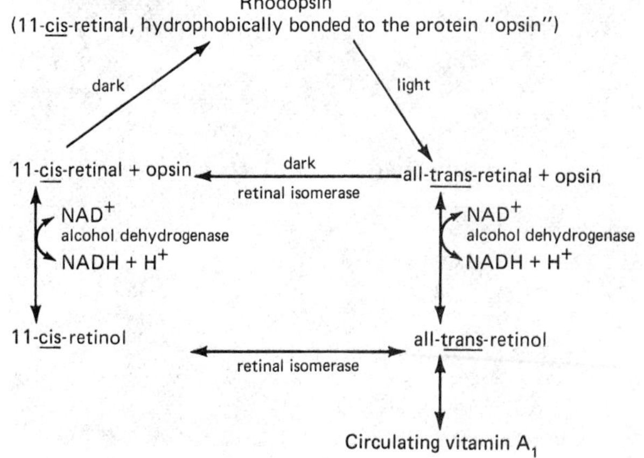

The ciliated epithelium of the respiratory tract is replaced by a keratinizing lining so that the important mechanical effects of the cilia are lost. However, the basal cells in all areas retain their potentiality for reverting to normal if their supply of vitamin A is restored.

How vitamin A maintains the integrity of epithelial structures remains a mystery. Vitamin A appears to be implicated in the metabolism of intracellular structures, the lysosomes, in mucopolysaccharide metabolism, and in steroid hormone formation.

Clinical findings The term *xerophthalmia* is used here in an inclusive sense to refer to certain structural abnormalities of the eye resulting from vitamin A deficiency. The lesions usually exhibit a definite sequence of stages in development. The initial change, which is called *xerosis* (*xerosis epithelialis conjunctivae*), consists of dryness and opacity of the bulbar conjunctiva. Secretion of tears is decreased. At the lateral margin of the cornea a triangular-shaped accumulation of sticky secretion may appear which projects onto the conjunctiva but not over the cornea. This is the Bitot spot, which resembles a plaque or pseudomembrane filled with bubbles (Fig. 80-2). While not pathognomonic, this lesion is highly suggestive of vitamin A deficiency. As the photograph indicates, the Bitot spot has the appearance of a fleck of meringue. This material is difficult to scrape off. Fine pigmentation may also be present throughout the conjunctiva. These alterations are either accompanied or soon followed by haziness and dryness of the cornea (*xerosis corneae*). The tarsal glands along the eyelid frequently are enlarged. Photophobia may be marked. The most serious consequence is the appearance of small, epithelial erosions on the cornea. These soon become infected and enlarged. If this ulceration continues, destruction of the cornea (*keratomalacia*) occurs, a process that may be extremely rapid. Thus a child with conjunctivitis and photophobia may open his eyes one morning to reveal the lens extruded, the bulb collapsed, and vision irrevocably lost (Fig. 80-3). Short of this, the cornea may heal but with a scar that greatly limits vision. In general, the severity of the eye lesions and the rapidity with which they occur are inversely proportional to age.

FIGURE 80-2
Bitot's spots showing the characteristic meringue texture. (Courtesy of DS McLaren and the American Journal of Clinical Nutrition*)*

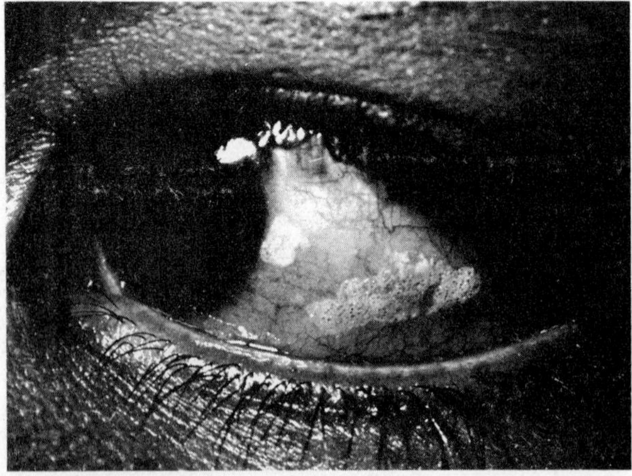

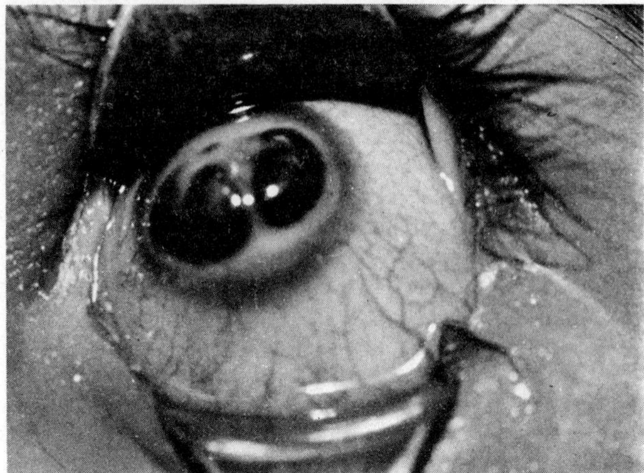

FIGURE 80-3
Destruction of the eye by colliquative necrosis of the cornea. The lense is about to drop out. (Courtesy of DS McLaren)

As already noted, *night blindness* is an early consequence of vitamin A deficiency. Two other terms, *nyctalopia* and *hemeralopia,* have been used to refer to this condition. *Nyctalopia* means an inability to see in subdued light. Hemeralopia refers to a decrease in vision that follows exposure to bright light. Defective ability to see in subdued light may be established by certain tests; however, these are difficult to perform under routine conditions and are particularly unsuited for children. The technique of electroretinography can be used to assess nyctalopia objectively in children as well as adults. Vitamin A deficiency is only one cause of night blindness, however; indeed, in the United States and other technically advanced countries diseases involving pigmentary degeneration of the retina remain the principal cause of nyctalopia.

The nonocular manifestations of vitamin A deficiency frequently are obscured by signs of general malnutrition or the presence of some conditioning disturbance, such as chronic obstruction of the pancreatic or biliary ducts, which may lead to poor absorption of the vitamin. Follicular hyperkeratosis often is found in association with vitamin A deficiency. Keratinization of the hair follicles and atrophy of the sebaceous glands result in the formation of dry papules with protruding cornified plugs. Characteristically, the lesions appear on the buttocks and on the extensor aspects of the legs and arms. Other cutaneous changes include dryness (xerosis) of the skin and acne. It must be emphasized that none of these skin manifestations is specific for vitamin A deficiency. Tracheitis, bronchitis, and pneumonia are complications sometimes associated with severe vitamin A deficiency.

Laboratory findings Laboratory values for vitamin A in serum or plasma are expressed in micrograms per 100 ml or, less commonly, in international units (IU) per 100 ml. One IU is equivalent to 0.3 μg vitamin A or 0.6 μg β-carotene. Serum values for vitamin A and carotene are usually considered to be normal if over 20 and 40 μg per

100 ml, respectively. When values for vitamin A and carotene fall to 10 and 20 μg per 100 ml, respectively, the deficient state is probably present. Vitamin A concentrations lower than 10 μg per 100 ml are diagnostic, but only if acute febrile illness, protein malnutrition, and liver disease have been ruled out. Carotene values may be misleading since the usual laboratory procedure nonspecifically measures all carotenoids and some interfering pigments. Also, carotene values tend to reflect the immediate dietary intake and do not necessarily parallel vitamin A status. Serum vitamin A levels in the range of 20 to 50 μg per 100 ml provide little information of value about vitamin A status except to indicate that the storage tissues are not totally depleted.

Valuable information on vitamin A nutriture among population groups has been obtained from postmortem analyses of liver tissue. For instance, among well-nourished groups in Canada, values averaging approximately 100 μg per g have been obtained. Liver reserves of vitamin A in people living in economically developed countries vary widely, and there is often a lack of correspondence between liver stores of vitamin A and plasma values. In conditions such as liver disease in which synthesis of retinol binding protein is decreased, plasma vitamin A concentration may be decreased while tissue reserves remain adequate. In cirrhosis of the liver, reserves of vitamin A also may be extremely low. Cancer, chronic nephritis, and a variety of infections appear to be associated with rapid depletion of vitamin A reserves.

Diagnosis The eye changes and biochemical findings in vitamin A deficiency often are poorly correlated. Diagnosis and treatment must not wait for all the confirmatory information. A dietary history suggesting a low carotene intake, especially if the diet is also low in fat with consequent poor absorption of carotene, should be suggestive. Protein deficiency appears to aggravate vitamin A deficiency by impairing transport of the vitamin in vivo. Malabsorption states will also predispose to vitamin A deficiency.

Vitamin A levels below 20 μg per 100 ml indicate the need for prompt therapy. Distinctive eye changes demand immediate therapy even without laboratory confirmation.

Therapy Oral administration of 25,000 IU vitamin A daily for 1 or 2 weeks is recommended for the treatment of conjunctival changes or night blindness. Corneal changes should be treated as an emergency, and for the first few days the water-dispersible form of vitamin A should be administered intramuscularly in daily doses of 100,000 IU. Subsequently, 25,000 IU should be given orally for several weeks to build up tissue reserves. When chronic malabsorption is present, a water-miscible preparation should be given orally. The diets of children with vitamin A deficiency are usually also lacking in other nutrients and hence should be improved, particularly with respect to protein. While the integrity of specialized epithelial structures does require vitamin A, it has not been shown that high intakes of vitamin A will prevent infections.

Prognosis The outcome as far as sight is concerned will depend on the degree of involvement of the ocular structures before therapy is instituted. If only clouding of the cornea has occurred, prognosis is excellent. However, if perforation and infection of the anterior chamber have taken place, restoration of sight is virtually unknown.

HYPERVITAMINOSIS A The ingestion by infants and adults of large amounts of vitamin A (doses ranging from 75,000 to 500,000 IU) results in a variety of signs and symptoms that sometimes may be extremely confusing, particularly if a history of ingestion has not been elicited. In adults, excessive amounts of the vitamin often are self-administered in the mistaken belief that such treatment can ward off respiratory infection or improve the appearance of the skin. Because preparations for young children containing vitamin A are usually highly concentrated, accidental overdosage is not uncommon.

In infants, the effects of acute toxicity are drowsiness, vomiting, and bulging of the fontanels as a result of increased intracranial pressure. More chronic evidences of toxicity include failure to gain weight, alopecia, coarseness of hair texture, hepatomegaly, and bone pain. X-ray examination of the skeleton reveals characteristic areas of periosteal new bone formation, particularly prominent in the shafts of the long bones.

In adults, symptoms of acute hypervitaminosis A appear within 4 to 8 hr following ingestion of toxic doses of the vitamin. Headache is the predominant manifestation, but blurred vision or diplopia, nausea, vomiting, vertigo, and drowsiness all may be present. In chronic hypervitaminosis A, bone pain and osseous changes similar to those occurring in children may be observed. In addition, calcification of ligaments, tendons, and subperiosteal tissues may be seen on x-ray examination. Peeling of the skin, neuritis, fissues and sores at the corners of the mouth, coarsening of the skin, alopecia, and localized areas of hyperpigmentation of the epidermis are common. As might be expected, the level of vitamin A in the serum is elevated; values up to 2,000 μg per 100 ml have been reported. However, plasma values of 165 μg per 100 ml and lower may accompany hypervitaminosis A. Plasma values cannot be relied upon to provide the diagnosis of either hypo- or hypervitaminosis A in every instance. Fortunately, the prognosis is good when vitamin A ingestion ceases.

Mention should be made of *carotenemia*, because it may be confused with jaundice. When large amounts of carotene-containing foods are ingested, the blood plasma may contain a high enough concentration of pigment to impart a yellowish color to the skin (especially the palms of the hands and the nasolabial folds) but not the conjunctivae (Chap. 42). *Carotenemia*, in turn, should be distinguished from *lycopenemia*, an analogous condition that results from excessive consumption of tomatoes or tomato juice.

VITAMIN E Vitamin E is the generic name for a group of closely related, naturally occurring, fat-soluble compounds, the tocopherols. Of these, α-tocopherol is biologically the most potent (1 IU = 1 mg *dl*-α-tocopherol acetate). Although they are active as antioxidants, the β, γ, and δ forms of tocopherol appear to be poorly absorbed and are often disregarded in dietary calculations. Vitamin E acts as an antioxidant in food and in animal tissues, inhibiting the peroxidation of unsaturated fatty acids and of such labile compounds as vitamin A. In the absence of vitamin E, rabbits and other herbivorous animals develop a nutritional form of muscular dystrophy, with degeneration and diffuse fibrosis of muscle fibers, deposition of ceroid in smooth muscle and creatinuria. Rodents appear to require vitamin E for normal reproduction, while vitamin E–deficient chicks develop an exudative diathesis and encephalomalacia. Monkeys rendered vitamin E–deficient exhibit a megaloblastic anemia which is reversed by α-tocopherol treatment. Certain synthetic antioxidants can replace α-tocopherol in preventing reproductive failure in rats, while selenium can substitute in part for vitamin E to prevent some of the manifestations of muscular dystrophy. Thus, it remains unclear whether vitamin E has any specific function beyond its role as a lipid antioxidant.

Erythrocytes from tocopherol-deficient laboratory animals and human subjects exhibit an increased in vitro susceptibility to hemolysis induced by dilute hydrogen peroxide, and this test has been used for the clinical estimation of vitamin E status. However, the hemolytic response to peroxide is not specific since it depends not only on the serum tocopherol concentration but on other variables, including the content of peroxidizable lipid in the erythrocyte membrane. Abnormal peroxide hemolysis usually does not occur when the serum tocopherol level exceeds 0.5 mg per 100 ml.

Infants are born with low serum levels of tocopherol and appear to be especially susceptible to vitamin E deficiency, particularly if they are fed diets relatively high in unsaturated vegetable oils that are unsupplemented with tocopherols. The vitamin E–deficiency syndrome that has been observed in premature infants is characterized principally by edema, anemia, thrombocytosis, and an erythematous papular eruption of the skin which is followed by desquamation. Children with cystic fibrosis and other forms of severe, chronic steatorrhea have been reported to have low serum levels of tocopherol, muscular lesions resembling those in experimentally induced nutritional muscular dystrophy, increased serum creatine phosphokinase (CPK) activity, and creatinuria that is reversed by administration of α-tocopherol.

Clinically manifest vitamin E deficiency is extremely rare in adults; however, it has been demonstrated in clinical studies that when the diet contains a high content of polyunsaturated fatty acids, more dietary vitamin E is needed to maintain a "normal" serum tocopherol concentration (usual range 0.6 to 1.4 mg per 100 ml) and a normal erythrocyte life span. Fortunately, most unsaturated margarines, shortenings, and salad oils also contain appreciable quantities of tocopherols, and the apparent absence of vitamin E deficiency in the general population suggests that the quantity of vitamin E in the United States diet is adequate. The recommended dietary allowance for adults is 25 to 30 IU per day.

A regrettable disparity exists between the wishful expectations of many individuals concerning the supposed health benefits of vitamin E and the existence of supporting experimental data. Reliable evidence is lacking that supplementary vitamin E, in whatever dose, can favorably affect physical endurance, cardiac status, potency, fertility, or longevity in individuals with normal serum levels of α-tocopherol.

VITAMIN K Vitamin K occurs in nature in at least two major forms: vitamin K_1 (*phylloquinone*) which is present in most edible vegetables, particularly in green leaves, and vitamin K_2 which is produced by intestinal bacteria. All the many compounds with vitamin K activity are structurally related to the simpler compound, 2-methyl-1,4-naphthoquinone (menadione). Menadione may be formed in the gut by the action of intestinal bacteria on vitamins K_1 and K_2. After absorption, menadione is converted in the body to the active *menaquinone*. Vitamin K is required by man and other animals to maintain prothrombin and clotting factors VII, IX, X, and possibly V. The vitamin appears to act at the ribosomal level, combining with a regulatory protein to control prothrombin synthesis.

Under ordinary circumstances, adequate amounts of vitamin K (judged to be about 0.03 g per kg for adults) are available from the diet and from intestinal bacteria that synthesize the vitamin. Because the naturally occurring forms of vitamin K are fat-soluble and are poorly stored in the body, a conditioned deficiency can occur in association with diseases that interfere with fat absorption. In addition, long-term treatment with certain antimicrobial drugs may temporarily eliminate intestinal bacteria as a vitamin K source. The coumarin anticoagulant drugs appear to induce hypoprothrombinemia by dissociating vitamin K from its regulatory protein. Atypical responses to treatment with coumarin drugs have been attributed to variations in dietary intake of vitamin K or, rarely, to a genetically determined resistance to their anticoagulant action.

Newborn infants tend to be deficient in vitamin K, exhibiting low plasma levels of several coagulation factors in the prothrombin complex. Such deficiencies result from minimal stores of vitamin K at birth, lack of an established intestinal flora, and a very limited dietary intake of the vitamin. The higher concentration of vitamin K in cow's milk (60 μg per liter) as compared with human milk (15 μg per liter) would seem to explain the greater incidence in the past of neonatal hemorrhage among breast-fed infants. Evidence has accumulated that the routine administration of vitamin K to neonates decreases the incidence of hemorrhage. Thus, all newborn infants should receive vitamin K prophylactically. A single intramuscular dose of 0.5 to 1.0 mg of the water-miscible form of vitamin K_1 should suffice for this purpose. Menadione and its water-soluble derivatives have been known to induce kernicterus in premature infants when given in relatively high doses (in excess of 5 mg). This toxic effect has been attributed to increased hemolysis and inhibition of glucuronide formation. Because vitamin K_1 is free of these side effects, its use is clearly preferable during pregnancy and for the neonate. Vitamin K_1 also is more effective than other vitamin K–active compounds in the treatment of coumarin overdosage.

REFERENCES

HOSSAN H et al: Syndrome in premature infants associated with low plasma vitamin E Levels and high polyunsaturated fatty acid diet. Am J Clin Nutr 19:147, 1966

HODGES RE, KOLDER H: Experimental vitamin A deficiency in human volunteers. Proceedings, workshop on biochemical and clinical criteria for determining human vitamin A nutriture, Washington: Food and Nutrition Board, National Academy of Sciences, 1971

HORWITT MK: Vitamin E and lipid metabolism in man. Am J Clin Nutr 8:451, 1960

KANAI M et al: Retinol-binding protein: The transport protein for vitamin A in human plasma. J Clin Invest 47:2025, 1968

MCLAREN DS: *Malnutrition and the Eye,* New York: Academic, 1963

OLSON RE: The mode of action of vitamin K. Nutr Rev 28:171, 1970

ROELS OA: Vitamin A physiology. JAMA 214:1097, 1970

STINSON WH: Vitamin A intoxication in adults. N Engl J Med 8:789, 1961

81
MACROELEMENT AND TRACE ELEMENT DEFICIENCIES

HAROLD SANDSTEAD

Syndromes observed in man which have been shown responsive to diet supplementation with sodium, potassium, magnesium, zinc, copper, chromium, and selenium are discussed here. Supplementation with iodine is discussed in Chap. 85, iron in Chap. 304, phosphorus in Chap. 354, and calcium in Chap. 349.

The factors which influence mineral element nutrition include the total content of the element in food, digestibility of the food, and the presence of ligands in the food which complex with mineral elements and thus increase or decrease their solubility and uptake by the intestinal mucosa. The physiologic status of the gastrointestinal tract also is important. Diseases which decrease intestinal absorption or increase enteric losses of other nutrients such as fat, protein, or water, have adverse effects on mineral element homeostasis. Urinary and/or sweat excretions are contributory factors in the pathogenesis of certain mineral element deficiencies, as is the inappropriate use of diuretic or cathartic drugs. Thus the evaluation of a patient's mineral element nutriture requires an understanding of the physiology of digestion, absorption, and excretion, and of the derangements which disease and drugs may produce in these processes.

SODIUM Under usual circumstances, sodium conservation in normal subjects is extremely efficient. Therefore, except in unacclimatized individuals, in patients with certain diseases or in those who are taking drugs which cause increased endogenous loss, sodium deficiency is rare. The clinical picture associated with sodium lack is nonspecific. Findings include weakness, leg cramps, confusion, apathy, and collapse. Azotemia and hyponatremia sometimes occur. The nonspecificity of these manifestations is indicated by the fact that patients with congestive cardiac failure, cirrhosis of the liver, and protein-calorie malnutrition may exhibit many of them at a time when their total body sodium is relatively increased, but diluted by an even greater increase in total body water (reduced *effective* plasma volume).

Sodium deficiency is best treated by the judicious administration of oral or intravenous sodium. Intravenously, isotonic saline usually is satisfactory, while hypotonic solutions are useful for maintenance therapy. Rarely is it necessary to give hypertonic saline; this should be done with extreme caution.

The consequences of excess dietary sodium are most often observed in patients with impaired myocardial, renal, or hepatic function. Congestive cardiac failure may be precipitated when the dietary sodium intake exceeds the renal excretory capacity; water retained because of the osmotic effect of sodium increases the workload of the heart to the point of failure.

When patients are given amounts of sodium which exceed their renal excretory capacity, acute sodium intoxication may result, with hypernatremia, hypertension, seizures, and cerebral hemorrhage.

POTASSIUM Potassium depletion may occur when enteric loss is excessive, when renal tubular conservation is impaired, when tissue catabolism is increased, and in chronic acidosis. In general, conditions which lead to potassium deficiency may also result in magnesium depletion.

Physiologically, potassium deficiency impairs neuromuscular function. Thus the clinical picture includes weakness, emotional lability, lassitude, ileus, polyuria, and electrocardiographic depression of the T wave and prolongation of the Q-S interval. The serum potassium concentration usually is depressed but may not be. The latter finding is perhaps more common in chronically depleted individuals. Measurement of the total body potassium content by whole-body gamma counting of ^{40}K, or chemical assay of the potassium concentration of muscle tissue, has been used to confirm the diagnosis of potassium deficiency in such patients.

Potassium deficiency may be treated by oral or intravenous administration of the cation or by a diet high in potassium. In general, the chloride salt is preferable because of the participation of chloride in the renal conservation of potassium. Enteric-coated pills of potassium chloride should be avoided as they have been implicated in the ulceration and stricture of the small intestine. In the patient who tends to be recurrently or chronically depleted, the inclusion of high-potassium foods in the diet is desirable.

Intravenously administered potassium should be given with care. Except under unusual circumstances, it is unwise to add more than 40 mEq of potassium per liter of intravenous fluid.

Potassium excess is uncommon. When it occurs, it is

often iatrogenic and is observed in patients with limited renal function or those who have been given drugs which limit potassium excretion. The most important manifestations of potassium excess involve cardiac function. Initially the T waves become "peaked." With increased serum levels, cardiac arrest may occur.

Emergency treatment of hyperkalemia includes the intravenous administration of 50% glucose and regular insulin, the oral or rectal administration of a cation exchange resin, and the administration of sodium chloride if not contraindicated by heart failure or edema. In some instances, hemodialysis may be necessary. Chronic therapy includes the use of diuretic drugs, cation exchange resins, and the avoidance of foods rich in potassium.

MAGNESIUM Primary magnesium deficiency of dietary origin is rare. It has been observed in small infants fed a diet limited to milk. When related to deficiency disease, it is most commonly associated with protein-calorie malnutrition. Other potential causes include malabsorption syndrome, alcoholism, cirrhosis of the liver, renal tubular necrosis in the diuretic phase, hypercalcinuria, diabetic acidosis, chronic diuretic therapy, acute pancreatitis, inappropriate secretion of antidiuretic hormone, and prolonged intravenous therapy with magnesium-free fluids. In many of these disorders the homeostasis of potassium and/or calcium also is abnormal. Hence, the clinical findings in magnesium-deficient patients may reflect combined deficiencies of these elements.

Magnesium deficiency causes an increase in neuromuscular reactivity. Thus the clinical signs include tremor, tetany, seizures, hallucinations, emotional lability, electroencephalographic abnormalities, and cardiac arrhythmias. The electrocardiogram often resembles that seen with hypokalemia; however, such need not be the case, as carefully done magnesium-deficiency experiments in monkeys have produced changes consistent with hyperkalemia. Some magnesium-depleted patients may not exhibit the hyperkinetic behavior noted above, but rather may be hyporeflexive or may have flaccid paralysis. This may be a consequence of associated electrolyte abnormalities. Such variability in manifestations may make the clinical assessment difficult. Magnesium-depleted patients may demonstrate low serum concentrations of the cation. However, as in potassium depletion, this is frequently not the case and establishment of the diagnosis of magnesium deficiency may require analysis of muscle tissue or a carefully controlled therapeutic trial.

Metabolically, magnesium, potassium, and calcium are closely interrelated. Experimental magnesium deficiency in man results in impaired urinary retention of potassium and calcium. With prolonged magnesium deprivation, hypokalemia and hypocalcemia occur. Because of this interrelationship, hypomagnesemia should be ruled out in the hypokalemic or hypocalcemic patient. Treatment of the patient with a combined deficiency with potassium and/or calcium alone may precipitate acute manifestations of magnesium deficiency of which the most serious are seizures and cardiac arrest.

In experimental animals, magnesium deficiency results in renal stones. Although a similar clear relationship has not been established for man, treatment of certain stone-forming individuals with magnesium will decrease the recurrence of stones.

Acute magnesium deficiency can be effectively treated by intramuscular administration of magnesium sulfate. Oral therapy with the chloride, citrate, acetate, or oxide salts is also effective. In some individuals, the cathartic effect of oral treatment may complicate the therapy. Magnesium may also be given intravenously. By this route, it is seldom necessary to give more than 50 mEq per day. During treatment care must be taken to avoid exceeding the renal excretory capacity, thereby inducing hypermagnesemia.

Magnesium excess is most frequently encountered in patients with renal failure. The excretion of magnesium is roughly proportional to the creatinine clearance. Hence if such individuals are given inappropriately large amounts of magnesium containing antacids or cathartics, hypermagnesemia may occur. If high blood levels occur, hypotension, nausea, vomiting, and central nervous system depression may result. Very high levels produce hyporeflexia, coma, respiratory depression, and cardiac arrest. Treatment includes the infusion of calcium and may require hemodialysis.

ZINC Disease in man responsive to zinc has been recognized. Manifestations include delayed sexual maturation, retarded growth, impaired wound healing, decreased sensitivity of taste (hypogeusia) and smell (hyposmia). The response of these disorders to zinc in patients with either low plasma or hair zinc concentrations indicates that zinc deficiency occurs not infrequently.

The total body content of zinc of adult man is 2 to 2.5 g, an amount roughly half that of iron (Chap. 73). Normal plasma zinc levels range from 80 to 120 μg per 100 ml. Experimental animal studies have shown that soft-tissue zinc is bound to intracellular proteins and nucleic acids, and is not found in a storage compound analogous to ferritin. Zinc in bone is relatively sequestered and is slowly exchanged with soft tissues. Thus animals depend on their daily intake to meet their requirement for zinc, and zinc deprivation even for a short time may result in signs of deficiency. Similar events are presumed to occur in man.

Zinc-responsive growth failure occurs in those populations whose intake of foods rich in available zinc (meat, fish, and dairy products) is low. Fruits and green vegetables contain little zinc, while that in grains and legumes is more plentiful. However, unrefined grains and legumes are rich in phytate, a potent chelator of zinc. Most of the zinc in grains is found in the husk. As a consequence, white flour and polished rice are poor sources of dietary zinc. Methods of bread preparation influence the amount of phytate present in the final product. Yeast produces an enzyme (phytase) which destroys phytate. Leavening therefore is thought to increase the availability of divalent cations including zinc from bread. Therefore, the degree of refinement of grains and the methods used in bread preparation are important factors influencing the zinc intake of populations which subsist primarily on foods derived from grains. Individuals who are most likely to be adversely affected by the above factors include rapidly growing children, adolescents, and pregnant women.

In economically advanced countries, a major factor in the occurrence of zinc deficiency is the nonconsumption of foods rich in available zinc. Those who for economic reasons, or because of preference, or for medical reasons habitually eat diets low in meat and other animal products are at risk. As the requirement for zinc is related to the physiologic state, persons consuming diets marginal in zinc may be expected to develop clinical deficiency when increased requirements for growth, tissue repair, or pregnancy are superimposed on the basal intake. Zinc-responsive hypogeusia in pregnancy and in patients subjected to the stress of disease may represent examples of such a phenomenon. Zinc-responsive growth failure in children who are "picky eaters" and zinc-responsive growth failure in young patients with intestinal malabsorption are other examples, as is zinc-responsive impaired healing. The increased excretion of zinc, which occurs in some patients with cirrhosis, alcoholism, chronic renal disease, recurrent febrile illness, and semistarvation, may be a contributory factor in the pathogenesis of zinc deficiency, particularly if the dietary intake of the patient is marginal.

At present, the diagnosis of zinc deficiency in man requires knowledge of the diet and of the contributing factors which may increase endogenous losses or requirements. This knowledge is helpful in the interpretation of plasma and/or hair concentrations. Finally, the diagnosis may be established by a carefully controlled therapeutic trial of zinc under conditions where the intake of other nutrients is adequate. Thirty milligrams of zinc twice daily as zinc sulfate is adequate for correcting deficiencies unless the patient has a disease which causes large endogenous loss. The response to therapy is often dramatic.

Poisoning with zinc may occur through inhalation in individuals working in brass foundries or from consumption of food or drink stored in zinc containers. Both conditions are infrequent. The quantities of zinc needed to produce toxicity are many times the requirements or usual therapeutic doses.

COPPER In contrast to zinc, copper deficiency in man occurs only under very unusual circumstances. For example, infants recovering from severe protein-calorie malnutrition who were maintained on the same milk formula developed hypochromic microcytic anemia, leukopenia, and thin bone cortices. One suffered a pathologic fracture similar to those observed in copper-deficient puppies. The anemia and other abnormalities responded to copper. The rarity of clinically evident copper deficiency is probably related to the wide distribution of copper in foods and the efficient mechanisms which maintain relatively large stores of copper within the body.

Copper intoxication is also unusual. As discussed in Chap. 103, individuals with impaired biliary secretion of copper, as in Wilson's disease, accumulate large amounts of copper in their livers and other tissues with adverse clinical effects.

OTHER TRACE ELEMENTS Deficiencies of other trace elements have not been unequivocally recognized in man (Chap. 73). The beneficial effect of trivalent chromium on the glucose tolerance of infants with severe protein-calorie malnutrition is consistent with the concept that the children were chromium-deficient. Evidence consistent with selenium lack also has been obtained in infants with protein-calorie malnutrition.

REFERENCES

HALSTEAD JA et al: Zinc deficiency in man. Am J Med 53:277, 1972

MERTZ W, CORNATZER WE (eds): *Newer Trace Elements*, New York: Marcel Dekker, 1971

O'DELL BL, CAMPBELL BJ: *Trace Elements: Metabolism and Metabolic Function in Comprehensive Biochemistry*, vol. 21, eds M Florkin, EH Stotz, New York: Elsevier, 1971, p. 179

SLINK EB, JONES E (eds): The pathogenesis and clinical significance of magnesium deficiency. Ann NY Acad Sci 162:705, 1969

THE NUTRITION FOUNDATION: *Present Knowledge in Human Nutrition*, 3d ed., New York: The Foundation, 1967

82
GENERAL CONSIDERATIONS AND MAJOR SYNDROMES

GEORGE W. THORN

INTRODUCTION It is now generally agreed that hormones do not initiate new events in the complicated biochemistry of metabolic processes, but rather produce their effects by regulating enzymatic and other chemical reactions already present. In view of the relatively large number of hormones, their diverse chemical structures, and their multiple sites of action, it may be assumed that scarcely a single important metabolic event can escape the effect of their primary or secondary action. From this one may conclude that a true understanding of any disease process or physiologic disorder must encompass an appreciation of the possible etiologic role of hormones and the factors regulating their synthesis, release, and degradation. In this regard, one may point to such widely diverse actions as the effect of catecholamines (adrenal medulla) on brain metabolism and psychologic behavior; the effect of adrenal steroids on the inflammatory reaction associated with infection, trauma, surgery, or burns; the effect of insulin on adipose tissue metabolism; and the importance of growth hormone on the fabrication of body proteins.

In this edition, the chapter on diseases of parathyroid function has been moved from the endocrinology section to a later section in which is presented a coordinated discussion on calcium and bone metabolism and diseases involving abnormalities in parathyroid function, vitamin D and calcitonin (see Chaps. 347 to 352).

MECHANISMS OF ENDOCRINOPATHIES Characteristically, endocrine abnormalities arise as a consequence of increased or decreased hormone secretion. In the majority of patients, the clinical manifestations derive from an excess of or deficiency of the *normally* secreted hormone. However, in certain syndromes, such as some cases of adrenal virilism, the endocrinopathy may result from secretion of an abnormal hormone. In addition, hormonal disorders may result from aberrations in the metabolism or degradation of hormones. For example, a deficiency of plasma proteins may decrease the quantity of hormone-carrying protein in the blood and hence modify significantly the balance between "free" and "bound" thyroid hormone; liver disease may alter the conjugation or degradation of steroid hormones, giving rise to abnormal blood and tissue hormone levels. In such types of abnormalities, however, serious endocrine disorders will result only if the "servo-regulating" mechanism, or feedback response, fails to stimulate the appropriate reaction in the trophic gland. Endocrine abnormalities may also develop when local tissues are unable to respond to a normal hormonal level. For example, localized myxedema over the tibia may occur in the presence of thyrotoxicosis or euthyroidism; in cases of pseudohypoparathyroidism, the abnormalities observed in hypoparathyroidism occur despite the presence of normal parathyroid glands. In some endocrinopathies, heightened tissue susceptibility to hormone action is the determining factor in the genesis of the syndrome, e.g., hirsutism in young women with a minimal abnormality in androgenic steroid secretion, or extreme degrees of hyperpigmentation observed in patients with early adrenal insufficiency and increased melanin pigmentation on a racial basis.

Hormonal secretions in general show wide fluctuations throughout the 24-hr period, periods of high activity often alternating with those of reduced secretion; e.g., in the early morning the level of adrenal cortical secretory activity is high. Evidence is accumulating that endocrinopathy may result from a loss of cyclic diurnal pattern due to a more or less constant hormonal elaboration throughout the day and night, resulting in only a slight increase, if any, in total secretion. Two important considerations have been derived from these observations: (1) Interpretation of single determinations of hormone content—of blood, tissues, or urine—reflecting instantaneous or relatively short collection periods may be unreliable; for final evaluation, repeated determinations, longer collection periods, or isotopic "turnover" studies may be required. (2) Clinical application of the cyclic method of hormone administration has been quite successful in minimizing undesirable hormone side effects while maintaining control of the underlying disease process.

DIAGNOSTIC APPROACH TO ENDOCRINE ABNORMALITIES The suspicion that an endocrine abnormality may play a role in a patient's illness will often derive initially from the gross physical appearance of the patient, as in myxedema, hyperthyroidism, pituitary dwarfism or gigantism, acromegaly, hypogonadism, carotenemia (diabetes mellitus or hypothyroidism), Addison's disease, Cushing's syndrome, and the adrenogenital syndrome. Although a careful history and physical examination will in most instances provide presumptive evidence of an underlying endocrine disorder, the definitive diagnosis will almost invariably depend upon the values obtained from laboratory examinations. Here, accuracy in diagnosis depends upon the specificity of the laboratory test, its precision and its reproducibility, the care and understanding with which specimens are collected, and the reliability of the laboratory that carries out the procedures. It is essential to realize, however, that a single determination of a specific hormone (in blood, urine, or tissue) does not necessarily establish or exclude an endocrine abnormality. The addition of hormonal "turnover" or "secretory" measurements by means of isotopic techniques represents a great step forward. The use of stressful situations or specific substances such as ACTH (adrenocorticotropin) for the adrenal, thyroid-stimulating hormone (TSH) for the thyroid, and glucose for the detection of early diabetes permits one to test the functional reserve of these endocrine systems and thereby facilitates the diagnosis of potential endocrine deficiency at a time when prophylactic measures may prove effective. In the evaluation of endocrine disorders associated with excessive secretion, suppressive-type tests are of greatest value; in deficiency states stimulatory tests often yield the most information. In the succeeding chapters, particular attention will be devoted to indicating the usefulness and limitations of diagnostic methods and the degree of specificity attached to the procedure. Because of its great practical importance, the source of common errors related to these determinations will also be emphasized.

ENDOCRINE SYNDROMES Although secretions of the endocrine glands govern widespread metabolic activities throughout the body, from the viewpoint of the internist, major endocrine disorders present over and over again as a limited number of syndromes. These will be reviewed briefly in relation to the cardinal manifestations of disease.

Weakness and increased fatigability (see also Chap. 15) These are without doubt the most frequent presenting symptoms of adult patients seeking assistance from the internist or general practitioner. Although in the majority of instances these complaints derive primarily from emotional or psychologic disturbances, underlying organic disease must always be considered. When endocrine abnormalities are suspected, one should inquire first whether the symptoms have been accompanied by *weight loss*—if so, adrenal cortical insufficiency, hyperthyroidism, and diabetes mellitus should be considered. Adrenal cortical insufficiency, if present, should be accompanied by some increase in pigmentation, hypotension, gastrointestinal disturbances, and perhaps salt craving. Hyperthyroidism would be suggested by goiter, eye changes, tremor, intolerance for heat, etc., and diabetes mellitus by polyuria and polydipsia.

Without weight loss, but with symptoms of weakness and fatigability, one would consider hypothyroidism, hypopituitarism, hyperparathyroidism, and hyperaldosteronism. The first of these is characteristically associated with delayed reflexes. intolerance to cold, dry skin, and carotenemia. Hypopituitarism is suggested by oligomenorrhea or amenorrhea in the female, impotence in the male, decreased tolerance to cold, hypoglycemic episodes, and hypotension. Hyperparathyroidism is suggested by the association of bone pain, renal calculi, and polyuria. Hyperaldosteronism might be accompanied by significant hypertension, demonstrable muscular weakness, polyuria, and electrocardiographic changes that suggest potassium depletion.

Menstrual irregularities (see also Chap 92) In addition to pregnancy and local disease of the uterus, menstrual irregularities are associated with four major endocrine disturbances: (1) *primary ovarian failure,* prior to natural menopause and characterized by hot flashes, gain in weight, increased emotional instability, and elevated urinary values of follicle-stimulating hormone; (2) *secondary ovarian failure,* associated with reduced or absent urinary gonadotropins and evidence of other target gland deficiencies, i.e., thyroid and adrenal; (3) *hypothyroidism,* in which menorrhagia as well as oligomenorrhea frequently occurs; (4) *adrenogenital syndrome,* in which oligomenorrhea or amenorrhea is seen in combination with increased muscular development, hirsutism, and other signs of masculinization.

Hirsutism (see also Chap 57) Increased body hair in females and decreased scalp hair in both sexes is a frequent disorder for which patients seek medical attention. Unfortunately, most female patients with increased hair do not have a demonstrable excess of adrenal or ovarian androgens. Increased androgenic secretion should be considered when *hirsutism* is associated with menstrual irregularities and amenorrhea, or with other evidence of virilism, i.e., increased muscular development and increased size of clitoris.

Although loss of scalp hair and baldness is almost never due to a specific endocrinopathy, a receding hair line in female patients associated with *increased* body hair should always suggest excessive androgenic hormone secretion of adrenal or gonadal origin. Thinning of the hair is frequent in patients with Cushing's syndrome, hypothyroidism, or hypopituitarism. It is rare, however, to observe disturbances in hair growth as a manifestation of serious endocrine abnormality in the absence of rather well-defined signs and symptoms of adrenal, pituitary, or gonadal dysfunction.

Impotence and decreased libido (see also Chap. 50) Although these cardinal manifestations of functional disorder are a frequent basis for medical consultation, they are rarely due primarily to endocrinopathies. In addition to primary disease of the generative organs, however, *anterior pituitary deficiency,* especially associated with chromophobe adenomas, should be considered. Evidence of local tumor (changes in vision, headache, etc.) and associated target gland deficiencies (adrenal, thyroid, and gonadal) should be sought. Patients with diabetes mellitus will often exhibit both impotence and decreased libido, but in most instances this occurs after the disease has been present for some time.

Obesity (see also Chap. 45) Obesity suggests the possibility of an underlying endocrine disturbance, which in practice rarely is causative. However, two serious disorders must be considered in patients with marked, generalized obesity. The first is diabetes mellitus, and this should be investigated with a postprandial glucose determination and a glucose tolerance test, if fasting blood glucose levels are within the normal range and if sugar is not present in the urine. The second serious disorder is insulinoma. Hunger, increased appetite, and weight gain are characteristic of patients with insulinoma as well as of those with "reactive" hypoglycemia. The former experience the greatest degree of hunger and symptoms after prolonged fast, the latter shortly after eating, particularly after a meal of high carbohydrate content. In both instances appetite and food intake are stimulated by absolute or relative hypoglycemia, and the vicious cycle is continued.

Hypothyroidism and mild hypopituitarism may be associated with moderate obesity. The final diagnosis of the former will require laboratory tests of thyroid function; the latter requires tests for the adequacy of target gland function.

Gross obesity in Cushing's syndrome is rare—what is more common is loss of adipose tissue in the extremities with an increase in abdominal fat pad, striae, and "buffalo hump."

There is no doubt that castration or ovarian failure predisposes to obesity. However, in young women there often occurs a reversal of this cycle; namely, rapid weight gain secondary to excess food intake, stress, and anxieties, which may be *followed* by oligomenorrhea or amenorrhea. Whether the weight gain itself is of primary importance in the genesis of the ovarian dysfunction, or whether weight gain and altered gonadal function are both secondary to changes in the hypothalamic centers is not known. However, it is well established that improvement in emotional status and with weight loss, normal ovulation and menstruation will often ensue.

Hypertension (see also Chaps. 86, 87, and 245) Hypertension is another frequent disorder that should suggest an underlying endocrine abnormality. The hypertensive patient with minimal abnormalities in urinary constituents but with polyuria and nocturia suggests hypokalemia (hyperaldosteronism) or hypercalcemia (hyperparathyroidism). Clinically the hypokalemic patient with *hyperaldosteronism* rarely presents with the malignant form of hypertension and characteristically exhibits neuromuscular weakness. The electrocardiogram will often reveal changes consistent with potassium depletion, whereas serum sodium concentration is usually *elevated.* The problem is to exclude hypokalemia induced by diuretic administration, especially the thiazides, and the ensuing secondary hyperaldosteronism.

The patient with hypertension, polyuria, and hypercalcemia associated with *hyperparathyroidism* will frequently give a history of urinary calculi or bone pain. He may also present the stigmas of psychoneurosis as a consequence of sustained hypercalcemia. Band keratopathy is rare except with long-continued elevated serum calcium level.

Two characteristic findings in patients with hypertension secondary to *pheochromocytoma* are the cyclic nature of hypertension in the classic syndrome and the absence of obesity. Unfortunately, most tumors secrete predominantly norepinephrine; hence, the textbook picture of tachycardia, nervousness, sweating, and glucosuria is infrequent.

Hypertension and moderate obesity, particularly of the truncal type, suggest *Cushing's syndrome.* This possibility is greatly increased if diabetes mellitus, easy bruisability, and pink abdominal striae are present. Every hypertensive patient with diabetes mellitus should be screened for adrenal overactivity.

Hypertension as an early manifestation of diabetes mellitus is uncommon. However, since hypertensive-vascular disease is such a frequent complication of diabetes mellitus, hypertensive patients—especially those who are obese—should have postprandial blood glucose determined and glucose tolerance test performed.

Hypertension as a manifestation of *adrenogenital syndrome* should be considered in young subjects with associated evidence of virilism.

Abnormalities in growth (see also Chaps. 83 and 85) Abnormalities in growth, particularly in children, are associated with *hyposomatotropism, gonadal dysfunction, hypothyroidism,* and *cretinism.* The latter must be detected within the first few weeks after birth if serious damage to the central nervous system is to be prevented. All babies with *persistent* umbilical hernia should be screened for possible *hypothyroidism.* Untreated diabetes mellitus will result in retarded growth, as will excess cortisol and androgen secretion. Long-standing renal disease will impair skeletal growth and mimic an endocrinopathy because of the frequent coexistence of secondary hyperparathyroidism.

Closely related to abnormalities in growth among adolescent boys is the problem of *undescended testes.* A conservative approach is urged, and the reader is referred to Chap. 91 for details as to the management of this important problem.

Other cardinal signs that should call attention to possible endocrine abnormalities include the following:

1 Changes in the skin (see also Chaps. 55 to 57). Dryness in hypothyroidism and Addison's disease; thin, atrophic skin with "wrinkles" in pituitary and gonadal failure; easy bruisability in Cushing's syndrome; moist, fine, warm skin in hyperthyroidism; coarse, reduplicated skin in acromegaly; hyperpigmentation in Addison's disease.

2 Arthropathies are not infrequent in acromegaly, gigantism, myxedema, and primary gonadal failure.

3 Tetany and convulsive seizures (see Chap. 24) may indicate hypoglycemia (insulinoma, reactive hypoglycemia, Addison's disease, hypopituitarism), hypocalcemia (hypoparathyroidism), or hypokalemia (hyperaldosteronism, Cushing's syndrome).

4 The presence of edema (see Chap. 30) should suggest hypothyroidism or myxedema as well as secondary hyperaldosteronism and Cushing's syndrome.

5 Psychologic abnormalities (see Chap. 14) are frequently observed in Addison's disease and Cushing's syndrome as well as in hypopituitarism, hypothyroidism, hyperthyroidism, hyperparathyroidism, and acromegaly.

IATROGENIC ENDOCRINOPATHIES With the widespread use of corticosteroids, thyroid, and sex hormones as nonspecific therapeutic agents, new and difficult problems present themselves to the internist and endocrinologist. One may be faced with iatrogenic Cushing's syndrome, hyperthyroidism, or virilism—or severe adrenal insufficiency or hypothyroidism if specific hormone therapy is discontinued rapidly or completely. Special problems relating to these phenomena will, because of their seriousness, be discussed at length in relation to each of the specific hormones so implicated. The use of hormones as nonspecific therapeutic agents, while offering great promise in many serious and often fatal diseases, is fraught with difficulties and requires, in addition to a thorough knowledge of the endocrine preparations a comprehension of their physiologic and pharmacologic effects.

83
DISEASES OF THE ANTERIOR LOBE OF THE PITUITARY GLAND

DON H. NELSON

The pituitary gland lies at the base of the brain in a bony cavity, the sella turcica, within the sphenoid bone. The normal gland measures 10 × 13 × 6 mm and weighs approximately 0.6 g. Anatomically it is divided into the anterior lobe, which constitutes three-quarters of the weight of the gland, a rudimentary intermediate lobe, and a posterior or neural lobe. The classic histology of the anterior lobe divides the cells into three types, depending on the presence and staining characteristics of the intracellular granules. These are the chromophobes, which are agranular, the eosinophils, and the basophils, in the proportions of approximately 52, 37, and 11 percent, respectively. More detailed studies suggest that some of the agranular cells may contain fine acidophilic and basophilic granules; hence the term "amphophils."

The anterior lobe secretes a variety of peptide hormones, of which six are clearly defined. Growth hormone (HGH) has a generalized somatic effect on growth; adrenocorticotropin (ACTH) stimulates the secretory activity of the adrenal cortex; thyroid-stimulating hormone (thyrotropin, TSH) stimulates the formation and release of thyroid hormones; follicle-stimulating hormone (FSH) stimulates growth of the graafian follicle and estrogen secretion in the female and spermatogenesis in the male; luteinizing hormone (LH) initiates ovulation and luteinization of the mature follicle in the female; in the male, this hormone is the testicular interstitial cell-stimulating hormone (ICSH), responsible for male hormone secretion. Prolactin or lactogenic hormone (LtH) is responsible for secretion of milk by the properly developed mammary gland. Although production of the melanocyte-stimulating hormone (MSH) is classically ascribed to the intermediate lobe, this hormone may also be a secretion of the anterior lobe.

According to classic concepts, the chromophobe cells are considered to be nonsecretory, the eosinophilic cells responsible for secretion of GH, LH, and LtH, and the basophilic cells producing ACTH, TSH, and FSH. Such a simple classification, however, does not now seem probable; some pituitary tumors associated with Cushing's syndrome have been found to be composed of chromophobe as well as eosinophilic cells, although the largest number are small basophilic tumors. Similarly, eosinophilic tumors are most often associated with increased growth hormone production, but tumors of other cell types may occasionally be responsible.

RELEASING FACTORS The isolation, identification, and synthesis of the gonadotropin-releasing factor and the thyrotropin-releasing factor have added a new dimension to the investigation of patients with hypothalamic pituitary disease. These small polypeptides cause release of the specific pituitary hormone but have also been found to have additional effects. TRH (thyrotropin-releasing hormone) produces an increase in prolactin as well as TSH. It is also of interest that the gonadotropin-releasing factor is effective in releasing both LH and FSH. Other hypothalamic hormones which have been identified include CRH (corticotropin-releasing hormone) and GRH (growth hormone–releasing hormone).

Administration of pharmacologic amounts of TRH to patients with hypothyroidism secondary to TSH deficiency has demonstrated that some of these patients have an increase in TSH. This would indicate that there is a primary deficit in TRH, rather than in TSH, in these patients. As the primary feedback control of TSH release is thought to be the "short loop" of thyroid hormone action on the pituitary gland, these results raise the possibility of some effect of TRH on this mechanism as well (see Chap. 85).

PITUITARY TUMORS

Pituitary tumors account for approximately 10 percent of all intracranial tumors. By far the commonest pituitary tumor is the *chromophobe adenoma,* which is usually nonsecretory in nature. Active pituitary tumors usually secrete only one pituitary hormone in excess. Tumors secreting GH, ACTH, MSH, TSH, and LtH have all been described, although the last three types of tumor are very rare. FSH- or LH-secreting tumors are notable by their absence.

In addition to producing the *signs and symptoms* of hormone excess, discussed in later sections on the specific hormones, these tumors may compress and destroy normal pituitary tissue within the sella turcica and produce hormonal deficiency states, or they may extend out of the sella turcica to compress the optic nerves, hypothalamus, and other nervous structures in the vicinity. Pressure on the optic chiasma most often involves the decussating nerve fibers supplying the nasal retinal fields and leads to loss of the temporal fields of vision and classical bitemporal hemianopsia. Further extension of the tumor may involve one or both optic nerves and result in loss of visual acuity and even in complete blindness. These tumors may also compress the hypothalamus and result in disturbances in sleep, temperature control, appetite, and autonomic nervous functions. Curiously, these tumors are not known to damage the supraopticohypophyseal tract to a degree to cause diabetes insipidus. Involvement of the third, fourth, and sixth cranial nerves is rare but may occur. Headache is a frequent complaint in patients with this condition and has no well-defined pattern.

Clinical evaluation of these patients should include roentgenograms of the skull and visual fields, ophthalmoscopic examination, spinal fluid examination (particularly for increased protein content), and pneumoencephalography, especially in patients with severe optic nerve compression, increased intracranial pressure, or signs of hypothalamic and brain involvement. Carotid angiography may also be useful in delineating any extension of a tumor out of the sella.

Therapy of pituitary tumors generally involves a choice between pituitary irradiation or surgery. Postponement of specific treatment is justifiable in occasional patients with small, localized chromophobe adenomas, in which case specific hormonal replacement therapy should be initiated and the patient carefully observed for signs of tumor growth and extension. Surgical resection of tumor tissue is indicated when there is rapid deterioration of vision, ventricular obstruction, or significant brain compression. Although surgery provides the greatest opportunity for arrest of tumor growth, it entails calculated morbidity and mortality rates, particularly with the large tumors extending outside the sella turcica.

Radiotherapy in tissue doses of 3,500 to 4,500 R is often associated with regression of the tumor and relief of local signs and symptoms. In these doses, normal pituitary tissue and surrounding nervous structures are unharmed. Some tumors recur and may require further x-ray therapy or surgery. Techniques such as cryohypophysectomy, proton-beam irradiation, and radioactive implantations have been found useful when applied by specific investigators but should still be considered experimental.

Hemorrhage into a tumor, so-called "pituitary apoplexy," may result in an acute catastrophe accompanied by severe headache, blindness, hypotension or shock, fever, and signs of meningeal irritation or brain involvement. Emergency treatment is required, which may include surgical aspiration of the sella turcica, use of adrenal-steroids, and other supportive measures. Pituitary apoplexy may occur spontaneously and is occasionally observed following irradiation.

The craniopharyngioma, which is usually suprasellar in position, is the most common type of tumor involving the pituitary gland in childhood and thus the most common cause of prepuberal hypopituitarism. The tumor represents a secretory vestige of Rathke's pouch cut off from its origin in the roof of the pharynx and carried cephalad by the migrating pituitary anlage. The viscous, cholesterol-containing fluid of such suprasellar cysts is liable to calcification, which provides a useful diagnostic sign on x-ray examination. Although these tumors are more frequent in the younger age group, occasionally they are slow-growing and may not be clinically apparent until adult life. These patients often mature normally and come to the physician with an adult form of hypopituitarism. These tumors usually require surgical intervention. *Other tumors* which may involve the pituitary or the suprasellar area include meningiomas, epidermoid or dermoid tumors, primary or metastatic carcinomas, and granulomatous disorders such as sarcoidosis, gummas, tuberculomas, and Hand-Schüller-Christian disease.

THE EMPTY SELLA SYNDROME It is common to equate enlargement of the sella turcica with an expanding intracranial lesion. At times, however, pneumoencephalography demonstrates that the sella is not occupied by a tumor mass but admits a significant amount of air (Neelon et al). Of 31 patients noted to have air within the sella, 27 were female. Headache was common but visual field disturbances attributable to lesions of the optic chiasm were absent. The dimensions of the sella were enlarged in 26 of the 31 patients, and endocrine disturbances were noted in eight. The primary empty sella is considered a benign condition probably caused by elevation of intracranial pressure that remodels the anatomy of the sella through a congenital incompleteness of the sellar diaphragm.

GROWTH HORMONE

Growth hormone, unlike the other anterior pituitary hormones, does not have a specific "target organ" but has a generalized effect on all tissues and organs. This hormone has a molecular weight of 22,000, although there is some indication that an "active core" may be considerably smaller. Though once thought to be solely concerned with growth in the early years of life, growth hormone has been found to exert significant physiologic functions throughout life. It has been shown to facilitate amino acid transport and incorporation into protein, to mobilize free fatty acids from peripheral fat stores, and to reduce lipid synthesis. Growth hormone also causes renal retention and body storage of calcium, phosphorus, sodium, potassium, and nitrogen as part of its generalized anabolic action. It has an anti-insulin or diabetogenic action and, in large doses, can produce glucosuria, impaired glucose tolerance, and insulin resistance. Growth hormone is responsible for the elevated level of serum inorganic phosphorus and alkaline phosphatase observed in growing children.

Growth hormone is species-specific, and only primate growth hormone has been found to have significant physiologic effects in man and to be capable of stimulating growth in pituitary dwarfs.

Plasma growth hormone levels are readily measured by radioimmunoassay, and elevated levels have been found in most patients with acromegaly. Significantly, growth hormone levels have been shown to increase following exercise, prolonged fast, and during hypoglycemia, which suggests a dynamic physiologic role for this hormone throughout life, in addition to its growth-promoting effects in childhood.

Other substances which may produce an increase in plasma growth hormone are arginine, vasopressin, pyrogens, and estrogens. The latter, because of their widespread use in contraceptive preparations, may give falsely high growth hormone values in patients suspected of having acromegaly.

Considerable evidence relates the action of growth hormone on bone to the production of a "plasma sulfation factor," which has been called *somatomedin.* This substance, presumably formed in the liver secondary to growth hormone action, has been related also to "plasma insulin-like activity" and has been shown to have antilipolytic and anabolic effects which are similar to those of insulin.

GROWTH HORMONE–SECRETING TUMORS Marie, in 1886, first described the classical clinical manifestations of acromegaly. One year later, Minkowski reported a case with a pituitary tumor, and Benda subsequently showed that such tumors were eosinophilic in nature. In 1895, Brissaud and Meige suggested an association between gigantism and acromegaly, and Hutchinson subsequently reported the pathologic findings in three cases of gigantism associated with pituitary tumors. Acromegaly and gigantism are now recognized as identical disturbances of growth hormone secretion, differing only in the age of onset of the disorder.

GIGANTISM Prior to puberty, excess growth hormone secretion results in a generalized overgrowth of the skeleton and soft tissues with resulting marked increases in height and size. Early in the course of the disorder, these patients are usually physically strong and alert. Later in the disease, however, pituitary insufficiency may develop, with its associated weakness and easy fatigability. Hypogonadism due to gonadotropin deficiency may develop late in the disease.

The underlying lesion is generally an *eosinophilic or mixed cell adenoma of the anterior lobe* which is usually visible radiologically. The condition, although rare, presents no difficulty in diagnosis and needs only to be differentiated clinically from the tall stature of primary gonadal failure. Persons with the latter condition exhibit the characteristic eunuchoid habitus and associated gonadal failure and, unlike the patient with gigantism, have increased titers of urinary follicle-stimulating hormone characteristic of primary hypogonadism. Treatment of pituitary gigantism is similar to that for acromegaly.

ACROMEGALY In adults, the same type of pituitary tumor producing excess growth hormone results in the clinical picture of acromegaly. The disease is usually first manifested by changes in facial features and overgrowth of the head, hands, and feet which may necessitate an increase in hat, glove, or shoe size (Fig. 83-1). In other instances, headache or visual disturbances from local effects of the expanding pituitary tumor may be the first indications of the disorder.

The fully developed syndrome is easily recognized, but in the earlier stages, comparison of serial photographs over a span of years may be extremely helpful in documenting a gradual and progressive change in features. The hands and feet are broad and greatly enlarged, the ends of the digits are square, and prognathism may be so marked as to interfere with mastication (Fig. 83-2). Arthritic manifestations are not unusual, and widespread osteoarthritic-like changes in the bones and joints are often demonstrable. Patients with acromegaly are particularly subject to psychologic disturbances and almost always exhibit considerable emotional instability.

Among the associated endocrine disturbances, enlargement of the thyroid and an increased basal metabolic rate are frequently found. Hyperthyroidism, however, occurs in only a small percentage of cases. Although frank diabetes mellitus is present in only 10 to 15 percent of these patients, glucose tolerance is impaired in the majority of patients during the active phase of the disease. Diabetes mellitus, when present, is typically mild but may be relatively resistant to insulin therapy. Libido may be increased at the onset but is lost subsequently, and gonadal atrophy may occur late in the disease. The course of the disease is usually one of benign chronicity, but fatal termination may occur as a result of cardiac failure, diabetic acidosis, local complications of the tumor, or unrecognized hypopituitarism.

Diagnosis Diagnosis is made by the typical changes in body configuration, possible demonstration of a pituitary tumor by x-ray or visual field defects, and most importantly, by an elevated basal plasma growth hormone level which does not decrease during a standard glucose tolerance test, although in some acromegalic patients a decrease has been seen. Because the skeletal changes are permanent, it is important in the treated as well as the untreated case to determine whether there is continual hypersecretion of growth hormone, or whether a deficiency of growth hormone and perhaps of other hormones has resulted from pituitary destruction from pressure, hemorrhage, or earlier x-ray therapy. Activity of the process is implied by continued skeletal and soft-tissue growth, by the presence of diabetes mellitus or a significantly impaired glucose tolerance test, by elevated levels of serum inorganic phosphorus and alkaline phosphatase, and by increased excretion of hydroxyproline in the

FIGURE 83-1
A forty-four-year-old woman with arrested acromegaly. Onset of the disease occurred when patient was twenty-four years of age, when enlargement of the sella turcica was demonstrated. Following x-ray therapy of the pituitary no further progression of the disease has been observed.

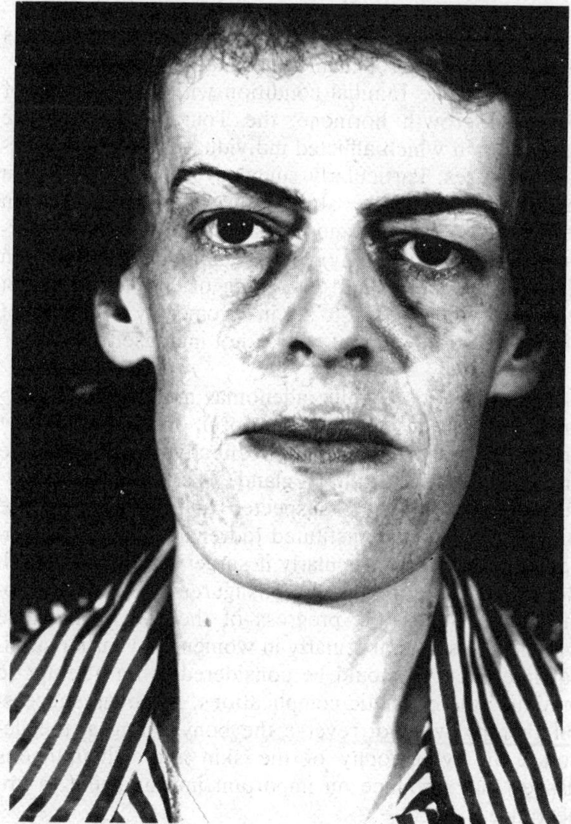

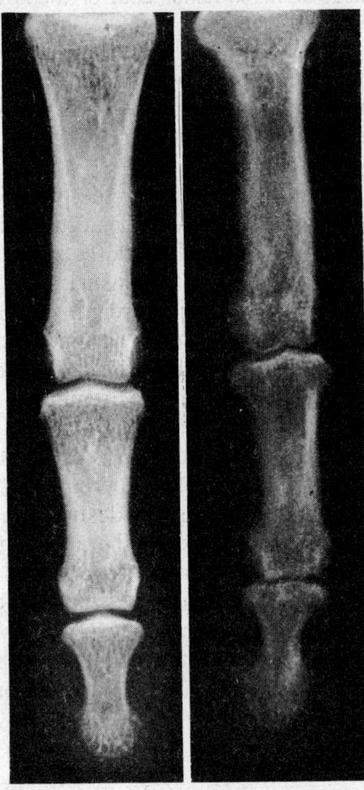

FIGURE 83-2
Characteristic tufting or "arrowhead" appearance of the terminal phalanx in acromegaly (right). Normal phalanx for comparison (left). Note also the thickness of the acromegalic finger.

urine. The basal plasma growth hormone determination is usually necessary for final determination of activity.

There is one familial condition without evidence of increased growth hormone, the Touraine-Solenti-Golé syndrome, in which afflicted individuals present acromegalic features. Particularly suggestive of acromegaly in this condition are the skin changes; thus its common designation, pachydermoperiostitis (idiopathic hypertrophic osteoarthropathy). Although the fingers are often clubbed, the periosteal thickening of the bones is not what one would expect to see in acromegaly. The amount of growth hormone is of course not increased.

Treatment Eosinophilic adenomas may respond to irradiation, but in general this form of therapy is not presently considered to be so effective as an ablative procedure of the pituitary gland. The presence of hypopituitarism must be suspected and the appropriate substitution therapy instituted (adrenal, thyroid, and gonadal hormones), particularly if surgery is contemplated. Because of the permanent disfigurement which acromegaly produces, the progress of the disease must be watched closely, particularly in women, and earlier surgical intervention should be considered in an attempt to minimize the cosmetic complications. Although successful therapy will not reverse the bony changes, the decrease in hypertrophy of the skin and subcutaneous tissues may produce an important improvement in appearance.

ADRENOCORTICOTROPIN (ACTH)

This hormone is a polypeptide composed of 39 amino acids with a molecular weight of approximately 4,500. The primary structure has been elucidated, and small quantities have been synthesized (Fig. 83-3).

The principal physiologic effect of this hormone is to stimulate the secretion of hydrocortisone from the adrenal cortex. Under the stimulus of ACTH, the adrenal gland also secretes corticosterone, aldosterone, estrogens, and certain so-called "adrenal androgens." In the case of aldosterone, ACTH is not the chief controlling factor regulating its secretion. As part of its adrenal-stimulating effect, ACTH promotes an increase in adrenal blood flow and hypertrophy of the gland. Certain extraadrenal actions of ACTH of obscure physiologic significance include a lipid-mobilizing effect and a hypoglycemic action. ACTH has intrinsic melanocyte-stimulating activity because of similarities between its N-terminal amino acid sequence and the structure of MSH (Fig. 83-3).

Secretion of ACTH is regulated by the concentration of hydrocortisone in plasma and by various parts of the brain, particularly the anterior median eminence of the hypothalamus. Nerve cells in this area are thought to produce one or more peptide neurohormones, termed corticotropin-releasing factors (CRF), which are released into the pituitary portal circulation and stimulate the secretion of ACTH by the anterior pituitary cells. Higher centers of the brain may act to stimulate or inhibit ACTH secretion.

Central nervous system activity maintains a diurnal rhythm of ACTH secretion, which results in highest levels in early morning and lowest levels at night. There is a considerable increase in plasma ACTH concentration in adrenal insufficiency because of loss of the normal reciprocal relationship between plasma hydrocortisone concentration and ACTH secretion. Substantial increases in ACTH secretion occur during stress irrespective of the plasma steroid level. Prolonged administration of corticosteroids depresses the secretion of ACTH and results in adrenal atrophy indistinguishable from that observed in spontaneous hypopituitarism.

CUSHING'S DISEASE
(See also Chap. 86)

In 1932, Cushing described the clinical disorder of pituitary basophilism associated with adrenocortical hyperplasia. This concept led to considerable controversy and a voluminous literature on the presence and significance of basophilic adenomas in patients with adrenocortical hyperfunction.

Relatively few patients with adrenocortical hyperfunction first come to the physician with definite enlargement of the pituitary gland; however, the incidence of pituitary tumor is significantly increased in those patients subjected to total adrenalectomy. Since bilateral total adrenalectomy has been widely practiced for less than two decades, it is possible that more patients will develop clinically evident pituitary tumors in due time. Curiously, most of the postadrenalectomy pituitary tumors have proved to be chromophobe adenomas. Eosinophilic and mixed-type tumors have also been found in Cushing's disease, but the largest number are associated with small basophilic tumors or hyalinization of the basophils.

Biologic tests for the measurement of ACTH in plasma, and more recently immunoassay techniques, may be of value in establishing the cause of adrenocortical hyperfunction. The finding of an elevated plasma ACTH level suggests a pituitary origin, but such an elevation may also be found in patients who have nonendocrine carcinomas that also secrete ACTH-like substances. In a series that we have undertaken, an elevated plasma ACTH level was found more often in those patients with a nonendocrine tumor, e.g., in the lung or pancreas, than in patients with Cushing's syndrome and adrenal hyperplasia. In an adrenalectomized patient with Cushing's disease, an abnormal elevation in ACTH, exceeding the level observed in Addison's disease or in patients adrenalectomized for other diseases, is highly suggestive of an ACTH-secreting pituitary tumor (Nelson's syndrome). These patients often show intense pigmentation of the skin, which is due to the MSH-like activity of ACTH referred to above but also to actual secretion of MSH by the tumor.

INCREASED PLASMA ACTH IN ADDISON'S DISEASE AND CONGENITAL ADRENAL HYPERPLASIA

Elevated plasma ACTH levels are apparent within 24 hr of steroid withdrawal in patients with Addison's disease and fall to normal several hours after a physiologic dose of steroid. This excess production of ACTH is not pathologic and has not been associated with pituitary tumors. It may be, at least in part, responsible for the hyperpigmentation which occurs in this disease.

Patients with congenital adrenal hyperplasia also have elevated plasma ACTH level, because of a similar mechanism, deficient secretion of hydrocortisone. As far as is known, the pituitary gland is normal in this disease. The excess secretion of ACTH is also easily suppressed by physiologic doses of corticosteroids (see Chap. 86).

FIGURE 83-3
Amino acid sequences of corticotropin and melanocyte-stimulating hormones. (Modified from I. Harris)

Corticotropin
1 2 3 4 5 6 7 8 9 10 11 12 13 39
H—Ser. Tyr. Ser. Met. Glu. His. Phe. Arg. Try. Gly. Lys. Pro. Val.···Phe.—OH

α-MSH (pig)
1 2 3 4 5 6 7 8 9 10 11 12 13
CH_3CO-Ser. Tyr. Ser. Met. Glu. His. Phe. Arg. Try. Gly. Lys. Pro. Val.—NH_2

β-MSH (pig)
1 2 3 4 5 6 7 8 9 10 11 12 13 14 15 16 17 18
H—Asp. Glu. Gly. Pro. Tyr. Lys. Met. Glu. His. Phe. Arg. Try. Gly. Ser. Pro. Pro. Lys. Asp.—OH

β-MSH (human)
1 2 3 4 5 6 7 8 9 10 11 12 13 14 15 16 17 18 19 20 21 22
H—Ala. Glu. Lys. Lys. Asp. Glu. Gly. Pro. Tyr. Arg. Met. Glu. His. Phe. Arg. Try. Gly. Ser. Pro. Pro. Lys. Asp.—OH

INCREASED ACTH SECRETION IN TUMORS OF NONENDOCRINE ORIGIN

A number of patients with Cushing's syndrome secondary to the release of ACTH-like substances from nonendocrine neoplasms has been reported. Carcinoma of the lung is the most frequent type of tumor associated with this syndrome. Of particular interest has been the association of Cushing's syndrome with benign bronchial adenomas as well as malignant tumors. In a few cases the substance produced by the tumor has been shown to be, in all probability, ACTH. It is possible that neoplastic tumors could also secrete an ACTH-releasing factor which would in turn stimulate the secretion or release of ACTH. The latter could be detected biologically by its effectiveness in the presence of an intact pituitary-adrenal system and its ineffectiveness in the absence of the anterior pituitary gland. To date, there is no evidence that these nonendocrine neoplasms secrete adrenal steroids; hence, removal of both adrenals should result in a cure of the Cushing's syndrome in circumstances which prevent the complete removal of the primary neoplasm.

THYROTROPIN (TSH)
(See also Chap. 85)

Thyrotropin is a glycoprotein of approximately 26,000 mol wt. It stimulates the uptake of iodide by the thyroid gland and the synthesis and release of thyroid hormones. Continued stimulation results in hypertrophy of the gland and an increase in the vasculature. Thyrotropin deficiency results in glandular atrophy and depressed thyroid function. The administration of thyroid hormone depresses the secretion of thyrotropin and produces similar changes in thyroid function. There is good evidence that the ventral medial nuclei and paraventricular nuclei of the hypothalamus are involved in the control of TSH secretion, and that destruction of these areas depresses thyroid hormone synthesis.

The role of the anterior pituitary in the causation of primary hyperthyroidism is not clear. Although elevated levels of TSH in the blood of patients with hyperthyroidism have been reported, the results have not been consistently reproducible. A long-acting thyroid stimulator (LATS) has been demonstrated in the plasma of a high proportion of patients with hyperthyroidism. Administration of synthetic TRF (thyrotropin-releasing factor) with measurement of serum TSH levels is a useful, sophisticated method of demonstrating the functional capacity of the pituitary gland to secrete TSH.

The occurrence of hyperthyroidism following hypophysectomy or pituitary stalk section suggests that TSH may not be essential for the development of hyperthyroidism. It does appear, however, that certain pituitary tumors may secrete excess TSH and result in thyroid hyperplasia and hypersecretion. Since TSH secretion may be increased by stimuli arising in the hypothalamus, it is thought that a mechanism acting through higher central nervous system centers may be related to the not-infrequent development of thyrotoxicosis following major emotional or psychic trauma. It is also probable that increased TSH secretion is involved in the hyperthyroidism associated with acromegaly.

GONADOTROPINS
(See also Chaps. 91 and 92)

The gonadotropins, FSH and LH, are large protein hormones of approximately 30,000 mol wt. These hormones regulate the development, reproductive functions, and hormonal secretions of the ovary and testicle. Prolactin (LtH) is also classed as a gonadotropin; however, its primary action is on the mammary gland and though it may be luteotropic (i.e., sustaining the function of the corpus luteum) in lower animal species, this action has not been shown to be of physiologic significance in man.

The secretion of gonadotropins is influenced by the rate of sex hormone production and by certain areas of the hypothalamus. Castration increases and estrogens decrease the secretion of FSH, probably by modifying the hypothalamic centers which control FSH secretion by the anterior pituitary. The secretion of LH is also increased by castration but is less sensitive to inhibition by estrogens. Progesterone depresses LH secretion in some species. Testosterone is a poor inhibitor of FSH secretion but does block the secretion of LH.

Secretion of LH has been clearly shown to be regulated by the posterior hypothalamus. This area is also important in prolactin secretion, probably by producing a hormone that inhibits the production and release of LtH by the anterior pituitary. Lesions in this area block LH secretion and result in enhanced secretion of prolactin and pathologic lactation.

Gonadotropins are not found in the urine until puberty. Thereafter, they are present in significant quantities throughout life, with peaks of excretion appearing at the time of ovulation and greatly increased levels occurring after the menopause or following castration. Although relatively crude, the bioassay for urinary gonadotropins (FSH assay) is widely used. The assay is not specific for FSH, since even small quantities of LH appear to be necessary for the biologic action of FSH. Low urinary FSH levels are occasionally found in normal persons, and several determinations are necessary for accurate clinical evaluation. Increasing availability of radioimmunassay of these and other pituitary hormones makes diagnosis of gonadotropin abnormalities much more reliable.

Chorionic gonadotropin (HCG) is derived from the placenta and appears in the urine in large quantities during pregnancy. Preparations from human pregnancy urine are available for clinical use. This hormone has predominantly an LH action and is used clinically to stimulate Leydig cell function and ovulation (Chap. 92).

SEXUAL PRECOCITY No definite pituitary disorders are associated with increased secretion of LH or FSH. There are cases of isosexual precocity, often familial, in which premature but normal sexual development occurs, probably on the basis of early maturation of central nervous system centers regulating gonadotropin formation and release. Lesions of the hypothalamus or pineal gland also may result in premature secretion of gonadotropic hormones and precocious puberty (Chap. 94).

GALACTORRHEA Abnormal lactation is sometimes observed in patients with acromegaly or chromophobe adenomas and also may occur after pituitary stalk section. A condition associated with persistent post-partum lactation and amenorrhea is referred to as the Chiari-Frommel syndrome. The galactorrhea in these disorders is most likely the result of excess prolactin secretion. If a pituitary tumor is found, it should be treated. In the absence of evidence of a tumor, galactorrhea may be suppressed by estrogen administration or by use of brom-ergocryptine, 3 mg daily, increasing after 2 days to 6 mg daily (see Chap. 93).

PANHYPOPITUITARISM

PREPUBERAL Prepuberal panhypopituitarism, which was first described in 1871 by Lorrain, is a rare condition usually associated with suprasellar cyst or craniopharyngioma. The disease is characterized by dwarfism and subnormal sexual development but normal mentality. The impairment of growth is symmetric, and the body proportions are normal. As in other cases of hypopituitarism, the skin often has a pale yellowish appearance and increased wrinkling. Sexual maturation is delayed, and in rare cases there may be obesity from hypothalamic involvement. Diabetes insipidus is not an infrequent accompaniment.

If the tumor is of sufficient size to affect the optic chiasma, there may be bitemporal hemianopsia or complete blindness. X-ray studies reveal delayed fusion of the epiphyses, supresellar calcification and, often, destruction of the sella turcica. The condition must be distinguished from genetic dwarfism and from hypothyroidism. Children with a familial type of dwarfism have isolated deficiency of growth hormone secretion but normal production of other pituitary hormones and development of epiphyses consistent with chronologic age.

Hypothyroid children have subnormal mentality, infantile body proportions, dwarfism, and the characteristic epiphyseal dysgenesis.

Treatment with cortisone, thyroid, and sex hormones, described in more detail in the next section, should be instituted, with dosage adjusted for body size and age. Although limited by the availability of material, human or monkey growth hormone in doses of 1 to 3 mg weekly has had considerable success in producing growth in these patients. Because of the psychologic and sociologic importance of reaching normal stature, every attempt should be made to obtain such therapy for these patients if the epiphyses have not closed. Growth hormone from nonprimate sources has had no effect on growth in human beings.

POSTPUBERAL PANHYPOPITUITARISM Panhypopituitarism designates total absence of all pituitary secretions and is synonymous with *Simmonds' disease.* Postpartum pituitary necrosis (Sheehan's syndrome) is due to extensive thrombosis of the pituitary circulation during delivery, usually associated with blood loss and hypotension. Other causes of panhypopituitarism in the adult include chromophobe adenoma, craniopharyngioma, and the end stages of acromegaly. Less common lesions include gliomas, basilar meningitis, head injuries, and granulomatous disorders such as sarcoid and Hand-Schüller-Christian disease.

Characteristically, patients with Sheehan's syndrome fail to lactate or to menstruate. The association of these signs should always suggest this diagnosis. There follows the insidious onset of a host of vague symptoms, including asthenia, lethargy, loss of libido, loss of axillary and pubic hair, and cold intolerance (Fig. 83-4). Some patients appear quite healthy and often are classified as psychoneurotic until the true diagnosis is revealed. Others gradually lapse into a far-advanced state of anterior pituitary insufficiency involving gonadal, thyroid, and adrenal function in approximately that order of development. Physical signs consist of bradycardia, hypotension, loss of axillary, pubic, and scalp hair, premature wrinkling and pallor of the skin, which is fine and atrophic, and a general loss of secondary sex characteristics, with atrophy of the breasts and genitalia.

FIGURE 83-4
Photographs of a forty-year-old woman when first seen for hypopituitarism (Simmonds' disease) and after 6 months' therapy.

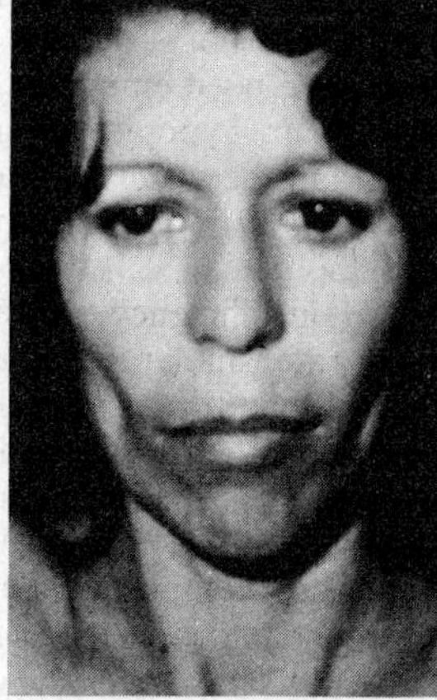
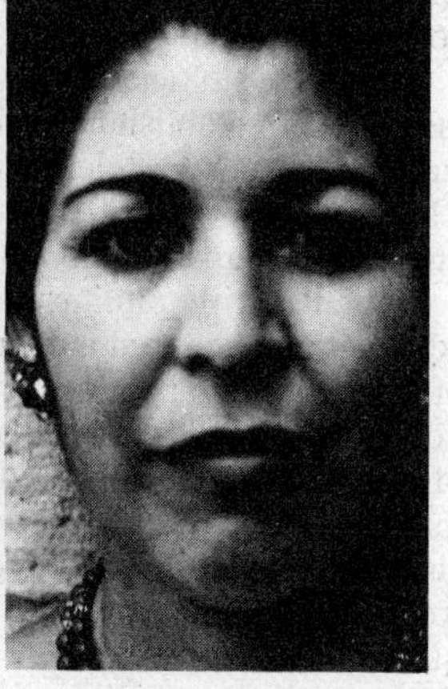

Irrespective of the cause of panhypopituitarism, the secondary effects on the endocrine glands are similar. There is marked atrophy of the thyroid, adrenals, and gonads. Interference with growth occurs if the lesion appears prior to epiphyseal closure. The pituitary gland has a large reserve, and substantial amounts of pituitary tissue must be damaged before significant hormone deficiency develops. Not all patients develop hypofunction of all three target glands; isolated gonadal failure is relatively common, or gonadal failure may be associated with either thyroid or adrenal insufficiency. Isolated growth hormone deficiency and TSH or ACTH deficiency may also be seen, although the latter is quite rare.

Laboratory findings Laboratory findings reflect decreased function of the target endocrine glands. Thus, the serum protein-bound iodine and thyroidal radioiodine uptake are low, and there is a decrease in the basal metabolic rate. The level of serum cholesterol, unlike that in primary myxedema, is rarely elevated, despite lowered thyroid function. Levels of urinary 17-ketosteroids, 17-hydroxycorticosteroids, and 17-ketogenic steroids are depressed, and urinary gonadotropins are subnormal or absent. Blood levels of ACTH and growth hormone are depressed. A normochromic anemia is often present, and there may be leukopenia and relative lymphocytosis in the presence of adrenal insufficiency. Fasting hypoglycemia is rarely found but may occasionally be severe enough to produce coma. The serum sodium concentration is usually normal, but hyponatremia may occur during periods of stress. The serum potassium level and BUN are usually normal, in contrast to increases seen in the patient with Addisonian crisis.

Diagnosis The diagnosis of hypopituitarism is generally not difficult to establish once it is suspected, but because of the insidious onset and the variable signs and symptoms, the disorder may escape detection for many years. These patients often come to the physician with acute medical emergencies associated with infection or trauma and fail to respond normally to the usual therapeutic measures. In such instances, clinical evidence of gonadal, thyroid, or adrenal insufficiency should be sought; if present, it will quickly suggest the diagnosis.

Patients with *pituitary myxedema* must be differentiated from those with primary thyroidal failure. Patients with the pituitary form often do not appear to be so myxedematous as those with primary hypothyroidism. An enlarged thyroid gland is indicative of primary hypothyroidism, since the thyroid is atrophic in hypopituitarism. In the absence of clear evidence of a primary thyroid disorder such as might result from radioiodine therapy, thyroidectomy, or thyroiditis, pituitary insufficiency should be ruled out in every patient with hypothyroidism. The response to TSH is helpful in differentiating primary from pituitary hypothyroidism. In contrast to the lack of response to TSH in the patient with primary hypothyroidism, a marked increase in the protein-bound iodine and the radioiodine uptake will be produced in the patient with the pituitary type of hypothyroidism by the administration of 10 units of TSH intramuscularly daily for 2 days. Some patients with pituitary myxedema may not respond to TSH, probably because of advanced thyroidal atrophy.

The patient with *adrenal failure* secondary to pituitary disease will usually show an increase in the 24-hr urinary excretion of 17-ketosteroids, 17-hydroxycorticosteroids, and 17-ketogenic steroids with administration of ACTH. These patients often do not respond to a single day's infusion of ACTH, but administration of 40 units intravenously over an 8-hr period on three or four successive days characteristically will reveal a stepwise increase in steroid excretion by the third or fourth day of administration. Hypopituitary patients secrete near-normal quantities of aldosterone and thus are usually in sodium balance. Hyponatremia, when it does occur, however, may be due to sodium depletion as well as to extracellular dilution. The hyponatremia seen secondary to hypopituitarism is easily corrected by the intravenous administration of cortisol, in contrast to hyponatremia secondary to the inappropriate secretion of antidiuretic hormone.

Measurement of urinary steroids following the administration of 2-methyl-1,2 bis-(3-pyridyl)-1-propanone (metyrapone) provides a particularly useful index of the ability of the pituitary gland to increase ACTH secretion. This compound inhibits the 11-hydroxylation of the steroid molecule in the adrenal gland and leads to decreased secretion of 17-hydroxycorticosterone (hydrocortisone) and increased secretion of 17-hydroxy-11-deoxycorticosterone (substance S). The hydrocortisone deficiency results in increased ACTH secretion from the anterior pituitary gland, a marked increase in the adrenal secretion of substance S, and a resultant increase in the urinary excretion of 17-hydroxycorticosteroids and 17-ketogenic steroids. Patients with normal pituitary-adrenal function will show an increase in these urinary steroids with this drug, but patients with either primary or secondary adrenal insufficiency will fail to demonstrate such an increase in urinary 17-hydroxycorticosteroids (Fig. 83-5). This test is of particular value in assessing pituitary ACTH reserve in patients who have normal or only slightly depressed basal urinary steroid levels. The urinary test, performed by administration of 500 to 700 mg metyrapone orally every 4 hr for 48 hr with measurement of urinary 17-ketogenic steroids, may produce adrenal insufficiency and should be performed only on hospitalized subjects. The single administration of approximately 30 mg per kg body weight at midnight with estimation of serum 11-deoxycortisol at 8 A.M. is less likely to produce insufficiency and is a useful screening test.

Hypogonadism secondary to pituitary disease is characterized by decreased or absent urinary gonadotropins, in contrast to the increased titers found in primary gonadal failure. The prolonged amenorrhea observed in many patients with chronic illness and especially in those with anorexia nervosa is often confused with that due to panhypopituitarism. Urinary gonadotropin concentration may be low in these patients, but adrenal and thyroid function is usually normal. The most useful single test in

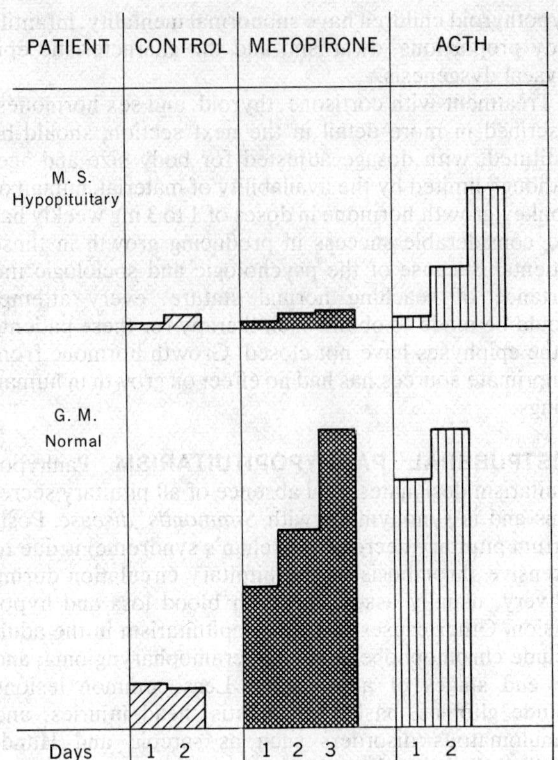

FIGURE 83-5
Response of urinary 17-ketogenic steroids in a hypopituitary patient (M.S.) and a normal subject (G.M.) to Metopirone (750 mg every 6 hr for 48 hr) and ACTH (40 units intravenously over 8 hr on two or three successive days). Note the lack of response to Metopirone (metyrapone) and delayed response to ACTH in the hypopituitary patient.

ruling out panhypopituitarism is a serum thyroxine determination. Almost all patients with pituitary deficiency will be found to have low values. If thyroid hormone levels are low, it is then necessary to determine the function of other target organs such as the adrenals and gonads. This can be done by estimation of plasma cortisol, plasma or urinary 11-deoxycortisol (substance S) after administration of metyrapone, or adrenal secretory response to ACTH. Ideally, when available, the serum levels of the pituitary hormones are measured after administration of the specific releasing factor of hypothalamic origin or appropriate stimulation of the endogenous hypothalamic hormone.

Other physiologic tests which have been employed in the past in establishing a diagnosis of hypopituitarism, such as the insulin tolerance test and the water test, are less specific and may be life-threatening if not carried out under close supervision.

Patients with pituitary-adrenal insufficiency excrete administered water at a depressed rate, similar to the rate of excretion in patients with primary adrenal failure; however, this test may be falsely positive in the presence of renal, hepatic, or cardiac disease. These patients may develop water intoxication during the test; they should be carefully observed for this complication and treated with intravenously administered cortisol if required.

Treatment The use of pituitary hormones would be true replacement therapy for panhypopituitarism. However, TSH and ACTH must be given daily by intramuscular injection, and pituitary gonadotropins cannot be used successfully for any prolonged period because of the tendency to antibody formation. In practice, excellent results are obtained by oral replacement therapy with the target gland hormones. Thyroxine should be given at first in a dose of 0.05 mg a day, with the amount gradually increased over a period of several weeks to a total daily dose of 0.2 to 0.3 mg. Cortisone acetate should be initiated at a level of 5 to 10 mg per day and increased to 15 to 30 mg as needed. Since the administration of thyroid hormone alone in a patient with associated pituitary-adrenal insufficiency may precipitate a serious adrenal crisis, it is important to initiate cortisone therapy prior to or at least simultaneously with thyroxine therapy in these patients. Salt-retaining hormone therapy is generally not needed, but if required, can be achieved with the oral administration of 0.05 to 0.1 mg fluorohydrocortisone daily.

A long-acting testosterone preparation should be given intramuscularly in doses of 100 to 200 mg every 2 to 4 weeks to male patients; proportionately smaller doses are often beneficial in female patients. In the female patient, estrogens may be given daily by mouth or at intervals of 2 to 4 weeks by injection. If desired, cyclic therapy with estrogens and progesterone may be given to induce artificial menstrual function.

Hormonal therapy is intended only to provide normal replacement of physiologic levels for proper body function. Although the harmful effects of large-dose corticosteroid administration may not be observed with this schedule, psychic disturbances of various kinds are occasionally noted in patients suddenly exposed to full replacement therapy after a long period of adrenal or thyroid hormone deficiency. Another problem often noted is that of excessive appetite in some patients receiving even small doses of cortisone. In this instance, it may be necessary to institute a restrictive diet or to decrease cortisone dosage.

Patients should be given careful instructions concerning their increased cortisol requirements if exposed to stress. They should be told to seek medical attention immediately if they develop fever or other signs of infection, and if traveling to areas in which such care is not available should be instructed on the intramuscular administration of the steroid.

OTHER SYNDROMES OF POSSIBLE PITUITARY ORIGIN

Froehlich's syndrome and the Laurence-Moon-Biedl syndrome are two disorders associated with failure of gonadal development in which disturbances in anterior pituitary gonadotropin secretion are postulated. However, no consistent lesions have been observed in the anterior pituitary, and it is thought that the primary disturbance is in the hypothalamus.

Froehlich's syndrome is associated with adiposity and sexual infantilism. Patients have truncal obesity, the gonads are underdeveloped, and the secondary sex characteristics are absent. The condition may be associated with mental retardation, visual disturbances, diabetes insipidus, and impaired skeletal growth. It is important to differentiate between cases of Froehlich's habitus (obesity and apparently delayed genital development) and true Froehlich's syndrome. The former condition is often observed in normal prepuberal boys who may have normal sex organs hidden in the adipose tissue. With the onset of puberty, these boys develop normally and often lose their adiposity and assume normal adolescent body proportions. Froehlich's syndrome may be associated with tumors or other disorders of the hypothalamic-pituitary area. The obesity may be caused by damage to hypothalamic centers regulating appetite.

The Laurence-Moon-Biedl syndrome is a hereditary disease characterized by adiposity, genital atrophy, mental retardation, skull deformities, retinitis pigmentosa, and associated congenital malformations such as polydactyly and syndactyly. Fewer than 100 cases have been reported, and there is no evidence of pituitary lesions in these patients. The adiposity and genital atrophy are assumed to be caused by hypothalamic-pituitary dysfunction.

INTERMEDIATE LOBE OF THE PITUITARY GLAND

The intermediate lobe of the pituitary gland is the probable site of production of melanocyte-stimulating hormone (MSH). Two types of MSH have been identified. Alpha-MSH is a polypeptide composed of the same 13 amino acids found in the N-terminal position of ACTH (Fig. 83-3). Human β-MSH contains 22 amino acids and is closely related structurally to α-MSH as well as to ACTH. Because of the common N-terminal sequence, ACTH preparations have intrinsic melanocyte-stimulating effects; however, pure MSH does not stimulate adrenal cortical secretion. It is of interest that cortisone administration may suppress MSH as well as ACTH secretion from the pituitary gland.

There have been descriptions of MSH-secreting tumors of the pituitary gland. These rare tumors are associated with a generalized increase in pigmentation similar to that observed in patients with pituitary tumors following adrenalectomy for Cushing's syndrome. The hyperpigmentation observed in patients with Addison's disease may be due to increased production of MSH as well as ACTH. Increased MSH secretion may also be responsible for the hyperpigmentation observed in some cases of hyperthyroidism, biliary cirrhosis, sprue, and other chronic diseases. Conversely, it is probable that the decreased pigmentation often apparent in patients with panhypopituitarism is due to decreased production of MSH.

REFERENCES

Besser GM et al: Galactorrhoea: Successful treatment with reduction of plasma prolactin levels by brom-ergocryptine. Br Med J 3:669, 1972

Brasel JA et al: An evaluation of seventy-five patients with hypopituitarism beginning in childhood. Am J Med 38:484, 1965

HARRIS GW, DONOVAN BT: *The Pituitary Gland,* London: Butterworth, 1966

KASTIN AJ et al: Release of LH and FSH after administration of synthetic LH-releasing hormone. J Clin Endocrinol Metab 34:753, 1972

MARTINI L, GANONG WF: *Neuroendocrinology,* vols. I and II, New York: Academic, 1966 and 1967

NEELON FA et al: The primary empty sella: Clinical and radiographic characteristics and endocrine function. Medicine 52:73, 1973

NELSON DH et al: ACTH-producing pituitary tumors following adrenalectomy for Cushing's syndrome. Ann Intern Med 52:560, 1960

ONTJES DA, NEY RL: Tests of anterior pituitary function. Metabolism 21:159, 1972

RABKIN MT, FRANTZ AG: Hypopituitarism: A study of growth hormone and other endocrine functions. Ann Intern Med 64:1197, 1966

RIMOIN DL et al: Growth hormone deficiency in man: An isolated recessively inherited defect. Science 152:1635, 1966

ROTH JS et al: Acromegaly and other disorders of growth hormone secretion. Ann Intern Med 66:760, 1967

SNYDER PJ, UTIGER RD: Response to thyrotropin releasing hormone (TRH) in normal man. J Clin Endocrinol Metab 34:380, 1972

UNDERWOOD LE et al: Human somatomedin, the growth hormone-dependent sulfation factor, is anti-lipolytic. J Clin Endocrinol Metab 35:194, 1972

84 DISEASES OF THE NEUROHYPOPHYSIS

JOSEPH F. DINGMAN
GEORGE W. THORN

Oliver and Schaefer in 1894 demonstrated a pressor effect of pituitary extracts, and in 1897 Howell showed that the pressor principle resided in the posterior lobe. The oxytocic action of posterior pituitary extracts was described by Dale in 1909 and the antidiuretic action by von den Velden in 1913. Fisher, Ingram, and Ranson in 1938 demonstrated a functional relationship between certain hypothalamic nuclei and the posterior pituitary. The studies of Scharrer and Scharrer since 1928 concerning the secretory activity of nerve cells (neurosecretion), the demonstration by Bargmann in 1949 of secretory granules in the neurons of the supraoptic and paraventricular nuclei of the hypothalamus, and the successful synthesis of oxytocin and vasopressin by du Vigneaud and coworkers represent important advances in current understanding of the endocrine functions of the neurohypophysis.

GENERAL CONSIDERATIONS

The principal effects of posterior pituitary extracts are to enhance the reabsorption of water by the renal tubules (antidiuretic effect); stimulate uterine contraction (oxytocic effect); promote the secretion of milk from the lactating breast (milk-ejecting effect); and, only in pharmacologic doses, produce a rise in blood pressure (vasopressor effect). The neurohypophyseal hormones are vasopressin (antidiuretic hormone, ADH) and oxytocin. The former is predominantly responsible for pressor and antidiuretic actions, whereas the latter is most potent in uterine stimulation and milk ejection. The neuroendocrine unit responsible for production and secretion of these hormones has been designated the neurohypophysis (Fig. 84-1), which includes the neurons of the supraoptic and paraventricular nuclei of the anterior hypothalamus, the axons that form the supraopticohypophyseal tract, and the posterior lobe of the pituitary body, the pars nervosa, in which the axon endings terminate.

Secretory granules can be demonstrated within the cytoplasm of these neurons, which migrate along the axons and accumulate as large aggregates known as Hering bodies in the perivascular axon end-plates of the posterior pituitary. There is some evidence that vasopressin and oxytocin are produced by separate neurons and that the secretory granules contain a specific carrier protein or neurophysin to which each hormone is bound. The bulk of neurohypophyseal hormone is contained in the posterior lobe, and only a small fraction of total activity is found in the tuber cinereum, stalk, and hypothalamic nuclei. The posterior pituitary, then, serves mainly as a reservoir of hormone readily available for rapid release into the systemic circulation.

Removal of the posterior lobe will lead to hormonal deficiency only if most of the axons of the hypothalamohypophyseal tract are severed and retrograde degeneration of the hypothalamic neurons occurs. With severance of the stalk close to the posterior pituitary body, short axons terminating at a higher level may escape injury and the remaining viable neurosecretory cells apparently can maintain secretion and release of hormones, probably into the vessels of the stalk and the hypothalamus.

The physiologic significance of the peculiar anatomic location of this neurosecretory organ, in which hypothalamic neurons extend their processes over relatively great distances into the posterior pituitary, is obscure. Such an arrangement may have been necessary, teleologically, in order to provide a ready route for hormone release into the systemic circulation through the highly vascularized posterior pituitary. In addition, posterior lobe extracts contain several hypothalamic neurohormones which regulate the release of anterior pituitary hormones. Thus, the neurohypophysis may provide an important link between the central nervous system and the secretion of anterior pituitary tropic hormones which so profoundly influence the body economy.

In view of this evidence, consideration of the posterior pituitary as an endocrine gland warrants revision, and reference should be made to the neurohypophysis when discussing this endocrine system. However, the terms posterior pituitary gland and posterior lobe hormone are still in common usage.

NATURE OF NEUROHYPOPHYSEAL HORMONES

Extracts of the neurohypophysis are assayed biologically with reference to oxytocic, vasopressor, and antidiuretic activities. One international USP or BP unit is defined as the activity of 0.5 mg of an international standard bovine posterior pituitary powder. In crude extracts of the posterior lobe the biologic activity is contained in a homogeneous protein or polypeptide fraction having a molecular weight of the order of 30,000 and an isoelectric point of pH 4.8. Such fractions show approximately equal vasopressor and oxytocic activities in terms of the reference powder, of the order of 16.6 IU per mg. It has not been conclusively established whether this protein-hormone complex represents the natural secretion of the neurohypophysis or whether vasopressin and oxytocin loosely bound to the protein by electrostatic forces are released in a free form into the circulation.

Highly purified preparations of vasopressin (600 IU per mg) and oxytocin (500 IU per mg) have been obtained from posterior lobe extracts. The peptide structure of each hormone has been determined, and both hormones have been successfully synthesized by de Vigneaud and his coworkers; this synthesis represents a milestone in peptide chemistry and hormone research. Both hormones are composed of five amino acids arranged in the form of a ring closed by the disulfide linkage of cystine, with a side chain of three amino acids. Oxytocin contains cystine, tyrosine, isoleucine, glutamine, and asparagine in the ring, with proline, leucine, and glycinamide in the side chain (Fig. 84-2). Vasopressin differs from oxytocin by only two amino acids. Phenylalanine replaces isoleucine in the ring, and leucine in the side chain is replaced by arginine (human, beef vasopressin, Fig. 84-3) or lysine (hog vasopressin). The molecular weight of oxytocin is 1,007 and of arginine vasopressin, 1,084. Both are ampholytes, oxytocin having an isolectric point of pH 7.7, and arginine vasopressin being considerably more basic, with an IP of pH 10.9.

Oxytocin has been shown to possess slight but definite pressor and antidiuretic effects, whereas vasopressin contains not only equal pressor and antidiuretic activities but also significant intrinsic oxytocic and milk-ejecting properties. Partially purified posterior pituitary preparations available commercially include Pitocin (oxytocin) and Pitressin (vasopressin), each fraction being slightly contaminated by the other in pharmaceutical preparations. Synthetic oxytocin and lysine vasopressin are also available for clinical use.

PHYSIOLOGY OF NEUROHYPOPHYSEAL SECRETION

Secretion of vasopressin is regulated by the total solute concentration or osmolality of plasma (osmoregulation), the intravascular or extracellular fluid volume (volume regulation), and by central nervous system activity (neural regulation). Secretion of oxytocin has been demonstrated during labor and milk release, consistent with the known uterotonic and milk-ejecting actions of the hormone. (Other factors regulating oxytocin secretion will be discussed below.)

The osmoregulatory mechanism controlling vasopressin release is exquisitely sensitive to slight changes in plasma osmolality. Dilution of the plasma solutes by administration of water inhibits the secretion of vaso-

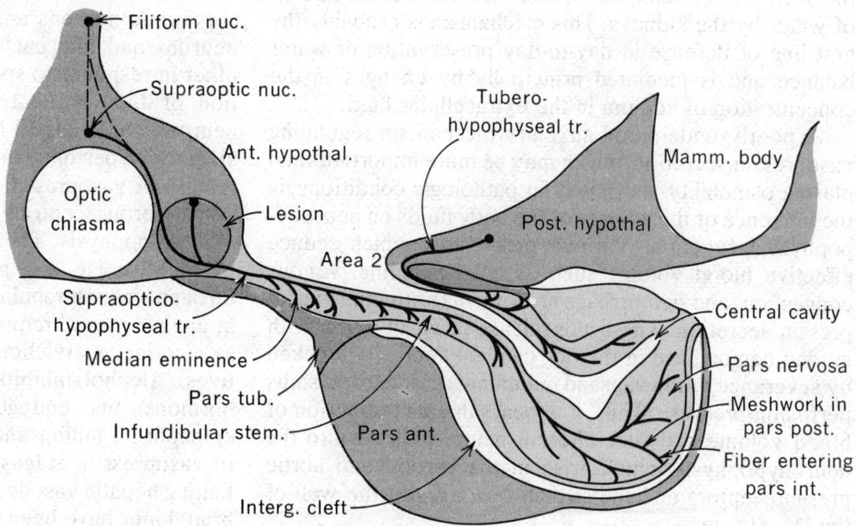

FIGURE 84-1
Diagram of a midsagittal section through the hypothalamus and hypophysis. The broken lines indicate proposed filiform-supraoptic connections and the tractus paraventricularis. The circled area indicates a typical lesion producing diabetes insipidus. (From Fisher et al, Diabetes Insipidus and the Neurohormonal Control of Water Balance, *Fig. 2, Ann Arbor, Mich.: Edwards, 1938)*

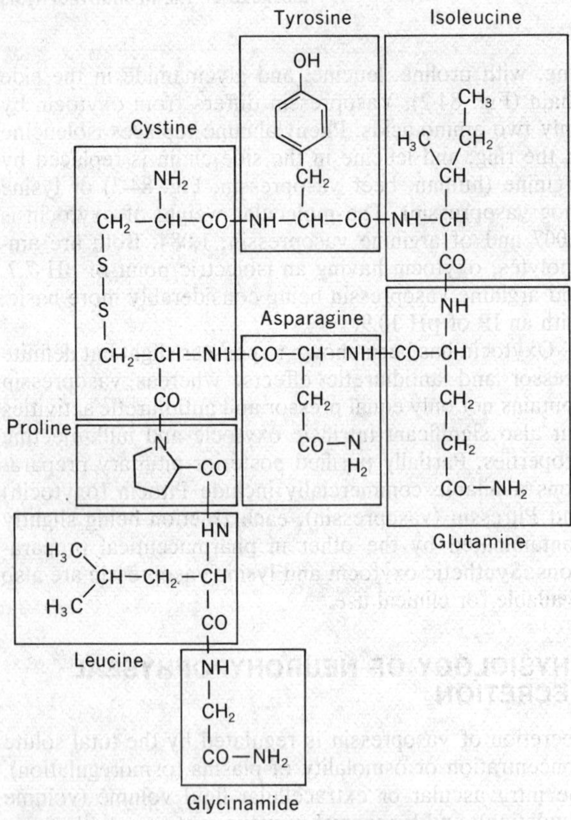

FIGURE 84-2
Oxytocin. (From B Berde, Recent Progress in Oxytocin Research, *Fig. 1, Springfield, Ill.: Charles C Thomas, 1959)*

pressin, and rapid excretion of water by the kidneys ensues; secretion is restored when plasma osmolality returns to normal. An increase in plasma osmolality resulting from a deficit of water or a relative increase in the ratio of extracellular to intracellular solutes stimulates the secretion of vasopressin and maximum conservation of water by the kidneys. This mechanism is probably the first line of defense in day-to-day preservation of water balance and is mediated principally by changes in the concentration of sodium in the extracellular fluid.

A poorly understood auxiliary mechanism regulating vasopressin secretion, which may be more important than plasma osmolality, especially in pathologic conditions, is the influence of the volume of the body fluids on neurohypophyseal function. Various procedures which reduce effective blood volume such as quiet standing, venous congestion, and hemorrhage are known to stimulate vasopressin secretion. The acute release of vasopressin with graded hemorrhage in the dog can be effectively blocked by severance of the vagi and maintenance of carotid sinus perfusion pressure. Thus, it appears that a contraction of blood volume activates afferent neural pathways to the neurohypophysis which arise in the carotid and aortic pressoreceptors and the stretch receptors in the wall of the left atrium.

Of the two vascular modalities, osmolality and volume, the former apparently operates effectively in most normal situations by retaining or releasing body water to suit the needs of the body. However, in pathologic conditions characterized by a decrease in intravascular or extracellular fluid volume or in cardiac output, volume regulation supersedes osmoregulation. In this situation, vasopressin secretion may persist despite the simultaneous occurrence of hypotonicity. A primary decrease in osmolality, such as that seen in the hyponatremia of Addison's disease, salt-losing nephritis, or long-standing congestive heart failure, would severely deplete body water if osmolality were the only factor governing vasopressin secretion. A regulator of secretion sensitive to the volume of the body water or the fullness of the vascular compartment or both would protect against desiccation and vascular collapse in these situations, the body giving up an optimal osmotic state for the vital requirements of the tissues for water. This antidiuretic mechanism, although protective in nature, may lead to serious complications, particularly in disorders already characterized by fluid retention and edema, since persistent water retention in patients in whom salt intake has been restricted may lead to severe hyponatremia, water intoxication, and further compromise of circulation and renal function (Chap. 264).

Since neurohypophyseal hormones represent secretions of the central nervous system, studies of the central neural control of the neurohypophysis have assumed great importance in neuroendocrine physiology. There is little doubt that the central nervous system has a dominant role in regulating vasopressin secretion. Release of vasopressin has been produced in man and monkeys by electrical stimulation of the hypothalamus and components of the "limbic system," including the hippocampus, the amygdala, the septal nuclei, and the mesencephalic reticular formation. Electrical stimulation of various areas of the cerebral cortex, however, has been shown not to evoke vasopressin release. These findings suggest that neural reflexes to the neurohypophysis may be transmitted primarily via the more primitive areas of the brain rather than through neocortical pathways.

There is evidence that vasopressin is secreted by the supraoptic neurons and oxytocin by the paraventricular neurons and that each is released independently of the other in response to specific physiologic stimuli. Stimulation of the genital tract activates the paraventricular neurons and leads to isolated release of oxytocin; infusions of hypertonic saline solution or nicotine stimulate release of vasopressin but not of oxytocin.

Numerous centrally acting substances stimulate the neurohypophysis. These include emotional stresses such as fright, noise, and pain; fainting, which may also act through volume regulators; coitus, suckling, and changes in environmental temperature; and numerous drugs such as nicotine, acetylcholine, and many hypnotics and sedatives. Alcohol inhibits ADH secretion. Of the various hormones and endogenous substances, small doses of epinephrine inhibit and large doses stimulate the release of vasopressin, at least in animals. Ferritin, the iron-containing hepatic vasodepressor substance, angiotensin, and bradykinin have been shown to be antidiuretic by virtue of stimulating the neurohypophysis, and the hydrocor-

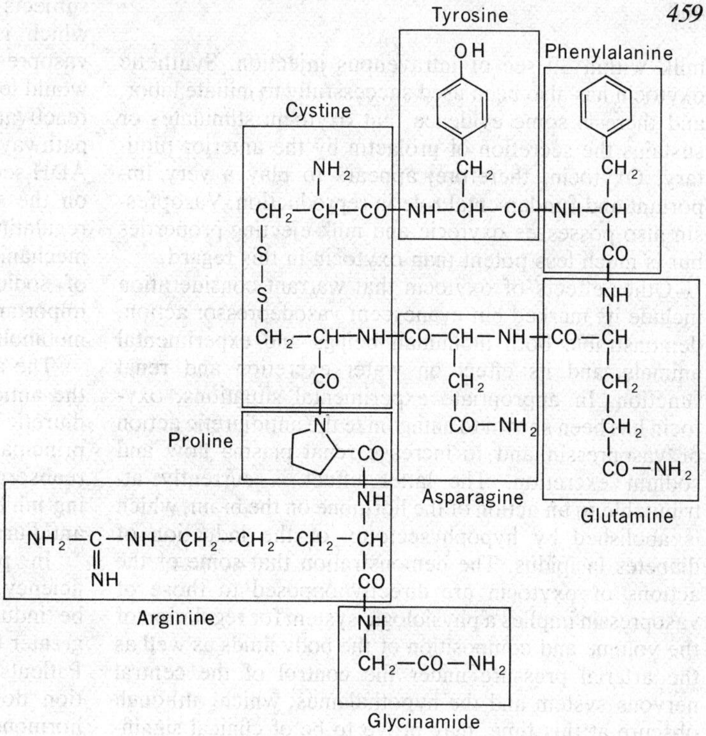
Tyrosine
OH
Phenylalanine
Cystine
NH2
CH2
CH2
CH2—CH—CO—NH—CH—CO—NH—CH
S
CO
S
NH
CH2—CH—NH—CO—CH—NH—CO—CH
CO
CH2
CH2
N
CO—NH2
CH2
Proline
CO
CO—NH2
NH
Asparagine
Glutamine
NH2—C—NH—CH2—CH2—CH2—CH
NH
CO
Arginine
NH
CH2—CO—NH2
Glycinamide

FIGURE 84-3
Vasopressin. (From B Berde, Recent Progress in Oxytocin Research, *Fig. 2, Springfield, Ill.: Charles C Thomas, 1959)*

tisone-like adrenal steroids have been shown to inhibit vasopressin secretion (see below).

PHYSIOLOGIC ACTIONS OF NEUROHYPOPHYSEAL HORMONES

VASOPRESSIN (ADH) The pressor and antidiuretic activities of vasopressin are properties of a single molecule. The antidiuretic action is of profound importance in regulating water balance. The current hypothesis as to the mechanism of action of vasopressin on water reabsorption by the kidney, based on experiments with various biologic membranes, such as frog skin and toad bladder, is that it acts on cyclic AMP in the medulla to render cells of the distal portions of the nephron permeable to water, permitting passive diffusion of tubular water along an osmotic gradient across the cell and into the peritubular vessels. The antidiuretic action of vasopressin is best demonstrated during water diuresis; *this effect represents the true physiologic role of the hormone on water metabolism, which is to prevent the bulk of the filtered water entering the distal tubular segment from escaping into the urine.* The effect of vasopressin during hypertonic urine flow is extremely variable and limited by the maximum rate of water reabsorption which the concentrating mechanism of the collecting tubules is capable of achieving.

An interesting aspect of the studies of the action of vasopressin on biologic membranes has been the demonstration that this hormone has a pronounced effect on transport of sodium as well as water across cell boundaries. The effect of vasopressin on sodium excretion by the kidney is, however, extremely variable and depends upon experimental conditions. It is probable that vasopressin does not have a direct effect on sodium excretion and that any observed change in sodium balance is secondary to the modifying influence of this hormone on the total volume and distribution of body water.

Vasopressin has been shown to exert a pressor effect in persons with postural hypotension, and large intravenous doses may also produce transient increases in blood pressure even in normal man. The significance of this observation in relationship to blood pressure regulation in normal persons is unknown. Generally, posterior lobe preparations used therapeutically in man have no consistent effect on blood pressure, probably because of compensatory adjustments elsewhere in the circulation.

Vasopressin has also proved to be of value as a means of assessing adrenocorticotropin secretion by the anterior pituitary. Although other corticotropin-releasing factors (CRF) differing from vasopressin have been extracted from the hypothalamus and posterior lobe, vasopressin itself has been shown to be a potent CRF. In clinical investigation, large intramuscular doses of 5 to 10 units are required to produce measurable increments in plasma steroid levels; however, intravenous doses as low as 50 to 80 microunits have been shown to produce significant increments in ACTH secretion in the rat. Since these vasopressin levels fall well within the physiologic range of stressed animals, it is possible that vasopressin may serve a physiologic role as an ACTH-releasing neurohormone in addition to its direct peripheral actions.

OXYTOCIN Studies with purified and synthetic oxytocin have significantly advanced understanding of the role of this hormone in uterine function and milk secretion. Oxytocin has been shown to be the hormonal substance of posterior lobe extracts responsible for release of milk from the lactating breast, as little as 0.5 unit, or 1 μg, synthetic hormone producing a copious flow of milk within 30 sec of intravenous injection. Synthetic oxytocin has also been used successfully to initiate labor, and there is some evidence that oxytocin stimulates or sustains the secretion of prolactin by the anterior pituitary. Oxytocin, therefore, appears to play a very important and fundamental role in reproduction. Vasopressin also possesses oxytocic and milk-ejecting properties but is much less potent than oxytocin in this regard.

Other effects of oxytocin that warrant consideration include its marked but evanescent vasodepressor action, demonstrable both in human beings and experimental animals, and its effect on water excretion and renal function. In appropriate experimental situations, oxytocin has been shown to antagonize the antidiuretic action of vasopressin and to increase renal plasma flow and sodium excretion. The latter effect is currently attributable to an action of the hormone on the brain, which is abolished by hypophysectomy or the induction of diabetes insipidus. The demonstration that some of the actions of oxytocin are directly opposed to those of vasopressin implies a physiologic system for regulation of the volume and composition of the body fluids as well as the arterial pressure under the control of the central nervous system and the hypothalamus, which, although obscure at this time, may prove to be of clinical significance in the future.

ADRENOCORTICAL-NEUROHYPOPHYSEAL RELATIONSHIPS

Patients with primary and secondary adrenocortical insufficiency characteristically show an increased amount of body water, hyponatremia, and an inability to excrete a water load. Studies in hydrocortisone-deficient patients maintained in normal sodium balance on mineral corticoid have shown abnormally elevated plasma vasopressin levels which remain above the normal range despite forced hydration. Administration of hydrocortisone-like steroids to dehydrated patients produces a fall in plasma vasopressin into the range of fasting normal subjects which is sufficient to maintain an antidiuretic state. Subsequent administration of a water load is accompanied by a normal osmoreceptor response to hemodilution with a fall in plasma vasopressin to immeasurable levels, and a normal diuretic response.

Hydrocortisone-deficient patients with associated mineral-corticoid deficiency, sodium depletion, and extracellular dehydration will show a persistent antidiuretic mechanism despite adequate hydrocortisone replacement, the volume deficit apparently blocking any inhibitory effect of hydrocortisone on vasopressin release. Thus it is apparent that the abnormal water metabolism of adrenocortical insufficiency is related to increased and sustained vasopressin secretion despite hypotonicity of the body fluids. Glucocorticoids can restore water metabolism to normal by a direct inhibition of vasopressin release and restoration of a normal osmoreceptor response to induced hypotonicity, provided that there is no severe deficit in the extracellular fluid volume capable of sustaining vasopressin secretion.

Hydrocortisone induces a transient water diuresis within the first few hours of administration even in subjects with normal adrenocortical function, an effect which is probably also due to an acute decrease in vasopressin secretion. The resulting loss of body water would lead to relative hypertonicity of the body fluids and reactivation of vasopressin release via osmoregulatory pathways, even though blockade of neural pathways for ADH secretion may persist. This effect of hydrocortisone on the secretion of a hormone of prime importance in regulating water metabolism may represent a hormonal mechanism for independently regulating the body content of sodium and water, which may be of fundamental importance in clinical disorders of sodium and water metabolism.

The adrenal steroids have not been shown to modify the antidiuretic effect of vasopressin in man. Thus, the diuretic effect of adrenal steroids is probably mediated principally not through a direct effect on the renal tubular reabsorption of water but by an indirect pathway involving inhibition of vasopressin secretion and a decrease in antidiuretic hormone action on the kidney.

In patients with partial neurohypophyseal insufficiency, a more complete state of diabetes insipidus can be induced with hydrocortisone administration, and a greater loss of solute-free water from the kidney occurs. Patients with a complete absence of vasopressin secretion do not have a true water diuresis with adrenal hormone administration. Since these hormones, at times, increase solute excretion by the kidney, there may be a concomitant increase in water excretion because of an inability of the kidney, in the absence of vasopressin, to increase the solute concentration of the urine.

Adrenal steroids affect water metabolism in several other ways. Prolonged steroid therapy may occasionally result in extensive potassium depletion and the development of kaliopenic nephropathy associated with isosthenuria and a two- to threefold increase in urine flow. Very rarely, adrenal steroids may produce a striking polydipsic syndrome with urine volumes as high as 15 to 20 liters per 24 hr. Steroid effects on thirst-regulating centers in the anterior hypothalamus or other parts of the brain may be implicated in this disorder.

The adrenal steroids thus appear to influence water metabolism in man (1) by inhibiting the central neural control of vasopressin secretion and decreasing vasopressin action on the kidney; (2) by increasing solute excretion and the obligatory excretion of water in patients with vasopressin deficiency; (3) by producing the sensation of thirst, possibly by an effect on hypothalamic and other central nervous system thirst centers; (4) by producing potassium deficiency and kaliopenic nephropathy.

The interrelationships between neurohypophyseal secretion and the adrenal secretion of aldosterone are not well defined. Patients with aldosterone-secreting tumors do not usually develop edema, and normal subjects treated with aldosterone have been shown to escape readily from sodium and water retention. Furthermore, patients with diabetes insipidus will retain sodium with aldosterone therapy but will not retain isosmotic quantities of water unless they receive vasopressin simultaneously.

Aldosterone secretion may be inhibited by expansion of body fluids despite the presence of hyponatremia. In this respect, the regulation of aldosterone secretion resembles that for vasopressin secretion, the influence of fluid volume having precedence over osmolal concentration. It is probable that there is an intimate physiologic interrelation between aldosterone, which governs sodium metabolism, and vasopressin, which regulates water metabolism. Both vasopressin and aldosterone are probably necessary for the isosmotic retention of fluid, and persistent secretion of both hormones could be responsible for the development of edema in patients with fundamental derangements in circulation.

VASOPRESSIN DEFICIENCY—DIABETES INSIPIDUS

Diabetes insipidus is a chronic symptom complex characterized by the passage of large quantities of pale, dilute urine, with secondary polydipsia. It results from a defect in the chain of events by which vasopressin is released from the neurohypophysis and acts on the cells of the renal tubules. The classic anatomic and physiologic studies of Fisher, Ingram, and Ranson revealed that the disease may be caused by interference with the functional integrity of the neurohormonal unit comprising the supraoptic and paraventricular nuclei of the hypothalamus, the supraopticohypophyseal tract, and the posterior lobe of the hypophysis. The full-blown disease occurs only when the tract is interrupted close enough to the hypothalamus to cause degeneration of at least 85 percent of the supraoptic and paraventricular neurons. There is also a relatively rare disorder, nephrogenic diabetes insipidus, which is mostly familial. This disorder is due to a hereditary refractoriness of the renal tubules to vasopressin.

The incidence of classic diabetes insipidus following hypophysectomy may be significantly diminished if damage to the supraoptic neurons is minimized by careful severance of the pituitary stalk as close to the pituitary gland as possible. The polyuria of hypophysectomized human beings has been shown to vary with the magnitude of vasopressin deficiency. Patients who lack this secretion demonstrate persistent polyuria despite withdrawal of adrenocortical replacement therapy. These observations illustrate the important role of vasopressin in determining the rate of water excretion and corroborate the concept that the diuretic effect of adrenal steroids is mediated indirectly through an effect on vasopressin secretion. The adrenal steroids may increase urine volume in such patients, however, by increasing solute excretion.

The thyrotropic and growth hormones of the anterior pituitary are necessary to maintain polyuria, probably by influencing the nutritional state and solute turnover as well as by sustaining renal function. A peripheral antagonism of vasopressin by thyroid hormone has been demonstrated, but this effect may not be a direct one.

INCIDENCE Diabetes insipidus is a rare disease, with a slightly greater incidence in youth and in males. In 1924 Rowntree reported 10 and 16 cases, respectively, in two series of 100,000 admissions to the Mayo Clinic. With the advent of hypophysectomy in recent years for the treatment of far-advanced breast carcinoma and other serious disorders, the disease is becoming much more prevalent in the general hospital population.

ETIOLOGY As shown by Fink's pathologic studies in 107 cases, the great majority of instances of this disease are due to anatomic lesions involving the hypothalamic-hypophyseal system and, hence, presumably interfering with vasopressin production. In clinical practice, it will often be impossible to elicit any other evidence of such a lesion; though the label *idiopathic* may be justifiable for such cases antemortem, the finding of an anatomic lesion at autopsy generally may be predicted.

PATHOLOGY The primary pathologic processes associated most frequently with the syndrome have been tumors of the diencephalopituitary region, basilar meningitis, sarcoidosis, and the histiocytic disorders. Transitory and occasionally permanent polyuria may follow severe head injuries. Pathologic changes consist of those due to the primary disorder, such as tumor, brain injury, and inflammation, and secondary changes in the urogenital tract, such as dilatation and hypertrophy of the bladder with megaloureter.

CLINICAL PICTURE The chief symptoms of diabetes insipidus are polyuria and polydipsia. The loss of large amounts of pale, dilute urine, occasionally as much as 15 to 29 liters per day, results in dehydration and, consequently, in such related symptoms and signs as dry skin, constipation, and an intense, almost insatiable thirst. Water deprivation to the limit of tolerance does not prevent polyuria, nor does it lead to a significant increase in urine concentration. Thus, in this disease, polydipsia is secondary to polyuria, in contrast to patients with psychogenic polydipsia, who pass large quantities of urine as an aftermath of a large fluid intake. In patients with diabetes insipidus, no consistent physical or chemical changes are noted other than those of dehydration. However, there may be symptoms referable to the localized disease process causing the syndrome.

The role of trauma in the production of diabetes insipidus deserves special comment, since the polyuria that sometimes follows head injury is not infrequently transient, as contrasted with the chronicity of most other forms of the disease. A similar syndrome may develop subsequent to cerebrovascular accidents or intracranial surgery, and in association with other forms of cerebral disease. When the full-blown syndrome develops under these conditions, serious dehydration may occur before the diagnosis is suspected, particularly in the incontinent patient or in the patient with clouded sensorium who is unable to request or partake of an adequate volume of fluids. The dehydration, which is due principally to water loss, may be accentuated by the administration of isotonic saline solution or solutions containing large amounts of protein. Such large solute loads will aggravate the renal loss of water in these patients because of an inability of the kidney to increase the solute concentration of the urine in the absence of vasopressin.

DIAGNOSIS The symptoms plus the large urine volume, with specific gravity below 1.010 and urinary osmolality less than that of plasma, unassociated with a history or other findings of diabetes mellitus or of chronic renal disease, will quickly suggest diabetes insipidus. Since this diagnosis commits the patient to sustained replacement therapy for an indefinite period, it is not to be made lightly, and the clinical impression should be supported by careful studies made under hospital conditions. All cases of diabetes insipidus, moreover, should be studied carefully for active intracranial lesions, which should be presumed to be present until proved otherwise. Thus, examination should include, in addition to the differential tests of water excretion outlined below, a study of the spinal fluid, roentgenograms of the skull and chest (metastatic disease), electroencephalogram, serologic test (syphilis), the serum protein level, sternal marrow aspiration (multiple myeloma), and visual fields.

DIFFERENTIAL DIAGNOSIS The syndrome must be differentiated from psychogenic polydipsia, chronic nephritis, and diabetes mellitus as well as from the polydipsia and polyuria so characteristically associated with the hypochloremic alkalotic syndrome and the hypercalcemia of hyperparathyroidism and vitamin D intoxication. Chronic nephritis may be excluded by the absence of protein or formed elements in the urine, a normal blood urea nitrogen level, and normal kidney function tests. Often the most difficult differential diagnosis is that between diabetes insipidus and psychogenic polydipsia. Other procedures helpful in making a differential diagnosis are the following:

Dehydration test The dehydration test is carried out as follows:

1 Begin test in the morning after a dry breakfast.
2 Weigh patient and obtain a blood sample for plasma osmolality at the beginning and end of the dehydration period.
3 Collect urine hourly for 6 to 12 hr or as long as the patient can tolerate fluid deprivation, maintaining the patient under constant surveillance to prevent surreptitious fluid ingestion.
4 Measure hourly urine volume and osmolality. From the minute urine flow and serum osmolality calculate free water clearance for each hourly period.[1]

INTERPRETATION Patients with normal ADH reserve will show a significant fall in urine flow, to less than 1 ml per min, and a negative free water clearance within 4 to 6 hr, even if they were overhydrated before the test; serum osmolality and body weight will change only slightly. Patients with hypophyseal or nephrogenic diabetes insipidus will continue to excrete hypoosmolal urine (positive free water clearance), despite a significant increase in serum osmolality and the loss of 1 to 3 kg body weight during the test. Patients with partial vasopressin deficiency will show significant weight loss and a subnormal increase in urinary osmolality, with failure to reach the isosmotic level (i.e., continued free water excretion). These findings reflect the release of small quantities of vasopressin which are insufficient to prevent the continued loss of solute-free water.

Vasopressin test If the patient is still polyuric at the end of the dehydration test, an intramuscular injection of 5 units aqueous vasopressin is given to test the renal sensitivity to ADH.

INTERPRETATION Vasopressin-deficient patients will show an antidiuretic response within 1 to 2 hr, reflected in a substantial increase in urinary osmolality and decrease in free water clearance; patients with nephrogenic diabetes insipidus do not respond to this dose, nor to as much as 0.5 unit given as a single intravenous injection.

Hypertonic saline test In place of the dehydration test, hypertonicity of the extracellular fluid can also be induced by administration of hypertonic saline solution. This stimulus is not as strong as dehydration, which produces a body water deficit as well as extracellular hypertonicity.

1 In the randomly hydrated patient, give a 20 ml water per kg load by mouth and collect urine samples every 15 to 30 min, preferably by having the patient void spontaneously. Insert a No. 18 needle or intravenous catheter into an antecubital vein using a slow drip of 5% dextrose in water to maintain patency.
2 When 50 percent of the water load has been excreted, administer 10 ml per kg of 3% sodium chloride solution as rapidly as possible, usually within a 20- to 30-min period.
3 Obtain serum for osmolality before and immediately after the saline infusion.
4 Collect urine for 90 to 120 min after the saline infusion.

INTERPRETATION Normal subjects will show a fall in urine flow and a sharp increase in urinary osmolality, until it is close to or above that of plasma, immediately after the infusion or within the period of observation. Massively overhydrated polydipsic patients may have a blunted response because of the excess body water which dilutes the hypertonic saline solution and lessens the increment in serum osmolality induced by the hypertonic infusion. Patients with diabetes insipidus do not show an antidiuresis and will often demonstrate an increase in urine flow and free water clearance because of the solute diuresis.

Nicotine test This drug, in sufficient dosage, stimulates the supraoptic neurons to secrete vasopressin. Enough nicotine must be administered to exceed the neuronal

[1] *The urine volume, V, is equal to the algebraic sum of the osmolal clearance, C_{osm}, and the free water clearance, C_{H_2O}.*

$$V = C_{osm} + C_{H_2O}$$

$$C_{osm} = V \frac{\text{total solute conc. urine}}{\text{total solute conc. plasma}}$$

C_{osm} represents the volume of water required to contain the urinary solutes in a solution isosmotic with plasma. C_{H_2O} represents the net excess or deficit of water beyond the osmolal clearance; it will be positive during a water diuresis and negative when urine is concentrated by the abstraction of solute-free water, as in antidiuresis. C_{H_2O} usually parallels urine flow during water diuresis studies, since osmolal clearance remains relatively constant. This index is particularly useful in determining the changes in water excretion occurring during the solute diuresis usually observed with hypertonic saline administration. Not infrequently, a large increase in C_{osm} may mask a concomitant decrease in C_{H_2O}. In this instance, urinary flow may fall only slightly or may actually increase, even though an increase in water reabsorption may be under way under the influence of released vasopressin.

threshold for excitation; this can usually be achieved if sufficient nicotine is given to induce nausea or vomiting. Ideally, nicotine should be used parenterally, but since this is an experimental drug, not freely available to the clinician, nicotine must be administered through the smoking of cigarettes.

1 Hydrate the patient with 20 ml water per kg, as in the preceding test.
2 When peak diuresis is achieved, usually within 30 to 60 min, the patient should smoke one to three unfiltered cigarettes as quickly as possible, inhaling the smoke deeply. The development of nausea indicates adequate nicotine administration.

INTERPRETATION Usually within 15 to 30 min after smoking there will be a sharp antidiuretic response in a normal subject or a patient with primary polydipsia, with excretion of hyperosmolal urine; patients with hypophyseal diabetes insipidus do not show any antidiuresis unless they become severely intoxicated with nicotine, and then it is a brief and subnormal response. Patients with nephrogenic diabetes insipidus do not respond.

FIGURE 84-4
Test of neurohypophyseal function. See text and footnote. Patient J. H., a nonsmoker, was given twice the usual dose of nicotine.

Combined test of neurophypophyseal function For convenience, a sequential test can be performed within a 4- to 6-hr period, combining nicotine, hypertonic saline solution, and vasopressin injection in one brief study (see Fig. 84-4).

1 The patient is hydrated with 20 ml water per kg, and urine is collected every 15 to 30 min. A constant state of hydration is maintained by oral or intravenous administration of a volume of fluid equal to that excreted during the preceding urine collection period.
2 When a sustained high rate of urine flow is reached (over 5 ml per min), one to three cigarettes are smoked, as in the preceding study. Additional fluid administration is stopped just prior to cigarette smoking.
3 If there is a normal antidiuretic response to nicotine the test can be terminated, but if antidiuresis does not ensue within 30 to 60 min, 15 to 50 milliunits aqueous vasopressin is injected intravenously.
4 After the vasopressin antidiuresis has dissipated, usu-

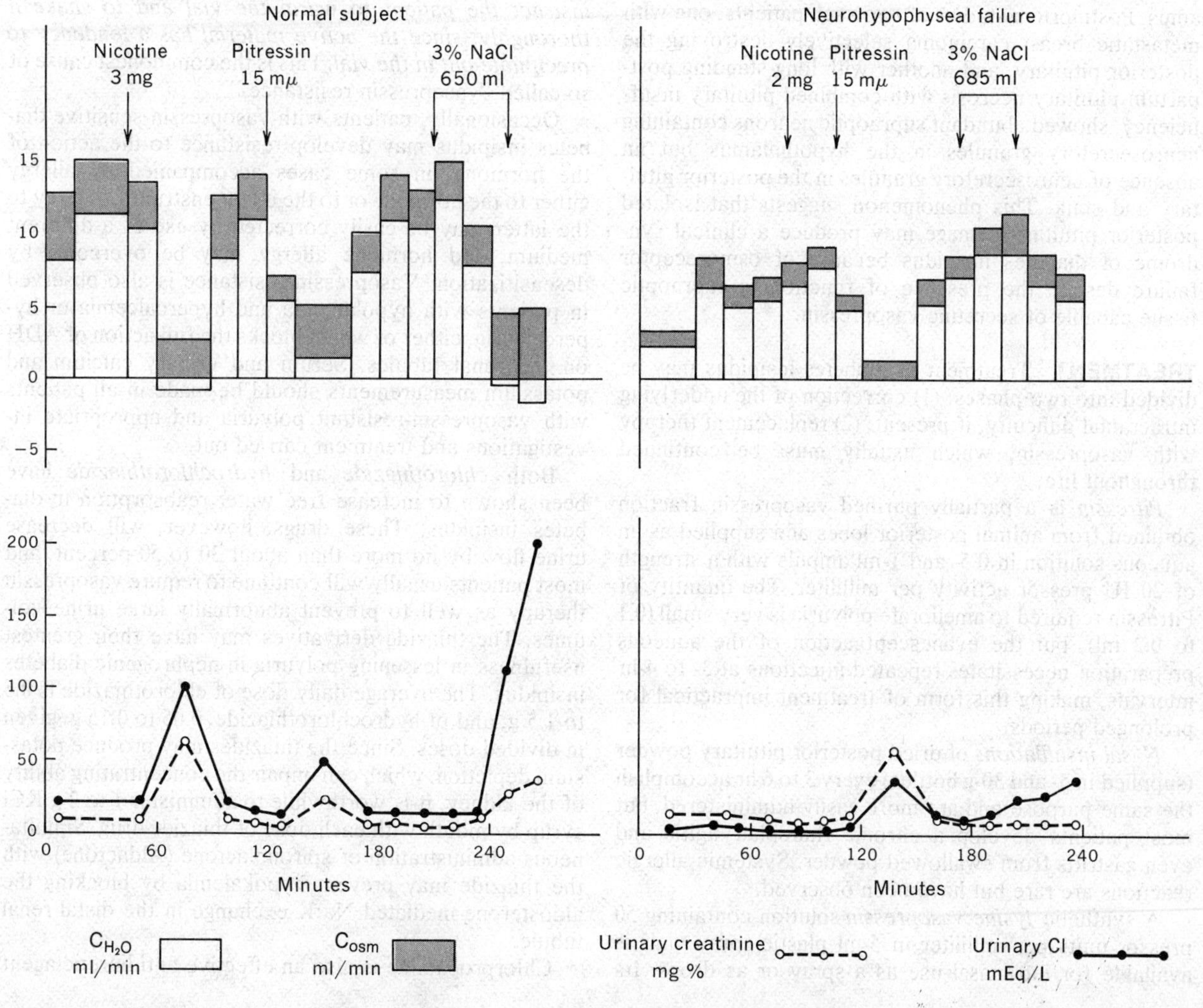

ally within the hour, the fluid balance is decreased to 10 ml per kg, following which the hypertonic saline test is performed.

INTERPRETATION This sequential test permits assessment of the neurogenic and osmolal control of vasopressin release and the renal response to vasopressin within a short period of time. Normal subjects and patients with primary polydipsia respond to all three stimuli; those with hypophyseal diabetes insipidus will show a response to vasopressin only; those with nephrogenic diseases do not respond to any stimulus. *Note*: When osmometry is not available, measurement of changes in urinary creatinine and chloride concentration will reflect the action of vasopressin on water reabsorption by the distal tubules.

Occasionally aberrations in the expected response may be observed. Some patients with primary polydipsia do not respond normally to nicotine even though they show a normal antidiuresis to dehydration or to hypertonic saline infusion. This phenomenon suggests that some derangement in the neural regulation of vasopressin release may exist in some patients. Several patients with vasopressin-deficient diabetes insipidus and no response to hypertonic saline solution have shown normal antidiuretic response to nicotine, suggesting the presence of functioning neurohypophyseal tissue in the hypothalamus. Postmortem studies of two such patients, one with metastatic breast carcinoma selectively destroying the posterior pituitary, and another with long-standing postpartum pituitary necrosis with combined pituitary insufficiency, showed abundant supraoptic neurons containing neurosecretory granules in the hypothalamus but an absence of neurosecretory granules in the posterior pituitary and stalk. This phenomenon suggests that isolated posterior pituitary damage may produce a clinical syndrome of diabetes insipidus because of osmoreceptor failure despite the presence of functioning supraoptic tissue capable of secreting vasopressin.

TREATMENT Treatment of diabetes insipidus may be divided into two phases: (1) correction of the underlying intracranial difficulty, if present; (2) replacement therapy with vasopressin, which usually must be continued throughout life.

Pitressin is a partially purified vasopressin fraction obtained from animal posterior lobes and supplied as an aqueous solution in 0.5- and 1-ml ampuls with a strength of 20 IU pressor activity per milliliter. The quantity of Pitressin required to ameliorate polyuria is very small (0.1 to 0.2 ml), but the evanescent action of the aqueous preparation necessitates repeated injections at 3- to 4-hr intervals, making this form of treatment impractical for prolonged periods.

Nasal insufflations of dried posterior pituitary powder (supplied in 5- and 30-g bottles) every 3 to 6 hr accomplish the same purpose and are more easily administered, but most patients develop a chronic rhinopharyngitis and even gastritis from swallowed powder. Systemic allergic reactions are rare but have been observed.

A synthetic *lysine vasopressin* solution containing 50 pressor units per milliliter in 5-ml plastic spray vials is available for intranasal use as a spray or as drops. Its activity is as rapid and as prolonged as posterior lobe powder, but this preparation has the decided advantage of eliminating the local or systemic allergic reactions to the foreign protein in posterior pituitary preparations of animal origin. Use of this material currently is the treatment of choice for ambulatory patients.

Pitressin tannate in oil is supplied in 1-ml ampuls with a strength of 5 IU per milliliter. This preparation provides relatively prolonged hormonal action; a single injection is usually effective for 24 to 72 hr. A test dose of 0.3 to 0.5 ml (1.5 to 2.5 IU) should be given initially to determine the effectiveness of treatment and to guard against the serious, but fortunately rare, occurrence of excess fluid retention and water intoxication in particularly sensitive individuals. For practical purposes chronic treatment with 1-ml doses of hormone should be tried and the frequency of injection gauged by the recurrence of polyuria. Most patients will retain 1 to 2 kg water following an injection, and the dissipation of effective hormone levels will be attended with a sudden polyuria and loss of body weight before onset of polydipsia. In general, injections should be timed to coincide with the onset of polyuria in order to prevent marked fluctuations in body water content and fluid compartmental shifts. Abnormal fluid retention may be mitigated by instructing the patient to guard against excessive fluid ingestion after treatment. The hormone is preferably given in the evening to ensure a restful night. *It is very important to instruct the patient to warm the vial and to shake it thoroughly, since the active material has a tendency to precipitate out in the vial.* This is the commonest cause of so-called "vasopressin resistance."

Occasionally, patients with vasopressin-sensitive diabetes insipidus may develop resistance to the action of the hormone, in some cases accompanied by allergy either to the hormone or to the oily menstruum. Allergy to the latter may be easily corrected by use of a different medium, and hormone allergy may be overcome by desensitization. Vasopressin resistance is also observed in patients with hypokalemia and hypercalcemia or hypercalcuria, either of which blocks the full action of ADH on the renal tubules. Serum and urinary calcium and potassium measurements should be made in all patients with vasopressin-resistant polyuria and appropriate investigations and treatment carried out.

Both *chlorothiazide* and *hydrochlorothiazide* have been shown to increase free water reabsorption in diabetes insipidus. These drugs, however, will decrease urine flow by no more than about 30 to 50 percent, and most patients usually will continue to require vasopressin therapy as well to prevent abnormally large urine volumes. The thiazide derivatives may have their greatest usefulness in lessening polyuria in nephrogenic diabetes insipidus. The average daily dose of chlorothiazide is 0.5 to 1.5 g, and of hydrochlorothiazide, 0.05 to 0.15 g, given in divided doses. Since the thiazides may produce potassium depletion, which can impair the concentrating ability of the kidney, it is worthwhile to administer 1 to 2 g KCl syrup by mouth with each dose of thiazide drug. Simultaneous administration of spironolactone (Aldactone) with the thiazide may prevent hypokalemia by blocking the aldosterone-mediated Na:K exchange in the distal renal tubule.

Chlorpropamide is also an effective antidiuretic agent

in some patients with hypophyseal diabetes insipidus but not in the nephrogenic variety. This drug apparently acts by potentiating the renal action of vasopressin, and there is some evidence that it may also increase the secretion of vasopressin from residual neurohypophyseal tissue. Patients who are capable of secreting trace quantities of hormone may show complete correction of the polyuria with this treatment; however, patients with complete vasopressin deficiency will not respond. The effective daily dose is between 100 and 500 mg per day, given in one or two doses. Above 250 mg per day the dangers of symptomatic hypoglycemia or polyphagia and weight gain are increased, and titrations should be carried out to determine the lowest possible dose which prevents nocturia and decreases daytime urine flow to tolerable levels. The value of this drug is that the volume depletion and hypokalemia from thiazides can be avoided.

The prognosis of diabetes insipidus is determined by the outcome of the primary disease process. With regular treatment, patients with isolated neurohypophyseal atrophy can lead normal lives.

EXCESS OF ANTIDIURETIC HORMONE

Abnormally elevated levels of antidiuretic substances in blood and urine have been reported in a variety of disease states associated with edema or defects in water diuresis, including cardiac failure, cirrhosis with ascites, and nephrosis. Though the hypothesis that excessive antidiuretic activity may be responsible for the water retention observed in edematous patients is quite attractive, proof has not been clearly established. It is generally agreed that patients with these disorders do not show excessive sensitivity to or delayed inactivation of administered vasopressin. Some studies with nicotine stimulation of endogenous vasopressin secretion in patients with edema have yielded normal results, but some patients whose disease is associated with severe hyponatremia have shown enhanced neurohypophyseal response to nicotine and other stimuli. Many of the studies that minimize a role of vasopressin in edema formation are based upon data observed in patients in equilibrium with their fluid retention who can excrete water loads, although at a somewhat depressed rate. It is obvious that vasopressin release mechanisms should be evaluated during the active phase of edema formation, but studies have been hampered by the fact that such patients frequently cannot excrete administered water, which automatically vitiates the only reliable biologic end point of vasopressin action, i.e., antidiuresis. Further advances in this field will depend upon the application of precise and reliable methods for measuring vasopressin levels in the plasma.

The level of vasopressin in the body fluids need not necessarily be increased to account for water retention, since even physiologic amounts effectively halt a water diuresis. The abnormality in water metabolism may be primarily related to a *persistence* of vasopressin secretion despite the presence of excess body water or hypotonicity, both of which normally should induce water diuresis. It appears that the distribution rather than the total quantity of body water may determine the secretory activity of the neurohypophysis, and more extensive studies of the precedence of volume versus osmolal regulation of vasopressin secretion should shed more light on the nature of fluid retention in these disorders.

INAPPROPRIATE ADH SYNDROME The above discussion is particularly pertinent in understanding the nature of the antidiuretic factors responsible for the *inappropriate ADH syndrome,* described in patients with oat cell carcinoma of the lung, acute intermittent porphyria, various central nervous system disorders, etc. Antidiuretic material indistinguishable from arginine vasopressin has been isolated from lung tumor extracts, and presumptive evidence for the synthesis of arginine vasopressin has been obtained in tissue culture of one such tumor. Assays of plasma for arginine vasopressin reveal values falling within or above the normal range, both in tumorous and nontumorous cases. Most patients show partial and incomplete suppression of plasma levels with forced hydration, suggesting that the plasma hormone concentration is responsive to some degree to osmoreceptor inhibition. The fact that an identical syndrome is observed in patients with and without malignant disease suggests that abnormalities in the neural or volume control of neurohypophyseal secretion may well prove to be a common denominator in these diverse clinical disorders.

REFERENCES

AHMED ABJ et al: Increased plasma arginine vasopressin in clinical adrenocortical insufficiency and its inhibition by glucosteroids. J Clin Invest 46:111, 1967

BARTTER FC, SCHWARTZ WB: The syndrome of inappropriate secretion of antidiuretic hormone. Am J Med 42:790, 1967

BAUMANN G et al: Plasma arginine vasopressin in the syndrome of inappropriate antidiuretic hormone secretion. Am J Med 52:19, 1972

DU VIGNEAUD V: Trail of sulfur research: From insulin to oxytocin. Science 123:967, 1956

MILLER M, MOSES AM: Urinary antidiuretic hormone in polyuric disorders and in inappropriate ADH syndrome. Ann Intern Med 77:715, 1972

Symposium on antidiuretic hormones. Am J Med 42:651, 1967

VERNEY EB: Absorption and excretion of water: Antidiuretic hormone. Lancet II:739, 1946

85 DISEASES OF THE THYROID

SIDNEY H. INGBAR
KENNETH A. WOEBER

The normal function of the thyroid gland is to secrete thyroxine (T_4) and 3,5,3′-triiodo-L-thyronine (T_3), iodinated amino acids that are the active thyroid hormones and that influence a diversity of metabolic processes (Fig. 85-1). Diseases of the thyroid gland are manifested by qualitative or quantitative alterations in hormonal secre-

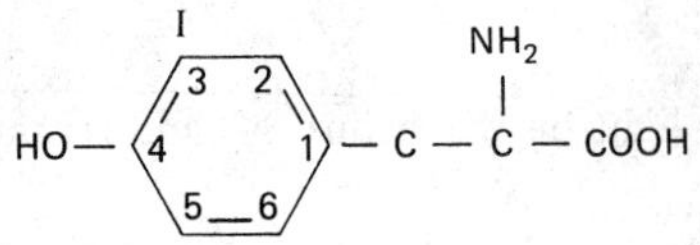

3 - Monoiodotyrosine

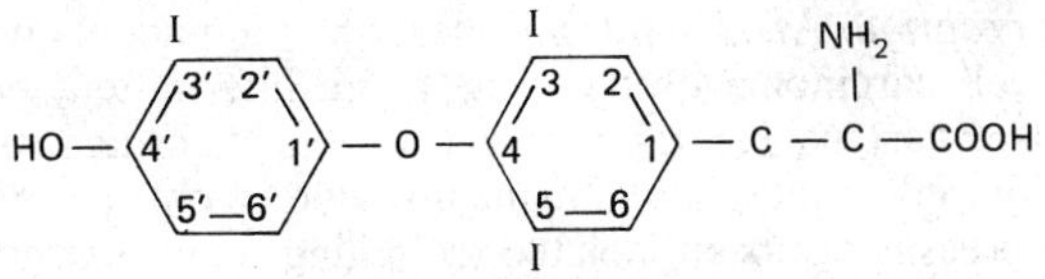

3, 5, 3' - Triiodothyronine (T_3)

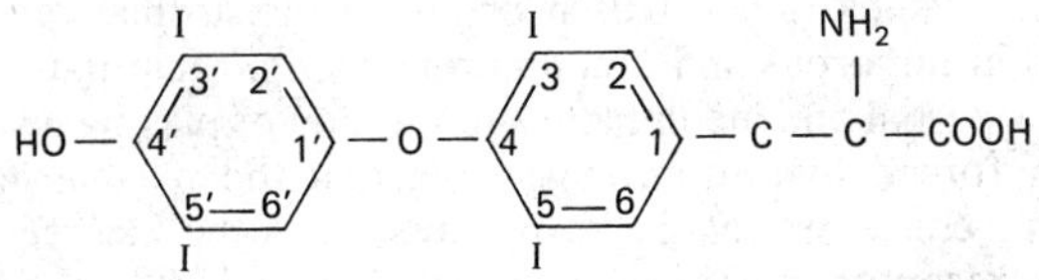

3, 5, 3', 5' - Tetraiodothyronine (thyroxine; T_4)

FIGURE 85-1
Structural formulas of the active thyroid hormones, thyroxine and triiodothyronine, and of the inactive precursor, monoiodotyrosine.

tion, enlargement of the thyroid (goiter), or both. Insufficient hormonal secretion results in the syndrome of hypothyroidism, in which decreased oxygen consumption (hypometabolism) is a classic manifestation. Conversely, excessive secretion of active hormone results in hypermetabolism and other features of a syndrome termed *hyperthyroidism*. Enlargement of the thyroid gland (normally 15 to 25 g in adults) may be generalized or focal. Generalized enlargements may not be absolutely symmetric, however, and they are associated with increased, normal, or decreased hormonal secretion, depending upon the underlying disturbance. Truly focal enlargement usually reflects neoplastic transformation, either benign or malignant, the former sometimes being responsible for hypersecretion of hormone and hyperthyroidism. Either type of goiter may result in compression of adjacent structures in the neck or mediastinum.

EMBRYOLOGY, ANATOMY, AND HISTOLOGY

The human thyroid originates embryologically from an evagination of the pharyngeal epithelium with some cellular contributions from the lateral pharyngeal pouches. Progressive descent of the midline thyroid anlage gives rise to the thyroglossal duct, which extends from the foramen cecum near the base of the tongue to the isthmus of the thyroid. Remnants of tissue may persist along the course of this tract as "lingual thyroid," as thyroglossal cysts or nodules, or as a structure contiguous with the thyroid isthmus called the *pyramidal lobe*. The latter is usually not discernible, except when the remainder of the gland is goitrous. In some individuals, lingual thyroid may be the sole functioning thyroid tissue. In such cases, its secretion may or may not be sufficient to maintain a normal metabolic (euthyroid) state.

Knowledge of the ontogenetic sequence in human thyroid development is limited by the availability of specimens for analysis. It is clear, however, that the fetal thyroid acquires the capacity to collect and organify iodine at about 10 weeks gestation. Both T_4 and thyroid-stimulating hormone (thyrotropin, TSH) are detectable in the blood soon thereafter. It is likely that the fetal pituitary-thyroid axis is a distinct functional unit, since little maternal TSH crosses the placenta and transplacental passage of T_4 and T_3 from mother to fetus appears similarly small. A thyroid stimulator termed *human chorionic thyrotropin* (HCT) has been extracted from placenta, but its role in maternal and fetal thyroid physiology is unknown.

The normal adult thyroid is a relatively vascular organ, comprising two lobes joined by an isthmus and lying just anterior and slightly caudad to the cartilages of the larynx. Fibrous septa divide the gland into pseudolobules which, in turn, comprise vesicles, called follicles or acini, surrounded by a capillary network. Normally, the follicle walls are composed of cuboidal epithelium. Their lumen is filled with a proteinaceous material, termed *colloid*, which contains a protein peculiar to the thyroid, thyroglobulin, within the peptide sequence of which T_4 and T_3 are stored.

HORMONAL SYNTHESIS, SECRETION, AND METABOLISM

SYNTHESIS AND SECRETION Thyroid hormone synthesis that is both qualitatively and quantitatively normal depends on entry into the thyroid of adequate quantities of iodine, a constituent of the active hormones, T_4 and T_3; normality of pathways for iodine metabolism within the gland; and concurrent synthesis of a normal receptor protein for iodine, thyroglobulin. Iodine enters the thyroid from the bloodstream in the form of inorganic or ionic iodide whose source is twofold: iodide derived either from the deiodination of thyroid hormones or from iodinated agents that the patient may have been given and iodide ingested in food, water, or medication. Formerly, a dietary iodine intake of approximately 200 μg was considered normal within the continental United States, and this was sufficient to sustain a plasma iodide concentration of approximately 0.5 μg per 100 ml. Recently, however, owing largely to enrichment of bread with iodine, the average iodine intake has increased substantially, to values as high as 1,000 μg daily, with corresponding increases in plasma iodide concentration. Iodide is removed from the plasma by the thyroid, kidneys, and salivary and gastrointestinal glands, but since iodide that enters gastrointestinal secretion is reabsorbed, net clearance is effected only by the thyroid and kidneys. In effect, the thyroid and kidneys compete for plasma iodide. However, since renal clearance is largely a function of glomerular filtration rate and is not influenced by humoral factors or plasma iodide concentration, the kidney is normally a passive participant in this competition. Hence, adjustments in the rate of entry of iodide into the thyroid relative to the rate of urinary excretion are mediated by changes in thyroid, rather than renal, avidity.

The reactions involved in the synthesis and secretion of the active thyroid hormones can be divided into four sequential steps (Fig. 85-2). The first involves active inward transport of iodide from the plasma into the thyroid cell and follicular lumen. This occurs at a rate that exceeds passive diffusion of iodide from the gland, with the result that the thyroid is capable of maintaining concentration gradients for iodide (thyroid/plasma concentration ratios) of substantial magnitude (up to 500, or more, under certain physiologic or pathologic conditions). Energy for iodide transport is phosphate bond–derived and therefore depends upon oxidative metabolism within the gland. The second step in hormonal biosynthesis involves oxidation of iodide to a higher valence form, as yet undetermined, that is capable of iodinating tyrosyl residues in thyroglobulin, a glycoprotein of approximately 650,000 molecular weight that is synthesized within the follicular epithelium. Oxidation of iodide is effected by an iodide peroxidase, which utilizes hydrogen peroxide generated during the course of oxidative metabolism within the gland. Organic iodinations, which occur at or near the apex of the cell, result in the formation of the peptide-bound, hormonally inactive precursors, monoiodotyrosine (MIT) and diiodotyrosine (DIT). Subsequently, these iodotyrosines undergo oxidative condensation, again through the mediation of peroxidase. This so-called "coupling reaction" occurs within the thyroglobulin molecule and yields a variety of iodothyronines, including T_4 and T_3. Although minute quantities of thyroglobulin are detectable in the blood of normal patients and those with thyroid disease, the vast bulk of thyroglobulin is retained for a time within the gland, serving as a storage form of thyroid hormone, or "prohormone." Liberation of the active hormones into the blood, forming the third step in hormonal synthesis and release, involves pinocytosis of follicular colloid at the apical margin of the cells to form colloid droplets. These fuse with thyroid lysosomes to form "phagolysosomes," in which thyroglobulin is hydrolyzed by proteases and peptidases. The final step is release of the now-free iodothyronines, T_4 and T_3, into the blood, while the inactive iodotyrosines are stripped of their iodine by an intrathyroidal enzyme, iodotyrosine dehalogenase. Normally, iodide liberated thereby is largely reutilized in the synthesis of hormone, but a small proportion is normally lost into the blood (iodide leak); this proportion may become very large in abnormal circumstances.

As with iodide, the thyroid is capable of concentrating other monovalent anions. Notable among these is the pertechnetate ion, which is available as the radioactive isotope, sodium pertechnetate Tc 99m. Unlike iodide, little pertechnetate is organically bound; hence, its duration of stay within the thyroid is short. This property, together with its short physical half-life, makes pertechnetate a highly valuable radionuclide for imaging the thyroid with scintillation scanning techniques.

The foregoing reactions are subject to inhibition by a variety of chemical compounds. Such agents are generally termed *goitrogens*, since, by virtue of their ability to inhibit hormonal synthesis and indirectly stimulate TSH secretion, they induce goiter formation. Certain inorganic anions, notably perchlorate and thiocyanate, inhibit the iodide transport mechanism and thereby reduce available substrate for hormone formation. The goiter and hypothyroidism that follow, however, can be prevented or relieved by doses of iodide sufficiently large to enable adequate quantities to enter the gland by simple diffusion. The commonly employed antithyroid agents, such as the derivatives of thiourea and mercaptoimidazole, exert more complex actions upon pathways of hormonal biosynthesis. These agents, as well as certain aniline derivatives, inhibit the initial oxidation (organic binding) of iodide, decrease the proportion of DIT relative to MIT, and block coupling of iodotyrosines to form the hormonally active iodothyronines. The latter reaction is the most sensitive. Thus, it is possible for the synthesis of hormonally active iodothyronines to be decreased greatly, although the total incorporation of iodine by the thyroid is inhibited but little. In contradistinction to the effect of the monovalent anions, the goitrogenic action of

FIGURE 85-2
Schema depicting pathways in the synthesis and secretion of thyroid hormones and mechanisms for the suprathyroidal and intrathyroidal regulation of thyroid function. Small, solid arrows indicate pathways of iodine metabolism; open arrows indicate stimulation; crosshatched arrows indicate inhibitory influences. TRH, thyrotropin-releasing hormone; TSH, thyroid-stimulating hormone; IPO, iodide peroxidase; prot., thyroid protease; peptid., thyroid peptidase; MIT, monoiodotyrosine; DIT, diiodotyrosine; T_4, thyroxine; T_3, 3,5,3′-triiodothyronine.

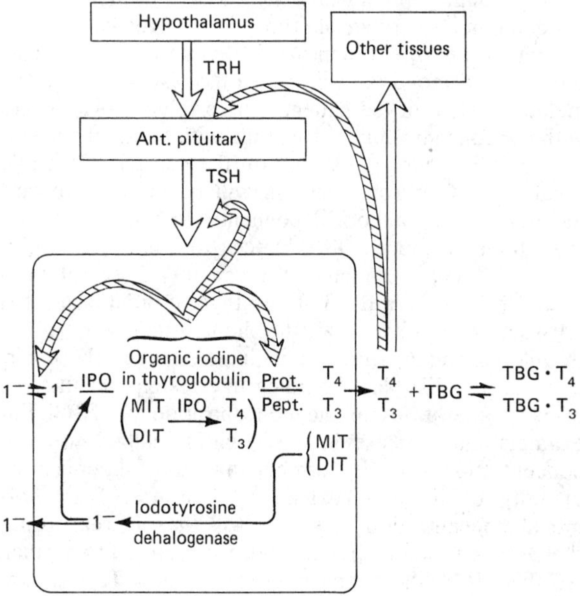

inhibitors of organic binding is not overcome by large quantities of iodine. Indeed, certain weak goitrogens, such as sulfonamides and antipyrine, are rendered more potent when given with iodide, an effect not clearly understood. Iodine itself, when given acutely in large doses, is capable of blocking the organic-binding and coupling reactions. This action (Wolff-Chaikoff effect) is normally transient. In a small proportion of seemingly normal individuals, however, prolonged administration of iodide is associated with continued inhibition of hormone synthesis and development of goiter, with (iodide myxedema) or without hypothyroidism. A large proportion of patients with Graves' disease treated with radioiodine or surgery and also patients with chronic thyroiditis are inordinately sensitive to the blocking effect of iodide and, when given iodides chronically, develop hypothyroidism. Iodides in large doses are capable of inhibiting proteolysis of thyroglobulin and hormonal release, an effect which is most readily demonstrable in hyperfunctioning thyroids and which is responsible for the rapid ameliorative action of iodides in patients with the diffuse toxic goiter of Graves' disease. Lithium, which is administered as the carbonate salt in some patients with depressive states, has a variety of effects on intrathyroidal iodine metabolism. Among these is an action to inhibit hormonal release. Thus, like iodides, it can be employed to effect a rapid reduction in the degree of thyrotoxicosis in patients with the hyperthyroidism of Graves' disease.

TRANSPORT AND METABOLISM In the blood, T_4 and T_3 are almost entirely bound to plasma proteins. Electrophoretic analyses indicate that T_4 is bound, in decreasing order of intensity, to an inter-alpha-globulin, termed thyroxine-binding globulin (TBG), to a T_4-binding prealbumin (TBPA), and to albumin. By virtue of its intense affinity for T_4, TBG is by far the major determinant of overall binding intensity. The interaction between T_4 and its binding proteins conforms to a reversible binding equilibrium in which the majority of the hormone is bound and a very small proportion (normally less than 0.1 percent) is free. It appears likely that only the free or unbound hormone is available to tissues; therefore, the metabolic state of the patient will correlate more closely with the concentration of free than with the total concentration of hormone in plasma. Furthermore, homeostatic regulation of thyroid function will be directed toward maintenance of a normal concentration of free rather than total hormone. Disturbances of the thyroid hormone–plasma protein interaction are of two general types (see Table 85-1). In the first, the thyroid-pituitary axis is intrinsically normal, and the homeostatic control of thyroid hormone secretion is intact. Under these circumstances, disordered binding interactions result from primary alterations in the concentration of TBG. For example, an increase in TBG will initially lower the concentration of free hormone and thus diminish the quantity of hormone available to tissues. Total hormonal concentration in serum will then increase until the concentration of free hormone is restored to normal. At this time, the proportions of T_4 and T_3 that are free will be decreased. The increase in total hormonal concentration counterbalances the decrease in the proportion free; as a result, the absolute concentration of free hormone is normal and the metabolic state of the patient is unchanged. Converse changes occur when the concentration of TBG declines. Table 85-2 summarizes those circumstances associated with primary alterations in the concentration of TBG.

The second type of disturbance of thyroid hormone–binding interactions results from a primary alteration in the concentration of thyroid hormones in the blood, such as occurs in hypothyroidism or thyrotoxicosis. Here, homeostatic control of thyroid hormone secretion is disrupted and pathologic factors determine the rate of hormone secretion independent of the thyroid-pituitary axis. Under these circumstances, the concentration of TBG is changed little, if at all, and the concentration of free hormone will vary directly with the total concentration of hormone. Since such changes in circulating hormone usually result from intrinsic disease of the pituitary or thyroid itself, homeostatic mechanisms cannot restore the concentration of free hormone to normal. Primary changes in thyroidal function are therefore associated with persistent changes in the concentration of both total and free hormone, and, consequently, with alterations in the metabolic state of the patient. In these disorders, the relative change in the concentration of free hormone is greater than the change in total hormonal concentration.

T_3 is not bound by TBPA and is bound by TBG less firmly than is T_4. As a consequence, the proportion of free T_3 is normally eight to ten times greater than that of T_4. As a result, T_3 is removed from the blood much more rapidly than is T_4. This accounts for its failure to contribute materially to the total hormonal iodine concentration in the blood and possibly for its more rapid onset and offset of action.

Following their penetration into the cell, T_4 and T_3 undergo a variety of reactions which lead ultimately to their excretion or inactivation. As judged from experiments with isotopically labeled hormones, the major

TABLE 85-1
Classification of the varieties of disordered thyroid hormone–plasma protein interactions

Type of abnormality	*Serum T_4*	*Percent free T_4 or resin T_3 uptake*	*Free T_4 conc. or T_4-RT_3 index*
1 Primary abnormality in thyroxine-binding proteins			
a Increased binding	↑	↓	N
b Decreased binding	↓	↑	N
2 Primary disorder of thyroid function			
a Hypothyroidism	↓	↓	↓
b Hyperthyroidism	↑	↑	↑

TABLE 85-2
Circumstances associated with altered concentration of TBG

Increased TBG	*Decreased TBG*
Pregnancy	Androgenic and anabolic steroids
Oral contraceptives and other sources of estrogen	Large doses of glucocorticoid
Acute intermittent porphyria	Chronic liver disease
Chronic liver disease	Active acromegaly
Acute hepatitis	Nephrosis
Genetically determined	Genetically determined

pathway of hormone metabolism is removal of iodine (deiodination). This general pathway is present in all tissues tested, leaves the diphenyl ether link of the thyronine nucleus intact, and accounts for approximately 80 percent of T_4 and T_3 disposal. Approximately 20 percent of labeled T_4 and T_3 is normally lost in the stool, principally in the form of conjugates with glucuronate or sulfate. Substantial quantities of labeled hormones are excreted in the bile and are presumably available for reabsorption, probably after hydrolysis of conjugates. However, the magnitude of the enterohepatic circulation of T_4 and T_3 in man is unknown. A small proportion of the hormones undergoes oxidative deamination and decarboxylation of the alanine side chain to yield the acetic acid analogues of T_4 and T_3, tetra- and triiodothyroacetic acids. A more important intermediate product of T_4 metabolism is T_3 itself. Since T_3 appears to be approximately three times more potent than T_4 in many metabolic respects, such monodeiodination of T_4, which can occur in many tissues, yields from T_4 a product of enhanced potency. Moreover, since approximately 30 percent of T_4 is metabolized via conversion to T_3, it would be possible to suggest that virtually all the metabolic potency of T_4 resides in the T_3 generated therefrom. Whether T_4 is in reality a "prohormone" in this manner is uncertain. In any event, it is likely that the majority of T_3 in the blood normally arises by peripheral conversion from T_4, rather than direct thyroidal secretion. An important corollary of the latter is that athyreotic or hypothyroid patients maintained with synthetic L-thyroxine to a normal value of serum T_4 concentration will have, in addition, nearly normal concentrations of T_3 in their blood.

Under certain circumstances, changes in the activity of cellular processes involved in hormone metabolism may be the major determinant of changes in the rates of metabolic clearance of T_4 and T_3. Both phenobarbital and diphenylhydantoin increase the metabolic clearance of thyroid hormones without increasing the proportion of free hormone in the blood. Indeed, in the case of diphenylhydantoin, both total and free T_4 concentrations are diminished. Nevertheless, a normal metabolic state is maintained, possibly owing to stimulation of the conversion of T_4 to T_3. The effects of these agents are doubtless related to the hypertrophy of smooth endoplasmic reticulum and increased activity of varied microsomal enzymes that they induce.

REGULATION OF THYROID FUNCTION Regulation of thyroid function is effected by two general mechanisms, one suprathyroidal and one intrathyroidal (Fig. 85-2). The proximate mediator of suprathyroidal regulation is thyrotropin or thyroid-stimulating hormone (TSH), a glycopeptide secreted by basophilic cells within the anterior pituitary gland. TSH stimulates thyroid hypertrophy and hyperplasia; accelerates most aspects of glandular intermediary metabolism; enhances synthesis of nucleic acid and protein, including thyroglobulin; and stimulates all steps in thyroid iodine metabolism leading to the synthesis and secretion of thyroid hormones. These actions are thought to be mediated, at least in large part, by increased synthesis of the "second messenger," cyclic 3′5′-adenosine monophosphate.

Regulation of TSH secretion, in turn, is effected by two opposing influences. TRH (thyrotropin-releasing hormone), a tripeptide amide (pyroglutamyl-histidylprolineamide) secreted in the ventromedial hypothalamus, reaches the pituitary via the hypophyseal portal capillary system and there stimulates synthesis and secretion of TSH. These effects of TRH are inhibited, however, by the extent of thyroid hormone action within the pituitary, and this is presumed to be closely related to the concentration of free thyroid hormones in the blood. Thus, negative feedback of thyroid hormones on TSH secretion occurs mainly in the pituitary gland itself; in what manner and to what extent thyroid hormones affect the secretion of TRH is unknown.

Intrathyroid regulation of thyroid function is less well understood, but is nevertheless important. In some manner as yet undetermined, changes in glandular organic iodine content are associated with reciprocal changes in thyroidal iodide transport activity, as well as in growth, glucose metabolism, and nucleic acid synthesis. Although these influences are evident in the absence of TSH stimulation, and hence may be termed *autoregulatory*, their most important role is to modify (iodine-enrichment inhibiting, and iodine-depletion enhancing) the response of these functions to TSH.

LABORATORY TESTS The availability of a variety of laboratory tests permits evaluation of many aspects of thyroid hormone economy. Such tests can be divided into five major categories: direct tests of thyroid function; tests related to the concentration and binding of thyroid hormones in blood; metabolic indexes; tests of the homeostatic control of thyroid function; and various tests that do not fit into other categories. A system of abbreviations to designate the various laboratory tests has been adopted by the American Thyroid Association and is used herein.

Direct tests of thyroid function The *thyroidal radioactive iodine uptake* (*RAIU*) is the most commonly used test for assessing glandular function per se. The administered radioiodine (^{131}I) mixes uniformly with the endogenous stable iodide and, in the steady state, indicates what percentage of the iodide entering and leaving the iodide space per unit time is accumulated by the thyroid. The RAIU is usually measured 24 hr after ^{131}I administration since it usually has reached a plateau value at this time. The RAIU varies inversely with the pool of endogenous stable iodide and directly with the functional state of the thyroid. Over the last decade, the widespread enrichment of bread and table salt with iodine has led to an increase in the endogenous iodide pool, with the result that the normal range for the 24 hr RAIU has declined to approximately 5 to 30 percent of the administered dose. Consequently, this test no longer discriminates between normal and hypothyroid states. Values above the normal range, however, indicate thyroid hyperfunction, and remain useful, therefore, in the diagnosis of hyperthyroidism. The RAIU is also used as part of the thyroid suppression test and the TSH stimulation test.

Tests related to hormonal concentration and binding in blood The *serum T_4 concentration* is measured by the ability of stable T_4 extracted from serum, as compared with known quantities of T_4, to displace labeled T_4 from a protein mixture containing TBG. By convention, this test has been designated T_4(D). This test is highly specific and is commonly known by the names of its developers (Murphy-Pattee). The normal range for T_4(D) is 4 to 11 μg per 100 ml. In some laboratories T_4(D) is expressed in terms of its iodine content as T_4I(D). This is derived by multiplying T_4(D) by 0.65, the value for the mole fraction of T_4 that is iodine. Thus, in interpreting values of serum T_4, it is important that one be aware of the manner in which the value is expressed. The *serum protein-bound iodine concentration (PBI)* was, until recently, the only method of estimating serum T_4, and such measurement was possible only by virtue of the iodine content of T_4. This test is much less specific than T_4(D), which has superseded it. It is occasionally useful in detecting the presence of abnormal iodoproteins in the blood arising as a result of an intrathyroidal biosynthetic defect, because here the PBI is disproportionately high in relation to the T_4(D). Normal values for the PBI range from 4 to 8 μg per 100 ml. The *serum T_3 concentration* can be measured by radioimmunoassay, abbreviated T_3(RIA); here, the ability of the stable T_3 in serum to displace labeled T_3 from anti-T_3 antibody is compared with that of known quantities of T_3. Normal values range from 100 to 170 ng per 100 ml.

As mentioned in the previous section, alterations in the concentration of TBG, as well as alterations in hormone secretion, will influence the total concentration of hormone in the blood. However, only alterations in hormone secretion will lead to steady-state alterations in the concentration of free hormone. The *percent of free hormone (percent FT_4* or *percent FT_3)* can be measured by equilibrium dialysis of serum enriched with a tracer quantity of the labeled hormone, and the product of this value and T_4(D) or T_3(RIA) yields the *concentration of free hormone (FT_4* or *FT_3)*. Measurement of percent FT_4 or percent FT_3 is a cumbersome procedure. Hence, for clinical purposes, the *in vitro uptake test* is employed, as it is simple to perform and yields qualitatively the same information. Here, the serum is enriched with labeled hormone and then incubated with an insoluble, particulate material, such as resin or charcoal, that binds hormone. The percent of labeled hormone taken up by the particulate material varies inversely with the concentration of unoccupied binding sites on TBG. Labeled T_3 is employed in preference to labeled T_4 since it is less strongly bound by the serum and hence yields higher and therefore more accurate uptake values. Normal values for the *resin-T_3 uptake (RT_3U)* range from 25 to 35 percent. Results may also be expressed as the quotient of the RT_3U value in the patient's serum and that obtained in a normal control specimen (*RT_3U ratio*). The product of T_4(D) and RT_3U ratio (*T_4-RT_3 index*) provides an index of FT_4. Primary alterations in the concentration of TBG (Table 85-2) produce *reciprocal* alterations in RT_3U and T_4(D), with the result that the T_4-RT_3 index remains normal. By contrast, primary alterations in T_4 secretion produce changes in RT_3U that are in the same direction as those in T_4(D). Hence, the T_4-RT_3 index affords a better discrimination from normal values than either of its component tests alone.

Metabolic indexes These tests measure the metabolic impact of thyroid hormone in the peripheral tissues. The *basal metabolic rate (BMR)* measures energy expenditure in terms of the amount of O_2 consumed in the basal state. Values are expressed as a percentage difference from the mean value for normal individuals of the same age, sex, and body surface area. The normal range is approximately −15 to +5 percent. Owing to the variety of nonthyroidal factors that affect the BMR, however, this test is of limited diagnostic value. Increases in the *serum cholesterol concentration* are suggestive of hypothyroidism of thyroidal origin; however, decreases in serum cholesterol concentration are of little value in the diagnosis of thyrotoxicosis. Prolongation of the *Achilles reflex time* as assessed by kinemometry or photomotography, though not pathognomonic, is suggestive of hypothyroidism, but the test has little discrimatory value in hyperthyroidism.

Tests of homeostatic control The measurement of *serum TSH* has become an important tool in the diagnosis of hypothyroidism and diminished thyroid reserve. The latter state represents a stage in the evolution of hypothyroidism in which a structural or functional abnormality that impairs hormonal synthesis is compensated for by hypersecretion of TSH and activation of the thyroid. Serum TSH is measured by radioimmunoassay; here, the ability of TSH in serum to displace labeled human TSH from anti-TSH antibody is compared with that of known quantities of human TSH. The normal range is less than 5 μU per ml; current sensitivity does not permit distinction between normal or low values. Measurement of serum TSH affords the best means of distinguishing between untreated hypothyroidism of thyroidal origin, in which the values are invariably increased, from pituitary or hypothalamic hypothyroidism, in which the values are usually undetectable but always within the normal range. In thyrotoxicosis, serum TSH is undetectable, except in rare cases of TSH-secreting tumors.

The *TSH stimulation test* is employed as a means of

assessing thyroid reserve. Here, the responses of the RAIU and T_4(D) to an intramuscular injection of bovine TSH are monitored. This test is of major value in the diagnosis of diminished thyroid reserve, in which the gland is under maximum stimulation by endogenous TSH and hence shows no further response to exogenous TSH, and in the differentiation of pituitary hypothyroidism from hypothyroidism of primary thyroidal origin. With the general availability of measurements of serum TSH, however, this test is now less frequently used.

The *thyrotropin-releasing hormone* (*TRH*) *stimulation test* is a test which may have value for diverse diagnostic purposes. Following the intravenous injection of TRH in normal subjects, the serum TSH begins to rise at 10 min, peaks between 20 and 45 min, and then falls rapidly. Subnormal response to a standard dose, therefore, may reflect diminished pituitary TSH reserve. The response to TRH within the pituitary is inhibited by thyroid hormone, with the result that a supranormal response occurs in patients with hypothyroidism of thyroidal origin, whereas little or no response occurs in patients with thyrotoxicosis. This lack of response serves as an excellent confirmatory test for thyrotoxicosis. This test is also of value in the recognition and differential diagnosis of pituitary and hypothalamic hypothyroidism; in the former, but not the latter, disorder, no response to TRH would be expected.

The *thyroid suppression test* is used to assess whether thyroid function is being controlled by normal homeostatic mechanisms. Normally, exogenous thyroid hormone suppresses pituitary TSH secretion, resulting in a decrease in the RAIU. Since liothyronine is usually employed (100 μg daily for 10 days), the resulting decline in T_4(D), as well as in the RAIU, can serve as an index of suppression. A normal suppressive response is a decrease of the RAIU to less than half of the control value and a decline of the T_4(D) to low normal or subnormal values. In patients with increased TBG, the decline in T_4(D) may be delayed. An abnormal suppression test is always present in hyperthyroidism, irrespective of the underlying cause; this indicates either autonomy of thyroid function, the presence of an abnormal stimulator, or, at least theoretically, unremitting hypersecretion of TSH. By universal agreement, a normal suppression test excludes the presence of hyperthyroidism. An abnormal suppression test does not necessarily indicate the presence of hyperthyroidism, however, since it is seen after treatment of hyperthyroidism in Graves' disease, in about half of the euthyroid patients with the ophthalmopathy of Graves' disease, and in seemingly euthyroid patients in whom an autonomous hyperfunctioning adenoma has suppressed the remainder of the gland.

Miscellaneous tests Tests for circulating antibodies directed against various glandular components are often of diagnostic value. For example, moderate to high titers of an *antithyroglobulin antibody* are found in the serum of most patients with Hashimoto's disease and in a high proportion of patients with primary thyroprivic hypothyroidism. In the active phase of Graves' disease, about 60 percent of patients have an abnormal thyroid stimulator in serum that differs from TSH in its longer duration of action in the mouse bioassay system; hence its designation *long-acting thyroid stimulator* (LATS). LATS is an immunoglobulin G of lymphoid origin and appears to be an antibody directed against some thyroid cell component.

Imaging by *scintiscanning* permits localization of sites of radioiodine or sodium pertechnetate Tc 99m accumulation. This technique is useful for defining areas of increased or decreased function within the thyroid and for detecting retrosternal goiter, ectopic thyroid tissue, and functioning metastases of thyroid carcinoma.

SIMPLE (NONTOXIC) GOITER

There is considerable confusion concerning the descriptive terms *endemic* and *sporadic* goiter. Endemic implies an etiologic factor or factors common to a particular geographic region. The term has been defined as the presence of generalized or localized thyroid enlargement in over 10 percent of the population. The connotation of sporadic is that goiter arises in nonendemic areas as a result of a stimulus that does not affect the population generally. Since these terms fail to define or distinguish the causes of such goiters and since thyroid enlargement of diverse etiology may exist in both endemic and nonendemic regions, it seems prudent to employ a general term such as simple or nontoxic goiter. This all-inclusive category can be further subdivided into specific etiologic groups as defined by objective procedures. Simple or nontoxic goiter may be defined as any enlargement of the thyroid gland that does not result from an inflammatory or neoplastic process and is not initially associated with thyrotoxicosis or myxedema.

ETIOLOGY Although the causes of simple goiter are manifold, their clinical manifestations are thought to reflect the operation of a common physiopathologic mechanism. Simple goiter results when one or more factors impair the capacity of the thyroid gland in the basal state to secrete quantities of active hormones necessary to meet the needs of the peripheral tissues. Although this has been presumed to lead to increased secretion of TSH, concentrations of TSH in the serum of patients with simple goiter are usually normal. Hence, some other mechanism of goitrogenesis may be operative. A likely possibility is that depletion of glandular organic iodine accompanying impaired hormone synthesis increases the responsiveness of thyroid structure and function to basal levels of TSH. The resulting increases in both functioning thyroid mass and cellular activity are sufficient to overcome mild or moderate impairment of hormone synthesis; thus, the patient remains metabolically normal, though goitrous. When, however, the underlying disorder is severe, compensatory responses, now including hypersecretion of TSH, are inadequate to overcome the impairment, and the patient is both goitrous and more or less severely hypothyroid. Thus, the entity simple goiter cannot be separated clearly, in the pathogenetic sense, from goitrous hypothyroidism. Specific causes of simple goiter are included in Table 85-3 and may exist with or without hypothyroidism.

PATHOLOGY The histopathology of the thyroid in simple goiter varies with the severity of the etiologic factor and the stage of the disorder at which the examination is made. In its initial stages, the gland reveals a uniform hypertrophy, hyperplasia, and hypervascularity. As the disorder persists or undergoes repeated exacerbations and remissions, uniformity of thyroidal architecture is usually lost. Occasionally, the greater part of the gland may display a reasonably uniform degree of involution or hyperinvolution with colloid accumulation. More often such areas are interspersed with patchy areas of focal hyperplasia. Fibrosis may demarcate a variable number of nodules, which may be hyperplastic or involuted. These may resemble, but do not really represent, true neoplasms (adenomas). Areas of hemorrhage and calcification may be present.

CLINICAL PICTURE In simple goiter, the clinical manifestations arise solely from enlargement of the thyroid since the metabolic state of the patient is normal. In goitrous hypothyroidism, symptoms caused by thyromegaly are similarly present, but are accompanied by signs and symptoms of hormonal insufficiency. Mechanical sequelae include compression and displacement of the trachea or esophagus, occasionally with obstructive symptoms if the goiter becomes sufficiently large. Superior mediastinal obstruction may occur with large retrosternal goiters. Signs of compression can be induced in the case of large retrosternal goiters when the patient's arms are raised above the head (Pemberton's sign); suffusion of the face, giddiness, or syncope may result from this maneuver. Compression of the recurrent laryngeal nerve leading to hoarseness is rare in simple goiter and suggests neoplasm. Sudden hemorrhage into a nodule may lead to an acute, painful swelling in the neck and may produce or enhance compressive symptoms. Hyperthyroidism not uncommonly supervenes in long-standing multinodular goiter (toxic multinodular goiter). It is not known whether this represents the superimposition of Graves' disease upon a chronic nontoxic goiter or a separate disease entity.

In geographic regions where iodine deficiency is severe, acquired goitrous enlargement may also be associated with varying degrees of hypothyroidism. Cretinism, both goitrous and nongoitrous, occurs with increased frequency in the children of goitrous parents, and contributes a significant sector of the socially dependent population in many countries where goiter is common. Although iodine deficiency is doubtless a necessary factor in the etiology of endemic goiter, the frequency of goiter may differ greatly among areas of equally severe iodine deficiency. In such instances, dietary or water-borne goitrogens appear to be important conditioning factors.

DIAGNOSIS The diagnosis of simple goiter requires, first, demonstration of a normal metabolic state and, second, differentiation of the goitrous condition from Hashimoto's disease or thyroid neoplasia. Physical examination alone cannot serve to make the diagnosis. A careful history is important, particularly with respect to the occurrence of thyroid pain or tenderness, rapid change in size, hoarseness, or previous drug ingestion. High titers of circulating antithyroglobulin antibodies (tanned red cell agglutinins > 1/25,000) indicate Hashimoto's disease. Needle biopsy may occasionally be indicated to make or exclude the diagnosis of Hashimoto's disease, but should not be performed where thyroid carcinoma is suspected. In areas where goiter is endemic, high values for the RAIU and low values for urinary iodine excretion are the common pattern. Low normal or subnormal values for T_4(D) are commonly found, even in the absence of hypothyroidism. In such cases, high values for serum T_3(RIA) apparently account for the normal metabolic (eumetabolic) state.

TREATMENT The object of treatment is to remove the thyroidal hyperplasia, either by relieving external encumbrances to hormone formation or by providing sufficient quantities of exogenous hormone to inhibit TSH secretion and thereby put the thyroid gland almost completely at rest. In disorders characterized by decreased thyroidal iodide stores, such as iodine deficiency or impairment of the thyroidal iodide-concentrating mechanism, small doses of iodide may prove effective. Occasionally, a known extrinsic goitrogen can be withdrawn. Most commonly, however, no specific etiologic factor can be detected, and suppressive thyroid therapy is required. For this purpose, sodium L-thyroxine (levothyroxine) in a dosage usually ranging from 200 to 300 μg is the agent of choice. Suppression of endogenous thyroid function is most readily assessed by serial measurements of the 24-hr RAIU. Functional suppression is indicated when the RAIU decreases to very low values. Lesser decreases indicate only partial suppression. In multinodular nontoxic goiter, lack of complete suppression usually indicates the presence of autonomously functioning foci, demonstrable by scanning techniques. RAIU tests can be performed at appropriate intervals, and the dose of exoge-

TABLE 85-3
Classification of the causes of hypothyroidism

I Thyroidal
- *A* Thyroprivic
  - *1* Congenital development defect
  - *2* Primary idiopathic
  - *3* Postablative (radioiodine, surgery)
- *B* Goitrous
  - *1* Heritable biosynthetic defects
  - *2* Maternally transmitted (iodides, antithyroid agents)
  - *3* Iodine deficiency
  - *4* Drug-elicited (para-aminosalicylic acid, iodides, phenylbutazone, iodoantipyrine, cobalt)
  - *5* Chronic thyroiditis (Hashimoto's disease)

II Suprathyroidal (trophoprivic)
- *A* Pituitary
- *B* Hypothalamic

nous hormone gradually adjusted as needed to achieve maximum suppression. Occasionally, physiologic replacement doses of exogenous hormones will induce mild, but usually transient, symptoms of thyrotoxicity. In such patients, more prolonged intervals between dosage changes will usually permit achievement of full thyroid suppression without inducing symptoms of toxicity.

Reported results of therapy vary widely. There is general agreement that the early diffuse, hyperplastic goiter responds well, with regression or disappearance in 3 to 6 months. In the authors' experience, the later, nodular stage responds less favorably, and significant reduction in gland size is achieved only in about half the cases. Internodular tissue regresses more often than do nodules themselves. The latter may therefore become more prominent during treatment. After maximum regression of the goiter, suppressive medication may be maintained for prolonged periods, reduced to minimal levels, or at times withdrawn. In an unpredictable manner, goiter will in some cases remain relieved while in others it will recur. In the latter instances, suppressive therapy should be reinstituted and should be continued indefinitely. When treatment is initiated in patients of childbearing age, it should probably be continued through the menopause.

In areas of endemic iodine deficiency, size and prevalence of goiter, and probably the frequency of cretinism, can be reduced by the infrequent injection of iodized oil.

Surgical therapy of simple goiter is physiologically unsound, but it may occasionally be necessary to relieve obstructive symptoms, especially those which persist after a conscientious trial of medical therapy. Surgical exploration of nodular goiter may be indicated in some individuals when evidence suggests carcinoma. However, the suggestion that subtotal resection of multinodular nontoxic goiter affords effective prophylaxis against the development of thyroidal carcinoma is unsound. If for some reason subtotal thyroidectomy has been performed, levothyroxine in a dose of 200 to 300 μg daily is recommended to inhibit regenerative hyperplasia and further goitrogenesis.

HYPOTHYROIDISM

Hypothyroidism is a clinical state that may result from any of a wide variety of structural or functional abnormalities that lead to insufficient synthesis of thyroid hormone. Hypothyroidism dating from birth and resulting in developmental abnormalities is termed *cretinism.* The term *myxedema* connotes a severe form of hypothyroidism in which there is accumulation of hydrophilic mucopolysaccharides in the ground substance of the dermis as well as other tissues, leading to thickening of the facial features and doughy induration of the skin.

ETIOLOGY A classification of the causes of hypothyroidism is presented in Table 85-3. In thyroprivic hypothyroidism, loss of thyroid tissue leads to inadequate synthesis of thyroid hormone, despite maximum stimulation of any thyroid remnant by TSH. The most common cause of thyroprivic hypothyroidism is surgical or radioiodine ablation of the thyroid gland in the treatment of Graves' disease. Thyroprivic hypothyroidism may also occur as a primary idiopathic phenomenon. The cause of this disorder is unknown, but the frequency of circulating thyroid antibodies and its coexistence with pernicious anemia and other diseases in which circulating antibodies are found suggest that it may belong to the autoimmune group of diseases. Finally, a developmental defect may result in failure of the gland to gain an adequate size, leading to sporadic nongoitrous cretinism or juvenile hypothyroidism.

Impaired functional ability to synthesize adequate quantities of thyroid hormone leads to hypersecretion of TSH and hence goiter. If this compensatory response is inadequate, goitrous hypothyroidism ensues. The commonest cause in North America is Hashimoto's disease, in which defective organic binding of iodide and abnormal secretion of iodoproteins are frequent biosynthetic abnormalities. Iodide-induced goiter with or without hypothyroidism appears to arise from an intrinsic defect in the organic binding mechanism which permits a persistent Wolff-Chaikoff effect. Patients with Graves' disease, especially after radioiodine treatment, and those with Hashimoto's disease are particularly susceptible to iodide-induced goiter. Less common causes of goitrous hypothyroidism are heritable defects in pathways of hormonal biosynthesis and ingestion of drugs which induce defects in hormonal biosynthesis, such as para-aminosalicylic acid, cobalt, and lithium carbonate. Finally, in many areas of the world where there is environmental iodine deficiency, goitrous cretinism and hypothyroidism occur on an endemic basis. Diminished thyroid reserve occurs as a stage in the evolution of both thyroprivic and goitrous hypothyroidism.

In hypothyroidism of suprathyroidal origin, the thyroid is instrinsically normal, but is deprived of stimulation by TSH. Deprivation of TSH, most commonly the result of post-partum pituitary necrosis or a tumor of the pituitary or adjacent regions, results in pituitary hypothyroidism. Hypothalamic hypothyroidism appears to be less common and results from inadequate secretion of TRH.

CLINICAL PICTURE The general appearance of children with hypothyroidism varies considerably, depending on the age at which the deficiency began and the promptness with which replacement therapy was instituted. Manifestations of cretinism may be present at birth, but are more commonly evident within the first several months, depending upon the extent of thyroid failure. During the neonatal period, the abnormally long persistence of physiologic jaundice, hoarse cry, constipation, somnolence, and feeding problems should call attention to the diagnosis. In later months, delay in reaching the normal milestones of development becomes evident, and the physical characteristics of the cretin appear. These include short stature, coarse features with protruding tongue, broad flat nose, widely set eyes, sparse hair, dry skin, and protuberant abdomen with an umbilical hernia. X-ray examination reveals retarded bone age, epiphyseal dysgenesis, and delayed dental development. Mental development is retarded; eventual intellectual attainment will depend upon how soon full replacement therapy is instituted.

In the older child with hypothyroidism, the clinical manifestations are intermediate between those of infantile and adult hypothyroidism. Retardation of linear growth results in shortness of stature, while retardation of sexual maturation results in delay in the onset of puberty. Poor performance at school may call attention to the diagnosis. The manifestations of adult hypothyroidism are present to a variable degree. X-ray examination reveals delayed union of the epiphyses.

In the adult, early symptoms of hypothyroidism are nonspecific and of insidious onset. They may include lethargy, constipation, cold intolerance, and menorrhagia. Over the succeeding months, slowing of intellectual and motor activity appears, appetite declines, and modest weight gain occurs. The hair becomes dry and tends to fall out. The patient may complain of dry skin and of stiff, aching muscles. The voice becomes deeper and hoarse and auditory acuity may deteriorate. Ultimately, the clinical picture of florid myxedema appears, with dull expressionless face, sparse hair, periorbital puffiness, large tongue, and pale, cool skin which feels rough and doughy. Thyroid tissue is not readily palpable, except in the goitrous variety of hypothyroidism. The heart is enlarged owing to both dilation and pericardial effusion; if the heart is small, pituitary hypothyroidism should be considered. Adynamic ileus may occur, producing the clinical picture of megacolon. Rarely, psychiatric reactions may dominate the clinical picture. The relaxation phase of the deep tendon reflexes is characteristically prolonged, the so-called "hung-up" reflex. If left untreated, the patient with severe long-standing hypothyroidism may pass into a hypothermic, stuporous state (*myxedema coma*), which is frequently fatal. Respiratory depression is an important component of this state, and hence an increased arterial P_{CO_2} is of premonitory value. Factors which predispose to myxedema coma include cold exposure, trauma, infection, and administration of central nervous system depressants. Dilutional hyponatremia is common in severe hypothyroidism and results from diminished renal perfusion leading to impaired water excretion.

LABORATORY TESTS A decrease in T_4(D) and in the T_4-RT_3 index is common to all varieties of hypothyroidism, as is a decrease in BMR. Because of the decline in the range of normal values, the RAIU is no longer of value in the diagnosis of thyroprivic hypothyroidism, unless it is used as a part of the TSH-stimulation test. In goitrous hypothyroidism, the RAIU may be increased or may display an abnormal pattern of accumulation. The serum TSH is invariably increased in the thyroprivic and goitrous varieties and is normal or undetectable in pituitary or hypothalamic hypothyroidism. In the latter varieties, in addition to possible evidence of intracranial disease, hyposecretion of TSH is accompanied by hyposecretion of other pituitary hormones; this is amenable to laboratory testing (see Chap. 83). A subnormal response of the serum TSH to the administration of TRH will confirm the presence of pituitary hypothyroidism.

Other frequent, but not invariable, manifestations of the hypothyroid state include an increased serum cholesterol in hypothyroidism of thyroidal (but not pituitary) origin, an abnormally prolonged relaxation time of the Achilles reflex, and increased concentrations in serum of creatine phosphokinase, glutamic oxalacetic transaminase, and lactic dehydrogenase. Electrocardiographic changes are common and include bradycardia, low amplitude, and flattened or inverted T waves. In primary thyroprivic hypothyroidism, overt pernicious anemia reportedly occurs in about 12 percent of patients; histamine-fast achlorhydria and the presence of circulating gastic parietal cell antibodies are even more common.

DIFFERENTIAL DIAGNOSIS Little difficulty will be experienced in diagnosing the classic picture of cretinism or juvenile and adult hypothyroidism. Occasionally, a mongoloid infant may be confused with a cretin. However, the characteristic mongoloid eyes, Brushfield's spots in the iris, hyperextensibility of the joints, and normal skin and hair texture distinguish the mongoloid imbecile from the hypothyroid cretin. Chronic nephritis and especially nephrosis may simulate myxedema, particularly because of the facial puffiness and pallor. The nephrotic patient may also display anemia, hypercholesterolemia, and anasarca. Since both the BMR and T_4(D) are often subnormal, the differential diagnosis may be confusing. However, the low T_4(D) is caused by a decrease in thyroxin-binding proteins in the blood, resulting from proteinuria; hence, the T_4-RT_3 index will be normal. Moreover, the RAIU is generally normal or increased.

Treatment Two general types of preparation are available for the treatment of hypothyroidism, either synthetic hormone or thyroprotein derived from animal thyroids. Synthetic hormones include L-thyroxine sodium (levothyroxine), L-triiodothyronine sodium (liothyronine), and a combination of the two (liotrix). The preparation of natural origin most commonly used is thyroid extract, USP. The approximate therapeutic equivalence of these drugs is presented in Table 85-4. Because of their uniform potency, the authors prefer the synthetic preparations, and of these the authors prefer levothyroxine. Unlike liothyronine, liotrix, and even thyroid extract, its ingestion does not lead to abrupt increases in serum T_3 concentration, which could be dangerous in the older patient or in the patient with coexisting heart disease.

In most instances, restoration of a normal metabolic state should be undertaken gradually, especially in the elderly or the patient with heart disease, since sudden increases in metabolic rate may tax cardiac reserve. In adults, an initial daily dose of 25 μg levothyroxine is recommended, and this can be increased by 25- to 50-μg increments at 2- to 3-week intervals, until a normal metabolic state is attained. The daily dose usually necessary to sustain a normal metabolic state is from 200 to 300 μg, and this is usually accompanied by a T_4(D) at the upper limit of the normal range. Because of its long half-life, levothyroxine is generally administered as a single daily dose. The optimum dose for the individual

TABLE 85-4
Approximate therapeutic equivalence of various thyroid hormone preparations

Preparation	*Average daily oral maintenance dose*	*Serum T_4*
Thyroid Extract, USP	120–180 mg	Normal
Levothyroxine	0.2–0.3 mg	Normal or slightly increased
Liothyronine	0.050–0.075 mg	Decreased
Liotrix (T_4/T_3 = 4/1)	1–3 units	Normal

patient should be based on clinical criteria, the T_4(D) being employed only as a confirmatory test.

In cretinism and juvenile hypothyroidism it is essential that full replacement therapy be begun as soon as possible; otherwise the chances of normal intellectual development and growth are poor. Infants and children require doses of levothyroxine that are disproportionately large in relation to body size. *In pituitary and hypothalamic hypothyroidism, thyroid replacement should not be instituted until treatment with cortisone acetate has been initiated,* since acute adrenocortical insufficiency may be precipated by an increase in metabolic rate.

In some cases, it is important that hypothyroidism be rapidly treated. These include patients with myxedema coma and, because of the extreme sensitivity to central nervous system depressants, hypothyroid patients being prepared for emergency surgery. Here, intravenous administration of levothyroxine or oral administration of rapidly acting liothyronine, both in conjunction with the use of glucocorticoids, is indicated.

GRAVES' DISEASE

Graves' disease, also known as Parry's or Basedow's disease, is a disorder of unknown etiology with a characteristic triad of major manifestations: hyperthyroidism with diffuse goiter, ophthalmopathy, and dermopathy. Although considered part of the same disease complex, the three major manifestations need not appear together. Indeed, one or two need never appear, and, moreover, the three tend to run a course independent of one another. Although hyperthyroidism is the most common manifestation of Graves' disease, it is important to be aware of the fact that this symptom complex, which merely reflects an excessive supply of thyroid hormone to the tissues, can also arise in a variety of other circumstances which are clearly distinct from Graves' disease, as is discussed below.

INCIDENCE Graves' disease is a relatively common disorder which may occur at any age, but occurs especially in the third and fourth decades. The disease is much more frequent in women than in men. In nongoitrous areas the ratio of predominance in females may be as high as 7:1. In endemic goitrous areas the ratio is lower. Hyperthyroidism is comparatively rare in children. When it occurs, there is usually a diffuse goiter free of nodules. There is a distinct familial predisposition to Graves' disease; in addition, among family members of patients with Graves' disease, a clinical and immunological overlap exists with respect to Hashimoto's disease, primary thyroprivic hypothyroidism, and pernicious anemia.

ETIOLOGY The etiology of Graves' disease is unknown. In view of the varied manifestations of Graves' disease and their differing courses, it is possible, and indeed likely, that no single etiologic factor is responsible for the entire syndrome. With respect to hyperthyroidism, it is apparent that central to this disorder is a disruption of homeostatic mechanisms that normally adjust hormone secretion to meet the needs of peripheral tissues; if such were able to operate, hyperthyroidism could not be sustained. In the past, it was suggested that this homeostatic disruption resulted from either overproduction of TSH or development of autonomous hyperfunction within the thyroid itself. More recently, attention has been focused on the etiologic role of a protein that under appropriate bioassay conditions can be demonstrated in the serum of approximately 60 percent of thyrotoxic patients with Graves' disease and to date has been convincingly demonstrated to be present only in this disorder. Like TSH, this protein stimulates hormonal release (a property employed in its assay), increases thyroidal ^{131}I uptake, stimulates several aspects of thyroid intermediary metabolism, increases the activity of thyroid adenyl cyclase, and is capable of inducing thyroid hyperplasia. As noted above, it is known as the *long-acting thyroid stimulator* (*LATS*), since, in the bioassay system employed in its measurement, its action is more prolonged than that of TSH. LATS is an immunoglobulin G, the activity of which is retained in the Fab fragment. It can be synthesized by the lymphocytes of patients with Graves' disease. Although the nature of the presumed thyroid antigen is unknown, these findings suggest that LATS is an antibody to some cytologic component of human thyroid. If so, Graves' disease should be included among those disorders associated with, if not necessarily caused by, autoimmune phenomena. Despite its capacity to reproduce in the thyroid of animals many of the features of diffuse toxic goiter, titers of LATS in patients' sera do not correlate well with the presence or absence of thyrotoxicosis or with its degree of severity. Moreover, significant titers of LATS are sometimes associated with normal suppressibility of thyroid function. The latter finding, in particular, makes it unlikely that LATS can alone account for the characteristic features of diffuse toxic goiter in man. Some authorities believe that LATS is an epiphenomenon, and that Graves' disease is caused by cell-mediated immunity, but evidence for this view is tentative.

Very little is known of the etiology of the ophthalmopathic component of Graves' disease. In many patients with progressive infiltrative ophthalmopathy, the serum contains one or more factors that cause exophthalmos in the recipient animal (goldfish or Atlantic minnow) or increased uptake of radioactive sulfate in the intraorbital Harderian gland of the guinea pig or mouse. Although distinguishable from LATS, the latter factor also may be an immunoglobulin. Nothing is known of the etiology of the dermopathy of Graves' disease.

PATHOLOGY In Graves' disease, the *thyroid gland* is diffusely enlarged, soft, and vascular. The essential pathology is that of parenchymatous hypertrophy and hyperplasia, characterized by increased height of the epithelium and redundancy of the follicular wall, giving the picture of papillary infoldings and cytologic evidence of increased activity. Such hyperplasia is usually accompanied by lymphocytic infiltration that may reflect the cell-mediated immune origin of the disease or may merely reflect associated chronic thyroiditis. Following iodine medication, there is colloid storage, which sometimes causes enlargement and increased firmness of the gland. Graves' disease is associated with generalized lymphoid hyperplasia and infiltration, and occasionally with enlargement of the spleen or thymus. Thyrotoxicosis may lead to degeneration of skeletal muscle fibers, enlargement of the heart, fatty infiltration or diffuse fibrosis of the liver, decalcification of the skeleton, and loss of body tissue (including fat deposits, osteoid, and muscle).

The *ophthalmopathy* of Graves' disease is characterized pathologically by an inflammatory infiltrate of the orbital contents, exclusive of the globe, with lymphocytes, mast cells, and plasma cells being the predominant cellular components. The orbital musculature is mainly involved and often is greatly enlarged, largely accounting for the increased volume of the orbital contents that causes the globe to protrude. Muscle fibers show degeneration and loss of striations, with ultimate fibrosis.

The *dermopathy* of Graves' disease is characterized by thickening of the dermis, which is infiltrated with lymphocytes and with hydrophilic, metachromatically staining mucopolysaccharides.

CLINICAL PICTURE The clinical picture of patients with Graves' disease varies according to the type of manifestations present and their individual severity. It is also modified by the age of the patient and the presence of underlying disease in other organs, particularly the heart.

Hyperthyroidism Common manifestations of hyperthyroidism in Graves' disease include goiter, fine tremor (especially of the extended fingers and tongue), increased nervousness, as well as emotional instability, excessive sweating and heat intolerance, palpitations, and hyperkinesis. Loss of weight and of strength usually exist, often despite increased appetite. Weakness is often manifested by difficulty in climbing stairs. When severe wasting of limb-girdle musculature is present, the condition is termed *thyrotoxic myopathy*. Hyperdefecation and occasionally anorexia, nausea, and vomiting may occur. Dyspnea, atrial arrhythmias, and, in individuals over the age of forty, cardiac failure occur not infrequently. Oligomenorrhea and amenorrhea are commoner than menorrhagia. In general, nervous symptoms dominate the clinical picture in younger individuals, whereas cardiovascular and myopathic symptoms predominate in older subjects.

The skin is warm and moist with a velvety texture, and palmar erythema is often found. The hair is fine and silky. Occasionally, increased loss of hair from the temporal aspects of the scalp may be noted. Excessive melanin pigmentation is not uncommon. *Ocular signs* include a characteristic stare with widened palpebral fissures, infrequent blinking, lid lag, failure of convergence, and failure to wrinkle the brow on upward gaze. These signs are thought to result from sympathetic overstimulation and usually subside when the thyrotoxicosis is corrected. The *infiltrative ophthalmopathy* characteristic of Graves' disease is discussed below.

The *diffuse toxic goiter* may be asymmetric and lobular. Often a bruit is heard directly over the gland. When heard, it usually signifies that the patient is thyrotoxic, but it may also rarely be present in association with other disorders in which the thyroid is markedly hyperplastic. Venous hums and carotid souffles should be distinguished from true thyroid bruits. A hyperplastic pyramidal lobe of the thyroid may often be palpable if carefully sought.

Cardiovascular findings include a wide pulse pressure, sinus tachycardia, atrial arrhythmias (especially atrial fibrillation), systolic murmurs, increased intensity of the apical first sound, cardiac enlargement, and at times, overt heart failure. A to-and-fro, high-pitched sound may be audible in the pulmonic area and may simulate a pericardial friction rub.

Ophthalmopathy The clinical signs associated with the ophthalmopathy of Graves' disease may be divided into two components: the spastic and the mechanical. The former includes the stare, lid lag, and lid retraction that accompany thyrotoxicosis and account for the "frightened" facies and classic eye signs previously described. These findings need not be associated with actual proptosis and usually return to normal after appropriate correction of thyrotoxicosis. The mechanical component includes proptosis of varying degrees with ophthalmoplegia and congestive oculopathy characterized by chemosis, conjunctivitis, marked periobital swelling, and the resultant complications of corneal ulceration, optic neuritis, and optic atrophy. When exophthalmos progresses rapidly and becomes the major concern in Graves' disease, it is usually referred to as *progressive*, and if severe, *malignant exophthalmos*. The term *exophthalmic ophthalmoplegia* refers to the ocular muscle weakness that so commonly accompanies this disorder and results in strabismus with varying degrees of diplopia. Exophthalmos may be unilateral early in the course of the disorder but usually progresses to symmetric involvement.

Dermopathy The dermopathy of Graves' disease usually occurs over the dorsum of the legs or feet and is commonly termed *localized myxedema* or *pretibial myxedema*. It occurs in patients with past or present Graves' disease and is not a manifestation of hypothyroidism per se. About half of the cases occur during the active stage of thyrotoxicosis; in the remainder the lesions develop after treatment. The affected area is usually well demarcated from normal skin by the fact that it is raised, thickened, has a peau d'orange appearance, and may be pruritic and hyperpigmented. The lesions are usually discrete, assuming a plaquelike or nodular configuration, but in some instances the lesions become widely confluent. Clubbing of the fingers and toes with characteristic bony changes differentiable from those of hypertrophic pulmonary osteoarthropathy may accompany the dermal changes (*thyroid acropachy*). Activity of this disorder is usually self-limited.

DIAGNOSIS When severe, Graves' disease presents

little difficulty in diagnosis. Florid thyrotoxicosis is manifested by weakness, weight loss despite good appetite, nervous instability, tremor, intolerance to heat, hyperhydrosis, palpitations, and hyperdefecation. When associated with diffuse thyroid enlargement, often accompanied by a bruit, and particularly when associated with ophthalmopathy, Graves' disease presents a clinical picture that is virtually unique. In such instances, laboratory tests, which reveal increased RAIU, T_4(D), T_3(RIA), RT_3U and T_4-RT_3 index, and increased BMR, serve mainly as base lines for evaluation of therapy, rather than necessary diagnostic aids.

In less severe cases, particularly when ophthalmopathy is lacking, the diagnosis may be substantially more difficult, since the symptoms of mild hyperthyroidism are similar to those of other disorders (see section on Differential Diagnosis below). Presence of a goiter makes the diagnosis of hyperthyroidism more likely, but careful palpation is necessary to determine whether toxic multinodular goiter or toxic adenoma is present, since treatment of these disorders may differ from that of diffuse toxic goiter. Absence of thyroid enlargement makes the diagnosis of Graves' disease unlikely, but does not exclude it absolutely. In mild cases, confirmatory laboratory tests assume great importance. Unfortunately, mild hyperthyroidism is often associated with only marginal abnormalities in laboratory tests, and values may, in fact, lie within the upper limit of the normal range. In instances like this, the thyroid suppression test, and perhaps the TRH stimulation test, assume crucial importance.

In a few patients, the clinical picture may be one of apathy, rather than hyperactivity, and evidence of hypermetabolism may be slight. In such patients, myopathic features may be pronounced. More often, cardiovascular manifestations predominate since, in patients with underlying heart disease, even mild hyperthyroidism may produce severe disability. Hence, *all patients with unexplained cardiac failure or irregularities in rhythm, especially if atrial in origin, should be examined for hyperthyroidism.* Clues to the diagnosis include a relatively rapid circulation time and resistance to the usual doses of digitalis, but laboratory confirmation will be required.

DIFFERENTIAL DIAGNOSIS Signs and symptoms in a number of nonthyroidal disorders may simulate certain aspects of the thyrotoxic syndrome. Anxiety is a prominent feature of hyperthyroidism, and there is thus some overlap in the symptomatology of this disorder with that of anxiety states of emotional origin. Such symptoms as tachycardia, tremulousness, irritability, weakness, and fatigue are common to the anxiety of both disorders. In anxiety of emotional origin, however, the peripheral manifestations of excessive thyroid hormones are absent; the skin of the extremities is usually cold and clammy rather than warm and moist. Weight loss, when present in emotional anxiety, is characteristically accompanied by anorexia, whereas in hyperthyroidism it is generally, but not invariably, accompanied by excessive appetite. Hyperthyroidism can occasionally be confused with such disorders as metastatic carcinoma, cirrhosis of the liver, hyperparathyroidism, sprue, and neuromyopathies, such as myasthenia gravis and muscular dystrophy. Hypokalemic periodic paralysis is more common in thyrotoxic patients, especially in the case of Oriental males. Signs and symptoms of hyperthyroidism may overlap with those of pheochromocytoma, which may present with heat intolerance, excessive perspiration, tachycardia with palpitations, and a hypermetabolic state that may often be severe. In all the above disorders, as well as other conditions considered in the differential diagnosis, judiciously applied laboratory tests will usually suffice to differentiate them from hyperthyroidism.

When bilateral ophthalmopathy is accompanied by goiter and thyrotoxicosis, the origin of the ophthalmopathy in the Graves' disease process is virtually assured. The presence of unilateral ophthalmopathy, even when associated with thyrotoxicosis, should alert the physician to the possibility of some other intraorbital or intracranial disease. In the patient who is not thyrotoxic, it is more difficult to ascribe ophthalmopathy to Graves' disease, and other causes must be actively excluded. Among the local causes of unilateral or bilateral exophthalmos are cavernous sinus thrombosis, sphenoidal ridge meningioma, and retrobulbar tumors, including leukemic deposits, as well as the rare granulomatous disorder, pseudotumor oculi. Exophthalmos may also be seen in some patients with certain systemic disorders, such as uremia, accelerated hypertension, chronic alcoholism, chronic obstructive pulmonary disease, superior mediastinal obstruction, and Cushing's syndrome. Ophthalmoplegia in the absence of overt infiltrative manifestations can be confused with that which occurs in diabetes mellitus, myasthenia gravis, and myopathies. When doubt exists concerning the cause of ophthalmopathy, the demonstration of an abnormal thyroid suppression test strongly suggests that the cause is Graves' disease.

When the diagnosis of thyrotoxicosis has been established in a patient lacking the ophthalmopathic manifestations of Graves' disease, other causes of thyrotoxicosis must be considered. Palpation of a symmetric, diffuse goiter, especially if associated with a bruit, excludes the diagnosis of *toxic multinodular goiter* or *toxic adenoma*, both of which disorders are discussed in later sections. Absence of a palpable thyroid gland raises the suspicion of ectopic thyroid tissue or, more commonly, self-administration of thyroid hormone (*thyrotoxicosis factitia*). Ectopic thyroid tissue producing thyrotoxicosis is rare and is most commonly located in the ovary (*struma ovarii*). RAIU, as measured over the thyroid, is low since TSH secretion is suppressed, but despite this, urinary excretion of the dose of ^{131}I is also low, owing to accumulation of ^{131}I by the ectopic tissue. Functioning ectopic tissue can be located by direct counting or scintillation scanning. Thyrotoxicosis factitia most frequently occurs in medical or paramedical personnel or in those who have easy access to thyroid hormone preparations. Physiologically, it resembles thyrotoxicosis caused by ectopic thyroid tissue in that the patient's thyroid gland is suppressed. By contrast, however, most of an administered dose of ^{131}I will be excreted in the urine. When the disorder is caused by ingestion of preparations containing T_4, such as levothyroxine or thyroid extract, the T_4(D) will be increased. On the other hand, when caused by liothyronine, the T_4(D) will be subnormal.

Irrespective of the preparation, the T_3(RIA) will be increased, but more so when liothyronine is the offending agent. Very rarely, thyrotoxicosis may be produced by *TSH-secreting tumors of the pituitary* or by *tumors of trophoblastic origin,* such as choriocarcinoma of the testis or hydatidiform mole, that elaborate thyroid-stimulating peptides. In these latter disorders, thyrotoxicosis is associated with hyperfunction of the thyroid gland.

TREATMENT Hyperthyroidism Hyperthyroidism in Graves' disease is a disorder often characterized by cyclic phases of exacerbation and remission, each of unpredictable onset and duration. Moreover, subtle tests of thyroid function indicate that long-standing disease is associated with progressive thyroid failure, probably consequent to chronic thyroiditis, with the result that hypothyroidism or decreased thyroid reserve supervenes. These characteristics of Graves' disease have important implications in the choice of and response to therapy, as is discussed below.

There are two major approaches to the treatment of hyperthyroidism; both are directed to limiting the quantity of thyroid hormones the gland can produce. The first major therapeutic modality, the use of antithyroid agents, interposes a chemical blockade to hormone synthesis, the effect of which is operative only as long as the drug is administered or until a spontaneous remission occurs. Thus, the agents can control successfully a given phase of active thyrotoxicity but probably will not prevent exacerbation at some subsequent period. The second major approach is ablation of thyroid tissue, thereby limiting hormone production. This may be achieved either surgically or by means of radioactive iodine. Since these procedures induce permanent anatomic alterations of the thyroid, they can control the individual active phase and are more likely to prevent recurrence of thyrotoxicity during a later exacerbation. On the other hand, the permanency of the effects of surgery or radiation makes these modes of therapy capable of leading to hypothyroidism, either shortly after treatment or with the passage of years.

Each major mode of therapy has advantages and disadvantages, indications and contraindications. The latter are more often relative than absolute. In general, a trial of long-term antithyroid therapy is desirable in children, adolescents, young adults, and pregnant women, but may also be employed in older patients. Indications for ablative procedures include relapse or recurrence following drug therapy, a large goiter, drug toxicity, and failure of the patient to follow a medical regimen or to return for periodic examinations. Subtotal thyroidectomy is usually elected for patients under the age of forty in whom ablative therapy is required; however, opinions differ, and some authorities employ radioactive iodine in the treatment of patients in the second or third decades. With older patients, radioactive iodine is clearly the ablative procedure of choice, as it is for patients who have had previous thyroid surgery or those in whom serious systemic disease contraindicates elective surgery.

In those patients selected for *long-term antithyroid therapy,* satisfactory control can almost always be achieved if a sufficient dosage of the drug is administered. Most patients can be managed successfully by propylthiouracil, 100 mg every 8 hr. Methimazole is at least as effective as propylthiouracil when administered in one-tenth the dosage. Once euthyroidism is achieved, the daily dosage may be reduced to the smallest doses that control the thyrotoxicosis fully. In many clinics, however, the initial dose is continued and is supplemented with levothyroxine. By this latter regimen, hypothyroidism resulting from overdosage of antithyroid drugs can be prevented. The undesirable consequences of hypothyroidism, such as enhancement of ophthalmopathy and enlargement of the goiter, may thereby be forestalled. The precise duration of therapy is difficult to predict in the individual patient and may be a function of the spontaneous course of the disease itself. If this is the case, the longer the course of therapy, the more likely it is that the patient will remain well when the drug is discontinued. In general, however, a 12- to 24-month course is usually employed. Following a regimen of this type, approximately half of the patients will remain well for a prolonged period or indefinitely. A normal suppressive response to exogenous thyroid hormone when withdrawal of antithyroid agent is contemplated increases the likelihood that the patient will remain in remission for some time. Decrease in goiter size during treatment has a similar connotation.

The *treatment of hyperthyroidism during pregnancy* is a subject of disagreement. Most physicians believe that antithyroid therapy is preferable to subtotal thyroidectomy, particularly during the first and third trimesters. The major disadvantage of antithyroid therapy is the possibility of inducing goiter and hypothyroidism in the fetus, since antithyroid agents readily traverse the placenta. Hence, a cardinal rule in the use of these agents during pregnancy is that the dosage of antithyroid agent should be the smallest necessary to control hyperthyroidism in the mother. Maintenance of normal values for FT_4 or T_4-RT_3 index will assist in this objective. Some authorities regularly supplement the antithyroid regimen with replacement doses of thyroid hormone. However, available evidence suggests that T_4 and T_3 traverse the human placenta from mother to fetus slowly, if at all. Supplemental thyroid hormone will produce no harm unless a false sense of assurance leads to administration of excessive doses of antithyroid agent or neglect of frequent observation of the patient. From the practical standpoint, pregnancy constitutes the sole indication for the assay of LATS in serum, since high titers in the mother are likely to be associated with thyrotoxicosis in the newborn.

Leukopenia is the principal undesirable side effect of antithyroid drugs. Mild transient leukopenia may occur in approximately 10 percent of patients treated and is not necessarily an indication for discontinuing therapy. When the absolute number of polymorphonuclear leukocytes reaches 1,500 or less, antithyroid medication should be discontinued. Allergic rashes and drug sensitivity develop in a small percentage of patients. These may disappear with antihistamine therapy at the same or reduced dosage of antithyroid agent, but it is probably preferable, when sensitivity reactions occur, to change to another drug. On rare occasions (in less than 0.2 percent), agranulocytosis may occur. This may be sudden in onset. Hepatitis, drug fever, and arthralgias are occasional adverse reactions to antithyroid agents.

Iodides inhibit the release of thyroid hormones from the thyrotoxic gland, and their ameliorative effects occur more rapidly than those of agents that merely inhibit hormone synthesis. Hence, their main use is in patients with actual or impending thyrotoxic crisis or in patients with severe thyrocardiac disease. However, the response to iodides is often incomplete and transient. Furthermore, by expanding the thyroidal stores of hormones, iodides may prolong greatly the latency of response to subsequently instituted antithyroid therapy. Therefore, iodides should be used in conjunction with other therapeutic measures. If the clinical course of the patient is sufficiently severe to require iodide administration, antithyroid drugs will usually be the primary therapeutic agents and should be given in large doses prior to iodides. Since iodides appear to synergize with radiation in the thyroid, they are also useful in controlling thyrotoxicosis following ^{131}I administration, during the period in which the therapeutic effect of radioiodine has not yet taken place.

Owing to the pronounced adrenergic component in thyrotoxicosis, various *adrenergic antagonists* have been employed in the management of this disorder. Of these, propranolol appears to be the agent of choice because of its relative freedom from side effects. In doses of 40 to 120 mg daily, propranolol alleviates such adrenergic manifestations as sweating, tremor, and tachycardia. However, propranolol should be used only as adjunctive therapy rather than sole therapy, as some have suggested, since the underlying metabolic abnormalities are essentially unaffected. Moreover, although the diminution in heart rate and cardiac work that propranolol induces may be beneficial, the withdrawal of adrenergic support of myocardial contractility contraindicates its use in the patient with coexisting heart disease.

Radioactive iodine (*^{131}I*) affords a relatively simple, effective, and economical means of treating thyrotoxicosis. Its major advantage is that it can produce the ablative effects of surgery without the immediate operative and postoperative complications. The principal disadvantage of ^{131}I therapy, in the dosage which has usually been employed, is its tendency to produce hypothyroidism with a frequency that increases progressively with time. As many as 40 to 70 percent of patients may develop this complication by 10 years after treatment. Although hypothyroidism is readily treated, once diagnosed, the insidious onset of the disorder may obscure the diagnosis until serious complications have developed. Hence, some recommend that all patients be treated with large doses of ^{131}I to ensure relief of thyrotoxicosis and then be placed on permanent physiologic replacement doses of thyroid hormone.

To date, studies have provided no evidence of significant carcinogenic or leukemogenic effect of radioiodine in those doses commonly used in treating hyperthyroidism. Nevertheless, many physicians prefer to reserve radioiodine therapy for patients over forty years of age, thinking that it is currently not justifiable to administer an agent of undetermined radiation potentialities to younger persons, particularly those of childbearing potential. Patients with recurrent thyrotoxicosis following surgery, those who refuse surgery, or those who have complicating illnesses contraindicating surgery are excellent candidates for radioiodine therapy.

The usual therapeutic dose of ^{131}I (approximately 160 μCi per g of estimated gland weight) is the dose that has led to the disturbingly high frequency of hypothyroidism. As a result, though continuing to use this dose, some authorities regularly administer prophylactic replacement doses of thyroid hormone. On the other hand, others have been led to administer smaller doses (approximately 80 μCi per g). Although this may diminish the frequency of late hypothyroidism, or merely delay its onset, such is by no means certain. The smaller dose is less likely to relieve thyrotoxicosis within a relatively short period. Antithyroid agents can be employed, however, to speed the attainment of a eumetabolic state while the effect of the ^{131}I is taking hold. There is general agreement that patients with thyrocardiac disease should receive ^{131}I in large doses in view of the hazard of recurrent thyrotoxicosis.

Radiation thyroiditis is an occasional immediate complication of ^{131}I therapy. When present, it commonly appears within 7 to 10 days and is associated with excessive release of hormone into the blood. For this reason, patients with severe hyperthyroidism or underlying heart disease should be rendered eumetabolic with antithyroid agents before ^{131}I is administered. Interruption of antithyroid therapy for several days before and after ^{131}I treatment will suffice to permit adequate accumulation and retention of administered ^{131}I. The swelling that accompanies radiation thyroiditis may contraindicate the use of large doses of ^{131}I in patients with large retrosternal goiters.

Before radioactive iodine was introduced, *subtotal thyroidectomy* was the classic form of ablative therapy, and it is still widely employed in younger patients in whom antithyroid therapy is unsuccessful. Although precise preoperative programs differ, several general principles should be emphasized. Patients should first be rendered fully euthyroid by means of antithyroid agents. Only then should iodides (5 drops Lugol's solution a day for approximately 10 days) be administered concomitantly to effect an involutional response in the gland. Antithyroid drugs should not be discontinued merely because treatment with iodides is instituted.

Hazards of subtotal thyroidectomy include immediate operative complications, such as anesthetic accidents, hemorrhage sometimes leading to respiratory obstruction, and damage to the recurrent laryngeal nerve leading to vocal cord paralysis. Later complications include wound infection, hemorrhage, hypoparathyroidism or hypothyroidism. In experienced hands, surgery is an effective and relatively safe mode of therapy. Postoperative recurrences are quite uncommon. However, carefully conducted follow-up studies reveal that hypothyroidism follows surgery more frequently than previously suspected, although not as commonly as following treatment with ^{131}I.

Ophthalmopathy, dermopathy When severe and progressive, ophthalmopathy is the most difficult component of Graves' disease to treat satisfactorily. Fortunately, however, in most patients the disorder runs a benign course that is largely independent of the course of the hyperthyroid component. In most instances, the activity of even moderately severe disease declines and disappears with time, although some exophthalmos and ophthalmoplegia may persist. In mild disease, considerable benefit may be obtained from simple measures, such as elevating the head at night, administering diuretics to reduce edema, and providing tinted glasses for protection from sun, wind, and foreign bodies. A 1% solution of methylcellulose or plastic shields may help to prevent corneal drying in patients unable to oppose the lids during sleep. In more severe cases, as evidenced by progressive exophthalmos, chemosis, ophthalmoplegia, or loss of vision, large doses of prednisone (120 to 140 mg daily) should be administered, since this is usually effective in reducing the edematous and infiltrative components. With improvement, the dosage is reduced to the lowest effective level, since prolonged administration of large doses will lead to adverse accompaniments of glucocorticoid excess. In those cases that progress despite these measures, orbital decompression, i.e., removal of part of the bony orbit to relieve intraorbital pressure, will usually halt progression of the disease. The management of the patient must always be conducted in concert with an ophthalmologist.

In general, treatment of associated hyperthyroidism should be carried out much as would be the case were ophthalmopathy not present, since there is no convincing evidence that the mode of treatment of the hyperthyroidism influences the course of the ocular disease. The suggestion that total thyroid ablation by surgery and large doses of ^{131}I are beneficial to the ophthalmic disease has not been borne out. It is agreed, however, that hyperthyroidism should be treated, but that hypothyroidism be avoided.

Severe dermopathy can be alleviated by the topical application of glucocorticoids.

TOXIC MULTINODULAR GOITER

Toxic multinodular goiter is a not infrequent consequence of long-standing simple goiter, although the exact proportion of cases in which this complication arises is uncertain. In areas of nonendemicity, the specific etiology of nontoxic multinodular goiter is usually indeterminate. Hence, it is unclear whether a specific etiologic factor underlies those cases of nontoxic multinodular goiter that progress to a thyrotoxic phase. Common to many nontoxic multinodular goiters, even in areas of iodine sufficiency, is a decrease in the iodine content of thyroglobulin, suggesting either a conditioned deficiency of iodine or an impairment of pathways for its normal incorporation into iodinated amino acids. Pathologically, there is nothing which serves clearly to distinguish the nontoxic from the toxic multinodular goiter. However, as judged from radioautographic and scintillation scanning studies, functional patterns may be of two types. In the first and most common, iodine accumulation occurs diffusely, but in patchy foci throughout the gland. Histologically, associated areas reveal cellular hyperplasia. Whether autonomy of function, a prerequisite for development of thyrotoxicosis, resides in these areas per se, or whether they are responding to an extrathyroidal stimulus, as is thought to be the case in Graves' disease, is uncertain. The second, less common, pattern is that of iodine accumulation in one or more discrete nodules within the gland, the remainder being essentially nonfunctional. Whether the former represent true adenomata or are merely colloid nodules that have developed functional autonomy is also uncertain. In both endemic and sporadic nontoxic multinodular goiter, administration of iodides may lead to the development of thyrotoxicosis, implying that areas of potentially autonomous function had been present.

Because it arises in long-standing simple goiter, toxic multinodular goiter is a disease of the aging or elderly. At least partly for this reason, and perhaps because of the nature of the underlying disease, the clinical presentation differs from that in the thyrotoxicosis of Graves' disease. Ophthalmopathy is rare, and would signal the emergence of Graves' disease superimposed on simple goiter. Some patients may present with quite typical thyrotoxicosis. Often, however, the degree of thyrotoxicosis is less severe than that seen in Graves' disease, although its physiologic impact upon specific organ systems may be great. Notable among these is the cardiovascular system, in which arrhythmias or congestive failure may be precipitated or accentuated by thyrotoxicosis that not infrequently is manifested by only subtle findings in other areas (apathetic hyperthyroidism). Weakness and wasting may often predominate, frequently with loss of appetite, rather than hyperphagia, suggesting the presence of a carcinoma.

A nodular goiter that is readily visible or palpable will establish the diagnosis of thyroid disease. In other instances, at least the upper margin of a gland that lies behind the manubrium becomes accessible to palpation during extension of the neck, swallowing, or a forced cough. Having detected a goiter, the physician is obligated to carry out those measures necessary to establish or to exclude the presence of thyrotoxicosis. This is often difficult, since results of conventional laboratory tests are frequently in the borderline range, consistent with the mild degree of thyrotoxicity. Despite their great value in situations such as this, thyroid suppression tests should be undertaken with great caution and reduced dosage of liothyronine, if at all, in the elderly patient because of the hazard of adverse cardiovascular response. As experience with the T_3(RIA) increases, it may well be that many of these patients can be shown to be thyrotoxic on the basis of hypersecretion of T_3 despite a normal or marginal T_4(D). The TRH test may also have value in suggesting the presence of thyrotoxicosis. When laboratory findings do not permit a clear diagnosis of thyrotoxicosis, but suggestive clinical findings are present, a therapeutic trial of antithyroid drugs is indicated.

Radioactive iodine is the treatment of choice for toxic multinodular goiter, once the diagnosis has been established. Large doses (20 to 30 mCi) are usually required, owing in part to the generally lower RAIU, and in part to the variable degree of function throughout the gland. Moreover, the physiologic instability of the elderly patient makes definitive treatment desirable. For the same reason, it is usually wise to initiate therapy with antithyroid agents, withholding radioiodine until a euthyroid state has been achieved, and thereby forestalling an exacerbation of thyrotoxicosis, should radiation thyroiditis occur. Hypothyroidism is only an uncommon consequence of radioiodine treatment of toxic multinodular goiter, owing to the variable activity of differing portions of the gland, which permits previously quiescent areas to replace functionally those that have been destroyed by ^{131}I.

T_3-TOXICOSIS T_3-toxicosis is a term employed to designate thyrotoxicosis in which $T_4(D)$ is normal or low in the absence of a deficiency of TBG, while the $T_3(RIA)$ is increased. Although the cause of the increased production of T_3 relative to T_4 is not known, the disorder may be seen in association with Graves' disease, multinodular goiter, or hyperfunctioning adenoma. The diagnosis should be suspected in a patient with clinical manifestations of thyrotoxicosis in whom the $T_4(D)$ and FT_4 are normal or low and the RAIU is normal or increased. This, together with the frequently palpable goiter, serves to differentiate this disorder from liothyronine-induced thyrotoxicosis factitia. In contradistinction to patients with nonthyroidal disorders mimicking thyrotoxicosis, patients with this disorder, as would be expected, demonstrate nonsuppressibility of thyroid function in response to exogenous T_3. In some patients, thyrotoxicosis with increased $T_3(RIA)$ and normal $T_4(D)$ antecedes emergence of typical increases in both, either during an initial episode of hyperthyroidism or during recurrence after previous treatment.

MAJOR COMPLICATIONS OF THYROTOXICOSIS

THYROCARDIAC DISEASE Thyrotoxicosis imposes a variety of burdens upon the heart. Hypermetabolism of the peripheral tissues increases both the metabolic and nonmetabolic (heat-loss) circulatory load, while direct effects of thyroid hormone on the myocardium increase the force, velocity, and rate of ventricular contraction. As a result, cardiac work and cardiac output are increased. Moreover, atrial irritability is enhanced, leading to tachydysrrhythmias, most importantly atrial fibrillation. In the patient with a normal heart, these burdens are usually, but not invariably, tolerated. In the patient with underlying heart disease, however, cardiac insufficiency may be precipitated or aggravated. As would be expected, this complication is more common in the elderly patient and is therefore usually seen in the patient with toxic multinodular goiter, not infrequently as the preponderant manifestation of thyrotoxicosis.

In patients with cardiac insufficiency, clues to the presence of thyrotoxicosis include atrial fibrillation, relatively rapid circulation time, increased cardiac output (high-output failure), and resistance to the usual therapeutic doses of digitalis.

Treatment is directed at both rapid alleviation of thyrotoxicosis and restoration of cardiac compensation. The former objective is best met by initiation of treatment with large doses of an antithyroid agent, followed by iodine if the clinical situation is urgent. Radioiodine, which is the ultimate therapy of choice, is withheld until a eumetabolic state has been achieved and the RAIU has returned to a satisfactory level as the stable iodine is excreted. In less severe cases, radioiodine treatment is anteceded by antithyroid drug treatment alone. Management of the cardiac decompensation is carried out in the usual manner, employing larger than usual doses of digitalis, but with care to avoid digitalis intoxication as the thyrotoxicosis is alleviated. Adrenergic antagonists should not be employed in the presence of cardiac failure.

THYROTOXIC CRISIS The clinical picture of thyrotoxic crisis or storm is that of a fulminating increase in all the signs and symptoms of thyrotoxicosis. In the past, this disturbance was most often observed postoperatively in patients poorly prepared for surgery. However, with the preoperative use of antithyroid drugs and iodide and with appropriate measures directed to control of metabolic factors, weight, and nutritional status, postoperative thyrotoxic crisis should not occur. At present, so-called "medical storm" is more common and occurs in untreated or inadequately treated patients. It is precipitated by surgical emergency or complicating medical illness, usually sepsis. The syndrome is characterized by extreme irritability, delirium, or coma, fever to 106°F or more, tachycardia, restlessness, hypotension, vomiting, and diarrhea. Rarely, the clinical picture may be more subtle, with apathy, severe prostration and coma, but with only slight elevation of temperature. Such postoperative complications as sepsis, septicemia, hemorrhage, and transfusion or drug reactions may mimic thyrotoxic crisis. It is thought that in some patients thyrotoxic crisis is associated with or precipitated by adrenocortical insufficiency. The possibility of this complication gains support from evidence indicating increased adrenocortical hormone requirements in thyrotoxicosis and from evidence of reduced adrenocortical reserve in this disorder.

Treatment of this most serious disorder consists in providing general supportive therapy while undertaking measures for the most rapid alleviation of thyrotoxicosis possible. Supportive therapy includes treatment of dehydration and provision of calories through the intravenous administration of glucose and saline, vitamin B complex, and glucocorticoids. Patients should be placed in a cooled, humidified oxygen tent, and, if hyperpyrexia is present, a cooling blanket should be used. Digitalization is required only in the presence of cardiac failure. If shock exists, intravenous pressor agents should be employed. Therapy of the hyperthyroidism consists of induction of blockade of hormone synthesis by the immediate and continued administration of large doses of an antithyroid agent (e.g., 100 mg propylthiouracil every 2 hr). If the patient is unable to swallow the medication, the tablets should be triturated and given by nasogastric tube, as parenteral preparations are unavailable. Following initiation of antithyroid therapy, inhibition of hormonal release is sought through the administration of large doses of iodine intravenously or by mouth. To alleviate some of the peripheral effects of thyrotoxicosis, adrenergic antagonists may be used. Propranolol given intravenously or orally appears to be the agent of choice in the absence of cardiac insufficiency. Antithyroid therapy and iodine must be continued until a normal metabolic state is restored, at which time iodine is progressively withdrawn and plans for a definitive regimen of treatment made.

NEOPLASMS

THYROID ADENOMAS True adenomas, as contrasted with localized adenomatous areas, are encapsulated and usually compress contiguous tissue. Adenomas vary greatly in size and histologic characteristics, and are often classified into three major types: papillary, follicular, and Hürthle cell. The follicular adenomas can be subdivided according to the size of the follicles into colloid or macrofollicular, fetal or microfollicular, and embryonal varieties. There is considerable variation in physiologic differentiation, as judged by their ability to concentrate radioiodine. The more highly differentiated adenomas (follicular) are by far the most common and are also the most likely to mimic the function of normal thyroid tissue. Unlike normal thyroid tissue, however, their function is independent of TSH stimulation (autonomous). They are usually unifocal, presenting as a solitary nodule. Often the patient reports that the nodule has been slowly growing over many years. Initially, their function is insufficient to disturb hormonal equilibrium, although their capacity to accumulate ^{131}I is apparent on scintiscanning ("warm" nodule). With the passage of time, the nodule grows larger, and its function increases until it is sufficient to suppress TSH secretion. Consequently, the remainder of the gland undergoes atrophy and loss of function, and the scintiscan then reveals ^{131}I accumulation only in the region of the nodule (*"hot" nodule*). At this time, the patient may or may not appear overtly thyrotoxic, but frank thyrotoxicosis will usually supervene in time (*toxic adenoma*). Relative to its overall rate of occurrence, hyperfunctioning adenoma is a frequent cause of T_3-toxicosis. Not infrequently, hyperfunctioning adenomas undergo hemorrhagic necrosis, resulting in loss of function and the appearance of a *"cold" nodule* on scintiscanning, since the remainder of the thyroid will have resumed function. Only very rarely are hyperfunctioning adenomas carcinomatous. Hyperfunctioning adenomas are readily amenable to ablation by surgery or ^{131}I; large doses of the latter are usually required (20 to 30 mCi). Prior to such treatment, it is desirable to administer exogenous TSH and repeat the scintiscan in order to demonstrate the capacity for function in the remaining tissue.

THYROID CARCINOMAS Thyroid carcinoma may be classified into two varieties, depending upon whether the lesion arises in thyroid follicular epithelium or whether it arises from the parafollicular or "C" cells. Since the latter disorder has distinctive physiologic and clinical characteristics, it will be discussed separately, below.

Carcinomas of follicular epithelium These are of three general histologic types which differ in their clinical course. The least common is *anaplastic carcinoma*, which is histologically undifferentiated, usually afflicts the elderly, and is highly malignant. Usually the lesion is rapidly fatal, owing to extensive local invasion which is refractory to radiation. The second type of tumor, *follicular carcinoma*, is also uncommon and histologically mimics closely normal thyroid tissue. This lesion usually undergoes early hematogenous spread, and hence the patient may present with a distant metastasis, usually in lung or bone. Follicular carcinoma or follicular elements in papillary carcinoma are responsible for those instances in which thyroid carcinoma, *in situ* or in metastases, accumulates significant quantities of ^{131}I. The third and most common type of tumor, *papillary carcinoma*, has a bimodal frequency, peaks occurring in the second or third decades and again in later life. This lesion is usually slowly growing and typically spreads to the regional lymph nodes, where it may remain indolent for many years. Although more common in the older patient, acceleration of the disease may take place at any time. Follicular elements are usually present in both the primary lesion and its metastases, accounting for those instances in which papillary tumors accumulate ^{131}I.

DIAGNOSIS AND MANAGEMENT The diagnosis and management of thyroid carcinoma is closely interwoven with the management of the nodular goiter. In the past, this subject has been one which evoked a wide disparity of views among authorities, stemming largely from seemingly contradictory data. On the one hand, surgically excised specimens of thyroid nodules, particularly solitary nodules, revealed a very high frequency of carcinoma (as much as 20 percent in some series). On the other hand, despite the frequency of nodular goiter in the general population (approximately 4 percent), the frequency of thyroid carcinoma, either newly diagnosed or as a cause of death, is very low. These respective data led to either very vigorous or very conservative approaches with respect to the management of nodular goiter. It now appears that this discordance can be explained, however, by the ability of the physician to select for surgery those patients who are at high risk of harboring thyroid carcinoma, with consequent weighting of statistics derived from surgical series.

The features which lead to a presumptive diagnosis of thyroid carcinoma are rather well defined. They include recent growth, especially if rapid and unaccompanied by tenderness, firm or hard consistency, and diminished or absent function or scintiscan. The presence of finely stippled calcification on x-ray examination suggests the presence of psammoma bodies within a papillary carcinoma. Hoarseness, fixation to adjacent structures, and regional lymphadenopathy are late features. Of particular importance is a history of x-ray irradiation to the head or neck in childhood, since this has been shown to be associated with a high incidence of thyroid carcinoma in later life. A nodule that is present in an otherwise normal gland (solitary nodule) is far more suspicious of thyroid tumor, while one nodule among many is much more likely to be part of a diffuse process, such as simple goiter.

The foregoing features permit the development of general guidelines for the management of nodular goiter. A solitary nodule, especially if nonfunctioning, should be promptly excised, particularly if it occurs in a young woman or in a man of any age, except the most elderly. This is true because multinodular goiter is a disease of older age and predominantly of women. Obviously, the presence of other features described above increase the likelihood of thyroid carcinoma. A prominent but functioning nodule within a multinodular goiter is of little concern. A nonfunctioning nodule within a multinodular goiter should be observed during suppressive therapy. Failure to regress, or particularly an increase in size, over a 3- to 6-month period strongly suggests that surgery is desirable. Needle biopsy is to be avoided when carcinoma is suspected.

At surgery, the nodule should be widely excised and subjected to frozen section examination. A diagnosis of carcinoma is an indication for near-total thyroidectomy in view of the evidence of frequent seeding of carcinoma throughout the gland as a result of transglandular lymphatic spread. Regional lymph nodes should be explored and removed if there is evidence of involvement. Radical neck dissection is no longer felt justified. If permanent sections reveal carcinoma when frozen sections had failed to do so, secondary surgery should be undertaken to remove residual thyroid tissue. Several weeks after surgery, a large scanning dose of ^{131}I is administered (approximately 2 mCi), and a whole-body scan and measurement of urinary ^{131}I excretion obtained. This serves to ablate any residual thyroid tissue and to demonstrate any functioning metastases. If functioning metastases are seen, a therapeutic dose of ^{131}I (approximately 50 mCi) is administered. Thereafter, the patient is given levothyroxine in fully suppressive dosage. At approximately yearly intervals, levothyroxine is replaced by liothyronine for approximately 3 weeks; this is then withdrawn to permit rapid resumption of TSH secretion and stimulation of any functioning residual tissue. If such is found, a further therapeutic dose of ^{131}I is administered. Discrete palpable lymph nodes which have emerged during suppressive therapy can often best be treated by surgical excision. The foregoing procedures are repeated during ensuing years until the disease appears to have been eradicated. Although suppressive therapy is physiologically sound and sometimes spectacularly successful, its general efficacy in the management of thyroid carcinoma is uncertain. Nevertheless, patients who have had carcinoma of the thyroid should be kept on suppressive therapy for the remainder of their lives, except for the brief interruptions described above.

MEDULLARY CARCINOMA This type, which accounts for 5 to 10 percent of cases of thyroid carcinoma, differs from the foregoing types in that it arises from the parafollicular cells and as a result is associated with high concentrations of calcitonin in the blood. Although the disease may occur sporadically, it is frequently familial and appears to be inherited as an autosomal dominant characteristic. Measurement of calcitonin is an excellent screening test for persons at high risk, since an increased serum calcitonin concentration antecedes the clinical expression of the disease. Despite the increased secretion of calcitonin, patients with this disease are almost invariably normocalcemic and display no bone changes, owing in all likelihood to a compensatory increase in parathyroid hormone secretion. In addition to calcitonin, these tumors may also secrete ACTH, serotonin, histaminase, and prostaglandins. Finally, these tumors may be associated with pheochromocytoma, which, when

present, is usually bilateral, hyperparathyroidism, multiple neuromas, and a marfanoid body habitus (see Chap. 351).

Apart from its functional potential and association with other disorders, this carcinoma has a distinctive histopathologic feature in that interspersed between the tumor cells is a stroma which has the properties of amyloid. This tumor metastasizes by both hematogenous and lymphatic spread and carries a prognosis that is worse than that for papillary or follicular carcinoma. Owing to the diffuse distribution of parafollicular cells, total thyroidectomy is indicated. This procedure should also be carried out in the absence of clinically overt disease when the serum calcitonin concentration is increased in family members of a patient with known medullary carcinoma.

THYROIDITIS

Thyroiditis is a generic term embracing several disorders of differing etiology. These are four general types, of which two are exceedingly uncommon, *pyogenic thyroiditis* and *chronic fibrosing (Riedel's) thyroiditis*. Pyogenic thyroiditis is usually anteceded by a pyogenic infection elsewhere and is characterized by tenderness and swelling of the thyroid, redness and warmth of the overlying skin, and constitutional signs of infection. Treatment consists of antibiotic therapy, along with incisional drainage if a fluctuant area within the thyroid should occur. Riedel's thyroiditis is a rare disorder in which intense fibrosis of the thyroid and surrounding structures, leading to induration of the tissues of the neck, may be associated with mediastinal and retroperitoneal fibrosis. The principal importance of this disorder is that it requires differentiation from thyroid neoplasia.

SUBACUTE THYROIDITIS This disorder, which is also termed *granulomatous, giant-cell,* or *de Quervain's thyroiditis,* is a distinct disorder of the thyroid that appears to be viral in origin.

Symptoms of thyroiditis usually follow those of an upper respiratory infection and most commonly comprise pronounced asthenia, malaise, and symptoms referable to stretching of the thyroid capsule, principally pain over the thyroid or pain referred to the lower jaw, ear, or occiput. Referred, rather than local, pain may predominate. These symptoms may smolder for many weeks before the correct diagnosis is suspected. Less commonly, the onset is acute, with severe pain over the thyroid, accompanied by fever and occasionally symptoms of thyrotoxicosis. Cardinal physical findings include exquisite tenderness and nodularity over the thyroid, which may be predominantly unilateral, but which usually migrates to other areas of the gland. Laboratory tests usually reveal an inordinately increased erythrocyte sedimentation rate and markedly depressed RAIU. Early in the disease, the PBI is usually increased, mainly as a result of iodoprotein release, although the $T_4(D)$ may be increased as well in some patients.

If left untreated, the disorder may smolder for

months, but eventually will subside with a return of normal thyroid function. In mild cases, aspirin suffices to control the symptoms. In more severe cases, glucocorticoid (prednisone, 20 to 40 mg daily) is generally effective. Return of the RAIU to normal indicates the time at which therapy can be withdrawn without recurrence of symptoms.

HASHIMOTO'S DISEASE This disorder, which is also termed *lymphadenoid goiter*, is a chronic inflammatory disease of the thyroid in which autoimmune factors are thought to play a prominent role. It is a common disorder, occurring most frequently in women of middle age. In all likelihood, it is, in addition, the most common cause of sporadic goiter in children. Evidence of the participation of autoimmune factors includes the lymphocytic infiltration of the gland, as well as the presence in the serum of increased concentrations of immunoglobulins and of antibodies directed against several components of thyroid tissue. Of these, the most important from the clinical standpoint are the antithyroglobulin antibody detected by the tanned red cell agglutination technique and the antimicrosomal antibody detected by immunofluorescence or complement fixation techniques. This disorder also coexists with inordinate frequency with other diseases of a presumed autoimmune nature, including pernicious anemia, Sjögren's syndrome, progressive hepatitis, systemic lupus erythematosus, rheumatoid arthritis, nontuberculous Addison's disease, and Graves' disease itself. These disorders, as well as Hashimoto's disease itself, also appear with unusual frequency in family members of patients with Hashimoto's disease.

Goiter is the outstanding feature of the disease. The enlargement involves the entire gland, but not necessarily symmetrically. Typically, the consistency is rubbery, the margins are scalloped, and the general outline of the gland is preserved. The pyramidal lobe may be prominent. Early in the disease the patient is metabolically normal; however, even then decreased thyroid reserve is often manifest in an increase in serum TSH. With the passage of time, hypothyroidism of increasing severity supervenes, owing to progressive replacement of thyroid parenchyma by lymphocytes or fibrous tissue. Early in the disease, the RAIU and PBI may be increased, reflecting the secretion of iodoproteins, but the T_4(D) is normal. With time, the RAIU, PBI, and T_4(D) decline as clinical hypothyroidism supervenes. Increased T_3(RIA) may herald the development of this sequence. High titers of antithyroglobulin antibody are usually, but not invariably, present. High titers may also occur in other thyroid disorders, particularly primary thyroprivic hypothyroidism and Graves' disease, but with lesser frequency. Patients lacking antithyroglobulin antibody almost always display antimicrosomal antibody. Although the foregoing findings usually suffice to permit a diagnosis, histologic confirmation by needle biopsy is occasionally required. In view of the frequency with which hypothyroidism is either present or eventually develops, treatment with replacement doses of levothyroxine is indicated. In some patients, such therapy is associated with regression of goiter.

REFERENCES

CHOPRA IJ et al: Thyroid gland in Graves' disease: Victim or culprit. Metabolism 19:760, 1970

HERSHMAN JM: The treatment of hyperthyroidism. Ann Intern Med 64:1306, 1966

——, PITTMAN JA: Control of thyrotropin secretion in man. N Engl J Med 285:997, 1971

INGBAR SH, WOEBER KA: The thyroid gland, in *Textbook of Endocrinology,* 4th ed., ed RH Williams, Philadelphia: Saunders, 1968

LEVEY GS: Catecholamine sensitivity, thyroid hormone and the heart: A re-evaluation. Am J Med 50:413, 1971

STANBURY JB: Familial goiter, in *The Metabolic Basis of Inherited Disease,* 3d ed., eds JB Stanbury et al, New York: McGraw-Hill, 1972

Symposium on Graves' Disease. Mayo Clinic Proc. vol. 47, Nov. and Dec., 1972

UTIGER RD: Thyrotrophin radioimmunoassay: Another test of thyroid function. Ann Intern Med 74:627, 1971

WERNER SC, INGBAR SH (eds): *The Thyroid: A Fundamental and Clinical Test,* 3d ed., New York: Harper & Row, 1971

86 DISEASES OF THE ADRENAL CORTEX

GORDON H. WILLIAMS
ROBERT G. DLUHY
GEORGE W. THORN

INTRODUCTION Thomas Addison's description in 1849 of a clinical syndrome resulting from destruction of the adrenal glands first attracted attention to these organs. Seven years later Brown-Séquard demonstrated that removal of both adrenals from experimental animals caused death soon after operation, whereas control animals subjected to a sham operation survived. Subsequent investigations established that the life-maintaining hormone was elaborated by cells in the cortex, since destruction of all medullary tissue was not accompanied by the classic signs and symptoms of adrenal insufficiency noted after complete removal of the glands.

Between 1927 and 1930, Hartman and his associates, Rogoff and Stewart, and Pfiffner and Swingle all independently described methods for preparing potent adrenocortical extracts. During the following decade, crystalline steroid substances were isolated from these extracts by Kendall, by Grollman, and by Reichstein. In 1937, Steiger and Reichstein synthesized the first natural corticosteroid, 11-deoxycorticosterone, a year before it was identified in adrenal extracts. From 1940 to 1950, the synthesis of several 11-oxygenated compounds was achieved, including cortisone and hydrocortisone. The contributions of Sarett and his collaborators, Reichstein et al., and Kendall and his coworkers were outstanding in this regard. In 1954 aldosterone, the principal salt-retaining hormone of the adrenal, was identified by Simpson and Tait in collaboration with the Swiss group under Reichstein.

Since 1954, a number of remarkable advances have occurred. ACTH has been isolated, its amino acid sequence determined, and the complete molecule synthesized. A number of substances which interfere with the action of adrenal steroids have also been synthesized. For example, amphenone and 2-methyl-1,2-bis-(3-pyridyl)-1-propanone (metyrapone) interfere with the synthesis of hydrocortisone. Spironolactone and 2,4,7-tri-amino-6-phenylpteridine (triamterene) block the physiologic effects of aldosterone. Among the most significant advancements have been the refinements in the ease and accuracy with which steroids and their metabolic products may be measured, e.g., by double isotope derivative, competitive protein-binding radioassay, and radioimmunoassay techniques.

BIOCHEMISTRY AND PHYSIOLOGY

STEROID NOMENCLATURE The adrenal steroids contain as their basic structure a cyclopentanoperhydrophenanthrane nucleus consisting of three 6-carbon hexane rings and a single 5-carbon pentane ring (D). The carbon atoms are numbered in a predetermined sequence beginning with ring A (Fig. 86-1). The Greek letter Δ indicates a double bond, as does the suffix -ene. The position of a substituent below or above the plane of the steroid molecule is indicated by the letters α and β respectively. The α-substituent is drawn with a broken line (- -OH), and the β-substituent is drawn with a solid line (—OH). The C_{19} steroids are those which have substituent methyl groups at positions C-18 and C-19. C_{19} steroids that also have a ketone group at C-17 are termed *17-ketosteroids.* These C_{19} steroids have predominant androgenic activity. The C_{21} steroids are those which have a 2-carbon side chain (C-20 and C-21) attached at position 17 of the D ring and, in addition, have substituent methyl groups at C-18 and C-19. C_{21} steroids that also possess a hydroxyl group at position 17 are termed *17-hydroxycorticosteroids* or *17-hydroxycorticoids.* The C_{21} steroids may have either predominant glucocorticoid or mineralocorticoid properties. *Glucocorticoid* signifies a C_{21} steroid with predominant action on intermediary metabolism, and *mineralocorticoid* indicates a C_{21} steroid with predominant action on the metabolism of the body minerals, sodium and potassium.

FIGURE 86-1
Basic steroid structure and nomenclature.

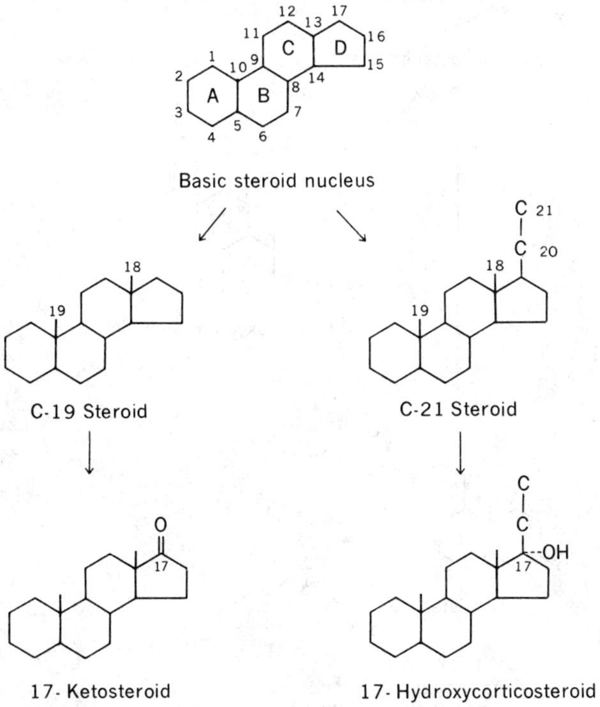

BIOSYNTHESIS OF ADRENAL STEROIDS Cholesterol, derived from the diet and from endogenous synthesis via acetate, is the principal starting compound in steroidogenesis. The three major adrenal biosynthetic pathways lead to the production of glucocorticoids (cortisol), mineralocorticoids (aldosterone), and adrenal androgens (dehydroepiandrosterone) (Fig. 86-2). Separate zones of the adrenal cortex have differing capacity to synthesize specific hormones. The two major divisions are the outer (glomerulosa) zone, mainly involved in aldosterone biosynthesis, and the inner (fasciculata-reticularis) zone, mainly involved in cortisol and androgen biosynthesis.

Glucocorticoid pathway Δ5-Pregnenolone is formed after cleavage of the side chain of cholesterol. Δ5-Pregnenolone is converted to progesterone by the action of the enzymes 3β-hydroxydehydrogenase and Δ5,Δ4-isomerase. These enzymes transform the 3β-hydroxy group of Δ5-pregnenolone to a C-3-ketonic group and transform the double bond between C-5:C-6 of Δ5-pregnenolone to position C-4:C-5 of progesterone. A series of hydroxylations mediated by specific hydroxylating enzymes then occurs in sequential fashion at C-17, then at C-21, and finally at C-11. With the introduction of a hydroxyl group at position C-17 of progesterone by the enzyme C-17 hydroxylase, 17α-hydroxyprogesterone is formed, which in turn has a hydroxyl group introduced at C-21 by the enzyme C-21 hydroxylase, producing 11-deoxycortisol (Compound S), the major precursor of cortisol. Finally, a third hydroxyl group is introduced at the C-11 position of 11-deoxycortisol by the enzyme C-11 hydroxylase, to produce cortisol (Compound F, hydrocortisone), the major glucocorticoid. The chemical name for cortisol is 11β,17α,21-trihydroxy-4-pregnene-3,20-dione.

Mineralocorticoid pathway Progesterone, after transformation from Δ5-pregnenolone, is hydroxylated at the C-21 position to form 11-deoxycorticosterone. This C-21 hydroxylase, rather than being identical to the enzyme used to form 11-deoxycortisol, may be an isoenzyme of it; 11-deoxycorticosterone is then hydroxylated at the 11 position to form corticosterone, compound B. A hydroxyl group is then introduced at the 18 position to form

FIGURE 86-2
Biosynthetic pathways for adrenal steroid production. Major pathways to mineralocorticoids, glucocorticoids, and androgens. Circled letters and numbers denote specific enzymes: DE = *debranching enzyme; 3β-3β-ol-dehydrogenase with Δ4-Δ5 isomerase; 11 = C-11 hydroxylase; 17 = C-17 hydroxylase; 21 = C-21 hydroxylase.*

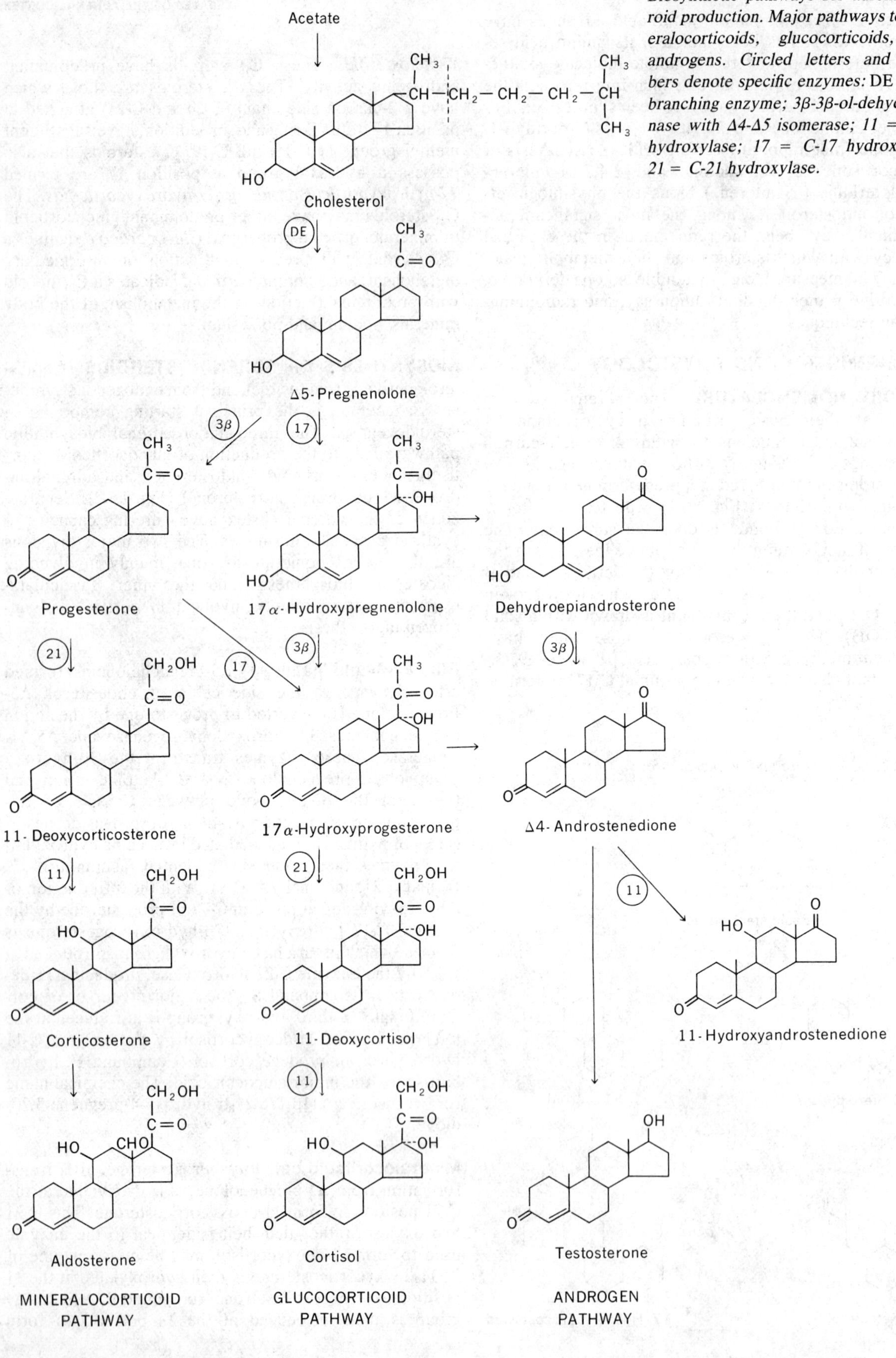

18-hydroxycorticosterone, the immediate precursor of aldosterone. With conversion of the hydroxyl group at C-18 to an aldehyde group, the major mineralocorticoid, *aldosterone*, is formed. The 18-aldehyde group exists free or in the hemiacetal form. The chemical designation for aldosterone is 11β,21-dihydroxy-18-aldo-4-pregnene-3, 20-dione.

Androgen pathway By the enzymatic action of 17α-hydroxylase, Δ5-pregnenolone is converted to 17α-hydroxypregnenolone, which on cleavage of its C-20:C-21 side chain forms the 17-ketosteroid dehydroepiandrosterone. The Δ5,-3 hydroxyl grouping of this compound is transformed to a Δ4,-3 oxo- grouping by the enzymes 3β-hydroxydehydrogenase and Δ5,Δ4 isomerase to produce the 17-ketosteroid androstenedione. Androstenedione can undergo direct transformation to testosterone as a result of hydrogenation at position C-17, and androstenedione also is converted to 11β-hydroxyandrostenedione by hydroxylation at position C-11. Note that the adrenal androgens require a preliminary hydroxylation at C-17 prior to their formation and, also, that 17-ketosteroids with an oxygen group at position C-11 are of adrenal origin.

It is unlikely that the normal adrenal gland can convert testosterone or androstenedione to estradiol and estrone, as had been previously thought. These conversions probably take place from adrenal precursors in the liver.

STEROID TRANSPORT In the analysis of the metabolic actions of steroids, an important feature is the mechanism of transport from origin to site of action. Many hormones, including some of the steroid hormones, e.g., testosterone and cortisol, appear to circulate to a considerable extent bound to plasma proteins. Aldosterone, however, seems to have a relatively poor binding affinity for any serum protein. Cortisol, after release into the systemic circulation, occurs in the plasma in three forms: free cortisol, protein-bound cortisol, and cortisol metabolites. *Free cortisol* refers to that quantity which is physiologically active but not protein bound and, therefore, represents a form of cortisol acting directly on tissue sites. Normally, less than 5 percent of circulating cortisol is free. *Protein-bound cortisol* is that portion of cortisol which is reversibly bound to circulating plasma proteins. There are two distinct cortisol-binding systems of plasma. One is a high-affinity, low-capacity globulin termed transcortin or cortisol-binding-globulin (CBG), and the other is a low-affinity, high-capacity protein, albumin. Cortisol-binding globulin in normal man can bind approximately 20 to 25 μg cortisol per 100 ml plasma. As the amounts of cortisol released by the adrenal gland exceed this level, the excess becomes bound in part to albumin. The CBG level may be increased by administration of natural or synthetic estrogens. This endogenous rise in CBG is accompanied by a parallel rise in protein-bound cortisol, with the result that the level of plasma 17-hydroxycorticosteroids is elevated. However, there is controversy as to whether or not the free-cortisol levels remain normal even though signs and symptoms of glucocorticoid excess are usually absent. This effect of estrogen on steroid binding is most evident in the third trimester of pregnancy or when estrogen-containing oral contraceptive medication is taken.

Cortisol metabolites such as tetrahydrocortisol also circulate in the plasma. These metabolites are biologically inactive and bind only weakly to circulating plasma proteins.

It is evident that the protein binding of steroids exerts a major influence on the equilibrium concentration of cortisol across membrane barriers. For example, by this mechanism, urine loss of steroids is minimized, since only the unbound cortisol and its metabolites are filtrable at the glomerulus. Furthermore, cortisol binding to proteins serves as a reserve buffer mechanism capable of binding excess cortisol when the plasma-free cortisol is high, and conversely, capable of releasing bound cortisol when the free-cortisol level is low.

Considerable evidence has accumulated for a testosterone-binding globulin with as strong an affinity for testosterone as cortisol-binding globulin has for cortisol. These two proteins are distinct, with the testosterone-binding protein being a β-globulin while the cortisol-binding protein is an α-globulin. The testosterone-binding globulin binds estradiol with equal affinity.

Aldosterone appears to be bound to proteins to a much smaller extent than either testosterone or cortisol. It has been shown that an ultrafiltrate of plasma probably contains as much as 50 percent of the circulating aldosterone. Aldosterone, like other steroids, is bound to albumin. There is also some evidence that a separate protein, other than albumin- or cortisol-binding globulin, may participate in partially binding aldosterone. The limited binding of aldosterone by plasma protein may be significant in the metabolism of this hormone.

STEROID METABOLISM AND EXCRETION Glucocorticoids The principal glucocorticoids secreted by the normal adrenal gland are cortisol and corticosterone. The daily adrenal secretion of cortisol ranges between 15 and 30 mg, with a pronounced diurnal cycle, and that of corticosterone between 2 and 4 mg. Cortisol is distributed in a volume of body fluids approximating the total extracellular fluid space. The total plasma concentration of cortisol in the morning hours is approximately 15 μg per 100 ml, with more than 90 percent of this cortisol appearing in the protein-bound fraction. The plasma concentration of cortisol is determined by the rate of secretion, the rate of inactivation, and the rate of excretion of free cortisol. The plasma half-life of cortisol is between 60 and 120 min. Cortisol is inactivated by means of six major biotransformations: (1) 11-dehydrogenation; (2) reduction of ring A; (3) reduction at C-20; (4) cleavage of the C-20:C-21 side chain; (5) 6β-hydroxylation; and (6) conjugation. The 11-dehydrogenase system converts cortisol to the inactive cortisone. This reversible system is one of the major factors in regulating the level of circulating cortisol under normal circumstances. The enzyme is strongly influenced by the level of circulating thyroid hormone, with hyperthyroidism markedly accelerating the oxidative reaction. The second mechanism is the reduction of ring A. The initial saturation of the C-4:C-5 double bond in ring A by the introduction of two hydrogen ions produces *dihydrocortisol* (Fig. 86-3). Next the

C-3 ketonic group of dihydrocortisol is reduced by further addition of two hydrogen atoms to form *tetrahydrocortisol* (THF). Furthermore, cortisone may go through a similar reduction process to produce tetrahydrocortisone (THE). The third mechanism of inactivation, C-20 hydroxylation, is brought into play by the addition of two hydrogen atoms at C-20. Further reduction elsewhere in the molecule is possible, and the products are the cortols and the cortolones. From 5 to 10 percent of the secreted cortisol is metabolized in the liver by cleavage of the C-20:C-21 side chain to form the corresponding 11-oxy-

FIGURE 86-3

Metabolism of cortisol to tetrahydrocortisol, tetrahydrocortisone, cortol, and cortolone. Conjugation occurs with glucuronic acid at C-3 position. Note interconversion of cortisol and cortisone.

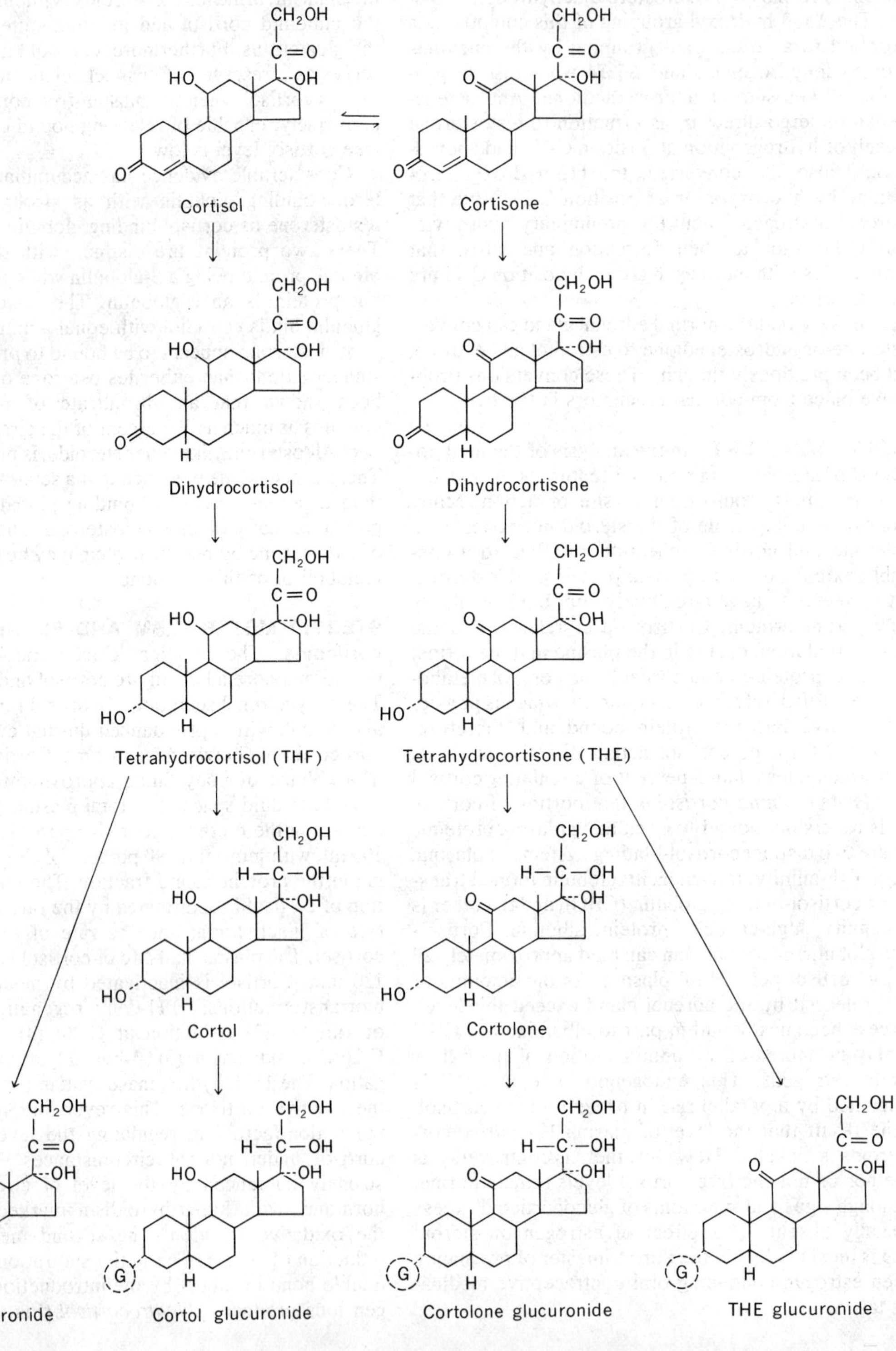

ketosteroid. Finally, in normal man, 6β-hydroxylation of cortisol represents a relatively minor metabolic transformation. However, under certain circumstances, in infancy and toxemia of pregnancy and with certain drugs, the formation of this product becomes important. The first four transformations produce compounds which are not water-soluble. These compounds are conjugated in the liver with glucuronic acid at position C-3 to produce water-soluble products. Sulfation appears to be a relatively minor process, except perhaps in infancy. The 6β-hydroxycortisol is sufficiently water-soluble that it can clear the kidney without conjugation.

Mineralocorticoids In normal subjects on a normal salt intake, the average daily secretion of aldosterone ranges between 50 and 250 μg, and the plasma concentration ranges between 5 and 15 mμg per 100 ml. Since aldosterone is only weakly bound to proteins, its volume of distribution is larger than that of cortisol and approximates 35 liters. Under normal circumstances, greater than 75 percent of circulating aldosterone is inactivated during a single passage through the liver. However, under certain conditions, such as congestive failure, this percentage is markedly reduced.

Under steady-state conditions, aldosterone exists as the 11-18-hemiacetal form rather than the 18-aldehyde form. Most transformations of this compound are reductive in nature. There has been no substantial evidence of oxidative reactions involving aldosterone, in contrast to cortisol metabolism. Of the numerous reductive metabolites that may be formed, 50 percent of aldosterone is transformed into the tetrahydro derivative produced by ring A reduction. This reaction appears to occur only in the liver, and because this metabolite is water-insoluble, it is conjugated with glucuronic acid before it is excreted in the urine. From 7 to 15 percent of aldosterone appears in the urine as a glucuronide conjugate, from which free aldosterone is released on standing at pH 1. This *acid-labile conjugate* appears to be formed both in the liver and in the kidney. The relative proportions appear to be related to relative blood flow to the two organs and the state of the general circulation. The acid-labile conjugate is also referred to as the *3-oxo conjugate,* because the 3-oxo grouping is not irreversibly reduced, as it is in tetrahydroaldosterone. Ninety percent of the acid-labile conjugate is excreted within 6 hr, whereas comparable tetrahydroaldosterone excretion requires 24 to 36 hr. For average salt intake, the 24-hr urine excretion of the acid-labile conjugate ranges from 2 to 20 μg, that of the tetrahydro derivative from 25 to 35 μg, and that of the nonconjugated, nonreduced free aldosterone from 0.2 to 0.6 μg.

Adrenal androgens The major androgenic compound secreted by the adrenal gland is dehydroepiandrosterone (DHEA) and its C-3 sulfuric acid ester. From 15 to 30 mg of these compounds is secreted daily. Much smaller amounts of Δ4-androstenedione and 11β-hydroxyandrostenedione and testosterone are secreted. The major fraction of dehydroepiandrosterone is found in the urine as the sulfate. However, only a small portion of the secreted compound reaches this stage without other metabolic alterations. The first step, which is irreversible, is the conversion to Δ4-androstenedione (Fig. 86-4). This compound is then interconvertible with testosterone and shares with testosterone a common group of metabolites, consisting of androsterone, epiandrosterone, and etiocholanolone. The second major route of transformation is the formation of the 16α-hydroxyl derivative of either dehydroepiandrosterone or its sulfate. In pregnancy, this compound performs a vital role as a precursor in the placental production of estriol.

Two-thirds of the urine 17-ketosteroids in the male are derived from adrenal metabolites, and the remaining one-third comes from testicular androgens. In the female, almost all urine 17-ketosteroids are derived from the adrenal gland. It is improbable that estrogens are synthesized by the normal adrenal gland. There has been no substantial proof of aromatic enzymes being present in adrenal tissue. The increased secretion of estrogens in ovariectomized patients and in feminizing adrenal tumors

FIGURE 86-4
Adrenal androgens. Δ-4 Androstenedione and testosterone contribute to the same metabolites.

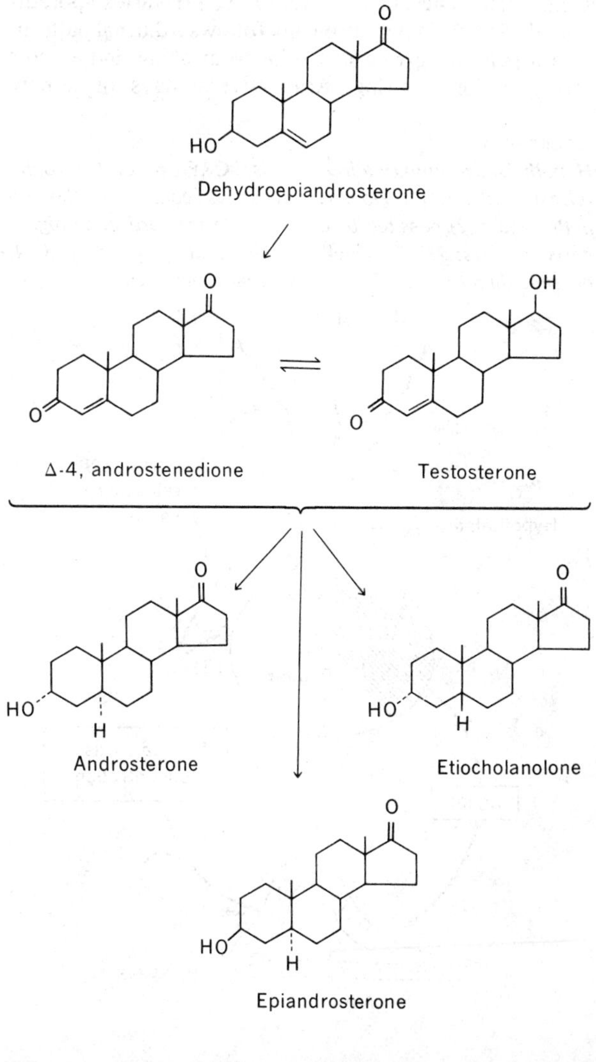

are probably secondary to the action of liver enzymes on androgenic precursors secreted by the adrenal gland.

ACTH PHYSIOLOGY The adrenocorticotropin hormone (ACTH) (see Chap. 83) is an unbranched long-chain polypeptide containing 39 amino acids. It is stored in and released from the anterior pituitary gland, where histologically it appears to be localized to basophil cells. Only 50 units, or roughly 0.25 mg, of the active peptide are stored in the anterior pituitary. Much of the potential for producing the corticotropic actions of ACTH is present in smaller polypeptide fragments. It appears that the significant structure necessary for high adrenocorticotropin activity is the unusual sequence of basic amino acids lys-lys-arg-arg occurring in the 15 to 18 position. The biologic half-life of ACTH is less than 10 min. The release of ACTH from the anterior pituitary gland is governed by a "corticotropin-releasing center" in the median eminence of the hypothalamus, which upon stimulation releases a chemical mediator (corticotropin-releasing factor, CRF) that travels via the pituitary-stalk portal bloodstream to the anterior pituitary gland, where it effects the release of stored ACTH (Fig. 86-5).

Three major factors control CRF and ACTH release: plasma free-cortisol concentration, stress, and the sleep-wake cycle. The plasma level of ACTH varies sporadically during the day but roughly follows a diurnal pattern, with a peak occurring just prior to awaking and a nadir shortly before retiring. After several days on a new sleep-wake cycle, the pattern will be altered to conform to the new cycle. However, an occasional deviation from the normal cycle does not produce an alteration. Stress can also affect ACTH release. When an individual is exposed to certain types of stress, e.g., pyrogens, surgery, severe emotional trauma, ACTH levels rise. Finally, the principal regulator of CRF and ACTH release is the plasma free-cortisol level, which by a negative feedback mechanism causes increased release of CRF when plasma cortisol level is low and a decreased release of CRF when plasma cortisol concentration is elevated. This servomechanism establishes the primacy of blood cortisol concentration and serves to buffer deviations in blood cortisol levels from a supposed optimal level. It also appears that cortisol feeds back directly on the pituitary gland and higher brain centers, and perhaps even on the adrenal cortex as well.

FIGURE 86-5
Hypothalamic-pituitary-adrenal axis. CRF = *corticotropin-releasing factor. (1) Dominant feedback control on the hypothalamus; (2) possible feedback of plasma cortisol on higher nerve centers; (3) feedback on the pituitary gland; and (4) possible direct feedback on the adrenal gland itself.*

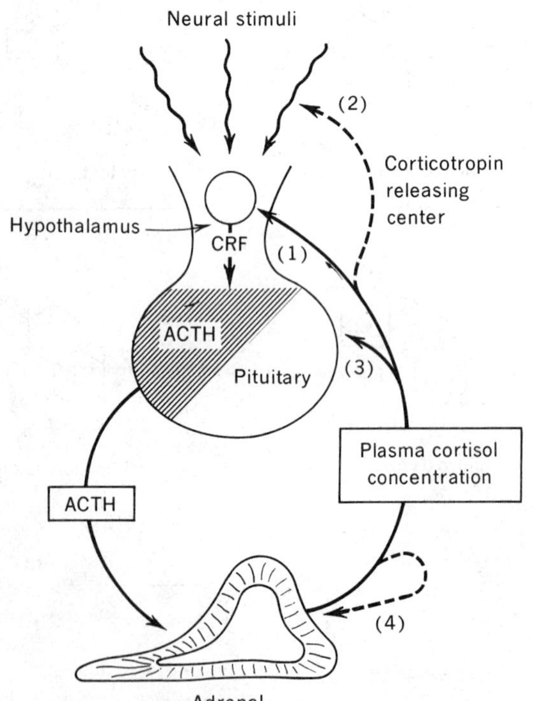

Besides its major action in stimulation of the biogenesis and release of steroid hormones by the adrenal gland, ACTH can stimulate melanocytes of amphibians and can increase adipokinetic activity in a number of species. Both these extraadrenal actions have been verified with synthetic ACTH molecules.

The action of ACTH on the adrenal gland itself is rapid; within minutes of its release, there is an increased concentration of steroids in the adrenal venous blood. It produces a number of biochemical changes: (1) an increase in adrenal weight; (2) a decrease in the amount of adrenal lipids, cholesterol, and ascorbic acid; (3) increase in adenyl cyclase activity and in adenosine-3′,5′-monophosphate (cyclic AMP concentration); (4) an increase in protein synthesis and oxidative phosphorylation; (5) an accelerated rate of glycogenolysis; and (6) increase in adrenal blood flow. The most likely mechanism by which ACTH stimulates steroidogenesis is via activation of the membrane-bound adenyl cyclase. This would increase the level of adenosine-3′,5′-monophosphate (cyclic AMP), which by a cascade effect would increase the synthesis of reduced coenzymes (NADPH) needed for steroid biosynthesis. Evidence has been obtained which suggests that activation of protein biosynthesis is an important if not an essential part of the action of ACTH and possibly of other tropic hormones. ACTH apparently increases protein biosynthesis either by stimulation of messenger ribonucleic acid or by enzyme activation.

RENIN-ANGIOTENSIN PHYSIOLOGY (see also Chap. 245) Renin is a proteolytic enzyme with an approximate molecular weight of 35,000 to 40,000. It has been semipurified. It is produced and stored in the granules of the juxtaglomerular cells surrounding the afferent arterioles of the cortical glomeruli. The juxtaglomerular apparatus consists of both the juxtaglomerular cells and the cells of the macula densa. The latter area also contains some renin. Renin acts on the basic substrate angiotensinogen (a circulating alpha$_2$-globulin) made in the liver, to form the decapeptide angiotensin-I. Various inhibitors of intrarenal renin formation are believed to exist (Fig. 86-6). Angiotensin-I is then enzymatically converted by converting enzyme to the octapeptide angiotensin-II by the splitting off of the two C-terminal amino acids. Angiotensin-II is the most potent pressor compound (on a milligram-for-milligram basis) made in

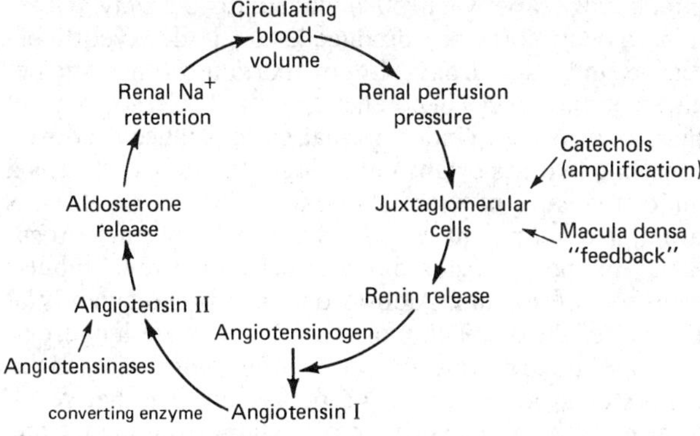

FIGURE 86-6
Renin-angiotensin-aldosterone volume regulation in normal man.

the body, and it exerts this pressor action by a direct effect on arteriolar smooth muscle. In addition, angiotensin-II is a potent direct stimulus to the production of aldosterone by the zona glomerulosa of the adrenal cortex. Various peptidases, collectively termed "angiotensinases," in organ tissue, vessel walls, and circulating plasma are responsible for the ultimate biochemical degradation of circulating angiotensin-II. Angiotensin-II may also play a role in modifying the renal tubular transport of sodium. Such a direct tubular effect, independent of its effect on renal hemodynamics, remains controversial.

Renin release is controlled by four major factors. For the most part, these are interdependent, and the amount of renin released is a composite of the input of all four. The *juxtaglomerular cells,* which are specialized myoepithelial cells cuffing the afferent arterioles, act as miniature pressure transducers, sensing renal perfusion pressure and corresponding changes in afferent arteriolar perfusion pressures. The changes in pressure are perceived as distortions in the existing stretch on the arteriolar walls. For example, under conditions of a reduction in circulating blood volume, there will be a corresponding reduction in renal perfusion pressure and, therefore, in afferent arteriolar pressure (Fig. 86-6). This will be perceived by the juxtaglomerular cells as a decreased stretch exerted on the afferent arteriolar walls. The juxtaglomerular cells will then release increasing quantities of renin within the kidney circulation, leading to the formation of angiotensin-I. Angiotensin-I leaves the kidney both by renal lymphatic and renal venous outflow. It is converted into angiotensin-II and directly stimulates the adrenal cortex to release increasing quantities of aldosterone. Increasing plasma levels of aldosterone lead to increasing renal sodium retention and thus result in expansion of extracellular fluid volume, which, as it is completed, dampens the initiating signal for renin release. Within this context, the renin-angiotensin-aldosterone system is subserving volume control by appropriate modifications of renal tubular sodium transport.

A second control mechanism for renin release centers in the *macula densa* cells. These are a group of special-staining distal convoluted tubular epithelial cells found in direct opposition to the juxtaglomerular cells. It has been suggested that they may function as chemoreceptors, monitoring the sodium load presented to the distal tubule, and that such information, while it is being monitored, is directly fed back to the juxtaglomerular cells, where appropriate modifications in renin release take place. Such an intrarenal renin-release mechanism is said to be capable of operating independently of changes in renal perfusion pressure. Under conditions of increased delivery of filtered sodium to the macula densa, feedback would occur to the juxtaglomerular apparatus, resulting in a release of increasing quantities of renin, which could then be capable of decreasing glomerular filtration rate, thereby reducing the filtered load of sodium. The evidence for this hypothesis is conflicting.

The *sympathetic nervous system* is also a significant factor regulating the release of renin. Infusion of catecholamines directly into the renal artery or electrical stimulation of renal nerves can increase renin release. Conversely, α- or β-adrenergic blockade can block the renin response to upright posture or acute volume depletion. The mechanism by which sympathetic activity alters renin secretion is not known. It may have a direct effect on the juxtaglomerular cell altering renin release or it may act indirectly on either the juxtaglomerular or macula densa cells or via a vasoconstrictive action on the afferent arteriole.

Finally, a number of circulating factors may alter renin release. Increasing dietary *potassium* can decrease renin release; decreasing potassium intake increases renin release. These effects are not secondary to a direct effect of potassium on aldosterone secretion with an alteration in sodium balance, since similar renin responses occur with subjects on a low sodium intake. In addition, direct infusion of potassium into the renal artery also decreases renin release. The significance of this potassium effect is unclear. *Angiotensin* itself can exert a negative feedback control on renin release independent of alterations in renal blood flow, pressure, or aldosterone secretion. There is also some evidence that both ACTH and vasopressin can increase renin release. Thus, the control of renin release is complex, consisting of both *intrarenal* (pressoreceptor and macula densa) and *extrarenal* (sympathetic nervous system, potassium, angiotensin, etc.) mechanisms. A given level of renin secretion probably reflects all these factors, with the intrarenal mechanism predominating.

GLUCOCORTICOID PHYSIOLOGY The division of adrenal steroids into glucocorticoids and mineralocorticoids is somewhat arbitrary in that most glucocorticoids have some mineralocorticoid-like properties, and vice versa. The descriptive term *glucocorticoid* is applied to those adrenal steroids having a predominant action on intermediary metabolism. The principal glucocorticoid is cortisol (hydrocortisone). The actions of the glucocorticoids on intermediary metabolism are predominantly anti-insulin and include the regulation of protein, carbohydrate, lipid, and nucleic acid metabolism. Their actions appear mainly to be catabolic in effect, with an increased protein breakdown and nitrogen excretion. Glucocorticoids increase hepatic glycogen content and promote the hepatic synthesis of glucose (gluconeogenesis). These actions of glucocorticoids are in part explained by the mobilization of glycogenic amino acid precursors from peripheral supporting structures, such as bone, skin, muscle, and connective tissue. In addition, glucocorticoids have a direct action on the liver to stimulate the synthesis of hepatic enzymes, such as tyrosine amino transferase and tryptophan pyrrolase. The elevated levels of these hepatic enzymes can "pull" precursors from the periphery, which in turn can diminish protein metabolism and produce cytolysis of lymphoid tissue and muscle. This inhibition of extrahepatic protein synthesis and stimulation of enzyme synthesis is reflected in the actions of glucocorticoids on nucleic acid metabolism. Corticoids inhibit the synthesis of nucleic acids in most body tissues, but in the liver ribonucleic acid (RNA) synthesis is stimulated. It is postulated that glucocorticoids interact with cytoplasmic and nuclear receptors to initiate the transcription of messenger RNA from chromosomal deoxyribonucleic acid (DNA). This action results in the increased synthesis of new enzyme protein in the liver. Glucocorticoids are necessary for fatty acid mobilization by permitting and enhancing activation of cellular lipase by lipid-mobilizing hormones (e.g., catecholamines and pituitary peptides).

The action of cortisol on structural protein and adipose tissue varies considerably in different parts of the body. For example, depletion of protein matrix of the vertebral column may be striking, whereas long-bone structure may be affected only minimally; peripheral adipose tissue may diminish, whereas abdominal and interscapular fat may accumulate. Glucocorticoids have anti-inflammatory properties, which are probably related to their actions on the microvasculature as well as to cellular effects. Cortisol maintains normal vascular responsiveness to circulating vasoconstrictor factors and opposes the increase in capillary permeability characteristic of acute inflammation. Glucocorticoids also impede endothelial sticking of leukocytes and diapedesis through the capillary wall. Glucocorticoids produce lysis of lymphoid tissue and diminish the number of circulating eosinophils. Glucocorticoids also stabilize lysosomal membranes, thereby suppressing the release of proteolytic acid hydrolases stored in these cytoplasmic organelles. Cortisol has a major effect on body water, in both its distribution and its excretion. It subserves the extracellular fluid volume by a retarding action on the inward migration of water into cells. It affects renal water excretion in a dual manner, by increasing the rate of glomerular filtration and by a direct action on the renal tubule, which actions summate to increase solute-free water clearance. Glucocorticoids, in general, will increase renal tubular sodium reabsorption and cause an increased urine potassium excretion. The integrity of personality is enhanced by cortisol, and emotional disorders are common with either excesses or deficits of cortisol. Lastly, cortisol is the major determinant of pituitary ACTH release by its direct effect on the hypothalamic corticotropin-releasing center.

MINERALOCORTICOID PHYSIOLOGY The major mineralocorticoid produced by the human adrenal cortex is aldosterone. Its production rate on a normal sodium intake varies between 50 and 250 μg per day. Other mineralocorticoids are produced, i.e., 11-deoxycorticosterone and 18-hydroxy-11-deoxycorticosterone, but because of differences in potency they are far less important than aldosterone. Under normal circumstances, aldosterone has two important physiologic functions: (1) it is a major regulator of extracellular fluid volume, and (2) it is a major determinant of potassium metabolism. It regulates volume through a direct effect on the renal tubular transport of sodium. Aldosterone acts predominantly at the site of the distal convoluted tubule, where it causes a decrease in the urine excretion of sodium with an increase in urine excretion of potassium. The net result appears to be a reabsorption of sodium from the filtrate, while potassium is secreted into the urine. The reabsorbed sodium ions are then transported out of the tubular epithelial cells into the interstitial fluid of the kidney and from there into the renal capillary circulation. Water will passively follow the aldosterone-mediated transported sodium. In effect, aldosterone can expand extracellular fluid by a mechanism analogous to an endogenous infusion of normal saline solution.

The above events are those that occur with the acute administration of aldosterone. When normal individuals are given a long-term course of aldosterone (or a comparable mineralocorticoid, such as parenteral deoxycorticosterone acetate), an initial period of sodium retention is followed by a natriuresis, and sodium balance is reestablished after 3 to 5 days. As a result, clinical edema formation does not develop. Thus, with continuous administration of the potent sodium-retaining hormone aldosterone, patients reachieve sodium homeostasis and do not continue to exhibit sodium retention. This phenomenon is referred to as the "escape phenomenon," signifying an "escape" by the renal tubules from the sodium-retaining action of chronically administered aldosterone. The mechanism responsible for the escape phenomenon has remained elusive. It appears to be dependent on normal renal hemodynamics, and it has been suggested that an as-yet-unidentified natriuretic principle may be involved. Such an "escape" phenomenon is exhibited by patients with hypertension but is characteristically absent in patients with edema disorders.

The action of aldosterone on the kidney is commonly referred to as the distal sodium-potassium exchange. A number of recent studies, however, cast doubt on the validity of this simplistic theory. Evidence from a number of sources suggests that potassium is not actively secreted by the tubular epithelium but rather simply follows a change in the transtubular electrical gradient. This relative electrical gradient is established by the active reabsorption of sodium by the epithelial cells of the distal tubule. In the resting state, the distal tubular cell membrane has a potential across it, with the luminal side positive and the intracellular side negative. The reabsorption of the positively charged sodium ion causes a fall in this transmembrane potential, thus producing an environment favorable for the flow of positive ions out of the cell into the lumen. The major singly charged positive ion present intracellularly is potassium. Since its concentration in the cell is forty- to eightyfold greater than in the lumen, it passively follows this relative electrical gradient in order to restore the normal positive charge to the lumen.

Hydrogen ion is also present in abundant concentration in the tubular epithelial cell. However, since its concentration in the lumen is greater than in the cell, it would still have to be actively secreted, but the reduced intraluminal positivity would allow more hydrogen to be secreted with the same amount of energy.

Aldosterone also acts indirectly on the epithelium of the salivary ducts and sweat glands and on the mucosal cells of the gastrointestinal tract to cause reabsorption of sodium in "exchange" for potassium ions. A direct cellular action, as on muscle cells, of aldosterone has been difficult to prove. It has been reported that in the absence of aldosterone, sodium tends to leave the extracellular fluid by migrating into cells, onto tendon and bone surfaces, as well as by increasing sodium wasting by the kidneys. Specific data on how aldosterone produces its effect are not presently available. However, enough information has been obtained to justify the assumption that it acts like other steroid hormones. Aldosterone probably enters the target cell by diffusion, combines with a specific cytoplasmic receptor protein, is transferred to a specific acceptor site on the chromatin tissue of the nucleus, which then produces an increase in RNA synthesis and later in protein synthesis.

There are three well-identified *control* mechanisms for aldosterone release—the renin-angiotensin system, potassium, and ACTH. The renin-angiotensin system is the major system for control of extracellular fluid volume, via regulation of aldosterone secretion. In effect, the renin-angiotensin system attempts to maintain the circulating blood volume constant by causing aldosterone-induced sodium retention during periods registered as volume deficiencies, and by decreasing aldosterone-dependent sodium retention under conditions in which volume is registered as being ample. In clinical medicine, volume deficits are much more common than volume excesses. Such deficits are repaired by stimulation of the renin-angiotensin system and its consequent effect on the renal retention of sodium and water. Volume regulation in the absence of the renin-angiotensin system (renoprival man) is extremely difficult and is characterized by marked oscillations of blood pressure. Furthermore, in normal man, studies of circadian secretion and acute and chronic sodium or volume repletion or depletion indicate that levels of renin, angiotensin-II, and aldosterone are always altered in parallel as long as other factors are kept constant. Such information documents that the renin-angiotensin system is the major control system for aldosterone-mediated volume regulation.

Potassium ions can regulate aldosterone secretion independently of the renin-angiotensin system. In normal man, oral potassium loading increases aldosterone excretion, secretion, and plasma levels. In addition, systemic infusion of potassium ions under certain circumstances significantly increases plasma aldosterone levels with as small as a 0.3 mEq per liter increase in serum potassium. That this effect is secondary to a direct action of the potassium ion is supported by a number of facts: potassium suppresses renin secretion; the effect of potassium on aldosterone excretion is independent of reciprocal changes in intravascular volume; the infusion of potassium ions directly into the adrenal artery produces an immediate increase in adrenal venous plasma levels; and finally, increasing the potassium content of incubation medium containing adrenal tissue results in an increase in aldosterone production. How potassium alters aldosterone secretion is not known. It may be related to small changes in serum potassium levels, to changes in intracellular potassium concentration, or to a change in the flux of potassium across the adrenal cortical cell membrane.

Potassium stimulation of aldosterone release may be a protective mechanism against potassium intoxication. When the human organism receives an acute load of potassium, aldosterone release will be stimulated, and the released aldosterone, by accelerating the potassium-sodium distal tubular exchange, will result in increased urinary loss of potassium, thus minimizing the increase in plasma potassium concentration. The magnitude of the aldosterone response to an acute potassium load is in part dependent on the prior potassium balance. During chronic potassium loading, the response is much greater than during chronic potassium restriction. This potassium-mediated control system for aldosterone release operates in parallel with the renin-angiotensin system and is probably of equal importance.

A number of facts support a role for ACTH in the control of aldosterone secretion. In supine normal man, plasma aldosterone has a rhythm parallel to that of cortisol and presumably ACTH. Hyponatremia and decreased aldosterone responsiveness to stress, ACTH infusion, and sodium restriction have also been reported in hypopituitary patients. However, several additional studies seem to relegate ACTH to a minor role in the control of aldosterone in normal man. Usually, only pharmacologic doses of ACTH can produce an increase in aldosterone release. Furthermore, subjects on high-dose steroid therapy for several years and with presumably complete suppression of ACTH have normal aldosterone-secretory responses to sodium restriction. Therefore, chronic ACTH deficiency per se does not alter glomerulosa cell responsiveness. Presumably, other pituitary factor(s) may be important in maintaining normal glomerulosa cell function. Thus, ACTH probably plays only a minor role in controlling aldosterone secretion.

Finally, the prior dietary intake of both potassium and sodium can alter the magnitude of the aldosterone response to acute stimulation. Increasing potassium intake or decreasing sodium intake will sensitize the response of the glomerulosa cells to acute stimulation. In vitro studies in animals indicate that aldosterone-stimulating substances may act on the late (corticosterone to aldosterone) as well as the early (cholesterol to pregnenolone) pathways for aldosterone biosynthesis. Since all acute stimuli increase the activity of the early pathway, an attractive unifying hypothesis that could explain the sensitizing effects of dietary sodium restriction and potassium loading is an increased activity of the final step of aldosterone biosynthesis.

In summary, while physiologic levels of ACTH under certain circumstances may stimulate aldosterone secretion, ACTH seems to be less important than potassium and the renin-angiotensin system in the control of aldosterone production. On the other hand, the renin-angiotensin system and potassium may be of equal importance in the regulation of aldosterone secretion in man (Fig. 86-7). Moreover, the interaction of dietary sodium and potassium can sensitize the response of aldosterone secretion following acute stimulation. Although the existence of early and late pathways for the control of aldosterone biosynthesis in man is speculative, evidence that diet can sensitize aldosterone secretion is consistent with this hypothesis. How dietary changes alter the late pathway, and whether sodium and potassium manipulations are acting on the same cells and/or receptor sites are not clear from the information presently available.

ANDROGEN PHYSIOLOGY Androgens are defined biologically as substances that stimulate male secondary sexual characteristics. The secondary sexual characteristics are affected through inhibition of the female characteristics (defeminization) and accentuation of the male characteristics (masculinization). These are seen clinically as hirsutism and virilization in the female with amenorrhea, atrophy of the breasts and uterus, enlargement of the clitoris, deepening of the voice, acne, increased muscle mass, increased heterosexual drive, and receding hairline. In the male there are increased body and sexual hair and enlargement of the sexual organs. Androgens also increase the synthesis of protein from amino acids, and this anabolic action leads to increased muscle mass and strength. Increased nitrogen retention may be used to assess androgenic biologic potency.

Steroids with predominant androgenic activity have 19 carbon atoms (Fig. 86-1). The principal adrenal androgens secreted are dehydroepiandrosterone (DHEA), androstenedione, and 11-hydroxyandrostenedione. DHEA and its sulfate are *quantitatively* the major androgens secreted by the adrenal cortex. The secretion of DHEA sulfate is approximately 10 mg per day; that of free DHEA is 2 mg per day. In the normal female, approximately 50 percent of the total secreted adrenal androgens are measured in the urine as 17-ketosteroids. DHEA, androstenedione, and 11-hydroxyandrostenedione, when assayed *biologically,* are weak androgens, but all are peripherally interconvertible with the potent androgen, testosterone. In normal women, only 40 percent of testosterone is directly secreted; 60 percent arises from androstenedione.

FIGURE 86-7
The interrelationship of the volume and potassium feedback loops on aldosterone secretion. Integration of signals from each loop determines the level of aldosterone secretion.

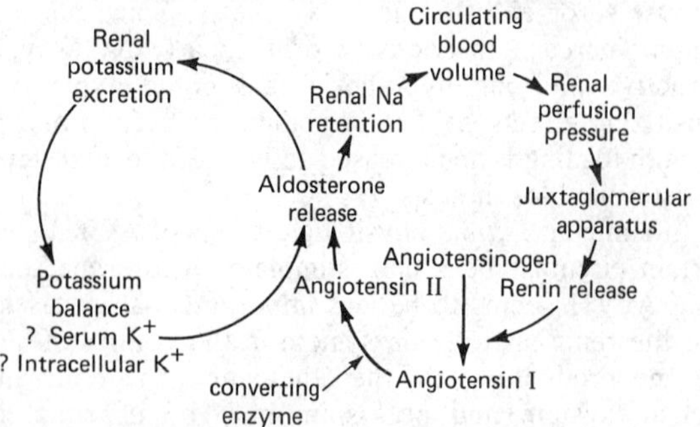

The release of adrenal androgens is stimulated by ACTH, not by gonadotropins. With ACTH stimulation, 17-ketosteroids increase but to a much lesser extent than do urine 17-hydroxycorticosteroids. Part of this increment in 17-ketosteroid excretion is due to the metabolism of increasing 17-hydroxycorticosteroids by the mechanism of C-20:C-21 side chain cleavage, producing 11-oxy-17-ketosteroids. Adrenal androgens are suppressed by exogenous glucocorticoid administration, as judged by decrements in urine 17-ketosteroid excretion.

LABORATORY EVALUATION OF ADRENOCORTICAL FUNCTION

Studies of adrenal function have been greatly facilitated by the development of sensitive radioimmunoassay procedures for a variety of steroid and polypeptide hormones. The essential elements of these procedures are (1) the development of a specific antibody which binds the hormone, and (2) competition between isotopically labeled and unlabeled hormone for the binding sites on the antibody. In practice, known amounts of *antiserum* specific for the hormone, *labeled* hormone, and plasma unknown are incubated together. At the completion of the incubation period, an equilibrium has occurred between labeled (H^*) and unlabeled hormone (H) and the specific antibody (Ab):

$$H + H^* + Ab \rightleftharpoons AbH^* + AbH$$

The bound hormone is then separated from the free hormone, and the amount of radioactivity bound to the antibody is compared to that remaining free. This ratio of bound to free is directly dependent upon the amount of unlabeled hormone present in the reaction mixture. By the preparation of standard curves, the unknown amount of the hormone can be determined. By such techniques, assays have been developed for plasma ACTH, angiotensin-I and -II, testosterone, cortisol, and aldosterone, as well as urine levels of the three steroids. The major problem with these assay systems resides in the specificity of the antibody. If it cross-reacts significantly with other substances, then a reliable answer will be achieved only if the plasma or urine is first processed to eliminate the cross-reacting substance.

A second major advance has been the clarification of the interrelation of plasma levels, secretion rates, and clearance rates of steroids. The basic assumption in the measurement of plasma levels or the urinary excretion of steroid metabolites is that they accurately reflect adrenal *secretory* rates of that steroid. A disadvantage of urine *excretion* values is that they may not truly reflect the secretion rate because of improper collection or altered metabolism. Measurement of the actual adrenal secretory rate of a given steroid would be preferable, and such methods are finding increasing clinical application. The adrenal secretory rate is calculated by the dilution that an administered radioactive steroid undergoes as a consequence of the admixture of endogenously secreted nonradioactive steroid hormone with the exogenous radioactive steroid. In practice, a major unique metabolite of the steroid is isolated and purified by chromatography; from a determination of its specific activity (counts per minute per microgram of steroid) and knowledge of the specific activity of the administered steroid one may calculate by the dilution principle the actual amount of the steroid secreted by the adrenal gland during the period of urine collection (usually 24 hr). In general, aldosterone and probably cortisol urine secretory rates closely reflect adrenal secretion of these hormones.

Plasma levels reflect the level of secretion only at the time of measurement. The plasma level (*PL*) is dependent on two factors: the secretion rate (*SR*) of the hormone and the rate at which it is metabolized, i.e., its metabolic clearance rate (*MCR*). These three factors can be related mathematically as follows:

$$PL = \frac{SR}{MCR} \quad \text{or} \quad SR = MCR \times PL$$

The secretion rate can also be estimated by determining the MCR and plasma levels of the steroid. When secretion is determined this way, it is called a *blood production rate.* Its accuracy is dependent on how closely the measured plasma levels and metabolic clearance rates reflect a 24-hr mean value. When no unique urine metabolite of the hormone exists or when there is significant peripheral interconversion of steroids (such as androgens in the female), then blood production rates more accurately reflect adrenal secretion than do urine secretion rates.

BLOOD LEVELS (see Table 86-1) **Peptides** ACTH and angiotensin-II can be measured by radioimmunoassay. There are still technical difficulties with both assays, related mainly to nonspecificity of the antibodies employed. ACTH is probably secreted episodically during the day, with a general trend for plasma levels to vary diurnally, with lower levels in the early evening than in the morning. Angiotensin-II levels also vary diurnally but are further influenced by dietary sodium intake and posture. Both upright posture and sodium restriction elevate angiotensin-II levels.

Measurements of the enzyme renin are made by several laboratories, utilizing a purified renin substrate. The majority of clinical determinations of the renin-angiotensin system, however, involve measurements of peripheral "plasma renin activity" (PRA) in which the renin activity is gaged by the generation of angiotensin during a standardized incubation period. This method depends on the presence of sufficient angiotensinogen in the patient's plasma as substrate. The generated angiotensin is then measured by radioimmunoassay. Plasma renin activity levels will depend on dietary sodium intake of the patient and whether or not the patient is ambulatory. In normal recumbent or upright man, a diurnal rhythm for plasma renin activity is characterized by peak values occurring in the morning, with decreases in activity in the afternoon.

Steroids The more cumbersome double-isotope derivative assay and less specific fluorometric method for adrenal steroids are being replaced by radioimmunoassay methods. Cortisol and aldosterone are both secreted episodically, but levels generally decline during the day, with peak values in the morning and low levels in the evening. In addition, the plasma level of aldosterone, but not of cortisol, is increased by increased potassium intake, sodium restriction, or assuming the upright posture. In contrast, plasma testosterone levels vary little during the day, although there is a tendency for the morning value to be higher. In the female, plasma testosterone is higher in the luteal than in the follicular phase of the menstrual cycle.

TABLE 86-1
Range of normal values for tests of adrenal function

Test		*Normal value, range*
Plasma cortisol, μg/100 ml	8 A.M.	9–24
	4 P.M.	3–12
Cortisol secretory rate, mg/24 hr		5–25
Urine free cortisol, μg/24 hr		20–100
17-hydroxycorticoids, mg/24 hr		2–10
17-ketogenic steroids, mg/24 hr:		
Males		5–23
Females		3–15
Plasma testosterone, μg/100 ml:		
Males		0.3–1.0
Females		0.01–0.1
17-ketosteroids, mg/24 hr:		
Males		7–25
Females		4–15
Plasma 11-deoxycortisol (S), μg/100 ml		<1.0
Urine tetrahydro 11-deoxycortisol (THS), mg/24 hr		0.1–1.0
Pregnanetriol, mg/24 hr:		
0–6 yr		<.2
7–15 yr		<1.2
Over 16 yr		0.5–2.5
Pregnanediol, mg/24 hr:		
Males		<1.0
Females		1.1–4.0
Plasma aldosterone, ng/100 ml (100 mEq Na, 60-100 mEq K, supine)		1–5
Aldosterone secretion, μg/24 hr (100 mEq Na, 60-100 mEq K, supine)		50–250
Aldosterone excretion, μg/24 hr (100 mEq Na, 60-100 mEq K, supine)		2–10
Plasma renin activity, ng/100 ml/3 hr (100 mEq Na, 60-100 mEq K, supine)		300–700
Plasma angiotensin II, pg/ml (100 mEq Na, 60-100 mEq K, supine)		10–30
Plasma ACTH (pg/ml) 8 A.M.		<150

URINE LEVELS The principal determinations are of urine 17-hydroxycorticoids, 17-ketosteroids, 17-ketogenic steroids, free cortisol, and aldosterone. The urine *17-hydroxycorticoids* are determined as Porter-Silber chromogens, i.e., these steroids react with the reagent phenylhydrazine to produce a characteristic color. This reaction is specific for steroids with a "dihydroxy acetone" C-17 side chain, i.e., with hydroxyl groups on C-17 and C-21 and a ketone group on C-20 (Fig. 86-8). Therefore, this determination will include cortisol, cortisone, tetrahydrocortisol, tetrahydrocortisone, and 11-dexoycortisol but not cortols, cortolones, and pregnanetriol. Normally, daytime (7 A.M. to 7 P.M.) excretion exceeds night values (7 P.M. to 7 A.M.) It is of extreme importance that the completeness of any and all urine steroid collections be checked by urine creatinine determinations.

The urine *17-ketosteroids* are those containing a ketone group at C-17; they originate either in the adrenal gland or the gonad. In the normal female, 90 percent or more of total urinary 17-ketosteroids is derived from the adrenal gland, while in the male, only 60 to 70 percent is of adrenal origin. Measurement depends on the Zimmermann reaction, whereby color is produced when 17-ketosteroids are condensed with *m*-dinitrobenzene. This reaction is specific for steroids with a ketone substituent with an adjacent unsubstituted carbon atom (Fig. 86-8). Urine 17-ketosteroid values are highest in young adults and decline with age.

The total urine 17-ketosteroids may be subdivided into those having either an oxygen or hydroxyl substituent at position C-11 (11-oxy-17-ketosteroids) and those having no such groups (11-deoxy-17-ketosteroids). These 11-oxy-17-ketosteroids are uniquely derived from the adrenal gland, since other tissues do not possess the enzymes for active C-11 hydroxylation, whereas the 11-deoxy-17-ketosteroids may arise from adrenal, testicular, or ovarian tissue.

Ketogenic steroids is a descriptive term for those C-21 hydroxycorticoids potentially capable of transformation into 17-ketosteroids in vitro. After the excreted 17-ketosteroids are reduced to noninterfering compounds, the side chains of C-21 hydroxycorticosteroids are oxidized to 17-ketonic groups, which then can be measured by the Zimmermann reaction as 17-ketosteroids. The Norymberski technique for ketogenic steroid analysis is specific for compounds containing the following groups: 17,21-dihydroxy-20-keto; 17,20,21-trihydroxy; and 17,20-dihydroxy-21-deoxy. It may be seen that the first of these groupings represents those compounds capable of reacting as *Porter-Silber chromogens;* the second, or trihydroxy, grouping would include the cortols and the cortolones; and the third, or 21-deoxy, grouping would include pregnanetriol. Thus, urine 17-ketogenic steroid determination includes all steroids determined as 17-hydroxysteroids by the Porter-Silber method and, in addition, includes the cortols, cortolones, and pregnanetriol (Fig. 86-8).

The determination of either urine *free cortisol* or *aldosterone* excretion is more difficult, usually requiring double-isotope derivative techniques or radioimmunoassay. Aldosterone excretion is measured by determining the excretion of a major metabolite, usually the acid-labile conjugate. A carefully timed urine collection is a prerequisite for all excretory determinations.

STIMULATION TESTS Stimulation tests are useful in documenting the existence of a hormonal deficiency state. A standardized and specific stimulus for the production and release of a given hormone is applied, and the quantity of the released hormone can then be measured.

Glucocorticoid stimulation tests Within minutes after initiating an infusion of ACTH, increased cortisol levels are noted in adrenal venous blood. This responsiveness of the adrenal gland to ACTH is utilized as an index of the "functional reserve" of the gland to produce cortisol. Under maximal ACTH stimulation the cortisol secretion increases tenfold to 300 mg per day. Such maximal stimulation is obtainable only with prolonged ACTH infusions. For clinical purposes, the functional adrenal

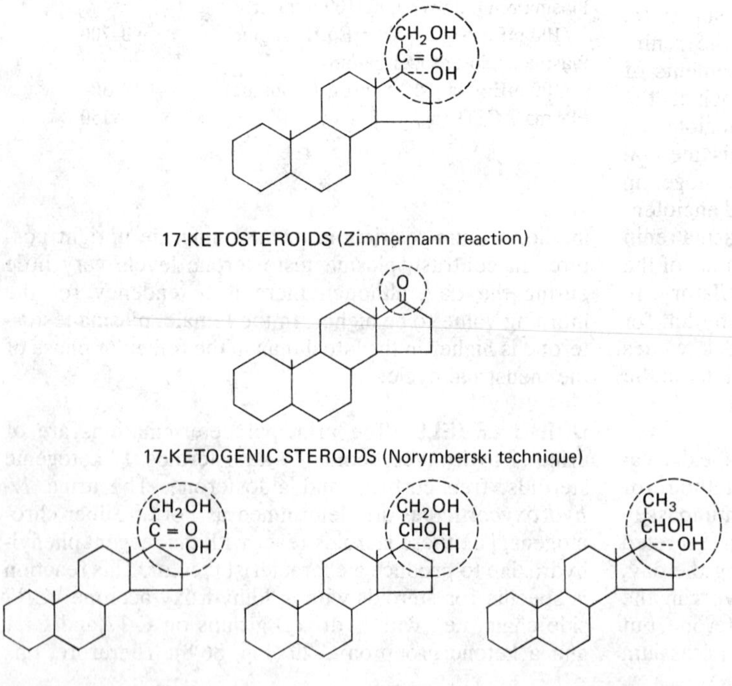

17-HYDROXYCORTICOIDS (Porter-Silber chromogens)

CH_2OH, C = O, OH

17-KETOSTEROIDS (Zimmermann reaction)

O

17-KETOGENIC STEROIDS (Norymberski technique)

CH_2OH, C = O, OH — CH_2OH, CHOH, OH — CH_3, CHOH, OH

FIGURE 86-8
Key reactive groups (enclosed by dashed circle) in urine steroid determinations.

reserve for cortisol production is standardized with a shorter infusion time (8 hr). The standard intravenous ACTH test is performed by administering 40 units of aqueous ACTH in 500 ml normal saline solution intravenously over an exact 8-hr interval (from 8 A.M. to 4 P.M.) on two successive days and collecting the complete 24-hr urine output for analysis of creatinine, 17-hydroxycorticoids (or 17-ketogenic steroids), and 17-ketosteroids. The patient may be ambulatory during this period. With such a method of testing, an average increment of 15 mg (range, 5 to 25) has been noted in urine 17-hydroxysteroids on the first day of testing and an average increment of 25 mg (range, 15 to 35) on the second infusion day, by one commonly used method. Much smaller rises in urine 17-ketosteroid excretion are noted, with average increments of 4 to 8 mg per day on the first and second day of testing, respectively. In the performance of the test the duration of the infusion must be strictly adhered to. Synthetic α 1–24 ACTH has become available as an alternative preparation. Because of its greater purity it has generally replaced the natural ACTH preparation. The standard infusion test would then be 25 units of the α 1–24 ACTH in 500 ml normal saline solution. A screening test for adrenal insufficiency utilizes the intramuscular administration of 25 units of synthetic ACTH with measurement of the rise in plasma cortisol levels. Normally, there will be a 50 percent increase within 1 hr. The test can give a false positive result for adrenal insufficiency, however, because of irregular absorption of the ACTH from the injection site.

Occasionally, it is necessary to prolong the ACTH infusion in order to separate primary from secondary adrenal insufficiency. This can be accomplished by using an 8-hr infusion on four or five consecutive days or by a continuous 24- or 48-hr infusion. The 48-hr test employs an infusion of 50 units of synthetic ACTH in 1,000 ml 5 percent dextrose in water or dextrose in normal saline solution over 24 hr for two consecutive days.

Mineralocorticoid stimulation tests Standardized aldosterone stimulation tests have been devised utilizing a protocol of programmed volume depletion, such as sodium restriction, diuretic administration, upright posture, or venesection. A simple potent stimulation test consists of severe sodium restriction and upright posture. After 3 to 5 days of a 10 mEq sodium intake, aldosterone secretion or excretion rates should exhibit a two- to threefold increase over control. Supine morning plasma aldosterone levels usually increase three- to sixfold. In addition, plasma levels increase two- to fourfold in response to 2 to 3 hr of upright posture.

Stimulation tests may also be carried out by the administration of a potent diuretic, such as ethacrynic acid of furosemide, or by venesection, with withdrawal of 400 to 600 ml venous blood over a period of 30 to 40 min. The normal response is a two- to fourfold rise in aldosterone secretion, excretion, or plasma levels. Because of adverse effects on the coronary circulation, angiotensin infusions have not found favor as a test of adrenal aldosterone responsiveness.

SUPPRESSION TESTS Suppression tests are used to document hypersecretion of adrenocortical hormones and are based on the demonstration of a decrease in the target hormone following standardized suppression of its tropic hormone. Thus, suppression testing for cortisol hypersecretion would involve suppression of ACTH release, with the documentation of an appropriately normal decrease in cortisol production, while suppression testing of aldosterone would involve demonstration of a decrease in aldosterone secondary to suppression of the renin-angiotensin system.

Glucocorticoid suppression tests The hypothalamic-pituitary ACTH release mechanism is sensitive to the circulating blood level of glucocorticoids. When such blood levels are increased in the normal individual, the corticotropin-releasing center decreases its production of the corticotropin-releasing factor (CRF), and consequently less ACTH is released from the anterior pituitary; secondarily, less steroid will be produced by the adrenal gland. The integrity of this feedback mechanism can be tested clinically by giving a potent glucocorticoid and judging suppression of the corticotropin-releasing center by analysis of urine steroid excretory values. A potent glucocorticoid such as dexamethasone is utilized in order that the administered compound may be given in such small amounts that it will not contribute significantly to the steroids to be analyzed.

One or more of the three standard tests are usually employed. The simplest is the overnight dexamethasone suppression test. This involves the measurement of plasma-corticoid levels at 8 A.M. and/or the urine 17-hydroxycorticoid and creatinine excretion between 7 A.M. and 12 noon following the oral administration of 1 mg dexamethasone the previous midnight. The 8 A.M. value for plasma corticoids in normal subjects should be less than 5 μg per 100 ml, and the ratio of urine Porter-Silber chromogens per milligram of creatinine in the 5-hr urine specimen should be less than 0.004.

The usual method of testing adrenal suppressibility is to administer 0.5 mg dexamethasone every 6 hr for two successive days while collecting urine over a 24-hr period for determination of creatinine, 17-hydroxysteroids, and 17-ketosteroids. In patients with a normal hypothalamic-pituitary ACTH release mechanism, a fall in the urine 17-hydroxycorticoids to less than 3 mg a day on the second day of dexamethasone administration is seen.

An intravenous dexamethasone suppression test is used less often. One milligram of dexamethasone is administered intravenously per hour for a total of 3 hr, and blood is collected for plasma glucocorticoid determinations. A 50 percent fall in plasma cortisol at the end of 3 hr of infusion is normally expected. Normal response to any of the suppression tests implies that the ACTH control of the adrenal glands is physiologically normal. However, an isolated abnormal result, particularly when the overnight suppression test is being used, does not in itself imply pituitary and/or adrenal disease.

Mineralocorticoid suppression tests Mineralocorticoid suppression testing procedures have been devised using saline infusions, oral salt loading, or DOCA administration as the means for expansion of the extracellular fluid volume. With expansion of extracellular fluid volume, there will be a decrease in renal renin release, a decrease in circulating plasma renin activity, and a decrease in aldosterone secretion and/or excretion. This would be the appropriate "normal" response. Varied tests differ in the rate at which extracellular fluid volume is expanded. The "normal saline suppression test" involves the intravenous administration of 2 liters of normal saline solution over a 4-hr period from 9 A.M. until 1 P.M. on two consecutive days. Aldosterone secretion or excretion rate is measured the day before and on the second day of saline loading; plasma aldosterone levels are measured before and at the end of the first day of infusion. The patient previously has been permitted to come into equilibration on a 10 mEq sodium and 100 mEq potassium constant diet. Normal response of suppression of aldosterone secretion by this maneuver is a value less than 200 μg per day (excretion < 15 μg per day and supine postinfusion plasma levels < 5 ng per 100 ml). The "oral salt-loading suppression test" is conveniently carried out by abruptly increasing the patient's sodium intake from a constant level of 10 mEq per day to 200 mEq per day for a period of 3 to 5 days, with measurement of aldosterone levels on the fourth or fifth day, at which time they should be similar to that for the saline suppression test. Potassium intake is held constant throughout the test, since potassium will cause aldosterone secretion to vary independently of the renin-angiotensin system. The "DOCA suppression test" is carried out by placing the patient on a normal (100 mEq) or high (200 mEq) sodium intake. After the patient is in sodium balance, deoxycorticosterone acetate is administered intramuscularly (10 mg every 12 hr) for a period of 3 to 5 days. Normal subjects on a sodium intake of 100 mEq daily demonstrate a 70 percent decrease in aldosterone levels when compared with control levels, which means that the aldosterone secretory value should be less than 250 μg per day (excretion < 15 μg per day and supine morning plasma levels < 5 ng per 100 ml).

TEST OF PITUITARY RESPONSIVENESS A number of stimuli, such as insulin hypoglycemia, arginine vasopressin, and pyrogen, will cause release of ACTH from the pituitary by an action on higher nerve centers, the hypothalamus, or the pituitary gland itself. By measuring plasma ACTH, or urine or blood glucocorticoids, the status of pituitary ACTH can be evaluated.

Metyrapone [SU4885 (Metopirone)] is a drug that selectively inhibits the enzyme action of 11-beta-hydroxylase in the adrenal gland. As a result, the conversion of 11-deoxycortisol (Compound S) to cortisol is interfered with and increased amounts of 11-deoxycortisol accumulate while blood levels of cortisol decrease (Fig. 86-2). Since 11-deoxycortisol is a weak suppressor of the hypothalamic-pituitary axis, the anterior pituitary responds to the declining cortisol blood levels by releasing larger quantities of ACTH in an attempt to stimulate the adrenal gland to release additional cortisol, which attempt, however, is thwarted by the metyrapone-induced enzymatic blockade. The metabolites of 11-deoxycortisol are excreted in increasing amounts in the urine, where they are measured as 17-hydroxycorticoids. *Note that the adrenal glands must be capable of being stimulated by ACTH, since assessment of the response depends on adrenal steroid production.*

The metyrapone response has been standardized for clinical evaluation of the reserve capacity of the anterior pituitary gland to release ACTH. Every 4 hr over a 24 to 48-hr period 750 mg metyrapone is administered orally, and daily urine collections for 17-hydroxycorticosteroids are obtained the day before testing, during the 2 days of testing, and the day after the last dose of metyrapone. The peak response of increased urine 17-hydroxysteroid excretion may be seen on the day after completion of metyrapone administration, and normal individuals will respond with at least a doubling of their basal 17-hydroxysteroid excretion.

TESTS FOR RENIN-ANGIOTENSIN RESPONSIVENESS Attempts have been made to standardize measurement of renin responsiveness by the acute induction of volume depletion and/or hypotension. Acute hypotension, induced either by diazoxide or by hydralazine, has been tried, but the results have been variable. Standardization has been improved by controlled volume depletion, induced by diuretics or by the assumption of the upright position.

The most widely accepted test, suggested by Conn, is based on postural augmentation of plasma renin activity. This test involves determination of plasma renin activity in the supine patient before and immediately following 3 hr of ambulation.

HYPERFUNCTION OF THE ADRENAL CORTEX

Distinct clinical syndromes are produced when excess amounts of the principal adrenocortical hormones are secreted. Thus, excess production of the principal glucocorticoid cortisol is associated with Cushing's syndrome; excess production of the principal mineralocorticoid aldosterone with clinical and chemical signs of aldosteronism; excess production of adrenal androgens with adrenal virilism. As would be expected, these syndromes do not always occur in the "pure" form but may have overlapping features.

CUSHING'S SYNDROME

ETIOLOGY From an analysis of the clinical and pathologic findings in a series of 12 patients, Harvey Cushing, in 1932, established a syndrome characterized by truncal obesity, hypertension, fatigability and weakness, amenorrhea, hirsutism, purplish abdominal striae, edema, glucosuria, and osteoporosis. As knowledge of this syndrome increased and as clinical tests of adrenocortical function became standardized and readily available, the diagnosis of Cushing's syndrome has been broadened into the classification shown in Table 86-2. It is apparent that, regardless of etiology, all cases of Cushing's syndrome are due to increased production of cortisol by the adrenal gland. The majority of cases are due to *bilateral adrenal hyperplasia,* in which the adrenal gland weight usually exceeds the normal combined total weight of 8 to 10 g. Harvey Cushing originally postulated that the adrenal hyperplasia in these patients was attributable to the

TABLE 86-2
Causes of Cushing's syndrome

I Adrenal hyperplasia
  A Secondary to hypothalamic dysfunction
  B Secondary to ACTH-producing tumors
    1 Pituitary tumors
    2 Nonendocrine tumors (bronchogenic carcinoma, thymoma, pancreatic carcinoma, bronchial adenoma)
II Adrenal nodular hyperplasia
III Adrenal neoplasia
  A Adenoma
  B Carcinoma
IV Exogenous, iatrogenic
  A Prolonged use of glucocorticoids
  B Prolonged use of ACTH

presence of pituitary basophilic adenomas. However, many cases are found without basophilic adenomas. Some are due to ACTH-producing chromophobe adenomas, but these cases represent a small fraction of the total. In the remaining cases attention has focused also on the elaboration of increased amounts of ACTH in the absence of pituitary tumors, possibly as a result of hypothalamic dysfunction, whereby the corticotropin-releasing center is reset to respond to a higher level of circulating cortisol. Measured plasma ACTH levels are usually normal or modestly elevated *or* fail to exhibit a normal decrease late in the day. However, normal plasma ACTH levels should be considered "inappropriately" high in the presence of hypercortisolism. In such cases of Cushing's syndrome due to adrenal hyperplasia, presumably due to excessive ACTH stimulation, both adrenal glands are always affected.

Adrenal adenomas are usually unilateral but on occasion may occur bilaterally. These adenomas may or may not function in autonomous manner; i.e., they may or may not be independent of ACTH stimulation and control. In addition, approximately 10 percent of cases of Cushing's syndrome are associated with *adrenal carcinomas,* most often unilateral and most often functioning autonomously. In those cases of Cushing's syndrome due to unilateral adrenal adenomas or carcinomas functioning independently of ACTH, atrophy of the contralateral gland is often found, attributable to suppression of ACTH release by the high levels of cortisol secreted by the tumors. A small number of patients with Cushing's syndrome are found to have *adrenal rest tumors,* i.e., aberrant adrenocortical tissue occurring outside the adrenal gland. These embryologic remnants may be in the perirenal area, ovaries, or testes and exhibit histologic features of hyperplastic or adenomatous changes.

Nonendocrine tumors secreting polypeptides biologically, chemically, and immunologically indistinguishable from ACTH are also occasionally responsible for Cushing's syndrome secondary to bilateral adrenal hyperplasia. These neoplasms also frequently synthesize melanocyte-stimulating hormone (MSH), with the result that patients frequently are hyperpigmented. The major association of a nonendocrine tumor has been with primitive "oat-cell" carcinomas of the lung; other ACTH-secreting tumors include malignant thymoma, pancreatic carcinoma, and bronchial adenoma. Hypokalemic alkalosis is often prominent in such cases, whereas many of the distinctive physical findings usually associated with Cushing's syndrome may be absent.

INCIDENCE Increasing numbers of patients with Cushing's syndrome are being detected among persons undergoing evaluation for such diverse entities as diabetes mellitus, hypertension, obesity, and osteoporosis. Many of these patients exhibit mild degrees of adrenal hyperfunction. The incidence of nontumorous adrenal hyperplasia in the female is three times that in the male, with the most frequent age of onset being the third or fourth decade. The incidence of Cushing's syndrome secondary to ACTH-secreting tumors will probably rise because of increased awareness of this syndrome.

CLINICAL SIGNS AND SYMPTOMS The frequency of clinical findings is listed in Table 86-3. Knowledge of the physiologic effects of glucocorticoids shows that many of the signs and symptoms logically follow. As a result of mobilization of peripheral supportive tissue, there are muscle weakness and fatigability, osteoporosis, and cutaneous striae. The latter involve a weakening and rupture of collagenous fibers in the dermis, so that the heavily vascularized subcutaneous tissues are exposed. Likewise, because of the loss of perivascular supporting tissue, there is easy bruisability, and ecchymoses often appear at sites of mild trauma. The osteoporosis may be so severe that collapse of vertebral bodies and pathologic fractures of other bones are frequently encountered. As a result of increased hepatic gluconeogenesis and insulin resistance, impaired glucose tolerance following a standard glucose load is common, occurring in 90 percent of patients. Frank diabetes occurs in less than 20 percent of patients, probably in individuals with a familial predisposition to this disorder. Hypercortisolism promotes the deposition of adipose tissue in characteristic sites. This is observed most notably in the upper part of the face, the classic "moon" facies; in the interscapular area, the "buffalo" hump; and in the mesenteric bed, where it produces the classic "truncal" obesity (Fig. 86-9). Rarely, there may be episternal fatty tumors and mediastinal widening secondary to fat accumulation. The reason for this peculiar distribution of lipid is not known. The face also appears plethoric, even in the absence of any increase in red blood cell concentration. Hypertension is most always present, and frequently there are profound emotional changes, ranging from irritability or emotional lability to severe depression, confusion, or even frank

TABLE 86-3
Incidence of signs and symptoms in 35 cases of Cushing's syndrome, percent

Typical habitus	97	Amenorrhea	77
Increased body weight	94	Cutaneous striae	67
Fatigability and weakness	87	Personality changes	66
		Ecchymoses	65
Hypertension (above) 150/90)	82	Edema	62
		Polyuria, polydipsia	23
Hirsutism	80	Hypertrophy of clitoris	19

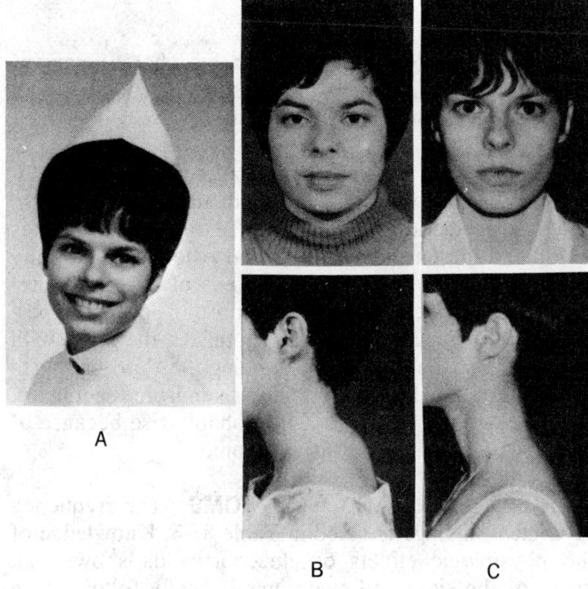

FIGURE 86-9
A twenty-year-old female with Cushing's syndrome due to a right adrenal cortical adenoma: A *Two years prior to surgery, age eighteen.* B *One month prior to surgery, age twenty.* C *One year after surgery, age twenty-one.*

psychosis. Acne and hirsutism are frequent in female patients, hirsutism often appearing as a fine "downy" coat over the face, forehead, and upper part of the trunk. Likewise in female patients, oligomenorrhea or amenorrhea is a frequent disturbance.

LABORATORY FINDINGS With rare exceptions, plasma and urinary 17-hydroxycorticoid levels are elevated. Circulating eosinophils are below 100 cells per mm^3 in 90 percent of cases, and patients characteristically show a mild neutrophilic leukocytosis. In spite of markedly plethoric facies, the hematocrit is usually within the normal range, but occasionally erythema with higher hematocrits is encountered, particularly when the syndrome is associated with excessive production of 17-ketosteroids. Serum sodium concentration is usually normal; however, with marked excess secretion of cortisol, there may be hypokalemia, hypochloremia, and metabolic alkalosis. More than three-fourths of patients exhibit intermittent glucosuria, and nearly all have a decreased rate of disappearance of infused glucose from the circulation. Some patients may have frank diabetes, necessitating insulin therapy. X-ray studies usually reveal generalized osteoporosis, most marked in the spine and pelvis, but also frequently found in the skull, with disappearance of the lamina dura, and fractures are often seen in the ribs and vertebras. Intravenous pyelography and laminograms with or without retroperitoneal insufflation may demonstrate adrenal enlargement, particularly when a carcinoma is the pathologic cause of the disease. More sophisticated x-ray techniques, such as selective adrenal arteriography or venography, may make the localization and diagnosis more specific but are not without risk. The increased friability of the adrenal veins in Cushing's syndrome makes retrograde venography particularly hazardous. The use of ^{131}I-tagged 19-iodocholesterol scintillation scanning is a promising technique that may be of considerable value in localizing adrenal tumors and differentiating them from bilateral hyperplasia.

DIAGNOSIS The diagnosis of Cushing's syndrome depends on the direct or indirect demonstration of increased cortisol production in the absence of stress. Once this is established, further testing is carried out to determine whether or not the excess cortisol is being produced in an autonomous manner, since such knowledge will permit a more specific etiologic diagnosis (see Fig. 86-10, Table 86-4).

For initial screening purposes, the rapid *overnight dexamethasone suppression test* is recommended. Baseline 24-hr urine 17-hydroxysteroid and 17-ketosteroid determinations may also be carried out, since values in excess of 10 mg per day for urine 17-hydroxysteroids (Porter-Silber) justify further evaluation. An ancillary screening procedure is to determine the diurnal excretion pattern for urine 17-hydroxysteroids by collecting urine between 7 A.M. and 7 P.M. and 7 P.M. to 7 A.M. The patient with Cushing's syndrome will generally excrete an equivalent or greater amount of the 17-hydroxysteroids in the night collection, in contrast to most normal subjects. Creatinine determinations are of critical importance to demonstrate the accuracy and adequacy of the collection procedure. An adult female excretes approximately 1,000 mg creatinine daily, with about 50 to 60 percent found in the daytime collection; an adult male excretes approximately 1,800 mg daily. Day-to-day variation in creatinine excretion by a patient should not exceed 20 percent. Adjustments for body size can be made; normal subjects excrete 3 to 7 mg 17-hydroxycorticosteroids per gram of creatinine. If it is demonstrated that the diurnal cycle for steroid excretion is "reversed," i.e., night urine 17-hydroxysteroids are almost equal to or greater than daytime excretion, one then knows that excessive cortisol is being released continuously "around the clock." These urine steroid determinations, which reflect the metabolites of cortisol, are indirect but adequate proof of excessive cortisol production. A direct method is available utilizing radioisotopic cortisol to determine the actual cortisol secretory rate, which in cases of Cushing's syndrome is in excess of 30 mg per day. Another method of direct confirmation of excess cortisol is the determination of the free cortisol in the urine, which reflects the active free cortisol in the blood. Normal persons excrete less than 100 μg daily of free cortisol. The sensitivity of this urine free cortisol test resides in the fact that only free cortisol of the plasma is freely filtrable at the glomerulus, and thus increments in the plasma level of this biologically active form are magnified in terms of urine excretory values.

Owing to a marked diurnal variability plasma 17-hydroxycorticoid determinations are not meaningful when performed in isolated fashion, but demonstration that the expected normal fall in late afternoon blood levels does not occur is increasingly used as a diagnostic measure. Normally, the plasma level declines by half or more; if such a decrease is not noted, one assumes that continuous hypersecretion of cortisol is occurring.

Specific diagnosis of the type of lesion causing Cushing's syndrome can usually be made by the combined use of ACTH-stimulation and dexamethasone-suppression tests. Adrenal hyperplasia, whether caused by hypothalamic dysfunction or by an ACTH-producing tumor, is characterized by hyperreactivity to exogenous ACTH. The continuous stimulation of the hyperplastic glands by endogenous ACTH appears to "prime" the adrenals to this hyperactive response to exogenous ACTH testing. This hyperactive response is evidenced in the parallel rise of both urine 17-hydroxy- and urine 17-ketosteroids. Whereas adrenal cortisol production is suppressed in normal subjects given dexamethasone 0.5 mg every 6 hr for 48 hr, no suppression occurs in patients with bilateral adrenal hyperplasia given this dosage. Suppression of cortisol production in normal subjects is judged by a decrease in urine 17-hydroxysteroids to less than 3 mg per day, demonstrating that the hypothalamic-pituitary axis is appropriately responsive to increases in blood glucocorticoid levels, with a resultant decline in ACTH release. Lack of suppression in patients with adrenal hyperplasia given 2 mg daily of dexamethasone suggests that their hypothalamic-pituitary axis is "reset" to a higher blood level of glucocorticoids. On higher doses of dexamethasone (2 mg every 6 hr) suppression of urine 17-hydroxysteroid levels to values less than half the baseline levels can be demonstrated, consistent with the view that the hypothalamic-pituitary axis in these patients is reset upward and is responsive only to higher blood levels of glucocorticoids, at which point an appropriate decline in ACTH release does occur. The finding of a normal plasma ACTH level in these patients is an abnormal sign, since with the elevated blood cortisol levels one would expect a decreased blood ACTH level. On metyrapone testing, patients with adrenal hyperplasia due to hypothalamic dysfunction will again demonstrate a hyperactive response. In patients with adrenal hyperplasia secondary to an *ACTH-producing tumor,* such as an oat-cell bronchogenic carcinoma, no suppression will occur after dexamethasone administration and an abnormally depressed metyrapone test results, since the ACTH production by the tumor functions in an autonomous manner.

In patients with Cushing's syndrome secondary to an *adrenal adenoma,* hyperreactivity to exogenous ACTH testing may or may not occur, depending on whether the adenoma is functioning in an autonomous manner; if it is, it will be found ACTH-insensitive and thus fail to demonstrate a brisk rise in urine 17-hydroxycorticoids on ACTH stimulation. The diagnosis of adrenal adenoma is suggest-

TABLE 86-4
Laboratory evaluation and testing of adrenocortical function in normal subjects and in patients with Cushing's syndrome*

	Plasma values		*Urine values*					
	Control		*Control*		*17-OH response to*			
	ACTH 8a pg/ml	*Cortisol 8a/4p μg/100 ml*	*17-OH mg/24 hr*	*17-KS mg/24 hr*	*25 units synthetic ACTH IV over 8 hr*	*Dexamethasone day 2, mg q.6h.* 0.5	2.0	*Metyrapone 750 mg q.4h. ×6 doses*
Normal values	<150	17/8	2–10	♀ 5–15 ♂10–25	↑3–5×	<3.0	<3.0	↑2×
Cushing's syndrome:								
I Hyperplasia with increased ACTH secretion								
A Secondary to hypothalamic dysfunction	50–400	30/25	15–25	20–35	↑4–7×	NR–↓	↓50%	↑3×
B Secondary to tumor secretion								
1 Pituitary	50–400	30/25	15–25	20–35	↑4–7×	NR	NR–↓50%	NR–↑
2 Nonendocrine	400–1,000	50/50	25–40	30–60	NR–↑	NR–↓	NR–↓	NR–↑
II Nodular hyperplasia	<150	30/25	15–25	20–35	NR–↑4–7×	NR	NR–↓	NR–↑
III Neoplasia								
A Adenoma								
1 Complete autonomy	<50	35/35	20–30	5–15	NR	NR	NR	NR
2 Incomplete autonomy	<50	35/25	15–20	5–15	↑3–5×	NR–↓	NR–↓	NR–↑
B Carcinoma	<50	35/35	20–40	50–80	NR	NR	NR	NR
IV Exogenous steroids (iatrogenic)	<50	2/2†	1–5†	5–10†	↑1–2×	NR	NR	NR

* *Abbreviations:* NR = *no response;* ↑ = *significant increase above control excretion;* ↓ = *significant decrease below control excretion;* NR–↑ = *no response or increase;* ↓50% = *decrease to 50% or more of control excretion value;* ↑2× = *increase 2× control excretion value.*

† *Absolute level dependent on steroid preparation.*

ed by the disproportionate elevation in base-line urine 17-hydroxycorticoids with only a modest rise in 17-ketosteroids. Those adenomas which function autonomously fail to suppress after administration of dexamethasone at either the 2- or 8-mg daily dosage schedule, whereas the ACTH-sensitive adenomas most often fail to suppress with the lower, 2-mg daily dosage but may demonstrate suppression at the higher, 8-mg daily dosage. The variability of dexamethasone suppression testing is greater at the higher dose levels, and the distinction between adenomas and carcinomas is as a result less decisive. Another entity in the differential diagnosis is multinodular ("adenomatous") adrenal hyperplasia, which is an uncommon condition characteristically having features of both hyperplasia and of adenomas. Response to ACTH stimulation is variable, but patients with multinodular adrenal hyperplasia most often do not show suppression with the standard doses of dexamethasone. However, with large doses, such as 4 to 8 mg every 6 hr, suppression often occurs.

Metyrapone testing is useful in differentiating adrenal tumors (adenoma or carcinoma) from adrenal hyperplasia, since the adrenal tumors by their autonomy suppress the ACTH-releasing capacity of the pituitary, with the result that on metyrapone challenge testing the pituitary fails to release ACTH in an appropriate manner and the

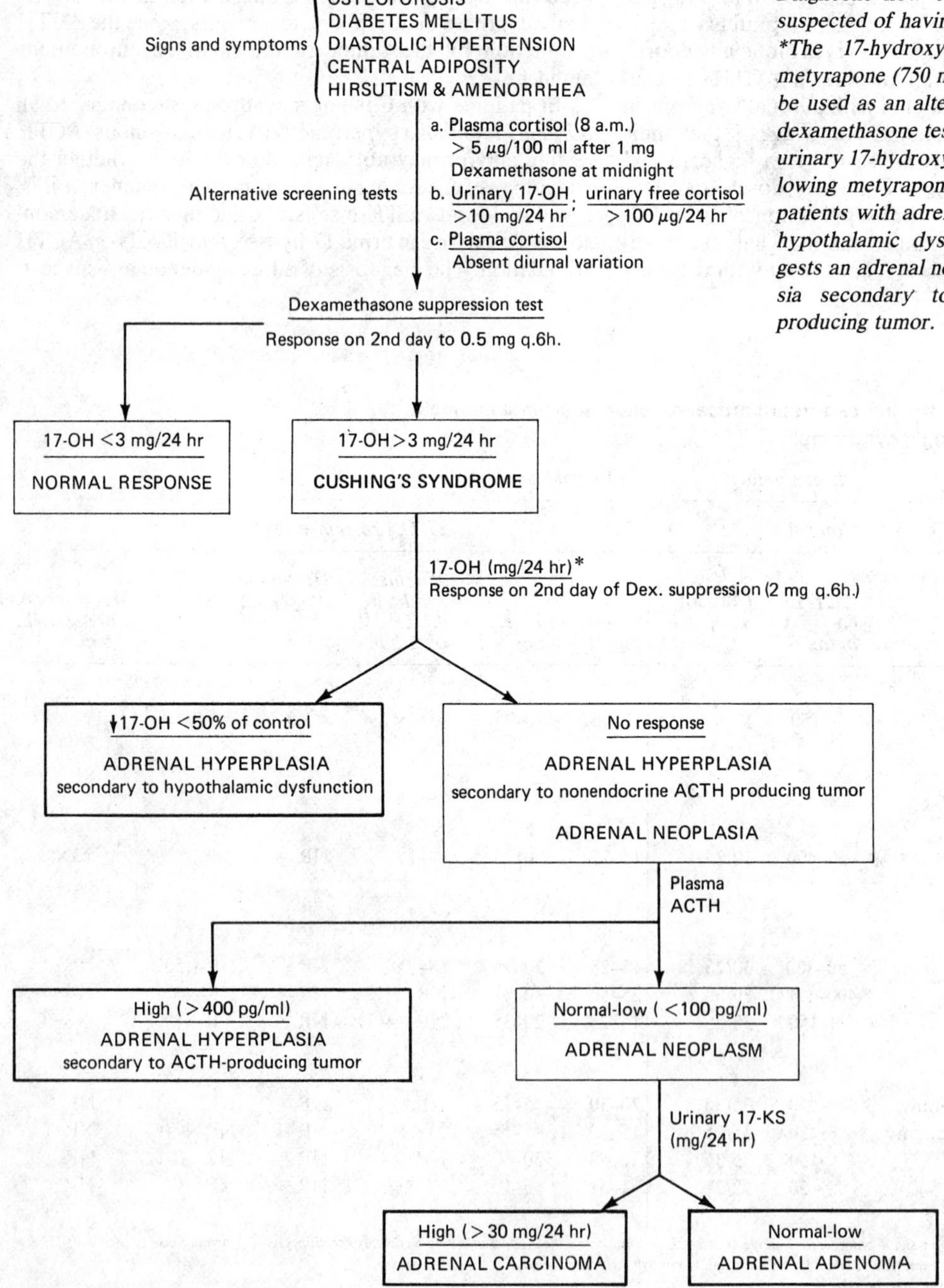

FIGURE 86-10
Diagnostic flow chart for evaluating patients suspected of having Cushing's syndrome.
**The 17-hydroxycorticosteroid response to metyrapone (750 mg p.o. q.4h. × 6 doses) may be used as an alternative test to the high-dose dexamethasone test (2 mg p.o. q.6h.). Increased urinary 17-hydroxycorticosteroid excretion following metyrapone occurs in the majority of patients with adrenal hyperplasia secondary to hypothalamic dysfunction; no response suggests an adrenal neoplasm or adrenal hyperplasia secondary to a nonendocrine ACTH-producing tumor.*

usual rise in urine 17-hydroxycorticoids fails to occur. This finding of impaired response to metyrapone challenge separates adrenal tumors from adrenal hyperplasia, in which normal or hyperactive responses occur.

The diagnosis of *adrenal carcinoma* as a cause of Cushing's syndrome is suggested by *markedly* elevated baseline values of *both* urine 17-hydroxycorticoids and urine 17-ketosteroids. Adrenal carcinoma is usually resistant to both ACTH stimulation and dexamethasone suppression because of the autonomy of the tumor tissue itself and because of extreme atrophy of the normal remaining adrenal tissue. Virilization is often present in the female; feminizing adrenocortical carcinoma in the male usually presents with gynecomastia. Functioning adrenal carcinomas that produce Cushing's syndrome are most often associated with elevated urine excretory values for the metabolites of the intermediates of steroid biosynthesis (such as tetrahydro-11-deoxycortisol and pregnanetriol) in addition to the cortisol metabolites, suggesting inefficient conversion of the intermediates to the final product. This is in contrast to Cushing's syndrome associated with adrenocortical hyperplasia, in which the elevation of urine steroids is largely accounted for by cortisol metabolites.

Cushing's syndrome is being reported with increasing frequency in association with the autonomous production of ACTH by *nonendocrine tumors,* with the resultant development of adrenal hyperplasia. The majority of these cases have been associated with the primitive small-cell type of bronchogenic carcinoma, and the remainder have been reported chiefly with tumors of thymus, pancreas, or ovary or with bronchial adenomas. The onset of Cushing's syndrome is distinctively sudden in these patients, and this partly accounts for their failure to exhibit all the classic physical findings of the syndrome. Extracts of some of these nonendocrine tumors have produced a compound that is biologically, physiochemically, and immunologically identical to pituitary ACTH. Since such tumors often produce large amounts of ACTH and MSH, base-line urine steroid values are usually markedly elevated, and increased skin pigmentation is usually present. A CRF-like material produced by the tumor has also been reported to cause hypercortisolism. Hypokalemic alkalosis, edema, and hypertension are much more common in these patients than in patients with Cushing's syndrome from other causes, and are attributed to extremely high levels of cortisol secretion. These patients will demonstrate a variable response to exogenous ACTH stimulation. A hyperactive adrenal response is seen unless endogenous ACTH levels have produced maximal adrenocortical activation. Similarly, *no suppression with dexamethasone* and no increment in urine 17-hydroxycorticoid excretion after metyrapone administration are the rule unless the endogenous secretion of cortisol is not sufficient to suppress ACTH secretion. Plasma ACTH levels are most often markedly elevated in these patients, a helpful diagnostic finding, since plasma ACTH levels in other categories of Cushing's syndrome are at most modestly elevated.

Hyperpigmentation in patients with Cushing's syndrome always points to an extraadrenal tumor, either in an extracranial location, as discussed in the previous paragraph, or within the cranium. In the first 100 cases reported of Cushing's syndrome associated with pituitary tumors the majority had associated basophilic adenomas; chromophobe adenomas were in a distinct minority. Since this original series, chromophobe adenomas and carcinomas are being reported in much greater frequency than are basophilic adenomas. Basophilic adenomas do not cause enlargement of the sella turcica, whereas chromophobe tumors are the commonest cause of ballooning of the sella. The chief complaint of patients with chromophobe tumors is decreasing visual acuity, often with blurred vision and always with headaches. The chromophobe adenomas are asymmetric in growth, and as they progress upward, pressure on the optic nerve tracts results in visual field defects in most patients, with earliest losses occurring in the superior temporal quadrants; later a full bitemporal hemianopsia results. Headaches would appear to be caused by traction on surrounding dural structures or on the diaphragma sella. This association of pituitary tumors with Cushing's syndrome has generated interest as to whether all cases of adrenal hyperplasia may be caused by extraadrenal tumors and has led further to the speculation that chronic hypothalamic dysfunction may lead to the development of anterior pituitary tumors. A limitation to such interpretation has been the finding that approximately one-tenth of patients undergoing bilateral adrenalectomy for Cushing's syndrome have developed enlarged sella turcica and pituitary tumors, clinically evident only after the surgery, strongly suggesting that the loss of adrenal tissue, and consequent loss of the usual negative cortisol feedback on ACTH release, may be instrumental in the genesis of such tumors. Since intrasellar tumors may be present at an early stage in many patients *without* sellar enlargement, a decisive opinion as to their role in the genesis of Cushing's syndrome, or in the sequelae of its surgical therapy, must be withheld for further investigation. Clinically, all patients suspected of having Cushing's syndrome must be carefully examined for visual field defects and enlargement of the sella turcica; if defects are found, further diagnostic procedures may be warranted, such as sellar tomography, pneumoencephalography, and angiography. A diagnostic flow chart for evaluation of patients suspected of having Cushing's syndrome is presented in Fig. 86-10.

DIFFERENTIAL DIAGNOSIS Patients with exogenous obesity, hypertension, and diabetes mellitus, occurring singly or in combination, present major problems in diagnosis. Extreme *obesity* is uncommon in Cushing's syndrome; furthermore, with exogenous obesity, the adiposity is generalized, not truncal. On adrenocortical testing, abnormalities, if noted in patients with exogenous obesity, are found never to be extensive but only modest. Basal urine steroid excretion levels in obese patients are either normal or slightly elevated, a finding similar to their cortisol secretory values. Some patients demonstrate an increased percentage of conversion of secreted cortisol into excreted metabolites. Blood cortisol levels are normal, and, of greater importance, a normal diurnal pattern in blood and urine levels is seen. On ACTH stimulation some of the patients will demonstrate a brisk response; however, in most cases this response is suppressed easily with dexamethasone. It would appear that exogenous obesity may *cause* alterations in the secretion and metabolism of steroids, pointing up the secondary nature of altered steroid testing patterns sometimes encountered. These patients are best treated by a concerted weight reduction program with periodic retesting of adrenal function.

Iatrogenic Cushing's syndrome, induced by the administration of either glucocorticoids or ACTH, is indistinguishable by physical findings from the endogenous forms of adrenocortical hyperfunction. On occasion one may wish to rule out an underlying endogenous form of Cushing's syndrome that may be clinically magnified by exogenous therapy. This is accomplished by changing the patient's therapy to 1 mg dexamethasone daily while collecting base-line and diurnal split urine output for corticosteroid analysis. Patients with a pure exogenous form of Cushing's syndrome due to prolonged suppression of their hypothalamic-pituitary axis by administered steroid will demonstrate low base-line steroid excretion, predominantly in the daytime, a finding in distinct contrast to that in patients with endogenous Cushing's syndrome. Patients receiving long-term ACTH therapy, in addition to the features of Cushing's syndrome, may also have melanodermia. The production of iatrogenic Cushing's syndrome is related both to the total steroid dose and to the duration of therapy. Also, patients on afternoon and evening doses of steroid develop Cushing's syndrome more readily and on smaller daily steroid doses than do patients on a steroid program limited to morning doses only. In addition, there appears to be a marked difference among patients in the enzymatic disposition of administered steroid. Several cases have been reported in which a spontaneous remission of Cushing's syndrome occurred; some have been characterized by intermittent abnormalities in adrenal testing. It is difficult to know whether such abnormalities are functional in nature or true pathophysiologic processes.

THERAPY When an adenoma or carcinoma is suspected, adrenal exploration is performed, with excision of the tumor. Since cortisol production by the tumor generally causes atrophy of the contralateral gland, if an atrophied gland is noted on the initial side of exploration, the tumor must be on the opposite side. Because of this probable atrophy of the contralateral adrenal, the patient is prepared and treated pre- and postoperatively for total adrenalectomy even when a unilateral lesion is suspected, the routine being similar to that for an Addisonian patient undergoing elective surgery (Table 86-9).

The principal antitumor drug used to chemically inhibit adrenal cortical function due to carcinoma is *o,p′*-DDD[2,2-bis-(2-chlorophenyl, 4-chlorophenyl)-1, 1-dichloroethane], an isomer of the insecticide DDT. This drug suppresses cortisol production and decreases plasma and urine steroid levels. Although its cytotoxic action is reported to be specific for the glucocorticoid-secreting zone of the adrenal cortex, the zona glomerulosa (site of aldosterone biosynthesis) may also be inhibited. *o,p′*-DDD also alters the extraadrenal metabolism of cortisol, resulting in a smaller percentage being excreted in the urine as 17-OHCS. Therefore, *plasma or urinary free-cortisol* levels must be followed to determine the effect of *o,p′*-DDD on the patient's hypercortisolism. *o,p′*-DDD is given in divided doses three to four times daily. The dose is gradually increased to 8 to 10 g daily or the highest dose tolerated by the patient. Almost all patients experience gastrointestinal (anorexia, diarrhea, or vomiting) or neuromuscular (lethargy, somnolence, dizziness) side effects. All patients should be placed on long-term maintenance glucocorticoid; in some instances mineralocorticoid replacement therapy should also be instituted. In some patients, dramatic regression of both tumor and metastases may occur, but long-term survival remains discouragingly limited. Predictability of expected response is poor. In many patients, *o,p′*-DDD only inhibits steroidogenesis and does not produce regression of tumor metastases. Osseous metastases are usually refractory to *o,p′*-DDD; radiation should be used to treat these lesions.

In patients with a severe form of Cushing's syndrome due to adrenal hyperplasia, with features of hypertension, overt diabetes, psychosis, and osteoporosis with pathologic fractures and in the absence of an enlarged sella turcica, a complete total bilateral adrenalectomy is preferred. Since, as mentioned earlier, one-tenth of these patients develop pituitary tumors after surgery, pituitary irradiation is also indicated in any patient who develops increased pigmentation or in whom the sella turcica size increases postoperatively. In patients past the reproductive years, pituitary irradiation may be carried out prophylactically in conjunction with complete adrenalectomy. It cannot be stressed too strongly that the status of all patients with bilateral adrenalectomy must be followed diligently with periodic reexaminations for evidence of increasing sellar size or pigmentary changes.

In severely debilitated patients who are not candidates for bilateral adrenalectomy, a chemical remission can be obtained with *o,p′*-DDD.

If patients with adrenal hyperplasia are noted to have signs of pituitary tumor (melanodermia, increased sellar size, visual field defects), specific therapy directed at the pituitary gland must be undertaken. In general, the type of therapy is either surgery or some form of radiation. Complications of surgical therapy include cerebrospinal fluid rhinorrhea, optic nerve and posterior pituitary injury, as well as removal of all tropic hormones. The morbidity and mortality rates are greater than with radiotherapy, and therefore surgery is often reserved for those cases not amenable to treatment with radiation. There are three major methods of directing radiotherapy at the pituitary gland. (1) The classical approach is the use of conventional external radiation at a dose of 3,000 to 5,000 R delivered over several weeks. The total dosage is limited by possible damage to surrounding neural structures and by the loss of additional pituitary tropic function. Treatment has been successful in fewer than one-third of the patients with Cushing's syndrome who were treated solely by this method. (2) The second method is internal pituitary irradiation by the stereotactic implantation of ^{90}Y pellets in the pituitary via the transnasosphenoid route. Possible limitation of this form of therapy may be found once long-term evaluation on the effects of the radiation on perisellar structures (such as the internal carotid artery) has been made. (3) The most recent development has been the use of the alpha particle or proton beam as a source of external radiation. By this method as much as 12,000 R can be directed at the pituitary gland without evident damage to surrounding structures. This is because the beam can be focused more sharply than the more commonly used gamma radiation and because multiple portals of entry can be used. Even with this therapy there is a significant incidence of ocular motor palsies. This form of therapy holds great promise because of its ease of application, insignificant mortality rate, and low morbidity rate. However, final evaluation awaits long-term follow-up studies on treated subjects.

In patients with milder forms of adrenal hyperplasia without serious steroid-induced complications, several methods of approach are available, such as unilateral adrenalectomy with or without pituitary irradiation, or external or internal pituitary irradiation. Patients with a severe form of Cushing's syndrome are not candidates for therapies such as external pituitary irradiation. The lag time between treatment and remission and a remission rate less than 50 percent contraindicate the use of external pituitary irradiation in the presence of rapidly progressing disease. Treatment of nonendocrine ACTH-producing tumors is surgical removal of the neoplasm. If the neoplastic disease is far advanced, bilateral total adrenalectomy or metyrapone may be indicated to correct the hypercortisolism.

If Cushing's syndrome redevelops after bilateral adrenalectomy, excessive stimulation of a remnant of adrenocortical tissue must be occurring. In very rare instances an embryologic extraadrenal remnant may be stimulated to produce excess cortisol. Surgical exploration is difficult because adrenocortical remnants are small. Measurement of cortisol levels preoperatively from various points along the inferior vena cava may locate the remnant tissue. The use of ^{131}I-tagged 19-iodocholesterol scintillation scanning offers interesting possibilities.

ALDOSTERONISM

Aldosteronism is a syndrome associated with hypersecretion of the major adrenal mineralocorticoid aldosterone. *Primary* aldosteronism signifies that the stimulus for the excessive aldosterone production resides within the adrenal gland; in *secondary* aldosteronism the stimulus is of extraadrenal origin.

PRIMARY ALDOSTERONISM Introduction The constellation of signs and symptoms of excessive inappropriate aldosterone production was first summarized by Conn in 1956. In the original case and in the majority of the subsequent cases, the disease was the result of an *aldosterone-producing adrenal adenoma* (Conn's syndrome). The majority of cases (75 percent) involved a unilateral adenoma, usually small and occurring with equal frequency on either side. Rarely primary aldosteronism has been reported in association with adrenal carcinoma. It is twice as common in women as in men, presenting between the ages of thirty and fifty. In recent years, a number of cases have been reported with clinical and biochemical characteristics previously considered diagnostic of primary aldosteronism, but a solitary adenoma was not found at surgery. Instead, these patients have *bilateral cortical nodular hyperplasia.* The cause of this hyperplasia is unknown. In the literature this disease has been alternatively termed "pseudo" primary aldosteronism (PPA), idiopathic hyperaldosteronism (IHA), or nodular hyperplasia.

Incidence Primary aldosteronism is an uncommon disease. The incidence in unselected hypertensive patients is between 0.5 and 2 percent. Because of special diagnostic procedures involved, diagnosis has been largely restricted to symptomatic patients. With greater availability of these procedures an increased incidence may be seen.

Signs and symptoms The continual hypersecretion of aldosterone increases the renal distal tubular exchange of intratubular sodium for secreted potassium and hydrogen ions, with progressive depletion of body potassium and development of hypokalemia. Almost all patients have diastolic hypertension, usually not of marked severity, and complain of headaches. The hypertension is related in some unknown manner to the increased sodium reabsorption. *Potassium depletion* is responsible for the major complaints of muscle weakness and fatigue and is related to the effect of intra- and extracellular potassium ion depletion on muscle membrane. The muscle weakness is most striking in the legs and may progress to transient paralysis. Muscles innervated by cranial nerves are usually spared. Most patients have nocturnal polyuria due to a vasopressin-insensitive, potassium-depletion-induced nephropathy. The polyuria results from impairment of concentrating ability and is often associated with polydipsia. These patients may have electrocardiographic and roentgenographic signs of left ventricular enlargement secondary to their hypertension, and hypertensive retinopathy is often seen but papilledema is absent. Electrocardiographic signs of potassium depletion such as prominent U waves are often present. In the absence of associated congestive heart failure, renal disease, or preexisting abnormalities (such as thrombophlebitis), edema is characteristically absent in these patients.

In cases of long duration, potassium-depletion nephropathy becomes manifest, with azotemia, often with superimposed bacilluria, and in some instances with congestive heart failure and edema.

Laboratory findings Laboratory findings are dependent on both the duration and the severity of the potassium depletion. On examination of the urine, negative to trace amounts of protein are found, sometimes with superimposed pyuria and bacilluria, presumably because of the predilection of potassium-depleted kidneys for infection. Urine specific gravity is low (less than 1.015), and an overnight concentration test with simultaneous vasopressin administration reveals impaired ability to concentrate the urine. Urine pH is often neutral to alkaline, because of excessive secretion of ammonium and bicarbonate ions; potassium depletion may lower the maximal tubular transfer rate for bicarbonate. Urine 17-hydroxycorticosteroid and 17-ketosteroid excretion levels are always within the normal range in patients with aldosteronomas but may occasionally be elevated in those rare instances of primary aldosteronism due to adrenal carcinoma. Mild azotemia is an inconstant finding.

Serial blood sampling usually reveals *hypokalemia* and sometimes hypernatremia. Serial blood sampling is stressed. The hypokalemia may be severe (less than 3 mEq potassium per liter) and reflects significant body potassium depletion, usually in excess of 300 mEq. *Hypernatremia* is due to both sodium retention and a concomitant water loss from polyuria. The serum bicarbonate level may be elevated as a result of hydrogen ion loss into the urine and migration into potassium-depleted cells, with alkalosis then developing. The alkalosis is perpetuated with potassium deficiency, since such deficiency increases the capacity of the proximal convoluted tubule to reabsorb filtered bicarbonate. This alkalosis predisposes to signs and symptoms of tetany. If hypokalemia is severe, serum magnesium levels will be reduced. In the absence of azotemia, serum uric acid concentration is normal.

Salivary sodium potassium ratios are reduced in the majority of cases, as is thermal sweat sodium concentration.

Total body sodium content is increased, but not to the degree seen in edematous states. Total exchangeable sodium is moderately elevated, and total exchangeable body potassium is usually, but not invariably, reduced. The volume of extracellular fluid is expanded in most cases, with expansion of plasma volume in many. The expanded extracellular fluid volume is thought to be responsible for the reversed diurnal excretory pattern for salt and water that many of these patients exhibit, with predominant salt and water excretion occurring during the night.

Diagnosis of primary aldosteronism The major criteria which permit the clinician to derive an unequivocal diagnosis of primary aldosteronism are (1) diastolic hypertension without edema; (2) hypersecretion of aldosterone which fails to be suppressed appropriately during volume expansion (salt loading); (3) hyposecretion of renin (as judged by low plasma renin activity levels) which fails to increase appropriately during volume depletion (upright posture); (4) hypokalemia and/or inappropriate urine potassium loss.

Diastolic hypertension is a prerequisite for the diagnosis of primary aldosteronism, even though transient periods of relative normotension may be observed during long-term evaluation. Diastolic hypertension exhibited by patients with primary aldosteronism does not differ from the labile variety of essential hypertension. Blood pressure readings characteristically become reduced after hospitalization, but moderate to severe rises may occur in hospital and are often related to emotional situations. Accelerated (sustained) diastolic hypertension is uncommon but has been reported.

Patients with primary aldosteronism characteristically *do not have edema,* since they are exhibiting a perpetuated "escape" phenomenon. Since they are in a chronic state of escape from the sodium-retaining aspects of mineralocorticoids, they characteristically excrete an administered salt load with a greater rapidity than do normotensive subjects, a characteristic which is shared by patients having essential hypertension. Only a limited sodium retention occurs when patients with primary aldosteronism are given sodium-retaining hormones parenterally. Rarely in patients with associated potassium-depletion nephropathy and azotemia, pretibial edema may be present.

Estimation of plasma renin activity has been valuable in separating patients with primary aldosteronism from those with other causes of hypertension. The failure of plasma renin activity to rise normally during volume-depletion maneuvers (e.g., sodium depletion, diuretic administration, hemorrhage, and/or ambulation) has been a major diagnostic criterion for primary aldosteronism. This is in contrast to what occurs in some hypertensive patients in whom hyperaldosteronism is secondary to *increased* renin levels. However, suppressed renin activity is not diagnostic of primary aldosteronism, as it occurs in about 25 percent of patients with essential hypertension, in patients with hyperaldosteronism secondary to idiopathic bilateral nodular adrenal hyperplasia, and in other mineralocorticoid excess syndromes, including deoxycorticosterone-secreting adrenal tumors.

Since the determination of plasma renin responsiveness is not sufficient, measurement of lack of suppression of aldosterone secretion is necessary to diagnose primary aldosteronism properly. The autonomy exhibited by aldosterone tumors in these patients refers only to their resistance to suppression of hypersecretion during volume expansion; such tumors can and do respond either in normal or supernormal fashion to the stimuli of potassium loading or ACTH infusion. Patients with primary aldosteronism do not respond to volume expansion since their renin-angiotensin system is already suppressed. Appropriate suppression testing may be carried out by saline loading, oral salt loading, or DOCA administration (see Mineralocorticoid Suppression Tests, earlier in this chapter). The autonomy of these tumors to volume expansion is not necessarily complete; many patients with primary aldosteronism will demonstrate some decrease of hypersecretion of aldosterone during volume expansion maneuvers, but such decreases are significantly less than the expected normal response. In some patients apparent suppression of plasma or urinary levels of aldosterone in response to saline loading may be produced by the associated kaliuresis and hypokalemia.

A major criterion for the diagnosis of primary aldosteronism is the demonstration of *hypokalemia* associated with an inappropriately high urine potassium excretion. Judgments as to the significance of a given degree of hypokalemia for a given rate of urine potassium excretion must take into account the patient's potassium and sodium intake. Patients with hypokalemia secondary to diuretics, laxatives, etc., will generally have a 24-hr urine potassium excretion of less than 40 mEq per day, and often the value is markedly less than this. Most patients with primary aldosteronism, on the other hand, with a potassium intake of 100 mEq per day will have a 24-hr urine potassium excretion of greater than 40 mEq per day. Since potassium excretion can be modified by manipulations in sodium intake, this latter factor must be taken into consideration. During periods of high sodium intake, delivery of sodium ions to the distal tubular sodium-potassium exchange site will be increased, resulting in a rise in potassium excretion over control values. Contrariwise, potassium excretion can be minimized for any degree of hypokalemia by restriction of sodium intake, which limits the amount of sodium reaching the distal tubular exchange site. Patients with primary aldosteronism will always exhibit inappropriate urine potassium losses during either saline or oral salt loading procedures.

Precise localization of aldosterone-producing adenomas may be determined preoperatively in many cases by the technique of percutaneous transfemoral bilateral adrenal vein catheterization with simultaneous adrenal arteriography and venography. Such a technique permits radiologic localization, and, in addition, the adrenal vein sampling may demonstrate a two- to threefold increase in plasma aldosterone concentration on the involved side compared with the uninvolved side. A flow chart for evaluation of patients with suspected primary aldosteronism is presented in Fig. 86-11.

Differential diagnosis All patients with *accelerated hypertension* and hypokalemia must be evaluated for unilateral renal disease. If such a diagnosis is confirmed, an additional diagnosis of primary aldosteronism is unlikely, although in rare instances both have been recorded

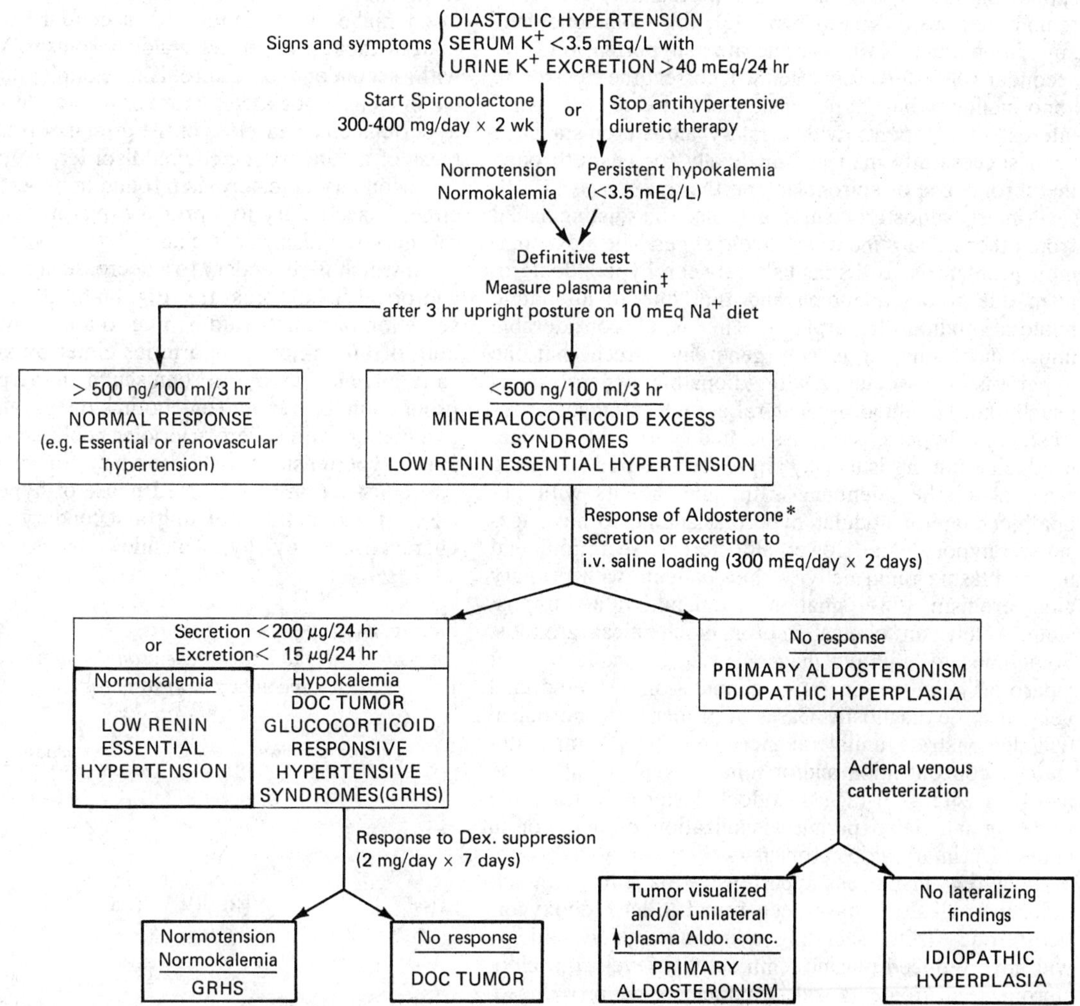

FIGURE 86-11
Diagnostic flow chart for evaluating patients with suspected primary aldosteronism. Identification of the hydroxylase deficiency in glucocorticoid-responsive hypertensive syndromes (GRHS) is the measurement of increased excretion of certain urinary metabolites of intermediates of cortisol biosynthesis (see Table 86-5).
** Alternative methods producing comparable suppression of aldosterone secretion include oral sodium loading (200 mEq per day × 5 days) or 10 mg deoxycorticosterone acetate (DOCA) intramuscularly q.12h. × 3 days.*
‡ An alternative outpatient method is the response of plasma renin activity to 3 hr of upright activity following 80 mg furosemide given the day before.

to occur simultaneously. A useful maneuver in distinguishing between secondary aldosteronism due to accelerated hypertension and primary aldosteronism is to monitor serum potassium levels and aldosterone secretion (or excretory rates) prior to and following therapeutic correction of the hypertension. In patients with accelerated hypertension and secondary aldosteronism, the aldosteronism will subside with successful antihypertensive therapy, i.e., aldosterone parameters will return to normal and the hypokalemia and/or alkalosis will disappear. In distinct contrast, patients with primary aldosteronism in whom successful blood pressure reduction is undertaken will continue to exhibit hypokalemic alkalosis with hypersecretion of aldosterone. An additional maneuver is sometimes useful. This is based on the observation of Melby that the majority of patients with primary aldosteronism become normotensive and normokalemic when treated with the aldosterone antagonist, spironolactone, when given in a dose of 50 to 100 mg every 6 to 8 hr daily over a period of 2 to 5 weeks. Some patients with essential hypertension also become normotensive, so a positive response to spironolactone is not diagnostic of primary aldosteronism. Most of these responsive patients with essential hypertension have "low-renin hypertension" (see Chap. 245). Spironolactone therapy in patients with accelerated hypertension and secondary aldosteronism often will correct the electrolyte abnormalities, but hypertension will persist. It is of interest that patients with primary aldosteronism have been successfully managed medically for years through the chronic use of spironolactone therapy.

Primary aldosteronism must also be distinguished from other *hypermineralocorticoid states.* The most common problem is to distinguish between hyperaldosteronism due to an adenoma and that due to idiopathic bilateral nodular hyperplasia. This is of considerable importance, since it is now generally agreed that the hypertension associated with idiopathic hyperplasia is usually not benefited by bilateral adrenalectomy. In contrast, the hypertension associated with aldosterone-producing tumors is usually improved or cured following removal of the adenoma. Although patients with idiopathic bilateral nodular hyperplasia tend to have less severe hypokalemia, lower aldosterone secretion, and higher plasma renin activity than patients with primary aldosteronism, differentiation is difficult, if not impossible, solely on clinical and/or biochemical grounds. Sometimes a definitive diagnosis can be made only at laparotomy, but preoperative cannulation of the adrenal veins may be diagnostic. Cases of primary aldosteronism will demonstrate unilateral increments in plasma aldosterone concentration and/or tumor visualization on the involved site. ^{131}I-tagged iodocholesterol scintillation scanning may also permit visualization of a tumor in cases of primary aldosteronism.

In a few instances, hypertensive patients with hypokalemic alkalosis have been found to have deoxycorticosterone (DOC)-secreting adenomas. Such patients will have reduced plasma renin activity levels, but aldosterone measurements will be either normal or reduced, suggesting the diagnosis of mineralocorticoid excess due to a hormone other than aldosterone. Rare cases of hypermineralocorticoidism due to a defect in cortisol biosynthesis, specifically 11 or 17 hydroxylation, have also been reported. ACTH levels are increased, with a resultant increase in the production of the mineralocorticoid 11-deoxycorticosterone. *Hypertension and hypokalemia can be corrected by glucocorticoid administration.* The definitive diagnosis is made by demonstrating an elevation of urinary metabolites of precursors of cortisol biosynthesis (Table 86-5). Occasionally, glucocorticoid administration will produce normotension and normokalemia although a hydroxylase deficiency cannot be identified (Fig. 86-11).

Licorice ingestion produces a syndrome mimicking primary aldosteronism. Licorice contains a sodium-retaining principle, glycyrrhizinic acid, which causes sodium retention, expansion of the extracellular fluid volume, hypertension, depressed plasma renin levels, and suppressed aldosterone levels. The diagnosis is excluded by a careful history.

SECONDARY ALDOSTERONISM Secondary aldosteronism refers to an appropriately increased production of aldosterone by the adrenal gland in response to stimuli originating outside the gland (Fig. 86-12). In all reported cases, the stimulus has been the renin-angiotensin system. The adrenal production rates of aldosterone are often higher in patients with secondary aldosteronism than in those with primary aldosteronism. Most patients with secondary aldosteronism exhibit this syndrome either as an associated feature of the accelerated phase of hypertension (regardless of the primary disease) or on the basis of an underlying edema disorder.

Secondary aldosteronism found in hypertensive states either is secondary to a primary overproduction of renin (primary reninism) or is caused by an overproduction of renin which is secondary to a decrease in renal blood flow and/or perfusion pressure (Fig. 86-6). Secondary hypersecretion of renin could be due to a narrowing of one or both of the major renal arteries either by an atherosclerotic plaque or by fibromuscular hyperplasia. Overproduction of renin from both kidneys also occurs in association with severe arteriolar nephrosclerosis (malignant hypertension) or secondary to profound renal vasoconstriction (accelerated phase of hypertensive disease). These patients exhibit a secondary aldosteronism characterized by hypokalemic alkalosis, absence of

FIGURE 86-12
Responses of the renin-aldosterone volume control loop in primary versus secondary aldosteronism.

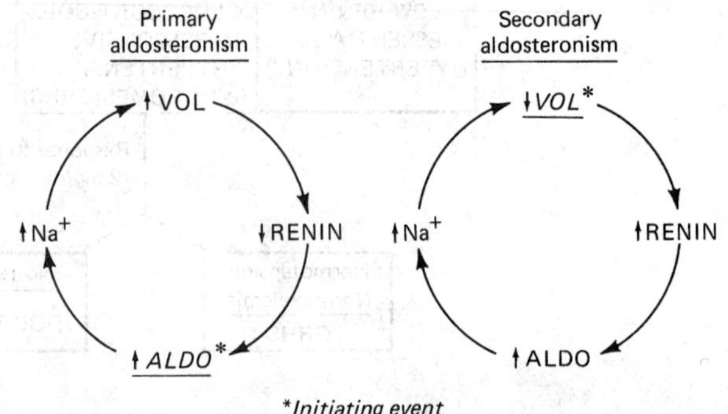

edema, moderate to severe increases in plasma renin activity, and moderate to marked increases in aldosterone secretion/excretion rates (see Chap. 245).

Secondary aldosteronism with hypertension is also associated with the rare renin-producing tumor, so-called primary reninism. These patients have all the biochemical characteristics of renal vascular hypertension; however, the primary defect is not a decrease in renal blood flow and/or perfusion pressure but a primary increase in renin secretion. The diagnosis can be made by the absence of changes in renal vasculature and/or the presence of a space-occupying lesion seen by renal arteriography, with unilateral increases in renal vein renin activity. A second differential test is the change in renin activity when the patient assumes the upright posture. Patients with primary reninism characteristically have a very brisk increase in renin activity in contrast to patients with other forms of secondary aldosteronism.

Secondary aldosteronism is present in most *edema* disorders. Edema may be said to be the cardinal finding on physical examination for the presence of secondary aldosteronism. Hypersecretion of aldosterone in such clinical states correlates best with the phases of rapid accumulation of edema fluid. During phases of stable body weight, aldosterone measurements are often reported to be within the normal range.

Increased aldosterone secretion rates have been amply documented in patients who form edema as a result of either cirrhosis or the nephrotic syndrome. In congestive heart failure, however, elevated aldosterone secretion is a variable finding. The stimulus for aldosterone release in these clinical conditions appears to be *arterial hypovolemia.* Arterial blood volume may be depleted in cirrhosis as a result of decreased hepatic protein synthesis and protein loss into ascitic fluid; likewise, urine protein losses in the nephrotic syndrome may lead to arterial hypovolemia. Despite venous congestion, arterial hypovolemia may occur in congestive heart failure as a result of a failing cardiac output. The finding of normal aldosterone secretory rates in some patients with congestive heart failure requires explanation. It has been shown that approximately 95 percent of the circulating blood aldosterone is removed from the plasma and metabolized or extracted by the liver during a single passage. The rate of removal of aldosterone from plasma is termed its *metabolic clearance rate,* and since aldosterone is almost exclusively "cleared" by the liver, hepatic blood flow will approximate the aldosterone clearance rate. Since the blood level of circulating aldosterone is presumed to be the critical factor in its biologic activity, it is to be appreciated that the blood level will be determined by both the aldosterone secretion rate and the rate of hepatic inactivation. Thus, in clinical states characterized by reduced hepatic blood flow, such as congestive heart failure, an increased blood circulating aldosterone level can occur and result in sodium retention, even though the secretion rate of the hormone is within the normal range. Patients with secondary aldosteronism due to edema disorders differ qualitatively from normal subjects and from patients with primary aldosteronism, in that they fail to exhibit a normal "escape" pattern in response to the chronic administration of DOC. These patients are exquisitely sensitive to the sodium-retaining properties of the mineralocorticoids and will exhibit a profound decrease in urine sodium excretion, often to barely detectable levels. They retain excess salt and water, but this retained fluid is ineffective in terms of reexpanding what is registered by the renin-angiotensin system as a deficient circulating blood volume. Instead, the excess salt and water that are retained accumulate in increasing quantities as edema fluid. Diuretic therapy often exaggerates the features of secondary aldosteronism via the mechanism of acute volume depletion; when this happens hypokalemia and on occasion alkalosis become prominent features.

Secondary hyperaldosteronism may rarely occur without edema or hypertension (Bartter's syndrome). This syndrome is characterized by the signs of severe hyperaldosteronism (hypokalemic alkalosis) with moderate to marked increases in renin activity but normal blood pressure and absence of edema. Renal biopsy shows juxtaglomerular hyperplasia. The pathogenesis of this syndrome is obscure, but many patients have a defect in the renal conservation of sodium. The renal loss of sodium is thought to stimulate renin secretion and subsequently aldosterone production. Hyperaldosteronism produces potassium depletion, with the hypokalemia further elevating plasma renin activity. In some cases, the hypokalemia may be potentiated by a defect in renal conservation of potassium. It has also been proposed that in some of these patients the lack of hypertension is due to vascular unresponsiveness to angiotensin. Whether this is a primary event or simply secondary to the altered metabolic state is unclear.

ADRENAL VIRILISM

INTRODUCTION The adrenal virilizing syndromes result from excessive productions of adrenal androgens, such as dehydroepiandrosterone and Δ4-androstenedione, which are converted to testosterone; the elevated testosterone levels account for most of the virilization. As in other states of adrenocortical hyperfunction, the syndrome may result from hyperplasia, adenoma, or carcinoma. It also may arise in a congenital form, termed *adrenogenital hyperplasia,* due to enzymatic deficits. The adrenal virilizing syndromes may be associated with secretions of greater or smaller amounts of other adrenal hormones and may, therefore, present as "pure" syndromes of virilization or as "mixed" syndromes associated with excessive production of glucocorticoid and some of the characteristics of Cushing's syndrome. In *congenital* adrenal hyperplasia the virilizing syndrome may be associated with either excessive or decreased secretion of mineralocorticoid or decreased production of glucocorticoid.

Since in man hydrocortisone is the principal adrenal steroid regulating ACTH elaboration, and since ACTH stimulates both hydrocortisone and adrenal androgen production, it stands to reason that an enzymatic interference with hydrocortisone synthesis may result in the enhanced secretion of adrenal androgens. In severe congenital virilizing hyperplasia, the adrenal output of hydrocortisone may be so compromised as to cause clinical evidence of glucocorticoid deficiency despite anatomic adrenal hyperplasia. Conversely, a high hydrocortisone output as the result of primary adrenal disease (adenoma) may inhibit ACTH secretion and thus result in a low adrenal androgen output.

INCIDENCE Congenital bilateral adrenocortical hyperplasia is by far the most common adrenal disorder of infancy and childhood. It has also been described later in life, predominantly in women. Its appearance in postpuberal men would obviously not be as clinically apparent; nevertheless, it has been reported. In its various forms, adrenogenital hyperplasia is thought to be related to a defective autosomal recessive gene. The most common form of significant "noncongenital" adrenal virilization is that seen with bilateral adrenocortical hyperplasia and is most frequently associated with various degrees of excessive production of glucocorticoid hormone and the clinical signs and symptoms of Cushing's syndrome.

CLINICAL SIGNS AND SYMPTOMS The congenital form of adrenal hyperplasia is secondary to a defect in steroid enzymatic activity. To date, defects have been described in the C-21, C-18, C-17, and C-11 hydroxylase enzymes, as well as in the 3β-ol-dehydrogenase enzyme. These enzyme deficits usually occur singly. The clinical expression of these enzyme deficiencies is variable, ranging from virilization of the female (C-21 deficiency) to feminization of the male (3β-ol-dehydrogenase deficiency).

Adrenal virilization in the female at birth is associated with ambiguous external genitalia (*female pseudohermaphroditism*). Adrenal virilism due to congenital adrenal hyperplasia in the male is manifested by premature virilization (*isosexual precocity*). The age of onset of virilization is most probably prenatal, after the fifth month of embryonic development. At birth there may be macrogenitosomia in the male infant, and in the female, enlargement of the clitoris, partial or complete fusion of the labia, and sometimes a urogenital sinus. If the labial fusion is nearly complete, the female infant will have external genitalia resembling a penis with hypospadias, changes consistent with female pseudohermaphroditism. Chromosomal sex can be determined by examination of oral mucosal smears or leukocyte cultures. In the *postnatal* period from infancy to adolescence, congenital adrenal hyperplasia will be associated with virilization in the female and isosexual precocity in the male. The excessive androgens produced will result in accelerated growth, with height age exceeding chronologic age. Since epiphyseal closure is hastened by excessive androgens, growth stops but truncal development continues, giving the characteristic appearance of a child of short stature with well-developed trunk. Incomplete variants of congenital adrenal hyperplasia sometimes become manifest only in adult life, with virilization or hirsutism occurring in the female.

In the adult female, regardless of the cause of the condition, the clinical signs and symptoms are those anticipated from excessive androgen production. These include hirsutism, acne, increased sebum production, temporal baldness, deepening of voice, increased muscle mass and strength, decreased breast size, atrophy of the uterus, amenorrhea, enlargement of the clitoris, increased heterosexual drive, and development of a male habitus. The clinical distinction between excessive hair growth (hirsutism) and virilization is useful. Virilization signifies that multiple signs of androgen excess are present in addition to hirsutism; one of the more easily recognized of these signs is hypertrophy of the clitoris. Hirsutism in the absence of other signs of virilization is uncommon in these patients. The virilizing syndromes are difficult to document in the *adult* male, for obvious reasons.

The most common form of congenital adrenal hyperplasia (95 percent of cases) is due to impairment of *C-21 hydroxylation.* There are reduced conversion of 17-hydroxyprogesterone to 11-deoxycortisol and thus reduced formation of cortisol from 11-deoxycortisol (Fig. 86-2). In addition to cortisol deficiency, in approximately one-third of the patients, there is an associated reduction in aldosterone secretion as a result of impaired C-21 hydroxylation of progesterone to 11-deoxycorticosterone, a precursor of aldosterone. Thus, with congenital adrenal hyperplasia secondary to C-21 hydroxylase deficiency, adrenal virilization will be present with or without an associated salt-losing tendency due to aldosterone deficiency. The accumulation of progesterone may also exaggerate any salt-losing tendency, since progesterone has an antialdosterone effect on renal tubular salt conservation. Since a cortisol deficiency exists, the adrenal glands become hyperplastic because of excessive ACTH stimulation. It is probable that the C-21 hydroxylase enzymes, rather than being identical, are isoenzymes. Rather than representing the severity of the enzyme deficiency, the difference between the salt-losing variety and the non-salt-losing variety may reside in whether the genetic abnormality involves one or both of these isoenzymes. As a result of the C-21 hydroxylase deficit, precursor products accumulate and are shunted into alternate pathways of metabolism, chiefly the androgen pathways, accounting for the hypersecretion of dehydroepiandrosterone and androstenedione and its 11 β-hydroxylated derivatives. The conversion peripherally of androstenedione to testosterone produces high levels of this potent androgen (Table 86-5).

With a *C-11 hydroxylase* deficiency a "hypertensive" variant of congenital adrenal hyperplasia develops with cortisol deficiency, since there is impaired conversion of 11-deoxycortisol to cortisol. Hypertension and hypokalemia occur because of the impaired conversion of 11-deoxycorticosterone to corticosterone, resulting in the accumulation of 11-deoxycorticosterone, a potent mineralocorticoid. Increased shunting again occurs into the androgen pathway.

The *C-17 hydroxylase* syndrome is characterized by hypogonadism and hypertension. In patients with this deficiency there is decreased production of cortisol with increased production of progesterone and its metabolite pregnanediol. There is shunting into the mineralocorticoid pathway with hypokalemic alkalosis, hypertension, and suppressed plasma renin activity. In most patients, 11-deoxycorticosterone and corticosterone productions are elevated, while aldosterone secretion is low. The subnormal production of aldosterone in some but not all patients with this syndrome may be related to an associated C-18 hydroxylase deficiency. However, in most patients, it is probably secondary to hypokalemia, intraadrenal regulation of aldosterone biosynthesis by precursor products, or the suppressed renin activity, since treatment restores aldosterone secretion to normal. Because C-17 hydroxylation is required for biosynthesis of adrenal androgens as well as gonadal testosterone and estrogen, this defect is associated with sexual immaturity, high urinary gonadotropin levels, and low urinary 17-ketosteroid excretion. Female patients have primary amenorrhea and lack of development of secondary sexual characteristics. Because of deficient androgen production, male patients have ambiguous external genitalia (male pseudohermaphroditism). Exogenous glucocorticoids can correct the hypertensive syndrome, but sex hormones are necessary to produce sexual maturation.

With the rare *3β-ol-dehydrogenase* deficiency, there is impaired conversion of pregnenolone to progesterone, with the result that pathways to both cortisol and aldosterone are "blocked," with shunting then occurring into the adrenal androgen pathway via 17α-hydroxypregnenolone to dehydroepiandrosterone. Since dehydroepiandrosterone is a weak androgen and because this enzyme deficiency is also present in the gonad, the genitalia of the male fetus may be ambiguous or feminized. Conversely, in the female, overproduction of dehydroepiandrosterone may produce virilization.

DIAGNOSIS The diagnosis of adrenal virilism due to *congenital adrenal hyperplasia* should be considered in all infants exhibiting "failure to thrive," particularly those having episodes of acute adrenal insufficiency or having sustained hypertension. The diagnosis is further suggested by the finding of hypertrophy of the clitoris, fused labia, or urogenital sinus in the female and isosexual precocity in the male infant. In infants and children with a *C-21 hydroxylation block,* increased urine 17-ketosteroid excretion is typically associated with an increase in the excretion of pregnanetriol, which is a metabolite of 17α-hydroxyprogesterone. These children will show low urine 17-hydroxycorticoid excretion levels and elevated levels of plasma ACTH. Ketogenic steroid excretion will be elevated, since the depressed 17-hydroxycorticoid excretion is more than offset by increments in pregnanetriol excretion, which metabolite is included in the analysis. On testing with ACTH, the altered metabolic pathways are exaggerated, with sharp rises occurring in 17-ketosteroid excretion and little or no rise in 17-hydroxycorticoid excretion (Table 86-5).

The diagnosis of a *salt-losing form* of congenital adrenal hyperplasia due to defects in both C-21 hydroxylase enzymes is suggested by episodes of acute adrenal insufficiency with hyponatremia, hyperkalemia, dehydration, and vomiting. These infants and children often "crave" salt and exhibit laboratory signs of concomitant deficits in both cortisol and aldosterone secretion.

With the *hypertensive form* of congenital adrenal hyperplasia due to impaired C-11 hydroxylation, the precursor 11-deoxycortisol will accumulate. As a result, both urine 17-keto- and 17-hydroxycorticoid excretion may be elevated, since 11-deoxycortisol would be included in the analysis of Porter-Silber chromogens. The diagnosis is secured by demonstrating increased amounts of tetrahydro-11-deoxycortisol in the urine with decreased amounts of tetrahydro metabolites of cortisol.

The finding of very high levels of urine dehydroepiandrosterone with low levels of pregnanetriol and of cortisol metabolites is characteristic of patients with congenital adrenal hyperplasia due to 3β-ol-dehydrogenase deficiency. These patients also exhibit marked salt wasting.

The *C-17 hydroxylase* deficiency results in the accumulation of progesterone and its metabolite, pregnanediol. The excretion of deoxycorticosterone and of corticosterone is increased, while aldosterone production is usually subnormal. In some patients aldosterone secretion is elevated.

The adrenal virilizing syndrome in adults is most often due to noncongenital causes—namely, tumor or adrenal hyperplasia. *Adrenal adenomas* and *carcinomas* may cause a pure or mixed virilizing syndrome. Since adrenal androgens are weak compared with gonadal androgens, adrenal virilization is characterized by *large increments in urine 17-ketosteroid excretion,* often with less impressive

TABLE 86-5
Urine excretory products in congenital adrenal hyperplasia

Deficiency	*17-KS*	*17-OH*	*THS*	*Pregnanetriol*	*Pregnanediol*	*THDOC*	*THB*	*Aldosterone*
C-21 hydroxylase deficiency:								
Salt-losing	I	N–D	N–D	I	I	D	D	D
Non-salt-losing	I	N–D	N–D	I	N–I	N–I	N–I	N–I
C-11 hydroxylase deficiency	I	I	I	I	N–I	I	D	D
C-17 hydroxylase deficiency	N–D	N–D	N–D	N–D	I	I	I	D–I
C-17 and C-18 hydroxylase deficiency	N–D	N–D	N–D	N–D	I	I	I	D
3β-ol-Dehydrogenase deficiency	I	N–D	N–D	N–D	N–D	N–D	N–D	N–D

Note: THS, tetrahydro 11-deoxycortisol; THDOC, tetrahydro 11-deoxycorticosterone; THB, tetrahydrocorticosterone; I, increased; N, normal; D, decreased.

clinical signs of virilism. Virilizing adrenocortical adenomas are rare. They produce very high levels of urinary 17-ketosteroids, often greater than 200 mg per day, and are associated with no rise or only a slight rise in urine 17-hydroxysteroids. They may or may not be sensitive to ACTH stimulation and likewise may or may not be sensitive to dexamethasone suppression. *Virilizing adrenal carcinomas* are the most common adrenal tumor causing virilization. They are associated with high urinary 17-ketosteroid excretion, reaching 100 mg or more per 24 hr, and may have normal or a moderate rise in 17-hydroxycorticosteroid excretion. They characteristically show no increase in steroid excretion upon stimulation with ACTH, and also characteristically fail to be suppressed with dexamethasone administration. These tumors are often associated with marked virilization of sudden onset. The very high ketosteroid excretion of both virilizing adenomas and carcinomas is made up in large part of the weak androgen dehydroepiandrosterone, which has approximately 5 percent of the androgenicity of testosterone. Functioning adrenocortical carcinomas are characteristically associated with elevated urinary excretion of metabolites of precursors of steroid biosynthesis (such as pregnanetriol and tetrahydro-11 deoxycortisol), probably representing inefficient conversion of intermediate compounds to the final product. The clinical differentiation between virilizing adrenal adenoma and carcinoma is tenuous and cannot be made with certainty preoperatively.

In adrenocortical hyperfunction of Cushing's syndrome, both urinary 17-ketosteroid and 17-hydroxycorticosteroid base-line values will be elevated. Adrenal hyperactivity associated with hirsutism but with normal 17-hydroxycorticosteroid base-line excretion (sometimes termed benign androgenic hyperplasia) represents an ill-defined, controversial, heterogeneous group of patients. Mild hirsutism usually appears after puberty and is characterized by normal or moderately elevated urinary 17-ketosteroids. With ACTH stimulation, there is a brisk rise in the urinary 17-ketosteroids when compared to the 17-hydroxycorticosteroids. Base-line 17-ketosteroids are easily suppressed by daily administration of 2 mg of dexamethasone. Some if not all of these patients may represent a mild form of congenital adrenal hyperplasia. A flow chart for evaluation of patients with excessive androgen production is presented in Fig. 86-13.

DIFFERENTIAL DIAGNOSIS In the female, the differential diagnosis of hirsutism and virilization is between adrenal and ovarian etiologies (Table 86-6; Fig. 86-13). *Sudden onset of progressive hirsutism and virilization* suggests an adrenal or ovarian neoplasm. Since adrenal tumors secrete weak androgens (such as DHEA), virilizing adrenal neoplasms are characterized by high urine 17-ketosteroid excretion, usually in excess of 30 to 40 mg per 24 hr. Failure to reduce 17-ketosteroid levels to normal following dexamethasone suppression (0.5 mg p.o. q.6h. × 7 days) supports a diagnosis of virilizing adrenal tumor and excludes congenital adrenal hyperplasia. The most common *ovarian tumor* causing virilization is the arrhenoblastoma, but other ovarian tumors, such as adrenal rest tumor, granulosa-cell tumor, hilar-cell tumors, and Brenner tumors have been associated with virilization. Virilization due to ovarian tumors is characterized by normal or moderate elevations of urinary 17-ketosteroids, since the neoplasm usually secretes the potent androgen testosterone. Moderate increases in 17-ketosteroid excretion occur in some patients with ovarian neoplasm, but base-line 17-ketosteroid excretion in excess of 30 mg per day is rare with the exception of adrenal rest tumors. Like adrenal neoplasms, ovarian tumors fail to be suppressed by dexamethasone. With the exception of adrenal rest tumors, they are largely independent of ACTH stimulation. Elevations of plasma testosterone or urinary testosterone excretion do not localize the neoplasm to the ovary, since testosterone can be elevated subsequent to peripheral conversion of adrenal precursors, such as DHEA (see Chap. 92).

Hirsutism without virilization beginning after puberty and associated with normal ovarian histology is diagnostic of idiopathic or familial hirsutism. In a second group of patients, hirsutism is seen in association with sclerocystic or polycystic ovaries. Oligomenorrhea, anovulatory bleeding, and/or amenorrhea commonly occur in these patients. The ovaries may be palpably enlarged bilaterally; unilateral enlargement suggests an ovarian neoplasm. Direct inspection of the ovaries by culdoscopy or laparoscopy is a valuable means of differentiating between ovarian and adrenal causes of hirsutism. If normal ovaries are found, an adrenal origin for the virilization is favored. Alternatively, the discovery of polycystic ovaries does not establish an ovarian causation since polycystic ovaries have been described in association with adrenal virilization. In 10 to 15 percent of patients with polycystic ovaries, hirsutism is associated with other signs of virilization. 17-ketosteroid excretion values in hirsute females with polycystic ovary disease or idiopathic hirsutism are usually normal or slightly elevated. *Plasma testosterone* levels tend to be higher in females with polycystic ovary disease than in normal females, but there is overlap. Studies indicate that some women with idiopathic hirsutism or polycystic ovaries probably have increased blood production rates of testosterone *(see p. 495).*

The differential diagnosis of isosexual precocity in young boys includes pineal tumors (Chap. 94), congenital adrenal hyperplasia, testicular neoplasia, hypothalamic-pituitary dysfunction, and hyperplasia of adrenal rest tissue occurring in the epididymis or testis. Testicular adrenal rests secrete high quantities of 17-ketosteroids and operate under ACTH control. Bilateral testicular enlargement occurs in association with hypothalamic-

TABLE 86-6
Causes of hirsutism in females

I Familial
II Idiopathic
III Ovarian
  A Polycystic ovaries; hilus cell hyperplasia
  B Tumor: arrhenoblastoma, hilus cell, adrenal rest
IV Adrenal
  A Congenital adrenal hyperplasia
  B Noncongenital adrenal hyperplasia (Cushing's)
  C Tumor: virilizing carcinoma or adenoma

pituitary lesions (because of stimulation of gonadotropin secretion), as well as with aberrant adrenal rest tissue. Unilateral testicular enlargement with contralateral atrophy usually is seen with true interstitial tumors. In congenital adrenal hyperplasia, the testes remain infantile although the patient is virilized.

TREATMENT Treatment of adrenal virilism is dictated by the type of lesion suspected. Patients with *congenital adrenal hyperplasia* have the fundamental defect of cortisol deficiency with resultant excessive ACTH stimulation, producing hyperplasia of the adrenal glands and causing additional "shunting" into the adrenal androgen pathway. Therapy in these patients consists of daily administration of glucocorticoids (dexamethasone, prednisone, cortisone, etc.) to suppress pituitary ACTH secretion. Because of its cost and intermediate half-life, prednisone has been the drug of choice except in infants, when hydrocortisone is usually used. The amount of steroid required to manage patients with congenital adrenal hyperplasia effectively is approximately 1.5 times the normal cortisol production rate of 12 to 13 mg cortisol per m^2 per day and is given in divided doses two or three times a day. As the patient grows, the maintenance dose obviously should be increased. The dosage schedule is governed by repetitive analysis of the urinary 17-ketosteroids and skeletal growth and maturation. In children, glucocorticoids not only suppress urinary ketosteroid excretion but also end virilization and the associated problems of hyperandrogenicity. Some infants and children with the associated defect of salt wasting require vigorous correction of salt deficits in conjunction with small doses of a potent mineralocorticoid such as 9α-fluorohydrocortisone. Children born with abnormalities of external genitalia may require surgical correction of labial fusion, urogenital sinus, etc. Diagnosis of the adrenogenital syndrome in the newborn with ambiguous external genitalia is crucial to avoid errors in the assignment of sex. Response of these children to steroid therapy is gratifying in that normal growth and development occur and the menarche and onset of spermatogenesis occur at the appropriate age. Many females with this disorder have married and have borne children. Steroid therapy is indicated throughout life.

In patients with adrenal virilization due to adrenal tumors, prompt surgical intervention with complete exci-

FIGURE 86-13
Diagnostic flow chart for evaluating the status of patients with suspected excess androgen production. Identification of the hydroxylase deficiency in congenital adrenal hyperplasia is the measurement of increased *excretion of certain urinary metabolites of intermediates of cortisol biosynthesis (see Table 86-5).*

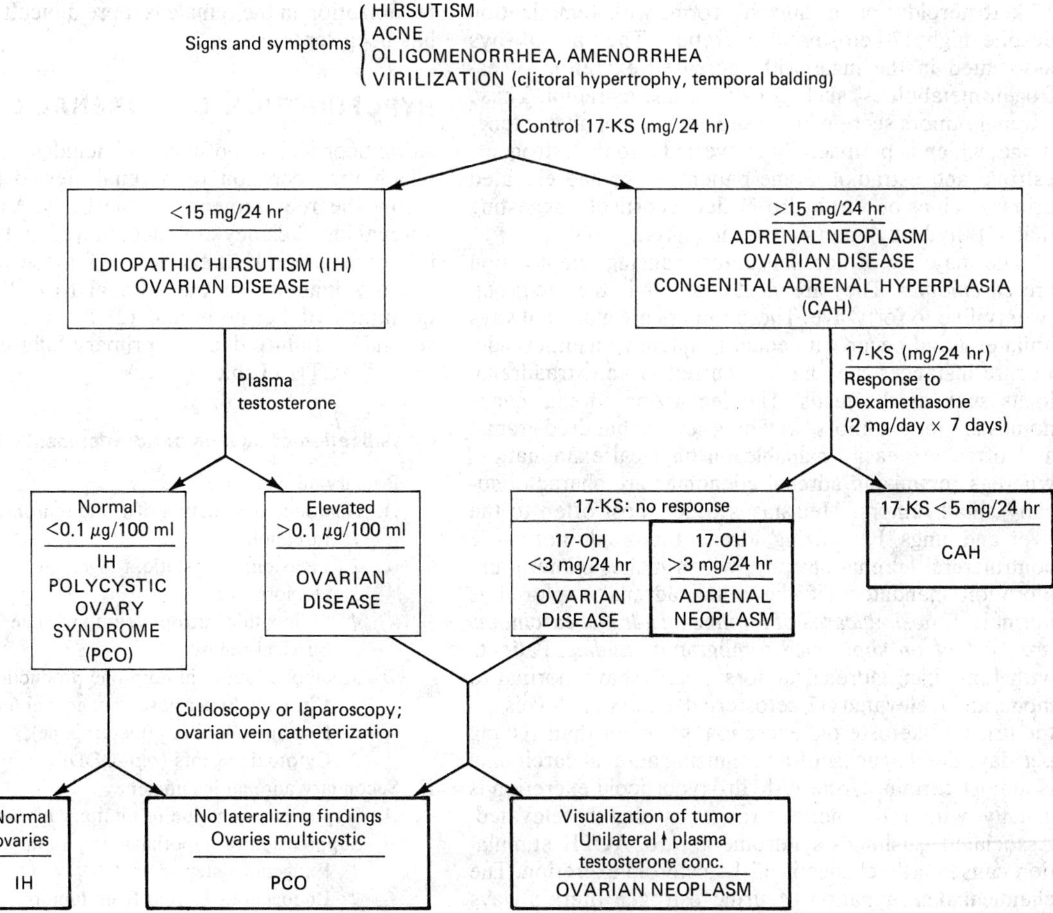

sion of the tumor is indicated. One cannot postpone surgical intervention in patients suspected of having virilizing adrenal adenomas, since such adenomas are practically indistinguishable from adrenal carcinomas, both clinically and biochemically. Preoperative localization of adrenal tumors can be attempted by renal tomography or adrenal angiography. Since "pure" virilizing adrenal tumors do *not* cause contralateral adrenal atrophy, thorough inspection and exploration of both suprarenal areas is mandatory. If metastases have occurred, one may consider the use of antitumor drugs, such as *o,p'*-DDD with or without local irradiation. *o,p'*-DDD in some patients has been associated with striking regression in peripheral metastases, paralleled by a decrease in urinary 17-ketosteroid and 17-hydroxycorticosteroid excretion; however, long-term survival is rare. In some patients given a trial of *o,p'*-DDD, regression of metastases is not seen but a fall in steroid biosynthesis occurs *(see p. 504).*

ADRENAL FEMINIZATION

Adrenal feminization is an exceedingly rare entity and, when present, is almost always due to adrenal tumor. These adrenal tumors will cause feminization in the male, with development of gynecomastia (often with breast tenderness), change in body habitus, testicular atrophy, feminizing hair changes, and loss of libido. They may occur in "pure" form, i.e., with normal levels of urine 17-ketosteroids, or in "mixed" form, with feminization despite high 17-ketosteroid excretion. They are always associated in the male with increased excretion of estrogen metabolites, such as estrone and estradiol. These adrenal tumors secrete increased amounts of androstenedione, which is peripherally converted into the estrogens, estrone and estradiol. Some patients have had elevated urinary values of tetrahydro 11-deoxycortisol, suggesting that 11β-hydroxylation may be impaired.

The majority of adrenal tumors causing feminization are *carcinomas.* They are most common in the age group twenty-five to forty-five. These tumors are almost always unilateral and occur with equal frequency on either side. In rare instances they have occurred in an extraadrenal locus such as the testis. The feminizing adrenal carcinomas are large tumors (weighing several hundred grams) and often are easily palpable on physical examination, whereas feminizing adrenal adenomas are characteristically small tumors. Metastases occur most often to the liver and lungs. Feminizing adrenal tumors do not cause contralateral adrenal atrophy, which makes bilateral exploration mandatory if the initial adrenal explored is normal. *Almost all cases of feminizing adrenal carcinoma are evident on suprarenal tomography studies.* Patients with feminizing adrenal tumors usually have normal to moderately elevated 17-ketosteroid excretion levels. If the urine 17-ketosteroid excretion is greater than 100 mg per day, the diagnosis of a feminizing adrenal carcinoma is almost certain. Urine 17-hydroxycorticoid excretion is usually within the normal range or slightly elevated. Associated Cushing's syndrome is rare. ACTH stimulation causes little change in 17-ketosteroid excretion. The chemical determination of urine estrogen titers always demonstrates an elevated value. The elevated urine estrogen excretion level is principally due to increased estriol and also to increments in estradiol and estrone. Since the estrogens produced by adrenal feminizing tumors are conversion products from androgen precursors, the amount of estrogens elaborated will depend both on the amount of androgen precursors formed and on the efficiency of the androgen-to-estrogen conversion process. Feminizing adrenocortical carcinomas have also been reported to produce gonadotropins (follicle-stimulating hormone and chorionic gonadotropin).

Radiotherapy has not been helpful in treatment. Despite operative intervention, most patients with adrenal feminizing carcinoma die within 3 years of diagnosis. With successful operative removal of feminizing tumors, the urine estrogen titer falls; a failure of the titer to fall or a recurrence of elevated urine titers indicates functioning tumor tissue.

The *diagnosis* of adrenal feminization in the male is strongly suggested by the onset of gynecomastia associated with a flank mass. The additional finding of increased urine estrogen titers confirms the diagnosis. Gynecomastia may also be seen with *testicular tumors* (chorioepithelioma, Sertoli cell, seminoma, interstitial-cell tumor) because of increased production of estrogen by the testes. Estrogen may be secreted by testicular neoplasms, or the tumor may produce chorionic gonadotropins, with an associated elaboration of estrogens by the testes. The course of feminizing adrenal and testicular neoplasms that also synthesize gonadotropins should be followed by urinary gonadotropin as well as estrogen titers. Adrenal feminization in the female is more difficult to detect, but it has been reported.

HYPOFUNCTION OF ADRENAL CORTEX

Adrenocortical hypofunction includes all conditions in which the secretion of adrenal steroid hormones falls below the requirements of the body. Various types of adrenal insufficiency are encountered and may be divided into two general categories: (1) those associated with primary inability of the adrenal to elaborate sufficient quantities of hormone and (2) those associated with a secondary failure due to a primary failure in the elaboration of ACTH (Table 86-7).

TABLE 86-7
Classification of causes of adrenal insufficiency

I Primary adrenal insufficiency
- *A* Anatomic destruction of gland (chronic and acute)
  - *1* Infection
  - *2* Invasion: metastatic, fungal, etc.
  - *3* Hemorrhage
  - *4* "Idiopathic" atrophy, autoimmune
  - *5* Surgical removal
- *B* Metabolic failure in hormone production
  - *1* Virilizing hyperplasia, congenital (certain types)
  - *2* Enzyme inhibitors (metyrapone)
  - *3* Cytotoxic agents (*o,p'*-DDD)

II Secondary adrenal insufficiency
- *A* Hypopituitarism due to pituitary disease
- *B* Suppression of hypothalamic-pituitary axis
  - *1* Exogenous steroid
  - *2* Endogenous steroid from tumors

PRIMARY ADRENOCORTICAL DEFICIENCY (ADDISON'S DISEASE)

This disorder is also called Addison's disease or chronic glucocorticoid deficiency. Addison's classic description in 1855, namely, "general languor and debility, remarkable feebleness of the heart's action, irritability of the stomach, and a peculiar change of the color of the skin," summarizes the dominant clinical features of the disease. Advanced cases usually cause little difficulty in diagnosis, but recognition of the disease in its earlier phases may present a real challenge. The disease, when unrecognized and untreated, carries an almost uniformly poor and frequently fatal prognosis. Early diagnosis is important, since present-day therapy provides complete correction of the metabolic derangement.

INCIDENCE Primary adrenocortical insufficiency is relatively rare. It may occur at any age in life and affects both sexes with equal frequency. Because of increasing therapeutic use of exogenous steroids, secondary adrenal insufficiency is seen with increasing frequency.

ETIOLOGY AND PATHOGENESIS Addison's disease results from progressive adrenocortical destruction, which must involve more than 90 percent of the glands before clinical signs of adrenal insufficiency appear. The adrenal is a frequent site for chronic infectious diseases of the granulomatous variety, predominately tuberculosis but also including fungal infections such as histoplasmosis, coccidioidomycosis, and cryptococcosis. In previous years, tuberculosis was found at postmortem examination in 70 to 90 percent of cases; however, the most frequent finding at present is *idiopathic* atrophy, and it has been suggested that an autoimmune mechanism may be responsible for this process. Rarely, other lesions are encountered, such as bilateral tumor metastases, amyloidosis, or sarcoidosis.

The possibility that some patients may have primary adrenal insufficiency on an *autoimmune basis* has been strengthened by the finding that one-half of patients with Addison's disease have complement-fixing and/or circulating adrenal antibodies, as tested by the indirect Coons' method. Certain of these patients also have additional circulating antibodies to thyroid or parathyroid tissue, a finding of interest because of the increased incidence of hypothyroidism and hypoparathyroidism in Addison's disease. It is not clear whether these antibodies cause adrenal atrophy or are secondary to the destruction of adrenal tissue.

In 1926, Schmidt described two patients with nontuberculous Addison's disease and chronic lymphocytic thyroiditis. Subsequent reports have documented association of thyroid insufficiency and Addison's disease, and the possibility of a common autoimmune process has been raised as the etiologic factor responsible for *Schmidt's syndrome.* More than 20 patients have been described with concomitant parathyroid and adrenal insufficiency. In most of these patients, autoantibodies have been discovered, raising the possibility that these two diseases may be related to a common event. Diabetes mellitus has now been reported as being associated with Addison's disease in more than 100 cases. Again, what role genetic predisposition and/or autoimmunity may play in the occurrence of these two diseases in the same individual is unknown. Rarely, the combination of Addison's disease, myxedema, and diabetes mellitus has been described. Between 3 and 4 percent of patients with Addison's disease have coexistent hyperthyroidism. The presence of both disorders in the same individual poses a difficult diagnostic problem, since many of the clinical manifestations are similar. Furthermore, the hyperthyroid state may change a subclinical insufficiency to complete adrenal insufficiency, because of the effect, mentioned above, of thyroid hormone on cortisol metabolism.

Further study of patients with combined endocrine dysfunction may prove valuable in revealing the cause of spontaneous adrenal destruction.

TABLE 86-8
Incidence of symptoms and signs in 125 cases of Addison's disease, percent

Weakness	99	Hypotension (below 110/70)	87
Pigmentation of skin	98	Abdominal pain	34
Pigmentation of mucous membranes	82	Salt craving	22
Weight loss	97	Diarrhea	20
Anorexia, nausea, and vomiting	90	Constipation	19
		Syncope	16
		Vitiligo	9

CLINICAL SIGNS AND SYMPTOMS Adrenocortical insufficiency is most frequently characterized by an insidious onset with slowly progressive fatigability, weakness, anorexia, nausea and vomiting, weight loss, cutaneous and mucosal pigmentation, hypotension, and occasionally hypoglycemia. These signs and symptoms compose the classic syndrome of Addison's disease; however, the spectrum may vary, depending on the duration and degree of adrenal hypofunction, from a complaint of mild chronic fatigue to the fulminating shock associated with acute massive destruction of the glands in the type of syndrome described by Waterhouse and Friderichsen. Table 86-8 lists the incidence of symptoms and signs noted in cases of Addison's disease.

Asthenia is the cardinal symptom of Addison's disease. Early it may be sporadic, usually most evident at times of stress; as adrenal function becomes more impaired, the weakness progresses until the patient is continuously fatigued, necessitating bed rest. Even the voice may fail, so that speech finally becomes listless and indistinct.

Pigmentation is the most striking sign of the disease. It commonly appears as a diffuse brown, tan, or bronze darkening of both exposed and unexposed points such as elbows or creases of the hand and in areas normally pigmented such as the areolas about the nipples. In many patients, bluish-black patches appear on the mucous membranes. Some patients develop dark freckles, and occasionally irregular areas of vitiligo may appear paradoxically. As an early sign, patients may notice an unusually persistent tanning following exposure to the sun.

Arterial hypotension is also extremely frequent, and in severe cases blood pressures may be in the range of 80/50 or less. Postural accentuation is common, and syncope may occur.

Abnormalities of gastrointestinal function are not only extremely frequent but often are the presenting complaint. Symptoms may vary from mild anorexia with weight loss to fulminating nausea, vomiting, diarrhea, and various types of ill-defined abdominal pain, which at times may be so severe as to be confused with an acute condition of the abdomen requiring surgery. Rarely a Landry's type of ascending paralysis with flaccid quadriplegia and mixed sensory defects accompanied by ascending muscular weakness has been noted in conjunction with a higher serum potassium level. In these instances, the electrocardiogram may reflect the hyperkalemia. In addition, patients with adrenal insufficiency frequently have marked personality changes, usually in the form of excessive irritability and restlessness. Enhancement of the sensory modalities of taste, olfaction, and hearing is often present and is reversible with therapy. A decrease in axillary and pubic hair is common in female patients due to loss of adrenal androgen production.

LABORATORY FINDINGS In the milder forms, sometimes called *partial* or *incomplete* Addison's disease, there may be no demonstrable abnormalities in any of the parameters measured in the routine laboratory, and even plasma and urinary steroid determinations may indicate values relatively low yet within normal range. However, definitive studies of adrenal stimulation with ACTH show abnormalities even in this stage of the disease. In the more advanced stages, levels of serum sodium, chloride, and bicarbonate are reduced while serum potassium is elevated. The hyponatremia is due to extravascular loss of sodium both into the urine (due to aldosterone deficiency) and from the vascular compartment into tendons, cartilage, and bone. This extravascular sodium loss depletes extracellular fluid volume and accentuates hypotension. Elevated plasma levels of vasopressin and angiotensin have been reported, and these may be contributing factors to hyponatremia through impairment of free-water clearance. The hyperkalemia is due to a combination of factors, including aldosterone deficiency, impaired glomerular filtration rate, and acidosis. These patients may show marked reduction in heart size, and in about one-quarter of the patients suprarenal calcification is seen but is unfortunately not pathognomonic. The electrocardiogram may show nonspecific changes, and the electroencephalogram a striking reduction and slowing of the predominant activity. The basal metabolic rate may be low, but other thyroid indexes are usually normal. There may be a normocytic anemia, a relative lymphocytosis, and usually a moderate eosinophilia.

DIAGNOSIS The diagnosis of adrenal insufficiency requires demonstration either directly or indirectly of decreased cortisol production by the adrenal in the basal state (*complete* adrenal insufficiency) or the unmasking of decreased cortisol production only in the stimulated state (*incomplete* adrenal insufficiency) (Fig. 86-14).

In all cases of *complete adrenal insufficiency* the cortisol secretory rate is markedly decreased, and this may be ascertained indirectly by the finding of low to absent 24-hr urine 17-hydroxycorticoids and urine 17-ketosteroids. Because of the contribution of the male gonads to urine 17-ketosteroids, basal excretory values in complete adrenal insufficiency will be higher for males than females. With incomplete adrenal insufficiency, urine steroid excretion values overlap into the normal range; because of this, a diagnosis of adrenal insufficiency cannot be made solely on the values of basal urine steroid determinations. Plasma cortisol values are from zero to the lower range of normal. Aldosterone secretion is very low judged by isotopic secretory rate determinations, as are aldosterone excretory values. In patients with primary adrenal insufficiency, plasma ACTH and MSH (melanocyte-stimulating hormone) levels are elevated because of loss of the usual cortisol-hypothalamic feedback relationship, whereas in secondary adrenal insufficiency, plasma ACTH values are low, a finding consistent with the absence of increased pigmentation in patients having the latter condition.

The specific and definitive diagnosis of adrenal insufficiency can be made only with the ACTH stimulation test to assay the adrenal reserve capacity for steroid production. In addition, ACTH testing is helpful in establishing whether adrenal insufficiency is primary or secondary. In patients undergoing ACTH testing as a diagnostic method for adrenal insufficiency, saline solution should be utilized as the diluent for the ACTH to be infused, since on occasion patients may experience water intoxication if a diluent of only glucose and water is used. An additional advantage of using saline diluent is that a clinical estimate of adrenal responsiveness may be made by the presence or absence of weight gain during the infusion period, weight gain commonly occurring when adrenocortical function is intact, because of the associated stimulation of aldosterone secretion. The potential dangers of ACTH testing in patients with limited adrenal reserves may be minimized by the prior administration of 1 mg of a potent steroid such as dexamethasone. The excretory products of 1 mg of this compound will not add appreciably to the amount of 17-hydroxycorticoids measured in the urine and therefore will not interfere with the test. For testing purposes, 40 units of ACTH (or 25 units α 1-24 corticotropin) is infused daily over 8 hr for 4 to 5 successive days, with daily urine collections tested for creatinine, 17-hydroxycorticoid, and 17-ketosteroid levels. Alternatively, a continuous 48-hr ACTH infusion may be used by giving 40 units of ACTH (or 25 units α 1-24 corticotropin) in 500 ml of 5 percent dextrose in normal saline solution every 12 hr for four consecutive 12-hr periods. In patients with complete primary adrenal insufficiency, ACTH stimulation by either method will cause a rise in steroid excretion of less than 2 mg per day.

In *incomplete adrenal insufficiency,* ACTH testing carried out by either method will result in subnormal increments in urinary 17-hydroxycorticoids. A variant of this response is sometimes seen in which small increments in steroid excretion occur on the first 3 days of the 5-day infusion test, while on the last 2 days, there is an actual decline in the level of steroids. Alternately, the last 12 hr of the continuous 48-hr infusion will show a decline in 17-hydroxycorticoid excretion. These results suggest that the limited adrenal tissue has been maximally stimulated and has insufficient steroid reserve capacity.

Indirect tests of adrenocortical hypofunction include (1) a delay in water excretion following an acute water load; (2) defective renal conservation of sodium when a low sodium diet is imposed; and (3) a tendency toward hypoglycemia during fasting. Since ACTH is available for direct evaluation of adrenocortical function, these procedures are not indicated; furthermore, in a patient with adrenocortical insufficiency, water intoxication, sodium deprivation, or hypoglycemia may all be life-threatening situations. A flow chart for evaluation of patients with suspected adrenal insufficiency is presented in Fig. 86-14.

DIFFERENTIAL DIAGNOSIS Since weakness and fatigue are such common complaints, clinical diagnosis of early adrenocortical insufficiency is frequently difficult (Fig 86-14). However, mild gastrointestinal distress with weight loss, anorexia, and a suggestion of increased pig-

FIGURE 86-14

*Diagnostic flow chart for evaluating the status of patients with suspected adrenal insufficiency. Plasma ACTH (and MSH) levels will be low in secondary adrenal insufficiency. In adrenal insufficiency secondary to pituitary tumors or idiopathic panhypopituitarism, other pituitary hormone deficiencies will be present. On the other hand, ACTH deficiency may be isolated, as seen following prolonged use of exogenous glucocorticoids. *An alternative test to the 8-hr infusion of ACTH for 3 or 4 days is a continuous infusion of 25 units of α 1–24 corticotropin q.12h. × 24 to 48 hr.*

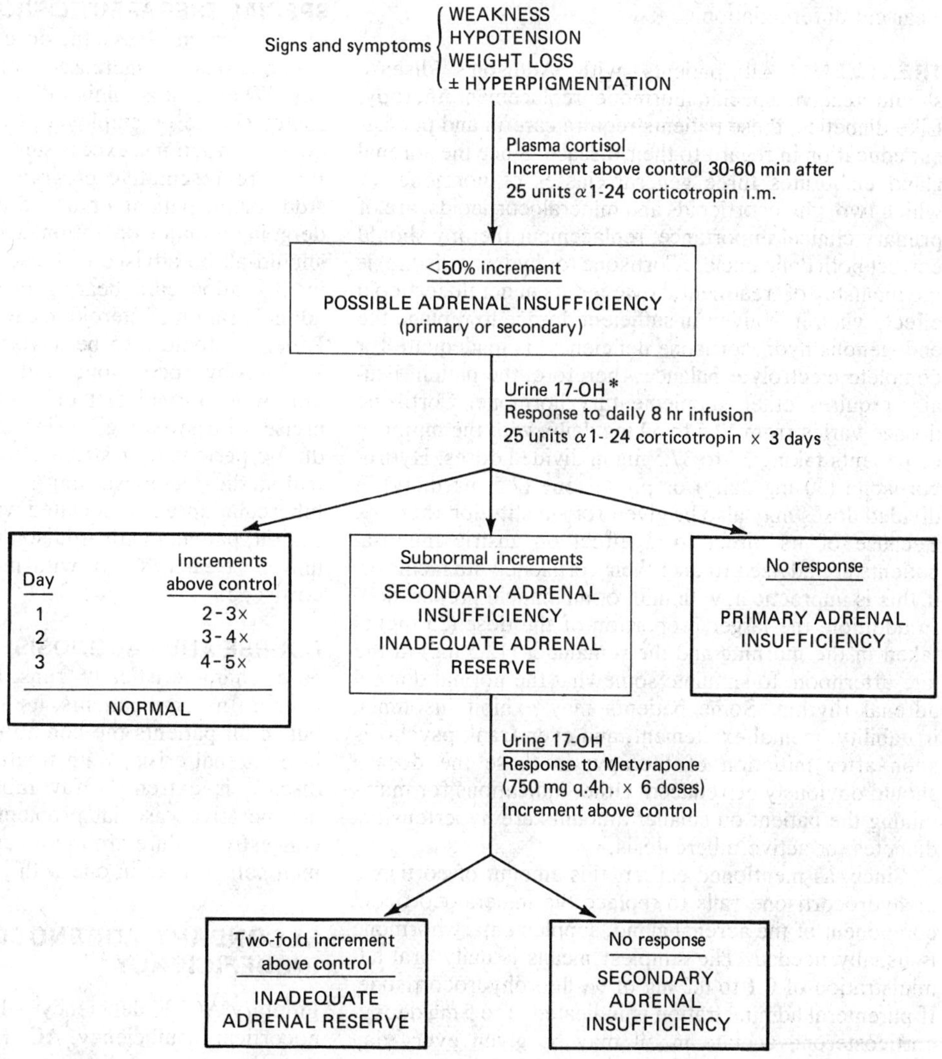

mentation make mandatory ACTH stimulation testing to rule out adrenal insufficiency, particularly before steroid treatment is begun. Weight loss is useful in evaluating the significance of weakness and malaise. Weight gain associated with lassitude is more characteristic of depressive syndromes. Racial pigmentation in Negroes, Orientals, Indians, Spanish Americans, and Latins may be a problem, but a *recent* and progressive *increase* is usually reported by the Addisonian patient. Hyperpigmentation in other diseases may also present a problem, but the appearance and distribution of pigment in Addison's disease are usually characteristic. Other diseases presenting with hyperpigmentation include hemochromatosis, acanthosis nigricans, porphyria, thyrotoxicosis, polyostotic fibrous dysplasia, chronic metal poisoning (bismuth, lead, arsenic, silver), chronic malnutrition (starvation, anorexia nervosa, sprue syndrome, pellagra), progressive malignancy, chronic anemia, salt-losing nephritis with hypotension, renal tubular acidosis, scleroderma, excess nicotinic acid, and hepatic cirrhosis. In most cases, differentiation from Addison's disease is not difficult, but when doubt exists, ACTH administration ordinarily provides clear-cut differentiation.

TREATMENT All patients with Addison's disease should receive specific hormone replacement therapy. Like diabetics, these patients require careful and persistent education in regard to their disease. Since the adrenal gland elaborates three general classes of hormone, of which two, glucocorticoids and mineralocorticoids, are of primary clinical importance, replacement therapy should correct both deficiencies. Cortisone (or hydrocortisone) is the mainstay of treatment; however, its mineralocorticoid effect, when it is given in sufficient dosage to replace the endogenous hydrocortisone deficiency, is inadequate for complete electrolyte balance; therefore, the patient usually requires other supplementary hormone. Cortisone dosage varies from 12.5 to 50 mg daily, with the majority of patients taking 25 to 37.5 mg in divided doses. Hydrocortisone (30 mg daily) or prednisone (7.5 mg daily) in divided doses may also be given for substitution therapy. Because of its direct local effect on gastric mucosa, patients are advised to take their cortisone with meals or, if this is impractical, with milk or an antacid preparation. In addition, the larger proportion of the dose (25 mg) is taken in the morning and the remainder (12.5 mg) in the late afternoon, to simulate somewhat the normal diurnal adrenal rhythm. Some patients may exhibit insomnia, irritability, mental excitement, and even frank psychosis soon after initiation of therapy; in these the dosage should obviously be reduced. Other indications for maintaining the patient on smaller amounts are hypertension, diabetes, or active tuberculosis.

Since, as mentioned earlier, this amount of cortisone or hydrocortisone fails to replace the mineralocorticoid component of the adrenal gland, supplementary hormone is usually needed. The simplest means is daily oral administration of 0.1 to 0.2 mg of 9α-fluorohydrocortisone. If parenteral administration is indicated, 2 to 5 mg deoxycorticosterone acetate in oil may be given every day intramuscularly. An alternative method of therapy is an injection of 25 to 50 mg deoxycorticosterone trimethylacetate in oil intramuscularly every 3 to 4 weeks, but as with the previous use of subcutaneous implantation of pellets of deoxycorticosterone which lasted for 8 to 10 months, most patients prefer the simplicity of daily oral administration of the 9α-fluorohydrocortisone.

Complications of cortisone therapy, with the exception of peptic disease, particularly ulcer or gastritis, are *extremely rare* in the dosage used in the treatment of Addison's disease. However, overtreatment with deoxycorticosterone preparations or 9α-fluorohydrocortisone is more frequent and may present as edema, hypertension, cardiac enlargement, or even congestive failure due to sodium retention. Overtreatment may also present as weakness, progressing to total paralysis, due to hypokalemia. In the management of patients with Addison's disease, regular measurements of body weight, serum potassium, heart size, and blood pressure, and serial electrocardiograms are useful.

All patients with adrenal insufficiency, including bilaterally adrenalectomized patients, should carry medical identification, should be educated and instructed in the parenteral self-administration of steroids, and should be registered with a national medical alerting system.

SPECIAL THERAPEUTIC PROBLEMS During periods of intercurrent illness, the dose of cortisone or hydrocortisone should be increased to levels of 75 to 150 mg per day. When oral administration is not possible, parenteral routes should be employed. Likewise, before surgery or dental extractions, excess steroid should be administered. For a representative program of steroid therapy for an Addisonian patient or an adrenalectomized patient undergoing a major operation, see Table 86-9. The patients should all be advised of these facts and should carry an identification card bearing detailed instructions for the administration of steroid in case of acute illness or injury. Patients should also be advised to increase the dose of 9α-fluorohydrocortisone and add excess salt to their otherwise normal diet during periods of excessive exercise with sweating, during extremely hot weather, or during periods of gastrointestinal upsets. In spite of animal studies demonstrating an increased susceptibility to tubercular spread associated with excess steroid administration, patients with Addison's disease and tuberculosis may be treated safely with maintenance daily doses of cortisone.

COURSE AND PROGNOSIS Untreated Addison's disease characteristically runs a chronic and relentless course. In some patients, its advance is relatively slow, but in all patients the condition may rapidly deteriorate into adrenal crisis. With treatment, the prognosis of the disease is extremely favorable. In fact, some of the degenerative vascular problems such as hypertension or congestive failure are more easily handled in an Addisonian patient than in one with intact adrenal glands.

SECONDARY ADRENOCORTICAL INSUFFICIENCY

Pituitary ACTH deficiency will produce *secondary* adrenocortical insufficiency. ACTH deficiency may be selective, as is seen following prolonged administration of excess glucocorticoids, or may occur in association with multiple pituitary tropic hormone deficiencies (panhypopituitarism) (see Chap. 83). Patients with secondary adrenocortical hypofunction may have many symptoms and signs in common with Addisonian patients but are *characteristically not hyperpigmented.* Patients with total pituitary insufficiency will also have signs and symptoms suggestive of multiple hormone deficiencies. An additional feature distinguishing primary from secondary adrenocortical insufficiency is the *near-normal levels of aldosterone secretion* seen in the presence of pituitary and/or isolated ACTH deficiencies. Patients with pituitary insufficiency may exhibit hyponatremia, which may be dilutional or secondary to subnormal increments in aldosterone secretion in response to sodium restriction. However, the findings of severe dehydration, *hyponatremia,* and *hyperkalemia* are characteristic of severe mineralocorticoid insufficiency and favor a diagnosis of primary adrenocortical insufficiency.

Patients receiving long-term steroid therapy, despite physical findings of Cushing's syndrome, develop adrenal insufficiency both because of prolonged suppression of the hypothalamic corticotropin-releasing center and because of actual adrenal atrophy. Adrenal atrophy results from the loss of endogenous ACTH stimulation, which stimulus is prerequisite for maintaining normal adrenal size. Thus, these patients acquire two deficits, a loss of adrenal responsiveness to ACTH and a failure of pituitary ACTH release. These patients are characterized by low blood cortisol and ACTH levels, low base-line steroid excretion, and abnormal ACTH and metyrapone test results. On testing these patients with ACTH, one looks for the "staircase" response, with successive daily increments in steroid excretion; however, *prolonged ACTH testing* may be needed to elicit such a response. The urine steroid pattern, when adrenal reactivation does occur, often reveals increments in 17-hydroxycorticoids without parallel increments in 17-ketosteroids. Practically all patients with steroid-induced adrenal insufficiency will eventually respond to ACTH testing, but individual response time is most variable, ranging from days to months. Once such patients are shown to have reacquired adrenal sensitivity to exogenous ACTH, their ability to release endogenous pituitary ACTH must be determined. The standard metyrapone test is utilized for this purpose. For a valid metyrapone test, it must be previously documented that the patient's adrenal glands are sensitive to ACTH, since the metyrapone test response depends on adrenal responsiveness to released ACTH. For this reason the test is *contraindicated* in patients with suspected or proved adrenal insufficiency. In patients with steroid-induced adrenal insufficiency, abnormal metyrapone tests usually continue for several months after the adrenal glands have regained responsiveness to ACTH. In interpreting the metyrapone test it is useful to consider it as an endogenous ACTH stimulation test and compare the peak urine 17-hydroxycorticoid excretion with the maximal values previously obtained with exogenous ACTH stimulation.

Plasma ACTH levels help distinguish between primary and secondary adrenal insufficiency, since they are elevated in the former and decreased to absent in the latter.

Substitution glucocorticoid therapy in patients with secondary adrenocortical insufficiency does not differ from that outlined for Addisonian patients. Mineralocorticoid replacement therapy is usually not necessary, since aldosterone secretion is preserved. Otherwise, it is stressed that the basic principles outlined for replacement should be applied to patients with secondary adrenocortical insufficiency.

ACUTE ADRENOCORTICAL INSUFFICIENCY

Acute adrenocortical insufficiency may result from several processes. One of these, usually termed *adrenal crisis,* is a rapid and overwhelming intensification of chronic adrenal insufficiency. Another process involves an acute hemorrhagic destruction of both adrenal glands, usually associated with an overwhelming septicemia. Adrenal

TABLE 86-9
Steroid therapy schedule for Addisonian patient undergoing a major operation*

	Cortisone acetate (intramuscularly)		*Hydrocortisone infusion*	*Cortisone acetate (orally)*				*Fluorohydrocortisone (orally)*
	7 A.M.	*7 P.M.*	*continuous*	*8 A.M.*	*12 Noon*	*4 P.M.*	*8 P.M.*	*8 A.M.*
Routine daily medication				25		12.5		0.1
Day before operation		50		25		12.5		0.1
Day of operation	100	50	200					
Postoperative day 1	50	50	100–150					
" 2	50	50	50–100					
" 3	50	50		25			25	
" 4	50			25	25	25		0.1
" 5				25	25	25	25	0.1
" 6				25	25	25		0.1
" 7				25	12.5	25		0.1
" 8				25	12.5	25		0.1
" 9–13				25		25		0.1
" 14				25		12.5		0.1

* *All steroid doses are given in milligrams.*

hemorrhage associated with anticoagulant therapy is being seen with increasing frequency. A third, and probably the most frequent, cause of acute insufficiency results from the rapid withdrawal of steroids from patients with adrenal atrophy secondary to chronic steroid administration. In the presence of severe stress, acute adrenocortical insufficiency may also occur in patients with congenital adrenal hyperplasia and those receiving pharmacologic agents which are capable of inhibiting steroid synthesis by the gland (such as *o,p'*-DDD).

ADRENAL CRISIS The long-term survival of patients with Addison's disease largely depends upon prevention and treatment of adrenal crisis. Consequently, the occurrence of infection, trauma (including surgery), gastrointestinal upsets, or other forms of stress requires an immediate increase in hormone. In previously untreated patients, preexisting symptoms are intensified. Nausea, vomiting, and abdominal pain may become intractable. Fever is frequently severe but may be absent. Lethargy deepens into somnolence, and the blood pressure and pulse fail as hypovolemic vascular shock ensues. In contrast, patients previously maintained on chronic glucocorticoid therapy may not exhibit severe dehydration or hypotension until preterminally, since mineralocorticoid secretion is usually preserved.

In all patients presenting in crisis a precipitating cause should be sought. Intercurrent infection associated with omission or failure to increase maintenance therapy is a common setting.

Treatment is primarily directed toward the rapid elevation of circulating adrenocortical hormone, in addition to the replacement of the sodium and water deficit. Hence, an intravenous infusion of 1,000 ml 5 percent glucose in normal saline solution containing 100 to 200 mg of any of several soluble hydrocortisone preparations is begun rapidly, with the first 250 ml infused in the first 1/2 to 1 hr and the remainder over the ensuing 4 to 8 hr. If the condition is extreme, immediate intravenous infusion of 100 mg hydrocortisone in the first few minutes is suggested, followed by a rapid infusion as described above. Epinephrine, 0.2 mg intravenously, may also be indicated. In any case, it is also advisable to administer 100 mg cortisone acetate intramuscularly in case the infusion becomes infiltrated or inadvertently stopped. If the crisis was preceded by prolonged nausea, vomiting, and dehydration, several liters of saline replacement is indicated. With large doses of steroid, as, for example, 200 mg cortisone or hydrocortisone, the patient receives a maximal mineralocorticoid effect, and supplementary deoxycorticosterone is superfluous. After the initial infusion, depending on the patient's condition, a second similar infusion may be given; if there has been marked improvement, the patient may be offered oral fluids and be given 50 mg cortisone acetate intramuscularly every 12 hr until gastrointestinal absorption is guaranteed, at which time the steroid can be given orally. Steroid dosage is then tapered over the next few days to maintenance levels, with reinstitution of supplementary mineralocorticoid if needed.

ADRENAL HEMORRHAGE Adrenal hemorrhage (adrenal apoplexy) is usually associated with overwhelming septicemia (Waterhouse-Friderichsen syndrome); however, it may also occur in the absence of sepsis. Occasionally, massive bilateral adrenal hemorrhage results from birth trauma. The infant may either be stillborn or die soon after birth of shock and hyperpyrexia. Adrenal hemorrhage also occurs during pregnancy, following idiopathic adrenal vein thrombosis, during convulsions in epilepsy or during electroconvulsive therapy, with excessive anticoagulant therapy, after trauma or surgery, and as a complication of adrenal venography (e.g., infarction of an adenoma). Pain in the flank and epigastrium is frequent, and if the hemorrhagic process ruptures into the abdomen, signs of peritoneal inflammation are present. Acute adrenal insufficiency should also be considered in the differential diagnosis of hypotension in patients maintained on anticoagulant therapy in the period immediately following a myocardial infarction.

The adrenal hemorrhage associated with septicemia is most frequent with meningococcemia but is also seen with overwhelming infections due to pneumococcus, staphylococcus, or *Hemophilus influenzae.* The onset is often explosive, with a shaking chill, violent headache, vertigo, vomiting, and prostration. A petechial rash appears on the skin and mucous membranes and progresses rapidly to a confluent, extensive purpura. Large areas of skin may become grossly hemorrhagic. Body temperature may be subnormal but is usually markedly elevated. Circulatory collapse rapidly ensues, and death may occur within 6 to 48 hr. Specific diagnosis requires immediate identification of the organism. Frequently, the septicemia is so massive that organisms may be seen in peripheral blood smears or petechial scrapings. Time is not sufficient for determination of adrenal function; however, a plasma sample for later determination of 17-hydroxysteroid level may be of academic interest.

Treatment must be immediate and intensive. Control of the infection by vigorous administration of parenteral, preferably intravenous, antibiotics is indicated in addition to the steroid schedule delineated for adrenal crisis. Intravenous norepinephrine (4 to 8 mg per liter) may also be required to maintain vascular tone. Since shock may also be associated with massive septicemia without adrenal hemorrhage, one is never completely certain whether adrenal insufficiency is contributing to the patient's decompensation; however, the authors think that because of the increasing frequency of survival of patients treated with steroid, some degree of adrenal insufficiency, whether relative or absolute, is present and that steroid treatment is therefore indicated in all patients in whom fulminating septicemia is associated with shock. The dose range administered in such patients is usually massive (e.g., 1,000 mg hydrocortisone daily).

HYPOALDOSTERONISM

Patients with *isolated* aldosterone deficiency are rare. Such a deficiency accompanied by normal cortisol production has been reported as a congenital biosynthetic defect; postoperatively following removal of aldosteronoma; during protracted heparin or heparinoid administration; in pretectal disease of the nervous system; in severe postural hypotension; and in association with complete heart block.

In severe cases urine sodium wastage is present on a normal salt intake, whereas in milder forms excessive urine sodium losses occur only during salt restriction. The patients always develop hyponatremia and hyperkalemia, the latter often to a severe degree.

A biosynthetic defect has been noted in some patients who are unable to transform the angular C-18 methyl group of corticosterone to the C-18 aldehyde grouping of aldosterone. This C-18 transformation requires first the formation of 18-hydroxycorticosterone from corticosterone, and then, secondly, dehydrogenation of the C-18 hydroxyl group to form the characteristic C-18 aldehyde group of aldosterone. These patients will manifest low to absent aldosterone secretion and excretion in association with elevated secretion and excretion values for corticosterone and 18-hydroxycorticosterone.

The feature common to all patients with hypoaldosteronism has been their inability to *increase* aldosterone secretion appropriately during severe salt restriction. An additional feature has been the reversal of the signs of salt wasting (hyponatremia and hyperkalemia) with the administration of potent mineralocorticoids. For practical purposes the oral administration of 9α-fluorohydrocortisone in a dose of 0.1 to 0.3 mg daily restores electrolyte balance.

NONSPECIFIC USE OF ADRENAL STEROIDS AND ACTH IN CLINICAL PRACTICE

The widespread utilization of glucocorticoids and ACTH in clinical practice emphasizes the need for a thorough understanding of the metabolic effects of these agents when used nonspecifically, if optimum effectiveness is to be obtained and if undesirable side reactions are to be minimized. Before instituting adrenal hormone therapy, a physician should weigh carefully the gains that can reasonably be expected versus the potentially undesirable metabolic actions of pharmacologic doses of hormone. Accurate appraisal will require familiarity with current medical literature, a critical evaluation of the significance of such reports, as well as a clear understanding of the chemical, physiologic, and psychologic changes that hormone preparations of this type are known to induce when used in pharmacologic dosage.

HOW SERIOUS IS THE DISORDER? Clearly, in the case of a patient whose life is threatened by unexplained shock, or in whom other measures have failed, the physician need not hesitate to employ large-dosage steroid therapy. On the other hand, one should exercise restraint in administering pharmacologic doses of steroids to a patient with early rheumatoid arthritis who as yet has not been exposed to the possible benefits of physiotherapy, analgesics, and a well-organized program of general medical care.

HOW LONG WILL GLUCOCORTICOID THERAPY BE REQUIRED? The use of intravenously administered steroids for a period of 24 to 48 hr in the treatment of such life-threatening situations as status asthmaticus or pseudotumor cerebri has little or no contraindication, in contrast to the initiation of a program of steroid therapy for chronic asthma, arthritis, or psoriasis. In the latter instances, the almost certain complication of a Cushing's syndrome of some degree must be weighed against the potential benefit to the patient. The need for minimizing these side effects by the use of shorter-acting steroid preparations, alternate-day or interrupted therapy programs, and the judicious use of supplementary adjuvants is evident.

WHICH ADRENAL PREPARATION IS PREFERABLE? Five considerations need to be taken into account in deciding which steroid preparation to use: (1) the biologic half-life of the particular compound. The rationale behind every-other-day therapy is to decrease the metabolic effects of the steroids for a significant amount of time over the 2-day period, yet at the same time to produce pharmacologic suppression of sufficient duration to maintain the disease in remission. Too long a half-life would defeat the first purpose, and too short a half-life would defeat the second. In general, the more potent the steroid, the longer its biologic half-life tends to be. (2) The importance of the mineralocorticoid effects of the steroid. The newer synthetic steroids have much less mineralocorticoid effect relative to their glucocorticoid effect than cortisol or cortisone (Table 86-10). This may be an important consideration in certain disease states. (3) The fact that cortisone and prednisone, in contrast to the other glucocorticoids, have to be converted to their bio-

TABLE 86-10
Adrenal preparations*

	Estimated potency†	
Commonly used name	*Glucocorticoid*	*Mineralocorticoid*
Short-acting		
Hydrocortisone	1	1
Cortisone	0.8	0.8
Intermediate-acting		
Prednisone	4	0.25
Prednisolone	4	0.25
Methylprednisolone	5	±
Triamcinolone	5	±
Long-acting		
Paramethasone	10	±
Betamethasone	25	±
Dexamethasone	30–40	±

* *The steroids are divided into three groups according to the duration of biologic activity. Short-acting preparations have a biologic half-life of less than 12 hr; long-acting, greater than 48 hr; and intermediate, between 12 and 36 hr. Triamcinolone has the longest half-life of the intermediate-acting preparations.*

† *Relative milligram comparisons to cortisol, setting the glucocorticoid and mineralocorticoid properties of cortisol as 1. Sodium retention is insignificant in usual doses employed of methylprednisolone, triamcinolone, paramethasone, betamethasone, and dexamethasone.*

logically active equivalents before any anti-inflammatory effects can occur. Because of this, in a clinical condition in which steroids are known to be effective and in which an adequate dose has been given without any response, one should consider substituting hydrocortisone or prednisolone for cortisone or prednisone. (4) The cost of the medication; this is a serious consideration if chronic administration is to be undertaken. Prednisone is the least expensive of available steroid preparations. (5) The appreciable variation among commercial preparations of glucosteroids in the manner in which the tablets are formulated. This factor may significantly modify absorption. Thus it is advisable for a patient whose steroid dosage has been standardized to continue to utilize the same pharmaceutical preparation to avoid relapse or overdosage.

ACTH VERSUS STEROIDS In most cases, the only decision of major consequence is whether to use ACTH rather than one of the adrenal steroid preparations. In general, adrenal steroid therapy is effective by mouth and can be regulated more accurately than ACTH therapy. The latter will fluctuate considerably in the amount of steroid produced from day to day, depending on the rate and extent of absorption of ACTH and on the state of the adrenal cortex. ACTH therapy does stimulate the secretion of adrenal androgens as well as hydroxysteroids. The former may have advantages in certain diseases, such as dermatomyositis, in which the adrenal androgens may prove helpful in maintaining the muscle mass while the inflammatory reaction is being suppressed by the 17-hydroxycorticosteroids. Combined androgen and corticoid therapy may, of course, attain the same objective. Sodium retention with ACTH has often been more marked than with cortisone or, particularly, with prednisone therapy.

ACTH therapy has proved useful in the treatment of neuromuscular disorders such as dermatomyositis and multiple sclerosis, particularly in female patients in whom the androgenic stimulation of ACTH may minimize the "muscle-wasting action" of glucocorticoids. Both ACTH and steroid therapy induce hypothalamic-pituitary suppression; however, in ACTH therapy adrenal gland size and activity are maintained, in contrast to the adrenal atrophy usually associated with steroid therapy. ACTH is often used, in small doses, to activate the adrenal cortex before steroid therapy is completely discontinued: however, this is rarely necessary when "every-other-day" short-acting steroid therapy has been utilized.

EVALUATION OF PATIENT PRIOR TO INITIATING STEROID THERAPY (Table 86-11) **Chronic infection** Three problems demand attention. (1) Any active infection, particularly tuberculosis, should be identified. If tuberculosis is present, steroid therapy can be employed, if indicated, in conjunction with antituberculous chemotherapy. (2) The chest film and tuberculin test will provide base-line information for future comparison. High-dosage steroids will minimize the tuberculin reaction. For this reason a chest roentgenogram should be carried out at 6 to 12-month intervals, or with evidence of unexplained fever or weight loss, in patients on long-continued steroid therapy. (3) Infection due to "opportunistic" low-virulence pathogens should be constantly considered in patients on high steroid dosage, especially when steroid therapy is combined with other immunosuppressive agents.

Diabetes mellitus Prolonged ACTH or cortisone-like steroid therapy may unmask latent diabetes mellitus and aggravate preexisting disease. For this reason a careful history is important to exclude familial incidence of diabetes. It is more valuable to carry out examinations of blood and urine following a test load of carbohydrate. A convenient method consists in measuring blood and urinary glucose 2 to 3 hr after the ingestion of a breakfast containing approximately 100 g carbohydrate (see Chap. 88). Obviously the presence of frank diabetes mellitus or the demonstration of impaired glucose tolerance will affect the physician's decision to institute adrenal hormone therapy. However, if such therapy appears necessary or desirable in the presence of latent diabetes, the judicious use of supplementary insulin therapy may be added to the therapeutic program. The insulin requirement of known diabetics will usually need to be increased with ACTH or cortisone-like therapy, except in those rare instances in which the diabetic patient is suffering from some degree of insulin resistance in which the anti-inflammatory or antiallergic effect of cortisone enhances the metabolic effectiveness of the insulin sufficiently to balance off the diabetogenic action of the former.

Osteoporosis All patients receiving long-continued steroid therapy are likely to develop some degree of osteoporosis. Obviously, considerable change in bone structure must occur before significant radiologic changes can be demonstrated. For patients at high risk (postmenopausal females, elderly individuals, and patients whose basic disease process results in restricted physical activity) initial films of the thoracolumbar segment of the spine are mandatory. Glucocorticoids decrease intestinal ab-

TABLE 86-11

A "check-list" for use prior to the administration of steroids in pharmacologic dosage.

1. Presence of tuberculosis or other chronic infection (chest x-ray, tuberculin test)
2. History of diabetes mellitus in family (postprandial blood glucose test, preferably after 100-g carbohydrate meal)
3. Evidence of preexisting osteoporosis (spinal x-ray in postmenopausal patients)
4. History of peptic ulcer, gastritis, or esophagitis (stool guaiac test)
5. Evidence of hypertension or cardiovascular disease
6. History or evidence of psychologic disorders
7. Base-line 24 hr urinary steroid excretion. (This measurement of the level of endogenous adrenal secretion may prove helpful in estimating the response to exogenous steroid therapy, as will the dose which may be required. Thus, patients with chronic illness and low endogenous steroid level may be expected to respond more favorably and to a lower steroid dosage than those with high endogenous levels of hormone.)

sorption of calcium, are collagenolytic, and may decrease growth hormone secretion. These combined actions make the vertebral column extremely vulnerable. Osteoporosis, with vertebral fractures or compression, is one of the most serious potential hazards of long-term steroid therapy. For this reason, it is urged that a program which includes large doses of vitamin D, fluoride, calcium, and anabolic hormones be prescribed in conjunction with "alternate-day" or interrupted steroid therapy (see below). Serum calcium levels should be monitored at monthly intervals to prevent hypercalcemia.

Peptic ulcer, gastric hypersecretion, or esophagitis Patients with a history of gastric hypersecretion or peptic ulcer are likely to experience aggravation of their symptoms while receiving adrenal hormone therapy. It is not known for certain whether aggravation of peptic ulceration and complicating gastrointestinal hemorrhage reflect the increased gastric secretory activity so frequently associated with adrenal hormone therapy or whether the nitrogen-depleting effect of these hormones accelerates the process of ulceration and perforation. Prophylactic antacid therapy and an ulcer diet are useful precautions in susceptible patients. *The development of anemia in a patient receiving ACTH or cortisone therapy should immediately suggest gastrointestinal bleeding,* and patients should be cautioned to note black or tarry stools. A clear-cut history of peptic ulcer constitutes a contraindication to ACTH and cortisone therapy, and steroid therapy, if required as a life-saving measure, should be accompanied by a vigorous "ulcer-combating" program.

Hypertension or cardiovascular disease In general, the sodium-retaining propensity of most adrenal steroid preparations requires that caution be used when they are given to patients with preexisting hypertension or cardiovascular or renal disease. Use of the now-available preparations in which sodium-retaining activity is minimal (triamcinolone and dexamethasone), restriction of dietary sodium intake, and the use of diuretic agents and supplementary potassium salts, will permit the safe use of steroid therapy where important indications exist. Sodium retention and edema are more marked with ACTH therapy than with glucocorticoid preparations. In some patients with congestive failure or pericardial effusion, steroid therapy may initiate a diuresis.

For all patients in whom prolonged steroid therapy is contemplated cardiovascular-renal status should be carefully evaluated, with a chest x-ray for *heart size* and an electrocardiogram included.

Psychologic difficulties From time to time steroid therapy may be complicated by severe psychologic disturbances; less severe abnormalities are relatively frequent. In general, serious psychologic disturbances are more closely related to the patient's personality structure than to the actual dose of hormone, although, as might be anticipated, larger doses of hormone will be associated with more frequent serious reactions. At present there is no reliable method of determining beforehand a patient's psychologic reaction to steroid therapy. Patients with known psychologic difficulties undoubtedly experience more frequent and more severe disturbances. Further difficulty arises because previous tolerance of steroids does not necessarily ensure immunity to subsequent courses of therapy, and untoward psychologic reactions on one occasion do not invariably mean that the patient will respond unfavorably to a second course of treatment. The physician must follow the course of his patient's condition carefully during the early period of steroid therapy and must take a responsible member of the patient's family into his confidence.

Sleeplessness is a well-known complication of glucosteroid therapy. This can be minimized by using the shorter-acting steroids and by prescribing the total dose as a single early-morning medication (Table 86-12).

"ALTERNATE-DAY" STEROID THERAPY Undoubtedly the single most effective measure in minimizing the Cushingoid effects of glucosteroid therapy is to administer the total dose for 48 hr as a *single* dose, of *intermediate-acting steroid* in the morning, *every other day!* If symptoms of the underlying disorder can be controlled by this technique, the physician can be assured that his therapeutic program is offering a distinct advantage to his patient. Three special considerations deserve mention. (1) The alternate-day schedule may be approached through a series of transition dose schedules which permit the patient an opportunity to adjust more successfully to the ultimate program. (2) The physician should make a conscientious effort to provide the patient with supplementary nonsteroid medications, if required, on the "off day" to minimize symptoms of the underlying disorder. (3) The physician and the patient should recog-

TABLE 86-12

Supplementary measures designed to minimize undesirable metabolic effects of glucocorticoids

1 Monitor caloric intake to prevent weight gain.
2 Restrict sodium intake to prevent edema, minimize hypertension and potassium loss.
3 Potassium supplement—a diet high in potassium and supplementary potassium as KCl elixir, 2–3 tsp three times daily with meals.
4 Antacid therapy—most patients will do well to receive regular antacid therapy between meals and at night. The antacid should be of the low-sodium variety.
5 Sodium fluoride, 6–9 mg daily (Luride tablets contain 2.2 mg NaF).
Calcium, 600 mg daily.
Vitamin D, 50,000 units twice weekly.
6 Estrogen and androgen therapy for postmenopausal females receiving steroid therapy; not necessary if ACTH is being used. 1.25-2.50 mg conjugated estrogens equine (Premarin) may be given "cyclically."
Oxandrolone (Anavar), 10-20 mg daily in divided doses.
7 "Alternate-day" steroid schedule if possible; if not, a single morning total-steroid dosage; in all instances use an "intermediate-acting" steroid preparation if possible (Table 86-10).
8 Patients maintained on steroid therapy over a prolonged period should be protected by an appropriate increase in hormone level during periods of acute stress. A rule of thumb is to *double* the maintenance dose.

nize that many of the symptoms which may be noted during the off day are really those of relative adrenal insufficiency, rather than an exacerbation of his underlying disease. Fatigue, joint pain, muscle stiffness or tenderness, and even fever, can be accounted for by the rapid fall in plasma cortisol level. Knowing this is of vital importance, since the physician can reassure his patient and will avoid giving up the program on the basis of a misconception.

The alternate-day concept capitalizes on the fact that normally cortisol secretion and plasma levels are highest in the early morning and lowest in the evening. The normal pattern is mimicked by administering steroids in the morning (7 to 8 A.M.), and preferably an intermediate-acting steroid, i.e., one whose hypothalamic-pituitary-suppressing effect lasts less than 1½ days (Table 86-10).

Initially the steroid program will usually require daily or more frequent doses of steroid in order to accomplish the desired anti-inflammatory or immunity-suppressing action. *Only after this desired effect has been achieved is an attempt made to switch over to an alternate-day program!* There are a number of programs which may be employed for transferring a patient from a daily to an alternate-day program. The key points to be considered are flexibility in arranging a program, and the use of supportive measures on the off day. One may attempt a transition by a series of gradations (Table 86-13), rather than by an abrupt complete changeover. In either case it is important to anticipate that the patient will experience some increase in pain or discomfort between the 36 to 48 hr following the last dose of steroid.

The general principles advocated in the long-term use of steroids and in implementing an alternate-day schedule are as follows:

1 Utilize intermediate-acting steroids such as prednisone or prednisolone.

2 As soon as possible give the total daily steroid dose as a single morning dose.

3 Begin a transition program just as soon as the clinical manifestations of the disease are under reasonable control.

4 If possible, ultimately eliminate entirely steroid medication on the alternate day.

TABLE 86-13
An outline of a schedule to taper patients off of pharmacologic doses of glucocorticoids

Day	*Prednisone, mg*	*Day*	*Prednisone, mg*
1	60	14	5
2	40	15	90
3	70	16	0
4	30	17	85
5	80	18	0
6	20	19	85
7	90	22	0
8	10	21	85
9	95	22	0
10	5	23	80
11	90	24	0
12	5		
13	90		

WITHDRAWAL OF CORTICOSTEROIDS FOLLOWING THEIR LONG-TERM USE AS PHARMACOLOGIC AGENTS

Complete withdrawal of steroids should not be contemplated until an Addisonian or normal replacement dosage has been reached, e.g., equivalent of 25.0 to 37.5 mg cortisone daily or 5.0 to 7.5 mg prednisone. Patients on an alternate-day program for a month or more will experience little difficulty as far as pituitary adrenal function is concerned when the dosage is gradually reduced and finally discontinued. Complications rarely ensue unless undue stress is experienced, and patients should understand that for 1 year or longer, after the complete withdrawal from long-term high-dosage steroid therapy, they should receive supplementary hormone in the presence of serious infection, operation, or injury.

If a patient in the final stage of steroid reduction cannot tolerate an alternate-day program, it is debatable as to whether complete discontinuance should be considered. Under these circumstances a daily dose of steroid could be continued, and at some future date another trial of gradual transition to the alternate-day schedule should be attempted. In patients with life-threatening disorders such as disseminated lupus erythematosus, or widespread skin disorders in which exfoliative dermatitis may complicate complete withdrawal of steroids, it may be desirable to consider life-long maintenance therapy at an Addisonian replacement dosage. These patients will not require mineralocorticoid therapy, as aldosterone secretion, in the absence of severe stress, is usually adequate.

REFERENCES

ADDISON T: *On the Constitutional and Local Effects of Disease of the Suprarenal Capsules,* London: D. Highley, 1855

AFIFI AK et al: Steroid myopathy. Clinical, histologic, and cytologic observations. Johns Hopkins Med J 123:158, 1968

BERSON SA, YALOW RS: Radioimmunoassay of ACTH in plasma. J Clin Invest 47:2725, 1968

BIGLIERI EG et al: Adrenal mineralocorticoids causing hypertension. Am J Med 52:623, 1972

BLIZZARD RM et al: Adrenal antibodies in Addison's disease. Lancet II:901, 1972

CAIN JP et al: The regulation of aldosterone secretion in primary aldosteronism. Am J Med 53:627, 1972

CONN JW, LOUIS IH: Primary aldosteronism, a new clinical entity. Ann Intern Med 44:1, 1956

CUSHING H: The basophil adenomas of the pituitary body and their clinical manifestations (pituitary basophilism). Bull Johns Hopkins Hosp 50:137, 1932

DAVIS WW et al: Bilateral adrenal hyperplasia as a cause of primary aldosteronism with hypertension, hypokalemia and suppressed renin activity. Am J Med 42:642, 1967

GRABER A et al: Natural history of pituitary adrenal recovery following long-term suppression with corticosteroid. Trans Assoc Am Physicians 77:296, 1964

HERRERA MG et al: Cushing's syndrome: diagnosis and treatment. Am J Surg 107:144, 1964

HUTTER AH JR, KAYHOE DE: Adrenocortical carcinoma: clinical features in 138 patients. Am J Med 41:572, 1966

NICHOLS T et al: Steroid laboratory tests in the diagnosis of Cushing's syndrome. Am J Med, 45:116, 1968

ODELL WD, DAUGHADAY WH: *Principles of Competitive Protein-binding Assays,* Philadelphia: Lippincott, 1971

ROSS EJ: Aldosterone and its antagonists. Clin Pharmacol Ther 6:65, 1965

THORN GW: Clinical considerations in the use of corticosteroids. N Engl J Med 274:775, 1966

WILLIAMS GH, DLUHY RG: Aldosterone biosynthesis: interrelationship of regulatory factors. Am J Med 53:595, 1972

—— LAULER DP: Water, electrolyte and acid-base disorders in congestive heart failure and hypertension, in *Clinical Disorders of Fluid and Electrolyte Metabolism,* 2d ed, eds MR Maxwell, CR Kleeman, New York: McGraw-Hill, 1972, p. 835

——, ——: Laboratory evaluation of adrenocortical function, chap. 4 in Tice's *Practice of Medicine,* vol II, Hagerstown, Md.: Harper & Row, 1970

87
PHEOCHROMOCYTOMA

ROGER B. HICKLER
GEORGE W. THORN

The first pheochromocytoma was described by Frankel in 1886, with the term subsequently given by Pick to describe tumors which are selectively colored by chromium salts. The syndrome of paroxysmal hypertension due to this tumor was first clearly described by Labbe, Tinel, and Coumier in 1922. In 1926 Roux and in 1927 Mayo performed the first successful surgical removals of the tumor. In 1936 Beer, King, and Prinzmetal determined that the characteristic paroxysmal rise in blood pressure was associated with the release of hormone from the tumor into the blood. *Persistent* hypertension was first attributed to the tumor in the same year by Kremer.

INCIDENCE It is estimated that over 1,000 cases of pheochromocytoma have been identified, the incidence rising with improved diagnostic techniques. Anatomic statistics from the Mayo Clinic showed 15 of these tumors in 15,984 autopsies, an overall incidence of 0.1 percent. Smithwick estimated the incidence in a hypertensive population explored for sympathectomy to be 0.5 percent.

ANATOMY Embryologically two cell types differentiate from a common stem cell, the sympathogonia of the primitive neuroectoderm, to form the adrenal medulla: the chromaffinoblast and the neuroblast, which mature into the chromaffin cell and the sympathetic ganglion cell, respectively. These medullary cells are richly supplied with preganglionic fibers from the splanchnic nerves.

The chromaffin cell is so named because of its capacity to show brown intracytoplasmic granules on treatment with chromium salts, a result of oxidation and polymerization of the catecholamine stored in the granules. Chromaffin cells are found in widely dispersed sites at birth: the adrenal medulla, the paraganglia (along the retropleural and retroperitoneal sympathetic chains), the organs of Zuckerkandl (paired structures lying anterior to the bifurcation of the abdominal aorta), chemoreceptor areas ("glomic tissue" at the carotid bifurcation, along the aortic arch, and at the jugular bulb), and the human dermis. Many of the extraadrenal sites undergo progressive involution until puberty, but remnants account for the extraadrenal occurrences of pheochromocytomas, reported in all of the areas cited with the exception of the skin.

PATHOLOGY Over 50 percent of pheochromocytomas occur in the region of the adrenals, sometimes bilaterally, and over 90 percent lie between the diaphragm and pelvic floor. As indicated by metastases, 6 percent are malignant, and 7 percent occur simultaneously in more than one focus. Metastases may be functional and have occurred in liver, lungs, and central skeleton, as well as paraaortic lymph glands. The tumor weight may vary from a gram to several thousand grams (averaging about 100) and correlates poorly with the severity of the symptomatology. The tumors are round, frequently lobulated, and highly vascular. They may show hemorrhagic and necrotic areas with cystic degeneration, particularly in large tumors. On section they appear brown or gray. Histologically they resemble the adrenal medulla; the nuclei are often multiple, cytoplasmic vacuolization is common, and dark staining with chromium salts is characteristic. Benign tumors may invade the capsule and are difficult if not impossible to distinguish from malignant forms on purely histologic grounds. Individual tumor cells usually contain both epinephrine and norepinephrine storage granules. After glutaraldehyde fixation, electron microscopic analysis shows the epinephrine granules as the gray core of round vesicles and the norepinephrine as the black core of oval vesicles. Cells from predominantly epinephrine-secreting tumors show mainly the former and norepinephrine-secreting tumors the latter, the concentration of each correlating with its granular density. There is no ultrastructural distinction between tumors from patients with differing symptoms, e.g., sustained versus paroxysmal hypertension, or a high versus a low rate of catecholamine turnover.

PHYSIOLOGY The sympathetic nerve terminals and the chromaffin cells of the adrenal medulla and pheochromocytomas synthesize norepinephrine according to the following enzymatic steps: hydroxylation of tyrosine to form dopa (3,4-dihydroxyphenylalanine), decarboxylation of dopa to form dopamine (3,4-dihydroxyphenylethylamine), the latter entering storage vesicles to undergo beta oxidation to form norepinephrine (Fig. 87-1). In the adrenal medulla and most pheochromocytomas a proportion of the norepinephrine undergoes N-methylation to form epinephrine. In the brain, dopamine as well as norepinephrine is stored, both serving as catecholamine neurotransmitters. Epinephrine is the major hormone of the adrenal medulla, constituting 80 percent of its stored content of catecholamine; the major

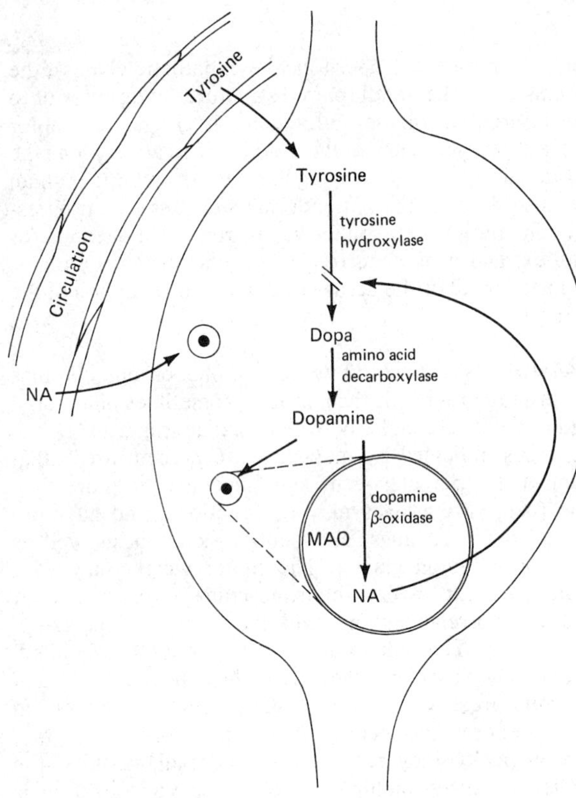

FIGURE 87-1
Biosynthesis of norepinephrine in the sympathetic neuron. NA, noradrenaline (norepinephrine); dopa, dihydroxyphenylalanine; MAO, monoamine oxidase. (Adapted from J Axelrod and IJ Kopin, The uptake, storage, release and metabolism of noradrenaline in sympathetic nerves. Prog Brain Res 31:21, 1969. By permission, from J Axelrod and R Weinshilboum: Physiology in medicine: Catecholamines. N Engl J Med 287:238, 1972)

source of norepinephrine is the postganglionic sympathetic neuron, where it acts as the neurotransmitter.

Adrenomedullary and presumably pheochromocytoma catecholamines are released in the process of *exocytosis,* the storage vesicle discharging its entire soluble contents (catecholamines, specific proteins such as dopamine-β-hydroxylase, and ATP) through the cell membrane (Fig. 87-2). In the adrenal medulla this is in response to cholinergic preganglionic sympathetic nerve stimulation and requires calcium ion. A number of agents can directly stimulate chromaffin cells or the adrenergic neurons to release catecholamines; these agents include acetylcholine, nicotine, histamine, 5-hydroxytryptamine, tyramine, and reserpine. An increase in the release of both epinephrine and norepinephrine is caused by a number of physiologic stimuli such as severe muscular work, asphyxia and hypoxia, and hemorrhagic hypotension. Insulin hypoglycemia causes a selective release of epinephrine alone, favoring the concept of separate control of the release of adrenomedullary epinephrine and norepinephrine.

The physiologic effects of the adrenomedullary hormones may be characterized as preparing the organism to meet an emergency situation. Both epinephrine and norepinephrine have a comparable direct beta-adrenergic (inotropic and chronotropic) cardiac effect. However, the predominant alpha-adrenergic (vasoconstrictor) peripheral effect of circulating norepinephrine results in diastolic and systolic hypertension, producing reflex slowing of the heart, so that cardiac output is generally unchanged or reduced. The net peripheral vasodilator (beta-adrenergic) effect of physiological doses of epinephrine (due primarily to vasodilatation of the resistance vessels of skeletal muscle), associated with its beta-adrenergic cardiac effects, produces a rise in cardiac output, with widening of pulse pressure through a rise in systolic pressure; diastolic pressure may fall slightly. Cutaneous and renal vasoconstriction is common to both hormones. Both increase the rate and depth of respiration and stimulate

FIGURE 87-2
Fate of norepinephrine at a varicosity of the sympathetic nerve terminal. Norepinephrine (NA) is stored in dense core vesicles together with the norepinephrine-forming enzyme dopamine β-hydroxylase (DBH). When the nerve is depolarized, the vesicle discharges norepinephrine and the soluble portion of dopamine β-hydroxylase into the synaptic cleft, by a process of exocytosis. Norepinephrine acts at the effector cell, and its actions are terminated by reuptake into the neuron, removal by circulation, and subsequent metabolism in the liver or by metabolism in the effector cell by catechol O-methyltransferase (COMT) and mitochondrial monoamine oxidase (MAO). Norepinephrine that leaks out of the vesicle is inactivated by intraneuronal monoamine oxidase. (By permission, from J Axelrod and R Weinshilboum: Physiology in medicine: Catecholamines. N Engl J Med 287:238, 1972)

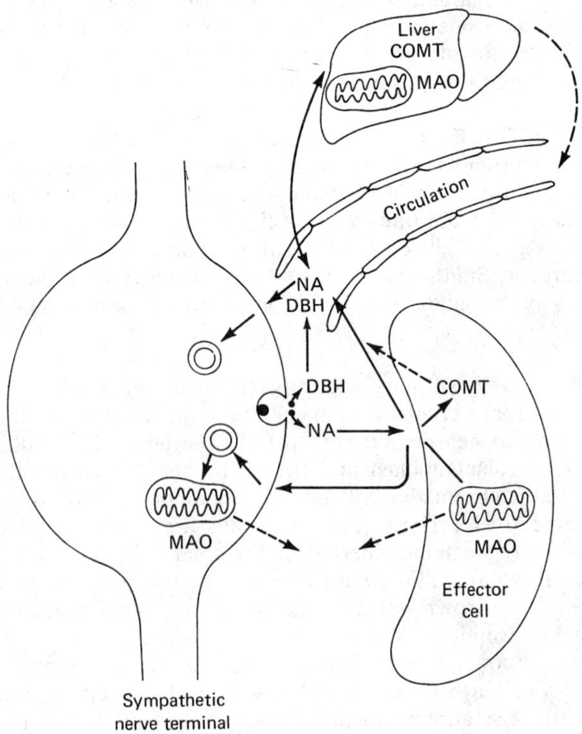

the release into plasma of nonesterified fatty acids from neutral fat depots. Another metabolic effect of epinephrine (and of norepinephrine in large doses), leading to an increased oxygen consumption and respiratory quotient, is the activation of hepatic and skeletal muscle phosphorylase by stimulating adenyl cyclase to increase the formation of cyclic AMP from ATP. This produces an accelerated glycogenolysis. The hepatic release of glucose 1-phosphate elevates blood glucose, and the release of glucose 6-phosphate from muscle elevates blood lactic acid.

CATECHOLAMINE METABOLISM Figure 87-2 shows the metabolic paths of norepinephrine derived from sympathetic nerve endings. The corresponding molecular transformation of released catecholamines of neural and adrenomedullary origin are detailed in Fig. 87-3. The major portion of neurally released norepinephrine is restored in neuronal vesicles in an economical process called "reuptake." Catecholamines released by the adrenal medulla (and pheochromocytomas) and part of the neurally released norepinephrine circulate to the liver. Hepatic catechol O-methyl transferase (COMT) inactivates the catecholamines by converting norepinephrine to normetanephrine and epinephrine to metanephrine. The subsequent action of hepatic monamine oxidase (MAO) converts both of these compounds into vanillylmandelic acid and 3-methoxy-4-hydroxyphenylglycol. The latter are the major urinary metabolites, although the metanephrines (normetanephrine and metanephrine) and unmodified catecholamine are also excreted. The effector cell also contains COMT and MAO, contributing to the pool of these inactive methoxylated metabolites of norepinephrine of neural origin. Finally, neuronal monamine oxidase inactivates excess norepinephrine that is outside of the storage vesicles, contributing to the circulating pool of metabolites. The concentration of the metanephrines in pheochromocytomas tends to be low, and constant over a wide range of active catecholamine concentration. This suggests that the rate of hormone turnover by the tumor is not modulated by variations in its content of catecholamine-metabolizing enzymes. Bilateral adrenalectomy results in only a minor depression of urinary catecholamines, since 80 percent is normally

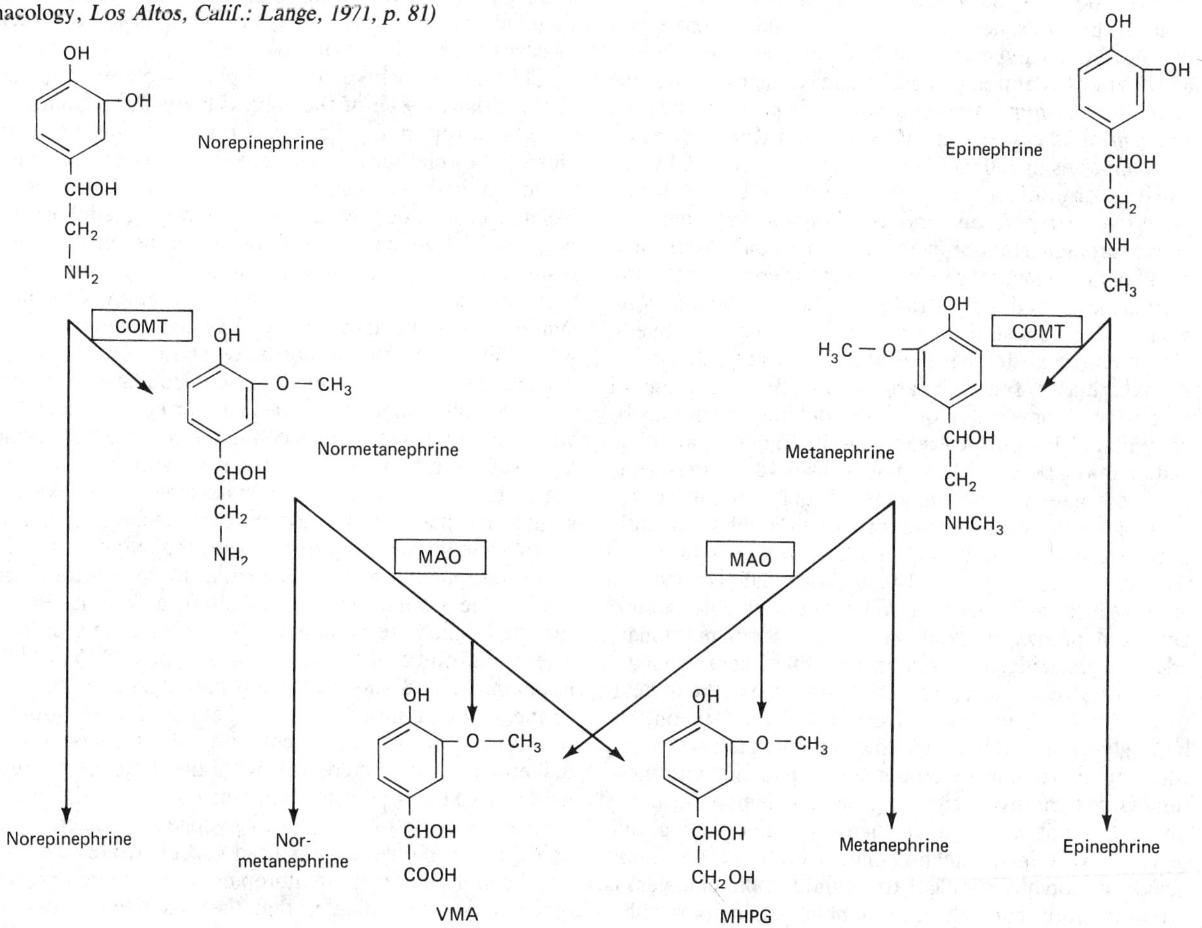

FIGURE 87-3
Metabolism of free catecholamines. Urinary excretion products appear on the lowest line. Excretion products may be conjugated with glucuronide or sulfate. COMT, catechol O-methyltransferase: VMA, 3-methoxy-4-hydroxymandelic acid; MHPG, methoxyhydroxyphenylglycol; MAO, monoamine oxidase. (By permission, from FH Myers et al: Review of Medical Pharmacology, *Los Altos, Calif.: Lange, 1971, p. 81)*

norepinephrine, largely derived from sympathetic nerve endings. The high activity of these two enzyme systems (MAO and COMT) is indicated by the fact that the daily urinary content, by weight, of the metanephrines (after hydrolyzing the major conjugated fraction free of its glucuronide or sulfate) is approximately seven times, and of VMA approximately thirty times, that of the total catecholamines. Half of the catecholamine is in the "free" form, and half is found as glucuronide or sulfate conjugates.

Increased sympathetic tone increases catecholamine synthesis and turnover, the rate-limiting step being the conversion of tyrosine to dopa by tyrosine hydroxylase. Tissue levels of catecholamines are kept fairly constant, since tyrosine hydroxylase is stimulated by low and inhibited by high catecholamine concentrations. Increased sympathetic nerve activity augments the activity of tyrosine hydroxylase and dopamine β-hydroxylase (Fig. 87-1), both of which enzymes require adrenocorticotropic hormone for functional integrity. Glucocorticoid activity has a potent stimulating effect on the adrenomedullary conversion of norepinephrine to epinephrine by phenylethanolamine-N-methyl transferase.

CLINICAL MANIFESTATIONS In a review of 507 cases of pheochromocytoma, Hermann and Mornex report that 26 percent of cases presented with paroxysmal hypertension and 60 percent with permanent hypertension; of the latter, nearly half had crises superimposed on their sustained hypertension. The remaining 14 percent had atypical features or absent clinical signs. Thus, *the characteristic hypertensive crisis is found in only about one-half of all cases.* Thomas, Rook, and Kvale reviewed the symptoms in 100 patients with the paroxysmal hypertensive form of the disease. The triad of headache, excessive perspiration, and palpitations was found in about three-quarters of instances. Commonly associated manifestations were pallor, nausea, tremor, weakness, nervousness, and epigastric pain. Less common complaints were chest pain, dyspnea, flushing, numbness, visual blurring, tightness of the throat, and dizziness. Bradycardia is found in approximately 20 percent of cases. Paroxysms are frequently spontaneous but may be precipitated by physical exertion, abdominal palpation, and emotional upset. They may occur several times a day or at rare intervals, and may last for only a minute or for as long as a week. Blood pressure levels frequently exceed 250/150 mm during an attack in association with the paroxysmal release of catecholamine. Shock and renal failure may attend or follow a paroxysmal attack. During a paroxysm death may occur from pulmonary edema, ventricular fibrillation, or cerebral hemorrhage.

Cases of *persistently* secreting tumors may be difficult to distinguish from cases of essential hypertension, but hyperglycemia and hypermetabolism (elevated BMR) are found in approximately 50 percent of patients with these tumors. Progressive weight loss and the demonstration of postural hypotension are further suggestive clinical evidence of sustained catecholamine secretion by a tumor. Frank retinopathy (grade 3 to 4 funduscopic changes) is found in more than half of these patients, an appreciably higher incidence than is found in the purely paroxysmal variety. This underscores the gravity of this form of hypertension and the importance of early clinical detection. Notable clinical features of the disorder that have been reported include intermittent claudication associated with tissue necrosis in the presence of palpable pulses, extensive necrosis of the tumor leading to shock, and a paralytic ileus that is frequently fatal associated with massive catecholamine discharge. Renal artery compression has been caused by the tumor.

Special features Several unique aspects of the disease deserve emphasis. The tumor may first appear in early childhood or old age, but the average age of onset is during the fourth decade. In childhood pheochromocytoma, the hypertension is almost always of the sustained variety, and the tumor is bilateral in 20 percent of cases and shows a higher incidence of malignancy than in the adult. Distinct genetic factors are implicated in some instances by the prevalence of the tumor in certain families, sometimes in association with other congenital disorders of the neuroectoderm such as neurofibromatosis and central nervous system hemangioblastoma. A number of reports deal with the familial coincidence of pheochromocytoma and thyroid cancer, which is usually the medullary or solid type with amyloid production. This complex also has been coupled with parathyroid hyperplasia and adenomas (multiple endocrine neoplasia, type 2), and has been associated with and could be secondary to a high level of thyrocalcitonin from the thyroid tumor. Familial pheochromocytomas are bilateral in 50 percent of cases (See chap. 351).

Chromaffin-positive norepinephrine-secreting tumors of the glomic tissue of the carotid body and jugular bulb have been reported. These may represent further examples of the relationship between dysplasia of the neuroectoderm and the paroxysmal syndrome. There is an isolated case report of unilateral adrenal medullary hyperplasia in which removal of the hyperplastic gland resulted in complete amelioration of the signs and symptoms of excessive catecholamine secretion. Cushing's syndrome may be associated with pheochromocytoma, in which instances the tumor may show mixed adrenal cortical and medullary cells (corticomedullary adenoma).

True polycythemia has been reported in association with the tumor, with return of the red cell mass to normal after successful surgery. Pheochromocytoma of the bladder wall produces a unique syndrome of paroxysmal symptoms, particularly throbbing headache, on micturition. While the majority of pheochromocytomas produce more norepinephrine than epinephrine (in contradistinction to the normal adrenal medulla), a few have been reported which are predominantly epinephrine secretors. These tend to be of the paroxysmal type and to produce hypotension and shock during a paroxysm, perhaps due to the vasodilating effect of the beta-adrenergic stimulation on the peripheral vasculature. The frequency of a diabetic tendency increases with the ratio of the epinephrine to the total catecholamine content of the tumor, perhaps because of the greater glycogenolytic activity of epinephrine. However, impaired carbohydrate tolerance has been found in pure norepinephrine secretors, and recent evidence indicates that the associated excessive alpha-adrenergic stimulation will inhibit insulin release to account for the impairment.

Over 50 percent of patients dying with a pheochromocytoma have an active myocarditis at autopsy. In the majority of these instances there was prior clinical evidence of left ventricular failure. In all probability this is a direct, "toxic" effect of the high levels of catecholamines on the myocardium.

Finally, a hypertensive response to smoking, to anesthesia, or to therapy with ganglionic blocking agents and guanethidine should raise the strong suspicion of a pheochromocytoma.

DIAGNOSIS The clinical picture of essential hypertension with marked vasomotor lability strongly suggests pheochromocytoma, but pheochromocytoma with sustained hypertension in the absence of paroxysms may be indistinguishable from essential hypertension. Thus, routine laboratory screening of all patients with significant hypertension is desirable for this potentially curable form of hypertension.

Urinary assay for catecholamines and their methoxy derivatives Modern chemical methods for the determination of 24-hr urinary catecholamines and their methoxy derivatives have largely replaced the older pharmacologic tests in routine screening because of their safety and greater accuracy. Current chemical methods for determining urinary free catecholamines involve modifications of the trihydroxyindole (THI) method of Lund. The urinary free catecholamines are adsorbed on an alumina or resin column, eluted with acid, oxidized to form "chromes," which, in turn, are tautomerized in alkali to form strongly fluorescent trihydroxyindoles. Free epinephrine and norepinephrine may be measured separately from fluorometric readings at different wavelengths. After acid hydrolysis to free the conjugated fractions, metanephrine (MN) and normetanephrine (NMN) may be isolated on resin and converted to trihydroxyindoles for fluorometric assay or oxidized to vanillin and read photometrically. VMA is measured by isolation and oxidation to vanillin, which may be read photometrically directly or after color development with added indole.

With these techniques Sjoerdsma and associates determined, simultaneously, the 24-hr urinary free catecholamines, metanephrines, and vanillylmandelic acid on 64 patients with proved pheochromocytoma. The results are shown in Fig. 87-4 and indicate that the values obtained for all three assays were above the upper limit of normal in all but a few instances, giving an overall diagnostic reliability in the range of 90 percent. The upper limits of normal are (1) free catecholamines (epinephrine plus norepinephrine), 100 μg; (2) metanephrine plus normetanephrine, 1.3 mg; (3) VMA, 6.5 mg. Therapy with alphamethyldopa will produce false elevations in the free catecholamines and, potentially, in the metanephrines. With methods that convert VMA to vanillin, dietary considerations may be disregarded in the determination of urinary VMA, but nonspecific chromatographic screening methods should be avoided. In general, *it is important to discontinue sympathomimetic agents and monamine oxidase inhibitors when performing these assays.* The relative diagnostic merits of the three different indices are debated, and it is probable that any one of them, carefully done, will serve as well as another.

The reliable measurement of plasma catecholamine levels requires highly sophisticated methodology and is not a practical approach. However, using an enzymatic double-labeled isotope assay, Engelman, Portnoy, and Sjoerdsma found the mean plasma catecholamine level in 10 patients with pheochromocytoma to be 5.0 mg per liter as compared with a mean of 0.24 mg per liter in 32 normal patients, with no overlap.

Pharmacologic tests for pheochromocytoma In the absence of facilities for these chemical determinations, reliance may be placed on the various intravenous pharmacologic tests. Along with the phentolamine (Regitine) test, which produces a precipitous fall in blood pressure in pheochromocytomas, there are now in use three "provocative" tests: the older histamine and the newer tyramine and glucagon tests. Unfortunately, deaths have occurred after both phentolamine and histamine in pheochromocytomas, and the pharmacologic approach probably fails to detect as many as 25 percent of cases. The matter is further complicated by the prevalence of false positive responses with these agents. This occurs frequently with phentolamine, occasionally with histamine (up to 11 percent) and tyramine (3 percent), and rarely, if at all, with glucagon. Other advantages of glucagon administration over histamine provocation are the absence of significant side effects, fewer false negative responses, and probable greater safety. The intravenous tyramine test has a higher incidence of false negatives in patients with *familial* pheochromocytoma than in sporadic cases. It has the advantage over histamine and glucagon of causing a milder rise in blood pressure in the presence of a pheochromocytoma, but, by the same token, the end point of a positive reaction is less succinct. It is strongly contraindicated in any patient receiving amine oxidase inhibitor therapy, where the administration of tyramine may precipitate a hypertensive crisis. Histamine and probably glucagon should not be used if the control pressure is 170/110 mm or above, and phentolamine should be ready for immediate administration in the advent of a precipitous rise in blood pressure when these tests are performed. With pressures in the range of 170/110 mm or above, the tyramine and phentolamine tests are the ones of choice.

In a small percentage of patients, particularly during a normotensive period in those with intermittently secreting tumors, 24-hr urinary assay for catecholamines (or derivatives thereof) may not be clearly elevated into a diagnostic range. If suspicion is still strong on clinical grounds, the tumor may be provoked to secrete with 0.01 to 0.025 mg histamine base, given intravenously. This should be followed by the rapid injection of 5 mg phentolamine intravenously, should an alarming rise in blood pressure ensue. Blood may be drawn during the control period and at intervals of 2 min in the immediate posthistamine period for plasma assay for catecholamines, or a timed urine specimen (after prior emptying of the bladder) may be collected for a period of 6 hr for analysis for catecholamines or methoxy derivatives, which may be expressed as amount excreted per milligram of creatinine.

The upper limit of normal for plasma epinephrine and norepinephrine varies with the method employed and must be established in a given laboratory to determine a diagnostic rise following histamine administration. The upper limit of normal for urinary catecholamines (epinephrine plus norepinephrine) is 0.05 μg per mg creatinine; for metanephrine plus normetanephrine, it is 2.1 μg per creatinine; for VMA, it is 9.5 μg per mg creatinine. Levels above these following histamine administration are diagnostic. If a spontaneous attack should occur while a patient is under observation, blood and urinary determinations should be made immediately. The plasma ethylenediamine condensation method for plasma catecholamines is invalid in the presence of uremia.

Localization of tumor While rarely palpable, a tumor mass may be detected on a plain film of the abdomen. A more specialized technique is an intravenous pyelogram with laminography, detecting *adrenal* pheochromocytomas in approximately 50 percent of cases. Another is abdominal filming of the contrast afforded by the presacral injection of carbon dioxide or nitrous oxide, which may detect relatively small tumors. However, variations in the suprarenal fat accumulation may render interpretation difficult. The advent of selective renal and adrenal angiography has afforded superb information in this regard; in some hands, these radiologic procedures are proving to be the ones of choice. Selective retrograde adrenal venography is the most sensitive approach, detecting tumors as small as 1 cm in diameter. The hazards attending these contrast techniques (including the potential for direct tumor stimulation) are apparent, and phentolamine should be ready for immediate administration during their performance. The analysis of catecholamines in plasma obtained by catheter at different levels in the

FIGURE 87-4

Urinary excretion of catecholamines and metabolites in 64 patients with proved pheochromocytoma. (By permission, from A Sjoerdsma et al: Combined clinical staff conference at the National Institutes of Health. Pheochromocytoma: Current concepts of diagnosis and treatment. Ann Intern Med 65:1306, 1966)

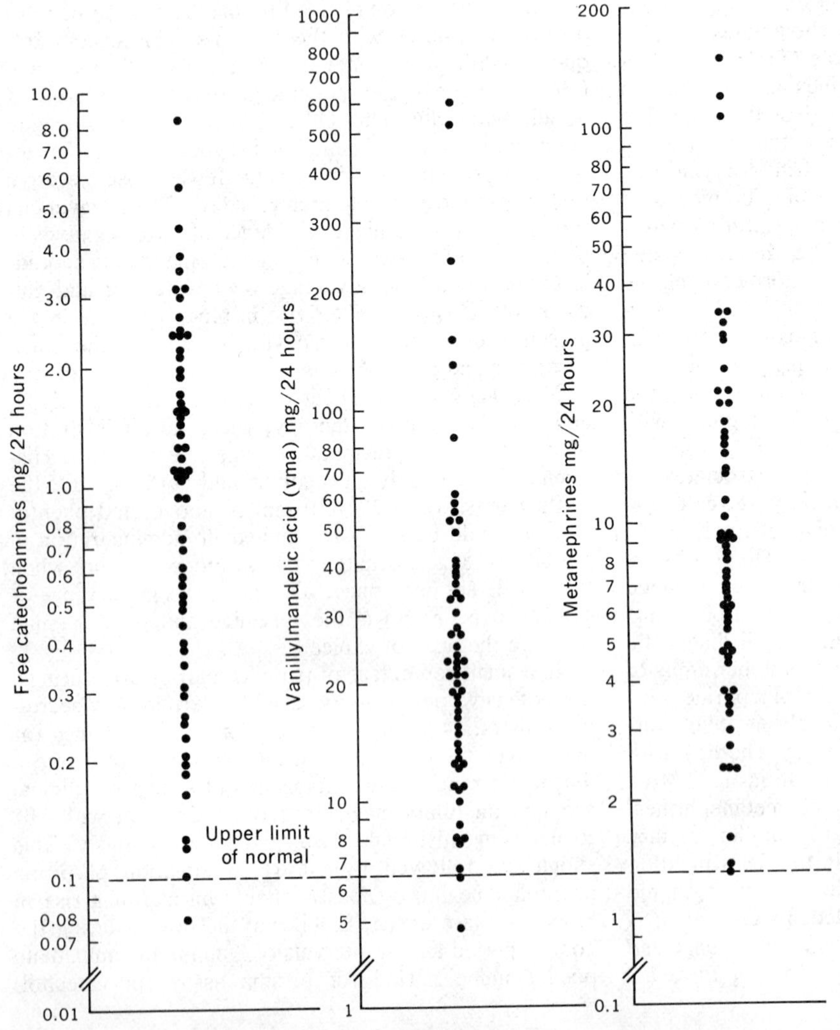

venous system under fluoroscopic control has also been useful. Thoracic tumors, while rare, may be seen on a plain chest film. Overexposure of the film enhances the chance of visualizing posterior masses along the sympathetic chains.

Crout and Sjoerdsma report that the separate determination of urinary epinephrine and norepinephrine is of predictive value in tumor localization. If there is a significant elevation of epinephrine as well as norepinephrine (42 percent of all cases), the tumor may be expected to lie in or adjacent to one of the adrenal glands or, rarely, in the organs of Zuckerkandl. If the urine contains elevated norepinephrine alone (58 percent of all cases), the tumor, of course, may still be found in one of the adrenal areas. Less than 10 percent of tumors are extraabdominal, and these will generally show only an elevation of urinary norepinephrine and probably reflect a deficiency of N-methylating enzyme, present in the normal adrenal medulla and necessary for the conversion of norepinephrine into epinephrine.

DIFFERENTIAL DIAGNOSIS False positive responses with pharmacologic testing and elevations in urinary levels of catecholamines and derivatives due to interfering substances and laboratory errors has led to unnecessary surgical exploration in many hypertensive patients. This problem is compounded by the elevated plasma levels (or excretion) of catecholamines frequently identifiable in essential hypertension, and in hypertension associated with such states as Guillain-Barré syndrome and intracranial tumors in the region of the posterior hypothalamus and medulla oblongata. Incorrect diagnoses in the presence of a pheochromocytoma have included diabetes mellitus, thyrotoxicosis, anxiety neurosis, "vascular" headache, epilepsy, and hypertensive crises due to lead poisoning and porphyria.

Patients with "nonchromaffin" sympathetic tumors, i.e., ganglioneuromas and, particularly, neuroblastomas, have shown elevated levels of norepinephrine in the urine as well as increased excretion of its precursors (dopa and dopamine) and of its methoxy metabolites (metanephrines and VMA). Since some of these patients have associated hypertension, these tumors are to be distinguished from true "chromaffinomas." Serum dopamine β-hydroxylase activity has been found to be elevated in over 50 percent of patients with neuroblastoma and may prove useful in the diagnosis of this disorder.

TREATMENT In patients in whom surgical resection of the tumor cannot be performed, as with functioning metastases, the regular oral administration of the alpha-adrenergic blocking agent phenoxybenzamine (Dibenzyline) has been reported to have controlled most of the disturbing signs and symptoms for a period of many months. This approach has also been recommended routinely for a period of several weeks in order to get patients into an optimum condition in preparation for surgery, as in the presence of malignant hypertension with congestive heart failure. The use of beta-adrenergic blockers, such as propranolol, may also be useful in protecting against beta-adrenergic–mediated cardiac arrhythmias from high circulating levels of catecholamines. The use of inhibitors of catecholamine synthesis is another approach to the pharmacologic treatment and preoperative control of patients with pheochromocytoma; preliminary reports of the use of alpha-methyl-para-tyrosine in this regard are very encouraging.

Surgical removal of the tumor is the treatment of choice for this potentially lethal disease. Since over 90 percent of all such tumors are located in the abdomen, a careful abdominal incision may be undertaken, even without the certain exclusion of a rare extraabdominal site. Halothane and fluroxene have been recommended as anesthetic agents of choice because of their relative lack of effect on stimulating sympathoadrenal activity, in contradistinction to ether and cyclopropane. To avoid extremes of hypertension during induction of anesthesia and surgical manipulation, an intravenous drip of phentolamine should be ready at all times. To avoid extremes of hypotension on clamping the blood supply of the tumor and following its removal, an intravenous drip of norepinephrine or other pressor amine should also be prepared in advance. *Administration of whole blood or plasma on removal of the tumor may be of paramount importance in preventing postoperative shock,* since the sudden relief of the prolonged vasoconstriction attending the disease produces a state of disparity between the vascular capacity and effective blood volume.

REFERENCES

Axelrod J, Weinshilboum R: Physiology in medicine: catecholamines. N Engl J Med 287:237, 1972

DeQuattro V: Evaluation of increased norepinephrine excretion in hypertension using L-dopa-^{3}H. Circ Res 28:84, 1971

Engelman K et al: Plasma catecholamine concentrations in patients with hypertension. Circ Res (suppl 1) 27:141, 1970

Hermann H, Mornex R: *Human Tumours Secreting Catecholamines: Clinical and Physiopathological Study of the Pheochromocytomas,* New York: Pergamon Press, 1964

Lauper NT et al: Pheochromocytoma: Fine structural, biochemical and clinical observations. Am J Cardiol 30:197, 1972

Packman RC et al: Pheochromocytoma: Therapeutic grand rounds no. 24. JAMA 212:780, 1970

Paloyan E et al: Familial pheochromocytoma, medullary thyroid carcinoma, and parathyroid adenomas. JAMA 214:1443, 1970

Thomas JD et al: The neurologist's experience with pheochromocytoma: A review of 100 cases. JAMA 197:754, 1966

88
DIABETES MELLITUS

JURGEN STEINKE
GEORGE W. THORN

Knowledge of diabetes is important because of its high prevalence. It has been estimated that there are 200 million diabetics in the world. After obesity and thyroid disorders, it is the third most common metabolic disorder. Diabetes consists of a metabolic and a vascular component, which are probably interrelated. The metabolic syndrome is characterized by an inappropriate elevation of blood glucose level, associated with alterations in lipid and protein metabolism, for which a relative or absolute lack of insulin is responsible. Its most severe manifestation is diabetic ketoacidosis. The vascular syndrome consists of accelerated nonspecific atherosclerosis (premature aging) and a more specific microangiopathy, particularly affecting the eye and kidney. Thus gangrene of the foot, arteriosclerotic heart disease, blindness, and uremia are the most frequent manifestations of the vascular syndrome. For this reason the long-term prognosis of severe diabetes is not bright, particularly if it is of juvenile-onset type. Statistically the diabetic is faced not only with a decrease in life expectancy but also with the ever-present possibility of disabling complications. Nevertheless, some patients with diabetes do very well for many decades.

HISTORY

Diabetes has been recognized from antiquity. Chinese medical writings mentioned a syndrome of polyphagia, polydipsia, and polyuria. Aretaeus (ca. A.D. 70) described the disease and, referring to the polyuria, gave it its name, which comes from a Greek root meaning "To run through."

The study of the chemistry of diabetic urine was initiated by Paracelsus in the sixteenth century. Some 100 years later, Thomas Willis described the sweetness of the diabetic urine, "as if imbued with honey" ("mellitus"), which Dobson proved to be sugar. This led to a rational dietary approach, introduced by Rollo 29 years later. Morton (1686) noted the hereditary character of diabetes. In 1859, Claude Bernard demonstrated the increased glucose content of diabetic blood and recognized hyperglycemia as the cardinal sign of the disease. In 1869, Langerhans, still a medical student, described the islets in the pancreas, which now bear his name. Kussmaul characterized the air hunger and labored breathing of the patient in diabetic coma in 1874. The careful work by clinicians such as Bouchardat, Naunyn, von Noorden, Allen, and Joslin led to a significant therapeutic success with diet. Von Mering and Minkowski carried out their studies in 1889, demonstrating that dogs could be made diabetic by pancreatectomy. However, it took more than 30 years before Banting and Best were able to prepare an extract from dog pancreas capable of reducing an elevated blood glucose level. In 1939, the first long-acting insulin was introduced by Hagedorn. The chemical structure of ox insulin was established by Sanger in 1953; Nicol and Smith described the chemical structure of human insulin in 1960. The basic unit contains two polypeptide chains united by disulfide bridges. In 1964, Katsoyannis in the United States and Zahn in Germany completed the synthesis of both the A and B chains of insulin and were able to combine both chains into biologically active material. In 1967 Steiner described a large "proinsulin" molecule which exhibits only little biologic activity. It is converted by enzymatic cleavage into the smaller biologically active insulin (Fig. 88-1). The experimental work of Loubatieres in France and the accidental discovery of the hypoglycemic action of carbutamide by Franke and Fuchs in Germany, in 1955, initiated the use of oral hypoglycemic agents of the sulfonylurea type. Recently the long-term safety of these drugs has been questioned.

PREVALENCE

Diabetes mellitus is a disease of worldwide distribution. If it is more frequent in some countries than in others, that will have to be established when diagnostic criteria are agreed upon and uniformly controlled detection drives are executed. In the United States there are approximately 4 million persons with diabetes. Diabetes is more frequent in older people. The U.S. Public Health Service estimates that there are 2 diabetics for every 1,000 persons up to age twenty-four, 10 between the ages of twenty-five and forty-four, 33 in the age group forty-five to fifty-four, 56 between ages fifty-five and sixty-four, and 69 between sixty-five and seventy-four years of age. Unless a cure or some preventive measure is found for diabetes, this number will continue to increase for the following reasons: (1) the population grows and becomes older; (2) the life expectancy of the treated diabetic is steadily increasing; (3) since more diabetics live long enough to have children, an increasing number of children will inherit the diabetic gene; and (4) obesity, which appears to precipitate diabetes among those predisposed to it, is also on the rise, thus allowing more potential diabetics to emerge.

Undiagnosed adult diabetes with few or no symptoms presents a major challenge to the practicing physician.

FIGURE 88-1
Synthesis of insulin from the single-chain, biologically less active precursor, proinsulin. Proteolytic enzymes within the beta cell split off the connecting peptide portion of proinsulin, resulting in the formation of double-chain insulin proper. The A and B chains are bound by disulfide bridges. (Reproduced with permission of W. B. Saunders Co.)

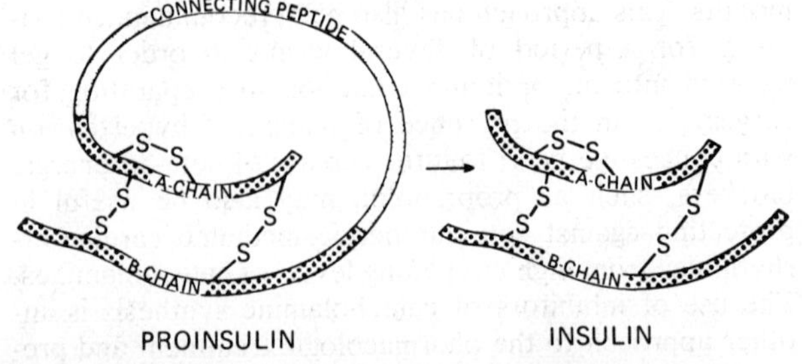

Because diabetic symptoms are minimal, the patient does not seek medical advice. In the United States, approximately 50 percent of the 4 million diabetics are unidentified. As it is not feasible to test the entire population, it is advisable to concentrate on those individuals with predisposition for the disease. They are (1) relatives of known diabetics, among whom diabetes is $2^1/_2$ times more frequent than in the general population; (2) obese persons, since 85 percent of diabetic patients are, or were at one time, overweight; (3) persons in the older age groups, as four out of five diabetics are over forty-five; and (4) mothers delivered of large babies, since the birth of a large infant may be an indication of maternal prediabetes.

Apart from these high-risk groups, routine testing for diabetes should be performed whenever patients are admitted to a hospital for elective surgery or seen for an annual checkup. Furthermore, it would be desirable to include testing for diabetes in preemployment examinations.

INHERITANCE

It is well established that diabetes mellitus is inherited; the mode of inheritance is still under discussion. The acceptance of heredity for diabetes is based on the greater frequency of diabetes among blood relatives of known diabetics. The pattern of inheritance is characterized by (1) a more frequent occurrence in the siblings of identical than nonidentical twins; and (2) the equilateral transmission of the trait by either affected parent (i.e., autosomal, non-sex-linked). However, genetic study is complicated by the fact that though susceptibility to diabetes is inherited, the disease itself may not become apparent clinically for years. Genetic studies are based on occurrence of clinical diabetes (phenotype), not on the presence of the genetic predisposition (genotype), for the latter cannot be detected at the present time. It is possible that the diabetic trait may be dominant and the manifest diabetic disease recessive. There is further confusion because diabetes is a syndrome; e. g. , chronic pancreatitis may be associated with hyperglycemia indistinguishable from that observed in genetic diabetes. This could lead to false designation of a person as affected with genetic diabetes. Diabetes has a variable age of onset (youth-onset and maturity-onset), each with a characteristic clinical pattern. This has led, on the one hand, to the hypothesis of multifactorial (polygenic) inheritance. There is also the hypothesis that the mode of inheritance in juvenile diabetes is homozygous, whereas the hereditary factor in maturity-onset diabetes is heterozygous. On the other hand, Rimoin has reviewed all available genetic data and expressed the belief that no simple hypothesis can explain all of it. It must be remembered that it is still not known what exactly is the genetic marker. Extensive studies in offspring of two diabetic parents have shown that no consistent abnormality could be detected at a time when glucose tolerance was still normal. Therefore an important role must be attributed to precipitating factors such as obesity, infections, and possibly even drugs. For these reasons accurate genetic counseling is impossible.

TABLE 88-1
Stages of diabetes mellitus

1 Clinical = overt = decompensated diabetes
2 Chemical = asymptomatic diabetes
3 Latent = stress diabetes
4 Prediabetes = potential diabetes

CLASSIFICATION

It is helpful to classify diabetic patients not only according to type of diabetes but also according to present stage of carbohydrate decompensation. The latter implies that progression or regression from one stage to the next occurs and may be very rapid, may proceed slowly, or may never take place. The following states of diabetes are almost universally accepted (Table 88-1): (1) Overt or clinical diabetes: this is frank diabetes either of the ketosis-prone (juvenile) or ketosis-resistant (adult) type. Fasting and random blood glucose levels are definitely elevated; symptoms related to hyperglycemia and glycosuria can usually be elicited. (2) Chemical or asymptomatic diabetes: the fasting blood glucose level is usually normal, but the postprandial level is frequently elevated. The result of an oral or intravenous glucose tolerance test performed in the absence of stress is clearly abnormal. There are no frank diabetic symptoms. If observed in children, this stage is usually of short duration, as the disease progresses rapidly to overt diabetes. There is however, a small group of asymptomatic, young, nonobese diabetic children whose condition appears to remain stationary for years. In adults this chemical stage may be present for years, and some patients never progress beyond it. Despite this, diabetic angiopathy may be present. (3) Latent or stress diabetes: present in a person who at the present time has a normal glucose tolerance but who is known to have been a diabetic at some previous time, i. e., during pregnancy (gestational diabetes), during infection, when obese, or when under stress, such as cerebrovascular accident, myocardial infarction, extensive burns, or endocrinopathies. The status of patients with such temporary carbohydrate intolerance should be watched closely, particularly when there is a family history of diabetes. (4) Prediabetes or potential diabetes: this is a conceptual term, a retrospective diagnosis, applied to the period of time preceding any glucose intolerance. By definition it cannot be diagnosed with certainty in the current state of our knowledge except possibly in the nondiabetic identical twin of a diabetic patient and in the offspring of two diabetic parents.

As to the *types* of diabetes, the following etiologic classification may be applied:

1 *Genetic (hereditary, idiopathic, primary, essential) diabetes*, subdivided according to the age of onset into juvenile and adult diabetes.
2 *Pancreatic diabetes*, in which the carbohydrate intolerance may be attributed directly to destruction of the pancreatic islets by chronic inflammation, carcinoma, hemochromatosis, or surgical removal.
3 *Endocrine diabetes*, in which the diabetes is associated with endocrinopathies such as hyperpituitarism (acro-

megaly, basophilism), hyperthyroidism, hyperadrenalism (Cushing's syndrome, primary aldosteronism, pheochromocytoma), and pancreatic islets–cell tumor of the A-cell type. Under this category may also be included the gestational diabetes and the various forms of stress diabetes listed above.

4 *Iatrogenic diabetes*, precipitated by administration of corticosteroids, certain diuretics of the benzothiadiazine type, and possibly also by estrogen-progesterone combinations, etc.

PATHOLOGY

PANCREAS With the use of special stains with the light microscope and with the availability of the electron microscope, it now appears very likely that almost all diabetic patients exhibit a correlation between severity of their diabetes, on the one hand, and reduced total mass of beta cells and degree of beta cell degranulation, on the other. These two factors correlate with the amount of extractable pancreatic insulin. In general, after several years of established clinical diabetes, the patient with youth-onset diabetes shows essentially no extractable pancreatic insulin, whereas the pancreas of the patient with adult-onset diabetes still contains some insulin, approximately half that found in control pancreases. Patients with maturity-onset diabetes studied at autopsy reveal a significant incidence of hyalinization of pancreatic islets.

Of special interest is the findings that some juvenile diabetics who come to autopsy shortly after clinical onset of diabetes show large islets of Langerhans. This would support the concept that the *initial* lesion is not necessarily decreased insulin production by the pancreas.

There is also the rare patient with recent onset of diabetes whose pancreatic islets indicate lymphocytic infiltration (insulitis), a lesion again found almost exclusively in young diabetics. This raises the possibility of an autoimmune mechanism or a specific infection restricted to the islets. Recently viruses of the picorna group have been implicated in such a role.

BLOOD VESSELS Atherosclerosis in the diabetic patient is not different from that commonly observed, but it is equally present in both sexes and occurs earlier in life. Coronary artery disease is a frequent cause of death, and cerebrovascular accidents are significantly more common. In addition, these patients usually have small-vessel disease, or microangiopathy, which has been found not only in the capillaries of the renal glomeruli and eye but also in skin and muscle. The initial lesion is a thickened basement membrane, which represents excess glycoprotein and which reacts with para-aminosalicylic acid (PAS) stain. It is likely that its biosynthesis is related to glucose metabolism.

Retina (see also Chap. 20) Microaneurysms, small hemorrhages, and exudates are often seen in patients after 10 to 15 years of diabetes. Frequently, there is also a striking dilatation of venules. If hypertension is present, its typical retinopathy may be superimposed, particularly segmental arterial constriction. Proliferative retinopathy is found frequently in juvenile diabetes of long duration. There is formation of new blood vessels around the optic disk. Hemorrhage into the vitreous may be the cause of sudden temporary loss of vision. If, in response to repeated extensive hemorrhages, scar tissue forms, it may upon retracting produce retinal detachment. In proliferative retinopathy, a secondary hemorrhagic glaucoma is often the final step leading to total blindness. At the present time, in the United States, diabetic retinopathy is the third most frequent cause of blindness, after cataracts and glaucoma.

A better understanding of the mechanism of early vascular changes has been made possible by the introduction of the in vitro trypsin digestion of the flattened retina. Two types of vascular cells have been described, the endothelial and the mural cell called pericyte. In diabetics, there is a specific loss of mural cells, resulting eventually in formation of microaneurysms, the specific diabetic eye lesion. In addition there is shunting of arterial blood, with consequent ischemia of adjacent areas. Finally there may be increased permeability of the blood vessel wall. These findings are supported by in vivo studies employing fluorescein, injected intravenously into the general circulation, followed by serial photographs of the fundus. In diabetics, one finds not only delayed emptying but also leakage of the dye from blood vessels in areas where exudates and hemorrhages are occurring. The earliest lesions are small areas of nonperfusion which can be visualized in life by fluorescence angiography.

KIDNEY The specific diabetic lesion is the nodular glomerulosclerosis described by Kimmelstiel and Wilson. The lesions consist of PAS-positive material, accumulating in the mesangial region and, in addition, in the basement membrane of the glomerular loops. The question has been raised if this is excess normally structured basement membrane or an abnormal glycoprotein. Experimental data support the latter. They found that the glycoprotein of diabetic human glomerular basement membrane contained less lysine but more OH-lysine. As both amino acids participate in the formation of cross links, a defect could contribute to increased permeability despite an anatomically thicker basement membrane. Pyelonephritis, a frequent complication, is a local manifestation of the generalized increased susceptibility to infection. The combination of these lesions constitutes diabetic nephropathy and manifests itself clinically with proteinuria, edema, and hypertension, usually an irreversible process.

LINK BETWEEN METABOLIC AND VASCULAR CHANGES

Some of the pathologic changes observed in diabetic patients are obviously secondary to hyperglycemia, such as deposition of glycogen in the loop of Henle, where it is directly correlated to the glucose concentration in the urine. Hyperglycemia also results in deposition of glycogen in non-insulin-dependent organs, such as skin, heart muscle, iris, and ciliary bodies of the eye. The liver of the diabetic patient, except in the terminal stages, contains normal amounts of glycogen; however, the distribution may be abnormal within the nuclei of the hepatic parenchymal cells. Occasionally the liver is enlarged and infiltrated with fat, mainly in untreated or poorly treated diabetics.

The relationship between derangement of intermediary carbohydrate metabolism and microangiopathy has not been clarified and is the subject of controversy.

Biochemically the glycoprotein nature of the basement membrane has been established. It contains about 7 percent carbohydrate, and thus it is possible that excessive glucose, via an insulin-independent pathway, leads to derangement of the basement membrane, with secondary infiltration by materials from the bloodstream. It has been questioned whether such a derangement is necessarily the consequence of only an abnormal glucose metabolism or if both the level of blood glucose and the state of the basement membrane could be influenced by a third factor. On the other hand, it is now well documented that all the complications of genetic diabetes may occur in secondary forms of diabetes in man and furthermore that they can be reproduced in animals with experimentally induced diabetes.

This somewhat philosophic discussion has practical consequences in the daily management of diabetes, as it will determine how well the status of the diabetic should be controlled. If one believes that the microangiopathy presents a true complication of the chronic hyperglycemia, then it is reasonable to aim at as close to normal blood sugars as possible. If on the other hand one believes that hyperglycemia is unrelated to the occurrence of the vascular syndrome, than one will reduce blood sugar only to such a level as to minimize signs and symptoms attributable to hyperglycemia.

It is obvious and does not need to be elaborated here that other factors also play a role, as they do in the general nondiabetic population, i.e., hypertension obesity, fat content of diets, smoking, etc.

PATHOPHYSIOLOGY

The diabetic syndrome is characterized by an absolute or relative lack of circulating insulin. It develops as a consequence of an imbalance between insulin production and release, on the one hand, and hormonal or tissue factors modifying the insulin requirement, on the other.

Insulin is absolutely lacking in those forms of secondary diabetes in which destruction or removal of the pancreas has taken place. Similarly overt growth-onset diabetes is characterized by insulin deficiency. One finds essentially no extractable pancreatic insulin, no response to oral hypoglycemic agents of the sulfonylurea type, a marked tendency to ketoacidosis, and therefore dependence on exogenous insulin for survival. It is assumed that diabetes in the child begins when the pancreatic production of insulin declines. However, this is not always irreversible, as at least one-third of all juvenile diabetics will develop a phase of remission, usually within 3 months after the acute onset of the disease. If present, the remission may last from several days to several months; it rarely exceeds 1 year. Often during such a remission no insulin treatment is necessary, and a glucose tolerance test result may be normal. Nevertheless, after this remission the juvenile diabetic progresses rapidly to a state of total insulin deficiency.

The patient with adult-onset diabetes develops his disease considerably more slowly. At the early stage no symptoms may be present, and diagnosis is suspected by discovery of elevated blood glucose levels 1 or 2 hr postprandially. Measurement of serum insulin may indicate close to normal fasting levels; however, the insulin response to administered glucose is abnormal in that it occurs late. This is responsible for the elevated blood glucose level 1 to 2 hr postprandially. As insulin release increases with the rising blood glucose, the blood glucose declines; with an excessive amount of insulin, the blood glucose level may fall precipitously, provoking the symptoms of reactive hypoglycemia between the *third and fifth hour* postprandially. As the disease progresses further, the insulin release becomes less pronounced and the episodes of reactive hypoglycemia tend to disappear; finally the amount of circulating insulin is insufficient to return the blood glucose to normal levels between meals. In maturity-onset diabetes the pancreatic insulin reserve is decreased but rarely totally absent. Thus the occurrence of diabetic ketoacidosis is uncommon.

Although in many patients the contrast between growth-onset and maturity-onset diabetes is, initially at least, quite sharp, there are crossovers between these two types, and the above comments must be considered only as generalizations.

Regardless of the type of diabetes, by definition, the cardinal sign is hyperglycemia, frequently associated with glycosuria. The hyperglycemia has two components: hepatic overproduction and peripheral underutilization. The source of the glucose released from the liver is dietary carbohydrate, liver glycogen, and gluconeogenesis from amino acids and glycerol. Underutilization of glucose in the peripheral tissue takes place mainly in adipose tissue and muscle, both of which are insulin-sensitive, and is attributed to a lack of circulating insulin. Impaired glucose uptake by muscle leads to loss of muscle glycogen and release of amino acids for gluconeogenesis. Impaired glucose uptake by adipose tissue causes impaired triglyceride synthesis. In addition, with lack of insulin, free fatty acids are released from adipose tissue into the bloodstream. In the liver, part of the fatty acids are metabolized to ketone bodies. Although the latter can be utilized by certain tissues such as muscle, they are formed in excess in the diabetic person. They accumulate in the blood and will spill over into the urine. As they are strong acids, it is necessary for the kidney to excrete a fixed base with them, leading to both sodium and potassium loss. Therefore, the diabetic organism loses glucose, water, ketone bodies, and base. This will result in dehydration, ketoacidosis, and weight loss, and in extreme cases may proceed to diabetic coma and death (Fig. 88-2).

The exact mechanism by which insulin acts remains unknown. However, it is well established that tissues vary widely in sensitivity and responsiveness to insulin. For example, in muscle and adipose tissue, insulin probably acts on cell membrane permeability and so facilitates the entry of glucose into the cell. On the other hand, liver cells exhibit no demonstrable permeability barrier to glucose. The insulin effect on liver appears to be on glycogen synthesis and on the phosphorylating mechanism. It has

TABLE 88-2
Work-up of the diabetic patient

History

Age	*Laboratory*
onset of symptoms	glycosuria
diagnosis established	blood sugar:
present age	fasting
	postprandial
	glucose tolerance test

General	*Weight*	*Cardiovascular*	*Feet*	*Neurologic*	*Vision*
polyuria	present	angina	claudication	paresthesia	blurriness
polydipsia	usual	infarction	ulcer	pain	hemorrhage
polyphagia	maximal	hypertension	gangrene	numbness	cataract
fatigue	marital	stroke	surgery	dizziness	glaucoma
ketoacidosis	or age 20		amputation		
hypoglycemia					

Sexual	*Drug intake*	*Kidney*
Male:		
impotence	steroids	proteinuria
balanitis	diuretics	infection
Female:		
birth weight of children	anticoagulants	neurogenic bladder
abortions	birth-control	
vulvar pruritus		

Previous treatment			*Urine testing*
Diet:	Tablets:	Insulin:	daily
calories	type	type	weekly or less
weighted	dose	dose	never
measured	duration	duration	results
free			

Complication of diabetic treatment		*Heredity*	
hypoglycemia:	insulin allergy	parents	relatives
insulin	insulin resistance	siblings	none
tablet	insulin dystrophy	offspring	

Physical examination—special reference to

Peripheral vessels	*Neurology*	*Eye grounds*	*Foot*
carotid	knee jerks	microaneurysm	muscle atrophy
femoral	ankle jerks	hemorrhages	temperature
popliteal	Babinski's reflex	exudates	hair growth
dorsalis pedis	pinprick	segmental constriction	pulses
posterior tibial	touch	neovascularization	blanching on elevation
edema	vibration	fibrous strands	rubor on dependency

Classification of diabetes

Stage	*Etiologic*
clinical	primary genetic
chemical	secondary:
latent	endocrine: obesity, pituitary, thyroid, adrenal
prediabetic	pancreatic: surgical removal, carcinoma, pancreatitis, hemochromatosis
	iatrogenic: steroids, diuretics, other

Concomitant:
- vascular disease: cardiac, brain, peripheral
- retinal disease
- neuropathy
- renal disease

recently been shown that the liver contains two enzymes for phosphorylation of glucose: hexokinase and glucokinase. Hexokinase is insulin-*independent*, and glucokinase is insulin-*dependent*. The effect of insulin on fatty acids has been mentioned above. It is noteworthy that this antilipolytic action requires a lower level of insulin than that for glucose uptake. Therefore an absolute deficiency of circulating insulin, as in juvenile-onset diabetes, will lead to hyperglycemia and marked lipolysis with resultant ketosis, whereas only a moderate decrease of circulating insulin, as in adult-onset diabetes, will lead to hyperglycemia without ketosis.

In diabetes the primary inherited defect responsible for the failing insulin production remains unknown. The recent discovery of proinsulin may be a step forward. Proinsulin is a larger molecule than insulin (molecular weight 9,000, versus 6,000) because of some 30 additional amino acids, but it exhibits considerably less biologic activity. It is converted into insulin by cleavage of the intermediate chain at the level of arginine. It is conceivable that in some diabetic patients there is a failure to activate proinsulin. As large quantities of proinsulin would be required to meet the body's insulin demand, this failure could eventually lead to pancreatic exhaustion and thus to frank diabetes. However, despite careful search, this mechanism has not been found to take place in human diabetes.

Recently the poly-ol *sorbitol* has received much attention, as its formation from glucose could be directly implicated in some of the diabetic complications. A new pathway of glucose has been discovered whereby it is not phosphorylated but rather is directly reduced by aldose reductase to sorbitol in the presence of a high NADPH/NADP ratio. Accumulation of sorbitol within the cells equipped to handle such an enzymatic process will lead to osmotic swelling. This reaction seems to be favored by a high concentration of blood glucose and is currently accepted as biochemical explanation for the occurrence of cataracts and neuropathy in poorly controlled diabetes.

PRECIPITATION OF DIABETES BY EXTRAPANCREATIC FACTORS

OBESITY Though it should not be inferred that all obese individuals are potential diabetics, obesity is frequently associated with diabetes. Biopsy studies have shown that adult-onset obesity is associated with hypertrophy of adipose cells and that the larger the cell, the less responsive to insulin it becomes. As less glucose can be disposed of, the resulting hyperglycemia will lead to hyperinsulinemia. In patients with a genetically predetermined susceptibility, this may lead to pancreatic exhaustion or at least to a relative insulin deficiency.

PREGNANCY In women so predisposed, pregnancy also exerts a definite diabetogenic action. Diabetes may become apparent only during pregenancy and disappear following delivery (gestational diabetes); rarely it remains; frequently, years or decades later, permanent diabetes develops. There is evidence that hormonal factors, such as placental lactogen and marked destruction of endogenous insulin by the placenta, may play a role in precipitating diabetes. It is speculated that the higher

FIGURE 88-2
Pathophysiology of diabetic ketoacidosis.

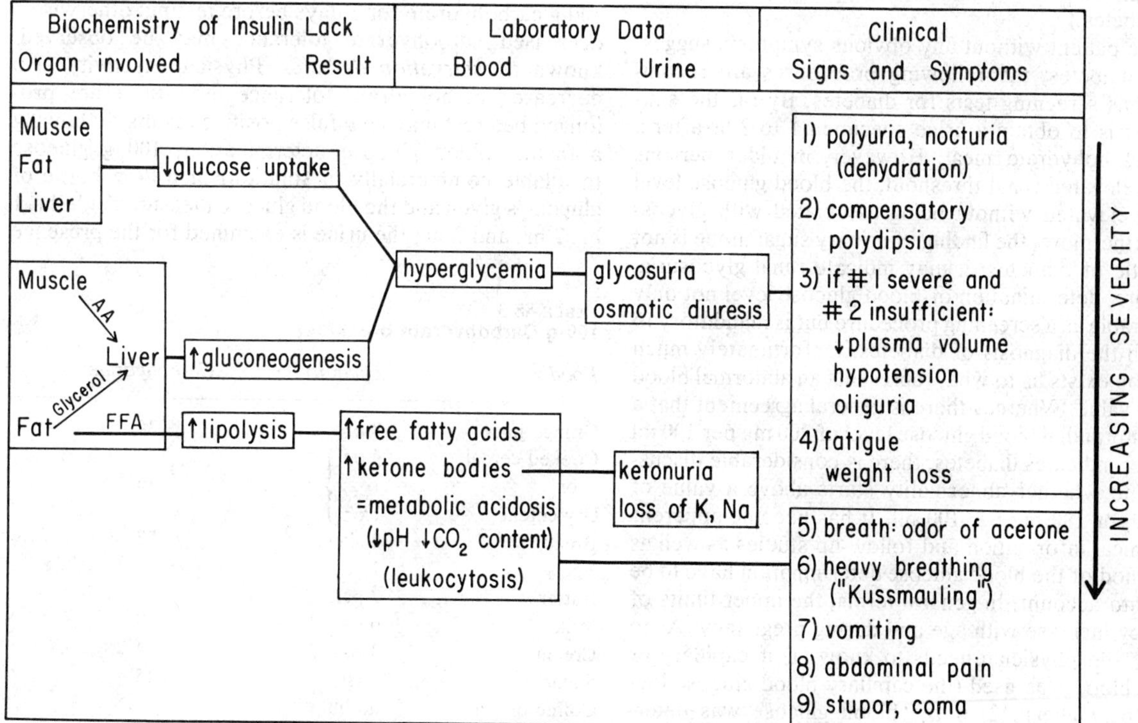

Abbreviations: AA = Amino Acids; FFA = Free Fatty Acids.

frequency of diabetes in adult females may be due to pregnancies and obesity. Contraceptive pills which contain estrogen may induce hyperglycemia in susceptible persons.

Recently, the diabetogenic action of certain *diuretics of the benzothiadiazine* type has been noted. There is evidence that these drugs mediate such a mechanism by inhibiting pancreatic insulin release. Diazoxide belongs to this group and is currently used for treatment of hypoglycemia. *Growth hormone* is diabetogenic by decreasing peripheral glucose utilization and by increasing release of free fatty acids. Excessive *epinephrine* causes increased hepatic glycogenolysis and, in addition, inhibits pancreatic insulin release (diabetes in pheochromocytoma). The *steroids* act by increasing hepatic gluconeogenesis and decreasing glucose uptake by adipose tissue. *Thyroxine* increases hunger and food intake and generally heightens the level of metabolic activity. *Infection* of any sort will impair glucose tolerance and may unmask the tendency to diabetes. The diabetogenic mechanism of infection is probably nonspecific and consists of elevated levels of corticosteriods and glucagon, fever that increases the general metabolic load, and possibly catecholamine release, all of which decrease the effectiveness of circulating insulin. In rare instances inflammation of the pancreatic islets takes place.

DIAGNOSIS

The diagnosis of diabetes mellitus is frequently suggested by a history of polydipsia, polyuria, and polyphagia, associated with weight loss. A clinical suggestion of diabetes is confirmed by finding glucose in the urine and by detecting an abnormally elevated blood glucose level. (See Table 88-2 for an outline of the workup of a patient with diabetes.)

In the patient without any obvious symptoms suggestive of diabetes, the following procedures are recommended as screening tests for diabetes. By far the simplest test is to obtain a urine specimen 1 to 2 hr after a heavy carbohydrate meal. However, in older persons with an elevated renal threshold, the blood glucose level may be elevated without being associated with glycosuria; furthermore, the finding of urinary sugar alone is not diagnostic of diabetes; it may indicate renal glycosuria. Therefore, determination of blood glucose level not only is preferable as a screening procedure but is mandatory to establish the diagnosis of diabetes. Unfortunately much confusion exists as to what represents an abnormal blood glucose value. Whereas there is general agreement that a 1-hr postprandial blood glucose level of 200 mg per 100 ml or higher indicates diabetes, there is considerable discussion as to whether abnormality starts above a value of 160, 170, or 180 mg per 100 ml. It has become apparent that clinical information and follow-up studies as well as the method of the blood glucose determination have to be taken into account. In general terms, the upper limits of normalcy increase with age and during pregnancy. As to method, the physician needs to know (1) if capillary or venous blood was used (the capillary blood glucose level will be higher); (2) if the blood glucose was determined on whole blood or plasma (plasma or serum will render higher values than whole blood; on the other hand, severe anemia will give falsely elevated values with whole blood); (3) which particular technique for measuring blood glucose was employed. A rather less specific method such as Folin-Wu will give the highest values, as it measures in addition to glucose also fructose, lactate, pyruvate, etc. The glucose oxidase method will reflect the "true" glucose content and therefore yield the lowest value. The autoanalyzer employs the ferricyanide method, which gives results slightly higher than the glucose oxidase technique. It is apparent that the possible variations are many; therefore the best advice is to be familiar with the methods and normal range in a given hospital. When blood glucose values are reported to outlying institutions or life insurance companies, the type of blood and the technique employed should be noted.

FASTING AND POSTPRANDIAL BLOOD GLUCOSE

The normal range for fasting blood glucose as measured by the autoanalyzer is between 70 and 110 mg per 100 ml whole blood. An elevated fasting blood sugar level is highly suggestive of diabetes; on the other hand, diabetes can never be ruled out by the presence of a normal fasting blood sugar level. Therefore, it is advisable to obtain a blood sugar determination 1 or 2 hr after a meal which has contained approximately 100 g carbohydrate, as indicated in Table 88-3 or a regular breakfast to which 50 g glucose have been added. A 1-hr value of 170 mg per 100 ml or higher is highly suggestive of diabetes, as is a 2-hr value above 120 mg per 100 ml. If the level is borderline, or especially if one wishes definitely to rule out diabetes, then a formal 3-hr glucose tolerance test is indicated.

ORAL GLUCOSE TOLERANCE TEST It is mandatory that the patient be on a preparatory diet containing 250 to 300 g carbohydrate for 3 days before testing; otherwise a decreased carbohydrate tolerance may be observed, known as *starvation diabetes*. Physical inactivity also decreases carbohydrate tolerance, and therefore prolonged bed rest may give false positive results. Following a fasting blood glucose determination, 100 g glucose (available commercially in solution) or a 7-oz bottle of glucola is given and the blood glucose measured at ½ hr, 1 hr, 2 hr, and 3 hr; the urine is examined for the presence

TABLE 88-3
100-g Carbohydrate breakfast

Food	*Quantity*	*Carbohydrate*
Orange juice	8 oz	24
Cooked cereal or Dry cereal	4 oz or 1 oz	16
Bread	2 slices	32
Egg	1	
Butter	2 pats	
Milk	6 oz	9
Cream	3 oz	4
Sugar	3 tsp	15
Coffee or tea	ad lib.	
Total		100

of sugar. The following are considered upper-normal values obtained with venous blood measured by the autoanalyzer method: fasting, 100 mg per 100 ml; 1/2 hr (or peak value), 170 mg; 1 hr, 170 mg; 2 hr, 120 mg; and 3 hr, 110 mg per 100 ml. There should be no glucose in the urine at any time. The result of the glucose tolerance test in an apparently healthy subject is influenced by at least three factors: diet, physical activity, and age. Age exerts an effect on glucose tolerance. Although standards are not available for individuals of different decades, especially over the age of fifty, it is suggested that between the ages of fifty and fifty-nine the 2-hr level may be considered normal up to 130; between the ages of sixty and sixty-nine, up to 140; between the ages of seventy and seventy-nine, up to 150; and above age eighty, above 160 mg per 100 ml. For the 1-hr value similar adjustments need to be made. As young healthy people rarely exceed 150 mg per 100 ml, one can allow 10 mg for each decade above 50 years of age. Additional factors known to affect glucose tolerance are fever, infection, endocrinopathies, liver disease, myocardial infarction, cerebrovascular accident, and certain medications such as diuretics of the benzothiodiazine type.

INTRAVENOUS GLUCOSE TOLERANCE TEST As intestinal absorption of glucose may interfere with a glucose tolerance test, it is occasionally desirable to perform an intravenous glucose tolerance test. This is especially indicated if there is a history of gastrointestinal surgery. Accelerated intestinal absorption of glucose, as in the "dumping syndrome," may result in a diabetic-type oral glucose tolerance curve; however, the intravenous glucose tolerance may be well within normal limits.

The dose of glucose is 0.5 g per kg body weight as a 25% solution. It is administered intravenously within 2 to 4 min, and blood is collected every 10 min for 1 hr. Under these conditions, the rate of blood glucose decreases in an exponential manner, and the glucose disappearance can be calculated. Disappearance rate $= 70/t^{1/2}$, where $t^{1/2} =$ number of minutes it takes for the blood glucose level to fall 50 percent. In normal individuals it usually exceeds 1.5 percent of the administered dose per minute, and values below 1 percent are clearly diabetic.

If glucose tolerance tests are performed routinely in a large hospital population, many patients afflicted with chronic diseases such as rheumatoid arthritis or cancer may exhibit an impaired glucose tolerance curve without any clinical evidence of diabetes. Because many of these cases of "chemical diabetes" will not progress to overt clinical diabetes, one has to be careful not to overdiagnose diabetes.

DIFFERENTIAL DIAGNOSIS OF GLYCOSURIA (See Chap. 89)

The presence of glucose in the urine should be considered to indicate diabetes until an alternate diagnosis can be definitely established. Glycosuria may indicate a low renal threshold, which is present in pregnancy, in some patients with chronic renal disease, and in patients with idiopathic renal glycosuria. In the latter, glucose is present in most urine specimens, including a second voided specimen after an overnight fast, but the glucose tolerance test result is normal. The transient glycosuria that occurs occasionally in apparently healthy persons under conditions of stress or infection or following ingestion of a high-carbohydrate meal is usually associated with an abnormal glucose tolerance test and, therefore, indicates chemical diabetes.

CLINICAL PICTURE

GROWTH-ONSET TYPE The growth-onset type of diabetes is characterized by a rapid onset, with symptoms such as polydipsia, polyuria, polyphagia, loss of weight and strength, marked irritability, and in children frequently, recurrence of bedwetting. The diabetes is apt to be of the unstable or brittle type, being quite sensitive to the administration of exogenous insulin and easily influenced by physical activity. The patient is liable to ketoacidosis. For adequate treatment, diet and insulin therapy are mandatory. Since the introduction of insulin therapy, diabetic ketoacidosis has been markedly reduced as a major cause of death; the primary causes of early death in diabetic patients are now cardiovascular and renal. Diagnosis of diabetes in the growth-onset type of patient is usually not difficult. However, occasional children and adolescents have asymptomatic diabetes demonstrable only by postprandial hyperglycemia or glucose tolerance test. In these patients the disease appears to progress very slowly.

MATURITY-ONSET TYPE Maturity-onset diabetes has a less stormy beginning; frequently symptoms are minimal or absent. The chief complaint may be moderate weight loss or, occasionally, weight gain. There may be some nocturia. A female patient might consult her gynecologist because of vulvar pruritus. Frequently, however, the patient seeks medical attention because of vascular complications. As a consequence of blurred or decreased vision, the patient may see an ophthalmologist first, who may diagnose diabetic retinopathy. Fatigue and anemia may be caused by fairly advanced diabetic nephropathy. Diabetic neuropathy may present as paresthesias, loss of sensation, impotence, nocturnal diarrhea, postural hypotension, or a neurogenic bladder. Not infrequently, the patient comes to the physician with an ulcer or gangrene of his toes or heel and on examination is found to have a pulseless or painless foot. Thus the patient with maturity-onset diabetes usually does not present the dramatic, acute metabolic syndrome observed in the juvenile-onset patient but rather a chronic vascular syndrome. It is therefore important to suspect diabetes as an underlying disease under a wide variety of circumstances.

TREATMENT

GENERAL PRINCIPLES The aims in managing diabetes are (1) to correct the underlying metabolic abnormalities in order to reduce diabetic symptoms; (2) to attain and maintain ideal body weight; (3) to prevent, or at least delay, specific complications commonly associated with the disease (disorders of eye, kidney, nerves); and (4) to stem the nonspecific accelerated atherosclerosis to which the diabetic is particularly liable.

Successful therapy will depend upon the thoroughness with which the physician understands the particular problems in each case, upon how well the patient has been instructed, and upon how conscientious he is about following instructions.

On initiating and during treatment of a patient with diabetes, it is essential to be certain that there is no active focus of infection, as it will aggravate the diabetic state. Infection of the urinary tract should be looked for particularly, and a chest x-ray is imperative. It is also advisable to obtain careful baseline evaluations of the state of the cardiovascular, nervous, and renal systems and of the eye grounds to serve as subsequent points of reference.

General advice should include regular exercise (as it lowers the blood sugar) and avoidance of cigarette smoking. Parameters to be monitored at regular intervals are urine and blood sugars, serum cholesterol and triglycerides, as well as renal function, blood pressure, and body weight.

DIET Dietary treatment of diabetes still constitutes the basis for management, although very often it is difficult to achieve adherence by the patient. The principal points to bear in mind in designing diabetic diets are the facts that the basic nutritional requirements of a patient with diabetes are the same as those of a nondiabetic patient, and that the diet should be varied and palatable.

Purpose The chief aims of a diabetic diet are:

1 Prevent excessive postprandial hyperglycemia and thus symptoms of diabetes
2 Prevent hypoglycemia if the patient is on exogenous insulin
3 Obtain ideal body weight
4 Normalize serum cholesterol and triglycerides
5 Prevent or delay premature atherosclerosis

TABLE 88-4
Food exchanges

Food	*Approx. meas. 1 exchange*	*Weight, g*
Bread: carbohydrate 15 g, protein 2 g, fat negligible		
Bread, baker's	1 slice	25
Biscuit, roll	2″ diameter	35
Muffin	2″ diameter	35
Cornbread	1 1/2″ cube	35
Cereals, cooked	1/2 cup, cooked	100
Cereals, dry (flakes, puffed, and shredded varieties)	3/4 cup, scant	20
Rice, macaroni, noodles, spaghetti	1/2 cup, cooked	100
Crackers:		
Graham	2 (2 1/2 × 2 3/4″)	20
Oyster	20 (1/2 cup)	20
Saltines	5 (2″ square)	20
Soda	3 (2 1/2 × 2 1/2″)	20
Round, thin varieties	6–8 (1/2″ diameter)	20
Vegetables:		
Beans, peas, dried (cooked) Includes limas, navy, kidney beans, black-eyed peas, cowpeas, split peas, etc.	1/2 cup, scant	100
Corn	1/3 cup or 1/2 ear	80
Parsnips	1/2 cup	125
Potatoes:		
White, baked	2″ diameter	100
White, boiled, mashed	1/2 cup	100
Sweet or yam	1/4 cup	50
Ice cream, vanilla (omit 2 fat exchanges)	1/8 qt	70
Sponge cake, no icing	1 1/2″ cube	25
Fruits: fresh, cooked, canned, or frozen unsweetened: carbohydrate 10 g per exchange; protein and fat negligible		
Apple, 1 small	2″ diameter	80
Applesauce	1/2 cup	100
Apricots, dry	4 halves	20
Apricots, fresh	2 medium	100
Banana	1/2 small	50
Berries (blackberries, raspberries, and strawberries)	1 cup	150
Blueberries	2/3 cup	100
Cantaloupe	1/2 (6″ diameter)	200
Cherries	10 large or 15 small	75
Dates	2	15
Figs, dried	1 small	15
Figs, fresh	2 large	50
Grapefruit	1/2 small	125
Grapefruit	1/2 cup	100
Grapes	12	75
Grape juice	1/2 cup	60
Honeydew melon	1/8 (7″ diameter)	150
Mango	1/2 small	70
Nectarines	1 medium	100
Orange	1 small	100
Orange juice	1/2 cup	100
Papaya	1/3 medium	100
Peach	1 medium	100
Pear	1 small	100
Pineapple	1/2 cup, cubed	80
Pineapple juice	1/3 cup	80
Plums	2 medium	100
Prunes, dried	2 medium	25
Raisins	2 tbsp level	25
Tangerine	1 large	100
Watermelon	1 cup diced 1 slice 3″ × 1 1/2″	175

Basic caloric requirement This is dictated by ideal weight, physical activity, and occupation of the patient. If he is obese, and most adult diabetics are, the diet should be restricted in total calories, yet be nutritionally adequate. With return to normal weight a marked improvement often will take place of hyperglycemia and glycosuria, frequently associated with a decline in serum triglyceride level. If the patient is undernourished, the initial diet has to exceed the basic caloric requirement. Particularly in children it should be sufficient to achieve desirable growth and development. The desired weight is calculated from the height, taking frame size into consideration. For an approximate calculation of the basic caloric requirement, the ideal weight in pounds is multiplied by 10, or 20 kcal per kg. Example: If a patient's ideal weight is 180 lb, his *basal* caloric requirement will be 1800 kcal. Additional calories are allowed according to the patient's occupation and activities. Calories may be reduced for patients over fifty years of age who are less active. Meals and snacks should be spaced to avoid intermittent hyper- or hypoglycemia, particularly if the patient receives exogenous insulin.

Partition of calories The average American diet consists of carbohydrate, 40 to 50 percent; protein, 15 to 20 percent; and fat, 35 to 40 percent. The diabetic diet can approximate this distribution. The caloric value of carbohydrate and protein is approximately 4 kcal per g, and of fat, 9 kcal per g. Alcohol contains 7 kcal per g, or 168 kcal per oz.

Carbohydrate Carbohydrate is contained in starches (polymer of glucose), milk (glucose, galactose), fruits, and refined sugar (glucose, fructose). To prevent acetonuria and protein catabolism a minimum of 1 g per lb body weight is necessary, or in the example of the patient weighing 180 lb, 180 g. If more carbohydrates are indicated, concentrated sugars should be avoided to prevent wide swings of blood glucose. Rarely should the total amount of carbohydrates exceed 250 g per day.

Protein Protein is contained in meat, fish, cheese, eggs, etc. A *minimum* of 0.5 g per lb body weight is indicated. This is further increased during pregnancy and during childhood.

TABLE 88-4 *(continued)*

Food	*Approx. meas. 1 exchange*	*Weight, g*
Fat: carbohydrate and protein negligible; fat, 5 g per serving. Fat exchanges used in cooking must be accounted for.		
Avocado	1/8 (4" diam.)	24
Butter or margarine	1 tsp level	5
Bacon, crisp	1 slice	10
Cream, light, sweet, or sour—20%	2 tbsp level	30
Cream, heavy—40%	1 tbsp level	15
Cream cheese	1 tbsp level	15
French dressing	1 tbsp level	15
Mayonnaise	1 tsp level	5
Nuts	6 small	10
Oil or cooking fat	1 tsp level	5
Olives	5 small	50

Vegetables: carbohydrate 7 g, protein 2 g, fat negligible. One exchange equals 1/2 cup.

Beets	Peas, green	Squash, winter
Carrots	Pumpkin	Turnip
Onions	Rutabaga	

Note: One or more fat exchanges from the diet allowance may be used to season the vegetables. All other vegetables, except those listed under Bread, contain negligible amounts of carbohydrate, protein, and fat. They may be used as desired.

Food	*Approx. meas. 1 exchange*	*Weight, g*
Milk: 170 kilocalories, carbohydrate 12 g, protein 8 g, fat 10 g per serving		
Milk, plain	1 cup (8 oz)	240
Milk, evaporated	1/2 cup	120
Milk, powder, skim*	1/3 cup (5 1/3 tbsp level)	48
Milk, powder, whole	1/2 cup (8 tbsp level)	35
Buttermilk*	1 cup	240
Milk, skim*	1 cup	240

Food	*Approx. meas. 1 exchange*	*Weight, g*
Meat (cooked weight): carbohydrate negligible, protein 7 g, fat 5 g per serving		
Meat: beef, fowl, lamb, veal (medium fat), liver, pork, ham (lean)	1 oz	30
Cold cuts: salami, minced ham, bologna, cervelat, liver sausage, luncheon loaf	1 slice 4 1/2" diam. × 1/8"	45
Frankfurters (8 to 9 per lb)	1	50
Fish:		
Cod, haddock, halibut, herring, etc.	1 oz	30
Salmon, tuna, crab-meat, lobster	1/4 cup	30
Shrimp, clams, oysters (medium)	5	45
Sardines	3 medium	30
Cheese:		
Cheddar type	1 oz	30
Cottage	3 tbsp level	45
Peanut butter (limit to one serving per day unless adjustment is made to balance carbohydrate content)	2 tbsp scant	30
Egg	1	50

* *Add 10 g fat (two fat exchanges). Most commercial buttermilk is skimmed. Check local supplies.*

SOURCE: *Modified from* Meal Planning with Exchange Lists, *obtainable from the American Diabetes Association, Inc., New York, N.Y.*

TABLE 88-5
An 1800-kilocalorie diabetic diet order (carbohydrate 181 g, protein 90 g, fat 80 g)

Exchange	*Break-fast*	*Lunch*	*Snack*	*Supper*	*Snack*
Milk	1/2	1			1/2
Bread	2	2	1	2	1
Meat	1	2	1	3	1
Fat	1	1		2	
Fruit	1	1		1	
Vegetable		1		1	
Partition in grams:					
Carbo-hydrate	46	52	15	47	21
Protein	15	26	9	27	13
Fat	15	25	5	25	10

Fat Fat is contained in butter, margarine, mayonnaise, cream, bacon, nuts, olives, and avocado, and meats in general.

Dietary fats, particularly those of animal origin, together with other factors, such as obesity, hypertension, smoking and decreased physical activity, seem to play an important role in the pathogenesis of atherosclerosis. Therefore fat intake should be kept to a minimum. The amount prescribed is calculated by subtracting calories allowed for carbohydrate and protein from the total caloric requirement. For example: Total calories based on an ideal weight of 180 lb = 1800. Assigned for carbohydrate: 180 × 4 = 720; for protein: 90 × 4 = 360; there remain 1800 − 720 − 360 = 720. These calories given as fat: 720 divided by 9 = 80 g fat. The final diet consists of carbohydrate 180 g, protein 90 g, and fat 80 g. It is advisable to reduce the total amount of cholesterol by avoiding eggs and to supply some of the fat as unsaturated fatty acids. Recently the American Diabetes Association has recommended decreasing fat further and making up calories by increasing carbohydrate. If fat is decreased by 20 g, 180 kcal carbohydrate (=45 g) have to be added. In above example, it would be changed to 235 carbohydrate, 60 fat, protein remaining at 90 g.

The American Diabetes Association and the American Dietetic Association have published a booklet on meal planning with exchange lists. In it all the available foods are divided into six types. Foods cannot be switched between the lists but can be interchanged within each list. Food is subdivided into (1) milk exchanges; (2) (*a*) essentially unlimited vegetables, (*b*) somewhat limited vegetables; (3) fruits; (4) bread exchanges which include apart from bread also cereal, rice, spaghetti, potato, etc.; (5) meat exchanges which include meat, cold cuts, egg, fish, cheese, and (6) fat exchanges. In Tables 88-4 and 88-5 these exchange lists are presented in more detail. Food can be weighed or measured with a standard 8-oz measuring cup, a teaspoon, and a tablespoon.

ORAL HYPOGLYCEMIC AGENTS They appear to have a place in the treatment of maturity-onset diabetes, provided it is of the nonketotic type and that dietary treatment alone is unsuccessful in achieving adequate control. The oral hypoglycemic agents are not related to insulin, nor can they replace it in conditions such as diabetic ketoacidosis. The agents presently in use are of two types: the sulfonylureas and the biguanides. However, the long-term cardiovascular safety of both types of oral hypoglycemic agents has been questioned (University Group Diabetes Program). The results of this study have stirred much controversy. The comments of rival clinicians and statisticians have become so complex that any practitioner may be excused for being uncertain as how to manage a particular case of diabetes. It must be stated, however, that the American Diabetes Association and the American Medical Association have endorsed the results of the UGPD study. Therefore, caution is urged in prescription of oral agents. At the moment they are recommended without reservation only if (1) dietary measures have failed, (2) the use of insulin is unacceptable to the patient, or (3) only a short-term use of an oral hypoglycemic agent is considered.

The condition of the patient with adult-onset diabetes can often be controlled by diet alone, and this should be given an *adequate* trial for several weeks, unless clinical circumstances such as acute infection dictate otherwise. The multitude of oral agents available, each with somewhat different dosage and duration of action, makes it difficult to master them all; therefore it is recommended that the physician become familiar with one or two. A summary of all the available agents is given in Table 88-6. Potentiation of their actions by other drugs, such as sulfisoxazole (Gantrisin), phenylbutazone (Butazolidin), and bishydroxycoumarin (Dicumarol), has been reported; therefore, the physician should be aware of such possibilities.

Sulfonylureas The sulfonylureas available by prescription are tolbutamide (Orinase), acetohexamide (Dymelor), chlorpropamide (Diabinase), and tolazamide (Tolinase). Although there is some evidence that they directly decrease hepatic glucose output, they act primarily by enhancing the secretion of endogenous insulin. Thus, for these drugs to be effective, at least residual function of the beta cells is necessary.

A patient can be started on sulfonylureas without the prior use of insulin, or he can be transferred from insulin

TABLE 88-6
Oral hypoglycemic agents

Generic name	*Available form, mg*	*Average dose, mg*	*Duration of action, hr*
Tolbutamide	500	500–1,000 b.i.d.	6–12
Acetohexamide	250	250–1,000 A.M.	12–24
	500		
Tolazamide	100	100–1000 A.M.	16–24
	250		
Chlorpropamide	100	100–750 A.M.	24–36
	250		
Phenformin	25 (tablet)	25 b.i.d.	4–6
	50 (capsule)	50 b.i.d.	8–12
	100 (capsule)	100 b.i.d.	

to sulfonylureas. The chance of therapeutic success with these agents is better when clinical diabetes has been present for a relatively short period of time, if the patient is over the age of forty, and if he or she is overweight. A large initial loading dose is not now considered necessary for the sulfonylureas. Side effects include increased chance of cardiovascular death of unknown mechanism; except for chlorpropamide in high doses, these agents have a good record with respect to hepatic function. Chlorpropamide has also been implicated in an occasional patient in the production of a state of water intoxication with hyponatremia. Thus it should be used with caution in patients with borderline heart failure. Alcohol intolerance has been observed under treatment with sulfonylureas. Occasionally, in elderly undernourished patients, severe hypoglycemia may follow their administration. Apart from this, prolonged hypoglycemia is frequently observed when a sulfonylurea is administered to a patient with uremia, as renal excretion of the drug will be delayed. This is the case particularly with chlorpropamide and acetohexamide, as the former is not metabolized to any significant extent and the latter is transformed by the liver to hydroxyhexamide, which also exhibits a potent hypoglycemic property. In both instances, elevated blood levels of the respective drug will lead to severe and protracted hypoglycemia. If this occurs, prolonged and intensive treatment with intravenous glucose (i.e., 200 g within 24 hr) and close medical supervision for at least 48 to 72 hr are mandatory.

From 20 to 30 percent of diabetic patients initially responding to treatment with sulfonylurea will fail to do so after several months or years. This *secondary failure* can often be attributed to poor adherence to a prescribed diet, the presence of infection, or the gradual progression of the diabetes to a more insulin-deficient state having the anatomic equivalent of further decrease in the number of functioning pancreatic islets.

Tolbutamide This is the most widely used oral hypoglycemic agent. Each tablet contains 500 mg. The biologic half-life is approximately 6 hr. It is administered before breakfast *and* before supper, the total daily dose ranging from 1 to 3 g. The excretory product in the urine may give a false positive test for albumin, since it is precipitated by acidifying the urine.

Acetohexamide Tablets are available in strengths of 250 and 500 mg. Its half-life is longer, and therefore a *single* dose may be effective.

Chlorpropamide Tablets are available containing 100 or 250 mg. The biologic half-life is approximately 36 hr, and daily administration may result in a cumulative effect. It is not metabolized and thus is almost completely excreted in the urine. The recommended daily dose is 100 to 250 mg before breakfast; it should not exceed 750 mg. Because of its long action, a bedtime snack containing carbohydrate, protein, and fat, e.g., milk with crackers, is advisable. As it has occasionally a slightly greater toxic effect on the liver than has tolbutamide or acetohexamide, and since its long half-life may occasionally result in hypoglycemia in the early morning, it is advisable to keep the daily dose as low as possible.

Tolazamide This is available in 100- and 250-mg tablets with a half-life of approximately 12 hr. It is administered in a single or divided dose, not exceeding 1,000 mg per day.

BIGUANIDES Phenformin Of the biguanides, phenformin, a phenethyl biguanide (DBI; Meltrol), is commercially available as a 25-mg tablet, with a biologic half-life of 3 to 4 hr, and as a 50-mg or 100-mg time-disintegration capsule of longer half-life. The mechanism of action differs fundamentally from that of the sulfonylureas in that phenformin can correct hyperglycemia in the pancreatectomized animal and the hypoglycemic effect cannot be produced in nondiabetic fed subjects. The mechanism of action is still poorly understood, but it appears that phenformin influences the anaerobic pathway of glucose and inhibits hepatic gluconeogenesis. As phenformin makes a diabetic patient occasionally more sensitive to exogenous insulin, it has been suggested that phenformin inhibits an insulin antagonist. Evidence indicates that phenformin decreases glucose uptake by the intestinal mucosa. It is likely that phenformin also interferes with absorption of some vitamins.

The sole use of phenformin as an antidiabetic agent is limited because the effective dose is frequently associated with gastrointestinal side effects such as anorexia, nausea, vomiting, and diarrhea. Furthermore, phenformin may contribute to excessive lactic acid; it should not be used in those circumstances in which marked tissue hypoxia might be expected to occur, i.e., myocardial infarction, hypotension, low arterial blood oxygen saturation, etc. Fatalities have been reported in which severe lactic acidosis, apparently facilitated by the administration of phenformin, constituted an important contributory effect. Apart from the general restrictions suggested by the UGDP study, indications for its use are (1) the very rare patient with maturity-onset diabetes who is allergic to the sulfonylureas (the daily recommended dose of phenformin ranges from 50 to 200 mg, to be given either as tablets t.i.d. or as capsules b.i.d.); (2) in combination with sulfonylurea in the elderly patient who fails to respond to a maximum dose of a sulfonylurea; (3) the patient with brittle diabetes on insulin with frequent hypoglycemic reactions, in whom the addition of phenformin might result in reduction of the insulin requirement and thus facilitate control (use of phenformin in this type of patient is often disappointing); (4) the obese overeating diabetic in whom diet and the sulfonylureas have failed and insulin is unacceptable.

INSULIN The use of insulin is clearly indicated in the youth-onset diabetic and in those patients with maturity-onset diabetes in whom diet has failed to maintain satisfactory levels of blood glucose in both the fasting and the postprandial state. Furthermore, the use of insulin is mandatory in diabetic ketoacidosis. Insulin is a potent hormone of short endogenous half-life once it is absorbed from its subcutaneous injection site.

Types of insulin In the United States the animal

sources for insulin are beef and pork. As human insulin has a structure similar to that of pork insulin, the use of pure pork insulin rather than a beef-pork mixture may be preferred. Apart from the species difference, seven types of insulin are commercially available. They may be divided into insulins of fast, intermediate, and long action. Their properties are summarized in Table 88-7.

Each of the insulins is available in three different strengths, namely, 40, 80, and 100 units per ml. The choice is governed by the amount of insulin required by the patient. If only a small amount is necessary, e.g., 20 units, the use of U 40 will allow a more accurate dosage; if a larger amount is required, U 80 has the advantage of a smaller volume. For example, 20 units of U 40 is 0.5 ml, whereas 20 units of U 80 is 0.25 ml. Many patients—and an occasional physician—find it difficult to understand that the difference between U 40 and U 80 is one of volume, not of units. A unit of insulin (there are 25 units to each milligram) always exhibits the same potency, regardless of whether it comes out of a U-40 or U-80 bottle. It is important, however, to measure U-80 insulin with a U-80 insulin syringe (labeled in green), and U-40 insulin with a U-40 syringe (labeled in red). Recently U 100 has become available. U 100 has the additional advantage of being essentially proinsulin free.

Choice of insulin *Crystalline insulin* is best for emergencies, such as the treatment of diabetic ketoacidosis or the achievement of fast control in the patient with marked hyperglycemia; it is also employed for daily use in combination with an intermediate insulin to bring on earlier action.

Intermediate insulins in a single dose injected before breakfast will control the majority of cases of diabetes. The dosage will be gaged by the prelunch, midafternoon, and fasting blood sugar values. The midafternoon blood glucose level corresponds to the peak of insulin action and will dictate the maximum morning dose. It is advisable that all patients receiving an intermediate insulin be given a midafternoon snack. If the midafternoon blood glucose level is between 80 and 120 mg per 100 ml, and the prelunch value is still unduly elevated, the addition of a small amount of crystalline insulin at breakfast time is indicated. It can be mixed with NPH (neutral protamine Hagedorn) or lente insulin in the same syringe. Almost all maturity-onset diabetes can be adequately controlled by intermediate insulins alone or in combination with crystalline insulin administered before breakfast.

The patient with youth-onset diabetes often develops nocturnal hyperglycemia because of very active gluconeogenesis and, consequently, will exhibit a high fasting blood glucose level associated with glycosuria. Further increase in the morning dose of intermediate insulin will often lead to hypoglycemia in the midafternoon. To reduce the fasting blood glucose to normal levels, a long-acting insulin can be tried, but often a second small dose of the intermediate insulin before supper or at bedtime is preferable. The latter regimen is eminently satisfactory in the 24-hr control of juvenile diabetes, and usually patients do not complain about the second injection because they feel so much better. Very rarely, sugar is spilled at bedtime but none before supper. Then the addition of a small amount of crystalline insulin to the evening dose of NPH is indicated, and both are given before supper. As a general rule, whenever insulin is given in the evening in addition to the morning dose, the latter should be reduced.

The use of *long-acting insulin* with the hope of establishing control with a single morning injection, in general, has been disappointing. The basic four insulin treatment patterns are summarized in Table 88-8.

Initiation of insulin therapy If the patient has massive glycosuria and elevated blood glucose level, insulin therapy is begun immediately with crystalline insulin. The following schedule is recommended: 20 units for a blood sugar above 300 mg per 100 ml or 4+ urine test; 10 units for a blood sugar between 200 to 300 mg per 100 ml or a 3+ or 2+ urine sugar. Once the acute syndrome is under reasonable control, or if the metabolic derangement is less dramatic, use of a longer-acting insulin can be started. It is best to start with 10 to 15 units of NPH or lente insulin and increase this by 5 units per day, as indicated by urine tests and blood glucose levels. Most diabetic patients will require between 30 and 50 units of insulin daily. For use in a general hospital or internist's office not catering to any special diabetic groups such as children or pregnant women, an approximate overall distribution of the above-described insulin treatment pattern would be as follows:

Pattern No. 1: 70 percent
Pattern No. 2: 20 percent
Pattern No. 3: 5 percent
Pattern No. 4: 5 percent

Obviously, the type of pattern employed will depend to a large extent on one's philosophy as to how strictly diabe-

TABLE 88-7
Insulin, types and action curves

Action	*Insulin*	*Modifier*	*Duration of action, hr*	*Peak effect, hr postinjection*
Fast	Crystalline zinc=clear =(regular)=soluble	None	6	2–3
	Semilente	Zinc	12	3–6
Intermediate	Globin	Globin	18	6–8
	NPH	Protamine	24	8–12
	Lente	Zinc	24	8–12
Long	Ultralente	Zinc	36	20–30
	Protamine zinc	Protamine	36	16–24

TABLE 88-8
Basic insulin treatment patterns

Pattern no.	*Before breakfast*	*Before supper*	*At bedtime*
1	NPH*		
2	NPH+CZI		
3	NPH+CZI		NPH
4	NPH+CZI	NPH+CZI	

* *Exchangeable with lente insulin.*
Note: CZI = crystalline zinc = regular insulin.

tes should be controlled. This, in turn, will determine how many blood sugar or urine tests are obtained.

Complications of insulin therapy INSULIN REACTIONS These are commonly caused by excessive insulin dosage, delayed food intake, or unusual physical activity. Very rarely, an increased sensitivity to insulin is due to early adrenal or pituitary hypofunction. Occasional insulin reactions are almost unavoidable, especially in the juvenile insulin-sensitive diabetic, but they are harmless if recognized and treated early. To reduce them to a minimum, it is essential that the patient know how to test his urine for glucose and, provided he does not have an elevated renal threshold for glucose, how to reduce his insulin dose when his urine tests indicate absence of glucose for several days. The patient also must be instructed to eat his meals on time and when unusual physical activity is anticipated, either to reduce his morning insulin dose or to ingest extra calories to compensate for the blood-sugar-lowering effect of exercise.

The signs and symptoms of an insulin reaction vary with the type of insulin used. *Crystalline insulin* produces a rapid fall in blood glucose level which is detected by the glucoreceptors in the hypothalamus and transmitted via neural pathways to induce release of epinephrine, with the purpose of elevating blood sugar level by glycogenolysis and inhibiting pancreatic insulin release. In the insulin-dependent diabetic person, insulin release cannot be inhibited, and thus if untreated, the hypoglycemia will continue to persist. The patient will be aware of symptoms of hyperepinephrinemia which enable him to diagnose his condition. It is a *characteristic reaction* of rapid onset consisting of hunger, a peculiar abdominal sensation, sweating, palpitation, tremor, tachycardia, weakness, irritability, and pallor. Patients usually recognize these symptoms early, and they are relieved within 10 to 20 min by ingestion of carbohydrate: sugar, orange juice, candy, etc. For protection, diabetic patients receiving insulin should carry several lumps of sugar with them at all times. A patient in insulin reaction may act as though he were intoxicated, and therefore *it is further recommended that everyone with diabetes carry a card identifying him as a diabetic.* This is especially important for patients with a long history of diabetes. Because of neuropathy, sympathetic nervous system signs may gradually be lost; the patient then lacks indications of impending reaction and may exhibit only impaired cerebral functions. *The intermediate and long-acting insulins produce a more gradual decline in blood glucose level,* with consequently less release of epinephrine; symptoms are produced by deficient glucose metabolism of the higher nervous centers. They consist of headache, blurred or double vision, fine tremor, uncontrollable yawning, hypothermia, mental confusion, incoordination, and eventually, unconsciousness. In elderly persons an insulin reaction may mimic a cerebrovascular accident. Treatment is administration of glucose by mouth or vein, or of glucagon if no vein can be found. Relatives of diabetic patients liable to severe insulin reactions, and especially parents of diabetic children, should be instructed in the use of glucagon. It can be injected subcutaneously, just as insulin is, and will lead to a transient rise in blood glucose level that is long enough to wake the patient up and enable him to receive some carbohydrate by mouth. Whereas the normal beta cell regulates insulin release according to the body's need on a minute-to-minute basis, the condition of the diabetic patient receiving subcutaneous administration of insulin mimics that produced by an autonomous "insulinoma" which does not respond to the patient's need but rather requires the patient to adjust to it with spaced meals and preplanned exercise. Recurrent hypoglycemic attacks, with their attendant anxiety, headache, loss of concentration power, etc., constitute a nuisance to the diabetic patient, but only *severe and prolonged* attacks of hypoglycemia will lead to intellectual deterioration as a result of irreversible damage to cortical neurons. It is unfortunate that the margin between the effective dose of insulin which produces euglycemia and the toxic dose which produces hypoglycemia is so small. However, there is hope of improving this situation with the development of artificial pancreases, which would consist of a glucosensor coupled to an insulin reservoir that would release insulin only in response to rising blood sugar level and would shut it off before hypoglycemia develops.

An insulin reaction initiates a counterregulatory mechanism characterized by release of epinephrine, adrenal corticosteroids, and growth hormone. This will result in a *rebound hyperglycemia,* for "hypoglycemia begets hyperglycemia." Knowledge of this physiologic defense mechanism will prevent the physician from administering extra insulin to combat this hyperglycemia. If the insulin reaction is due to excessive insulin, the patient will benefit from a reduced insulin dosage.

REACTIONS AT THE SITE OF INSULIN INJECTION Such reactions are not uncommon at the beginning of treatment. They are characterized by redness, swelling, pain, and nodule formation. As they usually disappear within a few days or weeks, the patient can be reassured, and no treatment is indicated. If the local reaction persists, it can be improved by changing to an insulin of the lente type, which does not contain protamine, or by switching to a pure pork insulin. Occasionally the simultaneous injection of an antihistamine in the same syringe is very helpful. Very rarely systemic allergic reactions occur, mediated by gamma-E globulin (IgE); desensitization may be necessary. Skin infections at the site of injection are extremely rare.

INSULIN LIPODYSTROPHY This reaction is characterized by either hypertrophy or atrophy of the subcutaneous adipose tissue at the site of insulin injection. This is frequent and affects children and females more than males. If the patient is bothered by the esthetic aspect of this complication, injection of insulin into other sites is recommended until the lesion improves; then the atrophic area may again be used in the hope of inducing lipogenesis.

INSULIN RESISTANCE Almost all diabetic patients treated with insulin for several months will develop circulating antibodies to insulin. However, only a few (approximately 1 in 1,000 insulin-treated diabetics) will develop insulin resistance. By definition it is present if the daily insulin requirement in the absence of ketoacidosis exceeds 200 units. Patients with insulin resistance may require several thousand units daily. When insulin resistance is associated with hemochromatosis, severe infections, Cushing's syndrome, acromegaly, or hyperthyroidism, it is secondary. Frequently, no obvious cause can be detected. Examination of serum will demonstrate the presence of large quantities of antibodies to insulin and an increased insulin-binding capacity. In such patients a trial with pure pork insulin is always justified, and very often a sizable reduction in insulin requirement can be achieved. A proinsulin-free single-peak insulin has been used with good results. If such measures fail, the use of steroids is indicated, for their anti-insulin effect is outweighed by their antiallergic effect. Rarely the addition of phenformin or sulfonylureas is helpful. The natural course of idiopathic insulin resistance is characterized by spontaneous remission within several weeks or months. Frequently, the resistance breaks abruptly and the patient exhibits episodes of severe hypoglycemia as the antibody-bound insulin is released and becomes suddenly available.

COMPLICATIONS OF DIABETES

DIABETIC KETOACIDOSIS AND COMA

Lack of insulin is the cause of diabetic ketoacidosis. The patient may have (1) undiagnosed diabetes, (2) known diabetes but fail to increase his insulin dose despite poor urine tests, or (3) known diabetes and suffer from nausea and vomiting but reason that he does not need his daily insulin because he does not eat. Omission of insulin probably constitutes the single largest cause of diabetic acidosis. Other common causes are infections and myocardial infarctions.

Diagnosis Among clinical signs and symptoms, vomiting is present in approximately two-thirds of patients with acidosis. Abdominal pain and tenderness may be related to nausea and vomiting or sodium depletion and may be so severe as to mimic an abdominal emergency ("pseudoappendicitis" of diabetic acidosis). Air hunger and heavy labored breathing as described by Kussmaul are expressions of the acidosis and correlate with the reduction in serum CO_2 content. There is dehydration as evidenced by soft eyeballs, dry skin, poor urinary output, and hypotension. Laboratory findings include the following: the urine usually contains massive amounts of glucose and acetone; frequently there is also transient albuminuria. The diagnosis of diabetic ketoacidosis is made, however, by finding hyperglycemia (usually between 300 to 600 mg per 100 ml), ketonemia, and reduction of serum CO_2 content (below 9 mEq per liter). The acidosis is metabolic and is caused by accumulation of ketone bodies associated with loss of sodium and potassium. The azotemia is due partly to dehydration and partly to tissue protein breakdown. Serum lipids are generally increased in number. The rise in hematocrit indicates dehydration; usually there is leukocytosis.

Differential diagnosis On clinical grounds alone it is sometimes difficult to distinguish between diabetic acidosis and an insulin reaction. If any doubt exists, blood should be drawn for laboratory tests and 50 ml of 50 percent glucose injected intravenously. If the coma is due to insulin reaction, the patient will wake up immediately; if he is in diabetic coma, no harm has been done. Among diagnoses to be considered are salicylate poisoning; lactic acidosis; hyperglycemic, hyperosmolaric, nonketotic coma; or far-advanced renal failure—all conditions which may occur in a diabetic patient.

Treatment Treatment will vary greatly from patient to patient; however, the general principles are as follows:

1 Through a large needle blood is withdrawn for laboratory tests (blood glucose, BUN, Na, K, C1, CO_2 content, pH, hematocrit, white blood cells, plasma acetone), and the vein is kept open with an infusion of normal saline solution. The rationale for this rests on the observation that patients in diabetic coma may decompensate very rapidly, and precious time will be lost in finding a vein and performing a venous cutdown.
2 Crystalline insulin is administered both subcutaneously and intravenously. The average total dosage of insulin required for patients in diabetic coma within the first 24 hr is 200 units. The dosage, of course, will vary from patient to patient; it may have to be larger for an obese diabetic and less in a frail, elderly diabetic. If the patient has been in diabetic coma previously and required 300 units to respond, chances are he may require a similar dose again. The initial dose of insulin will depend primarily on laboratory tests such as blood sugar and plasma ketone. An average initial dose would be 50 units intravenously and 50 units subcutaneously. Of the many schemes available, the most adequate is the one based on serial dilutions of plasma and testing for ketones (Table 88-9). Severe acidosis necessitates reevaluation of blood glucose, serum CO_2, and plasma acetone levels every 2 hr; if acidosis is less severe, reevaluation every 4 hr will suffice. If the blood glucose level remains above 500 mg per 100 ml and serum

TABLE 88-9
Treatment of ketoacidosis: tentative dosage of insulin based on presence of ketones in serial dilutions of plasma

Initial insulin dose, units	*Serum acetone positive at plasma dilution*
50	1:4
100	1:8
150	1:16
200	>1:16

acetone is positive at 1:4 dilution, another 100 units of insulin should be given. If the patient does not respond at all or if his condition deteriorates, successive doses are increased rapidly and given at hourly intervals. An occasional patient may require 5,000 or 10,000 units within the first 24 hr of treatment.

3 All patients in diabetic acidosis are severely dehydrated and depleted of sodium and potassium. They will require a large amount of fluid, usually a total of 4 to 8 liters during the first 24 hr. Many electrolyte formulas have been proposed for adequate replacement; though their value is not doubted, it is important to start fluid therapy *immediately*, which is best done with the universally available normal (0.9 percent) saline solution. Once treatment is under way and the laboratory has reported values for blood glucose, serum CO_2, and electrolytes, finer adjustments can be made. Part of the fluid may be given as $^1/_2N$ saline, particularly in older persons, in whom the central venous pressure should be monitored. The addition of bicarbonate is indicated only if the acidosis is very severe as bicarbonate may further lower serum K, produce relative spinal fluid acidosis (it does not cross the blood-brain barrier), and affect the hemoglobin oxygen dissociation curve. Once the blood glucose approaches 200 mg per 100 ml, intravenous fluid should be changed to 5% glucose in saline in order to avoid hypoglycemia and possible cerebral edema, as the patient responding to treatment will suddenly become more sensitive to insulin.

Usually there is also a deficiency of potassium; this should be replaced, once urine starts to flow, usually at the second or third hour. Potassium is administered at a rate not exceeding 20 mEq per hr; rarely more than 100 to 200 mEq is needed during the initial 24 hr of treatment. The need for and administration of potassium can be monitored with an electrocardiograph. Signs of hypokalemia are flattening or inversion of T waves, prolongation of the Q-T intervals, and appearance of u waves.

4 There are useful accessory procedures in the treatment of diabetic acidosis. If the patient is unconscious, gastric lavage should be performed to prevent aspiration pneumonia. If the patient is in obvious circulatory collapse, blood, plasma, or a plasma volume expander should be given. Finally, the precipitating cause for the development of diabetic acidosis has to be established for each patient so that specific treatment can be initiated. Errors frequently made are (*a*) not providing enough insulin soon enough, (*b*) not providing enough fluids, (*c*) not providing enough potassium, (*d*) providing too much bicarbonate.

5 The acute phase of diabetic acidosis is considered to be ended once the patient is completely responsive, the blood glucose level is below 200 mg per 100 ml, the serum diluted 1:1 shows no evidence of acetone, serum CO_2 is normal, and the urine shows minimal glycosuria. Ketonuria may persist for 24 to 48 hr. Now is the time to start the patient on intermediate insulin in a small dose to prevent a relapse into ketosis, and also, if needed, to give crystalline insulin in amounts dictated by urine sugar levels. A soft diet should be started. It is essential to begin with frequent small feedings. Intravenous fluid administration may be discontinued as soon as the patient is able to retain liquids by mouth. The overall mortality rate of patients with diabetic ketoacidosis is approximately 5 percent. It may be 10 to 20 percent in a city or county hospital because patients arrive late. A very rare but serious complication of diabetic ketoacidosis is facial mucormycosis (see Chap. 191).

HYPERGLYCEMIC NONKETOTIC COMA This entity is characterized by extreme elevation of blood glucose levels (values of 1,000 mg per 100 ml or higher are not rare; "syrupy" blood), and absent or only minimal ketonemia. The marked hyperglycemia and the associated hypernatremia secondary to water loss lead to an increase in extracellular fluid osmolarity with consequent intracellular dehydration, the effect of which on the central nervous system accounts for the neurologic symptoms and coma. Serum osmolarity can be estimated by multiplying the Na concentration times 2 and adding 5.5 for each 100 mg of glucose (molecular weight of glucose is 180, therefore $100/18 = 5.5$). Normal values range between 290 and 310 mOsm per liter. A patient with values of Na of 160 mEq per liter and of blood glucose of 1,000 mg per 100 ml exhibits an approximate serum osmolarity of $320 + 55 = 375$ mOsm per liter. The highest level recorded is 458 mOsm per liter. It remains a mystery why in these patients ketosis is minimal.

It is observed usually in the middle-aged or older person, frequently associated with corticosteroid or diuretic therapy or peritoneal dialysis, and may be the first indication of diabetes. Awareness of this syndrome is important, as the condition of a comatose patient seen for the first time may be misdiagnosed. He will show massive glycosuria but no acetone; therefore it is reasoned that the cause for his coma is not diabetic ketoacidosis, and no antidiabetic treatment will be initiated. Thus valuable time may be lost. Treatment consists of intravenous administration of fluid, preferably hypotonic saline solution and insulin. Some patients are markedly sensitive to insulin and may need only 25 to 50 units whereas others may require 200 or more units. According to the literature the mortality rate of this diabetic complication approximates 50 percent; however, in our personal experience it is much lower. After recovery not all patients will require insulin.

DIABETIC RETINOPATHY This can be detected in varying degrees in more than 90 percent of diabetic patients after 20 years of clinical diabetes.

The earliest recognizable lesions on fundoscopy are dilatation of veins and "microaneurysms," which actually consist of small punctate hemorrhages. Unless they occur within the macula, the vision will not be impaired. Other relatively early lesions are waxy exudates. This stage of the retinopathy can remain stationary for many years. It is the patient with long-term juvenile diabetes whose condition may progress to a more malignant stage, that of neovascularization and proliferative retinopathy. The new blood vessels usually emanate from the disk and grow toward the vitreous. If a preretinal hemorrhage occurs, organization takes place with formation of fibrous and collagenous tissue. Shrinkage of the scar tissue will produce retinal detachment (see color plate 8). Advanced diabetic retinopathy is frequently associated with retinal lesions caused by atherosclerosis, arterial hypertension, and renal insufficiency.

The appearance of retinopathy is fundamentally related to duration of diabetes. Controversy exists over whether strict chemical control of the metabolic component of diabetes will delay its onset or make it less severe. Poor vision in one eye and rapidly progressing retinopathy in the other eye constitute a major indication for pituitary ablation. However, this intervention should be performed only when the patient has emotional stability, long-term willingness to cooperate, and relative freedom from coronary artery disease or nephropathy. As hypoglycemia presents a major hazard after pituitary intervention, the patient should preferably not be living alone. The factor responsible for improvement has not been identified. Whereas pituitary manipulation represents a last effort to salvage vision, and is associated with the iatrogenic induction of thyroid, adrenal, and gonadal deficiency, newer forms of treatment are directed toward the affected eyes themselves. They are photocoagulation, introduced by Meyer-Schwickerath, and various green and red laser treatments of the retina. Preliminary results indicate that these procedures may be applied to *early* retinal lesions, and the results obtained are encouraging.

DIABETIC NEPHROPATHY See Chap. 279.

DIABETIC NEUROPATHY This is a common, distressing complication of diabetes which is difficult to treat at any stage. Although it most frequently involves peripheral nerves, it may involve any portion of the nervous system and, thus, has an almost unlimited range of manifestations (Table 88-10). The peripheral neuropathy is characterized by a nonsegmental distribution. An interesting differential diagnosis is presented by the patient with severe headache and ocular palsy. If an intracranial aneurysm can be ruled out by angiogram, diabetic neuropathy may be the underlying cause. The neuropathy may be primarily metabolic (sorbitol pathway), which is potentially reversible, or primarily vascular, which is less amenable to treatment.

Treatment of diabetic neuropathy consists of careful control of the diabetes; unfortunately, it is not specific, and weeks or months may pass before improvement, if any, takes place. Diphenylhydantoin (Dilantin), 100 mg three or four times daily, has provided some patients with relief. If improvement is not noted in 3 to 4 days, therapy should be discontinued.

GANGRENE OF THE FEET This is a serious and frequent complication of diabetes, especially in the older age group. It may be due to vascular lesions ("pulseless" foot) or to neuropathy ("painless" foot), usually with a superimposed infection or injury. Gangrene may also be associated with small-vessel disease in which pedal pulses are not decreased. Arterial insufficiency is diagnosed by a history of claudication, nocturnal cramps, or night pain. On examining the patient, one finds weak or absent pedal pulses, blanching of the foot when it is raised above a 45° angle, cyanosis, and delayed venous filling when the foot is dependent. There may be lack of hair growth and muscle atrophy. Diagnostic aids include oscillometry, arteriography, and ultrasonic flowmeter (Doppler). If arterial bypass operation fails or cannot be done, amputation is the treatment; unfortunately, in one-third of the patients amputation of one leg is followed by loss of the other leg within 3 years. Hence, prevention, or at least delay of onset, of gangrene is of paramount importance. Education of the patient to prevent injuries and infections is of the utmost importance. Simple rules for prevention include (1) washing the feet with warm but *never hot* water each evening; (2) applying lanolin two or three times weekly if the skin is dry; (3) inserting lamb's wool between overlapping toes; (4) avoiding injuries to feet (the patient should never go barefoot); (5) not cutting toenails if vision is poor; (6) treating of corns and calluses by a qualified podiatrist or surgeon; (7) stopping smoking.

TABLE 88-10
Diabetic neuropathies

Peripheral:
- Sensory: loss of vibratory sense, paresthesias, pain, loss of pain, usually subacute, symmetric, and distal
- Neuromuscular: weakness, paralysis, absent tendon reflexes, diabetic amytrophy (thighs), extraocular muscle palsies

Autonomic:
- Eye: pupillary changes
- Gastrointestinal: delayed gastric emptying, gallbladder dysfunction, nocturnal diarrhea
- Genitourinary: sexual impotence, atonic urinary bladder, retrograde ejaculation
- Vascular: orthostatic hypotension
- Bones and joints: neuropathic joint (Charcot)
- Skin: neurogenic ulcer, absent sweating, dependent edema

SURGERY AND DIABETES MELLITUS

Patients with diabetes mellitus may be affected by any surgical disease and on rare occasion may even be the object of spectacular surgical triumphs; the first successful heart transplant was performed in a diabetic. In addition, in the diabetic population-at-large conditions requiring surgery, such as peripheral vascular disease, gallbladder disease, and cancer of the pancreas, are more frequent.

The present surgical mortality in diabetics is approximately that of the general population. The surgical risk is increased in diabetics in the presence of poor metabolic control, obesity, arteriosclerosis, and cardiovascular-renal disease. However, even for the patient with uncomplicated diabetes, operation and anesthesia constitute an additional metabolic stress, which will accentuate the predisposition to hyperglycemia and ketosis. Nevertheless, diabetes constitutes no contraindication to surgery; and if the case is an emergency, only a few hours are generally needed to evaluate and prepare such a patient for operation.

On admission for elective or emergency surgery, the patient with diabetes presents either of two situations:

either he is a known diabetic under treatment with varying degree of metabolic control, or the diagnosis of diabetes is suggested by routine preoperative testing. If the scheduled surgery is elective in nature and the diabetes requires further regulation, surgery should be postponed until glycosuria is minimal, acetonuria absent, and the preprandial blood glucose level close to normal. If, on the other hand, surgery is urgent and marked hyperglycemia and ketosis are present, vigorous treatment is started immediately with intravenous fluid and insulin. The majority of diabetic patients will not present this dramatic problem. Their management during surgery will vary according to the severity of their condition. As a general principle, one should aim to prevent acetonuria and excessive protein breakdown by providing an adequate carbohydrate intake. This is done on the day of surgery by replacing the oral feedings with intravenous 5% or 10% glucose in water or saline solution, the volume being dictated by the cardiac state and fear of overhydration. Usually, 1,000 to 1,500 ml of 5% glucose in saline solution is sufficient. By history and laboratory evaluation three types of diabetes are encountered: (1) mild diabetes, treated with diet alone; only close surveillance with frequent urine testing and daily blood glucose is required. (2) Patients on oral hypoglycemic agents. As oral intake is usually impossible on the day of surgery, these patients are best changed to a small amount of intermediate-acting (lente or NPH) insulin, e.g., 10 to 20 units. Once oral feedings are resumed in the postoperative period, insulin is discontinued and the respective tablets are restarted at the former dose. (3) Patients previously on insulin and with well-controlled diabetes receive on the day of surgery two-thirds of their usual *total* dose, preferably divided into a preoperative and postoperative dose, and with crystalline insulin omitted. Example: Preoperative insulin dose = 10 units crystalline insulin, 35 units NPH, total dose 45 units. Therefore, on the day of surgery, one-third, or 15 units, of NPH is given preoperatively, and 15 units of NPH is given postoperatively. It is customary in some centers not to give any preoperative insulin, presumably because of fear of hypoglycemia, and only to administer crystalline insulin according to urine test in the postoperative period. In our experience, hypoglycemia occurs rarely if the preoperative insulin is only NPH or lente, provided the total dose is reduced by one-third and, furthermore, if glucose is administered intravenously throughout the operative period. The benefits of this regimen are that the patient does not escape into severe hyperglycemia or ketosis with resultant electrolyte imbalance during surgery or the immediate postoperative period. In summary, treatment of the diabetic during surgery will depend on previous diabetic management and on the extent of the surgical procedure, as outlined in Table 88-11.

PREGNANCY AND DIABETES MELLITUS

The problem of management during pregnancy has assumed increasing importance, as young diabetic patients now survive longer and are thus capable of procreation. Infertility in female diabetic patients, common before insulin therapy, is rarely seen with good control of the diabetes. The problems engendered by pregnancy in diabetics concern maternal survival, fetal salvage, and prevention of diabetes in the offspring.

Today pregnancy carries but slightly added risk to the mother with well-managed diabetes; the maternal survival is 99.7 percent (White). In contrast, fetal mortality is still high. Stillbirths among diabetics are six times as common as among nondiabetics. Fetal salvage ranges between 90 to 95 percent and will depend on the duration of the mother's disease and presence or absence of vascular lesions such as nephropathy.

DIAGNOSIS In patients not previously known to be diabetic, pregnancy may induce a temporary state of diabetes. The diagnosis may offer some difficulty, since with the lowered renal threshold of pregnancy, glycosuria is not uncommon even among nondiabetic pregnant women. If urinary glucose is found during pregnancy and there is, in addition, a history of frequent miscarriages, of babies with a birth weight exceeding 9 lb, or a family history of diabetes, diabetes should be suspected. The diagnosis can be firmly established only by abnormal blood glucose levels, whether fasting or postprandial. If they are borderline, performance of a glucose tolerance test is definitely indicated. Diagnostic criteria are slightly different during pregnancy. The upper limit of normal at the second hour is 145 rather than 120 mg per 100 ml.

TREATMENT The best results are obtained by close cooperation between the patient, the internist, and the obstetrician. The treatment of pregnant diabetic patients entails the same general health measures as those recommended for nondiabetic pregnant women. It is desirable to maintain a high intake of protein (i.e., at least 2 g per kg body weight per day) with a total caloric intake of 30 kcal per kg of body weight and an adequate intake of calcium and iron. To prevent edema and minimize hydramnios, a low-salt diet is indicated, and the liberal use

TABLE 88-11
Management of diabetes on the day of surgery

Surgical procedure	*Previous diabetic treatment*		
	Diet only	*Oral hypoglycemic agent*	*Insulin*
Minor	Observe	Withhold until after procedure	Withhold until after procedure
Major	Observe	Change to insulin (10-20 units NPH)	One-third of total dose preoperatively; one-third postoperatively; crystalline insulin only if needed

of diuretics is advisable. In most women, diabetes is regulated throughout pregnancy with insulin. Because of the lowered renal threshold for glucose one should not attempt to keep the urine sugar-free. It is admittedly often difficult to avoid excessive weight gain, but at least 200 g carbohydrate must be utilized to prevent ketosis.

Care of a diabetic patient through the first trimester may be difficult because of nausea and vomiting. In the last trimester the insulin requirement usually increases concurrently with a rise in adrenal cortical activity, the presence of placental lactogen, and placental destruction of insulin. It is of utmost importance to detect preeclamptic toxemia and hydramnios, since treatment will reduce fetal mortality. Timing of delivery is also important. The more advanced the diabetic state of the mother, the earlier the delivery should be attempted. Fetal viability can be monitored by determining estradiol levels in maternal urine. Patients with only chemical diabetes can be delivered at term; patients with vascular complications should be delivered at the thirty-sixth week. The child may be delivered vaginally or by section. Early delivery has the advantage of removing the infant before it becomes too large and before placental circulation is impaired. The latter may be either the cause or the effect of the tendency of toxemia. A sudden decrease of insulin requirement to prepregnancy level or even lower usually follows delivery, presumably because of removal of placental lactogen or possibly a temporary state of hypopituitarism. Thus, it is advisable to omit insulin altogether on the day of delivery and to administer only one-half the prepregnancy dose for 3 to 5 days following delivery. Similarly, any coverage with regular insulin should be reduced, i.e., 10 units for 4+ urine sugar, 5 units for 3+, and no coverage for 2+, 1+, or trace.

REFERENCES

BEIGELMAN PM: Severe diabetic ketoacidosis, 482 episodes in 257 patients. Diabetes 20:490, 1971

BIERMAN EL: Principles of nutrition and dietary recommendations for patients with diabetes mellitus. Diabetes 20:633, 1971

LUNDBARK K, KEEN H: *Blood Vessel Disease in Diabetes Mellitus*, Milano, Italy: Il Ponti, 1971

MCGARRY J, FOSTER DW: Regulation of ketogenesis and clinical aspects of the ketotic state. Metabolism 21:471, 1972

MARBLE A et al (eds): *Joslin's Diabetes Mellitus*, 11th ed., Philadelphia: Lea & Febiger, 1971

Proceedings Fiftieth Anniversary Insulin Symposium (Indianapolis, Indiana, Oct. 18–20, 1971). Diabetes 21:385, 1972

SPIRO RG: Chemistry and metabolism of the basement membrane, in *Diabetes Mellitus, Theory and Practice*, eds M Ellenberg, H Rifkin, New York: McGraw-Hill, 1970

SUSSMAN K: *Juvenile-onset Diabetes*, Springfield, Ill.: Charles C Thomas, 1971

University Group Diabetes Program: A study of the effects of hypoglycemia agents on vascular complications in patients with adult-onset diabetes. Diabetes 19 (suppl 2): 474, 1970

89 NONDIABETIC MELITURIAS

J. STUART SOELDNER

DEFINITION The nondiabetic meliturias comprise a group of diverse conditions in which sugar is detected in the urine by usual clinical testing in patients in whom diabetes mellitus is not suspected on other clinical grounds. In all cases of melituria, the clinical and laboratory work-up of the patient must include studies that rule out diabetes mellitus (see Chap. 88).

CLASSIFICATION The major distinction to make among meliturias is whether they are glucosurias or nonglucosurias. The readily available copper reduction type of tests (such as Clinitest, Ames Company), which detect any reducing sugar, and glucose-specific tests (such as Clinistix, Ames Company, or Tes-Tape, Eli Lilly and Company) permit easy and rapid differentiation of glucosuric from nonglucosuric meliturias. The general classification of the meliturias is outlined in Table 89-1. Only glucose will produce a positive glucose-specific test. Of all the other types of meliturias, *only sucrosuria* will not be detected by the copper reduction type of tests.

There are certain situations in which the conventional tests for melituria will be adversely affected. Some conditions, disease states, drugs, or poisons which might influence the conventional urine tests are outlined in Table 89-2. It is of more than passing interest that many situations result in both a false positive copper reduction test and a false negative (or delayed positive) glucose oxidase enzyme test.

PHYSIOLOGY The renal glomerular filtrate contains glucose in a concentration which equals that in plasma water. Glucose is reabsorbed in the proximal convoluted tubules by an energy-requiring active transport process. As the concentration of glucose in plasma water increases, the amount of glucose actively absorbed by the tubules reaches a transfer maximum (Tm) which in the normal adult is about 300 to 350 mg per min. When arterial blood glucose levels reach 150 to 180 mg per 100 ml, the amount of glucose presented to the tubules usually exceeds the Tm, and glucose begins to appear in the urine. Theoretically, as the glucose load delivered to the nephron increases, the amount reabsorbed by the tubules approaches a maximum Tm. In man, this theoretic situation is never quite achieved. Deviations from this ideal (or splay) occur in which glucose is excreted by the kidney before the Tm is reached. It is suspected that as the glucose load increases toward the Tm, some individu-

TABLE 89-1
The meliturias

Group	*Compounds*
Pentosurias	L-Xylulose, L-arabinose, D-ribose
Hexosurias	Glucose,* galactose, fructose
Heptosurias	Mannoheptulose
Dissaccharidurias	Lactose, sucrose,† maltose

* *The only sugar which produces a positive glucose oxidase test*
† *Will not produce positive copper reduction test*

al nephrons will achieve their Tm and excrete glucose. The blood glucose concentration which results in glucosuria is usually termed the *renal threshold*. Among the important factors that can vary this threshold are the glomerular filtration rate, variations in renal blood distribution, and minor alterations in the ratio of glomerular filtering surface to tubular absorptive capacity resulting in a normal distribution of slight glomerulo-tubular imbalances, physiologically expressed as "splay" about the mean Tm.

Some patients with diabetes mellitus may have a renal threshold lower than normal. Parallel studies of blood glucose and urine glucose will furnish a practical guide as to the significance of glucosuria in such patients.

GLUCOSURIC MELITURIAS

It should be assumed that any glucosuric melituria represents diabetes mellitus until proved otherwise. Following the detection of glucosuria (a positive glucose oxidase urine test), it is of prime importance to document the blood sugar level and the corresponding degree of glucosuria. A large number of conditions, some relatively infrequent, can produce both glucosuria and hyperglycemia in the absence of true idiopathic diabetes mellitus (Table 89-3). In many situations, the glucosuria may be present when only mild carbohydrate or glucose intolerance is present. Diseases of the pancreas (or the islet of Langerhans) resulting in a functional deficiency of beta cells are sometimes obvious (such as in pancreatitis), but may be geographically localized and/or rare (scorpion bite).

The relation between various hyperendocrinopathies and hyperglycemia, with resultant glucosuria, should be kept in mind as causes of *secondary diabetes mellitus*. In addition, a number of diseases involving the central nervous system have been shown to be related to hyperglycemia and/or glucosuria. Many varieties of gastrointestinal disease have also been implicated. Renal diseases, especially the uremic state, appear to be associated with glucosuria. A relatively large number of metabolic diseases and chronic diseases are also implicated as causes of nondiabetic glucosuria, again usually associated with hyperglycemia or carbohydrate intolerance.

Those conditions associated with clear-cut hyperglycemia or variable hyperglycemia are discussed in detail in Chap. 88. Those conditions mentioned in Sec. II of Table 89-3 represent a group in which care must be taken to document the presence of hyperglycemia. Temporary renal glucosuria may occur in pregnancy, especially in the latter half. If screening blood glucose tests (such as a blood glucose level determined 1 hr after a breakfast liberal in carbohydrate) are suspicious, then an oral glucose tolerance should be done. If this is not normal, repeat tests should be performed (see Chap. 88). Much the same approach should be used to exclude diabetes in chronic disease states. In these situations, however, the deleterious effect of age, poor nutrition, and inactivity per se upon the glucose tolerance test should be kept in mind. The following discussion deals primarily with those glucosurias not associated with hyperglycemia (Table 89-3).

RENAL GLUCOSURIA This is a benign condition characterized by the excretion of glucose in the urine in the presence of a normal concentration of blood glucose. The "true" type of renal glucosuria is rare. This is defined as persistent and constant glucosuria even in the fasting state with blood glucose levels below 100 mg per 100 ml. There are, however, other types of renal glucosuria in which the renal threshold is somewhat reduced so that glucosuria occurs after meals or glucose loads but not in

TABLE 89-2
Factors responsible for deviant urine tests for melituria

I	False positive copper reduction type tests	
	Condition:	*Compound:*
	A Unclean glassware	Some dentifrices, cleansers, and bleaches
	B Antibiotic therapy	Penicillin, streptomycin, cephalosporins, nalidixic acid, isoniazid, *para*-aminosalicylic acid, chloramphenicol, tetracyclines
	C Renal tubule transport blockers	Carinamide, probenecid
	D L-Dopa therapy	3,4-Dihydroxyphenylacetic acid
	E Alkaptonuria	Homogentisic acid
	F Miscellaneous drugs/poisons	Salicylates, ascorbic acid, chloral hydrate, chloroform, hippuric acid, amino acids, formaldehyde, oxalic acid, and phenols
	G Certain x-ray contrast media	Sodium diatrizoate (Hypaque), meglumine iothalamate (Conray), diatrizoate meglucamine (Renovist)
II	False negative copper reduction type tests	
	A Outdated reagents	
III	False positive glucose oxidase enzyme strips	
	A Unclean glassware	Certain cleansers and detergents
IV	False negative (or delayed positive) glucose oxidase enzyme strips	
	A Conditions above (I*D* to I*F*)	
	B Carcinoid syndrome	5-Hydroxyindoleacetic acid
	C Hepatic disease	Bilirubin glucuronide
	D Uremia	Indoles

the fasting state. A renal glucose titration test has been devised to quantify the Tm and to estimate the minimum threshold (F_{min}). By means of this technique, two types of abnormal curves have been described: type A in which there is a low threshold and a low Tm, and type B with a low threshold, an exaggerated splay to the curve, and a normal Tm.

Studies of families exhibiting renal glucosuria have shown that mild and severe types A and B can occur in the same pedigree, suggesting that familial renal glucosuria can be inherited as an autosomal recessive trait. Renal biopsy studies, few in number, have not revealed any specific or anatomic defect. Thorough evaluation of these patients by multiple blood glucose determinations, fasting or following meals, and oral glucose tolerance tests clearly rules out diabetes. Ketosis develops only during starvation rather than following dietary excess. Although this disease appears not to be related to diabetes, some studies have suggested that it may progress to true diabetes; however, the greater bulk of evidence suggests that the prevalence of diabetes in these patients is no greater than in the general population. Renal glucosuria, particularly the more severe type, appears to be a lifelong condition. Its severity may be reduced as the subject ages, probably because of arteriosclerosis. Hypertension or renal disease may also minimize the degree of glucosuria. In contrast to the frequent urinary tract infections seen in diabetic glucosuria, urinary tract infections appear not increased. Care must be taken at the time of diagnosis to identify those persons with borderline oral glucose tolerance tests. A regular follow-up program for at least the first few years should establish effectively the diagnosis of a benign condition.

FANCONI SYNDROME In addition to renal glucosuria, various other entities are related to glucosuria without hyperglycemia. The Fanconi syndrome with defective absorption of amino acids, phosphate, bicarbonate, and glucose is described in greater detail elsewhere (see Chaps. 97 and 98). This syndrome secondary to ingestion of outdated tetracyclines and multiple myeloma has also been described.

CHEMICAL AGENTS An increasing number of drugs,

TABLE 89-3
Nondiabetic glucosurias

I Usually not associated with hyperglycemia
- *A* Renal
  - *1* Renal glycosuria
  - *2* Fanconi syndrome
- *B* Drugs/chemical agents/poisons
  - *1* Phlorizin
  - *2* Heavy metal salts (chromium, mercury, uranium, ferric compounds, lead, cadmium, lithium)
  - *3* Curare
  - *4* Carbon monoxide
  - *5* Caffeine
  - *6* Morphine
  - *7* Strychnine
  - *8* Chloroform
- *C* Metabolic
  - *1* Glucoglycinuria (rare)

II Relation to hyperglycemia uncertain or variable
- *A* Metabolic
  - *1* Pregnancy
- *B* Chronic disease
  - *1* Rheumatoid arthritis
  - *2* Malignant disease
  - *3* Vascular hypertension
  - *4* Chronic nephritis and nephrosis
- *C* Chemical
  - *1* Organophosphorous compounds
  - *2* Pimozide

III Usually associated with hyperglycemia
- *A* Ablation of islets of Langerhans
  - *1* Surgical removal
  - *2* Pancreatitis, acute or chronic
  - *3* Carcinoma of pancreas
  - *4* Hemochromatosis
  - *5* Cystic fibrosis
  - *6* Scorpion bite pancreatitis
- *B* Endocrine hyperfunction
  - *1* Acromegaly
  - *2* Hyperthyroidism
  - *3* Hyperadrenocorticism
  - *4* Pheochromocytoma
  - *5* Functioning beta-cell tumor
  - *6* Functioning alpha-cell tumor
- *C* Nervous system diseases
  - *1* Hypothalamic damage
  - *2* Amyotrophic lateral sclerosis
  - *3* Severe emotional stress
  - *4* Brain tumors
  - *5* Brain trauma
  - *6* Cerebral hemorrhage
- *D* Gastrointestinal disease
  - *1* Severe hepatic disease
  - *2* Glycogen storage diseases
  - *3* Postgastrectomy syndrome
- *E* Renal disease
  - *1* Uremia
- *F* Metabolic disease
  - *1* Obesity
  - *2* Infections
  - *3* Poststarvation feeding
  - *4* Burns
  - *5* Physical inactivity
  - *6* Potassium deficiency
  - *7* Lipoatrophic diabetes
  - *8* Fractures
  - *9* Asphyxia
- *G* Drugs
  - *1* Oral antiovulatory steroids (progestational-estrogenic)
  - *2* Benzothiadiazine compounds (chlorothiazides, hydrochlorothiazides, diazoxide)
  - *3* Adrenocorticosteroids/adrenocorticotropic hormone
- *H* Miscellaneous/mixed
  - *1* Postmyocardial infarction

chemicals, poisons, and toxins have been related to defects of renal tubular absorption of glucose, particularly heavy metal salts.

METABOLIC A combined glucosuria/glycinuria has also been described, but is quite rare.

NONGLUCOSURIC MELITURIA

In patients with persistent normoglycemic melituria, identification of the type of sugar excreted is important. The vast majority prove to be glucose, but the number of nonglucosurias is sufficiently frequent to warrant special study. These nonglucosurias are for the most part benign and have no relation to diabetes. Their recognition may have important ramifications in regard to employment, military service, life insurance, etc. By employment of readily available testing materials, a preliminary diagnosis can often be made.

TEST PROCEDURES

1 Benedict's test, or a modification (Clinitest). This test is positive for all sugars found in urine, except sucrose. Fructose, L-xylulose, and mannoheptulose produce a positive reaction somewhat easier than does glucose (10 min at 55°C, or 3 hr at room temperature).
2 Glucose oxidase test (glucose specific). Paper strips (Tes-Tape and Clinistix) are available for quick testing. False negative or delayed positive results can occur (see Table 89-2).
3 Bial (orcinol hydrochloride) reaction. It is positive for pentose.
4 Seliwanoff (resorcinol hydrochloride) reaction. It is positive for fructose.
5 Paper chromatography systems can readily identify the sugar.
6 Osazone crystals. Characteristic crystals can be produced with phenylhydrazine (methylphenylhydrazine for fructose). In addition, glucose and fructose produce the same osazone but at slightly different rates. Melting point determinations show a characteristic 205°C for glucosazone and 157 to 160°C for pentosazone.
7 Fermentation with baker's yeast. Glucose and fructose are always, galactose usually, lactose occasionally, and pentose and mannoheptulose never, fermented.

PENTOSURIA Essential pentosuria, or chronic essential pentosuria, is a rare benign condition inherited as an autosomal recessive trait. Only 1 in 40,000 to 50,000 applicants for life insurance in the United States were found to have this condition. Most reported cases have been in Jewish or Lebanese families. It is characterized by the excretion of L-xylulose in the urine, 1 to 4 g per day. The Benedict's test usually shows a green end point. Paper chromatography easily demonstrates the L-xylulose. Current evidence suggests that this condition is produced by a deficiency of NADP-linked xylitol dehydrogenase, which is involved in the xylitol step in the glucuronic acid pathway (glucuronic acid to gulonic acid to L-xylulose to xylitol to D-xylulose to pentose phosphate pathway to hexose phosphate). The condition is harmless, asymptomatic, and unrelated to diabetes. It requires no treatment. The heterozygote can be identified by a glucuronolactone loading test.

Alimentary pentosuria in which the urine may contain small amounts (less than 0.1 g) of L-arabinose or L-xylose may follow the ingestion of large amounts of plums, cherries, fruit juices, or grapes. Ribosuria (D-ribose) in very small amounts may be found in the urine of some patients with muscular dystrophy.

FRUCTOSURIA **Essential fructosuria** This is a benign, asymptomatic metabolic defect which is rare and appears to be confined to Jewish people. Males and females are equally affected. Less than 100 cases appear in the world literature. Following fructose ingestion in these people, blood fructose levels reach higher values and remain higher for a longer period of time than in normal subjects. About 10 to 20 percent of a fructose load may appear in the urine. It is thought that there is a primary deficiency of hepatic fructokinase in these subjects, reducing the conversion of fructose to fructose 1-phosphate. No treatment is required in this condition.

Hereditary fructose intolerance This condition is a rare error of metabolism in which ingestion of fructose or foods high in fructose leads to symptomatic hypoglycemia and vomiting. In the very young, failure to thrive, hepatomegaly, jaundice, ascites, and plasma electrolyte imbalance may be seen. Occasionally, some degree of renal tubular dysfunction is noted. The metabolic defect is a deficiency of hepatic fructose 1-phosphate aldolase usually associated with a deficiency of hepatic fructose 1,6-diphosphate aldolase. It is thought to be inherited as an autosomal recessive trait. The mechanism responsible for the hypoglycemia is thought to be due to reduced gluconeogenesis and/or glycogenolysis rather than increased peripheral glucose utilization. Hepatic levels of adenosine triphosphate (ATP) and inorganic phosphorus are reduced, which may explain the defective hepatic glucose output.

Early recognition and treatment is mandatory if liver damage, renal dysfunction, and death are to be avoided. If fructose-containing foods are eliminated from the diet, the outlook is excellent. Interestingly, these patients usually have few or no dental caries, owing to their avoidance of foods containing fructose or sucrose.

GALACTOSURIA Galactosemia is a congenital and hereditary disease characterized by an inability to utilize ingested galactose or galactose-containing foods. Galactosuria is seen only when galactose is part of the diet (see Chap. 105).

HEPTOSURIA Mannoheptulose may appear in the urine after one eats large amounts of avocado. Although it is of no clinical importance, it is of interest that mannoheptulose inhibits insulin secretion by the beta cell.

DISACCHARIDURIA **Lactosuria** Lactose may appear in the urine toward the end of pregnancy and during lactation. During pregnancy, the finding of sugar in the urine should be followed up by a glucose tolerance test. Lactosuria can, of course, be a presumptive diagnosis on the basis of a positive copper reduction test but a negative glucose oxidase enzyme test.

Maltosuria Maltosuria and isomaltosuria are rare, but have been reported in the urine of severely injured patients.

Sucrosuria Alimentary sucrosuria has been noted in normal individuals ingesting large amounts of cane sugar. Small amounts of sucrose have been described in the urine of patients with cystic fibrosis. Endogenous sucrosuria, difficult to explain, has been noted rarely. In reported cases, specific gravity of the urine has been as high as 1.070, and up to 200 g sucrose has been detected in a 24-hr urine collection. One must keep in mind *cases of deception* in which patients bring in a urine sample to which they have added cane sugar, not realizing that sucrose will not produce a positive copper reduction test or a positive glucose oxidase enzyme test. *An unusually high specific gravity leads one to think of factitious sucrosuria.* A more difficult case of deception is the urine sample to which a reducing sugar has been added.

REFERENCES

ELSAS LJ, ROSENBERG LE: Familial renal glycosuria: A genetic reappraisal of hexose transport by kidney and intestine. J Clin Invest 48:1845, 1969

LEVIN B et al: Fructosaemia: Observations on seven cases. Am J Med 45:826, 1968

MARBLE A: Nondiabetic melituria, in Joslin's *Diabetes Mellitus*, 11th ed., eds A Marble et al, Philadelphia: Lea & Febiger, 1971, p. 818

STANBURY JB et al (eds): *The Metabolic Basis of Inherited Disease*, 2d ed., Pentosuria, HH Hiatt, p. 109; Fructosuria, ER Froesch, p. 124; The Fanconi syndrome, A Leaf, p. 1205; Renal glycosuria, SM Krane, p. 1221; New York: McGraw-Hill, 1966

WANG YM, VAN EYS J: The enzymatic defect in essential pentosuria. N Engl J Med 282:892, 1970

90
HYPERINSULINISM, HYPOGLYCEMIA, AND GLUCAGON SECRETION

STEFAN S. FAJANS

The maintenance of a constant blood glucose level is an essential part of homeostasis. The blood glucose level at any given time reflects the balance of two groups of physiologic processes: (1) those which add glucose to the blood, namely, (*a*) mobilization of glucose from glycogen stores, (*b*) formation of carbohydrate from nonglucose sources (gluconeogenesis), and (*c*) absorption of ingested carbohydrate; and (2) those which remove glucose from the blood, namely, utilization of glucose by liver, adipose tissue, muscle, brain, and other tissues.

A complete *classification* of hypoglycemia based on pathologic physiology is difficult, because hypoglycemia may be produced by a variety of factors and in some the mechanism is poorly understood. Nevertheless, the common causes of spontaneous hypoglycemia can be grouped as in Table 90-1. From the clinical view, patients with hypoglycemia can be divided into two groups, according to the usual relation of hypoglycemia to the fasting or postprandial (fed) state. Regardless of etiology, the conditions listed in Table 90-1 interfere with the homeostatic mechanism, which regulates the blood glucose level. Such interference may take place at different levels, even if the underlying cause of hypoglycemia is a single one. For example, in patients with functioning islet cell tumors, hypoglycemia is the result not only of increased glucose uptake in insulin-sensitive tissues and decreased hepatic glucose output but also of decreased inflow to the liver of substrates needed for gluconeogenesis. For example, the mobilization of amino acids from muscle is reduced.

The *clinical symptoms and signs* of hypoglycemia are the same regardless of the underlying cause. The symptoms which occur in any given patient vary with the degree and the rate of decline of blood glucose levels and with the variable and individual susceptibility of the underlying state of the central and autonomic nervous systems. Symptoms associated with a rapid decline in blood glucose levels are due in part to activation of the autonomic nervous system and the ensuing release of epinephrine. These symptoms are sweating, shakiness, trembling, tachycardia, anxiety, nervousness, weakness, fatigue, hunger, nausea, and vomiting. Other symptoms of hypoglycemia result from decreased uptake of glucose and decreased utilization of oxygen by the brain and usually occur when the decline in blood glucose levels is slow and/or when hypoglycemia is severe or prolonged. These symptoms are headache, visual disturbances, lethargy, yawning, faintness, restlessness, and difficulty with speech and thinking. Other manifestations may be agitation, mental confusion, somnolence, stupor, prolonged sleep, loss of consciousness, coma, and hypothermia. Twitching, convulsions, "epilepsy," and bizarre neurologic signs, motor as well as sensory in nature, may occur. Prominent signs observed in patients with alcohol-induced hypoglycemia are hypothermia, conjugate deviation of eyes, extensor rigidity of extremities, positive Babinski signs, and trismus. Repeated hypoglycemic episodes may lead to loss of intellectual ability and personality changes characterized by outbursts of temper or queer, bizarre, and psychotic behavior. Extensive and permanent mental or neurolgic damage may result from frequent and prolonged episodes of hypoglycemia.

PANCREATIC ISLET CELL DISEASE

Pathology Approximately 90 percent of functioning islet cell tumors are benign adenomas; approximately 10 percent are definitely malignant with identified metastases. Hyperplasia of the islet cells has not been proved to occur in adults. Functioning islet cell tumors may be diagnosed at any age, with a majority of cases occurring between thirty and sixty years. Benign islet cell adenomas vary in size from 0.14 to 15 cm in diameter, but the majority are between 0.5 and 3.0 cm. They are usually encapsulated, firmer than the normal pancrease, highly vascular, purplish and occasionally whitish in color, and they present an irregu-

TABLE 90-1
Classification of spontaneous hypoglycemia

I Organic hypoglycemia:* recognizable anatomic lesion
- *A* Pancreatic islet cell disease with hyperinsulinism
  - *1* Adenoma, single or multiple
  - *2* Microadenomatosis
  - *3* Carcinoma, with metastases
  - *4* Familial multiple endocrine adenomatosis
- *B* Nonpancreatic tumors associated with hypoglycemia
- *C* Anterior pituitary hypofunction
- *D* Adrenocortical hypofunction
- *E* Acquired extensive liver disease
- *F* Severe congestive heart failure

II Hypoglycemia due to specific hepatic enzyme defect
- *A* Glycogen storage diseases*
- *B* Fructose 1,6-diphosphatase deficiency*
- *C* Hereditary fructose intolerance (fructose 1-phosphate aldolase deficiency)
- *D* Galactosemia
- *E* Aglycogenosis
- *F* Familial fructose and galactose intolerance

III Functional hypoglycemia
- *A* Reactive functional
- *B* Reactive secondary to mild diabetes
- *C* Alimentary hyperinsulinism
- *D* Alcohol and poor nutrition*
- *E* Deficiency of glucagon*
- *F* Transient postnatal hypoglycemia in infant of diabetic mother*
- *G* Transient hypoglycemia in the newborn of low birth weight*
- *H* "Idiopathic hypoglycemia" of infancy and childhood*

IV Exogenous hypoglycemia*
- *A* Iatrogenic } insulin or sulfonylurea compounds
- *B* Factitious } insulin or sulfonylurea compounds

* *Fasting hypoglycemia*

lar surface. They are found to be equally distributed throughout the head, body, and tail of the pancreas. Benign adenomas of islet cell tissue rarely occur outside the pancreas. Multiple adenomas are found in approximately 10 percent of cases. Multiple adenomas of islet cells may be associated with adenomas of the pituitary, parathyroids, and other endocrine glands (familial multiple endocrine adenomatosis) and with peptic ulceration (ulcerogenic Zollinger-Ellison syndrome). Malignant islet cell tumor found in this syndrome, as well as sporadic ones, may secrete other polypeptide hormones as well, such as glucagon, gastrin, adrenocorticotropic hormone (ACTH), and melanocyte-stimulating hormone (MSH). Some tumors, including heteroptopic pancreatic islet cell tumors, may produce 5-hydroxytryptophan and/or serotonin, and are associated with the carcinoid syndrome. A family history of diabetes has been found in 25 to 30 percent of patients with functioning islet cell tumors.

Clinical picture Symptoms of hypoglycemia due to islet cell adenoma may develop insidiously, with periodic hypoglycemic attacks becoming more frequent and more severe. Fasting and exercise precipitate attacks. Attacks usually occur in the early morning hours before breakfast or during the longest daily fasting period, or they may occur in the late afternoon, especially if the noon meal is missed. Symptoms may also occur 2 to 5 hr after meals. Symptoms and signs secondary to decreased cerebral oxygen utilization usually predominate over symptoms secondary to hyperepinephrinemia. The pattern of symptoms is usually repetitive in the same patient, but it may differ from patient to patient. Many patients learn to avert symptoms by taking frequent feedings, including a feeding at 2 or 3 A.M. Obesity may thereby result but is not seen in the majority of patients. Symptoms are rapidly progressive in patients with malignant, metastatic tumors. Chronic hypoglycemia may not only produce profound personality changes but may result also in damage to anterior horn cells of the spinal cord, with progressive muscular atrophy.

Diagnosis A typical symptomatic attack with demonstrated hypoglycemia and relief of symptoms and signs by administration of glucose constitute the diagnostic criteria outlined by Whipple. This triad of Whipple is not specific for patients with functioning tumors of the pancreas, as it may occur in patients with other types of hypoglycemia. The level of the overnight fasting blood glucose is usually below 60 mg per 100 ml but may be normal in some patients. There may be fluctuation from normal to subnormal from day to day. More prolonged fasting is the most helpful diagnostic procedure and will cause a fall in blood sugar below 30 to 35 mg per 100 ml (true blood glucose method). In the majority of cases, hypoglycemia can be induced within the first 12 to 24 hr of fasting. If hypoglycemia and typical symptoms are not induced, fasting should be prolonged for up to 72 hr, at which time the patient should be exercised vigorously. In patients with insulinomas, or other types of fasting hypoglycemia, exercise produces a further fall in blood glucose levels, but it produces a rise in blood glucose in patients with functional hypoglycemia. On clinical grounds, other types of organic hypoglycemia and the exogenous hypoglycemias can usually be ruled out.

Assays of serum insulin (Chap. 88) performed in conjunction with fasting blood glucose levels are most reliable in confirming or establishing a diagnosis of insulinoma. Elevated fasting levels of serum insulin in peripheral blood (in absolute terms) are found in only two-thirds of patients with functioning islet cell tumors. Thus, diagnosis of insulinoma is confirmed by an elevated fasting insulin level, but a "normal" level does not rule out this diagnosis. When fasting insulin levels are measured daily for several days in the same patient, an elevated level can frequently be found in at least one specimen. A serum insulin level in the "normal range" associated with a fasting blood sugar level in the hypoglycemic range is also significant as it is inappropriately high for the existing level of blood glucose. In addition, when the overnight fast is prolonged for 4 hr or more in patients with fasting blood sugar levels in the borderline range, the blood glucose level may fall into the hypoglycemic range while the level of serum insulin remains constant or rises, indicating an abnormal glucose-insulin homeostatic relation (Fig. 90-1). This is good evidence for the presence of an autonomous insulin-producing tissue. An elevated fasting level of plasma insulin after an overnight fast is not specific for insulinoma as it is also seen in obese patients (without fasting hypoglycemia) and has been reported in patients with galactosemia and familial fructose and galactose intolerance. The estimation of fasting plasma levels of proinsulin may be helpful in the diagnosis of islet cell tumors when one cannot demonstrate definite increases in plasma levels of total immunoreactive insulin (IRI). In 82 percent of patients with islet cell tumors the proinsulin component was clearly elevated and exceeded 25 percent of fasting total IRI.

Provocative tests to insulin secretion may be used as adjuncts in the differential diagnosis of hypoglycemia. The intravenous tolbutamide test is one such aid. After

FIGURE 90-1

Decrease in blood glucose levels with inappropriate hyperinsulinemia during fasting in two patients with islet cell tumors. A *Levels of plasma insulin and blood glucose during the last 4 hr of a 12-hr fast. (From Excerpta Medica 172:894, 1969)* B *Levels of plasma insulin and blood glucose during 44-hr fast preoperatively, and normal levels during 72-hr fast postoperatively.*

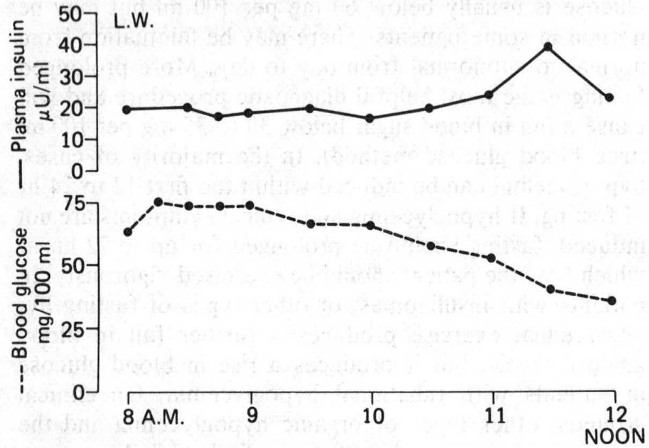

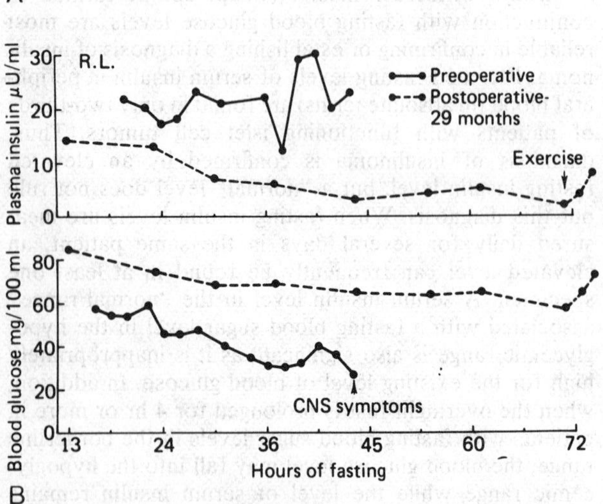

blood for a fasting blood glucose determination is obtained, 1 g sodium tolbutamide dissolved in 20 ml distilled water is injected intravenously over 2 min. Subsequently blood levels of glucose are determined every 15 min for the first hour and every 30 min during the second and third hours of the test. If plasma levels of insulin are obtained during the test (see below), blood samples for insulin assay should be obtained at least every 5 min during the first 15 min after administration of tolbutamide. A normal response to tolbutamide consists of a return of blood glucose to 70 percent or more of fasting levels after an initial drop in blood glucose. One use of the test is in obtaining evidence against a diagnosis of insulinoma in patients suspected of having functional hypoglycemia but whose history is unusual or in whom fasting blood glucose levels are in the lower range of normal. In such patients a normal 3-hr intravenous tolbutamide test may obviate hospitalization and determination of blood glucose during prolonged fasting. In patients with islet cell tumors tolbutamide induces a greater reduction in blood glucose and persistance of hypoglycemia. Tolbutamide-induced hypoglycemia persisted for 3 hr in 50 of 55 patients subsequently proved to have insulinomas. In these 55 patients fasting blood glucose levels were 50 mg per 100 ml or above. The lower the fasting blood glucose, the more frequently will the test have to be terminated early because of severe neurologic symptoms. False positive blood glucose responses can occur in association with severe liver disease, alcoholic hypoglycemia, idiopathic hypoglycemia of infancy, severe undernutrition, and azotemia. They also may occur in some patients with nonpancreatic tumors and associated hypoglycemia, particularly in those patients in whom blood sugar levels decrease rapidly on fasting. In contrast, no false positive responses have occurred in patients with functional hypoglycemia, diabetes mellitus with reactive hypoglycemia, or patients without spontaneous hypoglycemia. Obviously the test is of little help if the fasting blood glucose level is very low.

Assays of plasma insulin in conjunction with the intravenous tolbutamide test increase the value of the test. The finding of excessive increases in plasma insulin levels (above 195 μU per ml within the first 15 min after intravenous administration of tolbutamide and/or, more importantly, prolonged elevation of plasma insulin (increments above basal levels of 50 μU per ml at 30 min and/or of 25 μU per ml at 45 min and of 15 μU per ml at 60 min) thereafter (1) increases the specificity of this test in patients with insulinoma; (2) increases the usefulness of the test in patients with low fasting blood sugar levels, since it allows termination of the test when necessary; and (3) may differentiate insulinoma patients from patients with false positive blood glucose responses. Approximately 85 percent of patients with islet cell tumors exhibit an abnormal insulin response to intravenously administered tolbutamide. However, an increase in levels of insulin in the normal range after intravenous tolbutamide does not rule out the existence of hyperinsulism due to pancreatic islet cell disease.

Sensitivity to leucine may be useful diagnostically. In adult patients a large decrease in blood glucose (over 25 mg per 100 ml) and a large increase in plasma insulin (over 30 μU per ml) after administration of leucine strongly suggest diagnosis of an insulinoma. Approximately 80 percent of patients with functioning islet cell tumors exhibit an exaggerated response to leucine. In childhood, sensitivity to leucine does not differentiate between idiopathic hypoglycemia and insulinoma. Severe leucine-induced hyperinsulinemia and hypoglycemia will also be obtained in factitious hypoglycemia due to surreptitious administration of sulfonylureas, since profound sensitivity to leucine-hypoglycemia can be produced in normal subjects by pretreatment with such compounds. A negative response to leucine does not rule out the existence of an insulinoma.

An exaggerated increase in serum levels of insulin over 160 μU per ml after the intravenous administration of 1 mg glucagon is observed in 50 to 75 percent of patients with proven islet cell tumors. When this occurs, the hyperglycemic effect of glucagon may be subnormal and followed by a profound fall in blood glucose.

In patients with suspected islet cell disease all three provocative tests should be employed, since an abnormal response may be obtained with one but not another of these tests. Obese patients may have an exaggerated rise in plasma insulin with any of these stimuli to insulin secretion, but the hyperinsulinemia is not accompanied by abnormal secondary hypoglycemia.

The oral glucose tolerance test (Chap. 88) may give a relatively flat curve with rapid return of the blood glucose into the hypoglycemic range due to excessive insulin release from the tumor in response to a rising concentration of blood glucose.

Treatment When the diagnosis of functioning islet cell tumor is made, relief of hypoglycemia by early surgery is indicated to prevent any further damage to the central nervous system and to prevent obesity, which makes surgical management more difficult. Identification of the tumor at the time of surgery may present a problem, particularly in the case of a relatively small tumor not located on the anterior surface of the pancreas. Selective pancreatic (celiac and mesenteric) arteriography has made it possible to localize some of these tumors preoperatively. It was successful in locating a tumor radiographically in 15 of 28 patients with proven islet cell tumors. Of these 15 tumors several were located in the head of the pancreas and could not be palpated by the surgeon at the time of laparotomy.

The benzothiadiazine compound, diazoxide, particularly when used in conjunction with one of the diuretic thiazides, such as trichlormethiazide, has been useful to elevate blood levels of glucose into the normoglycemic or hyperglycemic range prior to operation. Diazoxide causes increases in blood glucose by decreasing the secretion of insulin. In addition, diazoxide and the diuretic thiazides elevate blood glucose by one or more extrapancreatic mechanisms. Effective dose ranges between 150 and 450 mg for diazoxide and 1 and 3 mg for trichlormethiazide. The drugs should be discontinued 2 days before surgery.

The surgical approach to insulinomas may be complicated by difficulty in identifying the tumor, by difficulty encountered in "shelling out" completely all tumor tissue, and by the fact that multiple tumors are not uncommon. In the absence of finding a definite insulinoma, resection of first the tail and then the body of the pancreas is justified, as a significant proportion of tumors are located in these areas. After excision of the adenoma or subtotal pancreatectomy to find the adenoma, the patient is usually cured except in cases of multiple tumors or unlocated tumors in the head of the pancreas. In the latter case treatment with diazoxide and trichlormethiazide has been successful for up to 6 years. In approximately 20 percent of cases diagnosed histologically as carcinoma, follow-up observations have failed to reveal a recurrence of symptoms or tumor for several years. Lethal hyperpyrexia has been reported in the first few postoperative days; a temperature of over 104°F warrants the intravenous administration of glucocorticoids.

Patients with nonresectable metastatic islet cell tumors present a management problem, as their hypoglycemia may be so severe as to respond only poorly to oral and even intravenous glucose administration. Since diazoxide is a potent inhibitor of pancreatic insulin release, it has proved to be an effective agent for the alleviation of symptomatic and biochemical hypoglycemia in many of these patients. To counteract the sodium-retaining effect of diazoxide administered in a dose of 600 to 1,000 mg per day, a naturetic thiazide, such as trichlormethiazide, should be used in a dose of 2 to 3 mg per day.

In patients with metastatic islet cell carcinoma, the careful use of streptozotocin may be indicated. Streptozotocin, an antibiotic and an experimental antitumor agent, is a highly effective cytotoxic agent for pancreatic beta cells. Although not devoid of renal and hepatic toxicity, it has considerably greater specificity for normal or abnormal beta cells than is true for alloxan. Several patients with metastatic islet cell carcinoma who were treated with streptozotocin have had complete relief from hypoglycemia and regression of tumor mass.

The use of glucocorticoids and injections of glucagon may also be valuable.

NONPANCREATIC TUMORS ASSOCIATED WITH HYPOGLYCEMIA Severe hypoglycemia has been reported in more than 200 patients harboring nonpancreatic tumors of mesothelial, epithelial, or endothelial origin. Most of these tumors are mesothelial in type and are classified as fibromas, sarcomas, or fibrosarcomas. They are usually situated in the thorax, the retroperitoneal space, or the pelvis. They may be attached to the diaphragm or found within the liver. Other cases of nonpancreatic tumors associated with severe hypoglycemia include more than 40 patients with primary hepatic carcinoma, 14 patients with carcinoma of the adrenal cortex, 5 patients with gastrointestinal carcinomas, 2 patients with pseudomyxoma peritonei, 2 patients with bronchogenic carcinoma, and 1 with a bronchial carcinoid tumor. The common clinical characteristics of these tumors, particularly of the fibrosarcomas, are their slow growth and their massive size (up to 10 kg). Hypoglycemia disappears after resection or occasionally after irradiation of the tumor. Many theories have been advanced to explain the mechanism by which these tumors cause hypoglycemia, but none of these is applicable to all patients. A block in hepatic glucose output, excessive glucose consumption by tumor tissue with a high rate of anaerobic glycolysis, and inhibition of lipolysis have been reported in some of these patients. In the majority of patients immunoreactive insulin and insulin-like activity in serum or extract of tumor tissue have been normal or subnormal. High levels of serum insulin have been reported in one patient with severe hypoglycemia due to a large fibrosarcoma and in another patient with a bronchial carcinoid tumor with metastases. Only rarely have tumor extracts contained immunologically recognizable insulin. Twelve reports indicate that extracts of tumors from some of these patients contain an insulin-like substance stimulatory in either isolated rat diaphragm or epididymal fat pad systems. It is possible that some of these tumors synthesize a polypeptide closely related to insulin, but which, in the majority of instances, is not recognized immunologically as insulin. It may suppress hepatic glucose output.

OTHER CAUSES OF FASTING HYPOGLYCEMIA
Although it is infrequent, fasting hypoglycemia may occur in patients with hypofunction of the anterior pituitary (Chap. 83) or hypofunction of the adrenal cortex (Chap. 86). Usually, other stigmas of these disorders enable one to make a diagnosis. In infants and children hypoglycemia due to isolated growth hormone deficiency has been reported. Occasionally, diffuse and extensive hepatic disease may be associated with hypoglycemia.

Fasting hypoglycemia due to a defect in a specific *hepatic enzyme* involved in glycogenolysis or gluconeogenesis is infrequent. Very seldom fasting hypoglycemia can be traced to a glycogen storage disease (Chap. 104) or to galactosemia (Chap. 105). A syndrome consisting of hypoglycemia and lactic acidosis in infancy due to a defect in hepatic fructose 1,6-diphosphatase activity has been described.

Alcohol ingestion superimposed upon an inadequate dietary intake can precipitate acute hypoglycemia. Blood glucose levels as low as 10 or 20 mg per 100 ml have been observed. Inhibition of gluconeogenesis is primarily responsible for hypoglycemia in conjunction with depletion of liver glycogen stores. In healthy subjects alcohol may precipitate hypoglycemia after fasting for 48 to 72 hr. In certain susceptible individuals (such as patients with ACTH deficiency) alcohol may precipitate hypoglycemia without prior deprivation of food intake. The blood glucose response to infused ethanol has been used as a test for gluconeogenetic reserve in patients in whom a susceptibility to alcohol hypoglycemia is suspected.

A young male has been reported who developed hypoglycemia on prolonged fasting (28 hr) as well as after protein meals. *Glucagon deficiency* was documented during fasting and after ingestion of protein meals and infusion of arginine (see p. 560).

In children the most common type of fasting hypoglycemia is that classified as *idiopathic hypoglycemia of infancy and childhood.* This entity is heterogeneous. It includes children with "ketotic hypoglycemia" precipitated by food deprivation (onset usually after eighteen months of age) and children with the leucine-sensitive type (onset before eighteen months of age). The hypoglycemia may be mild and intermittent or more persistent and severe. Usually by seven or nine years of age these children "outgrow" the occurrence of hypoglycemia. Differentiation from functioning islet cell tumor is most difficult although the occurrence of insulinoma is uncommon in this age group. Fasting hypoglycemia has also been reported in newborn infants with erythroblastosis fetalis and in infants with visceromegaly, giantism, microcephaly, macroglossia, and omphalocele.

In the leucine-sensitive type of idiopathic hypoglycemia, in erythroblastosis fetalis, and in the transient neonatal hypoglycemia in infants of diabetic mothers, plasma levels of insulin, although in the normal range, are inappropriately high in the presence of hypoglycemia.

POSTPRANDIAL HYPOGLYCEMIA Reactive functional hypoglycemia The most frequently encountered hypoglycemic disorder in the adult in whom no demonstrable anatomic lesion can be demonstrated is "functional" or "reactive" hypoglycemia. These patients have normal fasting blood glucose levels. Reactive functional hypoglycemia occurs almost uniformly in patients with emotional problems. Excessive secretion of insulin in response to the normal rise of blood glucose following meals is an infrequent finding. The mechanism involved in this type of hypoglycemia remains unclear. The diagnosis is suspected by a history of hypoglycemic symptoms occurring 2 to 3 hr after ingestion of a meal rich in carbohydrates, and it is confirmed by an oral glucose tolerance test extended for 4 hr, blood samples being obtained at half-hour intervals. After an initial normal rise in blood glucose, it is not unusual in such patients to find blood glucose levels of 30 or 40 mg per 100 ml between the second and fourth hour of the test with a spontaneous return of the blood glucose level toward fasting levels shortly thereafter.

The usual *symptoms* produced by reactive hypoglycemia are transitory and often subside spontaneously in 15 to 30 min. Weakness, hunger, inward trembling, sweating, and tachycardia are the most common symptoms in these patients. Loss of consciousness or convulsions do not occur, and the severity of symptoms is not progressive. In patients with functional hypoglycemia attacks are more frequent when emotional stress and anxiety are greater. A 72-hr fast is well tolerated, and the concentration of blood glucose rarely drops below 45 mg per 100 ml. The intravenous tolbutamide test is normal. A family history for diabetes mellitus is usually absent.

TREATMENT The distressing symptoms experienced by patients with functional hypoglycemia may be prevented by a diet low in carbohydrate (75 to 100 g) and high in protein, with adequate fat to maintain caloric requirements. The diet is divided into three to six feedings, with protein and carbohydrate proportions divided equally among the meals. In patients with a history suggestive of reactive hypoglycemia but in whom the diagnosis cannot be substantiated by a glucose tolerance test, diet therapy may be tried. An important approach is to improve the psychologic and emotional status of the patient with functional hypoglycemia. In this regard tranquilizers may prove useful. The prognosis is good, as usually the disease is self-limiting within a few months or years.

REACTIVE HYPOGLYCEMIA SECONDARY TO MILD DIABETES This condition has to be distinguished from reactive functional hypoglycemia, for both the underlying mechanism and the prognosis are different. Whereas in patients with reactive functional hypoglycemia the pancreatic insulin release is well-timed in response to the rising postprandial blood glucose, in patients with mild diabetes the insulin release is delayed. It is not until the blood glucose rises to frank diabetic levels that insulin is secreted in excess. Measurements of serum insulin during glucose tolerance tests in such patients have demonstrated that relatively large amounts of insulin are released, albeit late; the blood glucose then decreases from diabetic to normal levels and further to hypoglycemic levels. This type of hypoglycemic response is most likely to occur between the third and the fifth hours. It is apparent that these patients have only mild diabetes, as endogenous insulin is available and their fasting blood glucose is within normal limits. Their carbohydrate intolerance can be detected only by a postprandial blood glucose determination or an oral glucose tolerance test. Frequently there is a family history of diabetes mellitus.

Treatment consists of a diabetic diet with frequent feedings. Weight reduction in the obese patient may normalize glucose tolerance, with disappearance of reactive hypoglycemia. Contrary to the relatively benign prognosis of reactive functional hypoglycemia, this disorder is not self-limiting and some patients may eventually progress to a more advanced state of insulin deficiency and the clinical syndrome of diabetes mellitus (Chap. 88).

ALIMENTARY HYPOGLYCEMIA In patients with *gastroenterostomy* or *subtotal gastrectomy*, hypoglycemia is due to excessive insulin release in response to excessive postprandial hyperglycemia facilitated by accelerated absorption of glucose (alimentary hyperinsulinism). The diagnosis is made by history of abdominal surgery, an abnormal oral glucose tolerance test characterized by elevation of the peak blood glucose level, but not the 2-hr level, and a normal intravenous glucose tolerance test. In some patients alimentary hyperinsulinism and hypoglycemia are observed in the absence of gastric surgery.

OTHER CAUSES OF POSTPRANDIAL HYPOGLYCEMIA Some patients with islet cell tumors may have hypoglycemia postprandially due to excessive insulin release stimulated by ingestion of carbohydrate. Approximately 80 percent of patients with functioning islet cell tumors and 30 percent of patients with idiopathic hypoglycemia of infancy and childhood will demonstrate excessive insulin release after administration of leucine. In only the latter group of patients will the ingestion of protein high in leucine content precipitate symptomatic hypoglycemia. Hypoglycemia following the ingestion of fructose occurs in patients with hereditary fructose intolerance, because of an inborn error of metabolism in which there is a deficiency of the enzyme hepatic fructose 1-phosphate aldolase. It is very infrequent.

EXOGENOUS HYPOGLYCEMIA The possibility of factitious hyperinsulinism as a result of surreptitious administration of insulin or sulfonylureas should always be considered, particularly in nurses, other medical personnel, and relatives of diabetic patients. If self-administration of insulin is suspected, presence of insulin antibody in serum may disclose it, provided there is no history of previous insulin administration.

In the case of ingestion of tolbutamide (Orinase) in

TABLE 90-2
Work-up of adult patient with suspected hypoglycemia

I Careful history and physical examination.
II Laboratory tests and procedures.
- *A* Patient with suspected "reactive" or functional hypoglycemia.
  - *1* Glucose tolerance test to differentiate between:
    - *a* Reactive-functional hypoglycemia.
    - *b* Reactive hypoglycemia secondary to mild diabetes mellitus.
    - *c* Alimentary hyperinsulinism.
  - *2* If fasting hypoglycemia needs to be ruled out, proceed with B1. Fast up to 72 hr with exercise at end.
- *B* Patient with suspected fasting hypoglycemia.
  - *1* Fasting plasma glucose, insulin.
    - *a* After overnight fast.
    - *b* With 4-hr prolongation of overnight fast.
    - *c* During 12- to 72-hr fast if fasting blood sugar level is not diagnostic after (*a*) and (*b*); multiple determinations.
    - *d* After exercise at end of 72-hr fast. Blood specimens before and after exercise.
    - *e* Determine

$$\text{“amended } \frac{\text{IRI”}}{6} \left(\frac{\text{Plasma insulin } \mu\text{U/ml} \times 100}{\text{Plasma glucose mg/100 ml} - 30} \right)$$

  - *2* Provocative tests to insulin secretion. [Fasting hypoglycemia suspected or to be ruled out; insulin levels with (1) not yet available or not diagnostic. Islet cell tumor suspected because entities given in 4 to 7 have been ruled out; no, minimal, or moderate hypoglycemia after overnight fast.]
    - *a* Tolbutamide test
    - *b* Leucine test
    - *c* Glucagon test

    (*a*–*c*:) Serial plasma glucose and insulin determinations.
  - *3* Islet cell tumor diagnosed.
    - *a* Celiac and mesenteric angiography for localization.
    - *b* Liver scan if carcinoma suspected in view of rapid course, severe hypoglycemia.
    - *c* X-ray of skull, serum calcium, and phosphorus to rule out multiple endocrine adenomatosis.
  - *4* In older patient consider extrapancreatic neoplasm within thorax, liver, abdomen, retroperitoneal space, pelvis.
    - *a* X-ray chest.
    - *b* Flat film of abdomen.
    - *c* Gastrointestinal series.
    - *d* Intravenous pyelogram.
  - *5* If pituitary, adrenal, or pancreatic alpha-cell insufficiency suspected:
    - *a* Growth hormone levels after arginine infusion.
    - *b* Adrenal cortical function tests—metyrapone test.
    - *c* Glucagon levels after arginine infusion.
  - *6* Diffuse liver disease: liver function tests, response to glucagon.
  - *7* Rule out factitious hypoglycemia.
    - *a* Insulin antibodies to rule out factitious insulin administration.
    - *b* Check for sulfonylurea blood levels; urinary tolbutamide excretion product. Leucine sensitivity.
  - *8* Test for gluconeogenetic reserve if alcohol hypoglycemia suspected. Alcohol infusion. Pituitary and adrenal function tests.

large amounts, acidification of the urine will disclose a white precipitate which is a crystallization of the carboxylated excretion product of tolbutamide. In addition, plasma concentrations of sulfonylurea drugs may be determined.

Table 90-2 gives an outline of the work-up of an adult patient with suspected hypoglycemia.

REGULATION OF GLUCAGON SECRETION AND EFFECTS OF GLUCAGON

SOURCE AND CHARACTERISTICS Glucagon is a polypeptide hormone secreted by the alpha cells of the islet of Langerhans. The hormone is made up of 29 amino acids in a straight chain and has a molecular weight of 3,485. With a sensitive radioimmunoassay employing an antiserum specific for glucagon, its concentration can be assayed in pancreatic tissue and in blood. The plasma concentration of glucagon in peripheral blood is approximately 100 pg per ml in the basal state. From different portions of the gastrointestinal mucosa (stomach, but particularly small intestine) extracts have been prepared which have immunologic characteristics similar to but not identical with pancreatic glucagon. This immunoreactive material, called "gut glucagon," "enteroglucagon," or "glucagon-like immunoreactive material," has been found to be separable into two fractions, one of molecular weight of approximately 7,000 and the other with a molecular weight of 3,500. The former differs from glucagon in biologic activity (see the following).

FACTORS INFLUENCING SECRETION OF GLUCAGON Unger and associates have demonstrated that insulin-induced hypoglycemia is followed by increases in the concentration of glucagon in pancreatic and peripheral blood. Starvation is another stimulus to increased secretion of glucagon. On the other hand, hyperglycemia due to orally or intravenously administered glucose causes suppression of glucagon secretion. The ingestion of protein meals or the intravenous or oral administration of certain amino acids (arginine) are other potent stimuli to the secretion of pancreatic glucagon. Administration of pancreozymin, a gastrointestinal hormone released after protein ingestion, has also been found to increase plasma levels of glucagon and to augment the effect of amino acids on glucagon secretion.

The oral but not the intravenous administration of glucose is followed by a significant increase in immunoreactive glucagon in peripheral blood which is due to release of "gut glucagon."

METABOLIC EFFECTS OF GLUCAGON Glucagon exhibits a marked effect on carbohydrate, protein, and lipid metabolism in vivo and in vitro. Glucagon stimulates hepatic glycogenolysis by increasing cyclic 3′,5′-adenosine monophosphate (AMP) which leads to increased phosphorylase activity. Increased glycogenolysis and inhibition by glucagon of hepatic glycogen synthetase (also via cyclic AMP) cause hyperglycemia. Glucagon stimulates gluconeogenesis by promoting the hepatic uptake of amino acids. It inhibits the incorporation of amino acids into liver protein and increases excretion of nitrogen. Glucagon, by activating the adenyl cyclase systems, also promotes lipolysis in liver and adipose tissues. The resulting increased hepatic concentration and oxidation of free fatty acids stimulate hepatic gluconeogenesis and ketogenesis.

In addition to these effects of glucagon on hepatic and adipose tissues, glucagon has a direct effect on stimulating increased release of insulin from the pancreatic beta cells independent of the increases in blood glucose. Glucagon's effect on pancreatic beta cells may also be mediated by activation of the adenyl cyclase system. "Gut glucagon" of molecular weight 7,000 also increases the secretion of insulin but does not have the hepatic effects of pancreatic glucagon.

Other extrahepatic effects of glucagon are a positive inotropic effect upon cardiac muscle, a stimulation of adrenal medullary secretion, and a slight lowering of serum levels of calcium and phosphate.

PHYSIOLOGIC ROLE OF GLUCAGON The extreme sensitivity of hepatic and adipose tissues to glucagon and the fact that increased secretion of glucagon is stimulated by fasting and hypoglycemia suggest that glucagon is released in order to provide for increased distribution of energy substrates during periods of glucose need. Glycogenolysis and gluconeogenesis will lead to increased levels of blood glucose, and increased lipolysis will furnish free fatty acids for energy and will stimulate gluconeogenesis. In contrast to the effects of fasting and hypoglycemia, rapid increases in blood glucose inhibit the secretion of glucagon. In birds the removal of the pancreas, rich in alpha cells and glucagon, is followed by the development of severe hypoglycemia. This hypoglycemia can be alleviated by the injection of glucagon. Amino acid–induced glucagon release after protein feeding may be an important factor in preventing hypoglycemia which might otherwise occur during amino acid–induced insulin release.

Whether pancreatic glucagon plays a physiologic role in mediating increased release of insulin is still to be demonstrated.

ABNORMALITIES OF GLUCAGON SECRETION In a patient with a malignant tumor of the alpha cells of the pancreas (McGavran et al) who also exhibited diabetes, removal of part of the tumor resulted in decreased concentration of plasma levels of glucagon and in amelioration of the hyperglycemia. Abnormalities of glucagon secretion have also been reported in patients with diabetes of genetic origin. Thus high postprandial plasma levels of glucagon have been noted in overtly diabetic patients, and in contrast with normal subjects plasma levels of glucagon did not decrease after carbohydrate ingestion or glucose infusion (Muller et al, 1970). Protein ingestion or arginine infusion induced exaggerated increases in plasma glucagon. Although fasting levels of glucagon were in the normal range, they were inappropriately high for the degree of hyperglycemia. It was suggested that overt diabetes is characterized by a continuous state of relative or absolute hyperglucagonemia and that excess glucagon may exaggerate the metabolic consequences of insulin insufficiency. Patients with familial multiple endocrine adenomatosis have been shown to have elevated levels of plasma glucagon in addition to evidence of hyperinsulinism, hyperparathyroidism, and other hormonal hypersecretion.

A syndrome associated with decreased secretion of glucagon and hypoglycemia accentuated by a high-protein, low-carbohydrate diet has also been observed (Bleicher et al). The patient had a strong family history of diabetes and fasting hyperglycemia (fasting blood glucose level about 150 mg per 100 ml). Hypoglycemia was induced by a 28-hr fast, a high-protein diet, or an arginine infusion. Plasma levels of insulin were low during fasting. Plasma levels of glucagon were found to be either undetectably low or below the lower limits of normal fasting levels. Known potent stimuli of glucagon secretion, i.e., fasting, hypoglycemia, and arginine infusion failed to elevate levels of plasma glucagon. This patient appears to be the first well-documented case with an absolute glucagon deficiency. It can be anticipated that other hypoglycemic states due to glucagon deficiency will eventually be documented. Some infants and children with so-called "idiopathic hypoglycemia" may be found to be deficient of glucagon. Decreased plasma levels of glucagon and decreased glucagon reserve have been reported in some patients with severe chronic pancreatitis and associated diabetes. The plasma glucagon response to intravenously administered arginine should prove to be a valuable test for pancreatic glucagon reserve.

CLINICAL USEFULNESS OF GLUCAGON ADMINISTRATION In the presence of normal glycogen stores glucagon produces a hyperglycemic effect when given subcutaneously, intramuscularly, or intravenously. The acute administration of glucagon has been used clinically most frequently in the treatment of severe insulin-induced hypoglycemia of labile diabetics when oral or intravenous administration of glucose is not possible. More prolonged administration of a repository form of glucagon (zinc glucagon) has been of some help in the treatment of some patients with inoperable pancreatic islet cell tumors, but zinc glucagon is no longer available. Recently large amounts of glucagon have been administered to selected patients with severe heart failure and cardiogenic shock. Some patients have benefitted from the positive inotropic effect of glucagon.

GLUCAGON TESTS Several types of glucagon tests have been employed. One test takes advantage of the glycogenolytic properties of glucagon as a means for assessing adequacy of hepatic glycogen stores and the competency of enzymes in producing glycogenolysis. One milligram of glucagon is injected intravenously over 4 min and blood specimens are obtained at 0, 20, 30, 45, 60, 90, and 120 min. In healthy subjects the blood sugar level rises from 30 to 90 mg per 100 ml 20 to 30 min after injection of glucagon. In patients with cirrhosis or glycogen storage disease there is a subnormal or no rise in blood sugar.

Another glucagon test takes advantage of the insulin-releasing property of glucagon. In patients with functioning pancreatic islet cell disease, injection of 1 mg glucagon may be followed by excessive increases in plasma insulin. Blood samples are obtained at −15 min and 0 time, and again 3, 5, 10, 15, 30, 45, 60, 90, 120, 150, and 180 min after injection of glucagon. Excessive increases in plasma insulin (over 160 μU per ml) may occur during the first few minutes after injection of glucagon in 50 percent or more of patients with insulin-secreting tumors. This may be associated with a subnormal rise in blood glucose but may be followed by excessive secondary decreases in blood glucose. The test may have to be interrupted if severe hypoglycemic symptoms develop. Such patients should be treated with intravenous glucose.

Intravenous administration of 0.5 to 1.0 mg glucagon has also been used as a provocative test in patients suspected of harboring pheochromocytoma. In patients with pheochromocytoma, glucagon may evoke release of excessive quantities of pressor amines, resulting in a hypertensive paroxysm.

REFERENCES

BLACK J: Diazoxide and the treatment of hypoglycemia. Ann NY Acad Sci 150:194, 1968

BLEICHER SJ: Hypoglycemia, in *Diabetes Mellitus, Theory and Practice,* eds M Ellenberg, H Rifkin, New York: McGraw-Hill, 1970, p. 972

CARTER SK et al: Streptozotocin and metastatic insulinoma. Ann Intern Med 74:445, 1971

FAJANS SS: Diagnostic tests for functioning pancreatic islet cell tumors. Excerpta Med Int Cong Ser 172:894, 1969

MADISON LL: Ethanol-induced hypoglycemia. Adv Metab Disord 3:85, 1968

MCGAVRAN MH et al: Glucagonoma: The identification of a glucagon-secretion-alpha-cell carcinoma of the pancreas. N Engl J Med 274:1408, 1966

MULLER WA et al: Abnormal alpha-cell function in diabetes: Response to carbohydrate and protein ingestion. N Engl J Med 283:109, 1970

91
DISEASES OF THE TESTES

JOHN F. CRIGLER, JR.
LESLIE I. ROSE
EUGENIA ROSEMBERG

HISTORY Androgen deficiency resulting from loss of testicular tissue was undoubtedly recognized by prehistoric man, as was the associated sterility; indeed, testicular tissue was recommended for impotence over 30 centuries ago. This dual function of the testes, as both the site of spermatogenesis and the primary site of male hormone production, was clearly defined in the middle of the nineteenth century when Berthold returned to the capon the characteristics, both physical and behavioral, of the cockerel by testicular grafts, and when his contemporaries, the anatomists von Kolliker, Leydig, Sertoli, and Schweigger-Seidel, defined the morphologic characteristics of the gland. They recognized the spermatogonia, spermatids, the Sertoli (or sustentacular) cells, and cells located interstitially between the tubules (the Leydig or interstitial cells).

The tropic role played by the anterior pituitary gland in the development and maintenance of testicular function was demonstrated by Smith and Engle in 1927, and several years later Butenandt isolated androsterone from male urine. By 1935, testosterone had been synthesized from cholesterol and isolated in crystalline form from bull testes. In addition, it was conclusively shown to be the most significant natural androgenic material.

Early in the present century, experimental studies in certain animals indicated a role of the central nervous system in coitus-stimulated ovulation. Thus, luteinizing hormone was the first hormone of the anterior pituitary shown to be under hypothalamic control. In 1930, Popa and Fielding described the hypophyseal portal vessels, which subsequently were shown by Harris (1950) to be involved in mediating hypothalamic regulation of anterior pituitary–gonadal function in rats. Schally and coworkers (1971) have reported the structure and laboratory synthesis of the porcine LH[1]- and FSH[1]-releasing hormone (LH-RH/FSH-RH), a neurohumoral decapeptide active in man which was originally postulated to exist by Hinsey and Markee (1933), Friedgood (1936), Harris (1937), and Brooks (1938).

Embryologists had debated for many years the relative importance of sex chromosomal pattern, hormones, or "determiners" secreted by the embryonic gonads, and maternal hormones on sex differentiation. In 1917, Lillie described the role of sex hormones in the development of freemartins. Wiesner proposed in 1935 that there is an autonomous tendency which results in female development unless opposed by male hormone. However, it was not until the late 1940s and early 1950s that Alfred Jost (1947) and other experimental embryologists clearly demonstrated that secretions of the fetal testes are necessary for development of male genital ducts and external genitals and that female development occurs in the absence of gonads. About the same time, Barr and Bertram (1949) described sex chromatin masses at the periphery of the nucleus in resting ganglion cells of female cats, a distinguishing characteristic of the female sex subsequently shown to be present in the peripheral cells of most mammalian species. The application of this simple cytologic means of assessing the number of X chromosomes and of more sophisticated cytogenetic techniques to the study of patients with sexual abnormalities has added to our advances in the fields of embryology and cytogenetics, which have been of great importance in elucidating the pathophysiology of testicular disorders.

[1] *LH, luteining hormone; FSH, follicle-stimulating hormone.*

DEVELOPMENT

Embryogenic In the fourth to sixth weeks of fetal development, the primitive genital ridge differentiates into cortical and medullary components capable of becoming either a testis or an ovary. If the primordial germ cells which migrate from the dorsal endoderm of the yolk sac to the urogenital ridge have a Y chromosome, they become incorporated into testicular cords which differentiate *in situ* from the blastema of the indifferent genital ridge. The primary sex cords undergo proliferation to form seminiferous tubules which subsequently link up with convoluted tubules of mesonephric origin (rete testis and epididymis) and channel into the Wolffian duct. The cortex of the primitive gonad becomes isolated by the tunica albuginea and involutes. The histogenesis of testicular tunica albuginea and the regression of the Müllerian ducts are closely related, the latter apparently resulting from the local production of an "inhibitory substance" of unknown nature by the fetal testis. At approximately eight weeks, characteristic fetal Leydig cells appear and subsequently secrete fetal masculinizing hormones (androgens) necessary for the development of Wolffian duct structures (vas deferens, seminal vesicles), enlargement of the genital tubercle, and fusion of the labioscrotal and urethral folds to form male external genitalia. If the primordial germ cells have two X chromosomes and no Y chromosome, the medullary component of the primitive gonad involutes and the cortical component proliferates and persists as the future ovary. In the absence of masculinizing factors of the fetal testis (development presumably evoked by the presence of a Y chromosome), normal female development of genital ducts and external genitalia takes place, with the formation of the fallopian tubes, uterus, and upper vagina from the Müllerian ducts, regression of the Wolffian system, and persistence of the small genital tubercle and unfused urethral and labioscrotal folds.

Postnatal Shortly after birth the testes measure 1.5 to 2.0 cm in length and 0.7 to 1.0 cm in width and weigh approximately 0.5 g each. The interstitial cells, active during uterine life as a result of fetal pituitary and chorionic gonadotropins, undergo dedifferentiation and remain quiescent or semiquiescent until puberty. However, with current sensitive techniques, both gonadotropic and sex steroid hormones in blood have been demonstrated at all ages. It is recognized, also, that hypogonadal children show an earlier rise of gonadotropins than normal children, indicating a restraining influence of the prepuberal gonad upon the gonadotropic production of the pituitary. At birth, 10 percent of male infants have incompletely descended testes, but after the first year, this figure drops to 2 to 3 percent. Late prepuberal descent further decreases the number, so that only 0.3 to 0.4 percent of males have either unilateral or bilateral undescended testes, postpuberally, unilateral undescended testes being four to five times more frequent than bilateral.

During adolescence, each testis increases in size, as a result chiefly of changes in the seminiferous tubules under the stimulation of pituitary FSH and androgens produced locally by developing interstitial cells. The fully developed testis measures 3.5 to 5.5 cm in length and 2.1 to 3.2 cm in width, and weighs 15 to 20 g. Interstitial-cell–

stimulating hormone (ICSH) induces interstitial-cell differentiation, with the production of male sex hormones, genital enlargement, and the development of secondary sexual characteristics. Normal function, including demonstrated fertility, has been noted when testes were less than half the mean size.

Aberrations in embryonic development It is currently postulated that sex-determining genes on the X and Y chromosomes are responsible, through their effects on cellular function of the primitive gonad, for differentiation of these tissues into either a testis or an ovary. Embryologic studies have indicated that normally functioning fetal testes are required for male differentiation of genital ducts and external genitalia. The fetal testis appears to produce at least two types of substances: (1) a "duct-organizing substance," which stimulates development of the Wolffian system and involution of the Müllerian duct; and (2) an androgen, which may play a role in Wolffian duct development but is required for masculinization of the external genitalia. The correlation between chromosomal patterns, gonadal differentiation, and subsequent genital development in human beings has been quite consistent. Some cases, however, remain unexplained by the above-stated concepts, although they do not disprove the hypothesis, since current techniques do not detect all chromosomal anomalies (mosaicism, interchange of sex-determining factors between X and Y chromosomes, etc.) or measure directly fetal gonadal function.

If gonadal tissue does not develop (gonadal dysgenesis, genotypic XO, X isochromosome X, X deleted X, etc.) or fetal testicular cells are nonfunctioning before differentiation of genital ducts in a genotypic male (XY), *both internal and external genitalia are entirely female.* Partial failure in testicular development or in the elaboration of fetal masculinizing hormones (genotypic XY or mosaics having a cell line with a Y chromosome) results in ambiguous internal and external genital development, the type of abnormality reflecting the age of onset and degree of fetal gonadal dysfunction. Patients with abnormal fetal testes, therefore, may have genital development ranging from almost complete feminization through incomplete fusion of the labioscrotal and urethral folds with some enlargement of the genital tubercle and various degrees of development of the Müllerian ducts to mild degrees of hypospadias. In addition, if testicular tissue exists unilaterally (true hermaphrodite, mixed gonadal dysgenesis), male development of genital ducts occurs on the side of the testes and Müllerian duct structures develop on the side with the ovary or missing gonad. These findings are consistent with observations in other animal species which demonstrate a local effect by diffusion of fetal masculinizing hormones (Chap. 62).

Some genotypic males (XY) who have histologically normal-appearing testes before puberty show *total feminization of external genitalia although internal genitals are masculinized* (syndrome of testicular feminization). This abnormality is inherited as either a sex-limited recessive or a sex-limited autosomal dominant mutant gene, as half the genotypic males are affected. The lack of masculinization of external genitals (but not of internal genitalia), the absence of sexual hair (found in approximately one-third of the patients), and the occurrence of feminization at adolescence with normal plasma and urine testosterone concentrations for males indicate an abnormality in the response of tissues to androgens. Decreased reduction of testosterone to 17β-hydroxyandrostane urinary metabolites and activity of the steroid Δ^4-3-keto-5α-oxidoreductase of skin, which catalyzes the transformation of testosterone to 17β-hydroxy-5α-androstan-3-one (dihydrotestosterone), a metabolite with biologic activity comparable to testosterone, has been demonstrated in these patients. Intramuscular administration of dihydrotestosterone to a patient with testicular feminization, however, failed to produce the changes in urinary nitrogen, phosphorus, and citric acid excretion observed in a control individual. Nevertheless, these new biochemical observations are consistent with the hypothesis that the basic defect is an inability of end-organ tissues to metabolize testosterone in a normal manner. Feminization of the external genitals of these patients may be so complete that the abnormality is discovered only later in life when primary amenorrhea, the absence of sexual hair, or the appearance of inguinal masses makes the diagnosis apparent. Surgical exploration of these patients reveals the presence of vas deferens, epididymis, and testes, the latter showing variation in histologic findings with age and the completeness of the defect. After adolescence, tubular adenomas and hyperplasia of Leydig cells (often adenomatous) are common.

Occasionally, genotypic males (XY) and individuals with a mosaic cell line containing a Y chromosome with testes and female ambiguous (slight enlargement of the genital tubercle with or without partially fused labioscrotal folds) external genitals (male pseudohermaphrodites) have fallopian tubes, uterus, and vagina. These individuals have either unilateral or bilateral dysgenetic testes which presumably do not produce the "Müllerian inhibitory substance" or sufficient fetal androgens to totally masculinize the external genitals. Androgen insensitivity has not been demonstrated in these patients. In contrast to the testis of patients with the androgen-insensitive type of male pseudohermaphroditism, dysgerminomas, embryonal dysgerminomas, and gonadoblastomas commonly arise from dysgenic testis. For this reason, dysgenic testicular tissue should be surgically removed.

Finally, *masculinization of external genital development of a genotypic female* fetus (XX) may be induced by excessive fetal adrenal androgens (patients with congenital adrenal hyperplasia) or by excess androgens produced or taken (usually synthetic progestational steroid hormones) by the mother during pregnancy. Defects induced by these extragonadal androgens are limited to the external genitalia (hypertrophy of the genital tubercle with various degrees of fusion of the labioscrotal and urethral folds), so that if the condition is recognized, an appropriate female sex assignment can be made and the genital abnormality surgically corrected. The external genitals should be surgically corrected as soon after birth as possible.

PHYSIOLOGY The role of fetal testicular function on genital development has been described above. The precise interrelationships of hypothalamic-pituitary and testicular functions (Fig. 91-1) at adolescence and in adult life are not completely defined. A hypothalamic-releasing substance (LH-RH/FSH-RH) which stimulates secretion of pituitary gonadotropins has been isolated from porcine sources and found to be a decapeptide with the following amino acid sequence: (pyro)glu-his-trp-ser-tyr-gly-leu-arg-pro-gly-NH_2. Intravenous administration of the synthesized polypeptide to preadolescent boys and men increases serum ICSH(LH) and FSH levels. ICSH, reportedly identical to luteinizing hormone (LH) of females elaborated by the anterior pituitary gland, induces development and subsequently functional maintenance of the testicular interstitial (Leydig) cells. Pituitary FSH stimulates development of the seminiferous tubules. The role of ICSH and testosterone in seminiferous tubular development and spermatogenesis is not well defined. It is generally accepted that the Leydig cell is the principal site of synthesis of steroid hormones (testosterone, estrogens, and others). The probable role of ICSH and the Leydig cell in hormonal production in human beings is illustrated by observations on so-called "fertile eunuchs," patients who show spermatogenesis but lack masculine secondary changes and in whom testicular biopsies show a decrease in the number of mature Leydig cells.

FIGURE 91-1
Scheme showing hypothalamic-anterior pituitary-testes relationship.

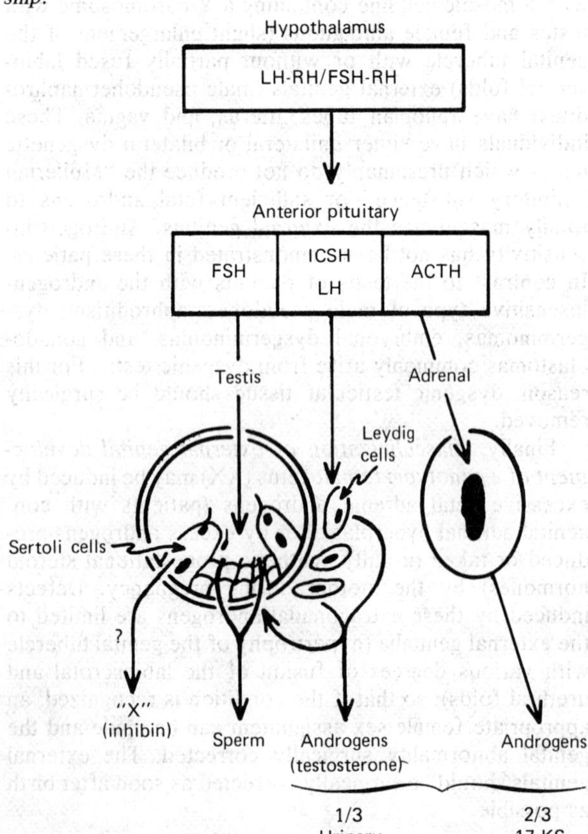

FSH and ICSH have been measured by bioassays and radioimmunoassays in the urine and serum of prepuberal children. Although it has been shown that sexual maturity is accompanied by a marked increase in the excretion of LH, with a relatively smaller increase in FSH, the factors, probably neural, initiating puberty are still unknown. Nevertheless, production of androgenic hormones by the testes at puberty effects the numerous somatic changes noted in the adolescent male. These include enlargement and increased pigmentation of the external genitalia, hypertrophy of the larynx with lowering of the voice, a generalized increase of amount of hair to hirsutism with growth of a beard and a typical masculine pelvic escutcheon and forehead hairline, enlargement of the prostate and seminal vesicles, and an overall increase in muscular development. Metabolic balance studies demonstrate retention of electrolytes, nitrogen, and phosphorus; and radiologic examination shows progression of osseous development with subsequent epiphyseal fusion.

The testes of the normal, young male secrete between 4 and 8 mg testosterone daily and approximately 10 μg of estradiol, another 25 to 35 μg of estradiol being formed from testosterone and androstenedione in other tissues. Approximately half the testosterone appears in the urine as measurable 17-ketosteroids, primarily androsterone and etiocholanolone, with a much smaller proportion (3 to 6 percent) as the androstane-3α,17β-diols (Fig. 91-2). The total 17-ketosteroid daily excretion for males is 8 to 18 mg, of which approximately 4 mg is derived from the testes and the remainder from the adrenals. Plasma testosterone concentrations in young adult males vary from 0.3 to 1.2 μg per 100 ml (mean 0.6 μg per 100 ml), whereas normal females of similar age have plasma concentrations between 0.02 and 0.07 μg per 100 ml. Studies of testosterone metabolism in normal men above sixty years of age indicate that with advancing years, there is a significant decrease in both total and free serum testosterone levels and metabolic clearance rate (thus a decrease in blood production rate) and a change in the extraglandular and extrahepatic metabolism similar to that observed in hypogonadal males. It is well known that urinary 17-ketosteroid excretion diminishes with increas-

FIGURE 91-2
Synthesis and metabolism of androgens. The broken line between cholesterol and pregnenolone signifies a series of reactions. The latter reactions and the conversion of pregnenolone to progesterone, 17-OH pregnenolone, 17-OH progesterone, dehydroepiandrosterone (D), androst-5-ene-3β,17β-diol, androst-4-ene-3,17-dione (Δ) and testosterone (T) occur in the testis. In addition, it is well recognized that D is irreversibly converted to Δ and that Δ and T are interconverted in peripheral tissue, a fact which permits the formation of small amounts of T from D, a major adrenal secretory product. Approximately 40 percent of T is metabolized to the major urinary 11-deoxy-17-ketosteroids, D, androsterone (A), and 5β-androsterone (E), and only 2 to 6 percent to 5α- and 5β-diols. The latter pathway of T metabolism, specifically, the conversion of T to 17β-hydroxy-5α-androstan-3-one (DHT), is recognized to be essential for the expression of androgen activity in certain androgen-sensitive tissues. The major T metabolites, A, E, 5α-and 5β-androstane-3α,17β-diols, are conjugated as glucuronides and sulfates, principally, by the liver, before excretion into the urine by the kidney.

ing age. Rarely, however, is sudden cessation in gonadal function, analogous to the process in the female, observed in the male.

Studies by Wilson and others have demonstrated that in some tissues the hormonal activity of testosterone is mediated by the intracellular reduction of testosterone to 17β-hydroxy-5α-androstan-3-one (dihydrotestosterone-DHT) (Fig. 91-2). The enzyme, Δ^4-3-keto-5α-oxidoreductase, required for this reaction has been demonstrated in male accessory sex tissues, skin, hair follicles, brain, and testes. DHT formed in the cells binds strongly to nuclear protein and is thought by this means to influence RNA synthesis and cellular function. A deficiency of this 5α-reductase in tissues from patients with the syndrome of testicular feminization has been described and thought to account for the lack of masculinization of these genetic males with normal testosterone secretion (see previous paragraph).

The principal abnormalities of testicular function, listed according to their effect on both interstitial and seminiferous tubular activity, are summarized in Table 91-1.

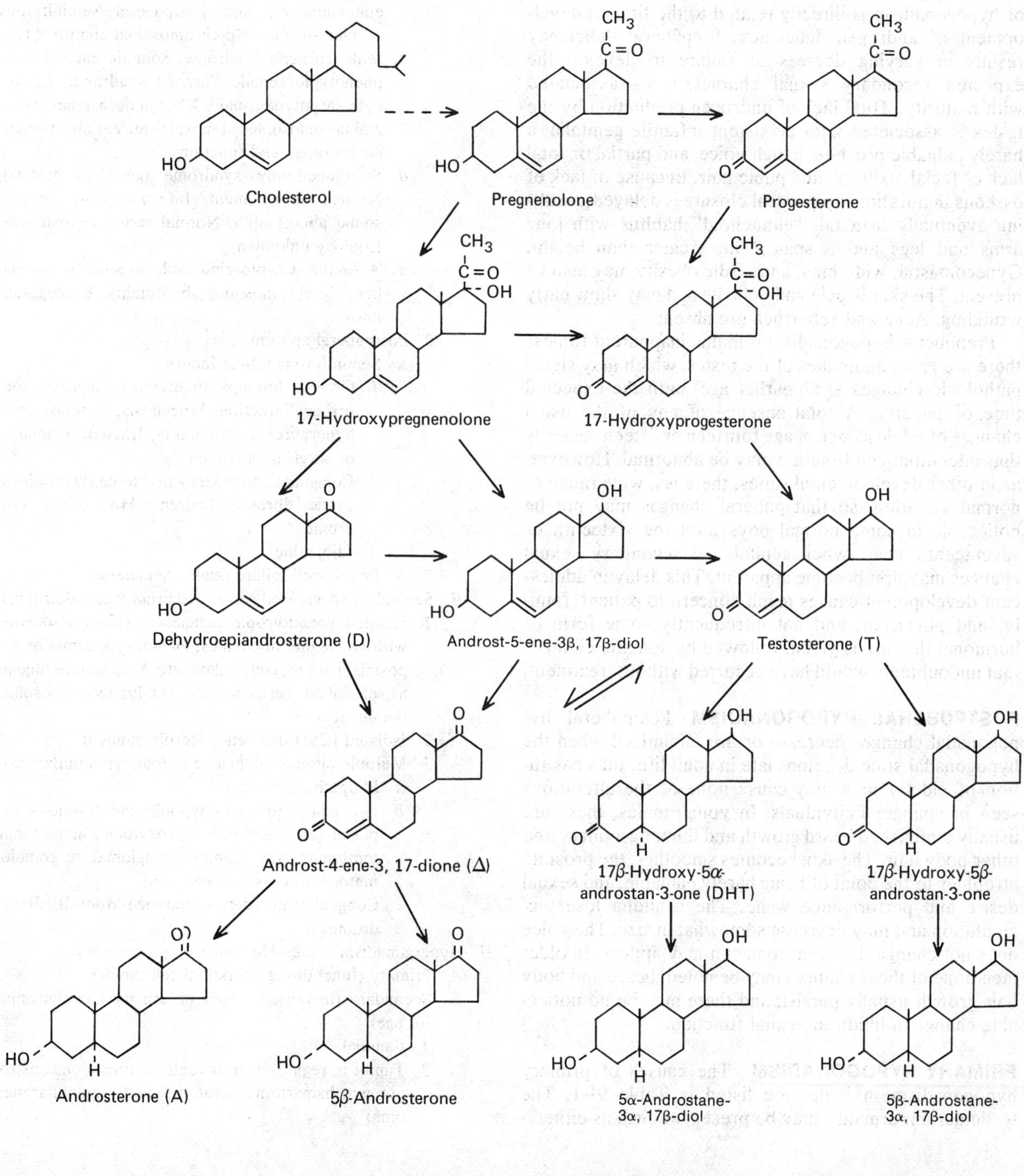

HYPOGONADISM

The clinical term *hypogonadism* as most often used refers to failure in interstitial-cell function which results in decreased or absent production of male sex hormones. Seminiferous tubular failure, however, often is associated and, indeed, may occur without significant changes in testicular hormonal production (Sertoli-cell-only syndrome and postpuberal abnormalities). Both testicular functions may be decreased either primarily by a developmental or destructive lesion of the testes or secondarily by failure in production of pituitary gonadotropins.

PREPUBERAL HYPOGONADISM The clinical picture of hypogonadism is directly related to the time of development of androgen deficiency. Prepuberal deficiency results in varying degrees of failure to develop the expected secondary sexual characteristics associated with maturity. Total lack of androgen production by the testes is associated with persistent infantile genitalia, a barely palpable prostate, a high voice, and partial or total lack of facial, axillary, and pubic hair. Because of lack of osseous maturation, epiphyseal closure is delayed, resulting eventually in a tall "eunuchoid" habitus with long arms and legs and a span 2 in. greater than height. Gynecomastia, wide hips, and girdle obesity may also be present. The skin is pale and delicate and may show early wrinkling. Acne and seborrhea are absent.

Prepuberal hypogonadism remains inapparent (unless there are gross anomalies of the testes, which may signal pathologic changes at an earlier age) until the expected time of puberty. A total absence of any of the usual changes of adolescence at age fourteen or fifteen suggests that interstitial-cell function may be abnormal. However, as in other developmental states, there is a wide range of normal variation, so that puberal changes may not be noticeable in some normal boys until the sixteenth or seventeenth year, when genital and secondary sexual changes may first become apparent. This delay in adolescent development causes much concern to patient, family, and physician, and not infrequently some form of hormonal therapy is given, followed by somatic changes that undoubtedly would have occurred without treatment.

POSTPUBERAL HYPOGONADISM Postpuberal hypogonadal changes decrease or are minimized when the hypogonadal state develops late in adult life; thus castration of elderly men may cause none of the alterations seen in younger individuals. In young males, there are usually diminished beard growth and thinning axillary and other body hair. The skin becomes smoother, the prostate atrophies to the point of being barely palpable, and sexual desire and performance wane. The genitalia lose pigmentation and may decrease somewhat in size. The voice does not change, but gynecomastia may appear. In older men none of these changes may be noted; beard and body hair growth usually persist, and there may be no noticeable change in libido or sexual function.

PRIMARY HYPOGONADISM The causes of primary hypogonadism in males are listed in Table 91-1. The testicular abnormality may be present at birth as either a

TABLE 91-1
Abnormalities of testicular function

- *I* Hypogonadism (decreased androgen production and/or spermatogenesis)
  - *A* Primary (increased serum and urinary gonadotropins)
    - *1* Developmental abnormalities
      - *a* Klinefelter's syndrome (seminiferous tubule dysgenesis). Classic form—eunuchoidism, gynecomastia, mental retardation, and small firm testes. Buccal smear—chromatin-positive. Leukocyte karyotype usually XXY or XXYY but may have other poly X and Y chromosomal constitution and mosaicism with combination of many cell lines
      - *b* Reifenstein's syndrome (male pseudohermaphroditism). Hereditary testicular disorder with hypospadias, varying degrees of gynecomastia and eunuchoidism, and postpuberal seminiferous tubular atrophy. No chromosomal abnormality
      - *c* Male Turner's syndrome. Somatic anomalies of phenotypic female Turner's syndrome. Leukocyte karyotype usually XY, but occasional abnormal chromosomes of mosaicism. Variable testicular histology and function
      - *d* Sertoli-cell-only syndrome (germinal aplasia). Normal development. Infertility. No chromosomal abnormality. Normal serum testosterone. Etiology unknown
      - *e* Anorchia. Cryptorchid with no somatic anomalies. No chromosomal abnormality. Etiology unknown
    - *2* Postpuberal abnormalities
      - *a* Seminiferous tubule failure
        - *1* Orchitis (mumps, tuberculosis, leprosy, gonorrheal infection, brucellosis, syphilis, etc.), hyperpyrexia, irradiation, trauma, neoplasm, or surgical castration
        - *2* Congenital disorders—myotonia dystrophica, cystic fibrosis, Laurence-Moon-Biedl syndrome
        - *3* Idiopathic
      - *b* Leydig-cell failure (male climacteric)
  - *B* Secondary (decreased serum and urinary gonadotropins)
    - *1* Isolated gonadotropin deficiency. Often associated with congenital anomalies, including anosmia or hyposmia, harelip, cleft palate, etc. May be inherited as a sex-linked recessive or sex-limited autosomal dominant trait
    - *2* Isolated ICSH deficiency (fertile eunuch)
    - *3* Multiple pituitary deficiencies (panhypopituitarism)
      - *a* Idiopathic prepuberal
      - *b* Secondary to neurohypophyseal lesions—neoplasm (chromophobe, astrocytoma, hamartoma, teratoma), cyst (craniopharyngioma), or granulomatous process (sarcoid, etc.)
      - *c* Congenital disorders—Laurence-Moon-Biedl syndrome
- *II* Hypergonadism (excessive androgen production)
  - *A* Primary (functioning interstitial-cell tumor)
  - *B* Secondary (increased serum or urinary gonadotropins for age)
    - *1* Familial
    - *2* Tumor in region of third ventricle (pinealoma, astrocytoma, hamartoma, teratoma, and craniopharyngioma)

genetic or an embryologic defect, or it may occur at any time later in life as a result of either testicular infections (such as mumps, tuberculosis, brucellosis, leprosy, syphilis) or following trauma, irradiation, neoplasm, or castration, either surgical or accidental. Beginning in early adolescence, even before the appearance of the obvious physical characteristics of hypogonadism, the patient may have increased serum concentrations of pituitary gonadotropic hormones (measured by radioimmunoassay) and may excrete excessive quantities in the urine. The immature mouse uterine weight assay, which measures both ICSH and FSH, is used most frequently for determination of total urinary gonadotropin content. In addition, because of lack of testosterone synthesis, plasma testosterone concentrations as well as urinary 17-ketosteroid excretion of adult patients are significantly decreased. It should be stated here with emphasis, however, that the patient's own tissues clinically observed frequently provide the most significant assay of androgen production. The following syndrome is an example of primary hypogonadism.

KLINEFELTER'S SYNDROME (seminiferous tubule dysgenesis) Klinefelter, Reifenstein, and Albright described in 1942 a clinical syndrome of hypogonadism that includes gynecomastia, eunuchoidism, elevated level of urinary gonadotropins, and decreased testicular size associated with hyalinization of the tubules. Barr demonstrated that many of these patients were *chromatin-positive*, exhibiting nuclei similar to those seen in females (see Chap. 62). Culture of leukocytes in vitro in the presence of colchicine has permitted direct chromosomal counting and classification; and, indeed, many patients with the triad described by Klinefelter et al. have been shown to possess an extra sex chromosome, resulting in a karyotypic classification of 22 autosomes plus 2 X chromosomes and 1 Y chromosome (see Chap. 62). Thus, they have 47 instead of 46 chromosomes, and it is therefore not surprising that many of these patients also have various degrees of mental deficiency. A clue to the diagnosis of this disorder, which has an incidence of approximately 1 in 400 males from studies performed in newborns, often lies in the behavior and personality of the Klinefelter patient. Talkativeness with little substance to the content is an outstanding behavioral trait. Klinefelter's syndrome in some patients who lack the classical clinical findings of gynecomastia, eunuchoidism, and small testes may be discovered only when they appear in an infertility clinic. In addition, Klinefelter's syndrome is not infrequently discovered when the patient seeks medical care for chronic pulmonary disease, obesity, diabetes mellitus, varicose veins, and thrombophlebitis, disorders which appear to be more prevalent in these patients; thus, the spectrum of Klinefelter's syndrome is broad, including obviously feminized males on one end and, on the other end, normally virilized men with only abnormal microscopic testicular anatomy but often with the associated diseases listed above.

SECONDARY HYPOGONADISM Secondary hypogonadism results from failure of pituitary elaboration of the necessary tropic hormones, specifically ICSH and FSH (Table 91-1, *I-B*). Isolated deficiencies of gonadotropic hormones without demonstrable loss of other pituitary hormones have been described in males in association with anosmia or hyposmia by Kallman. The condition is inherited either as a sex-linked recessive defect or as a sex-limited autosomal dominant one. Very rarely, an isolated ICSH deficiency occurs. In most cases, however, there is an associated loss of other pituitary tropic hormones, resulting in growth failure before adolescence and in decreased thyroid, adrenal, and gonadal function at all ages. When there is a progressive loss of hypothalamic-pituitary function because of a neoplasm (chromophobe adenoma, astrocytoma, hamartoma, teratoma), cyst (craniopharyngioma), or granulomatous process (sarcoid), a decrease of gonadotropins is at times the first deficiency observed, and the patient, therefore, may appear in the clinic with isolated hypogonadism. Prepuberal hypopituitarism is usually recognized because of the short stature that results from growth hormone deficiency. Occasionally, however, testes of preadolescent boys with other evidences of pituitary dysfunction are significantly small. Froehlich in 1901 described such an obese hypogonadal boy with signs of a tumor in the hypothalamic area. Since then, Froelich's name has been inappropriately applied to the condition of a large group of overweight boys with slightly retarded maturation but with normal linear growth and no demonstrated hypothalamic lesion; in such cases the delay in maturation is without any real clinical significance. Patients with the Laurence-Moon-Biedl syndrome have been described with both primary (germinal aplasia) and secondary (hypogonadotropic) hypogonadism.

The absence of serum and urinary gonadotropins after the age of adolescence in patients with diminished gonadal function is diagnostic of secondary hypogonadism. Studies of growth, thyroid, adrenal, and antidiuretic hormones may reveal clinically unsuspected deficiencies. Skull roentgenogram may also show intracranial calcification, enlargement of the sella turcica, or erosion of the clinoid processes, and visual field examination may demonstrate early involvement of the optic nerves.

EVALUATION OF HYPOGONADAL STATES An outline of principal clinical and laboratory information required for the diagnosis of the various hypogonadal states of males (Table 91-1) is listed in Table 91-2. A careful history and physical examination are of obvious importance, as they describe the biologic abnormality. The measurement of serum and urinary gonadotropins most often differentiates between the primary disorders of the testis and testicular deficiencies resulting from neuroendocrine dysfunctions, the latter due primarily to decreased production of either hypothalamic LH-RH/FSH-RH or pituitary ICSH and FSH. As synthetic releasing hormones become more available, differentiation between central nervous system (usually hypothalamic) and pituitary lesions will be possible. More readily available, specific techniques for measuring testosterone, 17β-estradiol, and other sex steroid hormones and their binding protein in serum make it possible now to diagnose significant abnormalities of hormone production more

TABLE 91-2
Clinical and laboratory diagnosis of hypogonadism in adolescent and adult males

I Clinical manifestations of hypogonadism in males

A Adolescence. Androgen deficiency–decreased rate of physical growth (absent growth spurt), eunuchoid body proportions, immature facies without change in voice or appearance of acne and seborrhea, small penis with or without small testes, decreased or absent (if also adrenal androgen deficiency) pubic and axillary hair, occasionally gynecomastia. Seminiferous tubules–lack of development resulting in small and, with tubular fibrosis firm, testes

B Adult. Androgen deficiency–decreased libido and sexual performance, diminished beard growth and decreased axillary and pubic hair, decreased pigmentation and size of penis and scrotum, atrophy of prostate, occasionally gyncomastia. Seminiferous tubular failure—infertility, decreased testicular size

II Primary testicular disorders (characterized by increased serum and urinary gonadotropin levels)

A History. Presence of development anomalies; behavior or personality disorder; associated illness (mumps, tuberculosis, venereal disease, chronic pulmonary disease, liver dysfunction, diabetes mellitus, etc.); family history of similar disorder

B Physical examination. Height, body proportions (span; *U*/*L*, *U* = height minus *L*, *L* = symphysis pubis to floor), weight, amount and distribution of sexual hair, presence of gynecomastia, size and pigmentation of penis and scrotum, size and consistency of testes (small, hard testes seen with tubular fibrosis)

C Laboratory

1 Serum LH, FSH, testosterone (T), and estradiol-17β (E_2) and urinary gonadotropin levels and their response to clomiphene citrate, LH-RH/FSH-RH, and human gonadotropins.

2 Evaluation of other neuroendocrine functions —thyrotropin (TSH), adrenocorticotropin (ACTH), growth hormone (GH), and vasopressin (ADH) production—either by direct measurement in serum before, during, and after appropriate stimuli (thyrotropin-releasing hormone, metyrapone, insulin-induced hypoglycemia, sleep, hypertonic saline solution, etc.) or by indirect measurement of thyroid (*l*-thyroxine and *l*-triiodothyronine levels, resin T_3-binding, etc.) and adrenal (serum cortisol response to insulin-hypoglycemia; serum cortisol and 11-deoxycortisol and urinary 17-KS and 17-OHCS response to metyrapone, excretion of water load, etc.) function and changes in serum osmolality and in urine specific gravity or osmolality after an appropriate tolerated water fast

3 X-ray—skull and hand and wrist (bone age)

4 Ophthalmologic examination with visual field determinations

5 Semen analysis and testicular biopsy (isolated LH or LH-RH/FSH-RH deficiencies, the so-called fertile eunuch; Klinefelter's syndrome)

6 Other neurologic studies (lumbar puncture, pneumoencephalogram, brain scans, electroencephalogram, etc.) as indicated

easily and to monitor the patient's response to therapeutic regimens.

TREATMENT OF HYPOGONADISM Patients with primary hypogonadism (increased serum and urinary gonadotropins) require testosterone replacement therapy. Preparations commonly used are listed in Table 91-3. The usual method of therapy is to start with relatively small doses of the long-acting depot preparations of testosterone, giving either 50 mg every 2 weeks or 150 mg every 3 to 4 weeks. The dosage subsequently (after epiphyseal fusion in adolescent boys) is increased to 200 mg every 2 weeks to obtain full androgen effect, including deepening of the voice and increased facial hair. Final adult maintenance requirements are usually satisfied by 200 mg of the depot preparations every 3 to 5 weeks. Excessive acne formation, edema from retention of sodium, and undesirable personality changes all indicate overtreatment, and the dosage should be diminished appropriately.

In patients with secondary hypogonadism, a trial on human chorionic gonadotropin (HCG) may be indicated. Usually HCG, 1,000 to 4,000 IU, every 3 to 5 days for 6 to 9 months, is given as a single course. If regression to a hypogonadal state occurs when HCG is discontinued, either a second course of HCG may be given or testosterone therapy as outlined above may be begun. In the past, long-term therapy with HCG has not proved practical. A gonadotropin preparation rich in FSH has been obtained from human menopausal urine. Experience with this preparation in gonadotropin-deficient postpuberal males indicates that it can restore spermatogenesis to normal. The prepuberal testes seem to require stimulation with ICSH before spermatogenesis can be induced by administration of the human menopausal gonadotropin preparation.

HYPERGONADISM

The production of excessive quantities of androgenic hormones in the adult male results in little, if any, morphologic or functional change. However, in the child, the somatic changes associated with puberty may be induced at an early age and therefore become clinically apparent (precocious puberty). The causes of hypergonadism and isosexual precocity in the male are listed in Table 91-1. Hypergonadism may be due to excessive androgen production from a functioning testicular tumor, the Leydig-cell, or interstitial-cell, carcinoma. Children with these tumors show all the changes associated with puberty, such as increased hair growth and phallic enlargement, and usually have a palpable testicular tumor. However, the presence of the tumor may be difficult to determine if the testes are undescended, or if the tumor is extremely active in producing hormone but is very small. Plasma testosterone concentrations are increased. Urinary 17-ketosteroids, however, may be normal or only slightly increased, because of the marked potency of testosterone. Urinary pituitary gonadotropins are usually absent. Hypergonadism may also result from an early onset of puberty due to altered hypothalamic-pituitary function. The sequence of development is similar to that observed in adolescence, with enlargement of genitalia, appearance of pubic and axillary hair, deepening of the voice, and appearance of acne and seborrhea occurring in that order

TABLE 91-3
Hormonal therapy for hypogonadism

Preparations	*Route and dosage*
Methyltestosterone (linguets)	Sublingual 5–10 mg, 4 times daily
Testosterone propionate	Intramuscular 25–50 mg, 3 times weekly
Testosterone enanthate Testosterone cyclopentyl-propionate Testosterone phenylacetate	Intramuscular 100–200 mg every 1–2 weeks for maximum effect, 200 mg every 3–5 weeks for maintenance
Human chorionic gonadotropin	Intramuscular 1,000–4,000 IU every 4–6 days for 6–9 months, with response monitored by measurement of serum testosterone levels. Repeated courses as required

and beginning as early as one to two years of age. The testes are large for the patient's chronologic age but are in accord with the size expected for the degree of maturity exhibited by the remainder of his somatic development. Gonadotropins may be present in the urine but are not invariably measurable by routine assay procedures. In the early stages, the level of 17-ketosteroids may not be significantly elevated for the patient's chronologic age (in contrast to virilism produced by adrenal abnormalities), but subsequently it rises to a degree appropriate for his developmental age. Isosexual precocity of this type in males, although uncommon, is often familial, in contrast to the more frequently occurring true precocity in females, from whom a family history of early puberty is seldom obtained. When true precocity occurs in males without a family history, it is almost always associated with space-occupying lesions in the region of the third ventricle (pinealoma, astrocytoma, hamartoma, and rarely a craniopharyngioma). The continued production of androgens excessive for their age in these patients results in accelerated skeletal growth and, especially, maturation during childhood, followed by early closure of the epiphyses, ending in an adult who frequently is smaller than his contemporaries.

Isosexual precocity in the male may also result from excessive quantities of adrenal androgens. The pattern of accelerated growth and development is similar to that produced by testicular hormones. The testes remain, however, prepuberal in size; and gonadotropins are invariably absent. The diagnosis is made on the basis of a markedly elevated level of urinary 17-ketosteroids. For further discussion, see Chap. 86.

NEOPLASMS OF THE TESTES

Neoplasms of the testes are the most common tumors of men twenty-nine to thirty-five years of age but may appear at any age. They occur more often in cryptorchid testis (1 in 2,000) than in descended testis (1 in 100,000), even when the cryptorchid testis is surgically placed in the scrotum. For this reason, frequent examination of the surgically corrected cryptorchid testis is recommended. The following classification of testicular neoplasms is given in their relative order of frequency:

1 Seminoma (germinoma)
2 Teratocarcinoma
3 Embryonal carcinoma
  a Chorioepithelioma
  b Others
4 Teratoma
5 Interstitial-cell tumor
6 Fibroma, lipoma, adrenoma, myxoma
7 Unclassified varieties

In addition, lymphoma, plasmacytoma, leukemia, and carcinoma of other tissues occasionally produce secondary tumors in the testes. The incidence of teratocarcinoma is roughly constant throughout life, whereas the incidence of seminoma tends to rise with age. One-year survival is rare for patients with embryonal carcinomas and chorioepitheliomas, not uncommon for those with teratocarcinomas and teratomas, and the rule for those with seminomas.

Endocrine changes (such as hyperestrogenism with gynecomastia and increased secretion of gonatropins with a positive test for chorionic gonadotropin) are occasionally seen with chorioepitheliomas, as well as with other embryonal carcinomas and teratocarcinomas. The endocrine effects of interstitial-cell tumors have been discussed.

Diagnosis The diagnosis is made by palpating a mass, usually firm, smooth, and painless. Neoplasms must be distinguished from the changes induced by tuberculosis or gonorrheal epididymitis, from syphilis (usually accompanied by a positive serologic test and a response to specific therapy), and from the various fluid-containing cysts (hydrocele, spermatocele), which may be transilluminated. The diagnosis may be aided also by increased urinary excretion of 17-ketosteroids, estrogens, or gonadotropins; the latter give a positive Aschheim-Zondek test result. When no testicular tumor can be palpated and adrenocortical disease has been excluded in a patient with a possible functioning testicular tumor, it may be necessary to catheterize selectively the spermatic veins and the inferior vena cava to obtain venous samples for determination of plasma estrogen and androgen concentrations in order to locate the tumorous testis. Rarely, tumor cells may be identified in the semen.

Treatment Surgical removal is indicated in any tumor of the testes and in seminomas; when surgery is accompanied by irradiation of the lymphatic drainage, a 10-year survival rate of 90 percent may be achieved. In metastatic seminoma, the addition of chlorambucil, 4{-*p*-[bis(2-chloroethyl)amino]-phenyl}butyric acid, to surgical and x-ray therapy has proved useful. A combined surgical and medical approach is often productive in the treatment of other malignant testicular tumors. The nature of the chemotherapy is dictated in part by the cell type of the tumor. In terato- and embryonal carcinomas, a combination of chlorambucil and dactinomycin may be tried. If this combination does not yield the desired results, methotrexate (4-amino-N^{10}-methylpteroylglutamic acid) or vincristine sulfate may be used. Mithramycin has been advocated also for treatment of widely metastatic embryonal carcinoma and in chorioepithelioma.

DISEASES OF THE PROSTATE

BENIGN PROSTATIC HYPERTROPHY This pathophysiologic disorder, which affects a high proportion of elderly men, is a significant cause of dysuria and incontinence (see Chap. 46) and urinary tract obstruction (see Chap. 274). It has been also considered a potentially precancerous lesion. Hormonally, the prostate is significant as a clinical indicator of androgen secretion, since appreciable reduction in prostatic size accompanies either primary or secondary hypogonadism as well as those disorders of liver function characterized by excessive estrogen activity. Tissue from hypertrophic prostates has been found to have an increased content of the biologically active testosterone metabolite, 5α-dihydrotestosterone.

CARCINOMA OF THE PROSTATE Adenocarcinoma of the prostate is one of the most common tumors of men. It is rare before the age of forty; the incidence rises rapidly with advancing age, with the condition occurring microscopically in 10 to 15 percent of men in the fifth decade and in as many as 60 percent of those in the eighth decade. However, only one-fourth of these cases may become clinically apparent before death. Three-fourths of these tumors arise in the posterior lobe. The majority are easily palpable; hence, frequent routine rectal examinations are indicated to demonstrate early, operable tumors. Although the whole gland need not be enlarged, the presence of stony, hard, indurated nodules or masses strongly suggests an adenocarcinoma. Frequently, there may be an elevation in the "prostatic" fraction of serum acid phosphatase while the tumor is still located within the prostatic capsule, and elevation of this enzyme may serve to differentiate a benign hypertropic nodule from a malignancy. Once the tumor has spread locally from the gland, particularly after it has metastasized, total serum acid and alkaline phosphatase levels may be greatly elevated.

Therapy consists of radical prostatectomy; irradiation by x-ray, radium, or radioactive isotopes (colloidal gold); and estrogen hormonal treatment (especially when metastatic disease develops). Androgens are decreased by orchidectomy and by adrenalectomy or adrenocortical suppression following dexamethasone administration (1 to 2 mg given orally in divided doses); estrogen levels are increased by administering diethylstilbestrol, 10 to 15 mg daily, or the equivalent dosage of other estrogenic products. Currently, antiandrogens (cyproterone acetate, etc.) are being evaluated also for their effectiveness in the treatment of this disorder.

REFERENCES

ALBERT A: Bioassay and radioimmunoassay of human gonadotropins. J Clin Endocrinol 28:1683, 1968

FEDERMAN DD: *Abnormal Sexual Development: A Genetic and Endocrine Approach to Differential Diagnosis*, Philadelphia: Saunders, 1967

GAY UL: The hypothalamus: physiology and clinical use of releasing factors. Fertil Steril 23:50, 1972

JIRASEK JE: *Development of the Genital System and Male Pseudohermaphroditism*, Baltimore: Johns Hopkins, 1971

PAULSEN CA: The testes, in *Textbook of Endocrinology*, ed RH Williams, Philadelphia: Saunders, 1968, p. 405

ROSEMBERG E, PAULSEN CA (eds): *The Human Testis: Advances in Experimental Medicine and Biology*, vol. 10, New York: Plenum, 1970

RUBIN P (ed): Current concepts in cancer. No. 29. Cancer of the urogenital tract: testicular tumors. JAMA 213:89, 1970

VERMEULEN A et al: Testosterone secretion and metabolism in male senescence. J Clin Endocrinol 34:370, 1972

WILSON JD, GLOYNA RE: The intranuclear metabolism of testosterone in the accessory organs of reproduction, in *Recent Progress in Hormone Research*, vol. 26, ed EB Astwood, New York: Academic, 1970, p. 309

92 DISEASES OF THE OVARY

JANET W. McARTHUR

HISTORY The ovulatory function of the ovaries was first described by a Dutch physician, Reinier de Graaf, in 1673. He recognized small fluid blisters, now known as *graafian follicles,* which had succeeded in reaching the surface of the ovaries before ovulation. The hormonal function of the ovaries was first demonstrated in 1896, by the German biologist Knauer, who showed that ovarian grafts in the dog would prevent the uterine atrophy that follows castration. It was next observed, by Marshall and Jolly, that the ovarian secretion which produced estrus differed from that which was formed by the corpus luteum. The presence of estrogens in the follicles was proved by R. T. Frank, and their occurrence in urine was established by Allen and Doisy, who demonstrated the effectiveness of potent urinary extracts in producing estrus in the vaginal mucosa of rodents. This relatively simple biologic assay method became of incomparable help in the isolation and synthesis of estrogenic compounds.

In 1929, Butenandt and Doisy and associates isolated estrone in a crystalline form from the urine of pregnant women. In 1930, estriol was identified by Browne in human placentas, and in 1936, MacCorquodale obtained estradiol, the most potent natural estrogen, from ovarian follicular fluid. The progestational activity of the corpus luteum hormone was first demonstrated by Corner and Allen in 1929. Five years later progesterone was isolated and identified simultaneously and independently by Butenandt, Allen, Slotta, and Hartmann. The chemical structure of the pituitary gonadotropic hormones, follicle-stimulating hormone (FSH), and luteinizing hormone (LH) is not yet known in comparable detail but is undergoing rapid elucidation. Like pituitary thyroid–stimulating hormone and human chorionic gonadotropin

(HCG), both are glycoprotein in nature and are composed of two similar but nonidentical subunits. The release (and perhaps also the synthesis) of the pituitary gonadotropins appears to be controlled by a single hypothalamic hormone, the FSH- and LH-releasing factor (FSH-LH-RF), a decapeptide which was isolated and synthesized by Schally in 1971 (Fig. 92-1).

INTRODUCTION The ovary is a specialized organ of reproduction which serves (1) as an exocrine gland which liberates gametes for fertilization, and (2) as a complex of endocrine glands which secretes hormones responsible for (*a*) the growth and cyclic function of the reproductive tract, and (*b*) a variety of metabolic effects in nongenital tissues. During mature reproductive life a new endocrine gland, the follicle, is activated each month. After ovulation the follicle undergoes transformation into a second gland of internal secretion, the corpus luteum. To the extent that the formation of the corpus luteum requires the prior existence of a follicle, the two structures are interdependent. Nevertheless, differences of fundamental significance obtain between their secretory products. Both structures are embedded in an interstitium, or stroma, which constitutes a third endocrine gland.

A major difference between the ovary and the testis is that the former is endowed with a finite stock of germ cells, whereas the latter proliferates gametes continuously. The number of ova reaches a maximum 5 months before birth. Thereafter the number declines, mainly as the result of atresia, until by the end of the fifth decade the original complement of germ cells is exhausted. An inexorable, though less-rapid, decline in follicular hormone secretion begins in the fifth decade. In addition, the secretion of luteal hormones becomes more and more erratic as the incidence of anovulatory cycles increases. By old age, only the ovarian stroma retains any semblance of functioning tissue.

DEVELOPMENT The formation of the gonads begins at a very early stage, when the embryo has attained a crown-rump length of 5 mm (twenty-one to twenty-eight days of age). The genetic sex of the conceptus is identifiable even earlier, at the age of fifteen days, by the presence of nuclear sex chromatin in the female. During the seventh week, the ovarian destiny of the "indifferent gonad" can be inferred histologically by the absence of the epithelial cords which characterize the developing testis.

Four major phases in the development of the ovary are recognized: (1) migration of primordial germ cells from their site of origin in the endoderm of the primitive gut to bilateral thickenings (the "germinal ridges") of the coelomic epithelium ventral to the developing mesonephros, (2) proliferation of the germinal and nongerminal cells in the genital ridges, (3) division of the gonads into a peripheral cortex and a central medulla, and (4) sex differentiation, consisting of proliferation of the cortex and involution of the medulla in the female, and the reverse process in the male. A complex sex-determining mechanism, the details of which are obscure, is responsible for the conversion of the "indifferent gonad" into an ovary or testis. The cortical germ cells (oogonia) increase rapidly in number as a result of mitotic division, whereupon they enter the meiotic prophase, to become, by definition, oocytes. Each is soon invested by a single layer of smaller supporting cells to form the primordial follicles. In this resting phase the oocytes remain throughout childhood and adult life until either preovulatory maturation or pseudomaturation with atresia occurs. The oocytes appear to exert an inductive influence upon the surrounding granulosa cells, since follicles fail to develop in ovaries which lack oocytes, and oocyte atresia is followed by granulosal degeneration.

COMPARTMENTS The complexity of the tasks devolving upon the ovary is reflected in the heterogeneity of

FIGURE 92-1
The structural formula of FSH-LH-RF.

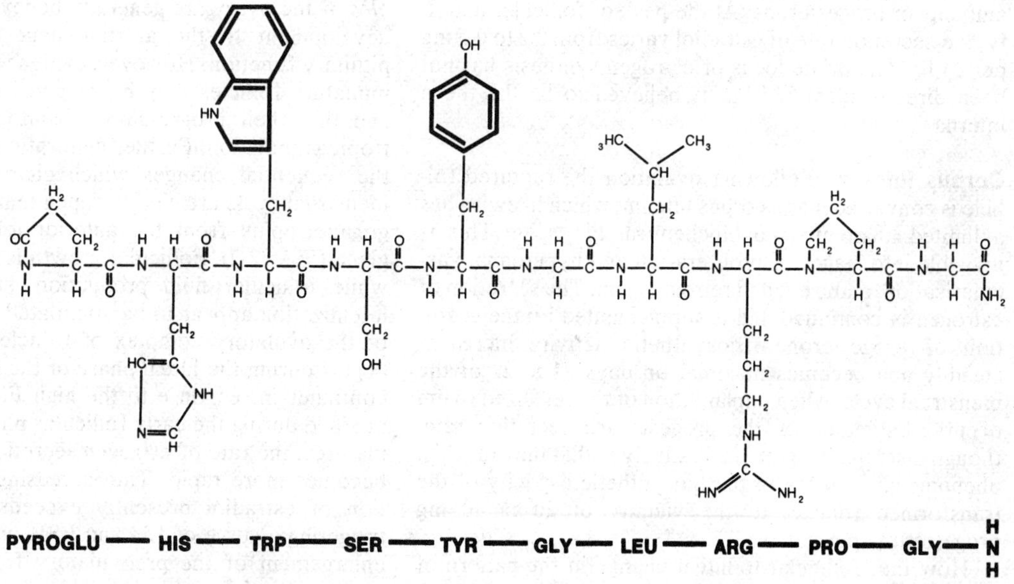

PYROGLU — HIS — TRP — SER — TYR — GLY — LEU — ARG — PRO — GLY — NH

its structure. Throughout active reproductive life, morphologic and biochemical events are occurring simultaneously in the follicular, luteal, and interstitial compartments. Anatomic specialization in the ovary is paralled by a degree of biochemical specialization. Thus, although in vitro studies reveal that upon incubation with acetate, each of the compartments is capable of synthesizing all the major categories of gonadal steroids, in vivo there is a preferential formation of estrogen by the follicle, of progestogens by the corpus luteum, and of androgens by the stroma.

Follicle Follicular growth comprises two phases. During the first, the oocyte enlarges rapidly to virtually adult dimensions while the investing cortical cells (the membrana granulosa), which convert the germ cell into a primordial follicle, grow very slowly. During the second phase, further growth of the oocyte is minimal but the follicle enlarges rapidly and develops an antrum, which fills with fluid secreted by the granulosa cells. The antrum first appears when the follicle attains a diameter two or three times that of the contained oocyte. Once a follicle has acquired an antrum it becomes, by definition, a graafian follicle.

Maturation falls short of completion in all but that minute proportion of graafian follicles destined to ovulate. Periodically, in response to gonadotropin stimulation (see below), the elected follicle exhibits an intense preovulatory growth spurt, accompanied by the increasing antral distention, the loosening of the cumulus oophorus (those granulosa cells which hold the egg in suspension), and the hypertrophy and hyperemia of the theca interna. As the follicle enlarges, its wall thins and presently ruptures, releasing the ovum into the peritoneal cavity. A complex of satellite follicles enlarges concomitantly, but to a lesser extent; and after ovulation they undergo rapid atresia.

Growth of the follicle is paralleled by biochemical processes resulting in the secretion of estrogen and, during the immediately preovulatory phase, of small amounts of progesterone. At the peak of follicular activity, the secretion rate of estradiol varies from 0.2 to 0.5 mg per 24 hr. The prime locus of estrogen synthesis has not been directly identified but is believed to be the theca interna.

Corpus luteum Following ovulation the ruptured follicle is converted into a corpus luteum, which likewise has a limited anatomic and biochemical life span. This is divisible into stages of proliferation and hyperemia, vascularization, maturity, and retrogression. The secretion of estrogen is continued and is supplemented by the secretion of progesterone. Biosynthetic activity increases steadily and becomes maximal on days 21 to 22 of the menstrual cycle, when implantation of the fertilized ovum occurs. Estimates of the progesterone secretion rate, though discrepant, agree qualitatively in that they reveal a phenomenal increase in the biosynthetic capacity of the transformed follicle, to the vicinity of 20 to 40 mg progesterone per day.

How the follicular-to-luteal change in the pattern of hormone synthesis is effected is the subject of much speculation. One view is embodied in the so-called "two-cell" theory. This postulates that the cells of the theca interna are endowed with the full enzyme complement required for the synthesis of estradiol-17β, whereas the cells of the granulosa possess little or no 17-desmolase activity and only weak 17-hydroxylase activity. During the follicular phase, the well-vascularized theca interna cells synthesize estrogens, which have ready access either to the follicular fluid or the systemic circulation, whereas the granulosa cells, lacking a blood supply, are presumably deprived of the nutrients required for hormone synthesis. After ovulation, the granulosa cells become richly vascularized, undergo enlargement, and form the corpus luteum. However, in consequence of their enzymic endowment, they are ill equipped to synthesize estrogen in quantity and secrete mainly progesterone.

Interstitium The interstitium, or stroma, acts as a supporting matrix for the follicles, corpora lutea, and corpora albicantia, and, in addition, it secretes steroids. Qualitative and quantitative changes in its structure occur in association with various reproductive processes. During pregnancy there is increasing luteinization of the stroma, and during the postmenopausal years stromal proliferation and luteinization are frequent. In extreme old age, the stroma tends to lose its stimulated appearance. The higher grades of stromal luteinization are sometimes associated with clinical indications of androgen hypersecretion.

The hilus may come eventually to be regarded as a fourth ovarian compartment, but at present it is generally treated as a specialized portion of the interstitium. It contains elements resembling testicular Leydig cells, which occur in nests, the size of which varies at different ages. Hyperplasia of these cells may occur during pregnancy, and the larger hilus cell complexes are more frequent in elderly women.

Androstenedione and dehydroepiandrosterone can be extracted from normal ovarian stroma, the highest concentrations being found in the hilus.

PHYSIOLOGIC CONTROL OF THE OVARY The *follicles* of the ovary are generally believed to be capable of development to the antrum stage in the absence of pituitary function. However, evidence suggests that more immature follicles may be responsive to gonadotropins and that their progression is contingent upon gonadotropic stimulation. Further maturation of the follicles and the sequential changes which characterize the normal menstrual cycle are clearly dependent upon the release of gonadotropins from the anterior lobe of the pituitary gland (Fig. 92-2). Follicular growth is stimulated by FSH, while follicular fluid production, steroidogenesis, and luteinization appear to be stimulated by LH. The growth of the ovulatory complex of follicles for a given cycle begins during the luteal phase of the preceding cycle and continues in response to the high FSH levels which are attained during the early follicular phase. As the complex matures, the rate of estrogen secretion, initially minimal, becomes more rapid. The increasing plasma concentration of estradiol presently exceeds a threshold level, triggering a surge of LH and FSH, which causes further enlargement of the preovulatory follicle, enhanced estrogen secretion, ovulation, and corpus luteum formation.

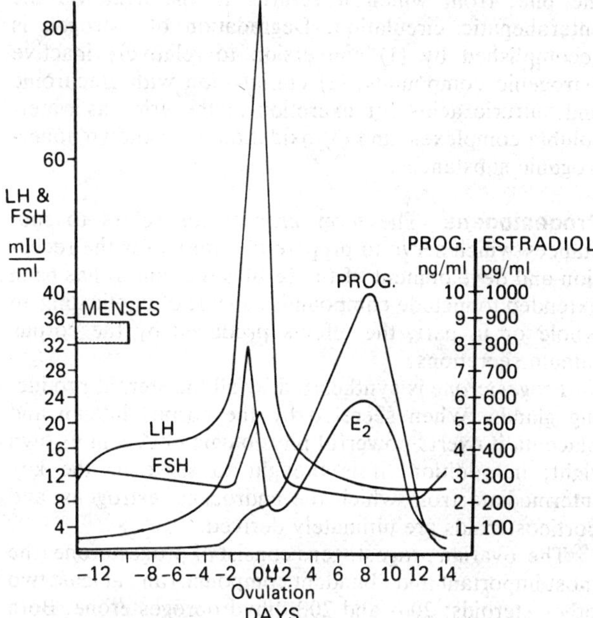

FIGURE 92-2
Plasma levels of FSH, LH, estradiol, and progesterone during the human menstrual cycle. The day of the midcycle LH peak is utilized as the central reference point for all data, and is designated as Day 0. (Adapted from L Speroff and R Vande Wiele, Am J Obstet Gynecol 109:234, 1971)

After cessation of the gonadotropin surge, the continued presence of low levels of LH in the circulation permits the *corpus luteum* to develop and to attain maximal capacity to synthesize estrogen and progesterone. However, unless supplementary luteotropic stimulation in the form of HCG secreted by the trophoblast of a conceptus embedded during the midluteal phase is delivered, the corpus luteum begins to regress within 9 to 11 days after ovulation and its secretory capacity rapidly diminishes. No uterine luteolytic factor such as that demonstrated in the sheep has as yet been isolated in the human being, and the mechanism responsible for the decline remains obscure. The in vitro synthesis of steroids by the *stroma* is increased by LH and HCG which, in the female as in the male, are interstitial cell–stimulating hormones.

The control of gonadotropin secretion is vested in the central nervous system. Regulation is effected by means of a vascular link between the hypothalamus and the pituitary, the hypothalamic-hypophyseal portal system. The neurohormone which regulates pituitary gonadotropin secretion is synthesized in the so-called hypophysiotropic area. This area occupies a medial position in the ventral hypothalamus, and extends from the median eminence to the optic chiasm. Neural inputs from other regions of the central nervous system (CNS) are received by the hypophysiotropic area, which translates them into neurohormonal signals to the pituitary. Biogenic amines acting as synaptic transmitters have the capacity to alter the level of activity of the FSH-LH-RF-secreting neurons in the hypophysiotropic area. In animals, dopamine exerts a stimulatory effect and serotonin an inhibitory effect upon the release of FSH-LH-RF. The areas of the human brain which are critically involved in reproduction are not yet accurately delineated. However, in rats a region of the medial basal hypothalamus which is responsive to the negative feedback action of estrogen and progesterone sustains acyclic gonadotropin release. A more rostral region which includes the suprachiasmatic area is responsive to the positive feedback action of estrogen. Under proper hormonal and environmental conditions, this region activates the terminal infundibular region and evokes the ovulatory gonadotropin surge.

HORMONES OF THE OVARY

The ovary secretes a water-soluble nonsteroid hormone or hormone complex known as relaxin and three types of steroid hormones: estrogens, progestogens, and androgens.

NONSTEROID (RELAXIN) Relaxin has not been isolated as a chemical entity, but its activity is associated with a water-soluble polypeptide structure. In conjunction with estrogens and progestogens, it facilitates parturition in certain mammals by loosening the symphysis pubis and sacroiliac joints. Relaxin has also been reported to soften the cervix, increase the uterine content of glycogen, nitrogen, and water, decrease the tone and motility of the uterus, increase uterine responsiveness to oxytocin, and promote tubuloalveolar growth of the mammary gland. In human pregnancy, blood relaxin values reach a maximum during the thirty-sixth week and remain high until delivery, whereupon a precipitous fall occurs. The cellular source in the ovary is unknown, and since the hormone can apparently be formed in other organs of the reproductive tract, its specificity as an ovarian secretion is in doubt.

STEROIDS The ovarian steroids are synthesized from acetate via cholesterol and pregnenolone by essentially the same pathways as exist in other steroid-producing organs—the testis, adrenal cortex, and placenta (Fig. 92-3).

Estrogens The term *estrogen* refers strictly to substances capable of inducing estrus, or sexual receptivity, in female mammals. However, it has been extended to include compounds which produce certain uterine changes and to the steroid metabolites of true estrogens, whether or not these possess biologic activity. In the nonpregnant female, the ovary is the principal site of estrogen formation; during pregnancy, estrogen formation by the fetoplacental unit gradually increases until, by the third trimester, it may exceed ovarian production by a thousandfold.

*Estradiol-17*β is believed to be the primary secretory product of the human ovary and to be interconvertible with estrone by dehydrogenases which are present in the ovary and in many other tissues. Estrone and estradiol are, in turn, irreversibly converted to estriol, an estrogen of human urine that is quantitatively important, especially during pregnancy. Additional estrogenic metabolites of low biologic activity have been isolated in great number

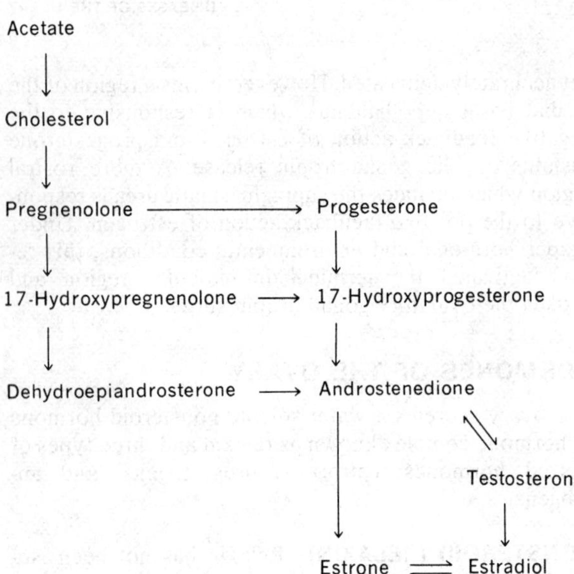

FIGURE 92-3
Biosynthetic pathways for the synthesis of ovarian estrogen in the human female. (Adapted from OW Smith and KJ Ryan, Am J Obstet Gynecol 84:141, 1962)

from human tissues and from the urine of pregnant and nonpregnant women.

The natural estrogens are all 18- or 19-carbon steroids which are characterized by the aromatic nature of ring A, the oxygen substituent at C-17, and the phenolic hydroxyl group at C-3. Many nonsteroidal estrogens have been synthesized for clinical use; they produce biologic effects resembling those of the natural estrogens. Representative examples from both the natural and synthetic categories are depicted in Fig. 92-4.

The liver is the principal site of the interconversion of estradiol and estrone, and is largely responsible for the inactivation of estrogen in the body. Protein-bound estrogen is abstracted from the plasma and excreted into the bile, from which it returns to the liver via the enterohepatic circulation. Degradation of estrogen is accomplished by (1) conversion to relatively inactive estrogenic compounds, (2) conjugation with glucuronic and sulfuric acids for excretion in the urine as water-soluble complexes, and (3) oxidation to unknown nonestrogenic substances.

Progestogens The term *progestogen* refers to substances which serve to prepare the uterus for the reception and development of the fertilized ovum. It has been extended to include compounds capable of duplicating, in whole or in part, the effects produced by the corpus luteum secretions.

Progesterone is synthesized by all the steroid-producing glands. When secreted by the corpus luteum and placenta it exerts powerful physiologic effects in its own right; in addition, it is thought to serve as the key intermediate from which the androgens, estrogens, and corticosteroids are ultimately derived.

The ovarian progestogens consist of progesterone (the most important and abundant compound) and at least two other steroids: 20α- and 20β-dihydroprogesterone. Both these partially reduced compounds have been detected in human follicular fluid and in the corpus luteum and placenta, the 20α isomer in higher concentration than the 20β. The basic molecule consists of 21 carbon atoms, two of which are contained in the side chain at C-17. These compounds are secreted by the follicle just prior to ovulation and are produced in much larger amounts by the corpus luteum. The quantity of progesterone which can be isolated from the corpus luteum is small compared with the amounts of progesterone secreted during the luteal phase of the cycle, indicating that progesterone is secreted almost as rapidly as it is produced.

A number of progestational steroids which mimic various facets of natural progesterone action have been synthesized. Many exhibit androgenic or estrogenic as well as progestational properties and, in these qualitative differences from the natural hormone, differ materially from the synthetic estrogen compounds. The short half-

FIGURE 92-4
The structural formulas of some important estrogens, natural and synthetic.

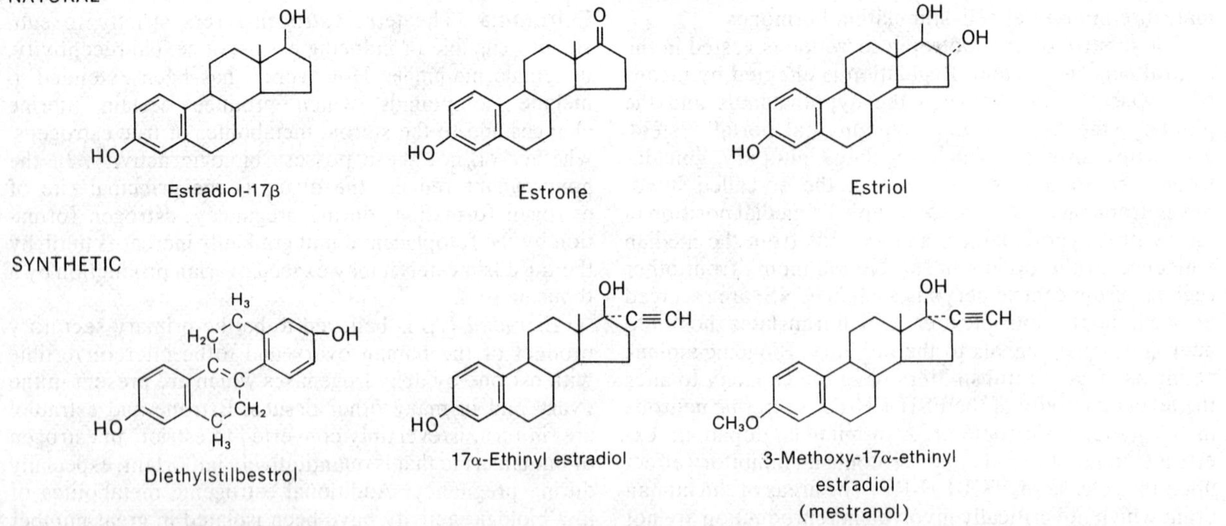

NATURAL

Estradiol-17β

Estrone

Estriol

SYNTHETIC

Diethylstilbestrol

17α-Ethinyl estradiol

3-Methoxy-17α-ethinyl estradiol (mestranol)

life of progesterone and the large doses consequently required to elicit biologic effects have prompted efforts to alter the progesterone molecule so as to increase its potency. Two groups of progestogens far surpassing the natural hormone in oral activity have been synthesized: (1) derivatives of testosterone (ethisterone) and of 19-nortestosterone (e.g., norethynodrel and norethindrone), the latter exhibiting the marked enhancement of oral potency which results from the removal of the angle methyl group C-19 attached to C-10 and (2) compounds derived from 17-hydroxyprogesterone [e.g., medroxyprogesterone (Provera), chlormadinone]. Esterification of 17α-hydroxyprogesterone by caproic or other long-chain fatty acids yields long-acting preparations useful for parenteral administration.

The structural formulas of some representative synthetic progestational steroids are shown in Fig. 92-5 together with allied natural compounds.

The liver is largely responsible for the inactivation of

FIGURE 92-5
The structural formulas of some important progestogens and allied compounds.

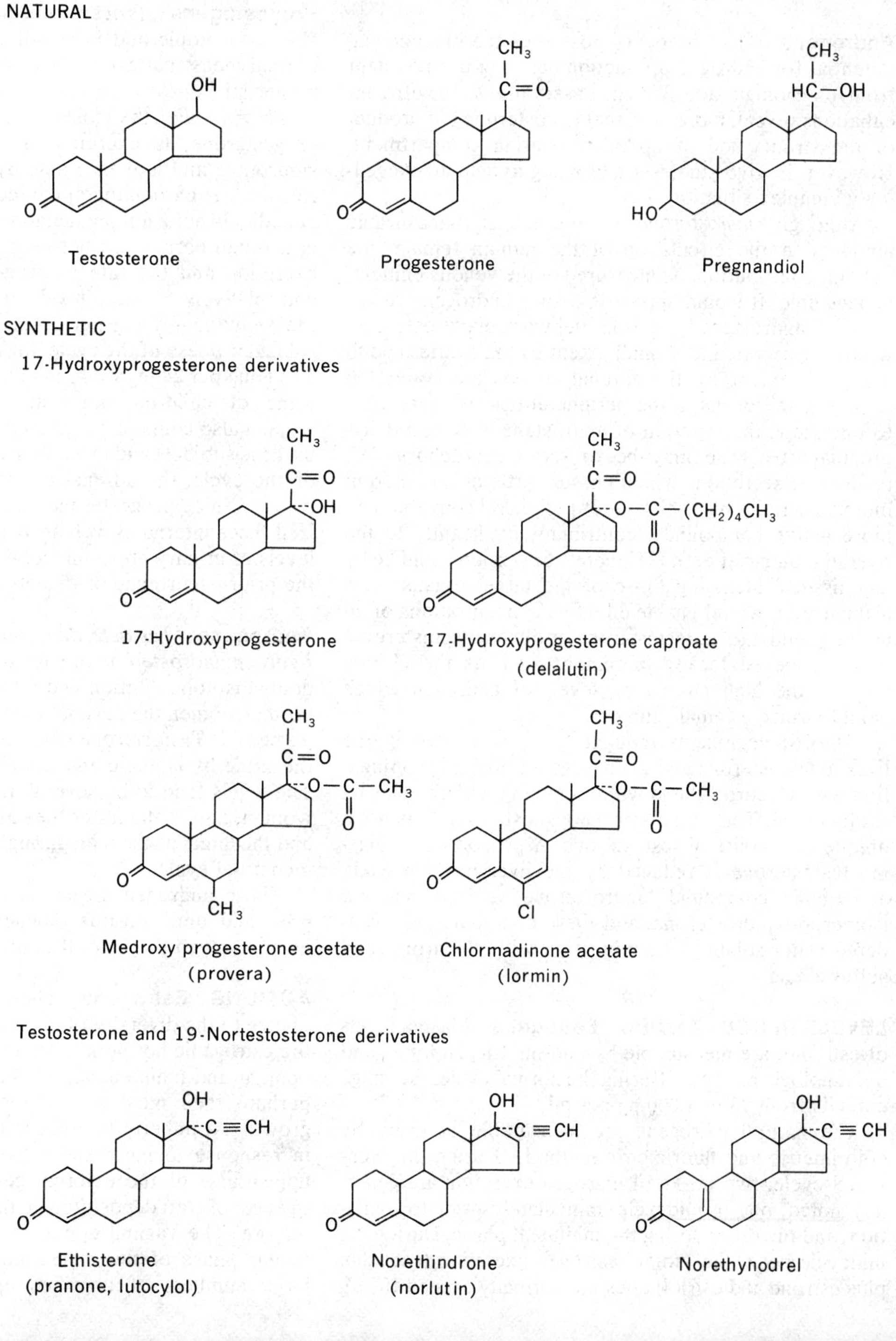

progesterone, which it first reduces to pregnanediol and then conjugates with glucuronic acid for excretion in the urine. These processes are aided by an enterohepatic circulation which differs from that of the estrogens in that approximately 30 percent of progesterone or its metabolites is lost in the feces, whereas the estrogens are almost completely absorbed from the intestine. Some 10 to 15 percent of exogenously administered progesterone can be accounted for by urinary pregnanediol, and a small additional percentage by several isomers and closely related pregnane derivatives. The major degradation products of progesterone are unknown.

Androgens That the ovary possesses the biochemical potential for androgen production has long been evident from physiologic and clinical observations. In vitro incubations reveal, moreover, that testosterone is a product of the stroma and of no other ovarian compartment. However, in vivo studies are bringing to light an exceedingly complex situation.

Although *testosterone* is present in measurable amounts in the circulation of the human female, the ovarian contribution, as measured in the venous effluent, is negligible. It would appear that such androgen precursors as androstenedione and dehydroepiandrosterone, which are secreted to a small extent by the ovaries and to a greater extent by the adrenal cortex, are converted to active androgens in the peripheral tissues. According to one view, the function of androstenedione and dehydroepiandrosterone may be to serve as prehormones (endocrine secretions which possess little or no inherent biologic activity but which, after peripheral conversion to more active compounds, contribute significantly to the overall biologic effect). Peripheral conversion could be by any tissues, including those of the target organs. This arrangement would enable effective concentrations of an active product (e.g., testosterone or dihydrotestosterone) to be achieved locally in regions such as the clitoris without the high circulating levels of androgen which would virilize a female subject.

Androstenedione is thought to be converted in the liver to testosterone and to undergo intrahepatic conjugation with glucuronic acid without mixing with the plasma testosterone. Thus, testosterone glucosiduronate is not a unique metabolite of testosterone. A proportion of plasma testosterone is reduced by the liver to the weakly androgenic compound, androsterone, and its inactive isomer, 5β-androsterone, and these compounds are rendered water-soluble by conjugation with glucuronic and sulfuric acid.

LEVELS IN BODY FLUIDS Estrogens Plasma levels of estradiol are measurable by fluorimetric, isotopic, and immunologic methods. During the normal cycle, the range extends from 75 to 1,000 pg per ml.

The natural estrogens are measurable in urine by colorimetric and fluorimetric methods. During the menstrual cycle, two peaks of estrogen excretion are generally noted, one in midcycle immediately prior to ovulation, and the other during the midluteal phase. During the midcycle peak, the "total" estrogen excretion (estradiol plus estrone and estriol) does not normally exceed 100 μg per 24 hr. In the fifth decade of life, the urinary estrogen levels of women commence a steady decline. The urinary estrogen level of postmenopausal women is low and is thought to be derived, in large part, from androstenedione secreted by the adrenal cortex.

Urinary levels of endogenous estrogen in patients with liver disease are variable, with only a proportion displaying the increased levels that might be anticipated.

Urinary estrogen determinations are sometimes helpful in detecting granulosa cell or theca cell tumors in postmenopausal women. The adrenogenital syndrome and occasional adrenocortical tumors are also associated with elevated levels of urinary estrogen.

Progestogens *Progesterone* plasma levels are measurable by isotopic and immunologic methods. During the normal menstrual cycle, the range extends from 0.5 to 20 ng per ml.

Pregnanediol, the most important reduction product of progesterone, is excreted in the urine as the glucosiduronate and is measurable by gravimetric, colorimetric, and gas chromatographic techniques. Although pregnanediol is not a unique metabolite of progesterone, there is a rough correlation between the rate of pregnanediol excretion and the rate of progesterone secretion. Low and relatively constant levels of urinary pregnanediol (in the vicinity of 1 mg per 24 hr) are detected during the follicular phase of the cycle; higher levels, with a range of 2 to 8 mg per 24 hr, are found during the luteal phase. The urine of children, adult males, and postmenopausal women also contains pregnanediol in low concentrations; in these subjects and in women during the follicular phase of the cycle, the adrenal cortex is presumed to be the source. Since progesterone can be secreted by a luteinized theca interna as well as by a corpus luteum, elevated levels of urinary pregnanediol do not necessarily connote the prior occurrence of ovulation.

Androgens *Testosterone, androstenedione,* and *dehydroepiandrosterone* are measurable in the plasma by double isotope dilution and by immunologic methods. In normal women the plasma testosterone level is below 0.1 μg per ml. *Testosterone glucosiduronate* is measurable in the urine by isotopic and gas chromatographic methods. The levels tend to be several times higher in men than in women, and in the latter they are higher during midcycle and the luteal phase than during the follicular phase of the menstrual cycle.

These androgen measurements are difficult to interpret, and until various biochemical complexities have been resolved they are of limited clinical usefulness.

ACTIONS Estrogens The name estrogen does scant justice to the diversity of physiologic effects produced by the estrogenic hormones. Their primary role is the development and maintenance of the female sex organs, and perhaps their most general effect is to promote tissue growth. At puberty the tubes, uterus, and vagina enlarge in response to increased estrogen stimulation, and the appearance of the external genitalia changes in consequence of fat deposition in the mons pubis and labia majora. The vaginal epithelium thickens during the follicular phase of the menstrual cycle, with shedding of large numbers of cornified epithelial cells containing pyknotic nuclei. The cervix is stimulated to secrete mucus of low viscosity and high permeability to spermatozoa. The uterine and tubal mucosa and their vasculature proliferate, and their musculature becomes contractile.

The estrogens exert direct effects on the ovary as well as indirect effects via the hypothalamic-pituitary system. Small amounts of estrogen promote the growth of vesicular follicles and increase their responsiveness to FSH. Puberal estrogen secretion causes the breasts to enlarge because of increased fat deposition, development of the supporting stroma, and ductal growth. The increased melanin pigmentation of the nipples and perineum is due, at least in part, to estrogen. There is a widespread deposition of fat in the subcutaneous tissues, particularly in the buttocks and thighs, leading to the characteristic rounding of the female figure.

The estrogens stimulate cell division in the deeper layers of the skin and gingivae, and in the mucosae of the oral cavity, nose, and urethra, causing a more rapid replacement of the outer cornified layers. Bone metabolism is significantly affected, with increased osteoblastic activity, a positive calcium and phosphorus balance, widening of the pelvic outlet, and accelerated epiphyseal closure. The composition of the circulating lipids is altered, with a fall in total cholesterol level and an increase in the α-lipoprotein fraction over the β fraction. Estrogens increase the levels of serum thyroxine-binding globulin, corticosteroid-binding globulin, ceruloplasmin, total copper, prothrombin, and AC-globulin. Antithrombin activity is decreased by estrogens.

Progestogens Although secreted in far greater amounts than estrogen, progesterone exerts only negligible effects on the general body economy. It produces few specific changes when present alone, acting ordinarily in conjunction with estrogen. Progesterone tends to encourage tissue differentiation, rather than growth. Its most important function is to induce secretory changes in the lining of the tubes and uterus, the endometrium being thereby adapted for the implantation of the fertilized ovum. The viscosity of the cervical mucus is increased during the postovulatory phase, rendering it impermeable to spermatozoa, and ferning disappears. Tubal and uterine contractility are altered to favor transport of the fertilized ovum and to prevent its expulsion from the uterus. Lobuloalveolar proliferation of the breast is stimulated. Progesterone exerts a thermogenic action, the basal body temperature increasing by approximately 1° in midcycle and remaining elevated during the luteal phase. A slightly negative nitrogen balance is induced by progesterone, and by antagonism to aldosterone, a negative balance of sodium, chloride, and water is favored. Progesterone acts as a mild respiratory stimulant, increasing minute ventilation while decreasing alveolar and arterial CO_2 tension and the respiratory quotient.

Androgens The physiologic role of the androgens in the human female has not been clearly delineated. However, it is probable that they act to promote a positive nitrogen balance and to increase libido and muscular strength. Experimental evidence suggests that by local action within the ovary small amounts of androgen hasten antrum formation by separating the granulosa cells; larger amounts cause destruction of ova and granulosa cell atrophy. It may be that atresia of those follicles not destined to ovulate is promoted by androgens. In excess, these compounds may blight the follicles of the ovary in the Stein-Leventhal syndrome, contributing to its polycystic structure.

ENDOCRINE DISORDERS OF THE OVARY

Diseases of the ovary may be classified as endocrine and nonendocrine, depending on the presence or absence of disturbances in hormonal secretion. Endocrine diseases of the ovary, because of the prominence of their systemic manifestations, are of concern to the internist as well as the gynecologist and will be considered here. Nonendocrine diseases, which comprise such entities as endometriosis, infections, and nonfunctioning tumors of the ovary, tend to produce localized effects and will not be treated in this chapter. The endocrine disorders of the ovary may be classified as (1) hypo-, hyper-, or dysfunctional, (2) primarily ovarian in origin or secondary to disturbances elsewhere, and (3) congenital or acquired. Some disorders, particularly those secondary to disturbances of hypothalamic or pituitary secretion, are general in that they affect follicular, luteal, and interstitial function. Others are compartmental in that they involve only one or two of the major subunits of the ovary (Table 92-1). Methodologic difficulties are responsible for the meager documentation of many ovarian syndromes. However, as these are overcome, a rational biochemical schema for classification is emerging.

TABLE 92-1
Classification of the endocrine disorders of the ovary

- *I* Ovarian hypofunction
  - *A* Primary
    - *1* General
    - *2* Gonadal dysgenesis (Turner's syndrome)
    - *3* Menopause
  - *B* Secondary
    - *1* General
      - *a* Hypothalamic disorders
      - *b* Hypopituitarism
      - *c* Constitutional and metabolic disturbances
    - *2* Compartmental
      - *a* Anovulatory bleeding
      - *b* Inadequate luteal phase
- *II* Ovarian hyperfunction
  - *A* Primary
    - *1* Feminizing tumors
    - *2* Masculinizing tumors
  - *B* Secondary
    - *1* General: true precocious puberty
    - *2* Compartmental
      - *a* Persistent follicle cyst
      - *b* Corpus luteum cyst
      - *c* Stein-Leventhal syndrome and hyperthecosis
- *III* Ovarian dysfunction
  - *A* Choriocarcinoma
  - *B* Struma ovarii
  - *C* Carcinoid

Because of the specialized role of the ovary as an *organ of reproduction,* its disturbances tend to give rise to more restricted symptoms than do those of many other endocrine organs. Unless the influence of a feminizing tumor, for example, is projected against the barren sexual background of childhood or the postmenopausal years, the manifestations may be so inconspicuous as to escape notice. Disorders heralded by infrequent menstruation, staining, or the disappearance of cramps may be trivial in systemic terms and yet have profound reproductive consequences. This is attributable to the fact that except during periods of temporary dissociation, such as adolescence and lactation, the exocrine and endocrine activities of the ovary are firmly integrated. Any deficiency in either results in impaired reproductive function.

OVARIAN HYPOFUNCTION

Although the suspension of established ovarian function is readily recognizable as pathologic, it may be less easy to determine whether delayed sexual maturation in a child reflects hypofunction of clinical significance. The *menarche* presently occurs at a mean age of 12.6 years; since its timing is significantly influenced by genetic factors, the family history as regards menarcheal age should be investigated. The menarche is ordinarily preceded by breast development, a spurt in skeletal growth, and the appearance of pubic hair (axillary hair tends to appear almost simultaneously with the menarche). The presence of any of the secondary sex characters, or of superficial cells in the vaginal smear or urinary sediment, constitutes presumptive evidence of incipient ovarian activation.

GONADAL DYSGENESIS (TURNER'S SYNDROME) Upon gaining the germinal ridges, the primordial germ cells may, for obscure reasons, degenerate without undergoing transformation into primordial follicles. A "streak gonad," incapable not only of ovulation but also of estrogen secretion, is thereby formed. In rare instances, the medullary stroma and hilus cells of such gonads secrete sufficient androgen to induce mild virilization.

In patients with this genetic disorder, the breasts fail to develop, sex hair growth is sparse, and the titers of FSH and LH early rise to menopausal levels. Although amenorrhea is the rule, the germ cell endowment is occasionally sufficient to permit menstruation for a few years, and one well-documented instance of pregnancy has been reported. The key genetic defect is an abnormality of the second X chromosome in some or all of the cells of the patient. Approximately one-half of the patients have a 45-X chromosome constitution, one-third have mosaicism (most frequently 45-X-46-XX), and a small proportion have a structural defect of the 1-X chromosome with the loss of a proportion of its genetic material. The presence of other congenital anomalies such as short stature, webbing of the neck, short metacarpals, and coarctation of the aorta often suggests the diagnosis during the prepuberal years.

Cyclic replacement therapy is indicated to prevent osteoporosis, premature aging of the skin, and other consequences of estrogen deficiency. Estrone sulfate 1.25 to 2.5 mg, or the equivalent dosage of other natural estrogenic preparations, should be given during the first 3 weeks of each month. Once withdrawal bleeding has begun to occur, medroxyprogesterone acetate 5 to 10 mg, or the equivalent dosage of other progestational agents, should be added during the last 5 to 10 days of each course to effect secretory differentiation of the endometrium, thereby preventing cumulative hyperplasia and functional bleeding.

MENOPAUSE The menopause, or final cessation of menses, occurs at a mean age of approximately forty-eight years and is frequently delayed until the early fifties. Termination of menstrual function before the age of forty may be considered premature. A small proportion of patients experiencing a precocious menopause have sex chromosomal mosaicism. Additional patients exhibit an unusual propensity to autoimmune disease, which may conceivably affect the ovaries. In the majority of instances, no explanation is available. The cause of the normally timed climacteric is also somewhat obscure. It appears to reflect an unduly rapid depletion of the oocytes, with the loss of their inductive effect upon the granulosa and theca cells. With a diminution of the steroid feedback influence upon the hypothalamus, the gonadotropin titer rises and the release of FSH and LH is no longer coordinated. Eventually, the stroma remains as the only functioning compartment.

The menopause is usually heralded by a period of menstrual irregularity. Amenorrhea tends to alternate with scanty periods or with bleeding which may be disconcertingly profuse. Hot flashes, the classic symptom of the climacteric, may begin at an early stage but tend to become more frequent after the periods have entirely ceased. They occur in approximately 85 percent of menopausal women and are brief in duration, lasting only a few minutes. The sensation of warmth is confined to the chest, neck, and face and may be accompanied by diffuse or patchy flushing of the skin and sweating. Hot flashes occur most frequently when heat production is increased (e.g., after meals or emotional stress) or when the dissipation of heat is impaired by bedclothes or by high ambient temperatures and humidity. Fatigue, arthralgias, insomnia, and emotional instability are common complaints in middle life; whether they are integral components of the climacteric or are only temporally related is in dispute. The rate at which involution of the ovary takes place affects the severity of menopausal symptoms. In women experiencing a sudden (not necessarily surgical) loss of ovarian function, hot flashes are likely to be severe and dyspareunia due to atrophy of the vagina may be troublesome. In women experiencing a gradual decline of ovarian activity, amenorrhea may be the sole symptom.

Treatment of the menopause comprises (1) the exclusion of organic causes of any associated menorrhagia, (2) explanation of the physiologic changes wrought by the climacteric, ventilation of the patient's anxieties, and reassurance, and (3) hormonal replacement. Estrogen therapy not only suppresses hot flashes, diminishes arthralgia, and relieves dyspareunia but also helps to prevent osteoporosis and may delay the onset of coronary arteriosclerotic heart disease. Sex steroid treatment should be administered indefinitely, as described in the section on gonadal dysgenesis. After a number of years, withdrawal bleeding will no longer occur and the progestational component can be omitted. Mild sedatives, such as phenobarbital 15 mg several times daily, are helpful in diminishing tension. Regular periodic examinations of the breasts and pelvis are essential, as are vaginal smears. The latter serve as a screening test for malignancy, particularly of the cervix. Smears are less reliable for the detection of carcinoma of the endometrium and, in the event of bleeding which is abnormal in timing or quantity, should be supplemented with endometrial biopsy and curettage. The maturation index obtainable from vaginal smears is useful for regulating estrogen dosage. If estrogen is given in amounts sufficient to maintain the superficial cells at a level of 10 percent, dyspareunia can be prevented.

HYPOTHALAMIC DISORDERS Ovarian hypofunction associated with congenital disorders affecting the hypothalamus, such as the *Laurence-Moon-Biedl syndrome,* has been described elsewhere (see Chap. 83). A different congenital disorder is believed to be responsible for the rare association of primary amenorrhea with anosmia or hyposmia.

Destructive lesions of the hypothalamus, such as those resulting from the expansion of tumors and cysts, may induce ovarian hypofunction. The *Frommel-Chiari syndrome* of continued lactation and genital atrophy following childbirth appears to be due to a lesion which somehow impairs the secretion of the prolactin-inhibiting factor and that of the FSH- and LH-releasing factors. In a high proportion of such patients, ovulation can be induced by treatment with clomiphene citrate (Clomid) in 5-day courses at a dosage of 50 to 100 mg per day (Fig. 92-6). This agent blocks the negative feedback action of estrogen at the hypothalamic level and evokes the release of FSH and LH from the pituitary.

Emotional strain which alters the afferent neural input to the hypothalamic centers controlling the secretion of the FSH-LH-RF is perhaps the commonest cause of amenorrhea, apart from pregnancy. The vulnerability of girls in the ten- to twenty-year age group to such stresses as attending school away from home has given rise to the term "boarding school amenorrhea." In older women the menstrual cycle is more resistant to disturbance, and either exceptional stress or frank emotional illness, such as depression, is required to suspend ovarian function. Treatment with Clomid will sometimes bring about ovulation, but in severe cases, psychotherapy may be needed to restore normal cyclicity.

HYPOPITUITARISM In early life, the commonest pituitary cause of sexual infantilism is a *craniopharyngioma;* in adult life, *chromophobe* or *eosinophil adenomas of the pituitary* and *necrosis resulting from post-partum hemorrhage (Sheehan's syndrome)* are the most frequent pituitary lesions resulting in ovarian insufficiency (Chap. 83). *Granulomatous diseases* (Hand-Schüller-Christian syndrome, sarcoid) and metastatic tumors or neoplasms arising in surrounding structures (meningioma) may diminish pituitary function at any age.

Headache, visual disturbances, or impaired growth suggest the possibility of a pituitary disorder in prepuberal girls, although failure of the menses to begin (primary amenorrhea) may be the sole manifestation. In adults, the cessation of menses previously present (secondary amenorrhea) and the coupling of lactation with amenorrhea should suggest the possibility of a chromophobe or acidophil tumor of the pituitary. X-ray visualization of the sella turcica is an essential component of the investigation of all patients with obscure amenorrheas. Sequential treatment with preparations of human menopausal urinary gonadotropin (as a source of FSH) and of human chorionic gonadotropin (as a source of LH-like activity) has, in occasional cases, resulted in ovulation and pregnancy. Pituitary enlargement sufficient to impair vision has occurred during the third trimester in some gonadotropin-treated patients with infertility due to pituitary tumor; such enlargement requires emergency measures.

FIGURE 92-6
The structural formula of Clomid.

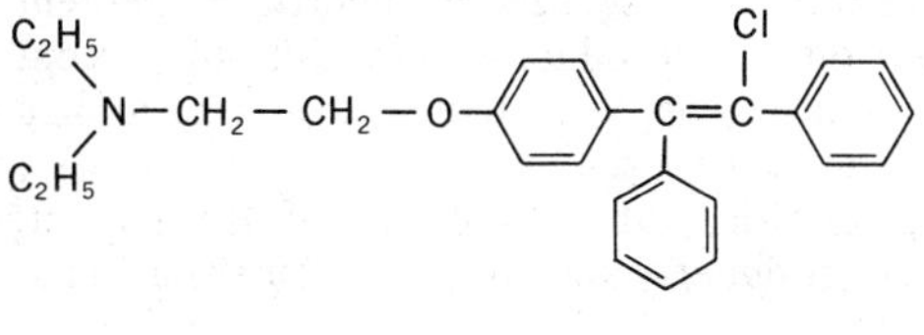

$(C_2H_5)_2N-CH_2-CH_2-O-C_6H_4-C(C_6H_5)=C(Cl)-C_6H_5$

CONSTITUTIONAL AND METABOLIC DISTURBANCES Severe constitutional illnesses such as *congenital heart disease, chronic renal disease,* or *rheumatoid arthritis* may delay the menarche and, in adult life, may cause amenorrhea and sterility. Injudicious dieting with too-rapid weight loss, anorexia nervosa, poorly controlled diabetes mellitus, and hyperthyroidism may also impair reproductive function. The point of impact of these different disorders upon the hypothalamic-pituitary-ovarian chain is poorly defined. A recovery of ovarian function generally follows successful treatment of the primary condition.

The adrenogenital syndrome (Chap. 86), a severe metabolic disorder commonly due to adrenocortical hyperplasia, is associated with pseudohermaphroditism and sexual infantilism. The adrenal cortex secretes estrogens as well as the "adrenal androgens" in greatly increased amounts, and the former, in particular, impair the hypothalamic control of FSH and LH release. Suppression of adrenal estrogen secretion by the administration of corticosteroids is speedily followed by sexual maturation and menstruation.

"Postcontraceptive amenorrhea" (i.e., that ensuing upon the suspension of a program of cyclic sex steroid treatment) is a not-uncommon iatrogenic state, which may or may not be accompanied by lactation. Omission of oral contraceptive preparations is generally followed by a prompt return of menstrual function. However, in some instances, prolonged and even seemingly permanent amenorrhea has followed omission. Anxiety and depression, sometimes associated with a significant loss of weight, may compound the problem. Women with previously irregular menses appear to be especially susceptible to this complication, and should be advised to employ nonhormonal means of contraception. In a proportion of the less severely affected patients,

the amenorrhea can be terminated by means of Clomid treatment.

ANOVULATORY (FUNCTIONAL) BLEEDING Puberty and the premenopausal years are epochs during which the sluggish waxing and waning of the ovarian follicles, with an abnormally prolonged secretion of estrogen and an absence of ovulation, are particularly likely to occur. A teetering level of circulating estrogen results and is likely to be accompanied by painless menorrhagia (excessive menstrual bleeding), metrorrhagia (intermenstrual bleeding), or both, interspersed with long periods of amenorrhea. Anovulatory (functional) uterine bleeding, or "metropathia hemorrhagica," is so common at the two extremes of reproductive life as to be virtually physiologic. During the postmenarcheal and adult years, the condition is traceable to an absence of the midcycle LH surge with abnormally low levels of estrogen in the circulation and an absence of progesterone.

On rare occasions, a persistent follicle cyst is large enough to be outlined on bimanual examination. However, the diagnosis must ordinarily be made by exclusion. The disorders requiring differentiation vary according to the age of the patient (Table 92-2).

Functional uterine bleeding is rarely fatal, but anemia is frequent and requires replacement treatment with iron. In younger patients, the oral progestational agents, fortified with estrogen, are exceedingly effective hemostatic agents. Doses of, for example, 2.5 to 10 mg daily of norethynodrel with mestranol (Enovid) may be given for a period of 3 weeks and then withdrawn to permit a "medical curettage." When the bleeding has been checked and the hemoglobin level restored, normal ovulatory menstrual function may resume spontaneously. If this does not occur, intermittent treatment with Clomid may establish a normal feedback mechanism, with cyclic release of the gonadotropic hormones.

The rare but grave occurrence of bleeding from carcinoma of the vagina in pubertal girls whose mothers were treated with diethylstilbestrol during pregnancy may be confused with functional bleeding. Inquiry concerning this possibility should be made routinely, and where a positive history is elicited gynecologic consultation for detailed inspection of the vagina (if necessary, under anesthesia), complemented if indicated with Schiller's staining and biopsy, should be obtained. Because of the frequent occurrence of necrosis in such tumors, a negative Papanicolaou smear cannot be relied upon to exclude the diagnosis of vaginal cancer. In older patients with bleeding which is seemingly functional in origin, pelvic examination under anesthesia and curettage to exclude organic lesions is mandatory.

TABLE 92-2
Some important causes of vaginal bleeding during different epochs of reproductive life

1 Adolescence
- *a* Functional uterine bleeding
- *b* Blood dyscrasias
- *c* Malignant tumors of the vagina

2 Maturity
- *a* Complications of pregnancy
- *b* Benign tumors (fibromyomas of the uterus, polyps of the endometrium and cervix)
- *c* Malignant tumors of the cervix and corpus of the uterus
- *d* Pelvic inflammatory disease

3 Premenopause
- *a* Functional uterine bleeding
- *b* Benign and malignant tumors of the uterus

4 Senescence
- *a* Estrogen treatment
- *b* Senile vaginitis
- *c* Malignant tumors of the uterus
- *d* Feminizing tumors of the ovary

INADEQUATE LUTEAL PHASE A clinically inconspicuous syndrome characterized by somewhat abbreviated menstrual cycles, infertility, and tendency to abortion is the so-called "inadequate luteal phase." In this disorder, the secretory activity of the corpus luteum is deficient and its term of activity is abbreviated.

A short luteal phase is physiologic (1) in the later phases of the postmenarcheal period, when it is an important cause of "adolescent sterility" (anovulation is the proximate cause of infertility during the immediately postmenarcheal years), and (2) in the puerperium, when menstrual periodicity is gradually being regained. At other times it is pathologic.

The diagnosis may be suspected from the character of the basal body temperature record, which is characterized by a slow rise to the luteal level and abbreviation of the luteal plateau. Confirmatory evidence may be obtained by histologic dating of appropriately timed endometrial biopsies or by demonstration of subnormal levels of plasma progesterone during the luteal phase. The cause of the condition is uncertain. However, there is evidence suggestive of a relative deficiency of FSH during the follicular phase, with impaired development of the follicle and subsequent inadequacy in corpus luteum formation or function.

OVARIAN HYPERFUNCTION

Ovarian hyperfunction may be relative or absolute. Thus, the elaboration of estrogen in amounts which are supraphysiologic for the reproductive age of the subject constitutes hyperfunction, even though the quantity secreted is less than that characteristic of mature reproductive life.

FEMINIZING TUMORS *Granulosa and theca cell tumors* and, on occasion, certain other ovarian neoplasms may secrete estrogen. The stromal elements of tumors in the latter category (e.g., cystadenofibroma and primary adenocarcinoma of the ovary) may resemble those of the thecoma or may contain elements resembling theca-lutein or stroma-lutein cells. The histogenesis of these tumors is uncertain. However, it would appear that granulosa and theca cell tumors arise from the stroma or its follicular wall derivatives and recapitulate the elements of the follicular wall. Approximately 5 percent of the reported granulosa cell tumors arise before puberty, 55 percent during the period of reproductive life, and 40 percent after the menopause. Theca cell tumors tend to occur in a slightly older age group.

The *symptoms* depend on the age of the patient. Precocious pseudopuberty and intermittent uterine bleeding result from the function of such tumors during the premenarcheal years; irregular uterine bleeding, frequently alternating with periods of amenorrhea, is common during active reproductive life; bleeding is the characteristic manifestation of these tumors during the postmenopausal years.

Granulosa cell tumors comprise approximately 10 percent of all primary ovarian carcinomas and are the most common hormone-secreting tumors of the ovary. From 10 to 15 percent of granulosa cell tumors exhibit a low degree of malignancy, in contradistinction to theca cell tumors, which are rarely, if ever, malignant. Both are almost invariably unilateral and tend at times to produce ascites. The Meigs syndrome of ascites and hydrothorax has been observed, especially with the theca cell tumor. Endometrial hyperplasia is a frequent concomitant, and the incidence of uterine leiomyoma, adenomyosis, and adenocarcincoma is increased.

The *diagnosis* is sometimes suggested by an unexpectedly high proportion of superficial cells in the vaginal smear. Urinary estrogen levels tend to be somewhat increased, and gonadotropin levels are occasionally depressed for a given age. Surgical removal is the treatment of choice.

MASCULINIZING TUMORS The *arrhenoblastoma* and the *hilus cell tumor of the ovary* are rare androgen-secreting lesions, the histogenesis of which is uncertain. The majority of arrhenoblastomas tend to occur in comparatively young women, while the hilus cell tumor is characteristically a neoplasm of the late reproductive or postmenopausal years. Both are ordinarily unilateral and benign. The clinical course is one of defeminization followed by masculinization. The 17-ketosteroid excretion tends to be normal or only slightly increased and to be refractory to dexamethasone suppression. Plasma testosterone levels are often elevated. The treatment is surgical.

The so-called *"lipoid cell tumor" of the ovary* is a lesion with an uncertain histogenesis, although in certain instances it appears to arise from the ovarian stroma. The large rounded polyhedral cells of which the tumor consists lack the pathognomonic crystalloids of Reinke but are otherwise identical with Leydig cells. The syndrome of masculinization resulting from the secretion of this tumor may be clinically indistinguishable from that produced by the arrhenoblastoma. The 17-ketosteroid excretion may assist in the differentiation in that it is generally elevated, sometimes to a marked degree. Both premenarcheal and postmenopausal cases have been reported, but twice as many tumors have occurred in premenopausal as in postmenopausal women.

TRUE PRECOCIOUS PUBERTY *Sexual precocity* associated with pituitary activation of graafian follicles is generally idiopathic or "constitutional" in origin. Constitutional precocity is presumed to be due to preternaturally early maturation of the hypothalamus, which escapes from the inhibition exerted by the small but physiologically significant amounts of estrogen secreted by the infantile ovary. Gonadotropin secretion can be materially reduced, with regression of the secondary sexual characteristics and protection from the hazard of pregnancy, by intramuscular injections of medroxyprogesterone ace-

tate. The dosage is easily monitored by periodic determinations of the maturation index, either from vaginal smears or from the sediment of freshly voided urine.

Sexual precocity is a cardinal feature of *Albright's syndrome* of *polyostotic fibrous dysplasia* (Chap. 354). There is no clear indication of the pathogenesis, and a genetic basis for the precocity has been postulated. In rare instances, the ovary is activated prematurely by gonadotropic hormones released in consequence of hypothalamic stimulation by cysts or tumors, and by postencephalitic or postmeningitic lesions.

An unusual form of precocity is that associated with *hypothyroidism,* which increases ovarian sensitivity to endogenous gonadotropins. The precocity can be reversed by the administration of desiccated thyroid in doses sufficient to provide physiologic replacement. These observations contrast with the effects of hypothyroidism on adult women, who commonly experience a failure of ovulation, with a tendency to functional bleeding.

PERSISTENT FOLLICLE CYSTS Follicle cysts which persist during the climacteric tend to differ from those of puberty and the reproductive years in that, because of the hypersecretion of FSH and LH, they are likely to secrete estrogen in amounts exceeding those which are physiologic during mature reproductive life. Massive estrogen treatment designed to inhibit the gonadotropic support of a palpable mass presumed to be a cystic follicle is warranted and is sometimes successful. However, because of the impossibility of distinguishing benign cysts from malignant tumors by palpation, the length of such trials should be carefully limited.

CORPUS LUTEUM CYSTS The classic instance of physiologic luteal hyperfunction is the first trimester of pregnancy. In response to stimulation by chorionic gonadotropin, the corpus luteum of pregnancy secretes estrogen and, to a lesser extent, progesterone in amounts which exceed those characteristic of the luteal phase of the menstrual cycle.

A biochemically similar, but pathologic, state results from the formation of corpus luteum cysts. These may arise spontaneously or iatrogenically as a result of the *administration of Clomid.* Those occurring in Clomid-treated patients may be multiple, giving rise to a severalfold enlargement of the ovary; those occurring spontaneously tend to be single, seldom exceeding a walnut in size.

The presenting complaint of patients with spontaneous cysts is often that of *sudden amenorrhea.* Such cases are frequently mistaken for ectopic pregnancy because of the adnexal enlargement, hyperemia of the vagina and cervix, and the swelling and tenderness of the breasts. The cysts are sensitive to touch, with fragile walls which are likely to rupture. The suspicion of ectopic pregnancy is therefore likely to be compounded by the occurrence of acute abdominal pain. So difficult is the clinical diagnosis that many patients are, in fact, operated upon to exclude the possibility of ectopic pregnancy.

The cysts resulting from Clomid treatment may enlarge with sufficient rapidity to induce lower abdominal discomfort. They are less fragile than the spontaneous variety and ordinarily regress spontaneously after the drug is discontinued.

STEIN-LEVENTHAL SYNDROME AND HYPERTHECOSIS OF THE OVARY These uncommon but important conditions reflect hypersecretion of androgens by the ovarian stroma and perhaps by the hyperplastic and luteinized theca interna enveloping the subcapsular cysts and atretic follicles. *Plasma levels of androstenedione and dehydroepiandosterone,* which may be converted peripherally to *testosterone,* are elevated, as, on occasion, are plasma levels of testosterone itself. The history is one of *irregular menstrual cycles,* generally experienced from puberty onward, and sometimes interspersed with long periods of amenorrhea and abnormal bleeding. Perhaps in consequence of erratic bursts of LH secretion (with an absence of the normal midcycle surge), the ovaries become polycystic, and, since ovulation occurs only rarely, there is associated sterility. Over a period of time the patients tend to develop hirsutism and, in occasional cases, frank virilism.

If the stroma contains nests of lipid-laden lutein cells, the term *hyperthecosis* is applied. Whether the Stein-Leventhal syndrome and hyperthecosis represent a pathologic continuum or distinct entities is uncertain. Hyperthecosis generally evolves in a manner similar to that described for the Stein-Leventhal syndrome. Occasionally, however, there is an abrupt onset in older women (sometimes after pregnancy), and there may be associated hypertension and impaired glucose tolerance.

There is much to suggest that an abnormal hypothalamic-ovarian feedback mechanism is responsible for the disorder. Prior to the introduction of Clomid treatment, *wedge resection of a substantial amount of ovarian tissue* was the treatment of choice for the induction of ovulation. It is still of value in those patients who prove to be refractory to Clomid. Because of the characteristic hyperresponsiveness of the polycystic ovary, *Clomid is best administered initially* in a dose of 25 to 50 mg daily for 3 to 5 days, which is somewhat lower than that ordinarily effective in patients with persistent anovulation due to other causes. Neither Clomid treatment nor wedge resection ameliorates the hirsutism, except in rare instances.

In a proportion of patients with menstrual irregularities, hirsutism, and a high-normal or slightly elevated 17-ketosteroid excretion, differentiation of mild adrenocortical hyperplasia from the Stein-Leventhal syndrome may be difficult (Chap. 86). Patients with this complex of findings should be given the benefit of a suppression test with small doses of a glucocorticoid, such as prednisone 2.5 mg three times a day.

OVARIAN DYSFUNCTION

In rare instances, bizarre dysfunction results from the presence of *ovarian teratomas. Choriocarcinoma,* a highly malignant tumor which secretes chorionic gonadotropin, may arise in the ovary of a prepuberal girl and induce sexual precocity. *Struma ovarii,* which is generally a benign neoplasm, may secrete thyroid hormone at any age. Occasionally, the rate of secretion is so rapid as to induce thyrotoxicosis. *Carcinoid tumors* are sometimes found in dermoid cysts containing intestinal or bronchial epithelium. They may induce the characteristic "carcinoid flush," together with cyanosis and diarrhea, and may, in rare instances, exhibit metastatic spread.

REFERENCES

Bogumil RJ et al: Mathematical studies of the human menstrual cycle. I. Formulation of a mathematical model. II. Simulation performance of a model of the human menstrual cycle. J Clin Endocrinol Metab 35:126, 1972; ibid 35:144, 1972

Morris JM, Scully RE: *Endocrine Pathology of the Ovary,* St. Louis: Mosby, 1958

Richardson GS: *Ovarian Physiology,* Boston: Little, Brown, 1967

Rogers J: *Endocrine and Metabolic Aspects of Gynecology,* Philadelphia: Saunders, 1963

Ross GT et al: Pituitary and gonadal hormones in women during spontaneous and induced ovulatory cycles. Recent Prog Horm Res 26:1, 1970

Savard K et al: Gonadotropins and ovarian steroidogenesis. Recent Prog Horm Res 21:285, 1965

Yates FE et al: Brain-adenohypophysial communication in mammals. Ann Rev Physiol 33:393, 1971

93 DISEASES OF THE BREAST

KENDALL EMERSON, JR.

APPROACH TO DISEASES OF THE BREAST For any physician providing primary care to adult women the examination of the organs of reproduction comprises the most important part of his task because they are the commonest source of fatal and preventable disease to which womankind is heir. Too often in this age of specialization the internist is apt to refer this task to a gynecologist, forgetting that the routine services of two doctors are a rare luxury today. This is not to say that every physician must be an expert in gynecology. It is his duty and responsibility, however, to be able to distinguish the abnormal from the normal in the breasts and pelvic organs, to be competent and thorough in examining them without allowing his judgment to be clouded by embarrassment, disinterest, or false optimism, and *never* to hesitate to call for assistance if he has the slightest doubt concerning the normality of his findings.

HISTORY The earliest description of cancer of the breast, and probably of cancer in any form, is credited to the Egyptian physician Imhotep in 3000 B.C. and is recorded in the Edwin Smith Surgical Papyrus under Case number 39, "Bulging Tumor of the Breast." The studies of Sir Astley Cooper in 1845 provided an adequate morphologic description of the breast and the first suggestion of its possible relationship to menstrual dysfunction. In the latter half of the nineteenth century German investigators discovered that normal breast development in animals depended upon intact ovarian function, and in 1896 Sir George Beatson first demonstrated the inhibition of the growth of mammary cancer by oophorectomy in human beings. The role of the corpus luteum and pituitary in the development of the breasts has been brought to light during the present century by the works of L. Loeb, Gardner, Riddle, Corner, Turner, and many others.

CONGENITAL ANOMALIES The occurence of aberrant breast tissue (polymastia) and supernumerary nipples (polythelia) situated along the so-called "milk-line" extending from the midclavicle to the inguinal ligament has been noted in art and legend since recorded time. Absence of one or both breasts (amastia) occurs very rarely.

ENDOCRINE RELATIONSHIPS The separation and isolation of *prolactin* from growth hormone, after four decades of effort, coupled with the ability to measure it quantitatively in human plasma, have clarified our knowledge of the endocrine relationships of the mammary gland. The growth of the normal nonlactating breast is directly dependent upon the synergistic action of three major hormones: estrogens, cortisol, and prolactin, not on growth hormone as was previously thought; in recent years the syndrome of congenital isolated growth hormone deficiency with normal reproductive and lactating ability has been described in human beings. Prolactin with progesterone is essential for the complete functional development of the alveolar lobules and the secretion of milk, whereas estrogens inhibit lactation by suppressing prolactin release from the pituitary. Prolactin with adrenal steroids can induce lactation in the absence of progesterone. In pregnancy a polypeptide hormone which has prolactin-like activity is secreted in large amounts by the placenta (chorionic somatomammotropin or placental lactogen) and may play an important role in preparing the breast, as well as maternal metabolism, for milk production.

Although the *thyrotropin*-releasing factor (TRF) of the hypothalamus has been shown also to cause the release of prolactin, the normal control of pituitary prolactin secretion appears to be a negative one through a prolactin-inhibitory factor (PIF) actively produced in the hypothalamus. The production of this factor is specifically stimulated by estrogens, which accounts for the suppression of lactation during pregnancy and its onset with the withdrawal of placental estrogens after delivery. Similarly, persistent lactation may occur in association with amenorrhea, low urinary follicle-stimulating hormones (FSH) and hypothyroidism following pregnancy, or the withdrawal after prolonged use of estrogen-containing contraceptives (Chiari-Frommel syndrome). In these instances the augmenting effect of TRF on prolactin release may play a role, since lactation may sometimes be interrupted by thyroid administration. Lactation may also occasionally be induced by nonspecific hypothalamic suppression with catecholamine-depleting drugs such as reserpine, the phenothiazines, and methyldopa. This effect can be countered by administration of the catecholamine precursor L-dopa or the ergot alkaloid, 2-Br-alpha-ergocryptine (CB 154). Finally, lactation may result directly from the excessive production of prolactin in eosinophilic or chromophobe adenomas of the pituitary, with growth hormone (acromegaly) or without it (Forbes-Albright syndrome), or without any demonstrable cause (Argonex-del Castillo syndrome) (see Chap. 83).

The hormones of greatest clinical importance in relation to the breast in man are the estrogens. Engorgement of the breasts may be seen as a transient phenomenon in newborn infants because of the high level of circulating estrogens of placental origin. The normal development of the female breast at puberty, which is sometimes accompanied by intermittent tenderness and edema, results from the rising levels of circulating estrogens secreted by the maturing ovarian follicles just prior to the menarche. Precocious breast development may occur as a result of inherited or constitutional factors; of abnormal pituitary, ovarian, or adrenal activity associated with functional tumors or hyperplasia of these organs; or of locally irritating lesions such as tumors of the pineal or fourth ventricle, fibrous dysplasia of the bones of the base of the skull, as in Albright's disease (polyostotic fibrous dysplasia), or rarely following viral encephalitis.

GYNECOMASTIA Gynecomastia occurs physiologically in normal males at puberty and may persist through adolescence. This breast enlargement usually subsides spontaneously, but if it presents a sufficiently serious psychologic problem, simple mastectomy with preservation of the nipples is justified since any reasonable hormonal treatment is ineffective. Gynecomastia should always raise the suspicion of seminiferous tubule dysgenesis with fibrosis, a variant of Klinefelter's syndrome, in which there is usually an elevated urinary excretion of follicle-stimulating hormone and a female pattern of sex chromatin (see Chap. 91).

Marked degrees of breast development in adolescent males or the onset of gynecomastia in later life may indicate the presence of an estrogen-secreting tumor of the adrenal gland. These tumors are usually associated with an elevation in level of the urinary 17-ketosteroids, the excretion of which is not further stimulated by ACTH or suppressed by adrenal steroids. Every effort should be made to locate such tumors by radiographic means and to remove them surgically because, though they are rare, a high percentage, if not all, are malignant.

Choriogenic tumors and, more rarely, interstitial cell and granulosa cell tumors of the testes may produce gynecomastia. This condition is also seen in males with cirrhosis of the liver and in states of severe malnutrition, presumably in both instances because of failure of inactivation of circulating estrogens. It regularly follows iatrogenic administration of estrogenic compounds in the treatment of carcinoma of the prostate and even occasionally occurs during testosterone therapy in eunuchoidism. Transient gynecomastia occurs as a normal physiologic phenomenon in elderly men and may be associated with the administration of common therapeutic agents having a basic steroid structure such as digitalis and spironolactone.

INFECTIONS OF THE BREAST Acute pyogenic infections of the breast are largely confined to the first 2 months of lactation and usually involve the staphylococcus, less often a beta-streptococcus. They should be prevented by proper hygiene and treated with appropriate antibiotics. Very rarely an acute mastitis unassociated with lactation may occur during the course of paratyphoid or typhoid fever, brucellosis, or mumps.

Chronic tuberculous mastitis is a rarity today. It usually results from the extension of tuberculosis of the underlying bone into the breast tissue and should be suspected from the presence of multiple sinus tracts and the finding of active tuberculosis elsewhere.

INFLAMMATORY LESIONS Mammary duct ectasia is a benign condition, usually seen in elderly women with atrophic breasts, in which the mammary ducts in or just beneath the nipple become dilated and filled with cellular debris and lipid-containing material. Intermittent pain and local inflammatory changes may be present, and because a discharge, at times bloody, and retraction of the nipple may occur, this condition must be differentiated from carcinoma. Excision of the nipple is usually indicated.

Fat necrosis is a common occurrence following trauma, which may be so slight as not to have been noticed. It presents as a painful lump usually associated with some ecchymosis and may be followed by local atrophy and dimpling of the skin, at which stage biopsy must be performed to distinguish it from carcinoma.

Thrombosis of the thoracoepigastric veins and sclerosing subcutaneous phlebitis (Mondor's disease) occur after trauma or for no apparent reason and are manifest by the appearance of long cordlike structures, initially tender, in the outer half of the breast, frequently extending up into the axilla or down toward the epigastrium. They may persist up to a year, but no treatment is indicated.

Sarcoid may very rarely involve the skin of the chest. Eosinophilic granuloma may occur in the submammary folds.

It must not be forgotten that carcinoma of the breast may rarely present as a subacute red, warm, indurated mass, resembling a bacterial cellulitis, the so-called "inflammatory carcinoma." This lesion may be suspected when the skin over it presents the characteristic *peau d'orange* appearance.

FIBROCYSTIC DISEASE With each menstrual cycle there is a recurring biphasic stimulation first of proliferation of breast tissue by estrogens, then of alveolar secretory activity by progesterone, followed by a period of involution. In most women these changes are of such slight degree as to cause few if any clinical symptoms. Not infrequently, however, well-marked inflammatory changes may occur preceding each menses, with tenderness, engorgement, and increasing nodularity of the breasts. This is more often seen in nulliparous women and may subside after childbearing and lactation. Methyltestosterone, 5 mg daily for 7 to 10 days before each menstrual period, will often provide relief.

In the later years of reproductive life the continued recurrent stimulation and involution of the breasts in the course of each menstrual cycle may result in diffuse and nodular fibrosis and the formation of cysts of varying sizes, so-called "chronic cystic mastitis." This condition may simulate carcinoma but is usually distinguishable by the fact that it is intermittently painful and may subside to some extent following menstruation. Nevertheless, carcinoma may coexist and be masked by the diffuse nodularity of the cystic disease. Moreover, the incidence of mammary carcinoma is greater in patients with fibrocystic disease of the breasts, and it is unwise to delay biopsy of suspicious areas in the hope that they may subside by the end of the next menstrual cycle. In severe cases simple mastectomy is fully justified.

TUMORS OF THE BREAST Benign fibroadenomas of the breast may occur at any age but are more common in women under the age of thirty. They may be distinguished from carcinomas by their mobility and well-defined margins, but biopsy is nonetheless imperative.

Benign intraductal papillomas may occur and cause a bloody discharge from the nipple. They are usually small and difficult to feel but may be located by noting that area of the breast on which pressure causes the bleeding. Excision is always advisable.

Sarcomas of all types make up less than 3 percent of all breast tumors. Fibrosarcomas are the most frequent; lymphosarcomas occasionally originate in the breast. Liposarcomas and hemangiosarcomas have been reported rarely. Cystosarcoma phyllodes is a curious, very large, relatively rapidly appearing tumor arising usually from a preexisting fibroadenoma. It presents as a tender, warm, cystic mass often replacing the whole breast. The skin over it is thinned, and the superficial veins are dilated. The tumor consists of fibrous cords covered with epithelium arising from the duct system. The cords are separated by cystic areas which become filled with leaflike (phyllodes) projections of epithelial tissue. Although these tumors are usually benign, blood-borne metastases have been reported and surgical removal of the tumor is always indicated.

CARCINOMA OF THE BREAST In Western civilization carcinoma of the breast is the more frequent malignant tumor to which the human female is subject and accounts for a greater number of deaths than any other single form of cancer in women. It occurs with increasing frequency from the age of twenty up to the menopause, when its incidence levels off until a second rise in frequency occurs after the age of sixty-five. For reasons as yet not entirely clear, breast cancer is very much less common in Japan and other oriental countries.

Etiology The cause of breast cancer, like that of most other forms of malignant disease, is unknown. A few factors affecting its incidence are, however, reasonably well established. The very strong hereditary influence seen in mice may be carried over, though in a much smaller degree, to human beings. A two- to sevenfold increase in the familial incidence of the disease is reported. In this connection renewed interest in a milk-borne virus, first proposed by Bittner in 1936, has been aroused by the finding of alleged virus particles and of virus-related information in the DNA of human breast cancer cells.

The role of the *estrogenic hormones* in the genesis of breast cancer in human beings in still controversial. The incidence of mammary cancer appears to be directly related to the duration of the period of ovarian activity. It is more common in childless women with a late menopause and less frequent in women with early and multiple pregnancies or who have undergone bilateral oophorectomy before the age of forty. The view most widely accepted at the present time is that estrogens do not initiate the cancer but may, nevertheless, hasten its development in genetically susceptible individuals. The prolonged use of these hormones, especially at or beyond the menopause in patients with a family history of cancer, should be discouraged. On the other hand, it must be said that estrogens inhibit the stimulating effect of prolactin on breast cancer in certain strains of rats and have no effect by themselves in the absence of prolactin. There is some evidence that these observations may be extended to certain types of human mammary cancer and that estriol may have an inhibitory action.

Recent observations on the epidemiology of breast cancer suggest that environmental influences may play a role. The disease is more common in Japanese women living in the United States than in Japan, in the women of Denmark than in their Scandinavian sisters in Finland, and in fat women than in thin. Wynder has gone so far as to speculate that one common variable, the quantity of saturated fat in the diet, might affect the growth of mammary cancer directly by providing precursors for the synthesis and/or a vehicle for the storage of the fat-soluble estrogens. Of particular interest is the high incidence of both breast cancer and polycystic ovaries among the Parsis in Bombay, more than twice that of the general population in India. This ancient religious sect comprises a closely interrelated and affluent community having access to a relatively rich diet, thus combining both genetic and environmental factors which might favor the growth of mammary cancer.

Pathology The primary site is usually in the ducts, less often in the alveoli. Multicentric origins are a frequent occurrence, and all gradations of differentiation may be observed. It is common to see a marked proliferation of dense connective tissue surrounding groups of malignant cells, whether primary or metastatic, the so-called "scirrhous carcinoma." Unfortunately all degrees of differentiation may be found in different portions of the same tumor and little prognostic value can be attached to the histologic appearance of any one area of such a malignancy.

Mammary carcinoma is likely to metastasize relatively early to the regional lymph nodes—axillary and supraclavicular if the primary site is in the outer half of the breast, the internal mammary chain if the disease arises in the inner quadrants of breast tissue. From thence spread occurs primarily to bone, lungs, liver, skin, and subcutaneous tissues generally, less frequently to the brain. Blood-borne metastases may occur even before lymphatic spread is clinically evident. It is interesting that there is a predilection for metastases to occur in the ovaries, adrenals, and pituitary—areas rich in the hormones stimulating the growth of this type of epithelial cell.

Diagnosis The diagnosis of breast cancer is facilitated by the fact that it is possible to palpate directly this type of neoplasm. Unfortunately, the diffuse nodularity of the adult female breast makes it difficult to detect early lesions. As a rule the physician must depend on such evidence as hardness, fixation to underlying structures, or dimpling of the overlying skin to distinguish a malignant mass from a benign nodule of breast tissue, and by the time these distinguishing signs have become apparent the cancer has all too often metastasized. Direct exposure of the breasts to irradiation with low-voltage x-rays in order to bring out contrasts in soft-tissue densities, so-called "mammography," has been of great value in screening for breast cancer and in discovering small lesions in large, fatty breasts. When secretions are obtainable from the nipple, cytologic examination may be helpful. The majority of patients with breast cancer suggest the diagnosis themselves because of their ready detection of abnormal lumps or masses during self-examination. Although the procedure of periodic self-examination of the breast may be decried as tending to encourage neuroticism and cancerphobia, it is the only practical way by which we can succeed in reducing the death rate from cancer of the breast until a final cure for cancer has been found.

Treatment Total *surgical excision* provides the only permanent cure for carcinoma of the breast, and x-ray therapy the best palliation for localized disease. The technical details of the surgical and radiologic treatment of breast cancer are beyond the scope of this chapter, as is the controversy over radical versus simple mastectomy with extensive local irradiation, as advocated by McWhirter and others. Because of the susceptibility of breast cancer to changes in its endocrine environment, however, every physician should be cognizant of the remarkable palliative effect which can be achieved in inoperable mammary cancer by intelligent hormonal manipulations.

The two most important factors governing the prognosis of disseminated breast cancer and the success of its treatment or palliation are (1) the age of the patient and (2) the length of the free interval between the discovery of the primary tumor and the appearance of metastases. As with neoplasia in general, the younger the age at which it occurs, the more rapid and malignant is its growth. The only exceptions to this rule are the rare cases of *juvenile breast cancer* reported in patients from three to fifteen years of age, which appear to have a more benign course. The length of the free interval is a rough measure of the balance between the biologic activity, or turnover rate, of tumor cells and the poorly understood factors of host resistance.

The rationale of the *endocrine treatment of breast cancer* is predicated on the assumption that in the total population of malignant cells some retain their metabolic dependency for growth upon estrogens for variable lengths of time before ultimately becoming autonomous. The first aim of therapy, therefore, is to remove all sources of estrogen from the afflicted subject. There is increasing evidence, but not universal agreement, that prophylactic oophorectomy and prednisone suppression of adrenal estrogen precursors at the time of initial mastectomy may significantly prolong the free interval, if not the total survival time of those patients with metastases ostensibly confined to axillary lymph nodes. Surgical or adequate x-ray castration will induce subjective and/or objective remissions in approximately 40 percent of patients with demonstrable metastases up to the menopause, the incidence of favorable responses tending to vary directly with age.

With cessation of ovarian activity the adrenal cortex takes over the function of supplying precursors for estrogen production, and *bilateral adrenalectomy* will then bring about a further remission in approximately 50 percent of subjects. The remissions following these procedures may last anywhere from 6 months to 5 years or longer. Although no statistics are currently available, some investigators believe that oophorectomy and adrenalectomy carried out simultaneously will bring about a more prolonged remission in a larger percentage of patients than when adrenalectomy is deferred until the remission following oophorectomy is ended or fails to occur. In particular, when the metastatic disease is far advanced, the condition of the patient may preclude the performance of a second operation.

Surgical *hypophysectomy,* or *pituitary stalk* section, induces a functional ovarian and adrenal abalation and results in a remission rate equal to but no greater than that brought about by the surgical extirpation of these target organs. The technical problems involved in total removal of the hypophysis and the degree of morbidity arising therefrom have tended to discourage this procedure. It has the theoretic advantage of eliminating the potential stimulating effect of prolactin on the tumor cells, and the longest reported remissions (10 years or more) have followed hypophysectomy. Pituitary ablation by roentgen or nuclear bombardment is too gradual to be of value in retarding the progress of a rapidly growing neoplasm.

Functional suppression of estrogen production by the ovaries may be achieved by the administration of depot progesterone, 200 mg intramuscularly, at monthly intervals, and simultaneously, the production of adrenal estrogen precursors can be inhibited by prednisone, 2.5 to 5 mg, at 8-hr intervals daily. Such measures may be successful in retarding mammary cancer growth when surgical procedures are unavailable or unwarranted, but they are less certain and suppression is rarely as complete.

As yet, no reliable means has been found to select beforehand those individuals who will respond favorably to endocrine ablative procedures. A marked stimulation of tumor growth by estrogen administration usually implies a favorable response to oophorectomy, and similarly, a suppression of growth by prednisone indicates that adrenalectomy will have a good effect. The converse is not always true, however, and even lack of response to oophorectomy does not necessarily preclude a favorable response to subsequent adrenalectomy. Bullbrook and associates have presented statistical evidence indicating that in women under sixty-five who excrete a low ratio of androgens (11-deoxy-17-ketosteroids) to 17-hydroxycorticosteroids in their urine, breast cancer has a poorer prognosis in terms of recurrence rate, 3-year survival, and response to adrenalectomy than in women of similar age with a higher androgen excretion rate. Moore and coworkers have noted a tendency for patients who respond favorably to adrenalectomy to show a greater rise in the urinary excretion of 17-keto- and 11-17-hydroxysteroids following ACTH stimulation than those who fail to respond. Statistical discriminants based on data derived from such urinary hormone measurements have been advocated for the preselection of patients for adrenalectomy, but have not yet found general applicability. The length of the free interval is still a much more reliable predictor of response. As a rule of thumb, a free interval of less than 12 months indicates a poor prognosis. More accurate predictions may result from studies which show that those cancer cells which respond to hormonal ablation have a higher intranuclear binding affinity for estradiol-17-beta and a greater capacity to sulfurylate dehydroepiandrosterone than estradiol.

Developments in *cancer chemotherapy,* however, have changed strikingly these predictions. The combination of ovarian and adrenal extirpation followed immediately by 5 fluorouracil (5-FU), 15 mg per kg body weight given as a daily intravenous infusion over 4 to 6 hr for 5 to 7 days has sharply increased the remission rate and extended it to include many patients with a free interval of less than 12 months. The 5-FU is well tolerated on this dosage schedule and should be continued as a single weekly intravenous injection or by mouth as long as the remission lasts, provided no evidence of bone marrow suppression intervenes. Many patients too sick for surgical procedures may show striking improvement for 1 to 2 years following combined administration of prednisone 20 to 40 mg daily and 5-FU in the aforementioned dosage schedule. Undoubtedly other chemotherapeutic agents will be found which are equally or more effective, but, hitherto, no agent has been shown to be effective in more than 20 percent of patients unless combined with simultaneous manipulation of the endocrine environment of the cancer cell.

In older patients, 15 years or more past the menopause, *large doses of estrogens* may provide remarkable palliation, and this is the treatment of choice. This paradoxic effect of estrogens, first clearly described by Nathanson, has never been fully explained.

The place of *androgens and estrogens* in the treatment of metastatic breast cancer has been well defined by a report of the American Medical Association's Council on Drugs, based on a 10-year nationwide cooperative study. In summary, androgens produced objective remissions in approximately 20 percent of patients both before and after the menopause. Estrogens, which should not be used before the menopause, will induce remissions in about 36 percent of patients during the first 8 postmenopausal years and in more than 38 percent in later years. Estrogens have a greater relative effect on soft tissue and visceral metastases than on bone but equal or exceed the effect of androgens on all types of tissue. Estrogens must be employed in large doses to achieve these results, e.g., stilbestrol, 15 mg, or ethinyl estradiol, 3 mg daily. Smaller amounts may adversely affect the tumor. Nausea and vomiting may occur at the onset of treatment but can be controlled by antiemetic agents and will disappear in time. Uterine bleeding may be troublesome but can usually be controlled by the cyclic administration of progesterone or methyltestosterone.

The optimum dose of *androgens* has been found to be equivalent to 100 mg testosterone propionate given intramuscularly three times weekly. Recent experience indicates that the newer anabolic androgens, such as 17-beta, 17-alpha dimethyltestosterone in oral doses of 50 mg four times daily, may be equally effective with much less tendency to produce the undesirable masculinizing side effects of testosterone.

All patients, but especially those within the first 8 postmenopausal years, should be observed carefully during the first few days and weeks of treatment because both androgens and estrogens may cause an exacerbation of their disease, estrogens by a direct stimulating effect and androgens presumably by being converted in small but effective amounts to estrogens. One of the most serious complications produced by administration of these hormones in patients who exhibit extensive skeletal metastases is calcium intoxication. This is presumed to result from the sudden stimulation of growth of the bony metastases by the hormone, with correspondingly rapid destruction of bone and flooding of the circulation with calcium. There is a marked increase in urinary calcium excretion, the serum calcium level may rise to as high as 15 to 20 mg per 100 ml, and drowsiness, coma, convulsions, and death from renal failure may ensue. It is important to distinguish this condition from cerebral or liver metastases or the terminal effects of widespread cancer because it can be reversed by forcing fluids, withdrawal of the offending hormone, and administration of large amounts of hydrocortisone, 200 mg daily by slow intravenous drip or in divided oral doses daily, until symptoms subside. The administration of neutral phosphate salts, in doses equivalent to 1.5 g phosphorus daily, may be of great value, presumably by redirecting the flow of calcium away from the kidneys back into bone.

Hypercalcemia may, of course, occur spontaneously in far advanced autonomously growing malignancy with widespread skeletal metastases but can still usually be controlled with the above measures plus the addition of a chemotherapeutic agent. Occasionally hypercalcemia may be found in the absence of demonstrable bony involvement. It has also been reported that a "calcium-mobilizing" steroid may be elaborated by breast tumors.

Carcinoma occurs in the male breast at least 100 times less frequently than in the female. Otherwise it behaves in exactly the same manner. The treatment is the same except that orchiectomy replaces oophorectomy. Prednisone and hypophysectomy have both been shown to induce remissions when the primary disease has metastasized, and progestational compounds may be of value.

REFERENCES

BARNES AB: Current concepts: Diagnosis and treatment of abnormal breast secretions. N Engl J Med 275:1184, 1966

BESSER GM, EDWARDS CRW: Galactorrhoea. Br Med J 2:280, 1972

BULLBROOK RD et al: Relation between urinary androgen and corticoid excretion and subsequent breast cancer. Lancet 2:395, 1971

HAAGENSEN CD: *Diseases of the Breast,* 2d ed., Philadelphia: Saunders, 1971

MOORE FD et al: Carcinoma of the breast. A decade of new results with old concepts. N Engl J Med 277:293, 343, 411, 460, 1967

WOLSTENHOLME GEW, KNIGHT J (eds): *Ciba Foundation Symposium on Lactogenic Hormones,* Edinburgh and London: Churchill-Livingstone, 1972

WYNDER EL et al: Correlation of international cancer death rates, an epidemiological exercise. Cancer 20:113, 1967

94 DISEASES OF THE PINEAL GLAND

RICHARD J. WURTMAN

INTRODUCTION Since the discovery of melatonin in 1958, compelling evidence has accumulated that the mammalian pineal is not a vestige but an important component of a neuroendocrine control system. This organ has been shown to function as a neuroendocrine transducer: it receives a cyclic input of sympathetic nervous "information" which is generated by retinal effects of environmental lighting. In response to this input, the pineal secretes a hormone, melatonin, into the bloodstream, much as the adrenal medulla releases epinephrine in response to cholinergic nervous stimulation. The synthesis and secretion of melatonin vary with a 24-hr periodicity, thereby providing the body with a circulating "clock" apparatus. Largely because of technical difficulties, few attempts have been made to exploit this new knowledge of pineal function in clinical medicine. Hence, the principal circumstance which forces the clinician to think about the pineal continues to be the rare case of a disorder with evidence of a pineal neoplasm. It can be anticipated that as information about pineal physiology increases, more situations will suggest themselves in which pineal malfunction might be a factor in causing a disease.

ANATOMY AND BIOCHEMISTRY OF THE PINEAL

The human pineal gland is a flattened, conical organ which lies beneath the posterior border of the corpus callosum and between the superior colliculi. It originates embryologically as an evagination of the ependyma which lines the roof of the third ventricle, and remains connected to this region by the pineal stalk. The adult gland weighs about 120 mg; its dimensions are 5 to 9 mm in length, 3 to 6 mm in width, and 3 to 5 mm in thickness. Most of the pineal is enveloped by pia mater, from which blood vessels, unmyelinated nerve fibers, and septums of connective tissue penetrate the gland, thereby dividing it into lobules. The pineal glandular or parenchymal cells on the periphery of the lobule are elongated; those in the central zone are ovoid. They contain numerous granular bodies (which might represent a stored secretion), and give rise to processes that terminate adjacent to the capillary endothelium.

In 1960, Kappers made the important discovery that the primary innervation of the mammalian pineal originates not within the brain but rather from sympathetic cell bodies in the superior cervical ganglions. Subsequent studies using the electron microscope revealed that the sympathetic nerve endings terminate directly on pineal parenchymal cells in an anatomic relationship that resembles the synapse. The sympathetic innervation of pineal glandular cells appears to be a new evolutionary adaptation. Such a parenchymal innervation may be unique in the body, and itself invalidates the vestige theory of pineal function.

In 1917, McCord and Allen showed that the pineal gland of the cow contained a factor which causes amphibian skin to blanch. When pineal homogenates were fed to tadpoles, the melanin granules within dermal melanophores aggregated around the cell nuclei, thereby lightening the skin. (This effect is opposite to that produced by the melanocyte-stimulating hormone, MSH, which is secreted by the pars intermedia of the pituitary gland.) Four decades later, Lerner and his colleagues identified this pineal factor as melatonin (5-methoxy-N-acetyltryptamine) (Fig. 94-1). Melatonin appears to have no effect on the melanocytes which are responsible for normal skin pigmentation in human beings.

Melatonin was shown to be a derivative of serotonin (Fig. 94-1), a widely distributed indole stored in very large quantities in mammalian pineals. It differs from all indoles previously identified in mammals in that it contains a methoxy group. The enzyme which catalyzes this methoxylation reaction (hydroxyindole-O-methyl transferase, HIOMT) was shown to be concentrated within the pineal gland in mammals. The high degree of localization of HIOMT has recently been used as a "marker" to differentiate true pinealomas from pineal tumors of glial or other origin.

PHYSIOLOGY OF THE MAMMALIAN PINEAL Environmental lighting conditions exert several important effects on the mammalian neuroendocrine apparatus. Light acts as an "inducer" that modifies the rate of sexual maturation; girls who have been deprived of light from birth may show early pubescence. The sequence of day and night also acts to generate some 24-hr biologic rhythms and to synchronize other rhythms which are produced by signals arising from within the body. There is evidence that one function of the mammalian pineal might be to mediate some of these endocrine effects of light. The "information" about light travels to the pineal by a route which involves (1) the inferior accessory optic tract, (2) centers in the brain and spinal cord that regulate the sympathetic nervous system, and (3) the sympathetic nerves to the pineal which originate in the superior cervical ganglions. The diurnal variation in pineal melatonin secretion provides the body with a circulating "clock" which is under the direct control of the lighting environment.

Less is known about which organs take cues from the pineal "clock" than about the mechanism responsible for its rhythmic changes. It seems likely that melatonin exerts physiologic inhibitory effects on gonadal and thyroid function and also modifies behavior and electroencephalographic activity. When tiny amounts of melatonin are implanted in the median eminence of the

FIGURE 94-1

Synthesis of melatonin in the pineal gland. The pineal takes up tryptophan from the circulation; the amino acid is hydroxylated to form 5-hydroxytryptophan; this is then converted to the amine serotonin (5-hydroxytryptamine) by the enzyme aromatic L-amino acid decarboxylase. Some of the serotonin synthesized in the pineal is destroyed by oxidative deamination, forming 5-hydroxyindole acetic acid. However, the major fraction of pineal serotonin is N-acetylated and O-methylated to form the hormone melatonin.

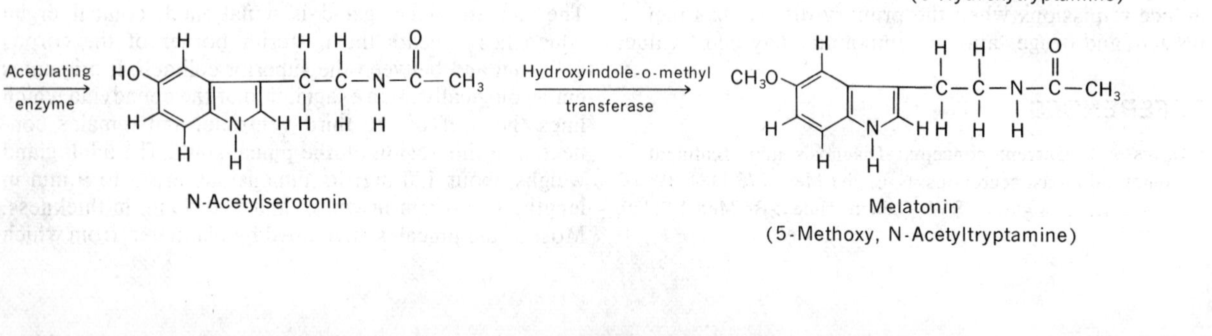

hypothalamus or the midbrain reticular formation, the increase in pituitary luteinizing hormone (LH) content which normally follows castration is blocked. Melatonin placed in the cerebrospinal fluid suppresses the secretion of pituitary LH and enhances the secretion of prolactin. Melatonin administration also changes the levels of serotonin in the brain.

PINEAL PATHOLOGY Two pineal lesions have been of interest to the clinician: pineal calcification, which is a universal autopsy finding, and pineal tumors, which are best known for their endocrine sequelae. In rare instances, pineal glands have also contained cancer metastases, gummas, tuberculous granulomas, or isolated segments of skeletal muscle.

Pineal calcification often first becomes visible on skull roentgenograms around the time of puberty, and it has been suggested that the gland degenerates at this time of life, and then becomes calcified. However, recent studies have not supported this hypothesis. If pineals are examined by appropriate microscopic techniques, evidence of calcification often is seen in patients who died long before the age of puberty. A ground substance believed to serve as the matrix for calcification was seen in 8 of 28 pineals taken from children under one year of age. Moreover, studies of pineal function have failed to show any differences between heavily calcified glands taken from aged subjects and pineals from young subjects with no gross evidence of calcification. The functional significance of pineal calcification remains entirely unexplained. The chemical identity of the calcified material appears to be hydroxyapatite; crystals of this compound taken from human pineals are similar to those prepared from bone or tooth.

Pineal tumors may be divided into several distinct categories by their microscopic appearance. Somewhat more than half of all pineal tumors may be classified as true pinealomas. These tumors contain clusters of two distinct types of cells: large, spheroidal, epithelial cells, and small, dark-staining cells with little cytoplasm and an ultrastructure indistinguishable from that of the lymphocyte. About 10 to 15 percent of all reported pineal tumors have been teratomas; these may contain mucus-secreting columnar epithelial cells, adenocarcinoma tissue, and areas resembling thyroid, muscle, cartilage, bone, and nerve. Like other midline teratomas, they are often malignant. The remainder of pineal tumors have been of vascular or glial origin.

Confirmation of pineal origin of the large pinealoma cells has been hampered by the lack of a specific pineal function which could be measured in these cells (such as the uptake of ^{131}I by thyroidal cells in follicular adenomas). However, studies suggest that assays for the melatonin-forming enzyme (HIOMT) may provide such a "marker." Two pineal tumors containing this enzyme have been described; one was a metastasis from a parenchymal pinealoma, and the other, a specimen from an ectopic pinealoma. Both tumors had the characteristic histologic appearance of the parenchymal pinealoma.

The natural history of a pineal tumor is related to its size and its histologic appearance. Tumors which originate within the pineal gland usually become clinically manifest because of symptoms which arise from their location (e.g., internal hydrocephalus, elevated cerebrospinal fluid pressure, and oculomotor signs such as paralysis of upward gaze, or Parinaud's syndrome); less frequently, the patient's family initially seeks medical attention because of the development of precocious puberty. About one-third of all boys below the normal age of sexual maturation who have pineal tumors develop precocious puberty. This neoplasm accounts for about 10 to 15 percent of all precocious sexual development in males. For unexplained reasons, pineal tumors are much less common among girls and are not associated with precocious menarche. Some investigators have suggested that the precocious sexual development in pinealoma patients is a nonspecific consequence of the pressure that these tumors exert on surrounding brain tissue. Kitay and others have summarized the evidence against this "pressure hypothesis": (1) Pineal tumors may produce precocious puberty, no gonadal signs, or even delayed pubescence. The endocrine effects of a particular tumor appear to be unrelated to its size. (2) Most cases of precocious puberty develop in patients with nonparenchymal tumors (frequently teratomas). An occasional parenchymal tumor leads to gonadal enlargement, but more commonly these neoplasms are associated with delayed pubescence or with secondary gonadal failure. (3) Gonadal abnormalities have been observed in a large number of pinealoma patients whose tumors had neither produced signs of a chronic elevation in cerebrospinal fluid pressure nor invaded other brain areas. The demonstration that a pineal hormone, melatonin, influences normal sexual maturation in rats supports the hypothesis that precocious puberty develops in pinealoma patients because the damaged pineal fails to release an inhibitory hormone. It has not been possible to test this hypothesis directly, because no assay is available which can be used to measure the level of melatonin or its metabolic products in blood or urine. It is noteworthy, perhaps, that both patients described above whose tumors contained melatonin-forming activity showed evidence of depressed sexual function.

Parenchymal pinealomas frequently show a good, if temporary, clinical remission following irradiation. Patients generally receive 3,000 to 5,000 rd; radiation is administered over a wide portal because pinealomas not infrequently metastasize throughout the ventricles and the subdural space. Japanese surgeons have reported encouraging results following the surgical extirpation of pinealomas; however, this method is complicated by the relative inaccessibility of the pineal, and consequently is used rarely in the United States. A patient with metastatic parenchymal pinealoma has been repeatedly treated during a 10-year period with x-ray and chemotherapeutic agents; each time an objective decrease in tumor mass occurred.

A small number of tumors with histologic appearance of pinealomas originate elsewhere in the brain at some distance from the normal pineal gland. These "ectopic pinealomas" generally arise in the hypothalamus in the region of the infundibulum. Hence, patients usually present a picture similar to that seen with craniopharyngioma with a clinical triad of bitemporal hemianopsia, hypopituitarism, and diabetes insipidus. Most ectopic pinealomas show a good clinical response to irradiation.

REFERENCES

RAMSEY HJ: Ultrastructure of a pineal tumor. Cancer 18:1014, 1965

WOLSTENHOLME GEW, KNIGHT J (eds): *The Pineal Gland*, Edinburgh: Churchill-Livingstone, 1971, p. 401

WURTMAN RJ et al: *The Pineal*, New York: Academic Press, 1968

——: The pineal gland, in *Endocrine Pathology*, ed JMB Woodworth, Baltimore: Williams & Wilkins, 1968, p. 117

section 4 | Errors of metabolism

95 INTRODUCTION

LLOYD H. SMITH, JR.

Few diseases are either wholly genetic or wholly environmental in their pathogenesis. The degree to which "environment" (microbiologic, physical, psychologic, chemical) is injurious depends on the genetic legacy of the host. This may represent a specific genetic defect phenotypically expressed as altered structure and function or inappropriate amount of a given protein, a group of disorders still often designated by Garrod's term as "inborn errors of metabolism." Perhaps more often the genetic propensity toward disease represents polymeric gene action, the summation of a number of genic expressions which can now be described only by statistical approaches. A number of factors have contributed to recent interest in genetic diseases: (1) With improved control of environment, disease is increasingly endogenous rather than exogenous. (2) Advances in molecular biology have elucidated the mechanisms of transmission and expression of genetic information, allowing the definition of certain diseases with increased precision. (3) Although genetic diseases cannot now be cured in the host, knowledge of the resulting biochemical derangements often allows rational means of treatment to be devised.

In this section major attention will be directed to individual genetic diseases rather than to broader topics in population genetics or molecular biology. It is not clear how many inborn errors of metabolism there are. By the use of current estimates of the number of different kinds of proteins in the body, the average number of amino acids per protein, and the possibility that at a given point any one of 20 amino acids might be substituted, it may be estimated that the possibilities for variation in structural genes alone are $>10^{10}$. Many factors reduce the number of diseases which are recognized. Certain variations are trivial, lead to no biologic disadvantage, and merely constitute the chemical basis of individuality. Other defects are intrinsically lethal and contribute to the high incidence of spontaneous abortions. Variations may occur not only among diseases but also within diseases, depending on the site of alteration in the protein and the degree of resulting dysfunction. More than 100 abnormal hemoglobins have been described. It may well be, by analogy, that there are more than 100 types of galactosemia or phenylketonuria. Individual genetic diseases vary widely in frequency, from diabetes mellitus (3 to 5 percent of the population) to sulfituria (a single case description). The variables in frequency—mutation rate and the balance of biologic advantage and disadvantage—are now the subject of considerable interest in human genetics.

The usual *inborn error of metabolism* results from the absence or severe reduction in catalytic activity of an enzyme, whether the protein is physically missing or is present but altered in a fashion which impairs its function. In microorganisms genetic disorders of too much enzyme activity occur. No examples of genetic diseases due directly to excessive enzyme activity have been found in man, although enzyme activities may be secondarily increased because of failure of control mechanisms (e.g., Δ-aminolevulinic acid synthetase in acute intermittent porphyria). *Genetic disorders* usually produce disease by the *accumulation of substrate of the abnormal enzyme or* by *absence or reduced availability of its product.* This concept is illustrated simply in diagrammatic form first introduced by Charles Dent:

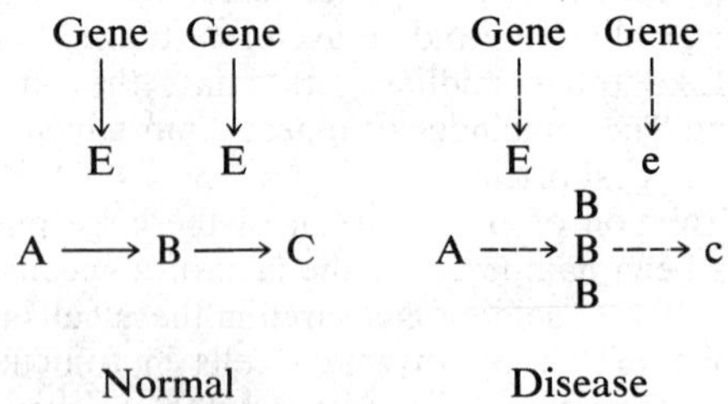

The accumulation of substrate *B* is the most frequently encountered abnormality productive of disease. This may be related to the fact that most genetic disorders so far discovered are in degradative pathways of metabolism. Some examples of substrate (and substrate by-product) toxicity are described in greater detail in subsequent chapters: phenylalanine and its by-products in phenylketonuria, galactose 1-phosphate in galactosemia, oxalate in primary hyperoxaluria, homogentisic acid and its pigment polymer in alcaptonuria. Such defects may result in storage diseases such as the lipidoses, cystinosis, and the glycogen storage diseases. The accumulated precursor may inhibit other metabolic pathways or interfere with amino acid transport into cells. Often the biochemical mechanism of injury is obscure.

Genetic disorders may lead to disease because of *absence* or *reduced availability of the product* rather than through accumulation of the precursor. Most of the recognized examples lie in defects in plasma protein synthesis or in the sequence of hormone synthesis, described elsewhere in this book. For example, deficiency of circulating thyroxine and triiodothyronine is the major defect in the various specific genetic forms of familial cretinism (Chap. 85), producing damage to the developing central nervous system, delayed maturation of the skeleton, hypometabolism, and failure of inhibition of TSH (thyroid-stimulating hormone) release, with resulting goiter. Similarly, deficiency of hydrocortisone in congenital adrenal virilism (Chap. 86) is the ultimate cause of adrenocortical hyperplasia (via ACTH) and of the excessive synthesis of steroidal precursors into adrenal androgens. A large number of genetic disorders of the synthesis of circulating proteins which participate in hemostasis have been described. In fact these proteins have been largely discovered in the study of patients with a hemorrhagic diathesis. The ultimate deficiency common to these disorders is that of appropriate formation of cross-linked fibrin polymer. The multiple types of genetic blocks in glycolysis associated with chronic nonspherocytic hemolytic anemia probably share a common deficiency of erythrocytic ATP (adenosine triphosphate). The defect in albinism is absence of melanin; and a major defect in the von Gierke form of glycogen storage disease is deficiency of circulating glucose secondary to loss of glucose 1-phosphatase activity. In hereditary orotic aciduria, uridine becomes an essential metabolite. In a sense these disorders represent analogs of auxotrophism in bacteria.

A number of *genetic diseases* have now been described in which there is a *defect* in the *active transport of metabolites across membranes,* as summarized in Chap. 98. Occasionally the physical properties of the abnormal protein may constitute the mechanism of disease, as in the propensity toward stacking and tactoid formation in sickle-cell anemia and the heritable disorders of connective tissue. Pharmacogenetics refers to inherited alterations in drug metabolism, sensitivity of response, and toxicity. As an example, pseudocholinesterase deficiency is innocuous except during the use of certain muscle relaxants in anesthesia, when prolonged paralysis may result. Immunogenetics refers not only to immunologic markers in gamma-globulins but also to the inherited basis of antigenic (chemical) individuality. It is apparent that genetic alterations may be productive of disease through a variety of mechanisms, both subtle and direct.

Genetic diseases cannot now be "cured" in the host, although current advances in molecular biology suggest that this limitation may eventually be removed. Knowledge of the mechanism of disease, however, often allows effective palliative measures to be instituted. Many of these are illustrated in the discussion of specific diseases in the chapters of this section. Some approaches which have been used may be summarized briefly:

1 *Replace the enzyme.* This could be done phenotypically or, in theory, genotypically. The latter would clearly be preferable if genotypic replacement, augmentation, or repair becomes feasible in multicellular organisms. Replacement now is largely limited to extracellular proteins such as coagulation factors, gamma-globulins, or hormones, of transient value only. Homotransplantation raises the possibility of localized extirpation and "cure" of genetic disease. The cystinuric kidney has been replaced. Drugs may alter the expression of genetic information. Phenobarbital has been used successfully to cause marked proliferation of the smooth-surfaced membranes of the endoplasmic reticulum in liver cells and thereby enhance pathways of bilirubin metabolism in certain cases of congenital hyperbilirubinemia.
2 *Reduce the accumulation of substrate.* This is usually carried out by dietary therapy, such as galactose-free diets in galactosemia or phenylalanine-restricted diets in phenylketonuria. The accumulation may be that of a by-product, such as uric acid or oxalate. In these cases new approaches to drug management are being pursued to inhibit the by-product formation or increase its excretion.
3 *Supply the product.* At the present time this approach is rarely employed except in endocrine replacement therapy, e.g., administration of a glucocorticoid in congenital adrenal hyperplasia or of thyroxine in the various forms of familial cretinism. The requirement for uridine in hereditary orotic aciduria is an exception, since this is replacement of an intermediate on a specific biosynthetic pathway.
4 *Miscellaneous.* A number of miscellaneous approaches have been successfully employed to compensate for errors of metabolism. Phlebotomy removes the excess iron of hemochromatosis, and D-penicillamine removes the excess copper of Wilson's disease. D-Penicillamine forms a more soluble mixed disulfide of cystine in cystinuria. Chlorothiazide reduces the diuresis of vasopressin-resistant diabetes insipidus. Other examples could be cited. In summary, the treatment of genetic diseases is a challenging and often rewarding category of therapeutics.

Garrod wrote in 1908, "The existence of chemical individuality follows of necessity from chemical specificity, but we should expect the differences between individuals to be still more subtle and difficult of detection." The molecular biology of genetic transmission and expression is perhaps the most important area of scientific advance in the past two decades. Application of these advances in man has elucidated a large number of genetic errors of metabolism, some of which are described in specific detail in the following chapters.

REFERENCES

HARRIS H: *Garrod's Inborn Errors of Metabolism,* New York: Oxford, 1963

Stanbury JB et al: (eds) *The Metabolic Basis of Inherited Diseases*, 3d ed., New York: McGraw-Hill, 1972

Wyngaarden JB: Human genetic disease: past, present, future. Trans Assoc Am Physicians 85:68, 1972

96 GENETIC DISORDERS OF AMINO ACID METABOLISM

LLOYD H. SMITH, JR.

In a sense, all genetic diseases represent disorders of amino acid metabolism in their phenotypic expression as protein synthesis. A large number of disorders represent specific defects in the synthesis, degradation, or membrane transport of individual amino acids. Three of Garrod's four original "inborn errors of metabolism" were those of amino acid metabolism (albinism, alcaptonuria, and cystinuria). The study of these disorders has greatly enhanced our understanding of normal pathways of amino acid metabolism and transport. In this chapter, only phenylketonuria, homocystinuria, and disorders of branched chain amino acids will be reviewed. Others have been classified as storage diseases (Chap. 97) or as errors in membrane transport (Chap. 98). In Table 96-1, a summary of genetic disorders of amino acid metabolism is presented with references for further information. The inclusion or omission of certain diseases is arbitrary in that they may represent defects in metabolism several steps removed from the parent amino acid.

PHENYLKETONURIA

DEFINITION Phenylketonuria, first described by Folling in 1934, is a metabolic disorder secondary to an inherited deficiency of phenylalanine hydroxylase. This results in the accumulation of phenylalanine and some of its metabolites (notably phenylpyruvate, phenyllactate, phenylacetate and O-hydroxyphenylacetate) and a syndrome of mental deficiency. Other neurologic deficits, epileptic seizures, and reduced pigmentation may also occur.

GENETICS AND PATHOGENESIS Phenylketonuria is transmitted as an autosomal recessive trait, occurring in its clinical (homozygous) form with a frequency of about 1 in 15,000 to 20,000 births in the United States. About 0.64 percent of the inmates in institutions for the mentally defective are patients with homozygous phenylketonuria. Heterozygotes usually exhibit slightly elevated fasting levels of plasma phenylalanine and reduced rates of plasma clearance of phenylalanine after its oral administration. Although some studies have suggested an increased incidence of mental deficiency or psychiatric disturbances in families of patients with phenylketonuria, the heterozygous state has not been demonstrated to be injurious.

In addition to classic phenylketonuria, there are several milder variants of the disorder in which there is greater tolerance for dietary phenylalanine. In these disorders, phenylalanine hydroxylase is also deficient in activity, although the genetic defects are presumably different mutations from that associated with the classic disease. Children born of mothers with phenylketonuria may also exhibit brain damage from intrauterine exposure to the deranged maternal metabolism of phenylalanine.

Phenylalanine is normally hydroxylated in the para position to form tyrosine, involving a complex biochemical reaction catalyzed by phenylalanine hydroxylase with an unconjugated pteridine, 7,8-dihydrobiopterin, as a cofactor. This enzyme is restricted to liver, where it exhibits increasing activity in the first few weeks after birth. Active enzyme fails to appear in the phenylketonuric infant. This results in accumulation of dietary phenylalanine in the plasma and presumably in cells, with secondary diversion (by transamination) into phenylpyruvate, phenyllactate, phenylacetate, and O-hydroxyphenylacetate, all four of these phenyl acids being excreted together with phenylalanine in the urine. Phenylalanine is a competitive inhibitor of tyrosinase on the pathway of melanin synthesis, which explains the decreased pigmentation of hair, eyes, and skin. High levels of phenylalanine in body fluids inhibit transport of amino acids into cells. The resulting deprivation of essential amino acids in the developing brain may be the immediate cause of cerebral damage, although this has not been established. Other explanations relate to altered patterns of synthesis of pharmacodynamic amines (serotonin, norepinephrine, phenylethylamine, etc.).

CLINICAL PRESENTATION AND DIAGNOSIS Retardation of mental development, usually of severe degree, is the major manifestation of phenylketonuria. Since the mental defect is stationary and not progressive in older children or adults, the brain injury appears to be limited to a particularly sensitive stage in brain development. Other neurologic abnormalities sometimes found are tremors, seizures, muscular hypertonicity, hyperkinesis, and EEG abnormalities. As noted, there tends to be reduced pigmentation of skin, hair, and eyes. Eczema has been commonly described.

Early diagnosis is essential for successful treatment since the neurologic abnormalities, once established, are largely irreversible. Diagnosis before one month of age requires the demonstration of grossly elevated levels of plasma phenylalanine. The excretion of the associated metabolites may not be remarkable at this time. Testing by screening for phenylketonuria of all newborn infants and of all infants of thirty days and under when admitted to a hospital is now mandatory in the majority of states. This routine blood testing can be carried out quite simply using the bacterial inhibition assay (Guthrie) or a fluorometric procedure. Positive tests must be carefully followed up with quantitative measurements of plasma phenylalanine and study of urinary metabolites to differentiate the disease from transient hyperphenylalaninemia related to prematurity, tyrosinemia, or heterozygosity. This is important because restrictive diets may be injurious in patients other than those with phenylketonuria. The ferric chloride test, a transient blue or olive-green color appearing on the addition of a few drops of 5% $FeCl_3$ to 5 ml urine, is still useful for

TABLE 96-1
Genetic disorders of amino acid metabolism

Disease	*Enzyme deficiency*	*Signs and symptoms*	*Laboratory abnormalities*	*Transmission*	*References*
Albinism:					
Ocular	Unknown	Absence or marked reduction of pigmentation in the eye, defects in vision	No changes in blood or urine	X-linked recessive	Fitzpatrick TB, Quevedo WC, Jr.,* p. 326
Oculocutaneous	Tyrosinase Tyrosine permease(?)	Hypopigmentation of eye and skin, defects in vision, sensitivity to actinic radiation in both tyrosinase-positive and-negative types	No changes in blood or urine	Autosomal recessive; two types are not allelic	
Alcaptonuria	Homogentisic acid oxidase	Pigmentation of cartilage and other connective tissues (ochronosis), degenerative arthritis, calcification of intervertebral disks	Homogentisic acid elevated in urine; serves as a reducing agent and also forms a dark pigment on standing, especially after alkalinization	Autosomal recessive	La Du BN,* p. 308
Argininosuccinic aciduria	Argininosuccinase	Severe mental retardation, ataxia, seizures, hepatic dysfunction, abnormally friable hair	Elevated plasma and CSF argininosuccinate, citrulline, and sometimes ammonia; argininosuccinate in urine	Autosomal recessive	Shih VE, Efron ML,* p. 370
Carnosinemia	Carnosinase (not established)	Mental retardation, seizures, spasticity, myoclonic jerks	Excessive plasma and urine carnosine and anserine	Probably autosomal recessive	Scriver CR, Perry TL,* p. 476
Citrullinemia	Argininosuccinic acid synthetase	Mental retardation, nausea, vomiting, tremors, hypotonicity, intermittent hyperammonemia	Citrulline elevated in blood and urine; blood NH_3 elevated postprandially; urea normal	Not established; probably autosomal recessive	Shih VE, Efron ML,* p. 370
Cystathioninuria	Cystathionase (pyridoxine dependency in most patients)	Mental deficiency may or may not be present; no other specific clinical picture has emerged	Excessive excretion of cystathionine in urine	Probably autosomal recessive	Frimpter GW,* p. 413
Cystinosis	Not established	Dwarfism, rickets, symptoms of acidosis and advancing renal failure, opacities from cystine deposits in corneas; a few patients have ocular cystinosis only	Renal tubular defects of the de Toni-Fanconi syndrome, uremia, cystine crystals in leukocytes	Autosomal recessive	Schneider JA, Seegmiller JE,* p. 1581
Histidinemia	Histidase (histidine α-deaminase)	Variable mental retardation, possibly a special tendency toward speech and language disorders	Increased histidine in blood and urine; increased excretion of imidazolepyruvate, imidazolelactate, and imidazoleacetate; low plasma glutamate; high blood and urine alanine	Autosomal recessive	La Du BN,* p. 338
Homocystinuria†	Cystathionine synthetase (Pyridoxine dependency?)	Mild mental deficiency (sometimes absent), ectopia lentis, osteoporosis, thromboembolic complications, skeletal deformities resembling Marfan's syndrome	Elevated plasma and urine methionine and homocystine	Autosomal recessive	Gerritsen T, Waisman HA,* p. 404
Hydroxyprolinemia (single patient)	Hydroxyproline oxidase	Severe mental retardation	Free L-hydroxyproline elevated in plasma and urine; bound hydroxyproline normal	Not established	Scriver CR, Efron ML,* p. 351
Hyper-β-alaninemia	β-Alanyl-α-ketoglutaric amino transferase (not established)	Failure of normal growth and development, seizures, somnolence	Increased plasma β-alanine and γ-aminobutyric acid (GABA); increased urine β-alanine, GABA, taurine, γ-aminoisobutyric acid	Not established	Scriver CR, Perry TL,* p. 476
Hyperammonemia (congenital):					
Type I	Carbamyl phosphate synthetase	Vomiting, lethargy, flaccidity	Hyperammonemia, metabolic acidosis, mild elevation of plasma and urinary glycine, cyclic neutropenia	Not established	Freeman JM et al, J Pediatr 65:1039, 1964
Type II	Ornithine transcarbamylase	Vomiting, lethargy, coma, especially after high protein ingestion; muscular rigidity, hepatomegaly, mental retardation	Hyperammonemia, increased plasma glutamine, increased urinary orotic acid and uridine	Not established	Shih VE, Efron ML,* p. 370
Hyperglycinemia (nonketotic)	Glycine decarboxylase (not established)	Mental retardation, seizures, spastic paraplegia	Increased plasma and urinary glycine	Probably autosomal recessive	Nyhan WL,* p. 464
Hyperlysinemia:					
Periodic	L-Lysine NAD oxidoreductase	Vomiting, spasticity, coma, mental retardation, exacerbation by protein ingestion	Hyperlysinemia and hyperargininemia with increase in blood ammonia intermittently, related to protein ingestion	Probably autosomal recessive	Ghadimi H,* p. 393

* *From JB Stanbury et al (eds):* The Metabolic Basis of Inherited Disease, *3d ed., New York: McGraw-Hill, 1972.*

† *This disease is discussed in more detail in the text.*

TABLE 96-1
Genetic disorders of amino acid metabolism *(Continued)*

Disease	*Enzyme deficiency*	*Signs and symptoms*	*Laboratory abnormalities*	*Transmission*	*References*
Hyperlysinemia: Persistent	Not established (block in saccharopine synthesis?)	Vomiting, spasticity, coma, mental retardation, exacerbation by protein ingestion	Hyperlysinemia and hyperlysinuria; no elevation of blood ammonia	Probably autosomal recessive	Ghadimi H,* p. 393
Hyperoxaluria (primary):					
Type I	2-Oxo-glutarate: glyoxylate carboligase	Symptoms and signs of kidney stones and advancing renal failure	Increase in urinary oxalate, glycolate, and glyoxylate	Autosomal recessive	Williams HE, Smith LH, Jr.,* p. 196
Type II	D-Glyceric dehydrogenase	Symptoms and signs of kidney stones and advancing renal failure	Increase in urinary oxalate and L-glyceric acid	Autosomal recessive	Williams HE, Smith LH, Jr.,* p. 196
Hyperprolinemia:					
Type I	Proline oxidase	Often no signs or symptoms; some increased linkage with renal disease	Hyperprolinemia, excess urinary excretion of proline, hydroxyproline, and glycine	Probably autosomal recessive	Scriver CR, Efron ML,* p. 351
Type II	Δ′-Pyrroline-5-carboxylate-dehydrogenase	Usually associated with mental retardation and a convulsive disorder	Same as in type I, but also excess excretion of Δ′-pyrroline-5-carboxylic acid	Probably autosomal recessive	Scriver CR, Efron ML,* p. 351
Hypersarcosinemia	Sarcosine dehydrogenase (not established)	Usually associated with mental deficiency	Increase in plasma and urinary sarcosine	Autosomal recessive	Gerritsen T, Waisman HA,* p. 459
Hypervalinemia†	Valine-α-ketoglutarate transaminase	Mental and somatic retardation, nystagmus, hypotonicity, unresponsiveness, vomiting	Valine elevated in plasma and urine	Presumed autosomal recessive	Dancis J, Levitz M,* p. 426
Isovaleric acidemia†	Probably isovaleryl-CoA dehydrogenase	Mild psychomotor retardation, intention tremor, attacks of acidosis, stupor, and coma; "sweaty-foot smell" of breath	Elevated plasma isovaleric acid	Not established; probably autosomal recessive	Budd MA et al, N Engl J Med 277:321, 1967
Maple syrup urine disease (branched chain ketoaciduria)†	Oxidases of α-ketoisocaproic acid, α-ketoisovaleric acid, α-keto-β-methylvaleric acid	Progressive deterioration of central nervous system function usually beginning shortly after birth and leading to early death; sweet, maple syrup-like odor to urine and sweat	Elevated levels of leucine, isoleucine, valine, and their corresponding keto acids in blood and urine	Autosomal recessive	Dancis J, Levitz M,* p. 426
β-Mercaptolactate-cysteine disulfiduria (single patient)	Not established	Slow development and history of seizures; "placid and hypokinetic"	Excessive urinary excretion of the mixed disulfide of β-mercaptolactate and cysteine	Not established	Crawhall JC et al, Am J Dis Child 117:71, 1969
Methylmalonic aciduria:					
Vitamin B_{12}-responsive	Synthesis of 5′-deoxyadenosylcobalamin (enzyme not established)	Signs and symptoms of recurrent ketoacidosis	Metabolic acidosis, hyperglycinemia and hyperglycinuria, hypoglycemia during attacks; marked methylmalonic aciduria	Probably autosomal recessive	Rosenberg LE,* p. 440
Vitamin B_{12}-unresponsive	Methylmalonyl CoA mutase	Signs and symptoms of recurrent ketoacidosis	Metabolic acidosis, hyperglycinemia and hyperglycinuria, hypoglycemia during attacks; marked methylmalonic aciduria	Probably autosomal recessive	Rosenberg LE,* p. 440
Phenylketonuria†	Phenylalanine hydroxylase	Severe mental deficiency, tremors, seizures, muscular hypertonicity, hyperkinesis, reduced pigmentation	Plasma phenylalanine elevated; phenylalanine, phenylpyruvate, phenyllactate, phenylacetate, and O-hydroxyphenylacetate elevated in urine	Autosomal recessive	Knox WE,* p. 266
Propionic acidemia	Propionyl CoA carboxylase	Developmental retardation, dehydration, lethargy, coma precipitated by high protein ingestion	Recurrent ketoacidosis, elevation of serum glycine and propionic acid; intermittent elevations of serum valine, leucine, and isoleucine	Autosomal recessive	Rosenberg LE,* p. 440
Sulfituria	Sulfite oxidase	Severe neurologic abnormalities at birth, deteriorating to an almost decorticate state; ectopia lentis in single described case	Excessive urinary excretion of sulfite, thiosulfate, and S-sulfo-L-cysteine; reduced urine sulfate	Not established	Laster L et al, J Clin Invest, 46:1082, 1967
Tyrosinemia	*p*-Hydroxyphenylpyruvic acid oxidase(?—not established)	Vomiting, diarrhea, rickets, failure to thrive, hepatosplenomegaly, sometimes mental retardation	Proximal tubular dysfunction with laboratory findings of Fanconi's syndrome; elevation of serum tyrosine and sometimes methionine; marked elevation of urinary excretion of *p*-hydroxyphenyllactic acid	Autosomal recessive	La Du BN, Gjessing LR,* p. 296
Tyrosinosis	Tyrosine transaminase(?) *p*-Hydroxyphenylpyruvic acid oxidase (?—not proved)	Single patient had myasthenia gravis	Excessive urinary excretion of *p*-hydroxyphenylpyruvic acid	Not established	La Du BN, Gjessing LR,* p. 296

screening older children or adults and is usually positive in infants.

TREATMENT The biochemical abnormalities can be corrected by preventing the accumulation of phenylalanine. This is done by a special diet in which protein is replaced by an amino acid mixture low in phenylalanine (Ketonil, Lofenolac). Supplementary foods are given to supply only the amount of L-phenylalanine needed for body growth. The program should attempt to maintain normal weight gain and near-normal plasma phenylalanine levels. The diet should be continued for as long as it is tolerated, with special emphasis on the first 4 years. Normal development has been obtained in some patients treated from early infancy. Little permanent improvement can be achieved by treatment begun later, the main effect being that of prevention of further intellectual deterioration.

HOMOCYSTINURIA

DEFINITION Homocystinuria is a genetic disease resulting from markedly reduced activity of cystathionine synthetase, an enzyme which catalyzes an important step in the transsulfuration pathway converting methionine to cysteine. It is characterized clinically by ectopia lentis, osteoporosis, thromboembolic phenomena, skeletal changes suggestive of Marfan's syndrome, and mental retardation (in approximately 50 percent of patients). There is excessive urinary excretion of homocystine and several other sulfur-containing compounds. Of the genetic disorders of amino acid metabolism, homocystinuria may rank second in frequency, following phenylketonuria. It occurs once in every 20,000 to 40,000 births (see also Chap. 62).

GENETICS AND PATHOGENESIS Homocystinuria is transmitted as an autosomal recessive trait. Heterozygotes have no stigmata of the disease, no detectable plasma homocystine, and no elevation of plasma methionine. They sometimes exhibit delayed plasma clearance of methionine loads given orally or intravenously. Assays of liver biopsy material from parents of homocystinurics (presumed heterozygotes) have revealed cystathionine synthetase activities intermediate between those of patients and controls. Homozygotes exhibit virtual absence of this enzyme activity in liver and brain. Some, but not all, patients have responded to large doses of pyridoxine with marked biochemical improvement. This suggests a defect in cofactor binding, a pyridoxine-dependency syndrome, although pyridoxal phosphate has not been shown to be required for cystathionine synthetase activity.

In the absence of cystathionine synthetase, homocystine and methionine accumulate and cysteine (or cystine) becomes an essential amino acid. There is no clear information about how these chemical derangements result in the diverse structural and functional manifestations of the disease. It has been suggested that the ability of homocystine to form mixed disulfides may inactivate critical sulfhydryl groups of enzymes or impair disulfide cross linkages in structural proteins. No role of cysteine deficiency has been established. Current studies are directed to other sulfur-containing metabolites in urine, such as the demonstration of 5-amino-4-imidazole-carboxamide-5′-S-ribonucleoside, S-adenosylhomocysteine, and homolanthionine.

CLINICAL PRESENTATION AND DIAGNOSIS Patients with homocystinuria often exhibit a superficial resemblance to those with Marfan's syndrome (Chap. 364). Some of the skeletal and connective tissue abnormalities which have been described are ectopia lentis, severe juvenile osteoporsis, kyphosis, scoliosis, genu valgum, deformities of the sternum such as pectus excavatum and pectus carinatum, abnormalities of the palate, and arachnodactyly. Mental deficiency is common, being found in approximately half these patients. When present, it is not usually as severe as that of phenylketonuria. Recurrent arterial and venous thromboses may complicate the course and lead to early death from pulmonary embolism or coronary or carotid occlusion. Patients with homocystinuria tend to resemble one another, with their skeletal deformities, light-colored hair, and coarse skin with malar flush and livido reticularis. Diagnosis is established by finding homocystine in the urine using paper or ion exchange column chromatography. As a disulfide, homocystine will also give a positive nitroprusside reaction in urine, but must then be differentiated from cystine by chromatographic techniques. Plasma methionine level is also elevated.

TREATMENT In the absence of clear evidence of the mechanism by which loss of cystathionine synthetase activity is injurious, current approaches to therapy are not firmly established. All patients should receive a trial with pyridoxine (250 to 500 mg per day). If biochemical improvement occurs, this form of treatment should be continued. Beneficial results may be obtained from the use of a diet low in methionine (20 to 40 mg per kg per day), supplemented by L-cystine. These programs may lead to improvement in the chemical derangements. Whether they will prolong life through reducing thromboembolic complications or will reduce disability has yet to be demonstrated.

MAPLE SYRUP URINE DISEASE (BRANCHED CHAIN KETOACIDURIA)

DEFINITION Maple syrup urine disease, so named because of the characteristic odor of the urine and sweat of affected patients, is a rare genetic disorder of the metabolism of branched chain amino acids and their corresponding keto acids. It is associated with severe neurologic damage and mental retardation occurring in the early neonatal period, usually leading to early death. A few atypical milder cases have been described in older children. Approximately 50 cases have been reported since its initial description in 1954. In two large surveys of newborn infants, the incidence was found to be between 1 in 100,000 and 1 in 250,000 births.

Two other disorders of branched chain amino acid metabolism have been discovered. One child with severe mental and physical retardation has exhibited persistent hypervalinemia in the absence of any abnormality of leucine or isoleucine metabolism. Three patients, two of whom were siblings, have been found with isovaleric acidemia associated with recurrent episodes of vomiting, acidosis, and coma and with mild mental retardation.

GENETICS AND PATHOGENESIS Leucine, isoleucine, and valine are normally metabolized to their corresponding keto acids (α-ketoisocaproic acid, α-keto-β-methylvaleric acid, and α-ketoisovaleric acid, respectively) by transamination. Previous biochemical studies suggested that a common enzyme catalyzed the transamination of all three amino acids, but the transamination defect for valine in leukocytes from the patient with hypervalinemia was specific for this amino acid alone. The branched chain keto acids formed from the corresponding amino acids then undergo oxidative decarboxylation in complex reactions comparable to those catalyzed by pyruvate and α-ketoglutarate oxidases, each keto acid having a specific oxidase. In maple syrup urine disease the activities of all three keto acid oxidases are markedly reduced or virtually absent in brain, kidney, liver, and peripheral leukocytes. The loss of activity of three analogous but seemingly distinct enzymes is unexplained. One postulate is that of a genetic defect in the synthesis of a common enzyme subunit. The disease is transmitted as an autosomal mendelian recessive trait. Some, but not all, presumed heterozygotes have reduced activities of the keto acid oxidases in their leukocytes, but otherwise exhibit no clinical or chemical stigmata of the disease. The metabolic block in these parallel degradative pathways leads to the accumulation of three branched chain keto acids and the corresponding amino acids in blood and their excessive excretion in urine. The mechanism of neurologic damage has not been established, although several hypotheses have been advanced. The keto acid derivatives of leucine and valine inhibit the activity of L-glutamic dehydrogenase in brain homogenates. Another suggestion relates to the inhibition of transfer of other essential amino acids into the central nervous system in the presence of elevated plasma levels of the branched chain amino acids.

In isovaleric acidemia there is deficient activity of isovaleric acid dehydrogenase, which normally converts this compound to β-methylcrotonic acid in the pathway of leucine metabolism. It is probably inherited as a rare autosomal recessive trait.

CLINICAL PRESENTATION AND DIAGNOSIS Infants with maple syrup urine disease are normal at birth but begin within a few days to exhibit progressive deterioration, with lethargy, poor feeding, diminished awareness, hypertonicity alternating with flaccidity, and convulsions. The characteristic urine odor from which the name derives is present. Death generally occurs within the first few weeks of life from severe neurologic damage with respiratory disturbances. If death is delayed, mental retardation becomes apparent. A few patients exhibit a milder form of the disease, with intermittent branched chain ketonuria. The diagnosis is usually first suggested from the odor of the urine, described as sweet, caramel-like, or like maple syrup. The urine gives a positive ferric chloride test and dinitrophenylhydrazine reaction for keto acids. The diagnosis is best established by ion exchange column chromatography of plasma to demonstrate elevated levels of leucine, isoleucine, and valine. Methods for demonstrating the enzyme defect in circulating leukocytes have been described.

The single Japanese child with hypervalinemia had vomiting, lethargy, and failure to thrive beginning soon after birth. There was severe retardation of physical and mental development at age three. The diagnosis was established by the finding of isolated elevation of valine in plasma and urine. The three patients with isovaleric acidemia had recurrent episodes of vomiting, acidosis, and coma accompanied by a characteristic offensive odor (which led to the discovery of the disorder), described as being like cheese or sweaty feet.

TREATMENT The treatment of maple syrup urine disease, like that of phenylketonuria, is based on the use of a diet restricted in the corresponding amino acids beginning early in life before the onset of permanent neurologic damage. In practice this has been very difficult because of the necessity to balance three different amino acids, the ubiquitous distribution of the branched chain amino acids in foods, and the large number of plasma chromatographic analyses required. A few encouraging results have been reported using strict dietary therapy. It is not clear whether such treatment can be omitted in later life. A selective restriction of valine and leucine should offer a rational approach to hypervalinemia and isovaleric acidemia, respectively.

REFERENCES

BUDD MA et al: Clinical features of a new genetic defect of leucine metabolism. New Engl J Med 277:321, 1967

DANCIS J, LEVITZ M: Abnormalities of branched-chain amino acid metabolism [hypervalinemia, branched-chain ketonuria (maple syrup urine disease), isovaleric acidemia], in *The Metabolic Basis of Inherited Disease,* 3d ed., eds JB Stanbury et al, New York: McGraw-Hill, 1972, p. 426

ELSAS LJ et al: Classical maple syrup urine disease: cofactor resistance. Metabolism 21:929, 1972

GERRITSEN T, WAISMAN HA: Homocystinuria, in *The Metabolic Basis of Inherited Disease,* 3d ed., eds JB Stanbury et al, New York: McGraw-Hill, 1972, p. 404

KNOX WE: Phenylketonuria, in *The Metabolic Basis of Inherited Disease,* 3d ed., eds JB Stanbury et al, New York: McGraw-Hill, 1972, p. 266

ROSENBERG LE, SCRIVER CR: Disorders of amino acid metabolism, in *Duncan's Diseases of Metabolism,* 6th ed., ed PK Bondy, Philadelphia: Saunders 1969, p. 366

SCHIMKE RN et al: Homocystinuria, in *Amino Acid Metabolism and Genetic Variation,* ed WL Nyhan, New York: McGraw-Hill, 1967, p. 297

WADA Y et al: Idiopathic hypervalinemia: probably a new entity of inborn error of valine metabolism. Tokoku J Exp Med 81:46, 1963

97 STORAGE DISEASES: ALCAPTONURIA AND OCHRONOSIS, PRIMARY HYPEROXALURIA WITH OXALOSIS, AND CYSTINE STORAGE DISEASE

LLOYD H. SMITH, JR.

A number of genetic diseases are characterized by excessive storage of metabolites in the host. Most often these represent blocks in degradative pathways. Examples may be cited in the glycogen storage disease (Chap. 104), the lipidoses (Gaucher's disease, Fabry's disease, Niemann-Pick disease, Tay-Sachs disease, Tangier disease, metachromatic leukodystrophy) (Chap. 106), certain amino acid degradative diseases (primary hyperoxaluria with oxalosis, alcaptonuria with ochronosis, possibly cystine storage disease), and possibly in some of the mucopolysaccharidoses (e.g., Hurler's syndrome) (Chap. 364). In addition excessive retention of dietary minerals may occur, as in hemochromatosis (Chap. 101) and Wilson's disease (Chap. 103). Tophaceous gout represents a special case, with excessive production and/or renal retention of a metabolic end product, uric acid (Chap. 100). Most of the above disorders have been described elsewhere in this book. This chapter will be concerned only with certain storage diseases of amino acid metabolism.

ALCAPTONURIA AND OCHRONOSIS

DEFINITION Alcaptonuria, one of the original inborn errors of metabolism studied by Garrod, is a rare disorder in the degradative pathway of phenylalanine and tyrosine metabolism. The genetic defect in the activity of the enzyme homogentisic acid oxidase leads to the accumulation and excessive urinary excretion of homogentisic acid. There is an associated deposition of dark pigment in connective tissues (ochronosis) and a particular form of degenerative arthritis. Over 600 cases have been reported.

GENETICS AND PATHOGENESIS Homogentisic acid, a normal intermediate in the metabolism of phenylalanine and tyrosine, is oxidized with opening of the phenyl ring to form maleylacetoacetic acid. The enzyme homogentisic acid oxidase, which catalyzes this step, has been found to be missing in activity in liver and kidney from patients with alcaptonuria. The disease seems to be transmitted as an autosomal mendelian trait, with a frequency of about one in 200,000 births. No biochemical method for detection of presumed heterozygotes has been devised, nor do they exhibit any of the clinical features of the disease. The renal excretion of excessive homogentisic acid (3 to 7 g per day) fully accounts for the reducing properties of urine, gentisic acid being the only other metabolite excreted in excess. At neutral pH or above, homogentisic acid is rapidly oxidized to a brown or black polymer, with darkening of the urine on standing and with staining of wet diapers or linen. The slower accumulation in the body of a similar polymer bound to cartilage and other connective tissues is presumably the origin of ochronosis. Recently an enzyme has been described in skin and cartilage which oxidizes homogentisic acid to a melanin-like polymer. The mechanism by which this oxidation produces cartilagenous degeneration and arthritis is not clear.

CLINICAL PRESENTATION AND DIAGNOSIS

Alcaptonuria is a benign disorder until middle life, when degenerative joint changes begin in the majority of cases. Prior to this time the darkening of urine is often unnoticed, although a positive but atypical Benedict's test for urine glucose may call it to one's attention. The increasing use of the glucose oxidase test will diminish the importance of this method of discovery. With the onset of arthritis, the large joints and the spine are affected with pain and stiffness, interspersed with periods of acute inflammation, which may resemble rheumatoid arthritis. Limitation of motion of the joints and ankylosis of the lumbosacral spine often occur later in the course of the disease. The roentgenogram of the spine is often almost pathognomonic, with degeneration and dense calcification of the intervertebral disks and resulting narrowing of the spaces. Ochronotic pigmentation may often be seen in the transmitted blueness of cartilages of the ear, nose, and costochondral junctions, and in brown areas in the sclerae, most frequently located at the insertions of the lateral rectus muscles. A high incidence of degenerative cardiovascular disease has been described in older ochronotic patients, but a cause-and-effect relationship has not been firmly established. The diagnosis is usually made from the triad of *arthritis, ochronotic pigmentation,* and *urine which darkens* on the addition of strong alkali. As noted, the urine reduces alkaline copper solutions, but since it turns black in the process, the erroneous diagnosis of glucosuria can be avoided. Homogentisic aciduria can be further identified by the ability of the urine to blacken undeveloped photographic film exposed to light. It may be conclusively demonstrated by chemical tests, chromatographic characteristics, or a specific enzymatic assay. Reversible acquired ochronosis has been described in the past after the prolonged use of carbolic acid dressings for cutaneous ulcers.

TREATMENT Alcaptonuria carries with it no metabolic disadvantage other than the deposition of polymerized pigment in connective tissues and the associated degenerative changes. Ascorbic acid, as a strong reducing agent, will impede the oxidation and polymerization of homogentisic acid in vitro. Its use in large doses has been suggested as a possible means of preventing pigment formation and deposition in ochronotics, but its efficacy has not been demonstrated. The long and relatively benign course of the illness discourages attempts at rigid control of phenylalanine or tyrosine in the diet. Symptomatic treatment is similar to that of osteoarthritis (Chap. 361).

PRIMARY HYPEROXALURIA AND OXALOSIS

DEFINITION Primary hyperoxaluria is a genetic disorder characterized biochemically by continued excessive urinary excretion of oxalic acid and clinically by calcium oxalate nephrolithiasis and nephrocalcinosis. At postmortem examination calcium oxalate is usually found to be widely deposited in the tissues, a condition called oxalosis. In its typical form primary hyperoxaluria generally leads to uremia and early death. A few milder cases have been described in adult life with recurrent calcium oxalate kidney stones.

GENETICS AND PATHOGENESIS Primary hyperoxaluria has been shown to represent two distinct genetic disorders, associated with glycolic aciduria (type I) and L-glyceric aciduria (type II), respectively. They are described here together, since they have similar levels of urinary oxalate and are indistinguishable clinically. The excessive synthesis of oxalate in glycolic aciduria results from a block in an alternate route of metabolism of its precursor, glyoxylic acid. The activity of the enzyme α-ketoglutarate:glyoxylate carboligase, which catalyzes the synthesis of α-hydroxy-β-keto adipic acid, has been found to be markedly reduced in liver, spleen, and kidney preparations. The resulting expansion of the glyoxylate pool behind the site of the metabolic block leads to its excessive oxidation to oxalic acid and reduction to glycolic acid. All three of these 2-carbon acids are excreted in increased amounts in the urine. The disease seems most likely to be transmitted as an autosomal mendelian recessive trait, but no means of detecting presumed heterozygotes has been found. In L-glyceric aciduria there is absent activity of D-glyceric dehydrogenase (demonstrated in leukocytes), an enzyme which catalyzes the reduction of hydroxypyruvic acid in the catabolic pathway of serine metabolism. The accumulated hydroxypyruvate is reduced by lactic dehydrogenase to the unnatural L isomer of glyceric acid, which is excreted in the urine. The reduction of hydroxypyruvate is coupled enzymatically to the oxidation of glyoxylate to oxalate, catalyzed by lactic dehydrogenase, as the probable explanation of the resulting hyperoxaluria. L-Glyceric aciduria is transmitted as an autosomal recessive trait, and partial reductions in D-glyceric dehydrogenase activity are found in heterozygotes. The pathogenesis of stone formation, nephrocalcinosis, and oxalosis seems to relate directly to the insolubility of calcium oxalate. The disease can be simulated in animals, and in man, by pyridoxine deficiency, which presumably inhibits the transamination of glyoxylate to glycine. It has been demonstrated that patients with ileal disease may have hyperoxaluria and calcium oxalate stones secondary to bacterial degradation of glycine-conjugated bile salts. These patients have normal or low urinary glycolate excretion and no detectable urinary L-glycerate.

CLINICAL PRESENTATION AND DIAGNOSIS

Primary hyperoxaluria usually presents in childhood with recurrent kidney stones, with or without radiographically demonstrable nephrocalcinosis (Chap. 275). Rarely renal failure secondary to nephrocalcinosis may be the initial finding. The course of the childhood form of the disease is usually that of progressive renal failure leading to death from uremia. In adults kidney stones are frequent and occasionally mild nephrocalcinosis is found, but renal function is usually well preserved. The diagnosis is established by demonstrating excessive excretion of oxalic acid in the absence of pyridoxine deficiency or ileal disease with altered metabolism of bile salts. The normal child or adult excretes less than 60 mg oxalic acid/1.73 m^2/24 hr. Patients with primary hyperoxaluria usually excrete at least two or three times that amount. The differential diagnosis of the glycolic aciduria (most frequent) and L-glyceric aciduria subvariants depends on specific measurements of those metabolites in urine.

TREATMENT There is no specific treatment for primary hyperoxaluria at this time. Large doses of pyridoxine (100 mg per day) may reduce urine oxalate, but the effect is not striking. Measures which may reduce the risk of stone formation are of use, such as forcing fluids, the use of a high phosphate regimen, and oral magnesium oxide (Chap. 275). Because of the seriousness of the disorder, attempts are being made to develop an inhibitor of oxalate synthesis, comparable to the use of allopurinol in gout.

CYSTINOSIS AND FANCONI'S SYNDROME

DEFINITION Cystine storage disease, or cystinosis (Lignac-de Toni-Fanconi syndrome), is a rare genetic disorder, usually found in childhood in association with Fanconi's syndrome. Rarely, ocular and systemic cystine storage occurs in an adult form in the absence of renal disease. Fanconi's syndrome is a descriptive phrase for a group of physiologic abnormalities which occur with proximal renal tubular dysfunction, notably glucosuria, generalized amino aciduria, phosphaturia, and renal tubular acidosis. Cystinosis is only one of many diseases which may be associated with Fanconi's syndrome, a classification of which is given in Table 97-1.

GENETICS AND PATHOGENESIS The metabolic defect resulting in cystine storage has not yet been discovered. A number of enzymes in cystine metabolism have been assayed without finding any consistent abnormality, and earlier claims of reduced levels of blood cystine reductase have not been confirmed. Marked increases in cystine have been found in circulating leukocytes and in fibroblasts grown in tissue culture from patients with cystinosis. The free cystine is compartmentalized within the lysosomes of the cell. The disease seems to be transmitted as an autosomal recessive trait, with heterozygotes demonstrating intermediate levels of intracellular cystine. Plasma cystine levels are usually normal or slightly elevated only. The biochemical link between cystine storage and proximal renal tubular dysfunction is obscure in the childhood form of the disease and missing in adults. Cystine has the ability to form mixed disulfides with sulfhydryl groups. It has been suggested that the injurious effect of cystine storage may result from inhibition of sulfhydryl-containing enzymes by the formation of half-cystine residues on the proteins. A number of the other agents which cause the tubular dysfunction of Fanconi's syndrome are known inhibitors of sulfhydryl-requiring enzymes.

As outlined in Table 97-1, Fanconi's syndrome may be of diverse origins, both inherited and acquired. It represents a nonspecific pattern of failure of proximal renal

TABLE 97-1
Classifications of Fanconi's syndrome

- *I* Idiopathic
  - *A* Sporadic
  - *B* Familial
- *II* As part of a genetic disease
  - *A* Cystinosis
  - *B* Wilson's disease
  - *C* Tyrosinemia
  - *D* Lowe's syndrome
  - *E* Hereditary fructose intolerance (with fructose)
- *III* Medullary cystic disease
- *IV* Acquired
  - *A* Abnormality of protein metabolism
    - *1* Nephrotic syndrome
    - *2* Multiple myeloma
    - *3* Sjögren's syndrome
    - *4* Amyloidosis
  - *B* Drugs
    - *1* Outdated tetracycline
    - *2* 6-Mercaptopurine
    - *3* Isophthalanilide
  - *C* Heavy metals
    - *1* Mercury
    - *2* Uranium
    - *3* Cadmium
  - *D* Malignancy
- *V* Experimental (animals)
  - *A* Maleic acid
  - *B* Malonic acid

SOURCE: *After RC Morris, Jr., The clinical spectrum of Fanconi's syndrome. Calif Med 108:225, 1968.*

tubular absorptive function, varying greatly in the degree of severity and the spectrum of functions impaired. The individual disease processes will not be discussed here. In idiopathic Fanconi's syndrome and that associated with cystinosis, microdissection studies have demonstrated a consistent structural change in the proximal tubule, the so-called "swan neck deformity." The proximal tubule is shortened and exhibits atrophy with flattened epithelium in the region adjacent to a normal-appearing glomerulus. These epithelial changes are not specific, however, and may merely represent the structural manifestations of injury.

CLINICAL PRESENTATION AND DIAGNOSIS

Cystine storage disease with Fanconi's syndrome is a serious disorder which usually leads to death from uremia by the age of ten. Failure to thrive and severe resistant rickets with stunting of growth develop in the first few months of life. Rickets results from several derangements: (1) failure of tubular reabsorption of phosphate with hypophosphatemia, (2) proximal renal tubular acidosis with bicarbonate wastage and chronic systemic acidosis, (3) hypercalcuria secondary to acidosis, and (4) the inhibition of osteoid calcification (vitamin D resistance) produced by azotemia. A more complete description of rickets and osteomalacia is presented elsewhere (Chaps. 347 and 350). Secondary hyperparathyroidism is a frequent complication. Glucosuria may be scanty and intermittent or profuse and constant at a normal blood glucose level; it is sometimes sufficient to produce ketosis and contribute to further exacerbation of acidosis. Excessive urinary loss of potassium associated with renal tubular acidosis may lead to hypokalemia with muscle weakness or paralysis. Potassium depletion may produce "clear-cell nephropathy" with further deterioration of renal tubular function, especially a renal tubular concentration defect productive of polyuria. Generalized amino aciduria occurs, with a nonspecific pattern. Although cystine is usually excreted in excess, the urinary concentration is not sufficient to lead to cystine kidney stones. Hypouricemia may result from failure of reabsorption of uric acid. It has been found that patients with Fanconi's syndrome excrete lysozyme and light chains of gamma-globulins in the urine as well. Pyelonephritis is frequent and may contribute, along with interstitial fibrosis, to the onset of renal failure. The idiopathic Fanconi's syndrome may occur in an identical clinical and pathologic combination except for the absence of cystine storage. Individual patients may exhibit some but not all of the proximal tubular defects. The clinical presentation may be dominated by other manifestations of the primary disease productive of Fanconi's syndrome (Table 97-1). Rarely, cystinosis may occur in the adult in the absence of renal dysfunction (Cogan's syndrome). Crystalline rods or plates of cystine are found in the cornea and conjunctiva as the only manifestation of adult cystinosis. Similar ocular cystinosis occurs in the infantile form of cystinosis, together with peripheral retinopathy characterized by patchy areas of depigmentation and pigment clumps.

The diagnosis of *Fanconi's syndrome* depends on the demonstration of the characteristic pattern of proximal renal tubular defects, of which the most important are phosphaturia, generalized amino aciduria, glucosuria, and renal tubular acidosis of the proximal (bicarbonate flooding) type. All these defects may be found individually or in various combinations, and may even vary with time in a given patient. It is therefore most useful to describe the actual physiologic derangements rather than to take refuge in the eponym. Cystinosis as cystine crystals may be demonstrated by slit-lamp examination of the eye, or may be found in bone marrow or circulating leukocytes. Cystinotic leukocytes have very high levels of cystine by chemical analysis, even in the absence of demonstrable crystals. The characteristic retinopathy may be one of the earliest manifestations.

TREATMENT Treatment would logically be directed toward the disease resulting in Fanconi's syndrome and toward replacement therapy to compensate for renal dysfunction. Some of the diseases listed in Table 97-1 can be treated (Wilson's disease, hereditary fructose intolerance, etc.); others cannot. In the absence of specific information about its biochemical defect, attempts to treat cystinosis have generally been unrewarding. The use of D-penicillamine or dimercaptopropanol has been advocated in an attempt to regenerate active sulfhydryl groups on enzymes (see Wilson's disease, Chap. 103). The use of these agents has not resulted in objective evidence of improvement. Cystine is synthesized from the essential amino acid methionine, so that specific dietary treatment has not been vigorously pursued. Renal transplantation has been carried out successfully in at least six children with cystinotic renal failure. Renal biopsies have demonstrated cystine accumulation in the donor kidneys, so that the long-term success of this procedure remains to be evaluated. Treatment of the secondary physiologic derangements has been more successful and has been directed toward replacement of calcium, phosphate, sodium, and potassium to reverse chronic acidosis, rickets (osteomalacia in the adult), and hypokalemia. Large amounts of vitamin D are required (usually 50,000 to 400,000 IU daily) to promote normal calcification of bone. It has been reported that vitamin D may improve certain parameters of tubular function as well, reducing amino aciduria, glucosuria, and bicarbonate wasting, possibly through reduction of the associated secondary hyperparathyroidism. Shohl's solution (98 g sodium citrate and 140 g citric acid per liter) is a suitable source of buffer base for chronic acidosis. Chronic potassium supplementation is not usually required after its initial repletion and the correction of acidosis. Improved healing of rickets may occur with supplemental phosphate if phosphaturia is severe. Despite considerable symptomatic improvement and healing of rickets, progressive renal damage in cystinosis leads to early death from uremia. Adult cystinosis is a benign disorder which does not require treatment. The treatment of adult Fanconi's syndrome is similar to that described for the infantile form, but the prognosis is much better.

REFERENCES

ADMIRAND WH et al: Hyperoxaluria and bowel disease. Trans Assoc Am Physicians 84:307, 1971

LA DU BN: Alcaptonuria, in *The Metabolic Basis of Inherited Disease,* 3d ed., eds JB Stanbury et al, New York: McGraw-Hill, 1972, p. 308

O'BRIEN WM et al: Biochemical, pathologic, and clinical aspects of alcaptonuria, ochronosis, and ochronotic arthropathy. Am J Med 34:813, 1963

SCHNEIDER JA, SEEGMILLER JE: Cystinosis and the Fanconi syndrome, in *The Metabolic Basis of Inherited Disease,* 3d ed., eds JB Stanbury et al, New York: McGraw-Hill, 1972, p. 1581

SCHULMAN JD et al: Cystine, cysteine, and glutathione metabolism in normal and cystinotic fibroblasts in vitro, and in cultured normal amniotic fluid cells. Clin Chim Acta 35:383, 1971

WILLIAMS HE, SMITH LH, JR.: Primary Hyperoxaluria, in *The Metabolic Basis of Inherited Disease,* 3d ed., eds JB Stanbury et al, New York: McGraw-Hill, 1972, p. 196

98 ERRORS IN MEMBRANE TRANSPORT: CYSTINURIA, RENAL GLYCOSURIA, AND RENAL TUBULAR ACIDOSIS

LLOYD H. SMITH, JR.

The transfer of metabolites across cell membranes is usually an active energy-requiring process of considerable specificity. The enzymology of these processes and the required structural characteristics of cell membranes are poorly understood, although this now represents an important area of biochemical and biophysical investigation. A number of diseases in man are best described as genetic defects in active transport of specific substances across epithelial cell membranes. In none of them has a specific enzymatic or structural defect been identified, other than in the description of the functional derangement. It is possible that defects may occur in the active transport of metabolites among the specific compartments or organelles within cells.

Some of the genetic diseases which might be classified as errors in membrane transport are cystinuria; Hartnup disease; hereditary renal tubular acidosis; renal glycosuria, familial renal gout; vasopressin-resistant diabetes insipidus; congenital hemolytic anemia with high sodium, low potassium in the red cells; familial goiter with iodide transport defect; methionine malabsorption syndrome; isolated tryptophan malabsorption (blue diaper syndrome); glucose and galactose malabsorption disease; congenital alkalosis with diarrhea (chloridorrhea); and hereditary intestinal malabsorption of vitamin B_{12}. Hemochromatosis might qualify in this category as an error excessive transport of iron. There are data which suggest that vitamin D–resistant rickets ("phosphate diabetes") represents a defect in vitamin D metabolism rather than a primary transport defect. Similarly cystinosis with the Fanconi syndrome seems to represent a disorder in cystine metabolism rather than a primary renal tubular defect. This section will be limited to brief presentations of cystinuria, Hartnup disease, renal glycosuria, and hereditary renal tubular acidosis.

CYSTINURIA

DEFINITION Cystinuria is a genetic disorder (or group of closely related disorders) characterized by continued excessive excretion of the dibasic amino acids cystine, lysine, arginine, and ornithine. This results from a transport defect for these amino acids in the renal tubule. Similar transport defects occur in the intestinal mucosa. The sole clinical manifestations are those of recurrent cystine kidney stones and their sequelae. Patients tend to be of short stature, which has been attributed, without supporting evidence, to lysine deficiency.

GENETICS AND PATHOGENESIS Cystinuria has been known to be a familial disease for almost a century. It was one of the four original "inborn errors of metabolism" studies by Sir Archibald Garrod, who demonstrated its transmission in a pattern consistent with autosomal recessive inheritance. Further advances awaited the application of modern methods of amino acid analysis and the study of tubular transport in the kidney and in intestinal mucosal biopsies in vitro. In approximately two-thirds of the families of affected patients the presumed heterozygotes have normal levels of urinary dibasic amino acids. In the remaining families heterozygotes excrete increased amounts of cystine and lysine. At least one additional phenotype can be identified on the basis of intestinal transport studies. Several families have been studied with different genetic types in conjugal heterozygotes of cystinuria. The resulting patterns of double heterozygote defects have been interpreted as evidence for multiple allelic mutations. The incidence of homozygous cystinuria is approximately 1:20,000.

For many years cystinuria was attributed to a defect in cystine metabolism and was often confused with cystine storage disease (cystinosis). Dent and Rose first demonstrated by clearance techniques that impaired renal tubular reabsorption of the specific amino acids cystine, lysine, and arginine was the explanation of aminoaciduria. Subsequent studies indicated similar defects in tubular reabsorption of ornithine and of the mixed disulfide cysteine-homocysteine. Clearance of cystine may significantly exceed glomerular filtration rate, indicating net tubular secretion of this amino acid. Plasma levels of the involved amino acids are reduced. A common renal tubular mechanism has been confirmed by competition of lysine, arginine, and ornithine for transport during infusion studies. A common transport mechanism for these three amino acids has also been found in tissue-slice preparations of kidney in vitro. It has not been possible to demonstrate a defect in cystine transport in vitro in renal biopsies from patients with cystinuria. Rarely, excretion of cystine or the other dibasic amino acids may occur as isolated defects. The interrelation of these transport defects at the level of the renal tubule remains to be clarified.

The transport defect for dibasic amino acids in cystinuria is also found in the intestine. This was first demonstrated by oral tolerance tests. It has been clearly confirmed in studies of active transport in jejunal mucosal biopsy specimens in vitro. At least three patterns of mucosal transport can be identified. With impaired absorption, lysine and ornithine are decarboxylated by intestinal bacteria to cadaverine and putrescine, respectively. These diamines are partially metabolized to pyrrolidine and piperidine, and all these compounds are excreted in increased amounts in cystinuric urine. No impairment of amino acid transport has been found in tissues other than the renal tubule and the intestinal mucosa in cystinuria.

Normal urinary excretion of cystine varies with size and diet, but has an upper normal range of about 18 mg per g creatinine. In homozygous cystinuria cystine excretion usually varies between 0.4 to 1.0 g per day, although values as high as 3.0 g per day have been found. The solubility of cystine in urine is approximately 350 to 400 mg per liter. Supersaturation and crystallization readily occur, particularly during nocturnal concentration of the urine. The accretion of such crystals as stones, with the resulting complications of obstruction and infection, is the direct cause of disability in cystinuria.

DIAGNOSIS The clinical manifestations of cystine kidney stones are indistinguishable from those of other kidney stones: flank pain, colic, hematuria, obstructive uropathy, infection. Cystine stones are as densely radiopaque as calcium-containing kidney stones. In overall incidence they constitute approximately 1 to 2 percent of all kidney stones. It is important to establish the composition of kidney stones in order to institute rational programs of stone prophylaxis (Chap. 275).

The most direct diagnostic procedure is that of stone analysis because cystine stones occur only in the genetic disorder cystinuria. The appearance of cystine crystals in the sediment of concentrated, acidified (addition of glacial acetic acid to pH 4.5), chilled urine specimens usually indicates a cystine concentration of greater than 200 to 250 mg per liter. The crystals are hexagonal plates resembling the formula of a benzene ring. The nitroprusside test for cystine is a nonspecific reaction for sulfhydryl groups after reduction of disulfides by sodium cyanide. It can be made semiquantitative for cystine in the absence of other sulfhydryl compounds.

The specific aminoaciduria of cystine, lysine, arginine, and ornithine can be directly demonstrated by paper or ion exchange column chromatography of urine. This pattern is diagnostic of genetic cystinuria. The urinary amino acid pattern of cystinuria may sometimes be found in the rare disorder of familial pancreatitis.

TREATMENT As a genetic disease cystinuria cannot be "cured" in the host (except by renal homotransplantation). In order to prevent formation and growth of stones, attempts are made to reduce the concentration of cystine in urine and to increase the solubility of cystine at a given urine concentration. Urinary excretion of cystine can sometimes be minimized by a diet low in methionine, the most important cystine precursor. Of greater practicality, cystine concentration can be reduced by increasing urine volume by forcing fluids, especially at night. Some increase in cystine solubility is obtained by alkalinizing the urine, but the solubility curve rises steeply only at pHs higher than 7.2.

A more direct approach is that of forming mixed disulfides of cysteine with other sulfhydryl compounds with enhancement of solubility. The use of D-penicillamine (1 to 2 g daily) leads to the excretion of a soluble cysteine-penicillamine disulfide (solubility fifty times greater than cystine) with reduction of cystine excretion below saturation concentrations. Pyridoxine supplementation (50 to 100 mg) should be given to prevent secondary deficiency of the vitamin, which forms a complex with penicillamine. Unfortunately, D-penicillamine is frequently toxic (causing fever, rash, arthralgias, nephrotic syndrome, pancytopenia), so that its use should be reserved for those patients who cannot be treated successfully by other means. Newer compounds, such as N-acetyl-D-penicillamine, may prove to be equally effective with less toxicity.

HARTNUP DISEASE

Hartnup disease (also called H disease) is a genetic disorder of the transport of a group of monoaminomonocarboxylic acids which share a common transport mechanism in the renal tubule and in the intestinal mucosa. The disease, so far described in about 43 patients, seems to be the homozygous manifestation of an autosomal recessive trait; the heterozygous state is not detectable by current techniques. Hartnup disease is characterized by massive aminoaciduria of alanine, serine, threonine, asparagine, glutamine, valine, leucine, isoleucine, phenylalanine, tyrosine, tryptophan, histidine, and citrulline. In contrast to what occurs in cystinuria, the associated intestinal defect is more important in producing the symptoms of the disease—intermittent pellagra-like rash appearing after exposure to sunlight, attacks of cerebellar ataxia often accompanying the skin manifestations, and psychiatric changes varying from emotional instability to dementia. Impaired absorption allows for bacterial degradation of amino acids which may (1) lead to nicotinamide deficiency from loss of precursor tryptophan, thereby producing pellagra, and (2) allow for the production and absorption of toxic metabolic products injurious to the central nervous system. The specific amino acid metabolites responsible for the signs and symptoms of cerebral and cerebellar dysfunction have not been identified. An isolated defect in tryptophan absorption, the blue diaper syndrome, does not result in a rash or in cerebellar dysfunction. The diagnosis can be established by the pattern of urinary amino acids, measured by paper or ion exchange chromatography. Most patients respond well to maintenance treatment with oral nicotinamide (50 to 200 mg per day). A high-protein diet is also recommended to counter the amino acid loss in the intestine and in the urine.

RENAL GLYCOSURIA

DEFINITION Renal glycosuria is a genetic disorder in which glucose is excreted in the urine at normal concentrations of blood glucose. In order to avoid confusion with other conditions associated with melituria, Marble's strict criteria should be followed (Chap. 89): (1) glycosuria occurs in the absence of hyperglycemia; (2) all specimens of urine should contain glucose with relatively little fluctuation in glycosuria related to diet; (3) the oral glucose tolerance test result is normal (sometimes slightly flat); (4) the reducing substance is specifically identified as glucose, ruling out other meliturias such as pentosuria, fructosuria, galactosuria, sucrosuria, maltosuria, mannoheptulosuria; (5) the storage and utilization of carbohydrates are normal. By these criteria, including the absence of other disorders of proximal renal tubular function, renal glycosuria can be identified as a rare (94 cases in 50,000 cases of melituria at the Joslin Clinic) isolated transport defect. Use of the more liberal criteria proposed by Lawrence, i.e., glycosuria which occurs with a normal glucose tolerance test result, will permit detection of many more abnormalities.

GENETICS AND PATHOGENESIS Current information is most consistent with the transmission of renal glycosuria as a mendelian dominant characteristic, although the suggestion has been made that the defect may be expressed in heterozygotes with homozygotes representing severer forms of the disease. Diabetes mellitus is frequently found in the families of patients with renal glycosuria. Whether renal glycosuria defined by the strict Marble criteria is a precursor of diabetes is disputed. Many patients with renal glycosuria by the Lawrence criteria will develop clinical diabetes mellitus within a few years of diagnosis.

No consistent structural alteration has been demonstrated in the renal tubule by light or electron microscopy. Most studies of the renal defect have been carried out by classical clearance techniques. Plasma glucose is completely filtrable in the glomerulus and is reabsorbed by an active process in the proximal tubule. The biochemical basis of active reabsorption of glucose has not been demonstrated; specifically, no intermediary product has been found. Reabsorption exhibits saturation kinetics with a transfer maximum (Tm) of about 325 ± 36 mg per min per 1.73 m^2 in the normal adult. Clearance studies in renal glycosuria have failed to yield a consistent pattern. In some patients a low Tm for glucose has been found; in others the Tm has been normal but there has been an increased splay in the curve describing the relationship of glucose reabsorbed to that filtered. Renal glycosuria could result from any one of the following defects: decrease in the anatomic mass of the proximal tubule in relation to its glomerulus (glomerulotubular imbalance), abnormal distribution of the transport system relative to glomerular filtration whether on a functional or anatomic basis, an abnormality in the presumed enzymatic step or steps (permeability, hypothetical membrane carrier, energy-yielding reactions) which constitute the active transport process. It is likely that there may be different genetic and pathogenetic forms of the disease.

DIAGNOSIS AND CLINICAL IMPLICATIONS The criteria for diagnosis have been included in the definition. It is important to identify the reducing substance as glucose (by glucose oxidase, for example) and also to rule out other primary or secondary renal tubular defects (e.g., aminoaciduria, phosphaturia, renal tubular acidosis). Most patients with renal glycosuria have no defect in intestinal transport of sugars. The related disorder of glucose and galactose malabsorption is characterized by impaired intestinal absorption of these monosaccharides and by renal glycosuria. In one family, renal glycosuria was coupled with hyperglycinuria (glucoglycinuria). The prognosis of renal glycosuria appears to be excellent except insofar as it may herald subsequent clinical diabetes. No treatment is required.

RENAL TUBULAR ACIDOSIS

DEFINITION Renal tubular acidosis (RTA) is a clinical disorder or group of disorders characterized by inability of the kidney to excrete an appropriately acid urine. This results in a persistent metabolic acidosis with hyperchloremia, and may be complicated by potassium depletion, hypercalcuria, or both. RTA may occur as an isolated tubular defect (sporadic or familial) or in association with dysproteinemic states, hyperthyroidism, vitamin D intoxication, and amphotericin B toxicity. The syndrome of RTA may be closely simulated by the chronic administration of potent carbonic anhydrase inhibitors. Its extracellular fluid pattern of hyperchloremic acidosis may be found following bilateral ureterosigmoid transplantations, during the ingestion of large amounts of ammonium chloride, or in some patients with chronic pyelonephritis.

GENETICS AND PATHOGENESIS Although often secondary to other metabolic disorders, RTA may occur with otherwise normal or nearly normal renal function and in the absence of associated diseases. Some of these cases have appeared to be sporadic; others have exhibited definite familial aggregation. The pattern of inheritance, including transmission in three successive generations, is consistent with a mendelian dominant trait. It seems unlikely that the transient infantile form of RTA, with a negative family history, represents the same disorder.

A complete discussion of the pathogenesis of RTA would demand a full treatment of the role of the kidney in the defense of acid-base balance. In brief, the kidney serves this homeostatic function in several closely related ways: by excretion of certain anionic products of metabolism (phosphate, sulfate), by conservation of filtered bicarbonate, by tubular secretion of hydrogen ions in exchange for sodium, and by tubular synthesis and excretion of ammonia. In RTA phosphate and sulfate excretions are not impaired in the absence of secondary renal failure. Normally, filtered bicarbonate is largely reclaimed in the proximal renal tubule by hydrogen ion exchange for sodium. This mechanism (as measured by the Tm for bicarbonate reabsorption) is usually unimpaired in RTA. The excretion of ammonia is often reduced, but only in proportion to the reduced urine acidity. The most plausible mechanism for RTA is that of inability of the distal renal tubule to develop a steep H^+ gradient between extracellular fluid and tubular urine. This transport defect or "gradient defect" for H^+ in the distal tubule results in reduced urine titratable acidity and ammonia, increased urinary loss of sodium and potassium (due to increased tubular exchange of potassium in lieu of H^+ for sodium), and systemic acidosis. Sustained acidosis results in mobilization of calcium from bone and hypercalcuria. A few patients have been described with "proximal RTA," i.e., a partial failure of bicarbonate reabsorption with flooding of the normal distal tubular acidification mechanism.

A second form of RTA has been described which is due to a defect in proximal tubular reabsorption of bicarbonate. In "proximal RTA," bicarbonate floods the normal distal H^+ secretory mechanism leading to impaired acidification. In contrast to what occurs in clasicial RTA, the Tm for bicarbonate is reduced. This disorder may occur as an isolated tubular defect or as part of the Fanconi syndrome. It has been described with heavy metal poisoning (cadmium, mercury), Wilson's disease, Lowe's syndrome, hereditary fructose intolerance, galactosemia, and also in some patients with dysproteinemic states.

DIAGNOSIS AND CLINICAL IMPLICATIONS The diagnosis of RTA depends upon demonstration of impaired acidification of the urine in the face of systemic acidosis and in the absence of uremia. In mild cases this may require a further acid challenge (0.1 g ammonium chloride per kg body weight). The serum chloride is usually elevated commensurate with the reduction in serum bicarbonate. Other disorders noted above which may lead to secondary impairment of renal tubular acidification must be excluded. The most important complications of RTA are potassium depletion (weakness, paralysis, secondary renal tubular dysfunction) hypercalcuria (nephrocalcinosis, nephrolithiasis, osteomalacia, or rickets), pyelonephritis, and renal failure secondary to these factors.

TREATMENT Acidosis, hypercalcuria, and potassium wasting are usually corrected by the oral administration of 1.0 to 1.5 mEq per kg per day of sodium bicarbonate, given in three divided doses. Alkali replacement may be better tolerated as Shohl's solution (140 g citric acid and 98 g hydrated crystals of sodium citrate per liter), given in a dosage of 50 to 100 ml per day in divided doses. The amount of alkali given should be sufficient to return the serum bicarbonate and pH to a normal range. Supplementary potassium and/or calcium and vitamin D may be required temporarily until body stores of these minerals have been repleted. In proximal RTA, larger amounts of sodium bicarbonate or citrate are often required to return extracellular fluid bicarbonate toward normal because of continued excessive urinary bicarbonate wastage.

REFERENCES

JEPSON JB: Hartnup disease, in *The Metabolic Basis of Inherited Disease*, 3d ed., eds JB Stanbury et al, New York: McGraw-Hill, 1972, p. 1486

KRANE SM: Renal glycosuria, in *The Metabolic Basis of Inherited Disease*, 3d ed., eds JB Stanbury et al, New York: McGraw-Hill 1972, p. 1536

MARBLE A: Non-diabetic melituria, in *The Treatment of Diabetes Mellitus*, eds EP Joslin et al, Philadelphia: Lea & Febiger, 1959

MILNE MD: Renal tubular dysfunction, in *Diseases of the Kidney*, 2d ed., eds MB Strauss, LG Welt, Boston: Little, Brown, 1971, p. 1071

MORRIS RC, JR: Renal tubular acidosis: mechanisms, classification and implications. N Engl J Med 281:1405, 1969

SELDIN DW, WILSON JD: Renal tubular acidosis, in *The Metabolic Basis of Inherited Disease*, 3d ed., eds JB Stanbury et al, New York: McGraw-Hill, 1972, p.1548

STEPHENS AD, WATTS RWE: The treatment of cystinuria with N-acetyl-D-penicillamine, a comparison with the results of

D-penicillamine treatment. Quart J Med 40:355, 1971
THIER SD, SEGAL S: Cystinuria, in *The Metabolic Basis of Inherited Disease*, 3d ed., eds JB Stanbury et al, New York: McGraw-Hill, 1972, p. 1504

99
THE CARCINOID SYNDROME

JOHN A. OATES

The association of carcinoid tumors with cutaneous flushes, telangiectasia, diarrhea, cardiac valvular lesions, and bronchial constriction eluded recognition until 1953. Once this connection was established by Thorson, Biörk, Björkman, and Waldenström, and independently by Isler and Hedinger, it was clear that the syndrome was mediated by release of one or more biologically active agents by the tumor. Serotonin was the first such agent to be discovered, and overproduction of this amine is the most consistent biochemical indicator of the carcinoid syndrome. Serotonin, however, is not the sole mediator of the clinical syndrome. These tumors vary in their synthesis of indoles and may elaborate chemically unrelated agents such as bradykinin, histamine, and adrenocorticotropic hormone (ACTH). Furthermore, evidence suggests that an additional unidentified substance participates in the production of flushing. Within the broad classification of carcinoid tumors there is great diversity in the production of biologically active substances and in the mechanisms for their storage and release. Accordingly, there is a varied spectrum of clinical manifestations.

PATHOLOGIC ANATOMY OF THE TUMOR Carcinoid tumors are slowly growing neoplasms of enterochromaffin cells. The metastatic tumors associated with carcinoid syndrome usually arise from small primary tumors in the ileum. The syndrome is also produced by neoplasms arising from the remainder of the small intestine, from organs derived from the embryonic foregut (e.g., bronchus, stomach, pancreas, and thyroid), and from ovarian or testicular teratomas.

Carcinoid tumors have an unusual proclivity for metastasis to the liver and may involve this organ extensively, with minimal metastatic disease elsewhere. Extrahepatic metastases occur in bone, where they are often osteoblastic, and in lung, pancreas, spleen, ovaries, adrenals, and other organs.

Primary carcinoid tumors of the appendix are common, but they rarely metastasize. Those from the large intestine may metastasize but do not exhibit an endocrine function.

The usual carcinoid tumor arising from the ileum has the classical histologic pattern of dense nests of cells with uniform size and nuclear appearance. Histochemically, they typically exhibit an argentaffin reaction in which the cells convert a silver salt to metallic silver. A positive argentaffin reaction is not required for the diagnosis, however, and carcinoid tumors arising from organs of the embryonic foregut do not usually contain many argentaffin cells. Tumors from these organs also have a broad histologic spectrum, which in the lung ranges from typical bronchial carcinoid to a form indistinguishable from oat-cell carcinoma.

CLINICAL FEATURES Unlike most metastatic neoplasms, carcinoid tumors have an unusually slow rate of growth; most patients survive for 5 to 10 years after the disease is recognized. For much of the duration of the illness, morbidity may result largely from the endocrine function of the tumor. Death results from cardiac or hepatic failure and from complications associated with tumor growth.

Vasomotor paroxysms The most common clinical feature is cutaneous *flushing.* The typical flush is erythematous and involves the head and neck (blush area). Some patients exhibit vivid color changes from red to violaceous to pallor during its course. Prolonged flushing attacks may be associated with lacrimation and periorbital edema. The systemic effects of the flush are variable. It may be accompanied by tachycardia, and the blood pressure usually falls or does not change. A rise in blood pressure during flushing is rare, and carcinoid syndrome is not a cause of sustained hypertension.

Flushing may be provoked by excitement, exertion, eating, ethanol ingestion, and epinephrine administration.

Telangiectasia In addition to paroxysms of cutaneous vasodilatation, some patients also develop purple telangiectasia, primarily on the face and neck and most marked in the malar area.

Gastrointestinal symptoms Intestinal hypermotility with borborygmi, cramping, and explosive diarrhea may accompany the episodic flushes. Chronic hypermotility with diarrhea is more common. When this is severe, malabsorption may occur.

Cardiac manifestations There is a unique deposition of fibrous tissue on the endocardium of the valvular cusps and cardiac chambers. It occurs primarily in the right side of the heart, but may involve the left side to a minimal degree. The fibrous deposition does not penetrate the internal elastic membrane. Distortion of the valve cusps, chordae tendineae, and papillary muscles interferes with valvular function in the right side of the heart and may lead to regurgitation, stenosis, or combined functional lesions. There is, however, a tendency for the fibrosing process to produce incompetence at the tricuspid valve and stenosis of the smaller pulmonary orifice, a deleterious hemodynamic combination. A high cardiac output, with its attendant imposition on cardiac function, may be found in some patients with carcinoid syndrome; this is due either to a continuing release of a vasodilator or to excessive flow in the metastatic tumors.

Pulmonary symptoms Bronchoconstriction is a less common feature of the syndrome, but it may be severe. It is usually most pronounced during flushing attacks.

General In addition to the endocrine effects, the tumors themselves may cause intestinal obstruction or bleeding. Necrosis of intestinal or hepatic tumor masses may produce abdominal pain, tenderness, fever, and leukocytosis. Hepatomegaly from the metastatic disease is usually present with the syndrome. Extensive metastatic involvement of the liver by these slowly growing tumors may occur before the liver function test results become abnormal.

Tryptophan ($CH_2-CH(NH_2)-COOH$)

↓ Tryptophan hydroxylase

5-Hydroxytryptophan (HO; $CH_2-CH(NH_2)-COOH$)

↓ Aromatic-L-amino acid decarboxylase

5-Hydroxytryptamine (Serotonin) (HO; $CH_2-CH_2-NH_2$)

↓ Monoamine oxidase

5-Hydroxyindoleacetaldehyde (HO; CH_2-CHO)

↓ Aldehyde dehydrogenase

5-Hydroxyindoleacetic acid (5-HIAA) (HO; CH_2-COOH)

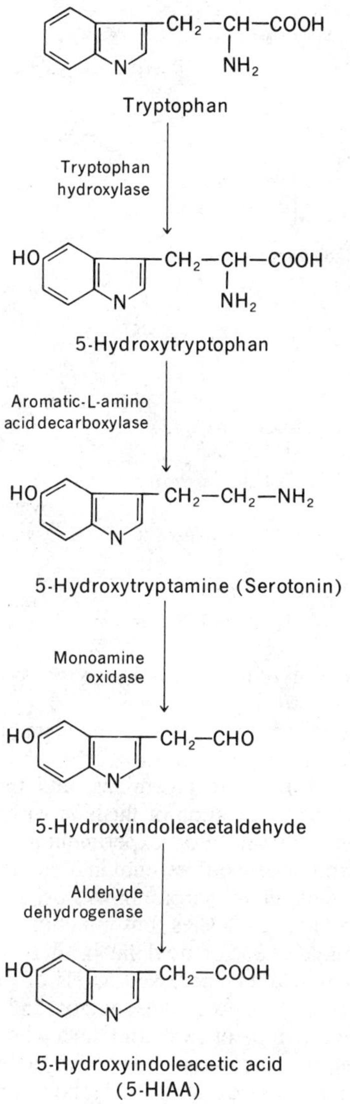

FIGURE 99-1
Metabolic pathway of serotonin.

ENDOCRINE FUNCTION OF THE TUMORS

Serotonin The most constant biochemical characteristic of carcinoid tumors is the presence of tryptophan hydroxylase, which catalyzes the formation of 5-hydroxytryptophan (5-HTP) from tryptophan (Fig. 99-1). Most tumors also contain the enzyme aromatic L-amino acid decarboxylase, which catalyzes the formation of 5-hydroxytryptamine (serotonin). Carcinoids from the stomach and from other organs derived from the embryonic foregut, however, are frequently deficient in this decarboxylase and release 5-HTP from the tumor.

Following its release from the tumor, serotonin is inactivated primarily by the enzyme monoamine oxidase; uptake into platelets also contributes to this inactivation. Monamine oxidase oxidizes serotonin to 5-hydroxyindoleacetaldehyde, which is rapidly converted to 5-hydroxyindoleacetic acid (5-HIAA) by aldehyde dehydrogenase. This acid is rapidly excreted in the urine, and almost all circulating serotonin can be accounted for as urinary 5-HIAA.

Carcinoid tumors vary widely in their capacity to store serotonin, with concentrations of the amine in tumors ranging from a few micrograms per gram to 3 mg per g. The concentration in the tumor appears unrelated to the rate of synthesis of serotonin as reflected by urinary 5-HIAA. Generally, tumors from the ileum have a much higher storage capacity for serotonin than do tumors from organs of the embryonic foregut.

Bradykinin A potent vasodilator peptide, bradykinin is released during flushes in some cases of carcinoid syndrome. In a few of these, excessive amounts continue to be released between flushes. Bradykinin and related kinins are formed by the action of a group of enzymes (kallikreins) which split these peptides from kininogen, a plasma globulin. It is thought that catecholamines and other stimuli initiate bradykinin formation, either by release of kallikrein from the tumor or by initiation of a sequence that leads to activation of the kallikrein normally present in plasma.

Other biologically active substances Some carcinoid tumors, particularly those of gastric origin, produce and release excessive amounts of histamine. This can be detected by an increased excretion of this amine in the urine.

Carcinoid syndrome has been associated with hyperadrenocorticism in a number of instances. This results from ectopic production of an adrenocorticotropic hormone by the tumors, which usually originate from sites other than the ileum (bronchus, pancreas, ovary, and stomach).

In a few cases, "multiple endocrine adenomas" have been seen in conjunction with carcinoids arising from organs of the embryonic foregut. The associated tumors have included parathyroid adenomas and pancreatic tumors, producing Zollinger-Ellison syndrome.

PATHOPHYSIOLOGY Serotonin can account for those aspects of the syndrome related to intestinal hypermotility, and there is evidence that the fibrous deposits on the endocardium also result from increased levels of circulating serotonin.

A secondary effect of serotonin overproduction occurs when a large fraction of dietary tryptophan is shunted into the hydroxylation pathway (Fig. 99-2), leaving less tryptophan available for the formation of niacin and protein. When urinary excretion of 5-HIAA exceeds 200 to 300 mg daily, low levels of plasma tryptophan and evidence of nicotinamide deficiency are seen.

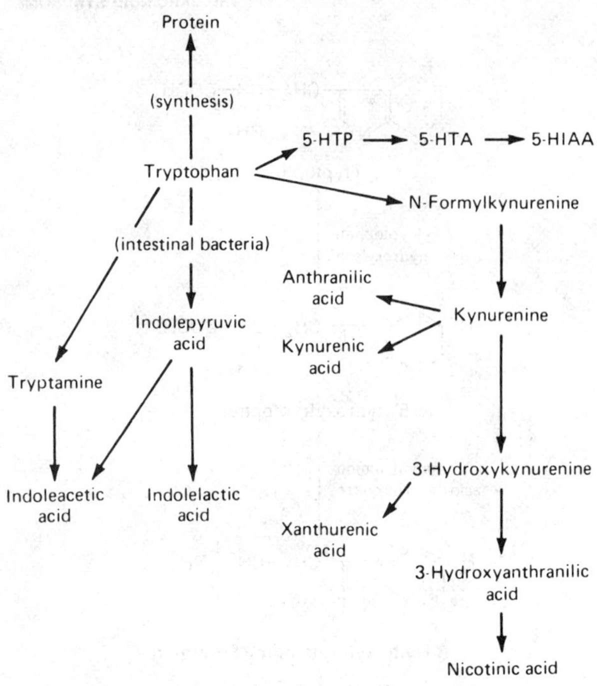

FIGURE 99-2
Metabolic pathways of tryptophan.

Mechanism of the flush The mechanism of the flush is unclear. Release of the flush-provoking substance(s) can be triggered by the catecholamines, and this probably accounts for the association of flushing with excitement and emotional stimuli. For experimental induction of flushing, injection of isoproterenol in amounts as little as 0.5 μg may be effective. Serotonin was originally thought to be the mediator of flushes, but injection of this amine does not mimic the carcinoid flush, and patients may exhibit flushes without increased levels of plasma serotonin. Bradykinin is a potent vasodilator, and its injection will simulate one type of carcinoid flush which is characterized by erythema in association with tachycardia and hypotension. Release of this peptide, however, could not be detected in a number of patients during flushing. While bradykinin, serotonin, and histamine may contribute to the varied types of flushes observed in the carcinoid syndrome, there appears to be an additional flush substance which has not yet been identified.

DIAGNOSIS With its full constellation of clinical features, carcinoid syndrome is easily recognized. The diagnosis also must be considered when any one of its features is present.

The diagnostic hallmark of carcinoid syndrome is *overproduction of 5-hydroxyindoles* with *increased urinary excretion of 5-hydroxyindoleacetic acid.* Normally, excretion of 5-HIAA does not exceed 9 mg daily. Ingestion of foods containing serotonin may complicate the biochemical diagnosis of carcinoid syndrome; both walnuts and bananas contain enough serotonin to produce abnormally elevated urinary excretion of 5-HIAA after their ingestion. Some drugs also interfere with the analysis of urinary 5-HIAA; cough syrups containing guaiacolate cause falsely elevated values, and phenothiazines interfere with the colorimetric test. When dietary 5-hydroxyindoles are excluded, a urinary excretion of more than 25 mg of 5-HIAA daily is diagnostic of carcinoid. Elevations in the range of 9 to 25 mg may be seen with carcinoid syndrome, nontropical sprue, or acute intestinal obstruction.

Measurement of *serotonin in blood* or platelets is of interest but has less diagnostic value than assay of the major metabolite of serotonin in the urine.

Measurement of an increased concentration of *serotonin in tumor tissue* is a useful and sometimes necessary supplement to histologic examination. A portion of suspected tumor should always be frozen for serotonin analysis (see Table 99-1).

VARIANTS OF THE SYNDROME: RELATION TO SITE OF TUMOR ORIGIN The origin of the tumor influences the biologically active substances produced and their storage and release. Carcinoid tumors arising from organs derived from the embryonic foregut (bronchus, stomach, and pancreas) tend to differ from those arising distal to the midduodenum (midgut). The typical carcinoid syndrome usually results from tumors of midgut origin, which almost invariably secrete serotonin with little or no 5-HTP. Tumor serotonin content is likely to be high, and the tumor usually contains dense nests of argentaffin-positive cells. Metastasis to bone and skin is infrequent.

In contrast, tumors arising from the embryonic foregut contain fewer argentaffin cells, have lower serotonin content, and may secrete 5-HTP. Hyperadrenocorticism and multiple endocrine adenomas are more likely to be associated with this group, and metastasis to bone and skin is more frequent.

In addition to the general characteristics of the foregut group, certain clinical and biochemical features have been associated with gastric and bronchial carcinoids. Patients with gastric carcinoids frequently exhibit unique flushing which begins as a bright-red patchy erythema with sharply delineated serpentine borders; these patches tend to coalesce as the blush heightens. Food ingestion is especially likely to produce flushes. The tumors usually are deficient in decarboxylase enzyme and secrete 5-

TABLE 99-1
Outline of diagnostic approach to a patient with suspected carcinoid syndrome

I Quantitative determination of 24-hr urinary excretion of 5-HIAA (5-hydroxyindoleacetic acid)
II When elevated 5-HIAA confirms clinical evidence for carcinoid syndrome, curable ovarian, testicular, or bronchial primary tumors should be sought
III Consideration of possible treatment of the syndrome by surgical resection of hepatic metastases or hepatic arterial perfusion of chemotherapeutic agents requires:
- *A* Assessment of the location and character of hepatic metastases with arteriography and scintillation scanning of the liver.
- *B* Evaluation of hepatic and cardiac function
- *C* A search for extrahepatic metastases in bone and other sites

IV In patients with substantial diarrhea, possible malabsorption of nutrients should be investigated

HTP; histamine secretion is also common, as is a high incidence of peptic ulceration. Diarrhea and heart lesions are not prominent features in the patients who secrete largely 5-HTP from the tumor without much preformed serotonin.

When the carcinoid tumor arises from the bronchus, attacks of flushing tend to be prolonged and severe and may be associated with periorbital edema, excessive lacrimation and salivation, hypotension, tachycardia, anxiety, and tremulousness. Nausea, vomiting, explosive diarrhea, and bronchoconstriction may progress to a severe degree. This group is therapeutically unique in that the severe flushes often can be prevented by corticosteroids, and chlorpromazine may be helpful in relieving the symptoms.

TREATMENT Recognition of the carcinoid syndrome has led to complete surgical cure of a few patients with tumors arising in ovarian or testicular teratomas or in the bronchus; by releasing their secretions directly into the systemic circulation, tumors from these locations can produce the syndrome before metastatic disease occurs. As the humoral substances released by tumors draining into the portal circulation are largely metabolized by the liver, tumors arising in this location produce the syndrome only after hepatic metastasis. Because of the relatively slow growth of carcinoid tumors, palliative resection of hepatic metastases is beneficial in carefully selected cases. Resection of large isolated hepatic metastases has led to relief of the symptoms of carcinoid syndrome and marked reductions in urinary 5-HIAA excretion for periods of several years. In some cases with multiple metastases, removal of as much as a hepatic lobe may be considered when these metastases are located primarily in the portion of the liver to be resected, as determined by arteriography, scintillation scanning of gamma-emitting colloidal particles taken up by the liver, and inspection of the hepatic surface at surgical exploration.

Of numerous approaches to chemotherapy of the tumor, the most promising appears to be regional arterial perfusion with agents such as 5-fluorouracil.

Pharmacologic therapy directed at the humoral mediators of the syndrome is useful in some cases. Methysergide, a serotonin antagonist, will improve the diarrhea, but prolonged therapy with this agent can produce retroperitoneal fibrosis. Blockade of serotonin synthesis with the tryptophan hydroxylase inhibitor *p*-chlorophenylalanine also ameliorates the diarrhea. The prevention of severe flushing by corticosteriods and amelioration of the syndrome by phenothiazines are limited largely to patients with tumors arising from the bronchus and other organs derived from the embryonic foregut.

Nicotinamide should be given to those patients who shunt a large fraction of dietary tryptophan into the hydroxyindole pathway.

Hypotensive episodes should not be treated with catecholamines; by stimulating the release of vasoactive substances from the tumor, norepinephrine, epinephrine, and other agents with adrenergic activity can exaggerate and prolong the circulatory disturbance. If pressor agents must be used, angiotensin or methoxamine is preferred.

REFERENCES

Oates JA, Butler TC: Pharmacologic and endocrine aspects of carcinoid syndrome. Adv Pharmacol 5:109, 1967

Robertson JIS et al: The mechanism of facial flushing in the carcinoid syndrome. Q J Med 31:103, 1962

Sjoerdsma A et al: A clinical, physiologic and biochemical study of patients with malignant carcinoid. Am J Med 20:520, 1956

Van Sickle DG: Carcinoid tumors; analysis of 61 cases, including 11 cases of carcinoid syndrome. Cleve Clin Q 39:79, 1972

100 GOUT AND OTHER DISORDERS OF URIC ACID METABOLISM

JAMES B. WYNGAARDEN

Primary gout is an inborn metabolic disorder manifested by hyperuricemia, recurrent attacks of a characteristic acute arthritis, and tophaceous deposits of sodium urate. Nephrolithiasis and parenchymatous renal disease commonly develop during the course of the illness. Gout is not a single disease, but rather a syndrome resulting from different biochemical abnormalities which lead to hyperuricemia. Secondary gout is an acquired form of the disease which supervenes in the course of a number of disorders in which hyperuricemia occurs.

A classification of gout is presented in Table 100-1.

HISTORY In the fifth century B.C., gout was described as podagra, cheiagra, or gonogra by Hippocrates, depending on whether the big toe, wrist, or knee was involved. Tophi were first described by Galen. The term *gout* is derived from the Latin *gutta*, a drop, and reflects an early belief that the disease was caused by a poison, falling drop by drop into the joint. A drug, probably identical with colchicine, was described in the Ebers Papyrus (1500 B.C.). The agent was known to Byzantine physicians in the fifth century A.D., and was brought to this country from Europe by Benjamin Franklin, who was himself a sufferer from gout. An astonishing list of men of royalty and genius have been afflicted with gout.

The modern clinical history of gout began in 1683 with Thomas Sydenham, whose surpassing description of the disease, based on 34 years of personal affliction, first clearly differentiated gout from other articular disorders. Uric acid was discovered in a kidney stone by Scheele in 1776. Twenty years later Wollaston and Pearson demonstrated urate in the tophi of patients with gout. Hyperuricemia was discovered by A. B. Garrod in 1848.

When the structure of uric acid was established by Emil Fischer in 1898, its relation to the purine bases of nucleic acids was at once apparent. The pathways of enzymatic synthesis of purine compounds were elucidated by Buchanan, Greenberg, and others during the 1950s.

The first specific enzymatic defect responsible for one subtype of adult primary gout was discovered by Seegmiller and associates in 1966, the second by Sperling and colleagues in 1971.

PREVALENCE AND INCIDENCE The prevalence of gout varies from about 0.3 percent in the population of Europe and the United States to 8 percent in adult male Maori of New Zealand. During World Wars I and II acute gouty arthritis was uncommon in Europe. When protein again became plentiful, the incidence returned to prewar levels. With the increase in protein consumption among the Japanese during the past two decades, gout has become a common disorder in that population. Although traditionally considered a disease of middle and upper social classes, gout involves all nationalities and income groups.

Primarily gout is a disease of the adult male. In large

TABLE 100-1
Classification of gout

Type	*Metabolic disturbance*	*Specific defect*	*Inheritance*
Primary gout			
Idiopathic adult primary gout			
Normal excreter of uric acid (75–80% of primary gout)	Overproduction of uric acid and/or underexcretion of uric acid (often both in same subject)	Undefined	Polygenic ?Autosomal-dominant forms
Overexcreter of uric acid (20–25% of primary gout)	Overproduction of uric acid	Undefined	Unknown
Gout associated with specific protein defects:			
Associated with glycogen storage disease, type I (von Gierke's disease) (juvenile gout)	Overproduction of uric acid, plus underexcretion of uric acid; excessive deposition of glycogen and lipids; hypoglycemia	Glucose 6-phosphatase: deficiency or absence	Autosomal-recessive
Associated with cerebral palsy, mental deficiency, and self-mutilation (Lesch-Nyhan syndrome) (childhood)	Overproduction of uric acid	Hypoxanthine-guanine phosphoribosyltransferase (HGPRT): deficiency (virtually complete)	X-linked
Associated with onset in early adult life, renal stones, occasionally with neurologic disease (<1% of primary gout)	Overproduction of uric acid	HGPRT: deficiency (partial)	X-linked
Associated with marked uric aciduria, stones in early adult life, and gout (rare)	Overproduction of uric acid	PP-ribose-P synthetase mutant: excessive activity	Unknown
Associated with tophaceous gout and minimally elevated plasma urate levels (rare)	Reduced binding of urate to plasma protein	α_1-α_2-Globulin: partial deficiency of urate-binding protein	Autosomal-recessive
Secondary gout			
Hematologic disorders			
Myeloproliferative diseases; chronic hemolytic anemia	Excessive production of uric acid	Accelerated turnover of nucleic acids	
Chronic renal diseases			
Glomerulonephritis, pyelonephritis, polycystic kidney disease	Reduced excretion of uric acid	Reduced renal functional mass	
Lead nephropathy	Reduced excretion of uric acid	?Acquired tubular lesion	
Hypertensive cardiovascular disease	Reduced excretion of uric acid	?Role of hyperlacticacidemia in suppression of tubular secretion of urate	
Hyperuricacidemogenic drugs	Reduced excretion of uric acid	?Suppression of tubular secretion of urate by drug or metabolite	
Starvation, especially in treatment of obesity	Reduced excretion of uric acid	Suppression of renal tubular secretion of urate by β-hydroxybutyric acid and other ketone bodies	

series, only 3 to 7 percent of cases are found in women, and these are chiefly in the postmenopausal group. Gout is very rare in prepubertal children and, when it occurs, may represent a specific form of gout associated with choreoathetosis, self-mutilation, and mental deficiency (Lesch-Nyhan syndrome), or with glycogen storage disease, type I (von Gierke's disease, Chap. 104).

Secondary gout generally constitutes 5 to 10 percent of cases of gout, and, especially in those instances complicating myeloproliferative disorders or hypertensive cardiovascular disease may involve women in as many as 30 percent of cases. In special circumstances secondary gout may be more common. In a 14-year period, one-half of new cases of gout in Framingham, Mass., occurred in subjects taking thiazide diuretics. In regions of the United States where bootleg whiskey is consumed, lead nephropathy is an important antecedent of gout. In one Southern Veterans' Administration hospital 37 of 43 male patients admitted with gout in 1 year showed evidence of lead intoxication.

INHERITANCE The familial incidence of gout is generally reported as 6 to 18 percent in the United States, but may be much higher as reflected in figures ranging up to 75 percent in English series. The incidence of hyperuricemia among asymptomatic blood relatives of gouty subjects is about 25 percent. The genetic determinants of hyperuricemia are multifactorial. Population studies suggest that some are autosomal dominant and others are sex-linked dominant factors. The metabolic and genetic heterogeneity of gout underscores the need for definition of specific subtypes so that patterns of transmission of each may be determined. In addition, serum urate values are positively correlated with surface area, obesity, and "ponderal index." Environmental factors, such as diet, alcohol, and drugs, operate in conjunction with genetic factors in determining hyperuricemia.

PATHOGENESIS OF HYPERURICEMIA The concentration of uric acid in body fluids is determined by the balance between rates of production and elimination of urate. Uric acid is formed by oxidation of purine bases, which are of both exogenous (dietary) and endogenous (biosynthetic) origins. After several days of reduced purine intake, the body contains about 1,200 mg uric acid and turns over about 700 mg per day. Two-thirds of this amount is excreted in the urine; one-third is excreted in bile, gastric, and intestinal secretions and is destroyed by colonic bacteria. The accumulation of excessive quantities of urate in the gouty subject could theoretically result from increased absorption of dietary purines, endogenous overproduction, diminished renal or gastrointestinal excretion, diminished endogenous destruction of urate, or a combination of these factors. Abnormalities of absorption or of intestinal uricolysis have been excluded, and endogenous uricolysis is not a significant process in human tissues because they lack uricase. In constrast, *abnormalities of endogenous purine production* and of *uric acid excretion* are important in the pathogenesis of hyperuricemia of both primary and secondary gout.

The normal range of uric acid excretion in American males is 250 to 600 mg per day on a restricted purine diet. About 20 or 25 percent of gouty subjects consistently excrete excessive amounts of uric acid. Tracer studies of the rate of turnover of the urate pool or of incorporation of labeled precursors, such as glycine, into urinary uric acid, indicate that these subjects synthesize abnormal amounts of purines. Such studies also disclose excessive purine production in about two-thirds of gouty subjects who excrete normal amounts of uric acid in the urine. A significant minority remains in whom present methods of study do not disclose excessive purine synthesis.

The structure of the purine ring and the metabolic precursors of individual atoms are shown in Fig. 100-1, and the major intermediates of nucleotide synthesis and uric acid production in Fig. 100-2. The key reaction is as follows:

$$\text{L-Glutamine} + \alpha\text{-phosphoribosylpyrophosphate} + H_2O \rightarrow \beta\text{-phosphoribosylamine} + \text{L-glutamic acid} + PP$$

This reaction is the site of a feedback regulatory process operated by the nucleotide products of the pathway. The amidotransferase catalyzing this first reaction has special inhibitor sites that are sensitive to adenylic and guanylic acids. Accelerated purine biosynthesis must involve an accelerated rate of this and subsequent reactions. The amidotransferase reaction is the rate-limiting step of the entire pathway. Therefore, the rate of purine biosynthesis will depend upon (1) the availability of the key substrates, glutamine and phosphoribosylpyrophosphate (PP-ribose-P), (2) the activity of the amidotransferase and the integrity of its regulatory mechanisms, and (3) the concentrations of regulatory nucleotides at the feedback control sites on the enzyme.

It is likely that examples of defects of each of these three classes of controls will be found in patients presently classified as having idiopathic primary gout, and thus allow more precise definitions of metabolic defects and subtypes of gout. In a few patients an understanding of the molecular defect leading to excessive purine biosynthesis has already been achieved.

Hypoxanthine-guanine phosphoribosyltransferase deficiency In 1 or 2 percent of adult gouty subjects with overproduction of uric acid, the responsible metabolic defect is a remarkable deficiency of activity of the enzyme which catalyzes the reconversion of hypoxanthine and guanine to their respective ribonucleotide forms by condensation with phosphoribosylpyrophosphate.

FIGURE 100-1
Metabolic donors of atoms of the purine ring.

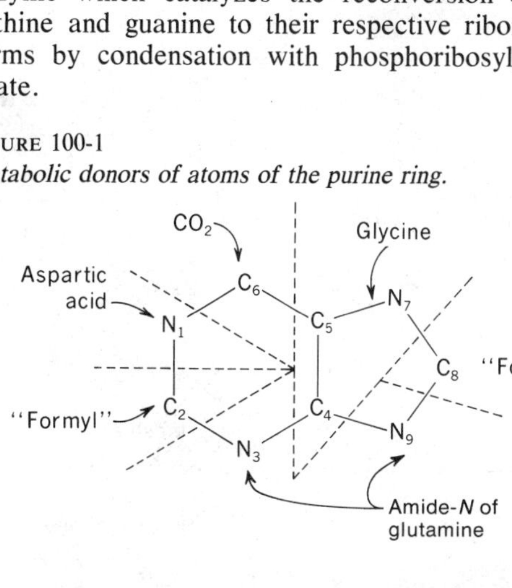

CO_2 Glycine Aspartic acid N_1 C_6 C_5 N_7 C_8 "Formyl" "Formyl" C_2 N_3 C_4 N_9 Amide-*N* of glutamine

Hypoxanthine + PP-ribose-P → inosinic acid + PP
Guanine + PP-ribose-P → guanylic acid + PP

Hypoxanthine-guanine phosphoribosyltransferase is the same enzyme in which activity is even more severely reduced in children with the Lesch-Nyhan syndrome. In all patients with phosphoribosyltransferase deficiency studied thus far, an approximately normal amount of enzyme protein is present, but the enzyme is structurally abnormal and functions poorly, if at all. A number of different types of abnormality of the enzyme have been demonstrated in different families with juvenile or adult forms of the deficiency.

Phosphoribosylpyrophosphate synthetase variants Recently a mutant form of PP-ribose-P synthetase has been identified in two gouty families. The enzyme is normally activated by inorganic phosphate and inhibited by nucleotides. The mutant enzyme exhibits markedly increased activity at low phosphate levels, resulting in increased intracellular concentrations of PP-ribose-P, accelerated purine biosynthesis, exceptionally high daily excretion values of urinary uric acid, and recurrent renal lithiasis as well as articular gout.

Other defects Two other enzymatic abnormalities have been described in gout which may result in increased synthesis of PP-ribose-P and of purines. These are *glucose 6-phosphatase deficiency* [von Gierke's (type I) glycogen storage disease] and *glutathione reductase variants* (with increased activity), both of which are thought to result in increased flux of the hexose monophosphate shunt and increased synthesis of ribose phosphate esters. A defect of glutamine metabolism has been proposed as the driving force of excessive purine biosynthesis in idiopathic primary gout, but the evidence on which this postulate was based has now been shown to be an isotope artifact. In addition, increased hepatic activity of *xanthine oxidase* has been reported in gouty overproducers of uric acid; this may represent secondary enzyme induction rather than a primary lesion. A partial deficiency of a *urate-binding* α_1-α_2-*globulin* has been described in a few gouty families without other known defects of purine metabolism. It is suggested that such a deficiency would favor tissue disposition of urate at lower than usual plasma values.

FIGURE 100-2
Purine biosynthesis and catabolism. The first reaction of the pathway is under inhibitory control of adenosine and guanosine 5′-phosphates. Key enzymes are indicated in parentheses.

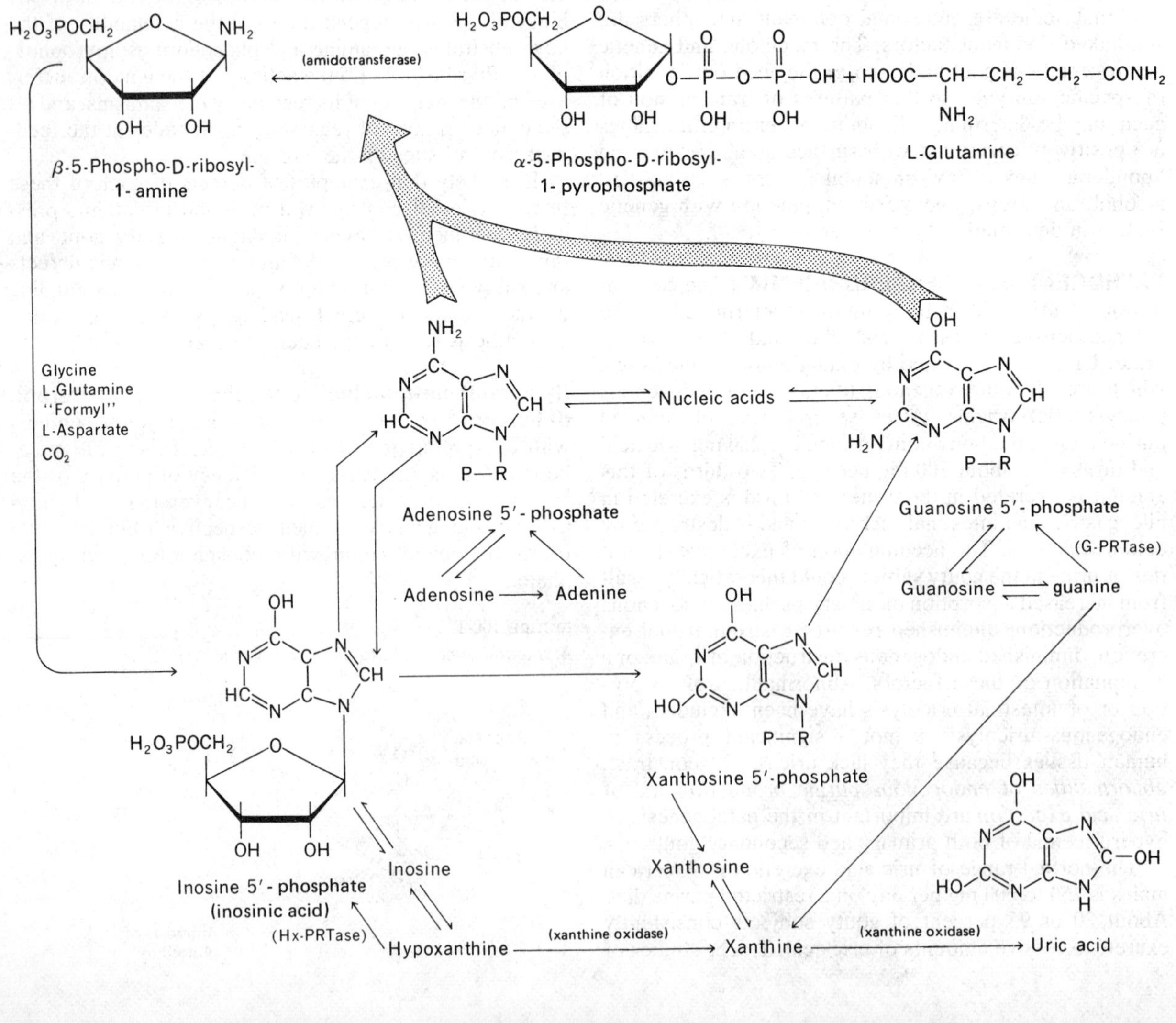

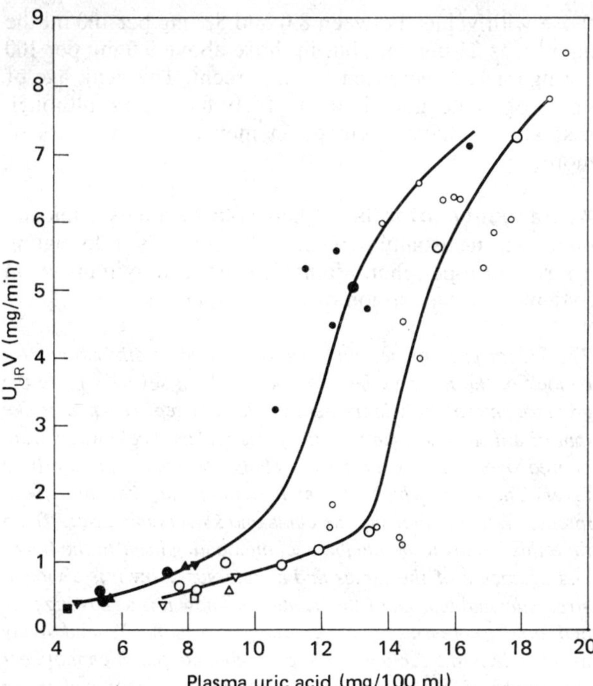

FIGURE 100-3
Rates of excretion of uric acid at various plasma urate levels in control and gouty subjects. The urate levels have been raised in both groups by feeding of RNA or by infusion of lithium urate. The gouty group (open symbols) includes asymptomatic hyperuricemic, normal excreter, and overexcreter subjects.

Renal handling of urate Excretion of urate is dependent on a three-compartment system: glomerular filtration, tubular reabsorption, and tubular secretion. A small percentage (0 to 4 percent) of plasma urate may be bound to nondiffusible elements, but the bulk of plasma urate is thought to be freely filterable. Most (98 percent) is reabsorbed, and the largest part of *excreted* urate (80 to 85 percent) derives from tubular secretion.

As pointed out above, evidence for overproduction of uric acid is equivocal or lacking in a substantial percentage of "normal-excreter" gouty subjects. These are the subjects whose urate excretion data often suggest most strongly the existence of a specific tubular defect in handling of urate. Figure 100-3 illustrates the tendency of gouty subjects to require a plasma urate value of 2 or 3 mg per 100 ml greater than the nongouty subject in order to achieve a given rate of urate excretion. This tendency is least evident in the flamboyant overexcreter, if at all, and most prominent in the gouty subject with normal turnover of the urate pool or normal values of incorporation of purine precursors into uric acid.

The pathophysiologic basis of this putative tubular defect is unknown. Among the possibilities are changes in renal tubular blood flow, changes in rate of transfer of urate into renal cells, or abnormalities of the secretory transport system itself. The latter mechanism presumably requires both a specific carrier and an energy-generating system. A number of chemical substances are known to inhibit urate excretion, presumably by blocking tubular secretion of urate. Some gouty patients with normal uric acid excretion and apparently reduced tubular secretion of urate may have gout secondary to unrecognized tubular damage, e.g., lead poisoning, rather than primary gout.

HYPERURICEMIA A satisfactory definition of hyperuricemia is difficult to offer, as serum urate values form a continuous distribution from low to high values. Statistical definitions depend on the populations examined and methods employed. In the United States normal ranges [mean ± 2 standard deviation (SD)] in males are approximately 2.2 to 7.5 mg per 100 ml and in females, 2.1 to 6.6 mg per 100 ml. In epidemiologic surveys, values of 7.0 and 6.0 mg per 100 ml, respectively, are often used as discriminants. The physicochemical solubility of uric acid in solutions having the sodium composition of body fluids is about 6.4 mg per 100 ml at pH 7.4. Protein binding of urate may account for an additional 0.4 mg per 100 ml of plasma at 37°C. Only a rare gouty subject will have serum urate values of less than 7 mg per 100 ml when reliable methods, such as the uricase differential spectrophotometric method, are employed.

HYPOURICEMIA Plasma urate values of <2.0 mg per 100 ml, unrelated to drug action, are rare. When encountered they may be due to a congenital deficiency of xanthine oxidase (xanthinuria) or to renal tubular lesions (idiopathic reabsorptive defect, Wilson's disease, Fanconi syndrome).

PATHOLOGY The pathognomonic lesion of gout is the *tophus*, a urate deposit surrounded by an inflammatory and foreign-body reaction. Because urate crystals are water-soluble, nonaqueous fixatives are necessary to preserve urate deposits in histologic sections. Urate crystals are brilliantly anisotropic when viewed with polarized light under the microscope. In gout, urates tend to deposit in cartilage, epiphyseal bone, periarticular structures, and kidneys.

Tophi commonly occur in the helix or antihelix of the ear, the olecranon and patellar bursas, and tendons. Less commonly, they occur in skin of fingertips, palms, or soles, the tarsal plates of the eyelids, the nasal cartilages, in the cornea or sclerotic coats of the eye, or along nerves, causing compression syndromes. Rarely they develop in the myocardium, aortic or mitral valves, vocal cords and arytenoid cartilages.

In the joint cartilaginous degeneration, synovial proliferation and pannus, destruction of subchondral bone, proliferation of marginal bone, and sometimes fibrous or bony ankylosis develop. The punched-out lesions of bone commonly seen in roentgenograms of gouty patients represent marrow tophus deposits, which may communicate with the urate crust on the articular surface through erosions and defects in articular cartilage (Fig. 100-4). In vertebral bodies, urate deposits are found in marrow spaces adjacent to intervertebral disks, as well as in disk tissue itself.

The only distinctive histologic feature of the *gouty kidney* is the presence of urate crystals in the medulla or pyramids and surrounding giant-cell reaction. These are

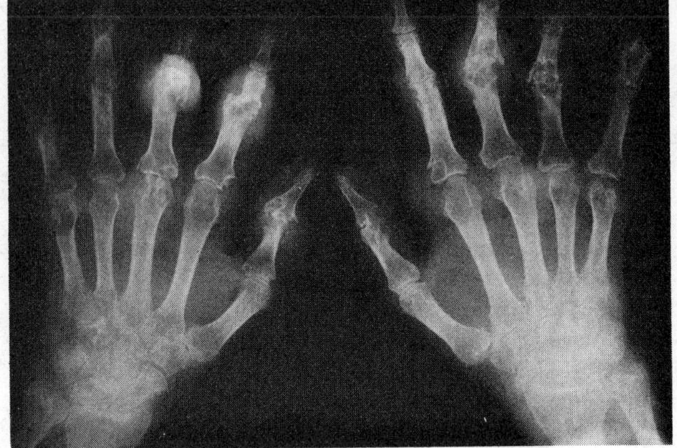

FIGURE 100-4
Advanced chronic gouty arthritis of the hands, showing extensive destruction of bone by urate deposits and large asymmetric soft-tissue tophi.

found in about 90 percent of gouty patients at autopsy and are associated with pyelonephritic or vascular changes. The pyelonephritic changes are both acute and chronic; the vascular changes include arterial and arteriolar sclerosis.

The earliest structural abnormality in the kidney is tubular damage associated with interstitial reaction. There is a distinctive glomerulosclerosis, with uniform fibrillar thickening of glomerular capillary basement membranes, different from that of nephrosclerosis or diabetic glomerulosclerosis. The Henle's loops show early atrophy and dilatation, occasionally associated with brown-pigment degeneration of epithelium. The interstitial reaction is maximal near the changes in the Henle's loops. In kidneys without tophi this reaction tends to spare the medulla and juxtamedullary cortex. The changes of chronic pyelonephritis do not appear to be of infectious origin. The vessels, both arteries and arterioles, show increased basophilia and degenerative changes which are out of proportion to the parenchymal changes.

CLINICAL MANIFESTATIONS The natural history of primary gout consists of three phases: asymptomatic hyperuricemia, acute gouty arthritis (characteristically recurrent with asymptomatic intervals), and chronic gouty arthritis.

Asymptomatic hyperuricemia In idiopathic gout this phase begins as an accentuation of the normal rise in serum urate value that occurs at puberty in the male and at the menopause in the female. Only a limited number of hyperuricemic subjects develop symptomatic gout, urolithiasis, or renal or vascular injury. The majority live their lifetimes with no detectable ill effects of this biochemical abnormality.

In the population study in Framingham, Mass., the likelihood of developing gout increased with the degree of hyperuricemia, and with age. Nevertheless, at mean age 58, only 17 percent of subjects with serum urate values between 7.0 and 7.9 mg per 100 ml had developed gout. In those with values between 8.0 and 8.9 mg per 100 ml the figure was 23 percent, but in those above 9.0 mg per 100 the figure had increased to 82 percent. The peak age of onset of acute gout is about forty-five years, although first attacks have occurred in men of eighty years or more.

Acute gouty arthritis When gout becomes clinically manifest, it usually appears abruptly, as fulminating arthritis of a peripheral joint. It is difficult to improve on Sydenham's description of the acute attack:

The victim goes to bed and sleeps in good health. About two o'clock in the morning he is awakened by a severe pain in the great toe; more rarely in the heal, ankle or instep. This pain is like that of a dislocation, and yet the parts feel as if cold water were poured over them. Then follow chills and shivers, and a little fever. The pain, which was at first moderate, becomes more intense. With its intensity the chills and shivers increase. After a time this comes to its height, accommodating itself to the bones and ligaments of the tarsus and metatarsus. Now it is a violent stretching and tearing of the ligaments—now it is a gnawing pain and now a pressure and tightening. So exquisite and lively meanwhile is the feeling of the part affected, that it cannot bear the weight of the bedclothes nor the jar of a person walking in the room. The night is passed in torture, sleeplessness, turning of the part affected, and perpetual change of posture; the tossing about of the body being worse as the fit comes on. Hence the vain effort, by change of posture, both in the body and the limb affected, to obtain an abatement of the pain.

The initial attack usually subsides spontaneously in a few days to a few weeks, and recovery is generally complete. About 50 percent of initial attacks involve the great toe (podagra), and occasionally the initial attack is bilateral. Ninety percent of gouty patients experience podagra during the course of their disease. Next as sites of initial involvement are the instep, ankle, heel, knee, and wrist. Recurring bursitis of shoulder or elbow may be a manifestation of gout. The more distal the site of involvement, the more typical is the character of the attack.

There are no characteristic changes of plasma urate levels that precede, accompany, or follow an acute attack of gouty arthritis. In some patients there may be an elevation of urinary uric acid excretion values during the acute attack, perhaps mediated by the uricosuric action of corticosteroids secreted during the stress of gouty inflammation. This sequence could explain the normal serum urate values occasionally observed during acute attacks. Garrod proposed in 1876 that the acute gouty paroxysm was triggered by precipitation of sodium urate crystals in the joint or neighboring tissues. In 1899, Freudweiler reproduced acute gouty attacks by injection of microcrystals of sodium urate, hypoxanthine, or xanthine. These observations have been confirmed by others with both purine and nonpurine microcrystals. A proposed pathogenetic mechanism involves crystallization of sodium urate from super-saturated body fluids, activation of Hageman factor by crystal surfaces, production of vasoactive kinin-like peptides in synovial fluid, induction of an inflammatory response involving leukotaxic factors, leukocytosis, ingestion of microcrystals by leukocytes, destruction of leukocytes, and release of lysosomal enzymes, with potential destruction of mucoproteins of cartilage (Fig. 100-5).

The events leading to the initial crystallization of monosodium urate, after an average of 30 years of asymptomatic hyperuricemia, are poorly understood. Attacks may be precipitated by stress of many kinds, dietary, physical, and emotional. One patient may indict fatiguing travel, another unusual walking or hiking (e.g., "pheasant hunter's gout"), or celebrations such as holiday dinners or alcoholic sprees. Ethanol intoxication may exacerbate hyperuricemia. Ethanol oxidation is coupled to pyruvate reduction (NAD-NADH–linked enzyme systems), and the lactate produced interferes with uric acid secretion in the renal tubule. Operative procedures are particularly prone to induce acute gout in hyperuricemic individuals, generally on the third to seventh postoperative day.

Interval gout The asymptomatic phase following the acute attack may last from a few weeks to many years. Generally in 6 months to 2 years the patient will suffer another episode in the same or another joint. With time, attacks tend to recur with increasing frequency. Later attacks are often polyarticular, more severe, longer, and accompanied by fever. Roentgenographic changes may develop, and the attacks may abate more gradually than before, but the joints may recover complete function.

Chronic gouty arthritis Before effective control of hyperuricemia became possible, 50 to 60 percent of gouty patients developed visible tophi, permanent joint changes, or chronicity of symptoms. The incidence of tophi now ranges from 13 to 25 percent. Development of tophi is correlated with height of serum urate concentration, severity of renal involvement, and duration of the disease. The time from initial attack to the beginning of chronic symptomatic or visible tophaceous involvement is usually many years, and ranged from 3 to 42 years in one large series, with an average of 11.6 years (Hench).

Chronic gouty arthritis is a consequence of the progressive inability to dispose of urate as rapidly as it is produced. The urate pool expands and crystalline deposits of urate appear in cartilage, synovial membranes, tendons, soft tissues, and elsewhere. In 1 or 2 percent of patients, tophi of the helix of the ear may be present at the time of the initial acute attack. Tophaceous deposits may produce irregular, asymmetric, moderately discrete tumescences over joints, requiring larger shoes or gloves. The classic gouty shoe is one with a window cut to accommodate an irregularly prominent joint, usually the first metatarsophalangeal. At later stages, tophaceous enlargements of Achilles tendons, or saccular distentions of olecranon bursas, are common and characteristic.

FIGURE 100-5
Crystals of sodium urate monohydrate in leukocytes of synovial fluid in acute gouty arthritis, as viewed under partially polarized light. (Courtesy Daniel J. McCarty, Jr.)

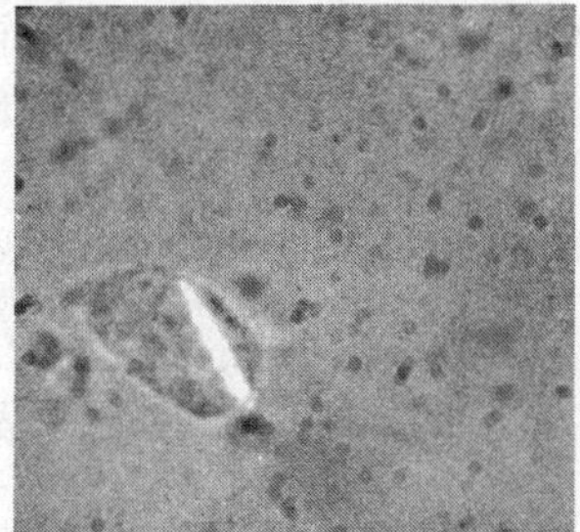

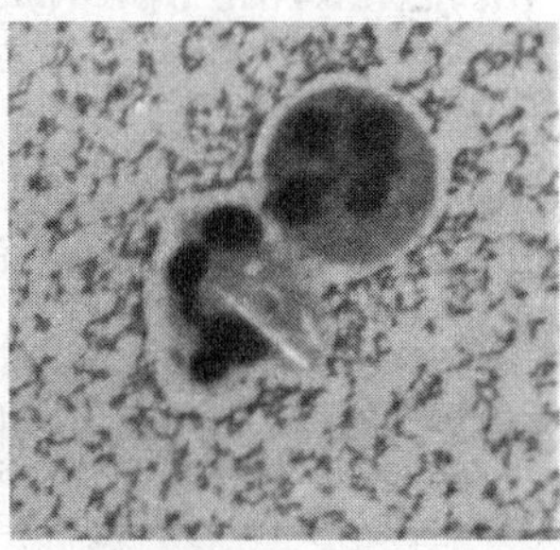

The process of tophaceous deposition advances insidiously, and although the tophi themselves are relatively painless, there is often progressive stiffness and persistent aching of affected joints. Eventually extensive destruction of joints and large subcutaneous tophi may lead to grotesque deformities, particularly of hands and feet, and to progressive crippling (Fig. 100-4). The tense, shiny, thin skin overlying the tophus may ulcerate and extrude white chalky or pasty material composed of myriads of fine, needlelike crystals.

As chronic gouty changes and renal disease advance, acute attacks occur less frequently and are milder; those that appear may be superimposed upon the indolent soreness of an involved joint, or may seek out new locations of previously uninvolved sites.

No joint is exempt from chronic gouty involvement, although those of the lower extremity and hand are most commonly involved. The hip and spinal joints are rarely affected by tophaceous changes in the absence of extensive disease elsewhere. Radiographic changes of the sacroiliac joint and aseptic necrosis of the hip are sometimes attributable to gout.

Urolithiasis The incidence of renal stone is about a thousandfold higher in gouty subjects than in the general population. Approximately 20 percent of gouty patients with normal urinary uric acid excretion values and 40 percent of those with elevated excretion values develop stones. Of those who pass stones about 20 percent have had their first episode of urolithiasis before the onset of gouty arthritis. The stones are composed of uric acid, not sodium urate, but in about 80 percent of instances they are mixed and contain in addition calcium phosphate, oxalate, or rarely carbonate. Such stones are radiopaque, whereas pure uric acid stones are radiolucent. Some gouty subjects pass uric acid sludge, gravel, or sand, occasionally almost daily.

Several factors have been implicated in the pathogenesis of stones. In 20 to 25 percent of gouty patients, urinary uric acid excretion values are excessive. Also, as a group, gouty subjects tend to produce acid urines, and do not show normal postprandial alkaline tides. Renal ammonia production is subnormal in response to a given acid load. The deficit in ammonia is compensated by an increase in titratable acidity.

Renal disease in gout Many gouty subjects show evidence of renal disease. Twenty to forty percent show albuminuria, which is rarely heavy in quantity and is often intermittent. Hypertension is frequent and is usually benign. Concentrating ability may be impaired. Mild degrees of nitrogen retention are common and often stable or only slowly progressive. Renal dysfunction does not shorten life expectancy in the average gouty subject, even though uremia is reported to be the eventual cause of death in 22 to 25 percent of gouty subjects. The majority of gouty patients die of cardiac or cerebral vascular disease or malignancies, which occur in about the same incidence and at about the same time of life as in nongouty American males.

Hyperlipoproteinemia in gout Both hypercholesterolemia and hypertriglyceridemia are common in primary idiopathic gout, although the relation between these abnormalities and hyperuricemia is unclear. In hyperuricemia and gout secondary to lead poisoning (saturnine gout) plasma lipoprotein values are normal, even though ethanol consumption may be excessive in both types of patients.

Gout associated with specific enzymatic defects Patients with virtually complete deficiency of hypoxanthine-guanine phosphoribosyltransferase (HGPRT) exhibit features of cerebral palsy, plus self-mutilation, mental deficiency, and marked hyperuricemia and uric aciduria (Lesch-Nyhan syndrome). The onset is within the first year of life. Renal stones and gout may supervene. Death occurs from renal failure, usually by age 10. Patients with partial deficiencies of HGPRT activity usually develop gout within the first two or three decades of life, show very high urinary uric acid values, and commonly develop stones. In about 20 percent of cases there is some neurologic abnormality, ranging from mild spinocerebellar ataxia to typical cerebral palsy.

All reported patients are males, although some abnormalities of purine metabolism may be present in the mothers. Phosphoribosyltransferase (PRT) deficiency obeys the laws of X-linked transmission with full expression only in hemizygous males. Patients with mutant forms of PP-ribose-P synthetase share the features of early onset of renal stones or gout and marked uric aciduria, but have not shown neurologic lesions.

Secondary gout Any acquired hyperuricemic state may be complicated by secondary gout. This disorder occurs in 5 to 9 percent of patients with polycythemia vera, especially those cases merging into the phase of myeloid metaplasia, occasionally in secondary polycythemia complicating congenital heart disease or chronic pulmonary disease, in chronic myelogenous leukemia, multiple myeloma, or chronic hemolytic anemias. In such instances the mean age of onset is later, women are more commonly involved, and both serum and urinary uric acid values tend to be higher than in idiopathic primary gout. Acute gouty arthritis may occasionally antedate evidence of the myeloproliferative disorder by many months, or even by several years.

In all the instances mentioned above, hyperuricemia appears to result from an increased turnover of nucleic acid. Hyperuricemia may also result from reduced renal excretion of urate, either because of chemical interference with tubular secretion of urate or because of reduced renal mass due to parenchymal disease.

Typical gouty attacks may occur in patients receiving such drugs as hydrochlorothiazide or pyrazinamide, which interfere with urate excretion. Extreme obesity may be associated with renal hyperuricemia. Total caloric restriction may result in extreme hyperuricemia, which is correlated with serum levels of β-hydroxybutyric acid and is not infrequently associated with severe attacks of acute gouty arthritis involving especially the knees and ankles. In patients with hyperlipoproteinemias there is a direct correlation between serum triglyceride and urate levels.

Chronic renal disease is a frequent cause of hyperuricemia, but apparently few patients with glomerulonephritis, pyelonephritis, or polycystic renal disease live long enough to develop gout. The number may increase with chronic dialysis programs, and acute gouty arthritis has complicated the course of patients so managed. Gout continues to be found in patients who survive lead exposure early in life and go on to develop the slowly progressive nephritis of plumbism.

Hyperuricemia complicates untreated benign essential and renal hypertension in 20 percent of cases and malignant hypertension in 65 percent of cases; it has been attributed provisionally to renal anoxia and local lactic acid excess. Gout occurs in 10 percent or more of patients previously subjected to sympathectomy or adrenalectomy for hypertension. In the absence of family data it may be difficult to distinguish between sporadic primary gout and gout secondary to hypertensive renal disease, or chronic lead intoxication.

DIAGNOSIS Acute gouty arthritis is readily diagnosed by its typical explosive onset, the characteristic severity of involvement of the peripheral joint, the presence of hyperuricemia, and the rapid response to treatment with colchicine. Less typical presentations may be difficult to distinguish from other arthritides on clinical grounds. If present, tophi or typical roentgenologic findings of punched-out, destructive lesions will suggest the correct diagnosis. In patients lacking such lesions, the only pathognomonic finding is the presence, in the leukocytes of synovial fluid, of urate crystals which are needlelike and birefringent under polarized light (Fig. 100-5). Valuable clues in the diagnosis are a history of renal stones or of antecedent mild trauma or surgery in the patient or a history of gout, arthritis, or renal stones in the family (see Table 100-2).

Chronic gouty arthritis may be diagnosed by the presence of urate deposits in or near the affected joints or bursas or of soft-tissue deposits in the helix of the ear, the fingertips, the Achilles tendon, or other locations. The diagnosis may be confirmed by removal of the chalky contents of a tophus, microscopic identification of sodium urate crystals by optical means, or chemical identification by the murexide test or, preferably, by ultraviolet spectrophotometry and degradation by uricase.

DIFFERENTIAL DIAGNOSIS Acute gout must be differentiated from acute rheumatic fever, rheumatoid arthritis, traumatic arthritis, osteoarthritis, pyogenic arthritis, sarcoid arthritis, cellulitis, bursitis, tendonitis, and thrombophlebitis. *Reiter's syndrome* in men and *palindromic arthritis* in women may present similar clinical manifestations of episodes of acute arthritis followed by periods of complete remission, but hyperuricemia will not generally be present, joint fluid will not contain urate crystals, and colchicine is ineffective. *Pseudogout,* which is chiefly a disorder of elderly persons and is manifested

TABLE 100-2
Outline of work-up of patient with suspected gout

History

Previous typical acute arthritic attacks or kidney stones, or family history of same or chronic tophaceous gout; history of use of diuretics (especially thiazide) or of unbonded alcohol.

Physical examination

Presence of acute monarticular arthritis, especially of first metatarsal phalangeal joint; or of asymmetric but polyarticular arthritis; or of tophi especially of helix of ear. Vascular status, especially B.P. Obesity.

X-rays

Of afflicted joints; of hands and feet; intravenous pyelogram for renal function and questions of stones.

Electrocardiogram

Chemistries

Serum urate (several), blood urea nitrogen (BUN) or creatinine, plasma lipids, lipoprotein phenotyping. Twenty-four-hour urinary uric acid × 2-3, after 3 to 5 days of low purine diet (of questionable value during acute attack or if patient receiving drugs which affect uric acid levels). Creatinine clearance.

If urinary uric acid values normal or low, and BUN normal or moderately elevated, check for lead intoxication: erythrocyte stippling, urinary lead determination, perhaps with use of EDTA.

If urinary uric acid values increased, check for occult myeloproliferative syndrome or chronic hemolysis; or for specific enzymatic subtype, by assay of erythrocyte enzymes (HGPRT activity: PP-ribose-P synthetase activation as function of inorganic phosphate concentration).

Diagnostic procedures

Arthrocentesis, examination of synovial fluid, especially for needlelike intracellular (WBC) crystals which are anisotropic under polarized light. With a first-order red compensator, urate crystals are yellow when oriented in parallel, blue when perpendicular to axis of compensator.

Aspiration or biopsy of tophi, and examination for urate crystals, as above.

Analysis of urinary stone. Uric acid stone (pure or mixed) in a hyperuricemic individual has same metabolic significance as articular gout.

by acute attacks of arthritis of knees and other joints, is always accompanied by calcification of joint cartilage; the synovial fluid contains nonurate crystals of calcium pyrophosphate or apatite. The patients are not usually hyperuricemic.

Chronic gouty arthritis must be differentiated from all other chronic arthritides which cause deformities of joints, chiefly rheumatoid arthritis, osteoarthritis, traumatic arthritis, and residua of pyogenic arthritis. The history of onset, progression, response to colchicine and demonstration of hyperuricemia, asymmetric tumescences, typical roentgenographic changes, and tophi or crystals of urate in synovial fluid and leukocytes should establish the diagnosis.

TREATMENT The therapeutic aims in gout are (1) to terminate the acute gouty attack as promptly as possible; (2) to prevent recurrences of acute gouty arthritis; (3) to prevent or reverse complications of the disease resulting from deposition of sodium urate in joints and kidneys; and (4) to prevent formation of uric acid kidney stones. Treatment depends on the stage at which the patient is seen.

Acute attack *Colchicine* is the only treatment for acute gout of specific diagnostic value. It should be given as soon as the diagnosis is suspected. The initial dose of 0.5 to 1.2 mg colchicine is followed by 0.5 or 0.6 mg every hour for 8 hr, then every 2 hr until pain is relieved or until nausea, vomiting, cramping, or diarrhea develops. Maximum tolerated doses range from 4 to 10 mg. In most patients dramatic relief of pain and gastrointestinal side effects occur simultaneously. The diarrhea may be treated with paregoric, 4 ml, or Kaopectate, 30 ml, after each loose stool. Colchicine should be discontinued until gastrointestinal symptoms subside. Since the effective dose of colchicine varies, each patient should learn his own tolerance dose and stop just short of this in treatment of subsequent attacks. Colchicine usually affords relief within 24 to 48 hr; a second full therapeutic dose should not be repeated sooner than 72 hr.

Colchicine may also be given intravenously. The usual initial dose is 1 to 2 mg in 20 ml saline solution given slowly, and if a single dose is not effective, the injection may be repeated once in 4 to 5 hr (maximum intravenous dose, 3 to 4 mg). Gastrointestinal symptoms are uncommon with intravenous administration.

Phenylbutazone is also effective in acute gouty arthritis, and may be preferred when the gouty attack has proceeded for some time, or when the attack does not abate completely with colchicine. The initial dose is 400 mg orally, followed by 100 mg every 4 to 8 hr for 2 to 3 days. Oxyphenbutazone, a metabolite of phenylbutazone, is also effective in acute gout. The dose is the same as that of phenylbutazone, and the same precautions should be taken.

Patients who recognize prodromal symptoms may abort acute attacks by prompt institution of colchicine or phenylbutazone therapy; they frequently require only a few tablets to achieve success.

Indomethacin is sometimes dramatically effective in acute gout. It is given orally in initial doses ranging from 50 mg three times a day to 100 mg every 4 hr. When pain is relieved, doses are tapered over another 48 to 72 hr. Large doses may cause severe headache, gastric distress, or a transient depersonalization reaction in some patients, but these side effects have been noted only rarely in gouty patients receiving short courses of the drug.

If full doses of colchicine, phenylbutazone, or indomethacin are contraindicated, or ineffective, ACTH gel may be employed. Doses of 40 to 80 USP units are given intramuscularly every 6 to 8 hr for 2 to 3 days, rarely longer, following which the doses are reduced in stepwise fashion and discontinued. To avoid rebound attacks of gout after ACTH therapy, 0.6 mg colchicine should be given two or three times daily during and after administration of ACTH for at least 7 days.

Hydrocortisone in a dose of 25 to 50 mg injected intraarticularly into the involved joint is useful in treating acute gout limited to a single joint or bursa, and relief from pain is usually prompt and complete within 24 to 36 hr. Steroid hormones are not recommended for parenteral use in acute gout, as the effects are inconsistent and rebound attacks frequent.

During the acute attack, bearing weight on the involved joints should be avoided. In severe attacks the patient will invariably immobilize himself voluntarily, but in milder attacks it is necessary for the physician to insist on this. Mobilization is permitted as soon as the joint is no longer painful.

Interval phase The patient with gout should avoid high purine foods so as to lessen the burden of uric acid excretion. A severe limitation of purine-containing foods is rarely indicated, unless renal function and the ability to excrete uric acid are reduced significantly. Many gouty patients are overweight, and gradual weight reduction is indicated. Sudden weight reduction may precipitate gouty attacks and should be avoided. In general, diets of moderate protein content, somewhat low in fat, are preferred.

A high fluid intake is advisable to maintain a urinary output of 2,000 ml per day. Uric acid excretion is thus promoted, and the dangers of crystal formation in the kidney or ureter are reduced. Alcoholic beverages, especially beer, ale, and wine, should be avoided if possible, as they may precipitate attacks. Distilled alcoholic beverages, in moderation, generally have little influence on the gouty process.

The daily ingestion of 0.6 to 1.8 mg colchicine is generally effective in reducing the number of acute gouty attacks in patients who are subject to frequent episodes. Maintenance colchicine therapy is particularly important during the first year or two after institution of uricosuric drugs, or of allopurinol.

Chronic gouty arthritis Use of a drug to lower the serum level of uric acid to 6 mg per 100 ml or less is indicated in all gouty patients with visible tophi, with roentgenographic evidence of urate deposits, with serum uric acid levels above 8.5 to 9.0 mg per 100 ml, or with a history of four or more major attacks of acute gouty arthritis per year. The drug of choice is allopurinol, but uricosuric agents may be used. None of these agents is of any value in the immediate treatment of the acute attack. With both types the number of acute gouty attacks may be increased during the first 6 months unless maintenance colchicine therapy is given, whereas after 12 to 18 months the number may be decidedly reduced. Uricosuric drugs block tubular reabsorption of filtered urate. Those of use in gout are probenecid, sulfinpyrazone, and salicylates.

Probenecid is given in doses of 0.5 to 3 g daily in two or three evenly spaced doses (average dose, 1 to 1.5 g). This drug may produce gastrointestinal upsets, headaches, or skin rash.

Sulfinpyrazone may be given in doses of 100 to 600 mg daily in three or four divided doses (average dose, 300 mg). This drug is related to phenylbutazone and can cause untoward reactions, but is generally somewhat better tolerated than probenecid.

Salicylates block the uricosuric action of both probenecid and sulfinpyrazone and must not be used concurrently. Salicylates are uricosuric when given in high doses (4 to 6 g daily), but few patients can tolerate these quantities.

With all uricosuric agents the doses should be low initially, so as to avoid sudden excretion of large quantities of urate. Fluids should be forced so as to prevent formation of concentrated urine, especially during the late hours of the night. During the first days or weeks of therapy the urine should be alkalinized; this may be difficult to achieve, as gouty patients tend to produce acid urine. In patients who are mobilizing urate, and especially those who form uric acid gravel, alkalinization during the night, when fluid intake is reduced, is important. A single 250-mg tablet of acetazolamide (Diamox) taken at bedtime will serve to keep the urine alkaline and dilute throughout the night.

A second approach toward controlling serum urate levels is that of regulating production of uric acid, rather than (or in addition to) augmenting its excretion. This is achieved by use of *allopurinol* or its derivative oxipurinol, both of which are potent inhibitors of xanthine oxidase. Allopurinol is converted to oxipurinol in the body, and the latter compound has a longer biologic half-life (28 hr), ultimately being largely excreted in the urine. Inhibition of conversion of hypoxanthine and xanthine to uric acid permits these uric acid precursors to be excreted instead. Use of allopurinol results in reduction of levels of uric acid in serum *and in urine.* The drug is effective even in the presence of renal failure, when uricosuric agents are generally ineffective. Its action is not blocked by salicylates. The usual dose is 100 mg, given orally two to four times a day. In the presence of moderate nitrogen retention the dose of allopurinol should be reduced as the biologic half-life of the active metabolite, oxipurinol, is prolonged. Allopurinol is usually well tolerated, but may cause gastric irritation, diarrhea, or skin rash, or induce an attack of gout. Uricosuric agents may be used concurrently to hasten mobilization of urate deposits. Since allopurinol decreases uric acid excretion, it is also very useful in controlling uric acid stone formation, especially in patients who are overproducers of uric acid.

In selected patients *surgical removal* of large extra-articular *urate deposits*, such as those in olecranon bursas, may be advisable. Occasionally amputation of irreparably damaged digits, especially those containing draining sinuses, is indicated. Physical therapy and appropriate self-help devices are valuable in patients who are partially disabled.

Asymptomatic hyperuricemia Asymptomatic hyperuricemia is frequently encountered in family members of patients with gout and in the general population. One must exclude hyperuricemia as a manifestation of reduced renal function or of action of certain drugs. Asymptomatic hyperuricemia generally requires no therapy, as only about one-third of patients will ever develop articular attacks, and adequate therapy can be instituted when these supervene. However, exceptions do exist, as in patients with serum levels of uric acid above 8.5 or 9 mg per 100 ml, especially if the urinary excretion levels are low and there is a family history of tophaceous involvement. In such circumstances the asymptomatic subject should be treated with allopurinol before articular or renal complications develop. It is essential that the physician maintain frequent close observation of the patient.

The role of diet It is not necessary to restrict purine intake severely in most gouty patients. However, weight reduction of the overweight patient and abstinence from alcohol may be markedly beneficial. In some patients who have achieved ideal weight and ceased use of alcohol, all clinical manifestations of gout have disappeared, and normal plasma and urinary urate levels, and normal values of the miscible urate pool and of glycine incorporation into urate have been reestablished. The analogy with dietary control of hyperglycemia and adult-onset diabetes is obvious, but the physiologic mechanisms of response are equally obscure.

Secondary gout Treatment of gouty arthritis occurring secondary to hematopoietic disturbances is the same as for primary gout except that one must be especially alert to potential complications. The basal uric acid excretion may be high, and use of uricosuric agents may intensify the risk of crystalluria and of tubular or ureteral blockage. High fluid intake and alkalinization are of great importance. The drug of choice for control of hyperuricemia for these patients is allopurinol.

XANTHINURIA

This is a rare genetic disorder, caused by a marked deficiency or absence of xanthine oxidase activity in liver and small intestinal mucosa. In the lactating female enzyme activity is deficient in breast milk or colostrum as well. Xanthinuria is probably transmitted as an autosomal recessive trait, but the heterozygote cannot be identified by present methods of study. A phenocopy of the genetic disorder is produced by allopurinol. Xanthine oxidase catalyzes the oxidation of hypoxanthine to xanthine, and of xanthine to uric acid. The disorder is characterized by the replacement of urinary uric acid by hypoxanthine and xanthine. When dietary purines are restricted, serum urate values are less than 1 mg per 100 ml, and urinary urate usually less than 30 mg per day. Only nine well-documented cases have been reported. In five the patients had no symptoms referable to the metabolic defect, and were diagnosed during study of hypouricemia. Two adult patients had muscle cramps on exercise, and a myopathy associated with crystalline deposits of hypoxanthine and xanthine in muscle. In three patients urinary xanthine stones developed at ages two, four, and six years. Xanthine stones, like urate, are radiolucent. They can be identified by spectrophotometric, chromatographic, or crystallographic methods. Urinary oxypurine (xanthine plus hypoxanthine) excretion values range from 100 to 600 mg per day of which 70 to 95 percent is xanthine, whose solubility in urine is less than that of uric acid at pH 5, and is increased very little in neutral or mildly alkaline urine. The lack of larger excretion values of hypoxanthine is attributed to its active reutilization by reconversion to inosinic acid in the reaction catalyzed by HGPRT, the enzyme which is deficient in the Lesch-Nyhan syndrome (see Gout, above). Xanthinuria must be differentiated from other causes of hypouricemia, the commonest of which are drugs (large doses of salicylates, other uricosurics, or allopurinol), or malignancies which may be associated with increased renal clearance of urate. Also to be considered are the renal tubular dysfunction of Wilson's disease and the Fanconi syndrome. In almost all these conditions serum urate values are above 1 mg per 100 ml, and the urine contains considerably more uric acid than does that of patients with xanthinuria.

Treatment is nonspecific. Maintenance of a high fluid intake and large urine volume is advised. Alkalinization is not indicated, as the high pK_{a_1} value of xanthine (7.7) allows only minimal increases in xanthine solubility at pH values that can safely be achieved and maintained. In one patient allopurinol resulted in a slight reduction in xanthine and increase in hypoxanthine excretion. Its use is logical in patients with low residual activity of xanthine oxidase, particularly if they have formed xanthine stones.

REFERENCES

Gout

KELLEY WN et al: Hypoxanthinequanine phosphyribosyltransferase deficiency in gout. Ann Intern Med 70:155, 1969

——, WYNGAARDEN JB: The drug therapy of gout, in *Seminars in Drug Treatment*, eds JR DiPalma, B Calesnick, New York: Henry M. Stratton, 1, 119, 1971

RUNDLES RW et al: Effects of xanthine oxidase inhibitor on clinical manifestations and purine metabolism in gout. Ann Intern Med 60:717, 1964

SEEGMILLER JE et al: An enzyme defect associated with an X-linked human neurological disorder and excessive purine synthesis. Science 155:1682, 1967

SPERLINE O et al: Evidence of molecular alteration of erythrocyte hypoxanthine-guanine phosphoribosyltransferase in a gouty family with partial deficiency of the enzyme. Rev Eur Etud Clin Biol 17:72, 1972

WYNGAARDEN JB: Gout, in *The Metabolic Basis of Inherited Disease*, 3d ed., eds JB Stanbury et al, New York: McGraw-Hill, 1972

YU TF, GUTMAN AB: Uric acid nephrolithiasis in gout: Predisposing factors. Ann Intern Med 67:1133, 1967

Xanthinuria

SEEGMILLER JE: Hereditary xanthinuria, in *Duncan's Diseases of Metabolism*, 6th ed., ed PK Bondy, Philadelphia: Saunders, 1969, p. 581

WYNGAARDEN JB: Xanthinuria, in *The Metabolic Basis of Inherited Disease*, 3d ed., eds JB Stanbury et al, New York: McGraw-Hill, 1972, p. 992

101 HEMOCHROMATOSIS

GEORGE E. CARTWRIGHT

DEFINITION Idiopathic hemochromatosis (bronze diabetes, pigment cirrhosis) is characterized pathologically by excessive deposits of iron in the body and clinically by hepatomegaly with eventual liver insufficiency, pigmentation of the skin, diabetes mellitus, and frequently cardiac failure.

HISTORY The first clinical description of the disease was given by Trousseau in 1865. In 1889 von Recklinghausen named the disease *hemochromatosis* and described the iron-containing pigment, hemosiderin. Sheldon, in a now-classic monograph, reviewed the world's literature in 1935. Finch and Finch in 1955 reviewed the literature since 1935 and added 80 cases of their own. More recently, MacDonald has made important contributions by emphasizing the role of excessive dietary iron and preexisting portal cirrhosis in the pathogenesis of acquired hemochromatosis.

INCIDENCE Hemochromatosis is a rare disease, recognized in approximately 1 in 20,000 hospital admissions, and 1 in 7,000 hospital deaths. It is observed ten times as frequently in males as in females. Nearly 70 percent of all patients with this disease develop their first symptoms between the ages of forty and sixty years. Hemochromatosis is rarely recognized below the age of twenty years.

PATHOGENESIS One of the earliest measurable alterations in iron metabolism in hemochromatosis is the elevation of the plasma iron and saturation of the plasma iron-binding protein, transferrin. As the disease progresses, the amount of storage iron increases. In advanced disease, the tissues contain over 20 g iron; total body iron in normal persons is in the range of 3 to 5 g. The excess iron is deposited primarily in parenchymal cells in the form of ferritin and hemosiderin. Increased amounts of iron are found in almost all body tissues, especially those in which there is organ dysfunction. Iron in the liver and pancreas is increased fifty to one hundred times; in the heart, ten to fifteen times; in the spleen, kidney, and skin, about five times.

Since iron is not excreted from the body in appreciable amounts even in normal persons, the conclusion that iron absorption is increased in idiopathic hemochromatosis is inescapable. There are two quite differing explanations as to why this occurs. The classic concept is that idiopathic hemochromatosis is due to an inherited inborn error in metabolism in which the basic abnormality is the increased absorption of iron. According to this view the excessive deposition of iron is the cause of the tissue damage. The other point of view is that hemochromatosis is a variant of portal cirrhosis of the liver. A high incidence (30 to 85 percent) of alcoholism has been observed in patients with idiopathic hemochromatosis, and it has been noted that the iron content of alcoholic beverages, particularly various wines, is high.

Hemochromatosis has been observed (1) as a familial occurrence without apparent cause other than an inherited inborn error of metabolism; (2) in alcoholic subjects with a high dietary intake of iron; (3) in malnourished Bantu subjects in South Africa secondary to long-term iron overload ("Bantu siderosis"); (4) in isolated instances of parenchymal iron overload following intake of medicinal doses of iron over many years; (5) in association with various types of refractory anemia; and (6) in a few patients given 100 or more transfusions of blood. Therefore, it would seem that hemochromatosis is a syndrome with several possible causes. The common denominator in all cases is the presence of excessive iron in parenchymal tissues.

PATHOLOGY At autopsy the enlarged, nodular liver and pancreas present a striking ochre color. Histologically, hemosiderin is deposited in many organs, particularly the liver and pancreas. The liver shows considerable fibrosis. Testicular atrophy is frequently present, both grossly and histologically. There are hemosiderin deposits in the myocardium, and they may be associated with myocardial edema, fibrosis, and necrosis. The epidermis of the skin is thin, and melanin pigment is found in the cells of the basal layer. Hemosiderin is deposited almost entirely in the corium.

CLINICAL MANIFESTATIONS The symptoms and signs of hemochromatosis are related to the *skin pigmentation, diabetes, liver impairment, and cardiac disease.* Of these the cirrhosis of the liver is the most constant abnormality.

The initial symptoms most frequently encountered are related to the onset of *diabetes.* Weakness, lassitude, weight loss, change in skin color, abdominal pain, dyspnea, edema, ascites, loss of libido, and peripheral neuritis are also frequent initial symptoms. Hepatomegaly, pigmentation, spider angiomas, splenomegaly, ascites, evidences of congestive failure or cardiac arrhythmias, loss of body hair, testicular atrophy, jaundice, and hypertension are the most prominent physical signs, given in decreasing order of frequency.

The liver is the first tissue known to be damaged, and hepatomegaly is present in about 93 percent of symptomatic cases. Hepatic enlargement may exist in the absence of symptoms or in the presence of normal liver function tests. Indeed, over half the patients with symptomatic hemochromatosis have little or no laboratory evidence of functional impairment of the liver in spite of hepatomegaly and proved fibrosis. Loss of body hair, palmar erythema, testicular atrophy, gynecomastia, spider angioma, and, particularly, loss of libido are often seen and are related to the severity of the liver damage. Manifestations of portal hypertension and esophageal varices may occur but are less commonly observed than in Laennec's cirrhosis. A nontender, slightly enlarged spleen is present in approximately half the cases. Primary carcinoma of the liver develops in about 14 percent. The incidence of this last complication increases greatly with age.

Excessive *skin pigmentation* is present in about 90

percent of the patients at the time the diagnosis is established. Pigmentation may be due to deposition of melanin or iron or both. In general, melanin deposition gives rise to bronzing, iron deposition to a metallic gray hue. Pigmentation usually is diffuse and generalized, but frequently it is deeper on the face, neck, extensor aspects of the lower forearms, dorsa of the hands, lower legs, genital regions, and in scars. In only 10 to 15 percent of cases is there demonstrable pigmentation of the oral mucosa.

About 82 percent of all patients develop *diabetes mellitus* and symptoms therefrom. The diabetes may appear rapidly, and insulin requirements may increase rapidly. About 72 percent of the patients require insulin for the control of the diabetes. In some instances severe insulin resistance develops, in others there may be sensitivity to insulin. In most instances, the diabetes is controlled with little difficulty. Since the diabetes is usually present for less than a decade, the late degenerative sequelae of the complication are not prominent.

Approximately one-third of patients with idiopathic hemochromatosis die of *cardiac failure.* The heart disease is extremely common in young adults, and symptoms may develop suddenly, with rapid progression to death. The most important manifestations of heart disease are congestive failure and cardiac arrhythmias, particularly ventricular extrasystoles and paroxysmal atrial tachycardia. Other arrhythmias may occur as well.

Patients with hemochromatosis may develop an arthropathy which differs from osteoarthritis and rheumatoid arthritis and is characterized by a progressive polyarthritis, often beginning in metacarpophalangeal joints and then involving other articulations. X-ray films show narrowing of joint space without osteophyte formation and without the marginal erosions of rheumatoid arthritis. Chondrocalcinosis is seen frequently, and the presence of calcium pyrophosphate deposits has been documented. The mechanisms of these abnormalities and their relation to iron metabolism are not known.

DIAGNOSIS The classic *triad of skin pigmentation, diabetes mellitus, and hepatomegaly,* especially in the presence of heart disease and evidence of hypogonadism, should always suggest the diagnosis. Confirmation of the presence of liver, pancreatic, heart, and gonadal disease should then be obtained by customary tests of the functions of these organs. It then remains to demonstrate that there is excessive storage iron.

The diagnosis is enhanced considerably if the plasma iron level is found to be elevated (above 150 μg per 100 ml) and the iron-binding protein of the plasma is 75 to 100 percent saturated. However, the only definitive test is liver biopsy. Other procedures which indicate an excess of body iron stores are bone marrow aspiration for hemosiderin, examination of the urine sediment for hemosiderin, skin biopsy, and gastric mucosal biopsy.

Finch and Finch state that there are no unique features in idiopathic hemochromatosis by which it may be distinguished pathologically from the terminal stage of other iron-storage diseases, such as dietary or transfusion hemochromatosis. They define *hemosiderosis* as a focal increase in tissue iron or a general increase in iron stores without associated tissue damage, and *hemochromatosis* as a general increase in body iron stores with resultant tissue damage. From these definitions, the differentiation of hemosiderosis from hemochromatosis can be easily made by the presence or absence of organ dysfunction. Dietary and transfusion hemochromatosis can be differentiated from idiopathic hemochromatosis on the basis of a history of excessive iron intake by mouth, by injection, or intravenously in the form of blood. In evaluating dietary iron exposure, the dietary iron content, type of diet, type of cooking utensils, intake of medicinal iron, and iron content of the drinking water or other beverages must be considered.

PROGNOSIS The life expectancy of patients after signs of clinical hemochromatosis have become manifest averages 4.4 years, but several instances have been recorded of patients living up to 20 or 30 years after manifestation of signs. The average duration of life after diabetes has developed is 3 years. The principal causes of death are cardiac failure (30 percent), hepatic coma (15 percent), hematemesis (14 percent), hepatoma (14 percent), and pneumonia (12 percent). The most recent advance in the therapy of this disease, the introduction of methods for the removal of iron, is expected to increase life expectancy further.

TREATMENT The therapy of idiopathic hemochromatosis involves removal of the excess body iron by phlebotomy and supportive treatment of damaged organs. The management of the hepatic failure, cardiac failure, and diabetes differs little from the conventional management of these conditions. Loss of libido and change in secondary sex characteristics are relieved by testosterone therapy. Iron is best removed from the body by a weekly or twice weekly phlebotomy of 500 ml. Since the average amount of iron in a patient with hemochromatosis is approximately 25 g, about 2 years of weekly bleeding will be required to deplete the iron stores. Chelating agents such as EDTA and desferrioxamine are of little or no practical value in the management of hemochromatosis.

REFERENCES

BOTHWELL TH, FINCH CA: *Iron Metabolism,* Boston: Little, Brown, 1962

CHARLTON RW, BOTHWELL TH: Hemochromatosis: Dietary and genetic aspects, in *Progress in Hematology,* eds EB Brown, CV Moore, vol. 5, New York: Grune & Stratton, 1966, p. 298

FINCH SC, FINCH CA: Idiopathic hemochromatosis: An iron storage disease. Medicine 34:381, 1955

HAMILTON E et al: The arthropathy of idiopathic hemochromatosis. Q J Med (n.s.) 37:171, 1968

MACDONALD RA: *Hemochromatosis and Hemosiderosis,* Springfield, Ill.: Charles C Thomas, 1964

——: Primary hemochromatosis: Inherited or acquired?, in *Progress in Hematology,* eds EB Brown, CV Moore, vol. 5, New York: Grune & Stratton, 1966, p. 324

102
DISORDERS OF PORPHYRIN METABOLISM

GEORGE E. CARTWRIGHT

DEFINITIONS *Porphyrins* are pigments that possess a basic structure of four pyrrole rings linked by methene (—CH—) bridges (Fig. 102-1). The individual porphyrins differ from each other according to the nature of the eight possible side chains. Each porphyrin has a number of stereoisomers. *Porphyrinogens* are colorless compounds (reduced porphyrins) with a basic structure of four pyrrole rings linked by methane (—CH_2—) bridges.

Porphyrin pigments are widely distributed throughout the plant and animal worlds in chlorophyll, hemoglobin, catalase, and a number of cytochrome and peroxidase enzymes.

The term *porphyrinuria* refers to excessive excretion of porphyrins in the urine. *Coproporphyrinuria,* the excretion of increased amounts of coproporphyrin, is not uncommon and occurs in a variety of conditions. The term *porphyria* embraces a group of diseases, each with unusual and characteristic manifestations, which have in common the excessive excretion of one or more of the porphyrins, porphyrinogens, and/or porphyrin precursors (Δ-aminolevulinic acid and porphobilinogen) in the urine and/or feces.

HISTORY Congenital porphyria was first described by Günther in 1911. Much of the knowledge of the chemistry of the porphyrins came from Hans Fischer and his school in Munich. In 1915, these workers described, named, and isolated in crystalline form the uroporphyrins and coproporphyrins from the urine of the patient in their famous case of congenital porphyria (Petry). Shemin and Granick and their groups in New York have made substantial contributions to knowledge of the biosynthesis of the porphyrins. Contributions to the understanding of the types and manifestations of porphyria have come from Waldenström in Sweden, Rimington in England, Barnes and Dean in South Africa, and Watson, Schwartz, and Schmid in the United States.

BIOSYNTHESIS The rather complex porphyrin molecule is synthesized in the body from two simple precursors, acetate and glycine (Fig. 102-2). Acetate enters the Krebs tricarboxylic acid cycle (Chap. 72) and is converted into succinate. Succinyl CoA (active succinate) is then formed in the presence of Mg^{++} ion, adenosine triphosphate (ATP), and coenzyme A (CoA). The activated form of succinate condenses with a pyridoxal phosphate-glycine enzyme (glycine-PE) to form the 5-carbon compound, Δ-aminolevulinic acid (Δ-ALA), and carbon dioxide by the decarboxylation of glycine. This step is enzymatically controlled (ALA synthetase), and several intermediate compounds have been suggested. Two molecules of Δ-aminolevulinic acid, in the presence of glutathione (GSH) and an enzyme, Δ-aminolevulinic acid dehydrase (Δ-ALA DH), condense to form a substituted monopyrrole, porphobilinogen, which contains acetic

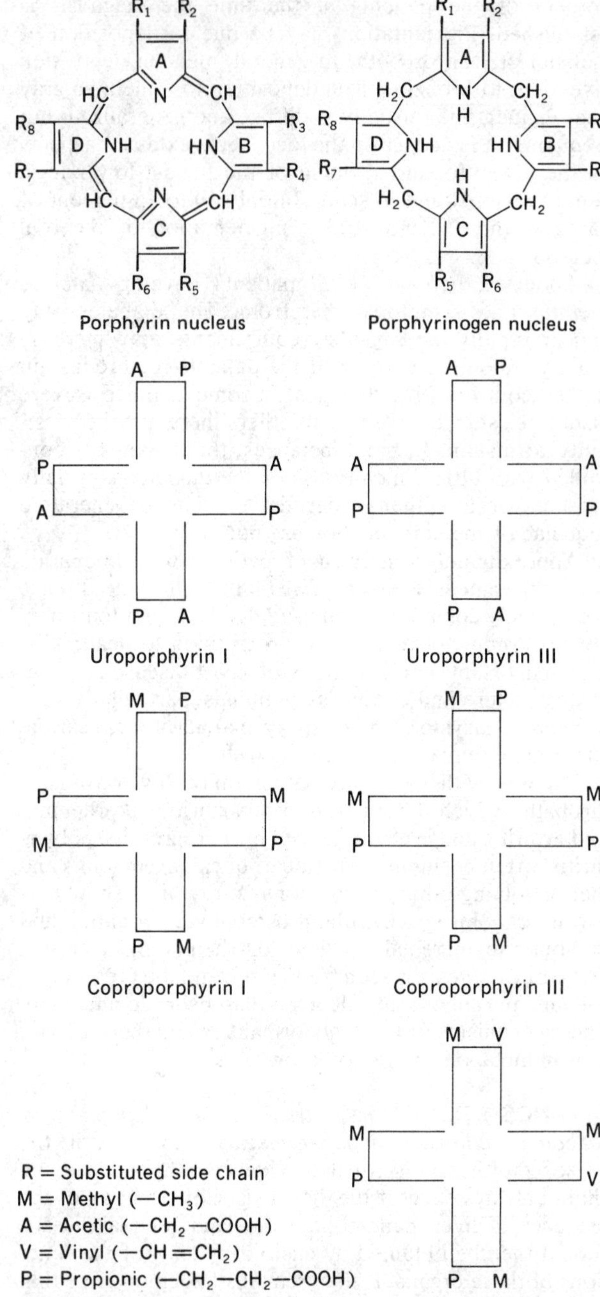

FIGURE 102-1
The structural formulas of the porphyrin and porphyrinogen nuclei and diagrammatic formulas of the important naturally occurring porphyrins.

acid (A) and propionic acid (P) side chains. In the next step in heme synthesis, four molecules of porphobilinogen condense to form the reduced tetrapyrrolic structure, uroporphyrinogen. This step is catalyzed by at least two enzymes, uroporphyrinogen synthetase (US) and uroporphyrinogen cosynthetase (UC). Details of the action of these enzymes and the sequence of reactions leading from porphobilinogen to uroporphyrinogen types I and III are not known. Uroporphyrin III is not in the direct pathway of heme synthesis, as was formerly assumed, but is a by-product. Uroporphyrinogen III (reduced uroporphyrin) is converted to coproporphyrinogen by the enzyme uroporphyrinogen decarboxylase (UD). Coproporphyrinogen III is then converted to protoporphyrin III in the presence of the enzyme coproporphyrinogen oxidase. Coproporphyrin III is a by-product, whereas the available evidence suggests that protoporphyrin III is in the direct pathway of heme synthesis. Protoporphyrin III is converted to hemoglobin in the presence of iron, glutathione, globin, and the enzyme heme synthetase (HS). The intermediate steps between protoporphyrin and hemoglobin have not been identified. It is not known whether heme or a porphyrin-globin compound is an intermediate in this reaction, although the former possibility seems more likely.

METABOLISM The most important of the naturally occurring porphyrins are uroporphyrin (isomer types I and III), coproporphyrin (types I and III), and protoporphyrin (type III).

Protoporphyrin III is present in hemoglobin and is, therefore, the most important of the porphyrins from the physiologic standpoint. It is absent from urine. The concentration of fecal protoporphyrin is related to the amount of blood in the gastrointestinal tract, the rate of liberation of protoporphyrin from hemoglobin by fecal bacteria, and the excretion of protoporphyrin by the liver.

Coproporphyrin is the predominant porphyrin in urine and feces under normal circumstances. Coproporphyrinuria occurs in a variety of clinical conditions, such as lead poisoning, poliomyelitis, liver disease, acute alcoholism, hemolytic anemia, and Hodgkin's disease. In all these disorders the increased coproporphyrinuria accompanies the underlying disease, and it is unlikely that the abnormality in porphyrin metabolism contributes significantly to the clinical picture. Coproporphyrinuria is also found in patients with certain types of porphyria. Abnormally high fecal coproporphyrin values are found in patients with hemolytic anemia, and low values occur in patients with liver disease.

Uroporphyrin is normally excreted in urine in only trace amounts. The urinary excretion of this porphyrin is moderately increased in lead poisoning and is greatly increased in patients with certain types of porphyria.

PORPHYRIA

Porphyria may be divided into two general groups (Table 102-1). In erythropoietic porphyria, excessive quantities of porphyrins accumulate in the normoblasts and erythrocytes. Under these circumstances, red fluorescence may be observed when the cells are exposed to ultraviolet light. The predominant porphyrin synthesized in erythropoietic uroporphyria (congenital porphyria) is uroporphyrin; in erythropoietic protoporphyria, protoporphyrin; and in erythropoietic coproporphyria, coproporphyrin. In porphyria hepatica, excessive porphyrin production occurs in the liver. Hepatic porphyria may be subdivided further into at least four different types: acute intermittent porphyria, porphyria cutanea tarda hereditaria (mixed porphyria, porphyria variegata, South African Caucasian porphyria, protocoproporphyria), porphyria cutanea tarda symptomatica, and hereditary coproporphyria.

This classification, although useful, is not entirely satisfactory. There is some overlap between the erythro-

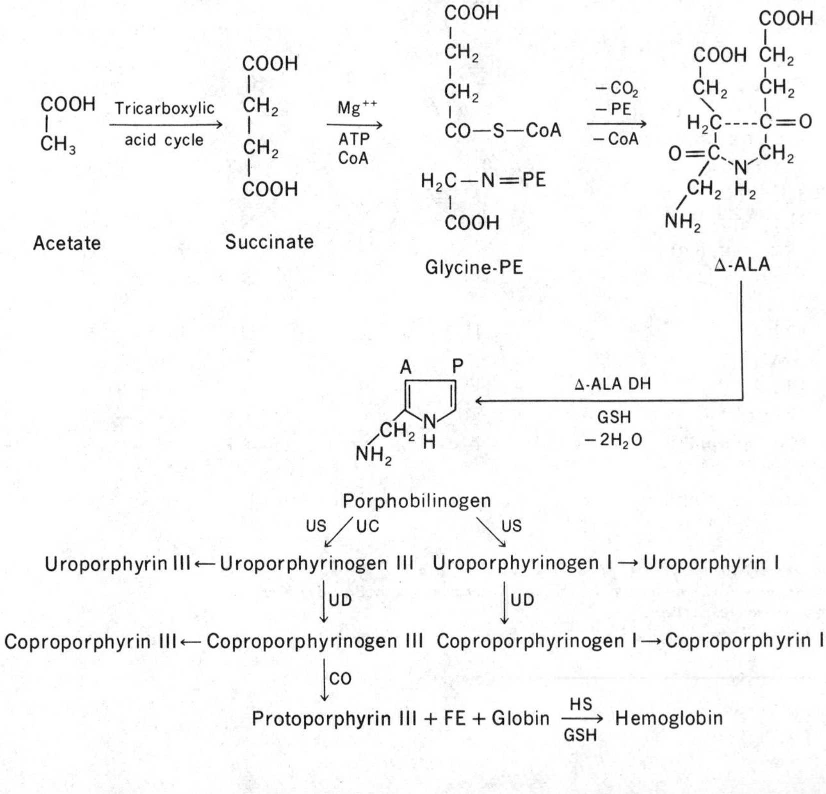

Acetate → (Tricarboxylic acid cycle) → Succinate → (Mg^{++}, ATP, CoA) → Glycine-PE → ($-CO_2$, $-PE$, $-CoA$) → Δ-ALA → (Δ-ALA DH, GSH, $-2H_2O$) → Porphobilinogen

Porphobilinogen → (US/UC) → Uroporphyrinogen III → Uroporphyrin III; Porphobilinogen → (US) → Uroporphyrinogen I → Uroporphyrin I

Uroporphyrinogen III → (UD) → Coproporphyrinogen III → Coproporphyrin III; Uroporphyrinogen I → (UD) → Coproporphyrinogen I → Coproporphyrin I

Coproporphyrinogen III → (CO) → Protoporphyrin III + FE + Globin → (HS, GSH) → Hemoglobin

FIGURE 102-2
The biosynthesis of the porphyrins from acetate and glycine and the biosynthetic pathway of hemoglobin. CoA, coenzyme A; ATP, adenosine triphosphate; PE, pyridoxal phosphate enzyme (ALA synthetase); Δ-ALA, delta-aminolevulinic acid; Δ-ALA DH, delta-aminolevulinic acid dehydrase; GSH, glutathione; US, uroporphyrinogen synthetase; UC, uroporphyrinogen cosynthetase; UD, uroporphyrinogen decarboxylase; CO, coproporphyrinogen oxidase; HS, heme synthetase; A, acetic acid; P, propionic acid.

poietic and hepatic groups, and not all patients with hepatic porphyria can be classified clearly into one of the four subgroups.

Porphyria erythropoietica

ERYTHROPOIETIC UROPORPHYRIA This is a very rare disorder, inherited probably as a recessive mendelian characteristic. The clinical manifestations occur very early in life, sometimes even a few days after birth, but often they are not observed until after an interval of a year or two. The disease is characterized by the excessive deposition of porphyrin in the tissues, leading to pronounced photosensitization. The early lesions of photodynamic origin are the blisters of hydroa estivale (hydroa vacciniforme) on skin surfaces exposed to light, especially of the face and hands. In time, scarring and mutilation occur. After years of continued photosensitivity, the mutilation becomes extensive, with loss of fingers, portions of the nose and ears, scarring of the cheeks and about the mouth, ectropion, or symblepharon. Skin not exposed to light remains unaffected. Hemolytic anemia and splenomegaly are an integral part of the disease. Erythrodontia may be observed in those cases in which sufficient porphyrin has been deposited in the teeth to make them grossly red or reddish brown. Teeth which do not show erythrodontia in ordinary light may exhibit red fluorescence in Wood's light. Red fluorescence may be seen in the phalangeal bones if a strong source of ultraviolet light is allowed to shine through the fingers. There is no marked disturbance of the nervous system, nor is there abdominal colic.

Because of the demonstration of large quantities of uroporphyrin and coproporphyrin in the normoblasts in the bone marrow, it has been suggested that in this type of porphyria the excessive quantities of uroporphyrin are formed in the marrow. It is for this reason that the disease had been called *erythropoietic uroporphyria* rather than congenital porphyria.

The color of the urine varies from pink to red. Uroporphyrin I and coproporphyrin I are the predominant porphyrins excreted. If the concentration of uroporphyrin is sufficiently great, the urine, on the addition of hydrochloric acid, exhibits an intense band at about 552 nm and a weaker band at 596 nm when viewed in a hand spectroscope. The excretion of porphyrin precursors, Δ-aminolevulinic acid and porphobilinogen, is not increased.

TABLE 102-1
Distinguishing features of the several types of porphyria

	Erythropoietic			*Hepatic*						
Characteristics	*Uro-porphyria*	*Proto-porphyria*	*Copro-porphyria*	*Acute intermittent*		*Cutanea tarda hereditaria*		*Cutanea tarda symptomatica*	*Hereditary coproporphyria*	
Inheritance	Recessive	Dominant	Dominant	Dominant		Dominant		Acquired	Dominant	
Sex	Both	Both		Both		Both		Both	Both	
Age of onset, years	0–5	0–5		15–40		10–30		Any age	Any age	
Phase of disease				*Latent*	*Acute*	*Latent*	*Acute*		*Latent*	*Acute*
Photosensitivity and cutaneous lesions	++++	++	++	0	0	0	+ or 0	++	0	0 or +
Abdominal, psychic, and/or neurologic symptoms	0	0	0	0	++	0	+	0	0	+
RBC:										
Uroporphyrin	++++	++	++	N	N	N	N	N	N	N
Coproporphyrin	+++	++	++++	N	N	N	N	N	N	N
Protoporphyrin	++	++++	+	N	N	N	N	N	N	N
Urine:										
Color*	Red*	N*	N*	N*	Red*	N*	N or red*	Red*	N*	N or red*
Δ-ALA†	N	N	N	+	++	N	++	N	+	++
PBG‡	N	N	N	++	++++	N	++	N	+	++
Uroporphyrin	++++	N	N	++	++	N	+++	++++	N	++
Coproporphyrin	++	N	N	++	++	N	+++	++	N or +	+++
Feces:										
Coproporphyrin	++	N	N	N	+	++++	+++	+++	++	++++
Protoporphyrin	++	N to ++	N	N	+	++++	+++	++	N	+

0, absent; N, normal; +, increased; ++++, greatly increased.
* *Freshly voided. On standing, the urine may become deep brownish-red or black.*
† *Δ-Aminolevulinic acid.*
‡ *Porphobilinogen.*

The disease is slowly progressive, and death is usually due to an intercurrent infection or severe hemolytic anemia. At autopsy there is extensive deposition of porphyrins in the skeleton and tissues. This may be so pronounced as to color the bones red. Erythroid hyperplasia of the bone marrow and splenomegaly are additional pathologic features.

Treatment Exposure to sunlight should be avoided. The harmful and disfiguring effects of light may be ameliorated by the use of an appropriate sunscreen preparation. Splenectomy is indicated if there is evidence of increased erythrocyte destruction. Splenectomy may be associated not only with amelioration of the hemolytic anemia but also with a reduction in photosensitivity and porphyrin excretion.

ERYTHROPOIETIC PROTOPORPHYRIA Erythropoietic protoporphyria, the most common form of erythropoietic porphyria, is transmitted as an autosomal dominant characteristic. The disease usually becomes manifest in childhood and is characterized clinically by *skin photosensitivity with intense, painful itching, edema, and erythema of the exposed parts.* Chronic skin changes may develop on the dorsa of the hands, especially over the knuckles, but may also be observed on the nose, cheeks, and lips. Biochemically, the disorder is characterized by an increase in the *protoporphyrin content of the normoblasts and erythrocytes,* an increased level of plasma protoporphyrin, and an increased excretion of protoporphyrin in the feces. The urinary excretion of Δ-ALA, porphobilinogen, coproporphyrin, and uroporphyrin is not increased. However, several patterns of chemical abnormality have been demonstrated in patients with the disease and in members of their families. Elevation of free erythrocyte protoporphyrin may occur with no increase in plasma or fecal protoporphyrin. Fecal protoporphyrin may be increased with no abnormalities of plasma or erythrocyte protoporphyrin. The complete biochemical stigmas of the disease have been observed in the absence of skin photosensitivity.

The metabolic defect consists of overproduction of protoporphyrin in erythroid cells leading to an increase in erythrocyte protoporphyrin and in the liver leading to greatly increased fecal excretion of the pigment. The nature of the metabolic defect in heme biosynthesis in protoporphyria is unknown.

Beta-carotene, 30 mg daily orally, may be of value in reducing dermal photosensitivity to sunlight.

ERYTHROPOIETIC COPROPORPHYRIA This disorder is less well defined than the two previous disorders, having been described in only two members of one family. Swelling of the skin and itching after exposure to sunlight were the only clinical manifestations in the propositus. The erythrocytes contained large amounts of coproporphyrin III, a moderate increase in protoporphyrin, and a relatively marked increase in uroporphyrin, in comparison with the normal. Urine and fecal porphyrin concentrations were within normal limits, and the excretion of porphyrin precursors was not increased.

Porphyria hepatica

ACUTE INTERMITTENT PORPHYRIA This is an uncommon disease which affects both sexes, with a slight predilection for the female. Young adults or the middle-aged are most frequently affected. Acute porphyria is extremely rare below the age of fifteen and after the age of sixty. The familial occurrence of the disease is marked. It is probably transmitted as a mendelian dominant characteristic. The disease is characterized clinically by (1) periodic attacks of intense abdominal colic, usually accompanied by nausea and vomiting; (2) obstinate constipation; (3) neurotic or even psychotic behavior; and (4) neuromuscular disturbances. The mortality rate is high.

Abdominal pain is frequently the presenting complaint. The pain is usually colicky in nature and may be extremely severe and associated with spasm without localizing signs but with fever, tachycardia, and leukocytosis. The abdominal signs may be, and frequently are, mistaken for manifestations of renal colic, acute appendicitis, cholelithiasis, or pancreatitis. It is not uncommon for patients with porphyria to have multiple surgical scars on the abdomen. The neurologic manifestations are quite varied and may include neuritic pain in the extremities, areas of hypesthesia and paresthesia, and foot and wrist drop. Paraplegia or a complete flaccid quadriplegia may ensue and may be followed by bulbar paralysis and death. Except for pain in the extremities, sensory changes are usually not prominent, and signs of upper motor neurone changes are usually absent. The neurologic manifestations may simulate a wide variety of conditions, including poliomyelitis, encephalitis, and arsenic or lead poisoning. A true ascending paralysis of the Landry type is not observed.

The patients frequently have many vague "neurotic" complaints, even when in remission from an attack. With an attack they may become confused or even psychotic. Hypertension may accompany an attack, there may be temporary loss of vision, and convulsions have been described.

The course of the disease is extraordinarily variable. Recurrent abdominal crises may be present for years, or the patient may die in the first attack. It is not at all uncommon to find in one parent or in several siblings of a patient with porphyria that porphobilinogen, the diagnostic feature of porphyria, is present in the urine, even though they have never had active symptoms of the disease. This condition is called *latent poryphyria.* In general, the neuromuscular and psychotic symptoms are late manifestations, and with their appearance the prognosis becomes more grave. Between attacks there may be no symptoms. The mechanism by which the latent disease is converted to manifest disease, i.e., an attack of acute porphyria, is unknown, but it is known quite definitely that attacks may be provoked by the administration of certain drugs, particularly barbiturates. Menstruation, pregnancy, infection, alcohol, or lead may be the precipitating factor in a few patients.

The freshly voided urine is frequently normal in color

and on standing in the sunlight turns to a Burgundy wine color or even black. This color change can be hastened by adding a small amount of acid to the urine and boiling for 30 min. The explanation for these color changes is that porphobilinogen (colorless) and not uroporphyrin (red) is excreted in the urine. Heating of porphobilinogen in an acid medium results in the nonenzymatic formation of uroporphyrin, together with a dark-brown or reddish-brown nonporphyrin pigment.

In acute intermittent porphyria during relapse the presence of porphobilinogen is a constant feature. During remission the porphobilinogen reaction is usually positive, but a negative test does not exclude the diagnosis of this type of porphyria. The qualitative determination of porphobilinogen by the Watson-Schwartz modification of the Ehrlich reaction is, therefore, a simple and valuable screening procedure. In this test 5 ml freshly voided urine is mixed with 5 ml Ehrlich's reagent (0.7g paradimethylaminobenzaldehyde, 150 ml concentrated hydrochloric acid, and 100 ml water). After mixing, 10 ml aqueous saturated sodium acetate is added. The solution is then extracted successively with 10 ml chloroform and 10 ml *n*-butanol. A positive test for porphobilinogen gives an intense red color remaining in the aqueous layer. This test is quite specific for acute intermittent porphyria. The test is negative in erythropoietic porphyria and in porphyria cutanea tarda symptomatica. It is positive in patients with porphyria cutanea tarda hereditaria during acute attacks but is negative in the interval between such episodes.

In addition to porphobilinogen, patients with acute intermittent porphyria excrete excessive quantities of uroporphyrin (types I and III), coproporphyrin (types I and III), and other as yet unidentified porphyrins. As mentioned previously, the porphyrins are formed in the renal tubules by the nonenzymatic transformation of porphobilinogen into uroporphyrin at an acid pH. Examination of the tissues of such patients, in contrast to the findings in erythropoietic porphyria, has revealed that the porphyrin content of the bone marrow is normal. The liver, on the contrary, regularly exhibits increased quantities of porphyrin, especially porphyrin precursors. For this reason, acute intermittent porphyria is classified among the hepatic porphyrias.

ALA synthetase is an inducible enzyme in both man and animals. Induction can be augmented by barbiturates, estrogens, certain 5β-H steroid metabolites, and a variety of chemical compounds. Induction can be inhibited by high carbohydrate intake. Thus, the major chemical manifestations of acute intermittent porphyria are best explained as resulting from overproduction of porphyrin precursors, secondary to induction of hepatic ALA synthetase. The precise metabolic lesion is not known. This could be in the operator gene mechanism for ALA synthetase or it could be due to a partial deficiency of the enzyme uroporphyrinogen synthetase.

Treatment Drugs such as barbiturates and estrogens which induce Δ-ALA synthetase must be avoided. In acute attacks, opiates such as meperidine (Demerol) or ganglioplegics such as tetraethylammonium may be used for relief of pain. Chloralhydrate or paraldehyde may be used for sedation. Neostigmine may be of value in treating severe constipation. Chlorpromazine, in doses of 50 to 100 mg, may affect rapid relief of acute symptoms, but without change in the underlying process. Hyponatremia and hypochloremia secondary to inappropriate secretion of antidiuretic hormone may occur in some patients during acute attacks and require therapy. Respiratory support may be needed in some patients. ACTH and corticosteroids and chelating agents such as BAL (2,3-dimercaptopropanol), EDTA (disodium ethylenediaminetetraacetate), and pencillamine have not been shown to be of value.

The most effective treatment of the acute attack is to provide a liberal intake of glucose, either orally or intravenously. A low carbohydrate intake enhances ALA induction and a high intake suppresses the induction of this enzyme, the so-called "glucose effect." Rapid remissions may be induced by a high carbohydrate intake.

PORPHYRIA CUTANEA TARDA HEREDITARIA Porphyria cutanea tarda hereditaria is characterized clinically by cutaneous lesions or acute attacks of abdominal colic and not infrequently by both. The disease is inherited as a non-sex-linked mendelian dominant. The onset of symptoms is usually between the ages of ten and thirty years. The outstanding biochemical feature of the disorder is the increased excretion of coproporphyrin and protoporphyrin in the feces *at all times* in the course of the disease.

During the latent phase of the disease the patients are entirely asymptomatic. Porphyrinuria is usually absent and the porphyrin precursors, Δ-aminolevulinic acid and porphobilinogen, are not excreted in increased amounts. The disease can be diagnosed only during the latent phase by examination of the stools for porphyrins. A simple screening test can be done by obtaining a small specimen of stool on a glove. The specimen is extracted with about 2 ml of solvent containing equal parts of glacial acetic acid, amyl alcohol, and ether. The supernatant solution is then extracted with 1.5 *N* HCl and viewed in a Wood's lamp. Red fluorescence in the acid layer is proportional to the porphyrin content.

In a number of patients, particularly males, the skin is unusually sensitive to light and blisters and abrades easily. Healed depigmented scars may be present over the exposed surfaces, particularly the hands. Hyperpigmentation of the skin may occur, and hirsutism has been observed in females. The photosensitivity and cutaneous deformities are not so great as in erythropoietic porphyria.

Acute attacks of jaundice and abdominal colic accompanied in some cases by psychotic manifestations and motor paralysis may intervene in the course of the disease. Indeed, any of or all the manifestations of acute intermittent porphyria may make their appearance. As in acute intermittent porphyria, death or recovery may occur. During the acute attacks the excretion of porphyrins in the feces frequently decreases, and the excretion of coproporphyrin and uroporphyrin in the urine increases. Both Δ-aminolevulinic acid and porphobilinogen are usually excreted in increased amounts in the urine during acute attacks. It has been suggested that the disease remains asymptomatic as long as the liver is capable of excreting the porphyrins in the bile (latent phase); when this capacity is impaired, bilirubinemia, porphyrinemia, porphyrinuria, and cutaneous lesions appear (cutaneous phase); and finally when porphyrin metabolism is greatly disturbed, Δ-aminolevulinic acid and porphobilinogen appear in the urine, and all the manifestations of acute intermittent porphyria may develop (acute phase). Porphyria cutanea tarda hereditaria is not an entirely suitable name for this disorder since not all patients develop cutaneous lesions. It is for this reason that the designation *porphyria variegata* has been suggested.

The treatment for this type of porphyria is the same as for acute intermittent porphyria. The "glucose effect" has been shown to operate in porphyria cutanea tarda hereditaria as well as in acute intermittent porphyria.

PORPHYRIA CUTANEA TARDA SYMPTOMATICA

This type of porphyria is characterized clinically by cutaneous lesions, hyperpigmentation of the skin, evidences of liver disease, and hypertrichosis, and chemically by the excretion of large amounts of uroporphyrin and lesser amounts of coproporphyrin in the urine. Abdominal pain and neurologic complications are conspicuously absent. The urine does not contain increased quantities of Δ-aminolevulinic acid or porphobilinogen. The excretion of protoporphyrin in the feces is normal; the excretion of coproporphyrin in the feces is usually increased.

The skin lesions are indistinguishable from those observed in porphyria cutanea tarda hereditaria. The skin is usually sensitive both to light and to mechanical trauma. Blisters appear on the exposed skin areas, frequently ulcerate, and finally lead to scar formation. The photosensitivity is similar to that in erythropoietic porphyria but not as marked.

This disorder has been described (1) in male subjects, forty to seventy years of age, with alcoholic cirrhosis of the liver; (2) in Bantu subjects in South Africa with nutritional cirrhosis of the liver; (3) in children and adults in Turkey who have ingested the fungicide hexachlorobenzene; (4) in three elderly subjects with a tumor of the liver; and (5) in an occasional young adult without a history of alcoholism or drug exposure. Porphyria cutanea tarda symptomatica is probably acquired, but constitutional factors may be involved in some cases.

Repeated phlebotomy has been established as an effective means of treatment of porphyria cutanea tarda secondary to alcoholism. The beneficial effect is probably related to removal of excess iron from the liver.

HEREDITARY COPROPORPHYRIA The unique feature of this disease is an increased excretion of coproporphyrin, isomer type III. In the latent phase, the patients are asymptomatic, and the only abnormality usually detectable is an increased excretion of coproporphyrin III in the urine and feces, particularly the latter. Urinary Δ-ALA and porphobilinogen may be normal or slightly increased. Acute attacks, similar to those which occur in acute intermittent porphyria, can be provoked by the ingestion of barbiturates and possibly by certain tranquilizers and anticonvulsants. During these attacks there is an excessive excretion of Δ-ALA and porphobilinogen in the urine, in addition to a massive excretion of coproporphyrin in both urine and stool. About 30 cases of this disorder have been reported. Psychiatric symptoms may be present without other

clinical manifestations of porphyria. Skin photosensitivity has been described in one case. The disease is inherited as a dominant characteristic and occurs in both sexes.

The neurologic and psychiatric aspects of porphyria are discussed further in Chaps. 323 and 26, respectively.

REFERENCES

DONALDSON EM et al: Erythropoietic protoporphyria: A family study. Br Med J 1:659, 1967

GOLDBERG A et al: Hereditary coproporphyria. Lancet 1:632, 1967

HEILMEYER L, CLOTTEN R: Congenital erythropoietic coproporphyria. Ger Med Mon 9:1, 1964

MARVER HS, SCHMID R: The Porphyrias, in *The Metabolic Basis of Inherited Disease,* 3d ed., eds JB Stanbury et al, New York: McGraw-Hill, 1972, p. 1087

MIESCHER PA, JAFFE ER (eds): Porphyria and disorders of porphyrin metabolism. Semin Hematol 5:293, 1968

103 HEPATOLENTICULAR DEGENERATION (WILSON'S DISEASE)

GEORGE E. CARTWRIGHT

DEFINITION Wilson's disease (hepatolenticular degeneration, progressive lenticular degeneration, pseudosclerosis of Westphal and Strümpell, tetanoid chorea of Gowers) is a rare, autosomal recessively inherited disorder, characterized by excess copper storage, particularly in the liver, kidneys, brain, and cornea, leading eventually to liver disease, proximal renal tubular reabsorption abnormalities, basal ganglion disease, and the characteristic rusty-brown corneal ring known as the *Kayser-Fleischer ring.*

HISTORY Kinnier Wilson, in 1912, in his classic monograph, "Progressive Lenticular Degeneration," defined this disease entity. A similar condition had previously been described in 1883 by Westphal and later by Strümpell. The symptoms resembled those of multiple sclerosis, but no demyelinative plaques were observed. For that reason it was called *pseudosclerosis.* The cirrhosis of the liver was overlooked until Spielmeyer reexamined the cases many years later. His studies and the clinical observations of Hall left little doubt that hepatolenticular degeneration and pseudosclerosis were the same disease. The corneal ring was described in 1902 by Kayser in a case diagnosed as "multiple sclerosis," but to Fleischer is due the credit for appreciating its significance in relation to the disease as it is now known.

A marked increase in the copper content of both the

brain and the liver was demonstrated by Haurowitz in 1930 and was later confirmed by Glazebrook and Cummings. Mandelbrote and his associates in 1948 observed by chance that the urinary output of copper was high and that this output is increased by the administration of BAL (British anti-lewisite). In the same year Uzman and Denny-Brown found that a persistent aminoaciduria is associated with the disease. Ceruloplasmin deficiency was recognized as a feature of the disease by Scheinberg and Gitlin in 1952. An effective treatment of the disease was introduced by Walshe in 1956.

INHERITANCE The condition is inherited as an autosomal recessive trait. The occurrence of Wilson's disease in the general population is about 1 in 200,000 persons. Heterozygotes are clinically well, although they may exhibit some of the biochemical abnormalities of the abnormal homozygotes. Since only about 1 in 200 persons in the general population is heterozygous for the Wilson's disease gene, most affected individuals are the products of consanguineous marriages.

PATHOGENESIS The clinical and pathologic manifestations are due to the toxic effects of the excessive amounts of copper on the tissues. Thus, Wilson's disease may be viewed as a copper storage disease. Patients with this disease ingest a normal amount of copper in the diet, but copper is retained in the liver, possibly because of an inability to excrete it at the normal rate in the bile.

During the first years after birth, copper accumulates progressively and primarily in the cytoplasm of hepatocytes. After some years the concentration of copper in the liver reaches values of 500 to 2,000 μg per g dry weight, necrosis of liver cells occurs, and copper is released into the serum and is deposited in other tissues. The copper which remains in the liver is sequestered in lysosomes in order to protect the cells from the toxic effects of the metal. In many patients this period of hepatic copper release and redistribution takes place slowly and in an orderly manner. In others the release of copper from the liver to the serum is more abrupt. Copper is then taken up by erythrocytes, and hemolytic anemia may occur as a consequence of oxidative damage to the red cells by the copper. In still others, the shift in copper is made with greater difficulty, and overt hepatic failure may ensue. If the patients survive this period of hepatic copper release and redistribution, they may again become asymptomatic while copper is accumulating in other tissues, particularly the kidneys, brain, and cornea. Accumulation of copper in the kidneys leads to damage to the proximal renal tubules. Neurologic disease results from the toxic effects of the copper on the brain. The deposition of copper in the cornea produces the characteristic Kayser-Fleischer ring.

Normally about 95 percent of the copper in serum is firmly bound to the serum enzyme ceruloplasmin. A deficiency of ceruloplasmin is one of the most characteristic biochemical abnormalities in this disease. The remainder of the copper in serum is bound to albumin and represents copper in the process of transport from the gastrointestinal tract and from one tissue to another. The amount of copper bound to albumin is increased in Wilson's disease, and since this copper is easily dissociable from the albumin, a portion is filtered by the kidneys, and this accounts for the hypercupriuria which is a feature of the disease. Since there is a greater reduction in ceruloplasmin than there is increase in albumin-bound copper, the total serum copper concentration is usually reduced.

It has been postulated that the inherited defect is an inability to synthesize ceruloplasmin. However, a mechanism whereby a deficiency of ceruloplasmin can lead to excessive tissue deposits of copper is not known. It would seem more likely that there is an intrahepatic defect in the metabolism of copper which leads to both impaired excretion of copper in the bile and impaired ceruloplasmin synthesis.

PATHOLOGY The histology of the liver varies considerably depending upon the stage of the disease. In the early, asymptomatic years, the liver appears grossly and histologically normal despite an increase in hepatic copper, or it may be enlarged by fatty infiltration. During the active hepatic stage, the changes are those of chronic active hepatitis: necrosis, erosion of the marginal plate, Councilman bodies, parenchymal collapse, polymorphonuclear and round-cell infiltration, proliferation of bile ducts, and Mallory's cytoplasmic hyalin. In patients with neurologic disease, the histology is that of postnecrotic cirrhosis with finely or coarsely nodular cirrhosis, bands of fibrous tissue of variable widths, round-cell infiltration, proliferation of small bile ducts, and glycogen-filled nuclei. Splenomegaly is a common finding.

The most striking gross finding in the brain is cavitation of the putamen on each side and rarely of cerebral cortex and white matter. In many cases, probably more than half, the putamen and caudate nuclei are atrophic and of light grayish-brown color, and there is no evidence of cavitation. Microscopic examination almost invariably reveals a remarkable hyperplasia of protoplasmic astrocytes in the cerebral cortex, lenticular and caudate nuclei, subthalamic nuclei of Luys, substantia nigra, and dentate and red nuclei. Nerve-cell loss is widespread but is most pronounced in the lenticular and dentate nuclei and cerebral cortex. The protoplasmic astrocytosis does not differ from that observed in hepatic coma.

CLINICAL MANIFESTATIONS The clinical manifestations of Wilson's disease usually first appear between the ages of six and twenty years. Rarely do they occur before the age of six years, but may be first noted as late as forty years of age. The mode of onset is extremely variable. Patients may present with symptoms and signs associated with liver disease, hemolytic anemia, or neurologic disease, less commonly with psychiatric, renal, or bone disease.

Liver disease is the most frequent mode of presentation, and it is usually noted between six and fifteen years of age. Clinically, the liver disease closely resembles chronic active hepatitis. The hepatic disease is frequently severe and progressive and accompanied by all the usual signs of liver insufficiency such as spider angiomas, jaundice, hepatomegaly, splenomegaly, ascites, hematemesis, anemia, leukopenia, and thrombocytopenia. Death may supervene from either hemorrhage or hepatic failure if the diagnosis is not established and appropriate specific therapy instituted.

The first clinical manifestation may be in the form of a Coombs negative hemolytic anemia in the absence of overt hepatic disease. The hemolytic episodes may be severe and recurrent but are usually transient and self-limited. Jaundice in some patients is due to concomitant hepatic failure and hemolytic anemia.

Neurologic disease appears at a somewhat later age than the hepatic and hematologic manifestations. A deteriorating performance at school, particularly in handwriting, and difficulty in speech are usually first noted. Tremor of one of or both the upper extremities, or of the head and trunk, may be an early as well as a prominent neurologic sign. The tremor is accentuated by excitement or attention being drawn to it. Abnormal movements of choreic or choreoathetoid type are present in some patients. Rigidity may be intermittent or constant. A mixture of parkinsonism and cerebellar ataxia is characteristic of the disease.

An occasional patient may present with psychiatric disturbances, renal disease, or bone disease. The proximal renal tubular defect may lead to aminoaciduria, peptidiuria, proteinuria, glycosuria, uricosuria, and phosphaturia. The uricosuria is associated with a diminished level of uric acid in the serum. The phosphaturia may result in hypophosphatemia and eventually in osseous change. Skeletal abnormality, manifested by osteomalacia, cartilage injury, or bone fragmentation, is a frequent finding in the disease. Azure lunulae, bluish crescent areas at the nail bases, have been observed in several patients.

The most remarkable and unique feature of the disease is the Kayser-Fleischer ring, a rusty-brown ring of pigment, located at the periphery of the cornea in Descemet's membrane. The pigment extends to the limbus and usually goes completely around the cornea; occasionally there may be only a crescent-shaped distribution. Although well-formed rings are easily visible in ordinary light, in the early stages of the disease or in patients in whom the color of the iris is brown, it may be necessary to use a slit lamp to visualize the rings. Under slit-lamp examination, the ring is seen to be composed of a multitude of granular specks. The rings are pathognomonic of the disease and are present in all patients with neurologic manifestations. Failure of an experienced observer to demonstrate rings by slit-lamp examination of a patient with neurologic abnormalities virtually rules out Wilson's disease. The rings may not be present in the early stages of the disease. They may be absent in children during the stage of acute hepatic disease and/or hemolytic anemia.

CLINICAL COURSE The course of the disease is extremely variable. Death occurs in about one-half of the patients who develop the severe, acute type of liver disease. The disease is frequently undiagnosed and untreated at this stage. The chronic active hepatitis may persist for months, or the jaundice and ascites may subside completely, never to recur during the course of the disease. A period in which the patients are asymptomatic not infrequently follows the acute hepatic or hemolytic anemia stage. About 40 percent of the patients enter the neurologic stage without a history of recognized acute hepatic decompensation or hemolytic anemia. Once the neurologic stage begins, it is usually progressive and invariably fatal if untreated. In the terminal stage, the facial muscles become set in a stiff, vacuous smile, permanent contractures and deformities are prominent, the neck and trunk become rigid, the upper extremities are held rigidly in flexion at the elbow, wrist, and metacarpal joints, and the lower extremities are held in a position of extension. Dysarthria or even anarthria is an almost constant finding in advanced cases. Cachexia and muscular wasting may be extreme. Terminally, marked mental deterioration may be present. The sensory system is intact and the reflexes are normal. Pyramidal signs are usually absent. This terminal stage is now rarely observed because of earlier diagnosis and effective therapy.

DIAGNOSIS The triad of Kayser-Fleischer rings, cirrhosis of the liver, and signs of basal ganglion disease is pathognomonic of this condition.

During the neurologic stage, the disease is relatively easy to diagnose. Kayser-Fleischer rings are present. Signs of liver disease are usually evident from the physical examination, but if not, the presence of liver disease may be established by liver function studies and/or by liver biopsy. The neurologic disorder may be confused with Parkinson's syndrome. Occasionally cerebellar ataxia, chorea, choreoathetosis, dystonia, or psychiatric disturbance predominates.

The diagnosis of Wilson's disease may be confirmed by finding one or more of the following four abnormalities in copper metabolism: (1) a serum copper concentration of less than 80 μg per 100 ml; (2) a serum ceruloplasmin concentration of less than 20 mg per 100 ml; (3) a urinary excretion of more than 100 μg of copper in 24 hr; or (4) a liver copper concentration of more than 250 μg per g of dried weight (see Table 103-1).

In the early asymptomatic stage during which copper is accumulating in the liver, neurologic signs are absent and Kayser-Fleischer rings are frequently not present. Liver function studies may be normal. The serum copper and ceruloplasmin concentrations are most commonly decreased. The urinary excretion of copper is usually increased, and the concentration of copper in the liver is increased (250 to 2,000 μg per g). The disease may be difficult to distinguish from the heterozygous condition. In some heterozygotes the serum copper may be decreased (60 to 80 μg per 100 ml), the serum ceruloplasmin

TABLE 103-1
Alterations in copper metabolism in Wilson's disease

Determination	*Normal subjects**	*Wilson's disease†*
Serum copper, μg/100 ml	114	
	81–147	10–110
Ceruloplasmin, mg/100 ml	33	
	25–43	1–20
Urine copper, μg/24 hr	15	
	5–25	100–4,000
Liver copper, μg/g, dry weight	31	
	18–45	250–2,000

* *Mean and range ±2 standard deviations.*
† *Expected range.*

decreased (5 to 20 mg per 100 ml), and the liver copper concentration increased (40 to 200 μg per g).

During the period of active liver disease, the disorder may be extremely difficult to diagnose. Kayser-Fleischer rings may or may not be present. Neurologic signs are usually absent. The diagnosis of Wilson's disease should be considered in all patients under the age of thirty years with a diagnosis of chronic active hepatitis. The serum copper and ceruloplasmin concentrations may be decreased, normal, or even increased during the period of active necrosis. The urinary excretion of copper is usually greatly increased and may be of the order of 1,000 to 4,000 μg in 24 hr. The concentration of copper in the liver is greater than 250 μg per g of dried weight and may be as much as 2,000 μg.

During the stage of hemolytic anemia, Kayser-Fleischer rings may not be present and the neurologic examination is usually normal. The serum copper is normal or increased, although the ceruloplasmin concentration is usually decreased. The concentration of copper in the liver is increased, as is the excretion of copper in the urine.

Hypocupremia and hypoceruloplasminemia are not specific for Wilson's disease. These two abnormalities are present in all normal newborn infants up to the age of four to six months and in some patients with kwashiorkor, sprue, celiac disease, and the nephrotic syndrome. Hypercupriuria may be observed in the nephrotic syndrome, in patients with alcoholic cirrhosis of the liver, and in patients with biliary cirrhosis. However, in the last two diseases mentioned, the serum copper and ceruloplasmin concentrations are normal or increased. In patients with biliary cirrhosis, the concentration of copper in the liver may be as great as in Wilson's disease.

TREATMENT The therapy of Wilson's disease is directed toward (1) the prevention of the continued accumulation of copper in the body and (2) the removal of copper already deposited.

Sulfurated potash, technical, 20 mg three times daily with meals, prevents the absorption of copper by the formation of insoluble unabsorbable copper sulfide in the gut. This therapy is continued for 6 to 12 months and then discontinued. No undesirable side effects have been observed from such therapy.

The administration of the copper chelating agent, D-penicillamine (β,β-dimethylcysteine), results in the mobilization of copper from the tissues and an increase in its excretion in the urine. Therapy consists of 0.5 g of the D isomer given orally three times daily for the lifetime of the patient. Acute "sensitivity" reactions manifested by fever, skin rash, adenopathy, arthralgia, severe leukopenia, or thrombocytopenia develop in about one-third of patients. Desensitization and therapy with corticosteroids are required in such cases. The occurrence of a lupus-like syndrome with a positive lupus erythematosus (LE) test and antinuclear binding antibodies has been reported. The chronic administration of less than 2 g D-penicillamine daily is rarely associated with toxicity other than minor skin changes. The occurrence of the nephrotic syndrome has been reported in a few patients receiving the DL isomer or more than 2 g per day of the D isomer. Reversible optic neuritis has followed the administration of the DL isomer but not the D isomer.

PROGNOSIS The disease is progressive and invariably fatal if untreated. Therapy is dramatically effective except in some patients with active liver disease in whom treatment is not begun sufficiently soon. After prolonged therapy, Kayser-Fleischer rings fade away, neurologic signs disappear, and liver function abnormalities revert to normal, even though hypocupremia, hypoceruloplasminemia, and hypercupriuria persist or become even more pronounced.

REFERENCES

DEISS A et al: Long-term therapy of Wilson's disease. Ann Intern Med 75:57, 1971

STERNLIEB I, SCHEINBERG IH: Chronic hepatitis as a first manifestation of Wilson's disease. Ann Intern Med 76:59, 1972

——, ——: Prevention of Wilson's disease in asymptomatic patients. N Engl J Med 278:352, 1968

WALSHE JN: Wilson's disease, a review, in *The Biochemistry of Copper*, eds J Peisach et al, New York: Academic, 1966

104 DISORDERS OF GLYCOGEN SYNTHESIS AND MOBILIZATION

RICHARD A. FIELD

The glycogen deposition diseases occupy a noteworthy place in the evolution of the conceptual approaches to the modern methods of study of disease. In 1952, Dr. Gerty T. Cori demonstrated by specific enzymatic studies of tissue from patients that von Gierke's disease is due to the loss of activity of a single tissue enzyme, and thus she provided a prototype for the study of genetically determined metabolic aberrations. Since the points of enzymatic abnormality of most of the syndromes to be discussed in this chapter concern the steps of synthesis and degradation between glucose 6-phosphate and glycogen, a working schema of these pathways is presented in Fig. 104-1. The Cori classification of glycogen deposition diseases is shown in Table 104-1.

GLUCOSE 6-PHOSPHATASE DEFICIENCY HEPATORENAL GLYCOGENOSIS First described pathologically by von Gierke in 1929, this condition, characterized by enlargement of liver and kidneys and bouts of severe hypoglycemia, is probably the most frequent form of glycogenosis. Symptoms and recognizable clinical signs usually appear in the first year of life, and hepatomegaly may be detectable at birth. The disorder is transmitted as an autosomal mendelian recessive characteristic.

Pathologic physiology Under normal conditions hepatic glycogen serves as the main reservoir compound in the overall economy of blood glucose homeostasis. During and after ingestion of carbohydrate foods, a major portion of the glucose arriving in the liver via the portal system is phosphorylated and, by several intermediary

TABLE 104-1
Disorders of glycogen deposition and mobilization

Cori type	*Enzyme defect*	*Organ*	*Glycogen structure*	*Eponymic name*	*Suggested clinical name*
1	Glucose 6-phosphatase	Liver, kidney, intestine (?)	Normal	von Gierke's disease	Glucose 6-phosphatase deficiency hepatorenal glycogenosis
2	α-Glucosidase (maltase)	Generalized	Normal	Pompe's disease	α-Glucosidase deficiency generalized glycogenosis
3	Amylo-1,6-glucosidase (debrancher)	Liver, heart, muscle, leukocytes	Abnormal; missing or very short outer chains	Forbes' disease	Debrancher deficiency limit dextrinosis
4	Amylo-(1,4:1,6) transglucosidase (brancher)	Liver, probably other organs	Abnormal; very long inner and outer unbranched chains	Andersen's disease	Brancher deficiency amylopectinosis
5	Muscle phosphorylase	Skeletal and cardiac muscle	Normal	McArdle-Schmid-Pearson disease	Myophosphorylase deficiency glycogenosis
6	Liver phosphorylase	Liver	Normal	Hers' disease	Hepatophosphorylase deficiency glycogenosis

steps, is stored as the regularly branched polysaccharide, glycogen (Chap. 72). During the postcibal period, peripheral utilization of glucose depletes circulating glucose, with the result that liver glycogen is depolymerized and free glucose is released into the hepatic vein (Chap. 72). The overall intracellular reactions in this process are called glycogenolyses, and the final enzymatic step is the hydrolytic dephosphorylation by the specific enzyme hepatic glucose 6-phosphatase (Fig. 104-1). Absence or marked reduction of this enzyme activity can be demonstrated by direct tissue assay in hepatorenal glycogenosis and accounts for most of, if not all, the metabolic disturbances noted in patients with this condition. The central feature of this limitation of hepatic glucose release is hypoglycemia, and it follows that little or no elevation of blood glucose concentration occurs following the injection of glucagon or epinephrine. Likewise, the normal expected rise in blood glucose level is not observed in patients with this hepatic enzyme deficiency following the intravenous administration of fructose or galactose. For all intents and purposes, these hexoses are metabolized solely by the liver and ultimately are converted intracellularly to glucose 6-phosphate, which, like the molecules of the same compound derived from glycogen depolymerization, cannot be dephosphorylated in the absence of glucose 6-phosphatase so as to appear in the bloodstream as free glucose. The administration of glycerol, another glucogenic substance, has been advocated in that it can be administered either parenterally or orally. As with fructose or galactose, there is no rise of blood glucose after glycerol. Apparently large quantities of glucose 6-phosphate are disposed of by increasing the amounts carried through the steps of anaerobic glycolysis resulting in an increased production and release of lactic and pyruvic acids; thus, hyperlacticacidemia is a characteristic finding in the syndrome and can be strikingly augmented by the administration of glucagon or other stimuli of hepatic glycogenolysis. Although ketonemia, lipemia, and ketonuria are frequently observed, because of the relative unavailability of glycogen stores and the resultant hypoglycemia which triggers mobilization of fat to meet energy requirements, marked and dangerous lactic acidosis is also frequent and may supervene precipitously. It is believed that the chronic hyperlacticacidemia is responsible for disturbance in renal clearance of water and accounts for the hyperuricemia seen in this condition. Chronic acidosis on a cellular level may play a role in the generally retarded growth, mild normochromic unresponsive anemia, hypophosphatemia, and generalized decreased bone density with mushrooming of the metaphyses and frequent fractures observed in these patients. Glycosuria and nonspecific aminoaciduria without aminoacidemia also occur and may be striking. It has been suggested that these findings correlate with the severity of glycogen infiltration and the hypothetically intracellular accumulation of phosphorylated hexoses in the renal tubular cells; but other impairments of renal function are not prominent.

Pathology In some cases a marked hemorrhagic diathesis occurs, characterized by prolonged bleeding time and an abnormal deficiency in platelet adhesiveness. Evidence indicates that this is not a primary platelet defect, but rather a result of the abnormalities of blood contents in this condition. The liver is markedly enlarged, smooth, firm, and brownish in color. Microscopic study shows the liver cells to be enlarged up to three times the normal size and to be filled with glycogen and at times excessive amounts of fat. In the kidneys, which are usually at least double normal size, intracellular excess of glycogen is found in the cells of the proximal tubules. That the excess of glycogen persists in these organs long after death is not surprising when the nature of the biochemical defect is recalled.

Clinical picture The child is pale and undersized, with a fat face and neck and a markedly distended abdomen containing a huge, easily palpable liver without associated ascites or splenomegaly. Xanthomas with prominent lipemia may be a feature. Occasionally, epileptiform seizures and vomiting occur; however, more often the gravity and prevalence of the low blood sugar level are not appreciated until serious central nervous system deterioration has resulted.

Laboratory examinations These examinations reveal fasting hypoglycemia, hyperlipidemia, hyperlacticacidemia, anemia, and, at times, ketonemia, and ketonuria. After glucose ingestion or infusion, the fall of blood levels may be delayed, yielding a pseudodiabetic curve. This may be explained as impaired capacity to increase the already superabundant stores of liver glycogen, rather than as a failure to utilize glucose at a normal rate in peripheral tissues. There is hypersensitivity to insulin, and severe prolonged hypoglycemia may follow its administration. Suspicion of this disorder is warranted when typical clinical characteristics are present and consonant results with glucagon or epinephrine challenge tests and of galactose, fructose, or glycerol infusion have been obtained. Final diagnosis, as with all glycogenoses, rests on biochemical assay of enzyme activity in biopsy material, in this instance, liver. In typical cases, liver glucose 6-phosphatase activity is found to be absent or reduced to less than 10 percent of normal. There is no ready explanation for the three cases reported in which glucose 6-phosphatase activity was either normal or only moderately reduced despite the careful characterization of the cases as clinically and pathophysiologically entirely consistent with the diagnosis.

Differential diagnosis The sporadic reports of cases of liver glycogenosis in which multiple enzymatic abnormalities in the glycogen pathways can be demonstrated and other cases in which members of the same kinship have

FIGURE 104-1
Pathways of glycogen synthesis and breakdown.

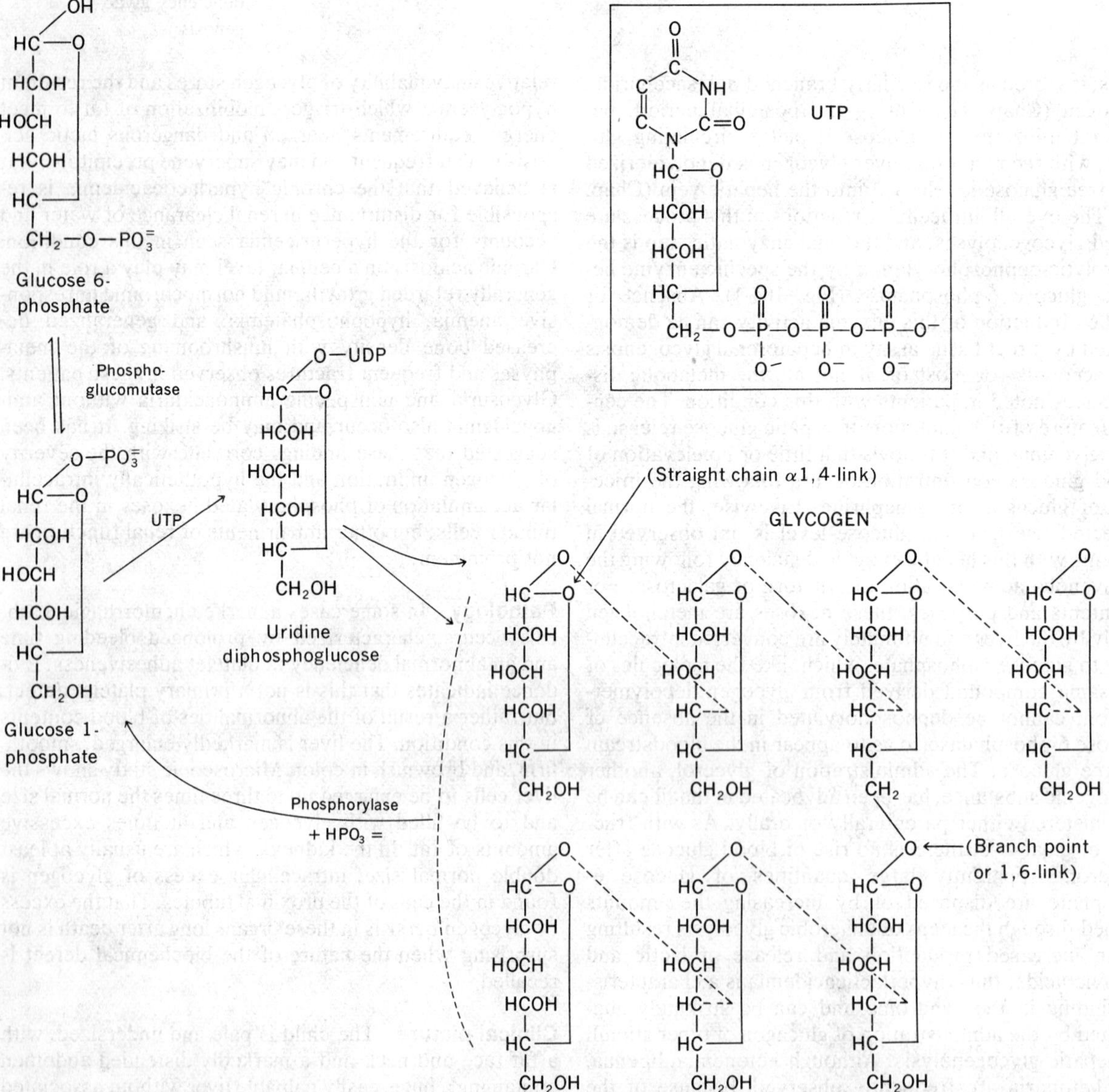

distinctly different enzymatic lesions have given rise to both diagnostic and conceptual confusion. At present, it is not clear whether such cases result from secondarily induced adaptations, a close relation of chromosomal genetic loci for determining and controlling the formation of the different enzymes, or from the influences of environmental factors. Until further investigations clarify these situations or augment the details of pathways of glycogen metabolism, the nonrestrictive labeling of cases that do not fit, either biochemically or functionally, into the classic groupings as simply "liver glycogen disease" seems wise.

Treatment Although no means of increasing tissue activity levels of glucose 6-phosphatase in typical cases is available, earlier diagnosis, combined with recognition of hypoglycemia, acidosis, and intercurrent infection as the causes of morbidity and mortality, has markedly improved the life expectancy in this disease. The observation that the disturbances in metabolism and function in patients who survive beyond the fifth year tend to ameliorate provokes inquiry into the biochemical mechanisms by which such could occur and points to the necessity for assiduous care of the afflicted infant. It appears that in cases with prolonged survival the hyperuricemia and urate deposition which result, especially in the kidneys, become the major causes of difficulties. For this the daily administration of 0.5 to 2.0 g probenecid (Benemid) may be employed (Chap. 100).

The use of allopurinol, an inhibitor of urate formation, can also be recommended when secondary complications of hyperuricemia are manifested.

In a small number of cases, surgical transposition of the vena cava and the portal vein has been performed with clinical improvement in hypoglycemia. Diazoxide, a thiazide compound with capability of inhibiting insulin release, has been shown to improve hypoglycemia in one case.

α-GLUCOSIDASE DEFICIENCY GENERALIZED GLYCOGENOSIS This disorder, the most devastating form of glycogenosis, causes death within the first two years of life. It is marked by a generalized deposition of glycogen and by striking cardiomegaly. Symptoms and signs appear within one or two months after birth and quickly produce an infant with marked muscular hypotonia, enlarged tongue, cretinoid appearance, cardiomegaly, and neurologic deficits. Increased susceptibility to recurrent respiratory infections is based on poor ventilative and tussive efforts.

The structure of isolated glycogen is normal, and hyperglycemia promptly follows glucagon or epinephrine administration or the infusion of galactose or fructose. Glycogen accumulation in vacuoles located in the cytoplasm of almost all body cells occurs to a variable degree and is a process in which the leukocytes participate. The principal mechanisms of death are cardiac failure and aspiration pneumonitis. The disease is familial in occurrence, and the mode of inheritance appears to be through a single recessive autosomal gene.

Hers has demonstrated in the tissues of five affected infants the absence of a normally ubiquitous α-(1 → 4) glucosidase which has optimum activity in the acid range. The enzyme characteristically hydrolyzes maltose and glycogen to glucose and can catalyze the transglucosylation from maltose to glycogen. Present hypotheses regarding glycogen metabolism do not provide a locus of influence at which this enzyme could effect glycogen deposition. Furthermore, spontaneous glycogenolysis occurs in excised tissues. Hers emphasizes the possible lysosomal nature of the enzyme and suggests that the polysaccharide accumulation is the result of a failure of physiologic digestion of areas of cytoplasm by the defective lysosomes. This interpretation is in agreement with the clinical observations of an absence of hypoglycemia, ketosis, and hyperlipidemia and the concept that the manifestations are the result of disruption of muscle fibers by the progressive glycogen accumulation. Although the clinical picture is highly characteristic, diagnosis depends on the demonstration of the absence of the acid α-(1 → 4)glucosidase in biopsy material.

Electron microscopic studies have demonstrated two forms of cytoplasmic glycogen aggregates, a monogranular and a multigranular. The ensacculated membrane-limited vacuoles found only in this condition probably represent lysosomes which have autophaged large amounts of monogranular glycogen and are unable to digest it because of their deficiency of acid maltase.

Treatment is unavailing, although chemotherapy of intercurrent bacterial respiratory infections appears to prolong life.

DEBRANCHER ENZYME DEFICIENCY (LIMIT DEXTRINOSIS) AND BRANCHER ENZYME DEFICIENCY (AMYLOPECTINOSIS) These two conditions are the result of defects of the enzymes concerned with the formation and the disengagement of the branch points of the typically arborized glycogen molecule (types 3 and 4 in Table 104-1). In the first instance, there is a deficiency of the specific enzyme required for cleavage of the branch point bond, and therefore glycogenolysis is interrupted as the first branch point is reached and a glycogen of abnormal structure with excessively frequent branch points and shortened inner and outer chains results. When the branching enzyme is deficient, an unusually structured glycogen which possesses excessively lengthened inner and outer chains and a paucity of branch points is produced. Apparently, this structure formation, which resembles that of plant starch, gives the polysaccharide the physical characteristics which lead to its sequestration within the cells, where it acts as an irritative nidus, producing a characteristic increase in periportal connective tissue.

Limit dextrinosis is a relatively frequent type of glycogenosis; amylopectinosis is exceedingly rare, only two cases having been recognized. Since the clinical picture of the debrancher deficiency disturbance (limit dextrinosis) so closely resembles a mild form of the glucose 6-phosphatase deficiency, many cases of the former were mistakenly diagnosed as the latter before precise enzymatic assay techniques were available. The confusion need no longer arise even on clinical grounds or on the basis of functional tests, for in limit dextrinosis infusions of galactose lead to prompt intrahepatic conversion to glucose, with prompt hyperglycemia, there being no impediment to dephosphorylation and release. In the differential diagnosis in cases with equivocal hyperglycemic responses to glucagon or epinephrine and in which hepatomegaly, growth retardation, and a tendency to hypoglycemia and ketonuria contribute uncertainty, a liver biopsy need not be done, since it has been demonstrated that the debrancher enzyme is also absent in leukocytes, muscle, and erythrocytes. Furthermore, fasting levels of lactate and pyruvate are likely to be normal, in contrast to the situation with the type 1 case (glucose 6-phosphatase deficiency), where they are distinctly elevated. In the type 3 case, erythrocyte glycogen content is elevated, but again this is not so in the type 1 individual.

Prognosis for the type 3 defect appears to be relatively good, and at least two patients with this condition have reached the fifth decade of life. Logical treatment consists of a high-protein, relatively low fat diet, with frequent feedings, prompt treatment of intercurrent infections, and prohibition of strenuous exercise, cardiodepressant drugs, and anesthetics, since the myocardium is involved.

GLYCOGEN DEPOSITION SYNDROMES DUE TO DEFICIENCIES OF GLYCOGEN PHOSPHORYLASES Glycogen phosphorylase (type 5, Table 104-1) catalyzes glycogen depolymerization by phosphorylytic cleavage to yield glucose 1-phosphate and thus mediates the major initiating step in making the glucose moieties available for metabolism. In the liver the bulk of the glucose derived from the action of this enzyme ultimately defends the level of blood sugar and maintains an adequate supply for the peripheral tissues, while in the muscle the phosphorylase-produced hexose phosphate provides an immediate fuel source for the energy demanded by quick, sharp increases in contractile activity. Muscle and liver phosphorylase are distinctly different proteins immunologically, structurally, and functionally, and it appears that each has its own genetic determinant. Both enzyme activities are enhanced by epinephrine, while only liver phosphorylase responds in vivo to injections of glucagon.

MYOPHOSPHORYLASE DEFICIENCY GLYCOGENOSIS (McARDLE) A group of patients consisting of members of several unrelated families have been shown to be lacking in muscle phosphorylase activity. None has any growth retardation, disturbance in carbohydrate economy, or abnormality of response to glucagon or epinephrine administration. However, they have in common an incapacity to perform prolonged or strenuous muscle work and are excessively sensitive to ischemic conditions in this regard because of the occurrence of weakness, pain, and spasm of the exercised muscle. The demonstration of the isolated absence of muscle phosphorylase adequately explains the clinical phenomena when the importance of brisk glycogenolysis in supplying substrate for anaerobic glycolysis during ischemic muscle work is recalled. The impediment limiting the acceleration and augmentation of anaerobic glycolysis thus curtails increased lactate production. The failure to detect a significant rise in lactate concentration in the venous return from a muscle working under imposed ischemic conditions is a useful diagnostic test. A modest excess of glycogen in the muscles has been described, and in some cases prolonged exercise may cause breakdown of muscle cells and myoglobinuria. Although it has been shown that cardiac muscle shares the defect, no cardiac disturbance on this account has been described.

Since liver phosphorylase is normal in amount and activity, patients do quite well provided they accept limitations in exertion, protect themselves from tight garments that produce muscle ischemia, and fortify themselves with exogenous carbohydrates before attempting unusual physical tasks.

HEPATOPHOSPHORYLASE DEFICIENCY GLYCOGENOSIS (HERS) Isolated development of hepatomegaly in infancy or childhood with a tendency to fasting hypoglycemia due to excessive accumulation of hepatic glycogen of normal structure characterizes this condition. Little in the way of other metabolic or developmental disturbance accrues as a consequence of the sluggish glycogenolysis which results from the absent or markedly reduced hepatophosphorylase activity. The deficiency of the enzyme can be demonstrated biochemically in hepatic tissue or in leukocytes. A possibly contingent deficiency of glucose 6-phosphate dehydrogenase has been described in some cases. No therapy beyond avoidance of prolonged fasting and the administration of a high-protein diet with frequent feedings appears to be necessary. The mechanism of failure of hyperglycemic response to glucagon or epinephrine is obvious, and the normal response to galactose infusion as well as the normal serum lactate level and lack of hyperlipemia allows easy differentiation of this disease from the more devastating glucose 6-phosphatase deficiency. Transmission appears to be by means of an autosomal recessive gene.

REFERENCES

DRASH A, FIELD JB: The glycogen storage diseases. Disease-a-Month Oct, 1971

STANBURY JB et al (eds): *The Metabolic Basis of Inherited Disease,* 2d ed., New York: McGraw-Hill, 1966

VAN CREVELD S: Glycogen disease. Arch Dis Child 34:298, 1959

105 GALACTOSEMIA

KURT J. ISSELBACHER

DEFINITION Galactosemia refers to an inborn error of metabolism associated with an impairment in the metabolism of galactose. Two disorders are currently recognized. "Classic" galactosemia is due to the deficiency of the enzyme galactose 1-phosphate uridyl transferase; it is typically associated with cataract formation, mental retardation, and cirrhosis. The second disorder, first described in 1965, is due to galactokinase deficiency and leads primarily to cataract formation.

PATHOGENESIS Lactose, the main carbohydrate in

milk, is a disaccharide containing galactose and glucose; when ingested it is hydrolyzed by intestinal lactase. Normally the absorbed galactose is converted in the liver to glucose. The first reaction in this pathway involves the phosphorylation of galactose to galactose 1-phosphate by galactokinase:

$$\text{Galactose} + \text{ATP} \xrightarrow{\text{galactokinase}} \text{galactose 1-phosphate}$$

The next step involves the conversion of galactose 1-phosphate to glucose-1-phosphate. This involves the participation of uridine diphosphate (UDP) sugars and the enzyme galactose 1-phosphate uridyl transferase as follows:

$$\text{Galactose 1-phosphate} + \text{UDP-glucose} \xrightarrow{\text{transferase}} \text{UDP-galactose} + \text{glucose 1-phosphate}$$

The UDP sugars can be reversibly interconverted by an epimerase reaction:

$$\text{UDP-galactose} \xrightleftharpoons{\text{epimerase}} \text{UDP-glucose}$$

Several alternate pathways of galactose metabolism appear to exist. Galactose can be converted (reduced) in the presence of NADPH (or NADH) to galactitol (dulcitol) by aldose reductase, an enzyme which occurs especially in the lens. Galactose can be oxidized to a limited extent by galactose dehydrogenase leading eventually to the formation of galactonic acid, xylulose, and CO_2. There is also a pyrophosphorylase reaction involving the interaction of galactose 1-phosphate with uridine triphosphate to form UDP-galactose. One or more of these pathways may account for a limited galactose metabolism in some patients with galactosemia.

In galactokinase deficiency, galactose accumulates in the blood and tissues. In the lens galactose is converted by aldose reductase to galactitol, a sugar to which the lens is impermeable. As a consequence, excessive hydration occurs which, together with a decrease in lenticular glutathione, leads to cataract formation.

In classic galactosemia, transferase deficiency leads to tissue accumulation of galactose 1-phosphate and galactose. As in galactokinase deficiency, cataracts develop secondary to galactitol accumulation in the lens. It is assumed but not proved that the cirrhosis and mental retardation of classic galactosemia are in some manner related to increased amounts of galactose 1-phosphate in these tissues. Elevated blood galactose levels may lead to a decreased hepatic output of glucose and hypoglycemia. In the kidney and intestine, accumulation of galactose and galactose 1-phosphate appears to lead to an inhibition of amino acid transport.

Both galactokinase- and transferase-deficiency galactosemia are transmitted as an autosomal recessive trait. Heterozygotes for these disorders have half-normal enzyme levels but are asymptomatic. However, not all persons with half-normal transferase enzymes in their cells are carriers of galactosemia. Some individuals homozygous for another gene, called the Duarte variant, normally have only half-normal transferase levels. This group can be differentiated from galactosemia heterozygotes on the basis of the electrophoretic properties of the mutant enzyme. In both types of galactosemia, the disorder is due either to the functional deficiency or absence of the involved enzyme. In the classic type of galactosemia there is evidence that the disorder may be due to a structural gene mutation and that the enzyme (transferase) protein is present but structurally altered and not functioning normally.

The exact incidence of classic galactosemia is still unclear. Estimates range from 1 in 18,000 to 1 in 100,000 births. Population studies indicate that 0.8 to 1.3 percent of the population are heterozygous for the galactosemia gene and about 10 percent carry the Duarte variant.

CLINICAL FEATURES Symptoms of classic galactosemia usually begin within days to several weeks after birth. The infant usually is reluctant to ingest breast milk or milk formulas, develops vomiting, shows poor nutrition, and fails to thrive. Jaundice, hepatomegaly, and evidence of liver disease may then develop. Cataracts are usually not present at birth but occur gradually over a period of weeks to months. Mental retardation may be difficult to detect but becomes evident after 6 or 12 months. The only recognized complication of galactokinase deficiency is cataract formation.

DIAGNOSIS Galactokinase deficiency should be suspected in infants or children with cataract formation who have non-glucose-reducing substances in their urine. The diagnosis is made by demonstrating the deficiency of galactokinase in red blood cells.

Classic galactosemia must be considered when one or more of the clinical features described above are found. If the patient is ingesting milk, reducing sugar may be found in the urine, which gives a negative glucose oxidase reaction (i.e., is not glucose) and is identified as galactose by other techniques, such as chromatography. If the child is vomiting, has a poor food intake, or is on intravenous glucose feedings, galactose may not be present in the urine. The definitive diagnosis consists of demonstrating a lack or deficiency of red cell galactose 1-phosphate uridyl transferase. A variety of assay techniques have been described.

The most important condition from which galactosemia needs to be differentiated in the neonatal period is primary liver disease. With liver damage, galactose removal from the blood is impaired, and elevated blood galactose levels as well as galactosuria may occur. However, in hepatitis or cirrhosis the transferase levels will be normal.

TREATMENT The treatment of galactosemia consists of the removal of galactose-containing foods from the diet, especially milk. In infants, milk substitutes such as Dextri-Maltose and Nutramigen are often used. Soybean preparations have also been used in the past, but their polysaccharides contain some galactose and should be avoided.

The institution of a galactose-free diet usually leads to a dramatic improvement in the patient; in fact, all clinical features except for mental retardation may improve or disappear. In general, patients are kept on galactose-free diets indefinitely or at least until they have reached adequate physical and neurologic development.

REFERENCES

HSIA DYY (ed): *Galactosemia,* Springfield, Ill.: Charles C Thomas, 1969

SEGAL S: Disorders of galactose metabolism, in *The Metabolic Basis of Inherited Disease,* eds JB Stanbury, et al, 3d ed., New York: McGraw Hill, 1972, p. 174

TEDESCO TA, MELLMAN WJ: Galactosemia: Evidence for a structural gene mutation. Science 172:727, 1971

106
DISORDERS OF LIPID METABOLISM AND XANTHOMATOSIS

DONALD S. FREDRICKSON

Lipidosis is a general term applied to disorders characterized by abnormal concentrations of lipids in tissues or in extracellular fluid. Sometimes it is restricted to only those abnormalities of lipid metabolism that are inheritable. *Xanthomatosis* is a morphologic term referring to lipid accumulation in tissues in association with large *foam cells.* The list of lipidoses and xanthomatoses in Table 106-1 encompasses most of the *primary* disturbances in lipid metabolism and includes some disorders in which secondary lipid storage is prominent and some of the disorders of adipose tissue. Omitted are several disorders in which lipids accumulate concomitantly with primary abnormalities in metabolism of other substances. Noteworthy among these are mucopolysaccharidoses (gargoylism) and the glycogen storage diseases.

PLASMA LIPOPROTEIN ABNORMALITIES

The commonest of the lipidoses are those that feature alterations in concentrations of the plasma lipids. These can usually be detected and diagnosed by measurements of cholesterol and triglyceride concentrations in plasma. It is easier to understand these disorders, however, when they are considered in terms of lipoproteins, the form in which nearly all lipids, except free fatty acids, are present in plasma. Both selective increases and severe deficiency or absence of some of the groups or classes of lipoproteins can occur. Abnormalities in the lipoproteins themselves may characterize a few disorders, but usually the lipoproteins are simply markers for intracellular abnormalities in lipid or carbohydrate metabolism that are reflected in abnormal plasma concentrations of lipids.

HYPERLIPOPROTEINEMIA

Increased concentrations of plasma lipids and lipoproteins represent metabolic problems that are difficult both to classify and to treat. Diagnosis proceeds in the following manner:

TABLE 106-1
Lipidoses and xanthomatoses

I Abnormal plasma lipoprotein concentrations
- *A* Hyperlipoproteinemia (HLP) or hyperlipidemia
  - *1* Hyperchylomicronemia (exogenous hyperglyceridemia; type I HLP)
    - *a* Primary
      - (*1*) Familial lipoprotein lipase deficiency
      - (*2*) Other
    - *b* Secondary, to
      - (*1*) Dysproteinemia
      - (*2*) Uncontrolled diabetes mellitus
  - *2* Hyperbetalipoproteinemia (hypercholesterolemia; type IIa HLP)
    - *a* Primary
      - (*1*) Familial monogenic disorders
        - (*a*) Familial hypercholesterolemia
        - (*b*) Familial combined hyperlipidemia, phenotypic variant of
      - (*2*) Other familial disorders
      - (*3*) Dietary-induced and other sporadic forms
    - *b* Secondary to other diseases
  - *3* Hyperbeta- and hyperprebetalipoproteinemia (mixed hypercholesterolemia and hyperglyceridemia; type IIb HLP)
    - *a* Primary
      - (*1*) Familial combined hyperlipidemia, phenotypic variant of
      - (*2*) Familial hypercholesterolemia, phenotypic variant of
      - (*3*) Other familial disorders
      - (*4*) Sporadic forms
    - *b* Secondary to other diseases
  - *4* Type III HLP ("Floating-beta" or "broad-beta" disorder; dysbetalipoproteinemia)
    - *a* Primary (usually familial)
    - *b* Secondary to hypothyroidism or uncontrolled diabetes mellitus
  - *5* Hyperprebetalipoproteinemia (endogenous hyperglyceridemia; type IV HLP)
    - *a* Primary
      - (*1*) Monogenic familial disorders
        - (*a*) Combined hyperlipidemia, phenotypic variant of
        - (*b*) "Pure" endogenous hyperglyceridemia
      - (*2*) Other familial forms
      - (*3*) Sporadic forms
    - *b* Secondary to other diseases

1 Measurement of plasma cholesterol *and* triglyceride concentrations after an overnight fast. For at least 2 weeks prior to the sample, the patient should be maintaining steady weight, eating the diet usual for the population, and not taking drugs known to affect plasma lipid concentrations. Table 244-4 gives age-adjusted values for cholesterol and triglycerides which, when exceeded, clearly indicate that *hyperlipidemia* is present. As discussed in Chap. 244, however, there are grounds for considering that children or young adults who have a cholesterol greater than 220 or a triglycer-

6 Hyperchylomicronemia and hyperprebetalipoproteinemia (mixed hyperglyceridemia; type V HLP: sometimes a variant expression of severe hyperprebetalipoproteinemia)
a Primary
(*1*) Familial form(s)
(*2*) Sporadic
b Secondary to dysproteinemia, uncontrolled diabetes mellitus, nephrotic syndrome, and other diseases
B Dyslipoproteinemia (circulation of abnormally lipidated lipoproteins)
1 Hyperlipidemia of obstructive jaundice
2 Familial lecithin: cholesterol acyltransferase (LCAT) deficiency
3 Type III HLP (see above)
C Hypolipoproteinemia
1 Primary
a Familial diseases
(*1*) Abetalipoproteinemia
(*2*) Hypobetalipoproteinemia
(*3*) Tangier disease (alpha-lipoprotein deficiency)
b Sporadic or subtle genetic variations?
2 Secondary to malabsorption, dysproteinemias, and possibly other diseases
II Lipid storage diseases due to deficient activity of a lysosomal enzyme
A Beta-galactosidase deficiencies
1 G_{M_1} gangliosidosis
a Generalized gangliosidosis (type I)
b Juvenile G_{M_1} gangliosidosis (type II)
2 Krabbe's globoid cell leukodystrophy
3 Lactosyl ceramidosis
B Alpha-galactosidase deficiency (Fabry's disease; angiokeratoma corporis diffusum universale)
C Beta-glucosidase deficiency (Gaucher's disease)
1 Nonneuronopathic ("adult")
2 Acute neuronopathic ("infantile")
3 Chronic neuronopathic ("juvenile")
D Cerebroside sulfatase deficiency (metachromatic leukodystrophy)
1 Late infantile form
2 Adult form
3 Variant with multiple sulfatase deficiencies
E Ganglioside G_{M2}-hexosaminidase deficiencies
1 Type 1, Tay-Sachs disease (hexosaminidase A deficiency)
2 Type 2 (hexosaminidases A and B deficiency)
3 Type 3 (lesser hexosaminidase A deficiency)
F Sphingomyelinase deficiencies
1 Clear-cut enzyme deficiency (massive sphingomyelin storage)
a Acute neuronopathic form (Type A; classic Niemann-Pick disease)
b Nonneuronopathic form (Type B)
2 Possible deficiency (mild sphingomyelin excess)
a Juvenile or delayed neuronopathic form (Type C)
b Nova Scotia variant (Type D)
G Probable acid cholesteryl ester hydrolase and triglyceride lipase deficiencies
1 Wolman's disease
2 Cholesteryl ester storage disease
III Phytanic oxidase deficiency (storage of 3,7,11,15-tetramethyl hexadecanoic acid; Refsum's disease; heredopathia atactica polyneuritiformis)
IV Granulomatous diseases with lipid storage
A Histiocytosis X (xanthoma disseminatum, eosinophilic granuloma, Hand-Schüller-Christian disease, Letterer-Siwe disease)
B Lipoid proteinosis (Urbach-Wiethe disease)
C Lipoid dermatoarthritis
D Disseminated lipogranulomatosis (Farber's disease)
V Other xanthomatoses
A Secondary to dysproteinemias (with macroglobulinemia, multiple myeloma, other paraproteinemias)
B With normolipoproteinemia
1 Cerebrotendinous xanthomatosis (cholestanol storage disease)
2 Simple xanthomas
3 Associated with trauma and chronic infections
VI Adipose tissue disorders
A Relapsing panniculitis (Weber-Christian disease)
B Lipodystrophy
1 Lipomas
2 Adiposis dolorosa (Dercum's disease)
3 Insulin lipodystrophy
C Lipoatrophy
1 Partial (progressive lipodystrophy)
2 Total (lipoatrophic diabetes mellitus)

ide greater than 150 may have hyperlipidemia with respect to excess risk of premature ischemic heart disease.

2 Screening for diseases to which hyperlipidemia may be *secondary* (hypothyroidism, obstructive liver disease, poorly controlled insulinopenic diabetes mellitus, plasma protein abnormalities); treatment of secondary hyperlipidemia is directed at the underlying disease.

3 Translation of *primary hyperlipidemia* to a particular lipoprotein pattern; for this purpose, the cholesterol and triglyceride determinations, observation of plasma after standing overnight at 4°C for a *chylomicron* layer at the top, and an estimation of low-density lipoprotein (LDL, beta-lipoprotein) concentration are the essential tests (Table 106-2). Lipoprotein electrophoresis, especially when quantitative, or ultracentrifugation is also useful but not essential.

4 Careful examination for xanthomas.

5 Examination of first-degree relatives. The last step is necessary to establish genetically determined hyperlipoproteinemia.

Classification of primary hyperlipidemia or hyperlipoproteinemia (HLP) continues to evolve. Nearly all hyperlipidemia can be converted to one of six abnormal lipoprotein patterns by arbitrary guides shown in Table 106-2. As Table 106-1 indicates, a given type of HLP does not signify a single disease. It also does not indicate

TABLE 106-2
Type of hyperlipoproteinemia as suggested by cholesterol (C) and triglyceride (TG) concentrations

C high; TG < 150	IIa
C high; TG 150–400	IIb, III*, or IV
C high; TG 400–1,000	III*, IV, or V†
C high; TG > 1,000	I†, or V†
C normal; TG > 150	IV

* Suggested by broad beta band on electrophoresis, but positive diagnosis requires demonstration of beta-migrating lipoproteins of density less than 1.006.
† Positive chylomicron tests.

whether the disorder is familial; and, in some familial disorders, a single abnormal genotype may be expressed in more than one lipoprotein or lipid pattern. For the practicing physician, the value of determining the type of hyperlipoproteinemia is its frequent association with certain clinical manifestations and its tendency to respond to relatively specific forms of therapy.

HYPERCHYLOMICRONEMIA (TYPE I HLP) DEFINITION This lipoprotein pattern reflects severe disability in removal of dietary triglycerides (in chylomicrons) from plasma without any marked increase in endogenous glycerides (pre-beta-lipoproteins). Normally, chylomicrons are not visible upon gross inspection or by electrophoresis of plasma drawn in the postabsorptive state. In type I HLP there is marked hyperchylomicronemia and a decrease in all other lipoproteins. The plasma is milky, and the triglyceride concentration ranges from 1,500 to 15,000 mg per 100 ml. Within 3 to 5 days of institution of a fat-free diet, chylomicrons disappear, a modest increase in pre-beta-lipoproteins occurs, and beta- and alpha-lipoproteins increase but remain low; the plasma clears, glycerides are in the range of 200 to 500, and cholesterol is lower than 200. Such "pure" hyperchylomicronemia occurs in a rare familial syndrome, and occasionally in association with dysglobulinemia or severe, uncontrolled diabetes mellitus.

Familial hyperchylomicronemia Hyperlipemia (lactescent plasma or serum due to hyperglyceridemia) dependent upon dietary fat intake was first reported in a child by Burger and Grutz in 1932; familial incidence was recorded by Holt, Aylward, and Timbres shortly thereafter. About 100 cases have since been discovered. The metabolic defect is believed to be deficient activity of the enzyme lipoprotein lipase. This enzyme facilitates removal of triglycerides at the capillary endothelial wall by promoting hydrolysis of the glyceride esters. The enzyme is "released" into plasma by heparin, and patients with this syndrome have uniquely low postheparin lipoprotein lipase activity.

CLINICAL PICTURE The disease is usually detected within the first decade, although sometimes not until early adulthood, usually when marked hyperlipemia is discovered during work-up for either sudden appearance of eruptive xanthomas, moderate hepatosplenomegaly, or bouts of severe abdominal pain. The latter usually follow a period of high fat intake. The pain is usually epigastric or midabdominal and rarely radiates to the back; it may be associated with signs of peritoneal irritation and fever and can mimic a number of acute abdominal emergencies. Recurrent pancreatitis is common and has been the cause of premature death in several patients. There is no evidence that familial hyperchylomicronemia is associated with accelerated vascular disease.

DIAGNOSIS In the untreated state, the triglyceride is greater than 1,000 mg per 100 ml, the chylomicron test is positive, and the heavy cream layer overlies a clear infranatant layer. The typical lipid and lipoprotein pattern and other manifestations in an otherwise healthy child or young adult provide a presumptive diagnosis if the acquired (secondary) form has been excluded. A fat-free diet should be administered for 1 week; the predicted changes in lipoproteins should occur rapidly. Familial hyperchylomicronemia is rare and sometimes is confused with more common mixed hyperglyceridemia (type V HLP). Patients with primary type V HLP differ in that (1) removal of fat from the diet is followed by rapid disappearance of chylomicrons from plasma, but pre-beta-lipoproteins tend to increase greatly, usually leaving plasma triglyceride concentrations well above 500 mg per 100 ml; (2) the protamine-sensitive (lipoprotein lipase) component of postheparin lipolytic activity is vanishingly small in familial hyperchylomicronemia, but usually normal in type V HLP; (3) the glucose intolerance and hyperinsulinemia that are very common in type V HLP are not characteristic of familial hyperchylomicronemia.

GENETICS The full-blown disorder appears in either sex. Vertical transmission has not been observed. The disorder(s) now perceived as familial hyperchylomicronemia usually appear to require a double dose of an abnormal allele for expression.

TREATMENT To avoid the crippling attacks of abdominal pain, pancreatitis, and foam-cell accumulation in liver, spleen, and bone marrow seen in most cases, it is recommended that the daily intake of fat be kept to 20 to 25 percent of calories or a maximum of 50 g fat per day. Both saturated and unsaturated fats are cleared poorly. Commercial preparations of medium-chain glycerides offer means of satisfying craving for fat without inducing chylomicronemia, since these glycerides go directly to the liver in the portal vein.

SECONDARY TYPE I HLP Phenocopies of familial hyperchylomicronemia are produced by systemic lupus erythematosus, myeloma, macroglobulinemia, lymphomas, or other diseases in which there are abnormal circulating globulins or other proteins. In such patients, heparin resistance, possibly due to heparin binding by the abnormal protein, is present and manifested by decreased prolongation of thrombin time. The hyperlipoproteinemia fluctuates with changes in the plasma protein abnormality. Depression of postheparin lipolytic activity also occurs in uncontrolled diabetes mellitus and may be associated with a type I pattern of hyperlipoproteinemia. Treatment is directed toward the underlying diseases.

HYPERBETALIPOPROTEINEMIA (TYPE II HLP)

DEFINITION Occasionally the concentration of alpha- or high-density lipoproteins may be uniquely elevated and produce hypercholesterolemia, with plasma cholesterol concentrations of 250 to 300 mg per 100 ml. This latter is not considered pathologic. It is perhaps most commonly seen in women receiving estrogens and can usually be detected from marked increase in staining of the alphalipoproteins on electrophoresis. Nearly always, however, hypercholesterolemia in the presence of a normal or modestly elevated triglyceride concentration means hyperbetalipoproteinemia (an increase in LDL concentrations). In the World Health Organization (WHO) classification, hyperbetalipoproteinemia alone is called type IIa HLP; when there is associated hyperglyceridemia, due to increased concentration of pre-beta- or very low density lipoproteins (VLDL), the pattern of hyperlipoproteinemia is called type IIb.

In simplest terms, hyperbetalipoproteinemia implies that the plasma pool of LDL is increased, either because of excessive production of LDL or abnormal limitation in removal or catabolism of these lipoproteins. Mechanisms regulating the synthesis of cholesterol, its removal from plasma and conversion to bile acids, which are the principal excretion products of cholesterol, are among some of the important determinants of LDL concentrations. "Pure" hyperbetalipoproteinemia is likely due to alterations in such regulators and tends to be responsive to reduced dietary intake of sterol or saturated fat content or to administration of bile acid sequestering resins. One of the major sources of plasma LDL is provided by catabolism of VLDL, the principal carriers of endogenous glycerides. Changes in VLDL turnover may lead to hyperbetalipoproteinemia and hyperglyceridemia. When VLDL metabolism is unstable, the VLDL and LDL concentrations may vary considerably over short periods of time. When this happens, the lipid pattern may shift variably between type IIa and type IIb HLP and simple endogenous hyperglyceridemia. Hyperbetalipoproteinemia is usually not present when triglycerides are greater than 400. In the presence of lesser glyceride concentrations, there is a convenient rule of thumb for estimating LDL concentrations in terms of the cholesterol content of these lipoproteins

$$(C_{LDL}):C_{LDL} = C - \left(\frac{TG}{5} + 45\right)$$

where C = plasma cholesterol
TG = plasma triglyceride concentration
45 = average for the cholesterol in HDL

A C_{LDL} exceeding 170 may be considered as hyperbetalipoproteinemia.

Mild primary hyperbetalipoproteinemia is most commonly sporadic and usually is ameliorated by reducing the amount of cholesterol and saturated fat ingested. It is very rarely associated with xanthomas. Familial hyperbetalipoproteinemia can be recognized reliably only by family screening. There are at least two forms, which are expressed when a single abnormal (dominant) allele is present: *familial hypercholesterolemia* and *combined hyperlipidemia.*

FAMILIAL HYPERCHOLESTEROLEMIA (HYPERCHOLESTEROLEMIC XANTHOMATOSIS) Definition

This is the oldest known form of familial HLP. The presence of a single gene leads to hyperbetalipoproteinemia that is easily detectable by one year of age, and often at birth. Type II HLP may be the only abnormality throughout life, but subcutaneous xanthomas, particularly in the Achilles and extensor tendons of the hands, the elbows, and over the tibial tuberosities, and cutaneous xanthomas begin to appear at about age twenty. This is often accompanied by early evidence of atherosclerosis, particularly involving the coronary arteries. By age fifty, the risk of premature ischemic heart disease is three to ten times normal. Corneal arcus is common. Diabetes, hyperuricemia, or other abnormalities seen in other forms of hyperlipoproteinemia do not seem to be unusually frequent. Offspring of two affected parents (homozygotes) tend to have more severe hyperbetalipoproteinemia; they may have xanthomas at birth, and atherosclerosis is particularly severe, often leading to acquired aortic stenosis and death from ischemic heart disease between ages one and thirty. Familial hypercholesterolemia affects both sexes and occurs in Caucasoids and black and Oriental races. The gene prevalence in the United States is of the order of 1:1000.

Diagnosis On the usual American diet, children with familial hypercholesterolemia nearly always have a C_{LDL} greater than 165 mg per 100 ml. This cutoff point corresponds to a plasma cholesterol of between 220 and 240. The cholesterol in heterozygotes is usually between 250 and 500, the mean value being slightly higher in adults than children. Triglyceride concentrations are normal in 95 percent of children below age 10 (type IIa HLP). The frequency of modest elevations up to 500 mg per 100 ml increases with age, and about one-third of adults have type IIb HLP. The diagnosis of familial hypercholesterolemia does not rest on any specific biochemical test; it is presumptive when hyperbetalipoproteinemia is also present in at least one parent or other first-degree relatives, and the likelihood of a correct diagnosis is enhanced when the patient or his affected relatives also have xanthomatosis. When the parental phenotypes are known, affected offspring can usually be diagnosed from values of C_{LDL} in cord blood. The homozygous phenotype is suspected when manifestations are severe and both parents have familial hyperbetalipoproteinemia. The metabolic defect has not been established.

Treatment The dietary content of cholesterol and saturated fat should be sharply reduced as soon as diagnosis is made. This will nearly always reduce the hyperlipidemia by 10 to 20 percent, often more dramatically in younger children. Cholestyramine, in four divided doses totaling 16 to 24 g per day, will further lower plasma cholesterol by 15 to 30 percent. Present practice dictates use of the drug in heterozygotes who are between fifteen and fifty-five years and whose plasma cholesterol remains above 300 despite stringent diet. Homozygotes sometimes respond to cholestyramine alone, or in combination with nicotinic acid. Xanthomas will soften and disappear if hyperlipidemia is successfully suppressed.

COMBINED HYPERLIPIDEMIA There are families in which hypercholesterolemia, hyperglyceridemia, or both may occur in different relatives at a frequency suggestive of determination by a single autosomal gene. In children, hyperglyceridemia is more common. Hyperbetalipoproteinemia (either type IIa or IIb HLP) occurs more frequently in the adults, and as a rule is less severe, and xanthomas less common, than in familial hypercholesterolemia. Other possible clinical differences have not yet been established, but premature ischemic heart disease probably is abnormally prevalent. The diagnosis cannot be established from lipid or lipoprotein analyses in a single patient. All available first-degree relatives must be screened. Half should theoretically be affected, and a majority of these should have hyperglyceridemia with or without hypercholesterolemia (type IIb or IV HLP). Therapeutic experience is limited, but inference that triglyceride or VLDL metabolism may be primarily affected directs attention to maintenance of ideal weight by avoidance of excess in either alcohol or other sources of calories. When dietary measurements fail to lower cholesterol below 300 or triglycerides below 250, therapeutic trial of clofibrate, nicotinic acid, or possibly *d*-thyroxine should be considered. The usefulness of cholestyramine is not yet established.

OTHER FAMILIAL OR SPORADIC FORMS Neither of these syndromes may be considered to represent single mutants. There also probably are polygenic forms of hyperbetalipoproteinemia. Familial involvement must always be sought in the absence of specific biochemical tests for phenotypes. The management of hyperbetalipoproteinemia of obscure origin proceeds empirically on the basis of distinctions already discussed for *familial hypercholesterolemia* and *combined hyperlipidemia.* It is also predicated on an unproved assumption that reduction in hyperlipidemia reduces the hazard of premature vascular disease, a premise that includes greater emphasis on younger patients.

TYPE III HYPERLIPOPROTEINEMIA

Definition This pattern is characterized by the presence of beta-migrating lipoproteins of density less than 1.006 ("floating beta"); performance of this test requires preparative ultracentrifugation. There are usually increased pre-beta-lipoproteins and often a positive visual test for chylomicrons. Half of patients have a broad beta band on electrophoresis, hence the synonym *broad-beta disease.* The cholesterol and glyceride concentrations tend to be similar, and fluctuate considerably between 200 and 1,000 mg per 100 ml. Type III hyperlipoproteinemia appears to be due to severe rate limitation in the conversion of VLDL to LDL; "intermediate" lipoproteins accumulate that are otherwise never seen in quantity. The anomalous lipoproteins may be seen transiently with severe hypothyroidism or uncontrolled diabetes mellitus. They are most strikingly evident in a rare familial disorder.

FAMILIAL TYPE III HLP Clinical picture The disorder is rarely detected before age twenty, and manifests later in women unless the menopause has been hastened or severe obesity is present. In addition to the typical lipoprotein pattern, two-thirds of patients have peculiar raised yellow plaques (plane xanthomas) in the palmar creases or on the fingers. Most of them also have soft, reddish yellow, single or confluent xanthomas on the elbows. Some have pedunculated xanthomas on the buttocks and elsewhere on the limbs; a few have tendon xanthomas. The majority of patients have intermittent claudication and evidence of decreased blood flow in the lower extremities; some have premature ischemic heart and cerebrovascular disease. Most have glucose intolerance, many are hypersecretors of insulin. Practically all are abnormally "carbohydrate-inducible," in terms of an exaggerated rise of plasma glycerides on high carbohydrate feeding. Hyperuricemia is common.

Diagnosis The ascertainment of the anomalous lipoprotein pattern is necessary for absolute diagnosis. Some observers report that "floating beta" is always present at any level of hyperlipidemia, others maintain it may come and go. The usual pattern of severe mixed hyperlipidemia, when combined with palmar xanthomas and severe vascular disease, allows a presumptive diagnosis. More than half of affected patients have a parent, sibling, or adult offspring with the same abnormalities. Some relatives have hyperglyceridemia without "floating-beta" lipoproteins, and both lipoprotein patterns possibly represent different phenotypic expression of an "incomplete dominant" mutant gene.

Treatment The hyperlipidemia in type III HLP nearly always can be returned to normal with appropriate treatment. The skin xanthomas also disappear, lending encouragement that treatment may desirably affect the hazard for premature vascular disease. Treatment consists sequentially of (1) reduction to ideal weight; (2) institution of a rigorous diet, with special attention to keeping carbohydrate intake below 5 g per kg per day by increasing the intake of polyunsaturated fat, if necessary, and elimination of alcohol; and (3) clofibrate, 2 g per day. The therapeutic effect of these steps is additive. Lipids should be monitored at least every 3 months. Nicotinic acid, 3 g per day, or *d*-thyroxine may be used in place of clofibrate.

HYPERPREBETALIPOPROTEINEMIA (ENDOGENOUS HYPERGLYCERIDEMIA; TYPE IV HLP)

Definition The plasma triglyceride concentration reflects mainly the transport of glycerides that come directly from the diet (in chylomicrons) and others that are secreted from the liver, intestine, and perhaps other tissues (in VLDL or pre-beta-lipoproteins). When chylomicrons are not visible—and the anomalous lipoproteins of type III HLP are not present—increased plasma triglycerides are equated with endogenous hyperglyceridemia (type IV HLP). The diagnosis is thus not difficult (Table 106-2), but this belies the many possible causes of endogenous hyperglyceridemia. The secretion of VLDL is influenced by many emotional and hormonal factors controlling release into plasma of free fatty acids, the major precursors of endogenous glycerides, their uptake by liver, oxidation or conversion to glycerides, and secretion as VLDL. The hydrolysis of VLDL glycerides and their uptake and reesterification in adipose tissue are also important regulators of the triglyceride concentration.

Among determinants acting on these metabolic pathways are caloric balance, supply and utilization of carbohydrate, insulin activity, alcohol intake, estrogen administration, physical activity, and stress. Moderate hyperglyceridemia may therefore be secondary to many diseases and have many primary causes. Evidence is accumulating that hyperglyceridemia in the presence of normal cholesterol concentrations increases risk of premature ischemic heart disease.

FAMILIAL TYPE IV HLP Endogenous hyperglyceridemia occurs in families in several disorders. These include the *combined hyperlipidemia* where it is one of the variant phenotypic expressions of a single gene. Hyperglyceridemia will be associated with significant hyperbetalipoproteinemia in some relatives. In *type III HLP* simple hyperglyceridemia also occurs in some relatives at a greater than expected frequency. The presence of anomalous lipoproteins in one or more relatives provides the diagnosis. There is also a *monogenic endogenous hyperglyceridemia* in which half of relatives have type IV HLP; expression is less frequent in children. This syndrome is not uncommon, and is frequently accompanied by glucose intolerance and hyperuricemia; it is worsened by obesity. A more severe form of this syndrome is described below as type V HLP. There are no specific biochemical tests to establish any of the above phenotypes in a given patient with endogenous hyperglyceridemia. It is desirable to have as much information about the family as possible.

Treatment Management of *primary* endogenous hyperglyceridemia is presently the same regardless of the cause. It consists of (1) maintenance of ideal weight; (2) avoidance of an excess contribution of carbohydrate to total calories (less than 45 percent); (3) restriction of alcohol intake; (4) in patients where the above measures fail to lower glycerides below 250 to 300 mg per 100 ml, a therapeutic trial of clofibrate or nicotinic acid may be justified. Avoid use of nicotinic acid in diabetes. Because triglycerides tend to be variable, their concentration should be followed weekly during any trial of therapy.

SECONDARY FORMS Endogenous hyperglyceridemia occurs in many other diseases such as poorly controlled diabetes mellitus, hypothyroidism, dysproteinemias, the nephrotic syndrome, idiopathic hypercalcemia, Werner's syndrome, Tangier disease, LCAT deficiency, and other lipidoses. Oral contraceptives and other estrogen-containing drugs may provoke hyperglyceridemia.

MIXED HYPERGLYCERIDEMIA (TYPE V HLP)

Definition Severe hyperglyceridemia, especially when the triglyceride concentration exceeds 1,000 (Table 106-2), usually implies chylomicronemia in addition to endogenous hyperglyceridemia. Upon standing, the turbid plasma separates into a cream layer overlying a turbid infranatant (VLDL). One of two general classes of defects is usually suspected. The plasma VLDL pool may be initially increased, perhaps because of oversecretion of endogenous glycerides. This taxes the normal glyceride removal mechanisms, and chylomicrons also accumulate. Alternatively, triglyceride clearance itself may be defective. It is difficult to distinguish between these situations by any widely applicable clinical tests. Postheparin lipolytic activity is not homogeneous and is, at best, an indirect measure of the functional capacity for triglyceride removal. The evidence is very suggestive that type V HLP secondary to uncontrolled diabetes mellitus is related to deficient maintenance of lipoprotein lipase activity by insulin. On the other hand, most patients with primary type V HLP do not have obvious deficiency in this enzyme activity. Other defects such as abnormal lipoproteins or inhibitors of hydrolysis have been proposed but not convincingly demonstrated.

FAMILIAL FORMS Patients with primary type V often come from families in which more than half of adult first-degree relatives have hyperglyceridemia, some with chylomicrons in the fasting state, others without them. It is probable that there are genetic differences between some of these families and many of the more common ones in which only lesser endogenous (type IV) hyperlipoproteinemia is present. There are no unique biochemical tests which segregate such families, however, or which allow one to determine whether primary type V HLP in a given patient is sporadic or familial. Most affected patients are adults.

Clinical features The majority of patients with primary type V HLP have glucose intolerance; many have hyperinsulinemia, and some complain of paresthesias ("diabetic neuropathy"?). Hyperuricemia and obesity are common, as is a history of excess ethanol intake. Bouts of abdominal pain, sometimes associated with chemical signs of pancreatitis, are typical and make this form of hyperlipoproteinemia potentially lethal. Hepatosplenomegaly, foam cells in bone marrow aspirates, lipemia retinalis, and eruptive xanthomas also may be present. There is probably an increased hazard of premature vascular disease.

Treatment All patients are benefited by some restriction in fat intake, but very severe restriction (below 40 g fat per day) is difficult to maintain, and the resultant increase in carbohydrate content of the diet sometimes causes marked increases in VLDL. Maintenance of ideal weight is usually helpful in suppressing the plasma glyceride elevations. Nicotinic acid (1.5 to 3.0 g per day) is sometimes very effective and may keep patients free of abdominal pain for years. Alcohol and estrogens are to be avoided.

SECONDARY TYPE V HLP All the diseases which may cause type IV HLP may sometimes give rise to this more severe form of hyperglyceridemia. The patient's fat intake may often determine whether chylomicronemia complicates lesser degrees of endogenous hyperglyceridemia. It is not known how often pancreatitis produces hyperglyceridemia; the reverse definitely occurs.

OTHER HYPERLIPOPROTEINEMIAS

All hyperlipidemia is not encompassed in these major lipoprotein patterns. Notable exceptions are hypercholesterolemia and massive hypercholesterolemia and massive hyperphospholipidemia associated with obstructive liver disease. This is accompanied by the presence of abnormal lipoproteins (Lp-X). It is detected by the combination of jaundice, hypercholesterolemia, and a great increase in *unesterified* plasma cholesterol, or by use of antiserums to Lp-X. Abnormally lipidated lipoproteins also accompany hyperlipidemia in familial LCAT deficiency, and possibly other lipidoses described below. *Autoimmune hyperlipoproteinemia* refers to hyperlipidemia due to interactions of various gamma-globins with lipoproteins and consequent interference with their metabolism. This is included in secondary hyperlipidemia due to paraproteinemia.

HYPOLIPOPROTEINEMIA

Beta- (low-density) lipoprotein deficiency

ABETALIPOPROTEINEMIA Abetalipoproteinemia is a rare familial disease, uniquely characterized by complete absence of beta-lipoproteins (LDL), pre-beta-lipoproteins, and chylomicrons, and of the apoprotein or apoproteins (apo-LDL) which form part of or all the polypeptide portions of these lipoproteins. The plasma contains only alpha-lipoproteins. The syndrome follows a fairly uniform course, beginning before the age of one year, with *malnutrition* and growth retardation, lordosis, abdominal distention, and steatorrhea. *Ataxia*, nystagmus, weakness and areflexia, and other signs of progressive neurologic dysfunction, particularly involving the posterolateral columns and spinocerebellar tracts, then appear. *Pigmentary retinal degeneration* develops during adolescence. The erythrocytes have a crenated appearance (acanthocytosis). The esterified lipids of these cells and of the plasma are deficient in both lecithin and lineoleic acid. Dietary fat is assimilated but is held up in the intestinal mucosal cells, creating a pathognomonic picture detectable by peroral biopsy. Some fat is absorbed, possibly by direct passage through the portal system into the liver.

The disease may occur in siblings and is likely due to a double dose of a mutant autosomal gene, since the consanguinity rate in affected families is high. Most relatives have normal concentrations of plasma lipoproteins. Whether the primary defect is related to formation of beta-apoprotein, beta-lipoprotein, or some other aspect of fat absorption is not known. The prognosis is guarded; patients may succumb relatively young, sometimes from cardiac arrhythmias. Familial instances of acanthocytosis and neurologic abnormalities without abetalipoproteinemia have also been reported.

Diagnosis The diagnosis is suspected when a plasma cholesterol concentration less than 100 mg per 100 ml is associated with the above clinical picture. It must be confirmed by immunochemical evidence of the absence of apo-LDL from plasma.

Treatment There is no definitive therapy. Medium-chain triglycerides may help provide some fat intake in the absence of chylomicron formation, and low vitamin A levels have been increased with supplements.

HYPOBETALIPOPROTEINEMIA Abnormally low cholesterol and glyceride concentrations with decreased, but not absent, beta- and very low density lipoproteins are common in malnutrition or malabsorption due to a variety of causes. Remissions are promptly associated with a rise in cholesterol and beta-lipoproteins. Rarely, patients with paraproteinemia may have severe hypolipoproteinemia, possibly due to autoantibodies to lipoproteins. There are also *heritable* forms of hypobetalipoproteinemia, at least one due to a dominant gene. Beta-lipoprotein levels down to 10 percent of normal occur, usually with no disability.

Alpha- (high-density) lipoprotein deficiency

Familial high-density lipoprotein deficiency is also called *Tangier disease*, after the island home in Virginia of the first recorded cases. The disease has been detected in other children and adults and must be suspected when hypocholesterolemia is associated with orange or yellowish gray discoloration of the tonsils and pharyngeal or rectal mucosa or *enlargement* of *spleen*, *liver*, or *lymph nodes*. Reticuloendothelial tissues are infiltrated with *foam cells* containing large amounts of cholesteryl esters. Corneal infiltration, hypersplenism, and severe, recurrent peripheral neuropathy also occur.

Parents and other relatives of patients with Tangier disease have lower than normal amounts of plasma high-density (alpha$_1$) lipoprotein. The propositi appear to have a double dose of a mutant allele at a locus directing synthesis of the major apoprotein of high-density lipoproteins (apoLP-Gln-I).

Diagnosis Diagnosis is suspected when plasma cholesterol is between 50 and 125 mg per 100 ml with normal or slightly elevated glycerides. It is established by immunochemical evidence that apoLP-Gln-I is present in only trace amounts. There is no definitive therapy.

PLASMA LECITHIN:CHOLESTEROL ACYLTRANSFERASE (LCAT) DEFICIENCY This is a rare familial disorder seen mainly in Scandinavians. The clinical manifestations include proteinuria, anemia with target-cell formation, and corneal infiltration. Plasma-esterified cholesterol and alpha-lipoproteins are markedly reduced, and unesterified cholesterol and lecithin are greatly increased. LCAT enzyme normally esterifies the plasma cholesterol, and activity of the enzyme is severely deficient in this disorder; there is no specific therapy.

LIPID STORAGE DISEASES

THE SPHINGOLIPIDOSES Many lipidoses are characterized by tissue rather than plasma lipid abnormalities. *In all it is exceedingly important that specimens of tissues* *obtained for diagnostic purposes be retained frozen without fixatives for chemical and enzymatic analyses. Histochemical diagnosis is usually not definitive.* The sphingolipidoses represent one group of these disorders; each member of this group is characterized by the accumulation of a specific (and different) derivative (—R) of ceramide (acylspingosine).

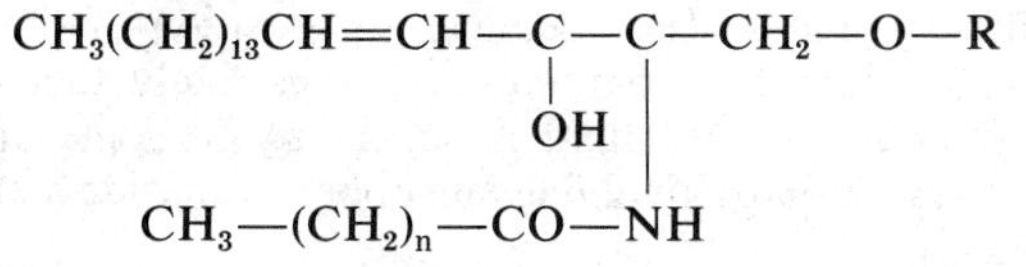

$$\begin{array}{l} CH_3(CH_2)_{13}CH{=}CH{-}\underset{\displaystyle OH}{\underset{|}{C}}{-}C{-}CH_2{-}O{-}R \\ \qquad\qquad\qquad\qquad\qquad\quad | \\ CH_3{-}(CH_2)_n{-}CO{-}NH \end{array}$$

Ceramide

These are all inheritable disorders; each may involve the nervous system. Most occur in several clinical forms or syndromes, possibly reflecting mutations at different loci. The underlying defect in each is deficiency of a specific lysosomal enzyme in the pathway of lipid catabolism (Table 106-1). They may also be grouped according to chemical similarities in the particular lipids that abnormally accumulate in the tissues.

GANGLIOSIDOSES (see also Chap. 332) *Gangliosidosis* is a generic term for several familial neurologic disorders associated with varying degrees of blindness and dementia. An older and somewhat misleading term for them is *amaurotic family idiocy.* Three of these diseases have been identified as characterized by defective metabolism and accumulation of different gangliosides, the major lipids in gray matter. *G_{M1} gangliosidosis, generalized gangliosidosis*, or *pseudo-Hurler's disease*, involves both brain and viscera. The tissues contain abnormal amounts of galactosylgalactosaminyl(*N*-acetylneuraminido)galactosylglucosyl ceramide. A galactosidase attacking the terminal glycosidic bond is deficient. *G_{M2} gangliosidosis* includes *Tay-Sachs disease*, which fatally involves only the central nervous system. The excess ganglioside is *N*-acetylgalactosaminyl(*N*-acetylneuraminido)galactosylglucosyl ceramide. Different phenotypic variants of G_{M1} and G_{M2} gangliosidoses are recognized (Table 106-1). A G_{M3} gangliosidosis has also recently been identified. Other forms of amaurotic idiocy, such as Batten-Mayou's disease (Vogt-Spielmeyer or juvenile amaurotic idiocy), and the Bielschowsky, Kufs, and Hallevorden types have not been chemically differentiated as lipidoses.

GLUCOSYLCEREBROSIDOSES (GAUCHER'S DISEASE) (see also Chap. 317) First described by Gaucher in 1882, these disorders represent storage of glucocerebrosides (glucosyl ceramide) in reticuloendothelial cells, producing marked splenomegaly and hepatomegaly. In adults there are often bone lesions, associated skin pigmentation, and characteristic pingueculae of the scleras. A genetic variant may cause progressive neurologic disturbances and a rapidly fatal course in infants. There is also a juvenile form. Deficient activity of glucocerebrosidase (a β-glucosidase) is present in all three forms.

GLUCOSYL CERAMIDE TRIHEXOSIDOSIS (FABRY'S DISEASE) (see Chap. 315) In this sex-linked disorder the manifestations are usually seen only in males and are due to deposition of glycolipids, mainly a trihexoside (galactosylgalactosylglucosyl ceramide), in blood vessels and nerves. Galactosylgalactosyl ceramide also accumulates. Because of its unusual skin lesions, this disease is also known as *angiokeratoma corporis diffusum universale.* The activity of an α-galactosidase is deficient.

GALACTOSYLSULFATIDOSIS (see also Chap. 332) *Metachromatic leukodystrophy* is a disorder that usually develops between 1 and 2 years of age. Abnormal amounts of sulfuric acid esters of galactosylceramide accumulate in the brain and kidney. The sulfatides are excreted in urine, making possible a provisional diagnosis. The disease is due to deficient cerebroside sulfatase activity.

GALACTOSYLCEREBROSIDOSIS (see Chap. 332) *Krabbe's globoid cell leukodystrophy* is a rapidly fatal, demyelinating disease of infants. Diagnosis is made by the finding of deficient activity of a β-galactosidase in leukocytes or serum.

PHOSPHORYLCHOLINECERAMIDOSES (NIEMANN-PICK DISEASE) (see Chap. 332) Several lipidoses are characterized by accumulation of massive amounts of sphingomyelin and cholesterol. They include disorders due to more than one mutation and may be partially distinguished by measurement of sphingomyelin-cleavage activity in liver, spleen, or fibroblasts in tissue cluture. The enzyme is severely deficient in both the classic infantile form of Niemann-Pick disease (type A) and in older children with visceral but not central nervous system involvement (type B). The enzyme has been normal or low normal in tissues examined from most of the older patients with late central nervous system involvement (type C) or those with the so-called "Nova Scotia" variant (type D).

CHOLESTERYL ESTER AND TRIGLYCERIDE HYDROLASE DEFICIENCIES

There are two inheritable disorders in which massive amounts of cholesteryl esters and triglycerides are stored in liver, spleen, lymph nodes, bone marrow reticulocytes (foam cells), intestine, and other tissues. This is associated with severe deficiency in lysosomal enzyme activity catalyzing hydrolysis of cholesteryl esters and triglycerides at acid pH. Diagnosis is made from enzyme assays on cultured skin fibroblasts or lipid measurements on a biopsy of the liver, coupled with the clinical picture.

WOLMAN'S DISEASE This disorder is manifested in infancy by failure to thrive associated with hepatosplenomegaly, gastrointestinal symptoms, and adrenal calcification demonstrable by x-ray. There is no treatment, and death usually occurs by six months of age.

CHOLESTERYL ESTER STORAGE DISEASE This disease has a more benign course, being compatible with adult life. Massive hepatomegaly, with or without splenomegaly, and hypercholesterolemia are common features. Hypertriglyceridemia and accelerated atherosclerosis also may occur. Much of the lipid stored in tissues is converted to insoluble ceroid pigment. There is no treatment.

PHYTANIC OXIDASE DEFICIENCY

REFSUM'S DISEASE In this condition there is accumulation of phytanic acid (3,7,11,15-tetramethyl hexadecanoic acid) in the esterified lipids present in both tissues and plasma. This familial disease is characterized by ataxic neuropathy, anosmia, retinitis pigmentosa, dry skin, skeletal deformities, and ichthyosis and is commonest in children or young adults of Scandinavian ancestry. Parents may have high levels of phytanic acid in plasma without other abnormalities. The prognosis is guarded, with the symptoms sometimes progressing to complete blindness and deafness, but often waxing and waning. Relapses are somewhat irregular, being correlated with the degree of increase in cerebrospinal protein. Phytanic acid, which is normally present only in trace quantities, constitutes 10 to 30 percent of total plasma fatty acids. The inherited defect is a block in the alpha oxidation of the phytanic acid derived from dietary phytols. The relation of phytanate accumulation to the nervous disorders is unknown. Diagnosis is usually made by chromatographic analysis of plasma. Therapy consists of a low-phytol diet.

CEROID STORAGE Ceroid and lipofuscin are insoluble pigments believed to arise from peroxidation of unsaturated fatty acids. They are identified histochemically by the combination of red periodic acid–Schiff stain, acid-fastness, and autofluorescence in ultraviolet light. Ceroid deposition is a feature of abetalipoproteinemia and many lipid-storage diseases and does not represent a specific disorder. The *syndrome of the sea-blue histiocyte* pertains to a diverse group of patients who have foam cells in bone marrow that appear light blue with Giemsa's stain. Identical-appearing cells occur in many of the known lipid-storage diseases, and their presence does not define a clear-cut or specific disease.

GRANULOMATOUS DISEASES WITH LIPID STORAGE

Frequently considered among the lipid storage diseases are certain tissue proliferative disorders sometimes accompanied by lipid deposition.

HISTIOCYTOSIS X (see also Chap. 317) This is the generic term for a group of disorders that affect the reticuloendothelial system and which may be either different stages or forms of the same disease. *Letterer-Siwe disease* and *xanthoma disseminatum* may be the two extremes of such abnormalities, with *eosinophilic granuloma* and *Hand-Schuller-Christian disease* representing intermediate and special forms. The usual order of progression of the pathologic lesions is reticuloendothelial cell proliferation and hyperplasia, granulomatous changes featuring eosinophils and giant cells, conversion of reticulum cells and histiocytes to foam cells or xanthomas, and finally, fibrosis. These disorders do not appear to be hereditary.

Several other uncommon diseases are associated with proliferation of histiocytes and deposition of material considered to represent both lipid and carbohydrate because it stains by both the Sudan and periodic acid–Schiff techniques. The chemical composition of the lesions has not been characterized. It is likely that any faulty metabolism of lipid is secondary to some other processes, perhaps involving mucopolysaccharide metabolism.

LIPOID PROTEINOSIS In *lipoid proteinosis* (cutaneous-mucosal hyalinosis; Urbach-Wiethe disease) the lesions share enough histologic features of *histiocytosis X* to suggest an etiologic relation. The skin and mucous membranes of the pharynx and larynx are infiltrated by extracellular deposits of hyaline material. Clinical manifestations include hoarseness or aphonia, widely distributed skin papules, dental anomalies, and symmetric calcifications in the region of the sella turcica as seen by x-ray. The disease is not incompatible with long life. This disorder may be heritable.

LIPOID DERMATOARTHRITIS In *lipoid dermatoarthritis* polyarthritis is associated with multiple nodular or papular skin lesions. In both skin and synovial tissues there is an infiltration of histiocytes, eosinophils, lymphocytes, red blood cells, and multinucleated giant cells. The joint changes may be extremely destructive, producing *arthritis mutilans*, or the "opera-glass hand." Serologic reactions for rheumatoid arthritis are negative. Familial occurrence has not been reported.

DISSEMINATED LIPOGRANULOMATOSIS (FARBER'S DISEASE) This is a rare disease that appears in infancy as generalized nodular periarticular swelling and dysphonia. There is progressive systemic involvement with widespread proliferation of histiocytes and neuronal abnormalities. Storage cells appear containing both mucopolysaccharide and lipids. The basic disorder probably involves the metabolism of certain acid mucopolysaccharides similar to those in Hurler's disease (Chap. 362).

OTHER XANTHOMATOSES

NORMOLIPOPROTEINEMIC XANTHOMATOSES

Many chronic infections, particularly accompanied by exudates, and other proliferative processes, such as osteitis fibrosa cystica or traumatic lesions, may be associated with collections of foam cells (*xanthomas*) and sometimes crystals of cholesterol. Most skin xanthomas are secondary to hyperlipoproteinemia, but *juvenile xanthomas* (nevoxanthoepithelioma) are benign skin lesions that can appear without abnormal plasma lipids. *Xanthelasmas* need not always be associated with hyperlipoproteinemia; very rarely they occur, along with Achilles tendon xanthomas, in family members who are normolipoproteinemic.

CEREBROTENDINOUS XANTHOMATOSIS An unusual example of normolipoproteinemic xanthomatosis is a familial disease in which large nodules appear on the upper portions of the Achilles tendons, often followed by pulmonary insufficiency and neurologic dysfunction, including dementia and progressive spastic ataxia. These signs are due to xanthomatous deposits in tendons, lung, and brain, which contain cholesterol and cholestanol (5α-cholestan-3β-o1). Cholestanol and other neutral and acidic sterols also appear in bile in abnormal amounts. The metabolic defect has not been established.

ADIPOSE TISSUE DISORDERS

Adipose tissue can be a site of expression of many disorders including those of connective tissue, lipid, and carbohydrate metabolism. There is therefore no simple classification of the adipose tissue diseases.

RELAPSING PANNICULITIS (WEBER-CHRISTIAN DISEASE) This classification may represent several diseases that share similar but rather nonspecific histologic changes (see Chap. 361).

LIPODYSTROPHY Although the term *lipodystrophy* is sometimes used to describe *lipoatrophy*, it also has a generic meaning that allows it to encompass several disorders in which adipose tissue is abnormal but not necessarily absent. Several abnormalities may properly be considered forms of lipodystrophy.

Lipomas These are benign mesenchymal tumors consisting of circumscribed masses of adipose tissue. There is usually a capsule, but the cells are histologically indistinguishable from ordinary fat. They may occur nearly anywhere in the body, singly or as multiple fatty growths (lipomatosis), most commonly in subcutaneous tissues. They also arise in retroperitoneal or peritoneal areas, in breast, mesentery, and mediastinum, and in other body cavities and organs. Lipomas have caused intestinal obstruction or dyspnea by superior mediastinal obstruction and may embarrass the function of other vital tissues. Rarely they may calcify, and it has been presumed that they may on occasion give rise to liposarcomas or other malignant tumors, but there is no general agreement on this. Multiple lipomas may be symmetrically placed and may run in families. The therapy is surgical excision; occasionally they will recur in the same site.

Adiposis dolorosa (Dercum's disease) *Adiposis dolorosa* refers to a poorly defined disorder in which painful subcutaneous lipomas, often widely and symmetrically situated, are sometimes associated with asthenia, decreased cutaneous sensation, motor weakness, or other evidence of peripheral neuropathy. Some patients have also had adenomas in the pituitary, thyroid, or adrenal glands. There may or may not be accompanying generalized obesity. Siblings may be similarly involved. The interstitial neuritis observed in the original adipose tissue nodules by Dercum has not been seen in many subsequent cases. There is no specific therapy.

Insulin lipodystrophy This term refers to changes in subcutaneous fat at the site of insulin injection (see Chap. 88) and may involve either localized hypertrophy or atrophy of adipose tissue.

LIPOATROPHY Lipoatrophy may be partial or complete.

Partial lipoatrophy Also called *progressive lipodystrophy*, partial lipodystrophy is characterized by the absence of subcutaneous fat over wide, symmetric areas of the body. The remaining parts of the body have normal or sometimes increased subcutaneous fat deposits. It occurs predominantly in females and often begins in childhood. The onset is usually insidious; the disease may begin with loss of subcutaneous fat in the face and subsequently involve that of the upper extremities and upper trunk. In other instances, the disorder may begin at the level of the iliac crest and extend downward. There are no subjective symptoms. The cause is unknown. There is no known therapy.

Total lipoatrophy In total lipoatrophy (lipoatrophic diabetes mellitus), generalized atrophy of body fat occurs gradually. In addition to subcutaneous fat deposits, nearly all other body fat, excepting that in the breasts, may disappear. This is usually but not always associated with diabetes, which may precede or follow the onset of lipoatrophy. There are also hyperlipoproteinemias with types IV or V patterns, decreased postheparin lipolytic activity, hepatomegaly, and sometimes acanthosis nigricans; serious nephropathy, including both nephritic and nephrotic manifestations, may occur whether the patient has diabetes or not. Some patients may also have hypermetabolism, others have features suggestive of "leprechaunism," and the syndrome undoubtedly results from several different causes. The diabetes is associated with high plasma insulin levels and may be very difficult to control. The course of the disease may be either indolent or rapidly progressive. No therapy is known.

REFERENCES

FREDRICKSON DS: *A Physician's Guide to Hyperlipidemia: Modern Concepts of Cardiovascular Disease*, New York: Am Heart Assoc, July, 1972

GOLDSTEIN JL et al: Genetics of hyperlipidemia in coronary heart disease. Trans Assoc Am Physicians 85:120, 1972

PISCATELLI RL et al: Partial lipodystrophy: Metabolic studies in three patients. Ann Intern Med 73:963, 1970

SALAN G: Cholesterol deposition in cerebrotendinous xanthomatosis. Ann Intern Med 75:843, 1971

STANBURY JB et al (eds): *The Metabolic Basis of Inherited Disease*, 3d ed, New York: McGraw-Hill, 1972, chaps. 26–35

107 AMYLOIDOSIS

EVAN CALKINS

INTRODUCTION Although amyloidosis has been recognized as a clinical and pathologic entity for over 100 years, our knowledge about the nature, pathogenesis, distribution, and possible clinical importance of amyloid has now entered a stage of rapid evolution.

Amyloidosis, defined most broadly, is the tissue accumulation of detectable amounts of extracellular hyaline material which has certain rather unique tinctorial characteristics and contains characteristic fibrils which can be identified by electron microscopy. Using this definition, the incidence of amyloidosis is probably extremely high, and the disorder may be almost universal in the aging human population.

A more practical clinical definition states that amyloidosis is the accumulation of amyloid in amounts that result in interference with normal body function. According to this definition the entity is probably quite rare, except in certain countries, such as Israel and Turkey, in which there appears to be a striking genetic predisposition. The remainder of this discussion will focus on amyloidosis as defined in this more restricted clinical sense.

Over the years, several types of clinical classification have evolved. The following may be of some help in understanding the disease:

1 Primary amyloidosis—no known predisposing factor
  a Familial forms
  b Sporadic form
2 Secondary amyloidosis
3 Amyloidosis accompanying multiple myeloma
4 Localized amyloid accumulations
5 Age-related amyloid accumulation

HISTOLOGICAL AND CHEMICAL CHARACTERISTICS Under the light microscope amyloid has a hyaline appearance and is eosinophilic with hematoxylin and eosin. Its most characteristic histologic reaction depends on its affinity for Congo red stain. An apparently specific reaction for amyloid, however, can be obtained by studying Congo red stained material with polarized light. Amyloid exhibits a positive birefringence in the direction of the long axis of the deposit and a color change, on rotation of the filter, between deep red and blue-green. Amyloid also stains positively with thioflavine T or S; this reaction is not specific but assists in localization of traces of amyloid. Every tissue which has shown these characteristic reactions has, when examined with the electron microscope, been shown to contain the typical amyloid fibrils.

It has been suggested that the site of involvement in amyloidosis varies, in a consistent manner, with the clinical type of amyloidosis. In secondary and familial Mediterrean fever–related amyloidosis, amyloid appears adjacent to reticular tissue or, in the case of blood vessels, in the subintimal layer; in most cases of primary or multiple myeloma–related amyloidosis, the amyloid is laid down more diffusely in the extracellular tissue matrix, adjacent to collagen.

On an ultrastructural level, amyloid has been shown to consist of a relatively amorphous ground substance containing a high concentration of characteristic fibrils. The fibrils measure approximately 85 A in width, are nonbranching, and may be of variable length. With special techniques the fibrils exhibit a beaded appearance. It is the fibril which is responsible for the Congo red staining property of amyloid, and this characteristic has aided in attempts to purify extracts of these structures. X-ray diffraction of purified amyloid fibrils is said to reveal a pattern charactristic of a beta-pleated sheet.

Over the past few years, techniques have been developed which permit the extraction and isolation of the amyloid fiber protein. Such protein, isolated from patients with multiple myeloma or with primary amyloidosis, has been shown to exhibit an amino acid sequence which is very similar to that of the variable portion of a type kappa light chain. Fibrils exhibiting Congo red staining, green birefringence under polarized light, and the ultrastructural and x-ray diffraction characteristics of amyloid have been produced in vitro by enzymatic digestion of certain Bence Jones proteins.

On the other hand, other investigators have shown that amyloid fiber proteins from patients with secondary and familial Mediterranean fever–related forms of amyloidosis contain, as their major ingredient, a component which is similar in all cases but whose partial amino acid sequence is distinct from any known immunoglobulin. The nature and source of this protein is unknown. So, too, is its relationship, if any, with the immunoglobulin-derived protein which constitutes the major form of primary and myeloma-related amyloid.

Extracts of amyloid-laden organs have shown, in addition to the fibrils, a relatively small concentration of a second, apparently unique globular component, 80 to 100 A in diameter, resembling and referred to as "doughnuts" or pentagonal structures. Preliminary analyses indicate that these structures have distinct chemical and immunologic characteristics from the amyloid fibril. Their nature and role is as yet unknown.

CLINICAL TYPES OF AMYLOIDOSIS Primary amyloidosis In the first and probably most common category of amyloidosis seen today the disease develops without any known predisposing disease. Clinical studies have provided increasing evidence that this so-called "primary" form of amyloidosis is, in turn, comprised of a number of relatively discrete syndromes, each with characteristic clinical expression and pattern of occurrence.

In at least one of these entities the involvement resembles that seen in the secondary form. This is the amyloidosis which often occurs in association with familial Mediterranean fever (FMF), primarily in members of the Sephardic and Iraqi Jewish races. The two disorders appear to be inherited as independent recessive traits; amyloidosis may be seen in members of a family who do not have FMF and vice versa (Chap. 225).

More commonly primary amyloidosis is manifested by more widespread evidence of the disease. One example is the primary familial amyloidosis described by Andrade. This entity, which occurs predominantly in individuals of Portuguese ancestry, is accompanied by severe impairment of the sensory function of the peripheral nerves, as well as less severe impairment of motor function. This is often accompanied by involvement of the sympathetic ganglions, with postural hypotension, impotence, absence of sweating, and intestinal hypermotility and malabsorption. Adie's pupil is apt to be present. The patients usually die from severe malnutrition and inanition. Another example of primary amyloidosis occurring in families is that described by Rukavina et al. in a family of Swiss ancestry. Although some members of the family resembled the patients described by Andrade, others exhibited a variety of different clinical manifestations. Other familial syndromes (family constellations, yielding a variety of syndromes) have also been described.

Despite the increasing awareness of the familial incidence of amyloidosis, many patients who develop the disease, without known predisposing cause, do not appear to have any genetic or familial predisposition. In some of these cases the distribution of the amyloid resembles that seen in the secondary form of the disease; others have diffuse involvement, especially of the skin or heart.

Secondary amyloidosis That form of the disease which occurs as a sequel of prolonged inflammatory or infectious disease is termed secondary amyloidosis. Although the pattern of organ involvement may vary, parenchymal involvement of the liver, spleen, and kidneys, with or without vascular infiltration elsewhere, is the most frequent presentation. Estimates relating the frequency of amyloidosis as a complication of a particular disease process must take into consideration the frequency with which amyloid accumulates in otherwise "normal" aged individuals (see below). One clue which may be of value in making this distinction is the fact that parenchymal infiltration of the spleen, liver, and kidney is not a feature of age-related amyloidosis.

Amyloidosis, in a pattern characteristic of secondary amyloidosis, occasionally occurs in patients with rheumatoid arthritis, ankylosing spondylitis, and Still's disease. Amyloidosis is a common cause of death in paraplegics who have developed decubitus ulcers and urinary tract infections. It is seen in approximately one-third of patients with leprosy at the U.S. Public Health Service Hospital in Carville, Louisiana, and is one of the chief causes of death at that hospital. It may also accompany ulcerative colitis and other prolonged inflammatory diseases.

Amyloidosis and multiple myeloma (see Chap. 65) Amyloidosis has been reported to complicate the course of multiple myeloma in 6 to 15 percent of the cases. Since myeloma tends to occur in the seventh and eighth decades of life, when the aging form of amyloidosis is also apt to occur, the frequency of amyloidosis, as a complication of multiple myeloma, may well be less than the highest published figures indicate. One controlled study showed that the pattern of myeloma-related amyloid was distinct from that in the nonmyelomatous controls in two respects: first, in the appearance of amyloid surrounding plasma cell infiltrates in the marrow, and, second, in the appearance of amyloid deposits around renal casts. Occasionally, the accumulation of renal tubular casts, many of which contain amyloid, may be sufficient to cause renal failure in the absence of demonstrable glomerular pathology. Clinical studies have shown, in a number of myelomatous patients, infiltration of amyloid in the carpal ligaments, a finding which has not been observed in the age-related form.

More telling evidence concerning the association of amyloidosis and plasma-cell dyscrasias is derived from careful immunodiffusion studies of the serum and urine of patients with the sporadic form of what appears, clinically, to be "primary" amyloidosis. It is now recognized that a considerable percentage, probably more than half, of these patients, if studied carefully, will be shown to have monoclonal light chains circulating in the blood or excreted in the urine. Occasionally, bone marrow aspiration and further clinical investigation of these patients suggests the presence of multiple myeloma. (In these cases, the prognosis is apt to be poor.) Most patients with the genetic forms of amyloidosis (including that associated with familial Mediterranean fever) or with amyloidosis secondary to an inflammatory condition do not exhibit abnormal circulating or urinary immunoglobulin fragments.

Localized accumulations Deposits of amyloid may occasionally develop in such organs as the skin, bones, or synovial tissue or in areas immediately adjacent to neoplasms, especially medullary carcinoma of the thyroid.

Amyloid and aging Sensitive histologic techniques, utilizing polarization and fluorescence microscopy, have permitted detection of what appears to be amyloid in a large number of persons over sixty years of age. In recent studies amyloid has been found in the small meningeal vessels and brain substance (senile plaques) of 64 percent of individuals over seventy years of age. Cardiac deposits, most commonly in the atrial endocardium, can be found in over 57 percent of such persons if carefully searched for. In perhaps 5 percent of aged individuals, the amount of cardiac amyloid deposition is sufficient to suggest possible clinical significance. Amyloid may also be found within the major blood vessels of elderly individuals, particularly within the aortic media and in the vicinity of atheromatous plaques. Pancreatic islet amyloid, a recognized accompaniment of diabetes, is also present in a large number of elderly individuals.

While further studies are required to determine whether all such deposits are indeed amyloid, electron microscopy has revealed characteristic amyloid fibrils in the pancreatic, cardiac, and cerebral lesions described above. Whether these deposits are of clinical significance is not yet known. Certain elderly patients with extensive cardiac infiltration appear to be symptomatic, presenting with either cardiac failure or arrhythmias. There is some evidence that so-called "senile dementia" may be associated in some way with large numbers of amyloid-containing senile plaques within the cerebral cortex. It is not clear whether amyloid infiltration of the meningeal vessels bears a similar relationship.

CLINICAL MANIFESTATIONS The clinical manifestations of amyloidosis depend on the organ or system involved. Since the symptoms may resemble those of a variety of other disorders, amyloidosis must frequently be considered in the differential diagnosis.

Amyloidosis of the skin is a fairly frequent concomitant of primary amyloidosis and amyloidosis accompanying multiple myeloma. The amyloid infiltration may be confined to the skin, or the dermatologic involvement may be part of generalized amyloidosis. Although several types of lesions may be seen, the most frequent are hyaline plaques, occurring chiefly in or near the folds of the skin in the neck and in the axillal, inguinal, or anal regions. Purpura may be seen in these areas or in a widespread distribution, and may be induced by gentle rubbing.

Although in most cases this purpura is thought to be due to involvement of the walls of small blood vessels, other mechanisms may be involved. These may include thrombocytopenia or deficiencies of several different clotting factors. As a result of the defects in hemostasis, prolonged bleeding may follow such minor surgical procedures as a gingival biopsy.

Amyloid *infiltration of the heart* classically results in congestive failure, often intractable to therapy, with either minimal or no murmurs. An enlarged cardiac silhouette may or may not be present. Arrhythmias are common. Electrocardiogram often reveals low voltage. Atrial ventricular block may also be seen, occasionally in association with amyloid infiltration of the cardiac nerves. Amyloid infiltration of the myocardium or pericardium leads to stiffening of the heart, sometimes resulting in a syndrome resembling constrictive pericarditis.

Amyloid involvement of *the liver* is characterized primarily by hepatomegaly. Clinical evidence of hepatic dysfunction and jaundice is rare, and patients with hepatic amyloidosis may live for a number of years. Liver function tests characteristically show minimal abnormalities, which are usually suggestive of biliary obstruction. Although liver biopsy has been recommended and often yields diagnostic information, it has been followed in a few instances by intractable bleeding and/or rupture of the liver. For this reason liver biopsy should probably be avoided when amyloidosis is suspected.

Renal amyloidosis may be manifested by mild proteinuria or by the nephrotic syndrome. The appearance of progressively severe proteinuria in patients with chronic inflammatory diseases such as rheumatoid arthritis should always lead to a suspicion of amyloidosis. In attempting to differentiate renal amyloidosis from other types of renal failure, the size of the kidneys, as seen on x-ray, may be helpful. In parenchymal renal disease the kidneys are usually reduced in size; amyloid-laden kidneys are likely to be normal in size. In addition, massive proteinuria is rare in chronic glomerular disease. Hypertension is not commonly observed in amyloidosis. Azotemia is a very late manifestation and indicates a grave prognosis. Kidney biopsy is a satisfactory method of confirming the diagnosis of renal amyloidosis in cases in which the clinical syndrome, plus rectal biopsy, has not already led to a definite diagnosis.

Amyloidosis may result in a variety of *neurologic lesions.* Diffuse motor and sensory neuropathy, together with interference with function of the sympathetic nervous system, is characteristic of several forms of primary amyloidosis. Sensory involvement may also be seen in amyloidosis secondary to multiple myeloma, because of diffuse involvement of the sheaths of the peripheral nerves. Ocular involvement may consist of diffuse infiltrates in the posterior chamber, discrete deposits of amyloid beneath the bulbar conjunctiva, and an Adie pupil.

Accumulations of amyloid in the *trachea* or *bronchi* may result in serious obstruction to the respiratory passages. Following excision, recurrences are frequent but by no means invariable. In addition, amyloid infiltration may occur in the lung itself. It may be accompanied by surprisingly little evidence of functional impairment, but some patients have severe restrictive lung disease.

Amyloid infiltration of the *gastrointestinal tract* occurs in both primary and secondary amyloidosis. Amyloid may infiltrate any portion of the gastrointestinal tract, resulting in a variety of syndromes, including decreased motility, bleeding, malabsorption, and, rarely, obstruction and the radiologic appearance of tumor masses. Resultant clinical syndromes may resemble sprue, carcinoma, tuberculosis, lymphoma, and Whipple's disease.

Infiltration of the *endocrine* organs may also ensue. This rarely results in insufficiency of function of the involved gland. Localized accumulations of amyloid frequently accompany medullary carcinoma of the thyroid gland.

DIAGNOSIS The first requisite to making the diagnosis of amyloidosis is to think of it. The manifestations of this disease may mimic, closely, many other far more common disorders, such as atherosclerotic heart disease, chronic renal disease, diabetic neuropathy, or cirrhosis. While the presence of an underlying inflammatory disease may add to the index of suspicion, most cases seen today in the United States are of the primary or myeloma-related varities. In this instance, clinical manifestations of amyloidosis usually precede those of multiple myeloma. Therefore, the clinician must rely, above all, on his clinical judgment and intuition to lead him to consider amyloidosis, especially in patients with a multisystem disease.

Confirmation of the diagnosis is best obtained by biopsy. Rectal biopsy has proved confirmatory in approximately 75 percent of cases. Skin biopsy may be positive in patients with primary amyloidosis, even in the absence of clinical evidence of dermatologic involvement. It is rarely positive in secondary amyloidosis. Renal and hepatic biopsy carry a higher risk of bleeding, and consideration should be given to this fact when such diagnostic studies are contemplated.

Histologic examination of biopsy specimens must be conducted with great care. Traces of amyloid should be sought in the walls of small blood vessels. In specimens of skin, deposits may also be seen in sweat glands, sebaceous glands, and surrounding the fat cells in the subcutaneous tissue (amyloid rings). Tissue should be fixed in formalin and stained with hematoxylin and eosin, crystal violet, Congo red (preferably the alkaline Congo red method of Puchtler), and thioflavine T or S. Sections should be examined under regular, ultraviolet, and polarized light.

Once the diagnosis of amyloidosis has been established, careful study should be undertaken to determine whether or not there is a familial tendency or an underlying disease, either an inflammatory disease or multiple myeloma. Studies should include bone marrow aspiration, bone survey, serum electrophoresis and total protein determination, and careful immunodiffusion studies of plasma and urine for immunoglobulin fragments.

COURSE AND TREATMENT The course of amyloidosis is usually progressively downhill, especially if the organs involved include the kidneys, heart, or gastrointestinal tract. Of the fifty-odd cases studied by the author, none has had a remission, except for those cases of localized amyloidosis in which surgical extirpation has been possible. The course may be prolonged, however, lasting many years. Patients with cardiac amyloidosis may be very sensitive to digitalis, and this drug should be administered with special care. If amyloidosis accompanies other inflammatory diseases, vigorous efforts to treat the underlying condition should be initiated. If these efforts are successful, remission of amyloidosis may ensue.

If multiple myeloma is demonstrated to be present, appropriate therapy should be undertaken. Unfortunately, immunosuppressive therapy has not been shown to be effective in the treatment of amyloidosis.

On a more encouraging note, it should be pointed out that amyloid infiltration of the spleen has been shown to be reversible, through the action of the multinucleated giant cells. This may be true of other areas as well. While renal amyloidosis has not proved to be reversible, renal transplantation has been carried out successfully in a few cases without redevelopment of amyloidosis in the transplanted kidney.

REFERENCES

Brownstein MH, Helwig EB: Systemic amyloidosis complicating dermatoses. Arch Dermatol 102:1, 1970

Buja LM et al: Clinically significant cardiac amyloidosis. Am J Cardiol 26:394, 1970

Cohen AS: Amyloidosis. N Engl J Med 277:522, 1967

Gilat T, Spiro HM: Amyloidosis and the gut. Am J Dig Dis 13(n.s.):619, 1968

Glenner GG et al: The immunoglobulin origin of amyloid. Am J Med 52:141, 1972

Levine RA: Amyloid disease of the liver: Correlation of clinical, functional, and morphologic features in forty-seven patients. Am J Med 33:349, 1962

Mandema E et al (eds): *Symposium on Amyloidosis*, Amsterdam: Excerpta Medica, 1968

Wright JR et al: Relationship of amyloid to aging. Medicine (Baltimore) 48:39, 1969

PART SIX | DISORDERS DUE TO CHEMICAL AND PHYSICAL AGENTS

section 1 | Chemical intoxications

108
GENERAL CONSIDERATIONS AND PRINCIPLES OF MANAGEMENT

JAN KOCH-WESER

Poisoning by chemical agents is a common and serious medical problem. In the United States accidental poisonings cause about 5,000 deaths each year. Suicides by chemical agents annually number more than 6,000. Malicious poisoning has become less common since the development of scientific toxicology, but toxic chemicals administered by homicides and abortionists are responsible for more deaths than is generally appreciated. In addition to fatal poisonings there is a much greater number of persons who are made seriously ill by chemical agents but recover after appropriate therapy. Unfortunately, some such victims are left with permanent sequelae of their intoxication. Finally, chemical agents impair the health of very many people by mechanisms not generally thought of as intoxications. Chemical carcinogenesis and mutagenesis, chronic alcoholic liver disease, allergic reactions, and chemical addiction and withdrawal syndromes are the most important examples.

Accidental poisonings may occur in the home or through industrial exposure. The former are far more frequent and usually acute; industrial intoxication is ordinarily the result of chronic exposure. Accidental poisoning is most commonly due to ingestion of toxic substances and involves children in the majority of cases. Each year 1 to 2 million American children accidentally swallow toxic materials, and approximately 1 ingestion in 1,000 is fatal. Aspirin is involved in 25 percent of all ingestions, other medicines in another 25 percent. Cleaning and polishing agents are ingested by 15 percent, while cosmetics, pesticides, petroleum products, and turpentine paints account for 6 percent each. Younger children tend to ingest household products, older children are more likely to choose drugs.

The frequency of accidental poisonings reflects the enormous number of toxic substances found in the American home. Many such accidents could be avoided by simple preventive measures. Physicians can play an effective role in safety education. All toxic substances must be kept out of the reach of small children. Household chemicals and medicines should be kept in the original containers, and all such containers should be labeled. Before taking or administering any medicine one should check the label carefully.

Despite all precautions, accidental, suicidal, and criminal poisonings will remain an important problem which every physician must be prepared to treat promptly and effectively. Besides their immediate therapeutic responsibilities, physicians have legal obligations in cases of attempted suicide, homicide, or criminal abortion and of industrial exposure. The physician should also obtain psychiatric care for any patient who has attempted suicide by poison.

DIAGNOSIS OF CHEMICAL POISONING

Optimal management of the poisoned patient requires a correct diagnosis. Unfortunately, in many such patients poisoning is initially not even considered as a possible cause of the clinical picture. The patient may be unaware of exposure to poison or, as after attempted suicide or abortion, he may be unwilling to admit it. Although the toxic effects of some chemical substances are quite characteristic, most poisoning syndromes can simulate other diseases.

Poisoning is usually included in the differential diagnosis of coma, convulsions, acute psychosis, acute hepatic or renal insufficiency, and bone marrow depression. It may not be considered when the major manifestation is a mild psychiatric disturbance or neurologic disorder, abdominal pain, bleeding, fever, hypotension, pulmonary congestion, or skin eruption. Chronic, insidious intoxications are much more frequently missed than acute poisonings whose symptoms appear suddenly and may be immediately related to a specific event. Physicians should always remember the variegated manifestations of poisoning and maintain a high index of suspicion.

In every case of poisoning, identification of the toxic agent should be attempted. Specific antidotal therapy is obviously impossible without such identification. In cases of homicide, suicide, or criminal abortion the identity of the poison may be of legal importance. When poisoning results from industrial exposure or therapeutic mishap, accurate knowledge of the responsible agents is essential for future prevention.

In acute accidental poisoning the offending substance

may be known to the patient. In many other cases information can be obtained from relatives or acquaintances, by a search for containers at the scene of the poisoning, or by questioning the patient's physician or pharmacist. Frequently such procedures yield only the trade name of a product, which gives no clue to its component chemicals. A number of books which identify the active ingredients of household products, agricultural compounds, proprietary medicines, and poisonous plants are listed in the references to this chapter. A small handbook of this type should be carried in every physician's bag. Poison control centers and manufacturers' representatives are other useful sources of such information. When poisoning is chronic, rapid identification of the toxic agent from the history is frequently impossible. It is therefore fortunate that the lesser therapeutic urgency of such cases usually permits the required painstaking exploration of the patient's habits and environment.

Some poisons can produce clinical features characteristic enough to strongly suggest the diagnosis. Careful examination of the patient may reveal the unmistakable odor of cyanide; the cherry-colored flush of carboxyhemoglobin in skin and mucous membranes; the pupillary constriction, salivation, and gastrointestinal hyperactivity produced by cholinesterase-inhibitor insecticides; or the lead line and extensor paralyses of chronic lead poisoning. Unfortunately, these features are not always present, and in any case telltales are the exception in chemical poisonings.

Chemical analysis of body fluids provides the most definite identification of the intoxicating agent. Some common poisons, such as aspirin, bromides, and barbiturates, can be identified and even quantitated by relatively simple laboratory procedures. Others require more complex toxicologic techniques, such as gas chromatography or bioassay, which are performed only in specialized laboratories. Furthermore, the results of toxicologic determinations are rarely available in time to guide the initial treatment of acute poisoning. Nevertheless, specimens of vomitus, gastric aspirate, blood, urine, and feces should always be saved for toxicologic study if diagnostic or legal questions are likely to arise. Chemical analyses of body fluids or tissues are of particular value in the diagnosis and evaluation of chronic intoxications. Finally, they are useful in following the success of some forms of therapy.

TREATMENT OF CHEMICAL POISONING

Although the physician should always try to identify the poison, such attempts must never delay vital therapeutic measures. Most poisons do not have specific antidotes. Essential supportive care must be given as indicated by the patient's clinical state and does not require knowledge of the toxic agent. Symptomatic treatment of circulatory, respiratory, neurologic, and renal function should be immediately administered as to any other seriously ill patient.

Correct treatment of the poisoned patients thus requires knowledge both of the general principles of management and of the details of therapy for specific poisons. Treatment may be divided into four approaches: (1) prevention of further absorption of the poison, (2) removal of absorbed poison from the body, (3) symptomatic or supportive therapy, and (4) administration of systemic antidotes (Table 108-1). The first three approaches are applicable to most types of poisoning, the fourth can be used only when the toxic agent is known and a specific antidote is available. Success often depends upon speed of treatment and, when indicated by the clinical situation, several approaches should be used simultaneously.

PREVENTION OF ABSORPTION OF INGESTED POISONS If appreciable amounts of a poison have been ingested, one should always attempt to minimize its absorption from the gastrointestinal tract. The success of such endeavors depends upon the time elapsed since ingestion and upon the site and speed of absorption of the poison. Prompt action is essential, and it is better to proceed with makeshifts than to waste time while waiting for special equipment or drugs. Conversely, it is unwise to temporize with unpredictable remedies when reliable and effective methods for removal of poison from the gastrointestinal tract are available. When skillfully applied, these methods do not lead to such complications as pulmonary aspiration, gastrointestinal perforation, or convulsions.

Evacuation of the stomach Attempts to empty the stomach are always worthwhile unless specifically contraindicated. They may be highly successful if made soon

TABLE 108-1
Treatment of acute chemical poisoning

I Prevention of further absorption of poison
- *A* Poisoning by ingestion
  - *1* Emptying the stomach
    - *a* Induction of vomiting
    - *b* Gastric lavage
  - *2* Minimizing gastrointestinal absorption
    - *a* Neutralization and precipitation
    - *b* Adsorption
    - *c* Catharsis
- *B* Poisoning by other routes

II Removal of absorbed poisons from body
- *A* Detoxification—enzyme induction?
- *B* Biliary excretion—interruption of enterohepatic circulation
- *C* Urinary excretion
  - *1* Forced diuresis
  - *2* Alteration of urinary pH
- *D* Dialysis
  - *1* Peritoneal dialysis
  - *2* Hemodialysis
- *E* Charcoal or resin hemoperfusion
- *F* Exchange transfusion
- *G* Chelation and chemical binding

III Supportive therapy

IV Administration of systemic antidotes
- *A* Chemical agents
- *B* Pharmacologic antagonists

after ingestion. Significant amounts of poison may be recovered from the stomach hours after ingestion because gastric emptying may be delayed by gastric atony or pylorospasm.

Emesis occurs spontaneously after the ingestion of many poisons. It may be induced in the home by mechanical stimulation of the posterior pharynx or by administration of gastric irritants such as a strong solution of salt or mustard. The emetic action of syrup of ipecac (not the fourteen times more concentrated fluid extract) in 10- to 20-ml dosage is more effective and is safe enough for home use. Regrettably its action has an average latent period of 20 min and depends in part on gastrointestinal absorption, so that it cannot be used in conjunction with other measures intended to minimize absorption of the poison. Apomorphine, 0.06 mg per kg intramuscularly, acts within 5 min but may cause prolonged vomiting. When given intravenously in doses of 0.01 mg per kg, apomorphine tends to produce almost immediate vomiting which is not followed by any other central nervous system effects. All attempts to induce emesis are more often successful if large amounts of fluid have been administered, but these may also hasten passage of the poison through the pylorus. Fluids with high fat content are preferable, since they enter the duodenum more slowly. Not uncommonly it is impossible to induce vomiting, and valuable time should not be lost with hopeful waiting. Induction of vomiting should not be attempted after ingestion of antiemetic drugs, in severely depressed or convulsing patients, or (because of the danger of gastroesophageal perforation or tracheal aspiration of vomitus) in patients who have ingested strong caustics or liquid hydrocarbons which are potent lung irritants (e.g., kerosene, furniture polish).

In comparison with emesis, *gastric lavage* is more predictably and immediately active but usually no more effective in removing poison from the stomach. It can be employed in unconscious patients, and removal of gastric contents reduces the risk of aspiration of vomitus in such patients. It is, however, contraindicated after the ingestion of strong corrosives because of danger of perforating injured tissues. When properly performed, gastric lavage carries little risk of aspiration of gastric contents into the lungs. The patient should be prone, with head and shoulders lowered. A mouth gag is placed and a gastric tube of sufficient diameter to permit withdrawal of particulate matter (size 30) is passed into the stomach. If central nervous system function is depressed and introduction of the tube produces retching, or if pulmonary irritants have been ingested, it is wise to place a *cuffed endotracheal tube* before lavaging. Gastric contents are withdrawn with a large syringe and usually contain most of the poison that will be removed. Thereafter 200 ml (less in children) of warm water or other lavaging solution is alternately instilled and withdrawn until the aspirate becomes clear.

Interference with gastrointestinal absorption

Since neither emesis nor gastric lavage empties the stomach completely, one should also minimize absorption by administering substances which inactivate or trap ingested poisons. If mineral acids, alkalies, or other corrosives have been swallowed, water, milk, or a neutralizer (aluminum hydroxide, milk of magnesia, dilute vinegar) is given. Some toxic alkaloids can be precipitated and rendered insoluble by the administration of sulfate. Many other poisons are effectively adsorbed by powdered, activated charcoal. A good grade of activated charcoal can rapidly adsorb as much as half its weight of many common poisons. It is more effective than the so-called "universal antidote," which should be relegated to oblivion. Administration of 100 to 200 ml of a slurry of activated charcoal should be alternated with evacuation of the stomach.

Adsorption by charcoal is reversible, and the effectiveness of adsorption of many poisons varies with the pH. Acidic substances are adsorbed better in acid solutions and may therefore be released in the small intestine. It is desirable to speed the charcoal with its adsorbed poison through the intestine as quickly as possible. This will also decrease intestinal absorption of any unadsorbed poison which has passed beyond the pylorus. It is best accomplished by oral or gastric administration of an osmotic cathartic. Sodium sulfate in 10 to 30 g dosage is the cathartic of choice, since, unlike magnesium sulfate, it produces no symptoms after systemic absorption. Cathartics are generally contraindicated after the ingestion of strong corrosives.

PREVENTION OF ABSORPTION OF POISON FROM OTHER SITES Most topically applied poisons can be removed by copious flushing with water. In certain instances weak acids or bases or appropriate organic solvents are more effective, but rapid and voluminous washing with water should always proceed while they are being obtained. Chemical antidotes can be hazardous because tissue injury may result from the heat of the chemical reaction.

The systemic distribution of injected poisons can be slowed by the application of cold to the injection site or by the proximal application of a tourniquet. Cruciate incision and suction is generally ineffective except after poisonous bites.

Following inhalation of toxic gases, vapors, or dusts, the victim should be removed into clean air and adequate ventilation maintained. If the patient cannot be moved, a protective mask should be applied.

REMOVAL OF ABSORBED POISON FROM THE BODY Unlike prevention or retardation of absorption, measures to speed removal of the toxic agent from the body rarely have much influence on the peak poison concentration. However, they can significantly abbreviate the time during which the concentration of many poisons remains above any given level and may thereby reduce morbidity, avoid complications, and save lives. In judging the need for such measures one must consider the patient's clinical state, the properties and metabolic fate of the poison, and the amount absorbed as judged by the history and the blood level. Removal of some poisons can be accelerated by several methods; selection depends on the clinical urgency, the amount in the body, and the skills and equipment available.

Detoxification Since many poisons are metabolically inactivated in the body, it is regrettable that no clinically effective measures to accelerate detoxification are known. Induction of hepatic enzymes would seem to hold some promise in the treatment of poisonings by certain long-acting drugs whose inactivation depends on the activity of inducible enzymes. The clinical usefulness of this approach remains to be shown. At present, therefore, one must rely on measures capable of accelerating excretion of the poison.

Biliary excretion Certain organic acids and active drugs are secreted into the bile against large concentration gradients. Again, this process cannot presently be accelerated. However, the intestinal resorption of substances already secreted into the bile can be decreased by duodenal suction or osmotic catharsis. These procedures may be useful in poisonings by substances such as glutethimide and chlortetracycline, the action of which is significantly prolonged by their enterohepatic circulation.

Urinary excretion Acceleration of renal excretion is applicable to a much larger number of poisons. Renal excretion of toxic substances depends on glomerular filtration, active tubular secretion, and passive tubular resorption. The first two processes should be protected by maintenance of adequate circulation and renal function, but for practical purposes they cannot be accelerated. On the other hand, passive tubular resorption of many poisons plays an important role in the prolongation of their action and can frequently be decreased by readily available methods.

Passive resorption of most filtered poisons occurs largely in the proximal tubules, because their concentration in the filtrate increases as salt and water are reabsorbed. It can be partly prevented by inhibiting water resorption at this site. This is best accomplished by the administration of osmotic diuretics such as mannitol or urea. By infusing 10 to 20 g per hr of mannitol or urea after a loading dose of 25 to 50 g, urine volumes up to 1 liter per hr can be achieved. Intravenous administration of 40 mg furosemide further increases urine flow. Great care must be used to supply water and electrolyte needs at the same time. Osmotic diuretics should not be used in the presence of congestive heart failure, shock, or renal failure. The effectiveness of forced diuresis in increasing renal excretion has been demonstrated for salicylates, barbiturates, meprobamate, and glutethimide but is potentially applicable to all ultrafiltered poisons which are passively reabsorbed.

Alteration of the urinary pH can also inhibit passive back-diffusion of some poisons and increase their renal clearance. The renal tubular epithelium is more permeable to uncharged molecules than to ionized solutes. Weak organic acids and bases readily diffuse out of the tubular fluid in their un-ionized form but are trapped in it when ionized. Acidic poisons are largely ionized only at pHs above their pK_a. Alkalinization of the urine greatly increases the ionization in the tubular fluid of such organic acids as phenobarbital and salicylate. In contrast, the pK_a of pentobarbital (8.1) and secobarbital (8.0) is so high that renal clearance is not greatly increased by raising the urinary pH into the physiologic alkaline range. Alkalinization of the urine is achieved by the infusion of sodium bicarbonate, sodium lactate, or tromethamine (which also acts as an osmotic diuretic) at a rate determined by the urinary and blood pH. Excessive systemic alkalosis or electrolyte disturbances must be carefully prevented. A combination of forced diuresis and alkalinization of the urine can raise the renal clearance of some acidic poisons tenfold or more and has been found highly effective in poisoning by salicylate and phenobarbital. The full range of its clinical applicability is undoubtedly much wider but remains to be established. Depression of the urinary pH beyond its usual range may increase the renal clearance of some weakly basic poisons, but clinical data are lacking.

Finally, the renal excretion of certain poisons can be increased in a highly specific fashion. An example is the removal of bromide by administration of chloride and chloriuretics. Such methods will be discussed with the individual poisons.

Dialysis The relative effectiveness of forced diuresis at favorable urinary pH and of dialysis must differ widely among drugs but has been established for very few. For barbiturates and some other poisons which are not actively secreted by the renal tubules, maximal clearance rates during extracorporeal dialysis are considerably greater than during peritoneal dialysis or forced diuresis. The latter two maneuvers appear about equally effective. Of course, a skilled team can proceed simultaneously with dialysis and solute diuresis. Dialysis has been found effective in the removal of barbiturates, borate, bromide, chlorate, dimercaprol, diphenylhydantoin, ethanol, ethchlorvynol, ethinamate, glutethimide, glycols, isoniazid, methanol, salicylate, sulfonamides, and thiocyanate. Beyond these, it should theoretically accelerate the removal from the body of any dialyzable toxin which is not irreversibly bound to tissues.

Peritoneal dialysis can be easily performed in any hospital and may be continued for long periods. It is particularly valuable for the removal of poisons if renal function is impaired. Obviously, its effectiveness does not extend to large-molecule, nondialyzable poisons and is decreased by a high degree of protein binding or lipid solubility of the toxic substance. Peritoneal clearance can be increased if the dialyzed poison can be trapped chemically in the dialysis fluid so that a high gradient of the dialyzable portion is maintained from blood to peritoneal cavity between fluid changes. A 5% concentration of albumin in the dialysis solution acts as an effective ligand during the dialysis of salicylate and should be similarly useful for the removal of other albumin-bound poisons. Another approach to prevent back-diffusion consists of making the pH of dialysis fluid sufficiently greater or less than 7.4 to ionize poisons which are dialyzable only in the undissociated form. Finally, the addition of various drugs to the dialysis fluid can increase peritoneal dialysis, presumably by increasing peritoneal blood flow or mesothelial permeability. The clinical value of this approach has not yet been defined.

Hemodialysis is unquestionably the most effective procedure for removing large amounts of dialyzable poisons. For barbiturates dialysance rates of 50 to 100 ml per min have been achieved, a removal rate two to ten times faster than during peritoneal dialysis or forced diuresis. Dialysis against solutions containing albumin or lipids can further speed removal of certain poisons. Extracorporeal dialysis is clearly the procedure of choice for the rapid removal of dialyzable poisons from patients who have absorbed amounts which make survival unlikely even under the best supportive care. Since the required equipment and skilled personnel are available only in a few hospitals, the possibility of transfer of such patients to one of these institutions should be considered.

Charcoal or resin hemoperfusion Perfusion of blood through activated charcoal or exchange resin columns achieves higher clearance rates for some poisons than hemodialysis. However, significant reductions in the formed elements of the blood may occur during the use of these techniques.

Exchange transfusion Withdrawal and replacement of blood is an effective procedure for the removal of those poisons which are not highly tissue-bound or lipid-soluble and therefore remain in the blood in appreciable concentration. It has obvious advantages in poisoning by nondiffusible and particularly by highly albumin-bound toxins. Though it requires little specialized equipment, its applicability to adults is limited by the requirement of large amounts of blood.

Chelation and chemical binding The removal of some poisons is accelerated by chemical interaction with other substances followed by renal excretion. These substances are usually considered specific antidotes and will be discussed with the individual poisons.

SUPPORTIVE THERAPY Most chemical poisonings are reversible, self-limited disease states. Skillful supportive therapy can keep many seriously poisoned patients alive and their detoxifying and excretory mechanisms functioning until the concentration of poison in the body has fallen to safe levels. Symptomatic measures are especially important when the poison is one of the many compounds for which no specific antidote is known. Even when an antidote is available, disturbances of vital functions must be prevented or controlled by appropriate supportive care.

The poisoned patient may suffer a variety of physiologic disturbances. Most of these are not peculiar to chemical intoxications, and their therapeutic management is described elsewhere in this text. Only those aspects of supportive therapy specially relevant to poisonings are briefly discussed here.

Central nervous system depression Specific therapy directed against the depressant effects of poisons on the central nervous system is usually both unnecessary and difficult. Most poisoned patients will emerge from coma as from a prolonged anesthesia. During the period of unconsciousness meticulous nursing care and close observation are essential. If depression of medullary centers results in circulatory or respiratory failure, these vital functions must be immediately and vigorously supported by chemical or mechanical means.

The use of analeptics in the treatment of poison-induced central nervous system depression has been largely abandoned, for the following reasons: (1) Their effect is unpredictable and their use in intoxicated patients produces an abnormal pattern of nervous activity in which paroxysmal excitation and convulsions may be superimposed on depression. (2) The availability of artificial ventilation and of effective measures to support the circulation has lessened the need for rapid restoration of normal medullary function. (3) It is doubtful that analeptics shorten the duration of coma sufficiently to justify their risks, and they have not been shown to improve prognosis. Certainly these agents should never be employed to restore consciousness, and it is doubtful whether their use to hasten the restoration of spontaneous breathing and active reflexes is ever justified. Picrotoxin, pentylenetetrazol, bemegride, and ethamivan are available analeptics.

Convulsions Many poisons (e.g., chlorinated hydrocarbons, insecticides, strychnine) cause convulsions by their specific excitatory effects. Poisoned patients may also have convulsions because of hypoxia, hypoglycemia, cerebral edema, or metabolic disturbances. In such cases these abnormalities should be corrected as far as possible. Regardless of the cause of the convulsions, anticonvulsant drugs are often required. Short-acting compounds, such as intravenously administered thiopental, may be preferable, because in poisoned patients profound depression may accompany or quickly follow convulsions. Intravenously administered diazepam has also been effective.

Cerebral edema Intracranial hypertension due to cerebral edema is also a characteristic effect of some poisons and a nonspecific result of other chemical intoxications. Cerebral edema is characteristically seen in poisoning by lead, carbon monoxide, and methanol. Symptomatic treatment consists of use of adrenocortical steroids and, when necessary, the intravenous administration of hypertonic solutions of mannitol or urea.

Hypotension The causes of hypotension and shock in the poisoned patient are legion, and often several of them coexist. Poisons can depress the medullary vasomotor centers, block autonomic ganglions or adrenergic receptors, directly depress the tone of arterial or venous smooth muscle, reduce myocardial contractility, or induce cardiac arrhythmias. Less specifically, the poisoned patient may be in shock because of tissue hypoxia, extensive tissue destruction from corrosives, loss of blood or fluids, or metabolic disturbances. When possible, these abnormalities should be promptly corrected. If the central venous pressure is low, fluid replacement should be the first therapeutic approach. Vasoactive drugs are often helpful and sometimes essential in the hypotensive poisoned patient, particularly in shock resulting from central depression. As in shock from other causes, choice of the most appropriate agent requires an analysis of the hemodynamic disturbance which goes beyond determination of the arterial pressure.

Cardiac arrhythmias Disturbances of cardiac impulse generation or conduction in the poisoned patient arise from the effects of certain poisons on the electrical properties of cardiac fibers or from myocardial hypoxia or metabolic disturbances. The latter should be corrected and antiarrhythmic agents administered as indicated by the nature of the arrhythmia.

Pulmonary edema The poisoned patient may develop pulmonary edema because of depressed myocardial contractility or because of alveolar injury from irritant gases or aspirated fluids. The latter type of edema is less responsive to treatment and may be associated with laryngeal edema. Therapeutic measures include suctioning, administration of high concentrations of oxygen under positive pressure, aerosols of surface-active agents, bronchodilators, and adrenocortical steroids.

Hypoxia Poisoning may cause tissue hypoxia by various mechanisms, and several of these may operate in one patient. Inadequate ventilation can result from central respiratory depression, from muscular paralysis, or from airway obstruction by retained secretions, laryngeal edema, or bronchospasm. Alveolar-capillary diffusion may be impaired by pulmonary edema. Anemia, methemoglobinemia, carboxyhemoglobinemia, or shock can interfere with oxygen transport. Cellular oxidation may be inhibited by cyanide, fluoroacetate, or general protoplasmic poisons. The highest priority in treatment must be given to maintenance of an adequate airway. The clinical situation and the site of obstruction may indicate frequent suctioning, insertion of an oropharyngeal airway or of an endotracheal tube, or a tracheotomy. If despite a clear airway ventilation remains inadequate, as judged by clinical appearance or by measurement of minute volume or blood gases, artificial ventilation by appropriate mechanical means is imperative. Administration of high concentrations of oxygen is indicated whenever tissue hypoxia occurs. When the central nervous system is severely depressed, oxygen administration often results in apnea and must be combined with artifical ventilation. Hyperbaric oxygen may be helpful in some situations. The treatment of methemoglobinemia, carboxyhemoglobinemia, and inhibition of cellular oxidation is discussed under the specific poisons which produce these changes.

Acute renal insufficiency Renal failure with oliguria or anuria may occur in the poisoned patient because of shock, dehydration, or electrolyte disturbances. More specifically, it may be due to the nephrotoxic potential of some poisons (e.g., mercury, phosphorus, carbon tetrachloride, bromate); many of which are concentrated and excreted by the kidney. Renal damage due to poisons is usually reversible. The management of acute renal insufficiency is outlined in Chap. 269.

Electrolyte and water disturbances Imbalances of fluid and electrolytes are common features of chemical poisoning. They may result from vomiting, diarrhea, renal insufficiency, or therapeutic maneuvers such as catharsis, forced diuresis, or dialysis. These disturbances are corrected or, ideally, prevented by appropriate therapy. Certain poisons produce more specific defects, such as metabolic acidosis (e.g., methanol, phenol, salicylate) or hypocalcemia (e.g., fluoride, oxalate). These abnormalities and any specific treatment will be described under the individual poisons.

Acute hepatic insufficiency The primary manifestation of some poisonings (e.g., chlorinated hydrocarbons, phosphorus, cinchophen, certain mushrooms) is acute hepatic failure. Its management is described in Chap. 294.

ADMINISTRATION OF SYSTEMIC ANTIDOTES

Specific antidotal therapy is available for only a few poisons. Some systemic antidotes are chemicals which exert their therapeutic effect by reducing the concentration of the toxic substance. They may do this by combining with the poison (e.g., ethylene diaminetetraacetate with lead, dimercaprol with mercury) or by increasing its excretion (e.g., chloride or mercurial diuretics in bromide poisoning). Other systemic antidotes compete with the poison for its receptor site (e.g., atropine with muscarine, nallorphine and naloxone with morphine, vitamin K_1 with coumarins). Specific antidotes will be discussed with the individual poisons.

REFERENCES

ARENA JM: *Poisoning,* 2d ed., Springfield, Ill.: Charles C Thomas, 1970

COLEMAN AB: Accidental poisoning. N Engl J Med 277:1135, 1967

CORBY DG et al: The efficiency of methods used to evacuate the stomach after acute ingestions. Pediatrics 40:871, 1967

DECKER WJ et al: Inhibition of aspirin absorption by activated charcoal and apomorphine. Clin Pharmacol Ther 10:710, 1969

DEICHMAN WB, GERARDE HW: *Toxicology of Drugs and Chemicals,* New York: Academic, 1964

DONE AK: Pharmacologic principles in the treatment of poisoning. Pharmacol Physicians 3(7):1, 1969

DREISBACH RH: *Handbook of Poisoning: Diagnosis and Treatment,* 7th ed., Los Altos, Calif.: Lange, 1971

GOSSELIN RE, SMITH RP: Trends in the therapy of acute poisonings. Clin Pharmacol Ther 7:279, 1966

HADDEN J et al: Acute barbiturate intoxication. JAMA 209:893, 1969

HENDERSON LW, MERRILL JP: Treatment of barbiturate intoxication. Ann Intern Med 64:876, 1966

IANZITO BM: Attempted suicide by drug ingestion. Dis Nerv Syst 31:453, 1970

KAYE S: *Handbook of Emergency Toxicology,* 3d ed., Springfield, Ill.: Charles C Thomas, 1970

LOCKET S: Haemodialysis in the treatment of acute poisoning. Proc Roy Soc Med 63:427, 1970

MATTHEW H, LAWSON AAH: *Treatment of Common Acute Poisonings,* 2d ed., Baltimore: Williams & Wilkins, 1970

MILNE MD: Potentiation of excretion of drugs. Proc Roy Soc Med 57:809, 1964

POLSON CJ, TATTERSALL RN: *Clinical Toxicology,* 2d ed., Philadelphia: Lippincott, 1969

ROSENBAUM JL et al: Resin hemoperfusion: a new treatment for acute drug intoxication. N Engl J Med 284:874, 1971

SCHREINER GE, TEEHAN BP: Dialysis of poisons and drugs—annual review. Trans Am Soc Artif Intern Organs 17:513, 1971

TEEHAN BP. et al: Acute ethchlorvynol (Placidyl[R]) intoxication. Ann Intern Med 72:875, 1970

THIENES CH, HALEY TJ: *Clinical Toxicology,* 5th ed., Philadelphia: Lea & Febiger, 1972

VERHULST HL, CROTTY JJ: Childhood poisoning accidents. JAMA 203:1049, 1968

Toxic product information

ADAMS WC: Poison control centers: their purpose and operation. Clin Pharmacol Ther, 4:293, 1963

BROWN RL: *Pesticides in Clinical Practice,* Springfield, Ill.: Charles C Thomas, Publisher, 1966

Drug Identification Guide, Oradell, N.J.: Medical Economics, Inc., 1973

GLEASON MN et al: *Clinical Toxicology of Commercial Products,* 3d ed., Baltimore: Williams & Wilkins, 1969

GOODMAN LS, GILMAN A: *The Pharmacological Basis of Therapeutics,* 4th ed., New York: Macmillan, 1970

KINGSBURY JM: *Poisonous Plants of the United States and Canada,* Englewood Cliffs, N.J.: Prentice-Hall, 1964

The Merck Index, 8th ed., Rahway, N.J.: Merck & Co., Inc., 1968

NATIONAL ACADEMY OF SCIENCES: *Toxicants Occurring Naturally in Foods,* publ. 1354, Washington: 1966

SAX NI: *Dangerous Properties of Industrial Materials,* 3d ed., New York: Reinhold, 1968

WILSON CO, JONES TE: *American Drug Index,* Philadelphia: Lippincott, 1973

109 COMMON POISONS

JAN KOCH-WESER

The poisons discussed in this chapter are those encountered by the general population such as commonly used drugs, household products, solvents, pesticides, and poisonous plants. It has been necessary to disregard many uncommon toxic materials as well as products to which exposure occurs only in specialized industrial environments. Details concerning poisoning by such compounds may be found in some of the references following Chap. 108. Toxic effects of many drugs are considered throughout this text in conjunction with their therapeutic use. Manifestations of hypersensitivity to chemicals are described in Chap. 68. The following discussions of specific poisons stress those details of their action which are pertinent to the recognition or treatment of clinical poisoning.

ACIDS Corrosive acids are used widely in industry and laboratories. Ingestion is almost always with suicidal intent. Death has occurred after an oral dose of 1 ml of a corrosive acid.

Toxic effects of corrosive acids are largely due to their direct chemical action. They convert tissue protein to acid proteinate which is soluble in the acid. Irritation, bleeding, sloughing, and perforation of the esophagus and stomach are common. Mouth and pharynx are brownish-black and may have a charred appearance. Yellow staining is seen after ingestion of nitric and picric acids. Severe pain in mouth, pharynx, chest, and abdomen is the rule and is soon followed by vomiting and diarrhea of coffee grounds appearance. Frequently profound shock develops. About half of those who ingest significant amounts of acid die from its immediate effects. The survivors often develop mediastinitis or peritonitis from esophageal or gastric perforation. Delayed perforation of the esophagus or stomach also occurs. Recovery from acid ingestion is often associated with esophageal stricture.

Ingested acid must be immediately diluted a hundredfold by water or milk or neutralized with weak alkali. Milk of magnesia or magnesium and aluminum antacids are excellent for the purpose. Sodium bicarbonate should be avoided because the evolved carbon dioxide may rupture an eroded viscus. The danger of perforation also contraindicates the use of emesis or gastric lavage except during the first 30 min after ingestion. Following the emergency measures, appropriate supportive therapy is administered for the relief of pain and the treatment of shock, perforation, and infection.

Certain gases found in industry may combine with water in the lungs to form corrosive acids. During rapid decomposition of plant material in silos, oxides of nitrogen are released which form nitric acid in the lungs. Inhalation of such gases causes coughing and choking sensations which are followed after a latent period of 6 to 8 hr by pulmonary edema. Treatment is supportive. Symptoms of dyspnea and hemoptysis may be prolonged, and frequent relapses may occur.

ALKALIES Strong alkalies such as ammonium hydroxide, potassium hydroxide (potash), potassium carbonate, sodium hydroxide (lye), and sodium carbonate (washing soda) are widely used in industry and in cleansers and drain cleaners. Sodium and potassium phosphates find use as water softeners. Strong alkalies form soaps with fats and proteinates with proteins, resulting in penetrating necrosis of tissues. Fatalities have occurred from the ingestion of 5 to 30 g of such compounds.

The toxic effects of alkalies are almost entirely due to irritation and destruction of local tissues. Ingestion is followed by severe pain in mouth, pharynx, chest, and abdomen. Vomiting of blood and sloughed mucosa and diarrhea are common. Reflex loss of vascular tone frequently leads to profound shock. Perforation of the esophagus or stomach may be immediate or delayed for several days. Mouth and pharynx show erythema and gelatinous necrotic areas. After ingestion of water softeners profound reduction in serum calcium may be seen and lead to tetany and hypotension. Ingestion of strong alkali is rapidly fatal in about 25 percent of cases. Survivors usually suffer from esophageal strictures.

Treatment consists of immediate administration of large amounts of water, milk, fruit juices, or 10 percent vinegar. The volume of liquids should exceed that of the ingested alkali a hundredfold. Vomiting should be allowed to occur, and gastric lavage may be performed during the first half-hour after ingestion. Because of the danger of perforation, both are contraindicated thereafter. After the ingestion of water softeners (phosphates), calcium gluconate should be administered intravenously as needed. Treatment is otherwise symptomatic and directed at the relief of pain, respiratory obstruction due to edema of the hypopharynx, fluid loss, and shock.

Inhalation of ammonia, which is used as a refrigerant, results in irritation of the upper and lower parts of the respiratory tract. Laryngeal and pulmonary edema may occur and must be treated symptomatically.

ANILINE This substance is used in printing and cloth-marking inks, crayons, paints, and paint removers. Both aniline and its derivatives, such as toluidine, nitroaniline, and nitrobenzene, are widely used in industrial synthesis. Aniline is absorbed from the gastrointestinal tract and through the lungs or skin. Ingestion of 1 g aniline has been fatal. Methemoglobinemia is the most important manifestation. Headache, dizziness, hypotension, convulsions, and coma may occur. If the acute period is survived, jaundice and anemia may appear. Treatment consists of correction of methemoglobinemia (see Chap. 58) and supportive measures.

ANTIHISTAMINES The common and unprescribed use of antihistamines makes them readily available for accidental overdosage and suicidal attempts. There is wide variation from patient to patient in tolerance to these drugs and in the manifestations of poisoning. A dose of 200 mg diphenhydramine has been fatal in one adult, whereas another tolerated 2 g. Manifestations of poisoning are central nervous system excitement or depression. In children the usual toxic manifestations are excitement, hyperthermia, hyperreflexia, tremors, and convulsions, followed by central nervous system depression. In adults depressive manifestations with drowsiness, stupor, and coma predominate, but convulsions followed by further depression may occur.

Treatment is supportive and directed toward removal of the unabsorbed drug and maintenance of vital functions. Stimulants should be avoided. Convulsions may be controlled with short-acting barbiturates, ether, or succinylcholine. Some antihistamines have prominent atropine-like properties. Patients poisoned with these drugs may show manifestations of atropine poisoning and are treated correspondingly.

ANTIMUSCARINIC COMPOUNDS Atropine, related belladonna alkaloids (hyoscyamine, scopolamine), and synthetic substitutes (e.g., benztropine, cyclopentolate, homatropine, methantheline, propantheline) are widely prescribed drugs and occur in many proprietary mixtures used in the treatment of gastrointestinal and upper respiratory diseases, asthma, and parkinsonism. Poisoning, especially in children, may also occur from the excessive use of ophthalmic solutions containing such compounds. Finally, children may be intoxicated by eating plants containing up to 0.5 percent of atropine or related alkaloids. Such plants are *Atropa belladonna* (deadly nightshade), *Hioscyamus niger* (henbane), and *Datura stramonium* (Jamestown or Jimson weed).

Individual sensitivity to the toxic effects of belladonna alkaloids varies widely; fatalities have occurred from as little as 10 mg atropine, but doses of 500 mg have been survived. Young children are particularly susceptible to poisoning with belladonna alkaloids. Old people appear to be more sensitive to the central nervous system effects of these drugs. Since atropine is both hydrolyzed in the liver and excreted unchanged in the urine, insufficiency of hepatic or renal function may lead to poisoning on therapeutic dosage.

The most characteristic manifestations of atropine poisoning are those of parasympathetic blockade: dryness of mucous membranes, thirst, dysphagia, hoarseness, xerophthalmia, dilated pupils, blurring of vision, rise in intraocular tension, flushing, dryness and increased temperature of the skin, fever, tachycardia, hypertension, urinary retention, and abdominal distention. This widespread parasympatholysis is almost diagnostic of belladonna poisoning, but the diagnosis can be further confirmed by the absence of any parasympathomimetic effects following the intramuscular injection of 10 mg methacholine.

Central nervous system symptoms are also very common during belladonna intoxication. Atropine and scopolamine produce similar toxic psychoses. Restlessness, excitation, confusion, and incoordination precede mania, hallucinations, and delirium. Patients intoxicated by scopolamine not infrequently show lethargy and somnolence rather than excitement. In severe intoxication with belladonna alkaloids, central nervous system depression and coma are the rule. When death results it is because of circulatory collapse and respiratory failure.

In the treatment of belladonna poisoning, gastric lavage with an aqueous slurry of activated charcoal should be initiated quickly. Symptomatic treatment is directed at the reduction of body temperature, the moistening of mucous membranes, and, when necessary, urethral catheterization. Excitement, convulsions, or depression may require appropriate pharmacotherapy. Parasympathomimetic agents, such as methacholine or pilocarpine, are of little value, since they cannot be given in concentrations sufficient to overcome the peripheral cholinergic blockade. Furthermore, they have no effect on the potentially lethal central nervous system toxicity of the belladonna alkaloids.

Death occurs in fewer than 1 percent of cases of atropine or scopolamine poisoning. No permanent sequelae have been observed, but manifestations may persist for several days.

BARIUM Poisoning may be due to the ingestion of rodenticides which contain soluble barium salts or of depilatories that contain barium sulfide. Intoxication may also occur in industry or from the accidental use of a soluble barium salt as a radiopaque contrast medium. Barium is extremely toxic, producing intense stimulation of muscles of all types. Its action on the gastrointestinal musculature causes vomiting, colic, and diarrhea. Skeletal muscle tremors and spasm are commonly seen. Arteriolar spasm results in marked hypertension. Cardiac arrhythmias may proceed to ventricular fibrillation. Anxiety, weakness, and convulsions may occur. Death is usually due to cardiac arrhythmia or respiratory arrest.

Treatment consists of the oral administration of 250 ml of 10% sodium sulfate or 5% magnesium sulfate. This will precipitate and remove any unabsorbed barium in the gastrointestinal tract. A dose of 10 ml of a 10% solution of sodium sulfate should be slowly administered intravenously every 30 min until symptoms subside. Procainamide may be used to reduce the danger of fatal cardiac arrhythmias. If necessary, pain should be relieved and artificial ventilation with oxygen administered.

BENZENE, TOLUENE These solvents are used in paint removers, dry-cleaning solutions, and rubber or plastic cements. Benzene is also present, to some extent, in most gasolines. Poisoning may result from ingestion or from the breathing of concentrated vapors. Toluene is the major ingredient in the cement used by teen-age glue sniffers.

Acute poisoning by these compounds causes central nervous system manifestations. With sufficient exposure, symptoms progress from an initial period of restlessness, excitement, euphoria, and dizziness to coma, convulsions, and respiratory failure. Ventricular arrhythmias may occur.

Chronic poisoning by benzene or toluene results from repeated exposure to their vapors in low concentration. Central nervous system symptoms include irritability, insomnia, headache, tremors, and paresthesias. Anorexia and nausea are also common. Fatty degeneration of the heart, liver, and kidneys may occur. By far the most important manifestation of chronic exposure to benzene is bone marrow depression, which may progress to aplastic anemia and complete aplasia of the bone marrow. Individual susceptibility to this effect varies greatly and may not become apparent for months after the initial exposure to the poison.

Treatment of both acute and chronic poisoning is symptomatic. After ingestion emesis must not be induced, and gastric lavage should await placement of an endotracheal tube with an inflatable cuff. Neurologic, pulmonary, or cardiovascular problems are treated as in poisoning by petroleum distillates.

BLEACHES Clorox, Purex, Sanichlor, and other bleaching solutions contain 3 to 6% sodium hypochlorite. Their corrosive action in mouth, pharynx, and esophagus is similar to that of sodium hydroxide. Acid gastric juice releases hypochlorous acid from such solutions. This compound is very irritating to mucous membranes, and inhalation of its fumes causes severe pulmonary irritation and pulmonary edema. However, the systemic toxicity of hypochlorous acid is low. Perforation and stricture formation are rare after the ingestion of bleaching solutions. The fatal dose is approximately 30 ml.

Treatment consists of emesis or gastric lavage with water, milk, milk of magnesia, aluminum hydroxide, or sodium bicarbonate solution. Acid antidotes should not be used. If available, 200 ml of a 5% solution of sodium thiosulfate should be administered by mouth, since this will immediately reduce hypochlorite to nontoxic products. Supportive measures may be needed as in alkali poisoning.

BORIC ACID This compound is a very weak germicide and has been widely employed in powders, lotions, solutions, and ointments. Though not highly toxic, boric acid is not nearly as benign as widely assumed. The lethal dose is approximately 15 g in adults and 5 g in infants. Such amounts can be easily absorbed through abraded skin, from serous cavities, and after ingestion. Furthermore, accumulation of the compound occurs because of slow renal excretion.

Regardless of the route of administration, the first symptoms of poisoning are nausea, vomiting, and diarrhea. This is followed by headache, weakness, restlessness, and an erythematous rash which may progress to desquamation of skin and mucous membranes. Renal toxicity and shock are common, and more than 100 fatalities have occurred. Treatment is entirely supportive. Boric acid should always be labeled as a poison and must not be applied to extensive skin lesions.

BROMATES These compounds are used as neutralizers in cold wave preparations. They produce widespread tissue injury, particularly in central nervous system and kidneys. The fatal oral dose of bromates is approximately 5 g. On contact of bromate with gastric acid, hydrogen bromate, an irritating acid, is formed. Ingestion of bromates is followed by vomiting, diarrhea, abdominal pain, drowsiness, coma, convulsions, hypotension, hematuria, oliguria, anuria, and hemolysis.

Treatment consists of emesis or gastric lavage with sodium bicarbonate solution followed by catharsis. A dose of 250 ml of a 1% sodium thiosulfate solution should be administered intravenously. Peritoneal dialysis or hemodialysis effectively removes bromate from the body. Appropriate supportive therapy should be given.

CANTHARIDIN This active principle of *Cantharis vesicatoria* (Spanish fly) is not a useful therapeutic agent. Poisoning is due to the unfortunate and wishful reputation of cantharidin as an abortifacient or aphrodisiac. The compound is a very potent irritant to all tissues, and ingestion of 10 mg may be fatal. Initial symptoms after ingestion are severe burning pain in the upper part of the gastrointestinal tract, hematemesis, and bloody diarrhea. These are rapidly followed by burning urethral pain, priapism, hematuria, oliguria, anuria, uremia, hepatic failure, myocarditis, shock, delirium, and coma. Death may occur within a few hours or up to 1 week after poisoning. Treatment is entirely symptomatic and supportive.

CARBON MONOXIDE Carbon monoxide is a colorless, odorless, tasteless, and nonirritating gas produced by the incomplete combustion of carbonaceous materials. Almost any flame or combustion device emits carbon monoxide. The gas is present in the exhaust of internal combustion engines in a concentration of 3 to 7 percent. Much higher concentrations are present in most illuminating and heating gases, but not in natural gas. Carbon monoxide is annually responsible for hundreds of accidental and suicidal deaths.

The toxic effects of carbon monoxide are the result of tissue hypoxia. Carbon monoxide combines with hemoglobin to form carboxyhemoglobin. Since carbon monoxide and oxygen react with the same group in the hemoglobin molecule, carboxyhemoglobin is incapable of carrying oxygen. The affinity of hemoglobin for carbon monoxide is two hundred times greater than for oxygen, and at equilibrium 1 part of carbon monoxide in 1,500 parts of air will result in 50 percent conversion of hemoglobin into carboxyhemoglobin. Carboxyhemoglobin also interferes with the release of oxygen from oxyhemoglobin. This further reduces the amount of oxygen available to the tissues and explains why tissue anoxia appears in the carbon monoxide–poisoned person at levels of arterial oxyhemoglobin concentration well tolerated by the anemic patient.

The extent of saturation of hemoglobin with carbon monoxide depends on the concentration of the gas in inspired air and on the time of exposure. The severity of hypoxic symptoms depends further on the state of activity of the individual, his tissue oxygen needs, and his hemoglobin concentration. As a general rule, no symptoms will develop at a concentration of 0.01 percent carbon monoxide in inspired air, since this will not raise blood saturation above 10 percent. Exposure to 0.05 percent for 1 hr during light activity will produce a blood concentration of 20 percent carboxyhemoglobin and result in a mild or throbbing headache. Greater activity or longer exposure to the same concentration causes a blood saturation of 30 to 50 percent. At this point headache, irritability, confusion, dizziness, visual disturbances, nausea, vomiting, and fainting on exertion may be observed. After exposure for 1 hr to concentrations of 0.1 percent in inspired air, the blood will contain 50 to 80 percent carboxyhemoglobin, which results in coma, convulsions, respiratory failure, and death. On inhalation of high concentrations of carbon monoxide, saturation of the blood proceeds so rapidly that unconsciousness may occur suddenly and without warning. When poisoning is more gradual, the individual may notice decreased exercise tolerance and dyspnea on exertion or even at rest. Excessive sweating, fever, hepatomegaly, skin lesions, leukocytosis, bleeding diathesis, albuminuria, and glycosuria have also been described. Cerebral edema and intracranial hypertension may result from the increased permeability of hypoxic capillaries. Myocardial hypoxia is reflected by electrocardiographic abnormalities.

The most characteristic sign of carbon monoxide poisoning is the cherry color of skin and mucous membranes, which is due to the bright red carboxyhemoglobin. If the characteristic flush is not present, 5 ml of 40% sodium hydroxide may be added to 5 ml of a 5% solution of blood in water. An oxyhemoglobin solution will turn brown, but a carboxyhemoglobin solution remains red.

Treatment of carbon monoxide poisoning requires effective ventilation in the presence of high oxygen tensions and in the absence of carbon monoxide. If necessary, ventilation should be supported artificially. Pure oxygen should be administered. This will result not only in the replacement of carbon monoxide by oxygen in the hemoglobin molecule but also in the partial relief of tissue hypoxia by oxygen dissolved in the plasma. For the same reasons hyperbaric oxygen is helpful in seriously poisoned patients. Transfusion of blood or packed cells is also of value. In order to reduce tissue needs for oxygen the patient must be kept absolutely quiet. The induction of hypothermia may further reduce oxygen requirements.

During the recovery from carbon monoxide poisoning symptoms regress gradually. If severe tissue hypoxia has obtained too long, neurologic symptoms such as tremors, mental deterioration, and psychotic behavior may persist. Histologic changes characteristic of hypoxia may be observed in cerebral cortex, medulla, myocardium, and other organs.

CASTOR BEANS The castor bean plant (*Ricinus communis*) is grown for commercial and ornamental purposes. The beans contain ricin, an extremely toxic albumin, which causes agglutination and hemolysis of red blood cells and injury to all other cells. After a delay of several hours to 2 days following ingestion, abdominal pain, vomiting, and profuse diarrhea appear and produce severe dehydration. Extreme weakness, drowsiness, disorientation, stupor, coma, convulsions, respiratory depression, and circulatory collapse may develop. Intravascular clotting and hemolysis have been observed. If the patient survives the acute symptoms, oliguria may progress to anuria and uremia, with death after several days. Treatment consists of fluid replacement, alkalinization of the urine with sodium bicarbonate to prevent precipitation of hemoglobin in the kidneys, and supportive measures.

CATHARTIC RESINS Colocynth, croton oil, gamboge, and podophyllum are drastic cathartics because of their content of highly irritating plant resins. These compounds have no therapeutic use; poisoning is usually the work of ignorant pranksters. Oral administration of 1 g of these substances has been fatal. Symptoms are burning pain in mouth, esophagus, and stomach, hematemesis, watery or bloody diarrhea, dehydration, shock, coma, and death. Treatment consists of removal of the irritant from the gastrointestinal tract and supportive measures. Large amounts of parenteral fluids, blood replacement, and morphine and atropine to quiet the intestinal tract may be required.

CHLORATES Sodium and potassium chlorates are strong oxidizing agents and are found in gargles, mouthwashes, matches, and weed killers. After oral ingestion, 2 g has been fatal for children and 10 g for adults. Chlorate ion acts as a catalyst in the production of methemoglobinemia, and absorption of a small amount can result in a high methemoglobin concentration. The symptoms of chlorate ingestion are those of local mucosal irritation and of methemoglobinemia (see Chap. 58). Renal toxicity is common. Treatment is directed at the methemoglobinemia and is otherwise supportive.

CHLORINATED INSECTICIDES These compounds are common ingredients of dusts, sprays, and solutions used as insecticides. The great majority of these compounds are chlorinated diphenyls (e.g., DDT, TDE, DFDT, DMC, Neotran) or chlorinated polycyclic compounds (e.g., Aldrin, Chlordane, Dieldrin, Endrin, Heptachlor). Lindane is a hexachlorobenzene. The toxic effects of all these agents are similar. The chlorinated insecticides are soluble in lipid and organic solvents but not in water. They are poorly absorbed unless dissolved in a vehicle such as kerosene, petroleum distillates, or other organic solvents. Under these circumstances they readily enter the body through the skin, lungs, or gastrointestinal tract. These compounds vary considerably in toxicity, and the toxicity of the dissolving vehicle must also be considered. The effects of the solvent may overshadow or modify those of the insecticide.

The initial symptoms of acute poisoning are nausea, vomiting, headache, dizziness, apprehension, excitement, and muscular tremors and weakness. These symptoms progress to generalized central nervous system hyperexcitability with delirium and clonic or tonic convulsions. This stage is in turn followed by progressive depression with paralysis, coma, and death. In chronically poisoned patients cerebellar symptoms and evidence of liver damage may develop. Hepatic toxicity is particularly prominent in poisoning by a hexachlorobenzene. Treatment consists of gastric lavage and catharsis, anticonvulsive therapy with short-acting barbiturates, artificial ventilation, and other supportive measures. Sympathomimetic compounds should be avoided, since chlorinated insecticides apparently increase susceptibility to ventricular fibrillation.

CHOLINESTERASE INHIBITOR INSECTICIDES

Many substances used in agriculture for control of soft-bodied insects are potent inhibitors of cholinesterase. Most of these compounds are organic phosphates (e.g., Parathion, Malathion, Systox, TEPP, HETP, OMPA), others are carbamates (e.g., Dimetan, Matacil). The toxicity of these compounds varies widely. They are usually prepared for use by dilution with powders, organic solvents, or water. Formulations containing 1 to 95 percent of the active ingredient are available. The cholinesterase inhibitor insecticides are rapidly absorbed through the intact skin and after inhalation or ingestion.

The organic phosphate esters act by combining with and inactivating acetylcholinesterase. Since this enzyme normally breaks down the acetylcholine liberated by the central nervous system, autonomic ganglions, parasympathetic nerve endings, and motor nerve endings, its inactivation allows the accumulation of large amounts of acetylcholine at these sites. In the central nervous system initial stimulation is followed by depression of cells, resulting in convulsions followed by coma and respiratory depression. Initial stimulation and later blockade of autonomic ganglions results in multiple and variable dysfunctions of structures innervated by the autonomic nervous system. Accumulation of acetylcholine at parasympathetic nerve endings produces pupillary constriction and blurring of vision; stimulation of intestinal muscle resulting in abdominal cramps, vomiting, and diarrhea; stimulation of secretory glands causing rhinorrhea, salivation, sweating, and bronchorrhea; constriction of the bronchial musculature with symptoms of respiratory distress; depression of the cardiac sinus pacemaker activity; and impairment of atrioventricular conduction. Persistence of acetylcholine at the neuromuscular junction results in muscular tremors, cramps, and fasciculations which are followed by neuromuscular block and flaccid paralysis. Other important clinical manifestations of these poisons are cyanosis and pulmonary edema.

Management consists of emesis or lavage, catharsis, and washing of contaminated skin with soap and water. Atropine should be given immediately to block the parasympathetic and central nervous system effects. A dose of 2 mg is injected intramuscularly and repeated every 10 min until parasympathetic manifestations are controlled and signs of atropinization appear. The same dosage must be repeated frequently to maintain xerostomia and mild tachycardia. Fatal respiratory failure or pulmonary edema may occur quickly upon cessation of atropine therapy. Atropine is virtually ineffective against the autonomic ganglionic actions of acetycholine and against the peripheral neuromuscular paralysis. Certain oximes act as cholinesterase reactivators. Pralidoxime is useful in the treatment of organic phosphate cholinesterase inhibition but should not be used if the inhibition is due to a carbamate. A dose of 1 g pralidoxime in aqueous solution is administered intravenously over a 5-min period and may be repeated twice each day. Supportive therapy includes administration of oxygen with artificial ventilation if necessary, removal of pulmonary secretions by suction, and treatment of convulsions with short-acting barbiturates. Energetic therapy with artificial ventilation, atropine, and pralidoxime allows survival after doses of organic phosphate esters vastly exceeding the usual fatal dose.

CYANIDE The cyanide ion is an exceedingly potent and rapid-acting poison, but one for which specific and effective antidotal therapy is available. Cyanide poisoning may result from the inhalation of hydrocyanic acid or from the ingestion of soluble inorganic cyanide salts or cyanide-releasing substances such as cyanamide, cyanogen chloride, and nitroprusside. Parts of many plants also contain substances such as amygdalin which release cyanide on digestion. Among these are the seeds of certain stone fruits (choke cherry, pin cherry, wild black cherry, peach, apricot, bitter almond), cassava roots, the berries of the jet berry bush, the leaves and shoots of elderberry, and all parts of hydrangea. Cyanides are widely used in industry and for fumigation and may reach the home in photographic chemicals or silver polishes. As little as 300 mg potassium cyanide may cause death.

The extreme toxicity of cyanide is due to its ready reaction with the trivalent iron of cytochrome oxidase. The role of the enzyme in cellular oxygen utilization is inhibited by the formation of the cytochrome oxidase–cyanide complex. The resultant cytotoxic hypoxia leads to cellular dysfunction and death.

Inhalation of hydrogen cyanide may cause death within a minute. Oral doses act more slowly, requiring several minutes for the appearance of symptoms and up to several hours for death. The first effect is an increase in ventilation because of the blockade of oxidative metabolism in the chemoreceptor cells. As more cyanide is absorbed, there are headache, dizziness, nausea, drowsiness, hypotension, profound dyspnea, characteristic electrocardiographic changes, coma, and convulsions. Death always occurs within 4 hr.

Cyanide poisoning is a true medical emergency. Treatment is highly effective if given rapidly. The chemical antidotes should be immediately available wherever emergency medical care is dispensed. The diagnosis may be made by the characteristic "bitter almond" odor on the breath of the victim, and physicians should familiarize themselves with this smell. Since the saturation of hemoglobin is not disturbed by cyanide, cyanosis is not seen until respiratory depression supervenes. The objective of treatment is the production of methemoglobin by the administration of nitrite. The trivalent iron of methemoglobin competes with cytochrome oxidase for the cyanide ion. The cytochrome oxidase–cyanide complex dissociates, and enzymatic function and cell respiration are restored. Further detoxification is then achieved by the administration of thiosulfate. Under the influence of the tissue enzyme rhodanese, thiosulfate reacts with cyanide liberated by the dissociation of cyanmethemoglobin to form thiocyanate. This substance is relatively nontoxic and readily excreted in the urine.

Since speed is of the essence, nitrite should be immediately administered by inhalation of amyl nitrite perles, one every 2 min unless blood pressure is below 80 mm. This is followed as soon as possible by the intravenous injection of 10 ml of 3% sodium nitrite over a 3-min period. An intravenous infusion of norepinephrine may be necessary to maintain blood pressure during this injection period. After the administration of sodium nitrite, 50 ml of 25% sodium thiosulfate should be administered intravenously over a 10-min period. Supportive measures, especially artifical respiration with 100% oxygen, should be instituted as soon as possible, but, unless methemoglobinemia is produced promptly, other forms of treatment are of no value. Administration of sodium nitrite and sodium thiosulfate may have to be repeated. If the patient survives 4 hr, recovery is likely but residual cerebral symptoms may persist.

DETERGENTS AND SOAPS These substances fall into the three groups of anionic, nonionic, and cationic detergents. The first group contains common soaps and household detergents. They may cause vomiting and diarrhea but have no serious effects, and no treatment is required. However, some laundry compounds contain phosphate water softeners whose ingestion may cause hypocalcemia. The ingestion of nonionic detergents is harmless and requires no treatment.

Cationic detergents, such as benzalkonium chloride (Zephiran) and many others, are commonly used for bactericidal purposes in hospitals and homes. These compounds are well absorbed from the gastrointestinal tract and interfere with cellular functions. The fatal oral dose is approximately 3 g. Ingestion produces nausea and vomiting, and shock, coma, convulsions, and death may occur in a few hours. Treatment consists of minimizing gastrointestinal absorption by emesis or gastric lavage with ordinary soap solution, which rapidly inactivates cationic detergents. If significant absorption has occurred, intensive supportive therapy may be required.

ERGOT This fungus *(Claviceps purpurea)* grows on rye and contains a number of highly toxic alkaloids (e.g., ergotamine, ergonovine) which are used in the treatment of migraine or as uterine stimulants. Poisoning may be due to therapeutic overdosage, particularly in patients with severe infections or liver disease, but more commonly results from the use of ergot as an abortifacient. The epidemic form of chronic ergot poisoning due to the ingestion of contaminated grain is now rarely seen. Ingestion of 1 g ergot has been fatal; ergotamine has caused gangrene in doses of 10 mg per day. Symptoms of acute or chronic ergot poisoning are vomiting, diarrhea, burning abdominal pain, severe muscle pains, ischemic peripheral gangrene, headache, psychotic behavior, muscle tremors, convulsions, and coma. Circulatory disturbances are due both to prolonged vasoconstriction and to intimal hyperplasia and thrombosis. Treatment of ergot poisoning is symptomatic. Vigorous vasodilator and analgesic therapy should be employed.

FLUORIDES Fluoride salts are widely used in insecticides. The gases fluorine and hydrogen fluoride are used in industry. The latter is a strong corrosive. Fluorine and fluorides are cellular poisons which block the glycolytic degradation of glucose. Fluorides also form an insoluble precipitate with calcium and cause hypocalcemia. Finally, in an acid medium fluorides form the corrosive hydrofluoric acid. Ingestion of 1 to 2 g sodium fluoride may be fatal.

Inhalation of fluorine or hydrogen fluoride produces coughing and choking. After an asymptomatic period of a day or two, fever, cough, cyanosis, and pulmonary edema may develop. Ingestion of fluoride salts is followed by nausea, vomiting productive of corroded tissues, diarrhea, and abdominal pain. Consequent to the decrease in serum calcium the victim develops muscular hyperirritability, fasciculations, tremors, spasms, and convulsions. Death is due to respiratory paralysis or circulatory collapse. If the patient survives the acute period, jaundice and oliguria may appear. Chronic fluoride poisoning (fluorosis) is characterized by weight loss, weakness, anemia, brittle bones, and stiff joints. Mottling of teeth is seen when exposure occurs during enamel formation.

Acute fluoride poisoning is treated by immediate administration of milk, lime water, calcium gluconate, or calcium lactate solution. Following lavage or emesis 10 g calcium gluconate and 30 g sodium sulfate should be administered to precipitate and remove fluoride from the intestine. Then 10% calcium gluconate or 1% calcium chloride should be slowly injected intravenously and repeated as needed to prevent a positive Chvostek's sign. Symptomatic and supportive therapy is administered as indicated.

FORMALDEHYDE This gas is available as a 40% solution (Formalin) which is used as a disinfectant, fumigant, or deodorant. Poisoning by Formalin may be diagnosed by the characteristic odor of formaldehyde. Formaldehyde reacts chemically with cellular constituents, depresses cellular functions, and causes cell death. The fatal dose of Formalin is about 60 ml.

Ingestion of Formalin immediately causes severe abdominal pain, nausea, vomiting, and diarrhea. This may be followed by collapse, coma, severe metabolic acidosis, and anuria. Death is usually due to circulatory failure.

Treatment consists of immediate administration of activated charcoal followed by emesis and gastric lavage with a solution containing 1% ammonium carbonate and 2% sodium bicarbonate. Parenteral administration of sodium bicarbonate is indicated to combat acidosis. The treatment is otherwise supportive.

GLYCOLS Ethylene glycol and diethylene glycol are commonly used in antifreeze solutions. The more than 50 annual deaths from these compounds usually result from intentional drinking of antifreeze by alcoholics. The fatal dose of ethylene glycol is about 100 g, that of diethylene glycol somewhat lower. Both compounds are metabolized to oxalate in the body.

The initial symptoms of acute poisoning by these glycols resemble those of alcoholic intoxication. They may progress to vomiting, stupor, coma with absent reflexes and anisocoria, and convulsions. Tachypnea, bradycardia, and hypothermia are commonly seen. After massive ingestion death may occur from respiratory failure within a few hours or from pulmonary edema within a day or two. If the patient survives the acute stage, hepatic and renal necroses manifest themselves with jaundice, anuria, and uremia.

Treatment is largely supportive. The administration of ethyl alcohol and of intravenous calcium gluconate may be helpful by slowing the oxidation to oxalic acid and by precipitating the acid. However, the effectiveness of these procedures has not been definitely established. Dialysis is highly successful in the removal of ethylene and diethylene glycol from the body.

HALOGENATED HYDROCARBONS Halogenated hydrocarbons (carbon tetrachloride, ethylene chlorohydrin, ethylene dichloride, methyl halides, tetrachloroethane, trichloroethylene) find wide industrial use as solvents, refrigerants, fumigants, and in chemical synthesis. They enter the home in household cleaners, floor waxes, fire extinguishers, and rubber or plastic cements. These compounds are highly fat-soluble and produce cell damage either directly or after conversion in the body to other compounds. Individual halogenated hydrocarbons differ considerably in the degree and the exact manifestations of their toxicity, but in sufficient concentration all these compounds are capable of inducing central nervous system depression and varying amounts of hepatic and renal toxicity. Myocardial depression, vascular damage, and pulmonary edema may also occur.

The most important halogenated hydrocarbon is carbon tetrachloride, widely employed as a nonflammable solvent and fire extinguisher fluid. Poisoning may occur from inhalation of the vapor, ingestion, or, rarely, percutaneous absorption. An oral dose of as little as 4 ml may be fatal. Absorption from the gastrointestinal tract is slow and unpredictable but is increased by the presence of fats and alcohol. Abdominal pain, hematemesis, and hepatic damage are more common and severe after ingestion than when the poison is inhaled. Inhalation may lead to irritation of the upper part of the respiratory tract.

Acute systemic absorption of carbon tetrachloride results in nausea, dizziness, confusion, and headache within a few minutes. Depending upon the quantity absorbed, the symptoms may quickly progress to stupor, coma, convulsions, respiratory failure, hypotension, or ventricular fibrillation. The patient may recover from these immediate manifestations until evidence of hepatic or renal toxicity appears several hours to several days after the exposure. Liver and kidney damage may also occur in the absence of any severe early central nervous system effects. Initially tender hepatomegaly may be present, jaundice may be rapidly progressive, and death due to severe centrilobular necrosis may occur within days. The renal lesion has the characteristics of acute tubular necrosis and manifests itself by proteinuria, hematuria, oliguria, or anuria. Uremia, acidosis, hypertension, and pulmonary edema may develop as complications of renal failure. Optic neuritis, pancreatitis, and adrenal cortical necrosis are less common manifestations of carbon tetrachloride intoxication.

Chronic poisoning may occur after repeated exposures to low concentrations of carbon tetrachloride and may also lead to liver or kidney damage. More usually it manifests itself by vague symptoms of fatigue, weakness, mental confusion, abdominal pain, anorexia, nausea, blurring of vision, and paresthesias.

Treatment of acute poisoning by halogenated hydrocarbons includes vigorous effects at minimizing gastrointestinal absorption by lavage or emesis and catharsis. Treatment is otherwise symptomatic. Sympathomimetic drugs should be avoided because of the danger of inducing ventricular arrhythmias in the sensitized myocardium. Acute renal and hepatic failure must be carefully managed. Hemodialysis is often required and may be lifesaving until kidney function returns three or more weeks after poisoning.

IODINE The traditional antiseptic iodine tincture is an alcoholic solution of 2% iodine and 2% sodium iodide. Strong iodine solution (Lugol's solution) is an aqueous solution of 5% iodine and 10% potassium iodide. Tincture of iodine is often taken for suicidal purposes. The fatal dose of iodine is approximately 2 g. Iodides are very much less toxic, and no fatalities have been reported.

The diagnosis of iodine poisoning is suggested by the brown staining of the oral mucous membranes. The effects are largely due to the corrosive effects of the compound on the gastrointestinal tract. Burning abdominal pain, nausea, vomiting, and bloody diarrhea may occur soon after ingestion. If the stomach contained starch, the vomitus is blue or black. Tissue trauma from corrosive gastroenteritis and fluid loss by vomiting and diarrhea may result in shock. Severe edema of the glottis, fever, delirium, stupor, and anuria have also been observed.

Treatment consists of gastric lavage with a starch solution made by adding 15 g flour or cornstarch to 500 ml water. Thereafter, catharsis should be induced, and milk should be given orally to relieve gastric irritation. Sodium thiosulfate will reduce iodine to less toxic iodide; 100 ml of a 5% solution should be given orally and 10 ml of a 10% solution intravenously every 4 hr. With appropriate treatment most patients poisoned by iodine survive, but esophageal strictures may complicate their recovery.

IPECAC, EMETINE Emetine is the major alkaloid of ipecac (dried roots or rhizomes of *Cephaelis ipecacuanha*) and is used for the treatment of amebiasis. Syrup of ipecac is used as an emetic or expectorant. Poisoning may be accidental or suicidal but most commonly results from overdosage during therapy, at times because of the erroneous substitution of the much more potent fluid extract of ipecac for syrup of ipecac. Emetine and other alkaloids of ipecac have serious toxic gastrointestinal, central nervous, and myocardial effects. The fatal oral dose of emetine is about 1 g.

Manifestations of poisoning begin with nausea, vomiting, diarrhea, and abdominal pain. Cardiac effects are heralded by electrocardiographic changes, and the depression of myocardial contractility leads to dyspnea, tachycardia, shock, and congestive heart failure. Coma and convulsions may occur, but death is usually due to heart failure. Treatment is symptomatic. Administration of digitalis may be of value.

IRON SALTS Ferrous or ferric salts produce gastrointestinal corrosive damage. Following mucosal damage, large amounts of iron may be absorbed, particularly in children. The fatal oral dose in children is 5 to 10 g.

Very soon after ingestion nausea, vomiting, diarrhea, and abdominal pain appear. Systemic effects include acidosis, shock, drowsiness, coma, and respiratory failure. These initial symptoms may partially clear but then recur with increased severity. In the later stages signs of hepatic and renal toxicity may appear.

The absorption of ingested iron should be minimized by the usual measures. Gastric lavage with a 10% sodium bicarbonate solution will precipitate the ferrous ion. Edetate calcium disodium 30 mg per kg daily in divided doses should be administered intravenously or orally. Deferoxamine methane sulfonate (Desferal) is even more effective as an iron-chelating agent than edetate. Use of chelating agents is guided by determinations of serum iron and iron-binding capacity. Peritoneal dialysis and hemodialysis effectively remove iron from the body. Acidosis, shock, and renal or hepatic toxicity must be treated supportively.

ISOPROPYL ALCOHOL This compound is used as a sterilizing agent or as rubbing alcohol. Ingestion produces gastric irritation and raises the danger of vomiting with aspiration. The systemic effects of isopropyl alcohol are similar to those of ethyl alcohol, but it is approximately twice as potent as the latter. Coma is readily produced but rarely lasts longer than 12 hr. Isopropyl alcohol is oxidized to acetone in the body, and transient acetonuria is common, but significant acidosis does not occur. Gastric lavage should always be performed to minimize the danger of aspiration following vomiting in the unconscious patient. Supportive therapy is required only after ingestion of massive amounts, and there are no sequelae other than transient gastritis.

MAGNESIUM Magnesium sulfate is used intravenously as a hypotensive agent and orally as a cathartic. The magnesium ion is a profound depressant of the central nervous system and of neuromuscular transmission. Poisoning after oral or rectal administration is unlikely in the presence of normal renal function, because the kidney removes magnesium more rapidly than it is absorbed by the gastrointestinal tract. In the presence of impaired renal function an oral dose of 30 g may be fatal. Symptoms begin at a serum magnesium level of 4 mEq per liter, and concentrations of over 12 mEq per liter may be fatal. Oral ingestion of concentrated solutions may cause gastrointestinal irritation. Manifestations of systemic poisoning are depression of reflexes, flaccid paralysis, hypotension, hypothermia, coma. and respiratory failure. Respiratory death usually precedes significant myocardial depression. The actions of magnesium on neurologic and neuromuscular function are antagonized by calcium. Treatment of magnesium poisoning therefore includes the intravenous administration of 10 ml of a 10% solution of calcium gluconate, which may be repeated as necessary.

METHYL ALCOHOL This simplest of the alcohols, also called wood alcohol or methanol, is used as a solvent, antifreeze, paint remover, and as a denaturant in ethyl alcohol. Denatured ethyl alcohol preparations, such as Sterno or Solox, contain 5 to 15 percent methyl alcohol as well as other denaturants. Methyl alcohol poisoning is due almost entirely to its ingestion as a substitute for ethanol or to the drinking of denatured ethyl alcohol. The toxic dose is very variable: death has occurred after a dose of 20 ml, but 250 ml has been ingested with survival. As little as 15 ml methanol has caused permanent blindness.

Methanol is less inebriating than ethyl alcohol, and inebriation is not a prominent symptom of methyl alcohol intoxication. Methanol is oxidized in the body to formaldehyde and to formic acid. The rate of its metabolism is independent of the concentration in the body and is only 15 percent that of ethanol. The enzyme alcohol dehydrogenase appears to be responsible for the first step in oxidation. The enzyme system will preferentially utilize ethyl alcohol if this compound is also available. Thus ethyl alcohol may depress the rate of metabolism of methanol. The manifestations of methanol poisoning are largely due to the accumulation of its toxic metabolites. These products, especially formaldehyde, have toxic actions on many cells, and the retina and optic nerve are specifically damaged. The toxic metabolites of methyl alcohol are also responsible for the severe acidosis, which is the most prominent feature of methyl alcohol poisoning. This acidosis is partly due to the accumulation of formic acid, but formate also appears to exert an inhibitory effect upon enzymes involved in the oxidation of carbohydrate with consequent accumulation of acid intermediates.

Symptoms of methanol poisoning usually do not appear until 12 to 24 hr after ingestion, when sufficient toxic metabolites have accumulated. Manifestations consist of headache, dizziness, nausea, vomiting, severe abdominal and back pain probably due to pancreatitis, vasomotor disturbances, central nervous system depression, and respiratory failure. Visual disturbance is almost universal and ranges from mild blurring of vision to total blindness. Impairment of vision may be transient, but permanent blindness may follow survival of the acute intoxication. The pupils are dilated and nonreactive, and there is hyperemia of the optic disk and retinal edema. Severe abdominal tenderness and spasm or nuchal rigidity may be present. Acidosis is commonly severe, but Kussmaul's respiration is absent in many severely acidotic patients (plasma carbon dioxide–combining power below 20 mEq per liter).

In the treatment of methyl alcohol intoxication gastric lavage is of use only during the first hour or two. The mainstay of treatment is intravenous administration of large amounts of sodium bicarbonate. Return of acidosis is frequent after initial correction, and additional alkali must be administered as indicated by close observation of the patient and laboratory determinations. Peritoneal dialysis and hemodialysis effectively remove methanol from the body and are useful in view of its slow oxidation. The administration of 0.5 ml per kg ethyl alcohol every 2 hr may inhibit the metabolism of methyl alcohol and is useful in conjunction with dialysis. Supportive therapy must be administered as required by the patient's clinical state.

MUSHROOMS There are many species of poisonous mushrooms, but in the United States most poisoning is due to *Amanita muscaria* (fly agaric) or *Amanita phalloides* (destroying angel). More than 100 deaths result each year from consumption of wild poisonous mushrooms, 90 percent are due to A. *phalloides.* Fatalities have occurred after ingestion of only part of one mushroom.

Amanita muscaria contains the parasympathomimetic alkaloid muscarine, as well as variable amounts of a substance active on the central nervous system and a parasympatholytic alkaloid. Symptoms are largely those of parasympathetic stimulation: lacrimation, pupillary constriction, perspiration, salivation, nausea, vomiting, diarrhea, abdominal pain, bronchorrhea, wheezing, dyspnea, bradycardia, and hypotension. Muscular tremors, confusion, excitement, and delirium are common in severe poisoning. Very rarely symptoms of atropine poisoning have predominated. After ingestion of *A. muscaria* symptoms appear within minutes to 2 hr. The patient may die within a few hours, but with appropriate therapy complete recovery in 24 hr is the rule.

Amanita phalloides, some other *Amanita* species, and *Galerina venenata* contain heat-stable polypeptide cytotoxins which are rapidly bound to tissues. Severe cell damage and fatty degeneration may occur in liver, kidneys, striated muscle, and brain. Ingestion of these dangerous mushrooms is followed by a latent period of 6 to 20 hr. Manifestations of cytotoxicity may then appear suddenly and consist of severe nausea, violent abdominal pain, bloody vomiting and diarrhea, and cardiovascular collapse. Headache, mental confusion, coma, or convulsions are common. Painful and tender hepatomegaly, jaundice, hypoglycemia, dehydration, and oliguria or anuria frequently appear on the first or second day after ingestion. The victim may die from acute yellow atrophy within 4 days. About one-half of all poisonings with *A. phalloides* have a fatal outcome in 5 to 8 days. Recovery tends to be slow.

Ingestion of other poisonous mushrooms may cause gastrointestinal symptoms, visual disturbances, ataxia, disorientation, convulsions, coma, fever, hemolysis, and methemoglobinemia.

Treatment of mushroom poisoning depends upon the species ingested. If parasympathomimetic manifestations are prominent, atropine in doses of 1 to 2 mg is given intramuscularly and repeated every 30 min until symptoms are controlled. Poisoning by cytotoxic mushrooms can only be treated symptomatically. Fluid and electrolyte balance must be carefully maintained. Hypoglycemia should be avoided; large quantities of carbohydrate may exert some protective effect on the liver. Excitement, convulsions, pain, hypotension, and fever may need symptomatic therapy. Hemodialysis is of no value in removing the toxin but may be required to maintain renal function until recovery occurs.

NAPHTHALENE Poisoning by this substance is almost always due to ingestion of moth repellents. An oral dose of 2 g has been fatal. Nausea, vomiting, and diarrhea are the initial symptoms. Larger doses may produce hepatic damage with jaundice and renal toxicity which may progress to hematuria, oliguria, or anuria. Depending upon the amount ingested, central nervous system manifestations may range from headache, mental confusion, and excitement to coma and convulsions. In persons with glucose 6-phosphate dehydrogenase–deficient red blood cells the ingestion of naphthalene will produce hemolysis. Treatment consists of emesis or gastric lavage and catharsis and supportive measures.

NICOTINE This alkaloid is an exceedingly potent and rapidly acting poison. It is a component of many insecticides. Nicotine is readily absorbed from the oral and gastrointestinal mucosa, from the respiratory tract, and through the skin. The lethal dose for an adult is approximately 50 mg, the quantity contained in two cigarettes. However, tobacco is much less toxic than would be anticipated on the basis of its nicotine content. Nicotine is poorly absorbed from ingested tobacco, and on smoking, most of the nicotine is burned. Nicotine acts on chemoreceptors, on synapses in the central nervous system and in autonomic ganglions, on the adrenal medulla, and on neuroeffector junctions. Furthermore, its initial stimulant effects are followed by a depressant phase of action. It is not surprising that the manifestations of nicotine poisoning are highly complex and somewhat unpredictable.

Small doses of nicotine produce nausea, vomiting, diarrhea, headache, dizziness, and neurologic stimulation manifested by tachycardia, hypertension, hyperpnea, tachypnea, sweating, and salivation. Larger doses also cause cortical irritability, progressing to convulsions, and myocardial arrhythmias. Finally coma, respiratory depression and arrest, and cardiac arrest or fibrillation may supervene. Severe poisoning may cause death within a few minutes.

Treatment consists of gastric lavage with activated charcoal or with a 1:10,000 solution of potassium permanganate, which oxidizes nicotine. Atropine, 2 mg, and phentolamine, 5 mg, may be given intramuscularly or intravenously and repeated as often as required to control signs and symptoms of parasympathetic or sympathetic hyperactivity. These compounds are ineffective in preventing paralysis of the respiratory muscles and disturbances in cardiac rhythm. Careful attention must be given to artificial ventilation with oxygen and to therapy of catecholamine-induced cardiac tachyarrhythmias. Propranolol is the drug of choice for the latter purpose. Nicotine is rapidly detoxified in the liver, and recovery will be prompt if the patient can be tided over the initial period.

NITRITES Poisoning by the nitrite ion may result from the ingestion of large amounts of drugs such as amyl nitrite or sodium nitrite. Nitrites are also used to preserve the color of meat, and amounts in excess of the allowable residue of 0.01 percent may appear in food. Ingested nitrates may be reduced to nitrite by intestinal bacteria, especially *Escherichia coli.* Except after the ingestion of very large amounts, adults usually absorb all nitrate before this reduction takes place. However, in children nitrite poisoning may result from the ingestion of nitrates or nitrate-containing well water. Fatalities have occurred from the oral ingestion of 2 to 4 g of nitrites.

Acute nitrite poisoning may lead to severe headache, flushing, dizziness, hypotension, and syncope. Usually the patient need only be positioned to facilitate venous return to the heart. Pressor agents are seldom required. The most important toxic effect of the nitrite ion is its ability to oxidize hemoglobin to methemoglobin (Chap. 58).

OXALIC ACID This acid is found in ink eradicators and stain removers. It is corrosive and combines with calcium to form insoluble calcium oxalate. Ingestion causes irritation and corrosion of mouth, esophagus, and stomach, followed by vomiting and abdominal pain. After absorption the reduction in serum calcium leads to muscular tremors, tetany, convulsions, and cardiovascular collapse. Ingestion of 5 g may cause death within minutes. Following recovery from the acute episode there may be renal failure due to blockage of renal tubules by calcium oxalate crystals.

Treatment consists of induction of emesis or gastric lavage with milk, limewater, chalk, or calcium salts. A dose of 10 ml of 10% calcium gluconate should be given intravenously and repeated as required to maintain normal serum calcium and prevent tetany. In supportive therapy the maintenance of a high urine output is essential.

PARAQUAT Paraquat is a dipyridilium compound which is used in 5 to 20% aqueous solutions as a herbicide. It is rapidly inactivated on contact with soil. It has been responsible for more than 20 accidental and suicidal deaths in recent years. An oral dose of 5 mg per kg may be fatal. Ingestion causes a burning sensation and vomiting. After a delay of 2 to 5 days ulcerations in the mouth and esophagus, oliguria, and hemoptysis appear. These may be followed in severe cases by jaundice, fever, respiratory distress, cardiovascular collapse, and death. Pathologic findings include characteristic pulmonary lesions, focal myocardial necrosis, and renal tubular necrosis.

Early administration of activated charcoal and gastric lavage with diluted bentonite magma can decrease absorption. Forced diuresis and hemodialysis are effective and should be started early. Treatment is otherwise supportive since no antidote is known.

PETROLEUM DISTILLATES Petroleum distillates (diesel oil, gasoline, kerosene, paint thinner, solvent distillate) are liquids with a boiling point between 50 and 325°C. They contain variable amounts of branched or straight-chain aliphatic and aromatic hydrocarbons. Kerosene is widely used as a fuel and as a vehicle for cleaning agents, furniture polishes, insecticides, and paint thinners. Not surprisingly, each year petroleum distillates cause about 100 accidental deaths in the United States, 90 percent of these in young children. Furthermore, these products are annually responsible for almost 20,000 hospitalizations. Ingestion of 10 ml kerosene has been fatal, but adults have recovered from as much as 250 ml. Petroleum distillates are central nervous system depressants; they damage cells by dissolving cellular lipids. Pulmonary damage manifested by pulmonary edema or pneumonitis is a common and serious complication.

Inhalation of gasoline or kerosene vapors induces a state resembling alcoholic intoxication. Headache, nausea, tinnitus, and a burning sensation in the chest may also be present. When aliphatic hydrocarbons are inhaled, these symptoms may progress to profound drowsiness or coma with absence of deep reflexes. If the distillate contains a high proportion of aromatic hydrocarbons, the coma is characterized by tremors, muscle jactitations, hyperactive reflexes, and convulsions. Death is usually due to respiratory depression, rarely to ventricular fibrillation.

The oral ingestion of petroleum distillates causes irritation of the mucous membranes of the upper part of the intestinal tract. When large amounts have been ingested, the same manifestations as after inhalation may appear. Frequently eructation or vomiting results in aspiration of petroleum distillates into the trachea. Because of their low surface tension, minute amounts of these substances may then spread widely throughout the lungs and produce pulmonary edema and pneumonitis. Pulmonary damage may also arise because of absorption of ingested petroleum distillates from the gastrointestinal tract. However, kerosene is at least one hundred times more toxic by the intratracheal route than when ingested.

In the treatment of poisoning by petroleum distillates extreme care must be used to prevent aspiration. When large amounts have been ingested, gastric lavage should be performed but only after insertion of an endotracheal tube with an inflatable cuff. A vegetable oil and a saline cathartic may be administered to decrease the absorption of the poison. All victims of kerosene poisoning should be hospitalized for at least 24 hr for observation. If signs or symptoms of pulmonary irritation appear, adrenal steroids, oxygen under positive pressure, and antibiotics to prevent bacterial pneumonia are often of value. Symptomatic therapy for central nervous system depression or convulsions may be necessary. Sympathomimetic amines should be avoided because of the danger of inducing ventricular fibrillation in the hydrocarbon-sensitized heart.

PHENOL Phenol and related compounds (creosote, cresols, hexachlorophene, hydroquinone, Lysol, resorcinol, tannic acid) are widely used as antiseptics, caustics, and preservatives. These substances poison all cells by denaturing and precipitating cellular proteins. The approximate fatal oral dose ranges from 2 ml for phenol and cresols to 20 ml for tannic acid.

Ingestion of phenolic compounds produces erosion of mucosa from mouth to stomach. The corroded areas may have a characteristic dead-white appearance. Hematemesis and bloody diarrhea may occur. After an initial phase of hyperpnea due to stimulation of the respiratory center, stupor, coma, convulsions, pulmonary edema, and shock are seen. The initial respiratory alkalosis is soon followed by a profound acidosis. The latter results from the renal excretion of base during the alkalotic stage, from the acidic nature of the phenolic radical, and from disturbances in carbohydrate metabolism presumably due to defects in enzymatic function. If the patient survives the acute stage, acute tubular necrosis may lead to oliguria or anuria and hepatic toxicity to jaundice.

Poisoning by phenolic compounds may often be diagnosed by their characteristic odor. Development of a violet or blue color of the urine after addition of a few drops of ferric chloride indicates the presence of a phenolic compound.

Treatment is directed at decreasing the absorption of ingested poison by administration of water, milk, or activated charcoal slurry and their removal by emesis or gastric lavage. Olive oil or castor oil dissolves phenol and retards its absorption. Supportive therapy consists of correction of the acidosis, the control of shock and convulsions, and the maintenance of a patent airway in the face of glottal edema by intubation or tracheotomy.

PHOSPHORUS Phosphorus occurs in two forms: a red, nonpoisonous form and a yellow, fat-soluble, highly toxic form. The latter is used in rodent and insect poisons and in fireworks. Yellow phosphorus and phosphides cause fatty degeneration and necrosis of tissues, particularly of the liver. The lethal ingested dose of yellow phosphorus is approximately 50 mg.

Ingestion of yellow phosphorus is followed within 1 hr by burning pain in the upper part of the gastrointestinal tract, vomiting, diarrhea, and a garlic odor of the breath and excreta. The patient may die in coma during the first day or two, or symptoms may subside after a few hours. Then, 1 to 2 days later, the victim may develop tender hepatomegaly, jaundice, hypocalcemia, hypotension, and oliguria, and may die following convulsions and coma. Death from acute yellow atrophy may occur in a few days.

Treatment consists of vigorous and repeated induction of emesis or gastric lavage. Calcium gluconate is given intravenously to maintain serum calcium level. Treatment is otherwise supportive, and a protective regimen for the liver should be instituted.

SALICYLATES Each year 30 million lb of aspirin is consumed in the United States, and salicylates can probably be found in every American household. It is therefore not surprising that salicylates (aspirin, methyl salicylate, salicylic acid, sodium salicylate) are more commonly involved in poisonings than any other agent. Aspirin is found in almost all compound analgesic tablets. Methyl salicylate (oil of wintergreen) is present in most skin liniments, and salicylic acid is used in ointments and corn plasters. The ingestion of 10 to 30 g aspirin or sodium salicylate may be fatal to adults, but survival has been reported after an oral dose of 130 g aspirin. On the other hand 3 g salicylate in a teaspoon of methyl salicylate has been fatal in children.

Salicylate intoxication may result from the cumulative effect of therapeutic administration of high doses. There is considerable individual variation: toxic symptoms may begin at dosages of 3 g per day or may not appear when 10 g per day is given. Toxic symptoms are also poorly correlated with the serum salicylate concentration, but few patients become intoxicated at levels less than 15 mg per 100 ml and most at levels over 35 mg per 100 ml. Therapeutic salicylate intoxication is usually mild and is called "salicylism." The earliest symptoms are vertigo, tinnitus, and impairment of hearing. Further overdosage causes nausea, vomiting, sweating, diarrhea, fever, drowsiness, headache, dimness of vision, and mental aberrations. The latter may be characterized by confusion, excitement, restlessness, and talkativeness; this "salicylate jag" resembles alcoholic intoxication without the euphoria. The central nervous system effects may progress to hallucinations, convulsions, and coma. Toxic doses of salicylates also have a direct stimulant effect on the respiratory center, resulting in hyperventilation, loss of carbon dioxide, and respiratory alkalosis. Renal excretion of bicarbonate may partially compensate for this.

In acute salicylate poisoning due to accidental or suicidal ingestion of massive amounts, the same manifestations may be seen in more rapid succession. However, they are usually overshadowed by severe disturbances in the acid-base balance which follow a definite sequence. Early in the course of intoxication there may be only hyperpnea, and the seriousness of the poisoning may not be appreciated at that time. The hyperventilation causes a fall in blood P_{CO_2} and an increase in pH. Renal excretion of bicarbonate, sodium, and potassium will bring the pH back toward normal and produce a compensated respiratory alkalosis. At that point the buffering capacity of the extracellular fluid will have been significantly decreased. In young children and after large doses in adults further developments may then produce a combination of respiratory acidosis and metabolic acidosis which stems from a number of factors. High concentrations of salicylate depress the respiratory center and cause CO_2 retention. Renal function becomes impaired because of dehydration and hypotension, and inorganic, metabolic acids accumulate. Furthermore, salicylic acid derivatives may displace several milliequivalents of blood bicarbonate. Finally, salicylates impair carbohydrate metabolism and cause accumulation of acetoacetic, lactic, and pyruvic acids. Severe acidosis and disturbances in electrolyte balance are most commonly seen in febrile young children.

Blood salicylate levels are of value in the estimation of the severity of poisoning. Serious poisoning is rare at levels less than 50 mg per 100 ml but usual at levels between 50 and 100 mg per 100 ml. Levels above 100 mg per 100 ml during the first 6 hr after poisoning signify severe intoxication and may be fatal. Excretion of salicylates is renal, and in the presence of normal renal function about 50 percent will be excreted in 24 hr. Addition of a few drops of ferric chloride solution to 5 ml boiled acidified urine containing salicylate yields a violet color and may aid in diagnosis.

Treatment of salicylate poisoning is largely supportive. In order to decrease absorption, activated charcoal is administered and emesis is induced or lavage with sodium bicarbonate solution is performed. Disturbances of acid-base or electrolyte balance and hypoglycemia are corrected by the intravenous administration of appropriate solutions. Respiratory depression may require artifical ventilation with oxygen. Convulsions may best be treated by the administration of succinylcholine and artificial ventilation with oxygen. Central nervous system–depressant agents should not be used. In order to increase renal excretion of salicylate, osmotic diuresis is induced and the urine is alkalinized. Peritoneal dialysis and hemodialysis are also highly effective in removing salicylate from seriously poisoned patients.

SMOKE Poisoning by smoke is usually due to carbon monoxide inhalation. However, burning material may also release irritant fumes. Many irritant gases combine with water to form corrosive acids or alkalies and cause chemical burns of exposed skin and of the upper part of the respiratory tract. Such gases (and the corrosives formed) are ammonia (ammonium hydroxide), nitrogen oxide (nitric acid), sulfur dioxide (sulfurous acid), and sulfur trioxide (sulfuric acid). These irritating gases as well as hydrogen sulfide may also be present in smog. Another highly toxic gas which may be inhaled by firefighters or victims is phosgene. This compound is formed by the high-temperature decomposition of chlorinated hydrocarbons and is released when carbon tetrachloride from fire extinguishers comes into contact with hot surfaces.

After inhalation of irritant gases the victim may notice burning pain in throat and chest and severe coughing. These symptoms may subside completely, but from several hours to a day after exposure dyspnea and cyanosis may appear and progress rapidly to severe pulmonary edema and death from respiratory and circulatory failure. Treatment consists of administration of oxygen and adrenal steroids and appropriate therapy of pulmonary edema, should that develop.

In many localities the term *smoke* is used to describe paint removers, lacquer thinners, antifreezes, and other solvent mixtures which are ingested for their supposed alcohol content. The toxicity of these compounds depends on their ingredients. Some such materials have caused profound hypoglycemia by a poorly understood mechanism. This possibility should be considered in the differential diagnosis of what appears to be alcoholic coma. Intravenous administration of glucose as a therapeutic test may be indicated.

SULFIDES Hydrogen sulfide is a gas released by the decomposition of organic sulfur compounds and is widely used in industry. Carbon disulfide is an industrial solvent. Other sulfides have industrial uses and release hydrogen sulfide in contact with water or acids. Significant concentrations of hydrogen sulfide may be present in smoke or smog. Inhalation of hydrogen sulfide in concentrations above 50 ppm (fifty times the minimum detectable by smell) causes conjunctivitis, headache, nausea, soreness of the upper respiratory passages, pulmonary edema, and drowsiness. Concentrations in excess of 300 ppm may cause coma, respiratory depression, and death. Ingestion of carbon disulfide or soluble sulfides is followed by vomiting, headache, hypotension, respiratory depression, tremors, coma, convulsions, and death. The fatal oral dose of carbon disulfide is approximately 1 g. Treatment of sulfide intoxication is supportive. Administration of sodium nitrite may promote the binding of sulfide in sulfmethemoglobin.

VOLATILE OILS The volatile or essential oils (citronella oil, eucalyptus oil, menthol, pine oil, turpentine) are colorless liquids which irritate all tissues. Poisoning may result from occupational exposure (painters) and accidental or suicidal ingestion. Unfortunately, some volatile oils also have an undeserved reputation as abortifacients. Absorption occurs from skin, intestine, or lungs; the less volatile oils are more slowly absorbed. Ingestion of 15 g turpentine has been fatal.

Ingestion is rapidly followed by abdominal burning, nausea, vomiting, and diarrhea. Inhalation produces severe bronchial irritation and may be followed by delirium, coma, and convulsions. If the patient survives the acute stage of poisoning, evidence of renal damage may appear and progress to acute tubular necrosis with anuria.

Treatment is entirely supportive. When gastric lavage is undertaken, aspiration must be prevented with extreme care. Since the renal lesion is reversible, treatment for renal failure should be vigorous and include dialysis if necessary.

REFERENCES

Antimuscarinic compounds

Hoefnagel D: Toxic effects of atropine and homatropine eyedrops in children. N Engl J Med 264:168, 1961

Weintraub S: Stramonium poisoning. Postgrad Med 28:364, 1960

Barium

Dean G: Seven cases of barium carbonate poisoning. Br Med J 2: 817, 1950

Benzene, toluene

Browning E: Toxic solvents: a review. Br J Ind Med 16:23, 1959

Brozovsky M, Winkler EM: Glue sniffing in children and adolescents. NY State J Med 65:1984, 1965

Glaser HH, Massengale ON: "Glue-sniffing" in children. Deliberate inhalation of vaporized plastic cements. JAMA 181:300, 1962

Boric acid

Valdes-Dapena MA, Arey JB: Boric acid poisoning. J Pediatr 61:531, 1962

Wong LC et al: Boric acid poisoning: report of 11 cases. Can Med Assoc J 90:1018, 1964

Cantharidin

Oaks WW et al: Cantharidin poisoning. AMA Arch Intern Med 105:574, 1960

Carbon monoxide

ANDERSON RF et al: Myocardial toxicity from carbon monoxide poisoning. Ann Intern Med 67:1172, 1967

COSBY RS AND BERGERON M: Electrocardiographic changes in carbon monoxide poisoning. Am J Cardiol 11:93, 1963

CRAIG TV et al: Hypothermia. Its use in severe carbon monoxide poisoning. N Engl J Med 261:854, 1959

LILIENTHAL JL JR: Carbon monoxide. Pharmacol Rev 2:324, 1950

MEIGS JW, HUGHES JPW: Acute carbon monoxide poisoning; an analysis of 105 cases. AMA Arch Ind Hyg 1:90, 1950

SMITH G et al: Treatment of coal gas poisoning with oxygen at 2 atmospheres pressure. Lancet I:816, 1962

Castor bean

BRUGSCH HG: The castor bean. N Engl J Med 262:1039, 1960

Caustics

HALLER JA, BACHMAN K: The comparative effect of current therapy on experimental caustic burns of the esophagus. Pediatrics 34:236, 1964

YARINGTON CT JR: Ingestion of caustic; a pediatric problem. J Pediatr 67:674, 1965

Chlorate

KNIGHT RK et al: Suicidal chlorate poisoning treated with peritoneal dialysis. Br Med J 3:601, 1967

Chlorinated insecticides

FINLEY AH, HAGGERTY RJ: Toxic hazards, insecticides. Chlorinated hydrocarbons. N Engl J Med 258:812, 1958

ZAVON MR: Chlorinated hydrocarbon insecticides. JAMA 190:595, 1964

Cholinesterase inhibitor insecticides

HEATH DF: *Organophosphorus Poisons,* Oxford: Pergamon, 1961

HOBBIGER F: Reactivation of phosphorylated acetylcholinesterase, in *Cholinesterases and Anticholinesterase Agents,* Handb Exp Pharmak Suppl 15:921, 1963

MANN JB: Diagnostic aids in organophosphate poisoning. Ann Intern Med 67:905, 1967

QUINBY GE: Further therapeutic experience with pralidoximes in organic phosphorus poisoning. JAMA 187:202, 1964

WYCKOFF DW et al: Diagnostic and therapeutic problems of parathion poisonings. Ann Intern Med 68:875, 1968

Cyanide

CHEN KK, ROSE CL: Treatment of acute cyanide poisoning JAMA 162:1154, 1956

COPE C: The importance of oxygen in the treatment of cyanide poisoning JAMA 175:1061, 1961

PIJOAN M: Cyanide poisoning from choke cherry seed. Am J Med Sci 204:550, 1942

Detergents

ARENA JM: Poisonings and other health hazards associated with use of detergents. JAMA 190:56, 1964

CANN HM, VERHULST HL: Toxicity of household soap and detergents and treatment of their ingestion. Am J Dis Child 100:287, 1960

Fluorides

PETERS JH: Therapy of acute fluoride poisoning. Am J Med Sci 216:278, 1948

Glycols

HAGGERTY RJ: Toxic hazards, deaths from permanent antifreeze ingestion. N Engl J Med 261:1296, 1959

HAGSTAM KE et al: Ethylene glycol poisoning treated by haemodialysis. Acta Med Scand 178:599, 1965

PETERSON DI et al: Experimental treatment of ethylene glycol poisoning. JAMA 186:965, 1963

PONS CA, CUSTER RP: Acute ethylene glycol poisoning: a clinicopathologic report of eighteen fatal cases. Am J Med Sci 211:544, 1946

Halogenated hydrocarbons

BAERG RD, KIMBERG DV: Centrilobular hepatic necrosis and acute renal failure in "solvent sniffers." Ann Intern Med 73:713, 1970

BROWNING E: Toxicology of organic compounds of industrial importance. Ann Rev Pharmacol 1:397, 1961

MYATT AV, SALMONS JA: Carbon tetrachloride poisoning. Arch Ind Hyg Occup Med 6:74, 1952

OETTINGEN WF von: *The Halogenated Hydrocarbons of Industrial and Toxicological Importance,* Amsterdam: Elsevier, 1964

Ipecac, emetine

SMITH RP, SMITH DM: Acute ipecac poisoning. N Engl J Med 265:523, 1961

WELCHMAN JM: The cardiac toxicity of emetine. J Trop Med Hyg 60:296, 1957

Iron salts

COVEY TJ: Ferrous sulfate poisoning: review, case summaries and therapeutic regimen. J Pediatr 64:218, 1964

JACOBS J et al: Acute iron intoxication. N Engl J Med 273:1124, 1965

LEIKIN S: Deferoxamine as a chelating agent. J Pediatr 72:148, 1968

Isopropyl alcohol

FREIREICH AW et al: Hemodialysis for isopropanol poisoning. N Engl J Med 277:699, 1967

Methyl alcohol

BENNETT IL JR et al: Acute methyl alcohol poisoning: a review based on experiences in an outbreak of 323 cases. Medicine 32:431, 1953

COOPER JR, KINI MM: Biochemical aspects of methanol poisoning. Biochem Pharmacol 11:405, 1962

SETTER JG et al: Studies on the dialysis of methanol. Trans Am Soc Artif Intern Organs 13:178, 1967

SMITH ME: Interrelations in ethanol and methanol metabolism. J Pharmacol 134:233, 1961

Mushrooms

BUCK RW: Mushroom toxins—a brief review of the literature. N Engl J Med 265:681, 1961

THÖLEN H et al: Early hemodialysis in poisoning by *Amanita phalloides.* Ger Med Mon 11:89, 1966

Naphthalene

HAGGERTY RJ: Naphthalene poisoning. N Engl J Med 255:919, 1956

Nicotine

OBERST BB, MCINTYRE RA: Acute nicotine poisoning. Pediatrics 11:338, 1953

Nitrites

BUCKLIN R, MYINT MK: Fatal methemoglobinemia due to well water nitrates. Ann Intern Med 52:703, 1960

Paraquat

HARGREAVE TB et al: Paraquat poisoning. Postgrad Med J 45:633, 1969

McDONAGH BJ, MARTIN J: Paraquat poisoning in children. Arch Dis Child 45:425, 1970

Petroleum distillates

BROWNING E: *Toxicity and Metabolism of Industrial Solvents*, Amsterdam: Elsevier, 1965

JACOBZINER H, RAYBIN HW: Kerosene and other petroleum distillate poisonings. N Y State J Med 63:3428, 1963

LAWTON JJ JR, MALMQUIST CP: Gasoline addiction in children. Psychiatr Q 35:555, 1961

MAYOCK RL et al: Kerosene pneumonitis treated with adrenal steroids. Ann Intern Med 54:559, 1961

SUBCOMMITTEE ON ACCIDENTAL POISONING: Cooperative kerosene poisoning study. Pediatrics 29:648, 1962

Phosphorus

ARENA JM: Phosphorus poisoning. Clin Pediatr (Phila) 2:132, 1963

DIAZ-RIVERA RS et al: Acute phosphorus poisoning in man; a study of 56 cases. Medicine 29:269, 1950

FLETCHER GF, GALAMBOS JT: Phosphorus poisoning in humans. Arch Intern Med 112:846, 1963

Salicylates

DONE AK: Salicylate intoxication; significance of measurements of salicylate in blood in cases of acute ingestions. Pediatrics 26:800, 1960

——: Salicylate poisoning. JAMA 192:770, 1965

——: Treatment of salicylate poisoning. Mod Treatment 4:648, 1967

LEVY G, TSUCHIYA T: Effect of activated charcoal on aspirin absorption in man. Clin Pharmacol Ther 13:317, 1972

MORGAN AG, POLAK A: Acetazolamide and sodium bicarbonate in treatment of salicylate poisoning in adults. Br Med J 1:16, 1969

PROUDFOOT AT, BROWN SS: Acidaemia and salicylate poisoning in adults. Br Med J 2:547, 1969

SEGAR WE, HOLLIDAY MA: Physiologic abnormalities of salicylate intoxication. N Engl J Med 259:1191, 1958

SUMMITT RL, ETTELDORF JN: Salicylate intoxication in children. Experience with peritoneal dialysis and alkalinization of the urine. J Pediatr 64:803, 1964

110
HEAVY METALS

DAVID C. POSKANZER
IVAN L. BENNETT, JR.

Three highly effective chemicals, BAL, Versene, and penicillamine, are now available for treatment of systemic poisoning with heavy metals by forming nontoxic, stable cyclic compounds with polyvalent metallic ions, thus permitting the offending material to be excreted safely in the urine.

The first to be developed was BAL (British antilewisite, 2,3-dimercaptopropanol, dimercaprol), which was originally intended as an antidote against the arsenical war gas, lewisite. Its tendency to combine with certain metallic ions such as arsenic, mercury, cobalt, nickel, antimony, and gold is so great that it can remove them from combination with the enzymes whose function they impair in the body. BAL is not useful in the treatment of lead poisoning. Because the effectiveness of BAL depends to some extent upon the speed with which its administration is begun, every attempt should be made to avoid delay in its use. For serious systemic intoxications, BAL should be given in doses of 4 mg per kg body weight intramuscularly as a 10% solution in oil and 20% benzyl benzoate. No single dose should exceed 300 mg. This dose should be repeated every 4 hr on the first day and every 6 hr on the second day. Thereafter, it should be given three times daily for several days; doses should then be tapered and discontinued about 10 days after acute poisoning. When the dose of poison has been relatively small, the schedule of BAL administration may be reduced by one-third. Because BAL is excreted in part by the kidneys, it can accumulate to toxic concentrations in anuric patients. Overdosage results in nervousness, hyperactivity, muscle twitching, and hyperreflexia. Large doses may produce convulsions. The presence of the material in tears sometimes causes blepharospasm. In patients with anuria or oliguria, therefore, BAL should be administered with caution and at a lower dosage than outlined above. If symptoms of overdosage occur, sedatives should be administered.

The second antidote to metal poisons is the chelating agent Versene (ethylenediaminetetraacetate, EDTA), which forms cyclic, stable, soluble, nontoxic compounds with most metals. Because Versene reacts with calcium in the same way as with other metals, it must be given as the calcium salt (Calcium Disodium Versenate; calcium disodiumedetate) to avoid hypocalcemia. The material has been used with notable success in the treatment of lead poisoning.

It is given in a dosage of 500 mg in 250 ml of 5% glucose intravenously every 12 hr for 5 days. After a pause to allow for further solution of metal from body stores a second and even a third course may be given.

Penicillamine (cuprimine; β,β-dimethylcysteine) is an excellent chelating agent for copper, mercury, and lead, promotes their excretion in the urine, and has the additional advantage of being well absorbed from the gastrointestinal tract. It may be given orally, while BAL and Versene require systemic injection. N-Acetyl-*dl*-penicillamine is even more effective than penicillamine in protecting against the effects of mercury, probably because it is more resistant to metabolic degradation, and it has the advantage of being less toxic. Penicillamine is administered orally in a dose of 1 to 4 g daily on an empty stomach to avoid chelation of dietary metals. It has much lower toxicity than BAL, the only other agent which is effective in the treatment of Wilson's disease (hepatolenticular degeneration), in which toxic amounts of copper are deposited in various tissues, but has the disadvantage of acute sensitivity reactions. It has also been shown to be useful in lead poisoning, but the excretion of urinary lead may not be as high after oral penicillamine as after intravenous Calcium Disodium Versenate.

N-Acetyl-*dl*-penicillamine, though still an investigational drug, has been demonstrated to be effective in mercury poisoning and has the advantage of allowing much higher doses with fewer toxic effects. It has less effect on copper levels than penicillamine and is therefore used in the treatment of mercury poisoning when one would wish to maintain copper levels. Courses of 10 days of 1 to 2 g daily in divided doses have been employed in patients with good results.

ANTIMONY Symptoms of poisoning after the ingestion of antimony may occur when an acid food is allowed to stand in cheap enamelware or "graniteware" for a sufficient time to allow solution of antimony, which is used in the manufacture of these products. The symptoms are similar to those produced by arsenic, except that antimony causes a more rapid onset of gastrointestinal symptoms. Treatment is the same as for arsenic, including use of BAL. Circulatory collapse occurs early and requires vigorous supportive treatment. The therapeutic injection of antimony (tartar emetic, etc.) may result in severe coughing, muscle and joint pains, or bradycardia. The last is an indication to stop medication.

ARSENIC Arsenic poisoning is usually the result of accidental or suicidal ingestion of insecticides or rodenticides containing Paris green (copper acetoarsenate) or calcium or lead arsenate. Pesticides containing arsenic are a frequent source of poisoning in rural areas of the United States. Medications such as Fowler's solution (potassium arsenite) and the organic arsenicals (arsphenamines and arsenoxides) were once common causes of intoxication.

The toxic dose of inorganic arsenic varies considerably and seems to depend upon individual susceptibility. Orchardists have been found to ingest as much as 6.8 mg arsenic a day without any signs of intoxication. On the other hand, as little as 30 mg arsenic trioxide has been fatal. Arsenic has a predilection for keratin, and the concentration of arsenic in the hair and nails is higher than that in other tissues. Arsenic reacts with the —SH groups in certain tissue proteins and thus interferes with a number of enzyme systems essential to cellular metabolism. Pathologic changes in fatal inorganic arsenical poisoning are fatty degeneration of the liver, hyperemia and hemorrhages of the intestine, and renal tubular necrosis. The peripheral nerves often show fragmentation and resorption of myelin, with disintegration of axis cylinders.

The symptoms of acute poisoning by the oral route are nausea, vomiting, diarrhea, severe burning of the mouth and throat, and agonizing abdominal pains. The vomitus often contains blood. Circulatory collapse is frequent, and death may ensue within a few hours. With chronic exposure, the first signs of poisoning are usually weakness, prostration, muscular aching, or nervous system involvement; gastrointestinal symptoms are minimal. In patients exposed to arsine gas (hydrogen arsenide), the outstanding features are hemolysis, chills, fever, and hemoglobinuria.

Patients who recover from acute poisoning and those with chronic intoxication usually develop skin and mucosal changes, peripheral neuropathy, and linear pigmentations in the fingernails (see Chap. 323). The *cutaneous manifestations* appear within 1 to 4 weeks and consist of a diffuse, dry, scaly desquamation, occasionally with hyperpigmentation, over the trunk and extremities. Hyperkeratoses of the palms and soles and edema of the face and extremities may also occur. The mucous membranes also show evidence of irritation, with conjunctivitis, photophobia, pharyngitis, or irritating cough. About 5 weeks after exposure to arsenic, a transverse white stria, 1 to 2 mm in width, appears above the lunula of each fingernail (*Mees lines*). Patients with more than one exposure to arsenic may show double lines several millimeters apart.

Symptoms of headache, drowsiness, confusion, and convulsions are seen in both acute and chronic intoxication. Evidence of peripheral neuropathy usually appears 1 to 3 weeks after exposure. There are numbness, tingling, and burning of the feet and hands, followed by muscular weakness. The extremities show a decrease in touch, pain, and temperature sensations, in a symmetrical "stocking-glove" distribution, and distal weakness with inability to walk or stand, weakness of grip, and wrist drop. Tendon reflexes are absent or diminished, and atrophy of the affected muscles develops rapidly.

The laboratory findings usually consist of moderate anemia and a leukopenia of 2,000 to 5,000 white blood cells with mild eosinophilia. There is slight proteinuria, and liver function tests show mild abnormalities. The spinal fluid is normal.

None of the clinical or laboratory manifestations of arsenic poisoning is specific, and the diagnosis depends upon analysis of the hair and urine for arsenic. Normal persons have an average concentration of 0.05 mg arsenic per 100 mg hair, with a range of 0.025 to 0.088 mg. Concentrations of arsenic greater than 0.1 mg per 100 mg hair are indicative of poisoning. The minimal level of arsenic in the urine indicating intoxication is difficult to establish. Normal persons have been found to excrete between 0.01 and 0.06 mg arsenic per liter, and a few individuals as much as 0.2 mg per liter. Although there is considerable overlap, most patients with evidence of arsenic intoxication will be found to excrete more than 0.1 mg per liter; soon after acute exposure, many will show levels greater than 1 mg per liter.

The treatment for acute ingestion is gastric lavage (see Chap. 108). Replacement of lost fluids and elevation of blood pressure by vasopressor agents is often indicated. Immediate treatment with BAL should be instituted. Patients with peripheral neuropathy rarely show significant improvement with BAL and continue to have sensory disturbances and weakness for many months. Dramatic responses, however, have been observed with the use of BAL in the treatment of exfoliative dermatitis, bone marrow depression, and encephalopathy caused by the arsphenamines and the organic arsenicals. BAL is of little value in the treatment of the hemolysis caused by inhalation of arsine.

BISMUTH Poisoning by bismuth is almost entirely a complication of antisyphilitic therapy. Toxic manifestations may appear in the mouth (gingivitis, followed by stomatitis), the kidneys (albuminuria and nephrotic syndrome), or the skin (exfoliative dermatitis), requiring immediate interruption of bismuth injections. The development of a bluish stippled line of pigmentation just at the margin of the gums is not dangerous but suggests that oral hygiene should be improved. Bismuth subnitrate occasionally gives rise to methemoglobinemia (Chap. 312).

CADMIUM Poisoning is likely to occur after ingestion of an acid food prepared in a cadmium-lined vessel. The classic example is lemonade served from metal cans. Symptoms of nausea, vomiting, diarrhea, and prostration usually develop within 10 min after ingestion. Treatment is symptomatic, and symptoms ordinarily subside within 24 hr. The short length of time after ingestion and the typical circumstances suggest the diagnosis. Inhalation of cadmium fumes in industry produces an acute, extremely severe pneumonitis. The use of BAL is not recommended for cadmium intoxication, as the BAL-cadmium complex dissociates in the kidneys and cadmium is nephrotoxic.

COPPER Acute poisoning due to ingestion of copper salts is rare. Copper sulfate (blue vitriol) is the chief offender, in which case the vomitus has a characteristic blue color. Manifestations are nausea, vomiting, bloody diarrhea, headache, severe thirst, and tachycardia. In fatal cases, death is preceded by convulsions. Treatment consists of gastric lavage with 1% solution of potassium ferrocyanide, fluid replacement, and control of pain and diarrhea with opiates.

GOLD Because practically all cases of poisoning by gold are associated with its use in the treatment of arthritis, diagnosis is usually easy. Manifestations are skin rashes of various types, bone marrow depression, icterus, oliguria, nausea, vomiting, and gastrointestinal bleeding. Treatment consists of symptomatic relief of discomfort and the use of BAL, an effective antidote.

LEAD Poisoning results from ingestion of lead-containing materials such as paint or water which has stood in lead pipes or from inhalation of fumes from burning storage batteries, solder, etc. Illicit whiskey contaminated by lead solder in the pipes of stills has been responsible for many cases of poisoning. Bullets or buckshot containing lead can cause poisoning years after becoming embedded in a serous cavity. The most common form of lead poisoning today is that encountered in children who ingest lead-containing outdoor paint, often used indoors in older houses. It has a sweetish, apparently attractive taste. Absorption is slow by any route, and prolonged exposure is required for the development of symptoms. Lead is a cumulative poison, excreted slowly. Acute poisoning is virtually nonexistent, although it was observed when lead was used for the treatment of malignant disease. Symptoms may develop suddenly after chronic exposure. Most of the absorbed lead is deposited in the bones; blood, urine, and feces contain only small amounts.

Manifestations of poisoning are colic, encephalopathy, peripheral neuritis, and anemia.

Lead colic, or painter's cramps, is characterized by agonizing, wandering, poorly localized abdominal pain, often with spasm and rigidity of the musculature of the abdominal wall. There is no fever or leukocytosis. Needless surgery has been carried out in these patients for supposed perforation of peptic ulcer or other catastrophe. Morphine has surprisingly little effect upon the pain; intravenous injection of calcium salts affords relief within a short time, although pain may recur. Attacks of colic seem to be brought on by intercurrent infection or alcoholic overindulgence.

Encephalopathy occurs chiefly in children and is manifested by convulsions, somnolence, mania, delirium, or coma. The mortality rate is high when convulsive seizures and coma occur. Mental enfeeblement is a common sequel.

Peripheral neuritis with paralysis, characteristically involving the muscles most used (e.g., wrist drop in painters, etc.), occurs in patients exposed to lead, often in the absence of other symptoms. It is rare in children. (See Chap. 323.)

Mild anemia, probably the result of increased brittleness of the erythrocytes as well as of a defect in cell maturation, is common. Pallor is out of proportion to anemia in patients with chronic plumbism and is attributed to spasm of small vessels in the skin. Anemia is almost never severe and is characterized by the presence of large numbers of erythrocytes with basophilic stippling. This is seen in other hematologic disorders, but a smear showing stippling should arouse suspicion of lead poisoning. In patients with poor oral hygiene a "lead line" of black lead sulfide may develop along the gingival margins. This is not seen in edentulous persons and is rare in children.

Patients with lead poisoning excrete increased amounts of coproporphyrin III in the urine (see Chap. 102). This is so consistent that examination of a urine specimen for porphyrin is the best screening test in suspected cases. A few milliliters of urine should be acidified with acetic acid and shaken with an equal volume of ether. Exposure of a specimen prepared in this manner under a Wood's lamp will reveal reddish fluorescence of the ether layer if coproporphyrin is present. A positive test result is strongly in favor of lead intoxication. Urinary lead determinations are of aid in confirming the diagnosis; a level of 0.2 mg per liter or more is usually regarded as significant, although interpretations vary. Diagnosis can be confirmed by precipitating lead excretion with three doses of Calcium Disodium Versenate (25 mg per kg) at 8-hr intervals. Excretion of over 500 μg in 24 hr is indicative of excessive lead burden.

Lead encephalopathy occurs chiefly in children, has a significant mortality rate, and causes severe permanent brain damage in 25 percent of survivors. Encephalopathy in adults is rare and usually results from consumption of lead-contaminated illicit liquor (moonshine). Once minor symptoms of poisoning are present, acute encephalopathy can develop with unpredictable rapidity. Any child with symptoms suggestive of lead poisoning should be considered to have a medical emergency and should be hospitalized immediately. The onset of encephalopathy is signaled by the development of gross ataxia, persistent vomiting, and intermittent lethargy and stupor. These symptoms are followed by convulsions, mania, and coma.

The most important single feature of treatment is removal of the patient from further exposure to lead. Once abnormal absorption is terminated, virtually all the lead in the body is shifted into bone. Chelating agents do not remove significant quantities of lead from bone. It takes approximately twice as long to excrete a given burden of lead as it does to accumulate it. As long as significant quantities of lead remain in bone, any intercurrent illness which causes demineralization can cause mobilization of toxic quantities of lead into soft tissues and exacerbate plumbism.

The treatment of lead encephalopathy is begun once adequate urine flow is established. A combination of BAL and Calcium Disodium Versenate is employed, and the Versene therapy continued for 5 to 7 days. If Calcium Disodium Versenate is given alone in the presence of very high tissue concentrations of lead, some of the toxic effects may be intensified. Acute symptoms usually subside within 48 to 72 hr after Versene is begun. Within 2 weeks urinary excretion of coproporphyrin ceases, and there is sometimes a dramatic improvement in neuritis.

Symptoms of acute increased intracranial pressure are best treated with repeated doses of mannitol given intravenously. Evidence for the use of high-potency steroids to relieve cerebral edema in patients with lead encephalopathy is incomplete. Treatment of increased intracranial pressure by surgical decompression is no longer indicated.

The problem of lead poisoning in children is so significant that many health departments are carrying out extensive programs for removal of lead-containing paints in old low-income housing areas.

In adults combined therapy with BAL and Calcium Disodium Versenate followed by oral penicillamine is probably indicated whenever blood levels exceed 100 mg lead per 100 g blood, even in the absence of symptoms. Evidence of lead toxicity is usually present at this level, and the risk of symptomatic episodes is considerable. The use of oral penicillamine alone in a dose of 1 to 1.5 g daily for 3 to 5 days in mildly symptomatic cases has been suggested and has the advantage of easy administration and the avoidance of painful injections.

MERCURY Poisoning occurs chiefly as a result of the acute ingestion of a soluble salt, usually mercuric chloride (bichloride of mercury). Toxic symptoms may occur with 0.1 g and 0.5 g is almost always fatal unless immediate treatment is instituted. The mercuric ion is corrosive and produces severe local inflammation. Oral, pharyngeal, and laryngeal pain are severe; abdominal cramps with nausea and vomiting occur within 15 min. As mercury is absorbed, it is concentrated in the kidneys, where it poisons the tubular cells, producing a tendency to diuresis within the first 2 to 3 hr. The combination of vomiting, dehydration, shock, and progressive tubular damage, however, soon leads to anuria and uremia. The poison is also excreted into the colon and produces severe enteritis, with bloody diarrhea and tenesmus. Death is usually from uremia. The chief objectives of treatment are to prevent the shock of dehydration and to remove mercury from the body. Early in treatment, copious quantities of fluid should be infused intravenously to prevent dehydration and to reduce the concentration of mercuric ion in the renal tubules. That the patient is anuric early is often simply the result of dehydration and shock. In such instances, forcing fluids is advisable. However, the gradual development of oliguria and anuria in a hydrated patient indicates renal damage by mercury, and at this stage a regimen for acute renal shutdown should be instituted (Chap. 269).

Chronic poisoning from metallic mercury vapor occurs in persons exposed to large amounts of the metal in laboratories or in industry and occasionally as a result of prolonged therapeutic use, as in vaginal douches. Manifestations may be those of subacute poisoning, with salivation, stomatitis, and diarrhea or primary neurologic signs, including tremors of the extremities, tongue, and lips, ataxia and dysarthria, erethism, a state of easy embarrassment, irritability, apprehension, withdrawal, and depression.

Some poison can be removed from the body by gastric lavage, but more important in treatment is the binding of the mercuric ion in a harmless compound by BAL. The therapeutic usefulness of BAL depends on its immediate administration. In chronic mercury poisoning, N-acetyl-*dl*-penicillamine may well be the drug of choice. It can be administered orally and appears to chelate mercury selectively, with considerably less effect on copper, which is essential to many metabolic processes.

SILVER Most poisoning by silver involves silver nitrate, a caustic salt. There are intense nausea, vomiting, and diarrhea after swallowing nitrate (lunar caustic), and death from shock may occur within a few hours. The mouth is usually deeply stained by silver nitrate. Treatment is entirely supportive, with fluid replacement and control of pain.

Chronic exposure (usually to nose drops) produces a peculiar bluish skin discoloration (argyria).

THALLIUM Thallium is a component of certain rodenticides and depilatories, and clinical poisoning is usually a result of accidental ingestion of these materials. The fatal dose is approximately 1.0 g. Manifestations are vomiting, diarrhea, and leg pains, followed by weakness and paralysis of the legs. There may be visual and mental disturbances. About 3 weeks after poisoning, the patient's hair falls out, providing a strong diagnostic clue if the cause has not previously been determined. Treatment is symptomatic. The alopecia is temporary if the patient recovers.

REFERENCES

LEVINE WG: Heavy-metal antagonists, in *The Pharmacological Basis of Therapeutics*, 4th ed., eds LS Goodman, A Gilman, New York: Macmillan, 1970, pp. 944-957

Arsenic

JENKINS RB: Inorganic arsenic and the nervous system. Brain 89:479, 1966

KEUSLER CJ et al: Arsine poisoning, mode of action and treatment. J Pharmacol Exp Ther 88:99, 1946

LONGCOPE WT, LUETSCHER JA: The use of BAL (British antilewisite) in the treatment of the injurious effects of arsenic, mercury, and other metallic poisons. Ann Intern Med 31:545, 1949

Bismuth

HEYMAN A: Systemic manifestations of bismuth toxicity; observations on 4 patients with pre-existent kidney disease. Am J Syph Gonor Vener Dis 28:721, 1944

Cadmium

KENDREY G, ROE FJC: Cadmium toxicology. Lancet 1:1206, 1969

Lead

AUB JC et al: Lead poisoning. Medicine 4:1, 1925

CHISOLM JJ JR: Treatment of lead poisoning. Mod Treatment 4:710, 1967

Mercury

ARENA JM: Treatment of mercury poisoning. Mod Treatment. 4:734, 1967

DOOLAN PD et al: Acute renal insufficiency due to dichloride of mercury: observations of gastrointestinal hemorrhage and BAL therapy. N Engl J Med 249:273, 1953

KARK RAP et al: Mercury poisoning and its treatment with N-acetyl-D,L-penicillamine. N Engl J Med 285:10, 1971

Thallium

BANK WJ et al: Thallium poisoning. Arch Neurol 26:456, 1972

111 ALCOHOL

MAURICE VICTOR
RAYMOND D. ADAMS

Intemperance in the use of alcohol creates many problems in modern society, the importance of which can be judged by the repeated emphasis they receive in contemporary writings, both literary and scientific. These problems may be divided into three categories—psychologic, medical, and sociologic. The main psychologic problem is why a person drinks excessively, often with full knowledge that such action will result in physical injury to himself and irreparable harm to his family. The medical problem embraces all aspects of alcoholic habituation as well as the diseases which result from overindulgence in alcohol. The sociologic problem comprises the effects of sustained inebriety on the family and community.

The various problems raised by excessive drinking cannot be separated from one another, and the physician must therefore be conversant with all sides of the subject. He may be asked to help the patient conquer his alcoholic tendency or to diagnose and to treat the numerous diseases to which he is subject; often he must admit or commit the patient to a general or mental hospital, according to the nature of the presenting clinical disorder; and lastly, he may be required to enlist the aid of available social agencies when their services are needed by either the patient or his family.

Alcoholism has been defined as both a chronic disease and a disorder of behavior, characterized in either context by the repeated drinking of alcoholic beverages to an extent that exceeds customary dietary use or surpasses the social drinking customs of the community and that interferes with the drinker's health, interpersonal relations, or economic functioning. Reduced to pharmacologic terms, it is alcoholic addiction. The precise number of such persons, commonly called alcoholics, in the United States is not known. The estimate is 8 to 9 million—approximately 5 percent of the total adult population. It requires little projection of the imagination to conceive the havoc wrought by alcohol in terms of decreased productivity, accidents, crime, mental and physical disease, and disruption of family life.

PHARMACOLOGY AND METABOLISM OF ALCOHOL

Ethyl alcohol, or ethanol, is the active ingredient in beer, wine, whiskey, gin, brandy, and other less common alcoholic beverages. In addition, the stronger spirits contain enanthic ethers, which give the flavor but have no important pharmacologic properties, and impurities such as amyl alcohol (fusel oil) and acetaldehyde, which act like alcohol but are more toxic. Contrary to prevailing opinion, the content of B vitamins in American beer and other liquors is so low as to have little nutritional value.

Alcohol is absorbed unaltered from the gastrointestinal tract, about 80 percent from the intestine and the remainder from the stomach. Its presence may be detected in the blood within 5 min after ingestion, and the maximum concentration is reached in ½ to 2 hr. The ingestion of milk and fatty foods impedes and water facilitates its absorption. In habituated persons the blood alcohol concentration rises somewhat faster and reaches a higher maximum than in abstainers.

Alcohol is carried chiefly in the plasma and enters the various organs of the body, as well as the spinal fluid, urine, and pulmonary alveolar air, in concentrations which bear a constant relationship to that in the blood. It is eliminated chiefly by oxidation, 5 percent or less being excreted chemically unchanged in the urine, sweat, and breath. The energy liberated by the oxidation of alcohol (7 kcal per g) can be utilized as completely as that of fats, sugars, and proteins, which it replaces isodynamically. It should be emphasized that alcohol cannot be stored in the body or used in the replacement of destroyed tissue. Unless, therefore, the protein intake is adequate, a state of negative nitrogen balance will develop, a common finding in chronic alcoholics.

The first step in the metabolism of alcohol is accomplished mainly in the liver, where alcohol dehydrogenase oxidizes alcohol to acetaldehyde. The latter substance may be further metabolized in the liver or carried to other tissues, where it is converted, possibly via the stage of free acetate, to acetyl coenzyme A, of which the acetate portion can be oxidized completely to carbon dioxide and water.

For all practical purposes it may be accepted that once absorption is ended and an equilibrium established with the tissues, ethyl alcohol is oxidized at a constant rate, independent of its concentration in the blood. Actually, slightly more alcohol is burned per hour when the initial concentrations are very high, but this increment is of little clinical significance. On the other hand, the rate of oxidation of acetaldehyde does depend on its concentration in the tissues. This fact is of importance in connection with the drug disulfiram (Antabuse), which raises the tissue concentration necessary for the metabolism of a certain amount of acetaldehyde per unit of time. The patient taking both Antabuse and alcohol will accumulate an inordinate amount of acetaldehyde, resulting in nausea, vomiting, and hypotension, sometimes pronounced and even fatal in degree. This pharmacologic principle underlies the treatment of alcoholism with Antabuse.

Very few factors are capable of increasing the rate of alcohol metabolism. There is some evidence that repeated ingestion facilitates its metabolism in both normal and alcoholic subjects. Insulin and probably amino acids have similar effects, but neither of these has proved to make a significant difference in the treatment of intoxication. On the other hand, starvation slows the rate of alcohol metabolism in the liver, although this varies greatly in degree from one person to another.

PHYSIOLOGIC AND PSYCHOLOGIC EFFECTS OF ALCOHOL The immediate effects of alcohol on organs other than the central nervous system are relatively unimportant. There appears to be a direct action on the excitability and contractility of heart muscle. With intoxicating doses there is a rise in cardiac rate and output and in systolic and pulse pressures, and a cutaneous vasodilatation at the expense of splanchnic constriction. Some authors have stated that prolonged intoxication may have a damaging effect on cardiac and skeletal muscle, a degeneration of fibers supposedly due to suppression of myophosphorylase activity. Increased sweating and vasodilatation cause a loss of body heat and a fall in temperature. In low concentrations, by whatever route it is administered, alcohol is capable of stimulating the gastric glands to produce acid, apparently by causing the tissues to form or release histamine. With the ingestion of alcohol in concentrations of over 10 to 15 percent the secretion of mucus is increased, the stomach mucosa becomes congested and hyperemic, and the secretion of acid then becomes depressed. This is a state of acute gastritis, from which recovery is relatively rapid. The increase in appetite following ingestion of alcohol is due to the stimulation of the end organs of taste and to a general sense of well-being. Similarly, the reviving effect of alcohol in fatigue states is a cerebral one, not due to a direct stimulating effect on muscle or other organs.

Alcohol has an effect on intermediary metabolism in the liver cells, particularly lipid metabolism (see Chap. 291), and also exerts a distinct effect on the renal excretion of water and electrolytes. The ingestion of 4 oz 100-proof bourbon whiskey, for example, results in a diuresis qualitatively indistinguishable from that which follows the drinking of large amounts of water. This diuresis is most likely due to the transient suppression of the release of antidiuretic hormone (ADH) from the supraopticohypophyseal system, since a relatively small amount of alcohol injected directly into a carotid artery evokes a prompt diuresis without a detectable rise in the concentration of alcohol in the systemic blood. Alcohol does not alter the sensitivity of the kidney tubules to endogenous or exogenous ADH (Pitressin) and has no discernible effect on renal hemodynamic function in normal persons. The degree of diuresis seems to be more closely related to the duration of the rising blood alcohol level than to the rate of increase or the absolute level attained if the period of alcohol intoxication is sustained. Diuresis occurs only during the initial phase of alcohol administration and does not persist during prolonged drinking. There are also an increased urinary excretion of ammonium and a titratable acidity following alcohol ingestion, owing to a mild degree of both metabolic and respiratory acidosis. The former is presumably due to an accumulation of acid metabolites and the latter to the direct action of alcohol on the respiratory center.

Apart from the derangements noted above, the obvious effects of acute, nonlethal doses of alcohol are those exerted on the nervous system, constituting the characteristic symptoms and signs of alcohol intoxication. A large body of data has accumulated regarding the psychomotor effects of alcohol, the nature of tolerance, and the relation of blood alcohol levels to various manifestations of intoxication. Only the most pertinent data are presented here.

It is now generally accepted that alcohol is not a stimulant of the central nervous system, but a depressant. Some of the early effects of alcohol, manifested by garrulousness, aggressiveness, and excessive activity and increased electrical excitability of the cerebral cortex, which suggest stimulation, are due to the inhibition of certain subcortical structures (high brainstem reticular formation?) which ordinarily modulate cerebral cortical activity. Similarly, the initial hyperactivity of tendon reflexes may represent a transitory escape of spinal motor neurons from higher inhibitory centers. With increasing amounts of alcohol, however, the depressant action spreads to involve the cerebral cortical neurons directly, as well as other brainstem and spinal neurons.

All manner of motor performance, whether simply the maintenance of a standing posture, the control of speech and eye movements, or highly organized and complex motor skills—is adversely affected by alcohol. The movements involved in these acts are not only slower than normal but also more inaccurate and random in character and therefore less adapted to the accomplishment of specific ends.

Alcohol also impairs the efficiency of mental function by interfering with the learning process, which is slowed and rendered less effective. The facility of forming associations, whether of words or of figures, tends to be hampered, and the power of attention and concentration is reduced. The person is not as versatile as usual in directing thought along new lines appropriate to the problems at hand. Finally, alcohol impairs the faculties of judgment and discrimination and, all in all, the ability to think and reason clearly.

A scale relating the various degrees of clinical intoxication to the blood alcohol level in nonhabituated persons has been constructed. It has been found that at blood alcohol levels of 30 mg per 100 ml, a mild euphoria was detectable, and at 50 mg per 100 ml, a mild incoordination. At 100 mg per 100 ml, ataxia was obvious; at 300 mg per 100 ml, the patient was stuporous; and a level of 400 mg per 100 ml was accompanied by deep anesthesia and could prove fatal. These figures are valid, provided that the alcohol content rises steadily over a 2-hr period.

It should be emphasized, however, that such a scale has virutally no value in the chronic alcoholic patient, for it does not take into account the adjustment which the organism makes to alcohol, i.e., the phenomenon of tolerance. It is common knowledge that a habituated person can drink more and show fewer effects than the moderate drinker or abstainer. Even with blood alcohol levels as high as 200 mg per 100 ml there may be little decrement in performance.

This phenomenon of tolerance accounts for the surprisingly large amounts of alcohol that can be consumed by the chronic inebriate without significant signs of drunkenness. In such patients, there is a very narrow margin between the doses associated with low blood alcohol levels and sobriety and the doses associated with high blood levels and drunkenness. One must question the validity, therefore, of a single estimation of alcohol concentration as a reliable index of drunkenness. The organism is obviously capable of adapting to alcohol after a very short exposure. If the alcohol concentration in the blood is raised very slowly, no symptoms appear, even at quite high levels. It would appear that the important factor in this rapid adaptability is not so much the rate of increment or the height of the blood alcohol level, but the length of time the alcohol had been present in the body. It has also been shown that if the dosage of alcohol which just causes blood levels to be high is held constant, the blood alcohol concentration falls and clinical evidence of intoxication disappears. The cause of this fall in alcohol concentration is not clear. This type of tolerance has been referred to as "metabolic" and refers to the adjustments made by the nervous system to long-continued exposure to alcohol. There must be a subtle alteration in the metabolism of the neurons such that they can function in the face of high tissue alcohol levels. This alteration requires some time for its establishment. Removal of alcohol from the habituated nervous system results in another disturbance in neuronal function, presumably an overactivity.

A rhythmic need for alcoholic depression is easily induced and may depend on biochemical as well as psychologic factors. The unusual susceptibility of certain persons to alcohol is probably determined by some inborn idiosyncracy.

CLINICAL MANIFESTATIONS OF ALCOHOLISM

The clinical effects of alcohol are mainly on the digestive organs and on the nervous system. Each of these will now be considered.

Effect on digestive organs Symptoms of disordered gastrointestinal function are particularly common in alcoholics; of these the most distinctive are *morning nausea and vomiting.* Characteristically, the patient can suppress these symptoms by taking a drink or two, after which he is able to consume large quantities of alcohol without their recurrence until the following morning. Since sufficient alcohol actually relieves these symptoms, they are probably due to the local effects of alcohol on the stomach, but have a "central" origin and represent the mildest manifestations of the withdrawal syndrome (see below).

Other complaints referable to the gastrointestinal system are abdominal distention, epigastric distress, belching, typical or atypical ulcer symptoms, and hematemesis. The most common pathologic basis for these symptoms is a superficial *gastritis,* which is an almost invariable sequel to prolonged drinking. Most instances of gastritis are benign, and the symptoms subside after a few days of abstinence, but more severe forms are associated with mucosal erosions or ulcerations and may be the source of serious bleeding. The incidence of *peptic ulcer* is exceptionally high in the alcoholic population. A less frequent but serious cause of hematemesis is the so-called *Mallory-Weiss syndrome,* which is characterized by lacerations of the gastric mucosa, occurring at or just below the gastroesophageal junction. In many of these cases bleeding is preceded by an episode of forceful vomiting or protracted retching; in others, a hiatus hernia or mucosal atrophy appears to be the predisposing factor. The typical lesions appear to depend upon raising the intragastric pressure to 100 to 150 mm Hg, i.e., to the range of pressure attained by normal subjects during a period of induced straining and retching.

Patients admitted to the hospital following a period of prolonged drinking and severe dietary depletion almost invariably show enlargement of the liver because of infiltration of the parenchymal cells with fat. Fatty hepatosis, as this is called, is essentially a reversible state, provided that the patient remains abstinent and receives a nutritious diet. About 10 percent of patients with severe alcoholism develop a permanent form of liver disease, i.e., cirrhosis, in which a diffuse proliferation of fibrous tissue replaces the normal lobular architecture of the organ. The alcoholic variety of cirrhosis (also referred to as Laennec's or portal cirrhosis) is discussed in Chap. 296.

The excessive use of alcohol is also a significant factor in the causation of pancreatitis. The mildest form of this disorder may be attributed to gastritis or may go unnoticed, unless revealed by a transient elevation of the serum amylase level. In more severe form pancreatitis presents as an acute abdominal catastrophe, i.e., with epigastric pain, vomiting, and rigidity of the upper abdominal muscles. These symptoms closely simulate those of perforated peptic ulcer, so that an operation may be performed needlessly. In these circumstances the pancreas appears tense and edematous, often with a serosanguineous exudation of fluid on its surface. The most severe form of acute pancreatitis is characterized by widespread necrosis and hemorrhage (see Chap. 302).

It is generally believed that acute pancreatitis is caused by the activation of proteolytic enzymes, with consequent autodigestion of the pancreatic tissue. Two factors are probably important in the pathogenesis: (1)

the powerful stimulating effect of alcohol on the gastric acidity, which stimulates the production of secretin and in turn provokes an increase in the formation of pancreatic enzymes; (2) obstruction to the flow of pancreatic enzymes, the result of inflammatory changes in the duodenum, with edema and spasm of the sphincter of Oddi.

Alcoholics are also likely to develop a chronic relapsing form of pancreatitis. The type associated with irregular calcification of the pancreas is practically confined to alcoholics. The cause of this disorder is obscure, but the occurrence of chronic pancreatic changes in patients with kwashiorkor, as well as in rats given a methionine-deficient diet, suggests that it may be due to nutritional deficiency. This subject is discussed further in Chap. 74.

[The *management* of the various gastrointestinal complications of alcoholism is considered in the section dealing with these diseases (Chaps. 280 and 283).]

Effect on nervous system A large number of neurologic disorders are associated with alcoholism. The factor common to all of them, of course, is the abuse of alcohol, but the mechanism by which alcohol produces its effects varies widely from one group of disorders to another. The classification which follows is based for the most part on known mechanisms.

I Alcohol intoxication—drunkenness, coma, excitement ("pathologic intoxication")
II The abstinence or withdrawal syndrome—tremulousness, hallucinosis, "rum fits," delirium tremens, and auditory hallucinosis
III Nutritional diseases of the nervous system secondary to alcoholism
  A Wernicke-Korsakoff syndrome
  B Polyneuropathy
  C Retrobulbar neuropathy ("tobacco-alcohol amblyopia")
  D Pellagra
IV Diseases of uncertain pathogenesis, associated with alcoholism
  A Cerebellar degeneration
  B Marchiafava-Bignami disease
  C Central pontine myelinolysis
  D Cerebral atrophy
  E "Alcoholic" cardiomyopathy and myopathy
V Neurologic disorders consequent upon Laennec's cirrhosis and portal-systemic shunts
  A Hepatic stupor and coma
  B Chronic hepatocerebral degeneration

Alcohol intoxication Drunkenness is such a common phenomenon that its psychologic and physical manifestations require little elaboration. The signs consist of varying degrees of exhilaration and excitement, loss of restraint, irregularity of behavior, loquacity, slurred speech, incoordination of movement and gait, irritability, drowsiness, and, in advanced cases, stupor and coma. On rare occasions acute intoxication is characterized by an outburst of irrational, combative, and destructive behavior, which terminates when the patient falls into a deep stupor and of which he may later have no memory. This state has been referred to as "pathologic intoxication" or "acute alcoholic paranoid state." Allegedly this reaction may follow the ingestion of small amounts of alcohol, and it has been variously ascribed to constitutional differences in susceptibility to alcohol, previous cerebral injury, and "an underlying epileptic predisposition." However, there are no critical data to support any of these contentions. An analogy may be drawn between this state of alcoholic excitement and a similar reaction which occasionally complicates the administration of barbiturates.

The symptoms of intoxication caused by alcohol acting on nerve cells resemble those of general anesthetics. The margin of safety, i.e., the difference in dose levels required for surgical anesthesia and that which dangerously depresses respiration, is very narrow, a fact which accounts for the occasional fatality in cases of alcoholic narcosis.

The signs of alcohol intoxication are distinctive and as a rule present no problem in diagnosis or management. On the other hand, coma due to alcohol may present difficulties in differential diagnosis. It should be stressed that the diagnosis of alcoholic coma is made not merely on the basis of a flushed face, stupor, and the odor of alcohol, but only after the careful exclusion of all other causes of coma (see Chap. 22). Furthermore, alcoholic coma is not always benign, as are the more common manifestations of intoxication. Serious depression of respiration, heralded by a loss of corneal and pupillary reflexes, calls for the use of respiratory stimulants and the treatment of peripheral vascular collapse, if this should manifest itself.

TREATMENT OF ALCOHOL INTOXICATION Mild to moderate degrees of intoxication require no special treatment. Certain time-honored remedies such as a cold shower, strong coffee, forced activity, or induction of vomiting may be helpful, but there is no evidence that any of these methods influences the rate of disappearance of alcohol from the blood. *Alcoholic stupor* is also a short, self-limited state, and if the vital signs are normal no special therapeutic measures are necessary. *Pathologic intoxication* may require the use of restraints and the parenteral administration of phenobarbital sodium (200 mg subcutaneously) or amobarbital sodium (500 mg intramuscularly), repeated once in 30 to 40 min if necessary.

Coma due to alcohol intoxication represents a medical emergency. The main object of treatment is to prevent respiratory suppression and the complications which it engenders. The management of the comatose patient is described in Chap. 22. One should like to be able to lower the blood alcohol level as rapidly as possible. The administration of insulin and glucose for this purpose is not of proved value. Analeptic drugs such as amphetamine, pentylenetetrazole (Metrazole), and various mixtures of caffeine and picrotoxin are antagonistic to alcohol only insofar as they are powerful cerebral cortical stimulants and overall nervous system excitants; they do not hasten the combustion of alcohol.

THE ABSTINENCE OR WITHDRAWAL SYNDROME

A second category of alcoholic neurologic disease comprises the tremulous, hallucinatory, epileptic, and delirious states. Although a sustained period of chronic intoxication is the underlying factor in each of these disorders, the symptoms become manifest only after a period of relative or absolute abstinence from alcohol—hence the designation *abstinence* or *withdrawal syndrome*. Each of the major manifestations of the withdrawal syndrome may occur distinct from the others and will be so described; more frequently, however, they occur in various combinations. The prototype of the patients afflicted with these symptoms is the spree or periodic drinker, although the steady drinker is not immune if, for some reason, he or she stops drinking.

Tremulousness By far the most common manifestation of the abstinence syndrome is a state of tremulousness, commonly referred to as "the shakes" or "the jitters," combined with general irritability and gastrointestinal symptoms, particularly nausea and vomiting. The symptoms first show themselves after several days of drinking, usually in the morning, after the short period of abstinence that occurs during sleep. The patient then needs to "quiet his nerves" by a few drinks. Indeed his symptoms are relieved by alcohol, only to return on successive mornings with increasing persistence and severity. The usual spree lasts about 2 weeks, but the duration varies greatly. It is terminated not only because of recurrent tremor and vomiting, but for one or more other reasons such as lack of funds, weakness, self-disgust, injury, illness or collapse. The symptoms then become greatly augmented, reaching their peak intensity 24 to 36 hr after the complete cessation of drinking.

At this stage, the patient presents a distinctive clinical picture. He is alert and startles easily. His face is deeply flushed, the conjunctivas are injected, and there is usually a tachycardia. Anorexia, nausea, and retching are always in evidence. He may complain of insomnia and craves rest and sleep. Preoccupied with his misery, inattentive, and disinclined to answer questions, he may respond in a rude or perfunctory manner. The patient may be mildly disoriented in time and have a poor memory for events of the last few days of his drinking spree but shows no serious confusion, being generally aware of his surroundings and the nature of his illness.

Generalized tremor is an outstanding feature of this illness. It is of fast frequency (6 to 8 tremors per sec), slightly irregular, and variable in its severity, tending to diminish when the patient is in quiet surroundings and increasing with motor activity or emotional stress. The tremor may be so violent that the patient cannot stand without help, speak clearly, or feed himself. Sometimes there is little objective evidence of tremor, and the patient complains only of being "shaky inside."

Although the flushed facies, anorexia, tachycardia, and tremor subside to a large extent within a few days, the patient does not regain his full composure for a much longer time. The overalertness, tendency to startle easily, and jerkiness of movement may persist for a week or longer; the feeling of uneasiness may not leave the patient completely for 10 or 14 days, and only at the end of this time is he able to sleep undisturbed, without sedation. An attempt should be made to keep the patient in the hospital for this length of time. To discharge him after a few days increases the likelihood that he will turn to alcohol to suppress his still-present tenseness and sleeplessness.

Hallucinosis Symptoms of disordered perception occur in about one-quarter of the tremulous patients. The patient may complain of "bad dreams"—nightmarish episodes associated with disturbed sleep, which are difficult to separate from real experience. Sounds and shadows may be misinterpreted, or familiar objects may be distorted and assume unreal forms. Although these are not hallucinations in the strict sense of the term, they represent the most common forms of disordered sense perception in the alcoholic. Hallucinations may be purely visual or auditory in type, mixed visual and auditory, and occasionally tactile or olfactory. There is little evidence to support the popular belief that certain visual hallucinations are specific to alcoholism. They are more commonly animate than inanimate and may comprise various forms of human, animal, or insect life. They may occur singly or in panoramas; they may appear shrunken or enlarged; they may be natural in appearance or take distorted and hideous forms (see Chap. 26).

Acute and chronic auditory hallucinosis This phenomenon merits separate consideration. For many years, an alcoholic psychosis has been recognized in which vivid auditory hallucinations are the major abnormality. Kraepelin referred to this as the *hallucinatory insanity of drunkards or alcoholic mania*. The central feature of the illness, in the beginning, is the occurrence of auditory hallucinations despite an otherwise clear sensorium, i.e., the patients are not confused, disoriented, or obtunded and have an intact memory. The hallucinations are almost always vocal in nature, although there may be other auditory phenomena, such as the sound of running motors, buzzing, music, ringing of telephones, or dogs barking. When the voices can be identified, they are attributed to the patient's family, friends, or neighbors, rarely to God, radio, or radar. The voices may be addressed directly to the patient, but more frequently they discuss him in the third person. In the majority of cases the voices are maligning, reproachful, or threatening in nature and are disturbing to the patient; a significant proportion, however, are not unpleasant and leave the patient undisturbed. The voices are intensely real and vivid, and they tend to be exteriorized; i.e., they come from behind the door, from the corridor, or through the floor. Another quality of these hallucinations (and of visual ones) is the appropriateness of the patient's emotional response to them. He may call on the police for protection or barricade himself against invaders; he may even attempt suicide to avoid what the voices threaten. The hallucinations are most prominent during the night, and their duration varies greatly—they may be momentary, or they may recur intermittently for days on end and, in exceptional instances, for weeks or months.

Most patients, while hallucinating, have no appreciation of the unreality of their hallucinations. As improvement occurs, the patient begins to doubt their reality, is reluctant to talk about them, and may even question whether he had been sane during the episode. Full recovery is characterized by the realization that the voices were imaginary and by the ability to recall, sometimes with remarkable clarity, the abnormal thought content of parts of the psychotic episode.

A unique feature of this psychosis is the evolution of a chronic auditory hallucinosis in a small proportion of the patients. The patient becomes quiet and resigned, even though the hallucinations remain threatening and derogatory. Ideas of reference and influence and other poorly systematized paranoid delusions become prominent. At this stage these patients show many of the symptoms of schizophrenia—illogical thinking, vagueness, tangential associations, and a dissociation of affect and of thought content. There is some evidence that repeated attacks of acute auditory hallucinosis render the patient more vulnerable to this paranoid schizophrenic syndrome.

Withdrawal seizures ("rum fits") In this particular setting (i.e., where relative or absolute abstinence follows a period of chronic inebriation) there is a marked tendency to develop convulsive seizures. Over 90 percent of seizures occur during the 7- to 48-hr period following the cessation of drinking, with a peak incidence between 13 to 24 hr after, and they continue for a few days. During the period of seizure activity the electroencephalogram may be abnormal, but it reverts to normal in a matter of days, even though the patient may go on to develop delirium tremens. Also during the period of seizure activity the patient is unusually sensitive to stroboscopic stimulation. About half these patients respond to this activating procedure with generalized myoclonus (photomyoclonus) or a convulsive seizure (photoconvulsion). In contrast, patients with idiopathic epilepsy rarely show this type of response to photic stimulations.

Seizures occurring in the abstinence period have a number of other distinctive features. There may be only a single seizure, but in the majority of cases they occur in short bursts of two to six, or even more, and an occasional patient develops status epilepticus. The seizures are grand mal in type, i.e., major generalized convulsions with loss of consciousness. They may, however, be multifocal in nature, particularly under the influence of anticonvulsant medication. A single unilateral patterned seizure suggests that a focal lesion (usually traumatic) will be found. Almost one-third of the patients with generalized seizure activity go on to develop delirium tremens, in which case the seizures invariably precede the delirium. The postictal confusional state may blend imperceptibly with the onset of the delirium, or there may be a clearing of the postictal state, over several hours or even a day or two, before the delirium sets in. Seizures of this type occur in patients who have been drinking for many years, so that they have to be distinguished from other forms of epilepsy beginning in adult life.

It is suggested that the term *rum fits,* i.e., the words used by the alcoholic himself, be reserved for seizures which possess the attributes described above. This would serve to distinguish this form of seizure activity, which occurs only in the immediate abstinence period, from that which occurs in the interdrinking period, long after withdrawal has been accomplished. This is not to deny that the "idiopathic" or posttraumatic forms of epilepsy may be influenced by alcohol. In patients with idiopathic or posttraumatic epilepsy, a seizure or seizures may be precipitated by only a short period of drinking (e.g., a weekend, or even one evening of heavy social drinking); interestingly, in these circumstances, the seizures occur not when the patient is intoxicated, but usually the morning after, in the "sobering-up" period.

Electroencephalographic (EEG) findings in alcoholic subjects with "rum fits" do not support the notion that the seizures merely represent latent epilepsy made manifest by alcohol. Instead, the EEG reflects a sequence of changes induced by alcohol itself—a decrease in the frequency of brain waves during the period of chronic intoxication; a rapid return of the EEG to normal immediately after cessation of drinking; the occurrence of a brief period of dysrhythmia (sharp waves and paroxysmal changes) which coincides with the flurry of convulsive activity; and again, a rapid return of the EEG to normal. Except for the transient dysrhythmia in the withdrawal period, the incidence of EEG abnormalities in patients who have had "rum fits" is not greater than in the normal population, in sharp contrast to patients who are indeed subject to seizures (see Chap. 322).

Delirium tremens This is the most dramatic and grave of all the alcoholic complications. It is characterized by profound confusion, delusions, vivid hallucinations, tremor, agitation, and sleeplessness, as well as by increased activity of the autonomic nervous system, i.e., dilated pupils, fever, tachycardia, and profuse perspiration. The clinical features of delirium have been presented in detail in Chap. 26.

Delirium tremens develops in one of several settings. The patient, an excessive and steady drinker of many years' duration, may have been admitted to the hospital for an unrelated illness, accident, or operation, and 3 to 4 days later becomes delirious. Or, following a prolonged spree, he may have already experienced several days of tremulousness and hallucinosis, or one or more seizures, and may even be recovering from these symptoms, when he suddenly develops delirium tremens.

In the majority of cases delirium tremens is benign and short-lived, ending as abruptly as it begins. Consumed by the relentless activity and wakefulness of several days' duration, the patient falls into a deep sleep; he awakens lucid, quiet, and exhausted, with virtually no memory for the events of the delirious period. Less commonly, the delirious state subsides gradually; more rarely still, there may be one or more relapses, several discrete episodes of delirium being separated by lucidity, the entire process lasting for as little as several days or as long as 4 to 5 weeks. The recurrent type presents the most confusing picture of all, for the delirious periods may be of varying severity and duration, and the lucid intervals of varying degrees of completeness. When the delirium occurs as a single episode, the duration is 72 hr or less in over 80 percent of the cases.

About 15 percent of cases of delirium tremens, as defined above, end fatally. In the majority of these there is an associated infectious illness or injury, but in a few no other discernible complicating illness. Frequently, these latter patients die in a state of hyperthermia or peripheral circulatory collapse; in some, death comes so suddenly that the nature of the terminal events cannot be determined.

Closely related to typical delirium tremens and about as common are the *atypical delirious-hallucinatory* or *confusional states,* in which one facet of the delirium tremens complex assumes prominence to the practical exclusion of the other symptoms. The patient may simply exhibit a transient state of quiet confusion, agitation, and peculiar behavior that may last several weeks (simulating Korsakoff's psychosis), or he may become violent and disturbed. Other patients present a vivid delusional state and abnormal behavior, consistent with their false beliefs. Unlike typical delirium tremens, the atypical states always present as a single circumscribed episode without recurrences, are only rarely preceded by epilepsy, and do not end fatally. This may be another way of saying that they are a partial or less severe form of the disease.

Pathologic examination is singularly unrevealing in patients with delirium tremens. Edema and brain swelling have been absent in the authors' pathologic material except when there was shock, terminal hypoxia, or electrolyte imbalance, and there have not been any significant microscopic changes in the brain. Abnormalities of the blood nonprotein nitrogen, carbon dioxide, spinal fluid, serum sodium, chloride, sugar, potassium, and calcium occur unpredictably. The electroencephalographic findings have been discussed in relation to alcoholic epilepsy.

The *pathogenesis* of the tremulous-hallucinatory-delirious state has been a matter of considerable controversy. The idea that it simply represents the most severe form of alcohol intoxication is not tenable. It is obvious that the symptoms of toxicity, consisting of slurred speech, uninhibited behavior, staggering gait, stupor, and coma, are distinctive and different from the symptom complex of tremor, hallucinations, fits, and delirium. The former symptoms are associated with an elevated blood alcohol level, whereas the latter become evident only when the blood alcohol is reduced. Finally, the toxic symptoms increase in severity as more alcohol is consumed, whereas tremor and hallucinosis and even full-blown delirium tremens may be nullified by the administration of alcohol.

Although much discussed in the past, there is no evidence that endocrine abnormality or nutritional deficiency plays a role in the abstinence syndrome. Instead, it is of neural origin—the parts of the nervous system which became habituated to alcohol appear to overact when it is withdrawn. The duration of the illness seems to correspond to the time required for neuronal excitability to return to normal. The lesion is a biochemical one, of obscure nature, still.

It has been shown that the early phase of alcohol withdrawal (beginning 7 to 8 hr after cessation of drinking) is regularly attended by a drop in serum magnesium levels and a rise in arterial pH values, on the basis of respiratory alkalosis. Indeed it is possible that the compounded effect of these two factors, both of which are associated with hyperexcitability of the nervous system, might be responsible for seizures and perhaps for other symptoms which characterize the early phase of withdrawal. The elevation in pH is explained as withdrawal release of the neurons of the "respiratory center," which had been previously rendered insensitive to circulating CO_2. In the "rebound" phase these cells become more sensitive than normal to CO_2, with resultant hyperventilation and respiratory alkalosis. But as an explanation of delirium tremens, hypomagnesemia is probably not important, since the serum magnesium level has frequently been restored to normal before the onset of the delirium.

Treatment of the alcoholic withdrawal syndrome The general aspects of management of the delirious and confused patient have been described in Chap. 26.

More specifically the treatment of delirium tremens begins with a careful search, followed by appropriate treatment, for associated injuries or infections, particularly head injury with cerebral lacerations or subdural hematoma, and pneumonia or meningitis. Because of the frequency and seriousness of these complications, skull and chest roentgenograms should be obtained and lumbar puncture should be performed routinely. In severe forms of delirium tremens, the temperature, pulse, and blood pressure should be recorded at 30-min intervals in anticipation of peripheral circulatory collapse and hyperthermia, which, added to the effects of injury and infection, are the usual causes of death in this disease. In the case of shock, one must act quickly, utilizing whole-blood transfusions, fluids, and vasopressor drugs. The occurrence of hyperthermia demands the use of a cooling mattress in addition to specific treatment for any infection that may be present.

A very important element in treatment is the correction of fluid and electrolyte imbalance. Severe degrees of agitation and perspiration may require the administration of 6,000 ml fluid daily, of which 1,500 ml should be normal saline solution. The specific electrolytes and the amounts in which they are added are governed by the laboratory values for these electrolytes. Occasionally, the withdrawal syndrome is characterized by hypoglycemia, in which case the administration of glucose becomes of prime importance.

A special danger attends the use of glucose solutions in alcoholic patients. Usually these persons have subsisted on a diet disproportionately high in carbohydrate (alcohol is metabolized almost entirely as carbohydrate) and low in thiamine, and their reserves of B vitamins may have been further reduced by gastroenteritis and diarrhea. The administration of intravenous glucose may serve to consume the last available stores of thiamine and precipitate Wernicke's disease. For this reason it is good practice to add B vitamins in all cases requiring parenterally administered glucose, even though the alcoholic disorder under treatment, i.e., delirium tremens, is not primarily due to vitamin deficiency.

In respect to the use of drugs, it is important to distinguish between mild withdrawal symptoms, which are essentially benign and responsive to practically all sedative drugs, and delirium tremens, which has a serious mortality and is relatively unresponsive to drugs. In the case of minor withdrawal symptoms, the purpose of medication is to ensure rest and sleep. In delirium tremens, the object of drug therapy is to blunt agitation and prevent exhaustion and facilitate the administration of parenteral fluid and nursing care; one does not attempt to suppress agitation at all costs, since to accomplish this requires an amount of drug that might seriously depress respiratory function.

A wide variety of drugs is effective in controlling withdrawal symptoms. Some of the more common ones are prochlorperazine (Compazine), chlorpromazine (Thorazine), promazine (Sparine), promethazine (Phenergan), meprobamate, reserpine, chlordiazepoxide (Librium), and benactyzine. There is little difference in the therapeutic efficacy of these drugs, and it is not certain that any of them can prevent hallucinosis or delirium tremens, or shorten the duration or alter the mortality rate of the latter disorder. In general, phenothiazine drugs should be avoided because of their epileptigenic properties. Furthermore, the advantages of these drugs over paraldehyde have not been proved by controlled studies; in fact, there is some evidence that in the more severe forms of the withdrawal syndrome paraldehyde is superior to both chlorpromazine and promazine. Paraldehyde has the additional advantage of being extremely safe provided it is freshly prepared and kept in brown, tightly stoppered bottles to prevent deterioration and the accumulation of acetaldehyde. If the patient can take paraldehyde by mouth, doses of 8 to 12 ml in orange juice should be given. It may also be administered rectally, but the intramuscular route should be avoided if possible, since it may damage nerves, and it should be given intravenously only with caution because of the danger of respiratory depression. If parenteral medication is necessary, sodium phenobarbital or sodium amytal in doses of 120 ml, repeated at 3- to 4-hr intervals, may be given, provided there is no serious liver disease. Adrenal corticotropic hormone (ACTH) and cortisone have no place in the treatment of the withdrawal syndrome. These hormones do not significantly modify the course of the abstinence syndrome and in addition have many serious disadvantages, namely, the masking of infection, a deleterious effect on tuberculosis and peptic ulcer, and a tendency to produce a negative nitrogen balance and excessive excretion of potassium. All these complications are of more than theoretical interest in the alcoholic patient.

Treatment of "rum fits" In most cases the type of convulsive seizures that occur in the withdrawal period ("rum fits") does not require the use of anticonvulsant drugs. In this setting there may be only a single seizure or a brief flurry of seizures which usually have ceased by the time that certain medicines, such as diphenylhydantoin (Dilantin), become effective. The parenteral administration of sodium phenobarbital early in the withdrawal period could conceivably prevent "rum fits" in patients with a previous history of this disorder or in those who might be expected to develop seizures on withdrawal. Also, the long-term administration of anticonvulsants is not practical; if the patient remains abstinent, he will be free of seizures, and if he resumes drinking he usually abandons his medicines. In rare instances, withdrawal seizures take the form of status epilepticus; such cases should be managed as are seizures of any other type (see Chap. 336). Alcoholics with a history of idiopathic or posttraumatic epilepsy should drink only in moderation or not at all, because of the deleterious effects of relatively short periods of drinking on their epilepsy, and they should be maintained on anticonvulsant drugs.

NUTRITIONAL DISEASES OF THE NERVOUS SYSTEM Nutritional diseases of the nervous system comprise a relatively small but serious group of illnesses in chronic alcoholics. In contrast to the role of alcohol in intoxication and abstinence syndromes, its role in these nutritional diseases is purely secondary, serving mainly to displace food in the diet. These illnesses, the role of alcohol in their production, and their treatment, are discussed in Chap. 332, Metabolic and Nutritional Diseases of the Nervous System, and Chap. 323, Diseases of the Peripheral Nervous System.

ALCOHOLIC DISEASES OF UNCERTAIN PATHOGENESIS Included in this category are several diverse disorders which are practically always encountered in alcoholic patients. Their relationship to the excessive use of alcohol is not fully understood and probably is not crucial, since all of them have been described in nonalcoholic patients. There is a considerable amount of indirect evidence that these disorders are nutritional in origin, but as yet this relationship must be regarded as unproved.

Alcoholic cerebellar degeneration This term is applied to a nonfamilial type of cerebellar ataxia which occurs in adult life against a background of prolonged ingestion of alcohol. The symptoms may progress slowly over a long period, but more frequently they evolve in a subacute fashion (several weeks or months), after which they remain stationary for many years. The signs are those of cerebellar dysfunction, affecting stance and gait predominantly. The legs are involved more frequently and severely than the arms, and nystagmus and speech disturbances are rare. Once established, the signs change very little, although some improvement of gait (due mainly to recovery from complicating polyneuropathy) may follow cessation of drinking. The essential pathologic changes consist of degeneration of varying severity of all the neurocellular elements of the cerebellar cortex, particularly of the Purkinje cells, with a striking topographic restriction to the anterior and superior aspects of the vermis and hemispheres. The disorder of stance and gait seems to be related to the lesion in the vermis, and the ataxia of the limbs to the anterior lobe of the cerebellum. A similar clinical syndrome has been observed in a few nutritionally depleted nonalcoholic patients.

It is likely that the cerebellar lesions in this disorder and in Wernicke's disease represent the same disease process. The latter designation is used when the cerebellar abnormalities are associated with the characteristic ocular and mental disorders, and the term "alcoholic" cerebellar degeneration when only the cerebellar signs are clinically manifest.

Marchiafava-Bignami disease (primary degeneration of the corpus callosum) This is a rare complication of alcoholism originally described in Italian men addicted to crude red wine. The symptoms are diverse and include psychic and emotional disorders, delirium and intellectual deterioration, convulsive seizures, and varying degrees of tremor, rigidity, paralysis, apraxia, aphasia, and sucking and grasping reflexes. The duration is variable, from several weeks to months, and recovery is possible. The pathologic picture is more constant than the clinical one. It consists of symmetrically placed areas of demyelination in the corpus callosum, particularly the middle lamina, and less consistently of the anterior commissure and other parts of the white matter. Axis cylinders are better preserved than medullated fibers in these areas, and there are appropriate reactions in the macrophages and astrocytes. Various degrees of recovery may occur if alcoholic abstinence and good nutrition are established and maintained.

Pontine myelinolysis This term refers to a unique pathologic change affecting the center of the basis pontis, in which the medullated fibers are destroyed in a single symmetric focus of varying size. In contrast, the axis cylinders, nerve cells, and blood vessels are relatively well preserved. The disease may manifest itself by pseudobulbar palsy and quadriplegia, but usually the lesion is so small that it causes no symptoms and is found only at postmortem examination. The relationship of this condition to either alcoholism or malnutrition is obscure, but most of the cases have occurred in patients with prolonged and severe nutritional depletion.

Cerebral atrophy The pathologic examination of relatively young alcoholic patients not infrequently discloses an unexpected degree of convolutional atrophy, most prominent in the frontal lobes, and a symmetric enlargement of the lateral and third ventricles. The ventricular enlargement may also be found on pneumoencephalography. In some patients these findings are associated with overt complications of alcoholism, such as the Wernicke-Korsakoff syndrome, but in many of them no other abnormalities can be found, and the history discloses no symptoms of neurologic disease. The nature of this disorder is quite unclear.

"Alcoholic" myopathy Attention has been drawn to several disorders of skeletal and cardiac muscle, apparently primary in nature, in association with chronic alcoholism. One type of myopathic syndrome, which may be generalized or focal, is characterized by the acute onset of severe pain, tenderness, and edema of muscles, accompanied by myoglobinuria, renal damage, and hyperpotassemia in severe cases. In other cases, diffuse muscle weakness is associated with hypopotassemia and vascular necrosis of muscle. Yet another type is characterized by the subacute development of weakness and atrophy of the proximal limb and girdle muscles, with "myopathic" changes in the electromyogram and elevated creatine phosphokinase levels in serum, but without local pain or edema. Muscle power is slowly restored in these patients following abstinence from alcohol and improvement in nutrition. That this disorder represents a primary affection of muscle has not been established beyond doubt. Muscle biopsies that we have examined from such patients suggest that it may represent a proximal form of polyneuropathy, despite relatively mild clinical signs of peripheral nerve disease. "Alcoholic cardiomyopathy" is the name given to a nonspecific affective of cardiac muscle which has a higher incidence in patients with chronic alcoholism than in the nonalcoholic population. The role of alcohol, malnutrition, or some hitherto unsuspected factor in the genesis of these disorders is not known, and their structural and biochemical basis requires further study (see Chap. 341).

NEUROLOGIC DISORDERS CONSEQUENT UPON CIRRHOSIS AND PORTAL-SYSTEM SHUNTS *Hepatic coma* refers to an episodic disorder of consciousness which frequently complicates (or terminates) advanced liver disease and/or portal-system shunts. It is associated with typical electroencephalographic abnormalities and intermittency of sustained muscular contraction which presents as an irregular flapping movement of the outstretched limbs (asterixis). Patients dying in hepatic coma consistently show an increase in the number and size of the protoplasmic astrocytes throughout the central nervous system, particularly in the deep layers of the cerebral and cerebellar cortex, the basal ganglions, and the dentate nuclei.

Less frequently, cirrhosis is complicated by a chronic and largely irreversible form of hepatocerebral disease, the main symptoms of which are dementia, dysarthria, ataxia, and athetosis. The brain in such cases shows not only an astrocytic hyperplasia but also a degeneration of nerve cells and fibers, the distribution of the destructive lesions following closely that of the astrocytic changes. Both hepatic coma and the chronic form of hepatocerebral disease are characterized by hyperammonemia, which is probably important in their pathogenesis. Ammonium is derived from the bacterial action on intestinal proteins and normally is converted to urea in the liver. A failure to metabolize ammonium, or perhaps some other substance absorbed from the bowel, may be the result of either hepatocellular disease or of shunting of blood around the liver. Presumably, the acute and rapidly developing effect of this toxin on the brain is episodic stupor or coma, which is reflected pathologically by a diffuse astrocytic hyperplasia; a prolongation of this effect may lead to irreversible neurologic symptoms and parenchymal lesions.

The treatment of recurrent hepatic stupor and coma consists essentially of the use of a low-protein diet and neomycin. Intractable cases of coma and protein intolerance, as well as the chronic form of hepatocerebral disease cannot, as a rule, be controlled by these medical means alone; such cases have been treated by surgical means, either by colectomy or by exclusion of the colon. Undoubtedly some patients have been helped by these surgical measures, but their precise indications and effectiveness remain to be determined. The neurologic complications of liver disease are considered further in Chaps. 291 and 332.

TREATMENT OF ALCOHOL ADDICTION. Following recovery from the acute medical and neurologic complications of alcoholism, the underlying problem—that of alcohol dependence—remains. To treat only the medical complications and to leave the management of the drinking problem to the patient himself is indeed shortsighted. Almost always drinking is resumed, with a predictable recurrence of medical illness. For this reason the physician must be prepared to deal with the addiction or at least to initiate treament.

The problem of excessive drinking is formidable but not necessarily as hopeless as it is made out to be. A common misconception among physicians is that specialized training in psychiatry and an inordinately large amount of time are required to deal with the addictive drinker. Actually, a successful program of treatment can be initiated by any interested physician, using the standard techniques of history taking, establishing rapport with the patient, and seeing him frequently, though not necessarily for prolonged periods. A useful point at which to undertake this task is during convalescence from a serious medical or neurologic complication of alcoholism or in relation to loss of employment, arrest, or threatened divorce. Such a crisis may help convince the patient, better than any argument presented by family or physician, that his drinking has reached serious proportions.

The requisite for successful treatment is total abstinence from alcohol, and for all practical purposes, this represents the only permanent solution. It is generally agreed that any attempts to curb the drinking habit will fail if the patient continues to drink. There are said to be cases in which the patient has been able to reduce his intake of alcohol and eventually to drink in moderation, but they must be extremely rare. Also, it is frequently stated that the patient must recognize that he is an alcoholic, i.e., that his drinking is beyond his control, and he must express willingness to be helped. Undoubtedly there is truth in both these statements, but they should not be interpreted to mean that the patient must gain this recognition and willingness entirely on his own initiative and that he will be helped only after he does so. Actually, the physician can do a great deal to help the patient understand the nature of his problem and thus to motivate him to accept treatment. Logic and reasoning must be used to convince the patient that abstinence is preferable to chronic inebriety. The patient must be made fully aware of the medical and social consequences of continued drinking and must also be made to understand that because of some constitutional peculiarity (like that of the diabetic, who cannot handle sugar) he is incapable of drinking in moderation. These facts should be presented in much the same way as one would explain the essential features of any other disease. There is nothing to be gained from adopting a punitive or moralizing attitude; nor should the patient be given the idea that he is in no way blameworthy for his illness. There appears to be an advantage in making the patient feel that he is responsible for doing something about his drinking.

The prevalent belief that an alcoholic will not stop drinking under duress also requires qualification. In fact, one of the few careful studies of this matter disclosed that relatively few patients would have sought help unless pressure had been exerted by family or employer; furthermore, patients who came to the clinic under duress of this sort did just as well as those who came voluntarily.

If an earnest and sustained effort by the physician fails to convince the patient that alcohol offers a problem, it is usually impossible to modify his alcoholic tendency. The only way to make such an individual discontinue drinking is to commit him to a psychiatric hospital or special institution for the management of alcoholism in the hope that with forced abstinence and improvement in his physical state he will gain insight and later accept psychiatric or other forms of therapy.

On the other hand, if the patient comes to realize that his drinking is beyond control and that he needs to do something about it, his chances of being helped are raised considerably. Indeed, under these circumstances, many persons stop drinking of their own volition. Some of these patients, despite the best of intentions, will relapse. This should not serve as an excuse to abandon treatment; many patients have attained a state of prolonged sobriety after several false starts. A number of methods have proved valuable in the long-term management of patients. The most important of these are the use of Antabuse, aversion treatment, psychotherapy, and the participation in social organizations for combating alcoholism.

Antabuse (tetraethylthiuram disulfide, disulfiram) interferes with the metabolism of alcohol, so that a patient who takes both alcohol and Antabuse accumulates an inordinate amount of acetaldehyde in the tissues, resulting in nausea, vomiting, and hypotension, sometimes pronounced in degree. It is no longer considered necessary to demonstrate these effects to the patient; it is sufficient to warn him of the severe reactions that may result if he drinks while he has the drug in his body. Treatment with Antabuse is instituted only after the patient has been sober for several days, preferably longer. It should never be given to patients with cardiac or liver disease. The drug is taken each morning, or at another suitable time daily, in a dosage of 0.5 g, preferably under supervision. This form of treatment is of particular value in the spree or periodical drinker, in whom relapse from abstinence usually represents an impulsive rather than a carefully planned or premeditated act. The patient taking Antabuse, aware of the dangers of mixing liquor and the drug, is "protected" against the impulse to drink, and this protection may be renewed every 24 hr by the simple expedient of taking a pill. The willingness with which the patient accepts this form of treatment also serves as a rough index of his motivation. Should the patient drink when he is taking Antabuse, the ensuing reaction is usually severe enough to require medical attention, and a protracted spree can thus be prevented. Antabuse may lead to a mild polyneuropathy if continued over a period of months or years.

The aversion treatment consists of the simultaneous administration of a drink of alcohol and an injection of emetin. The violent nausea and vomiting which ensue are intended to create in the patient a strong revulsion for alcohol. This form of treatment, as well as other types of conditioned reflex treatment, has been successfully employed in special clinics but has not gained widespread popularity.

Alcoholics Anonymous (AA), an informal fellowship of former alcoholics, has proved to be the single most effective force in the rehabilitation of alcoholic patients. The philosophy of this organization is embodied in their so-called "twelve steps," a series of propositions about alcohol and alcoholism which guide the patient to recovery. The AA philosophy stresses in particular the practice of making restitution, the necessity to help other alcoholics, trust in God, the group confessional, and the belief that the alocholic is powerless over alcohol. AA philosophy also embodies the 24-hr plan, in which the alcoholic strives for just 24 hr of abstinence (a concept inspired by the Sermon on the Mount) as a means of facilitating the maintenance of sobriety. Although accurate statistics are lacking, it is stated that about half the members who express more than a passing interest in the program have no relapses, and that a significant additional number relapse but eventually recover.

The methods used by AA are not suited to every patient; some prefer the more personalized approach offered by special clinics and centers for the treatment of alcoholism. The physician should, therefore, be fully aware of all the community resources which are available for the management of this problem, and should be prepared to take advantage of them in appropriate cases.

Finally, it should be noted that alcoholism is frequently associated with psychiatric disease of some other type. There is among alcoholics an increased frequency of schizophrenia, psychoneurosis, sociopathy, and particularly manic-depressive disease. In the latter case, the prevailing mood is far more often one of depression than of mania, and is more often encountered in the female who is more apt to drink under these conditions than the male. The presence of concomitant psychiatric disease complicates the management of the alcoholism, and in these circumstances expert psychiatric help should be sought.

REFERENCES

Alcohol and Health. U.S. Department of Health, Education, and Welfare Publication (HSM) 72-9099, 1971

Isbell H et al: An experimental study of the etiology of "rum fits" and delirium tremens. Quart J Stud Alcohol 16:1, 1955

Meldelson JH: Medical progress. Biologic concomitants of alcoholism. N Engl J Med 283:24, 71, 1970

Victor M: The pathophysiology of alcoholic epilepsy, in "The Addictive States." Res Publ Assoc Res Nerv Ment Dis 46:431, 1968

——: Treatment of alcoholic intoxication and the withdrawal syndrome. A critical analysis of the use of drugs and other forms of therapy. Psychosom Med 28 (4, pt. 2): 636, 1966

——, Adams RD: The effect of alcohol on the nervous system, in "Metabolic and Toxic Diseases of the Nervous System." Res Publ Assoc Res Nerv Ment Dis 32:526, 1953

——, Hope J: The phenomenon of auditory hallucinations in chronic alcoholism. J Nerv Ment Dis 126 (5,6):451, 1958

—— et al: A restricted form of cerebellar cortical degeneration occurring in alcoholic patients. AMA Arch Neurol 1:577, 1959

Wolfe SM, Victor M: The relationship of hypomagnesemia and alkalosis to alcohol withdrawal symptoms. Ann NY Acad Sci 162: 973, 1969

—— et al: Respiratory alkalosis and alcohol withdrawal. Trans Assoc Am Physicians 82:344, 1969

112 OPIATES AND OTHER SYNTHETIC ANALGESIC DRUGS

MAURICE VICTOR
RAYMOND D. ADAMS

The drugs included in this category are morphine, opium, heroin (diacetylmorphine), dihydromorphinone (Dilaudid), codeine (methylmorphine), Pantopon, dihydrocodeinone (Hycodan), dihydroxycodeinone (Eucodal), and 14-hydroxydihydromorphinone (Numorphan). The synthetic analgesics meperidine (Demerol), the meperidine derivatives, anileridine and alphaprodine (Nisentil), methadone (Dolophine or amidone), metopon (6-methyldihydromorphinone), racemorphan (Dromoran), levorphan, (*l*-Dromoran), *d*-propoxyphene (Darvon), diphenoxylate (the main component of Lomotil), and phenazocine (Prinadol) possess properties similar to those of the opiates, both in their pharmacologic effects and in the patterns of abuse, the differences being mainly quantitative. In fact, *d*-propoxyphene and Lomotil have such low addictive liabilities that they are not controlled by the federal narcotic laws. The same statement applies to the synthetic analgesic pentazocine (Talwin), and although its overall addictive quality is low, rare cases of physical dependency have been reported.

As in the case of alcohol and the barbiturates, the opiates will be considered from two points of view: (1) acute poisoning, and (2) addiction.

OPIATE POISONING Because of the high incidence of addiction, which leads to irregular and nonmedical usage of opiates, poisoning is not an infrequent accident. This may happen as a result of ingestion with suicidal intent, errors in the calculation of dosage, or unusual sensitivity. Children may exhibit an increased susceptibility to opiates, so that relatively small doses prove toxic. This is true also in adults who have myxedema, Addison's disease, chronic liver disease, or pneumonia. Acute poisoning may also overtake addicts who are unaware that tolerance for opiates declines quickly after the withdrawal of the drug: upon resuming the habit, a formerly well-tolerated dose can be fatal.

Varying degrees of unresponsiveness, shallow respirations, slow respiratory rate (e.g., two to four per minute), or periodic breathing, miosis, bradycardia, and hypothermia are the well-recognized clinical manifestations of acute poisoning. In the most advanced stage the pupils dilate, the skin and mucous membranes become cyanotic, and the circulation fails. The immediate cause of death is usually respiratory depression, with consequent asphyxia. Patients who have a cardiorespiratory arrest are sometimes left with a residuum of anoxic encephalopathy. Others recover from coma revealing in rare instances a hemiplegia, presumably due to vascular occlusion. In the stage of mild intoxication anorexia, nausea, vomiting, constipation, and loss of sexual interest are the only symptoms.

Treatment consists of gastric lavage if the drug was taken orally. This procedure may be efficacious many hours after ingestion, since one of the toxic effects of opiates is severe pylorospasm, which may cause much of the drug to be retained in the stomach. Other measures must be directed toward the maintenance of an adequate airway and oxygenation, as described in the section dealing with barbiturate intoxication below. If the patient does not respond rapidly to these measures, *N*-allylnormorphine (Nalline) should be administered. This is a specific antidote to the opiates and also to the synthetic analgesics. It is given in doses of 5 to 10 mg subcutaneously or intravenously. The improvement of circulation and respiration is usually dramatic; in fact, failure of Nalline to produce a striking improvement in respiration should cast doubt on the diagnosis of opiate intoxication. Nalline does little to restore consciousness, however, and the patient may remain drowsy for many hours. This is not harmful, provided respiration is well maintained. Since the duration of action of Nalline is shorter than that of all the analgesics except Dilaudid and meperidine, respirations may again become depressed an hour or so after the administration of the antidote. It should then be given a second time, in smaller dosage.

Once the patient regains consciousness, usually in about 8 hr, other complaints such as severe pruritus, sneezing, persistent obstipation, and urinary retention may necessitate symptomatic treatment. Nausea and severe abdominal pain, due presumably to pancreatitis (from spasm of the sphincter of Oddi), are other troublesome symptoms. The antidote must be used with great caution in an addict who has taken an overdose of opiate, because in this circumstance it may precipitate withdrawal phenomena.

In addition to the toxic effects of opiate itself, the addict is exposed to a variety of neurologic and infectious complications, resulting mainly from the injection of crude adulterants (mainly quinine, lactose, powdered milk, fruit sugars) and various infectious agents (injections often administered by unsterile methods). Amblyopia, due probably to the toxic effects of quinine in the heroin mixtures, has been reported, as well as transverse myelopathy and several types of peripheral neuropathy. The spinal cord disorder expresses itself clinically by the abrupt onset of paraplegia with a sensory level on the trunk. Pathologically, there is an acute necrotizing lesion involving both grey and white matter over a considerable vertical extent of the thoracic and occasionally the cervical region. In some cases the myelopathy has followed the first intravenous injection of heroin after a prolonged period of abstinence. Involvement of single peripheral nerves, particularly of the radial nerve, and painful affection of the branchial plexus, independent of compression and remote from the site of injection, have been observed. There are probably pressure palsies (see Chap. 323) of an unusual sequel in acute and subacute symmetric neuropathies.

An acute generalized myopathy with myoglobinuria and renal failure has been ascribed to the intravenous injection of adulterated heroin. Brawny edema and fibrosing myopathy are the sequelae common to venous obliteration resulting from the administration of heroin and its adulterants by the intramuscular and subcutaneous routes. Occasionally there may be an inexplicable swelling of an extremity (sometimes massive) into which heroin had been injected subcutaneously or intramuscularly. Infection and venous thrombosis appear to play parts in its causation.

The diagnosis of drug addiction or the suspicion of this diagnosis should always encourage surveillance for infectious complications, particularly abscesses and cellulitis at injection sites, septic thrombophlebitis, hepatitis, and periarteritis. Tetanus, endocarditis (due mainly to *Staphylococcus aureus*), spinal epidural abscess, meningitis and brain abscess, and tuberculosis are found less frequently.

OPIATE ADDICTION Just over a decade ago there were about 60,000 persons addicted to narcotic drugs in the United States, not including those who were receiving drugs because of hopeless medical diseases. This represented a relatively small public health problem, in comparison with the large numbers of patients that abused barbiturates and alcohol; and the addiction problem was confined mainly to a few cities—New York, Chicago, Los Angeles, Washington, and Detroit. In the past 10 years a remarkable increase in opiate (principally heroin) addiction has taken place. The number of addicts in the United States has risen severalfold, and in New York City alone it is estimated that there are more than 400,000.

Etiology and pathogenesis A number of factors, socioeconomic, psychologic, and pharmacologic, all contribute to the genesis of opiate addiction. In our culture, the most susceptible subjects are young men or delinquent youths living in the economically depressed areas of large cities. The onset of opiate use is usually in adolescence, with a peak at seventeen to eighteen years. Fully two-thirds of addicts start using the drug before the age of twenty-one. A disproportionately large number are American Negroes and persons of Puerto Rican or Mexican descent. Almost 90 percent of addicts engage in criminal activity, often necessary to obtain their daily ration of drug, and many of them show psychiatric disorders, psychoneurosis and psychopathy being the most common. However, the precise "personality" factor which renders them vulnerable to addiction has not been defined. Association with addicts is the chief reason for beginning addiction. A small, almost insignificant, proportion of addicts are introduced to drugs by physicians in the course of an illness.

The abuse of opiate drugs evolves in three successive phases: (1) episodic intoxication, or euphoria, (2) pharmacogenic dependence, or addiction, and (3) the propensity to "relapse after cure," or inhibition.

Some of the symptoms of opiate intoxication have already been considered. Of equal importance are the symptoms designated as *morphine euphoria,* a term which refers to the pain- and anxiety-reducing abilities of this drug, as well as to the state of elation or sense of unusual well being which it produces and which is much sought after by psychopathic thrill-seekers. Individuals who take opiates for their euphoria-producing effects quickly discover the need to increase the dose in order to obtain an effect which approaches that given by the original dose. Although the intensity of the initial euphoria is not fully recaptured, the progressively increasing dose of drug does abate the discomforts which arise as the effects of each injection wear off. In this way the use of opiates becomes self-perpetuating. At the same time a marked degree of tolerance is produced, so that enormous amounts of drugs, e.g., 5,000 mg morphine daily, have been administered without the development of toxic symptoms. The mechanism of tolerance is not understood. There is some experimental evidence that during addiction there is a progressive decrease in the capacity of the liver to demethylate morphine and other opiates.

The altered physiologic state that develops with continued use of the drug is manifested in another dramatic way at the time of withdrawal. This constitutes a specific illness, termed the *abstinence syndrome.* Strictly speaking, addiction is defined as physical or pharmacologic dependence. This definition distinguishes between *addicting drugs* (opiates, alcohol, barbiturates) and *habit-forming drugs* (bromides, cocaine, and marijuana), since no consistent abstinence symptoms follow the discontinuation of the latter group, even after prolonged exposure. Stated in another way, all addicting drugs are habit-forming, but the opposite is not true. The place of amphetamines in this scheme is uncertain. Undoubtedly they are habit-forming drugs, but chronic use is believed by some to be associated with physical dependence, evidenced by prolonged sleep [mostly rapid eye movement (REM)] followed by voracious appetite and then affective depression upon withdrawal.

The intensity of the opiate abstinence syndrome depends mainly on the dose of the drug and duration of addiction, but also on individual factors. In respect to morphine it has been found that the majority of individuals receiving 240 mg daily for 30 days or more will show moderately severe abstinence symptoms following withdrawal, whereas mild grades of abstinence may be detected following as little as 80 mg daily for a similar period.

The abstinence syndrome which occurs in the morphine addict may be taken as the prototype of the opiate group. The first 8 to 16 hr of abstinence usually pass asymptomatically. At the end of this period yawning, rhinorrhea, sweating, and lacrimation become manifest. At first mild, these symptoms increase in severity over a period of several hours and then remain constant for several days. The patient may be able to sleep during this early period but is restless, and thereafter insomnia remains a prominent feature. Dilatation of the pupils, recurring waves of gooseflesh, and twitchings of the muscles appear. The patient complains of severe aches in the back, abdomen, and legs and of hot and cold "flashes" so that he covers himself with blankets. By the end of about 36 hr the restlessness becomes more extreme, and nausea, vomiting, and diarrhea usually develop. The temperature, respiration, and blood pressure are slightly elevated. All these symptoms reach their peak intensity 48 to 72 hr after withdrawal, and then gradually decline. The abstinence syndrome is rarely fatal. After 7 to 10 days, all clinical signs of abstinence have disappeared, although the patient may complain of insomnia, nervousness, weakness, and muscle aches for several more weeks, and a small deviation of a number of physiologic variables can be detected with refined techniques for up to 10 months (protracted abstinence).

There are two types of abstinence changes—*nonpurposive* and *purposive.* The former comprise the various autonomic and neuromuscular signs and are relatively transient in nature. That these symptoms represent an altered physiologic state and are not psychic in origin has been clearly demonstrated experimentally. Physical dependence on morphine and other opiate drugs develops even in the lower limbs of dogs whose spinal cords have been transected; the flexor and crossed extensor spinal reflexes that are depressed or abolished by the opiate become remarkably exaggerated when the drug is withdrawn. The purposive changes refer to the patient's craving for the drug and the manipulative activity directed toward obtaining it. These symptoms may persist indefinitely and are important in relation to that characteristic of addiction referred to as *habituation, emotional dependence,* or *psychologic dependence.* These terms are used interchangeably and refer to the substitution of drug-seeking activities for all other aims and objects in life.

Habituation is regarded as the most important quality of addiction, since it is this feature which governs the initial use of the drug and relapse following apparent cure of addiction. An individual takes drugs initially not because he needs the drug to prevent withdrawal symptoms but because of its euphoria-producing effect, i.e., the relief of pain and emotional discomfort. Similarly, relapse to the use of the drug may occur long after the nonpurposive abstinence changes seem to have disappeared. The cause for relapse is imperfectly understood. It has been theorized that fragments of the abstinence syndrome may remain as a conditioned response, and that these abstinence signs may be evoked by the appropriate environmental stimuli. Thus, when a "cured" addict finds himself in a situation where narcotic drugs are readily available, or in circumstances that were responsible for the initial use of drugs, the incompletely extinguished drug-seeking behavior reasserts itself.

The characteristics of addiction and of abstinence are qualitatively similar with all the drugs of the opiate group as well as the related synthetic analgesics. The differences are mainly quantitative and are related to the differences in dosage, potency, and length of action. Heroin is two to three times more potent than morphine but otherwise the same; nevertheless, the heroin withdrawal syndrome encountered in hospital practice is usually mild in degree because of the low dosage of this drug in the product sold in the street. Dilaudid and metopon are more potent than morphine and have a shorter duration of action; hence the addict requires more doses per day, and the abstinence syndrome comes on and subsides more rapidly. The length of action of Dromoran is somewhat longer than that of morphine, but withdrawal phenomena are similar to those of morphine in temporal course and intensity. Abstinence symptoms from codeine, while very definite, are less than those from morphine. The addiction liabilities of Darvon are even less than those of codeine. Abstinence symptoms from methadone are less intense than those from morphine and do not become evident until 3 or 4 days after withdrawal; furthermore, this drug is qualitatively different from morphine insofar as autonomic signs are less severe in the abstinence period. For these reasons methadone is used in the treatment of morphine addiction. Demerol addiction is of particular importance because of the high incidence among doctors and nurses and because there is still a widespread belief that this drug is nonaddicting. Tolerance to the toxic effects of Demerol is not complete, so that the addict may show tremors, twitching of the muscles, confusion, hallucinations, and at times convulsions. Signs of abstinence appear 3 to 4 hr after the last dose and reach maximum intensity in 8 to 12 hr, at which time they may be worse than those of morphine abstinence. Examples are seen, however, in which the interval between withdrawal and symptoms is 7 to 8 days.

Diagnosis of addiction This is usually made by the patient's statement that he is using and needs drugs. Should he decide to conceal this fact, one must rely on collateral evidence such as miosis, needle marks, emaciation, or abscess scars. Demerol addicts are likely to have dilated pupils and muscles that twitch. A method for the testing of the urine for opiates is now generally available. The finding of morphine or other opiates (heroin is excreted as morphine) in the urine would confirm the suspicion that the patient has taken or has been given a dose of such drugs within 24 hr of the test.

Formerly it was necessary to isolate questionable cases and to observe the patient over a period of at least 2 days for signs of abstinence. Through use of the specific antagonist *N*-allylnormorphine (Nalline), a diagnosis of addiction to opiates and related analgesic drugs can be made within an hour. The Nalline should be administered only in the presence of another physician or nurse, with the full understanding and permission of the patient. A dose of 3 mg of the antagonist is given subcutaneously, and if no signs of abstinence have appeared in 20 min, an additional 5 mg is given. If no signs have appeared in another 20 min, a final dose of 8 mg is given. If the patient has taken more than occasional doses of the drug within a week of the test, the administration of Nalline will precipitate symptoms of abstinence. These become evident within 5 min of the first injection, reach their peak intensity in 20 min, begin to decline in 60 min, and disappear after 3 hr. Nalline does not precipitate abstinence symptoms in Demerol addiction, unless the patient has been taking more than 1,600 mg daily. Another morphine antagonist, naloxone hydrochloride (Narcan), is much more potent than Nalline and lacks the agonistic action of the latter drug, so that it will probably become the drug of choice where an opiate antagonistic effect is required.

Management and avoidance of addiction The ambulatory treatment of addiction never succeeds and should therefore not be undertaken, except in special settings, such as a carefully supervised methadone treatment program (see below). Addicts who are refused opiates may ask for methadone, Demerol, or Dromoran, on the ground that these drugs are synthetic and nonaddicting. These drugs are addicting and have been legally defined as opiates. The physician should also be aware that he is breaking both the letter and the spirit of the regulations if he prescribes narcotics for an addict merely for the purpose of preventing abstinence changes. Occasional exceptions may be made in cases of seriously ill addicts who are awaiting treatment in a hospital or methadone program, or of patients who are suffering from incurable, painful disease.

An alternate method, and one that is used now almost exclusively, is to substitute methadone for opiate, in the ratio of 1 mg methadone for 3 mg morphine, 1 mg heroin, or 20 mg meperidine. Since methadone is long-acting and effective orally, it need be given only twice daily by mouth—10 to 20 mg per dose being sufficient to suppress abstinence symptoms. After a stabilization period of 3 to 5 days on this dosage of methadone alone, the drug may be reduced rapidly and withdrawn over a similar period of time.

Regardless of the method of drug withdrawal employed, treatment is best carried out in an institution with proper facilities for postwithdrawal rehabilitation in a drug-free environment. If such institutional facilities are not available locally (private, municipal, or state), the patient may apply to the U.S. Attorney in his community for commitment to a Federal institution (Lexington, Kentucky, or Fort Worth, Texas) under the Narcotic Addict Rehabilitation Act (NARA) of 1966. Acceptance of the patient under the provisions of this act entails institutional treatment for up to 6 months after admission, followed by aftercare in the patient's community for 3 years.

The physician must be constantly alert to the dangers of addiction, particularly in susceptible individuals, i.e., in those with psychoneurosis, psychopathic personality, or alcoholism. The use of opiates should be limited to cases where pain is the chief problem; they should not be used primarily as sedatives, for the relief of asthma, or even in chronic pain until all other measures have been exhausted. It follows that it is most important to make a precise diagnosis of the cause of pain, since in some cases measures other than opiates will suffice, while in others, such as hysteria and depression, narcotics are contraindicated.

If narcotics have to be used for the relief of pain, consideration should be given to the choice of the appropriate drug and to the mode of administration. Morphine is still the drug of choice for most patients requiring relief of severe pain for short periods. Demerol may be useful in patients who cannot tolerate morphine. Patients with chronic pain should be managed with the least potent and smallest dosage of drug that will do the job; doses should be spaced as far apart as possible and discontinued as soon as the need for pain relief has passed. In general, the opiates should be administered orally whenever possible, and the intravenous route should be avoided, since this method produces maximum euphoria and, hence, the greatest danger of addiction. The oral administration of codeine and aspirin is a useful way to begin treatment of the patient with chronic pain. If these drugs fail to control the pain, the parenteral administration of codeine should be tried. If the more potent opiates are needed, methadone and levorphan should be used, because of their effectiveness by the oral route and the relatively slow development of tolerance. Should long-continued injections of morphine or meperidine become necessary, maximum analgesic effect is obtained with 10 mg morphine rather than with 15 mg, as is often prescribed, and with 60 to 70 mg rather than with 100 mg meperidine. In these cases, use of the narcotic antagonist pentazocine (Talwin) might be considered. It is claimed that this drug, administered parenterally in doses of 40 to 60 mg, has analgesic effects comparable with morphine and other opiates, but has few of the addicting properties. However, the respiratory depression produced by pentazocine is not counteracted by Nalline, a serious disadvantage in some patients.

Ambulatory treatment of opiate addiction The most significant development in the treatment of opiate (almost exclusively heroin) addiction has been the establishment and growth of ambulatory methadone maintenance clinics. The scope of this activity, like the incidence of addiction, cannot be stated precisely, but can be judged roughly by the fact that 50,000 addicts were participating in such programs in 1973 in New York City alone.

The method of treatment consists of the oral administration of methadone, once daily, in doses sufficient to suppress the craving for heroin and to abolish the euphoria-producing effects of that drug given intravenously (heroin blockage). The daily dosage of methadone required to achieve these effects varies between 60 and 100 mg; some patients can be maintained on as little as 40 mg per day, and with higher dosage they need take the drug only once in 48 hr. In principle, these effects could be achieved by multiple daily injections of heroin or morphine, but the effectiveness of methadone orally, its prolonged duration of action, and the fact that it precludes the desire and need for taking other opiates make methadone far more practical.

Methadone is no longer dispensed in tablet form but only as a liquid (dissolved in fruit juice), which is taken under supervision. The collection of urine samples is also supervised, and these are analyzed for opiates and other drugs, to monitor the patient's adherence to the program. Once this has been established, the patient is allowed to take home a 1- to 3-day supply. These measures are designed to prevent the diversion of methadone into illicit channels. Various forms of individual psychotherapy, group psychotherapy, social service counseling, and vocational guidance are included in most programs. The use of former heroin addicts (who are themselves on methadone treatment) as counselors is considered to be a particularly important adjunct to methadone treatment.

The results of methadone treatment are difficult to assess and vary considerably from one program to another. Even the best programs suffer an attrition rate of about 25 percent after several years. Of the patients that remain, between 80 and 95 percent achieve a high degree of social rehabilitation, i.e., they are gainfully employed and no longer engage in criminal behavior or prostitution. This has been the very notable achievement of the methadone maintenance programs.

Although the effectiveness of methadone treatment in the social rehabilitation of many addicts cannot be doubted, a number of questions about this method remain. The usual practice of methadone programs is to accept only adult addicts with a history of heroin addiction for several years. This leaves unanswered the problem of the adolescent addict. Although some individuals have been withdrawn from methadone, this has been accomplished so far in only a small number, and their capacity to maintain a drug-free existance remains to be determined. This means that the large majority of addicts now enrolled in methadone programs are committed to an indefinite period of methadone maintenance, and the effects of such a regimen are uncertain.

An alternate method of ambulatory treatment of the opiate addict centers about the use of the narcotic antagonist cyclazocine. After withdrawal of the opiate, cyclazocine is administered orally, in increasing amounts over a period of 2 to 6 weeks, until a dosage of 2 mg per 70 kg is being taken twice daily. The cyclazocine-stabilized individual is highly refractory to the euphoria-producing and pharmacologic effects of opiates. The idea of treatment is to continue the administration of cyclazocine until all drug-seeking behavior is extinguished, after which it is withdrawn. The value of this kind of "extinction therapy" has not yet been determined, but the results in some patients have been encouraging, and the search for improved methods of using opiate antagonists continues.

REFERENCES

Ball JC, Chambers CK (eds): *The Epidemiology of Opiate Addiction in the United States,* Springfield, Ill.: Charles C Thomas, 1970

Dole VP, Nyswander ME: Methadone maintenance and its implication for theories of narcotic addiction. Res Publ Assoc Res Nerv Ment Dis 46:359, 1968

Isbell H: Perspectives in research on opiate addiction. Br J Addict 57:17, 1961

Martin WR: The basis and possible utility of the use of opioid antagonists in the ambulatory treatment of the addict. Res Publ Assoc Res Nerv Ment Dis 46:367, 1968

Richter RW et al: Neurological complications of heroin addiction. Bull NY Acad Med 49:3, 1972

Wikler A: Narcotics: The effect of pharmacologic agents on the nervous system. Res Publ Assoc Res Nerv Ment Dis 37:334, 1959

———: Drug dependence, p. 1, in *Clinical Neurology,* eds AB Baker, LH Baker, Hagerstown, Md.: Harper & Row, 1971

113 BARBITURATES

MAURICE VICTOR
RAYMOND D. ADAMS

The high incidence of addiction, suicides, and accidental deaths attributable to the improper use of the barbiturate drugs is a matter of continuing concern to the medical profession. The production of barbiturates greatly exceeds the amount needed for therapeutic purposes; almost 500,000 kg is produced each year in the United

States, enough to supply thirty 60-mg barbiturate capsules for every person in the country. It is estimated that barbiturates account for 20 percent of acute poisonings admitted to general hospitals and that they are responsible for 6 percent of suicides and 18 percent of accidental deaths, figures exceeded by no other single poison. Despite an estimated mortality rate of only 8 percent of hospitalized cases, barbiturates reportedly cause about 1,500 deaths annually in the United States. This figure is probably a gross underestimation, since in 1964 there were over 2,200 registered deaths in Great Britain due to barbiturate poisoning and for the period 1957 to 1963, an average of 166 fatalities occurred yearly in New York City alone.

About 50 barbiturates have been marketed for clinical use, but only the following are encountered with any frequency: barbital (Veronal), phenobarbital (Luminal), diallylbarbituric acid (Dial), amobarbital (Amytal), aprobarbital (Alurate), pentobarbital (Nembutal), secobarbital (Seconal), and thiopental (Pentothal). In the United States, pentobarbital, secobarbital, and amobarbital are the most commonly abused barbiturates. These drugs are similar pharmacologically and differ only in their speed of onset and duration of action.

In addition to the barbiturates, a number of nonbarbiturate sedative and hypnotic drugs have to be considered, since they have been shown to possess very much the same intoxicating and addicting properties as the barbiturates.

The clinical problems posed by the barbiturates differ considerably, however, depending on whether the intoxication is acute or chronic, and these two types will be treated separately.

ACUTE BARBITURATE INTOXICATION Acute barbiturate intoxication results from the ingestion of large amounts of the drug either accidentally or with suicidal intent, the incidence of the two types being about equal. An uncommon form of accidental poisoning occurs in individuals who are intoxicated with barbiturates or with alcohol and who, being confused, ingest more of the drug than was intended. This type of poisoning has been termed *involuntary suicide.*

The ingestion of barbiturates with suicidal intent is most frequently the act of a depressed person. An individual with hysteria or psychopathic personality may take an overdose as a suicidal gesture and sometimes become seriously intoxicated because of a miscalculation or ignorance of the toxic dosage. At times, no psychiatric disease is present, the drug being taken impulsively or while the patient is inebriated. The combination of alcohol and barbiturate intoxication is frequent and particularly dangerous, since these drugs have an additive effect.

Site and mode of action of barbiturates Barbiturates decrease the excitability of nerve cells, although the mechanism is not fully understood. Attempts have been made to localize the action of barbiturates to certain anatomic regions, or even to specific nuclei within the nervous system, but it would appear that all parts are to some extent sensitive to the drug. Nevertheless, the reticular formation of the thalami and midbrain are particularly susceptible. There is little experimental evidence to support the clinical impression that with the administration of barbiturates the cerebral cortex is affected first and then the lower centers. Reflex and other activity of the nervous system are probably depressed, although in some cases the spinal reflexes appear to be accentuated in the early stages of poisoning.

Symptoms and signs The symptoms and signs of acute barbiturate intoxication vary with the type and the amount of drug, as well as with the length of time that has elapsed since it was ingested. Pentobarbital and secobarbital produce their effects quickly, and recovery is relatively rapid. Phenobarbital induces coma more slowly, and its effects tend to be prolonged. The duration of action of these drugs can be judged from the hypnotic effect of an average oral dose. In the case of the long-acting barbiturates, such as phenobarbital, barbital, and diallylbarbituric acid, it lasts 6 hr or more; with the intermediate-acting drugs, amobarbital and aprobarbital, 3 to 6 hr; with the short-acting drugs, secobarbital and pentobarbital, less than 3 hr.

In general, much larger doses of long-acting barbiturates are required to produce a depth of unconsciousness comparable with that produced by the short-acting ones. The ingestion by adults of more than 3.0 g secobarbital, pentobarbital, amobarbital, or diallybarbituric acid at one time may be fatal unless intensive and skillful treatment is applied promptly; it has been estimated that to produce a comparable effect, the following amounts of long-acting barbiturates would have to be ingested: 6.0 to 9.0 g phenobarbital, 5.0 to 20.0 g barbital, and 15.0 g aprobarbital. Because of the serious complications of prolonged coma, the fatalities are greater with the long-acting than with the short-acting drugs.

Clinically, it is useful to recognize three grades of severity of acute barbiturate intoxication, particularly in regard to prognosis and treatment. Mild intoxication follows the ingestion of approximately 0.6 g pentobarbital or its equivalent. The patient is drowsy or asleep, a state from which he is readily roused by calling his name loudly or by shaking him. The symptoms resemble those of alcohol intoxication, except that the face is not flushed, the conjunctivas are not suffused, and there is no odor of alcohol. The patient thinks slowly, and there may be mild disorientation, lability of mood, impairment of judgment, slurred speech, drunken gait, and nystagmus. Reflex activity and vital signs are not affected.

Moderate intoxication follows the ingestion of five to ten times the oral hypnotic dose. Here the state of consciousness is more severly depressed and is usually accompanied by depressed or absent deep reflexes and slow but not shallow respiration. Corneal reflexes are retained, with occasional exceptions. At times the patient can be roused by vigorous manual stimulation; when awakened, he is confused and dysarthric, and after a few moments he drifts back into coma. At other times the patient cannot be roused by any means. In the latter case the depth of coma and seriousness of the respiratory depression may be roughly judged by the response of respiration to painful stimulation such as the application of firm pressure to the sternum or supraorbital ridge or to the inhalation of 10% carbon dioxide. If these stimuli cause an increase in the depth and rate of respiration, the outlook for recovery is good, and only symptomatic treatment is indicated.

Severe intoxication occurs with the ingestion of fifteen to twenty times the oral hypnotic dose. The patient cannot be roused by any of the means indicated. Respiration is slow and shallow or irregular, and pulmonary edema and cyanosis may be present. The deep tendon reflexes are usually but not invariably absent. Most often, the patients show no response to plantar stimulation, but in those who do, the plantar responses are extensor. In the most advanced cases the corneal and gag reflexes may also be abolished. Ordinarily the pupillary light reflex is retained in severe intoxication and is lost only if the patient is asphyxiated. In the early hours of coma, there may be a phase of rigidity of the limbs, hyperactive reflexes, ankle clonus, extensor plantar signs, and decerebrate posturing; persistence of these signs indicates a severe degree of anoxia. The temperature may be subnormal, the pulse thready and rapid, and the blood pressure at shock levels.

Diagnosis The diagnosis of barbiturate intoxication is made from the history and physical findings. If a reasonable suspicion of the diagnosis exists, then a careful search for drugs or their containers may be rewarding. One should also examine the mouth and gastric contents for any characteristically colored capsules. Acute barbiturate intoxication which presents as a state of coma must be distinguished from other forms of coma by the method outlined in Chap. 22, Coma and Related Disturbances of Consciousness. Actually there are few conditions other than barbiturate intoxication which cause a flaccid coma with reactive pupils, hypothermia, and hypotension. Glutethimide poisoning may produce an identical clinical picture, excepting that the pupils are fixed (a parasympathomimetic action). In the differential diagnosis, hysteria presents the main problem.

The use of gas chromatography has provided a reliable means of identifying the type and amount of barbiturate in the blood. The major virtue of this method is in determining the precise cause of coma when this is in question. The blood level also helps to identify the drug as long- or short-acting, thus giving information as to whether the therapeutic problem will be short or prolonged. A blood barbiturate level of 2 mg per 100 ml in a *comatose* patient is usually due to poisoning with secobarbital or pentobarbital; although the immediate mortality is high in such instances, the therapeutic problem will be short. A level of 11.5 to 12.0 mg per 100 ml is usually due to poisoning with barbital or phenobarbital, and the comatose state will be prolonged. Because of the potentiating effects of alcohol, a patient who has ingested both drugs may be comatose with relatively low blood barbiturate levels. For this reason, and also because of differences in individual tolerance, the correlation between blood barbiturate levels and depth of coma is not entirely dependable.

The *electroencephalogram* may also be useful in diagnosis, since characteristic patterns accompany barbiturate intoxication. In mild intoxication, the normal activity is replaced by fast activity, in the range of 20 to 30 cycles per sec, and is most prominent in the frontal regions. In more severe intoxication, the fast waves become less regular and interspersed with 3- to 4-per-sec slow activity. In the most advanced cases, there are short periods of suppression of all activity, separated by bursts of slow (delta) waves of variable frequency.

Management The management of acute barbiturate intoxication depends on its severity. In mild or moderate intoxication, recovery is the rule, and no vigorous treatment is required. The mildly intoxicated patient should be watched closely for signs of deepening coma, and analeptics such as coffee or parenteral caffeine sodium benzoate may be used. If the patient is unresponsive, special attention should be given to maintaining respiration and urinary excretion and to the prevention of infection. It is most important to maintain a patent airway, at first by the insertion of an endotracheal tube; suctioning should be used when necessary, and the patient should be turned frequently. Tracheotomy and bronchoscopic suctioning usually become necessary if atelectasis becomes manifest, or if intubation must be maintained for longer than 48 hr. If there is any risk of respiratory depression or underventilation, it is advisable to support respiration, so as to provide adequate oxygenation and minimize the risk of atelectasis.

Cases of severe respiratory depression, with cyanosis and pupillary dilatation, represent a serious medical emergency. A clear airway should be secured immediately and some form of assisted respiration begun with an automatic intermittent positive-pressure respirator. If the patient is in shock, the foot of the bed should be elevated, and norepinephrine and whole blood or plasma administered. Catheterization is required to determine the adequacy of urinary output, to obtain samples for laboratory examination, and to prevent distention of the bladder. Since the amount of barbiturate cleared by the kidney is directly proportional to the amount of urine formed, 8 to 10 liters of 5% glucose in saline solution should be given daily. Forced diuresis is also important because toxic amounts of barbiturate have an antidiuretic effect. Coma of any significant duration requires the administration of other electrolytes as well, the amounts being governed by their serum and urinary values. The occurrence of pulmonary and urinary infections calls for the use of appropriate antibiotic treatment.

If ingestion has been recent, gastric lavage may be a therapeutic as well as a diagnostic measure. It must be performed within several hours of ingestion of the drug, since barbiturates are absorbed rapidly and completely. Laryngospasm may complicate this procedure but can be avoided by preliminary endotracheal intubation; the stomach must be entirely emptied to prevent aspiration.

Dialysis of the blood by means of the artificial kidney has proved to be an effective form of therapy. This measure should be reserved for cases of profound intoxication due to long-acting barbiturates, in which a trial of symptomatic measures has failed, and in which uremia or anuria develops.

The treatment of severe barbiturate intoxication with analeptic drugs (Metrazol, picrotoxin, Megimide), which enjoyed a brief period of popularity, has been generally abandoned. These drugs are antagonistic to barbiturates only insofar as they are powerful cortical stimulants as well as overall nervous system excitants; they do not affect the rate of metabolism or excretion of barbiturate. Recent reports have stressed the value of alkalinization of the blood, by the use of large amounts of bicarbonate solution, as a means of mobilizing the barbiturate and increasing its rate of excretion. This method of therapy does seem to be useful, particularly where phenobarbital is the responsible agent.

Occasionally, in the case of a barbiturate addict who has taken an overdose of the drug, recovery from coma is followed by the development of an abstinence syndrome, which has to be managed by the methods outlined below.

CHRONIC BARBITURATE INTOXICATION Barbiturate addiction The problem of chronic barbiturate intoxication is quite different from that of acute intoxication, because of such phenomena as tolerance and addiction as well as the effects of withdrawal of the drugs. In these respects there is a remarkable similarity to the problem of chronic alcoholism.

Chronic barbiturate intoxication, like other addictions, usually develops on a background of some psychiatric disorder, most commonly depression or psychoneurosis with symptoms of anxiety and insomnia, or so-called "character disorder." The drug is usually prescribed for nervousness and insomnia; as the desired effects are lost, the patient increases the dose gradually until he is taking an amount sufficient to produce symptoms when it is withdrawn. Individuals with character disorders are usually introduced to the drug by associates; since the drug is taken for its intoxicating effect, the dose tends to be increased rapidly. Addiction to alcohol or to opiates may predispose to barbiturate addiction. Alcoholics find that barbiturates effectively relieve their nervousness and tremor; then they may continue to take both alcohol and barbiturates, or the barbiturate may replace the alcohol. Heroin and morphine addicts may turn to barbiturates when they are unable to obtain opiates. As with other addicting drugs, the incidence of barbiturism is particularly high in individuals with ready access to drugs, such as physicians, pharmacists, and nurses.

The symptoms and signs of chronic barbiturate intoxication may be described in relation to (1) the toxic effects of the drug, (2) the development of tolerance, and (3) the effects of sudden withdrawal of the drug after a period of prolonged intoxication.

The toxic symptoms of chronic barbiturism are much the same as those of mild acute intoxication or of alcoholic inebriation. The barbiturate addict thinks slowly, shows an increased emotional lability, and becomes untidy in his dress and personal habits. The neurologic signs are quite characteristic and include dysarthria, nystagmus, and cerebellar incoordination. Both the mental and neurologic signs fluctuate greatly in the same individual, being more severe if the drug is taken in the fasting state and tending to increase during the day as more of the drug is ingested. If the dosage is elevated rapidly, the signs of moderate or severe intoxication become manifest.

A characteristic feature of chronic barbiturate intoxication is the development of tolerance, sometimes striking in degree. The average addict will ingest about 1.5 g daily of a potent barbiturate and will not develop signs of severe intoxication unless this amount is exceeded. Tolerance to barbiturates does not develop as rapidly as to opiates. Daily doses of 2 g have been reached, but this takes many months. Individual variations in the degree of tolerance make it difficult to state precisely the minimal amount of drug which must be ingested before the resulting condition is designated as chronic barbiturate intoxication. Most persons can ingest 0.4 g daily for as long as 3 months without developing major withdrawal signs (seizures or delirium). With a dosage of 0.8 g daily, the efficiency at all tasks is greatly reduced, and after a period of 2 months on this dosage, abrupt withdrawal will result in serious symptoms in the majority of patients. Even after 2 weeks of this dosage, some patients will show mild withdrawal symptoms and paroxysmal electroencephalogram changes with photic stimulation. Individuals taking 0.4 to 0.7 g daily fall into an intermediate category; practically all show some mental dulling, and episodes of forgetfulness and occasionally severe withdrawal symptoms may occur.

Abstinence or withdrawal syndrome Following the withdrawal of barbiturates from addicted individuals, a characteristic sequence of symptoms occurs. Immediately following withdrawal the patient seemingly improves over a period of 8 to 12 hr as he loses the symptoms of intoxication. After this short period a new group of symptoms appears, consisting of nervousness, tremor, postural hypotension, and weakness. Generalized seizures, with loss of consciousness, may then occur, usually between the second and fourth days of abstinence, occasionally as long as 6 or 7 days after withdrawal. There may be a single seizure, several, or rarely status epilepticus. A varying degree of improvement follows the convulsive phase, to be followed by a delusional-hallucinatory state or a full-blown delirium, almost indistinguishable from delirium tremens. Death has been reported under these circumstances. The abstinence syndrome may occur in varying degrees of completeness; some patients have seizures and recover without developing delirium and others have a delirium without preceding seizures. The abrupt onset of seizures or an acute psychosis in adult life should always raise the suspicion of addiction to barbiturates or other sedative-hypnotic drugs.

The electroencephalogram shows a number of changes in chronic barbiturate intoxication and following withdrawal. During chronic intoxication, the predominant pattern is that of fast activity of moderate voltage, interspersed with some 6- to 8-cycles per sec activity chiefly in the frontal and parietal regions. The electroencephalogram does not correlate closely with the degree of intoxication, but some subjects do develop "EEG tolerance," i.e., a disappearance of the rapid pattern described above, while receiving moderate doses of barbiturate (400 mg daily for 90 days). On withdrawal of barbiturates the fast activity diminishes. Also in the first few days of abstinence, paroxysmal bursts of mixed spike and slow waves or 4-cycles per sec "spike and dome" paroxysmal discharges occur, and these may or may not be associated with seizures. Most of these abnormalities disappear after 4 or 5 days, the record returning to a completely normal pattern in 2 weeks as a rule. The most characteristic electroencephalographic findings which follow the withdrawal of barbiturates are paroxysmal changes evoked by photic stimulation.

INTOXICATING AND ADDICTING EFFECTS OF OTHER SEDATIVE-HYPNOTIC DRUGS In recent years a large number of nonbarbiturate sedative-hypnotic drugs have been introduced into medical practice. At least eight of them have the same intoxicating and addicting effects as barbiturates. These drugs are meprobamate (Miltown, Equanil), glutethimide (Doriden), ethinamate (Valmid), ethchlorvynol (Placidyl), methyprylon (Noludar), chlordiazepoxide (Librium), diazepam (Valium), methaqualone (Quaalude), and perhaps oxazepam (Serax). Like the barbiturates, each of these drugs can cause slurred speech, nystagmus, ataxic gait, drowsiness, confusion, and coma. Furthermore, if the daily dose exceeds a minimal safe range, a state of physical dependence develops, so that abstinence symptoms appear. These include hallucinations, seizures, and delirium and closely resemble those observed with barbiturates and alcohol. The seriousness of the abstinence syndrome in these cases is emphasized by reports of death following withdrawal of meprobamate, methyprylon, and diazepam. In view of these observations, physicians must exercise caution in prescribing the new sedative drugs which are continually being introduced and which are said to possess no addicting or habit-forming properties. Treatment of the symptoms which result from withdrawal of the nonbarbiturate sedative drugs requires barbiturate substitution, followed by its gradual withdrawal at a rate not to exceed 0.1 g daily. It should be noted that diphenylhydantoin (Dilantin) and phenothiazine derivatives are not effective against abstinence convulsions.

TREATMENT OF CHRONIC BARBITURATE INTOXICATION This treatment should always be carried out in the hospital. If the diagnosis of addiction is made before signs of abstinence have appeared, the first step in treatment should be the determination of the "stabilization dosage." This is the amount of short-acting barbiturate required to produce mild symptoms of intoxication (nystagmus, slight ataxia, and dysarthria). Usually 0.2 g pentobarbital given orally every 6 hr is sufficient for this purpose. The patient is examined 1 hr after each dose. If the signs of intoxication are severe, the next scheduled dose is reduced or omitted. If, instead, tremulousness and postural tachycardia appear, an additional 0.1 g of pentobarbital is given and the next scheduled dose is increased. This method is preferable to a blind reduction of dosage, since patients frequently underestimate the amount of drug taken. In such patients, establishment of the "stabilization dosage" may have diagnostic as well as therapeutic value. A patient who can take 0.8 g or more of pentobarbital daily, without developing signs of intoxication, is probably physically dependent on drugs of this type. Then a gradual withdrawal of the drug is undertaken, 0.1 g daily, the reduction being stopped for several days if abstinence symptoms appear. In this way a severely addicted person can be withdrawn in 14 to 21 days. Patients undergoing withdrawal treatment require careful observation of symptoms of abstinence, and special precautions have to be taken to prevent the smuggling or concealment of drugs.

If the patient comes to the physician with severe symptoms of abstinence, such as seizures, he should be given 0.3 to 0.5 g Luminal Sodium intramuscularly and then enough to maintain mild intoxication. Most anticonvulsant medicines have been shown, both in animals and in man, to be ineffective against barbiturate withdrawal convulsions. Withdrawal should then be carried out as indicated above. If the abstinence symptoms are not severe, it is not necessary to reintoxicate the patient, but treatment can proceed along the lines laid down for the delirious and confused patient (Chap. 26).

The same principles of treatment apply to patients who are addicted to nonbarbiturate hypnotic-sedative drugs. Thus, if the drug and its dosage can be determined, it should be withdrawn at the rate of one therapeutic dose per day. Should abstinence symptoms appear, the reduction in dosage is stopped for several days. If the offending drug cannot be identified, a barbiturate such as Seconal can be administered to the point of mild intoxication and then withdrawn, in the manner indicated above.

After recovery has taken place, whether from the symptoms of chronic intoxication or of abstinence or from acute intoxication due to attempted suicide, the psychiatric problem requires evaluation and an appropriate plan of therapy. Many of the considerations in the management of alcoholism are equally applicable to the patient addicted to barbiturate or nonbarbiturate hypnotic drugs (Chap. 111, Alcohol).

BARBITURATE PROVOCATION OF OTHER DISEASES At times the administration of one of the barbiturates may induce an attack of another disease. The most striking example of this is in hereditary porphyria where a severe and sometimes fatal outbreak of abdominal pain, psychosis, and polyneuropathy may follow the ingestion of a few capsules of Seconal (see Chap. 102). With severe liver disease, detoxification of barbiturates may be impaired, as is discussed in Chap. 291.

REFERENCES

Clemmesen C, Nilsson E: Therapeutic trends in the treatment of barbiturate poisoning: The Scandinavian method. Clin Pharmacol Ther 2:220, 1961

Essig C: Chronic abuse of sedative-hypnotic drugs, in *Drug Abuse* (proc int conf), ed CJD Zarafonetis, Philadelphia: Lea & Febiger, 1972, p. 205

Fraser HF et al: Degree of physical dependence induced by secobarbital or pentobarbital. JAMA 166:127, 1958

Isbell H et al: Chronic barbiturate intoxication: An experimental study. Arch neurol Psychiat 64:1, 1950

Plum F, Swanson AC: Barbiturate poisoning treated by physiological methods. JAMA 163:827, 1957

Wulff MH: The barbiturate withdrawal syndrome: A clinical and electroencephalographic study. Electroencephalog Clin Neurophysiol (suppl) 14:173, 1959

114
DEPRESSANTS, STIMULANTS, AND PSYCHOTOGENIC DRUGS

MAURICE VICTOR
RAYMOND D. ADAMS

DEPRESSANT DRUGS

These drugs may be divided into two main classes. The first, which may be designated *general depressants,* includes the barbiturates (discussed in Chap. 113) and other sedative-hypnotic drugs, the most important of which are meprobamate (Miltown) and the benzodiazepine derivatives—chlordiazepoxide (Librium) and diazepam (Valium). Their pharmacologic actions are to produce muscle relaxation and depression of central nervous system excitability in proportion to increasing dosage but modified by tolerance, habituation, and abstinence. A second class of *special depressants,* commonly referred to as tranquilizers, includes chlorpromazine and other phenothiazine antipsychotics, the sedative antihistaminics, such as hydroxyzine (Atarax) and diphenhydramine (Benadryl), the butyrophenones, and the rauwolfia alkaloids. The special depressants, in contrast to the general ones, increase muscle tone, lower the seizure threshold, and do not produce tolerance or physical dependance. They also reduce hyperexcitability of certain parts of the nervous system, but the sedative-hypnotic effects fail to keep pace with the increase in dosage, and excitability may remain at relatively normal levels over a wide range of dosages. Thus, the special depressants have the capacity to suppress symptoms of anxiety, irritability, and so forth, leaving the patient alert enough to work and function in an acceptable manner. An added advantage of these drugs is that large single doses, ingested with suicidal intent, may cause no serious depression of nervous system function. The phenothiazines and their derivatives have a strong adrenergic and weaker cholinergic and ganglionic blocking actions, so that they are sometimes referred to as *sedative-autonomic* drugs, in distinction to the general depressants, which are sedative-hypnotic.

GENERAL DEPRESSANTS The most important members of this group, the barbiturates, have been fully discussed in the preceding chapter. Other general depressants of clinical importance are the bromides, chloral hydrate, paraldehyde, and some of the newer drugs being used for the treatment of anxiety—chlordiazepoxide (Librium), diazepam (Valium), and meprobamate (Miltown).

Bromides are seldom prescribed by physicians at the present time, but are contained in many "nerve tonics" and proprietary remedies (Bromo-Seltzer, Nervine, Neurosine), so that cases of bromide intoxication are encountered with some regularity. Acute poisoning with bromide is rare because large doses of the drug are irritating to the gastric mucosa and vomiting prevents the attainment of significant blood levels. Taken in smaller doses, however, bromide tends to accumulate in the body because of its slow excretion by the kidney, and toxic symptoms may appear in a matter of weeks. These symptoms are caused by the bromide ion itself and are not simply a reflection of a decrease in chloride due to the displacement of the chloride by the bromide ion.

The symptoms of chronic bromide intoxication are predominantly in the mental sphere and range from dizziness, drowsiness, irritability, and emotional lability to a quiet confusional state, with impairment of thinking and memory, and in severe cases, to delirium and mania or to stupor and coma. Skin manifestations are associated in many cases, taking the form usually of an acne-like eruption and less frequently of proliferative nodular lesions, resembling those of tertiary syphilis. Headache, mild conjunctivitis, gastric distress, anorexia, and constipation may be associated as well. The blood bromide levels and the severity of toxic symptoms do not necessarily correspond. As a general rule, levels of 75 mg per 100 ml (9 mEq per liter) or more are considered abnormal and diagnostic of bromism, if the clinical picture suggests it. However, higher levels are sometimes well tolerated, and symptoms of bromism may persist for some days even after the blood levels have been reduced to normal or near-normal levels.

Treatment consists of removing the source of the bromide and administering sodium chloride (at least 6 g daily, in divided doses). Ammonium chloride may be substituted if an accumulation of sodium is to be avoided and if there is no danger of an uncompensated acidosis or hepatic failure. Confused or delirious patients require sedation, paraldehyde being the drug of choice, and anorectic and emaciated patients need careful nursing care and special attention to diet. The administration of a mercurial or thiazide diuretic serves to promote a bromide diuresis. Hemodialysis is an effective means of removing bromide and should be utilized in the most severe cases of intoxication.

Chloral hydrate is the oldest and at the same time one of the safest, most effective, and cheapest of the sedative-hypnotic drugs. After oral administration, chloral hydrate is reduced rapidly to trichloroethanol, which is the agent responsible for the depressant effects on the central nervous system. A significant portion of the trichloroethanol is excreted in the urine as the glucuronide, which may give a false positive test for glucose.

In large doses, chloral hydrate is toxic to the heart, kidneys, and liver, but only in the presence of preexisting disease in these organs. Chloral hydrate is a strong gastric irritant, so that it requires dilution and should not be taken on an empty stomach. Tolerance and addiction to chloral hydrate develop only rarely, and for these reasons it is an appropriate medication for the management of insomnia, particularly the type which is associated with depression. Poisoning with chloral hydrate is a rare occurrence and resembles acute barbiturate intoxication, except for the finding of miosis, which is said to characterize the former. In combination with alcohol, the well-known "Mickey Finn" or "knockout drops," its effects are additive, leading to a rapid onset of coma. Death from poisoning is due to respiratory depression and hypotension; patients who survive these events may show signs of liver and kidney disease.

Paraldehyde is also an effective and safe hypnotic, providing that certain precautions are taken in its preparation and administration. On exposure to light, paraldehyde decomposes to acetaldehyde, which is very toxic, and oxidizes to acetic acid. It must be freshly prepared, therefore, and stored in tightly stoppered, amber-colored bottles. Paraldehyde is unique in that a significant proportion is excreted unchanged through the lungs; the remainder is detoxified in the liver, so that it should be used cautiously in patients with liver disease.

Paraldehyde has a wide margin of safety when administered orally (or rectally), and even three or four times the usual dose (8 to 10 ml) causes no more than prolonged sleep or mild stupor. Intramuscular use of the drug should be avoided because of its propensity to produce sterile abscesses and to damage the sciatic nerve if injected too close to it. Intravenous injections should be made with caution and only in a hospital, because of their unpredictable effects on respiration. The main objections to this drug are its bitter taste (this can be obviated by diluting in fruit juice) and its lingering, unpleasant odor.

Paraldehyde is very effective in suppressing the tremulousness, restlessness, and insomnia that characterize the early phase (6 to 60 hr) of the alcohol withdrawal period. The use of paraldehyde in the alcoholic patient allegedly carries the risk, albeit small, of replacing an addiction to alcohol with one to paraldehyde. Patients with symptoms of alcohol withdrawal make repeated demands for the drug, which is not surprising, in view of the pharmacologic similarities between paraldehyde and alcohol and the effectiveness of both drugs in suppressing withdrawal symptoms. This should not present a problem in management, however, if the need for the drug is determined before each dose is given and the drug is withdrawn as soon as the agitation and tremor are under control. Should a relapse from abstinence then occur, substitution of paraldehyde for alcohol rarely if ever occurs.

Two agents of the benzodiazepine group, chlordiazepoxide (Librium) and diazepam (Valium), have been used extensively to control anxiety (also overactivity and destructive behavior in children) and the symptoms of alcohol withdrawal. These drugs possess anticonvulsant properties, and the intravenous use of diazepam is a very effective means of controlling status epilepticus. In addition, diazepam has been used with moderate success in the treatment of extrapyramidal movement disorders and dystonic spasms. The benzodiazepine drugs, while comparatively safe in the recommended dosages, frequently cause unsteadiness of gait and drowsiness and at times hypotension and syncope, particularly in the elderly. In severely disturbed schizophrenic patients, rage, hostility, uncontrollable excitement, confusion, and depersonalization may develop. Nausea, diminished libido, headache, skin rashes, leukopenia, eosinophilia, agranulocytosis, and enhancement of the effects of alcohol have all been reported but are rare. Additional central nervous effects are slurred speech, dysphagia, ataxia, confusion, and faulty memory.

The carbonic acid derivatives are capable of modest depressant action and are appropriate for relieving mild degrees of nervousness, anxiety, and muscle tension. Maximal action occurs with relatively small doses of these drugs. Meprobamate (Equanil, Miltown) is the best-known member of this group. With average doses (400 mg, three or four times a day) the patient is able to function quite effectively; large doses cause ataxia, drowsiness, stupor, coma, and vasomotor collapse. Hypersensitivity reactions in the form of fever, pruritis, and erythematous, maculopapular, and occasionally urticarial or bullous eruptions have been reported. Cutaneous petechiae or ecchymoses may also occur, without thrombocytopenia. Diplopia, syncope, menstrual irregularities, angioneurotic edema, peripheral edema, leucopenia, thrombocytopenia, and pancytopenia are other rare complications.

It is important to note that addiction to meprobamate does occur and if four or more times the daily recommended dose is administered over a period of weeks to months, withdrawal symptoms (including convulsions) may appear, resembling those which follow withdrawal of barbiturate in a chronically intoxicated patient. Several other nonbarbiturate sedative-hypnotic drugs, listed in Chap. 113, have the same liability.

SPECIAL DEPRESSANTS Since the mid-1950s, a large new series of pharmacologic agents, generally referred to as tranquilizers, has come into prominent use, mainly for the control of nervousness, agitation, apprehension, anxiety, and depression. Their application in medical practice, which has been on an enormous scale, is fraught with difficulty. Since the symptoms for which they are prescribed are manifestations of many conditions, some of them being normal reactions to trying environmental circumstances and others being symptoms of a disease state such as anxiety neurosis or depression, the physician should be certain of the diagnosis before using them. These drugs are not curative, but only suppress or partially alleviate the symptoms, and they should not serve as a substitute for, or divert the physician from, the use of other measures for the relief of the abnormal mental state. They are so toxic and expensive that they should not be used indefinitely.

There are an unnecessarily large number of tranquilizing agents on the market. No attempt will be made here to describe or even list all of them. Some have had only an evanescent popularity, and others have yet to prove their value. Chemically these compounds form a heterogeneous group, three categories being of particular clinical importance: (1) the ethylamine group of drugs (including the phenothiazines), (2) the butyrophenones, and (3) the rauwolfia alkaloids.

The phenothiazines comprise some of the most widely used tranquilizers such as chlorpromazine (Thorazine, Largactil), promazine (Sparine), triflupromazine (Vesprin), prochlorperazine (Compazine), perphenazine (Trilafon), fluphenazine (Permitil, Prolixin), thioridazine (Mellaril), and trifluoperazine (Stelazine). In addition to sedative effects, this group of drugs has a number of other actions, so that derivatives of these compounds are used as antiemetics (prochlorperazine) and antihistaminics (promethazine).

The phenothiazines have had their widest application in the treatment of the psychoses (schizophrenia and manic-depressive psychosis). Under the influence of these drugs, many patients who would otherwise be hospitalized are able to live at home and even work productively; the hospital care of hyperactive and combative patients has been greatly facilitated.

Side effects of the phenothiazines are frequent and often serious. All of them may cause a cholestatic type of jaundice, agranulocytosis, convulsive seizures, orthostatic hypotension, skin sensitivity reactions, mental depression, and disorders of the extrapyramidal motor system. Jaundice and blood dyscrasias have occurred less often with prochlorperazine, perphenazine, and fluphenazine than with other members of the group, but the extrapyramidal side effects have been relatively more pronounced. Several types of extrapyramidal symptoms have been noted: (1) A parkinsonian syndrome—masklike facies, tremor, generalized rigidity, shuffling gait, and slowness of movement; these symptoms usually appear after several weeks of drug therapy. (2) Muscle spasms and dystonia, taking the form of involuntary movements of face, protrusion of the tongue, dysphagia, torticollis and retrocollis, oculogyric crises, and tonic spasms of a limb (dyskinesias); these complications usually occur early in the administration of the drug, sometimes after the initial dose, and often can be improved dramatically by the intravenous administration of diphenhydramine hydrochloride (Benadryl). (3) An inability to sit still and an inner restlessness, so that the patient paces the floor constantly (akathisia); involuntary movements of a choreoathetotic type may be added.

These reactions must be recognized at once and the medication discontinued, but even then the extrapyramidal disorder may persist for weeks or months, *and exceptionally, even for years.* Administration of antiparkinsonian drugs (trihexyphenidyl, procyclidine, benztropine) may hasten the recovery of some of the symptoms. Oral, lingual, and laryngeal dyskinesias are affected relatively little by antiparkinsonian drugs. Sometimes, however, one such medication has better effect than another. Amantadine (Symmetrel) in doses of 50 to 100 mg t.i.d. has been especially useful in some of the postphenothiazine dyskinesias. Chlorprothixene (Taractan), a thioxanthene drug with effects similar to the phenothiazines, and thioridazine (Mellaril), although not the best tranquilizing agents, are favored by some because of their lesser tendency to produce symptoms of extrapyramidal motor disorder. The latter drug, however, if given in large doses over a period of time, may cause deposits in the maculae of the retina with resulting visual impairment.

The butyrophenones (haloperidal, trifluperidol) have much the same antipsychotic effects as the phenothiazines, as well as the same side effects. Unlike the phenothiazines, they have little or no adrenergic blocking action. The butyrophenones are effective substitutes for the phenothiazines in patients who are intolerant to the latter drugs, particularly to their autonomic effects.

Reserpine is the prototype of the rauwolfia alkaloids. It was in relation to the sedative effects of these drugs that the term *tranquilization* was used for the first time. These drugs, so effective in controlling hypertension, are no longer recommended for the treatment of emotional disorders, except perhaps in patients who cannot tolerate phenothiazines. When given in therapeutic doses, the rauwolfia alkaloids often provoke a parkinsonian syndrome or a serious depression of mood, which may prove more troublesome than the disorder for which they were prescribed.

Meprobamate, chlordiazepoxide, and diazepam have been referred to as "minor tranquilizers," the implication being that these drugs share the antipsychotic properties of the phenothiazines. This is not the case. In fact, the pharmacologic effects of the minor tranquilizers resemble those of the barbiturates and for this reason are more appropriately considered as general depressants (see above).

It hardly need be pointed out that the tranquilizing drugs have been much abused. This would be suspected just from the frequency with which they are being prescribed. It is stated that in the decade 1955 to 1965, 50 million patients in the United States received chlorpromazine alone; the minor tranquilizers are probably prescribed as frequently.

STIMULANTS

Drugs that act primarily as stimulants of the central nervous system can be divided into two general groups on the basis of difference in their pharmacologic actions and clinical use. (1) The first group is exemplified by analeptics such as amphetamine and picrotoxin; the latter produces a prompt and short-lived effect on the nervous system and a grossly recognizable increase in motor and electrical activity, often taking the form of convulsive seizures. (2) The monoamine oxidase inhibitors and dibenzazepine compounds, which make up the second group of stimulant drugs, have considerable clinical usefulness, mainly in elevating mood and ameliorating the symptoms and signs of mental depression. The effects of these drugs on the nervous system, in contrast to the more direct-acting stimulants, are slow to appear, persist for long periods after their administration has been stopped, and cannot be assessed in animals.

Such a division, though clinically useful, requires qualification. Certain of the direct-acting stimulants, e.g., amphetamine, may have a beneficial effect on the low energy of mental depression and in other fatigue states. Also, certain drugs that are useful in the treatment of depression (e.g., amobarbital) are not central nervous system stimulants but depressants. In the latter case, a depressant acts as a mood elevator. These commonly used terms must not be confused—the former referring to a drug that reduces nervous system excitability and the latter to the capacity of the drug to ameliorate the symptoms of mental depression.

DIRECT-ACTING STIMULANTS Amphetamine (benzedrine) and its *d*-isomer, dextroamphetamine, are powerful analeptics and in addition have significant hypertensive, respiratory-stimulant, and appetite-depressant effects. These drugs are useful in the management of narcolepsy, but they are much more widely and indiscriminately used for the control of obesity and the abolition of fatigue. Undoubtedly, they are able to reverse fatigue, postpone the need for sleep, and elevate mood, but these effects are not entirely predictable and certainly not indefinite, and the user must pay for the period of wakefulness with even greater fatigue and often with depression. Because of the popularity of the amphetamines and ease with which they can be procured, instances of acute and chronic intoxication are observed frequently. Nonetheless dextroamphetamine in doses of 5 mg morning and noon is a valuable therapy in many reactive depressions, such as following myocardial infarction or stroke. The toxic signs of large dosages are essentially an exaggeration of the analeptic effects —restlessness, excessive speech and motor activity, tremor, and insomnia. In severe cases, hallucinations, delusions, and changes in affect and thought processes may occur, a state that may be indistinguishable from paranoid schizophrenia. Treatment consists of removal of the offending drug and the administration of barbiturates. Nitrites may be useful if the blood pressure is markedly elevated. Ritalin has much the same type of action as amphetamine and is also useful in the treatment of narcolepsy.

Picrotoxin is a powerful nervous system excitant, the main effects being to produce convulsive seizures and to reverse respiratory depression induced by drugs, particularly by barbiturates. However, the modern treatment of barbiturate intoxication does not include the use of picrotoxin or other analeptics, because of their epileptogenic properties and because barbiturate intoxication can be managed successfully by other means (see Chap. 113).

It has been shown by Eccles and his colleagues that picrotoxin increases neuronal activity by blocking presynaptic inhibition, i.e., blocking the action of inhibitory fibers that synapse with the presynaptic terminals of excitatory fibers. Strychnine, on the other hand, increases neuronal excitability by interfering with postsynaptic inhibition. The therapeutic value of strychnine is negligible, but in children accidental poisoning may occur from ingestion of "A.S. & B." cathartic pills or "rat biscuits." Very rarely, strychnine is taken with suicidal intent. After a period of heightened irritability and muscle twitching, tonic seizures occur, characterized by opisthotonus, rigid extension of the legs, facial tetanus, and apnea due to spasm of the muscles of respiration. Death from anoxia may follow several seizures.

The immediate need, in the treatment of strychnine poisoning, is to control the convulsions. This calls for the intravenous administration of a short-acting barbiturate or the application of inhalation anesthesia if the appropriate drug is not immediately available; endotracheal intubation is an important safeguard. The patient must then be observed carefully, and if any signs of irritability recur, more sedative should be given. During this period, supportive care is indicated, as for any comatose patient. Morphine, which is principally a medullary depressant, is contraindicated.

Pentylenetetrazol (Metrazol, Cardiazol) is a potent stimulant of all parts of the nervous system. For a number of years it served as the convulsive agent in "shock treatment" of depression and schizophrenia but was abandoned in favor of less dangerous and more effective forms of convulsive therapy. The use of this drug to activate latent epileptogenic foci or to reproduce convulsions, with the purpose of studying the underlying cerebral mechanisms, is restricted to a few clinical centers.

The actions of bemegride and nikethamide (Coramine) are much like those of pentylenetetrazol. For many years it was common clinical practice to administer nikethamide as a final therapeutic gesture in patients dying of cardiac and respiratory failure, but there is little evidence that this drug has a significant stimulant effect on either heart or respiration. Poisoning with these drugs, which is usually due to parenteral overdosage, is best treated with barbiturates.

Caffeine and other xanthine derivatives do have therapeutic value, by virtue of their diuretic effects and their ability to stimulate the heart and nervous system. The major use of these agents is to abolish fatigue and maintain wakefulness, and the usual mode of administration is in coffee, a cup of which contains 100 to 150 mg caffeine. Overdosage leads to insomnia, mild delirium, tinnitus, tachycardia, prominent diuresis, and cardiac arrhythmias. The excitatory effects are easily controlled with barbiturates, and fatalities due to caffeine poisoning are extremely rare.

Camphor (camphorated oil) was formerly a popular stimulant, but is now rarely used therapeutically; however, occasional cases of poisoning are still seen as a result of ingestion of liniment or moth flakes. The manifestations of poisoning are headache, sensation of warmth, confusion, clonic convulsions, and terminal respiratory depression; the characteristic odor of camphor facilitates the diagnosis. Treatment consists of supportive care and the cautious use of barbiturates to combat convulsions.

INDIRECT-ACTING STIMULANTS Monoamine oxidase inhibitors The observation that iproniazid, an inhibitor of monoamine oxidase (MAO), has a mood-elevating effect in tuberculous patients initiated a great deal of interest in compounds of this type, and led quickly to their exploitation in the treatment of depression. Iproniazid (Marsilid) proved exceedingly toxic and was soon taken off the market, as have several more recently developed MAO inhibitors; but other drugs, much better tolerated, have become available. These include isocarboxizid (Marplan), nialamide (Niamid), phenelzine (Nardil), and tranycypromine (Parnate), the latter two being the most frequently used. Tranylcypromine has proved to be the most potent of these agents, but it has also produced the most serious toxic effects.

The exact mode of action of the MAO inhibitors has not been determined. They have in common the ability to block the oxidative deamination of naturally occurring amines (norepinephrine, epinephrine, and serotonin), and it has been suggested that the accumulation of these neurohormonal substances is responsible for the antidepressant effect. However, these drugs inhibit many enzymes other than monoamine oxidases and have numerous actions unrelated to enzyme inhibition. Furthermore, many agents with antidepressant effects like those of the monoamine oxidase inhibitors do not inhibit this enzyme. At the present time, one cannot assume that the therapeutic effect of these drugs has a direct relation to the property of MAO inhibition.

These drugs must be dispensed with great caution and

a constant awareness of their potentially serious side effects. (Orthostatic hypotension of a serious degree may also develop.) Patients taking the drugs must be warned against the use of sympathomimetic amines and tyramine, for this may induce a severe hypertensive episode and cerebral vascular accident, headache, atrial and ventricular arrhythmia, pulmonary edema, and even death. Sympathomimetic amines are contained in some of the commonly used nasal sprays, nose drops, and in so-called "coryza" tablets and the common tyramine-containing compounds, in cheeses, yogurt, beer, and wine.

The MAO inhibitors may at times cause excitement, restlessness, agitation, insomnia, and anxiety; occasionally, with the usual dose and more often with an overdose, mania and convulsions may occur (especially in epileptic patients). Other side effects are increased neuromuscular activity in the form of muscle twitching and involuntary movement of an extremity, urinary retention, skin rashes, tachycardia, hepatic disturbance, jaundice, visual impairment, enhancement of glaucoma, impotence, sweating, muscle spasms, and a variety of paresthesias.

Since the MAO inhibitors have such widespread possibilities of causing toxic effects and potentiating the effect of other drugs, it is wise not to give them with other medications. In particular, the phenothiazines and other powerful central nervous system stimulants should not be given with the MAO inhibitors, since occasional fatalities and severe reactions have followed their concomitant use. Exaggerated responses to the usual dose of meperidine (Demerol) and other narcotic drugs have also been observed; respiratory function may be depressed to a serious degree, and hyperpyrexia, agitation, and pronounced hypotension may occur as well, sometimes with fatal issue. Unpredictable side effects may also accompany the simultaneous administration of barbiturates.

Dibenzazepine derivatives Soon after the first convincing successes in the treatment of depression with MAO inhibitors, a new class of tricyclic antidepressant compounds appeared. The first of this group was imipramine (Tofranil), which was soon followed by amitriptyline (Elavil), and then by desipramine (Norpramin) and nortriptyline (Aventyl). The first two members of this group have proved to be the most popular.

The exact mode of action of these agents is unknown, but they produce a central stimulating effect. In the absence of other considerations, they are presently the most effective drugs for the treatment of depressive illnesses that are associated with anxiety and agitation. Persistence of their pharmacologic effects after the drug is stopped is very short in comparison with the MAO inhibitors, and their side effects are far less frequent and serious.

All the tricyclic or dibenzazepine compounds are capable of causing orthostatic hypotension, urinary bladder weakness, dizziness, and, occasionally, ataxia and blood dyscrasias. They may produce central nervous system excitement, leading to insomnia, agitation, and restlessness, but usually these effects are controlled readily by the use of phenothiazines or chlordiazepoxide given concurrently or in the evenings. The dibenzazepine drugs should never be given with an MAO inhibitor, since the reactions which may occur are frequently serious; hypertensive crises and lethal hyperpyrexia have been reported. These reactions have allegedly occurred when small doses of imipramine were given to patients who had discontinued the MAO inhibitor 1 week previously.

PSYCHOTOGENIC DRUGS

Included in this category are a heterogeneous group of drugs, the primary effect of which is to alter perception, mood, and thinking out of proportion to other aspects of cognitive function and consciousness. This group of drugs comprises lysergic acid derivatives, e.g., lysergic acid diethylamide (LSD); phenylethylamine derivatives (mescaline or peyote); psilocybin; certain indolic derivatives, cannabis (marihuana), and a number of less important compounds. They are also referred to as psychotomimetic drugs, hallucinogens, and psychedelics, but none of these names is entirely suitable.

Tolerance to these drugs develops rapidly, even on a once-daily dosage of LSD, mescaline, or psilocybin. Furthermore, subjects tolerant to any one of these three drugs are cross-tolerant to the other two. Tolerance is lost rapidly when these drugs are discontinued abruptly, but no abstinence syndromes ensue. In this sense, addiction does not develop, although users may become dependent upon them for emotional support. In the case of marihuana, "reverse tolerance" (i.e., increasing sensitization) may be observed initially, but on continued use, tolerance to the "euphoriant" effects of the drug has been observed in one of the few "chronic" experimental studies that have been made, and the subjects reported "jitteriness" during the first 24 hr after abrupt cessation of marihuana cigarette smoking, although no objective withdrawal signs could be detected.

LSD, mescaline, and psilocybin produce much the same clinical effects if given in comparable amounts. The perceptual changes are the most dramatic—the user describes vivid visual hallucinations, alterations in the shape and color of objects, unusual dreams, and feelings of depersonalization. An increase in auditory acuity has been described, but auditory hallucinations are rare. Cognitive functions are difficult to assess because of inattention, drowsiness, and inability to concentrate and to cooperate in mental testing. The somatic symptoms consist of dizziness, nausea, drowsiness, paresthesias, and blurring of vision. Sympathomimetic effects—pupillary dilation, piloerection, hyperthermia, and tachycardia—are prominent, and the user may also show hyperreflexia, incoordination of the limbs, and ataxia.

The effects of marihuana, when taken by inhaling the smoke from cigarettes, are prompt in onset and evanescent. In low doses the symptoms are like those of mild intoxication with alcohol. With increasing amounts of drug, the effects are similar to those of LSD, mescaline, and psilocybine, and they may be quite disabling for many hours. Very large doses result in severe depression and stupor, but death is unusual.

The fact that small quantities of these drugs can produce gross mental aberrations has stimulated the search for similar but endogenous substances that may be responsible for schizophrenia and other psychoses. The mechanisms involved in producing and antagonizing the "psychotomimetic" effects are also being studied intensively, in the hope of elucidating the mechanisms of the psychoses and finding improved psychotherapeutic agents. Doubtless these studies are adding greatly to our knowledge of abnormal behavior, but the fundamental problems remain to be solved.

Numerous claims have been made that LSD and related drugs are effective in the treatment of mental disease and a wide variety of social ills and that they have the capacity to increase one's intellectual performance, creativity, and self-understanding. At this time, there are no acceptable studies that validate any of these claims.

LSD is not yet an approved drug, and marihuana falls under the Federal narcotic laws. Nevertheless, these drugs are very widely used. They are taken by narcotic addicts as a temporary substitute for more potent drugs, by "drug heads," i.e., individuals who use literally any agent that alters consciousness, and by many troubled, unhappy college and high-school students, often for reasons that they cannot ascertain. The unsupervised use of these drugs is attended by a number of serious adverse reactions, taking the form of acute panic attacks, long-lasting psychotic states resembling paranoid schizophrenia, or serious physical injury, consequent upon impairment of the user's critical faculties. Whether prolonged usage leads to permanent damage to the nervous system

is not certain; there are some data suggesting that this may happen. The reports claiming that LSD may cause chromosomal damage remain to be validated. A discussion of the legal implications of the illicit use of these drugs and their social impact is beyond the scope of this chapter, but can be found in the appended references.

REFERENCES

HOLLISTER LE: *Chemical Psychoses: LSD and Related Drugs,* Springfield, Ill.: Charles C Thomas, 1968

——: Mental disorders—antianxiety and antidepressant drugs. N Engl J Med 286:1195, 1972

JARVIK ME: Drugs used in the treatment of psychiatric disorders, in *Pharmacological Basis of Therapeutics,* 4th ed., eds LS Goodman, and Alfred Gilman, New York: Macmillan, 1970, p. 151

Psychopharmacology. A Review of Progress, 1957–1967, ed DH Efron, U.S. Public Health Service, no. 1836, Washington, D.C.: 1968

WIKLER A: Drug dependence, in *Clinical Neurology,* eds AB Baker, LH Baker, Hagerstown, Md.: Harper & Row, 1971

section 2 | Disorders caused by venoms, bites, and stings

115 DISORDERS CAUSED BY VENOMS, BITES, AND STINGS

JAMES F. WALLACE
ROBERT G. PETERSDORF

INTRODUCTION Man has the propensity to come into contact with a great variety of venomous animals. These contacts occur with many zoologic classes including snakes, lizards, sea animals, spiders, scorpions, and numerous species of insects. In general two types of injuries result: those due to the direct effect of venom on the victim, as exemplified in snakebite, and those due to indirect effects of the poison, of which hypersensitivity reaction to beestings is an example. Each year in the United States at least 50 persons die as the result of venomous injuries. Three groups of animals—hymenopterous insects, snakes, and spiders—account for over 90 percent of the fatalities.

SNAKE AND LIZARD BITES **Epidemiology** Fewer than one-tenth of the nearly 3,500 known species of snakes are venomous. These poisonous varieties belong to five families or subfamilies: Elapidae (cobras, kraits, mambas, and coral snakes) found in all parts of the world except Europe; Viperidae (true vipers) found in all parts of the world except the Americas; Hydrophidae (sea snakes); Crotalidae (pit vipers) found in Asia and the Americas; and Colubridae (boomslangs, bird snakes) of the African continent. The poisonous varieties of the United States, with the single exception of the coral snake, are pit vipers and include rattlesnakes, the water moccasin, and the copperhead. Although this discussion centers around these species, the therapeutic measures outlined are applicable to snakes in all parts of the world.

The number of individuals bitten by poisonous snakes in the United States is estimated at 6,000 to 7,000 per year, with a relatively large number occurring in the Southeastern and Gulf states, particularly Texas. Deaths are not reported separately but are undoubtedly rare, numbering fewer than 20 per year, and most are due to bites of various species of rattlesnake. In many European countries deaths from snakebite have averaged only one every 3 to 5 years for the last half-century. In contrast, the estimate of annual deaths from snakebite throughout the world is between 30,000 and 40,000, with the largest number occurring in the countries of Burma and Brazil, where 2,000 deaths are estimated to occur each year.

Etiology The *coral snake* is found in the Southern states from Florida to Arizona. It is usually marked by alternating red and black bands separated by yellow rings; however, black and albino forms exist. Coral snakes are generally nocturnal in their activities, shy and elusive, and rarely bite man. Their fangs are short and permanently erect; the highly toxic venom is injected into multiple puncture wounds produced by a series of chewing movements.

The *pit vipers* are so named because of a small pit between the eye and the nostril. Large venom glands in the temporal regions give the head a triangular appearance. They are generally aggressive and likely to strike if disturbed. The fangs are long and hinged, folding posteriorly when the mouth is closed. Pit vipers strike suddenly with a forward thrust of the head. The instant that the erect fangs make contact, venom is expressed by sudden muscular contraction.

The *rattlesnakes*, recognized by the horny rattle on the tail which buzzes when the snake is disturbed, are widely distributed. The diamondbacks (*Crotalus adamanteus* in the Southeast and *C. atrox* in the Southwest) are the largest and most dangerous snakes in this country. Others include the prairie rattler (*C. confluentus*), the timber rattler (*C. horridus*), and the pigmy rattlers.

The *water moccasin*, or cottonmouth (*Agkistrodon piscivorus*), is found in swampy areas or along the banks of streams. It is a strong swimmer and can bite under water. This snake is notorious for inflicting severe facial bites when disturbed in the branches of small trees. The copperhead, or highland moccasin (*A. mokasen*), is a closely related species. Its bite is painful but rarely fatal.

Pathogenesis SNAKE VENOMS The venoms of most species which have been analyzed have been found to be mixtures of several toxic proteins and enzymes with diversified and complicated pharmacologic effects. As an example, the venom of the Indian cobra (*Naja naja*) contains these distinct and separate substances: a neurotoxin, a hemolysin, a cardiotoxin, a cholinesterase, at least three phosphatases, a nucleotidase, and a potent inhibitor of cytochrome oxidase. Several venoms, including those of the pit vipers, contain hyaluronidase and numerous proteolytic enzymes. Although the exact roles of these components in toxicity are incompletely understood, the venom of a given species is usually predominantly neurotoxic or necrotizing, and frequently associated with hemolysis, abnormalities of blood coagulation, changes in cardiac dynamics, and alterations in vascular resistance. The venom of elapids, including the coral snake, is neurotoxic, with death resulting from respiratory paralysis probably caused by damage to brain centers and a curariform interference with transmission at the neuromuscular junction. The venom of crotalid snakes produces local tissue injury, hemorrhage, and hemolysis; death is often preceded by circulatory collapse associated with a marked fall in circulating blood volume resulting from pooling of blood in the microcirculation, and loss of plasma due to increased capillary permeability. Systemic absorption of venom occurs through the lymphatics, and therapeutic measures designed to reduce lymphatic function are helpful in controlling symptoms.

FACTORS AFFECTING SEVERITY OF SNAKE BITE Several factors affect the outcome of snake bite:

1 The age, size, and health of the patient. Envenomation in children is usually serious, and a fatal outcome more likely, since a relatively larger dose of poison is injected into a small victim.
2 Location of bite. Bites on extremities or into adipose tissue are less dangerous than those on the trunk, face, or directly into a blood vessel. A direct strike of the fangs is more dangerous than a scratch, a glancing blow, or one hitting a bone. The discharge orifice of a fang is well above its tip so that the point of the fang can penetrate the skin without envenomation; even a thin layer of clothing may afford great protection. Because of the superficial nature of the wound as many as one-fifth of patients bitten by venomous snakes will have no evidence of envenomation, even though the fangs have penetrated the skin.
3 The size of the snake (a large pit viper can inject over 1,000 mg venom, six times a lethal dose for an adult), the extent of its anger or fear (if hurt it may inject a larger amount of venom), the condition of the fangs (broken or recently renewed), and the condition of the venom glands (recently discharged or full). All these factors are important. Contrary to popular belief, the bite of a snake which has recently killed and fed is not necessarily less venomous for man; the snake usually does not exhaust its venom in a single bite.
4 The presence of various bacteria, particularly clostridia and other anaerobic organisms, in the mouth of the snake or on the skin of the victim. This may lead to serious infection in the necrotic tissues at the local site.
5 Exercise or exertion, such as running immediately after the bite. This speeds systemic absorption of toxin.

Manifestations Following the bite of a pit viper, severe burning pain develops within a few minutes at the site of the wound. Local swelling rapidly develops and spreads in all directions, accompanied by the appearance of ecchymoses and bullae over the involved area. As the edema spreads, serosanguinous fluid oozes from the puncture wounds. Later gangrene of the skin and subcutaneous tissues may develop. Systemic effects resulting from the absorption of venom and local tissue destruction may include fever, nausea and vomiting, circulatory collapse, bleeding into the skin and from all body orifices, low-grade jaundice, neuropathic muscle cramping, pupillary constriction, disorientation, delirium, and convulsions. Death may occur after 6 to 48 hr. Survival may be attended by massive local tissue loss from gangrene or secondary infection, or may be complicated by acute renal failure, secondary to disseminated intravascular clotting and cortical necrosis, or by tubular necrosis following circulatory collapse.

The bite of the coral snake causes little pain and local swelling. There are usually multiple fang marks. Within 10 to 15 min numbness and weakness begin in the region of the bite followed by ataxia, ptosis, pupillary dilatation, palatal and pharyngeal paralysis, slurring of speech, salivation, and occasionally nausea and vomiting. The patient becomes comatose, develops respiratory paralysis and seizures, and dies within 8 to 72 hr.

Cobra bites are painful and are often accompanied by severe hemolysis, local necrosis, and sloughing in addition to their more widely appreciated neurotoxic effects. Sea snake bites are mainly myotoxic and neurotoxic, while coagulopathic manifestations predominate following Viperidae and Colubridae envenomation.

Laboratory abnormalities In severe cases, laboratory abnormalities may include progressive anemia, polymorphonuclear leukocytosis of 20,000 to 30,000 cells per mm^3, thrombocytopenia, hypofibrinogenemia, disordered tests of coagulation, proteinuria, and azotemia.

Treatment An attempt should be made to determine with certainty that the patient has been bitten by a poisonous snake. Absence of distinct fang punctures and failure of local pain, edema, numbness, or weakness to appear within 20 min are strong evidence against a bite having been inflicted by a venomous species.

FIRST AID This consists of reassuring and calming the victim and instituting measures to retard the absorption of venom and to remove it from the tissues as quickly as possible after the bite. The patient should be promptly placed at rest and his bitten extremity immobilized to reduce the rate of spread of the venom. If anatomically feasible, a wide tourniquet should be placed a few centimeters above the bite and made tight enough to allow one finger to pass beneath with difficulty. The purpose is to impede lymph flow; it is not necessary to obstruct venous return. The tourniquet should be loosened and moved proximally at hourly intervals when local swelling causes it to tighten. Unless the victim can be transported to a hospital within less than 15 min, incision and suction of the wound should be started prior to his evacuation. By use of whatever antisepsis is available, 1.0 cm *linear* (not cruciate) incisions about 0.5 cm deep should be carefully made through each fang mark and suction applied. A rubber bulb, breast pump, or heated jar are all preferable to mouth suction, but if other means are not available and no oral lesions are present, this method may be employed. Suction should be continued for at least an hour; as the swelling progresses, successive rings of radiating linear, shallow incisions at the advancing edge of edema are useful, particularly if early evacuation to a hospital cannot be accomplished. *Incision and suction are extremely important and should be diligently carried out in every poisonous snake bite.* When begun promptly, they may result in the removal of up to 50 percent of subcutaneously injected venom.

As soon as possible, the patient should be transferred to a hospital. Immobilization of the affected part during transportation is important in controlling lymph flow and is best achieved by splinting. Although ice packs relieve pain and slow lymphatic drainage, they do not neutralize venom, and their use can result in irreparable damage to already injured tissue through freezing.

IMMEDIATE HOSPITAL CARE This should include appropriate treatment for shock and respiratory difficulty, antivenin, measures to combat infection, and general supportive care.

Antivenin is the only specific treatment of snake venom poisoning, and its use in severe bites is vital. In the United States polyvalent antivenin effective against all American pit vipers is commercially available, and antivenin for coral snake poisoning has also been released. Both products are a lyophylized powder of refined horse serum. Kits are available containing antivenin powder (reconstituted by diluting with water to 10 ml per ampul), syringe, normal horse serum for prior sensitivity testing of the patient, and detailed instructions. Intravenously administered antivenin leads to the most rapid and effective response. It is not advisable to infiltrate antivenin at the local site. The initial dose should depend upon the amount of envenomation; for severe bites 5 to 10 vials (50 to 100 ml) may be required. When progressive swelling in the bitten part ceases, an adequate dose has generally been achieved; improvement in the victim's clinical signs is often extremely rapid.

In the patient with severe envenomation who is allergic to horse serum, the relative risks of death from anaphylaxis rather than from venom poisoning should be carefully weighed before undertaking desensitization with small doses of diluted horse serum.

No antivenin for other snakes is manufactured in the United States, but antiserum for various types is usually kept on hand at large zoos all over the world.

Maintaining *respiration* by mechanical or other means is important. In patients bitten by elapid snakes, respiratory failure is usually reversible. *Tetanus toxoid* or *tetanus immune globulin* of human origin should be given. If wound infections appear, antibiotics should be used with the knowledge that the predominant microorganisms in the mouths of snakes are gram-negative pathogens. Treatment should be preceded by appropriate aerobic and anaerobic cultures. *Fasciotomy* may be necessary to prevent further ischemic injury to a massively swollen limb. *Surgical debridement* of vesicles and superficial necrotic tissue should be done near the end of the first week following the bite. *Relief of pain* with salicylates or meperidine, moderate sedation, maintenance of fluid balance, measures to combat shock and hemorrhagic diathesis, and appropriate management of coma or convulsions are all important.

The usefulness of corticosteroids to prevent tissue damage or systemic intoxication has not been convincingly demonstrated. However, these drugs may be of value in the management of severe shock associated with envenomation and for allergic reactions following the administration of antivenin.

Prevention In snake-infested regions long trousers, high shoes, boots or leggings, and gloves should be worn. Most important of all is to look where one steps or reaches. A sharp knife or lacet, tourniquet, suction bulb, and antiseptic suffice for an emergency kit, and in inaccessible areas, antivenin should also be carried.

GILA MONSTER BITE The Gila monsters include the large orange and black lizard (*Heloderma suspectum*) of the arid Southwest and *H. horridum,* a closely related Mexican species. These reptiles are not aggressive, and virtually every instance of their attacking man has involved teasing or handling the animals in captivity. The venom is elaborated in eight glands in the floor of the mouth and secreted directly into the oral cavity, where it bathes the teeth, which are grooved posteriorly. The lizard clings tenaciously and is often dislodged only after considerable effort; envenomation occurs by contamination of the wound. The venom contains a potent neurotoxin which is undoubtedly responsible for its lethal effect in experimental animals. Death in man has been reported as occurring within a few hours after a bite. The venom also produces local tissue injury, excruciating pain, massive edema, and patchy erythema. In recovered patients, acute symptoms have lasted for 3 to 4 days and include nausea, vomiting, hematemesis, blurred vision, dyspnea, dysphonia, and profound weakness. Intense hyperesthesia of the bitten extremity may persist for several weeks. There is no antivenin available. Treatment should consist of tourniquet, incision, suction, cooling of the bitten area, measures to prevent or combat infection, including tetanus, and supportive measures. Because meperidine has been shown to potentiate the venom's action in animals, some other analgesic should be used to relieve pain.

ENVENOMATION BY SPIDERS, SCORPIONS, INSECTS, AND OTHER ARTHROPODS The bite of many spiders is locally irritating, and several species can cause severe, even fatal systemic poisoning in man. The most numerous and important of the venomous spiders are members of the genus *Latrodectus*, widely distributed throughout the world. In the United States and Canada, *Lat. mactans*, the black widow or shoe-button spider, causes a majority of clinically significant arachnidism. In Florida, *Lat. bishopi*, the red-legged widow spider, has been reported to produce human poisoning resembling mild black widow bite. From the Southern and Midwestern states, there are increasing numbers of reports of poisoning from the bite of common brown spiders, including *Loxosceles reclusa* and *Lox. unicolor*. These bites are characterized by intense local pain and ischemic necrosis at the site, often followed by deep ulceration. Hemolysis occasionally is seen, and in severe cases hemoglobinuria and acute renal failure may occur.

The symptoms and mortality from bites of large, hairy spiders, the tarantulas, such as *Lycosa raptoria* and *Phoneutria fera* in Brazil or *Glyptocranium gasteracanthoides* in Peru, and of such spiders as *Loxosceles laeta* in Chile are similar, with severe ulceration, necrosis, and hemolysis. Neurotoxic manifestations of the type produced by *Latrodectus* are sometimes admixed with local necrosis and hemolysis.

It is the female *Lat. mactans*, the black widow, that bites man. She is glossy black with a body 1 cm in diameter, a leg span of 5 cm, and a characteristic red "hourglass" mark on her abdomen. She spins her web in woodpiles, sheds, basements, or outdoor privies, is very aggressive, and will bite on slight provocation. The venom produces diffuse central and peripheral nervous excitement, autonomic activity, muscle spasm, hypertension, and vasoconstriction.

In the United States, most black widow bites occur between April and October, and many patients are males bitten on the genitalia or buttocks while using a privy. After a momentary sharp pain at the site, there is cramping pain that begins locally within 15 to 60 min and gradually spreads. It may involve all extremities and the trunk. The abdomen is boardlike, and the waves of pain become excruciating, causing the patient to turn, toss, and cry out. Respirations are often labored and grunting. There are also nausea, vomiting, headache, sweating, salivation, hyperactive reflexes, twitching, tremor, paresthesias of hands and feet, and occasionally, systolic hypertension. A mild polymorphonuclear leukocytosis is usual, and many patients have slight fever. After several hours, the pains subside, although mild recurrences for 2 or 3 days are common. It may be a week before well-being is restored. Deaths due to cardiac or respiratory failure have occurred, mostly in children and the aged.

Because the bite itself is not prominent, patients are often thought to have some abdominal catastrophe such as perforated ulcer, pancreatitis, or volvulus. Renal colic, coronary occlusion, tetanus, strychnine poisoning, tabetic crisis, lead colic, and porphyria are other conditions to be ruled out. The abdomen is not tender to palpation in arachnidism, and pains in the extremities are not typical of most of these other disorders.

Treatment For *Latrodectus* poisoning, treatment consists of measures to relieve pain and administration of antiserum. Initial treatment should include a hot tub bath which affords prompt, although temporary, relief. An intravenous injection of calcium gluconate or magnesium sulfate usually produces dramatic, but transient, cessation of cramps. Opiates are sometimes necessary. When available, a single intramuscular injection of 1 ampul (2.5 ml) reconstituted antiserum usually is quite effective within a few hours. If the cramps return, administration of antiserum can be repeated.

Treatment of *Loxosceles* bites consists mainly of local wound management and treatment of secondary infection if it occurs. The ulcer usually heals spontaneously, although skin grafting may be required on occasion. Renal failure should be treated as advised in Chap. 269.

SCORPION STING Scorpions are eight-legged arthropods. Glands in the terminal segment produce venom, which is injected into the victim by a stinger located on the tip of the tail. Scorpions often enter dwellings. During the day they retreat into crevices; emerging at night, they often get into shoes and clothing and even into bedding. They do not deliberately attack man, but accidental contact results in a sting.

Of about 650 species, roughly 40 occur in the United States, distributed over three-fourths of the nation. They are most numerous in the South from Florida to California, but the only two lethal species, *Centruroides sculpturatus* and *C. gertschi*, are limited to Arizona and portions of neighboring states.

Dangerous species found in the United States, *C. sculpturatus and C. gertschi*, reach a maximal length of about 7 cm. Their sting may be fatal to young children or old people, but seldom to a healthy adult.

Most of the nonlethal species of scorpions in the United States cause only minor reactions, like a beesting. Some in the Southwest, however, produce local edema and ecchymosis, with burning pain. In contrast, many species whose venom has potentially dangerous systemic effects, including the Arizona *Centruroides*, evoke little or no visible reaction at the site of the sting. There is an immediate burning sensation followed by local paresthesia ("pins and needles"), hyperesthesia, or numbness.

These sensations spread to involve the whole extremity, and within an hour or two, malaise, restlessness, lacrimation, rhinorrhea, salivation, perspiration, nausea, and vomiting appear.

The patient passes from an agitated state with hyperactive reflexes into coma; convulsions follow. In addition to these neurotoxic symptoms, cardiovascular effects due to myocarditis may be seen and include various arrhythmias and intractable heart failure. Death usually occurs within 12 hr, but sometimes as late as 2 days after the sting.

Treatment This consists of immediately placing a tight ligature on the extremity just proximal to the sting, followed by application of ice and, as soon as possible, immersion of the involved member above the ligature in ice water. The ligature must be removed in 5 to 10 min, but the limb is kept cool for at least 2 hr. After this time, if treatment has been applied promptly, no serious effects are experienced following the sting of *C. sculpturatus* or *C. gertschi*. If the sting is on the head, trunk, or genitalia, of course, the ligature cannot be used, but the area may be cooled.

Although tourniquet, incision, and suction as in the treatment of snake bite have been recommended, the amount of venom is minute; it produces no local necrotizing effect and is absorbed very rapidly.

Specific antivenin, reconstituted from lyophilized cat serum, is available and should be employed if the victim develops signs of central nervous system or cardiac involvement. Supportive therapy is directed at combating shock and dehydration. Barbiturates in large doses are useful in reducing restlessness. Morphine or meperidine should not be used for pain since these drugs may convert a sublethal dose of scorpion venom into a lethal one.

Prevention This depends upon alertness in avoiding contact with scorpions in infested areas. Clothing and shoes should be well shaken before being put on in the morning. Towels and bedclothes should be inspected. A house infested with scorpions can in time be rid of them by closing all obvious ways of ingress; picking up debris in the environment, such as piles of brush, logs, stones; introducing a mixture of fuel oil or kerosene, containing a small amount of creosote, between the earth and the house foundation; and spraying with a mixture of 2% chlordane, 10% DDT, and 0.2% pyrethrins in an oil base.

HYMENOPTERA STINGS Each year in the United States, nearly twice as many people die as a result of bites by hymenopterous insects (including bees, wasps, hornets, and fire ants) than from poisonous snake bites. Occasionally, multiple stings in man in enormous numbers (500 to 1,000) are the cause of death. However, the majority of systemic reactions and deaths are due to allergic reactions to the venoms of these insects.

Hymenopteran venoms contain histamine, various kinins, and other vasoactive substances, phospholipases, and hyaluronidase. They are hemolytic and neurotoxic in addition to being effective hypersensitizing agents. The usual reaction to a single wasp sting or beesting is sharp pain, local wheal and erythema, intense itching, and in loose tissues such as the eyelid or genitalia, considerable edema which subsides in a few hours. Only in the rare case when a bee is swallowed or inhaled and edema of the laryngopharynx or glottis develops is there danger. A sting directly into a peripheral nerve can destroy its function for a time, much as does an injection of alcohol. Bell's palsy has followed a sting into the trunk of the facial nerve.

In hypersensitive individuals, a single sting may produce serious anaphylaxis with urticaria, nausea, abdominal cramps, asthma, massive edema of the face and glottis, dyspnea, cyanosis, hypotension, coma, and death. Sensitization is usually the result of previous stings. Beekeepers who develop allergic rhinitis followed by asthma when near bees or objects that have been in contact with bees are likely to have serious reactions to stings. It has been estimated that nearly 1 percent of the general population in this country has hymenoptera allergy.

Many ants can produce stinging bites with local redness and swelling, including the notorious fire ant whose bite may result in vesiculation.

Treatment The usual sting is treated by local cool application and antipruritic lotions or oral antihistamines. Epinephrine, 0.3 to 0.5 ml of a 1:1,000 aqueous solution subcutaneously repeated every 20 to 30 min, may be lifesaving in patients with an allergic reaction to a bee sting or wasp sting. Oxygen, endotracheal intubation, vasopressors, and other supportive measures should be used as needed. In addition, corticosteroids should be employed in severe cases.

Prevention Desensitization by injection of extracts of whole bees and wasps is effective and should be considered for any patient who has had a systemic or generalized reaction to hymenopterous insect stings. In addition, contact with these insects should be avoided, and if exposure seems likely, patients should carry an antihistamine or ephedrine for immediate oral use in case of a sting without waiting for symptoms to develop.

TICK BITE AND TICK PARALYSIS The local reaction to the bite of a tick may be nothing more than an itching papule which subsides within a few days unless there is secondary bacterial infection. However, incomplete removal of a tick, with retention of the mouthparts, may result in the local formation of a nodule which continues to grow and is sometimes annoyingly pruritic. The definitive treatment is surgical excision of the nodule. Histologically, the nodule is a granuloma, but the inflammatory response is sometimes so bizarre and changes in the overlying epithelium are so striking that, in the absence of a history of tick bite, a mistaken diagnosis of malignant tumor may be made.

Removal of a tick by steady pulling is preferable to crushing. Touching with a glowing cigarette, freezing, or application of a drop of oil facilitates removal without leaving embedded remnants.

Tick paralysis Tick paralysis is a reversible disorder of the nervous system which sometimes develops in the host while a tick is engorging. It occurs in man and animals. The disease has been reported from many countries and has long been recognized in the northwestern United States and Western Canada, where the wood tick, *Dermacentor andersoni* Stiles, is responsible. The dog tick, *D. variabilis* Say, has been identified in a number of cases occurring in the Eastern states. *Amblyomma americanum*, the lone star tick, and *A. maculatum*, the Gulf Coast tick, have also been incriminated.

While engorging, the tick apparently injects a neurotoxin which acts upon the spinal cord and bulbar nuclei, causing incoordination, weakness, and paralysis. There is failure of neuromuscular transmission and striking impairment of stretch reflexes. The toxin appears to be destroyed or excreted rapidly, for when the tick is removed the nerve cells soon regain normal function.

The tick must feed for several days before symptoms develop. Female ticks commonly remain attached for 7 to 9 days or longer. Paralysis is seen in experimental animals after 5 to 7 days of engorgement. Male ticks feed for a shorter period, a fact which may explain why they are less likely to cause paralysis. In short, the nature, site of production, and mode of action of the toxin are still unknown.

Most human cases occur in children, generally in young girls. The tick is usually attached to the scalp and hidden by the hair, but may be found on any part of the body, especially the ear, axilla, groin, vulva, or popliteal region.

The patient may be irritable and have mild diarrhea for 24 hr before frank motor involvement appears. There are weakness and poor control of the legs, the tendon reflexes in the legs are diminished or absent, and the Romberg sign is positive. Temporary improvement may occur, and if the tick is removed at this stage, true paralysis may never develop. Otherwise the symptoms recur within 24 hr, with flaccid paralysis which extends in 24 to 48 hr to involve the trunk, arms, neck, tongue, and pharynx. Sensory changes are usually absent, but there may be paresthesia and hyperesthesia in the affected extremities. Nystagmus, strabismus, and facial paralysis are sometimes noted. The respirations become shallow, rapid, and irregular. The patient sinks into stupor, cyanosis appears, and death results from respiratory paralysis or from obstruction of the airway by aspirated material. There is little or no fever unless a secondary infection is present. The leukocyte count is usually not elevated, but moderate leukocytosis may occur. The spinal fluid is almost always normal.

Tick paralysis is apt to be confused with poliomyelitis, the more so because ticks are active in warm weather when poliomyelitis is most prevalent.

Among other diseases which might be considered in differential diagnosis are polyneuritis, transverse myelitis, and Guillain-Barré syndrome.

Definitive treatment is removal of the tick. Mouthparts retained in the skin should be promptly excised. The patient's body should be searched for other ticks. There is striking improvement within a few hours after removal of ticks.

If the tick is removed before bulbar involvement develops, the paralysis subsides, and recovery is complete in a few days, sometimes within 24 hr. The patient should be observed until the recovery trend is established, because if other ticks or retained mouthparts have been overlooked, the paralysis may progress. When bulbar or respiratory paralysis is present, death may occur if the tick is not removed in time. Other treatment is supportive.

OTHER ARTHROPOD BITES **Flea bite** There are many fleas that attack man, including *Pulex irritans* and chicken fleas. In sensitive individuals, the salivary secretion of these bloodsuckers produces large, itching papules. Treatment is symptomatic only. Elimination of fleas from the environment may be very difficult, but persistent treatment of animals and of premises with appropriate insecticides is usually successful.

Centipede bite Local irritation is the usual reaction to centipede venom, although extensive necrosis and systemic illness have followed severe poisoning by tropical species. Treatment is purely symptomatic.

Caterpillar urticaria Contact with hairy caterpillars of many species produces irritation of skin or mucous membranes. The type of venom involved is not known, but severe pain, erythema, urticaria, and even blister formation may come on rapidly after direct contact with caterpillars,.after handling cocoons, or on being exposed to windblown fuzz. There are often a regional lymphangitis and transient eosinophilic leukocytosis. The discomfort subsides within 24 hr, but local soaks, oral antihistaminics, and when pain is severe, oral codeine are often indicated.

Bedbug bite Members of the genus *Cimex* inflict bites that leave reactions varying from a simple puncture to large urticarial lesions, apparently depending on the sensitivity of the bitten individual. There is no specific treatment.

Chiggers or redbugs These are tiny mites which are commonly found in foliage, grass, etc., in many parts of the world. In the United States, the larval form of *Eutrobicula alfreddugesi* attacks the skin by secreting a substance which digests tissue, creating a red papule that itches intensely. The tiny reddish larva can be seen in the center of the lesion. Treatment is palliative and consists of antipruritic applications.The use of insect repellents, appropriate protective clothing, and prompt bathing after exposure reduce the risk of infestation considerably.

Myiasis There are, generally speaking, three ways in which human tissues may become infested by maggots. Species of flies which usually deposit eggs in carrion, feces, or garbage may lay eggs in an open wound or ulcer, usually a lesion that is necrotic and suppurating. When the larvae hatch, they feed upon the dead tissue, and despite the unesthetic aspects, the deliberate introduction of maggots has been used to supplement surgical debridement.

Occasionally, food containing fly eggs will be ingested, and when the larvae hatch, *intestinal myiasis* can result in nausea, cramps, and diarrhea. The larvae are passed in the feces.

Finally the larvae of many flies, including the sheep fly and horsefly, will attack living, viable tissue. If eggs are laid in the eyes, nose, ears, mouth, or vagina, an event that usually occurs in sleeping infants, the larvae hatch out and can produce extensive destructive lesions; indeed, fatalities have been reported.

The treatment for maggot infestation is surgical removal by irrigation and mechanical extraction. Obviously, control of fly populations by appropriate sanitary precautions is the important step in prevention. Protection of infants by screening and of wounds by bandaging is indicated in infested areas.

MARINE ANIMAL STINGS The venoms of certain marine animals are known to cause illness in man after injection or inoculation under naturally occurring conditions. Information concerning these toxins is limited; most appear to be composed of proteins and peptides as well as other substances that are pharmacologically active. Although probably less complex than the venoms of reptiles, many marine animal venoms are capable of causing several pathologic effects including neurotoxicity as well as local necrosis.

Sea anemone sting (sponge diver's disease) Contact with certain sea anemones (especially *Sargatia elegans*) in Mediterranean and African waters produces extensive dermatitis with chronic ulceration. Occasionally, especially during August and September, systemic symptoms of headache, sneezing, nausea, chills, fever, and collapse are noted. Rare fatalities have occurred. No specific therapy is known; the skin lesions have been thought to benefit from local x-ray irradiation. The disease confers no immunity.

Sponge poisoning Direct contact with several species of sponge results in a painful dermatitis. Dilute acetic acid ameliorates local pain strikingly, and alkali will intensify it. The lesions are self-limited.

Portuguese man-o-war and jellyfish stings The burning discomfort induced by contact with "sea nettles" or jellyfish is familiar to most surf bathers. Contact with the tentacles of the colorful Portuguese man-o-war (*Physalia* species), which is found mainly in the Gulf of Mexico area, or more toxic jellyfish (*Chiropsalmus* of the Indian Ocean and *Rhizostoma* of the Atlantic) is followed by severe pain, swelling, and erythema. Muscle pain, weakness, abdominal cramps, nausea, dyspnea, cyanosis, and collapse may persist for several days, and fatalities have occurred, sometimes within hours after contact.

Treatment consists of local application of alkaline substances such as ammonia which neutralize the toxin, analgesics for the pain, and calamine lotion or antihistamines orally if there is an accompanying pruritic rash. Corticosteroids may be helpful in severe cases.

Cone shell poisoning The colorful cone shells are highly prized by collectors. Many species in the Pacific are venomous, a great danger to unwary hobbyists who pick them up. The poison is delivered into a wound inflicted by pointed hollow teeth resembling darts in the long proboscis of the animal. Local manifestations include sudden intense pain, swelling, and cyanosis followed by numbness. The venom is apparently a neurotoxin and produces muscular incoordination, weakness, confusion, tachycardia, and dyspnea. Death may occur within 3 to 5 hr, but recovery within 24 hr is the rule. Recommended treatment is the use of tourniquet, incision, and suction (as for snake bite) and supportive measures which may include artificial respiration and administration oxygen.

Sea urchin sting Contact with the spines of some species of sea urchin results in painful erythema and ulceration, occasionally accompanied by neurotoxic symptoms of weakness and frank paralysis of lips, tongue, and face lasting for several hours. Treatment is purely symptomatic and supportive. The toxins isolated from sea urchins have produced paralysis in animals and are notably resistant to heat. Deaths from paralysis and drowning have been reported.

Venomous fish stings The dorsal fins or spines of bullhead sharks, dogfish, and ratfish and the dorsal and other fins of the scorpion fish, weeverfish, toadfish, and catfish are grooved, and at their bases are found venom glands. Injury by these spines results in severe pain and swelling and, in some instances, neurotoxic manifestations. Local gangrene with extensive tissue loss is a complication of catfish stings that may prolong convalescence. Little or nothing is known of the venoms involved. Suction and hot applications are advocated immediately after injury. Tetanus toxoid or antitoxin should be given also. Narcotics are often required to control the pain. Secondary pyogenic infection is a frequent complication.

Probably the most frequent type of venomous fish injury in the United States is that produced by the lashing tail of the stingray of the California coast (*Urobatis halleri*). The bony spine is encased in a sheath of epithelial cells containing venom which is expressed into the puncture wound. The wound may be several centimeters deep; portions of the bony spine may break off in it, or, more often, the integumentary sheath remains in the wound. The venom is a circulatory depressant in animals, but local injury predominates in man. There are immediately severe pain and cyanosis followed by erythema and edema. Weakness, rarely, convulsions, and death may ensue. Treatment consists of application of a tourniquet (the vast majority of these injuries occur on the legs) and copious syringing of the wound with salt water to remove fragments of sheath followed by immersion in water as hot as the patient can stand for 1 hr. The venom is heat-labile, and extensive trials have indicated the usefulness of this last procedure. Tetanus toxoid or antiserum is indicated; as with other fish stings, pyogenic infection is a frequent complication.

REFERENCES

Hymenoptera bites

BEARD RL: Insect toxins and venoms. Annu Rev Entomol 8:1, 1963

FAVORITE FG: The imported fire ant. Pub Health Rep 73:445, 1958

MARKS MB: Stinging insects: Allergy implications. Pediatr Clin N Am 16:177, 1969

MCLEAN JA: Management of insect sting reactions. Mod Treat 5:814, 1968

Marine toxins and venoms

KEEGAN HL, MACFARLANE WV (eds): *Venomous and Poisonous Animals and Noxious Plants of the Pacific Region*, Oxford: Pergamon, 1965

NIGRELLI RF (ed): Biochemistry and pharmacology of compounds derived from marine organisms. Ann NY Acad Sci 90:615, 1960

RUSSELL FE: Marine toxins and venomous and poisonous marine animals. Adv Marine Biol 3:255, 1965

Other arthropod bites

HANEVELD GT: Centipede bites. Br Med J 2:592, 1952

JAMES MT: The flies that cause myiasis in man. U.S. Dept of Agriculture Misc Publication no. 631, 1947

MCMILLAN CW, PURCELL WR: Health hazard from caterpillars. N Engl J Med 271:147, 1964

Scorpion stings

BARTHOLOMEW C: Acute scorpion pancreatitis in Trinidad. Br Med J 1:666, 1970

HOREN WP: Insect and scorpion sting. JAMA 221:894, 1972

SITA DEVI S, et al: Defibrination syndrome due to scorpion venom poisoning. Br Med J 1:345, 1970

Snake bite and gila monster bite

COMBINED STAFF CLINIC: Poisoning by venomous animals. Am J Med 42:107, 1967

NATIONAL RESEARCH COUNCIL: Ad hoc committee report on snake bite therapy. Toxicon 1:81, 1963

PARRISH HM: Analysis of 460 fatalities from venomous animals in the United States. Am J Med Sci 245:129, 1963

PARRISH HM, HAYES RH: Hospital management of pit viper venenations. Clin Toxicol 3:501, 1970

RUSSELL FE: Clinical aspects of snake venom poisoning in North America. Toxicon 7:33, 1969

RUSSELL FE, PUFFER HW: Pharmacology of snake venoms. Clin Toxicol 3:433, 1970

SHANNON FA: Case reports of the gila monster bites. Herpetology 9:127, 1953

SPARGER CF: Problems in the management of rattlesnake bites. AMA Arch Surg 98:13, 1969

Spider bites

EDITORIAL: Spider bites. Lancet 2:509, 1969

GORHAM JR: The brown recluse spider, loxosceles reclusa and necrotic spider bite—A new public health problem in the United States. J Environ Health 31:138, 1968

HOREN WP: Arachnidism in the United States. JAMA 185:839, 1963

Tick paralysis

CHERINGTON M, SNYDER RD: Tick paralysis: Neurophysiologic studies. N Engl J Med 278:95, 1968

EDITORIAL: Tick paralysis. Br Med J 3:314, 1969

section 3 | Physical agents

116
DISORDERS DUE TO ENVIRONMENTAL TEMPERATURES

GEORGE W. THORN

Three clinical syndromes are associated with high environmental temperature: *heat cramps, heat exhaustion,* and *heat pyrexia.* These disorders are discussed in Chaps. 11 and 12.

For the internist *cold injuries* involve primarily peripheral tissues and peripheral vascular changes. *Frostbite, immersion foot,* and the prevention of cold injury by *cold acclimatization* are discussed in Chap. 247. In present day medical practice, the use of hypothermia is limited to cardiovascular surgery.

117
DISORDERS DUE TO ALTERATIONS IN BAROMETRIC PRESSURE

ALBERT R. BEHNKE

INTRODUCTION Man can perform efficiently for periods of weeks in the pressure-reduced (0.33 atm) oxygen atmosphere of space capsules or altitude chambers. In the open sea, he has descended to a depth of 1,000 ft (31 atm), and he has endured pressurization in chambers to 61.6 atm, equivalent to a depth of 2,001 feet. Saturation diving, which entails prolonged exposures in high-pressure habitats and slow decompression in submersible chambers, is now routine in the recovery of oil from the sea bottom. Pressurized (air) tunneling is employed extensively in the installation of sewage conduits and the construction of vehicular tunnels and underground transit systems. The recreational and exploratory facets of diving with scuba (Self-Contained Underwater Breathing Apparatus) claim the interest of several million enthusiasts. Numerous investigators and technicians conduct experiments in altitude and pressure chambers. In medicine, hyperbaric oxygen has been strikingly effective as an adjuvant in the treatment of gas gangrene, carbon monoxide poisoning, and other acute hypoxic conditions. These accelerating developments require the attention of the physician to the physiologic problems and measures to be employed in handling the usually dramatic accidents connected with dysbarism.

Injury arises from too rapid ascent (aeroembolism, decompression sickness); indirectly from cold, hypoxia, nitrogen narcosis, hyperventilation tetany, and overexertion; and in closed breathing systems from oxygen toxicity and carbon dioxide excess. Mishaps are caused by logistic failure (the empty gas bottle); equipment deficiencies, notably lack of recompression chambers; and casual organization. Always in imminent danger of drowning, the scuba diver (breathing unnaturally through a mouthpiece and with head surrounded by water) often complicates the environmental hazard with his obsession to establish new records with diving gear which for the novice should be restricted to "free ascent" depths (without need for recompression). The practice, particularly among adolescents, of breath holding under water is conducive to hypoxic heart failure, especially during the course of heavy exertion required in swimming. Too rapid ascent of scuba divers may overexpand the lungs and give rise to air embolism, pneumothorax, and subcutaneous emphysema. "Squeeze" effects may involve the eye, middle ear and mastoid cells, and paranasal sinuses, and occasionally produce minute gas aggregates in pulp of diseased teeth. Rapid decompression after sojourn at diving depths, and even following rapid ascent to simulated or actual high altitude, may initiate bubble evolution and decompression sickness.

Diving tables evolved on an empirical basis, for the most part from fragmentary tests, afford high (96 to 99 percent) but no complete protection against decompression sickness. Oxygen inhalation provides a reliable safeguard. It is likely that all decompressions (not attended by oxygen inhalation) conducted in accord with current diving tables are associated with some degree of nascent bubble evolution in circulating blood. Of importance is the abrupt onset, following a latent period of well-being, of postdecompression malaise, which may be related to liberation of painless "silent bubbles," detected by the Doppler ultrasonic technique. Such bubbles may be conducive to tissue hypoxia and liberation into the circulation of proteolytic enzymes, peptides, and potassium ions.

Decompression sickness in man in the majority of cases (type I, bends) readily responds, without complications, to recompression therapy. In severe decompression sickness (type II), substantial observations in animals show that intravascular bubbles are complicated by fat embolization of the lungs and disseminated microemboli consisting of aggregates of platelets and cells, in conjunction with hemoconcentration.

Advances in recompression therapy emphasize the value of oxygen inhalation at tolerance pressures (27 psi) without resorting to high air atmospheres except in unusual circumstances. Dramatic recoveries have occurred when prompt treatment has been accorded seemingly moribund divers. Even divers rendered paraplegic as a result of delay in treatment due to lack of on-site pressure chambers nevertheless may recover motor function following prolonged pressurization and appropriate follow-up hospital therapy. Promising advances in treatment relate to the value of fluid (dextran) administration to counteract hemoconcentration frequently observed in serious cases, notably in aviation personnel who have not been recompressed to hyperbaric atmospheres.

Important is the role of the physician in administrative leadership. In cooperation with the well-qualified members of the National Association of Underwater Instructors (NAUI) who are available in every community, he should prepare a chart of emergency procedures which (1) establishes lines of communication, (2) outlines measures to handle near-drowning accidents, air embolism, and decompression sickness, and (3) nominates persons qualified to handle "on-the-spot" emergencies.

HYPERBARIC CHAMBERS Catastrophic fires have occurred in oxygen-enriched atmospheres at normal and even hypobaric pressures, but the hazard is compounded in the hyperbaric chamber. *In an oxygen-enriched atmosphere, in contrast with air atmospheres, there are no immediately effective measures to quench a fire.* In large chambers in which attending personnel are present, it is mandatory that oxygen be administered to patients by means of closed systems which cannot enrich the ambient air. There is danger of implosion if sealed capsules or containers are brought into the pressurized chamber.

The National Research Council brochure provides guidelines for safe operation of hyperbaric chambers, but indoctrination at successfully operating installations is strongly recommended.

PRIMARY PRESSURE PHENOMENA

EFFECT OF PRESSURE PER SE AND OF BAROTRAUMA Normally some tissues of the body are subjected to compressive or distending pressure (the arteries, vertebras, and lower extremities) of the order of 100 to 200 mm Hg (1 to 2 psi). Pressure gradients also exist in an individual who is immersed in water up to his neck. In this condition, cardiac output (heart rate unchanged) may increase 32 percent (1.8 liters per min), accompanied by a decrease in vascular resistance (30 percent) and an increase of central blood volume of 0.7 liter. By contrast, the pressure of the atmosphere (sea level, 760 mm Hg, 14.7 psi, equivalent to 33 ft of seawater) can be increased at a moderate rate to 60 atm in the hyperbaric chamber without appreciable impairment. Rapid compression (3 atm per min) followed by prolonged residence at depths deeper than 300 ft is associated frequently with *arthralgia*, which was not recognized in a previous era of relatively short surface-depth and return dives. The joint pain does not supervene if descent is slowed to about 50 ft per hr. An explanatory hypothesis underlying this phenomenon is that initially, during the course of rapid compression, equilibrium is incomplete between inert gas tension in blood and in tissue. Hence, there may be an "osmotic" effect which serves to shift fluid from cartilage. Another pressure phenomenon, distinct from the narcosis induced by nitrogen, is the *high-pressure hyperexcitability syn-*

drome manifest in man at simulated depths of about 1,100 ft and characterized by tremors and somnolence. Various mammalian species are susceptible at deeper depths to pressure-induced tremors and convulsive seizures.

Density of inhaled gases increases linearly with pressure, but the work of breathing is roughly proportional to the square root of pressure. Compared with air, the equivalent pressure while breathing helium-oxygen at 10 atm is reduced by a factor of three. Test data show that man can remain for days in a chamber–wet pot complex and perform moderate work without respiratory impairment at simulated depths of 1,000 feet (31 atm).

In air (3 atm), despite the increased density, emphysematous patients may report improvement during and following sojourn under pressure. However, in respiration conducted with valvular systems there may be distress. Hence, it is mandatory *that there be physician-technician trial of all respiratory equipment at all pressures prior to use by the patient.*

In contrast to innocuous application of great external forces equally distributed over the body is the small pressure difference (50 to 100 mm Hg) which serves to distend blood vessels and induce edema in occluded sinal (aerosinustis) and aural (aerotitis media) spaces. Following hyperbaric oxygen therapy, patients may experience this cupping effect during sleep, when the auditory tubes are not opened periodically by swallowing and negative pressure is created by oxygen absorption. The most frequent cause of blockage of auditory tubes (which usually is only relative in relation to rate of pressure application) is acute and chronic infection of the nasopharynx. At any one time as many as one-third of submarine personnel may show varying grades of barotrauma. A convenient classification is grade 0 (normal), 1 (redness of Shrapnell's membrane and along the manubrium), 2 (redness of entire membrane), 3 (same as grade 2 plus fluid or fluid and bubbles in the middle ear), and 4 (blood in the middle ear, perforation of the tympanic membrane, or both). These changes are clearly apparent on routine otoscopic inspection. Remarkably there is no residual impairment of auditory acuity in the speech range incurred by this type of trauma. Deafness for higher tones is frequent in divers, with noise implicated as the etiologic factor. *Specific therapy is not required for barotrauma;* healing in the author's experience is spontaneous and rarely complicated by secondary infection. In grade 4 (blood in middle ear) the otologist should be consulted.

COMPLICATIONS ARISING FROM OVERINFLATION OF THE LUNGS If a diver holds his breath on ascent to the surface, the intrapulmonic pressure tends to increase relative to hydrostatic pressure. Excess pressures of 80 mm Hg or higher overinflate the lungs, rupture blood vessels, and force gas along dissecting planes. With the first inhalation of air by the diver on reaching the surface, gas is aspirated into pulmonary veins and disseminated to the central nervous system to bring about collapse. This type of accident has occurred 23 times in 150,000 submarine training escapes. In one instance death followed a too rapid ascent from the shallow depth of 15 ft. It is not an uncommon accident in scuba diving. Acute collapse during decompression has been reported in tunnel workers. The signs and symptoms were those of aeroembolism, not of decompression sickness. In several of the patients lung cysts were identified. Treatment of aeroembolism calls for immediate recompression with oxygen inhalation. This disability can be minimized by physical examination to exclude pulmonary pathologic change (cysts, costophrenic adhesions, bronchiolitis) and by proper training. Routine free ascents can be made from depths of 100 ft if exhalation is continuous. The practice, however, is not encouraged.

SECONDARY PRESSURE PHENOMENA RELATED TO INCREASED PARTIAL PRESSURE OF GASES

NARCOTIC ACTION OF NITROGEN When the air pressure in a chamber is raised above 3 atm, the increased partial pressure of nitrogen is associated with changes in mood, notably euphoria, and impaired judgment and motor performance. The effects are similar to those induced by intoxicants, such as alcohol. Although all individuals are in varying degrees narcotized at diving depths, emotionally stable persons react to the stress by compensatory effort and are able to carry out an assigned task (slowly at high pressures) until consciousness is lost. The unstable person is incapable of purposeful effort and gives way to emotional aberrations characteristic of some alcoholics. Sophisticated studies havé provided quantitative assessment of the impairment. If, for example, the elctroencephalogram is recorded at normal pressure when a subject is attempting to solve an arithmetical problem, there is a blocking of occipital alpha rhythm which at increased pressure ("nitrogen threshold") disappears after a latent period. The period of latency is inversely proportional to the square of the pressure. Of interest is the fact that at relatively low pressures (2.5 atm, 50 ft) not associated with overt impairment, a nitrogen effect on the brain may be detected. The nitrogen narcotic phenomenon, as an innocuous stress without residual impairment, may be applied in psychic evaluation of individuals. The lack of narcotic effect of helium makes diving to depths of 2,000 ft feasible.

OXYGEN POISONING Although inhalation of oxygen at high pressures (OHP) may give rise to limiting pulmonary and CNS alterations, it has been breathed routinely up to 3 atm during decompression of divers, in the treatment of decompression sickness, and in hyperbaric chambers in hospitals. Oxygen (OHP) therapy is possible because there is a latent period preceding overt signs and symptoms, during which cardiac function is not impaired, and initial untoward reactions are reversible when air breathing is resumed. Tolerance time for inhalation of oxygen at higher pressures is greatly extended by short intervals of air inhalation in accord with the outline in Table 117-1.

In man, pulmonary (and tracheal) irritation is elicited at lower pressure levels (0.6 to 2 atm), while neurotoxic effects are observed at higher pressures. In carefully monitored studies, it was found that healthy men could breathe oxygen (2 atm) for about 8 hr before significant (5 to 10 percent) decreases in vital capacity occurred. After 8 to 12 hr of inhalation, the symptoms, progressive in

TABLE 117-1
Guide for administration of hyperbaric oxygen during decompression and in recompression therapy*

Pressure, psi	*Unit exposure (U.E.) intervals, min* — *Oxygen*	*Air*	*No. of U.E. for routine inhalation*†
27	20	5	1, 2, 3
27–13	40		1
13	20	5	1, 2, 3
13–0	40		1

* *Based on U.S. Navy experience.*
† *Depending upon duration of previous hyperbaric air exposure (decompression) or the condition of the patient during recompression.*

intensity, were burning sensation on deep inspiration, carinal irritation, cough, and dyspnea. At higher pressures, the pulmonary limit for oxygen inhalation has not been determined. Despite edema and hemorrhagic consolidation observed chiefly in the lungs of small animals exposed to hyperbaric O_2, there has been in man a virtual absence of pulmonary complications. No exacerbation of subclinical respiratory infection has been reported in divers who inhaled O_2 for periods of several hours or longer (up to 3 atm) in the treatment of decompression sickness. In over 1,000 experiments (1.9 to 4.68 atm) reported by Donald, the endpoint was anchored to signs and symptoms referable to the nervous system. Data compiled by Goodman from 1951 to 1961 at the U.S. Navy Deep Sea Diving School summarize 1,388 exposures of 30-min duration to O_2 inhalation at 2.82 atm (27.8 psi, 60 ft equivalent). There were adverse reactions in 14 examinees, 5 of whom had seizures. Subsequently, in accord with the "low-pressure" O_2 treatment tables, 20-min periods of O_2 inhalation interspersed with 5-min intervals on air have been well tolerated during the course of hundreds of treatments. In the author's series of 135 cases of decompression sickness treated with hyperbaric O_2 with air-spaced intervals, there have been no adverse reactions. Notably, cardiac function is not impaired, despite the inhibitory action of OHP on many enzyme systems, particularly those containing essential sulfhydryl groups. Thus the heart in anesthetized dogs may beat for periods of 1 hr or longer following respiratory paralysis, and succumbs only after asphyxial concentrations of CO_2 (+100 to 200 mm Hg) have accumulated in the lungs.

Limitations to O_2 hyperbaric therapy pertain not only to deficiencies in our knowledge as to etiology but also to the variability of individual response and unpredictability of tissue O_2 tensions. At 3 atm (oxygen) arterial blood may contain 6 vol percent of oxygen in solution (P_{O_2} 2,000 mm Hg). As a result of vasoconstriction (a direct oxygen effect) or vasodilatation (a CO_2 effect), there may be widely fluctuating tensions (70 to 1,400 mm Hg) of oxygen in mixed venous blood withdrawn from the right ventricle. The inference is that O_2 tensions at the cellular level also fluctuate widely.

Neurotoxic effects terminate the relatively benign latent period after about 2 hr of oxygen inhalation at 3 atm. Underlying individual variability of response are such factors which shorten the latent period of comparative well-being as adrenal, thyroid, or pituitary hormones, exercise, increased CO_2 tensions, elevated metabolism, and apprehension. On the other hand, individuals at rest, following overnight fast, and phlegmatic in disposition have tolerated inhalation of O_2 (99 percent) for periods of 30 min at the usually convulsive level of 4 atm. Untoward responses in susceptible individuals at from 3 to 4 atm are twitching or tremors of facial muscles (notably lips and eyebrows), restlessness, anxiety, periodic waves of nausea, occasional vomiting, diminished visual acuity, narrowing of visual fields, numbness of fingers and toes, reversal of pulse rate, sharp rise in diastolic pressure, auditory hallucinations and other aura, fainting (occasionally), and violent convulsive seizures. Residual effects following seizures have not been observed in man. In regard to pharmacologic protective agents, succinate and gamma-aminobutyric acid have been highly effective in animals. Coupled with newer knowledge of membrane transport, the pharmacologic approach holds promise for man.

ALTERATION OF CARBON DIOXIDE TENSION Carbon dioxide enhances not only the toxicity of oxygen (a specific CO_2 effect independent of the lowering of pH) but the narcotic effect of nitrogen and other inert gases as well. An elementary assessment of this phenomenon relates CO_2 enhancement to increased cerebral blood flow. During rapid descent in deep sea diving, momentary vertigo and confusion are in part attributed to inadequate exhalation of CO_2 as a result of rapid compression. The effective CO_2 percentage should not exceed 1.5 percent, although percentages of CO_2 up to 5 are fairly well tolerated in submarines for at least 60 hr. There are no reliable data for extended periods of inhalation of high concentrations of CO_2 (+3 percent).

In the presence of elevated concentrations of CO_2 during inhalation of oxygen at 1 atm or higher pressures, consciousness may be lost suddenly (oxygen blackout) without onset of dyspnea. Divers working in air at high pressures have tolerated some remarkably high P_{CO_2} levels (e.g., 57 mm Hg) in arterial blood without distress when using breathing apparatus which prevented adequate pulmonary ventilation. A critical consideration is that warning signs of CO_2 excess at normal pressures may be absent in the pressurized environment. Hyperventilation may induce respiratory alkalosis and tetany. The danger of hypoxemia is greatly enhanced when hyperventilation in air removes the CO_2 stimulus during breath holding.

UPTAKE OF NITROGEN AT INCREASED PRESSURE At atmospheric pressure (P_{N_2}: 570 mm Hg) about 9 ml of nitrogen is dissolved per kilogram of body fluid, and about 55 ml per kilogram of body fat. In a lean, 70-kg man (7 kg fat) about 400 ml of nitrogen is in body fluids, 100 ml in bone and spinal cord, and 400 ml in fat. About 5.2 liters of blood per minute perfuses the nonlipid cellular mass, and only about 0.7 liter of blood perfuses bone and adipose tissue. The half-time for N_2 uptake of various nonlipid tissues varies from 2 to 20 min (98.5 percent saturation in 12 to 120 min), and for organs containing large amounts of lipid (adipose tissue, long bones, spinal cord), half-time uptake may vary from 60 to 120 min (1 to 2 hr) in a lean man. In men with more fat (20 to 30 percent of body weight), half-time for saturation of adipose tissue may be increased two- to threefold. In the United States the worktime in tunnel operations is limited to men with a tissue half-time of usually not more than 120 min. In England operational schedules are more rigorous and the incidence of avascular bone necrosis is high.

DECOMPRESSION PROCEDURES It is evident that decompression time following prolonged exposures will be greatly influenced in air dives by the amount of fat in the body. If exposures are of short duration, the amount of fat is not important as a decompression hazard. Haldane's ratio principle applies to short exposures in compressed air, and it is relatively safe to halve the absolute pressure to permit rapid ascent to the first stop. However, after prolonged (saturation) exposures in the hyperbaric environment, it is becoming increasingly evident that the ratio principle does not apply to *successive stages* of decompression and that only a small pressure head (ΔP) governs inert gas transport from tissues to lungs. In accord with the isobaric ("oxygen window") principle of decompression, ΔP is the difference between arterial and venous oxygen pressures. Hence safe decompression following helium-oxygen saturation exposures at deep depths requires from 10 to 15 min per ft of ascent. The time required for decompression is measured not in hours, but in days. Based on the hypothesis that ΔP can be appreciably elevated above isobaric tissue levels (i.e., inert gas pressure in tissue is never allowed to exceed ambient pressure during decompression), diving tables become in effect "treatment" tables applicable to a state of gas transport not in solution but, in part at least, in bubble form.

FACTORS AFFECTING BUBBLE FORMATION After exposure to high pressure or high altitudes (in chambers, unpressurized aircraft), factors conducive to decompression sickness fall into two groups. In the first are conditions which increase gas content of tissues, namely, the amount of fat, degree and duration of exposure, intensity of work, and, in rapid ascent to high altitudes, exercise, which expands the gaseous reservoir with CO_2 accretion and facilitates cavitation. In the second group are variables affecting tissue perfusion and diffusion of gas in transport from tissue as well as surface tension and other biophysical factors affecting blood. Thus age, time of day, disruption of circadian rhythms, dehydration, fright, injury, and postalcoholic residuum seemingly affect gas transport.

ACCLIMATIZATION Divers subjected to older decompression schedules for tunnel workers developed a high incidence of bends. It appears that men who expose themselves regularly to compressed air day after day become less susceptible to attacks of decompression sickness. About 14 days are required for maximal effect. Acclimatization is gradually lost when men cease to work in compressed air. The recognition of this phenomenon by Paton and Walder is of practical importance.

DECOMPRESSION SICKNESS

ETIOLOGY The preponderance of experimental data implicates intravascular bubbles as the initiating causal agent. In rapidly decompressed animals circulating bubbles can be observed in arteries and veins; subsequently sequestered bubbles accumulate in veins. Secondary phenomena complicate the simple etiology. Newer knowledge of the role of platelets in arterial thrombosis has been applied to the decompression complication. Thus, intravascular bubbles serve not only to free lipid by disruption of lipoprotein linkages but to form aggregates of platelets and red blood cells incident to release of serotonin and adenosine diphosphate (ADP). It is evident that in severe decompression sickness both the bubble formation and the particulate aggregate precipitate stasis and hemoconcentration.

SIGNS AND SYMPTOMS Sequestration of nascent gas bubbles in vascular beds of tissues and organs gives rise to a remarkable array of dissimilar syndromes (Table 117-2). In British classification, pain in the region of joints (bends) is designated type I (mild); respiratory, cardiovascular, and neurologic involvement is designated type II (serious), which includes *aeroembolism* arising, as explained previously, from gas introduced extraneously into the circulation. Type I cases may progress to type II. The chief problem concerns the early recognition of signs and symptoms and application of recompression therapy.

Bends The bends may be described as an aching, radiating type of pain, occasionally synchronous with pulse beat, of gradual onset, progressive in intensity, and felt in the joints, muscles, and bones of the extremities. Response to recompression therapy is immediate (occasionally there is exacerbation of pain if pressure is applied too rapidly), and there is no residual disability, with the reservation that the relationship of bends to aseptic bone necrosis remains to be clarified.

TABLE 117-2
Signs and symptoms of decompression sickness

Central nervous system	*Cardio-respiratory*	*Extremities*	*Skin; systemic*
Loss of consciousness	Substernal distress	Pain	Pruritus
Scintillating scotomata	Paroxysmal coughing	Paresthesia	Mottling
Ménière's syndrome	Tachypnea	Numbness	Rash
Vertigo, aphasia	Asphyxia (chokes)	Weakness	Pallor
Staggering gait	Shock	Bone necrosis	Lowered temperature
Spastic paralysis	Hemoconcentration	Cartilage destruction	Fever, sweating, malaise
Sensory loss	Platelet–RBC aggregates	Edema	
Bladder, bowel paralysis			

Chokes and the shock syndrome A type of asphyxia referred to by early workers as "chokes" may be preceded by several hours of well-being following decompression. An early symptom is a sensation of substernal soreness elicited by deep inspiration which may provoke paroxysmal coughing. Inhalation of cigarette smoke aggravates the untoward reaction. Hemoconcentration and classical signs of circulatory shock are associated with this disability, particularly if onset is gradual.

Neurologic involvement (CNS) Scintillating scotomata and transient episodes of vertigo and dizziness are not uncommon. The staggering gait and slurred speech simulate drunkenness, and recompression must be resorted to for differential diagnosis. Ménière's syndrome, presumably resulting from infarction of blood supply to the inner ear, was not uncommon in early tunnel workers. In recent decompressions following saturation dives, nerve deafness has been reported. Aeroembolism usually can be recognized as distinct from the neurologic sign of decompression sickness, by abrupt onset, unconsciousness with convulsion (usually focal), and independence of duration of exposure.

Paralysis of spinal cord origin, manifest as a spastic monoplegia or paraplegia, is usually confined to the lower extremities. Areas of hypersensitivity are present above the site of the cord lesion, and paresthesia of sensory paralysis occurs below. *An early premonitory sign is numbness,* which should alert the physician to anticipate a type II condition rather than bends. There is incontinence of urine and feces following involvement of the lower part of the spinal cord. The imperative requirement to catheterize the bladder in the acute condition may be overlooked. Recovery or at least considerable improvement may occur following prolonged recompression with oxygen, even though many hours may elapse between onset of disability and recompression therapy. Prognosis for ultimate restoration of function cannot be made early since improvement may continue over a 2-year period following injury. Gas bubbles impair blood supply but do not transect the spinal cord!

Bone lesions A serious complication associated with work in pressurized tunnel operations is aseptic bone necrosis, and as many as 75 percent of oldtime workmen show radiographic bone disease. Lesions have also been observed in divers. Aseptic bone necrosis is related to the number of times a man has been decompressed, to the pressure level at which he has worked, and to the number of reported bends. Accepted decompression procedures in England, where hours of work are relatively long, are not adequate to prevent bone lesions. Innovations in decompression practice as incorporated into Washington State Tables (1963) greatly extend decompression time by stage rather than uniform decompression. There is good reason to believe that the extended decompression time and *shorter daily exposures* will prevent occurrence of crippling lesions.

Crippling lesions which are the result of juxtaarticular infarction and subsequent deformity and destruction of the joint surface are confined to shoulder and hip joints. By contrast, the knee joint, which is the most common site of bends, is not disabled. *A prime consideration is that the lesions are asymptomatic unless joint surfaces are involved.* The vivid x-ray visualized lesions in the medullary shaft of long bones are innocuous. An impediment in diagnosis is a latent period of a year or longer before pathologic change becomes manifest. Our lack of definitive knowledge of aseptic bone necrosis is reflected by inability to explain why similar workmen in the same environment remain free from joint and medullary lesions. An essential part of the physical examination *prior to work in compressed air* and at yearly intervals during work in compressed air is radiologic survey of the long bones.

RECOMPRESSION TREATMENT OF DECOMPRESSION SICKNESS AND AIR EMBOLISM The value of oxygen therapy without the need for higher air or oxygen pressures has been confirmed for type I cases (bends), and shows promise also in management of type II cases, including aeroembolism (Workman 1968). However, with availability of proper gas mixtures, in the author's opinion, high pressures should be utilized for treatment of serious cases. The outline of oxygen decompression and recompression procedures (Table 117-1), adapted from earlier and current U.S. Navy experience, is a guide for employment of hyperbaric oxygen inhalation. Recompression procedure in the U.S. Navy Diving Manual is to be regarded as standard practice. Occasionally long periods of time measured in days are required for compression therapy to be fully effective. Patients can be kept for weeks (if necessary) at 2.52 atm (50 ft) if there is indication that pressure decrement will cause further deterioration. Occasionally a puzzling relapse may occur during the course of treatment which is not responsive to additional pressure (occasionally to 10 atm). Errors in treatment relate to (1) inadequate time spent at peak pressure when patients are seriously ill—*the condition of the patient must regulate decompression therapy,* (2) failure to apply the compression test to doubtful cases, (3) inadequate medical monitoring during the recompression period, (4) failure to keep the treated patient near the recompression for a 24-hr period, and (5) overzealous fluid and drug therapy in type I and uncomplicated cases which respond solely to oxygen recompression therapy.

Other therapeutic measures Adjuvant therapy depends upon whether a patient is in a recompression chamber or in an intensive care unit. With oxygen recompression and recourse to high pressure, one can anticipate immediate recovery in type I cases, and in the absence of shock, a reversal of circulatory and pulmonary derangements without additional supportive treatment except administration of fluids by mouth and sedation. A problem area centers in the relapse of the neurologic patient who fails to respond to additional recompression. Plasma has proved to be restorative when administered to divers who were not revived by additional recompression. In animals administration of low molecular weight dextran has been strikingly effective in the absence of recompression. Pauley and Cockett have outlined the merits of dextran administration and more extensive adjuvant therapy than that presented by this author.

The treatment of traumatic injuries under pressure poses difficult and unresolved problems. An emergency tray should provide a selection of items outlined in the National Research Council brochure.

DERANGEMENTS AT HIGH ALTITUDE

ALTITUDE LIMITS About 600 million persons live at altitudes above 6,500 ft (0.79 atm); although remarkable adaptation is seen in the Andean at 15,000 ft (0.57 atm), permanent residence is restricted to about 18,000 ft (0.5 atm). At higher altitudes, cold and inadequate food and shelter are supplementary to the severe hypoxia which in itself forfends adaptation. However, the mountaineer acclimatizes sufficiently in 1 to 3 months at intermediate altitudes so as to enable him to climb Mt. Everest (29,002 ft) with the aid of supplemental oxygen, and Nanga Parbat (26,660 ft) without added oxygen. These feats represent exceptional acclimatization and endurance but are limited to no more than about 10 days, since rapid deterioration ensues after longer periods at elevations above 25,000 feet. Physicians and physiologists, despite extreme conditions, have spent more than 5 months conducting tests at 19,000 ft. Noteworthy is the persistent loss of weight in climbers above 22,000 ft, explained in part by depression of appetite attending a diet adequate in nutrients but consisting of highly concentrated, processed foods. "In contrast, fresh foods of any description including tough goat meat that would have been rejected as inedible under normal conditions, were eagerly consumed at all altitudes"(Siri).

ACCLIMATIZATION The newcomer to altitude is affected both by hypoxia and the respiratory alkalosis that attends compensatory hyperventilation. These physiologic stresses account for the initial dyspnea, tachycardia, malaise, headache, and insomnia, which are intensified relative to level of altitude and activity. The acute symptoms subside in 2 to 3 days, and the most important physiologic adjustments take place within 2 to 3 weeks. The opportunity to study Olympic athletes in preparation for the 1968 Games in Mexico City (altitude, 7,500 ft, 0.75 atm) afforded highly reliable data. Noteworthy in trained men whose performance at sea level is within a fractional second was the individual variation at the moderate altitude in such tests as maximal O_2 consumption even after altitude training. Compensating mechanisms tending to restore normal aerobic activity were increase in pulmonary ventilation, alteration in cardiac output for any given work intensity, an initial hemoconcentration incident to reduction in plasma volume, gradual increase in red blood cells and hemoglobin content, increase in myoglobin, and vasodilatation in tissues supporting optimal function.

The striking response to arterial hypoxemia of altitude is the compensatory linear response of erythropoiesis to decreasing arterial saturation. Iron supplementation may augment this response. This is exemplified by the study of Hannon et al. of college women resident at 700 ft altitude who worked in the summer in a tourist concession at the top of Pike's Peak (14,110 ft). During March, the women (at 700 ft) were conditioned by sports activity and their diet was supplemented by 5-gr tablets daily of ferrous sulfate. This supplementation prior to the altitude sojourn was accompanied by an increase in mean hematocrit from 40.3 to 43; after 2½ months at Pike's Peak, hematocrit level increased to 49.6 percent. Subjects who did not receive the iron supplement had a mean altitude hematocrit of 44.6 A reliable index of acclimatization was the resting pulse rate, which declined from over 100 initially, to the control level of about 75 at the end of the altitude tests. Plasma volume decreased about 20 percent. Of more than passing interest is the more rapid acclimatization to altitude of the college women than of soldiers previously tested at Pike's Peak.

ADAPTATIONS IN THE ANDEAN At a somewhat higher altitude than Pike's Peak (Morococha, 14,900 ft), the Andean, descended from generations of inhabitants living continuously at high altitude, has adjusted completely to an alveolar P_{O_2} as low as 50 mm Hg. In performance of the hard labor required to cultivate the slopes of the Andes, his high degree of efficiency well exceeds that of the sea-level worker. His pulmonary ventilation is greater, oxygen consumption is less for a given work load, pulse rate and blood pressure are lower, and he has a smaller rise in lactic and pyruvic acid levels, which compensates for a decreased buffer base.

Hurtado as well as Hultgren and Grover has enumerated morphologic and functional characteristics of the resident reared at high altitudes, namely, (1) decreased weight relative to stature; (2) increased vital capacity and pulmonary ventilation; (3) increased red blood cell volume and myoglobin; (4) elevated pulmonary arterial pressure; (5) hypertrophy of the right ventricle and of the median muscular coat of the smaller pulmonary vessels, and (6) sustained, hypoxic arteriolar vasoconstriction.

The data from Hurtado afford a comparison of several parameters for the sea-level resident (S.L.) and the Andean (Table 117-3). These values are all the more remarkable in that the mean weight of the lean Andean was 52.7 kg (height, 159 cm), and that of the S.L. resident, 63.3 kg (height, 168 cm). Scaled to the same leanness as the shorter Andean, the S.L. resident would weigh 57.8 kg, or 5.5 kg (presumably fat) less than the recorded mean weight. Despite the arduous life and deprivations, it is uncommon to find peripheral hypertension, coronary thrombosis, myocardial infarction, or peripheral arteriosclerosis. The compensatory polycythemia of altitude is

TABLE 117-3
Some comparisons between sea-level resident (S.L.) and Andean

	Blood vol., liters	*Pulmon. vent., liters*	*Hct., %*	*Hemoglobin g/100 ml*	*Hemoglobin Total, g*	*Alveolar P_{O_2}*	*Alveolar P_{CO_2}*
S.L.	4.77	2.52	46.6	15.6	679	104	39
Andean	5.70	2.23	59.5	20.1	1,146	51	29

stabilized and differs from the erythremia and attendant thrombocytosis of polycythemia vera. However, the pathognomonic implications of pulmonary hypertension and the associated structural changes in the pulmonary arterioles and right ventricle remain to be evaluated.

CHRONIC MOUNTAIN SICKNESS (SOROCHE, MONGE'S DISEASE)

The Andean is affected by a clinical condition which represents a breakdown in compensation and adaptation to low oxygen tension. Loss of tolerance to the altitude environment, as pointed out by Monge in 1928, may be observed in the striking accentuation of the "normal" erythrocytosis. The hematocrit is markedly elevated, usually in excess of 70 percent, and there is an abnormal rise in pulmonary arterial pressure and resistance. Clinical symptoms are manifest as fatigue, dyspnea, and somnolence, and physical findings are marked cyanosis, plethora, and clubbing of the digits. Oxygen administration brings about improvement, and symptoms as well as characteristic features disappear upon return to sea level. Etiology of the derangements (which have not been systematically examined) is linked to hypoventilation which permits CO_2 level to rise. A comparison has been made with the idiopathic hypoventilation syndrome seen at sea level, often in association with obesity. The fundamental defect may be diminished chemoreceptor response to hypoxia (Hultgren and Grover).

Some features of Monge's disease (cyanosis, clubbing of the fingers, polycythemia) are observed in Ayerza's syndrome (cardiacos negros), in which pulmonary hypertension is associated with pulmonary fibrosis and sclerosis of arterioles, and emphysema with congestive failure of the right side of the heart.

HIGH-ALTITUDE PULMONARY EDEMA The resident in high altitudes who lives with a moderate degree of pulmonary hypertension is liable to development of pulmonary edema, notably on return to altitude after two or more weeks sojourn at sea level. Ominous also is the circumstance that the healthy but unacclimatized person who travels within a day or two to elevations of over 9,000 ft may develop cough, dyspnea, and substernal pain some 6 to 36 hr after arrival at altitude. Findings in severe cases are tachycardia, rapid, shallow respiration, cyanosis, and rales, and x-ray reveals confluent or nodular densities throughout the lung fields. Treatment includes immediate removal to lower elevation and oxygen inhalation. Prevention requires that adequate time be taken in ascent to high altitude, with care taken to avoid overexertion.

CONCLUDING REMARKS

More than intrinsic interest centers in derangements associated with pressurized and high-altitude atmospheres which are potentially injurious for large numbers of persons. The adverse symptoms mimic those in clinical syndromes pertaining to circulatory, pulmonary, and nervous system disease. Not only would systematic studies of dysbarism enhance clinical knowledge, but we have much to learn from the lean Andean whose fitness to work and cope with hardship is commensurate with a frugal, monotonous diet.

REFERENCES

BEHNKE AR: Medical aspects of pressurized tunnel operations. J Occup Med 12:101, 1970

——: Decompression sickness: Advances and interpretations. Aerosp Med 42:255, 1971

BENNETT PB, ELLIOTT DH (eds): *The Physiology and Medicine of Diving,* London: Baillière, 1969

HANNON JP et al: High altitude acclimatization in women, in *Effects of Altitude on Physical Performance* (international symposium), Chicago: Lovelace Foundation, The Athletic Institute, 1967

HULTGREN HN, GROVER RF: Circulatory adaptation to high altitude. Ann Rev Med 19:119, 1968

HURTADO A: Adaptation to the environment, sec 4 in *Handbook of Physiology,* ed DB Hill, Washington: American Physiology Society, 1964

LAMBERTSEN CJ (ed): *Underwater Physiology,* 4th Symposium, New York: Academic, 1971

LANPHIER EH: Medical aspects of diving, in *The New Science of Skin and Scuba Diving,* New York: Association Press, 1968

NATIONAL ACADEMY OF SCIENCE, NATIONAL RESEARCH COUNCIL: *Fundamentals of Hyperbaric Medicine,* Washington: 1966

PAULEY SM, COCKETT ATK: Role of lipids in decompression sickness. Aerosp Med 41:56, 1970

PHILP RB et al: Platelets and microthrombi in decompression sickness. Aerosp Med 42:494, 1971

SIRI WE: Physiological studies on Mt. Everest climbers. Report of Donner Laboratory, University of California (Berkeley), June, 1965, p. 58

US Navy Diving Manual, NAVSHIPS 250–538, Navy Dept., Washington, 1963

WORKMAN RD: Treatment of bends with oxygen at high pressure, in *Modern Aspects of Treatment of Decompression Sickness* (a symposium). Aerosp Med 39:1076, 1968

118 PROBLEMS OF AIR AND SPACE TRAVEL

STUART BONDURANT

Ordinary air travel imposes so little physiologic stress that most patients who can be moved at all can be moved by air if proper equipment and attendants are available. Medical problems unique to air travel may be caused by unusual environmental conditions which may be encountered because of limitations of equipment or abnormal operating circumstances.

Many modern aircraft fly at altitudes of 20,000 to 40,000 ft, with cabins pressurized to maintain an effective cabin altitude of less than 7,500 ft (jets) or 9,000 ft (reciprocating engines). Unusual accelerations may be encountered, and the normal metabolic diurnal rhythm may be disturbed by rapid movement between time zones.

ALTITUDE An increase in altitude is equivalent to a decrease in barometric pressure. There is a consequent reduction in the partial pressure of oxygen and an increase in the volume of any gas trapped within the body (Table 118-1). The normal person acclimatized to sea level tolerates oxygen tension equivalent to that at altitudes of 10,000 to 12,000 ft with little change in arterial oxygen saturation. At altitudes above 12,000 ft, hypoxia becomes more marked and supplementary oxygen is usually used. By breathing 100 percent oxygen, one can maintain normal oxygen saturation at altitudes of 30,000 to 35,000 ft.

A second consequence of decreased barometric pressure is expansion of gas trapped in body cavities. In the normal person, intestinal gas is passed as it expands, and middle-ear and sinus air escapes without difficulty during ascent. Gas which cannot escape (as in the case of pneumothorax or pneumoperitoneum) may cause pain, injury, or death. Patients with intracranial gas from wounds or diagnostic procedures in body cavities should not be exposed to a significant decrease in barometric pressure.

ACCELERATION Acceleration is the instantaneous rate of change of velocity. The unit of acceleration, *g*, is the acceleration of a body which is falling freely *in vacuo* due to earth's gravity. It represents a change in velocity of 32.2 feet per sec each second. Most of the physiologic consequences of acceleration are due to the force (inertia) which is equal in magnitude but opposite in direction to that causing the acceleration. Thus, headward acceleration causes footward displacement of soft tissues and blood. Duration, magnitude, direction, and rate of onset of acceleration determine the physiologic effects. In general, the longer and greater the acceleration, the less well it is tolerated. Prolonged forward or backward acceleration is tolerated better (approximately 14 to 20*g*, limited by apnea) than headward acceleration (4 to 7*g*, limited by blackout and cerebral ischemia); footward acceleration (3 to 5*g*, limited by asystole and conjunctival and mucous membrane bleeding) is tolerated least well. Brief headward accelerations of 25*g* and backward accelerations of 40*g* are tolerated by normal subjects when well positioned and supported. In ordinary flight, linear accelerations greater than 1*g* are not encountered. Turbulent flight may cause brief linear accelerations of 10 to 12*g*, which are great enough to cause fractures in persons who are not restrained. Angular accelerations of turn and the linear-angular accelerations of turbulent flight are important causes of motion sickness.

TABLE 118-1
Representative values of arterial oxygen and the relative volume of gas at various altitudes

Altitude, ft	Pressure, mmHg	Arterial blood: Oxygen tension, mmHg	Arterial blood: Oxygen saturation, %	Relative volume of gas
0	760	94	98	1.0
5,000	632	66	92	1.2
8,000	564	60	89	1.25
10,000	523	53	86	1.5
14,000	446	44	79	1.7
18,000	379	36	71	2.0
37,500 with 100% O_2	159	74	94	4.8
44,000 with 100% O_2	116	36	72	6.5

DIURNAL RHYTHMS A dissociation between metabolic diurnal rhythms and actual local time may occur following longitudinal flight or flight over the poles. From 3 to 5 days may be required for diurnal metabolic rhythms to come into phase with the new local time. There are no proved adverse clinical or physiologic effects of changing the diurnal rhythm. However, the management of diseases with diurnal manifestations, such as peptic ulcer, and the scheduling of all-important medications, such as insulin, should be carefully planned in preparation for a trip to another time zone.

MISCELLANEOUS Some fuels and lubricants and their combustion products are toxic and may, with equipment failure, become concentrated in closed cabins. Reciprocating engines produce large quantities of carbon monoxide. Jet engines use fuels which are vesicants, with fumes that may cause nausea, vomiting, and headache. Pyrolysis of lubricating oils produces fumes which cause conjunctival irritation. Ozone has not accumulated in toxic quantities.

Flight line personnel develop hearing loss after prolonged exposure to jet noise unless protected by position or by mechanical devices. Noise levels inside aircraft are very low, and those in terminals and around airfields are apparently insufficient to cause hearing loss.

SUPERSONIC TRANSPORT Supersonic transports cruise at speeds of Mach 2 to Mach 3 (1,300 to 1,800 mi per hr) at altitudes of 50,000 to 70,000 ft. Flight characteristics are well known from extensive experience in military aircraft. Cabin pressure, oxygen content, and temperature will be similar to those of current jet aircraft. There are two potential environmental hazards which are not present in ordinary subsonic air travel: ozone and radiation.

Ozone is present in the toxic concentration of 6 to 9 ppm at the operational altitude of the supersonic transport. For this reason, the cabin atmosphere control system includes thermal or catalytic devices for the dissociation of ozone to maintain concentrations below 0.2 ppm.

Passengers and crew will be exposed to galactic cosmic radiation and to solar flare radiation. Under the most adverse ordinary circumstances galactic cosmic radiation, composed of protons, alpha particles, and a few heavy nuclei, will be less than 2 millirem (mrem) per hr or approximately 6 mrem for a single intercontinental flight. The aircrew may receive 2 rem per year from this source. Solar flares produce protons and heavy nuclei. During a major solar flare, the dose rate for a passenger may reach 2 millirads (mrd) per hr. For this reason, the aircraft will carry radiation monitoring equipment and will descend to lower altitudes when major solar flares occur.

The supersonic transport will cause a sonic boom, or wave of overpressure, of approximately 2.0 lb per ft^2 at ground level along a corridor of 25 miles on each side of the flight path. Overpressure of this magnitude does not cause physical or physiologic damage but does cause psychologic reactions.

AIRCREW SELECTION Physical requirements for aircrews are described in appropriate governmental and airlines literature. Absence of circulatory, pulmonary, neurologic, visual, and auditory defects is of particular importance.

AIR TRANSPORTATION OF PATIENTS Since it is now possible to fly without experiencing physiologically significant departure from the usual environmental conditions, there are no absolute medical contraindications to moving patients by air. However, in many instances patients should not be moved at all, and in others, adequate aircraft with pressurized cabin and attending personnel may not be available. Commercial airlines will carry many patients subject to the discretion of the airline medical director. In addition to the condition of the patient, the comfort and convenience of other passengers must be a major factor in the decision of the commercial airlines. The following points apply to air transportation in general. Specific advice concerning commercial air transportation should be obtained from the appropriate airline medical director.

Circulatory disease The lower partial pressure of oxygen which may be encountered constitutes the major deterrent to flight for patients with circulatory diseases. With oxygen breathing, normal arterial oxygen saturation can be maintained at all altitudes encountered in routine flight (Table 118-1). There is no evidence that ordinary flying is associated with an increased incidence of angina, myocardial infarction, or cerebral vascular accidents.

Coronary artery disease manifested by occasional angina or old myocardial infarction, minimal cerebral or peripheral vascular disease, hypertension, and compensated congenital or rheumatic heart disease appear to entail no added risk in flying. Patients with angina related to emotional stress may benefit from preflight sedation.

Patients with severe or frequent angina, severe hypertension, recent vascular accidents, or cardiac decompensation at rest or with moderate exercise should fly only when a pressurized aircraft or supplementary oxygen is available to maintain ambient oxygen tension at levels of 150 mmHg (sea level equivalent) or more. It is generally considered preferable to forego unnecessary flying for 6 weeks after a myocardial infarction or a cerebral infarction or hemorrhage.

Pulmonary disease Persons with pulmonary decompensation at rest or with very mild exercise should fly only if ambient oxygen tension is maintained at levels of 150 mmHg or more and facilities and personnel are available to treat acute ventilatory decompensation. Persons with pulmonary decompensation with moderate (two flights of stairs) or severe exercise usually fly without difficulty to altitudes of 10,000 ft. Asthmatic patients who do not respond well to self-administered treatment should not fly unattended during acute episodes. The likelihood of rupture of an emphysematous bleb does not appear to be increased by ordinary flight. Because of the increase in volume of bullae as altitude increases (Table 118-1), patients with marked bullous emphysema are advised not to fly above 6,000 ft. Individuals with pneumothorax should not fly unless the cabin pressure is maintained at ground-level equivalent. Expansion of the trapped gas causes, in effect, a tension pneumothorax. Several patients with therapeutic pneumothorax have died in flight.

Hematologic disease In the absence of cardiopulmonary disease, patients with a hemoglobin of 7 to 9 g per 100 ml usually tolerate flight at 4,000 to 6,000 ft without difficulty. If greater cabin altitudes are to be encountered, hemoglobin should be above 10 g per 100 ml.

Hypoxia causes increased sickling of erythrocytes containing hemoglobin S. There have been many well-documented reports of splenic infarction in patients with hemoglobin S during flights which usually exceeded 10,000 ft and lasted for several hours. Two patients with SC hemoglobin have had splenic infarctions during flights which did not exceed 6,000 ft. If ambient oxygen tension cannot be maintained at 150 mmHg, flying is contraindicated for patients with SS (sickle-cell anemia) and SC hemoglobin and for those with SA (sickle-cell trait) who have large quantities of hemoglobin S. Others with hemoglobin S should be restricted to cabin altitudes below 10,000 ft. Symptoms of splenic infarction, nausea, vomiting, left upper quadrant pain, and shock should be treated with supplemental oxygen and immediate return to ground level.

Pregnancy A large amount of experience has accumulated which suggests that ordinary flying has no adverse effects on the normal pregnant woman or fetus. Pregnant women should sit, when possible, facing the rear of the plane and should place the seat belt over the upper thighs and hips rather than around the abdomen. When pregnancy is complicated by preeclampsia or cardiopulmonary or hematologic disease, considerations similar to those discussed above for the nonpregnant patient apply.

Ear, nose, and throat disease Acute infections of the upper respiratory tract and chronic sinusitis may obstruct the eustachian tubes or sinus ducts, with barotitis or barosinusitis resulting when external pressure is increased during descent. If it is necessary for a person with acute upper respiratory infection to fly, use of a nasal spray containing ½% phenylephrine (Neo-Synephrine) 6, 3, and ½ hr before flight and ½ hr before descent may help to maintain patency of the ducts. A swallow or a Valsalva maneuver with the nose occluded will usually open the ducts. Children may be fed during descent to encourage swallowing. The treatment of barotrauma depends on its severity and the underlying cause. Intubation of the eustachian tubes is not advised. In most instances, conservative treatment with decongestants will suffice. Severe barotitis may be associated with hemorrhage into the middle ear, requiring myringotomy and aspiration of blood to prevent ossicular ankylosis. Plastic repair of the ducts may be required to prevent recurrence.

Metabolic disease Control of diabetes may be complicated by rapid movement from one time zone to another and by motion sickness. Careful planning of the flight in terms of elapsed rather than local time, with consideration of the meals to be served and appropriate management of motion sickness, should enable the patient with well-controlled diabetes to fly without difficulty. Patients in diabetic acidosis may be transported after treatment is started if in-flight medical facilities are adequate.

Communicable disease Persons known to have a communicable disease may not enter a state or nation without the consent of the local health department.

Postoperative conditions Because of the expansion of abdominal gas with decrease in barometric pressure, it is generally considered preferable to forego flying for 10 days after abdominal or other major surgery. However, experience with air evacuation of military casualties suggests that, with proper facilities and personnel, practically all patients whose condition is stable can be moved by air if necessary. Most persons with fractures are flown without difficulty. Fracture of the mandible, particularly when the mandible is immobilized, constitutes a special problem because of the possibility of vomiting and aspiration. A quick-release wire support has been designed for in-flight use.

Epilepsy Most patients with well-controlled epilepsy fly to altitudes of 10,000 ft without difficulty. Flight to greater altitude in unpressurized aircraft may precipitate seizures.

MOTION SICKNESS The use of modern aircraft has considerably reduced the incidence of motion sickness. The problem remains because of occasional turbulent flights and persons who are extremely susceptible to motion sickness. Such persons should sit over the wings of the aircraft, where motion is least. Cyclizine (Marezine) 50 mg, meclizine (Bonine) 25 mg, and dimenhydrinate (Dramamine) 50 mg are effective prophylactic agents.

SPACE TRAVEL The medical problems of space flight relate in part to the design of spacecraft and propulsion systems and in part to the characteristics of the space environment.

With design and engineering improvements it will be possible to build spacecraft which require only a small departure from man's ordinary environment. For example, the accelerations of launch and reentry which are of the order of 4 to 8*g* in present systems could be reduced to a fraction of a *g* by prolonging the time of acceleration. Present Soviet manned space systems operate with a cabin atmosphere which is very near to that at sea level on earth. To avoid the effects of weightlessness, an acceleration equivalent to that of the earth's gravity can be produced by rotating the spacecraft, if this should prove necessary. Radiation shielding can be provided, albeit with a weight penalty. Present space systems represent a series of engineering compromises which are necessary largely because of the limitations of the propulsion systems.

During the flights of the Mercury, Gemini, and Apollo series, several adaptations were observed. Human performance, eating, drinking, urination and defecation, respiration, heart rate, and blood pressure showed no important changes. Weight loss occurred predominantly during the first few days of orbital flight. It was related in part, at least, to negative water balance associated with decreased fluid intake. Several astronauts had leukocytosis, that is, 20,000 to 30,000 leucocytes per cubic millimeter of blood, upon return to earth, presumably due to stress and immobilization. There is evidence of a reduction in red blood cell mass during orbital flight, possibly related in part to the high ambient oxygen tension. Astronauts manifest orthostatic hypotension after return to gravitational field. This may be due to reduced blood volume as well as impaired cardiovascular response to gravity. Weightlessness is expected to be associated with a negative calcium balance. There is evidence that negative calcium balance and bone demineralization occur, but the effect has not been important in flights of less than 2 weeks' duration.

REFERENCES

ARMSTRONG HB: *Aerospace Medicine,* Baltimore: Williams & Wilkins, 1960

GAUER OH, ZUIDEMA GW: *Gravitational Stress in Aerospace Medicine,* Boston: Little, Brown, 1961

GERATHEWOHL SJ: Aeromedical aspects of the supersonic transport. Aerosp Med 38:1225, 1967

SHAEFER HJ: Radiation exposure in air travel. Science 173:780, 1971

SIEGER PV et al: Time zone effects. Science 164:1249, 1969

119 RADIATION INJURY

EUGENE P. CRONKITE

TYPES OF RADIATION The types of ionizing radiation most often causing injury are x-rays, gamma rays, alpha and beta rays, protons, and neutrons. X-rays and gamma rays are identical; a separate name was given because of their difference in origin. The former are produced by x-ray machines and as secondary emissions from particle accelerators or electron tubes. The latter are produced by radioactive decay. In general, gamma radiations are more energetic than x-rays; however, the energy spectrum of x-rays is continuous. Beta rays are electrons. Ordinary electrons originate from the shells surrounding the atomic nucleus, and beta rays originate only from within the nucleus. Alpha rays are the stripped nuclei of the helium atom with a mass of 4 and a charge of 2+. Protons are stripped nuclei of hydrogen atoms with a mass of 1 and a charge of 1+. Protons are becoming of more interest because of their common use as primary particles in accelerators and their prevalence as an extraterrestial space radiation as described by Van Allen. Protons are of additional interest since they are usually the secondary damaging particle produced by neutron interaction with tissue or other materials. Neutrons have a mass of 1 and charge of 0. Biologic injury is produced primarily by ionization from secondary charged particles. Neutrons produce the secondary charged particles in diverse ways. Fast neutrons react principally with the hydrogen atoms, and as a result of the collision a portion of the energy is imparted to the hydrogen atom and a proton is ejected which does the damage. With thermal or slow neutrons the damage is done by actual capture of the neutrons and a secondary emission of ionizing radiation as the transmuted hydrogen, nitrogen, or other substance in tissue decays and emits radioactivity. These are the basic types of radiation with which a physician may be concerned.

MECHANISM OF ACTION Historically the theories and concepts for mechanism of action of ionizing radiation on living things are discussed in the classic volume by Lea. The concepts of direct hits on the target molecules versus the indirect action mediated through products of reaction with the protoplasmic solvent water are analyzed lucidly. The most acceptable current view to account for a major part of the biologic effects of radiation may be divided into three interlinked steps. First, photons, or particles, penetrate the protoplasm, interacting to produce ion pairs. This reaction takes of the order of 10^{-13} sec. The second step is a primary radiochemical reaction of these ions primarily with water, producing free radicals such as H and OH. These reactions take about 10^{-9} sec. These free radicals produce a further chain of reactions with themselves and tissue water to produce further reactive forms such as H_2O_2 and HO_2. These products persist for microseconds or in part a few seconds. The last reaction is between these products and critical protoplasmic molecules. The nature of this last reaction is not known, but since the actual amount of energy imparted to the system is small, it is generally thought that the damage must involve substances of low concentration but major importance to the living system, for example, nucleic acids or enzymes. It is of interest that the amount of energy deposited to produce 100 percent mortality in animals will raise the body temperature only 0.001°C. Whatever the mechanism may be, it sets into motion a series of observable histologic or chemical lesions that unfold with time. In addition to the effects observable within days, "bad invisible information" may be stored in the proliferative or nonproliferative cells, presumably in DNA, that may not be manifested as a disease process for several years.

DOSE UNITS In pharmacology, standardization of drugs becomes scientific only when the structure is known and one can measure the drug in an appropriate unit such as a milligram. With ionizing radiation one is concerned not with the mass of the agent administered but with the *amount* and the distribution of energy that has been absorbed by tissue at the *point of interest* (tumor, tissue essential for life, gonads, etc.).

Two dose units are essential for the understanding of the quantitative effects of radiation. The *roentgen* (R), a measure of total dose in air, is defined as the quantity of x-ray or gamma radiation such that the associated corpuscular emission per 0.001293 g of air at standard conditions produces in air ions carrying one electrostatic unit of either sign. For energy to be deposited, there must be an interaction with matter. Hence, with x-rays passing through a vacuum, no radiation dose is delivered. In practice we are interested in the energy imparted to various tissues from a number of different types of radiation, and it is therefore essential to have a second unit of radiation which overcomes the limitation of the roentgen. This second unit, the *rad* (rd), is a unit of absorbed dose equal to 100 ergs per g of absorbed energy which applies to any type of radiation in any tissue. For small pieces of tissue in an x-ray beam of 1 R per min, the absorbed dose is very close to 1 rd per min. However, as irradiated objects become larger and change in composition, one must consider the diminution in intensity due to the interaction of radiation with matter (buildup and then exponential attenuation) and the changing types of interaction (photoelectric effect, Compton effect, etc.). In tissue of uniform density this leads to a decreasing absorbed dose at successive levels after equilibrium is attained. However, at interfaces such as soft tissue and bone, the absorbed dose may sharply increase. Thus, in addition to the exposure dose in roentgens and the absorbed dose in rads, one must be concerned with the distribution of the absorbed dose in the areas of interest. For example, if there is sufficient protection of bone marrow by shielding of one's own tissues to permit marrow regeneration and survival from what is considered an otherwise fatal *exposure dose,* one may ascribe incorrectly some great benefit to a procedure used therapeutically. Unfortunately, failure to consider the critical influence of the distribution of absorbed dose at the site of interest on the outcome of radiation injury has resulted in ascribing therapeutic benefit to various agents of no value at all.

The *density of ionization* in tissue varies with the energy and type of radiation as well as the tissue composition. The density of ionization is referred to as *specific ionization* (ions per unit track length) or as *linear energy transfer* (LET, kiloelectron volts deposited per unit track length). Among other factors, the density of ionization influences the biologic effect for equivalent amounts of energy deposited, in general the effect being greater with more densely ionizing radiation. This leads to consideration of the relative biologic effectiveness (RBE), which is defined as the ratio of the dose in rads of standard radiation (usually x-ray or gamma radiation of 250 to 400 kV energy) to produce a given degree of biologic effect, to the dose in rads of an unknown radiation to produce the same degree of biologic effect. For example, if the median lethal dose (LD_{50}) of x-rays is 600 rd and for neutrons 300 rd, the RBE will be 2. The RBE may vary with the biologic response or the conditions of irradiation. For example, when the same radiations are used, a different value may be obtained for mortality, cataract, or tumor development. Another useful unit is the rem, which stands for roentgen equivalent mammal. Numerically, rem = rads × RBE.

Also of importance is the *dose rate.* In general, the lower the dose rate, the less will be the acute somatic effect. In a crude sense, dose rates in excess of approximately 5 R per min give essentially the same result. However, as the dose rate falls below 5 R per min, the effect per unit of radiation becomes less. In the past, genetic effects were believed independent of dose rate. This implies that all increments of radiation received by the gonads, irrespective of when or how, would add up directly as mutations, to give a total effect ultimately to be measured as detectable effects in succeeding generations. However, it is now known that there is a dose-rate dependence in respect to the production of mutations by irradiation of spermatogonia in mice and also for leukemogenesis in mice, which is considered to be a somatic genetic effect of bone marrow irradiation.

If the dose of radiation is sufficiently high, actual death of any living cell can be observed promptly in terms of classic pathologic criteria of cell necrosis. However, after lower doses of radiation (precise values vary with the tissue), only disturbances in cell proliferation are seen. The rate at which cells divide is decreased. DNA synthesis is impaired in two manners: (1) the rate of synthesis is slower; (2) cells may continue DNA synthesis and become polyploid. It is reasonably certain that radiation has effects other than the outright killing of cells and the interference with mitosis and DNA synthesis. Among the less well understood manifestations of radiation exposure are those dealing with the effects of rather small doses of radiation on the nondividing central nervous system. This work, pioneered in the U.S.S.R., has in recent years received more attention from Western radiobiologists. However, it is still not completely understood.

The diminution in the production of new cells in these tissues that are undergoing continual renewal (mucosa, blood, gonads, etc.) results in a progressive hypoplasia to total atrophy, depending on dose. Some cells still capable of mitosis that are not killed outright may be so injured that they will go through one or two generative cycles, producing abnormal progeny, such as giant metamyelocytes and hypersegmented neutrophils, before dying. The atrophy of these steady-state cell renewal systems and direct injury of other tissues produce clearly defined clinical syndromes.

CLINICAL PHENOMENA IN RELATION TO DOSE AND TIME AFTER EXPOSURE Human experience is based on the effects of atomic bombs; accidental exposure to fallout from a hydrogen bomb; laboratory and reactor accidents in the United States, U.S.S.R., and Yugoslavia; and on *whole-body* clinical radiotherapy. After any radiation accident close cooperation of the physician and health physicist is essential to obtain the best estimate of the radiation dose and to evaluate its probable effect in terms of the likely *distribution of the absorbed dose* in rads. However, clinical signs and symptoms remain paramount in the management of human disease and injury. Physical estimates of dose never substitute for clinical judgment and experience.

For teaching purposes three acute radiation syndromes may be classified generally as *cerebral, gastrointestinal,* and *hematopoietic.*

The *cerebral* syndrome is produced by extremely high doses of radiation, i.e., following exposure to several thousand roentgens. It is always fatal, whether the radiation is delivered to the brain alone or to the whole body. Three processes have been described: a prodromal phase of nausea and vomiting; then listlessness and drowsiness ranging from apathy to prostration (probably traceable to nonbacterial inflammatory foci in the brain); and finally, a more generalized component characterized by tremors, convulsions, ataxia, and death. This sequence was observed in an industrial accident, death occurring 36 hr after exposure.

The *gastrointestinal* syndrome occurs when the dose of radiation is lower, in the range of 600 to 1,500 R. It is characterized by intractable nausea, vomiting, and diarrhea; these lead to severe dehydration, diminished plasma volume, vascular collapse, and death. The syndrome is initiated by a pronounced "intoxication," arising presumably from diffuse necrosis of tissue throughout the body; it is extended by severe injury to the gastrointestinal tract. The latter development is caused by two factors: direct killing of a fraction of the crypt cells and inhibition of mitosis. The mature epithelial cells continue to migrate out on to the villus in an orderly fashion, eventually being lost from the tip of the villi; this produces a progressive diminution in the number of cells covering the villi. The epithelial cells progressively become cuboidal and then squamous in appearance, and ultimately the intestinal villi become denuded, with massive loss of bloody plasma into the intestine. The usual 3- to 4-day death from the gastrointestinal syndrome can be prevented by massive plasma replacement during the first 4 to 6 days after irradiation. After doses greater than circa 1,300 R regeneration is poor and slow. After doses below roughly 1,300 R, regeneration commences around the sixth day with complete restoration of the gastrointestinal epithelium. However, the respite is only temporary, since hematopoietic failure will ensue, commencing within 2 to 3 weeks.

The *hematopoietic syndrome* which occurs following whole-body exposure in the midlethal range is accompanied by temporary anorexia, nausea, and vomiting which is maximal between 6 and 12 hr after exposure to doses of radiation between 600 and 800 R. Thereafter, the gastrointestinal symptoms rapidly subside so that within 24 to 36 hr after exposure the subject is usually asymptomatic. These symptoms have been correlated with a period of rapid necrosis of radiosensitive tissues. The prodromes must be distinguished from the gastrointestinal syndrome described earlier and from that which occurs later on. After subsidence of the prodromes, a period of relative well-being is experienced, during which atrophy of lymph nodes, spleen, and bone marrow progresses, leading to a pancytopenia. This atrophy is the result of two clearly defined processes—direct killing of radiosensitive cells and inhibition of new cell production. In the peripheral blood, lymphopenia commences immediately, becoming maximal within 24 to 36 hr. Thereafter, the lymphocytes remain at low levels for weeks and recover over several months. Within a few hours after irradiation a neutrophilic leukocytosis appears. Following this an oscillation in the neutrophil count occurs, the rate at which it falls to the minimum being a function of the dose of radiation. After sublethal and low lethal doses, the minimal values occur in 4 to 6 weeks; after high lethal doses granulocytes diminish more rapidly, and minimal values approaching zero appear within 7 to 10 days.

Thrombopenia and its relation to radiation bleeding have been studied exhaustively. After single doses of radiation a close correlation with the decrease in the platelet count and the tendency to bleed is evident. In animals and after various accidents, significant purpura was seen only when the platelet counts fell below 20,000 per mm^3. The platelets remain steady or increase for 2 to 3 days after irradiation and thereafter diminish more or less linearly with time, the ultimate minimum and the rate attained being dose-dependent. After about 200 rd, it takes about 30 days for minimum platelet levels to develop. After 600 to 800 rd, minimal levels were observed within 10 to 12 days. Earlier observations in which bleeding in radiation injury was attributed primarily to hyperheparinemia have been refuted. Today there is no evidence of hyperheparinemia; consequently the use of antiheparin agents in the therapy of bleeding induced by radiation is not indicated. Fresh viable platelet transfusions will stop bleeding, and maintenance of platelet levels by platelet transfusions will prevent development of bleeding in animals.

Decreases in the red blood cell count are prominent only after large doses of radiation that significantly interfere with new cell production and produce bleeding.

Studies of *decreased resistance to infection* have resulted in the conclusion that there are (1) a dose-dependent decrease in circulating granulocytes and lymphocytes; (2) a dose-dependent impairment of antibody production; (3) impairment of granulocyte migration and phagocytosis; (4) decreased ability of the reticuloendothelial system to kill phagocytized bacteria; (5) diminished resistance to diffusion in subcutaneous tissues; and (6) hemorrhagic areas of the skin and bowel that present foci for entrance and growth of bacteria. Obviously an increased susceptibility to infection by both commensals and pathogens must be present.

The preceding syndromes may be produced when the whole body is uniformly exposed to radiation or if there is a substantial inhomogeneous exposure of the whole body. An expression of the lethal dose range for man is desirable to assist in the management of casualties. In the case of inhomogeneous exposure, one can see how misleading any single air or exposure dose may be. There is a hierarchy of effects that vary with time, dose, and organs involved. Although 10,000 rd to the brain will be fatal, 10,000 rd to a hand may only necessitate amputation. Since the bone marrow is somewhat more sensitive than other tissues, ultimate survival is determined in large part by the dose to this tissue. For uniform whole-body exposure *without therapy* it has been estimated that the lethal dose curve will commence at about 200 rd and that survivals will be rare after doses in excess of 800 rds. Between these limits the percentage mortality dose curve is sigmoid. Even if the dose to an individual is known with precision, the prognosis must remain probable because one can never predict whether an individual belongs on the sensitive or resistant portion of the curve.

INHOMOGENEOUS EXPOSURE TO RADIATION The preceding description of radiation injury was based primarily on human clinical experience and animal experimentation in which the distribution of dose absorbed by tissues was relatively uniform. However, in actuality, conditions of exposure may be such that there are marked inhomogeneities in absorbed dose. For example, the geometry of an exposure may result in almost no exposure to the lower part of the body and very heavy exposure to the abdomen and hands, resulting in extensive necrosis of the skin of these areas in addition to the fatal injury to deeper tissues. In one accident, the direction of the beam resulted in severe exposure to the head, but the low energy permitted marked attenuation of the beam within the head, so that the absorbed dose through the brain decreased markedly from the side closest to the beam to the side farthest from it. The superficial layers of the brain were injured badly, but death did not ensue because vital centers were not destroyed. In evaluating any radiation accident, one must reconstruct the geometry and consider the probable distribution of absorbed dose within the body. What may initially appear as a fatal accident in terms of air exposure dose may turn out to be sublethal when effects of distribution of the absorbed dose are considered.

MANAGEMENT OF ACUTE HUMAN RADIATION INJURY Presumptive evidence of exposure to radiation and signs or symptoms described earlier must be recognized before there need be cause for concern. No therapy is available for the cerebral form of radiation injury after uniform brain exposure. Whereas a small percentage of persons with the gastrointestinal syndrome may be kept alive until the affected tract regenerates, they must also face the hematopoietic syndrome; hence that is the real therapeutic problem. Therapy rests on the control of the sequelae of marrow aplasia and thus is similar to management of drug-induced and idiopathic marrow aplasia, suggesting that combined use of antibacterials and transfusions would be useful. The spontaneous course of radiation injury in man has clearly shown that signs and symptoms develop at different times in different subjects after identical doses of radiation. Accordingly, the time of institution and type of therapy should be individualized. The following general therapeutic regimen is outlined.

1 *Maintain rigid asepsis* until one is confident that a sublethal exposure to radiation has been experienced. All medical staff involved in the care of irradiated individuals must have negative cultures of the nasopharynx for pathogenic organisms. Physicians and nursing staff with any evidence of respiratory or other infections are forbidden entrance to the rooms of irradiated patients. If at all possible, reverse isolation should be instituted to prevent introduction of pathogens into the environment of the patient. This requires either the use of plastic rooms in which the patient is placed or the sterilization of a room and the institution of laminar flow air barriers and appropriate ultraviolet

light sources to prevent the introduction of pathogens into the patient's environment.

2 Observe *fluid and electrolyte balance* closely and restore as necessary with appropriate replacement solutions.

3 *Provide sterile, bland diet* prepared in the patient's room.

4 Administer *nonabsorbable intestinal antibiotics* such as neomycin to sterilize the gastrointestinal tract and minimize the probability of invasion by commensal organisms in the gastrointestinal tract.

5 *Treat infection* when it develops or relapses, using various antibiotics sequentially in doses two to three times the usual size. Use sulfonamides when antibiotics are exhausted. One is fighting for additional time to permit spontaneous regeneration.

6 *Use fresh whole blood* to control bleeding and/or to restore adequate red cell levels. Fresh blood is defined as that which has been taken from the donor not more than 1 hr previously and placed in plastic bags with Na_2EDTA. When the hematocrit is returned to normal range, to control bleeding use fresh platelet-rich plasma as clinically indicated, not on an inflexible schedule. Despite many claims concerning the value of lyophilized and frozen platelets, radiation bleeding has been successfully managed to date only by the use of fresh viable platelets that circulate in adequate numbers.

The preceding therapy has increased the survival rate of animals. Unless infection or serious hemorrhage develops, therapy is not needed. Prophylactic therapy other than the use of nonabsorbable intestinal antibiotics is believed to be contraindicated. Many human beings with epilation, severe pancytopenia, and purpura have recovered without therapy from doses of radiation ranging from 200 to 300 R. Recently individuals who received 400 to 500 R inhomogeneous irradiation have recovered when treated in accordance with this therapeutic regimen despite near-zero granulocyte and platelet counts.

Syngenesious and autologous bone marrow transplantation will prevent death in almost all otherwise fatally irradiated animals up to doses of about 1,200 R. In fatally irradiated animals saved by allogenic bone marrow transplantation, the transplanted marrow may eventually produce a reaction (presumably against the host) of immunologic nature, resulting in a severe late degenerative disease of the skin, kidneys, liver, and lymph nodes. A similar late fatal effect has been observed in children treated for leukemia with extensive chemotherapy and whole-body irradiation in whom allogenic marrow transplantation was successful.

Although marrow transplantation has been widely acclaimed as the solution to fatal whole-body radiation, the results in human beings so far do not warrant optimism. This author believes it should be reserved for patients in whom there is a progressive deterioration of the hematopoietic system with granulocytes falling below 500 per mm³ in the first 2 weeks after exposure and an early rapid decline in the platelet count. The profile scoring method of Thomas and Wald may be useful on a day-to-day basis for evaluating the severity and may give some indication of when one may have to resort to allogenic marrow transplantation. In the rare case in which there is an identical twin, bone marrow transplantation should be lifesaving following fatal radiation injury up to a maximum exposure of about 1,200 R. Rigid rules cannot be formulated in advance. Decisions can be made only at the bedside.

PREVENTION Nothing can substitute for prevention. Shielding, distance, and limiting of exposure time are the only effective preventive measures against exposures from radiation sources, whether in industry, medical practice, military action, or civil defense. A series of drugs, primarily sulfhydryl groups, that will protect against radiation by an effective dose reduction up to 50 percent are available. However, these must be administered within minutes preceding exposure. Accidents and warfare are not predictable. The severe toxic effects of these drugs prevent continuous prophylactic administration.

LONG-TERM EFFECTS Radiation alters the "information system" of proliferating somatic and germ cells. Thus the perpetuating cells of the blood, gastrointestinal tract, skin, lens, gonads, and other areas pass on either "bad or inadequate information," presumably in altered DNA, to their progeny, resulting in late somatic disease, e.g., cancer, cataracts, degenerative disorders, or nonspecific shortening of life. Leukemia yield from radiation in human groups has been quantified. It is asserted, but not proved, that there is no threshold and that the yield of leukemia increases with dose. However, the greatest exposure of the American public comes from the medical uses of diverse types of radiation (predominantly diagnostic x-rays). If the assumption of no threshold dose for leukemia is correct, the medical uses of radiation are producing their small toll in an additional burden of leukemia and probably other disease also. Therefore, it behooves the practitioner to be exceedingly cautious and to expose patients to radiation only when it is clearly indicated and needed for diagnosis.

Radiation can produce mutation of genes, the information and transmission centers for heredity. Of this there is no doubt. Not all mutations are harmful, but the chances are overwhelming that a change will be detrimental to the species. Not all mutations produce visible, immediately detectable effects. The concern is not only with an increase in the number of obvious freaks or cripples but with changes that will lead to such undesirable characteristics as lowered life expectancy, decreased fertility, a general increase in physical and mental disease, and an increase in fetal or neonatal death rates. It is the less obvious changes that are of the greatest importance. The more obvious changes usually lead to early death in the individual and reduced fertility in those that survive. Thus the harmful mutant is relatively quickly deleted from the population. The more subtle changes, however, are propagated longer and affect a very large number of persons. The mutation may be dominant or recessive. Most dominant mutations are also lethal, and many such mutations may be missed because the fertilized egg never develops far enough to be recognized as a new individual. If the mutation is recessive, the mutant will not become evident unless both parents of the individual have the same mutant genes and transfer these to the individual concerned. It is extremely difficult to quantify these considerations. If the mutation rate were increased by a single exposure of the population to radiation, the effects would be spread through many generations. Half the total damage produced would not be observed until some 30 to 50 generations had been born. These are the practical considerations that make the problem particularly difficult to analyze. Damage that is inflicted now cannot be detected now and will only become evident many generations hence. These considerations also indicate why it is not possible to take negative evidence in populations that have been exposed to date as an indication that the degree of genetic damage is small. If, for instance, an effect were already obvious in the children born of individuals irradiated in Japan by the atom bombs, it would mean that the total genetic effect would be great indeed. These are sobering considerations for thoughtful persons. Since exposure to irradiation cannot be avoided in our modern industrial society and in the practice of medicine and because of the uncertainty about the quantitative effect in producing somatic or genetic effects, it is mandatory that exposure be minimal and rigidly controlled in order to protect the present generations from somatic effects and future generations from genetic effects.

RADIUM POISONING Today it appears strange that radium water was used as a therapeutic agent only three decades ago and resulted in poisoning. In addition, radium watch dial painters were poisoned during World War I. The radium (often mesothorium) is deposited primarily on the surface of the bones, and its distribution changes with the slow rebuilding of the osseous structure. Histologically one sees haversian systems plugged with highly calcified material; gross regions of resorption; and osteocyte death as evidenced by empty and highly calcified lacunae. Autoradiographs show both a "diffuse" distribution and "hot spots" of radioactivity. Pathologists consider the characteristic bony injury almost pathognomonic of chronic radium poisoning. Many of the effects are due to direct radiation injury; some are secondary to vascular injury. Bone necrosis and interference with normal processes of internal reconstruction of bone result in the formation of small and large cavities, which give the characteristic radiolucency in radiographs of bone. Fibrosis of the bone is a constant feature, usually limited to the endosteal surfaces of cortical and trabecular bone. The marrow may be spottily fibrotic. The disturbed structure of bone may so weaken it as to permit pathologic fractures. The long-term irradiation is carcinogenic. Malignant bone tumors arise. The induction time is long—greater than 10 years, with an average of about 20 years. The types of tumors are not different from human bone tumors in general. In addition to bone tumors, carcinomas of the sinuses and nasopharynx have been seen in greatly increased numbers over the rare expected incidence. Leukemias have been conspicuous by their almost total absence. Aplastic anemia has also been observed as a cause of death. There is no satisfactory treatment of early or late radium poisoning. Prevention is the cure. Although these cases are mainly of historical interest, many elderly persons are still alive with significant body burdens of radium from therapy and employment in the watch dial industry. It is not possible to construct a dose-effect curve for radium poisoning. An estimate of the numerator of the incidence ratio is possible, since the diseases are brought to the attention of physicians. However, the denominator is sadly lacking since those who did not develop a disease that necessitated medical care are absent from most serious studies of the problem.

MICROWAVES Microwave frequency extends from 300 to 200,000 MHz, with wavelengths from about 1 to 50 cm.

Microwaves are the output of radars; they are used to accelerate nuclear particles in accelerators, for cooking, for industrial heating problems, and in medical diathermy for local heating of tissue. A common diathermy today utilizes a magnetron tube which operates at 2,450 MHz and 12 cm wavelength. Numerous applicators are available for heating surfaces, within the rectum, vagina, etc. Medically the local heating of tissue at depths apparently increases blood flow and promotes more rapid healing of traumatized or inflamed areas.

Harmful effects are produced from deposition of energy too rapidly, producing excessive local heating of tissue. Deposition of energy varies with the type of tissue and the reflection from interfaces. Experimentally, bone growth has been impaired, testicles have been destroyed, and cataracts have been produced. Very high intensity radar exposure for 1 min 10 ft from the antenna resulted in sufficient injury to the bowel to produce an acute abdominal emergency, necessitating laparotomy and followed later by intestinal perforations, peritonitis, and death. Presumably the bowel was "cooked" in part. A few servicemen looked down the wave guide of a radar and later developed cataracts. Cataracts also developed in an employee who worked near an operating microwave antenna. A hazard is known to exist. Injuries can be avoided by educating those who work near and plan the propagation of microwaves so that the beam is directed away from human beings.

ULTRASOUND Ultrasound consists of sound waves from a few hundred hertz to many megahertz. The passage of the sound wave through tissue produces successive positive and negative pressures which increase molecular motion and then generate heat via frictional forces. With large intensities (greater than 1 watt per cm^2), cavities are produced during the negative phase which become filled with gas dissolved in the medium. Cavitation produces large local temperatures, electrical discharges, and intense mechanical movement. Chemical reactions involving "free radicals" produced by the electrical discharges may occur, depending on the chemical nature of dissolved gases which may enhance or suppress the free radicals.

Ultrasound can kill cells, disrupt bacteria, etc., but local heat may inactivate enzymes and disturb subsequent chemical studies.

Ultrasound has been used in therapy, with some success, to produce local heating, as in diathermy for the treatment of arthritis, painful neuromas, and myositis. There is little danger since destruction of tissue takes about fifty times as much energy as production of pain; hence there is a built-in physiologic safeguard.

Unique ingenious multiple-port focusing devices have been built to focus ultrasonic energy in distinctly circumscribed volumes to destroy tissue. Such devices are being developed for neurosurgical work. Bone overlying the area at which the sound is focused must be removed. It is possible to destroy all neural components in a specific region without interrupting the capillary network. Ultrasonic neurosurgery is being evaluated in the treatment and relief of the hyperkinetic, hypertonic, and intractable pain disorders. It has also been used for prefrontal lobotomy instead of the usual surgical approach.

Ultrasound can also be used to localize foreign bodies and some tumors.

See also Chap. 56, Photosensitivity and Other Reactions to Light.

REFERENCES

BOND VP et al: *Mammalian Radiation Lethality,* New York: Academic, 1965

CASARETT AP: *Radiation Biology,* Englewood Cliffs, N.J.: Prentice-Hall, 1968

CRONKITE EP, BOND VP: *Radiation Injury in Man,* Springfield, Ill.: Charles C Thomas, 1960

——et al: Radiation leukemogenesis. Am J Med 28:673, 1960

ELKIND MM, WHITMORE GP: *The Radiobiology of Cultured Mammalian Cells,* New York: Gordon and Breach, 1967

HEMPELMANN LH: The acute radiation syndrome: A study of 9 cases and a review. Ann Intern Med 36:279, 1952

KNAUFF GM: Biological effects of microwave radiation on Air Force personnel. AMA Arch Ind Health 17:48, 1958

LEA DE: *Actions of Radiation on Living Cells,* New York: Macmillan, 1947

MCLAUGHLIN JT: Tissue destruction and death from microwave radiation (radar). Calif Med 86:336, 1957

Report of U.N. Scientific Committee on the Effects of Atomic Radiation, 19th Session, suppl. 14 (A/5814), chap. 3: Radiation carcinogenesis in man, 1964

RUBIN PR, CASARETT GW: *Clinical Radiation Pathology,* Philadelphia: Saunders, 1968

SCHWAN HP: Biophysics of diathermy, in *Therapeutic Heat,* ed S. Licht, New Haven, Conn.: S. Licht, Publisher, 1958

120 ELECTRICAL INJURIES

JAMES F. WALLACE
ROBERT G. PETERSDORF

EPIDEMIOLOGY Electrical injury has become progressively more common since the first human fatality from accidental electrocution was reported in 1879. In the United States, approximately 1,000 deaths occur annually from electric-current accidents, while another 200 persons die as a result of being struck by lightning. In addition, major electrical burns presently constitute nearly 3 percent of all admissions to burn centers in this country. Electrical injuries occur most commonly among utility pole linemen and construction workers who come into contact with high-tension current, but nearly a third result from accidents in the home or other settings including the hospital with its many electrically powered instruments and appliances.

PATHOGENESIS In understanding the fundamental aspects of electric-current injury, it is helpful to consider some electrophysical principles. For an electric current to flow, there must be a closed pathway or circuit, and a difference in potential or voltage must exist between two points in this completed circuit. The flow of current is directly related to the voltage difference and inversely proportional to the electrical resistance between two points in the circuit (Ohm's law). High-resistance paths allow relatively small currents to flow, while low resistances permit large currents to flow. When voltage is very high, flow of current will likewise be relatively great, unless the resistance is increased proportionally to the voltage; however, if the potential difference between two points can be minimized, the current flow can also be minimized regardless of the resistance.

Although the end result of passage of an electric current through the human body is unpredictable in the individual case, many factors are known to influence the nature and severity of electrical injuries. Body tissues vary considerably in their *resistance* to the flow of current, with conductivity being roughly proportional to water content. Bone and skin offer relatively high resistance, while blood, muscle, and nerve are good conductors. The resistance of normal skin can be lowered by *moisture*, and this factor alone can convert what might ordinarily be a mild injury to a fatal shock. Of importance at the time of contact is *grounding* which, if effective, can minimize the voltage difference between two points in the electric circuit and thus lower the intensity of current passing through the body. The *pathway of the current through the body* is also crucial. An accident involving passage of a current between a point of contact on the leg and the ground is less likely to be injurious than one between the head and the foot, in which the heart lies between the two poles of the circuit. Similarly, a small current leak which would be innocuous when applied to the surface of the intact body may result in a fatal arrhythmia when conducted directly to the heart via a low-resistance intracardiac catheter. *Duration of contact* also influences the outcome of electrical injury. Current can cause tetanic muscular contractions that prevent the victim from being able to release his contact with the circuit. This is usually accompanied by sweating, which lowers skin resistance, allowing current of still greater intensity to pass into the body until fatal cardiac arrhythmia results.

The pathophysiologic effects of electricity on the body are incompletely understood, but, in general, low voltage produces ventricular fibrillation and death from circulatory failure, while high voltage produces cardiac asystole and respiratory arrest, probably as a result of injury to the medullary centers of the brain. In addition, contact with high-intensity current causes several types of thermal injuries. As it traverses the skin, the energy from electric current is converted into heat, producing coagulation necrosis at the points where it enters and exits from the body as well as in the striated muscle through which it passes. Current coursing external to the body from the contact point to the ground may generate temperatures as high as 10,000°C and cause extensive carbonification of skin and immediately underlying tissues, termed *arc burns*. In addition, flame burns caused by ignition of clothing or environmental objects by the current may also occur.

PATHOLOGY In patients who die immediately, autopsy findings are limited to burns and generalized petechial hemorrhages. If patients survive for a period of days or longer, postmortem examination reveals focal necrosis of nerve, spinal cord, or brain, involving both neurons and white matter, with appropriate glial and vascular reactions. Renal tubular necrosis may be seen when acute renal failure follows extensive tissue destruction.

CLINICAL MANIFESTATIONS Immediately after a severe electrical shock, patients are usually comatose, apneic, and in circulatory collapse from ventricular fibrillation or cardiac standstill. Surviving this stage, they often are disoriented, combative, and frequently may have seizures. Often they will be found to have fractures of bone caused either by convulsive muscular contractions accompanying the shock or from falls at the time of the accident. Hypovolemic shock often appears soon after high-tension electrical injury and is due to the rapid loss of fluid into areas of tissue damage, and from body surface burns. Hypotension, along with renal tubular damage from myoglobin and hemoglobin pigments liberated during massive muscle necrosis and hemolysis, may lead to acute renal failure.

Besides the extensive destruction of tissue occurring instantly in electrical burns, additional injury from ischemia produced by swelling of damaged tissues may appear later. Both anaerobic and aerobic infections originating in inadequately debrided necrotic muscle masses often are serious early complications.

Late effects include various neurologic disabilities, visual disturbances, and the residual damage left by burns. Nervous system injuries are frequent and include peripheral neuropathies, incomplete transection of the spinal cord, and reflex sympathetic dystrophies, as well as late convulsive disorders and intractable headache. The development of cataracts of one or both eyes has been reported to occur up to 3 years following electrical injury.

LABORATORY FINDINGS Immediately following major electrical injury the hematocrit is commonly elevated and the plasma volume reduced, reflecting sequestration of fluid in the wound. Unless extensive flame burns are also present, serial determinations of either of these parameters provide a good means of monitoring the adequacy of fluid replacement therapy. Myoglobinuria is seen frequently in association with severe shocks, and when it persists following establishment of urine flow, usually indicates massive muscle injury. In many patients, profound metabolic acidosis is also present. Lumbar puncture may show elevated pressure associated with cerebral edema or bloody spinal fluid as a result of intracerebral hemorrhage. The electrocardiogram not infrequently shows tachycardia and minor S-T segment alterations which can persist for several weeks following injury. Unexplained acute hypokalemia leading to respiratory arrest and cardiac arrhythmias has developed in some patients between the second and fourth weeks following injury.

TREATMENT Removal of the victim from contact with the current should be accomplished immediately without touching him directly. Rescuers should use a rubber sheet, wooden pole, or other nonconductive material to detach him, and this should be preceded by cutting off the source of current when possible. If the victim is not breathing, mouth-to-mouth ventilation should be instituted at once. Although most cases who survive develop spontaneous respiration within half an hour, complete recovery after longer periods occurs often enough so that respiratory support should be continued for at least 4 hours. If there is no evidence of heartbeat, external cardiac massage should accompany ventilatory resuscitation. Persons struck by lightning frequently have cardiac asystole which responds to a manual blow to the chest, while victims of low-voltage shocks will usually require defibrillation to restore heart action. During cardiopulmonary resuscitation and evacuation to the hospital, attention should be paid to possible broken bones and spinal cord injuries incurred at the time of the accident.

Subsequent hospital care of electrical injuries is mainly supportive. With major electrothermal trauma, rapid institution of fluid and electrolyte therapy for hypovolemic shock is essential, with guidelines being the patient's urine output, hematocrit, and plasma volume. If myoglobinuria persists after adequate urine flow has been established, the use of furosemide or an osmotic diuretic such as mannitol along with alkalinization of the urine is frequently indicated. Management of the electrical wound should include adequate debridement of necrotic tissue and often will require fasciotomy to prevent further ischemic injury. Topical antimicrobial chemotherapy with Sulfamylon or silver nitrate may be useful in preventing or delaying infections in extensive surface burns. Survivors of the acute episode often require extensive treatment for infection, cerebral edema, and delayed hemorrhage as devitalized tissues slough. If acute renal failure occurs, it should be managed as described in Chap. 269.

PREVENTION Proper installation of appliances, grounding of telephone lines and radio and television aerials, and the use of rubber gloves and dry shoes when working with electric circuits should be routine. Unused wall sockets should be kept plugged and live extension cords not left unattended, particularly in households when there are young children. During a severe thunderstorm, refuge near hilltops, riverbanks, hedges, telephone poles, and trees should be avoided. The safest shelter is the closed house while an automobile, cave, ditch, or even lying flat on the ground are relatively secure. In hospitalized patients, the hazard of ventricular fibrillation precipitated by minute current leaks conducted directly to the myocardium from monitoring equipment via pacemakers or intravascular manometric catheters should be more widely appreciated. Hospital personnel should be aware that in addition to medical instruments, patient contact with two or more other power line–operated devices such as television sets, radios, electric razors, lamps and especially electric beds can also result in electrocution if the heart lies within the current path through the patient. These hazards can be minimized by proper grounding of equipment *before* a patient is connected to the instrument, periodic measurement for leakage of current supplied by each device, and by instruction in the principles of electrical safety for hospital personnel who use the complex and dangerous equipment that is so much a part of modern medical practice.

REFERENCES

Baxter CR: Present concepts in the management of major electrical injury. Surg Clin North Am 50:1401, 1970

DiVincenti FC et al: Electrical injuries: A review of 65 cases. J Trauma 9:497, 1969

Fischer H: Pathologic effects and sequelae of electrical accidents. J Occup Med 7:564, 1965

Kilpatrick DG: The electrical environment. Med Clin North Am 55:1095, 1971

Starmer CF et al: Electrical hazards and cardiovascular function. N Engl J Med 284:181, 1971

Taussig HB: Death from lightning—and the possibility of living again. Ann Intern Med 68:1345, 1968

121 IMMERSION INJURY AND DROWNING

RUSSELL S. FISHER

About 7,000 deaths by drowning occur in the United States each year. This is the fourth leading cause of death and represents about one-fifteenth of the total number of fatal accidents.

DIAGNOSIS The term *drowning* is used to categorize a series of related phenomena resulting from submersion in a liquid medium that is per se innocuous. It, therefore, includes asphyxial changes as well as complex acute hemodynamic alterations and disturbances of the biochemical equilibrium of the blood.

PATHOGENESIS Knowledge of the sequence of phenomena that occur in drowning is based upon a number of observations on humans and on experimental drowning in animals. Submersion is usually followed by an intensive and panicky struggle in an effort to reach the surface. Breath holding for varying lengths of time has been recorded to occur in the next stage, possibly lasting until the accumulating CO_2 in blood and tissues stimulates the respiratory center sufficiently to lead to an inevitable inhalation of considerable volumes of water. Swallowing of water, coughing and vomiting, loss of consciousness, and terminal gasping with flooding of the lungs and death then take place in rapid succession. When the process is interrupted before terminal gasping has set in, spontaneous recovery sometimes occurs. It has commonly been asserted that drowning essentially involves asphyxia resulting from obstruction of the airway by the drowning fluid. More recent investigations, however, show that asphyxial death in drowning is limited to between 10 and 15 percent of all cases and is due to laryngospasm and closure of the glottis. Moreover comparative enzymologic studies in rats of fresh and salt water drowning and asphyxia by exclusion of air indicate significant statistical differences between test and control groups. This seems to further stress the distinction between the mode of death in asphyxia versus that of drowning. In the majority of fatalities, death results from complex pathophysiologic events differing widely according to the chemical composition of the submersion liquid. For purposes of illustration, drowning in fresh water and sea water may be considered as separate entities.

Drowning in fresh water Large amounts of water enter the lungs, and due to the hypotonicity of fresh water, rapid absorption into the circulating bloodstream takes place. This results in a sudden and violent increase in blood volume with hemodilution and hypervolemia. Using deuterium oxide in the water as a tracer, Swann and Spafford have demonstrated that after 2 min submersion, a dog's blood may be diluted by as much as 51 percent of its original volume. This hemodilution is associated with massive hemolysis and an inevitable upset of the normal balance of the blood constituents. Sodium, chloride, calcium, proteins, and hemoglobin are all diluted, and the level of potassium rises. Ventricular fibrillation is often considered to be a characteristic feature of fresh water drowning. When it occurs, expulsive heartbeats are arrested at once. Ventricular fibrillation is believed to be directly related to the dilution of the blood electrolytes, in particular sodium. It cannot, however, be produced experimentally by injecting large volumes of water intravenously. The precedent condition is anoxia; the animal must be anoxic for an experimental hydremic plethora to cause fibrillation. The original hypothesis, based upon animal experiments, of "potassium intoxication" secondary to massive hemolysis as the underlying factor causing ventricular fibrillation has proved erroneous. The main intracellular cation in dog erythrocytes is not potassium as in man, but sodium, and fresh water drowning and hemolysis in the dog does not release a flood of potassium ions. The slight increase observed in plasma potassium after fresh water drowning may be accounted for by prolonged anoxia, as described by Fenn. These speculations do not answer the question of whether ventricular fibrillation occurs in fresh water drowning in man, but it would appear desirable to include defibrillation in the emergency treatment of a drowning victim.

Drowning in sea water Sea water is strongly hypertonic. Its salt concentration, mainly sodium chloride, is over 3.0 percent. Submersion in sea water results in a rapid diffusion of salts into the bloodstream. The concentration of sodium, chloride, magnesium, etc., in the plasma rise conspicuously, while water moves from the circulation into the pulmonary alveoli—thus reestablishing the osmotic equilbrium. The consequences are marked hemoconcentration and fulminant pulmonary edema. Hypotension and hypovolemia accompanied by considerable bradycardia develop, and death supervenes within a few minutes. Ventricular fibrillation is not usually observed in experimental salt water drowning in spite of the adverse prevailing electrolyte environment, probably because the plasma sodium level is elevated rather than low.

Death associated with diving (see also Chap. 117) In the case of divers, death is often the result of underwater asphyxia following hyperventilation; the latter leads to a sharp fall in blood carbon dioxide and to vasconstriction, which in turn brings about a decrease of the cerebral circulation. Diminished cerebral blood flow is followed by loss of consciousness, which leads to inhalation of water. Involuntary exhalation against a closed glottis results in hypotension and diminished cardiac output, further aggravating the condition. In diving with a scuba (self-contained underwater breathing apparatus), the cause of death is usually closely associated with the overconfidence of the diver in his breathing machine. Nitrogen narcosis occurs commonly, resulting from the increase of nitrogen concentration in the tissues as evident from Henry's law, according to which the solubility of a gas is directly proportional to the absolute pressure upon it. There is an increase of 1 atmosphere (atm) of pressure for each 33 ft of water depth. Barotrauma and air embolism are second in frequency and occur during the ascent of the diver, when the air inhaled from the scuba expands proportionately as the pressure decreases (Boyle's law). An ascent, for instance, from 33 ft results in a twofold increase in volume due to the decrease in pressure from 2 to 1 atm. At this point any interference with expiration prevents release of this increased volume and results in acute pulmonary emphysema with tears in the lungs, hemoptysis, hemothorax, air embolism, and often death.

Careful investigation of the circumstances of submersion is mandatory to rule out cervical spinal trauma in those cases where the victim dove into the water and impacted the bottom.

RESUSCITATION FROM DROWNING The main objective of adequate resuscitation in drowning is to institute such measures before circulatory failure sets in. Resuscitative procedures currently employed consist of clearing the airway by postural drainage, suction, etc., and giving artificial respiration, supplemented by closed-chest cardiac massage if no heart sounds are obtainable and the pulse is absent. Intermittent positive-pressure breathing with air, or preferably with oxygen, should be employed when such is available, and external electrical defibrillation should be carried out as soon as feasible after the condition arises. Plasma infusion to correct hemoconcentration is often thought to be of great value in salt water drowning, while in fresh water drowning it may be expected that an exchange transfusion, which in itself is a relatively harmless procedure, will be effective in reestablishing a normal circulating blood volume and in correcting an upset electrolyte balance. So-called "semi-" or "near drowning" in which death occurs suddenly several hours or longer after submersion has been repeatedly reported, but the mechanism of death in such cases remains obscure. Treatment should be directed to maintaining high cerebral oxygen supply and preventing pneumonia. Lower nephron nephrosis may also be anticipated in survivors of fresh water submersion due to hemoglobinemia; if oliguria or anuria develops, appropriate therapy should be initiated. Methylprednisolone therapy has been suggested for pulmonary edema following near drowning (Sladen and Zauder).

REFERENCES

Denny MK, Read RC: Scuba-diving deaths in Michigan. JAMA 192:220, 1965

Kvittingen TD, Naess A: Recovery from drowning in fresh water. Br Med J 1:1315, 1963

Sladen A, Zauder HL: Methylprednisolone therapy for pulmonary edema following near drowning. JAMA 215:1793, 1971

Spitz WU: Drowning. Hosp Med 5:8, 1969

Swann HG: Mechanism of circulatory failure in fresh and sea water drowning. Circ Res 4:241, 1956

PART SEVEN DISORDERS CAUSED BY BIOLOGIC AGENTS

section 1 Basic considerations

122 AN APPROACH TO INFECTIOUS DISEASES

ROBERT G. PETERSDORF

INTRODUCTION The vast majority of human and animal diseases of known etiology are produced by biologic agents: viruses, rickettsias, bacteria, mycoplasma, fungi, protozoa, or nematodes. No small part of the past and present importance of infectious diseases in medical practice is attributable to their enormous frequency and the public health implications of the contagiousness of many of them. However, developments in sanitary engineering, vector control, techniques of immunization, and specific chemotherapy have modified the situation favorably. Although important exceptions remain, infectious diseases as a class are more easily prevented and more easily cured than any other major group of disorders. Despite the virtual elimination of certain infectious diseases and profound reduction in the morbidity and mortality of many, man is by no means free of infection. In fact, the total human load of disease produced by microbial parasites has decreased only modestly, primarily through smallpox and malaria control and better health care in developing countries. As certain specific microbial infections have been controlled, others have emerged as troublesome therapeutic and epidemiologic problems. With the introduction of cytotoxic drugs, massive x-ray irradiation in the treatment of malignant diseases, and immunosuppressive agents to control the rejection of transplanted organs, infections due to organisms previously considered saprophytic or commensal have increased. As Dubos has pointed out, microbial infections appear to form an inherent part of human life.

Because of better environmental sanitation and other measures that now prevent contact with many microbial agents, and the development of acquired immunity early in childhood, certain infections have been seen more frequently in adults. For example, as contact with poliomyelitis virus in childhood declined in many countries, paralytic poliomyelitis became more common in young adults. *Hemophilus influenzae* meningitis is being reported more frequently in adults than heretofore, and decreasing infection with the tubercle bacillus raises questions about the status of antituberculous immunity in adults.

As antimicrobial agents reduce the mortality associated with certain common infections, other microbes emerge as important causes of human disease. It is relatively unusual nowadays for patients to die of uncomplicated pneumococcal pneumonia, a disease readily handled with available antimicrobials. However, it is common to see serious disease produced by microorganisms which form part of man's normal microbial flora. These include infections produced by staphylococci, enteric bacilli, and fungi (see Chap. 123).

THE PARASITE AND THE HOST The complex interaction between microorganism and man that results in infection and disease has been subjected to extensive study. Much has been learned about the initiation of the process, the ways in which microbes produce tissue injury, the influence of specific immunity and "nonspecific" resistance of the host, and the mechanisms of recovery. Unfortunately, it is not yet possible to transfer in any specific way much of the information that has been acquired to the individual patient with an infection. In this presentation those general aspects of the host-parasite relation that form the basis for diagnostic procedures, that are of importance in deriving therapeutic principles, or that help explain the epidemiology of infection are stressed.

Infection and clinical disease It is well known that microorganisms of different species or different strains of the same species vary widely in their capacity to produce disease and that human beings are not equally susceptible to the disease caused by a given bacterium or virus. Furthermore, while a specific infectious disease will not occur in the absence of the causative organism, the mere presence of the organism in the body does not lead invariably to clinical illness. Indeed, the production of symptoms in man by many parasites is the exception rather than the rule, and the *subclinical infection* or the "carrier state" is the usual host-parasite relation. *Disease* in a clinical sense is not synonymous with the presence of the organism or *infection* in a microbiologic sense. The ratio of subclinical infection to overt clinical disease varies widely for different microbial species. For example, subclinical infections with the agent causing infectious hepatitis are the rule. In contrast, active human infection with the rabies virus nearly always produces progressive fatal disease, and subclinical infections with rabies have not been observed.

Mechanisms of injury It is customary to refer to bacteria or other microorganisms that are capable of producing disease as *pathogenic*. *Virulence*, the *degree* of pathogenicity, should be distinguished from *invasiveness*, the ability to spread and disseminate in the body. For example, *Clostridium tetani* is pathogenic and, by virtue of its exotoxin, highly virulent, but it is almost completely lacking in invasiveness. These distinctions are valuable in microbiology and experimental pathology, but they often mean relatively little at a clinical level. Under certain circumstances and in certain anatomic locations, mildly "pathogenic" organisms can produce fatal disease, or highly "pathogenic" species can multiply without producing any harmful effect.

A few parasites produce *toxins* that account for the tissue damage and physiologic alterations of infection. *Hypersensitivity* to components of the parasite is demonstrable in several infections to account for the manifestations of disease. For many pathogenic agents, an explanation of their damaging effects upon the host is incomplete or wholly lacking. Generally, therefore, the aim of therapy is to stop multiplication or to kill the parasites with appropriate drugs; in diseases caused by toxin-producing organisms, the use of antiserum (as in tetanus or diphtheria) is the definitive procedure, and chemotherapy is secondary.

The tendency of certain pathogenic organisms to *localize in certain cells or organs* and to produce damage is also unexplained. Clinically, however, the presence of disease in a specific anatomic site or a combination of symptoms referable to certain organs often suggests the identity of the causative organism. For example, the pneumococcus usually causes infection in the lung but almost never in the kidney, and *H. influenzae* infections are confined almost solely to the respiratory tract and meninges. Similarly, in the presence of disease known to be caused by a given agent, complicating involvement of other tissues can be anticipated or predicted. Examples include the multiple lung abscesses which are so characteristic of hematogenously disseminated staphylococcal disease and metastatic skin lesions which complicate *Pseudomonas* bacteremia.

Frequently, the proper management of infectious disease involves the use of techniques completely unrelated to microbiology or chemotherapy, in an effort to support the function of damaged organs. Survival in poliomyelitis may depend upon treatment of respiratory failure, the management of heart failure in endocarditis is sometimes a greater problem than the eradication of the causative organism, and in epidemic hemorrhagic fever, or Weil's disease, maintenance of fluid and electrolyte balance, with peritoneal dialysis or hemodialysis during the stage of acute renal failure, is the important therapeutic objective.

Resistance and susceptibility Many so-called "host factors" are known to influence the likelihood that disease will occur if organisms enter the tissues, or, if infection becomes established, to play a determining role in the outcome of infection—recovery or death. These include natural antibodies, interferon, phagocytic activity, and the level of the general inflammatory response.

In experimental animals, sex, microbial strain, age, route of infection, the presence of specific antibody, other diseases, nutritional state, and the use of such procedures as exposure to ionizing radiation or high environmental temperature or administration of mucin, nitrogen mustard, adrenal steroids, epinephrine, xerosin, and metabolic analogues can be shown to exert a profound effect upon infection by bacteria, viruses, and other agents.

In man, these factors are no less important, although controlled studies are lacking for many. Alcoholism; diabetes; deficiency or absence of immunoglobulins (Chap. 64); defects in cellular immunity (Chap. 64); malnutrition; chronic administration of adrenal hormones; chronic lymphedema; ischemia; the presence of foreign bodies such as bullets, calculi, or bone fragments; obstruction of a bronchus, the urethra, or any hollow tube; agranulocytosis; various blood dyscrasias, and many other circumstances influence susceptibility to systemic or local infection. Furthermore, in those instances where the extenuating condition is remediable, the probability of recovery is enhanced.

Racial differences in susceptibility, such as the poor resistance of dark-skinned people to tuberculosis, their predilection for developing disseminated coccidioidomycosis, and the resistance of Negroes to malaria caused by *Plasmodium vivax* are well established. Resistance to infection may be determined genetically. The relation of sickle-cell trait to malaria is one example. The increased frequency and severity of some infections in children, of others in pregnant women, and still others in the aged are familiar.

Prior contact with an organism or its products, whether by active infection or by artificial immunization, increases resistance to some infection, such as measles, diphtheria, and pertussis by stimulating antibody production, but seems to have little influence on resistance to others, such as gonorrhea.

Present knowledge of the factors involved in human resistance and susceptibility is incomplete. Explanations such as changes in physical or chemical activity of phagocytes; antibacterial substances such as lysozyme, phagocytin, or lysozomal enzymes; qualitative or quantitative alterations in serum proteins; disordered metabolism at the cellular level, "products of tissue injury" that influence vascular permeability, and the effects of tissue pressure remain to a considerable extent in the realm of hypothesis.

The profound influence of host factors upon the infectious process makes it clear, however, that their understanding is probably essential for the control of infections in predictable fashion. The understanding and study of these host factors remain a fertile field for investigation.

PATHOGENESIS OF INFECTION With relatively minor variations, the development of an infectious disease follows a consistent pattern. The parasites enter the body through the skin, nasopharynx, lung, intestine, urethra, or other portal, and a regular sequence ensues. Once established in the host, the organisms can multiply and, in so doing, establish a local or primary lesion. From this site, there may be local spread along fascial planes or tubular structures, such as a bronchus or ureter. The next step is systemic spread of the microorganisms via the circulating blood. Bacteria may enter the bloodstream by direct invasion of vessels, a relatively unusual occurrence, or more commonly by traversing peripheral lymph nodes to enter the thoracic duct lymph and thence the venous system. In the bloodstream, they spread to other tissues and can produce distant or secondary lesions. In infections such as tetanus and diphtheria, distant lesions are produced by toxins elaborated at the primary site without systemic spread of the parasites. The infectious process may terminate in recovery or death at any stage: the local lesion, systemic spread, or distant lesion.

The apparent inconsistency of this pattern in clinical medicine is attributable to the fact that the infection is recognized as a clinical entity only at the stage when symptoms are most likely to appear. For example, pneumococcal pneumonia is a local lesion, and the distant lesion, pneumococcal meningitis, is referred to clinically as a complication. In the meningococcal infections, the local lesion, a nasopharyngitis, is rarely symptomatic and has no status as a clinical entity, but the stage of spread, meningococcemia, and the commonest distant lesion, meningitis, are clinical entities. A rarer distant lesion, arthritis, is called a complication. In a patient who has osteomyelitis, a clinical entity, a recent furuncle may be referred to as a predisposing factor. In another patient with extensive furunculosis who develops osteomyelitis, the infection in bone may be regarded as a complication of the superficial infection. The stages mentioned are in no way limited to bacterial diseases; the primary lesion of poliomyelitis is intestinal, viremia may occur without neurologic involvement, or a distant lesion, the classic "infantile paralysis," may be established.

Because of established clinical usage and terminology based upon the symptomatic illness that leads patients to seek medical aid, the consistency of this general sequence in the pathogenesis of infection is often not recognized. However, the concept is useful and offers some basis for systematizing what may otherwise seem to be a miscellaneous collection of unrelated clinical signs and symptoms.

CLINICAL MANIFESTATIONS OF INFECTIONS So varied are the disorders attributable to infection or infestation of man by lower organisms that generalizations about them are difficult. The clinical manifestations of infection can duplicate those of diseases of any other etiology. However, certain clinical features are highly suggestive of infection, including abrupt onset, fever, chills, myalgia, photophobia, pharyngitis, acute lymphadenopathy and splenomegaly, gastrointestinal upset, and leukocytosis or leukopenia. It is obvious that the presence of one, several, or all of these features does not constitute proof of the microbial origin of illness in a given patient. Conversely, serious, even fatal, infectious disease may exist in the absence of fever or other signs and symptoms.

Although there is no infallible clinical criterion of infection, it is still possible to recognize accurately many specific infectious diseases from information obtained by *history, physical examination, blood count, and urinalysis.* The importance of interrogation about past illness, predisposing factors such as alcoholism, familial disease, exposure to ill persons, contact with animals or insects, ingestion of contaminated food, type and order of onset of symptoms, and recent or remote residence in endemic areas is discussed in subsequent chapters for specific diseases, and etiologic agents. Cardinal physical signs are also described for each entity.

The mechanisms that produce most of the signs and symptoms of human infection are unknown. The pathogenesis of fever is discussed in Chap. 12. The physiologic alterations underlying "malaise," "postinfectious asthenia," "toxicity," and other common complaints are completely mysterious. The factors responsible for leukocytosis or leukopenia are only partially understood (Chap. 61). Why the rash of typhus begins on the trunk while that of another rickettsiosis, Rocky Mountain spotted fever, begins on the extremities is unanswered. Failure to understand these manifestations does not impair their clinical usefulness, although it is probable that understanding them might lead to more accurate diagnosis and better management.

DIAGNOSTIC PROCEDURES When dealing with diseases produced by living agents, it is evident that confirmation of a presumptive diagnosis, or sometimes the first suggestion as to the etiology of illness, depends upon laboratory procedures. The availability of a multitude of laboratory tests in the modern hospital has not made it possible to substitute a "routine laboratory work-up" for history, physical examination, and observation of a patient's course. Indeed, the information derived from these procedures is the only reasonable basis for selecting the tests to be performed by the laboratory.

The importance of roentgenographic changes, alterations in chemical constituents of the blood, and tests of the functional capacity of organs such as the liver and kidney is as great in infectious disease as in illnesses of other etiologies and needs no discussion here.

The specific procedures for the diagnosis of infectious disease involve *direct demonstration of the causative organism or proof of its presence by indirect means.*

Demonstration of the organism In bacterial disease, it is often possible to find the causative organism by *microscopic examination of properly stained preparations of sputum, spinal fluid, and other body fluids.* This simple procedure is often neglected as an unnecessary bother when material is being sent for bacteriologic culture, but it is a most valuable source of immediate information. In some diseases, the etiologic agent cannot be cultured (bartonellosis), and in others isolation is time-consuming (tuberculosis, blastomycosis). In some patients with systemic candidiasis, an increasingly important problem in patients with compromised host resistance, *Candida* blastospores and pseudohyphae have been found in blood smears several days before the blood culture became positive. The diagnosis of meningococcal infection by finding the organism in fluid from skin lesions or in the buffy coat, the diagnosis of staphylococcal sepsis by finding organisms in their leukocytes, or the discovery of *H. influenzae* in stained smears of cerebrospinal fluid permits the initiation of specific chemotherapy immediately with the assurance that the regimen is the proper one.

Direct examination of bone marrow is a useful method for demonstrating organisms in some diseases such as kala azar, histoplasmosis, and tuberculosis. In protozoan (amebiasis, malaria) and parasitic diseases (schistosomiasis, filariasis), *direct examination of blood, feces, or urine* is the only feasible method for establishing a diagnosis.

There are also infections in which the detection of characteristic cytologic changes or the causative organism itself in smears or histologic sections of biopsy material may be the quickest method for diagnosis. Tubercles and tubercle bacilli in lymph nodes or liver biopsies, *Mycobacterium leprae* in skin or nasal scrapings, inclusion bodies in the skin lesions of varicella or variola and the exudate of inclusion blenorrhea, "Warthin" cells from the nasal or pharyngeal mucosa in measles, schistosome ova in punch biopsies of rectal mucosa, and the Councilman bodies of yellow fever in the liver are examples. In addition, characteristic histologic changes make it feasible to identify the lesions of chancroid, syphilis, lymphogranuloma venereum, or viral hepatitis in biopsy specimens. Indeed, even in diseases where other reliable tests are available, diagnosis by histologic examination is sometimes the most rapid method available; the characteristic muscle lesion of Weil's disease is an example (Chap. 161).

Special microscopic techniques *Dark-field examination* of material from genital lesions for the spirochete of syphilis is a well-known but often neglected procedure. In several other spirochetal diseases, including leptospirosis, the dark-field technique can be useful, but experience in recognition of the organisms is necessary for correct interpretation of findings.

Fluorescence microscopy in which the causative organisms can be recognized and identified rapidly by the use of fluorescent antibody preparations (Coons' technique) is being used in the diagnosis of syphilis, gonorrhea, pertussis, streptococcal pharyngitis, and a number of other bacterial, viral, fungal, and parasitic infections. The final role of this procedure remains to be established, but with increasing availability of specific serums and continuing technical refinement, it will certainly be of increasing value in the future.

The nitroblue tetrazolium (NBT) test is based on the increased intracytoplasmic reduction of NBT by actively phagocytic segmented neutrophils. It has been shown to be valuable in differentiating systemic bacterial infections from nonbacterial inflammatory states. In normal hosts bacterial infection results in more than 10 to 15 percent of polymorphonuclear leukocytes containing reduced NBT (formazan pigment). The test rapidly reverts to normal following treatment with appropriate antibiotics. It depends upon functionally intact leukocytes, opsonins, and an intact complement system. Nonbacterial causes of positive tests include neonates, Nocardia infection, candidemia, malaria, typhoid vaccination, and contraceptive pills. Negative tests occur in complement-deficient states, agammaglobulinemia, infections in patients with sickle-cell disease, and chronic granulomatous disease. The test is negative in mycobacterial infections. While the NBT test is useful in the presumptive diagnosis of bacterial infection, care must be taken in its interpretation because in inexperienced hands, errors are common.

Culture and animal inoculation Specimens for bacteriologic culture should be collected *before the initiation of chemotherapy*. The material to be cultured—sputum, pus, blood, or bone marrow—should be selected on the basis of the suspected infections, and the precise cultural techniques employed—media, CO_2 incubation, anaerobic incubation—must be determined in similar fashion. There are new developments in identification of a wide range of viruses in tissue culture, and refinements in these techniques are increasing the value of tissue culture in clinical diagnosis.

In several infections, including Weil's disease, rat-bite fever, certain mycoses, tuberculosis, and the rickettsioses, the etiologic organism can be isolated by *inoculation of appropriate material into mice or guinea pigs*. This is a cumbersome procedure for routine use, but should be employed in selected instances. Many viruses can also be isolated by inoculation of appropriate animals. This is rarely feasible for ordinary clinical diagnosis and, for several agents, is hazardous.

Blood cultures and bacteremia Because of the peculiar clinical importance of demonstrating bacteria in the bloodstream and because there are varying opinions about optimal timing and sites of sampling for blood cultures, it is of practical importance to understand something about the mechanisms of bacteremia.

Excepting intravascular infections (bacterial endocarditis or endarteritis, mycotic aneurysm, suppurative thrombophlebitis), bacteria usually enter the circulation through the lymphatic system. Consequently, when bacteria multiply at a site of local infection in the tissues, the likelihood of bacteremia parallels the occurrence of local conditions that favor drainage of lymph from the infected area to the thoracic duct and eventually to the venous blood. These factors include the number and anatomic arrangement of local lymph vessels, accumulation of fluid, increase in tissue pressure, and manipulation of the part.

Once bacteria enter the blood, they are removed rapidly by the fixed phagocytes of the reticuloendothelial system in the liver, spleen, and bone marrow and by engulfment in polymorphonuclear leukocytes in capillaries, especially those of the lung.

Clinically, bacteremia can be transient, intermittent, or continuous. Many transient bacteremias result from manipulation of infected or contaminated tissues, common examples being instrumentation of the genitourinary tract, tonsillectomy, dental procedures, and massage or surgical incision of furuncles or abscesses. In the vast majority of instances, the sudden discharge of bacteria into the blood produces no symptoms or, at most, a rigor and brief fever, and the organisms are promptly removed. The great danger of these "man-made" bacteremias is their role in producing bacterial endocarditis in patients with endocardial damage.

Transient bacteremia accompanies the early phase of many infections. In pneumococcal pneumonia, the typical rigor at the onset is a result of transient bacteremia. In most cases, with localization of the pulmonary lesion, blood cultures rapidly revert to negative. The poor prognosis of patients with pneumonia who continue to have positive blood cultures is not due to the presence of organisms in the blood but reflects spreading infection in the lung itself.

A sudden single influx of microorganisms into the bloodstream may be followed by a shaking chill and fever. However, there is a "lag period" of 30 to 90 min before the febrile response (Chap. 12). During this delay, the bacteria are usually promptly removed from the circulation by phagocytosis; consequently, a blood culture taken at the time of the rigor may be negative.

Continuous bacteremia is a feature of the first several days of typhoid fever, of brucellosis, and of intravascular infections such as endocarditis or endarteritis.

Blood cultures should be taken at frequent intervals in patients with febrile disease of unknown cause; in general, an attempt should be made to obtain blood *before* an expected rise in fever or chill. When a patient is suspected of bacterial endocarditis, or another of the diseases in which bacteremia is constant, two to four cultures daily for 2 to 3 days are more than sufficient to establish the diagnosis, and treatment in such cases should not be withheld for a longer period.

There is no evidence that arterial blood cultures possess any advantage over venous cultures. Suspected bacteremia is sometimes mentioned as a contraindication to diagnostic lumbar puncture because of the possible development of meningitis, but clinical evidence does not support this idea. Culture of bone marrow is occasionally superior to peripheral blood for recovery of organisms in typhoid, brucellosis, and rare cases of subacute bacterial endocarditis. It is common practice to make pour plates of blood and to quantify bacteremia in terms of a certain number of colonies per milliliter of blood. Although this procedure may seem cumbersome, colony counts are of value in distinguishing contaminating organisms. Colony counts may also be of prognostic value because a large number of organisms in the absence of severe clinical disease almost always means that bacteria are entering the bloodstream from a contaminated extracorporeal focus such as an infusion or an arteriovenous shunt. When blood cultures are taken for diagnostic purposes, some should be incubated in carbon dioxide, and a sample of blood should also be cultured in thioglycollate broth or some other anaerobic medium. Anaerobic cultures are especially important in women with puerperal or postabortal infections.

Immunologic methods These diagnostic methods are intended to supply evidence of past or present infection by demonstrating antibodies in serum or other body fluids, by indicating changed reactivity of the host (hypersensitivity, allergy) to products of the organism, or rarely to detect components of the causative organism in the body.

SEROLOGIC TESTS The finding on a single occasion that a patient's serum contains antibody that reacts with a certain antigen merely indicates that the patient has had previous contact with the antigen or a closely related substance. For this reason, with rare exceptions, the clinical interpretation of serologic tests depends on serial determinations. If the antibody titer is found to *rise or fall significantly*, it is likely that the response is a result of recent contact with the antigen. In subsequent chapters, the need for serologic testing of acute phase and convalescent serum is emphasized repeatedly. *In any patient with a puzzling illness, a sterile specimen of serum should be preserved in a frozen state so that it can, if necessary, be studied and compared with serum collected at a later date.*

Prior contact with an antigen may be the result of past immunization with vaccines; interpretation of serum agglutinin titers for typhoid bacilli is often made difficult by prior immunization. The so-called "anamnestic reaction," a nonspecific stimulation of antibody formation by an acute illness (e.g., a rise in *Brucella* agglutinins in a patient with acute tularemia), occurs only when the two organisms are antigenically related, and rarely presents a serious problem.

The methods employed for detecting antibody rises in various infections have been selected empirically on the basis of the ease with which the test can be performed and careful study to correlate the results of the test with other diagnostic criteria in patients. Therefore, the fact that antibodies against one agent are detected by a precipitin technique, another by agglutination of whole organisms or the production of capsular swelling, another by indirect fluorescent-antibody methods, and still another by complement fixation is a practical matter and bears no necessary relation to the agent, the type of infection, or its pathogenesis. By coating some particulate material, such as erythrocytes or latex, with antigen derived from a certain organism, antibody can sometimes be demonstrated by an agglutination test rather than by some more complex method.

Particular properties of the causative organism can sometimes be utilized to devise a simplified clinical test for antibody. Two striking instances of this are widely used. The ability of influenza and related viruses to clump erythrocytes makes possible the demonstration of antibody to virus by merely testing the capacity of a patient's serum to prevent the agglutination of red cells by suspensions of virus, the so-called "hemagglutination-inhibition" reaction. Similarly, because many microorganisms possess hemolytic components or toxins, the assay of a patient's serum for capacity to prevent lysis of red cells is a convenient and simple clinical test for antibody. The anti-streptolysin O test in group A beta-hemolytic streptococcal infections is an example of this.

In a few infections, predominantly those caused by viruses, the only reliable serologic test is a *neutralization or protection* test, an assay of the protection afforded by the patient's serum against active infection in tissue culture or in experimental animals. This technique is time-consuming and is usually performed only in diagnostic virology laboratories.

Some mention of "nonspecific" serologic changes may serve to emphasize again that clinical laboratory tests have come into use *only because they have been found to correlate reasonably well with clinical findings.* In several diseases, it has been found, often accidentally, that serum antibody develops that will react with antigens derived from sources other than the etiologic agent (which may actually be unknown). Common examples are heterophil agglutinins in infectious mononucleosis, cold agglutinins in mycoplasma pneumonia, and the agglutination of certain strains of *Proteus* bacilli by serum of patients with rickettsial diseases. The Wassermann test for syphilis and related flocculation tests are performed with antigens derived from sources completely unrelated to *Treponema pallidum.*

The results of serologic tests must be interpreted in the light of other information about the patient, including such factors as previous immunizations and illnesses, the possibility of exposure to chemically but etiologically unrelated antigens, and the importance of a changing titer in serial tests as opposed to a single isolated observation.

SKIN TESTS Exposure to antigens of certain types, by various routes, and under circumstances not completely understood often results in the development of immediate (anaphylactic, atopic) hypersensitivity or delayed (bacterial, tuberculin) hypersensitivity.

Active infection with some, but not all, bacteria and viruses results in delayed hypersensitivity to the infecting agent in some, but not all, individuals. Clinically, this allergic state is detected by intradermal injection of the organism or one of its components; in a sensitive individual, induration and erythema will appear at the local site within 24 to 48 hr. If an individual is highly "sensitive" or if the amount of antigen injected is excessive, there may be extensive local inflammation with necrosis, vesicle formation, edema, regional lymphadenopathy, and even malaise and fever. Antigens prepared in concentrations unlikely to provoke severe reactions are generally available for intradermal testing for tuberculosis, leprosy, mumps, lymphogranuloma venereum, cat-scratch disease, chancroid, brucellosis, tularemia, glanders, toxoplasmosis, blastomycosis, histoplasmosis, coccidioidomycosis, and many other infections. The immune reaction to vaccination (Chap. 198) is also an example of delayed dermal hypersensitivity.

The reliability, specificity, and usefulness of the individual tests differ and are discussed in the chapters on specific infections. However, certain general principles apply to their use and interpretation:

1 They are highly useful in epidemiologic surveys as indicators of the incidence of infection in a population.

2 In most individuals, dermal reacticity persists for many years or for life. A single positive test means only that at some past time the individual was infected with the organism (or a closely related one). Unless supplementary information in the form of clinical findings, cultural studies, or more specific serologic data bear out the presence of active infection, a diagnosis of the disease is not justified.

3 The appearance of a positive dermal reaction in an individual known to have been nonreactive a short time before is good evidence of recent infection; this is a useful method for detecting tuberculosis.

4 *A negative intradermal test does not rule out past or present infection.* For unknown reasons, patients with measles, Hodgkin's disease, or sarcoidosis often develop a state of *anergy*, or inability to react to intradermally injected antigens. In several diseases, dermal sensitivity develops after weeks or months of infection; an important example is acute histoplasmosis, in which patients can be ill for many weeks without showing a positive skin test. The skin test to coccidiodin is always negative in disseminated coccidioidomycosis; in far-advanced or miliary tuberculosis in elderly patients, failure to react to intradermal tuberculin in the usual amounts employed for testing occurs in as many as 10 to 15 percent of the cases.

Intradermal injection of antigens derived from sources other than microorganisms usually produces an immediate *wheal and erythema* reaction which subsides promptly. The greatest clinical usefulness of this type of reaction is in the detection of allergy to foreign serums, pollens, and animal dander (Chap. 67). The skin tests for demonstrating infestation with helminths (trichinosis, filariasis) produce reactions of the immediate type in allergic individuals, but many of the antigens employed are so nonspecific that they are of little use in diagnosis.

IMPORTANCE OF SPECIFIC DIAGNOSIS IN INFECTIOUS DISEASES **Medicine and microbiology** The diagnostic procedures employed for infectious diseases are no more absolute than those in other diseases; they cannot be blindly equated with the science of microbiology. The responsibility for interpreting the facts supplied by the bacteriologist, immunologist, and virologist in the total context of a patient's illness remains that of the physician. A positive tuberculin skin test certainly does not indicate that a patient has active tuberculosis. The finding of *Candida albicans* (*Monilia*) in a stool culture does not necessarily mean that a patient's diarrhea is caused by intestinal moniliasis. The presence of staphylococci in nasal cultures from a patient with headaches does not establish a diagnosis of staphylococcal sinusitis. A throat culture containing beta-hemolytic streptococci does not rule out diphtheria, nor does such a culture establish that a febrile illness in a patient with mitral stenosis is a recurrence of acute rheumatic fever rather than bacterial endocarditis. A positive serologic test for syphilis, which measures Wassermann-type antibodies, may be the first sign of incipient lupus erythematosus.

The etiologic agent From a practical point of view, two important steps are vital to the correct diagnosis of infection: (1) The organ(s) or organ systems involved must be found; (2) the etiologic agents causing the infections must be identified precisely. A previous section has dealt with the diagnostic approaches that are available, and the following three chapters describe some important problems in infectious diseases, namely infections that occur in debilitated patients in the hospital, endotoxin shock, and antimicrobial therapy. The remaining chapters take up the specific bacteria, spirochetes, fungi, rickettsias, viruses, mycoplasma, and protozoa which cause infections. The common syndromes caused by these agents are described in the individual chapters. For example, bacterial pneumonia is discussed in detail in the chapter on pneumococcal infections (Chap. 128), osteomyelitis is described with staphylococcal infections (Chap. 129), the manifestations of bacteriuria are described in Chaps. 133 and 273, and those of meningitis in Chaps. 128, 131, and 329. Nevertheless, when confronted with specific organ involvement, it is important to know the most common pathogens which cause disease in the involved organ. Table 122-1 provides a listing of those pathogens. Used in conjunction with the individual chapters dealing with specific agents and the summary of chemotherapy (Chap. 125), the table should provide a rational guide to treatment which often must be instituted before the results of antimicrobial sensitivity tests are available.

Chemotherapy The impact of chemotherapy upon mortality and morbidity from infection and upon epidemic disease is now a matter of record. These therapeutic agents, however, have in no way lessened the importance of specific diagnosis; indeed, their availability has increased the need for obtaining exact etiologic information. It requires but a moment's reflection to realize that the substitution of a prescription for a broad-spectrum antibiotic or a quick injection of penicillin for the systematic collection of facts and thoughtful consideration of diagnostic possibilities is a fallacious, unwise, and dangerous practice. Numerous antibiotics with overlapping spectra are now available, dosages for different

TABLE 122-1
The syndromic approach to infection

	Etiologic agents		
Type of infection	*Common*	*Relatively common*	*Unusual but important*
Skin and subcutaneous tissue	*Staphylococcus aureus*	Group A streptococcus, *candida* and superficial fungi	Gram-negative bacilli (burns, wounds)
Sinusitis	*Staph. aureus*	Group A streptococcus, *Diplococcus pneumoniae*	Mucor
Pharyngitis	Respiratory viruses, Group A streptococcus	Gonococcus	*Corynebacterium diphtheriae*
Epiglottitis	*Hemophilus influenzae*		
Otitis, mastoiditis	*D. pneumoniae, H. influenzae* (children)	*Staph. aureus*, Group A streptococcus	*Pseudomonas, Proteus*
Pneumonitis	*D. pneumoniae, Mycoplasma pneumoniae, Mycobacterium tuberculosis*	*Staph. aureus, Klebsiella*, respiratory viruses	Group A streptococcus, gram-negative enteric bacilli, psittacosis, systemic mycoses, pneumocystis, *H. influenzae, Pasteurella multocida*
Empyema and lung abscess	*Staph. aureus*, anaerobic streptococcus, *Bacteroides*	*Klebsiella* (abscess)	
Bacterial endocarditis	*Streptococcus viridans, Staph. aureus*, enterococcus	*D. pneumoniae*, anaerobic streptococcus	Gram-negative bacilli, *Candida*
Gastroenteritis	*Salmonella, Shigella*	*Staph. aureus, Escherichia coli* (infants), *Clostridia*	*Pseudomonas, Entamoeba histolytica, Vibrio-cholerae, V. parahemolyticus*
Peritonitis, cholangitis, intraabdominal abscess	*E. coli*, enterococcus, *Bacteroides*	*Klebsiella-Enterobacter, Proteus* species, anaerobic streptococcus	*Clostridia, Staph. aureus*
Urinary infection (cystitis, pyelonephritis)	*E. coli, Klebsiella-Enterobacter* paracolon, *Proteus*, enterococcus	*Pseudomonas*	*Staph. aureus*
Urethritis	Gonococcus, ?*Mycoplasma*, ?*Mima-Herellea, Chlamydia*	*Treponema pallidum*	
Pelvic inflammatory disease	Gonococcus, *E. coli*	*Klebsiella-Enterobacter, Bacteroides*, anaerobic streptococcus, enterococcus	*Clostridia, Staph. aureus*
Bones (osteomyelitis)	*Staph. aureus*	*Salmonella*	Group A streptococcus
Joints	*Staph. aureus*, gonococcus, *D. pneumoniae, H. influenzae*	Group A streptococcus, *Neisseria meningitidis*	*E. coli, Proteus, Pseudomonas*
Meninges	*D. pneumoniae, H. influenzae* (children), *N. meningitidis*, echo and mumps viruses	*E. coli, Klebsiella-Enterobacter, Proteus, Pseudomonas*	Group A streptococcus, *M. tuberculosis, Cryptococcus, Staph. aureus, Listeria monocytogenes*

infections vary widely, the drugs themselves are potentially dangerous, and their administration entails considerable expense. They should never be prescribed as placebos, antipyretics, or substitutes for diagnosis. In the vast majority of instances in which this is done, patients recover just as they would if no "therapy" had been given and the drugs are wasted. More importantly, an inadequate dosage of a drug or the wrong agent may suppress symptoms temporarily without achieving cure and may make isolation of the etiologic agent difficult, delay recognition of the true nature of an illness, and postpone the institution of curative treatment. Furthermore, antibiotics may select out resistant variants or facilitate the transfer of R factors between both pathogenic and commensal enterobacteria. Resistant variants can then replace sensitive strains and pose the additional hazard of spread to others. Finally, to expose a patient to the risk of drug reaction without proper indication is inexcusable, whether the drug is an antibiotic, a sedative, a laxative, or a narcotic.

Epidemiologic and other considerations Just as the decision to administer antibiotics to a patient with a febrile illness of presumed infectious etiology must be made on an individual basis, the selection of cases in which extensive cultural and serologic testing is required is a matter of judgment. The majority of common grippe-like illnesses subsides spontaneously, and symptomatic treatment is sufficient. However, because of this tendency toward spontaneous recovery and also because the results of serologic tests may not be available until after recovery has taken place, the effort to determine the specific etiology of illness is often considered an impractical, "academic" procedure. Such an attitude fails to recognize that in addition to the individual patient, the welfare of the community must be considered. For example, a clinical diagnosis of "virus pneumonia" may turn out, following serologic tests, to be psittacosis. Although the "index" patient may have recovered completely, others in the community may be at risk until the "pet parakeet" which was the source of the illness has been eliminated.

Pursuing the diagnosis of obscure, often self-limited, illnesses may be academic, but this approach has led to clarification of some important etiologic relations. For example, the syndrome of infectious mononucleosis has been linked with development of antibody to a herpes-like virus, the EB virus (Chap. 224); some cases of erythema multiforme may be due to herpes simplex virus; several patients with encephalitis have been found to have central nervous system infections with myxoviruses. Some congenital anomalies have been related to prenatal viral infections; most of these relations remain to be clarified. The finding of bacteria-like bodies in the intestinal mucosa of patients with Whipple's disease and the improvement of these patients with tetracycline therapy provides another example of an entity of unknown etiology entering the realm of infectious diseases. Patients with sarcoidosis have been shown to have high titers against herpes-like virus, similar to patients with infectious mononucleosis, Burkitt's lymphoma, and carcinoma of the posterior nasal space. The relation of these viruses to these diseases is not clear; suffice it to say, these associations raise some interesting possibilities concerning the lymphocytic system and virus infections. Along the same vein, the possibility has been raised that the Chédiak-Higashi syndrome, a rare familial disorder characterized by albinism, photophobia, nystagmus, anomalous cellular granules, marked susceptibility to infection, and development of lymphoma, is caused by a virus. This association, among others, relates the field of infection to that of oncogenesis.

These discoveries clearly are the result of academic procedures which might have little immediate applicability to infection in a particular patient; yet few can question their fundamental biologic importance. Moreover, it is conceivable that they will assume practical importance in the future.

REFERENCES

Bennett IL Jr, Beeson PB: Bacteremia: A consideration of some experimental and clinical aspects. Yale J Biol Med 26:241, 1954

Burnet M: *Natural History of Infectious Disease*, New York: Cambridge, 1953

Cluff LE, Johnson JE III: *Clinical Concepts of Infectious Diseases*, Baltimore: Williams & Wilkins, 1972

Davis BD et al: *Microbiology*, New York: Harper & Row, 1968

Dubos RJ: *Biochemical Determinants of Microbial Diseases*, Cambridge: Harvard, 1954

——: *The Evolution of Microbial Diseases: Bacterial and Mycotic Diseases of Man*, 4th ed., Philadelphia: Lippincott, 1965, p. 20

Hirshaut Y et al: Sarcoidosis, another disease associated with serologic evidence for herpes-like virus infection. N Engl J Med 283:502, 1970

Horsfall FL Jr: Cancer and viruses. Bull NY Acad Med 42:167, 1966

——, Tamm I: *Viral and Rickettsial Diseases of Man*, 4th ed., Philadelphia: Lippincott, 1965

MacLeod CM, Cluff LE: Symposium on non-specific resistance to infection. Bacteriol Rev 24:1, 1960

Matula G, Paterson P: Spontaneous in vitro reduction of nitroblue tetrazolium by neutrophils of adult patients with bacterial infection. N Engl J Med 285:311, 1971

White JG: Virus-like particles in the peripheral blood cells of two patients with Chédiak-Higashi syndrome. Cancer 19:877, 1966

Wilson GA, Miles AA: *Topley and Wilson's Principles of Bacteriology and Immunity*, 5th ed., Baltimore: Williams & Wilkens, 1965

Wood WB Jr: Studies on the cellular immunology of acute bacterial infections. Harvey Lect 47:72, 1951-1952

123 NOSOCOMIAL INFECTIONS

ROBERT G. PETERSDORF

DEFINITION A nosocomial infection is an infection occurring during hospitalization, usually in a patient with a defect in host resistance.

EPIDEMIOLOGY Hospital-acquired infections occur in approximately 5 percent of all patients admitted to a general hospital. The prevalence of hospital infection is approximately 12 percent in large tertiary-care hospitals and 6 percent in community hospitals, and the incidence figures are 6 percent and 3.5 percent, respectively. In numeric terms, there are approximately 1.5 million hospital infections in the United States annually. The most common nosocomial infections encountered are urinary tract infections (40 percent), surgical wound infections (25 percent), respiratory infections (15 percent), and infections in skin and subcutaneous tissues, septic thrombophlebitis, and bacteremia.

PREDISPOSING FACTORS Defects in host resistance Certain infections occur with increased frequency with particular diseases. For example, patients with diabetes mellitus are prone to development of cutaneous infections, bacteriuria, tuberculosis, moniliasis, and, when ketoacidosis is uncontrolled, mucormycosis. Patients with hypoparathyroidism have a predilection for *Candida* (formerly *Monilia*) infections; nocardiosis is more common in alveolar proteinosis; *Salmonella* infections are more prevalent in patients with sickle-cell disease, schistosomiasis, malaria, and bartonellosis; pneumococcal infections occur often in very young children who have undergone splenectomy, in individuals with hypogammaglobulinemia, and in association with multiple myeloma; cryptococcosis tends to infect patients with Hodgkin's disease and sarcoidosis; and a variety of bacterial infections complicate illnesses associated with granulocytopenia. The reasons for the coexistence of these infections and the underlying diseases are largely unknown. In a sense, however, these associations represent peculiar experiments of nature and are overshadowed by infections resulting from the iatrogenic alterations in host resistance that follow the use of *corticosteroids, antimetabolites*, and *radiomimetic, immunosuppressive*, and *antimicrobial drugs*. Chronic therapy with corticosteroids not only favors acquisition of new infections but may result in reactivation and dissemination of latent disease. Why these hormones increase susceptibility to infection is unknown; perhaps they depress the reticuloendothelial system, impair the development of immunity by decreasing antibody formation, and suppress other host-defense mechanisms. Usually steroids produce infections in patients with those underlying diseases for which they were given, but because of their anti-inflammatory effects, the hormones may mask the signs and symptoms of the complicating infections until they are relatively far advanced. The increased incidence of infection following cytotoxic drugs is probably a consequence of these agents' ability to produce granulocytopenia and lymphopenia and to decrease antibody production.

Superinfections Superinfections may be defined as infections which occur while a course of antimicrobial therapy is administered for either therapeutic or prophylactic purposes. They are seen in approximately 2 percent of all patients treated with antibiotics, and are more common when antimicrobials are given in large doses, when several antimicrobials are administered concurrently, or when broad-spectrum agents are employed.

Clinical superinfections must be distinguished from the normal ecologic change in bacterial flora which accompanies all antimicrobial therapy. Most antibiotics lower the number of resident microorganisms and occasionally eradicate them entirely; the normal flora is then replaced by resistant exogenous or more commonly endogenous bacteria. In the vast majority of instances the number of bacteria replacing those eradicated by the drug is small, and clinical disease does not take place. However, when the concentration of the superinfecting organisms is high, and anatomic conditions are favorable, clinical superinfection is likely to occur.

Superinfections are particularly common following administration of certain drugs; the tendency for *Pseudomonas* to colonize and infect patients receiving one of the cephalosporins is a notable example. Clinically significant superinfections usually appear 4 to 5 days after chemotherapy is instituted and must be watched for, especially in patients being treated for pneumonia, chronic obstructive lung disease, otitis, and urinary tract infection, or when a urethral catheter is in place. They often complicate the course of patients with respiratory viral diseases, particularly influenza, who are given antibiotics to prevent bacterial complications. As a rule, superinfections are caused by organisms that are resistant to the drug the patient is receiving; penicillinase-producing staphylococci were until recently the most common offenders, but gram-negative enteric bacilli and fungi are now the most common superinfecting microorganisms. The usual clinical manifestations include recrudescence of fever and other signs and symptoms at the site of the initial infection.

Other diagnostic and therapeutic measures resulting in infections The hospitalized patient is subjected to a variety of diagnostic and therapeutic procedures which predispose to infection. These include insertion of intravenous catheters and urethral catheterization, particularly if an indwelling catheter is left in place; less commonly, injections, thoracenteses, paracenteses, aspiration of joints, lumbar punctures, and tissue biopsies may be incriminated. At least 2 to 3 percent of operative procedures are complicated by infections; the rates vary with the type of operation. Large surgical wounds associated with prolonged operative procedures are the most likely to become infected. Infections are common in association with the use of equipment for inhalation therapy, and may be spread in the hospital by a variety of inanimate vehicles. The risk of a complicating infection depends on the underlying disease as well as on the number and complexity of therapeutic or diagnostic manipulations, and is enhanced by the concomitant indiscriminate use of antibiotics.

ETIOLOGY The bacteria most commonly responsible for complicating infections are *Escherichia coli, Klebsiella-enterobacter,* and *Proteus* sp. (Chap. 133), *Pseudomonas* and *Mima-Herellea* (Chap. 134), *Serratia* (Chap. 133), and less commonly penicillinase-producing staphylococci (Chap. 129), group D streptococci, enterococci (Chap. 130) and *Clostridia* (Chap. 154). Among the fungi, *Candida* (*Monilia*) (Chap. 171), *Mucor* (Chap. 172), *Nocardia* (Chap. 173), and *Aspergillus* (Chap. 174) are frequent pathogens implicated in secondary infections. Cytomegalovirus (Chap. 206), disseminated herpes zoster (Chap. 194), and pneumocystis (Chap. 214) are common causes of complicating infections in patients with depressed host resistance.

MANIFESTATIONS The clinical picture of a complicating infection will vary with its site and, to a lesser extent, the microorganisms causing it. In most instances, the major sign is fever, which usually occurs after patients have been in the hospital 4 to 5 days or longer. However, in some patients the diagnosis rests only on signs of local inflammation such as phlebitis, cellulitis, or evidence of a deep-seated infection. Sometimes a complicating infection may be heralded by no more than unexplained hyperventilation, confusion, or disorientation. Specific types of infection are considered below.

Postoperative infections These consist primarily of wound infections or collections of pus which form in and around the operative site. Although urinary tract infections and pneumonia are common in patients who have undergone surgery, postoperative infections are usually related to the surgical locus rather than an unrelated site. The majority of wound infections are caused by only a relatively few surgical procedures; these infections are particularly likely to occur when operations are long or require extensive resection and when contamination is unavoidable. Abdominal perineal resections, wounds involving arterial bypass grafts, insertion of cardiac protheses, and portacaval shunts are associated with a relatively high rate of complicating infections. Most postoperative wound infections are caused by staphylococci and gram-negative enteric bacteria. Although group A streptococcal infections are averted with most chemoprophylactic regimens, wound infections which develop in patients receiving postoperative chemoprophylaxis usually are caused by organisms resistant to the drug being given. In general, chemoprophylaxis has not been successful in preventing wound infections, although one regimen which involves the administration of 10 million units of penicillin G at 2-hr intervals, beginning immediately prior to and continuing throughout the operation, has been shown to reduce postoperative wound sepsis.

Cutaneous, subcutaneous, and soft-tissue infections While wound sepsis constitutes the major part of superficial infections, other sites are involved. These include abscesses in the skin, subcutaneous tissues and muscle, cellulitis, decubitus ulcers, vascular stasis ulcers, and lesions secondary to diminished arterial blood supply. Most often staphylococci are the causative organisms, but group A and anaerobic streptococci, gram-negative enteric bacilli, and even clostridia may be pathogenic under these circumstances. These infections may follow subcutaneous or intramuscular injections or extravasation of intravenous infusions. Soft tissue infections involving the perineal and perianal areas are common in acute leukemias. Although the infections usually remain localized, they may involve contiguous structures and may produce bacteremia. Gas in soft tissues should call to mind infection with *E. coli* as well as anerobic organisms. Antimicrobial therapy should be directed at the specific organism. Staphylococcal infections should be treated with penicillinase-resistant penicillin unless the organism is shown to be sensitive to penicillin G. Surgical drainage and debridement are often essential to recovery.

Burns regularly become infected secondarily. Most of these patients are receiving systemic or local chemoprophylaxis, and usually infection develops after the gram-positive flora has been replaced by gram-negative organisms, particularly *Pseudomonas.* These organisms are usually acquired from the environment and have been shown to survive on the floors, walls, and equipment used in burn wards. The sudden development of shock in a patient with a burn is almost certain evidence that *Pseudomonas* bacteremia is present. Treatment is discussed in Chaps. 124 and 134.

Urinary tract infections Urinary tract infections usually are associated with instrumentation of the urethra, bladder, or ureters and most often are due to insertion of an indwelling urethral catheter which permits entry of bacteria from the external environment to the bladder. Nosocomial urinary infections do not occur without predisposing instrumentation. The organisms are usually *E. coli, Klebsiella-enterobacter, Serratia, Proteus, Pseudomonas,* and enterococci and tend to be resistant to one or several antibiotics. Epidemics of *Klebsiella-enterobacter* and *Pseudomonas* urinary infections following spread of bacteria from contaminated equipment have been reported. Most patients with hospital-acquired bacteriuria are asymptomatic, some have cystitis, and others have clear-cut evidence of pyelonephritis which may be associated with bacteremia. Treatment should be reserved for patients with symptoms and for those suspected of bacteremia. Patients with indwelling catheters who have asymptomatic bacteriuria should not receive antibiotics because it is unlikely that the organisms will be eradicated; instead, superinfections will develop.

Considerable progress has been made in preventing hospital-acquired urinary infections by maintaining a system of closed drainage. In this fashion, the urine can be kept sterile for 5 to 7 days after insertion of the catheter. Failure to maintain closed drainage will result in infection in almost all patients within 48 hr after catheter drainage is instituted.

Pneumonia Pulmonary infections are common in hospitalized patients with a variety of severe medical or surgical diseases. They may follow aspiration from any cause, atelectasis, heart failure, tracheostomy, and therapy with drugs that depress respiration. In a general hospital, pneumonia occurs commonly as a complication of cardiac or neurosurgery, but these infections are also seen in debilitated general medical patients, particularly when respiratory assistance devices have been employed. Mainstream reservoir nebulizers containing saline solutions are often heavily contaminated with *Pseudomonas*, flavobacteria, *Herellea*, and *Achromobacter* and are capable of producing severe pulmonary infections when nebulized directly into the tracheobronchial tree. This risk can be reduced sharply by bubbling a 0.25% acetic acid solution through the nebulizing equipment for 5 min prior to use. Gram-negative enteric bacteria usually are implicated in complicating pulmonary infections, particularly when patients have received antimicrobials. Although tracheostomies are sometimes necessary to maintain adequate ventilation, they are almost invariably associated with infections. Pulmonary infections are less common in association with tracheal intubation, which is preferable to tracheostomy. However, when tracheostomy is necessary, infection can be prevented only by meticulous aseptic technique during suctioning and the use of sterile suction catheters. The major therapeutic problem in many patients with complicating infections of the lung is mechanical; positive pressure breathing, postural drainage, frequent suctioning, and sometimes bronchoscopy are at least as important in the treatment of these infections as appropriate antibiotics.

Bacterial endocarditis Patients undergoing open-heart surgery have a relatively high incidence of wound, urinary, and pulmonary infections, but the most dreaded complication of open-heart surgery is endocarditis on a prosthetic valve. It occurs predominantly in patients whose operation is conducted on cardiopulmonary bypass, and surgery on the aortic valve is complicated by endocarditis much more frequently than surgery on the mitral valve. *Staphylococcus aureus* and *S. albus* are the most common pathogens. Clinical signs of endocarditis are often absent, and fever during the first four postoperative weeks provides the best clue to infections which follow in the wake of surgery. However, in some instances the prosthetic valve becomes infected years after its insertion, emphasizing the importance of preventing bacteremia in these patients. The prophylactic regimens for preventing endocarditis are detailed in Chap. 127. The diagnosis depends upon isolation of the organism from blood cultures. Treatment of endocarditis on intracardiac prostheses has been notoriously unsuccessful, and although the infection may be suppressed with antibiotics, reoperation, which often has a fatal outcome, is usually necessary. Therefore, to prevent endocarditis, antimicrobial administration to patients undergoing open-heart surgery has become routine practice. It is clear that administration of a penicillinase-resistant penicillin or a cephalosporin will prevent postoperative pneumococcal endocarditis, but the efficacy of these drugs in preventing endocarditis with other organisms, including staphylococci, is less certain. Bacterial endocarditis, usually with organisms found in the skin, is a rare but well-documented complication of chronic hemodialysis.

Bacteremia Invasion of the bloodstream can occur in any nosocomial infection, and among the various foci, the urinary tract predominates. However, the *indwelling venous catheter* is fast becoming the most common source of bacteremia in hospitalized patients, particularly when it is left in place longer than 48 hr. Many of these patients develop phlebitis before bacteremia, and the catheter should be removed from all patients with inflammation at the catheter site. Staphylococci are implicated most often in catheter-associated infections, but *Mima-Herellea* and other gram-negative organisms have been cultured from both the local site and the bloodstream.

Treatment of catheter-induced bacteremia requires removal of the catheter and systemic antimicrobial therapy; the treatment of staphylococcal bacteremia is discussed in Chap. 129 and that of gram-negative sepsis in Chap. 124. These infections can be prevented by (1) use of the catheter only when absolutely necessary; (2) strict aseptic technique during placement of the catheter; (3) application of bacitracin-neomycin-polymyxin ointment at the catheter site; and (4) removal of the catheter within 48 hr, or sooner if phlebitis or cellulitis is present.

Patients receiving parenteral *hyperalimentation* appear to be at particular risk for developing *Candida* septicemia. The reason for this complication is not clear, but prolonged intravenous catheterization is probably the most important factor in the pathogenesis of this syndrome.

A number of cases of bacteremia emanating from *intravenous infusion* sets have been reported. Usually contamination occurs after the set has been placed into use, and the screw cap appears to be the most vulnerable site for introducing exogenous bacteria. The organisms that have been incriminated in clinical bacteremia usually have been *Escherichia* or *Klebsiella-enterobacter*, but in addition to these, other gram-negative enteric organisms, staphylococci, and corynebacteria have been cultured from infusion sets. In most instances, contamination could be traced to faulty technique involved in changing bottles, adding medications, adjusting air filters, etc., and attention to the details of handling these materials by *all hospital personnel* is essential if this complication is to be prevented. Finally, the storage of blood products at room temperature has also been implicated in bacteremia. *Enterobacter* sepsis was induced in several patients transfused with pooled platelets, and a significant number of other bacteria including staphylococci, streptococci, *Sarcina*, *Herellea*, *Pseudomonas*, and flavobacter have been recovered from packed pooled platelets.

Miscellaneous nosocomial infections *Staphylococcal parotitis* is common in debilitated patients with a variety of medical diseases; it often follows in the wake of dehydration. *Septic arthritis* is not uncommon in patients with antecedent rheumatoid or degenerative joint disease who are subjected to diagnostic aspiration of the joint or who are treated with intraarticular drugs, usually corticosteroids. Pneumococcus, group A streptococcus, and staphylococcus are the most common pathogens. Septic arthritis of the sternoclavicular joint has also been described following placement of an intravenous catheter into the subclavian vein. *Iatrogenic meningitis* is a rare complication of spinal anesthesia, epidural block, injection of the stellate ganglion, diagnostic lumbar puncture, and myelography. Pneumococcus, staphylococcus, and

Pseudomonas have been cultured from these patients. *Staphylococcal enterocolitis* occurs primarily in patients who have had gastrointestinal surgery who were given antibiotics preoperatively. It is also common in patients with liver disease who are treated with neomycin to reduce ammonia production by the bowel flora. Oral vancomycin (0.5 g every 6 to 12 hr for four doses), systemic penicillinase-resistant penicillins, or cephalosporins are all effective modes of treatment.

Infections occurring during organ transplantation Aside from host-versus-graft reactions (Chap. 66), infections pose the most serious threat to patients undergoing organ transplantation. These patients all receive immunosuppressive drugs and large quantities of adrenal cortical hormones and have readily available portals of entry for a variety of microorganisms. Multiple infections are common. Coagulase-positive staphylococci, *Pseudomonas,* gram-negative enteric bacilli, and enteric (non–Group A) streptococci are the usual offending bacteria. These organisms are often present in the nasopharynx or on the skin of patients prior to transplantation, and for this reason it is recommended by some authorities that all staphylococcal carriers be treated with a penicillinase-resistant penicillin for several days prior to the procedure and afterward until the wound has healed. Likewise, bacteriuria should be eradicated before surgery. When transplantation is performed for pyelonephritis, the ureters should be excised in their entirety along with kidneys.

Patients who have undergone transplantation are particularly susceptible to fatal pulmonary infections which may produce few symptoms and signs. In addition to the bacteria mentioned above, cytomegalovirus, *Candida, Aspergillus,* and *Pneumocystis* are found at autopsy. These infections are characterized by little in the way of an inflammatory response, and the fungi, in particular, tend to produce a necrotizing reaction. Although no definitive information is available, it is likely that pulmonary superinfections with fungi or cytomegalovirus in these patients have an almost uniformly fatal prognosis.

LABORATORY FINDINGS Cultures of pus, appropriate body fluids, and blood form the cornerstone of treatment and always should be obtained even in patients receiving chemotherapy. Antimicrobial sensitivity tests should be performed when indicated. Gram stains of pus or secretions are helpful when only one or two types of bacteria are present in large numbers, but may be misleading and should be interpreted with caution. Superinfections usually are accompanied by leukocytosis, but granulocytopenia may be seen because of previous drug therapy or underlying disease. Moreover, many patients have a leukocytosis to begin with, and an elevated leukocyte count is of value as a clue to a complicating infection only if it was normal previously.

THERAPEUTIC CONSIDERATIONS Because most nosocomial infections are caused by bacteria, treatment depends upon identification of the organism but must not be delayed until the results of cultures and sensitivity tests are at hand. Hence, the antibiotic must be chosen on the basis of previous cultures, the gram-stained smear, and the clinical picture. For example, patients with subcutaneous and soft-tissue infections should be treated with a penicillinase-resistant penicillin and those with bacteriuria with a drug active against enteric bacteria or enterococci. Patients with pneumonia or sepsis may require treatment with several drugs pending identification of the pathogen. The appropriate regimens are found in chapters dealing with the specific organisms and in the chapter on chemotherapy (Chap. 125). A general approach to therapy of undiagnosed bacteremia is provided in Chap. 124. Removal of the mechanical factors which are often the basis for complicating infections is as important as chemotherapy. This may involve withdrawing intravenous or urethral catheters, drainage of pus, debridement of a burn eschar, removal of sutures, aspiration of bronchial secretions, a change in inhalation equipment, and even, occasionally, removal of a cardiac prothesis.

PREVENTION A number of steps can be taken to diminish the prevalence of hospital infections, and to eliminate some altogether. These include the following:

Surveillance Many hospitals have found a full-time or part-time nurse-epidemiologist useful in monitoring the prevalence of hospital infections, their relation to antibiotic usage, the location of infection, etc. In addition to providing early clues about the presence of infections, the epidemiologist can maintain a high index of awareness among hospital personnel, and perhaps indirectly reduce the prevalence of infection.

Isolation of infected patients Patients with untreated staphylococcal wound or pulmonary infections, pulmonary tuberculosis, and hepatitis should be isolated. However, it is important not to maintain isolation after it is no longer required. Too rigid adherence to isolation procedures may interfere with essential patient care.

Control of personnel Hospital personnel with purulent draining lesions should be removed from patient contact, but those with minor infections should not. Routine screening of hospital personnel for carriage of staphylococci is not useful. It is important to maintain the immune status of hospital workers against smallpox, poliomyelitis, diphtheria, and tetanus. Early detection of tuberculosis is essential, and periodic chest x-rays and tuberculin skin tests need to be encouraged. Tuberculosis poses a serious hazard to hospital workers as well as patient contacts. Likewise, hospital personnel must guard closely against infection with hepatitis B virus; dialysis units and blood processing areas pose particular risks.

Control of the environment Needless to say, cleanliness should be the hallmark of every hospital. Particular care needs to be observed in certain patient care areas in which the prevalence of nosocomial infections is high—nurseries, operating rooms, and intensive care units. All these must have ample facilities for hand-washing, and hand-washing must be enforced rigidly. Routine sampling of air or fomites in patient care areas is wasteful, although this procedure is useful for spot-testing air nebulizers, fluids for soaking surgical instruments, and ethylene oxide sterilizers, and for monitoring potential common source outbreaks of infection.

Control of patient care procedures Indwelling intravenous and urethral catheters, respiratory assistance devices, and intravenous infusion sets are probably the four procedures that are employed in all patients at risk of developing nosocomial infections. In them the appropriate measures for preventing these infections described above are absolutely essential.

Antimicrobial prophylaxis While prophylactic antibiotics have been useful when aimed at a single organism such as the group A streptococcus to prevent rheumatic fever, the meningococcus, and occasionally other pathogens, nosocomial infections are usually caused by one or more of several strains, species, and genera of microorganisms. In this situation, the attempt to place an "antibiotic umbrella" over the infection-prone patient has been futile; in fact, the use of antibiotics prophylactically has generally resulted in superinfection with endogenous or exogenous organisms resistant to the drug being administered.

PROGNOSIS Most nosocomial infections occur in patients being treated for another disease which is often chronic, disabling, and potentially fatal. While these secondary infections demand vigorous treatment, they may be only incidental to the patient's primary problem. For example, a patient with disseminated carcinomatosis will die even if his complicating infection is contained; and conversely a complicating infection often will not respond to therapy unless a remission is produced in the underlying disease. However, in many instances, nosocomial infections could have been prevented by more attention to meticulous technique or by greater restraint in the use of manipulative procedures, antibiotics, and other potent drugs.

REFERENCES

BENTLEY DW, LEPPER MH: Septicemia related to indwelling venous catheter. JAMA 206:1749, 1968

BUCHHOLZ DH et al: Bacterial proliferation in platelet products stored at room temperature. N Engl J Med 285:429, 1971

CURRY CR, QUIE PG: Fungal septicemia in patients receiving parenteral hyperalimentation. N Engl J Med 285:1221, 1971

DUMA RJ et al: Septicemia from intravenous infusions. N Engl J Med 284:257, 1971

EICKHOFF TC: Hospital infections. Disease-a-Month Sept, 1972

—— et al: Current problems and approaches to diagnosis of infection in renal transplant recipients. Transplant Proc 4:693, 1972

FEINGOLD DS: Hospital-acquired infections. N Engl J Med 283:1384, 1970

MOSER RH: *Diseases of Medical Progress*, Springfield, Ill.: Charles C Thomas, 1969

REINARZ JA et al: Potential role of inhalation therapy equipment in nosocomial pulmonary infection. J Clin Invest 44:831, 1965

RIFKIND D et al: Infectious diseases associated with renal homotransplantation. JAMA 189:397, 1964

THOBURN R et al: Infections acquired by hospitalized patients. Arch Intern Med 121:1, 1968

THORNTON GF, ANDRIOLE VT: Bacteriuria during indwelling catheter drainage: II. Effect of a closed sterile drainage system. JAMA 214:339, 1970

TILLOTSON JR, FINLAND M: Bacterial colonization and clinical superinfections of the respiratory tract complicating antibiotic treatment of pneumonia. J Infect Dis 119:597, 1969

124 SEPTIC SHOCK

ROBERT G. PETERSDORF

DEFINITION Septic shock is characterized by inadequate tissue perfusion, usually following bacteremia with gram-negative enteric bacilli. This circulatory insufficiency is a consequence of increased peripheral vascular resistance, pooling of blood in the microcirculation, diminished cardiac output, and tissue anoxia.

ETIOLOGY Shock is sometimes associated with gram-positive infections, but in them there is usually hypotension, low peripheral resistance, peripheral vasodilatation, normovolemia, and normal cardiac output—so-called warm shock—which is readily corrected with fluids and appropriate antibiotics. For practical purposes, septic shock follows bacteremia with gram-negative bacilli: the *Enterobacteriaceae* (Chap. 133) and *Pseudomonas* and related organisms (Chaps. 134 and 146). Furthermore, the vasoactive phenomena collectively termed *septic shock* are probably not only due to the gram-negative bacteremia but are primarily related to release into the circulation of endotoxin, the lipopolysaccharide moiety of the organisms' cell walls.

EPIDEMIOLOGY Gram-negative bacteremia and septic shock occur primarily in hospitalized patients who usually have an underlying disease which renders them susceptible to bloodstream invasion. Predisposing factors include diabetes mellitus; cirrhosis; leukemia, lymphoma, or disseminated carcinoma; transplantation and its associated immunosuppression; childbirth; a variety of surgical procedures and antecedent infections in the urinary, biliary, or gastrointestinal tracts. Most adults with gram-negative sepsis are elderly males, but neonates and child-bearing women are also prone to develop this syndrome. There has been an appreciable increase in the prevalence of serious gram-negative infections among hospitalized patients since 1935. For example, in 1958, the diagnosis of gram-negative sepsis was 0.8 per 1,000 hospital admissions; in 1968, this had risen to 8.0 per 1,000, and in one recent series it was 10 per 1,000. In addition to the predisposing factors mentioned above, the widespread use of antibiotics, immunosuppressive and cytotoxic agents, adrenal steroids, intravenous catheters, humidifiers, and other hospital equipment (Chap. 123), and the increasing longevity of patients with chronic diseases, has given momentum to this upward trend.

PATHOGENESIS AND PATHOLOGY With the exception of *Pseudomonas* and *Mima-Herellea,* which are ubiquitous in the hospital environment, most of the bacteria causing gram-negative sepsis are normal commensals in the gastrointestinal tract. From there they may spread to contiguous structures as in peritonitis following appendiceal perforation, or migrate from the perineum into the urethra or bladder. Gram-negative bacteremia follows infection in a primary focus, usually the genitourinary tract, biliary tree, gastrointestinal tract and adjoining structures or lungs, and, less commonly, the skin, bones, and joints. In patients with leukemia, the skin and subcutaneous tissues are often a portal of entry, as is also the case in burn patients. In many instances, however, notably in patients with debilitating diseases, cirrhosis, and cancer, no primary focus is apparent. When bacteremia is followed by metastatic lesions in distant sites, classic abscess formation occurs. More often, however, the autopsy findings in gram-negative sepsis are scanty or nonspecific and reflect primarily the infection at the primary locus. This lack of concrete morphologic data has led some investigators to question the role of endotoxin in gram-negative shock in man. On the other hand, damage to the endothelial lining of capillary walls has been demonstrated early in experimental endotoxin shock, and many patients who die with gram-negative shock have been treated intensively. This treatment tends to obfuscate the pathologic findings which are often clear-cut in experimental animals.

PATHOPHYSIOLOGY General considerations Endotoxin exerts its major effects on small blood vessels with sympathetic (alpha-receptor) innervation. The toxin causes intense arteriolar and venospasm leading to significant immobilization of blood in the pulmonary, splanchnic, and renal capillaries, and to stagnant anoxia in these tissues. Local acidosis develops and promotes relaxation of the arteriolar sphincters while the venules remain constricted. Blood pools in the capillary bed, and the increased hydrostatic pressure, results in leakage of plasma into the interstitial fluid. This, in turn, results in a sharp decrease in effective circulating blood volume, lowered cardiac output and systemic arterial hypotension, which stimulates the baroreceptors and results in further sympathetic activity, vasoconstriction, and selective reduction of blood flow to visceral organs and skin. If ineffective perfusion of vital organs is permitted to continue, metabolic acidosis and severe parenchymal damage ensue, and shock is then irreversible. In man, the kidneys and lungs are the organs particularly susceptible to endotoxin; oliguria as well as tachypnea and, in some instances, pulmonary edema develop early. On the other hand, the heart and brain are spared early in shock, and myocardial failure and coma are late and often terminal manifestations of the shock syndrome. There is also experimental evidence that, following the administration of live gram-negative bacteria, significant arteriovenous shunting occurs around the capillary beds of susceptible organs. This intensifies tissue anoxia. These findings suggest that septic shock is a consequence both of the presence of bacteria as well as endotoxin. Other experiments have shown that endotoxin must be activated by components of plasma, including but not only complement, in order to exert its pathophysiologic effects.

Hemodynamic alterations in man Many of the observations dealing with the pathophysiology of endotoxin shock were made in animals, and the hemodynamic data often varied according to the species studied and the dose of endotoxin administered. The establishment of centers for the study of shock has permitted detailed pathophysiologic studies in man. The results of these studies may vary with the time at which they are performed. For example, early in septic shock, the picture is one primarily of vasodilatation with an increase in cardiac output, a decrease in systemic vascular resistance, a decrease in central venous pressure, and an increase in stroke volume. In contrast, later in septic shock, the predominant picture is one of vasoconstriction with an increase in systemic vascular resistance, a decrease in cardiac output, a decrease in central venous pressure, and a decrease in stroke volume. Despite these differences, certain patterns of septic shock have emerged when large groups of patients have been studied. These may be summarized as follows:

1 Shock characterized by a normal cardiac output, normal blood volume, normal circulation time, normal or high central venous pressure, normal or high pH, and *reduced* peripheral resistance. These patients have warm, dry skin. Their prognosis is generally good. Hypotension, oliguria, and lactic acidemia are present. Shock in this group has been attributed to shunting of blood through arteriovenous communications, making it unavailable for perfusion of vital organs.

2 Shock characterized by normal blood volume, high central venous pressure, normal or high cardiac output, reduced peripheral resistance but *marked metabolic acidosis*, oliguria, and very high blood lactate indicating ineffective tissue perfusion or impaired oxygen utilization. Despite the presence of warm, dry extremities in these patients, the prognosis is extremely poor.

3 Patients with low blood volume, low central venous pressure, high hematocrit, increased peripheral resistance, low cardiac output, hypotension, oliguria, but only a moderate elevation of blood lactate and normal or slightly high pH. These patients may be hypovolemic prior to bacteremia, and their prognosis is reasonably good provided blood volume is restored, bacteremia is treated with appropriate antibiotics, septic foci are removed or drained, and vasoactive drugs are given.

4 Shock characterized by low blood volume, low central venous pressure, low cardiac output, marked decompensated metabolic acidosis, and lactic acidemia. In these patients the extremities are cool and cyanotic. The prognosis is very poor.

Although these observations suggest that there are various forms of septic shock, for the most part the data are consistent with the hypothesis that the most common abnormality in endotoxin shock is *vasoconstriction, reduction in cardiac output, hypotension,* and *oliguria.* Low peripheral resistance and normal or high cardiac output can generally be ascribed to arteriovenous shunts that occur in cirrhosis or in the inflamed peritoneum or lung and prevent perfusion and oxygenation of vital organs. Therefore even the seemingly high cardiac output is insufficient to meet the needs of the body because arteriovenous shunting precludes oxygen utilization at the cellular level.

Coagulation defects in shock In most patients with septic shock there is a deficiency in several clotting factors, due to consumption of these factors, a syndrome termed *disseminated intravascular coagulation.* The pathogenesis of this syndrome is complicated and probably involves the vasoactive peptide system as follows: endotoxin leads to activation of factor XII (Hageman factor), which in turn leads to activation of kallikrein from its inactive precursors. Kallikrein then activates bradykinin, a potent local vasodilator which promotes the pooling of blood in peripheral tissues as well as increased capillary permeability and localized tissue damage. In addition, endotoxin per se, by a mechanism analogous to the generalized Shwartzman reaction, produces fibrin thrombi in capillaries, and these form the nidus of the fibrin-platelet aggregates which are typical of disseminated intravascular coagulation (DIC), which is characterized by a decrease in factors II, V, and VIII, fibrinogen, and platelets. There may be some degree of fibrinolysis, with appearance of split products (positive Fi test). These clotting abnormalities are present to some degree in most patients with septic shock, but usually there is no clinical bleeding, although hemorrhagic phenomena due to thrombocytopenia or deficiency in clotting factors occur occasionally. A more important effect of disseminated intravascular coagulation is development of capillary thrombi, particularly in the lung. Unless there is bleeding, the coagulopathy requires no therapy and disappears spontaneously as shock is treated.

The lung in septic shock Respiratory failure is the most important cause of death in patients with shock, particularly after the hemodynamic aberrations have been corrected. The respiratory lesion has been called the "shock lung" and is characterized by pulmonary congestion, hemorrhage, atelectasis, edema, and formation of capillary thrombi. This lesion may develop and progress even as other abnormalities return to normal. Pulmonary surfactant decreases, and pulmonary compliance becomes progressively compromised.

Renal failure Oliguria occurs early in shock and is probably due to inadequate renal perfusion. If renal perfusion remains inadequate, acute renal failure, which is characterized by cloudy swelling of renal tubules, develops. In an occasional patient, renal cortical necrosis, as occurs in the generalized Shwartzman reaction, is seen.

CLINICAL MANIFESTATIONS Usually gram-negative bacteremia begins abruptly with chills, fever, nausea, vomiting, diarrhea, and prostration. When septic shock develops, there are, in addition, tachycardia, tachypnea; hypotension; cool, pale extremities, often with peripheral cyanosis; mental obtundation, and oliguria. When present in its full-blown form, gram-negative shock is detected readily, but occasionally the findings are quite subtle, particularly in old, debilitated patients or in infants. Unexplained hypotension, increasing confusion, and disorientation or hyperventilation may be the only clues to gram-negative shock. Some patients are hypothermic, and in the absence of fever the diagnosis is often missed. Jaundice occurs occasionally and signifies infection in the biliary tree, intravascular hemolysis, or "toxic" hepatitis. As shock progresses, oliguria persists, and heart failure, respiratory insufficiency, and coma supervene. Death usually occurs from pulmonary edema, generalized anoxemia secondary to respiratory insufficiency, cardiac arrythmias, disseminated intravascular coagulation with bleeding, cerebral anoxia, or a combination of these factors.

LABORATORY FINDINGS The laboratory data in septic shock vary greatly and depend in many instances on the cause of the shock syndrome and on the stage of shock. The volume of packed red cells is often elevated and falls to below normal as the volume deficit is repaired. There usually is *leukocytosis* between 15,000 and 30,000 per mm^3 with a shift to the left. However, the white blood cell count may be normal, and some patients have leukopenia. The *platelet count* is usually decreased, and the prothrombin consumption and partial thromboplastin times may be abnormal, reflecting a deficiency of *clotting factors.*

The *urinalysis* shows no specific abnormalities. Initially, the specific gravity is high; as oliguria persists, isosthenuria develops. The *blood urea nitrogen* and *creatinine* are elevated, and creatinine clearance is reduced.

Simultaneous measurements of urine and plasma osmolalities are a useful clue to impending renal failure. If the urinary osmolality is greater than 400 mOsm and the ratio of urine to plasma osmolality is greater than 1.5, renal function is preserved and oliguria is probably due to volume depletion. On the other hand, a urine osmolality of less than 400 and a urine/plasma ratio less than 1.5 signify renal failure. Electrolyte patterns vary considerably, but there is a tendency to *hyponatremia* and hypochloremia. The serum potassium may be high, low, or normal. The *bicarbonate concentration* is usually low and *blood lactate* is elevated.

Early in endotoxin shock there is *respiratory alkalosis* manifested by a low P_{CO_2} and high arterial pH, probably an attempt to blow off CO_2 to compensate for developing lactic acidemia and because of progressive anoxemia. As shock progresses, *metabolic acidosis* develops. There often is striking *anoxemia,* and P_{O_2} values below 70 mm Hg are common. Hemodynamic measurements usually show a low *central venous pressure,* low *pulmonary artery and wedge pressures, low cardiac output* and cardiac index, high *peripheral resistance,* and slow circulation time. Occasionally cardiac output is hypernormal, and systemic vascular resistance low. *Blood volume* is usually low, but this determination is notoriously unreliable in septic shock and should not be trusted. The *electrocardiogram* generally shows depression of the S-T segment, inversion of the T waves, and a variety of arrhythmias, and may mistakenly suggest the diagnosis of myocardial infarction.

In untreated gram-negative shock, the blood cultures should reveal the causative pathogens, but bacteremia is often intermittent and the blood cultures may be negative. Furthermore, many patients will have received antimicrobial agents when they are first seen, masking the bacteriologic diagnosis. *A negative blood culture does not exclude the diagnosis of septic shock.* Culture of the primary septic focus may aid in the diagnosis, but the bacteriology may have been altered by prior chemotherapy. The ability of endotoxin to coagulate the blood of the horseshoe crab *Limulus* is the basis of a test for endotoxemia, which may be of value because it is usually positive in patients with the clinical picture of septic shock in whom blood cultures are negative. It may also provide a clue to the outcome because patients with a positive *Limulus* test and positive blood cultures have a worse prognosis than patients with gram-negative bacteremia in whom the test is negative.

DIAGNOSIS The diagnosis of septic shock is not difficult in the presence of chills, fever, and an overt focus of infection. However, none of the obvious clues may be present. Elderly, debilitated patients, in particular, may have severe infections in the absence of fever. Unexplained confusion and disorientation and hyperventilation without abnormal chest x-rays should call the diagnosis to mind. Pulmonary embolism, myocardial infarction, cardiac tamponade, aortic dissection, and silent hemorrhage are entities often confused with septic shock.

COURSE The rational treatment of septic shock depends upon careful monitoring of patients. Specifically, four parameters need to be followed at the bedside:

1 The *central venous pressure* (CVP) should be measured. Insertion of a catheter into the great veins or right atrium provides an accurate index of the relation between right ventricular competence and effective blood volume and should be used as a guide to fluid replacement therapy. When the CVP exceeds 12 to 14 cm water, there is some danger of overloading the circulation and precipitating pulmonary edema. It is important to be sure that the flow through the catheter is free and that the catheter is not in the right ventricle. *The CVP is the cornerstone of managing shock and should be measured in every patient.* Many investigators feel that the pulmonary artery and wedge pressures are better guides of fluid overload and incipient pulmonary edema than the CVP. The ready availability of the Swan-Ganz catheter has made this measurement feasible in many hospitals. However, correct placement is as important with the Swan-Ganz catheter as with the CVP line.
2 The *pulse pressure* serves as an estimate of stroke volume.
3 *Cutaneous vasoconstriction* provides a clue to peripheral resistance, although it does not reflect accurately blood flow to kidney, brain, or gut.
4 Hourly *urine output* should be used to monitor splanchnic blood flow and visceral perfusion. Usually this requires placement of an indwelling urethral catheter.

By means of these four measurements the patient with shock can be followed carefully and managed intelligently. Indirect arterial blood pressure does not provide an accurate picture of the hemodynamic situation, and perfusion of vital organs may be adequate in patients with hypotension; conversely, some patients with normal blood pressures may have marked pooling and inadequate visceral blood flow.

In units organized for treatment of shock, frequent measurements of pulmonary artery and wedge pressures, direct measurement of systemic arterial pressure, arterial and venous pH, blood gases, blood lactate, sophisticated renal function tests, and electrolyte measurements should be performed.

TREATMENT **Support of respiration** In many patients with septic shock arterial P_{O_2} is markedly depressed. It is essential to establish an airway at the outset and to administer oxygen nasally or by mask. Tracheal intubation usually suffices; tracheostomy is rarely necessary. However, a positive pressure-volume cycled respirator should be employed early to achieve proper ventilation and to overcome the severe hypoxia.

Volume replacement With the CVP or pulmonary wedge pressure as a guide, blood volume should be replaced with blood (if anemia is present), plasma, dextran (molecular weight 70,000 or 40,000), human serum albumin, and appropriate electrolyte solutions, primarily dextrose-saline and bicarbonate (which is preferable to lactate for treating the acidosis). The quantity of fluid required may be in excess of "normal" blood volume and may amount to 8 to 12 liters in only a few hours. Large quantities may be required even when the cardiac index is normal. *Oliguria in the presence of hypotension is not a contraindication to continued vigorous fluid therapy.* In order to guard against pulmonary edema, diuresis with furosemide should be attempted when the CVP reaches a level of approximately 10-12 cm and the pulmonary artery pressure 16-18 cm of water.

Antibiotics Blood cultures and cultures of relevant body fluids or exudates should be taken before instituting antimicrobial therapy. Drugs should be given intravenously, and bactericidal agents used when possible. When the results of blood cultures and sensitivities are known, one of the appropriate drugs recommended in the chapters dealing with the specific infections and discussed in Chap. 125 should be given. Usually cultures and sensitivities are not at hand at the onset of shock, and the etiologic diagnosis entails an educated guess based upon culture from the primary focus—urine, bile, pus, or sputum, or on the setting in which the infection occurs. For example, a young woman with dysuria, chills, and flank pain and septic shock is likely to have *Escherichia coli* bacteremia, while gram-negative sepsis in a burn patient is probably caused by *Pseudomonas*. The drugs of choice for gram-negative bacteremia are:

E. coli:	Ampicillin or cephalothin
Klebsiella-Enterobacter:	Gentamicin
Proteus mirabilis:	Ampicillin or cephalothin
Pr. rettgeri, morganii, or vulgaris:	Gentamicin
Mima-Herellea:	Gentamicin
Pseudomonas:	Gentamicin

The dosages and routes of administration for these agents are detailed in Chap. 125. Cephalothin can be substituted for ampicillin in patients with a history of penicillin allergy. Because of its toxic effect on the vestibular portion of the eighth nerve, gentamicin must be given cautiously to oliguric patients; a single dose of 80.0 mg achieves blood levels which should suffice throughout the period of oliguria. Similar precautions should be taken with kanamycin, where the loading dose is 1.0 g.

When the cause of septic shock is unknown, therapy should be initiated with both gentamicin and cephalothin or a penicillinase-resistant penicillin. If *Bacteroides* is suspected, chloramphenicol or 7-chlorlincomycin (clindamycin) can be added. As soon as culture results become available, the unnecessary drugs can be deleted.

Surgical intervention Many patients with septic shock have an abscess, infarcted or necrotic bowel, an inflamed gallbladder, infected uterus, pyonephrosis, or other local situations which lend themselves to surgical drainage or excision. As a rule, successful treatment of shock requires surgical intervention even if the patient is desperately ill. Operations should not be postponed "to get the patient in shape" because these patients' condition will continue to deteriorate unless the septic focus is removed or drained.

Vasoactive drugs Septic shock is accompanied by maximal stimulation of alpha-adrenergic receptors, and pressor agents which act by stimulating these receptors such as norepinephrine, levarterenol, and metaraminol are contraindicated. The two groups of drugs which have been of value in septic shock are alpha-receptor blocking agents exemplified by phenoxybenzamine and phentolamine (Regitine) and beta-receptor stimulants, notably isoproterenol. *Phenoxybenzamine* (Dibenzylene), an adrenolytic agent, effects a central phlebotomy by reducing resistance and increasing intravascular capacity. Hence there is a redistribution of blood. Blood leaves the lungs, relieving pulmonary edema and enhancing gas exchange. Central venous pressure and left ventricular end-diastolic pressure fall, cardiac output rises, and peripheral venous constriction regresses. The recommended dose is 0.2-2.0 mg per kg intravenously. Small doses can be injected instantaneously and large doses over a period of 40 to 60 min. Fluids must be given simultaneously to compensate for the increment in venous capacitance; failure to do so aggravates shock. Dibenzylene is not available for general use, and experience with phentolamine has not been great enough to recommend it. *Chlorpromazine* in multiple small doses of 2.5 to 5 mg also relieves vasoconstriction through its direct adrenolytic effect and by ganglionic blockage.

Isoproterenol (Isuprel) counteracts arteriolar and venous constriction in the microcirculation by its direct vasodilating effect. In addition, the drug exerts a direct inotropic effect on the heart. Cardiac output is increased by stimulation of the myocardium and by reduction of cardiac work as peripheral resistance decreases. The dose of isoproterenol is 2 to 8 μg per min for the average adult. Ventricular arrhythmias may result from this drug, and shock may be made worse if fluid administration does not keep pace with relieved vasoconstriction.

Digitalis and diuretics A rapidly acting preparation of digoxin or Cedilanid should be given when the CVP or pulmonary artery pressure remains high in the face of systemic hypotension. In addition, the urine output of these patients should be increased, preferably with intravenous furosemide.

Adrenal cortical hormones In very large doses these agents overcome increased peripheral resistance, mitigate the cellular injury evoked by endotoxin, prevent platelet aggregation, and have a variety of other actions which may be beneficial to the host. The only way that these hormones are effective in septic shock is in dosages of 30 mg methylprednisolone per kg given as a single dose and repeated for two or three doses. Usually by that time the issue has been decided and the drug can be discontinued without tapering. While these high-dose steroid regimens have been controversial, the evidence that they are effective is mounting.

Other measures Hemorrhage as a consequence of clotting-factor deficiencies has been controlled with fresh frozen plasma, but when thrombocytopenia is the cause of bleeding, whole blood transfusions must be given. Hyperbaric oxygen has been tried in gram-negative bacteremia with indifferent results.

PROGNOSIS The measures described above usually will resuscitate most patients, at least temporarily. Indicators of a favorable response are:

1 Improved sensorium and general appearance
2 Decreased peripheral cyanosis
3 Warming of the skin over the extremities
4 Urine output of 40 to 50 ml per hr
5 Increased pulse pressure
6 Return of CVP to normal
7 Increased blood pressure

The ultimate outcome, however, is dependent upon several other factors:

1 Ability to eliminate the source of infection with surgery or antibiotics. The prognosis of urinary tract infections, septic abortions, abdominal abscesses, gastrointestinal or biliary fistulas, and subcutaneous or anorectal abscesses is better than that of primary foci in the skin or lungs.
2 Previous contact with the organism. Patients with chronic urinary tract infections who develop bacteremia rarely have severe gram-negative shock, perhaps

because they have become tolerant to the endotoxin.

3 Underlying disease. Patients with lymphoma or leukemia who develop septic shock while their hematologic disease is out of control rarely recover; conversely, if hematologic remission is achieved, the shock is more likely to respond to therapy.
4 Metabolic status; the development of severe metabolic acidosis and lactic acidemia—irrespective of cardiac output—is associated with a poor prognosis.
5 Development of pulmonary insufficiency even after the hemodynamic abnormalities have been corrected.

The overall mortality of septic shock remains 50 percent; however, with better monitoring and more physiologic treatment, the outcome should improve.

PREVENTION The poor results in the treatment of septic shock are not due to lack of potent antibiotics or vasoactive agents. Rather, failure to institute therapy sufficiently early is a major roadblock to success. Septic shock usually is recognized too late, all too often after irreversible changes have taken place. Because many patients who are likely to develop septic shock are in the hospital *before* signs and symptoms of shock appear, it is essential to watch patients who are candidates for development of shock assiduously, to treat their infections vigorously and early, and to perform appropriate surgery before catastrophic complications occur. There is some preliminary evidence that early therapy of septic shock improves the ultimate outcome.

REFERENCES

BLAIN CM et al: Immediate hemodynamic effects of gram-negative vs gram-positive bacteremia in man. Arch Intern Med 126:260, 1970

BRYANT RE et al: Factors affecting mortality of gram-negative rod bacteremia. Arch Intern Med 127:120, 1971

CHRISTY JH: Treatment of gram-negative shock. Am J Med 50:77, 1971

CLAUSS RH, RAY JFR: Pharmacologic assistance to the failing circulation. Surg Gynecol Obstet 126:611, 1968

CORRIGAN JJ JR et al: Changes in the blood coagulation system associated with septicemia. N Engl J Med 279:851, 1968

HARDAWAY RM et al: Intensive study and treatment of shock in man. JAMA 199:799, 1967

JONES LW, WEIL MH: Water, creatinine and sodium excretion following circulatory shock with renal failure. Am J Med 51:314, 1971

LEVIN J et al: Gram-negative sepsis: Detection of endotoxemia with the Limulus test. Ann Intern Med 76:1, 1972

LILLEHEI RC et al: Treatment of septic shock. Mod Treat 4:321, 1967

MACLEAN LD et al: Patterns of septic shock in man—A detailed study of 56 patients. Ann Surg 166:543, 1967

MYEROWITZ RL et al: Recent experience with bacillemia due to gram-negative organisms. J Infect Dis 124:239, 1971

125 CHEMOTHERAPY OF INFECTION

WILLIAM M. M. KIRBY
ROBERT G. PETERSDORF

INTRODUCTION From the standpoint of overall reduction in morbidity and mortality rates, the greatest impact of drug therapy has been in the field of infectious diseases. Modern chemotherapy of infectious diseases dates from the mid-1930's when the sulfonamides were introduced. Penicillin G, the first of the antibiotics to be used systemically, came into widespread use in the early 1940's, and since then several dozen chemotherapeutic agents have appeared that are effective in a wide variety of bacterial, rickettsial, fungal, and parasitic infections. The efficacy of antimicrobial agents is due to their action in inhibiting growth of the parasite rather than to an enhancement of defense mechanisms, and it is remarkable that such a large number of substances can interfere effectively with multiplication of invading organisms without seriously damaging the cells of the host. Effective new agents continue to appear in surprising numbers, both from large-scale screening programs in which samples of organic matter are tested for antimicrobial activity and from chemical modifications of the known chemotherapeutic drugs. Specific recommendations for therapy are made in chapters dealing with individual diseases; this section is devoted to general principles of chemotherapy and to a consideration of individual therapeutic agents.

FACTORS INFLUENCING SELECTION OF ANTIMICROBIAL AGENTS AND THE OUTCOME OF THERAPY

SUSCEPTIBILITY OF THE INFECTING MICROORGANISMS No antimicrobial agent is effective against all pathogenic microorganisms; each has its own spectrum of activity against one or a variety of species, within which the majority of strains have been found to be susceptible. There are a few instances, such as the susceptibility of group A streptococci and pneumococci to penicillin G, in which resistant strains occur rarely if at all, and where in which treatment with penicillin can be given without concern about resistance. With the majority of chemotherapeutic agents, however, a variable percentage of strains of each susceptible species is resistant, i.e., they are not inhibited by concentrations of the drug attainable in the patient's blood and tissues with the usual dosage schedules. It is customary, therefore, to determine the susceptibility of most pathogens to a variety of chemotherapeutic agents, and this has become one of the most important functions of clinical microbiology laboratories. *Dilution methods* of susceptibility testing, considered to be the most accurate, involve adding serial dilutions of each agent to be tested to agar or broth containing a standardized inoculum of the infecting organisms and determining the smallest amount (the minimal inhibitory concentration, or MIC) of the drug that inhibits growth after overnight incubation. These procedures are too time-consuming for most routine laboratories, however, and the much simpler *agar diffusion method*, which is accurate and reliable when properly performed, is the one usually used. Zones of inhibition of growth of a standardized inoculum of the infecting organism around filter paper disks impregnated with antibiotics are measured, and the zone sizes reflect the inhibitory concentrations of drug, which are in turn related to the blood levels usually attained. Susceptibility of 8 to 10 chemotherapeutic agents can be tested on a single large agar plate, and a report of susceptible, intermediate, or resistant can be made. Disk testing has a number of limitations; it is applicable chiefly to rapidly growing pathogens, and the results are usually not reported until 24 hr after the pathogen is isolated.

BACTERICIDAL VERSUS BACTERIOSTATIC AGENTS Although these are relative terms, some chemotherapeutic drugs can be clearly shown to have a killing (bactericidal) action at or near the minimal inhibitory concentration, while others simply inhibit bacterial growth (bacteriostatic), leaving the host to strike the *coup de grâce*. Bactericidal agents include the penicillins, cephalosporins, polymyxins, and vancomycin, while examples of bacteriostatic agents are the tetracyclines, sulfonamides, chloramphenicol, erythromycin, and lincomycin. Bactericidal agents give definitely superior results in diseases such as bacterial endocarditis and pneumococcal meningitis, and are more likely to give a favorable response in life-threatening infections, particularly when there is impairment of the host's defense mechanisms. In mild infections in otherwise healthy individuals, on the other hand, there is little to choose between "-cidal" and "-static" agents. In uncomplicated urinary tract infections, for example, the clinical results are as good with sulfonamides as with broad-spectrum penicillins or cephalosporins.

CLINICAL PHARMACOLOGY Knowledge of the clinical pharmacology of antimicrobial agents is helpful in prescribing therapy that is both safe and effective. Important information includes details of absorption and excretion, blood and urine levels with various routes of administration, protein binding, renal clearance, half-lives of drugs, stability in solutions and within the body, and the conversion to metabolic breakdown products. With some agents, such as ampicillin, much higher blood levels are obtained with the same doses given parenterally than orally, whereas with others such as dicloxacillin and doxycycline, where there is complete absorption from the intestinal tract, the oral and parenteral doses are the same. Because of possible incompatibilities, *it is advisable never to administer more than one agent at a time by the intravenous route.* Absorption from the intestinal tract is impaired by a variety of foods and chemicals, and in general antimicrobials should be administered temporally as far removed from food and other drugs, such as antacids, as possible.

Antimicrobials are bound to a varying extent to serum proteins, especially albumin. Although the significance of protein binding is uncertain and controversial, it is clear that the bound antibiotic has no antimicrobial activity, and it is probable that the concentration of free, unbound antibiotic in the tissues is no greater than the peak level of free antibiotic in the blood. All other features being equal, antimicrobials with relatively low binding should be preferable to those with a high degree of binding. In general this point of view is reflected in the dosages of antimicrobial agents that are commonly recommended.

Renal clearance is one of the most important determinants of antibiotic blood levels and is mainly responsible, for example, for the much higher levels attained with the same dose of cephaloridine than of cephalothin, and of carbenicillin than of ampicillin. Antibiotics with a high renal clearance such as penicillin G and cephalothin have a large component of tubular secretion, and their blood levels are elevated to a greater degree by probenecid than those of ampicillin and cephaloridine, where the tubular contribution is less important. Plasma half-life, the time required for a blood level to fall by one-half, is also determined primarily by renal clearance mechanisms and is much shorter for those penicillins and cephalosporins that are secreted by the renal tubules than for antibiotics such as the aminoglycosides with little or no tubular component. Protein binding also has an important influence on the half-life of antibiotics, particularly those that are excreted mainly or entirely by glomerular filtration. Thus, the plasma half-life of gentamicin, which is not bound by proteins, is 2 hr, whereas that of doxycycline, which is over 90 percent protein-bound, is about 16 hr. Antibiotics with little or no protein binding have a much larger apparent volume of distribution (AVD) than those with a high degree of binding; i.e., the AVD of gentamicin is 30 percent of body weight compared with 14 percent for cefazolin. Cephalothin has a high plasma clearance with a high rate of nonrenal clearance due to its partial conversion in the body to a less active metabolic breakdown product. These are a few examples of the pharmacologic features of individual antimicrobial agents; others will be mentioned as the individual drugs are considered.

DOSE, ROUTE, AND DURATION OF THERAPY In prescribing dosages of antimicrobial agents, the objective is to deliver a concentration in excess of that needed to inhibit and/or kill the infecting organism at the site of infection. Since it is not feasible to measure tissue concentrations, a blood level that exceeds the MIC two- to eightfold is a commonly accepted guideline. This is an arbitrary concentration of drug and obviously does not take into account all the variations in penetration into different tissues, or the role of host defense mechanisms. These variations may be very important because in many instances, infections have been cured with antibiotics such as the tetracyclines where the concentration of free, active drug in the blood is not much greater than the MIC. The relation between blood levels and MIC does not hold in urinary tract infection, where the concentration of drug cleared by the kidney usually far exceeds the MIC. In this situation, an excess of drug in the urine is obviously important.

The route of administration, as well as the dose, is important in achieving appropriate drug levels. In general, parenteral therapy should usually be given in severe infections to be certain that high, effective blood levels are attained. The *intravenous route* is especially indicated initially in meningitis, endocarditis, and osteomyelitis, where barriers to penetration of the antimicrobial agent can be overcome by high blood levels. Intravenous therapy is also indicated when there is hypotension, and when bleeding diatheses are present. For milder infections, *intramuscular administration* is often an acceptable or preferable alternative, particularly with antibiotics such as procaine penicillin that cause relatively little pain and produce prolonged, effective blood levels. With gentamicin, blood levels are the same with an intramuscular injection as with an intravenous infusion given over a period of 30 min, so that the route can be chosen on the basis of comfort for the patient and the need for other intravenous medications. The *oral route* is used chiefly for mild to moderate infections, and for completion of therapy of severe infections after they have been brought under control with parenteral therapy. Absorption from the intestinal tract is variable even in the fasting state, and all oral antibiotics should be taken at least 1 hr before and 3 hr after food and other medications. This presents difficulties with drugs such as antacids that need to be taken frequently and that are especially likely to interfere with absorption of antimicrobial agents. Parenteral administration is often the only solution to this problem.

The optimal duration of antimicrobial treatment is unknown for many infections, and there is considerable variation from one medical center to another in the length of time antimicrobial therapy is given. In bacterial endocarditis, for example, the usual course of parenteral therapy may vary from 2 to 8 weeks with an average of about four weeks. For most acute infections a good general rule is to continue therapy for 2 to 3 days after the temperature has returned to normal and all signs of infection have subsided. However, fever can continue for weeks from sterile effusions complicating pneumonia, and cerebrospinal fluid abnormalities can persist for considerable periods in bacterial meningitis, leading to a continuation of chemotherapy for much longer than is necessary. Empiricism needs to be tempered with reason and experience, and in actual practice the guidelines for duration of therapy must be sufficiently flexible to be appropriate for the patient being treated.

ALLERGY AND TOXICITY The patient's allergic history should always be explored before prescribing antimicrobial agents. In addition to allergic manifestations in general, a report of previous drug allergies is of particular importance, and agents that have caused clear-cut reactions should be avoided. Unfortunately, no reliable test is available to determine the presence of allergy to the penicillins, and they may or may not be well tolerated by patients with a history of a previous reaction. The possibility of a severe anaphylactic reaction can be reliably excluded by skin tests containing major and minor determinant mixtures, but these reagents are not generally available. When administration of a penicillin is considered essential, one approach is to begin with a very small dose intravenously and increase the amount every few minutes until it is learned whether the patient can tolerate the antibiotic. Specifically, with an intravenous infusion running 1 unit penicillin diluted in 3 to 5 ml saline or glucose solution is injected slowly into the tubing, and 5 min is allowed to elapse to see if an untoward reaction occurs. A solution of adrenalin is available in another syringe to be injected if needed. If no reaction occurs, 2, 5, 10, 25, and 50 units, etc., are injected at 5-min intervals, and within an hour or so it either becomes apparent that the patient can tolerate a full therapeutic dose, or he develops a reaction that is readily controlled by epinephrine. If a reaction occurs, administering another antibiotic is usually best, although in mild reactions, continuing the penicillin along with antihistamines and/or steroids is possible in some instances. Such a program can be quite troublesome as well as risky, requiring frequent adjustments to suppress urticaria and itching. The number of alternative antibiotics available is large enough that switching to another agent is usually the best course to follow.

Drug toxicity related to renal function is of particular importance. Some antimicrobials, such as the penicillins, cephalothin, chloramphenicol, erythromycin, and lincomycin, are relatively safe at normal or only slightly reduced dosage in the presence of impaired renal function. Other agents, such as the aminoglycosides, are potentially quite toxic but can be administered at reduced dosage if proper guidelines, based on serial determinations of the serum creatinine, are followed, and particularly if blood levels can be monitored. Certain toxic agents should be avoided if at all possible in the presence of renal insufficiency. These include most of the tetracyclines, streptomycin, cephaloridine, the sulfonamides, the nitrofurans, and nalidixic acid. One of the long-acting tetracyclines, doxycycline, has the same half-life in healthy and uremic subjects, and can be administered to patients with impaired renal function either orally or intravenously. A number of patients with chronic renal failure are being maintained on dialysis programs, and may require antimicrobials for a variety of infections. Table 125-1 summarizes adult dosage schedules for various antibiotics for patients with renal failure, on or off dialysis.

SITE OF INFECTION Soft-tissue infections in sites with a good blood supply and a minimum of tissue necrosis, are, in general, easily treated. In meningitis and endocarditis, on the other hand, penetration into the site of the infection presents formidable problems and is not infrequently responsible for treatment failures. Penetration across the blood-brain barrier is a complex phenomenon involving protein binding, lipid solubility, and ionization of the drug being administered. In addition, the permeability of this barrier to drugs depends on the degree of inflammation. Because of their low toxicity the penicillins can be administered in doses large enough to provide therapeutic concentrations in the spinal fluid, whereas more toxic drugs such as the aminoglycosides and polymyxins must be injected intrathecally to be effective clinically in meningitis. On the other hand, agents such as the sulfonamides, chloramphenicol, and the tetracyclines appear in the spinal fluid in amounts adequate for the treatment of some types of meningitis when they are given in doses appropriate for the treatment of systemic infections.

Other examples of problems of penetration, and of the influence of localized physiologic conditions, may be cited. The sulfonamides are excreted in the saliva in amounts adequate to eradicate the meningococcal carrier state, whereas most penicillins and tetracyclines are not. As a result, these drugs are not effective in the eradication of meningococci because most of the strains encountered at the present time are sulfonamide-resistant. In urinary infections, erythromycin and the aminoglycosides are relatively ineffective at an acid pH, whereas a pH of less than 5.5 is essential for the acitivity of mandelamine. The lack of efficacy of sulfonamides in the presence of pus, due to the competition for binding sites by the large amounts of *p*-aminobenzoic acid present, greatly limits the usefulness of this class of drugs.

Foreign bodies, abscesses, and obstruction to normal pathways of drainage almost always interfere with the response to chemotherapy and usually prevent cure until they are removed, drained, or relieved. Suture materials, prostheses, sequestrations, and calculi are examples of foreign bodies that interfere with drug therapy and usually, but not always, need to be removed. In many abscesses, bacteria tend to be in a metabolically inactive state in which they are not actively synthesizing cell wall and are not susceptible to the damaging effects of antimicrobial drugs; hence drainage plus chemotherapy is necessary to eradicate the infection. Obstruction to bronchial, biliary, and renal drainage interferes seriously with the response of bacterial infections to antibiotics, and these infections generally cannot be cured with these drugs until the obstruction is relieved. A thorough knowledge of mechanical, metabolic, and physiologic factors is essential in planning therapy that will bring about optimal results in infections located in different parts of the body.

COMBINATION THERAPY, SYNERGISM, ANTAGONISM Once the etiologic agent is known, most bacterial infections can be treated successfully with a *single* antimicrobial agent. Combination therapy is used frequently, however, to broaden the antibacterial spectrum while awaiting the results of cultures, and also to cover the possibility that a mixed infection might be present. For example, in a hospitalized patient who suddenly becomes ill with presumed sepsis, cephalothin and gentamicin may be given empirically to provide antibacterial activity against a variety of gram-positive and -negative pathogens that might be fatal if therapy were delayed (Chap. 124). Until recently over 100 fixed-dose combinations were available commercially in the United States for oral or parenteral therapy, but virtually all have been ordered off the market by the Food and Drug Administration on the grounds that it has not been shown in controlled studies that both agents contribute to the claimed therapeutic effects, that the amounts of each agent present were often not appropriate, and that patients were often being exposed to the potential hazards of two drugs when only one was needed. When combination therapy is

TABLE 125-1
Recommended dosages of antimicrobials in oliguric patients (creatinine clearance less than 10 percent of normal)

		Dosage significantly affected by dialysis?	
Agent	*Dosage off dialysis**	*Hemodialysis*	*Peritoneal dialysis*
Penicillin G	0.5–2 million units q.6–8h.		No
Ampicillin	1 g; then 0.5 g q.8h.	Yes (0.5–1 g q.6h.)	No
Methicillin	1 g q.8–12h.	No	No
Oxacillin	1 g q.8–12h.	No	No
Dicloxacillin	0.5 g q.8h.	No	Yes (25 μg/ml)†
Carbenicillin	2 g; then 1 g q.8–12h.	Yes (1 g q.4h.)*	Yes (100 μg/ml)†
Cephalothin	1 g q.8–12h.	Yes (1 g q.6h.)*	Yes (20 μg/ml)†
Cephaloridine‡	1 g q.24h.	Yes (0.5g q.4h.)*	Yes (20 μg/ml)†
Chloramphenicol	0.5 g q.6h.	No	No
Erythromycin	0.5 g q.6h.	No	No
Lincomycin	250 mg q.12h.	No	No
Kanamycin	0.5 to 1 g; then 0.5 g q.3–4d. (or 7 mg/kg body weight q. third half-life)§	Yes (250 mg after each dialysis)*	Yes (20 μg/ml)†
Gentamicin	80 mg; then 40 mg q.2d.	No	
Colistin (polymyxin E)	200–300 mg; then 100–150 mg q.2–4d.	No	No
Polymyxin B	100–150 mg; then 50–100 mg q.2–4d.	No	No
Vancomycin	1 g q.10–14d.	No	

* *Dosages for intramuscular or intravenous administration.*

† *When antibiotic blood levels are affected significantly by peritoneal dialysis, the agents should be added to the dialysate at the desired serum concentration, with continuation of the usual intramuscular or intravenous administration. Figures in parentheses represent suitable concentrations when adding to peritoneal dialysis fluid.*

‡ *Not used because of nephrotoxicity; may prove useful in patients on chronic dialysis programs to whom nephrotoxicity is of no significance.*

§ *Plasma half-life (hours)* $= \dfrac{\text{(3.6) (body weight in kilograms)}}{\text{creatinine clearance (milliliter/minute)}}$ *This formula may be applied to patients with normal renal function as well as to patients with renal insufficiency. Thus a man weighing 50 kg whose kanamycin plasma half-life is calculated to be 12 hr would receive 350 mg every 36 hr.*

SOURCE: *Bulger RJ, Petersdorf RG, Postgrad Med 47:160, 1970*

indicated, it is most rational to prescribe separately the indicated drugs in doses that take into the account the patient's age, weight, and physiologic status.

Another indication for giving two antimicrobial agents simultaneously is to prevent the emergence of resistant mutants. An example is the administration of aminosalicylic acid or ethambutol in conjunction with isoniazid in tuberculosis. In some instances, a second agent is given to avoid superinfections; the use of nystatin together with tetracycline to prevent an overgrowth of *Candida albicans* that causes disorders such as thrush and vaginitis is an example. In general, this is a questionable practice.

A significant enhancement of antibacterial activity from exposing microorganisms to two or more drugs is rare. Usually the two drugs have an indifferent effect, but sometimes additive action can be demonstrated. True synergism occurs with penicillin and streptomycin against many strains of enterococci, and with gentamicin and carbenicillin against *Pseudomonas* and some other gram-negative bacilli. In severe *Pseudomonas* infections, it should be theoretically possible to reduce the dose and thus the cost and toxicity of gentamicin and carbenicillin because of their synergistic action, but in actual practice the extent of the reduction that would be compatible with maximal efficacy is unpredictable, and it is safer to administer full doses and not risk compromising the therapeutic result. With enterococci, penicillin disrupts the cell wall and permits streptomycin to gain access to the ribosomes, to which it is lethal. Strains with ribosomes that are resistant to streptomycin do not manifest synergism in vitro between penicillin and streptomycin, and treating infections by these strains with a penicillin-streptomycin combination is probably no better than using penicillin alone. Penicillin or ampicillin plus kanamycin or gentamicin also has shown significant synergism against enterococci. Clinically significant antagonism between antimicrobial agents is also rare, a prime example being a higher mortality rate in pneumococcal meningitis treated with penicillin and tetracycline compared with penicillin alone. The rate of killing by penicillin is decreased by the presence of the bacteriostatic agent, tetracycline, and this can alter the outcome when survival depends on rapid killing of the pneumococci.

DEVELOPMENT OF RESISTANCE DURING ANTIMICROBIAL THERAPY A number of microorganisms are genetically resistant to one or more antimicrobials, and they obviously will not be affected by antibiotic therapy. Most antibiotics will alter the host's normal flora by removing those organisms which are sensitive to the drug. In most cases this ecologic change is of little consequence, but occasionally the commensal bacteria of the host set up infection in the same location as the original infection, a state termed *superinfection* (Chap. 123). The superinfecting organism is resistant to the drug being administered, and in order to eradicate it, its susceptibility must be determined. Some superinfecting organisms, particularly gram-negatives, acquire resistance to multiple drugs by an episomal transfer mechanism (R factors). For example, multiple resistant *E. coli* and *Klebsiella-Enterobacter* pose a particular hazard to hospitalized patients.

Comparatively few organisms become resistant to the antibiotic being given during therapy. Some that do develop resistance are *E. coli* to streptomycin and nalidixic acid, occasional strains of staphylococci to erythromycin, and *Pseudomonas* to carbenicillin. In general, however, sensitive organisms are supplanted by resistant ones, rather than acquiring resistance themselves. From a practical point of view, it is important to know which agents are likely to induce resistance, and to look for this phenomenon clinically.

SPECIFIC ANTIMICROBIALS

PENICILLINS Penicillinase-susceptible *Penicillin G* (benzyl penicillin), the prototype, is still widely used, especially parenterally, when high blood levels are desirable as in meningitis and endocarditis. Large doses are necessary either continuously or at 3- to 4-hr intervals because of problems of penetration into vegetations and across the blood-brain barrier, and also because of its high renal clearance, which is due chiefly to rapid tubular excretion. Blood levels can be doubled by the concomitant administration of probenecid, 0.5 g every 6 hr, but since penicillin G is now quite inexpensive and the optimal blood levels are not precisely known, it is customary in most instances simply to give more penicillin. *Procaine penicillin* is well tolerated intramuscularly and is quite slowly absorbed, so that injections need to be given only every 12 to 24 hr for the treatment of many infections due to susceptible bacteria. In dosage of 300,000 to 600,000 units every 12 hr, it is the drug of choice for most patients with pneumococcal pneumonia. *Benzathine penicillin* provides a depot in the muscle that releases penicillin so slowly that low blood levels are present for 2 or 3 weeks. These low levels are adequate for the therapy and prevention of streptococcal pharyngitis and for the treatment of some forms of syphilis.

Penicillin G given orally in doses of 250,000 units once or twice daily is also effective in preventing streptococcal sore throats, but less so than benzathine penicillin (Chap. 238). Because of its instability in the presence of acid, however, it is less reliable for therapy than the acid-stable penicillin V (phenoxymethyl penicillin), and attempts to overcome this disadvantage by giving larger amounts of penicillin G are associated with an increased incidence of nausea and diarrhea. A number of dosage forms of penicillin G are available; an important feature of their continued usefulness is the fact that very little resistance has developed among penicillin G-susceptible microorganisms.

Broad-spectrum penicillins *Ampicillin* differs from penicillin G only in the presence of an amino group in the side chain, but this minor chemical difference is responsible for some unique features that have led to the widespread use of this antibiotic. Ampicillin is active in low concentrations against a number of gram-negative bacteria causing respiratory (*Hemophilus influenzae*), intestinal (*Shigella, Salmonella*), and urinary (*E. coli, Proteus mirabilis*) infections. When it is given orally, the peak blood level occurs later (2 to 3 hr versus 1/2 to 1 hr) and is lower than with penicillin V, and the ampicillin blood level then declines more slowly. This more prolonged blood level, along with its greater in vitro activity, is probably responsible for the greater efficacy of ampicillin, compared with penicillin V, in the oral therapy of gonococcal urethritis.

When given in an intravenous infusion, blood levels are more than 80 percent higher with ampicillin than with penicillin G, chiefly because of its much higher rate of renal clearance (390 versus 210 ml per min per 1.73 m^2). When the in vitro activity of the infecting organisms is the same for the two antibiotics, this difference can mean equal efficacy with smaller doses of ampicillin, or higher blood levels with the same dose when maximum serum concentrations are considered necessary. Ampicillin is also more stable in the body, with a serum half-life twice as long as penicillin G, due chiefly to slower breakdown by the liver. Serum protein binding of amipicillin is approximately 20 percent compared with 60 percent for penicillin G and 80 percent for penicillin V; this may mean that with ampicillin there is a higher concentration of free, active antibiotic at the site of the infection. All these features contribute to the efficacy and widespread use of ampicillin, and in the United States, competition has led to a marked decrease in the cost in the last few years.

Hypersensitivity reactions occur with about the same frequency with ampicillin as with penicillin G and V, and with all three are much more frequent and severe when the drug is given parenterally and topically than by the oral route. About 5 to 10 percent of patients develop skin rashes with oral ampicillin, but the incidence is as high as 90 percent when patients with infectious mononucleosis take this drug. This remarkably high incidence, which does not occur with penicillins G and V, does not represent true penicillin allergy, and its exact nature is not known.

Hetacillin, a penicillin with a complex side chain, is hydrolyzed rapidly in the body to ampicillin, and for practical therapeutic purposes can be regarded the same as ampicillin. Indeed, because of its larger molecule, a 250-mg capsule is converted to only 225 mg ampicillin in the body and therefore provides 10 percent less antibiotic activity.

Although acid-stable, ampicillin is not very well absorbed when taken orally, giving peak blood levels only one-sixth as high as dicloxacillin and cephalexin. Two derivates of ampicillin, *pivampicillin* and *amoxicillin*, give blood levels and urinary excretion over twice as great as ampicillin, and these better-absorbed preparations, now undergoing clinical trials, may extend the range of infections that can be treated orally.

Carbenicillin is a broad-spectrum penicillin similar chemically to ampicillin, except that the amino group in the side chain is replaced by a carboxyl group. As a result, carbenicillin is active in vitro against *Pseudomonas*, indole-positive *Proteus*, and some strains of *Enterobacter*, in addition to the other gram-negatives that are susceptible to ampicillin. The MIC for *Pseudomonas* is much higher than that usually considered within the therapeutic range for other antibiotics, i.e., about 75 to 100 μg per ml. However, extraordinarily high blood levels can be readily attained, in the range of 200 to 400 μg per ml., so that carbenicillin provides the safety and bactericidal activity of a penicillin for an organism that has been notably refractory to most other antibiotics. The much higher blood levels that can be readily attained with carbenicillin as compared with ampicillin are due chiefly to its much lower renal clearance (100 versus 210 ml per min per 1.73 m^2). In addition, carbenicillin is much more stable in the body, so that blood levels obtained with 30 g a day in patients with normal renal function can be achieved with only 3 or 4 g a day in patients with no renal function. Since many patients with severe gram-negative infections have considerable renal impairment, reduced doses can be administered with the knowledge that full therapeutic blood levels will be achieved. To give 30 g daily for the therapy of severe *Pseudomonas* infections in patients with normal renal function, it is customary to administer 5 g intravenously every 4 hr, diluting each dose in 100 to 200 ml fluid and allowing it to drip into the vein within 1 to 2 hr. Except for severe *Pseudomonas* infections, 30 g daily is not necessary, and much smaller doses, 10 or 15 g daily, are adequate for the therapy of other gram-negative infections, including those caused by indole-positive *Proteus* and *Enterobacter*. Urinary concentrations in excess of 1,000 μg per ml are attained with 0.5- or 1.0-g doses intramuscularly, so that doses comparable to those used with ampicillin are appropriate for urinary tract infections, including those due to *Pseudomonas*. An oral form of carbenicillin, the indanyl salt of the sodium ester, has recently become available, and one or two 0.5-g tablets (each equivalent to 382 mg carbenicillin) every 6 hr produce urinary concentrations well in excess of MICs for susceptible gram-negative bacilli, including *Pseudomonas*.

An increase in bacterial resistance has been noted in some patients with severe gram-negative infections treated with carbenicillin, but the frequency and extent of the resistance has varied in different reports. The concomitant administration of gentamicin has tended to delay the development of resistance to carbenicillin, and in addition a synergistic action has been found to occur with these two antibiotics against many gram-negative bacilli. It has therefore become customary in severe infections to give both of these antibiotics, to enhance antibacterial activity and to delay the emergence of resistance as well. Since there is inactivation of the antibiotics, especially gentamicin, when the two are present in the same solution for several hours, it is preferable to administer them separately, either intramuscularly or intravenously, and under these circumstances the blood levels of each are the same as if they were being given alone.

Penicillinase-resistant penicillins The advent of these antibiotics in the early 1960s greatly enhanced the ability to cope with severe staphylococcal infections, because at that time over three-fourths of strains causing infections in hospitals were penicillinase producers. Furthermore, the number of strains resistant to these new penicillins has remained very small, especially in the United States. This is probably due to the low incidence of naturally occurring methicillin-resistant strains, and the fact that only a small proportion of the cells in a "resistant" culture are actually lacking in susceptibility. In many hospitals during the last decade there has also been a marked decline in infections caused by penicillinase-producing staphylococci, due in part at least to the widespread use of effective bactericidal agents such as the penicillinase-resistant penicillins and the cephalosporins.

Five penicillinase-resistant penicillins are currently marketed in the United States: *methicillin, oxacillin, nafcillin, cloxacillin,* and *dicloxacillin.* The first three are available for parenteral administration. Methicillin is less active when tested in broth cultures than are oxacillin and nafcillin, but this is probably offset by its much lower protein binding, 40 percent as compared with 90 percent or more for the other two. Clinical studies do not provide convincing evidence of superiority of any of these three penicillins for the parenteral therapy of severe staphylococcal infections. Methicillin is given in the same dose as, or in twice the dose of, the other two because of its lower in vitro activity, i.e., 1 or 2 g every 4 to 6 hr in adults. For intravenous administration, each dose is diluted in 50 to 100 ml fluid, and is infused over a period of 30 min to minimize phlebitis. Intramuscular injections are painful and are poorly tolerated for more than a few days. Methicillin nephritis, an uncommon but important allergic reaction, has been reported rarely with oxacillin and nafcillin; it is not known whether this is due simply to the fact that methicillin is more widely used. Nafcillin has been found by many observers to give lower blood levels than equal doses of oxacillin; this appears to be due to sequestration of nafcillin in the liver and possibly in other tissues so that less is available to circulate in the blood. The therapeutic implications of this phenomenon are unknown.

With oral administration both nafcillin and oxacillin give low blood levels, and for this reason their use is avoided by some. Cloxacillin gives blood levels twice as high, and dicloxacillin four times as high, as oxacillin when the same doses are given orally. However, there is also a progressive increase in serum protein binding (92 percent for oxacillin, 94 percent for cloxacillin, and 96 percent for dicloxacillin), so that the differences in free, active antibiotic may offset the blood level differences. In general cloxacillin or dicloxacillin in doses of 0.5 g and 0.25 g four times daily respectively, is preferred for oral administration. The efficacy of these antibiotics, either initially in mild to moderate soft-tissue infections, or for completion of therapy following administration of one of the three parenteral preparations described above, is well established by clinical experience.

The chief indication for the penicillinase-resistant penicillins is the therapy of infections caused by penicillinase-producing staphylococci, but they are often administered empirically before the etiologic organism is known. Pneumococci and most streptococci are more susceptible to penicillin G and ampicillin, but blood levels are sufficiently high with the penicillinase-resistant penicillins, especially when given parenterally, so that it is not necessary to give both types of penicillins to provide coverage for these organisms. However, infections caused by enterococci and *Neisseria* cannot be expected to respond to therapy with a penicillinase-resistant penicillin given alone, and if these organisms are suspected, ampicillin should be used.

CEPHALOSPORINS The cephalosporins differ from the penicillins in having a six-membered dihydrothiazine ring, instead of a five-membered thiazolidine ring, fused to the beta-lactam ring. As a result of this chemical difference there is no true cross-allergenicity, and most patients who are allergic to penicillins can be treated with cephalosporins without hypersensitivity reactions. The small number in whom this is not possible seem to be highly allergic individuals who react separately to the two groups of antibiotics.

Most bacteria susceptible to the penicillins are also susceptible to the cephalosporins, including group A and viridans streptococci, pneumococci, penicillin G–sensitive and –resistant *Staphylococcus aureus, Neisseria,* clostridia, *Actinomyces,* and *Corynebacterium diphtheriae.* Among the gram-negatives most strains of *E. coli, P. mirabilis, Klebsiella* but not *Enterobacter, Shigella, Salmonella,* and most strains of *H. influenzae,* are susceptible. The cephalosporins act on the cell wall in a manner similar to the penicillins, and are bactericidal. As with the penicillins, there has been little tendency for susceptible species to become resistant despite widespread use of the cephalosporins for more than a decade.

Of the four cephalosporins marketed in the United States, cephalothin, cephaloridine, cephaloglycin, and cephalexin, the first two are effective only when given parenterally, and the last two are available only as oral preparations. Because of its broad spectrum of activity, *cephalothin* is used widely in hospitals, often in conjunction with other antibiotics, for initial therapy in seriously ill patients while awaiting the results of cultures. It is usually administered intravenously in doses of 1 or 2 g every 4 or 6 hr; each dose is diluted in 50 to 100 ml fluid and infused over a period of 20 to 30 min to minimize the phlebitis that occurs frequently with more concentrated solutions. Convincing evidence of nephrotoxicity is lacking, and only a moderate reduction in dosage is necessary in the presence of uremia. Cephalothin is partially converted in the body to a metabolic breakdown product, desacetylcephalothin, that is less active than the parent compound, particularly against gram-negative bacteria. This partial breakdown is relatively small in extent, usually not more than 25 percent, and for the most part is of no importance clinically because of the large quantity of the parent compound present. Meningococcal meningitis may be a possible exception; in this disease relapses and failures to eradicate the infecting organism have been described. Meningococci have been observed to be only about one-fifteenth as susceptible to desacetylcephalothin, which has been found to be present in the spinal fluid in significant amounts. *Cephaloridine* has three potential advantages over cephalothin because it is less painful on intramuscular injection, is less avidly bound to protein (15 versus 70 percent), and achieves much higher and more prolonged blood levels with the same dose. The blood level differences favoring cephaloridine are due to lower renal clearance and greater stability in the body. However, cephaloridine is nephrotoxic, causing renal tubular damage when blood levels are excessive, and the recommended dose is limited to no more than 4 g daily in adults with normal renal function.

Reduced doses are necessary in patients with impaired renal function; precise recommendations are available in the labeling that accompanies the antibiotic. Because of its nephrotoxicity, cephaloridine should be restricted for the most part to patients in whom it is necessary to administer a cephalosporin intramuscularly. However, intravenous administration is warranted in a few patients with meningitis or endocarditis who are allergic to the penicillins and in whom high blood levels are considered important. Cephaloridine is less stable in the presence of staphylococcal penicillinase than cephalothin, but it has not been possible clearly to relate this characteristic to inferior clinical results. Cephalothin, on the other hand, has definitely been shown to be as effective as the penicillinase-resistant penicillins for the treatment of severe infections due to penicillinase-producing staphylococci.

Cephaloglycin is poorly absorbed orally, giving low blood levels, but provides urinary concentrations adequate for the therapy of some urinary infections. However, its usefulness has practically disappeared with the advent of *cephalexin*, a well-absorbed oral cephalosporin that gives high blood levels, has low serum protein binding, is over 90 percent excreted in the urine without nephrotoxocity, and has no adverse metabolic breakdown product. A 0.5-g dose of cephalexin orally gives an average peak blood level in adults of about 18 μg per ml, six times as high as that produced by the same dose of ampicillin. Cephalexin has the same antibacterial spectrum as the other cephalosporins, although it is somewhat less active against some organisms in vitro, and it has not been clearly established that it is effective in infections caused by *H. influenzae.* Because of its broad spectrum of activity and its high blood levels, cephalexin is widely used for initial treatment of a variety of infections, and for continuation of therapy following the administration of cephalothin or cephaloridine.

Several new cephalosporins are under active clinical investigation and will become available in the next year or two. *Cephapirin* is almost identical in antibacterial spectrum and pharmacologic characteristics to cephalothin. *Cefazolin*, although quite highly protein bound (about 85 percent), produces high blood levels because of its low renal clearance and has a longer half-life than cephalothin and cephaloridine. Whether any of these new cephalosporins will be superior clinically to the four now available is not known as yet.

AMINOGLYCOSIDES *Streptomycin*, one of the first antibiotics available for systemic administration, was widely used during the late 1940s and the 1950s. For a number of years it was given almost routinely in conjunction with penicillin in surgical cases of the prophylaxis and treatment of postoperative infections. Because of the tendency for highly resistant organisms to appear within 2 or 3 days, and its potential for causing vestibular damage and deafness, streptomycin has been largely supplanted by kanamycin and gentamicin, although it is still in use for certain specific purposes. Tuberculosis is still treated with streptomycin, particularly when triple drug regimens are used for the first few weeks; 1 g intramuscularly each day is the usual dose. Streptomycin is also used in conjunction with penicillin to treat enterococcal infections and for the treatment of certain less common infections such as brucellosis and tularemia. In addition to vestibular nerve toxicity, other adverse reactions of streptomycin include rashes, fever, contact dermatitis, pancytopenia, anaphylaxis, and renal irritation.

Neomycin, another aminoglycoside that appeared in the 1940s, is no longer used parenterally because of its nephro- and neurotoxicity. Respiratory arrest is a serious adverse reaction that has occurred when neomycin is instilled topically in the peritoneal cavity in anesthetized patients, and deafness has resulted from the topical application of neomycin soaks injudiciously in burns and wounds. Neomycin is useful and relatively safe when given orally in doses of 4 to 6 g daily to "prepare" the bowel preoperatively, and in patients with hepatic insufficiency where inhibition of bacterial growth in the intestine is necessary to reduce the absorption of nitrogenous substances. However, the amount of neomycin absorbed from the intestine is variable, and toxic levels have been demonstrated in some patients. Neomycin is also used as a spray and an ointment to decrease the bacterial count in individuals who are nasal carriers of staphylococci.

Kanamycin is similar in structure to neomycin but is sufficiently less toxic that it is widely used parenterally for the therapy of infections caused by most of the commonly encountered gram-negative bacilli except *Pseudomonas.* It is also active against staphylococci, but not against the other common gram-positive pathogens such as streptococci and pneumococci. Kanamycin should be administered intramuscularly or by slow intravenous infusion in doses not larger than 0.5 g every 8 hr, and the total dose should not exceed 15 g in patients with normal renal function. Kanamycin is not protein-bound, and is excreted by glomerular filtration; over 80 percent of a dose appears in the urine within 24 hr. In contrast to the penicillins, the toxic blood level is not greatly above the therapeutic blood level, and the dose needs to be decreased when there is impaired renal function. The best way to accomplish this is by measuring blood levels once or twice a day; this can be done by bioassay within 3 or 4 hr. Blood level determinations are not widely available, however, and dosage is usually adjusted on the basis of the serum creatinine. The full therapeutic dose is given every three half-lives, and the serum half-life has been shown to be about three times the serum creatinine. Thus, if the serum creatinine is 7, the half-life is 21, and this means that the usual dose of 0.5 g should be administered every 63 hr. An alternative plan is to administer half the usual dose every half-life; this has the advantage that the drug concentration in the blood does not reach as low a level prior to each succeeding dose. There has been little tendency for pathogens to become resistant to kanamycin despite its widespread use in hospitals. Kanamycin is administered alone to treat specific infections, and is used even more widely in conjunction with other antibiotics in seriously ill patients where the exact etiologic diagnosis is pending, or remains indeterminate.

Gentamicin is similar to kanamycin in its antibacterial spectrum, and in addition is active against *Pseudomonas.* Its toxicity is similar to that of kanamycin except that it is more likely to cause *vestibular* damage rather than deafness. Most gram-negative pathogens are highly susceptible to gentamicin, although MICs vary considerably depending on the medium used for in vitro testing. Human serum potentiates the action of gentamicin against most gram-negative organisms but inhibits its action against *Pseudomonas*; this is related to the presence of calcium. Gentamicin is given in much smaller doses than kanamycin, i.e., 80 versus 500 mg every 8 hours, and a representative peak blood level is 3 to 4 μg per ml, both with intramuscular injections and with slow intravenous infusions. Its basic pharmacology is nearly the same as for kanamycin, and the same principles and detailed procedures that were described above for modifying dosage in the presence of impaired renal function are applicable.

TETRACYCLINES Since they first appeared in the late 1940s, the tetracycline antibiotics have been very widely used because of their broad spectrum of activity against many gram-positive and gram-negative bacteria, and also other microorganisms such as *Mycoplasma, Rickettsia,* and *Bedsonia.* They have been effective, although not necessarily the drugs of choice, in the treatment of common venereal diseases including gonorrhea, syphilis, lymphogranuloma venereum, and granuloma inguinale. Their use has become more restricted during the last decade because of the advent of bactericidal antibiotics such as the cephalosporins, the penicillinase-resistant penicillins, and gentamicin, and increasing awareness of the limitations of the tetracyclines. These limitations include the appearance of resistant strains of commonly encountered pathogens such as Group A streptococci and pneumococci, the primarily bacteriostatic action of the tetracyclines, the occurrence of hepatotoxicity with high blood levels, the relatively high incidence of superinfections, and the common occurrence of side effects such as nausea, diarrhea, and photosensitivity reactions. Despite these limitations, the tetracyclines are still widely used for respiratory, urinary, soft tissue, and venereal infections.

Chlortetracycline (Aureomycin) and *oxytetracycline* (Terramycin), the two original compounds, have been largely replaced by *tetracycline,* which is marketed by a number of companies, and competiton has led to a marked reduction in its price. The usual adult dose is 1 to 2 g daily in two to four equally divided doses. Intramuscular preparations are not very satisfactory, but the intravenous form is well-tolerated and gives relatively high blood levels with doses of 0.5 g every 12 hr. Excessive blood levels occur with renal insufficiency unless the dose is decreased, and can cause fatty degeneration of the liver, which may be fatal because tetracycline persists in the body for many days when its normal route of excretion through the kidneys is blocked.

Four long-acting tetracyclines have been introduced in the last few years: *demeclocycline, methacycline, doxycycline,* and *minocycline.* They have high protein binding (over 90 versus 70 percent for tetracycline) and a prolonged plasma half-life, so that blood levels are well maintained when they are administered orally only every 12 or 24 hr. However, the half-life of tetracycline is sufficiently prolonged so that blood levels with administration only every 12 hr are similar to those of the smaller doses recommended for the long-acting tetracyclines. Unfortunately, the reduction in dose is not matched by a proportionate decrease in price. Thus, the potential advantages of the long-active tetracyclines, i.e., greater convenience from less frequent administration and decreased cost from lower doses, have not been entirely realized, and these preparations cannot be recommended as possessing clear-cut advantages over tetracycline. Doxycycline is the single exception to this because it does not give excessive blood levels in the presence of renal insufficiency following either oral or intravenous administration, and provides a safety feature when the exact status of the patient's renal function is uncertain or unknown.

ERYTHROMYCIN, LINCOMYCIN, CLINDAMYCIN
Erythromycin is primarily a bacteriostatic antibiotic that is active against the commonly encountered gram-positive bacteria, and is used chiefly for the oral therapy of respiratory and soft-tissue infections, particularly in patients thought to be allergic to penicillin. The susceptibility of *Mycoplasma pneumoniae* to erythromycin enhances its usefulness in respiratory infections. Erythromycin base is absorbed in an erratic manner and cannot be relied upon. Erythromycin estolate has been thought to give much higher blood levels than erythromycin stearate, but the difference may be not as great as was once postulated because the estolate needs to be hydrolyzed in the body to the active form, and the hydrolysis is not as complete as during the blood level assay procedure. The estolate salt is associated with a low incidence of cholestatic hepatitis, which is readily reversible and rarely serious. The usual oral dose is 1 or 2 g daily. Intramuscular preparations are irritating, and intravenous administration is not used widely, partly because the preparations are not entirely satisfactory but chiefly because oral therapy is adequate for most infections treated with erythromycin.

Lincomycin and *clindamycin* are similar in antibacterial activity and clinical usefulness to erythromycin. Clindamycin gives somewhat higher blood levels and has less gastrointestinal side effects than lincomycin. An excellent parenteral preparation of both is available. Clindamycin is considerably more active against *Bacteroides fragilis,* and intravenous administration of this antibiotic in abdominal and pelvic infections is widely advocated for this reason.

CHLORAMPHENICOL This antibiotic has a broad spectrum of activity similar to the tetracyclines and during the 1950s was very widely used. However, the occurrence of aplastic anemia, even though quite uncommon (about 1 in 25,000 persons exposed) has led to a restriction of chloramphenicol to those serious infections in which it is quite clearly the drug of choice. Typhoid fever is the principal example, and there are occasionally other severe gram-negative infections where the etiologic agent is susceptible only to chloramphenicol. With increasing interest in anaerobic infections, it is now realized that *B. fragilis* is the commonest of the anaerobic pathogens and that over half the strains are resistant to the penicillins and tetracyclines. This has led to an increase in the use of chloramphenicol since almost all *Bacteroides* strains are susceptible to it. As pointed out above, however, clindamycin is also very active against *B. fragilis*, and since a parenteral preparation has become available, it may largely replace chloramphenicol for the treatment of patients with proved or presumed *Bacteroides* infections. Clindamycin lacks the broad gram-negative spectrum of chloramphenicol, and for this reason, the latter may be preferred under certain circumstances.

Chloramphenicol is well absorbed by the oral route, and the usual adult dose is 0.5 g every 6 hr. The parenteral preparation, chloramphenicol succinate, needs to be hydrolyzed in the body to the active form, and this conversion is incomplete so that the blood levels with intravenous administration are not much higher than when the antibiotic is taken by mouth. With intramusuclar administration, blood levels are considerably lower than with the oral route, and although the drug was widely used by this route for a number of years, the present labeling does not authorize intramuscular injections.

In addition to aplastic anemia, which may be an allergic or "idiosyncratic" reaction that usually occurs with prolonged and repeated administration, chloramphenicol inhibits protein synthesis, especially with doses larger than 2 g a day, an effect that is reversible. Clinically this is manifested by leukopenia, inadequate erythopoiesis (anemia), and thrombocytopenia as well as absence of reticulocytosis, high serum iron, and full saturation of transferrin. To monitor toxicity, blood counts should be performed at least twice weekly and the antibiotic should be stopped if there is significant hematologic toxicity. The gray syndrome, consisting of pallor, listlessness, and often death, occurs in neonates who have inadequately developed hepatic and renal mechanisms for metabolizing chloramphenicol; this can be prevented by restricting the dose to 25 mg per kg per day.

POLYMYXINS Polymyxin B and E (colistin) are polypeptide antibiotics that are active against most gram-negative bacteria except for the *Proteus* group. They have been of importance chiefly because of their action against *Pseudomonas aeruginosa*. However, their use systemically has decreased markedly since the advent of gentamicin and carbenicillin, which appear to be superior.

Polymyxin B is administered intramuscularly every 8 hr, or as a continuous intravenous infusion, in doses no larger than 2.0 mg per kg per day. It is effective in treating urinary infections, but its efficacy in systemic infections is uncertain. Polymyxin B is also administered topically for eye and ear infections, and intrathecally for *Pseudomonas* meningitis. Colistin is available as the sodium salt of colistimethate and is administered in doses of 3.0 to 5 mg per kg per day intramuscularly or intravenously as described for polymyxin B.

Polymyxin B and colistimethate both cause perioral paresthesias and other neurotoxic manifestations with excessive blood levels; of these, apnea is the most life-threatening. Renal irritation and azotemia, which are usually reversible, may also occur. It is important to monitor renal function and to decrease the dose in the presence of renal insufficiency.

VANCOMYCIN Vancomycin is a relatively toxic but highly effective antibiotic that warrants special consideration because of its occasional usefulness in treating certain specific infections. Vancomycin is bactericidal and is effective against gram-positive bacteria including penicillinase-producing staphylococci and enterococci. It is particularly useful in treating severe staphylococcal infections when penicillins and cephalosporins cannot be given, and in the treatment of infections caused by viridans streptococci and enterococci, including endocarditis, under the same circumstances. It can be given only by the intravenous route, and 0.5 g every 6 hr for 2 or 3 weeks is the usual dose. Thrombophlebitis is the principal side effect; it can be minimized by diluting each dose in 100 ml fluid and administering it over a period of at least 1 hr. Chills, fever, renal irritation, and deafness are other adverse reactions that have been described, and these can be minimized by slow administration and by reduction of the dose if renal function is impaired.

SULFONAMIDES The sulfonamides have been used clinically since 1937, and were the principal drugs administered for systemic antibacterial chemotherapy before penicillin and the other antibiotics became generally available. Their role has declined steadily, and they now occupy an important although relatively small place in clinical therapy since they are less active than the antibiotics, they are primarily bacteriostatic, resistant organisms occur frequently, and adverse reactions are common. Uncomplicated urinary tract infections are the principal indication for sulfonamides because of their efficacy, relative safety, and low cost. In addition, sulfonamides are drugs of choice for the therapy of nocardiosis and trachoma. They are no longer the preferred agents for the treatment of bacillary dysentery, meningococcal infections, and *H. influenzae* meningitis. Sulfonamides are still prescribed on a large scale for upper respiratory infections, but their efficacy in this area is highly questionable since the majority of such infections is caused by viruses.

Sulfadiazine, once widely used as an all-purpose sulfonamide, tends to produce crystalluria and has been largely replaced by the more soluble *sulfisoxazole* (Gantrisin) and its close congener, *sulfamethoxazole* (Gantanol). Mixtures of three sulfonamides (trisulfapyrimidines) are also widely used since they are associated with a low incidence of crystalluria. The sulfonamides are usually administered orally, although very satisfactory intravenous preparations of the sodium salts are available. Orally, an initial dose of 2 to 4 g is followed by 1 g every 4 or 6 hr.

Long-acting sulfonamides have also been used widely, and their only advantage is that they can be administered orally only once or twice daily. Examples are sulfamethoxypyridazine and sulfadimethoxine. The primary clinical indication for these long-acting compounds has been urinary tract infections, in instances where the convenience of taking only one dose a day has been considered important. However, it is undesirable to use a drug that leaves the body slowly, because this may prolong adverse reactions. Moreover, certain severe toxic reactions such as erythema multiforme or myocarditis have been reported to occur more commonly with long-acting sulfonamides. It is probably best not to use this class of compounds at all.

There are also some poorly absorbed sulfonamides, succinylsulfathiazole (Sulfasuxidine) and phthalysulfathiazole (Sulfathalidine), that are used principally to decrease the number of bacteria in the colon prior to certain types of abdominal surgery. These agents are of doubtful value. The drug Azulfidine (Chap. 288) is of value in ulcerative colitis.

Adverse reactions caused by the sulfonamides include erythema multiforme, serum sickness, hemolytic and aplastic anemias, arthralgias, hepatitis, nausea, vertigo, and lesions resembling those of polyarteritis nodosa.

ANTIFUNGAL AGENTS *Amphotericin B* is a highly toxic antibiotic that is effective in the treatment of deep-seated mycotic infections. It produces marked improvement and sometimes cures in cryptococcosis, histoplasmosis, blastomycosis, disseminated candidiasis, and coccidioidomycosis, and it has a beneficial effect in at least some cases of aspergillosis and mucormycosis. It is administered intravenously in 5% dextrose solution over a period of 5 or 6 hr. The safest procedure is to administer 1 mg on the first day, 5 mg on the second, and 10 mg on the third. The dose is then increased by 5 to 10 mg each day until 1 mg per kg is being administered daily. The dose may then be changed to 1.5 mg per kg every other day, and treatment is continued for 2 to 4 months, depending on the severity of the infection and upon the patient's response. In patients with severe infections where intensive therapy is considered essential, it may be necessary to assume the risk of administering 15 mg very cautiously as the initial dose, with the addition of antihistamines and/or steroids to help ameliorate the chills and fever, which are quite variable from patient to patient. In some debilitated patients who develop *Candida* infections with oral or esophageal lesions, or bacteremias secondary to intravenous catheters, 10 or 15 mg amphotericin B daily for only 3 or 4 days may be adequate to bring the infection under control.

Some degree of renal impairment invariably occurs when amphotericin B is administered for several weeks; this is manifested during therapy by a rise in the blood urea nitrogen (BUN) and serum creatinine. Renal function may return to normal following therapy if attention is devoted to giving the minimum amount of drug that is compatible with a satisfactory therapeutic response, and if particular attention is directed to lowering the dose and frequency of administration when the creatinine becomes markedly elevated. Many patients have permanent renal damage; this poses special problems when relapses occur and subsequent courses of therapy are needed. Other adverse effects of amphotericin B include anemia, hypokalemia, thrombocytopenia, and hepatitis.

Nystatin (Mycostatin) is another antifungal antibiotic that is less potent than amphotericin B and is too toxic for systemic administration. It is applied topically in ointments, tablets, and suspensions. It is used particularly for oral, intestinal, skin, and vaginal lesions due to *Candida*, and the best results are obtained when applications are made several times a day. The individual dose varies from 100,000 to 1 million units, depending on the location of the lesion.

Flucytosine (Ancobon) is an oral antifungal agent that is relatively nontoxic and has been used successfully in cryptococcal, *Candida*, and *Torulopsis* infections. The dose is 150 mg per kg per day administered in divided doses at 6 hourly intervals. Some cases of cryptococcal meningitis and pulmonary disease have seemed to respond as well as to amphotericin B. Flucytosine is probably less potent than amphotericin. For example, an appreciable percentage of initial isolates of *Candida* is resistant to the drug, and resistance also occurs during therapy. Adverse effects have consisted chiefly of nausea, vomiting, diarrhea, and rashes, but pancytopenia and abnormal liver function tests have also been reported.

Flucytosine is not effective in histoplasmosis, blastomycosis, and coccidiomycosis. It is indicated chiefly in patients with severe cryptococcal, *Candida*, and *Torulopsis* infections who cannot tolerate amphotericin B. It can also be used for *Candida* infections of the bladder and for superficial lesions that do not respond to topical therapy. There is in vitro evidence of synergism between flucytosine and amphotericin B, and it is possible that clinical results in some severe systemic infections may be improved by administering these two antifungal agents together.

ANTITUBERCULOSIS DRUGS *Isoniazid* remains the most important single agent for the treatment of tuberculosis. After years of being considered virtually free from adverse reactions, hepatotoxicity has been reported on a number of occasions, although not sufficiently frequently to make routine liver function tests in individuals receiving prolonged therapy mandatory. *Ethambutol* is replacing aminosalicylic acid (PAS) as the usual companion drug for isoniazid because it avoids the necessity of taking large numbers of tablets and also avoids the gastrointestinal side effects associated with PAS. *Rifampin* is another new, important drug that is comparable with isoniazid in activity against tuberculosis; it should also be used in combination with other drugs to prevent the emergence of rifampin-resistant tubercule bacilli. Streptomycin is still used to some extent, particularly for triple drug therapy in seriously ill, hospitalized patients. The secondary drugs, used chiefly in cases that have failed to respond to initial therapy, are cycloserine, pyrazinamide, ethionamide, and viomycin. These drugs are all associated with significant toxic side effects and should be administered and monitored by experts who are familiar with their use. A more detailed consideration of the antituberculosis drugs and the present treatment regimens is given in Chap. 156.

TABLE 125-2

Conventional antibiotic regimens for adults with normal renal and hepatic function

Organism	*Disease*	*Drug*	*Dosage*	*Route*	*Duration*
Pneumococcus	Lung	Penicillin G	600,000 U q.12h.	IM	5–7 days[1]
	Meningitis	Penicillin G	20 million U/day	IV	7–10 days
	Joints	Penicillin G	20 million U/day	IV	7–10 days
	Endocarditis	Penicillin G	20 million U/day	IV	4–6 weeks[2]
Group A *Streptococcus*	Pharyngitis	Penicillin G	600,000 U/day	IM	10 days[3]
	Erysipelas	Penicillin G	600,000 U/day	IM	10 days[3]
	Other sites	See Pneumococcus			
Coagulase-positive *Staphylococcus*[4]	Furunculosis, cellulitis, abscess	Erythromycin *or*	500 mg q.6h.	PO	7–10 days
		7-chlorlincomycin	500 mg q.6h.	PO	7–10 days
		or cloxacillin	500 mg q.6h.	PO	7–10 days
		or cephalexin	500 mg q.6h.	PO	7–10 days
	Pneumonia	Methicillin *or*	1.0 g q.4h.	IM,IV	10–14 days
		cloxacillin *or*	500 mg q.4h.	PO	10–14 days
		cephalothin	1.0 g q.4h.	IV	10–14 days
	Arthritis	Methicillin *or*	1.0 g q.4h.	IV	10–14 days
		cephalothin	1.0 g q.4h.	IV	10–14 days
Coagulase-positive *Staphylococcus*	Meningitis, endocarditis	Methicillin *or*	1.0 g q.2h.	IV	4 weeks
		cephalothin	1.0 g q.2h.	IV	4 weeks
	Enterocolitis	Vancomycin	500 mg q.6h.	PO	Until diarrhea ceases
Streptococcus viridans	Endocarditis	Penicillin G, *then*	6-12 million U/day	IV	14 days
		penicillin V	500 mg q.4h.	PO	14 days
Strep. fecalis (enterococcus)	Genitourinary infection	Ampicillin	500 mg q.6h.	PO	10-14 days
	Surgical wound	Ampicillin	4.0 g/day	IM or IV	7-10 days
	Endocarditis	Ampicillin *or*	8-12 g/day	IV	4 weeks
		penicillin G plus	20 million U/day	IV	4 weeks
		streptomycin *or*	500 mg q.12h.	IM	2 weeks
		kanamycin	500 mg q.8h.	IM	2 weeks
Neisseria meningitidis	Meningitis, meningococcemia	Penicillin G	20 million U/day	IV	7-10 days
N. gonorrheae	Urethritis	Penicillin G *or*	4.8 million U/day	IM	1-2 doses
		spectinomycin[5]	2 g/day	IM	1 dose
	Arthritis	Penicillin G	6 million U/day	IV	7-10 days
Hemophilus influenzae	Bronchitis and pneumonia	Ampicillin *or*	500 mg q.4h.	PO	5-7 days
		tetracycline	500 mg q.4h.	PO	5-7 days
	Meningitis	Ampicillin *or*	8–12 g/day	IV	7-10 days
		chloramphenicol	25–50 mg/kg/day (given q.6h.)	IV	7–10 days
Brucellosis		Tetracycline *and*	500 mg q.6h.	PO	14 days
		streptomycin	500 mg q.12h.	IM	14 days
Salmonella typhosa		Chloramphenicol[6] *or*	1.0 g q.8h.	IV, PO	14 days
		ampicillin[6]	3.0 g/day	PO, IM IV	14 days
Salmonella	Abscess, bacteremia	Ampicillin	6 g/day	IV	2-4 weeks
Shigella	Stool	Ampicillin	500 mg q.4–6h.	PO, IM IV	7 days
Klebsiella pneumoniae	Genitourinary infection	Gentamicin *or*	40 mg q.8h.	IM	10-14 days
		cephalothin *or*	500 mg q.6h.	IM, IV	10-14 days
		kanamycin	500 mg q.8h.	IM	10-14 days

[1] *Last 3-4 days can be given orally as penicillin V 2 g/day in many cases.*

[2] *Last 2 weeks can be given as penicillin V 4-6 g/day orally.*

[3] *Penicillin V 1-2 g/day for 10 days or a single shot of 1.2 × 10^6 U benzathine penicillin are acceptable alternates.*

[4] *Appropriate doses (see Pneumococcus and Streptococcus) of penicillin G (parenteral) or penicillin V (oral) if organism is sensitive to penicillin G.*

[5] *For patients allergic to penicillin.*

[6] *Start with parenteral but switch to oral as soon as possible.*

[7] *Early follow-up cultures are essential to be sure resistance has not developed.*

[8] *Uncomplicated infections only.*

Organism	*Disease*	*Drug*	*Dosage*	*Route*	*Duration*
K. pneumoniae	Pneumonia, bacteremia	Cephalothin *or*	1.0 g q.4h.	IV	7 days
		kanamycin *or*	500 mg q.8h.	IM	7 days
		gentamicin	5 mg/kg/day in 3 equal doses	IM	7 days
Tularemia		Streptomycin	1.0 g q.12h.	PO	10-14 days
Enterobacter aerogenes	Genitourinary infection	Nalidixic acid[7] *or*	500 mg q.6h.	PO	10-14 days
		kanamycin *or*	500 mg q.8h.	IM	7 days
		gentamicin	40 mg q.6-8h.	IM	7 days
	Bacteremia	Kanamycin *or*	500 mg q.8h.	IM	7 days
		gentamicin	5 mg/kg/day in 3 equal doses	IM	7 days
Escherichia coli	Genitourinary infection	Sulfisoxazole[8] *or*	1 g q.6h.	PO	10-14 days
		tetracycline *or*	500 mg q.6h.	PO	10-14 days
		ampicillin *or*	500 mg q.6h.	PO	10-14 days
		nitrofurantoin	100 mg q.6h.	PO	10-14 days
	Bacteremia, arthritis, peritonitis	Ampicillin *or*	6–12 g/day	IV	7-10 days
		kanamycin *or*	500 mg q.8h.	IM	7-10 days
		gentamicin *or*	5 mg/kg/day in 3 equal doses	IM	7-10 days
		cephalothin	1–2 g q.4h.	IV	7-10 days
	Meningitis	Ampicillin *or*	8–12.0 g/day	IV	7-10 days
		chloramphenicol	25–50 mg/kg/day (q.6h.)	IV	7-10 days
Proteus mirabilis	Urine	Ampicillin *or*	500 mg q.6h.	PO	10-14 days
		cephalexin	500 mg q.6h.	PO	10-14 days
	Blood	Ampicillin *or*	6.0 g/day	IV	7-10 days
		kanamycin *or*	500 mg q.8h.	IM	7-10 days
		cephalothin *or*	6.0 g/day	IV	7-10 days
		gentamicin	5 mg/kg/day in 3 equal doses	IM	7-10 days
Indole-positive *Proteus*	Urine	Kanamycin *or*	500 mg q.8h.	IM	10-14 days
		carbenicillin *or*	1 g q.6h.	IV	10-14 days
		nalidixic acid *or*	500 mg q.6h.	PO	10-14 days
		gentamicin	40 mg q.8h.	IM	10-14 days
	Blood	Kanamycin *or*	500 mg q.8h.	IM	7-10 days
		carbenicillin *or*	2 g q.2h.	IV	7-10 days
		gentamicin	5 mg/kg/day in 3 equal doses	IM	7-10 days
Pseudomonas	Blood, joint	Gentamicin *or*	5 mg/kg/day in 3 equal doses	IM	7 days
		carbenicillin *or*	1.5 g/hr	IV	7 days
		colistin *or*	75 mg q.6h.	IM	7 days
		polymyxin B	30–35 mg q.6h.	IM, IV	7 days
	Meningitis, brain abscess	Gentamicin *or*	5 mg/kg/day in 3 equal doses	IV, IM	5-7 days
		carbenicillin and	1.5 g/hr	IV	5-7 days
		polymyxin B *or*	2 mg	Intrathecally	
		gentamicin	5 mg	Intrathecally	
	Urine	Colistin *or*	75 mg q.6h.	IM	10-14 days
		carbenicillin *or*	2 g q.6h.	IM, IV	10-14 days
		polymyxin B *or*	30 mg q.6h.	IM, IV	10-14 days
		oxytetracycline *or*	500 mg q.6h.	PO	10-14 days
		gentamicin	40 mg q.8h.	IM	10-14 days
Bacteroides	Abscess, bacteremia	Chloramphenicol *or*	0.5 g q.4h.	IV, PO	10-14 days
		Clindamycin	0.5 g q.6h.	IV, PO	10-14 days
Mycoplasma	Sputum	Erythromycin *or*	250–500 mg q.6h.	PO	7 days
		tetracycline	500 mg q.6h.	PO	7 days

MISCELLANEOUS ANTIBACTERIAL AGENTS *Spectinomycin* (Trobicin) is an antibiotic that is effective in single 2- to 4-g doses intramuscularly for the treatment of gonorrhea. Side effects are minimal, and it is useful to have an agent similar in effectiveness to penicillin available for the treatment of patients who are allergic to penicillin or who have failed to be cured by penicillin.

Nitrofurantoin (Furadantin) is an antibacterial agent that is effective in treating urinary tract infections although susceptibility of the *Proteus* group is variable and *Pseudomonas* is resistant. It is administered orally in doses of 100 to 200 mg four times a day. In addition to treating acute uncomplicated urinary tract infections, it is widely used to suppress symptoms of infection in patients with prostatism and other chronic obstructive uropathies. Nausea is sometimes troublesome, and pulmonary hypersensitivity and peripheral neuropathy may occur. The latter is especially likely to occur with renal insufficiency, and nitrofurantoin should be used very cautiously in the presence of uremia.

Nalidixic acid (NegGram) is another drug used orally for urinary tract infections. Its principal defect lies in the rapidity with which bacteria become resistant to it. This means that cultures should be made during, as well as following, therapy to be sure that bacteria are being cleared from the urinary tract. The usual dose is 4 g daily in divided doses for 1 to 2 weeks. Nausea, vomiting, and rashes are the chief adverse reactions. Other agents are usually selected in preference to nalidixic acid because of the problem of resistance.

Troleanodomycin (TAO) is an antibiotic similar to, although less active than, the erythromycins. It is an ester and occasionally causes cholestatic jaundice. In general, erythromycin, lincomycin, and clindamycin are preferable to troleandomycin because of their greater antibacterial activity.

DRUGS OF CHOICE

It is quite clear from reading about the pharmacology of individual agents, as well as about their indications and uses in individual diseases, that many agents are available for the treatment of these diseases. Table 125-2 presents a summary of drugs, indications, dosage schedules, routes of administration, and duration of therapy. The table presents only a limited number of drugs, and many equally acceptable regimens are available. Moreover, while these treatment programs are appropriate for the present, changes in them should be expected as new drugs come on the market and as more experience with the newer agents is gathered.

CHEMOPROPHYLAXIS OF INFECTION

Much of the time antimicrobial agents are directed at *preventing* infection rather than treating it. While it should be possible on theoretic grounds to keep an organism from entering a potential site of infection if that site contains a concentration of antibiotic greater than the minimum inhibitory concentration, in actual fact this does not occur. Instead, most of the time the sensitive flora is eradicated and replaced by a resistant species. However,

TABLE 125-3
Chemoprophylaxis of infections

Usually effective		*Sometimes effective*		*Ineffective*	
Disease or organism	*Drug*	*Disease or organism*	*Drug*	*Disease or organism*	*Drug*
Group A streptococcus (rheumatic fever)	Penicillin G, sulfonamides	Shigellosis	Ampicillin, neomycin	Viral respiratory diseases	
Neisseria meningitidis	Rifampin, minocycline	Gonococcal urethritis	Penicillin	Viral exanthems	
N. gonorrheae (ophthalmia)	Penicillin, silver nitrate	Chronic bronchitis (*Hemophilus influenzae* or *Diplococcus pneumoniae*)	Ampicillin, tetracycline	Clean abdominal surgery	Penicillin and streptomycin
Enteropathic *Escherichia coli* diarrhea	Neomycin, kanamycin	Prolonged labor	Ampicillin, tetracycline	Gynecologic surgery	
Streptococcus viridans (SBE)	Penicillin, vancomycin	Short-term urethral catheterization (< 24 hr)	Ampicillin, tetracycline	Burns Coma Shock	
Congenital syphilis	Penicillin	Cardiac surgery	Methicillin	Congestive heart failure	
Tuberculin contacts	Isoniazid	Large-bowel surgery (preoperative) Cystic fibrosis	Neomycin, kanamycin Tetracycline	Prematurity Prolonged urethral catheterization (> 24 hr) Prolonged intravenous catheterization High-dose steroid therapy	

under certain specific circumstances, when antibiotic prophylaxis is directed at a *single sensitive* pathogen, it may be effective; most of the time these circumstances do not obtain. Table 125-3 summarizes situations in which the efficacy of antimicrobial prophylaxis has been examined. This table is by no means complete; in addition, antibiotics are used prophylactically "by custom"; examples include in skull fractures to prevent meningitis, arterial grafting, lung surgery, major osseous trauma, etc. In these situations the effectiveness of prophylaxis is based on hearsay and "clinical impressions."

DISADVANTAGES OF ANTIBIOTIC PROPHYLAXIS

Even if it is not effective, antimicrobial prophylaxis is unlikely to be harmful if it is maintained for only a short period of time, less than 5 days, and if only a single drug is used in comparatively low doses. On the other hand, prophylaxis with multiple drugs, administered in high doses and for relatively prolonged periods, is much more likely to be harmful. Adverse effects include: (1) superinfections (see above and Chap. 123); (2) increased incidence of toxic or allergic reactions to drugs (Chap. 68); (3) increased cost; and (4) last, but not least, a sense of false security on the part of some physicians. In some instances, antimicrobial prophylaxis tends to promote laxity in the careful observation of the patient. However, many of the patients who are given antibiotics prophylactically are precisely the ones who are susceptible to complicating infections, and in them particular care must be taken to watch assiduously for the development of infection and to treat it promptly when it occurs. Such policy is often superior to the use of antimicrobial prophylaxis.

REASONS FOR FAILURE OF CHEMOTHERAPY

This chapter as well as others dealing with specific disease entities has documented that there are few organisms not sensitive to some antibiotic. Despite this seemingly salutary observation, a large number of patients develop infections and many continue to die from them. In these patients antibiotics appear to have failed. Often this failure of chemotherapy is more apparent than real and may be attributed to one of several reasons.

Failure to adjust the dose of the antibiotic Different doses of antibiotics are required in different locations. For example, 600,000 units penicillin G is more than adequate to cure pneumococcal pneumonia, but as much as 20 million units may be required to cure pneumococcal meningitis and more than 50 million units to treat pneumococcal endocarditis. The pneumococcus in each of these locations remains exquisitely sensitive to penicillin, nor is the penetration of the drug inadequate. However, the host's environment is such that higher doses are required to cure the infections in different locations. Failure to appreciate this phenomenon may lead to inadequate doses.

Treatment of nonbacterial infections Viral infections do not respond to the drugs generally considered as antibiotic agents, and these drugs must not be expected to exact a therapeutic effect in these situations. Similarly, antibiotics do not prevent bacterial complications of viral infections.

Failure to drain purulent material or to remove obstruction Antimicrobial drugs work well only in an environment free of obstruction. Infections will not respond optimally unless obstructions such as a plug of mucus or an enlarged prostate, or a foreign body such as a suture or splinter, are removed, or unless purulent material is drained. It is particularly important to drain an abscess cavity because antibiotics do not kill bacteria enmeshed in pus.

Superinfections The role of antibiotics in promoting superinfections is mentioned above and in Chap. 123. In 2 to 3 percent of patients seeming failure of antimicrobials is a consequence of superinfection.

Drug reaction The development of drug fever without rash or any other manifestation of hypersensitivity may make it appear as if the infection were not responding to therapy, when instead the fever is due to the very drug being given to cure the infection. Drug fever is extremely common with certain antimicrobials, particularly penicillin. The best way to make the diagnosis is simply to discontinue therapy. If fever disappears, the diagnosis is established. A second challenge with the suspected drug is neither necessary nor safe.

Incorrect drug Only rarely does chemotherapy fail because the incorrect drug has been administered. Most drugs have a sufficiently broad spectrum, and combinations of drugs are administered with sufficient frequency, whether indicated or not, to make it highly unlikely that the patient is not given an agent active against the etiologic pathogen. One of the most common errors, when the patient is not responding, is to add more antimicrobials indiscriminately, when the correct course should be to discontinue therapy and to watch the patient.

Defects in host resistance The type of patient requiring antimicrobial therapy has changed from a young or middle-aged individual to an elderly one with degenerative and debilitating disease or one whose host defenses have been compromised by neoplastic disease, large doses of antimicrobials, antineoplastic or immunosuppressive drugs, x-ray therapy, major surgical procedures, or transplants. For a variety of reasons, this type of patient does not, and should not be expected to, respond to antimicrobials as does a normal individual. This factor is often ignored in gauging the results of chemotherapy. It does not mean that antibiotics should not be used when indicated; rather, no miraculous results should be expected in patients with severe associated disease of noninfectious origin.

REFERENCES

The choice of systemic antimicrobial drugs. Med Lett Drugs Ther vol. 14, 1972

CLUFF LE, JOHNSON JE (eds): *Clinical Concepts of Infectious Diseases*, Baltimore: Williams & Wilkins, 1972

GARROD LP, O'GRADY F: *Antibiotic and Chemotherapy*, 3d ed., Baltimore: Williams and Wilkins, 1971

Second International Symposium on Gentamicin. J. Infect Dis 124:S1-300, 1971

SWENSON RM, SANFORD JP: Clinical implications of the mechanisms of action of antimicrobial agents. Adv Intern Med 16:373, 1970

Symposium on Carbenicillin: A clinical profile. J Infect Dis 122:S1-116, 1970

Symposium on Cephalosporin Antibiotics. Postgrad Med J 47:S1-142, 1971

WEINSTEIN L: Chemotherapy of microbial diseases, in *The Pharmacological Basis of Therapeutics*, eds LS Goodman, A Gilman, New York: Macmillan, 1970

section 2 | Infections of specific tissues and anatomic sites

126 LOCALIZED INFECTIONS AND ABSCESSES

ROBERT G. PETERSDORF
IVAN L. BENNETT, JR.

GENERAL CONSIDERATIONS

INTRODUCTION In contrast to most bacterial diseases, which can be conveniently described in terms of their specific etiologic pathogens, there are some in which the clinical picture is determined primarily by their location. Examples of such infections include abscesses, soft-tissue infections, bacterial endocarditis (Chap. 127), pyogenic infections of the central nervous system (Chap. 329), urinary tract infections (Chap. 273), lung abscess (Chap. 253), mediastinitis (Chap. 261), liver abscess (Chap. 298), appendicitis and appendiceal abscess (Chap. 287), diverticulitis (Chap. 288), osteomyelitis (Chap. 129), and infections on the pericardium (Chap. 241). Infections in these sites can be caused by many pathogens, and although their bacteriologic identification may be time-consuming, knowledge of the usual flora causing infection in certain anatomic loci should permit institution of therapy before the results of cultures are available. Although treatment of these infections is usually surgical, the internist may be the first one to see these patients and may also be the one to prescribe chemotherapy on the basis of the presumed pathogen.

ETIOLOGY Localized pyogenic infection can develop in any region or organ of the body, and may be initiated by *trauma* and secondary bacterial contamination, by some *alteration in local conditions* that renders a tissue susceptible to infection with organisms already present as part of the "normal flora" to which it is ordinarily resistant, by *contiguous spread* from a nearby lesion, or by *metastatic implantation* of microorganisms carried in blood or lymph.

Under appropriate conditions of lowered tissue resistance, almost any of the common bacteria can initiate an infectious process. Cultures from open lesions such as those of the skin or from intraabdominal foci arising from perforations of the gastrointestinal tract frequently contain several bacterial species; as might be expected, the organisms found most frequently are the "normal flora" of these regions.

Infection in some areas is more likely to be caused by certain organisms, staphylococci in the skin and coliform bacteria in the urinary tract, and special features of the tissue reaction produced by some bacterial species make it possible to recognize infection by them with considerable accuracy. The *staphylococci* produce rapid necrosis and early suppuration with large amounts of creamy yellow pus (Chap. 129). Group A beta-hemolytic streptococcal infections (Chap. 130) tend to spread rapidly through tissues, causing intense edema and erythema but relatively little necrosis and thin, serumlike exudates; anaerobic streptococci (Chap. 130) and members of the *Bacteroides* group (Chap. 135) produce necrosis and profuse, brownish, foul-smelling pus. *Pseudomonas* infections (Chap. 134) are often rather indolent, with thick, bluish-green exudate; the *pneumococcus* (Chap. 128) stimulates the production of viscid greenish pus containing large plaques of fibrin and denatured protein.

The causative agents of many other diseases are capable of producing localized infection in tissues that are not usually involved in the specific "clinical entities" ascribed to them. An example is the cutaneous ulcer caused by *Corynebacterium diphtheriae*.

The identification of infecting organisms is important in the choice of local or systemic chemotherapy. However, when infection occurs in a certain area, as in paranasal sinuses or cutaneous ulcers, or shows up in sputum, it is unlikely that sterility can ever be achieved. In these locations, serial cultures during therapy must be interpreted in the light of this knowledge.

PATHOGENESIS Factors predisposing to the initiation and persistence of infection in a tissue include trauma, obstruction of normal drainage (sweat glands, biliary tract, bronchial tree, urinary tract), ischemia (infarction, gangrene), chemical irritation (by gastric contents, bile, or intramuscularly injected drugs), hematoma formation, accumulation of fluid (lymphatic obstruction, cardiac edema), foreign bodies (bullets, splinters, sutures), and others such as the occurrence of stasis or turbulence in the vascular system.

Infection in soft tissue usually begins as a *cellulitis*, a diffuse acute inflammation with hyperemia, edema, and leukocytic infiltration but little or no necrosis and suppuration. With some organisms, this is followed by necrosis, liquefaction, accumulation of leukocytes and debris, suppuration, loculation and walling off of the pus, and formation of one or more *abscesses*. Abscess formation is particularly likely to follow infection in a preexisting space or cavity, examples being the fallopian tubes or lung cysts.

The local spread of infection generally follows the path of least resistance along fascial planes; proper surgical treatment is based upon a knowledge of these routes, which will be described for specific infections later in this chapter. Lymphatic spread may lead to lymphangitis, lymphadenitis, or, if the regional nodes suppurate, to the formation of a *bubo*. Involvement of local venules or large veins may lead to infective thrombophlebitis with resulting bacteremia, septic embolization, and systemic dissemination of infection. Staphylococci, streptococci, and bacteroides are notorious for the frequency with which they produce vascular lesions of this type.

Depending upon the infecting organism and the anatomy of the affected region, a small abscess may subside completely; there may be gradual encapsulation of the accumulated pus and persistence of the focus in a quiescent state; or the lesion may "point" and rupture into adjacent tissues or to the outside surface of the body, as usually happens with furuncles. Spontaneous drainage ordinarily leads to subsidence and healing of a superficially situated suppurative focus. However, if the abscess is deeply situated and well encapsulated, there are often persistence of a fistulous tract and the formation of a chronic, draining sinus. *The development of persistent sinuses over an area of suppuration produced by ordinary pyogenic bacteria should always suggest involvement of underlying bone or the presence of a foreign body.* Fistulas that open onto the skin are, of course, soon colonized by microorganisms from the external environment. Ordinary bacterial cultures of drainage fluid almost invariably show a mixed flora and should not be relied upon for the etiologic diagnosis of the underlying disease. This is particularly important in disorders that characteristically lead to persistent sinus formation: tuberculosis, actinomycosis, blastomycosis, melioidosis and glanders, tularemia, and, rarely, amebic abscess of the liver or cecum. In these situations, superficial organisms about the opening of the sinus tract may mask the true nature of the lesion by obscuring the real pathogen.

MANIFESTATIONS Secondary infection of wounds and cutaneous ulcers is usually recognizable by inspection. Infections of the skin and subcutaneous tissues almost invariably produce the classic manifestations: *redness, tenderness, heat,* and *swelling.* Reddish streaks extending proximally and associated with tender enlargement of regional lymph nodes indicate lymphangitis. Systemic symptoms may be absent or mild, or there may be fever, malaise, prostration, and leukocytosis.

Infection and suppuration in deeper tissues or in body cavities are often manifested by local pain and tenderness, but the task of locating and determining the exact nature of the lesion may be difficult. The palpation of a tender mass is helpful, but muscle spasm and intervening structures often interfere. Abdominal or pelvic examination under anesthesia is sometimes useful in these circumstances.

Auscultation may reveal a friction rub over an abdominal viscus, the pleura, or the pericardium. The rapid development of an effusion in the pericardium, pleura, abdomen, or a joint should suggest infection. Similarly, fluid detected by transillumination of paranasal sinuses or inspection of the tympanic membrane may be the first sign of infection.

Depending on the location of an abscess, symptoms and signs referable to encroachment upon adjacent structures may dominate the picture. Respiratory obstruction may be the first sign of mediastinal abscess; dysphagia often first calls attention to peritonsillar or retropharyngeal abscesses; and tamponade is sometimes the initial clue to pericardial infection. Localizing signs of dysfunction are especially striking and important with brain and spinal cord abscesses, although brain abscesses may be clinically silent (Chap. 329). In some patients local pain and tenderness or signs of dysfunction are mild or equivocal, and fever, prostration, and weight loss dominate the picture. The fever may be low-grade but is often hectic, with repeated rigors and drenching night sweats. Fatigue and anemia are frequent, and weight loss may be so rapid as to result in emaciation within a few weeks. A patient with these symptoms and signs may have chronic subphrenic, perinephric, or other abscess in the complete absence of any detectable physical sign pointing to the location of a large accumulation of pus. With the advent of antibiotics some deep-seated abscesses present the picture of a chronic illness manifested by no more than malaise, easy fatiguability, low grade fever, mild anemia, and an elevated sedimentation rate.

Fluctuation of a mass on palpation is a reliable sign that it contains fluid, perhaps pus, but failure to detect this sign when deeper structures are examined is no guarantee that suppuration is absent and should not be taken by itself to indicate that the mass is noninfectious in origin or that drainage is not required.

LABORATORY FINDINGS Peripheral polymorphonuclear leukocytosis is frequent with abscesses, and unexplained elevation of the white blood cell count in any patient should lead to a search for localized suppuration. Depending on the severity and duration of infection, there may be a chronic normocytic, normochromic anemia. The sedimentation rate is almost always rapid. Mild albuminuria, occasionally noted in febrile patients, has no diagnostic import.

Pus or fluid obtained by needle aspiration or incision

of a suspected lesion should *always* be stained and examined directly in addition to being cultured aerobically and anaerobically. Pus is a poor metabolic substrate, and bacteria may fail to grow in cultures from an abscess of long standing. In such instances, the findings on microscopic examination may be the only guide in choosing proper chemotherapy. *Failure to examine exudates with Gram's stain is the single greatest deterrent to appropriate antimicrobial therapy*; it is the responsibility of the internist as well as the surgeon to see that this procedure is performed.

Blood cultures are often positive in intravascular infections such as endocarditis (Chap. 127) and in pyogenic infections in which localized abscesses are metastatic, as in staphylococcal, streptococcal, and *Salmonella* bacteremias. Moreover, manipulation, including surgical incision, of any localized infection may be followed by transient bacteremia.

X-ray examinations may be of considerable help in detecting localized collections of pus when they show atypical collections of gas, displacement of organs, and tissue densities in abnormal locations. Angiography of visceral organs and scintiscans using radioactive materials are also helpful in localizing abscesses.

THERAPEUTIC CONSIDERATIONS Recognition of the striking symptomatic improvement that follows spontaneous evacuation of a suppurative focus led long ago to the adoption of *surgical incision* for the treatment of abscesses. The exact reasons for the amelioration of local and constitutional manifestations that results from drainage of pus are unknown, but, clinically, the benefits of adequate incision and drainage are unequivocal.

Incision of infected tissue before the stage of liquefaction and accumulation of pus is often deleterious and fails to relieve discomfort. Premature incision may even at times facilitate spread of infection. For this reason, it is sometimes necessary to wait until an abscess "ripens," i.e., localizes and "comes to a head." The *application of heat* to an area of inflammation will relieve pain and often speed the subsidence of cellulitis without suppuration. If necrosis of tissue is already under way, hot applications appear to facilitate localization of the process and accumulation of pus, making incision and drainage feasible at an earlier time. Another procedure that aids in reduction of swelling and relief of pain is *elevation of the affected part*.

The availability of specific chemotherapeutic drugs has modified the need for heat, elevation, and incision surprisingly little. The early administration of chemotherapeutics has reduced the incidence of suppurative complications in many disorders, but once suppuration has appeared, antimicrobial drugs become remarkably incapable of eradicating the infecting organisms, although they may mask the classical clinical features of abscess formation.

Some antimicrobials, notably the penicillins, appear to retain their antibacterial activity in the presence of pus, while others, exemplified by the aminoglycosides and the polymyxins, are at least partially inactivated in purulent exudates. However, inability of the drug to penetrate into an area of suppuration is rarely the reason for therapeutic failure. Although this possibility exists in some infections, such as osteomyelitis, it is usually overcome by increasing dosage. Because direct instillation of the antibiotic into an infected area is not, by itself, a curative procedure, other factors are probably more important than faulty diffusion of the agent into the focus. Nevertheless, in some infections, such as empyema or pyarthrosis, and with some agents which provide poor tissue levels, such as the polymyxins, direct instillation of an antimicrobial into an area of suppuration is distinctly worthwhile.

It has been shown clearly that an established inflammatory exudate is a relatively poor environment for bacterial multiplication. Because the bactericidal action of the penicillins and the cephalosporins is exerted only against multiplying organisms, it is believed that failure of these antibiotics to eradicate bacteria in an abscess is related to the organisms' inactive metabolic state. Although the mechanism of their antibacterial action differs from that of the penicillins, bacteriostatic agents such as tetracycline or chloramphenicol also are incapable of eradicating bacteria in the static phase of growth. Furthermore, by definition, these drugs are capable only of inhibiting multiplication of bacteria and usually exert no direct lethal action; the death of organisms in any infection treated with bacteriostatic agents is dependent on other mechanisms. For most pyogenic bacteria, phagocytosis is one of the most important of these mechanisms (although there must be others that have not been studied so carefully), and it is known that, in the absence of phagocytes or in circumstances which inhibit their activity, bacteriostatic drugs are relatively ineffective. In fluid-filled cavities, particularly in the metabolically unfavorable milieu of an abscess, phagocytosis is greatly reduced. Consequently, despite inhibition of bacterial multiplication, organisms can remain dormant and survive for long periods of time. It is probably a combination of these two circumstances, decreased multiplication of bacteria and decreased phagocytosis, that makes infection on the heart valves, in the kidney, or in the meninges so relatively resistant to antimicrobial therapy. Large doses of bactericidal drugs for long periods are needed to achieve cure.

Antimicrobial drugs may be expected to prevent suppuration if given early or to prevent spread of an existing abscess, but cannot be substituted for surgical drainage. Indeed, their use in the face of a lesion requiring evacuation of pus is one of the most common serious errors in treating infections.

In empyema, suppurative pericarditis, or pyarthrosis, excellent therapeutic results are sometimes achieved by aspiration of pus and instillation of antibiotics into the infected area. The success of this procedure, however, is fully as dependent on the adequacy of drainage as it is upon the instillation of the antibiotic, and if there is loculation or if the exudate becomes too viscid to allow removal, surgical incision becomes mandatory.

In the presence of infective thrombophlebitis, surgical interruption of the veins by ligation or, in certain instances, by total excision of an infected segment is often indicated to prevent seeding of other organs by infected emboli.

CLINICAL FEATURES OF INFECTIONS IN VARIOUS REGIONS

Superficial abscesses

SKIN AND SUBCUTANEOUS TISSUES *Impetigo* is a superficial infection caused by hemolytic staphylococci and group A hemolytic streptococci. It is primarily a disease of children, common in warm weather, characterized by multiple erythematous lesions which vesiculate and are intensely pruritic. Local spread occurs through scratching and release of infected vesicle fluid. Serious complications are metastatic abscesses and hemorrhagic nephritis. Treatment consists of local and general cleansing of the skin, application of bacitracin-neomycin ointment, covering with a loose dressing to prevent further contamination, and appropriate systemic antibiotics.

Deeper infections of the skin are almost invariably staphylococcal in origin and are described in Chap. 129. Erysipelas, a characteristic dermal lesion produced by group A streptococci, is described in Chap. 130.

Lymphadenitis with or without suppuration may complicate any pyogenic skin lesion and is often striking with superficial streptococcal infections. Specific diseases characterized by suppurative regional lymphadenitis include lymphogranuloma venereum (Chap. 203), cat-scratch disease (Chap. 204), tularemia (Chap. 141), and bubonic plague (Chap. 142).

INFECTIONS OF THE HAND These are almost invariably secondary to trauma and are very common. Because of the rapidity with which infection can spread through the complex fascial spaces of the hand, wrist, and forearm, with the production of irreparable functional damage, *any deep infection in this area should receive expert surgical attention immediately.* The importance of such care has in no way been lessened by the availability of antibiotics.

The ordinary *paronychia,* or "run-around," is a superficial infection of the epithelium lateral to a nail, usually a result of tearing a hangnail and most frequently caused by staphylococcus. Hot applications will lead to subsidence of paronychial cellulitis, but often a superficial blister of pus appears or the infection burrows beneath the nail to form a painful *subungual abscess.* Incision and drainage with partial or complete removal of the nail are then necessary. Recurrence is common, especially in nail biters, and this seemingly trivial infection can cause painful disability. Chronic paronychial inflammation produced by various fungi occurs in diabetics, and a similar lesion is seen in psoriasis and some types of pemphigus.

What appears to be a small furuncle of the webs of the fingers sometimes produces a *collar-button abscess,* consisting of a superficial and a deep compartment connected by a narrow tract. Evacuation of the shallow pocket without emptying the deeper abscess can lead to puzzling persistence of infection. Sometimes a foreign-body granuloma forms in the skin of the digital webs. This is most common in barbers, in whom a hair is the core of the foreign-body granuloma, the "barber's interdigital pilonidal sinus."

Infection of the distal phalanx of a finger, usually acquired by pinprick, thorn prick, etc., may lead to the formation of a *felon,* or *whitlow.* This is a suppurative infection in the tightly enclosed fibrous compartments of the finger pulp, the "anterior closed space," which can compromise the distal blood supply by compression of the digital arteries, with consequent necrosis of bone and the development of osteomyelitis. The manifestations are swelling, extreme pain, and tenderness of the palmar surface of the finger tip. The treatment is immediate incision, using a lateral approach and cutting all the fibrous septums that radiate from the periosteum to the subcutaneous fascia.

Suppurative tenosynovitis, usually a complication of a puncture wound, is an even more serious infection of the hand from the point of view of functional damage; early diagnosis and treatment are mandatory to prevent permanent disability from destruction of the tendon or its sheath. The three cardinal manifestations of tenosynovitis are (1) exquisite tenderness limited to the course of the sheath; (2) the fingers held in flexion; and (3) extension of the involved finger, producing excruciating pain, most marked at the base of the digit. *Immediate incision* of the sheath is indicated, not only to prevent damage to the tendon itself but to avoid proximal extension of the process into the major fascial spaces of the hand or forearm. Vigorous antibiotic treatment should accompany surgery. The definitive treatment of any serious infection of the hand is a matter for a skilled surgeon, but the early recognition of the need for surgery often falls to other physicians.

Human bites lead to very important hand infections, which, if neglected almost invariably produce a highly destructive, necrotizing lesion contaminated by a mixture of aerobic and anaerobic organisms. A deliberately inflicted bite on the hand or elsewhere is usually recognized as dangerously contaminated, but wounds on the knuckles produced by striking an opponent's teeth with the fists may not be recognized as potentially dangerous. In general, bite wounds should be cleaned thoroughly and not sutured. Patients should be given prophylaxis for tetanus and antibiotics, preferably both a penicillinase-resistant penicillin and ampicillin.

CHRONIC CUTANEOUS ULCERS A partial list of the causes of chronic ulcers of the skin includes circulatory disturbances, such as varicose veins and obliterative arterial disease, extensive injury from frostbite or burns, trophic changes accompanying many neurologic disorders, bedsores or decubiti, systemic diseases such as sicklemia and myxedema, neoplasms, and various infections. No matter what the underlying disease, secondary infection is very likely to occur and to interfere with healing, complicate grafting or other restorative procedures, or produce extension of the process.

The management of secondary bacterial infection in skin ulcers associated with obliterative arterial disease, a common problem in diabetics, is especially important, because infection is frequently the factor that precipitates spreading gangrene and makes amputation necessary.

Studies of the microflora of chronic cutaneous ulcers have almost invariably shown bacteria of many species, including staphylococci, aerobic and anaerobic streptococci, coliform bacilli, and members of the *Proteus* and *Pseudomonas* groups. Depending on the patient's environment and on systemically or locally administered antimicrobial drugs, the predominating bacterial species show great variation when lesions are cultured serially. Particularly noteworthy is the replacement of sensitive organisms by resistant strains or species during the course of chemotherapy.

Treatment of chronic dermal ulcers should be directed toward the underlying disorder but should also include *local debridement* and *chemotherapy.* Debridement by surgical excision is often needed, but the local application of proteolytic enzymes such as Varidase, a mixture of streptokinase and streptodornase, or trypsin, so-called "chemical or medical debridement," is sometimes sufficient. Intensive systemic administration of antibiotics should be carried out only in conjunction with definitive surgical procedures or when infection can be controlled in no other way. The prevention of infection by "prophylactic" administration of antimicrobial drugs is futile because it results in the development of a flora resistant to the drugs being used. The *local application of antibiotics* is sometimes highly effective, and it is in the management of chronic mixed infections of this type that several potent but toxic antibiotics have great value. An ointment or solution containing neomycin, bacitracin, and polymyxin exerts a bactericidal effect against a wide variety of organisms and will sometimes temporarily sterilize a chronic lesion. Other useful topical medications are furacin and 3 percent acetic acid, which is especially helpful in *Pseudomonas* infections.

Diphtheritic ulcer of the skin is discussed in Chap. 151.

INFECTIONS OF THE HEAD AND NECK Pustules of the nose and upper lip may be particularly dangerous, because they are likely to extend intracranially through the angular vein to the cavernous sinus. These lesions should be treated conservatively, manipulation or incision should be avoided if possible, and systemic antibiotics should be used if local swelling or redness appears.

Suppurative parotitis, which is usually a complication of chronic debilitating disease or blockage of Stensen's duct by a calculus, is largely avoidable by maintenance of hydration and oral hygiene. Its onset is heralded by local pain and swelling; fever and chills are frequent. Frank pus can sometimes be expressed from the duct, and the gland itself is firm and tender, often with pitting edema of the overlying skin and facial palsy. Most cases of suppurative parotitis are caused by hemolytic *Staphylococcus aureus.* Treatment consists of removal of obstructing calculi, but its mainstay is antimicrobial therapy with a penicillinase-resistant penicillin, cephalothin or vancomycin. Incision and drainage of a septate gland such as the parotid has not been particularly effective. Despite chemotherapy and drainage, the mortality rate of suppurative parotitis is 30 to 50 percent, perhaps because this infection occurs in patients with debilitating disease.

The use of penicillin and other antibiotics has reduced the incidence of many formerly common suppurative complications of streptococcal pharyngitis. However, as a result of streptococcal sore throat, *Bacteroides* infections of the pharynx, or introduction of infection by trauma to the floor of the mouth or the pharyngeal wall, abscesses of the deep cervical structures still occur. *Suppurative cervical adenitis,* once an all-too-common sequel to streptococcal pharyngitis in children, is now rare. *Peritonsillar abscess (quinsy)* is manifested by fever, sore throat, unilateral pain radiating to the ear on swallowing, and enlargement of the tonsil with redness and swelling of the adjacent soft palate. Treatment with penicillin and irrigations of warm saline solution sometimes lead to subsidence of the process, but if digital palpation reveals fluctuation, surgical drainage with or without tonsillectomy is indicated.

The course of *deep cervical infections* is fully as dependent upon the anatomic arrangement of fascial planes as is that of infections of the hand. Infection in this area is serious and is attended by fever, prostration, and leukocytosis. A tender mass may be palpated, but *surgical evacuation of such an infection should not be delayed because of failure to detect fluctuation,* which is usually absent because of the dense fascial layers.

Infection of the *sublingual space,* so-called "Ludwig's angina," is characterized by brawny induration of the submaxillary region, edema of the floor of the mouth, and elevation of the tongue. There are severe pain, dysphagia, and, within hours, dyspnea from respiratory obstruction. The usual causative organism is a *Streptococcus.* Mortality was formerly about 50 percent. *Treatment* consists of large doses of penicillin and careful observation. If there is significant progression of obstruction during the 4 to 6 hr after treatment is instituted, wide incision is indicated and tracheostomy may need to be performed.

The retropharyngeal space lies between the muscles anterior to the cervical vertebrae and the pharyngeal mucosa. *Retropharyngeal abscess,* formerly common in children, is manifested by dysphagia, progressive stridor, pain, and fever. The bulging mass is easily seen and can completely occlude the airway within hours. Incision and drainage are mandatory; spontaneous rupture may lead to death by aspiration. Tuberculous abscess, secondary to spinal disease, occasionally appears in the retropharyngeal space; it is painless, and relief of obstruction follows surgical incision.

Submastoid abscess, or suppuration in the submastoid space, known as *Bezold's abscess,* is usually secondary to otitis and produces nuchal rigidity, which may lead to a mistaken diagnosis of otogenous meningitis. Infection can extend down the carotid sheath to the mediastinum. A suppurative thrombophlebitis of the jugular vein usually accompanies this infection, and the vessel is easily felt as a tender cord. Bacteremia and systemic spread of infection are common, and the involved venous segment may need to be excised. Spontaneous rupture of the carotid artery with rapid death from exsanguination is a rare complication.

Deep-seated infections

SPLENIC ABSCESS Splenic abscess occurs by several mechanisms: (1) dissemination via the bloodstream during bacteremia; primary foci include the endocardium, lung (lung abscess or pneumonia), pleural cavity (empyema), skin and soft tissues, ear and nasopharyngeal structures, and pelvis (pelvic inflammatory disease and septic abortion); (2) infection in a spleen damaged by bland infarcts (sickle-cell disease, leukemia) or, more rarely, by other diseases such as malaria, typhoid, hydatid or dermoid cysts, and ameboma or by trauma (following subcapsular hematoma formation); (3) extension from a perforated or diseased stomach, colon, or tail of the pancreas, as in carcinoma; and (4) rarely, without apparent cause. Onset is sudden, with chills, fever, and left upper quadrant pain. There are tenderness and muscle spasm, and the skin and subcutaneous tissues overlying the spleen may be edematous. Involvement of the upper pole commonly leads to left pleuritic pain, radiating to the shoulder, with elevation of the diaphragm or left pleural effusion. Lower pole abscess gives signs of tender splenomegaly and peritoneal inflammation. Splenic friction rub is often audible. Disorders to be considered in differential diagnosis are subphrenic abscess, infection of the left lower lobe, bland infarction of the spleen, pancreatic pseudocyst, pyelonephritis, and abscess secondary to perforation of the transverse colon. X-ray examinations are an important adjunct in the diagnosis. Abnormal radiographic findings include (1) soft-tissue mass in left upper quadrant; (2) extraintestinal gas, which may occur even in the absence of gas-forming bacteria but which is probably due to perforation of an adjacent hollow viscus; (3) downward displacement of the splenic flexure of the colon; (4) inferior displacement of the left kidney, best visualized on an intravenous pyelogram; (5) displacement of the stomach bubble medially; (6) elevation of the left hemidiaphragm; and (7) left pleural effusion. Spleen scan is also of great value in localizing the mass.

Treatment consists of administering antibiotics and performing splenectomy. The splenic artery and vein should be ligated prior to splenectomy. Small or multiple metastatic abscesses may subside with antibiotics alone, and abscess in a very ill patient may require splenotomy and drainage, with more definitive surgery at a later time. Splenic abscess is particularly common in patients with sickle-cell disease, but splenic infarction in subacute bacterial endocarditis caused by *Streptococcus viridans* almost never suppurates. Infected splenic infarcts are a rare cause of continued bacteremia in acute bacterial endocarditis, even in the face of massive chemotherapy, and splenectomy may then be necessary to achieve the final eradication of the organism.

SUBPHRENIC ABSCESS Peritoneal infections show a striking tendency to localize in the upper part of the abdomen between the transverse colon and the diaphragm. True subphrenic abscesses are located between the liver and diaphragm on the left or right, and many so-called "subphrenic infections" are, in fact, subhepatic. Most of these infections are related to perforations in the gastrointestinal or biliary tracts, and over half of them follow operations on the gallbladder, duodenum, or stomach. Subphrenic abscesses following perforated appendicitis occur rarely nowadays. Closed blunt trauma following laceration of the liver is an important cause, and a few abscesses occur without predisposing neighborhood infection. These may occur on the left and may be caused by *Salmonella*. The most common organisms are *Escherichia coli*, non–group A streptococci, staphylococci, and *Klebsiella*-enterobacter; mixed infections are common. About 60 percent of abscesses occur on the right, 25 percent on left, and 15 percent are bilateral. They are more common in males and elderly patients, who often have a debilitating disease such as cancer. *Any patient with persistent fever and a history of recent intraabdominal sepsis should be suspected of having a subphrenic abscess.*

Manifestations include fever, upper abdominal pain, and tenderness, usually along the costal margin. Shoulder pain, dyspnea, dullness, and rales at the lung base are more common than abdominal signs and symptoms, and emphasize the location of a true abscess between the liver and the diaphragm. Foul sputum connotes perforation of the abscess into the lung. The localizing signs are by no means striking in all cases, however. The widespread practice of "covering" postoperative patients with antibiotics prophylactically can attenuate subphrenic infection without eradicating it and may result in an insidiously progressive illness with weight loss, malaise, fatigue, and low-grade fever beginning weeks or months after a laparotomy, a syndrome termed *chronic subphrenic abscess.* Roentgenograms may show gas, sometimes with an air-fluid level beneath the diaphragm. The gas is usually from a perforated viscus or enters through an external sinus; it is only rarely the result of bacterial multiplication.

Other radiographic findings include pleural effusion, which is usually sterile, basilar infiltrates, and elevation —but not necessarily fixation—of the diaphragm. Barium meal with the patient in the head-down position may show indentation of the gastric fundus in left subphrenic abscess, a lesion that is often notoriously difficult to localize. Combined lung-liver scintiscan is a considerable advance in the diagnosis of subphrenic abscess.

The outlook in subphrenic abscess is poor because so many patients have cancer as an underlying cause. As to benign predisposing causes, patients who develop subphrenic abscess in the wake of a perforated gastric ulcer seem to do poorly. Even with surgical drainage, the mortality rate approaches 30 to 35 percent; without it, nearly 75 percent of patients die. Drainage should be extraperitoneal, usually through the bed of the twelfth rib. Appropriate antibiotics should be given, both locally and systemically.

RETROPERITONEAL INFECTIONS Strictly speaking, all perinephric and many subphrenic abscesses are located outside the peritoneum, but the term *retroperitoneal abscess* usually refers to infection in the lumbar and iliac regions. Suppuration in these areas is relatively rare, but the importance of recognizing its existence in patients with fever and pain in the lower part of the back is great. In one series, the average duration of illness in 65 patients before diagnosis was approximately 1 month.

Infection in the retroperitoneal space usually reflects extension from posterior perforations of the appendix, small bowel or colon, renal or spinal infections, and occasionally suppurative lymphadenitis in the iliac area, usually secondary to streptococcal infections of the lower extremities in children.

Lumbar abscess is characterized by tenderness and spasm of the back muscles on the affected side, and a mass is usually palpable in the lumbar region; or there may be a prominent, tender abdominal mass without lumbar pain or spasm. Infection in the wall of an abdominal aneurysm, often with *Salmonella*, may present as a lumbar abscess. Flexion of the hip (psoas sign) occurs in a few cases but is more often present with infections lower in the retroperitoneal area. *Fever, leukocytosis*, and *lumbar spasm* should suggest the diagnosis. The absence of a palpable mass may lead to protracted observation, and it is in these instances that palpation under anesthesia is often helpful.

Psoas (iliac) abscess is typically attended by abdominal pain in the iliac or inguinal region, and, particularly when the psoas muscle is involved, severe pain may be referred to the hip, thigh, or knee. Careful palpation of the lower part of the abdomen or groin usually reveals a mass, and fullness and tenderness on rectal examination are common. Hip spasm (psoas sign) is often present. Although psoas abscesses characteristically occur in association with tuberculosis of the spine, the acute bacterial form has been reported in perforation or fistula formation of the bowel in Crohn's disease (regional enteritis). Roentgenograms may delineate the inflammatory mass; pyelography shows displacement of the kidney or ureter in some cases, scoliosis with concavity on the side of the infection, and blurring of the psoas shadow. When regional enteritis is suspected, a small-bowel x-ray and barium enema should be performed. Treatment consists of surgical drainage and appropriate antibiotic therapy.

RENAL ABSCESS Single or multiple abscesses of the renal *cortex* are almost invariably the result of metastatic implantation of staphylococci from another focus. There is no relationship to previous renal disease; the infection occurs in younger individuals, is usually unilateral, and occurs on the right side oftener than on the left. Many patients give a history of recent skin infection such as furuncle. Although acute pyelonephritis is a diffuse disease with foci of cellular infiltrates in the interstitium of the renal medulla, these inflammatory foci may coalesce to form a distinct abscess cavity. This situation probably ensues more frequently than is generally appreciated.

The onset of renal abscess is abrupt, with chill and fever, followed by costovertebral pain and tenderness. If the abscess is cortical, the urine contains *no white blood cells*; medullary abscesses are usually accompanied by pyuria. The stained urinary sediment will show myriads of gram-positive cocci in cortical abscesses, and gram-negative organisms in medullary abscesses. Transient gross or microscopic hematuria may occur at the onset. The white blood cell count is usually elevated and may exceed 30,000 cells per mm^3. Physical signs are usually localized to the region of the kidney, but abdominal spasm may lead to confusion with appendicitis, cholecystitis, or pancreatitis. Early in the disease, ureteral calculus or acute hydronephrosis may be considered as possible diagnoses. Sudden onset of *fever, leukocytosis, and renal pain in the absence of pyuria* should suggest the diagnosis of renal abscess, especially in a patient with infection elsewhere. Obstruction of the ureter by pus or cellular debris may also yield a urine sediment sparse in white blood cells and bacteria. *Treatment* consists of appropriate antibiotics, adequate fluids, and relief of pain. An abscess may suddenly discharge into the renal pelvis, with relief of pain and the passage of cloudy urine containing enormous numbers of leukocytes and bacteria. *Complications* include formation of a thick-walled chronic renal "carbuncle," requiring surgical removal, rupture into the perirenal space, and secondary pyelonephritis, usually produced by coliform bacilli. Recovery is ordinarily prompt, and chronic sequelae are rare.

Perinephric abscess in the past was most often due to hematogenous dissemination during streptococcal or staphylococcal infection, but at present it more often follows calculi in the ureter and hydronephrosis, noncalculous renal infection, tuberculosis, and actinomycosis. Diabetics are particularly susceptible. The causative organisms are those which are primarily responsible in acute pyelonephritis—*E. coli, Proteus* species, and *Klebsiella-enterobacter*. Flank pain with radiation to the upper part of the abdomen, back, or even the shoulder, nausea, vomiting, fever, malaise, leukocytosis, tenderness with spasm of flank and upper abdominal muscles, and a palpable mass which moves with respiration are the main manifestations. Symptoms referable to the urinary tract are present when perinephric abscess is associated with pyelonephritis or stone. In a few patients, elevation of the diaphragm on the diseased side occurs and leads to confusion with subphrenic infection. The psoas muscle is involved by the inflammatory process, and patients are frequently more comfortable with the thigh held in flexion. The roentgenogram occasionally will reveal a mass; there is usually blurring of the renal silhouette; and the psoas shadow is indistinct on the involved side. There may also be scoliosis to the side of the lesion, fixation of the kidney, anterior displacement of the organ on lateral pyelograms, and gas formation within the perinephric mass, or total nonvisualization of the kidney. Chest roentgenograms often show basal infiltrates and pleural effusions. Complications include perforation into adjacent organs, particularly the colon. *Treatment* by surgical drainage and systemic administration of antibiotics (*not* urinary antiseptics) is usually followed by dramatic subsidence of pain and fever, and unless intrinsic renal disease is present, recovery is complete. Nevertheless, the overall outcome is poor, in part because the diagnosis is often made too late or is missed altogether, and also because of the generally poor condition of many of these patients.

RECTAL ABSCESS Suppurative diseases of the anorectal region have been classified in several ways, most of the classifications being based on the surgical approaches required for drainage. Infection in the apocrine glands (hidradenitis) or folliculitis in the perianal region, extension of cryptitis or obstructions in the "anal glands" which open into the crypts of Morgagni, and contamination of submucosal hematomas, sclerosed hemorrhoids, or anal fissures may lead to abscess formation. These are usually painful, easily palpable, often visible on inspection. Superficial rectal abscesses may be confused with Bartholin's cysts, sebaceous cysts, tuberculosis, actinomycosis, urethroperineal fistulas, carcinoma of the anus, foreign body, and pilonidal sinus. Treatment is application of heat and appropriate drainage or excision. Antibiotics may be indicated in some instances.

Difficulties in diagnosis are likely to arise with infections higher in the rectum, especially those above the pelvic diaphragm, the so-called *supralevator abscess.* Patients with this type of infection often have fever, malaise, and leukocytosis for several days or even weeks before any symptoms referable to the rectum develop. There is vague pelvic discomfort, relieved by defecation, and constipation punctuated by short episodes of diarrhea is common. In males, the inflammation often involves the base of the bladder, and urinary urgency or retention is not infrequent, falsely centering attention on the urinary tract as the source of fever and malaise. Eventually, the abscess produces severe pain, chills, and fever; palpation and instrumentation will reveal the swelling in the rectal ampulla. Such an abscess may surround the rectum and produce narrowing that is differentiated from that caused by neoplasm by the fact that the mucosa remains intact. A useful sign of deep rectal abscess is eliciting of severe pain by pressure in the region between the anus and the coccyx. The supralevator space is continuous with the ischiorectal space, with both the gluteal and obturator regions, and with the retroperitoneal space. In neglected cases, the abscess may drain through the skin of the perineum, the groin, or the buttock or may extend as high as the perirenal areas. Rectal abscesses are not uncommon in patients with diabetes, and infections in this area are also peculiarly frequent in patients with acute leukemia, especially when the white count is severely depressed. Because the clinical picture may be that of "fever of unknown origin" for a long period, it is important that thorough digital and endoscopic examination of the rectum be carried out in febrile patients. A rectal examination should be made in all patients with diabetes, especially if ketosis is present; failure to observe this rule has more than once led to delay in detecting the infection responsible for diabetic ketosis or coma.

A rectal abscess may be a forerunner of both ulcerative colitis and regional enteritis, and may occur months and even years before other overt manifestations of these diseases. For this reason, proctosigmoidoscopy, barium enema, and, often, upper gastrointestinal roentgenograms are indicated in nonhealing rectal lesions.

Treatment of high rectal abscesses consists of incision and drainage, hot sitz baths, analgesics, and antibiotics as indicated by culture of the exudate.

REFERENCES

Deep abscesses

BARNHILL JF: Deep abscess of the neck: Surgical treatment. Am J Surg 42:207, 1938

BURGER RH et al: Perinephric abscess with gas formation. Am Surg 30:302, 1964

CURRERI WP et al: Subphrenic abscess secondary to salmonellosis. Arch Surg 95:189, 1967

EISENHAMMER S: The internal anal sphincter and the anorectal abscess. Surg Gynecol Obstet 103:501, 1956

FRANKEL A et al: Splenic abscess. J Mt Sinai Hosp NY 33:404, 1966

GASTON EA, WARREN LO: Supralevator abscess. N Engl J Med 229:613, 1943

JANKE WH, BLOCK MA: Chronic retroperitoneal pelvic abscesses. Arch Surg 90:389, 1965

JOHNSON TH JR: The subdiaphragmatic abscess in the antibiotic era. South Med J 61:455, 1968

KYLE J: Psoas abscess in Crohn's disease. Gastroenterology 61:149, 1971

MAGILLIGAN DJ JR: Suprahepatic abscess. Arch Surg 96:14, 1968

OZERAN RS: Subdiaphragmatic abscess. Am Surg 33:64, 1967

PETERSDORF RG et al: Staphylococcal parotitis. N Engl J Med 259:1259, 1958

RICHARDS L: Retropharyngeal abscess. N Engl J Med 215:1120, 1936

ROSENBERG M: Chronic subphrenic abscess. Lancet II:379, 1968

SALVATIERRA O JR et al: Perinephric abscess. J Urol 98:296, 1967

Superficial abscesses

BUNNELL S: *Surgery of the Hand,* 4th ed., ed TH Boyes, Philadelphia: Lippincott, 1964

127 BACTERIAL ENDOCARDITIS

LEIGHTON E. CLUFF

DEFINITION Bacterial endocarditis is a microbial infection of the heart valves or of the endocardium in proximity to congenital or acquired cardiac defects. A similar clinical illness develops when there is infection of arteriovenous fistulas or aneurysms. The infection may develop abruptly or insidiously, may pursue a fulminant or prolonged course, and is fatal unless treated. The infection caused by indigenous microorganisms with low pathogenicity is ordinarily subacute, whereas infection by microorganisms with high pathogenicity is often acute. Fever, cardiac murmurs, splenomegaly, anemia, hematuria, mucocutaneous petechiae, and embolic manifestations are characteristic of the disease. *Streptococcus viridans* is the commonest cause of bacterial endocarditis when superimposed upon congenital or acquired endocardial lesions and usually is associated with a subacute course.

ETIOLOGY AND EPIDEMIOLOGY *Acute bacterial endocarditis* is caused by relatively pathogenic microorganisms, exemplified by *Staphylococcus aureus,* pneumococcus, group A streptococcus, gonococcus, and less often *Histoplasma capsulatum, Brucella,* and *Listeria.* Endocarditis attributed to these organisms usually follows dissemination from an infected focus, which is often insignificant. Gonococcal, staphylococcal, and monilial endocarditis has been described frequently in narcotic addicts. Staphylococcal, monilial, and coliform bacilli infection of the heart resembling endocarditis has become a serious complication of surgery in which sutures or prostheses are placed in the heart or peripheral arteries. Endocarditis is sometimes observed in association with pneumococcal meningitis and bacteremia (Chap. 128). Staphylococcal endocarditis can result from bacteremia associated with septic thrombophlebitis or complicating a cutaneous, bone, or pulmonary infection. Group A streptococcal endocarditis is probably never a complication of septic sore throat, but it may follow the bacteremia of streptococcal skin or puerperal infection.

Subacute bacterial endocarditis develops usually in persons with acquired valvular or congenital cardiac lesions. It is most commonly caused by S. *viridans,* which is part of the normal upper respiratory bacterial flora. *Streptococcus faecalis* (enterococcus), indigenous to the fecal and perineal flora, is also an important cause of subacute bacterial endocarditis, particularly in elderly men, and often occurs in association with prostatism or other genitourinary conditions. *Staphylococcus aureus* may produce subacute as well as acute bacterial endocarditis. Suppuration, cellulitis, or other infected foci may precede subacute bacterial endocarditis but are recognized infrequently. *Streptococcus viridans* is commonly found in the blood immediately after dental extractions. Tonsillectomy is also occasionally associated with transient bacteremia. Chewing of food may result in bacteremia in patients with gingival disease or dental infection. Transient bacteremia of this sort is probably an important initiating factor in subacute bacterial endocarditis.

PATHOGENESIS Subacute bacterial endocarditis occurs most frequently in persons with preexisting heart disease in the absence of congestive cardiac failure or chronic atrial fibrillation. Valvular stenosis without insufficiency is infrequently associated with bacterial endocarditis. Infection most commonly involves the left side of the heart. The mitral, aortic, pulmonary, and tricuspid valves may be involved, in the order of frequency as listed. Valves damaged by rheumatic fever are most commonly involved, but valves damaged by syphilis and arteriosclerosis are also susceptible to bacterial endocarditis. Enterococcal endocarditis in elderly men is associated with involvement of the aortic valve, and frequently results rapidly in marked valvular damage. Subacute bacterial endocarditis rarely involves interatrial septal defects. Infection in patients with interventricular septal defects often involves the endocardium opposite the septal defect in the direction of the shunt. Infection associated with patent ductus arteriosus develops in the pulmonary side of the ductus. Valvular infection in association with rheumatic heart disease is usually on the valve edge along the line of closure.

Hemodynamic events are important in the pathogenesis of the disease. Alterations in blood flow can cause marked changes in vascular endothelium. It has been demonstrated experimentally that bacteria are deposited on the endothelium in areas of high flow with decreased lateral pressure. These factors are undoubtedly important in determining the situations and location where bacterial endocarditis develops. Infection in the heart is most often at a site of a structural change or abnormality. Thrombi developing on endocardial irregularities have been implicated as foci for bacterial implantation, and infection has been shown in thrombotic endocardial lesions. It seems likely that a sterile vegetation consisting of platelets and fibrin is the nidus on which bacteria become implanted.

Serum antibody in high titer against the infecting microorganism is often found in patients with bacterial endocarditis. However, the role of immunity in bacterial endocarditis of man is not known.

Bacterial endocarditis leads to deposition of fibrin and platelets at the site of infection, producing a *vegetation.* Highly pathogenic microorganisms often cause valvular destruction and ulceration. Less pathogenic microorganisms usually cause less valvular destruction or ulceration but can lead to development of large polypoid vegetations. The infection may extend from the valve to the mural endocardium. Involvement of chordae tendineae may lead to rupture and profound valvular insufficiency. Acute bacterial endocarditis, particularly when caused by *Staph. aureus,* often is associated with abscesses in the valve ring. Vascularization of involved valves may increase during endocarditis but rarely extends into the area of infection. Phagocytes are not prominent in the area of bacterial growth, which may explain why infection by microorganisms of low pathogenicity progresses uncontrolled without bactericidal antimicrobial therapy. The lack of vascularization of the granulation tissue in the vegetation also may account for ineffectiveness of host defenses and the requirement for intensive and prolonged treatment.

The bacteremia of bacterial endocarditis is ordinarily continuous. For this reason few blood cultures are required to demonstrate the microorganisms. The microorganisms are primarily cleared from the blood by the reticuloendothelial cells of liver and spleen. There is no obvious reduction in the number of bacteria in the blood during circulation through the extremities. Arterial blood cultures, therefore, are no more likely to show bacteremia than are venous blood cultures.

Embolization is a characteristic feature of bacterial endocarditis. The friable fibrin vegetations may separate from the site of infection and be propelled as emboli into the systemic or pulmonary circulation, depending on whether the endocarditis involves the left or right side of the heart. Emboli vary in size but may involve the brain, spleen, kidney, gastrointestinal tract, or extremities. Pulmonary infarction is common in right-sided endocarditis. Septic infarction is uncommon in subacute bacterial endocarditis caused by microorganisms of low pathogenicity, and suppurative complications are rarely seen at these sites when *S. viridans* is the offending agent. Osteomyelitis has been described, however, as an embolic complication of endocarditis due to *S. viridans* and enterococci. Septic infarction is common in acute bacterial endocarditis attributable to bacteria of high pathogenicity, as are metastatic abscesses. Involvement of vasa vasorum in major arteries by emboli produces mycotic aneurysms, which may rupture. Myocardial infarction may develop after coronary embolization. In addition, focal myocarditis is common in subacute bacterial endocarditis and may be embolic.

The spleen is almost always enlarged, particularly in subacute cases. Three types of renal lesions may be produced. When large emboli find their way into the kidney, infarction may develop. Smaller emboli may produce a focal glomerulitis. In most instances there is a diffuse glomerulonephritis that is difficult to distinguish from other types of immune complex glomerulonephritis. Petechial skin lesions, characterized histologically by acute vasculitis, are probably not embolic and may be immunologic in origin. Other skin lesions associated with pain, tenderness, and cellulitis, however, may be embolic.

MANIFESTATIONS **Subacute bacterial endocarditis** Patients ordinarily cannot date the onset of the infection. Symptoms begin insidiously, and gradually the illness becomes apparent. In some individuals, however, the onset of infection can be related to a recent dental extraction, urethral instrumentation, tonsillectomy, acute respiratory infection, or abortion.

Weakness, fatigability, weight loss, feverishness, night sweats, anorexia, and arthralgia are the usual symptoms of subacute bacterial endocarditis. Emboli may produce paralysis, chest pain, acute vascular insufficiency with pain in the extremities, hematuria, acute abdominal pain, or sudden blindness. Painful fingers or toes and painful skin lesions may also be important symptoms. Chills are not common.

Physical examination may reveal a variety of findings, none of which alone is pathognomonic of subacute bacterial endocarditis. The association of the different manifestations, however, usually provides a characteristic picture of the disease. The patient usually appears chronically ill and pale and has an elevated temperature. The fever is most often remittent, with afternoon or evening peaks. The pulse is usually rapid, and if cardiac failure complicates the infection, it may be greater than expected with the degree of fever.

Mucocutaneous lesions are common and vary in type. Petechiae are most frequent and may be found in the mucosa of the mouth, pharynx, or conjunctivas. These small, red hemorrhagic-appearing lesions do not blanch on pressure and are not tender or painful. On the mucous membranes or conjunctivas these petechiae may have a pale center (Fig. 127-1). Small, occasionally flame-shaped, hemorrhages are found in the retina, and may also have pale centers (Roth's spots). Petechiae may be found anywhere on the skin but are most common over the upper trunk anteriorly. They are frequently difficult to distinguish from angiomas, but they gradually become brownish and disappear. Frequently, petechiae continue to appear, even during convalescence. Linear hemorrhages (splinter hemorrhages) may be found under the nails, but these are difficult to differentiate from traumatic lesions, particularly in manual laborers. These mucocutaneous lesions are not specific for bacterial endocarditis but may be found in patients with other diseases such as profound anemia, leukemia, trichinosis, and sepsis without endocarditis.

The pulp of the fingers may show tender subcutaneous papules which are purplish or erythematous (Osler's nodes). Larger erythematous, painful, and tender nodules may develop on the palms of the hands or soles of the feet. These are probably embolic lesions. Emboli to larger peripheral arteries may result in gangrene of fingers, toes, or larger portions of the extremities.

Clubbing of the fingers is observed in long-standing or prolonged bacterial endocarditis. Mild jaundice is found occasionally.

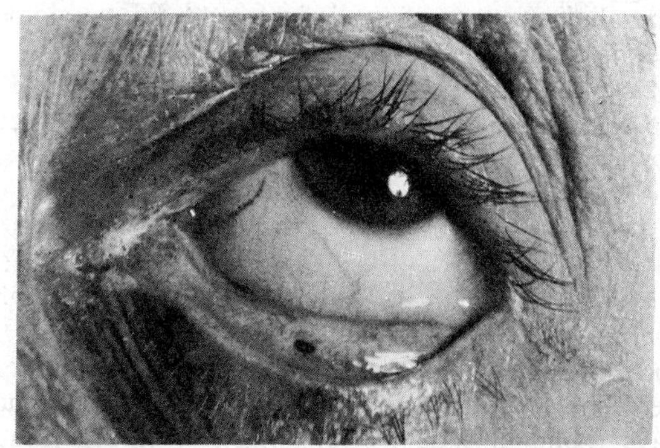

FIGURE 127-1
White-centered conjunctival petechia in a patient with subacute bacterial endocarditis. (Courtesy Dr. John Wedgwood, Cambridge, England)

Findings in the heart are usually those of underlying heart disease. Major changes in cardiac murmurs, primarily a development of a new diastolic murmur, may be attributable to ulceration of a valve, dilatation of the heart or valve ring, rupture of chordae tendineae, or development of a very large vegetation. Minor changes in systolic bruits are usually of little significance. In rare instances, no cardiac murmurs are detected. In this situation, right-sided endocarditis or an infected pulmonary or peripheral arteriovenous fistula should be suspected.

Splenomegaly is common in subacute bacterial endocarditis. Rarely is the spleen tender, but a friction rub may be heard over it when there is infarction. Hepatomegaly is not characteristic unless heart failure develops.

Arthralgia is relatively common, and arthritis resembling acute rheumatic fever may occur.

Embolic phenomena may precipitate awareness of the infection. Sudden development of hemiplegia, flank pain with hematuria, abdominal pain with melena, pleuritic pain and hemoptysis, left upper abdominal pain with splenic friction rub, blindness, or monoplegia in a patient with fever and cardiac murmurs makes bacterial endocarditis suspect. Pulmonary emboli in right-sided endocarditis may be confused with pneumonia.

Acute bacterial endocarditis Infectious endocarditis caused by highly pathogenic microorganisms usually begins abruptly. Suppurative infection commonly antedates the onset of endocarditis. For example, infection of the heart may develop as a complication of pneumococcal meningitis, septic thrombophlebitis, group A streptococcal cellulitis, or staphylococcal abscesses. The source of cardiovascular infection, therefore, is often evident.

Acute bacterial endocarditis often involves the normal heart, in contrast to the subacute infection, which almost invariably involves the abnormal heart. It is particularly common in intravenous drug users. The acute infection is fulminant and pursues a rapid course. Fever is often greater, may be intermittent, and in certain instances (as in gonococcal endocarditis) may be characterized by a double quotidian temperature curve. Chills are common. Petechiae may be numerous, and embolic phenomena are prominent. Osler's nodes and painful erythematous nodules of palms and soles are uncommon. Hematuria is seen with embolic lesions of the kidney, and diffuse glomerulonephritis may occur. Destruction of the cardiac valves can be complicated by rupture of chordae tendineae or perforation of cusps, leading to rapidly progressing cardiac failure. Metastatic abscesses are frequent following septic emboli.

LABORATORY FINDINGS Leukocytosis with neutrophilia is the rule but is by no means an invariable finding. Macrophages (histiocytes) may be found in the blood, particularly in the first drop of blood obtained from the earlobe. Normocytic, normochromic anemia is almost always found in subacute bacterial endocarditis, but it may not be present early in acute bacterial endocarditis. The erythrocyte sedimentation rate is increased. Serum immunoglobulins are increased but return to normal during convalescence. The anti-gamma-globulin latex fixation test is commonly positive, and the Rose-Waaler test is negative. Mild bilirubinemia is detected occasionally. Proteinuria is common, and microscopic hematuria is frequent.

Blood cultures are positive in the majority of cases. Three to five cultures of 10 ml blood taken at short or long intervals, depending on the patient's clinical status, are usually adequate to demonstrate the bacteremia, if it is demonstrable at all. Blood cultures may not become positive for several days, however, in patients who have been receiving penicillin prophylactically for rheumatic heart disease. Similarly, the cultures may be temporarily negative or growth may be delayed in patients who have received antibiotics prior to the time when cultures are obtained. Failure to demonstrate bacteremia also may be attributable to infection by unusual microorganisms such as *H. capsulatum, Brucella, Pasteurella,* or anaerobic streptococci which require special nutrient media or culture methods. Endocarditis of the right side of the heart is as likely to produce bacteremia as endocarditis involving the left side of the heart.

DIFFERENTIAL DIAGNOSIS When several of the manifestations of bacterial endocarditis occur together, the diagnosis is not difficult. In particular, the presence of fever, petechiae, splenomegaly, microscopic hematuria, and anemia in a patient with cardiac murmurs is most suggestive of infection. When only a few manifestations are present, however, the diagnosis is not simple. Prolonged fever in a patient with rheumatic heart disease is particularly troublesome, but the diagnosis of bacterial endocarditis should be considered in every patient with fever and a heart murmur. The diagnosis becomes even more difficult when blood cultures show no growth.

Acute rheumatic fever with carditis is often difficult to distinguish from bacterial endocarditis, and in a few instances, active rheumatic fever has been found to coexist with the valvular infection. The diagnosis of rheumatic carditis hinges on a combination of clinical and laboratory criteria (Chap. 238).

Subacute bacterial endocarditis is a common cause of "fever of undetermined origin" (Chap. 12). It may be mistaken for a hidden neoplasm, systemic lupus erythematosus, periarteritis nodosa, poststreptococcal glomerulonephritis, and intracardiac tumors such as myxoma of the atrium. Dissecting aneurysms with acute aortic insufficiency also may mimic bacterial endocarditis. Drug fever may be erroneously diagnosed as bacterial endocarditis. Postoperative endocarditis should be suspected in patients who develop fever, anemia, and leukocytosis after cardiovascular surgery. These intracardiac infections tend to develop about a suture or prosthesis. Symptoms and signs may be indistinguishable from bacterial endocarditis, but may be sparse and consist only of fever or a change in cardiac sounds. "Nonpathogenic" organisms such as *Staph. albus,* diphtheroids, and other micrococci may be cultured. The infection usually cannot be controlled unless the foreign body is removed. In these postoperative patients, the various postthoracotomy and postcardiotomy syndromes must also be considered.

PROGNOSIS Recovery from untreated bacterial endocarditis is rare. With appropriate antibiotic therapy, however, over 70 percent of patients survive the infection. The infection has a poor prognosis when complicated by congestive heart failure, when unassociated with demonstrable bacteremia, when produced by antibiotic-resistant microorganisms, or when therapy is delayed. Acute bacterial endocarditis is associated with the poorest prognosis.

The commonest cause of death in treated endocarditis is congestive heart failure, attributable either to valve destruction or myocardial damage. Additionally, death may be precipitated by embolization to vital organs, by renal insufficiency, or by rupture of a mycotic aneurysm. Many patients recover completely without apparent worsening of the underlying cardiovascular disease. When recurrent endocarditis develops, it usually involves the same valve and is due to failure to kill microorganisms in an environment of suboptimal host resistance.

PROPHYLAXIS Patients with congenital, syphilitic, arteriosclerotic, or rheumatic valvular heart disease should be given antibiotics before and immediately after dental manipulation, urethral catheterization, or other forms of intubation. The rationale for this practice is that when these patients get bacteremia they are more prone to develop endocarditis. The best experimental evidence available holds that for prevention of *S. viridans* endocarditis with penicillin, both a high concentration and prolonged duration of action are necessary. This can be achieved with a single dose of 2 million units of aqueous and 600,000 units of procaine penicillin administered within 30 min of dental surgery. A single dose of 1.2 million units of procaine penicillin plus 1.0 g streptomycin or 1.0 g vancomycin are equally effective. The best regimen for preventing *S. fecalis* endocarditis is ampicillin plus streptomycin. *The prophylactic doses of penicillin used to prevent group A streptococcal infection and recurrent rheumatic fever will not prevent bacterial endocarditis,* although these doses of penicillin (200,000 units once or twice daily) rarely predispose to bacterial endocarditis caused by penicillin-resistant microorganisms.

TREATMENT Successful therapy of bacterial endocarditis is ensured when treatment is begun early in the illness, when an effective *bactericidal* antimicrobial is selected, and when treatment is continued over a long period of time.

Selection of the most effective antibiotic for treatment of bacterial endocarditis depends on the sensitivity of the infecting microorganism. When bacteremia is not demonstrated, selection of the therapeutic agent depends on understanding the probable infecting bacteria and their probable antibiotic sensitivity.

Bacterial endocarditis in young persons with rheumatic or congenital heart disease is most often due to *S. viridans*. These microorganisms are usually very sensitive to penicillin G. Administration of 2.4 to 6 million units of penicillin daily to these patients is usually effective in eliminating the infection when therapy is continued for 4 weeks. The penicillin should be given parenterally for 2 weeks but for the second two weeks may be oral (phenethicillin or V-cillin). There is a synergistic effect of streptomycin with penicillin on *S. viridans*, and streptomycin in a dose of 0.5 g twice a day may be administered in addition to penicillin. Streptomycin should be given for no longer than 2 weeks.

Bacterial endocarditis in older men and in women after abortion or endometritis is often due to *S. faecalis* (enterococci). These microorganisms are relatively resistant to penicillin alone. The combination of penicillin with streptomycin is synergistic against these bacteria, however, and administration of these two antibiotics together is the treatment of choice in the infection. Penicillin G should be given parenterally in a dose of 6 to 20 million units a day, together with streptomycin in a dose of 0.5 to 1.0 g twice a day. Ampicillin in dosage of 6 to 12 g a day may be substituted for penicillin G. Treatment must be continued for a minimum of 4 weeks.

Penicillin G, 6 to 12 million units a day given parenterally, is satisfactory for treatment of pneumococcal and group A streptococcal endocarditis. Treatment should be continued for 4 weeks. Penicillinase-resistant penicillin analogues should be used in the initial treatment of staphylococcal endocarditis, because of the possibility that the infection is due to a penicillin-resistant organism. Methicillin should be given parenterally in a dose of 12 g per day, intramuscularly in divided doses or intravenously. If injected intravenously, the antibiotic should be given in divided doses in 50-ml volumes injected over 5 to 10 min. Oxacillin, cloxacillin, nafcillin, cephalothin, and vancomycin may be administered in lieu of methicillin. If the staphylococcus is found to be sensitive to penicillin G, this antibiotic should be given rather than methicillin, in a dose of 6 to 10 million units per day. Treatment should be continued for at least 4 weeks. In staphylococcal endocarditis, in particular, attention must be given to possible metastatic abscesses requiring surgical drainage.

In patients allergic to penicillin, cephalothin, vancomycin, lincomycin, and erythromycin are alternative drugs. If an allergic reaction to penicillin develops during the course of therapy, antihistamines may be used to alleviate the manifestations of the reaction. In several instances, corticosteroids have been employed to suppress allergic drug reactions during treatment of bacterial endocarditis without deleterious consequences, as long as an effective antimicrobial drug is used to treat the infection.

At times, probenecid, in dosage of 0.5 g twice daily, may be given with penicillin or its analogues to slow renal excretion of the antibiotic and to increase blood levels. This regimen may be employed to provide a margin of safety but should not be substituted for adequate doses of the antibiotic.

Fever begins to disappear usually within 3 to 7 days after the start of treatment of bacterial endocarditis. Embolic complications of the disease, heart failure, and infection by insusceptible microorganisms, however, may delay defervescence. Drug fever may occasionally supervene and complicate the febrile course. Cessation of all therapy for 72 hr is not hazardous and may identify such a drug reaction readily.

Some patients with arteriovenous fistulas and infected cardiac prostheses may require surgical intervention before the infection can be controlled. In addition, early valve replacement should be considered in patients who develop marked valvular damage (particularly aortic regurgitation) as a consequence of bacterial endocarditis. Valve replacement has been lifesaving and must be effected before intractable heart failure ensues.

When bacterial endocarditis recurs, it usually develops within 4 weeks after treatment is terminated. Reinstitution of antibiotic therapy will be required, but the sensitivity of the microorganism to the antibiotic must be reevaluated. Relapse may indicate inadequate or inappropriate therapy. If bacterial endocarditis develops more than 6 weeks after cessation of treatment, it usually is a new infection.

REFERENCES

BRANIFF BA et al: Valve replacement in active bacterial endocarditis. N Engl J Med 276:1464, 1967

CHERUBIN CE et al: Infective endocarditis in narcotic addicts. Ann Intern Med 69:1091, 1968

——, NEU HC: Infective endocarditis at the Presbyterian Hospital in New York City from 1938–67. Am J Med 51:83, 1971

DURACK DT, PETERSDORF RG: Chemotherapy of experimental streptococcal endocarditis: I. Comparison of commonly recommended prophylactic regimens J Clin Invest 52:592, 1973

GOODMAN JS et al: Infection after cardiovascular surgery: Clinical study including examination of antimicrobial prophylaxis. N Engl J Med 278:117, 1968

GREEN GR, et al: Treatment of bacterial endocarditis in patients with penicillin hypersensitivity. Ann Intern Med 67:235, 1967

GUTMAN RA et al: The immune complex glomerulonephritis of bacterial endocarditis. Medicine 51:1, 1, 1972

HOOK EW, KAYE D: Prophylaxis of bacterial endocarditis. J Chronic Dis 15:635, 1962

KERR AJ JR: *Subacute Bacterial Endocarditis*, Springfield, Ill.: Charles C Thomas, 1955

LERNER PI, WEINSTEIN L: Infective endocarditis in one antibiotic era. N Engl J Med 274:199, 1966

MANDELL GL et al: Enterococcal endocarditis. Arch Intern Med 125:258, 1970

RODBARD S: Blood velocity and endocarditis. Circulation 27:18, 1963

128
PNEUMOCOCCAL INFECTIONS

ROBERT AUSTRIAN
IVAN L. BENNETT, JR.

ETIOLOGY The pneumococcus is a gram-positive encapsulated coccus that usually grows in pairs or short chains. In the diplococcal form, the adjacent margins are rounded and the opposite ends slightly pointed, giving the organisms a "lancet" shape. In stained preparations of exudate, gram-negative forms are sometimes present. Because pneumococci produce greenish discoloration of blood agar, they are sometimes confused with alpha-hemolytic streptococci, to which they are closely related. The two organisms can be distinguished by the bile solubility and mouse virulence of the pneumococcus or by serologic typing. Another method, utilizing inhibition of pneumococci by Optochin-impregnated paper disks, is less cumbersome and very effective, but standard zones of inhibition determined for aerobic cultures cannot be applied to cultures grown under 5 percent carbon dioxide for the identification of pneumococcus.

The capsular substances are complex polysaccharides and are the basis for dividing pneumococci into serotypes. Organisms exposed to type-specific antiserum show a positive capsular precipitin reaction, the *Neufeld quellung reaction;* by this means, 82 serotypes have been identified. All are pathogenic for man, but types 1, 3, 4, 7, 8, and 12 are encountered most frequently in clinical practice. Types 6, 14, 19, and 23 often cause pneumonia in children but are less common in adults.

Specific typing of pneumococci remains of great clinical importance if pneumococcus is to be identified with regularity, but has been largely abandoned since the introduction of sulfonamides and antibiotics which are effective against pneumococci of all types. Recognition of pneumococcus has decreased significantly since the abandonment of pneumococcal typing by many clinical laboratories.

EPIDEMIOLOGY Pneumococci are normal inhabitants of the human upper respiratory tract in 5 to 60 percent of the population, depending upon the season. Pneumococcal infection occurs predominantly during the winter and early spring; the ratio of infection in males and females is 3:2, and morbidity and mortality are higher for Negroes than whites. Person-to-person transmission by droplets is undoubtedly common, but true epidemics of pneumococcal pneumonia are rare, even in closed populations. Patients with pneumococcal infection need not be isolated because the risk of cross infection is relatively small.

PATHOGENESIS The mechanism by which pneumococci damage tissue is obscure. It is conceivable that toxic substances may be elaborated, but no such toxin has been demonstrated. It has been suggested that rapid growth of pneumococci interferes with essential metabolic processes in the host, but this hypothesis is not supported by firm evidence. The capsular substances, though nontoxic, are known to be necessary factors in virulence, and protect the organism to a certain extent from engulfment by phagocytes.

Invasion of the tissues of the nasopharynx rarely, if ever, occurs, and "pneumococcal pharyngitis" is a doubtful entity. The organisms multiply readily in vivo, however, and may produce acute inflammation in the lungs, serous cavities, and the endocardium.

The normal human respiratory tract is provided with a variety of mechanisms which act to protect the lungs from infection. The lower respiratory tract is protected by the glottis and larynx and material passing these barriers stimulates the expulsive cough reflex. Removal of small particles impinging on the walls of the trachea and bronchi is facilitated by their mucociliary lining; and growth of bacteria reaching normal alveoli is inhibited by their relative dryness and by the phagocytic activity of alveolar macrophages. Any anatomic or physiologic derangement of these coordinated defenses tends to augment the susceptibility of the lungs to infection. Anesthesia, alcoholic intoxication, convulsions, and disturbed innervation of the larynx depress cough reflex and may permit aspiration of infected material. Alterations in the tracheobronchial tree leading to anatomic changes in the epithelial lining or to localized obstruction increase the vulnerability of the lungs to infection. Pulmonary edema, local or generalized, resulting from viral infection, inhalation of irritant gases, cardiac failure, or contusion of the chest wall, provides a fluid menstruum in the alveoli for the growth of bacteria and their spread to adjacent areas of the lung. Viral infection of the respiratory epithelium with concomitant disruption of its component cells interferes significantly with the clearance of bacteria from the lungs, an observation in accord with the high incidence of pneumococcal pneumonia during epidemics of viral influenza and its frequent clinical association with sporadic viral respiratory infections.

Pneumonia begins usually in the right lower, right middle, or left lower lobe, those areas to which gravity is most likely to carry upper respiratory secretions aspirated during sleep. Bronchial embolization with infected mucinous secretions during the course of an upper respiratory infection appears to be the initiating factor in many cases of pneumococcal pneumonia. Protected initially from phagocytosis by mucinous material, the bacteria multiply and, in infected alveoli, evoke the outpouring of proteinaceous fluid which serves both as a nutrient and as a vehicle for spread to adjacent alveoli. Soon thereafter, polymorphonuclear leukocytes migrate from the pulmonary capillaries to phagocytize a part of the pneumococcal population before the appearance of detectable antibody. Delay in the polymorphonuclear leukocytic response occurs during alcoholic intoxication and certain forms of anesthesia, permitting spread of infection. Adrenocortical steroids and their congeners may also interfere with leukocyte migration. Later, as the pneumonic lesion evolves, macrophages appear in the exudate and remove the debris of fibrin and cells. It is probable that antibody to the capsular polysaccharide of the invading pneumococcus makes its appearance locally in the lung before being detectable in the circulation. Such antibody increases the efficiency of phagocytosis approximately twofold and causes agglutination of the organisms and their adherence to alveolar walls, thereby slowing their dissemination in the lung. The outcome of infection depends, therefore, on the rate at which bacteria can multiply in the edema fluid and spread, and on the host's ability to immobilize and destroy them by phagocytosis. Individuals with hypogammaglobulinemia and patients with multiple myeloma incapable of producing anticapsular antibody are prone to recurrent attacks of pneumococcal pneumonia. Repeated infection with the same pneumococcal type should always prompt a search for dysgammaglobulinemia.

Failure of local defense mechanisms in the lung results in lymphatic spread of pneumococci to the hilar lymph nodes. In the sinusoids of these organs, a sequence of events not unlike that in the lung ensues. If infection is not checked in this secondary line of defense, organisms find their way into the thoracic duct and then into the circulation. Although transient bacteremia may occur at the onset of many cases of pneumococcal pneumonia, it is detectable in only 25 to 30 percent of cases. Bacteremia, which reflects the body's inability to localize the pulmonary infection, is a poor prognostic sign and carries with it the danger of metastatic infection. The mortality of treated or untreated bacteremic pneumococcal pneumonia is four times that resulting from comparably managed nonbacteremic infections. Metastatic infection secondary to bacteremia may occur in the meninges, joints, or peritoneum or on the endocardium. Direct spread from the infected lung may give rise to pleural empyema or to pericarditis.

Natural recovery from pneumococcal infection coincides usually, but not invariably, with the appearance of detectable type-specific antibody in the circulation and is often accompanied by a dramatic and abrupt fall in temperature, the so-called "crisis." Antibody aids recovery by increasing the efficiency of phagocytosis and by limiting dissemination of the organisms. Bacteriostatic drugs, such as sulfonamides, facilitate control of the infection by limiting the size of the pneumococcal population, but the host's defense mechanisms are still required for the elimination of the bacteria. Bactericidal agents, such as penicillin, cause the death of pneumococci in the lung and are effective when some of the host's defense mechanisms are inoperable. With the arrest of infection, the alveolar exudate undergoes liquefaction, the inflammatory debris is removed by expectoration and via the lymphatic channels, and the lung is restored to its normal state. Necrosis of pulmonary tissue as a result of pneumococcal infection is distinctly uncommon. Primary pneumococcal lung abscess is a rare clinical entity, although the diagnosis is mistakenly made at times when pneumococcal infection complicates lung abscess of other origins.

In addition to causing pneumonia and its metastatic sequelae, pneumococcus can extend from the nasopharynx to its adjacent structures, giving rise to otitis media, mastoiditis, paranasal sinusitis, or conjunctivitis.

PNEUMOCOCCAL PNEUMONIA

Pneumococcal pneumonia is a disease remarkable for its uniformity, in contrast to other infections such as typhoid fever and tuberculosis. The diseases produced by different pneumococcal serotypes show little variation in severity or in clinical manifestations. The prognosis in type 3 pneumococcal pneumonia is usually regarded as poor, probably because type 3 infections occur frequently in the aged and in patients with other debilitating diseases such as diabetes and congestive heart failure. The usual lesion in adults is lobar in distribution, but in children and the aged, bronchopneumonia, characterized by patchy involvement, is frequent.

MANIFESTATIONS Pneumonia is often preceded for a few days by coryza or some other form of common respiratory disease. The onset is usually so abrupt that patients frequently can state the exact hour that illness began. There is a sudden *shaking chill* in more than 80 percent of the cases, a rapid rise in temperature, and a corresponding tachycardia. Most patients with pneumococcal pneumonia have a single rigor unless antipyretic drugs are administered, and repeated chills should suggest another etiologic agent.

About 75 percent of patients develop severe *pleuritic pain* and *cough,* productive of pinkish or "rusty" mucoid sputum within a few hours. The chest pain is agonizing, and respirations become rapid, shallow, and grunting as the patient tries to splint the affected side. Many patients are mildly cyanotic as a result of reduced alveolar ventilation, which accompanies altered respiration, and show dilatation of the alae nasi when first seen. Patients appear acutely ill; but nausea, headache, and malaise are not prominent, and most individuals are alert. Pleuritic pain and dyspnea are the dominant complaints.

In the untreated disease, there are sustained fever of 102.5 to 105°F, continued pleuritic pain, cough, and expectoration; and *abdominal distention* is frequent. *Herpes labialis* is a common complication. After 7 to 10 days, there are diaphoresis, abrupt defervescence, and dramatic improvement in well-being, the "crisis."

In cases which terminate fatally, there is usually extensive pulmonary involvement, and dyspnea, cyanosis, and tachycardia are prominent. Circulatory collapse or a picture resembling heart failure is common. Death in a few patients is associated with empyema or some other suppurative complication such as meningitis or endocarditis.

Physical examination reveals restricted motion of the affected hemithorax. Tactile fremitus may be decreased during the initial day of illness but is usually increased when consolidation is fully established. Deviation of the trachea away from the affected lung suggests pleural effusion or empyema. The percussion note is dull, and if the lesion is in an upper lobe, impaired motion of the diaphragm can be detected on the affected side. Very early in the course of infection, breath sounds are diminished, but as the lesion evolves, they become tubular or bronchial in quality, and bronchophony and whispered pectoriloquy can be elicited. These findings are accompanied by fine crepitant rales.

EFFECT OF SPECIFIC CHEMOTHERAPY Pneumococcal pneumonia usually improves promptly when an appropriate antimicrobial drug is given. Within 12 to 36 hr after initiation of treatment with penicillin, temperature, pulse, and respiration begin to fall and may reach normal values, pleuritic pain subsides, and the spread of the inflammatory process is halted. The temperature of approximately half the patients, however, requires 4 days or longer to become normal, and failure of the patient's temperature to reach normal in 24 to 48 hr should not prompt a change in antibacterial therapy in the absence of other indications.

COMPLICATIONS The typical course of pneumococcal pneumonia can be modified by the development of one or more local or distant complications:

In the lung ATELECTASIS Atelectasis of all or part of a lobe may occur during the active stage of pneumonia or after treatment has been instituted. The patient may complain of sudden recurrence of pleuritic pain and show rapid respirations. Small areas of atelectasis are often detected by x-ray in the absence of symptoms. These areas usually clear with coughing and deep breathing, but bronchoscopic aspiration is occasionally necessary. If atelectasis is allowed to persist, the affected area becomes fibrotic and functionless.

DELAYED RESOLUTION The removal of exudate from the lung following pneumococcal infection is usually complete within 2 to 3 weeks, at which time the x-ray of the chest appears normal; but, occasionally, especially in elderly individuals and in alcoholics, consolidation persists for longer periods. Sometimes the involved area never becomes reaerated, and fibrosis results.

ABSCESS Lung abscess is a rare sequel to pneumococcal infection, although pneumococcal pneumonia is a not uncommon complication of lung abscess of other origins. It is manifested by continued fever and profuse expectoration of purulent sputum. X-ray shows one or more cavities. This complication is exceedingly rare in patients who receive penicillin therapy and is most likely to follow infection with pneumococcus type 3.

In adjacent structures PLEURAL EFFUSION Pleural effusion occurs in about 5 percent of patients with pneumococcal pneumonia, even with specific therapy. The amount of fluid is usually not sufficient to cause obvious displacement of mediastinal structures. Usually the effusion is sterile and is reabsorbed spontaneously within a week or two. Sometimes, however, the effusion is large and requires aspiration.

EMPYEMA Prior to the introduction of effective chemotherapy, empyema occurred in 5 to 8 percent of patients with pneumococcal pneumonia; it is now observed in less than 1 percent of treated cases. It is manifested by persistent fever or pleuritic pain, together with signs of pleural effusion. In the early stages, the gross appearance of infected fluid may not differ from that of a sterile pleural effusion; later, there is a profuse outpouring of polymorphonuclear leukocytes and fibrin, resulting in an exudate of thick greenish pus containing large clots of fibrin. The quantity of exudate may become large enough to displace mediastinal structures. In neglected cases, this process leads to extensive pleural scarring, with limitation of thoracic movement. Rupture and drainage through the chest wall (*empyema necessitatis*) occurs but is rare. Metastatic *brain abscess* is an occasional complication of chronic empyema.

PERICARDITIS A particularly serious complication is spread of infection to the pericardial sac. This lesion is characterized by pain in the precordial region, a friction rub synchronous with the heartbeat, and distension of cervical veins, although one or all of these findings may be absent. The possibility of coexisting purulent pericarditis should be considered whenever a very ill patient with pneumonia develops empyema.

Metastatic infections *Arthritis* occurs more often in children than in adults. The affected joint is swollen, red, and painful, with a purulent effusion. It usually subsides promptly with systemic administration of penicillin, although aspiration and intraarticular injection of penicillin may be necessary in adults.

Acute bacterial endocarditis complicates pneumococcal pneumonia in less than 0.5 percent of cases. Its manifestations and treatment are discussed below. *Meningitis,* another complication of pneumococcal pneumonia, is also discussed subsequently.

Paralytic ileus Gaseous abdominal distention is commonly present and in severely ill patients may assume such serious proportions that the term *paralytic ileus* is justified. This complication further impairs respiratory movement by elevation of the diaphragm and constitutes a difficult problem in management. A rarer and more serious gastrointestinal complication is acute gastric dilatation.

Impaired liver function Alterations in liver function are very common during the course of pneumococcal pneumonia, and mild jaundice is not at all rare. The pathogenesis of the jaundice is not entirely clear.

LABORATORY FINDINGS *X-ray of the chest* reveals a homogeneous density in the affected area of lung. In well-established cases, the density may occupy one or more entire lobes. The white blood count usually shows a polymorphonuclear *leukocytosis* ranging from 12,000 to 25,000 cells per mm^3. A normal leukocyte count or leukopenia is sometimes observed in patients with overwhelming infection and bacteremia, in the aged, and in alcoholics. The *blood culture* is positive for pneumococci during the first 3 or 4 days of the untreated illness in 20 to

25 percent of cases. The *sputum,* when stained by Gram's method, shows polymorphonuclear leukocytes and variable numbers of gram-positive cocci, singly and in pairs. These can be typed directly, by the Neufeld quellung, or capsular precipitin reaction technique, and this procedure should be employed to facilitate diagnosis whenever possible.

DIFFERENTIAL DIAGNOSIS OF PNEUMONIA Fever, cough, and pulmonary consolidation form a symptom complex that can be produced by many diseases of infectious, toxic, or other origin.

Staphylococcal pneumonia (Chap. 129) is encountered most often in infants, in adults during an epidemic of influenza, and in debilitated individuals as a nosocomial infection. The clinical picture is less uniform than that of pneumococcal pneumonia. Multiple chills, early formation of lung abscess or pneumatoceles, and empyema suggest the diagnosis. Stained smears of sputum contain myriads of staphylococci.

Hemolytic streptococcal pneumonia (Chap. 130) may occur in association with influenza or measles or following streptococcal sore throat. Toxemia is often profound, and empyema is a common complication. The diagnosis is confirmed by cultures of sputum, blood, and pleural fluid.

Friedländer's (Klebsiella) pneumonia (Chap. 133) is commonest in adults, and about half such infections occur in alcoholics. Sputum is tenacious and contains large numbers of gram-negative bacilli. Recovery may be accompanied by residual pulmonary scarring and cavitation, and relapses are not uncommon.

Tularemia (Chap. 141) is often accompanied by pulmonary lesions of varying clinical prominence. A cutaneous lesion or a history of contact with the vectors of the disease assist in making the diagnosis.

Other bacterial pneumonias: Other bacteria can produce pneumonia. Pneumonia caused by enterobacteria (*Escherichia coli, Proteus* species, *Pseudomonas*) occurs usually in the debilitated and aged, in alcoholics, in those with deranged defenses against infection, and following the administration of antimicrobials (Chap. 123). Of infections caused by salmonellas, those with *Salmonella chloraesuis* are most often complicated by pneumonia. *Bacteroides* species may give rise to necrotizing pneumonia (Chap. 136). *Hemophilus influenzae* is a common cause of pulmonary infection in children and may be an occasional cause of pneumonia in adults (Chap. 138). Pulmonary lesions occur in melioidosis (Chap. 143) and predominate in pneumonic plague (Chap. 142).

Mycoplasma pneumoniae infection (Chap. 187) is usually more insidious in onset than bacterial pneumonia and affects primarily children and young adults. It is rarely fatal.

Viral pneumonias (Chap. 186) may result from infection with a variety of agents including myxoviruses, respiratory syncytial virus, adenoviruses, rhinoviruses, Coxsackie, ECHO, and rheoviruses and the viruses of measles and varicella. Although many of these illnesses are mild and resemble that caused by *Mycoplasma pneumoniae,* occasional infections caused by influenza virus may be difficult to distinguish from bacterial pneumonia. Secondary bacterial pneumonia may complicate viral pneumonia, especially in influenza and measles.

Psittacosis (ornithosis) (Chap. 189) may follow contact with any infected avian species.

Differential diagnosis of *Q fever* is discussed in Chap. 182.

Acute tuberculous pneumonia (Chap. 156) may be difficult to recognize because tubercle bacilli may not be demonstrable in the sputum early in the disease. Many patients with tuberculous pneumonia feel surprisingly well, despite consolidation of an entire lobe. *Pleurisy with effusion* is seldom abrupt in onset, cough (when present) is nonproductive, and the physical and x-ray findings are those of pleural fluid rather than of consolidation.

Mycotic infections: Histoplasmosis (Chap. 169), blastomycosis (Chap. 167), and coccidioidomycosis (Chap. 168) may present initially as acute pneumonic processes. Infections with actinomycetes (Chap. 165) are more likely to be confused with tuberculosis or lung tumor.

Lung abscess (Chap. 253) may have an abrupt onset resembling that of pneumonia. A history of epilepsy, alcoholic intoxication, tonsillectomy, or aspiration of a foreign body suggests the diagnosis. The development of cavitation accompanied by expectoration of large amounts of foul-smelling sputum makes the diagnosis clear. Pneumococcal pneumonia at the site of the lesion may complicate the illness at any stage prior to treatment.

Atelectasis (Chap. 253) may occur in bedridden patients or following surgery when respiratory motion is limited and when the cough reflex is depressed. Infection of the collapsed pulmonary segment may lead to pneumonia. Diagnosis is facilitated when the mediastinum is shifted toward the affected side.

Neoplasms are considered in Chap. 260.

Pulmonary adenomatosis (Chap. 260) is an uncommon neoplasm that may at first be mistaken for bacterial pneumonia.

Pulmonary infarction (Chap. 256) is especially frequent in patients with congestive heart failure and after surgical procedures. It may be asymptomatic or present many of the features of pneumonia, though true chills are rare. Septic pulmonary infarcts may be complicated by abscess and cavitation and, in women, suggest the diagnosis of septic abortion or puerperal sepsis.

Other points in differential diagnosis Pulmonary infiltrates may be seen in the lungs of patients with *uremia* and of those with *acute pulmonary edema* and *heart failure.*

The inhalation of noxious materials, irritants, allergenic substances, or lipids can lead to pulmonary infiltrates and clinical symptoms that may at times be mistaken for bacterial pneumonia. The diagnosis rests on an accurate history of occupation, habits, and exposure.

Pneumonitis may occur as a feature of erythema multiforme, lupus erythematosus, rheumatic fever, or intestinal helminthiasis. Infectious mononucleosis and lymphocytic choriomeningitis are sometimes accompanied by pulmonary infiltrations. Pulmonary lesions of viral origin occur in a small proportion of patients with smallpox, chickenpox, or measles. Rupture of an amebic abscess into the pleural cavity can be mistaken for acute pneumonia; and, in a patient with estivoautumnal malaria, blockage of pulmonary capillaries by parasites can lead to confusion with respiratory infection.

EXTRAPULMONARY PNEUMOCOCCAL INFECTIONS **Pneumococcal meningitis** The pneumococcus is second only to the meningococcus as a cause of purulent meningitis in adults; in children, meningitis caused by *H. influenzae* is also more frequent than pneumococcal infection.

Pneumococcal meningitis can develop as a "primary" disease without preceding signs of infection elsewhere; as a complication of pneumococcal pneumonia; by extension from otitis, mastoiditis, or sinusitis; or following a skull fracture which creates an opening between the subarachnoid space and the nasal cavity or paranasal sinuses. Patients with pneumococcal endocarditis frequently develop meningeal infection. Patients with multiple myeloma seem to be prone to pneumococcal infection of the meninges, just as they are to pneumonia.

The *manifestations* are of those of any acute pyogenic meningitis (Chap. 329) and include chills, fever, headache, nuchal rigidity, Kernig's and Brudzinski's signs, delirium, and cranial nerve palsies. Evidence of otitis, sinusitis, or pneumonia should be carefully sought by physical and roentgenographic examination in all patients.

The *spinal fluid* is under increased pressure, appears cloudy, often with a greenish tint, and shows a high protein and low glucose content. Stained smears usually reveal gram-positive diplococci and polymorphonuclear leukocytes; in some patients, the number of cells in the spinal fluid is surprisingly small, and much of the cloudiness is produced by the bacterial content. The diagnosis can be established rapidly by identification of pneumococci in the spinal fluid by Gram's stain and by direct typing with the Neufeld quellung reaction.

With appropriate chemotherapy, recovery can be expected in 50 to 70 percent of cases; the prognosis is better in children than in infants or in adults. Relapse may occur but is unusual if adequate treatment is carried out. Subarachnoid block, the result of accumulation of large amounts of thick exudate in the meningeal space and at the base of the brain, is now an unusual complication.

Pneumococcal endocarditis Endocarditis is usually a complication of pneumonia or meningitis. The clinical picture is that of acute bacterial endocarditis (Chap. 127), with remittent fever, splenomegaly, and metastatic infection of the lungs, meninges, joints, eye, and other tissues. Petechiae are uncommon. The infection can attack normal valves and is particularly likely to occur on the aortic valve. The valvular infection is destructive, and loud murmurs and heart failure develop rapidly. Rupture or perforation of cusps or even rupture of the aorta may occur. The blood culture is consistently positive for the pneumococcus in the absence of treatment with antimicrobial drugs; yet at the same time antibodies to the infecting organism may be demonstrable in the blood, a combination of findings seldom observed except in endocarditis or brucellosis. Although the infection is relatively easy to cure with penicillin, damage to valve leaflets, especially to the cusps of the aortic valve, may be followed by rapidly progressive heart failure. Surgical repair or replacement of damaged valvular structures should be carried out early, before heart failure becomes intractable.

Pneumococcal peritonitis Pneumococcal peritonitis is a rare disease which occurs in young girls; presumably the vagina and fallopian tubes are the portal of entry. Symptoms are fever, pain, abdominal distention, vomiting, and accumulation of peritoneal fluid. The diagnosis is made by examination of the purulent ascitic fluid; blood cultures are often positive, and a polymorphonuclear leukocytosis is the rule. In adults, the disease may occur in association with cirrhosis or with carcinoma of the liver. Peritonitis used to be a common complication of the nephrotic syndrome, particularly in children, but is rare nowadays.

TREATMENT **Specific antimicrobial therapy** Penicillin G (benzyl penicillin) is the drug of choice for all manifestations of pneumococcal infection. Although mutants of pneumococcus resistant to this drug can be selected in the laboratory, evidence that they may occur in the respiratory flora of man has been lacking until recently. Strains of pneumococcus manifesting a modest increase in resistance to penicillin have now been recovered infrequently from humans outside the United States; and although the level of such resistance does not preclude treatment with this antibiotic, awareness of the phenomenon is necessary. The minimum curative dose for *pneumonia* caused by strains of usual sensitivity to penicillin G is less than 60,000 units daily, and a total dose of 600,000 units daily provides a good margin of safety for bacteremic and nonbacteremic pulmonary infection in adults in the absence of an extrapulmonary focus. Treatment may be administered at 12-hr intervals in doses of 300,000 units aqueous crystalline penicillin G or procaine penicillin. Therapy should be continued until the patient has been afebrile for 48 to 72 hr. The response is usually dramatic, and relapse is extremely uncommon. Pneumococcal pneumonia can be treated adequately with oral penicillin (preferably one of the drugs resistant to gastric acid, see Chap. 125) in dosage of 1.2 to 2.4 million units daily. *Peritonitis* usually responds within 36 to 48 hr to 2 to 4 million units of penicillin daily.

Pneumococcal *meningitis* should be treated with 12 to 20 million units aqueous penicillin G daily intravenously in adults. In many clinics, even larger amounts are used, though care must be taken to avoid neurotoxicity from excessive dosage. Intrathecal administration of penicillin is of no value. The addition of sulfadiazine to this regimen affords no advantage, and supplementary administration of chlortetracycline (and presumably, of other broad-spectrum drugs) actually exerts a deleterious effect. In the presence of sinusitis, otitis, or mastoiditis, surgical drainage should be carried out as soon as is feasible. The response of meningitis is usually less dramatic than that of pneumonia; patients often remain febrile and disoriented, and signs of meningeal irritation may persist for several days, but improvement becomes gradually evident with continued treatment.

Large doses are required in pneumococcal endocarditis also—12 to 20 million units daily by intravenous injection. Rapidly developing heart failure in these patients and the tendency to form myocardial abscess, however, often lead to a fatal outcome despite large doses of antibiotics. Surgical repair or replacement of damaged heart valves should be considered when cardiac failure develops.

Cephalosporins in parenteral doses of 1.0 to 2.0 g daily are effective in pneumococcal pneumonia but must be administered with caution to those hypersensitive to penicillin. *Cephalothin* should not be used in the treatment of pneumococcal meningitis because of its poor ability to penetrate the blood–cerebrospinal fluid barrier; cephaloridine is superior for achieving therapeutic CSF levels. The *tetracyclines* in doses of 1.0 to 2.0 g daily, *erythromycin* in doses of 1.6 g daily, or *lincomycin* in doses of 1.2 g daily are effective treatment for pneumococcal pneumonia but are recommended only for patients who have had untoward reactions to penicillins or cephalosporins. Mutants of pneumococcus resistant to each of these antibiotics have been isolated from man; and if one of these drugs is to be employed, it is essential to ascertain that the organism is sensitive to it. Despite its efficacy, chloramphenicol should not be used to treat pneumococcal infections other than meningitis in the patient hypersensitive to penicillin. *Sulfonamides* have little place in the present-day treatment of pneumonia and are useless in endocarditis and meningitis. Aminoglycosides, such as gentamicin, kanamycin, and streptomycin, should not be employed to treat pneumococcal infections.

Pneumococcal arthritis responds to systemic penicillin, but aspiration and intraarticular instillation of the drug may be necessary.

Empyema should be detected and treated as early as possible. When an effusion is found, the fluid should be examined for organisms; and if they are present, 50,000 to 200,000 units of penicillin G should be injected intrapleurally. In addition, the same antibiotic should be administered systemically in doses of 6 to 8 million units a day. Aspiration of fluid and instillation of penicillin should be carried out at 1- to 2-day intervals until cultures are persistently negative and fever disappears. Fluoroscopic guidance may be needed for aspiration of small empyema pockets. If the exudate is especially thick or viscid, streptokinase-streptodornase (Varidase) may facilitate its withdrawal. When definite improvement is not evident in 4 to 6 days or when the empyema is of long duration, a large-lumen intercostal tube should be placed in the pleural cavity to facilitate drainage. Failure to effect prompt cure of empyema may be followed by pleural fibrosis and necessitate subsequent surgical decortication of the lung to restore pulmonary function.

PROGNOSIS AND PREVENTION Although the mortality from pneumococcal pneumonia has diminished significantly since the advent of antimicrobial drugs, available evidence indicates that the incidence of the disease has changed little, if at all. The fatality rate in patients over the age of twelve years with bacteremic pneumococcal pneumonia treated with an antibiotic is 18 percent; and, in patients over the age of fifty and in those with underlying systemic illness, it is significantly higher.

Signs of poor prognosis in pneumonia include leukopenia, bacteremia, multilobar involvement, any extrapulmonary focus of pneumococcal infection, presence of preexisting systemic disease, circulatory collapse, and occurrence of the infection in the first year of life or after the age of fifty-five. Infection with pneumococcus type 3 has a higher mortality than that caused by other pneumococcal types. Death is most likely to occur in individuals sustaining irreversible physiologic damage early in the course which is unaltered by antimicrobial therapy. Until the nature of the injury produced by pneumococcus is understood and ways devised to repair it, vaccination will remain the only means of protecting those at high risk of a fatal outcome.

Despite the large number of pneumococcal serotypes, most of the serious infections are caused by a limited number; organisms of capsular types 1 through 8 account for 60 percent of such infections in adults. The efficacy of prophylactic vaccination with 50 μg each of the capsular polysaccharides of pneumococcal types 1, 2, 5, and 7 was demonstrated convincingly by MacLeod et al. in 1946, and the properties of hexavalent vaccines were studied later by MacLeod, Heidelberger, and their associates. Most individuals receiving such vaccines showed an antibody response to all six antigens, and half maximal levels of antibody persisted for 5 to 8 years following a single injection of vaccine. Preparations of pneumococcal vaccines were available commercially for a short period but were removed from the market because their use was considered unnecessary by most physicians. This view has been challenged by more recent clinical and epidemiologic studies, and efforts are currently in progress to make vaccines of capsular types 1 through 9 and types 12, 14, 18, 19, and 23 available for those at high risk of infection and death. Relicensure of such vaccines prior to 1975 is unlikely. The potential utility of similar vaccines in the prevention of pneumococcal otitis media in infancy and early childhood remains to be determined. Should they prove effective in preventing this pediatric disorder, they would be of significant value in lessening the impairment of hearing in certain segments of the population.

REFERENCES

Austrian R: Pneumococcal endocarditis, meningitis, and rupture of aortic valve. AMA Arch Intern Med 99:539, 1957

——, Gold J: Pneumococcal bacteremia with especial reference to bacteremic pneumococcal pneumonia. Ann Intern Med 60:759, 1964

Bisno AL, Freeman J: The syndrome of asplenia, pneumococcal sepsis, and disseminated intravascular coagulation. Ann Intern Med 72:389, 1970

Hansman D et al: Increased resistance to penicillin of pneumococci isolated from man. N Engl J Med 284:175, 1971

Heffron R: *Pneumonia with Special Reference to Pneumococcus Lobar Pneumonia,* New York: Commonwealth Fund, 1939

Lepper MH, Dowling HF: Treatment of pneumococci meningitis with penicillin compared with penicillin plus aureomycin. AMA Arch Intern Med 88:489, 1951

MacLeod CM et al: Prevention of pneumococcal pneumonia by

immunization with specific capsular polysaccharides. J Exp Med 82:445, 1945

Ragsdale AR, Sanford JP: Interfering effect of incubation in carbon dioxide on the identification of pneumococci by optochin discs. Appl Microbiol 22:854, 1971

Shulman JA et al: Errors and hazards in the diagnosis and treatment of bacterial pneumonias. Ann Intern Med 62:41, 1965

Wood WB Jr: Studies on the mechanism of recovery in pneumococcal pneumonia: 1. The action of type specific antibody upon the pulmonary lesion of experimental pneumonia. J Exp Med 73:201, 1941

Zinneman HW, Hall WH: Recurrent pneumonia in multiple myeloma. Ann Intern Med 41:1152, 1954

129
STAPHYLOCOCCAL INFECTIONS

DAVID E. ROGERS
MARVIN TURCK

INTRODUCTION Staphylococci most commonly produce superficial suppurative infections in man which are relatively harmless. They also produce certain serious infections of the lungs, pleural space, endocardium, myocardium, long bones, kidneys, and surgical wounds.

The majority of life-threatening staphylococcal infections arise within hospitals, and these infections are considered among the "diseases of medical progress." Although staphylococcal cross infection in hospitals may be less frequent now than 10 to 15 years ago and although various gram-negative rods challenge the staphylococcus as the most common nosocomial pathogens, there is good evidence that the problem has not disappeared.

ETIOLOGY Staphylococci are members of the genus *Micrococcus*. This genus includes many morphologically similar saprophytic microorganisms which do not cause human infection. The parasitic micrococci of primary concern in medicine are grouped in the species *M. pyogenes*. Through established usage, these pathogenic micrococci are termed *staphylococci*.

Staphylococci are spherical gram-positive cells. On solid agar media, staphylococcal colonies develop characteristic pigmentation by which three species can be differentiated: *M. pyogenes* var. *aureus* (*Staphylococcus aureus*), golden yellow; *M. pyogenes* var. *albus* (*S. albus*), ivory white; and *M. citreus*, lemon yellow. Most human infections are caused by *S. aureus*, a few by *S. albus*. The name "staphylococcus" derives from the characteristic grapelike clusters of organisms seen in stained smears prepared from colonies on solid media. In stained smears obtained from pus, smaller clusters, diploids, and short chains are seen. In such preparations, staphylococci characteristically retain their uniform round shape, in contrast to the boatlike forms assumed by pneumococci. Staphylococci may be seen within the cytoplasm of polymorphonuclear cells in pus, a rare finding in other gram-positive coccal infections.

In general, pathogenic strains possess a broader complement of biochemical activity than do nonpathogenic strains. Most staphylococci isolated from human infections produce yellow pigment and hemolyze blood cells. The ability to produce coagulase, a substance which clots the plasma of certain animals and man, the elaboration of *alpha toxin*, and the fermentation of *mannite*, are characteristics of infection-producing strains. The ability of a given strain to produce coagulase is generally considered the best single evidence of pathogenicity. Staphylococci that are coagulase-positive and ferment mannitol are classified by bacterial taxonomists as *S. aureus*, whether they produce the "aureus" pigment or not.

Different strains of pathogenic staphylococci can be recognized by the patterns of lysis produced by staphylococcal bacteriophages. Although the technique is cumbersome, phage typing of staphylococci has allowed more precise strain characterization and is commonly used in studies of intrahospital disease and epidemics of staphylococcal infection.

PATHOGENESIS Little is known of the events which allow staphylococci to invade host tissues. While strains of staphylococci capable of producing infection are common skin and mucous membrane inhabitants, an enormous number of bacteria must be used to establish experimental infections in animals or man, and more than a million organisms are necessary to produce serious infection in most laboratory animals. Over 50 percent of serious staphylococcal infections of deep tissues arise from cutaneous foci and a smaller number originate in the respiratory or genitourinary tract. Direct inoculation of staphylococci into the bloodstream also is a route of infection amongst drug addicts.

Staphylococcal disease is more common in patients with *diabetes, liver disease, renal failure*, severe *debilitation* and/or *malnutrition*, or when skin continuity is broken. *Abrasions, wounds, burns*, and skin areas denuded by *exfoliative dermatitis* are commonly infected with staphylococci. *Influenza, measles*, and *mucoviscidosis* appear to predispose to primary staphylococcal invasion of the lung. Patients receiving *broad-spectrum antimicrobial therapy* also appear to have a higher incidence of staphylococcal disease.

Staphylococci invade the integument via hair follicles and sebaceous glands. When skin continuity has been breached, local microbial multiplication is accompanied by inflammation and tissue necrosis at the site of infection. Polymorphonuclear leukocytes rapidly enter the area and ingest large numbers of staphylococci. Thrombosis of surrounding capillaries occurs, fibrin is deposited about the periphery; and, later, fibroblasts create a relatively avascular wall about the area. The fully developed staphylococcal lesion consists of a central core of dead and dying leukocytes and bacteria which gradually liquefies to form characteristic thick, creamy pus, surrounded by a fibroblastic wall.

When host mechanisms fail to contain the cutaneous or subcutaneous infection, staphylococci may enter the bloodstream. Common sites of metastatic seeding are the diaphyseal ends of long bones in children, lungs, kidneys, endocardium, myocardium, liver, spleen, and brain.

Certain biologic properties of staphylococci appear to contribute to pathogenicity. Many pathogenic strains elaborate an *exotoxin* (alpha toxin) capable of causing dermal necrosis in animals. Fever, tachycardia, cyanosis, shock, and death ensue when exotoxin is administered to experimental animals, a picture similar to that seen occasionally in certain fulminating cases of staphylococcal bacteremia in man. A delta toxin also has been incriminated in pathogenesis of severe staphylococcal infection. However, it is conjectural that any of these toxins have any role in the circulatory disturbances seen prior to death.

The high correlation between *coagulase* production and virulence suggests that this substance is important in the pathogenesis of staphylococcal infections. Coagulase has been said to protect staphylococci from phagocytosis by polymorphonuclear leukocytes, to promote abscess formation in man and in animal species which have coagulable plasmas, or to protect staphylococci from bacteriostatic substances present in normal serum. However, none of these postulates has shown that coagulase per se is a determinant of pathogenicity, and its precise role has not been established.

Certain pathogenic staphylococci produce a *leukocidin* which destroys human and rabbit leukocytes in vitro. Some strains elaborate *hyaluronidase*. Many staphylococci produce an *enterotoxin* which produces nausea, vomiting, and diarrhea in certain experimental animals and man.

In vitro and in vivo studies have indicated that pathogenic staphylococci can survive within human leukocytes, whereas nonpathogenic strains do not. Such intracellular survival may be a means of transporting staphylococci and spreading them to distant tissues. This intracellular survival may also account for the relative refractoriness of staphylococcal infection to antibiotic treatment.

IMMUNITY Some degree of resistance to staphylococcal infections develops with age. For example, primary staphylococcal pneumonia is common in infants, but rare in adults. Acute staphylococcal osteomyelitis is almost exclusively a disease of children. Abscess formation appears less common and bacteremia more frequent in infants than in adults.

Coagulase-positive staphylococci have a characteristic cell wall teichoic acid, which may be antiphagocytic. Certain unusual strains possess a definite capsular structure which impedes phagocytosis, and specific opsonizing antibody is required for the ingestion of these unusual strains. A number of antistaphylococcal antibodies have been shown to pass from mother to fetus, and the incidence of a variety of antibodies rapidly rises with age. Virtually 100 percent of adults possess antibodies to several staphylococcal antigens in their serum. Nevertheless, the role of humoral immunity in modifying or protecting against staphylococcal infection is uncertain. Immunization of animals with alpha toxin, toxoids, coagulase, or whole staphylococci may prolong experimental staphylococcal infection, but does not protect against eventual death. At present there has been no satisfactory demonstration that human staphylococcal disease is followed by immunity or that infection can be modified significantly by vaccination.

EPIDEMIOLOGY Pathogenic strains of staphylococci reside in the anterior nares and upon the skin of a significant number of people. Hospital patients and personnel have significantly higher staphylococcal carrier rates than the general population.

While staphylococci remain viable for long periods in dust, blankets, or clothing, and viable staphylococci are often demonstrable in the environment by air-sampling techniques, the significance of airborne transmission remains uncertain, and the best evidence suggests that direct person-to-person contact is the most important means of transmission of staphylococci. Active staphylococcal infections are probably a more serious source of cross infection than the simple carrier state. For example, discontinuation of the use of hexachlorophene in hospital nurseries has been associated with an increase in infection in some hospitals, and it is apparent that continued surveillance in hospitals is necessary to thwart the development of epidemics of staphylococcal infection.

Certain phage types of staphylococci have been associated with a majority of intrahospital infections. Some strains, particularly antibiotic-resistant strains in phage group III, appear to have greater "epidemic virulence" than other staphylococci. In specific hospitals, one phage type often emerges to prominence and may cause most of the serious intrahospital infections. Such "epidemic strains" have shifted from time to time and vary from hospital to hospital. The high incidence of active staphylococcal disease in carriers of certain strains (for example, the 80/81 strains) suggests that some staphylococci may possess higher virulence for humans than others. Some of the decrease in the frequency of staphylococcal infection in hospitals during the past decade has been attributed to the disappearance of 80/81 strains.

ANTIMICROBIAL RESISTANCE In the past, the introduction of new antibiotics active against staphylococci has generally been followed by the appearance of staphylococci specifically resistant to that agent. When penicillin was first introduced, less than 10 percent of staphylococcal strains isolated from patients or carriers were resistant to penicillin. Now 60 to 90 percent of staphylococci isolated from hospitalized patients throughout the Western world are resistant to penicillin G, and the incidence of infection due to penicillinase-producing strains in nonhospitalized individuals is almost as high as in hospitalized patients. The incidence of resistance to a specific antimicrobial has correlated closely with the frequency of its administration, and the emergence of resistant strains has followed the use of most antibiotics. Vancomycin, first employed in 1958, and the penicillinase-resistant penicillins and the cephalosporins, both introduced in the 1960s, have been exceptions to this rule. Although some strains of *S. aureus* resistant to the penicillinase-resistant penicillins, such as methicillin, have produced infections in England, France, and the United States, such strains have been unusual in this country, and, in general, these agents have retained a high degree of activity against both penicillin-sensitive and penicillin-resistant staphylococci. However, methicillin resistance may emerge as a problem in the future.

Most observations on the incidence of antimicrobial-resistant strains have been made within hospitals where antimicrobial use is heaviest. It has been shown that drug-susceptible strains carried by patients may be replaced by drug-resistant phage group III staphylococci present in the hospital environment during antimicrobial treatment. These strains are in turn acquired by hospital personnel who serve as reservoirs of potentially pathogenic, antimicrobial-resistant strains. Staphylococci isolated from population groups outside the hospital have shown a slower increase in the incidence of antimicrobial-resistant strains, but in some communities the incidence of extra-hospital infections caused by penicillin-resistant strains is similar to that found in hospitalized patients.

MANIFESTATIONS **Superficial infections** Simple infection of hair follicles manifested by a minute erythematous nodule without involvement of the surrounding skin or deeper tissues is termed *folliculitis*. A more extensive and invasive follicular or sebaceous gland infection with some involvement of subcutaneous tissues is termed a *furuncle*, or *boil*. Itching and mild pain are followed by progressive local swelling and erythema, and the overlying skin becomes exquisitely painful on pressure or motion. Relief of pain occurs promptly after spontaneous or surgical drainage.

Furuncles occur most commonly on the face, neck, axillas, forearms, buttocks, thighs, breast, upper back, and labia. The acne of adolescence is frequently complicated by secondary furunculosis. Staphylococcal infection may involve the sweat glands in the axillas (*hidradenitis suppurativa*). These infections may be deep-seated, slow to localize and drain, and are prone to recurrence and scarring.

Staphylococcal infections within the thick, fibrous, inelastic skin of the back of the neck and upper part of the back lead to formation of a *carbuncle*. The relative thickness and impermeability of the overlying skin lead to lateral extension and loculation, and a large indurated, painful lesion with multiple ineffective drainage sites results. These extensive lesions appear more frequently among diabetics. Carbuncles produce fever, leukocytosis, extreme pain, and prostration. Bacteremia is common.

Osteomyelitis Staphylococci are responsible for the majority of cases of *acute osteomyelitis*. This infection occurs most commonly in children under the age of twelve, but adults also are susceptible to acute osteomyelitis, especially of the spine. There appears to have been a sharp decrease in the incidence of acute osteomyelitis since the introduction of antibiotics. Approximately 50 percent of patients give a history of a furuncle or superficial staphylococcal infection preceding osteomyelitis. Bone involvement follows hematogenous dissemination of bacteria. The frequent localization in the diaphyseal end of long bones is thought to be due to the endarterial circulation of the diaphysis. Many patients give a history of preceding trauma to the involved area.

Once established, infection spreads through the newly formed juxtaepiphyseal bone to the periosteum or along the marrow cavity. If the infection reaches the subperiosteal space, the periosteum is lifted, a subperiosteal abscess forms, and rupture with infection of the subcutaneous tissues may occur. Rarely, the joint capsule is penetrated, producing a pyogenic arthritis. There is death of bone, producing a *sequestrum*, followed by new bone formation, the *involucrum*.

Occasionally indolent staphylococcal infections of bone remain localized within dense granulation tissue about a central necrotic cavity. Such a local infection may persist for years as a so-called "Brodie's abscess."

Osteomyelitis in children usually begins abruptly with chills, high fever, nausea, vomiting, and progressive pain at the site of bony involvement. Muscle spasm about the affected bone is a common early sign of osteomyelitis, and the child may refuse to move the affected limb. Leukocytosis is the rule. Blood cultures are positive for staphylococci in 50 to 60 percent of cases early in the disease. The tissues overlying the involved bone become edematous and warm, and the skin becomes erythematous and shiny. Anemia develops during the course of untreated disease. Roentgenograms are usually normal during the first week. Bony rarefaction, local periosteal elevation, and new bone formation can frequently be seen during the second week.

Staphylococcal spinal infection in the adult differs considerably from acute osteomyelitis in the child. The onset is less abrupt, and there is a greater tendency for bony fusion with obliteration of the disc space.

DIAGNOSIS Osteomyelitis should be suspected in any child with fever, limb pain, and leukocytosis. Similarly, neck or back pain in an adult, when accompanied by fever, should raise the possibility of acute osteomyelitis or a disk space infection. History of a preceding cutaneous infection, local tenderness over the bone, and the finding of *S. aureus* in blood cultures are confirmatory. In early stages, osteomyelitis must be differentiated from acute rheumatic fever and pyogenic arthritis.

PROGNOSIS Prior to the advent of antimicrobials, the overall mortality was approximately 25 percent. Death was more common in individuals with demonstrable bacteremia. Chronic osteomyelitis with recurrent activation and metastatic foci in other bones was common. However, acute staphylococcal osteomyelitis is declining in incidence, death is rare, and chronic osteomyelitis is also becoming less frequent.

Staphylococcal pneumonia Staphylococci are the cause of approximately 1 percent of bacterial pneumonias. This disease occurs sporadically except during epidemics of influenza, when staphylococcal pneumonia is more common, although even then it is not as frequent as pneumococcal infection.

Primary staphylococcal pneumonia in infants and young children is a frequent cause of pyopneumothorax and pneumatocele. This complication occurs early and should suggest *S. aureus* infection. In older children and adults, primary staphylococcal pneumonia may be secondary to influenza or measles. In addition, staphylococcal pneumonia has been seen in hospitalized patients with mucoviscidosis, leukemia, collagen disease, or other chronic debilitating disease.

In healthy adults, staphylococcal pneumonia is generally preceded by an influenza-like respiratory infection. Onset of staphylococcal involvement is abrupt, with chills, high fever, progressive dyspnea, cyanosis, cough, and pleural pain. Early peripheral vascular collapse is common, and examination frequently reveals a patient who seems sicker than his physical findings would suggest. Sputum in the early phases is not characteristic, but may be bloody or frankly purulent. Admixture with blood may produce a thick, creamy pink sputum.

Staphylococcal pneumonia in hospitalized patients usually begins more insidiously. Increasing fever, tachycardia, and an elevated respiratory rate may be the only indications of infection. Typical pneumonic symptoms may be absent. The disease is also less abrupt when pulmonary involvement occurs during the course of staphylococcal bacteremia, as may be the case in drug addicts or in patients with endocarditis. Staphylococci generally produce patchy, centrally located areas of pneumonia. Pleural involvement and empyema are common.

Because of the central pulmonary involvement, chest findings are variable. Signs of frank consolidation are rare. Scattered fine to coarse rales and rhonchi may be heard over the involved areas. Empyema produces typical signs of pleural fluid. Signs of abscess may appear late in the course of the disease. Bacteremia is unusual in primary staphylococcal pneumonia (less than 20 percent of patients), and *its presence should suggest that the pneumonic involvement is metastatic and secondary to foci of infection elsewhere.*

The course of staphylococcal pneumonia may be stormy despite adequate antimicrobial therapy. Gradual defervescence starting 48 to 72 hr after the initiation of therapy is the rule. Pulmonary abscesses or empyema cavities may require surgical treatment.

DIAGNOSIS Staphylococcal pneumonia must be differentiated from other pneumonias. The preceding influenza-like illness, rapid onset of pleural pain, cyanosis, and prostration out of proportion to physical findings should suggest primary staphylococcal pneumonia. The finding of masses of polymorphonuclear leukocytes and gram-positive intraleukocytic cocci strongly suggests the diagnosis. The blood leukocyte count is generally above 15,000. Pneumonia developing suddenly or insidiously, with higher fever, tachycardia, and leukocytosis, in debilitated hospitalized patients receiving antimicrobials should be considered to be staphylococcal in origin.

PROGNOSIS Prior to 1942, mortality ranged from 50 to 95 percent. The presence of bacteremia was almost invariably associated with a fatal outcome. The prognosis has improved with the use of antimicrobials, but some patients continue to die with staphylococcal pneumonia, especially debilitated individuals acquiring staphylococcal pneumonia in the hospital. Abscess formation and pleural involvement often prolong convalescence.

Staphylococcal bacteremia Staphylococcal bacteremia may arise from any local staphylococcal infection. Infections of the skin (including infections about inlying venous cutdowns or catheters), respiratory tract, bones, or genitourinary tract precede bacteremia. Trauma to local lesions, such as pinching, or surgical drainage before adequate localization may precipitate bacteremia.

Rarely, patients with bacteremia die in 12 to 24 hr, with high fever, tachycardia, cyanosis, gastrointestinal symptoms, and vascular collapse. Commonly, the disease progresses more slowly, with hectic fever and metastatic abscess formation in the skin, bones, kidneys, brain, lungs, myocardium, spleen, or other tissues. *Meningitis* is an occasional complication.

Endocarditis may occur in patients with protracted bacteremia. Normal heart valves are frequently involved, the aortic being the most frequent. Typically, staphylococcal endocarditis runs an acute course with high fever, progressive anemia, and metastatic abscesses in the skin and deeper structures. Rupture of the valve leaflets and valve ring abscesses are common. Specific diagnosis of endocardial involvement is difficult; because of its frequency, it should be assumed to be present in patients with staphylococcal bacteremia with demonstrable cutaneous lesions (petechiae or cutaneous pustules) and a significant heart murmur. At times, especially among addicts with right-sided valvular lesions, a significant heart murmur may not be demonstrable. Both coagulase-positive and coagulase-negative staphylococci have been a major cause of endocarditis in patients undergoing cardiac surgical procedures, particularly valve replacement, and both coagulase-positive and coagulase-negative staphylococci occasionally produce a subacute endocarditis indistinguishable from that produced by *Streptococcus viridans.* Persistent *Staphylococcus albus* bacteremia has also been common after ventriculoatriostomy.

Staphylococcal bacteremia is generally accompanied by a polymorphonuclear leukocytosis of 12,000 to 20,000, but a normal leukocyte count or leukopenia is occasionally seen. Diagnosis of bacteremia can be facilitated by doing a Gram stain of the buffy coat, which may show staphylococci within the cytoplasm of polymorphonuclear cells. Anemia develops rapidly during the course of the illness. Cyanosis and hypoxemia may be seen with staphylococcal bacteremia, even in the absence of significant pulmonary lesions on chest roentgenogram.

PROGNOSIS Staphylococcal bacteremia is an extremely serious disease. Prior to the development of antimicrobials, over 80 percent of individuals died, the majority within 10 days of the onset of illness. The development of endocarditis or meningitis during bacteremia was almost invariably fatal. The sulfonamides produced little alteration in this mortality. With the administration of effective antibiotics and appropriate surgical treatment of local sites of infection, 50 to 70 percent of patients survive. However, when staphylococcal endocarditis has occurred on a prosthetic cardiac valve, the outcome has been almost invariably fatal unless reconstructive surgery can be performed.

Staphylococcal food poisoning Certain strains of staphylococci produce an enterotoxin which is responsible for many outbreaks of acute gastroenteritis. Foods are commonly contaminated from superficial infections in food handlers or by nasal droplets containing pathogenic staphylococci. Cream-filled pastries, custards, cottage cheese, milk products, or meats subjected to improper refrigeration, allowing staphylococcal multiplication, are the common offenders.

Symptoms typically appear 1 to 6 hr after ingestion of enterotoxin-contaminated food. Onset is usually abrupt, with severe nausea, vomiting, cramping abdominal pain, diarrhea, and prostration. The disease is brief and requires only rest and sedation. Rare fatalities have occurred in the aged. The diagnosis is based on the short incubation period, the epidemic nature of the disease, the short duration of symptoms, and the lack of fever. The etiology can be established only if specimens of ingested food can be shown to contain large numbers of enterotoxin-producing staphylococci. Staphylococcal food poisoning should not be confused with staphylococcal enterocolitis, an illness associated with actual proliferation and overgrowth of viable staphylococci in the gut.

Miscellaneous infections Staphylococci may cause otitis, sinusitis, or mastoid infections as well as infection in and around the orbit. Certain strains elaborate an erythrogenic toxin that results in a rash indistinguishable from that of streptococcal scarlet fever. Epidemics of staphylococcal pyoderma in newborn infants and maternal breast abscesses are a recurring problem in maternity units, but appear to be decreasing in frequency.

TREATMENT Features of staphylococcal infection which influence therapy While the development of penicillinase-resistant penicillins and cephalosporins has simplified treatment, certain characteristics of staphylococcal disease should be borne in mind in designing therapy.

1 The host setting in which infection occurs. Acute staphylococcal infections arising outside the hospital in otherwise healthy adults have a better prognosis than intrahospital infections arising in sick individuals with compromised host defense mechanisms.
2 The rapid necrosis of tissues produced by staphylococci. Delays in effective therapy may allow a progressing infection to advance to frank abscess formation. While many antimicrobials reach abscess cavities in adequate concentrations, the physiologic insusceptibility of microorganisms residing in areas of extensive necrosis or suppuration renders antibiotic therapy quite ineffective in this situation. Surgical drainage of such lesions is often required.
3 The sluggish response to therapy. Staphylococci are killed slowly by antimicrobials and relapses are frequent. Hence antimicrobial therapy must be continued longer than in many bacterial infections.
4 The problem of antimicrobial resistance. While treatment must be initiated empirically when serious staphylococcal infection is suspected, rational therapy requires that the antibiotic susceptibility of the infecting strain be known.

Treatment of serious staphylococcal infections The effectiveness of the penicillinase-resistant penicillins has simplified the approach to life-threatening staphylococcal disease. However, two methods of initiating treatment when serious staphylococcal disease is suspected have been proposed.

In the *first method,* following appropriate cultures, treatment with large doses of both aqueous penicillin *and* methicillin (or parenteral oxacillin or nafcillin) should be instituted immediately. In adults, aqueous penicillin, 20 million units, should be given by continuous intravenous drip. The companion penicillinase-resistant penicillin can be given intravenously or intramuscularly. Methicillin is rapidly eliminated from the body, and initial doses of 2 g every 4 hr are indicated. Parenteral oxacillin or nafcillin in doses of 1 or 2 g every 4 hr can be substituted for methicillin.

If in vitro sensitivity studies show the infecting strain to be sensitive to penicillin G, therapy with methicillin can be discontinued and treatment maintained with aqueous penicillin alone. If the strain is penicillin-resistant, the penicillinase-resistant penicillins alone should be continued.

The above regimen may be theoretically advantageous because penicillin-sensitive strains of staphylococci are twenty- to fiftyfold more susceptible to penicillin G than to methicillin. However, in fact, there is little clinical proof that this regimen is necessary even in patients with severe life-threatening staphylococcal infection.

In the *second method* a penicillinase-resistant penicillin is used alone. All strains of staphylococci are susceptible to penicillinase-resistant penicillins, and because of the high incidence of penicillinase-producing staphylococci as causes of infection, some authorities initiate treatment with methicillin, oxacillin, or nafcillin alone, shifting to aqueous penicillin G if the strain is subsequently proved to be susceptible to that drug.

Despite differences in structure, the major allergenic properties of the penicillins reside in the 6-aminopenicillanic acid molecule. There is significant cross allergenicity between penicillins, and patients who have had well-established allergic reactions to penicillin G should not receive penicillinase-resistant penicillins. Further, there is increasing evidence that a significant number of these individuals may react to the cephalosporin derivatives as well. These agents, which are good antistaphylococcal drugs, have a 7-aminocephalosporanic acid nucleus quite similar to that of penicillins and should be used with caution in patients with prior reaction to penicillin.

Cephalothin and *cephaloridine* are semisynthetic derivatives of cephalosporin C. Cephalothin is highly active against both penicillin-sensitive and penicillin-resistant strains. Cephaloridine appears more susceptible to staphylococcal penicillinase and should not be used in treatment of severe infections by penicillin-resistant strains unless the organism is shown to be sensitive to it. Intramuscular or intravenous doses of 1.0 to 2.0 g cephalothin every 4 hr are recommended; the dose of cephaloridine is limited to 1.0 g every 6 hr by regulation because of its potential for nephrotoxicity.

Vancomycin is uniformly active against coagulase-positive staphylococci regardless of their sensitivity to penicillin. It should be given intravenously in doses of 1.0 to 1.5 g over a 30- to 40-min period every 12 hr.

The development of these new agents has relegated several antibiotics formerly used in treatment to minor or secondary roles. Lincomycin and erythromycin are still useful in certain circumstances, but are not frontline agents in staphylococcal bacteremia. They are used primarily in patients allergic to penicillin.

Changes in therapy Established staphylococcal infections respond slowly even to the most effective antimicrobial regimens, making it difficult to know when therapy should be considered inadequate. Characteristically, 24 to 48 hr elapse before a decline in fever is noted, and recovery is accompanied by slow return of the temperature to normal in 7 to 10 days. Treatment should be continued for a minimum of 4 to 6 weeks if endocarditis is suspected.

Special therapeutic situations ASYMPTOMATIC NASAL CARRIER STATE The role of asymptomatic carriers in hospital transmission of infection remains controversial. Hospital personnel are carriers if they harbor, in their anterior nares, coagulase-positive staphylococci which are producing intrahospital disease, and it is generally agreed that they must be removed from nursery units, operating theaters, delivery rooms, and surgical floors. Although no method of treatment has been uniformly satisfactory, the following regimens have had limited success in treatment of nasal carriers.

1 Simple removal from the hospital environment for 3 to 4 weeks
2 Frequent baths with germicidal soaps
3 The use of topical antibiotics of low sensitizing potential in a water-soluble base (i.e., bacitracin, neomycin, or a combination of these agents) four to five times daily for 2 weeks

If the carrier state returns, a second course of treatment is indicated. In infants, colonization with disease-producing strains may be prevented by deliberate implantation of a staphylococcal strain of low virulence. This approach has been applied to adult carriers in a limited way, but evidence regarding its efficacy is not yet available.

SUPERFICIAL INFECTIONS Superficial infections frequently do not require the use of antibiotics. There is no adequate therapy for recurrent furunculosis, but if the disease is severe, antimicrobial treatment may be attempted. Antibiotics to which the strain is susceptible should be administered systemically for a minimum of 10 to 14 days. Local moist heat, immobilization of the infected part, and incision and drainage should be utilized. The surrounding skin should be protected with a coating of zinc oxide to prevent maceration. Treatment of the nasal carrier state by the local application of topical antibiotics (see above) may be advisable. Careful daily baths with germicidal soaps, attention to personal and family hygiene, and the passage of time appear to be measures most likely to interrupt the process. Attempts to prevent recurrence by autogenous or other vaccines have not been effective.

EMPYEMA Empyema should be treated by aspiration, generally with a large-bore tube since loculation and thick exudate may prevent adequate needle drainage. Direct instillation of penicillin or methicillin into the pleural space may be beneficial, and this procedure is employed in some instances. Similarly, while the local instillation of proteolytic enzymes may occasionally aid in liquefying the exudate, surgical drainage is generally necessary and should be performed promptly.

OSTEOMYELITIS The initial regimen already outlined for other serious infections is recommended, and treatment should be continued for 14 to 28 days in acute osteomyelitis. Local drainage of abscess cavities in soft tissues or bones should be considered in all patients in whom severe pain persists or when response to antimicrobials is inadequate. If sequestration occurs, devitalized bone should be removed. Lincomycin has been reported to be superior to other agents in the treatment of chronic osteomyelitis, but the evidence for this is not convincing. The optimal duration of treatment in established chronic infection is not known, but frequently several months of antimicrobial therapy are recommended.

NURSERY EPIDEMICS The hazards of epidemic staphylococcal disease in newborn nurseries are well recognized. Pediatric texts should be consulted for full discussion of the special techniques employed in prevention and management of nursery infections. The use of deliberate colonization of newborns with a staphylococcus of low disease potential to prevent colonization with more pathogenic strains has important biologic implications.

REFERENCES

EICKHOFF TE: Hospital infections. Disease-a-Month (Chicago), 1, September, 1972

JESSEN O et al: Changing staphylococci and staphylococcal infections. N Engl J Med 281:627, 1969

KOENIG MG: Staphylococcal infections: Treatment and control. Disease-a-Month (Chicago), April, 1968

NAHMIAS AJ, EICKHOFF TC: Staphylococcal infections in hospitals. N Engl J Med 265:74,120, 177, 1962

SMITH IM: Death from staphylococci. Sci Am 218:83, 1968

130 HEMOLYTIC STREPTOCOCCAL INFECTIONS

CHARLES H. RAMMELKAMP, JR.

INTRODUCTION

Streptococci are probably the most important bacterial pathogens of man. They can invade any tissue, and depending on the site of invasion and the host-parasite relationship, produce different clinical syndromes. They cause such common, dramatic, acute septic illnesses as sore throat, scarlet fever, lymphangitis, puerperal fever, and erysipelas. In addition, certain serologic strains are capable of producing serious late complications, including acute rheumatic fever and acute glomerulonephritis.

ETIOLOGY

Streptococci are gram-positive and tend to form chains. Cultured on sheep blood agar they produce three types of reactions. *Alpha* colonies exhibit a zone of incomplete hemolysis with greenish discoloration; they are termed *viridans* streptococci. *Beta*-hemolytic colonies exhibit complete clearing of sheep red cells because of the action of hemolysins, including streptolysins O and S. *Gamma* colonies are nonhemolytic.

On the basis of specific carbohydrates, 13 serologic groups of streptococci have been identified; they are designated A through O. All groups may infect man, but respiratory infections are caused by group A and only rarely by groups C and G streptococci. Groups A and B cause neonatal and post-partum sepsis. Group D, or enterococci, both hemolytic and nonhemolytic varieties, are found in the intestine and are responsible for infections of the urinary tract and abdominal cavity. There are over 50 specific types of group A streptococci which are identified by a precipitin test for M protein or by an agglutination reaction to the T antigen. The M protein is responsible for type-specific immunity in man and is probably responsible for the virulence of group A organisms. Glossy forms of group A which contain no M protein are avirulent.

Several extracellular products are produced by streptococci. *Streptolysin O* is produced by groups A, C, and G, and antibody develops following infection. Approximately 85 percent of group A respiratory infections result in a measurable increase in antistreptolysin O. *Streptolysin S* is nonantigenic.

Scarlatinal or *erythogenic toxin* is responsible for the rash of scarlet fever. Toxigenic strains are lysogenic and vary in the amount of toxin produced. There are three immunologically distinct toxins which may account for second attacks of scarlet fever. Injection of toxin into the skin of susceptible children causes erythema, which reaches its maximum in 24 hr; this is termed a *positive Dick test.* The test reverts to a negative reaction following infection.

Streptokinase is an enzyme that catalyzes the conversion of plasminogen to plasmin, causing the lysis of fibrin. It is produced by strains of groups A, C, and G and occasionally in small amounts by groups B and F streptococci. Group A strains vary in the amount produced. Two distinct streptokinases, A and B, are produced by group A streptococci, and antibodies develop following infection; however, this antibody is not widely employed as a diagnostic test. *Diphosphopyridine nucleotidase* is produced by certain strains of group A streptococci, especially type 12, a nephritogenic strain. When leukocytes ingest such strains, a leukocytotoxic effect is immediately apparent. Antibody develops which inhibits the action of the enzyme.

Four specific immunologic *deoxyribonucleases*, A, B, C, and D, are produced by group A streptococci. These enzymes depolymerize the viscous deoxyribonucleoprotein present in thick pus and have been used clinically to liquefy exudates.

Hyaluronidase, or spreading factor, attacks the polysaccharide gel of the capsule of the streptococcus and the ground substance of connective tissue. It is produced by group A streptococci and in large amounts by types 4 and 22. Antibodies develop following infection. Whether or not hyaluronidase is responsible for the tendency of streptococci to spread rapidly in tissues is not known. Other substances produced by streptococci include *leukocidin, proteinase*, and *amylase.*

EPIDEMIOLOGY

Aerobic streptococcal infections are observed in all races, in both sexes, and at all ages and occur during any season of the year throughout the world. Streptococcal respiratory infections, including scarlet fever, are encountered especially during the colder months of the year. Scarlet fever is rare in the tropics. Under the age of three months, streptococcal infections are rare. Between the ages of six months and ten years, scarlet fever occurs frequently. Tonsillitis and pharyngitis are especially prevalent throughout childhood and early adult life. In women during the childbearing period, puerperal infections caused by streptococci occur occasionally. Finally, erysipelas, which may occur at any age, appears to be more prevalent in infants and the older age groups.

Soon after birth, alpha streptococci appear in the upper part of the respiratory tract and may be isolated therefrom throughout life. Streptococci of Lancefield groups C and G and, more rarely, organisms of groups other than A may be isolated from the oropharynx of 5 percent or more of the normal population.

The group A flora of the oropharynx is made up of many different specific types, but usually several types predominate. In general, at least 5 percent of the people of any community harbor group A streptococci. The prevalence varies and depends upon the cultural methods used as well as upon environmental, host, and bacterial factors. Persons under twenty years of age are most likely to harbor group A streptococci, especially if the tonsils are present.

Following either apparent or inapparent infection, the carrier state usually persists for several months and occasionally for longer periods. Throat cultures inoculated directly on blood agar plates during the first, fourth, eighth, and eleventh weeks following infection show 10 or more colonies of streptococci in 90, 65, 25, and 10 percent of patients, respectively. Carriers of non-group A streptococci usually show only a few colonies on culture. In addition, as the carrier state progresses, the streptococci lose their ability to produce M protein, so that by the eleventh week, about 40 percent of strains cannot be typed. Quantitative examination of cultures and typing provide important data regarding the possible duration of the carrier state, and this information is valuable in determining whether or not therapy should be instituted.

Ability to spread disease appears to be an attribute of individuals who have been infected recently. Whether such persons harbor numerous streptococci in the nose and throat or whether the organisms are especially capable of parasitizing another person cannot be determined from the available evidence. It is established that nasal carriers of group A streptococci are likely to spread disease. The spread of streptococci in any population group is related to the degree of exposure, and, during the winter months when people are confined to enclosed areas, and under crowded conditions, dissemination of bacteria is especially likely to occur.

Group A streptococci naturally deposited in dust and on blankets will not produce respiratory infections in man. The evidence implicates the direct mode of transfer as primarily responsible for dissemination of such infections.

Outbreaks of streptococcal infection occasionally occur following the contamination of food. These outbreaks are dramatic because a large number of persons are affected almost simultaneously.

Primary infection of the upper part of the respiratory tract is undoubtedly the most common form of streptococcal infection in man. It is doubtful whether anyone in the United States escapes one or more of these infections. In most areas the disease is endemic. Epidemics are usually due to one or, at the most, several types of group A streptococci, while many different types are responsible for cases of pharyngitis and tonsillitis occurring sporadically.

Tonsillitis and pharyngitis are characterized by an acute sore throat which may or may not be accompanied by a cutaneous rash. If a rash is observed, a diagnosis of *scarlet fever* is made. The severity of scarlet fever is decreasing; the reason for this is not entirely clear.

Bacterial pneumonia caused by aerobic streptococci accounts for less than 5 percent of all cases of pneumonia. The disease is almost invariably caused by group A streptococci and may arise secondarily to an infection of the upper part of the respiratory tract. Epidemics have been observed following influenza and measles.

Formerly it was thought that *erysipelas* was caused by a specific strain of beta-hemolytic streptococcus, but it is now known that group A, C, or G streptococci may be isolated from the skin lesions. Group A organisms are responsible for the majority of infections, and the organisms may belong to any of the various types in this group. Erysipelas tends to occur in the older age groups, especially in those individuals with chronic disabling diseases. Immunity does not develop; in fact, individuals who have had one attack are more susceptible than the normal population. In some of the recurrences, however, the organisms cannot be isolated from the skin lesions but may be found in the oropharynx. In these instances the disease may be due to absorption of some streptococcal toxin, which, in turn, causes the local inflammatory lesion in the skin that has altered its reactivity.

Wounds may be infected by droplet contamination at the time of dressing. *Lymphangitis* may arise from a minute abrasion.

Numerous studies have indicated that either aerobic or anaerobic streptococci cause *puerperal sepsis*, but approximately 70 percent of fatal cases are due to beta-hemolytic streptococci. Because the group A streptococcus is rarely isolated from the genital tract either before or after labor, infection probably is contracted from an outside source and occasionally from the respiratory tract of the patient herself.

In contrast to streptococcal pharyngitis, *impetigo* occurs most frequently during the summer and early fall months and in most tropical climates. Minor skin trauma, insect bites, and poor personal hygiene predispose to infection, especially in infants and young children. Modes of infection are not well defined, but physical contact with infected children, deposits in the environment, or transfer by flies probably play a role. Primary respiratory spread is not required. Impetigo is especially likely to be caused by M types 8, 11, 22, 33, 41, 43, 52 to 54, 56, 59, 61 and in addition by the nephritogenic skin M types 2, 49, 55, 57, and 60. Rheumatic fever, rarely, if ever, follows such skin infections.

PATHOGENESIS

Streptococci gain entrance into the body through inhalation and are usually cleared away rapidly by normal defense mechanisms. Multiple factors determine whether or not infection occurs. The *dosage* of streptococci is important; infection usually results when there is exposure to large numbers of group A streptococci, as occurs in food-borne outbreaks. The *virulence* of streptococci is decisive, since non-group A streptococci and nontypable group A organisms rarely produce recognizable respiratory disease. Rapid passage of typable group A organisms in man is thought to increase virulence, but there is no good evidence to support this hypothesis.

Perhaps as important as the organism itself is the susceptibility of the host. Immunity to group A infection is type-specific and, once acquired, lasts for years. In the absence of type-specific antibody, phagocytosis is markedly suppressed and invasion and spread of organisms can occur rapidly. Recovery in 5 to 7 days is assumed to be due to the development of type-specific antibodies, with attending phagocytosis and killing of the bacteria. Little is known concerning immunity in group A skin infections or infections with other groups of streptococci. Indeed, streptococci of groups A, B, C, and D, as well as *anaerobic* streptococci and *streptococcus viridans*, are opportunistic, invading the uterus after abortion, infecting wounds, causing endocarditis, peritonitis, urinary tract infections, meningitis, and metastatic abscesses. In addition to these suppurative complications, immediate and delayed allergy to group A streptococcal products develops in early life, which may be responsible for the pathogenesis of some cases of *erythema nodosum*. *Rheu-*

matic fever and *acute glomerulonephritis* are extremely unique complications of only group A infections. Evidence is accumulating to support the concept of the possible role of cross-reactive antigen-antibody systems in the pathogenesis of rheumatic fever and rheumatic valvular disease. Less clearly defined immune mechanisms appear to be important in acute poststreptococcal glomerulonephritis. Why only certain types of group A streptococci cause nephritis is unknown, nor is there an explanation for the clinical observation that rheumatic fever seldom, if ever, follows a skin infection.

MANIFESTATIONS

ACUTE TONSILLITIS, PHARYNGITIS, AND SCARLET FEVER

Symptoms The incubation period is usually 3 to 5 days. The illness begins abruptly with symptoms of feverishness, chilliness, headache, and sore throat. Nausea and vomiting are especially common in children. A few patients complain of diarrhea. Within a period of 24 to 48 hr the disease reaches its maximum intensity. Chilliness is a constant symptom, but true rigors are rare. Approximately 75 percent or more of the patients complain of headache, malaise, and loss of appetite.

Sore throat is almost constantly present within 24 hr of onset. The soreness is aggravated by swallowing and may be referred to the neck, so that even turning of the head is accompanied by pain. Nasal obstruction and discharge are minor complaints but occur in 60 percent of patients. About half the patients develop very mild symptoms referable to the lower part of the respiratory tract, including cough and hoarseness. The cough is not productive and is rarely associated with chest pain. Loss of voice due to laryngitis does not occur. Earache is common and may last a few hours to several days. Occasionally, epistaxis is observed.

During the period of maximum temperature there may be a diffuse blush of the skin. In some cases it becomes more pronounced, and a diagnosis of *scarlet fever* is made. The rash appears 1 to 5 days after onset of illness and is first noticed over the neck and upper part of the chest. It spreads rapidly to include the skin over the abdomen and upper and lower extremities. The face appears flushed, and circumoral pallor is prominent. Itching occasionally occurs but is rarely severe.

Physical signs The degree of prostration varies, but the majority of patients appear mildly or moderately ill. The temperature is usually elevated to 102 to 104°F; occasionally it may be as high as 106°F. A few patients have no fever. In children the pulse rate is between 140 and 160, in adults between 120 and 140 per min.

Various degrees of diffuse redness of the mucous membranes of the posterior pharynx, faucial tonsils, and soft palate are invariably present. The uvula is frequently edematous, as are the tonsils and pharynx. Lymphoid hyperplasia and edema give the posterior pharynx a cobblestone appearance. Characteristically there is discrete to confluent exudate on the tonsils, and variable numbers of pinhead-size areas of exudate appear on the pharynx. In severely ill patients these are seldom seen, because nasal secretions cover the posterior wall. The exudate is often yellow, sometimes gray or white, and is relatively easily removed by swabbing. In about 20 percent of adults, and more frequently in infants, exudative lesions on the mucous membranes do not develop. If sinusitis and rhinitis are present there is a thick mucopurulent nasal discharge which may be tinged with blood. In children the nares may be excoriated. The cervical lymph nodes are swollen and frequently tender. The lymph nodes just below the angle of the jaw are the first to enlarge; rarely they attain such size that the head is thrown back. Marked adenopathy is frequently followed by suppuration.

In those patients with *scarlet fever* the signs include both an enanthem and an exanthem. The appearance of the throat is similar to that seen in tonsillitis and pharyngitis without rash, except that diffuse redness is more intense and has been described as "boiled-lobster" red. There may be punctate redness of the soft and hard palate. The buccal mucous membranes appear red and swollen, as do the lips. About the second to fifth day, small milk-white patches may be seen on the buccal mucous membranes. They represent desquamation of the epithelium and are easily peeled off.

Early in the course of the infection the tongue is heavily coated and grayish. Soon the tip and edges become an angry red. Fungiform papillae become swollen and emerge through the gray surface of the tongue. By the fourth to fifth day there is complete lingual desquamation, which leaves multiple papillary elevations, the so-called "strawberry tongue."

The color of the exanthem varies and has been described as scarlet, bright red, rose-colored, or dull, dusky red. At a distance there appears to be a uniform blush, but upon close inspection innumerable small reddish points are seen. Because of pinpoint elevations at the site of the hair follicles, the skin may feel like sandpaper. This sign is of special importance in races where the skin is heavily pigmented. When the eruption is intense, there may be many small miliary vesicles over the chest and abdomen. The face may be free of rash, but ordinarily the temples and cheeks are deep red, leaving an area of pallor around the mouth and nose. The rash is due to hyperemia, and pressure causes it to fade. In some areas there may be punctate hemorrhages which do not fade; these are commonly seen in the creases at the elbow flexure (Pastia's sign), groin, and axillary folds.

Course of illness The majority of upper respiratory illnesses caused by group A streptococci are self-limited. In adults the temperature usually returns to normal by the third to fourth day; in children fever may persist for 5 to 9 days. The temperature curve is not characteristic, although there is usually a slight morning remission. In patients with scarlet fever the temperature remains elevated until the rash has reached its maximum intensity. Fever may last for several weeks, but in such instances it is well to search for some suppurative complications. The constitutional symptoms, as well as the localizing symptom of sore throat, usually disappear shortly after the fever subsides.

The edema, redness, and exudate disappear rapidly, and except for a few small isolated spots of exudate and a slight degree of redness, the throat appears normal shortly after the fever subsides. The lymphoid tissues of the posterior pharynx as well as the tonsils decrease in size and by the third to sixth week appear to be normal. The lymph nodes may not return to normal size for 6 weeks.

When rash does occur, it usually makes its appearance on the second day, reaches its maximum intensity shortly thereafter, and then begins to fade. The exfoliation of the epithelium begins during the decline of the eruption and is seen first in those areas where the rash originally appeared. By the sixth to seventh day it is more or less generalized. On the hands and feet the skin sheds in flakes or, more rarely, as an entire cast of the hand or foot. The skin in these areas becomes dry, hard, and wrinkled. The most typical form of desquamation is seen beneath the free edge of the fingernails. A fissure appears under the edge of the nail and then widens, revealing the soft, pinkish underlying skin.

Laboratory findings In 80 percent of patients the total leukocyte count is increased. During the first 2 days of disease the average count is 14,000, and as the illness progresses, it returns to normal values. If the number of leukocytes remains elevated after 1 week, evidence of a complication may be found. During the first 2 days of illness eosinophils are rarely seen, but convalescence is characterized by an increase in number of these cells. Patients with scarlet fever are especially likely to have eosinophilia. Not frequently a trace of albumin may be found in the urine during the acute phase of the illness, and rarely, such specimens show a few red cells or casts. Proteinuria during the first 5 days of illness is transient and is not attended by serious sequelae.

Diagnosis Important features in the diagnosis of streptococcal pharyngitis and tonsillitis are the history of an acute onset of soreness on swallowing, associated with feverishness and other constitutional symptoms. The physical signs of diffuse redness and edema of the mucous membranes of the oropharynx, tonsils, and soft palate, the presence of discrete to confluent exudate, and the enlargement and tenderness of the lymph nodes at the angle of the jaw are especially helpful. These findings, together with a leukocyte count of at least 12,000, suggest a streptococcal infection. If the culture of the local lesion shows a predominant growth of beta streptococci, the diagnosis is established with certainty. When only a few colonies grow on the blood agar plate, it is impossible to be sure whether the patient is a carrier or actually has an infection due to the streptococcus. In such cases it is of considerable help to obtain acute and convalescent blood specimens for determination of antistreptolysin titers.

When a rash is associated with the above clinical and laboratory findings, the diagnosis is scarlet fever. Confirmation is obtained if the skin desquamates.

Differential diagnosis of sore throat *Nonbacterial exudative tonsillitis and pharyngitis* must be differentiated from streptococcal infections of the oropharynx (Chap. 186). Adenoviruses will produce respiratory infections associated with exudative lesions, and in some outbreaks the conjunctiva is involved. In general the onset of illness is not rapid, sore throat is seldom marked, and constitutional symptoms are mild. Hoarseness and cough are likely to occur several days after the onset. The exudate is rarely confluent. The lymph nodes may be slightly enlarged but are not remarkably tender.

The leukocyte count is usually normal, although in a few cases it may be slightly elevated. Cultures of the throat fail to show beta-hemolytic streptococci. Occasionally a few streptococci are recovered, but these organisms usually belong to groups other than A and occur only in small numbers.

Infectious mononucleosis is most frequently observed in young adults and, because of the local reaction in the throat, is likely to be confused with streptococcal pharyngitis (Chap. 224). The onset may be insidious, and malaise is prominent. Sore throat with exudative lesions of the tonsils is observed in over half the cases. Fever is more prolonged than is usual in streptococcal infections. Lymph node enlargement is more generalized, but suppuration is not observed. The spleen may be palpable. In 10 to 15 percent of cases a fleeting skin rash occurs, which may be identical with that seen in scarlet fever. The blood changes are characteristic, and a positive heterophil antibody test is usually obtained.

Vincent's angina (Chap. 150) is not easily confused with streptococcal infections. The disease is characterized by insidious onset without constitutional symptoms. Fever is rare. The area surrounding the exudate shows little inflammatory reaction, generally only one tonsil is involved, and cervical adenopathy is usually unilateral.

In contrast to streptococcal pharyngitis, the onset of *diphtheria* is rarely sudden and the symptoms are not severe (Chap. 151). Sore throat is not a constant feature of the disease. The exudate is smooth and cream-colored and appears to be incorporated in the mucous membranes. The membrane is removed with difficulty, leaving a bleeding bed. Cutaneous rashes are absent. Cultures show *Corynebacterium diphtheriae.*

In patients with a rash, the disease must be differentiated from *rubella* (Chap. 196) and *rubeola* (Chap. 195). In German measles the posterior cervical lymph node enlargement is helpful, as well as the fact that the rash tends to be macular and discrete. The tongue never peels, and a leukopenia is characteristic. In measles there are prodromal respiratory symptoms, and the maculopapular rash occurs chiefly on the face and neck. The presence of Koplik's spots aids in establishing the diagnosis.

Streptococcal infections without exudate or a cutaneous rash must be differentiated from *influenza virus infection* (Chap. 188) and *common respiratory diseases* (Chap. 186). In general, this differentiation cannot be made on clinical evidence alone, and the leukocyte count, culture studies, and serologic tests must be employed.

Primary *herpes simplex pharyngitis* (Chap. 200) and *herpangina* (Chap. 190) are characterized by vesicles which rupture and produce small ulcers covered with exudate. Herpetic lesions are scattered over all mucous membranes of the mouth, and the kissing ulcer under the tip of the tongue is typical. The ulcers of herpangina, caused by Coxsackie A viruses, are observed on the anterior pillars and the soft palate. In both diseases the leukocyte count is usually normal.

Sinusitis, otitis media, mastoiditis, and peritonsillar abscess Infection of the paranasal sinuses probably occurs to a minor degree in all patients with streptococcal respiratory infections. Sinusitis and otitis media presenting overt clinical signs develop in approximately 3 percent of patients whose tonsils and adenoids are intact. Mastoiditis is observed in less than 1 percent of patients. Peritonsillar cellulitis is observed in 2.5 percent of patients with tonsils, but it rarely occurs in those whose tonsils have been removed or in those patients who receive proper therapy with antibiotics. The diagnosis and management of these suppurative complications are described in Chap. 251.

PNEUMONIA AND EMPYEMA Primary group A streptococcal pneumonia is rare in the absence of influenza, but many cases may occur during an influenza epidemic. The onset of pneumonia tends to be abrupt, with symptoms of chills, fever, anorexia, and vomiting. Cough, sputum that is pink and thin, and chest pain are characteristic. The temperature is usually high (104°F), and fever is intermittent. Examination reveals scattered fine rales, but signs of lobar consolidation are rare.

The leukocyte count is high (20,000 to 30,000), and large numbers of group A organisms are cultured from the sputum. Usually the blood cultures are sterile. With proper therapy with penicillin, recovery is rapid. Empyema is a frequent complication in patients who receive no therapy. The pleural fluid is pink and thin; it thickens only when infected with other organisms.

PERICARDITIS, ARTHRITIS, PERITONITIS, AND MENINGITIS Streptococcal infections of the various body cavities result from bacteremia or from extension from a local lesion. *Pericarditis*, a rare complication, is especially likely to occur during the course of pneumonia or empyema. The diagnosis is difficult, because the symptoms arising from pericarditis are overshadowed by the primary disease. The first sign may be a sudden increase in pulse rate and the development of an audible pericardial friction rub.

Suppurative arthritis is secondary to bacteremia or to extension of a local cellulitis. It is a rare complication of streptococcal sore throat. Pain is the most common symptom, and usually only one joint is involved. The pain is first noticed on motion, but within a short period redness, swelling, and tenderness develop and the pain becomes intense. Aspiration reveals a fluid containing polymorphonuclear leukocytes and streptococci. Nonsuppurative arthritis seen in patients with scarlet fever during the first week of illness indicates the onset of rheumatic fever and should not be considered a manifestation of erythrogenic toxin.

Infection of the peritoneum with the hemolytic streptococcus is rare but is especially apt to be associated with such local infections as erysipelas and scarlet fever. In these cases the organism belongs to Lancefield group A. Symptoms develop rapidly, and in addition to fever and other constitutional symptoms, prostration, abdominal pain, and vomiting are prominent. The pulse is rapid and weak. The abdomen is distended, tender, and rigid to palpation.

Streptococcal *meningitis* is usually caused by group A organisms, but occasionally members of other groups may be isolated from the spinal fluid. In most instances the meningitis arises by extension from otitis media, mastoiditis, or petrositis, which are especially likely to develop following infection of the respiratory tract and are seen most frequently in the young. Prior to the introduction of specific therapy these infections were always fatal. The symptoms are not distinguishable from those of other types of bacterial meningitis. All patients, especially infants, with infections of the middle ear should be watched for signs of meningeal irritation.

WOUND AND SKIN INFECTIONS, LYMPHANGITIS, PUERPERAL FEVER, AND ERYSIPELAS Wounds, small abrasions, and children with chickenpox and other skin lesions may become infected with group A or C streptococci. *Impetigo* in children caused by group A streptococci is common. The initial lesion is a papule which then becomes vesicular with a small surrounding area of erythema. The vesicles rupture early so that they may not be observed by the physician, who sees instead small crusted lesions. Regional adenopathy is usually present. Pure cultures of streptococci are obtained from the vesicle, but, in addition, staphylococci may be present in the crusted stages. Bullous impetigo is primarily staphylococcal in origin.

Hemolytic streptococci are responsible for the majority of cases of *lymphangitis*, characterized by the rapid development of one or more fine red streaks extending upward from the hand or foot. Usually the process continues up to the axilla or groin, and the lymph nodes in these areas become enlarged and tender. Associated with the spread of the infection in the lymphatics, such symptoms as rigor, fever, malaise, headache, and vomiting occur. Occasionally the bloodstream is invaded. The original site of infection in these cases of lymphangitis may not be apparent. Although these infections may be serious, the course of the illness is usually short, and suppuration along the course of the lymphatics seldom occurs. Within 2 weeks after a streptococcal respiratory infection, some children develop persistent *lymphadenitis*. In children with enlarged cervical nodes 75 percent of the cases are secondary to a streptococcal infection. In these patients aspiration of the node will usually reveal the organism.

Puerperal infection may be caused by group A streptococci, but group B has assumed the predominant role in both puerperal infection in the mother and neonatal sepsis and meningitis in the infant. In approximately one-third of pregnant women harboring group B streptococci in the genital tract, childbirth will be complicated by neonatal sepsis, meningitis, prematurity, or abortion. In the mother, the streptococci invade the endometrium and lymphatics and may result in bacteremia. A high, irregular fever, rapid pulse, leukocytosis, and a foul-smelling discharge yielding group B streptococci are characteristic.

Erysipelas is an acute streptococcal infection of the skin and, to a lesser extent, of the mucous membranes. Group A streptococci are the usual cause, but other streptococci may cause this syndrome. The onset is usually abrupt, after an incubation period of 1 to 4 days. A history of preceding respiratory infection is sometimes obtained. The initial symptoms include chilliness, feverishness, headache, malaise, anorexia, and vomiting. At the onset the local cutaneous lesion may not be apparent. The skin may itch and feel sore around the point of entry of the organisms. Within a few hours, the cutaneous lesion becomes obvious.

The face is most commonly involved, but any area of the body may be infected. The point of entry may be just anterior to the ear, at the inner canthus of the eye, around the lips and nose, or over the cheeks. From these points the lesion spreads rapidly, reaching its maximum extent within 3 to 6 days. Erysipelas frequently involves the butterfly area of the cheeks and nose. The lesion consists of an advancing border which is raised from the surrounding normal skin and may be purple. Within this border the skin is tense and usually a dark dull red. If the infection occurs in areas where the skin is lax, such as around the eyes, edema is pronounced. The eyelids frequently become so swollen that they cannot be opened. Blebs or necrotic areas may appear as the disease progresses.

At the height of the infection the temperature is usually high (104 to 105°F), although occasionally the febrile response is slight. The bloodstream is not uncommonly invaded during this period. In most instances recovery is apparent by the sixth to seventh day. The local lesion begins to fade in the center, with some desquamation and pigmentation. No scarring results unless abscesses develop.

Before the introduction of chemotherapy, the fatality rate was about 15 percent. During the first 6 months of life approximately 65 percent of patients die, while in older children and young adults the death rate is low. In patients with fatal infections the lesion is likely to involve the trunk.

BACTEREMIA Streptococci are a common cause of bacteremia, but in uncomplicated tonsillitis and pharyngitis the organisms rarely invade the bloodstream. Bacteremia occurring under the age of twenty usually is secondary to otitis media, mastoiditis, or thrombosis of the lateral or cavernous sinuses. In adults, invasion of the bloodstream is especially likely to occur in puerperal infections, whereas after the age of forty bacteremia is usually secondary to cellulitis and erysipelas. Metastatic abscesses are infrequent.

The diagnosis of bacteremia is difficult and can be made only by culturing the organisms from the blood. The sudden development of chills and high fever suggests invasion of the bloodstream. There may be arthritis, signs of pneumonia, petechiae, or skin eruptions. In fulminating cases, anemia develops rapidly and jaundice may occur. Without specific therapy the mortality rate is 70 percent.

OTHER STREPTOCOCCAL INFECTIONS Non-group A and *anaerobic streptococci* as well as *streptococcus viridans* cause a wide variety of infections in man. Since these organisms are carried in the upper respiratory and the gastrointestinal tracts, they are opportunistic, invading tissues when resistance is lowered.

Group D streptococci, or enterococci, are a frequent cause of urinary tract infections and peritonitis; less frequently they cause bacterial endocarditis. In this instance, small metastatic abscesses may be observed which rarely develop when the endocarditis is caused by streptococcus viridans. Group D organisms cause some urinary tract infections in women and in men with prostatic obstruction. Treatment with ampicillin is effective, but in treating endocarditis penicillin combined with streptomycin or kanamycin is usually employed (Chap. 127).

Group C streptococci may infect burns and wounds, but they rarely cause pharyngitis or endocarditis. Streptococci of most groups have been isolated from such infections as endocarditis, meningitis, and abscesses in various tissues.

Anaerobic streptococci along with bacteroides (Chap. 135) may be cultured from the mouth, intestinal tract, and vagina, and therefore one or both of these organisms are frequently cultured from septic foci. The majority of infections occur in the perineal and inguinal regions. Thus perirectal, pilonidal, and sebaceous cyst abscesses are commonly associated with this organism. Aspiration of oral debris may result in an abscess in the lung and empyema. Brain abscess arises secondary to infections of the lungs or nasal sinuses. The fact that the brain is relatively avascular may predispose to infections with anaerobic bacteria.

A number of characteristic infections caused by anaerobic streptococci have been described. *Streptococcal myositis* develops slowly and is characterized by marked edema, crepitant myositis, and pain. Many leukocytes and chains of gram-positive cocci are seen in the seropurulent exudate. *Chronic burrowing ulcers* and *progressive synergistic gangrene* are two primarily surgical infections. The former usually develops following surgery and progresses over several months; sinus tracts develop, but pain and systemic reactions are minimal. *Synergistic gangrene*, in contrast, is painful. It develops around stay sutures and gradually spreads, presenting as an ulcer surrounded by gangrenous skin.

TREATMENT

There are now several agents which may be employed in the therapy of aerobic streptococcal infections. The sulfonamides exert a bacteriostatic effect against all Lancefield groups except D. However, some strains of group A streptococci have acquired resistance. Most antibiotics have some antistreptococcal activity, but penicillin clearly is the best antistreptococcal drug because it kills group A organisms. If it is administered for at least 10 days, in most instances all streptococci are eliminated. Therapeutic measures which do not result in the eradication of the infecting organism do not alter the attack rate of rheumatic fever.

The administration of penicillin or other antibiotics within 24 hr of the onset of streptococcal respiratory infections results in definite improvement of the symptoms and signs. When therapy is instituted after 48 hr, a favorable effect is difficult to demonstrate, but suppurative complications, including sinusitis, otitis media, and peritonsillar cellulitis are prevented. The time that treatment is started is not decisive in the reduction of rheumatic fever; however, early therapy may be important in the prevention of nephritis. In general, proper therapy instituted during the first 24 hr of illness will reduce the predicted rheumatic fever attack rate by 95 to 98 percent. If therapy is started 1, 2, or 3 weeks after the onset of sore throat, the reduction in attack rates is 90, 67, and 42 percent, respectively. Therefore to prevent rheumatic fever, a full course of therapy should be given to those who have recovered from acute-phase symptoms and received no therapy even though the onset was 3 weeks previously.

In the average case of streptococcal infection, whether scarlet fever, tonsillitis, or erysipelas, sufficient concentration of antibiotic can be maintained readily by a single injection of 600,000 to 1,200,000 units of benzathine penicillin. In patients with rheumatic heart disease who develop a streptococcal infection, it is advisable to administer 600,000 units of procaine penicillin twice daily for 2 weeks.

Oral therapy may be prescribed, but many patients discontinue the medication when the acute symptoms subside. Under these circumstances, the organism frequently invades the tissues again, and a clinical relapse occurs. More important, the attack rate of the nonsuppurative complications is not altered. All forms of oral medication must be taken in full doses for at least 10 days and preferably for 2 weeks. Oral penicillin G should be given in doses of at least 250,000 units four times daily. Penicillin V in dosage of 1 to 2 g daily or phenethicillin may be preferable because these agents resist degradation by gastric acid. Patients sensitive to penicillin may be given erythromycin in doses of 0.25 g every 6 hr. Tetracycline drugs should not be employed because of the high prevalence of resistant strains.

The *sulfonamides* should never be employed in the treatment of streptococcal infections because they fail to eliminate the infecting organism and do not alter the subsequent attack rate of rheumatic fever. Penicillin decreases the incidence of suppurative complications of tonsillitis and pharyngitis.

Infections of the mastoid and paranasal sinuses should be treated by the parenteral administration of 1.2 to 2.4 million units penicillin G every day. Streptococcal pneumonia should be treated with somewhat larger amounts of penicillin. Empyema, purulent pericarditis, and arthritis are treated best by local instillation of 10,000 to 50,000 units penicillin G every 48 to 72 hr until cultures are sterile. In addition, full doses of parenteral penicillin should be administered. In these infections early treatment is required if surgical drainage is to be avoided.

Treatment of streptococcal infections caused by groups other than A with penicillin is usually effective, although some strains of groups D and F are relatively resistant. In treating anaerobic infections, drainage of abscesses, debridement, and supportive measures are important. Cultures and smears of exudate or aspirate from patients with cellulitis or streptococcal myonecrosis will assist in the selection of the proper antibiotics to be used in addition to penicillin.

PREVENTION

There is no completely adequate method for the prevention of streptococcal infections. A number of procedures will limit the spread of the organism. The problem is exceedingly complicated because group A streptococci occur in the upper part of the respiratory tract of many individuals.

In the past it was customary to isolate all patients with scarlet fever, but this seems unwarranted, particularly because no precautions are taken for sore throat without a rash caused by the same bacterium. Any patient with a streptococcal infection of the upper part of the respiratory tract may be a source of infection. During the acute stage of all such illnesses the patient should be advised against intimate contact with others.

Approximately 90 percent of patients with untreated streptococcal infections continue to carry the organism in the pharynx 3 months after the acute infection. Usually the number of organisms is small. Individuals with suppurative sinusitis are likely to harbor large numbers of streptococci and are a dangerous source of infection. Proper therapy of acute infections with penicillin prevents the development of the carrier state and promptly eliminates the organism.

Individuals or groups can be protected from streptococcal infections by the prophylactic use of sulfonamides. For this purpose 1 g sulfadiazine or sulfisoxazole is administered daily. When given to populations already experiencing an epidemic, this prophylactic measure will control the outbreak as long as the drug is administered. When therapy is discontinued, streptococcal infections again occur because of the failure of sulfonamides to eliminate the infecting organism. For this reason, oral penicillin in doses of 250,000 units two or three times daily for 10 days or a single injection of 1,200,000 units of benzathine penicillin is a preferred form of prophylaxis in large groups. Benzathine penicillin in doses of 600,000 and 1,200,000 units will protect the individual from new infections for 3 or 4 to 6 weeks, respectively.

Tonsillectomy has been employed widely as a prophylactic measure against streptococcal infections because tonsillitis cannot occur if the organ is removed. However, no protection is afforded against streptococcal pharyngitis. Indeed, tonsillectomy makes subsequent recognition of the cause of the respiratory illness more difficult.

REFERENCES

BORNSTEIN DL et al: Anaerobic infections—review of current experience. Medicine 43:207, 1964

DAJANI AS et al: Etiology of cervical lymphadenitis in children. N Engl J Med 268:1329, 1963

REINARZ JA, SANFORD JP: Human infections caused by non-group A or D streptococci. Medicine 44:81, 1965

STOLLERMAN GH: Nephritogenic and rheumatogenic group A streptococci. J Infect Dis 120:258, 1969

WANNAMAKER LW: Differences between streptococcal infections of the throat and of the skin. N Engl J Med 282:23, 1970

——, MATSEN JM: *Streptococci and Streptococcal Diseases: Recognition, Understanding and Management*, New York: Academic, 1972

131 MENINGOCOCCAL INFECTIONS

HARRY N. BEATY

DEFINITION The meningococcus *Neisseria meningitidis* is the causative organism of a variety of infections, notably meningitis and bacteremia.

ETIOLOGY The organism responsible for "cerebrospinal fever" was first described by Weichselbaum in 1887. It was subsequently assigned to the genus *Neisseria,* and is now designated by the binomial *Neisseria meningitidis* and the common name meningococcus. In stained smears, meningococci are gram-negative and characteristically appear as single cocci or diplococci with flattened adjacent sides. They grow well on solid or semisolid media containing blood, serum, or ascitic fluid, and thrive best at temperatures between 35 and 37°C in an atmosphere reduced in oxygen and containing 5 to 10 percent CO_2. The organism is recovered readily from biologic fluids when fresh specimens are inoculated on warm chocolate agar plates which are incubated 18 to 24 hr in a candle jar or in a more sophisticated apparatus that provides a suitable environment.

The biochemical reactions of the *Neisseria* are relatively limited, but they contain cytochrome oxidase, which is responsible for the positive "oxidase" test, and clinically significant species usually are differentiated by their ability to produce acid in glucose, maltose, or sucrose. Typically the meningococcus ferments both glucose and maltose, but on occasion maltose-negative strains have been isolated.

Meningococci can be divided into serologic groups on the basis of agglutination reactions with immune serum. The present classification into groups A, B, C, and D was agreed upon in 1950, but since 1960, new groups including X, Y, and Z have been identified. The major groups are remarkably heterogeneous, but subclassification with bacteriocin typing or additional serologic markers has been possible.

EPIDEMIOLOGY The natural habitat of meningococci is the nasopharynx of man, and no other reservoir or vector has been recognized. The principal means of spread is through inhalation of droplets of infected nasopharyngeal secretions, and it is unlikely that the disease is spread by contact with contaminated fomites. Meningococci cause either epidemic or sporadic disease, and there is a cyclic variation in the prevalence of meningococcal infection with peaks of increased frequency occurring every 8 to 12 years and lasting 4 to 6 years. A minor upward trend in this cycle began in the United States in 1962 and reached a peak in 1965. For the epidemic years 1967 through 1971, the attack rate of meningococcal disease was somewhat lower and constant. The prevalence of meningococcal infection is also subject to seasonal influences; the lowest attack rate occurs in midsummer and the highest in late winter and early spring. This seasonal variation follows that of other bacterial and viral respiratory infections and may reflect crowded indoor living conditions encountered during the winter months.

The attack rate of meningococcal disease is highest for children between six months and one year of age. A second, much lower, peak in incidence occurs among adolescents, and the lowest attack rate occurs in individuals over twenty-five. There is no clear-cut tendency for racial or sexual predominance, but presumably because of an increased opportunity to acquire infection, males develop meningitis and meningococcemia more frequently than females. Military recruits are particularly susceptible, and worldwide epidemics of meningococcal disease have occurred during most major wars. These outbreaks usually parallel less apparent trends in the civilian population.

Since 1915, most epidemics of meningococcal disease have been caused by group A meningococci, and strains of groups B and C have been associated with sporadic, interepidemic infections. However, in the outbreaks of 1963 and 1964 a major shift in the pattern of meningococcal infection became apparent as group B meningococci were isolated from the majority of clinical infections in both civilian and military populations. In 1967, over 70 percent of meningococci isolated were group B. However, early in 1968, another shift began, and in the epidemic year 1971, 63 percent of the meningococcal strains submitted to the Center for Disease Control were group C. The significance of these epidemiologic shifts is enhanced by the fact that a high proportion of the meningococci in groups B and C are resistant to 1 mg per 100 ml sulfadiazine, and prophylaxis with this drug, which was successful in aborting epidemics during World War II, has been relatively ineffective since 1960. The few group A meningococci recovered in this country since 1967 remain sensitive to sulfonamides, but in Africa sulfonamide-resistant strains have been isolated.

Carriers Between epidemics, 2 to 15 percent of the individuals in urban centers harbor meningococci in the nasopharynx. When sporadic cases of meningococcal disease occur, the carrier rate in close contacts may rise to 25 percent, and in closed populations or during epidemics, may approach 100 percent. Although some individuals harbor meningococci for months or years, nasopharyngeal infection is usually transient, and in 75 percent of carriers the organism disappears within a few weeks. The relation between the proportion of carriers in a population and the occurrence of meningococcal disease is unclear. Case-to-case transmission of infection is documented rarely, and carriers, not patients, are the foci from which disease is spread. It appears that the prevalence of meningococcal disease can be attributed to the prevailing carrier rate only in a general way, and that the occurrence of clinical disease is most dependent on unknown circumstances within the host which lead to spread of infection beyond the nasopharynx.

Immunity The fact that meningococcal meningitis is primarily a disease of childhood has long suggested that natural immunity develops in most individuals within the first two decades of life. There is a correlation between susceptibility to meningococcal disease and absence of bactericidal antibody in the serum, and the serum of most adults contains antibodies to pathogenic strains of meningococci. Natural immunization appears to result from asymptomatic carriage of meningococci in the nasopharynx. Not only does the carrier state produce antibodies to the infecting strain, but cross-reacting antibodies may develop, even after colonization with avirulent nongroupable organisms. The immunity conferred by meningococcal meningitis or meningococcemia is usually group-specific, and second episodes of meningococcal disease have been encountered.

PATHOGENESIS The primary focus of meningococcal infection is in the nasopharynx. In most instances, this infection is subclinical, but occasionally localized inflammation occurs and mild symptoms develop. Dissemination of meningococci from the nasopharynx occurs via the bloodstream, and generally is followed by clinical manifestations of meningococcal disease. *Purulent meningitis* is the most common form of metastatic infection encountered and is either associated with signs and symptoms of meningococcemia or constitutes the predominant clinical expression of illness. Organisms in the meninges induce an acute inflammatory reaction, and purulent exudate spreads across the surface of the brain. Rarely, a more extensive inflammatory reaction produces an acute diffuse encephalitis.

Although the mechanisms responsible for the pathologic changes associated with meningococcal infection have not been explained entirely, the tissue injury observed in laboratory animals appears to be caused by a toxic substance liberated from dead bacteria. This substance is presumed to be an endotoxin which has not been characterized biochemically, but which is biologically similar to endotoxins of other gram-negative bacteria. It may be responsible for hypotension and vascular collapse observed in fulminant meningococcemia and may also play a role in the pathogenesis of the purpura and visceral hemorrhages associated with meningococcal bacteremia. Thrombosis of dermal venules, adrenal sinusoids, and renal glomerular capillaries is commonly seen in patients who die of fulminant meningococcemia and is strikingly similar to the pathologic changes observed in the experimental Shwartzman reaction. It is postulated that endotoxin either induces a Shwartzman reaction directly or effects the release of clotting factors which initiate intravascular coagulation and produce these characteristic pathologic changes.

CLINICAL MANIFESTATIONS Ninety to ninety-five percent of patients with meningococcal disease have meningococcemia and/or meningitis.

Meningococcemia Thirty to fifty percent of patients who develop overt disease have meningococcemia without meningitis. The onset of clinical illness may be abrupt, but patients usually have nonspecific prodromal symptoms of cough, headache, and sore throat followed by the sudden development of spiking fever, chills, arthralgia, and muscle pains which may be particularly severe in the lower extremities and back. Patients usually appear acutely ill with an inordinate degree of prostration. In addition to high fever, tachycardia, and tachypnea, mild hypotension may be present. However, clinical shock does not occur unless fulminant meningococcemia supervenes. In the course of meningococcal bacteremia, about three-fourths of the patients develop a characteristic petechial rash. Lesions are frequently sparse, and the axillas, flanks, wrists, and ankles are the most commonly involved sites. Often petechiae are located in the center of lighter-colored macules, and they may become nodular as the disease progresses. The diagnosis of meningococcemia occasionally can be established by demonstrating gram-negative diplococci in scrapings from these nodular lesions. In severe cases, purpuric spots or large ecchymoses develop, and a widespread petechial or purpuric eruption suggests fulminating disease. However, the absence of rash does not necessarily indicate that the illness will be mild.

Fulminant meningococcemia, or the Waterhouse-Friderichsen syndrome, is meningococcemia associated with vasomotor collapse and shock. It occurs in 10 to 20 percent of patients with generalized meningococcal infection, and is associated with a high fatality rate. The onset is abrupt, and profound prostration frequently occurs within a few hours. Petechiae and purpuric lesions enlarge rapidly, and hemorrhage into the skin may be extensive. Early in the preshock stage, there is generalized vasoconstriction; patients are alert and pale, with circumoral cyanosis and cold extremities. Upon entering the shock stage, however, coma develops, the cardiac output decreases, and the blood pressure drops. Unless incipient shock is recognized and appropriate therapy instituted early, death from cardiac and/or respiratory failure almost invariably occurs. Patients who recover may have extensive sloughing of skin lesions and even loss of digits because of gangrene.

Chronic meningococcemia is a rare form of meningococcal infection which lasts for weeks or months and is characterized by fever, rash, and arthritis or arthralgia. Typically, the fever is intermittent, and during afebrile periods, which may last several days, patients appear remarkably well. The usual rash is a maculopapular or polymorphous eruption which waxes and wanes with the fever, but petechial or nodular lesions may be seen. Joint involvement is present in two-thirds of the patients, and splenomegaly is detected in about 20 percent. If the diagnosis is not suspected or treatment is otherwise delayed, complications such as meningitis, carditis, or nephritis may occur.

Meningitis Meningitis is a common form of meningococcal disease which occurs primarily in children over six months of age and in adolescents. Fever, vomiting, headache, and confusion or lethargy are the commonest symptoms; in about one-fourth of the patients, symptoms begin abruptly and rapidly increase in severity. The more typical patient, however, has symptoms of an upper respiratory tract infection followed by an illness which progresses over several days. Twenty to forty percent of patients have meningitis without clinical evidence of meningococcemia, and the diagnosis depends upon bacteriologic examination of the cerebrospinal fluid. However, when meningitis occurs in association with a petechial or purpuric rash, a presumptive diagnosis of meningococcal disease is warranted, because this pattern of illness is seen only rarely in other infections.

Rarer manifestations The meningococcus is a rare cause of purulent conjunctivitis or sinusitis, and it has been reported to cause lobar or bronchopneumonia in patients without evidence of meningitis or meningococcemia. Bacterial endocarditis also has been reported. On rare occasion, meningococci have produced genital infections clinically indistinguishable from gonococcal disease.

LABORATORY FINDINGS Aside from bacteriologic data, laboratory studies are of little value in establishing the diagnosis of meningococcal infection. Polymorphonuclear leukocyte counts usually range from 12,000 to 40,000 cells per mm^3, but in meningococcemia, normal or low leukocyte counts may be encountered. Anemia is uncommon, and levels of serum electrolytes and blood urea nitrogen are normal unless shock develops. Patients with prominent hemorrhagic manifestations may have low platelet counts and decreased levels of circulating clotting factors as a result of intravascular coagulation. In meningitis, the cerbrospinal fluid pressure is increased, and the fluid usually contains from 100 to 40,000 polymorphonuclear leukocytes per mm^3. The protein content is increased, and the concentration of glucose is almost always less than 35 mg per 100 ml and often is between 0 and 10 mg per 100 ml.

Meningococci can be recovered readily from cultures of blood or spinal fluid, and, on occasion, material aspirated from skin lesions or joints yields the organism. In addition, gram-negative diplococci may be seen in stains of nodular petechiae or the buffy coat of blood from patients with meningococcemia. In meningococcal meningitis, a smear of the spinal fluid is diagnostic in about half the patients but often shows only a few intracellular bacteria which are located with difficulty.

COMPLICATIONS Herpes labialis occurs in 5 to 20 percent of patients with meningococcal disease. Other complications, which result from neurologic damage or secondary foci of infection, are uncommon following appropriate treatment and are often transient. Seizures or deafness occurs in 10 to 20 percent of patients during the acute stages of meningitis, but postmeningitic epilepsy is rare, and the frequency of permanent eighth nerve damage is probably less than 5 percent. Peripheral neuropathy, cranial nerve palsies, and hemiplegia are seen occasionally, but usually clear completely within 2 to 4 months. Hydrocephalus and thrombosis of venous sinuses, once frequent sequelae of meningococcal meningitis, are encountered rarely. A number of patients complain of recurrent headache, emotional lability, insomnia, backache, memory loss, and difficulty in concentrating for months after an episode of meningitis. The organic basis for these symptoms is obscure, but they usually disappear a year or two after the infection.

Arthritis is a common metastatic complication of meningococcemia and occurs in 2 to 10 percent of patients. As a rule, multiple joints are involved, and signs and symptoms may not appear until after treatment of meningitis or meningococcemia has been instituted. Joint fluid usually contains many granulocytes, but meningococci are recovered infrequently. Antibiotic therapy does not appear to influence the course of the arthritis, and permanent joint changes are rare. Other purulent complications have become extremely uncommon since antibiotics have gained widespread use. Pneumonia occurs occasionally, but it is uncertain whether it is caused by the meningococcus or coincident infection with other bacteria. Bacterial endocarditis is quite rare, but *a high proportion of patients who die of meningococcal infection have myocarditis.* The etiology of these myocardial changes is uncertain, but cardiac failure may be an important factor in the pathogenesis of the shock syndrome in meningococcemia. A pericardial friction rub or electrocardiographic change of pericarditis is seen in about 5 percent of patients.

DIAGNOSIS The diagnosis of meningococcal disease depends upon recovering *N. meningitidis* from cultures of blood, spinal fluid, or petechial scrapings from patients with a typical clinical picture. Recovery of meningococci from the nasopharynx does not, in itself, establish the diagnosis.

Few diseases need to be considered seriously in the differential diagnosis of meningococcal disease. If meningococcal meningitis is not accompanied by manifestations of bacteremia, it is indistinguishable from meningitis caused by other common pathogens. Occasionally, the common viral exanthems, Rocky Mountain spotted fever (Chap. 176), and vascular purpuras (Chap. 313) may be confused with meningococcemia, and their differentiation depends upon demonstration of the organism and knowledge of the epidemiology and clinical manifestations of each disease.

TREATMENT Antimicrobial therapy of suspected or documented meningococcal disease should be instituted as early as possible. Penicillin G is the drug of choice, and should be administered intravenously. The dosage for the treatment of meningitis in adults is 12 to 24 million units per day, and in the pediatric age group, 16 million units per square meter (day). Meningococcemia can be treated with 5 to 10 million units a day, because it is not necessary to achieve high levels of antibiotic in the spinal fluid. If treatment with these doses is continued for a minimum of 7 days, or 4 to 5 days after the patient becomes afebrile, relapse is extremely rare. Ampicillin in doses of 200 to 300 mg per kg (day) is as effective as penicillin G, and has been recommended for initial treatment of meningitis in children because it is effective against *Hemophilus in-*

fluenzae. When bacteriologic confirmation of meningococcal disease is available, however, treatment should be switched to penicillin G because it is less costly. Meningococci are susceptible to other antimicrobial agents such as chloramphenicol and tetracycline, but they should not be used unless a patient is allergic to penicillin. Under these circumstances, chloramphenicol hemisuccinate 4.0 to 6.0 g per day in divided doses (in adults) is an acceptable alternate. Sensitivity tests usually indicate that cephalothin could be a suitable alternative to penicillin, but treatment failures with this drug have been reported. *Because a significant proportion of meningococci isolated are resistant to sulfonamides, these drugs should not be used alone in the treatment of meningococcal infections,* and their use in combination with penicillin offers no advantage.

Patients with meningococcal infections require supportive treatment as well as antimicrobial therapy. Maintenance of fluid and electrolyte balance and prevention of respiratory complications in comatose patients are of primary concern. When shock occurs, visceral perfusion must be improved by maintenance of an adequate intravascular volume, treatment of heart failure, and support of the blood pressure. Vasopressors may produce temporary improvement, but agents which block alpha-adrenergic receptors (Dibenzylene) or which stimulate beta-adrenergic receptors (isoproterenol) may be more physiologic. This can be determined best by carefully monitoring the blood pressure, pulse, arterial blood gases, cardiac output, peripheral resistance, pulmonary artery wedge pressures, and arteriovenous oxygen differences. When heart failure is present, diuretics and digitalis should be given. When intravascular coagulation is recognized, treatment with heparin, whole blood, or fibrinogen can be tried, but dramatic results should not be expected. Massive doses of adrenal cortical steroids as used in the treatment of septic shock (Chap. 124) may be helpful, but lower "replacement" doses are of uncertain value.

PREVENTION With the widespread emergence of sulfonamide-resistant meningococci, alternate methods of preventing meningococcal disease in closed populations were sought. High molecular weight polysaccharide antigens from organisms of serogroups A and C have been shown to induce a group-specific bactericidal antibody response after subcutaneous injection. Large-scale field trials with the group C vaccine led to a 90 percent reduction in group C disease among vaccinated recruits. Similar results are expected with the group A vaccine, and when a suitable antigen from group B organisms is available, it is likely that a highly effective polyvalent vaccine can be developed.

For intimate contacts of sporadic cases of meningococcal disease, chemoprophylaxis should be considered. If the organism isolated from the patient is sensitive to sulfonamides, these drugs are preferred for prophylaxis. When sensitivities are not known or the organism is resistant to sulfonamides, rifampin in dosage of 600 mg a day for 4 days or minocycline in dosage of 100 mg every 12 hr for 5 days can be expected to temporarily eradicate the carrier state and minimize spread of meningococci.

PROGNOSIS Before the introduction of antibiotics, meningococcal meningitis and meningococcemia were almost invariably fatal. With prompt and appropriate chemotherapy, the mortality rate of meningitis without fulminant meningococcemia has dropped to less than 10 percent in the United States, and neurologic sequelae are rare. The mortality of fulminant infection remains high primarily because patients are often in irreversible shock when treatment is instituted. Most deaths occur within 24 to 48 hr of admission, and the capacity of the meningococcus to kill a perfectly healthy individual within a few hours remains one of the most awesome characteristics of this disease.

REFERENCES

ARTENSTEIN MS et al: Prevention of meningococcal disease by group C polysaccharide vaccine. N Engl J Med 282:417, 1970

GOLDSCHNEIDER I et al: Human immunity to the meningococcus: I. The role of humoral antibodies. J Exp Med 129:1307, 1969

——: Human immunity to the meningococcus: II. Development of natural immunity. J Exp Med 129:1327, 1969

MANIOS SG et al: Fulminant meningococcemia. Scand J Infect Dis 3:127, 1971

The clinical spectrum of meningococcal disease (medical staff conference). Calif Med 113:36, 1970

132 GONOCOCCAL INFECTIONS

KING K. HOLMES
HARRY N. BEATY

DEFINITION Gonorrhea, an infection of columnar and transitional epithelium caused by *Neisseria gonorrhoeae*, is the most common reportable communicable disease in the United States. Anatomic sites which can be infected directly by the gonococcus include the urethra, anal canal, conjunctivae, pharynx, and endocervix. Local complications include salpingitis, endometritis, peritonitis, and bartholinitis in the female, and periurethral abscess and epididymitis in the male. Systemic manifestations of gonococcemia include arthritis, dermatitis, endocarditis, and meningitis, as well as myopericarditis and "toxic" hepatitis.

ETIOLOGY *Neisseria gonorrhoeae* is a gram-negative diplococcus which forms oxidase-positive colonies and is differentiated from other *Neisseria* by its ability to ferment glucose, but not maltose, sucrose, or lactose. Occasionally, fastidious strains of *N. gonorrhoeae* repeatedly fail to ferment glucose but can be identified by specific immunofluorescent staining.

At least four morphologically distinct colony types of gonococci occur when the organism is passed in vitro. Colony types 1 and 2 predominate on primary isolation, retain virulence during repeated selective subculture in vitro, and are covered by surface projections called pili, which are visible on electron microscopy. Spontaneous transition to colony types 3 and 4 in vitro results in some loss of virulence together with the disappearance of pili.

EPIDEMIOLOGY An estimated two and one-half million cases of gonorrhea were treated in the United States in 1972. Teen-agers comprise nearly 25 percent of cases, while 90 percent are under age thirty-five. The annual incidence of reported gonorrhea in the United States, corrected for population growth, increased by only 10 percent during the 5-year period 1957–1962, then rapidly climbed by over 150 percent during the decade 1962–1972. The sudden upward trend followed the introduction of oral contraceptives in 1960 and the availability of the intrauterine device in 1963. These new methods of contraception have resulted in the abandonment of mechanical prophylactics, such as the condom, and in increased sexual promiscuity among adults of all ages. Use of subcurative therapy and inadequate tracing of infected contacts have also contributed to the current gonorrhea pandemic.

The only natural host for *N. gonorrhoeae* is man, although chimpanzees have been inoculated experimentally and have subsequently transmitted the infection during intercourse. Since most individuals with symptomatic gonorrhea seek treatment, it is axiomatic that asymptomatic men and women who are chronic or incubating carriers of *N. gonorrhoeae* comprise the remaining reservoir of gonococcal infection in the community. When patients with acute symptomatic gonorrhea are interviewed to determine their source contacts, it is essential to remember that these source contacts, whether male or female, are frequently without symptoms. The prevalence of gonorrhea in United States servicemen has recently been found to be 2.5 percent, and two-thirds of those infected have been asymptomatic carriers. Among women, the prevalence of asymptomatic endocervical infection ranges from 1 percent of young married women of middle income to nearly 10 percent of young single women of low income.

Transmission of *N. gonorrhoeae* among adults occurs only during sexual activity. The risk of transmission of gonorrhea from an infected woman to a man during intercourse has ranged from 5 percent to 20 percent in separate studies. The risk of infection of women by men has not been studied.

CLINICAL MANIFESTATIONS The clinical spectrum of gonococcal infections depends upon the site of inoculation, the temporal stage of the disease, and the presence or absence of local or systemic spread of the organism.

Gonorrhea in the male The usual incubation period of gonococcal urethritis ("clap") in the male is 2 to 6 days following exposure, although longer intervals are not infrequent, and perhaps 10 to 20 percent of men who become infected never develop symptoms. Symptoms include a profuse purulent urethral discharge, usually associated with dysuria and frequent urination. Before antibiotic treatment became available for gonorrhea, these symptoms persisted for an average of 8 weeks, and unilateral epididymitis occurred in 5 to 10 percent of untreated men. Epididymitis is now a rare complication of gonorrhea, and most cases of epididymitis in young men are nongonococcal. Other local complications which are now unusual include inguinal lymphadenitis, edema of the penis due to dorsal lymphangitis or thrombophlebitis, periurethral abscess or fistula, cowperitis, and seminal vesiculitis. The existence of gonococcal "prostatitis" is putative, although gonococcal prostatic abscess has been described.

In homosexual men, anorectal and pharyngeal gonococcal infection are common. Anorectal infection may be asymptomatic from the outset, or may produce anorectal burning or pruritus, tenesmus, and a bloody, mucopurulent rectal discharge. Proctoscopy is essential in such men, to exclude syphilis, lymphogranuloma venereum, granuloma inguinale, and other conditions which cause similar symptoms. These symptoms may subside without treatment, leaving a chronic asymptomatic carrier state. Pharyngeal gonococcal infection occurs in approximately 20 percent of homosexual men or heterosexual women who engage in fellatio with men who have urethral infection. Pharyngeal infection may produce exudative tonsillitis, but frequently is asymptomatic.

Nongonococcal urethritis (NGU) Approximately one-half of all young men with urethritis examined in practice or public clinics do not have gonorrhea. The etiology of nongonococcal urethritis in the male is uncertain, although urethral infection with *Chlamydia* species (TRIC agent) is found in 50 percent of cases. Both the patient with NGU and his sexual contact should be treated with tetracycline, 2 g daily for 1 to 3 weeks.

Gonorrhea in the female Acute uncomplicated gonorrhea in the female often causes dysuria, frequency, increased vaginal discharge, and anorectal discomfort. While dysuria and frequency in young men arouse the suspicion of gonococcal urethritis, the same symptoms in a young woman are often automatically attributed to "cystitis." Actually only about one-half of young women with these symptoms are found to have at least 10^5 coliform bacteria per ml of clean voided midstream urine, while many of those without significant bacteriuria have gonococcal infection of the urethra and of Skene's glands. Acute symptoms of gonococcal urethritis in the female may subside spontaneously or following subcurative therapy with sulfonamides or other urinary antiseptics. The proportion of women with gonorrhea who never develop symptoms is undefined.

Asymptomatic gonococcal infection in the female involves the endocervix, urethra, anal canal, and pharynx, in decreasing order of frequency. Extension of infection from the endocervix to the fallopian tubes occurs in 10 to 15 percent of women with gonorrhea. This tends to occur soon after acquisition of infection or during menstruation and results in *acute salpingitis*, the major complication of gonorrhea. Approximately half of all women with acute salpingitis have gonorrhea. The clinical diagnosis of salpingitis is imprecise; at laparoscopy, only 60 to 70 percent of clinically suspected cases are confirmed, while 15 percent have other findings such as appendicitis, ectopic pregnancy, diverticulitis, endometriosis, or hemorrhagic ovarian cyst, and the remainder have no abnormal findings. True salpingitis is nearly always associated with lower abdominal pain, cervical motion tenderness, adnexal tenderness, and elevation of the erythrocyte sedimentation rate above 15 mm per hr Westergren; it usually is bilateral and is associated with fever. Chills, adnexal swelling, and leukocytosis occur in half of all cases of salpingitis. Extension of infection to the pelvis may produce signs of pelvic peritonitis, accompanied by nausea and vomiting, and may lead to pelvic abscess with bulging into the posterior cul-de-sac, requiring drainage by posterior colpotomy. Early antibiotic treatment, before development of adnexal masses, restores normal tubal function and fertility in nearly all cases of salpingitis. However, if prominent adnexal swelling has occurred before treatment is begun, bilateral tubal dysfunction occurs in 15 to 25 percent.

Spread of gonococci into the upper abdomen may cause *gonococcal perihepatitis* (Fitz-Hugh-Curtis syndrome) manifested by right upper quadrant or bilateral upper abdominal pain and tenderness, and occasionally by a hepatic friction rub. Gonococcal perihepatitis may mimic acute cholecystitis, with transient nonvisualization of the gallbladder and mild liver function abnormalities. Perihepatitis should be distinguished from toxic hepatitis resulting from gonococcemia.

Acute inflammation of Bartholin's gland is usually unilateral and frequently is due to gonococcal infection. The acutely infected duct is surrounded by a red halo and exudes pus at the posterior aspect of the labium majus. Occlusion of the duct results in formation of a Bartholin's abscess. Chronic Bartholin cysts are rarely caused by active gonococcal infection.

There is suggestive but inconclusive evidence that endocervical gonococcal infection is associated with prematurity and with prolonged labor following rupture of membranes, both of which may produce increased perinatal morbidity.

Gonorrhea in children During childbirth, the gonococcus may infect the conjunctivae, pharynx, respiratory tract, or anal canal of the newborn. The risk of contamination apparently increases with prolonged rupture of membranes. Prevention of gonococcal ophthalmia by prophylactic use of 1 % silver nitrate eyedrops has led to the emergence of inclusion conjunctivitis caused by *Chlamydia* as a more common form of ophthalmia neonatorum. During the first year of life, infection of the infant usually results from accidental contamination of the eye or vagina by an adult. Between one year of age and puberty, most cases of gonorrhea involve vulvovaginitis in females who have been molested by a relative, and medicolegal considerations necessitate a complete bacteriologic diagnosis.

Disseminated gonococcal infection From 1 to 3 percent of adults with gonococcal infection develop gonococcemia. Approximately two-thirds of such patients are women. Just as the majority of men and women with gonococcal infection at any point in time are asymptomatic carriers, the majority of men and women with gonococcemia lack any symptoms of urogenital, anorectal, or pharyngeal gonococcal infection. Gonococcemia may occur soon after acquisition of new infection or later, during menstruation or pregnancy. The onset of gonococcemia is characterized by fever, polyarthralgias, and papular, petechial, or hemorrhagic pustular skin lesions. Approximately 3 to 20 such lesions appear, usually on the distal extremities. The initial joint involvement is characteristically limited to tenosynovitis involving several joints asymmetrically. The wrists, fingers, knees, and ankles are most often involved. Without treatment, the duration of gonococcemia is variable; the systemic manifestations of the bacteremic stage may subside within a week, or a *septic joint stage* may ensue. Pain and swelling then increase in one or more joints, with accumulation of purulent synovial fluid, leading to progressive destruction of the joint if treatment is delayed.

Other common manifestations of disseminated gonococcal infection include mild myopericarditis and "toxic" hepatitis, while endocarditis and meningitis are infrequent but severe complications. Endocarditis is suggested by pathologic or changing heart murmurs, major embolic phenomena, severe myocarditis, deterioration of renal function, or by an unusually large number of skin lesions.

DIAGNOSIS The demonstration of gram-negative intracellular diplococci warrants a presumptive diagnosis of gonococcal infection only in the examination of urethral exudate. Isolation of *N. gonorrhoeae* by culture is required when other sites are examined and when Gram's stain of urethral exudate is negative. Thayer-Martin (TM) medium, which contains antibiotics to inhibit most other organisms selectively, is most useful for recovering the gonococcus from the endocervix, anal canal, and pharynx, which are always heavily colonized by a mixed bacterial flora. After inoculation, the TM medium should be placed in an atmosphere containing sufficient carbon dioxide to permit growth of the gonococcus. This can be accomplished in a candle jar, or by packaging the TM medium in sealed vials to which carbon dioxide was added before sealing (Transgrow medium), or by generation of carbon dioxide chemically within tubes of media which are sealed after inoculation.

In men with incubating or chronic asymptomatic urethral infection without exudate, or as a test of cure following treatment, a very thin cotton swab or wire bacteriologic loop should be inserted 2 to 5 cm into the anterior urethra and used to inoculate TM medium. Cultures of the pharynx and anal canal should be obtained from all homosexual men with suspected gonorrhea.

The most efficient screening test for gonorrhea in women is the endocervical culture, which is positive on a single examination in up to 80 percent of those with asymptomatic infection. In young women with symptoms of cystitis or urethritis, cultures for *N. gonorrhoeae* should be obtained from both the endocervix and the urethra. A culture of the anal canal is most useful as a test of cure in women, since persistent infection is limited to the anal canal in 25 percent of those who remain infected after unsuccessful treatment.

Demonstration of *N. gonorrhoeae* by culture or by specific immunofluorescent stain of blood, synovial fluid, cerebrospinal fluid, or skin lesions constitutes proof of disseminated gonococcal infection. The diagnosis of gonococcemia is almost as certain in a patient with typical skin lesions or tenosynovitis if gonococcal infection is proved by recovery of *N. gonorrhoeae* from anogenital or pharyngeal sites from the patient or his sex partner. Therefore, when disseminated gonococcal infection is suspected, cultures of the genitalia, anal canal, and pharynx are indicated, and the patient's sex partner should also be examined by culture. *Neisseria gonorrhoeae* can be recovered from the blood of most patients seen very soon after the onset of gonococcemia, and from the synovial fluid of at least half of those patients seen during the septic-joint stage of infection. Standard blood culture broth medium containing liquoid and 3 to 10 percent carbon dioxide should be used in culturing blood and is also recommended for culturing synovial fluid. In pus from skin lesions, *N. gonorrhoeae* is more often demonstrable by Gram's stain or immunofluorescent staining than by culture. A fourfold or greater rise in gonococcal antibody can be demonstrated in many patients with gonococcal arthritis, using complement fixation, immunofluorescent, or gonococcal pili antigen-binding assays.

TREATMENT The preferred drug for gonococcal infection is penicillin or ampicillin, despite increasing resistance of *N. gonorrhoeae* to these antibiotics. For uncomplicated urethral, cervical, rectal, or pharyngeal gonococcal infection, the regimen recommended for both men and women is aqueous procaine penicillin G, 4.8 million units, divided into at least two injections given intramuscularly at different sites at one visit, together with 1 g oral probenecid, preferably given at least 30 min prior to the injections. An effective alternative regimen is ampicillin, 3.5 g given as a single oral dose, with probenecid, 1 g administered simultaneously. For patients who are allergic to penicillin, ampicillin, or probenecid, either spectinomycin or tetracycline can be used. A single intramuscular dose of 2 g spectinomycin is adequate for both sexes. However, spectinomycin does not seem to be very effective in the treatment of pharyngeal gonococcal infection. The tetracyclines are no longer effective in a single dose. The recommended dose of tetracycline hydrochloride is 1.5 g initially as a loading dose, followed by 0.5 g four times a day for 4 days, a total of 9 g. Other tetracyclines are not more effective. Patients with known exposure to gonorrhea should receive the same treatment as those known to have gonorrhea.

As a test of cure, follow-up cervical and anal canal cultures should be obtained from women 7 to 14 days after completion of treatment, and follow-up urethral specimens should be obtained from men 7 days after treatment. An interesting phenomenon known as postgonococcal urethritis (PGU), consisting of either asymptomatic pyuria or symptomatic urethral discharge, may persist for several weeks in men after eradication of the gonococcus with penicillin treatment. When PGU is symptomatic, it can be managed, like NGU, with tetracycline therapy.

All patients with gonorrhea should have a serologic test for syphilis at the time of diagnosis. Those treated with the recommended procaine penicillin G regimen need not have later follow-up tests for syphilis, since this regimen cures incubating syphilis. In geographic areas where syphilis is endemic, and in all homosexual males, a follow-up serologic test for syphilis is recommended 6 weeks and 3 months after treatment of gonorrhea, if ampicillin, spectinomycin, or tetracycline was used.

Treatment of disseminated gonococcal infection and gonococcal salpingitis must be individualized. Gonococcal isolates from patients with disseminated infection appear to be significantly less resistant to penicillin G than isolates from patients with uncomplicated gonorrhea. However, because of the threat of endocarditis, meningitis, and joint sepsis, patients with disseminated infection should preferably be hospitalized and treated with aqueous crystalline penicillin G intravenously, 10 million units per day until clinical improvement occurs, usually within 2 days. Treatment can then be completed on an outpatient basis with ampicillin, 2 g per day orally to complete a 10- to 14-day course of therapy. Failure to improve with this regimen strongly suggests a diagnosis other than disseminated gonococcal infection. Repeated joint aspiration is occasionally required to reduce inflammation, and, rarely, closed irrigation of the joint with sterile saline is of benefit. Open drainage is seldom if ever required for gonococcal arthritis. Temporary immobilization of the joint may reduce discomfort for the patient and may be useful during initial ambulation in patients with persistent effusions of the knee or ankle. Antibiotics should not be injected directly into the joint. Patients with gonococcal salpingitis who require hospitalization respond well to this same regimen. Those who are less ill should receive the initial loading dose of antibiotic recommended for uncomplicated gonorrhea (e.g., 4.8 million units procaine penicillin G parenterally or 3.5 g ampicillin orally, together with 1 g oral probenecid) followed by ampicillin, 2 g per day orally for an additional 10 to 14 days. A 2-week course of tetracycline, 2 g per day, can be used in nonpregnant patients with gonococcal arthritis or salpingitis who are allergic to penicillin.

Gonococcal conjunctivitis in the adult or newborn should be managed as a medical emergency by irrigation of the conjunctiva with penicillin, together with penicillin G given intravenously.

PREVENTION AND CONTROL There is probably no more striking illustration than gonorrhea of the failure of specific treatment alone to eradicate a communicable disease. Vaccination is not available, and there is some doubt as to whether any resistance to reinfection occurs during natural infection, although humoral, local, and cellular immune responses have all been demonstrated during acute or recurrent gonococcal infection. Use of the condom can prevent transmission. Prophylactic antibiotics are also effective but are not recommended for general use. The efficacy of local vaginal antiseptic and spermicidal preparations for prevention of venereal disease requires further study. The most effective additional measures now available for control of gonorrhea include diagnostic screening for asymptomatic disease and tracing sexual contacts of infected patients. Experienced interviewers are able to identify and bring to treatment an average of 1.5 additional cases for every patient interviewed.

REFERENCES

FALK V: Treatment of acute nontuberculous salpingitis alone and in combination with glucocorticoids. Acta Obstet Gynecol Scand XLIV (Suppl 6):1965

HARKNESS AH: The pathology of gonorrhea. Br J Vener Dis 24:137, 1948

HOLMES KK et al: Disseminated gonococcal infection. Ann Intern Med 74:979, 1971

JACOBSEN L, WESTROM L: Objectivized diagnosis of acute pelvic inflammatory disease. Am J Obstet Gynecol 105:1088, 1969

SCHROETER AL, PAZIN GJ: Gonorrhea. Ann Intern Med 72:553, 1970

section 5 | Diseases caused by enteric gram-negative bacilli

133 INFECTIONS DUE TO ENTEROBACTERIACEAE

MARVIN TURCK

ESCHERICHIA COLI INFECTIONS

ETIOLOGY *Escherichia coli* is a group of gram-negative nonsporing rods which belong to the tribe Enterobacteriaceae. They generally ferment lactose, as opposed to the medically significant non-lactose-fermenting organisms, *Salmonella, Shigella,* and *Proteus.* The so-called "paracolon" bacilli are organisms which ferment lactose late, irregularly, or not at all, and on more careful biochemical and antigenic testing are found to belong to one or another of the genera of the tribe Enterobacteriaceae, which comprises *Salmonella, Arizona, Citrobacter, Shigella, Escherichia, Klebsiella, Enterobacter, Hafnia, Serratia, Proteus,* and *Providence.* All these organisms are readily culturable on ordinary media and are aerobic and facultatively anaerobic. All species ferment glucose, reduce nitrates to nitrites, and are oxidase-negative and catalase-positive. They are differentiated among members of their own tribe by biochemical and serologic tests. It is important to make this differentiation, not only from the point of view of taxonomy, but also because of epidemiologic and therapeutic implications.

PATHOGENESIS *Escherichia coli* is regarded generally as a normal commensal in the gastrointestinal tract, from which it may spread to infect contiguous structures if normal anatomic barriers are interrupted, as occurs in appendiceal perforation. It is believed that the urinary tract is infected from without via urethral contamination, but direct hematogenous spread may also account for renal infection. Once infection has occurred in a primary focus, further spread to distant organs may occur via the bloodstream. There is experimental and clinical evidence that *E. coli* tends to settle in avascular or necrotic tissue. In more than 50 percent of *E. coli* infections the urinary tract is the portal of entry; infections of the hepatobiliary tree, peritoneal cavity, skin, and lung are not uncommon. A number of patients with *E. coli* bacteremia have no demonstrable portal of entry; they often have neoplastic and hematologic diseases, and *E. coli* is considered an "opportunistic" invader. There may be other defects in host resistance, including diabetes mellitus, cirrhosis, and sickle-cell anemia, or recent administration of irradiation, cytotoxic drugs, adrenal steroids, or antibiotics. There also is epidemiologic evidence that *E. coli* and other Enterobacteriaceae tend to avidly colonize the skin and mucous membranes of debilitated patients, possibly accounting for the increased frequency of these infections in patients with advanced illness. Morphologically the lesions produced in various tissues show typical acute inflammation with pus and abscess formation. There is a common misconception that *E. coli* bacterial infections are characterized by a foul-smelling, feculent exudate. Such an odor is caused by anaerobic streptococci or *Bacteroides* species, which are often associated with coliform bacteria in mixed infection. In fact, organisms of the genus *Bacteroides* frequently far outnumber *E. coli* as the most prevalent gram-negative flora in the intestine.

EPIDEMIOLOGY Strains of *E. coli* are characterized by their somatic (O), flagellar (H), and capsular (K or B) antigens, and there are hundreds of different serologic varieties. Any of the strains is capable of causing disease. Clinical and epidemiologic studies have demonstrated that certain specific *E. coli* serotypes are more frequently incriminated in diarrheal disease of the infant and newborn, that is, 026:B6, 055:B5, 0111:B4, and 0127:B8. Strains incriminated in infantile diarrhea probably are disseminated within nurseries by symptomatic or asymptomatic infant carriers, mothers, and nurses. Although fecal contamination is the usual mode of spread, airborne contamination and fomite spread may also occur.

Some epidemiologic studies have suggested that *E. coli* 04, 06, and 075 are responsible for most *E. coli* infections other than infantile diarrhea. It is unclear whether these strains actually are more virulent or merely are more prevalent than other somatic types. In fact, virulence factors may be associated more closely with the K than with the somatic antigen, and may account for the frequency in which certain strains cause parenchymal infection.

MANIFESTATIONS **Urinary tract infections** *Escherichia coli* accounts for well over 75 percent of urinary tract infections, including cystitis, pyelitis, pyelonephritis, and asymptomatic bacteriuria. Strains cultured from patients with acute, uncomplicated urinary tract infections are almost invariably *E. coli,* whereas other Enterobacteriaceae and strains of *Pseudomonas* become prevalent among patients with chronic infection. Urinary tract infections are discussed in Chap. 273.

Peritoneal and biliary infections *Escherichia coli* can usually be cultured from a perforated or inflamed appendix or from abscesses secondary to perforated diverticula, peptic ulcers, subphrenic or lesser sac abscesses, mesenteric infarction, etc. Often, other organisms, including anaerobic streptococci, clostridia, and bacteroides, are found along with *E. coli.* Acute cholecystitis with gangrene and perforation is often associated with *E. coli* infection. An air-fluid level associated with stones or a circumferential layer of gas in the wall of the gallbladder may be detectable by x-ray and is characteristic of acute emphysematous cholecystitis. From the gallbladder, infection may ascend via the biliary tree to produce cholangitis and multiple liver abscesses. More rarely *E. coli* infection in the peritoneal cavity may produce a septic thrombophlebitis of the portal vein (pylephlebitis), which in turn is followed by liver abscesses.

Bacteremia Invasion of the bloodstream is the most serious manifestation of *E. coli* infection; it is characterized usually by the sudden onset of fever and chills, but sometimes only by mental confusion, dyspnea, or unexplained hypotension. It is most common in patients with urinary tract infection and biliary or intraperitoneal sepsis, and following abortions or pelvic surgery. In some patients no portal of entry is evident. Most cases occur in elderly males, presumably because of the high incidence of urethral instrumentation and catheterization in this group. Fever ranges between 100 and 106°F and is higher in younger patients. Hyperventilation may be an early sign. Hypotension may be present from the onset but usually occurs within 12 to 16 hr after bacteremia; if it is persistent, it is accompanied by oliguria and often by mental confusion, stupor, and coma. The skin is warm and dry initially, but most patients develop some evidence of peripheral vasoconstriction characterized by cold and cyanotic extremities. Fortunately hypotension is transient and self-limited in most patients with *E. coli* bacteremia and is absent altogether in some. However, about 25 percent of patients with bacteremia develop more prolonged hypotension, a syndrome known as *gram-negative* or *endotoxin shock,* which is discussed in Chap. 124.

Occasionally *E. coli* bacteremia develops in patients with cirrhosis without an overt portal of entry. This has been variably attributed to portosystemic shunts both in and around the liver, impaired reticuloendothelial function, and diminution in humoral and cellular defense mechanisms.

Other manifestations *Escherichia coli* may produce abscesses anywhere in the body. Subcutaneous infections are found at the site of insulin administration in diabetics, in extremities with ischemic gangrene, or in surgical wounds. Perirectal phlegmons are not uncommon in patients with leukemia. Subcutaneous abscesses are often characterized by formation of gas in tissue, especially among diabetics, which may be detected by crepitation or by x-ray and which must be differentiated from clostridial infection. From 5 to 10 percent of patients with *E. coli* bacteremia develop metastatic infection in bone, brain, liver, and lung. *Escherichia coli* may cause pneumonia *de novo;* also, coliform bacilli are often cultured from sputum in pulmonary superinfections.

Neonatal infection Neonates, particularly premature infants, often develop *E. coli* bacteremia associated with meningitis and bloodborne pyelonephritis. Fecal soiling and absence of maternal gamma-G-globulin (IgM) antibody are two of the factors which render this group particularly susceptible to coliform infections.

Gastroenteritis Children under two years of age develop gastroenteritis, typified by nausea, vomiting, and diarrhea. Most outbreaks have occurred in nurseries and have been due to specific strains of enteropathogenic *E. coli* (EPEC). These particular strains may produce a toxin similar to the toxin elaborated by *Vibrio cholerae.* Fluorescent antibody techniques have been most useful in the rapid identification of these organisms. The rapid dehydration, with its attendant high mortality, demands prompt recognition of this condition, isolation of the infants, and treatment of both patients and contacts with the appropriate antibiotic. *Escherichia coli* per se has rarely been incriminated in diarrheal disease in adults, although certain strains of *Arizona* have presumably been responsible for benign outbreaks of gastroenteritis.

LABORATORY FINDINGS There are no characteristic laboratory abnormalities. The white blood cell count is usually elevated, and there is a preponderance of granulocytes. At times, however, the white count is normal or low. When *E. coli* infection occurs in previously healthy individuals, anemia is absent, but more commonly there is anemia which is usually related to the patient's underlying disease. *Escherichia coli* grows readily in a variety of bacteriologic media and should be cultured from appropriate secretions and blood. In the presence of gram-negative shock, there are often profound metabolic derangements, including azotemia, metabolic acidosis, hypokalemia, and hyperkalemia, as well as a variety of coagulation defects (Chap. 124).

DIAGNOSIS *Escherichia coli* cannot be differentiated from most other gram-negative bacteria on gram stain, and culture followed by appropriate biochemical characterization is necessary to identify the organism precisely. Fluorescent antibody techniques are valuable for identifying EPEC. In addition, serologic typing of *E. coli* may be useful in individual patients with recurrent urinary tract infections in order to help differentiate between relapse and reinfection.

TREATMENT As with other infections, drainage of pus and removal of foreign bodies are essential. If *E. coli* is suspected as the etiologic agent in a particular infection, choice of an appropriate antimicrobial will depend upon the site and type of infection as well as upon its severity. Often the outcome of the infection depends upon the status of the associated disease, rather than on eradication of bacteria. For example, in acute, uncomplicated urinary tract infection in females, the disease is frequently self-limited even without antimicrobial therapy, and there is no evidence that antibiotics are superior to sulfonamides. Conversely, *E. coli* bacteremia in a patient with leukemia may not respond to antimicrobials unless a hematologic remission is achieved simultaneously.

In most situations, antibiotics should be selected, when possible, on the basis of their in vitro sensitivity tests. Although no drug is uniformly active against all strains of *E. coli,* a number of agents are effective against the majority of clinical isolates. If average obtainable plasma concentrations become the criteria for in vitro susceptibility, approximately 75 percent of *E. coli* strains are likely to be sensitive to the tetracyclines, 85 to 90 percent to chloramphenicol or ampicillin, and 90 percent to gentamicin, kanamycin, polymyxin B, or colistin; 50 percent of *E. coli* isolated from hospitalized patients will be inhibited by streptomycin, and 75 to 90 percent by cephalothin or cephaloridine. Many strains of *E. coli* are sensitive to high concentrations of penicillin G (50 to 100 μg per ml), and this drug may be used in dosage of 10 to 40 million units intravenously daily, particularly if probenecid is given concomitantly. This regimen has been largely superseded by ampicillin, 2 to 4 g per day intravenously or intramuscularly; in some instances the dose can be raised to 6 to 12 g per day. The antibacterial spectrum of ampicillin against *E. coli* is probably identical to that achieved with very high concentrations of penicillin G, and to the spectrum covered by the tetracyclines or chloramphenicol. However, the bactericidal properties of ampicillin may be a distinct advantage over these two drugs, particularly in deep-seated infections. Kanamycin sulfate is most useful for the initial treatment of serious *E. coli* infections. Severe urinary tract infections refractory to other antimicrobials have responded to 15 mg per kg per day, intramuscularly, in divided doses every 6 to 8 hr. In life-threatening infections, kanamycin can probably be used for 24 to 48 hr with little hazard of ototoxicity or nephrotoxicity, even in patients with concomitant renal impairment, pending results of in vitro sensitivity tests. However, some recent isolations of specific serologic strains of hospital-derived *E. coli* from newborn with diarrheal disease have been resistant to kanamycin and neomycin. More recently, gentamicin has been employed in the initial treatment of severe *E. coli* infections in doses of 3 to 5 mg per kg per day in divided doses every 8 hr. This drug probably has superseded kanamycin in the treatment of many patients. Cephalothin in concentration of 25 μg per ml is effective against many *E. coli* strains. This serum concentration can be obtained only with 1.5- to 2.0-g dosages at 3- to 4-hr intervals. Although cephalothin is highly effective against many common pathogens, peak serum concentrations after standard doses barely reach or may fall short of requirements for *E. coli.* Another cephalosporin antibiotic, cephaloridine, has become available for the treatment of *E. coli* infections. This agent yields higher and more sustained levels than does a comparable amount of cephalothin and is more active against *E. coli* in vitro. However, because of potential nephrotoxicity, the total daily dose of cephaloridine is limited to 4.0 g per day by law. Tetracyclines and chloramphenicol are still widely used in the treatment of *E. coli* infection, but better drugs are now available. Polymyxin B and colistin are also highly effective in vitro against the majority of *E. coli.* However, it is difficult to obtain adequate tissue and serum concentrations with these agents, and they should probably not be used for treatment of systemic *E. coli* infections. Although combinations of antimicrobials, i.e., streptomycin and tetracycline or streptomycin and chloramphenicol, have been recommended, there is little need to employ more than one agent in most situations. Nitrofurantoin (400 mg) and nalidixic acid (2 to 4 g) are reserved for treating patients with *E. coli* bacteriuria, and are not employed when infection is suspected outside the urinary tract.

PREVENTION Isolation and antimicrobial therapy of infants and contacts are essential to abort epidemic infantile diarrhea. In adults, many *E. coli* infections are hospital-associated, and their incidence can be reduced by limiting use of indwelling urinary catheters, by careful surgical aseptic technique, by appropriate isolation of infection-prone patients, and by judicious use of antibiotics, steroids, and cytotoxic agents. There is mounting evidence that the promiscuous use of antibiotics may propagate the transfer of resistance factors among intestinal *E. coli.* These organisms may in turn transmit their resistance to other virulent Enterobacteriacae, such as *Salmonella.*

KLEBSIELLA-ENTEROBACTER-SERRATIA INFECTIONS

ETIOLOGY Next to *E. coli,* strains of *Klebsiella, Enterobacter,* and *Serratia* are the most important enteric organisms infecting man. In many laboratories *Klebsiella* species are not differentiated from *E. coli.* This is potentially a serious error because strains of *Klebsiella* are, in general, more resistant to antibiotics, and their isolation from blood, purulent exudates, and urine is of more serious epidemiologic and prognostic significance. The Friedländer bacilli (*K. pneumoniae*) are encapsulated gram-negative bacilli, found among the normal flora of the mouth and intestinal tracts. *Klebsiella pneumoniae* has been considered to be a virulent respiratory pathogen since first described by Friedländer in 1882. *Klebsiella* is closely related to the genera *Enterobacter* and *Serratia* and may be differentiated only by certain amino acid decarboxylase tests. In addition to differentiation by these biochemical tests, which group *Klebsiella, Enterobacter,* and *Serratia,* strains of *Klebsiella* usually are nonmotile and form large mucoid colonies on solid media, whereas the other species are typically motile. Klebsiellas also are usually sensitive to concentrations of cephalothin, to which *Enterobacter* and *Serratia* are resistant. These characteristics, however, are not invariable enough to differentiate various isolates from clinical sources. Strains of *Klebsiella* can be further distinguished on the basis of type-specific capsular antigens; more than 75 known capsular types have been identified. There is little evidence that certain types are more virulent than others, and the main role of capsular typing of *Klebsiella* is as an epidemiologic tool in nosocomial outbreaks of infection. The significance of *Enterobacter* and *Serratia* in human infections has been less well clarified than of infections secondary to *Klebsiella,* but all are potential pathogens, especially as opportunistic invaders in the compromised host.

Klebsiella rhinoscleromatis is probably the causative agent of rhinoscleroma, and *K. ozenae* has been isolated occasionally from the nose of patients with ozena, a chronic severe rhinitis associated with turbinate atrophy and progression to anosmia.

PATHOGENESIS *Klebsiella, Enterobacter,* and *Serratia* are all capable of causing disease in diverse anatomic sites. However, results of clinical and epidemiologic studies suggest that differences in pathogenicity may exist among these genera and that precise taxonomic identification is of value. Although infections of the respiratory tract with *K. pneumoniae* have been emphasized most in the past, the urinary tract presently accounts for the majority of clinical isolates. In this site clinical manifestations and pathogenesis are similar to infections produced by *E. coli,* but klebsiellas are more frequently found in patients with complicated and obstructive urinary tract disease. Infections of the biliary tract, the peritoneal cavity, the middle ear, mastoids, paranasal sinuses, and meninges also are not uncommon. In these locations, *Klebsiella* is more frequent than either *Enterobacter* or *Serratia* and is more likely to produce an illness of greater severity. The apparent increased frequency of infection by serratias represents an increase primarily due to nosocomial spread of this organism.

MANIFESTATIONS Symptoms and signs of common infections caused by *Klebsiella*—namely, those involving the urinary tract, biliary tree, and peritoneal cavity—are indistinguishable from those caused by *E. coli.* These infections commonly occur in diabetics and in the form of superinfections in patients who have received antimicrobials to which these organisms are resistant. *Klebsiella* infection is also an important etiologic factor in septic shock (Chap. 124).

Pneumonia *Klebsiella* is well recognized as a pulmonary pathogen, but probably accounts for less than 1 percent of all cases of bacterial pneumonia. The disease is most common in men over forty years of age and is more frequently found in alcoholics. Other factors associated with increased susceptibility include diabetes mellitus and chronic bronchopulmonary disease. Aspiration of oropharyngeal secretions containing *Klebsiella* organisms is the likely inciting factor among alcoholic patients. The clinical manifestations are indistinguishable from those of pneumococcal pneumonia (Chap. 128), with sudden onset of chills, fever, productive cough, and severe pleuritic chest pain. Patients are frequently delirious and prostrated, but this may also occur with pneumococcal infection. A "characteristic" clinical feature, which occurs in only 25 to 50 percent of patients, is the dark-brown or red currant-jelly sputum which may be so tenacious that the patient has difficulty in expelling it from his mouth and lips. The pulmonary lesion is most frequent in the right upper lobe but often rapidly progresses and, if untreated, may spread from lobe to lobe. Cyanosis and dyspnea develop rapidly, and jaundice, vomiting, and diarrhea may be present. Physical findings consist primarily of signs of consolidation unless pleural effusion or necrotizing pneumonitis with rapid cavitation has intervened. The blood leukocyte count may be elevated but is often low, which probably is merely a reflection of severe infection in an alcoholic patient with poor bone marrow reserve and folate deficiency. Lung abscess and empyema are much more frequent than in pneumococcal pneumonia and are related to the destructive capabilities of this organism. So-called "characteristic" radiographic features such as bulging fissures and loss of lung volume occur only occasionally, and also may be found in pneumococcal infection, as well as in necrotizing pneumonia caused by other gram-negative species.

Chronic infection of the lung Rarely, infection with *Klebsiella* may progress, often in indolent fashion, to a chronic necrotizing pneumonitis resembling tuberculosis. It may follow acute *Klebsiella* pneumonia but is also seen in patients who give no history of an acute onset. The principal symptoms are productive cough, weakness, and anemia. Hemoptysis, chronic empyema, or sterile serous effusions are also encountered. Cavitation, frequently with thin walls, occurs primarily in the upper lobes.

DIAGNOSIS Diagnosis is established by an awareness of the clinical setting in which *Klebsiella* infections occur and by isolation of the organism. A presumptive diagnosis of *Klebsiella* pneumonia should be made on the basis of gram stain of the sputum which shows a predominance of short, plump, gram-negative bacilli, frequently surrounded by a clear space because of the capsule. Often these gram-negative organisms occur together with gram-positive cocci, and because the gram-positives are easier to see, the gram-negative bacteria may be ignored and the diagnosis may be missed, which, in turn, may lead to potentially serious delays in instituting therapy. Additional proof of *Klebsiella* infection in the lung is afforded by isolation of the organisms from blood and pleural exudate. In extrapulmonary infections, the organisms are readily seen in and cultured from pus or secretions of involved organs.

TREATMENT *Klebsiella, Enterobacter,* and *Serratia* have variable susceptibility to antimicrobial drugs, and cultures of these organisms need to be tested in vitro. Frequently, however, antimicrobial therapy needs to be instituted before results of antibiotic susceptibility tests become available. In general, the majority of strains of *Klebsiella* is susceptible to gentamicin, kanamycin, cephalothin, chloramphenicol, and polymyxin B or colistin. *Klebsiella* isolates do not respond to penicillin and its analogues, although many isolates of *Enterobacter* are inhibited by 25 μg per ml carbenicillin. The antimicrobial regimen of choice in the treatment of *Klebsiella, Enterobacter,* and *Serratia* infection will vary from one institution to another and upon the degree of clinical severity of infection. In severely ill patients, the combination of an aminoglycoside such as gentamicin (5 mg per kg per day) or kanamycin (15 mg per kg per day) with cephalothin (6 to 12 g per day) is usually preferred. Because of the relatively poor blood and tissue levels with the polymyxins, they should probably not be employed as first-line agents in the treatment of severe *Klebsiella* infections despite apparent in vitro susceptibility. Regardless of the antimicrobial regimen employed, treatment should be continued for a minimum of 10 to 14 days and prolonged if there is extensive cavitation. Pleural effusions must be drained; antibiotic therapy alone is not sufficient treatment for closed-space infections of the pleural cavity. At times, rib resection with open drainage may be necessary, and should be considered if effusions recur.

PROGNOSIS Prior to the introduction of antimicrobials, the fatality rate reported in different clinics varied from 50 to 80 percent, and death within 48 hr was not infrequent. Even with antimicrobial treatment the course of the disease is quite variable and the prognosis must be guarded. For the most part, this prognosis reflects the age group involved and the frequent association of *Klebsiella* infection with alcoholism, malnutrition, and severe underlying disease.

PROTEUS INFECTIONS

ETIOLOGY The genus *Proteus* consists of gram-negative bacilli which do not ferment lactose and are characterized by their active motility and spreading growth on solid media. There are four pathogenic species: *P. mirabilis, P. vulgaris, P. morganii,* and *P. rettgeri. Proteus mirabilis* causes 75 to 90 percent of human infections and is distinguishable from the other three species by its inability to form indole. All four split urea, with production of ammonia. Some strains of *P. vulgaris* share a common antigen with certain rickettsia, accounting for the appearance of antibodies against *Proteus* organisms (Weil-Felix reaction) in typhus, scrub typhus, and Rocky Mountain spotted fever. The *Providence* group of organisms resembles those of the genus *Proteus* closely except that it fails to produce a urease.

EPIDEMIOLOGY AND PATHOGENESIS Members of the genus *Proteus* are normally found in soil, water, and sewage and are part of the normal fecal flora. Occasionally, they have been implicated as a cause of epidemic diarrhea in infants, but the evidence for this is inconclusive. The organism is frequently cultured from superficial wounds, draining ears, and sputum, particularly in patients who have received antibiotics, and replaces the more susceptible flora eradicated by these drugs. *Proteus* organisms often localize in already damaged tissues, where they produce a typical exudative inflammatory reaction.

MANIFESTATIONS *Proteus* organisms are rarely primary invaders but produce disease in locations previously infected by other organisms. These locations include the skin, ears and mastoid sinuses, eyes, peritoneal cavity, bone, urinary tract, meninges, lung, and bloodstream.

Cutaneous infections *Proteus* organisms are frequently isolated from surgical wounds, particularly following antimicrobial therapy, but they do not interfere with normal wound healing provided that the tissues are viable and foreign bodies are not present. Burns, varicose ulcers, and decubiti may become contaminated with *Proteus* organisms, often in company with other gram-negative organisms or staphylococci.

Infections of the ears and mastoid sinuses Otitis media and mastoiditis in which *Proteus* organisms are present can result in extensive destruction of the middle ear and mastoid sinuses. Fetid otorrhea, cholesteatoma, and granulation tissue constitute a chronic focus of infection in the middle and inner ears and mastoid, and deafness ensues. Paralysis of the facial nerve is an occasional complication. The great danger of these infections lies in intracranial extension, leading to thrombosis of the lateral sinus, meningitis, brain abscess, and bacteremia.

Ocular infections *Proteus* infection may cause corneal ulcers, usually following trauma to the eye, which occasionally terminate in panophthalmitis and destruction of the eyeball.

Peritonitis Being part of the normal intestinal flora, *Proteus* organisms may be isolated from the peritoneal cavity following perforation of viscera or mesenteric infarction.

Urinary tract infections *Proteus* organisms are a common cause of urinary tract infections, usually in patients with chronic bacteriuria, many of whom have had obstructive uropathy, a history of instrumentation of the bladder, and repeated courses of chemotherapy. The organism is rarely a pathogen in anatomically normal urinary tracts except occasionally in patients with diabetes mellitus. *Proteus* organisms are also often cultured from bacteriuric patients with renal or bladder calculi. This fact may be related to the ammoniagenic property of this organism, which renders the urine alkaline and provides a fertile medium for formation of ammonium-magnesium-phosphate stones.

Bacteremia Bloodstream invasion is the most serious manifestation of infection with this organism. In 75 percent of cases, the urinary tract serves as the portal of entry; in the remainder, the biliary tree, gastrointestinal tract, ears and sinuses, and skin are the primary foci. *Proteus* bacteremia is frequently preceded by cystoscopy, urethral catheterization, transurethral prostatic resection, or other operative procedures. Clinically, the signs, symptoms, and laboratory findings of *Proteus* sepsis—high fever, chills, shock, metastatic abscesses, leukocytosis, and rarely thrombocytopenia—are indistinguishable from those of bloodstream infections with other gram-negative bacteria.

DIAGNOSIS The diagnosis of *Proteus* infection depends on culture of the organism from blood, urine, or exudate and its identification by appropriate biochemical tests. It is especially important to separate *P. mirabilis,* the indole-negative species, from *P. morganii, rettgeri,* and *vulgaris,* which are indole-positive, because only *P. mirabilis* is susceptible to the action of penicillin and many other antibiotics. *Proteus* organisms are often present in mixed infections with other pathogens. Particular care should be exercised in the isolation of other organisms growing in the same medium with members of the genus *Proteus* lest they be masked by its spreading growth. The spreading character of this organism may also make antibiotic sensitivity tests difficult to interpret.

TREATMENT Most strains of *P. mirabilis* are sensitive to penicillin in high concentration (10 units per ml or greater), ampicillin, carbenicillin, kanamycin, gentamicin, cephalothin, and chloramphenicol. *Proteus* bacteriuria can be readily eradicated with any of these drugs during treatment; ampicillin in dosage of 0.5 g every 4 to 6 hr is highly effective. In severe infection, therapy should be parenteral: 6 to 12 g ampicillin or 20 million units of penicillin G plus kanamycin 1.0 to 1.5 g per day, if renal function is adequate. There is good evidence that kanamycin is synergistic with ampicillin and penicillin G in *Proteus* infections, and that chloramphenicol may be ineffective despite the results of in vitro tests. In view of the numerous more effective agents, there is no reason to use chloramphenicol in *Proteus* infections. In general, all strains of *P. mirabilis* are resistant to tetracycline. Most strains other than *P. mirabilis* and *Providence* bacilli are sensitive only to kanamycin. A newer aminoglycoside, gentamicin, appears to be very effective against indole-positive *Proteus* organisms in vitro and in vivo. In addition, although ampicillin and penicillin G alone are ineffective against indole-positive *Proteus,* a combination of either drug and kanamycin or gentamicin displays synergism. Carbenicillin, a semisynthetic penicillin, is also effective against the majority of indole-positive *Proteus* species. As with all other gram-negative infections, appropriate attention must be given to drainage of pus, maintenance of fluid and electrolyte status, and treatment of circulatory collapse.

REFERENCES

Escherichia coli infections

CONN HO, FESSEL JM: Spontaneous bacterial peritonitis in cirrhosis. Medicine 50:161, 1971

FIELDS BN et al: The so-called paracolon bacteria. Am J Med 42:89, 1967

TILLOTSON JR, LERNER AM: Characteristics of pneumonia caused by escherichia coli. N Engl J Med 277:115, 1967

TURCK M et al: Studies on the epidemiology of escherichia coli 1960–1968. J Infect Dis 120:13, 1969

Klebsiella-Enterobacter-Serratia infections

EDMONDSON EG, SANFORD JP: The klebsiella-enterobacter (aerobacter)-serratia group. Medicine 46:323, 1967

EICKHOFF TC et al: The klebsiella-enterobacter-serratia division: Biochemical and serologic characteristics and susceptibility to antibiotics. Ann Intern Med 65:1163, 1966

MANFREDI F et al: Clinical observations of acute Friedländer pneumonia. Ann Intern Med 58:642, 1963

PIERCE AK et al: An analysis of factors predisposing to gram-negative bacillary necrotizing pneumonia. Am Rev Resp Dis 94:309, 1966

PRICE DJE, SLEIGH JD: Control of infection due to klebsiella aerogenes in neurosurgical unit by withdrawal of all antibiotics. Lancet 2:1213, 1970

Proteus infections

LEWIS J, FEKETY FR: Proteus bacteremia. Johns Hopkins Med J 124:151, 1969

SERIFF NS: Lobar pneumonia due to proteus infection in a previously healthy adult. Am J Med 46:480, 1969

TILLOTSON JR, LERNER AM: Characteristics of pneumonia caused by bacillus proteus. Ann Intern Med 68:287, 1968

TURCK M et al: The role of carbenicillin in treatment of infections of the urinary tract. J Infect Dis 122:529, 1970

134 PSEUDOMONAS AND MIMA-HERELLEA INFECTIONS

MARVIN TURCK

PSEUDOMONAS INFECTIONS

ETIOLOGY *Pseudomonas aeruginosa* is a gram-negative motile rod which generally is not encapsulated and forms no spores. It grows readily in all ordinary culture media, and on agar it forms irregular, soft, irridescent colonies which usually have a fluorescent yellow-green color because of diffusion into the medium of two pigments, pyocyanin and fluorescin. *Pseudomonas* produces acid but no gas in glucose, and it is proteolytic. It is oxidase-positive and produces ammonia from arginine. A number of different strains have been identified by immunofluorescent techniques or bacteriophage typing. There is no evidence that these strains vary in their virulence for man.

EPIDEMIOLOGY *Pseudomonas* organisms are present on the skin of some normal persons, particularly in the axilla and anogenital regions. They are uncommon in the stools of adults not receiving antibiotics. In the majority of instances, *pseudomonas* organisms are cultured as avirulent secondary contaminants in superficial wounds, or from the sputum of patients treated with antibiotics. Ordinarily this is of little consequence because the organisms merely fill the bacteriologic vacuum left by the elimination of more sensitive bacteria. Occasionally, however, superinfections with *Pseudomonas* organisms occur in the ear, lung, skin, or urinary tract of patients whose primary pathogen has been eradicated by antibiotics. Serious infections are almost invariably associated with damage to local tissue or with diminished host resistance. Premature infants; children with congenital anomalies and patients with leukemia, usually receiving antibiotics, adrenal steroids, or antineoplastic drugs; patients with burns; and geriatric patients with debilitating diseases are likely to develop *Pseudomonas* infections. Most often these infections occur in the hospital environment, and the organisms have been cultured from a variety of sources in hospitals, including water from laboratory sinks and washbasins, antiseptic solutions, including benzalkonium chloride (Zephiran) and hexachlorophene soap, ophthalmic fluorescein and contact lens solution, saline, penicillin, procaine, and a variety of other medications. Other sources are incubators, humidifying equipment, air-cooling systems, forceps, and syringes. The organism is prevalent in urine receptacles and catheters, and on the hands of orderlies, nurses, and surgeons on urologic wards; in several outbreaks, *Pseudomonas* urinary tract infections have presumably been transmitted from patient to patient by human carriers. Similar epidemics have been reported in nurseries among premature infants, and cross infection on burn wards is also common.

PATHOGENESIS The portal of entry of *Pseudomonas* organisms varies with the patient's age and underlying disease. In infancy and childhood, the skin, umbilical cord, and gastrointestinal tract predominate; in old age, the urinary tract is more often the primary focus. Often the infections remain localized in the skin or subcutaneous tissues. In burns the region below the eschar may become massively infiltrated with bacteria and inflammatory cells, and usually serves as the focus for bacteremia, the single most lethal complication. Hematogenous dissemination is characterized by hemorrhagic nodules in many areas, including the skin, heart, lungs, kidneys, and meninges. The histologic picture is one of necrosis and hemorrhage. Typically the walls of arterioles are heavily infiltrated with bacteria, and the vessels are partially or wholly thrombosed.

MANIFESTATIONS *Pseudomonas* infections occur in many locations, including the skin, subcutaneous tissue, bone and joints, eyes, ears, mastoid and paranasal sinuses, meninges, and heart valves. Bacteremia without a detectable primary focus may also occur.

Infections of the skin and subcutaneous tissues *Pseudomonas* organisms are frequently cultured from surgical wounds, varicose and decubitus ulcers, and burns, particularly following antibiotic therapy. Draining tuberculous or osteomyelitic sinuses may become secondarily infected. The mere presence of *Pseudomonas* in these sites is of little significance provided that bacterial multiplication deep in subcutaneous tissues does not occur and bacteremia does not ensue. Cutaneous infections usually heal after removal or slough of devitalized tissue. *Pseudomonas* organisms may be responsible for green nails in persons whose hands are excessively exposed to water, soap, and detergents, who have onychomycosis, or whose hands are subject to mechanical trauma. The organism can usually be cultured from the nail plate.

Infections of the ear, mastoid, and paranasal sinuses Otitis externa is the most common form of *Pseudomonas* infection involving the ear. It is particularly troublesome in tropical climates and is characterized by chronic serosanguineous and purulent drainage from the external auditory canal. Otitis media or mastoiditis usually occurs as a superinfection following eradication of pneumococci, streptococci, or staphylococci by antimicrobial agents. Frequently *Pseudomonas* organisms are present in association with other gram-negative or gram-positive organisms.

Infection of the eye Corneal ulceration is the most severe form of ocular *Pseudomonas* infection. It usually follows a traumatic abrasion and may terminate in panophthalmitis and destruction of the globe. Purulent conjunctivitis occurs as a manifestation of *Pseudomonas* infection in premature infants. Contamination of contact lenses or lens fluid may be an important means of infecting the eyes with *Pseudomonas* organisms.

Urinary tract infections *Pseudomonas* organisms are common pathogens in the urinary tract and are usually found in patients with obstructive uropathy who have been subjected to repeated urethral manipulations or to urologic surgery. They are rarely cultured from the urine of patients who have not seen a urologist. At times *Pseudomonas* is one of several pathogenic bacteria in the urine, the others being *Escherichia coli, Klebsiella, Proteus,* and enterococci. *Pseudomonas* bacteriuria is in no way unique and cannot be distinguished from infection with other organisms on clinical grounds.

Gastrointestinal tract *Pseudomonas* organisms have been implicated as a cause of epidemic diarrhea of infancy. In addition, a number of infants dying from neonatal sepsis have the classic necrotic, avascular ulcers of *Pseudomonas* bacteremia in the bowel at autopsy. A "typhoidal" form of *Pseudomonas* infection characterized by fever, myalgia, and diarrhea occurs predominantly in the tropics. This illness, also called 13-day fever or Shanghai fever, is self-limited, and the prognosis is good.

Respiratory tract Primary *Pseudomonas* pneumonia is infrequent, and culture of this organism from the sputum usually is indicative of aspiration of oropharyngeal contents with secondary infection or of superinfection following eradication of a more sensitive flora with antibiotics. Pulmonary infection is often associated with microabscesses. The organism is often isolated from the sputum of patients with bronchiectasis, chronic bronchitis, or cystic fibrosis who have lingering infections punctuated by multiple courses of chemotherapy and is recovered frequently from the stomata of tracheostomy sites. *Pseudomonas* bronchitis and bronchiolitis may be the terminal event in cystic fibrosis.

Meningitis Spontaneous *Pseudomonas* meningitis is most unusual, but the bacilli may be introduced into the subarachnoid space by lumbar puncture, spinal anesthesia, intrathecal medication, or head trauma. Ventriculomastoid or ventriculoatrial shunts performed for hydrocephalus may become contaminated with *Pseudomonas* organisms. Usually revision or removal of the shunt offers the best hope of cure. Meningitis may be a terminal phenomenon in *Pseudomonas* bacteremia and in this instance represents a metastatic infection in the meninges.

Bacteremia Bloodstream invasion tends to occur in debilitated patients, premature infants, children with congenital defects, patients with lymphomas, leukemias, or other malignant tumors, and elderly patients who have undergone surgery or instrumentation of the biliary or urinary tract. *Pseudomonas* bacteremia is an important cause of death in patients with severe burns. In adults, *Pseudomonas* bacteremia is indistinguishable from bloodstream infection with other bacterial species except for two findings: (1) Ecthyma gangrenosum, the classic skin lesion, often located in the anogenital or axillary region as a round, indurated, purple-black area about 1 cm in diameter with an ulcerated center and a surrounding zone of erythema; and (2) the passage rarely of green urine, presumably due to the hemoglobin pigment, verdoglobin. Other features of *Pseudomonas* sepsis include hectic fever, shaking chills, hyperventilation, confusion, delirium, and circulatory collapse. Hypothermia, leukopenia, and thrombocytopenia are more common in *Pseudomonas* bacteremia than in other gram-negative bacteremia but are often related to an underlying blood dyscrasia. In addition to ecthyma gangrenosum, other skin lesions consist of hemorrhagic cellulitis and macular lesions on the trunk similar to "rose spots." Organisms usually can be cultured from cutaneous lesions and may provide an early clue to the diagnosis. *Pseudomonas* organisms may be in the bloodstream concomitantly with other organisms, notably Enterobacteriaceae or staphylococci. More often, however, *Pseudomonas* bacteremia follows staphylococcal sepsis in patients with burns.

Bacterial endocarditis A number of cases of *Pseudomonas* subacute bacterial endocarditis have followed open-heart surgery. Usually the organisms become implanted on a silk suture or a synthetic patch employed for closure of septal defects. Reoperation with removal of the vegetation and foreign bodies offers the best hope of cure. *Pseudomonas* endocarditis has been found on normal heart valves in patients with burns or in drug addicts; it has been postulated that staphylococcal endocarditis develops first and that the vegetation is secondarily infected with *Pseudomonas* organisms. Metastatic abscesses in bone, joints, brain, adrenal glands, and lungs are frequent consequences of *Pseudomonas* endocarditis.

TREATMENT Localized infections should be treated by irrigation with 1% acetic acid or topical therapy with colistin or polymyxin B. The administration of colistin subconjunctivally has been of value in ocular infections. Drainage of purulent material and removal of devitalized tissues are essential. The outcome of *Pseudomonas* bacteremia is more dependent on the underlying disease than on the chemotherapy. For example, in patients with leukemia, remission generally must be attained before sepsis can be controlled. In burns, wound infection must be eradicated before the bloodstream can be cleared of organisms. Most strains of *Pseudomonas* are sensitive to polymyxin B and colistin, and a number of strains respond to oxytetracycline. These drugs should be used in full dosage of 30 to 50 mg every 6 hr for polymyxin B (in adults) and 75 to 100 mg every 6 hr (in adults) for colistin in life-threatening *Pseudomonas* bacteremia. Both drugs are excellent for eradicating bacteriuria, but because blood levels exceed minimal inhibitory concentrations only two- or threefold, the results in bacteremia and deep-seated tissue infection are inconsistent. Gentamicin, an aminoglycoside antibiotic, inhibits most strains of *Pseudomonas* and presently has superseded the polymyxin-type antibiotics for systemic infection with *Pseudomonas*. The dose for severe infection in patients with normal renal function is 3 to 5 mg per day in divided doses. Carbenicillin, a new semisynthetic penicillin, is also active against many isolates and may be useful. However, carbenicillin must be used in doses of 24 to 30 g per day for control of severe infection. The combination of gentamicin and carbenicillin is frequently employed to delay emergence of resistance during therapy. Asymptomatic bacteriuria, particularly when confined to the bladder, should be treated with the least toxic and least painful agent, which, at times, may be a sulfonamide or a tetracycline.

The prognosis has been improved in burned patients with *Pseudomonas* sepsis as well as in a few other patients with endocarditis and with necrotizing papillitis by the use of large doses of hyperimmune γ-globulin in addition to antimicrobials.

PROPHYLAXIS *Pseudomonas* cross infections in hospitals can be reduced by careful attention to aseptic techniques, particularly in nurseries for premature infants, operating rooms, and urologic wards; avoidance of cold sterilization procedures wherever possible; and scrupulous attention to clean plumbing fixtures, humidifying equipment, etc. Judicious use of antibiotics, steroids, and cytotoxic agents should also diminish the incidence of *Pseudomonas* infections. Systemic antibiotic prophylaxis aimed at preventing colonization and infection with *Pseudomonas* organisms has been notoriously unsuccessful and should be interdicted.

PROGNOSIS The mortality rate in *Pseudomonas* bacteremia is 75 percent and is highest in patients with shock or severe associated disease such as massive third-degree burns, leukemia, or prematurity. When bacteremia originates in the urinary tract and is not accompanied by shock, the prognosis is considerably better. Localized *Pseudomonas* infections do not present a threat to life unless hematogenous dissemination occurs.

MIMA-HERELLEA INFECTIONS

DEFINITION Organisms of the tribe Mimae are pleomorphic, gram-negative bacilli which are easily confused with members of the genus *Neisseria.* Severe infections with these organisms, including meningitis, bacterial endocarditis, pneumonia, and bacteremia, are being described with increasing frequency.

ETIOLOGY *Mima polymorpha,* described by DeBord in 1939, is one of two well-characterized species within the tribe Mimae, the other being *Herellea vaginicola.* Organisms formerly described as *Bacterium anitratum* and B5W are synonymous with *H. vaginicola.* These organisms are pleomorphic, gram-negative, encapsulated, and nonmotile. They grow well on ordinary media, forming white, convex, smooth colonies. Diplococcal forms predominate in colonies grown on solid media; rods and filamentous forms are more common in liquid media. The species can be differentiated from the Enterobacteriaceae by their negative nitrate reaction and from members of the genus *Neisseria,* which they may resemble morphologically, by their simple growth requirements, their bacillary form in liquid media, and their usually negative oxidase reaction. *Herellea vaginicola* may be distinguished from *M. polymorpha* by its capacity to ferment 10 percent lactose.

EPIDEMIOLOGY AND PATHOGENESIS Mimae are ubiquitous and have been cultured from a variety of human sources, including urethral, vaginal, and conjunctival secretions, sputum, pleural fluid, blood, cerebrospinal fluid, feces, cutaneous ulcers, abscesses, chancroid lesions, joint fluid, ascitic fluid, and bone marrow. In addition, these organisms have been found in river water, humidifiers, and oxygen tents. Recent observations indicate that 25 percent of normal subjects are skin carriers of *H. vaginicola,* and 10 percent of *M. polymorpha.* The striking association of mima-herellea bacteremia with cutdowns or indwelling intravenous catheters favors the skin as a major portal of entry in man. The increasing incidence of mima-herellea pneumonia, both as a primary infection and as a superinfection, also points to the respiratory tract as an important portal of entry. It is most likely that the *Mima* organisms are normal human commensals of relatively low virulence which produce serious infections under conditions of decreased host resistance, or in the presence of local tissue trauma, and in this way resemble the Enterobacteriaceae. Although members of the Mimae tribe have been implicated as an important cause of penicillin-resistant venereal urethritis, the evidence for this relation is not convincing. Similarly, the role of these organisms as a cause of conjunctivitis and vaginitis requires documentation.

MANIFESTATIONS Serious infections caused by *Mima* organisms include (1) meningitis, (2) subacute and acute bacterial endocarditis, (3) pneumonia, (4) urinary tract infections, and (5) bacteremia. Usually, the signs and symptoms associated with infections in these sites are no different from those produced by other pathogens. For example, subacute bacterial endocarditis has usually been reported in patients with congenital or rheumatic heart disease and pursues an indolent course, while urinary tract infections may be manifested by asymptomatic bacteriuria, cystitis, or pyelonephritis. Pneumonia often occurs in the form of a superinfection in patients who have received antibiotics, but occasionally herelleae may be primary pathogens in the lung. Occasionally, *M. polymorpha* may be the cause of a fulminating bacteremia, with high fever, vascular collapse, petechiae, and ecchymoses, indistinguishable from fulminant meningococcemia. More often, however, bacteremia is associated with an overt portal of entry, such as infected cutdowns or indwelling intravenous catheters, surgical wounds, or burns, or it may follow urethral or other surgical instrumentation. These patients usually have severe debilitating disease or have undergone surgery. Many times they have received antibiotics, adrenal cortical hormones, irradiation, or tumor chemotherapy and have had infections with other organisms, usually gram-positive, prior to development of sepsis with Mimae. The clinical picture presented by these patients is dominated by endotoxemia, and the prognosis is very poor.

DIAGNOSIS The diagnosis of herelliosis is usually missed because the clinical bacteriology laboratory is unfamiliar with these organisms and reports them incorrectly or because they are considered contaminants. The confusion attending the taxonomic classification of these organisms has not simplified matters. For practical purposes, isolation of mimae-herelleae (or their synonyms, *B. anitratum,* B5W, *Diplococcus mucosus,* or *Neisseria winogradskyi*) from blood, spinal fluid, sputum, urine, or pus should be considered significant unless there is no evidence of infection on clinical grounds. Since Mimae are resistant to penicillin and members of the genus *Neisseria* are sensitive, differentiation of these organisms is of obvious importance.

TREATMENT Antibiotic sensitivities of *Mima* and *Herellea* strains vary, but most strains are inhibited by kanamycin, gentamicin, colistin, or polymyxin B. Sensitivity to the tetracyclines is unpredictable, and most strains are also resistant to penicillin, ampicillin, cephalothin, erythromycin, and chloramphenicol. For serious systemic infections, kanamycin should be administered in doses of 0.5 g intramuscularly every 8 to 12 hr (in adults). Since these organisms may produce localized abscesses, surgical drainage may be necessary.

REFERENCES

Mima-Herellea infections

Inclan AP et al: Organisms of the tribe mimeae: Incidence of isolation and clinical correlation. South Med J 58:1261, 1965

Reynolds RC, Cluff LE: Infections of man with mimae. Ann Intern Med 58:759, 1963

Pseudomonas infections

Alexander JW et al: Immunologic control of pseudomonas infection in burn patients: Clinical evaluation. Arch Surg 102:31, 1971

Bodey GP: Epidemiologic studies of pseudomonas species in patients with leukemia. Am J Med Sci 260:82, 1970

Curtin JA et al: Pseudomonas bacteremia: Review of 91 cases. Ann Intern Med 54:1077, 1961

Fierer J et al: Pseudomonas aeruginosa epidemic traced to delivery room resuscitators. N Engl J Med 276:991, 1967

Grieble HG et al: Fine particle humidifiers: Source of pseudomonas aeruginosa infections in a respiratory disease unit. N Engl J Med 282:531, 1970

Stone HH: Review of pseudomonas sepsis in thermal injury. Ann Surg 163:297, 1966

Tillotson JR, Lerner AM: Characteristics of non-bacteremic pseudomonas pneumonia. Ann Intern Med 68:295, 1968

135
BACTEROIDES INFECTION

EDWARD W. HOOK

ETIOLOGY The genus *Bacteroides* includes a group of gram-negative, non-spore-forming, strictly anaerobic bacilli that are normal inhabitants of the mouth, intestinal tract, and vagina. These organisms are found in large numbers in human feces in an average concentration of about 10^{11} viable units per gram, outnumbering other bacteria by a hundredfold or more.

Anaerobic gram-negative bacilli are grouped into genera on the basis of the production of short-chain fatty acids. In general, members of the genus *Bacteroides* do not produce significant quantities of butyric acid, in contrast to members of the genus *Fusobacterium*, which form butyric acid as a major fermentation product.

Members of the genus *Bacteroides* are the anaerobes most frequently isolated from clinical specimens, and *B. fragilis* and *B. melaninogenicus* are the species most often responsible for infection in man. *Bacteroides fragilis* strains can be divided into at least five subspecies: *fragilis, distasonis, ovatus, thetaiotamicron*, and *vulgatus*. *Fragilis* is the most common subspecies from clinical specimens but the least common subspecies in the normal intestinal flora.

PATHOGENESIS Species of *bacteroides* are not highly invasive microorganisms, and infection is usually secondary to an underlying disease, a surgical procedure, or drug or radiation therapy which impairs the normal defenses of the host. The initial reaction to infection results in a localized suppurative lesion characterized by the formation of fetid pus. The characteristic odor is caused by certain metabolic end products of bacterial origin, primarily short-chain fatty acids and volatile amines. Infection usually remains localized, but bloodstream invasion may occur. In instances of bacteremia, suppurative thrombophlebitis adjacent to the site of initial infection is a frequent occurrence, and emboli harboring viable bacilli are occasionally dislodged, resulting in septic pulmonary infarction. Organisms of the genus *Bacteroides* elaborate a heparinase, but the role of this enzyme in the formation of thrombi is unknown. Localization of bloodborne organisms at distant sites is not unusual and may result in abscess formation in brain, lung, liver, joints, kidneys, or other organs.

Although *Bacteroides* may be isolated in pure culture from infected tissue or pus, other organisms are present in the majority of cases, usually anaerobic or aerobic streptococci, coliform species, staphylococci, or *Fusobacterium* species. *Bacteroides* and anaerobic streptococci have been shown to act synergistically in the induction of abscesses in mice.

MANIFESTATIONS Local infections Species of *Bacteroides* are frequently isolated from local suppurative lesions of any tissue liable to contamination with the flora of the mouth, intestinal tract, or vagina. For example, members of this genus have been isolated from peritonsillar, appendiceal, ischiorectal, or pelvic abscesses, and from infected Skene's or Bartholin's glands. These organisms may be associated with sinusitis and otitis media, and can also be cultured from the surfaces of acutely inflamed appendixes, from exudate in localized or generalized peritonitis, and from purulent discharge in patients with endometritis. Surgical wounds of the gastrointestinal or genitourinary tract may be complicated by *Bacteroides* infection. The bacterial flora of bronchiectatic cavities frequently includes these organisms.

Local infection is usually manifested by pain and tenderness, and the course and outcome depend on the site of involvement and extent of infection. Necrosis of blood vessels in an abscess cavity occasionally results in severe hemorrhage.

Systemic infection Invasion of the bloodstream by *Bacteroides* organisms is usually secondary to local infection of the tonsils, female genital tract, or peritoneum. The initial manifestations are determined by the portal of entry and may be those of peritonsillar abscess, endometritis, or appendicitis. When bloodstream invasion occurs, the patient may become extremely ill. Severe chills, hectic fever ranging from 101 to 106°F, and marked diaphoresis are common. When bacteremia complicates tonsillar infection, the internal jugular vein may be the site of suppurative thrombophlebitis, and in pelvic infections the iliac and femoral veins may be involved. Palpation along the course of an involved vein, such as the internal jugular, may disclose a firm, tender cord, indicating the presence of a thrombus. Emboli may be dislodged, resulting in multiple septic pulmonary infarcts manifested by rales, dyspnea, cough, hemoptysis, pleurisy, and roentgenographic evidence of consolidation. Lung abscess and empyema often complicate septic pulmonary infarction. Metastatic infection at other sites is not unusual, and may be manifested as brain abscess, liver abscess, or septic arthritis. A diffuse hepatitis may develop, leading to enlargement and tenderness of the liver and jaundice. The prognosis in systemic *Bacteroides* infection is grave, and death may occur in a few days.

The genus *Bacteroides* has also been implicated in certain other systemic infections. These organisms, often mixed with another bacterial species, appear to be responsible for one-third or more of the cases of brain abscess. Meningitis or brain abscess may result from direct extension of infection from the middle ear or sinuses, or from hematogenous spread from the lungs or other sites.

Bacteroides species play an important etiologic role in pleuropulmonary disease caused by anaerobic bacteria. These anaerobic organisms may cause lung abscess, necrotizing pneumonia, and empyema, and are second only to the pneumococcus as a cause of acute bacterial infection of the lungs. Infection usually results from aspiration of secretions or vomitus harboring anaerobes, most often various combinations of *Fusobacterium* species, *Bacteroides* species, and anaerobic cocci. Common predisposing conditions include altered consciousness, regurgitation, oral sepsis, and stasis or obstruction in the lower respiratory tract. These infections are frequently slow to respond to appropriate therapy and are associated with considerable morbidity and mortality.

Nonclostridial anaerobes, principally *Bacteroides* species and anaerobic streptococci, are the major invasive pathogens in septic abortion. Bacteremia, often transient and frequently polymicrobic, can be demonstrated in 50 to 60 percent of these patients. Improved techniques for transport and culture of specimens have shown that anaerobic organisms, including *Bacteroides* species, also can be implicated in the etiology of 40 to 50 percent of the cases of pyogenic liver abscess. Bacteremia is frequently demonstrable in these patients. Transient *Bacteroides* bacteremia may occur after dental extraction, and a few cases of subacute bacterial endocarditis have been described. These organisms occasionally cause infection of the urinary tract.

LABORATORY FINDINGS Leukocytosis of 12,000 to 25,000 cells per mm^3 may occur in localized *Bacteroides* infections and is almost always present in systemic infection. Patients with liver abscesses or hepatitis have elevated serum bilirubin values and other aberrations of hepatic function. Gas formation at sites of infection occasionally results in air-fluid levels detectable by roentgenography.

Bacteroides infection should be considered whenever pus with an extremely foul odor is encountered, and anaerobic cultures should be made. A smear of the pus reveals slightly elongated gram-negative bacilli, and often another organism. Definitive diagnosis depends on isolation of the organisms from infected tissue or blood. Bacteroides grow slowly and may be difficult to detect when associated with another organism. Specimens for culture should be collected to avoid "contamination" with *Bacteroides* species normally present in the oropharynx, genital or intestinal tracts, and on all mucosal surfaces. Anaerobic cultures should not be performed on expectorated sputum, bronchoscopic aspirates, or secretions from mucosal surfaces which normally harbor anaerobes. Acceptable materials for culture include blood, pleural fluid, transtracheal aspirates, and other tissues or fluids which are sterile under normal conditions. Agglutinins against the strain responsible for an infection develop during the second or third week of infection, but because of the variable antigenic composition of these organisms, serologic methods are not helpful in the diagnosis.

TREATMENT Surgery is of prime importance in the management of patients with *Bacteroides* infections. Drainage of abscess cavities should be carried out as soon as fluctuation and localization occur; perforations must be closed promptly, and devitalized tissues or foreign bodies should be removed. Antimicrobial therapy is indicated when infection is not localized, especially if systemic manifestations are present. In patients proved or suspected to have a severe systemic *Bacteroides* infection, either clindamycin, 1.2 to 1.8 g per day divided into three equal doses in adults, or chloramphenicol, 3 g per day divided into three equal doses in adults, is the antimicrobial drug of choice. Chloramphenicol is preferred for patients with infections of the central nervous system because clindamycin does not effectively penetrate the blood-brain barrier. Both antibiotics can be administered orally, but parenteral therapy is advisable for patients with severe infection. Almost all *Bacteroides* strains are susceptible in vitro to concentrations of clindamycin or chloramphenicol readily obtainable in the blood of patients treated with full doses of the antibiotics. Hematologic parameters should be monitored carefully during chloramphenicol therapy because of the dose-related marrow-suppressive effect as well as the more serious complication of aplastic anemia.

Although tetracyclines and penicillin G have been considered to be effective agents for treatment of *Bacteroides* infections, a large proportion of strains of *B. fragilis*, the most common isolate, are resistant in vitro. The use of these antibiotics in patients with severe *Bacteroides* infections is inadvisable unless it has been determined by in vitro tests that the causative organism is sensitive. Many strains of *Bacteroides* are highly resistant to the penicillinase-resistant penicillins, cephalothin, carbenicillin, or ampicillin, and the vast majority of isolates are resistant to streptomycin, kanamycin, neomycin, and gentamicin.

Bacteroides species frequently coexist at infected sites with other anaerobic or aerobic bacteria. Although clindamycin or chloramphenicol shows excellent activity against almost all anaerobes of clinical importance, the occurrence of polymicrobic infection may necessitate administration of another antibiotic in some patients.

Anticoagulant therapy and venous ligation should be considered in patients with thrombophlebitis and multiple septic pulmonary infarctions.

REFERENCES

ANAEROBE LABORATORY: Outline of clinical methods in anaerobic bacteriology, 2d revision, Blacksburg, Va.: Virginia Polytechnic Institute and State University, 1970

BARTLETT JG, FINEGOLD SM: Anaerobic pleuropulmonary infections. Medicine 51:413, 1972

—— et al: Treatment of anaerobic infections with lincomycin and clindamycin. N Engl J Med 287:1006, 1972

BODNER SJ et al: Bacteremia bacteroides infections. Ann Intern Med 73:537, 1970

BORNSTEIN DL et al: Anaerobic infections—Review of current experience. Medicine 43:207, 1964

CHOW AW, GUZE LB: Treatment of bacteroidaceae bacteremia: Clinical experience with 112 patients. Proceedings of the

Anaerobic Bacterial Conference, Atlanta, Georgia, November 27–29, 1972

HEINEMANN HS, BRAUDE AI: Anaerobic infection of the brain. Am J Med 35:682, 1963

MARTIN WJ et al: In vitro antimicrobial susceptibility of anaerobic bacteria isolated from clinical specimens. Antimicrob Agents Chemother 1:148, 1972

ROTHERAM EB JR, SCHICK SF: Nonclostridial anaerobic bacteria in septic abortion. Am J Med 46:80, 1969

SABBAJ J et al: Anaerobic pyogenic liver abscess. Ann Intern Med 77:629, 1972

WILKINS TD et al: Standardized single-disc method for antibiotic susceptibility testing of anaerobic bacteria. Antimicrob Agents Chemother 1:451, 1972

136 SALMONELLA INFECTIONS

EDWARD W. HOOK

INTRODUCTION The genus *Salmonella* consists of more than 1,400 different serologic types which can be distinguished one from the other on the basis of specific antigens. Striking variation in pathogenicity of the serotypes occurs, but almost all are pathogenic for animals and man. Certain serotypes are characterized by specific host preferences. The best example of a serotype adapted to a specific host is *S. typhi* which under natural conditions of transmission produces disease only in man. *Salmonella* infections of man are *acute gastroenteritis*, *enteric fever* (*typhoid or paratyphoid fever*), *bacteremia*, and *localized infection* which may occur at almost any site. In addition, *asymptomatic intestinal infections* and *convalescent intestinal carriers* are common. A *chronic carrier* state with a focus of persistent infection in the gallbladder or urinary tract also occurs occasionally.

ETIOLOGY The salmonellas are motile gram-negative bacilli that do not ferment lactose or sucrose but ferment glucose and a number of other sugars. Almost all serotypes produce gas, although *S. typhi* is a notable exception. Presumptive identification of these organisms is established by fermentation and other metabolic reactions in differential media and by relatively simple agglutination tests performed with group-specific antiserums. *Salmonella* groups are designated by letters of the alphabet, and the vast majority of strains isolated from natural sources fall into the first five groups (A to E). Final identification of individual sterotypes is based on highly specific differences in structure of O or somatic and H or flagellar antigens and is accomplished routinely only in large *Salmonella* typing centers which have the necessary collection of antiserums required for such work. Certain serotypes, for example *S. typhi* or *S. typhimurium*, can be further subdivided on the basis of susceptibility to lysis by specific bacteriophages. Serotyping is an important epidemiologic tool and should be carried out on all isolates.

The Salmonella Surveillance Unit of the Center for Disease Control has reported that 305 different salmonella serotypes were recovered from human beings in the 7-year period 1965 to 1971. The most frequently reported serotypes in descending order were *S. typhimurium*, *S. enteritidis*, *S. heidelberg*, *S. newport*, *S. infantis*, *S. saint paul*, *S. thompson*, *S. typhi*, *S. blockley*, *S. derby*, *S. javiana*, *S. oranienberg*, and *S. montevideo*. Year after year, *S. typhimurium* accounts for about 25 percent of the isolates, and the 10 or 12 most frequently isolated serotypes account for about 70 percent of the total isolates from human sources.

TYPHOID FEVER

DEFINITION Typhoid fever is an acute systemic disease resulting from infection with *S. typhi*. The disease is unique to man. It is characterized by malaise, fever, abdominal discomfort, transient rash, splenomegaly, and leukopenia. The most prominent major complications are intestinal hemorrhage and perforation. The disease is the classic example of enteric fever caused by *Salmonella* species. However, enteric fever, similar to typhoid, can also be caused by other *Salmonella* serotypes and is termed *paratyphoid fever*.

EPIDEMIOLOGY *Salmonella typhi* gains access to the body by the oral route in almost all cases as a consequence of the ingestion of contaminated food, water, or milk. Man is the only true reservoir of *S. typhi* in nature, and persons with typhoid fever or convalescent or chronic carriers always serve as the ultimate source of infection. Infected individuals can excrete millions of viable typhoid bacilli in the feces, which is the usual source of contamination of food or drink. Patients with active disease also occasionally have organisms in respiratory secretions, vomitus, or other body fluids and may be responsible for spread of infection. Flies or other insects can carry organisms in feces or other infected material to food or drink and have been implicated in a few outbreaks. Oysters or other shellfish are contaminated at times in polluted waters and occasionally serve as sources of typhoid.

The incidence of typhoid fever has steadily decreased in the United States during the past century to the present relatively low level of less than 400 cases per annum. The decrease in incidence has been coincident with improvement in socioeconomic conditions and is specifically related to development of pure water supplies, effective sewage disposal, pasteurization of milk, and methods to detect and control spread of organisms from persons with active disease or from carriers. Typhoid continues to occur on a large scale in countries where sanitation is suboptimal. It is not at all unusual to find that patients with typhoid fever in the United States have acquired the infection in another area of the world.

Typhoid can be eradicated ultimately because the infection is confined to man and both the disease and the carrier state can be controlled by appropriate therapy. The importance of sewage disposal, a pure water supply, and control of carriers is highlighted repeatedly by the occurrence of small outbreaks which develop when defects in sanitation develop during natural disasters such as flood.

The sex distribution of patients with typhoid fever in the United States shows no significant predilection. In recent years, about 75 percent of cases have occurred in persons less than 30 years of age. In contrast, the chronic carrier state is much more common in females than males (the female/male ratio is 3:1) and in older individuals (88 percent over 50 years of age).

There is no seasonal variation in incidence of typhoid fever in the United States. However, in areas of the world where the disease is endemic, the incidence increases in the summer months.

PATHOGENESIS The outcome of the interaction between the typhoid bacillus and man is determined during the early hours after ingestion of the organisms. Typhoid bacilli reach the upper small intestine shortly after ingestion and may multiply there. The organisms may then invade the mucosa and enter intestinal lymphatics to be carried via the thoracic duct to the bloodstream. This initial early bacteremia apparently occurs within 24 to 72 hr after ingestion of organisms and is rarely detected in natural infections because patients are usually asymptomatic at this early stage. The bacteremia is transient and is rapidly terminated as bacilli are phagocytized by cells of the reticuloendothelial system. Nevertheless, viable bacilli are disseminated throughout the body and apparently persist within reticuloendothelial cells. If multiplication at the intracellular site takes place, organisms reenter the bloodstream, producing a continuous bacteremia for days or weeks. The reappearance of bacteremia corresponds with the onset of manifestations of the disease. Intracellular organisms are eventually destroyed as manifestations of disease subside and recovery ensues. Enhanced intracellular killing and recovery appear to be related to the onset of delayed hypersensitivity. Recovery is unrelated to the appearance, even in high titer, of agglutinins against the somatic, flagellar, or Vi antigens of the typhoid bacillus.

The number of organisms ingested is of obvious importance in determining whether typhoid fever results from exposure to *S. typhi.* Studies in volunteers have shown that about 10^7 typhoid bacilli of the Quarles strain must be taken orally to produce typhoid fever in 50 percent of normal volunteers. The number of organisms ingested also influences the incubation period, and short incubation periods, in general, correspond with large doses of organisms. The volunteer studies have also demonstrated that different strains of typhoid bacilli vary considerably in their capacity to produce disease in man.

The normal flora of the upper intestinal tract is an important protective mechanism against invasion by *S. typhi.* Volunteer studies have demonstrated that antimicrobial therapy a day or so before oral challenge with *S. typhi* markedly decreases the number of viable bacilli required to produce disease. It is possible that certain factors known to be associated with typhoid outbreaks, such as malnutrition, enhance susceptibility to typhoid infection by alterations in the intestinal flora.

During the phase of persistent bacteremia, all organs are repeatedly exposed to typhoid bacilli. Abscess formation may occur but is unusual. However, localization does occur in the gallbladder in almost all cases. Organisms multiply in the bile to high titer, usually without manifestations of cholecystitis, and are excreted with bile into the intestinal tract. Stool cultures, which are usually negative for *S. typhi* during the incubation period and early phases of the disease, become positive in a large proportion of cases during the third or fourth week of the disease, when excretion of organisms multiplying in bile reaches a peak.

The factors responsible for the fever, leukopenia, and other manifestations of typhoid fever have been inadequately defined. Typhoid bacilli contain biologically active lipopolysaccharides or endotoxins which produce fever, leukopenia, thrombocytopenia, and hyperplasia of reticuloendothelial cells when injected into animals or man. It has been assumed for years that these materials play an important role in the pathogenesis of the signs and symptoms of typhoid fever. However, the evidence regarding the role of endotoxin in the genesis of the manifestations of typhoid is confusing and inconclusive. For example, tolerance to the pyrogenic effects of endotoxins can be demonstrated during convalescence from typhoid fever, which suggests release of endotoxins during infection. Nevertheless, other studies show that typhoid fever follows a normal course in volunteers rendered tolerant to endotoxins prior to challenge, indicating that mechanisms other than endotoxemia are responsible for the sustained fever and toxemia.

PATHOLOGY The most prominent microscopic lesion in typhoid fever is proliferation of large mononuclear cells in many different tissues. Mononuclear hyperplasia leads to lymphadenopathy, splenomegaly, and impressive enlargement of lymphoid tissues in the intestines, especially in the terminal ileum (Peyer's patches). Proliferating mononuclear cells may also be observed in bone marrow, liver, and lung. Studies in volunteers using ^{131}I-tagged aggregated albumin have shown increased phagocytic activity of the reticuloendothelial system by the third to fifth days after onset of symptoms. Necrosis in hyperplastic Peyer's patches may be associated with erosion of blood vessels in the lesions in the intestinal tract, which leads to oozing of blood or massive hemorrhage. Lesions may extend deep into the intestinal wall and cause perforation of the bowel, an event which characteristically occurs late in the disease, most often in the third febrile week. The site of perforation is usually in the distal 24 in. of the ileum.

The gallbladder and bile ducts are routinely infected during the disease. As a rule, this biliary infection is asymptomatic, although acute cholecystitis may occur occasionally. Biliary infection terminates spontaneously during convalescence in the vast majority of patients, but about 3 percent of adults continue to harbor organisms in the gallbladder and become chronic carriers of the typhoid bacillus.

MANIFESTATIONS The incubation period averages about 10 days but may vary from extremes of 3 to 60 days depending on the infecting dose.

The clinical manifestations and duration of illness vary markedly from one patient to another. Mild forms of the disease, characterized primarily by fever, may last only a week, or illness may be prolonged, lasting 8 weeks or more if untreated.

In a typical patient not treated with antimicrobials, the illness lasts about 4 weeks. The onset is insidious with headache, malaise, anorexia, and fever. Headache may be the first manifestation of disease and is usually generalized and severe. Chilly sensations are common, and frank chills may be observed. The fever is remittent, frequently increasing in a steplike manner from day to day as the illness develops. Abdominal discomfort, bloating, and constipation are common during the early phase of illness. A dry cough is observed in about two-thirds of the patients and occasionally may be so prominent as to direct attention away from the generalized nature of the infectious process. Nosebleeds may occur during the early phase of illness.

The temperature gradually increases for 5 to 7 days and then plateaus as a continuous or mildly remittent fever in the range of 39 to 40°C. The temperature may be sustained at these levels with little variation for 2 or 3 weeks. A relative bradycardia occurs in 30 to 40 percent of the patients. The prolonged persistent fever leads to general debility; patients are weak and anorectic. Mental dullness is common and delirium may occur. Abdominal pain and marked distention are usual. Constipation, so common during the early phase of illness, may give way to frank diarrhea which occurs in about one-fifth of the patients. Toward the end of the third week or in the fourth week the fever begins to abate and the symptoms of the disease subside.

The characteristic rash (rose spots) is most often observed during the second week of the disease. The lesions are small, 2- to 4-mm, erythematous macules which occur in small numbers on the upper abdomen and anterior thorax. The lesions blanch on pressure and last only 2 to 3 days. Some reports describe rose spots in as many as 90 percent of patients, whereas other reports indicate a frequency of only 10 percent or even less. The evasive nature of the rash and the difficulties encountered in detecting lesions in highly pigmented individuals probably account for the marked variation in incidence reported in the literature.

The liver and spleen are frequently enlarged and palpable from the end of the first week of illness. The spleen is palpable in about three-quarters of the patients. The liver may be tender, and occasionally a friction rub is audible over the spleen.

Abdominal tenderness is frequent and distention occurs in the majority of cases. Marked abdominal pain with signs of peritonitis should call attention to the possibility of perforation of the bowel.

After the third week, the symptoms slowly abate, and the temperature returns to normal over a period of days.

Jaundice secondary to extensive mononuclear cell infiltration in the liver and hepatic cell necrosis is a rare complication of typhoid. Acute renal failure also is observed rarely; the pathogenesis of this so-called "typhoid nephritis" has not been adequately defined. Disseminated intravascular coagulation may develop in severe typhoid and lead to additional clinical manifestations secondary to thrombosis or hemorrhage.

Complications Prior to the introduction of chloramphenicol, the prolonged febrile course of typhoid often led to profound debility, weight loss, and multiple nutritional deficiencies. Intestinal hemorrhage and bowel perforation, the most feared complications, were common causes of death. The frequency of complications in typhoid fever has been reduced since the advent of effective chemotherapy.

INTESTINAL HEMORRHAGE Erosion of blood vessels in hyperplastic and necrotic Peyer's patches or in other mononuclear cell accumulations in the wall of the intestine leads to bleeding into the intestinal tract. Occult blood in feces is quite common during the course of the disease, occurring in 20 percent or more of patients. Gross blood is present in feces in about 10 percent of patients, and massive hemorrhage occurs occasionally. Major hemorrhage is usually a late complication, occurring most often during the second or third week of disease. A sudden drop in blood pressure or temperature may be the first manifestation of hemorrhage.

INTESTINAL PERFORATION The pathologic process in the lymphoid tissues of the intestine may also penetrate the muscular and serosal layers of the bowel and lead to perforation. Prior to the advent of chloramphenicol, perforation occurred in about 3 percent of patients with typhoid. The incidence has been reduced by antimicrobial therapy to about 1 percent. Perforation is most common in the distal 24 in. of ileum and is observed most frequently during the third week of the disease. The onset of perforation may be quite unexpected during an otherwise uncomplicated convalescence. Pain in the right lower quadrant of the abdomen is the most frequent initial manifestation, but signs of localized or generalized peritonitis develop rapidly.

OTHER COMPLICATIONS Typhoid bacilli may localize in any tissue in the body with the production of localized suppurative infection. Meningitis, chondritis, periostitis, osteomyelitis, arthritis, and pyelonephritis are examples of localized infections that may be observed occasionally. Pneumonia is not unusual and may be related to a secondary bacterial invader, such as the pneumococcus, or to the typhoid bacillus. Severe deep thrombophlebitis may occur during the febrile period. Late complications also include peripheral neuritis, deafness, and alopecia. Hemolytic anemia may be observed, especially in infected individuals deficient in glucose 6-phosphate dehydrogenase.

Relapse After illness has subsided for a variable period, usually about two weeks, all the manifestations which characterized the initial infection may recur. Blood cultures, negative during convalescence, may become positive again. Although relapse may be severe, it is usually milder and of shorter duration than the original illness. The incidence of relapse was about 5 to 10 percent prior to the introduction of effective chemotherapy. Chloramphenicol has not decreased the frequency of relapse; in fact, the relapse rate in chloramphenicol-treated patients is higher than in patients not receiving the drug. Periods of antimicrobial therapy longer than 2 weeks do not seem to alter the incidence of relapse. Relapse cannot be correlated with the titer of agglutinins against the flagellar, somatic, or Vi antigens of the typhoid bacillus.

Chronic carriers Although the vast majority of patients with typhoid fever eradicate the site of infection in the gallbladder during convalescence, about 3 percent of adults do not, and these individuals become chronic typhoid carriers who continue to excrete organisms in feces for years, usually for life. A chronic carrier is defined as a person documented to have been excreting typhoid bacilli in the stool for a period of at least 1 year. In the United States, almost all chronic carriers have a persistent site of infection in the gallbladder from which organisms reach the intestinal tract in bile. Chronic carriers may be detected by follow-up of patients with typhoid fever, but many carriers give no history of typhoid. In these patients, it is assumed that the initial illness was so mild as to go unrecognized or undiagnosed. Once organisms have been demonstrated in the stools for as long as a year, it is quite unlikely that the focus of infection in the gallbladder will terminate spontaneously. The chronic carrier state is rare in children and occurs more commonly with increasing age and is about three times more common in women than men. It is possible that these age and sex characteristics are related to the greater prevalence of gallbladder disease in older women, a factor which would favor persistence of organisms in the biliary tract.

The chronic biliary carrier is usually asymptomatic. Despite millions of organisms entering the intestine in each milliliter of bile, patients show no systemic manifestations. Gallstones and dysfunction of the gallbladder on cholecystogram can be demonstrated in a large proportion of chronic carriers, and carriers occasionally develop acute cholecystitis.

In areas of the world where *Schistosoma haematobium* infections are common, a chronic urinary carrier state results from localization of typhoid bacilli or other *Salmonella* serotypes in the obstructed urinary tract or adjacent lesions resulting from the schistosomiasis. These chronic urinary carriers not only excrete *Salmonella* in the urine but also may have intermittent bacteremic episodes which are not necessarily accompanied by fever.

LABORATORY FINDINGS Leukopenia of 3,000 to 4,000 cells per mm^3 is characteristic of the febrile phase of typhoid fever. A sudden increase in leukocyte count to 10,000 cells per mm^3 or higher should suggest the possibility of intestinal perforation, hemorrhage, or a pyogenic complication, but these complications may occur in the absence of leukocytosis. A normocytic normochromic anemia develops during the course of the disease and may be aggravated by blood loss from intestinal lesions. Occult blood in feces is common from the second week of disease. Urine is usually normal except for transient albuminuria during the febrile period.

The most dependable way to establish a definitive diagnosis of typhoid fever is by blood culture. Organisms can be recovered by culture of blood in 70 to 90 percent of patients during the first week of disease. Bacteremia is continuous and prolonged. Positive blood cultures are obtained in as many as 30 or 40 percent of patients during the third week of disease, but the incidence of bacteremia rapidly decreases after this time. Blood cultures frequently are positive during relapse.

Only about 10 to 15 percent of patients have positive stool cultures during the first week of disease. However, the frequency of positive stool cultures increases as the disease progresses, reaching a maximum of about 75 percent during the third or fourth week of illness. The frequency of positive cultures then begins to decline so that only about 10 percent of patients have positive stool cultures by 8 weeks after onset of illness. Most of these patients' cultures become negative over the next several weeks or months, but about 3 percent of adults continue to excrete organisms even after 1 year. Persistent excretion in these chronic carriers is secondary to infection in the gallbladder and biliary tract.

The incidence of positive urine cultures varies markedly during the course of typhoid fever and parallels the frequency of positive stool cultures. At least some of the positive cultures represent contamination of urine with feces harboring typhoid bacilli.

The majority of patients, but by no means all, develop a fourfold or greater rise in agglutinins against the somatic or O antigens of the typhoid bacillus during the course of the disease. A significant fourfold or greater increase in titer in the absence of recent typhoid immunization is compatible with infection with *S. typhi* but is by no means specific. All the group D organisms, one of which is *S. typhi*, as well as organisms in groups A and B, have certain common antigens which can evoke the formation of antibodies reactive with the O antigen used in the Widal test. Agglutinins against flagellar or H antigens also appear, frequently in higher titer than agglutinins against the O antigens. However, the H agglutinins are even more subject to nonspecific variation than O agglutinins and are of no value in diagnosis. Agglutinins begin to appear after about one week of illness and reach a peak titer during the fifth or sixth week. Early antimicrobial therapy may dampen the immunologic response in patients with typhoid fever. Relapse bears no relation to agglutinin titer. Rheumatoid factor activity in high titer can be detected in a large proportion of patients with typhoid or paratyphoid fever.

DIFFERENTIAL DIAGNOSIS The clinical features of typhoid fever, while characteristic and suggestive of the diagnosis, are certainly not pathognomonic. Many other diseases give a clinical picture which may be confused with typhoid; these include the rickettsioses, brucellosis, tularemia, leptospirosis, psittacosis, infectious hepatitis, infectious mononucleosis, primary atypical pneumonia, miliary tuberculosis, malaria, lymphoma, and rheumatic fever. Typhoid should be considered in any patient with unexplained fever, especially if there is a history of recent foreign travel to endemic areas.

TREATMENT Antimicrobial therapy Chloramphenicol is the antibiotic of choice for the treatment of typhoid fever. Despite the fact that a number of antimicrobial agents show excellent in vitro activity against *S. typhi*, chloramphenicol has consistently been shown to be more effective in terminating the febrile toxic course of the disease in the greatest proportion of patients in the shortest period of time. Nevertheless, the response to chloramphenicol is not dramatic or rapid. Subjective improvement usually occurs within about 48 hr after beginning therapy, but the temperature usually does not return to normal for 2 to 5 days after initiating treatment. Bacteremia usually clears within hours after therapy is instituted, but occasionally organisms can be recovered from the blood 24 or 48 hr after beginning treatment. The dose of chloramphenicol should be 50 mg per kg body weight per day divided into three or four equal doses given orally at intervals of 6 or 8 hr. After the patient has become afebrile, the dose may be reduced to 30 mg per kg per day. Therapy should be continued for 2 weeks. If chloramphenicol cannot be given by the oral route, comparable doses should be given parenterally.

Ampicillin in doses of 80 mg per kg per day or 6 g per day for adults divided into four or six doses given parenterally or a combination of trimethoprim and sulfonamide is effective in the treatment of typhoid, but the response is not as predictable or as prompt as with chloramphenicol. If there is a contraindication to therapy with chloramphenicol, ampicillin is recommended.

Occasional patients with typhoid without evidence of suppurative complications do not respond clinically even after 4 or 5 days of antimicrobial therapy, even though blood cultures become negative. Delayed responses of this type occur in only about 1 percent of patients treated with chloramphenicol, in contrast to 5 or 10 percent of patients treated with ampicillin.

Sporadic chloramphenicol-resistant strains have been reported rarely, but the first epidemic due to a resistant strain occurred in Mexico in 1972. Antimicrobial resistance in this strain was due to a transferrable R factor which was associated with resistance to chloramphenicol, sulfonamides, tetracycline, and streptomycin. If chloramphenicol resistance is encountered, ampicillin should be used if the organism is sensitive to that agent.

Adrenal hormones The administration of prednisone or steroids with similar activity can terminate within a matter of hours the severe febrile toxemic state seen in some patients. Because of the lag in time between institution of antimicrobial therapy and evidence of response, patients with life-threatening toxemia should be treated with a brief course of adrenal corticosteroids in addition to chloramphenicol. An appropriate regimen is 60 mg prednisone the first day, 40 mg the second day, and 20 mg the third day; no additional steroid therapy should be administered. Hypothermia and hypotension occasionally occur within hours after initiation of steroids.

Supportive treatment Nursing care and attention to nutritional requirements are important. Laxatives and enemas should be avoided despite constipation because of the danger of precipitating hemorrhage or perforation. Salicylates should not be used, because in addition to their effects on blood platelets and irritating action on the bowel, these compounds can induce wide swings in temperature with very uncomfortable chills and sweats. Hypothermia and hypotension occur in some patients after administration of salicylates.

Hemorrhage and perforation Patients should be observed carefully to detect these complications at an early stage. Typing and cross matching should be carried out at the time of initial diagnosis of typhoid, and transfusion is indicated in the event of significant hemorrhage. Patients with typhoid are poor surgical risks. If perforation is suspected, emphasis should be placed on efforts to combat shock and decompress the bowel. Additional antimicrobials may have to be added to control peritonitis. Small perforations may localize and can be managed without surgical intervention. However, if evidence of localization does not develop, surgical intervention may be required.

Relapse The therapy of relapse is identical to that for the primary episode.

Chronic carriers Chronic carriers should be investigated for the presence of gallstones or a nonfunctioning gallbladder. Carriers without evidence of gallstones or gallbaldder disease on cholecystogram usually can be cured with a prolonged course of ampicillin. One program which has been found to be effective consists of 6 g ampicillin divided into four equal oral doses each day with probenecid for a period of 6 weeks. If gallstones or a nonfunctioning gallbladder are demonstrated on cholecystogram, antimicrobial therapy is unlikely to be effective in terminating the carrier state. These patients should have cholecystectomy, which cures the chronic carrier state in about 85 percent of patients. Ampicillin may be used in conjunction with cholecystectomy. Therapy should be started a few days prior to the procedure and continued for 2 or 3 weeks.

PREVENTION AND CONTROL Although immunization with typhoid vaccine affords significant protection against typhoid infection, the degree of immunity is not great and can be readily overcome with a large dose of organisms. Nevertheless, immunization is recommended for individuals living or traveling to areas where the disease is endemic and for persons working with the organism in laboratories. Adults should receive 0.5 ml vaccine on two occasions separated by a period of 1 or 2 weeks. A yearly booster is required to maintain immunity. Immunization with typhoid vaccine causes a transient elevation for several months in titer of agglutinins against typhoid O antigens and a persistently elevated titer for H antigens.

All typhoid patients should be reported to local health authorities, and stool specimens should be cultured during convalescence. Three consecutively negative stool cultures obtained at weekly intervals indicate that a carrier state has not developed.

Caution should be observed to prevent spread of infection from persons with active disease or from carriers. Chronic or convalescent carriers should not be allowed to prepare food until clear documentation shows that at least three or more stool cultures are negative for typhoid bacilli. Carriers should be cautioned regarding routine sanitary techniques.

PROGNOSIS The mortality rate of typhoid fever prior to the introduction of chloramphenicol was about 12 percent. Death was associated with toxemia, inanition, pneumonia, bowel perforation, and intestinal hemorrhage. The mortality rate is still 2 or 3 percent; deaths are observed primarily in infants, the aged, or individuals with malnutrition or other underlying diseases.

OTHER SALMONELLA INFECTIONS

DEFINITION Bacteria of the genus *Salmonella* may produce asymptomatic infection of the intestinal tract in man or several different clinical syndromes including acute gastroenteritis (or enterocolitis), bacteremia, paratyphoid fever, or localized infections ranging from osteomyelitis to endocarditis. The clinical syndromes resulting from infection with *Salmonella* cannot always be sharply differentiated and sometimes overlap.

Salmonella infections are among the most prevalent communicable diseases caused by bacteria in the United States today. These infections are transmitted in the vast majority of cases from animals to man and occasionally from man to man and are usually brief, self-limited, and mild.

EPIDEMIOLOGY Salmonellas can be isolated from the intestinal tracts of man and many lower animals. The incidence of asymptomatic excretors of these organisms in the general population is about 0.2 percent, but the most important reservoir of salmonellas is in domestic and wild animal species in which infection rates vary from less than 1 to more than 40 percent. An incomplete list of animals from which *Salmonella* species have been isolated includes chickens, turkeys, ducks, pigs, cows, dogs, cats, rats, parakeets, as well as certain cold-blooded animals and insects. Animals sold as pets, especially baby chicks, ducks, and turtles, may also harbor *Salmonella* and serve as sources of infection.

Salmonella infection is almost always acquired by the oral route, usually by ingestion of contaminated food or drink. Any food product is a potential source of human infection. The source of contamination of food or drink may be asymptomatic human carriers or persons with active clinical disease, but the greatest single source of human infection in the United States is the vast reservoir of *Salmonella* in lower animals. The high incidence of infection in domestic animals used as a source of food for man and present methods of processing foods and food products in bulk result in the availability of foods for human consumption with a potentially high incidence of contamination with *Salmonella*. For example, a significant proportion varying from 1 to more than 50 percent of raw meats purchased in retail markets is contaminated with *Salmonella*. Meat is contaminated by many routes, but the most common are natural infection of the animal used as a source of meat and contamination of the carcass during slaughter and processing. Eggs or egg products, including dried or frozen eggs, are also very common sources of *Salmonella* infection. Of the various animal species, domestic fowl, including chickens, turkeys, ducks, and eggs and egg products, constitute the single largest reservoir of infection and the source most often responsible for infection of man. Cooking of food prior to human consumption serves to decrease the possibility of infection. However, salmonellas may survive cooking at low temperature, or food may be recontaminated after cooking by organisms from kitchen equipment or personnel.

Food or drink may also be contaminated by rats, mice, insects, or other vermin harboring these organisms. Cross infection occurs occasionally by the airborne route from dried foods such as egg whites or dust which contain viable *Salmonella*. *Salmonella* contamination of a large variety of processed foods has also been documented. Some of these foods contain ingredients of animal origin such as eggs, whereas others contain contaminated products of vegetable origin such as coconut or yeast. A variety of pharmaceutical products of animal origin have been shown to be responsible for *Salmonella* infections of man; these products include carmine dye, pancreatin, bile salts, and extracts of various organs such as thyroid, adrenal, and stomach.

Pet turtles may be an important source of *Salmonella* infection in man, especially in children, accounting for perhaps as many as 10 to 20 percent of reported *Salmonella* infections in certain areas. Turtles are infected on breeding farms and continue to excrete organisms in feces into tank water for long periods of time. Although knowledge of the manner of transmission to man is incomplete, it is likely that turtle feces or tank water harboring salmonellas contaminate hands of handlers, from which organisms are passed to the mouth or to food or drink.

Salmonella species may also be transmitted directly from man to man or from animals to man without the intervention of contaminated food or drink, but this method of spread is not common. Cross infection of this type has been shown to be responsible for a number of outbreaks of salmonellosis among patients in nurseries and hospitals.

Fish meal, meat meal, bone meal, and other by-products of the meat-packing industry are often contaminated with *Salmonella* organisms. These products are incorporated in animal and poultry feeds and apparently play an important role in the perpetuation of infection among domestic animals.

The true incidence of *Salmonella* infection is difficult to determine. The number of reported isolations of salmonellas from humans in the United States from 1964 to 1971 was about 20,000 to 25,000 per year, or about 10 cases per 100,000 population. However, reported cases represent only a small proportion of the actual number because bacteriologic studies are usually performed only on patients with severe or protracted diarrhea, and many outbreaks are not investigated. Although *Salmonella* infection occurs throughout the year, the Salmonella Surveillance Unit of the National Communicable Disease Center has observed a distinct seasonal pattern with the greatest number of isolations reported from July through October for each year.

A close correlation exists between the *Salmonella* serotypes most often responsible for human infection and those isolated from animals in any specific geographic area. The similarities document the importance of nonhuman reservoirs of *Salmonella* in the epidemiology of *Salmonella* infection in man.

PATHOGENESIS The course of events after *Salmonella* organisms have gained access to the gastrointestinal tract is determined by the dose, serotype, and invasive potential of the organism, and by the resistance of the host. Multiplication of ingested organisms in the intestinal tract may be followed by symptoms of gastroenteritis. The intestinal irritation and inflammation are produced by a true infection of the mucosa; ingestion of billions of dead organisms causes no ill effects. Bloodstream invasion may occur as a complication of gastroenteritis but usually develops without preceding intestinal symptoms. Bacteremia may be transient or prolonged, and may be accompanied by recurrent chills and fever or manifestations of paratyphoid fever. Bloodborne bacteria may localize at any site and lead to suppuration in bone, joints, meninges, pleura, or other tissues.

Studies in volunteers indicate that large numbers of viable organisms must be ingested to produce clinically apparent disease. However, a transient carrier state can be produced with doses 10 or 100 times smaller than those required to evoke symptoms of infection. The minimal infectious dose varies markedly among different serotypes.

Salmonella serotypes also show marked variation in invasive potential and capacity to produce disease. For example, *S. anatum* characteristically produces asymptomatic intestinal infection and rarely invades the bloodstream. In contrast, *S. choleraesuis*, the most invasive serotype, frequently produces bacteremia and metastatic infection.

The bacterial flora of the intestine is important in determining the fate of ingested salmonellas. Administration of certain antibiotics by the oral route to mice results in a 10,000-fold increase in susceptibility to infection with *S. enteritidis*. Somewhat similar observations have been made in experimental typhoid fever in volunteers. In these studies the dose of *S. typhi* required to initiate infection by the oral route in man can be reduced sharply by giving certain antimicrobials orally prior to challenge. Epidemiologic studies have also shown that prior antimicrobial therapy alters the capacity of the human intestinal tract to eradicate *Salmonella* acquired naturally. The effect of antibiotic therapy may be related to a marked diminution in number of bacteroides or other organisms which produce antimicrobial substances such as short-chain fatty acids which are active against *Salmonella*. Alteration in intestinal flora also has been suggested as a mechanism of the increased susceptibility of patients with previous major gastric surgery, especially gastrectomy and gastroenterostomy, to intestinal infection with salmonellas. However, reduced acidity or rapid emptying time consequent to gastric surgery also may play a role by increasing the number of viable organisms reaching the small intestine.

About one-third of patients who are hospitalized because of salmonellosis have some type of major underlying disease, such as leukemia, lymphoma, lupus erythematosus, or aplastic anemia. This may be coincidence but more often reflects a decrease in resistance to bacterial infection in general. In a few diseases there is evidence to indicate an almost specific predisposition to infection by salmonellas that exceeds susceptibility to other bacterial species. Patients with sickle-cell anemia and other sickle hemoglobinopathies are unusually susceptible to bloodstream invasion by salmonellas. In these patients there is a strong tendency for localization in bone, and salmonellas, not staphylococci, are the most common cause of osteomyelitis in patients with sickle-cell diseases. *Salmonella* bacteremia is also an unusually frequent complication of the acute hemolytic phase of bartonellosis (Chap. 146).

Infants are more susceptible to *Salmonella* infection and remain convalescent carriers for a longer period of time than adults. The mortality rate from the disease is also higher in infants than in adults.

CLINICAL MANIFESTATIONS Gastroenteritis Although gastroenteritis often occurs in large epidemics among individuals who have eaten the same contaminated food, family outbreaks and sporadic cases are even more common. After an incubation period of 8 to 48 hr, there is sudden onset of colicky abdominal pain and loose, watery diarrhea, occasionally with mucus or blood. Nausea and vomiting are frequent but are rarely severe or protracted. Fever of 38 to 39°C is common, and there may be an initial chill. Patients usually have mild to moderate abdominal tenderness on palpation, but severe tenderness, even with rebound, occurs in occasional patients. Peristalsis is usually hyperactive. Abdominal findings may be prominent in some patients and lead to confusion with certain intraabdominal emergencies, such as acute appendicitis or acute cholecystitis. Symptoms usually subside promptly within 2 to 5 days and recovery is uneventful. However, the illness is occasionally more protracted, with persistence of diarrhea and low-grade fever for 10 to 14 days. Fatalities rarely exceed 1 percent of the affected population and are limited almost entirely to infants, the aged, and debilitated patients.

The causative organism can often be isolated from the suspected food and from feces during the acute illness. Stool cultures usually become negative for salmonellas within 1 to 4 weeks, but occasional patients continue to excrete organisms for months. Organisms tend to persist in the stools of infants and young children for longer periods than in older children or adults. The blood leukocyte count is usually normal. The blood culture is usually negative.

Enteric or paratyphoid fever Certain species can produce an illness clinically indistinguishable from typhoid fever, with prolonged fever, rose spots, splenomegaly, leukopenia, gastrointestinal symptoms, and positive blood and stool cultures. The organisms most likely to produce this picture are *S. paratyphi* A, *S. paratyphi* B, (*S. schottmülleri*), and *S. choleraesuis* (*S. suipestifer*). Occasionally a typical attack of food poisoning is followed in a few days by manifestations of paratyphoid fever. Generally, paratyphoid fevers tend to be milder than *S. typhi* infections, but differentiation on clinical grounds is not possible in the individual case. Recovery may be followed by continued excretion of the causative organism in the stools for several months, but the chronic carrier state is less frequent than in typhoid fever.

Bacteremia *Salmonella* species may produce a syndrome characterized primarily by prolonged fever and positive blood cultures. Although symptoms of gastroenteritis can precede bacteremia, they are usually lacking, and most cases arise sporadically. In many instances, the only manifestations are prolonged fever, which is usually spiking and is accompanied by repeated rigors, sweats, aching, anorexia, and weight loss. The characteristic features of typhoid and paratyphoid fever, such as rose spots, persistent leukopenia, and sustained fever, are absent. Stool cultures are usually negative. In contrast to the constant bacteremia of typhoid fever, discharge of organisms into the bloodstream is intermittent, and repeated blood cultures may be required to demonstrate the causative organism. At some time in the course of the illness, localizing signs of infection appear in about one-fourth of the cases. Pulmonary infection in the form of bronchopneumonia or abscess, pleurisy, empyema, pericarditis, endocarditis, pyelonephritis, meningitis, osteomyelitis, and arthritis are relatively common. The blood leukocyte count is usually normal, but with the development of focal lesions, polymorphonuclear leukocytosis as high as 20,000 to 25,000 cells per mm^3 occurs. *Salmonella* bacteremia can be a very puzzling disorder, especially before localization takes place, and should be considered in cases of fever of unknown origin.

A prolonged febrile illness lasting weeks or months and characterized by weight loss, marked anemia, hepatosplenomegaly, and bacteremia with *Salmonella* has been described in Brazil and other areas of the world in patients with hepatosplenic schistosomiasis due to *Schistosoma mansoni.* Intermittent bacteremia with *Salmonella* also occurs in patients with *Schistosoma haematobium* infection who are also urinary carriers of *Salmonella.*

Local pyogenic infections *Salmonella* organisms can produce abscesses in almost any anatomic site, and these can occur independently of previous symptoms of gastroenteritis or other systemic illness, or as complications of bacteremias. There is nothing characteristic about the suppurative lesions, and the correct etiologic diagnosis is rarely made on the basis of clinical findings alone. There is a strong tendency for salmonellas to localize in tissues that are the site of preexisting disease. Localization has been described in aneurysms, bone adjacent to aortic aneurysms, hematomas, and many different tumors, including hypernephroma, ovarian cyst, and pheochromocytoma. Meningeal localization of infection is common in newborns and infants, and occasional small outbreaks of *Salmonella* infection in nurseries have consisted almost entirely of meningitis.

DIAGNOSIS Febrile gastroenteritis produced by presumed viral agents and shigellosis can be distinguished from *Salmonella* gastroenteritis only by appropriate stool cultures, especially in sporadic cases. Staphylococcal food poisoning usually is not associated with fever, and vomiting is a more prominent feature than in most *Salmonella* infections. Systemic manifestations are usually absent in patients with gastroenteritis caused by *Clostridium welchii.* Many toxic agents and drugs can produce diarrhea, nausea, and abdominal pain, but fever is rarely a feature of these disorders, and the diagnosis depends upon a history of exposure or ingestion. The diagnosis of paratyphoid fever or *Salmonella* bacteremia depends upon isolation of the causative organism. Agglutination tests with acute and convalescent serums as performed in the usual clinical laboratory are not very helpful. The possibility of an underlying disease should be considered in every patient with a severe *Salmonella* infection.

TREATMENT The treatment of *Salmonella* gastroenteritis is supportive. Dehydration should be corrected by parenteral administration of fluids and electrolytes. Abdominal cramps and diarrhea can be alleviated by diphenoxylate hydrochloride combined with atropine sulfate (Lomotil), paregoric, or small doses of morphine and often are much improved if the patient takes nothing by mouth for 8 to 12 hr. Antimicrobial therapy, irrespective of type, does not appear to exert a beneficial effect on the clinical course of *Salmonella* gastroenteritis or decrease the duration of excretion of organisms in the stools. In fact, recent studies show that the period of excretion of *Salmonella* in stools during convalescence is actually longer in patients who have been treated with antimicrobial drugs during the acute illness than in patients who received no antimicrobial therapy.

Chloramphenicol in doses of 3 g daily in adults is the antibiotic of choice in systemic infections including *Salmonella* bacteremia, metastatic infection, and paratyphoid fever. The response is characteristically slow, and the temperature rarely returns to normal until 3 to 4 days after beginning therapy. Therapy should be continued for at least 2 weeks, but in certain infections, such as osteomyelitis or meningitis, the duration may have to be extended.

Ampicillin is also effective in systemic infections caused by *Salmonella* strains sensitive to the action of this antibiotic. However, a significant proportion of *Salmonella* strains are highly resistant to ampicillin in vitro. For this reason, ampicillin should not be used in therapy of serious infections unless it is known that the causative organism is sensitive. The tetracycline derivatives have sometimes appeared to exert a beneficial effect, but streptomycin, polymyxin, neomycin, kanamycin, and the sulfonamides are generally ineffective. Antimicrobial resistance is usually related to transferable resistance factors.

Antimicrobial therapy is usually not indicated in convalescent or asymptomatic transient carriers of *Salmonella* species. The carrier state will spontaneously cease in 1 to 3 months in the vast majority of individuals.

The chronic carrier state with localization of infection in the gallbladder and positive stool cultures for a period of time exceeding 1 year is rarely caused by *Salmonella* serotypes other than *S. typhi* and *S. paratyphi* A and B. Its treatment has been discussed. Surgically accessible suppurative lesions should be drained.

REFERENCES

BENNETT IL JR, HOOK EW: Some aspects of salmonellosis. Ann Rev Med 10:1, 1959

BLACK PH et al: Salmonellosis—A review of some unusual aspects. N Engl J Med 262:811, 864, 921, 1960

Center for Disease Control: *Salmonella surveillance—Annual Summary 1971*, Atlanta: The Center, 1972

Dinbar A et al: The treatment of chronic biliary salmonella carriers. Am J Med 47:236, 1969

Edwards HR, Galton MM: Salmonellosis. Adv Vet Sci Comp Med 11:1, 1967

Freitag JL: Treatment of chronic typhoid carriers by cholecystectomy. Public Health Rept. US 79:7, 1964

Gezon HM: Salmonellosis. Disease-a-Month July, 1959

Hook EW: Salmonellosis: Certain factors influencing the interaction of salmonella and the human host. Bull NY Acad Med 37:499, 1961

Hornick RB et al: Typhoid fever: Pathogenesis and immunologic control. N Engl J Med 283:686, 739, 1970

Kaye D et al: Treatment of chronic enteric carriers of salmonella typhosa with ampicillin. Ann NY Acad Sci 145:429, 1967

Lamm SH et al: Turtle-associated salmonellosis. Am J Epidemiol 95:511, 1972

Proceedings of the National Conference on Salmonellosis, March 11–13, 1964. Washington, D.C., Public Health Service Publ. no. 1262, 1965

Reynolds DW et al: Diagnostic specificity of Widal's reaction for typhoid fever. JAMA 214:2192, 1970

Robertson RP et al: Chloramphenicol and ampicillin in salmonella enteric fever. N Engl J Med 278:171, 1968

van Oye E (ed): *The World Problem of Salmonellosis*, The Hague: W Junk Publishers, 1964

Wicks ACP et al: Endemic typhoid fever. A diagnostic pitfall. Q J Med 40:341, 1971

Woodward TE, Smadel JE: Management of typhoid fever and its complications. Ann Intern Med 60:144, 1964

137 SHIGELLOSIS

HARRY N. BEATY

DEFINITION Shigellosis is an acute, self-limited infection of the intestinal tract of man which is characterized by diarrhea, fever, and abdominal pain. The disease is frequently called *bacillary dysentery*, but the term *shigellosis* is preferred.

ETIOLOGY The genus *Shigella* of the family Enterobacteriaceae includes a group of closely related species which are nonmotile, nonencapsulated, slender, gram-negative rods. They are aerobes or faculative anaerobes and grow best at 37°C. Nutritional requirements are relatively simple, and the ability of these organisms to grow in the presence of bile salts is used in devising selective media which facilitate their isolation. However, *S. dysenteriae* type 1 may be inhibited by these media, and growth may not be apparent for several days. Fermentation of carbohydrates differs according to species, but all strains produce acid in glucose and either fail to ferment lactose or do so only slowly. The shigellas are classified into subgroups A, B, C, or D on the basis of biochemical and antigenic characteristics. The clinically important species within the respective groups are *S. dysenteriae, S. flexneri, S. boydii,* and *S. sonnei.* While these shigellas share antigens among themselves and with other enteric bacilli, serologic classification is not difficult, and with the exception of *S. sonnei* a number of serotypes of each species has been recognized.

The somatic antigen of the shigellas is an endotoxin which is chemically and biologically similar to the endotoxins of other gram-negative bacilli. *Shigella dysenteriae* type 1 (Shiga bacillus) also produces an exotoxin which causes neurologic abnormalities in experimental animals. The role of this neurotoxin in the pathogenesis of shigellosis is unknown, and there is no evidence that other species of *Shigella* produce a similar substance.

EPIDEMIOLOGY The principal habitat of the shigellas is the gastrointestinal tract of higher primates. Natural disease is limited almost entirely to man, and the convalescent or asymptomatic carrier is the only recognized reservoir. In 1972 a family outbreak of the disease was attributed to a pet monkey. Spread of infection from person to person occurs primarily when organisms on hands and inanimate objects contaminated with infected feces are ingested. In the United States, common source outbreaks usually involve food which has been contaminated by careless handlers. Waterborne outbreaks are rare. In regions where sanitation is poor, flies which have been in contact with infected human feces may serve as an important vector in the transmission of this disease.

Shigellosis is worldwide in distribution, and is particularly common in countries where effective sanitation is lacking. Around ten thousand cases are reported annually in the United States, but many more undoubtedly occur. *S. sonnei* is responsible for about three-fourths of the infections encountered in this country; *S. flexneri* is isolated from all but a small percentage of the rest. *S. dysenteriae* type 1, which formerly produced disease predominately in Asia, has been responsible recently for large outbreaks of diarrhea in Central America. The few cases encountered in the United States, however, have occurred almost exclusively among foreign travelers or their contacts. Major epidemics of shigellosis are uncommon in the United States, but high-risk groups do exist in the inner cities, in mental or penal institutions, and on Indian reservations. Poor sanitation, low standards of personal hygiene, crowded conditions, and a high proportion of children in a population favor spread of the infection. Infected persons may excrete organisms intermittently during convalescence, but the carrier state rarely persists longer than 3 months.

Humoral antibodies frequently develop in response to clinical infection, but there is no evidence that they influence the course of the disease or protect against reinfection. However, persons living in endemic areas seem to develop immunity to recurrent episodes of clinical disease, and volunteers infected with a specific strain are resistant to rechallenge with that strain for weeks to months. This immunity may be mediated by coproantibody, which has been identified in the stool of patients with shigellosis, or by cellular defense mechanisms in the wall of the bowel. In any event, it has led to the development of live, attenuated vaccines which, given orally, induce the same degree of immunity as natural infection. Parenteral vaccines are of no value.

PATHOGENESIS AND PATHOLOGY The major pathologic feature of shigellosis is mucosal inflammation which usually involves the entire colon and may extend into the terminal ileum. A fibrinous exudate often develops, and necrosis of the mucosa produces shallow ulcers which bleed readily. Microscopic examination shows that the submucosa and muscularis are infiltrated with bacteria and polymorphonuclear leukocytes. Ulcers are sharply demarcated and are not undermined. These lesions are produced only by organisms which can transmigrate through intact epithelial cells and multiply in the lamina propria. Avirulent strains multiply in the lumen of the bowel, elaborate endotoxin, and induce intestinal immunity, but without the capability of penetrating the mucosa, they cannot produce disease. Unlike members of the genus *Salmonella* which require a large inoculum to produce infection, as few as 200 virulent *Shigella* can cause disease. This probably explains why person-to-person spread of this infection is so common.

The systemic manifestations of shigellosis are primarily due to the fluid and electrolyte disturbances consequent to the diarrhea. Bacteremia is rare, and fever is often attributed to "toxins" which presumably are absorbed from the intestinal tract.

CLINICAL MANIFESTATIONS *Shigella* infections are characterized by fever, abdominal pain, and diarrhea. However, mild diarrhea alone or asymptomatic infection occurs in a significant proportion of individuals infected. The incubation period is usually 24 to 48 hr, and the first symptom is often colicky abdominal pain which is followed within an hour by high fever and diarrhea, often accompanied by tenesmus. Other symptoms include nausea, vomiting, headache, myalgia, and convulsions in children. The stools are liquid, greenish in color, contain shreds of mucus, and in 20 to 30 percent of cases various amounts of gross blood. Depending upon the severity of diarrhea and the height of fever, patients may become profoundly dehydrated, and circulatory collapse can occur. Lower abdominal tenderness and hyperactive bowel sounds are common, but there is no peritoneal irritation. Splenomegaly has been reported, but is rare. Sigmoidoscopic examination reveals diffuse mucosal inflammation, often with multiple ulcerations.

LABORATORY FINDINGS Blood leukocyte counts usually range between 5,000 and 15,000 per mm^3, and anemia is uncommon. Microscopic examination of the stool reveals shreds of mucus, erythrocytes, and many polymorphonuclear leukocytes. Stool culture is positive, but blood cultures rarely are. Electrolyte abnormalities depend upon the degree of vomiting and diarrhea.

COURSE Shigellosis is generally a self-limited disease, and patients usually become afebrile in about four days. Diarrhea and abdominal cramps may continue a few days longer, but within a week most patients have recovered. However, a significant proportion of untreated patients continue to shed organisms in the stool for two or more weeks. In about 10 percent of cases a clinical or bacteriologic relapse occurs unless antibiotics are given. In the United States, the overall mortality rate associated with shigellosis is less than 0.1 percent. However, among young children and elderly patients, the illness is often more severe and the prognosis poorer. *Shigella dysenteriae* type 1 produces particularly severe infections, and mortality rates of 25 to 50 percent have been recorded in epidemics produced by this species.

Complications of *Shigella* infections are encountered infrequently. An uncommon but significant problem is perforation of the colon. Hematogenous dissemination of the shigellas is also rare, but these organisms have been encountered in metastatic foci of infection such as abscesses and meningitis. In some series, bacteremia due to other gram-negative bacilli has been seen in association with shigellosis. An acute, nonsuppurative arthritis involving large, weight-bearing joints may occur during convalescence, but in patients given chemotherapy this complication is unusual. Conjunctivitis, iritis, and peripheral neuropathy accompany shigellosis on rare occasions.

DIAGNOSIS A definitive diagnosis can be established only when pathogenic members of the genus *Shigella* are isolated from cultures. These organisms survive for only a short time in feces, and fresh stool specimens or rectal swabs should be cultured promptly. Recovery of the shigellas is facilitated if saline suspensions of stool are streaked directly onto selective media such as SS agar or desoxycholate citrate agar. Agglutinating antibodies can be detected in the serum of a majority of patients with positive cultures, but serologic tests are of little value in establishing the diagnosis of shigellosis. Immunofluorescent techniques have been developed, however, which allow rapid detection of organisms in the stool.

Shigellosis infection should be considered in every febrile illness associated with diarrhea. Occasionally, children with infections such as tonsillitis or otitis have diarrhea, but the major differential diagnosis of shigellosis includes acute ulcerative colitis, viral enteritis, amebic dysentery, salmonellosis, and clostridial or staphylococcal food poisoning. Shigellosis can closely mimic acute ulcerative colitis, and should be excluded with cultures in patients thought to have this disease. In viral infections, fever is uncommon, and the stool usually does not contain gross blood or pus. The onset of amebic colitis is gradual, and the diarrhea is relatively mild. Staphylococcal food poisoning is associated with more nausea and vomiting, and usually is not associated with fever. *Salmonella* infections can be differentiated with certainty only by bacteriologic studies.

TREATMENT The treatment of shigellosis is primarily supportive, and the major goal is correction of fluid and electrolyte abnormalities. Antibiotics are of secondary importance, and are used chiefly to shorten the duration of illness and to prevent relapse. Sulfonamides formerly were effective in the treatment of bacillary dysentery, but almost 90 percent of *S. sonnei* isolated in the United States are resistant to these drugs. More significantly, since 1955 epidemics of shigellosis in various parts of the world, including the United States, have been caused by organisms resistant to multiple antibiotics. The molecular basis for multiple drug resistance involves the episomal transfer (R factor) of drug resistance determinants between enteric bacilli.

In the United States about 16 percent of isolates are resistant to antimicrobials other than sulfonamides. Ninety-five percent are sensitive to ampicillin and 85 percent to tetracycline, however, and these drugs are preferred for the treatment of shigellosis. In adults they should be given in a dosage of 2.0 g per day for 5 to 7 days. Kanamycin, neomycin, and colistin administered orally may be effective in shigellosis, but they should be given only for 2 or 3 days because longer treatment can produce malabsorption and increased diarrhea.

PREVENTION The most important prophylactic measures are the maintenance of proper sanitation and adequate sewage disposal. The detection and elimination of carriers are difficult and rarely practical. Methods for increasing resistance with oral vaccines may be useful in preventing outbreaks among susceptible populations.

REFERENCES

DuPont HL et al: Immunity in shigellosis: I. Response of man to attenuated strains of *Shigella.* J Infect Dis 125:5, 1972

—— et al: Immunity in shigellosis: II. Protection induced by oral live vaccine or primary infection. J Infect Dis 125:12, 1972

Farrar WE Jr, Eidson M: Antibiotic resistance in *Shigella* mediated by R factors. J Infect Dis 123:477, 1971

Reller LB et al: Shigellosis in the United States: Five-year review of nationwide surveillance, 1964–1968. Am J Epidemiol 91:161, 1970

Tong JM et al: Clinical and bacteriological evaluation of antibiotic treatment in shigellosis. JAMA 214:1841, 1970

section 6 | Diseases caused by other gram-negative bacilli

138
HEMOPHILUS INFECTIONS

LOUIS WEINSTEIN

The genus *Hemophilus* consists of nonmotile, gram-negative rods or coccobacilli which require specific growth factors (X and V) for multiplication. The organisms of importance in human disease are *H. influenzae, H. pertussis, H. ducreyi, H. aphrophilus,* the Koch-Weeks bacillus, and *Moraxella lacunata.* Two other species are found in the pharynges of normal individuals and, rarely, may produce pharyngitis (*H. hemolyticus*) or endocarditis (*H. parainfluenzae*). The site invaded most frequently is the respiratory tract, and the organism responsible for the bulk of infections is *H. influenzae.*

HEMOPHILUS INFLUENZAE INFECTIONS

Hemophilus influenzae produces a wide variety of diseases in many organ systems. The organism was first isolated by Pfeiffer during a pandemic of influenza in 1890 and was thought to be the causative agent of this disease. During the 1918 influenza pandemic, extensive bacteriologic investigations revealed a high incidence of *H. influenzae* in the nasopharynges and lungs of patients in many parts of the world.

ETIOLOGY *Hemophilus influenzae* is a gram-negative, nonsporulating, pleomorphic rod. In exudates, the organisms are usually predominantly coccobacillary and can be mistaken for pneumococci or meningococci. Some strains demonstrate biopolar staining and bacillary forms that vary from short rods to long filamentous ones.

Hemophilus influenzae grows well on chocolate agar and Levinthal's medium, which has the advantage of being transparent. On Levinthal's agar, typical colonies are iridescent when viewed by obliquely transmitted light when they are about 4 to 6 hr old; this property disappears after 24 hr.

Although it had been thought that strains without capsules were nonpathogenic, such strains have been implicated in infections of the respiratory tract. On the basis of specific capsular polysaccharides, *H. influenzae* may be classified into six types. Type B produces about 95 percent of human infections.

EPIDEMIOLOGY *Hemophilus influenzae* infects only man naturally. It is not ordinarily invasive for any of the smaller animals, although monkeys can be infected experimentally.

The incidence of *H. influenzae* infections is greatest in the winter and early spring. Nose and throat cultures during these seasons reveal the organisms in many asymptomatic individuals. Penicillin therapy increases the incidence of positive throat cultures.

Children in the first 2 months of life have a high level of passively transferred bactericidal antibody. Between the ages of two months and three years, most children show little antibody, but with aging the levels increase.

PATHOLOGY The characteristic tissue response to *H. influenzae* is acute suppurative inflammation. Infections of the larynx, trachea, and bronchial tree are characterized by edema of the mucosa and thick exudate, and invasion of the lungs results in a bronchopneumonia. A severe, diffuse bronchiolitis may develop in young children. In influenzal meningitis, the brain is covered with thick, greenish yellow exudate.

Microscopic examination of the lesions produced by *H. influenzae* reveals an exudate consisting primarily of polymorphonuclear leukocytes and large numbers of organisms enmeshed in fibrin.

CLINICAL MANIFESTATIONS Severe *H. influenzae* infections are usually accompanied by high fever, usually without rigors, and generalized malaise. In milder infections, fever is inconstant. The commonest diseases produced by this organism are pharyngitis, epiglottitis, laryngotracheitis, pneumonia, bronchitis and bronchiolitis, otitis media, and meningitis. The symptoms and signs of invasion of the respiratory tract or meninges are similar to those of infection of these areas by other organisms, and differential etiologic diagnosis depends upon epidemiologic background, the age of the patient, and demonstration of the causative agent.

Pharyngitis *Hemophilus influenzae* is a relatively common cause of pharyngitis in children; acute influenzal pharyngitis is now being observed more often in adults, where it may develop as a complication of chemotherapy for other infections. Examination of the throat often reveals no remarkable findings. Rarely, however, the pharyngeal mucosa is reddened; patchy, soft, yellow exudate may be present. The pharyngitis tends to persist for many days unless properly treated. Dissociation between the appearance of the pharynx and the intensity of local discomfort is common in adults. The pharyngeal mucosa frequently appears normal or shows only slight diffuse redness at the same time that pain is so severe that swallowing of saliva is difficult and eating impossible.

Epiglottitis Disease of the upper part of the respiratory tract produced by *H. influenzae* is sometimes limited to the epiglottis, which becomes reddened, swollen, and stiff. Discomfort in the hypopharynx and "croupy" breathing may progress to a point at which tracheostomy becomes necessary. This disease is rare in adults.

Laryngotracheobronchitis This is most common in young children. The entire laryngotracheobronchial tree may be infected, with resulting rapidly progressive obstruction of the airway. "Croupy" cough is accompanied by increasing signs of respiratory embarrassment, and tracheostomy is sometimes necessary. Influenzal laryngotracheitis is very rare in adults. The disease can lead to death in children within 18 to 24 hr.

Pneumonia Primary pneumonia due to *H. influenzae*, with rare exceptions, is a disease of children. In adults, it is usually secondary to viral influenza, measles, or bacterial pneumonitis. It may complicate rubeola or pertussis in the young. Bacteremia occurs in approximately one-third of the cases.

Bronchitis and bronchiolitis Severe, diffuse bronchiolitis characterized by persistent nonproductive cough, wheezing, and dyspnea occurs primarily in children. Physical examination usually reveals depression and fixation of the diaphragms, prolonged expiration, and typical asthmatic breathing. Roentgenographic examination of the chest discloses increased radiolucence and flattening of the diaphragms consistent with emphysema. This is an extremely serious illness and unless promptly recognized and treated may be rapidly fatal.

Superimposed bacterial infection contributes significantly to the clinical manifestations and progressive deterioration in established chronic bronchitis or "senile emphysema" in adults. Among the bacteria involved, the pneumococcus and *H. influenzae* are the commonest; the latter has been isolated from the respiratory tracts of 80 to 90 percent of patients in Europe. It is recovered much less frequently in the United States.

Otitis media *Hemophilus influenzae* is a common cause of suppurative otitis media in children; the infection is uncommon in adults. In many instances, middle ear disease due to this species is indistinguishable from that produced by *Staphylococcus aureus*, *Diplococcus pneumoniae*, or group A *Streptococcus pyogenes*. In many cases, however, the appearance is that of serous otitis media and leads to a misdiagnosis of nonbacterial disease. Paracentesis, or aspiration of fluid from the middle ear, and culture are required in such cases to establish the presence of *H. influenzae* and to guide appropriate chemotherapy.

Meningitis *Hemophilus influenzae*, type B, is the commonest cause of meningitis between the ages of six months and two years and is frequent in later childhood. There has been a recent increase in the frequency of this disease in otherwise healthy adults of any age. Next to the pneumococcus, *H. influenzae* is the organism most likely to cause recurrent bacterial meningitis. Ninety-five percent of the cases are produced by type B organisms, a few by type A, and a rare one by nonencapsulated strains. About two-thirds of patients have a preceding infection of the upper part of the respiratory tract or otitis media, and about one-third have bronchopneumonia. Signs of meningeal irritation are usually prominent, except in very young babies in whom bulging of the fontanels may be the only sign. The diagnosis should be suspected because of the age of the patient and the frequent prodrome of respiratory infection.

Other diseases Subacute and acute bacterial endocarditis may be produced by *H. influenzae* or *H. parainfluenzae*. The influenza bacillus is a rare cause of suppurative pericarditis. In the winter, acute conjunctivitis may be due to *H. influenzae*. No clinical features distinguish this from "pinkeye" produced by the Koch-Weeks bacillus; however, epidemics of conjunctivitis due to the latter are most common in the summer. Although it has been suggested that *H. influenzae* and the Koch-Weeks bacillus are identical, recent studies indicate that, although antigenically related, they are distinct species. *Moraxella lacunata* is also an occasional cause of acute purulent conjunctivitis. Acute pyogenic arthritis due to *H. influenzae* has been reported. Among other diseases produced by this organism are osteomyelitis, paranasal sinusitis, appendicitis, cellulitis, and infections of the liver, genital tract, and skin.

LABORATORY FINDINGS As a rule, infections due to *H. influenzae* are accompanied by polymorphonuclear leukocytosis ranging from 15,000 to 30,000 per mm^3. In young children with severe disease, leukopenia (2,000 to 3,000 leukocytes per mm^3) with a deficiency of polymorphonuclear leukocytes can occur. Bacteremia occurs irregularly in influenzal infections of the respiratory tract but is demonstrable in about 50 percent of cases of meningitis.

COURSE AND COMPLICATIONS The course of *H. influenzae* infections is influenced completely by the location of the disease. Epiglottitis, laryngotracheobronchitis, bronchiolitis, or pneumonia may be fulminating. Some patients succumb to the uncontrolled infection, but in many the cause of death is obstruction of the airway. This cannot always be relieved by surgical methods, because impediment to flow of air is most marked in the smaller radicles of the bronchial tree. Virtually 100 percent of untreated cases of influenzal meningitis terminate fatally. Internal and external hydrocephalus, brain abscess, subdural empyema, diffuse cortical necrosis, and, rarely, shock (the Waterhouse-Friderichsen syndrome) are possible complications. With specific therapy, the incidence of complications is generally sharply reduced. However, if subdural aspiration is carried out routinely in children with influenzal meningitis which is responding to antibiotics, sterile fluid is demonstrable in about half the cases. Neurologic disturbances from subdural effusions are uncommon. Epileptiform seizures due to discrete thrombosis of cerebral veins may occur while the disease is responding favorably to chemotherapy.

TREATMENT *Hemophilus influenzae* is susceptible in vitro to several antimicrobial agents including streptomycin, the tetracyclines, chloramphenicol, and the sulfonamides. Most strains are inhibited by penicillin G in concentrations of 0.6 μg per ml or less. All appear to be highly sensitive to ampicillin, a drug which has greatly simplified the management of disease produced by this organism. The dose of ampicillin in *H. influenzae* meningitis is 300 to 400 mg per kg per day, given in equal-sized and -spaced quantities. The management of otitis media or pharyngitis often requires no more than 100 to 150 mg per kg per day given by mouth. For adults with these infections, 2 to 4 g per day orally for 7 to 10 days usually suffices. Diarrhea is not infrequent in patients treated with ampicillin. Ampicillin therapy may fail in influenzal meningitis when complications, e.g., subdural empyema, supervene. Although the organism has rarely been thought to be resistant to ampicillin, this remains to be substantiated and should be the subject of continuous observation because of the increasing frequency with which other gram-negative bacilli insensitive to this agent are being recovered. Despite the fact that practically all strains of *H. influenzae* are sensitive to very small quantities of penicillin G, the therapeutic effects of this antibiotic are poor, and it must not be used as the sole agent for the treatment of meningitis due to this organism. The results with the tetracyclines are too variable to recommend their use. An alternate regimen useful in influenzal meningitis is chloramphenicol (50 mg per kg per day) in equal-sized and -spaced doses intramuscularly plus sulfisoxazole or sulfadiazine (100 mg per kg per day). Regardless of the drug used, therapy should be continued for 2 weeks. Chloramphenicol or tetracycline is usually sufficient to treat upper respiratory tract infections, pneumonia, or otitis media in patients who are "sensitive" to penicillin.

HEMOPHILUS PERTUSSIS

Whooping cough (pertussis) occurs in about 85 percent of all unimmunized children. It is characterized by an inflammation of the entire respiratory tract which produces paroxysmal cough and the typical inspiratory stridor, or "whoop."

ETIOLOGY The causative agent is *Hemophilus pertussis* (*Bordetella pertussis*), a short or ovoid, gram-negative, nonmotile, nonsporulating, facultatively anaerobic bacillus. Bipolar staining is frequent, and encapsulation can be demonstrated by special stains.

The organism multiplies best on Bordet-Gengou medium. It contains two antigens. The heat-stable O antigen is common to all strains. Five varieties of a heat-labile specific agglutinogen K (1,2,3,4,5) are also present. All strains contain two or more of these antigens. This is of clinical importance because, in some areas of the world, the infecting strain has been found to have different K agglutinogens than those present in the vaccine being used to prevent the disease, resulting in failure of immunization.

Other infectious agents may rarely produce the syndrome of whooping cough. Among these are *B. parapertussis* and *B. bronchiseptica.* Several types of adenovirus (1,2,3,5,12) have been reported to produce a syndrome identical in all respects to that due to *B. pertussis.*

EPIDEMIOLOGY Pertussis is worldwide. Where the disease has not been present for several years, it tends to assume epidemic proportions when it reappears. In some areas, it is most common during the winter; in others it is seen with greatest frequency in the late summer and fall. The index of contagion is 80 to 100 percent; about 200,000 cases occur in the United States each year.

Approximately 40 percent of episodes of pertussis occur in the first 2 years of life; the same number is observed between the ages of two and five. At least 50 percent of all children have had whooping cough before they reach the age of five and 75 percent by the age of seventeen.

Pertussis is spread by droplets from the respiratory tract. Rarely, the organisms may be transmitted by fomites. Infectivity during the incubation period is questionable; the disease is most contagious during the catarrhal stage. Healthy carriers play no role in dissemination, but mild or missed cases are of great importance.

PATHOLOGY The initial lesion in whooping cough is hyperplasia of the peribronchial and tracheobronchial lymphoid tissue. The bronchi, trachea, larynx, and nasopharynx are soon involved in a necrotizing inflammatory reaction. The organisms are present in large numbers between the cilia of the trachea and following desquamation of the alveolar epithelium.

CLINICAL MANIFESTATIONS The incubation period of whooping cough averages 12 to 15 days but may be as long as 20 days. The first clinical manifestations (catarrhal stage) are slight nasal discharge, conjunctivitis, and mild cough without fever; these persist for 7 to 14 days.

The paroxysmal phase of pertussis follows and is characterized by paroxysms of coughing ending in a loud, crowing inspiratory noise (the whoop), the expulsion of varying quantities of thick, mucoid sputum from the respiratory tract, and vomiting. Episodes of cough may vary from 1 or 2 to 40 to 50 per day. Children under the age of six months frequently do not whoop. The mere presence of a whoop is in itself not diagnostic of pertussis. Rarely, the paroxysms of coughing are preceded by or replaced completely by sneezing.

Fever does not occur in the paroxysmal phase unless complications are present. Soreness over the trachea and main bronchi is common. Spasm, ulcer, or edema of the glottis sometimes occurs. In cases with severe vomiting and inability to retain food, serious inanition, wasting, and tetany may appear.

There is a bleeding tendency in pertussis. This is not associated with detectable defects in the clotting mechanisms; it has been suggested that it may be related to increased fragility of small blood vessels. Hemoptysis, epistaxis, purpura, and subconjunctival or intestinal hemorrhages occur but are usually of little clinical significance.

Physical examination in pertussis is often entirely normal, but there may be injection of the blood vessels of the nose and pharynx. Although there are usually no abnormal findings in the lungs, fine, crackling, "sticky" rales are sometimes present. There are ulcers of the frenum of the tongue in about 20 percent of cases; these occur only in children in whom the lower central incisor teeth are present.

The paroxysmal stage of pertussis usually lasts from 1 to 6 weeks. When coughing persists beyond 6 weeks, it is usually due to the development of a so-called "habit whoop," not to continuation of the disease.

LABORATORY FINDINGS The total peripheral leukocyte count may be over 100,000 cells per mm^3, and mature lymphocytes may constitute 90 percent of the cells. This helps to distinguish the blood picture from that of acute leukemia but not from acute lymphocytosis. The lymphocytosis appears to be induced by a constituent of the organism, most of the cells being released from lymphoid tissue including the thymus. Blood cultures are sterile. Nasopharyngeal cultures or "cough plates" on Bordet-Gengou agar are helpful in recovering the organism. X-ray study of the lungs in the uncomplicated case usually reveals only hilar lymphadenopathy and increase in the density of the bronchovascular markings.

COMPLICATIONS Bronchopneumonia occurs in from 1 to 10 percent of cases of pertussis; the organisms most frequently involved are group A. *S. pyogenes*, *D. pneumoniae*, *S. aureus*, *H. influenzae*, and *B. pertussis*. Pneumonitis appearing during the course of chemotherapy is most often due to *Escherichia coli*, *Proteus* strains, *Klebsiella aerogenes*, or *Pseudomonas aeruginosa*. Another important complication is atelectasis; small areas of collapse are an almost constant finding, but major portions or a whole lung may be involved. Pneumothorax is rare.

The severe coughing of pertussis may lead to several complications. Hemorrhage may appear in the anterior chamber of the eye or in the retina. Detachment of the retina and blindness develop in rare cases. Prolapse of the rectum and inguinal or umbilical hernias have been noted.

Nervous system manifestations are not rare in pertussis. The commonest is convulsions; these often appear as fever develops rapidly during secondary bacterial infection. Other causes of seizures are encephalopathy (1 to 14 percent of cases), multiple petechial or gross hemorrhages of the brain, and cerebral hypoxia due to the combined effect of anoxic anoxia and venous stasis. The encephalopathy is characterized by an increase in the protein and cell content of the spinal fluid. Its etiology is unknown. Hyperreflexia, nuchal rigidity, cranial nerve palsies, areflexia, extensor plantar responses, flaccid hemiplegia, spasticity of the extremities, opisthotonus, difficulty in speaking, twitching, papilledema, nystagmus, blindness, strabismus, and dysphagia may occur. Some of the more important residua are mental retardation, recurrent convulsions, personality disorders, amnesia, aphasia, diffuse cerebral atrophy, chorea, and athetosis.

DIAGNOSIS The diagnosis of pertussis can frequently be made on clinical grounds alone. Knowledge of contact is helpful, but the appearance of paroxysms of typical coughing and whooping, after a short period of upper respiratory symptoms, is strongly suggestive of pertussis. It must be stressed, however, that in babies under the age of six months there is usually only paroxysmal coughing, without the characteristic whoop. An increased number of circulating lymphocytes is characteristic.

Isolation of *B. pertussis* from the respiratory tract establishes the diagnosis. Using "cough plates," nasopharyngeal swabs, and Bordet-Gengou medium, positive cultures can be obtained in 90 percent of patients in the catarrhal stage of the disease. The incidence of positive cultures is lower after paroxysmal coughing appears, and decreases with the duration of symptoms. The incidence of positive cultures in the catarrhal stage is about 90 percent. In the first week of the paroxysmal phase it is 75 percent; in the second week, 60 percent; in the third week, 45 percent; in the fourth week, 40 percent; in the fifth week, 10 percent.

Serologic studies are of little or no help in establishing the presence of pertussis.

PREVENTION Active immunization is effective in preventing pertussis in the majority of individuals. This may be started at the age of three months; both antibody production and protection against invasion by *B. pertussis* result. If the procedure is carried out at this early age, a "booster" injection should be administered at the end of the first year of life, and again just before the child starts school. Vaccine should not be given in the presence of the active disease; not only is it useless, but it may provoke serious neurologic reactions. There is evidence that the administration of "quadruple" vaccine—poliomyelitis virus, tetanus and diphtheria toxoids, and *H. pertussis*—leads to some degree of suppression of the response to the pertussis bacillus. For this reason, when poliomyelitis vaccine (formalinized) is used, it should be given separately from the "triple" vaccine.

In children who have been exposed to pertussis but have not been actively immunized, passive protection may be given by the injection of 20 to 30 ml of human hyperimmune pertussis antiserum or 2 ml of immune γ-globulin as soon as possible after exposure, and again 1 week later. Such prophylaxis is 75 to 85 percent effective. The use of hyperimmune serum should be avoided if possible because it has been associated with the subsequent development of infectious hepatitis.

TREATMENT Although most of the antimicrobial drugs have been employed in the treatment of pertussis, there is no good evidence that they are beneficial. Chlortetracycline, chloramphenicol, oxytetracycline, erythromycin, and other antibiotics have been used, but the results obtained in controlled studies are not convincing.

There are few controlled studies of serum therapy in whooping cough, but in many clinics it is the practice to administer human hyperimmune serum (20 ml every 48 hr for three doses), or immune γ-globulin (2 ml every 48 hr for three doses) to all children with pertussis under the age of two.

Most important in therapy of pertussis is repair of the water and salt loss which follows severe and frequent vomiting. If failure to retain food is combated by prompt refeeding, patients can be made to maintain or gain weight.

Early detection and treatment of complications is one of the most important factors in the reduction of mortality. The prompt recognition of secondary bacterial infections of the lungs or middle ear, and therapy with a properly selected antibiotic agent lead to cure in practically all cases. When gross atelectasis occurs, correction by tracheal catheter suction or bronchoscopy may be lifesaving. Little can be done to influence the course or outcome of such complications as cerebral hemorrhage or encephalopathy.

Proper management of whooping cough has made the outlook for complete recovery excellent.

HEMOPHILUS APHROPHILUS

Human infections due to *H. aphrophilus*, although uncommon, are being reported with increasing frequency. This species differs from *H. influenzae* in some biochemical characteristics and requires the X but not the V factor for growth in an atmosphere containing 10 percent CO_2, but needs neither factor, in most instances, when incubated in moist air. The diseases produced by *H. aphrophilus* include endocarditis, brain abscess, bacteremia, acute and chronic sinusitis, otitis media, cervical abscess, pneumonia, meningitis, wound infection, and septic arthritis. Most strains of the organism appear to be fairly sensitive to penicillin G, cephalothin, gentamicin, chloramphenicol, and rifampin.

REFERENCES

Hemophilus influenzae

COLLIER AM et al: Systemic infection with *Hemophilus influenzae* in very young infants. J Pediatr 70:539, 1967

FEINGOLD M, GELLIS SS: Cellulitis due to *Hemophilus influenzae* type B. N Engl J Med 272:788, 1965

GOLDSTEIN E et al: *Haemophilus influenzae* as a cause of adult pneumonia. Ann Intern Med 66:35, 1967

HOLDAWAY MD, TURK DC: Capsulated *Haemophilus influenzae* and respiratory tract disease. Lancet 1:358, 1967

NORDEN CW et al: Immunologic responses to *Hemophilus influenzae* meningitis. J Pediatr 80:209, 1972

PATTERSON RL JR, LEVINE DB: *Hemophilus influenzae* pyarthrosis in an adult. J Bone Joint Surg [Am] 47A: 1250, 1965

TURK DC, MAY JR: *Hemophilus influenzae. Its Clinical Importance*, London: English Universities Press, 1967

Hemophilus pertussis

BROOKSALER F, NELSON JD: Pertussis. A reappraisal and report of 190 confirmed cases. Am J Dis Child 114:389, 1967

CONNOR JD: Role of adenoviral infection in pertussis syndrome. N Engl J Med 283:390, 1970

MORSE SI: Studies of the lymphocytosis induced in mice by *Bordetella pertussis*. J Exp Med 121:49, 1965

PEREIRA MS, CANDEIAS JAN: The association of viruses with clinical pertussis. J Hyg (Camb) 69:399, 1971

PRESTON NW: Type-specific immunity against whooping cough. Br Med J 2:724, 1963

WHITE R et al: The modern morbidity of pertussis in infants. Pediatrics 33:705, 1964

WILSON AT et al: Whooping cough: Difficulties in diagnosis and ineffectiveness of immunization. Lancet 2:623, 1965

Hemophilus aphrophilus

SUTTER VL, FEINGOLD SM: *Haemophilus aphrophilus* infections: Clinical and bacteriologic studies. Ann NY Acad Sci 174:468, 1970

139 CHANCROID

KING K. HOLMES

DEFINITION Chancroid, or soft chancre, is an acute, sexually transmitted infection characterized by painful genital ulcerations usually associated with inflammatory, often suppurative, inguinal adenopathy. A presumptive diagnosis is supported by exclusion of syphilis, genital herpes, and other specific causes of genital ulceration, together with improvement following sulfonamide therapy. A specific diagnosis is proved only when *Hemophilus ducreyi* is isolated from the lesion or suppurative node.

ETIOLOGY The specific microbial etiology of chancroid has repeatedly been supported by isolation of Ducrey's bacterium, *H. ducreyi*, in mixed culture from chancroidal ulcers and in pure culture from bubos. However, anaerobic bacteria are also universally present in chancroidal ulcers, and spirochetal forms which can be confused with *Treponema pallidum* are occasionally seen as well. The role of such organisms as synergistic or independent pathogens remains undefined. The reported frequency of recovery of *H. ducreyi* from typical chancroid ulcers ranges from 30 to 90 percent. *Hemophilus ducreyi* is one of the most poorly characterized of all aerobic pathogens, and isolates from suspect lesions are identified principally by the requirement for whole blood for optimal growth, and by the formation of parallel chains of small gram-negative rods in blood. Organisms which possess these rather nonspecific properties have also been recovered from smegma of normal men and from the vagina of normal women.

INCIDENCE The incidence of chancroid is unknown, since accurate bacteriologic diagnosis is seldom attempted and reporting is incomplete. Thus, only 1,520 cases of chancroid were reported in the United States during 1971, compared with 23,783 cases of infectious syphilis. However, in military personnel, chancroid is as common as syphilis, and currently is most frequent among troops stationed in Southeast Asia.

CLINICAL MANIFESTATIONS After an incubation period of 3 to 5 days, a small inflammatory papule appears, which becomes pustular or occasionally vesiculopustular and ulcerative within 2 to 3 days. The classical chancroid is superficial and shallow, ranging from a few millimeters to two centimeters in diameter. The edge usually appears ragged or scalloped and is surrounded by an inflammatory red halo. The base is covered by a necrotic exudate and bleeds easily when the exudate is removed. In contrast with syphilitic chancre, the chancroidal ulcer is extremely painful and tender, and is not indurated. In men, the most frequent locations are the preputial orifice or internal surface of the prepuce, and the frenulum; and in women, the labia and fourchette. Multiple ulcers are more common than single ulcers.

Acute, painful, tender, inflammatory inguinal adenopathy accompanies over 50 percent of cases, and is unilateral in about two-thirds. In untreated patients, the involved nodes become matted, forming a unilocular suppurative *bubo*. The overlying skin becomes erythematous, tense, thinned, and finally ruptures, forming a large single ulcer.

DIAGNOSIS Other diseases which may be confused with chancroid, in decreasing order of frequency, are genital herpes, primary syphilis, and lymphogranuloma venereum (LGV). The clinical diagnosis of chancroid often depends upon exclusion of these three diseases, together with response to sulfonamide therapy. Primary genital infection with *herpesvirus hominis type* 2 may be associated with tender inguinal lymphadenopathy, but, unlike chancroid, primary herpes often produces fever and other constitutional symptoms, has a characteristic initial vesicular stage, and causes acute, transient, necrotizing cervicitis in females. A localized cluster of vesicles characterizes the onset of secondary (recurrent) genital herpes. In *primary syphilis*, the chancre is indurated, and the associated adenopathy is bilateral, nontender, and nonsuppurative. However, at least three dark-field examinations should be performed on separate days, together with monthly serologic tests for syphilis for 3 months, in order to exclude syphilis. The typical genital lesion of LGV is an evanescent papule rather than a painful ulcer, and the associated adenopathy is multinodular rather than unilocular. However, a form of chancroid resembling LGV has been described in which a small ulcer heals in 4 to 6 days, to be followed 10 to 20 days later by inguinal lymphadenopathy. A negative Frei skin test and LGV complement fixation test provide evidence against LGV.

The only reliable method for diagnosis of chancroid consists of isolation of *H. ducreyi* from the ulcer or bubo. One recommended method of culture consists of inoculation of pus into tubes containing slants of 1.5 percent nutrient agar, overlain with 2 ml of coagulated or defibrinated rabbit blood. The stained smear of exudate from lesions and the histologic appearance of biopsy material may suggest chancroid but are not specific.

TREATMENT Chancroid is one of the few remaining infections for which a sulfonamide is the drug of choice. Sulfisoxazole (Gantrisin) is usually effective in a dose of 4 g daily, and should be continued until the lesion and adenopathy have healed, which usually requires about 2 weeks. Sulfonamide therapy alone will not interfere with dark-field examination or with development of reaginic or treponemal antibody in patients with syphilis or mixed infections. However, if the response to sulfisoxazole alone is unsatisfactory, tetracycline hydrochloride should be added in a dose of 2 g daily. Tetracycline alone is frequently inadequate. Alternative antibiotics include streptomycin, erythromycin, and chloramphenicol. Circumcision is now required only rarely in the acute management of chancroid complicated by phimosis or paraphimosis. Needle aspiration of tensely fluctuant nodes is useful to prevent spontaneous rupture.

REFERENCES

Kerfer RE et al: Treatment of chancroid. A comparison of tetracycline and sulfisoxazole. Arch Dermatol 100:604, 1969

Sullivan M: Chancroid. Am J Syph Gonor Vener Dis 24:482, 1940

140 BRUCELLOSIS

WESLEY W. SPINK

DEFINITION Brucellosis (undulant fever) is caused by microorganisms belonging to the genus *Brucella* and is transmitted to man from lower animals. The acute illness is frequently characterized by fever without localized findings, while the chronic form consists of fever, weakness, and vague complaints, which may persist for months and years.

HISTORY The first clear-cut picture of the disease was presented in 1863 by Marston, and the etiologic agent (*Brucella melitensis*) was discovered by Bruce in 1886. In 1897, Bang reported that *Br. abortus* was the cause of contagious abortion in cattle in Denmark. In 1911 brucellosis was found to be endemic in the goats of Texas, and Gentry and Ferenbaugh traced human cases to this source. Traum first identified *Brucella* organisms (*Br. suis*) from aborting sows in 1914. New species include *Br. canis* causing abortions in dogs, especially the beagle breed, and *Br. ovis* causing epidemics that result in sterility in rams.

ETIOLOGY Human brucellosis is primarily due to one of three species: *Br. melitensis* (goats), *Br. suis* (hogs), and *Br. abortus* (cattle). Several subtypes have been described under each of these three main categories. Brucellae are small, nonmotile, non-spore-forming, gram-negative rods. Growth is best at 37°C in trypticase soy broth or tryptose phosphate broth having a pH of 6.6 to 6.8, under conditions in which 10 percent of the air is displaced by carbon dioxide. The differentiation of the three species is dependent upon biochemical and serologic reaction.

EPIDEMIOLOGY The natural reservoir of brucellosis is in domestic animals, particularly cattle, swine, goats, and sheep. The disease is very rarely transmitted from man to man.

Studies in the United States and elsewhere indicate that the majority of cases are acquired through contact, and fewer cases are caused by the ingestion of milk or milk products. This trend is due to the enactment of local and state ordinances requiring all milk sold for human consumption to be pasteurized. There is some evidence that brucellosis may be airborne, with the disease resulting from the inhalation of *Brucella*. Infections caused by *Br. abortus* are spread through cow's milk or through dermal contact with *Brucella*. Contact with infected porcine tissue is a common cause of infections due to *Br. suis*. Thus, brucellosis is primarily an occupational disease of rural areas, involving primarily meat-packing plant employees, farmers, veterinarians, and livestock producers. Disease due to *Br. melitensis* rarely occurs in the United States, but it is the most common cause of brucellosis on a worldwide basis.

PATHOGENESIS Following invasion of the body by brucellae through the oropharynx or through the skin, the organisms tend to localize in tissues of the reticuloendothelial system, such as the bone marrow, lymph nodes, liver, spleen, and also the kidneys. A characteristic but nonspecific reaction of these tissues to the brucellae is the appearance of epithelioid cells, giant cells of the foreign body and Langhans' types, and lymphocytes and plasma cells. Necrosis and caseation rarely occur in these granulomatous areas. When caseation is encountered, it is usually caused by *Br. suis*. The granulomas are similar to those of sarcoidosis and tuberculosis. Other, less frequent, sites of localization of *Brucella* organisms are the bones, especially the spine, the endocardium, and the testes. Although the central nervous system and peripheral nerves are commonly affected deleteriously by brucellae, the mechanism whereby this takes place is not known. Like other bloodborne bacilli, brucellae may on occasion localize in any tissue or organ in the body. Though brucellosis is a common cause of abortions in cattle, swine, and goats, authentic human abortions occur no more frequently with this disease than with other bacteremias. Orchitis in the male is rarely the cause of subsequent sterility.

MANIFESTATIONS The incubation period varies between 5 and 21 days, though many months may elapse between the time of infection and the first appearance of symptoms. The onset in many instances may be insidious; patients have a low-grade fever with no localized findings and complain of headache, weakness, insomnia, sweats, anorexia, constipation, pain over the spine, and generalized aches and pains. Less frequently, the disease may be ushered in by chills, high fever, and prostration, but, again, localizing abnormal physical findings may be absent. An enlarged and tender spleen is usually associated with the more severe cases. Pain on pressure over the vertebras occurs occasionally, and pain along the course of peripheral nerves, particularly the sciatic nerve, is encountered. Orchitis appears after several days of illness and, like the orchitis of mumps, is ushered in with a chill or chilliness, high fever, and tender and enlarged testes. Painful and swollen joints are seen occasionally, but persistent and deforming arthritis is not specific for the disease. Signs and symptoms referable to the lungs and pleurae are uncommon. A rare but serious complication is subacute bacterial endocarditis. Ocular disorders are associated with the more chronic forms of the disease.

The initial febrile stage of the illness may last from a few days up to several weeks. The persistence of fever and symptoms is definitely related to physical activity. Rest in bed during the acute illness is frequently associated with prompt improvement. The natural course of the disease in the majority of patients is marked by a permanent remission of fever and symptoms within 3 to 6 months, or sooner. A small number of patients with bacteriologically proved cases may have an illness that persists for a year or more.

The status of chronic brucellosis is extremely difficult to assess. There is no doubt that the infection may persist in a relatively small number of individuals for months and years. Such patients are in a state of ill health manifested by weakness, fatigue, mental depression, vague aches and pains, and no abnormal physical findings. Intermittent fever may occur. Of considerable importance in the suspected chronic case is the investigation of possible sites of chronic suppuration manifested by calcified caseating areas in the liver and spleen that can be detected by careful x-ray films of the abdomen. Abacteriuric pyuria should suggest, among other causes, renal suppuration due to brucellae.

LABORATORY FINDINGS A precise diagnosis of brucellosis is dependent upon the results of laboratory procedures.

Blood The total leukocyte count is usually normal, or slightly reduced but is rarely over 10,000 cells per mm^3. The differential count reveals a relative lymphocytosis. The erythrocyte sedimentation rate is of no specific diagnostic aid, being normal or accelerated.

The most practical method for screening suspected cases of brucellosis is the agglutination reaction. Agglutinins usually appear during the second or third week of illness. If proper techniques and antigens are employed, agglutinins are demonstrated in the vast majority of bacteriologically proved cases. Active brucellosis is usually associated with titers of 1:100 or above. On rare occasions, the titer may be depressed by "blocking antibodies" in chronic illness. Only very rarely are agglutinins absent in patients with bacteriologically proved disease. Agglutinins for brucellosis are not always specific, since cross-reactions occur with the cholera vibrio and with *Pasteurella tularensis*. Agglutinins may persist in the blood long after the patient has recovered. One of the most critical diagnostic problems in the sporadic case of brucellosis is the interpretation of an agglutination titer of 1 to 100 or lower in the absence of definitive bacteriologic data and localizing signs. *Brucella*-agglutinating immunoglobulins in serum consist of both 7S and 19S globulins, but only 7S globulins have been associated with active disease in acute and chronic cases, providing a stimulating dose of antigen (skin test) has not been given prior to obtaining blood from the patient.

At least one, and preferably more, cultures of blood should be carried out in every suspected case of brucellosis. Brucellae have been isolated from aspirated sternal bone marrow when simultaneous blood cultures are sterile. It is too impractical for routine purposes to attempt to isolate brucellae from the urine, bile, or feces.

Intradermal tests A positive reaction to *Brucella* antigen has no more significance than that obtained with tuberculin in suspected cases of tuberculosis. A positive reaction indicates previous invasion of the body by brucellae and does not mean that active disease is present. When agglutinins are absent and cultures remain sterile, considerable caution must be exercised before making a diagnosis of brucellosis, even though the skin test is positive.

DIFFERENTIAL DIAGNOSIS Brucellosis must be differentiated from other acute febrile illnesses such as influenza and other upper respiratory diseases of doubtful etiology. Other diseases from which it must be differentiated include malaria and typhoid fever. Brucellosis may be confused with infectious mononucleosis.

Chronic brucellosis simulates psychoneurosis, anxiety states, and chronic nervous exhaustion. Indeed, a patient with brucellosis may also have these nervous disorders.

TREATMENT Patients with acute brucellosis should be reassured that a large majority of those with the disease recover spontaneously. Rest and psychotherapy are important during the febrile illness.

The course of acute brucellosis can be shortened and complications prevented by the prompt use of tetracycline, in dosage of 0.5 g four times daily orally for at least 3 weeks. In case of a relapse, this dose schedule can be repeated. Except in rare instances there is no advantage in more than two courses of tetracycline therapy. For more seriously ill patients streptomycin in dosage of 0.5 g twice daily may be used in addition to tetracycline. Tetracycline therapy, with and without streptomycin, is also effective in proved chronic brucellosis.

Febrile patients with either acute or chronic brucellosis sometimes have severe anorexia, depression, and generalized debilitation. Such individuals should receive an adrenocorticoid steroid preparation in addition to antibiotic therapy. Prednisone in oral dosage of 20 mg can be given twice daily for 72 to 96 hr, or 100 mg hydrocortisone can be administered intravenously, followed by 50 mg orally twice daily.

A therapeutic practice in the more chronic cases is to attempt desensitization to *Brucella* organisms by treating patients with one of the several antigenic preparations, such as heat-killed *Brucella* cells or filtrates of *Brucella* cultures. Such therapy is seriously questioned and cannot be recommended.

For the relief of headache and the generalized aches and pains, salicylates may be prescribed; the occasional use of barbiturates is desirable for the insomnia which is so commonly a part of the disease.

PROGNOSIS Although brucellosis may be a chronic and disabling disease, the overall mortality rate is very small. Even without the aid of effective drug therapy, only 15 percent of patients have an illness exceeding 3 months.

Cases of bacteriologically proved brucellosis in which the disease has continued for up to 25 years have been studied at the University of Minnesota Hospitals, but such cases are rare. So-called "chronic brucellosis" is diagnosed all too often on the basis of procedures of doubtful value, especially the intradermal test with *Brucella* antigen.

Relapses can occur in some chronic cases of brucellosis. These recurrences are not common and are manifested by fever, mental and physical disability, and generalized aches and pains. Too little attention has been given to the problem of reinfections. Clinical observations in meat-packing plant employees have confirmed studies made in experimentally infected animals, showing that the immunity induced by one attack of brucellosis is only relative and that second and third infections do take place. In individuals who continue to be exposed to the disease, it may be quite difficult to differentiate between relapses and reinfections. Furthermore, patients who have recovered from brucellosis have an acquired *Brucella* hypersensitivity that may render them extremely susceptible to the effects of contact with *Brucella* antigen. This is particularly applicable to veterinarians who have accidentally injected viable *Brucella* antigen into their skin while immunizing animals. Violent local and systemic febrile reactions follow such an incident within a few hours.

PREVENTION As long as a reservoir of brucellosis persists in domestic animals, human brucellosis will occur. The only practical means of eliminating the disease in human beings is to eradicate the disease from cattle, hogs, sheep, and goats. Control measures in animals are being worked out in several areas in the United States. Since human brucellosis may be contracted through the ingestion of contaminated milk and milk products, it is essential that only properly pasteurized milk be utilized for human consumption. Brucellosis is an occupational disease involving farmers, livestock workers, veterinarians, and those working in meat-packing plants, and there is no entirely safe means for immunizing these groups against the disease.

REFERENCES

Busch LA, Parker RL: Brucellosis in the United States. J Infect Dis 125:289, 1972

Hall WH: Epidemic brucellosis in beagles. J Infect Dis 124:615, 1971

Reddin JL et al: Significance of 7S and macroglobulin brucella agglutinins in human brucellosis. N Engl J Med 272:1263, 1965

Reports of the Commission for the Investigation of Mediterranean Fever, parts 1 to 7, London: Harrison & Sons, Ltd., 1905–1907

Spink WW: *The Nature of Brucellosis,* Minneapolis: University of Minnesota Press, 1956

141 TULAREMIA

LEIGHTON E. CLUFF

DEFINITION Tularemia (rabbit fever, deer-fly fever, Ohara's disease) is an infectious disease of animals transmitted to man by direct contact or by insect vectors. A cutaneous or mucous membrane lesion at the site of inoculation and regional lymph node enlargement are the characteristic manifestations of the disease in man.

HISTORY The microorganism responsible for tularemia was identified by McCoy and Chapin in 1912 among infected ground squirrels in Tulare County, California. The first description of tularemia in man was by Wherry and Lamb in 1914.

ETIOLOGY *Pasteurella* (*Francisella*) *tularensis* is a pleomorphic, nonsporulating, gram-negative bacillus. It can be cultured only on media containing glucose, cystine, and serum. Thorough cooking renders meat from infected animals safe for consumption, but tularemia can develop in persons handling carcasses that have been frozen for many days. *Pasteurella tularensis* is related antigenically to the causative organisms of brucellosis and plague and possesses an endotoxin similar to those of many other gram-negative bacteria.

EPIDEMIOLOGY AND PATHOGENESIS Contact with infected animals is the commonest source of tularemia in man, but the disease also may be acquired from insects or by exposure to the organism in the laboratory. A variety of rodents, carnivores, ungulates, birds, and arthropods is naturally infected by *P. tularensis,* including rabbits, squirrels, woodchucks, muskrats, skunks, coyotes, foxes, opossums, mice, rats, quail, chickens, pheasants, snakes, ticks, and flies. The Rocky Mountain tick, western wood tick, eastern dog tick, and the Lone Star tick (*Dermacentor andersoni, D. variabilis, D. occidentalis,* and *Amblyomma americanum*) may act as reservoirs of infection. One species of deer fly (*Chrysops discalis*) and, in Sweden, a mosquito (*Aëdes cinereus*) can transmit tularemia to man. Ticks are an important reservoir of the disease because the microorganism is transferred transovarially from the female to her progeny. Sporadic episodes and epidemic tularemia have occurred among human beings following contact with water and fish contaminated by infected animal carcasses. However, human-to-human transmission of infection does not occur. Wild cottontail rabbits are the principal source of tularemia in the United States. A large-scale epidemic, presumably transmitted by infected muskrats, occurred in Vermont in 1968.

Man is highly susceptible to tularemia; the organism usually invades through the skin, mucous membrane, gastrointestinal tract, or respiratory tract. Hunters, butchers, and housewives are most often affected.

PATHOLOGY Microscopically, the primary cutaneous lesion shows neutrophilic infiltration, granulomatous reaction, and necrosis. The regional lymph nodes develop similar changes and often suppurate. The granulomatous reaction in tularemia resembles tubercles in liver, spleen, lung, and kidney. *Pasteurella tularensis* has been recovered from lymph nodes many days after apparent subsidence of the disease.

MANIFESTATIONS The incubation period is 3 to 7 days. Because a typical lesion of skin or mucous membranes is not invariably present, tularemia classically has been separated into several clinical types.

More than 80 percent of infections by *P. tularensis* produce a lesion of the skin or mucous membranes which begins as a reddened papule that may be pruritic and soon ulcerates. The primary lesion in this *ulceroglandular* form of the disease is rarely very painful, is usually present before onset of systemic symptoms, and may not heal until convalescence is well under way. Frequently it is overlooked, or its relation to severe systemic symptoms is not recognized. Regional lymph node enlargement is usually more prominent than that accompanying infections of similar severity produced by other microorganisms. The involved nodes are often exquisitely tender, fluctuant, hot, and reddened. Drainage can occur spontaneously. Generalized lymphadenopathy is present in some cases, but the regional nodes are most prominently involved. There is considerable variation in the intensity of the systemic symptoms of ulceroglandular tularemia; the patient may be almost asymptomatic or severely prostrated. Clinical and roentgenographic evidence of pneumonitis may accompany this form of the disease, illustrating its disseminated character, but bacteremia is rarely demonstrable.

Localized lymph node enlargement without a detectable skin lesion is referred to as *glandular* tularemia. The pathogenesis of this form of the disease is probably identical with that of ulceroglandular tularemia, and the features of the illness are also the same.

Rarely, the portal of entry of the organism is the conjunctiva, where there develops an ulcer, with edema, congestion, lacrimation, photophobia, and pain. In this *oculoglandular* type of tularemia the preauricular, submaxillary, and anterior cervical lymph nodes may enlarge. Corneal ulceration and scarring or perforation of the globe may occur.

Ingestion of contaminated meat or water may result in primary lesions in the gastrointestinal tract. This rare form of the disease produces diarrhea, abdominal pain, nausea, vomiting, melena, and hematemesis, but otherwise differs little from tularemia introduced through other portals. Ulcerative lesions are often found in the buccal mucosa, pharynx, or intestine, and the mesenteric or cervical lymph nodes are involved early in the disease.

Tularemia without obvious primary ulcer or localized lymphadenitis is referred to as *typhoidal.* Constitutional symptoms in typhoidal tularemia differ in no way from those in other types of the disease, although there is usually more prostration. In the absence of localized manifestations, the diagnosis of tularemia is more difficult and depends on serologic tests, isolation of the organism, or a strong epidemiologic history.

Pneumonia may accompany tularemia. Involvement of the lung is secondary to hematogenous dissemination, even when infection is acquired by inhalation of the organism (as in bacteriology laboratories). Pneumonitis in tularemia may cause cough, mucoid sputum, hemoptysis, pleuritic pain, dyspnea, and cyanosis, but extensive x-ray evidence of pneumonitis is sometimes present in the absence of any symptoms of pulmonary disease. Physical findings often correlate poorly with the roentgenologic changes, which consist of diffuse patchy or lobar infiltrations and inconstant hilar adenopathy. Pleural effusion may occur, but lung abscess is rare.

Rarely *P. tularensis* causes endocarditis, pericarditis, peritonitis, appendicitis, osteomyelitis, or meningitis.

Fever in tularemia develops abruptly, often with rigors, and in untreated patients may persist with temperatures of 104 to 106°F for as long as 4 weeks. The fever is sustained or mildly remittent, and defervescence is by lysis.

Splenomegaly is detectable in many patients. An evanescent macular or papular rash is sometimes present on the trunk and extremities early in the disease.

Convalescence in untreated tularemia is prolonged, and fever, lassitude, fatigability, myalgia, irritability, or anorexia may persist or recur for many months. Recovery is usually prompt if acute tularemia is treated with antibiotics. When therapy is delayed, however, patients are more likely to be left with mild debilitation that is unresponsive to further administration of antimicrobial drugs.

Recovery from tularemia is usually followed by immunity to recurrence of disease. However, immunity is not complete, and several instances of second, even third, attacks of tularemia have been recorded. Almost invariably, they have consisted of the development of a local lesion and mild regional adenopathy without systemic symptoms and with little or no fever.

LABORATORY FINDINGS Serum agglutinins for *P. tularensis* are present after the second week of illness. Cross agglutination may occur with antigens of *Brucella,* but this is not a constant finding.

Pasteurella tularensis can be recovered by appropriate cultures or animal inoculation. It is rarely found in blood but can be isolated from the mucocutaneous ulcer or regional lymph nodes with regularity. The organism has been cultured from the sputum and gastric washings even in patients without roentgenographic evidence of pneumonitis. Accidental infection of personnel in diagnostic laboratories may occur.

Skin test with a diluted suspension of killed *P. tularensis,* or purified antigen, becomes positive during the first week of disease. The cutaneous hypersensitivity response is "delayed" and resembles the tuberculin reaction. The skin test may become positive earlier and persist longer than the agglutination test.

The total blood leukocyte count is usually normal. The erythrocyte sedimentation rate is normal in ulceroglandular or mild disease but is frequently elevated in severe typhoidal tularemia.

DIFFERENTIAL DIAGNOSIS Brucellosis, typhoid fever, disseminated tuberculosis, the early stage of several rickettsial diseases, and infectious mononucleosis may closely resemble typhoidal tularemia. History of possible contacts is important, and appropriate serologic and cultural studies are usually successful in differentiating these infections. Pneumonic tularemia must be distinguished from viral, mycotic, and other bacterial infections of the lung. The differential diagnosis of pneumonia is discussed in Chap. 128. Oculoglandular syndromes likely to be confused with tularemia are described in Chap. 204.

Ulceroglandular tularemia must be distinguished from a variety of infections in which a *local cutaneous ulcer with regional lymphadenopathy* may occur. Besides pyoderma caused by streptococci or staphylococci, these infections include lymphogranuloma venereum, cat-scratch fever, rat-bite fever, bubonic plague, anthrax, glanders, several rickettsioses of which the important one in this country is rickettsialpox, several viral infections of the skin such as orf and cowpox, and inoculation syphilis or tuberculosis. In all these, with the exception of lymphogranuloma venereum and cat-scratch fever, the regional lymph node involvement is usually proportional to the size of the cutaneous ulcer. Extragenital lymphogranuloma is rare; fever and systemic symptoms in cat-scratch fever are rarely severe for more than a few days.

TREATMENT Streptomycin is the antibiotic of choice for tularemia. The dosage is 0.5 to 1.0 g every 12 hr for 10 days. *Pasteurella tularensis* cannot be recovered from lymph nodes or skin lesions after 24 to 48 hr of therapy. However, the regional lymph nodes may continue to enlarge and suppurate for several days. Pulmonary lesions usually subside rapidly, although the evolution of the cutaneous lesion is not interrupted. The tetracycline antibiotics and chloramphenicol also are effective, although fever and other manifestations may recur 7 to 14 days after cessation of therapy. Recrudescent illness, however, responds rapidly to readministration of the antibiotic. Aspiration of pus from suppurating nodes rarely is necessary; but if fistulas persist, total surgical removal of the involved tissue can be carried out. Surgery may be followed by transient recurrence of fever despite failure to demonstrate the organism in excised tissues.

PROPHYLAXIS A killed bacterial vaccine developed by Foshay has been shown to stimulate serum agglutinins and induces positive skin reactions to the bacterial antigens, but it produces little immunity to infection with *P. tularensis*. An attenuated live bacterial vaccine has been developed, however, and is effective in inducing protection against infection.

Antibiotic prophylaxis with streptomycin following exposure to tularemia will protect against infection. Chloramphenicol and tetracycline, however, only prolong the incubation period of the disease and do not prevent its occurrence.

Avoidance of contact with possible sources of infection is important in prevention, and the incidence of tularemia in several localities has fallen sharply with the introduction of laws prohibiting the sale of wild rabbits by butchers.

PROGNOSIS The mortality rate in untreated tularemia is 6 to 7 percent. With antimicrobial therapy, death is rare.

REFERENCES

BUCHANAN TM et al: The tularemia skin test. 325 skin tests in 210 persons: Serologic correlation and review of the literature. Ann Intern Med 74:336, 1971

FRANCIS E: Tularemia, in *Oxford Medicine,* Fair Lawn, N.J.: Oxford University Press, 1948

MCCRUMB FR JR et al: Studies on human infection with *pasteurella tularensis:* Comparison of streptomycin and chloramphenicol in the prophylaxis of clinical disease. Trans Assoc Am Physicians 70:74, 1957

STUART BM, PULLEN RL: Tularemic pneumonia: Review of American literature and report of fifteen additional cases. Am J Med Sci 210:233, 1945

YOUNG LS et al: Tularemia epidemic: Vermont 1968. Forty-seven cases linked to contact with muskrats. N Engl J Med 280:1253, 1969

142 PASTEURELLA INFECTIONS INCLUDING PLAGUE

JOSEPH E. JOHNSON

Gram-negative bacilli of the genus *Pasteurella* have been reclassified recently in accordance with increasing knowledge about the characteristics of the bacteria. *P. pestis* (the plague bacillus) and *P. pseudotuberculosis* are now included in the genus *Yersinia* along with a third closely related organism, *Y. enterocolitica. Pasteurella multocida* (formerly *P. septica*) initially included a group of several closely related species producing hemorrhagic septicemia in animals and man. Related species with at least potential pathogenicity for humans include *P. urae, P. haemolytica,* and *P. pneumotropica.*

PLAGUE Definition Plague is an infectious disease of animals (principally wild and domestic rodents) which is transmitted to man through the bite of infected ectoparasites (especially the rat flea). Disease in man is usually characterized by the abrupt onset of high fever, lymphadenopathy and suppuration of regional lymph nodes draining the exposure site, bacteremia, and prostration. This clinical form of the disease is known as *bubonic* plague because of the presence of enlarged suppurating lymph nodes, or *buboes*. Secondary pneumonia may occur and lead to direct respiratory transmission by infectious aerosols from man to man. This primary *pneumonic* type of human disease is highly fatal.

History Plague was known and feared in ancient times and has been the subject of dread as well as a source of literary stimulation to authors from Dionysius in the third century to Camus in the present. At least three major pandemics have occurred in which large segments of the population were destroyed. The first authentic pandemic was recorded in the sixth century A.D.; the second great pandemic occurred in the fourteenth century and was known as the "Black Death," and the last major pandemic originated in China in 1894, spread eventually to all continents, and was first recognized in the United States in 1900. It is likely, however, that the disease was present in the wild rodent population (sylvatic plague) in California long before this. The disease is now well established in wild rodents in many parts of the world, including the western United States. It is present on every continent except Australia. Human disease is endemic in parts of Asia, Africa, and South America, and sporadic human cases still occur in the United States.

Etiology The causative agent, *Yersinia pestis*, is a gram-negative, nonmotile, and non-spore-forming bacillus which grows both aerobically and anaerobically. It is pleomorphic in exudate or sputum, and may appear bacillary, ovid, or coccal. When stained with Giemsa's or Wayson's stain, it displays a bipolar "safety pin" structure. *Yersinia pestis* grows readily although somewhat slowly on ordinary culture media, forming small, round, transparent colonies which assume a "beaten-copper" appearance after 48 hr. At least two types of toxins have been identified, including a soluble exotoxinlike protein and an insoluble endotoxic lipopolysaccharide. Although readily killed by sunlight, organisms have been shown to survive in sterile soil for 16 months and in nonsterile soil for as long as 7 months, and it is likely that organisms may be present in rodent burrows in the absence of fleas and rats for long periods.

Epidemiology Plague is firmly entrenched as an enzootic among approximately 200 species of rodents in many parts of the world. While the disease in wild rodents (sylvatic plague) is not usually a direct threat to man, it nevertheless serves as a vast reservoir for infection of domestic rats (murine or rat plague) which, along with their ectoparasites, live in close association with man. The endemic reservoir of sylvatic plague includes wild rats, ground squirrels, mice, marmots, owls, gophers, badgers, rabbits, prairie dogs, and chipmunks; in the Western Hemisphere the disease is firmly entrenched in the wild rodent population of California, Oregon, Washington, Utah, Idaho, Nevada, New Mexico, Texas, Louisiana, Florida, Michigan, Arizona, Colorado, Montana, Wyoming, Kansas, North Dakota, Hawaii, western Mexico, and western Canada. The principal murine hosts are the domestic rats, *Rattus rattus* and *R. norvegicus*, which are found throughout the world. Although ticks, lice, and bedbugs may occasionally serve as vectors, the principal ectoparasite vector is the oriental rat flea, *Xenopsylla cheopis*.

Between epidemics the infection persists as a chronic disease of wild rodents which is maintained by the insect vector. Although occasionally acquired through contact with wild rodents and their parasites, human disease is usually a result of association with domestic rats and occurs in urban areas in the wake of rat epizootics. When the concentration of people and of rats under circumstances of poor sanitation provides opportunity for the migration of fleas from rats to man, an outbreak is likely to occur. Because sylvatic plague appears virtually impossible to eradicate, it will continue to pose a constant threat of extension into urban rat populations and thence to man. Infection of the flea takes place through ingestion of blood of a bacteremic animal. After multiplication in the intestinal tract of the flea, the organisms are regurgitated when the flea attempts to ingest another blood meal. Because rat fleas will attack man if rats are not immediately available, the infection is likely to be transmitted as the rat population decreases and the fleas transfer from dead hosts to human beings. Plague can be acquired by direct contact with the tissues of an infected animal, by its bite, or by scratching of infected material into the skin.

The bubonic form of the disease rarely results in transmission from man to man because bacteremia in human disease is rarely of a level sufficient to allow infection of fleas. The principal mode of spread from man to man is by the pulmonary route, which occurs when a patient with bubonic disease develops secondary plague pneumonia and thereafter excretes large quantities of organisms in the sputum. Airborne infection by droplet nuclei is highly contagious, and primary pneumonic plague is common among those attending such a patient. Although asymptomatic oropharyngeal carriers have been identified among healthy family contacts of bubonic plague patients in Vietnam, the role of these carriers in the transmission of the disease has not been determined.

Pathogenesis In the more common bubonic form of disease, *Y. pestis* gains entry into the human host through the bite of an infected flea. Organisms are carried to the local lymphatics, then to the bloodstream and finally are disseminated. The prominent clinical manifestations are usually in the lymphatic system. In bubonic plague, a hemorrhagic zone of edema surrounds an inflamed and suppurating group of regional lymph nodes. The glands are hyperplastic and show multiple areas of necrosis, in which there are swarms of organisms. Metastatic lesions sometimes develop in other lymphatics or in the viscera. Particularly likely is the occurrence of secondary pneumonia, which constitutes a potential source of pneumonic spread. Hemorrhages are numerous, probably as a result of a toxin produced by *Y. pestis*, and it is not unusual for individuals given chemotherapy at a late date to die of toxemia when plague bacilli can no longer be cultured from any organ. Primary pneumonic spread occurs through the inhalation of infectious aerosols emanating from another case or, rarely, from infected fomites. It is apparent that the tonsils and/or oropharyngeal mucous membranes may occasionally serve as portals of entry resulting in a cervical bubonic-septicemic form of the disease. Rarely a skin papule forms at the site of entry of the bacillus, and may develop into a pustule or a carbuncle.

Bacteremia is a constant feature of bubonic and pneumonic plague. The precise mechanisms by which the plague bacillus and its toxic factors produce severe tissue injury are not understood completely.

Manifestations After an incubation period of 1 to 12 days (usually 2 to 4 days), the patient develops an acute and often fulminant illness. In the more common *bubonic* variety, symptoms begin abruptly with chills, a rise in temperature to 102 to 105°F, tachycardia, headache, vomiting, uncertain gait, marked prostration, and delirium. The spleen is sometimes palpable. The fleabite at the portal of entry rarely can be seen; if present, it is marked by a papule or vesicle which ultimately becomes pustular. Pain and tenderness are present in the infected regional lymph nodes. Of the buboes, 60 to 75 percent are in the inguinal or femoral regions because the lower extremities are more commonly the site of the initial fleabite. Less often, especially in children, buboes are found in the axillary or cervical regions. Infection may extend to other superficial or deeply situated groups of glands. The bubo consists of a firm, matted group of glands measuring 2 to 5 cm in diameter and is surrounded by a boggy and frequently hemorrhagic zone of edema. It usually suppurates and drains spontaneously after 1 or 2 weeks, although in some instances there is complete resorption.

There is a marked hemorrhagic tendency, presumably because of the effect of plague toxin on blood vessels.

Petechiae or ecchymoses occur often. Bleeding may occur into a viscus or a serous cavity, or from the nose and alimentary, respiratory, or urinary tracts.

The course of bubonic plague is marked by an irregular or remittent fever, which often drops at the time of appearance of the bubo, only to rise again. In favorable cases, the temperature falls gradually during the second week concomitant with improvement in the general clinical condition. A rise to hyperpyrexic levels or a precipitous fall to normal or to subnormal frequently heralds approaching death. Most fatalities occur during the first week of illness. Although bubonic plague is usually severe, mild cases called *pestis minor* are sometimes seen during epidemics.

The "primary septicemic" form of plague is actually a variant of bubonic disease. The patient experiences a sudden and overwhelming systemic illness. There is a marked constitutional reaction, with chills, fever, rapid pulse, severe headache, nausea, vomiting, and delirium. Death ensues within a few days, before localizing lesions become clinically apparent. Nevertheless, autopsy usually reveals inflammation in some part of the lymphatic system.

Plague also may take the form of pneumonia. The initial cases appear in patients with bubonic plague, of whom as many as 5 percent develop secondary lesions in the lungs. These individuals may provide the starting point for a man-to-man epidemiologic cycle of airborne primary pneumonic plague. It is a fulminating infection accompanied by great prostration, cough, dyspnea, and in the later stages, cyanosis. The sputum is abundant, blood-stained, and teeming with *Y. pestis*. Often there are no clear-cut pulmonary signs, though scattered rales or areas of dullness may be found. In the absence of specific therapy, plague pneumonia invariably ends fatally within 1 to 5 days.

Infection may localize in other regions of the body. Subcutaneous abscesses and cutaneous ulcerations sometimes occur, and occasionally the meninges are involved.

Laboratory findings Laboratory confirmation of plague is relatively simple, although the disease is often misdiagnosed in the United States because of its rarity. Consideration of epidemiologic and clinical features provide highly characteristic leads, and once a suspicion of plague is entertained, it can readily be verified by smear, culture, and animal inoculation of appropriate specimens. The technique of staining a suspected specimen with fluorescent specific antiserum provides an elegant method for rapid identification of *Y. pestis*. If a bubo is present, a small quantity of interstitial fluid should be aspirated from its center. Large numbers of morphologically characteristic bacilli are usually seen in a stained smear. Infected sputum likewise contains many organisms. Bacteremia of varying degrees occurs at some time during the course of the disease in nearly all cases. Pus and sputum should be cultured on blood agar plates, while blood is inoculated into nutrient broth. Organisms are identified by their morphologic and colonial characteristics and by agglutination with specific antiserum. Guinea pig inoculation is the final step in identification. In this animal the gross and microscopic lesions are highly characteristic. Caution should be observed in handling infected materials or animals, because of the great danger of infection to laboratory workers.

Specific antibodies appear in the serum of patients convalescing from the disease and can usually be detected early in the second week by complement fixation, agglutination, passive hemagglutination, or immunoelectrophoretic agar-gel precipitation methods. A passive mouse-protective test serves to indicate the immune status of a convalescent or vaccinated individual.

The white blood cell count is elevated to levels often above 20,000 cells per mm^3, and there is a predominance of polymorphonuclear leukocytes. The red blood cell count usually is normal.

Diagnosis Early in the acute phase of illness, before the appearance of localizing signs, plague may be confused with severe systemic illnesses such as typhoid, typhus, or malaria. The presence of buboes may suggest other forms of infectious lymphadenitis, including tularemia, syphilis, and lymphogranuloma venereum, as well as lymphadenitis of staphylococcal or streptococcal origin. Pneumonic plague must be distinguished from tularemic, pneumococcal, and other gram-negative pneumonias as well as from anthrax, psittacosis, and mycoplasma pneumonia. The consideration of epidemiologic factors, plus bacteriologic studies, will aid in the differentiation. Serologic diagnosis is of aid only for retrospective confirmation. When plague is suspected, it is imperative to begin treatment as soon as adequate specimens have been taken for culture because early institution of therapy is essential to ensure recovery. To delay treatment may risk toxemic death in the face of a bacteriologic cure.

Treatment When antibiotic treatment is instituted early in the course of the disease, the response is usually dramatic and complete. Even patients with pneumonic or septicemic disease can be cured if treatment is initiated within the first 15 to 20 hr after onset. Streptomycin and tetracycline are the drugs of choice. Streptomycin is given intramuscularly in doses of 0.5 g every 4 hr for 48 hr followed by 0.5 g every 6 hr for a total of 7 to 10 days or until the patient has been afebrile at least 3 days. Tetracyclines are given in initial doses of 2 to 3 g daily intravenously, and the dose is reduced to 2 g daily orally when improvement occurs. Chloramphenicol is also a potent antiplague agent and should be given in initial doses of 6 to 8 g daily intravenously (100 mg per kg) and the dose reduced to 3 g (50 to 75 mg per kg) daily orally for a total dose of 20 to 25 g. Sulfonamides are less effective, especially in pneumonic plague, and should be used only when the other agents are not available. Buboes are treated with hot, moist applications. Incision and drainage should be postponed until the lesion becomes well localized and the patient has been treated with antibiotics.

Control Prevention of plague must be directed toward elimination of endemic rodent foci, and in endemic urban areas constant vigilance is required in detecting and combating rodent epizootics. Prevention includes extermination of rats, eradication of ectoparasite vectors, and sometimes the immunization of the human population. Rats are attacked by poisoning and trapping, by elimination of harborage areas, and by separating them from their food supplies. Unfortunately, rodent control has proved to be most difficult in the endemic areas because of generally poor living standards. Vector control with DDT has been used with brilliant success in diminishing the flea population infecting both rodents and human beings, but recent studies in Southeast Asia show a significant incidence of DDT-resistant fleas; however, these may yield to other insecticides such as aldrin, dieldrin, and chlordane. The complete elimination of sylvatic plague appears to be impossible in the foreseeable future, and the control program must be aimed at eradicating foci of wild rodent infection around areas of human habitation. In these peripheral zones, the wild and the domestic rodents live commensally, exchange fleas, and threaten the human community.

Patients must be disinfested and carefully isolated, while other intimately exposed persons should be quarantined. Prophylaxis has been achieved effectively in the past by administering sulfadiazine in a dose of 3 g per day for 1 week. However, there is now significant in vitro resistance to sulfadiazine. Alternatively, prophylaxis with streptomycin in a dose of 1 g per day or with tetracycline is often effective.

Vaccines have been used for many years and apparently provide limited and transitory immunity. Three types of vaccines have been available. A Formalin-killed vaccine approved for use in the United States has been advised for all persons traveling to Vietnam, Cambodia, and Laos, for those whose vocations bring them into frequent and regular contact with wild rodents in plague enzootic areas, and for all laboratory personnel working with *Y. pestis* or with plague-infected rodents. Although the precise effectiveness of this vaccine has not been measured satisfactorily, it appears to reduce the incidence and severity of the disease. A second promising vaccine is a living attenuated strain of the organism which may be particularly suitable for endemic areas in Asia. Studies in the U.S.S.R. indicate that the attenuated vaccine administered by the aerosol route may be especially valuable in prevention of pneumonic plague. A third vaccine consisting of a chemical extract has been effective in experimental laboratory infections. Immunity is relative, and protection is not always conferred by the active disease, since a number of reinfections have been described. Although general vaccination may be worthwhile in an area threatened by an epidemic, the results are too slow for immediate prophylaxis. In such epidemic situations, combined use of all available control measures is indicated.

Prognosis The availability of effective antibiotic therapy has improved the prognosis in this formerly highly fatal disease. In the past the mortality rate of bubonic plague varied from 50 to 90 percent, and the pneumonic, septicemic, and meningitic forms were almost invariably fatal. In treated cases the mortality is 5 to 10 percent, and even the gravest varieties of infection respond to chemotherapy if treated early enough.

YERSINIA INFECTIONS (Y. PSEUDOTUBERCULOSIS AND Y. ENTEROCOLITICA)

Yersinia pseudotuberculosis is a gram-negative, non-spore-forming bacillus which is nonmotile at 37°C but usually motile at 22°C. It has frequently been identified as a pathogen in animals, especially rodents and birds, and now is increasingly being implicated as a cause of human disease.

The organisms have been identified as the cause of several hundred cases of mesenteric lymphadenitis in Europe, and, recently, similar cases have been found in the United States.

Human infection may present as a mild, benign, and usually self-limited form of mesenteric lymphadenitis or as a more severe and often fatal septicemia. Cervical and other nonmesenteric adenitides as well as erythema nodosum have also been described. Patients usually present the clinical picture of acute appendicitis with mid- or right-lower-quadrant abdominal pain, fever, and leukocytosis. At laparotomy, the appendix is usually normal, but large, inflamed, mesenteric lymph nodes are found, sometimes with associated terminal ileitis.

Diagnosis may be confirmed by culture of lymph nodes or by serologic titers, which have been reported in the range of 1:80 to 1:1,200 in clinical infections. Histologic examination of inflamed nodes has revealed reticulogranulocytic infiltration with or without small abscess formation.

Antibiotic treatment, especially indicated with sepsis, has been successful with streptomycin or tetracycline. Kanamycin and ampicillin have also been effective.

It is likely that *Y. pseudotuberculosis* will be more frequently identified as a cause of acute mesenteric lymphadenitis and terminal ileitis, when cultures and examination of mesenteric lymph nodes, as well as serologic testing, are carried out.

Yersinia entercolitica, a closely related organism, has also been associated with abdominal symptoms, including abdominal pain, fever, and diarrhea, and with a nonpurulent form of polyarthritis resembling rheumatic fever or Reiter's syndrome. Erythema nodosum has also been described.

PASTEURELLA MULTOCIDA INFECTION

Definition *Pasteurella multocida* (formerly *P. septica*) is a gram-negative nonsporulating bacillus which differs from *Yersinia* organisms in cultural characteristics, antibiotic sensitivity, and pattern of animal parasitism. For example, all strains of *P. multocida* are sensitive to penicillin. *Pasteurella multocida* is frequently identified as a commensal in cattle, horses, swine, sheep, fowl, dogs, cats, and rats, and on occasion causes hemorrhagic septicemia, or chronic pulmonary infiltrates, in these species. Human infection with *P. multocida* is uncommon and usually related to animal contact. Related species which have occasionally been identified as human pathogens include *P. urae*, *P. haemolytica*, and *P. pneumotropica*.

Manifestations Human disease due to *P. multocida* is usually a consequence of a dog or cat bite and appears as a localized wound infection with cellulitis, suppuration, and adenitis. Osteomyelitis sometimes ensues. Rarely, in patients with bronchiectasis, *P. multocida* is isolated from sputum, and animal handlers are sometimes identified as asymptomatic respiratory carriers. Empyema has occasionally been associated with the organisms. Bacteremia with fever and chills may develop after an animal bite, occasionally without an apparent local lesion. Meningitis, brain abscess, pyogenic arthritis, endocarditis, and pyelonephritis may occasionally complicate the bacteremia.

Not all *P. multocida* infections follow documented animal bites or animal contact.

Diagnosis Except for the association with animal (especially cat) bites, local infections with *P. multocida* show no unique characteristics, and may resemble cat-scratch fever, tularemia, or staphylococcal or streptococcal infection. Leukocytosis, uncommon in tularemia and cat-scratch fever, is the rule in *P. multocida* infection.

Gram stain of infected material shows pleomorphic gram-negative bacilli, usually extracellular. The bacteria may have bipolar staining and may be mistaken for gram-negative diplococci prior to cultural identification.

Treatment Penicillin in a dosage of 600,000 to 1,200,000 units daily is the preferred antibiotic, but a variety of other antibiotics may be effective.

REFERENCES

Plague

CAVANAUGH DC et al: Some observations on the current plague outbreak in the Republic of Vietnam. Am J Public Health 58:742, 1968

GILBERT DN et al: Potential medical problems in personnel returning from Vietnam. Ann Intern Med 68:662, 1968

GIRARD G: Plague. Annu Rev Microbiol 69:253, 1955

HIRST LF: *The Conquest of Plague: A Study of the Evolution of Epidemiology.* Fair Lawn, N.J.: Oxford, 1953

REED WB et al: Bubonic plague in the southwestern United States. Medicine 49:465, 1970

WHO EXPERT COMMITTEE ON PLAGUE: Fourth report, WHO Tech. Rept. Ser. 447, Geneva, 1970

P. Multocida

BEARN AG et al: *Pasteurella multocida* septicemia in man. Am J Med 18:167, 1955

MORRIS AJ et al: *Pasteurella multocida* and bronchiectasis. Bull Johns Hopkins Hosp 91:174, 1952

SWARTZ MN, KUNZ LJ: *Pasteurella multocida* infections in man: Report of two cases—meningitis and infected cat bite. N Engl J Med 261:888, 1959

Yersinia

ARVASTSON B et al: Clinical symptoms of infection with *Yersinia Enterocolitica.* Scand J Infect Dis 3:37, 1971

HUBERT WT et al: *Yersinia Pseudotuberculosis* infection in the United States: Septicemia, appendicitis and mesenteric lymphadenitis. Am J Trop Med 20:679, 1971

WEBER J et al: Mesenteric lymphadenitis and terminal ileitis due to *Yersinia Pseudotuberculosis.* N Engl J Med 283:172, 1970

143 MELIOIDOSIS AND GLANDERS

JAY P. SANFORD

MELIOIDOSIS Definition Melioidosis is a glanders-like infection of man and animals with a protean clinical spectrum. Melioidosis, which means "a resemblance to distemper of asses," bears a striking resemblance to glanders both clinically and pathologically, but is epidemiologically dissimilar.

Etiology Melioidosis is caused by a gram-negative motile bacillus, *Pseudomonas pseudomallei*, which can be differentiated from *Malleomyces mallei* by bacteriologic and serologic means. *Pseudomonas pseudomallei* (also known as Whitmore's bacillus, *Malleomyces pseudomallei*, or *Pfeifferella whitmori*) is a small, gram-negative, motile, aerobic bacillus. When stained with methylene blue, Wayson's, or Wright's stain, marked irregularities with a bipolar "safety pin" pattern are observed. It grows well on standard bacteriologic media with a characteristic wrinkling of colony surfaces after 48 to 72 hr of incubation.

Epidemiology The disease is endemic in Southeast Asia, with the greatest concentration of cases reported from Vietnam, Cambodia, Laos, Thailand, Malaysia, and Burma. Cases in human beings have also been reported from adjacent areas including India, Borneo, the Philippines, Guam, Indonesia, Ceylon, New Guinea, and North Queensland. Cases in man or animals have been reported from Madagascar, Chad, and Turkey. Human melioidosis has been described only rarely in the Western Hemisphere (Panama, Ecuador), and confirmed melioidosis has occurred in United States or European residents only when they have traveled in endemic areas. From April, 1965 through December, 1969, there have been 187 cases with 13 deaths reported in United States Army personnel who were or had been in Vietnam. Since that time through 1971, approximately three cases per month have been recorded. The majority of these cases occurred in individuals without intercurrent illness, although patients who sustained burn injuries in Vietnam account for a disproportionately high number of the cases.

Pseudomonas pseudomallei is a saprophyte which can be isolated from soil, stagnant streams, ponds, rice paddies, and market produce in endemic areas. Its ubiquitous nature is illustrated by its isolation as a laboratory contaminant. *Pseudomonas pseudomallei* is capable of causing disease in epizootic form among sheep, goats, swine, and horses. Occasional isolates have also been reported from cows, rodents, dogs, and cats. Although animals are susceptible to the disease, they apparently do not represent a reservoir for human disease. Attempts to culture *P. pseudomallei* from the urine and feces of a large variety of healthy animals have been unsuccessful. Arthropod-borne infection does not occur naturally. Man contracts melioidosis by soil contamination of skin abrasions. Ingestion, nasal instillation, or inhalation are other probable methods of spread. In contrast to glanders, infections have been uncommon in laboratory workers. Man-to-man transmission of melioidosis has not been documented, although the development of melioidosis in a 2-day-old newborn in Hawaii and demonstration of a significant antibody titer in a nurse who had never been in an endemic area but who had worked on wards with melioidosis patients raises the question of man-to-man spread within the hospital.

Pathology In acute infections, the majority of lesions occur in the lungs with occasional abscesses in other organs. In subacute infections, lung abscesses tend to be more extensive, and lesions are found throughout the body, in the skin, subcutaneous tissue, meninges, brain, eye, heart, liver, kidney, spleen, bone, and lymph nodes. The acute abscesses are characterized by an outer border of hemorrhage, a medial zone heavily infiltrated with polymorphonuclear leukocytes, and an inner core of necrotic debris containing large histiocytes with two or three nuclei that have been termed *giant cells.* As in glanders, a striking histologic feature has been the marked karyorrhexis. In chronic infections, the lesion consists of a central area of caseation necrosis, mononuclear and plasma cells, and granulation tissue. Calcification does not occur.

Clinical manifestations The clinical manifestations of melioidosis are variable. The illness can present as an acute, subacute, or chronic process. The incubation period has not been defined; however, based upon the development of infection following injury, it may be as short as 2 days. Following a laboratory accident, an incubation period of 3 days ensued. Clinically inapparent infections may remain latent for a number of years after an individual leaves an endemic area, with an interval of 9 years reported in one patient. Men are more often affected than women, a finding which is thought to represent occupational exposure. Melioidosis may be recognized as inapparent infection, asymptomatic pulmonary infiltration, acute localized suppurative infection, acute pulmonary infection, acute septicemic infection, or chronic suppurative infection.

INAPPARENT INFECTION In Thailand, Vietnam, and Malaysia, 6 to 8 percent of healthy adult men have significant antibody titers against *P. pseudomallei,* with the prevalence reaching 20 percent in a group of Army recruits from the rice-growing states of Western Malaysia. Only 1 percent of Thai women had positive reactions. None of the serums from a control group from the United States was positive. The prevalence of significant antibody titers has been reported as 2 percent for Europeans living in Vietnam and 1 to 2 percent in unselected patients in United States Army hospitals and in a group of normal uninjured soldiers who had served in Vietnam. Occasionally, asymptomatic infections have been discovered by routine chest x-ray.

ACUTE LOCALIZED SUPPURATIVE INFECTION Infection by inoculation of a break in the skin usually results in a nodule with an area of acute lymphangitis and regional lymphadenitis. There is usually fever and generalized malaise. This form of infection may rapidly progress to the acute septicemic form.

ACUTE PULMONARY INFECTION The most common form of the disease has been pulmonary infection, which may represent a primary pneumonitis or hematogenous spread. The acute pulmonary infection can vary in severity from a mild bronchitis to overwhelming necrotizing pneumonia. The onset may be abrupt without prodromal symptoms or more gradual with headache, anorexia, and generalized myalgia. Fever occurs in almost all patients, is often in excess of 102°F, and may be associated with rigors. Dull or pleuritic chest pain is common. Cough, with or without sputum, occurs. There may be mild pharyngitis. Tachypnea may be out of proportion to the fever and findings on physical or x-ray examination. Chest findings may be minimal but usually consist of rales in the area of pneumonitis. In the absence of dissemination, the spleen and liver are not palpable. Laboratory findings include total leukocyte counts ranging from normal to 20,000 per mm^3. Mild normochromic, normocytic anemia may appear during the illness. The pneumonia usually involves the upper lobes with the radiographic appearance of consolidation. Cavitation frequently occurs. Without specific therapy, the temperature may become normal within a few days; however, the upper lobe cavitation persists, resulting in a radiographic appearance of tuberculosis. In some instances there is progressive pulmonary spread or hematogenous dissemination with the development of septicemic manifestations.

ACUTE SEPTICEMIC INFECTION This is the form originally described primarily among narcotics addicts. Subsequent reports, however, have not shown a predilection for debilitated patients. The onset may be abrupt with the dominant symptoms depending upon site of major involvement. In individuals with bacteremia complicating pneumonitis, symptoms may include disorientation, extreme dyspnea, severe headache, pharyngitis, diarrhea, and development of cutaneous pustular lesions on the head, trunk, or extremities. There is high fever, extreme tachypnea, a flushed skin, and cyanosis. Muscle tenderness may be striking. On examination of the chest, signs may be absent or rales, rhonchi, and pleural rubs may be heard. The liver and spleen may be palpable. Signs of arthritis or meningitis may appear. Patients with the septicemic form usually have a rapidly progressive fatal course which in some instances may be too fulminant to be altered by therapy. The leukocyte count may be normal or slightly increased. Chest radiographs most commonly show irregular nodular densities 4 to 10 mm in diameter disseminated throughout the lungs. These enlarge, coalesce, and often undergo cavitation as the disease progresses. Pleural effusion is rare. Other radiographic patterns include unilateral irregular mottled densities which become confluent.

CHRONIC SUPPURATIVE INFECTION In some patients secondary abscesses develop which dominate the clinical picture. Organs involved include skin, brain, lung, myocardium, liver, spleen, bones, joints, lymph nodes, and even the eye. These patients may be afebrile.

RECRUDESCENT INFECTION Disease may present as acute localized suppurative, acute pulmonary, acute septicemic, or chronic suppurative infection remote from the probable time of exposure (up to 9 years having been reported). In 6 of 10 reported cases, surgery, trauma, or intercurrent illness appeared to act as triggering events.

Diagnosis Melioidosis should be considered in the differential diagnosis of any febrile illness in an individual who has been in an endemic area, especially if the presenting features are those of fulminant respiratory failure, if multiple pustular or necrotic skin or subcutaneous lesions develop, or if there is a radiographic pattern of tuberculosis in a patient from whom tubercle bacilli cannot be isolated.

Microscopic examination of exudates will reveal poorly staining, small, gram-negative bacilli which show the characteristic staining irregularities and "safety pin" bipolar staining with methylene blue. *Pseudomonas pseudomallei* will grow on most laboratory media, including eosin-methylene blue agar (EMB) or MacConkey's agar, in 24 to 48 hr. The organisms can be readily differentiated from *M. mallei* and *P. aeruginosa* by standard bacteriologic procedures. The characteristic wrinkling of the colonies may require 72 hr or longer. The hemagglutination, direct agglutination test, and complement fixation test are an aid in diagnosis if a fourfold or greater rise in titer is demonstrated in paired serums. Single low titers are difficult to interpret because of nonspecific responses. The complement fixation test is said to be specific with titers above 1:8 during the acute illness, but may cross-react with *M. mallei.* A negative complement fixation test does not exclude disease. The hemagglutination and agglutination tests show more cross-reactions. Titers of 1:40 or more suggest infection.

Treatment The treatment regimen should vary with the form of the disease. Individuals with low-titer positive serologic tests but with no clinical evidence of infection do not require therapy. The choice of antibiotics in active infection should be based upon sensitivity studies, and therapy should be given for a minimum of 30 days. *Pseudomonas pseudomallei* is usually sensitive in vitro to the tetracyclines, chloramphenicol, novobiocin, kanamycin, sulfadiazine or sulfisoxazole, and trimethoprim-sulfamethoxazole, and in most instances is resistant to penicillin G, ampicillin, carbenicillin, dicloxacillin, streptomycin, gentamicin, cephalosporins, vancomycin, lincomycin, rifampin, nalidixic acid, and colistin. In patients with pneumonitis or chronic suppurative lesions who are not too ill, effective therapy has included tetracycline, 2 to 3 g daily (40 mg per kg); chloramphenicol, 3 g daily (40 mg per kg); or sulfisoxazole, 4 g daily (70 mg per kg). If the patient is severely ill, two of these antimicrobials in combination have been recommended for 30 days followed by another 30 to 60 days of tetracycline alone. In patients with extrapulmonary suppurative lesions, prolonged therapy for 6 months to 1 year should be considered. In addition, the usual principles of surgical drainage should be followed. In desperately ill patients with severe pneumonitis or the septicemic form of melioidosis, multiple antibiotics should be administered by the parenteral route. One such regimen has included the use of chloramphenicol, 12 g per day; novobiocin, 6 g per day; and kanamycin, 4 g per day. In view of the severe potential toxicity of this regimen, its use should be considered only in extremely ill patients, and then only on a short-term basis. Current recommendations for antibiotics in the septicemic form of melioidosis are tetracycline, 4 to 6 g per day (80 mg per kg); chloramphenicol, 4 to 6 g per day (80 mg per kg); and one of the following: sulfisoxazole (140 mg per kg), kanamycin (30 mg per kg), or novobiocin (60 mg per kg). In vitro studies have revealed antagonism between the following pairs of drugs: chloramphenicol-kanamycin; tetracycline-kanamycin; and sulfadiazine-chloramphenicol. While the significance of such antagonism in clinical therapy has not been assessed, the data would favor selection of novobiocin as the third drug. The dosage should be tapered rapidly as clinical improvement occurs.

Prognosis Prior to antimicrobials, the mortality of apparent infection was 95 percent. With better diagnosis and more prolonged appropriate therapy, the mortality in all except the septicemic form is low. Even with vigorous appropriate antibiotics and supportive therapy, the mortality rate in patients with melioidosis septicemia is greater than 50 percent. Very few patients have had long-term follow-up, and the incidence of late relapses cannot be predicted.

Prevention There is no means of active immunization. In endemic areas, vigorous cleansing of abrasions and lacerations is recommended.

GLANDERS

Definition Glanders is a serious infection of equine animals caused by *M. mallei,* which is transmitted occasionally to other domestic animals and to man.

Etiology *Malleomyces mallei* is a small, slender, nonmotile, gram-negative bacillus. When stained with methylene blue, marked irregularities in staining are observed. Organisms grow on most common meat infusion media, but require glycerol for optimum growth.

Epidemiology Glanders was at one time widespread throughout Europe, but owing to the introduction of control measures, its incidence has decreased steadily in most countries. The disease still occurs in Asia, Africa, and South America, but not in the United States. Glanders has never been common in man; the occasional infection, however, may be very serious. There have been no naturally acquired infections in the United States since 1938, but with increasing international travel, patients with glanders may be encountered.

Glanders is primarily a disease of horses, mules, and donkeys, although goats, sheep, cats, and dogs sometimes naturally contract the disease. Pigs and cattle are said to be absolutely resistant. In horses, the disease may be systemic with prominent pulmonary involvement, *glan-*

ders, or may be characterized by subcutaneous ulcerative lesions, and lymphatic thickening with nodules, *farcy*. The route of infection in animals remains controversial; inhalation, ingestion, and inoculation through breaks in the skin have been suggested. In man, the disease occurs primarily in individuals with close contact with horses, mules, or donkeys through inoculation of or a break in the skin or by exposing the nasal mucosa to contaminated discharges. A number of instances of airborne infection have been reported in laboratory workers.

Pathology The acute lesion is characterized by nodules consisting of polymorphonuclear leukocytes surrounded by a zone of congestion. A characteristic histologic feature is a peculiar nuclear degeneration known as *chromatotexis* which occurs early and is extensive. Small foci of deeply staining detritus within the abscess result from this degeneration. In older nodules, the reaction is characterized by epithelioid cells surrounding an area of central necrosis. Giant cells may be present. Virtually any organ may be involved.

Clinical manifestations The manifestations which frequently overlap may be categorized as (1) acute localized suppurative infection, (2) acute pulmonary infection, (3) acute septicemic infection, and (4) chronic suppurative infection. Nearly 60 percent of patients have been between the ages of 20 and 40 years. The disease has been rare in women, probably because of less opportunity for contact.

Infection acquired by inoculation through an abrasion in the skin usually results in a nodule with an area of acute lymphangitis. The incubation period is probably 1 to 5 days. In all types of acute glanders, there is usually fever, generalized malaise, and prostration.

Infection of the mucous membranes may result in a mucopurulent discharge involving the eye, nose, or lips followed by extensive ulcerating granulomatous lesions which may or may not be associated with systemic reactions. With systemic invasion, a generalized papular eruption which may become pustular is frequent. This septicemic form of disease is usually fatal in 7 to 10 days.

Infection by inhalation is followed by an incubation period of 10 to 14 days. The more common symptoms include fever, occasionally associated with rigors, generalized myalgia, fatigue, headache, and pleuritic chest pain. Other symptoms consist of photophobia, lacrimation, and diarrhea. Examination is usually normal except for fever and occasional lymphadenopathy, especially in the cervical chain, and splenomegaly. Laboratory findings include mild leukocytosis with 60 to 80 percent neutrophilic leukocytes, but leukopenia with relative lymphocytosis has been recorded. In the acute pulmonary form, chest radiographs characteristically reveal circumscribed densities which suggest early lung abscesses. Other findings may include lobar or bronchopneumonia. In the chronic suppurative form of the disease, the most frequent finding is multiple subcutaneous and intramuscular abscesses which most often involve the arms or legs. Approximately one-half of the patients will have associated fever, lymphadenopathy, and nasal discharge or ulceration. Visceral involvement including pulmonary or pleural, ocular, skeletal, hepatic, splenic, and meningeal or intracranial involvement occurred in some patients.

Diagnosis Microscopic examination of exudates may reveal small gram-negative bacilli which stain irregularly with methylene blue; however, organisms generally are very scanty, and it is often difficult to find them even in acute abscesses. Giemsa or other modifications of the Romanowski stain may be the best way to identify organisms. *Malleomyces mallei* and *P. pseudomallei* cannot be distinguished morphologically from one another. Culturing is often avoided because of the hazard to laboratory personnel; however, if cultures are made, growth occurs on most meat infusion nutrient media. The material is often contaminated with other microorganisms, and incubation with penicillin G (1,000 units per ml) prior to culturing may be helpful. Subcutaneous inoculation of material into a guinea pig or hamster affords an alternative means of isolation. Blood cultures are usually negative except in the terminal stages of disease. Serologic tests show a rapidly rising agglutination titer, which reaches levels of 1:640 within 2 weeks. Serum from normal persons has been reported to show agglutination titers in dilutions up to 1:320. The complement fixation test is less sensitive but more specific and usually becomes positive during the third week; it is considered positive in dilutions of 1:20 or greater. The mallein skin test is of help diagnostically; 0.1 ml of a 1:10,000 dilution of commercial mallein is injected intradermally. Erythema exceeding 10 mm in 48 hr is considered to represent a specific test. The test becomes positive in most patients by the third or fourth week of disease and remains positive for years.

Treatment The limited number of infections in man has precluded evaluation of most of the antibiotic agents. Sulfadiazine has been found to be an effective agent in experimental animals and in man. The dosage utilized has been approximately 100 mg per kg administered in divided doses. In experimental infections, 3 weeks of therapy gave better results than 1 week. Benzyl penicillin is ineffective in vitro and in experimental infections. Streptomycin is bacteriostatic in vitro but was ineffective in experimental infections in hamsters. Broad-spectrum antibiotics such as tetracycline, chloramphenicol, and kanamycin have not been evaluated. In the acute infections, appropriate supportive measures are essential, and in chronic suppurative infections, the usual principles of surgical drainage should be followed.

Prognosis The prognosis depends upon the type of infection. The acute septicemic form has been uniformly fatal. The localized or chronic forms have a much better prognosis.

Prevention Next to acquisition from diseased horses, the commonest source of natural disease in man has been contact with human glanders. Isolation is indicated.

REFERENCES

EICKHOFF TC et al: Pseudomonas pseudomallei: Susceptibility to chemotherapeutic agents. J Infect Dis 121:95, 1970

HOWE C, MILLER WR: Human glanders: Report of six cases. Ann Intern Med 26:93, 1947

——et al: The pseudomallei group: A review. J Infect Dis 124:598, 1971

JACKSON AE et al: Recrudescent melioidosis associated with diabetic ketoacidosis. Arch Intern Med 130:268, 1972

KISHIMOTO RA et al: Melioidosis: Serologic studies on U.S. Army personnel returning from Southeast Asia. Milit Med 136:694, 1971

SPOTNITZ M et al: Melioidosis pneumonitis. JAMA 202:950, 1967

144
VIBRIO FETUS INFECTIONS

MARVIN TURCK

DEFINITION *Vibrio fetus* infection is economically the most important cause of infectious abortion in cattle. In man, this organism may be associated with obscure febrile illnesses, subacute bacterial endocarditis, meningoencephalitis, and perhaps abortion.

ETIOLOGY *Vibrio fetus* is a motile, comma-shaped or spirillar, gram-negative rod with a single unipolar flagellum. It is best identified by its appearance in smears made from cultured material. The organism is slow-growing and microaerophilic, and grows best in liquid media incubated under increased CO_2 tension. Several serotypes have been isolated by agglutination with antiserums from human and bovine strains. Cross-agglutination reactions occur with other bacterial species, particularly *Brucella abortus.*

EPIDEMIOLOGY AND PATHOGENESIS Vibriosis is a venereal infection of cattle, sheep, and goats; when transmitted to gravid heifers or ewes, it results in abortion. The male acts as an asymptomatic carrier of the infection, and the organism has been isolated from the genitalia and semen of bulls. Although vibriosis has been thought to occur only rarely in man, reports of this disease are appearing with increasing frequency. Vibriosis in man may result from direct contact with the organism, as happens in laboratory-acquired infection, or from direct contact with infected cattle. Food and water have been implicated, without convincing evidence, as vehicles for infection. The mouth has been postulated as a portal of entry because cases of *V. fetus* endocarditis have followed dental extractions. Because *V. fetus* has been isolated from several aborted fetuses and has been the cause of neonatal meningitis, a venereal route of infection has been postulated. It is presumed that, as in cattle, the male acts as an asymptomatic carrier who transmits the infection to a pregnant partner. The relation of *V. fetus* to prematurity, abortion, and neonatal meningitis requires further documentation. In most instances of vibriosis, the portal of entry is not known.

MANIFESTATIONS Fever is the only characteristic sign of vibriosis in adults, and may be relapsing in character. Thrombophlebitis involving both arms and legs is not uncommon. The disease may also present as classic subacute bacterial endocarditis; septic arthritis or osteomyelitis; chronic, indolent meningoencephalitis; and fever and abortion in pregnant women. A number of patients have had coexisting disease, including cirrhosis, cardiac amyloidosis, and chronic lymphatic leukemia, or antecedent gastric surgery. Several neonates with fulminating, lethal meningoencephalitis have been reported. It has been postulated that infection was transmitted to these infants via the placenta. A mild, self-limited diarrheal disease in which vibrios closely related but not identical to *V. fetus* have been isolated from the stool has also been reported in infants.

DIAGNOSIS Lack of awareness of vibriosis by both the bacteriologist and the clinician has resulted in mistaken diagnosis in most instances. The organisms have been erroneously described as "fastidious strains of *Hemophilus.*" Recovery of spirillar organisms in blood cultures should suggest the diagnosis because other spirochetes causing relapsing fever usually do not grow in artificial media. Failure to incubate blood cultures under increased CO_2 tensions may delay growth. Identification of the organisms in smears of cultures is the only definitive method of making the diagnosis, which should then be confirmed by agglutinating the vibrios with specific antiserums. Complement-fixing antibody may be present in high titers in the active phase of the disease. Clinically, vibriosis should be suspected in obscure febrile illnesses associated with thrombophlebitis or abortion and premature delivery in pregnant women.

TREATMENT There are few reports of antibiotic sensitivity of the organisms, and various antibiotics, alone or in combination, have been used. A 10-day course of tetracycline or chloramphenicol in dosage of 2.0 g per day, alone or coupled with streptomycin, 1.0 g per day, should eradicate the organisms in most instances. In cases of endocarditis antimicrobial therapy should be extended to 6 weeks. Kanamycin and erythromycin have also been effective in vitro. Penicillin, novobiocin, vancomycin, and polymyxin B are ineffective.

REFERENCES

KILO C et al: Septic arthritis and bacteremia due to vibrio fetus: Report of unusual case and review of literature. Am J Med 38:962, 1965

LAWRENCE GD et al: Infection caused by vibrio fetus. Arch Intern Med 120:459, 1967

RUBEN FL, WOLINSKY E: Human infection with vibrio fetus. Antimicrob Agents Chemother 1967–1968, p. 143

WHITE WD: Human vibriosis: Indigenous cases in England. Br Med J 2:283, 1967

145
STREPTOBACILLUS MONILIFORMIS INFECTION

ROGER BULGER

DEFINITION *Streptobacillus moniliformis* is a gram-negative organism which can produce an acute febrile disease, characterized by skin and joint manifestations, and, rarely, leading to endocarditis. Most recently cases of *Strep. moniliformis* infection have been associated with the bite of a rat and may be designated as "rat-bite fever," a term which also refers to infections with *Spirillum minus* (Chap. 163).

ETIOLOGY AND EPIDEMIOLOGY *Streptobacillus moniliformis* is a pleomorphic, microaerophilic, gram-negative bacterium, which may yield long, filamentous forms or chains of beaded or fusiform bacilli when grown on artificial media. Although primary isolation is best achieved in specialized fluid media, precise bacteriologic diagnosis is often delayed because isolation from routine blood cultures may require from 2 to 7 days of incubation.

This organism has an unusual capacity to produce stable L-forms during routine growth of the bacterial phase; these L-forms can be maintained in pure culture indefinitely and then may revert to the bacterial phase. The L-form has been isolated from the blood of man as long as 10 weeks after the onset of infection.

In some studies, *Strep. moniliformis* has been isolated from the nasopharynx of as many as half of the rats investigated. Human infection most often follows exposure to wild rats, but cases have also been reported following bites by a variety of other rodents. Three cases have been traced to bites by laboratory rats in a single institution within a 6-month period, making this disease an important consideration in febrile illnesses among laboratory workers.

Strep. moniliformis infection has occurred in epidemic proportions in association with ingestion of contaminated food or milk. The outbreak which occurred in 1926 at Haverhill, Massachusetts is the most famous of these; it involved 86 persons, was related to contamination of raw milk or ice cream with streptobacilli, and led to the disease becoming known as *Haverhill fever* when it is not associated with a rodent bite. Turkeys are also widely infested with streptobacilli, presumably secondary to rat bites, suggesting other potential sources for human infection.

CLINICAL MANIFESTATIONS The incubation period is short, usually 1 to 2 days, although extremes have been described ranging from a few hours to 22 days. The onset of disease is sudden, and may resemble a viral syndrome, with fever, headache, myalgia, malaise, and occasionally vomiting. Chills occur in more than half the patients. Usually the local puncture site will be healed, but it may be ulcerated with associated regional lymphadenopathy.

A discrete macular rash which fades on pressure develops in 75 to 80 percent of the patients 1 to 3 days after the onset of symptoms. This rash is most marked on the extremities, often involving the palms and soles, but may become generalized. In some patients, the cutaneous lesions become purpuric and may become pustular, confluent, or papular.

Involvement of multiple joints appears in about half the patients during the first week. Large joints are usually involved, asymmetrically, but fingers and toes may also be affected. The joint involvement may simply be an arthralgia, but arthritis is also common, particularly affecting the knees; swelling, heat, redness, and effusion may be present.

Clinical signs and symptoms usually regress after 1 to 2 weeks, although without appropriate antimicrobial therapy convalescence may be prolonged because of recurrent fever and arthritis. Abscesses in the brain or other tissues have been rare but serious complications. Bacterial endocarditis is the most feared and potentially fatal complication. Fortunately, it is rare; only 1 of the 337 cases of bacterial endocarditis at the Boston City Hospital during 12 selected years between 1933 and 1965 was due to streptobacillus.

When the infection is food-borne, its clinical manifestations are the same except for the absence of the local lesions.

LABORATORY FINDINGS The blood leukocyte count ranges from 6,000 to 30,000 per mm^3, with an average of only 12,000. Although the total count may be below 10,000, there is usually an increase in the proportion of polymorphonuclear neutrophils with a shift to the left. The organism can usually be isolated from the blood, joint fluid, or pus during the acute febrile phase, but often only after prolonged incubation and occasionally for 1 to 2 weeks after subsidence of fever. Agglutinins against the organism develop during the second or third week and are of diagnostic importance if an increase in titer is demonstrated.

DIFFERENTIAL DIAGNOSIS Infection due to *Strep. moniliformis* must be differentiated from that due to *Spirillum minus* because both occur following rat bites (Chap. 163). Although the manifestations of these two infections can be remarkably similar, the clinical presentations are fairly characteristic of one or the other. The characteristics of *Strep. moniliformis* infections are as follows: Latent period usually less than 10 days; prompt healing of the bite site without flare-up at the onset of systemic symptoms; sudden onset of chills and fever followed by a macular rash on the palms and soles; and a high incidence of arthralgias and arthritis; a relapsing febrile course is uncommon. Infections caused by *spirillum minus* tend to have the following characteristics: Prolonged latent period (from 1 to 4 weeks); recurrence of a marked inflammatory response at the site of the rat bite and lymphangitis accompanying the onset of systemic symptoms; sudden onset of fever usually without joint symptoms and often without skin lesions; commonly, a relapsing febrile course.

A clinical picture of sudden onset of fever, nausea, vomiting, myalgias, arthralgias, macular purpuric rash, minimal leukocyte response, and a lack of a focus of infection should also suggest infection with *Rickettsia rickettsi* or Coxsackie B virus.

Streptobacillus moniliformis infection must also be

differentiated from other forms of acute infectious arthritis, rheumatic fever, and meningococcemia.

TREATMENT AND PROGNOSIS Before effective antimicrobial therapy was available, the mortality rate in cases of *Strep. moniliformis* infection was approximately 10 percent; death usually was associated with the development of bacterial endocarditis. Prompt treatment with an effective antimicrobial agent should prevent fatalities due to this infection.

A suitable dosage schedule for the most infections is 1,200,000 units procaine penicillin intramuscularly or 2 g penicillin V orally in divided doses for 7 to 10 days. Erythromycin is acceptable as an alternative in patients with penicillin allergy.

REFERENCES

Cole JS et al: Rat-bite fever. Ann Intern Med 71:979, 1969

McCormack RC et al: Endocarditis due to *Streptobacillus moniliformis*. JAMA 200:77, 1967

Roughgarden JW: Antimicrobial therapy of rat-bite fever: A review. Arch Intern Med 116:39, 1965

Wilson GS, Miles AA: *Topley and Wilson's Principles of Bacteriology and Immunity*, Baltimore: Williams & Wilkins, 1964, p. 1128

146 BARTONELLOSIS

JAMES J. PLORDE

DEFINITION Bartonellosis (Carrión's disease) is an infection with *Bartonella bacilliformis*. Two well-defined clinical stages occur: an acute febrile anemia of rapid onset and high mortality, designated *Oroya fever*, and a benign eruptive form with chronic cutaneous lesions, called *verruga peruana*. Either of these types may be mild, and asymptomatic cases constitute the greatest epidemiologic hazard.

ETIOLOGY *Bartonella bacilliformis* is a small, motile, aerobic, pleomorphic, gram-negative bacillus which stains reddish violet with Giemsa's stain. It can be cultured on enriched media and does not produce a hemolysin. The organisms are sensitive to several antibiotics in vitro.

EPIDEMIOLOGY The disease is limited to certain valleys in the Andes Mountains comprising parts of Peru, Ecuador, and Colombia. It occurs in regions between the altitudes of 2,400 and 8,000 ft where the sandfly vector, *Phlebotomus*, propagates. Although only *P. verrucarum* has been shown to transmit the disease, other species are undoubtedly involved. Asymptomatic cases and convalescent carriers are the only known reservoir of infection. A low-grade bacteremia may persist for years following resolution of symptoms, and *B. bacilliformis* can be recovered from the blood of 5 to 10 percent of the apparently normal population in an endemic area. Epidemics often coincide with immigration of workers from uninfected areas.

PATHOLOGY AND PATHOGENESIS The manifestations of the disease are thought to reflect the immune status of the host. In nonimmune individuals Oroya fever develops. Large numbers of the *Bartonella* bacteria enter the bloodstream, adhere to erythrocytes, and invade the endothelial cells of the capillaries and lymphatics. The presence of the organisms on the surface of the red cell results in their phagocytosis and destruction by the liver and spleen. The red cell life span is greatly shortened, and anemia develops. This is accentuated by a defective erythropoietic response early in the course of infection. The pathogenesis of the hemolytic anemia remains unknown. Agglutinins and hemolysins have not been found, and tests for mechanical fragility of red cells have given variable results. Invasion and swelling of capillary endothelial cells may lead to vascular occlusion and tissue infarcts. It is possible that an impairment of reticuloendothelial function secondary to massive phagocytosis of red cells is responsible for the frequency with which *Salmonella* and other coliform bacteremias are seen in Oroya fever.

With developing immunity, the bacteria nearly disappear from the peripheral blood and capillary endothelium. After a latent period they reappear in the skin and subcutaneous tissue where they are apparently responsible for the development of the hemangioid lesions of verruga peruana. Second attacks of Carrión's disease are very unusual. When they occur, they almost invariably present as verruga.

CLINICAL MANIFESTATIONS The incubation period is approximately three weeks but may be longer. The initial symptoms are fever and pains in the bones, joints, and muscles. At this point the disease often resembles influenza or malaria, but blood cultures are positive. After these prodromes, the patient usually develops one of the two classic forms of the infection.

Oroya fever This form is characterized by sudden onset of high fever, extreme pallor, weakness, and a precipitous drop in the number of red blood cells. The count may fall from normal to 1 million per mm^3 within 4 or 5 days. The anemia is characterized by normochromic macrocytes in the peripheral blood, striking polychromasia and polychromatophilia, nucleated red cells, Howell-Jolly bodies, Cabot rings, and basophilic stippling. There may also be a mild leukocytosis with a shift to the left. Organisms are numerous in the blood, and stained smears may show 90 percent of the erythrocytes heavily invaded. Salmonellosis, malaria, amebiasis, tuberculosis, and other intercurrent infections may occur and are an important factor in fatal cases.

Muscle and joint pain and headache are severe, and insomnia, delirium, and coma are the terminal manifestations. In untreated patients, mortality may exceed 50 percent; death occurs within 10 days to 4 weeks. With treatment, or sometimes spontaneously, recovery results if the organisms decrease and fever abates. The red cell count stabilizes and approaches normal values in about 6 weeks, when convalescence begins.

Verruga peruana This form of the disease, characterized by a profuse skin eruption, may follow the anemic form or may occur in patients without previous symptoms. The verrugas vary in color from red to purple. They may be miliary, nodular, or eroding, and they range in size from 2 to 10 mm up to 3 or 4 cm in diameter. The three types of verrugas may occur together; since eruption takes place in successive crops, verrugas of all types and in all stages of development may be found on the same patient. The chief sites involved are the limbs and face, and less frequently the genitalia, scalp, and mucosa of the mouth and pharynx. They may persist for 1 month to 2 years. The eruption is accompanied by pain, fever, and moderate anemia. Bartonellas may be demonstrated in the lesions and cultured from the blood.

DIAGNOSIS A clinical diagnosis can be made with accuracy in endemic areas. During Oroya fever the organism is easily seen on peripheral blood smears. It may be recovered from blood cultures in all stages of the disease.

TREATMENT Oroya fever responds dramatically to a number of antibiotics including tetracycline and chloramphenicol. The latter in a dose of 2 g per day for 7 days is often preferred because of the frequency with which *Salmonella* infections complicate this disease. Fever disappears within 48 hr and the patient recovers rapidly. Transfusions may be required when the anemia is severe. Antibiotic therapy of the verrugal stage may hasten the involution of these lesions. The use of DDT in both the interior and exterior of human dwellings is highly effective in controlling the night-biting sandflies. Insect repellents and bed netting afford personal protection.

REFERENCES

CAUDRA MC: Salmonellosis complication in human bartonellosis. Tex Rep Biol Med 14:97, 1956

KAYE D et al: Factors influencing host resistance to salmonella infections: The effects of hemolysis and erythophagocytosis. Am J Med Sci 254:205, 1967

RICKETTS WE: Clinical manifestations of Carrión's disease. AMA Arch Intern Med 84:751, 1949

SCHULTZ MG: Daniel Carrión's experiment. N Engl J Med 278:1323, 1968

URETEAGA OB, PAYNE EH: Treatment of the acute febrile phase of Carrión's disease with chloramphenicol. Am J Trop Med 4:507, 1955

WEINMAN D: The bartonella group, in *Bacterial and Mycotic Infections of Man,* eds RJ Dubos, JG Hirsch, 4th ed., Philadelphia: Lippincott, 1965, p. 775

147 GRANULOMA INGUINALE

KING K. HOLMES

DEFINITION Granuloma inguinale is a mildly contagious, chronic, indolent, progressive, autoinoculable, ulcerative disease involving the skin and lymphatics of the genital or perianal areas. The disease may be sexually transmitted and is associated with the presence in affected tissues of an intracellular microorganism, identified morphologically as the Donovan body.

ETIOLOGY Granuloma inguinale was described by McLeod in India in 1882, and in 1905 Donovan described the intracellular bodies which are thought to cause the disease. Granuloma inguinale has been reproduced in humans by inoculation of pus containing Donovan bodies but no other bacteria. Similar attempts to reproduce the disease in experimental animals have been unsuccessful. Encapsulated bacteria resembling Donovan bodies have repeatedly been recovered from lesions and pseudobuboes of granuloma inguinale by inoculation of chick embryo yolk sacs or yolk-agar medium. These bacteria, which are known as *Calymmatobacterium granulomatis*, are antigenically related to *Klebsiella* species but do not reproduce the disease when inoculated intradermally in humans. It is uncertain whether these bacteria are responsible for the disease or represent secondary invaders. Similar bacteria have been isolated from feces. Recent electron microscopic studies of Donovan bodies confirm their morphologic resemblance to gram-negative bacteria and show bacteriophage attached to the bacterial cells.

EPIDEMIOLOGY Granuloma inguinale is endemic in the tropics, particularly in New Guinea and among Hindus in India. In the United States, only 103 cases were reported in 1971. Most cases occur in the southeastern states and involve male homosexuals. The disease is uncommon in Caucasians. The role of sexual transmission is unclear, since the reported frequency of granuloma inguinale in conjugal partners of chronically infected patients ranges from 1 to 64 percent. The predilection for anorectal infection in male homosexuals, together with the reported isolation of *Calymmatobacterium granulomatis* from feces, suggests an intestinal source of contamination in some cases.

CLINICAL MANIFESTATIONS The incubation period is uncertain but appears to range from 8 days to 12 weeks. Following experimental inoculation, a typical ulcerative lesion develops within 50 days.

Granuloma inguinale begins as a papule, which ulcerates and develops into a painless elevated zone of clean, beefy-red, friable granulation tissue. The edges are irregular and spread by continuity or by autoinoculation of approximated skin surfaces. Secondary anaerobic infection may produce pain and a foul-smelling exudate. In men, the lesions are usually located on the glans, prepuce, or shaft of the penis, or the perianal area, while infection of the labia is most common in women. The chronicity of the disease is of diagnostic importance, since several months often elapse before patients seek treatment. Extension to the inguinal region by autoinoculation or via the lymphatics results in diffuse intradermal and subcutaneous swelling or suppuration, known as "pseudobubo," because involvement of the underlying lymph nodes is minimal. Locally destructive lesions and secondary infection may produce severe morbidity or death. Fatal disseminated disease, involving the bones or joints, has been reported after several years of chronic local infection. The relationship of granuloma inguinale to subsequent carcinoma of the genitalia is uncertain.

DIAGNOSIS Granuloma inguinale of the penis, labia, cervix, or perianal region may be mistaken for carcinoma. Epithelial proliferation resembling neoplasia in the genital region in a young subject should always raise the suspicion of granuloma inguinale. Histologic studies in granuloma inguinale reveal marked acanthosis and pseudoepitheliomatous hyperplasia. Because Donovan bodies are seldom detectable in sections stained with hematoxylin and eosin, these changes may lead to an erroneous diagnosis of carcinoma and to unnecessary, destructive surgery. Although silver impregnation techniques are useful for demonstration of Donovan bodies in sections, the diagnosis is best made by examination of a specimen obtained by punch biopsy from the periphery of a lesion; the deep portion of the specimen is removed, crushed between two slides, air dried, and stained with Wright-Giemsa stain. With this method, Donovan bodies appear as very rounded coccobacilli, 1 by 2 μm in size, which lie within cystic spaces in the cytoplasm of large mononuclear cells. The capsule stains as a dense acidophilic zone surrounding the bipolar basophilic bacterium, which resembles a closed safety pin. The pathognomonic mononuclear cell is 25 to 90 μm in diameter and has many cystic areas containing Donovan bodies.

Perianal granuloma inguinale may resemble condylomata lata of secondary syphilis. Other venereal diseases, particularly syphilis, very frequently coexist with granuloma inguinale. Repeated dark-field examinations of lesions before treatment and a serologic test for syphilis should therefore be performed.

TREATMENT The treatment of choice is tetracycline, 2 g daily, continued for at least 10 days, or until healing occurs. Healing is usually complete within 3 weeks. If tetracycline cannot be given, streptomycin may be used in a dose of 1 g intramuscularly every 12 hr for 10 to 15 days.

REFERENCES

Beerman H, Sonck CE: The epithelial changes in granuloma inguinale. Am J Syph Gonor Vener Dis 36:501, 1952

Davis CM: Granuloma inguinale. A clinical, histological, and ultrastructural study. JAMA 211:632, 1970

Lal S: Continued efficacy of streptomycin in the treatment of granuloma inguinale. Br J Vener Dis 47:454, 1971

——, Nicholas C: Epidemiological and clinical features in 165 cases of granuloma inguinale. Br J Vener Dis 46:461, 1970

U.S. Public Health Service: Management of chancroid, granuloma inguinale, lymphogranuloma venereum in general practice. USPHS Publ. 255:15, 1964

section 7 | Miscellaneous bacterial diseases

148 ANTHRAX

LEIGHTON E. CLUFF

DEFINITION Anthrax (also called malignant pustule, charbon, splenic fever, milzbrand, woolsorters' disease) is a disease of wild and domesticated animals that is transmitted to man by contact with infected animals or their products and, rarely, by insect vectors which act as mechanical carriers of the etiologic organism. The characteristic lesion of human anthrax is a necrotic cutaneous ulcer, the *malignant pustule.*

HISTORY The classic studies of Robert Koch in 1877, showing that *Bacillus anthracis* was the cause of anthrax, serve as the prototype for the establishment of causation of infectious diseases.

ETIOLOGY *Bacillus anthracis* is a large, encapsulated, gram-positive, aerobic, spore-forming microorganism that grows well in most nutrient media. Its pathogenicity for laboratory animals differentiates it from *Bacillus subtilis,* which it closely resembles. The spores are killed by boiling for 10 min but can survive for many years in soil and animal products, an important factor in persistence and spread of the disease. The anthrax bacillus possesses a capsule of glutamyl polypeptide, which interferes with phagocytosis of the microorganism. In addition, it contains an anticomplementary substance and elaborates a "protective" antigen and a toxin which is probably of importance in determining virulence.

EPIDEMIOLOGY Anthrax is worldwide; repeated outbreaks have occurred in Southern Europe, Africa, Australia, Asia, and on both American continents.

Cattle, horses, sheep, goats, and swine are most commonly infected. There have been outbreaks of anthrax among animals in the United States, centering mostly in South Dakota, Nebraska, Arkansas, Mississippi, Louisiana, Texas, and California. The disease tends to occur in animals in late summer and early fall.

The disease in man is acquired by butchering, skinning, or dissecting infected carcasses or by handling contaminated hides, wool, hair, or other materials. It is seen principally in agricultural and industrial employees. The majority of cases of human anthrax involves workers handling imported and unprocessed wool, hair, or hides. The disease usually follows inoculation of bacilli or spores into the skin, often through a wound or abrasion. Intestinal infection has followed ingestion of contaminated meat, and anthrax may develop after inhalation of spores.

PATHOGENESIS The malignant pustule which follows cutaneous inoculation of anthrax organisms is characterized by vesiculation, neutrophilic infiltration, gelatinous edema, and necrosis. Suppuration is rare in the absence of secondary pyogenic infection. Spread of the bacilli to the regional lymph nodes may be followed by systemic dissemination. Examination of tissues from fatal human cases reveals masses of the bacteria in blood vessels, lymph nodes, and the parenchyma of various organs. There is scanty or absent cellular exudation at these foci, but hemorrhage and edema are widespread. So-called "anthrax pneumonia" and "anthrax meningitis" are, in all probability, an expression of this generalized hemorrhage and edema.

The blood of fatally infected experimental animals contains a lethal toxin, which can be neutralized by specific antiserum. This toxin has been isolated in vitro and is important in the pathogenesis of some of the manifestations of the disease.

MANIFESTATIONS The malignant pustule of human anthrax begins usually on an exposed body surface, as a painless, pruritic, erythematous papule, which vesiculates and ulcerates to form a black eschar. Tiny satellite vesicles are frequent. The ulcer may be surrounded by extensive edematous swelling, which is nontender, nonpitting, and so characteristic of anthrax that it is a valuable diagnostic sign. After about 5 days the ulcer begins to subside, but edema may persist for many days or weeks. Mild tenderness and enlargement of regional lymph nodes are frequently present. Constitutional symptoms are often absent despite extensive local changes, but there may be mild fever, headache, and malaise. In disseminated anthrax, high fever, prostration, and a rapidly fatal course are seen. So-called "woolsorters' disease," a highly fatal disseminated infection, is characterized by cyanosis, dyspnea, mediastinitis, and hemoptysis and is probably dependent on the pulmonary route of inoculation. Human infection may occur from ingestion of the uncooked meat of infected animals; however, enormous numbers of organisms are probably necessary to produce disease by this route.

LABORATORY FINDINGS The fluid from the cutaneous lesion frequently contains many bacilli, demonstrable by Gram's stain and culture. Bacilli may be found on direct examination or culture of the blood of patients with bacteremia. The blood leukocyte count is normal in mild cases, but there is polymorphonuclear leukocytosis in severe disease. Similarly, the erythrocyte sedimentation rate may be increased. Patients with meningeal involvement show bloody spinal fluid in which the organisms are easily found by direct examination or culture.

DIAGNOSIS A serologic agar-gel precipitin inhibition test has been devised which has proved useful in epidemiologic studies of anthrax, showing that subclinical infection may occur in persons exposed to the microorganism in industry and demonstrating increasing serum antibody titers following vaccination. A positive diagnosis of anthrax can be made by isolation of the organism in culture. A history of occupational exposure and characteristic eschar and edema should suggest the proper diagnosis. Pyogenic infections of the skin are usually painful; the malignant pustule is not. In addition, cutaneous anthrax is rarely purulent. The differential diagnosis of other diseases characterized by local ulceration at the portal of entry is discussed in Chap. 141.

TREATMENT AND PROPHYLAXIS Many antibiotics are effective in the treatment of human anthrax, including penicillin, chloramphenicol, tetracycline, erythromycin, and streptomycin. A dosage of 600,000 units of penicillin should be given once or twice daily until the local edema subsides. The eschar goes through its natural evolution in spite of treatment, and lymph node enlargement may persist for several days. *Bacillus anthracis* cannot be recovered from the skin lesion after 24 to 48 hr of penicillin therapy, but it may persist for a longer period when chloramphenicol or tetracycline is used.

Infection of personnel in industrial plants where contaminated animal products are handled still occurs. An outbreak of inhalation anthrax with a high mortality rate was reported in a goat hair processing mill in the United States in the late 1950s. Sterilization of all raw wool, mohair, etc., would probably remove this hazard but has had only limited use. A vaccine prepared from the "protective" antigen of *B. anthracis* is available and is effective in reducing the incidence of infection in an exposed population. Spore vaccines of various types are used with good effect in domestic animals in endemic areas but are not suitable for use in human beings.

Transmission of anthrax from one human being to another has never been recognized. The cutaneous disease was fatal in 20 to 30 percent of cases before antimicrobial drugs were available. The mortality now is less than 1 percent with proper treatment.

REFERENCES

BRACHMAN PS et al: An epidemic of inhalation anthrax: II. Epidemiologic investigation. Am J Hyg 72:6, 1960

GOLD H: Anthrax: Report of 117 cases, AMA Arch Intern Med 96:387, 1955

HOWE C: Anthrax, in *Oxford Medicine*, New York: Oxford, 1950

NORMAN PS et al: Serologic testing for anthrax antibodies in workers in a goat hair processing mill. Am J Hyg 72:32, 1960

SMITH H, KEPPIE J: Observations on experimental anthrax: Demonstrations of a specific lethal factor produced in vivo, by *Bacillus anthracis*. Nature 173:869, 1954

149 INFECTIONS CAUSED BY LISTERIA AND ERYSIPELOTHRIX

PAUL D. HOEPRICH

LISTERIA MONOCYTOGENES INFECTIONS

DEFINITION Listeriosis—disease caused by *L. monocytogenes*—consists of many clinical syndromes. Perinatal infection, acquired either transplacentally or during parturition, is the most nearly unique form of listeriosis.

ETIOLOGY *Listeria monocytogenes* is a gram-positive, microaerophilic, motile bacillus that forms smooth colonies. Seven serotypes have been defined; the epidemiologically essential aid of typing is available from the Center for Disease Control in Atlanta, Georgia. Type 1b is currently most common in the United States, with type 4b second in frequency. Weakly hemolytic gram-positive bacilli are presumed to be listerias if they are motile, reduce 2,3,5-triphenyltetrazolium chloride, and display characteristic animal pathogenicity. The Anton test is classical: 3 to 5 days after inoculation into the conjunctival sac of a rabbit or a guinea pig, *L. monocytogenes* causes a keratoconjunctivitis. Also, general listeriosis in the rabbit typically provokes a monocytosis, and focal hepatic necrosis is usual in lethal murine listeriosis.

EPIDEMIOLOGY AND PATHOGENESIS Found on every continent, save the Antarctic, *L. monocytogenes* appears to be saprophytic as well as parasitic and is readily isolated from mud, stream water, sewage, silage, and dry vegetation. Despite this, listeriosis in man is uncommon and occurs sporadically; moreover, it is actually more common in urban than rural dwellers. The reservoir from which man becomes infected is frequently occult and the mode of transmission often obscure. Direct transmission from an infected nonhuman animal via contaminated secretions has been documented only rarely. On the other hand, transmission from the infected pregnant female to her offspring is well established as a route of infection.

Transplacental perinatal infection results in disseminated fetal listeriosis. The fetus is usually stillborn or is prematurely ejected, virtually always with lethal listeriosis. Fetal listeriosis that is acquired during delivery is typically not clinically evident for 1 or 2 weeks postpartum and usually presents as a meningitis.

Listeriosis is preponderantly a disease of persons under one month (about 27 percent) and over forty years (about 56 percent) in age.

Although persons in apparent good health may contract listeriosis, infection appears to be facilitated by neoplasia (particularly of the lymphoreticular system), alcoholism, cardiovascular disease, diabetes mellitus, tuberculosis, and any condition requiring treatment with pharmacologic doses of glucocorticoids, with irradiation, or with cytotoxic agents.

MANIFESTATIONS *Meningitis* accounts for about three-fourths of the cases verified by culture and is the predominant clinical form of listeriosis in the United States. Clinically, meningitis caused by *L. monocytogenes* cannot be distinguished from meningitis caused by other kinds of bacteria.

Listeriosis of the newborn, the most nearly unique clinical form of listeriosis, ranges from meningitis that is clinically apparent within 1 month postpartum to diffuse disseminated disease in aborted, premature, and stillborn infants and neonates, who die within minutes to days after birth. In newborns listeriosis becomes overt 1 to 4 weeks postpartum. They, like children one month to six years of age, generally have listeriosis localized in the central nervous system.

Infants born alive with listeriosis may or may not have fever; yet these babies are critically ill with cardiorespiratory distress, vomiting, and diarrhea. Dark-red skin papules are frequent, particularly on the lower extremities. Hepatosplenomegaly may be present. This form of listeriosis is also known as septic or miliary granulomatosis, granulomatosis infantiseptica, argentophil-rod infection, or pseudotuberculosis. The findings at postmortem examination are characteristic and mimic those seen in listeriosis of rodents: widely disseminated abscesses varying in size from grossly visible to microscopic, involving, in order of decreasing frequency, liver, spleen, adrenal glands, lungs, pharynx, gastrointestinal tract, central nervous system, and skin. Typically, the lesions are abscesses, but classic granuloma formation may be seen, depending principally on the duration of infection before death. Microscopic examination of a gram-stained smear of meconium from the normal newborn infant does not disclose bacteria; fetal listeriosis results in meconium laden with gram-positive bacilli. For this reason, examination of meconium by Gram's stain and by culture should be carried out whenever there is gross soiling of the amniotic liquid with meconium, prematurity, or unexplained fever in the mother before or at the onset of labor. This is particularly important because listeriosis in the pregnant woman may be asymptomatic. At some time, a week to a month prepartum at most, there may have been malaise, a shaking chill, diarrhea, pain in the back or flanks, and itching of the skin. Even when symptomatic, the disease is benign and self-limited in the mother; however, as symptoms subside, a decrease or cessation of fetal movement may be noted. Infection of the fetus may occur as early as the fifth month of gestation. Following delivery of infants with proved fetal listeriosis, cervical cultures are, or soon become, negative for *Listeria*; subsequently, conception, gestation, and delivery of normal offspring are usual.

Oculoglandular listeriosis is the rare human analogue of the illness initiated in the rabbit by conjunctival inoculation of *Listeria*. There is a purulent conjunctivitis, which may lead to corneal ulceration. Regional-node involvement usually limits the spread from the eye. However, listerial meningitis has been reported as a complication of oculoglandular listeriosis.

Other rare syndromes caused by *Listeria* include general illness with bacteremia and high fever, endocarditis, polyserositis, and cutaneous infection.

LABORATORY FINDINGS Although *L. monocytogenes* grows well on the usual culture media, etiologic diagnosis by isolation and identification may be hampered by failure of differentiation from *Corynebacterium* sp., *Erysipelothrix insidiosa*, and *Streptococcus* sp. Recognition of listerial colonies in a mixed culture, like those obtained with vaginal or cervical specimens, is difficult and may be aided by using selective media and/or enrichment procedures.

Serodiagnosis has not been useful because of the high frequency of so-called natural antibodies. Because such nonspecific reactions are due to IgM, a test based on IgG may be of value to diagnosis.

Monocytosis is not common in human listeriosis. Leukocytosis with neutrophilia, as in any acute bacterial infection, is seen in listerial meningitis, oculoglandular infection, bacteremia, and endocarditis. The cerebrospinal fluid in meningitis is compatible with that in other purulent meningitides.

DIFFERENTIAL DIAGNOSIS Abortion, premature delivery, stillbirth, and neonatal death are more often due to causes other than listeriosis: Rh incompatibility, syphilis, or toxoplasmosis.

In patients with leptomeningitis, conjuctivitis, endocarditis, bacteremia, or polyserositis, reports of isolation of "diphtheroids" or "nonpathogens" must always be challenged. A statement that *L. monocytogenes* has been excluded should be required.

TREATMENT *Listeria monocytogenes* is susceptible to several antimicrobials in vitro, including penicillin G, tetracyclines, and erythromycin. Dosage and duration of therapy should vary according to the kind of listerial infection under treatment.

In fetal listeriosis, therapy must be rapidly effective and should be bactericidal to be of value. A regimen of proved value has yet to be devised. Penicillin G in a dose of 100 mg (160,000 units) per kg body weight per day given by continuous intravenous injection along with erythromycin (25 to 30 mg per kg body weight per day also by intravenous injection) merits trial.

Listerial meningitis will usually respond to treatment with penicillin G in a dose of 150 mg (240,000 units) per kg of body weight per day, given by continuous intravenous infusion. Cephalothin is not an acceptable alternative. Erythromycin as the gluceptate or lactobionate can be given in a dose of 60 to 75 mg per kg body weight per day as four equal portions given intravenously every 6 hr. Tetracycline is effective—15 mg per kg body weight per day as four equal portions given intravenously every 6 hr. Treatment should be continued in full dosage by intravenous injection for seven days after defervesence.

Listeriosis in the pregnant female and oculoglandular listeriosis can be treated with a 2-week course of either erythromycin (25 to 30 mg per kg body weight per day given as four equal portions, every 6 hr by mouth) or tetracycline, in the same dosage as erythromycin.

Endocarditis and bacteremia from an unknown site require vigorous therapy: penicillin G [150 mg (240,000 units) per kg body weight per day by continuous intravenous injection]. The addition of erythromycin (dose as given for meningitis) should be evaluated by assay of serum bactericidal activity against the patient's isolate.

PROGNOSIS Prompt, vigorous antimicrobial treatment of the acute forms of listeriosis, excepting fetal listeriosis, is usually curative. On the basis of agglutinin titers (IgG), specific antibody disappears during the months following cure. However, reinfection has not been reported.

ERYSIPELOTHRIX INFECTIONS

DEFINITION Erysipeloid is the commonest and most nearly unique form of human *Erysipelothrix* infection. Infective endocarditis and septic arthritis are rare forms of *Erysipelothrix* in man.

ETIOLOGY As gram-positive, microaerophilic bacilli, *E. insidiosa* may be confused with nontoxinogenic *Corynebacterium* sp. and *Listeria monocytogenes*. However, *E. insidiosa* is nonmotile and fails to grow on media selective for *Corynebacterium* sp. Also, unlike *L. monocytogenes*, *E. insidiosa* only rarely causes conjunctivitis, following conjunctival inoculation, and monocytosis, after intravenous inoculation, in the rabbit. Isolates of *E. insidiosa* appear to be serologically homogeneous. Although serodifferentiation from other gram-positive bacilli is possible, few laboratories are capable of definitive serodiagnosis.

EPIDEMIOLOGY AND PATHOGENESIS Primarily a saprophyte, *E. insidiosa* is worldwide in distribution. Man is virtually always infected by traumatic dermal inoculation; erysipeloid is the usual result. The disease is almost wholly restricted to persons who in their occupations handle edible or nonedible dead animal products. If the organism does not remain confined to skin, bacteremia in persons with preexisting valvular heart disease may lead to infective endocarditis.

The seasonal incidence of erysipeloid parallels that of swine erysipelas, being highest in summer and early fall. Yet persons who tend pigs, even pigs ill with porcine erysipelas, do not commonly develop erysipeloid.

MANIFESTATIONS Erysipeloid begins 2 to 7 days after injury, often after the initial lesion has healed. An itching, burning, painful irritation may precede, and always accompanies the appearance of the maculopapular, nonvesiculated, sharply defined, raised, purplish-red zone surrounding the site of entry. There is local swelling, and when, as is usual, a finger or the hand is involved, nearby joints may become stiff and painful. Centrifugal spread from the site of inoculation is apparent in a day or so. Movement is slow, 1 to 2 cm per 24 hr maximally, and more rapid proximally than distally; involvement of the terminal phalanx of a finger is rare, while spread to other fingers and the hand below the wrist is common. With extension, the original center subsides without desquamation or suppuration. There are usually no systemic signs or symptoms; regional lymphangitis and lymphadenitis are rare. Untreated, the disease heals within three weeks in most patients, although relapse has been observed.

The manifestations of *Erysipelothrix* endocarditis may be either acute or chronic, depending on the virulence of the infecting strain and on the state of resistance of the host. Usually, there are no classic erysipeloid skin lesions to suggest the disease at the time that endocarditis is clinically evident. However, a history of recent erysipeloid may be helpful.

Erysipelothrix arthritis is not clinically characteristic but usually can be related to erysipeloid or *Erysipelothrix* bacteremia. Isolation of *Erysipelothrix* from synovial fluid has not been reported.

LABORATORY FINDINGS The usual culture media are adequate for the growth of *E. insidiosa.* However, differentiation from diphtheroids and listerias depends primarily on the clinician's alerting the laboratory to the possibility of erysipelothrix.

In erysipeloid, *E. insidiosa* are best recovered by incubating, in broth containing glucose, a full-thickness biopsy of skin removed from the advancing edge of a lesion. Culture of an aspirate obtained after injection of sterile, 0.9 % NaCl solution into the periphery of a lesion may also yield *Erysipelothrix.*

With endocarditis and arthritis, the findings are in keeping with the respective clinical syndromes and are in no way characteristic for *E. insidiosa.*

DIFFERENTIAL DIAGNOSIS The appearance and location of erysipeloid, its slow and limited spread, the lack of constitutional reaction, the history of occupation and injury, all serve to identify this disease. The afflicted skin in *erysipelas* is very erythematous, and the face and scalp are affected; there are regional lymphangitis and lymphadenitis, leukocytosis, fever, and malaise. Eczematous lesions may itch, but they display vesicles and little abnormal color. The various erythemas have a different location and do not usually itch or burn; they are more apt to be chronic and nonmigratory.

TREATMENT Penicillin G, tetracyclines, chloramphenicol, erythromycin, and novobiocin inhibit *E. insidiosa* in vitro at concentrations practical in therapy. Penicillin G is the agent of choice. Erysipeloid is adequately treated by injection of 1,200,000 units of benzathine penicillin G. Erythromycin (15 mg per kg body weight per day, as four equal portions taken orally for 5 to 7 days) is an alternative. Cure of *Erysipelothrix* endocarditis has followed the daily injection of 2,000,000 to 20,000,000 units of penicillin per day for 4 to 6 weeks; the dose should be monitored by determination of the bactericidal activity of serum from the patient against his infecting strain.

PROGNOSIS Penicillin therapy is highly effective in curing *Erysipelothrix* infections. As with infective endocarditis from any cause, the prognosis after eradicating the infecting microorganism is primarily a function of the residual valvular damage.

REFERENCES

GRAY ML (ed): Second Symposium on Listeria Infection. Aug. 29-31, 1962, Bozeman, Mont.: Montana State College

HOEPRICH PD: Listeriosis, chap. 46, and Erysipeloid, chap. 79, in *Infectious Diseases,* ed PD Hoeprich, New York: Harper & Row, 1972

NELSON E: Five hundred cases of erysipeloid. Rocky Mt Med J 52:40, 1955

SEELIGER HPR: *Listeriosis,* Basel: Karger, 1961

150 FUSOSPIROCHETAL INFECTIONS

JOHN C. RIBBLE

Fusospirochetal infections are characterized by gangrenous, foul-smelling ulcers containing large numbers of spirochetes and bacteria. The lesions are usually located in the mouth and pharynx but may occur in the respiratory tract, the genitalia, surgical wounds, or human bites.

ETIOLOGY The term fusospirochetal infection has been used to indicate that both fusobacteria and spirochetes are found in the lesions. In addition to these organisms, common mouth bacteria such as bacteroides, anaerobic streptococci, anaerobic vibrios, and spirilla are also present. It is probable that fusospirochetal disease results from synergistic action of several organisms.

The bacteria and spirochetes associated with fusospirochetal disease are found as normal flora in the mouths of most adults and grow best under anaerobic conditions. Fusobacteria are gram-negative, unencapsulated, nonmotile, spindle-shaped bacilli. The spirochetes associated with the disease are identifiable by a rapid, characteristic motility and can be cultured in artificial media under strict anaerobiasis.

CLINICAL MANIFESTATIONS **Acute ulcerative gingivitis (trench mouth, Vincent's stomatitis)** The onset of disease is usually sudden and is associated with tender bleeding gums, fetid breath, and a bad taste. The gingival mucosa, especially the papillae between the teeth, becomes ulcerated and may be covered with gray exudate which is removable with gentle pressure. Although involvement of the gums is usually patchy, the process may extend to most of the gingival tissue. If the ulceration is extensive, there are fever, cervical lymphadenopathy, and leukocytosis. The disease may spread to involve other tissues of the oropharynx; it may become less severe and chronic; or it may subside spontaneously. Recurrent ulceration has been described. Most patients who develop fusospirochetal infection have poor oral hygiene. Tartar deposits and eruption or extraction of teeth may damage the gums and allow for bacterial invasion. Edentulous persons almost never develop the disease. Ulcerative gingivitis is prevalent in wartime when nutritional deficiency, crowding, and emotional upsets are common, but the role of these factors in pathogenesis is not known.

Cancrum oris (noma) Occasionally, ulcerative gingivitis spreads to involve the buccal mucosa, the cheek, and the mandible or maxilla, resulting in widespread destruction of bone and soft tissue. The first indication of cancrum oris is usually slight inflammation of the skin of the cheek. The destruction of tissue proceeds very rapidly. The teeth may fall out, and large areas of bone, even the whole mandible, may be sloughed. A strong putrid odor is present. The lesions are not usually painful, and children may push their fingers through the necrotic areas. The gangrenous lesions eventually heal, but large disfiguring defects are left. Cancrum oris is seen most commonly in severely malnourished children in underdeveloped areas of the world.

Fusospirochetal pharyngitis (Vincent's angina) Fusospirochetal infections of the pharynx may occur alone or in association with ulcerative gingivitis. The main complaints are an extremely sore throat, foul breath, bad taste in the mouth, sensation of choking, and fever. The pharynx in the area of the tonsillar pillars is swollen, red, and ulcerated and is covered with a grayish membrane which peels easily. Lymphadenopathy and leukocytosis are common. The disease may last for only a few days or may persist for weeks if not treated. The lesion begins unilaterally but may spread to the other side of the pharynx or to the larynx. Aspiration of infected material may result in lung abscess.

Infections of human bites Gangrenous lesions resulting from human bites commonly contain fusospirochetal flora, and fusobacterial septicemia following an infected human bite has been reported. Human bites are much more likely to become infected than dog bites, possibly because of the large number of bacteria and spirochetes surrounding the teeth of human beings and the relative lack of the organisms in dogs and other animals with widely spaced teeth.

Infection of genitalia Gangrenous balanitis and ulcers and gangrene of the vulva have been associated with the fusospirochetal flora.

DIAGNOSIS The diagnosis can be made with certainty only by demonstrating the typical bacteria and spirochetes in sections of necrotic lesions. In clinical practice the diagnosis is made by the appearance and putrid odor of the lesions. Smears of material from mouth ulcers are not usually helpful because fusospirochetal flora are found in the mouths of healthy persons. Ulcerative gingivitis can be distinguished from herpetic gingivostomatitis by the absence of vesicles and the tendency to involve mainly the gingival papillae. In suspected cases of fusospirochetal pharyngitis, diphtheria and streptococcal pharyngitis must be excluded by appropriate cultures.

TREATMENT Treatment of ulcerative gingivitis consists of local measures and antibacterial therapy if the disease is severe and painful. During the acute phase the patient should avoid brushing his teeth or causing trauma to the gums. A 3 % solution of hydrogen peroxide diluted with equal amounts of warm water should be used as a mouthwash several times a day. Tartar and necrotic debris should be removed from the gum margins by a dentist. In severe painful cases of gingivitis 600,000 units procaine penicillin twice a day or 1.0 g tetracycline a day should be used until improvement is evident. Metronidazole, a drug with some activity against spirochetes and fusobacteria, administered in dosage of 200 mg three times a day for 3 to 7 days is as effective as penicillin in promoting healing of gingival lesions and is considered by some to be the most satisfactory drug for the treatment of fusospirochetal gingivitis. Patients with fusospirochetal pharyngitis or infections of the genitalia should receive 600,000 units procaine penicillin twice a day or 1.0 g per day of tetracycline. The treatment of cancrum oris consists of antibiotic therapy with penicillin or tetracycline, debridement of necrotic tissue, and eventual repair of damaged structures. Human bites should be cleansed thoroughly, and obviously necrotic tissue should be removed. The wounds should not be sutured but should be left open and irrigated frequently. Antibiotic therapy should be given to all patients with human bites.

REFERENCES

Glenwright HD, Sidaway DA: The use of metronidazole in the treatment of acute ulcerative gingivitis. Br Dent J 121:175, 1966

Uohara GI, Knapp MJ: Oral fusospirochetosis and associated lesions. Oral Surg 24:113, 1967

section 8 | Diseases caused by toxin-producing bacteria

151 DIPHTHERIA

LOUIS WEINSTEIN

DEFINITION Diphtheria is an acute infectious disease produced by *Corynebacterium diphtheriae.* It is characterized by a local inflammatory lesion, usually in the upper part of the respiratory tract, and by remote effects resulting from toxin, which affects particularly the heart and peripheral nerves.

ETIOLOGY *Corynebacterium diphtheriae* is a gram-positive, nonsporulating, nonmotile rod. There is a characteristic swelling at one end of the bacillus, which gives it a club shape. Diphtheria bacilli have been classified into *mitis, gravis,* and *intermedius* groups on the basis of colonial morphology, appearance on tellurite medium, fermentation reactions, and ability to produce hemolysis. European workers have suggested that there is a significant difference in the clinical manifestations and in the severity of disease related to the strain; gravis and intermedius infections are thought to be accompanied by more severe toxic manifestations and a higher death rate. In the United States, the gravis strain is comparatively uncommon, and less significance is attached to the relationship of the type of organism and the clinical form of the disease.

Corynebacterium diphtheriae produces a protein exotoxin which is responsible for many of the clinical manifestations; as little as 0.0001 mg is lethal for guinea pigs. Strains of diphtheria bacilli which elaborate exotoxin are lysogenic. Absence of lysogeny generally is associated with lack of toxin formation and virulence. However, diphtheria may also follow invasion by strains of *C. diphtheriae* that cannot be shown to produce toxin.

EPIDEMIOLOGY Diphtheria occurs primarily in the Temperate Zone and is still very common in some parts of the world. In general, the number of cases of diphtheria in the United States and the British Isles has been decreasing steadily. In 1959 and 1960, however, this trend was reversed, and 1,741 cases were recorded from 45 states in the United States. The largest number was observed in the South, and more than 80 percent of the patients had never received primary immunization. The highest frequency has been in children over six years of age, and adults have been involved with increasing frequency. Another striking change has been a decrease in the incidence of laryngeal involvement. Diphtheria is acquired by droplet transmission from active cases or carriers and fomites play little role in spread of the infection.

PATHOGENESIS AND PATHOLOGY The commonest portal of entry for the diphtheria bacillus is the upper respiratory tract. The skin, genitalia, eye, or middle ear may also be sites of invasion. Growth of the organism is superficial in most cases, and there is little tendency to invade the lymphatics or bloodstream except in the terminal stages. The exotoxin elaborated in the local lesion is absorbed and carried by the blood to all parts of the body. The intensity of the toxic effects is greatest when the primary lesion is in the pharynx, less when it is in the larynx, and least when it is on the nasal mucosa. Simultaneous involvement of the pharynx, larynx, trachea, and bronchial tree is associated with most severe intoxication.

The *membrane,* the primary lesion of diphtheria, is thick, leathery, and blue-white and is composed of bacteria, necrotic epithelium, phagocytes, and fibrin. It is surrounded by a narrow zone of inflammation and is firmly adherent to the underlying tissues; bleeding follows its forcible removal. Ulceration is not a regular feature. Regional lymphadenitis is frequent, especially with gravis infections.

The *toxic manifestations* involve primarily the heart, kidneys, and peripheral nerves. The brain is rarely affected. Cardiac enlargement is frequent; this appears to be related to myocarditis rather than hypertrophy. The kidneys may be enlarged and reveal cloudy swelling and interstitial changes. Bronchopneumonia due to *C. diphtheriae* or to secondary invading organisms occurs in some patients, especially those with laryngeal involvement. Membrane is present throughout the bronchial tree when the diphtheria bacillus is responsible for the pulmonary infection. The peripheral nerves may reveal fatty degeneration, disintegration of the medullary sheaths, and involvement of the axis cylinder. Both motor and sensory fibers are affected, but the main impact is on motor innervation. The anterior horn cells and the posterior columns of the spinal cord may be damaged. Other central nervous system involvement includes cerebral hemorrhage, meningitis, and encephalitis. Petechial and purpuric lesions are occasionally present in the kidneys, skin, or adrenals. Endocarditis due to *C. diphtheriae* is rare.

Death results from respiratory obstruction by membrane or edema, or from the effects of toxin on the heart, nervous system, or other organs.

IMMUNITY Susceptibility to diphtheria is related to the presence or absence of circulating antibody to exotoxin. The Schick test yields a rough estimate of the quantity of antitoxin in the circulation. This test is carried out in the following manner: 0.1 ml purified diphtheria toxin (one-fiftieth the minimum lethal dose) dissolved in buffered human serum albumin is injected intradermally on the volar surface of the forearm; 0.1 ml purified diphtheria toxoid is injected into the other arm as a control. These areas are examined at 24 and 48 hr and between the fourth and seventh days and interpreted in the following way:

1 *Positive reaction:* The site of injection of toxin begins to redden in 24 hr; this increases and reaches a maximum in about a week, at which time the lesion may be as large as 3 cm in diameter and moderately swollen and tender. There is usually a small (1 to 1.5 cm) dark-red central zone which gradually turns brown, desquamates, and leaves a pigmented area. The area of toxoid injection shows no reaction. A positive test indicates little or no circulating antitoxin and no immunity.
2 *Negative reaction:* There is no reaction at the site of injection of either toxoid or toxin. This is consistent with a blood antitoxin level of 1/30 to 1/100 unit and immunity to ordinary exposure.
3 *Pseudoreaction:* Inflammation at both sites of injection within 12 to 14 hr, which reaches a maximum in 48 to 72 hr and then fades. This usually indicates immunity plus hypersensitivity to the toxin or other materials in the solution.
4 *Combined reaction:* This begins like the pseudoreaction, but the inflammatory response at the toxin site persists after that in the area of toxoid injection has faded. It indicates delayed sensitivity to toxin or other proteins and either low levels or no antitoxin. The incidence of combined reactions increases with age and is highest in unimmunized groups living in areas where diphtheria is prevalent.

Individuals with negative Schick tests occasionally contract diphtheria, and some persons with positive Schick reactions do not develop the disease after exposure. In some parts of the United States fewer than 50 percent of adults have "protective" levels of circulating antitoxin.

Second attacks of diphtheria are rare despite the fact that about 10 percent of patients who have had the disease remain Schick-positive. This suggests that factors other than antitoxin may play a role in protection against infection. In general, immunized patients have a milder illness than unimmunized ones when the initial clinical picture and level of circulating antitoxin are the same. Early therapy of diphtheria with antibiotics may lead to recurrence of the disease if exposure to fresh infections occurs shortly after discontinuation of treatment, suggesting that the development of antitoxic immunity is suppressed in these cases.

CLINICAL MANIFESTATIONS The incubation period of diphtheria is 1 to 7 days. The local symptoms vary with the site of the primary lesion. Constitutional reactions usually are of only minor to moderate severity in uncomplicated disease. Fever is usually low (100 to 101°F), unless infection with another organism (often group A *Streptococcus pyogenes*) supervenes. When toxic manifestations are absent, patients feel well except for a varying degree of discomfort at the site of the local lesion. Pallor, listlessness, tachycardia, and weakness are common in more severe cases. Peripheral vascular collapse often develops in the terminal stages of the disease.

Nasal diphtheria Diphtheria is occasionally restricted to the nasal mucosa. It is usually localized to the septum or turbinates in the anterior portion of one side of the nose, does not extend, and may persist for a long time. A foreign body is frequently present. A unilateral serosanguineous discharge is characteristic. When the disease is located in the posterior nasal areas, it commonly extends to the pharynx, from which toxin is absorbed.

Pharyngeal diphtheria The early diphtheritic membrane in the pharynx consists of small areas of soft exudate which wipe off easily and leave no bleeding points. As the disease progresses, the discrete exudate coalesces to form an easily removable thin sheet which spreads to cover tonsils or pharynx, or both. Later, it becomes thicker, bluish-white, gray, or black, depending on the degree of hemorrhage, and is so firmly attached to the underlying tissues that attempts to remove it result in bleeding. If infection with group A *S. pyogenes*, is superimposed, the pharynx is diffusely red and edematous. There is very little pharyngeal discomfort in the average case of diphtheria; in some cases, however, this may be severe. There is usually a moderate leukocytosis with 15,000 or fewer white blood cells per mm^3.

Local spread of the pharyngeal membrane may occur, and the throat, tonsils, and soft and hard palates become completely covered. Patients with severe disease may develop so-called "malignant" diphtheria, characterized by marked edema of the submandibular areas and the anterior neck, giving the characteristic "bullneck" appearance. Respiration is noisy, the tongue protrudes, the breath is foul, and the speech thick. The pharyngeal tissues are red and edematous, and the cervical lymph nodes are enlarged. The skin is pale and cool. The patient complains of overwhelming weakness. Purpuric eruptions of the skin, particularly on the neck and anterior chest wall, may appear occasionally. Drowsiness and delirium are common.

Laryngeal diphtheria Involvement of the larynx is usually the result of extension of the diphtheritic membrane from the pharynx. The infection may rarely be limited to the larynx or trachea. This possibility must be considered in the differential diagnosis of all cases of "croup"; it can be ruled out only by direct examination of the airway. The clinical features of this type of disease are described below.

Cutaneous diphtheria Although diphtheria of the skin is a problem primarily in tropical areas, where it is responsible for some cases of "jungle sore" and may be epidemic, it occurs occasionally in the Temperate Zone. *Corynebacterium diphtheriae* is unable to penetrate unbroken skin and invades wounds, burns, etc. Although the lesions develop most often on the lower extremities, they may appear at any site, including the perianal region. The typical lesion is a round, deep, "punched-out" ulcer, 0.5 cm to several centimeters in diameter. In the early stages, it is covered by a gray, yellow, or gray-brown membrane which strips off easily to reveal a clean hemorrhagic base that dries quickly and becomes covered by thin, leathery, dark-brown or black, adherent membrane. This separates spontaneously 1 to 3 weeks after infection. The margin of the fully developed ulcer is usually slightly undermined, purple, rolled, and sharply defined. Breakdown, either after minor trauma or spontaneously, is frequent, and the development of anesthesia, after a few weeks, is characteristic. Healing is usually slow. Scarring is the rule. Myocarditis occurs in about 5 percent and peripheral neuritis in about 20 percent of cases of cutaneous diphtheria; the Landry-Guillain-Barré syndrome may develop occasionally.

Diphtheritic lesions in other areas Diphtheria may involve the uterine cervix, vagina, vulva, bladder, urethra, or penis (after circumcision). Toxic manifestations are common. The tongue, buccal mucous membrane, gums, and esophagus may also be affected. Infection of the conjunctiva occurs rarely. Otitis media may occur as an isolated syndrome or secondary to diphtheria in the upper part of the respiratory tract; the aural infection may become chronic; virulent organisms may be isolated from the discharge for many months.

COMPLICATIONS OF DIPHTHERIA The complications of diphtheria are of two types: (1) those that result from spread of the membrane in the respiratory tract, and (2) those due to the effects of the toxin.

Extension and spread of membrane The membrane of diphtheria may spread from the fauces over the posterior pharyngeal wall into the larynx, trachea, and, uncommonly, the bronchial tree, leading to severe illness and a high incidence of toxic manifestations. Occlusion of the airway is manifested by tachypnea and, as obstruction increases, restlessness, use of accessory muscles of respiration, cyanosis, and finally death. In some cases, the membrane extends diffusely into the bronchial tree and produces clinical manifestations of pneumonia. Bronchopulmonary diphtheria is very serious, not only because of obstruction but also because of the large surface from which toxin can be absorbed; the death rate is very high. When the pulmonary lesion regresses, pieces of membrane may break off and produce sudden occlusion of the airway; a cast of the bronchial tree may be coughed up. On occasion, pharyngeal membrane has extended into the esophagus and cardia of the stomach.

Toxic complications of diphtheria Studies of the mechanisms of action of diphtheria toxin suggest that it inhibits the transfer of amino acids from soluble RNA to growing polypeptide chains, resulting in failure of the amino acids to be incorporated into the polypeptide; a cofactor, nicotinamide-adenine dinucleotide, is required for activity of the toxin. The effects of the toxin on the myocardium are thought to result from its ability to decrease the rate of oxidation of long-chain fatty acids by interfering with the metabolism of carnitine. Because of this, triglycerides accumulate in the myocardium and cause fatty degeneration of muscle.

Myocarditis develops in about two-thirds of patients with diphtheria. However, it is clinically evident in only about 10 percent of cases; alterations in the intensity of the heart sounds, systolic murmurs, bundle branch block, incomplete or complete heart block, atrial fibrillation, ventricular premature beats or tachycardia, or both, are common. Ventricular fibrillation is a constant threat and is frequently responsible for sudden death. Ninety percent of patients with atrial fibrillation, ventricular tachycardia, or complete heart block die. Overt congestive cardiac failure is uncommon. Evidence of decompensation of the right side of the heart usually develops first; the most common symptom is pain in the right upper quadrant of the abdomen due to rapid engorgement of the liver. Failure of the left side of the heart may appear later. Diphtheritic heart disease is not necessarily "benign" in survivors of the disease; permanent cardiac damage may occur. Fibrosis of the myocardium has been observed in patients who have expired several weeks after "mild" myocarditis was detected in the electrocardiogram. The degree and extent of fibrotic change has often been greater than could have been predicted on the basis of the type of abnormality present in the ECG.

Peripheral neuritis may occur in the course of diphtheria. Paralysis of the soft palate and posterior pharyngeal wall occasionally appears very early in the disease (2 to 3 days). A more common neuritis (10 percent of cases) usually develops 2 to 6 weeks after onset of the disease. It is characterized by cranial nerve dysfunction; the third, sixth, seventh, ninth, and tenth nerves are most commonly involved. Loss of accommodation, nasal voice, and difficulty in swallowing are the most frequent manifestations. However, any of the peripheral nerves may be affected, with resulting paralysis of the extremities, diaphragm, or intercostal muscles; death may occur from failure of respiration. The peripheral neuritides which appear in the second to the sixth week of the disease are characterized primarily by motor loss; sensory changes are uncommon and, when present, are minor. Peripheral neuritis may not appear until 2 to 3 months after the onset of diphtheria. In these cases, the clinical picture and course resemble infectious polyneuritis. The outstanding findings are loss of sensation in the "glove-and-stocking" distribution and albuminocytologic dissociation in the cerebrospinal fluid identical with that observed in the Landry-Guillain-Barré syndrome. Motor weakness and areflexia may develop with progression of involvement. Facial diplegia may accompany the other neurologic manifestation. A fatal, rapidly ascending paralysis of the Landry type may develop rarely. Complete recovery is the rule in this late peripheral neuritis, although it may require as long as a year. Encephalitis is a rare toxic complication of diphtheria.

Shock, which develops suddenly and without warning, is an occasional cause of sudden death in this disease. In some instances, this may be a consequence of myocarditis; in others, no cause can be discovered.

Other complications Cerebral infarction with hemiplegia occurs rarely; it is probably due to embolization from atrial thrombi in patients with myocarditis and cardiac dilatation. Superinfection of the lungs is a risk in all patients with diphtheria who are given antimicrobial agents. Purpuric skin eruptions may be seen in severe, malignant cases; thrombocytopenia occurs rarely. A mild morbilliform rash may be present during the early stage of diphtheria. Secondary invasion of the pharynx by group A *S. pyogenes* may take place in patients who have not received an antibiotic. Serum sickness occasionally follows the use of antitoxin. Relapses of diphtheria may occur when patients given antimicrobial agents are exposed to fresh cases soon after therapy has been discontinued. Bacteremia, endocarditis, and meningitis are rare complications.

COURSE AND PROGNOSIS The diphtheritic membrane may be present for only 3 to 4 days in mild cases, even when no antitoxin is given; it usually lasts for about a week in cases of moderate severity. Commonly, the pharyngeal lesion increases in extent and thickness during the first 24 hr after the administration of antitoxin. As the disease begins to recede, the exudate softens, wipes off easily, leaving no bleeding areas, becomes patchy so that it resembles the picture of "follicular" tonsillitis, and finally disappears, leaving normal underlying mucous membrane.

The fatality rate of diphtheria prior to the use of specific antitoxin was about 35 percent in average cases and 90 percent in those with laryngeal involvement. Since specific serotherapy has been employed, this has been reduced to a range of 3.5 to 22 percent, but it is still highest when the larynx is affected. The overall death rate in the United States is about 10 percent and may be related primarily to cardiac involvement and infection with one mitis strain. Death is most frequent in the very young and the old. Immunization is a factor of great importance in prognosis. The fatality rate in immunized individuals is one-tenth that in the unimmunized population. Paralysis is five times and "malignant" disease fifteen times less common in immune than in nonimmune individuals. As a rule, the longer the delay in the administration of antitoxin, the greater the incidence of complications and death. However, antitoxin is ineffective in reducing risks of complications and death if it is given much later than 48 hr after diphtheria begins.

A white blood cell count higher than 25,000 per mm^3 is associated with a higher risk of complications and death. This is possibly related to simultaneous infection of the portal of entry of the diphtheria bacillus by other organisms, especially group A *S. pyogenes*.

DIAGNOSIS The clinical features of the fully developed diphtheritic membrane, especially in the pharynx, are sufficiently characteristic to suggest the possibility of the disease in most instances. However, the appearance of the pharyngeal exudate alone does not clinch the diagnosis. There are a number of other infections in which pseudomembranes resembling those of diphtheria are present; among these are infectious mononucleosis, streptococcal pharyngitis, viral exudative pharyngitis, fusospirochetal infection, and acute pharyngeal candidiasis.

The specific diagnosis of diphtheria depends completely on demonstration of the organism in stained smears and their recovery by culture. Methylene blue-stained preparations are positive, in experienced hands, in 75 to 85 percent of cases. Diphtheria bacilli can be recovered by culture on Loeffler's medium in 8 to 12 hr if patients have not been receiving antimicrobial agents. *Corynebacterium diphtheriae* also multiplies, but more slowly, on ordinary blood agar. If an antibiotic, especially penicillin or erythromycin, has been administered prior to obtaining cultures, the organisms may not grow for as long as 5 days, or may fail to grow at all.

Staining of suspected material with fluorescein-labeled diphtheria antitoxin may allow rapid diagnosis.

TREATMENT Patients with diphtheria should be isolated and kept at strict bed rest; physical effort should be reduced during the early convalescent stages. Local therapy of the diphtheritic lesion is useless. The only specific treatment for diphtheria is antitoxin. Antiserum must never be given until the patient's sensitivity to horse serum, using the eye and skin tests, has been determined. Despite a negative test for hypersensitivity, it is probably best to administer antitoxin in divided doses to all adults, using the following schedule: When exudate is present on only one tonsil, 5,000 units; for lesions covering both tonsils, 10,000 units; when the entire pharyngeal wall and the tonsils are involved, 20,000 to 50,000 units; for laryngeal disease, 50,000 to 100,000 units. Because of the length of time required for antibody to reach maximal levels in the blood after intramuscular injection, one-half the calculated dose is given by this route. If no reaction occurs, the rest of the antitoxin is infused slowly by vein. Desensitization should be attempted if the initial skin or eye test is positive. A rare patient may be sensitive to such a high degree that the antiserum cannot be administered without the risk of death.

Antitoxin should be given as early in the course of diphtheria as possible. Antimicrobial agents do not alter the course, incidence of complications, or outcome of diphtheria.

Patients with laryngeal obstruction should be watched very carefully. In mild cases, inhalation of warm or cool steam may be beneficial. If advancing signs of airway obstruction develop, intubation or tracheostomy is indicated. These procedures must never be delayed until cyanosis appears, because, at this point, stimulation of the pharynx or trachea may produce cardiac standstill and death. Sedative or hypnotic agents should never be given because they may obscure increasing respiratory difficulty.

The pulse and blood pressure should be measured frequently. Little can be done to alter the course of the myocarditis. Quinidine has been tried to prevent and treat arrhythmias, but appears to be of no value; there is some suspicion that it may produce deleterious effects. The use of procaine amide when ventricular premature beats or tachycardia supervene has been suggested, but no documented observations of its effect have been recorded. The administration of digitalis for cardiac failure in diphtheria is controversial. Some consider this drug to be completely contraindicated; others feel, however, that, used carefully, digitalis may be given safely and with beneficial effects. Shock should be treated, depending on its etiology (Chaps. 33 and 124). There is no evidence that corticosteroids or corticotropin are of any value in the treatment of diphtheria or any of its complications.

Treatment of carriers *Corynebacterium diphtheriae* usually disappears from the upper part of the respiratory tract after 2 to 4 weeks in patients who do not receive antimicrobial drugs; in a small number of individuals the organism may persist for a long time or be present permanently. The most effective treatment of the acute and chronic carrier state is erythromycin. A dose of 2 g per day orally for 2 weeks appears to be adequate. Retreatment is indicated for carriers whose organisms do not disappear on the first trial. This is preferable to tonsillectomy, which may be considered as a last resort should the carrier state persist despite repeated courses of antibiotic.

PREVENTION Diphtheria is, for the most part, a preventable disease. Immunization at the age of three months should be routine. Diphtheria toxoid is best given together with tetanus toxoid and pertussis vaccine (DPT), because antibody titers are higher with combined immunization than with either agent alone. "Booster" doses should be administered at the age of one year and again just before a child goes to school. Although it has been suggested that Schick testing is not necessary in those who have been immunized, many physicians still carry this out to determine the status of antitoxic immunity. A Schick test acts as a "booster." A negative reaction does not indicate absolute protection. The development of highly purified toxoid has made it possible to protect adults with little or no risk of untoward sequelae. The usual procedure is to inject 0.1 ml purified toxoid subcutaneously (Moloney test). If there is no reaction in 24 to 48 hr, the regular immunization procedure is carried out.

Unimmunized persons exposed to an active case of diphtheria should be given 3,000 units of antitoxin intramuscularly, after appropriate skin and eye tests. In those who have been previously immunized, a "booster" dose of toxoid is usually sufficient. Patients with diphtheria should be quarantined until three successive cultures of the nose, throat, or other infected areas, taken at 24-hr intervals, are negative. If antibiotics have been administered, cultural studies should not be initiated until at least 24 hr after cessation of therapy.

REFERENCES

DOEGE TC et al: Diphtheria in the United States, 1959–1960. Pediatrics 30:194, 1962

GOOR RS, PAPPENHEIMER AM JR: Studies on the mode of action of diphtheria toxin. J Exp Med 126:899, 913, 923, 1967

GORE I: Myocardial changes in fatal diphtheria: A summary of observations in 221 cases. Am J Med Sci 219:257, 1948

HOLLANDER MH: Diphtheria of the skin. US Air Force Med J 2:229, 1951

IPSEN J: Circulating antitoxin at the onset of diphtheria in 425 patients. Medicine (Baltimore) 251:459, 1954

——: Immunization of adults against diphtheria and tetanus. N Engl J Med 251:459, 1954

NAIDITCH MJ, BOWER AG: Diphtheria: A study of 1,433 cases observed during a ten-year period at the Los Angeles County Hospital. Am J Med 17:229, 1954

SCHEID W: Diphtherial paralysis: An analysis of 2,292 cases of diphtheria in adults which include 174 cases of polyneuritis. J Nerv Ment Dis 116:1095, 1952

WITAKER JA et al: The fluorescent antitoxin test for the immediate diagnosis of diphtheria. Pediatrics 27:214, 1961

WITTELS B, BRESSLER R: Biochemical lesion of diphtheria toxin on the heart. J Clin Invest 43:630, 1964

152 TETANUS

HARRY N. BEATY
ROBERT G. PETERSDORF

DEFINITION Tetanus is an acute, often fatal, disease caused by an exotoxin produced in a wound by *Clostridium tetani.* It is characterized by generalized increased rigidity and convulsive spasms of skeletal muscles.

HISTORY Accurate clinical descriptions of tetanus date back to antiquity. However, the infectious nature of the disease was not recognized until 1884 when Nicolaier produced tetanus in animals by injecting them with samples of soil. In 1889, Kitasato isolated the organism, showed that it produced disease when injected into animals, and reported that the toxin could be neutralized by specific antibodies. In 1897, Nocard demonstrated the protective effect of passively transferred antitoxin, and passive immunization in man was used on a massive scale during World War I. Tetanus toxoid was developed by Ramon in the early 1920s, and the effectiveness of active immunization was demonstrated unequivocally in World War II.

ETIOLOGY *Clostridium tetani* is a strictly anaerobic, gram-positive rod which is motile and readily forms endospores. In stained preparations, organisms may occur singly, in pairs, or in long chains. Spore-bearing bacilli usually contain a single, spheric, terminal endospore which swells the end of the organism and produces a characteristic "clubbed" appearance.

The organism grows well on blood agar at 37°C under anaerobic conditions. Slight hemolysis is usually apparent, but isolated colonies are rare because the organism tends to swarm. *Cl. tetani* is relatively inert biochemically, with no proteolytic activity and no fermentation of carbohydrates. Vegetative forms of the tetanus bacillus are no more resistant to adverse conditions than other bacteria, but spores are highly resistant to antiseptics and moderately resistant to heat.

Ten distinct types of *Cl. tetani* can be distinguished on the basis of flagellar antigens. All these types have one or more common somatic antigens, and are capable of producing at least two exotoxins. One, a hemolysin, is relatively unimportant clinically. The other, tetanospasmin, generally referred to as tetanus toxin, is a protein with a molecular weight of approximately 67,000, and is responsible for the clinical manifestations of tetanus. The tetanospasmins produced by the various types of *Cl. tetani* are essentially identical antigenically, and only one antitoxin is needed to neutralize the tetanus toxins produced by all strains.

EPIDEMIOLOGY The tetanus bacillus is found in the superficial layers of soil and as a saprophyte in the intestinal tract of man and certain animals. It is most frequently encountered in densely populated regions in hot, damp climates and in soil which is rich in organic matter. This explains, in part, why the disease is rare in the polar regions and relatively uncommon in North America, the U.S.S.R., and most of Europe. Urbanization, mechanization of agriculture, and socioeconomic factors such as poverty and lack of availability of health services also significantly influence the occurrence of this disease.

Worldwide, there are probably 300,000 to 500,000 cases of tetanus each year with a mortality rate of roughly 45 percent. There is no racial predilection, but the male-to-female ratio is 2.5:1, even among neonates where the opportunity for infection is presumably equal. In the United States, there are less than 200 reported cases each year, and these occur almost exclusively in nonimmunized or only partially immunized individuals. The highest incidence of disease is among nonwhites in the southern states. However, spores of *Cl. tetani* are distributed widely throughout urban centers and rural areas of the entire country, and are found commonly on clothing and in house dust, placing the nonimmune individual at risk following relatively minor household injuries. Tetanus has been known to follow surgery and innocuous procedures such as skin testing or intramuscular injection of medication. The disease is inordinately common in narcotics addicts, perhaps because heroin is frequently "cut" with quinine which drastically lowers the redox potential at the site of injection and favors the growth of *Cl. tetani.*

Tetanus neonatorum is a major cause of infant mortality in developing countries and is directly related to poor obstetric conditions. In Japan, the disease was virtually eliminated well before extensive active immunization programs were instituted, by improving obstetric facilities.

PATHOGENESIS AND PATHOLOGY *Clostridium tetani* is a noninvasive organism. Therefore, tetanus can occur only after spores or vegetative bacteria gain access to tissues and produce toxin locally. The usual mode of entry is through a puncture wound or laceration on the hand, foot, or leg. However, tetanus may follow elective surgery, burn wounds, otitis media, dental infection, abortion, and pregnancy. Neonatal tetanus usually follows infection of the umbilical stump. The disease not infrequently follows injuries too trivial to be seen by a physician, and in 20 percent of cases there is neither a history of injury nor a detectable lesion.

Wounds are undoubtedly contaminated frequently with spores of *Cl. tetani,* but tetanus develops rarely because germination of spores occurs only when the oxygen tension is much lower than that of normal tissue. Spores may survive in the body for months to years and finally produce disease at some later date after minor trauma which alters local conditions. Toxin production in wounds is favored by necrotic tissue, foreign bodies, calcium salts, and associated infections which establish low oxidation-reduction potentials. Infection caused by the tetanus bacillus remains strictly localized, but the toxin produced is disseminated through the bloodstream and lymphatics to the central nervous system where it binds to gangliosides. Retrograde spread through perineural interstitial spaces probably occurs also, but there is little support for the hypothesis that spread occurs through the neuronal axon itself.

The typical clinical manifestations of tetanus are caused by the effect of tetanospasmin on the central nervous system. The toxin acts at the synapse of interneurons of inhibitory pathways and motor neurons to produce blockade of spinal inhibition. Generalized muscle rigidity arises from uninhibited afferent stimuli entering the central nervous system from the periphery. When the stimuli become more vigorous, spasms occur. Emotional and, to a lesser extent, visual stimuli can also cause muscle spasm. Tetanus toxin also has other, apparently minor, effects. Peripherally it produces neuromuscular blockade similar to that of botulinum toxin, and it acts directly on muscle to produce contraction which is unaccompanied by an action potential in nerves. Certain clinical observations have raised the possibility that tetanus toxin also has an effect on the sympathetic nervous system.

Both the major and minor effects of tetanus toxin appear to be self-limited and completely reversible, because patients who recover from the disease have no residual defect. Likewise, there are no distinguishable pathologic changes which are characteristic of tetanus.

CLINICAL MANIFESTATIONS The incubation period of tetanus, i.e., the time between injury and the appearance of unmistakable symptoms, ranges from 2 to 56 days. However, over 80 percent of patients become symptomatic within 14 days. A short incubation period indicates severe disease, and when symptoms occur within 2 or 3 days of injury, the mortality rate approaches 100 percent.

Nonspecific premonitory symptoms such as restlessness, irritability, and headache are encountered occasionally, but the commonest presenting complaints are pain and stiffness in the jaw, abdomen, or back and difficulty in swallowing. As the disease progresses, stiffness gives way to rigidity, and patients often complain of difficulty in opening their mouths. In fact, trismus is the commonest manifestation of tetanus and is responsible for the familiar descriptive name of *lockjaw.* As more muscles are involved, rigidity becomes generalized, and sustained contractions of facial muscles produce a characterisitic expression called *risus sardonicus.* The intensity and sequence of muscle involvement is quite variable. In a small proportion of patients, only local signs and symptoms develop in the region of the injury. In the vast majority, however, most muscles are involved to some degree, and the signs and symptoms encountered depend upon the major muscle groups affected.

Reflex spasms usually occur within 24 to 72 hr of the first symptoms, an interval referred to as the *onset time.* As in the case of the incubation period, a short onset time is associated with a poor prognosis. Spasms are caused by sudden intensification of afferent stimuli arising in the periphery, which increases rigidity and causes simultaneous and excessive contraction of muscles and their antagonists. Spasms may be both painful and dangerous. As the disease progresses, minimal or inapparent stimuli produce more intense and longer-lasting spasms with increasing frequency. Respiration may be impaired by laryngospasm or tonic contraction of respiratory muscles which prevents adequate ventilation. Hypoxia may then lead to irreversible central nervous system damage and death.

Patients are almost invariably conscious and mentally alert at the time of admission. Low-grade fever, profuse sweating and tachycardia are common. Deep tendon reflexes are hyperactive, and there may be labile hypertension. The physical examination should be undertaken with care, because reflex convulsive spasms may be precipitated easily. The wound through which *Cl. tetani* was introduced should be evaluated, and the examination should determine the extent of rigidity; the severity of trismus; the presence or absence of dysphagia and respiratory embarrassment; the frequency, intensity, and duration of convulsive spasms; and the presence of complications such as respiratory infection.

Characteristically, the manifestations of tetanus increase in severity for about 3 days after the first sign, and then remain stable for the next 5 to 7 days. After about 10 days, spasms begin to occur less frequently, and by the end of 2 weeks, they disappear altogether. Although residual stiffness may persist for a prolonged period, most survivors recover completely in 4 weeks.

Tetanus neonatorum is a severe form of the disease which usually occurs within 10 days of birth. Early signs include difficulty in sucking, irritability, and excessive crying associated with peculiar grimacing. Intense rigidity characteristically produces opisthotonus, flexion of the arms, clenched fists, extension of the legs, and plantar flexion of the toes. Typical spasms occur with minimal stimuli.

Complications Complications contribute significantly to the morbidity and mortality of tetanus. Some result from overly vigorous therapy and prolonged bed rest, while others are attributed to the action of tetanus toxin. Inadequate ventilation, either from laryngospasm or spasm of respiratory muscles, is a constant threat. In addition to hypoxia, atelectasis is a common consequence of impaired respiration. Difficulty in swallowing leads to aspiration of secretions, which may also cause atelectasis and initiate pulmonary infection. Thrombophlebitis is occasionally encountered, but bland venous thrombosis is more common and may lead to pulmonary embolization. Cardiovascular complications thought to be due to hyperactivity of the sympathetic nervous system include tachycardia, with heart rates over 180 beats per min, severe vasoconstriction, and hypertension. Pulmonary edema may occur either as a consequence of myocarditis or excessive fluid replacement. High fever usually signifies secondary infection. Pneumonia is a common late complication of tetanus, and is found in 50 to 70 percent of autopsied cases. Other frequent sites of secondary infections include the original wound, decubitus ulcers, and the urinary tract of patients with indwelling bladder catheters. Fractures of midthoracic vertebras are probably due to severe spasms, and are particularly common among children and adolescents. Gastrointestinal complications include acute peptic ulceration, paralytic ileus, and constipation. Hemolysis is seen in a small proportion of patients.

Pneumonia is the major cause of death. Other autopsy findings in early deaths include intense congestion of viscera and, occasionally, intracranial hemorrhage or thrombosis. In about 20 percent of cases, no obvious pathology is identified, and death is attributed to the direct effects of tetanus toxin.

LABORATORY FINDINGS There are no laboratory findings characteristic of tetanus. Granulocytosis is seen in about one-third of patients, but anemia is rare. Blood chemistries are almost always normal initially, but various fluid and electrolyte disturbances may arise in the course of the disease. The electrocardiogram usually shows only sinus tachycardia, but occasionally T-wave inversion is seen. Roentgenograms are not helpful except in the evaluation of complications.

The diagnosis of tetanus is entirely clinical and does not depend upon bacteriologic confirmation. *Clostridium tetani* is recovered from the wound in only 30 percent of cases, and not infrequently it is isolated from patients who do not have tetanus. Laboratory identification depends on cultural and morphologic characteristics, absence of fermentative activity, and, most importantly, demonstration of toxin production in mice.

DIFFERENTIAL DIAGNOSIS With the exception of strychnine poisoning, no disease resembles fully developed tetanus. Early on, it may be difficult to exclude local causes of jaw pain, and the combination of neck stiffness and fever may suggest meningitis. However, this can be excluded by lumbar puncture, because in tetanus the spinal fluid is normal. When there is doubt about the diagnosis, clinical observation usually settles the issue within a matter of hours.

TREATMENT In order to formulate a rational plan of therapy, it is useful to assess the severity of tetanus. *Mild tetanus* is characterized by an incubation period of at least 14 days and an onset time of more than 6 days. Trismus is usually present, but dysphagia is absent, and generalized spasms are brief and mild. *Moderately severe tetanus* has a somewhat shorter incubation period and onset time; trismus is marked, dysphagia and generalized rigidity are present, but ventilation remains adequate even during spasms. The criteria for *severe tetanus* include a short incubation time, an onset time of 72 hr or less, severe trismus, dysphagia and rigidity, and frequent, prolonged, generalized convulsive spasms. Because of the poor prognosis of tetanus in older individuals, the disease should be considered moderate to severe in all patients over 50.

General measures Patients should be hospitalized in an *intensive care unit.* After initial evaluation, necrotic tissue and foreign bodies should be removed from the infected wound, and abscesses should be drained. Patients should be placed in a quiet room and observed closely for development of complications or unexpected changes in the course of the disease. While it is a good general principle to disturb patients as little as possible, vital signs must be monitored and aspiration must be averted by positioning the patient carefully and by aspirating nasopharyngeal secretions frequently. Care must be taken to prevent development of decubitus ulcers or contractures, but many routine nursing procedures should be omitted because they may precipitate uncomfortable or dangerous spasms. Initially, nutrition is not a major consideration, and fluid and electrolyte balance should be maintained over the first several days by administration of appropriate solutions intravenously, accompanied by careful recording of intake and output. After the patient's condition has been stabilized and the threat of aspiration has been minimized, adequate nutrition can be given through a nasogastric tube. Intravenous hyperalimentation may be used in patients with an unusually severe and prolonged illness.

Antiserum Antiserum does not neutralize tetanus toxin fixed in the central nervous system, and does little to ameliorate symptoms already present at the time of admission. However, it has been the practice for many years to give antitoxin to patients with tetanus, and it is likely that the case-fatality ratio in mild to moderately severe disease is reduced significantly when antiserum is administered early. Human tetanus immune globulin (TIG) is generally available in the United States, and is far superior to equine antiserum. Because its half-life is about 25 days, only one dose of 250 to 3,000 units intravenously is recommended. Local infiltration at the site of the wound is of no proven value. Hypersensitivity reactions do not occur with TIG, obviating the need for pretreatment testing.

If human antitoxin is not available, a single dose of equine antiserum should be given after the patient has been tested for hypersensitivity to horse serum. Although the dosage of heterologous antitoxin often recommended for adults is 100,000 to 200,000 units, studies have shown that 10,000 units is probably optimal. Anaphylaxis can occur despite negative sensitivity tests, and patients must be observed carefully to institute treatment at the first sign of an anaphylactic reaction. Up to 25 percent of patients develop delayed reactions including serum sickness after equine antitoxin. Occasionally, serious neurologic complications accompany other manifestations of serum sickness (Chap. 69).

Active immunization of patients with tetanus is necessary, because the disease does not confer natural immunity. However, there is no need to begin primary immunization until the patient has recovered.

Management of muscle spasms Muscle relaxation is the key to therapy, but mild sedation is also desirable because it reduces the effect of sensory stimuli. Ideally, this should be accomplished without significantly affecting respiration. Although a variety of agents have been used in the treatment of tetanus, none has achieved universal acceptance. However, two groups of drugs, barbiturates and phenothiazines, have been particularly useful. Among the barbiturates, phenobarbital, in adult doses of 50 to 100 mg every 3 to 6 hr, produces adequate sedation which may suffice in the management of mild tetanus. When rapid action is required, amylbarbital or pentobarbital, 50 to 200 mg intravenously, may be used. Frequent and severe spasms cannot be managed with barbiturates alone, because the dosage required for control leads to unconsciousness and suppressed respiration. For this reason, muscle relaxants usually are used, either alone or in combination with barbiturates, in the treatment of moderate or severe tetanus. Electromyographic studies have shown that the phenothiazines effectively produce relaxation while sparing the sensorium and respirations. Chlorpromazine, in doses of 200 to 300 mg a day, minimizes rigidity and decreases the frequency of spasms. Diazepam, in adult dosages of 40 to 120 mg a day, is also useful; it acts quickly, relieves rigidity, and has significant sedative effect without depressing respiration. Other drugs which have been employed extensively in the past include mephenesin, meprobamate, paraldehyde, and chloral hydrate.

Another approach to the management of muscle spasms involves the use of neuromuscular blocking agents such as tubocurare. This method can be used only where facilities and personnel are available to provide controlled mechanical ventilation for the paralyzed patient. This limits its application and increases the possibility of pulmonary complication.

Tracheostomy Tracheostomy has an important role in the management of tetanus. It protects against suffocation due to laryngospasm, reduces the risk of aspiration, and facilitates mechanical assistance of ventilation. While most patients with mild tetanus and some with more severe disease can be managed without it, all patients should be considered candidates for tracheostomy, and the necessary equipment should be at the bedside. Where secretions are copious or respiration has been compromised, the need for tracheostomy should be recognized early, and whenever possible it should be performed electively rather than as an emergency.

Other measures Although antibiotics are frequently prescribed to treat the infected wound and prevent toxin production, there is no indication that they influence the disease favorably. If antibiotics are used, penicillin G is the drug of choice because it is highly effective against the tetanus bacillus, and its limited spectrum is less likely to predispose patients to superinfections. Appropriate cultures to detect complicating infections should be obtained periodically throughout the course of the disease, and specific antibiotics prescribed when indicated. Adrenocortical steroids have been used empirically in the treatment of tetanus, but there is no experimental or clinical evidence to support their effectiveness. Likewise, beneficial results have been claimed for hyperbaric oxygen, but insufficient information is available to evaluate its potential.

PREVENTION *Clostridium tetani* is so ubiquitous in nature that the only hope for prevention of tetanus lies in massive immunization programs. Effective active immunization is possible, and if applied universally, according to recommendations, tetanus could be virtually eliminated. Even tetanus neonatorum could be prevented, because infants are protected by antibody which passes the placental barrier. Two types of tetanus toxoids are available for immunization, a fluid and an adsorbed form. The adsorbed toxoid is preferred because it produces higher antitoxin titers and longer-lasting immunity. Immunization failures are exceedingly rare.

According to current recommendations, children two months to six years of age should be immunized with diphtheria and tetanus toxoids and pertussis vaccine (DPT). Ideally, the first dose should be administered within 2 or 3 months of birth, the second and third should follow at 4- to 6-week intervals, and the fourth dose should be given 1 year after the third. Schoolchildren and adults should be immunized with three doses of adult type tetanus and diphtheria toxoids (Td). The second dose should be given 4 to 6 weeks after the first, and the third 6 months to 1 year after the second. A booster of DPT is recommended for children at the time of entrance into kindergarten or elementary school. Thereafter and for everyone else who has received a primary immunization series, routine boosters of Td should be given every 10 years. Side effects are uncommon after the primary series, but occur more frequently in persons who have received an excessive number of booster injections. Reactions usually take the form of local swelling, erythema, lymphadenopathy, and fever, but on rare occasions more severe hypersensitivity reactions occur.

In the management of wounds, the question of prophylaxis against tetanus frequently arises. Because active immunization is so effective, a reliable immunization history can greatly simplify the problem. If a patient has received three or more doses of toxoid, antiserum need not be given, and a toxoid booster is required only if more than 5 or 10 years has elapsed since the last dose. The shorter interval pertains for all but clean, minor wounds. With a history of two previous doses of tetanus toxoid, a booster is indicated, but antitoxin should be used only if a significant wound is more than 24 hr old. For patients who have received fewer than two doses of toxoid or have an uncertain immunization history, a dose of Td is required for all wounds, and the primary immunization series should be completed in the succeeding weeks to months. Antiserum is also indicated for these patients unless the wound is clean and minor.

When passive immunization is contemplated, TIG is preferred to horse serum because it offers longer protection and freedom from serious reactions. The currently recommended prophylactic dose for adults is 250 units intramuscularly. If TIG is not available, equine antitoxin in doses of 3,000 to 6,000 units should be administered after careful screening for sensitivity to horse serum. When both toxoid and antitoxin are indicated, they can be given simultaneously, but separate syringes and separate injection sites should be used.

Prompt and adequate care of wounds is also important in preventing tetanus. They should be cleaned carefully, and foreign bodies or necrotic, devitalized tissue should be removed. Administration of tetracycline or penicillin is advocated by some to prevent multiplication of *Cl. tetani*, but tetanus may occur in spite of prophylactic antibiotics, and their role in the prevention of tetanus has not been established. However, severe wounds should be examined regularly and treated promptly with antimicrobials if infection develops.

PROGNOSIS The overall case-fatality ratio of tetanus is variable, but in the United States it ranges between 50 to 60 percent. This reflects the fact that the incidence of tetanus is eight to ten times greater among people over 60 compared with people 10 to 20 years of age, and the mortality rate is twenty-five to fifty times greater in the elderly. Neonatal tetanus is uncommon in this country but is fatal in more than 60 percent of cases. The shorter the incubation period and onset time, the poorer the prognosis in tetanus. Three-fourths of the deaths occur within the first week, primarily from pulmonary infection or aspiration. Survivors recover completely, but remain susceptible to the disease unless actively immunized with tetanus toxoid.

REFERENCES

Adams EB et al: *Tetanus*, Oxford: Blackwell Scientific Publications, Ltd., 1969

Brooks GF et al: Tetanus toxoid immunization of adults: A continuing need. Ann Intern Med 73:603, 1970

Cole L, Youngman H: Treatment of tetanus. Lancet 1:1017, 1969

Eckmann L (ed): *Principles of Tetanus: Proceedings of the 2nd International Conference on Tetanus*, Berne: Hans Huber Publications, 1967

Young LS et al: An evaluation of serologic and antimicrobial therapy in the treatment of tetanus in the United States. J Infect Dis 120:153, 1969

153 BOTULISM

M. GLENN KOENIG
HARRY N. BEATY

DEFINITION Botulism is an acute form of poisoning which results from ingestion of a toxin produced by *Clostridium botulinum.* The illness is characterized by progressive descending bulbar and skeletal muscle paralysis, and is often fatal.

HISTORY The disease was first recongnized over 200 years ago by South German physicians who adopted the term *botulismus* for the often fatal syndrome which sometimes followed the consumption of spoiled sausage (*botulus* is Latin for sausage). Botulism was rare in the United States prior to World War I. The growth of commercial and home canning at this time led to a great increase in cases. A series of studies by K. F. Meyer and his associates in the early 1920s defined the habitat of *Cl. botulinum*, the foods often incriminated, and the conditions necessary for the destruction of *Cl. botulinum* spores. This knowledge led to the virtual elimination of botulism from the commercial canning industry, and most cases of clinical botulism now follow consumption of improperly canned, home-preserved foods. However, the need for constant surveillance is emphasized by periodic outbreaks of botulism caused by commercially processed foods.

ETIOLOGY *Clostridium botulinum* is a strictly anaerobic, spore-forming, gram-positive rod which elaborates a potent exotoxin during growth and autolysis. Morphologically and culturally similar strains are differentiated into types A, B, C, D, E, or F on the basis of antigenic characteristics of the toxin each produces. Type A, B, and E toxins have been implicated most frequently in human disease in the United States. Only two outbreaks of type F botulism have been reported. Types C and D produce disease almost exclusively in animals, including wild waterfowl, cattle, horses, and mink.

Type A and B spores are widely distributed in soil throughout the world. Type A spores are most common in the United States, especially along the Pacific Coast and the Rocky Mountain states. Type B spores have been found more frequently in the Eastern states and in Europe. Type E spores have been demonstrated in lakeshore mud, coastal sand, and sea-bottom silt in northern latitudes. Fish apparently contaminate their intestinal tracts with these spores, which accounts for the high incidence of type E strains in fish-borne botulism. Type F spores have been found in marine sediments collected off the coast of California and Oregon and in salmon taken from the Columbia River.

Botulinum toxins are the most potent poisons known. Types A through E have been highly purified and identified as simple proteins. Although they differ in terms of antigenicity, molecular size, electrophoretic mobility, and amino acid content, they appear to have an identical effect on neuromuscular transmission. Pharmacologic differences are manifested by the variable susceptibility of specific animal species to the different toxins.

Spores of *Cl. botulinum* can withstand 100°C for several hours. Moist heat at 120°C for 30 min will destroy spores of all types, but the toxins are considerably more heat-labile. All varieties of toxin are destroyed by boiling for 10 min, or by temperatures of 80°C for 30 min.

PATHOGENESIS Most human botulism follows the ingestion of foodstuffs contaminated with preformed botulinus toxin. Rarely, wounds secondarily infected with *Cl. botulinum* have been the portal of entry of the toxin. There is no convincing evidence that the botulinus bacillus produces toxin in the human gastrointestinal tract, and no cases of disease have been recognized following the ingestion of fresh food. Clinical botulism can occur only when the following conditions are met: (1) a food product is contaminated with viable *Cl. botulinum* bacilli or spores; (2) proper conditions for germination of the spores exist; (3) time and conditions permit production of toxin prior to eating; (4) the food is not heated or is heated insufficiently to destroy botulinus toxin, (5) the toxin-containing food is ingested by a susceptible host (Table 153-1). Though a relatively anaerobic environment and temperatures above 80°F are optimal for toxin production, strict anaerobic conditions are not necessary and toxin production by some type E strains has been observed at temperatures as low as 6°C (42.8°F).

Although a variety of home-processed foods have been sources of botulism in the United States, certain foods seem to be safer than others. This may be because low pH (acidity) inhibits germination of spores and, therefore, of toxin production. Between 1941 and 1971, commercially processed liver paste, cheese, smoked fish, tuna, and soup (vichyssoise) have been implicated in outbreaks of botulism. Contaminated foods often appear putrefied, perhaps because many type A and B strains of *Cl. botulinum* are proteolytic. However, type E strains do not elaborate proteolytic enzymes, and foods containing type E toxin may look and taste perfectly normal.

TABLE 153-1
Important factors in the pathogenesis of botulism

Spores	*Toxin production*	*Toxin*
1 Survive at 6°C (42.8°F) for several months	*1* Strict anaerobic conditions not always required	*1* Destroyed at 80°C (176°F) after 30 min or 100°C for 10 min
2 Can withstand boiling for several hours	*2* Can occur at 6°C (42.8°F)	*2* Unstable at high pH
3 Destroyed at 120°C (248°F) after 30 min	*3* Optimal temperature 30°C (86°F)	*3* Type E toxin activated by trypsin
	4 Reduced at low pH	

Botulinus toxin is absorbed primarily in the stomach and upper part of the small intestine. The toxins are large protein molecules which are absorbed intact after they have been reduced in size by proteolytic enzymes which do not destroy activity. In fact, the toxicity of type E toxin may be enhanced by tryptic digestion. Either absorption is incomplete or toxins are inactivated partially by digestion, because the amount of toxin which appears in the bloodstream is variable, and in animals the lethal dose orally is 1,000 times greater than the lethal dose intravenously. Toxin which reaches the lower part of the small intestine and colon may be absorbed slowly, which probably accounts for the delayed onset and the prolonged symptoms observed in many patients.

Botulinus toxins exert their major effect by blocking neuromuscular transmission in cholinergic nerve fibers while sparing adrenergic fibers. They either inhibit the release of acetylcholine or bind with it at or near its site of release within presynaptic clefts. Muscle reactivity to acetylcholine applied directly to the motor end plate is unimpaired. Some studies have suggested that botulinus toxins exert an inhibitory effect on cholinergic internuncial neurons in the spinal cord, but the clinical importance of this central action is uncertain.

CLINICAL MANIFESTATIONS Botulism may vary from a mild illness for which patients seek no medical advice to a fulminant disease which ends in death within 24 hr. Symptoms usually begin 12 to 36 hr after ingestion of toxin, although extremes of 3 hr to 14 days are recorded. In general, the earlier the symptoms appear, the more serious the disease. Nausea and vomiting occur in approximately one-third of patients with type A or B disease and are very severe with type E intoxication. Weakness, lassitude, dizziness, and vertigo are early complaints. Severe dryness of the mouth and throat, sometimes associated with pharyngeal pain, is also noted. Neurologic symptoms may occur at the same time as these complaints, or they may be delayed for 12 to 72 hr.

Blurred vision, diplopia, dysphonia, dysphagia, and weakness are followed by involvement of the muscles of respiration.

On examination, patients are usually alert, oriented, and afebrile, even with severe disease. Rarely, marked somnolence is noted. Difficulties in speech and deglutition may be obvious. The pupils may be dilated and fixed but in many cases are normal. Extraocular palsies may be present. The mucous membranes of the mouth and tongue are dry and crusted. Weakness of striated muscle groups (particularly of the neck and proximal extremities and the muscles of respiration) appears as the disease progresses, but superficial and deep-tendon reflexes remain intact. Abdominal distention with absent bowel sounds is sometimes marked, and urinary retention may be present.

Respiratory paralysis may occur with startling swiftness. Failure of respiration, airway obstruction, and secondary pulmonary infection are the major causes of death. Sudden cardiac arrest has occurred in some patients with severe respiratory involvement, but whether this is secondary to anoxia or a primary action of botulinus toxin is unknown.

In patients recovering from botulism, return of function of the muscles of respiration, deglutition, and speech may be rapid, and improvement is often apparent within a week. General weakness, constipation, and ocular abnormalities may persist for weeks and sometimes for several months.

LABORATORY FINDINGS Routine laboratory studies do not aid in diagnosing clinical botulism. The cerebrospinal fluid is normal. Electrocardiographic abnormalities, including minor disturbances in conduction, nonspecific T-wave and S-T segment changes, and various disorders of rhythm, have been described. The diagnosis of botulism rests on clinical grounds and can be established only by the identification of botulinus toxin in suspected food or in patients. If available, portions of the suspected food should be suspended in saline solution and injected intraperitoneally into mice. If toxin is present, the animals will develop typical botulism and usually die within 24 hr. Mice protected with specific antiserums survive. Fresh serum from patients suspected of having botulism should be obtained prior to administration of antitoxin, and should be injected intraperitoneally into mice with and without added type A, B, E, and F antiserums. Detection of circulating toxin in this manner has been useful in diagnosing type B and E intoxications and at least one outbreak of type A disease.

DIFFERENTIAL DIAGNOSIS When the full clinical syndrome is evident, the symptoms and signs of botulism are sufficiently characteristic to lead to prompt diagnosis. In many instances the sequential appearance of findings may be confusing, particularly when no clear-cut history of ingestion of home-canned foods has been elicited.

The cranial nerve palsies, muscle weakness, and respiratory paralysis may lead to confusion with myasthenia gravis, Guillain-Barré syndrome, acute poliomyelitis, or stroke. A negative Tensilon test, normal cerebrospinal fluid, lack of sensory abnormalities, preservation of deep-tendon reflexes, mental clarity, and absence of corticospinal tract signs in patients with botulism help to exclude these other possibilities.

Certain nonneurologic phenomena also have led to misdiagnosis. The pharyngeal pain, erythema, and dysphagia seen in some patients may suggest streptococcal or viral pharyngitis. The widely dilated pupils plus a dry mouth and mucous membranes resemble signs found in atropine, belladonna, or Jimson weed poisoning. The lack of nervous system excitement and hallucinations and the delay in onset of symptoms observed in botulism should exclude these possibilities. Nausea, vomiting, abdominal distention, constipation, and ileus may lead to consideration of intestinal obstruction. The dilated pupils and general paralytic phenomena should aid in differentiation.

Unexplained postural hypotension; dilated, unreactive pupils; extremely dry mucous membranes; and progressive muscle paresis occurring in a previously healthy afebrile patient should suggest botulism.

TREATMENT The most immediate threat to the survival of patients with botulism is respiratory failure. Early elective tracheostomy and mechanical assistance of ventilation may be lifesaving. Cathartics and cleansing enemas should be administered to remove any unabsorbed toxin from the bowel. Fluid and electrolyte balance should be maintained by intravenous fluid administration, and a bladder catheter should be inserted if urinary retention occurs. Good nursing care is essential to combat development of aspiration pneumonia and decubitus ulcers, and passive range-of-motion exercises should be instituted early to counteract thromboembolic complications or contractures. As soon as the clinical diagnosis of botulism is suspected, patients should be tested for hypersensitivity to horse serum and treated with trivalent antitoxin which contains antibodies to type A, B, and E toxins (Connaught). Those who react to initial testing must be desensitized before treatment. Because antitoxin remains in the circulation for over 30 days, the manufacturer's recommended dose should be given immediately, rather than in multiple small doses administered over a longer period. The effectiveness of antitoxin in type A botulism has not been established, although some animal studies indicate that the course of the disease is modified dramatically when antitoxin is given promptly after the appearance of neurologic signs. In contrast, the use of type-specific antitoxin has reduced the mortality rate significantly in several outbreaks of type E disease. Nonfatal hypersensitivity reactions occur in 15 to 20 percent of patients receiving equine antitoxin, and may require treatment with adrenal corticosteroids. Otherwise, these drugs are not indicated.

A number of reports have appeared since 1967 describing the use of *guanidine hydrochloride* in the treatment of botulism. This drug presumably acts by binding toxin presynaptically or enhancing the release of acetylcholine from nerve terminals. Most reported cases have shown improvement with oral doses of 35 to 50 mg per kg per day, and in some instances the salutary effect of the drug has been documented with neurophysiologic studies. However, failures also have been reported with guanidine, and its role in the management of botulism remains to be defined. Dose-related side effects of treatment, which include gastrointestinal upset, hyperirritability, tremors, and muscle twitching, may limit the usefulness of the drug.

Because there is no evidence to suggest that *Cl. botulinum* can multiply in the gastrointestinal tract of man, antibiotics should be reserved for specific infectious complications.

PROGNOSIS Type A strains have been the most frequent cause of botulism in the United States. Mortality rates of 60 to 70 percent have been reported in most outbreaks. Type B disease, which has been more common in Europe, has had consistently lower fatality rates, i.e., 10 to 30 percent. Type E botulism has produced outbreaks in northern latitudes among people eating raw fish (Japanese, Canadian Eskimos), with mortality rates ranging from 30 to 50 percent in large series. With more rapid diagnosis, aggressive management of respiratory paralysis, and use of polyvalent antitoxin, it seems likely that these figures will be improved. Once the patient has survived the paralytic illness, the outlook for complete recovery is excellent.

REFERENCES

Cherington M: Botulism: Clinical and therapeutic observations. Rocky Mt Med J 69:55, 1972

Donadio JA, Gangarosa EJ: Surveillance for botulism in the United States, 1968–1969. J Infect Dis 122:122, 1970

Faich GA et al: Failure of guanidine therapy in botulism A. N Engl J Med 285:773, 1971

Koenig MG et al: Type B botulism in man. Am J Med 42:208, 1967

Ryan DW, Cherington M: Human type A botulism. JAMA 216:513, 1971

154
OTHER CLOSTRIDIAL INFECTIONS

EDWARD W. HOOK

INTRODUCTION Bacteria of the genus *Clostridium* are normal inhabitants of soil and the gastrointestinal tracts of man and animals. Most of the species that have been described are saprophytic, but some are infectious for man and animals, usually under conditions of lowered host and tissue resistance. Infections with these organisms are often associated with profound systemic manifestations, and all pathogenic clostridia, except *Clostridium tetani* and *C. botulinum*, are capable of causing extensive tissue destruction. Diseases caused by these other clostridia are gas gangrene, cellulitis, postabortal and puerperal sepsis, and on occasion pneumonia, pleurisy, peritonitis, meningitis, endocarditis, cystitis, or bursitis. In addition, ingestion of food contaminated with *C. perfringens* Type A is a common cause of enterocolitis.

ETIOLOGY Wounds complicated by gas gangrene usually contain a mixture of pathogenic and saprophytic clostridia, often including *C. tetani*, as well as a variety of other bacteria. *Clostridium perfringens* (*welchii*), *C. novyi* (*oedematiens*), or *C. septicum* (*Vibrion septique*) can be cultured from most cases of gas gangrene and clostridial cellulitis, and *C. perfringens* causes virtually all clostridial infections of the uterus. *Clostridium bifermentans*, *C. histolyticum*, and *C. fallax* are less virulent organisms that occasionally cause gas gangrene but are more commonly associated with localized cellulitis. Proliferation of *C. botulinum* in wounds occasionally leads to clinical manifestations of botulism (Chap. 153).

The clostridia of gas gangrene and related infections are anaerobic or microaerophilic gram-positive bacilli that produce abundant gas in artificial media and form subterminal endospores. *Clostridium perfringens* is encapsulated and nonmotile, rarely sporulates in artificial media, and produces spores that can usually be destroyed by boiling.

EPIDEMIOLOGY AND PATHOGENESIS Clostridia do not penetrate intact skin or mucous membranes, but frequently gain access to tissues through wounds or perforated abdominal viscera. Although these organisms can be cultured from one-third to two-thirds of severe traumatic wounds, gas gangrene develops in only an occasional case. The most important prerequisite for the conversion of clostridial contamination of a wound to a progressive infection is an environment with low oxidation-reduction potential, which permits spore germination and anaerobic growth. Local oxidation-reduction potential can be reduced by failure of the blood supply to a contaminated area, by the presence of foreign bodies such as clothing, dirt, or fragments of metal or wood, or by the multiplication of other bacteria in the wound. Once multiplicaton and toxin production are established, rapid invasion and destruction of healthy tissue follow.

The pathogenicity of clostridia is related to the capacity of these organisms to form exotoxins which destroy tissue cells. The nature and amount of toxins vary considerably for different species and strains. For example, at least 12 different extracellular *toxins* are produced by *C. perfringens*. Alpha toxin, a lecithinase, is clearly the most important and is the principal tissue-destroying, hemolytic, and lethal toxin. Other *C. perfringens* products include collagenase, hyaluronidase, hemolytic theta toxin, leukocidin, deoxyribonuclease, and fibrinolysin.

Gas gangrene is characterized by marked systemic symptoms and a local reaction with extensive necrotizing myositis, edema, thrombosis of small vessels, interstitial gas bubbles, and minimal infiltration of leukocytes. The local reaction in infected tissue can be explained by the action of clostridial toxins, especially alpha toxin, but the factors responsible for the general reaction are unknown. Alpha toxin, or other clostridial toxins, have not been demonstrated in circulating blood during the course of severe clostridial myonecrosis.

CLINICAL MANIFESTATIONS Clostridial myonecrosis (gas gangrene, clostridial myositis) Gas gangrene develops in anoxic devitalized tissues in which the arterial circulation has been compromised by trauma, constricting tourniquets or casts, or obliterative arterial disease. Infection is most frequent after extensive injury to skeletal muscle, particularly of the thigh and buttock, and is more common in wounds complicated by compound fractures or lodgment of foreign bodies. Once infection is established, it rapidly spreads to involve healthy muscle undamaged by previous trauma or ischemia.

The incubation period is usually 1 to 4 days but may vary from 3 hr to 6 weeks or longer. The earliest symptom is sudden, severe pain in the injured part. The distal portion of an involved limb becomes cold and edematous within a few hours, and eventually pulseless and gangrenous. The wound drains a watery, brown or hemorrhagic material which may have a peculiar sweet odor. The appearance of the wound is usually not that of a pyogenic inflammatory lesion. Depending on the duration of the process, the surrounding skin may be normal, white, and tense, or dusky brown and reddish. Vesicles or hemorrhagic bullae may develop, particularly in *C. septicum* infections. Gas is usually not detectable in the tissues by palpation except in advanced lesions, although it may be visible easily by x-ray. Occasionally, tiny bubbles may be seen in the discharge from the wound; rarely, crepitation can be detected at an early stage by auscultation. The involved muscle appears dark red or black, may herniate through the wound, and is noncontractile when stimulated.

Systemic manifestations developing shortly after onset of severe pain and swelling of an injured extremity strongly suggest gas gangrene. The patient is prostrated, pale, and motionless but is usually well oriented, alert, and extremely apprehensive. The temperature usually does not exceed 101°F and may be normal. As the illness progresses, there may be anorexia, vomiting, profuse watery or bloody diarrhea, and eventually circulatory collapse. The pulse rate usually exceeds 120 beats per min and is elevated out of proportion to the temperature. Massive intravascular hemolysis is rare in patients with clostridial myositis. Pericardial effusion is sometimes noted. Delirium and coma may precede death, but more commonly the patient dies suddenly several days after onset of illness, often during surgery or anesthesia. Acute renal failure is occasionally a late complication.

Gas gangrene has been described after hypodermic injection, especially injection of epinephrine. Minor trauma also occasionally activates clostridial spores dormant in scar tissue and leads to development of myonecrosis years after original injury.

Gas gangrene must be differentiated from nonclostridial infections of gangrenous limbs caused by anaerobic streptococci, aerobic gas-forming coliform bacilli, *Bacteroides* species, and group A streptococci.

Clostridial cellulitis This is a relatively benign infection of skin and subcutaneous tissues that occurs in a small proportion of wounds contaminated with pathogenic clostridia. The disease is characterized by spreading necrosis of superficial tissues and a profuse, foul-smelling, brown, seropurulent exudate. Gas, which crepitates on palpation, invariably forms in the subcutaneous tissues and may involve an entire limb or form a localized gas pocket. In clostridial cellulitis, the underlying skeletal muscle is not involved, pain is not severe, and the only systemic manifestations are slight fever and moderate tachycardia. It can usually be differentiated from group A streptococcal cellulitis by the presence of subcutaneous gas and the absence of erythema.

Postabortal and puerperal sepsis Uterine infections with *C. perfringens* usually occur after incomplete abortions induced under unsterile conditions and occasionally after spontaneous abortions, prolonged labor at term, ruptured membranes, or operative interference with pregnancy. The organisms presumably invade the damaged endometrium through the retained products of conception. The earliest symptoms may be related to instrumentation and consist of metrorrhagia, suprapubic and back pain, chills, and fever. Fever of 100 to 103°F, often with chills, usually recurs several days after abortion, but the incubation period can be as short as 6 hr. Vaginal bleeding is almost invariably present, and there is often a brown, foul-smelling, vaginal discharge containing necrotic tissue. The cervix is soft and patulous, and the uterus and adnexae are usually very tender. The lower abdominal wall is often tense, or signs of generalized peritonitis may be present, secondary to perforation of the uterus or parametrial extension of infection. Nausea, vomiting, and profuse diarrhea are often prominent.

Systemic manifestations may appear with dramatic suddenness. Massive intravascular hemolysis, accompanied by hemoglobinemia, hemoglobinuria, and jaundice, may be the most striking feature of the disease. Icterus may appear within hours after onset of illness. As in gas gangrene, the clinical picture may be dominated by circulatory collapse with hypotension, extreme tachycardia, cyanosis, hyperpnea, and pulmonary edema. Despite severe prostration, the patient is frequently well oriented, alert, and apprehensive. The mortality rate in postabortal or puerperal sepsis caused by *C. perfringens* and associated with intense hemolysis is 40 to 70 percent. Death may occur a few hours after onset or may be delayed for days. Acute renal failure secondary to shock, dehydration, or hemolysis occurs frequently.

Unusual local complications of the uterine infection are gas gangrene of the vagina and rectum and clostridial cellulitis of the anterior abdominal wall following cesarean section or hysterectomy. At times, the infectious process is confined to the endometrium and myometrium with intrauterine gas formation (physometra).

Septic abortion with *C. perfringens* bacteremia without overt hemolysis is a more common occurrence than bacteremia with gross hemolysis, as described above. Death is unusual in the absence of hemolysis.

Diseases to be considered in the *differential diagnosis* include perforated uterus, ruptured ectopic pregnancy, ingestion of toxic abortifacients, streptococcal or staphylococcal puerperal sepsis, pelvic thrombophlebitis with septic pulmonary emboli, acute hepatic necrosis of pregnancy, and sickle-cell crisis.

Clostridium perfringens food poisoning Meat and meat products contaminated with *C. perfringens* type A are frequently responsible for outbreaks of acute gastroenteritis. In 1971 in the United States, *C. perfringens* accounted for 16 percent of reported foodborne outbreaks.

Most outbreaks of *C. perfringens* food poisoning have been associated with the ingestion of meat or poultry dishes. Most market meats and poultry are heavily contaminated, and the organism can be isolated with ease from soil, water, air, and human or animal feces. The usual story is that the food has been prepared and cooked 24 hr or more before consumption, allowed to cool slowly at room temperature, and then served either cold or warmed. During this period of incubation, contaminating clostridia grow to large numbers sufficient to constitute an infectious inoculum. *C. perfringens* food poisoning can be reproduced experimentally in man by feeding the actively growing organisms which apparently multiply and sporulate in the small intestine. Sporulation is associated with the production of an enterotoxin *in situ*.

Typical symptoms of diarrhea with abdominal pain and cramps develop 6 to 24 hr after ingestion of meat, stew, or soup which has been stored at a warm temperature for several hours after cooking. Nausea occurs occasionally, but vomiting is rare. Systemic manifestations are usually absent, and recovery is uneventful after 12 to 24 hr.

A severe form of clostridial infection termed *enteritis necrotans* was observed in Germany after World War II. This disease was characterized by hemorrhagic necrosis of the small intestine, bloody diarrhea, severe dehydration, shock, and death. A similar infection termed *necrotizing jejunitis* has been described in natives of New Guinea who had eaten inadequately cooked pork.

Miscellaneous clostridial infections Clostridia can be isolated from bile obtained at elective cholecystectomy in patients without symptoms of clostridial infection. Clostridial cellulitis or myonecrosis may occasionally follow surgical procedures, particularly surgery on the gastrointestinal tract or gallbladder. Pathogenic clostridia are occasionally introduced into the abdomen, thoracic cavity, or cranium through penetrating wounds. Primary pneumonia in the absence of a penetrating wound or distant focus has been described. Clostridial pleurisy may involve the underlying lung but is usually an indolent localized infection with minimal systemic manifestations. Meningitis is usually secondary to a puncture wound of the skull and is often associated with a necrotizing cerebritis. Clostridial peritonitis may follow perforation of the gallbladder, appendix, or other viscus and is usually rapidly fatal.

More than 70 cases of clostridial septicemia have been reported in patients with far-advanced neoplastic disease, including leukemias, lymphomas, and metastatic solid tumors. Over two-thirds of these patients had been receiving antineoplastic chemotherapy or radiation therapy. The primary site of invasion is usually the gastrointestinal tract which is frequently extensively involved by the neoplastic process. Abdominal surgical procedures, endoscopy, small bowel series, and paracentesis have been reported to predispose to sepsis in these patients. The course of the disease is rapid, death often occurring within 24 hr after onset of recognizable infection. Hypotension, hyperpyrexia, and dyspnea are the most common clinical manifestations of infection. Jaundice and hemolysis occur occasionally. Cellulitis, with or without crepitation, may appear in the flanks and should suggest the diagnosis, especially in patients with leukemia or lymphoma.

Cystitis with pneumaturia, gaseous cholecystitis, endocarditis, and bursitis after needle aspiration are other examples of rare clostridial infections.

LABORATORY FINDINGS The diagnosis of gas gangrene, clostridial cellulitis, postabortal sepsis, or other clostridial infections is based primarily on clinical criteria. Smears of wound exudate, uterine scrapings, or cervical discharge may show abundant large gram-positive rods, as well as other organisms. Spores are rarely observed in smears of exudates. Thioglycollate broth, deep meat broth, and blood-agar plates incubated in an anaerobic jar should be inoculated for definitive identification of specific clostridia. However, interpretation of positive wound cultures is difficult because clostridia are frequent contaminants. *Clostridium perfringens* bacteremia is common in postabortal infections but rare in gas gangrene.

Polymorphonuclear leukocytosis occurs frequently in gas gangrene and invariably in postabortal sepsis; total blood leukocyte counts range from 15,000 to 40,000 cells per mm^3 and occasionally exceed 60,000 cells per mm^3. Marked thrombocytopenia develops in about 50 percent of patients with clostridial sepsis. The urine frequently contains protein and casts. Renal insufficiency may lead to severe uremia.

X-ray examination sometimes provides the first clue leading to the correct diagnosis by revealing the presence of gas in muscle, subcutaneous tissue, or uterus; however, demonstration of gas in tissues is not diagnostic of clostridial infection. Other bacteria, especially *Enterobacter* or *Esherichia*, may be responsible for gas production, and occasionally air is sucked into a wound at the time of penetrating injury.

Profound alterations of circulating erythrocytes are common in postabortal sepsis but are much less frequent in other clostridial infection. Hemolytic anemia may develop with almost unbelievable rapidity; the red blood cell count occasionally decreases by 2 million cells per mm^3 in less than 24 hr and is associated with hemoglobinemia, hemoglobinuria, and elevated levels of serum bilirubin. Spherocytosis, increased osmotic and mechanical red cell fragility, erythrophagocytosis, and methemoglobinemia have also been described. Abnormalities of the clotting mechanism characteristic of intravascular coagulation may be observed in patients with severe clostridial infections.

TREATMENT The traditional therapeutic approach to serious clostridial infection, such as diffuse, spreading myositis, is immediate surgical intervention with wide radical debridement followed by open drainage without closure or open amputation when necessary. Early surgery not only aids diagnosis, but permits decompression of fascial compartments and excision of devitalized muscle and may obviate amputation. A number of authorities feel that hyperbaric oxygen therapy has modified this traditional approach to gas gangrene by assuming priority over radical surgical debridement. Proponents report that hyperbaric oxygenation produces impressive, almost immediate improvement in patients with gas gangrene, with rapid disappearance of systemic toxicity and prompt arrest of local spread of the gangrenous infection. Opinion differs about whether conservative debridement should be carried out before or after hyperbaric oxygen therapy, but no one advocates hyperbaric oxygen alone for gas gangrene. Oxygen toxicity consequent to hyperbaric oxygenation may lead to convulsions in some patients.

Curettage of the uterus should be performed for diagnosis and treatment of postabortal clostridial infections. In the absence of hemolysis, standard therapy for septic abortion with antibiotics and uterine curettage usually produces rapid improvement, even in patients with bacteremia. The mortality rate in patients with abortion, *C. perfringens* bacteremia, and intense hemolysis is high irrespective of the therapeutic approach. The role of hysterectomy is controversial and ill-defined; some surgeons strongly advocate hysterectomy, whereas others feel that the potential benefits of the procedure do not outweigh the risks. Heparinization, exchange transfusion, and hyperbaric oxygen have been utilized but are not of established benefit.

Simple excision and adequate drainage usually suffice for treating clostridial cellulitis.

Penicillin is the antibiotic of choice for all clostridial infections and should be administered in doses of 20 million units a day by continuous intravenous infusion. Tetracycline is also active against most strains of *Clostridium* and has been recommended as an adjunct to penicillin therapy. Clostridia are also susceptible in vitro to cephalothin, chloramphenicol, and clindamycin.

The efficacy of polyvalent gas gangrene antitoxin is controversial. Many centers have discontinued the use of antitoxin in the management of patients with suspected gas gangrene or clostridial postabortal sepsis.

Intravenous infusions of blood, plasma volume expanders, fluids, and electrolytes are required to combat shock, anemia, and dehydration. Renal insufficiency should be treated in the same manner as acute tubular necrosis from other causes.

The most reliable protection against gas gangrene is early and adequate wound debridement. Antitoxin is ineffective as a prophylactic agent. The use of clostridial toxoids for prophylactic immunization of individuals in hazardous occupations awaits evaluation.

REFERENCES

ALTEMEIER WA, FULLEN WD: Prevention and treatment of gas gangrene. JAMA 217:806, 1971

CENTER FOR DISEASE CONTROL: *Foodborne Outbreaks—Annual Summary 1971,* Atlanta: The Center, 1972

HAUSCHILD AHW: *Clostridium perfringens* enterotoxin. J Milk Food Tech 34:596, 1971

HITCHCOCK CR et al: Treatment of clostridial infections with hyperbaric oxygen. Surgery 63:759, 1967

MACLENNAN JD: The histotoxic clostridial infections of man. Bacteriol Rev 26:177, 1962

MAHN E, DANTUONO LM: Postabortal septicotoxemia due to *Clostridium Welchii:* Seventy-five cases from the maternity hospital, Santiago, Chile 1948–1952. Am J Obstet Gynecol 70:604, 1955

MURRELL TGC et al: Pig-Bel: Enteritis necroticans: A study in diagnosis and management. Lancet 1:217, 1966

NAKAMURA M, SCHULZE JA: Clostridium perfringens food poisoning. Annu Rev Microbiol 24:359, 1970

PRITCHARD JA, WHALLEY PJ: Abortion complicated by clostridium perfringens infection. Am J Obstet Gynecol 111:484, 1971

TRIPPEL OH et al: Hyperbaric oxygenation in the management of gas gangrene. Surg Clin N Am 47:17, 1967

WYNE JW, ARMSTRONG D: Clostridial septicemia. Cancer 29:215, 1972

155 CHOLERA

CHARLES C. J. CARPENTER

DEFINITION Cholera is an acute illness which results from colonization of the small bowel by *Vibrio cholerae.* The disease is characterized by its epidemic occurrence and the production in the more severe cases of massive diarrhea with rapid depletion of extracellular fluid and electrolytes.

ETIOLOGY AND EPIDEMIOLOGY *Vibrio cholerae* is a curved, aerobic, gram-negative bacillus with a single polar flagellum. It is rapidly motile and possesses both O and H antigens. Serologic identification is based on differences in the polysaccharide O antigens.

Cholera has been endemic in the Gangetic Delta of West Bengal and Bangladesh and is often epidemic throughout South and Southeast Asia. The most recent pandemic spread of this disease, from 1961 to 1972, extended from the Celebes northward to Korea and westward to the whole of North and West Africa and certain Western European nations. The last major epidemic of cholera in the Western Hemisphere occurred during 1866–1867.

The majority of major epidemics have clearly been waterborne, but direct contamination of food by infected feces probably contributes to spread during major outbreaks. Poor sanitation appears to be primarily responsible for the continuing presence of cholera, but host factors, such as relative or absolute achlorhydria, may also play an important role.

A chronic gallbladder carrier state has been observed in a small percentage of convalescent cholera patients, largely limited to older individuals. These chronic *Vibrio* carriers may provide a vehicle for spread outside of endemic areas. The basis for the annual cholera epidemics throughout the Gangetic Delta, for the periodic outbreaks throughout the remainder of South and Southeast Asia, and for the occasional global pandemics has, however, not been clearly delineated.

PATHOGENESIS *Vibrio cholerae* produces an enterotoxin which appears to be responsible for all known pathophysiologic aberrations in cholera. This enterotoxin stimulates adenyl cyclase in the gut epithelial cells, and the resultant increase in intracellular cyclic adenosine 3′,5′-monophosphate leads to secretion of isotonic fluid by all segments of the small bowel. The enterotoxin-induced electrolyte secretion occurs in the absence of any demonstrable histologic damage to gut epithelial cells or to the capillary endothelial cells of the lamina propria. Precise studies have demonstrated that the adult cholera stool is nearly isotonic, with sodium and chloride concentrations slightly less than those of plasma, a bicarbonate concentration approximately twice that of plasma, and a potassium concentration three to five times that of plasma. Disease caused by all known strains of *V. cholerae* results in the same stool electrolyte pattern. The pathophysiologic defect in cholera is extracellular fluid depletion with resultant hypovolemic shock, base-deficit acidosis, and progressive potassium depletion. There is no convincing evidence that the cholera *Vibrio* invades any tissue, nor has the enterotoxin been shown, in human disease, to have any direct effect on any organ other than the small intestine.

MANIFESTATIONS The incubation period is generally from 6 to 48 hr. This is followed by the abrupt onset of watery, generally painless diarrhea. In the more severe cases, the initial diarrheal stool may be in excess of 1,000 ml, and several liters of isotonic fluid may be lost within hours, leading rapidly to profound shock. Vomiting generally follows, but occasionally precedes, the onset of diarrhea; the vomiting is characteristically effortless and not preceded by nausea. As saline depletion progresses, severe muscle cramps, commonly involving the calves, occur.

When first seen, the typical severely ill cholera patient is cyanotic, with pinched facies, scaphoid abdomen, poor skin turgor, and thready or absent peripheral pulses. The voice is faint, high-pitched, and often inaudible, and there are tachycardia, hypotension, and varying degrees of tachypnea. In all epidemics there are mild cases in which gastrointestinal fluid loss is not severe enough to require hospitalization.

The disease runs its course in 2 to 7 days, and subsequent manifestations depend on the adequacy of electrolyte repletion therapy. With prompt fluid and electrolyte repletion, physiologic recovery is remarkably rapid, and mortality exceptionally rare. However, if therapy is inadequate, the mortality is quite high. The important causes of death, in inadequately treated patients, are hypovolemic shock, metabolic acidosis, and uremia resulting from acute tubular necrosis.

LABORATORY FINDINGS In epidemics or in endemic areas, the clinical picture should arouse strong suspicion immediately. The most reliable technique for identification of *V. cholerae* consists of direct plating of a sample of cholera stool on bile salt, gelatin-tellurite-taurocholate (GTT), or thiosulfate-citrate-bile salt-sucrose (TCBS) agar. On bile salt or GTT agar the organisms appear as typical translucent colonies within 24 hr. On TCBS agar, *V. cholerae* appears at 24 hr as distinct, large yellow colonies. Further classification requires agglutination with type-specific antiserums. In mild or convalescent cases, recovery of vibrios may be enhanced by initial enrichment for 6 hr in alkaline peptone water followed by subculture on bile salt, GTT, or TCBS agar. Rapid diagnosis is possible either by directly observing immobilization of vibrios by type-specific antiserums, using dark-field or phase microscopy, or by identifying the organisms by immunofluorescent methods.

TREATMENT Successful therapy requires only prompt and adequate replacement of gastrointestinal losses of saline and alkali. A uniformly satisfactory solution for intravenous fluid therapy can be simply prepared by the addition of 5 g sodium chloride, 4 g sodium bicarbonate (or acetate), and 1 g potassium chloride to 1 liter of pyrogen-free distilled water. If commercially prepared fluids are available, a combination of isotonic sodium bicarbonate (or acetate or lactate) and isotonic sodium chloride, infused in a 2:1 ratio may be employed. The intravenous fluids are initially infused at 50 to 100 ml per min, until a strong pulse has been restored. The same fluids should subsequently be infused in quantities equal to the gastrointestinal losses. If losses cannot be measured accurately, intravenous fluids should be given at a rate sufficient to maintain a normal radial pulse and normal skin turgor. Overhydration can be avoided by careful observation of neck venous filling and auscultation of the lungs. Close observation is mandatory during the acute phase of the illness, because the cholera patient can lose as much as 1 liter of isotonic fluid per hour during the first 24 hr of the disease. Inadequate or delayed restoration of fecal fluid losses may result in a very high incidence of acute renal failure. Serious hypokalemic symptoms are rare in adults, and potassium repletion can be carried out orally if potassium-containing intravenous fluids are not available. Hypokalemia contributes significantly, however, to the morbidity in inadequately treated pediatric cholera, and potassium, 10 to 13 mEq per liter, should be included in the intravenous fluids administered to pediatric patients.

Although adequate intravenous saline and alkali repletion alone results in rapid recovery of virtually all adult cholera patients, a dramatic reduction in the duration and volume of the diarrhea, and early eradication of vibrios from the stool, may be effected by antibiotic therapy. Oral tetracycline, 500 mg every 6 hr for the first 48 hr of treatment, has been most successful. Other antibiotics, including chloramphenicol and furazolidone, are also of value, but both appear to be slightly less effective than tetracycline.

Oral therapy Since the cholera enterotoxin does not alter glucose-facilitated sodium absorption, fluid repletion can be effected by the oral administration of glucose-containing electrolyte solutions. Since the limiting factor in treatment of cholera in both epidemic and endemic situations is often the lack of adequate quantities of intravenous fluids, the availability of an oral treatment regimen has greatly reduced the mortality from cholera outbreaks during the most recent pandemic spread of this disease. A solution containing glucose 20 g per liter, sodium bicarbonate 4 g per liter, sodium chloride 4 g per liter, and potassium chloride 1 g per liter can be readily prepared and should be satisfactory for treatment of all age groups. This solution, administered orally at a rate equal to the stool losses, can be given to milder cholera cases throughout the course of illness and is satisfactory in the more severe cases, once the hypovolemic shock has been corrected by intravenous fluid therapy. Oral therapy does not decrease the rate of gut fluid loss but provides an electrolyte solution which can be absorbed at a rate sufficient, in most cases, to counterbalance the continuing fluid losses. Therefore, successful management of the cholera patient with oral therapy requires just as close supervision, with careful monitoring of pulse volume, skin turgor, and neck veins, as does management with intravenous solutions. Supplemental intravenous fluids must be administered whenever clinical signs of saline depletion recur.

PROGNOSIS Under ideal conditions and with prompt and adequate fluid replacement, mortality approaches zero, and significant sequelae are rare. Unfortunately, death rates as high as 60 percent still occur, especially during the initial phases of certain outbreaks. This high mortality reflects lack of pyrogen-free intravenous fluids in remote areas, the difficulties of initiating treatment promptly when large numbers of cases are occurring in poverty-stricken populations, and the compromises which may have to be made under emergency conditions.

PREVENTION Immunization by standard commercial vaccine, containing 10 billion killed organisms per ml, provides significant protection for a limited (4- to 6-month) period. Immunization with toxoid provides significant protection in experimental animals, but toxoid has not yet been tested in man. Careful hygiene provides the only sure protection against cholera.

ENTEROTOXIGENIC ESCHERICHIA COLI

Enterotoxin-producing *E. coli* may cause a diarrheal disease which is similar at time of onset to that produced by *V. cholerae,* with the rapid development of profound saline depletion, hypotension, and metabolic acidosis. Like the cholera enterotoxin, the *E. coli* enterotoxin causes loss of isotonic fluid from the small bowel, in the absence of any morphologic damage to the gut mucosa. The diarrhea caused by the enterotoxin-producing *E. coli* differs from that caused by *V. cholerae*, however, in that it is characteristically of much shorter duration. There are at least two reasons for this difference: colonization of the upper small bowel by *E. coli* is characteristically of much shorter duration, and the effect of *E. coli* on gut fluid secretion is of much shorter duration than that of cholera enterotoxin.

Since the intestinal fluid losses caused by the *E. coli* enterotoxin are quantitatively identical to those produced by cholera enterotoxin, the same principles of intravenous and oral fluid therapy which pertain to the treatment of cholera are followed in the treatment of diarrhea caused by enterotoxin-producing *E. coli.* The average patient requires, however, a smaller quantity of intravenous and/or oral fluids than the average cholera patient because of the much shorter duration of diarrheal fluid loss. Antibiotic therapy has not been shown to be of significant value in the management of this disease.

VIBRIO PARAHEMOLYTICUS INFECTION

Vibrio parahemolyticus is one of the leading causes of diarrheal diseases in Japan and recently has been responsible for several outbreaks in this country. The organism is ingested with fresh or steamed crabs or shrimp. The incubation period ranges from 15 to 24 hours, and symptoms consist of weakness, nausea, vomiting, abdominal pain, diarrhea, and tenesmus. There may be low-grade fever. The stools may be bloody and contain numerous polymorphonuclear leukocytes. Sigmoidoscopy shows shallow ulcerations of the rectosigmoid. The diagnosis is made by culturing the organism from stool on thiosulfate-citrate-bile salt medium. Contaminated seafoods usually also yield positive cultures. The illness usually lasts 2 to 5 days, and with appropriate supportive treatment complete recovery occurs.

REFERENCES

Cholera

CARPENTER CCJ et al: Clinical studies in Asiatic cholera I–VI. Bull Johns Hopkins Hosp 118:165, 1966

GANGAROSA EF et al: The nature of the gastrointestinal lesion in Asiatic cholera and its relation to pathogenesis: A biopsy study. Am J Trop Med Hyg 9:125, 1960

GORBACH SL et al: Acute undifferentiated human diarrhea in the tropics. I. Alteration in intestinal microflora. J Clin Invest 50:881, 1971

WALLACE CK et al: Optimal antibiotic therapy in cholera. Bull WHO 39:239, 1968

WATTEN RH et al: Water and electrolyte studies in cholera. J Clin Invest 38:1879, 1959

Vibrio parahemolyticus

THATCHER FS, CLARK DS (eds): *Microorganisms in Foods: Their Significance and Methods of Enumeration*, Toronto: University of Toronto Press, 1968, p. 14

156 TUBERCULOSIS

WILLIAM W. STEAD

DEFINITION Tuberculosis is a necrotizing bacterial infection with protean manifestations and wide distribution. The lungs are most commonly affected, but lesions may occur also in the kidneys, bones, lymph nodes, or meninges or be disseminated throughout the body. There are two stages in which the infection may cause clinical disease: (1) Primary tuberculosis, in which tubercle bacilli invade a host having no specific immunity; at this stage the disease most commonly heals spontaneously, but it may progress to clinical disease if immune mechanisms fail. (2) Postprimary, or adult, tuberculosis (often erroneously called "reinfection tuberculosis"), which is the result of progression of infection years later in spite of specific immunity. In the Western world where bovine tuberculosis has been controlled, the portal of entry in man is almost exclusively the lung.

HISTORY Some of the races of man (Caucasian, Mongolian) have lived with tubercle bacilli throughout much of their history. African, American Indian, and Eskimo peoples have had contact with tuberculosis over a much shorter period. Tuberculosis was named to indicate its formation of firm nodules, or "tubercles." For many years the chronic form (then often called phthisis or consumption) was considered a degenerative or hereditary disease, quite separate from primary tuberculosis which occurred in childhood and was obviously infectious. Laennec (1819) was the first to recognize the chronic form as merely a later development in the same infection. Koch identified (1882) the causative organism. There has been a great drop in prevalence of tuberculosis in the economically developed countries. The death rate from tuberculosis had already begun to fall by 1900, coincidently with improvement in nutrition and standard of living. For the person with active tuberculosis, however, the most important development occurred in 1944 with the discovery of streptomycin. With the introduction of para-aminosalicylic acid (PAS) in 1947, isoniazid (INH) in 1952, ethambutol (EMB) in 1967, and rifampin (RFN) in 1971, specific therapy has become excellent and easy to administer.

ETIOLOGY *Mycobacterium tuberculosis* is a rod of 2 to 4 μm in length and 0.3 μm in thickness. Its distinguishing staining property, i.e., resistance to decolorization by acid alcohol when stained with basic fuchsin, is related to the waxy component of the cell wall, probably specifically to its content of mycolic acid. This "acid-fastness" is dependent in some way upon the structural integrity of the bacillus; it is lost when the organisms are damaged by grinding but is not affected by prolonged extraction with fat solvents.

Tubercle bacilli are strict aerobes and thrive best when there is a P_{O_2} of 100 mm Hg or more and a P_{CO_2} of about 40 mm Hg. The organs most commonly affected by tuberculosis are those with relatively high oxygen tension; metastatic foci are most common in the apices of the lungs where the P_{O_2} is in the range of 120 to 130 mm Hg in the upright position, followed by the kidney and the growing end of bones, where the P_{O_2} approaches 100 mm Hg. The liver and spleen, where the P_{O_2} is quite low, are rarely affected, except in overwhelming disseminated infection.

Two strains of *M. tuberculosis* affect man: human and bovine. By far the greatest number of cases in the United States are caused by the human strain. Programs for eradication of bovine tuberculosis have been so effective that the disease now appears only sporadically in this country. Avian bacilli have little invasiveness for man.

Several other species of mycobacteria have been noted to cause chronic pulmonary infection (Chap. 158). The most common are the avian-Battey group (*Mycobacterium intracellulare* or Runyon's group III) and *Mycobacterium kansasii* (Runyon's group I). Clinical infection due to Runyon's groups II and IV is rare. These mycobacteria appear not to be transmissible, and the epidemiology of the respective infections remains obscure. They tend to infect lungs that have been damaged by silicosis or chronic obstructive lung disease. *Mycobacterium kansasii* responds well to antituberculous drugs in high dosage, but *M. intracellulare* is quite resistant to all drugs presently in use.

TRANSMISSION Most cases of contagious tuberculosis among adults develop because of a late recrudescence of dormant infection with no history of recent exposure. The liquid caseum from a cavity in such a case abounds in tubercle bacilli which are excreted in aerosolized droplets during coughing, sneezing, and speaking. Droplets larger than 10 μm are usually caught on the mucociliary blanket and cleared from the lung without harm, but droplets of smaller size may reach the respiratory bronchiole and deposit bacilli beyond the protective mucus blanket. There, in a susceptible host, the organisms may invade tissue and establish an infection. Persons who have been infected previously are largely protected from reinfection by specific immunity which is mediated by "T cells" (thymus lymphocytes).

In a susceptible host infection may result from inhalation of tubercle bacilli in *fresh* droplet nuclei from a person with cavitary tuberculosis and can be blocked effectively in hospital by ultraviolet light and exhaust ventilation. While tubercle bacilli can often be cultured from dust in a room of a tuberculous person, they constitute no hazard to others because the irregular shape and electrostatic charge of the attached dust particles prevent them from carrying bacilli beyond the mucociliary protective mechanism. Persons with primary tuberculosis are rarely infectious because they expel so few organisms. Tuberculosis is not spread on hands, dishes, glasses, or utensils or by fomites.

In milk tubercle bacilli are killed readily by boiling and by pasteurization. In countries where bovine tuberculosis is still prevalent, pasteurization is particularly important, since milk from a tuberculous cow often contains millions of bacilli per milliliter when the udder is involved.

The small numbers of organisms sprayed on food by a tuberculous food handler are inadequate to transmit infection. The danger from the diseased food handler is the same as from any other person excreting tubercle bacilli into the air.

PREVALENCE AND INCIDENCE There has been a great fall in prevalence of tuberculosis in the United States since 1900. Early in this century over 80 percent of the population was infected *before* the age of twenty. In an autopsy study in 1946, there was evidence of tuberculosis in 80 percent of the persons over the age of fifty. In 1972, only 3 to 5 percent of young adults react to tuberculin (except in some urban areas), whereas about 30 percent of persons over the age of fifty react. The decline in incidence of the infection is most apparent among children and young adults and is due to a reduction in the number of open infectious cases, which, in turn, is attributable to an improved standard of living, reduced risk of late progression of infection, and prompter recognition and treatment of infectious cases.

LATENT INFECTION The great majority of persons who harbor tubercle bacilli have latent or dormant ("healed") tuberculosis. Apical scars may remain dormant for many years and then reactivate and produce clinical tuberculosis. Other sites in which tubercle bacilli may lie dormant for years and then reactivate include the kidney (from which bacilli may spread to the genital tract in the male), spine, long bones, fallopian tubes, brain, and lymph nodes in the hilum and in the neck.

MORBIDITY AND MORTALITY In 1971 there were about 34,000 new cases of clinical tuberculosis in the United States, an incidence of 17 per 100,000, down from 24 in 1966 and 53 in 1953. There were about 16,000,000 tuberculin reactors, indicating a prevalence of infection of 8,000 per 100,000. Of these, 68,000 were classified as having active tuberculosis and 600,000 as having healed or "inactive" tuberculosis. The remainder had never developed clinical tuberculosis but simply harbored foci of latent infection. It is toward this latter group that programs of prophylactic therapy with INH are directed.

Mortality has fallen steadily over the past 70 years. Tuberculosis has dropped from the leading cause of death, with over 200 deaths per 100,000 in 1906 to 2.1 per 100,000 in 1971. This figure may be somewhat low, because residual pulmonary scarring may lead to cor pulmonale.

IMMUNITY **Natural resistance** The Caucasian and Mongolian races have a distinct natural resistance to tuberculosis consisting of an ability to develop an immune response to the infection which enables recovery from primary infection. In them, primary infection usually subsides spontaneously; late reactivation may produce chronic disease characterized by cavitation and scarring. Africans, American Indians, and Eskimos were spared tuberculous infection until extensive contact began with members of the white race in which chronic tuberculosis was common. These peoples have less ability to develop an effective immune response to primary infection, and in them the infection tends to be more rapidly progressive.

Specific (acquired) immunity Immunity to tuberculosis is mediated largely by T lymphocytes, which, in response to specific antigenic stimulation, develop an ability to activate macrophages to lyse ingested mycobacteria. The role of immunoglobulins in the process is less clear, although IgA is often increased in patients with active tuberculosis and drops as the infection is controlled by therapy.

The mechanism by which latent infection becomes active is not completely understood. From the fact that it occurs more commonly in old age and during other forms of illness, it appears likely that reactivation is due to reduced immunologic surveillance by T lymphocytes.

Tuberculin hypersensitivity The most readily obtained evidence of a past or present infection with tubercle bacilli is the finding of hypersensitivity to tuberculin, a protein derivative of the broth in which tubercle bacilli have been grown. Epidemiologic evidence strongly suggests that tuberculin hypersensitivity indicates the presence of living tubercle bacilli. The larger the skin reaction, the greater the chance that the infection is active.

PATHOGENESIS AND PATHOLOGIC ANATOMY
Primary tuberculosis In the nonimmune subject tubercle bacilli can gain entrance to the body by several routes: lung, gastrointestinal tract, and by direct cutaneous or percutaneous inoculation (as in an accident at the autopsy table). For practical purposes, the only route that is of importance in the United States is the lung. The majority of primary lesions are in the lower two-thirds of the lungs, where ventilation is best and exposure to contaminated inspired air is the greatest. Because they produce no toxins and thus no tissue reaction, tubercle bacilli initially are free to multiply without deterrence. They reach regional (hilar) nodes and even the bloodstream before their progress is inhibited by the gradual development of specific immunity over a period of several weeks. At this time, the characteristic tissue reaction develops, with epithelioid cell granulomas and caseation necrosis in the primary lesion, regional lymph nodes, and any site to which the bacilli have spread. The number of bacilli drops drastically with the appearance of caseation necrosis, suggesting that the process of caseation is important in the defense of the host by producing a milieu which is deleterious to the organisms. Thereafter, the infection in the primary site usually heals by a combination of resolution, fibrosis, and calcification. Occasionally defenses fail and the infection may overwhelm the host or enter a chronic stage directly.

Secondary stage In the course of primary infection tubercle bacilli reach the general circulation in varying numbers. This event is marked only by fever and mild symptoms and is recognized as tuberculosis only when a patient is being observed closely because of a known recent exposure to tuberculosis. This stage is important in the pathogenesis of tuberculosis, because it is the time when bacilli reach distant sites to establish metastatic foci of infection which are the seeds from which postprimary chronic tuberculosis may develop.

While bacilli presumably reach all organs in the secondary stage, they establish lesions with frequency in only a limited number of sites, which have one feature in common: high tissue oxygen tension. In the upright position the apex of the lung has the highest oxygen tension in the body and is the most frequent site for the development of significant metastatic foci. It seems paradoxic that such a high P_{O_2} should exist in the poorly ventilated apices, but this is because of a paucity of pulmonary circulation to that region when the body is in the upright position, resulting in a high ventilation:perfusion ratio. Occasionally such metastatic foci progress and produce destructive tuberculosis in a short time, but more commonly the development of specific immunity causes the lesions to regress, scar, and become dormant. Such localized apical scars are often referred to as *Simon's foci.*

Latent (dormant) infection Whenever a tuberculous lesion regresses and heals, the infection enters a latent phase in which it may persist without producing illness. Though the infection may remain dormant for life, it may become active at any time.

Tertiary stage (post-primary tuberculosis) Chronic fibrocaseous tuberculosis may develop wherever there is a dormant lesion. The most common site is the apical portion of the lung. An old caseous hilar lymph node occasionally liquefies and spills its contents into a bronchus, to produce a segmental or lobar tuberculous pneumonia. Massive bloodstream invasion (miliary tuberculosis) may also occur in this stage. Chronic tuberculosis is characterized by localized nodular infiltrations, fibrosis, and cavitation.

OUTLOOK FOR PERSONS INFECTED WITH TUBERCULOSIS Of new tuberculous infections revealed by conversion of tuberculin reaction from negative to positive, 5 to 15 percent progress to serious disease within 5 years if left untreated. The risk of direct progression varies with age: it is greatest when infection begins in the first year of life and next greatest in young adults and adolescents. Among those remaining well for 5 years, a further 3 to 5 percent may develop late recrudescence at some time during life. The total morbidity rate in persons infected with *M. tuberculosis* is 8 to 20 percent. Both the early and late appearance of chronic tuberculosis can be prevented if prompt treatment with INH is given when tuberculin "conversion" is discovered.

MANIFESTATIONS

Primary infection

Uncomplicated primary tuberculosis often produces no significant clinical illness. It is usually diagnosed only when contacts of an open case are examined or when it progresses to a serious form of disease. The incubation period is 4 to 8 weeks from inoculation to appearance of mild fever and malaise and tuberculin hypersensitivity. Symptoms usually subside without specific therapy because of the appearance of adequate specific immunity. Occasionally, however, the infection progresses, either in the lung or by dissemination through the bloodstream. This turn of events is extremely serious unless detected and treated promptly.

Massive hematogenous dissemination is most common in very young children. For this reason any child under the age of three years who reacts to tuberculin should be given appropriate long-term antituberculosis chemotherapy. In older children primary infection only rarely progresses to a fatal form and often passes completely unnoticed. The principal danger arises later during adolescence or early adulthood when the infection may undergo late progression.

Primary tuberculosis may produce pleurisy with effusion, cervical lymphadenitis, miliary tuberculosis, and meningitis. In addition, allergic manifestations, erythema nodosum, and phlyctenular conjunctivitis occasionally develop.

PRIMARY TUBERCULOSIS IN THE ADOLESCENT AND ADULT In the United States, 90 to 98 percent of young adults have never been infected with tuberculosis. There have been several "epidemics" of tuberculosis among young persons. For example, sailors aboard ships were infected when late progression of infection developed in a shipmate who had been infected years before. Persons working in the Peace Corps, Armed Forces, or State Department who are assigned to countries where the prevalence of tuberculosis is high may be heavily exposed to open cases of tuberculosis. If never previously infected or vaccinated with BCG (bacillus Calmette-Guérin) they may become infected as adults. As in children, primary tuberculosis usually produces only mild and nonspecific symptoms, but in the young adult it has a greater tendency to progress to a chronic phase. There may be an area of pneumonitis in any portion of the lung, but hilar adenopathy is not common. *Whenever a young adult has a pleural effusion or a parenchymal infiltrate in the lung, a tuberculin test should be performed.* If the skin test is positive, the possibility of primary tuberculosis should be considered strongly because of the low incidence of positive reactions among young persons. The source of infection is usually an adult with cavitary tuberculosis.

Postprimary tuberculosis

OF THE LUNGS Chronic pulmonary tuberculosis may follow the primary infection directly or after a short or long period of dormancy (see Tertiary Stage, under Pathogenesis and Pathologic Anatomy, earlier in this chapter). Progressive disease has been observed to develop after 60 years of clinical dormancy. The most striking features of postprimary tuberculosis are (1) absence of recent exposure to an open case of tuberculosis (except in cases of direct progression from primary infection in adolescents and young adults), (2) tendency to chronicity and cavitation, and (3) production of fibrous tissue of repair. The last two phenomena are characteristic of the responses in persons sensitized to tubercle bacilli. While the solid caseation necrosis of the primary stage contains few bacilli, the liquid caseum in a tuberculous cavity contains abundant bacilli and may spread infection to other portions of the lungs and into the environment.

Symptoms In most instances, the onset of chronic pulmonary tuberculosis is insidious, and the patient may be entirely asymptomatic. Many cases are discovered because a routine roentgenogram is taken upon admission to hospital for some other illness.

The earliest symptoms are constitutional and probably result chiefly from the absorption of tuberculoprotein from the active lesion by the hypersensitive host. Abdominal symptoms may dominate the clinical picture. Fever is often present in the late afternoon or evening; its only manifestations may be profuse sweating during sleep ("night sweats"). It is common for a patient with tuberculosis to be unaware of a fever as high as 40°C. General malaise may be present, but often there is nothing more than irritability, depression, and an increased need for rest at the end of the day.

Weight loss may precede symptoms but is often passed off as being due to overwork or to voluntary caloric restriction. Often weight is well maintained until late in the course of the illness. When abdominal symptoms predominate, loss of weight may be rapid.

Headache may be noted occasionally, especially in the evening. Palpitation may occur during mild exertion. Menstruation is usually not disturbed until the disease is far advanced, when amenorrhea may develop.

Cough is frequent but not invariable and is often passed off as a "cigarette cough." When sputum is produced it is usually odorless, green or yellow in color, and raised principally upon arising in the morning. Hemoptysis may accompany the cough and usually consists of streaking of the sputum with small amounts of blood. In some patients the onset of pulmonary tuberculosis is relatively sudden, with fever, productive cough, or pleuritic pain suggestive of bacterial pneumonia.

PHYSICAL AND ROENTGEN EXAMINATIONS Early asymptomatic infiltrations due to tuberculosis are usually undetectable by physical examination, even though obvious by x-ray. Crepitant inspiratory rales may be present, especially when inspiration is preceded by full expiration and a small cough (posttussive rales).

Long-standing tuberculosis with extensive fibrosis causes contraction and distortion of pulmonary tissue and of bronchi. In such instances, a wide variety of physical signs may be present, such as apical dullness and bronchial breath sounds, coarse rales, deviation of the trachea, and diminished mobility of one hemithorax.

Because findings on examination of the lungs in the early stages are so frequently unremarkable, *the importance of the chest roentgenogram in diagnosis of tuberculosis cannot be overemphasized.*

Of particular importance is the comparison of the x-ray film with one made months or years earlier, so that subtle changes can be detected in clinically dormant lesions. Because fibrous tissue does not change appreciably with time, any change in the lesions on serial films must be taken to indicate activity of the disease. Among 90 patients over the age of fifty with newly active chronic pulmonary tuberculosis, over 70 percent showed evidence of preexisting tuberculous scars. Comparison of abnormal films with those made in previous examinations makes it possible to detect and treat early active lesions before liquefaction and spread of bacilli to other portions of the lungs and into the environment occur.

Complications of pulmonary tuberculosis CAVITATION When nodular lesions of tuberculosis become active and coalesce, liquefaction necrosis develops, from which liquid material escapes, leaving a cavity within the parenchyma of the lung. The sputum then often abounds with organisms, making the patient highly infectious.

HEMOPTYSIS In the majority of instances of bleeding from the lungs in tuberculosis, the blood arises from ulceration of the bronchial mucosa and presents as streaks of bright red blood on the sputum. Bleeding usually subsides spontaneously if the patient lies quietly. One type of hemoptysis has a very serious prognosis. When the blood is copious and dark (bluish red), its source is more likely a branch of the pulmonary artery within the wall of a cavity. The branches of the pulmonary artery in the vicinity of tuberculous cavities are usually thrombosed, but occasionally one remains open, is eroded by the infection (Rasmussen's aneurysm), and may rupture, causing death from exsanguination or drowning.

PLEURISY WITH EFFUSION A superficial tuberculous lesion may involve the overlying pleura and give rise to "dry" pleurisy, attended by localized pleuritic pain on deep inspiration. However, when a small caseous pulmonary focus actually erodes through the visceral pleura and extrudes a small amount of liquid caseum, the immune response to the pleural contamination is a vigorous inflammatory reaction with formation of considerable pleural exudate. Although such a pleural effusion may develop at any stage of tuberculosis, it is most common in the early postprimary stage, particularly in young adults (age fifteen to thirty-five years). The fluid is usually clear and light yellow. Its exudative nature is identified by a high protein content (>3 g per 100 ml), an elevated LDH, and a lymphocytic cell response.

The importance of recognizing the probable tuberculous nature of such a pleural exudate is indicated by the fact that 65 percent of untreated cases are followed sooner or later by overt tuberculosis. The diagnosis must often be clinical, because smears of the pleural fluid rarely reveal tubercle bacilli, and even the culture is positive in only 20 to 25 percent of cases. Percutaneous needle biopsy may reveal granulomatous pleuritis, but organisms are often not demonstrable. Thus, in most instances proof of tuberculosis is lacking at the time antituberculous treatment must be given if development of manifest tuberculosis is to be prevented. Fortunately, the intermediate tuberculin skin test is so regularly negative in healthy young adults that a positive reaction in a patient with a lymphocytic pleural exudate constitutes adequate evidence of tuberculous causation to warrant initiation of two-drug therapy. However, it is not uncommon for the intermediate-strength PPD (Purified Protein Derivative) test to be negative in patients with large tuberculous effusions, probably because of mobilization of the available small lymphocytes in the pleural reaction, leaving too few to give a positive skin reaction. A second-strength PPD will almost always be positive if the effusion is of tuberculous etiology.

TUBERCULOUS PNEUMONIA The onset of tuberculosis occasionally is quite acute, resembling that of bacterial pneumonia. This picture is seen most often in Negroes, persons with diabetes, children with overwhelming primary infection, and elderly persons in whom the lungs are flooded with bacilli discharged from an area of liquid necrosis in the lung or hilar nodes. Chills, fever, productive cough, pleuritic chest pain, and leukocytosis may be noted. Smear of the sputum usually reveals numerous tubercle bacilli.

BRONCHOPLEURAL FISTULA AND EMPYEMA Though minimal pleural contamination from a small superficial caseous focus produces only a clear exudate, massive contamination from rupture of a large caseous lesion produces pneumothorax (bronchopleural fistula) and tuberculous empyema. This is one of the most dreaded complications of pulmonary tuberculosis. Tubercle bacilli are usually easily found in the purulent exudate. Management is largely surgical and consists of establishing adequate drainage, in combination with the administration of three effective antituberculosis drugs.

TUBERCULOSIS OF BRONCHI, TRACHEA, AND LARYNX These organs are all protected from implantation of *M. tuberculosis* by a covering of secreted mucus but may become involved in advanced cavitary pulmonary tuberculosis with excretion of numerous tubercle bacilli. Bronchial ulceration may result in hemoptysis and a localized wheeze during respiration. The bronchial lumen also may be compromised by pressure of enlarged hilar lymph nodes during primary infection.

In a patient with cavitary pulmonary tuberculosis, hoarseness and pain in the throat accentuated by swallowing suggest tuberculous laryngitis. The diagnosis can be confirmed by indirect laryngoscopy. It is important to exclude cavitary tuberculosis before a laryngectomy is performed for carcinoma of the larynx, because tuberculous laryngitis is occasionally mistaken for carcinoma, even on histologic examination. Antituberculous chemotherapy is highly effective for tuberculosis of any of the mucous membranes.

Smaller bronchi which lie within tuberculous lesions are regularly weakened by the inflammatory process and dilated by contraction of fibrous tissue in healing. In the upper lobes this is rarely clinically significant, but in portions of the lung which are dependent when the patient is upright, it may lead to secondary infection, producing a chronic productive cough and sporadic hemoptysis (see Bronchiectasis, further on).

GASTROINTESTINAL TUBERCULOSIS The gastrointestinal tract is resistant to tuberculosis, but in cavitary pulmonary tuberculosis associated with excretion of numerous bacilli, it may become involved, usually in the ileocecal region. The symptoms consist chiefly of intermittent abdominal pain, cramping, and diarrhea. Occasionally the infection spreads through the wall of the intestine, to produce tuberculous peritonitis (see further on).

Differential diagnosis The clinical picture presented by pulmonary tuberculosis varies widely and may simulate a great number of other diseases.

CARCINOMA OF THE LUNG (Chap. 260) Tuberculosis is commonly confused with carcinoma of the lung because the highest incidence of both diseases is in the upper lobes and in older men. Both cause loss of weight, chronic cough, blood-streaked sputum, and mild fever. In addition to bacteriologic studies for tubercle bacilli, sputum cytology, bronchial brushing, and bronchoscopy should be employed to aid in the differentiation. Comparison of prior roentgenograms may be of considerable help, but in many instances nothing short of a diagnostic thoracotomy will serve to make the distinction. When tuberculosis is considered among the diagnostic possibilities, therapy with two antituberculous drugs should be instituted a few days before thoracotomy in order to avoid infectious complications in the event the lesion is tuberculous.

MYCOTIC INFECTIONS (Chaps. 164 to 174) Whenever tubercle bacilli cannot be isolated from a patient suspected of having tuberculosis, appropriate tests should be made for the various fungous infections, which may present a clinical picture indistinguishable from pulmonary tuberculosis. Reliable skin and serologic tests are available for coccidioidomycosis and histoplasmosis, but blastomycosis, aspergillosis, mycormycosis, cryptococcosis, and sporotrichosis can be diagnosed only by demonstrating the organisms in a biopsy specimen or on culture.

ACTINOMYCOSIS AND NOCARDIOSIS (Chaps. 165 and 173) Although usually referred to as fungous diseases, these infections are actually caused by bacteria. Diagnosis is made by culture.

SARCOIDOSIS (Chap. 223) The typical patient with sarcoidosis is afebrile and has a negative tuberculin test and a roentgen picture of diffuse pulmonary infiltrations and hilar adenopathy, but the disease is protean in its manifestations and may mimic tuberculosis. Scalene node and liver biopsies, as well as determination of serum protein and serum calcium, are of value in establishing this diagnosis. The Kveim test may be helpful.

ASPIRATION PNEUMONIA, LUNG ABSCESS Pulmonary infection which is introduced by the drainage of contaminated saliva from a focus of pyorrhea during sleep occurs predominantly in the upper and midposterior portions of the lung and can mimic tuberculosis. The distinction can usually be made eventually, but much valuable time may be lost while the patient is treated for the wrong disease. The presence of foul sputum, hemoptysis, fever, and leukocytosis in a patient who has pyorrhea and has recently undergone surgery or who drinks to excess strongly suggests a pyogenic abscess. If the differentiation cannot be made readily, it is advisable to treat with antimicrobials in addition to antituberculosis medications.

OTHER FORMS OF PNEUMONIA Bacteria or mycoplasma (Chap. 187) may present with clinical and roentgen appearances which at first are indistinguishable from pulmonary tuberculosis. Cultures, cold agglutinins, precipitin, and complement fixation tests often establish the correct diagnosis. Cavitation is rare, and sputum examination does not yield tubercle bacilli. Primary tuberculosis may present with localized infiltrate in the lung and slowly subside spontaneously or coincidently with tetracycline therapy in the manner of mycoplasma pneumonia. If clearing is incomplete, tuberculosis should be strongly considered. A tuberculin skin test should be performed in all patients with "viral pneumonia," particularly if a pleural effusion, which is rare in viral pneumonia, is present. A positive tuberculin skin test result in an adolescent or young adult with pneumonitis strongly suggests tuberculosis because of the infrequency of reactors in this age group.

PNEUMOCONIOSIS Pulmonary infiltrations associated with exposure to silicon dioxide, asbestos, ferrous oxide, and beryllium as well as hypersensitivity reactions to various organic inhalants may present a roentgenographic appearance suggestive of tuberculosis. Silicosis may present great difficulty in diagnosis because it may produce conglomerate masses and even cavitation that mimic tuberculosis. When the tuberculin skin test is positive in a patient with silicosis, smoldering tuberculosis is so likely that two-drug therapy is indicated if activity is suggested by x-ray, and prophylaxis with isoniazid is justified if there is no evidence of activity.

BRONCHIECTASIS A productive cough due to chronic infection in dilated bronchi occurs much less frequently than formerly because of more effective antibiotic therapy for necrotizing pneumonias of childhood and the reduction in the number of children whose bronchi have been damaged by primary tuberculosis. The lower and middle lobes (or lingula on the left) are most often involved, and a bronchogram effectively demonstrates the pathologic condition. Tuberculosis should be considered as one possible cause of bronchiectasis. If the tuberculin skin test is positive, isoniazid should be administered prophylactically to prevent late progression of tuberculosis from coexistent foci in apices, whether or not they are visible radiographically.

CONFUSION CAUSED BY SYSTEMIC EFFECTS OF TUBERCULOUS INFECTION Because of the insidious nature of tuberculosis, the clinical picture may be mistaken for that produced by several other disorders. Malaise, easy fatigability, inability to concentrate, anorexia, and loss of weight may be mistaken for *psychoneurosis*. The symptoms may suggest *hyperthyroidism* or *diabetes mellitus*, but with a little care the distinction can be made. Tuberculosis should always be considered in the differential diagnosis of *fever of unknown origin* (Chap. 12). If the roentgenogram reveals a pulmonary infiltrate, the possibility of tuberculosis is increased, but in cases of disseminated or extrapulmonary tuberculosis, the chest roentgenogram may be normal. In these cases biopsy of an enlarged lymph node, bone marrow, or liver may be of help. Formerly, tuberculosis was overdiagnosed in patients presenting with general systemic symptoms. Today, however, because of a lessening awareness of tuberculosis, the principal danger is that tuberculosis will be overlooked. Furthermore, it is important to realize that *tuberculosis may appear without reexposure in anyone who has ever been infected with in.*

CHRONIC TUBERCULOSIS OF OTHER ORGANS

Localized tuberculous infection may occur in a number of other organs, notably, the lymph nodes, kidney, long bones, genital tract, brain, and meninges. Organisms reach these sites from the primary lesion, either by lymphatic spread or by way of the bloodstream.

Tuberculosis of lymph nodes The most common involvement of lymph nodes occurs in the hilus draining the lung involved with a primary infection. The enlargement is usually modest but may be massive and give rise to obstruction and even ulceration of a major bronchus. The prognosis is good with proper chemotherapy, but the nodes may continue to enlarge even after therapy is started and then resolve slowly.

Cervical adenitis (scrofula) This disease has become uncommon in the United States as a result of the elimination of tuberculous cattle and pasteurization of milk, but it occasionally occurs during primary tuberculosis. In Negroes, tuberculous cervical lymphadenitis occasionally appears as a late manifestation. The nodes may be large (several centimeters in diameter) and matted together in a mass with an area of soft fluctuation. Signs of acute inflammation are rarely present. Swelling begins insidiously without systemic symptoms. Spontaneous rupture may occur, with drainage of caseous material. In some cases the offending organism is *Myeobacterium scrofulaceum,* and for this reason culture of the pus is necessary for accurate diagnosis.

Tuberculosis of the kidney Second to the upper lobes of the lungs, the kidney is the most common site for the late appearance of localized tuberculous infection. The mechanism of implantation is the same as that in the pulmonary apices, namely, by hematogenous spread during the primary infection. The oxygen tension in the cortical portion of the kidney approaches that in arterial blood, which enhances the growth and persistence of tubercle bacilli. As in the lungs, foci of tuberculosis may remain dormant for many years and produce clinical disease late in life. The pathologic process is essentially the same as in the lung: inflammation, followed by caseation, liquefaction, and discharge of contaminated material into the collecting system and down the ureter to the bladder and, in the male, to the genital tract.

Symptoms of renal tuberculosis are usually insidious and may be overlooked completely until the appearance of cystitis or epididymitis. Gross or microscopic hematuria and pyuria with a "sterile" urine on culture for bacteria should always call tuberculosis to mind and lead to the performance of a tuberculin skin test and culture of urine for tubercle bacilli. Intravenous pyelography may reveal a cortical cavity communicating with the caliceal system. Therapy consists of a multiple-drug regimen and should be continued for 18 to 24 months. Symptoms usually subside promptly with chemotherapy. Resection of residual areas of destruction is only rarely necessary.

Genital tuberculosis, male Infection of the genital tract in the male is secondary to renal tuberculosis. Bacilli discharged from a caseous lesion in the kidney may reach the seminal vesicles, prostate gland, and epididymis through their connections with the excretory tract. Symptoms begin insidiously, most commonly with scrotal pain due to inflammation of the epididymis and vas deferens. Tenderness and swelling may be found in the vas, seminal vesicles, and/or the prostate gland.

Genital tuberculosis, female When primary infection occurs after puberty, tuberculosis occasionally spreads hematogenously to the highly vascular fallopian tube. Infection may then spread into the uterus and give rise to endometritis. Symptoms are usually mild and of insidious onset, with abdominal pain, white vaginal discharge, metromenorrhagia, and dyspareunia. Systemic symptoms and signs are uncommon, probably because the infection is indolent and localized. The most common manifestation is sterility, but tubal scarring may cause pregnancy to be ectopic. Tuberculosis of the fallopian tube may also spread to the peritoneum and produce either a tuberculous pelvic abscess or generalized peritonitis.

Osseous tuberculosis Hematogenous spread of tuberculosis to the long bones and vertebras is most common when primary infection occurs in childhood, because of the high P_{O_2} associated with the vascularity at the epiphyseal plates during active bone growth. It usually occurs within 3 years of the primary infection, but dormant lesions may be reactivated by trauma years later. Infection begins in the ends of the long bones but becomes obvious when it involves the adjacent joint: hip, knee, elbow, or wrist. Tenosynovitis is most common at the wrist.

Tuberculous spondylitis (Pott's disease) This disease may result from hematogenous seeding or from spread of infection from paravertebral lymph nodes draining a tuberculous pleurisy. Spondylitis may develop in childhood or be delayed until later in life. Localized pain in the back may be present for months before x-rays reveal an abnormality. Though infection begins in the body of the vertebras, the first radiographic sign is usually destruction and narrowing of the intervertebral disk. A paravertebral abscess may be seen as a fusiform density extending the length of several vertebras and occasionally dissects and ruptures in the inguinal area. Appropriate orthopedic management (immobilization, fusion, etc.) must be combined with prolonged multiple-drug chemotherapy.

Tuberculous peritonitis The peritoneum may be implanted with tubercle bacilli by any of at least four mechanisms. Bacilli may spread (1) through the wall of infected intestine; (2) from a mesenteric lymph node; (3) from an infected fallopian tube; or (4) from hematogenous seeding in the course of disseminated tuberculosis. Symptoms are insidious, with increasing abdominal girth, but ultimately the patient has fever, night sweats, weakness, diarrhea, and abdominal pain. As with other forms of tuberculosis, there is an increased frequency among alcoholics. Tuberculosis should be strongly considered whenever ascitic fluid contains protein in excess of 3 g per 100 ml, with an LDH over 200 units and abundant lymphocytes. Diagnosis may be made by open or needle biopsy.

Tuberculous pericarditis Tuberculous infection may spread from the mediastinal lymph nodes or contiguous segments of lung to the pericardium in the same manner as to the pleura. The pathologic process is the same as in tuberculous pleurisy, with outpouring of a clear exudate, formation of granulomas, and subsequent fibrosis. The clinical picture is that of chronic pericardial tamponade, with hepatomegaly, edema, friction rub, and enlargement of the cardiac shadow during the active phase, and constriction during the phase of fibrosis. When such an illness is accompanied by afternoon fever or night sweats and a positive tuberculin reaction, tuberculosis should be strongly considered. The diagnosis is usually made by study of aspirated fluid or by open pericardial biopsy. A tuberculous effusion contains more than 3 g per 100 ml protein, an LDH over 200 units, and lymphocytes. Early in the disease, multiple-drug chemotherapy is usually sufficient, but surgical resection of the pericardium is occasionally necessary when the process is well established before therapy is begun.

If tuberculous pericarditis has undergone spontaneous healing, the patient may present years later with the picture of constrictive pericarditis (Chap. 241). Pericardiectomy is often desirable at this stage to improve cardiac function but may be technically difficult because of extensive calcification extending into the myocardium.

Tuberculosis of the adrenals Occasionally hematogenous tuberculosis localizes in the adrenal glands and may result in their total destruction, giving rise to adrenal cortical insufficiency (Addison's disease, Chap. 86). This must be differentiated from adrenal cortical atrophy, which is more common, and from other causes of adrenal destruction, such as histoplasmosis. Therapy consists of the use of three antituberculosis agents plus physiologic doses of adrenal steroids.

Tuberculous meningitis Tuberculosis may involve the meninges, either as a part of miliary tuberculosis or as extension of infection from a focus within the brain. In areas with a high incidence of tuberculosis, tuberculous meningitis is seen most commonly in young children during the first year of infection. In areas of low incidence such as the United States, meningitis is more common among older adults as a result of late reactivation of dormant infection. Pathologically, the meninges contain small tubercles and a fibrinous exudate over the base of the brain.

Symptoms consist of headache, restlessness, and irritability, usually accompanied by fever, malaise, night sweats, and loss of weight. Nausea and vomiting may be prominent. Stiffness of the neck and Brudzinski's sign are usually present. Spinal puncture usually reveals increased pressure, clear fluid containing an increased amount of protein, reduced glucose (less than half the blood glucose), and 100 to 1,000 white blood cells, 80 to 95 percent of which are lymphocytes.

The differential diagnosis includes partially treated pyogenic meningitis, fungal meningitis, and carcinomatosis of the meninges. There is considerable urgency in establishing the correct diagnosis because specific therapy is most effective when instituted early in the course of the illness. Irreversible brain damage may result from waiting 6 to 8 weeks for cultural proof of diagnosis. For this reason it is occasionally advisable to begin therapy for tuberculosis on the basis of a presumptive clinical diagnosis while awaiting results of bacteriologic studies. Therapy consists of at least two drugs, including isoniazid. Steroids are indicated when there is an impending subarachnoid block or cerebral edema. Intrathecal therapy is not indicated.

Inappropriate secretion of antidiuretic hormone (ADH) Older persons with tuberculous meningitis or overwhelming pulmonary tuberculosis occasionally present with somnolence or coma associated with a very low serum sodium concentration (110 to 125 mEq per liter), because of inappropriate secretion of ADH. This must be distinguished from adrenal insufficiency, which depresses the serum sodium concentration modestly in concert with an elevated serum potassium level. In addition to use of three antituberculosis agents, adequate sodium chloride should be administered and water intake restricted.

Disseminated tuberculosis

SILENT DISSEMINATION Hematogenous dissemination of small numbers of tubercle bacilli is common during the primary infection but usually produces little clinical illness. The principal importance of the event is the seeding of bacilli in sites far removed from the primary infection.

MASSIVE DISSEMINATION (MILIARY TUBERCULOSIS) When a liquid caseous focus empties its contents into a vein, there is a massive dissemination of tubercle bacilli throughout the body. Defense mechanisms are overwhelmed, and tubercles become established in all organs of the body. Without specific therapy, death is almost a certainty.

Miliary tuberculosis is the most dreaded manifestation of tuberculosis. It may arise shortly after primary infection (progressive primary tuberculosis) or by reactivation of a dormant focus years or decades later. Because the resistance of the body is overwhelmed, lesions are not limited to those organs with an elevated P_{O_2} but are often found in the liver, spleen, bone marrow, and meninges. The best way to make the diagnosis of miliary tuberculosis is to perform a biopsy of the liver, lymph node, or bone marrow in search of caseating granulomas and tubercle bacilli.

Symptoms are usually nonspecific and consist of weight loss, weakness, gastrointestinal disturbance, fever, and sweats. The patient has usually had a course of penicillin or broad-spectrum antibiotics without control of the fever before the diagnosis comes to mind. Cough is not a prominent feature, but dyspnea may be. The correct diagnosis is often not suspected until the typical "miliary" pattern is noted on the chest roentgenogram. The white blood count may be normal or low, or may show a leukemoid pattern suggesting leukemia. There may be a monocytosis. An identical clinical picture can be presented by histoplasmosis, coccidioidomycosis, blastomycosis, cryptococcosis, and other chronic infections. Therefore, it is imperative to obtain any material possible by biopsy or aspiration to establish a correct diagnosis on which to base therapy.

SUBACUTE AND CHRONIC HEMATOGENOUS TUBERCULOSIS Instead of a single massive invasion of the bloodstream, smaller numbers of tubercle bacilli may escape intermittently into the circulation and give rise to a variety of clinical manifestations, including myelophthisic anemia, low-grade fever, lymphadenopathy, effusion into pleural and peritoneal cavities, and splenomegaly. There may be destructive lesions of bones, kidneys, subcutaneous tissue, or skin. Such a clinical picture is most common among Negroes of any age and in elderly Caucasians, in whom the process usually represents an overwhelming of immunity during reactivation of tuberculosis after years of dormancy.

The protean manifestations and bizarre clinical pictures caused by subacute and chronic forms of hematogenous tuberculosis provide tremendous diagnostic challenges. To add to the confusion, the tuberculin reaction is often suppressed in persons with overwhelming infection. The intermediate-strength tuberculin test is often negative and the PPD No. 2 (see Diagnosis, below) occasionally so. The solution to the clinical problem most commonly comes when the possibility of tuberculosis is belatedly considered. Confirmation must be sought from appropriate histologic and bacteriologic studies. Prognosis is uniformly bad without specific therapy, but good with a multiple-drug regimen including INH.

DIAGNOSIS

TUBERCULIN SKIN TEST Tuberculin is a protein fraction of tubercle bacilli. When introduced into the skin of a person with tuberculous infection, whether active or dormant, it triggers release of migratory inhibitory factor (MIF), which over the next 24 to 72 hr causes a localized thickening of the skin because of accumulation of sensitized small lymphocytes. Though there are several methods for testing healthy populations with tuberculin for evidence of unsuspected infection, the method preferred in clinical practice is to inject 0.1 ml of a solution containing 5 tuberculin units of Purified Protein Derivative stabilized with Tween 80 (5 TU of PPD-T) into the skin of the volar aspect of the forearm with a small needle—an "intermediate-strength tuberculin test." The test is read 48 to 72 hr later and is considered positive if the diameter of skin thickening measures 10 mm or more, doubtful if 5 to 10 mm, and negative if less than 5 mm.

Intermediate-strength PPD produces a positive reaction in the majority of persons infected with tubercle bacilli. However, it is a biologic test which is dependent upon the presence of adequate circulating sensitized T lymphocytes. For this reason, false negative results may occur even in the presence of active tuberculosis whenever sensitized T lymphocytes are temporarily depleted, as in persons who are clinically ill, febrile, or have a large pleural effusion. In persons who are ill enough to be admitted to hospital, false negative results may run as high as 15 to 30 percent. If the intermediate PPD is negative in a patient in whom tuberculosis is suspected, the test should be repeated using "second-strength" PPD (100 or 250 TU). If this is also negative, tuberculosis can be dismissed with considerable certainty, although persons who are moribund from tuberculosis may fail to react even to PPD No. 2.

A positive reaction to intermediate-strength PPD indicates the presence of a tuberculous infection but does not help in distinguishing active from dormant infection. This distinction must be made on clinical, bacteriologic, and radiographic grounds. A positive reaction which is elicited only by PPD No. 2 in a patient who is clinically ill means that active tuberculosis cannot be dismissed as a diagnostic possibility. In healthy persons, however, it usually signifies only healed tuberculosis or infection with one of the other mycobacteria.

RADIOGRAPHY While never providing an etiologic diagnosis, x-rays of the chest provide most valuable information. The abnormality which is most suggestive of tuberculosis is a multinodular infiltrate with cavitation in one or both of the upper lobes of the lung. Because of the propensity of active tuberculosis to spread to other parts of the lungs, the basilar areas may also be involved. Occasionally, especially in the elderly, the lesions are limited to the lower lobe(s). Multiple infiltrates, especially if bilateral, are most suggestive of tuberculosis, because pyogenic pneumonia and carcinoma are much more likely to produce single lesions. Carcinoma usually produces a solid lesion, in contrast to the multinodular infiltrate of tuberculosis. Planigrams (laminograms) are particularly valuable in making such distinctions and in detecting cavitation. Lateral, lordotic, and oblique films are also of value in defining the location and character of lesions. Primary tuberculosis is not usually apical in location but may involve any other segment of the lungs. Hilar adenopathy is common in primary tuberculosis, but may not be obvious by x-ray in adults. Large pleural effusions are easily detected, but for small ones it may be necessary to lay the patient on the involved side to permit the fluid to be seen along the lateral chest wall (lateral decubitus film).

BACTERIOLOGIC DIAGNOSIS The only absolute proof of active tuberculosis is the cultural identification of *M. tuberculosis* from tissue or body fluid: sputum, gastric washing, urine, cerebrospinal fluid (CSF), serous effusion, or pus from an abscess or sinus. A useful preliminary examination, however, is to make a smear of the material and stain it for microscopic examination. Kenyon or Ziehl-Nielsen stain is used for standard microscopy or auromine-rhodamine stain for the more sensitive fluorescence microscopy. The smear is not a very sensitive method at best, but it has the virtue of quickly identifying the highly infectious patient who is excreting great numbers of organisms into the environment. For positive identification cultures must be made either on solid egg medium (Lowenstein-Jensen) or Middlebrook 7H-11 medium using 20 to 40 mm Hg CO_2 to speed growth.

The most commonly examined material is sputum. When it can be produced spontaneously (usually in the early morning), it makes the most satisfactory material for both smear and culture. If none can be produced spontaneously, the patient may be asked to inhale a heated aerosol containing 10 percent each of glycerine and sodium chloride, which stimulates production of bronchial secretions. Bacteriologic specimens may also be collected by bronchial washing, bronchial brushing, or tracheal aspiration. Sputum should never be collected over a 24-hr period because of the increased contamination associated with such prolonged collections. Guinea pig inoculation is no longer widely used for identification of *M. tuberculosis* because of the economic and technical advantages of the culture methods.

When no sputum can be collected, as in young children or senile or psychotic persons, morning gastric contents may be aspirated and cultured. Diagnosis by smear of this material is less reliable than examination of sputum because of the frequency of saprophytic acid-fast bacteria in the stomach.

Multiple specimens may be needed before the organisms are recovered. This is particularly true in cases of primary tuberculosis, tuberculous pleurisy with effusion, and minimal chronic tuberculosis. Also, old chronic tuberculous lesions may shed organisms only intermittently.

HEMATOLOGY The white blood cell count is usually not significantly elevated, except in tuberculous pneumonia (when it may suggest a pyogenic infection) and in miliary tuberculosis (when a leukemoid reaction may be mistaken for leukemia). Hemoglobin and hematocrit are usually normal unless a prolonged period of active disease has produced anemia of infection.

URINALYSIS There are no specific changes except when a urinary lesion is present. Renal tuberculosis is not rare; it most often presents with microscopic hematuria and pyuria with negative cultures for pyogens. Cultures may have to be repeated several times before revealing *M. tuberculosis*.

OTHER TESTS Despite great efforts to develop one, there is no specific serologic test to distinguish active from dormant tuberculosis. Biopsy of the liver, bone marrow, or lymph node can be of great aid in reaching a presumptive diagnosis of disseminated tuberculosis by revealing caseating granulomas. This finding may enable initiation of specific therapy in time to save a life; awaiting the results of culture may allow the situation to pass beyond the point of no return before the diagnosis is made and therapy is initiated.

TREATMENT

GENERAL Treatment of tuberculosis is based upon intensive and prolonged use of specific bacterial antagonists. If properly managed, tuberculosis can be controlled in more than 95 percent of patients, but accompanying diseases often are the limiting factor. Because healing depends upon body defenses aided by specific drug therapy, the total period of therapy must be prolonged, i.e., from 18 to 24 months, although a shorter period of very intensive therapy may be effective in some cases. With excellent oral drugs, most of the therapy may be accomplished while the patient is ambulatory and even at work.

PRINCIPLES OF THERAPY Chemotherapeutic agents owe their effectiveness to specific interference with various vital functions of the microorganisms without harming the host: isoniazid inhibits DNA (deoxyribonucleic acid) synthesis and intermediary metabolism of *M. tuberculosis,* and ethambutol and rifampin interfere with RNA (ribonucleic acid) synthesis. The first principle of therapy is to *choose drugs to which the organisms are susceptible.* Fortunately, this presents little difficulty in the United States, where the vast majority of new cases are caused by *M. tuberculosis,* which is susceptible to all the major drugs. The reason for this lies in the natural history of tuberculosis in man: most cases develop from infections that were implanted years before, and most primary infections are acquired from such reactivated cases before any therapy has been administered. In a new case therapy with two or three drugs may be initiated without awaiting the results of susceptibility studies, though such studies should be performed as a guide to rational choice of drugs if resistance should be found to one or more of the drugs used.

The second principle is always to *inflict multiple "biochemical lesions"* on the bacilli simultaneously at the outset. Even in a population of organisms that is susceptible to a given drug, about 1 in 100,000 is resistant. Active tuberculous lesions frequently contain many times this number of organisms and thus enough resistant mutants to permit the emergence of clinical resistance to any single drug. This can be avoided only by using several drugs in concert at the outset.

The third principle is *never to add a single drug* to a regimen that appears to be failing.

The fourth is that *therapy must be continued long enough* to permit the body's slow healing processes to proceed to completion; this appears to require 18 to 24 months. If therapy is discontinued as soon as the patient feels well, bacteriologic tests are negative, and the x-ray shows improvement, the likelihood of reactivation is great, because anatomic healing lags far behind these favorable signs.

Lastly, a *single peak concentration of drugs is preferred* over an attempt to maintain a blood level throughout the day. Where possible drugs should be given simultaneously in the full daily dose, preferably before breakfast when intestinal absorption is the most rapid.

MAJOR DRUGS **Isoniazid** INH remains the most effective antituberculosis drug. It is relatively nontoxic and is well accepted by patients because of ease of administration and freedom from annoying side effects. It acts through interference with DNA synthesis and intermediary metabolism of tubercle bacilli. It is acetylated in the liver and excreted by the kidney. Because of its great effectiveness, it should always be included in the original regimen.

DOSE The usual dose for adults is 5 mg per kg per day, usually 300 mg per day given as a single dose. In children the dosage is higher—10 to 15 mg per kg per day, because of more rapid excretion. Dosage should be reduced in the presence of renal insufficiency. It is safe to use in pregnancy. In infections with *M. kansasii* a dose of 10 mg per kg per day is recommended because of the incomplete susceptibility of this organism. Although some persons inactivate INH more rapidly than others, this has not proved to be of clinical significance.

TOXICITY Toxicity from INH is not common, but two types do occur: (1) Direct toxicity consists of peripheral neuropathy and anemia due to competition of INH with pyridoxine. Pyridoxine in a dose of 50 mg per day effectively combats this problem, which is most common when a large dose is used and in alcoholics whose nutrition is impaired. (2) Allergic reactions consist of skin rash, fever, general malaise, anorexia, nausea, vomiting, and *hepatitis.* Allergic reactions usually appear within the first 2 months of therapy, are accompanied by elevation in level of SGOT (serum glutamic oxalacetic transaminase), and require withdrawal of the drug. Surveillance for these reactions is best accomplished by clinical observation and close communication with each patient. Since the symptoms of INH allergy resemble those of influenza, the greatest confusion occurs during the winter months. When such symptoms develop, INH should be discontinued promptly and tests of liver function performed. When all symptoms have cleared, a small challenge dose of INH, 50 mg, may safely be administered. If this causes a mild recurrence of symptoms, INH allergy is confirmed and the drug must be discontinued. If it does not, the drug may be resumed gradually, reaching full dosage in a few days. Surveillance on the basis of symptoms of nausea and anorexia is preferred to frequent determination of SGOT. The only therapy needed for INH hepatitis is withdrawal of the drug before hepatitis becomes full-blown. If allowed to progress to the development of jaundice the reaction may be fatal.

Rifampin (rifampicin) This drug is the most recent addition to therapy. Its mode of action lies in inhibiting RNA polymerase. Emergence of resistance is rapid when the drug is used alone. The dose is about 10 mg per kg per day, or 600 mg, for adults and about 15 mg per kg per day for children. It is not recommended during pregnancy. Toxicity and side effects are mild, although hypersensitivity with thrombocytopenia may develop when it is resumed after an interruption. It regularly colors the urine and other body fluids a bright orange, about which the patient should be told in advance.

Ethambutol In conjunction with other drugs, ethambutol is a very effective drug against tuberculosis. Its mode of action is inhibition of RNA synthesis and phosphate metabolism. It has largely replaced PAS in routine treatment because of better acceptance by patients and fewer toxic reactions. Dosage should be about 25 mg per kg for the first 2 months and 15 mg per kg thereafter in a single daily dose. It is not recommended for use in pregnancy or in children who are too young to report changes in vision. Toxicity is almost inconsequential but consists of occasional reduction of visual acuity and temporary reduction of color vision (green). Periodic examination of the visual field and acuity has been recommended, but asking the patient to report any reduction in visual acuity when reading newsprint appears to be an adequate guide to the development of toxicity.

Aminoglycosides: streptomycin and capreomycin These drugs inhibit protein synthesis in tubercle bacilli. Since their toxic effects are similar (vestibular apparatus and renal tubular effects), they should not be employed simultaneously. Capreomycin is effective against organisms which are resistant to streptomycin. The dosage for both drugs is 1 g per day for adults, but this should be reduced to 0.5 g per day in persons over the age of sixty or when renal impairment is present. In children the dosage is 20 mg per kg per day. Streptomycin is safe during pregnancy, but capreomycin has not been approved for pregnant women. After daily use for 2 months, injections should be reduced to twice a week for an additional period of 2 to 4 months. Slight dizziness and circumoral paresthesia are common immediately after injections of streptomycin but are usually harmless. In addition to direct toxicity to the eighth cranial nerve and kidney, allergic reactions may occur, with fever, rash, and general malaise.

Para-aminosalicylic acid (PAS) Although there has been a wide and favorable experience in treatment of tuberculosis with this drug, it has lost favor because other effective agents which produce fewer side effects and allergic reactions are now available. However, it remains a valuable drug in young children and in pregnancy, where there is limited experience with the newer drugs. Its activity is through interference with intermediary metabolism of the organisms; it potentiates the effects of INH. Side effects consist of anorexia, nausea, vomiting, and diarrhea. Allergic reactions are common, with chills, fever, skin rash, and general malaise, which preclude continuation of therapy.

MINOR DRUGS Pyrazinamide The mechanism of action of this drug is unknown, and there is no way to determine susceptibility to it in vitro. Nevertheless, pyrazinamide is an effective drug, particularly for inclusion in a regimen of drugs for use in re-treating a patient in whom previous therapy has failed and in whom resistance to some of the major drugs has developed. Its toxicity is to the liver, and it regularly causes an elevation of serum uric acid level. It may be given in a single daily dose of 30 mg per kg.

Cycloserine This is a drug of modest efficacy as an inhibitor of cell wall synthesis, again principally for use in retreatment problems. Dosage is 500 to 750 mg per day for adults. Neurotoxicity may result in psychotic behavior or generalized seizures, both of which are largely prevented by pyridoxine in a dosage of 100 to 200 mg per day.

Ethionamide This drug inhibits protein synthesis and is of value in retreatment cases. Its use is limited by its gastric irritation. Dosage is 750 to 1,000 mg per day in adults.

Aminoglycosides: kanamycin and viomycin These injectable agents have limited effectiveness but may be useful in retreatment of resistant cases.

Thiocetazone and isoxyl These drugs are in common use in developing countries, because of moderate effectiveness and low cost, but are not available for use in the United States.

Choice of therapy in active tuberculosis

ORIGINAL TREATMENT The principles of therapy of active tuberculosis are the same regardless of the organ involved. Therapy should be initiated with at least two effective drugs, even when activity of the infection is uncertain. When the disease is overtly active, as in cavitary disease or in patients with a positive sputum smear, three drugs should be employed at the outset. It is easy to withdraw drugs as the situation becomes clarified with time, but it is impossible to restore susceptibility of organisms which has been lost because of use of inadequate drugs initially.

Although not mandatory, it is usually desirable to initiate therapy in the hospital, partly to facilitate accurate diagnosis and to ensure an adequate assessment of the patient's general status. Enough bacteriologic specimens should be obtained for culture to enable identification of the organisms and to determine their in vitro susceptibility.

Now that three very effective oral agents of low toxicity are available, it is not usually necessary to use streptomycin or capreomycin in the original regimen. In the uncomplicated case with little or no systemic illness and negative smears, two drugs suffice, most commonly isoniazid-ethambutol or isoniazid-rifampin. The latter combination is slightly better, but this is outweighed by the much greater cost of rifampin. Isoniazid is so effective that it should always be included. The second drug should be continued until the disease appears well controlled radiographically and bacteriologically; isoniazid should be continued until 18 to 24 months of therapy has been completed.

When clinical illness is prominent, a large cavity is present, or the sputum smear is positive, the addition of a third drug is advisable. For this, rifampin is usually employed, despite its expense, because it permits hospitalization to be shortened. Streptomycin is equally effective, but the daily injections may prolong the hospital stay. The third drug should be continued until bacteriologic cultures are negative, the x-ray shows improvement, and the patient feels clinically well. A second drug may be withdrawn when x-ray stability is achieved if repeated sputum cultures have been negative (usually 6 to 8 months). INH should be continued for a total of 18 to 24 months. A recent report suggests that intensive therapy with rifampin, isoniazid, and ethambutol for 6 months may be quite effective.

It is no longer necessary to keep most patients in hospital very long. Modern chemotherapy reduces infectiousness promptly, and cooperative patients may be permitted to take their drugs at home. For home therapy to be successful, the patient must comprehend enough of the nature of tuberculosis and the importance of chemotherapy that his cooperation can be assured. Irregularity in taking drugs and premature discontinuance when symptoms subside are the major dangers. The booklet *Understanding Tuberculosis Today,* by W. W. Stead, Milwaukee, Central Press, 1971 (revised frequently), available from local Christmas Seal associations, explains tuberculosis and its therapy in terms most patients can comprehend.

It is imperative that early discharge not result in inferior medical care. Patients with active tuberculosis who are discharged on therapy should be seen weekly for clinical evaluation and bacteriologic examination until cultures have been negative on three consecutive occasions. X-rays should be taken every month or two. If such a program is not instituted, failure of therapy and emergence of resistant organisms will occur in some patients. After cultures are negative, the interval between visits may be lengthened to a month and later to 3 and then to 6 months. Follow-up with x-ray and bacteriologic examinations should be continued for 4 to 5 years to assure successful therapy. If sputum conversion is delayed, a change in therapy may be indicated. The assistance of the health department may be needed to enlist cooperation of some patients.

RETREATMENT OF "RESISTANT CASES" Failure of initial treatment may result from an inadequate use of drugs at the outset or from premature discontinuance of medication. The skill required to manage a retreatment case is much greater than for initial therapy, and advice should always be sought from a physician who is skilled in this aspect of tuberculosis. Retreatment does not mean the addition of a drug to a regimen that has failed. It must *always* involve the use of three or more drugs which the patient has not received before. Where the patient has received several drugs in the past, it is necessary to await the results of in vitro susceptibility tests before instituting therapy. The drugs employed must be given in maximum tolerated dosage, and for this reason it is advisable for much of the therapy to be given in hospital.

CORTICOSTEROIDS The use of cortisone and its derivatives has been shown to increase the chance of reactivation of dormant tuberculosis. Despite this, in some patients who are very seriously ill with active tuberculosis, these agents may be lifesaving. They should be used only when there is an immediate threat to life, such as hypotension, debilitating fever, dyspnea, or an impending blockage of the subarachnoid space in tuberculous meningitis. Prednisone may be used in a dosage of 40 mg per day for 1 to 2 weeks and then 20 mg for another 8 weeks before gradual withdrawal. The effect upon the temperature and the general well-being of the patient may be dramatic, but there is no decrease in residual fibrosis. The frequency of side effects makes the routine use of steroids in conjunction with chemotherapy very unwise. An increase in the disease may be seen radiographically when steroid therapy is withdrawn (steroid rebound phenomenon).

The role of surgery in pulmonary tuberculosis

Surgical exploration and resection may be indispensable in establishing a diagnosis when bacteriologic and cytologic means have failed in making a diagnosis.

A few years ago it was common practice to remove localized fibrocaseous residuals of active tuberculosis on the premise that they were likely to reactivate if not removed. However, modern chemotherapy, with a multilateral initial attack on the organisms followed by prolonged suppression to permit complete healing, has all but eliminated the need for surgical resection of such fibrocaseous residuals. The chance of late reactivation of well-healed lesions is very small. However, the rigorous demands that successful use of modern chemotherapy place upon the physician and patient are not always met. It is usually possible to achieve success after initial failure if the patient will cooperate fully in a program of intensive retreatment. But when this, too, has failed, it is desirable to remove the cavitary or bronchiectatic area which is either bleeding periodically or shedding bacilli. It is desirable to make this decision before susceptibility to all drugs has been lost, in order to permit sufficient suppression of the organisms prior to resection. Such a patient should be given several drugs to which his organisms remain susceptible before, during, and following surgical intervention.

The mere persistence of a thin-walled cavity in the lung after otherwise successful chemotherapy no longer constitutes an indication for resection. When the sputum remains free of tubercle bacilli for a long period, such cavities become epithelialized and appear to present little risk of reactivation.

PREVENTION OF TUBERCULOSIS

BIOLOGIC PROPHYLAXIS BCG vaccine (bacillus Calmette-Guérin) is a live attenuated strain of bovine tubercle bacilli which has been used widely in many countries to induce specific immunity against tuberculosis. Although it reduces the chance of natural infection, it is most notable for preventing the development of serious forms of tuberculosis when natural infection occurs. There has been great controversy on the effectiveness of BCG, but most authorities agree that it affords about 80 percent protection. Its greatest value is in infants in countries of high prevalence where exposure of children is common. In the United States today vaccination is indicated only for nonreactors who cannot avoid exposure, as when assigned to countries of high prevalence in the Peace Corps, State Department, or Armed Forces or when working with patients in large city hospitals where tuberculosis is still fairly common.

CHEMOPROPHYLAXIS OF TUBERCULIN REACTORS Chemotherapy with isoniazid for a year has been shown to reduce the risk of the development of a dormant infection into active tuberculosis by as much as 75 percent. Though some recommend treating all who react to a 5-TU dose of tuberculin, it should be borne in mind that INH is not completely harmless. The indications for prophylactic INH for tuberculin reactors on which most authorities[1] would agree include:

1 All close contacts of a patient with an infectious case
2 Persons whose tuberculin conversion has occurred within the previous year or two
3 Persons with inactive tuberculosis who have never been treated with INH
4 Persons with abnormal but stable chest scars suggestive of old tuberculosis
5 Those whose health and defenses may be compromised by any of the following: diabetes, alcoholism, gastrectomy, silicosis, malignancy, prolonged corticosteroid therapy, or poor nutrition

Whenever INH is prescribed prophylactically it should be with the informed consent of the patient after a discussion of its toxicity. Toxic reactions are uncommon and need not progress to serious effects if early symptoms are heeded.

ERADICATION OF TUBERCULOSIS The decline in mortality rate from tuberculosis early in this century led some to predict the eradication of the disease in the United States by 1945. This prediction was based on the idea that infection with tubercle bacilli was harmless and that only reinfections were dangerous. It was reasoned that tuberculosis would disappear when reinfections could be prevented by isolating all infectious cases. It is now clear, however, that clinical tuberculosis develops largely from reactivation of dormant infections and that eradication must await the natural disappearance of tubercle bacilli from the population. It is hoped that this process can be accelerated by the wise use of INH as prophylactic therapy, but clinical tuberculosis will continue to occur for many years.

IMPLICATIONS OF A POSITIVE TUBERCULIN REACTION In the United States today, the chance of a tuberculin reactor's developing active tuberculosis from a dormant infection is greater than of a nonreactor's acquiring a new infection; thus it is preferable to be tuberculin-negative, unless the positive reaction is induced by vaccination. On the other hand, if exposed to tuberculosis in a country of high prevalence, a nonreactor would be more likely to become infected than a healthy reactor, and it would be preferable then to be tuberculin-positive, particularly if the positive reaction was induced by vaccination.

[1] *American Thoracic Society: Preventive treatment of tuberculosis. Am Rev Resp Dis 104:460, 1971*

REFERENCES

HEFFERMAN et al: East African/British Medical Research Councils: Controlled clinical trial of short-course (6-month) regimens of chemotherapy for treatment of pulmonary tuberculosis. Lancet I: 7760, 1972

LESTER W: *Treatment of Drug-resistant Tuberculosis,* Disease-a-Month, Chicago: Year Book, April, 1971

PAGEL W et al: *Pulmonary Tuberculosis,* London: Oxford, 1964

RALEIGH JW: Rifampin in treatment of advanced pulmonary tuberculosis. Am Rev Resp Dis 105:397, 1972

STEAD WW: *Tuberculosis and Atypical Mycobacterioses, Current Therapy,* 25th ed, Philadelphia: Saunders, 1973

——: Evidence of "silent" bacillemia in primary tuberculosis. Ann Intern Med 74:559, 1971

——: *Fundamentals of Tuberculosis Today, for Students in the Health Professions.* Milwaukee: Marquette University Press, 1971

——: The new face of tuberculosis. Hosp Practice 4:62, 1969

——: Pathogenesis of a first episode of chronic pulmonary tuberculosis in man: Recrudescence of residuals of the primary infection or exogenous reinfection? Am Rev Resp Dis 95:729, 1967

——: Pathogenesis of the sporadic case of tuberculosis. New Engl J Med 277:1008, 1967

—— et al: The clinical spectrum of primary tuberculosis in adults: Confusion with reinfection in the pathogenesis of chronic tuberculosis. Ann Intern Med 68:731, 1968

157 LEPROSY

CHARLES C. SHEPARD

DEFINITION Leprosy (Hansen's disease) is a chronic granulomatous infection of man, which, in its various clinical forms, attacks superficial tissues, especially the skin, peripheral nerves, and nasal mucosa. The two major clinical types are *lepromatous* and *tuberculoid;* when the disease has features of both these types, it is called *borderline.* In addition an early *indeterminate* form is seen, which may later develop into one of the three types mentioned.

ETIOLOGY *Mycobacterium leprae,* or Hansen's bacillus, is the causal agent of leprosy. It is an acid-fast rod, found in enormous numbers in lepromatous lesions. Although it has not been cultivated in artificial media, nor convincingly in tissue, it can be propagated in cooler tissues of small rodents, most consistently in the foot pads of mice. This development has made possible much recent experimentation, especially on drugs. The organism grows very slowly, and experiments usually require 6 to 12 months. Estimates of bacillary viability are also made microscopically by determination of the "solid ratio" or "morphologic index"; only viable bacilli are thought to stain solidly.

Lepromin is a suspension of killed *M. leprae* prepared from the tissues of lepromatous patients. Intradermal injection elicits, somewhat irregularly, a tuberculin-like reaction at 48 hr (Fernandez' reaction) and, more consistently, a papular reaction at 4 weeks (Mitsuda's reaction). The Mitsuda reaction is usually positive in tuberculoid patients and negative in lepromatous patients and is therefore an aid in clinical classification. However, because it is also positive in nearly all normal adults, it has no diagnostic value.

EPIDEMIOLOGY At present there are probably 10 to 20 million patients with leprosy in the world. The disease is more common in tropical countries, in many of which 1 to 2 percent or more of the population is affected. It is also common in certain regions with cooler climates, such as Korea, China, and central Mexico. In the United States the chief leprosy areas are Texas, California, Hawaii, Louisiana, Florida, and New York. Some of the cases are acquired domestically, some are acquired abroad.

Leprosy is frequently a family infection. Many patients give a history of prolonged exposure, and in close family contacts (spouse-spouse) of untreated lepromatous patients the attack rate is 5 to 10 percent. Among young children of untreated lepromatous parents, 30 to 50 percent develop a mild, single-lesion type of leprosy which heals spontaneously. After the index case is under treatment, spread within the family apparently does not occur. Transmission from patients with tuberculoid leprosy is uncommon. The portal of entry is a matter of conjecture, but it is probably either the skin or the nasal mucosa. The chief portal of exit is thought to be the ulcerated nasal mucosa of lepromatous patients.

The *incubation period* is frequently 3 to 5 years, but it has been reported to range from 6 months to several decades.

CLINICOPATHOLOGIC CLASSIFICATION As is true of other chronic infections, such as syphilis and tuberculosis, the manifestations of leprosy are many and variable. The classification now in general use is based on clinical findings, histopathologic changes, and the lepromin test.

Lepromatous leprosy is one of the polar forms. The involvement is extensive, diffuse, and bilaterally symmetric. Histologically, there is a diffuse granulomatous reaction with macrophages, large foam (Virchow's) cells, and many intracellular bacilli, frequently in spheroidal masses ("globi"). The lepromin reaction is usually negative.

Tuberculoid leprosy is the other polar type. Skin lesions are usually much fewer, and are sharply demarcated. Neurologic involvement is relatively pronounced and may be severe. The histologic picture consists of lymphocytes and epithelioid cells, and bacilli are few and sometimes difficult to demonstrate. The lepromin reaction is usually positive.

Borderline, or *dimorphous*, leprosy is a form in which the clinical features and histologic changes are a combination of the two polar types. The disease may change to the lepromatous or to the tuberculoid form. Change from one polar type to the other is exceedingly rare, however.

In all types of leprosy peripheral nerve involvement is a constant feature. In any histologic section involvement of nerves will tend to be more severe than involvement of other tissues, and in some sections the nerves may be the only tissues involved.

PATHOGENESIS *Mycobacterium leprae* probably enters the body through the skin or the mucosa of the upper part of the respiratory tract. The early stages of infection have not been described accurately. In lepromatous leprosy bacillemia is frequent and often so profuse that the organisms can be stained in smears of peripheral blood. Even in the most advanced lepromatous cases, destructive lesions are limited to the skin, peripheral nerves, anterior portion of the eye, upper respiratory passages above the larynx, testes, and structures of the hands and feet. The probable reason for the predilection of the disease for all these tissues is that they are all usually several degrees cooler than 37°C. Two sites of preferential involvement are the ulnar nerves near the elbow and the peroneal nerves where they pass around the head of the fibula; above and below these levels where these nerves take deeper courses, they are much less severely involved. In mice that have been experimentally infected in the foot pads, bacillary multiplication is maximal when the mice are kept at air temperatures at which the foot pad tissues are about 30°C; this is also the usual temperature of the most severely involved tissues of human beings. In patients with lepromatous leprosy, collections of bacilli are also found in the liver, spleen, and bone marrow, but these are probably scavenged from the blood.

Lepromatous leprosy is thought to be the result of a poor immune response and tuberculoid leprosy the result of a stronger immune response, but whether these different immune states precede the infection is not clear. Lepromatous patients have been shown to be deficient in the ability to develop delayed hypersensitivity, their lymphocyte transformation in response to general stimulants is weak, and the paracortical areas of their lymph nodes are depleted of lymphocytes. Furthermore mice that have been rendered immunologically deficient by thymectomy and irradiation with bone marrow replacement respond to inoculation of *M. leprae* by developing heavy bacilliferous infections which are histologically identical to lesions of lepromatous leprosy in man (and which spread to the ears, nose, and uninoculated feet, i.e., the cooler tissues).

CLINICAL MANIFESTATIONS Early leprosy The first signs of leprosy are usually cutaneous. One or more hypopigmented or hyperpigmented macules or plaques may be seen. There is little to distinguish them from other conditions, but they are frequently anesthetic. Often an anesthetic or paresthetic patch is the first symptom noted by the patient, but on careful examination skin involvement can also be found. When contacts are being examined, a single skin lesion is often noted, especially in children; usually a hypesthetic macule, the lesion is reported to clear in a year or two without treatment, but specific treatment is usually recommended. The earliest loss of sensation is that of temperature, followed by light touch (wisp of cotton) and then by pain (sharp or dull end of pin).

Tuberculoid leprosy Early tuberculoid leprosy is frequently manifested by a hypopigmented macule, sharply demarcated and hypesthetic. Later the lesions are larger, and the margins are elevated and circinate or gyrate. There are peripheral spread and central healing. The lesions are usually few and not symmetric. Nerve involvement occurs early, and the nerves leading from the lesions may be enlarged. The larger peripheral nerves may be palpably and visibly enlarged, especially the ulnar, peroneal, and greater auricular nerves. There may be severe neuritic pain. Neural involvement leads to muscle atrophy, especially of the small muscles of the hand. Contractures of the hand are frequent; so is foot drop. Trauma, especially from burns and splinters and from excessive pressure, leads to secondary infection of the hands and to plantar ulcers. Later resorption and loss of phalanges is frequent. When the facial nerves are involved, there may be lagophthalmos, exposure keratitis, and corneal ulceration leading to blindness.

Lepromatous leprosy The skin lesions are macules, nodules, or papules. The macules are more often hypopigmented. The borders of the lesions are not sharp, and the centers of raised lesions are convex (rather than concave as in tuberculoid disease). There is also diffuse infiltration between the lesions. The sites of predilection are the face (cheeks, nose, brows), ears, wrists, elbows, buttocks, and knees. Involvement with little or no nodulation may progress so subtly that the disease goes unnoticed. Loss of the eyebrows, especially the lateral portions, is common. Much later the skin of the face and forehead becomes thickened and corrugated ("leonine facies"), and the earlobes become pendulous.

Nasal symptoms (nasal "stuffiness," epistaxis, and obstructed breathing) are common early symptoms. Complete nasal obstruction, then laryngitis and hoarseness, are also frequent. Septal perforation and nasal collapse lead to saddle nose.

In adult males infiltration and scarring of the testes lead to sterility. Gynecomastia is common. Invasion of the anterior portion of the eye leads to keratitis and iridocyclitis. Painless inguinal and axillary lymphadenopathy occurs.

Neurologic involvement, of the same type as that seen in tuberculoid disease, tends to be less prominent in the lepromatous form. A diffuse hypesthesia involving the peripheral portions of the extremities is common in advanced lepromatous disease.

Reactional states The general course of leprosy is leisurely, but it may be interrupted by two types of reaction, which tend to complicate chemotherapy.

Erythema nodosum leprosum (ENL) occurs in lepromatous patients, most frequently toward the end of the first year of treatment. Tender, inflamed subcutaneous nodules develop, usually in crops. Each nodule lasts a week or two, but more develop. ENL may last only a week or two or it may continue for long periods. Low-grade fever accompanies severe ENL, and lymphadenopathy and arthralgia may appear. Even in untreated patients with ENL the bacilli have greatly reduced viability, as indicated by low infectivity for mice and by low "solid ratios." Histologically ENL is characterized by polymorphonuclear infiltration and deposits of IgG and complement; thus it resembles an Arthus reaction.

Reversal reaction is also seen during treatment, but less often than ENL. Existing skin lesions develop erythema and swelling, and new lesions may appear. An early influx of lymphocytes is followed by edema and a shift toward tuberculoid histology. Cellular immunity apparently has increased. Reversal reactions can be differentiated from frank progression, such as occurs when drug-resistant bacilli appear, by mouse inoculations to test bacillary viability and by histologic studies.

The *Lucio phenomenon* is limited to patients with a diffuse nonnodular lepromatous disease; it is seen more often in Mexico, especially in Sinaloa. Arteritis leads to ulceration of the skin, in a characteristic angular shape, and subsequently to angular thin scars.

Complications The crippling that follows involvement of the peripheral nerves has been mentioned. Leprosy is probably the most frequent cause of crippling of the hand in the world. Blindness also is common.

Amyloidosis is a frequent complication of lepromatous disease in the United States but is less common elsewhere.

Patients with leprosy are said to be likely to develop other chronic infections. Tuberculosis was the chief cause of death in many leprosariums.

DIAGNOSIS The demonstration of acid-fast bacilli in the skin smears made by the scraped-incision method is strong evidence for leprosy, but in tuberculoid disease bacilli may be too few for demonstration. Wherever possible, a skin biopsy specimen confined to the affected area should be sent to a pathologist or dermatopathologist knowledgeable in leprosy. The histologic involvement of peripheral nerves is pathognomonic.

The lepromin reaction has no diagnostic value. No diagnostic blood changes occur. Lepromatous patients frequently have mild anemia, elevated erythrocyte sedimentation rate, and hyperglobulinemia. From 10 to 40 percent of lepromatous patients have false positive serologic tests for syphilis.

The combination of a chronic skin disease and peripheral nerve involvement should always lead to the consideration of leprosy.

The differential diagnosis includes conditions such as lupus erythematosus, lupus vulgaris, sarcoidosis, yaws, dermal leishmaniasis, and the host of banal skin diseases. The skin lesions of leprosy, especially of tuberculoid disease, are characterized by hypesthesia, however, and peripheral nerve involvement can always be demonstrated. Peripheral neuropathy from other causes and syringomyelia are often confused with leprosy.

TREATMENT The treatment of leprosy is largely in the hands of specialists, and hospitalization is advantageous for the first few months while the treatment is being established.

Specific chemotherapy Dapsone (4,4′-diaminodiphenylsulfone, DDS, diaphenylsulfone) is effective and inexpensive. Oral treatment is begun with small doses and raised during the first few weeks to a maintenance dose of about 50 mg a day in adults. In a few months enough bacilli are killed to render mouse inoculations negative. However, in lepromatous disease nonviable bacilli in large numbers (and a few viable bacilli) persist for many years, and treatment should be continued for several years after the bacilli are no longer demonstrable in skin smears. Often this amounts to 6 to 10 years. In tuberculoid disease, especially in the milder cases, treatment is often discontinued after 3 years if the disease is clinically quiescent. Regularly scheduled follow-up is needed to detect possible relapses of lepromatous cases.

If dapsone is given in the dosage mentioned, toxicity is rare. Dermatitis and hepatitis occur. With higher doses, anemia and methemoglobinemia are seen regularly.

Other sulfones, such as sulfoxone or Sulphetrone, are still used at times. Use of acedapsone (DADDS), a repository sulfone given only five times a year, is under study.

Sulfone resistance has been demonstrated in mice on isolates from patients who are unresponsive after many years of sulfone therapy. In these patients the initial response was apparently favorable, but in many of them treatment was interrupted or irregular. After seven or more years there is no longer any response to therapy. The frequency of sulfone resistance in patients initially treated with dapsone is not yet known because resistance develops slowly. Patients with sulfone-resistant bacilli are best treated with clofazimine(B663), a riminophenazine compound.

The clinical response to adequate therapy is gradual, and the picture may be confused by reactional conditions. However, progression of the basic disease ceases and there is gradual improvement of skin lesions. Recovery from neurologic impairment is limited.

Among nonsulfone drugs that have been recommended in leprosy are thiambutosine, Etisul, and ethionamide. When used alone, these other drugs are less effective than dapsone. Rifampin has recently been found to be much more rapidly bactericidal than dapsone, at least initially.

Treatment of reactional states Moderate ENL is managed by antipyretics and analgesics. If severe, it can be treated with corticosteroids or ACTH; the dosage is adjusted to alleviate severe distress but not to eliminate all signs of reaction. Sulfone therapy should be continued, if necessary in reduced dosage. In the past some leprologists have discontinued sulfone therapy at the first signs of ENL, but most now feel that such action is not warranted because it allows bacillary multiplication. Corticosteroid therapy promotes the viability of *M. leprae* in mice not given antileprosy drugs.

Corticosteroids are helpful in severe reactional tuberculoid states, but analgesics and antipyretics may suffice.

Thalidomide is the most effective drug and in appropriate dosage can completely suppress ENL. Because of its teratogenicity, however, its use is severely restricted and it can be used only when its administration can be strictly controlled.

Other measures Many of the deformities and disabilities of leprosy are preventable through proper attention from the beginning of treatment. Plantar ulcers, which are very common, may be prevented by rigid-soled footwear or walking plaster casts, and contractures of the hand may be prevented by physical therapy and application of casts. Reconstructive surgery is frequently necessary. Nerve and tendon transplants and release of contractures can give patients much more functional ability. Vocational retraining is often necessary for those with permanent disability. Plastic repair of facial deformities assists acceptance of patients in society. The psychologic trauma which resulted from prolonged segregation is now minimized by permitting patients to continue therapy at home as soon as possible.

CONTROL Early detection and treatment of the disease, which prevents the further development of deformities and which simplifies sulfone therapy, can be aided by education of physicians and laity in endemic areas. Because the disease is best treated by specialists, the establishment of clinics is helpful. Regular and complete skin examination of family contacts is essential. Field trials of BCG vaccination in endemic areas have shown contradictory results. Chemoprophylaxis with low dosages of dapsone or with acedapsone injections may be considered for family contacts and groups with high attack rates. Removal of patients from their families and normal environment is probably not necessary, except perhaps in the first few months when therapy is being established, unless the patient does not follow regular treatment.

REFERENCES

Cochrane RG, Davey TF (eds): *Leprosy in Theory and Practice*, 2d ed., Baltimore: Williams & Wilkins, 1964

Fasal P: A primer in leprosy. Cutis 7:525, 1971

Ridley DS, Jopling WH: Classification of leprosy according to immunity. A five-group system. Int J Leprosy 34:255, 1966

Shepard CC: The first decade in experimental leprosy. Bull WHO 44:821, 1971

WHO Expert Committee on Leprosy: *Fourth Report*, WHO Tech Rep Ser, No. 459, 1970

Wolstenholme GEW, O'Connor M: *Pathogenesis of Leprosy*. Boston: Little, Brown, 1963

158

OTHER MYCOBACTERIAL INFECTIONS

CHARLES C. SHEPARD

EXTRAPULMONARY DISEASE PRODUCED BY "ATYPICAL" MYCOBACTERIA

Species of acid-fast bacteria morphologically similar to tubercle bacilli are widely distributed in nature as saprophytes or as pathogens of lower animals. Many examples are known of parasitism of amphibians and fishes by mycobacteria that cannot multiply at mammalian body temperatures. Among mammalian diseases that have been studied extensively are a chronic enteritis in cattle and sheep caused by *Mycobacterium paratuberculosis* (Johne's bacillus), a leprosy-like disease of water buffalo and oxen called *lepra bubalorum* or *lepra bovinum*, and murine leprosy (of wild rats). The long-standing view that all other acid-fast bacilli are of importance in clinical medicine only because they might be confused with *M. tuberculosis* or *M. leprae* in smears or cultures has gradually given way to the realization that many other mycobacterial species are pathogenic for man, producing chronic *cutaneous disease*, *pulmonary disease*, or *lymphadenitis*.

MYCOBACTERIUM MARINUM (BALNEI) ("SWIMMING-POOL BACILLUS") This acid-fast organism inhabits swimming pools and gains entry to the human body through cutaneous abrasions on rough concrete. A few weeks later papules or nodules develop at the site and frequently ulcerate and enlarge to form superficial granulation tissue. The involved area usually is not extensive. Originally confused with cutaneous tuberculosis, "swimming-pool granuloma" has now been described in many parts of the world including the United States. In Hawaii a much more chronic form lasting many years has been reported; exposure to swimming pools had usually not occurred. *Mycobacterium marinum* grows optimally at 25 to 35°C and poorly, if at all, at 37°C. This temperature range probably accounts for the lack of systemic spread; regional lymph nodes remain uninvolved unless secondary pyogenic infection occurs.

The diagnosis is made by culturing the organism, usually from biopsy material on mycobacterial media at appropriate temperatures. Although it grows slowly on primary isolation, on transfer the organism grows more rapidly and is photochromogenic (develops pigment only after exposure to light). Histologically the lesion is a nonspecific granuloma in which acid-fast bacilli can often be detected. Many, but not all, patients become tuberculin-positive.

Treatment with antituberculous drugs, especially streptomycin, appears to speed healing. Most strains are sensitive to rifampin in dosage of 600 mg per day. Tests of antibiotic sensitivity are helpful in selecting drugs.

Prevention of the swimming-pool outbreaks requires disinfection of the pool. The pool may have to be reconstructed to eliminate rough surfaces.

MYCOBACTERIUM ULCERANS This acid-fast organism produces extensive granulomatous ulceration which destroys subcutaneous tissue down to the muscle or fascia and extends peripherally under a characteristic undermined edge. Extensor surfaces of arms and legs are most often affected, but the trunk may also be involved. Histologically necrosis is prominent, and epithelialization of the ulcer floor extends under the overhanging margins. Systemic dissemination does not occur, although new lesions may develop at distant sites. In its natural course the disease may heal spontaneously in a year or two or may persist for many years with extensive ulcerations and contractures. Originally observed in Southern Australia, the disease has since been described in Central Africa and Southeast Asia. Isolated cases and localized outbreaks, especially near rivers, have been described, but little is known of the distribution of the organism in nature.

Mycobacterium ulcerans grows optimally at 30 to 33°C and poorly, if at all, at 37°C. The organism grows very slowly, and colonies require 7 weeks to develop at optimal temperatures. Inoculation of mouse foot pads is helpful in the isolation and identification of the organism. *Mycobacterium marinum* is easily differentiated on bacteriologic media because it is photochromogenic, grows rapidly, and, when inoculated into foot pads of mice, produces disease much more rapidly than does *M. ulcerans*.

Treatment has been carried out with antituberculous drugs, such as streptomycin and isoniazid. However, experimental results indicate that rifampin and clofazimine (B663) are now considered the most active. Surgical extirpation of the necrotic tissue and overlapping margins of the ulcer, followed by skin grafting, has usually been required.

PULMONARY DISEASE PRODUCED BY "ATYPICAL" MYCOBACTERIA

DEFINITION Mycobacterial species other than *M. tuberculosis* are capable of causing chronic progressive pulmonary disease with fibrosis and cavitation closely resembling pulmonary tuberculosis.

ETIOLOGY The nontuberculous mycobacteria isolated from clinical sputum and lung specimens can be divided into four groups. Group I, which is photochromogenic, is given the species name *M. kansasii.* Group II, the scotochromogens, which produce pigment when grown in the dark, contains at least two species: *M. scrofulaceum*, which produces cervical and occasional pulmonary infections, and one or more species commonly isolated from tap water. Group III, the nonchromogens, includes *M. intracellulare* (Battey bacilli), the closely related *M. avium*, and several nonpathogenic species. Group IV contains *M. fortuitum*, which occasionally causes human disease, and several nonpathogens. Isolation of nontuberculosis mycobacteria from clinical specimens does not have the same etiologic significance as the isolation of *M. tuberculosis*, because similar organisms can be isolated from sputum, saliva, etc., of healthy persons. Therefore, before a nontuberculosis mycobacterium is accepted as the cause of disease, it should be isolated from more than one specimen or in significant numbers (more than 10 colonies per culture). However, when *M. kansasii* and *M. intracellulare* are identified by appropriate additional tests, single isolations have etiologic significance.

EPIDEMIOLOGY The mode of transmission is unsettled. There is a cross-sensitization between antigens of tubercle bacilli and other mycobacteria, but sensitization to the etiologic organism is usually greater. Comparative skin tests with antigens from *M. intracellulare* and tuberculin indicate that many healthy individuals in the southeastern United States have been infected by organisms related to Battey bacilli, and in these areas chronic pulmonary disease that is not caused by *M. tuberculosis* is usually caused by *M. intracellulare.* In Texas and in Chicago *M. Kansasii* is a more frequent causative agent than *M. intracellulare.* The proportion of new cases of chronic pulmonary disease caused by mycobacteria other than *M. tuberculosis* varies in different locations and is not more than 5 to 10 percent but may be expected to increase as the number of infections due to *M. tuberculosis* decreases. In contrast to tuberculosis, multiple cases in the same family are very rare, and enforced isolation is not indicated.

PATHOLOGY Comparative studies of pulmonary tissue have failed to reveal consistent and reliable features distinguishing these infections from those due to *M. tuberculosis.* Extrapulmonary lesions are rare. Cervical adenitis due to *M. kansasii* or *M. scrofulaceum* is seen in children.

MANIFESTATIONS AND DIAGNOSIS The symptoms and signs are those of pulmonary tuberculosis (Chap. 156), although there is some tendency for the infection to be more indolent. The disease, especially that due to *M. intracellulare,* is more frequent in older adults and in males. Underlying chronic obstructive pulmonary disease is often present and is associated with a poorer chemotherapeutic response. The diagnosis is established only by isolation and identification of the mycobacteria from the sputum. The laboratory should carry out tests for the production of nicotinic acid, at least on all isolates from new patients, because only *M. tuberculosis* consistently produces it. Differentiating tests can then be carried out in nicotinic acid–negative cultures.

TREATMENT *Mycobacterium kansasii* infections usually respond to intensive antituberculous chemotherapy with isoniazid, streptomycin, and paraaminosalicylic acid. The cultures should be studied for drug susceptibility because many organisms are also susceptible to rifampin, viomycin, and ethionamide, and treatment can be adjusted appropriately. *Mycobacterium intracellulare* infections usually do not respond to antituberculosis chemotherapy. With both infections, if a 6-month trial with chemotherapy is not successful, resection of the involved lung can be expected to give good results without undue risk of complication.

REFERENCES

Clark HF, Shepard CC: Effect of environmental temperatures on infection with *Mycobacterium marinum* (Balnei) of mice and a number of poikilothermic species. J Bacteriol 86:1057, 1963

Johanson WG Jr, Nicholson DP: Pulmonary disease due to *Mycobacterium kansasii,* an analysis of some factors affecting prognosis. Am Rev Resp Dis 99:73, 1969

Linell F, Norden A: Mycobacterium balnei: A new acid-fast bacillus occurring in swimming pools and capable of producing skin lesions in humans. Acta Tuberc Scand suppl no. 33, 1954

Mollohan CS, Romer MS: Public health significance of swimming pool granuloma. Am J Public Health 51:883, 1961

Uganda Buruli Group: Clinical features and treatment of preulcerative Buruli lesions (*Mycobacterium ulcerans* infections): Report II of the Uganda Buruli group. Br Med J 1:390, 1970

Wayne LG et al: Mycobacteria: A guide to nomenclatural usage. Am Rev Resp Dis 100:732, 1969

159
SYPHILIS

KING K. HOLMES

The great ailment of modern syphilological practice is a lack of comprehension of the why and wherefore, rather than the what to do. J. H. Stokes

DEFINITION Syphilis is a chronic systemic infection caused by *Treponema pallidum*, is usually sexually transmitted, and is characterized by an incubation period averaging 3 weeks, followed by a primary lesion associated with regional lymphadenopathy; a secondary bacteremic stage associated with generalized mucocutaneous lesions and generalized lymphadenopathy; a latent period of subclinical infection lasting many years; and, in 30 to 50 percent of untreated cases, a tertiary stage characterized by progressive destructive mucocutaneous or parenchymal lesions, aortitis, or central nervous system disease.

ETIOLOGY The discovery of *Treponema pallidum* in syphilitic material was made by Schaudinn and Hoffman in 1905. *Treponema pallidum* is one of the many spiral-shaped microorganisms which are propelled by spinning around their longitudinal axis. The spiral organisms of medical significance, the *Treponemataceae*, includes three groups which are pathogenic for man and for a variety of other animals: the *Leptospira*, which cause human leptospirosis; the *Borrelia*, including *B. recurrentis* and *B. vincentii*, which cause relapsing fever and Vincent's angina, respectively; and the *Treponema*, responsible for the diseases known as treponematoses. The *Treponema* include *T. pallidum*; *T. pertenue* and *T. carateum*, the organisms which cause yaws and pinta (Chap. 160); and *T. cuniculi*, the cause of rabbit syphilis. Other treponema include nonpathogenic species found in the human mouth, and several species of anaerobic saprophytic genital treponemes of low pathogenicity which often coexist with anaerobic gram-negative rods in ulcerative genital lesions (so-called "fusospirochetal" infections). These can also be confused with *T. pallidum* on dark-field examination by inexperienced individuals.

T. pallidum is a thin, delicate, spiral organism with 6 to 14 spirals and tapered ends, measuring 6 to 15 μm in total length and 0.2 μm in width. The cytoplasm is surrounded by a delicate inner mucopeptide layer, the periplast, which provides some structural rigidity, while an outer lipoprotein membrane is selectively permeable and osmotically sensitive. The unique spiral structure of *T. pallidum* is maintained by six fibrils, three arising at each end of the organism, which wind around the cell body in a groove between the inner cell wall and the outer cell membrane, and may be the contractile elements responsible for motility. None of the four pathogenic treponemes has yet been cultured in vitro, and no convincing morphologic, antigenic, or metabolic differences between them have been discerned. They are distinguished primarily according to the clinical syndrome they produce. Limited animal inoculation studies also indicate some differences in host range and virulence. However, variation in virulence even among different strains of *T. pallidum* has also been noted. The only known natural hosts for pathogenic treponema are man, higher apes, and rabbits, but all warm-blooded animals so far tested can be successfully infected with *T. pallidum*. Lesions can be regularly produced in rabbits, and virulent strains of *T. pallidum* are usually maintained in that species.

HISTORY The first clear descriptions of syphilis were recorded at the end of the fifteenth century, when a pandemic known as the great pox, as distinguished from smallpox, swept over Europe and Asia. The pandemic began soon after the return of Columbus from Haiti in 1493, and also coincided with the invasion of Italy by the army of Charles VIII of France in 1494. Severe morbidity or death often occurred during the secondary stage, indicating an unexplained virulence then which is almost unknown today, except in congenital syphilis. The source of the European pandemic 500 years ago is controversial. The sudden appearance and high morbidity of syphilis in 1494 led to the theory of the importation of a highly virulent strain of *Treponema pallidum* from America. However, many historians discern earlier references to syphilis in various writings from Hippocrates on through the middle ages.

The sexual mode of transmission of syphilis was recognized early during the European pandemic, and description of the three cutaneous stages of the disease followed. The major cardiovascular and neurologic complications of late syphilis were recognized during the eighteenth and nineteenth centuries. However, the erroneous concept that gonorrhea, chancroid, and syphilis were produced by the same organism was strengthened by John Hunter, who developed syphilis following self-inoculation with gonorrheal pus in 1767. These three diseases were finally distinguished by Ricord and his students in the mid-1800s.

A rapid series of important advances began in 1903 with the successful inoculation of syphilis into primates by Metchnikoff and Rowe. The discovery of *Treponema pallidum* in serum from secondary lesions was made by Schaudinn in 1905, and was confirmed by Landsteiner by dark-field microscopy in 1906. In 1910, Wasserman introduced the complement fixation test for the diagnosis of syphilis, and in the same year, Ehrlich and Hata introduced an arsenic derivative, arsphenamine (Compound 606, Salvarsan), which was effective in treatment.

The present era of syphilology began with the first use of penicillin for syphilis by Mahoney in 1943. Subsequent advances have included the development of specific antitreponemal antibody tests for the diagnosis of syphilis.

EPIDEMIOLOGY The recent demonstration of naturally occurring pathogenic treponemal infection in subhuman primates, together with the close relation of the various human treponematoses, suggests the long existence of a large common reservoir of closely related treponemal infections of humans and animals. The "unitarian" hypothesis suggests that the epidemiology and manifestations of the human treponematoses are influenced by environment, and that improved sanitation and living conditions in advancing societies have eliminated the chain of infection responsible for perpetuation of yaws or endemic syphilis in childhood. Consequently, the development of a population of nonimmune adults has led to the perpetuation of treponemal infection as a venereal disease. Nearly all cases of syphilis are now acquired by sexual contact with infectious lesions (i.e., the chancre, mucous patch, or condyloma latum). Uncommon modes of transmission include nonsexual personal contact, contact with contaminated fomites, or infection *in utero* or following blood transfusions.

The annual incidence of syphilis in the United States has been recorded since 1941. Infant deaths due to syphilis and new admissions of patients with syphilitic psychoses have fallen by 98 to 99 percent since 1940. The number of new cases of infectious syphilis reached a peak in 1947, then fell steadily to about 6,000 in 1957. Since 1957, the annual incidence of syphilis has varied in inverse proportion to the federal expenditures on syphilis control. The incidence of congenital syphilis in infants has increased progressively during the past several years. In 1972, approximately 24,000 cases of primary and secondary syphilis and 68,000 other cases of untreated syphilis were reported. The actual occurrence of primary and secondary syphilis was estimated to be about 80,000 new cases in 1972. The discrepancy between reported and estimated cases is based on the fact that private physicians who treat most cases of early syphilis, report only 12 to 19 percent of such cases. *Inadequate tracing of sexual contacts of unreported cases is the major factor responsible for resurgence of syphilis in this country.*

Experience has shown that interviewing of patients with early syphilis discloses an average of three sexual contacts at risk per patient, and the recent innovation of "cluster" tracing may disclose additional associates of the patient or his contacts who are also at risk. Approximately one of two individuals exposed to infectious syphilis become infected, and tracing of sexual contacts of infectious patients is essential for control of the disease. Many contacts will have already developed manifestations of syphilis when they are first seen, and about 30 percent of apparently uninfected contacts of infectious syphilis who are examined within 30 days of exposure will actually be in the incubation stage, and will themselves go on to develop infectious syphilis if not treated. Because of this, the identification and treatment of all recently exposed contacts has become an important aspect of syphilis control in the United States. Equally important is the identification of syphilitics by routine serologic screening of premarital applicants, pregnant females, blood donors, hospital admissions, military inductees, and persons undergoing examination in physicians' offices. Of 38,000,000 blood specimens examined annually in the United States, 1,100,000 tests are reactive, representing untreated syphilis, previously treated syphilis, or false positive tests. Approximately 40 percent of all cases of primary and secondary syphilis and 80 percent of early latent cases of less than 1 year's duration are detected as a direct result of either contact tracing or serologic screening tests.

Syphilis actually is now under control in some states in which new cases are limited to sporadic outbreaks which tend to involve homosexual men and are contained by aggressive contact tracing. Unfortunately, despite the availability of the necessary tools for control of syphilis, they are not being applied in the most effective manner.

Although the reported incidence of syphilis at present is nearly twenty times as great in nonwhites as in whites, and is higher in urban than in rural areas, these differences partly reflect the fact that indigent urban nonwhites are treated at public clinics, where case reporting is complete. The peak incidence of syphilis, like that of gonorrhea, occurs in the age group 20 to 24 years, followed by ages 25 to 29, then 15 to 19. The incidence of infectious syphilis is higher in males than in females, particularly in the primary stage, when primary lesions may be hidden in the female. However, a very significant new aspect of syphilis epidemiology is the growing incidence among male homosexuals, who account for approximately two-thirds of all cases of infectious syphilis in many areas.

NATURAL COURSE OF UNTREATED SYPHILIS
Treponema pallidum can rapidly penetrate intact mucous membranes or abraded skin, and within a few hours enters the lymphatics and blood to produce systemic infection and metastatic foci long before the appearance of a primary lesion. Thus, blood from a patient with incubating syphilis is infectious. The median incubation period is 21 days, but may vary from 10 to 90 days. The generation time of *T. pallidum* in man is 30 to 33 hr, and the incubation period of syphilis is inversely proportional to the number of organisms inoculated. The concentration of treponemes generally reaches 10^7 per g tissue before the appearance of a clinical lesion. In experimental infection of rabbits or man, a single treponeme can initiate infection which leads to a discernible lesion only after many weeks, although histopathologic changes are evident earlier, while intradermal injection of 10^7 organisms usually produces a lesion within 72 hr.

The *primary* lesion appears at the site of inoculation, persists for 2 to 6 weeks, then heals spontaneously. *Treponema pallidum* is demonstrable in the chancre and in the regional lymph nodes at this time. The generalized parenchymal, constitutional, and mucocutaneous manifestations of *secondary* syphilis usually appear about 6 weeks after healing of the chancre, although the secondary rash may appear while the chancre is still present, or only after several months have passed. The secondary rash subsides within 2 to 6 weeks, and the patient enters the latent stage, which is detectable only by serologic testing. Approximately 25 percent of patients will experience one or more subsequent generalized or localized mucocutaneous relapses at some time during the first 2 to 4 years after infection. Since 90 percent of such infectious relapses occur during the first year, identification and examination of sexual contacts is most important for patients with syphilis of less than 1 year's duration. However, because relapse may occur at any time up to 4 years after infection, latent syphilis is arbitrarily divided by the World Health Organization into early latent (less than 4 years' duration) and late latent (over 4 years' duration) stages. About one-third of patients with untreated latent syphilis develop clinically apparent tertiary disease. The most common type of tertiary disease is the gumma, a usually benign granulomatous lesion. The remaining tertiary lesions are caused by obliterative small-vessel endarteritis which usually involves the vasa vasorum of the ascending aorta and less often involves the central nervous system.

The course of untreated syphilis has been studied retrospectively in a group of nearly 2,000 patients with primary or secondary syphilis diagnosed clinically, before the dark-field and Wasserman tests came into use (the *Oslo Study*, 1891–1951); and prospectively in 431 Negro men with seropositive latent syphilis of three or more year's duration (the *Tuskegee Study*, 1932–1972).

In the *Oslo Study*, 24 percent of the patients developed relapsing secondary lesions within 4 years, and 28 percent eventually developed one or more manifestations of late syphilis. Cardiovascular syphilis, including aortitis, was detected in 10.4 percent, with no cases occurring in those infected before age 15; symptomatic neurosyphilis occurred in 6.5 percent and 16 percent developed benign tertiary syphilis (gumma of the skin, mucous membranes, and skeleton). Syphilis was the primary cause of death in 15.1 percent of males and 8.3 percent of the females. However, many patients alive when the Oslo Study was completed remained at risk for developing complications, while tuberculosis and other infections prematurely eliminated others before complications of syphilis occurred, so the Oslo figures probably represent minimum estimates of the risk of late complications. Cardiovascular syphilis was found in 35 percent of men and 22 percent of women who eventually underwent autopsy. In general, serious late complications were nearly twice as common in men as in women.

The *Tuskegee Study* showed that the death rate of syphilitic Negro men, 25 to 50 years of age, was 75 percent greater than that of a group of controls, and cardiovascular or central nervous system syphilis was the primary cause of death in 30 percent. By far the most important factor in increased mortality was cardiovascular syphilis. Anatomic evidence of aortitis was found in 40 percent to 60 percent of autopsied syphilitics (versus 15 percent of controls), while central nervous system lues was found in only 4 percent. Hypertension was also increased in the syphilitics. Thus, the incidence of cardiovascular syphilis was higher and central nervous system syphilis lower in the prospective Tuskegee Study, as compared with the Oslo Study. Part of the increased mortality among the Tuskegee patients was not attributable to specific discernible anatomic syphilitic lesions, a phenomenon which has also been noted in experimental syphilis.

MANIFESTATIONS **Primary syphilis** The typical primary chancre usually begins as a single painless papule which rapidly becomes eroded and usually, but not always, is indurated, with a characteristic cartilaginous consistency on palpation of the edge and base of the ulcer. Histologic examination of the ulcer shows mononuclear and histocytic infiltrates with obliterative endarteritis and periarteritis of small vessels. *Treponema pallidum* is seen by electron microscopy to lie in interstitial perivascular spaces and within invaginations or phagosomes of neutrophils, macrophages, endothelial cells, and plasma cells.

The chancre is usually located on the external genitalia, but it may occur on any site on the body. Other primary sites which are commonly overlooked include the cervix and mouth of the female and the perianal area, anal canal, and mouth of the male homosexual. Regional lymphadenopathy accompanies the primary lesion, appearing within 1 week of the onset of the lesion. The nodes are firm, nonsuppurative, and painless. Inguinal lymphadenopathy is bilateral. The chancre heals within 4 to 6 weeks (range 2 to 12 weeks), but the lymphadenopathy may persist for months.

Atypical primary lesions are common. The clinical appearance depends upon the number of treponemes inoculated and upon the preinfection immune status of the patient. A large inoculum produces a dark-field positive ulcerative lesion in nonimmune human volunteers, but in individuals with a previous history of syphilis produces either a small dark-field negative papule, an asymptomatic but seropositive latent infection, or no response at all. A small inoculum usually produces only a papular lesion, even in nonimmune humans. Thus, syphilis should be considered even in the evaluation of trivial or atypical, dark-field negative, genital lesions. The most common genital lesions which must be differentiated from primary syphilis include traumatic, superinfected lesions, genital *Herpesvirus hominis* type II infection (Chap. 200), and chancroid (Chap. 139). *Primary genital herpes* may produce inguinal adenopathy, but is initially characterized by multiple painful vesicles which later ulcerate, and with systemic symptoms including fever; *recurrent genital herpes* typically begins with a cluster of painful vesicles without associated adenopathy. *Chancroid* produces painful, superficial exudative, nonindurated, usually multiple ulcers; adenopathy is either unilateral or bilateral, tender, and may suppurate.

Secondary syphilis The manifestations of the secondary stage are protean but usually include symmetric mucocutaneous lesions and generalized nontender lymphadenopathy. The remnant of the healing primary chancre is still present in many cases. The skin rash consists of macular, papular, papulosquamous, and occasionally pustular syphilides, often with one or more forms present simultaneously. Initial lesions are bilaterally symmetric, pale red or pink, nonpruritic, discrete, round macules, 5 to 10 mm in diameter, distributed on the trunk and proximal extremities. After 1 to 2 months, red, papular lesions 3 to 10 mm in diameter also appear which are associated with increasing endarteritis and perivascular mononuclear infiltration. These are distributed widely and may occur on the palms, soles, face, and scalp. Tiny papular *follicular syphilides* involving hair folicles may result in patchy alopecia and loss of eyebrows or beard.

Progressive endarteritis obliterans and ischemia result in superficial scaling of papules (*papulosquamous syphilides*) and eventually may lead to central necrosis (*pustular syphilide*). In warm, moist, intertriginous areas, including the perianal area, vulva, scrotum, and inner thighs, axillas, and the skin under pendulous breasts, papules enlarge and become eroded, to produce broad, moist, pink or grey-white highly infectious lesions called *condyloma lata*. Superficial mucosal erosions, called *mucous patches*, occur in about a third of patients, and may involve lips, oral mucosa, tongue, palate, pharynx, vulva and vagina, glans penis, or inner prepuce. The typical mucous patch is a silver-grey erosion surrounded by a red periphery, and is usually painless.

During relapses of secondary syphilis, condyloma lata are particularly common, and skin lesions tend to be asymmetrically distributed and more infiltrated, resembling skin lesions of late syphilis, perhaps reflecting increasing cellular immunity.

Constitutional symptoms which may accompany secondary syphilis include fever, weight loss, malaise, and anorexia. Headache and meningismus are common. Acute meningitis occurs in only 1 to 2 percent of patients, but increased cells and protein have been found in the cerebrospinal fluid in 5 percent or more of patients. *Treponema pallidum* has also been recovered by rabbit inoculation from cerebrospinal fluid during secondary syphilis even in the absence of other cerebrospinal fluid abnormalities.

Other less common complications described in secondary syphilis include hepatitis, nephropathy, arthritis and periostitis, and iridocyclitis. It is uncertain whether the association between secondary syphilis and hepatitis is causal or coincidental. *Syphilitic hepatitis* is distinguished by an unusually high serum alkaline phosphatase and by a nonspecific histologic appearance which is unlike viral hepatitis and includes moderate inflammation with polymorphonuclear leukocytes and lymphocytes, some hepatocellular damage, and no cholestasis. The *renal involvement* is associated with proteinuria, an acute nephrotic syndrome, or rarely with hemorrhagic glomerulonephritis, and which is characterized by subepithelial electron-dense deposits and glomerular immune complexes, suggesting that this complication is a form of immune complex glomerulonephritis. Anterior uveitis has been reported in 5 to 10 percent of patients with secondary syphilis, and *T. pallidum* can be demonstrated in the aqueous humor in such cases. Posterior uveitis occurs rarely.

Latent syphilis A diagnosis of latent syphilis is established by the finding of a positive specific treponemal antibody test for syphilis, together with a normal cerebrospinal fluid examination, the absence of clinical manifestations of syphilis on physical examination and chest films, and a history of primary or secondary lesions, history of exposure to syphilis, or delivery of an infant with congenital syphilis. *Early latent* syphilis encompasses the first 4 years after infection, during which relapse of mucocutaneous lesions may occur, while *late latent* syphilis, beginning 4 years after infection, in the untreated patient, is associated with immunity to infectious relapse and with resistance to reinfection. *Treponema pallidum* may still intermittently seed the bloodstream during this stage, pregnant women with latent syphilis may infect the fetus *in utero*, and transfusion syphilis has been transmitted from patients with latent syphilis of many years duration. Until recently it was thought that untreated late latent syphilis had three possible outcomes: (1) It could persist throughout the life of the infected individual; (2) it could end in development of late syphilis; (3) it could end with spontaneous cure of infection, with reversion of serologic tests to negative. It is now apparent, however, that the more sensitive antitreponemal antibody tests rarely if ever become negative. Thus, 50 to 70 percent of untreated patients with latent syphilis never develop clinically evident late syphilis, but the occurrence of spontaneous cure is in doubt.

Late syphilis The onset of slowly progressive inflammatory disease of the aorta or central nervous system begins early during latent syphilis. Pathogenic studies have shown evidence of early syphilitic aortitis soon after the secondary lesions subside, while asymptomatic neurosyphilis can be detected readily during life by cerebrospinal fluid examination.

ASYMPTOMATIC NEUROSYPHILIS In patients with untreated latent syphilis, if the cerebrospinal fluid (CSF) is normal 2 years or more after infection, there is probably no future risk of subsequent development of neurosyphilis, except for the purely vascular type. The diagnosis of asymptomatic neurosyphilis is made in patients with cerebrospinal fluid abnormalities, including pleocytosis, elevated protein, or positive cerebrospinal fluid Wasserman or VDRL test. One or more of these findings are present in 20 percent of patients with untreated syphilis after 2 years. In patients with untreated asymptomatic neurosyphilis, the overall cumulative probability of progression to clinical neurosyphilis is about 20 percent in the first 10 years, but increases with passing time, and is highest in those who show the greatest degree of pleocytosis or protein elevation. The fluorescent treponemal antibody (FTA) test on undiluted cerebrospinal fluid has been found to be reactive far more often than the VDRL test in cases of latent syphilis. It is possible that passive transfer of serum antibody may produce a positive CSF-FTA test. Since the prognosis of patients with a positive CSF-FTA test without other cerebrospinal fluid abnormalities is unknown, the significance of this finding is uncertain. Similarly, the finding of a positive CSF-FTA test without other cerebrospinal fluid abnormalities in patients with a positive serum FTA-ABS (fluorescent treponemal antibody-absorption) associated with nonspecific neurologic findings does not necessarily prove a diagnosis of "atypical" neurosyphilis. However, a therapeutic trial of penicillin in doses adequate for neurosyphilis is warranted in any patient with a positive serum treponemal antibody test who also has unexplained neurologic findings.

SYMPTOMATIC NEUROSYPHILIS The risk of neurosyphilis is two or three times greater in Caucasians than in Negroes, and is twice as common in men as in women.

Although mixed features are common, the major clinical categories of symptomatic neurosyphilis include meningovascular and parenchymatous syphilis. The latter category includes general paresis and tabes dorsalis. The average interval from infection to onset of symptoms is 5 to 10 years of meningovascular syphilis, 20 years for general paresis, and 25 to 30 years for tabes dorsalis. However, many patients with symptomatic neurosyphilis do not present a classic picture, but have mixed or incomplete syndromes. *Meningovascular syphilis* is associated with inflammation of the pia and arachnoid, together with evidence of focal or widespread cerebrovascular disease or often only with pupillary or reflex changes. The manifestations of *general paresis* reflect widespread parenchymal damage, and include abnormalities corresponding to the mnemonic "paresis": *p*ersonality, *a*ffect, *r*eflexes (hyperactive), *e*ye (e.g., Argyll Robertson pupils), *s*ensorium (illusions, delusions, hallucinations), *i*ntellect (decreased recent memory orientation, calculations, judgment, insight), and *s*peech. *Tabes dorsalis* presents symptoms and signs of demyelinization of the posterior columns, dorsal roots, and dorsal root ganglia. Symptoms include ataxic, wide-based gait and footslap, paresthesias, bladder disturbances, impotence, and signs including areflexia, loss of position, deep pain, and temperature sensation. Trophic joint degeneration (Charcot's joints) and perforating ulceration of the feet may result from loss of pain sensation. The Argyll Robertson pupil, seen in both tabes dorsalis and paresis, is a small, irregular pupil which reacts to accommodation but not to light. *Optic atrophy* also occurs frequently in association with tabes.

CARDIOVASCULAR SYPHILIS Cardiovascular manifestations are limited to the large vessels in which the blood supply is provided by vasa vasorum. Endarteritis obliterans of the vasa vasorum produces medial necrosis with destruction of elastic tissue, particularly in the ascending and transverse segments of the aortic arch, resulting in uncomplicated aortitis, aortic regurgitation, saccular aneurysm, or coronary ostial stenosis. These complications do not occur following congenital syphilis or syphilis acquired before age 14, indicating some unexplained resistance of the large blood vessels in youth to invasion by *T. pallidum*. The onset of symptoms occurs from 10 to 40 years after infection, and the rate of progression is said to be increased in individuals involved in strenuous labor. Thus, cardiovascular complications are commoner and occur at an earlier age in men than in women, and in Negroes than in Caucasians. The incidence of symptomatic cardiovascular complications in late untreated syphilis is approximately 10 percent, with aortic regurgitation being two to four times as common as aneurysm. However, syphilitic aortitis can be demonstrated at autopsy in about one-half of Negro males with untreated syphilis, according to the pathologic criteria used in the Tuskegee Study.

Asymptomatic syphilitic aortitis may be suspected in life if linear calcification of the ascending aorta is demonstrated on chest x-ray films, since arteriosclerotic disease seldom produces this sign. Aortic dilatation and a tambour quality of the sound of aortic closure are unreliable signs of aortitis. Syphilitic aneurysms are usually saccular, occasionally fusiform, and do not lead to dissection. Approximately 1 in 10 aortic aneurysms of syphilitic origin may involve the abdominal aorta, but tend to occur above the renal artery, whereas arteriosclerotic abdominal aneurysms usually are found below the renal artery. The nervous system is also affected in 40 percent of patients with cardiovascular syphilis.

LATE LESIONS OF THE EYES Iritis associated with pain, photophobia, and dimness of vision or chorioretinitis, occurs not only during secondary syphilis, but also as a relatively common manifestation of late syphilis. Adhesions of the iris to the anterior lens may produce a fixed pupil, not to be confused with Argyll Robertson pupil.

LATE BENIGN SYPHILIS (GUMMA) Gummas may be multiple or diffuse, but are usually solitary lesions which range from microscopic size to several centimeters in diameter, and histologically consist of nonspecific granulomatous inflammation with central necrosis surrounded by mononuclear, epithelioid, and fibroblastic cells, occasional giant cells, and perivasculitis. Although *T. pallidum* cannot be demonstrated microscopically, it can be recovered from the lesions by rabbit inoculation. The most commonly involved sites are the skin and skeletal systems, mouth and upper respiratory tract, larynx, liver, and stomach. Virtually any organ may be involved. Gummas of skin produce painless nodular, papulosquamous, or ulcerative lesions, which are indurated, and form characteristic circles or arcs, with peripheral hyperpigmentation. The lesions are usually indolent, and may heal spontaneously with scarring, but may also be explosive in onset and are often destructive. These lesions may resemble many other chronic granulomatous conditions, including *tuberculosis* and *sarcoidosis* of skin, leprosy, and *deep fungal infections*. Skeletal gummas involve long bones of the legs with greatest frequency, although any bone may be affected. Trauma may predispose to involvement of a specific site. Presenting symptoms usually include focal pain and tenderness. When sufficiently advanced to produce radiographic abnormalities, the findings may include periostitis or destructive or sclerosing osteitis. Gummas of the upper respiratory tract can lead to perforation of the nasal septum or palate. Gummatous hepatitis may produce epigastric pain and tenderness and low-grade fever, and may be associated with splenomegaly and anemia.

The histopathology and extensive tissue necrosis associated with gummas suggest that cellular hypersensitivity to relatively few treponemes produces these lesions. This response might result from transient treponemia with seeding of sensitized tissues, or from reinfection of a previously sensitized individual. This has been reported in areas where syphilis is endemic in childhood; when one member of a household acquires a fresh infection, other members of the household who then become reinfected develop gummas. Experimental inoculation of *T. pallidum* into individuals with latent or late syphilis also sometimes results in gumma formation at the site of inoculation.

Since the histologic changes may be suggestive but are nonspecific, the diagnosis of late benign syphilis is confirmed by serologic testing and by therapeutic trial.

Treatment with penicillin results in rapid healing of active gummatous lesions.

Congenital syphilis The fetus becomes susceptible to congenital syphilis only after the fourth month of gestation, when atrophy of the Langhans' cell layer of the placenta is completed, and also when immunologic competence begins to develop. This suggests that the pathogenesis of congenital syphilis may depend upon the immune response of the host rather than upon a direct toxic effect of *T. pallidum.* The risk of infection of the fetus during untreated early maternal syphilis is estimated to be 80 to 95 percent, decreases to about 70 percent at 4 years, and is still lower during late latent maternal syphilis. Adequate treatment of the mother before the sixteenth week of pregnancy prevents infection of the fetus. The later treatment is begun during pregnancy, the greater the likelihood of development of stigmas of congenital syphilis, particularly of dental abnormalities. Untreated early maternal infection may result in up to 40 percent fetal loss (stillbirth is more common than abortion, because of the late onset of fetal infection), prematurity, neonatal death, or in nonfatal congenital syphilis. The manifestations of *early congenital syphilis* develop within the first 2 years of life and consist of rash, which may include extensive superficial desquamation, vesicles, bullae, petechiae, and, later, papulosquamous lesions; oral mucous patches; rhinitis, sometimes with hemorrhagic mucoid nasal discharge; hepatosplenomegaly; hemolytic anemia; jaundice; and osteochondritis of long bones which may produce "pseudoparalysis." Thrombocytopenia and leukocytosis are frequent. There is no primary stage, since the infection is initiated by direct bloodstream infection *in utero.* Neonatal congenital syphilis must be differentiated from other generalized congenital infections, including rubella, cytomegalovirus infection, and toxoplasmosis, and also from erythroblastosis fetalis. Neonatal death is usually due to pulmonary hemorrhage, secondary bacterial infection, or severe hepatitis. Pathologic findings include interstitial and perivascular inflammation followed by variable fibroblastic proliferation, involving skin, bones, liver, kidneys, pancreas, spleen, lungs, and intestines, with extramedullary hematopoiesis.

Late congenital syphilis is defined as congenital syphilis which remains untreated after 2 years of age. In perhaps 60 percent of cases, the infection remains latent, while the clinical spectrum in the remainder differs in certain respects from that of acquired late syphilis in the adult. For example, cardiovascular syphilis rarely develops in late congenital syphilis, whereas *interstitial keratitis* is much more common in late congenital syphilis, occurring between ages 5 and 25 in from 10 to 50 percent of cases. The onset is acute with symptoms of iritis, followed by corneal clouding with superficial and deep vascularization of the stroma which progresses despite antibiotic therapy, but which is suppressed by corticosteroid therapy. Characteristic dental abnormalities include *Hutchinson's teeth,* the centrally notched, widely spaced upper central incisors which are barrel or screwdriver-shaped, and "mulberry" molars, sixth-year molars which have multiple, poorly developed cusps, rather than the usual four. The abnormal facies, which include frontal bossing, saddlenose, and poorly developed maxilla, may also be seen in congenital ectodermal dysplasia. *Saber shins,* or anterior tibial bowing, are rare, but were probably more common in the past when syphilitic periostitis of the anterior tibia was associated with vitamin D deficiency. Neurologic findings include eighth-nerve deafness, usually appearing around the time of puberty, juvenile paresis, appearing at the same time, and tabes dorsalis, which occurs later and is less common than in acquired late syphilis.

LABORATORY DIAGNOSIS Diagnostic tests for syphilis include serologic tests and methods for demonstration of *T. pallidum* in lesions by dark-field or phase contrast microscopy or by staining the treponemes with various silver impregnation techniques or with fluorescent antibody.

Dark-field examination technique Dark-field examination is essential in evaluating moist lesions, such as the chancre of primary syphilis, or condyloma lata of secondary syphilis. Although it is difficult to demonstrate *T. pallidum* in dry maculopapular lesions in secondary syphilis by dark-field examination, the organism may be demonstrated by saline aspiration of lymph nodes during this stage. The surface of the suspected ulcerated lesion should be cleaned with saline and gauze, then gently abraded further with dry gauze, without production of bleeding. The lesion is then squeezed to express a serous transudate, and a drop of the transudate is picked up on the surface of a glass slide. A drop of saline (without bacteriostatic additives) may be mixed with the transudate if necessary, and this is then covered with a cover slip and examined for *T. pallidum* with a dark-field or phase contrast microscope by an experienced individual. A single negative examination does not exclude syphilis, since at least 10^4 treponemes per milliliter transudate must be present to be detected, and prior use of topical antiseptic or cleansing by the patient may obfuscate the examination. Cleansing or use of topical medication should, therefore, be avoided, and the dark-field examination should be repeated on three successive days before being considered negative.

Serologic tests for syphilis The profusion of serologic tests for syphilis causes much unnecessary confusion. Syphilitic infection produces two types of antibodies, the *nonspecific reaginic antibody* and *specific antitreponemal* antibody.

The term *reagin* is unfortunate, since the unrelated gamma-E globulin (IgE) antibody involved in certain allergic phenomena is also known as *reagin.* The nontreponemal reaginic antibodies produced in syphilis contain both IgG and IgM immunoglobulins directed against a lipoidal antigen that results from the interaction of *T. pallidum* with host tissues, and possibly against a lipoidal antigen of *T. pallidum* itself. The cardiolipin antigens initially used in the detection of reaginic antibody were relatively crude extracts of beef heart, and it is not surprising that false positive reactions were extremely common in many conditions other than syphilis. The cardiolipin-cholesterol-lecithin antigen now in use in a variety of tests for reaginic antibody (Table 159-1) is more purified and gives fewer false positive reactions than did earlier antigens. The tests for treponemal antibody employ antigens derived from *T. pallidum*, rather than from tissues, and detect antibody related only to past or present treponemal infections.

The most widely used reagin antibody tests are the sensitive rapid plasma reagin (RPR) tests, which can be automated and are used to screen large numbers of serums, and the VDRL slide flocculation test, which is used to determine quantitatively the exact titer of serum reagin antibody. The reagin titer reflects the activity of the disease: false positive VDRL titers usually do not exceed 1:8; a fourfold or greater rise in titer may be seen during the evolution of primary syphilis; VDRL titers usually reach 1:32 or higher in secondary syphilis; a persistent fall in titer following treatment of early syphilis provides essential evidence of an adequate response to therapy.

The standard antitreponemal antibody test is the FTA-ABS test. The patient's serum is first absorbed with a nonpathogenic treponemal antigen (sorbent) to remove group-specific antibody which may be produced by the human beings against saprophytic oral and genital treponemes. The patient's absorbed serum is then placed on a slide which contains dried *T. pallidum*. If specific antibody to *T. pallidum* remains in the patient's serum after the absorption step, it is fixed to the dried treponemes, and then is detected by the addition of fluorescein-labeled antihuman gamma-globulin and subsequent examination of the slide by fluorescence microscopy. The *Treponema pallidum* immobilization (TPI) test, in which immobilization of live *T. pallidum* is produced by immune serum plus complement, is more laborious, but still is occasionally used in reference laboratories in this country in problem cases. The *T. pallidum* hemagglutination assay (TPHA) is a convenient test for treponemal antibody but is not yet widely used in this country. The relative sensitivities of the VDRL, FTA-ABS, and TPI tests in the various stages of syphilis are shown in Table 159-2.

The VDRL is negative in nearly one-third of patients with primary, latent, or late syphilis. It is therefore not sufficient to obtain a reagin antibody test alone in evaluating very early, latent, or late syphilis; the more sensitive FTA-ABS test should be routinely obtained at these stages. However, both tests are always positive during

TABLE 159-1
Common serologic tests for syphilis

Nonspecific (reagin) antibody tests
- Flocculation: VDRL
- Complement fixation: Kolmer
- Agglutination: rapid plasma reagin (RPR)

Specific treponemal antibody tests
- Immunofluorescence: fluorescent treponemal antibody–absorption (FTA-ABS)
- Immobilization: *Treponema pallidum* immobilization (TPI)
- Hemagglutination: *T. pallidum* hemagglutination assay (TPHA)

TABLE 159-2
Frequency of positive tests in untreated syphilis

	VDRL, %	*TPI, %*	*FTA-ABS, %*
Primary syphilis	70	50	85
Secondary syphilis	100	95	100
Latent or late syphilis	70	95	98

secondary syphilis, and a negative VDRL or FTA-ABS virtually excludes syphilis in a patient with otherwise compatible mucocutaneous lesions. (An estimated 1 percent of patients with secondary syphilis have a negative VDRL test with undiluted serum which becomes positive in higher dilutions—the *prozone* phenomenon.)

False positive serologic tests for syphilis An estimated 20 to 40 percent of all positive reagin tests are false positive tests, depending upon the population being examined. False positive reagin tests are classified as acute if they become negative within 6 months. Acute false positive reagin tests occur during atypical pneumonia, malaria, and various acute bacterial or viral infections, and following smallpox vaccinations. Chronic reactions, which persist 6 months or longer, can be remembered as occurring in conditions beginning with *A*, including *a*ddiction, *a*utoimmune diseases, and *a*ging. False positive reagin tests occur in 25 percent of narcotics addicts, and in 10 to 20 percent of patients with active systemic lupus erythematosus. Other antibodies which have been found with great frequency in serums from chronic false positive reactors include antinuclear, antithyroid, and antimitochondrial antibodies, as well as rheumatoid factor and cryoglobulins. The Donath-Landsteiner antibody responsible for paroxysmal cold hemoglobinuria is a hemolysin which appears in syphilis. The autoimmune nature of the false positive reagin test is further suggested by the occurrence of systemic lupus erythematosus or other connective tissue diseases in 15 to 45 percent of chronic false positive reactors. The incidence of false positive reagin tests increases with advancing age, and 10 percent of people over 70 years of age have false positive reactions. Other diseases associated with hyperglobulinemia, such as leprosy, may also produce chronic false positive reactions.

In the patient with a false positive reagin test, syphilis is readily excluded by obtaining an FTA-ABS or TPI test, which is negative in such cases. Most individuals who have a typical positive FTA-ABS but a negative TPI test have evidence of past or present syphilis, indicating lack of sensitivity of the TPI, rather than lack of specificity of the FTA-ABS. The results of the FTA-ABS test are reported as negative, borderline, or positive. *Borderline* results occur in less than 1 percent of a normal population, but are more common in patients who are pregnant or have diseases associated with abnormal or increased globulins, and are frequently not associated with either clinical, historical, or other serologic evidence of syphilis. Borderline results should, therefore, always be repeated in questionable cases, and interpreted with caution. A typical "positive" FTA-ABS occurs infrequently in conditions other than syphilis. Although false positive FTA-ABS tests have been reported in 15 percent of patients with active systemic lupus erythematosus, the fluorescent staining is "borderline" or has an atypical "beaded" appearance in most cases (thought to be due to attachment of antinuclear antibody to treponemal DNA or nucleoprotein leaked through breaks in the outer treponemal membranes). However, because of the occasional occurrence of false positive FTA-ABS tests, only a positive TPI provides conclusive proof of past or present treponemal infection. Both the FTA-ABS and TPI tests are positive in patients who have had yaws or pinta.

For practical purposes, most clinicians need to be familiar with the three serologic tests used by their laboratories: (1) For screening large numbers of serums for reaginic antibody (e.g., RPR); (2) for quantitative measurement of reaginic antibody titer in order to assess the clinical activity of syphilis, and to follow the reagin titer in response to therapy (e.g., VDRL); and (3) to confirm the diagnosis of syphilis in a patient with a positive reagin antibody test or with a suspected clinical diagnosis of syphilis (e.g., FTA-ABS).

IgM-FTA-ABS test for active congenital syphilis in the newborn All newborn infants of mothers with reactive VDRL or FTA-ABS tests will themselves have reactive tests whether or not they have become infected, because of passive transplacental transfer of maternal IgG immunoglobulins which are reactive in these tests. However, if IgM antitreponemal antibody is present in the infant's serum, it reflects fetal antibody production in response to intrauterine infection, particularly if there is a rise in titer, since maternal IgM antibody does not cross the intact placental barrier. Neonatal IgM antibody is detected in cord or neonatal serums in a modified FTA-ABS test, employing fluorescein-labeled antihuman IgM to detect antitreponemal IgM antibody. Similar tests have been developed for detection of congenital toxoplasmosis, rubella, and cytomegalovirus infections. The IgM-FTA-ABS test is sensitive and is positive in all infants with active congenital syphilis, except when the mother and fetus become infected very late during pregnancy. Occasional positive IgM-FTA-ABS tests may occur in normal infants, due to leakage of maternal blood into the fetal circulation. This should also produce detectable elevation of ceruloplasmin in the infant's serum.

TREATMENT AND FOLLOW-UP MANAGEMENT

Arsenic and heavy metal therapy was suppressive or curative in many cases of early syphilis or asymptomatic neurosyphilis, but not in parenchymal neurosyphilis. However, *T. pallidum* is very temperature-sensitive, and fever therapy, produced deliberately with *Plasmodium vivax* malaria, was found to be effective in the treatment of some cases of general paresis.

Following the introduction of penicillin therapy for syphilis, these formerly used toxic regimens were gradually abandoned, and benzathine penicillin G eventually became the drug of choice for most forms of syphilis. *T. pallidum* is killed by very low concentrations of penicillin G, although a long period of exposure to penicillin is required for treatment because of the unusually slow rate of multiplication of the organism. The efficacy of penicillin for syphilis remains undiminished after 30 years of use. Other antibiotics which are effective in syphilis include the tetracyclines, erythromycin, chloramphenicol, and the cephalosporins. Streptomycin inhibits *T. pallidum* only in very large doses, and the sulfonamides are inactive. The treatment schedules currently recommended by the United States Public Health Service for the various stages of syphilis are summarized in Table 159-3.

Infectious syphilis In experimental syphilis in rabbits, the minimum curative dose of penicillin G is proportional to the size of the inoculum and to the duration of the

TABLE 159-3
Treatment schedules recommended by the U.S. Public Health Service for syphilis

For patients without penicillin allergy	*Early congenital syphilis*	*Early or latent* syphilis and exposed contacts*	*Late syphilis (acquired or congenital) and asymptomatic neurosyphilis*
Benzathine penicillin G (Bicillin)	50,000 units/kg, single dose	2.4 million units single dose (1.2 million units in each hip)	6.0–9.0 million units (3.0 million units at 7-day intervals)
Aqueous procaine penicillin G	100,000 units/kg total dose (10,000 units/kg/day for 10 days)	4.8 million units total dose (600,000 units/day for 8 days)	6.0–9.0 million units (600,000 units/day for 10–15 days)
For patients with penicillin allergy			
Tetracycline HCl	Not recommended for children	30–40 g total oral dose (2–3 g/day for 10 to 15 days)	No USPHS recommendations. Some syphilologists advise doubling the dose and duration of therapy when using tetracycline or erythromycin for late syphilis
Erythromycin	No USPHS recommendation 400 mg/kg total oral dose over 10 days probably effective	30–40 g total oral dose (2–3 g/day for 10 to 15 days)	

* *If no spinal fluid examination is done, treatment for possible asymptomatic neurosyphilis is recommended.*

infection. Thus, in incubating preprimary, or seronegative, syphilis in human beings, the recommended dose of 2.4 million units of benzathine penicillin G exceeds the minimum necessary, and even a single injection of procaine penicillin G, in the dose currently recommended for gonorrhea, appears to be 100 percent effective in curing incubating seronegative syphilis. For this reason, follow-up serologic testing for syphilis is unnecessary in patients treated for gonorrhea with the recommended dose of procaine penicillin G. In primary and secondary syphilis, each of the four regimens listed in Table 159-3 is associated with less than 5 percent failures; the recommended tetracycline and erythromycin regimens are based upon studies in which increasing doses were evaluated, and the recommendations represent minimum effective doses. Erythromycin estolate may be more effective than erythromycin base in early syphilis.

Jarisch-Herxheimer reaction A dramatic reaction, consisting of fever (average temperature elevation 1.5°C), chills, myalgias, headache, tachycardia, increased respiratory rate, increased circulating neutrophil count (average 12,500 total white blood count per ml), and vasodilation with mild hypotension, may occur following initiation of treatment of syphilis. This reaction occurs in approximately 50 percent of patients with primary syphilis, 90 percent with secondary, and 25 percent with early latent syphilis. The onset occurs within 2 hours after treatment, with peak temperature occurring at about 7 hr, and defervescence takes place within 12 to 24 hr. In patients with secondary syphilis, an increase in erythema and edema of the mucocutaneous lesions occurs; occasionally subclinical or early mucocutaneous lesions may first become apparent during the reaction. The pathogenesis of this reaction may involve release of endotoxin in tissues. Patients should be warned to expect such symptoms, which can be managed by bedrest and aspirin.

The response of early syphilis to treatment should be determined by following the quantitative VDRL titer 1, 3, 6, and 12 months after treatment. Because the FTA-ABS test remains positive after 2 years in approximately 95 percent of patients treated for seropositive early syphilis, this test is not useful in following the response to therapy. Following successful treatment of seropositive primary or secondary syphilis, the VDRL titer progressively declines, becoming negative within 3 to 12 months in about 75 percent of seropositive primary cases and 40 percent of secondary cases. After 2 years, nearly all patients with primary syphilis have a negative VDRL, although 25 percent of secondary cases and a higher proportion of those treated for early latent syphilis still maintain low titers of reagin. If the VDRL becomes negative or reaches a fixed low titer within 1 or 2 years, it is unnecessary to perform a lumbar puncture at that time, since the spinal fluid examination is invariably normal and there is no risk of subsequent neurosyphilis. However, if the VDRL titer fails to become negative, does not reach a fixed low titer, or actually increases, treatment failure should be suspected. Because asymptomatic neurosyphilis is frequently present in such patients, spinal fluid examination is indicated, and retreatment should be based upon the presence or absence of asymptomatic neurosyphilis.

Latent syphilis Treatment of early latent syphilis prevents infectious relapses, and treatment of latent syphilis prevents the subsequent development of late complications and conceivably may prevent the additional unexplained reduced life expectancy of untreated latent syphilis. In the case of the infected female, treatment also prevents the occurrence of congenital syphilis in her offspring. Spinal fluid examination should be done before treatment of latent syphilis, because approximately 20 percent of patients will have asymptomatic neurosyphilis after 2 years of infection. Whereas 2.4 million units benzathine penicillin G is effective therapy for uncomplicated latent syphilis of any duration, spinal fluid abnormalities dictate higher doses of penicillin, and also provide a base line for evaluation of serial improvement in the spinal fluid in response to therapy.

Asymptomatic neurosyphilis The activity of asymptomatic neurosyphilis is correlated best with the degree of cerebrospinal fluid pleocytosis. Changes in the cerebrospinal fluid cell count, and to a lesser extent, in cerebrospinal fluid protein concentration, provide the most sensitive index of response to treatment. Spinal fluid examination should be performed every 3 to 4 months for 2 years after treatment of asymptomatic neurosyphilis. An elevated cerebrospinal fluid cell count falls to 10 or less per mm^3 within 3 to 12 months in 95 percent of adequately treated cases, and becomes normal in all cases within 2 to 4 years. Elevated levels of cerebrospinal fluid protein fall more slowly, and the cerebrospinal fluid reagin titer declines slowly over a period of several years. Asymptomatic neurosyphilis has been found to relapse in nearly one-quarter of patients treated with 2.4 million units benzathine penicillin, whereas progression to symptomatic neurosyphilis has rarely, if ever, occurred in patients who received a total dose of 6,000,000 units or more.

Late syphilis Lumbar puncture should be performed even in the evaluation of late complications other than symptomatic neurosyphilis, since asymptomatic neurosyphilis may coexist with other late complications, and abnormal cerebrospinal fluid findings can then be followed serially as a guide to therapy. The response of cardiovascular syphilis to penicillin is seldom dramatic because aortic aneurysm and aortic regurgitation cannot be repaired by antibiotic treatment, although further progression of these lesions may be arrested by treatment. In contrast, the response of benign tertiary syphilis and of meningovascular syphilis to penicillin G is usually impressive. The response of parenchymal neurosyphilis has been variable. In a cooperative study of the treatment of 1,086 general paretics with penicillin, the frequency of clinical improvement or termination of progression ranged from 38 percent of those with severe involvement to 81 percent of those with mild involvement. All patients who relapsed following initial improvement in cerebrospinal fluid pleocytosis had received less than 6,000,000 units of penicillin, and all improved with subsequent therapy. Tabes dorsalis or optic atrophy respond less often. In general, treatment of inactive neurosyphilis in which permanent neurologic damage has already occurred may not produce any clinical change, and retreatment of such cases is not warranted. However, persistence of cerebrospinal fluid pleocytosis, or recurrence following initial response to treatment, indicates continuing active infection, which should respond to additional treatment. The optimal dose and duration of penicillin in such cases has not been determined, but administration of 900,000 units procaine penicillin G daily for 10 days has been effective in the past. If this is ineffective, more prolonged courses of procaine or benzathine penicillin G are certainly indicated.

Persistence of treponemal forms The persistence of treponemes in tissues following treatment of syphilis with arsenicals or bismuth has been documented in the past. The persistence of *T. pallidum* in the aqueous humor, cerebrospinal fluid, lymph nodes, brain, inflamed temporal arteries, and other tissues following "adequate" penicillin treatment of latent or late syphilis has also been suggested by dark-field microscopy and by immunofluorescent antibody and silver staining techniques. Treponemal forms have also been demonstrated in patients with various clinical findings suggestive of syphilis, but in whom serologic tests, including the FTA-ABS test, were negative. Although many of these findings could be explained by artifact or by the coincidental presence of nonpathogenic treponemes, in a few cases the persistence of pathogenic *T. pallidum* after antibiotic treatment was proved by rabbit inoculation experiments. The question has been raised as to whether the life-long persistence of antitreponemal antibody measured in the TPI and FTA-ABS tests following treatment of latent or late syphilis represents prolonged immunologic memory or actually represents continued antigenic stimulation by persisting treponemes in lymph nodes and other tissues.

It is not surprising that *T. pallidum* might persist in the aqueous humor or cerebrospinal fluid despite penicillin treatment, because of poor penetration of the antibiotic, but persistence in lymph nodes and other sites remains unexplained. Limited evidence indicates no increase in resistance to penicillin of such persistent treponemes. At present, no modification of the treatment recommendations for latent or late syphilis seems warranted, but further studies on the nature of persistent treponemal forms and their relation to the persistence of positive treponemal antibody tests are required.

IMMUNITY AND PREVENTION OF SYPHILIS Only about 50 percent of the named contacts of primary and secondary syphilis become infected. The relative importance of variations in sexual and hygienic practices, inoculum size, body and environmental temperature, and other local and systemic factors affecting transmissibility of syphilis remains undefined. Studies of experimental syphilis showed that the risk of infection by *T. pallidum* was reduced following exposure by topical application of 30 percent calomel ointment or of a detergent surfactant-mepharsen preparation, whereas simple washing with soap and water was ineffective. The use of calomel in the military "pro kit" was never evaluated in controlled field trials, but was generally believed to reduce the incidence of syphilis. There is currently some interest in the possible efficacy of intravaginal contraceptive gels as prophylactics against venereal diseases including syphilis, since many available preparations have bacteriostatic as well as spermicidal properties.

Man has no natural resistance to infection by pathogenic treponemes. The rate of development of acquired resistance to *T. pallidum* following natural or experimental infection is quantitatively related to the amount of antigenic stimulus, which depends upon both the size of the infecting inoculum and the duration of infection prior to treatment.

Resistance to reinfection or superinfection by challenge inoculation develops about three months after the primary (immunizing) infection in animals with experimental syphilis. Resistance of human beings to reinfection by intradermal inoculation of *T. pallidum* was studied in volunteers. Those who had previously been treated for *early* syphilis developed a primary lesion and a serologic response, while the majority of those who had previously been treated for *late latent* syphilis and all those with *untreated latent* syphilis developed neither primary lesions nor serologic response following inoculation. Two patients treated for late latent or late congenital syphilis developed gummas at the site of inoculation.

The role of serum antibody in conferring immunity to syphilis remains controversial. Reagin antibody is not protective, and the evidence is equivocal that antibody directed against specific treponemal antigens confers immunity. Delayed hypersensitivity to *T. pallidum* has been demonstrated by skin test in late syphilis, and lymphocytes from patients with syphilis have been demonstrated to undergo blast transformation when exposed to treponemal or cardiolipin antigen. Passive transfer experiments in syngeneic animals suggest that development of cellular immunity contributes to resolution of the early lesions and to resistance to infection, while the histopathology of gummas suggests that the cellular immune response is somehow involved in the pathogenesis of these lesions.

Inability to cultivate pathogenic treponemes in vitro has hindered analysis, purification, and concentration of treponemal antigens, and attempts to induce immunity to syphilis by vaccination have shown limited promise. Injection of rabbits with motile strains irradiated with x-rays or with strains of *T. pallidum* inactivated during cold storage have conferred limited immunity, but many injections over long periods of time were required. Attempts to provide cross-resistance by immunization of rabbits with cultivated nonpathogenic treponemes have been unsuccessful. Experiments in man have shown that varying degrees of cross-immunity exist in patients infected with *T. pallidum*, *T. pertenue*, and *T. carateum*, but chimpanzees with experimental pinta have not developed cross-resistance to syphilis. These findings indicate that the prospects for a syphilis vaccine are still remote, and the prevention of syphilis still depends upon use of mechanical or antiseptic prophylactic agents, and upon detection and treatment of infectious cases.

REFERENCES

BHORADE MS et al: Nephropathy of secondary syphilis: A clinical and pathological spectrum. JAMA 216:1159, 1971

BROWN WJ: Status and control of syphilis in the United States. J Infect Dis 124:428, 1971

CLARK EG, DANBOLT N: The Oslo study of the natural course of untreated syphilis. Med Clin North Am 48:613, 1964

MAGNUSON HJ et al: Inoculation syphilis in human volunteers. Medicine 35:33, 1956

PREWITT T: Cardiovascular syphilis. Med Aspects Hum Sexuality 12:68, 1972

SCHROETER AL et al: Treatment for early syphilis and reactivity of serologic tests. JAMA 221:471, 1972

SHERLOCK S: The liver in secondary (early) syphilis. N Engl J Med 284:1437, 1971

SHORT DH et al: Neurosyphilis, the search for adequate treatment: A review and report of a study using benzathine penicillin G. Arch Dermatol 93:87, 1966

SMITH JL: *Spirochetes in Late Seronegative Syphilis, Penicillin Notwithstanding.* Springfield, Ill.: Charles C Thomas, 1969

SPARLING PF: Diagnosis and treatment of syphilis. N Engl J Med 284:642, 1971

TURNER TB: *Syphilis and the Treponematoses, Infectious Agents and Host Reaction,* ed S Mudd, Philadelphia: Saunders, 1970, p. 346

WORLD HEALTH ORGANIZATION: Treponematosis research: Report of a WHO scientific group. WHO Tech Rept Ser 455, 1970

160
NONVENEREAL TREPONEMATOSES

KING K. HOLMES
JAMES P. HARNISCH

GENERAL CONSIDERATIONS Nonvenereal treponematoses are endemic in certain rural, remote, and isolated areas of the world between the Tropic of Capricorn and the Tropic of Cancer. Yaws, pinta, and bejel are produced by treponemes which are morphologically and antigenically identical to *Treponema pallidum* but are distinguished from syphilis by clinical and epidemiologic features. Pinta involves the skin alone, yaws affects skin and bones, and bejel involves the skin, bone, and mucous membranes. Prenatal infections and cardiovascular and central nervous system involvement occur rarely in the nonvenereal treponematoses but are common in syphilis. In yaws as in syphilis, treponemes resembling *T. pallidum* have been demonstrated in the aqueous humor with fluorescent antibody staining.

EPIDEMIOLOGY The nonvenereal treponematoses are primarily contagious diseases of childhood. Environmental factors favoring transmission of yaws by close personal contact include warmth, humidity, scanty clothing, and poor personal and community hygiene associated with a low standard of living. Biting insects have also been implicated in the transmission of pinta, and domestic utensils such as cooking vessels may be involved in the spread of bejel. In areas of Africa where yaws is endemic, treponemes have been discovered in the lymph glands of asymptomatic cynomolgus monkeys, and these treponemes have resembled *T. pertenue*, the causative agent of yaws. Since 1949 mass campaigns for the eradication of endemic nonvenereal treponematoses have been launched under the auspices of WHO in 46 countries. Approximately 50 million cases or contacts have been treated, and the prevalence of these diseases has fallen markedly. During 1971 only 782 new cases of yaws were reported in the Americas, and pinta was even less common.

IMMUNOLOGIC RELATIONS Specific anti-*T. pallidum* humoral antibodies are produced in individuals with yaws, pinta, or bejel, but the time of appearance of antibodies after onset of infection is variable. Seroreactivity with nontreponemal antibody tests may take four times longer to develop in pinta than in syphilis. The fluorescent treponemal antibody absorption (FTA-ABS) test is a sensitive and specific diagnostic measure during all stages of the nonvenereal treponematoses but cannot differentiate the specific clinical diseases.

Cross-immunity between the various treponematoses exists, and individuals who have had yaws or pinta are considered to be relatively immune to syphilis. However, under experimental circumstances this immunity has been overcome.

CLINICAL MANIFESTATIONS Yaws Yaws (pian, framboesia, buba, bouba) is a chronic infectious disease of childhood caused by *T. pertenue.* The disease is characterized by an initial skin lesion and relapsing, nondestructive, secondary lesion of skin and bone. In the late stages destructive lesions of bone and joints take place.

The incubation period following experimental inoculation of susceptible human beings is 3 to 4 weeks. Disruption of the skin by insect bites, abrasions, or injuries promotes acquisition of natural infection from infected contacts. The initial early lesion is a single papule which is usually located on a leg. The lesion enlarges and becomes papillomatous, superficially eroded, and covered by a thin, yellow crust. Erythema and induration are not common. The lesion is pruritic, and regional lymphadenopathy occurs. The initial lesion usually heals in 6 months. A generalized secondary eruption of similar lesions appears either before or after the initial lesion has healed and is most extensive on the exposed surfaces of the body. These early cutaneous lesions of yaws have a variety of forms including desquamative macular and papular as well as papillomatous types. Painful papules on the soles of the feet result in a crablike gait referred to as *crabyaws.* Early lesions are infectious and heal slowly; they may result in scarring, hyperpigmentation, or depigmentation. Histologically there is mononuclear-cell infiltration, acanthosis, hyperkeratosis, and many treponemes are present. Other manifestations of early yaws include lymphadenopathy and nocturnal bone pain due to periostitis. Fever and other constitutional symptoms may occur. Infectious cutaneous relapses may occur any time during the first 5 years after infection. Late yaws lesions occur 5 years or more after infection and differ histologically from early lesions in showing endarteritis. Late lesions include gummas of the skin and long bones, particularly of the legs, hyperkeratoses of the soles and palms, osteitis, periostitis, juxta-articular fibromatous nodes, and hydrarthrosis.

Treponema pertenue can be demonstrated by darkfield examination in early cutaneous lesions but should not be confused with other spirochetes found in tropical ulcers. The serum reagin antibody tests become positive after 1 month, and the FTA-ABS test is also positive.

Pinta Pinta (mal del pinto, carate, azul, purupuru) is an infectious disease of the skin caused by *T. carateum*. This disease has three cutaneous stages characterized by marked changes in skin color, does not involve the viscera, and causes no disability other than that associated with cosmetic disfigurement. Pinta is confined to tropical regions of Central and South America.

The initial lesion is a small papule which appears 7 to 30 days after exposure and is located most often on the extremities, face, neck, or buttocks. It increases in size slowly by peripheral extension and by coalescing with smaller satellite papules. Regional lymphadenopathy occurs. A secondary eruption appears 1 month to 1 year after the appearance of the initial lesion. The secondary lesions are termed *pintides*, may be numerous, and evolve into a psoriatic, circinate, or scaly erythematous macular configuration. These pintides are initially red but become deeply pigmented, reaching a slate-blue color after a period of time which is related to exposure to sun. Pigmentation occurs most rapidly on the exposed parts of the body. These pigmented lesions are known as *dyschromic macules* and contain treponemes which are located principally in the epidermis in older lesions. Histologically there is deposition of pigment in the dermis with decreased melanin pigment in the basal cell layer. Within 3 months to a year, most of the pintides show varying degrees of depigmentation, becoming brown and finally white and giving the skin a mottled appearance. The porcelain white achromic lesions represent the "late" stage of the disease in which the epidermis is atrophic and melanocytes and melanin are absent. *Treponema carateum* can be demonstrated in transudates from initial, early secondary, or late dyschromic lesions; serologic reaginic and antitreponemal antibody tests are positive.

Bejel Bejel is a chronic, nonvenereal, treponemal infection of childhood characterized by early mucous membrane or mucocutaneous lesions, a latent period of indeterminate duration, and late complications including gummas of bone and skin. The causative organism is indistinguishable from *T. pallidum*. Whereas yaws is endemic in humid tropical climates, endemic foci of bejel exist throughout the arid areas of the Arabian peninsula, North Africa, and Middle Eastern countries. Bejel has not been found in the Western Hemisphere.

Primary cutaneous lesions are infrequent. The initial manifestation is usually a mucous patch or a mucocutaneous lesion resembling the split papules or condylomata of secondary syphilis. Regional lymphadenopathy occurs but generalized lymphadenopathy is unusual. Treponemes are abundant in the moist early lesions and in aspirates from regional lymph nodes. After a variable latent period, late lesions may develop. These resemble lesions of late benign syphilis and include osseous or cutaneous gummas. Gummas, osteitis, or periostitis of nasopharyngeal structures are particularly common. Other complications of late venereal syphilis such as cardiovascular or central nervous system syphilis occur rarely if at all in bejel.

TREATMENT Treatment is similar for all the treponematoses. Intramuscular injection of 2.4 million units benzathine penicillin G in adults and half this dose in children results in rapid resolution of lesions and in prevention of recurrence. Procaine penicillin in oil and 2 percent aluminum monostearate (PAM) has been used extensively. In persons who are allergic to penicillin, tetracycline hydrochloride in a dose similar to that used for infectious syphilis (Chap. 159) is effective. In areas where less than 5 percent of the population has active disease, cases are managed on an individual basis, and all contacts of infected persons are treated with antibiotics.

REFERENCES

Guthe T: Clinical, serological and epidemiological features of framboesia tropica (yaws) and its control in rural communities. Acta Derm Venereol 49:343, 1969

Marquez F et al: Mal del pinto in Mexico. Bull WHO 13:299, 1955

Taneja BL: Yaws: Clinical manifestations and criteria for diagnosis. Indian J Med Res 56:100, 1968

World Health Organization: Treponematoses research: Report of a WHO scientific group. WHO Tech. Rept. Ser. no. 455:1, 1970

161 LEPTOSPIROSIS

JAY P. SANFORD

DEFINITION Leptospirosis is a term applied to disease caused by all leptospiras regardless of specific serotype. Correlation of clinical syndromes with infection by differing serotypes leads to the conclusion that a single serotype of *Leptospira* may be responsible for a variety of clinical features; conversely, a single syndrome, e.g., aseptic meningitis, may be caused by multiple serotypes. Hence there is a preference for the general term leptospirosis rather than the synonyms such as Weil's disease and canicola fever.

ETIOLOGY The genus *Leptospira* contains only one species, *L. interrogans*, which may be subdivided into two complexes, interrogans and biflexa. The interrogans complex includes most of the pathogenic strains, while the biflexa complex includes saprophytic strains with no recognized hosts. Within each complex the organisms show wide antigenic variations that are stable and allow them to be classed as serotypes. Certain serotypes with common antigens are arranged in serogroups. Despite contrary common usage, an example of the correct designation of *Leptospira* is as follows: pomona serogroup of *L. interrogans,* not *L. pomona.* The interrogans complex now contains about 130 serotypes arranged in 16 serogroups (the number in parentheses refers to number of serotypes within the serogroup): icterohemorrhagiae (13), hebdomadis (28), autumnalis (13), canicola (11), australis (10), tarassovi or hyos (10), pyrogenes (9), bataviae (8), javanica (6), pomona (6), ballum (3), cynopteri (3), celledoni (2), grippotyphosa (2), panama (2), and shermani (1). At least 22 serotypes of *Leptospira* occur naturally in the United States.

EPIDEMIOLOGY Although leptospirosis is not a common disease, it has been reported from all regions of the United States. Between 1960 and 1971, 70 to 80 cases have been reported annually. Occasional upswings in number of cases have been the result of common source outbreaks. Infection of man is an incidental occurrence and is not essential to the maintenance of leptospirosis. Leptospirosis occurs in a wide range of domestic and wild animal hosts. In many species, such as opossums, skunks, raccoons, and foxes, infectivity ratios in the range of 10 to 50 percent are not unusual. Interspecies spread of specific serotypes of leptospiras between animal hosts is frequent, e.g., pomona, a serotype principally associated with livestock, has been demonstrated in dogs. The infection in animals may vary from inapparent illness to severe fatal disease. The carrier state may develop in many animals wherein the host may shed leptospiras in its urine for months to years.

It has not been established that pathogenic leptospiras are capable of multiplication outside a host. Survival in nature is governed by factors including pH of the urine of the host, pH of soil or water into which they are shed, and ambient temperature. Acid urine permits only limited survival; however, if the urine is neutral or alkaline and is shed into a similar moist environment which has low salinity, is not badly polluted with microorganisms or detergents, and has a temperature above 22°C, leptospiras may survive for several weeks. Human infections can occur either by direct contact with urine or tissue of an infected animal or indirectly through contaminated water, soil, or vegetation. The usual portals of entry in man are abraded skin, particularly about the feet, and exposed conjunctival, nasal, and oral mucous membranes. The previously held concept that organisms could penetrate intact skin has been questioned. While leptospiras have been isolated from ticks, these arthropods appear to be unimportant in transmission.

With the ubiquitous infection of animals, leptospirosis in man can occur in all age groups, at all seasons, and in both sexes. However, it is primarily a disease of teen-age children and young adults (54 percent of patients are between ages 10 and 39 years), occurs predominantly in males (80 percent), and develops most frequently in hot weather (in the United States two-thirds of infections occur from June to October). The wide spectrum of animal hosts results in both urban and rural human disease. Leptospirosis has been considered an occupational disease; however, improved methods of rat control and better standards of hygiene have reduced the incidence among occupational groups such as coal miners and sewermen. Currently less than 20 percent of patients have direct contact with animals; they are mostly farmers, abattoir workers, or veterinarians. In the majority of patients exposure is incidental; two-thirds of cases occur in children, students, or housewives. Swimming or partial immersion in contaminated water has been implicated in one-fifth of patients and has accounted for most of the recognized common source outbreaks.

PATHOLOGY In patients who have died with either hepatic involvement (Weil's syndrome), renal involvement, or both, the significant gross changes include hemorrhages and bile staining of tissues. The hemorrhages, which vary from petechial to ecchymotic, are widespread and are most prominent in skeletal muscle, kidneys, adrenals, liver, stomach, spleen, and lungs.

In skeletal muscle, focal, necrotic, and necrobiotic changes thought to be rather typical of leptospirosis occur. Biopsies early in the illness demonstrate swelling, vacuolation, and subsequently hyalinization. Leptospiral antigen has been demonstrated in these lesions by the fluorescent antibody technique. Healing ensues by the formation of new myofibrils with minimal fibrosis. The renal lesions in the acute phase involve predominantly the tubules and vary from simple dilatation of distal convoluted tubules to degeneration, necrosis, and basement membrane rupture. Interstitial edema and cellular infiltrates consisting of lymphocytes, neutrophilic leukocytes, histiocytes, and plasma cells are uniformly present. Glomerular lesions either are absent or consist of mesangial hyperplasia and focal foot process fusion which are interpreted as representing nonspecific changes associated with acute inflammation and protein filtration. Microscopic alterations in the liver are not diagnostic and correlate poorly with the degree of functional impairment. The changes include frequent double nuclei and cloudy swelling of parenchymal cells, disruption of liver cords, enlargement of Kupffer cells, and bile stasis in biliary canaliculi. The changes in the brain and meninges are also minimal and are not diagnostic. Thickening of the meninges with a polymorphonuclear leukocytic infiltration has been observed. Microscopic evidence of myocarditis including focal hemorrhages, interstitial edema, and focal infiltration with lymphocytes and plasma cells has been recorded. Pulmonary findings consist of a patchy, localized hemorrhagic pneumonitis. Special staining techniques utilizing silver impregnation methods have demonstrated organisms in the lumina of renal tubules but rarely in other organs.

CLINICAL MANIFESTATIONS General features The incubation period following immersion or accidental laboratory exposure has shown extremes of 2 to 20 days, the usual range being 7 to 13 days and the average, 10 days.

Leptospirosis is a typically biphasic illness. *During the leptospiremic* or *first phase* leptospiras are present in the blood and cerebrospinal fluid. The onset is typically abrupt, and initial symptoms include headache, which is usually frontal, less often retroorbital, but occasionally may be bitemporal or occipital. Severe muscle aching occurs in most patients, the muscles of the thighs and lumbar areas being most prominently involved and often accompanied by severe pain on palpation. The myalgia may be accompanied by extreme cutaneous hyperesthesia. Chills followed by rapidly rising temperature are prominent. Following the abrupt onset, the leptospiremic phase typically lasts 4 to 9 days. Features during this interval include recurrent chills, high spiking temperatures (usually 102°F or greater), headache, and continued severe myalgia. Anorexia, nausea, and vomiting are encountered in one-half or more of the patients. Pulmonary manifestations, usually either cough or chest pain, have varied in frequency of occurrence from less than 25 to 86 percent. Hemoptysis occurs but is rare. Examination during this phase reveals an acutely ill febrile patient, with a relative bradycardia and normal blood pressure, although European authors comment on early hypotension. Disturbances in sensorium may be encountered in up to 25 percent of patients. The most characteristic physical sign is conjunctival suffusion, which usually first appears on the third or fourth day but has been lacking in some patients. This may be associated with photophobia, but serous or purulent secretion is unusual. Less common findings may include pharyngeal injection, nuchal rigidity, cutaneous hemorrhages, and skin rashes that are usually macular, maculopapular, or urticarial and usually occur on the trunk. Uncommon findings are splenomegaly, hepatomegaly, lymphadenopathy, or jaundice. The first phase terminates after 4 to 9 days, usually with defervescence and improvement in symptoms. This coincides with the disappearance of leptospiras from the blood and cerebrospinal fluid.

The second phase has been characterized as the "immune" phase and correlates with the appearance of circulating IgM antibodies. The concentration of C3 in serum has remained within normal range during this phase. The clinical manifestations of this phase show greater variability than those during the first phase. After a relatively asymptomatic period of 1 to 3 days, the fever and earlier symptoms recur and meningismus may develop. The fever rarely exceeds 102°F and is usually of 1 to 3 days' duration. It is not uncommon for fever to be absent or quite transient. Even when symptoms or signs of meningeal irritation are absent, routine examination of cerebrospinal fluid after the seventh day has revealed pleocytosis in 80 to 90 percent of patients. Less common features include iridocyclitis, optic neuritis, and other nervous system manifestations including encephalitis, myelitis, and peripheral neuropathy.

Some clinicians recognize a third or convalescent phase. During this period and usually between the second and fourth weeks, both fever and aching may recur. The pathogenesis of this stage is poorly understood.

Leptospirosis during pregnancy may be associated with an increased risk of fetal loss.

Specific features WEIL'S SYNDROME Weil's syndrome, which may be due to serotypes other than icterohemorrhagiae, is defined as severe leptospirosis with jaundice, usually accompanied by azotemia, hemorrhages, anemia, disturbances in consciousness, and continued fever. There is uncertainty as to the pathogenesis of the syndrome, i.e., whether it represents direct toxic damage due to leptospiras or whether it is the consequence of immune response to leptospiral antigens. The consensus favors toxic damage.

The onset and first stage are identical with the less severe forms of leptospirosis. The distinctive features of Weil's syndrome appear from the third to the sixth days but do not reach their peak until well into the second stage. As in the other forms of leptospirosis, there is a tendency for the fever to lyse about the seventh day; however, it recurs and may then persist for several weeks. Either renal or hepatic manifestations may predominate. Hepatic disturbances include tenderness in the right upper quadrant and hepatic enlargement, both of which are common when jaundice is present. Abnormalities of liver function involve primarily tests of hepatocellular function such as the thymol turbidity. Serum glutamic oxaloacetic acid transaminase values are only moderately elevated.

Renal manifestations consist primarily of proteinuria, pyuria, hematuria, and azotemia. Dysuria is rare. Serious renal damage usually occurs in the form of acute tubular necrosis associated with oliguria. Hemorrhagic manifestations are most prevalent in this group of patients; epistaxis, hemoptysis, gastrointestinal bleeding, hemorrhage into the adrenal glands, hemorrhagic pneumonitis, and subarachnoid hemorrhage have all been described. These have been explained on the basis of capillary injury. In addition, in some patients hypoprothrombinemia and thrombocytopenia have been observed.

ASEPTIC MENINGITIS The syndrome of aseptic meningitis is characterized by cerebrospinal fluid pleocytosis, usually with tens to hundreds of leukocytes that are predominantly mononuclear cells, normal sugar, i.e., greater than 60 percent of the concomitant blood sugar, and protein of less than 100 mg per 100 ml. A leptospiral etiology has been ascribed to 6 percent of sporadic cases of aseptic meningitis. An observation causing difficulty in differential diagnosis has been the infrequent but definite demonstration of lowered cerebrospinal sugar levels. Xanthochromic cerebrospinal fluid has been observed in the presence of jaundice. Each of the serotypes of leptospiras that are pathogenic for man is probably capable of causing aseptic meningitis. The most prevalent serotypes have been canicola, icterohemorrhagiae, and pomona.

PRETIBIAL (FORT BRAGG) FEVER An illness was observed in the summer of 1942 that had an onset identical with that of the first phase of leptospirosis. The most distinctive feature was the development on about the fourth day of a rash, characterized by 2- to 5-cm, slightly raised, erythematous lesions that were usually symmetrically distributed over the pretibial areas. In contrast to other leptospiral syndromes, splenomegaly occurred in 95 percent of these patients. This outbreak was shown to be due to the autumnalis serogroup. Subsequently, pomona has been observed in association with rashes, which are usually truncal but which have also been pretibial.

MYOCARDITIS Cardiac arrhythmias including paroxysmal atrial fibrillation, atrial flutter, ventricular tachycardia, and premature ventricular contractions have been described but are usually of little clinical significance. However, on rare occasions definite cardiac dilatation with acute left ventricular failure has been observed. Associated manifestations have included jaundice, pulmonary infiltrates, arthritis, and skin rashes. The serogroups thus far incriminated have included icterohemorrhagiae and pomona.

LABORATORY FEATURES Leukocyte counts vary from leukopenic levels to mild elevations in the anicteric patients. In patients with jaundice, leukocytosis as high as 50,000 cells per mm^3 may be present. However, regardless of the total leukocyte count, neutrophilia of greater than 70 percent is almost always encountered during the first stage.

Hemolytic substances have been demonstrated in cultures of pathogenic leptospiras. In contrast to many hemolysins of bacterial origin, which are not hemolytic in vivo, the leptospiral hemolysins appear to be active in vivo. In patients with jaundice, anemia may be severe and is most characteristically due to intravascular hemolysis. Other mechanisms of anemia include azotemia and blood loss secondary to hemorrhage. Anemia due to leptospirosis is unusual in anicteric patients.

Rarely thrombocytopenia sufficient to be associated with bleeding is encountered. Additional hematologic abnormalities include almost uniform elevation of the erythrocyte sedimentation rate.

Urinalysis during the leptospiremic phase reveals mild proteinuria, casts, and an increase in cellular elements. In anicteric infections, these abnormalities rapidly disappear after the first week. Proteinuria and abnormalities in the urine sediment usually are not associated with elevations in blood urea nitrogen. Since the anicteric form of the disease often has gone undiagnosed, estimates of the frequency of azotemia and jaundice are probably high. Azotemia is usually associated with jaundice. The serum bilirubin levels may reach 40 mg per 100 ml; however, in two-thirds of patients the levels are less than 20 mg per 100 ml.

DIAGNOSIS Diagnosis is based upon culture of the organism or serologic proof of its existence. The most common initial diagnostic impressions in patients with leptospirosis are meningitis, hepatitis, nephritis, fever of undetermined origin (F.U.O.), and influenza. Leptospiras may be isolated quite readily during the first phase from blood and cerebrospinal fluid or during the second phase from the urine. Leptospiras may be excreted in the urine for up to 11 months after the onset of illness. Whole blood should be inoculated immediately into tubes containing semisolid medium, such as Fletcher's medium. If culture medium is not available, leptospiras reportedly will remain viable up to 11 days in blood to which anticoagulants, preferably sodium oxalate, have been added. Animal inoculation (preferably either suckling hamsters or guinea pigs) may be used and is of particular value if specimens, such as urine, are contaminated. Direct examination of blood or urine by dark-field methods has been employed; *however, this method so frequently results in failure or misdiagnosis that it should not be employed as the only diagnostic test.* Serologic methods are applicable during the second phase; antibodies appear from the sixth to the twelfth days of illness. Four serologic tests are available: macroscopic plate agglutination test (easy to perform but not very sensitive), hemolytic test (complex but requires only a single antigen), microscopic agglutination test (complex but most specific), and complement fixation tests. Serologic criteria for diagnosis include a fourfold or greater rise in titer during the course of illness. Crossagglutination reactions between various serotypes commonly occur so that the infecting serotype often cannot be determined with certainty without isolation of leptospiras.

PROGNOSIS The prognosis is dependent upon both the virulence of the organism and the general condition of the patient. Between 1965 and 1968, there were 10 deaths (4 percent) in the 277 patients reported in the United States. Age is the most significant host factor related to increased mortality. In a representative series, the mortality rose from 10 percent in men less than 50 years of age to 56 percent in those over 51 years of age. The virulence of the infecting leptospiras correlates best with the development of jaundice. In anicteric patients, mortality does not occur, but with the development of jaundice, mortality in various series has ranged from 15 to 40 percent. The long-term prognosis following the acute renal lesion of leptospirosis is good. Glomerular filtration rates have returned to normal; however, a few patients exhibit residual tubular dysfunction, e.g., a defect in renal concentrating capacity.

TREATMENT A variety of antimicrobial drugs, including penicillin, streptomycin, the tetracycline congeners, chloramphenicol, erythromycin, and oleandomycin, have been effective in vitro and in experimental leptospiral infections. Data concerning the efficacy of antibiotics in man are conflicting. If antimicrobial drugs have any beneficial effect, they must be administered within 4 days, and preferably within 2 days, of the onset of illness. Of the agents studied, penicillin G and various tetracyclines have been most effective. There is general agreement that antimicrobials administered after the fifth day of illness have no beneficial effect. There exists the clinical impression that early bedrest may minimize subsequent morbidity. Azotemia and jaundice require meticulous attention to fluid and electrolyte therapy.

REFERENCES

ALSTON JM, BROOM JC: *Leptospirosis in man and animals*, Edinburgh: E & S Livingstone, 1958

BUSCH LA: Leptospirosis 1965–1968. J Infect Dis 121:458, 1970

EDWARDS GA, DOMM M: Human leptospirosis. Medicine 39:117, 1970

HEATH CW JR, ALEXANDER AD: Leptospirosis in the United States: Analysis of 483 cases in man, 1949–1961. N Engl J Med 273:857, 915, 1965

KOCEN RS: Leptospirosis: A comparison of symptomatic and penicillin therapy. Br Med J 1:1181, 1962

MEYER HJ et al: Central nervous system syndromes of "viral" etiology: Study of 713 cases. Am J Med 29:334, 1960

Ooi BS et al: Human renal leptospirosis. Am J Trop Med Hyg 21:336, 1972

Tong MJ et al: Immunological response in leptospirosis. Am J Trop Med Hyg 20:625, 1971

Turner LH: Leptospirosis. Br Med J 1:231, 1969

World Health Organization: Current problems in leptospirosis research: Report of a WHO Expert Group. Tech. Rept. Ser. 380, Geneva, 1967

162
RELAPSING FEVER

JAMES J. PLORDE

DEFINITION Relapsing fever refers to a group of acute infectious diseases that are characterized clinically by cyclic periods of fever and apyrexia. They are caused by spirochetes of the genus *Borrelia* and occur in two epidemiologic varieties, louse-borne and tick-borne.

ETIOLOGY Borreliae are slender helical organisms which measure 10 to 20 μm in length. They have 3 to 10 irregular coils, move in a corkscrew fashion, and divide by longitudinal fission. Unlike other spirochetes, they readily stain with aniline dyes. *Borrelia recurrentis* is the causative agent of louse-borne relapsing fever. Many strains of *Borrelia* have been found in tick-borne disease, and they are generally known by their vector (e.g., *B. hermsi* is transmitted by *Ornithodoros hermsi*). The organisms have been cultured on artificial media.

EPIDEMIOLOGY Louse-borne relapsing fever is transmitted from man to man by the human body louse. Spirochetes that are ingested by the vector during feeding penetrate the gut wall and multiply in the body cavity. Infection of man occurs when the louse is crushed against an abrasion or wound. There is no known animal reservoir. The disease persists in endemic focuses in Ethiopia and probably South America and the Far East. Like typhus, it occurs in epidemic form during war and famine. Major epidemics involving millions of people occurred in Europe and Africa after both the First and Second World Wars. A third, much smaller outbreak, was seen at the time of the Korean conflict.

The tick vectors of relapsing fever belong to several species of the genus *Ornithodoros*. Like lice, they ingest the borreliae during feeding. The organisms may remain viable in the ticks for several years and can be passed transovarily to the next generation, making the tick a major reservoir of the disease. It is likely that rodents and other small animals act as vertebrate reservoirs in some locales. Man is involved when he comes into contact with an infected tick in its natural habitat. Transmission occurs if the tick's saliva or coxal fluid contaminates the feeding site. The tick-borne disease is found in localized areas throughout the world, and occurs sporadically in the western United States. In 1968 an outbreak of 11 cases occurred in a Boy Scout troop after a camping trip in northeastern Washington State.

PATHOGENESIS AND PATHOLOGY After inoculation into man, the borreliae reach the bloodstream producing spirochetemia and a febrile illness. After several days immobilizing and borrelicidal antibodies appear, the organisms are cleared from the peripheral blood, and the fever resolves. Following a latent period of approximately one week, during which the spirochetes are sequestered in the body, a new antigenic variant of the organism arises. There is reinvasion of the bloodstream causing a second paroxysm of fever and eventually, with the formation of specific antibodies, a second defervescence by crisis. The continued sequential production of new antigenic variants and specific antibodies results in the characteristic relapsing febrile course.

At autopsy follicular splenic abscesses, interstitial myocarditis, intracranial hemorrhage, and hepatitis with focal necrosis may be seen. Spontaneous splenic rupture and hemorrhagic gastrointestinal lesions have been noted occasionally. Borreliae have been recovered from the brain, heart, spleen, liver, and skin.

MANIFESTATIONS Clinical manifestations vary from outbreak to outbreak and between the tick- and louse-borne varieties of the disease. Generally, patients with louse-borne relapsing fever are more seriously ill but have fewer relapses than those with tick-borne illnesses. After an incubation period of 4 to 18 days, the disease begins abruptly with rigors, headache, anorexia, nausea, vomiting, photophobia, and pain in the muscles and joints. The temperature rises rapidly reaching 39 to 40°C, where it remains until the time of the crisis. The patient appears dull, apathetic, and is uncomplaining. He may have conjunctival suffusion and a macular or petechial rash. Cough, tachypnea, and rhonchi are common. A gallop rhythm and premature ventricular beats may occur in the louse-borne variety. Cardiac enlargement and heart failure are more uncommon. Upper abdominal tenderness is frequent. The liver and spleen are palpable and tender in 20 to 80 percent of cases, and may enlarge 6 to 10 cm during the course of fever. Jaundice secondary to hepatocellular destruction is present in 7 to 36 percent of patients. It is usually seen in louse-borne disease, occurs relatively late in the illness, and if severe, is often associated with purpura.

Bleeding is common in louse-borne relapsing fever. Petechiae develop in the skin and serous membranes, apparently as a result of damage to the capillary endothelium by clumps of spirochetes. Mild epistaxes and microscopic hematuria are present in many patients early in the disease. Later, with the development of liver disease, severe prolonged epistaxes and widespread ecchymoses occur. Infrequently, there may be massive gastrointestinal, urinary, or intracranial hemorrhage. Disseminated intravascular coagulation has been described. Neck stiffness, confusion, and transient focal neurologic signs may be seen even without intracranial bleeding. Patients with tick-borne disease with repeated relapses may develop iritis or iridocyclitis with permanent visual impairment. Pregnant women with relapsing fever often abort.

Three to six days after the onset of illness, the attack

ends in a crisis. Clinically this is characterized by a chill and an abrupt but transient rise in temperature, heart rate, respiratory rate, and arterial blood pressure. As the spirochetes disappear, the patient becomes flushed, diaphoretic, and hypotensive. Occasionally, cardiovascular collapse and death may occur at this point. More frequently the blood pressure and temperature return to normal over several hours, leaving the patient comfortable but exhausted. After 7 to 10 afebrile days, a relapse occurs which mimics the original illness. In the louse-borne disease there is usually only a single relapse, but in tick-borne relapsing fever there may be several, each somewhat briefer and milder than the preceding one.

LABORATORY FINDINGS A moderate anemia is common. The leukocyte count is usually normal or slightly elevated. During the crisis, a marked leukopenia occurs which may be followed by a transient rebound leukocytosis. A consumptive thrombocytopenia is seen in most cases, and the prothrombin and partial thromboplastin times may be prolonged. Fibrinogen levels are increased. Liver function tests reveal disturbed hepatocellular function. In severe cases, the total serum bilirubin level may reach 16 mg per 100 ml. Azotemia unrelated to extracellular fluid depletion is common among jaundiced patients. Electrocardiogram abnormalities including a prolonged Q-Tc interval and ST-T wave changes may occur. Reagin tests for syphilis are positive in 5 to 10 percent of cases. Patients with louse-borne relapsing fever frequently develop agglutinins to *Proteus* OXK antigens.

The definitive diagnosis is made by demonstrating borreliae in the peripheral blood during a febrile episode. This is most easily accomplished by examining thick and thin films stained with Wright's and Giemsa's stains. Repeated examinations may be required, especially in tick-borne disease. Spirochetes may also be seen in wet mounts with phase-contrast microscopy. When the direct methods are negative, blood may be injected into mice or rats and their blood examined frequently for the presence of borreliae.

DIFFERENTIAL DIAGNOSIS Many acute febrile illnesses including malaria, salmonellosis, typhus, dengue, rat-bite fever, and Weil's disease must be considered. Practically, there is seldom confusion if blood films are examined carefully.

TREATMENT The peripheral blood is quickly cleared of spirochetes by a variety of drugs including penicillin, tetracycline, and chloramphenicol. Treatment with these antimicrobial agents, however, is accompanied by a Jarisch-Herxheimer–like reaction which contributes to the morbidity, and perhaps mortality, of the disease. The reaction appears both clinically and pathophysiologically to be an exaggeration of the spontaneously occurring crisis. Its mechanism is unknown, but it may be related to release of endotoxin liberated during destruction of spirochetes. It is certainly related temporally to disappearance of spirochetes from the blood, and its severity appears to depend upon the speed with which they are removed.

In louse-borne relapsing fever, where the spirochetemia is often intense and the Jarisch-Herxheimer reaction severe, the drug of choice is a repository penicillin such as penicillin aluminum monostearate (PAM). Unlike tetracycline, this drug achieves a very gradual clearing of the spirochetes and a correspondingly mild reaction. The drug is given intramuscularly in a dose of 600,000 units. If the shorter-acting procaine penicillin is used, the dose should be repeated in 12 to 24 hr to prevent relapse. In epidemics, a single 0.5 to 1.0 g oral dose of chloramphenicol can be used with good results.

In tick-borne disease where penicillin is not effective in terminating relapses, tetracycline is most rapidly borrelicidal. This drug should be given in dose of 0.5 g four times a day for 5 to 10 days. The Jarisch-Herxheimer reaction tends to be less severe in this form of the disease.

PROGNOSIS When epidemics strike a nonimmune population, the high mortality rate due to the louse-borne disease shows the potential menace of this disease. Most patients, however, recover quickly and completely; relapses do not occur if antibiotic therapy is adequate. Adverse signs are deep jaundice, uncontrolled bleeding, and a grossly prolonged Q-Tc interval.

Typhus and enteric fever may occur simultaneously with louse-borne relapsing fever, and they probably contribute to the mortality rate, particularly during epidemics.

REFERENCES

Bryceson ADM et al: Louse-borne relapsing fever: A clinical and laboratory study of 62 cases in Ethiopia and a reconsideration of the literature. Q J Med 39:139, 1970

Felsenfeld O: *Borrelia: Strains, Vectors, Human and Animal Borreliasis*, St. Louis: Warren H. Green, 1971

Kelly R: Cultivation of *Borrelia hermsi.* Science 30:443, 1971

Southern PM Jr, Sanford JP: Relapsing fever. Medicine 48:129, 1969

163
RAT-BITE FEVER (SPIRILLUM MINUS INFECTION)

ROGER BULGER

DEFINITION The acute infection caused by *Spirillum minus* follows the bite of a rodent, usually a rat, and is characterized by a prolonged incubation period, followed by relapsing fever, recurrence of local inflammation at the puncture wound site with lymphangitis, and skin lesions. The term *rat-bite fever* refers to infection with either *S. minus* or *Streptobacillus moniliformis* (see Chap. 145).

ETIOLOGY AND EPIDEMIOLOGY *Spirillum minus* is a rigid spiral organism 2 to 5 μm in length, with polar flagella and from two to five spirals. It has never been cultivated on artificial media; animal inoculation is required for its isolation from patients. These organisms are readily recognized with dark-field microscopy by their quick, darting motility; they may be seen also in Wright-stained smears of blood from infected animals and patients.

Infection with *S. minus* in man almost always follows a rat bite, although examples of infection from the bite of a mouse are known. The disease is most common in people who live or work in rat-infested areas and in laboratory workers who handle rats. It is useful to remember that rats can bite babies or sleeping or inebriated people without their realizing it.

CLINICAL MANIFESTATIONS The incubation period is usually from 1 to 4 weeks and occasionally longer. If the original bite has healed completely, the patient may neglect to associate the bite with the illness. Usually, however, after initial healing, the wound site becomes swollen, and pain returns before or at the time of the onset of systemic symptoms of infection. Lymphangitis and swollen, tender regional lymph nodes are also usually found when chills and fever commence. During febrile periods, which usually last from 2 to 4 days, there may also be malaise, headache, photophobia, nausea, and vomiting. In more than half the cases, an asymmetric rash occurs, usually on the extremities; the rash is usually macular and the lesions may become confluent. Arthritis is uncommon. Afebrile periods are from 2 to 4 days in length, alternating with periods of fever, and the course is protracted, usually lasting from 4 to 8 weeks. Cases have been reported in which signs and symptoms persisted for more than a year; rarely, subacute bacterial endocarditis due to this organism has been reported.

LABORATORY FINDINGS The blood leukocyte count may be normal or may be as high as 20,000 per mm^3. The organism cannot be cultured on artificial media, but can be seen in the blood of patients by dark-field microscopy or on Wright-stained smears. When this disease is suspected, the patient's blood must be inoculated introperi-

toneally in mice or guinea pigs; 5 to 15 days later, *S. minus* will be found in the animal's blood or peritoneal fluid. In about half the patients, there are biologic false positive serologic tests for syphilis.

DIFFERENTIAL DIAGNOSIS It is important to inquire about rat bite in all patients with a relapsing type of fever. In patients with a history of rat bite, the principal problem is in differentiating between *S. minus* and *Strep. moniliformis* infections. This cannot be done with certainty on clinical grounds (Chap. 145), but a prolonged incubation period, relapsing instead of sustained fever, and few or no manifestations of arthritis suggest a diagnosis of *S. minus* infection. Laboratory tests should be made for both organisms. The significance of a previous rat bite may not be appreciated in cases with a long incubation period, and the disease may be confused with other infections characterized by relapsing fever, such as malaria, meningococcemia, and *Borrelia recurrentis* infection.

TREATMENT AND PROGNOSIS Penicillin, in dosage of 600,000 units twice a day intramuscularly, is the drug of choice. In patients allergic to penicillin, tetracycline in dosage of 2 g a day for 7 days may be used.

Patients treated with penicillin become afebrile within 24 to 72 hr, and complete recovery is the rule. Prior to the availability of effective antibiotics, fatality was estimated to occur in 2 to 10 percent of those with clinical infection.

REFERENCES
(See also Chap. 145)

COLE JS et al: Rat-bite fever. Ann Intern Med 71:979, 1969

section 11 | Diseases caused by fungi

164
INTRODUCTION

ABRAHAM I. BRAUDE

Except for their etiology, fungous infections differ little from bacterial infections. The close relationship between bacteria and fungi is apparent from transitional forms connecting the two classes, and from the similarity of the pathologic changes and clinical manifestations induced by them.

The intermediate, or transitional, forms are represented by the *Actinomycetes.* These possess the branched mycelium of fungi but divide into gram-positive bacillary or coccoid forms. The acid-fast property of one species, *Nocardia asteroides,* indicates a relationship to the tubercle bacillus. The *Actinomycetes* also differ from fungi in their susceptibility to phages, their unorganized nuclei, and their sensitivity to antibiotics, which attack bacteria, but not to the antifungal polyene antibiotic amphotericin B. The *Actinomycetes* do not possess the sterols which complex with polyene antibiotics and injure the cell membranes of fungi. Finally, actinomyces, like bacteria but unlike fungi, contain neither chitin nor cellulose in their cell walls. *Although actinomycosis and nocardiosis are placed among the fungous diseases in this book, the causative agents are bacteria.*

An important characteristic of pathogenic fungi is dimorphism, growth in two distinct forms under different environmental conditions. The fungi responsible for blastomycosis, sporotrichosis, and histoplasmosis assume unicellular "yeast" forms in infected tissues but grow as mycelia and produce asexual spores on Sabouraud's agar. The reverse is true for the fungus causing moniliasis. Another type of dimorphism is found in coccidioidomycosis. The organism responsible for this infection is multicellular in vivo and in vitro, but its form differs under the two conditions. In tissues it is a sac filled with spores, but on agar it grows as a segmented mycelium. *Cryptococcus neoformans* is one pathogenic fungus that fails to change form when the environment varies.

Mycotic diseases are not transmitted from one person to another. Many fungous infections are acquired by inhalation of spores growing freely in nature. These spores may be rectangular unicellular mycelial fragments known as *chlamydospores,* or spherical bodies borne on thin mycelial stalks and called *conidia.* Some infections, such as sporotrichosis, result from inoculation of spores directly into the skin.

A few fungous diseases are endogenous in origin. *Actinomyces israeli* and *Candida albicans* are normal residents of the intestine and mouth. When resistance is lowered, endogenous infection with either agent may develop. Actinomycosis often follows tooth extraction, and overgrowth of normal saprophytic bacteria by *C. albicans* in the course of antibiotic therapy can lead to moniliasis.

The mechanisms whereby fungi produce disease are obscure. *Cryptococcus neoformans* has a polysaccharide capsule similar to that of the pneumococcus which seems to protect the yeast from phagocytosis. This capsular material also produces mechanical injury in the nervous system. It is possible that the thick walls of other fungi such as *Blastomyces dermatitidis* and *Coccidioides immitis* also protect against leukocytes. Some fungi are ingested by phagocytes but seem to flourish within them. In histoplasmosis, for example, the parasites are found in enormous numbers within reticuloendothelial cells. The endothelium of small vessels can become so packed with histoplasma organisms that blood flow is compromised.

Another possible factor in the pathogenesis of these infections is hypersensitivity. In most fungous diseases there is marked local or even systemic reactivity to intradermal injection of the causative organism. In coccidioidomycosis this type of reaction is closely associated with the development of erythema nodosum and pleural effusions. In allergic pulmonary aspergillosis, the disease results from both reaginic and precipitating antibodies against aspergillus antigens. The occurrence of necrosis at the site of injection of fungous antigens suggests that hypersensitivity may be responsible for necrosis of infected tissues. In other patients, however, widespread destruction of tissue may occur despite absence of dermal sensitivity.

Despite the differences in structure and life cycle of fungi and bacteria, both elicit similar pathologic changes and clinical manifestations. For this reason, specific diagnosis can seldom be made without demonstration of the causative organism. Fortunately, most pathogenic fungi are easily seen in infected tissues or exudates. In a few circumstances, however, it is necessary to rely upon epidemiologic and immunologic methods for diagnosis.

The following chapters deal only with those infections in which fungi penetrate beneath the skin and mucous membranes to involve the underlying tissues and viscera.

165 ACTINOMYCOSIS

ABRAHAM I. BRAUDE

DEFINITION Actinomycosis is a noncontagious infection produced by an anaerobic organism normally resident in the mouth. The disease is characterized by chronic inflammatory induration and sinus formation.

ETIOLOGY The causative agent is a branching gram-positive filamentous organism. Two separate pathogenic anaerobic species of the genus *Actinomyces* have been recognized: *Actinomyces bovis* is responsible for actinomycosis in cattle, and *A. israeli,* for human actinomycosis.

Actinomyces israeli and *A. bovis* differ from other actinomyces in their intolerance of free oxygen and failure to grow on Sabouraud's medium. On blood agar, colonies require 4 to 6 days of anaerobic incubation at 37°C to reach a size of 1 to 2 mm. Although most strains require anaerobic conditions for isolation, some can be subcultured aerobically in 10 to 20 percent carbon dioxide. *Actinomyces israeli* has never been found outside man or animal, and case-to-case transmission is unknown.

PATHOGENESIS The oxidation-reduction potential of normal tissues is probably too high for multiplication of *A. israeli,* but devitalized tissues allow it to reproduce and spread. The frequency of actinomycosis of the face and neck may be explained by the greater population of *A. israeli* on teeth, in carious teeth, and in tonsillar crypts and by trauma from eating, dental procedures, or infection with oral bacteria. Anaerobic conditions also prevail in atelectatic areas of the lung after aspiration of *A. israeli* so that pulmonary actinomycosis can develop. It is also possible that pulmonary actinomycosis may arise hematogenously from an infected focus in the mouth. Mediastinal actinomycosis probably spreads from the esophagus into the superior or posterior mediastinum, quickly involving the pleura to produce early pleural effusion or empyema, and then tends to attack the adjacent ribs and vertebral bodies. Eventually mediastinal actinomycosis produces abscesses which point in the paravertebral region. Ileocecal actinomycosis is the most common intestinal form, occurring after appendiceal rupture and the escape of actinomyces to form an inflammatory mass in the right iliac fossa. The liver is the solid abdominal viscus most frequently attacked by actinomycosis.

From foci in the jaw, lung, or intestine, actinomycosis may spread by contiguity or through the bloodstream to the liver, spine, brain, kidneys, genitalia, spleen, and subcutaneous tissues. Lymphatic spread is rare.

The inflammatory reaction to *A. israeli* is characterized by three features: (1) chronic suppuration, (2) extensive necrosis, and (3) intense fibrosis. The so-called "sulfur granules" in the inflammatory lesion are composed of intertwined mycelial filaments.

CLINICAL MANIFESTATIONS The essential feature of actinomycosis is a painful, indurated swelling. This lesion may appear over the jaw a week or more after such trauma as tooth extraction or compound fracture of the mandible. As it increases in size, points of suppuration, the openings of fistulas, appear on the bluish-red surface of the edematous skin. Trismus is prominent early. Cervical lymphadenopathy is rare.

The lower lobes of the lung are frequently affected; then the disease suddenly becomes evident when the pleura and chest wall are involved by direct extension from the lung. Until then the patient may notice only fever, cough, and expectoration. Physical examination at this time reveals a diffuse, tender, indurated swelling of the chest wall with pulmonary consolidation and empyema.

Abdominal actinomycosis is often mistaken for appendicitis, carcinoma of the cecum, tuberculosis, or amebiasis. Patients with abdominal actinomycosis are subjected to surgery for drainage of a supposed appendiceal abscess, and the true nature of the disease is recognized only when an indurated draining sinus stubbornly refuses to heal. Actinomycosis may also be mistaken for tumor of the reproductive organs in women or for tuberculous psoas abscess. Peritonitis is rare.

In the rare case of hematogenous disseminated actinomycosis, lesions appear in all parts of the body. Painful indurated nodules under the skin of the legs, arms, back, and scalp are prominent, and nonsuppurative effusions of the pleura or pericardium develop.

DIAGNOSIS The disease is easily recognized by detecting *A. israeli* in pus obtained from sinuses, empyema fluid, or abscess cavities. Interpreting actinomyces in sputum is difficult because the organisms are normal inhabitants of the mouth. Sulfur granules vary in size from several microns to 3 mm in diameter. Large granules are found if a thorough search is made by diluting the pus with saline solution and filtering through gauze. They are white, yellow, or brown and stand out sharply against the background of blood-tinged pus. Gram-positive filaments or bacilli which fail to grow aerobically are key findings. Granules of other organisms (staphylococci, nocardias, monosporia), fragments of caseous material, and clumps of pus cells or fibrin may be confused with actinomycotic granules. Sabouraud's medium will not support its growth. Cultural isolation of *A. israeli* is not difficult if anaerobic methods are used. A small microaerophilic gram-negative bacillus, *Actinobacillus actinomycetemcomitans,* is often associated with *A. israeli* in actinomycosis. Anaerobic streptococci, *Bacteroides,* and other anaerobes are also present frequently. Hence *actinomycosis is characteristically a mixed anaerobic infection.*

Biopsy may establish the diagnosis if the actinomycotic colony ("ray fungus") is observed microscopically. Demonstration of the organism may be difficult, requiring careful search of many sections.

Intradermal or serologic tests with *A. israeli* or its fractions are of no diagnostic aid. Radiologic examination may suggest actinomycosis if consolidation of the lungs and periosteal proliferation of the ribs are found, because this combination rarely occurs in other conditions. The appearance of the spine in lateral views may be almost pathognomonic, because the areas of absorption and newly formed bone give a picture of a coarse sieve not seen in any other vertebral disease.

TREATMENT Penicillin and the tetracycline antibiotics are so effective that the disease is disappearing through the wide use of these drugs in conditions that would otherwise evolve into actinomycosis. When either is administered in large doses over long periods of time, remarkable improvement may be expected even when the purulent foci are inaccessible to surgical drainage. Many reports indicate that the tetracycline drugs (chlortetracycline, oxytetracycline, tetracycline) are superior to penicillin. When the tetracyclines are given in doses of 500 mg every 6 hr, there is a reduction in pain and swelling within a few days as well as gain in strength, increase in weight, and prompt defervescence. Treatment should be continued for several weeks after the patient appears cured. Because penicillin is no more effective than the tetracyclines and because it requires repeated intramuscular or intravenous injection of large doses for long periods of time, it should be reserved for patients who cannot tolerate tetracycline drugs. The optimum dose of penicillin is not known, but at least 4 million units daily should be given intramuscularly.

Surgical drainage is a valuable adjunct to chemotherapy and may occasionally lead to spontaneous cure. Older treatments such as iodides, irradiation, or the sulfonamides have no place in the treatment of actinomycosis, and amphotericin B is of no value.

REFERENCES

Cope VZ: *Actinomycosis,* London: Oxford, 1938

Flynn MW, Felson B: The roentgen manifestations of thoracic actinomycosis. Am J Roentgenol 110:707, 1970

Garrod LP: Actinomycosis of the lung: Etiology, diagnosis, and chemotherapy. Tubercle 33:258, 1952

McVay LV Jr, Sprunt DH: A long-term evaluation of aureomycin in the treatment of actinomycosis. Ann Intern Med 38:995, 1953

Nichols DR, Herrell WE: Penicillin in the treatment of actinomycosis. J Lab Clin Med 33:521, 1948

166 CRYPTOCOCCOSIS

ABRAHAM I. BRAUDE

DEFINITION Cryptococcosis is a pulmonary infection caused by *Cryptococcus neoformans,* an encapsulated yeast with a special predilection for the central nervous system. It occurs with increased frequency in patients with leukemia or lymphoma.

ETIOLOGY Members of the genus *Cryptococcus,* to which *C. neoformans* belongs, form neither mycelia nor spores and reproduce entirely by budding. The cells of *C. neoformans* are spherical, measure 5 to 15 μm in diameter, retain the Gram stain, and are surrounded by a capsule which may have a diameter three times that of the cell. The capsular material contains a polysaccharide which is responsible for the slimy appearance of the yeast in culture, for the myxomatous character of cryptococcal lesions, and for the serologic type. Of the four serotypes, type A is by far the commonest recovered from human infections, except in California where the majority appear to be types B and C.

The organisms grow readily on various media at room temperature and at 37°C. On Sabouraud's glucose agar, visible growth appears within a few days at 37°C and gradually becomes brownish and slimy. Unlike other pathogenic yeastlike fungi, cryptococci never form mycelia. Most cells of *C. neoformans* are killed in 24 hr at temperatures of 40.6°C or higher.

PATHOGENESIS AND PATHOLOGY Cryptococci resembling *C. neoformans* have been isolated from soil, the surface of fruit, and the skin and intestinal tract of normal man. The most constant sources of virulent strains, however, are pigeon droppings. These cryptococci are unencapsulated but can rapidly develop capsules upon contact with human beings. Hence it is possible for infections to be of either endogenous or exogenous origin. Although neurologic disturbances overshadow others, there is good evidence that infection is usually established in the lung and other viscera before dissemination to the brain and the meninges occurs. Often the pulmonary foci give rise to no clinical findings, although they can be detected if a careful search is made postmortem.

The cryptococcus does not evoke the active inflammatory response observed with other fungi or bacteria. The cellular reaction is very slow to develop and is seldom intense. The cryptococcus seems to meet little resistance and frequently proliferates so freely that macroscopic masses of gelatinous yeasts fill the lesions. Older lesions occasionally show granulomatous reactions. The small number of cryptococci observed within granulomas suggests that mononuclear cells can destroy the organism. This may account in part for the fact that lymphomatous diseases involving the mononuclear cells lower resistance to cryptococcal infection. At other times, however, many cryptococci are present within mononuclear and giant cells. It is unusual to see necrosis in cryptococcosis.

Granulomas or gelatinous cryptococcal masses may appear in the nervous system, lungs, bones, or skin. In the nervous system, lesions usually develop in the meninges at the base of the brain with involvement of the brainstem, cranial nerves, and cerebellum. Large masses of yeast in the subarachnoid space may extend diffusely along perivascular spaces into the brain to produce cystic nodules. Because the fungal masses shrink after fixation of the brain in formalin, cystlike spaces remain. In the lung, scattered miliary nodules, diffuse pneumonic infiltrations, or solitary masses easily mistaken for pulmonary neoplasms may occur. Calcification or hilar lymphadenopathy is extremely rare. These characteristics of the cryptococcal pulmonary lesions are helpful in distinguishing the disease from tuberculosis, sarcoidosis, and other mycoses. In contrast to cryptococcal meningoencephalitis, serious predisposing diseases accompany pulmonary cryptococcosis in only 10 percent of patients.

CLINICAL MANIFESTATIONS Most patients with cryptococcal infection consult a physician only after the onset of neurologic manifestations. Complaints of severe headache, diplopia, dizziness, ataxia, vomiting, tinnitus, memory disturbances, or Jacksonian convulsions are common. Fever is usually absent. Many patients die within a few months, but some have lived for many years as the disease undergoes remissions and relapses.

When pulmonary infection is present in the absence of meningoencephalitis, the patient is generally free of constitutional symptoms. The disease is detected when roentgenographic examination of the chest shows a dense, usually solitary infiltration of the lower portions of the lung. Cough may be a prominent feature of diffuse cryptococcal pneumonia. Cavities are not rare.

Involvement of bones in the absence of disseminated disease is rare, and cryptococcosis of joints is almost always secondary to adjacent osseous lesions.

Disseminated infection may also produce multiple nodules or papules in the skin. These range from a few millimeters in diameter to masses resembling strawberries in size and color.

The possibility of underlying Hodgkin's disease, lymphosarcoma, leukemia, or diabetes should be considered in every patient with cryptococcosis.

DIAGNOSIS Cryptococcal meningitis must be distinguished from other diseases which present as aseptic meningitis, including brain abscess, tuberculous meningitis, coccidioidal meningitis, and carcinomatous meningitis. In each of these, the spinal fluid is sterile by ordinary cultural methods and may contain from a few to several hundred mononuclear cells, increased protein, and reduced glucose. Because *C. neoformans* is recovered with much greater ease than the etiologic agents of the other diseases, culture of the spinal fluid is the decisive procedure in differential diagnosis. The cryptococcus is isolated on Sabouraud's agar at room temperature and usually grows after 1 to 2 weeks. In tuberculous and coccidioidal meningitis positive cultures are much less common, and in uncomplicated brain abscess the spinal fluid is sterile. Cryptococcal cells may also be found by direct microscopic examination of sediment from centrifuged spinal fluid. Mixing a drop of sediment with India ink facilitates the recognition of the mucinous capsule. The organism can be cultured from the blood and urine in 25 to 35 percent of patients with cryptococcal meningitis. Specimens obtained via bronchoscopy or transbronchial brush biopsy may contain cryptococci in pulmonary cryptococcosis when sputum cultures are negative. Biopsy is essential for diagnosis in most cases of pulmonary infection. In tissue, intracellular forms with small capsules may resemble *Histoplasma capsulatum* but can be differentiated by mucicarmine, which stains the capsular mucopolysaccharide peculiar to *C. neoformans*. Biopsied material should also be inoculated onto Sabouraud's glucose agar. In many cases, the patients' serums give positive tests for either cryptococcal antigen or antibody. Circulating antigens appear to indicate continuing disease, while antibodies are found only after treatment, when the cryptococcus and its antigens are disappearing from the body fluids.

TREATMENT All forms of cryptococcosis usually improve after intravenous infusions of 0.75 to 1 mg per kg amphotericin B daily. These maximum daily doses are reached only after gradual increments of the initial dose of 1 mg. When maintenance levels are reached, the drug should be given every other day. Patients without meningoencephalitis can be cured with total doses of less than 1.5 gm, but 3.0 gm is probably required for infections of the nervous system. If relapse occurs after intravenous treatment, amphotericin B may be dissolved in the spinal fluid and 0.5 mg injected intrathecally on alternate days in conjunction with intravenous administration. Strict precautions must be taken during intrathecal injection to avoid bacterial contamination and drug overdosage. One milligram amphotericin B intrathecally may cause fever, temporary paralysis of the bladder and legs, and arachnoiditis. The chief dangers of intravenous amphotericin B are anemia, hypokalemia, and renal damage characterized by renal tubular acidosis. The anemia frequently occurs after prolonged treatment and is normocytic, normochromic, and reversible. The hypokalemia develops with or without impaired renal function and requires prophylactic potassium supplements. Disturbances in renal function should be expected. Azotemia, impaired urine concentration, and microscopic hematuria with granular casts are the main findings but are reversible if caught in time. Treatment should be discontinued if the blood urea nitrogen exceeds 40 mg per 100 ml and resumed when it approaches normal levels. Serious and permanent renal damage with nephrocalcinosis has occurred in patients given a total dosage greater than 5 g. In cryptococcal meningitis, sterility of the spinal fluid is probably the best endpoint of successful treatment. Dead cryptococci may be visible for years after the disease is cured and do not require more treatment.

Flucytosine (5-fluorocytosine) is also successful in some patients with cryptococcal infections. It is given orally in doses of 150 mg per kilogram per day, with little toxicity and a success rate of about 50 percent in cryptococcal meningitis. Treatment failures result from the development of drug resistance during treatment, a phenomenon not seen with amphotericin B.

Diamox in doses of 500 mg twice daily is valuable for lowering the cerebrospinal fluid pressure during and after antifungal therapy.

REFERENCES

LITTMAN ML, WALTER JE: Cryptococcosis: Current status. Am J Med 45:922, 1968

UTZ JP: Flucytosine. N Engl J Med 286:777, 1972

WALTER JE, JONES RD: Serodiagnosis of clinical cryptococcosis. Am Rev Resp Dis 97:275, 1968

167 BLASTOMYCOSIS

ABRAHAM I. BRAUDE

DEFINITION Blastomycosis is a fungous infection of the skin and viscera, caused by *Blastomyces dermatitidis* in North America and by *Paracoccidioides brasiliensis* in South America. South American blastomycosis is also termed paracoccidioidomycosis.

ETIOLOGY In infected tissues *B. dermatitidis* has the appearance of a yeast, forming single buds from 3 to 24 μm in diameter. Two features aid in recognition: (1) its thick wall, spoken of as "double-contoured," because the inner and outer margins can be seen, and (2) the wide opening between parent cell and bud at the base of attachment.

In culture, *B. dermatitidis* is dimorphic and appears as the wrinkled, waxy yeast form on blood agar incubated at 37°C, or as a mold with branching hyphae on Sabouraud's agar at room temperature. On microscopic examination the cultured yeast may be found to be identical with that in the infected lesions or may have abortive mycelia. The mycelia give rise to oval or pear-shaped exogenous spores.

Multiple buds on the yeastlike cell of *P. brasiliensis* distinguish it morphologically from *B. dermatitidis.* The tiny multiple buds have the appearance of a crown of small beads attached to the cell wall. The fungus reproduces by budding both in tissues and when cultured at 37°C. At room temperature it produces mycelia but not true spores.

PATHOGENESIS AND PATHOLOGY The skin has been proposed as a portal of entry in North American blastomycosis because cutaneous lesions are prominent and because infections may follow injury to the skin. The lung is also a likely portal, but the fungus has seldom been cultured from the soil and soon disappears from natural soils into which it is introduced.

The fungus of the South American blastomycosis is probably harbored in the soil of the warm, wet forest areas of Colombia, Venezuela, and Brazil. The portal of entry is debatable. Some feel that man is infected by inhalation, with the primary lesion being in the lung and with the ulcerative lesions appearing in the oral cavity, nasopharynx, and larynx as a consequence of disseminated disease. Alternatively, the fungus may penetrate the buccal, pharyngeal, or nasal mucosa and then be carried to the lymph glands, lungs, and other viscera via the lymph channels or the bloodstream.

Characteristic pathologic features are found in the lung and skin in both North and South American forms. Pulmonary lesions vary in size from miliary granulomatous nodules to confluent areas of pneumonia involving an entire lobe with a combination of suppuration and epithelioid-cell granulomatous reactions. The granulomas may undergo caseation and fibrosis but rarely, if ever, calcification. Differentiation from tuberculosis is facilitated by finding the yeast in giant cells or other phagocytes.

In the skin, microabscesses lie just beneath the epidermis and are surrounded by a granulomatous reaction. The epidermis itself often becomes so hyperplastic that it resembles an epithelioma.

In both North and South American varieties, the infection may spread to the lymph nodes, brain, bones, urogenital tract, liver, spleen, and adrenals.

CLINICAL MANIFESTATIONS In the typical case of systemic North American blastomycosis the onset is insidious. The patient may seek medical attention because of a persistent "chest cold," low-grade fever, weight loss, or progressive disability. Physical examination and a roentgenogram of the chest disclose evidence of pneumonia, which may involve any segment or lobe of the lung. Cavitation is frequent, and mediastinal lymph nodes may be prominent. Hemoptysis, purulent sputum, chest pain, and dyspnea appear as the disease progresses. Although the pulmonary infection may subside spontaneously, extrapulmonary lesions of the skin, bones, joints, and viscera eventually call attention to dissemination. These metastatic suppurative lesions are accompanied by an increase in fever, sweats, chills, and weakness. Death in the untreated infection sometimes occurs in less than 6 months, but most patients live for a year or two. The overall mortality rate in systemic blastomycosis is said to be 92 percent in patients whose cases have been followed for 2 years or longer without specific therapy.

Primary infection of the skin by *B. dermatitidis* (Gilchrist's disease) first appears on unclothed areas such as the hands, face, or forearm but not the scalp, palms, or soles. The infection begins as a firm nodule surrounded by similar lesions which tend to coalesce. Suppuration in the center of the nodule is followed by partial healing and fibrosis as extension occurs peripherally. The hyperplastic epithelium gives these lesions a hard, raised, wartlike margin. When fully developed, blastomycosis of the skin presents the appearance of one or more ragged ulcers with partially healed centers and thick raised margins. The primary cutaneous infection may be confined to the skin for months or years.

South American blastomycosis may be present in a *pulmonary* or *disseminated* form. Symptoms of the pulmonary form include productive cough, hemoptysis, dyspnea, fever, fatigue, malaise, and weight loss. Dissemination is characterized by painful ulcers of the mouth and nose, hoarseness, dysphagia, cervical lymphadenopathy which may be massive and which is occasionally accompanied by sinus formation, inability to eat, abdominal pain, and cachexia. The disease may spread to viscera, bones, and central nervous system, and, if left untreated, is fatal after a few months or several years.

DIAGNOSIS Pulmonary blastomycosis closely resembles tuberculosis, carcinoma of the lung, aspiration pneumonitis, and other fungous infections, including coccidioidomycosis, actinomycosis, nocardiosis, and histoplasmosis. Differentiation must be based on the recovery of the etiologic agent, because neither clinical nor epidemiologic features are specific. Most cases of North American blastomycosis are found in the Southeastern United States and in the Mississippi River Valley, but the disease occurs throughout the United States and Canada.

It is usually possible to find either *B. dermatitidis* or *P. brasiliensis* by microscopic examination of biopsied material, sputum, or pus. The yeastlike forms can be observed if a drop of purulent material is first mixed on a slide with a drop of 10% potassium hydroxide and kept at room temperature for 30 min. The multiple buds covering the entire surface of *P. brasiliensis* are connected by a narrow neck to the parent cell, while buds of *B. dermatitidis* are connected by a wide communication. *Blastomyces dermatitidis* is isolated by culturing pus on Sabouraud's agar at room temperature and on blood agar at 37°C. *Paracoccidioides brasiliensis* can also be isolated on blood agar at 37°C but grows so slowly that more than a month may elapse before colonies appear.

The diagnostic value of the skin test for blastomycosis is limited. The complement fixation test in both North and South American blastomycosis is positive in high titer with serums of patients who have systemic infections. The results of intradermal and serologic tests may be of prognostic value. Patients with marked dermal hypersensitivity and low serum titers of complement-fixing antibody are said to have a better prognosis in North American blastomycosis than those with negative skin tests and high complement fixation titers.

TREATMENT Amphotericin B is curative in both North and South American blastomycosis. North American blastomycosis also responds, but less favorably, to 2-hydroxystilbamidine, while South American blastomycosis is resistant to it. Either drug is given daily or every other day by slow intravenous drip in increasing doses. The maximum adult daily dose of amphotericin B is 75 mg, and that of 2-hydroxystilbamidine is 250 mg. Complete arrest of North American blastomycosis has been observed after a total of 1 g amphotericin B; 4 to 10 g of 2-hydroxystilbamidine may be required. Anesthesia over the distribution of the trigeminal nerve is the main untoward reaction from 2-hydroxystilbamidine; it persists after treatment. Surgical excision of pulmonary cavities or destroyed tissues is sometimes necessary in addition to chemotherapy.

In South American blastomycosis the sulfonamide drugs produce dramatic clinical remissions of most forms of the disease, but relapses invariably occur unless the patient is maintained on continuous therapy. Sulfadiazine in doses of 4 to 6 g daily or sulfisoxazole in dosage of 6 to 8 g per day has been successful in arresting the disease. In severe cases both amphotericin and sulfonamides should be used.

REFERENCES

Chick EW: Blastomycosis—the enigma of systemic mycoses. Chest 60:2, 1971

Lontero AT, Ramos CD: Paracoccidioidomycosis. Am J Med 52:771, 1972

Restrepo A et al: Paracoccidioidomycosis (South American blastomycosis). Am J Trop Med Hyg 19:68, 1970

Witorsch P, Utz JP: North American blastomycosis: A study of 40 patients. Medicine 47:169, 1968

168 COCCIDIOIDOMYCOSIS

ABRAHAM I. BRAUDE

DEFINITION Coccidioidomycosis is an infection acquired by inhalation of *Coccidioides immitis*, a fungus existing only in the mycelial phase in nature and converted to a spherule in tissues. Although most infections are mild or inapparent, *C. immitis* may produce a fatal disseminated disease with destructive lesions in the lungs, lymph nodes, spleen, liver, bones, kidneys, and brain.

ETIOLOGY *Coccidioides immitis* grows readily at room temperature or at 35°C and produces white, cottony mycelia. As the culture ages, the segmented mycelium breaks up into thick-coated rectangular *arthrospores*, 2 × 4 μm in size. These arthrospores can survive in stored cultures and are highly infectious for laboratory personnel. The mycelium and its spores are pathogenic for various laboratory animals. The mycelial form is converted to a thick-walled spherule filled with endospores in animal tissues and under special cultural conditions.

PATHOGENESIS AND PATHOLOGY Coccidioidomycosis is acquired by inhalation of *chlamydospores* in endemic areas in the semiarid regions of the Southwestern United States and the Chaco district of Argentina. The majority of infections occur during the dry seasons, particularly after exposure to dust storms. The fungus grows in the soil in rainy weather and becomes disseminated in dust during dry weather. *Coccidioides immitis* is isolated from soil and from desert rodents.

The inhaled spores are carried to the terminal bronchioles and alveoli, where the first reaction is an outpouring of polymorphonuclear leukocytes, fluid, and a few mononuclear cells. In most cases, the organism is probably killed or arrested. In others, the organisms proliferate and elicit an inflammatory response which appears to depend on their multiplication. Rapid multiplication is manifested by frequent discharge of endospores from spherules and an exudate rich in polymorphonuclear leukocytes. The phase of slow multiplication, with infrequent rupture of spherules, produces a granulomatous reaction in which epithelioid cells and giant cells predominate. Although polymorphonuclear leukocytes congregate about the point of rupture of a spherule and invade the broken capsule, phagocytosis by these cells is unsuccessful. As the released endospores develop into spherules, the neutrophilic reaction gives way to proliferating mononuclear cells which ingest the fungus.

Either phase of this inflammatory cycle may predominate, or a mixture of the two may be found. Rapidly progressive infections produce large areas of confluent suppurative pneumonia and necrosis. In contrast, granulomatous lesions contain exudates composed almost exclusively of mononuclear cells and giant cells which fill alveoli but leave their walls intact. Both reactions are accompanied by involvement of the overlying pleura and of the hilar and mediastinal lymph nodes. Ultimately the bronchopneumonia in most patients resolves or heals by fibrosis; in others, the lesions are permanently arrested but persist as cavities or solid nodules.

Recovery is accompanied by the development of hypersensitivity to the fungus. This hypersensitivity is apparently responsible for at least two special manifestations: (1) *erythema nodosum*, a sterile, focal, nodular granulomatous reaction usually limited to the skin of the lower extremities and characterized by extravasation of red cells into the lesion; (2) *pleural effusion*. It is believed that rupture of a pleural granuloma discharges antigenic material onto the sensitized pleural membranes.

In patients who do not develop dermal hypersensitivity, the infection spreads to lymph nodes, spleen, bones, liver, kidney, meninges, skin, adrenals, and pericardium. In the meninges, the reaction may take two forms: (1) the granulomatous reaction is commoner and produces a firm plastic lesion which encloses the brainstem and other structures in a rigid mass of tissue; (2) the suppurative reaction results in outpouring of polymorphonuclear leukocytes with little granulomatous change. In either type, but especially in the granulomatous, involvement of the brainstem may lead to severe hydrocephalus.

CLINICAL MANIFESTATIONS The infection may be either benign or disseminated. The benign infection, so-called "desert fever," is self-limited, and as many as 50 percent of benign infections are asymptomatic. The remainder have influenza-like symptoms. After an incubation period of 1 to 3 weeks, the patient has fever, chills, fatigue, headache, severe arthralgia, a maculopapular pruritic eruption, erythema nodosum, and symptoms of respiratory infection. The most frequent complaint is poorly localized chest pain, aggravated by breathing or coughing. A nonproductive cough is common, but hemoptysis is infrequent. Although hydrothorax may be massive and require repeated thoracenteses, it eventually resorbs without further difficulty.

Despite the paucity of signs in the chest, prominent abnormalities are found in roentgenograms. These include focal areas of infiltration, hilar and mediastinal lymphadenopathy, nodules or cavities, and pleural effusion. The commonest are single or multiple infiltrates in any segment that simulate tuberculosis if the upper lobe is involved. They usually resolve after several weeks.

In about 2 percent of benign infections a solid or cavitary pulmonary lesion remains. The typical cavity of coccidioidomycosis is peripheral, has a thin wall, and gives a cystlike appearance in roentgenograms. The cavitary disease may also be indistinguishable from chronic pulmonary tuberculosis and produce chronic cough, weight loss, fever, hemoptysis, chest pain, and dyspnea. Residual solid lesions may be as large as 3 cm in diameter. Both solid and cavitary lesions are commoner in the upper lobes.

In a few individuals (0.05 to 0.2 percent), the primary infection progresses to the disseminated form of the disease, usually within a few months of infection. Dark-skinned persons and pregnant women are more vulnerable. Among Negroes and Filipinos, 85 to 90 percent with dissemination die, as compared to 50 percent of whites. Patients who develop progressive coccidioidomycosis do not give a history of erythema nodosum.

The course of disseminated infection is marked by fungating or ulcerating skin lesions, multiple pulmonary nodules or cavities, widespread destructive lymphadenopathy, osteomyelitis, and meningitis. Weight loss, fever, and weakness are the outstanding systemic manifestations, and the course is often rapid, with death occurring in less than a year. If vital organs are spared, however, patients with disseminated coccidioidomycosis may feel surprisingly well, continue to work, and even gain weight despite the presence of large numbers of *C. immitis* in the sputum or subcutaneous abscesses. The meningeal form is invariably fatal, but even it is compatible with survival for several years. In the presence of meningitis with progressive hydrocephalus, patients experience severe headaches, cranial nerve palsies, memory disturbances, and disorientation. The spinal fluid shows 100 to 200 cells, mostly mononuclear, elevated protein levels, and frequently a reduction in glucose concentration.

DIAGNOSIS Except in meningitis, *C. immitis* is easily recovered from the lesions of disseminated coccidioidomycosis by direct examination and cultures of exudates or biopsied tissues. The characteristic spherule is seen best in purulent material treated with 20% potassium hydroxide. Occasionally, in biopsied tissue, spherules may all be immature and contain no endospores, making them indistinguishable from *B. dermatitidis.* Cultural identification becomes essential for diagnosis. On Sabouraud's agar, mycelial growth appears in 4 to 8 days, and diagnostic spherules develop when the mycelia are incubated in Converse medium at 40°C in 20% CO_2. In meningitis, only a few spherules appear in the spinal fluid, despite the presence of large numbers in the granulomatous exudate around the brainstem. Occasionally, the culture of 20 to 30 ml of spinal fluid yields positive results, but sometimes the diagnosis can be based only on a positive coccidioidin complement fixation test with spinal fluid.

Serologic tests are performed with coccidioidin, a filtrate from cultures of *C. immitis.* By the third week of primary infection, precipitins are found in the serum of 91 percent of patients with symptomatic infection but in only 7 percent of asymptomatic individuals. Complement-fixing antibodies appear later and persist longer than precipitins in nondisseminated coccidioidomycosis; they are almost always present in the disseminated disease and in the spinal fluid in meningitis. The simpler serum immunodiffusion test gives nearly identical results to the complement fixation test. Intradermal tests with coccidioidin are of value in the recognition of primary benign infections because they become positive before precipitins appear, but in disseminated infection the skin test is frequently negative.

The x-ray suggests pulmonary coccidiodomycosis if hilar lymphadenopathy progresses while the parenchymal infiltrate is subsiding or if the adenopathy is associated with multiple areas of pneumonitis. A smooth, thin-walled cavity without surrounding infiltration is also characteristic of residual primary disease. Other residual lesions include calcified or noncalcified nodular foci and localized bronchiectasis. In disseminated pulmonary infection the commonest picture is that of multiple infiltrates accompanied by pleural involvement and prominent hilar or mediastinal lymphadenopathy. Acute miliary coccidioidomycosis cannot be distinguished radiographically from acute miliary tuberculosis, while chronic pulmonary coccidioidomycosis can resemble tuberculosis, with chest films showing soft confluent infiltrates and single or multiple apical cavities.

The only remarkable hematologic finding is eosinophilia, which may reach 35 percent of the total leukocyte count in the primary disease, especially if erythema nodosum is present.

TREATMENT Intensive intravenous treatment with amphotericin B in daily doses of 1 mg per kg body weight appears to be effective in some cases of extrameningeal coccidioidomycosis. Coccidioidal meningitis should be treated with repeated intrathecal injections of 0.5 mg amphotericin B, as well. The total dose varies from less than 1 g to more than 10 g intravenously. Severe nausea, venous thrombosis, and reversible impairment of renal and hepatic function often interrupt the treatment schedule, but persistent administration of amphotericin B in the face of troublesome side effects has occasionally produced improvement. A fall in titer of complement-fixing antibodies and a return of coccidiodin skin sensitivity are evidence of effective treatment. Drug therapy may have to be supplemented by surgical removal of peripheral granulomas.

Primary surgical excision of residual pulmonary foci is indicated because of secondary infection or hemoptysis. Dissemination from these foci almost never occurs.

REFERENCES

Ajello L: *Coccidioidomycosis*, Tucson: University of Arizona Press, 1967

Fiese MJ: *Coccidioidomycosis*, Springfield, Ill.: Charles C Thomas, 1958

Smith CE et al: Pattern of 39,500 serologic tests in coccidioidomycosis. JAMA 160:546, 1956

169 HISTOPLASMOSIS

ABRAHAM I. BRAUDE

DEFINITION Histoplasmosis is caused by the dimorphic fungus *Histoplasma capsulatum*, found as a tiny body within reticuloendothelial cells. The disease varies from mild or unnoticed respiratory infection to widely disseminated lethal disease.

ETIOLOGY Although *H. capsulatum* grows on Sabouraud's agar at room temperature as a spore-bearing mold, it is transformed after animal inoculation into nonencapsulated oval yeastlike cells measuring 2×4 μm. In histologic section the protoplasm is shrunken so that the unstained space beneath the cell wall has the appearance of a capsule. The fungus also grows in the yeastlike phase if incubated at 37°C in sealed tubes of blood agar. The most distinctive cultural feature, however, is the tuberculate *chlamydospore* found only on mycelia; it is round, 10 × 20 μm in diameter, and covered with warty projections. Another smaller spore, not distinguishable from that of *Blastomyces dermatitidis*, is also present on the mycelium. A recently recognized species, *Histoplasma duboisii*, resembles *B. dermatitidis* and is responsible for an infection in Africa that involves the skin and bones but not the lung.

PATHOLOGY AND PATHOGENESIS Infections with *H. capsulatum* are prevalent in the great river valleys of South America, Africa, India, Burma, Thailand, Cambodia, and Indonesia, but are rare in Europe. In the United States it is highly prevalent in the Mississippi River Valley and its tributaries. The source of human infection is probably soil containing spores of *Histoplasma.* Several studies have emphasized the isolation of the fungus from soil in areas inhabited by chickens, birds, and bats. City dwellers are often exposed to histoplasma growing in soil under trees which shelter starlings or blackbirds. The portal of entry is the lung, where a primary complex may be formed by extension of infection from the pulmonary focus to the regional lymph nodes. Most primary infections have benign self-limited dissemination, as evidenced by hepatic and splenic calcifications.

The basic pathologic process is multiplication of *H. capsulatum* in reticuloendothelial cells of the liver, lymph nodes, lung, spleen, adrenal glands, intestine, and marrow. In addition to diffuse lesions, the reticuloendothelial tissues contain nodular accumulations of epithelioid cells and giant cells of the Langhans type. Histoplasma organisms are difficult to demonstrate in the epithelioid cells of the noncaseous granuloma.

Caseous necrosis may accompany both diffuse lesions and granulomas. The adrenals, which are involved in nearly all disseminated infections, are often massively enlarged. Caseous necrosis is usually present in the center of the pulmonary granulomas, which resemble those of cavitary pulmonary tuberculosis. Necrotizing histoplasmosis may also take the form of renal papillitis. Extracellular forms of histoplasma are readily found in the necrotic areas of all organs by special stains (periodic acid–Schiff, Gridley). These extracellular organisms may be much larger than the intracellular ones, appear distorted, and occasionally assume the mycelial form.

CLINICAL MANIFESTATIONS The signs and symptoms of histoplasmosis range from those of a slight self-limited infection to fatal disseminated disease. The high incidence of positive intradermal reactions to histoplasmosis in healthy persons in many parts of the world indicates that most infections by *H. capsulatum* are inapparent or very mild. This variability in severity is observed among different persons in the same outbreak. Severe infections are characterized by prolonged fever, dyspnea, chest pain, weight loss, prostration, widespread pulmonary infiltrates, hepatomegaly, and splenomegaly. Other infected persons may have only a benign acute pneumonitis lasting a week or less, while still others are entirely free of symptoms. Widespread ill-defined noncalcified pulmonary infiltrates of miliary size or larger are found in symptomatic infections and may also be present, although less extensively, in the asymptomatic ones. Eventually, pulmonary lesions either disappear or calcify. In the east central part of the United States there is a high incidence of pulmonary calcification in persons who have negative tuberculin and positive histoplasmin skin tests. In some epidemics of acute histoplasmosis, erythema nodosum and erythema multiforme have been prominent in middle-aged women.

Least resistance to histoplasmosis is encountered in young infants and in adults after the fifth decade. Most cases of disseminated infection have occurred at these extremes of life. In the infant there are fever, emaciation, anemia, and leukopenia, and evidence of widespread involvement of many viscera, including the liver, spleen, lung, intestine, lymph nodes, adrenals, skin, kidney, brain, eye, and endocardium. In the adult, visceral involvement is usually less widespread. Unlike the disease in infancy, adult histoplasmosis shows a marked predilection for males. Histoplasmosis of the lips, mouth, nose, and larynx occurs almost exclusively in adults and is the initial manifestation in about one-third of the fatal cases. Among the various syndromes encountered are subacute vegetative endocarditis, massive lymphadenopathy resembling tuberculosis or lymphoma, various forms of pneumonia, cerebral histoplasmoma, and meningitis. The last is characterized by signs of basilar localization with spinal fluid findings and a clinical course identical with those of tuberculous meningitis.

In addition to the acute benign and disseminated infections, chronic localized histoplasmosis occurs in adults. Two main clinical types of chronic localized histoplasmosis are encountered: (1) *Pulmonary.* This may resemble pulmonary tuberculosis in all respects. The patient may be asymptomatic or may complain of a chronic and occasionally productive cough. Roentgenograms will show lesions identical to those of reinfection tuberculosis, sometimes with cavitation, and accompanied by consistently positive cultures of sputum for *H. capsulatum.* (2) *Mucocutaneous.* Ulcers of the mouth, tongue, pharynx, gums, larynx, penis, or bladder are rare lesions found only in adults. Regional lymphadenopathy is common in these types.

In African histoplasmosis, the predominant lesions are in the skin. These may rupture through the epidermis or encroach on underlying bone. In the disseminated form, multiple lesions involve the lymph nodes, bone, skin, liver, and spleen, but, in contrast to what happens in *H. capsulatum* infections, the lungs are spared.

DIAGNOSIS Isolation of *H. capsulatum* is not difficult in disseminated or chronic localized infections if cultures are made of bone marrow, blood, biopsied lesions, sputum, or exudate from an ulcer. After incubation of infected material on Sabouraud's agar at room temperature there appears a white cottony colony which later turns brown and produces the diagnostic tuberculate chlamydospores. Isolation from sputum is best accomplished in mice, because contaminants are suppressed and the mouse is extremely susceptible to infection by histoplasmas. The animal does not die, but subculture of the spleen 1 month later on Sabouraud's agar yields the organism. Histoplasmas may also be seen in bone marrow, material from open or biopsied lesions, and occasionally in blood smears of terminally ill patients. Special fungous stains (periodic acid–Schiff, Gridley) should be used. Certain intracellular forms of *Cryptococcus neoformans* may be indistinguishable from histoplasma in histologic sections, unless stains for the cryptococcal mucinous capsule are employed.

In cases from which *H. capsulatum* cannot be isolated, indirect clues to identification are (1) history of exposure to soil or dust in an endemic area, (2) positive complement fixation tests, (3) positive histoplasmin skin tests, and (4) development of miliary calcifications in the lung and spleen. Although these criteria are not dependable individually, they are reliable when used together. The serologic and skin tests are frequently negative in culturally proved cases of histoplasmosis, and their specificity is not fully established. Histoplasmin skin tests may confuse the serologic picture by producing complement-fixing antibodies to mycelial antigens but not to yeast-phase antigens.

Histoplasmosis must be differentiated from tuberculosis, sarcoid, leukemia, infectious mononucleosis, Hodgkin's disease, brucellosis, and kala-azar. Because cortisone is frequently of value in sarcoid but can cause dissemination in histoplasmosis, differential diagnosis between these two diseases is critical and diagnosis of sarcoid should be withheld until tissues have been examined with special fungous stains. In kala-azar the intracellular Leishman-Donovan body bears a close resemblance to *H. capsulatum*, and cultural isolation of the fungus may be important in distinguishing between the two.

TREATMENT Amphotericin B in intravenous doses of 0.75 to 1.0 mg per kg per day is of some value in all forms of histoplasmosis, including African histoplasmosis due to *H. duboisii*. In progressive disseminated histoplasmosis caused by *H. capsulatum*, a minimal total of 40 mg per kg amphotericin should be given. But even with this dosage a low survival rate (37 percent) is to be expected unless fatal Addison's disease can be averted by early recognition and treatment of this complication. In chronic pulmonary histoplasmosis the infection is controlled in two-thirds of patients given only 0.5 g over 3 to 5 weeks, and retreatment is uniformly successful in the other third.

REFERENCES

Sarosi G et al: Disseminated histoplasmosis: Results of long-term follow-up. Ann Intern Med 78:511, 1971

Sellers TE Jr et al: Epidemic of erythema multiforme and erythema nodosum caused by histoplasmosis. Ann Intern Med 62:1244, 1965

Sutliff W: Histoplasmosis Cooperative Study V. Amphotericin B dosage for chronic pulmonary histoplasmosis. Am Rev Resp Dis 105:60, 1972

Sweany Henry C: *Histoplasmosis*, Springfield, Ill.: Charles C Thomas, 1960

170 SPOROTRICHOSIS

ABRAHAM I. BRAUDE

DEFINITION Sporotrichosis is a chronic infection due to *Sporotrichum schencki*. It is characterized by the formation of suppurating nodules along the lymphatics of the skin and subcutaneous tissues. Hematogenous dissemination is rare.

ETIOLOGY The fungus *S. schencki* is dimorphic. On Sabouraud's agar at room temperature its growth is mycelial, but in the tissue it takes the form of tiny, cigar-shaped yeast cells. The yeast phase also develops in vitro by incubation at 37°C on blood agar containing cystine.

PATHOGENESIS AND PATHOLOGY The fungus lives as a saprophyte on vegetation and penetrates the hands when the skin is broken. Many cases have followed injury by thorns; sporotrichosis is primarily an occupational disease in people working with plants. Sphagnum moss is an important source of infection, and its increased use as mulch may lead to a greater occurrence of sporotrichosis.

From 7 to 40 weeks after penetrating the skin, the fungus produces at the inoculation site a reddish-purple necrotic nodule, the sporotrichotic chancre. Occasionally the lesion at the inoculation site remains confined to the skin or epidermis without lymphatic involvement, but in the vast majority of cases the fungus spreads from the chancre up the extremities and evokes nodular lesions along the thickened lymphatics. Microscopically the nodules are granulomas with central necrosis. In rare infections the organism may become disseminated throughout the subcutaneous tissues, the liver, testicles, bone, and kidney. Disseminated disease is not usually accompanied by primary infections of the extremities, and its portal of entry is believed to be the gastrointestinal tract.

CLINICAL MANIFESTATIONS There is a marked disproportion between symptoms and findings. A chain of hard, reddened discrete lumps extends up the arm or leg to the axilla or groin, and the intervening lymphatics are red and thickened, but there is no pain, fever, or other constitutional symptom. Older nodules may rupture to produce fistulas or ulcers. In the rare patient with disseminated sporotrichosis, constitutional symptoms may be marked and the disease is rapidly fatal. Unlike other disseminated mycoses, sporotrichosis seldom involves the lungs or central nervous system. Instead, it has a predilection for bone, joints, periosteum, and muscle.

Without treatment, sporotrichosis does not heal, and the lesions often become secondarily infected with bacteria.

DIAGNOSIS The fungus cannot be seen upon microscopic examination of biopsied material or pus in most cases. Cultural isolation is invariably successful, however, if pus is aspirated from an unbroken nodule and inoculated onto Sabouraud's agar. The growth at first has the soft creamy character of bacterial colonies and later develops a wrinkled dark-brown appearance without the cottonlike filament of most molds. Microscopically, typical clusters of pear-shaped spores are found at the tips of conidiophores arising from the tangled mass of delicate branched mycelia. If the mold or the pus is inoculated intraperitoneally into mice or rats, numerous yeast forms will be seen in lesions of the peritoneal cavity or testicle, where they take the form of gram-positive cigar-shaped rods within polymorphonuclear leukocytes.

Recovery of the organism by these techniques permits ready differentiation of sporotrichosis from other chronic infections of the subcutaneous tissues such as syphilis, tularemia, blastomycosis, coccidioidomycosis, and mycobacterial infections. The lymphangitic forms of *Mycobacterium marinum* and *Mycobacterium kansasii* infections cannot be distinguished from sporotrichosis clinically, but skin injuries in an aquarium or swimming pool point to *M. marinum*.

TREATMENT The common lymphangitic form of sporotrichosis is almost invariably dramatically cured by saturated potassium iodide. This should be given orally in starting doses of 10 drops t.i.d. after meals and gradually increased to the point of maximum tolerance. Treatment should be continued for a month after lesions disappear. Additional local therapy may be required for cutaneous ulcers, which should be painted with tincture of iodine. It may also be necessary to excise the epidermal lesions, because these may not subside with oral iodides. Systemic sporotrichosis is resistant to iodides, but it responds well to intravenous treatment with amphotericin B, given in a total dose of 1.5 to 2.0 g over a period of 6 to 8 weeks.

REFERENCES

DICKEY RF: Sporotrichoid mycobacteriosis caused by *M. marinum* (balnei). Arch Dermatol 98:385, 1968

KEDES LH et al: The syndrome of the alcoholic rose gardener: Sporotrichosis of the radial tendon sheath. Ann Intern Med 61:1139, 1964

WILSON DE et al: Clinical features of extracutaneous sporotrichosis. Medicine 46:265, 1967

171 MONILIASIS (CANDIDIASIS)

ABRAHAM I. BRAUDE

DEFINITION Moniliasis is a common mild mucocutaneous infection due to *Candida albicans*. This fungus also causes widespread visceral infection.

ETIOLOGY Among the many species of *Candida*, only *C. albicans* is a common pathogen for man. On the usual nutrient laboratory media *C. albicans* grows as a budding yeast in creamy white colonies, but it produces both mycelia and yeastlike cells in infected tissues. *Candida parapsilosis* is important only as a cause of endocarditis. *Candida guilliermondii* and *Candida tropicalis* have also been isolated rarely in endocarditis.

PATHOGENESIS *Candida albicans* resides normally on the mucous membranes and is frequently cultured from the mouth and feces of persons in good health. The rate of cultural isolation from feces in numerous surveys has ranged from 14 to 19 percent. In debilitated infants, and sometimes in adults, the fungus may produce white patches on the buccal mucosa and initiate mild inflammatory reaction in the underlying tissues. At times chronic moniliasis of the oral mucosa induces chronic hyperplastic changes that resemble leukoplakia. In pregnancy and diabetes, *C. albicans* frequently causes a mild superficial infection of the vagina. Presumably, the high glycogen content of the vaginal mucosa in pregnancy and the glycosuria of diabetes favor its growth. Although *Candida* multiplies excessively in the intestine or mouth if the normal bacterial flora is suppressed by antibiotics, true infection seldom accompanies this overgrowth. Membranous esophagitis is probably the best-defined *Candida* infection of the intestine. *Candida* is usually introduced directly into the bloodstream by intravenous catheters or injections of narcotics, but *Candida* septicemia may also develop from infected burns or wounds. The kidney and brain bear the brunt of hematogenous infection, but lesions also occur in the thyroid, myocardium, endocardium, pancreas, adrenals, and liver. The visceral lesions are granulomatous nodules or abscesses containing both mycelia and yeastlike cells.

A striking susceptibility to moniliasis of the skin and nails is seen in children with congenital hypoparathyroidism. Extensive cutaneous moniliasis occurs in infants with the Swiss type of agammaglobulinemia (alymphocytosis), but not in those with the Bruton form (Chap. 64). Chronic mucocutaneous candidiasis is also seen in other patients with diseases or therapy that depress cellular immunity.

CLINICAL MANIFESTATIONS No systemic disturbances accompany the local signs of mucocutaneous infection. Infection of the mucous membranes, known as *thrush*, gives rises only to soft white patches on the tonsils, cheeks, gums, and tongue. These patches are easily removed and leave a reddened surface. Although usually self-limited, the disease may become chronic and spread to other mucosal surfaces or intertriginous areas in the groins, the antecubital fossae, the interdigital folds, the inframammary areas, the umbilicus, and the axillas. Eczematoid lesions and vesicles are also found in vulvovaginal moniliasis of pregnancy or diabetes. Bladder thrush may cause cystitis.

Painful swallowing or chest pain is the main symptom of *Candida* esophagitis. In some patients the pain may simulate myocardial infarction. This syndrome should be kept in mind in myeloproliferative diseases and during intensive courses of immunosuppressive drugs and antibiotics. Patients with esophogeal moniliasis may have no oropharyngeal thrush.

Bloodstream infections are seen in the late stages of severe debilitating disease and seem to occur most commonly in children and debilitated adults given prolonged parenteral feeding or antibiotic therapy through intravenous catheters. Clinical signs range from fever alone to azotemia, depressed sensorium, and shock. *Candida* endocarditis may also develop from intravenous catheters, but most *Candida* endocarditis is seen in narcotic addicts and affects the aortic or mitral valve. Meningitis is a rare form of moniliasis; it produces a clinical syndrome similar to tuberculous meningitis.

DIAGNOSIS In thrush, the organisms are seen upon microscopic examination of the white patches as a tangled mass of mycelia and yeastlike cells. They grow readily on Sabouraud's agar. In fungemias the fungus can be isolated repeatedly from the blood and can be seen in a direct smear of the catheter tip. Diagnosis of candidemia may also be aided by finding retinal lesions that look like colonies of *C. albicans* and often produce visual blurring and pain. *Candida* esophagitis is recognized roentgenographically by characteristic signs of mucosal irregularities, submucosal edema, and ulcerations. Endoscopy discloses a yellow-white friable pseudomembrane from which candida are obtained.

TREATMENT Oral and vaginal thrush are best treated topically. Nystatin oral suspension is used in the mouth and nystatin or candicidin tablets in the vagina. Topical therapy with nystatin ointments, amphotericin B lotion, or alcoholic solutions of gentian violet is effective in cutaneous moniliasis. Nystatin oral suspension also produces marked improvement in *Candida* esophagitis. Candidemia usually disappears within several days after removing the contaminated intravenous catheters. Otherwise the disease is best treated with oral 5-fluorocytosine in doses of 150 mg per kg body weight daily. The heavy urinary excretion of this drug produces remarkable reversal of severe renal moniliasis not seen with other therapy. *Candida* endocarditis is best treated by surgical replacement of the infected aortic or mitral valve.

REFERENCES

Braude AI, Rock J: The syndrome of acute disseminated moniliasis in adults. AMA Arch Intern Med 104:91, 1959

Curry CR, Quie PB: Fungal septicemia in patients receiving parenteral hyperalimentation. N Engl J Med 285:1221, 1971

Fishman L et al: Hematogenous candida endophthalmitis—a complication of candidemia. N Engl J Med 286:675, 1972

Kirkpatrick C et al: Chronic mucocutaneous candidiasis: Model-building in cellular immunity. Ann Intern Med 74:955, 1971

172 PHYCOMYCOSIS

ABRAHAM I. BRAUDE

DEFINITION Phycomycosis is the general name given to two entirely different infections by two orders of the class Phycomycetes: (1) Mucormycosis is a malignant infection of cerebral, pulmonary, and abdominal blood vessels due to Mucorales. (2) Tropical subcutaneous and nasal phycomycosis is a benign chronic infection due to Entomophthorales.

ETIOLOGY The etiologic agent of cerebral mucormycosis has rarely, if ever, been cultured from the brain or spinal fluid even when expert mycologic techniques were used with fresh cerebral tissues known to harbor the characteristic mycelium. The mycelium is broad, branching, and aseptate, with a diameter of 6 to 15 μm. The fungus *Rhizopus oryzae,* a species of the order Mucorales, has been recovered from the paranasal sinuses of patients with fatal mucormycosis, and the mycelia in culture were identical in appearance with those in the brain. In addition to *R. oryzae,* it has been possible to isolate *Absidia corymbifera, Rhizopus arrhizus,* and *Mucor pusillus* from infected foci outside the nervous system. The Entomophthorales responsible for tropical phycomycosis are curious fungi capable of shooting off their conidia. Rhinoentomophthoromycosis is caused by the genus *Entomophthora coronata,* and subcutaneous phycomycosis by *Basidiobolus ranarum,* a phycomycete with septate mycelia.

PATHOGENESIS The Mucorales abound in soil, manure, and starchy foodstuffs, but become pathogenic for man only in rare cases of diabetic acidosis and even less commonly in patients debilitated by uremic acidosis, leukemia, irradiation, or radiomimetic drugs. The usual portal of entry appears to be the nasal turbinates or paranasal sinuses; from there the organism is thought to extend along the invaded vessels to the retroorbital tissues and cerebrum. Thrombosis of arteries and veins leads to multiple infarcts throughout the brain, but only a minimal inflammatory response is found. Cerebral mucormycosis may be associated with hematogenous spread to pulmonary and intestinal vessels. Pulmonary and intestinal infarction may also develop as a primary infection apparently after inhalation or ingestion of the fungus. Organisms probably penetrate the walls of bronchi or intestine and infect the adjacent hilar or mesenteric vessels. Intestinal mucormycosis takes the form of hemorrhagic segmental infarction of the ileum or colon. Invasion of coronary arteries may produce myocardial infarction.

CLINICAL MANIFESTATIONS Cerebral mucormycosis is characterized by: (1) uncontrolled diabetes with acidosis, (2) ophthalmoplegia, and (3) signs of acute diffuse cerebrovascular disease. If the portal of entry is the nose, further features consist of a black nasal turbinate, malar anesthesia, and a necrotic palatal ulcer. When the patient is first seen, drowsiness and semistupor are usually attributed to the metabolic disturbance, but the cerebral manifestations persist and progress after the acidosis is corrected. Headache and fever are prominent, and paranasal sinusitis is frequently present.

In addition to complete internal and external ophthalmoplegia, there may be edema of the eyelids and retina, proptosis, and signs of retinal vascular occlusion. Nuchal rigidity and mild mononuclear pleocytosis in the spinal fluid have also been described. Pulmonary mucormycosis may start gradually or suddenly with chest pain, fever, hemoptysis, and a friction rub. A few cases have been described in which the orbit or sinuses were infected without extension to the brain. In contrast to nasal mucormycosis, the African form of nasal phycomycosis does not invade blood vessels. Instead *E. coronata* causes a submucosal granuloma near the inferior turbinate that spreads along fascial planes and through sutures and foramens to produce progressive nasal obstruction and firm irregular swellings of the face without breaking through the skin. The other African phycomycete, *B. ranae* produces a woody-hard, freely movable lump in the thighs, buttocks, and forearms, with no constitutional disturbances. Most patients are children. The Sassoon Hospital syndrome, a remarkable disorder attributed to the toxin of *Rhizopus nigricans*, is characterized by epidemic polyuria and polydipsia.

DIAGNOSIS The syndrome of cerebral mucormycosis is so characteristic that it can be recognized by its clinical features alone. The fungus can be found in sections and cultures of the infarcted nasal turbinate or paranasal sinus.

PROGNOSIS Untreated cerebral mucormycosis is almost invariably fatal. Rare cases of recovery have followed control of diabetic acidosis.

TREATMENT A few patients with cerebral mucormycosis have recovered after treatment with amphotericin B in doses of 50 to 70 mg intravenously daily. The total doses were approximately 2.2 g. Treatment should also be directed toward rapid correction of the hyperglycemia and acidosis as well as local excision of infected tissue in the nose, paranasal sinuses, or orbit. Surgical removal of infected lung has been successful. Subcutaneous and nasal types of African phycomycosis improve with oral potassium iodide.

REFERENCES

AMBRAMSON E, ARKY R: Rhinocerebral phycomycosis in association with diabetic ketoacidosis. Ann Intern Med 66:735, 1967

BURKITT DP et al: Subcutaneous phycomycosis: A review of 31 cases seen in Uganda, Br Med J 1:1669, 1964

173
NOCARDIOSIS

ABRAHAM I. BRAUDE

DEFINITION Nocardiosis, an infection caused by an aerobic actinomycete, may produce lung abscesses and spread to the brain and elsewhere; or it may appear as a chronic deforming granulomatous infection limited to the foot (maduromycosis).

ETIOLOGY Pulmonary and disseminated nocardiosis usually results from infection with *Nocardia asteroides.* This organism is relatively acid-fast, and its bacillary form resembles the tubercle bacillus, but *N. asteroides* is easily differentiated from the tubercle bacillus by rapid growth on Sabouraud's medium or 10 percent blood agar at room temperature, and by the presence in exudates of long-branched, gram-positive mycelial forms.

PATHOGENESIS *Nocardia asteroides* can be recovered readily from soil. Nocardiosis appears, therefore, to be an exogenous infection usually having its portal of entry in the lungs. In almost every patient with nocardiosis (other than maduromycosis) the earliest and most extensive lesions are pulmonary acute suppurative foci. A well-defined wall is absent, a fact which probably accounts for the marked tendency of nocardial abscesses to spread to the brain and to a lesser extent to the spleen, skin, peritoneum, and kidney. Occasionally noncaseating granulomas are found. Susceptibility to nocardiosis is increased in Cushing's syndrome, in pulmonary alveolar proteinosis, and in some patients with lymphomas or leukemia after antitumor chemotherapy.

CLINICAL MANIFESTATIONS The chief symptom is cough, usually productive of a thick, sometimes bloody, sputum. Chest pain and dyspnea are common, as are fever, sweats, chills, leukocytosis, weakness, anorexia, and weight loss. The illness may be prolonged and present the picture of chronic pulmonary tuberculosis, lung abscess, or unresolved suppurative pneumonia. In nearly one-third of the patients this syndrome is interrupted suddenly by the acute neurologic changes of metastatic brain abscess. At this time the patient may have severe headache and focal sensory or motor disturbances. The protein, cells, and pressure of the spinal fluid are increased, but the concentration of glucose is not reduced unless the meninges are also infected. Occasionally, abscess is the first clinical manifestation of nocardiosis, especially in Cushing's syndrome secondary to adrenal steroid therapy. Infection of the skin is frequent and produces numerous scattered abscesses or single draining sinuses of the hand, chest wall, or buttocks.

The disease is usually fatal, after months to years.

DIAGNOSIS Because patients with nocardiosis are suspected of having tuberculosis, their sputums are examined for tubercle bacilli. The usual methods for concentrating tubercle bacilli often kill *N. asteroides. Nocardia asteroides* may also be overlooked in smears stained by the Ziehl-Neelsen method, because it is less resistant than the tubercle bacillus to decolorizing by alcohol. Killing the organism can be avoided by concentrating with trisodium phosphate, and overdecolorizing can be avoided by using 1% sulfuric acid.

Although sulfur granules are not found in pulmonary or disseminated nocardiosis, the gram-positive filamentous organisms in nocardial exudates often resemble *Actinomyces israeli.* The two pathogens can be distinguished, however, by the ease with which *N. asteroides* is cultivated on Sabouraud's medium or blood agar aerobically, and by its acid-fast staining characteristics. In biopsy material the nongranulomatous and minimally fibrotic character of the nocardial suppurative reaction also helps to distinguish it from infections due to *A. israeli.* The absence of tubercles is valuable in differential diagnosis from tuberculosis.

TREATMENT Administration of sulfadiazine is sometimes successful treatment. Penicillin and tetracycline appear ineffective, and resistance of nocardiosis to these drugs may be used in distinguishing it from actinomycosis due to *A. israeli* and from other pulmonary infections which respond to these antibiotics. Patients with nocardiosis should receive 8 to 12 g sulfadiazine daily. Cycloserine shows promise for patients allergic to sulfonamides.

REFERENCES

ANDRIOLE VT et al: The association of nocardiosis and pulmonary alveolar proteinosis. Ann Intern Med 60:266, 1964

DANOWSKI TS et al: Cushing's syndrome in conjunction with *Nocardia asteroides* infection. Metabolism 11:2, 1962

WEED LA et al: Nocardiosis: clinical, bacteriologic and pathologic aspects. N Engl J. Med 253:1138, 1955

174
OTHER DEEP MYCOSES

ABRAHAM I. BRAUDE

ASPERGILLOSIS

DEFINITION Aspergillosis is an infection produced by *Aspergillus fumigatus* and other species of *Aspergillus*, a group of fungi of low pathogenicity for man unless resistance is overcome by an overwhelming inoculum or debilitating illness. The disease may become disseminated or remain localized to the lung, ear, orbit, or paranasal sinuses.

ETIOLOGY Aspergilli assume the mycelial form both in culture and in infected tissues. They are hardy, widely prevalent organisms and grow rapidly on all culture media at room temperature or 35°C as colored woolly colonies peppered with dark dots. They are composed of segmented mycelia that bear masses of small round spores on a knoblike swelling at the end of specialized mycelial stalks known as conidiophores.

PATHOGENESIS AND PATHOLOGY Primary infection of the lung sometimes develops after inhalation of massive numbers of spores from mycelia growing on grain. Secondary pulmonary infection may be superimposed on tuberculous cavities, bronchiectasis, and bronchogenic carcinoma or may become established after resistance is lowered by leukopenia, Hodgkin's disease, irradiation, and other debilitating processes. Excessive use of adrenal steroids or antibiotics is also thought to favor secondary invasion by *Aspergillus.* The most distinctive pulmonary lesion is the aspergilloma, a mycelial mass in a fibrous cavity lined with bronchial epithelium. Aspergillomas (fungus balls) often form in the upper-lobe cystic cavities of sarcoidosis and in patients with ankylosing spondylitis. Chronic granulomatous lung lesions resembling tuberculosis have also been described. More destructive infections take the form of bronchopneumonia and lung abscesses. Thrombosis of pulmonary vessels by invading mycelia leads to local necrosis with hemorrhage and to hematogenous abscesses in the brain, lung, kidney, spleen, heart, and thyroid. Primary infections of the ear, orbit, and nasal sinuses may also be invasive and extend locally into the middle ear and brain.

CLINICAL MANIFESTATIONS In pulmonary aspergillomas the chief symptom is hemoptysis. *Aspergillus* lung abscesses and granulomas are associated with cough and fever. In fulminating disseminated infections, pulmonary manifestations are often overshadowed by coma and other signs of cerebral infection. Fever, joint pains, and skin eruptions lasting for a few weeks or months may also accompany disseminated aspergillosis. A syndrome of *allergic aspergillosis* occurs in asthmatics who develop hypersensitivity to *Aspergillus* antigens. These patients are subject to recurrent episodes of localized pulmonary infiltrations with blood eosinophilia, increased wheezing, cough, fever, and pleuritic pain. The allergic process may lead to bronchiectasis and aspergilloma. Both reaginic and precipitating antibodies are considered responsible for the pulmonary and systemic responses. Allergic aspergillosis is said to be the most frequent cause in Great Britain of transient lung infiltrates with eosinophilia. A form of allergic aspergillosis, known as hemp disease, produces asthma in people working in rope factories.

DIAGNOSIS Cultures of aspergilli have no diagnostic value unless they are obtained directly from infected tissues. They may be present in the mouth and in sputum cultures in the absence of *Aspergillus* infection, and they may contaminate uninfected biopsy specimens unless strict sterile precautions are observed. Cultural findings should be confirmed by demonstration of mycelia in biopsy material. In chronic aspergillomas the sputum cultures may sometimes become negative after the fungus loses its ability to sporulate.

Aspergillomas of the lung can usually be recognized by the unique appearance in roentgenograms of a crescentic radiolucency surrounding a circular mass. In other forms of pulmonary aspergillosis the roentgenogram is not diagnostic and may resemble that of bronchogenic carcinoma, bacterial lung abscess, and tuberculosis. In allergic aspergillosis, the sputum may contain small plugs of eosinophilic and mycelial fragments. *Aspergillus* antigens produce immediate intradermal wheals followed by Arthus phenomena, and serum precipitins against *Aspergillus* antigens are found by double diffusion in agar gel. These precipitins are also present constantly in pulmonary aspergillomas but not in invasive disseminated aspergillosis.

TREATMENT Localized lesions have been successfully excised from both the lung and the brain. Endobronchial infusion of amphotericin B is effective in properly selected patients with aspergillomas. The value of chemotherapy has not been established in systemic infections, but intravenous amphotericin B shows enough promise to warrant its use. Corticosteroids may cure allergic pulmonary aspergillosis by suppressing the bronchial edema and secretions so that the fungus can be eliminated from the respiratory tract.

GEOTRICHOSIS

DEFINITION Geotrichosis is the name given to certain disorders of the mouth, bronchi, and intestinal tract from which *Geotrichium candidum* has been isolated. This fungus has not been established as a human pathogen, and the validity of geotrichosis as a disease entity remains questionable.

ETIOLOGY The fungus *G. candidum* may resemble *Coccidioides immitis* in culture because its septate mycelium fragments into large square-ended arthrospores. *Geotrichium candidum* does not form sporangia in vivo, however, and its soft creamy colonies on solid medium are easily distinguished from those of *C. immitis*.

PATHOGENESIS Geotrichium is a normal inhabitant of the pharynx and intestine and may proliferate locally to produce visible white colonies on the mucous membranes. It may also appear in devitalized tissues and secretions of the nasopharynx, bronchopulmonary tree, and colon but probably not as a primary pathogen.

CLINICAL MANIFESTATIONS Geotrichosis is reported to cause pulmonary cavities and colitis. In bronchopulmonary geotrichosis, the patient coughs up gelatinous sputum tinged with blood, and in rare cases thin-walled cavities like those of coccidioidomycosis have been described.

DIAGNOSIS In secretions and exudates, *G. candidum* has the appearance of oval or barrel-shaped spores measuring up to 8 to 10 mm in diameter. They are easily recovered on Sabouraud's agar at room temperature.

TREATMENT Lesions resembling thrush respond to local application of 1:10,000 solution of gentian violet. Bronchopulmonary geotrichosis is said to respond to oral treatment with potassium iodide, and intestinal geotrichosis is treated by oral administration three times daily of capsules containing 0.32 mg gentian violet.

MYCETOMA

DEFINITION Mycetoma is a chronic destructive infection of the skin, subcutaneous tissues, fascia, and bone. The infection produces a localized swelling containing multiple fistulas which extrude mycotic granules.

ETIOLOGY The most frequent cause of mycetoma in the United States is a higher fungus known as *Monosporium apiospermum*, the "imperfect" form of the ascomycete *Allescheria boydii*. It grows rapidly on Sabouraud's agar as a cottony mycelium bearing asexual spores either singly or in small groups at the tips or sides of conidiophores. Other higher fungi isolated in mycetoma include members of such diverse genera as *Aspergillus, Penicillium, Madurella, Cephalosporium,* and *Phialophora*.

Streptomyces and *Nocardia* are important causes of mycetoma outside the United States. *Streptomyces madurae* is found in southeastern Asia and *Nocardia brasiliensis* in South America and Mexico.

PATHOGENESIS AND PATHOLOGY The fungi found in mycetoma are inhabitants of the soil and enter the tissues of the bare foot and leg, presumably after trauma. The chest wall is infected by sacks, contaminated with soil, carried over the shoulder. The buttocks, abdomen, and arm are also infected.

The infection begins in the outer tissues and burrows through to destroy bone, muscle, and connective tissue indiscriminately. The areas of destruction show chronic suppuration with fibrosis and are connected by multiple fistulas which rupture to the outside. Mycotic granules are seen in the suppurative foci. The prolonged proliferation of granulation and scar tissue leads to enlargement of the affected part.

CLINICAL MANIFESTATIONS The earliest sign is usually a small swelling on the sole or dorsum of the foot which undergoes a recurring cycle of swelling, suppuration, and healing. Later, similar lesions appear on other parts of the foot, and over a period of months destruction of deeper tissues is manifested by slight or moderate pain, generalized swelling, and redness. The course is intermittently progressive, and there may be periods of remission. Ultimately the foot becomes a swollen, deformed mass of destroyed tissue with many fistulous openings through which mycotic granules are discharged. The infection does not spread hematogenously to other parts, but in rare instances there is direct extension along lymphatics. Death may occur from secondary bacterial infection.

DIAGNOSIS The characteristic granules are 0.5 to 2 mm in diameter and may be white, yellow, black, or red. Nocardial granules are easily distinguished from those of *Aspergillus boydii* and other higher fungi by direct microscopic examination. They are masses of radiating gram-positive filaments; those of higher fungi contain large segmented hyphae and numerous chlamydospores. Either type of granule grows rapidly on Sabouraud's agar.

Roentgenograms disclose destruction of bone which is more extensive than the external appearance and pain might indicate.

TREATMENT Nocardial and streptomycotic mycetomas should be treated with oral sulfonamides, and those due to higher fungi with intravenous and local amphotericin B. Antibacterial chemotherapy is valuable in arresting secondary infection. There is no dependable cure, however, and many cases eventually require amputation.

CHROMOBLASTOMYCOSIS

DEFINITION Chromoblastomycosis is an infection of the skin produced by several species of the genus *Phialophora* and characterized by slowly progressive cauliflower-like lesions of the skin of agricultural workers in tropical or subtropical regions.

ETIOLOGY The three species *P. pedrosi, P. compactum,* and *P. verrucosa* cannot be distinguished upon microscopic examination of infected tissue, in which all appear as small clusters of spores with thick, dark-brown walls. On culture, however, the three differ in their methods of sporulation. On Sabouraud's agar all three grow very slowly and will produce deeply pigmented olive or black colonies.

PATHOGENESIS AND PATHOLOGY The fungi live in the soil or vegetation and enter the skin of agricultural workers. The disease occurs mostly on the lower extremity of barefoot workmen, but sometimes on the upper extremity or buttocks.

Three pathologic processes are found: (1) microabscesses in the dermis containing numerous fungi, (2) extensive fibrosis, and (3) epidermal hyperplasia and hyperkeratosis. The lesions progress along the lymphatics but only rarely beyond them, and they do not penetrate deeply to involve bone.

CLINICAL MANIFESTATIONS The earliest lesion is a papule, which develops into a well-circumscribed bluish lesion with a warty, raised margin. Although it resembles the cutaneous form of North American blastomycosis at this early stage, it does not spread peripherally. Instead, adjacent new lesions appear over a period of years and, as the epithelial hyperplasia and hyperkeratosis increase, the entire area assumes a cauliflower-like appearance. Eventually the whole extremity is covered. Pain and constitutional symptoms are absent unless secondary bacterial infection occurs or elephantiasis develops as a result of lymphatic scarring.

DIAGNOSIS The typical dark-brown septate bodies are seen in large numbers in biopsied tissue or pus, and brown hyphae can be found in crusts treated with 10% potassium hydroxide. For specific identification, however, it is necessary to culture the slowly growing fungus on Sabouraud's agar.

TREATMENT Early in the disease, the lesions may be destroyed by electrocoagulation or removed by surgical excision. Later in the course, excision of the larger nodules leaves indolent ulcers which heal very slowly.

Saturated solution of potassium iodide, given to tolerance orally, as in sporotrichosis, is said to be effective when combined with weekly injections of calcipherol. Local injection into the lesions of 0.035 mg amphotericin B in 7 ml of 2% procaine solution at weekly intervals has been used because the organisms are resistant to the levels achieved after intravenous injection. This local treatment produced complete resolution of lesions in a limited trial and should be tried. Oral and topical 5-fluorocytosine is the latest treatment to show promise. In general, the treatment of chromoblastomycosis has been disappointing. The disease is never fatal, however, and the usefulness of the limb is retained despite its unsightly appearance.

RHINOSPORIDIOSIS

DEFINITION Rhinosporidiosis produces small tumorlike masses usually confined to the nose and nasopharynx. An endosporulating fungus seen in the tissues cannot be cultured on laboratory media.

ETIOLOGY The fungus *Rhinosporidium seeberi* is placed in the class Phycomycetes and family Coccidioidaceae because characteristic giant sporangia develop in the tissues. These thick-walled endospore-filled sporangia resemble the smaller spherules of *Coccidioides immitis.*

PATHOGENESIS AND PATHOLOGY The disease is probably acquired by bathing or diving into infected water. In India, where rhinosporidiosis reaches endemic proportions, its rarity in women is attributed to social taboos that prohibit their bathing in open places. The characteristic lesion is a vascularized papillomatous proliferation of the nasal or pharyngeal mucous membrane containing sporangia in various stages of maturity. Red cells, inflammatory cells, and extruded endospores fill the interstitial tissue. As sporangia enlarge they compress the columnar epithelium of the nose or the squamous epithelium of the pharynx and allow endospores to escape and reinoculate the adjacent tissue.

CLINICAL MANIFESTATIONS Single or multiple pedunculated fleshy red masses appear in the nares or pharynx and produce symptoms of rhinitis, epistaxis, and nasal obstruction. In exceptional cases hoarseness may develop from laryngeal infection. The conjunctivas and lacrimal sac may also be involved.

DIAGNOSIS The characteristic sporangia are easily identified in biopsied tissue section. Because the only endemic foci are in India, most patients are Asiatic.

TREATMENT The lesions can be completely removed surgically or by electrocautery. Electrocautery is preferred because surgery leaves open incisions in which spores can be implanted.

REFERENCES

Barwasser NC: Chromoblastomycosis: Thirteenth reported case in the United States. JAMA 153:566, 1953

Finegold SM, Well D: Aspergillosis: A review and report of twelve cases. Am J Med 27:463, 1959

Gilbert T, Patterson R: Pulmonary allergic aspergillosis. Ann Intern Med 72:395, 1970

Grcevic N, Mathews WF: Pathologic changes in acute disseminated aspergillosis. Am J Clin Pathol 35:536, 1959

Israel H, Ostrow A: Sarcoidosis and aspergillomas. Am J Med 47:243, 1969

Lopez C et al: Treatment of chromoblastomycosis with 5-fluorocytosine. O Hosp (Brazil) 75:1335, 1969

Murray IG: *Laboratory Aspects of Mycetoma, in Systemic Mycoses,* A Ciba Foundation Symposium, eds G. Wolstenholme, R. Porter, Boston: Little, Brown, 1967

Purandare NM, Deoras SM: Rhinosporidiosis in Bombay. Indian J Med Sci 7:603, 1953

Scadding JG: The bronchi in allergic aspergillosis. Scand J Resp Dis 48:372, 1967

Smith DT: Geotrichosis. J Chronic Dis 5:532, 1957

section 12 | The rickettsioses

175 GENERAL CONSIDERATIONS

THEODORE E. WOODWARD

The rickettsial diseases of man consist of a variety of clinical entities caused by microorganisms of the family *Rickettsiaceae.* The rickettsias are obligate intracellular parasites about the size of bacteria and are usually seen microscopically as pleomorphic coccobacilli. Each of the rickettsias pathogenic for man is capable of multiplying in one or more species of arthropod as well as in animals and man. Indeed, the majority of the rickettsias are maintained in nature by a cycle which involves an insect vector and an animal reservoir, and infection of man is unimportant in the cycle. Epidemic typhus presents a number of points of dissimilarity to most of the other rickettsioses, because the natural cycle of the infection involves only man and the louse.

A compendium of information on the rickettsial diseases is given in Table 175-1. Because each of the rickettsioses responds therapeutically to tetracyclines or chloramphenicol, the table mentions no therapy. Procedures for diagnostic isolation of the rickettsias are omitted because they generally are less useful than serologic methods, and the techniques which they require are highly specialized and hazardous. Information on isolation may be found in textbooks devoted to viral and rickettsial diseases.

HISTORY OF THE RICKETTSIAL DISEASES Of all the afflictions of mankind the rickettsial diseases, particularly epidemic typhus, rank among the foremost as a cause of human suffering and death.

The record of deaths from epidemic typhus in this century in the Balkan countries and in Poland and Russia reaches astounding figures. Typhus ravaged Russia and eastern Poland from 1915 to 1922, infecting 30 million of the inhabitants and causing an estimated 3 million deaths.

The past two decades have seen the development of excellent methods for the prevention and treatment of the rickettsioses of man. In fact, these measures have been so successful that the rickettsioses have become of minor importance in the United States and in many other countries. Although conquered, the rickettsioses have not been eliminated, and they could again become rampant if the will to control them, the present high standards of sanitation, and the necessary industrial capacities for production of effective insecticides and therapeutic agents should be decreased through war or disaster.

Gerhard in 1836 differentiated typhoid fever from louse-borne typhus fever. In 1899, Maxcy described the clinical manifestations of Rocky Mountain spotted fever. In a series of studies from 1906 to 1909, Ricketts, for whom the rickettsial microorganisms are named, successfully transmitted this disease to guinea pigs, incriminated the wood tick as a vector, and observed rickettsias in smears prepared from tick tissues.

Nicolle in 1909 reproduced typhus fever in monkeys and demonstrated transmission by the body louse. Von Prowazek in 1914 and Da Rocha-Lima in 1916 demonstrated small microorganisms in the tissues of lice taken from typhus patients.

Brill in 1910 recognized a febrile disease in patients in New York City as an example of mild epidemic typhus unassociated with lousiness. Zinsser in 1934 postulated that this disease was a recurrent form of typhus occurring in patients during periods of stress or waning immunity. Subsequent studies have confirmed Zinsser's hypothesis. This entity is now called Brill-Zinsser disease.

Weil and Felix, working with typhus patients in Poland in 1915, recognized that agglutinins for certain *Proteus* organisms appeared in the serum of convalescent patients. The Weil-Felix reaction, although nonspecific, affords a simple and valuable screening method for several rickettsioses.

In 1926 Maxcy, on purely epidemiologic evidence,

surmised that typhus in the United States had its reservoir in rodents and was transmitted to man by ticks or fleas. Confirmation of Maxcy's hypothesis was obtained in Baltimore in 1930 by Dyer and others when they isolated rickettsias from the brains of rats and shortly thereafter incriminated the flea as a vector. This disease, caused by *Rickettsia mooseri* and now designated endemic or murine typhus, is distinct from epidemic typhus and Brill-Zinsser disease.

The development of suitable vaccines and specific diagnostic antigens was impeded until it was possible to prepare appreciable quantities of highly infectious rickettsial material in the laboratory. The most important steps were (1) the Weigl vaccine (1930), a phenolized suspension of gut tissue obtained from body lice which had been injected intrarectally with the rickettsias of

TABLE 175-1
Rickettsial diseases

Disease			*Natural cycle*			*Serologic diagnosis*	
Type	*Agent*	*Geographic distribution*	*Arthropod*	*Mammal*	*Transmission to man*	*Weil-Felix reaction*	*Complement fixation*
Spotted fever group							
Rocky Mountain spotted fever	*R. rickettsii*	Western hemisphere	Ticks	Wild rodents; dogs	Tick bite	Positive OX-19 OX-2	Positive group- and type-specific
Boutonneuse fever	*R. conorii*	Africa, Europe, Middle East, India	"	"	"	"	"
Queensland tick typhus	*R. australis*	Australia	"	Marsupials, wild rodents	"	"	"
North Asian tick-borne rickettsiosis	*R. sibirica*	Siberia, Mongolia	"	Wild rodents	"	"	"
Rickettsial-pox	*R. akari*	United States, Russia, Africa(?)	Blood-sucking mite	House mouse, other rodents	Mite bite	Negative	"
Typhus group							
Endemic (murine)	*R. mooseri*	Worldwide	Flea	Small rodents	Infected flea feces into broken skin	Positive OX-19	Positive group- and type-specific
Epidemic	*R. prowazeki*	Worldwide	Body louse	Man	Infected louse feces into broken skin	Positive OX-19	"
Brill-Zinsser disease	*R. prowazeki*	Worldwide	Recurrence years after original attack of epidemic typhus			Usually negative	"
Scrub	*R. tsutsugamushi*	Asia, Australia, Pacific islands	Trombiculid mites	Wild rodents	Mite bite	Positive OX-K	Positive in about 50% of patients
Other rickettsial diseases							
Q fever	*R. burnetii*	Worldwide	Ticks	Small mammals, cattle, sheep, goats	Inhalation of dried infected material	Negative	Positive
Trench fever	*R. quintana*	Europe, Africa, North America	Body louse	Man	Infected louse feces into broken skin	Negative	None available

epidemic typhus; (2) the killed murine typhus vaccine prepared by Casteneda (1939) from lung tissues of rats injected intranasally; and (3) the inactivated Rocky Mountain spotted fever vaccine obtained by Cox (1941) from infected yolk sacs of embryonated hen eggs. The low cost and relative simplicity of the egg techniques have led to their general use for preparation of vaccines and diagnostic antigens.

The years of World War II saw many strides in the conquest of the rickettsioses; perhaps greatest among these were the highly successful attacks on the arthropod vectors. The lousicide DDT proved to be ideal for control when dusted on the clothes of infested persons. The epidemic at Naples during the winter of 1943 to 1944 established a milestone, because it was the first to be suppressed by the use of insecticides. Scrub typhus (mite-borne typhus) was creating a major problem in the Pacific area. Here, too, the major contributions to successful control were concerned with application of miticidal chemicals to the person and his clothes.

The advent of broad-spectrum antibiotics—first chloramphenicol, then chlortetracycline in 1948, and later oxytetracycline—provided dramatic therapeutic results in each of the rickettsioses.

PATHOGENESIS Rickettsial diseases of man develop following infection through the skin or the respiratory tract. Agents of the typhus and spotted fever group are introduced through the bite of the infected arthropod vector. Ticks and mites, which transmit the agents of spotted fever and scrub typhus, inoculate the rickettsias directly into the dermis during feeding. The louse and flea, which transmit epidemic and murine typhus, respectively, deposit infected feces on the skin; infection occurs when organisms are rubbed into the puncture wound made by the arthropod. The rickettsia of Q fever gain entry through the respiratory tract by inhalation of infected dust; moreover, the respiratory route is occasionally implicated in epidemic typhus when infection results from inhalation of dried infected louse feces.

Although organisms probably multiply at the original site of entry in all instances, local lesions appear with regularity only in certain diseases, namely, the initial cutaneous lesions of scrub typhus, rickettsialpox, and boutonneuse fever, and the pneumonitis which develops in about half the persons infected with Q fever.

Volunteers infected with either scrub typhus or Q fever develop rickettsemia late in the incubation period, often some hours before the onset of fever. Similar events probably occur in all the rickettsial diseases; circulating rickettsias can be detected during the early febrile period in practically all patients. Little is known about the pathogenesis of infection during the midportion of the incubation period. However, it is reasonable to assume that during this time in patients with typhus or spotted fever, a transient low-grade rickettsemia results from release of organisms multiplying at the initial site of infection and that this seeds infection in the endothelial cells of the vascular tree. Vascular lesions developing at such sites account for the pathologic changes, including the rash.

Rickettsias apparently invade and proliferate in the endothelial cells of small blood vessels. Endothelial cell destruction occurs from the proliferation of organisms and eventual disruption. Rickettsia may exert a cytotoxic effect on endothelial cells; in mice the rickettsial toxin causes remarkable increase in capillary permeability, independent of proliferation. Later manifestations in rickettsial diseases may result from immunopathologic mechanisms, since humoral antibodies are present during the second febrile week, when increases in capillary permeability and vascular thrombosis and ecchymoses are greatest. Also, a delayed type of hypersensitivity occurs during infection.

The underlying cause of the toxic-febrile state which characterizes the rickettsial diseases remains unknown. Several rickettsial species contain type-specific toxins which are lethal for mice; these may play a role.

PATHOLOGIC PHYSIOLOGY Peripheral vascular collapse results in death in fulminating cases during the first week, with capillary dilatation and pooling of blood without increased capillary permeability or loss of fluid into extravascular spaces. As proliferative and thrombotic lesions develop in small vessels, anoxia occurs in the areas supplied, resulting in necrosis and increased capillary permeability, with loss of water, electrolytes, proteins, and erythrocytes. This, in turn results in a decrease in blood volume, together with an increase in extravascular space (thiocyanate space) and clinical edema. Edema and anoxia of the myocardium are indicated by electrocardiographic changes. Liver function is impaired. The azotemia which develops in seriously ill patients appears to be prerenal. Clinical manifestations resulting from the peripheral vascular collapse are oliguria and anuria, azotemia, anemia, hypoproteinemia, hyponatremia, edema, and coma. In spotted fever and typhus patients with hemorrhagic skin lesions, consumptive coagulopathy is manifested by thrombocytopenia, hypofibrinogenemia, and other coagulation abnormalities. All these alterations are absent or minimal in mild cases or in those who are given specific treatment early.

PATHOLOGY The basic changes in the spotted and typhus fever groups are vascular, with resultant widespread lesions in adjacent parenchymatous tissues throughout the body. They are most common in the skin, muscles, heart, lung, and brain. The most conspicuous and diverse of these are found in Rocky Mountain spotted fever. Here swelling, proliferation, and degeneration of the endothelial cells occur, frequently with thrombus formation which partially or completely occludes the lumen. The muscle cells of the arterioles undergo swelling and fibrinoid changes. The adventitial tissues are infiltrated with mononuclear leukocytes, lymphocytes, and plasma cells. The vascular damage is scattered along the arteries, veins, and capillaries, with normal architecture prevailing throughout most of the vascular bed. The changes in murine, epidemic, and scrub typhus fevers resemble those in Rocky Mountain spotted fever, but thrombosis is uncommon and involvement of the musculature is rare.

Interstitial myocarditis occurs in each of these diseases but is usually most extensive in Rocky Mountain spotted fever and in scrub typhus. In the brain glial nodules are found in all members of the group, but microinfarcts in the brain tissue or in the myocardium are most often observed in spotted fever.

A rickettsial pneumonitis occurs, at least to some extent, in many patients with spotted or typhus fever and is the characteristic pathologic change in patients with Q fever. The process is patchy and consists microscopically of areas of congestion and edema with gray granular consolidation. Microscopically, within the consolidated areas the alveoli are filled with compact fibrinocellular exudate containing lymphocytes, plasma cells, large mononuclear cells, and erythrocytes but few, if any, polymorphonuclear leukocytes.

Rickettsias can occasionally be observed microscopically in sections of tissue. Failure to demonstrate them is of no diagnostic significance.

LABORATORY DIAGNOSIS Diagnostic procedures which depend on isolation of the etiologic agent from blood or other clinical material are expensive, time-consuming, and hazardous to laboratory personnel. Except in unusual circumstances, currently available serologic tests are adequate for laboratory confirmation of the clinical diagnosis in each of the rickettsial diseases. The demonstration of a rise in titer of specific antibody during convalescence is of prime importance in establishing the laboratory confirmation. Table 175-2 summarizes the serologic results usually encountered in persons who have rickettsial diseases in the United States. The Weil-Felix test employing *Proteus* strains OX-19 and OX-2 gives positive results in patients with spotted fever and murine typhus and negative results in those with rickettsialpox and Q fever. It is useful as a screening procedure but cannot be relied upon to differentiate spotted fever from murine typhus. In patients with Brill-Zinsser disease the *Proteus* OX-19 reaction is usually negative or low in titer.

Complement fixation tests employing group-specific rickettsial antigens provide data which clearly differentiate the most common infections, i.e., murine typhus, Rocky Mountain spotted fever, and Q fever. Moreover, if type-specific rickettsial antigens are employed, it is generally possible to distinguish rickettsialpox from spotted fever and Brill-Zinsser disease from murine typhus.

Antibodies during response to a primary infection of epidemic typhus or Rocky Mountain spotted fever are usually 19S globulins. In patients with Brill-Zinsser disease, which is a recrudescence, antibodies occur more quickly (within several days after onset of illness), rise to a higher titer, and are 7S globulins.

Specific antibiotic therapy has little effect on the time of appearance of antibodies or on their ultimate titer, provided treatment is instituted some days after onset of the illness. However, if the illness is cut short by early and vigorous treatment, antibody production may be delayed for a week or so, and also the maximal titers attained may be below those illustrated in Table 175-2. Under these circumstances a sample of blood taken 4 to 6 weeks after onset of illness should also be tested.

An additional serologic test is based on the agglutination of sheep or human O erythrocytes after sensitization with a serologically active fraction of rickettsias designated ESS (erythrocyte-sensitizing substances). Erythrocytes exposed to the typhus ESS are specifically agglutinated by serums of patients as early as the eighth febrile day. The ESS test is simple and inexpensive.

The immunofluorescent antibody test is a very useful procedure for detecting rickettsia in the tissues of patients with the typhus group of rickettsioses, the spotted fevers, and Q fever. The technique also visualizes rickettsia in ticks and the tissues of animals.

Normochromic anemia occurs in patients severely ill with rickettsial diseases. The white blood cell count in Rocky Mountain spotted fever, rickettsialpox, murine and epidemic typhus, Brill-Zinsser disease, Q fever, and other rickettsial diseases is usually within the normal range: 6,000 to 10,000 cells per mm^3. Leukopenia is occasionally observed, and in the presence of complications, such as superimposed infections and extensive vascular lesions, moderate leukocytosis occurs. The differential blood cell count is usually normal.

Thrombocytopenia occurs in severely ill spotted and scrub typhus fever patients with extensive vascular lesions; hypofibrinogenemia, prolonged prothrombin time, partial thromboplastin times, and other clotting abnormalities occur.

REFERENCES See end of Chap. 183.

TABLE 175-2
Serologic diagnosis of rickettsial diseases of the United States

		Weil-Felix reaction				*Complement fixation tests with type-specific antigen*				
			Illustrative titer				*Illustrative titer*			
Group	*Disease*	*Proteus*	*10th day*	*20th day*	*Cases with diagnostic titer*	*Rickettsial antigen*	*10th day*	*20th day*	*30th day*	*Cases with diagnostic titer*
Spotted fever	Rocky Mountain spotted fever	OX-19	40	320	Most	*R. rickettsii*	20	160	80	Most
		OX-2	20	160						
	Rickettsialpox	OX-19	0	0	None	*R. akari*	0	64	128	Most
		OX-2	0	0						
Typhus	Murine typhus	OX-19	160	640	Most	*R. mooseri*	0	160	160	Most
		OX-2	10	40						
	Brill-Zinsser disease	OX-19	160	20	Infrequent	*R. prowazeki*	1,280	640	320	Most
		OX-2	0	0						
	Q fever	OX-19	0	0	None	*R. burnetii*	10	80	160	Most
		OX-2	0	0	None					

176 ROCKY MOUNTAIN SPOTTED FEVER

THEODORE E. WOODWARD

DEFINITION Rocky Mountain spotted fever is an acute febrile illness caused by *Rickettsia rickettsii*, transmitted to man by ticks. The disease is characterized by sudden onset with headache and chills and by fever which persists for 2 to 3 weeks. A characteristic exanthem appears on the extremities and trunk about the fourth day of illness. Delirium, shock, and renal failure occur in the severely ill.

ETIOLOGY AND EPIDEMIOLOGY The causative microbe *R. rickettsii* is the prototype for the rickettsial group of agents. The minute organisms are purple when stained by Giemsa's method or red by Macchiavello's technique; most of them are gram-negative. These organisms often occur in pairs and possess a cell wall similar in structure and chemical composition to that of gram-negative bacteria; one finds a cell membrane, cytoplasmic granules corresponding to ribosomes, and prokaryotic organization of nuclear material. The cell membrane is selectively permeable; the cell wall is the focus of important antigens and an endotoxin-like substance.

The rickettsias grow in the nucleus and the cytoplasm of infected cells of ticks, mammals, and embryonated eggs; the intranuclear situation of the organisms is shared by the other members of the spotted fever group, but not by rickettsias of the typhus group. *Rickettsia rickettsii* is readily distinguishable from the agents of the typhus fevers by cross-immunity tests in guinea pigs and by complement fixation tests employing antigens prepared from infected yolk sac tissues. The differentiation of *R. rickettsii* from closely related members of the spotted fever group frequently requires elaborate procedures. Strains of the agent of Rocky Mountain spotted fever vary considerably in their virulence for man and animals.

The first reports of spotted fever in Idaho and Montana during the final decade of the last century led to the name Rocky Mountain spotted fever. However, the disease has been reported in all states except Maine and Vermont, as well as in Canada, Mexico, Colombia, and Brazil. Although related diseases are found on other continents, this particular infection is limited to the Western Hemisphere. Currently about 200 cases of spotted fever occur annually in the United States. The mortality rate in the days before specific therapy was about 20 percent but has decreased to about 5 percent. Although the attack rate per unit of population is highest in Wyoming, almost half the cases occur in the South Atlantic states, with the greatest number of these in Virginia, North Carolina, Georgia, and Maryland.

A number of species of ticks are found infected with *R. rickettsii* in nature, but only two are important in transmitting spotted fever to man. These are *Dermacentor andersoni*, the wood tick, which is the principal vector in the West, and *D. variabilis*, the dog tick, which assumes this role in the East. Infected female ticks transmit the agent transovarially to at least some of their offspring. Ticks which become infected, either through the egg or at one of the stages during their development cycle by feeding on an infected mammal, harbor the rickettsias throughout their lifetime, which may be several years. Thus, the tick serves as a reservoir in addition to being a vector. Small wild mammals are suspected of playing an important role in spreading the rickettsias in nature by infecting ticks which feed on them during rickettsemia.

Disease in man is generally acquired from the bite of an infected tick. Transmission is unlikely unless the tick remains attached for a number of hours. Infection may also be acquired through abrasions in the skin which become contaminated with infected tick feces or tissue juices; hence, the hazard associated with crushing ticks between the fingers when removing them from persons or animals.

There are seasonal variations in the incidence of cases of spotted fever, as well as differences in age and sex distribution of cases. In each instance these differences are related to exposure to ticks. Most cases are seen during the period of maximal tick activity, i.e., late spring and early summer. About half the cases in the Western states occur in men over forty, whereas half those in the Eastern states are in children under fifteen. This age distribution is undoubtedly influenced by propinquity to the wood and dog ticks, respectively. Mortality increases with age of the patient.

CLINICAL MANIFESTATIONS Incubation period and prodromata A history of tick bite is elicited in approximately 80 percent of patients. The incubation period varies between 3 and 12 days, with a mean of 7. A short incubation period usually indicates a more serious infection.

Onset In nonvaccinated persons, the onset is usually abrupt, with severe headache, a sudden shaking rigor, prostration, generalized myalgia, especially in the back and leg muscles, nausea with occasional vomiting, and fever which reaches 103 to 104°F within the first 2 days. Pain in the abdominal muscles may be severe, and arthralgia is not uncommon. Deep muscle palpation often elicits tenderness. Occasionally the debut of illness in children and adults is mild, accompanied by lethargy, anorexia, cephalgia, and low-grade fever. These symptoms are similar to those of many acute infectious diseases, making specific diagnosis difficult during the first few days.

Pyrexia Fever continues for approximately 15 to 20 days in untreated cases. The febrile course in children may be shorter. Hyperthermia of 105°F or greater is of unfavorable prognostic significance, although fatalities may occur when the patient is hypothermic, with concurrent vasomotor collapse. Fever generally terminates by lysis over a period of several days, but rarely does so by crisis. Recurrent fever is uncommon except in the presence of secondary pyogenic complications.

The *headache* is generalized and excruciating, and frequently more intense over the frontal area. It persists throughout the first and second week of illness in untreated cases. Malaise continues for the first week; irritability is notable, and the patient shuns distractions such as questioning and examination.

Cutaneous manifestations The rash which is present in practically all cases is the most characteristic and helpful diagnostic sign. It usually appears on the fourth febrile day; the range is 2 to 6 days. The initial lesions are on the wrists, ankles, palms, soles, and forearms. The first lesions are macular, nonfixed, pink, irregularly defined, and measure 2 to 6 mm. A warm compress applied to the extremity accentuates the rash in the early stages. The exanthem is most prominent when the temperature is elevated. After 6 to 12 hr, the rash extends centripetally to the axilla, buttocks, trunk, neck, and face. (This is in contrast to the eruption of typhus fever, which begins on the trunk and spreads centrifugally, rarely involving the face, palms, or soles.) The rash becomes maculopapular after 2 to 3 days (it may be felt by light palpation) and assumes a deeper red hue. By about the fourth day it is petechial and fails to fade on pressure. Not uncommonly, the hemorrhagic lesions coalesce to form large ecchymotic blemishes; these lesions tend to form over bony prominences and may ultimately slough to form indolent, slow-healing ulcers. Patients who have had the typical rash show brownish discolorations at the site for several weeks during convalescence. In milder cases, the rash does not become purpuric and may disappear within a few days. Antibiotic therapy may abort the early exanthem; the later fixed lesion fades less rapidly with specific therapy.

The application of tourniquets for several minutes, or the occasional taking of the blood pressure, may provoke additional petechiae (Rumpel-Leede phenomenon), further evidence of capillary abnormalities.

Cardiovascular and respiratory features During the early stages, the pulse is full and regular but accelerated in proportion to the height of the temperature, and the blood pressure is well sustained. During the peak of illness in seriously ill patients, the pulse is rapid and feeble, and hypotension of 90 mm Hg is common. If circulatory failure is sustained, the resultant hypoxia and shock lead to agitation and delirium and contribute to the formation of ecchymoses and gangrene of fingers, toes, genitalia, buttocks, earlobes, and nose. Cyanosis of the peripheral parts of the body is common. Venous pressure determinations show no elevation. A reduction of the total blood volume is occasionally found, as are evidences of myocardial impairment as shown by low voltage of ventricular complexes, minor S-T segment deflections, and occasionally delay in atrioventricular conduction on the electrocardiogram. These changes are transient and nonspecific. Severely ill patients have a puffy appearance of the face, hands, ankles, feet, and lower sacrum.

Respirations are either normal or slightly accelerated. Cough may be harassing and nonproductive, and localized pneumonitis may occur, but pulmonary consolidation is extremely rare. Pulmonary edema may develop after injudicious use of intravenous fluids.

Hepatic and renal manifestations In the majority of patients, there is little alteration in renal or hepatic function. The liver may be enlarged, but jaundice is unusual. Oliguria commonly occurs in the seriously ill, and anuria may mark the critically ill patient. Azotemia is common and when marked, is a very unfavorable sign. Abnormalities in liver function are probably responsible for the hypoproteinemia, with reduction in the albumin fraction.

Neurologic manifestations The principal neurologic manifestations are headache, restlessness, and varying degrees of insomnia. Stiffness of the back is common. The cerebrospinal fluid is clear, with normal dynamics and normal chemical constituents. Coma and muscular rigidity may occur. Athetoid movements, convulsive seizures, and hemiplegia are grave manifestations. Deafness during the active stages of the disease is not uncommon. As a rule, all neurologic signs abate without residua. Findings based upon follow-up examinations and electroencephalograms may be interpreted as indicative of minor residual brain damage for a year or more following recovery of certain patients from Rocky Mountain spotted fever.

Other physical manifestations Patients become dehydrated, with extreme dryness of lips, gums, tongue, and pharynx. The skin is hot and dry, the conjunctivas are frequently injected, and the eyes suffused. Photophobia is common in the early stages of illness. Petechial hemorrhages may be noted in the conjunctivas or in the retina. The spleen is enlarged in approximately one-half the cases and is firm and nontender. Abdominal distention is frequent, and occasionally some degree of intestinal ileus is observed. Constipation is usual.

COURSE In mild and moderately severe cases given no specific antibiotic therapy, the disease abates within 2 weeks, and convalescence is rapid. In fatal cases death usually occurs during the latter part of the second week as a result of toxemia, vasomotor weakness, and shock or renal failure.

In vaccinated individuals who contract the disease, the illness is mild, with a short febrile course and an atypical rash.

COMPLICATIONS AND PROGNOSIS If the serious manifestations of spotted fever mentioned above are regarded as intrinsic parts of the disease, then complications are uncommon and consist mainly of secondary bacterial infections, namely, bronchopneumonia, otitis media, and parotitis. Thrombosis of major blood vessels may result in gangrene of a portion of an extremity. Hemiplegia and peripheral neuritis are rare sequelae.

The overall mortality rate for spotted fever was formerly about 20 percent. Death occurred in more than half of persons over forty years of age, but the mortality rate was much lower in children and young adults. Since the introduction of the broad-spectrum antibiotics and the development of more precise knowledge regarding correction of the physiologic abnormalities which develop during the disease, fewer deaths occur from this infection. Some of the fatalities can be attributed to failure to consider spotted fever in the differential diagnosis.

DIFFERENTIAL DIAGNOSIS During the early stages of infection before the rash has appeared, differentiation from other acute infections is difficult. History of tick bite while living or traveling in a highly endemic area is helpful. The rash of menigococcemia (Chap. 131) resembles Rocky Mountain spotted fever in certain aspects, because it is macular, maculopapular, or petechial in the chronic form, and petechial, confluent, or ecchymotic in the fulminant type. The meningococcic skin lesion is tender and develops with extreme rapidity in the fulminant form, whereas the rickettsial rash occurs on about the fourth day of disease and gradually becomes petechial. *Spotted fever is often confused with measles.* The exanthem of rubeola rapidly becomes confluent, while that of rubella *usually remains discrete.*

Murine typhus is a milder disease than Rocky Mountain spotted fever; the rash is less extensive, nonpurpuric, nonconfluent; and renal and vascular complications are uncommon. Not infrequently differentiation of these two rickettsial infections must await the results of specific serologic tests. Epidemic typhus fever is capable of causing all the pronounced clinical, physiologic, and anatomic alterations seen in patients with Rocky Mountain spotted fever, i.e., hypotension, peripheral vascular collapse, cyanosis, skin necrosis and gangrene of digits, renal failure with azotemia, and neurologic manifestations. However, the rash of classical typhus is noted initially in the axillary folds and on the trunk and later extends peripherally, rarely involving the palms, soles, or face. The serologic patterns in these two diseases are distinctive when specific rickettsial antigens are employed in tests. Moreover, louse-borne typhus is not recognized in the United States except in the form of Brill-Zinsser disease (recurrent typhus fever). Rickettsialpox, although caused by a member of the spotted fever group of organisms, is usually readily differentiated from Rocky Mountain spotted fever by the initial lesion, the relative mildness of the illness, and the early vesiculation of the maculopapular rash. The Weil-Felix reaction is positive in Rocky Mountain spotted fever and in murine and epidemic typhus, but is negative in rickettsialpox. Agglutinins against *Proteus* OX-19 and OX-2 appear in the serum of patients with spotted fever, but only those against OX-19 are generally found in murine and epidemic typhus.

THERAPY Certain physiochemical changes occurring in the patient seriously ill with one of the diseases of the typhus–spotted fever group should be understood before a therapeutic regimen is outlined. These changes are circulatory collapse, coma, oliguria and anuria, azotemia, anemia, hypoproteinemia, hypochloremia and hyponatremia and edema of the underlying tissues. These alterations are often absent in the mildly ill, and in them management is much less complicated. The therapeutic principles necessary for treatment of all rickettsioses are (1) specific chemotherapy and (2) supportive care. Attention to both is mandatory for the seriously ill patient first recognized late in the disease. During the first week in the moderately ill patient, supportive therapy may be less energetic, because specific chemotherapy usually suffices. The early mild case may be successfully treated at home; the later cases should receive hospital care.

Therapeutic measures advisable for the management of Rocky Mountain spotted fever will be described in detail. Variations of this regimen which apply to the other rickettsioses are described in subsections dealing with other diseases of the typhus–spotted fever group and Q fever.

Specific therapy Specific therapy is most effective when initiated during the early stages of disease coincident with the appearance of the rash. When therapy is delayed until the rash has become hemorrhagic and widespread, the response is less dramatic. The antibiotics of choice are chloramphenicol and the tetracyclines, which are effective because of their rickettsiostatic properties. They are not rickettsiocidal.

The following antibiotic regimen is considered optimal: for chloramphenicol, an initial dose of 50 mg per kg body weight, and for tetracycline, 25 mg per kg body weight. Subsequent daily doses are the same as the initial loading dose, with the requirement divided equally and given at 6- to 8-hr intervals. Antibiotic treatment is continued until the patient has improved and has been afebrile approximately 24 hr. In patients too ill to take oral medication, an intravenous preparation of one of the antimicrobials may be employed for the loading dose.

Adrenal cortical hormones may need to be utilized for their antitoxemic effects, in patients first observed late in the course of severe illness. Large doses for brief periods (5 to 7 days) are recommended.

Therapy with antibiotics is continued until the toxemia has abated, the general condition has markedly improved, and the temperature has remained at normal levels for 24 hr. In uncomplicated cases of spotted fever, there is symptomatic improvement within 24 hr and temperature becomes normal in 60 to 72 hr.

Supportive care Frequent turning of the patient relieves pressure from prominent bony parts and also militates against the development of aspiration pneumonia. Proper mouth care, with frequent swabbing of the oral cavity, may avert the development of parotitis and gingivitis. Sucking of the juice of a lemon or the oral use of glycerin or mineral oil is helpful.

A generous intake of protein should be provided by frequent feedings as soon as the disease is suspected, in order to avoid subsequent protein deficiency. Usually food is well tolerated by patients with rickettsial disease, and the daily diet should provide 3 to 5 g protein per kg normal body weight, with adequate carbohydrate and fat to make it palatable. When the patient is uncooperative, the diet may be supplemented by hourly liquid protein feedings via stomach tube, provided that there is no abdominal distention.

At the critical stage, when hypoproteinemia is present and changes in capillary permeability lead to edema and vascular embarrassment, careful attention must be given to parenteral hyperalimentation. When indicated by hematologic studies, whole-blood transfusions given slowly are helpful. Intravenous albumin may be particularly useful, because it aids in the reduction of tissue edema. The judicious administration of one of the plasma expanders at this stage may have a definite favorable effect upon impending circulatory collapse. If the patient is anuric and azotemia is pronounced, overloading the circulation with fluids should be avoided. The type and amount of parenteral therapy should be governed by clinical judgment and very careful laboratory studies. Frequent determinations of hemoglobin, hematocrit, electrolytes, and protein, sometimes at intervals of a few hours during crucial periods, are necessary in order to ascertain abnormalities and to permit institution of corrective measures. Dialysis is indicated when there is clear-cut evidence of acute tubular necrosis (Chap. 269).

COMPLICATIONS *Pyogenic complications*, including otitis media and parotitis, are encountered in patients severely ill with Rocky Mountain spotted fever and other rickettsioses. These localized infections respond to therapy with appropriate antibiotics combined with ordinary supplemental surgical measures.

Pneumonitis usually develops as a result of specific rickettsial action. The sputum is scant but should be examined to determine whether superimposed bacterial infection is present. Specific therapy is guided by the results of these laboratory studies. The pneumonitis generally responds to the antibiotic therapy the patient is receiving, but if staphylococcal pneumonia is suspected, a penicillinase-resistant penicillin should be added to the broad-spectrum drug.

Circulatory failure of peripheral or central origin is combated by careful administration of plasma expanders and fluids. Heart failure may develop from the disease or as a result of overzealous intravenous alimentation and is recognized by common signs of rapid pulse, gallop rhythm, and increase in venous pressure. When the clinical signs reveal unmistakable evidence of cardiac failure, digitalis should be employed. Oxygen therapy improves the cardiac and circulatory status and is helpful in hypoxic patients with involvement of the central nervous system.

PREVENTION Prevention is attained primarily by avoidance of tick-infested areas. When this is impractical, prophylactic measures include (1) spraying the ground with dieldrin or Chlordane for area control of ticks, (2) application of repellents such as diethyltoluamide or dimethylphthalate to clothing and exposed parts of the body, or in very heavily infested areas the wearing of clothing which interferes with attachment of ticks, i.e., boots and a one-piece outer garment, preferably impregnated with repellent, and (3) daily inspection of the entire body, including the hairy parts, to detect and remove attached ticks. In removing attached ticks great care should be taken to avoid crushing the arthropod, with resultant contamination of the bite wound; touching the tick with gasoline or whisky encourages detachment but gentle traction with tweezers applied close to the mouth parts may be necessary; the skin area should be disinfected with soap and water or other antiseptics. Similarly, precautions should be employed in removing engorged ticks from dogs and other animals, because infection through minor abrasions on the hands is possible. Vaccines containing *R. rickettsii* are available commercially and should be used for those exposed to great risk, namely, persons frequenting highly endemic areas and laboratory workers exposed to the agent. Because the broad-spectrum antibiotics are such excellent therapeutic agents in spotted fever, there has been less impetus for vaccination of persons who run only a minor risk of infection.

REFERENCES See end of Chap. 183.

177
OTHER TICK-BORNE RICKETTSIAL DISEASES

THEODORE E. WOODWARD

DEFINITION Boutonneuse fever, North Asian tick-borne rickettsiosis, and Queensland tick typhus, three diseases occurring in the Eastern Hemisphere, are caused by rickettsias closely related to one another and to the agent of Rocky Mountain spotted fever. Each is transmitted by the bite of an ixodid tick. These mild to moderately severe illnesses are characterized by an initial lesion (called *tache noire* in boutonneuse fever), a fever of several days to 2 weeks, and a generalized maculopapular erythematous rash which appears on about the fifth day and usually involves the palms and soles. Specific complement-fixing antibodies appear in the patients' serums during convalescence, but agglutinins to *Proteus* OX-19 (Weil-Felix reaction) are frequently found only in low titer.

ETIOLOGY AND EPIDEMIOLOGY The etiologic agents of these three diseases are all members of the spotted fever group of rickettsias. Together with *Rickettsia rickettsii* and *R. akari* they possess common group antigens which are readily demonstrated by agglutination and complement fixation.

Boutonneuse fever, which may be regarded as the prototype of the three, is caused by *R. conorii.* Modern serologic methods employing specific rickettsial antigens have shown this rickettsia to be the causative agent for a single widely disseminated disease known by various local names. Information on the distribution and etiology of the various tick-borne rickettsial diseases is contained in Table 175-1.

In general, the epidemiology of these tick-borne rickettsioses resembles that of spotted fever in the Western Hemisphere. Ixodid ticks and small wild animals maintain the rickettsias in nature; man, if he intrudes accidentally into the cycle, is a dead end in the transmission chain. In certain areas, the cycle of boutonneuse fever involves domiciliary environments, with the brown dog tick *Rhipicephalus sanguineus* as the dominant vector.

CLINICAL MANIFESTATIONS These three tick-borne rickettsioses, which occur in different parts of the Eastern Hemisphere, resemble one another closely. The clinical course is usually milder than that of spotted fever, with a shorter febrile period and fewer severe complications; fatalities are rare and generally limited to the aged and debilitated. The initial lesion, which is present in most cases at the onset of fever, heals slowly; the regional lymph nodes are enlarged. The rash usually remains papular and only in severe cases becomes hemorrhagic.

The clinical picture (including the primary lesion), the geographic location, and epidemiologic considerations are helpful in establishing the diagnosis. The typhus fevers, meningococcal infections, and measles must be considered in the differential diagnosis; the serologic reactions, i.e., Weil-Felix and complement fixation tests, are of value here.

TREATMENT AND PREVENTION Chloramphenicol and the tetracyclines are effective therapeutic agents for boutonneuse fever. Patients generally become afebrile after 2 to 3 days of treatment, and recovery is rapid. The therapeutic procedures are comparable to those used in spotted fever. Presumably these measures are also applicable to North Asian tick-borne rickettsiosis and Queensland tick typhus.

The major effective methods of control are concerned with avoidance of tick bites; these include application of newer repellents and prompt removal of attached ticks. Effective vaccines are not available commercially.

REFERENCES See end of Chap. 183.

178 RICKETTSIALPOX

THEODORE E. WOODWARD

DEFINITION Rickettsialpox is a mild, nonfatal self-limited, febrile illness caused by *Rickettsia akari,* which is transmitted from mouse to man by mites. It is characterized by an initial skin lesion at the site of the mite bite, a week's febrile course, and a papulovesicular rash.

ETIOLOGY AND EPIDEMIOLOGY Rickettsialpox was first recognized in New York City in 1946, and about 180 cases were reported annually for several years thereafter. It has been diagnosed in several other areas of the United States, and outbreaks have been reported in European Russia. The vector is a small, colorless mite, *Allodermanyssus sanguineus* (Hirst), which infests small mice and rodents. House mice serve as the reservoir of infection.

Rickettsia akari is morphologically and biologically similar to other rickettsias and is antigenically related to, but distinct from, *R. rickettsii,* the cause of Rocky Mountain spotted fever. Mice, guinea pigs, and fertile hen eggs are susceptible to experimental infection. Diagnostic antigens prepared from infected yolk sacs are used in complement fixation tests.

CLINICAL MANIFESTATIONS The initial skin lesion appears about 7 to 10 days after the mite bite as a firm red papule 1 to 1.5 cm in diameter. In a few days, the center vesiculates, and the papule is surrounded by an area of erythema. The regional lymph glands are moderately enlarged. The primary lesion, which is never painful, becomes covered with a black scab; it heals slowly, and a small scar is visible on separation of the crust.

The febrile phase begins 3 to 7 days following the initial lesion, and exanthem may accompany the fever or begin several days later. The onset of fever is sudden, with chilly sensations or frank chills, headache, sweats, myalgia, anorexia, and photophobia. The pyrexia ranges from 103 to 104°F and continues for about a week, occasionally with morning remissions.

The exanthem is maculopapular-vesicular, generalized in distribution, and may be abundant or scant. The lesions may involve the oral cavity but not the palms or soles. In a week, the vesicles dry and form scabs which eventually scale but leave no scar.

The constitutional symptoms are generally mild, and the course of illness is uncomplicated. No fatal cases have been reported.

The disease may be confused with chickenpox, which is different because it occurs usually in childhood and has no initial lesion and the papular cutaneous lesion is entirely transformed into a vesicle. Variola (smallpox) is accompanied by a more severe constitutional reaction, and the vesicles become pustules. The skin lesions of the other rickettsioses differ in their lack of vesiculation. The Weil-Felix reaction is usually negative in this rickettsial disease, but the specific complement fixation test is a useful laboratory diagnostic aid even though there is considerable crossing with materials from Rocky Mountain spotted fever.

TREATMENT AND PREVENTION Chloramphenicol and the tetracycline antibiotics are all effective for treating patients with rickettsialpox. The temperature reaches normal levels in about 2 days, and recovery is rapid.

Control measures should be directed toward elimination of house mice and the vector mites responsible for transmitting the disease.

REFERENCES See end of Chap. 183.

179 MURINE (ENDEMIC) TYPHUS FEVER

THEODORE E. WOODWARD

DEFINITION Murine typhus fever is an acute febrile disease caused by *Rickettsia mooseri* and transmitted to man by fleas. The clinical illness is characterized by fever of 9 to 14 days, headache, a maculopapular rash appearing on the third to fifth day, and myalgia.

ETIOLOGY AND EPIDEMIOLOGY *Rickettsia mooseri* resembles other rickettsias in morphologic properties, staining characteristics, and intracellular parasitism. Under the electron microscope *R. mooseri* contains dense masses of nuclear material in a less dense homogeneous protoplasmic substance, the whole of which is surrounded by a limiting membrane. It differs from *R. rickettsii* in that it always multiplies within the cytoplasm of cells, in contrast to the intranuclear and cytoplasmic positions of spotted fever rickettsias.

Invasion of the body by *R. mooseri* provokes specific and nonspecific immunologic responses. Utilizing highly purified antigens, specific antibodies may be demonstrated readily by complement fixation and agglutination reactions. The positive Weil-Felix reaction which occurs in this disease is nonspecific, because it is attributable to the presence of a common carbohydrate antigen in *Proteus* OX-19 and *R. mooseri* and because the reaction is also positive in epidemic typhus and spotted fever. Group-specific rickettsial antigens are common to both *R. mooseri* and *R. prowazeki*. Furthermore, both murine and epidemic rickettsias possess toxic factors which are lethal to mice and rats and can be neutralized by convalescent serum from man or lower animals.

The common vector of *R. mooseri* for rats and man is the rat flea (*Xenopsylla cheopis*). In nature, the rat louse (*Polypax spinulosis*) may transmit the agent among rodents. Customarily, rat fleas become infected on ingestion of blood from diseased rats; the rickettsias multiply within the intestinal cells of the arthropod and are excreted in the feces. Infection in man occurs following the flea bite and contamination of the broken skin by rickettsia-laden feces. Dried flea feces may also infect via the conjunctivas or the upper part of the respiratory tract.

Rats and mice are naturally infected with murine typhus, and although the rodent disease is nonfatal, viable rickettsias persist in the brain for variable periods.

Murine typhus is one of the most benign and widespread of the rickettsioses in the United States. Prevalent in the Southeastern and Gulf Coast states, it has been identified in most of the other states and in harbor centers throughout the world wherever rats and fleas abound. Through control of rats and their fleas a sharp decline in incidence has occurred since 1951, particularly in the Southern United States. In urban areas the disease is more prevalent during the summer and fall months and occurs predominantly among persons working in proximity to granaries or food depots. There has been an extension to certain rural areas when changing agricultural practices have provided rats with ready access to adequate food supplies.

CLINICAL MANIFESTATIONS **Incubation period and prodromata** The incubation period ranges from 8 to 16 days, with a mean of 10. Common prodromata are headache, backache, arthralgia, and chilly sensations. Nausea, malaise, and transient temperature rises may precede the true onset of disease.

Onset and general symptoms A frank shaking chill and repeated rigors are present at the onset, associated with a severe frontal headache and fever. This triad of headache, chill, and pyrexia is usually followed within a few hours by nausea and vomiting. Prostration, malaise, and weakness are sufficient to enforce cessation of activity in adults, in contrast to children, whose illness is less severe. Occasionally, mild symptoms make it difficult to define the actual onset.

Pyrexia The usual febrile course in murine typhus lasts for about 12 days in adults; the temperature ranges from 102 to 104°F but may reach 105 to 106°F in children. The temperature may reach high levels abruptly after onset or ascend in a stepwise manner during the first few days. With the appearance of the rash, fever is usually sustained, with partial daily remissions which occasionally reach normal levels in the morning. Defervescence is generally by lysis over several days but sometimes occurs by crisis. Transient mild fever of 100°F is not uncommon during early convalescence. A few patients experience only low-grade fever throughout, but this does not necessarily connote a mild illness.

Cutaneous manifestations The early lesions, which are sparse and discrete, are hidden in the axillas and inner surface of the arm. Most patients then develop with surprising suddenness a generalized, dull red macular rash of the upper part of the abdomen, shoulders, chest, arms, and thighs. The individual lesions are discrete and pea-size, with an ill-defined border, and fade on pressure during the first 24 hr. They later become maculopapular, in contrast to the exanthem of epidemic typhus, which is persistently macular. The distribution over the trunk with sparse involvement of the extremities, palms, soles, and face differs from the peripheral distribution and facial involvement of Rocky Mountain spotted fever. The murine rash generally appears initially on the fifth febrile day, but rarely it is seen concurrently with the onset of fever or developing as late as the seventh day.

Eighty percent of patients develop a rash which persists for 4 to 8 days and fades before defervescence. The cutaneous manifestations vary greatly in intensity and duration and may be fleeting. They are readily overlooked in dark-skinned patients, in whom they should be searched for by light palpation and indirect lighting.

Cardiovascular and respiratory features An irritating, nonproductive cough is frequent and is occasionally associated with moderate hemoptysis. Early in the second week, rales may be detected in the basilar lung areas. These changes are generally rickettsial rather than bacterial in origin and respond to the broad-spectrum antibiotics. Pulmonary congestion occurs in extremely ill and elderly patients.

Accelerated pulse, hypotension, and general circulatory weakness occur in this disease, although less frequently than in patients with epidemic typhus or Rocky Mountain spotted fever.

Neurologic manifestations Headache is the most common neurologic manifestation of murine typhus and may dominate the clinical picture. It is frontal and continues into the second week of illness. Stupor and prostration may occur in the second week, and in severe cases, there may be muttering delirium, extreme agitation, or coma. Coma in elderly patients after 2 weeks of illness presages death. Nuchal rigidity and general spasticity often suggest meningitis, although the spinal fluid is normal except for slight increases in pressure and lymphocytes (5 to 30 per mm^3). Transient partial deafness occurs occasionally, but rarely is there localized neuritis or hemiplegia. Neurologic sequelae are unusual. Children experience minimal neurologic changes.

Other physical manifestations During the first 2 days of illness the patient may be nauseated and vomit, but vomiting later in the illness should arouse suspicion of an intercurrent complication. Abdominal pain is bothersome; when associated with diarrhea it responds to intravenous alimentation. Hepatomegaly and jaundice are unusual. There is splenomegaly in approximately 25 percent of patients.

Photophobia, retroocular pain, suffusion of the eyes, and congestion of the conjunctivas are common but are less severe than in the other typhus and spotted fevers.

Renal function is usually unaltered except in elderly patients with prolonged hypotension. Under these circumstances, azotemia may develop to the degree observed in epidemic typhus. In severe murine typhus, as in the epidemic typhus, hyponatremia and hypoalbuminemia are encountered.

COURSE After defervescence, murine typhus patients recover rapidly. Fatalities occur between the ninth and twelfth days in elderly or debilitated patients, usually as a result of circulatory and renal failure or intercurrent bacterial infection.

PROGNOSIS The mortality rate in murine typhus was low even before the introduction of modern specific therapy. Only one death occurred in 114 cases studied by Maxcy and none in the 180 reported by Stuart and Pullen.

DIFFERENTIAL DIAGNOSIS Because murine typhus and Rocky Mountain spotted fever occur in many of the same states, the problem of differential diagnosis often arises. Flea-borne murine typhus, which is predominantly an urban disease, is more likely to occur in late summer and autumn. In contrast, spotted fever is a rural and suburban disease in which exposure to ticks is important. Most cases occur in the spring and summer.

TREATMENT AND PREVENTION The therapeutic procedures are comparable to those used in spotted fever. Both chloramphenicol and the tetracycline antibiotics have controlled the disease.

Prevention of murine typhus in man is attained by reducing the natural reservoir and vector by applying measures for eliminating rodents and employing DDT in rat-infested areas to control fleas.

REFERENCES See end of Chap. 183.

180
EPIDEMIC TYPHUS FEVER AND BRILL-ZINSSER DISEASE

THEODORE E. WOODWARD

EPIDEMIC (LOUSE-BORNE) TYPHUS FEVER

DEFINITION The classical epidemic form of typhus is a severe, febrile disease caused by *Rickettsia prowazeki* and transmitted to man by the body louse. Intense headache, continuous pyrexia of about 2 weeks, a macular skin eruption appearing on about the fifth febrile day, malaise, and vascular and neurologic disturbances represent the principal clinical features. Confirmation of the diagnosis is made by demonstration of *Proteus* OX-19 agglutinins and of specific complement-fixing antibodies in convalescence. The broad-spectrum antibiotics are specific therapeutic agents.

ETIOLOGY AND EPIDEMIOLOGY The causative microbe, *R. prowazeki*, is closely related to *R. mooseri*, which causes murine typhus; indeed, the two have a number of common antigens.

Man generally is infected when rickettsia-laden louse feces are rubbed into the broken skin; scratching the louse bite facilitates this process. *Pediculus humanus corporis*, which is peculiarly adapted to man, is the only important vector of epidemic typhus. It dies of its infection and fails to transmit rickettsias to its offspring. There is no known animal habitat of *R. prowazeki*; it is maintained by a cycle involving man-louse-man. New epidemics apparently originate from patients with Brill-Zinsser disease (recurrent epidemic typhus). Inhalation of dust containing dried louse feces may rarely cause infection.

Epidemic typhus, if uncontrolled, behaves as a cyclic disease in a susceptible population, extending over a 3-year period. During the first year there is a gradual seeding of cases throughout the group; during the second there is epidemic spread; and during the third the epidemic tapers off, because the majority of persons have become immune. Outbreaks of epidemic typhus last occurred in the United States in the nineteenth century, and its presence is now recognized only in the form of Brill-Zinsser disease.

CLINICAL MANIFESTATIONS Epidemic typhus resembles murine typhus but is more severe. After an incubation period of about 7 days an abrupt onset of headache, chill, and rapidly mounting fever ushers in the illness. Headache, malaise, and prostration continue unabated until the rash appears on the fifth febrile day. It is initially macular in the axillary folds but ultimately invades the trunk and extremities as a pink, irregular macular lesion which becomes fixed, petechial, and confluent in the later stages.

Neurologic features range from headache and general spasticity to extreme agitation, stupor, and coma. Circulatory disturbances consisting of tachycardia, hypotension, and cyanosis are more profound than those observed in murine typhus and are almost as severe as in Rocky Mountain spotted fever. Ultimately, in untreated cases azotemia often reaches high levels as a result of vascular and renal failure, and death occurs late in the second week of illness. Furthermore, thrombosis of major blood vessels and cutaneous gangrene develop in a manner similar to that seen in the virulent form of Rocky Mountain spotted fever.

The complications and sequelae of epidemic typhus are more severe than those in murine typhus, but not as severe as those in Rocky Mountain spotted fever. However, during certain outbreaks, epidemic typhus was fatal in 60 percent of those infected, and convalescence in survivors was prolonged. Broad-spectrum antibiotics have eradicated mortality in this dread disease, provided therapy is instituted before irreversible changes have been established in the tissues.

DIFFERENTIAL DIAGNOSIS Differentiation of epidemic typhus from the various rickettsioses and other diseases with which it may be confused is described in Chap. 176. The disease in epidemic form never occurs in the absence of lousiness in the general population. Under the conditions in which typhus epidemics are likely to occur, other diseases which may cause confusion include malaria, relapsing fever, pneumonia, and tuberculosis. Classic typhus contracted by a previously vaccinated person is usually mild and may be clinically indistinguishable from murine typhus except by serologic methods.

TREATMENT AND PREVENTION Both chloramphenicol and the tetracycline antibiotics have been found to be highly efficient therapeutic agents in epidemic typhus. Usually the patient becomes afebrile after 2 days of treatment. The therapeutic procedures are comparable to those used in spotted fever.

The most effective measures for controlling epidemic typhus are those which eliminate lousiness. DDT or lindane powder when dusted into clothing is suitable for this purpose. If resistant lice are found, malathion may prove effective.

A commercially available vaccine prepared from formalin-treated suspensions of infected yolk sac tissue is an effective immunizing agent. A viable vaccine utilizing an attenuated strain of *R. prowazeki* is under development.

BRILL-ZINSSER DISEASE (RECRUDESCENT TYPHUS)

DEFINITION Brill-Zinsser disease is a recrudescent episode of epidemic typhus fever which occurs years after the initial attack, in persons who had recovered from the epidemic disease acquired while residing in countries where it was prevalent. *Rickettsia prowazeki* have been isolated from lice fed on patients during the active stages of illness.

CLINICAL MANIFESTATIONS The clinical entity, not always mild, resembles epidemic typhus in the character of the rash, circulatory disturbances, and hepatic, renal, and nervous system changes. Recovery is the rule. The Weil-Felix reaction with the various *Proteus* antigens is usually negative, or positive in very low titer. The specific complement fixation reaction is valuable in establishing the diagnosis. In Brill-Zinsser disease the specific complement-fixing antibodies appear as early as the fourth day after the onset of illness; the peak response is attained by the eighth to tenth days. Specific antibody titers in the primary attack of epidemic typhus begin later, about the eighth to twelfth day, with maximum titers on about the sixteenth day after onset. Antibodies in Brill-Zinsser disease and the primary attack are associated with 7S and 19S globulins, respectively. Therapy is like that used in spotted fever.

REFERENCES See end of Chap. 183.

181 SCRUB TYPHUS

THEODORE E. WOODWARD

DEFINITION Scrub typhus is limited to eastern and southeastern Asia, India, northern Australia, and the adjacent islands. It is caused by *Rickettsia tsutsugamushi* and characterized by a primary lesion at the site of the bite of an infected mite, a fever of about 2 weeks' duration, a cutaneous rash which develops about the fifth day, and the appearance late in the second week of agglutinins against the OX-K strain of *Proteus* bacillus. The broad-spectrum antibiotics are specific therapeutic agents.

ETIOLOGY The agent of scrub typhus resembles other rickettsias in its physical properties but differs from them in antigenic structure, vector, and reservoir. The disease is transmitted by larvae of several species of mites, especially *Trombicula akamushi* and *T. deliensis.* These tiny chiggers attach themselves to the skin and during the process of obtaining a meal of tissue juice may acquire infection from the host or transmit rickettsias to the vertebrate. The infection is maintained in nature by a cycle involving mites and small rodents and by transovarial transmission in mites; human infection represents an accident attributable to propinquity.

CLINICAL MANIFESTATIONS About 10 to 12 days after infection, illness begins abruptly with chilliness, severe headache, fever, conjunctival injection, and moderate generalized lymphadenopathy which is most prominent in the nodes draining the area of the primary lesion. The initial lesion at the beginning of fever is evidenced by an erythematous indurated area 1 cm in diameter, surmounted by a multiloculated vesicle; within a few days the vesicle ulcerates and becomes covered with a black crust.

Fever increases progressively during the first week, generally reaching 104 to 105°F, but the pulse remains relatively slow, 70 to 100 per min. The red macular rash, which begins on the trunk about the fifth day and spreads to the extremities, sometimes becomes maculopapular but usually fades in a few days. The course of the disease and the complications resemble those of endemic and epidemic typhus; however, interstitial myocarditis is more prominent than in the other typhus fevers.

PROGNOSIS Prior to the introduction of the broad-spectrum antibiotics the mortality rate varied from 1 to 60 percent, depending on the geographic area and the virulence of the local strains of *R. tsutsugamushi*, and convalescence was prolonged. With modern therapeutic methods, deaths are extremely rare and convalescence is short.

DIFFERENTIAL DIAGNOSIS Scrub typhus is to be differentiated from the other members of the typhus and the spotted fever group of diseases as well as from measles, typhoid fever, and the meningococcal infections. The geographic localization of scrub typhus, the primary lesion, and the occurrence of OX-K agglutinins are especially useful in establishing the diagnosis.

TREATMENT AND PREVENTION Chloramphenicol and the tetracycline antibiotics are valuable specific therapeutic agents in scrub typhus. The therapeutic procedures are comparable to those used in spotted fever. In fact, scrub typhus is more amenable to drugs than are the other rickettsial infections, and patients with this disease regularly become afebrile and are decidedly improved within 24 to 36 hr after beginning treatment, irrespective of the stage of disease.

Prevention of disease in the individual is accomplished by the application of miticidal chemicals (dibutyl phthalate, benzyl benzoate, diethyltoluamide, and others) to clothing and the skin. There is no satisfactory vaccine.

REFERENCES See end of Chap. 183.

182 Q FEVER

THEODORE E. WOODWARD

DEFINITION Q fever is an acute infectious disease caused by *Coxiella burnetti* and characterized by a sudden onset of fever, malaise, headache, weakness, anorexia, and interstitial pneumonitis. Rickettsemia occurs during the febrile period, and specific complement-fixing antibodies are present during convalescence. In contrast to the other rickettsioses, the disease is not associated with a cutaneous exanthem or agglutinins for the *Proteus* bacteria (Weil-Felix reaction).

ETIOLOGY AND EPIDEMIOLOGY *Coxiella burnetii* possesses the general properties of other rickettsias but is somewhat more resistant to inactivation in unfavorable environments and more pleomorphic than the others. Its infectivity after drying under natural conditions is of importance in the spread of infection to man. *Coxiella*

burnetii has a wide host range in nature, but guinea pigs and embryonated eggs are the common laboratory hosts employed for its propagation.

Human cases of Q fever are contracted by inhalation of infected dusts, by handling infected materials, and possibly by drinking milk contaminated with *C. burnetii.* The disease in Australia is enzootic in animals, especially bandicoots, and is transmitted in nature by ticks. Rickettsia-laden tick feces may contaminate cattle hides, and inhalation of this material has caused infection in man. In the United States, a number of species of ticks are naturally infected, among them *Dermacentor andersoni* and *Amblyomma americanum*, and in North Africa transovarial transmission of the agent in indigenous ticks has been demonstrated. Sheep, goats, and cows have been found to be naturally infected in North America and in Europe, and *C. burnetii* has been recovered from the milk of such animals. Milk, as well as infected excretions from livestock, probably accounts for certain outbreaks of human disease following inhalation by cows of infected dust from barns and pens. The airborne route of dried contaminated material is the most likely method of spread. A number of epidemics have occurred among laboratory workers engaged in studies on *C. burnetii.* The disease is not transmitted from man to man.

CLINICAL MANIFESTATIONS After incubation of approximately 19 days (the range is 14 to 26), the disease begins with headache, chilly sensations, fever, malaise, myalgia, and anorexia. For several days, the temperature ranges from 101 to 104°F; the entire course rarely exceeds 2 weeks and usually ranges from 3 to 6 days. There may be wide fluctuations in the fever. Respiratory and gastrointestinal symptoms are not conspicuous in the early stages. Headache and fever predominate. A dry cough and chest pain occur after about 5 days, when rales are usually audible. Roentgenographic findings indistinguishable from those of primary atypical pneumonia are present usually by the third to fourth day of disease, first as patchy areas of consolidation involving a portion of one lobe, giving a homogeneous ground-glass appearance. These manifestations persist beyond the febrile period and may appear in patients who are unaware of pulmonary involvement. Complications are rare, and coincident with defervescence the appetite begins to return. Convalescence progresses slowly for several weeks, during which time the principal disability is weakness. It is not uncommon for patients to lose 15 to 20 lb during the active stages of disease. The disease may be protracted in approximately 20 percent of cases, with fever persisting for longer than 4 weeks, particularly in elderly patients. Occasionally relapse occurs, especially in patients treated with antibiotics during the first several days of disease.

Hepatitis, with the development of clinically detectable icterus, occurs in approximately one-third of patients with the protracted form. This form of Q fever is characterized by fever, malaise, absence of headache or respiratory signs, and hepatomegaly with right upper quadrant pain. Liver biopsy specimens show diffuse granulomatous changes with multinucleated giant cells and scattered infiltrations of polymorphonuclear leukocytes, lymphocytes, and macrophages. *Coxiella burnetii* may be demonstrated in such specimens with the fluorescent antibody technique. Therefore, Q fever must be included in the differential diagnosis of liver granulomas such as tuberculosis, sarcoidosis, histoplasmosis, brucellosis, tularemia, syphilis, and others.

Endocarditis also has been reported, and *C. burnetii* has been identified by smear and isolation in vegetations on the heart valves obtained at operation or autopsy. The aortic valve is most commonly involved. It is important, therefore, to suspect the possibility of Q fever in cases of apparent subacute bacterial endocarditis with persistently negative blood cultures. Operative intervention with replacement of damaged valves may be necessary for recovery because the available antibiotics are not rickettsicidal. A high complement-fixing antibody titer is present in both endocarditis and granulomatous hepatitis.

PROGNOSIS Few fatalities have been recorded and, except for the patient with protracted illness and hepatic involvement or endocarditis, the course of disease is generally uncomplicated and benign.

TREATMENT AND CONTROL The tetracycline antibiotics and chloramphenicol are effective in the treatment of patients with Q fever. Most patients, when treated early in the course of disease, respond promptly and recover without relapses. The therapeutic procedures are comparable to those used in spotted fever.

Control of Q fever depends primarily on immunization of susceptible persons with specific vaccines. Vaccines made from phase I rickettsias are potent and afford considerable protection to slaughterhouse and dairy workers, herders, rendering-plant workers, woolsorters, tanners, laboratory workers, and others at risk. Measures should be taken to avoid exposure to infected aerosols; milk from infected domestic livestock must be pasteurized or boiled.

REFERENCES See end of Chap. 183.

183
TRENCH FEVER

THEODORE E. WOODWARD

DEFINITION Trench fever is a febrile disease transmitted from man to man by the body louse, *Pediculus humanus corporis.* It is characterized by a sudden onset with headache and severe pain in the muscles, bones, and joints. In most cases, the fever and other symptoms assume a relapsing character. Fatalities are rare. The disease is also known as shin bone fever, Volhynia fever, His-Werner disease, and Quintan fever.

ETIOLOGY AND EPIDEMIOLOGY *Rickettsia quintana*, the etiologic agent, grows extracellularly in the louse gut, in contrast to other pathogenic rickettsias which can multiply only within cells. A European strain of *R. quintana* has been cultivated on blood agar, and typical trench fever has been induced in volunteers.

Man is the only known reservoir of infection. The louse does not transmit the organism transovarially but acquires its infection by ingesting the blood of a person with rickettsemia. The organisms multiply extracellularly in the louse gut, without injury to this host, and are excreted in large numbers with the feces. Man becomes infected by the inoculation of the contaminated feces into his abraded skin or conjunctivas. *Rickettsia quintana* may be recovered periodically from human blood for several years after convalescence from an acute attack. Trench fever is known to exist in Mexico, Tunisia, Eritrea, Poland, the U.S.S.R., and possibly China.

PATHOLOGY Since there have been no recorded fatalities, histologic examination has been confined to excised macules of the skin, which have shown nonspecific perivascular infiltrates without the involvement of the vessel walls that is seen in typhus fever.

CLINICAL MANIFESTATIONS A variety of clinical manifestations is displayed in trench fever, ranging from a mild afebrile disease to a debilitating illness with a protracted clinical course involving numerous relapses. Following an incubation period of 10 to 30 days the onset may be insidious or dramatically abrupt. The acute disease is characterized by malaise, headache, fever, and bone and body pain, especially severe in the shins. In some cases only one fever peak occurs; in others the fever continues for 5 to 7 days; and in others there is an initial febrile episode lasting 1 to 3 days followed by relapses which characteristically occur at 4- to 5-day intervals. In some cases the fever and symptoms are continuous for 2 or 3 weeks. Enlargement of the spleen and a red macular rash occur in 70 to 80 percent of the cases. Pain and soreness in the muscles usually recur with each febrile relapse.

The disease is marked by a persistent rickettsemia, which is present during the initial attack and which continues during the relapses, throughout the asymptomatic periods between relapses, and for months or even years after cessation of physical symptoms. A relapse has been reported 10 years after the original attack.

PROGNOSIS The disease causes no known deaths, but its duration is variable. About 85 percent of patients are able to return to work within 2 months of onset, but about 5 percent of all cases become chronic. Recovery is even more delayed in the aged and debilitated.

DIFFERENTIAL DIAGNOSIS During epidemics, typical cases are easily diagnosed on the basis of symptoms. The disease may be differentiated from influenza, typhoid, typhus, dengue, and relapsing fever by the specific laboratory tests available for the diagnosis of each of these diseases.

TREATMENT AND PREVENTION *Rickettsia quintana* is highly sensitive in vitro to the broad-spectrum antibiotics, but no reliable information has been obtained about the value of these drugs in treating trench fever. The treatment is symptomatic. Aspirin is used to control pain and discomfort, but codeine may be necessary. The patient should remain in bed for a week or more after complete cessation of subjective and objective evidence of infection. He should be kept under observation for several months and returned to bed at the first sign of relapse.

The methods employed to control epidemic typhus should be equally efficacious in controlling trench fever. These are based on the elimination of lousiness and the improvement of living conditions with provision for frequent bathing and washing of clothing. DDT or lindane powder should be applied by hand or power duster at appropriate intervals to clothes and persons of populations living under conditions favoring lousiness. If resistant lice are found, malathion or other effective lousicides may be substituted as a dusting powder.

REFERENCES
(Chaps. 175 to 183)

ANDREW R et al: Tick typhus in North Queensland. Med J Aust 2:253, 1946

BLAKE FG et al: Studies on tsutsugamushi disease (scrub typhus, mite-borne typhus) in New Guinea and adjacent islands: Epidemiology, clinical observations and etiology in the Dobadura area. Am J Hyg 41:243, 1945

DERRICK EH: The epidemiology of Q fever: A review. Med J Aust 1:245, 1953

FERGUSON IC et al: Clinical, virological and pathological findings in a fatal case of Q fever endocarditis. Brit J Clin Pathol 15:235, 1962

GEAR J: The rickettsial diseases of Southern Africa: A review of recent studies. S Afr J Clin Sci 5:158, 1954

GREENBERG M: Rickettsialpox in New York City. Am J Med 4:866, 1948

HARRELL GT: Rocky Mountain spotted fever. Medicine 28:333, 1949

——: Rickettsial involvement of the nervous system. Med Clin North Am 37:395, 1953

LENNETTE EH: Epidemiology of Q fever. Arch Inst Pasteur (Tunis) 36:521, 1959

MARMION BP, STOKER MGP: The epidemiology of Q fever in Great Britain: An analysis of the findings and some conclusions. Br Med J 2:809, 1958

MAXCY KF: Typhus fever in the United States. Public Health Rep (Washington) 44:1735, 1929

MOHR CO, SMITH WW: Eradication of murine typhus fever in a rural area. Bull WHO 16:255, 1957

MOULTON FR (ed): *The Rickettsial Diseases of Man*, Washington: American Association for the Advancement of Science, 1948

MURRAY ES et al: Brill's disease: I. Clinical and laboratory diagnosis. JAMA 142:1059, 1950

——, SNYDER JC: Brill's disease: II. Etiology. Am J Hyg 53:22, 1951

ORMSBEE RA et al: The influence of phase on the protective potency of Q fever vaccine. J Immunol 92:404, 1964

PRATT HD: The changing picture of murine typhus in the United States. Ann NY Acad Sci 70:516, 1958

ROSE HM: The clinical manifestations and laboratory diagnosis of rickettsialpox. Ann Intern Med 31:871, 1949

SCHAFFNER W, KOENIG MG: Thrombocytopenic Rocky Mountain spotted fever. Arch Intern Med 116:857, 1965

SMADEL JE: Influence of antibiotics on immunologic responses in scrub typhus. Am J Med 17:246, 1954

——: Status of the rickettsioses in the United States. Ann Intern Med 51:421, 1959

——(ed): *Symposium on Q Fever*, Med Sci Publ 6, Washington: Walter Reed Army Institute of Research, 1959

——, JACKSON EB: Rickettsial infections, in *Diagnostic Procedures for Viral and Rickettsial Diseases*, 3d ed, New York: American Public Health Association, 1964, p. 743

SNYDER JC: Typhus fever rickettsiae, in *Viral and Rickettsial Infections of Man*, 4th ed., eds FL Horsfall, Jr., I Tamm, Philadelphia: Lippincott, 1965, p. 1059

STRONG RP: Trench fever, in *Stitt's Diagnosis, Prevention and Treatment of Tropical Diseases*, 7th ed., New York: McGraw-Hill, 1944, p. 984

STUART BM, PULLEN RL: Endemic (murine) typhus fever: Clinical observations of one hundred and eighty cases. Ann Intern Med 23:520, 1945

VINSON JW: Etiology of trench fever in Mexico in *Industry and Tropical Health*: *V*, Boston: Harvard School of Public Health, 1964, p. 109

WOODWARD TE: Rickettsial diseases in the United States. Med Clin North Am 43:1507, 1959

184
INTRODUCTION TO VIRAL DISEASES

A. MARTIN LERNER

An introduction to viral diseases in a field advancing so rapidly is difficult. Animal models suggest that a number of degenerating diseases of the central nervous system, certain "collagen diseases," and some malignancies may be virus-induced. A more complete view of causes and manifestations of the usual viral diseases is unfolding. Attenuated vaccines against measles, rubella, mumps, and poliomyelitis are available. The era of antiviral prophylaxis and chemotherapy is dawning.

Though viruses may be cultured or seen by electron or fluorescent microscopy during some phases of viral illness, these techniques are usually not readily available, and to the physician caring for a patient, retrospective diagnoses based upon fourfold or greater rises in humoral antibodies are academic. The compelling need is for development of rapid means of virologic diagnosis.

GENERAL PROPERTIES AND CLASSIFICATION Viruses are grouped according to their biophysical characteristics: (1) nucleic acid, (2) size, (3) sensitivity to ether, (4) presence of an envelope, and (5) symmetry (cubic or helical). They contain macromolecular cores of ribonucleic acid (RNA) or deoxyribonucleic acid (DNA). They do not contain both types of nucleic acid or ATP-generating enzymes, as do chlamydozoaceae (psittacosis, lymphogranuloma, trachoma, inclusion conjunctivitis) and rickettsia. They exhibit marked species and organ specificity. Viruses infecting plants, insects, rickettsia, bacteria, other animals, and man have been found.

Human viruses range in size from 17 nm (picornavirus) to 300 nm (poxvirus). They may be naked and contain only nucleic acid (genome) which is protected by a closed shell or tubing, the capsid. Other viruses contain a lipid envelope, acquired during maturation as virus evaginates from the nucleus (*Herpesvirus hominis*) or cytoplasm (influenza, *H. hominis*). The capsid consists of protein and is composed of repeating subunits, capsomeres. Mature virus particles are called virions (Fig. 184-1).

The nucleic acid contains all the genetic material necessary to reproduce itself (transcription) and the code for structural proteins and enzymes (translation) important in synthesis and attachment to susceptible cells. The nucleic acid core plus the capsid is known as the nucleocapsid (Fig. 184-1). When the virion is stripped of its capsid, nucleic acid may enter a host of foreign species and produce a single cycle of mature virus (e.g., poliovirus in mouse renal cells). Species and organ specificities of virus-cell union are functions first of complementary physical characteristics and then of covalent union between proteins of the virus and susceptible cell membranes. For instance, molecules of neuraminic acid act as receptors on human red cells, allowing hemagglutination by influenza virus. Within several hours after virus adsorption, neuraminidase, one of the proteins of the influenza capsid, digests the neuraminic acid. Elution of influenza virus from red cells follows.

At present there are seven known groups of RNA viruses (picornavirus, reovirus, arbovirus, myxovirus, rhabdovirus, coronavirus, arenovirus) and four groups of DNA viruses (papovavirus, adenovirus, herpesvirus, poxvirus) (Table 184-1).

Nucleic acids of infectious and serum hepatitis viruses have not yet been identified. By electron microscopy these agents are seen to have cubic symmetry and are about 20 nm in diameter. Other viruses belonging to the parovirus and leukovirus groups have not been shown to affect man.

VIRUS MULTIPLICATION Virus adsorption is a specific physical and then chemical reaction. Capsids of reoviruses and enteroviruses may contain glycoproteins. Attachment involves free carbonyl groups. Sulfhydryl groupings on enteroviruses need to be intact. After absorption, virus enters the cell by pinocytosis and is uncoated; i.e., nucleic acid is stripped from the capsid. With DNA viruses, specific virus DNA strands are transcribed into specific mRNA, which is, in turn, translated to synthesize virus-specific proteins and enzymes necessary for biosynthesis of virus DNA. In the case of virus RNA, single-stranded RNA serves as its own messenger. The mRNA is translated, resulting in the formation of an RNA polymerase. Synthesis of host cell protein and nucleic acid is suppressed to variable degrees. Assembly of protein subunits around virus DNA results in formation of complete virions which may be released by cell lysis or budding from the cytoplasm. Recently, virions of RNA tumor viruses have been found to contain an

FIGURE 184-1
Components of a complete virus particle (virion).

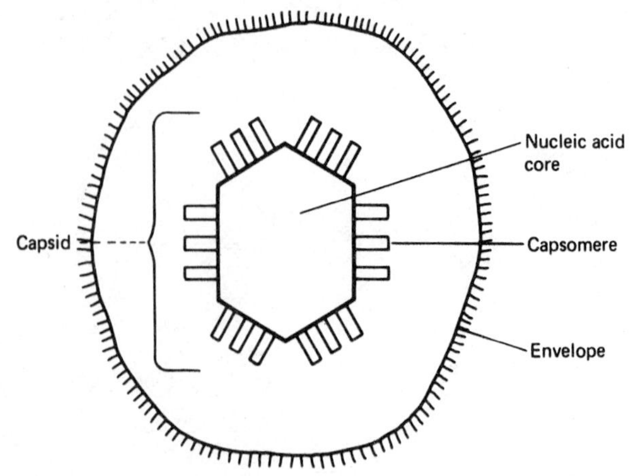

enzyme which is able to catalyze synthesis of DNA. The product consists of small fragments of DNA, most of which are complementary in base sequence to 70S RNA of the virion. Thus, information can travel not only from DNA to RNA but also, at least in certain cases, in the reverse direction.

ROUTES OF INFECTION Viruses, like fungi, bacteria, parasites, or rickettsia, infect man by respiratory, enteric,

TABLE 184-1
Major groups of viruses infecting man

Nucleic acid	*Size, nm*	*Ether sensitivity**	*Presence of envelope*	*Symmetry*
RNA				
Picornavirus	17–30	–	–	Cubic
Coxsackie virus A				
Coxsackie virus B				
Echo virus				
Poliovirus				
Rhinovirus				
Reovirus	74	–	–	Cubic
Arbovirus	20–100	+	?	
Group A (equine encephalitis, Semliki Forest)				
Group B (Japanese B, Russian tick-borne, yellow fever, dengue)				
Group C (Morituba, Oriboca)				
Ungrouped (Rift Valley, Colorado tick fever, sandfly)				
Myxovirus and paramyxovirus	80–200	+	+	Helical
Influenza A, influenza B, influenza C				
Parainfluenza				
Mumps				
Rubeola				
Respiratory syncytial				
Rhabdovirus: rabies	65–180	+	+	
Coronavirus		+	+	
Arenovirus				
Togavirus: rubella (most arboviruses of groups A and B)	50	+	+	
Tacaribe-LCM	50–300	+	+	
Lymphocytic choriomeningitis				
South American hemorrhagic fevers (Junin, Machupo)				
DNA				
Papovavirus	40–55	–	–	Cubic
"Warts"				
Simian virus 40				
Adenovirus	65–85	–	–	Cubic
Herpesvirus	120–180	+	+	Cubic
Herpesvirus hominis				
Monkey B				
Varicella–herpes zoster				
Cytomegalovirus				
Epstein–Barr				
Poxvirus	150–300	+ or –	+	Cubic
Variola				
Vaccinia				
Molluscum contagiosum				
Orf—milker's nodules				
Unclassified				
Human hepatitis				
Infectious hepatitis				
Serum hepatitis				

* +, yes; –, no.

or contact mechanisms. Coughs, sneezes, or ordinary speech give rise to infectious units. From human respiratory reservoirs droplets of water over 10 μm in diameter containing virus travel short distances, or droplet nuclei, minus moisture and less than 10 μm in diameter, are wafted in air over greater distances. Infection depends upon the number of virions circulating per cubic foot of air and the time of exposure. For instance, if an aerosol contains four virions per liter of air, and 30 virions are required for infection, then persons breathing this air will inspire an infectious dose within a half-hour. The paucity of respiratory infections, usually caused by rhinoviruses, during summer may, in part, be due to open windows and frequent exchange of air.

Fecal-oral contamination is usual with enteroviruses (Coxsackie viruses A and B and polioviruses). Occasionally, they, too, are spread by droplets or their nuclei. On the other hand, rabies virus in the saliva of a rabid dog reaches the victim's brain after a bite exposes peripheral nerve endings. Contaminated urines disseminate rubella or cytomegaloviruses. Blood, plasma, or buffy coat transmits herpesviruses and viruses of infectious or serum hepatitis. Insect vectors (arboviruses) or life cycles in other animal species may be important (arboviruses, lymphocytic choriomeningitis). Infection via ovum or sperm is possible but has not been demonstrated in man.

PATHOGENESIS OF DISEASE The primary site of virus multiplication depends upon the route of acquisition. Respiratory viruses (rhinovirus, myxovirus, coronavirus, rubella, adenovirus, herpesvirus) multiply in upper respiratory epithelium, injuring, denuding, and slowing ciliary movements. Respiratory viruses in the nasopharynx may involve the conjunctivas via connecting lymphatics, producing serous conjunctivitis, as in the pharyngoconjunctival fever of adenovirus, type 3. Rhinoviruses and coronaviruses usually remain within the nasopharynx. Parainfluenza viruses involve larynx and trachea. Influenza A, adenoviruses, varicella-zoster, cytomegaloviruses, and enteroviruses may produce pneumonias. Adjacent areas of atelectasis and emphysema, mixed cellular infiltrates, and thickening of alveolar septums are common. Alveoli may be free or contain edema amid red cells, a modest number of mononuclear cells, and a few polymorphonuclear leukocytes. Virus-specific structures (inclusion bodies) may be present within the cytoplasm (variola), nucleus (*H. hominis*, varicella-zoster, adenovirus), or both (measles). Viremia may or may not occur. In many virus infections, in distinct contrast to bacteremias, viremia occurs during the incubation period when the patient is well. Viremia is usual with the exanthems of enteroviruses, rubeola, and varicella-zoster viruses. Herpesviruses may multiply within lymphocytes sequestered from antibodies and phagocytes.

Enteric viruses multiply in epithelium and lymphoid tissues first in the pharynx and later in the intestine. Lysis of affected cells (polioviruses) may follow. On the other hand, a slowly destructive, relatively symbiotic relationship ensues in subacute sclerosing panencephalitis (measles virus) and progressive multifocal leukoencephalopathy (papovavirus).

With enterovirus infections, viremia occurs early. Secondary sites of infection are the heart, liver, pancreas, kidneys, and brain. Echo and Coxsackie viruses multiply in the choroid plexus and seed cerebrospinal fluid; polioviruses do not grow within the choroid plexus. Therefore, echo and Coxsackie viruses are regularly isolated from cerebrospinal fluid, but polioviruses are rarely isolated from it.

RESPONSES OF THE HOST At sites of virus multiplication extracellular virus often abounds, and interferon and B and T lymphocytes are activated.

Interferon Viruses, endotoxin, certain parasites, double-stranded RNA of reoviruses, synthetic polyribonucleotide complexes such as poly rI:rC (polyinosinic polycytidilic ribonucleic acid) and synthetic anionic polymers stimulate interferon. Within several hours after onset of virus infection, and days before humoral antibodies can be measured by ordinary methods, interferon is found in tissues where virus is synthesized, and in the blood. Interferons of two classes are produced. The first, a high molecular weight protein (i.e., 8.5×10^4 daltons), is preformed and released within 2 hr. At 18 hr serum contains proteins with biologic activity of interferon with molecular weights of 3 to 4×10^4 daltons. Interferon is acid-stable (pH 2), trypsin-sensitive, nondialyzable, and nonsedimentable by ultracentrifuge forces sufficient to pellet viruses. Most cells tested produce interferon, but those of the reticuloendothelial system and lymphocytes are most important.

Interferon has no effect upon extracellular virus. Following entry of virus nucleic acid into a susceptible cell, the cell nucleus is stimulated to produce interferon, which is released through the cytoplasm of the infected cell to induce a second noninfected cell to release an antiviral protein distinct from interferon. This second protein is translational inhibitory protein (TIP). The TIP binds to cellular ribosomes and alters them so that virus RNA is not translated. Cellular messenger RNA is probably translated normally, permitting normal cell functions, but synthesis of virus-directed coat proteins and enzymes is prevented. New virus is not formed.

Interferons have activity against a wide variety of viruses and are not virus-specific. However, interferon is an effective antiviral substance only in cells of the same species in which it is produced. For instance, anti-influenza A interferon produced in hamster tissue cultures is effective against influenza in hamsters but not in man.

Viruses vary greatly in their sensitivity to interferon. Myxoviruses are sensitive, while herpesviruses are much more resistant. Likewise, the importance of interferon in recovery from virus infection varies. With Coxsackie virus B-3, interferon titers actually parallel virus titers. In patients with immunosuppressed herpes zoster, a delay in the appearance of interferon in vesicular fluids is associated with dissemination.

Antibodies Proteins of the virus capsid stimulate B lymphocytes to synthesize humoral and secretory antibodies. Immunoglobulins are produced in local lymph nodes, at body surfaces (saliva, respiratory secretions, colostrum), and in inflammatory exudates within organs (kidney, brain, cervix). During the first 3 to 10 days after the onset of virus infections, IgM antibodies predominate. Later, IgG antibodies usually prevail. Immunoglobulin M is important in clearing viremias, and remains within vascular spaces; IgG antibodies enter interstitial spaces. At surfaces, IgA antibodies contain an added secretory piece, allowing functional integrity in the presence of hydrolytic enzymes of the secretions. Many molecules of antibody combine with a single virion. Covering a critical number of essential sites on the virion renders an antigen-antibody complex noninfectious. Antigen-antibody complexes attract components of complement which are mediators of polymorphonuclear leukocytes. Immune complexes may be fixed in tissues, circulate, or precipitate at the glomerulus.

Secretory IgA antibodies in respiratory secretions are primary in defense against infection with respiratory viruses such as influenza and rhinoviruses. During rhinovirus infection of the nasopharynx, viremia does not occur regularly. Humoral antibodies persist only for months. Immunity is transient; reinfections with the same virus at a later time are possible. On the other hand, after systemic infections, humoral antibodies and immunity persist. Likewise, after killed virus vaccines immunity is briefer than with attenuated viruses. Antigenic mass and persisting virus may be important.

Antibodies to viruses are measured by neutralization of cytopathic effects in tissue cultures or by protection tests using embryonated eggs or animals. Complement fixation, precipitin, or radioimmunoassay techniques are also used. Certain viruses such as *H. hominis*, type 1, and cytomegalovirus form complement-requiring neutralizing antibodies early after infection. Myxoviruses, some enteroviruses, and reoviruses hemagglutinate several species of red blood cells. In these cases antibodies can be measured by inhibition of hemagglutination. Virus capsids of nonhemagglutinating viruses may be adsorbed to the surface of tanned sheep red blood cells. Antibodies are assayed by passive hemagglutination. Kinetics of rises and falls of the several antibodies suggest that different assays test separate immunoglobulin responses to distinct proteins of the capsid.

Cell-mediated immunity Thymic-derived T lymphocytes confer delayed immune functions. T lymphocytes are important in infections with some viruses (herpesviruses) but are less vital with others (picornaviruses). In most virus infections, both T and B lymphocytes participate in the containment of virus replication. After a latent period, stimulated human T lymphocytes transform to lymphoblasts. They release a number of nonspecific, nondialyzable effector molecules which migrate with albumin on electrophoresis. Among these effector molecules are lymphocyte-transforming factor, migration inhibitory factor, cytotoxin factor, and possibly interferon. Components of complement react with the surface of sensitized lymphocytes, releasing a chemotactic factor to monocytes, the phagocytes of cellular immunity.

Lysates of human lymphocytes release transfer factor, a dialyzable nonantigenic macromolecule (mol wt, approximately 10,000) which endows specific and prolonged delayed hypersensitivity. Transfer factor may be a double-stranded polynucleotide or polypeptide; it has been used experimentally in treatment of several diseases where cell-mediated immunity is deficient, such as disseminated vaccinia or mucocutaneous candidiasis. Inadvertently, transfer factor is passaged from donor to recipient during blood transfusions, relaying cellular immunity and hypersensitivity. When viruses multiply within lymphocytes, transient hypofunction probably ensues.

DIAGNOSIS Detection of virus infection depends upon isolation of the virus or recognition of virus antigen or of its immune response. Etiologic associations are more secure if virus is isolated or demonstrated by electron or fluorescence microscopy in diseased tissues. For instance, a definitive diagnosis of herpes simplex virus encephalitis is possible when *H. hominis*, type 1, is recovered from a brain biopsy. Isolations of Coxsackie virus B-5 from throat or feces in a case of acute myopericarditis are suggestive but insufficient to relate the disease in question to the recovered agent. A fourfold rise in specific antibodies in convalescent serum is also suggestive but, likewise, insufficient for definitive diagnosis. The finding of antibodies at the site of disease is a rapid means of stronger association. Antibodies are synthesized in B lymphocytes of inflammatory exudates in the brain. Spinal fluids from patients with subacute sclerosing panencephalitis or herpes simplex virus encephalitis often contain measles or *H. hominis* antibodies, respectively.

When diagnosis is required, acute specimens are obtained by swabbing the nasopharynx, throat, conjunctiva, or cervix. Urine, feces, respiratory secretions, vesicular fluids, blood, buffy coat, and cerebrospinal fluid may be collected. Swabs are transferred to the laboratory in balanced salt solution containing antibiotics to inhibit bacteria. Optimally, specimens are inoculated promptly into tissue cultures for incubation at 35°C. Recognition of virus particles by electron microscopy, or antigens by fluorescence microscopy by using specific antiserums allows immediate presumptive diagnosis. Sometimes specimens may be held for 24 to 48 hr prior to processing (echo viruses), but this is hazardous with many respiratory or herpesviruses. Concomitant use of human foreskin and rhesus kidney tissue cultures offers a broad spectrum of isolation media. Cell cultures must be observed for cytopathic effects daily for a minimum of 14 days. In other cases, inoculations into suckling mice (Coxsackie viruses, group A) or embryonated eggs (influenza) are required.

In contrast to most antibodies, complement-requiring neutralizing antibodies peak early, and fall during convalescence. Current antibody responses may be noted in single acute-phase serums by finding complement-requiring or 2-mercaptoethanol-sensitive (IgM) specific immunoglobulins. Types of antibodies usually measured have been discussed above.

PROPHYLAXIS AND THERAPY Vaccine prophylaxis with live or inactivated vaccines is available for poliomyelitis, measles, smallpox, mumps, rubella, influenza, rabies, and yellow fever. Under special circumstances inactivated vaccines against adenovirus and Japanese B, equine, and Russian spring-summer encephalitis are available. Vaccinia immune globulin (VIG) is effective in reducing the risk of smallpox in exposed susceptibles: VIG is also indicated when a person, at increased risk of generalized vaccinia, is given smallpox vaccine. Persons at increased risk of generalized vaccinia are those with eczema, burns, neurodermatitis, pyoderma, immunologic defects, white cell defects, malignancy, neurologic disease, and undiagnosed febrile illness.

Chemoprophylaxis against smallpox with oral N-methylisatin β-thiosemicarbazone (Marboran) is effective. Amantadine hydrochloride (Symmetrel) taken by mouth throughout the period of exposure to certain strains of influenza A is prophylactic. Amantadine is not effective against strains of influenza B. Topical idoxuridine (5-iodo-2′-deoxyuridine) and cytosine arabinoside (ara-C) are therapeutic in herpes simplex virus keratitis. These two agents and adenine arabinoside (ara-A, 9-β-D-arabinofuranosyladenine) are likely to be useful in disseminated herpes zoster in patients with immunosuppressed disease. Parenteral idoxuridine, ara-C, and ara-A are being tested experimentally in the treatment of *H. hominis*, type 1, encephalitis, and disseminated infections of the newborn with *H. hominis*, type 2, and cytomegalovirus. Corticosteroids suppress both T and B cells as well as chemotaxis, and should not be given during active virus multiplication.

REFERENCES

DAVIS BD et al: *Microbiology*, New York: Hoeber-Harper, 1967

HORSFALL FL JR, TAMM I: *Viral and Rickettsial Infections of Man*, 4th ed., Philadelphia: Lippincott, 1965

HOSKINS JM: *Virological Procedures*, New York: Appleton-Century-Crofts, 1967

JAWETZ E et al: *Review of Medical Microbiology*, 9th ed.; Los Altos, Calif: Lange, 1970

LAWRENCE HS: Transfer factor and cellular immune deficiency disease. N Engl J Med 283:411, 1970

TOMASI T: The gamma A globulins: The first line of defense. Hosp Prac 2:26, 1967

section 14 | Viral diseases of the respiratory tract

185 GENERAL CONSIDERATIONS OF RESPIRATORY VIRAL DISEASE

VERNON KNIGHT

The viral respiratory diseases as a group are responsible for one-half or more of all acute illnesses, and although influenza virus is the only agent among them which causes significant mortality in adults, several different viruses make a large contribution to the 20 percent of childhood mortality due to respiratory disease. Respiratory disease morbidity, due primarily to virus infections, causes 30 to 50 percent of time lost from work in adults, and from 60 to 80 percent of time lost by children from school. These diseases are worldwide, and although studies in many areas are scanty, reports from Great Britain, Western Europe, U.S.S.R., Czechoslovakia, Latin America, and the Orient indicate many common denominators in the problems of etiology, prevalence, and severity.

Viral respiratory diseases are associated with a spectrum of host responses ranging from asymptomatic carriers to severe and sometimes fatal pneumonias. There is a recurring pattern of severe illness in infants and young children and milder disease with increasing age. A few clinical and epidemiologic entities can be recognized without laboratory aids, such as acute respiratory disease (ARD) in military recruits, caused by adenovirus type 4, and rhinovirus coryza in adults. The causative agent in a large proportion of cases, however, cannot be identified without virologic study.

EPIDEMIOLOGY IN THE UNITED STATES There are at present more than 150 serotypes, representing 12 groups of viruses, which have been or may be associated with acute respiratory illness in man. With the capacity to isolate this large group of agents and with the recognition of the importance of the pleuropneumonia-like organism (PPLO), *Mycoplasma pneumoniae* (Chap. 187) in respiratory illness, it has been possible to define the cause of many respiratory illnesses. In all studies, a majority of illnesses was caused by viruses. It seems probable that the inability to identify etiologic agents is greater than can be accounted for by lack of efficient application of known diagnostic methods and that additional viral and possibly other causes of respiratory illness remain to be discovered. The recent identification of coronaviruses as a cause of respiratory illness increases the potential for diagnosis, but other etiologic agents undoubtedly remain to be discovered.

FREQUENCY AND SEVERITY There has also been considerable progress in determining the frequency of respiratory disease, chiefly as a result of the National Health Survey, which, since 1957, has made annual estimates from selected population samples of the incidence of acute respiratory illness in the United States. These studies were designed to measure the socioeconomic impact of illness, and cases were reported only if they caused restriction of daily activity or required medical care. There were 259 million cases of acute respiratory illness in the United States between July 1, 1961, and June 30, 1962, an average of 1.4 illnesses per person per year. A similar incidence has been noted in

TABLE 185-1
Percentage distribution by diagnosis of 259 million acute respiratory conditions: United States, July 1961 to June 1962

Condition	*Percentage of total*
Common cold	43.1
Influenza	28.6
The "virus"	9.6
Sinusitis, pharyngitis, tonsillitis, laryngitis, etc.	11.3
Pneumonia; Bronchitis; Influenza with digestive manifestations; Other	6.1
Streptococcus sore throat	1.3
Total	100.0

SOURCE: *Condensed from National Health Survey.*

every year of the survey. The percentage distribution of these illnesses according to clinical diagnosis (International Classification of Diseases, 1955 revision) is shown in Table 185-1.

Except for streptococcal sore throat, some cases of bacterial pneumonia, sinusitis, etc., the remaining cases were undoubtedly largely of viral origin. It seems that some illnesses were incorrectly reported as influenza, but in other respects, the diagnostic categorization correlates well with that in smaller studies in which the specific cause of respiratory disease has been determined.

As already indicated, the National Health Survey included only cases in which there was an appreciable severity of illness. For example, in the National Health Survey in the period of July 1961 to June 1962, loss of time from work or school averaged 4.2 days for the 80 percent (207 million) of cases in which some restriction of activity was reported. About 50 percent, or 130 million, of persons sought medical attention although at least 52 million reported no restriction of activity.

In other studies, milder illness has been included, with a corresponding rise in annual frequency of reported cases. The Cleveland Family Study found an annual rate of illness of 6.2 per person per year, amounting to an estimated more than 1 billion cases annually in the United States. The greatest proportion of these illnesses were so mild that they constituted no hazard to health, but they are of significance in the spread of infection. In addition, it is known that wholly asymptomatic virus infections occur.

AGE, SEX, AND SEASONAL VARIATION All studies have been in agreement that infants and young children have the greatest number of viral respiratory infections and that children under six may have twice as many illnesses per year as the average of the population. Females have more illness than males; the excess is most marked during adult years and amounts to about 25 percent.

There are prominent seasonal differences in the frequency of acute respiratory illnesses; the rates are highest in winter, with values approximating 30 cases per 100 persons per quarter. Illness is least frequent during the summer—about one-third of the maximum. Epidemics of influenza cause pronounced increases in wintertime frequency of respiratory illness and are the most significant cause of mortality among the respiratory viruses. In 1957, during the Asian influenza pandemic there were almost 50 cases of acute respiratory illness per 100 persons in the October to December quarter, the great majority of which were influenza.

ETIOLOGY The known viral causes of acute respiratory disease and their estimated relative frequency in adults

TABLE 185-2
Patterns of illness with respiratory viruses in older children and adults

Agent	*Relative frequency of occurrence*	*Rhinitis*	*Pharyngitis*	*Tracheobronchitis*	*Pneumonia*	*Constitutional*
Rhinoviruses	40	++	±	+	Rare	± (usually afebrile)
Influenza A, B	10	+	+	++	Severe when present	++ (high fever common)
Parainfluenza viruses	8	+	++	++*	Rare	+ (low or no fever)
Respiratory syncytial virus	6	++	+	+†	?	+ (usually afebrile)
Adenoviruses	2	+	++	++	Severe, when present	++ (high fever)
Coxsackie and echo viruses	<1	±	+	+	?	++ (fever, visceral and CNS complications)
Coronaviruses	33 (Coronaviruses, Herpesviruses, Other)	++	+	±	?	±
Herpesviruses		++	+	?	?	?
Other		?	?	?	?	?

Note: ++ = severe; + = moderately severe; ± = mild; ? = unknown or uncommon.
* Laryngeal involvement common.
† Especially in older patients.

and older children in relation to their common patterns of illness are shown in Table 185-2.

Viruses, as a group, probably cause three-fourths or more of acute respiratory illness, and nearly one-half of these illnesses are due to one of the rhinoviruses. The principal nonviral causes of respiratory illness are *M. pneumoniae* and hemolytic streptococci. In infants and young children most illnesses are due to respiratory syncytial virus, parainfluenza viruses, influenza A and B, and rhinoviruses. The proportion of illness caused by viruses as a group and individually is uncertain; but among the agents listed, all but coronaviruses are of known significance, and their role in infection is not yet defined.

In Table 185-3 is shown a current classification of the respiratory viruses based on size, structure, and biochemical and other properties. Adenoviruses and herpesvirus, which is an infrequent cause of respiratory illness, are DNA viruses, while the remainder possess RNA cores. Respiratory tract disease is not known to be associated with particular properties of the viruses except that the long incubation period of adenovirus infection may be related to its long cycle of replication. The relatively nonspecific response of the respiratory tract to virus infection probably indicates that the target cells of the respiratory tract (i.e., the respiratory epithelium), when damaged by infection, have a limited variability of pathologic response. Classification of viruses will certainly assume greater importance, however, as new chemotherapeutic agents are developed, since many of them will act on specialized viral functions unique to single or related groups of viruses.

CLINICAL SYNDROMES OF VIRAL RESPIRATORY DISEASE INCLUDING THE COMMON COLD

The descriptive term "common cold" was coined to describe the coryzal syndrome before its diverse causes were known. It refers to illness characterized by nasal obstruction and discharge, sneezing, moderate sore throat, and mild constitutional reaction, usually without fever. Patterns of illness shown in Table 185-2 demonstrate that most respiratory viral infections may produce this picture. However, in adults and older children, syndromes more or less restricted to these manifestations are caused by infection with rhinoviruses, respiratory syncytial virus, and coronaviruses. These three groups of viruses may account for as much as two-thirds of cases of acute respiratory viral disease. The other agents listed, while causing coryzal syndrome, also cause varying degrees of involvement of the lower part of the respiratory tract, with additional symptoms.

In the following chapter (Chap. 186) consideration is given to five of the seven groups of viruses chiefly responsible for respiratory disease, i.e., rhinoviruses, adenoviruses, respiratory syncytial viruses, parainfluenza viruses, and coronaviruses. Included also is a description of the small contribution to respiratory illness of the enteroviruses, Coxsackie viruses A and B, and echo viruses, which are discussed in detail in Chap. 190. Influenza is described in Chap. 188. Pneumonia due to *M. pneumoniae* and psittacosis, are included in this section because of their similarity to respiratory viral diseases, although neither is carried by a virus.

REFERENCES

DINGLE JH et al: A study of illness in a group of Cleveland families: I. Plan of study and certain general observations. Am J Hyg 58:16, 1974, 1953

U.S. PUBLIC HEALTH SERVICE: Acute Conditions, Incidence and

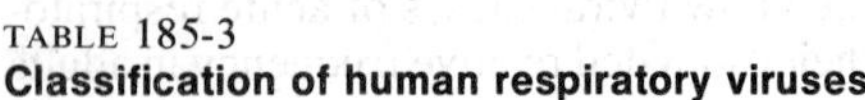
TABLE 185-3
Classification of human respiratory viruses

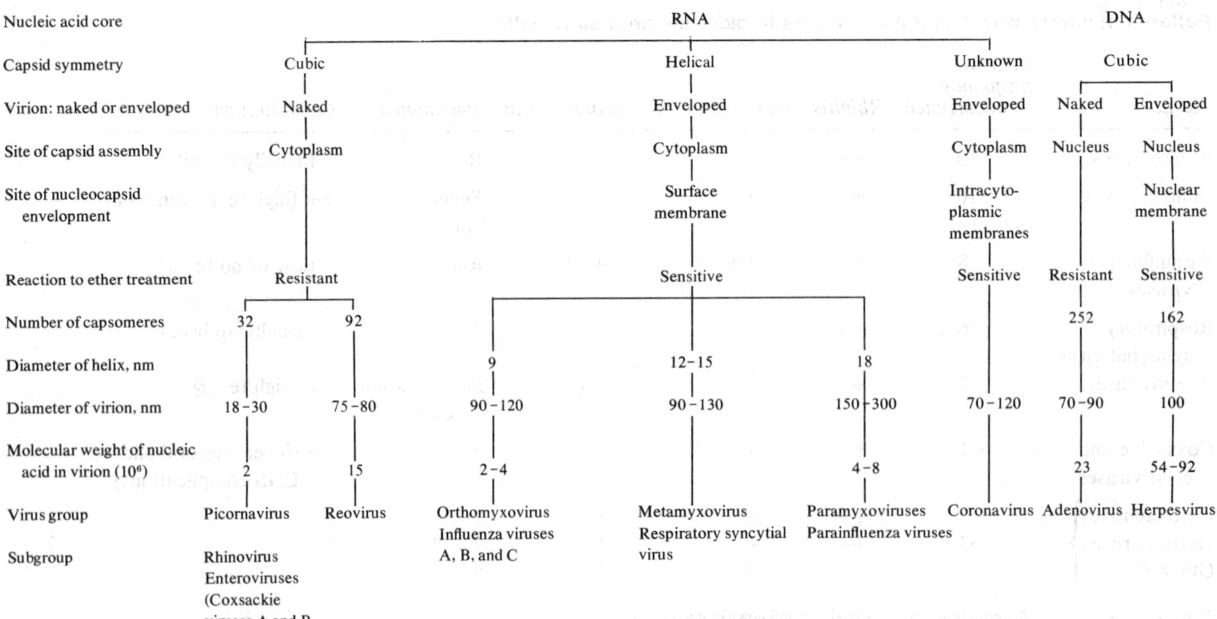

SOURCE: *Condensed from J. L. Melnick, Classification and nomenclature of viruses, 1972, vol. 14 in* Progress in Medical Virology, *Basel: Karger, 1972, p. 327.*

Associated Disability, United States, July 1961–June 1962, National Health Survey, USPHS Publ. 1000, ser. 10, no. 1, 1963

WORLD HEALTH ORGANIZATION: Technical Report Series 408:1, 1969

186
COMMON VIRAL RESPIRATORY ILLNESSES:
RHINOVIRUSES, ADENOVIRUSES, RESPIRATORY SYNCYTIAL VIRUS, PARAINFLUENZA VIRUSES, COXSACKIE VIRUSES, ECHO VIRUSES, AND CORONAVIRUSES

VERNON KNIGHT

RHINOVIRUS INFECTIONS

ETIOLOGY Nearly 100 types of rhinovirus are known, and others are certain to be found. Some of the properties of rhinoviruses are shown in Table 185-3. Some rhinoviruses produce cytopathic effects in monkey kidney cell culture (M strains); others are not cytopathic for monkey cells but will grow in cells of human origin (H strains).

EPIDEMIOLOGY As much as 40 percent of acute respiratory illness in adults may be caused by rhinoviruses. Infections occur throughout the year but are most frequent in the late winter and early spring. Multiple serotypes circulate simultaneously. Individual types usually persist for only a few months, however, and do not recur during succeeding seasons. Adults commonly have antibody against several serotypes, whereas young children (except for the very young with maternal antibody) are relatively free of antibody. A small percentage of non-ill controls have yielded positive cultures for rhinoviruses, but in the main, the presence of rhinoviruses in the respiratory tract is associated with illness.

Most patients develop appreciable titers of type-specific antibody, and measurable levels persist for 2 to 4 years. In screening of prisoner volunteers for participation in experiments with rhinoviruses, it was found that only one-third of men were entirely free of antibody to four rhinovirus serotypes. However, illness and virus shedding can be readily induced in volunteers unless very high titers of antibody are present.

CLINICAL MANIFESTATIONS The incubation period for rhinovirus infections in volunteers is 1 to 2 days. The common cold syndrome induced in volunteers resembles naturally occurring cases in adults. Within 24 hr of inoculation there are scratchy throat, nasal congestion and discharge, malaise, and mild headache. There is usually no fever. Nasal secretions increase sharply between days 1 and 2 and then as promptly return to pre-illness values. Recovery is rapid and complete. Virus shedding begins a few hours after inoculation and continues for almost 2 weeks. Type-specific neutralizing antibody rises to 1:128 at 21 days.

Table 186-1 summarizes clinical experience with naturally occurring rhinovirus infections in adults and children and artificial infection in volunteers. Most adults have only a common cold syndrome, with a rare case of bronchitis the only other form of illness. In contrast, more than one-half of children develop bronchitis, bronchiolitis, or bronchopneumonia. Although these findings resemble those of respiratory syncytial (RS) virus infection, rhinovirus disease is generally milder than that due to RS virus.

LABORATORY FINDINGS In illness with rhinovirus there is usually slight neutrophilia. About one-third of volunteers develop moderate elevations in sedimentation rate.

COMPLICATIONS No serious complications have been reported with rhinovirus infections.

DIFFERENTIAL DIAGNOSIS Among the respiratory viruses, rhinovirus infection most consistently causes coryzal illness. In any one case, however, the illness cannot be distinguished from coryza due to other agents. Except for rare confusion with an atypical case of streptococcal sore throat, only respiratory viral diseases and *Mycoplasma pneumoniae* infection need be considered in differential diagnosis.

TREATMENT AND PREVENTION There is no specific treatment, and no vaccines are currently available for rhinovirus infections. Rest, analgesics, antihistamines, and nose drops are advised.

Adenovirus infections

ETIOLOGY The adenovirus group contains 31 human and 17 animal serotypes. Strains of types 3, 7, 11, 12, 14, 16, 18, 21, and 31 have been shown to cause sarcomas when injected into newborn hamsters.

Adenoviruses share a common antigen. An antigenic

TABLE 186-1
Illness association with rhinovirus infections

Diagnosis	*Adults (61)*	*Children (32)*	*Adult volunteers with nasopharyngeal inoculation (31)*
	%	%	%
Common cold	58 (92)	14 (44)	26 (84)
Croup		1 (3)	
Bronchitis	1 (2)	7 (23)	2 (6)
Bronchiolitis		3 (9)	
Bronchopneumonia		3 (9)	
No disease	2 (3)	4 (12)	3 (10)

SOURCE: *Hamparian et al, Proc Soc Exp Biol Med 117:469, 1964; and Cate et al, J Clin Invest 43:56, 1964*

determinant on this protein is the basis for a diagnostic complement fixation test. Type specificity in neutralizing antibody tests depends on antigenic determinants present and on other protein determinants. Except for types 12 and 18, hemagglutination inhibition (HI) tests also permit type-specific identification. Adenovirus hemagglutinins, the basis for the HI test, are variably associated with protein subunits and with the intact virion. Human adenoviruses grow well in continuous cell lines of epithelial origin.

EPIDEMIOLOGY Even though serologic surveys suggest an appreciable prevalence of infection with many serotypes, definite virus-associated illness is now limited to about 10 serotypes. These serotypes produce five major patterns of illness, all of which occur in epidemics. A summary of these is presented in Table 186-2.

Acute respiratory disease (ARD), a respiratory illness of military recruits, has been shown to be caused by adenoviruses. Later it was shown that regular winter and spring outbreaks of ARD in military recruits in the United States were caused by adenovirus types 4 and 7, and with lesser frequency by type 3. Types 14 and 21 have caused similar outbreaks in military personnel in the Netherlands and elsewhere. In military groups, 15 to 50 percent of acute respiratory illness is caused by adenoviruses, but in civilian adults, only about 2 percent of respiratory illnesses are due to adenoviruses, and in children about 6 percent.

Febrile pharyngitis due to adenoviruses is usually a disease of civilians, often occurring sporadically or in small outbreaks in children. Its manifestations are summarized in Table 186-2. *Pharyngoconjunctival fever* is febrile pharyngitis associated with acute follicular conjunctivitis. This disease occurs as summer epidemics, frequently among children in relation to exposure in swimming pools. Although it is not limited to swimming pool exposure, it is believed that eye irritation from water, sun, or chlorine may be a factor in its initiation. Conjunctivitis may occur without pharyngitis.

Pneumonia due to adenovirus infection is rare in civilian adults, but it now seems certain that an atypical pneumonia due to adenovirus infection occurs in military recruits, usually as an extension of ARD. In infants and

TABLE 186-2
Illness associated with adenovirus infection

		Order of association (serotypes)		*Respiratory tract involvement*					
Disease	*Occurrence*	*Common*	*Less common*	*Common cold*	*Pharyngitis*	*Bronchitis*	*Pneumonia*	*Constitutional reaction*	*Other*
Acute respiratory disease (ARD)	Epidemic in winter and spring in military recruits	4, 7	3, 14, 21	Often present	*Most frequent,* usually with fever, often with laryngitis	Frequent, usually with fever and laryngitis	Infrequent complication of ARD, but adenovirus pneumonia is an important type of pneumonia in recruits	Headache, malaise, often high fever for several days	Usually no other involvement
Pharyngoconjunctival fever	Summer epidemics in civilians, often in school-age children, related to swimming pools. Sporadic cases of conjunctivitis may occur without pharyngitis.	3, 7	4, 14	Often present	*Most frequent,* usually with fever and cervical lymphadenopathy, hoarseness	Uncommon	Rare	Headache, malaise, high fever for several days	Acute follicular conjunctivitis, usually unilateral, occurs with varying frequency. Preauricular lymphadenopathy common with conjunctivitis
Febrile pharyngitis	Sporadic or epidemic, resembles ARD, often in children	3, 7	1, 2, 5	Often present	*Most frequent,* usually with fever	Frequent, especially in older children	Infrequent but severe complication	High fever, malaise, headache	Nausea, vomiting and diarrhea may occur, especially in infants
Pneumonia in children	Highly fatal illness in infants, sporadic or epidemic	3, 7		Occurs	Very frequent	Very frequent	Primary, with acidophilic necrosis of tracheal and bronchial mucosa resembling tissue culture CPE	High fever, prostration	Conjunctivitis, skin rash, diarrhea, intussusception, and CNS invasion in some cases
Keratoconjunctivitis (EKC)	Epidemic disease in shipyard workers; also spread from infected eye solutions	8	11	Unusual	Uncommon	Not reported	Not reported	Usually afebrile	Usually unilateral severe, acute conjunctivitis followed by corneal subepithelial keratosis; preauricular lymphadenopathy common

children, sporadic and epidemic occurrence of highly fatal adenoviral pneumonia has been described in several parts of the world. Such outbreaks have been principally caused by types 3 and 7. The severity of disease in this young age group may reflect the lack of prior experience with these agents, but other factors such as size and route of inoculation, general health, or greater susceptibility due to immaturity may be important.

Epidemic keratoconjunctivitis due to type 8 and less often to type 11 or other serotypes is described in Chap. 202.

Incubation period The period of incubation for pharyngoconjunctival fever and ARD is 5 to 10 days. A similar incubation period has been noted for induced disease in volunteers. Incubation periods for the other naturally occurring syndromes have not been established but are probably similar.

PATHOGENESIS Illness in volunteers is produced when the conjunctival sac is swabbed with suspensions of adenovirus. In these cases, conjunctivitis occurs and there is sometimes respiratory involvement. The initiation of illness appears to require a significant degree of conjunctival irritation. A second method of producing illness is administration of virus aerosol by inhalation. Volunteers inoculated in this way have developed ARD and primary atypical pneumonia.

These observations suggest the existence of at least two routes of inoculation for naturally occurring respiratory illness with adenoviruses: (1) ocular inoculation associated with eye irritation such as may occur in outbreaks around swimming pools, with the development of *pharyngoconjunctival fever;* (2) inoculation through inhalation of infectious aerosol generated by sneezing and coughing of ill recruits under the crowded circumstances incidental to recruit training. The route of inoculation of infants is less likely to be limited to aerosolized virus, and the occurrence of pneumonia may represent primarily a lack of resistance in this young age group.

The regular production of virus infection without illness by nasopharyngeal inoculation in volunteers suggests that a similar circumstance may occur naturally as an explanation for the high frequency of antibody to many serotypes in the population. This antibody may also result from intragroup cross reactions among serotypes in the three broad immunologic groups of adenovirus.

CLINICAL MANIFESTATIONS *Acute respiratory disease* is an acute febrile illness lasting about 1 week and characterized by fever, cough, hoarseness, and sore throat. Fever has gradual onset and reaches a maximum of 103 to 104°F on the second or third day. There are associated malaise and often headache. Pharyngitis, the most prominent localized manifestation of the disease, reaches maximum severity after about 3 days. There may also be regional lymphadenopathy, pharyngeal injection, some edema, frequent lymphoid follicular hyperplasia, but little or no faucial exudate. Nasal obstruction and discharge occur in almost one-half of cases, but these abnormalities are not usually conspicuous. Cough is almost always present, and hoarseness is also frequent.

Pharyngoconjunctival fever is usually a milder respiratory illness than ARD, although fever may be high for 5 or 6 days. Nontender submandibular lymphadenopathy is common even in the absence of sore throat. Lower respiratory tract involvement has not been described. Conjunctivitis is mild to moderate but may last longer than respiratory symptoms. It is an acute, nonpurulent, follicular conjunctivitis. In most cases, it is unilateral, and preauricular lymphadenopathy is rare. There is usually no involvement of the cornea or uveal tract.

Febrile pharyngitis without conjunctivitis resembles the foregoing illness, except for the absence of conjunctivitis.

Adenoviral pneumonia in children occurs as a primary illness and is associated with as much as 15 percent mortality. Pediatric texts should be consulted for further details.

DIFFERENTIAL DIAGNOSIS The differential diagnosis of ARD should include the respiratory viral diseases described in the present chapter and influenza (Chap. 188), nonpneumonic forms of *M. pneumoniae* infection (Chap. 187), streptococcal sore throat, and purulent sinusitis. Pharyngitis and upper respiratory illness may also accompany the onset of infections hepatitis and infectious mononucleosis.

Differential diagnosis of *pharyngoconjunctival fever*, when conjunctivitis is prominent, includes leptospirosis, influenza, measles, herpangina, and the nonpurulent conjunctivitides, such as inclusion conjunctivitis and physical or chemical trauma to the eye.

TREATMENT There is no specific treatment for adenovirus infection. Treatment is limited to alleviation of general discomfort, headache, and coughing with analgesics, cough syrup containing terpin hydrate, codeine, antihistamines, or other antitussives.

PREVENTION Communicability of adenovirus infection probably extends from a day or so before onset of illness to recovery, and conventional precautions against respiratory spread should be employed during acute illness for patients in the hospital and to the extent reasonably possible in care of patients at home. Avoidance of swimming pools during outbreaks of pharyngoconjunctival fever is recommended.

Formalin-treated vaccines against types 3, 4, and 7 afford significant protection against infection and illness, but these vaccines were withdrawn from civilian use when it was discovered that some serotypes of adenoviruses produced tumors in hamsters. A live adenovirus vaccine given orally in enteric-coated capsules has been highly effective in preventing infection with adenovirus types 3, 4, and 7 in military recruits. More recently, purified preparations have demonstrated a high degree of protection against experimental infections in volunteers. No vaccine is now marketed for civilian use.

RESPIRATORY SYNCYTIAL VIRUS INFECTION

ETIOLOGY Respiratory syncytial virus (RS) is classified as a subgroup of the myxoviruses (Table 185-3). In tissue culture, it causes formation of giant cells, or syncytia, from which its name was derived. It grows well in several human primary and continuous cell lines and in primary rhesus monkey kidney culture. There is a soluble complement-fixing antigen which, with the neutralization test, permits virus identification and serologic studies. Respiratory syncytial virus contrasts with other myxoviruses because it does not grow or cause detectable changes in mice, guinea pigs, rabbits, or chick embryos and does not cause hemagglutination or hemadsorption.

EPIDEMIOLOGY Epidemiologic studies have delineated a very substantial role of this agent in acute respiratory disease in children. Illness in young children occurs most commonly in epidemics in the late winter and early spring. Attack rates are nearly 100 percent among susceptibles, who are mostly children under four years of age. In older children and adults, the disease appears in nonepidemic patterns. The limitation of epidemic disease to the younger age group is also evidence for unchanging antigenicity of the agent, in contrast to the situation with influenza virus, in which antigenic shifts are associated with recurrent epidemics in persons of all ages. In serologic surveys of several hundred Federal prisoners for selection as volunteers, all were found to possess a measurable titer of neutralizing antibody to RS virus. Mild upper respiratory illness appears to be the principal form of the disease in adults, but the virus has been isolated from cases of acute flare-ups of bronchitis in older people with chronic pulmonary disease.

It is probable that RS virus is transmitted by means of infected respiratory secretions. The incubation period of naturally occurring disease in children is about 4 days, and in adult volunteers who developed common cold syndromes, the average incubation period was approximately 5 days. Virus was generally recovered from volunteers a day or so before the onset of illness, and throat swabs yielded a higher proportion of positive cultures than nasal swabs. Virus shedding continues for 3 to 4 days after onset of illness.

CLINICAL MANIFESTATIONS Somewhat less than one-half of children have symptoms defined as a common cold; the remainder have bronchiolitis or bronchopneumonia. Fever is present in 91 percent of all children, with an average elevation of 102°F. Cough is almost invariably present, and severe malaise is frequent. Pharyngitis is not usually severe. Fatalities have been reported in infants.

In contrast, naturally occurring illness or induced disease in adult volunteers is a mild syndrome characterized by rhinitis and pharyngitis. Intranasal inoculation of virus into a normal volunteer was followed in 4 days by an afebrile illness consisting of nasal obstruction, clear, profuse nasal discharge, headache, malaise, and slight cough. Improvement was rapid, and recovery was nearly complete 8 days after inoculation. Virus shedding preceded symptoms by 2 days and continued during the first 4 days of illness.

LABORATORY FINDINGS In children, leukocytosis occurs with some frequency, but no significant hematologic changes were observed in adult volunteers. Bacterial flora of the nasopharynx and other laboratory indices show no significant alterations in either age group.

COMPLICATIONS Except for progression to overwhelming lower respiratory tract disease in a few young children, no special complications are known. There is no evidence of secondary bacterial infection or systemic invasion by the virus in children. In adults, bacterial sinusitis is occasionally encountered.

DIFFERENTIAL DIAGNOSIS The resemblance of this disease in children to influenza has been suggested. In adults, the differential diagnosis should include rhinovirus and parainfluenza infection and, less often, other respiratory viral diseases and *M. pneumoniae* infection.

TREATMENT As with the other respiratory viral diseases, treatment should include rest and palliative medications such as aspirin, nose drops, and medication for sleep when restlessness occurs. The possibility of bacterial sinusitis in adults should be kept in mind and an-

TABLE 186-3
Respiratory illness associated with Coxsackie viruses A and B, and echo viruses

Diagnosis	*Description*	*Associated viruses*
Herpangina	Febrile pharyngitis, anorexia, and discrete vesicular eruption on anterior faucial pillars. Occurs chiefly in children in summer and early fall outbreaks. Similar illnesses without eruption caused by the same viruses probably occur. An illness with nonulcerating nodules on anterior pillars caused by Coxsackie virus A-10 has also been described.	Coxsackie virus A-1 through 6, 8, 10, and 12
Febrile respiratory illness ("summer grippe")	Undifferentiated febrile illness marked by headache, sore throat, and anorexia occurring in summer or early fall. Includes epidemics in recruits with Coxsackie virus A-21 infection, in which illness patterns have been confirmed by experimental inoculation of volunteers	Coxsackie virus A-21, 24, B-2, 3, 5 (?), and echo virus 1, 3, 6, 19, 20
Upper respiratory illness associated with gastroenteritis	Cases occurring largely in infants and exposed mothers	Echo virus 1, 11, 19, 20
Acute laryngotracheobronchitis (croup)	Winter outbreaks in nurseries and institutions. Association less definite than with other syndromes	Coxsackie virus A-9, B-5, and echo virus 11
Pneumonitis and pleuritis	Largely confined to young infants and children; uncommon	Coxsackie virus A-9, B-4, 5, and echo virus 9, 19, 20

timicrobial treatment, drainage procedures, or other therapy instituted when necessary.

PREVENTION A formalin-inactivated RS vaccine elicited a high frequency of antibody, but a few months later vaccinated children experienced more severe illness than nonvaccinated children in the same population. This paradoxic effect of vaccination is a major contraindication for further attempts to develop a vaccine. The infection spreads rapidly among children in institutions and poses a threat to debilitated or very young children.

PARAINFLUENZA VIRUS INFECTIONS

ETIOLOGY On the basis of antigenic differences, parainfluenza viruses are divided into four types, of which type 4 is divided into two subtypes. They agglutinate avian and mammalian erythrocytes and grow slowly in tissue culture; only type 2 produces readily visible cytopathic effects. Growth of these agents in tissue cultures is detected by addition of guinea pig erythrocytes, which absorb on the surface of infected cells to form rosettes, a process known as hemadsorption. Parainfluenza viruses have antigens common to Newcastle disease and mumps viruses, but influenza virus does not share these. Parainfluenza serotypes are distinguished by complement fixation, hemagglutination-inhibition, or tissue culture neutralization tests.

Primary monkey or primary human embryonic kidney cell cultures are suitable for isolation. They grow slowly or not at all in embryonated chicken eggs.

EPIDEMIOLOGY The first three types of parainfluenza viruses have been found in many parts of the world; type 4 has so far been isolated only in the United States. Infection with parainfluenza viruses occurs early in life. By the age of eight years, a majority of children show antibody to types 1 to 3, and it appears that most adults have antibody to all four types.

In children, illness with parainfluenza viruses occurs throughout the year, with seasonal increases in the winter and spring. Type 3 virus spreads more rapidly than types 1 and 2. Heterotypic rises are frequent, with antibody to type 3 developing in half the cases with type 1 infection. In both children and adults, reinfection is frequent. In one outbreak, 96 percent of children without antibody, 67 percent with low levels, and 33 percent with high levels of antibody became infected. In adults, the disease is almost invariably a reinfection and is much milder than in children.

The total contribution of parainfluenza infections to respiratory illness is variable, its frequency increasing in institutions in which general health status is lower than average and levels of sanitation and personal hygiene are less than optimum. In the United States, the percentage contribution of parainfluenza infections in several studies of children has varied from 4.3 to 17. The milder illness which occurs in adults has usually constituted less than 5 percent of respiratory illnesses.

CLINICAL MANIFESTATIONS In all age groups, the incubation period appears to be 5 to 6 days. The disease is most serious in infants and children, the characteristic syndrome being laryngotracheobronchitis, or croup. Much of the bronchiolitis, bronchitis, and bronchopneumonia in children is also caused by parainfluenza infections. In older children the disease is less serious, usually without evidence of pulmonary involvement, and in adults, the virus produces a common cold syndrome with hoarseness and cough.

Fever is a constant feature of illness in children but is less frequent in adults. Nasal discharge is a common occurrence at all ages. Cough and hoarseness are common, and stridor, indicative of croup, is present in many of the cases among infants and children.

Physical findings are not distinctive. The throat is reddened, with little or no exudate. There may be tender submandibular lymphadenopathy.

LABORATORY FINDINGS In adult volunteers given type 2 virus, leukocyte counts were not abnormal. In children there is a considerable variation in leukocyte counts early in illness, making it difficult to distinguish this disease from pneumococcal and other bacterial infections. No characteristic alterations have been reported in other laboratory indices such as liver or renal function tests, electrocardiograms, and urinalyses.

COURSE AND COMPLICATIONS In children, *otitis media* has occurred as a complication more often with parainfluenza than with the other respiratory viral infections. It may be caused by pneumococci, streptococci, or *Hemophilus influenzae*. The illness is characterized by slow resolution of pulmonary involvement and long persistence of cough and other symptoms. In very young or debilitated children, the outcome can be fatal. In adults, bacterial sinusitis may occur, and in persons with chronic bronchitis, emphysema, or bronchiectasis, the possibility of pulmonary bacterial superinfections should be considered.

TREATMENT There is no specific treatment. Therapy is limited to symptomatic measures and efforts aimed at early detection and treatment of bacterial complications such as otitis media or pneumonia. Nursing care is important in pediatric cases, especially children with croup.

In adults, analgesics, antihistamines, and small doses of codeine for cough are generally sufficient.

PREVENTION Vaccines against parainfluenza virus infections are not available. In hospitals, respiratory precautions should be carried out. At home, bed rest or room isolation during acute illness is advised, with special effort to avoid contact with very young or aged persons.

COXSACKIE VIRUS AND ECHO VIRUS INFECTIONS

Diseases produced by these agents are described in Chap. 190. Table 186-3 summarizes the respiratory illnesses sometimes seen in infections by these viruses.

CORONAVIRUSES

ETIOLOGY Most of the human agents were first isolated in organ cultures (explants of fetal trachea), although one group of these agents (229E) was isolated in human embryo kidney culture.

EPIDEMIOLOGY The disease, characteristically a common cold syndrome, occurs in winter and spring outbreaks that vary from year to year, with maximum attack rates in the fifteen- to nineteen-year-old age group, but it may involve adults of forty years of age and older. The incubation period is 3 to 5 days.

CLINICAL FEATURES The disease closely resembles that caused by rhinoviruses, with profuse watery and later mucopurulent nasal discharge and mild constitutional symptoms. It is of short duration. Diagnosis is based on isolation of the agent in organ culture or human embryo kidney culture. The neutralizing antibody test is more sensitive than the complement fixation test, and rises in titer persist for a longer time. Both tests, however, will provide adequate diagnostic information.

TREATMENT AND PREVENTION Treatment is symptomatic, and no preventive measures are available.

REFERENCES

Adenoviruses

BELL, JA et al: Pharyngoconjunctival fever: Epidemiological studies of a recently recognized disease entity. JAMA 157:1083, 1955

KASEL JA et al: An immunologic classification of heterotypic antibody responses to adenoviruses in man. Proc Soc Exp Biol Med 119:1162, 1965

Coronaviruses

CAVALLARO JJ, MONTO AS: Community-wide outbreak of infection with 229E-like coronavirus in Tecumseh, Michigan. J Infect Dis 122:27, 1970

HAMRE D, PROCKNOW JJ: A new virus isolated from the respiratory tract. Proc Soc Exp Biol Med 121:190, 1966

TYRELL DAJ, BYNOE JJ: Cultivation of a novel type of common cold virus in organ cultures. Br Med J 1:1467, 1965

Coxsackie and echo viruses

SPICKARD A et al: Acute respiratory disease in normal volunteers associated with Coxsackie A-21 viral infection. III. Response to nasopharyngeal and enteric inoculation. J Clin Invest 42:840, 1963

Parainfluenza virus

CHANOCK RM et al: Newly recognized myxoviruses from children with respiratory disease. N Engl J Med 258:207, 1958

JOHNSON KM, CHANOCK RM: Studies of a new human hemadsorption virus. I. Isolation, properties, and characterization. Am J Hyg 71:81, 1960

Respiratory syncytial virus

AHERNE W et al: Pathological changes in virus infections of the lower respiratory tract in children. J Clin Pathol 23:7, 1970

KAPIKIAN AZ et al: An epidemiologic study of altered clinical reactivity to respiratory syncytial (RS) virus infection in children previously vaccinated with an inactivated RS virus vaccine. Am J Epidemiol 89:405, 1969

Rhinoviruses

CATE T et al: Studies with rhinoviruses in volunteers: Production of illness, effect of naturally acquired antibody, and demonstration of a protective effect not associated with serum antibody. J Clin Invest 43:56, 1964

HAMPARIAN V et al: Epidemiologic investigations of rhinovirus infections. Proc Soc Exp Biol Med 117:469, 1964

187
PNEUMONIA CAUSED BY MYCOPLASMA PNEUMONIAE

VERNON KNIGHT

SYNONYMS Primary atypical pneumonia, Eaton's agent pneumonia, cold agglutinin-positive pneumonia, "virus" pneumonia.

DEFINITION Pneumonia caused by *Mycoplasma pneumoniae* is characterized by fever, pharyngitis, cough, and pulmonary infiltration, often multilobular, in which roentgenographic signs are more extensive than indicated by physical examination. This organism is also the cause of upper respiratory illness without pneumonia and of asymptomatic infection.

ETIOLOGY *Mycoplasma pneumoniae*, one of several species of human and animal pleuropneumonia-like organisms (PPLO), is one of the smallest organisms (150 to 250 nm) capable of replication in cell-free media. It lacks a cell wall, requires cholesterol for development of its limiting membrane, and has exacting nutritional requirements. It grows on or beneath the surface of agar slants in a small, round, granular colony without the "fried egg" peripheral zone characteristic of many other PPLO. It is inhibited in vitro by tetracycline derivatives, streptomycin, kanamycin, erythromycin, oleandomycin, chloramphenicol, and gold salts. It is not inhibited by penicillin, sulfonamides, or thallium acetate. It is distinguished from other human mycoplasmas by rapid hemolysis of guinea pig erythrocytes and utilization of glucose and other sugars. It also hemolyzes human and rat erythrocytes. It may also be distinguished from other mycoplasmas by fluorescent antibody, complement fixation, growth inhibition, and indirect hemagglutination tests, all of which are useful for serologic diagnosis of human infection. In addition to growing on agar, the organism grows on the surface of cells of embryonated eggs and monkey kidney cell culture with little evidence of cytopathic effect. In human cell cultures, however, there is intracellular growth with cytopathic effects.

EPIDEMIOLOGY In the general population *M. Pneumoniae* infection is characterized by intrafamily spread. In most cases the infection is introduced into the family by a schoolchild. Once it is introduced, most family members become infected. In family outbreaks, pneumonia occurs with greatest frequency among school-age children, with a predominance in males. The disease is rare above age forty. *Mycoplasma pneumoniae* pneumonia occurs throughout the year, although prolonged wintertime outbreaks may occur in college groups or communities. The total incidence of *M. pneumoniae* pneumonia in a study in Seattle was 1.3 per 1,000 per year, which constituted about 10 percent of pneumonia from all causes.

In the military, *M. pneumoniae* infections account for a small proportion of upper respiratory illness in recruits —in one study, 6.3 percent. However, it accounted for almost one-half of cases of pneumonia in the same military population. The disease appears to be endemic at military bases.

Mycoplasma pneumoniae is probably spread by means of infected respiratory secretions. The organisms can be cultured from sputum of naturally occurring cases and from volunteers inoculated artificially. Primary atypical pneumonia has been induced in volunteers both by nasopharyngeal inoculation and by inhalation of a small-particle aerosol containing the agent. In volunteers naturally acquired antibody is associated with a high degree of resistance to infection.

CLINICAL MANIFESTATIONS The incubation period is from 9 to 12 days. Illness usually begins with symptoms of upper respiratory illness, which in a small percentage of cases, progresses to bronchitis and pneumonia. Cough is almost universal in pneumonia and is frequent in cases without pulmonary involvement. Blood-flecked sputum may occur in the more severe cases, but gross hemoptysis is rare. A variety of other respiratory and systemic complaints may occur. Fever, nasal congestion, and sore throat are common. In pneumonia, harsh or diminished sounds are frequent but bronchial breathing is uncommon. Fine inspiratory rales are found in most patients but are not impressive. Pleural rubs and pleural effusion are infrequent. Studies on the distribution of pneumonia show frequent bilateral involvement in the lower lobes. Involvement of a single lower lobe is less common, and upper lobe involvement is rare. Pulmonary infiltrates may occur as an isolated area in the lung periphery but more often spread from the hilum.

The disease is variable in severity, but high fever may persist for 1 to 2 weeks in untreated cases. X-ray changes last for as long as 3 weeks in untreated cases, but for 7 to 10 days in treated cases. Even in untreated cases, complications are rare and consist of occasional purulent sinusitis, persistent cough, and, rarely, pleurisy. Prolonged weakness and malaise follow the untreated illness in adults.

Ear involvement consisting of congestion of the tympanic membrane and of bullous and, rarely, hemorrhagic myringitis may occur in as many as 10 percent of cases, most often in children.

Studies with volunteers have revealed, in addition to pneumonia, the occurrence of febrile and afebrile upper respiratory illness characterized by nonexudative pharyngitis and tracheobronchitis, often associated with cough, headache, and nasal congestion. Recovery occurred without complications in about 2 weeks. Upper respiratory disease occurs more commonly than pneumonia with infection in children and adults.

LABORATORY FINDINGS During acute illness leukocytosis in the range of 10,000 to 15,000 per mm^3 occurs in about 25 percent of cases. Increase in sedimentation rate above 40 mm per hr occurs in at least two-thirds of cases. Urinalysis, electrocardiograms, and fluid and electrolyte and liver function studies show no characteristic changes. The complement fixation, fluorescent antibody, indirect hemagglutination, and growth inhibition tests all yield highly specific diagnostic information. The simplicity of the complement fixation test recommends it for general use. Fourfold rises in titer often occur within 2 weeks, and maximum rise is achieved in 4 weeks. In atypical pneumonia, agglutinins to *Streptococcus MG* have been reported to develop in varying frequency. Higher titers are correlated with more severe illness. Of probably greater diagnostic value than *Streptococcus MG* agglutination is the appearance late in illness of cold agglutinins for human, type O red cells. The test may be positive in as high as 90 percent of severely ill patients but is less often positive in nonpneumonic cases.

DIFFERENTIAL DIAGNOSIS Pneumonia due to *M. pneumoniae* needs to be distinguished from pneumonia of all other types. It is usually less severe and is associated with less dense pulmonary infiltration than pneumococcal and other bacterial pneumonias. The discovery of pulmonary infiltrate in the absence of symptoms or physical signs may initially suggest acute pulmonary tuberculosis. In military populations adenovirus pneumonia must be excluded. Pneumonic involvement as a direct result of influenza viral infection or its complication by pneumococcal, streptococcal, staphylococcal, or *H. influenzae* infection may cause difficulty in diagnosis. Q fever, psittacosis, and tularemia are less frequent causes of pneumonia which may be difficult to distinguish from *M. pneumoniae* infection. In children, especially young infants, pneumonia due to respiratory syncytial, parainfluenza, adenovirus, and influenza viruses may resemble *M. pneumoniae* infection. Cases of undiagnosed pneumonia, despite careful workup, are a regular finding in both military and civilian populations, suggesting that other causes of pneumonia remain to be discovered.

TREATMENT Tetracycline derivatives and erythromycin are effective in treatment of pneumonia due to *M. pneumoniae.* Demethylchlortetracycline may be given to adults in daily doses of 0.9 g; tetracycline, 1.5 g; erythromycin stearate or ethyl succinate, 1.5 and 1.2 g per day, respectively. Response to treatment is characterized by prompt defervescence, rapid clearing of x-ray signs of pneumonia, and disappearance of malaise and weakness. Persistent cough, despite treatment, is a relatively common finding, especially in women.

Treatment temporarily reduces the frequency of positive cultures from the respiratory tract, but shedding may continue for several weeks after treatment, a finding similar to that in psittacosis pneumonia. Relapse of *M. pneumoniae* pneumonia occurs occasionally, but such cases respond to retreatment. In cases in which there is doubt between *M. pneumoniae* and pneumococcal infection, erythromycin should be used in preference to a tetracycline.

PREVENTION Although antibody is apparently highly protective, effective vaccines are not available. Acutely ill patients should be isolated from very young children and persons in whom a complicating respiratory illness would constitute a special hazard.

REFERENCES

CLYDE WA, DENNY FW: Mycoplasma infections in childhood. Pediatrics 40:669, 1967

SHAMES JM et al: Comparison of antibiotics in the treatment of mycoplasmal pneumonia. Arch Intern Med 125:680, 1970

RIFKIND D et al: Ear involvement (myringitis) and primary atypical pneumonia following inoculation of volunteers with Eaton agent. Am Rev Resp Dis 85:479, 1962

188 INFLUENZA

VERNON KNIGHT

DEFINITION Influenza is an acute respiratory infection of specific viral etiology characterized by sudden onset of headache, myalgia, fever, and prostration. The terms *influenza* and "flu" should be restricted to those cases with clear-cut epidemiologic or laboratory evidence of infection with influenza viruses.

HISTORY According to the best available records, influenza was uncommon in Europe during the nineteenth century until the pandemic of 1889. Subsequently, the frequency and severity of epidemics increased, culminating in the disastrous pandemic of 1918, which caused an estimated 20 to 40 million deaths. The isolation of the causative virus in 1933 led to the development of simple diagnostic tests, which have greatly advanced knowledge of the disease.

ETIOLOGY There are three distinct antigenic types of influenza virus, designated A, B, and C. Infection with one type confers no immunity to infection with the other two. They are all approximately 100 nm in diameter, visible as spheres or filaments by electron microscopy, and are biologically related by their infectivity for chick embryos, capacity to agglutinate erythrocytes, and affinity for the respiratory epithelium of various mammals. Influenza viruses are the prototypes of the myxovirus group and are related to the larger paramyxoviruses, which include mumps, Newcastle disease, measles, and the parainfluenza viruses. Influenza viruses are composed of a helical ribonucleoprotein core with a lipid-containing envelope from which protrude protein spikes. The protein spikes, or coat proteins, are of two types, hemagglutinins and neuraminidase. The former are responsible for attachment of the virus to cell receptors; the latter enzymatically inactivate neuraminic acid, the active receptor substance. Enzyme activity frees virus from attachment sites if cell penetration is unsuccessful. Hemagglutinins and neuraminidase are antigenic and elicit protective antibody.

EPIDEMIOLOGY Influenza B usually occurs sporadically or in localized outbreaks, particularly in schools and military camps. Illness with influenza C is rarely detected, although antibody surveys indicate a wide prevalence of infection with this agent. Influenza A viruses are the cause of major epidemics that tend to recur at intervals of 2 to 4 years in the winter months. The factors responsible for this periodicity are the decline in effective immunity of a population in interepidemic periods and the emergence every few years of new strains of virus. Antigenic shifts in influenza viruses are due to changes in the coat proteins, hemagglutinins (H), and neuraminidase (N). The designation of antigenic changes, and the major occurrences of influenza for which they were responsible are described below.

Pandemic 1918	Swinelike agent
Epidemics 1933	H0N1, formerly A_0
Epidemics 1947	H1N1, formerly A_1
Pandemic 1957	H2N2, formerly A_2 (Asian)
Pandemic 1968	H3N2 (Hong Kong)

Hemagglutinins and neuraminidase of some equine, swine, and avian strains of influenza share antigenic properties with some human influenza viruses. It is not known whether the animal viruses interact in some way with human viruses, possibly by exchange of genetic material (recombination), to account for new antigenic variants. Against this possibility is the lack of evidence of natural spread of infection between human and animal hosts.

The next major occurrence of influenza of pandemic proportions will involve further changes in H or N antigens. The degree of change will determine the severity of the pandemic. Some observers feel that the next pandemic will occur before the end of the 1970s.

Influenza A epidemics start abruptly, reach a peak in 2 to 3 months, and subside almost as rapidly. The attack rate is variable but was noted in 1957 to exceed 50 percent of urban populations. An additional 25 percent of individuals may show serologic evidence of infection without clinical manifestations. Experiences in 1957 proved conclusively that crowding, even in summer months or in tropical countries, is the major factor predisposing to epidemics. Schoolchildren, in particular, are the primary focus and disseminators of infection in the United States. The end of summer recess in September brings a highly susceptible population into close proximity and facilitates rapid spread. If the general immunity of a population is at low levels, community-wide epidemics may occur within a few weeks of the opening of schools. If, on the other hand, immune individuals predominate, the case rate will rise slowly and may not reach epidemic proportions, or may do so later in the winter.

PATHOGENESIS Influenza is primarily an infection of the respiratory epithelium that is transmitted from man to man by inhalation of infective droplet nuclei. Detailed experimental studies of the pathogenesis of the disease have been made in ferrets and mice. After intranasal inoculation, the virus multiplies to maximum titers in 24 to 48 hr and rapidly involves the entire tracheobronchial tree. At first, the mucosa becomes boggy and hyperemic and loses its normal ciliary activity. This may shortly be followed by necrosis of respiratory epithelium, invasion by leukocytes, pulmonary consolidation, and abnormal regeneration of metaplastic squamous epithelium in the bronchi and bronchioles. The infection is largely confined to the respiratory tract and hilar lymph nodes of adult animals; viremia is a transient and inconstant feature. However, virus has been isolated from heart, kidney, and other extrapulmonary tissues in fatal human infections, suggesting that virus products can enter the circulation and may account for systemic manifestations of the disease.

The findings at autopsy are pulmonary hemorrhages, necrosis of bronchial epithelium, bronchiolitis, squamous metaplasia of respiratory epithelium, and marked edema of alveolar septums and spaces. Human fatalities can be caused by the influenza virus itself or by combined viral and bacterial infections.

MANIFESTATIONS The disease assumes its typical form during major epidemics of influenza A, but clinical differentiation between influenza A and B is not possible in localized outbreaks. Sporadic infections with either influenza A or B are likely to result in relatively minor illnesses, with predominantly respiratory symptoms, similar to those of common respiratory disease. Influenza C is particularly difficult to recognize because of its mildness. Although the manifestations and severity of influenza A vary from year to year, cases in a single epidemic often follow a remarkably similar pattern. The clinical description that follows is a composite picture of epidemic influenza A of the past three decades.

The *incubation period* is usually 18 to 36 hr but may be as long as 3 days. Mild prodomal symptoms of cough, malaise, and chilliness are sometimes present, but extremely sudden onset is often such a characteristic feature that many patients can recall its exact time. The most common initial symptom is severe generalized or frontal *headache*, frequently accompanied by stabbing retroorbital pain that is accentuated by lateral or upward gaze. Diffuse *myalgia*, particularly marked in the legs and over the lumbosacral area, occurs in more than half the cases. Pain and spasm of the abdominal muscles may simulate acute peritonitis, and incapacitating periarticular pains are sometimes confused with acute arthritis. *Feverishness* and *chilliness*, or occasionally true rigors, may be the first manifestations, but more often they are preceded by headache and myalgia. The temperature rises abruptly to a maximum of 100 to 103°F several hours after onset; rarely it may reach 106°F. Thereafter, the fever and pain usually subside over a 2- to 3-day period but may persist for as long as a week. A common variant in the temperature course is rapid defervescence after the initial peak, with a secondary rise to the original level on the following day. In general, severity of illness parallels the height and duration of the fever. The pulse rate is usually slow in relation to the fever, but marked tachycardia may occur in severely ill patients.

Prostration of some degree is almost invariable and is often the most prominent and alarming manifestation. The face is flushed, and the skin is hot and dry; however, profuse sweating and cold, mottled extremities are sometimes noted. Anorexia, nausea, and constipation are frequent secondary symptoms, but vomiting and diarrhea are rare. There is no evidence that influenza viruses infect the gastrointestinal tract, and the term *intestinal flu* is a misnomer. Meningoencephalitis, polyneuritis, cranial nerve palsies, transient nerve deafness, aphasia, hemiplegia, psychoses, and other neurologic disorders have been described in association with influenza but are very unusual. Hypotension, heart block, peripheral vasoconstriction, and fatal myocarditis have also been reported in a few cases. The exact relationship of these neurologic and cardiovascular disorders to influenza viral infection has not been determined.

Respiratory symptoms may be present at the onset but become most prominent when the systemic manifestations and fever begin to subside. They are frequently less pronounced than in common respiratory disease and may be entirely absent. Sneezing, water nasal discharge, and stuffy nose occur in most cases; hoarseness and epistaxis are less frequent. Conjunctival suffusion and burning, itching, watery eyes are often noted. The throat may feel dry, and the pharynx often appears slightly injected. *Cough* develops during the course of the illness in more than three-fourths of the cases, and in about a third of these it is productive of small amounts of tenacious, mucoid sputum. *Chest pain*, usually substernal in location and accentuated by coughing but not by breathing, is present in almost half the patients. Pleurisy and pleural effusion are uncommon. Slight hyperpnea is often noted, but the most ominous, although infrequent, signs are dyspnea and cyanosis, which signal bronchiolar or pneumonic involvement. Findings on physical examination of the lungs are often negative in uncomplicated influenza, but scattered rhonchi, wheezes, and showers of moist rales have been reported in 5 to 40 percent of cases in different epidemics. These changes may persist for several days after apparent recovery. Patients with uncomplicated influenza may have restrictive ventilatory defects and increased alveolar-capillary oxygen tension gradients, suggesting the regular occurrence of lower pulmonary tract involvement in the disease. Influenzal bronchiolitis should be suspected if rales persist in the absence of x-ray evidence of pneumonitis and if the patient raises mucopurulent or blood-tinged sputum.

COMPLICATIONS The chief complications of influenza are pneumonia, either primary (due to influenza virus infection alone) or secondary bacterial pneumonia superimposed on the lesions produced by the influenza virus. In addition, bacterial infections of the paranasal sinuses and middle ear may occur. The incidence of bacterial pneumonia is greatly increased during influenza epidemics; even mild or asymptomatic infections with influenza viruses predispose to pneumococcal and other types of pneumonia. The most serious complication is staphylococcal pneumonia, which tends to follow a fulminant, often fatal, course. Primary influenza virus pneumonia typically has its onset about 1 week after onset of influenza, often following a period of apparent improvement. The disease is characterized by severe dyspnea and cyanosis, scanty sputum containing gross blood, leukopenia, few physical findings in the lung, and perihilar infiltrates. The disease has a rapid course, and fatality, when it occurs, results from acute pulmonary insufficiency. Secondary bacterial pneumonia responds less well to antimicrobial treatment than pneumonia that occurs in the absence of influenza, presumably because of underlying pulmonary damage from the influenza virus infection. Superinfection with *Hemophilus influenzae*, so common in the pandemic of 1918, is rarely encountered now.

Recovery from uncomplicated influenza is often complete in 2 to 3 days or, occasionally, in a week, but convalescence may be prolonged by "postinfectious asthenia" and depression, particularly in elderly persons. Minor relapses with fever may occur but are uncommon.

The *mortality* rate from all causes always increases markedly during epidemics of influenza. In the fall and winter of 1957-1958 it was estimated that 40 million persons in the United States became ill with influenza and the total numbers of influenza-associated deaths was reported to be in excess of 8,000. In addition, approximately 60,000 more deaths from various causes occurred during this period than would be expected under normal conditions. The greatest incidence of excessive mortality occurred among infants under one year of age and adults over sixty years of age. Data from small series of cases clearly indicate that influenza is frequently fatal in individuals with preexisting pulmonary or cardiac disease, regardless of age. Chronic rheumatic heart disease with mitral stenosis, in particular, appears to predispose to fatal influenzal pneumonia.

LABORATORY FINDINGS Virus is isolated most readily during the acute phase of the disease by inoculation of broth garglings into the amniotic cavity of chick embryos or into tissue cultures of monkey kidney or human cells. Serologic diagnosis can be made most reliably by hemagglutination-inhibition or complement fixation tests, using paired serum samples obtained in both the acute and convalescent phases. However, type-specific antibody against soluble complement-fixing antigens of influenza A virus often appears in the circulation of patients during the acute illness.

X-ray of the lungs in uncomplicated influenza is usually normal but occasionally reveals increased vascular markings, basilar streaking, small areas of patchy infiltration, atelectasis, nodular densities, or pleural effusion. The blood leukocyte count may be low 2 to 4 days after onset of illness, but is often normal or slightly elevated. Leukocytosis with counts above 15,000 cells per mm^3 indicates secondary bacterial infection, but leukopenia may occur in severe staphylococcal pneumonia. Slight proteinuria is common during the height of the febrile illness.

DIFFERENTIAL DIAGNOSIS Many bacterial and viral infections simulate influenza at their onset, but few febrile diseases have such a self-limited course. The pattern of clinical manifestations becomes readily apparent during an epidemic. Noninfluenzal respiratory diseases are generally characterized by more gradual onset, milder systemic manifestations, and predominant symptoms of coryza, rhinorrhea, pharyngitis, and conjunctivitis.

TREATMENT Antibiotics do not affect the course of uncomplicated influenza, nor is there any evidence that they prevent complications. Specific chemotherapy should be reserved for secondary bacterial infections. Clinical trials have shown some effectiveness of amantadine, a symmetric amine that inhibits cellular penetration of influenza virus, as a chemoprophylactic and therapeutic agent, but the results are not impressive. Codeine affords relief from incapacitating cough and is more effective than salicylates for symptomatic treatment of headache and myalgia; salicylates often increase discomfort by causing drenching sweats and chills. Bed rest and gradual return to full activity are advisable.

PROPHYLAXIS Formalinized egg vaccines purified by zonal ultracentrifugation or other methods and containing a mixture of influenza A(H3N2) and B viruses are available commercially in the United States. Present purified vaccines contain larger amounts of virus than in previous years, with resulting increased potency. Current vaccines can be expected to be effective when given in suitable dosage at an interval of several weeks to several months before exposure, and when the antigens of the vaccine are still closely related to the epidemic strain.

The U.S. Public Health Service strongly recommends routine yearly immunization with polyvalent influenza vaccine for high-risk groups, including persons of all ages who suffer from chronic rheumatic heart disease, other cardiovascular diseases, chronic bronchopulmonary diseases, diabetes mellitus, or Addison's disease; also pregnant women and persons sixty-five years of age, or older, regardless of their previous state of health. For initial immunization it is advisable to administer the vaccine subcutaneously in two divided doses of 1 ml each, the first injection in September and the second several weeks or months later. A single subcutaneous dose of 1 ml given each autumn is satisfactory as a yearly booster. Intradermal injection of vaccine is far less satisfactory because a sufficient antigenic mass cannot be administered by this route.

Influenza vaccination is generally safe but not completely innocuous. Fatal anaphylactic reactions and purpura have been reported in individuals sensitive to egg proteins, and inactivated virus itself is pyrogenic and can sometimes produce an illness similar to active influenza. Influenza vaccine should be administered only advisedly and in much smaller doses to infants and young children, in whom severe febrile reactions may result in convulsions and deaths. Most influenza vaccines are contaminated with bacterial pyrogens. Large-scale purification of virus by zonal centrifugation shows considerable promise for production of vaccines from pure viral antigens.

REFERENCES

CHANOCK RM et al: A revised system of nomenclature for influenza viruses. WHO Bull 45:119, 1971

International conference on influenza. WHO Bull 41:335, 1969

JOHANSON WG, JR et al: Pulmonary function in uncomplicated influenza. Am Rev Resp Dis 100:141, 1969

KNIGHT V et al: Serological responses and results of natural infectious challenge of recipients of zonal ultracentrifuged influenza A21/Aichi/2/68 vaccine. WHO Bull 45:767, 1971

REIMER CB et al: Purification of large quantities of influenza virus by density gradient centrifugation. J Virol 1:1207, 1967

189
PSITTACOSIS

VERNON KNIGHT

DEFINITION Psittacosis is an infectious disease of birds caused by an organism that has a number of properties in common with gram-negative bacteria. Transmission of infection from birds to man results in a febrile illness characterized by pneumonitis and systemic manifestations. Inapparent infections or mild influenza-like illnesses may also occur. The term *ornithosis* is sometimes applied to infections contracted from birds other than parrots or parakeets, but *psittacosis* is the preferred generic term for all forms of the disease.

ETIOLOGY The causative agent *Chlamydia psittaci* is a gram-negative obligate intracellular parasite, formerly classified as a virus. Now chlamydias, along with the rickettsias, may be considered specialized bacteria. Both synthesize ribonucleic acid (RNA) and deoxyribonucleic acid (DNA), reproduce by binary fission, and are susceptible to antimicrobial drugs. In contrast to rickettsias, the chlamydias are dependent on their hosts for metabolic energy. Slight but definite homology of the DNA of members of the *Chlamydia* genus with the DNA of *Neisseria meningitidis* has been shown. The psittacosis agent is the prototype of a biologically and antigenically homogeneous class of microorganisms that includes the causative agents of lymphogranuloma venereum, trachoma, and 30 or more mammalian parasites which rarely produce human disease.

EPIDEMIOLOGY Psittacosis is widely distributed throughout the world, and almost any avian species can harbor the agent. Psittacine birds are most commonly infected, but human cases have been traced to contact with pigeons, ducks, turkeys, chickens, and many other birds. Psittacosis may be considered an occupational disease of pet-shop owners, poultry raisers, pigeon fanciers, taxidermists, and zoo attendants. The incidence of human infection in the United States rose steadily from 1930, owing in large measure to the increasing popularity of parrots and parakeets as pets and, as subsequently recognized, transmission of infection by barnyard fowl and pigeons. The number of reported cases reached a peak in 1956 and gradually declined thereafter. By 1963, with acceptance of control measures such as incorporation of tetracyclines in poultry feed, the disease had again become relatively uncommon. In contrast, the disease appears to be more common in England, where budgerigars are common household pets and where restrictions on the importation of these birds have been eased.

The agent is present in nasal secretions, excreta, tissues, and feathers of infected birds. Although the disease can be fatal, infected birds frequently show only minor evidence of illness such as ruffled feathers, lethargy, and anorexia. Asymptomatic avian carriers are common, and complete recovery may be followed by continued shedding of the organism for many months.

Psittacosis is almost always transmitted to man by the respiratory route. On rare occasions the disease may be acquired from the bite of a pet bird. Intimate and prolonged contact is not essential for transmission of the disease; a few minutes spent in an environment previously occupied by an infected bird has resulted in human infection. The severity of the disease in man bears no apparent relationship to closeness or duration of contact, although sick birds are more likely to transmit infection than healthy ones. Human-to-human transmission of a psittacosis-like agent has occurred among hospital personnel, with severe and sometimes fatal infections. There is evidence that these "human" strains are more virulent than native avian organisms. There is no record of infection acquired by eating poultry products.

PATHOGENESIS The psittacosis agent gains entrance to the body through the upper part of the respiratory tract and eventually localizes in the pulmonary alveoli and in the reticuloendothelial cells of the spleen and liver. Invasion of the lung probably takes place by way of the bloodstream rather than by direct extension from the upper air passages. A lymphocytic inflammatory response occurs on both the interstitial and respiratory surfaces of the alveoli as well as in the perivascular spaces. The alveolar walls and interstitial tissues of the lung are thickened, edematous, necrotic, and occasionally hemorrhagic. Histologically, the affected areas show alveolar spaces filled with fluid, erythrocytes, and lymphocytes. The picture is not pathognomonic of psittacosis unless macrophages containing characteristic cytoplasmic inclusion bodies (LCL bodies) can be identified. The respiratory epithelium of the bronchi and bronchioles usually remains intact.

MANIFESTATIONS The clinical manifestations and course of psittacosis are extremely variable. After an *incubation period* of 7 to 14 days, or longer, the disease may start abruptly with shaking chills and high fever, but the onset is often gradual with increasing fever and malaise over a 3- to 4-day period. Headache is almost always a prominent symptom; it is usually diffuse and excruciating and often the patient's chief complaint. Generalized myalgia is also common. Spasm and stiffness of the muscles of the back and neck may lead to an erroneous diagnosis of meningitis. A faint, macular rash (Horder's spots) simulating the rose spots of typhoid fever has been described. Lethargy, mental depression, agitation, insomnia, and disorientation have been prominent features of the illness in some epidemics, but not in others; delirium and stupor occur near the end of the first week in severe cases. Occasional patients are comatose when first seen, and the diagnosis of psittacosis may be missed. Gastrointestinal complaints such as abdominal pain, nausea, vomiting, or diarrhea are present in some cases; constipation and abdominal distention sometimes occur as late complications. Icterus, the result of severe hepatic involvement, is a rare and ominous finding. Symptoms of upper respiratory tract infection are not prominent, although mild sore throat, pharyngeal infection, and cervical adenopathy are often present; on occasion they may be the only manifestation of illness. Epistaxis is encountered early in the course of nearly one-fourth of the cases. Photophobia is also a common complaint.

A dry, hacking cough is characteristic; it is usually nonproductive, but small amounts of mucoid or bloody sputum may be raised as the disease progresses. Cough may appear early in the course of the disease or as late as 5 days after the onset of fever. Chest pain, pleurisy with effusion, or a friction rub may all occur but are rare. Pericarditis and myocarditis have been reported. Most patients have a normal or slightly increased respiratory rate; marked dyspnea with cyanosis occurs only in severe psittacosis with extensive pulmonary involvement. In psittacosis, as in most nonbacterial pneumonias, the physical signs of pneumonitis tend to be less prominent than symptoms and x-ray findings would suggest. The initial examination may reveal fine, sibilant rales, or clinical evidence of pneumonia may be completely lacking. Rales usually become audible and more numerous as the illness progresses. Signs of frank pulmonary consolidation are usually absent.

Patients without cough or other clinical evidence of respiratory involvement come to the physician with fever of unknown origin. The pulse rate is slow in relation to the fever. When splenomegaly is present in a patient with acute pneumonitis, psittacosis should be considered; the reported incidence of splenomegaly ranges from 10 to 70 percent. Nontender hepatic enlargement also occurs, but jaundice is rare. Thrombophlebitis is not unusual during convalescence; indeed, pulmonary infarction is sometimes a late complication and may be fatal.

In untreated cases of psittacosis, sustained or mildly remittent fever persists for 10 days to 3 weeks, or occasionally as long as 3 months. Defervescence is by lysis and is accompanied by abatement of respiratory manifestations. Psittacosis contracted from parrots or parakeets is more likely to be a severe, prolonged illness than infections acquired from pigeons or barnyard fowl. Relapses occur but are rare. Secondary bacterial infections are uncommon. Immunity to reinfection is probably permanent.

LABORATORY FINDINGS The x-ray of the lungs in psittacosis mimics a great variety of pulmonary diseases. The pneumonic lesions are usually patchy in appearance but can be hazy, diffuse, homogeneous, labar, atelectatic, wedge-shaped, nodular, or miliary. The white blood cell count is normal or moderately decreased in the acute phase of the disease but may rise in convalescence. The erythrocyte sedimentation rate is frequently not elevated. Transient proteinuria is common. The cerebrospinal fluid sometimes contains a few mononuclear cells but is otherwise normal. Cold agglutinins are rarely present.

The diagnosis can be confirmed only by isolation of the causative microorganism or serologic studies. The agent is present in the blood during the acute phase of the disease and in the bronchial secretions for weeks or sometimes years after infection, but it is difficult to isolate. Psittacosis is most readily diagnosed by the demonstration of a rising titer of complement-fixing antibody in the patient's blood. An acute and convalescent specimen should always be tested. Even a low titer of antibody during the acute febrile phase constitutes presumptive evidence of psittacosis. The prompt initiation of treatment with tetracycline has been shown to delay antibody rise in convalescence for several weeks or months. Interpretation of a single complement fixation test may sometimes be difficult because of the antigenic cross reaction between the agent of psittacosis and that of lymphogranuloma venereum.

DIFFERENTIAL DIAGNOSIS A history of exposure to birds may be the only clinical basis for differentiating psittacosis from a great variety of infectious and noninfectious febrile disorders. A partial list of pneumonic diseases that may be confused with psittacosis includes mycoplasma pneumonia, Q fever, coccidiodomycosis, tuberculosis, carcinoma of the lung with bronchial obstruction, and bacterial pneumonias. In the early stages, before pneumonitis appears, psittacosis may be mistaken for influenza, typhoid fever, miliary tuberculosis, and infectious mononucleosis.

TREATMENT The tetracyclines are consistently effective in the treatment of psittacosis. Defervescence and alleviation of symptoms usually occur in 24 to 48 hr after instituting therapy with 2 g daily. To avoid relapse, treatment should probably be continued for at least 7 days after defervescence. In severe cases, oxygen and other supportive measures are indicated.

REFERENCES

CUNNINGHAM AI, WALKER WJ: Psittacosis in Hamilton: A case report and epidemiological study. Can Med Assoc J 102:69, 1970

EDITORIAL: Psittacotic references. Lancet 2:72, 1972

MEYER KF: Psittacosis-lymphogranuloma venereum agents, in *Viral and Rickettsial Infections of Man*, 4th ed., eds FL Horsfall, Jr., I Tamm, Philadelphia: Lippincott, 1965, p. 1006

MOULDER JW: The life and death of the psittacosis virus. Hosp Practice, June 1968

190
ENTERIC VIRUSES:
COXSACKIE VIRUSES, ECHO VIRUSES, REOVIRUSES

A. MARTIN LERNER

GENERAL CONSIDERATIONS It has been over 20 years since Dalldorf and Sickles isolated the first Coxsackie viruses by inoculating suspensions of feces from two children with signs of clinical paralytic poliomyelitis into suckling mice. Subsequently, some 67 enteroviruses, including poliovirus and Coxsackie and echo viruses (Table 190-1) have been shown to multiply at various times in the gastrointestinal tracts of man. Enteroviruses have been recovered wherever attempts have been made; their distribution appears global. With notable exceptions such as Coxsackie virus, type A-21, and echo virus 28, which are predominantly respiratory pathogens and are only incidentally isolated from feces, enteroviruses such as *Salmonella* periodically multiply within the human alimentary canal and sometimes concomitantly produce disease. Available information suggests that there is no normal enteric virus flora. In addition to enteroviruses, adenoviruses (Chap. 186) and reoviruses are commonly recovered from stools.

Coxsackie viruses are named for their site of origin, the village of Coxsackie on the banks of the Hudson River in the state of New York. Echo viruses were descriptively named: *E*, for their *enteric* residence; *C*, the filtrable agents produced *cytopathic* effects in tissue cultures of rhesus kidney; *H*, *human*; *O*, *orphan*, indicating that their relationship to disease remained to be established. They were viruses "in search of a disease." It is increasingly evident that a wide but definite variety of illnesses may result from enterovirus infections. As observations accumulate, these illnesses (Table 190-2) are continually being defined.

Etiologic associations are difficult to establish and usually require virologic, serologic, epidemiologic, and volunteer studies. It is especially useful if viruses are isolated from sites other than the pharynx or anus, where they often multiply without causing significant injury to tissues. More meaningful are isolations from blood, vesicular fluids of patients with rashes, urine, cerebrospinal fluid, or from tissues at biopsy or autopsy. Coxsackie or echo viruses have been recovered from lung, heart, pericardial fluid, liver, spleen, testicle, kidney, muscle, and brain. Dual virus infections and possible bacterial-virus synergisms are being defined. Until enteroviruses had been repeatedly documented in infants by isolations from pneumonic lungs, prevalent opinion was that they did not produce pneumonias. The same skepticism must remain concerning etiologic associations of enterovirus infections and chronic myocardiopathies, nonrheumatic valvular deformities, subendocardial fibroelastosis, and other congenital malformations.

TABLE 190-1
Classification of enteroviruses

I Picornaviruses of human origin
- *A* Enteroviruses
  - *1* Polioviruses (3 types)*
  - *2* Coxsackie virus A (24 types)
  - *3* Coxsackie virus B (6 types)
  - *4* Echo viruses (34 types)†
- *B* Rhinoviruses (see Chap. 186)
- *C* Unclassified

II Picornaviruses of lower animals

* *Typing is by neutralization of infectivity with immune serums either in suitable tissue cultures or in suckling mice.*

† *Echo virus, type 10, has been reclassified as belonging to another taxonomic group, now known as reoviruses.*

Characteristics of the viruses Enteroviruses consist of a ribonucleic acid (RNA) core surrounded by a capsid of protein. The subunit structure of the capsomeres determines species, tissue, and age specificities as well as antigenicity. The RNA of the virus within infected cells transcribes and translates its own genetic information independent of DNA (deoxyribonucleic acid) of the host. Particle diameters are 17 to 30 nm. Enteroviruses are quite stable in acid and lipid solvents. They can be protected from thermal inactivation by certain cations.

When inoculated into suckling mice, group A Coxsackie viruses induce primarily inflammation and necrosis of skeletal muscle, whereas group B viruses cause lesions of the central nervous system and other viscera, but only focal muscular involvement. Coxsackie viruses B and echo viruses are cytopathogenic for cultures of monkey kidney cells, but this is not the case for Coxsackie viruses of group A. These distinctions are not without exception. Some strains of echo viruses, types 6 and 9, have been adapted to produce lesions in baby mice, the former in viscera and the latter in skeletal muscles. Some strains agglutinate human erythrocytes obtained from adults or umbilical cords at the time of delivery. None of the Coxsackie or echo viruses has been adapted to grow in embryonated eggs.

Epidemiology Fecal-oral contact is the usual method of transmission. Personal hygiene inhibits the infectious cycle. Toddlers often bring enteroviruses into a household. Insects, including flies and mosquitoes, may act as passive vectors. Echo virus, type 6, may multiply in the gastrointestinal tracts of dogs. This has not been noted with other Coxsackie or echo viruses, and with echo virus 6 canine-to-human transmission has not been demonstrated. Respiratory transmission by droplets or their nuclei also occurs.

The incubation period is 2 to 5 days. Multiple concurrent infections within a family are not unusual. Clinical manifestations of infection vary within the family and community. Thus a two- to three-year-old child may have a mild fever with rash, while an older sibling may have pleurodynia, myocarditis, or one of a number of syndromes heralding involvement of the central nervous system (Table 190-2). The mechanism of the varied expression of enterovirus disease is not well understood but may relate to developmental changes in the number or availability of specific receptors at the surfaces of susceptible cells.

Enterovirus infections are most common during the summer. Prevalence is mirrored by virus isolations from samples of sewage. Serotypes present in a community vary from year to year. The level of immunity of a population as reflected by the prevalence of type-specific neutralizing antibodies in serums apparently determines the likelihood of infection by a particular enterovirus. In an individual usually one enterovirus multiplies within the intestine at any time. Vaccination with attenuated polioviruses has virtually eliminated these interfering agents, and there may be a real increase in infections due to Coxsackie or echo viruses. Improved hygiene and urbanization has led to an "epidemiologic shift" from infants to adults. On the basis of intrahousehold spread, infectivity of Coxsackie viruses is fairly high (76 percent of exposed susceptibles and 25 percent of immunes). For echo viruses, apparent infectivity is substantially lower (43 percent of susceptibles) and immune contacts are rarely infected. At least 49 percent of Coxsackie virus and 55 percent of echo virus infections are subclinical.

An interesting correlate has been a seasonal incidence of new cases of insulin-dependent diabetes mellitus in patients under thirty years old. This autumn peak has been correlated with an annual prevalence for Coxsackie virus B 4, but does not relate to other virus infections.

TABLE 190-2
Illnesses (or syndromes) associated with Coxsackie or echo virus infections

	Viruses (not inclusive)		
	Coxsackie virus group		
	A, types	*B, types*	*Echo virus, types*
I No illness (probably 75% of cases)	1–24	1–6	1–8,* 11–34
II Mild or moderate illness			
A Undifferentiated mild febrile illness (nonspecific)	1–24	1–6	1–8, 11–34
B Upper respiratory syndromes (rhinitis, pharyngitis, including herpangina and lymphonodular pharyngitis, conjunctivitis)	1–10,16,21,22,24†	1–5	1,3,6,9,16,19,20,28
C Laryngotracheitis	9	5	11
D Exanthems (various)	5,9,16	3,5	2,4,5,9,11,16
E Lymphadenitis, with or without splenomegaly	5,6,9	5	4,9,16,20
F Pleurodynia (sometimes with pleural effusion)	4,6,10	1–5	1,6,9
G Orchitis		1–5	9
H Gastroenteritis		3,4	2,3,6–9,11–14,18,19,22–24
III Severe or life-threatening illness			
A Hepatitis	4,9	5	4,9
B Hemolytic-uremic syndrome	4	4	
C Pneumonia	9	1,4	3,8,9,19,20
D Diabetes mellitus‡		4	
E Cardiac			
1 Myocarditis/pericarditis	1,2,4,5,8,9,16	1–5	1,4,6,8,9,14,19,22,25,30
2 Chronic myocardiopathy		2,4,5	
3 Subendocardial fibroelastosis‡		3	
4 Endocardial deformities		4	
5 Constrictive pericarditis		1,2	
6 Congenital malformations‡	9	3,4	
F Neurologic			
1 Aseptic meningitis/encephalitis including variants (b–f)	7,9,16	1–5	1–9,11–23,25,30–32
2 Acute cerebellar ataxia	3,4		
3 Benign intracranial hypertension			
4 Transverse myelitis			
5 Postencephalitic parkinsonism			
6 Guillain-Barré syndrome‡			

* *Asymptomatic infection is common with echo virus, type 9. Variation in attack rates among types (and strains of a single type) occurs.*
† *Coxsackie virus A, type 21, is also known as Coe virus.*
‡ *Suggested (and probable), but cause not established.*

Virus isolation Primary multiplication occurs in epithelial and paraepithelial lymphatic cells of the pharynx. During this early period of infection the patient may be asymptomatic or have mild malaise, sore throat, or low-grade fever. Slightly later virus multiplies in the intestines. If a critical virus concentration within the pharynx results, viremia follows. During the viremic phase the patient is asymptomatic. Secondary foci of virus multiplication may occur in various tissues (skin, muscle, heart, nervous system, etc.). Major illness of moderate to serious severity sometimes results (Table 190-2). Occasionally (especially during infancy) aspiration of pharyngeal virus leads to lower respiratory infection.

Virus may be isolated from the throat during the minor illness and for as long as a week thereafter. Virus shedding persists in feces for a longer interval. Viremia can be documented during the incubation period until type-specific neutralizing antibodies appear.

Protective responses and serologic diagnosis Intracellular virus multiplication stimulates interferon production within the infected cell (Chap. 184). At about 3 days after the onset of infection specific antibodies appear in saliva and serum. These immunoglobulins combine with extracellular virus to limit spread of virus. Virus-antibody complexes are eliminated by phagocytosis or, conceivably, could be fixed to tissues.

Secretory immunoglobulins in saliva and succus entericus are in the IgA class, while the earliest antibodies to appear in serum are IgM. Both species of macromolecules have complement-fixing and neutralizing qualities. Within 3 to 4 weeks complement-fixing antibodies reach their peak and decline. Neutralizing antibodies of higher avidity (IgG) replace the IgM molecule at about 2 weeks after the onset of infection. IgG antibodies persist and provide permanent type-specific immunity.

This information is important in diagnosis, because IgM molecules are susceptible to reduction and resultant biologic inactivation with sulfhydryl active compounds such as 2-mercaptoethanol (2-ME). IgG immunoglobulins are resistant to 2-ME.

IgG antibodies to Coxsackie and echo viruses traverse the placenta freely. IgM immunoglobulins do not. IgA antibodies in colostrum and milk are not absorbed, but apparently provide some local protection in the intestines of nursing babies. Passively acquired antibodies in serums protect the newborn from viremia for 3 to 6 months. Since the half-life of IgG immunoglobulins is about 3 weeks, durations of firm neonatal immunity depends upon initial titers of the transferred antibodies. Passively acquired antibodies inhibit active synthesis of immunoglobulins, and also may not protect the respiratory tract. Active synthesis of secretory antibody in saliva and nasal secretions seems required. The role of cellular immunity in enterovirus infections remains to be fully defined.

A fourfold rise in neutralizing antibodies or a titer which is similarly diminished by 2-ME indicates recent infection. When applicable, hemagglutination inhibition tests are simpler, and the results parallel those obtained in more cumbersome neutralization tests. Complement-fixing antibodies to enteroviruses are not type-specific. Many cross-reactions render these tests less useful.

The neutralizing antibody response is highly type-specific in primary or initial enterovirus infections. In subsequent infections heterotypic responses occur with increasing frequency; they presumably arise from a booster effect of the current infecting virus on the level of antibodies to other types with which the individual has previously been infected. Levels of heterotypic antibody frequently exceed the level of homotypic antibody. Neutralizing antibodies to group B Coxsackie virus, types 1 to 5, are frequently found in titers of 1/64 to 1/512 in patients without evidence of current Coxsackie virus infections.

Other laboratory findings Enterovirus infections are acute processes, and the existence of persistent or chronic infections has not been documented. Hence, changes in concentrations of hemoglobin, albumin, or globulins are unusual. Occasionally hemolysis occurs (see Coxsackie virus A and echo virus infections). White blood cell counts and the erythrocyte sedimentation rates are only mildly elevated. If there is necrosis (e.g., liver, lung), a neutrophilic leukemoid reaction may be noted. Hyperbilirubinemia, elevated transaminase and alkaline phosphatase levels, and delayed excretion of Bromsulphalein may be seen in cases of hepatitis. Albuminuria often occurs transiently, but hematuria is rare.

Treatment and prophylaxis Antiviral chemotherapy is not available. The 64 antigenic varieties of Coxsackie and echo viruses make vaccine prophylaxis impractical. Pooled human gamma-globulin contains enterovirus antibodies, but during serious infections administration is not helpful. Most human enterovirus infections are mild, and gamma-globulin prophylaxis is not often warranted. As with poliomyelitis, tonsillectomy and other inoculations are probably best delayed during an outbreak of enterovirus disease. In a murine model of Coxsackie virus B-3 myocarditis, virus was isolated in higher titer from hearts of mice vigorously exercised daily by swimming, and a benign myocarditis was transformed into a lethal infection. Rest is the cornerstone of symptomatic therapy.

It has been repeatedly shown in experimental animals that during the acute phase of infection administration of steroids appreciably increases the quantity of virus in tissues and the degree of ensuing injury. Corticosteroids also depress cell-mediated immune functions, interferon and antibody synthesis, and leukocyte migration to the area of injury. Therefore, at least during the acute phase of enterovirus infections, steroids are contraindicated. Pregnancy, with its associated increased levels of circulating steroids, may be associated with enhanced susceptibility to these and other infections. Alcohol, cold temperature, and chronic undernutrition are also associated with an increased virulence of Coxsackie virus and perhaps other virus infections. Alcohol depresses phagocytic function. Malnutrition suppresses T and B lymphocytes, early mononuclear cell migration, and interferon.

GROUP A COXSACKIE VIRUS INFECTIONS Group A Coxsackie viruses cause herpangina, lymphonodular pharyngitis, upper and lower respiratory disease, cutaneous eruptions, hepatitis, aseptic meningitis, paralytic disease, myopericarditis, and some sudden unexpected deaths in infancy. Diarrheas are also probably caused by Coxsackie virus A infections. Pharyngeal multiplication may induce infection of superficial vessels or diffuse moderate erythema. Purulent exudate is not seen. More characteristic is *herpangina*, a common febrile illness characterized by small papular, vesicular, or ulcerative lesions on the anterior pillars, soft palate, tonsils, pharyngeal mucous membrane, and posterior part of the buccal mucosa. Herpangina has been seen during infections with Coxsackie viruses, group A, types 1 to 10, 16, and 22. Vesicular lesions of herpangina have also been described in patients with illnesses due to Coxsackie viruses, group B, types 1 to 5, and echo viruses, types 9 and 17. Coxsackie virus A-10 may induce *acute lymphonodular pharyngitis*. Lesions here are raised, discrete, white to yellow 3- to 6-mm papules surrounded by a zone of erythema. All the papules appear at the same time; they do not ulcerate, and they occur on the uvula, anterior pillars, and posterior pharynx.

Coxsackie virus A-21 (Coe virus) is predominantly a respiratory pathogen, being regularly isolated from the throat and occasionally from feces. It has been associated with several outbreaks of a common cold-like illness in military recruits.

The first enterovirus etiologically implicated in causation of pneumonia was Coxsackie virus A-9. Subsequently, a number of other enteroviruses have been implicated (Table 190-2). Fatal cases have occurred in infants or young children. Hyperpnea, cyanosis, hyperpyrexia, leukocytosis (or leukemoid reactions), and subsequently coma have been characteristic. Interstitial diffuse polylobed bronchopneumonia with alternate areas of atelectasis and emphysema have been found. Microscopically mixed alveolar septal infiltration without necrosis or formation of giant cells is seen.

A striking cutaneous vesicular eruption, *hand-foot-and-mouth disease* (Chap. 201), has repeatedly been associated with infections due to Coxsackie virus, group A, type 16. Recently infants and children with Coxsackie virus, group A, type 4 (also Coxsackie virus B-4) infections have been described with respiratory or gastrointestinal symptoms, acute renal disease, thrombocytopenia, and hemolytic anemia. Reticulocytosis, albuminuria, and hematuria accompany this constellation of findings, which has been described as the *hemolytic-uremic syndrome*. Aseptic meningitis with occasional paralytic disease (especially with A-7) also occurs. Acute myopericarditis has been associated with infections with Coxsackie virus A, types 1, 2, 5, 8, and 9; there are firmer etiologic data for Coxsackie virus, types 4 and 16. One estimate suggests that 23 percent of acute virus cardiomyopathies may be caused by Coxsackie virus A. A significantly greater incidence of infection with Coxsackie virus, group A, type 9, has been reported in mothers of infants with congenital heart disease.

GROUP B COXSACKIE VIRUS INFECTIONS Infections with group B Coxsackie viruses cause a number of upper respiratory syndromes, exanthems, diarrheas, pleurodynia, orchitis (with subsequent atrophy), pneumonia, hemolytic-uremic syndrome, and cardiac and central nervous system disease. Pleurodynia and cardiac disease due to enteroviruses were first associated with this group of enteroviruses (Table 190-2). In 1965 the Public Health Service (Britain) reported 1,160 Coxsackie virus B-5 infections. Gastroenteritis (90 percent), aseptic meningitis (31 percent), myalgia and Bornholm's disease (23 percent), respiratory disorders (15 percent), and cardiomyopathies (5 percent) were included. There were 41 patients with pericarditis and 5 with myocarditis. Of 6 deaths, 2 each were due to neurologic, respiratory, or cardiac cause. During infancy, mortality of acute infectious myocarditis approaches 50 percent.

Pleurodynia (epidemic myalgia, Bornholm's disease, devil's grip) Prodromal symptoms of malaise, sore throat, and anorexia are interrupted by increasing debility, fever, and sudden onset of muscle, pleuritic, and abdominal pain. Pain is sharp, severe, and paroxysmal over the lower ribs or substernal area. It is accentuated by moving, breathing, coughing, sneezing, and hiccuping, and may be referred to the shoulders, neck, or scapulae. Pain and spasm of anterior abdominal muscles occur in about half the cases, often in combination with chest pain. Muscle tenderness is usually not prominent, but some patients complain of intense cutaneous hyperesthesia and paresthesia over the affected area. The illness usually lasts 3 to 7 days, but relapses may occur. Among differential diagnoses are myocardial infarction and acute surgical conditions of the abdomen. Coxsackie viruses B have been isolated from striated muscle of patients with pleurodynia during epidemics. Occasionally pleuritis is accompanied by effusion, and virus has been isolated from pleural fluid. Bornholm's disease may occur at any age, but is commonest in children and young adults.

Early in the course of illness meningitis, myocarditis, or hepatitis may ensue. Liver biopsy in patients with complicating jaundice shows subacute portal triaditis and intense cloudy swelling of central-zone hepatocytes. A late complication is orchitis, occurring in 3 to 5 percent of cases of pleurodynia during relapse.

Cardiac disease Acute idiopathic myocarditis may be caused by Coxsackie viruses of groups A and B as well as echo viruses. Infections with strains of Coxsackie virus, group B, have been most frequent. When congenital or neonatal infection occurs, the course is often rapidly fatal, with concomitant myocarditis, encephalitis, hepatitis, and sometimes adrenal necrosis. Later in childhood or in adult life the heart and pericardium more frequently are involved as the single site of disease. Cardiac inflammation varies in intensity and degree of muscle necrosis. Pericarditis may dominate the clinical presentation, with myalgia, fever, precordial pain, friction rub, and even cardiac tamponade. There may be prominent signs of myocarditis, with myocardial failure or arrhythmias. Illnesses may be self-limited and recovery complete. However, of 22 episodes of acute virus cardiomyopathies associated with infections due to Coxsackie viruses, group B, 12 patients developed chronic heart disease. Strict bed rest until all electrocardiographic changes have reverted to normal (or are stationary) is indicated. This may require 4 to 6 weeks. Since steroids increase virulence of Coxsackie B myocarditis in mice, they are contraindicated. Some infections may heal with significant myocardial scarring.

Coxsackie virus particles have been localized along tubules of the sarcoplasmic reticulum in infected mice with myocarditis, and Coxsackie virus B-4 has been shown to cause experimental murine valvulitis and mural endocarditis. These findings may prove to be pertinent to man. Of 40 hearts from autopsies of patients dying before age 30, 17 were positive by fluorescent antibody staining for Coxsackie virus antigen in the myocardium. Chronic focal interstitial myocarditis was present in each of the positive cases and viral antigens were found both in the myocardium and mitral valve in 3 cases. Similarly, there is epidemiologic evidence implicating Coxsackie virus B, types 3 and 4, and congenital heart disease. Most infections in pregnant mothers are subclinical and occur in the first trimester. There are other data associating group B Coxsackie viruses with congenital subendocardial fibroelastosis. These findings need confirmation, particularly because a similar study failed to demonstrate an association of echo virus, type 9, infection and congenital malformations. After experimental Coxsackie virus B infections in mice and monkeys, Aschoff bodies and Anitschkow myocytes, as well as valvular deformities, are seen. At this time strong or suggestive evidence indicates that the following conditions may be caused by infections with Coxsackie viruses belonging to group B: chronic continuing cardiomyopathies (B-2, B-4, B-5); congenital calcific pancarditis (B-3); aortic/mitral valvular incompetence (B-4); and constrictive pericarditis (B-1, B-2), with or without superior or inferior vena caval obstruction.

ECHO VIRUS INFECTIONS Echo virus infections may be asymptomatic or mild, moderate, or life-threatening (Table 190-2). Mild to moderate are undifferentiated fevers, upper respiratory infections, various rashes (Chap. 197), pleurodynia, and diarrheas. Pneumonia, myopericarditis, hemolytic-uremic syndromes, and neurologic involvement may be quite serious. They do not differ from similar illnesses caused by Coxsackie viruses.

Viral gastroenteritis Sporadic endemic cases of nonbacterial diarrheas, as well as acute outbreaks in summer or winter, occur. The latter have been termed *winter vomiting diseases* or *intestinal flu.* Gastrointestinal symptoms are not caused by influenza virus. Diarrhea may occur as a minor manifestation of enterovirus disease during a summer outbreak, but this is not usually the case. In individuals and in epidemiologically controlled series Coxsackie virus, types B-3 and B-4, as well as echo viruses, types 2, 3, 6 to 9, 11 to 14, 18, 19, and 22 to 24, have been implicated etiologically as a cause of gastroenteritis, as has oral attenuated poliovirus vaccine.

Attacks of vomiting and diarrhea occurring in winter outbreaks due to echo viruses are brief but debilitating illnesses. Malaise and several watery stools herald their onset. Fever is not invariably present. Typically, within 24 hr repeated vomiting, retching, and chilliness ensue. Abdominal cramps and myalgia may occur. The disease is highly contagious, with multiple cases within the family at one time or following closely one upon another. Similar spread results in the adjoining community. Recovery from this acute but severe episode usually occurs within 48 hr, but mild diarrhea and a malabsorption syndrome may persist for several weeks. During initial chilliness and cramping, echo viruses have been isolated from the blood, posterior pharyngeal wall, and rectal swabs. Shedding of virus is brief, and virus isolation is often unsuccessful by 36 hr after onset. Reoviruses and adenoviruses have been implicated in similar gastroenteritides.

Aseptic meningitis There may be a mild prodromal malaise, but major illness usually begins with fever, headache, and stiff neck. Papilledema and Kernig's, Brudzinski's, and Babinski's signs may be present. Localizing sensory or motor deficits are unusual. Confusion and delirium are common. These acute findings may persist for 4 to 7 days. Cerebrospinal pleocytosis is usually less than 500 cells per mm^3. Early there may be as many as 90 percent polymorphonuclear leukocytes, but within 48 hr the cellular response becomes completely mononuclear. Persistence of polymorphonuclear leukocytes in the cerebrospinal fluid suggests pyogenic meningitis or intracerebral, subdural, or epidural abscess. Gram stain and appropriate spinal fluid cultures must be done to exclude bacterial meningitis, tuberculosis, or mycotic meningitis. Protein concentration in the cerebrospinal fluid is moderately elevated, but glucose is normal. Early in the illness echo viruses may be isolated from spinal fluid. It usually takes several weeks before the cerebrospinal fluid reverts to normal.

For attempts at virus isolation, throat and rectal swabs, serum, and cerebrospinal fluid should be collected as early in the course as possible. Acute and convalescent serums should be studied for rises in type-specific neutralizing antibody.

It is not possible to distinguish clinically between aseptic meningitis due to various enteroviruses and mumps. Localizing findings, hemiplegia, prolonged fevers, oculogyric crises, coma, and bloody spinal fluid favor the diagnosis of herpes simplex virus encephalitis. Although echo virus aseptic meningitis most often is self-limited and recovery complete, about 10 percent of patients have more serious involvement of the central nervous system. Minor muscle weakness with reflex changes may persist for weeks to months, but over 90 percent of patients recover completely within a year. Occasionally, choreiform movements, ataxia, nystagmus, transverse myelitis, Guillain-Barré syndrome, coma, bulbar involvement, and death result.

REOVIRUS INFECTIONS Reoviruses were discovered inadvertently in studies of the intestinal viral flora of healthy children and adults. They were initially classified as echo virus, type 10, but were later reclassified. They were named to emphasize their (1) *respiratory* or (2) *enteric* human origins, and their (3) *orphan* status.

Reoviruses are quite different from picornaviruses (Table 190-1). They are about 2½ times larger (70 nm in diameter) and show icosohedral symmetry. Their RNA is unique in that it consists of 10 discrete segments and is resistant to ribonuclease. The protein capsid consists of an inner core and 92 outer shell capsomeres. The capsid is composed of 7 species of polypeptides. Unlike that of enteroviruses, reovirus cytopathic effects are nonlytic. Reoviruses multiply in primate and nonprimate tissue cultures. The particles hemagglutinate human or avian erythrocytes. On the basis of tests of hemagglutination inhibition antibodies (HIA) with type-specific serums, there are three serotypes.

Human infections with reoviruses are common, and their distribution is worldwide. Like Coxsackie and echo viruses, reoviruses spread by enteric and respiratory routes. Fifty to eighty percent of adults in the Western Hemisphere have had reovirus infections, as measured by the presence of persisting neutralizing or hemagglutinating antibodies. Infections are more frequent in winter but occur in every season. Reoviruses have been isolated from human nasal secretions, posterior pharyngeal and rectal swabs, spinal fluid, brain, and lung. They have been recovered from tissues of Burkitt's lymphoma. In addition, reovirus isolations or serologic data indicate that natural infections occur in cattle, dogs, cats, mice, horses, swine, birds, and monkeys. Although animal-to-human transmission has never been demonstrated, its possibility is likely.

Widespread evidence of infection and few associations with disease indicate that most infections with reoviruses are asymptomatic. Isolations of virus and fourfold rises in HIA in individual patients with common colds, nonspecific febrile illness, exanthem, and diarrhea suggest an etiologic role in some instances. Provocative data came from three thoroughly studied fatal cases of encephalitis, myocarditis, hepatitis, or interstitial pneumonias. In these patients reoviruses and no other bacterial or viral pathogens have been isolated.

REFERENCES

General

GELFAND HM: Occurrence in nature of coxsackie and ECHO viruses. Prog Med Virol 3:193, 1961

HORSTMANN DM: Clinical virology. Am J Med 38:738, 1965

KIBRICK S: Current status of coxsackie and ECHO viruses in human disease. Prog Med Virol 6:27, 1964

KOGON A et al: The virus watch program: A continuing surveillance of viral infections in metropolitan New York families. VII. Observations on viral excretion, seroimmunity, intrafamilial spread and illness association in Coxsackie and echovirus infections. Am J Epidemiol 89:51, 1969

Coxsackie A virus infection

HUEBNER RJ et al: Herpangina: Etiological studies of a specific infectious disease. JAMA 145:628, 1951

LERNER AM et al: Infections due to coxsackievirus, group A, type 9, in Boston, 1959, with special reference to exanthems and pneumonia. N Engl J Med 263:1265, 1960

Coxsackie B virus infection

BAIN HW et al: Epidemic pleurodynia (Bornholm's disease) due to coxsackie B 5 virus: The interrelationship of pleurodynia, benign pericarditis and aseptic meningitis. Pediatrics 27:889, 1961

BROWN GC, EVANS TN: Serologic evidence of coxsackievirus etiology of congenital heart disease. JAMA 199:151, 1967

BURCH GE et al: Coxsackie B viral myocarditis and valvulitis identified in routine autopsy specimens by immunofluorescent technique. Am Heart J 74:13, 1967

——, COLCOLOUGH HL: Progressive Coxsackie viral pancarditis and nephritis. Ann Intern Med 71:963, 1969

JOHNSON RT et al: Acute benign pericarditis: Virologic study of 34 patients. Arch Intern Med 108:828, 1961

KIBRICK S: Viral infections of the fetus and newborn. Perspect Virol Symp NY 2:140, 1961.

LERNER AM, WILSON FM: Virus myocardiopathy. Prog Med Virol 15:63, 1973

SAINANI GS et al: Adult heart disease due to Coxsackievirus B infection. Medicine 47:133, 1968

Echo virus infection

BEHBEHANI AM, WENNER HA: Infantile diarrhea (a study of the etiologic role of viruses). Am J Dis Child 111:623, 1966

GOODWIN MH JR et al: Observations on the association of enteric viruses and bacteria with diarrhea. Am J Trop Med 16:178, 1967

HORSTMANN DM, YAMADA N: Enterovirus infections of the central nervous system. Res Publ Assoc Res Nerv Ment Dis 44:236, 1968

Reovirus infection

EL-RAI FM, EVANS, AS: Reovirus infections in children and young adults. Arch Environ Health 7:700, 1963

JOKLIK WK: The molecular biology of reovirus. J Cell Physiol 76:289, 1970

ROSEN L: Serologic grouping of reoviruses by hemagglutination-inhibition. Am J Hyg 77:29, 1963

——, et al: Reovirus infections in human volunteers. Am J Hyg 77:29, 1963

TILLOTSON JR, LERNER AM: Reovirus, type 3, associated with fatal pneumonia. N Engl J Med 276:1060, 1967

section 16 | Viral diseases of the central nervous system

191
LYMPHOCYTIC CHORIOMENINGITIS

HARRY N. BEATY

DEFINITION Lymphocytic choriomeningitis (LCM) is an acute systemic viral infection which is frequently accompanied by the clinical syndrome of aseptic meningitis in man.

ETIOLOGY The agent responsible for LCM is a small RNA virion which morphologically and serologically resembles the Machupo, Lassa, and similar viruses. Many different strains of the virus have been identified on the basis of tissue tropism and pathogenicity, but none is antigenically distinct. The agent can be propagated readily in many mammalian cell cultures, but it produces little or no cytopathic effect.

EPIDEMIOLOGY The virus of LCM is probably worldwide in distribution, but is an uncommon cause of human disease. Although infection can be induced in a variety of animals, mice are the major natural reservoir as well as the primary host in which latent, asymptomatic infection occurs. The latency of mouse infection depends upon immunologic tolerance, and animals infected *in utero* or shortly after birth excrete the virus for life without overt disease. In man, LCM has followed direct contact with wild mice or infected rodents in experimental laboratories, and it is assumed that contact with contaminated mice or their excreta is the major mechanism for spread of this infection to human beings. LCM occurs throughout the year, but is somewhat more frequent in the colder months when human contact with wild rodents is greatest. Transmission of the virus by arthropod vectors has been accomplished experimentally, but has never been demonstrated to occur naturally. Man-to-man transmission is extremely rare.

PATHOGENESIS In natural infection, the portal of entry of the LCM virus is probably through the respiratory tract. Virus multiplication occurs initially in the respiratory epithelium, and in some patients symptoms of an upper respiratory tract infection or influenza-like illness develop. Dissemination of virus to secondary extraneural sites of growth, possibly in reticuloendothelial cells, may be an important step in the pathogenesis of central nervous system disease. The virus multiplies in these sites, and when sustained viremia develops, crosses the blood-brain barrier and infects meningeal cells. In mice, the resulting meningitis, which is characterized by lymphocytic infiltration, is attributed to an immunologic reaction. It is postulated that this immune response is mediated by lymphocytes rather than antibody and is directed against host cells which are no longer recognized as self because of membrane alterations induced by the virus. Support for this hypothesis derives from observations that disease but not infection can be prevented in experimental animals by neonatal thymectomy, irradiation, or immunodepressant drugs. Similar pathogenetic mechanisms may operate in human beings.

CLINICAL MANIFESTATIONS Infection of man by the LCM virus produces a variety of clinical manifestations. Serologic surveys indicate that inapparent or unrecognized infection is common. It is also clear that symptomatic infection ordinarily consists of a clinically nonspecific upper respiratory tract infection which may resemble influenza. Neurologic manifestations appear only infrequently, and take the form of aseptic meningitis or encephalitis.

The exact incubation period is not known, but it is probably only a few days. Initially, symptoms consist of remittent fever, anorexia, malaise, generalized aching, headache, and respiratory manifestations ranging from pharyngitis, cough, and bronchitis to frank pneumonia. Fever and discomfort often vary in intensity, abating somewhat and then recurring over a period of 1 to 3 weeks. Many patients then recover completely. In others, however, apparent convalescence is interrupted by a recurrence of fever and the abrupt onset of headache, photophobia, and signs of meningeal irritation. This second stage of the disease ordinarily lasts 7 to 10 days, but relapses or recurrences of meningeal symptoms are seen occasionally. A few patients have transient erythematous or papular rashes during the meningeal phase.

Patients with aseptic meningitis almost always recover without sequelae. With encephalitis, however, 25 to 30 percent of patients have neurologic abnormalities, and convalescence may be prolonged. Arthralgia and frank arthritis may be seen during recovery from the acute systemic illness, and in a few well-documented cases of infection with the LCM virus, orchitis has been observed.

LABORATORY FINDINGS Leukopenia with granulocytopenia and relative lymphocytosis is commonly seen in the acute systemic illness. If meningitis develops, the leukocyte count is often normal, but may be elevated with a predominance of polymorphonuclear leukocytes. Typically, cerebrospinal fluid pressure is elevated, and protein concentration increased. The glucose concentration is usually normal, but levels of 35 to 40 mg per 100 ml have been observed. The cell count in the spinal fluid usually ranges from 100 to 3,000 cells per mm^3 with 90 percent lymphocytes.

DIAGNOSIS The diagnosis of LCM can be established with certainty by recovery of the virus from blood or spinal fluid, or by serologic studies. Complement-fixing antibodies are usually detectable 1 to 2 weeks after the onset of infection, and neutralizing antibody appears after 6 to 8 weeks. Immunofluorescent studies have detected antibody to the LCM virus earlier in the course of the illness, and its appearance seems to parallel the development of the neurologic phase. The clinical manifestations of LCM cannot be differentiated from those produced by infections with numerous other viruses. A detailed discussion of aseptic meningitis appears in Chap. 330

TREATMENT The management of infections with the LCM virus is purely supportive and symptomatic.

REFERENCES

Baum SG et al: Epidemic nonmeningitic lymphocytic choriomeningitis virus infection. N Engl J Med 274:937, 1966

Hotchin J: Virus, cell surface, and self: Lymphocytic choriomeningitis of mice. Am J Clin Pathol 56:33, 1971

Johnson RT, Mims CA: Pathogenesis of viral infections of the nervous system. N Engl J Med 278:23, 1968

Meyer HM Jr et al: Central nervous system syndromes of viral etiology. Am J Med 29:334, 1960

192
POLIOMYELITIS

LOUIS WEINSTEIN

DEFINITION Poliomyelitis is a common acute viral infection which occurs naturally only in man and produces a wide variety of clinical manifestations. In its most severe form, it involves parts of the central nervous system. In most instances, the nervous system is not invaded; infection may take place without apparent illness, or it may result in the production of nonspecific syndromes or in invasion of the nervous system with or without the development of dysfunction.

ETIOLOGY The causative agent of poliomyelitis is an RNA virus of the picorna group, 8 to 30 nm in diameter, pathogenic for man and primates. Three antigenically distinct types have been defined: type 1 (Brunhilde), type 2 (Lansing), and type 3 (Leon). Cross neutralization is demonstrable in highly immunized experimental animals, but infection in man with one type does not protect against invasion by another. Poliomyelitis virus grows well in tissue culture.

Under proper conditions, the virus may remain viable in water or sewage for as long as 4 months. It is not killed by ether, Merthiolate, tincture of Zephiran, ethyl alcohol, low concentrations of mercury, oxidizing agents, 2% tincture of iodine, ultraviolet light, and 10-min exposure to a chlorine concentration of 0.05 ppm.

EPIDEMIOLOGY Poliomyelitis is worldwide, but epidemics have been limited to a relatively small number of areas. That infection is much more prevalent than is suggested by the number of clinically recognized cases is proved by the widespread distribution of neutralizing antibody in population groups all over the world. Poliomyelitis occurs with the highest frequency from July through September in the North Temperate Zone, although it may appear as early as April or as late as December. In tropical or subtropical regions, the "season" may be prolonged.

In areas of poor sanitation, most individuals develop neutralizing antibodies in early childhood, whereas, in other localities, the peak of immunity is not reached until fifteen years of age or older. Urban dwellers become immune earlier than those who live in rural areas. In lower-income groups, evidence of contact with poliomyelitis virus appears at a younger age than in individuals whose financial status is good.

PATHOGENESIS Man is the sole reservoir of poliomyelitis virus. Carriers with inapparent infection are most important in transmission of the virus. A history of contact with recognized cases is uncommon. Milk was incriminated as the source of infection in one epidemic.

Virus is recoverable from pharyngeal secretions for only a few days but is demonstrable in the feces for several weeks. The intestinal tract is the main source from which virus is disseminated. Therefore, the route of infection, fecal-oral, is the same as that in salmonellosis, shigellosis, and other enteric infections. Large quantities of virus are present in sewage drained from areas in which the infection is present. Poliomyelitis is as highly communicable as measles or varicella. In individuals under fifteen years of age, infection, with or without clinical manifestations, occurs in 100 percent of household and 87 percent of daily contacts.

The following sequence of events has been postulated for the pathogenesis of poliomyelitis: (1) The virus enters the body by way of the mouth and begins to multiply in the oropharynx and lower part of the intestinal tract. Virus is present in pharyngeal secretions and stool during the incubation period; it has been demonstrated in the feces as long as 19 days prior to onset of the disease. (2) The phase of "minor illness" (described below) develops in association with the presence of the virus in the blood, throat, and feces; the viremia persists for only a few days, until antibodies make their appearance. Virus in the intestinal tract penetrates the lymphatic channels and enters the bloodstream, from which it is disseminated. (3) The final stage is invasion of the nervous system. It has been suggested that the virus enters the nervous system from the blood in the area postrema of the medulla oblongata; it has also been postulated, however, that viral invasion of the nervous system occurs at many points by direct passage of virus from capillaries to neurons. Once the infectious agent has reached the nervous system, it spreads along nerve fibers.

Strains of poliomyelitis virus vary greatly in their ability to invade nervous tissue and to destroy neurons. The early presence of detectable antibody results from multiplication of virus in nonnervous tissue and accounts for the short persistence of the agent in the pharynx and blood, sites in which antibody is demonstrable. The persistence of virus in the nervous system and intestine is probably due to the difficulty which antibody has in reaching these areas.

The most important determinant of human susceptibility to poliomyelitis is serum antibody. Previous inapparent infection and illness without invasion of the nervous system are common. Many children and most adults possess neutralizing antibody for all three types of virus; this probably accounts for the relative infrequency of the disease in older age groups. Infants under six months old rarely get poliomyelitis because immunity is passively transferred from the mother. Babies born to women in the acute phase of poliomyelitis can develop the disease shortly after birth. Among children, males are affected more often than females; the opposite is true in adults. Pregnancy increases the risk of clinically apparent poliomyelitis, and multiparous females are more susceptible than primiparas. The disease is somewhat more frequent in the second than in the first or third trimesters of pregnancy. Menstruation or ovulation appears to heighten susceptibility. Absence of the tonsils and adenoids, regardless of the time of their removal, is associated with a marked increase in incidence of bulbar poliomyelitis. Chilling or physical exertion after invasion by the virus leads to more frequent development of paralytic poliomyelitis, especially in adults.

CLINICAL MANIFESTATIONS The incubation period of poliomyelitis varies from 3 to 35 days; about 80 percent of cases occur 6 to 20 days after contact with the virus. The infection may assume one of four forms: (1) inapparent infection, (2) "minor illness," (3) nonparalytic poliomyelitis, (4) paralytic poliomyelitis.

Inapparent infection The bulk of infection with the virus of poliomyelitis (95 percent) occurs in this form. There are no symptoms, but the virus is present in the pharynx and intestine and probably also in the blood. Type-specific neutralizing antibody usually develops.

"Minor illness" The entire course of poliomyelitis may consist of a nonspecific illness without clinical or laboratory evidence of central nervous system invasion; this is "abortive" poliomyelitis. Three syndromes have been observed: (1) upper respiratory manifestations, consisting of fever of varying degree, pharyngeal discomfort, with or without coryza, and reddening and swelling of the lymphoid tissues of the throat; (2) gastrointestinal disturbances, with nausea, vomiting, diarrhea or constipation, and abdominal discomfort, accompanied by moderate fever; (3) grippelike disease with fever and symptoms resembling influenza. Virus can be demonstrated in the pharynx, feces, and blood in the early stages of these "minor" illnesses. Type-specific neutralizing and complement-fixing antibodies develop during convalescence.

Nonparalytic poliomyelitis Nonparalytic poliomyelitis consists of prodromal manifestations, signs of meningeal irritation, and abnormalities of the spinal fluid. The prodrome is similar to that of the "minor" illnesses and is usually present for several days before the onset of other signs. Stiffness of the neck and back, positive Kernig's sign, and, with severe meningeal irritation, Brudzinski's sign are present. The tripod (patient extends arms behind back with hands on bed for support when sitting up) and Hoyne's signs (head falls back when, with patient in supine position, shoulders are elevated) can be elicited in paralytic or nonparalytic poliomyelitis but are not pathognomonic. The spinal fluid usually contains between 25 and 500 cells, rarely as many as 1,000 to 2,000. Very early in the disease, there is often a preponderance of neutrophils (up to 80 percent); within a few days, however, mononuclear cells predominate. The protein is normal or slightly elevated at the beginning of the illness but may increase to between 50 and 100 mg per 100 ml. The sugar content is normal. These findings are not diagnostic of poliomyelitis. They are also present in all of the entities classified as aseptic meningitis (Chap. 330). The diagnosis of nonparalytic poliomyelitis is impossible on clinical grounds alone, because the signs, symptoms, and laboratory findings are completely nonspecific. Viral and immunologic studies suggest that fewer than 40 percent of patients in whom "nonparalytic poliomyelitis" is diagnosed actually have the disease.

The course of nonparalytic poliomyelitis is benign. Defervescence occurs in 3 to 5 days, but meningeal irritation may persist for 2 weeks. No change in muscle and nerve function is detectable. The white blood cell count may be as high as 15,000 in the early stage of the disease but is usually normal within a week.

Paralytic poliomyelitis The syndrome of paralytic poliomyelitis consists of prodromal manifestations ("minor illness"), signs of meningeal irritation, abnormal spinal fluid, and involvement of motor nerve cells in the spinal cord, brain, or cranial nerve nuclei, resulting in paresis or paralysis of various muscles. Lesions may also be present in parts of the nervous system other than anterior horn cells; the precentral gyrus, the reticular formation in the medulla, the roof nuclei and vermis of the cerebellum, Auerbach's and Meissner's plexuses, and sympathetic ganglions are usually found to be involved in fatal cases. Seldom, however, are there clinical signs pointing to disease of these parts. "Skip" areas are common in spinal paralytic disease; e.g., involvement of the cervical and lumbar cords is often present with no dysfunction of the thoracic portion.

Paralytic poliomyelitis may be subdivided into the following types:

- *I* Spinal
  - *A* Cervical
  - *B* Thoracic
  - *C* Lumbar
  - *D* Any combination of A, B, and C
- *II* Bulbar
  - *A* Upper cranial nerve involvement—III, IV, V, VI, VII, VIII
  - *B* Lower cranial nerve involvement—IX, X, XI, XII
  - *C* Involvement of cardiorespiratory centers
- *III* Bulbospinal
- *IV* Polioencephalitis, paralytic or nonparalytic
  - *A* Diffuse encephalitis
  - *B* Focal encephalitis
  - *C* Cerebellar involvement (?)
  - *D* Bulboencephalitic disease
  - *E* Spinal-encephalitic disease

Prodromal manifestations are often absent in paralytic poliomyelitis. In some cases, the illness is biphasic in character. The disease starts with fever and manifestations of one of the "minor" illnesses. After several days, all symptoms disappear; in 5 or 10 days, there is recrudescence of fever, the development of signs of meningeal irritation, and the appearance of paralysis. The commonest prodromal symptoms in adults are generalized muscle and bone discomfort. In children, upper respiratory tract syndromes are most frequent. The spinal fluid findings in paralytic poliomyelitis are the same as those in the nonparalytic disease. A completely normal spinal fluid may be present initially and, rarely, throughout the entire course of the disease.

SPINAL PARALYTIC POLIOMYELITIS In the early stages of spinal paralytic poliomyelitis, severe cramping pain in the muscles innervated by the affected neurons and hyperesthesia of the overlying skin are present. Muscle "spasm," the exact mechanism of which is not clear, is usually detectable. In some instances, progression of muscle weakness is very slow; in others, it becomes widespread within 48 hr. A rapidly ascending paralysis of the Landry type may develop rarely. Age is determinant of the extent of involvement. In children less than five years old, paresis of one leg is most common. In patients between five and fifteen years of age, weakness of one arm, or paraplegia, is most frequent, while in adults (sixteen to sixty-five years old), quadriplegia is observed most often. Dysfunction of the urinary bladder is ten times more frequent in adults than in children. Paralysis of the muscles of respiration is most common in those older than sixteen years of age. Infants younger than one year are subject to very extensive involvement. Among adults, men develop quadriplegia, respiratory paralysis, and loss of bladder function more frequently than do women. Pregnancy does not increase the severity of the disease unless parturition takes place during the acute phase. There is a definite association of inoculation of antigenic materials ("triple vaccine," for example) with involvement of the muscles around the site of injection.

When the cervical cord is involved, there is paresis or paralysis of the muscles of the shoulders, arms, neck, and diaphragm. Very early in the disease, the reflexes in the arms remain lively; they diminish rapidly, however, and are usually absent by the time paralysis has become established. Coarse twitching of the affected muscles is common. There is always danger of respiratory paralysis when the cervical cord is involved; this is related to spread of the infection to the motor nuclei of the phrenic nerves and medulla.

Weakness of the muscles of the chest, upper portion of the abdomen, and spine follows involvement of the thoracic portion of the spinal cord. Difficulty in breathing results from dysfunction of the intercostal and other thoracic muscles. The chest wall may be in "spasm" and may appear rigid despite the presence of only a minor degree of paresis.

Disease of the lumbar portion of the spinal cord produces weakness of the legs and inferior portions of the abdomen and back. Pain, tenderness, "spasm," and twitching herald the oncoming paralysis, and the reflexes are abolished with the development of flaccid paralysis. In adults, complete paraplegia is not infrequent. Paralysis of the urinary bladder, usually temporary, occurs in about one-third of patients over sixteen years of age and is rarely observed in the absence of weakness of the legs.

The abdominal and cremasteric reflexes usually disappear before muscle weakness is marked in paralytic poliomyelitis and may be absent during the entire course of the disease. An extensor plantar response is a rare finding; its persistence is incompatible with poliomyelitis. Hyperesthesia of the skin is frequent, but sensory loss does not occur. Constipation, abdominal cramps, and meteorism are common and are due to ileus resulting from involvement of the autonomic nervous system and weakness of the abdominal muscles. When the disease is severe, sympathetic nervous system disturbances are present: tachycardia, hypertension, abnormal sweating, and cyanosis and coldness of the involved extremities.

Fever in spinal paralytic poliomyelitis is usually present for the first few days of the disease and disappears by lysis. In about 90 percent of cases, there is little or no extension of paralysis after defervescence has been established for 48 hr. In about 10 percent, however, noticeable progression of weakness may continue for as long as a week or more.

BULBAR POLIOMYELITIS The incidence of bulbar poliomyelitis differs from one epidemic to another and varies between 6 and 25 percent. About 85 percent of patients subjected to tonsilloadenoidectomy within 30 days of onset of the disease as well as others who have had this operation years before develop the bulbar form of infection. Pure bulbar involvement, without any signs of spinal cord involvement, is commonest in children; adults with bulbar disturbances usually have associated spinal paralysis. The syndromes which develop depend on the area of the brainstem involved, and result from damage to the medulla, pons, and midbrain. Signs and symptoms are produced by (1) dysfunction of the upper cranial nerve nuclei, (2) damage to the lower cranial nerve nuclei, and (3) disturbances of the respiratory and vasomotor regulating centers in the medulla. Combined bulbar and diffuse or focal encephalitis or spinal involvement may occur.

Upper cranial nerve nuclei—III, IV, V, VI, VII, VIII. Isolated ocular nerve palsies, total external ophthalmoplegia, pupillary disorders, and Horner's syndrome occur. There may be unilateral or bilateral involvement of the fifth nerve. Paralysis of the seventh cranial nerve is common and usually unilateral; the entire face or only the upper or lower parts may be affected. Disturbances of vestibular function and deafness resulting from damage to the nucleus of the eighth nerve occur infrequently.

Lower cranial nerve nuclei—IX, X, XI, XII. Life may be endangered when the muscles of deglutition are paralyzed because of involvement of the nucleus ambiguus. Hoarseness and laryngeal stridor follow weakness or paralysis of the vocal cords. Unilateral or bilateral weakness of the tongue and of the sternocleidomastoid and trapezius muscles may be present. Inability to swallow results in pooling of saliva and food in the pharynx, with obstruction of the airway. Aspiration into the larynx, reflex spasm of the glottis, and abductor paralysis of the vocal cords constitute very serious threats to life. Minor or major pareses of the soft palate and pharyngeal muscles are detectable by a nasal quality of the voice.

Disease of the medullary respiratory center This produces irregularity of the rhythm, depth, and rate of breathing. Respirations are shallow, and as the disease progresses, there are longer and longer periods of apnea until breathing stops completely. The thoracic muscles and diaphragm are not weak, unless spinal involvement is present. Hiccuping is frequent in the early phase of respiratory center dysfunction. Hypoxia, without visible cyanosis, is common and contributes to the intensity of the manifestations. In the late stages, cyanosis, not responsive to oxygen administration, is common, and temperature, pulse rate, and blood pressure are elevated. The final event is usually irreversible shock.

The manifestations of involvement of the circulatory regulating center are a cherry-red color of the lips, flushed skin, rapid, irregular pulse, small pulse pressure when the blood pressure is normal, and moderate to severe hypotension. Hyperthermia, cold, mottled, clammy skin, shallow respiration, and anxiety, restlessness, and confusion appear as the circulation becomes progressively impaired.

POLIOENCEPHALITIS Encephalitic symptoms occur as isolated syndromes or together with bulbar or spinal poliomyelitis. The incidence of polioencephalitis is variable. The diffuse form is characterized by confusion, agitation, anxiety with a feeling of impending doom, or somnolence. Quivering and jerking of the facial muscles and extremities, flushing of the face, tremor of the hands, and restless movements occur. Insomnia may be severe. In fatal cases, the confusion is marked and progresses to lethargy and death.

In focal polioencephalitis, there may be clinical evidence of brain damage, or the lesions may be silent and demonstrable only at necropsy. Visual-verbal agnosia, myoclonic jerks, grand mal convulsions, which occasionally persist for a long time after recovery, spastic hemiparesis, ataxia of one arm or leg, and hydrocephalus have been described.

DIAGNOSIS The diagnosis of paralytic poliomyelitis can usually be made on clinical grounds. The outstanding manifestation is rapidly developing lower motor neuron dysfunction resulting in flaccid weakness and hypo- or areflexia. Signs of upper motor neuron disease or decreased sensation are not compatible with poliomyelitis. A number of other forms of encephalitis may present with similar manifestations. The only positive method of establishing the diagnosis of paralytic poliomyelitis is the isolation of the virus from the stool or pharyngeal secretions (spinal cord or brain at necropsy) and the demonstration of a rise in the level of neutralizing antibody to the isolated strain in acute- and convalescent-phase serums. The three type strains maintained in tissue culture may be used for serologic tests. A significant rise in titer of neutralizing antibody against a specific serotype is diagnostic.

COMPLICATIONS Complications occur most frequently when the respiratory muscles are involved. Disturbances in water and electrolyte balance are common in patients receiving continuous artificial respiration. Fever and the sweating which follows enclosure in a tank during the summer months, together with vomiting, diarrhea, inability to take food, and disturbances in blood gases due to improperly regulated ventilation, may produce severe chemical disturbances. Edema and low electrolyte levels often follow overenthusiastic hydration. *Myocarditis*, probably the result of viral invasion of the heart, is not uncommon in poliomyelitis. Changes in the ECG, mainly T and ST-T and P-R abnormalities, are present in from 10 to 20 percent of cases. Interstitial infiltration of the myocardium with round cells, and mild muscle changes are not infrequent. Cardiomyopathy has been thought to be responsible for death in some cases. *Hypertension* may develop by two mechanisms: (1) transient elevation of blood pressure due to hypoxia, and (2) persistent hypertension secondary to hypothalamic involvement, which may become "malignant" and lead to retinopathy, convulsions, and mental deterioration.

Pulmonary edema and *shock*, the exact pathogenesis of which is not known, are usually the terminal events in fatal cases of poliomyelitis. Although relatively young adults are involved, phlebothrombosis of the legs with or without pulmonary embolism is not uncommon. When patients are placed in respirators under negative tank pressure (positive intratracheal pressure) after hypotension and impending shock have developed, the peripheral vascular collapse often is intensified. Acute and severe dilatation of the stomach and large bowel, perforation of the cecum, acute ulceration of the duodenum, stomach, and esophagus, and multiple erosions of the entire gastrointestinal tract with considerable bleeding and paralytic ileus have been observed. Marked depression of prothrombin, with massive spontaneous hemorrhage, may result from the administration of large doses of broad-spectrum antibiotics orally. Severe bulbar (ninth and tenth cranial nerves) or bulbospinal disease with paralysis of the respiratory muscles is accompanied by the risk of atelectasis. Pneumonia is quite common in patients with paralysis of the muscles of respiration or deglutition. Its incidence is greatly increased by tracheostomy and is highest in the respirator patient subjected to this operation. The organisms involved most often are *Staphylococcus aureus* and gram-negative bacilli, many strains of which are not sensitive to the commonly used antimicrobial agents. Chemoprophylaxis is of no value in preventing secondary bronchopulmonary bacterial invasion.

A common site of infection in poliomyelitis is the urinary tract; this is usually related to the presence of an indwelling urethral catheter; chemoprophylaxis, even when given together with tidal drainage, is usually ineffective. Renal lithiasis, with infection, is common and is due to immobility, with mobilization of calcium, infection, stasis, dehydration, and calcium intake. Liberal administration of fluids, decreased calcium intake, acidification of the urine, administration of salicylate, and early mobilization may reduce the incidence of stone formation.

A syndrome resembling rheumatoid arthritis, with redness, swelling, pain, and tenderness of the larger joints, may occur in the convalescent phase of paralytic poliomyelitis. Markedly paralyzed patients, especially those whose life is threatened by respiratory difficulty, frequently experience very difficult emotional problems. Disorientation, acute panic states, Korsakoff-like syndromes, and acute psychoses have been noted. Chronic anxiety and depression are almost universal in adults with severe disease, and probably reflect the sudden impact of a crippling disease, rather than brain damage due to viral invasion.

IMMUNITY One attack of poliomyelitis usually confers lifelong immunity against the same serotype. Both neutralizing and complement-fixing antibodies appear early in the disease; the latter persist for several years after infection, while the former persist throughout life. Theoretically, an individual could develop three episodes of the disease, because immunity is strictly type-specific. Most adults and many children have poliomyelitis, without nervous system invasion, two or three times, as shown by the presence in their serums of neutralizing antibody for more than one virus type. There are, however, well-documented instances of two episodes of paralyzing infection separated by a number of years in the same individual.

TREATMENT Cases of abortive poliomyelitis require no therapy. The management of nonparalytic poliomyelitis involves primarily the relief of the headache, pain in the back, and "spasm" of the legs. Rest in bed with the mattress supported by a board may be valuable in preventing paralysis and is helpful in reducing the back discomfort. The application of wet heat, in the form of "hot packs," to the affected muscles produces considerable relief. Analgesics such as Demerol and codeine are very useful and are preferable to other morphine derivatives. Antimicrobial agents are useless, because they have no effect on the primary disease and do not decrease the risk of secondary infection. Neuromuscular examination should not be carried out more often than every 3 to 4 days. Bed rest is terminated as soon as severe discomfort is absent, in order to reduce the risk of phlebothrombosis and pulmonary embolism. Every patient thought to have nonparalytic poliomyelitis should have careful assessment of muscle function for 2 to 3 months after recovery. The purpose of this is to detect and correct minor degrees of weakness which may become apparent only when muscles which appear normal at rest are taxed by the exertion of normal physical activity.

The treatment of paralytic poliomyelitis involves (1) the use of all measures to spare the life of the patient threatened by involvement of vital areas, (2) relief of discomfort, (3) maintenance of weak muscles in as good a condition as possible, (4) immediate recognition and treatment of medical complications, (5) prophylaxis and therapy of emotional disorders, (6) surgical treatment of correctable defects, and (7) social, economic, occupational, and physical rehabilitation.

Patients with paralysis of swallowing or respiratory muscles, pulmonary edema, or shock are in great danger of death. Dysfunction of the ninth and tenth cranial nerves is most important because of the danger of fatal airway obstruction. For this reason, it has been suggested that tracheostomy be performed in all such cases. However, this procedure is followed by a much higher incidence of bronchopulmonary infections due to organisms difficult to eradicate with antibiotic agents than occurs when the procedure is not carried out. In some cases, nevertheless, tracheostomy becomes necessary, despite the risks. The indications for this operation are (1) abductor paralysis of the vocal cords; (2) pneumonia with inability to clear the lungs of exudate; (3) repeated bouts of major atelectasis requiring tracheal catheterization or bronchoscopy; (4) inability to keep the airway relatively free of secretions (this is often purely a matter of availability of experienced personnel).

Decreased function of the diaphragms or intercostal muscles necessitates frequent determination of vital capacity. When this is reduced to 50 percent of normal or less, respiratory assist devices must be used (Chap. 263). An electrophrenic respirator is indicated when the respiratory center is involved.

Shock is easier to prevent than to treat. Assurance of adequate oxygen saturation, prevention of dehydration, and early treatment of superimposed bacterial infection are of prophylactic value. When marked hypotension and clinical evidence of shock develop, treatment is similar to that employed in other situations in which infection is responsible for the syndrome (Chap. 124). However, treatment may not be effective because of failure of the neurologic control of blood pressure and oxygen perfusion. Hypotension appearing during artificial respiration may respond to alternating positive and negative tank pressures of approximately the same magnitude.

Relief of discomfort is the same as for nonparalytic disease. Changing the position of paralyzed limbs and moving the patient about in bed are effective in reducing pain.

Weak muscles must be maintained in as good condition as possible until neural function returns; the time, degree, and extent of resumption of function are unpredictable, but treatment should be continued for at least 2 years. Daily physiotherapy is usually started 3 to 4 days after complete defervescence, and when extension of weakness has ceased.

The prevention and treatment of the emotional disorders which accompany severe paralytic poliomyelitis are often best carried out by the attending physicians and nurses. Although the help of the psychiatrist is necessary in difficult situations, the physicians, nurses, and attendants who are in constant contact with the patient and are properly oriented toward his problems should play the major role.

Maximal return of muscle function usually is established at the end of 2 years following the onset of paralysis. If there is a considerable degree of residual paralysis after this time, a program of surgical rehabilitation should be initiated.

The impact of paralytic poliomyelitis on the social and economic status of adults is often very severe. Every effort must be made to enlist the cooperation of social service agencies to minimize the disruptive effects of the disease. Many patients require occupational rehabilitation because of inability to perform the work in which they were engaged prior to being crippled. For others, the use of devices such as movable splints, hooks, etc., is very helpful in physical rehabilitation.

PROGNOSIS The overall mortality rate for poliomyelitis is about 5 percent. Patients with abortive or nonparalytic disease recover completely. About 2 to 5 percent of children and 15 to 30 percent of adults (increasing with age) with paralyzing infection die. When bulbospinal involvement, especially with medullary or phrenic and intercostal nerve dysfunction, is present, the fatality rate varies between 25 to 75 percent; in these cases, it is greatly influenced by age and the presence of shock, pulmonary edema, superimposed infection, or other medical complications.

Many persons with paralytic poliomyelitis recover completely, and in most muscle function returns to some degree. Only a few remain totally paralyzed. The more life-threatening the disease in the acute stage, the more frequent is complete functional recovery, if the patient survives; paralysis of the respiratory center usually disappears completely. Similarly, dysfunction of the ninth and tenth cranial nerves is followed by total recovery in most instances, although mild palatopharyngeal weakness may occasionally persist for life. Paralysis of the muscles of respiration often disappears completely, and in most cases the final vital capacity is adequate to maintain ventilation. In a very few instances chronic respirator care is necessary. Weak extremities regain about 60 percent of the total strength that they will ever recover in 3 months, and 80 percent within 6 months, but improvement may continue for as long as 2 years.

PREVENTION Because 90 to 95 percent of cases of poliomyelitis are inapparent, or "minor" infections, and are not diagnosed, the prevention of the disease by isolation is very difficult. The common practice of isolating clinically evident cases is of much greater individual than public health benefit. The usual period of isolation is about 2 weeks, although virus may be present in the feces for a much longer period. Contact with known cases should be avoided. Restriction of community activities such as swimming, gathering of people, etc., is not indicated except with large epidemics, when it is more effective in allaying panic than in reducing infection. Pregnant women should take special precaution because of the increased susceptibility to the disease during pregnancy. Tonsillectomy is contraindicated in areas where poliomyelitis is present. All individuals with "minor" illnesses during the poliomyelitis season should limit their physical activity and avoid chilling until all symptoms have disappeared.

Active immunization against paralytic poliomyelitis has been successfully produced by parenteral administration of formalin-inactivated strains of the three viral serotypes grown in monkey kidney tissue culture. The vaccine is 60 to 70 percent effective against type 1 and 85 to 90 percent against types 2 and 3. A booster dose should be given within 2 years after initial injection series. The effectiveness of this type of vaccine is evidenced by the fact that, in the year (1955) in which it was introduced, there were 28,985 cases of poliomyelitis in the United States. Two years later, only 2,218 cases were reported. However, this vaccine does not appear to decrease the incidence of nonparalytic poliomyelitis and has no effect on the intestinal phase of the disease. It has been practically completely replaced by "live vaccines."

Oral administration of attenuated strains of poliovirus is highly effective in stimulating antibody production and preventing infection and is the method of choice for protecting a population. The virus preparations are easily handled and are stable. They may be stored in a conventional refrigerator for up to 30 days. Once a vial has been used in part, the rest of its contents should be discarded after 7 days.

Vaccine virus multiplies in the intestinal tract and remains at this site. Viremia occurs rarely, and then only with some strains. Live vaccine virus spreads and infects contacts of vaccinated individuals. This type of immunization in the presence of epidemic poliomyelitis may lead to replacement of the "wild" paralytogenic strain by the one in the vaccine, actually aborting spread of the disease.

Significant levels of antibody develop in 90 to 100 percent of persons receiving live virus vaccine; they develop more rapidly and persist longer than those which follow the use of formalinized vaccines. Intestinal immunity is present after feeding of the "live" preparations so that minimal or no multiplication in the bowel occurs on exposure to "wild" strains of virus.

The highest levels of poliomyelitis-neutralizing antibody appear when monovalent oral vaccines are administered. The recommended order of administration is type 1, followed after no less than 8 weeks by type 3, and at 6 or more weeks later by type 2. If the polyvalent vaccine (all three types) is given to adults, two doses are fed 8 weeks apart. If newborns are given vaccine, the viruses should be refed at a later date, because about 50 percent of neonates fail to develop significant levels of immunity if treated shortly after birth. Immunization of breast-fed infants is best delayed until they are taking regular diets. It has been suggested that a community-wide program of vaccine virus feeding followed by routine immunization of infants in the first year of life may result in eradication of poliomyelitis. Immunization with live vaccine is best carried out during the colder months of the year. The widespread prevalence of other enteroviruses in the intestinal tract, especially in children, in the summer may result in a low level of immunization because these other viruses may interfere with the implantation of the vaccine strains. Although the necessity for "booster" doses of this preparation in older children and adults has not been proved, many physicians are administering the triple vaccine 1 to 2 years after primary immunization; some are giving a second "booster" 1 to 2 years after the first.

The administration of live poliomyelitis virus vaccines to millions of persons in many areas of the world has demonstrated very convincingly the very high degree of protection (over 90 percent) against paralytic poliomyelitis conferred by this preparation and a tendency for epidemic strains to be replaced by those present in the vaccine. The vaccines are remarkably safe. Although instances of the disease are thought to have been associated with feeding of each of the three strains (0.4 cases per million doses for type 3, 0.16 per million doses for type 1, and 0.02 per million doses for type 2), it has been suggested that the greatest risk of developing active disease produced by the vaccine strain is related to the administration of the type 3 preparation to individuals in the age range of twenty to thirty-nine years of age. Some observers have pointed out that firm proof of the association of vaccine virus and the development of poliomyelitis is lacking. Type 1 vaccine strain has been incriminated in a case of paralytic poliomyelitis in a young child with marked hypogammaglobulinemia. Children known to have this defect probably should not receive this agent.

REFERENCES

HENDERSON DA et al: Paralytic disease associated with oral polio vaccines. JAMA 190:41, 1964

SABIN AB: Commentary on report on oral poliomyelitis vaccines. JAMA 190:52, 1964

——: Poliomyelitis. Accomplishments of live virus vaccine. First international conference on vaccines against viral and rickettsial diseases. Bull WHO 171, 1967

SPECIAL ADVISORY COMMITTEE TO THE SURGEON GENERAL: Oral poliomyelitis vaccines. JAMA 190:49, 1964

Symposium on poliomyelitis. Pediatr Clin North Am 1:1, 1953

WEINSTEIN L: Diagnosis and treatment of poliomyelitis. Med Clin North Am September: 1377, 1948

——: The influence of muscular fatigue, tonsilladenoidectomy and antigen injections on the clinical course of poliomyelitis. Boston Med Q 3:11, 1952

——: Influence of age and sex on susceptibility and clinical manifestations in poliomyelitis. N Engl J Med 254:47, 1957

——: Cardiovascular disturbances in poliomyelitis. Circulation 15:735, 1957

193 RABIES

ROBERT H. RUBIN

DEFINITION Rabies is an acute viral disease of the central nervous system that affects virtually all mammals, and is transmitted from one to another by infected secretions, usually saliva, or tissue. The common mode of transmission is by the bite of an infected animal.

ETIOLOGY The rabies virus is a bullet-shaped RNA virus belonging to the rhabdovirus group, with a diameter of 750 to 800 A and varying lengths. Excrescenses, 60 to 70 A long, each with a knoblike structure at the distal end, cover the surface of the virion. The virus can be grown in tissue culture and avian embryos. A soluble complement-fixing antigen and a nonsoluble hemagglutinating antigen have been defined. Only one serologic type has been identified, but multiple passages of the virus through animals or tissue culture can change tissue infectivity. Interferon is induced by rabies virus, but only in those tissues with high concentrations of the virus. There is some question whether interferon plays any role in host defense.

EPIDEMIOLOGY Rabies exists in two epidemiologic forms: *urban*, propagated chiefly by unimmunized domestic dogs, and *sylvatic*, propagated in skunks, foxes, raccoons, mongooses, wolves, and bats. Infection in domestic animals usually represents a "spillover" from sylvatic reservoirs of infection, and man can be infected by either. Hence, human infection tends to occur in locales where rabies is enzootic or epizootic, where there is a large population of unimmunized domestic animals, and where human contact with the outdoors is common. Approximately one thousand human cases are reported to the World Health Organization each year, with many times that number believed to go unreported. Southeast Asia, the Philippines, Africa, and the Indian subcontinent are areas with an especially great problem. In contrast, the United States has noted only one to three cases per year for the last decade.

In most areas of the world the dog is the important vector of rabies virus, but the wolf (Eastern Europe, Arctic regions), the mongoose (South Africa, the Caribbean), the fox (Western Europe), and the vampire bat (Latin America) have an even greater impact in some places. In the United States skunks, raccoons, and domestic dogs are of greatest potential danger to man since their behavior patterns bring them into proximity with human populations. They are quite aggressive when ill, and they tend to have higher titers of virus in their saliva than other species. Aerosol transmission of the disease has been clearly demonstrated, but only in the unique ecologic conditions of the bat caves of Texas.

PATHOGENESIS The essential first event is the introduction of live virus into intimate contact with nerve tissue. Virus may persist at the inoculation site for up to 96 hr, but then spreads centripetally up the nerve to the central nervous system. Experimentally, viremia has been shown to occur, but it is not thought to play a role in naturally acquired disease. The exact site of transmission within the nerve fasciculus is not clear, but the tissue spaces appear to be more important than the Schwann cells, endoneurium, or axon cylinder. Once the virus reaches the central nervous system, it replicates almost exclusively within the gray matter, and then passes centrifugally along autonomic nerves to reach other tissues—the salivary glands, adrenal medulla, kidney, and heart. Passage to the salivary glands allows for further communication of the disease through infected saliva. The amount of time this process takes is exceedingly variable, with incubation periods of 10 days to 1 year (mean 1 to 2 months). This time period appears to depend more upon the amount of virus introduced, the type of tissue and tissue injury involved, and host defense mechanisms than the actual distance from site of inoculation to central nervous system that the virus has to travel.

The important point about the neuropathology of rabies is that it resembles that of any other viral encephalitis. These nonspecific findings include hyperemia; varying degrees of chromatolysis, nuclear pyknosis, and neuronphagia of the nerve cells; infiltration by lymphocytes and plasma cells of the Virchow-Robin spaces; and parenchymal areas of nerve cell destruction. The pathognomonic lesion of rabies is the Negri body, which is an eosinophilic mass approximately 10 μm in size, found in relatively undamaged nerve cells and distributed particularly in Ammon's horn, cerebral cortex, medulla, and the Purkinje cells of the cerebellum. Electron microscopic studies have demonstrated that the Negri body is the site of virus replication. The absence of the Negri body on light microscopy of brain material from at least 20 percent of rabies victims has been correlated with a higher degree of cellular damage and degeneration than occurs in cells that show the characteristic Negri bodies. The absence of Negri bodies does not rule out the diagnosis of rabies.

MANIFESTATIONS The clinical manifestations of rabies can be divided into three stages: a nonspecific prodrome; an encephalitis similar to other viral encephalitides; and a profound dysfunction of brainstem centers. It is this last which causes the classic features of rabies encephalitis.

The prodromal period usually persists for 1 to 4 days and is marked by fever as high as 102°F, headache, malaise, increased fatigability, anorexia, nausea and vomiting, sore throat, and a nonproductive cough. Characteristically, there are paresthesias at or about the site of inoculation of the virus in over 80 percent of cases during this period.

The encephalitic phase is usually ushered in by periods of excessive motor activity, excitation, and agitation. Quickly, confusion, hallucinations, combativeness, bizarre aberrations of thought, muscle spasms, meningismus, opisthotonic posturing, seizures, and focal paralysis appear. Characteristically, the periods of mental aberration are interspersed with completely lucid periods, but as the disease progresses, the lucid periods get shorter until the patient lapses into coma. Hyperesthesia, with sensitivity to bright light, loud noise, touch, and even gentle breezes, is very common. On physical examination the temperature may be as high as 105°F. Abnormalities of the autonomic nervous system, with dilated, irregular pupils, increased lacrimation, salivation, and perspiration, and postural hypotension may be seen. Evidence of upper motor neuron paralysis with weakness, increased deep tendon reflexes, and extensor plantar responses is the rule. Paralysis of the vocal cords is common.

The manifestations of brainstem dysfunction begin shortly after the onset of the encephalitic phase. Cranial nerve involvement causes diplopia, facial palsies, optic neuritis, and the characteristic difficulty with deglutition. The combination of excessive salivation and difficulty in swallowing produces the traditional picture of "foaming at the mouth." The first manifestation of difficult swallowing is usually painful spasms of the muscles of deglutition, rapidly progressing to frank paralysis. If the patient is still lucid during this period, he avoids swallowing water and manifests classic hydrophobia. From this point the patient quickly lapses into coma, and involvement of the respiratory centers produces an apneic death. The prominence of early brainstem dysfunction distinguishes rabies from other viral encephalitides and accounts for the rapid downhill course. The median survival after the onset of symptoms is 4 days, with a maximum of 20, unless artificial supporting measures are instituted.

An atypical form of rabies, resembling the Landry-Guillain-Barré syndrome has been described, and has been especially correlated with illness occurring after the bite of the vampire bat.

LABORATORY FINDINGS The hematocrit, urinalysis, and routine blood chemistries are usually normal. The white cell count is typically moderately elevated (12 to 17,000 per mm^3), but may be normal or as high as 30,000. The electrocardiogram may show evidence of a myocarditis. Cerebrospinal fluid findings include normal pressures, a few hundred cells (usually less than 100) with a predominance of lymphocytes, a normal sugar, and a moderately increased protein (60 to 85 mg per 100 ml). Virus has rarely been isolated from the cerebrospinal fluid, but not uncommonly from saliva.

Specific diagnosis of rabies depends on either serologic testing or examination of brain material. If the patient has not received antirabies immunization, then a greater than fourfold change in neutralizing antibody titer in serial specimens, as in any viral disease, is diagnostic of rabies. If the patient has received antirabies immunization, a clue to the diagnosis of rabies may be the absolute titer of neutralizing antibody found; immunization rarely produces titers greater than 1:1,000, while clinical rabies characteristically produces titers greater than 1:5,000. Obviously, this does not permit a definitive diagnosis, and specific diagnosis rests upon examination of brain material.

Samples of brain, obtained either at postmortem or at brain biopsy, are tested in three ways: special histologic staining for Negri bodies, fluorescent antibody staining for viral antigen, and mouse inoculation tests. If any one of these is positive, a definitive diagnosis can be made. Negri body tests have an incidence of 20 percent false negatives. Mouse inoculation tests and fluorescent antibody staining are quite reliable in the usual case of rabies, but if the patient's life is prolonged for a long period of time, "auto-sterilization" may occur and these tests become negative.

DIFFERENTIAL DIAGNOSIS There is little to distinguish rabies from other viral encephalitides, and the most helpful point in diagnosis is the history of exposure. Other problems to be considered include hysterical reactions to animal bites (pseudohydrophobia), Landry-Guillain-Barré syndrome, poliomyelitis, and allergic encephalomyelitis to rabies vaccine. The latter condition occurs most commonly after use of nervous tissue–derived vaccine, and usually begins 1 to 4 weeks after vaccination.

PREVENTION AND TREATMENT Approximately thirty thousand people in the United States and approximately one million in the world are given postexposure therapy for rabies each year. This therapy is based upon the concept that the level of neutralizing antibody can be correlated with immunity to the disease. The general principle in postexposure therapy is to minimize the amount of virus at the site of inoculation with local treatment of wounds, and then to have as high a titer of neutralizing antibody present as early and as long as possible. To this end, the following therapeutic regimen is employed:

1 Local wound therapy with generous scrubbing with soap and then flushing the wound with water or ethyl alcohol. This is followed by a second scrubbing with a quaternary ammonium compound such as 1 to 2% benzalkonium chloride (Zephiran) or 1% certrimonium bromide (Cetavlon). Local anesthesia is not contraindicated, but lacerations should not be sutured primarily.

2 Active immunization with either nervous tissue–derived vaccine (NTV) or duck embryo–derived vaccine (DEV). This consists of 14 to 21 daily injections of 1 ml vaccine subcutaneously, followed by boosters 10 and 20 days after the initial series.

3 Passive immunization with antirabies antiserum. At present, only equine-derived antiserum, with its risk of serum sickness, is available, and this is given in a dose of 40 units per kg, with 50 percent administered, if possible, by local infiltration of the wound, and the rest intramuscularly.

The critical problem with antirabies treatment is the reactions to therapy. Because of the exceedingly rare occurrence of the dreaded neuroparalytic reaction when DEV is used, this is the vaccine favored by the United States Public Health Service (USPHS), and this is the vaccine used approximately 85 percent of the time in the United States. Less serious reactions seen with DEV include the following: rare anaphylaxis, occasional gastrointestinal upset, and very common (up to 50 percent) local skin reactions with or without adenopathy, fever, chills, and myalgias. Treatment of such reactions is symptomatic with salicylates and antihistamines. Life-threatening neurologic reactions should be treated with steroids, but the use of steroids must be tempered by the evidence that they interfere with immunologic defenses and may activate latent rabies infection.

Although the therapy of a bona fide rabies exposure is relatively simple, the major difficulty is in deciding whether therapy is indicated. Table 193-1 presents the guidelines suggested by the USPHS. In making this decision, the following points should be kept in mind: What is the status of animal rabies in the locale where the exposure took place; was the attack provoked or unprovoked; what is the immunization status of the animal involved; what species inflicted the injury; is the animal available for examination; and what is the state of health of the animal? Most animals can transmit rabies virus in their saliva only a few days before becoming ill (the dog 5 days, the cat 1 day, the skunk 5 days, the fox 3 days), although bats may do so for months. Bites of wild animals, especially skunks, foxes, raccoons, and bats, should always be regarded as highly suspect. Local health authorities can be invaluable in helping with this decision, especially in assisting with veterinary aspects of the exposure.

TABLE 193-1
Postexposure antirabies prophylaxis guide of the United States Public Health Service

Animal		*Treatment*		
Species	*Status at time of attack*	*No lesion*	*Mild exposure**	*Severe exposure†*
Dog or cat	Healthy	None	None‡	S‡
	Signs suggestive of rabies	None	V§	S + V§
	Escaped or unknown	None	V	S +V
	Rabid	None	S + V	S + V
Skunk, fox, raccoon, coyote, or bat	*Regard as rabid in unprovoked attack*	None	S + V	S + V
			V	
Other		Consider individually; see Prevention and Treatment in text		

* *Scratches, lacerations, or single bites on areas of the body other than the head, face, neck, hands, or fingers. Open wounds, such as abrasions, suspected of being contaminated with saliva also belong in this category.*
† *Multiple or deep puncture wounds, or any bites on the head, face, neck, hands, or fingers.*
‡ *Begin vaccine at first sign of rabies in biting dog or cat during holding period (preferably 7–10 days).*
§ *Discontinue vaccine if biting dog or cat is healthy 5 days after exposure, or if acceptable laboratory negativity has been demonstrated in animal killed at time of attack. If observed animal dies after 5 days and brain is positive, resume treatment.*
V = Rabies vaccine.
S = Antirabies serum.

The availability of the relatively safe DEV has permitted the initiation of preexposure therapy for individuals with a high risk of exposure to rabies virus: veterinarians, spelunkers, residents of highly endemic areas of the world, and animal handlers. Such preexposure therapy consists of two 1-ml subcutaneous injections of DEV given 1 month apart, followed by a 1-ml booster 7 months later. At the completion of the three-shot series a neutralizing antibody titer should be checked through the state health department.

Until recently, rabies in humans had been regarded as being 100 percent fatal. However, since abortive rabies infection with full recovery was recognized in animals, and since neuropathologic changes from the virus itself are relatively minor, it was suggested that survival might be possible if prolonged intensive cardiorespiratory assistance were employed to counteract brainstem dysfunction. There has now been a human survivor of clinical rabies as a result of this mode of therapy. For the first time in history there is now hope in this dread disease.

REFERENCES

CAMPBELL JB et al: Present trends and the future in research. Bull WHO 38:373, 1968

CENTER FOR DISEASE CONTROL: Morbidity and mortality weekly report. 50(19):479, 1970

MATSUMATA S: Rabies virus. Adv Virus Res 16:257, 1970

PLOTKIN SA, CLARK HF: Prevention of rabies in man. J Infect Dis 123:227, 1971

RUBIN RH et al: A case of human rabies in Kansas: Epidemiologic, clinical and laboratory considerations. J Infect Dis 122:318, 1970

WHO Expert Committee on Rabies: Fifth report, WHO Tech. Rept. Ser. 321, 1966

194 DISEASES CAUSED BY SLOW VIRUSES

DONALD H. HARTER

Slow virus diseases are characterized by a long asymptomatic period, often of the order of months or years, between the introduction of the infectious agent and the appearance of clinical illness.

The factors responsible for this protracted incubation period have not been defined. Viruses causing slow infections do not appear to have any unique or common features, and the slowness of the disease may be due in large measure to the manner in which the host reacts or accommodates to the virus.

Some slow viruses provoke a conventional inflammatory response during the time they are clinically silent; others are able to reside within cells for long periods without causing detectable cytopathic changes. The role of immunity in slow virus infection is largely unknown. Some slow virus infections occur in the presence of elevated levels of circulating antibodies; in others, there may be no detectable immune response.

In animals, slow viruses are known to produce a variety of pulmonary, hepatic, renal, and neurological disorders. At present, there are only four definitely identified slow virus infections of man. These are four infrequently encountered neurological diseases: *kuru, Creutzfeldt-Jakob disease, progressive multifocal leukoencephalopathy*, and *subacute sclerosing panencephalitis*. Kuru and Creutzfeldt-Jakob disease share common neuropathological features and are referred to as the *transmissible spongiform encephalopathies*. Although these diseases have been shown to be of infectious etiology by the transmission of neurological illness to higher primates, little is known about the nature of the causative agents. Viruses have been recovered from the nervous system of patients with subacute sclerosing panencephalitis and progressive multifocal leukoencephalopathy, but the pathogenesis of these disorders is still largely unknown.

KURU Kuru, or "trembling with fear," is a progressive and fatal neurologic disorder which occurs exclusively among natives of the New Guinea Highland.

Difficulty in walking is usually the first sign of kuru. This usually progresses from a minor disturbance in gait rhythm to marked side-to-side lurching and staggering. Eventually, ambulation becomes incoordinated, and the patient is unable to use his limbs. As the disease progresses, cerebellar involvement (intention tremor, inability to perform rapid alternating movements, slurring of speech, hypotonia), abnormal involuntary movements resembling myoclonus, athetosis, or chorea, and convergent strabismus appear. Dementia develops in the later phases of the disease. The illness terminates fatally in 4 to 24 months, usually from decubitus ulcers or bronchopneumonia. Approximately 80 percent of adults afflicted with the disease are women.

Pathologic changes are limited to the central nervous system and include widespread neuronal loss, intense astrocytic and microglial proliferation, loss of myelinated fibers, and the presence of plaque-like bodies. Perivascular cuffing by lymphocytes and mononuclear cells has been observed occasionally.

It was the close similarity between the neuropathologic and clinical findings found in kuru and in scrapie, a slow infectious disease of sheep, that suggested the possibility that kuru was caused by a virus or other infectious agent. The infectious origin of kuru was confirmed subsequently by the appearance of a kuru-like syndrome in chimpanzees 18 to 21 months after intracerebral inoculation of suspensions of brain from human cases. Furthermore, the kuru syndrome has been transmitted from chimpanzee to chimpanzee by intracerebral passage with shortening of the incubation period to 12 months. The chimpanzee has been the only animal found to be susceptible to experimental kuru. Although a number of known and novel viruses have been recovered from tissue explants prepared from chimpanzees with the kuru syndrome, the specific agent responsible for the disease has not yet been characterized.

Cannibalism has been considered as a possible mode of transmission of kuru. Native custom in New Guinea dictates that marrow, viscera, and brain be cooked and eaten. The marked predilection of kuru for the adult female may be explained by the observation that cannibalism appears more prevalent among women and that males who practice cannibalism seldom eat the bodies of women. The recent influx of foreign settlers into the kuru area has led to increasing rejection of cannibalistic practices, and this, in turn, may be responsible for the progressive decline in the number of cases of kuru since 1960.

CREUTZFELDT-JAKOB DISEASE Creutzfeldt-Jakob disease is a fatal degenerative disease of the central nervous system which appears in middle or late middle age, most commonly as a rapidly evolving dementia with myoclonic seizures. Unlike kuru, the disease is not geographically limited.

Although Creutzfeldt-Jakob disease may have a diverse clinical presentation, it is usually first manifested by organic mental changes similar to those seen in the presenile dementias. The earliest changes include impairment of reasoning and judgment, memory disturbances, and bizarre behavior. The patient may complain of distortions in the shape and appearance of objects. Hallucinations, delusional ideas, and confusion occur as the disease progresses, and myoclonic movements and convulsive episodes develop. Ataxia, dysarthria, muscular atrophy, and other signs of anterior horn cell damage may be noted in some cases. Spasticity and rigidity appear later. The disease progresses rapidly to death within 3 to 12 months, often from intercurrent infection. There are no abnormalities in the cerebrospinal fluid, but the electroencephalogram is usually abnormal.

The cerebrum and cerebellum are affected predominantly. There is a marked proliferation of astrocytes and disappearance of nerve cells. Cytoplasmic vacuoles are found in glial cells. There is virtually no evidence of inflammatory changes. In the spinal cord, anterior horn cells may be damaged or lost, and there may be degeneration of the corticospinal tracts.

A neurological disease with the clinical and pathological features of Creutzfeldt-Jakob disease occurs in chimpanzees 12 to 14 months after inoculation with brain suspensions from patients with Creutzfeldt-Jakob disease. It is also possible to retransmit the disease to other chimpanzees. Neutralizing antibodies to the Creutzfeldt-Jakob agent have not yet been demonstrated in the serums of patients with the disease or of chimpanzees with the experimental disease.

PROGRESSIVE MULTIFOCAL LEUKOENCEPHALOPATHY This rare neurological condition, first described in 1958, usually occurs in patients who have leukemia, malignant lymphomas, carcinomatosis, or a variety of other chronic disease processes.

The disease affects adults of both sexes, and its duration from onset of symptoms to death is 1 to 4 months. The neurological signs and symptoms show diffuse, asymmetrical involvement of the cerebral hemispheres. Hemiplegia, hemianopsia, aphasia or dysarthria, and organic mental changes are frequent, and complete or incomplete transverse myelitis may develop. Headache and convulsive seizures are rare, but electroencephalographic abnormalities consisting of diffuse or focal abnormalities are often present. Cerebrospinal fluid is normal in most cases.

The pathologic changes consist of multiple areas of demyelination with little or no perivascular infiltration. The presence of distinctive intranuclear inclusions in oligodendrocytes first suggested that the disease was of a viral etiology. Electron microscopic observations show the intranuclear inclusion bodies to be composed of closely packed spheres, which have the physical dimensions and properties of members of the polyoma, SV-40, and K virus subgroups of the papovaviruses. The papova group consists of several tumor-producing viruses, including the human wart virus. A papova-like virus has been isolated by inoculating tissue cultures with suspensions prepared from the brains of patients with the disease.

The disease has not been transmitted to animals.

It has been postulated that the patient's initial underlying illness so alters immunologic responsiveness that the papovavirus is able to enter and multiply within the central nervous system. The demyelination which occurs may be related to virus-induced damage of oligodendroglia, cells which appear to be required for the normal maintenance of myelin.

SUBACUTE SCLEROSING PANENCEPHALITIS (INCLUSION-BODY ENCEPHALITIS) This progressively fatal disease of children and adolescents has been suspected to be of viral origin since its initial description by Dawson in 1932. Recently measles virus or a virus very closely related to measles virus has been recovered from the brains of patients with the disease. The disorder may be considered to be a "slow" form of measles encephalitis.

Subacute sclerosing panencephalitis occurs between four and twenty years of age; 80 percent of patients are under eleven. The disease affects boys three to ten times as frequently as girls. Most patients are from rural areas or small towns. Onset is usually insidious, and mental deterioration, often expressed by a decline in the patient's schoolwork, is the presenting symptom. Incoordination, ataxia, and myoclonic jerks develop along with abnormalities of the pyramidal and extrapyramidal motor systems. Cortical blindness, papilledema, and optic atrophy may be present, and focal chorioretinitis has been described.

The patient becomes bedridden within 6 to 9 months. Death occurs from superimposed pulmonary or urinary tract infections or from decubiti. Neither fever nor signs of meningeal irritation occur.

The cerebrospinal fluid gamma-globulin, as determined by electrophoresis, quantitative immunochemical assay, or colloidal gold curve is elevated, but the fluid is otherwise normal. The electroencephalogram typically shows a "burst suppression" pattern characterized by synchronous and symmetrical spike and high-voltage slow wave activity. Elevated levels of measles antibody are often found in serum and cerebrospinal fluid. Brain biopsy may be required to make a definitive antemortem diagnosis.

There is no effective treatment for the disease.

Pathologic findings include round-cell infiltration about small cerebral arteries and veins, intranuclear and intracytoplasmic inclusions in neurons and glial cells, and varying degrees of demyelination.

Measles virus is now considered to be the etiologic agent. Electron microscopic studies show that the intranuclear inclusions in brain cells are composed of hollow tubular filaments resembling paramyxovirus internal nucleocapsid component. Staining of brain tissue from patients with the disease demonstrates measles virus antigen in the inclusions. An agent serologically identical to measles virus and having measles virus properties has been recovered from brain by cocultivating cell cultures originated from brain tissue with established laboratory cell lines.

Attempts to transmit the disease to animals have met with variable results. Ferrets inoculated with suspensions of brain from patients with the disease develop a nonfatal neurological disorder with electroencephalographic changes.

Subacute sclerosing panencephalitis appears many years after the patient's initial experience with rubeola. There is evidence that subacute sclerosing panencephalitis patients have clinical measles at an unusually early age. A few reported cases may have been related to measles vaccination. The disorder appears to represent an unusual response of the nervous system to measles infection. It is possible that the virus is present in a defective form or that a carrier state is produced wherein cells may continue to elaborate intracellular viral antigen without producing detectable amounts of mature infective virus. One can speculate that similar virus-cell interactions may be important in the development of other diseases of the central nervous system such as parkinsonism and multiple sclerosis.

REFERENCES

ABINANTI FR: Further evidence to support the role of infectious agents and/or immunologic sequelae in the causality of the chronic and degenerative diseases of man. Ann NY Acad Sci 174:967, 1970

FREEMAN JM: The clinical spectrum and early diagnosis of Dawson's encephalitis. J Pediatr 75:590, 1969

GIBBS CJ JR, GAJDUSEK DC: Transmission and characterization of the agents of spongiform virus encephalopathies: Kuru, Creutzfeldt-Jakob disease, scrapie and transmissible mink encephalopathy. Res Publ Assoc Res Nerv Ment Dis 49:383, 1971

RICHARDSON EP: Progressive multifocal leukoencephalopathy. N Engl J Med 265:815, 1961

SIEDLER H, MALAMUD N: Creutzfeldt-Jakob's disease: Clinicopathologic report of 15 cases and review of literature. J Neuropathol Exp Neurol 22:381, 1963

TER MEULEN V et al: Subacute sclerosing panencephalitis: A review. Curr Top Microbiol Immunol 57:1, 1972

THORMAR H: Slow infections of the central nervous system. Z Neurol 199:1, 151, 1971

ZURHEIN GM: Association of papova-virions with a human demyelinating disease (progressive multifocal leukoencephalopathy). Prog Med Virol 11:185, 1969

section 17 | Diseases with lesions of skin or mucous membranes

195 MEASLES (RUBEOLA)

JOHN C. RIBBLE

DEFINITION Measles, or rubeola, is an acute febrile eruption which has been one of the most common diseases of civilized man. With the development of effective prophylactic measures it promises to become a rarity.

HISTORY Measles probably did not exist before the building of large cities. Rhazes wrote about the disease in the tenth century, and Sydenham in the seventeenth century wrote a full account of the disease and differentiated it from other exanthems. In 1905 measles was transmitted by the blood of infected persons to human volunteers and in 1911 to monkeys by both blood and nasopharyngeal secretions that had previously been passed through bacteria-retaining filters. Enders and Peebles in 1954 obtained from patients with measles an agent that produced cytopathic changes in cell cultures. This achievement has allowed the investigation of the characteristics of the measles virus and of the pathogenesis of the disease and has established means for the development of diagnostic and prophylactic measures.

ETIOLOGY The measles virion is composed of a central core of ribonucleic acid with a helically arranged protein coat encased in a lipoprotein envelope with small, spikelike structures. The virion is 1200 to 2500 A in diameter, and in structure and size resembles some of the myxoviruses.

The measles virus is isolated most easily from infected persons by utilizing primary cultures of monkey or human kidney, although primary isolations have been accomplished by using human amnion or chorion or dog kidney. After several passages, the virus can be propagated on a number of stable cell lines of human origin, human leukocytes, and primary cultures from other animals, including chick embryo cells upon which many of the vaccine strains are grown.

Measles virus infection of cells in culture results in the formation of multinucleated giant cells, many with eosinophilic intranuclear, and intracytoplasmic, inclusions. The number of infectious particles of measles virus can be determined by visible plaque formation in suitably prepared cell layers or by use of immunofluorescence techniques.

EPIDEMIOLOGY Measles occurs naturally only in human beings, although infection with the virus can be demonstrated in laboratory colonies of monkeys exposed to infected individuals. Before active immunization became widespread, epidemics of measles occurred every 2 or 3 years, and about 95 percent of town and city dwellers developed the disease before the age of fifteen years. The virus is transmitted by transfer of nasopharyngeal secretions, either directly or in airborne droplets, to the respiratory mucous membranes or conjunctivas of susceptible individuals. Persons infected with the virus may transmit the disease during a period which extends from 4 days before until 5 days after skin lesions have appeared. Measles is a disease of childhood in populous areas, but may occur at any age in remote isolated communities if the disease is introduced. Infants are uncommonly affected under the age of six to eight months because of the persistence for this period of time of antibody acquired by transplacental transmission from the mother.

PATHOGENESIS AND PATHOLOGY It is probable that after infection, measles virus multiplies in the epithelium of the respiratory tract and is disseminated by way of the blood to distant sites. For a few days before, and for 1 or 2 days after, the rash appears, the virus can be isolated from blood or washed white cells, conjunctiva, lymphoid tissue, and respiratory mucous membranes and secretions. The virus can be obtained from urine for as long as 4 days after the onset of the eruption.

The skin and mucous membrane lesions (Koplik's spots) consist of vesicle formation and epithelial necrosis and may be due either to direct infection of these areas or, as suggested by Enders, to the action of complexes of measles antigen and antibody. Large multinucleated cells (Warthin-Finkeldey cells) are characteristic of measles virus infection and can be found in hyperplastic lymphoid tissues, respiratory epithelium and secretions, and in urine. An unusually high number of white cells from patients with the disease contain broken chromosomes. The epithelium of the respiratory passages may become necrotic and slough, leading to secondary bacterial infection; in addition, interstitial pneumonia with giant-cell infiltration may be observed. Changes in the brain of patients with encephalitis resemble those seen in other postviral encephalitides and consist of focal hemorrhage, congestion, and demyelinization.

MANIFESTATIONS The time from exposure to the development of the first symptoms of measles infection is usually 9 to 11 days, and from exposure to the appearance of rash is about 2 weeks. The initial manifestations of the disease are malaise, irritability, fever as high at 105°F, conjunctivitis with excessive lacrimation, edema of the eyelids and photophobia, moderately severe hacking cough, and nasal discharge. Koplik's spots, small red irregular lesions with blue-white centers, appear 1 or 2 days before the onset of the rash on the mucous membranes of the mouth and occasionally on the conjunctiva or intestinal mucosa. The findings of the prodromal illness subside or disappear within 1 or 2 days after the outbreak of skin lesions, although the cough may persist throughout the course of the disease.

The red maculopapular rash of measles breaks out first on the forehead, spreads downward over the face, neck, and trunk, and appears on the feet on the third day. The density of lesions is greatest on the forehead, face, and shoulders, where coalescence of individual spots usually occurs. The lesions in each area persist for about 3 days and disappear in the same order in which they appeared, resulting in total duration of rash of about 6 days. As the maculopapules fade, a brown discoloration of the skin may be noticed, and finely granular skin may be desquamated. In adults the duration of fever may be longer, the rash more prominent, and the incidence of complications higher.

The course of measles can be altered by the administration of gamma-globulin soon after exposure. The incubation period may be prolonged for as long as 20 days. The prodromal period of the modified disease may be shorter, the fever, respiratory symptoms, and conjunctivitis milder, and the rash less marked; Koplik's spots may not be present. An atypical, severe form of measles is seen in some persons who have received inactivated measles vaccine several years before exposure. The prodromal period with prominent fever, headache, myalgias, and abdominal symptoms lasts for 2 or 3 days and is followed by an eruption of maculopapules, vesicles, and petechiae. In contrast to natural measles, the rash begins on the feet and progresses toward the head and is especially prominent on the legs and in body creases. Peripheral edema and pneumonia have been prevalent in this form of atypical measles. The pneumonia is lobar or segmental; hilar lymphadenopathy and pleural effusion are frequent. Ill-defined nodular shadows may persist at the periphery of the lung for as long as 1 to 2 years.

COMPLICATIONS Measles, usually a benign self-limited disease, may be associated with a number of complicating illnesses. Viral involvement of the respiratory tract may lead to croup, bronchitis, bronchiolitis, or rarely to *interstitial pneumonia*, which is seen most often in children suffering from severe systemic disease such as leukemia and which is characterized by severe respiratory symptoms, pulmonary infiltrations, and the presence in the lungs of giant cells. It may occur in the absence of the typical measles exanthem. *Conjunctivitis*, which is seen regularly in the course of uncomplicated measles, may occasionally progress to permanent corneal ulceration, keratitis, and blindness. *Myocarditis* characterized by transient changes in the electrocardiogram occurs in about 20 percent of patients with measles, but clinical evidence of cardiac dysfunction is rare. Viral involvement of the mesenteric lymph nodes and appendix may result in abdominal pain and signs of peritoneal inflammation so severe that surgical exploration is considered. The situation is especially confusing if the evidence of appendiceal involvement becomes manifest during the preeruptive phase of the disease. Measles infection of pregnant women results in death of the fetus in about 20 percent of the cases; however, a teratogenic effect such as that observed in rubella has not been demonstrated.

Superimposed bacterial pneumonia caused by streptococci, pneumococci, staphylococci, or *Hemophilus influenzae* is considerably more common than giant-cell pneumonia and may progress to formation of empyema or lung abscess. Bacterial otitis media is a frequent sequel of measles infection in children. In tropical areas stomatitis, probably of bacterial etiology, progressing to cancrum oris may be encountered during the course of the disease.

In addition to conditions associated with consequences of viral infection and the complications resulting from superimposed bacterial infection, there are several situations which may arise after measles infection which are of uncertain pathogenesis. Clinically apparent *encephalomyelitis* occurs in 1 of 1,000 patients with measles. It begins 4 or 5 days after the appearance of the eruption and is characterized by return of high fever, headache, drowsiness, and coma, and in some patients by focal brain or spinal cord involvement. Death occurs in about 10 percent of affected individuals, and persistent signs of central nervous system damage including mental changes, epilepsy, and paralysis are encountered. Electroencephalographic abnormalities without other signs of central nervous system dysfunction may be demonstrated in 50 percent of patients with otherwise uncomplicated measles. There is no evidence that encephalomyelitis is due to direct invasion of the nervous system by measles virus, and it is postulated that the disease has an allergic origin. An extremely rare condition, *subacute sclerosing panencephalitis* (Chap. 194), is now thought to be a late complication of measles. *Thrombocytopenia* may occur 3 to 15 days after the onset of the rash and results in purpura as well as bleeding from mouth, intestine, and genitourinary tract. Measles is associated with disappearance of delayed hypersensitivity to tuberculin, exacerbation of existing tuberculosis, and an increased incidence of new tuberculous infections.

LABORATORY FINDINGS Leukopenia is frequent in the prodromal phase of measles, and the appearance of leukocytosis suggests bacterial superinfection or another complication. During the prodrome and in the early eruptive phase, Warthin-Finkeldey cells can be identified in stained preparations of sputum, nasal secretions, or urine, and the measles virus can be isolated by inoculation of the same materials into appropriate cell cultures. Complement fixation, neutralization, and hemagglutination-inhibition tests are available for serologic confirmation of measles. Spinal fluid of patients with encephalomyelitis may contain increased protein and 500 to 1,000 lymphocytes per mm^3. Bacterial infection can be identified by appropriate cultures.

DIFFERENTIAL DIAGNOSIS Measles with its prodrome, Koplik's spots, and characteristic rash, is infrequently confused with other diseases. Rubella is a shorter, milder disease with more prominent lymphadenopathy. Infectious mononucleosis and toxoplasmosis can be identified by the presence of atypical lymphocytes and by a serologic test, respectively. Drug reactions and secondary syphilis may display skin lesions similar to the measles rash. The atypical form of measles in patients previously immunized with inactivated vaccine may suggest Rocky Mountain spotted fever.

PROPHYLAXIS Measles can be prevented by the administration of 0.25 mg per kg gamma-globulin within 5 days of exposure. Passive immunization should be considered for any susceptible person exposed to the disease, but is especially important for children under three years of age, for pregnant women, for patients with tuberculosis, and for those patients in whom immune mechanisms are impaired. A modified, less severe form of the disease which results in some degree of active immunity may be observed if 0.05 mg per kg gamma-globulin is given within 5 days of exposure (see Manifestations above). Administration of antibiotics does not decrease the frequency or severity of bacterial superinfections.

Active immunity can be induced by the use of live, attenuated measles virus without spread to contacts of vaccinated individuals. The administration of Edmonston strain vaccines, prepared either in chick embryo or dog kidney cells, frequently results in a febrile illness beginning about 6 days after vaccination, a mild rash, and occasionally respiratory symptoms and Koplik's spots. To modify these manifestations of disease, gamma-globulin, 0.01 mg per kg in a separate syringe and at different site, may be given concomitantly. A further attenuated vaccine (Schwarz) and a more attenuated Edmonston strain are associated with fewer manifestations of disease and are administered without gamma-globulin. Vaccination with these preparations induces antibody formation in more than 95 percent of susceptible individuals. The magnitude of serologic response following use of the Edmonston strain approximates that seen after natural measles and is slightly greater than that induced by the further attenuated strains or Edmonston strain vaccine plus gamma-globulin. Vaccination results in protection for at least 8 years, but the total duration of immunity is not known. Live measles vaccine should not be given to pregnant women, to those sensitive to egg proteins or dog dander, to patients with tuberculosis, to patients with leukemia or lymphoma, or to those who are receiving therapy which depresses immune response. Measles vaccination has been very effective in decreasing the incidence of measles in the United States without producing serious side effects. Measles occurs almost exclusively among the unvaccinated who, for the most part, are members of low socioeconomic groups. The disease rarely occurs in those who have been vaccinated, although there have been a few vaccine failures. These are related, in part, to early vaccination of infants who still have maternal neutralizing antibody or to the use of improperly stored vaccine.

There is no indication for the use of *inactivated* vaccine because of severe atypical measles which has been observed in persons immunized with it (see Manifestations above).

TREATMENT No therapy is indicated for uncomplicated measles. Gamma-globulin, although effective in prophylaxis, is of no value once symptoms are evident. Bacterial infections should be treated with appropriate antibiotics.

REFERENCES

ENDERS JF, PEEBLES T: Propagation in tissue cultures of cytopathogenic agents from patients with measles. Proc Soc Exp Biol Med 86:277, 1954

FULGINITI VA et al: Altered reactivity to measles virus, atypical measles in children previously immunized with inactivated measles virus vaccines. JAMA 202:1075, 1967

KATZ SL: Measles, its complications, treatment, and prophylaxis. Med Clin N Am 46:1163, 1962

KRUGMAN S: Present status of measles and rubella immunization in the United States: A medical progress report. J Pediatr 78:1, Jan 1971

196 GERMAN MEASLES (RUBELLA)

JOHN C. RIBBLE

DEFINITION Rubella, or German measles, a febrile disease with rash and lymphadenopathy, is usually a benign condition, but when it occurs in pregnant women it may lead to infection and serious disorders of the fetus.

ETIOLOGY In the late 1930s and 1940s rubella was transmitted to humans and monkeys, and in 1962 a viral agent was recovered in cell cultures inoculated with nasopharyngeal secretions of infected persons. Human primary amnion cells infected with rubella virus display rounding, clumping of nuclear chromatin, and eosinophilic intranuclear inclusions. Rabbit kidney and some other cell lines also display cytopathic effects. Rubella virus can be detected indirectly in monkey kidney cells by the interference or exclusion method. In this system, cells infected with rubella appear normal, but are resistant to viruses such as echo 11 or Coxsackie A9 that ordinarily produce cytopathic effects in monkey kidney cells. Complement-fixing antigen, and a hemagglutinin against red cells from young chickens, have been identified.

The rubella virion is a 70- to 75-nm spheroid that contains a core of RNA.

PATHOGENESIS AND PATHOLOGY Rubella can be induced in susceptible persons by the instillation of infected materials into the nasopharynx, and natural infection is probably induced in the same way. Virus is present in blood, throat washings, and stools for several days before the exanthem becomes apparent. It can be detected in blood for 1 or 2 days, and in throat washings and stools for as long as 2 weeks after appearance of rash. Lymph nodes show edema, hyperplasia, and loss of follicles.

Congenital rubella results from transplacental transmission of virus to the fetus from an infected mother, and may be associated with growth retardation, infiltration of liver and spleen by hematopoietic tissue, interstitial pneumonia, decreased number of megakaryocytes in the bone marrow, and various structural malformations of the cardiovascular and central nervous systems. The virus may persist in the fetus during intrauterine life and for many months, perhaps years, after birth.

EPIDEMIOLOGY Rubella is not as contagious as measles, and immunity to the disease is not so widespread. Epidemics occur at 6- to 9-year intervals; in 1964 more than 1.8 million cases of rubella were reported in the United States. Rubella is most frequent among children five to nine years of age, but a significant number of cases occur in younger children, adolescents, and young adults.

MANIFESTATIONS The time from exposure to the appearance of the rash of rubella is 14 to 21 days, usually about 18 days. In adults there may be a prodromal illness preceding the exanthem by 1 to 7 days and consisting of malaise, headache, fever, mild conjunctivitis, and lymphadenopathy. In children the rash may be the first manifestation of disease. It is apparent from serologic studies that rubella infection may be associated with no signs or symptoms, or may result in lymph node enlargement without skin lesions; however, rash without lymphadenopathy is uncommon. Respiratory symptoms are mild or absent. Small, red lesions (Forcheimer spots) occasionally may be seen on the soft palate, but are not pathognomonic of the disease.

The rash begins on the forehead and face and spreads downward to the trunk and extremities. The small, pink, maculopapular lesions, of lighter hue than those of measles, are usually discrete but may coalesce to form a diffuse erythema suggestive of scarlet fever. The rash may last from 1 to 5 days, but is most commonly present for 3 days. Enlarged, tender lymph nodes appear before the rash, are most impressive during the early eruptive phase, and may persist several days after the rash has disappeared. Splenomegaly or generalized lymphadenopathy may occur, but the postauricular and suboccipital nodes are most strikingly involved. Arthralgias and slight joint swellings may be a complication of rubella, especially in young women. The pain and swelling, usually in the small joints, are most marked during the period of rash and may persist for several days after other manifestations of rubella have disappeared. Purpura with or without thrombocytopenia may occur and be associated with hemorrhage. Encephalomyelitis following rubella resembles other postinfectious encephalitides and is much less common than encephalitis following measles.

Congenital rubella The syndrome of congenital rubella has conventionally been thought to consist of heart malformations—patent ductus arteriosus, interventricular septal defect, or pulmonic stenosis; eye lesions—corneal clouding, cataracts, chorioretinitis, and microphthalmia; microcephaly, mental retardation, and deafness. In the American epidemic of 1964 thrombocytopenic purpura, hepatosplenomegaly, intrauterine growth retardation, interstitial pneumonia, and metaphyseal bone lesions were encountered frequently in association with the previously recognized manifestations, leading to the term *expanded rubella syndrome.* Any combination of lesions may be seen in an individual infant.

Congenital rubella is usually the result of maternal infection during the first trimester of pregnancy, although well-documented cases have resulted from infection several days prior to conception; deafness may occur as a result of infection in the fourth month. In the 1964 epidemic, about 10 percent of women with clinically recognized rubella during the first trimester gave birth to infants with the rubella syndrome. Serologically identified, asymptomatic maternal rubella can also result in fetal disease. If exposure of a pregnant woman occurs in the first trimester, rubella antibody levels should be obtained immediately and 2 or 3 weeks later. The combination of determinations may allow the detection of seroconversion occurring in subclinical infection, aid in the diagnosis of rubella if an exanthematous disease develops, or suggest remote postinfection and immunity to the disease.

DIAGNOSIS Rubella is frequently confused with other

mild diseases, such as those described in Chap. 197, and with infectious mononucleosis (Chap. 224). A certain diagnosis of rubella can be made by virus isolation and identification, or by changes in antibody titers. Rubella antibodies may be present by the second day of rash and increase in quantity over the next 2 or 3 weeks. Patients with the congenital rubella syndrome may lose hemagglutinin-inhibiting antibodies at age 3 or 4 years. Therefore a negative serologic test in a child over 3 does not exclude the possibility of congenital rubella. There are no other laboratory findings helpful in the diagnosis of rubella, although lymphocytosis with atypical lymphocytes may occur. Congenital rubella should be differentiated by appropriate serologic tests from congenital syphilis, toxoplasmosis, and cytomegalic inclusion virus disease.

PREVENTION In adults and children rubella is usually a mild disease with infrequent complications. However, the severity of congenital infection has prompted efforts to prevent the disease. Administration of gamma-globulin to exposed persons can abort the clinical disease, but seroconversion and transmission of the disease from mother to fetus may occur despite the administration of large amounts of gamma-globulin soon after exposure.

Active immunization with live attenuated rubella vaccines prepared in duck, dog, or rabbit cells has been practiced in this country since 1969, especially among young children. The aim has been to decrease the frequency of the disease in the population, thus decreasing the chance that susceptible pregnant women will be exposed.

The attenuated virus can be detected in the secretions of vaccinees for as long as 4 weeks after immunization, but transmission to other susceptible individuals almost never occurs. The vaccine induces antibodies in about 90 percent of recipients, but the degree and duration of protection it affords are still being evaluated. After heavy exposure in closed populations, vaccinated individuals develop subclinical cases of rubella (diagnosed by antibody rises and virus isolation) with some frequency. However, viremia does not occur in immunized persons, which suggests that vaccinated pregnant women will not infect their fetuses even if they acquire subclinical rubella.

Side effects of fever, rash, lymphadenopathy, or joint pains occur very seldom in vaccinated children, but joint pain and swelling are seen in more than 25 percent of women who are immunized. The joint symptoms may begin as long as 2 months after vaccination, and they may be confused with other forms of arthritis. *Rubella vaccine must never be given to pregnant women or to those who may become pregnant within 2 months of immunization.* This precaution is necessary because the vaccine virus is capable of infecting and possibly damaging the fetus of susceptible women.

REFERENCES

Cooper LZ et al: Loss of rubella hemagglutination inhibition antibody in congenital rubella. Am J Dis Child 122:397, 1971

Horstmann D: Rubella: The challenge of its control. J Infect Dis 123:640, 1971

Krugman S: Present status of measles and rubella immunization in the United States: A medical progress report. J Pediatr 78:1, Jan 1971

Sever JL et al: Rubella epidemic, 1964: Effect on 6,000 pregnancies. Am J Dis Child 110:395, 1965

197 OTHER VIRAL EXANTHEMATOUS DISEASES

JOHN C. RIBBLE

In addition to the diseases such as measles, rubella, and chickenpox which historically have been associated with prominent skin lesions, there are other virus infections in which skin manifestations may occur. A transient maculopapular eruption may be seen during the course of infectious mononucleosis, cytomegalic inclusion disease, cat-scratch fever, psittacosis, and illnesses caused by arboviruses. Exanthem subitum and erythema infectiosum are mild exanthematous diseases which have been recognized by their distinctive clinical features and which are presumably of viral origin. The study of epidemics using techniques of virus isolation has identified exanthematous diseases associated occasionally with adenovirus and reovirus infection, and more frequently with illnesses caused by enteroviruses.

EXANTHEM SUBITUM (ROSEOLA INFANTUM) Exanthem subitum is a benign disease of infants six to twenty-four months of age that is characterized by a high fever and rash. The disease can be transmitted to humans and monkeys by the transfer of blood obtained from a patient during the first few days of illness. The infectious agent is probably a virus, although it has not been isolated. The first manifestation of disease, after an incubation period of 10 days, is the abrupt onset of fever which lasts for 3 to 5 days and may be as high as 105°F. There may be mild pharyngitis, slight lymph node enlargement, and convulsions may occur during the height of the fever. On the fourth or fifth day of illness, there is a sudden drop in temperature to normal or below normal. Several hours after defervescence the rash suddenly and surprisingly appears. It is characterized by faint maculopapules over the neck and trunk and may extend to the thighs and buttocks; it may last for only a few hours or may be present for a day or two. Leukopenia is frequent during the febrile period. The disease is benign and not associated with complications, although occasionally an infant may show sequelae as a result of febrile convulsions.

ERYTHEMA INFECTIOSUM (FIFTH DISEASE) Erythema infectiosum is a mild febrile exanthematous disease without a prodrome. The incubation period is probably 5 to 10 days, but it has not been ascertained precisely. The first manifestations are low-grade fever and the appearance of a rash on the cheeks, giving a "slapped face" appearance. A day or so later, a bilaterally symmetrical eruption is seen on the arms, legs, and trunk, but rarely on the palms or soles. The lesions are maculopapular and tend to be confluent, forming slightly raised blotchy areas and reticular or lacy patterns. The rash usually lasts about a week, and during this time it may disappear, only to reappear in the same areas a few hours later. The waxing and waning eruption may occasionally persist for several weeks, and can be brought on by fever, heat, or emotional stress. Mild joint pain and swelling have been observed in a large proportion of adults with the disease. Erythema infectiosum affects all ages but is most common in children of school age and may occur in epidemic form. The mode of transmission of the disease is not known, and an infectious agent has not been recovered.

ENTEROVIRAL EXANTHEMS Many individual enteroviruses have been associated with rash-poliomyelitis virus only rarely, Coxsackie B5, A2, A4, and A9, and echo viruses 2, 3, 4, 5, 6, 11, 14, 18, 19, occasionally. Three enterovirus infections are frequently associated with rashes and have been studied extensively enough to warrant individual description.

Hand-foot-and-mouth disease (Coxsackie A16 infection) See Chap. 190.

Boston exanthem (infection with echo virus 16) This is probably a common infectious disease of childhood. It was described first and most extensively during an epidemic in Boston in 1951 in many patients with echo virus type 16 infection. Children who were infected usually had a disease characterized by exanthem and low-grade fever, while adult family contacts developed high fever, prostration, and signs of aseptic meningitis with absent or fleeting rash. The first manifestation of the disease in children was fever of 101 to 102°F, lasting for a day or two, pharyngitis with ulcerated lesions resembling herpangina, and slight enlargement of the cervical and postauricular lymph nodes. The rash appeared during or after defervescence and consisted of small pink maculopapules on the face, upper chest, and occasionally on the whole body, including the palms and soles. The rash lasted for 1 to 5 days, and there were no important complications or sequelae. The disease resembled exanthem subitum but occurred in children of all ages and in adults.

Infection with echo virus 9 Infection with this virus has occurred in epidemics among children and adults and has been characterized by a febrile disease with a high incidence of aseptic meningitis. The incubation period is 5 to 8 days. About 30 percent of patients have a rash, which may occur with or without meningitis, is usually maculopapular, presents at the onset of the disease, appears first on the face and neck, spreads to the trunk and extremities, may involve the palms and soles, and persists for 3 to 5 days. Petechiae with or without maculopapules have been recognized, and when seen in association with meningitis, there may be confusion with meningococcal meningitis. Vesicular eruption with crusting lesions has been seen occasionally. An exanthem on the buccal mucosa and soft palate occurs in about 30 percent of patients and consists of small red areas with white centers which resemble Koplik's spots. The disease is usually benign, but rarely has been associated with permanent central nervous system damage.

REFERENCES

BALFOUR HH: Erythema infectiosum: Clinical description of 91 cases seen in an epidemic. Clin Pediatr 8:721, 1969

LERNER AM et al: New viral exanthems. N Engl J Med 269:678, 1963

MILLER GD, TINDALL J: Hand, foot and mouth disease. JAMA 203:827, 1968

NEVA FA et al: Clinical epidemiological features of unusual epidemic exanthem. JAMA 155:544, 1954

WENNER HA, LOU T: Virus diseases associated with cutaneous eruptions. Progr Med Virol 5:219, 1963

198 SMALLPOX, VACCINIA, AND COWPOX

JOHN C. RIBBLE

Poxviruses are a group of large (200 to 320 nm), brick-shaped, DNA-containing viruses that possess a common antigen and have a predilection for skin. Many of the poxviruses, such as myxoma and fowl pox agents, cause disease mainly in lower animals. Smallpox (variola major), alastrim (variola minor), vaccinia, and cowpox agents are closely related members of the poxvirus group that causes human disease. All these viruses grow and produce pox on the chorioallantoic membrane of chick embryos incubated at 37°C and can be cultivated in cells from various mammalian tissues with formation of intracytoplasmic inclusions, rounding, fusion, and heaping up of cells, and eventual degeneration of the infected area. The poxviruses responsible for human disease may be distinguished from each other by minor antigenic differences and by the type and severity of lesions they induce in experimental animals and man. Smallpox and alastrim viruses produce smaller pox on the chorioallantoic membrane than vaccinia, and there are differences in incubation temperatures at which pox viruses produce lesions.

SMALLPOX (VARIOLA)

DEFINITION Smallpox is a severe, contagious, febrile disease characterized by a vesicular and pustular eruption. Alastrim is a similar but milder illness.

PATHOGENESIS AND PATHOLOGY The virus gains access to the body by the respiratory tract and multiplies in unidentified sites, probably in lymph nodes or liver. After several days, during which there is no evidence of infection, viremia ensues, with production of swelling of the endothelium of blood vessels in the corium and perivascular inflammation. Loculated vesicles are the result of cellular destruction and exudation of serum. The infected epithelial cells are swollen and contain intracytoplasmic inclusions surrounded by a halo (Guarnieri bodies). The extent of skin involvement is greater in smallpox than in chickenpox and reaches into the corium. Pitting, most commonly seen on the face, is said to result from destruction of sebaceous glands which are abundant in this area. The liver, spleen, and lymph nodes may be enlarged and may show focal accumulations of large mononuclear cells.

EPIDEMIOLOGY Smallpox is not as contagious as measles or influenza, and ordinarily face-to-face contact with an infected person is required to transmit the disease. Aerial dissemination may have been responsible for a recent epidemic in a German hospital. A patient with smallpox is infectious from a day before the rash appears until the lesions have healed and the scabs have fallen off. During the early phase of the illness, the virus is transmitted in nasopharyngeal secretions; when the eruption is fully formed, the lesions themselves are a major source of infectious material. Variola virus may contaminate clothing, bedding, dust, or other inanimate objects and remain infectious for months, necessitating disinfection of articles in the patient's environment. Although smallpox is usually disseminated by a patient with recognizable disease, it is possible that the virus may be transmitted by an individual, especially a partially immune person, who has an inapparent or very mild infection. The World Health Organization's program to eradicate smallpox has resulted in marked decrease in the incidence of the disease since 1966. In 1970, endemic smallpox was limited to Brazil, several countries in East Africa, Nigeria, Indonesia, and the Indian subcontinent.

MANIFESTATIONS The incubation period of smallpox from the time of exposure to the onset of the prodrome is about 12 days with extremes of 9 to 15 days. The disease can be divided into a prodrome, an early eruptive phase, and a period of vesiculation and pustule formation. The prodrome is characterized by fever of 102 to 106°F, headache, myalgia especially in the back, abdominal pain, vomiting, and in some patients by a transient, blotchy, erythematous eruption. After 3 or 4 days the fever subsides, the symptoms decrease, and the patient seems to recover. It is at this time, when the patient is afebrile, that the focal eruption begins. Early manifestations are painful ulcers on the buccal mucosa and macules which appear first on the face and forearm, and rapidly become firm, shotty papules. The papules increase in number and spread from the face and distal extremities to involve the trunk. The individual lesions may remain discrete and scattered or they may become confluent and involve most of the body. They are most concentrated on the face and distal extremities including the palms and soles and are relatively sparse in the axilla. On the third or fourth day after the appearance of the focal rash, the papules progress to vesicles containing clear fluid, which, over the next few days, become cloudy because of infiltration by pus cells and desquamated epithelial cells; hemorrhage into the vesicles surrounding skin may also be seen. During the course of smallpox, the lesions at any one time, in one area, are all at the same stage of evolution. At the time the vesicles become pustular, there is recurrence of fever, which may persist until healing occurs. The pustules umbilicate and form crusts and scabs which usually fall off 3 weeks after the beginning of illness, leaving small scars or deep pits.

The above description applies to disease of moderate severity. A milder illness may occur in previously immunized persons or in some who have no history of vaccination. It is characterized by the usual incubation period and prodrome, but is followed either by focal eruption of fewer than 100 papules, or by a rash resembling chickenpox. Smallpox with prodrome, but no eruption of any kind, has been recognized (variola sine eruptione). The disease may also occur in a rapidly fulminating form ("sledgehammer" smallpox). After the usual incubation period, the patient develops an initial illness characterized by severe prostration, fever, bone-marrow depression, hemorrhagic skin lesions, bleeding from the mouth and intestine, shock, coma, and death. The disease progresses from inception to death within 3 or 4 days without evidence of the typical focal skin lesions.

Alastrim is similar to mild and moderate forms of variola major in that it has the same incubation period and prodromal illness, but the skin eruption is less extensive, and fatalities are extremely rare and are related to secondary infections.

COMPLICATIONS Bacterial superinfections of the lesions, usually with *Staphylococcus aureus*, may occur in the late pustular stage. Viral infections of the trachea, pharynx, and larynx, and superimposed bacterial pneumonia, may be seen in severe forms of smallpox. Mild conjunctivitis is quite common, and iritis and keratitis have been recognized. Encephalomyelitis may occur in the late stage of the disease and is similar to other postinfectious encephalitides. Osteomyelitis and joint effusions may complicate the disease.

LABORATORY FINDINGS Leukopenia is present during the prodromal illness, and there is usually leukocytosis during the pustular stage. Rapid diagnosis of poxvirus infection can be made by finding of characteristic brick-shaped particles in preparations of vesicle fluid examined by electron microscopy. Specific precipitation in agar by use of antigen prepared from lesions and antivariola or antivaccinia immune serum may also allow detection of poxvirus within a few hours. These tests do not distinguish variola from vaccinia or other poxviruses but do allow rapid differentiation from herpes simplex and varicella-zoster viruses. For definitive identification the virus must be grown in cell culture or on the chorioallantoic membrane and examined for its biologic characteristics.

DIFFERENTIAL DIAGNOSIS The major problem in differential diagnosis is in distinguishing smallpox from chickenpox. Smallpox is preceded by a longer prodrome than chickenpox, and its eruption vesiculates over a period of days instead of hours. The smallpox lesions are all characteristically in the same stage of development, whereas those of chickenpox may, in one area, display all stages of evolution. Electron microscopy and agar precipitation techniques (see above) are especially useful in distinguishing between smallpox and chickenpox.

PROPHYLAXIS Smallpox may be prevented among the patient's contacts by vaccination. Because this procedure is most successful if carried out during the early part of the incubation period, all exposed persons, regardless of previous immunization, should be vaccinated immediately upon recognition of exposure. Large, controlled, clinical trials have demonstrated that oral administration of *N*-methylisatin 3-thiosemicarbazone (methisazone), a drug which interferes with poxvirus multiplication, can prevent smallpox and alastrim in patients exposed to these diseases. The use of the drug together with prompt vaccination results in greater chance of protection than either measure alone. A drawback to the use of methisazone is its tendency to induce vomiting. The combined use of vaccination and parenteral administration of vaccinia immune globulin early in the incubation period is effective in the prevention of smallpox in exposed individuals. It is now usual to apply these control measures selectively to the primary and secondary contacts of a patient rather than to all the inhabitants of a city or town.

TREATMENT There is no specific therapy for smallpox. Thiosemicarbazone, although effective in prophylaxis, has not been shown to be of value in the treatment of established cases. Fluid deficits incurred by lack of intake and by loss from affected areas should be replaced by the administration of appropriate solutions. During the vesicular and pustular phases of the disease, an attempt should be made to prevent bacterial infection by the use of sterile sheets and sterile nursing procedures. Antihistamines may be helpful in decreasing pruritus. Bathing and application of lotions or ointments should be avoided. Later in the course of the illness, when desquamation has begun, showers or baths may be helpful in removing desquamating tissue.

Administration of parenteral penicillin, beginning on the fifth day of rash, has been reported to decrease the incidence of infection of skin lesions and the formation of boils and abscesses due to penicillin-sensitive bacteria. Inasmuch as penicillin-resistant staphylococci are frequently responsible for bacterial infections, the use of penicillinase-resistant penicillin may be of value, but its efficacy as a prophylactic agent in smallpox has not been evaluated. If bacterial infection is demonstrated, an antibiotic active against the infecting organism should be given by the parenteral route. Topical antibiotics should be avoided.

VACCINIA

Vaccinia is a virus disease of the skin which is induced by inoculation for the prevention of smallpox. The exact origin of the vaccinia virus is obscure. The material used by Jenner for vaccination was derived from cowpox lesions, and the infectious agent was propagated for many years by successive passage from person to person through use of exudate from fresh skin lesions. The original agent possibly became contaminated with variola virus during the period when transfer was being carried out without strict controls. It has been suggested that vaccinia virus is a hybrid of cowpox and variola agents, a contention supported by the finding that laboratory-induced hybrids of variola and cowpox viruses have many of the characteristics associated with vaccinia.

VACCINATION Live, lyophilized vaccinia virus prepared from vesicle fluid of infected calves is commercially available and maintains potency for 18 months at 46°F. It is dissolved in a diluent solution just prior to use. The usual method for vaccination is to apply a small drop of vaccine to the skin over the deltoid muscle and to press a sterile needle through the vaccine several times in such a way that only the superficial layer of skin is entered. Vaccination should always induce some form of skin reaction; complete absence of any kind of lesion indicates that the vaccine was not viable or was not administered properly. The reaction which occurs in nonimmune individuals is characterized by a red papule at the site of inoculation 3 to 5 days after vaccination. The papule becomes vesicular on about the fifth or sixth day and pustular by the ninth or eleventh day after inoculation. The vesicle and pustule may be surrounded by a large area of erythema. About two weeks after vaccination, the pustule dries and develops a crust which falls off by the end of the third week, leaving a scar. Fever, malaise, and irritability are common in children during the vesicular and pustular phases, and axillary lymphadenopathy may develop and persist for several months. In the partially immune person, a modified reaction develops without fever or constitutional symptoms. A papule appears on the skin within 3 days, vesiculates in 5 to 7 days, and heals without much scarring. In an immune person a small papule forms in 3 days, but it does not vesiculate or result in scarring.

COMPLICATIONS Healing of the primary vaccinal lesion may not occur, and there may be during a period of weeks or months progressive necrosis with destruction of large areas of skin, subcutaneous tissue, and underlying structures (*vaccinia gangrenosum*). In addition to the local destruction, there may be metastatic lesions on other parts of the skin surface and in bone and viscera. Vaccinia gangrenosum occurs most frequently in persons with disorders of immunity and, if untreated, is nearly always fatal. *Eczema vaccinatum* is a serious complication that is seen in persons with eczema or other type of chronic dermatosis. Widespread infection in the previously affected areas, as well as in normal skin, may result from direct vaccination of an eczematous patient or from exposure to a recently vaccinated individual. *Generalized vaccinia* in patients without preexisting skin disease is characterized by a few satellite lesions surrounding the inoculation site or by widely disseminated pox resembling the primary vaccination lesion. This condition may be mild, and recovery is to be expected. Vaccinia virus may be transferred from the primary inoculation site to the eye or other sites by scratching. *Postvaccinal encephalomyelitis* appears from 2 to 25 days after vaccination. The patient becomes severely ill quite suddenly, with nuchal rigidity, drowsiness, vomiting, convulsions, coma, and signs suggesting disease of the spinal cord. The period of coma lasts for a few days, and in those who recover there are usually no permanent sequelae. Death occurs in about half of the patients with encephalomyelitis. Erythema multiforme bullosum or diffuse blotchy erythema may occur in vaccinated patients 7 to 10 days after vaccination, and is thought to be an allergic reaction to the virus or other components of the vaccine.

The incidence of complications has been compiled for 1968 by the Center for Disease Control. The frequencies of adverse effects per million primarily vaccinated persons were vaccinia gangrenosum, 0.9; eczema vaccinatum, 10.4; generalized vaccinia, 23.4; vaccinal lesions resulting from accidental implantation of virus, 25.4; postvaccinal encephalitis, 2.9; other complications, 11.8; death rate was one per million. Because of the severe complications of vaccination and because smallpox incidence has decreased so markedly in most parts of the world making it extremely unlikely that the disease will be introduced into this country, it has been recommended by the Public Health Service that routine vaccination be discontinued in the United States. It is imperative that immunization be continued on a regular basis among hospital workers, travelers to endemic areas, and military personnel.

COWPOX

Cowpox is primarily a disease of the teats and udders of cows. Man is almost always infected by milking, but occasional spread to contacts may occur from an infected person. The human disease is characterized by low-grade fever and by small papules on the fingers and hand which go through vesicular and pustular stages resembling the course of vaccinia infection. The lesions may be ruptured by trauma and spread to immediately adjacent areas on the hand and continue to ulcerate for several weeks. Edema, lymphangitis, and axillary lymph node enlargement are common. Very rare cases of postcowpox encephalitis and serious infections of eczematous persons have been reported. In general, the disease is benign, heals without scarring, and is usually uncomplicated.

REFERENCES

Bedson HS, Dumbell K: Smallpox and vaccinia. Br Med Bull 23:119, 1967

Brown GC (ed): Symposium: Is routine smallpox vaccination necessary in the United States? Am J Epidemiol 93:221, 1971

Dixon CW: *Smallpox*, London: J. & A. Churchill Ltd., 1962

Joklik WK: The poxviruses. Bacteriol Rev 30:33, 1966

Lane JM et al: Smallpox and smallpox vaccination policy. Annu Rev Med 22:251, 1971

199

CHICKENPOX (VARICELLA) AND HERPES ZOSTER

JOHN C. RIBBLE

DEFINITION Chickenpox is a contagious disease characterized by fever and a disseminated vesicular eruption. Herpes zoster, or shingles, is characterized by unilateral, segmental inflammation of the spinal or cranial nerves and their ganglions, and by a painful localized vesicular eruption of the skin along the distribution of the involved nerve. Chickenpox and herpes zoster are different manifestations of infection with the same viral agent.

ETIOLOGY In 1953 a virus was recovered from patients with chickenpox and herpes zoster that produced intranuclear, eosinophilic inclusions and multinucleated giant cells in lines of cells derived from various monkey and human tissues. The varicella-zoster virus in culture spreads from cell to adjacent cell by direct invasion, rather than by way of suspending medium, and ordinarily can be passed to other tissue cultures only by transfer of infected cells. The structure of the varicella-zoster virion resembles that of herpes simplex.

PATHOGENESIS AND PATHOLOGY Varicella is presumably transmitted by the respiratory route, although the virus has only rarely been isolated from nasopharyngeal secretions of infected persons. Virus multiplication occurs at some unidentified site and probably results in intermittent viremia, as suggested by the successive crops of widely spaced lesions. Focal viral infection of blood vessels in the corium, with intranuclear inclusions in endothelial cells, results in degeneration of epidermis and formation of vesicles containing serum, epithelial and inflammatory cells, and multinucleated giant cells. Virus can be isolated from vesicle fluid, but not usually from crusting lesions or scabs, for several days after eruption. In patients with varicella pneumonia of the tracheobronchial mucosa, the alveolar septums, and the interstitial areas of the lungs are edematous and contain monocytic inflammatory cells, cells with intranuclear inclusions, and giant cells. The nodular areas of pneumonia may eventually become calcified. The changes in the central nervous system in patients with postinfectious varicella encephalomyelitis resemble those seen in measles. Rarely, encephalomyelitis with inclusion bodies resembling herpes simplex infection may occur, and varicella-zoster virus can be recovered from the central nervous system.

The pathogenesis of herpes zoster is not clear (see Epidemiology, below), but the tissue changes are well documented. The dorsal root ganglion of the affected nerve is swollen and hemorrhagic; the edema spreads along the peripheral nerve and may reach the spinal cord. The nerve tissue shows hemorrhagic infarction, inflammation, and necrosis of many of the ganglion cells, some of which contain intranuclear inclusions. The microscopic appearance of zoster skin lesions is almost identical to that described for chickenpox vesicles. Virus can be cultured from the lesions for as long as 5 days after onset.

EPIDEMIOLOGY Chickenpox is a highly contagious disease with attack rates of 70 percent or more among susceptible persons exposed to a patient with the disease. The infectious period extends from a day or two before the rash until as long as 6 days after the appearance of new skin lesions. Patients with herpes zoster may be the source of an outbreak of chickenpox among susceptible contacts. Children from five to eight years of age are most commonly affected, but younger children, including newborn infants, and adults may develop chickenpox; an estimated 2 to 20 percent of cases occur in persons over the age of 15 years. In the United States the disease is endemic, with superimposed epidemics every 2 to 5 years, usually in the winter or spring.

Herpes zoster is mainly a disease of adults who have previously had chickenpox. It has been suggested but not demonstrated that herpes zoster results from reactivation of virus that has lain dormant in spinal nerves since an episode of chickenpox. Alternatively the disease may be due to reinfection of a partially immune person from an exogenous source. Epidemiologic evidence favors the reactivation theory. Most patients with zoster have no recent exposure to patients with zoster or varicella, and the incidence of the disease does not increase during seasonal chickenpox epidemics. Probably reactivation accounts for zoster in most patients, whereas reinfection may be responsible for the disease in some.

Zoster occurs commonly in patients with neoplasms, most frequently in those with lymphomas, especially Hodgkin's disease, where the incidence may be as high as 25 percent. Advanced disease, cutaneous anergy, recent radiation of affected nodes, and possibly splenectomy predispose patients with Hodgkin's disease to zoster. In patients with neoplastic disease herpes zoster recurs at least once in about a fifth of those who have had one bout.

MANIFESTATIONS The incubation period from the time of exposure to the appearance of varicella rash is 10 to 21 days, most often 14 to 17 days. There may be a 1- or 2-day prodrome with fever and malaise, but these symptoms usually begin when the rash appears. The first skin manifestations are pruritic maculopapules that evolve in a few hours to thin-walled vesicles which contain clear fluid and are surrounded by a red border. During the next day the erythema diminishes and the vesicles collapse in the center, forming annular or umbilicated lesions which dry further and form scabs that fall off after several days without scarring. New maculopapules continue to erupt during the first 3 or 4 days of illness and go through a similar evolution. The findings at one time, in one area, of skin lesions in all stages of development—maculopapules, vesicles, umbilicated lesions, and scabs—is characteristic of chickenpox. The rash is most concentrated on the trunk, but pox are frequently seen on the face and scalp, occasionally on the mucosal surface of the mouth or conjunctiva, and rarely on the palms or soles.

Chickenpox in adults is often more severe than the disease in children, with more profuse rash, higher fever, and greater incidence of pneumonia.

Herpes zoster Herpes zoster is a disease of nerves of the skin and other tissues they supply. It affects the thoracic (55 percent of cases), cervical (20 percent), and lumbar and sacral nerves (15 percent), and ophthalmic division of the trigeminal nerve (15 percent).

The incubation period is not known. Fever and pain that is localized to the areas served by the affected nerves may begin 4 or 5 days before or be concomitant with the appearance of the skin eruption. Rarely characteristic pain and serologic evidence of zoster occur with no clinical involvement of the skin (zoster sine eruptione). The discomfort is mild to severe and can be sharp, burning, or dull. In addition to disorders of sensation, herpes zoster is occasionally associated with motor paralysis of arms, legs, intercostal muscles, or muscles innervated by cranial nerves. The skin lesion starts with local redness followed by red papules that progress over the next 2 weeks through vesicular, pustular, and crusting stages that resemble the evolution of individual pox of varicella. The lesions are arranged unilaterally in characteristic bandlike clusters which follow radicular lines. They may run transversely along the hemithorax or vertically over the arm or leg.

Disease of the individual cranial nerves leads to characteristic groups of symptoms. If the trigeminal (Gasserian) ganglion is affected, there will usually be pain in the distribution of the nerve, headache, weakness of the eyelid muscles, and possibly Argyll Robertson pupil. Lesions appear on the face, in the mouth, and frequently on the cornea. Iridocyclitis, anesthesia of the cornea, and scarring may result. If the geniculate ganglion is involved, there may be Bell's palsy, disorders of hearing, and vertigo, with unilateral herpetic lesions of the external ear and canal and of the anterior portion of the tongue. Central nervous system inflammation is prominent when herpes zoster attacks the cranial nerves, and meningeal signs and symptoms are frequent.

COMPLICATIONS Hemorrhage into vesicles and surrounding skin may be seen in adults with severe chickenpox or in children receiving adrenal steroids. Infection of the varicella lesions by bacteria, most commonly *staphylococcus* aureus, results in delayed healing and scarring of skin, and occasionally in bacteremia.

Of adults with chickenpox, 15 percent develop primary *varicella pneumonia,* and adult patients account for 90 percent of the patients who develop this complication. Pneumonia is invariably associated with skin lesions and appears 1 to 6 days after onset of rash. The degree of pulmonary involvement correlates to some extent with the severity of the rash; patients may be virtually asymptomatic or may develop serious, life-threatening disease. Tachypnea, dyspnea, cough, and fever of 102°F or more are present in most patients with symptomatic pneumonia; cyanosis, pleuritic chest pain, and hemoptysis each occur in 20 to 40 percent of the recorded cases. The physical examination may disclose no abnormalities, or there may be intercostal retractions, a few rhonchi, wheezes, scattered rales, and rarely evidence of pleural effusion. In contrast to the paucity of physical signs, roentgenograms demonstrate widespread nodular infiltration of both lungs, most prominent at the hila and least evident at the apexes. Vital capacity is decreased, arterial oxygen saturation is diminished, and the airways may be blocked by tenacious bronchopulmonary secretions. Most patients with varicella pneumonia show symptomatic improvement at the time the rash begins to wane; however, seriously ill patients can remain febrile and dyspneic for as long as 2 weeks. Roentgenographic evidence of disease diminishes at the time of clinical improvement, but may persist for several weeks. Abnormalities of pulmonary gas diffusion have been demonstrated several months after apparent recovery.

Encephalomyelitis is a less frequent complication of chickenpox than of measles and occurs predominantly in children. It begins 3 to 14 days after the onset of rash with drowsiness and irritability progressing to vomiting, convulsions, and coma which last 4 or 5 days. As the patient regains consciousness, evidence of central nervous system abnormalities may be apparent. Varicella encephalomyelitis is frequently associated with cerebellar dysfunction either isolated or associated with other nervous disorders such as hemiparesis, athetosis, cranial nerve abnormalities, and various spinal syndromes.

Patients who contract *varicella while receiving steroids* may have recurrent crops of new skin lesions for as long as 3 weeks. They have a higher incidence of hemorrhagic and progressive gangrenous lesions and occasionally develop a fatal disseminated disease with viral infection in all the viscera. The fatal form of the disease has been encountered most frequently in children being treated with steroids for leukemia or other disease of the hematopoietic system, but it has also been seen in those receiving therapy for rheumatic fever and allergic disorders. Children with the rare syndrome of cartilage-hair hypoplasia may suffer from unusually severe and perhaps fatal chickenpox. *Other complications of chickenpox* such as myocarditis, corneal lesions, iritis, nephritis, orchitis, and appendicitis have been recognized but are rare. Congenital infection with varicella can occur, and infants born of mothers with chickenpox may display the typical skin lesions. Evidence of congenital malformations as a result of infection in early pregnancy is not convincing.

Postherpetic neuralgia may last for several months or years and become the most troublesome part of the disease. In nearly all patients with zoster, healing with loss of scab is complete within 2 to 3 weeks. In the young, pain persists for only a week or two after healing and then usually disappears, although hypo- or hyperesthesia may remain. However, in patients over sixty years of age moderate to severe pain persists for more than 2 months in as many as 70 percent, even though the skin lesion has healed normally.

Zoster skin lesions do not always remain localized. *Generalized zoster* occurs in 5 percent of zoster patients with no underlying disease and in as many as 70 percent of those with Hodgkin's disease, and is characterized by dissemination to all parts of the skin, producing a picture similar to that of chickenpox. The scattered lesions last 6 to 9 days in normal hosts, but they may persist for 3 to 4 weeks in those with serious underlying disease. In these patients dissemination may also involve the visceral

organs (including the lungs) and frequently results in death.

LABORATORY FINDINGS Multinucleated giant cells and epithelial cells with eosinophilic intranuclear inclusions can be identified in material scraped from the base of a vesicular lesion or in sputum from patients with varicella pneumonia. For specific diagnosis, virus can be isolated from vesicular fluid, and antigens can be demonstrated in vesicular fluid and in crusts of lesions by the use of a simple gel-precipitin technique. The white blood count in patients with uncomplicated chickenpox or zoster is normal. Mononuclear pleocytosis is present in the cerebrospinal fluid of patients with herpes zoster especially those with involvement of the cranial nerves. The spinal fluid in varicella-zoster encephalomyelitis contains increased protein and as many as 3,000 lymphocytes per mm^3.

DIFFERENTIAL DIAGNOSIS Chickenpox can usually be diagnosed by the history of recent exposure and the character of the rash. In situations where smallpox is a possibility, differentiation from chickenpox can be attempted by noting the distribution and evolution of the rash and by examining the cells from vesicles, but definitive diagnosis can be made only by identification of the virus. Disseminated vaccinia lesions similar to chickenpox may occur in patients, especially those with disorders of immunity or eczema, who have recently been vaccinated or exposed to a vaccinated person. Herpes simplex infection in patients with chronic eczema or neurodermatitis may present as as varicelliform eruption confined to previously involved areas of skin. The diagnosis can be confirmed by virus isolation. Rickettsialpox can be differentiated from chickenpox by the presence of an eschar in the area of mite bite, prominent headache, and specific complement-fixing antibodies to *Rickettsia akari.*

In the preeruptive stage, the diagnosis of herpes zoster is difficult, and the disease is usually confused with other causes of pain, such as pleurisy, appendicitis, pleurodynia, or collapsed intervertebral disk. After the unilateral eruption appears, the clinical features are so characteristic that the diagnosis is simple. Occasionally, localized herpes simplex along the distribution of a segmental nerve may simulate zoster, including the localized pain and tenderness. The diagnosis of herpes simplex infection can be confirmed in the laboratory by virus isolation.

PROPHYLAXIS Chickenpox can be prevented by the administration of specific zoster immune globulin (ZIG) derived from the serum of patients recovering from herpes zoster. It should be given within 72 hr of exposure to susceptible individuals who are receiving large doses of adrenal steroids or immunosuppressive drugs. Its use may also be justified in pregnant women and newborn infants who are exposed to chickenpox. This material should not be used for healthy children who are exposed to the disease. ZIG has not been evaluated in the treatment of chickenpox after lesions have developed, nor is its usefulness in prevention or treatment of herpes zoster known.

TREATMENT The patient with uncomplicated chickenpox should receive local applications for the relief of itching. Secondary bacterial infections should be treated with appropriate antibacterial agents. Patients with varicella pneumonia require skillful nursing care, removal of bronchial secretions, administration of oxygen, and on occasion ventilatory assistance, such as positive pressure breathing. Adrenal steroids have been considered by some to be beneficial in the treatment of varicella pneumonia, but convincing evidence of their efficacy in this condition is not available. Patients suspected of having varicella-zoster infection of the eye should be promptly treated by an ophthalmologist. The therapy consists of analgesics for severe pain and the use of atropine to prevent synechiae. Some ophthalmologists recommend the use of adrenal steroids if uveitis is present.

The use of cytosine arabinoside should be considered for the treatment of patients whose lives are threatened by severe chickenpox, inasmuch as this drug has apparently had beneficial effects on the outcome of the disease in seriously ill individuals. It is possible that cytosine arabinoside also has a beneficial effect on the course of serious disseminated herpes zoster.

It has been claimed that in patients with herpes zoster and no underlying disease, the administration of adrenal steroids by mouth during the early eruptive phase of the disease reduces the incidence and duration of postherpetic neuralgia without inducting dissemination or other complications. Steroids should *not* be used for this purpose in patients with neoplasms or other underlying disease.

REFERENCES

BRUNELL PA et al: Prevention of varicella by zoster immune globulin. N Engl J Med 280:1191, 1969

EAGLESTEIN WH et al: The effects of early corticosteroid therapy on the skin eruption and pain of herpes zoster. JAMA 211:1681, 1970

GOFFINET DR et al: Herpes zoster-varicella infections and lymphoma. Ann Intern Med 76:235, 1972

HALL TC et al: Treatment of varicella-zoster with cytosine arabinoside. Trans Assoc Am Physicians 82:201, 1969

TRIEBWASSER JH et al: Varicella pneumonia in adults: Report of seven cases and a review of literature. Medicine 46:409, 1967

WELLER TH: Varicella-herpes zoster virus, in *Viral and Rickettsial Infections of Man*, eds FL Horsfall, Jr., I Tamm, 4th ed., Philadelphia: Lippincott, 1965

200 INFECTIONS WITH HERPESVIRUS HOMINIS (HERPES SIMPLEX)

A. MARTIN LERNER

Herpesvirus hominis, types 1 and 2, formerly known as herpes simplex virus, establishes diverse relations with man. Acute disseminated primary infection (gingivostomatitis), chronic infection with continual virus shedding (herpes keratitis and herpes labialis), and clinical reactivation occur. Virus multiplies within lymphocytes, probably impairing T- and B-cellular functions, and by its intracellular locus escapes antiherpesvirus antibodies. Herpesvirus antibody complexes may be infectious, and when this is the case, are called "sensitized virus." Interactions with the complement system are important in neutralizing sensitized virus. Since the decline of poliomyelitis with the development of an effective vaccine, herpes simplex virus encephalitis is the most frequent endemic encephalitis in this country. Type 2 *Herpesvirus hominis* (HVH) has been associated with carcinoma of the cervix.

ETIOLOGY The virus particle consists of DNA, protein, lipid, and carbohydrate. On an average there are 100 parts DNA, 25 parts carbohydrate, and 320 parts phospholipid to 1,000 parts protein. Virus DNA is double-stranded with densities of 1.727 (type 1) and 1.729 (type 2). The base composition (guanine plus cytosine per 100 ml) of HVH, type 1, is 68.3, and that for HVH, type 2, is 70.4. The molecular weight of the virion is about 100×10^6 daltons. On phosphotungstic acid staining by electron microscopy the virion consists of a roughly spheric central area or "core" of DNA which measures 75 nm in diameter, a stable "capsid" which measures 100 nm in diameter, and appears to be an icosahedron with a 5:3:2 axial symmetry consisting of 162 capsomeres (9 to 10 nm by 12 to 13.5 nm) of which 150 are hexagonal and 12 pentagonal in cross section, and a surrounding envelope derived from host cell membranes, 145 to 200 nm. Particles appear with or without envelopes [enveloped and/or with or without cores ("full" or "empty")].

Although complete virions are more efficient, both "enveloped" and "naked" particles can infect cells. Phagocytosis of virions by susceptible cells, viropexis, precedes the digestion of virus envelopes and proteins. After initiation of infection, virus absorption is complete in 3 hr. New virus infectivity rises sharply from the sixth to the ninth hour, when it levels off. Viral DNA enters the nucleus where new virus DNA is synthesized. Virus proteins are synthesized in the cytoplasm and migrate to the nucleus. To date, from 9 to 24 distinct proteins (or polypeptides) are identified. The complete virion has a triple-layered envelope. The inner envelope is made within the nucleus, while the second and third are formed by evagination processes at the nuclear and cytoplasmic membranes, respectively. Host materials make up major portions of the envelope. Virus envelope contains adenosine triphosphatase (ATPase), which also is present in host membranes. Antihost serum agglutinates "enveloped," but not "naked," particles. An infected cell produces about 1,000 virus particles, but only 5 to 10 percent are infectious.

BIOLOGIC CHARACTERISTICS By means of neutralization kinetics, hyperimmune unitypic serums in conventional neutralization tests or direct immunofluorescent methods, strains of *H. hominis* can be readily typed. Type 1 strains are recovered from the nasopharynx, skin (other than thigh or buttocks), and brain in cases of postnatal encephalitis. Type 2 strains are uniformly related to the adult genital tract. Isolates have been recovered from the penis, cervix, endocervix, vagina, vulva, skin, and spinal fluid. In infections of the newborn *H. hominis*, type 2 (HVH-2), has been recovered from brain, liver, adrenal, and lung.

Optimal virus isolation occurs in rabbit or baby hamster kidney and human foreskin tissue cultures. Cytopathic effects are usually evident within 72 hr after inoculation. However, when isolation of virus by brain biopsy is attempted, trypsinized suspensions of cells, rather than ground tissue suspensions, should be planted both for primary growth as well as for cocultivation with herpesvirus-susceptible tissue cultures. Typical of in vitro and in vivo cytopathic effects is the type A inclusion of Cowdry, an eosinophilic mass surrounded by a halo in a nucleus with marginated chromatin (Fig. 200-1). After infection of rabbit kidney cells with *H. hominis*, a cell factor is released which, upon incubation with serum, cleaves the fifth component of complement. The product of this cleavage, C5a, is chemotactic for polymorphonuclear leukocytes which accumulate at the site of herpetic lesions.

In addition to site of recovery, a number of other properties separate type 1 from type 2 *H. hominis*: type 2 HVH produces (1) larger pocks on the chorioallantoic membrane of embryonated eggs, (2) greater virulence for female mice which have been infected by the genital route, and (3) greater tendency toward formation of giant cells in tissue cultures. These strains also exhibit (4) difference in density and base composition of DNA and (5) antigenic distinctiveness. Likewise, (6) minimal inhibitory concentrations (MIC) of idoxuridine (IDU; 5-iodo-2′-deoxyuridine) versus type 1 strains are 2.5 to 10 μg per 0.4 ml, while similar values for type 2 herpesviruses are 25 to 50 μg per 0.4 ml.

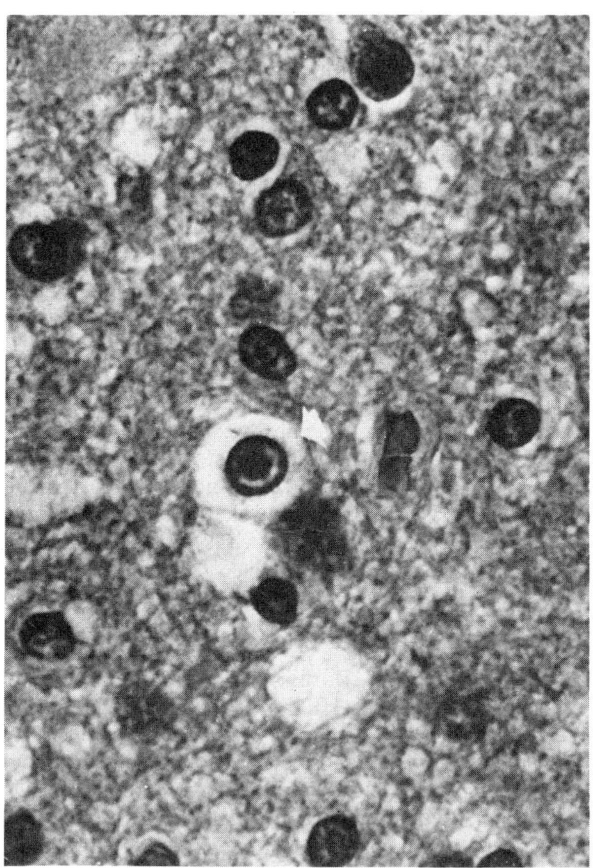

FIGURE 200-1
Cowdry, type A (owl-eye) intranuclear inclusions are seen in this hematoxylin and eosin section (855) obtained at biopsy from the right temporal lobe of a 57-year-old woman in coma. Herpesvirus hominis *(4,000 fifty-percent tissue culture doses) was recovered from the specimen.*

IMMUNOLOGY Following primary exposure to *H. hominis*, humoral antibodies appear. Different polypeptides of the virus capsid probably stimulate distinct antibodies which rise and fall describing separate kinetic curves. In contrast to other antibodies (conventional neutralizing, complement-fixing, passive hemagglutinating), complement-requiring neutralizing antibodies peak during the acute phase of primary infections with HVH-1 and fall during convalescence. Complement apparently enhances the immunoaggregation of herpesvirus. In early immune serum complement-requiring antibody behaves like monovalent antibody sensitizing virus to the action of complement. Immunoaggregates form when complement is added. Each virus-antibody-complement aggregate functions as a single infectious unit. Late immune serum is polyvalent, and convalescent serum alone aggregates and neutralizes virus. IgM and early IgG antibodies to type 1 *H. hominis* may be complement-requiring. Several strains of HVH-2 have been tested and have not been shown to stimulate homotypic complement-requiring neutralizing antibodies.

After initial exposure immunoglobulin M antibodies appear in serum within 1 week. In respiratory secretions IgA antibodies form. In cases of encephalitis, passive hemagglutinating antibodies can be measured in cerebrospinal fluid. Seven days after infection IgG antibodies appear and antiherpesvirus IgM synthesis decreases. Complement-fixing antibodies appear in 14 days.

Antiherpesvirus IgM antibodies may be measured by conventional or complement-requiring neutralization techniques, fluorescent microscopy, or passive hemagglutination.

After an initial exposure, complement-fixing antibodies fall to low levels within several months, while neutralizing antibodies persist for many years. Reactivations of infection evoke variable rises in sera of conventional neutralizing or complement-fixing IgG antibodies. Low titers of heterologous antibodies to HVH-1 and

HVH-2 are also found by complement-fixing and passive hemagglutination tests. There are some low-titered cross-reactions when anti-HVH antibodies are measured against varicella-zoster or cytomegalovirus.

By means of the passive hemagglutination technique, herpesvirus protein is indiscriminately adsorbed to the surface of tannic acid–treated sheep red blood cells, providing a comprehensive measure of several antibodies and increasing sensitivity. For strains of HVH, type 1 and type 2, respectively, titers of passive hemagglutinating antibodies are 2.6 to 14 times and 4 to 22 times greater than conventional neutralizing antibodies.

HVH-1 IgA complexes are generally noninfectious, while HVH-1 IgC complexes (sensitized virus) are infectious. Complete covering of the virion and a resulting steric hindrance to absorption may be important in order to neutralize sensitized virus. Thus, antibody to gammaglobulin, papain-derived Fab fragments of IgG anti-HVH-1 serums, IgM rheumatoid factor, and components of complement (C1 plus C4) can neutralize sensitized virus. There is every likelihood that during herpesvirus infections of man, sensitized virus is present in the circulation and is fixed in tissues. It remains to be determined what role these infectious antigen-antibody complexes have in disease.

MANIFESTATIONS Herpesvirus hominis, type 1 Primary infection with HVH-1 causes *acute gingivostomatitis, rhinitis, keratoconjunctivitis, meningoencephalitis, eczema herpeticum* (Kaposi's varicelliform eruption), and *traumatic herpes*, including *herpetic whitlow* and *generalized herpes simplex* in burned patients or wrestlers. In immunosuppressed patients initial infection or clinical reactivation may induce esophageal ulceration or interstitial pneumonia.

The incubation period is 2 to 12 days, averaging 6 or 7 days. The route of infection is usually respiratory. During acute herpetic gingivostomatitis there is fever, irritability, red swollen gums, a vesicular eruption on the mucous membranes of the mouth, oral fetor, and local submaxillary adenopathy. A visit to the dentist may precede an attack. Any portion of the oral mucosa may be affected. Viremia may occur. A generalized vesicular eruption may follow and appear in crops. Lesions are generally smaller than those of varicella. In the eczematous infant (Kaposi's varicelliform eruption) large quantities of fluid, electrolytes, and protein may be lost.

Within the tense vesicles is a clear fluid. An impression smear of an opened vesicle demonstrates syncytial giant cells undergoing ballooning degeneration. Intranuclear inclusions are seen. Virus can readily be isolated from the fluid; no bacteria are seen by Gram's stain and none may be cultured. Later, vesicles collapse and ulcerate. Sometimes the nose is the site of primary infection. Tiny vesicles surrounding reddened areolae appear in the nostrils. Usually, there is fever and the anterior cervical lymph nodes enlarge.

Infected secretions from patients contaminate the fingers of hospital personnel through unnoticed abrasions, producing *herpetic whitlow*. Painful deep vesicles appear suddenly and spread locally for about a week. The nail may be separated from its matrix by a lesion at its base.

Follicular conjunctivitis (often unilateral) with chemosis, edema of the lids, and conjunctival ulcers may be seen. The cornea may be involved in primary or recurrent infections. When the cornea is affected, a diffuse epitheliolitis develops with superficial punctate erosions which extend into small dendritic ulcers. If untreated, this ulcer increases in size to form a large, anesthetic "geographic" ulcer. Erosions of the cornea recur. *Deeper interstitial keratitis* with secondary bacterial invasion, hypopyon, iridocyclitis, synechia, and opacification of the lens follows.

Others with preexisting neutralizing antibodies in serums may suffer *recurrent attacks of herpes labialis* or trigeminal neuralgia. Pneumococcal and meningococcal, but not gram-negative infections; menstruation; emotional upset; and other little-understood events seem to trigger recurrent localized episodes. Recurrences are associated with continued virus shedding, rather than reactivation of latent infection. An occasional patient develops encephalitis.

Encephalitis Occasionally, and for as yet ill-defined reasons, *H. hominis*, type 1, begins an ascent from the respiratory epithelium of the nose up the olfactory tract to reach the frontal and temporal areas of the brain. An often fatal or severely damaging necrotizing encephalitis results. Immediate mortality of patients with seizures who are in coma is about 38 percent, but the majority of the survivors are markedly impaired.

Postnatal patients of any age, either sex, and of any socioeconomic status may be affected. About 15 percent of patients who develop herpes simplex virus encephalitis have histories of recurrent herpes labialis. Prodromal illnesses begin 3 to 4 days before admission to the hospital. Various combinations of headache, rhinorrhea, sore throat, fever, nausea, or vomiting are noted. Less frequently photophobia, vertigo, insomnia, or anorexia occurs. One-third of the patients have concurrent fever blisters during the course of their illness. Neurologic symptoms necessitate hospitalization. In order of frequency, disorientation, personality change, hallucinations, photophobia, ataxia, facial weakness, incontinence of stool or urine, tremors, and amnesia appear. Patients with proven herpes simplex virus encephalitis have been mistaken as inebriates or psychotics. Neurologic signs include stupor, seizures (Jacksonian or generalized), coma, extensor plantar reflexes, nuchal rigidity, motor deficit, cranial nerve palsies, sensory deficit, decorticate and decerebrate posture, abnormal conjugate deviation of eyes, frontal lobe signs (glabella, snout, sucking), asymmetric deep tendon reflexes, and dysphasia.

Leukocyte counts average 13,000 per mm^3 with concomitant "shifts to the left." Cerebrospinal fluid samples are completely normal or contain only a few to several hundred leukocytes which may be predominantly mononuclear or polymorphonuclear. Grossly bloody spinal fluid is an ominous sign. Cerebrospinal fluid protein is normal or elevated as high as 250 mg per 100 ml. Glucose in cerebrospinal fluid is usually normal, but may be low. In every case electroencephalograms are diffusely abnormal, or show focal lesions in the temporal or frontal regions. The abnormal electroencephalogram is an especially important finding particularly in cases in which the cerebrospinal fluid is normal. Bilateral carotid angiograms are indicated to rule out an epidural, subdural, or intracerebral hematoma, abscess, or tumor. In a few cases of HVH-1 encephalitis, the focal hemorrhagic necrotic mass deviates carotid vessels, and craniotomy is necessary for diagnosis.

The following criteria are used to make a presumptive or definitive diagnosis of *H. hominis* encephalitis: (1) Encephalitis is present clinically and confirmed by an abnormal electroencephalogram, often with focal changes in the frontal or temporal lobes. (2) Cerebrospinal fluid is sterile for bacteria (including *Mycobacterium tuberculosis*), fungi, and other viruses. (3) Carotid angiograms are done when focal signs persist. When cerebral vessels are displaced at angiography, craniotomy is done to exclude a diagnosis of subdural, epidural, or intracerebral abscess, hematoma, or tumor. (4) A fourfold rise (or occasionally fall) in complement-fixing, conventional neutralizing, or passive hemagglutinating antibodies is demonstrated in acute and convalescent phase specimens of serum in all the survirors. In addition, a single serum with a ratio of complement-requiring to conventional neutralizing antibodies to *H. hominis*, type 1, of 4 or more is considered equal to information gleaned through retrospective rises in complement-fixing, conventional neutralizing, or passive hemagglutinating antibodies. In every patient with a presumptive diagnosis of herpesvirus encephalitis, the same serums are tested for concomitant rises in complement-fixing antibodies to mumps or rubeola viruses; they must be negative. Passive hemagglutinating antibodies have been found in cerebrospinal fluids of several patients with definitive *H. hominis* encephalitis. To date, these antibodies have not been found in cerebrospinal fluids of controls. (5) Isolation of *H. hominis* from the brain at biopsy or autopsy is diagnostic. Cowdry, type A (owl-eye) intranuclear inclusions may be demonstrated from the brain (Fig. 200-1). (6) Cases are excluded if the course suggests another diagnosis or if the above criteria are not met. Attempts at isolation of viruses from throat or rectal swabs, urine, and cerebrospinal fluid as well as from brain, spinal cord, and vesicular fluid, when available, should be made.

Herpesvirus hominis, type 2 Infection with *H. hominis*, type 2, is a venereal disease. In one study seven of eight female contacts of men with penile herpetic infection showed evidence of current HVH genital infection. Similarly, 63 of 64 HVH isolates from male genitalia and 155 of 162 from the female genital tract were HVH-2. This infection is the most common cause of genital vesicles and/or ulcers found in women, and is second only to primary syphilis as the cause of such lesions in males. Teen-agers make up one-fourth to one-half of patients with genital herpetic infections.

Neutralizing antibodies to HVH-2 are reported to be present in 35.7 percent of patients who subsequently develop carcinoma *in situ* of the cervix, but are found in 7.1 percent of matched controls. However, an etiologic relation between carcinoma of the cervix and infection with HVH-2 is not established.

During primary infections fever, malaise, and inguinal adenopathy may be seen and viremia may follow. A benign aseptic meningitis has resulted. In the male there may be tiny vesicles on the glans or shaft of the penis, burning, urgency, frequency, and watery discharge. Herpesvirus is easily cultivated from vesicular fluids.

In women there are tiny vesicles on the labia minora and inner surfaces of the labia majora and cervix. They rapidly ulcerate to round and oval, discrete, and coalescent gray-white lesions. Typical cytologic changes of infection with herpes simplex virus, which may be recognized with a Papanicolaou preparation, occur. If initial infection occurs during pregnancy, transplacental infection of the fetus may ensue.

Recurrent attacks may be associated with neurologic pain and vesicles on the penis or vulva, thighs, or buttocks. If the cervix or vulva is affected at the time of delivery, perinatal infection of the infant may occur during transit through the birth canal. The newborn infant may show signs of illness by the fourth to seventh day of life. Viremia is usual. Cutaneous vesicles may occur at diverse sites. The lungs, liver, brain, and adrenals are also affected. A diffuse encephalitis, respiratory failure, diffuse hepatic destruction with increasing jaundice, and adrenal insufficiency may follow. Most cases are fatal.

TREATMENT Neither killed nor attenuated vaccine has been shown to be effective. When there is a history of recurrent herpetic vulvovaginalis coupled with a clinical exacerbation at term, delivery by cesarean section must be considered. If primary herpetic vulvovaginitis is documented during gestation, the fetus may be infected during the mother's viremia, and the indication for cesarean section is less clear.

Idoxuridine, a metabolic analogue of thymidine, is effective topically in *H. hominis* keratitis. This drug is being evaluated in disseminated perinatal infections and encephalitis. It competes with deoxythymidine triphosphate in the biosynthesis of DNA, and exhibits feedback inhibition of deoxycytidylate deaminase, thymidine kinase, and ribonucleoside diphosphate reductase. Cytosine arabinoside (ara-C) and adenine arabinoside (ara-A) are also being used experimentally. Interferon, interferon inducers, and corticosteroids are not useful. For herpetic keratitis topical IDU is applied in a 0.1% solution every hour during the day and every 2 hr during the night. A simpler means of application is a 0.5 percent ointment four or five times a day. Patients have used this ointment locally in recurrent herpes labialis and progenitalis. Although there are no controlled data, pain and morbidity may be shortened. Several patients with herpetic vulvovaginitis have been treated with idoxuridine (100 μg per ml) in water as a sitz bath four times a day with rapid relief of fever and pain, and healing of lesions.

When IDU is given intravenously as a rapid infusion (50 mg per min), antiviral concentrations in serum (10 to 36 μg per 0.4 ml), cerebrospinal fluid (up to 833 μg per 0.4 ml), and urine (45 to 1,040 μg per 0.4 ml), are attained. When IDU is given as a slow intravenous infusion, no IDU is found in serum, cerebrospinal fluid, or urine.

Idoxuridine is not inactivated to its inactive metabolites (iodouracil, uracil, and iodide) in serum, urine, or cerebrospinal fluid. It is not bound to serum proteins. Inactivation occurs in tissues. Present recommendations for use of IDU are 60 mg per kg intravenously per day for 5 days. No more than 20 g should ever be given to a single patient. In a 70-kg patient 2 g IDU in 200 ml, 5% glucose in water is infused by vein over a 45-min interval every 12 hr. Treatment is continued for 5 days. When this regimen is used, stomatitis, diarrhea, leukopenia, thrombocytopenia, secondary bacterial infections, alopecia, and loss of nails have not occurred.

REFERENCES

CATALANO LW, JOHNSON LD: Herpesvirus antibody and carcinoma *in situ* of the cervix. JAMA 217:447, 1971

Dowdle WR et al: Association of antigenic type of *Herpesvirus hominis* with site of viral recovery. J Immunol 99:974, 1967

KAUFMAN HE: Clinical cure of herpes simplex keratitis by 5-iodo-2′-deoxyuridine. Proc Soc Exp Biol Med 109:251, 1962

LERNER AM, BAILEY EJ: Concentrations of idoxuridine in serum, urine, and cerebrospinal fluid of patients with suspected diagnoses of *Herpesvirus hominis* encephalitis. J Clin Invest 51:45, 1972

NAHMIAS AJ et al: Genital infection with type 2 *Herpesvirus hominis*: A commonly occurring venereal disease. Br J Vener Dis 45:294, 1969

NOLAN DC et al: *Herpesvirus hominis* encephalitis in Michigan: Report of 13 cases, including 6 treated with idoxuridine. N Engl J Med 282:10, 1970

TERNI M et al: Aseptic meningitis in association with herpes progenitalis. N Engl J Med 285:503, 1971

WHEELER CE, HUFFINES WD: Primary disseminated herpes simplex of the newborn. JAMA 191:455, 1965

201 MINOR VIRAL DISEASES OF THE SKIN AND MUCOSAL SURFACES

ALVIN E. FRIEDMAN-KIEN

HERPANGINA Herpangina is a specific, benign, infectious disease of childhood, although it is not uncommon in young adults. It is caused by group A Coxsackie viruses types 2, 3, 4, 5, 6, 8, and 10. It occurs throughout the world in epidemic form, usually in the summer and early fall. Similar disorders have been attributed to echo and Coxsackie B viruses (Chap. 190).

The incubation period for herpangina is about 4 to 6 days. Children between the ages of one and seven are most commonly afflicted. Immunity persists for at least 1 year; reinfection with another strain of the virus may occur.

Herpangina is characterized by sudden onset of fever, temperatures often rising to 104°F, severe sore throat, nausea, and vomiting. Anorexia, dysphagia, excessive salivation, and severe malaise are common. The throat and posterior portions of the mouth are usually quite red and injected and are covered with numerous minute vesicles (1 to 2 mm in diameter), which quickly rupture, erode, and enlarge to form 3- to 4-mm punched-out, shallow ulcers with grayish centers surrounded by deep red areolas. The number and size of the lesions increase for 2 to 3 days; lesions heal within 4 or 5 days. The anterior faucial pillars of the pharynx, the tonsils, and the soft palate are usually involved. Occasionally, similar vesicles are found in the vaginal mucosa.

The systemic and local symptoms begin to regress within 4 to 5 days, and total recovery occurs within 7 days. Headache, coryza, and other respiratory tract symptoms are absent. Myalgia and arthralgia are rare. Mild cervical lymphadenopathy is sometimes noted. Parotitis and aseptic meningitis have been reported.

Recovery from the illness is always uneventful. Treatment is confined to topical symptomatic measures; frequent mouthwashes and gargles with topical anesthetics such as Benadryl elixir or butacaine are soothing. A fluid or soft diet is advisable. Demonstration of a Coxsackie virus from one of the vesicles or isolation from pharyngeal washing and/or stool may be helpful, especially when combined with a demonstrable rise in antibody titer in the convalescent as compared to the acute serum.

Differential diagnosis should include a primary herpes simplex infection, which may produce a severe oropharyngeal eruption. However, herpes does not usually occur in epidemics, and the herpetic lesions are more typically confined to the anterior portions of the mouth, such as the lips and tongue. With herpes, the gingiva are typically red and edematous. Aphthous stomatitis, bacterial pharyngitis, and the oropharyngeal lesions of viral exanthems, such as chickenpox and measles, may be confused initially with herpangina. The natural course of the disease will help clarify the diagnosis.

FOOT-AND-MOUTH DISEASE Foot-and-mouth disease is a fairly common epidemic viral disease of farm animals in Europe, Asia, and Africa. It is rarely known to affect man. The causative agent is the smallest virus known to infect animals. A few cases have been reported in children and adults who had had contact with an infected stock of animals, had ingested contaminated meat or dairy products, or had been exposed to the hides or excretions of sick animals. The incubation period seems to range between 2 to 18 days. Multiloculated vesicles appear on the skin and mucous membranes. Intranuclear inclusion bodies have been observed in the epidermal cells at the base of the vesicles and in the surrounding tissue.

The onset of the infection is characterized by fever, headache, malaise, and dryness and burning sensation of the oral mucosa. Within 2 to 3 days loculated vesicles develop on the lips, tongue, and buccal mucosa. The palms and soles and interdigital skin may also show such lesions. Generalized pruritus may occur. The vesicles go on to develop into irregularly shaped, painful ulcers which may become edematous and bleed easily. At times either the mouth or the hands alone may be involved. Rarely, other areas of the skin may be affected. The course of the disease is usually mild; the temperature falls rapidly, and the lesions begin to heal after 6 or 7 days. Total healing is complete by 2 to 3 weeks, leaving no scars.

Diagnostic confirmation depends upon demonstration of a rise in specific complement-fixing antibody titers. The virus can be isolated in tissue cultures, guinea pigs, and chick embryos. In the United States, strict regulations of quarantine and meat inspection have limited the occurrence to a few outbreaks near the Mexican border. Treatment is symptomatic.

HAND-FOOT-AND-MOUTH DISEASE Hand-foot-and-mouth disease is a syndrome characterized by a vesicular eruption of the skin and the mouth. It has been reported to occur in epidemics in the United States, England, and Australia. Laboratory studies suggest that the disease is associated with Coxsackie A viruses, types 16, 5, and others. The infection occurs primarily in children. The disease is mild, running its course in 4 to 8 days. A transient, low-grade fever may be present at the onset. The most troublesome symptom is stomatitis. Initially vesicles appear in random distribution on the tongue, buccal mucosa, gingiva, and palate, usually sparing the pharynx. These vesicles are few in number, are somewhat larger than those seen in herpangina, and quickly develop into shallow, whitish ulcerations with red areolas.

Lesions on the skin are not always present but are typically vesicular, approximately 4 or 5 mm in size. They are characteristically few in number, ovoid or elongated in shape, grayish in color, surrounded by a fine, red margin. These vesicles appear on the dorsum of the fingers and especially about the periungual region and the heel margin. Occasionally vesicles may be found on the palms or soles. They usually start to disappear within a few days after onset. On rare occasions a more diffuse, vesicular eruption and exanthematous rash have been reported, with particular concentration of such lesions on the buttocks.

The differential diagnosis includes herpangina, aphthous stomatitis, and other Coxsackie and echo virus infections. The confirmation of the exact diagnosis depends upon viral and serologic studies.

VESICULAR STOMATITIS Vesicular stomatitis is a viral illness of horses, cattle, and pigs, but it occasionally affects man. The disease occurs in the United States and South America. The mode of natural spread among livestock is unknown, but the disease is probably transmitted by direct and indirect contact. Epidemics do not occur in freezing weather, and it is therefore assumed that the virus is arthropod-borne in nature. The virus has been isolated from flies and mosquitoes. Two antigenically distinct viruses are known to cause the disease in the United States, the Indiana type and the New Jersey type. The incubation period is 2 to 6 days. In man the disease is mild and self-limited; the symptoms are similar to those of influenza. The virus has been studied and used extensively in experimental laboratories. Consequently, several cases have been reported in laboratory personnel as well as farm workers.

The sudden onset is characterized by fever up to 104°F lasting 24 hr, chills, and profuse sweating. Myalgias, malaise, headache, and aching of the eyes are common. The symptoms are worse on the second day. One-third of the patients develop sore throats with cervical and submandibular adenopathy. The tongue and mucous membranes may become sore as well, and conjunctivitis may occur. In a few cases, small, subcorneal, intraepithelial vesicles appear on the fingers. Symptoms last only 3 to 4 days, but relapses may occur. Inapparent infections have been demonstrated by a rise of both complement-fixing and neutralizing serum antibodies in laboratory workers. Differential diagnosis must include hand-foot-and-mouth disease, herpangina, and other mucocutaneous syndromes. Viral isolation from patients is rare, but the comparison of acute and convalescent serums in a suspected case will help to confirm the diagnosis.

WARTS (VERRUCAE) Warts are an infectious disease of the skin and contiguous mucous membrane. The etiologic agent is a member of the papova group of viruses, which includes the animal papilloma viruses, the polyoma, and the simian vacuolating viruses, such as SV_{40} and SV_5. These viruses have been shown to induce tumors in experimental animals and to cause in vitro transformation of tissue cultures.

The human wart virus, which is a DNA virus measuring about 45 nm in diameter, has been extracted from human lesions and has been used experimentally to induce the formation of warts at inoculated sites in the skin of human volunteers. The incubation period, based on the experimental inoculations, varies between 1 to 20 months, averaging about 4 months. The virus has been shown electronmicroscopically to parasitize the nuclei of epidermal cells. The successful isolation of the human wart virus in tissue culture has not been accomplished conclusively.

The skin lesions induced by the wart virus are due to an abnormal proliferation of epidermal cells. The lesions, which are skin-colored, may occur as single lesions or in multiples widely disseminated over the entire body. Although the same virus is thought to cause all varieties of human warts, the character of the lesion depends upon the local response of the affected skin to the virus host. Immunity may also play a role. For convenience, lesions are classified according to location and structure.

Common warts (*verrucae vulgares*) are usually seen on the hands or under and about the fingernails. These lesions are rough-surfaced, horny papules which vary in size from 1 mm to 2 cm in diameter. Confluency of clustered lesions occurs frequently. The lesions are asymptomatic.

Plantar warts occur mostly beneath pressure points on the soles of the feet and are frequently quite painful. The surface lesions are flat, firm, stippled, and horny. They may occur individually or in a mosaiclike cluster. The mass of plantar warts is beneath the skin surface. These warts are generally larger than one might expect. They have a conical shape, the pointed end projected inward. This configuration is probably due to the pressure imposed by walking. Plantar warts are most common in teenagers; females seem slightly more susceptible than males.

The differential diagnosis of plantar warts includes calluses and corns. The normal epidermal ridges are continuous across the surface of calluses and corns, whereas the surface of warts disrupts the normal pattern. Local foreign-body reactions and congenital keratotic lesions of the palms and soles also have to be ruled out.

Flat warts (*verrucae planae*) are skin-colored, smooth, flat or slightly elevated, round or polygonal papules that vary between 1 and 5 mm in diameter. They almost always occur in multiples, up to several hundred. The common sites are the face, neck, chest, dorsum of the hands, flexor surface of the forearms, and shins. The mucous membranes are rarely involved. The surface of these lesions shows a stippled appearance when examined under a magnifying glass. Flat warts are most frequently confused with the lesions of lichen planus. Multiple lesions on the dorsum of the hands may be mistaken for one of the inherited disorders known as acrokeratosis verruciformis, epidermodysplasia verruciformis, or Darier's disease.

Filiform warts are most frequently seen in adult males and usually occur in the bearded area of the face. The lips and eyelids are often involved. The lesions are horny, fingerlike projections which may grow to considerable length if left unattended. They occur in multiples but are seen occasionally as individual lesions. Differential diagnosis includes cutaneous horns.

Digitate warts are seen on the scalp of adults as clusters of fleshy fingerlike projections. They must be differentiated from epidermal nevi.

Condylomata accuminata (*moist warts*), also known as venereal or fig warts, are the lesions which occur at the mucocutaneous junctions of the skin in the genital and perianal areas. Rare cases have been seen about the areola of the nipple in females, the margins of the mouth, both the inguinal and axillary folds, and in the interdigital skin between the toes.

These warts are pink to red in color and moist and soft. They may be pedunculated or elongated. Clusters of these warts may resemble a cauliflower in appearance. They may occur in great numbers and can become macerated and malodorous because of their location. These warts are most often seen in young adults, but children as well as adults are affected. The eruption of moist warts is frequent and more severe in pregnancy. Although the lesions have been known to be transmitted between sexual partners, it is a misconception that these lesions are usually venereal in origin.

Condylomata accuminata, unlike other warts, are most effectively treated with the repeated topical application of a 25 percent podophyllum resin in tincture of benzoin. A single, persistent, fungating lesion on the penis, resistant to this treatment, should be biopsied to rule out a malignancy, such as squamous-cell carcinoma or a rare, abnormal growth, known as the Buschke-Lowenstein tumor. The more sessile condylomata lesions of secondary syphilis may be confused with viral-induced and genital warts.

Warts often tend to recur, even after apparently adequate treatment. The variety of methods used for removal are primarily destructive, such as electrodesiccation and curettage, surgical excision, x-ray, or cryosurgery by applying liquid nitrogen or dry ice. Repeated paring of warts, followed by the application of caustic agents such as mono- or trichloracetic acid, salicylic acid, phenol, or silver nitrate is very helpful. It is important to avoid radical means of therapy, because all warts will eventually disappear spontaneously, leaving no scar, suggesting the development of an immune response. However, warts may persist and spread within the same host for several years.

ORF (ECTHYMA INFECTIOSUM) Orf is an infectious disease which primarily affects the mouth and lips of sheep. It is caused by a specific virus which has been isolated in tissue culture. The disease is transmitted between animals and also from virus-contaminated, dried crusts of lesions found in grazing pastures. The virus may remain in an infective state for several months or years. The disease has a worldwide distribution. The mouths of young lambs are most often affected; infection confers lifelong immunity. Human infection occurs in shepherds, butchers, veterinarians, and children who play with sheep.

In man, the incubation period is about 5 to 6 days. The eruption may occur as single or multiple lesions on the hands and other exposed parts of the body. Initially, a small, reddish-blue papule appears and rapidly enlarges to form a 2- to 3-cm hemorrhagic bulla. Itching is intense, and the bulla ruptures to form an umbilicated, erythematous ulcer which develops a gray-white crust. Systemic manifestations are rare, except for occasional low-grade fever and mild regional lymphangitis and lymphadenopathy. A transient macular and papular red rash may occur on the trunk during the second week of the disease. Spontaneous healing occurs within 3 to 6 weeks.

The disease should be suspected when the characteristic lesions develop in individuals exposed to sheep. The diagnosis can be confirmed by virus isolation in the laboratory as well as by a comparative rise of antibody titers in acute and convalescent serums.

Differential diagnosis must include milkers' nodule, anthrax, tularemia, primary inoculation tuberculosis, and cowpox.

MILKERS' NODULE (PARAVACCINIA, MILKERS' WARTS) Milkers' nodule is a benign, poxvirus disease contracted from infected cows. The disease has a worldwide distribution. Nodules and ulcers occur on the teats of infected dairy cattle. In man, lesions appear within 5 to 7 days after milking an infected cow. They usually occur on the hands, but other exposed parts of the body, such as the face, may be inoculated. The virus has been isolated in bovine kidney tissue culture and resembles the orf virus. The early, flat, dark red papules enlarge up to 1 to 2 cm in diameter within a week and develop into solid, elastic, shiny, brownish-purple, highly vascular nodules. No pus or fluid accumulates. The nodules may be slightly tender, and mild regional lymphadenopathy may occur. Mild temperature elevations have been reported. Gradually an opaque, gray, slightly depressed eschar develops over the surface of the nodules' red granulation tissue. The lesion is surrounded by an areola of erythema.

Resolution occurs within 5 to 6 weeks without scarring. One infection provides permanent immunity. The virus can be isolated in tissue culture, but this is not a practical routine procedure. There is no cross immunity between milkers' nodule, cowpox, and vaccinia.

Differential diagnosis between milkers' nodule and warts may not be possible on clinical grounds. Pyogenic granuloma and cowpox should also be considered.

MOLLUSCUM CONTAGIOSUM Molluscum contagiosum is an infectious disease of the skin and mucous membranes caused by one of the largest known viruses. It is limited to man and most frequently occurs in childhood. Although the virus has not been grown in the laboratory, it has been classified morphologically on the basis of electronmicroscopy with the pox group of viruses. No cross-antigenicity with other pox viruses has yet been demonstrated. The mode of transmission is unknown. The disease has a worldwide distribution and has occurred in epidemics within children's institutions, between wrestlers, and members of the same family. Infections have been transmitted between genitalia during sexual intercourse and from the mouth of a suckling baby to its mother's breast. Successful experimental inoculation of lesion extracts to the skin of human volunteers has been reported. The incubation period varies between 2 weeks and 2 months. Fluorescent-antibody and gel-diffusion immunologic studies have shown demonstrable antibody in the serum of infected individuals.

The lesions may vary in number and size, ranging from 1 mm up to "giant" lesions of 1 to 2 cm in diameter, and average about 4 mm. They are elevated, waxy, pearly white papules which show an umbilicated central pore. By squeezing such a papule, one can express from the pore a curdlike, cheesy material, which, upon electronmicroscopic examination, proves to be loaded with virus particles. Ordinary light microscopy smears of the curd show a specific diagnostic picture of clusters of cells containing eosinophilic, giant cytoplasmic inclusion bodies. The papules may appear alone or in groups. Autoinoculation is frequent; the lesions are usually present for 6 months to a year, but may persist and spread for 3 to 4 years. The face, especially the eyelids, the trunk, and anogenital areas are most commonly involved. The conjunctiva, lips, and buccal mucosa may rarely be involved. Molluscum lesions are frequently traumatized and become secondarily infected, but injury seems to cause individual lesions to resolve. Spontaneous regression eventually occurs without scarring.

Treatment by sharp curettage clears up the lesions with little, if any, scarring.

Diagnosis of multiple lesions is fairly simple. A single lesion may be confused with a keratoacanthoma, basal-cell epithelioma, or pyogenic granuloma. The diagnosis can be made histologically.

REFERENCES

Friedman-Kien AE et al: Milkers' nodule: Isolation of a virus from a human case. Science 140:1335, 1963

——, Vilcek J: Induction of interference and interferon synthesis by non-replicating molluscum contagiosum virus. J Immunol 99:1092, 1967

Kibrick S: Current status of coxsackie and ECHO viruses in human disease. Prog Med Virol 6:27, 1964

Nagington J, Whittle CH: Human orf: Isolation of the virus by tissue culture. Br Med J 2:1324, 1961

Patterson WC et al: A study of vesicular stomatitis in man. J Am Vet Med Assoc 133:57, 1958

Rowson KEK, Mahy WJ: Human papova (wart) virus. Bacteriol Rev 31:100, 1967

Tindall JP, Miller GD: Hand-foot-and-mouth disease. Cutis 9:457, 1972

section 18 | Viral diseases of the eye

202
VIRAL INFECTIONS OF THE EYE

J. THOMAS GRAYSTON
CHANDLER R. DAWSON

INTRODUCTION The eye and its adnexa may be infected during the course of many cutaneous and systemic viral diseases. Sometimes these ocular infections produce minor manifestations, such as the transient loss of accommodation in dengue and the milder forms of conjunctivitis in systemic adenovirus infections. Other virus infections, however, such as herpes simplex (Chap. 200), herpes zoster (Chap. 199), measles (Chap. 195), and vaccinia or smallpox (Chap. 198), occasionally produce serious and permanent visual loss. In addition, congenital viral infections are an important cause of blindness, particularly rubella, which leads to cataracts and microphthalmus, and cytomegalic inclusion disease with retinal involvement.

The diseases described in this chapter are caused by microorganisms that produce localized eye disease. Although they are mainly of concern to ophthalmologists, these diseases are important in the differential diagnosis of systemic disorders involving the eye. Knowledge of the epidemiology of the diseases will aid in their recognition.

TRACHOMA AND INCLUSION CONJUNCTIVITIS (INCLUSION BLENNORRHEA) Definition Trachoma is a chronic conjunctival infection. It is still the most important cause of visual loss, having produced an estimated 20 million cases of blindness throughout the world. Inclusion conjunctivitis is a closely related acute ocular inflammation in sexually active adults and in their newborn offspring.

Etiology The microorganisms that cause trachoma and inclusion conjunctivitis (TRIC) and lymphogranuloma venereum (LGV) are very closely related. Along with the psittacosis organisms they form the *Chlamydia* group. *Chlamydia* are obligate, intracellular microorganisms; they are not viruses, being more closely related to bacteria, because they have cell walls with chemical and metabolic properties similar to bacteria and are affected by broad-spectrum antibiotics. TRIC agents grow primarily in the epithelium of the conjunctiva, urethra, and cervix. They can be identified by the typical cytoplasmic inclusion bodies in Giemsa-stained smears of cells from these sites. The agents may be isolated and grown in yolk sacs of embryonated hens' eggs or now, more easily, in special tissue culture cells. Primates are the only laboratory animals susceptible to eye infections with TRIC organisms. TRIC and LGV agents have been serologically classified into 12 types by an immunofluorescent technique.

Epidemiology In the United States a mild form of trachoma still occurs in American Indians and in Mexican Americans as well as in immigrants from endemic trachoma areas. Acute relapse of old trachoma may be seen occasionally following treatment with cortisone eye ointment. The worldwide incidence and severity of trachoma have decreased dramatically during the past 25 years in areas with improving hygienic and economic conditions. The disease is still highly prevalent in North Africa, the Middle East, and Northern India. Transmission of the disease occurs primarily through close personal contact, particularly among young children. Development of the chronic disease usually requires repeated infections.

Inclusion conjunctivitis in adults or newborn infants is an occasional manifestation of what is becoming better recognized as frequent genital tract infection with TRIC agents. These microorganisms are now known to cause considerable venereal disease (urethritis and cervicitis) in the United States and Europe and probably throughout the world.

Clinical manifestations Initial TRIC eye infection is a follicular conjunctivitis that is not different from many other types of follicular conjunctivitis. The syndrome of trachoma presents as a chronic follicular conjunctivitis with involvement of the cornea. As the disease progresses, scarring of the conjunctiva occurs, as well as corneal vascularization and leukocytic infiltration (pannus formation). If the scarring of the conjunctiva is severe enough, distortions of the lid result, with inversion of the entire lid margins (entropion) or of individual lashes (trichiasis). Destruction of the lacrimal glands may produce keratitis sicca and xerosis (abnormal dryness). Complete corneal pannus may occur as part of the primary disease process or as a result of secondary complications. Visual loss or complete blindness frequently occurs as a result of bacterial corneal ulcers late in the course of the disease.

Diagnosis The diagnosis of trachoma or inclusion conjunctivitis should be considered in all cases of follicular conjunctivitis persisting for more than 3 weeks. Trachoma is usually a clinical diagnosis. However, laboratory diagnosis has been greatly improved. The presence of the typical cytoplasmic inclusion bodies in Giemsa-stained or fluorescent antibody–stained smears of the conjunctival epithelium is considered adequate proof of TRIC infection. Such inclusions are sometimes difficult to demonstrate, particularly in milder disease or chronic disease. Isolation in eggs and cell cultures and the direct immunofluorescent test to detect serum antibodies provide evidence of infection, but these procedures are limited to a few research laboratories. Follicular conjunctivitis in Americans or Europeans exposed in countries where trachoma is endemic is only very rarely trachoma.

Treatment Sulfonamides, tetracycline, and erythromycin are effective in vitro and are reported to be effective in vivo. In the absence of bacterial superinfection, mild chronic trachoma such as that found in American Indians responds to 3 to 6 weeks of full courses of these chemotherapeutic agents. Where trachoma is more severe and complicated by secondary bacterial conjunctivitis, particularly with *Hemophilus*, local treatment with tetracycline eye ointments has been used most extensively. In mass therapy campaigns, treatment for 60 days with tetracycline or erythromycin ointment locally has produced marked clinical improvement. The World Health Organization has suggested intermittent therapy consisting of topical application twice daily for 1 week each month for 6 months. In countries where mass treatment programs have not been accompanied by a rise in the standard of living, trachoma and its blinding complications have not been markedly reduced. In such endemic areas, control programs frequently have provision for surgical repair of entropion and trichiasis to prevent visual loss later in the course of the disease.

Prevention Efforts to develop a practical vaccine following the initial isolation of the agent in 1957 have not been successful. General hygienic measures associated with improved living standards are effective in the elimination of trachoma. Adequate water supply for personal cleanliness may be a key factor. In order to prevent spread of the disease to uninfected family members, treatment of healthy contacts with antibiotic ointment once daily is an effective procedure.

INCLUSION CONJUNCTIVITIS In contrast to trachoma with its eye-to-eye transmission, inclusion conjunctivitis, or inclusion blennorrhea, is transmitted as a venereal infection with occasional involvement of the eye. In the newborn, inclusion blennorrhea can be differentiated from gonococcal ophthalmia by its longer incubation period (5 to 14 days versus 1 to 3 days). Neonatal inclusion blennorrhea has an acute onset and produces a profuse mucopurulent discharge with membrane formation and occasional scar formation on the conjunctiva. Adult inclusion conjunctivitis usually presents as an acute or chronic follicular conjunctivitis with keratitis. Infection occurs by accidental infection of the conjunctiva with genital secretions. If untreated or mistakenly treated with corticosteroids, adult inclusion conjunctivitis may be associated with significant although transient visual loss and corneal vascularization. Untreated cases may persist for several months to 2 years. Administration of systemic tetracycline, erythromycin, or sulfonamide controls the symptoms of the disease within 48 hr but should be continued for at least 3 weeks.

EPIDEMIC KERATOCONJUNCTIVITIS (EKC) EKC typically occurs in epidemics; the etiologic agent found in most outbreaks is adenovirus type 8, although minor forms of EKC occur with the other adenovirus types. Adenovirus spread occurs when medical personnel manipulate the eye, e.g., for foreign-body removal in industrial dispensaries or during eye examinations by an ophthalmologist. The virus, which is unusually resistant to inactivation, is transmitted on the fingers, by instruments, or in solutions. EKC presents as a moderate to severe follicular conjunctivitis which subsides spontaneously within 10 to 18 days. The incubation period varies from 5 to 12 days.

The disease is usually unilateral at onset. The more severe cases may be associated with conjunctival membrane formation and subsequent conjunctival scarring and with subconjunctival hemorrhages. Mild systemic manifestations such as low-grade fever, headache, and malaise may occur. A preauricular lymph node on the side of the affected eye is usually enlarged. With corneal involvement, about 7 days after onset, there is often a marked increase in pain (foreign-body sensation), lacrimation, and photophobia. The typical punctate corneal opacities appear to progress as the conjunctivitis subsides. These opacities may persist for as long as 2 years. If visual acuity is impaired, treatment with topical corticosteroids will temporarily suppress the opacities. There is no specific treatment. In epidemics, milder episodes of disease in adults are often recognized. In children, adenovirus type 8 infections may present as upper respiratory disease, often with otitis media, and may be overlooked as a source of infection for the eye disease. Explosive epidemics in industrial dispensaries and ophthalmologists' offices can be controlled by scrupulous hand washing and adequate cleansing of instruments to break the chain of infection.

NEWCASTLE DISEASE Human infection with this avian virus, which is related to influenza, occurs mainly in poultry workers, veterinarians, and virologists. In man, accidental introduction of contaminated material from naturally infected animals or from live virus (e.g., vaccines) is followed in 24 to 72 hr by conjunctivitis, edema of the lids, and tearing. Systemic symptoms occur very rarely, and recovery is complete in 10 to 14 days. The diagnosis may be confirmed by virus isolation in embryonated eggs.

REFERENCES

Dawson CR et al: Infections due to adenovirus type 8 in the United States. III. Epidemiological, clinical and microbiological features of epidemic keratoconjunctivitis. Am J Ophthalmol 69:473, 1970

Grayston JT et al: Epidemic keratoconjunctivitis on Taiwan. Am J Trop Med 13:492, 1964

Hanna L: Conference on trachoma and allied diseases. Am J Ophthalmol 63:1027, 1967

Jawetz E, Thygeson P: Trachoma and inclusion conjunctivitis agents, in *Viral and Rickettsial Infections of Man,* 4th ed., eds FL Horsfall, I Tamm, Philadelphia: Lippincott, 1965, p. 1042

Nelson CB et al: Outbreak of conjunctivitis due to Newcastle disease virus (NDV) occurring in poultry workers. Am J Public Health 42:672, 1952

Nichols RL (ed): *Trachoma and Allied Diseases,* Amsterdam, New York: Excerpta Medica, 1971

203
LYMPHOGRANULOMA VENEREUM

KING K. HOLMES

DEFINITION Lymphogranuloma venereum (LGV) is a venereally transmitted infection caused by small intracellular bacteria known as *Chlamydia.* It is characterized by a transient primary genital or anorectal lesion followed by multilocular suppurative regional lymphadenopathy in heterosexual men, or by proctocolitis with perianal lymphadenitis in homosexual men and women. Acute LGV is associated with nonspecific constitutional symptoms and occasionally with systemic complications such as meningoencephalitis. After a latent period of years, late complications may include genital elephantiasis or rectal stricture.

ETIOLOGY The agents responsible for LGV, trachoma, inclusion conjunctivitis, psittacosis, and probably some cases of nongonococcal urethritis are all members of the genus *Chlamydia.* Although the chlamydiae are obligate intracellular organisms, with a distinctive life cycle and are grown by virologic methods, they are considered to be small bacteria rather than viruses because they divide by binary fission, possess cell walls and ribosomes, contain both DNA and RNA, and are sensitive to various antibiotics in concentrations which are not toxic for mammalian cells. The individual organisms are only 300 nm in diameter but produce inclusions containing many individual organisms in epithelial cells; these are visible in Giemsa-stained preparations. The chlamydiae which cause trachoma, inclusion conjunctivitis, and LGV are closely related and are best distinguished by immunofluorescent serotyping. Although chlamydiae isolated from bubo pus of patients with LGV have occasionally resembled isolates associated with inclusion conjunctivitis or even psittacosis, the majority of LGV-associated chlamydiae fall into two distinct serotypes which have not been identified with any other syndrome and which produce meningoencephalitis in mice and monkeys.

EPIDEMIOLOGY Lymphogranuloma venereum is usually sexually transmitted, but occasional transmission by nonsexual personal contact, fomites, or laboratory accidents has been documented. The worldwide incidence of LGV is falling, but the disease is still endemic in certain developing countries. The annual incidence of LGV in United States servicemen stationed in Vietnam was 1 to 2 percent. In the United States, only 828 cases were reported in 1972, most from the southeastern states. The early manifestations are recognized far more often in men than in women. The majority of cases in the United States involve travelers, seamen, or servicemen returning from abroad; male homosexuals; or individuals of low socioeconomic status living in areas of low endemicity in the southeast. The reservoir of infection may be the female or homosexual male with chronic subacute asymptomatic infection. The prevalence of LGV has been studied by use of the complement fixation test, the Frei skin test, and attempted isolation of the organism. Unfortunately, the complement fixation test and the Frei test may remain positive long after treatment of LGV and may be positive in patients with *Chlamydia* infection other than LGV. Although trachoma and psittacosis are rare in the United States, genital infection with strains of *Chlamydia* other than those serotypes usually associated with LGV is extremely common. For example, approximately 40 percent of men with nongonococcal urethritis have urethral *Chlamydia* infection, and approximately one-third of unselected women examined in venereal disease clinics have endocervical *Chlamydia* infection. Approximately 10 percent of these endocervical isolates from asymptomatic women have been the same serotype as those isolated from a minority of patients with clinical LGV, but none of the genital isolates has been of the same serotype as "classic LGV" strains found in the majority of patients with LGV. Although the reported frequency of isolation of organisms thought to be LGV from asymptomatic prostitutes has occasionally ranged as high as 20 percent, the identity of these *Chlamydia* as LGV strains has not been confirmed by newer techniques of serotyping. In summary, the true prevalence of the asymptomatic carrier state of clinical LGV strains is unknown but is probably lower than previously estimated.

CLINICAL MANIFESTATIONS A *primary genital lesion* occurs in about one-third of heterosexual male patients but is rarely detected in women. It is a small, painless vesicle or nonindurated ulcer or papule located on the penis in the male or on the labia, posterior vagina, or fourchette in the female. It occurs from 3 days to 3 weeks after exposure, and healing takes place within a few days.

The organism spreads via the regional lymphatics, leading to inguinal, deep iliac, perirectal, or femoral lymphadenopathy. The most common presenting picture in men is the *inguinal syndrome.* This is characterized by painful inguinal lymphadenopathy beginning 2 to 6 weeks after presumed exposure; the onset rarely occurs after a few months. The inguinal adenopathy is unilateral in two-thirds of cases, and palpable enlargement of the iliac and femoral nodes is often present on the same side as the enlarged inguinal nodes. The nodes are discrete initially, but progressive periadenitis results in an extensively matted mass of nodes which become fluctuant and suppurative. The overlying skin is fixed, inflamed, and thin and finally leads to multiple draining fistulas. Extensive enlargement of chains of inguinal nodes above and below the inguinal ligament is characteristic, but is present in only a minority of cases. Histologic involvement of nodes initially shows characteristic small *stellate abscesses* surrounded by histiocytes. These abscesses coalesce to cause large, necrotic, suppurative foci. Untreated inguinal adenopathy often progresses to multiple fistula formation. These heal spontaneously in several months.

Constitutional symptoms are common during the stage of regional lymphadenopathy and include fever, chills, headache, meningismus, anorexia, myalgias, and arthralgias. The frequency of other systemic complications is low, but those which have been reported occasionally include arthritis with sterile effusion, aseptic meningitis and meningoencephalitis, hepatitis, and erythema nodosum. Chlamydiae have been recovered from the cerebrospinal fluid and in one case from the blood in patients with severe constitutional symptoms, indicating the occurrence of disseminated infection. Associated laboratory findings during this stage include leukocytosis, marked elevation of the sedimentation rate, abnormal liver function tests, and hyperglobulinemia. The immunoglobulin abnormalities in subacute or chronic LGV include rheumatoid factor activity, elevated IgG, IgA, and IgM and mixed cryoglobulinemia. In women and homosexual males, the *anorectal syndrome* occurs, and the onset of symptoms is noted after an unknown period of infection. In homosexual men and some women the anorectal syndrome presumably results from direct inoculation during rectal intercourse. In most women, anorectal infection is probably secondary to spread via the pelvic lymphatics, or due to direct spread of infection from the genitalia along the perineum to the anal canal. In some women the occurrence of large perirectal nodes or perirectal lymphangitis in the absence of proctitis favors the former route. On the other hand, the possibility of direct extension is supported by the observation that rectal colonization by *Chlamydia* occurs in nearly half of all women with genital infection due to non-LGV strains of these organisms. The earliest manifestations of anorectal infection include proctocolitis associated with mucopurulent or bloody anal discharge, tenesmus, and diarrhea. Sigmoidoscopy reveals diffuse proctitis or discrete ulcerations. Complications include perirectal abscess, fistula in ano, rectovaginal, rectovesical, and ischiorectal fistulas, and, late in the course of the disease, rectal stricture. This usually occurs 2 to 6 cm from the anal orifice and may extend proximally for several centimeters. Perianal excrescences of a granulomatous or a smooth nature (lymphorrhoids) are also seen. A higher frequency of positive LGV complement fixation reactions and Frei tests have been observed among male and female patients of low socioeconomic status who have perirectal abscess or fistula in ano than among controls. Rectal LGV may be treatable if detected early and should be excluded in patients with perirectal disease.

An uncommon late complication of LGV is *genital elephantiasis*, a chronic induration or edema of the penis or vulva caused by chronic lymphatic obstruction. Polypoid swelling of the skin and large stellate hyperplastic keloidal scars of the genitalia may be associated with this complication. A variety of subacute or chronic ulcerating lesions of the female genitalia may be associated with vulvar induration or lymphedema and are difficult to distinguish clinically from granuloma inguinale. The *urethral syndrome* is produced by infiltrative lesions in the posterior urethra which may produce stricture or fistula formation. The significance of reports of malignant changes associated with chronic anorectal or genital LGV is uncertain.

LABORATORY FINDINGS The most reliable method of diagnosis is isolation of an LGV strain of *Chlamydia* from aspirated pus from a bubo. Isolation can be accomplished in the chick embryo yolk sac or in special tissue cell culture systems. Cultures rapidly become negative after appropriate antibiotic therapy. The most practical but least specific diagnostic test is the LGV complement fixation test which becomes positive (titer greater than 1:16) earlier than the Frei test, probably within 1 to 3 weeks after infection. The LGV complement fixation test is positive in 85 to 90 percent of patients with LGV but also may be positive in patients with other *Chlamydia* infections. Because most patients have already been infected for several weeks when they are first seen, fourfold rises in complement fixation antibody titer are uncommon. The immunofluorescent antibody test is currently being evaluated for the serodiagnosis of LGV. The Frei skin test is not as sensitive as the LGV complement fixation test and is probably positive in only 35 to 70 percent of patients with LGV. The test should be repeated after 2 to 3 weeks if initially negative, but most tests which are initially negative remain so on repeated testing. *A negative Frei test does not exclude the diagnosis of LGV.* The histopathology of excised nodes or of rectal biopsy specimens is usually not specific, but suggestive features may raise the question of LGV and lead to more specific tests.

TREATMENT Chlamydiae associated with LGV are susceptible to the tetracyclines, sulfonamides, erythromycin, rifampin, and chloramphenicol and are moderately sensitive in vitro to the penicillins. They are resistant to the aminoglycosides such as streptomycin. A few isolates have been resistant to sulfonamides. Despite this, treatment with a sulfonamide is effective in over 95 percent of the cases, and tetracycline is always effective. Therapy terminates the acute constitutional symptoms and significantly shortens the duration of the bubo. It is usually not helpful in inducing significant improvement and late complications such as rectal stricture or genital elephantiasis unless active LGV or secondary infection is also present. The recommended regimen is 0.5 g tetracycline hydrochloride four times a day for 21 days. There is some evidence that 4 g per day of triple sulfonamide preparation is more effective than the same dose of a more rapidly excreted sulfonamide. A fourfold or greater fall in the complement fixation titer occurs in most treated patients. Failure of the LGV titer to fall should raise consideration of retreatment. Aspiration of fluctuant nodes rather than incision or excision is indicated.

REFERENCES

ABRAMS AJ: Lymphogranuloma venereum. JAMA 205:199, 1968

GREAVES AB et al: Chemotherapy in bubonic lymphogranuloma venereum. Bull WHO 16:277, 1957

SCHACHTER J et al: Lymphogranuloma venereum: I. Comparison of the Frei test, complement fixation test, and isolation of the agent. J Infect Dis 120:372, 1969

SIGEL MM: *Lymphogranuloma Venereum*, Coral Gables, Fla.: University of Miami Press, 1962

SONCK CE: Lymphogranuloma inguinale: Clinical, epidemiological, and immunological aspects. Hautarzt 23:280, 1972

204 CAT-SCRATCH DISEASE

ROBERT G. PETERSDORF

DEFINITION Cat-scratch disease is an infection characterized by indolent, occasionally suppurative, regional lymphadenitis, secondary to a primary cutaneous lesion at the site of inoculation, usually a cat scratch. Because more than 90 percent of the reported cases have originated from cat scratches and a history of close contact with cats is often elicited, the name *cat-scratch disease* has become popular. However, rarely a similar disorder has been acquired from splinters, thorns, beef-bone fragments, and dog and monkey scratches, and in some patients no inciting trauma is recalled.

ETIOLOGY A specific etiologic agent has not been identified. Among agents that have been incriminated are atypical acid-fast bacteria, organisms of the psittacosis-lymphogranuloma group, and herpes-like (EB) virus. The evidence to ascribe a definitive causative role to any of these is not convincing.

EPIDEMIOLOGY Cats act only as vectors for the disease. They are not ill, and have negative skin tests. The disease occurs mostly in children (75 percent), and several cases have been described in siblings, due to contact with the same cat. The disease is most common in fall and winter. Cats may act as long-term carriers, a hypothesis supported by the familial occurrence of several infections interspersed by months or years.

PATHOLOGY The histopathologic appearance of lymph nodes is not specific. Three stages have been described: (1) Early lesions show reticulum-cell hyperplasia; (2) intermediate lesions show granuloma formation; and (3) late lesions show microabscesses. These reactions are not readily distinguished from those induced by the tubercle bacillus. However, acid-fast bacilli are invariably absent.

MANIFESTATIONS The incubation period lasts a few days to several weeks, with an average of 3 to 10 days. In a typical case the primary lesion consists of a raised, slightly tender, nonpruritic papule crowned by a small vesicle or eschar; it often resembles an indolent furuncle or insect bite. Multiple primary lesions have been described. In some patients a primary lesion cannot be found.

Regional lymphadenopathy becomes evident in a few days or as long as 6 weeks after infection. Adenopathy is unilateral and asymmetric; in most instances only one node is involved. The axillary, cervical, preauricular, submandibular, epitrochlear, femoral, or inguinal nodes (in decreasing order of frequency) on one side become visibly swollen and tender, often with redness of the overlying skin. The nodes occasionally suppurate, soften, and drain spontaneously; fistulas heal completely with only slight scarring. Usually the tenderness subsides gradually, and nontender, firm, enlarged nodes remain palpable for some weeks or even months. There is no generalized glandular enlargement, and the spleen is not palpable.

Systemic symptoms are usually mild and consist of headache, fever, and malaise, which subside within a few days. Shaking chills and fever as high as 104°F can occur but are unusual. Many patients are entirely symptom-free. A transient macular or vesicular rash which subsides within 48 hr is rarely present during the early stages. Erythema nodosum and multiforme have been reported.

Clinical forms of this disease other than that described above may be delineated. These include: (1) encephalitis characterized by fever, convulsions, alterations in consciousness, mild cerebrospinal fluid pleocytosis and elevation in protein, and complete recovery; (2) Parinaud's oculoglandular syndrome characterized by granulomatous conjunctivitis and enlargement of the homolateral preauricular node; more rarely, mesenteric lymphadenitis; osteolytic bone lesions, which subside spontaneously, and thrombocytopenic purpura. In all of these syndromes the diagnostic criteria for cat-scratch disease must be present before the illness can be ascribed to cat-scratch disease.

DIAGNOSIS The following criteria should be fulfilled before a diagnosis of cat-scratch disease is established: (1) history of contact with cats, (2) finding of a primary lesion, (3) regional lymphadenopathy, (4) positive intradermal skin test, (5) biopsy of lymph node with demonstration of histopathologic changes consistent with cat-scratch disease (this may not be necessary if the skin test is positive), and (6) failure to demonstrate other causative agents.

The specific diagnosis is made by means of a skin test. Antigen for this is prepared by mixing one part pus aspirated from infected lymph nodes with three parts saline, and inactivating the mixture by heating. A positive reaction is of the delayed, tuberculin type, consisting of 5 mm induration and 1.0 cm erythema, that appears in 24 to 48 hr. Although batches of antigen vary in potency, in general, patients reacting to one batch react to another. Skin test material can be preserved by freezing. The test becomes positive within 30 days after infection and may persist for many years. Each batch of antigen must be tested against patients known to have had the disease. A well-standardized batch should provide highly reliable results. Approximately 10 percent of normal individuals have false positive reactions. The chance of carrying hepatitis virus in the antigen is remote.

Other laboratory abnormalities include mild leukocytosis (up to 15,000 cells per mm^3), occasional mild eosinophilia, and an elevated sedimentation rate. The Frei test is negative.

Cat-scratch disease is a benign illness, and the prognosis is uniformly good. Its main clinical importance lies in its possible confusion with other more serious diseases of the lymphatics. Diseases to be considered are tularemia, lymphatic tuberculosis, sporotrichosis, histoplasmosis, coccidioidomycosis, toxoplasmosis, and bacterial adenitis. Because of the indolent character of the adenopathy, Hodgkin's disease or other lymphomas may be suspected. Neck masses may be confused with thyroglossal duct cysts, bronchial cleft cysts, dermoids, cystic hygromas, thyroid and parathyroid adenomas, salivary gland tumors, carotid body tumors, aneurysms, pharyngeal or esophageal diverticula, and mesodermal tumors, as well as lymphomas. Appropriate serologic and cultural tests serve to rule out other infections; biopsy may be needed to exclude tumor, but a positive skin test with cat-scratch antigen effectively rules out the necessity for biopsy.

TREATMENT In instances of node suppuration, aspiration of accumulated pus affords relief of pain (and incidentally, serves as a source of material for the preparation of skin-test antigen). Aspiration is required in only a few cases. Antibiotics and steroids are ineffective.

REFERENCES

CARITHERS HA et al: Cat-scratch disease: Its natural history. JAMA 207:312, 1969

FUTRELL JW et al: Unsuspected etiology of lateral neck masses. Arch Otolaryngol 95:277, 1972

LYON LW: Neurologic manifestations of cat-scratch disease. Arch Neurol 25:23, 1971

MARGILETH AM: Cat-scratch disease: Nonbacterial regional lymphadenitis. The study of 145 patients and a review of the literature. Pediatrics 42:803, 1968

WARWICK WJ: The cat-scratch syndrome: Many diseases or one disease? Prog Med Virol 9:256, 1967

section 20 | Other systemic viral diseases

205 MUMPS

ROBERT G. PETERSDORF

DEFINITION Mumps is an acute communicable disease of viral origin characterized by painful enlargement of the salivary glands and, sometimes, particularly in adults, by involvement of the gonads, meninges, pancreas, and other organs.

ETIOLOGY The causative agent of mumps is a myxovirus of intermediate size. It has a tight helical inner core (RNA) enclosed in an outer shell of lipid and protein. Serologic cross reactions have been demonstrated between it and some other members of this group. The virus of mumps causes agglutination of erythrocytes of fowl, man, and some other species, produces hemolysis, and has two components capable of fixing complement, the soluble, or S, and the viral, or V, antigens. It elicits a delayed allergic reaction when used as an antigen in persons who have mumps. The virus can be cultivated in the chick embryo and propagated in tissue cultures of HeLa cells and monkey kidney cells.

EPIDEMIOLOGY Man is the only natural host for mumps. The disease is worldwide and is endemic in urban communities. Epidemics are relatively infrequent and are confined to closely associated groups who live in orphanages, army camps, or schools. The disease is most frequent in spring, and occurrence is highest in April and May. Although mumps is generally considered less "contagious" than measles and chickenpox, this difference may be more apparent than real because many mumps infections (at least 25 percent) tend to be inapparent clinically. In some surveys, 80 percent of an adult population had serologic evidence of previous infection with mumps.

Infections are rare before the age of two and then increase rapidly in frequency, reaching a peak at ages six to ten. Clinical mumps may be more common in males than in females. Adults are usually infected through direct contact. In North American cities, most infections are contracted from schoolmates and infected family members. The virus is transmitted in infected salivary secretions, although its isolation from urine suggests that the virus may spread via this route. Mumps virus is rarely cultured from stools. The saliva is infectious for approximately 6 days prior to the onset of parotitis, and virus has been cultured for as long as 2 weeks after onset of swelling. Viruria also persists for several weeks in some patients. Despite this prolonged secretion of virus, the peak of infectivity occurs a day or two before onset of parotitis and subsides rapidly after appearance of glandular enlargement.

One attack of clinical or subclinical mumps confers lasting immunity, and second attacks are most unusual.

Unilateral parotitis affords protection just as effectively as does bilateral disease.

PATHOGENESIS The virus enters via the oral route; during the incubation period of 18 to 21 days, it presumably multiplies in the salivary glands, from which it is disseminated via the bloodstream to other organs, including the meninges, gonads, pancreas, breasts, thyroid, heart, liver, kidneys, and cranial nerves. An alternative, but less likely, hypothesis is that salivary adenitis is secondary to viremia and that the primary locus of multiplication is elsewhere in the respiratory tract.

MANIFESTATIONS **Salivary adenitis** The onset of parotitis is usually sudden, although it may be preceded by a prodromal period of malaise, anorexia, chilly sensations, feverishness, sore throat, and tenderness at the angle of the jaw. In many cases, however, parotid swelling is the first indication of illness. The swollen gland extends from the ear to the lower portion of the mandibular ramus and to the inferior portion of the zygomatic arch. The skin over the gland may be red, hot, and taut, and there may be reddening and pouting of the orifice of Stensen's duct. Usually, pain and tenderness are marked, although at times they are absent. The edema of mumps has been described as "gelatinous," and when the involved gland is tweaked, it rolls like jelly. Swelling may involve the submaxillary and sublingual glands and may extend over the anterior part of the chest, presenting as *presternal edema.* Swelling of the glottis occurs rarely but may require tracheostomy. Parotitis is bilateral in two-thirds of cases and remains confined to one side in the remainder. The second gland tends to swell as the first is subsiding, usually 4 to 5 days after onset. In general, parotitis is accompanied by fever of 100 to 103°F, malaise, headache, and anorexia, but systemic symptoms may be virtually absent, particularly in children. In most patients, the chief complaints refer to difficulty in eating, swallowing, and talking.

Epididymoorchitis Mumps is complicated by orchitis in 20 percent of postpubertal males. Testicular involvement usually appears 7 to 10 days after onset of parotitis, although it may precede it or appear simultaneously. Occasionally, orchitis occurs in the absence of parotitis. Gonadal involvement is unilateral in approximately 75 percent of patients. Orchitis is heralded by recrudescence of malaise and appearance of chilly sensations, headache, nausea, and vomiting. Shaking chills and high fevers, with temperatures between 103 and 106°F, are frequent. The testicle becomes greatly swollen and exquisitely painful. The epididymis is often palpable as a swollen tender cord. Occasionally there may be epididymitis without orchitis. Swelling, pain, and tenderness persist for 3 to 7 days and gradually subside; lysis of fever usually parallels abatement of swelling. Occasionally, the temperature falls by crisis. Mumps orchitis is followed by progressive atrophy of the testicle in one-half the cases. Even after bilateral orchitis, sterility is unusual, provided no significant atrophy has taken place. However, if bilateral testicular atrophy occurs after mumps, sterility or subnormal sperm counts are quite common. *Pulmonary infarction* has been noted to follow mumps orchitis. This may be the result of thrombosis of the veins in the prostatic and pelvic plexuses in association with the testicular inflammation. Priapism is a rare but painful complication of mumps orchitis.

Pancreatitis Pancreatic involvement is a potentially serious manifestation of mumps, which may rarely be complicated by shock or pseudocyst formation. It should be suspected in patients with abdominal pain and tenderness, and clinical or epidemiologic evidence of mumps. It is difficult to document, since hyperamylasemia, the hallmark of pancreatitis, is also often present in parotitis. Many times the symptoms resemble those of gastroenteritis, and it is conceivable that the high incidence of gastrointestinal symptoms seen in association with the mumps epidemic in Great Britain in 1961 was due to involvement of the pancreas. Although diabetes or pancreatic insufficiency rarely follows mumps pancreatitis, several children have developed "brittle" diabetes a few weeks after mumps.

Central nervous system involvement Nearly half the patients with mumps have an increased number of cells, usually lymphocytes, in the cerebrospinal fluid (CSF), although symptoms of meningitis, stiff neck, headache, and drowsiness are less common. The CSF protein is moderately elevated, and CSF glucose tends to be normal, although in as many as 10 percent of patients low CSF glucose concentrations, in the range of 20 to 50 mg per 100 ml, may be seen. True encephalitis is very unusual, although it is responsible for most of the central nervous system sequelae, including behavioral disturbances, headaches, seizures, deafness (usually unilateral), and visual disturbances. One case of aqueductal stenosis and hydrocephalus has been reported. Mumps also should be recognized as capable of presenting a picture of mild paralytic poliomyelitis; definition of the cause depends on isolation of virus from the CSF or serologic confirmation of mumps in the absence of changing antibody titers to poliomyelitis viruses. Rarely mumps may produce a transverse myelitis or the Guillain-Barré syndrome. Although mumps meningitis may occur in association with parotitis, it is often the sole manifestation of mumps virus infection, and some 10 to 15 percent of cases of aseptic meningitis in the United States are caused by mumps virus. Mumps meningitis, without clinical encephalitis, is benign and leaves no residua.

Other manifestations Mumps virus tends to involve glandular tissues; inflammation of the lacrimal glands, thymus, thyroid, breasts, and ovaries occurs occasionally. *Oophoritis* may be recognized by persistence of pain in the lower part of the abdomen and fever. It does not result in sterility. Mumps virus has been implicated in the causation of subacute thyroiditis; the diagnosis can be made serologically, and occasionally the virus can be isolated from the thyroid gland. A case of myxedema following mumps thyroiditis has been reported. Ocular manifestations of mumps include dacryadenitis, optic neuritis, keratitis, iritis, conjunctivitis, and episcleritis. Although these conditions interfere with vision transiently, complete resolution is the rule. Mumps *myocarditis* evidenced primarily by transient abnormalities in the electrocardiogram is relatively common but does not produce symptomatic disease or impair cardiac function. Similarly, *hepatic* involvement may be manifested by mild abnormalities in liver function, but icterus and other clinical signs of hepatic damage are extremely rare. *Thrombocytopenic purpura* as a complication of mumps has been described, and an occasional patient has a leukemoid reaction involving predominantly lymphocytes.

A rare but interesting manifestation of mumps is *polyarthritis*. It is most common in males between the ages of twenty and thirty. Joint symptoms begin 1 to 2 weeks after subsidence of parotitis, and usually the large joints are involved. The illness lasts about 6 weeks, and complete recovery is the rule. It is not clear whether arthritis is due to viremia or whether it is a "hypersensitivity reaction."

Acute hemorrhagic glomerulonephritis in the absence of streptococcosis has been reported after mumps. The relationship of these two diseases is not clear.

Late complications With the exception of the rare central nervous system sequelae which follow mumps encephalitis, and the occasional patient who is sterile following bilateral testicular involvement, mumps leaves no sequelae. There is no firm evidence that stillbirths and offspring with congenital defects are more common among mothers who have mumps during pregnancy. Likewise, the causal relationship between intrauterine mumps infection and endocardial fibroelastosis has not been clearly established.

LABORATORY FINDINGS In uncomplicated parotitis, the blood leukocyte count is normal, although there may be mild leukopenia with relative lymphocytosis. Patients with mumps orchitis, however, may have a marked leukocytosis with a shift to the left. In meningoencephalitis, the white blood cell count is usually within normal limits. The erythrocyte sedimentation rate is usually normal but may rise with testicular or pancreatic involvement. The serum amylase level is elevated both in pancreatitis and in salivary adenitis. It may also be elevated in some patients in whom the sole evidence of mumps is meningoencephalitis, and probably reflects subclinical involvement of the salivary glands. In contrast to the amylase, serum lipase level is elevated only in pancreatitis, in which hyperglycemia and glucosuria, also may occur. The cerebrospinal fluid contains 0 to 2,000 cells per mm^3, almost all mononuclears. The pleocytosis in mumps meningitis tends to be greater than in aseptic meningitides caused by the poliomyelitis, Coxsackie, and echo viruses. There is no relationship between the cell count and the severity of central nervous system involvement. Transient hematuria and mild reversible abnormalities in renal function, including inability maximally to concentrate the urine and to clear creatinine, occur in association with the viruria of mumps.

DIAGNOSIS The definitive diagnosis of mumps depends on isolation of the virus from blood, throat swabs, secretions from Stensen's duct, cerebrospinal fluid, or urine. However, even with the simplification of viral isolation by means of tissue culture techniques, culture of the virus is rarely necessary. When an etiologic diagnosis is needed, as in aseptic meningitis or in atypical cases of parotitis, the complement fixation test is highly reliable, simple, and inexpensive. It becomes positive during the second week of the disease, and titers remain elevated for at least 6 weeks. Paired serums should be obtained, and a fourfold rise in titer is necessary to confirm recent infection. The hemagglutination inhibition reaction is demonstrable somewhat later and persists for several months. The serum neutralization test is the most sensitive indicator of previous mumps infection, although it is more complicated to perform. However, it is a much better indicator than the skin test of previous mumps infection, and individuals with a significant amount of neutralizing antibody are highly unlikely to contract mumps. The *skin test* consists of intradermal injection of killed mumps virus; previous exposure will result in a delayed reaction of the tuberculin type. The skin test is of value only in large-scale epidemiologic studies; it is unreliable in the individual case and is useless in the diagnosis of acute mumps.

The diagnosis of mumps during an epidemic is usually obvious. Sporadic cases, however, must be distinguished from other causes of parotid enlargement. Parotitis may be caused by other viruses, notably parainfluenza. *Bacterial parotitis* usually occurs in debilitated patients with severe underlying diseases such as uncontrolled diabetes mellitus, cerebrovascular accidents, or uremia. It may also follow surgical operations. The parotid glands are swollen and tender, and pus can be expressed from the orifices of Stensen's ducts. Marked polymorphonuclear leukocytosis is present. The disease is usually acquired in the hospital, and *Staphylococcus aureus* is the causative organism. Dehydration followed by inspissation of secretions in the salivary ducts is an important predisposing factor. *Calculus* in a salivary duct is usually detectable by palpation or by injection of radiopaque media into Stensen's duct. *Drug reactions* may produce tender swelling of the parotid and other salivary glands. "Iodine mumps" is the commonest type; it may follow such procedures as intravenous urography. Mercurialism and the antihypertensive agent, guanethidine, may also cause parotid enlargement and tenderness. Careful history usually serves to clarify the cause of these reactions. *Cervical adenitis* caused by streptococci, "bull-neck" diphtheria, infectious mononucleosis, cat-scratch disease, sublingual cellulitis (Ludwig's angina), and cellulitis of the external auditory canal are usually easy to distinguish from mumps by careful examination. Parotid tumors and chronic infections such as actinomycosis tend to follow a more indolent course, with slowly progressive swelling. The common "mixed tumor" of the parotid is well circumscribed, nontender, and very firm, almost cartilaginous on palpation. Parotid swelling and fever, often accompanied by lacrimal adenitis and uveitis (Mikulicz's syndrome), may occur in tuberculosis, leukemia, Hodgkin's disease, and lupus erythematosus. The onset may be sudden, but the process is usually painless and of long duration. "Uveoparotid fever" of similar type may be the first manifestation of sarcoidosis; in this disease parotid swelling is frequently accompanied by single or multiple palsies of cranial nerves, particularly the facial nerve, and is referred to as Heerfordt's syndrome. Presternal edema may also be a manifestation of malignant lymphoma involving retrosternal lymph nodes. Bilateral painless parotid swelling unassociated with fever is found in patients with Laennec's cirrhosis, chronic alcoholism, malnutrition, diabetes mellitus, pregnancy and lactation, and hypertriglyceridemia.

Sjögren's syndrome (Chap. 363) is a chronic inflammation of the parotid and other salivary glands which is often associated with atrophy of the lacrimal glands and occurs most commonly in women past the menopause. With cessation of lacrimal and salivary function, there may be striking dryness of the conjunctiva and cornea (keratoconjunctivitis sicca) and of the mouth (xerostomia). These patients may also have a variety of systemic manifestations, including arthritis of the rheumatoid type, splenomegaly, leukopenia, and hemolytic anemia. The chronicity of the process and its occurrence in elderly women make confusion with mumps unlikely. Finally, benign hypertrophy of both masseter muscles, presumably due to habitual clenching and grinding of teeth, may be confused with painless parotid swelling. The causes of aseptic meningitis are listed in Chap. 330.

Orchitis occurring in the absence of parotitis is likely to remain undiagnosed. Serologic testing may later confirm the diagnosis of mumps. Orchitis may occur in association with acute bacterial prostatitis and seminal vesiculitis. It is a rare complication of gonorrhea. Occasionally testicular inflammation accompanies pleurodynia, leptospirosis, melioidosis, relapsing fever, chickenpox, brucellosis, and lymphocytic choriomeningitis.

TREATMENT There is no specific treatment for infections with the mumps virus. Patients with parotitis should receive mouth care, analgesics, and a bland diet. Bed rest is advisable only as long as the patient is febrile; contrary to popular belief, physical activity has no influence on the development of orchitis or other complications. Patients with epididymoorchitis may be acutely ill and in great pain. Many forms of treatment, including surgical decompression of the testicle, infiltration of the spermatic chord with local anesthetics, estrogens, convalescent serum, and broad-spectrum antibiotics, have not been regularly effective. Despite failure to document their effectiveness in controlled studies, adrenal steroids have been of considerable benefit in diminishing fever, as well as testicular pain and swelling, and in restoring the sense of well-being in a number of patients. It is important to give a single large dose corresponding to 300 mg cortisone or 60 mg prednisone, initially. During the ensuing 24 hr the same quantity should be given in divided doses. Subsequently, administration of the hormone can be tapered over 7 to 10 days. Adrenal steroids have not exerted an adverse effect on concomitant pancreatitis or meningitis, although they have not benefited patients with meningeal involvement, and their withdrawal has usually been accompanied by a sharp recrudescence of symptoms. Adrenal steroids have not prevented the appearance of parotid involvement on the contralateral side. Mumps arthritis is usually mild and requires no treatment. Mumps thyroiditis may subside spontaneously, but excellent relief has been obtained with adrenal hormones.

PREVENTION A live attenuated mumps virus vaccine (Jeryl Lynn strain) has been highly effective in producing significant rises in mumps antibody in individuals who are seronegative prior to vaccination. The vaccine also has boosted antibody levels in seropositive vaccines, and has afforded 95 percent protection to individuals exposed to mumps. The vaccine produces an inapparent, noncommunicable infection which is not associated with fever or mumpslike symptoms. It has conferred excellent protection for at least 5 years and has not interfered with vaccines against measles, rubella, and poliomyelitis or with smallpox vaccination given simultaneously. Protection has been demonstrated in both children and adults.

Live mumps vaccine should be given to children approaching adolescence, adolescents, and adults, especially men who have not had mumps. Individuals living in groups or in institutions should be vaccinated, particularly because it has been shown that physical isolation of mumps patients does not prevent transmission of the infection. Mumps is a mild infection in young children, and most authorities do not recommend vaccination of all children. The vaccine should be given in dosage of 0.5 ml subcutaneously. A single dose suffices; simultaneous administration of gamma-globulin does not interfere with development of mumps antibody.

Vaccination is contraindicated in babies under the age of one because of the interfering effect of maternal antibody; in individuals with a history of hypersensitivity to egg proteins; in patients with febrile illnesses, leukemia, lymphoma, or generalized malignancies; and in those receiving steroids, alkylating drugs, antimetabolites, or irradiation.

It is not known whether the vaccine will prevent infection when administered after exposure, but no contraindication to its use in this situation exists. Specific mumps-immune globulin has been effective in aborting orchitis when given 1 to 2 days after exposure, although it may not prevent parotitis. Ordinary gamma-globulin is not effective in preventing mumps.

REFERENCES

Brunell PA et al: Ineffectiveness of isolation of patients as a method of preventing the spread of mumps. N Engl J Med 279:1357, 1968

Caranasos GJ, Felker JR: Mumps arthritis. Arch Intern Med 119:394, 1967

Kaltreider HB, Talal N: Bilateral parotid gland enlargement and hyperlipoproteinemia. JAMA 210:2067, 1969

Karchmer AW et al: Simultaneous administration of live virus vaccines. Am J Dis Child 121:382, 1971

Kocen RS, Critchley E: Mumps epididymo-orchitis and its treatment with cortisone. Brit Med J 2:20, 1961

Lerner AM: Guide to immunization against mumps. J Infect Dis 122:116, 1970

Levitt LP et al: Central nervous system mumps: A review of 64 cases. Neurology 20:829, 1970

Stokes J Jr et al: Trivalent combined measles-mumps-rubella vaccine: Findings in clinical-laboratory studies. JAMA 218:57, 1971

UTZ JP et al: Studies of mumps: IV. Viruria and abnormal renal function. N Engl J Med 270:1283, 1964

WEIBEL RE et al: Persistence of immunity four years following Jeryl Lynn strain live mumps virus vaccine. Pediatrics 45:821, 1970

WILFERT CM: Mumps meningoencephalitis with low cerebrospinal fluid glucose, prolonged pleocytosis and elevation of protein. N Engl J Med 280:855, 1969

206
CYTOMEGALIC INCLUSION DISEASE (SALIVARY GLAND VIRUS DISEASE)

WALTER H. SHELDON

DEFINITION Cytomegalic inclusion disease (CID) is a viral infection which affects man at all ages beginning with the time of conception. In adults the manifestations may be those of an illness like infectious mononucleosis, or may represent a terminal complication of chronic debilitating disease.

ETIOLOGY Cytomegalovirus (CMV) belongs to the herpes virus family and produces large, intranuclear (10 to 15 nm) and inconspicuous cytoplasmic (2 to 4 nm) inclusions which occur in all types of normal and neoplastic tissues including white blood cells. The agent is affected by temperature and other environmental factors. For shipment and storage low temperatures (−80°C) and stabilizers are needed. Several antigenically heterogenous strains have been isolated which are largely species-specific for man and grow in human fibroblast cultures. Of the various immunologic procedures available for diagnosis the complement fixation test is most widely used, since the different human strains share a common complement-fixing antigen. Species-specific CMV occurs in many different animals and animal models. The mouse CMV systems are particularly important in the experimental study of the infection.

EPIDEMIOLOGY The infection is worldwide and in this country affects children of low economic background. It may be congenital but is often acquired during the first year of life. Complement-fixing antibody is relatively infrequent at birth, increases during childhood, and is present in about 80 percent of adults (in some areas, in all adults). The virus persists in the host for a long time, perhaps indefinitely, and is excreted in saliva and urine even in the presence of antibody. Breast milk and feces may also transmit the infection. Close and prolonged contact appears necessary for transmission of the infection. Carriers with latent infection may massively contaminate the environment. Transplacental transmission produces congenital infection, and perinatal infection may follow exposure to the virus in the infected cervix uteri during delivery. In adults CID may represent either activation of latent infection or may be newly acquired. It may be transmitted by transfusion of fresh blood.

PATHOGENESIS Localized or systemic CID which may be latent or active occurs in hematopoietic and lymphocytic-reticular disorders (various anemias, leukemias, lymphomas), other chronic debilitating diseases, and often during immunosuppression. It is a complication of therapy which results in an impairment of humoral and/or cellular immunity. Physiologic factors related to age or pregnancy favor viral proliferation and dissemination. CID may be associated with stillborn, premature, or low-birth-weight infants. Self-limited forms with generally mild clinical manifestations are being increasingly recognized in apparently normal persons.

PATHOLOGY Enlarged cells, 25 to 40 nm in diameter, with the distinctive nuclear inclusions, are the morphologic hallmark of the infection, and are similar in all forms and sites of infection. Infected cells elicit an inflammatory cell response only after cell death. In adults localized infection most commonly consists of interstitial pneumonitis and gastrointestinal ulcers. Less frequently affected are the nasal mucosa, salivary glands, liver, and adrenals. Hepatitis without the distinctive inclusions has been related to CID by serologic studies. In the disseminated form nearly every tissue may be affected except for the central nervous system. Involvement of the latter, however, has been noted in the immunosuppressed adult. In infancy the localized form is largely confined to the salivary glands, hence the original designation of salivary gland virus disease. In disseminated disease the more common sites are salivary glands, kidney, liver, lung, pancreas, gastrointestinal tract, thyroid, adrenal, and central nervous system. Multiple infections are frequently associated with CID. Bacterial, fungal, and various forms of herpes virus infections are common. Concomitant infection with pertussis, toxoplasmosis, and *Pneumocystis carinii* are frequent. Interesting interactions between CMV and toxoplasmosis and Newcastle-disease virus have been noted experimentally. Particles consistent with CMV have been seen within *P. carinii* organisms in electron micrographs from the lung lesions of a patient with combined CID and *P. carinii* infection.

CLINICAL MANIFESTATIONS In adults CMV infection is generally latent. It becomes clinically manifest mostly in chronic disorders with impaired host resistance, but has been encountered in the absence of demonstrated underlying disease. The manifestations are nonspecific and vary according to the principal organ involved. Acute pneumonia is the most common presentation, but chronic lung disease and gastrointestinal disorders have been noted. The course of disseminated CID is generally fatal.

Congenital CMV infection produces the constellation of hepatosplenomegaly with hepatitis and cirrhosis, purpura, and encephalitis with microcephaly and microgyria. Despite the common occurrence of viruria and inclusion-bearing cells in the kidney, progressive renal disease has not been noted at any age.

CMV mononucleosis is an acute febrile illness with relative or absolute lymphocytosis and many atypical lymphocytes. The patient complains of headache and back and abdominal pain. Icteric hepatitis and hemolytic episodes have sometimes been the presenting feature. Myocarditis, pericarditis, and a rubelliform rash occur. Polyneuritis has been attributed to the syndrome. Tonsillitis and significant lymphadenitis and hepatosplenomegaly are lacking. The heterophil antibody test is negative, but liver function tests are commonly abnormal. Rising CMV antibody titers, viruria, and virus isolation establish the etiology. The disease occurs spontaneously or after perfusion with fresh whole blood, the postperfusion syndrome, and resolves without residua in 3 to 6 weeks.

CID in infancy presents quite consistently with hepatitis, hemolytic anemia, thrombocytopenia, interstitial pneumonia, and meningoencephalitis. In older children a relation of CMV infection with lymphadenitis and an acquired hemolytic anemia has been described. The effects of congenital CMV infection range from asymptomatic viruria to crippling brain damage and diffuse injury incompatible with life.

DIAGNOSIS Demonstration of rising antibody titers are most useful. Virus isolation from blood, body fluids, or tissues establishes the presence of active infection but cannot be equated with disease. Morphologic demonstration of CMV inclusions is not a reliable diagnostic tool. Roentgenographic and laboratory findings are nonspecific except for the lymphocytosis and atypical lymphocytes in CMV mononucleosis.

TREATMENT No specific therapy is available. No clearly beneficial results have been obtained with interferon or with viral antagonists such as floxuridine or indoxuridine.

REFERENCES

HANSHAW JB: Congenital cytomegalovirus infection: A fifteen year perspective. J Infect Dis 123:555, 1971

WELLER TH: The cytomegaloviruses: Ubiquitous agents with protean clinical manifestations. N Engl J Med 285:203 and 269, 1971

207 ARBOVIRUS AND ARENOVIRUS INFECTIONS

JAY P. SANFORD

Most viral infections in man are either asymptomatic or present as undifferentiated grippelike illnesses characterized by fever, malaise, headaches, and generalized myalgia. The similarities in clinical features between infections caused by viruses as dissimilar as the myxoviruses (e.g., influenza, rubella), the enteroviruses (e.g., poliovirus, Coxsackie virus, echo virus), some of the herpesviruses (e.g., cytomegalovirus), and the arboviruses usually preclude an etiologic diagnosis based entirely on clinical manifestations without ancillary information regarding epidemiologic features and serologic findings. The purpose of this chapter is to direct attention to the ever-expanding list of viruses, with particular attention to the arboviruses, which produce febrile disease in man. Because the number of agents is large, mention will be made of those which have been best documented, have demonstrated unusual features, or seem to be of greatest potential significance.

DEFINITION AND CLASSIFICATION

It has not always been easy to determine that an agent is an arbovirus; hence with further characterization some agents which were initially registered as arboviruses have been reclassified, e.g., the zoonotic agents, Junin virus (Argentinian hemorrhagic fever) and Machupo virus (Bolivian hemorrhagic fever) have been shown to be morphologically and serologically related to lymphocytic choriomeningitis virus and are now classified as arenoviruses. Similarly, vesicular stomatitis virus and Lagos bat virus, provisionally registered as arboviruses, were found to be related to rabies virus morphologically or serologically, and both are now classified as rhabdoviruses. The currently accepted definition of an arthropod-borne virus was published in 1967 by the World Health Organization:

Arboviruses are viruses which are maintained in nature principally, or to an important extent, through biological transmission between susceptible vertebrate hosts by hematophagous arthropods; they multiply and produce viremia in the vertebrates, multiply in the tissues of arthropods, and are passed on to new vertebrates by the bites of arthropods after a period of extrinsic incubation.

There are more than 250 distinct arboviruses, which have been subdivided into groups based upon antigenic differences. Originally the groups were designated A, B, and C, but with the recognition of multiple antigenically distinct agents, groups are now named after the first-discovered virus of a new antigenic cluster. There currently are 23 groups, one supergroup which contains 11 groups, and an ungrouped category (Table 207-1). The characteristics of individual members of this large group of viruses are not uniform; those in group A are 40 to 60 nm in diameter, those in group B about 30 nm, and those of the Bunyamwera supergroup are about 100 nm. The majority of agents contains single-stranded RNA, although some, such as Colorado tick fever, contain double-stranded RNA.

Arboviruses are distributed widely throughout the world and are of importance in both temperate and tropical zones. Representative viruses have been isolated in almost every geographic area outside the polar regions.

Arbovirus infection of vertebrates is usually asymptomatic. The viremia which develops stimulates an immune response which sharply limits the duration of the viremia. In arbovirus infections other than urban yellow fever, phlebotomus fever, and dengue, infection of man represents an incidental occurrence which is tangential to the basic maintenance cycle of the virus. Hence, the isolation of virus from arthropod vectors or the detection of infection in the natural vertebrate host may provide a

TABLE 207-1
Antigenic classification of arboviruses by groups

A	Changuinola
African horsesickness	Congo
Anopheles A	Epizootic hemorrhagic disease
Anopheles B	Ganjam
B	Hughes
Bakau	Kaisodi
Bluetongue	Kemerovo
Bunyamwera supergroup	Mapputta
Bunyamwera	Mossuril
Bwamba	Nyando
C	Phlebotomus fever
California	Qalyub
Capim	Quaranfil
Guama	Timbo
Koongol	Turlock
Patois	Uukuniemi
Simbu	Ungrouped
Tete	
Unassigned	

means for early detection and enable the control of epizootic infection before significant spread to man occurs.

As determined by serologic evidence of host responses, at least 80 immunologically distinct arboviruses are capable of infecting man, while somewhat fewer have been incriminated as causing clinical disease. The spectrum of clinical illness produced by the arboviruses is varied both in predominant features and in severity. Five broad, often overlapping, and somewhat arbitrary clinical syndromes may be delineated (Table 207-2).

ARBOVIRUS INFECTIONS CHARACTERIZED PREDOMINANTLY BY FEVER, MALAISE, HEADACHES, AND MYALGIA

Phlebotomus fever

Phlebotomus (sandfly, pappataci, or 3-day) fever is an acute, relatively mild, self-limited infection caused by at least two immunologically distinct arboviruses, the Sicilian and Naples strains, but there may be additional immunologically distinct strains. The viruses have been adapted to white mice, but there is no evidence of an animal reservoir in nature.

PREVALENCE The disease occurs throughout the Mediterranean Basin, the Balkans, the Near and Middle East, the eastern part of Africa, the Soviet republics of Central Asia, West Pakistan, and possibly certain parts of southern China. In highly endemic areas, native populations acquire the disease at an early age and with repeated exposure develop and maintain high levels of immunity. The apparent absence of phlebotomus fever in indigenous adult populations residing in areas where sandflies are abundant may present a deceptive picture of the actual risk to susceptible persons.

EPIDEMIOLOGY The disease occurs during the hot, dry seasons (summer or autumn months) and is transmitted to human beings by the bite of infected sandflies *(Phlebotomus papatasii). Phlebotomus papatasii* is a small fly which can penetrate ordinary house screens. Only the female bites and usually does so during the night. In persons who are not sensitive there is neither pain nor local irritation after the bite; hence only about 1 percent of patients will remember having been bitten. Approximately 7 days after feeding on an infected individual, the insect acquires the capacity to transmit infection. The sandflies continue to be infectious for their life span. Transovarial transmission of the virus to the next generation of insects has been demonstrated and offers the best explanation for the mechanism of overwinter survival of the virus. In man, the incubation period may be as short as 3 days. Viremia is present for at least 24 hr before and after the onset of fever, but is not detectable for more than 2 days after the onset of illness.

CLINICAL MANIFESTATIONS The onset of symptoms is abrupt in over 90 percent of patients, with the temperature rapidly rising to its highest point, which may vary from 100 to 105°F. Headache is nearly always present and often is accompanied by pain on moving the eyes and by retroorbital pain. Myalgia is common and may be localized to the chest, resembling pleurodynia, or to the abdomen. Other symptoms which occur include vomiting, photophobia, giddiness, neck stiffness, alteration or loss of taste, and arthralgia. Physical signs include conjunctival injection in approximately one-third of patients. Small vesicles may be seen on the palate, and macular or urticarial rashes occur. The spleen is rarely palpable, and lymphadenopathy is absent. The pulse rate may be elevated in proportion to the temperature on the first day; thereafter bradycardia is often present. The fever persists 3 days in most patients, with gradual defervescence. Giddiness, weakness, and feelings of depression are frequently encountered during convalescence. Second attacks 2 to 12 weeks after the first occur in 15 percent of cases.

In common with other arbovirus infections, phlebotomus fever may be associated with *aseptic meningitis.* In one series, 12 percent of patients had symptoms and signs sufficient to warrant a lumbar puncture. Findings in these patients included pleocytosis, with an average cell count of 90 per mm^3 and a predominance of either polymorphonuclear or mononuclear leukocytes. Spinal fluid protein concentration ranged from 20 to 130 mg per 100 ml. In another series mild papilledema was observed in a few patients with severe illness.

LABORATORY FINDINGS The changes in leukocyte count constitute the only positive laboratory findings. Total leukocyte counts of less than 5,000 per mm^3 are observed in 90 percent of patients if daily counts are done during the febrile period and convalescence. The leukopenia may not appear until the last day of fever or even after defervescence. The differential leukocyte count will reveal an absolute decrease in lymphocytes on the first day, accompanied by an increase in nonsegmented neutrophils. During the second or third day, the number of lymphocytes begins to return to normal and may constitute 40 to 65 percent of the total count. At the same time,

TABLE 207-2
Summary of clinical and epidemiologic features of arboviruses and arenoviruses associated with disease in man

Syndrome	*Virus*	*Vector*	*Known geographic range of infection*
Fever with malaise, *headaches,* and *myalgia*	Mayaro	Mosquito	Trinidad, Colombia, Brazil
	Mucambo	Mosquito	Brazil
	Uruma		Lowland forest, Bolivia
	Venezuelan equine encephalitis	Mosquito	Florida, Texas, Louisiana, Mexico, Central America, Ecuador, Colombia, Venezuela, Brazil, Trinidad, Surinam, Guyana, French Guiana
	Kunjin	Mosquito	Northern Australia
	Spondweni	Mosquito	South Africa, Mozambique, Nigeria
	United States bat salivary gland	?	California, Texas, Sonora in Southwest North America
	Wesselsbron	Mosquito	South Africa, Bechuanaland
	Yellow fever	Mosquito	Africa, Central and South America
	Zika	Mosquito	Uganda, Nigeria
	Apeu	Mosquito	Brazil
	Caraparu	Mosquito	Brazil, Panama, Trinidad
	Itaqui	Mosquito	Brazil
	Madrid	?	Panama
	Marituba	Mosquito (?)	Brazil
	Marutucui	Mosquito (?)	Brazil
	Oriboca	Mosquito	Brazil
	Ossa	?	Panama
	Restan	Mosquito	Trinidad
	Calovo	Mosquito	Czechoslovakia
	Germiston	Mosquito	South Africa, Angola
	Ilesha	Mosquito (?)	Nigeria
	Guaroa	Mosquito	Colombia, Brazil
	Tahyna	Mosquito	Czechoslovakia, Yugoslavia
	Catu	Mosquito	Brazil, Trinidad
	Guama	Mosquito	Brazil, Trinidad
	Oropouche	Mosquito	Brazil, Trinidad
	Bwamba	Mosquito	Uganda
	Phlebotomus, Naples	Sandfly	Italy, Egypt, Iran, West Pakistan
	Phlebotomus, Sicilian	Sandfly	Italy, Egypt, Iran, Pakistan, Yugoslavia
	Chagres	?	Panama
	Candiru	?	Brazil
	Punta Toro	?	Panama
	Colorado tick fever	Tick	Western United States
	Nairobi sheep disease	Tick	Kenya, Congo
	Rift Valley fever	Mosquito	Africa
	Quaranfil	Tick	Egypt, South America
	Dugbe	Tick	Nigeria
Fever with malaise, headaches, myalgia, *arthralgia,* and *rash*	Chikungunya	Mosquito	South, East, West, Central Africa; India, Thailand, Vietnam, Malaya
	Mayaro	Mosquito	Brazil, Trinidad
	O'nyong-nyong	Mosquito	East Africa, Senegal
	Sindbis	Mosquito	South and East Africa; Egypt, Israel, India, Malaya, Philippines, Australia
	Bunyamwera	Mosquito	South, East, West Africa
	Changuinola	Phlebotomus	Panama
Fever with malaise, headaches, myalgia, rash, and *lymphadenopathy*	Dengue 1	Mosquito	Hawaii, Oceana, New Guinea, Japan, Malaysia, Thailand, India
	Dengue 2	Mosquito	Circumglobal
	Dengue 3	Mosquito	Caribbean, Oceana, Philippines, Thailand
	Dengue 4	Mosquito	Philippines, Thailand, India
	West Nile	Mosquito	South and West Africa, Rhone delta, Near East, Israel, India, Malaysia, Borneo

TABLE 207-2 *(continued)*

Syndrome	*Virus*	*Vector*	*Known geographic range of infection*
Fever with *central nervous system involvement* (meningitis to encephalitis)	Eastern equine encephalitis	Mosquito	Eastern Canada, United States, Mexico, Dominican Republic, Jamaica, Panama, Trinidad, Brazil, Colombia, Argentina
	Western equine encephalitis	Mosquito	Canada, United States, Mexico, Brazil, Argentina
	Venezuelan equine encephalitis	Mosquito	Florida, Texas, Louisiana, Mexico, Central America, Ecuador, Colombia, Venezuela, Brazil, Trinidad, Surinam, Guyana, French Guiana
	Apoi	?	Hokkaido, Japan
	Ilheus	Mosquito	Northern South America, Trinidad, Central America, Florida
	Japanese encephalitis	Mosquito	Japan, China, Malaya, Taiwan, Thailand, Vietnam, Burma, Guam, Philippines, Korea, Australia, New Zealand
	Kyasanur Forest disease	Tick	India
	Louping ill	Tick	Great Britain, Eire
	Medoc		United States
	Murray Valley encephalitis	Mosquito	Australia, New Guinea
	Negishi	?	Japan
	Powassan	Tick	Canada
	St. Louis encephalitis	Mosquito	United States, Caribbean Islands, Panama, Brazil, Argentina
	Tick-borne encephalitis	Tick	Central and Eastern Europe, U.S.S.R.
	West Nile	Mosquito	South and West Africa, Rhone delta, Near East, Israel, India, Malaysia, Borneo
	California encephalitis	Mosquito	United States
	Phlebotomus, Naples	Sandfly	Italy, Egypt, Iran, West Pakistan
	Congo	Tick	Central Africa, West Pakistan, Bulgaria, U.S.S.R.
Fever with malaise, headaches, myalgia, and *hemorrhagic signs*	Chikungunya	Mosquito	Thailand, Malaysia, India, Vietnam
	Dengue 1	Mosquito	Thailand, India
	Dengue 2	Mosquito	Philippines, Vietnam, Thailand, Malaysia, India
	Dengue 3	Mosquito	Philippines, Thailand
	Dengue 4	Mosquito	Philippines, Thailand
	Kyasanur Forest disease	Tick	India
	Omsk hemorrhagic fever	Tick	Western Siberia, U.S.S.R.
	Yellow fever	Mosquito	Africa, Central and South America
	Central Asian hemorrhagic fever	Tick (?)	Central Asia, U.S.S.R.
	Crimean type hemorrhagic fever	Tick	Southern U.S.S.R.
	Congo	Tick	Central Africa, West Pakistan, Bulgaria, U.S.S.R.
	Junin (Argentinian hemorrhagic fever)*	Rodent	Argentina
	Machupo (Bolivian hemorrhagic fever)*	Rodent	Eastern Bolivia
	Lassa*	Rodent (?)	Nigeria, Guinea
	Far Eastern or Korean hemorrhagic fever (hemorrhagic nephrosonephritis)*	Rodent, mite (?)	U.S.S.R., Manchuria, China, Korea

* *Members of the arenovirus group.*

the number of segmented neutrophils decreases, and the number of immature cells increases sharply until they outnumber the segmented forms. The differential count usually returns to normal within 5 to 8 days after defervescence. Erythrocyte values and urinalyses are usually normal.

DIAGNOSIS In the absence of a specific serologic test, the diagnosis must be made on clinical and epidemiologic grounds.

TREATMENT The disease is self-limited, and no specific therapy is available. Symptomatic care, including bed rest, adequate fluid intake, and analgesia with aspirin, is recommended. Convalescence may require a week or longer.

PROGNOSIS No fatalities have been recorded among the tens of thousands of cases.

Colorado tick fever

Colorado tick fever is the only tick-transmitted virus disease of man that is recognized in the Western Hemisphere. Though "mountain fever" had been described ever since the advent of immigrants to the Rocky Mountain region, Becker in 1930 differentiated it from mild Rocky Mountain spotted fever, established the clinical picture of disease, and renamed it Colorado tick fever.

ETIOLOGY The causative agent in Colorado tick fever is classified as an arbovirus because it replicates in ticks. Recent ultrastructural studies have demonstrated that the virus resembles reovirus both in structure and in containing double-stranded RNA.

PREVALENCE The disease has been contracted only in Colorado, Idaho, Nevada, Wyoming, Montana, Utah, and the eastern portions of Oregon, Washington, and California. However, the virus of Colorado tick fever has been reported to have been isolated from the dog tick, *Dermacentor variabilis*, obtained from Long Island. This observation has not been confirmed, but suggests the possibility that Colorado tick fever may occur over a wider geographic area. The actual prevalence is difficult to assess, but the disease is relatively common. Mild and clinically inapparent forms of the disease occur, but its frequency has never been determined. The number of cases of Colorado tick fever reported in Colorado is twenty times greater than that of Rocky Mountain spotted fever.

EPIDEMIOLOGY Colorado tick fever is transmitted to man by the adult hard-shelled wood tick, *Dermacentor andersoni*. The virus has been found in as many as 14 percent of this species of ticks collected in endemic areas. Transovarial transmission of the virus in the tick has been established. Illness occurs primarily in the spring and summer months, with a predilection for April and May at lower altitudes and for June and July at higher altitudes. Virus has been obtained from both the blood and the spinal fluid of patients during the acute illness.

CLINICAL MANIFESTATIONS The incubation period is usually 3 to 6 days, and in most cases a history of tick bite can be obtained. Persons affected usually are those whose occupational or recreational activities bring them in contact with ticks. The disease may occur at any age. The clinical picture is characterized by the sudden onset of severe aching of the muscles of the back and legs, chilliness without true rigors, a rapid increase in temperature, which usually reaches 102 to 104°F, headache with pain on ocular movement, retroorbital pain, and photophobia. Occasionally nausea and vomiting occur. The physical findings are not specific. Tachycardia in proportion to the temperature, flushed facies, and variable conjunctival injection may be present. Occasionally the spleen is palpable. A rash is usually not present, but on occasion a petechial rash involving primarily the arms and legs or a maculopapular rash over the entire body may occur. Rarely, punched-out ulcers may form at the site of tick bite. The fever with the associated symptoms lasts about 2 days, then abruptly lyses to normal or subnormal, leaving the patient very weak. After an afebrile period of about 2 days, the temperature recurs, may be higher than in the first phase, and may last as long as 3 days. Over 90 percent of patients show this saddleback pattern of temperature. Rarely there may be three febrile phases. The febrile episode may be followed by a period of weakness of several weeks' duration.

Evidence of central nervous system involvement has been recorded in a few patients. The findings are those of either an aseptic meningitis with stiffness of the neck or encephalitis with clouding of the sensorium, delirium, and coma.

LABORATORY FINDINGS The most important laboratory feature is moderate to marked leukopenia. On the first day of illness, the total leukocyte count may be at normal levels, but usually by the fifth or sixth day there has been a decrease to 2,000 to 3,000 per mm^3. Characteristically there is a proportionate decrease in lymphocytes and granulocytes. A moderate "left shift" in the neutrophilic series is usually apparent. Toxic changes in neutrophils are often conspicuous, and "virocyte" types of lymphocytes are frequently observed. Bone marrow examination reveals "maturation arrest" in the granulocytic series. Erythrocyte values remain normal. Thrombocytopenia has been recorded in an isolated case report. The blood picture returns to normal within a week after the fever subsides.

DIAGNOSIS The diagnosis of Colorado tick fever is suspected on the basis of the epidemiologic history and clinical findings. The diagnosis can be established by the isolation of the virus from blood obtained during the febrile phase. Specific neutralizing and complement-fixing antibodies appear in the blood between the eighth and fourteenth days of illness. Because neutralizing antibodies persist for many years, demonstration of a rise in titer is required.

TREATMENT Treatment is entirely symptomatic.

PROGNOSIS The prognosis is excellent.

PREVENTION No patients have been reported as having the disease twice. Active immunity with an attenuated virus has been produced, but the immunization itself frequently produced mild disease. Colorado tick fever is best prevented by avoiding contact with the wood tick.

Venezuelan equine encephalitis

Venezuelan equine encephalitis was first noted in equines in Colombia in 1935.

ETIOLOGY Like other group A arboviruses, VEE is a relatively small, 40 to 45 nm, RNA virus. On the basis of serologic tests, differing serotypes have been identified, IA-E, II, III, and IV. Strains ID, IE, II, III, and IV have remained sylvatic in distribution. IA was the original epidemic strain which occurred in Venezuela, and IB, which was recognized in Ecuador in 1963, spread through Central America into Mexico and was responsible for the epidemic in Mexico in 1971 which spread into southern Texas, with the occurrence of at least 76 laboratory-confirmed human cases.

EPIDEMIOLOGY VEE has been primarily a disease of equines and other mammals, although occasionally the agent has infected man. Evidence of human infection (virus isolation or specific neutralizing antibodies) has been found in Colombia, Ecuador, Panama, Surinam, Guyana, French Guiana, Mexico, Brazil, Curacao, Trinidad, Argentina, Florida, and Texas. The VEE virus complex in nature has been associated with numerous mosquitoes (at least 9 genera and 37 species), including *Aëdes*, *Mansonia*, *Psorophora*, and *Culex*. In this respect it differs markedly from other mosquito-borne encephalitogenic arboviruses, which usually are associated with only one to three vector species. VEE apparently has different vectors for its endemic-epizootic and its epidemic-epizootic cycles. The virus has a wide host range in wild mammals, with at least 20 genera, including capuchin monkeys, rats, mice, oppossum, jackrabbit, fox, and bats being naturally infected. Domestic animals other than equines which have been shown to be infected include cattle and pigs in Mexico and goats and sheep in Venezuela. VEE appears to multiply well in mammals with high titers of virus in the blood, e.g., infected horses may have titers of up to $10^{7.5}$ mouse intraperitoneal lethal doses per milliliter of blood. Though 29 species of wild birds have been shown to be naturally infected with VEE (20 percent of which are colonial nestling herons and related species), whether the VEE-viremia levels in birds are high enough to infect vector mosquitoes is not yet known. During the initial 3 days of illness, viremia has been detected in approximately two-thirds of patients. The levels of viremia are sufficiently high that man also could serve as a reservoir. VEE virus also has been isolated by pharyngeal swab in a few patients, suggesting the potential for person-to-person transmission. The available observations make it reasonable to consider that the natural vector is a mosquito, with the primary reservoir being either wild or domestic terrestrial mammals. However, natural infection can probably take place without an arthropod vector. Laboratory infections have occurred and are probably due to inhalation of aerosols.

CLINICAL MANIFESTATIONS In man, infection with VEE virus usually results in a mild acute febrile illness without neurologic complications. No age is spared, and there is no sex preponderance. The incubation period is 2 to 5 days, followed by the abrupt onset of headache, fever often associated with rigors, malaise, and myalgia. Other common symptoms may include nausea, vomiting, diarrhea, and sore throat. Uncommon features include seizures, mental confusion, coma, tremors, and diplopia. On laboratory examination the cerebrospinal fluid may reveal pleocytosis with modest increases in protein concentration and normal glucose concentration. Virus may be isolated both from blood and from cerebrospinal fluid. The symptoms usually last 3 to 5 days in mild cases and up to 8 days in more severe cases, although one patient reported from Florida was febrile for 3 weeks. A biphasic course of illness may be encountered, with recrudescence of symptoms at the sixth to the ninth day. In one case report, palatine petechiae were noted and the patient vomited "coffee-grounds" material. In an epidemic in Venezuela in 1962, almost 16,000 cases of acute disease were evaluated; 38 percent were classified as encephalitis, but only 3 to 4 percent had severe neurologic abnormalities: convulsions, nystagmus, drowsiness, delirium, or meningitis. The mortality rate was estimated to be less than 0.5 percent, and nearly all deaths occurred in young children.

Rift Valley fever

Rift Valley fever is an acute disease principally of sheep and cattle and first described in man during an investigation of an extensive epizootic of hepatitis in sheep in the Rift Valley in East Africa. During this epizootic in 1930, workers associated with the investigations contracted a severe but limited febrile disease. A similar syndrome was common among the herders of infected flocks. More than 200 cases of human disease were originally recognized. The infection is widespread throughout East and South Africa. During an epizootic in South Africa in 1950–1951, an estimated 20,000 human beings became infected.

Virus has been found in several species of mosquitoes: *Eretmapodites chrysogaster*, *Aëdes caballus*, *Aëdes circumluteolus*, and *Culex theileri*. Antibodies to Rift Valley fever have been found in wild field rats in Uganda. Man appears to be incidentally infected during the course of an epizootic. Although man presumably can be infected by arthropods, many human infections occur as a result of handling infected animal tissues. In addition, laboratory-acquired infections have been common, which suggests a respiratory route.

The incubation period is usually 3 to 6 days. The onset is usually abrupt, with malaise, chilly sensation or rigors, headache, retroorbital pain, and generalized aching and backache. The temperature rises rapidly to 101 to 104°F. Later complaints include anorexia, loss of taste, epigastric pain, and photophobia. Findings on examination are usually unremarkable except for flushing of the face and conjunctival injection. The temperature curve is often saddleback in type, with an initial elevation lasting 2 to 3 days, followed by a remission and second febrile period. Convalescence is typically rapid. Complications are rare; jaundice has not been seen in man. Macular exudates, with decreased vision, have been reported. One of the most characteristic findings is the initial normal total leukocyte count followed by leukopenia with a decrease in neutrophils associated with an increase in band forms. The diagnosis is made by isolating the virus from the blood by inoculation of mice. In human beings, viremia is present during the first 3 days. Neutralizing antibodies have been demonstrated as early as 4 days after onset. There is no specific treatment. The prognosis in human infections is good. Only one fatality has been recorded, and in this instance death was not due directly to the infection.

Semliki Forest–Mayaro virus disease

Mayaro virus was initially isolated from man in Trinidad in 1954. Outbreaks involving a number of persons subsequently have occurred in Brazil and Bolivia. Mayaro virus has been isolated from a wild mosquito, *Mansonia venezuelensis*, and can be maintained serially in *Aëdes aegypti* and *Anopheles quadrimaculatus*. Semliki Forest virus has been isolated from *Aëdes abnormalis* mosquitoes in Uganda and from various *Eretmapodites* mosquitoes in West Africa. Serologic surveys in man document widespread virus activity, although naturally occurring acute illness has not been described. Antigenically these two group A arboviruses are very closely related, suggesting that these two viruses may have been derived from one strain, with geographic separation having led to some antigenic variation. The mechanism of spread has not been determined, but the presence of viremia favors a biting arthropod vector. The predominance of illness and greater incidence of immunity in males suggests a forest infection.

Symptoms include fever of several days' duration, which may be marked during the first 1 to 2 days. Systemic complaints include severe frontal headache, epigastric pain, backache, nausea, photophobia, and vertigo. Signs have included conjunctival injection, mild icterus in a few patients, and arthritis in at least one patient. The leukocyte count is in the range of 5,000 to 8,000 per mm^3. The fever lasts 3 to 5 days in most patients. Recovery is usually complete, although in Bolivia the illness was more severe, and several fatalities were reported.

Bat salivary gland virus

During the course of a survey of rabies infection in bats, an agent was obtained from the salivary glands of Mexican free-tailed bats in Texas. The virus is related to the St. Louis encephalitis complex of viruses (group B). It is not known how the virus is maintained in nature. Five laboratory-acquired human infections have been recorded. The illnesses were characterized by fever associated with headache, myalgia, and a mild nonproductive cough. In two patients, there was evidence of central nervous system involvement with encephalitis and aseptic meningitis. One patient had oophoritis, and two developed orchitis. By the sixth to seventh day of illness, leukopenia in the range of 2,000 to 3,000 per mm^3 was observed in two individuals.

Zika virus

Zika virus was first isolated from a captive rhesus monkey in Uganda and subsequently from wild mosquitoes. On the basis of serologic surveys, it is known to infect man in Uganda and Nigeria. During investigation in eastern Nigeria of an outbreak of jaundice that was suspected of being yellow fever, physicians isolated Zika virus from one patient and noted that two others had a rise in neutralizing antibodies. The symptoms in these patients included fever, arthralgia, and headache with retroorbital pain. Jaundice was present in one, and bile was demonstrated in the urine of another. Albuminuria was noted in one patient. Prothrombin times were normal. The clinical syndrome appears to simulate mild yellow fever.

Group C arboviruses

Currently 11 viruses are classified in group C, of which 9 have been isolated from blood obtained from man. The geographic distribution includes Brazil (Apeu, Caraparu, Itaqui, Marituba, Murutucui, Oriboca), Trinidad (Caraparu, Restan), and Panama (Madrid, Ossa). Several of these viruses have been isolated from Culicine and Subethine mosquitoes, as well as from several species of rodents. Isolates have been obtained mostly from forest workers and laboratory technicians. Epidemics have not been recognized. The disease begins with headache, fever (with temperature up to 105°F), and myalgia. Additional symptoms include malaise, photophobia, vertigo, and nausea. Illness is generally mild, lasting 2 to 4 days, and is occasionally followed by a relapse. No fatalities have been reported. Occasionally a prolonged period of convalescence ensues. Leukopenia, with total leukocyte counts as low as 2,600 per mm^3, is a common finding. Diagnosis has been established mainly by virus isolation.

Bunyamwera group

Representative viruses of this group are found in all inhabited continents except Australia. Only four viruses of the group—Bunyamwera itself, Germiston, Ilesha, and Guaroa—have been associated with clinical disease. Serologic surveys give evidence of a high prevalence of inapparent infection in some areas. The clinical patterns of infection due to Germiston, Ilesha, and Guaroa viruses seem similar, while infection due to Bunyamwera virus is associated often with arthralgia and sometimes with a rash. The mild clinical illness is characterized by low-grade fever, headache, and myalgia which last several days, and it may be followed by weakness during convalescence.

ARBOVIRUS INFECTIONS CHARACTERIZED PREDOMINANTLY BY FEVER, MALAISE, ARTHRALGIA, AND RASH

Chikungunya

In 1952 an epidemic of a disease similar to dengue occurred in Tanganyika, an area in which dengue had never been observed. The disease was given the name *chikungunya* ("that which bends up") because of the local description of the sudden onset of distinctive joint pains. A group A arbovirus was isolated in 1956 both from serum of patients ill with the disease and from a pool of *Aëdes aegypti* mosquitoes.

Chikungunya virus is responsible for a dengue-like illness in South Africa, India, and Southeast Asia, as well as for a rather mild form of hemorrhagic fever in Asiatic children. Outbreaks have been associated with high attack rates, with as many as 80 percent of the inhabitants in some settlements becoming ill. It is not known definitely what vertebrates and arthropods are involved in the wild transmission cycle. Because the virus has been isolated from *Aëdes africanus* and because antibodies against the virus can be detected in chimpanzees, it appears that these may play a role in the natural cycle in Africa.

After an incubation period estimated at no less than 8 days, the onset is typically abrupt, with a rapid rise in temperature to 102 to 105°F, often associated with a rigor and headache. Pain in large joints occurs early, incapacitating some individuals within a few minutes of onset. The pain is frequently severe enough to prevent sleep. The arthralgia is often associated with objective arthritis. Sites of involvement include knees, ankles, shoulders, wrists, or proximal interphalangeal joints. Myalgia, especially backache, and malaise occur frequently. In 60 to 80 percent of patients a maculopapular eruption, which may appear at any time during the febrile course, is noted on the trunk or on the extensor surfaces of the extremities. Mild lymphadenopathy, predominantly in the axillary or inguinal areas, may be evident. Pharyngitis and conjunctival suffusion may be observed in a few patients. Elevated temperatures continue for 1 to 6 days, and in some patients an afebrile interval of 1 to 3 days is followed by a secondary rise in temperature. The joint pains sometimes continue after the temperature has returned to normal. In a few individuals joint pains have persisted for up to 4 months. Hematocrit values remain normal. Total leukocyte counts may be less than 5,000 per mm^3 in some patients, while in others they remain normal. Urinalyses are normal. There is no specific antiviral treatment. Anti-inflammatory agents such as aspirin or indomethacin have been utilized. No second attacks have been recognized, and in the absence of the hemorrhagic fever syndrome, no deaths have been described.

O'nyong-nyong fever

O'nyong-nyong fever was first noted as an epidemic illness characterized by joint pains, rash, and lymphadenopathy in the northern province of Uganda in 1959. The agent is a group A arbovirus which shows close antigenic relationships with chikungunya and Semliki Forest viruses. The original outbreak was associated with an explosive epidemic which spread to Tanzania and other areas in East Africa. By 1961, 2 million cases were recorded. In some areas, 91 percent of the population had either clinical disease or inapparent infection. Local outbreaks extended over the entire year. All age groups were affected. The most likely vector is *Anopheles funestus.* The clinical features are similar to those of chikungunya virus infection.

Sindbis virus

Sindbis virus infection in man rarely presents as a clinical disease. Of five cases from Uganda, one patient gave a history of joint pain. In the only well-studied clinical illness, a South African woman had arthritis as a prominent finding. Two days after a headache she noted swelling in her hands and feet. Soon thereafter she developed a confluent macular rash, followed by vesicle formation. The small joints of the hands and feet were swollen at the time of examination. Slight swelling of the fingers was present at 10 weeks, although she had otherwise recovered.

Other arboviruses

Epidemics of polyarthritis associated with rashes have been observed in Australia since 1928. The clinical and epidemiologic features of each outbreak were quite uniform, and therefore the name *epidemic polyarthritis* was applied. More recently, a presumed etiologic agent (designated as Ross River virus) has been isolated. The clinical features include development of a rash on the cheeks and the forehead which occasionally spreads to the trunk and lasts 2 to 10 days. Mild joint pain occurs in two-thirds of patients. Temperature elevations are rarely recorded, but a few patients give a history of feverishness.

In addition, Mayaro and Bunyamwera viruses have been associated with the syndrome of rash and arthralgia.

ARBOVIRUS INFECTIONS CHARACTERIZED PREDOMINANTLY BY FEVER, MALAISE, LYMPHADENOPATHY, AND RASH

Dengue fever

Dengue is endemic over large areas of the tropics and subtropics. From 1963 to 1964 epidemic dengue occurred in the Caribbean, and a number of travelers returned to the United States with clinical illness. In these areas a high proportion of infections are inapparent or represent undifferentiated febrile illnesses. It is now recognized that the dengue syndrome can be caused by other arboviruses; hence the exact etiology of some of the earlier epidemics is uncertain.

ETIOLOGY There are four distinct serogroups of dengue viruses, types 1, 2, 3, and 4, all of which are group B arboviruses. The existence of at least two further antigenic types has been suggested. They are transmitted solely by mosquitoes of the genus *Aëdes.*

EPIDEMIOLOGY So far as is known, dengue infections in nature involve only man and *Aëdes* mosquitoes. Attempts have been made to implicate lower vertebrates, especially monkeys, as reservoir sylvatic hosts, but the data are inconclusive. *Aëdes aegypti* is the most important worldwide vector species. This species, as well as the less common vector species, bite man readily or even preferentially, breed in small collections of water such as cisterns and backyard litter, and are peridomestic in nature. They fly during the day. Man appears to be uniformly susceptible, and susceptibility is not influenced by age, sex, or race. The disappearance of dengue from an area may be the result either of elimination of the vector or of exhaustion of the susceptible population. During outbreaks, attack rates may be very high: in Louisiana in 1922 the attack rate was estimated to be 1,740 per 100,000 (1.74 percent).

PATHOLOGY The skin lesions in nonfatal uncomplicated disease produced in volunteers have been studied by biopsy. The chief abnormality occurred in small blood vessels and consisted of endothelial swelling, perivascular edema, and infiltration with mononuclear cells. Since the disease is self-limited, other studies have not been made.

CLINICAL MANIFESTATIONS Dengue viruses frequently produce inapparent infections in man. When symptoms develop, three broad clinical patterns may be encountered: classical dengue, hemorrhagic fever, and a mild atypical form. Classical dengue (breakbone fever) occurs primarily in nonimmune individuals, specifically nonindigenous adults and children. The usual incubation period is 5 to 8 days. Prodromal symptoms such as mild conjunctivitis or coryza may occur, followed in hours by the abrupt onset of a severe splitting headache, retroorbital pain, backache, especially in the lumbar area, and leg and joint pains. The headache is aggravated by movement. At least three-fourths of patients have ocular soreness, with pain on moving the eyes. A few have mild photophobia. Though true rigors are common during the course, they are usually not present at the onset. Additional symptoms include insomnia, anorexia with a loss of taste or bitter taste, and weakness. Mild transient rhinopharyngitis occurs in as many as one-quarter of individuals. Epistaxis has been observed. Examination reveals scleral injection (90 percent), tenderness upon pressure on the ocular globe, and nontender posterior cervical, epitrochlear, and inguinal lymphadenopathy. Over one-half of patients have an enanthem characterized initially by pinpoint-sized vesicles over the posterior half of the soft palate. The tongue is often coated. Skin rashes, varying from diffuse flushing to scarlatiniform and morbilliform, are frequently present over the thorax and inner aspects of the arms. These are transient and fade, only to be followed by a more apparent maculopapular rash which appears on the trunk on the third to the fifth day and spreads peripherally. The rash may be pruritic and generally terminates with desquamation. Extreme bradycardia is not observed. Within 2 to 3 days after the onset, the temperature may decrease to nearly normal and other symptoms disappear. The remission typically lasts 2 days and is followed by return of fever and the other symptoms, although they are generally less severe than during the initial phase. This "saddleback" diphasic febrile course is considered characteristic, but often is not encountered. The febrile illness usually lasts 5 to 6 days and terminates by crisis. Complaints of fatigue for several weeks after infection are common.

In addition to this "classical" syndrome, an atypically mild illness may occur. Symptoms include fever, anorexia, headache, and myalgia. On examination, evanescent rashes may be seen, but lymphadenopathy is usually absent. The course is usually less than 72 hr in duration.

At the onset both in classical and in mild dengue, the leukocyte counts may be low or normal; however, by the third to the fifth day, leukopenia, usually with counts of less than 5,000 per mm^3, and neutropenia are usually seen. Occasionally albuminuria of moderate degree occurs.

DIAGNOSIS Virus isolation in tissue culture of serum obtained during the first days of illness is definitive. Diagnosis can be made by serologic tests employing paired serums for hemagglutination inhibition tests and complement fixation tests. Specific serologic diagnosis is complicated by cross reactions with other group B arbovirus antibodies such as those following immunization with yellow fever vaccine.

TREATMENT The treatment is entirely symptomatic.

PROGNOSIS Mortality is nil.

PREVENTION Attenuated vaccines are undergoing experimental evaluation but are not available. The hypothesis of "second infections" being responsible for the dengue hemorrhagic fever syndrome raises further questions about a program of active immunization. Control depends upon mosquito abatement.

West Nile fever

West Nile virus is distributed from South Africa to southeastern India, but has been shown as a cause of significant disease only in the Near East, where it can produce a clinical picture closely resembling dengue.

ETIOLOGY West Nile virus is a group B arbovirus with pathogenicity for common laboratory animals. The virus multiplies and causes cytopathic effects in a variety of cells in tissue culture.

PREVALENCE In 1940 the virus was isolated from the blood of a febrile patient. Subsequent serologic surveys demonstrated neutralizing antibodies against the virus to be widely prevalent in the native populations of Uganda, Kenya, the Congo, and the Sudan. However, the clinical manifestations were unknown until the virus was isolated from the blood of a child during an epidemic of febrile disease in Israel in 1951. Outbreaks of disease involving several hundred patients occurred in Israel in 1950 to 1952. In one outbreak, over 60 percent of the population developed overt disease.

EPIDEMIOLOGY The disease is highly endemic in Egypt but goes largely unrecognized. Presumably the adult population is for the most part immune, and the infection in childhood is an undifferentiated mild febrile illness. The infection occurs in the summer both in Israel and in Egypt. The transmission cycle in Egypt is believed to be bird-to-mosquito-to-bird, with *Culex univittatus* as the principal vector. Although man and a variety of other vertebrates are infected by the virus, their involvement is believed to be tangential. In Israel, the most probable vectors are *Culex molestus* and *C. univittatus*.

CLINICAL MANIFESTATIONS Most of the patients in Israel have been young adults, with neither sex predominating. The onset is usually abrupt and without prodromal symptoms. The temperature quickly rises to 101 to 104° F, with chills occurring in one-third of patients. Symptoms include drowsiness, severe frontal headache, ocular pain, and pain in the back. A small number of patients have anorexia, nausea, and dryness of the throat. Cough is uncommon. Signs observed include flushing of the face, conjunctival injection, and coating of the tongue. The prominent finding is general enlargement of lymph nodes, which are of moderate size but are not hard and are only slightly tender. Occipital, axillary, and inguinal nodes are usually involved. The spleen and liver are slightly enlarged in a small proportion of patients. In one-half the patients a rash may appear from the second to the fifth day of illness and may persist for several hours or until defervescence. The rash occurs predominantly over the trunk and consists of pale roseolar maculopapular lesions. The illness is self-limited and lasts 3 to 5 days in 80 percent of patients.

In a few patients, transitory meningeal involvement may be encountered. Spinal fluid examinations may reveal a pleocytosis and some increase in protein concentration.

Leukopenia occurs in the majority of patients, and total leukocyte counts are lower than 4,000 per mm^3 in one-third. Differential counts vary from a moderate shift to the left to a slight lymphocytosis.

Convalescence is often prolonged, lasting 1 to 2 weeks, with prominent symptoms of fatigue. Enlargement of lymph nodes subsides over several months. Only rarely have complications, sequelae, or fatalities been seen in natural infections, although in one outbreak in a group of elderly patients a high proportion of patients developed meningoencephalitis, and four fatalities ensued.

Accurate diagnosis rests on virus isolation, which can be accomplished because viremia persists for as long as 6 days, or the demonstration of a rising specific antibody titer.

The treatment is symptomatic.

ARBOVIRUS INFECTIONS CHARACTERIZED PREDOMINANTLY BY CENTRAL NERVOUS SYSTEM INVOLVEMENT

Four arboviruses are presently recognized as numerically important causes of central nervous system disease in the United States: St. Louis encephalitis virus, Eastern equine encephalitis virus, Western equine encephalitis virus, and the California encephalitis group of viruses. The spectrum of infection caused by these agents includes inapparent infection, fever with headache, aseptic meningitis, and encephalitis. Of the more than 1,950 patients reported with encephalitis during 1970, 19 percent were classified as postinfectious. This is a broad category which includes measles, mumps, chickenpox, rubella, and cytomegalovirus. An enteroviral etiology (poliovirus, Coxsackie virus, and echo virus) was confirmed in 2.7 percent of cases, while 5.6 percent were due to arboviruses. In 69.7 percent, the etiology was unknown. For 8 of the 12 years from 1955 to 1966, St. Louis encephalitis virus was the most common cause of arboviral encephalitis in the United States. In contrast, from 1967 through 1970, the California encephalitis group of viruses accounted for 50 to 81 percent of the reported cases of human arthropod-borne encephalitis.

ETIOLOGY Despite the diversity of specific viral etiologies (Table 207-2), in individual patients the clinical manifestations of aseptic meningitis and encephalitis are very similar, and preclude an etiologic diagnosis without ancillary information regarding epidemiologic and serologic features. The clinical features of aseptic meningitis due to arboviruses are indistinguishable from those due to the more prevalent enteroviruses, which are discussed in Chap. 190. The broad clinical picture of arbovirus encephalitis will be discussed; then the specific epidemiologic and prognostic features which characterize the major types will be presented.

CLINICAL MANIFESTATIONS The clinical features of arbovirus encephalitis differ among age groups. In infants under one year of age, the only consistently noted symptoms are sudden onset of fever, which is often accompanied by convulsions. Convulsions may be either generalized or focal. Typically the fever ranges between 102 and 104°F. Other physical findings may include bulging of the fontanelle, rigidity of the extremities, and abnormalities in reflexes.

In children between five and fourteen years of age, subjective symptoms are more easily elicited. Headache, fever, and drowsiness of 2 to 3 days' duration before medical attention is sought are common. The symptoms may then subside or become more intense and may be associated with nausea, vomiting, muscular pain, photophobia, and, less frequently, convulsions (less than 10 percent). On examination, the child is found to be acutely ill, febrile, and lethargic. Nuchal rigidity and intention tremors are often present, and on occasion muscular weakness can be demonstrated.

In adults, the initial symptoms commonly include the fairly abrupt onset of fever, nausea with vomiting, and severe headache. The headache is most often frontal but may be occipital or diffuse in location. Mental aberrations, represented by confusion and disorientation, usually appear within the subsequent 24 hr. Other symptoms may include diffuse myalgia and photophobia. The abnormalities found on physical examination predominantly relate to the neurologic examination, although conjunctival suffusion is frequently seen and skin rashes may occur. Disturbances in mentation are among the most outstanding clinical features. These range from coma through severe disorientation to subtle abnormalities detected only by cerebral function tests such as the subtraction of serial 7s. A small proportion of patients show only lethargy, lying quietly, apparently asleep unless stimulated. Tremor is common and is observed more frequently in individuals over forty years of age. The tremors vary in location and may be continuous or intention in type. Cranial nerve abnormalities resulting in oculomotor muscle paresis and nystagmus, facial weakness, and difficulty in deglutition may occur, and are usually present within the initial several days. Objective sensory changes are unusual. Hemiparesis or monoparesis may occur. Reflex abnormalities are also common; these include exaggerated palmomental reflexes, and suck and snout reflexes. Superficial abdominal and cremasteric reflexes are usually absent. Changes in the tendon reflexes are variable and inconstant. The plantar response may be extensor and fluctuates almost hourly. Dysdiadochokinesia often exists.

The duration of the fever and neurologic symptoms and signs varies from several days to a month but usually ranges from 4 to 14 days. Clinical improvement generally follows the subsidence of the fever within several days unless irreversible anatomic changes have occurred.

LABORATORY FINDINGS Erythrocyte values are usually normal. Total leukocyte counts often reveal both a slight to moderate leukocytosis (occasionally greater than 20,000 per mm^3) and neutrophilia. Examination of the cerebrospinal fluid usually reveals several hundred cells per cubic millimeter but on occasion cloudy cerebrospinal fluid with cells in excess of 1,000 per mm^3 may be seen. Within the first several days of illness, polymorphonuclear neutrophils may predominate. The initial cerebrospinal fluid protein is usually only slightly elevated but on occasion may exceed 100 mg per 100 ml. The level of spinal fluid sugar is normal; a significant decrease should raise serious consideration of an alternative diagnosis. As the illness progresses, mononuclear cells in the cerebrospinal fluid tend to increase so that they predominate and the protein concentration may increase. Other laboratory studies have been performed only sporadically, but abnormalities may include hyponatremia, often due to the inappropriate secretion of antidiuretic hormone, and elevations in serum creatine phosphokinase.

DIAGNOSIS Specific diagnosis requires the isolation of the virus or detection of antibodies with a rising titer between the acute phase of disease and convalescence. Antibodies can be detected by hemagglutination inhibition, complement fixation, or virus neutralization techniques.

TREATMENT Treatment is entirely supportive and requires meticulous attention in the comatose patient.

Eastern equine encephalitis

Eastern equine encephalitis, a group A arbovirus, was first isolated in 1933 from the brain tissue of horses during an outbreak of equine illness in New Jersey. The first recognized human outbreak occurred in Massachusetts in 1938.

EPIDEMIOLOGY The virus is distributed along the eastern coast of the Americas from Northeastern United States to Argentina. Viral isolations also have been reported in the Philippines, Thailand, Czechoslovakia, Poland, and the U.S.S.R., but the question of type specificity has not been resolved. In the Northeastern United States, epidemics occur in the late summer and early fall. Epizootics in horses precede the occurrence of human cases by 1 to 2 weeks. The disease affects mainly infants, children, and adults over fifty-five years of age. There is no sex preponderance. Inapparent infection occurs in all age groups, suggesting that the decreased likelihood of developing overt infection in the fifteen- to fifty-four-year age group is not the result of decreased exposure. The ratio of inapparent infection to overt encephalitis approximates 25:1.

The natural reservoir is unknown. Isolations have been made from numerous species of wild birds and also from amphibians, reptiles, and mammals. The natural vector is the mosquito, including *Aëdes sollicitans* and *Culiseta melanura. Aëdes sollicitans*, a salt-marsh mosquito which is an avid human feeder, has been postulated as the epidemic vector, while *C. melanura* is important in bird-to-bird transmission. Equine animals and man are probably "dead ends" in the transmission cycle, and infection in them is accidental.

PATHOLOGY An outstanding feature is the predominance of neutrophilic leukocytes in the infiltrates. Foci of tissue damage represented by rarefaction necrosis are common. Neuronolysis also is very common. Large perivascular collections of neutrophils and activated histiocytes are frequently detected in the white matter of the cortex. Other sites of predilection are the thalamus, putamen, substantia nigra, and pons.

CLINICAL MANIFESTATIONS Though human infections have been thought usually to result in serious, if not fatal, central nervous system involvement, the detection of inapparent infection as well as relatively mild disease establishes the occurrence of milder forms. In many patients, the cerebrospinal fluid is cloudy and contains in excess of 1,000 cells per mm^3.

DIAGNOSIS The hemagglutination-inhibition or neutralization tests are the serologic methods of choice. The complement fixation test may be negative in patients with confirmed infections.

PROGNOSIS The mortality rate in clinical infection exceeds 50 percent. In the most severe cases, death occurs between the third and fifth days. Children under ten years of age have a greater likelihood of surviving the acute illness, but they also have a greater likelihood of developing severe disabling residuals: mental retardation, convulsions, emotional lability, blindness, deafness, speech disorders, and hemiplegia.

Western equine encephalitis

Western equine encephalitis (WEE) virus is a group A arbovirus which was isolated in 1930 in California from horses with encephalitis. In 1938 it was recovered from a fatal human infection.

EPIDEMIOLOGY WEE virus has been isolated in the United States, Canada, Brazil, Guyana, and Argentina. Human disease has been diagnosed only in the United States, Canada, and Brazil. In the United States, the virus is found in virtually all geographic areas. The central valley of California represents an important endemic area. The disease occurs mainly in early summer and midsummer. Wild birds, which develop viremia of sufficiently high titer to be able to infect mosquitoes that feed on them, are the basic reservoir, although nonavian vertebrate hosts may be important. *Culex tarsalis* is the principal vector in the Western United States. In areas east of the Appalachian Mountains, another vector must be operative. The virus has been repeatedly isolated from *Culiseta melanura*; however, the importance of this species has been questioned, since it is not primarily a man-biting mosquito. The ratio of inapparent infection to disease, as evidenced by serologic survey studies, varies from 58:1 in children to 1,150:1 in adults. Approximately one-fourth of patients are less than one year of age. The highest attack rates occur in persons fifty years or older.

PATHOLOGY The outstanding feature is the presence of many foci of rarefaction necrosis, which are most numerous in the striatum, then the globus pallidus, cerebral cortex, thalamus, and pontine tegmentum. A number of foci contain neutrophils and resemble abscesses. Perivascular collections of lymphocytes and ameboid cells are common. Occasional chronic cases have been characterized by severe cystic transformation in the basal ganglions, cerebral white matter, and cerebral cortex.

PROGNOSIS The fatality rate approximates 2 to 3 percent in laboratory-confirmed cases. The incidence and severity of sequelae are related to age. Sequelae among very young infants are frequent (appearing in 61 percent of a group of patients less than three months old) and severe; they consist of upper motor neuron impairment, involving the pyramidal tracts, extrapyramidal structures, and cerebellum, and result in behavioral problems and convulsions. Both the incidence and severity of sequelae diminish rapidly after one year of age. Adults may complain of nervousness, irritability, easy fatigability, and tremulousness for 6 months or longer after the acute illness. Probably not more than 5 percent of adults have sequelae which are sufficiently severe to be of practical significance. Postencephalitic seizures are rare.

Japanese encephalitis

The name Japanese B encephalitis was employed during an epidemic which occurred in 1924 to distinguish it from von Economo's disease, which was designated as type A encephalitis (see Chap. 330). The designation as Japanese B no longer seems useful, and the term Japanese encephalitis will be employed.

EPIDEMIOLOGY Japanese encephalitis virus infection is known to occur in eastern Siberia, China, Korea, Taiwan, Japan, Malaya, Vietnam, Singapore, Guam, and India. In temperate climates, the disease shows a late-summer, early-fall seasonal incidence. In tropical climates there is no seasonal variation. The mosquito *Culex tritaeniorhynchus* is the major vector species. It is a rural mosquito which breeds in rice fields and preferentially bites large domestic animals, such as pigs, but also feeds on birds and man. Man is an accidental host in the transmission cycle. In several outbreaks, a higher incidence of cases has been reported in children than in adults.

PATHOLOGY Japanese encephalitis is characterized by intense neuronophagia. Gliomesenchymal nodules are found in the cerebral cortex and the molecular and Purkinje cell layers of the cerebellum. In the thalamus and substantia nigra, foci of tissue breakdown are found. Perivascular infiltration adjacent to damaged nerve tissue occurs. Relatively severe involvement of the spinal cord also may occur.

CLINICAL MANIFESTATIONS The occurrence of severe rigors at the onset has been noted in almost 90 percent of patients. Localized paresis is found more often than with other arboviral encephalitides, e.g., in 31 percent of cases, with predominantly upper extremity involvement. Weight loss has been very striking, averaging 26 lb in one report. The failure of the temperature to lyse, appearance of diaphoresis, tachypnea, and the accumulation of bronchial secretions are grave prognostic signs.

PROGNOSIS The immediate mortality rate has varied from 7 to 33 percent or higher. The rate of occurrence of sequelae varies inversely with the fatality rate; in those series with high fatality rates (33 percent), sequelae occurred in 3 to 14 percent. In another series with a fatality rate of 7.4 percent, the sequelae rate was 32 percent. Sequelae consisted of neurologic or intellectual defects and psychiatric complaints.

St. Louis encephalitis

St. Louis encephalitis was first recognized as an entity during a major outbreak in St. Louis, Mo., and the surrounding area in 1933. St. Louis encephalitis (SLE) has been the most common type of arbovirus encephalitis in the United States.

EPIDEMIOLOGY In the United States, epidemics of SLE fall into two epidemiologic patterns. One pattern is found in the West, where mixed outbreaks of Western equine encephalitis and SLE have occurred primarily in irrigated rural areas. The vector has been *Culex tarsalis*. The second pattern occurred in the original St. Louis outbreak and the numerous subsequent epidemics in the Midwest, New Jersey, and Florida. These outbreaks have been more urban in location and are characterized by a marked tendency for the development of encephalitis in older persons. In such urban-suburban epidemics, the epidemic vectors have been mosquitoes of the *Culex pipiens-quinquefasciatus* complex, with the exception of the Florida epidemic, in which *Culex nigripalpus* was incriminated. The presence of SLE virus outside the United States has been proved by isolations in Trinidad, Panama, and Jamaica. However, except in Jamaica, no case of encephalitis due to this virus has been reported outside the United States. The basic transmission cycle is that of wild bird–mosquito–wild bird. The mechanism by which the virus overwinters has not been defined. The disease in man usually appears in midsummer to early fall. There is no sex preponderance. Man represents an accidental host and plays no role in the basic transmission cycle. Serologic studies following most urban epidemics indicate that infection rates are similar in all age groups, and that the increasing age-specific attack rate for clinical encephalitis which is typical of urban St. Louis encephalitis is probably due to age differences in host susceptibility to overt disease rather than to a higher rate of infection.

PATHOLOGY The basic lesions are small perivascular hemorrhages and cuffs of round cells. Nerve-cell damage occurs in small clusters of cells in the gray matter. The lesions of SLE predominate in the thalamus and substantia nigra, but the cerebral cortex may be slightly to moderately affected. There is usually little neuronophagia.

CLINICAL MANIFESTATIONS Infection with SLE virus most commonly results in an inapparent infection. Of the patients with confirmed disease, approximately three-fourths have clinical encephalitis; the remainder present with aseptic meningitis, febrile headaches, or nonspecific illness. Virtually all patients over forty years of age have encephalitic manifestations. Urinary frequency and dysuria have been symptoms in approximately 20 percent of patients despite sterile routine aerobic urine cultures. The basis for the urinary tract symptoms is not understood.

DIAGNOSIS The occurrence of either encephalitis or aseptic meningitis as manifested by febrile illness with cerebrospinal fluid pleocytosis in the months of June through September in an adult, especially over thirty-five years of age, should raise the suspicion of St. Louis encephalitis. Because appproximately 40 percent of patients with SLE have antibodies detectable by hemagglutination inhibition at the onset of illness, acute serum for serologic studies should be submitted promptly to a competent laboratory.

PROGNOSIS The case fatality ratio in the original St. Louis epidemic was 20 percent. In most subsequent outbreaks the mortality rate has varied from 2 to 12 percent. Subjective nervous complaints, including nervousness, headaches, and easy fatigability and excitability, appear to be the most common residuals. Late organic defects such as speech defects, difficulty in walking, and disturbances in vision were demonstrated in approximately 5 percent of patients 3 years following infection.

California encephalitis

A neurotropic virus which was named the California virus was isolated in 1943 and 1944 from three separate pools of mosquitoes in Kern County in the San Joaquin Valley of California. In 1945, serologic evidence of infection by this virus was demonstrated in three patients. Since 1963, a large number of isolations of what is now known to be the California group of viruses have been made. Cases of encephalitis and inapparent infection have been discovered, and the California group of viruses is now well established as a significant cause of encephalitis in the United States, being the single most common laboratory-confirmed cause since 1966.

EPIDEMIOLOGY The epidemiology has not been fully elucidated. Infection has been demonstrated to occur in the Midwest, especially in Ohio, Indiana, and Wisconsin, as well as in wooded areas in eastern Texas and along the Eastern Seaboard. Birds do not appear to be an important host of the California viruses. Most of the potential host isolations have been from mammals. Virus has been isolated from *Aëdes triseriatus* mosquitoes. Some tick isolations also have been made. A basic transmission cycle involving small mammalian hosts and *Aëdes* species of mosquitoes has been suggested. Most of the illnesses have occurred in the late summer and early fall. One-half the patients are children six years of age and younger. The home or recreational area of patients has been found to be in areas of high mosquito incidence.

DIAGNOSIS Neutralizing and hemagglutination-inhibition antibodies are usually present a few days after the reported onset of disease. Complement-fixing antibodies usually are detectable 10 to 12 days after the onset of illness.

PROGNOSIS The case fatality ratio is low, and most patients recover. Follow-up studies have not been underway for sufficient time to evaluate sequelae; however, complaints of emotional lability, difficulty in learning in school, and personality problems have been frequent.

Other arboviruses with central nervous system involvement

A large group of additional arboviruses have been associated with encephalitis or aseptic meningitis. Some of these agents are listed in Table 207-2. Though the epidemiologic picture of each of these agents is unique, the general features are sufficiently similar to require laboratory support for their differentiation.

ARBOVIRUS AND ARENOVIRUS DISEASES PRESENTING PRIMARILY WITH HEMORRHAGIC MANIFESTATIONS

For 300 years, yellow fever was the only epidemic viral disease known to be accompanied by grave hemorrhagic manifestations. Since the 1930s diverse viral etiologies of the hemorrhagic fever syndrome have been recognized and are now known to be responsible for the variety of epidemiologic situations in which this syndrome occurs (Table 207-2). One or more illnesses so named occurs on three continents. Despite the diverse viral etiology, there are many similar clinical manifestations. The onset is usually sudden, with headache, backache, generalized myalgia, conjunctivitis, and prostration. From approximately the third day, the initial stage is followed by hypotension, and hemorrhagic manifestations may occur; these are characterized by bleeding gums, epistaxis, hemoptysis, hematemesis, melena, petechiae, ecchymoses, and hemorrhages into most visceral organs. Early mild leukopenia develops, but with the appearance of hemorrhagic manifestations, leukocytosis may occur. The pathophysiology of the cardinal signs is attributable to hematopoietic and capillary damage, with variable localization of lesions. On the basis of limited confirmatory observations, variable degrees of disseminated intravascular coagulation may be responsible for a significant part of the pathophysiology of the hemorrhagic fever syndromes. Death usually occurs in the second week of disease, at which time a high titer of antibody has developed and the patient may have become afebrile. Death is usually associated with coma, which is due not to encephalitis but to an encephalopathy. The pathologic changes may be similar despite diverse viral etiologies, with midzonal hepatic necrosis and acidophilic cytoplasmic inclusions similar to the Councilman bodies of yellow fever.

Yellow fever

Yellow fever is an acute infectious disease of short duration and extremely variable severity; it is caused by a group B arbovirus and is followed by lifelong immunity. The classic triad of symptoms—jaundice, hemorrhages, and intense albuminuria—is present only in severe infections, which now comprise only a small proportion of the total.

PREVALENCE Yellow fever remains the most dramatically serious arbovirus disease of the tropics. For more than 200 years, after the first identifiable outbreak occurred in Yucatan in 1648, it was one of the great plagues of the world. As late as 1905, New Orleans and other Southern United States ports experienced at least 5,000 cases and 1,000 deaths. Because of the existence of the sylvatic form of the disease, protective measures must be maintained against human disease, as demonstrated by recent outbreaks in Trinidad in 1954, Central America in 1948 to 1957, the Congo in 1958, and Sudan and Ethiopia in 1959 to 1962, Senegal in 1965, and central West Africa in 1969.

EPIDEMIOLOGY Human infection results from two basically different cycles of virus transmission, urban and sylvatic. The urban cycle is man-mosquito-man, i.e., *Aëdes aegypti*-transmitted yellow fever. After a 2-week extrinsic incubation period, mosquitoes can transmit infection. Sylvan yellow fever differs under various ecologic circumstances. In the rain forests of South and Central America, species of tree-top *Haemagogus* or *Sabethes* mosquitoes maintain transmission in wild primates. Once infected, the mosquito vector remains infectious for life; hence it may serve as a reservoir as well as a vector. When man comes into proximity with the forest-canopy mosquitoes, sporadic cases or focal outbreaks may occur. In East Africa, the mosquito-primate cycle is maintained by the forest-canopy mosquito *Aëdes africanus*, which seldom feeds on man. The peridomestic mosquito *Aedes simpsoni* feeds upon primates entering the village gardens and can then in turn transmit the virus to man. Once yellow fever is reintroduced into urban areas, the urban cycle can be reinitiated, with the potential for epidemic disease. Why yellow fever has never invaded Asia despite widespread distribution of man-biting *A. aegypti* mosquitoes has never been satisfactorily explained.

PATHOLOGY The lesions are predominantly visceral. The diagnosis of yellow fever in the experimental animal may be suspected by the presence of acidophilic degeneration in Kupffer's cells of the liver within 24 hr after inoculation. By the fourth day necrobiosis and acidophilic necrosis of the parenchymal cells of the liver with the formation of Councilman bodies may occur in a characteristically discontinuous fashion in the midzones of the liver lobules. In the kidney, the virus produces fatty changes, necrobiosis, and necrosis of the tubular epithelium. Multiple minute hemorrhages occur in the gastrointestinal tract. In the brain, the chief lesion is perivascular hemorrhage, which is most frequently found in the subthalamic and periventricular regions at the level of the mammillary bodies.

CLINICAL MANIFESTATIONS The incubation period is usually 3 to 6 days. In accidental laboratory- or hospital-acquired infections longer incubation periods (10 to 13 days) have been reported. In considering the clinical features it is advantageous to classify the illness as to severity: inapparent, mild, moderately severe, and malignant. In mild yellow fever the only symptoms may be the abrupt onset of fever and headache. Additional symptoms may include nausea, epistaxis, relative bradycardia known as Faget's sign (e.g., with a temperature of 102°F the pulse may be only 48 to 52 beats per min), and slight albuminuria. The mild illness lasts only 1 to 3 days and resembles influenza except that coryzal symptoms are lacking.

Moderately severe and malignant attacks of yellow fever are characterized by three distinct clinical periods: the period of infection, the period of remission, and the period of intoxication. Prodromal symptoms are usually absent. The onset is characteristically sudden, with headache, dizziness, and temperature elevations to 104°F without a relative bradycardia. Young children may have febrile convulsions. The headache is followed quickly by pains in the neck, back, and legs. Often there is nausea with vomiting and retching. Examination reveals a flushed face and injection of the conjunctiva. The congestion of the eyes persists until the third day. The tongue characteristically shows bright red margins and tip and a white furred center. Faget's sign appears by the second day. Epistaxis and gingival bleeding are common. On the third day of illness, the fever may fall by crisis and the patient enters remission, or, in the malignant form, copious hemorrhages, anuria, or delirium may occur. The stage of remission lasts from several hours to several days. In the third stage, the "classic" symptoms develop; the fever returns but the pulse remains slow. Jaundice becomes detectable about the third day; however, jaundice often is not prominent even in fatal illnesses. Increased epistaxis, melena, and uterine hemorrhages are common, but gross hematuria is rare. Of the "classic" signs, "black vomit" is more characteristic than is jaundice. Hematemesis usually does not occur before the fourth day and is often associated with a fatal outcome. Albuminuria, which rarely develops before the third day, occurs in 90 percent of patients and may be quite marked

(3 to 20 g albumin per liter). In spite of this massive albuminuria, edema or ascites has not been reported. In malignant infections, coma frequently occurs 2 or 3 days before death. Shortly before death, which usually occurs between the fourth and the sixth days, it is not uncommon for the patient to become delirious and wildly agitated. Though the duration of fever in the third stage is usually 5 to 7 days, the period of intoxication is the most variable of the stages and may last up to 2 weeks. Clinical yellow fever is relatively free from complications, suppurative parotitis being the most striking of those which do occur. Clinical relapses are not characteristic of yellow fever.

LABORATORY FINDINGS Early in the disease, progressive leukopenia may occur. By the fifth day, total leukocyte counts of 1,500 to 2,500 cells per mm^3 often are found, the decrease being due mostly to a decrease in neutrophils. Total leukocyte counts return to normal by the tenth day, and in fatal cases there may be a marked terminal leukocytosis. Hemoglobin values remain normal except terminally, when hemoconcentration or bleeding may occur. Platelet counts are reported to be normal. Detailed coagulation studies have been performed only in rhesus monkeys experimentally infected with yellow fever. Within 72 hr after viral inoculation and prior to apparent clinical illness, a coagulation defect was observed. This was characterized by a prolonged one-stage prothrombin time and a prolonged partial thromboplastin time, reflecting measured deficiencies in factors II, V, VII, VIII, IX, X, and XI. Both the euglobulin lysis time and the thrombin time were prolonged, suggesting a depression of plasminogen activation and accumulation of fibrinogen degradation products. At this time platelet counts and chemical measurements of fibrinogen were normal. During the subsequent 48 hr, these coagulation defects worsened as the monkeys developed clinical illness; terminally, depression of platelet counts and fibrinogen levels occasionally was observed. The disturbances in coagulation occurred during the stage of viremia and existed before the stage of hepatic necrosis in liver biopsy specimens. These data suggest that the *hemorrhagic manifestations are primarily caused by a disseminated intravascular coagulation rather than by hepatic failure.* Also, in experimental infections in primates, modest increases in total bilirubin and alkaline phosphatase levels and marked increases in serum glutamic oxalacetic transaminase occur. Electrocardiograms may show T-wave changes. Clinical examinations of cerebrospinal fluid have not revealed abnormalities.

DIAGNOSIS There are three established procedures for the laboratory diagnosis of yellow fever: (1) Isolation of the virus from blood. This must be done early, preferably during the first 3 days. Caution must be exercised to avoid autoinoculation. (2) Demonstration of increase in neutralizing antibody. (3) Demonstration of the typical, although not completely specific, histopathologic lesions on liver biopsy.

TREATMENT The management has been symptomatic and supportive. Current management should be based upon assessment and correction of the circulatory abnormalities. If evidence of disseminated intravascular coagulation is present, the administration of heparin should be considered. Close attention to fluids and electrolytes is essential.

PROGNOSIS The overall fatality rate in yellow fever is between 5 and 10 percent of clinical cases; it may be less now since many infections are mild or inapparent.

PREVENTION Effective control measures are available. Immunization has been effective in the prevention of outbreaks. With the occurrence of sylvatic outbreaks, work in the area of epizootic activity should be discontinued and intensive mosquito abatement measures should be instituted. These measures may provide the time necessary for a mass immunization program.

Mosquito-borne hemorrhagic fevers

The term "hemorrhagic fever" was first applied to illness in Southeast Asia in the Philippines in 1953. Subsequently the hemorrhagic fevers have grown steadily as a disease problem. Initially they were classified on the basis of geography as Philippine, Thai, and Southeast Asian hemorrhagic fevers. With further study it appeared more rational to classify the syndromes as hemorrhagic dengue or chikungunya, depending upon the etiology. These diseases are caused by viruses transmitted by *A. aegypti.*

ETIOLOGY At least four (dengue types 1, 2, 3, 4) and possibly six types of dengue and chikungunya virus have been isolated from arthropods and man during outbreaks of hemorrhagic fever.

PREVALENCE The reasons for the apparent sudden "appearance" of the syndrome in the past 15 years are completely obscure. However, during the 1922 epidemic of dengue fever in Louisiana, hemorrhagic manifestations, including epistaxis, bleeding gums, melena, menorrhagia, and even "black vomit," were observed. Hemorrhagic disease with dengue also was seen in Durban in 1927 and in Athens in 1928. Yet no deaths were attributed directly to the dengue, which is at variance with the observations in Southeast Asia. Outbreaks have tended to recur at the original site and to spread to other *A. aegypti*-infested areas. Outbreaks have occurred in the Philippines, Vietnam, Cambodia, Thailand, Malaysia, Singapore, and India. Hemorrhagic fever is a disease of children, with virtually all cases occurring in children under age fourteen years. In 1962 in Bangkok and Thonburi, an estimated 10 to 20 percent of children under age fifteen had illness due either to dengue or to chikungunya virus. Approximately 5 percent of children with dengue or chikungunya had hemorrhagic fever. Dengue hemorrhagic fever occurs almost exclusively in indigenous populations; it has been observed only once in Caucasians of European descent despite the frequent occurrence of classic dengue in this group.

EPIDEMIOLOGY *Aëdes aegypti* is the vector of both dengue and chikungunya viruses. It is an urban mosquito which breeds in artificial containers and receptacles. Outbreaks are confined to the rainy season, although in areas without marked seasonal rainfall cases may occur throughout the year. Man-mosquito-man transmission of dengue is responsible for urban epidemics. Recent isolates of chikungunya virus from *Culex tritaeniorhynchus* in Thailand where human population densities are low suggest a nonhuman reservoir for this virus.

PATHOLOGY The reported pathologic studies are based primarily upon clinical and epidemiologic diagnoses, rather than on virologic confirmation. There are no pathognomonic findings. Focal subserosal hemorrhage, gastrointestinal hemorrhage, tissue edema with effusions in serosal cavities, and patchy areas of pneumonitis are common. Microscopically, the most common findings include maturation arrest of megakaryocytes or hypocellularity of bone marrow, focal areas of necrosis of individual hepatic parenchymal cells with the formation of Councilman-like bodies, infiltration of portal areas and sinusoids by lymphoid cells, and interstitial pneumonitis. Involvement of the kidneys, adrenals, pituitary, or central nervous system is rare.

CLINICAL MANIFESTATIONS The hemorrhagic dengue syndrome is almost exclusively a disease of children. There is no sex predominance. Illness begins abruptly with a minor stage characterized by fever, cough, pharyngitis, headache, anorexia, nausea, vomiting, and abdominal pain. This continues for 2 to 4 days. In contrast to what occurs in classic dengue, myalgia, arthralgia, and bone pain are unusual. Physical signs include fever varying from 101 to 105°F, injection of the tonsils and pharynx, and palpable lymph nodes and liver. The initial state is followed by abrupt deterioration, with the rapid onset of lassitude and weakness. On examination the child is found to be restless and to have cold clammy extremities with a warm trunk and flushing of the face. Petechiae, most frequently located on the forehead and distal extremities, are seen in half the cases. Occasionally there may be a macular or maculopapular rash. The extremities are frequently cyanotic. Hypotension, with narrowing of the pulse pressure, and tachycardia occur. Pathologic reflexes may be observed. Most fatalities occur on the fourth or fifth day of illness, melena, hematemesis, coma, or unresponsive shock being poor prognostic signs. Cyanosis, dyspnea, and convulsions are terminal manifestations. Following this critical period, survivors show steady and quite rapid improvement.

LABORATORY FINDINGS In one study, hemoconcentration was found in one-fifth of the children. The majority had leukocyte counts between 5,000 and 10,000 per mm^3, with one-third showing a leukocytosis. Only 10 percent of children had a true leukopenia. The most characteristic findings were thrombocytopenia, rarely with blood platelets under 75,000 per mm^3, positive tourniquet test, and prolonged bleeding time. Prothrombin time and partial thromboplastin times were usually near normal values. Depression of clotting factors V, VII, IX, and X may be present. Bone marrow examination may reveal maturation arrest of megakaryocytes. Urinalyses are usually normal, as are cerebrospinal fluid examinations. Other abnormal laboratory findings may include hyponatremia, acidosis, elevated blood urea nitrogen levels, elevation in serum glutamic oxalacetic transaminase levels, mild hyperbilirubinemia, and hypoproteinemia. Electrocardiograms may reveal diffuse myocardial abnormalities. Two-thirds of patients have radiologic evidence of bronchopneumonia, with many showing pleural effusions.

DIAGNOSIS Specific virologic diagnosis of dengue virus infection by serologic means often is difficult because broad antibody responses to group B arboviruses occur. Virus isolation may provide the only means of identifying the specific agent. Chikungunya virus diagnosis poses less difficulty, since it can be isolated from acute serum in suckling mice or hamster kidney cells. Serologic responses can also be demonstrated.

PATHOPHYSIOLOGY Recent correlations of clinical, epidemiologic, and serologic observations suggest that the severe form of dengue hemorrhagic fever occurs in persons previously infected by dengue virus and may represent an "immune-complex" disease (Chap. 69). If confirmed, this hypothesis may account for the rarity of the syndrome in nonindigenes.

TREATMENT The treatment is primarily supportive with correction of dehydration and avoidance of fluid overload. Adrenocorticosteroids have been used in patients with thrombocytopenia, regardless of the clinical severity, and have been considered beneficial. In a group of Filipino children with hemorrhagic fever due to dengue 3 virus, administration of heparin (1 mg sodium heparin per kilogram) was associated with a dramatic rise in number of platelets and level of plasma fibrinogen.

PROGNOSIS Mortality has varied from 6 to 23 percent. Deaths have been most common in infants under one year of age.

PREVENTION At present, vector control is the only method available to prevent hemorrhagic fever.

Tick-borne hemorrhagic fevers

CRIMEAN HEMORRHAGIC FEVER At the close of World War II, a new disease entity was recognized in the Crimea region of the U.S.S.R. Retrospective studies demonstrated that an almost identical syndrome had been recognized in the south central Asian republics of the U.S.S.R. for many years. Soviet workers repeatedly isolated virus strains during 1967 to 1969.

Etiology The virus of Crimean hemorrhagic fever (CHF) has been shown to be antigenically identical with Congo virus, which has been isolated from patients, cattle, and ticks in Africa (Kenya, Uganda, Congo, and Nigeria). CHF-Congo isolates now have been made from an area extending from southwestern and central U.S.S.R. to Pakistan and across central Africa from Nigeria to Kenya.

Epidemiology Approximately 30 cases of CHF have

been recorded annually in each of the known areas of occurrence in the U.S.S.R. The cases occur between April and September. The sex distribution of CHF is equal, and 80 percent of the cases occur in the twenty- to sixty-year age group, with the majority occurring in milkmaids and agricultural workers. The major arthropod vectors for transmission to man are ticks which belong to the genus *Hyalomma*. Cattle and wild hares appear to be important reservoirs, and rooks and other birds have been implicated, although the detailed epidemiology has yet to be defined.

Clinical manifestations The onset is abrupt, with temperatures to 104°F, dizziness, headache, and diffuse myalgia. The course of fever is occasionally biphasic, with an average duration of 8 days. Physical signs include flushing of the face, conjunctival injection, vomiting, and, on occasion, epigastric pain. Hepatomegaly is found in half the patients. Splenomegaly has been reported in 2 to 25 percent of patients. Respiratory symptoms or signs are unusual. Hemorrhagic manifestations generally begin on the fourth day with petechiae on the oral mucosa and skin, epistaxis, gingival bleeding, hematemesis, and melena. Neurologic abnormalities, seen in 10 to 25 percent of patients, include nuchal rigidity, excitation, and coma. Laboratory findings include leukopenia, with the number of white blood cells falling as low as 1,000 per mm^3, and thrombocytopenia, which is often severe. Proteinuria and microscopic hematuria are common, but azotemia and oliguria are not. Convalescence may be prolonged. Death is usually attributed to shock or intercurrent infection. Sequelae include transient alopecia and mononeuritis or polyneuritis. Although the clinical disease seen in Africa due to Congo virus generally has not been associated with hemorrhagic manifestations, one fatal case with gastrointestinal bleeding has been reported from Uganda.

Treatment The major approach to therapy has been transfusions of blood or plasma. The clinical similarities to other hemorrhagic fever syndromes in which the phenomenon of intravascular coagulation seems to occur are sufficient to suggest that appropriate studies should be done. If evidence of disseminated intravascular coagulation is demonstrated, treatment with heparin should be considered. In view of the clinical impressions of the value of corticosteroids in treating the hemorrhagic fevers of Southeast Asia, their administration also should be considered.

Prognosis The reported mortality rate has shown variation between 9 and 50 percent.

OMSK HEMORRHAGIC FEVER OHF is an acute febrile disease which occurs in the Omsk and Novosibirsk oblasts in the U.S.S.R. and is caused by a group B arbovirus of the Russian spring-summer complex.

Epidemiology The seasonal occurrence of OHF shows a biphasic pattern with peaks in May and August. OHF is transmitted to man either by the bite of infected ticks of the genus *Dermacentor* or by the handling of infected muskrats. The natural reservoir includes muskrats, other rodents, and ticks. Epidemics occurred from 1945 to 1948, and limited numbers of cases (~ 15 per year) recently have been recorded.

Clinical manifestations Following an incubation interval of 3 to 8 days, illness begins abruptly with fever, headache, and hemorrhagic manifestations, which include epistaxis and gastrointestinal and uterine bleeding. Rarely, neurologic abnormalities may occur. Laboratory features include the occurrence of leukopenia. In contrast to many of the other hemorrhagic fevers, OHF has a low case fatality rate (0.5 to 3.0 percent).

KYASANUR FOREST DISEASE Kyasanur Forest disease was first recognized in south India in 1957 as a discrete clinical entity shown to be due to an arbovirus.

Etiology The virus is a group B arbovirus immunologically related to the Russian spring-summer complex.

Epidemiology Kyasanur Forest disease occurs following occupational exposure to *Haemaphysalis spinigera* ticks in the tropical forests of western Mysore in southern India. The silent reservoir cycle which infects the primate- and bird-feeding *Haemaphysalis* ticks is now believed to be *Ixodes* ticks transmitted among small forest mammals, especially the shrew. The virus is highly infectious for man, and laboratory-associated infections are common.

Clinical manifestations The major symptoms include the abrupt onset of fever, headache, fatigue, myalgia (especially of the lumbar area and calf muscles), and retroorbital pain. Cough and abdominal pain occur in half the patients. Additional symptoms may include photophobia and polyarthralgia. Epistaxis and hematemesis are observed in some patients. On examination, findings include relative bradycardia, conjunctival injection, and generalized lymphadenopathy. Fine and coarse rales are frequently heard. Hepatosplenomegaly has been encountered occasionally. During the initial phase, generalized hyperesthesia of the skin occurs occasionally. The fever usually lasts from 6 to 11 days. After an afebrile period of 9 to 21 days, approximately half the patients may develop a second phase, which lasts from 2 to 12 days. This phase is manifested by recurrence of fever, severe headache, neck stiffness, mental disturbance, coarse tremors, giddiness, and abnormalities in reflexes, as well as by recurrence of many of the initial symptoms. No sequelae have been observed, but convalescence is often prolonged.

Only limited laboratory studies have been performed. During the initial phase, leukopenia is a constant feature, with a total leukocyte count of fewer than 3,000 per mm^3 by the fourth to sixth day. The leukopenia is associated with neutropenia. During the second phase there is a mild leukocytosis. Lumbar puncture during the second phase has shown a pattern of aseptic meningitis in the cerebrospinal fluid.

Diagnosis Diagnosis is based upon virus isolation from blood; this is readily accomplished, since viremia is prolonged. Serologic tests of paired serums also can be performed.

Treatment The management is supportive.

Prognosis The mortality rate is approximately 5 percent.

Arenovirus hemorrhagic fevers (zoonotic hemorrhagic fevers)

ARGENTINIAN AND BOLIVIAN HEMORRHAGIC FEVERS The first cases of a new American hemorrhagic disease were seen near the Argentinian town of Junin near Buenos Aires in 1953. A virus was isolated from patients' blood and from local rodents and their mites. In 1959, cases of a disease thought to resemble severe epidemic typhus were noted among rural workers in northeastern Bolivia. The similarity between these syndromes was recognized. In 1963, the causal virus was isolated from patients and rodents and named the Machupo virus. Machupo virus is serologically related to but distinct from Junin virus.

Etiology Junin and Machupo viruses are antigenically related to Tacaribe virus. There is no antigenic relationship between these agents and the etiologic agents of the other viral hemorrhagic fevers.

All viruses in the Tacaribe group, except for Tacaribe itself, have been isolated from rodents in the Western Hemisphere (Table 207-2). Recently the Tacaribe complex of viruses has been shown to be morphologically related to lymphocytic choriomeningitis virus. The name arenoviruses has been suggested for this group of ribonucleic acid–containing lipid-solvent susceptible viruses which are antigenically related and have a distinctive appearance on electron microscopy.

Prevalence Junin virus infections have been observed annually in epidemic form since 1958. In these outbreaks, between 300 and 1,000 cases have been reported annually. The hemorrhagic disease in Bolivia has been particularly severe. Of a total population of 4,000 to 6,000 in the endemic area, 750 persons were affected between 1959 and 1963.

Epidemiology Argentinian hemorrhagic fever occurs in sharply epidemic seasonal form (March to August), mostly among male rural workers, especially those exposed to fields at the time of the maize harvest. The vector and reservoir are unknown; however, the virus has been isolated from mites and wild rodents in the endemic zone. The natural cycle has not been reproduced under controlled conditions, but there is little evidence that vectors play a major, if any, role in transmission.

Bolivian hemorrhagic fever appears to be a rodent-transmitted disease. Infection of *Calomys callosus* with Machupo virus in the epidemic area was widespread, prevalent, and persistent. Direct human-to-human transmission is possible but does not appear to be the principal method of dissemination. Disease has not occurred in medical personnel attending patients with the disease.

Clinical features Argentinian hemorrhagic fever presents manifestations of renal, cardiovascular, and hematologic involvement. The incubation period is estimated to be 7 to 16 days, followed by a gradual onset of chills, fever, headache, malaise, myalgia, anorexia, nausea, and vomiting. The temperature reaches 102 to 104°F, facial flushing may be prominent, and there is a painless enanthem of the pharynx. Lymphadenopathy and splenomegaly are not present. From 3 to 5 days after onset, the signs and symptoms worsen, with the appearance of signs of dehydration, hypotension to 50 to 100 mm Hg, oliguria, and relative bradycardia. In the more severe cases, hemorrhagic manifestations, including bleeding from the gums, hematemesis, hematuria, and melena, occur. Progressive oliguria and tremor of the tongue and extremities may develop. Some patients develop psychic manifestations, with agitation, delirium, or stupor. Progressive shock, hypothermia, gallop rhythm, or gastrointestinal bleeding may occur from the seventh to tenth days. In fatal cases, pulmonary edema usually is the cause of death. During convalescence a temporary alopecia has been noted. Erythrocyte counts are normal or elevated. The total leukocyte count drops to 1,200 to 3,400 white blood cells per mm^3. Thrombocytopenia may occur. The urine is dark and may approach the color of mahogany, with intense albuminuria. Blood urea nitrogen levels rise rapidly.

The clinical picture of Bolivian hemorrhagic fever is similar to Argentinian, although epistaxis and hematemesis at the onset is more common.

Diagnosis Complement-fixing antibodies appear in 15 to 30 days in about 75 percent of the clinically diagnosed cases.

Treatment Available reports do not provide details as to therapy. Supportive measures, including peritoneal dialysis to correct both the azotemia and the pulmonary edema, would seem to offer the most reasonable approach.

Prognosis The mortality rate among patients with clinically diagnosed cases approximates 30 percent.

Prevention In Bolivia, rodent control measures directed primarily against *C. callosus* populations in the houses resulted in a prompt and dramatic cessation of human cases.

LASSA FEVER A new virus disease, which is both highly contagious and virulent, occurred in a missionary nurse in Lassa, a town in northeast Nigeria, in 1969.

Etiology A series of isolates were recovered in cell tissue cultures from specimens of serum, pleural fluid, urine, and throat washings. The agent probably contains ribonucleic acid, is susceptible to sodium deoxycholate, is spherical in shape, and cross-reacts to a low degree with lymphocytic choriomeningitis virus and possibly with some members of the Tacaribe group. It appears that this agent, designated Lassa virus, is an arenovirus.

Epidemiology The original patient was flown from

Lassa to Jos, Nigeria, where two nurses who cared for her subsequently became ill; one was transferred to New York City. Later an investigator working with Lassa virus became ill. In January 1970 a number of patients were hospitalized in Jos with an unidentified acute febrile illness. By mid-February there had been 26 suspected cases with 10 deaths in Jos and 6 additional suspected cases in another hospital, 13 miles from Jos. The data from serologic surveys indicate that antibody to Lassa virus is distributed over a wide area of Nigeria and as far west as Guinea. No information is available on the natural reservoir or the mode of transmission. Since Lassa virus is a member of the arenovirus group, it is likely that there is a rodent reservoir.

Clinical features The incubation period appears to be 7 to 17 days. In 1970 in Jos, the patients ranged from five months to forty-six years of age; 17 were women and 9 were men. Initial symptoms may be gradual in onset or associated with rigors, and include severe myalgia, weakness, and headache. Early examination reveals fever, flushing of the face and V area of the neck, and mild erythema of the pharynx. Over several days, the temperature rises and pharyngeal symptoms increase, with the development of severe dysphagia. Petechiae and small vesicles occur on the tonsillar pillars, soft palate, and buccal mucosa. Cervical adenopathy and puffiness of the neck occur. Petechial and ecchymotic lesions occurred on the extremities of one patient. By the end of the week, there are likely to be clouding of the sensorium, pulmonary rales, signs of pleural effusion, peripheral edema, and evidence of renal involvement. In one of the initial patients, the febrile course lasted 4 weeks. In the patients in Jos in 1970, illness lasted from 1 to 4 weeks. During convalescence occasional flurries of rapid involuntary eye movements (oculogyric crises) occurred. A number of milder illnesses also were encountered. The patients who died, and the mortality rate has approximated 50 percent, did so between 1 and 2 weeks after onset of symptoms. The immediate cause of death seemed to be cardiac failure.

Laboratory features The hematologic findings include relatively normal hematocrit values and early leukopenia with a relative neutrophilia and immature forms of leukocytes. Strikingly, in two cases in which it was recorded, the erythrocyte sedimentation rate was normal. Urinalyses revealed proteinuria, which was often massive. Chest radiographs may suggest basilar pneumonitis and pleural effusions. Electrocardiographic abnormalities compatible with diffuse myocardial disease have been encountered. Levels of serum enzymes, serum glutamic oxaloacetic transaminase (SGOT), creatinine phosphokinase (CPK), and lactic dehydrogenase (LDH) have been elevated.

Treatment The management has been supportive. Fever subsided in one patient who received convalescent plasma from an earlier case. In view of the hospital association and the presence of virus in pharyngeal secretions and urine, strict isolation is required.

Hemorrhagic fever with renal syndrome

Synonyms for this disease include Korean hemorrhagic fever, Far Eastern hemorrhagic fever, endemic or epidemic nephrosonephritis, Manchurian epidemic hemorrhagic fever, Songo fever, and Churilov's disease.

Epidemic hemorrhagic fever (EHF) is an acute febrile, often fatal, otherwise self-limited, illness of unknown etiology characterized by severe toxemia, widespread capillary damage, hemorrhagic phenomena, and renal insufficiency. In 1932, the Russians first observed a disease in southeastern Siberia along the Amur River, which forms the boundary between Manchuria and the Soviet Far East. On the basis of extensive clinical, pathologic, and epidemiologic studies, Smorodintsev, who led the Soviet research group, provisionally classified EHF as one of the zoonotic hemorrhagic fevers. In April 1951, a previously unknown illness, subsequently recognized as EHF, broke out among the United Nations forces in Korea.

ETIOLOGY The causative agent of EHF has not been definitively isolated in either culture or lower animal hosts, and immunologic or serologic diagnostic procedures have not been developed.

PREVALENCE In Korea between April 1951 and January 1953, 2,070 cases of EHF were reported among United Nations personnel. The disease usually occurs as an isolated event; hence, overall attack rates have relatively less meaning. With this reservation, attack rates in two United States Army divisions stationed in an area of Korea varied between 1.9 and 2.9 cases per 1,000 men per epidemic season. Sporadic cases have continued to occur in United States military personnel assigned to endemic areas of Korea. The Soviet Union reports 500 to 2,000 cases yearly.

EPIDEMIOLOGY In Korea, although sporadic cases may occur throughout the year, the majority of cases occur in May to June and in October to November. These peaks coincide with the dry seasons in Korea. Geographically, EHF occurred among troops stationed in the vicinity of Seoul to north of the 38th parallel, with only rare cases reported from the southern portion of the Korean peninsula. The epidemiology of EHF observed in Korea is compatible with the assumption that EHF is transmitted by some arthropod and that the reservoir of disease is a member of the local fauna. Trombiculid mites (chiggers), bloodsucking mites (laelaptids), fleas, and ticks may all be regarded as potential vectors, but chiggers, especially *Trombicula pallida*, correlate most closely with the epidemiology of EHF in Korea.

Since World War II, rather remarkable outbreaks have occurred in northeast Asia between November and January. In these outbreaks, the peak of the epidemic was preceded by a marked increase in forest rodent populations (usually the red-backed vole *Clethrionomys glariolus*), which migrated into the fields, barns, and even houses near the forest. On the basis of these data, Soviet investigators now believe that EHF is transmitted directly from asymptomatically infected rodents to man by means of virus-contaminated rodent excreta, an epidemiologic pattern analogous to that demonstrated for Bolivian hemorrhagic fever. Thus, EHF may represent either a zoonotic hemorrhagic fever, as postulated by Soviet investigators, or an arthropod-borne infection involving one or more species of mites.

CLINICAL MANIFESTATIONS The incubation period in EHF is usually 10 to 25 days, with possible extremes of 7 and 36 days, and individuals who contract the disease in an endemic area may easily not develop illness until their return to the United States. Inapparent or mild disease is less common than typical EHF.

The clinical course of EHF may be divided into phases on the basis of the underlying physiologic aberrations: febrile, hypotensive, oliguric, diuretic, and convalescent. There is considerable variation among patients in the severity of the illness. In one study two-thirds of the 264 cases studied were classified as mild, while 14 percent were termed severe. The illness in most patients was of comparable severity in each phase.

Febrile phase (invasive phase) From 10 to 20 percent of patients describe vague prodromal symptoms resembling mild upper respiratory infections. The onset is then usually abrupt, often initiated by a chill and accompanied by fever, headache, backache, abdominal pain, and generalized myalgia. Anorexia and thirst are almost universal, while nausea and vomiting are common although not constant symptoms. The headache is most commonly frontal or retroorbital. Eye symptoms, especially mild photophobia and pain on movement of the eyes, are characteristic. Diarrhea is not a feature. Fever is present in almost all patients; the temperature ranges from 100 to 106°F, reaches a peak on the third or fourth day after onset, and falls by lysis on the fourth to seventh day. There is a relative bradycardia. Initially the blood pressure is normal. One of the most typical early findings is a diffuse reddening of the skin, most marked over the face and V area of the neck. It may resemble a severe sunburn. The erythema blanches on pressure. Dermographism can be demonstrated in over 90 percent of patients at the same time as the flush. Slight edema of the upper eyelids causes a bleary-eyed appearance. Bulbar and palpebral conjunctivas show injection and look as if the patient had measles without lacrimation. Conjunctival petechiae may develop by the third to fifth day of illness. Subconjunctival hemorrhages may be striking. Intense pharyngeal reddening without significant sore throat is typical. The first location for petechiae is usually the palate, where they occur in half the patients. Within 12 to 24 hr, petechiae appear at pressure areas such as the axillary folds, lateral chest wall, belt line, hips, and thighs. Retinal hemorrhages occur rarely. Cervical, axillary, and inguinal nodes are moderately enlarged but nontender. Abdominal and costovertebral tenderness is almost a constant finding. Splenomegaly is unusual and in Korea was generally attributable to malaria with which EHF coexisted in about 1 percent of patients. The degree of flush, fever, and conjunctival injection and the number of petechiae correlate quite well with the overall severity of illness.

Laboratory studies during this phase are often not striking. Initial hemoglobin and hematocrit values are usually normal. Prior to the fourth day, leukocyte counts range from 3,600 to 6,000 per mm^3 but are associated with a left shift in the neutrophilic series. Early in the course urine specific gravity may be high. Albuminuria, which is an almost universal finding, appears, often abruptly, between the second and fifth days of illness. The urinary sediment reveals microscopic hematuria and hyaline, granular, red blood cell casts and/or white blood cell casts. Erythrocyte sedimentation rates are normal during the first week. Capillary fragility tests are usually positive at the time of admission and become most abnormal by the ninth day. Electrocardiographic abnormalities may be seen in 15 to 30 percent of patients; these include sinus bradycardia and low or inverted T waves. Lumbar punctures may reveal gross blood in the spinal fluid.

Hypotensive phase On about the fifth day of illness, during the last 24 to 48 hr of the febrile phase, hypotension or shock may occur. In mild cases, only a transient fall in blood pressure occurs; among moderately and severely ill patients shock may persist for 1 to 3 days. In 828 patients, 16.5 percent had clinical shock, and another 14 percent had hypotension without shock. Headache often diminishes, but thirst persists. In the beginning of the hypotensive phase most patients have warm, dry skin and extremities. As the hypotensive phase progresses and the systolic blood pressure decreases and pulse pressure narrows, the skin becomes cool and moist. Tachycardia replaces the relative bradycardia.

At this stage of EHF, an increase in hematocrit with no change in total serum protein level is found. This is thought to reflect a loss of plasma through damaged capillaries. On about the fifth day, all patients develop marked proteinuria. The previously normal urine specific gravity begins to fall and in 2 to 3 days is usually around 1.010. Blood urea nitrogen concentrations begin to increase. Other laboratory findings include leukocytosis, with white blood cell counts of 10,000 to 56,000 per mm^3 and a left shift in the neutrophilic series, and toxic granulation. The number of blood platelets decreases, with levels often being less than 70,000 per mm^3. In a single patient who became ill 30 days after leaving Korea and who was studied on the fourth day of illness (i.e., in the hypotensive phase), there were marked thrombocytopenia, hypofibrinogenemia, and hypoprothrombinemia with a prolonged thrombin time. The deficiency of multiple blood coagulation factors suggests that the bleeding defect was due to disseminated intravascular coagulation.

Oliguric phase (hemorrhagic or toxic phase) About the eighth day of illness, blood pressure returns to the normal range and in some instances increases to hypertensive levels. While oliguria may have appeared during the shock phase, it now becomes a prominent feature. Oliguria develops even though shock or hypotension was not recognized. Symptomatically patients continue to feel weak and thirsty and have more severe backache. Protracted vomiting and hiccoughs may ensue.

Blood urea nitrogen levels increase rapidly and are associated with hyperkalemia, hyperphosphatemia, and hypocalcemia. Of note is the observation that the metabolic acidosis which develops is rarely severe. Although platelets begin to return to normal, hemorrhagic manifestations become more prominent. Excluding petechiae, hemorrhagic manifestations include hematemesis (analogous to "black vomit" in yellow fever), melena, hemoptysis, gross hematuria, and hemorrhages into the central nervous system. The enlarged lymph nodes may now become tender.

With the onset of diuresis on about the seventh day in moderately ill patients and the ninth to eleventh day in severely ill patients, symptoms of fluid and electrolyte abnormalities and central nervous system or pulmonary complications may appear. Central nervous system symptoms include disorientation, extreme restlessness, lethargy, paranoid delusions, and hallucinations. Grand mal seizures occur in some patients, as do pulmonary edema and pulmonary infection.

Diuretic phase With the onset of diuresis, progressive improvement is the rule. Most patients begin to eat and regain their strength. In fatal cases the diuretic phase is associated with a daily urine output of less than 4 liters and often less than 2 liters, in contrast to larger volumes in surviving patients.

Convalescent phase The convalescent phase lasts 3 to 6 weeks. Weight is regained slowly. Complaints include muscular weakness, intention tremor, and lack of stamina. Inability to concentrate the urine and polyuria are present; however, within 2 months most patients are able to concentrate their urine to a specific gravity of 1.023 or greater after a 12-hr period of water deprivation.

DIAGNOSIS In the absence of both techniques for isolation and identification of the causative agent or agents and specific serologic methods, the diagnosis of EHF is one of exclusion. The following criteria are necessary for diagnosis: the patient must have been in the endemic area within the limits of the incubation period, and there must be a characteristic history, hemorrhagic findings, and evidence of renal involvement. In addition, studies to exclude other forms of the hemorrhagic fever syndrome must be undertaken, particularly in the sporadic cases.

PATHOLOGY The most characteristic fundamental alteration is widespread capillary and endothelial damage, with all subsequent manifestations being the result of this damage. This is manifested by dilatation of all small vessels in tissues, congestion, plasma transudation, and multiple small hemorrhages. Three features are prominent and characteristic: hemorrhage, particularly in the renal medulla, right atrium, and gastrointestinal submucosa; a peculiar type of necrosis of the renal pyramids, anterior lobe of the pituitary body, and adrenal gland; and a mononuclear cellular infiltration of the myocardium, spleen, and liver. Moderate to severe retroperitoneal edema was present in three-fourths of patients who died in the hypotensive phase of EHF.

PATHOPHYSIOLOGY Many of the clinical features of the febrile as well as subsequent phases could be the consequence of generalized capillary dysfunction. By direct microscopy of the capillary nailbed in patients with EHF, Greisman observed a pattern of sequential changes. During the febrile and hypotensive phases, decreased vasomotor activity, refractoriness to *l*-norepinephrine, dilatation, and hemorrhagic diathesis were the outstanding features.

These physiologic changes correlate with the clinical features, flushing of the face, and injection of the conjunctiva and pharynx. During the early febrile phase, the cardiac index is normal. Late in the febrile phase widespread capillary dysfunction becomes evident. This is manifest by loss of protein-rich plasma through damaged capillaries and results in hemoconcentration and a progressive fall in cardiac output. Measured total peripheral resistance is low, a finding compatible with the observed capillary dilatation and refractoriness to *l*-norepinephrine. During the hypotensive phase, the increases in hematocrit values and decreases in plasma volume are accentuated. These findings have the pathologic corollary of marked retroperitoneal edema. The hypotensive phase is associated with a reduction in cardiac output and an increase in peripheral vascular resistance. The reduced cardiac output is probably the result of multiple factors: reduction in circulating blood volume, inadequate vasoconstriction, and possibly myocardial damage. Although adrenal hemorrhages can be seen at necropsy, adrenal insufficiency does not seem to be a contributing cause of shock. The initial pathophysiologic changes may result in impairment of circulation through various organs, with the development of functional and morphologic changes secondary to inadequate perfusion with its attendant hypoxemia. The hemorrhagic manifestations appear to be the result of capillary damage, with diapedesis of erythrocytes and the development of disseminated intravascular coagulation.

The plasma loss and arteriolar dysfunction are limited in duration, and, for unknown reasons, the sequestered plasma rather abruptly returns to the vascular system at the time of the oliguric phase. During this phase, examination of nailbed capillaries revealed increased vasomotor activity and vasoconstriction. When patients who became hypertensive were divided on the basis of the presence or absence of diuresis, the clinical and hemodynamic differences became more apparent. During the hypertensive phase in anuric or oliguric patients, some individuals presented with full veins, an exaggerated cardiac apical thrust, and wide pulse pressure. In this group the cardiac index was high, and the peripheral resistance and hematocrit were low. This state was termed "relative hypervolemia"; other terms include "hyperdynamic state" and the "venous congestive state." Hypertensive patients who had begun to have diuresis had normal cardiac outputs and significantly elevated values for peripheral vascular resistance.

Although diuresis is a harbinger of convalescence, a daily urine output of 3 to 8 liters contributes to further serious fluid and electrolyte imbalances. If fluid output exceeds intake, low cardiac indices may be seen and shock may ensue. Conversely, if fluid intake exceeds output, hypertension and pulmonary edema may develop.

TREATMENT Clinical management primarily revolves around meticulous supportive care. Trials with a variety of agents including antibiotics, adrenocortical steroid hormones, antihistamines, and convalescent serum were without significant beneficial effect during the Korean epidemics.

Early hospitalization with a minimum of physical trauma is important. Accurate and prompt recording of temperature, pulse, blood pressure, and intake-output is necessary. During the febrile phase, bed rest and adequate sedation are essential. In the initial 8-hr interval after admission, 500 ml of 5 percent glucose in water is administered. In each succeeding 8-hr interval, the total output (urine, vomitus, stool) plus 250 ml is replaced with 5 percent glucose in water. Salt-poor human albumin (50 g in 200 ml) is given in volumes sufficient to maintain the systolic blood pressure above 90 mm Hg, the pulse below 120 beats per minute, and the hematocrit below 50 percent. The goal of therapy during this phase is to sustain circulation, yet avoid overhydration. Management during the oliguric phase is essentially that of the patient with acute renal tubular necrosis (Chap. 269).

PROGNOSIS The Soviet experience indicates a mortality rate of 3 to 32 percent; in other early reports the mortality has ranged from 10 to 15 percent. Between April 1951 and January 1953, the overall case fatality ratio in Korea was 5.9 percent; however, during 1967–1968, there were no fatalities among 44 patients admitted to the Hemorrhagic Fever Center.

Residua are uncommon. Of 783 surviving patients cared for at the Hemorrhagic Fever Center in Korea between April and December 1952, only 16 were unable to return to duty within a period of 4 months. Fifteen of these individuals still had hyposthenuria. Follow-up studies on former EHF patients 3 to 5 years later showed that they had many more subsequent hospital admissions for urologic problems than did a control group and that the relative frequency correlated with the severity of the acute episode of EHF. Asymptomatic residual renal tubular dysfunction may be more common than generally has been appreciated.

REFERENCES

Definition and classification

THE SUBCOMMITTEE ON INFORMATION EXCHANGE OF THE AMERICAN COMMITTEE ON ARTHROPOD-BORNE VIRUSES: Catalogue of arthropod-borne and selected vertebrate viruses of the world. Am J Trop Med 20:1018, 1971

WHO STUDY GROUP: *Arthropod-borne viruses*, WHO Tech Rep Ser. 219, Geneva, 1961

WHO SCIENTIFIC GROUP: *Arbovirus and Human Disease*, WHO Tech Rep Ser 369, Geneva, 1967

Arbovirus infections characterized by fever, malaise, headaches and myalgia

BECKER FE: Tick-borne infections in Colorado. Colorado Med 27:36, 1930

BRICENO ROSSIE AL: Rural epidemic encephalitis in Venezuela caused by a group A arbovirus (VEE). Prog Med Virol 9:176, 1967

DAUBNEY R et al: Enzootic hepatitis or Rift Valley Fever. J Pathol Bacteriol 34:545, 1931

DIASIO JS, RICHARDSON FM: Clinical observations on dengue fever. Milit Surg 94:365, 1944

ECKLUND CM et al: Distribution of Colorado tick fever and virus-carrying ticks. JAMA 157:335, 1955

EHRENKRANZ NJ et al: Natural occurrence of Venezuelan equine encephalitis in USA. N Engl J Med 282:298, 1970

FLEMING J et al: Sandfly fever. Review of 664 cases. Lancet 1:443, 1947

FLORIO L et al: The etiology of Colorado tick fever. J Exp Med 83:1, 1946

LENNETTE EH, KOPROWSKI H: Human infection with Venezuelan equine encephalomyelitis virus. JAMA 123:1088, 1943

LLOYD LW: Colorado tick fever. Med Clin North Am, March 1951

SABIN AB: Research on dengue during World War II. Am J Trop Med 1:30, 1952

—— et al: Phlebotomus (Papataci or sandfly) fever; disease of military importance: Summary of existing knowledge and preliminary report of original observations. JAMA 125:603, 693, 1944

SCHERER WF et al: Ecologic studies of Venezuelan encephalitis virus in Southeastern Mexico. VII. Infection of man. Am J Trop Med 21:79, 1972

SCHRIRE L: Macular changes in Rift Valley fever. S Afr Med J 25:926, 1951

SIDWELL RW et al: Epidemiological aspects of Venezuelan equine encephalitis virus infections. Bacterial Rev 31:65, 1967

SILVER HK et al: Colorado tick fever. Am J Dis Child 101:30, 1961

SMITHBURN KC et al: Rift Valley fever. J Immunol 62:213, 1949

SULKIN SE et al: Bat salivary gland virus: Infections of man and monkey. Tex Rep Biol Med 20:113, 1962

Arbovirus infections characterized by fever, malaise, arthralgia, and rash

ANDERSON SG, FRENCH EL: An epidemic exanthem associated with polyarthritis in the Murray Valley, 1956. Med J Aust 2:113, 1957

DELLER JJ JR., RUSSELL PK: Chikungunya disease. Am J Trop Med 17:107, 1968

DOHERTY RL et al: Studies of epidemic polyarthritis: The significance of three group A arboviruses, isolated from mosquitoes in Queensland. Aust Ann Med 13:322, 1964

MALHERBE H et al: Sindbis virus infection in man. Report of a case with recovery of virus from skin lesions. S Afr Med J 37:547, 1963

ROBINSON MC: An epidemic of virus disease in Southern Province, Tanganyika territory in 1952–53. I. Clinical features. Trans R Soc Trop Med Hyg 49:28, 1955

SHORE H: O'nyong-nyong fever: An epidemic virus disease in East Africa. III. Some clinical and epidemiological observations in the Northern Province of Uganda. Trans R Soc Trop Med Hyg 55:361, 1961

SMORODINTSEV AA et al: *Haemorrhagic Neophrosonephritis*, London: Pergamon, 1959

Arbovirus infections characterized predominantly by fever, malaise, lymphadenopathy, and rash

Marberg K et al: The natural history of West Nile fever. I. Clinical observations during an epidemic in Israel. Am J Hyg 64:259, 1956

Taylor RM et al: A study of the ecology of West Nile virus in Egypt. Am J Trop Med 5:579, 1956

Arbovirus infections characterized predominantly by central nervous system involvement

Altman R et al: The impact of vector-borne viral diseases in the middle Atlantic States. Med Clin N Amer 51:661, 1967

Center for Disease Control: Neurotropic viral diseases surveillance, encephalitis. Annual Encephalitis Summary-1970, January 1972

Cramblett HG et al: California encephalitis virus infections in children. Clinical and laboratory studies. JAMA 198:108, 1966

Dickerson RB et al: Diagnosis and immediate prognosis of Japanese B encephalitis. Observations based on more than 200 patients with detailed analysis of 65 serologically confirmed cases. Am J Med 12:277, 1952

Feemster RF, Haymaker W: Eastern equine encephalitis. Neurology 8:882, 1958

Finley KH et al: Western equine and St. Louis encephalitis. Preliminary report of a clinical follow-up study in California. Neurology 5:223, 1955

Luby JP et al: The epidemiology of St. Louis encephalitis (SLE): A review. Ann Rev Med 20:329, 1969

Thompson WH, Inhorn SL: Arthropod-borne California group viral encephalitis in Wisconsin. Wis Med J 66:250, 1967

Weaver OM et al: Japanese encephalitis: Sequelae. Neurology 8:887, 1958

Arbovirus and arenovirus diseases presenting primarily with hemorrhagic manifestations

Buckley SM, Casals J: Lassa fever, a new virus disease of man from West Africa. III. Isolation and characterization of the virus. Am J. Trop Med 19:680, 1970

Casals J et al: A current appraisal of hemorrhagic fevers in the USSR. Am J Trop Med 15:751, 1966

Dennis LH, Conrad ME: Accelerated intravascular coagulation in a patient with Korean hemorrhagic fever. Arch Intern Med 121:449, 1968

——— et al: The original hemorrhagic fever: Yellow fever. Blood 30:858, 1967

Frame JD et al: Lassa fever, a new virus disease of man from West Africa. I. Clinical description and pathological findings. Am J Trop Med 19:670, 1970

Giles RB et al: The sequelae of epidemic hemorrhagic fever: With a note on causes of death. Am J Med 16:629, 1954

Greisman SE: Capillary observations in patients with hemorrhagic fever and other infectious illnesses. J Clin Invest 36:1688, 1957

Halstead SB: Mosquito-borne haemorrhagic fevers of South and Southeast Asia. Bull WHO 35:3, 1966

Johnson KM et al: Hemorrhagic fevers of Southeast Asia and South America. A comparative approach. Prog Med Virol 9:105, 1967

Kerr JA: Clinical aspects and diagnosis of yellow fever, *Yellow Fever,* ed GK Strode, New York: McGraw-Hill, 1951, p. 389

Kirk R: An epidemic of yellow fever in the Nuba Mountains, Anglo-Egyptian Sudan. Ann Trop Med Parasitol 35:67, 1941

Low GC, Fairley NH: Laboratory and hospital infections with yellow fever in England. Br Med J 1:125, 1931

MacKenzie RB et al: Epidemic hemorrhagic fever in Bolivia: I. A preliminary report of the epidemiologic and clinical findings in a new epidemic area in South America. Am J Trop Med 13:620, 1964

Nelson ER: Hemorrhagic fever in children in Thailand: Report of 69 cases. J. Pediatr 56:101, 1960

Powell GM: Hemorrhagic fever: A study of 300 cases. Medicine 33:97, 1954

Rubini ME et al: Renal residuals of acute epidemic hemorrhagic fever. Arch Intern Med 106:378, 1960

Sheedy JA et al: The clinical course of epidemic hemorrhagic fever. Am J Med 16:619, 1954

Troup JM et al: An outbreak of lassa fever on the Jos Plateau, Nigeria, in January-February, 1970; A preliminary report. Am J Trop Med 19:695, 1970

208 OTHER VIRAL FEVERS

JAY P. SANFORD

RHABDOVIRUS INFECTIONS OTHER THAN RABIES

The rhabdoviruses consist of a group of RNA viruses which previously were ungrouped or grouped with the arboviruses but which do not meet the revised criteria established for arboviruses, and which share a characteristic morphology. On electron microscopy, these agents are bullet-shaped, one of the extremities being pointed and the other flattened. Members of the rhabdovirus group which infect vertebrates include rabies, vesicular stomatitis virus, and Marburg virus which produce disease in man and Lagos bat, Cocal, Chandipura, Mount Elgon bat, Flanders, Hart Park, Kern Canyon, and Piry viruses which have not been recognized as producing human disease.

VESICULAR STOMATITIS VIRUS This virus disease of animals, which chiefly affects cattle, horses, swine, and wild animals, including deer, raccoons, skunks, and bobcats, appears in man as an acute, self-limited infection with signs and symptoms similar to those of influenza. Two distinct serotypes, New Jersey and Indiana, have been recognized. Most of the outbreaks, especially in North America, have been due to the New Jersey strain. Although most commonly occurring as a laboratory infection in man, this infection is transmissible under natural conditions. In one report, three-fourths of the laboratory personnel handling experimentally infected animals or manipulating the viruses developed neutralizing antibodies. In nature, the virus has been isolated from *Phlebotomus* sandflies collected in a tropical rain forest in Panama and from a pool of *Aëdes* sp. (probably *dorsalis*) mosquitoes during an epizootic in New Mexico. In the areas of Panama which were involved, 17 to 35 percent of the population had neutralizing antibodies against vesicular stomatitis virus (VSV). Of the laboratory workers with serologic evidence of infection, approximately one-half reported clinical symptoms. In the majority of cases the incubation period has been 2 to 6 days, although symptoms have developed within 30 hrs of accidental inoculation. The onset usually is sudden, with chills, fever, profuse diaphoresis, and generalized myalgia including pain on ocular movement. One-third to one-half of patients have sore throats, and 20 percent have coryza. Physical signs include a temperature of 102 to 104°F in severe cases; fever is absent in mild cases. Conjunctivitis is noted in 20 percent, and in some patients (10 percent), small, raised vesicles may be present on the buccal mucosa. Submaxillary and cervical lymphadenitis is seen in approximately one-third of patients. A diphasic course is noted in approximately 10 percent of patients. Treatment is symptomatic.

MARBURG VIRUS DISEASE From the middle of August through September 1967, 31 individuals developed a febrile illness characterized by rash and hemorrhagic manifestations. Twenty-five of the patients had direct contact with African green monkeys (*Cercopithecus aethiops*) or tissue culture cells derived from them. The cases occurred in Marburg (23 cases) and Frankfurt (6 cases), Germany, and Belgrade, Yugoslavia (2 cases). The illness was clinically dramatic. It was associated with a 23 percent mortality, and evoked immediate worldwide concern and investigation, since thousands of monkeys are used in virologic studies and vaccine production.

Etiology The agent was propagated in guinea pigs, in which electron microscopy of liver revealed spheric particles 80 to 100 nm in diameter, filamentous forms, rods, and bullet-shaped organisms. It can be propagated in several primate tissue culture systems and has the characteristics of an RNA virus. While morphologically similar to rabies and VSV, it is serologically unrelated to 200 agents including other rhabdoviruses.

Epidemiology The outbreak related to vervet monkeys from the Lake Kyoga area of Uganda, which were shipped to London and then distributed to Europe. While there were no unusual illnesses or deaths among monkeys in the Lake Kyoga area, complement-fixing antibodies were demonstrated in up to 36 percent of *C. aethiops* trapped near Lake Kyoga; they were also present in three monkey trappers. Twenty of twenty-nine persons who had contact with blood or organs of this batch of vervet monkeys became ill, while 4 of the 13 persons exposed to tissue cultures prepared from these monkeys became ill. Infection from monkey to man occurred through direct contact with blood or organs, with no evidence for airborne spread. Secondary cases occurred reflecting man-to-man transmission, again probably through direct contact with blood or possibly body secretions (semen) from primarily infected patients.

Clinical manifestations After an incubation of 5 to 9 days, patients suddenly developed prostration, headache, myalgia, especially in the lumbar area, nausea, and vomiting. Initially the temperature rose to 103 to 104°F and often was associated with relative bradycardia. Other initial signs included conjunctivitis in at least three-fourths of patients and occasionally pharyngitis. One to two days after the onset, patients developed watery diarrhea, drowsiness, and changes in mentation. At about the fourth day of illness, an enanthem was noted, and lymphadenopathy was observed in some patients. The most reliable clinical feature was an erythematous rash which began on the fifth to seventh days on the buttocks, trunk, and outer surfaces of both upper arms. During the first week the temperatures continued in the range of 104°F, falling by lysis during the second week, to increase again between the twelfth and fourteenth days. Other clinical signs which were observed in some patients in the second week included splenomegaly, hepatomegaly, facial edema, and scrotal or labial reddening. Gastrointestinal hemorrhages occurred in approximately one-third of patients. After the sixteenth day, desquamation occurred and involved especially the palms and soles. Complications included orchitis in at least three patients, two of whom developed late testicular atrophy, and myocarditis with irregular pulse and electrocardiographic abnormalities. Fatalities occurred between the eighth and sixteenth days of illness, with an overall fatality rate of 23 percent. Late sequelae included myelitis and possible psychosis.

Laboratory findings Leukopenia was detected as early as the first day, with leukocyte counts as low as 1,000 per mm^3, with a neutrophilia by the fourth day. Subsequently between the fourth and nineteenth days, atypical lymphocytes appeared. At the end of the first week, a leukocytosis supervened. Thrombocytopenia appeared early and was most marked (often less than 10,000 cells per mm^3) between the sixth and twelfth days. In fatal cases evidence of disseminated intravascular coagulation was demonstrated. Several patients had proteinuria and azotemia. At the end of the first week, elevations in serum glutamic oxaloacetic transaminase (SGOT) were usual. Lumbar punctures performed on five patients revealed minimal pleocytosis in two.

Diagnosis The diagnosis was based upon the characteristic clinical course and epidemiologic features. With the preparation of antigens, serologic diagnosis is now possible.

Treatment The patients received a multiplicity of drugs without apparent influence on the course of the illness. Convalescent serum was administered to four patients, whose subsequent disease followed a mild course. However, similarly benign courses were observed in patients who did not receive serum.

ENCEPHALOMYOCARDITIS VIRUSES The encephalomyocarditis (EMC) viruses, Columbia S-K, MM, Mengo, are a group of small RNA viruses which are immunologically indistinguishable from each other. Rodents, in particular certain species of wild rats, constitute the major reservoir for EMC viruses. Strains also have been isolated from primates, swine, and other rodents from many parts of the world. Strains of Mengo virus have been isolated from mosquitoes (*Taeniorhynchus fuscopennatus*) in Uganda, but the epidemiologic evidence does not suggest that EMC viruses are arboviruses. The prevalence of neutralizing antibodies in surveys of healthy individuals in the United States, Germany, Sweden, and Mexico ranges up to 7 percent.

Human infections vary from inapparent to mild febrile illness to severe encephalomyelitis. Study of an outbreak of aseptic meningitis characterized by chills, fever, headache, stiff neck, and cerebrospinal fluid pleocytosis of 50 to 500 cells per mm^3, which involved a group of 44 U.S. Army personnel in the Philippine Islands, revealed that during convalescence 39 percent of the individuals had high titers of specific neutralizing antibodies. In this outbreak fever lasted 2 to 3 days, and all patients recovered promptly without sequelae. Sporadic EMC virus isolates have been made from adults and children with illnesses diagnosed as paralytic poliomyelitis, the Guillain-Barré syndrome, and severe meningoencephalitis. Myocarditis has not been a feature of EMC virus infection in man. Nothing is known of the pathologic findings in man. The diagnosis of human EMC virus infection depends upon isolation of the virus from blood, cerebrospinal fluid, or stool or the demonstration of a rising titer of specific antibodies during convalescence. Treatment is symptomatic and supportive.

REFERENCES

Encephalomyocarditis viruses

GAJDUSEK DC: Encephalomyocarditis infection in childhood. Pediatrics 16:902, 1955

WARREN J: Encephalomyocarditis viruses, in *Viral and Rickettsial Infections of Man*, 4th ed., eds FL Horsfall Jr, I Tamm, Philadelphia: Lippincott, 1965

Marburg virus disease

MARTIN GA, SIEGERT R (eds): *Marburg Virus Disease*, New York: Springer-Verlag, 1971

Vesicular stomatitis virus

FIELDS BN, HAWKINS K: Human infection with the virus of vesicular stomatitis during an epizootic. N Engl J Med 277:989, 1967

SUDIA WD et al: Isolation of vesicular stomatitis virus (Indiana strain) and other viruses from mosquitoes in New Mexico, 1965. Am J Epidemiol 86:598, 1967

section 21 | Diseases caused by protozoa

209 AMEBIASIS

JAMES J. PLORDE

DEFINITION Amebiasis is an infection of the large intestine produced by *Entamoeba histolytica*. It is an asymptomatic carrier state in most individuals, but diseases ranging from chronic, mild diarrhea to fulminant dysentery may occur. Among extraintestinal complications, the commonest is hepatic abscess, which may rupture into peritoneum, pleura, lung, or pericardium.

ETIOLOGY There are seven different species of ameba that naturally parasitize the mouth and intestine of man, but of these only *E. histolytica* causes disease. *Entamoeba coli* and *E. hartmanni* are the two species with which it is most likely to be confused in examination of stools.

Entamoeba histolytica exists in two forms: the motile trophozoite and the cyst. The trophozoite is the parasitic form and dwells in the lumen and/or wall of the colon, divides by binary fission, grows best under anaerobic conditions, and requires the presence of either bacteria or tissue substrates to satisfy its nutritional requirements. When diarrhea occurs, the trophozoites are passed unchanged in the liquid stool, where they can be distinguished by their size (10 to 20 μm in diameter), directional motility, clear pseudopodia, and finely granular cytoplasm. In dysentery, the trophozoites are larger (up to 50 μm in diameter), and often contain ingested erythrocytes. In the absence of diarrhea, the trophozoites usually encyst before leaving the gut. The cysts are highly resistant to environmental changes and are responsible for transmission of disease. The cysts of *E. histolytica* can be distinguished from those of *Entamoeba coli* by their nucleus with a small centric karyosome and fine peripheral chromatin and by their thick chromatoid bodies with round ends.

Entamoeba histolytica had been classified into large and small races depending upon whether they form cysts measuring more or less than 10 μm in diameter. Strains of the small race, however, are not pathogenic for man and are now considered as a distinct species, *Entamoeba hartmanni.*

Entamoeba histolytica-like amebas are organisms isolated from man that are morphologically indistinguishable from true *E. histolytica*. However, unlike *E. histolytica* they are nonpathogenic, grow best at 20°C, and can multiply indefinitely in hypotonic solutions.

Entamoeba histolytica occurs normally in the intestines of a few cats, dogs, primates, and rats. A number of animals can be infected experimentally. Amebas can be cultivated in artificial media, a procedure that is useful in direct diagnosis and in the preparation of purified antigens for serologic testing.

EPIDEMIOLOGY Infection with *E. histolytica* is worldwide. Stool surveys indicate that the prevalence of infection in the United States is between 1 and 5 percent. Much higher rates occur in areas where the level of sanitation is low. Reports of amebic liver abscess suggest that invasive amebiasis is concentrated in comparatively few parts of the world, most notably Mexico, Western South America, South Asia, and West and Southwestern Africa. In this country, the incidence of amebiasis has decreased sharply in the past 20 years. Furthermore, an increasing proportion of reported cases are now acquired outside the United States. Cases of dysentery and liver abscess still occur, however, in institutions for the mentally retarded. Cases of amebic dysentery are usually sporadic, but epidemics, that are sometimes waterborne, have occurred. Outbreaks of amebiasis are never explosive, as are those produced by pathogenic intestinal bacteria. Symptomatic amebiasis is unusual below the age of ten years in temperate climates, and both intestinal and hepatic lesions predominate in adult males to an extent that is not readily explainable on the basis of different rates of exposure to infection.

PATHOGENESIS AND ANATOMIC CHANGES

After ingestion, cysts pass through the stomach unchanged. In the small intestine, the cyst wall disintegrates, and eventually four to eight trophozoites result. Because trophozoites die rapidly after leaving the intestine, patients with amebic dysentery do not play a major role in transmission of the disease. Asymptomatic cyst passers are the source of new infections. The cysts are usually spread through contaminated food or water. Direct fecal spread may occur in situations where there is massive contamination of the environment. The immature amebas are carried to the large intestine where they live in the lumen of the gut as commensals feeding on bacteria and superficial mucosal cells. On occasion the amebas may invade the mucosa causing ulcerations that are sufficiently extensive to produce symptoms. The factors responsible for this are not completely understood, but the state of the host and the virulence of the infecting organism both play roles. Epidemiologic evidence suggests that amebic strains indigenous to temperate climates are usually avirulent. It has also been shown, however, that invasiveness is not a stable strain characteristic. It can either be lost after continued cultivation in vitro or enhanced by rapid animal passage. The virulence of various strains of *E. histolytica* is dependent upon the association with living bacteria. This suggests that an episome-like factor provided by certain strains of bacteria may be required to maintain virulence of *E. histolytica.*

Amebic ulceration of the intestinal wall is characteristic. A small mucosal defect overlies a larger, burrowing area of necrosis in the submucosa and muscularis, producing a bottle-shaped lesion. There is little acute inflammatory response, and in contrast to the picture in bacillary dysentery, the mucosa between ulcers is normal. The sites of involvement in order of frequency are cecum and ascending colon, rectum, sigmoid, appendix, and terminal ileum. In the cecum and elsewhere, chronic infection leads to the formation of large masses of granulation tissue or *amebomas.* Amebas can enter the portal circulation and lodge in venules; liquefaction necrosis of liver tissue leads to the formation of an abscess cavity. Rarely, embolization results in lung, brain, or splenic abscess.

CLINICAL MANIFESTATIONS

Asymptomatic cyst passer In the majority of patients with this common form of amebiasis, *E. histolytica* probably lives as a commensal in the bowel lumen. Individuals infected in temperate climates are unlikely to develop significant tissue invasion. However, invasion does occur occasionally, so treatment of cyst passers is warranted.

Symptomatic intestinal amebiasis In some patients there is intermittent diarrhea consisting of one to four foul-smelling loose or watery stools daily. The stools sometimes contain mucus and blood. Loose stools alternate with periods of relative normality and may persist for months or years. Flatulence and abnormal cramping are frequent. The only physical findings are occasional tender hepatomegaly and slight pain when the cecum and ascending colon are palpated. Sigmoidoscopy sometimes reveals typical ulcerations with areas of normal mucosa interspersed. The diagnosis depends upon finding the organism in the feces.

Fulminating attacks of amebic dysentery are less common. Waterborne outbreaks may occur, but fulminating dysentery is more likely to occur spontaneously in debilitated individuals. Attacks may be precipitated by pregnancy or corticosteroids. The onset in half the cases is abrupt with high fever, between 104 and 105°F, severe abdominal cramps, and profuse, bloody diarrhea with tenesmus. There is diffuse abdominal tenderness, often so severe that peritonitis is suspected. Hepatomegaly is very frequent, and sigmoidoscopy almost always demonstrates extensive rectosigmoid ulceration. Trophozoites are numerous in stools and in material obtained directly from the ulcers.

In some cases there may be extensive destruction of the colonic mucosa and submucosa, massive hemorrhage or perforation of the bowel wall, with resultant peritonitis. Repeated severe attacks of intestinal amebiasis can lead to an ulcerative postdysenteric colitis. Amebas can usually not be demonstrated in this condition, but serologic tests are strongly positive. Invasion of the appendix may lead to a clinical picture of *appendicitis.* Penetration of trophozoites through the muscle wall of the bowel may result in the development of large masses of granulation tissue. When the entire circumference of the intestine is involved, there may then be partial obstruction, and a tender, sausage-shaped mass is often palpable. This lesion or ameboma is most frequently seen in the cecum where a palpable mass and radiologic demonstration of a ragged encroachment on the lumen may lead to a mistaken diagnosis of adenocarcinoma.

Hepatic amebiasis The parasites usually reach the liver through the portal vein; rarely, they may traverse the lymphatic vessels. It has been believed for a long time that amebas which lodged in the liver could produce a diffuse hepatitis. Careful postmortem and biopsy studies indicate that the syndrome of tender hepatomegaly, right upper quadrant pain, fever, and leukocytosis in patients with amebic colitis is not a result of the presence of amebas in hepatic tissues, is accompanied by nonspecific periportal inflammation, and is rarely, if ever, a prelude to hepatic abscess. It is evident, then, that these manifestations are best regarded as an accompaniment of colitis and do not merit a separate diagnosis of "diffuse amebic hepatitis."

Hepatic abscess may develop insidiously, with fever, sweats, weight loss, and no local signs other than painless or slightly tender hepatomegaly. In other patients, there is abrupt onset, with chills, fever to 105°F, nausea, vomiting, severe upper abdominal pain, and polymorphonuclear leukocytosis. Initially, cholecystitis, perforated ulcer, or acute pancreatitis may be suspected.

Most commonly, the abscess occurs singly and is localized in the posterior portion of the right lobe of the liver, because this lobe receives most of the blood draining the right colon through the "streaming" effect in portal vein flow. This location is responsible for several features that aid in diagnosis. *Point tenderness* in the posterolateral portion of a lower right intercostal space is frequent even in the absence of diffuse liver pain. Most abscesses enlarge upward, producing a bulge in the diaphragmatic dome, obliteration of the costophrenic gutter, small hydrothorax, basilar atelectasis, and pain referred to the right shoulder. Liver function tests may be mildly to moderately disturbed but are of little diagnostic aid. Jaundice is uncommon. Radiologically, unruptured abscesses do not show a fluid level, and calcification of the liver parenchyma is very rare. Isotope liver scan utilizing two, or preferably three, projections is invaluable in confirming both the presence and location of a liver abscess. Serologic tests are positive in over 90 percent of patients.

Needle puncture results in the withdrawal of "pus" which consists of liquefied, necrotic liver, the classic "chocolate syrup" or "anchovy paste" exudate; the pus contains no polymorphonuclear leukocytes (barring secondary bacterial infection) and, usually, no amebas. The parasites are localized in the cyst wall and may be demonstrated at times by a Vim-Silverman needle biopsy of the cyst wall following aspiration of the abscess.

Hepatic abscess complicates asymptomatic infection of the colon more often than symptomatic intestinal disease, another factor making recognition difficult. Trophozoites or cysts are demonstrable in the feces of only about one-eighth of patients with abscess, and fewer than one-half can recall significant diarrheal illness.

Pleuropulmonary amebiasis The right pleural cavity and lung are involved by direct extension from the liver in 10 to 20 percent of patients with liver abscess. Rarely, amebic lung abscess has resulted from embolization rather than direct extension.

Manifestations are those of massive pleural effusion; aspiration of chocolate fluid is diagnostic, or if the lung parenchyma is involved and perforation into a bronchus occurs, patients expectorate large amounts of the typical exudate, some patients even commenting that the sputum "tastes like liver." Cough, pleural pain, fever, and leukocytosis are the rule, and secondary bacterial infection is frequent.

Other extraintestinal lesions Rupture of liver abscess into the *pericardium* has occurred; these patients are often thought initially to have tuberculous pericarditis. *Peritonitis* is a result of perforation of colonic ulcer or rupture of liver abscess. Painful ulcers of the genitalia, perianal skin, or abdominal wall (draining sinuses), vaginitis, urethritis, and prostatitis are unusual complications resulting from extension of intestinal disease. Metastatic brain abscess is rare, and an etiologic diagnosis is seldom made clinically. Splenic abscess has been reported but is very unusual.

DIAGNOSIS The diagnosis of intestinal amebiasis depends upon *identification of the organism in the stool or tissues.* Formed stools are examined initially in saline and iodine mounts for amebic cysts; concentration methods such as the formalin-ether technique greatly increase the yield. Liquid or semiformed stools must be examined immediately in saline solution if motile trophozoites are to be detected; a second preparation stained with buffered methyline blue can help in distinguishing morphologic characteristics. If there is any delay in examination of the stool, a portion of the specimen should be placed in a fixative solution. Polyvinyl alcohol and 10 percent formalin not only preserve amebas for better identification but permit preparation of permanently stained smears. Careful examination of four to six stool specimens may be required for diagnosis. If possible, the stool should be examined before the administration of antimicrobial, antidiarrheal, or antacid preparations because all these agents may interfere with the recovery of amebas. Likewise, enemas and radiographic procedures utilizing barium sulfate are best postponed until after a thorough search for *E. histolytica* has been made.

Sigmoidoscopy is of value in symptomatic cases. The mucosal lesions should be aspirated and the material examined for trophozoites. Stained sections of biopsy material obtained from such lesions also will frequently reveal trophozoites.

The diagnosis of extraintestinal amebiasis is difficult. The parasite usually cannot be recovered from stool or tissue. Cultivation of amebas from feces or pus is possible but is not practical in most laboratories. The most important diagnostic procedure in suspected liver abscess is a *therapeutic trial of antiamebic drugs.* The response is often dramatic within 3 days. In the event that demonstrating parasites is difficult, the therapeutic trial should be instituted without hesitation.

Serologic tests employing purified antigens are positive in nearly all patients with proved amebic liver abscess and in a great majority of those with acute amebic dysentery. However, the persistence of significant antibody titers for months to years after complete cure makes serology, particularly in endemic areas, of more value in excluding the diagnosis than in confirming it. The tests are generally negative in asymptomatic cyst passers, suggesting that a tissue invasion is required for antibody production. Of the available tests, the indirect hemagglutination appears to be the most sensitive. Intradermal tests have been shown to correlate well with serologic tests for amebiasis. However, their value in the diagnosis of amebiasis remains to be determined.

TREATMENT Treatment should be aimed at relief of symptoms, replacement of fluid, electrolyte, and blood losses, and eradication of the organism. Amebas may be found in the lumen of the bowel, in the intestinal wall, or extraintestinally. Most amebicides are not effective at all sites or when used alone, and a combination of drugs is often necessary to achieve cure. The available drugs based on their site of action fall into several different categories, as described below.

Luminal amebicides These oral agents act by direct contact with trophozoites dwelling in the bowel lumen but are ineffective against amebas in tissue. Of the large number of available drugs, diloxanide furoate (0.5 g three times daily for 10 days) is one of the most effective and well tolerated but is not presently available in the United States. Diodoquin, a halogenated hydroxyquinoline, is used most frequently in this country. It is given in dosage of 0.65 g three times daily for 21 days. Side effects are rare and are related to its iodine content.

Antibiotics Tetracycline, chlortetracycline, and oxytetracycline, when given in dosage of 2.0 g daily for 10 days, are effective against amebas residing in the intestinal wall as well as in the lumen. They probably act indirectly by altering the bacterial flora of the intestine.

Tissue amebecides *Chloroquine diphosphate* (Aralen) is a systemic amebecide which is useful in hepatic disease because of its high concentration in the liver. It has little activity elsewhere. The dose is 0.6 g base initially, 0.36 g base 6 hr later, and then 0.5 g base twice daily for 14 to 28 days.

Emetine is an alkaloid derivative of ipecac. When given intramuscularly (1 mg per kg with a maximum of 65 mg daily for 10 days), it is highly effective in destroying trophozoites in tissue including those in the wall of the intestine. It is ineffective against luminal amebas. Emetine is relatively toxic and may produce vomiting, diarrhea, abdominal cramping, weakness, muscle pain, tachycardia, hypotension, precordial pain, and electrocardiographic abnormalities. The common ECG changes include T wave inversion and prolongation of the Q-Tc interval. Rarely arrhythmias and prolongation of the QRS complex are seen. A synthetic derivative, dehydroemetine, is thought to be less toxic by virtue of its more rapid excretion and lower concentration in myocardial tissue. This drug is given intramuscularly in twice the dose of emetine. It is not free of toxicity, however, and patients treated with either drug should be at bed rest with ECG monitoring. Neither drug should be used in patients with renal, cardiac, or muscle disease, during pregnancy, or in children unless other drugs fail.

Amebicides effective at multiple sites Metronidazole (Flagyl) is unique because it is both safe and effective against trophozoites at all sites, intestinally and extraintestinally. It is the drug of choice in most forms of amebiasis. For intestinal amebiasis it is given in dosage of 800 mg three times daily for 5 days. Smaller doses are effective in hepatic amebiasis. Metronidazole has an Antabuse-like action, and alcohol should be avoided during its administration.

In asymptomatic or mildly symptomatic patients, stools should be examined monthly for 6 months to detect relapse. If relapse recurs, retreatment should consist of a combination of Diodoquin and tetracycline. Chloroquine can be added for its potentiating effect on tetracycline as well as its ability to eradicate subclinical hepatic infection. Although probably effective, the role of metronidazole in symptomless amebiasis is still uncertain.

Treatment of acute dysentery involves control of symptoms as well as eradication of the organism. A number of regimens can be used:

1 Emetine or dehydroemetine given intramuscularly rapidly controls the acute attack and destroys trophozoites in the intestinal wall as well as any that may have reached the liver. Because of their toxicity, these drugs should be discontinued once symptoms abate. Usually they need to be given for only 3 to 5 days. Agents active against luminal trophozoites must be given concurrently to effect a cure. A combination of tetracycline and either Diodoquin or diloxanide furoate is satisfactory.
2 In mild or moderate cases of amebic dysentery, emetine is not required. Tetracycline together with a luminal amebicide is adequate to bring the acute attack under control and to terminate the intestinal infection. A 2-week course of chloroquin should be given to eradicate subclinical hepatic infection.
3 For both mild and severe dysentery, metronidazole given in a dose of 800 mg three times daily for 5 days is the simplest and least toxic regimen. This drug will cure more than 90 percent of cases and by virtue of its multiple sites of action, does not need to be combined with other agents. Of some concern is the occurrence of amebic liver abscess in a few patients treated for dysentery with metronidazole.

If hepatic abscess is suspected, chloroquine is the drug of choice. It is effective, nontoxic, and produces symptomatic relief in 48 to 72 hr. Even larger abscesses subside, but relapse is relatively frequent. If aspiration or a dramatic response to chloroquine proves that a hepatic abscess is of amebic etiology, the drug should be continued for 3 or 4 weeks. In addition, emetine or dehydroemetine should be given for 10 days to prevent relapse. Alternatively, metronidazole may be administered. In dosage of 800 mg three times daily for 5 days, it is less toxic and probably just as effective as the chloroquine-emetine combination. Although lower doses have been shown to be effective in hepatic amebiasis, they are not consistently effective in eradicating intestinal trophozoites that might lead to relapse. If the drug is employed in lower dosage, it should be combined with a luminal amebicide. Luminal amebicides must always be given with the chloroquine-emetine regimen.

A diagnostic trial of metronidazole in patients with suspected amebic liver abscess may lead to serious error because this drug readily inhibits anaerobic bacteria, common causes of pyogenic liver abscess.

Drainage of an amebic abscess usually is not necessary and should be performed only if there is localized swelling over the liver, marked elevation of the diaphragm, severe localized liver tenderness, and failure to respond to systemic amebicides. Adequate drainage can usually be accomplished by needle alone, and surgical drainage is rarely necessary. The greatest hazard in needling an abscess is secondary bacterial infection.

Amebiasis in locations other than the intestine and liver should be treated with emetine or dehydroemetine and a luminal amebicide.

PROGNOSIS Intestinal amebiasis usually responds readily and completely to appropriate drugs. Parasitologic relapses sometimes occur, and posttreatment stools should be checked monthly for 6 months. Repeated relapses, however, are usually a manifestation of reinfection, complicating illness, inadequate therapy, or incorrect diagnosis. The fatality rate is less than 5 percent.

Hepatic and pulmonary amebiasis are still accompanied by an appreciable mortality, but no reliable figures are available.

PREVENTION For the individual, avoidance of contaminated food and water, scalding of vegetables, and the use of iodine-releasing tablets in drinking water (chlorine, in the form of halazone, is ineffective) are important measures. Globaline tablets, containing tetraglycine hydroperiodide, are convenient and effective.

Improvements in general sanitation and the detection of cyst passers and their removal from food-handling duties are general measures in prophylaxis, but such segregation of carriers is rarely practiced.

PRIMARY AMEBIC MENINGOENCEPHALITIS

Primary amebic meningoencephalitis is caused by free-living amebas, usually of the genus *Naegleria.* It most often affects children and young adults, appears to be acquired by swimming in fresh warm water, and is almost invariably fatal.

Free-living amebas are ubiquitous in nature where they are commonly found in soil and water. Although generally considered harmless, some varieties are clearly pathogenic for the central nervous system of mammals. Early reports incriminating *Hartmanella* and *Acanthamoeba* in human meningoencephalitis were based on the morphologic appearance of the trophozoites in histologic preparations. In those instances where the responsible organism has been isolated and cultured, however, it has, with a single exception, been identified as an amoeboflagellate, and has been assigned to the genus *Naegleria.* One isolate has been classified as a slime mold of the order Myxomycetale.

Over 50 cases have been reported from different parts of the world including Australia, Czechoslovakia, Great Britain, New Zealand, and the United States. Most of the cases recognized in this country have occurred in the Southeastern states particularly Florida, Georgia, and Virginia. Characteristically the patients have fallen ill during the summer months approximately one week after swimming in fresh or brackish water. The 16 Czechoslovakian cases followed swimming in an indoor pool with chlorinated water maintained at 24°C, and five cases have been acquired apparently after bathing in hot mineral water. Histologic evidence suggests that the amebas reach the central nervous system directly via the nasal mucosa at the level of the cribriform plate. Clinically, the illness is rapid in onset, brief in duration, and inexorable in course. The initial symptom is a severe, persistent, frontal headache followed by nausea, vomiting, fever, and nuchal rigidity. Unusual tastes or smells may be noted. Later, drowsiness, confusion, convulsions, and coma appear. Focal neurologic findings may occur late in the course of the illness.

A careful examination of the cerebrospinal fluid is the single most helpful diagnostic procedure. The fluid is usually bloody or sanguinopurulent and demonstrates an intense neutrophilic response. The protein is elevated and the glucose diminished. No organisms are demonstrated on Gram's stain or routine culture. Early examination of a wet preparation of unspun spinal fluid will usually reveal viable trophozoites. They are 10 to 20 μm in diameter, possess a granular cytoplasm, a distinct ectoplasm, and bulbous pseudopodia. If the specimen is allowed to cool, the trophozoites may become immobile and more difficult to recognize. Although the amebas may be easily grown on ordinary culture media which have been seeded with coliform bacteria, this is not helpful in clinical management, so rapidly progressive is the disease. Treatment with standard antiprotozoal agents seems completely ineffective. *Naegleria,* however, is highly sensitive to amphotericin B in vitro, and to date the only patient who has survived a *Naegleria* infection was diagnosed early and treated with this agent. Intracisternal, as well as intravenous, administration of amphotericin is probably essential to rapidly obtain effective levels in the cerebrospinal fluid. The intraventricular dose is 0.5 to 1.0 mg for the first few days. The intravenous dose is similar to that for cryptococcal meningitis (Chap. 166).

If the souce of the infection can be determined, further cases might be prevented by closing the area to further bathing.

REFERENCES

Amebiasis

ELSDON-DEW R: The epidemiology of amebiasis. Adv Parasitol 6:1, 1968

HEALY GR: Laboratory diagnosis of amebiasis. Bull NY Acad Med 47:478, 1971

JUMPER K JR et al: Serologic diagnosis of amebiasis. Am J Trop Med Hyg 21:157, 1972

LAMONT NMcE, POALER NR: Hepatic amebiasis. Q J Med 27:389, 1958

MOST H: Drug therapy: Common parasite infections of man. N Engl J Med 287:698, 1972

NEAL RA: Pathogenesis of amebiasis. Bull NY Acad Med 47:462, 1971

WHO EXPERT COMMITTEE: Amebiasis, WHO Tech. Rept. Ser. 421, Geneva, 1969

WILMOT AJ: *Clinical Amebiasis,* Philadelphia: Davis, 1962

Primary amebic meningoencephalitis

BUTT CG: Primary amebic meningoencephalitis. N Engl J Med 274:1473, 1966

CARTER RF: Sensitivity to amphotericin B of a *Naegleria* sp. isolated from a case of primary amebic meningoencephalitis. J Clin Pathol 22:740, 1969

CERVA L, NOVAK K: Amebic meningoencephalitis: Sixteen fatalities. Science 160:92, 1968

DUMA RJ et al: Primary amebic meningoencephalitis caused by

Naegleria. Ann Intern Med 74:861, 1971

GILBERTSON CG et al: Pathogenic *Naegleria* sp.—Study of a strain isolated from human cerebrospinal fluid. J Protozool 15:353, 1968

210 MALARIA

JAMES J. PLORDE

DEFINITION Malaria is a protozoan disease transmitted to man by the bite of *Anopheles* mosquitoes. It remains the major infectious disease problem in the world. The increased import of malaria into the United States by travelers and military personnel in recent years has caused a resurgence of interest in this disease. Malaria is characterized by *rigors, fever, splenomegaly, anemia*, and *a chronic relapsing course*.

ETIOLOGY *The causative organisms are protozoa of the genus Plasmodium.* The four species known to infect man do not produce disease in lower animals, although many species affecting animals and birds are known. *Plasmodium vivax* causes tertian malaria; *P. malariae* causes quartan malaria; *P. falciparum* causes malignant tertian malaria; *P. ovale* causes ovale tertian malaria, a relatively rare and mild illness.

Man is the intermediate and the mosquito the definitive host. In man, after a stage of exoerythrocytic development in the liver, the parasites invade circulating erythrocytes where they reproduce asexually. They first appear in the red cells as ring-shaped trophozoites which later enlarge and assume an irregular or amoeboid shape. Following mitotic division of the nucleus, the organism is known as a *schizont. After several divisions, daughter cells (merozoites) fill the corpuscle, which ruptures and releases them (sporulation) to parasitize additional erythrocytes.* With repetition of this cycle, some of the red cells become filled with *sexual forms (gametocytes)*; these do not induce cell lysis and are unable to undergo further development unless ingested by an appropriate mosquito during a blood meal. In the stomach of the mosquito fertilization occurs, and the resulting *ookinete* encysts on the outer surface of the stomach and releases myriads of *sporozoites*. These migrate to the salivary glands and, if inoculated into a human subject, lead to repetition of asexual multiplication.

The asexual cycle in the erythrocyte requires 36 to 48 hr for *P. falciparum*, 48 hr for *P. vivax* and *P. ovale*, and 72 hr for *P. malariae*. The periodicity of febrile paroxysms in infections by the different species coincides with the cyclic discharge of merozoites. The incubation period between the bite of an infected mosquito and onset of symptoms is 10 to 14 days in vivax and falciparum malaria and 18 days to 6 weeks in quartan infections. The incubation period may be prolonged for weeks or months with certain strains of *P. vivax* and in persons who have taken antimalarial suppressants. Occasionally the infection may remain asymptomatic. There is good evidence of the existence of several strains of each species of human malarial *Plasmodium*, and greater virulence of some strains is suggested by the consistent severity of clinical illness which they produce.

EPIDEMIOLOGY Malaria survives only in areas where the mosquito and the infected human populations remain above a *critical density* for each. These critical densities are interdependent, but either may fluctuate in a given area. Control measures are directed toward reducing both populations to levels that are too low for the infection to survive. Important procedures include drainage or filling of breeding areas, use of residual insecticide sprays (this has largely replaced the use of oil or other antilarval measures), screening, use of skin repellents, effective treatment of cases, and large-scale suppressive drug programs in some human populations.

An active international cooperative program aimed at the eradication of malaria has resulted in a significant decline in the incidence of the disease since 1945. In over three-quarters of the original malarial areas of the world, the disease has been eradicated or active eradication programs have been instituted. The presence of mobile populations, outdoor biting mosquitoes, and high levels of disease transmission make successful eradication in the remaining areas less certain. Furthermore, the emergence of insecticide-resistant mosquitoes and drug-resistant parasites as well as a variety of administrative and socioeconomic problems has produced serious setbacks to several previously successful eradication programs. The demonstration of naturally occurring simian malaria in man has raised the question of an animal reservoir of the disease. Although this may not prove to be a major problem, the global eradication of malaria remains today a distant goal.

Endemic malaria did not disappear from the United States until the 1950s. Imported cases and occasional outbreaks of malaria acquired by mosquito transmission from imported infections (*introduced malaria*) continued to occur, but until 1966 the total never exceeded 200 cases a year. This number rapidly increased with the return of infected military personnel from Southeast Asia, reaching a peak of over 4,000 in 1970. Associated with this wave of imported malaria was a smaller increase in the number of infections induced by blood transfusion and intravenous heroin use. Fortunately this epidemic has now waned, but the continued increase in international travel will ensure the presence of this disease in the United States until malaria is eradicated on a worldwide basis.

PATHOGENESIS AND PATHOLOGY The invasion, alteration, and destruction of red cells by malaria parasites, systemic and local circulatory changes, and immune phenomena are probably all important in the pathophysiology of malaria. Malaria species differ significantly in their ability to invade red cells. *Plasmodium vivax* and *P. ovale* attack only immature erythrocytes; *P. malariae*, only senescent ones. During infection with these species, therefore, no more than 1 or 2 percent of cells are involved at any one time. *Plasmodium falciparum* invades red cells regardless of age and may cause extremely high levels of parasitemia. Only the presence of certain abnormal hemoglobins, notably S, is capable of limiting parasitemia produced by the species. Whether the same protective effect is exerted in hemoglobin C, thalassemia, and glucose 6-phosphate (G-6-PD) deficiency awaits confirmation.

Once parasitized, the cells may be destroyed at the time of sporulation or phagocytosed in the liver or spleen. In the spleen the parasites are also removed from some cells, and the intact erythrocytes are returned into the circulation. However, anemia usually develops, and in the case of falciparum malaria, may be severe. This species also induces physical changes in parasitized cells resulting in intravascular agglutination and sludging.

Although paroxysms of fever coincide with sporulation and the destruction of red cells, the cause of the fever remains obscure and may be related to release of an endogenous pyrogen from injured cells.

The circulatory changes in malaria are characterized by vasoconstriction during the "cold" stage followed by vasodilation during the "hot" stage. In falciparum malaria vasodilation in the skin is accompanied by hypotension, decreased central venous pressure, increased radioiodinated serum albumin space, and increased excretion of aldosterone, suggesting a decrease in effective circulating blood volume due to enhanced vascular permeability and/or capacitance. On the other hand, there may be localized vasospasm, increased capillary permeability with a resulting increase in blood viscosity, obstruction of capillaries with agglutinated red cells, and intravascular coagulation which may compromise perfusion to vital organs such as the kidney, brain, liver, and lung.

Normal as well as parasitized red cells are destroyed in malaria. The explanation for this phenomonon is unknown although immunologic mechanisms have been suggested. The destruction is most profound in blackwater fever where there is massive intravascular hemolysis. More commonly, however, the red cells are sequestered and destroyed in the reticuloendothelial system of the liver and spleen. Immune mechanisms may also be operative in platelet destruction and in renal disease where host gamma- and beta-1C-globulin deposits have been noted along the glomerular capillary basement membrane of patients with the nephrosis of quartan malaria.

Negroes seem to be peculiarly resistant to *P. vivax* infection; the mechanism for this is unknown.

Immunity in malaria is mediated by species-specific IgG and IgM antibodies which appear early in malaria infection in response to the erythrocytic phase of parasitemia. These antibodies have an antiplasmodial effect. The relative rarity of malaria in young infants has been attributed to transplacental passage of IgG antibodies. While immunity in malaria has been thought to be strain specific, different strains appear to share common antigens. Furthermore, there appear to be antigenic changes in the parasites during chronic simian malaria which may provide an explanation for the relapsing course of malarial infection.

MANIFESTATIONS General There is some variation in malaria produced by the different plasmodia, but in all, chills, fever, headache, muscle pains, splenomegaly, and anemia are common. Herpes labialis is frequent and usually appears after the infection is well established. Hepatomegaly, mild icterus, and edema are often observed, especially in falciparum infections. Urticaria is common in patients with chronic malaria.

The hallmark of the disease is the malarial *paroxysm*, which recurs regularly in all but falciparum infections. The typical paroxysm begins with a rigor that lasts 20 to 60 min—the "cold stage"—followed by a "hot stage" of 3 to 8 hr with temperature of 104 to 107°F. The "wet stage" consists of defervescence with profuse diaphoresis and leaves the patient exhausted.

First attacks are often severe, but repeated episodes become milder, although debilitation may be progressive. In untreated cases, the attacks may persist for weeks. The paroxysms eventually become more irregular and less frequent and finally cease, corresponding with the disappearance of parasites from the blood and marking the end of the primary attack. Relapses occur when exoerythrocytic parasites persisting in the liver reinvade the bloodstream.

Tertian malaria (P. vivax or P. ovale) This infection is rarely fatal, although relapses are common, and it is the most difficult to cure. A prodrome of myalgia, headache, chilliness, and low-grade fever for 48 to 72 hr heralds the onset of the acute illness. Initially, the fever may be irregular because the maturation cycle of the parasite is not synchronized. Synchronization usually occurs toward the end of the first week, and typical paroxysms then occur on alternate days. The spleen becomes palpable at the end of the second week. Infections with *P. ovale* tend to be milder, and primary attacks shorter than those caused by *P. vivax*.

Quartan malaria (P. malariae) Paroxysms occur every third day and tend to be regular. The disease is usually more disabling than tertian but responds well to treatment. Edema, albuminuria, and hematuria (*not* hemoglobinuria), a clinical state similar to acute hemorrhagic nephritis, occasionally appear during the course. This complication should not be confused with *black-water fever*. Chronic *P. malariae* infection may be associated with a clinically and histologically unique nephrosis.

Falciparum malaria (P. falciparum) Because of an asynchronous cycle of multiplication, the onset may be insidious and fever continuous, remittent, or irregular. Typical paroxysms occur in a minority of patients. Splenomegaly occurs rapidly and mental confusion, postural hypotension, edema, and gastrointestinal symptoms are common. If the acute attack is treated rapidly, the disease is usually mild and recovery uneventful. If left untreated anemia becomes severe, and the decreased effective circulating blood volume results in capillary blockage that can give rise to serious complications. This feature of *P. falciparum* infections accounts for the protean manifestations of this form of malaria, and the high morbidity and mortality associated with it. Depending upon the organ system involved, several so-called *pernicious syndromes* are seen. *Cerebral malaria* can lead to hemiplegia, convulsions, delirium, hyperpyrexia, coma, and rapid death. When the *pulmonary* circulation is involved, there may be cough and blood-streaked sputum, leading to confusion with many other diseases of the lung. Severe pulmonary insufficiency closely resembling the "shock lung" syndrome frequently accompanies cerebral malaria. The splanchnic capillaries can be obstructed, with consequent vomiting, abdominal pain, diarrhea, or melena. Such patients are sometimes thought to have bacillary dysentery or cholera. Fever in these disorders may be low or absent. Indeed, in patients with predominantly gastrointestinal manifestations, there are usually cold clammy skin, hypotension, profound weakness, and repeated syncopal attacks, so-called *algid malaria.* Tender hepatomegaly, with or without jaundice, and acute renal failure are common. The pernicious syndromes should be anticipated if more than 5 percent of red cells are parasitized.

Blackwater fever This is a disorder that occurs in association with malaria, particularly and perhaps only with *P. falciparum* infections. The usual attack begins with a rigor and fever followed by massive intravascular hemolysis, icterus, hemoglobinuria, collapse, and often acute renal failure and uremia. The pathologic findings in the kidney are necrosis of tubules and occasionally hemoglobin casts. The mortality is 20 to 30 percent, and survivors are very likely to experience hemolytic episodes with subsequent malarial infections.

Although blackwater fever is often classified as one of the "pernicious" complications of falciparum malaria, its etiology is obscure. In many patients, parasitemia is absent at the time hemolysis occurs. Because blackwater fever has usually occurred in patients with chronic falciparum infections who were treated with quinine, it was suggested that the hemolysis results from an autoimmune reaction to the red cells that have been altered by the drug, parasite, or both. However, blackwater fever can occur in patients not given drugs. The institution of an appropriate regimen for acute renal failure (Chap. 269) will reduce the fatality rate considerably.

Complications In addition to the several complications already mentioned, others deserve comment. Rupture of the spleen is relatively rare, but malaria is by far the commonest cause of spontaneous rupture and predisposes to traumatic rupture of this organ.

Chronic malaria or repeated infection in an endemic area leads to anemia, debility, and cachexia. Secondary bacterial infection is often the immediate cause of death. Bacillary dysentery, cholera, and pyogenic pneumonia are common. Tuberculous foci often extend in malarial patients, and miliary tuberculosis is occasionally observed.

Patients living in endemic malarious areas commonly present with chronic hepatosplenomegaly of unknown etiology. In some of these, liver biopsies reveal sinusoidal lymphomatosis, and serologic tests for malaria are positive. Long-term antimalarial therapy leads to a decrease in spleen size and a disappearance of hepatic sinusoidal lymphocytosis. It has been suggested that this syndrome represents an abnormal immune response to malaria. The epidemiologic evidence implicating malaria as a contributory factor in the etiology of Burkitt's lymphoma has increased. It has been suggested that continuous stimulation of the lymphoid system in chronic malaria makes it more susceptible to neoplastic transformation in the presence of EB virus.

LABORATORY FINDINGS The blood leukocyte count is low or normal. The platelet count is often reduced, especially in falciparum malaria. The erythrocyte sedimentation rate is elevated. Plasmodia are demonstrable in smears of peripheral blood from the vast majority of patients with symptomatic malaria. When the disease is suspected, appropriately stained blood films should be examined diligently. For the inexperienced examiner, a thin smear of fingertip blood on a clean glass slide should be stained with Wright's or Giemsa's stain. Parasitized erythrocytes are most frequent at the edges of a smear; extracellular parasites are not found. Thick smears should be thoroughly dried and stained with diluted Giemsa's or Field stain. This method has the advantage of concentrating the parasites, but artifacts are numerous, and correct interpretations of these preparations require much experience.

The morphology of the four species of plasmodia that infect man is specific enough to allow identification in blood smears. The parasitized red cells in *P. vivax* infections are enlarged, pale, and may contain diffuse bright red dots (Schaffner's dots), and the parasite presents in a wide variety of shapes and sizes; in *P. ovale* infections, the red cells containing parasites are oval but otherwise resemble those in *P. vivax*; in *P. malariae* the red cells are of normal size and do not contain dots. The parasites often present in "band" forms and the merozoites are arranged in a rosette around central pigment; in *P. falciparum* infections the rings are very small, may contain two rather than one chromatin dot, and often are found lying flat against the margin of the cell. Only the ring stages of the asexual forms are found in the peripheral smear, and there may be more than one ring in a single red cell. The gametocytes are distinctively large and banana-shaped.

There is no advantage of blood over material obtained by splenic or sternal puncture. The administration of epinephrine with the idea of dislodging parasites by producing contraction of the spleen has been advocated, but results are irregular. Serologic tests are used primarily for epidemiologic rather than diagnostic purposes, but are also helpful in speciation of the infecting organism and in detection of occult malaria in the bloodstream.

DIAGNOSIS The most important diagnostic test is the search for parasites in peripheral blood. Because the intensity of parasitemia varies greatly from hour to hour, particularly in *P. falciparum* infections, blood smears should be examined repeatedly and at frequent intervals. History of residence in an endemic area, previous attacks of malaria, typical malarial paroxysms, or some artificial exposure (blood transfusion, narcotic injections in an addict) should suggest the disease. Splenomegaly is an almost invariable finding during the second week of illness. Leukocytosis is *not* a feature of malaria.

While final cure of malaria may be difficult, particularly in *P. vivax* infections, almost all cases will respond symptomatically to quinine or one of the newer antimalarial drugs, and failure of response to a therapeutic trial argues strongly against the diagnosis.

TREATMENT The use of appropriate chemotherapy can suppress symptoms in individuals exposed in endemic areas or cure malarial infection completely. The emergence of drug-resistant falciparum malaria in Southeast Asia, South America, and adjacent areas of Central America, however, necessitates the use of drug combinations in the treatment of this infection.

Treatment of acute attack Treatment of an acute attack can be accomplished with chloroquine for all types of malaria except drug-resistant falciparum infection. Administration of 0.6 g chloroquine base (four tablets) followed by 0.3 g 6 hr later and then 0.3 g daily for 2 days usually produces complete subsidence of symptoms and destruction of the erythrocytic forms of the parasite. If vomiting is present, chloroquine hydrochloride should be given intramuscularly in dosage of 0.2 to 0.3 g base every 6 hr. Oral therapy should be resumed as soon as possible.

If the patient has contracted malaria in an area known to harbor drug-resistant *P. falciparum*, he should be treated with a combination of quinine, pyrimethamine, and one of the sulfonamides or sulfones. *Quinine sulfate*, 0.6 g orally three times a day, should be given for 10 days. If nausea and vomiting preclude oral therapy, quinine dihydrochloride diluted in saline or glucose can be given very slowly intravenously. The dose may be repeated every 6 hr, but oral therapy should be instituted as soon as possible. In the presence of renal failure, the dose of quinine should be limited to 0.6 g a day. An overdose of quinine produces cinchonism of which tinnitus is an early manifestation. The drug may also cause mild hemolysis, allergic purpura, and drug fever. Pyrimethamine should be given orally in dosage of 25 mg two times daily for 3 days. This is an antifolate agent and may cause megaloblastic anemia. Sulfisoxazole or sulfadiazine, 2.0 g initially and then 0.5 g every 6 hr for 5 days, should be given concurrently with the other two drugs. A variety of other combinations of antifolate agents with sulfonamides or sulfones have also been used alone or with quinine to good effect. The combination of tetracycline (1.0 g per day for 10 days) and quinine has been suggested for the treatment of drug-resistant malaria.

Patients should be followed for 1 month to detect recrudescence of the infection, and if there is evidence of recurrence, retreatment with pyrimethamine and a sulfonamide should be instituted.

Radical cure *Plasmodium vivax, P. ovale*, and *P. malariae* all persist in the liver in the exoerythrocytic stage and in this form are not affected by drugs used in the treatment of the acute attack. Unless destroyed, they will eventually reinvade the bloodstream. Primaquine base 15 mg by mouth daily for 14 days will effect a radical cure in most cases. If relapse occurs after primaquine therapy, a second course of the drug should be given. This agent may cause hemolysis in patients with G-6-PD deficiency, but in the dosage recommended hemolysis is rare and usually mild.

Treatment of complications This includes careful attention to fluid and electrolyte balance, prevention of fluid overload in patients with oliguria, and early diagnosis and treatment of renal failure. In severe hemolysis large doses of steroids may be helpful in combating hemolysis. Transfusions should be given in severe hemolysis, care being taken to match the patient's cells and plasma with those of the recipient. Intravenous, low-molecular weight dextran may be helpful in increasing capillary blood flow in cerebral malaria. Dexamethasone is used in management of cerebral edema. The value of heparin in this syndrome, even when evidence suggestive of intravascular coagulation is present, remains controversial.

Suppressive therapy Although it is not possible to prevent infection with chemotherapeutic agents, it is possible to suppress symptoms while residing in an endemic area by the administration of chloroquine base in dosage of 300 mg weekly (2 tablets Aralen). If the medication is continued for 1 month after leaving the area, sensitive strains of *P. falciparum* will be eradicated. *Plasmodium ovale, P. malariae*, and *P. vivax* will produce clinical manifestations some weeks or months after chloroquine is discontinued because of their persistence outside red cells. This can be circumvented by administration of primaquine after chloroquine is discontinued. Chloroquine is not effective in suppressing drug-resistant *P. falciparum*.

REFERENCES

BLOUNT RE: Management of chloroquine-resistant falciparum malaria. Arch Intern Med 119:557, 1967

CAHILL KM (ed): Symposium on malaria. Bull NY Acad Med 45:997, 1969

HEINEMAN HS: The clinical syndrome of malaria in the United States. Arch Intern Med 129:607, 1972

HENDRICKSE RG et al: Quartan malarial nephrotic syndrome. Lancet 1:1143, 1972

HUNTER GW et al: *A Manual of Tropical Medicine*, 4th ed., Philadelphia: Saunders, 1966

KAGAN IG: Malaria: Seroepidemiology and serologic diagnosis. Exp Parasitol 31:126, 1972

McGREGOR IA: Immunology of malarial infection and its possible consequences. Br Med Bull 28:22, 1972

NEVA FA: Malaria—Recent progress and problems. N Engl J Med 277:1241, 1967

PETERS W: Advances in malariology relating to control and eradication. Br Med Bull 28:28, 1972

211 LEISHMANIASIS

JAMES J. PLORDE

DEFINITION Leishmaniasis designates three separate disorders of man that are produced by protozoa of the genus *Leishmania*. All are transmitted by the bite of sandflies (*Phlebotomus*).

ETIOLOGY AND PATHOGENESIS There is confusion over speciation of *Leishmania*. These organisms appear morphologically identical and must be differentiated by serologic techniques which are not entirely satisfactory. There are antigenic differences among various strains of *Leishmania* species, but the significance of these differences is not known. Four species are generally recognized: *L. donovani*, *L. tropica*, *L. mexicana*, and *L. brasiliensis*. Two others, *L. peruviana* and *L. pifanoi*, are considered by some to be variations of *L. brasiliensis* and *L. mexicana*, respectively.

Leishmania donovani is the cause of kala azar, the visceral form of leishmaniasis.

Leishmania tropica causes Old World cutaneous leishmaniasis or oriental sore, also known as Delhi boil, Bagdad boil, Aleppo button, and Salek and Pendeh sore.

Leishmania mexicana produces a cutaneous leishmaniasis known as forest yaws, bay sore, and *chiclero ulcer*. *Leishmania brasiliensis* is the cause of American mucocutaneous leishmaniasis also known as *espundia*. *Leishmania brasiliensis* (var.) *peruviana* produces *uta*, another type of cutaneous leishmaniasis, and disseminated cutaneous leishmaniasis is caused by *L. pifanoi* in Venezuela and by *L. tropica* in Ethiopia.

In the sandfly, the parasites assume the flagellated leptomonas form, but in man, the organisms lose their flagella, enter mononuclear phagocytes, and multiply as small, rounded leishmanial forms 2 to 3 μm in diameter, the pathognomonic Leishman-Donovan bodies.

In man continued intracellular multiplication of the parasite leads to rupture of the affected phagocyte and invasion of other cells, resulting in extensive histiocytic proliferation which is followed by infiltration with plasma cells and lymphocytes. The course of the disease from this point is apparently determined by the host's immunologic reaction, which is still poorly understood. In cutaneous leishmaniasis the secondary cellular infiltration is associated with a reduction in the number of parasites, the development of a delayed skin (leishmanin) reaction, and spontaneous cure. In the mucocutaneous form, the spontaneous disappearance of the primary lesion may be followed by destructive metastatic mucocutaneous lesions at some later date. An interesting exception to the general pattern in cutaneous disease is disseminated cutaneous leishmaniasis (*leishmaniasis tegumentaria diffusa*) in which there is no infiltration of lymphocytes and plasma cells, the leishmanin reaction is negative, and the skin lesions become chronic, progressive, and disseminated. In visceral leishmaniasis, the cellular changes are similar to those seen in cutaneous disease. However, the skin test remains negative, and the parasites spread to reticuloendothelial cells throughout the body. This spread is associated with development of marked hyperglobulinemia. As in the mucocutaneous form of the disease, circulating antibodies are detectable but do not seem to have a protective function. A positive skin test develops in the visceral form after successful treatment.

KALA AZAR

DISTRIBUTION AND EPIDEMIOLOGY Kala azar occurs in China, Russia, India, the Middle East, Egypt, Sudan, East Africa, several Mediterranean countries, including Greece, Crete, and Malta, and a few areas of South and Central America. Although the manifestations of the disease throughout this area, which touches all continents but Australia, are basically similar, certain definite peculiarities in its behavior justify classification of visceral leishmaniasis into at least three main types. These differences are attributed to variations in the strains of *L. donovani* in a given area and, perhaps more important, to the length of time that the disease has been endemic in a population. It is believed that kala azar (and also infection by *L. tropica*) is introduced into a new area from animal reservoirs and that this "primitive" or zoonotic infection is likely to result in many cases of acute, rapidly fatal illness among the population coming into contact with the parasites for the first time. After generations, kala azar becomes endemic, the disease assumes a more chronic form, and the domestic dog becomes an important reservoir.

Mediterranean, or *infantile, kala azar* is primarily a disease of children under the age of two years and has its reservoir in dogs, but in some areas jackals and foxes also play a part. Adults are by no means spared, but the preceding sentence describes the predominant pattern of the disorder as it occurs in the Mediterranean area, China, Russia, and Latin America.

Indian kala azar shows no special predilection for infants and has never been found in dogs or other animals in India, indicating that the human reservoir is responsible for perpetuation of the disease.

African kala azar shows no predilection for children, is endemic in gerbils and other rodents in many areas, and is more resistant to therapy with antimony compounds than that found in the rest of the world.

MANIFESTATIONS The incubation period varies from 10 days to 1 year but is usually about 3 months. No lesion appears at the site of the infecting bite in most cases, but a primary "chancre" which heals with scarring before the onset of systemic symptoms is commonly noted in the African disease. The organisms multiply extensively in the macrophages of spleen, liver, bone marrow, lymph nodes, and small intestine, accounting for many of the manifestations of the disease. Organisms may be found in the blood for several months before the onset of symptoms.

Fever, which is characterized at times by two daily spikes, may be abrupt or gradual in onset. It persists for 1 to 6 weeks and then disappears, only to reappear at irregular intervals during the course of the illness. Although prostration is absent even during periods of high fever, there is progressive weakness, pallor, weight loss, and tachycardia. Gastrointestinal disturbances are frequent in Indian cases. Physical findings include enormous splenomegaly, lymphadenopathy, hepatomegaly, and often edema, which tends to conceal the extent of the wasting. Mucocutaneous lesions similar to those seen in espundia occur in the African form of the disease. Anemia is the rule, and thrombocytopenia with gingival and other mucosal bleeding is common. The peripheral leukocyte count is low (usually less than 4,000 per mm^3); in children, agranulocytosis with cancrum oris (noma) and secondary pulmonary or intestinal infections contribute to the high mortality. The presence of a short erythrocyte life span, anti–red cell antibodies, positive Coombs test, and antibody against white cells and platelets suggests an autoimmune basis for the pancytopenia.

Hypergammaglobulinemia is universally present. Proteinuria and hematuria are frequent in the course of kala azar, and symptoms of heart failure can occur terminally; uremia due to renal amyloidosis may complicate chronic cases.

DIAGNOSIS The diagnosis is made by finding *leishmania* organisms in stained preparations of blood (often possible in Indian but rarely so in other forms), bone marrow, lymph nodes, or material obtained by splenic puncture. The last is the best source of organisms, but the spleen should be needled only when it is firm and enlarged well below the left costal margin. The organisms will grow out as flagellated forms in Nicolle-Novy-MacNeal (NNN) medium containing defibrinated rabbit blood incubated at 22°C.

A complement fixation test using an antigen from *Mycobacterium phlei* gives positive results in 95 percent of patients with kala azar, but tuberculosis gives positive test results also. Fluorescent antibody and indirect hemagglutination tests with leishmanial antigens are more specific but are not generally available. The leishmanin skin test is negative during active kala azar but becomes positive several months after successful treatment of the disease.

TREATMENT Rest, good diet, transfusions, and treatment of complicating infections, of which tuberculosis, bacterial pneumonia, amebiasis, and bacillary dysentery are the more important, must supplement or precede specific therapy. Pentavalent antimony compounds are highly effective against the parasites. Owing to its lack of toxicity, Pentostam (sodium antimony gluconate) given intravenously or intramuscularly is the drug of choice. The adult dose is 0.6 g (6 ml) daily for 6 days in Indian kala azar and for 30 days in other forms. Neostibosan (ethylstibamidine) can also be used. Urea stibamine is popular in India.

More than 90 percent of cases respond promptly to antimony, except in Africa, where the cure rate is as low as 70 percent. Resistant cases can be treated with the more toxic diamidines. Pentamidine is given intramuscularly in the dose of 4 mg of base per kg body weight dissolved in 3 to 4 ml water daily for 10 days. The course may be repeated twice after intervals of 10 days. Hypotension, hypoglycemia, and diabetes mellitus can complicate therapy with this drug. The more effective hydroxystilbamidine is given intravenously in 10 daily injections of a fresh solution in dosage of 0.25 g daily. The course may have to be repeated in African kala azar. Amphotericin B has been effective in some cases.

POST–KALA AZAR DERMAL LEISHMANIASIS Patients treated successfully with antimony compounds for kala azar may later develop cutaneous lesions called *leishmanoids*, in which *Leishmania* are demonstrable. These are rare in Mediterranean or Chinese kala azar. They occur after a latent period of 1 to 2 years in as many as 10 percent of Indian cases, and in 30 percent of Sudanese cases, they occur almost immediately after systemic symptoms subside. The lesions range from patchy areas of depigmentation to erythematous papules and confluent nodules which may involve the ears and mucous membranes and have been mistaken for leprosy.

Antimony will cure these dermal leishmanoids, but the response is slow.

PROGNOSIS AND CONTROL The mortality in untreated kala azar is 95 percent in adults and 80 percent in children. This has been greatly reduced by treatment with antimony and the aromatic diamidines. Relapses, occasionally several in number, occur in 5 to 15 percent of African and Mediterranean cases up to 2 years after treatment. They should be re-treated in the same fashion as the initial illness.

The treatment of the disease in man, the elimination of diseased dogs, and the use of DDT residual sprays against sandflies are the important preventive measures. Incidence of the disease has diminished greatly in many areas where DDT has been used to eradicate malaria—an unexpected added benefit of this program. When the vectors are exophilic, control is difficult. Attempts at vaccination with avirulent strains of *L. donovani* have been unsuccessful.

AMERICAN CUTANEOUS LEISHMANIASIS

These diseases occur in every country of Central and South America except Chile. In some areas, 10 to 20 percent of the population are infected. There are four varieties of American cutaneous leishmaniasis. All begin with a local lesion at the site of the infecting sandfly bite after an incubation period of from 10 days to 3 months.

Chiclero ulcer, which is found in Mexico, Guatemala, British Honduras, and possibly other parts of Central America, is a zoonosis caused by *L. mexicana*. The disease occurs naturally in several arboreal rodents. It is occasionally transmitted to men entering forests to harvest chicle. In immunocompetent individuals, it is a relatively mild infection characterized by a single cutaneous lesion on the ear, face, or hand which is chronic and shows little tendency to ulceration. The leishmanin skin test is positive. Spontaneous healing usually occurs within 6 months. The parasites are never numerous in the lesions. Mucosal ulceration does not occur. Ear lesions cause extensive destruction of the pinna and should be treated with a single 350 mg intramuscular dose of cycloguanil pamoate. Immunization with live cultures of *L. mexicana* has been effective in forest workers.

Uta, which occurs in cooler climates and at altitudes of more than 2,000 ft, consists of single or multiple skin ulcers in which parasites are readily demonstrable. Spontaneous healing within 3 months to a year is the rule, and mucosal spread is unusual. The etiologic agent is *L. peruviana*, and the reservoir is the domestic dog. With widespread use of insecticides in Peru, the disease has almost disappeared.

In tropical Latin America, *L. brasiliensis* causes the better-known and more serious *espundia*. The organism causes a natural infection in large forest rodents and is transmitted to man by sandflies when new settlements are made in jungle areas. The initial skin lesion enlarges progressively, and secondary bacterial infection is frequent. The disease may spread by direct extension or by lymphatics to the mucosal surfaces of the mouth and nose where, after the primary lesion has healed, painful, destructive, and multilating erosions scar and distort the involved structures. Fever, anemia, and weight loss accompany these mucosal complications. Destruction of the nasal septum produces a characteristic deformity called *tapir nose* or *camel nose*. The hard palate may be destroyed, and largyngeal erosion can lead to aphonia. In Negroes, the lesion is often hypertrophic, and large polypoid masses deform the lips and cheeks, perhaps representing a type of keloid reaction. This can be mistaken for South American blastomycosis (Chap. 167). Secondary bacterial infection, inanition, and respiratory obstruction lead to death.

The diagnosis is made by finding the organisms in scrapings or by culture. The leishmanin skin test is specific and highly useful. Treatment consists of antibiotics for bacterial infections and pentavalent antimonials used as in kala azar. Cases that fail to respond to antimonials often respond to pyrimethamine, 25 mg by mouth daily for 2 weeks. The course may be repeated twice after an interval of 1 week. Folic acid should be given concurrently. Amphotericin B has also been used with some success in resistant infections.

The early lesions respond well, but even with repeated courses of antimony the mucosal complications of the espundia type heal slowly. In advanced cases, the prognosis is very poor. Diffuse cutaneous leishmaniasis apparently results from a specific deficiency of cell-mediated immunity to leishmanial antigen. In South America it is most commonly caused by *L. pifanoi*, but other New World *Leishmania* organisms have occasionally been implicated. In Ethiopia, the disease is caused by *L. tropica*. This remarkable disease is characterized by massive dissemination of skin lesions without visceral involvement. The clinical picture often bears a striking resemblance to lepromatous leprosy (Chap. 157). The diagnosis is not difficult because the lesion contains a large number of organisms. In contrast to all other types of cutaneous leishmaniasis, the leishmanin skin test is negative. The disease is progressive and very refractory to treatment. Amphotericin B and pentamidine have been used to reduce remissions, but cure is rare.

OLD WORLD CUTANEOUS LEISHMANIASIS: ORIENTAL SORE

This, the least serious form of human leishmaniasis, consists of localized cutaneous ulceration which heals spontaneously and is endemic in the European countries bordering the eastern Mediterranean, in North Africa, Asia Minor, Southwest Asia, and India. Two major strains of the causative organism, *L. tropica*, produce similar but distinctive clinical syndromes. Homologous immunity after recovery from infection by either strain is solid and lifelong. Infection with *L. tropica* (var.) *major* protects against *L. tropica* (var.) *minor*, but the opposite is not the case. The rural or moist type, caused by (var.) *major*, has its reservoir in gerbils and other small rodents; the ulcers usually appear on the extremities 2 to 6 weeks after the bite of the sandfly and are accompanied by regional lymphadenopathy in a majority of cases. Spontaneous healing occurs within 3 to 6 months, leaving a depigmented, pitted scar.

The incubation period in the *urban*, or *dry*, type ranges from 2 months to more than a year. The lesion is usually facial and begins as a pruritic, purplish nodule (the Aleppo button), which slowly enlarges and finally breaks down after 3 or 4 months. Healing of the indolent, granulomatous ulcer may require a year or more; lymphatic involvement is uncommon. Man and the domestic dog serve as the reservoirs of infection.

The typical oriental sore is a sharply punched-out, ragged ulcer about 1 in. in diameter, surrounded by an erythematous rim. Satellite lesions which fuse with the original are not rare. The center of the granulating base of the ulcer frequently contains a hard excrescence called the *Montpellier sign* or the *rake* beneath which the parasites are most likely to be found when scrapings are examined.

The wet and dry types occur together in Asia Minor; indeed, it is not rare to find simultaneous infections in the same patient. In Africa, Southeastern Europe, and India, only the dry type is prevalent.

Diagnosis is usually made on clinical grounds and is confirmed by finding the parasites, which occur both intra- and extracellularly. Pyogenic infection makes direct visualization difficult, but *L. tropica* can be cultured in NNN medium at room temperature, and a skin test using *L. tropica* antigen becomes positive in the vast majority of patients with the disease.

Treatment should include vigorous measures for bacterial infection, such as hot soaks and appropriate systemic antibiotics. Infrared heat treatment has also been suggested, as the leishmanial organisms are very heat sensitive. Systemic antimonials may be required where ulceration is extensive or multiple. Pentostam is used as in kala azar in a course of 10 daily injections totaling 6 g. It may be injected locally in dosage of 0.6 g three to four times on alternate days. In endemic areas the custom is to withhold treatment directed against the parasite until the initial nodule ulcerates, to assure the development of immunity against reinfection.

Prevention consists of use of insect repellents on exposed parts of the body, residual DDT sprays, and fine-mesh screening for dwellings. The lesions should be covered to prevent infection of vectors and, of course, contact with the lesion or its discharges should be avoided.

In Asia Minor, a relapsing form known as *leishmaniasis recidiva* is common. Nodules appear at the periphery of the scarred area and mimic lupus vulgaris so closely that errors in diagnosis are very frequent.

REFERENCES

BRAY RS: Leishmaniasis in the Old World. Br Med Bull 28:39, 1972

BRYCESON ADM: Diffuse cutaneous leishmaniasis in Ethiopia. Trans R Soc Trop Med Hyg 64:369, 1970

CONVIT J, KERDEL-VEGAS F: Disseminated cutaneous leishmaniasis. Arch Dermatol 91:439, 1965

HUNTER GW et al: *A Manual of Tropical Medicine*, 4th ed., Philadelphia: Saunders, 1966

LAINSON R, SHAW JJ: Leishmaniasis of the New World: Taxonomic problems. Br Med Bull 28:44, 1972

MAEGRATH BG, GILES HM: *Management and Treatment of Tropical Diseases*. Oxford: Blackwell Scientific Publications, Ltd., 1971

WOODRUFF AW et al: The anemia of kala azar. Br J Haematol 22:319, 1972

212 TRYPANOSOMIASIS

JAMES J. PLORDE

SLEEPING SICKNESS

DEFINITION African trypanosomiasis or sleeping sickness is a disease caused by the hemoflagellate *Trypanosoma brucei*, which is transmitted to man by several species of tsetse fly belonging to the genus *Glossina*. Clinically, the untreated disease is characterized by an acute febrile lymphadenopathy followed, after a variable period, by a chronic lethal meningoencephalomyelitis. It occurs in two principal epidemiologic patterns: Gambian or Mid- and West African sleeping sickness, and Rhodesian or East African sleeping sickness.

ETIOLOGY Trypanosomes are fusiform protozoa recognized by an undulating membrane which extends along the length of the cell and terminates in an anterior flagellum. The morphologic characteristics of many varieties are so nearly identical that they are distinguishable only by their pathogenicity for certain animals, differences in biochemical requirements, and ability to multiply in insects. *Trypanosoma brucei* strains are polymorphic organisms varying in shape from slender to stumpy and in length from 8 to 30 μm. The slender forms have a long flagellum that in the shorter types is rudimentary or absent. The Gambian and Rhodesian forms of sleeping sickness were previously thought to be caused by two distinct species of trypanosomes, *T. gambiense* and *T. rhodesiense*. It is felt now, however, that they, along with the animal trypanosome responsible for *nagana* in cattle, are all variants of a single species. The individual varieties are referred to as *T. brucei gambiense*, *T. brucei rhodesiense*, and *T. brucei brucei*.

Trypanosomiasis in animals is a great economic problem in many parts of the world. It is probable that an area of approximately 4 million square miles in Africa is not populated because of the impossibility of keeping animals in sites where tsetse flies are infected with trypanosomes.

EPIDEMIOLOGY Gambian sleeping sickness occurs in tropical, West, and Central Africa extending from the Sahara to the Kalahari Deserts and east to the Rift Valley. Rhodesian trypanosomiasis is found in tropical East Africa from Ethiopia in the north to Botswana in the south.

Transmission of the trypanosomes of sleeping sickness occurs by what is referred to as the "anterior station." After ingestion by a feeding tsetse, the parasites first develop in the intestine of the fly and then migrate to the salivary glands where they are discharged when the host is bitten. In some situations it is possible that the trypanosomes can be mechanically transmitted from host to host by the tsetse and other hematophagous arthropods. This may be of importance during epidemics.

The Gambian strains of *T. brucei* are transmitted mainly by *G. palpalis* and *G. tachinaides*. These species live in shaded areas near water. Less than 5 percent of the flies are infected even in the most notorious endemic focuses. Although *G. palpalis* and *G. tachinaides* are not exclusively anthropophilic, man is thought to be the only reservoir for Gambian sleeping sickness.

Rhodesian sleeping sickness, on the other hand, is primarily a zoonosis. It is transmitted to man from antelope by the bite of *G. morsitans*, a savannah tsetse. It is seen typically in men who travel away from their villages to hunt or fish. Domestic cattle and sheep may also serve as reservoirs, and man-fly-man transmission can occur.

PATHOLOGY AND PATHOGENESIS The tsetse fly inoculates the organism into the subcutaneous pool of blood that forms during its feeding. Some of the parasites may reach the bloodstream directly, but most remain at the site of inoculation where they multiply to produce a local chancre. Following the appearance of this lesion, the trypanosomes spread through tissue spaces and lymphatics, eventually spilling over into the general circulation where they continue to multiply by longitudinal fission. The parasitemia is of low intensity and typically occurs in waves; each wave disappears with the production of antibody to an exoantigen of the protozoan and reappears when a new antigenic variant arises. These waves of parasitemia, which are accompanied by fever and a mononuclear leukocytosis, tend to become more infrequent and irregular in the later stages of the disease. At some time during this stage of dissemination, trypanosomes localize in the tissues of the central nervous system. This is first manifested as a diffuse leptomeningitis and later by a perivascular cerebritis. If untreated, this parenchymal inflammation gives rise to a demyelinating panencephalitis. Leishmanial or short forms have been demonstrated in experimental *T. brucei* infections suggesting that this organism has an intracellular tissue phase in its developmental cycle. This could be of significance in occult infections.

The mechanism by which the trypanosome elicits tissue damage is unknown. It has been suggested that antigen-antibody reactions lead to the release of kinins. The release of proteolytic enzymes by degenerating phagocytes may be important. The parasitemia stimulates the production of large quantities of IgM immunoglobulin, perhaps in response to the rapid antigenic variation of the parasite.

CLINICAL MANIFESTATIONS The Gambian and Rhodesian forms of sleeping sickness differ somewhat in symptoms, severity, and duration. Rhodesian trypanosomiasis is the more acute and severe of the two forms, usually terminating fatally within a year. Fever is higher, emaciation more rapid, and lymphatic involvement less evident. Death from intercurrent infections or myocarditis usually occurs before the typical sleeping sickness syndrome appears. In the Gambian variety there are often successive bouts of clinical activity with intervening latent periods that persist for a number of years. The early stages may be mild and the disease may go unrecognized until the central nervous system is involved. In both forms of the disease, however, an entry lesion, a febrile period of dissemination, and a stage of central nervous system involvement are found to some degree. The *trypanosomal chancre* appears as an erythematous nodule at the site of inoculation 2 or 3 days after the bite of an infected fly. It may occur anywhere in the body but is most commonly seen on the head or limbs and is accompanied by regional lymphadenopathy. The lesion, which subsides spontaneously, is noted more frequently in Rhodesian sleeping sickness, perhaps because of the acute nature of the disease.

The incubation period is usually about two weeks, but in *T. brucei gambiense* infections may be several years. Systemic manifestations generally become apparent during the hematogenous dissemination of the trypanosomes. In the usual case the patient develops a high remittent fever, severe headache, insomnia, and inability to concentrate. In Caucasians a characteristic circinate erythema resembling erythema marginatum is frequent. Transient firm areas of painful subcutaneous edema localized to the hands, feet, and periorbital tissues may appear. All these signs and symptoms may disappear and reappear intermittently over a period of months to years. Tender lymphadenopathy with gradual induration of the nodes and splenomegaly are almost invariably present in Gambian sleeping sickness. The lymph nodes of the posterior cervical triangle are frequently prominent. This is referred to as *Winterbottom's sign.* Eventually the parasites enter the central nervous system. This may occur early in the course of the disease or may be delayed for as long as 8 years. Cerebral trypanosomiasis can be explosive, causing repeated convulsions or deep coma and death within a few days. Most patients show gradual progression to the classic picture of *sleeping sickness.* The patient develops a vacant expression, the eyelids droop, the lower lip hangs loosely, and it becomes more and more difficult to gain his attention or prod him to any activity. Patients will eat when offered food, but they never ask for it or engage in spontaneous conversation, and speech gradually becomes blurred and indistinct. Tremors of the hands and tongue, choreiform movements, seizures with transient paralysis, loss of sphincter control, ophthalmoplegia, extensor plantar responses, and finally death in coma, status epilepticus, or from hyperpyrexia follows inexorably.

Death may also occur from intercurrent infection, of which bacillary and amebic dysentery, malaria, and bacterial (often pneumococcal) pneumonia are the most important.

DIAGNOSIS AND LABORATORY FINDINGS *Anemia* and *hypermacroglobulinemia* are invariably present, and spontaneous clumping of erythrocytes in blood specimens is grossly evident in many cases. The sedimentation rate is rapid, and peripheral monocytosis is frequent. When there has been invasion of the central nervous system, the *cerebrospinal fluid* shows mononuclear pleocytosis and increased protein concentration. The protein concentration is a better index of severity of disease and therapeutic response than the number of cells. The presence of IgM in the spinal fluid is almost pathognomonic of cerebral trypanosomiasis.

The definitive diagnosis depends upon finding the trypanosomes in the blood, aspirate of lymph node, or cerebrospinal fluid. These should be examined first in wet mounts; actively motile organisms are seen easily under high power. For final identification thin and thick blood films should be stained with Wright's or Giemsa's stain. If the blood smears are negative, citrated blood should be centrifuged at 1,000 rpm for 10 min, the supernatant (including the leukocytes) recentrifuged at 2,000 rpm for 15 min, and the sediment examined. Cerebrospinal fluid should be centrifuged at 2,000 rpm for 15 min before examination. Alternatively the blood and spinal fluid may be centrifuged in a heparinized capillary tube at 12,000 rpm for 4 min and the tubes examined under a microscope using a 10-power objective. The trypanosomes are found at the junction of the plasma and buffy layer in centrifuged blood and near the sealed end of the tube in centrifuged spinal fluid. If these methods are negative, rats or mice may be inoculated and examined after several weeks. A severalfold increase in IgM globulins in the serum is of confirmatory value. Complement fixation and indirect fluorescent antibody tests utilizing stable antigens are useful in endemic areas.

TREATMENT *Suramin* (Bayer 205, Antrypol) is the most effective agent before central nervous system involvement has occurred. The initial dose should be limited to 0.2 g intravenously because of possible idiosyncrasy. If there is no evidence of sensitivity, a full course of therapy can be instituted the following day. One gram (10 ml of a fresh 10% solution) is given intravenously on the first, third, seventh, fourteenth, and twenty-first days for a total of 5 g. If red cells, casts, or significant amounts of protein occur in the urine, therapy should be discontinued. Pentamidine given in water intramuscularly each day for 10 injections is also effective in early disease. The dose is 3 to 4 mg pentamidine base per kg for each injection. When the agent is given too rapidly by the intravenous route, it may cause hypotension.

Lumbar puncture should always be performed in patients who are about to undergo therapy for trypanosomiasis. If the central nervous system is involved, agents that will penetrate the blood-brain barrier must be used; for this purpose the most effective agent is *melarsoprol* (Mel B). This drug, an arsenic derivative of British anti-lewisite (BAL), is effective at all stages of the disease but is more toxic than suramin. It is given intravenously in a 3.6 percent solution. The initial dose is 0.5 ml. Each subsequent dose is increased by 0.5 ml until the maximum single dose of 5.0 ml is reached. The first three doses are given at daily intervals followed by a

7-day rest. This schedule is repeated until a total of 37.5 ml has been given over a period of 1 month. If signs of arsenic toxicity occur, the drug should be discontinued. A reactive encephalopathy, probably due to the release of trypanosomal antigen, may occur early in the course of treatment. Pretreatment with suramin may help avert this complication. A hemorrhagic encephalopathy, a direct arsenic toxic reaction, may also occur and is usually fatal. BAL may be of some use in this situation.

Nitrofurazone can also be given for cerebral trypanosomiasis in an oral dose of 0.5 g three times a day for 7 days, but is more toxic than melarsoprol, and it should not be used unless the patients have failed to respond to this drug. The increasing incidence of drug-resistant parasites has limited the usefulness of *tryparsamide* in the treatment of certain *T. brucei gambiense* infections.

PROGNOSIS The disease is probably always fatal if untreated. If the infection is treated with suramin prior to central nervous system involvement, the cure rate is high and recovery is rapid and complete. When the nervous system becomes involved, the prognosis is less bright, and in far-advanced disease the survivors may suffer neurologic damage. Relapses may occur, particularly following treatment with suramin, if the central nervous system was already involved at the time therapy was instituted. Less commonly they may be the result of drug resistance. Examination of the spinal fluid 6 and 12 months after therapy, or earlier if symptoms recur, is helpful in detecting relapse. Such patients must be retreated with a second therapeutic agent.

PREVENTION Personal protection is best achieved by the use of repellents and protective clothing. A single intramuscular injection of pentamidine in dosage of 3 to 4 mg base per kg (maximum 300 mg) will protect against the Gambian form of disease for 6 months or more; its usefulness in Rhodesian trypanosomiasis is controversial. Because of the danger of cryptic infections occurring during chemoprophylaxis, it has been generally restricted to mass prophylactic campaigns. Other methods of disease control include clearing vegetation and the use of insecticides.

CHAGAS' DISEASE

DEFINITION American trypanosomiasis is an infection caused by *Trypanosoma cruzi* that is characterized by chronic cardiac and gastrointestinal sequelae.

ETIOLOGY *Trypanosoma cruzi* circulates in the blood as a slender, fusiform hemoflagellate measuring 20 μm in length. In stained preparations, its narrow undulating membrane, large kinetoplast, and characteristic C shape are easily recognized. Unlike the trypanosomes of sleeping sickness, it does not multiply within the bloodstream. After invading tissue cells, it loses its undulating membrane and flagellum, assumes its leishmania form, and divides by binary fission. Eventually, new flagellated forms are produced which reenter the general circulation to initiate another cycle.

EPIDEMIOLOGY This infection is found from Chile and Argentina to Mexico, where it affects more than 7 million people. *Trypanosoma cruzi* has been found in insect vectors and wild animals in several areas of the southern United States, but few authenticated cases are known in which the disease was acquired in this country.

The disease is transmitted to man by reduviid ("assassin" or "kissing") bugs, primarily those of the genera *Triatoma, Panstrongylus*, and *Rhodnius*. These winged, hematophagous insects can be found in the burrows of animals and in the cracks and thatch of poorly constructed rural dwellings. The insect attacks man at night, usually biting the face at the mucocutaneous junction (most frequently the lip or outer canthus of the eye). The flagellated trypanosomes are ingested by the bug while feeding, and after multiplying and developing in the midgut of the insect for 8 to 10 days, are discharged in the feces; infection in man occurs through contamination of the bite wound. This is referred to as transmission by the "posterior station." The reduviid may remain infected as long as 2 years.

Man, domestic animals (cats and dogs), and wild animals, especially the opossum and armadillo, may serve as reservoirs for the infection. The close association of man, domestic animals, and the vector within human dwellings is of prime epidemiologic importance, but the disease is occasionally transmitted by a blood transfusion and via the placenta to newborns.

PATHOGENESIS AND CLINICAL MANIFESTATIONS A local inflammatory reaction, manifested clinically as an erythematous nodule or *chagoma*, appears within a few days at the site of inoculation of the protozoan. If, as is commonly the case, the portal of entry has been the conjunctiva, the presenting manifestations are a unilateral, painless conjunctivitis, palpebral edema, and preauricular lymphadenopathy (Romaña's sign). This primary complex may persist for 1 to 2 months during which parasites can be demonstrated in the lesion.

Following an incubation period of 2 weeks, trypanosomal forms reach the general circulation, producing a parasitemia and initiating the acute phase of the illness. After circulating in the blood for some time, the trypanosomes invade tissue cells, and, in the leishmanial form, multiply, producing intracellular pseudocysts. In 4 to 6 days these pseudocysts rupture, releasing both leishmanial and newly formed trypanosomal organisms. The leishmanial forms disintegrate, eliciting an intense inflammatory reaction, while the trypanosomal forms regain the bloodstream to maintain the infection and invade new tissues, particularly the heart, skeletal muscle, smooth muscle, and nervous system.

Clinically, the patient experiences a continuous or recurrent fever, generalized lympadenopathy, hepatosplenomegaly, and in some cases extensive gelatinous edema of the face and trunk. A transient morbilliform or urticarial skin eruption may occur early in the acute phase. Rarely, in newborns and young children, an acute meningoencephalitis may complicate the acute illness. Myocarditis characterized by tachycardia and electrocardiographic changes is very common. In severe cases, there may be conduction disturbances, cardiac dilatation, and heart failure. The duration of the acute illness is variable. When meningoencephalitis or severe heart disease is present, the outcome may be fatal in a few days or weeks. Most often it resolves slowly over a period of several weeks. Parasites become extremely scanty in both the tissues and blood, and the patient remains asymptomatic until the onset of the chronic phase 1 or 2 years later. Most patients presenting with late manifestations, however, deny a history of acute illness, suggesting that subclinical infections often result in chronic disease. It is generally thought that late manifestations are neuropathies caused by the destruction of ganglionic nerve cells during the acute phase of the disease and resulting in the dilatation and malfunction of the affected organs.

The most important late manifestation is heart disease which may affect as many as 10 percent of the rural population in endemic areas. Symptoms and signs range from arrhythmias and heart block to chronic congestive heart failure (predominantly right sided). Thromboembolic phenomena and sudden cardiac arrest are relatively common. At autopsy the hearts of patients with Chagas' disease may show a peculiar herniation of the endocardium through the apical muscle bundles. Megacolon and megaesophagus are sequelae frequently seen in southern South America, but they are less common in Central America and in northern South America.

DIAGNOSIS The diagnosis depends on the demonstration of *T. cruzi* in the patient or upon serologic tests. In the acute phase of the disease the parasite may be seen in the peripheral blood by means of the same direct methods described for African trypanosomiasis. If these are negative, blood may be cultured in Nicolle-Novy-MacNeal (NNN) medium or inoculated into rats, mice, or guinea pigs.

Trypanosoma cruzi is easily grown in blood broth incubated at 28°C. The technique of *xenodiagnosis* is often used in endemic areas; a laboratory-reared vector, known to be parasite-free, is allowed to feed on suspected cases, and 2 weeks later, the insect's intestinal contents are examined for parasites. Confusion sometimes arises from the finding of trypanosomes in blood. Many children in Venezuela and other South American countries are infected with a harmless species, *T. rangeli,* which produces no symptoms but may be present in the blood for many months. By utilization of both culture and xenodiagnosis repeatedly, organisms can be recovered from most acute cases and from up to 40 percent of chronic ones. Biopsy of an involved lymph node or calf muscle may reveal the organism during the initial illness when the parasites cannot be recovered from the blood. The Machado-Guerreiro test (a complement fixation reaction) is most helpful in the diagnosis of chronic cases and in survey work. Fluorescent antibody and hemagglutination inhibition tests appear useful.

TREATMENT AND PREVENTION There is *no specific treatment* for Chagas' disease. Prevention consists of using residual insecticide sprays—of which benzene hexachloride (BHC) is the most effective—on the walls of houses, the main habitat of the vectors. Reinfestation, however, may occur within a year or two of spraying.

REFERENCES

Barrett-Connor E: Chemoprophylaxis of amebiasis and African trypanosomiasis. Ann Intern Med 77:797, 1972

Goodwin LG: The apthology of African trypanosomiasis. Trans R Soc Trop Med Hyg 64:797, 1970

Hunter GW et al: *A Manual of Tropical Medicine,* 4th ed., Philadelphia: Saunders, 1966

Kaberle F: Chagas' disease and Chagas' syndromes: The pathology of American trypanosomiasis. Adv Parasitol 6:63, 1968

Maegrath BG, Giles HM: *Management and Treatment of Tropical Diseases,* Oxford: Blackwell Scientific Publications, Ltd., 1971

Mulligan HW (ed): *The African Trypanosomiasis,* London: Allen & Irwin, 1970

Tumsden WHR: Trypanosomiasis. Br Med Bull 28:34, 1972

WHO: Comparative studies of American and African trypanosomiasis, Tech. Rept Ser. 411, Geneva, 1969

213 TOXOPLASMOSIS

HARRY A. FELDMAN

DEFINITION Toxoplasmosis is caused by *Toxoplasma gondii,* an obligate intracellular protozoan parasite which is widely distributed among mammals and birds. In man it produces either acquired (usually asymptomatic) or congenital infections.

HISTORY Although *Toxoplasma* was first demonstrated in 1908, it was not proved to cause human disease until 1939 when several cases of fatal neonatal encephalomyelitis were shown to have resulted from congenital infections with this parasite. The development of the dye, complement fixation, and other serologic procedures as well as the skin test led to the observation that *Toxoplasma* frequently infects man and animals and that human congenital toxoplasmosis represents only one segment of this disease.

ETIOLOGY *Toxoplasma gondii,* a protozoon, is a coccidian of cats. All strains are antigenically similar, and there is only one species. Trophozoites measuring about 2 by 5 μm and appearing crescentic, oval, or round may be found free in tissues, but usually move through the host within cells. They divide by endogamy and are best stained with either Wright's or Giemsa's stain. Toxoplasma is unique in that it can infect any nucleated cell of any warm-blooded animal. Parasites can be maintained in mice, tissue cultures, or embryonated eggs, but require living cells in whose cytoplasm they multiply. Under special conditions toxoplasma can be frozen and stored, but ordinary freezing kills them. They remain alive in cysts in any tissue, but especially muscle and the central nervous system. These cysts do not calcify, have a sharply demarcated elastic surrounding membrane, and may reach 100 μm in size with thousands of zoites.

Following the ingestion of toxoplasma cysts in meat or oocysts from cat feces, susceptible cats acquire infections, antibodies, and immunity. Such material is infective for other animals as well, but in the cat (and at least some other Felidae) schizogonic and gametogonic cycles follow in their intestinal epithelium. Subsequently, oocysts containing two sporocysts are excreted which on maturation develop into four sporozoites resembling trophozoites. Sporocysts are shed for about one to two weeks but are not infectious until exposed to temperature, air, and moisture conditions which permit sporulation. This usually requires 1 to 5 days. Under suitable humidity and temperature, oocysts can retain their infectivity for a year or more, but they are killed by drying, boiling water, and certain chemicals. Oocysts have not been identified in animals other than Felidae.

EPIDEMIOLOGY Serologic surveys indicate that toxoplasma infections are worldwide in distribution. With the dye test, the most sensitive indicator of specific antibody, it was demonstrated that approximately 33 percent of the inhabitants of several American cities, 63 percent of Hondurans, and 70 percent of Tahitian natives had positive tests as compared with 1 percent of residents of several islands off the northern coast of Australia and 4 percent of Navajo Indians. Among American military recruits, marked differences were found in the prevalence of antibodies among those originating in different areas of the United States. While 20 percent of East Coast recruits were positive, only 3 and 8 percent, respectively, from the Mountain and Pacific Coast regions reacted similarly. Overall, 14 percent of the American recruits had antibodies in comparison with 51 and 56 percent, respectively, of Colombian and Brazilian recruits.

Two longitudinal studies of seroconversion in American families were especially informative. In a Cleveland population, it was found during a 10-year observation period that only four individuals who had no indirect hemagglutinating antibodies at the start acquired them subsequently. During a 4-year period, three persons in a group of Syracuse families had seroconversions (dye test), or 1 in 2,392 person-months of observation. In neither study was an associated clinical illness identified.

In animal surveys, cats, dogs, goats, guinea pigs, sheep, swine, rabbits, pigeons, and many others have been found to have different prevalences of positive tests. Many wild animals are infected. These surveys show that *Toxoplasma* infections are frequent in man and animals, but that their prevalence varies considerably from place to place and in different species in the same general locale.

The pathways whereby man and animals acquire *Toxoplasma* generally are unknown. Human-to-human transfer seems not to occur except from mother to fetus. Rarely, it has followed organ transplantation or the transfusion of fresh blood. It long has been known that animals can acquire parasites by cannibalizing others which are infected. This also may apply to man because children without antibodies frequently acquire them following the ingestion of undercooked mutton and beef; no clinical illnesses were noted. However, this would not explain the route by which herbivores acquire *Toxoplasma*. Human infections are contracted in all seasons, usually with equal frequency by the two sexes. High infection rates have been noted in some areas where there are no cats, pointing again to the multiplicity of sources of infections for human beings.

CLINICAL MANIFESTATIONS **Congenital toxoplasmosis** Congenitally infected infants may be born prematurely or at term and stillborn or alive with active disease, which can be expressed by fever, icterus, hepatomegaly, rash, splenomegaly, chorioretinitis, convulsions, and xanthochromic spinal fluid in various combinations. The newborn infant may have none of these signs, but subsequently hydrocephaly or microcephaly, chorioretinitis, psychomotor retardation, cerebral calcifications, and convulsions may appear, either singly or in combination. The most common residuals in congenitally affected children are chorioretinitis, cerebral calcifications, psychomotor retardation, hydro- or microcephaly, and convulsions. Any of or all these may follow other congenital infections, especially those due to cytomegalic virus (Chap. 206). The mothers of congenitally damaged offspring ordinarily are unaware of having had specific illness during the pregnancy. They should be advised that future pregnancies can be undertaken with confidence since the risk of producing a second such baby is nil. This complication occurs only in a female who happens to be pregnant when she has a parasitemia with her initial, usually asymptomatic, *Toxoplasma* infection. Congenital cases should be most rare in those areas where childhood infection rates are high. A study of pregnant women found to be free of antibodies early in pregnancy has shown that the offspring of 60 percent of more than 100 such women were found not to be infected at all and of those that were, more than two-thirds were normal. Most of the others had only isolated areas of chorioretinitis. It appears, therefore, that better than 80 percent of such pregnancies end in uninfected or unaffected offspring. Elevated IgM levels in neonates have been noted in congenital toxoplasmosis.

Acquired toxoplasmosis Although the clinical features show great variability, certain manifestations may be suggestive of this disease. Maculopapular rashes often appear soon after the clinical onset of the illness but tend to disappear in 3 to 4 days. Lympadenopathy is common and may be present alone or in combination with other signs. Myalgias, arthralgias, myocarditis, and pneumonitis also have been noted. The disease may resemble infectious mononucleosis or cytomegalovirus disease because lymphadenopathy and lymphocytosis with atypical lymphocytes are present, but splenomegaly and positive heterophil tests are absent. Parasites have been demonstrated in lymph nodes removed from such patients, some of whom were afebrile.

Toxoplasma has been isolated from several cases of posterior granulomatous uveitis, the result of either congenital or acquired infections. The proportion of such cases which is caused by *Toxoplasma* has not been established. In contrast to congenital chorioretinitis which is usually bilateral, the acquired form more often is unilateral.

The incubation period, recovery and mortality rates, average duration of illness, and the residual defects resulting from acquired toxoplasmosis remain undefined. Cerebral calcifications are not found in postnatally acquired infections.

LABORATORY DIAGNOSIS A specific diagnosis may be made by serologic methods, by demonstrating the organism in smears, or by their cultivation in mice. *Toxoplasma* can be identified in cerebrospinal fluid sediments with Wright's or Giemsa's stain, or occasionally in biopsied lymph node or muscle. Laboratory-reared mice are best for isolation trials from fresh spinal fluid sediment (when acute central nervous systems signs are present) or suspensions of tissue.

Serum antibodies can be detected with the dye, complement fixation, indirect hemagglutination, and immunofluorescence tests. The results are most helpful when they are negative or when a rising titer is demonstrated. Dye test antibodies appear early and persist for many years. They seem to be paralleled most closely by the immunofluorescent antibody test. Complement-fixing antibodies are slower to develop and disappear more rapidly. A high dye test titer (1:256 or more) and a negative complement fixation reaction in the same serum suggest either very recently acquired infection or the serologic residual of a previous one. Hemagglutinating antibodies often follow dye test antibodies, but on occasion the results of the two are quite divergent.

Antibodies of the IgM class are demonstrable by immunofluorescence and should be indicative of a recent, active infection. This reaction is especially useful in the differentiation of passively transferred antibody from congenital infection in newborns.

Skin test antigens prepared from mouse peritoneal fluid or embryonated eggs have been used and yield reactions of the delayed type. While still popular in some parts of the world, they are quite insensitive and their use is not recommended.

TREATMENT There is evidence from the treatment of experimental infections that a combination of sulfonamide and 5-*p*-chlorophenyl-2,4-diamino-6-ethylpyrimidine (Daraprim) is more effective than sulfonamide alone. Combinations of sulfadiazine or triple sulfonamides (not sulfisoxazole) and Daraprim have been reported to yield excellent results in some cases of uveitis but have not affected the course of others at all. Information on the effectiveness of this regimen in systemic toxoplasmosis is inadequate; it does appear to control acute symptoms but does not eradicate encysted organisms. This combination of drugs is not specific for toxoplasmosis so that the patient's favorable response does not prove the diagnosis. The sulfonamide should be administered in dosage of 2 to 4 g daily with 50 mg Daraprim daily in adults. Since Daraprim is an antifolic agent, leukocyte counts should be determined at least twice weekly. The dosage of Daraprim probably should be halved after 2 weeks, and 1 month of treatment certainly constitutes an adequate trial. The leukopenia and thrombocytopenia which may result from Daraprim administration can be corrected by the simultaneous administration of leucovorin calcium and yeast cakes without interfering with the antitoxoplasmic effect of the drug.

REFERENCES

Feldman HA: Medical Progress: Toxoplasmosis. N Engl J Med 279:1370 and 1431, 1968

Hentsch D (ed): *Toxoplasmosis*, Bern: Hans Huber Publishers, 1971

Maumenee AE, Silverstein AM: *Immunopathology of Uveitis*, Baltimore: Williams & Wilkins, 1964

Siim J Chr: *Human Toxoplasmosis*, Baltimore: Williams & Wilkins, 1960

214
PNEUMOCYSTIS CARINII PNEUMONIA (PNEUMOCYSTOSIS, INTERSTITIAL PLASMA CELL PNEUMONIA)

WALTER H. SHELDON

DEFINITION In general, *Pneumocystis carinii* pneumonia occurs in patients with impaired antibody and/or cellular immune responses. Pulmonary insufficiency is the cardinal clinical manifestation.

ETIOLOGY *Pneumocystis carinii* has not been cultured, and its taxonomic position remains uncertain; some consider it a protozoan, others a fungus. The consistent presence of the agent in the lesions is the primary evidence for its causative role which is supported by similar findings in experimentally induced disease and by serologic studies. The organisms are best seen in smears as 2 to 4 nm oval or crescentic structures with a single nucleus-like body or as 5 to 10 nm cysts containing two to eight bodies. Electron microscopic studies reveal a complex structure and suggest the capacity for protein synthesis and oxidative metabolism, while structures usually associated with phagocytosis are lacking. The agent can be visualized with many dyes (but not with hematoxylin-eosin stain), with phase microscopy, and with fluorescent antibody. The organism seen in man is morphologically similar to that in animals but species-specific serologic differences may exist.

EPIDEMIOLOGY Lacking in vitro culture and readily applicable serologic tests, the incidence of *P. carinii* infection is uncertain, and epidemiologic data are based on indirect evidence. It appears that latent infection is not rare in man and is frequent in many wild, domestic, and laboratory animals. In man the disease is worldwide and occurs in all age groups either as epidemics in nurseries or as isolated cases. Clinical observations suggest that the disease is contagious and is acquired by inhalation from asymptomatic carriers, persons with clinically inapparent infection, and perhaps also from infected rodents. Intrauterine *P. carinii* pneumonia acquired probably by transplacental transmission has been reported. The incubation period is 1 to 2 months.

PATHOGENESIS The organism is of low virulence, proliferates slowly, and may require the presence of another living agent for multiplication. The disease occurs in patients with primary or acquired defects of antibody formation and/or cellular immunity. It is a complication of neoplasia, particularly of malignant lymphocyte-reticular disorders, cyclic neutropenia, various anemias, collagen-vascular and autoimmune diseases, renal failure, and in patients with transplants who are receiving immunosuppressive drugs and adrenal steroids. *P. carinii* pneumonia has also been reported in the absence of demonstrated underlying disease. In general, however, it is seen during prolonged survival in states of impaired humoral or cellular host defenses. Progressive *P. carinii* infection has been produced in various laboratory animals.

The largest group of patients with *P. carinii* pneumonia are premature or debilitated newborns in whom the disease, first described as interstitial plasma cell pneumonia, occurs about the age of three to four months, often in nursery epidemics. In this group the pathogenesis has remained unclear. Age-related or as yet undefined deficits of antibody formation and of the lymphocyte-monocyte cell function during the inflammatory response have been suggested as an explanation. Increased susceptibility has also been attributed to preexisting chronic lung disease and to previous antimicrobial therapy which in animals activates latent *P. carinii* infection.

Many infections occur together with *P. carinii* pneumonia, and these are often multiple. Acute and chronic bacterial infections are common. Localized and disseminated cytomegalic inclusion disease is particularly frequent. Particles interpreted as cytomegalovirus have been reported in *P. carinii* organisms of two adults with combined *P. carinii* and cytomegalovirus infection. This finding may explain the frequent combined infection by these two agents. A wide range of concurrent viral, fungal, and some protozoan infections has been observed.

PATHOLOGIC FINDINGS In widespread disease the lungs are massively consolidated. The consolidation may be focal and confined to the central or dorsal lung areas. The alveoli are distended by a foamy material which suggests the diagnosis and, when stained, appropriately shows the organisms. Hyaline membranes may be present. The sparse cellular response consists of mononuclear cells. Alveolar septal infiltration with plasma cells is prominent in many cases and absent in others. Septal fibrosis is generally slight. The changes appear reversible. Granuloma formation, calcification, and focal and diffuse persistent fibrosis have been noted. Fragments of the alveolar contents in the bronchi may account for dissemination throughout the lung. In latent infection the lesions are few and minute, organisms are scanty, the foamy intraalveolar material is lacking, and the cellular response is sparse. The infection is confined to the lung, but organisms have been seen in the regional lymph nodes. Pleuritis is characteristically absent, and systemic dissemination with focal lesions in distant sites is extremely rare.

CLINICAL MANIFESTATIONS Generally the onset is insidious. The fully developed clinical picture shows severe dyspnea and tachypnea. The patient displays all signs of extreme air hunger and is anxious and cyanotic. There may be a dry cough which, together with the cyanosis, is aggravated by any movement. Fever is absent or slight. Pulmonary physical findings are scanty in contrast to the grave clinical state and the extensive lung involvement seen roentgenologically. Roentgenograms show soft infiltrates spreading from the hilum and eventually affecting most of the lung. Pleural effusions are unusual but focal emphysema may be present. Laboratory studies reveal no consistent abnormalities, and pulmonary function tests indicate impaired diffusion. Complications include pneumothorax from a ruptured emphysematous bleb and rib fractures from forced respiratory movements. After relentless progression death occurs by asphyxia or cardiac failure after 6 to 10 weeks.

COURSE Morbidity and mortality figures are uncertain. Beyond doubt *P. carinii* infection is not rare at any age and seems likely to become more frequent. The prognosis of *P. carinii* pneumonia is grave since it is generally a complication of a severe underlying disorder. A mortality of 40 to 50 percent has been suggested. Remissions and spontaneous cures have been reported. The outcome may be heavily dependent on the course of the underlying disease.

DIAGNOSIS The diagnosis depends on the morphologic demonstration of the organism. Bronchial secretions, tracheal lavage, and various biopsy techniques have been used. Examination of secretions has, in general, yielded poor results but may be improved by fluorescent antibody methods. Needle or open lung biopsy are often diagnostic but carry a considerable risk. Endobronchial brush biopsy has been reported as a simple, frequently successful procedure. The complement fixation test widely used in Europe has not become established in this country.

TREATMENT Pentamidine isethionate appears to be effective in the treatment of *P. carinii* infection, and clinical recovery has been reported in a substantial number of patients. The drug may be obtained from the Parasitic Disease Drug Service of the National Communicable Disease Control Center in Atlanta, Georgia. The recommended daily dose is 4 mg per kg body weight given by a single intramuscular injection for 12 to 14 days. Daily doses of 150 mg per m^2 body surface area have been used successfully in children with leukemia. In desperately ill patients the drug has been given intravenously. The drug is toxic and may produce abscesses and ulcers at the site of injection as well as serious systemic effects including azotemia, hypoglycemia, changes in liver function, and pulmonary fibrosis. Pyrimethamine (25 to 75 mg) and sulfadiazine (2 to 6 g) per day given orally may be beneficial. Antibiotics, convalescent serum, and commercial immunoglobulin have no effect. Symptomatic treatment with oxygen and digitalis may be indicated.

REFERENCES

BURKE BA, GOOD RA: *Pneumocystis carinii* infection. Medicine 57:23, 1973

KIRBY HB et al: *Pneumocystis carinii* pneumonia treated with pyrimethamine and sulfadiazine. Ann Intern Med 75:505, 1971

RUSKIN J, REMINGTON JS: The compromised host and infection: *I. Pneumocystis carinii* pneumonia. JAMA 202:1070, 1967

WESTERN KA et al: Pentamidine isethionate in the treatment of *Pneumocystis carinii* pneumonia. Ann Intern Med 73:695, 1970

215 MINOR PROTOZOAN DISEASES

JAMES J. PLORDE

TRICHOMONIASIS Trichomoniasis is a venereal infection caused by the protozoan *Trichomonas vaginalis*. Of the many members of the genus *Trichomonas*, three are parasites of man: *T. hominis* in the intestine, *T. tenax* in the oral cavity, and *T. vaginalis*, the only one capable of producing disease, in the vagina, urethra, and prostate. All three exist only in the trophozoite stage and resemble one another morphologically. *Trichomonas vaginalis* is the largest, however, and confusion in diagnosis is rare because of the anatomic specificity of their habits.

Trichomonas vaginalis is transmitted by sexual intercourse. Although the organism may survive on moist washcloths for a few hours, transmission by fomites has not been convincingly demonstrated and is probably rare. Newborn children of infected mothers have, on occasion, acquired the infection. The parasite is cosmopolitan in its distribution, and estimates hold that up to 25 percent of the sexually active population may be infected.

In the female, trichomoniasis usually presents as a persistent vaginitis. Initial manifestations include itching, burning, and profuse, creamy yellow, frothy leukorrhea. This acute stage may persist for a week or months, often fluctuating in intensity; it may worsen following menstruation. Eventually the discharge and other symptoms subside and may actually disappear completely, even though the patient still harbors trichomonads. Examination shows inflammation ranging from mild hyperemia of the vaginal vault to extensive erosion, petechial hemorrhages, and perianal intertrigo.

The prostate and urethra are the usual sites of infection in the male. It may present as persistent or recurring nonspecific urethritis, or, more commonly, be completely asymptomatic. Occasionally an acute purulent urethritis occurs.

The diagnosis is made by examining vaginal, prostatic, or urethral secretions for the presence of *Trichomonas*. The organism may also be found in the sedimented urine. A wet mount will usually reveal numerous motile organisms. A Giemsa-stained preparation is confirmatory. *Trichomonas vaginalis* may be grown in culture, but this technique is not generally available. A variety of serologic tests, including a complement fixation, an indirect hemagglutination, and an immunofluorescent reaction, have been described, but are not generally available or completely reliable.

Trichomonas is sometimes responsible for confusing changes in the cytologic pattern of exfoliated vaginal cells. Moreover, ordinary Papanicolaou preparations are not well suited to the diagnosis, and when trichomoniasis is suspected, fresh material should be looked at immediately.

Treatment consists of oral metronidazole (Flagyl) in dosage of 250 mg three times daily for 5 days. In vaginitis local therapy may be added. Sexual partners should be treated concurrently to prevent reinfection.

GIARDIASIS *Giardia lamblia* is a pear-shaped multiflagellar protozoan that parasitizes the human duodenum and jejunum where it multiplies by longitudinal fission. Under a microscope, its two nuclei give the organism the appearance of a face with two large eyes. It is actively motile but may attach itself to the intestinal mucosa by means of a large ventral sucker. Encystation occurs in transit through the colon. The resulting ovoid cysts are the infective form of the parasite and are transmitted by the fecal-oral route. A waterborne outbreak of giardiasis has been reported.

The response to infestation is highly variable and seems related at least in part to host factors. Children are three times more likely to be parasitized than adults and probably have more prominent clinical manifestations. Gastrectomy or decreased gastric acidity in adults may increase their susceptibility. Giardiasis also has been reported frequently in patients with immunoglobulin deficiencies, and may be a major cause of intestinal abnormalities in these patients. Similarly, *G. lamblia* infections appear to be a significant cause of travelers' diarrhea. Unlike the typical syndrome seen in travelers, however, the diarrhea usually begins late in the course of travels and may persist for several weeks.

Most often the infection is asymptomatic, but in some patients nausea, flatulence, epigastric pain, abdominal cramps, distention, and watery diarrhea occur. After a few days the stools may become semisolid, bulky, and malodorous. Symptoms and accompanying weight loss may persist for several weeks. These symptoms are more common in children and are usually self-limited. Rarely, fulminating and extensive duodenal ulceration has been described. Radiographically, asymptomatic carriers may show irritability of the duodenal bulb. Chronic giardiasis may lead to malabsorption of carbohydrate, fat, and vitamin B_{12}. Lactase intolerance and disaccharidase deficiencies have been described. The pathogenesis of these abnormalities is poorly understood. Mechanical blockage of microvilli by the parasites, competition between the organisms and host for nutrients, altered motility, and mucosal invasion have been suggested as possible mechanisms. Jejunal biopsy of patients infested with *Giardia* sometimes shows flattening of the microvilli and an inflammatory infiltrate. Both malabsorption and the jejunal lesions have been reversed with specific treatment.

The diagnosis is made by finding the trophozoite stage of the parasite in duodenal washings, jejunal biopsies, or diarrheal stools. Cyst forms are often passed in solid stool; they contain two to four nuclei and are readily identified when stained with iodine.

Treatment consists of the administration of 0.1 g Atabrine Hydrochloride three times daily for 3 days, a regimen which eliminates the organisms in 90 percent of the cases. Metronidazole (Flagyl) 250 mg three times daily for 10 days is tolerated better but may be slightly less effective.

COCCIDIOSIS This is an infrequently recognized disease characterized by fever, diarrhea, abdominal pain, and weight loss which results from ingestion of the oocysts of coccidia belonging to the genus *Isospora*. Coccidia are widespread in the animal kingdom; each vertebrate host harbors a specific species. *Isospora hominis* and *I. belli* are the two that most commonly infect man. Parasitization is much more common in children and is worldwide in distribution, particularly in tropical areas.

Like the related plasmodia, there is both an asexual and sexual stage of multiplication. Unlike plasmodia, however, both occur within a single host. Following the ingestion of an oocyst, *sporozoites* are released which invade the epithelial cells of the intestine to become trophozoites. These multiply asexually producing a large number of *merozoites*, which in turn invade other epithelial cells to continue the cycle. In some cells sexual gametocytes are produced. With the fertilization of the female gametocyte, an oocyst is formed which is then passed in the stool. Transmission is by the fecal-oral route. Volunteers develop symptoms about one week after the ingestion of viable oocysts. The illness usually has an acute onset with fever, headache, abdominal cramps, and diarrhea. Stools are often fatty and weight loss is common. Coccidiosis may be associated with a malabsorption syndrome and abnormalities of the mucosa in the small bowel. Symptoms, which presumably continue as long as the asexual cycle of multiplication continues, usually subside spontaneously within a few weeks. In some cases, however, they may persist for months or even years, eventually resulting in death.

A peripheral eosinophilia occurs in approximately half of the infected patients. The diagnosis can be made by examination of stool for oocysts. These are often scanty, and concentration techniques such as zinc sulfate flotation or the formol-ether method must usually be employed. Incubation of the stool for 2 days at room temperature improves the recovery rate. Duodenal aspiration and jejunal biopsy are less cumbersome and more reliable.

BALANTIDIASIS *Balantidium coli*, the largest protozoon of man, inhabits the large intestine. In addition to producing an asymptomatic carrier state, it elicits disease ranging from mild recurrent diarrhea to fulminant ulceration with perforation and death. In many respects the disease is similar to amebiasis in its range of manifestations, exclusive of spread to the liver.

The illness has been reproduced by feeding the organism to volunteers. The diagnosis is made by finding the trophozoite or cyst in the stool, but repeated examinations may be required because shedding of *Blantidium* is intermittent. The disease is more likely to occur in tropical areas, but at least 60 cases have been reported in the United States. Swine are frequent carriers of *B. coli* and may play an important role in the spread of the disease to man.

The tetracyclines in ordinary doses are highly effective in treatment, as is Diodoquin in a dosage of 0.65 g three times daily for 3 weeks. Metronidazole given in dosage of 750 mg three times daily for 5 or 6 days is also effective.

REFERENCES

General

FAUST EC et al: *Craig and Faust's Clinical Parasitology*, Philadelphia: Lea & Febiger, 1970

Coccidiosis

BRANDBORG LL et al: Human coccidiosis—A possible cause of malabsorption. N Engl J Med 283:1306, 1970

SMITSKAMP H, OEY-MULLER E: Geographical distribution and clinical significance of human coccidiosis. Trop Geogr Med 18:133, 1966

Giardiasis

AMENT ME, RUBIN CE: Relation of Giardiasis to abnormal intestinal structure and function in gastrointestinal immunodeficiency syndromes. Gastroenterology 62:216, 1972

BABB RR et al: Giardiasis: A cause of traveler's diarrhea. JAMA 217:1359, 1971

HOSKINS LC et al: Clinical Giardiasis and intestinal malabsorption. Gastroenterology 53:265, 1967

MOORE GT et al: Epidemic Giardiasis at a ski resort. N Engl J Med 281:402, 1969

Trichomoniasis

JIROVEC O, PETRU M: *Trichomonas vaginalis* and trichomonas, in *Advances in Clinical Parasitology*, vol. 6, ed B Dawes, London: Academic, 1968, p. 117

KEIGHLEY EE: Trichomonas in a closed community: Efficacy of metronidazole. Br Med J 1:207, 1971

section 22 | Diseases caused by worms

216 INTESTINAL NEMATODES

JAMES J. PLORDE

HOOKWORM DISEASE Hookworm disease is a symptomatic infection caused by *Ancylostoma duodenale* or *Necator americanus.* Asymptomatic infection may be termed simply *hookworm infection,* and the individual with such infection is called a *carrier.*

Etiology *Ancylostoma duodenale,* also known as the "Old World" hookworm, possesses four prominent hooklike teeth in its adult stage. The adults are about 1 cm long and inhabit the upper part of the small intestine of man, where they attach to the mucosa by means of the mouth parts and suck blood. Each adult extracts approximately 0.20 ml blood daily. The adults migrate within the small intestine, and each site of attachment persists temporarily as a bleeding point. Following fertilization, the female liberates eggs which measure about 40 by 60 μm and are usually in the two- to four-celled stage when discharged in the feces.

Necator americanus, the "New World" hookworm, has a buccal capsule containing dorsal and ventral plates rather than teeth. It is slightly smaller and causes much less blood loss than *A. duodenale. Ancylostoma ceylonicum,* a hookworm of cats, found in the Far East, may occasionally reach maturity in man.

The life cycles of both hookworms are similar. Under appropriate conditions, the eggs hatch in 24 to 48 hr, releasing free-living or rhabditiform larvae. Within a few days, these develop into infective or filariform larvae which may remain viable in the soil for several weeks. These, in turn, penetrate the skin to enter vessels which carry them to the lungs. The larvae leave the alveolar capillaries, enter the alveoli, ascend the respiratory tree, enter the pharynx, and are swallowed. They reach the intestine about 1 week after penetration of the skin, and mature within 5 weeks. Adults have been known to survive in the human intestine for as long as 15 years.

Epidemiology It has been estimated that one-quarter of the world's population has hookworm infection. *Necator americanus* is found predominantly in the tropical areas of Africa, Asia, and the Americas, while *A. duodenale* occurs in the Mediterranean Basin, the Middle East, northern India, China, and Japan. In many areas both species are seen. In general, *Ancylostoma* presents a greater public health hazard than *N. americanus,* the species which is most prevalent in the southern United States, because it is most persistent in the environment, more harmful to the host, and less amenable to treatment. Conditions conducive to the development of the hookworm egg into infective filariform larvae are a warm climate with abundant rainfall, shade, and well-drained, sandy soil. Hookworm infection occurs where there is opportunity for contact of the skin with contaminated soil. The disease may also be acquired by oral ingestion of infective larvae, particularly those of *A. duodenale.* Probably because of greater exposure, males show a higher incidence of infection than females.

Repeated infections of hookworm in dogs result in immunity and elimination of the parasite. It seems probable that a similar phenomenon occurs in human infections. When the possibility of reinfection is eliminated, the majority of worms is eliminated spontaneously within 1 or 2 years.

Pathogenesis and clinical manifestations During the invasion of the exposed skin by the larvae, there may be an erythematous maculopapular skin rash and edema with severe pruritus. These manifestations, which may persist for several days, are more marked in *N. americanus* infection. The lesions are most common about the feet, particularly between the toes, and have been termed "ground itch."

During migration through the lungs, cough and, in severe infections, fever are common. Usually, however, pulmonary involvement does not give rise to clinical symptoms.

Various gastrointestinal symptoms, ranging from vague epigastric distress and pica to typical ulcer pain, have been reported in association with hookworm infection. Roentgenographic studies may reveal nonspecific changes such as excessive peristalsis and "puddling," particularly in the proximal jejunum. However, gross and microscopic examination of the bowel itself reveals conspicuously little damage. Previous reports of absorptive abnormalities in hookworm infection have not been supported.

The major clinical manifestations of hookworm disease clearly are those of iron-deficiency anemia and hypoalbuminemia consequent to chronic intestinal blood loss. Whether anemia develops and how severe it becomes depend on the balance between iron lost in the gut and iron absorbed from the diet. In many endemic areas, dietary iron is largely of vegetable origin and is absorbed poorly. General dietary deficiency also may lower resistance to parasitic infections. The severity of the disease and the prognosis depend on such factors as the age of the patient, the magnitude of the worm burden, the duration of the disease, and diet. Young children often have extreme anemia, with cardiac insufficiency and anasarca. Those who survive to puberty show retarded physical, mental, and sexual development. Milder degrees of the disease, as seen in older children and adults, are characterized by lassitude, dyspnea, palpitation, tachycardia, constipation, and pallor of the skin and mucous membranes.

Asymptomatic infections outnumber symptomatic infections, considering all age groups, twenty to forty times in endemic areas. The worm burden is small in asymptomatic infections, and the carrier state may be indicative of some degree of acquired host resistance.

Laboratory findings In symptomatic infection, hookworm eggs are usually numerous enough to be detected by microscopic examination of a direct or concentrated fecal smear. A quantitative egg count, using the Stoll or Beaver technique, allows an estimation of the intensity of infection. If a stool specimen is allowed to stand for several hours before examination, the eggs may hatch, releasing larvae which are easily confused with those of *Strongyloides*. Abdominal and pulmonary symptoms appear before eggs are discharged, although a presumptive diagnosis may be made on the basis of the clinical history and the eosinophilic leukocytosis.

The feces seldom contain gross blood in hookworm disease, although tests for occult blood are usually positive. *Trichostrongylus* eggs are larger and in a later stage of maturation when observed in a fresh fecal specimen than are those of *Necator* or *Ancylostoma*.

Generally, the leukocyte count is normal. However, in some early cases, leukocytosis may be marked, with an eosinophilia as high as 70 or 80 percent. The anemia is characteristically hypochromic and microcytic.

Differential diagnosis Since hookworm disease occurs in areas in which beriberi and malaria are also more common, these diseases must be differentiated from hookworm disease, or their coexistence must be established.

Treatment Specific therapy for the infection and that directed toward improvement of nutrition and the anemia should be considered simultaneously. In the usual case, anthelmintics may be administered immediately, followed by iron therapy and a high-protein diet. A number of satisfactory anthelmintic agents are available, but the drug of choice is tetrachlorethylene (TCE). (The USP tetrachlorethylene available to veterinarians may be used.) In most instances a single dose of this agent will decrease the worm load substantially. Complete cure may require several courses of treatment but is not necessary in endemic areas; the aim of therapy is reduction of the worm load to an asymptomatic level. Tetrachlorethylene is administered as a single 5-ml oral dose. Children should receive 0.12 ml per kg (to a maximum of 5 ml) by the same route. The night before treatment, the patient is permitted a light, fat-free meal. The following morning, breakfast is omitted and the drug is administered. No food is permitted for 4 hr and no alcohol for 24 hr. Purgation following administration of the drug is no longer recommended. Treatment can be repeated in a week if complete cure is desired and has not been accomplished. The drug is inexpensive, nontoxic, and ideal for mass therapy. If ascariasis is also present, it should be treated first with piperazine citrate (see Ascariasis below).

Biphenium hydroxynaphthoate (Alcopar) is also a drug of low toxicity which is said to be more effective than TCE against *A. duodenale* but possibly less effective against *N. americanus*. In mixed infections with *Ascaris* it can be used alone because it is active against both types of parasite. A single dose of 5 g biphenium hydroxynaphthoate is dispersed in water and ingested in the morning on an empty stomach. No food is permitted for 2 hr, and no purgation is recommended. The dose for children is the same as for adults. In *N. americanus* infections, treatment should be repeated on three consecutive days. Another drug which has been introduced for treatment of hookworm infections is thiabendazole (Mintezol). This is a broad-spectrum drug which is effective against *Ascaris*, *Trichuris*, and *Strongyloides* as well as hookworm. The dose is 25 mg per kg twice a day for 2 or 3 days. Twenty-five percent of patients treated with this agent develop nausea and vomiting. Bitoscanate (Jonit), a new anthelmintic, has been introduced. Given in oral dosage of 100 mg every 12 hr for three doses, it is equally effective against *N. americanus* and *A. duodenale*. It is not available in the United States.

The anemia requires iron replacement.

When anemia is severe and there is malnutrition with anasarca, blood transfusions and a high-protein diet should be given before drug treatment is begun. Blood should be given in an amount sufficient to raise the hemoglobin level to 10 g per 100 ml. In advanced cases it may be necessary to delay drug treatment for 2 to 3 weeks.

Prognosis Generally, the immediate prognosis is good. When opportunity for reinfection persists and nutrition cannot be maintained, a state of chronic debility develops. Maturation of children is impaired, and intercurrent disease is a serious problem in adults.

Prevention Many of the measures required are obvious but difficult to apply on a large scale. Even if facilities for proper disposal of feces are provided, it is no simple matter to educate the population in their use. Soil pollution must be eliminated. Avoidance of direct skin contact with the soil (by wearing shoes) is often not practical in endemic areas. Periodic mass treatment of the population has been used in some hookworm control programs.

CUTANEOUS LARVA MIGRANS (CREEPING ERUPTION)

Definition Creeping eruption is an infection of the skin in man caused by the larvae of the dog and cat hookworm, *A. brasiliense*. The other dog hookworms, *A. caninum* and *Uncinaria stenocephala*, and the horse botfly, *Gasterophilus*, in their larval stage may produce a similar cutaneous infection.

Etiology *Ancylostoma brasiliense* reaches adulthood regularly only in the dog and cat. The larvae emerging from eggs discharged in the feces develop to the filariform stage and then are capable of penetrating the skin. In man, the larvae usually remain in the skin and migrate, producing an irregular erythematous tunnel visible on the skin surface.

Epidemiology and distribution Transmission to man requires environmental temperature and humidity appropriate for development of the egg to the infective filariform larva stage. Beaches and other moist, sandy areas are hazardous, because animals choose such areas for defecation, and the *A. brasiliense* eggs develop well in such soil.

Pathogenesis and clinical manifestations The site of penetration of the skin by the larva becomes apparent in a few hours. The migration of the larva in the skin is accompanied by severe itching. Scratching may lead to bacterial infection. In the course of 1 week, the initial red papule develops into an irregular, erythematous, linear lesion which may attain a length of 15 to 20 cm.

Wright and Gold have observed Loeffler's syndrome in 26 of 52 cases of creeping eruption. Transient, migratory pulmonary infiltrations associated with an increased number of eosinophils in the blood and sputum were interpreted as an allergic reaction to the helminthic infection.

Laboratory findings Eosinophils occur in the lesion, but eosinophilic leukocytosis is slight, except when Loeffler's syndrome appears. The percentage of eosinophils in the blood may then rise to 50 percent, and in the sputum to 90 percent.

Treatment Thiabendazole is the drug of choice; it should be given orally in the dosage suggested for hookworm, or it may be applied topically as a 10 percent aqueous suspension. Topical administration avoids systemic toxicity. Superficial bacterial infections are improved by the application of wet dressings and elevation of the extremity. For intense itching, oral antihistaminics may be of aid.

Prognosis Untreated infections last several months. Treatment, which is usually sought because of severe pruritus, is usually successful.

Prevention Dogs and cats should be prevented from contaminating recreation areas.

STRONGYLOIDIASIS **Definition** Strongyloidiasis is an intestinal infection of man and other mammals caused by *Strongyloides stercoralis.*

Etiology The tiny (2 mm in length) adult female resides and lays her eggs in the mucosa of the upper part of the small intestine. The eggs quickly hatch, releasing rhabditiform larvae which enter the lumen of the bowel and are passed in the feces. On reaching the soil, the larvae develop into the infective filariform stage. There, as in the case of the filariform larvae of hookworm, they penetrate the skin and small blood vessels of man. They are then carried to the lungs where they leave the alveolar capillaries, ascend the respiratory tree, enter the pharynx, and are swallowed. On reaching the small intestine, they mature and copulate. The fertilized female burrows into the jejunal mucosa, while the male is excreted in the stool. It is likely that the females also reproduce parthenogenetically. In addition to the *direct* host-soil-host cycle, *Strongyloides* has two alternative cycles. In the first or *indirect* cycle, the rhabditiform larvae, after passing from the host, develop into free-living adults which reside and reproduce in the soil, thus creating a reservoir of infection independent of the human host. Under certain environmental conditions, the free-living larvae are capable of transforming back into filariform larvae which initiate a new cycle in man. In the second, or *autoinfection* cycle, the rhabditiform larvae develop into filariform larvae before they are passed in the stool. They may then invade the intestinal mucosa or perianal skin of the same host without first going through a soil phase. This may explain the long persistence (20 to 30 years) of strongyloidiasis in patients who have left endemic areas and may also account for the extremely heavy worm loads in some individuals. The early transformation of the filariform larvae is probably also responsible for the frequency with which strongyloidiasis is seen in crowded, unsanitary institutions for the mentally retarded.

Epidemiology The usual mode of infection is the penetration of the skin by larvae. Some infections may result from ingestion of contaminated food and drink, and some are believed to be transmitted by contact. This disease is endemic in the tropics, where the warmth, moisture, and lack of sanitation favor its spread. Sporadic cases appear throughout the world.

Pathogenesis and clinical manifestations The initial cutaneous penetration of the filariform larvae usually produces no symptoms. However, transitory skin eruptions characterized by blotchy erythema, serpiginous lesions, and urticaria may recur at irregular intervals and may be related to episodes of autoinfection. Cough, dyspnea, and gross hemoptysis occasionally accompany migration through the lungs. Chest x-rays may show pulmonary infiltration at this time. The intestinal infestation is usually asymptomatic or productive only of vague abdominal complaints. In heavier infections, epigastric pain and tenderness, nausea, flatulence, vomiting, and diarrhea alternating with constipation may be observed. The mucosal inflammation may be severe enough to produce subacute obstruction, segmental ileus, and impaired absorption. A severe form of ulcerative colitis, accompanied by intestinal perforation and peritonitis, has been encountered. In debilitated, immunodepressed, or steroid-treated patients massive autoinfection with widespread dissemination of larvae to the intestinal organs may occur. This hyperinfection is often associated with severe enterocolitis and gram-negative bacteremia. Unrecognized, it may lead to death.

Laboratory findings Although clinical findings may be suggestive, the definitive diagnosis can be made only in the laboratory. Fresh fecal specimens should be examined to avoid confusion with hookworm infection; generally, fresh specimens contain *larvae* in strongyloidiasis infections, while in hookworm infection they contain *eggs.* Since the number of larvae in the stool is small and varies from day to day, several samples should be checked, using concentration and cultural techniques. If pulmonary involvement is present, the sputum should be examined for larvae. Microscopic examination of the duodenal washings and jejunal biopsies may also establish the diagnosis. The filarial complement fixation test is positive in approximately 75 percent of patients and may be helpful in the diagnosis of light infections.

Eosinophilic leukocytosis is common, except in very severe cases. When eosinophilia occurs in association with peptic ulcer symptoms, strongyloidiasis should be suspected.

Treatment The drug of choice is thiabendazole, which should be given orally in dosage of 25 mg per kg twice a day for 2 or 3 days. Light-headedness, nausea, and vomiting are common accompaniments of therapy with this agent. Hypersensitivity reactions may occur but usually respond to treatment with antihistamines.

Prognosis In the usual case, the prognosis is good. Since the occurrence of hyperinfection is unpredictable, every effort should be made to eradicate the infection in each case. In severe cases with hyperinfection, the prognosis is poor.

Prevention In general, the measures are those for the control of hookworm infection. In addition, it is well to remember that infection may be contracted by ingestion of contaminated food (especially uncooked vegetables) or of contaminated drinking water and by contact.

ASCARIASIS Definition Ascariasis is an infection of man caused by *Ascaris lumbricoides* and characterized by an early pulmonary phase related to larval migration and a later, prolonged intestinal phase. It is estimated that 25 percent of the world's population is infested with this nematode.

Etiology The adult ascarids are large (15 to 40 cm in length), cyclindric worms with blunt ends which maintain themselves in the lumen of the jejunum by virtue of their muscular activity. Despite a life span of only 6 to 18 months, the female releases millions of eggs, both fertile and infertile, into the fecal stream; the daily output is estimated to be 200,000 per worm. Fertilized eggs are elliptic (30 to 40 μm by 50 to 60 μm) and have an irregular, dense outer shell and a regular, translucent inner shell. They require a period of soil incubation before they become infective. Under optimum conditions of warmth and moisture this occurs in 9 to 13 days. The eggs may then remain viable for several months. When an infective egg is ingested, the larva is liberated in the small intestine. It migrates through the wall and is carried by the bloodstream or lymphatics to the lung. After about 10 days in the pulmonary capillaries and alveoli, the larvae pass in turn up the bronchioles, bronchi, trachea, and epiglottis, are swallowed, and return to the jejunum. There they develop into mature adult worms within 2 to 3 months of ingestion. *Ascaris suum,* a roundworm of pigs, may occasionally complete a similar life cycle in man.

Epidemiology Infection follows the ingestion of the embryonated egg contained in contaminated food, or, more commonly, the introduction of the eggs into the mouth by the hands after contact with contaminated soil. In endemic areas, the infection is maintained primarily by ...ll children who defecate indiscriminately in the area ... home. In dry, windy climates, eggs may become ... get into the mouth, and be swallowed. Since the eggs are resistant to desiccation and wide variations in temperature, the disease is worldwide.

Pathogenesis and clinical manifestations Because of the extensive migration of which both the larvae and adults are capable, the manifestations may be diverse. Bronchopneumonia characterized by fever, cough, wheeze, eosinophilic leukocytosis, and migratory pulmonary infiltrates may occur during the passage of the larvae through the lungs. Severity of symptoms is apparently related to both intensity of infection and the degree of sensitization resulting from previous exposures. Significant arterial oxygen desaturation and rarely, death may occur. Adult worms may cause no symptoms if the infection is light and may be detected accidentally when an adult worm is vomited or passed in the stool. Heavier infections may cause abdominal pain, and occasionally a bolus of worms may result in partial or complete intestinal obstruction in the ileocecal area. Obstruction often follows febrile illnesses which stimulate the worms to increased motility. Rarely an adult will migrate into the appendix, bile ducts, or pancreatic ducts, causing obstruction of the organs, or penetrate the intestinal wall producing peritonitis. Biliary tract obstruction may be associated with a bacterial cholangitis and liver abscess.

Laboratory findings The diagnosis is usually made by finding the ova in the feces. The fertilized eggs are usually numerous, characteristic, and not easily confused with those of other helminths. The occasional unisexual infection may pose diagnostic problems. The male produces no eggs, and the unfertilized ova produced by a single female may be atypical and difficult to recognize. Ascaris pneumonia may be diagnosed by finding larvae in the sputum or gastric aspirate. Eggs will usually not be found until after the larvae have matured in the intestine.

Treatment Only symptomatic treatment can be used during the period of pulmonary involvement by the migrating larvae. For removal of the adult worms from the intestines, piperazine citrate, as a flavored syrup administered in a single dose after breakfast on two successive days, will cure the majority of cases. The drug acts by paralyzing the ascarids, which are then passed in the stool. The dose of piperazine is 75 mg per kg, with a maximum of 4 g. No particular dietary regulation is necessary. The drug must be administered with caution to patients with renal insufficiency, because impaired elimination may produce neurotoxic signs. In intestinal obstruction, nasogastric suction should be initiated. After vomiting is controlled, piperazine should be given through the nasogastric tube every 12 to 24 hr in dosage of 65 mg per kg (maximum 1.0 g) for six doses. Surgery usually is not required.

While piperazine citrate is the treatment of choice, pyrantel in a single dose of 10 mg per kg (maximum 1.0 g) is also very effective. Thiabendazole (see Strongyloidiasis, above) or biphenium hydroxynaphthoate (see Hookworm Disease, above) may be used. When both ascariasis and trichuriasis are present, treatment with thiabendazole is effective. When both ascariasis and infection with *A. duodenale* are present, treatment with biphenium hydroxynaphthoate is recommended.

Prognosis The prognosis in intestinal infection is generally good. When acute or chronic obstruction of ducts of hollow viscera has occurred, the immediate prognosis is determined by the promptness of diagnosis and treatment.

Prevention Ascariasis is primarily a household infection of rural areas. All infections should be treated, personal hygiene stressed, and adequate toilet facilities provided.

TOXOCARIASIS (VISCERAL LARVA MIGRANS)

Definition This is a human infection with *Toxocara canis* or *T. cati.* The animal ascarids are usually unable to complete their life cycle in man, but they may be widely disseminated in the body, producing a variety of clinical manifestations, collectively referred to as *visceral larva migrans.*

Etiology and epidemiology The large adult toxocaral worms live in the intestine of cats and dogs. Their eggs must be passed in the stool and incubate in soil for 2 to 3 weeks before they become infective. If the ova are then ingested by man, larvae are liberated in the intestine, penetrate the wall, and are carried in the blood to the liver and lung. At the time the larvae reach the pulmonary capillaries, they are still very small (approximately one-half the size of *A. lumbricoides*), and many pass through the lungs to reach the systemic circulation. Larvae penetrate into the tissues where their gradually increasing size approaches the diameter of the vessel through which they are traveling. Rarely the organisms break into the alveoli, ascend the respiratory tract, and are swallowed to reach the small intestine where they mature into adult worms. *Toxocara* infections of cats and dogs are common and widespread. Although most human infections have been reported from the United States and Europe, it seems likely that the disease is present in other areas of the world as well. Children, because of their sanitary habits and intimate association with domestic pets, are most frequently involved.

Pathogenesis and clinical manifestations The larvae migrate freely in tissues, causing hemorrhage, necrosis, eosinophilic inflammatory reaction, and eventually granuloma formation. The most frequently involved organs are in the liver, lungs, brain, eye, heart, and skeletal muscles. Symptoms and signs are related to the number and location of the granulomas as well as sensitization to the parasite antigen. Most frequently patients present with fever and tender hepatomegaly. Splenomegaly, skin rash, and recurrent pneumonitis with wheezing respirations may occur in more severe infections. There is often a history of dirt eating and contact with cats and dogs. Leukocytosis with eosinophilia to high levels (over 60 percent) and hypergammaglobulinemia are common. Anti-IgG factors have been reported in the serum of children with this syndrome. These manifestations may persist for several months. A granulomatous endophthalmitis, which may be mistaken for retinoblastoma, convulsions, and myocarditis, may also be observed. Asymptomatic infection is probably common.

Diagnosis The clinical diagnosis can usually be made on the basis of clinical findings. *Ascaris lumbricoides* and *S. stercoralis* infections may also on occasion present as visceral larva migrans, making the etiologic diagnosis difficult. Open biopsy of a granulomatous lesion followed by serial section of the specimen may reveal a characteristic *Toxocara* larva. A standardized skin test and indirect hemagglutination and fluorescent antibody tests are available. While other helminthic diseases may cause cross reactions, these tests are often very helpful.

Treatment No uniformly effective therapy is available. Diethylcarbamazine as used in bancroftian filariasis (Chap. 219) is probably the drug of choice. Thiabendazole in dosage of 25 to 50 mg per kg for 7 to 10 days may be helpful. Adrenocortical steroids may be beneficial when respiratory difficulty is pronounced. Control measures are directed toward preventing ingestion of eggs. Removal and repeated worming of infected cats and dogs must be considered.

ANISAKIASIS *Anisakis marina* is an ascarid of seals, whales, and other large sea mammals. Its larval stages are found in the flesh of several marine fish including cod, salmon, and herring. Man is infected by eating raw or inadequately pickled fish. The larva burrows into the mucosa of the stomach and small intestine, producing an eosinophilic granulomatous tumor which may be mistaken for gastric carcinoma. Colicky abdominal pain, intestinal obstruction, and perforation have been reported. The definitive diagnosis can be made only by the identification of the larvae in tissue. The disease usually subsides spontaneously. Cases have been recognized in Northern Europe and Japan.

ENTEROBIASIS Definition Enterobiasis (pinworm, seatworm, or threadworm infection; oxyuriasis) is an intestinal infection of man caused by *Enterobius vermicularis* and characterized by perianal pruritus.

Etiology The female averages 10 mm in length, the male 3 mm. They live with their heads attached to the mucosa of the cecum, appendix, and adjacent parts of the bowel. The gravid female migrates through the anal canal at night and deposits eggs on the perianal skin. In female patients the worm may enter the vagina and occasionally gains access to the peritoneal cavity through the fallopian tubes. Each egg contains an embryo which, within a few hours, develops into the infective larva. After the egg has been ingested, the larva is released in the small intestine and migrates down the bowel lumen to the cecum. In less than 1 month from the time of ingestion, newly developed gravid females are again discharging eggs. They are planoconvex and measure approximately 20 by 50 μm. The shell is clear and doubly contoured.

Epidemiology Man is usually infected by the direct transfer of eggs from the anus to the mouth by the way of contaminated fingers. Retroinfection may occur when the eggs hatch in the perianal area and the larvae migrate back into the bowel to become mature adults. The eggs, which are relatively resistant to desiccation, also contaminate night clothes and bed linen, where they remain viable and infective for 10 to 20 days. Airborne transmission is possible, and spread within family and children's groups occurs readily. Enterobiasis is found in all climates and is probably the most common helminthic infection of man. Its low incidence in some tropical areas, however, defies explanation.

Clinical manifestations The most common symptom is pruritus ani, which is most troublesome at night, being related to the migration of the gravid female worms. Scratching may lead to perineal eczema or pyogenic infection. Vaginal discharge has been reported, and rarely a chronic granulomatous salpingitis or endometritis results from the presence of ectopic adults.

Laboratory findings Examination for ova of material obtained from the perineal skin by means of a cellophane or Scotch brand cellophane tape swab is the preferable method for the detection of enterobiasis. Searching for ova in the feces is rarely helpful. Scrapings from under the nails may reveal ova. The diagnosis is sometimes made by finding adult worms in feces following a laxative or an enema. Eosinophilic leukocytosis is not a typical finding.

Treatment All infected individuals in a family or communal group should be treated simultaneously. The frequently recommended sanitary measures aside from hand washing before meals and after stools are of dubious benefit. It is relatively easy to eradicate the worms, but reinfection is frequent. Retreatment does not appear necessary unless symptoms recur.

Pyrvinium pamoate (Povan) is the drug most frequently used. A single dose of 5 mg per kg is given orally, in tablet or liquid form. This compound turns the stool red and may stain bedclothes or undergarments. An acceptable alternative is pyrantel (Banminth). It is given in a single oral dose of 10 ml per kg (maximum 1.0 g) and does not cause staining. Piperazine citrate given in dosage of 65 mg per kg (maximum 2.5 g) once daily for 8 days is very effective. When renal insufficiency is present, the dose should be reduced to avoid neurotoxicity. In heavily contaminated environments, treatment with the above drugs may be repeated after an interval of 2 weeks to eliminate any new infections. Thiabendazole in dosage of 25 mg per kg twice a day for 1 day may also be used. This is repeated in 7 days.

Prevention Methods of preventing autoinfection and dissemination within a group involving children are extremely difficult to enforce. Personal environmental hygiene should be stressed, and anthelmintic and symptomatic treatment of pruritus ani should be instituted. To control infection within a group, simultaneous treatment of all cases is mandatory.

TRICHURIASIS Definition Trichuriasis (whipworm infection, trichocephaliasis) is an intestinal infection of man caused by *Trichuris trichiura* and is characterized by invasion of the colonic mucosa by the adult trichuris.

Etiology The adult whipworms are found in the large intestine with their anterior ends deeply embedded in the mucosa. They are 30 to 50 mm in length and possess a threadlike anterior two-thirds with a stouter posterior third, giving them a whiplike structure. The female produces about 5,000 eggs each day. They are characteristically barrel-shaped (20 by 50 μm), brown, thick-walled, and translucent with knoblike ends. The eggs, like those of *ascaris*, must incubate at least 2 to 3 weeks in soil before they become infective. After ingestion, the egg hatches in the small intestine and the larvae become attached to the intestinal villi. After several days they migrate to the large intestine where they mature in about three months.

Epidemiology Whipworm is a cosmopolitan parasite but is most commonly found in the tropics where the level of sanitation is low and environmental conditions necessary for the incubation of the eggs are optimal. Its distribution is similar to that of *Ascaris* and hookworm, but the eggs are less resistant than those of *Ascaris* to sunlight and drying.

Pathogenesis and clinical manifestations Symptomatic infection generally requires the presence of large numbers of adult whipworms and may be correlated in part with the degree of mucosal involvement. Heavy infections usually occur only in children and may be accompanied by nausea, abdominal pain, diarrhea, and dysentery. It has been estimated that infected patients lose 0.005 ml blood per worm per day. Infection with more than 800 worms often results in anemia. Heavier infections may result in rectal prolapse.

Laboratory findings In symptomatic infection, large numbers of eggs are present in the feces and there may be eosinophilic leukocytosis and anemia. In light infections, concentration techniques may be necessary to recover the eggs.

Treatment Treatment is unsatisfactory. Patients who have severe symptoms should be given a hexylresorcinol enema. The bowel is first cleansed with a saline enema, and the buttocks and perianal area are then coated with petrolatum to protect the skin from the effects of the drug. The colon is filled with a 0.3% aqueous solution of hexylresorcinol. The buttocks may be taped to help retain the enema for 20 to 30 min. The enemas can be repeated at weekly intervals in severe infections. Thiabendazole, 25 mg per kg twice daily for 2 to 3 days, will cure a small percentage of cases. A single dose of 25 mg per kg per day for 11 to 30 days may be more effective.

Prognosis Whipworm infection, unless characterized by severe diarrhea, blood loss, and systemic reaction, usually responds well to treatment. Serious infections may require supportive treatment as well as chemotherapy.

Prevention Measures recommended for ascariasis apply also to trichuriasis.

TRICHOSTRONGYLIASIS Definition Trichostrongyliasis is an intestinal infection of man and other mammalian hosts, including sheep, goats, and cattle.

Etiology Almost a dozen species of *Trichostrongylus* are known to have infected man. Few human infections have been reported in the United States. In view of the high frequency of animal infections here, the low incidence of human infections is difficult to understand. The possibility exists that some such infections are mistaken for hookworm infection.

The ova resemble those of the hookworm but are larger and, when observed in a fresh fecal specimen, show a more advanced stage of segmentation (16- to 32-celled stage).

Pathogenesis Infection is acquired by ingestion of the larvae, rather than by their penetration of the skin. On reaching the small intestine, they attach themselves to the mucosa and develop into adult worms within 4 weeks. The adult maintains residence in the intestine for long periods. Sandground, who infected himself, observed infection to last more than 8 years.

Manifestations Diarrhea is observed occasionally when infection is massive, but most infections are asymptomatic. The parasite owes its importance primarily to the resemblance of its ova to those of the hookworms. Moreover, because the trichostrongylidae do not respond to anthelmintics effective in hookworm infection, it may be assumed incorrectly that one is dealing with refractory hookworm infection.

Laboratory diagnosis The diagnosis depends on the finding of the ova in the feces. Since they are few, they are usually found only when a concentration method is used. In symptomatic infections, there may be leukocytosis with marked eosinophilia (e.g., 80 percent).

Treatment These infections do not respond to tetrachloroethylene. Thiabendazole, 25 mg per kg twice daily for 2 or 3 days, or piperazine citrate as used against enterobiasis, is effective in symptomatic infections.

Prevention Contamination of the hands is to be avoided, as well as food grown in contaminated soil.

INTESTINAL CAPILLARIASIS Definition Intestinal capillariasis is an infection of man caused by the roundworm *Capillaria philippinensis*. This species of *Capillaria* was first discovered in 1963 from a fatal human infection occurring in the Philippines. The infection results in intractable diarrhea with a high mortality rate. Clinical studies have shown a severe protein-losing enteropathy and malabsorption of fats and sugars.

Etiology Capillaria are nematodes of the family Trichuroidea, and are closely related to comembers Trichuris and Trichinella. Adult *C. philippinensis* are small, measuring 2 to 4 mm in length. The peanut-shaped eggs have flattened bipolar plugs and an average size of 42 by 20 μm. The adults inhabit the mucosa of the small intestine, especially the jejunum. Adults, larval forms, and eggs are found in the stool.

Epidemiology The infection has been found only in persons residing in the Ilocano ethnic region in Northwest Luzon, Philippines. Since 1966 the disease has occurred in epidemic form, and more than 1,000 cases and 100 deaths have been reported. Males are infected more frequently than females, perhaps because of occupational exposure. Prior to the discovery of an effective chemotherapeutic agent, the mortality rate in untreated cases was about 30 percent. With chemotherapy, the case fatality rate has been reduced to 6 percent.

The mode of transmission and life cycle of the parasite are not established. The presence of many adult worms, larviparous females, embryonated eggs, and all larval stages in human intestinal contents suggests that autoinfection may be part of the life cycle. In addition, indirect evidence indicates that man-to-man transmission occurs. The mechanism by which man originally became infected remains obscure. Because the Ilocano people of the region eat many animal foods raw or semicooked, numerous species of local fauna have been examined for *Capillaria*, but without success. Developing larvae have been recovered from experimentally infected fish.

Pathogenesis and manifestations Adult worms in large numbers invade the small-intestinal mucosa and cause a severe protein-losing enteropathy and malabsorption. Hypokalemia, hypocalcemia, and hypoproteinemia are the rule. Autopsy studies have failed to show extraintestinal spread of the parasite. Initial symptoms of intestinal "gurgling" (borborygmi) and recurrent vague abdominal pain are followed, usually within 2 to 3 weeks, by a voluminous watery diarrhea. Other findings, consistent with the basic pathophysiologic process, are anorexia, vomiting, weight loss, muscle wasting and weakness, hyporeflexia, and edema. Abdominal tenderness and distention may occur. The period between onset of symptoms and death is usually 2 to 3 months. Subclinical infection has not been noted.

Diagnosis The diagnosis is made by finding ova in the stool. *Capillaria philippinensis* ova must be differentiated from those of *Trichuris trichiura*, which are similar. Care must be taken that capillaria are not overlooked in patients with *Trichuris* infections because in the endemic area most patients with capillariasis have coexistent *Trichuris* infection.

Treatment Administration of thiabendazole, combined with fluid and electrolyte replacement, leads to dramatic improvement. Thiabendazole therapy must be given over a prolonged period to prevent relapse. A divided dose of 25 mg per kg body weight per day is given for 1 month, followed by a maintenance of 1 g every other day for 6 months. On this schedule ova disappear from the stool within 2 weeks.

REFERENCES

AUR RJA et al: Thiabendazole in visceral larva migrans. Am J Dis Child 121:226, 1971

Aziz MA, Seddiqui AR: Morphological and absorption studies of small intestine in hookworm disease (Ancyclostomiasis) in West Pakistan. Gastroenterology 55:242, 1968

Beaver PC: The nature of visceral larva migrans. J Parasitol 55:3, 1969

Chitwood MB et al: *Capillaria philippinensis* N. (Nematoda: Trichinellida) from the intestine of man in the Philippines. J Parasitol 54:368, 1968

Davis CM, Israel RM: Treatment of creeping eruption with topical thiabendazole. Arch Dermatol 97:325, 1968

Faust EC et al: *Craig and Faust's Clinical Parasitology*, 8th ed., Philadelphia: Lea & Febiger, 1970

Franz KH et al: Clinical trials with thiabendazole against intestinal nematodes infecting humans. Am J Trop Med 14:383, 1965

Kanani SR, Rees PH: The diagnosis of strongyloidiasis with special reference to the value of the filarial complement-fixation test as a screening test. Trans R Soc Trop Med Hyg 64:246, 1970

Layrisse M et al: Blood loss due to infection with *Trichuris trichuria*. Am J Trop Med Hyg 16:613, 1967

Maegraeth BG, Gilles HM (eds): *Management and Treatment of Tropical Diseases*, Oxford: Blackwell Scientific Publications, Ltd., 1971

Mak CH: Visceral larva migrans: A discussion based on a review of the literature. Clin Pediatr 7:565, 1968

Markett EK: Pseudohookworm infection—Trichostrongyliasis: Treatment with thiabendazole. N Engl J Med 278:831, 1968

Matsen JM, Turner JA: Reinfection in Enterobiasis (Pinworm infection): Simultaneous treatment of family members. Am J Dis Child 118:576, 1969

Most H: Drug therapy: Common parasitic infections of man. N Engl J Med 287:495, 1972

Neva FA: Parasitic diseases of the GI tract in the United States. DM June, 1972

Phills JA et al: Pulmonary abnormalities and eosinophilia due to *Ascaris suum*. N Engl J Med 286:965, 1972

Piggott J et al: Human ascariasis. Am J Clin Path 53:223, 1970

Rivera E et al: Hyperinfection syndrome with *Strongyloides stercoralis*. Ann Intern Med 72:199, 1970

Roche M, Layrisse M: The nature and causes of hookworm anemia. Am J Trop Med Hyg 15:1029, 1966

Stemmerman GN: Strongyloidiasis in migrants: Pathological and clinical considerations. Gastroenterology 53:59, 1967

Whalen GE et al: Intestinal capillariasis. Lancet I:13, 1969

Yokogawa M. Yoshimura H: Clinicopathologic studies on larval anisakiasis in Japan. Am J Trop Med Hyg 16:723, 1967

217
TISSUE NEMATODES

JAMES J. PLORDE

ANGIOSTRONGYLIASIS Definition *Angiostrongylus cantonensis*, the rat lungworm, is the etiologic agent of the common form of *eosinophilic meningitis* found in Southeast Asia in the tropical areas of the Pacific.

Etiology The delicate filariform adults (20 mm in length) reside and lay their eggs in the lungs of rats and certain other rodents. After hatching, the larvae migrate up the respiratory tract, are swallowed, and pass in the feces. They develop into infective third-stage larvae within snails and slugs, their natural intermediate host. Viable third-stage organisms may also be found in land planarians, crabs, and freshwater prawns. These carriers or parasitic hosts appear to acquire the larvae by feeding on the tissues of infected mollusks. Man, like rodents, becomes parasitized when he ingests raw intermediate or carrier hosts containing the infective stage. In rodents the larvae migrate to the brain where they grow into young adults. After a period of further maturation, the worms travel to the lungs and begin to deposit eggs. The nematode does not complete its life cycle in man and dies after reaching the central nervous system.

Epidemiology Human infections with *A. cantonensis* have been found in Thailand, Vietnam, Indonesia, the Philippines, Taiwan, Hawaii, and several smaller Pacific islands from Okinawa in the north to New Caledonia and Tahiti in the south. In addition, rodent infections have been found in the islands of East Africa, Ceylon, India, and China. The rat lungworm may have been spread from Madagascar to Asia and to the Pacific by the recent dispersal of the giant African land snail, *Achatina fulica*.

Pathology and pathogenesis The nematode can produce extensive tissue damage by moving through the brain when alive and provokes a marked inflammatory reaction when dead. The pathologic lesions are characterized by (1) marked lymphocyte and eosinophilic infiltration of the meninges, (2) hemorrhagic and nonhemorrhagic worm tracts through the brainstem and spinal cord, (3) granuloma formation around dead parasites and necrotic debris which sheathes the worm; and (4) engorgement of almost all blood vessels, particularly the veins. Necrosis of vessel walls, aneurysmal dilatation of arteries, and perivascular hemorrhages have been noted. Living worms have been removed from the eyes of patients without central nervous system involvement.

Clinical manifestations The eosinophilic meningoencephalitis is characterized by a relatively mild fever, headache, and neck stiffness. Paresthesias of the trunk and lower extremities are a common complaint, and paralysis of the sixth and seventh nerves is seen in 3 to 7 percent of cases. Paralysis of the limbs, convulsions, and loss of consciousness are rare. The disease usually ends in complete spontaneous recovery. The cerebrospinal fluid contains several hundred cells per cubic millimeter and many eosinophils, and the cerebrospinal fluid protein is elevated. There may or may not be an eosinophilia in the peripheral blood.

The second clinically distinct form of eosinophilic meningitis has been reported from Thailand. This presents as a radiculomyeloencephalitis with limb pain and paresis and is thought to be caused by the nematode *Girathostoma spinigerum*. The cerebrospinal fluid eosinophilic leukocytosis is less marked than in *angiostrongylus* infections. The fluid is often xanthochromic. Death may occur from cerebral hemorrhage or destruction of vital centers.

Treatment and prevention There is no effective treatment. Prevention depends upon avoidance or proper cooking of such foods as snails, prawns, and crabs. Raw vegetables should be carefully inspected for the presence of planarians and mollusks before they are eaten. Freezing of crustaceans and mollusks at −15°C for 12 hr will destroy infective larvae of *A. cantonensis.*

DRACUNCULIASIS Definition Dracunculiasis is an infection of the connective and subcutaneous tissues of man by the guinea worm, *Dracuncula medinensis.* The gravid female produces symptoms when she ruptures the skin to discharge her eggs.

Etiology and epidemiology Dracunculiasis affects about 50 million people in West, Central, and Northeast Africa, the Middle East, Iran, Pakistan, and India. Man acquires the parasite when he ingests raw drinking water containing infected copepods (*Cyclops* sp.) which serve as the intermediate host. Shallow ponds, cisterns, and wells are the usual habitat of these crustaceans. In the stomach the copepod is digested and the larvae are released. The larva penetrates the intestinal wall and matures in the connective tissue of the retroperitoneal space. The adult male is small, seldom seen, and presumably dies after mating. In contrast, the female *Dracunculus* is one of the largest nematodes known—1 to 2 mm in diameter and 300 to 800 mm in length. The female reaches gravidity in approximately one year and then migrates to the subcutaneous tissue of the lower extremities. When the anterior end of the worm approaches the skin, a blister forms. This breaks down in a few days, forming a superficial ulcer. When the protruding portion of the worm comes in contact with water, the uterus prolapses through the body and discharges large numbers of motile rhabditiform larvae. Following ingestion by one of several species of *Cyclops*, the larvae undergo further development, becoming infective in 10 to 12 days. Mammals other than man may be infected, but their importance as a disease reservoir is uncertain.

Pathogenesis and manifestations The infection is asymptomatic until the gravid female appears in the subcutaneous tissues where it may, on occasion, be palpable. A few days before the formation of the blister, the patient frequently has fever, generalized urticaria, periorbital edema, and wheezing. Blister formation is accompanied by intense local pain and pruritus; like the systemic manifestations, this is thought to represent an allergic reaction to prematurely liberated larvae. The local lesion is usually found over the feet and ankles but may occur on the trunk or upper extremities. Multiple infections are common. With the rupture of the blister and the release of embryos, the systemic manifestations abate, and the worm is slowly extruded over a period of 4 to 5 weeks. Secondary infection and cellulitis are common, particularly if the worm is ruptured during the process of extraction. In Nigeria, guinea worm ulcers are a common portal of entry for the spores of *Clostridium tetani.* The female worm often fails to reach the surface and discharge her larvae. In most of these cases, it dies without producing symptoms. The calcified appearance on roentgenograms is characteristic. Occasionally the worm may invade the deep tissues, causing serious symptoms, and sterile abscesses may follow the release of embryos. Invasion of joint spaces by the adult worm or larvae results in arthritis.

Diagnosis The clinical picture is characteristic. Placing a small amount of water on the worm results in discharge of larvae which can then be examined microscopically. A fluorescent antibody test may permit the diagnosis to be made prior to emergence of the gravid female.

Treatment and prevention If the outline of the worm can be clearly seen or palpated, it may sometimes be completely removed with a single incision. The gradual extraction of the worm can be accomplished by winding a few centimeters onto a stick each day. Administration of niridazole (Ambilhar) results in prompt remission of symptoms and extrusion of the adult worms. The dose is 25 mg per kg body weight given in three divided doses for 7 days. Thiabendazole in dosage of 75 mg per kg for 2 days is also effective. Dracunculiasis can be prevented by the chemical treatment of drinking water.

REFERENCES

ALICATA JE: Present status of *Angiostrongylus cantonensis* infection in man and animals in the tropics. J Trop Med Hyg 72:53, 1969

MULLER R: Dracunculus and dracunculiasis, in *Advances in Parasitology*, vol. 9, ed B Dawes, London: Academic, 1971, p. 73

NYE SW et al: Lesions of the brain in eosinophilic meningitis. Arch Pathol 89:9, 1970

PUNYAGUPTA S et al: Eosinophilic meningitis in Thailand. Am J Trop Med 19:950, 1970

218 TRICHINOSIS

JAMES J. PLORDE
IVAN L. BENNETT, JR.
ROBERT G. PETERSDORF

DEFINITION Trichinosis is caused by the intestinal nematode *Trichinella spiralis.* The disease is characterized by diarrhea during the development of the adults in the intestine and by myositis, fever, prostration, periorbital edema, and, occasionally, evidence of myocarditis or encephalitis during the stage of larval migration and invasion.

ETIOLOGY Trichinosis in man is contracted by ingestion of meat containing the encysted larvae of *T. spiralis.* The meat is almost always pork, although a number of infections from bear meat have been observed, particularly in Canada, Alaska, and the northeastern and western United States. There are no intermediate hosts, and both the adult and larval stages develop in the same host. Infection has been produced or observed in the bear, wild boar, wolf, coyote, fox, muskrat, horse, cow, dog, cat, rabbit, guinea pig, mouse, and marine mammals, in addition to the rat and the pig. Man is particularly susceptible; most fowl are resistant. Among pigs, infection is contracted following feeding of uncooked pork scraps, less often by eating infected rats. The incidence of infection in pigs has been reduced by laws requiring that garbage be cooked thoroughly before being fed. Rats also feed on uncooked pork scraps and, in addition, maintain a high incidence of infection by their cannibalism.

Soon after ingestion, the larvae are liberated from their cysts by gastric digestion and migrate into the intestinal mucosa, where copulation takes place. The male dies, and within a week, the viviparous female is discharging larvae (100 × 6 μm), which enter vascular channels and are distributed throughout the body. Larviposition continues for about 4 to 6 weeks. The larvae enter skeletal muscle and encyst. The muscles of the diaphragm, tongue, and eye, and the deltoid, pectoral, and intercostal muscles are most often affected. Larvae carried to sites other than skeletal muscles do not encyst but disintegrate. The life cycle can be carried further only if a new host ingests the encysted larvae.

EPIDEMIOLOGY Trichinosis is common in Europe and North America and uncommon in other parts of the world, including the Tropics. In the United States its prevalence by finding cysts in human diaphragms at autopsy has declined from 16.1 to 4.2 percent over the past 30 years. This decline has been accompanied by a similar reduction of trichinosis in pigs. In 1971, 115 cases with 3 deaths were reported in this country. Large outbreaks are usually caused by a consumption of ready-to-eat pork sausage prepared in noninspected facilities.

PATHOLOGY The most striking lesions are in the skeletal muscles, where there is a severe myositis with basophilic granular degeneration of the invaded muscle fiber. Adjacent fibers exhibit hyaline or hydropic degeneration, and the focus becomes infiltrated with neutrophilic and eosinophilic leukocytes, some lymphocytes, and mononuclear macrophages. Hyperemia, edema, and hemorrhages are constant features.

Larvae do not encyst in cardiac muscle, but an intense myocarditis has been observed in fatal cases.

In cases of central nervous system involvement, there may be granulomatous nodules, and vasculitis involving small arterioles and capillaries of the brain and meninges. Encystment of larvae in the brain is unusual.

CLINICAL MANIFESTATIONS The first symptoms usually appear within 1 to 2 days after ingestion of the uncooked or undercooked meat containing encysted larvae. At that time diarrhea, abdominal pain, nausea, and sometimes prostration and fever develop. The next stage, that of muscular invasion, begins about the end of the first week and may last as long as 6 weeks. During this period, patients have fever, edema of the eyelids, conjunctivitis and subconjunctival hemorrhages, muscle pain and tenderness, and often severe weakness. There may be a maculopapular rash which lasts for several days and subungual "splinter hemorrhages." Central nervous system involvement may be evident as polyneuritis, poliomyelitis, myasthenia, meningitis, encephalitis, focal or diffuse pareses, delirium, psychosis, and coma. Despite the severity of central nervous system involvement in some patients, the cerebrospinal fluid remains normal.

Myocarditis is characterized by persistent tachycardia or development of congestive heart failure. There may be marked electrocardiographic alterations, including ST-T wave changes and conduction abnormalities.

LABORATORY FINDINGS The most constant finding, and one of significance early in the course of the disease, is the eosinophilic leukocytosis (over 500 eosinophilic leukocytes per mm^3) which generally appears before the end of the second week. In cases of moderate severity, the proportion of eosinophilic leukocytes ranges between 15 and 50 percent. In severe cases, particularly terminally, the eosinophilic leukocytosis may disappear entirely.

The skin test to larval antigen becomes positive early in the third week of infection, and may remain so for up to 20 years. The usual positive response is a wheal of 5 mm or more appearing within 30 min, but early in the infection (before the seventeenth day) the response may be of the delayed type. The antigens vary in their sensitivity, and care must be taken to employ a potent preparation.

There is a variety of serologic tests for trichinosis, including the precipitin reaction, the complement fixation test, the indirect fluorescent antibody test, and the bentonite flocculation test, which is probably the best. These serologic tests all become positive by about the third week of the disease and may remain positive for a few years. The serologic tests are most valuable if they are negative initially and then in turn positive or if there is a change in titer.

Muscle biopsy when carried out during the fourth week of infection remains the most useful test for demonstration of larvae or cysts. Myositis is a significant finding even in the absence of larvae or cysts.

In severe trichinosis there may be marked hypoalbuminemia, probably because of protein leakage from damaged capillaries. During the fourth, fifth, and sixth weeks of the disease, concomitant with a rise in antibody, diffuse hypergammaglobulinemia occurs. Elevated levels of circulating IgE have been reported. There may be moderate rises in SGOT, serum aldolase, and creatininephosphokinase, probably related to myositis; the sedimentation rate is characteristically slow.

DIFFERENTIAL DIAGNOSIS Trichinosis must be differentiated from diseases which are characterized by eosinophilia (such as Hodgkin's disease, eosinophilic leukemia, and periarteritis nodosa) and from entities which are characterized by myopathy, such as dermatomyositis. When the central nervous system is involved, the diagnosis may be very difficult.

TREATMENT Thiabendazole, in dosage of 25 mg per kg b.i.d. for 5 to 7 days has resulted in apparent improvement in a number of patients, with relief of muscle pain, and tenderness and with lysis of fever. The results have not been uniform, however, and the use of this drug in trichinosis has been associated with nausea, vomiting, abdominal discomfort, dermatitis, and drug fever.

Patients with "allergic" manifestations of trichinosis, including angioedema and urticaria as well as myocardial or central nervous system involvement, should be treated with prednisone in dosage of 20 to 60 mg per day. Response to steroids usually has been prompt, particularly in central nervous system trichinosis. Not all focal lesions have resolved, however.

Other measures should be directed at relief of pain and maintenance of adequate caloric and fluid intake.

PROGNOSIS The prognosis in trichinosis has improved markedly, and even when the central nervous system is involved, the mortality rate has fallen to under 10 percent. The overall mortality rate is probably less than 5 percent.

PREVENTION The responsibility for control rests with the consumer. Adequate cooking of pork involves heating all portions of the meat to 60°C. Freezing procedures to kill the larvae require a temperature of −15°C for 20 days or −18°C for 24 hr. Proper smoking and pickling will also destroy the larvae. Important in control is the cooking of garbage fed to hogs. There is no practical method of inspection which will detect trichinous pork.

REFERENCES

DALESSIO DJ, WOLFF HG: *Trichinella spiralis* infection of the central nervous system. Arch Neurol 4:407, 1961

GRAY DF et al: Trichinosis with neurologic and cardiac involvement. Ann Intern Med 57:230, 1962

HALL WJ III, MCCABE WR: Trichinosis: Report of a small outbreak with observations of thiabendazole therapy. Arch Intern Med 119:65, 1967

RACHÓN K et al: Serum proteins in human trichinosis. Am J Med 44:937, 1968

ROSENBERG EB et al: Increased circulating IgE in trichinosis. Ann Intern Med 75:575, 1971

SULZER AJ, CHISHOLM ES: Comparison of the IFA and other tests for *Trichinella spiralis* antibodies. Public Health Rep 81:729, 1966

WAND M, LYMAN D: Trichinosis from bear meat. JAMA 220:245, 1972

ZIMMERMAN WJ: Prevalence of *Trichinella spiralis* in commercial pork sausage. Pub Health Rep 85:717, 1970

——— et al: The changing status of trichiniasis in the U.S. population. Pub Health Rep 83:957, 1968

219 FILARIASIS

JAMES J. PLORDE

DEFINITION Filariasis is a group of disorders produced by infection with nematodes of the superfamily Filarioidea. These worms invade the subcutaneous tissues and lymphatics of man, producing reactions ranging from acute inflammation to chronic scarring. The clinical pictures produced by various species in this group are more or less specific. The term *filariasis* is commonly used to designate the disease produced by *Wuchereria bancrofti* or *Brugia malayi*, the organisms responsible for elephantiasis. The disorders associated with infection by *Loa loa* or *Onchocerca volvulus* are usually referred to as *loiasis* and *onchocerciasis*.

FILARIASIS (BANCROFTIAN AND MALAYAN)

ETIOLOGY AND EPIDEMIOLOGY The threadlike adult worms live coiled together in the lymphatics of man. The male *W. bancrofti* measures 35 mm and the female 80 to 100 mm. The *B. malayi* adults are about one-half as long. Gravid females release microfilariae in large numbers into the lymphatics. These embryos, which are sheathed, measure approximately 200 to 300 μm. They eventually reach the peripheral blood, where further development depends on their ingestion by a proper mosquito vector. Species of *Culex*, *Aëdes*, and *Anopheles* transmit Bancroftian filariasis; *Mansonia* and *Anopheles* serve as vectors in Malayan disease. After further development in the vector, larvae migrate to the mouthparts. If the mosquito feeds on a human host, they penetrate the puncture site and reach maturity in about a year. In the absence of reinfection, man harbors microfilariae for 5 to 10 years, the reproductive life of the adult worms. In most *W. bancrofti* and *B. malayi* infections, the microfilariae are found in the blood in greatest numbers between 9 P.M. and 2 A.M. During the day, apparently in response to changes in oxygen tension, they accumulate in the pulmonary vessels and disappear from the peripheral blood. However, in Polynesia there is a variety of *W. bancrofti* that displays a diurnal periodicity in which the peak occurs in the early evenings (subperiodic form). Periodicity is of epidemiologic significance because it determines which species of mosquito serves as the vector. Furthermore, several subperiodic forms of *B. malayi* have been found in animals, suggesting the possibility that this disease has an animal reservoir. Man is the only known vertebrate host for *W. bancrofti.*

Wuchereria bancrofti infection is endemic between latitudes 41°N and 30°S. Distribution is irregular, and there are many peculiar "skip areas" in this geographic pattern, presumably because the endemic disease can be maintained only where human infection and mosquitoes are prevalent. *Brugia malayi* infection is much more restricted in its distribution and occurs in India, Ceylon, Burma, Thailand, Vietnam, China, South Korea, Japan, Malaysia, Indonesia, Borneo, New Guinea, and the Philippines.

Two new types of microfilaria have been described recently. One, found in Brazil, has been named *W. lewisi,* while the taxonomic status of the strain from Portuguese Timor has not been settled.

There were approximately 15,000 *W. bancrofti* infections among American military personnel in World War II. A small endemic focus of *W. bancrofti* once existed near Charleston, South Carolina, but no new cases have been observed since 1930.

PATHOGENESIS Pathologic changes are caused primarily by the presence of the adult worm in the lymphatics and may be divided into inflammatory and obstructive. The inflammatory response, most marked around molting larvae and dead or dying adult worms, consists of infiltration with lymphocytes, plasma cells, and eosinophils. This is followed by a granulomatous reaction which may lead to lymphatic obstruction. There are hyperplasia of lymphatic endothelium, acute lymphangitis, and thrombosis. Repetition of this process over a period of years leads to permanent lymphatic obstruction. The tissues become edematous, thickened, and fibrotic. Secondary streptococcal infections are common. Dilated lymphatics may rupture into surrounding tissue. Elephantiasis is actually a relatively unusual complication of filarial infections. If repeated reinfections do not occur, the disease is self-limited.

MANIFESTATIONS The clinical manifestations vary with the geographic area, species of parasite, and intensity of infection. Light infections may be completely asymptomatic. Symptoms may occur within 3 months of infection, but ordinarily the incubation period is 8 to 12 months. The clinical findings closely reflect the pathologic changes, with inflammation early in the disease followed by obstruction later. Inflammatory filariasis consists of a series of brief febrile attacks occurring over a period of weeks. Fever is usually low grade but may reach 104°F and be accompanied by chills and sweats. Other symptoms include headache, nausea and vomiting, photophobia, and muscle pain. If the involved lymphatics lie close to the surface, the local symptoms dominate the clinical picture. Lymphangitis is very common, involving the legs more frequently than the arms. It often begins as a tender spot in the region of the malleoli or femoral area and spreads centrifugally. The involved vessels are palpably tender and painful. The overlying skin is red and swollen. When abdominal lymphatics are involved, the picture may simulate that of an acute condition of the abdomen. In Bancroftian filariasis the vessels of the spermatic cord and testes may be involved, resulting in painful orchitis, epididymitis, or funiculitis. Lymphadenitis almost always accompanies and may sometimes precede lymphangitis. The inguinal, femoral, and epitrochlear nodes are involved. Abscesses which may form about involved lymphatics and lymph nodes may discharge to the surface, resulting in persistently draining sinus tracts. The acute manifestations last only a few days and then subside spontaneously, only to recur at irregular intervals over a period of weeks or months. Recovery finally ensues. With repeated infections, slowly progressive lymphatic obstruction may develop in areas where the inflammatory reactions have occurred previously. Edema, ascites, lymph scrotum-hydrocele, pleural effusion, or joint effusion may appear as a result of interference with lymphatic drainage. Lymphadenopathy persists. The lymphatic vessels become palpably enlarged as tense elastic masses beneath the skin, especially in the femoral, inguinal, and scrotal areas. They may rupture and form draining sinuses. Internal rupture of lymphatics may give rise to chylous ascites or chyluria. In a small percentage of cases elephantiasis develops. This complication is rare below the age of twenty even in natives of heavily infested areas. The chronic obstructive phase of the disease often is punctuated by acute inflammatory episodes.

Attention has recently been focused on an aberrant type of filariasis which is characterized by hypereosinophilia, the presence of microfilariae in tissue but *not in the blood*, and a chronic clinical course that can be terminated with specific antimalarial treatment. These amicrofilaremic forms were originally thought to be caused by zoontic parasites, but it is more likely that they represent an atypical host response to various filariae including *W. bancrofti* and *B. malayi*. Experience with filariasis in American servicemen during World War II suggests that this response is the rule in individuals who have their first contact with the disease. Clinically there may be marked enlargement of the lymph nodes and spleen (Meyers-Kouwenaar syndrome) and/or chronic cough, nocturnal bronchospasm, and miliary pulmonary infiltrates.

DIAGNOSIS A history of exposure, the long incubation period, the occurrence of typical inflammatory episodes, and the finding of regional lymphadenopathy, thickening of the spermatic cord, or swelling of an extremity should suggest the diagnosis. There is usually eosinophilia during acute episodes. Lymphangiography may reveal dilated afferent and small efferent lymphatics. The definitive diagnosis depends on demonstration of the parasite. Although adult worms can be demonstrated in biopsied lymph nodes, biopsy is not recommended because it may interfere further with lymphatic drainage. Microfilariae are found in the blood during intermediate stages but not early or late in the disease. As in malaria, they are demonstrated best in thick smears. Concentration methods may be used if the parasite is not found in thick smears. Microfilariae are motile and sometimes may be seen in wet mounts. Because the appearance of microfilariae in peripheral blood is periodic, it is essential to obtain blood at appropriate times. Microfilariae may also be found in lymphatic fluid, hydrocele fluid, ascites, and pleural fluid. Skin tests as well as complement fixation, bentonite flocculation, and soluble antigen fluorescent antibody tests are available and, although not completely reliable, are helpful when microfilariae cannot be demonstrated.

TREATMENT Diethylcarbamazine (Hetrazan) rapidly eliminates microfilariae from the blood. It probably also kills or injures adult worms, impairing their ability to reproduce, and clears microfilariae permanently from the bloodstream of many patients. The drug is given in dosage of 2 mg per kg three times a day for 3 or 4 weeks. Treatment with this agent is often followed by allergic reactions to the dying parasite. These reactions may be quite severe, especially in Malayan filariasis. They can be controlled with aspirin, antihistamines, or steroid hormones. In heavy infections, it may be desirable to begin treatment with antihistamines before administration of Hetrazan.

Antimony compounds have no place in the treatment of filariasis.

Reassurance of the patient is very important in this disease. Vaccines and antiserums are valueless. Pressure bandages and surgery sometimes benefit elephantiasis. The prognosis for life is excellent, particularly if infected individuals leave endemic areas or otherwise avoid reinfections. Disease control is accomplished by combining mass treatment with mosquito control measures.

ONCHOCERCIASIS ("RIVER BLINDNESS")

DEFINITION Onchocerciasis is a cutaneous filariasis caused by *Onchocerca volvulus.* It is characterized by subcutaneous nodules, a pruritic skin rash, and ocular lesions.

ETIOLOGY AND EPIDEMIOLOGY The disease is found in focal areas within Mexico, Guatemala, and Venezuela and throughout tropical Africa. New focuses have been discovered in Yemen and Colombia. It is estimated that at least 20 million individuals are infected and that about five percent of these are blind as a result of the disease.

The infection is transmitted by flies of the genus *Simulium,* which breed along fast-moving streams. An inoculated larva matures into a single male or female in approximately one year. Since larvae do not multiply within the human host, heavy parasite loads are the result of repeated infections. The adult worms are found coiled together in fibrous subcutaneous nodules. The gravid females, which may live as long as 15 years, release unsheathed microfilariae that are actively motile and migrate in the skin, subcutaneous tissue, and eye until they die or are ingested by a feeding *Simulium.*

PATHOGENESIS AND CLINICAL MANIFESTATIONS The subcutaneous nodules which enclose the adult worms are usually 2 to 3 cm in diameter when fully developed. Their location on the body is related to the biting habits of the vector. In Central America, where the fly bites on the upper part of the body, the nodules are frequently over the head; in Africa they are primarily on the trunk. They may number from 1 to more than 100.

The important pathologic changes occur as a result of a hypersensitivity reaction to the dead or dying microfilariae. The skin lesion may appear as an erysipelas-like reaction over the face or a pruritic papular rash over one extremity. In chronic cases lichenification and depigmentation may be present. In Africa gross skin lesions are common and may be associated with large folds of skin called *hanging groins.* The most serious complications of onchocerciasis are eye lesions which are usually found in patients repeatedly infected on the upper part of the body. A punctate keratitis, iridocyclitis, or less commonly a chorioretinitis may eventually lead to blindness.

DIAGNOSIS The diagnosis is made by demonstrating microfilariae in a skin snip taken from an involved area. A thin sliver of superficial skin is removed with a razor or punch. Care must be taken to prevent bleeding and possible contamination with blood microfilariae. The skin is placed in saline, teased with a pair of sharp dissecting needles, and observed for emerging microfilariae over the next hour. Multiple skin snips may be necessary. In patients with eye lesions, microfilariae can sometimes be seen in the anterior chamber with a slit lamp. If organisms cannot be detected by the above methods, the patient may be given 50 mg diethylcarbamazine orally. The occurrence of a pruritic papular rash within 24 hr strongly suggests the presence of cutaneous microfilariae (Mazzotti's test). One of the filarial serologic tests may also be helpful.

TREATMENT AND PREVENTION Diethylcarbamazine is effective in destroying microfilariae but has little effect on the adult worm. The drug must be used with great care as rapid destruction of the parasites may cause a severe allergic reaction. If the eye is involved, this can result in further ocular damage. The initial adult dose is 50 mg orally. It is increased to 50 mg three times daily on the second day, 100 mg three times daily on the third day, and finally 200 mg three times a day for an additional 7 days. Antihistamines, or in rare cases steroids, can be used to control allergic reactions. In ocular reactions, the pupil should be dilated and topical steroids applied.

The adult worms may be eliminated by excision of nodules on the head and neck, a procedure which is useful in preventing ocular complications, or by chemotherapy with suramin. Details of the administration and toxicity of this drug are given in Chap. 212. The dosage is 0.1 g given intravenously to detect drug idiosyncrasy, followed by 1.0 g intravenously once weekly for five to six doses.

Chemoprophylaxis is not practical, and personal protection depends upon the use of protective clothing. Insecticides, mass therapy, and nodulectomies have been used but have not been very satisfactory.

LOIASIS

This form of filariasis is produced by *Loa loa* and is prevalent in West and Central Africa. The infection is transmitted by flies of the genus *Chrysops.* The adult worms, which like the other filariae may live for 10 to 15 years, migrate continuously through the subcutaneous tissue. The resulting localized areas of allergic inflammation known as *Calabar swellings* are the hallmark of the disease. Occasionally the adult worms are visible beneath the conjunctiva, and *Loa loa* is often called the *eye worm.* Infestation may, however, be completely asymptomatic. An association between loiasis and endomyocardial fibrosis has been reported. The diagnosis can be made by finding the adult worm or by demonstrating the distinctive sheathed microfilariae in contents of the Calabar swellings or in the bloodstream which they eventually reach. Diethylcarbamazine, administered for 2 or 3 weeks in the manner described for onchocerciasis, will kill both adult worms and microfilariae. This drug taken in a dose of 200 mg twice daily for 3 days each month is also effective as a chemoprophylactic agent.

REFERENCES

AKISADA M, TANI S: Lymphangioadenopathy of filariasis. Trans R Soc Trop Med Hyg 64:885, 1970

BEAVER PC: Filariasis without microfilaremia. Am J Trop Med 19:181, 1970

DUKE BOL: Onchocerciasis. Br Med Bull 28:66, 1972

EDESON JFB: Filariasis. Br Med Bull 28:60, 1972

HAWKING F: The 24-hour periodicity of microfilariae: Biological mechanisms responsible for its production and control. Proc R Soc Lond [Biol] 169:59, 1967

HUNTER GW et al: *A Manual of Tropical Medicine*, 4th ed., Philadelphia: Saunders, 1966

IVE FA et al: Endomyocardial fibrosis and filariasis. Q J Med 36:495, 1967

MAEGRAETH BG, GILLIS HM: *Management and Treatment of Tropical Diseases*, Oxford: Blackwell Scientific Publications, Ltd., 1971

WHO EXPERT COMMITTEE ON FILARIASIS: Wuchereria and Brugia infections, 2d report, Tech. Rept. Ser. 359, Geneva, 1967

220 SCHISTOSOMIASIS (BILHARZIASIS)

JAMES J. PLORDE

DEFINITION Schistosomiasis (bilharziasis) designates a group of diseases produced by three closely related species of digenetic trematodes, or blood flukes, belonging to the family Schistosomatidae—*Schistosoma mansoni*, *S. haematobium*, and *S. japonicum*. These flukes inhabit the circulatory system of man and animals living in tropical and subtropical countries. The organs and tissues most frequently affected are the colon, urinary bladder, liver, lungs, and central nervous system.

ETIOLOGY AND LIFE CYCLE The adult worms, which grow and mature within the portal venous system of the liver, measure 1 to 2 cm in length. The male has a central trough, the gynecophoral canal, that enfolds the longer slender female during most of its life. After copulation the male carries the female against the flow of portal blood to the small mesenteric vessels. *Schistosoma japonicum* ascends the superior mesenteric vein and *S. mansoni*, the inferior mesenteric vein. Both eventually reach the submucosal vessels of the intestine; *S. japonicum* ends up in the small intestine and ascending colon and *S. mansoni*, in the descending colon and rectum. *Schistosoma haematobium* finds its way through the hemorrhoidal anastomoses to the systemic capillaries of the bladder and other pelvic organs. When they can travel no further, the females deposit their eggs one by one, slowly retreating down the vessel in front of them. The eggs, which remain viable for 3 weeks, secrete an enzymatic substance which destroys the surrounding tissue. If the eggs lie close to the mucosal surface, they rupture into the lumen of the gut (or bladder in the case of *S. haematobium*) and are carried to the outside in the urine or feces. On reaching fresh water, the eggs quickly hatch, liberating ciliated *miracidia*. These miracidia have a life span of 6 to 8 hr in which to search out and penetrate the specific snail host appropriate to the species. Within the snail the miracidia are transformed by a process of asexual reproduction into thousands of infective larvae called *cercariae*. When cercariae are released 1 to 2 months after the original penetration of the snail, they swim around vigorously, and if they contact human skin within 2 days, they penetrate it and become *schistosomulae*. Within 24 hr the schistosomulae work their way into the peripheral venules and are carried to the right side of the heart and then to the pulmonary capillaries. After some delay, they enter the systemic circulation. Those parasites that survive the passage through the mesenteric capillary bed finally reach the portal venous system, where they mature into adult flukes in 4 to 10 weeks.

EPIDEMIOLOGY AND CONTROL Schistosomiasis is possibly the most important of the helminthic diseases because of its worldwide distribution and the extensive pathologic changes produced by the parasites. It is believed that about 150 million persons are affected by this condition. It is likely that increasing use of land irrigation in endemic areas will increase this number substantially. Control measures have been relatively ineffective.

The continuing presence of schistosomiasis depends on the disposal of human excrement into fresh water, the presence of suitable snail hosts, and the exposure of persons to water infested with cercarias. Promiscuous defecation, latrine drainage, and unsanitary sewage disposal are the more important sources of pollution of streams and rivers. The disease is contracted by persons washing clothes, bathing, wading, or working in contaminated water. There is a close correlation between the degree of water contact and infection rates in endemic areas. The infection rates and intensity of infection decrease with advancing age. This might be explained in part by reduced exposure to contaminated water but also may reflect slowly developing immunity. In animal models, immunity develops to reinfection with *S. mansoni* but does not seem to affect already established infections. The major stimulus to the development of this immunity seems to be the presence of live adult worms.

Of these three disease-producing blood flukes of man, *S. mansoni* is the most common in the Western Hemisphere. It was brought to the Caribbean area and South America by African slaves. In South America it is present in Venezuela, Surinam, and Brazil. In Africa, it occurs in the Nile Delta, limited areas of North and South Africa, tropical Africa, and the Middle East.

Schistosoma japonicum affects the agricultural population in Japan, China, the Philippines, Thailand, and Laos. Men are more frequently infected than women. An important source of infection in the Orient is the use of human excreta as a fertilizer in vegetable gardens.

Schistosoma haematobium is distributed widely throughout the African continent and is found in several countries of the Middle East. In Africa, it is highly prevalent among the agricultural population of the Nile Valley.

The best attack on schistosomiasis is preventive. Public health measures, including proper disposal of human excrement, provision of pure water supplies, and antihelmintic therapy, should be carried out in endemic areas. The effectiveness of these measures is diminished if there are significant animal reservoirs of the disease, as in *S. japonicum* and possibly in *S. mansoni* infections. Extermination of the mollusk intermediate host by chemical agents in areas where the infestation rate is high is an extremely costly undertaking. Available molluscicides include copper sulfate, pentachlorophenate, and niclosamide (Bayluscid). This drug appears to be the most effective, but the selection of an agent is determined in large part by the nature of the habitat. Biologic snail control methods, although showing promise, have not yet been demonstrated to be effective in the field. Careful attention to the design of irrigation systems in endemic areas can prevent further spread of snail hosts.

SCHISTOSOMIASIS MANSONI (INTESTINAL BILHARZIASIS, SCHISTOSOMAL DYSENTERY)

ETIOLOGY *Schistosoma mansoni* is distinguished from the two other major species by the structure of its eggs and the adult flukes. The eggs are bluntly oval, have a lateral spine, and measure about 140 by about 60 μm. They are passed in feces and, rarely, in the urine. The intermediate snail hosts belong to the genera *Biomphalaria*. Man is thought to be the principal host, but baboons in Kenya have been found to be infected naturally. It is not known as yet whether they constitute an important reservoir of the disease independent of man.

PATHOLOGY AND PATHOGENESIS Schistosomiasis mansoni is divisible into three stages: (1) an early stage of migration, during which the schistosomulae are carried by the blood to the liver and mature into adult parasites within intrahepatic portal veins; (2) an intermediate stage, during which ova are accumulating in various viscera; and (3) a late stage, characterized by scarring and fibrosis.

The greatest damage to man is caused by the eggs or their secretions. Reactions may take the form of a hypersensitivity reaction, granuloma formation, intravascular obstruction, and eventual fibrosis. However, the secretions, metabolic products, and toxins of the adult worms are believed by some investigators to play an important role. As long as they are living, the adult parasites apparently produce no reaction, but when they die numerous eosinophils gather about them.

Eggs that are passed into the lumen of the bowel cause little tissue damage, but if retained, they elicit an eosinophilic and mononuclear cell infiltration followed by granuloma formation. This has been demonstrated to be a delayed hypersensitivity reaction to a soluble antigen secreted by the egg. Healing occurs by formation of fibrous tissue and calcification.

In the bowel, congestion of the colonic mucosa, punctate hemorrhages, and thickening of the wall due to edema and fibrosis of the submucosa are the main findings; in Egypt, pedunculated or sessile polyps were commonly found in the rectum, but this is now unusual. Ova transported from the colon by venous blood are retained in the hepatic portal spaces, where they may produce an endophlebitis. Pseudotubercles form around them, accompanied by eosinophils. The organ is enlarged during the intermediate stage but later contracts as a characteristic periportal fibrosis develops. The larger portal veins are surrounded by collars of fibrous tissue, resulting in a severe presinusoidal form of portal hypertension which frequently leads to marked splenic enlargement. With the development of portacaval anastomoses, some eggs are carried past the liver to the vessels of the lung, where they may produce an inflammatory endarteritis with deposition of hyaline, granuloma formation, and obstruction of pulmonary arterioles. There may be interstitial fibrosis and destruction of pulmonary capillaries. On roentgenogram the granulomas may resemble miliary tuberculosis. In time cor pulmonale may develop. Occasionally ova are carried to the spinal cord through anastomotic venous channels or are deposited there by ectopic adults. The resulting inflammatory reaction may lead to various neurologic manifestations.

MANIFESTATIONS The finding of schistosome ova in the stools of apparently healthy individuals is a relatively frequent occurrence in endemic areas, and heavy worm loads are necessary for the development of severe disease. Because the parasites do not multiply within the human host, symptomatic disease is dependent on the continued exposure to infection.

Itching and urticaria, sometimes with fever, are common but not invariable after exposure. Anorexia, headache, generalized aches and pains, and diarrhea accompanied by abdominal discomfort soon follow and last 1 to 2 weeks. These symptoms occur after invasion of the parasite and during the periods of migration of the larvae. From 30 to 70 days following exposure, when the schistosomulae have become adult males and females and oviposition has occurred, more severe symptoms may appear. These apparently are caused by an allergic response to the growing antigenic mass of ova and adult parasites and consist of high fever, chills, cough, urticaria, abdominal pain, diarrhea, and occasionally melena. Physical examination shows lymphadenopathy, an enlarged tender liver, and fine scattered rales. Sigmoidoscopy reveals an inflamed, engorged mucosa with small areas of ulceration and hemorrhage. The peripheral blood shows an eosinophilic leukocytosis. Ova may not be present in the stool initially but usually appear within a few weeks. The clinical picture in severe infections resembles that of typhoid except for the eosinophilia. This acute illness may last as long as 3 months and subsides gradually. When the initial infection is not severe or when antihelmintic treatment is given, the patient may recover rapidly.

Deposition of eggs continues during the life of the female worm (which may be as long as 30 years) and recurrence of these acute symptoms is common.

The late clinical manifestations are related to granuloma formation, vascular obstruction, and fibrosis elicited by ova in the tissues. Abdominal pain, diarrhea with or without blood, intestinal obstruction, and rectal prolapse reflect the pathologic changes in the colon. The periportal fibrosis in the liver and resulting portal hypertension cause splenomegaly, anemia, leukopenia, and thrombocytopenia. Massive hematemesis from ruptured gastroesophageal varices is a common cause of death. The liver is enlarged, but hepatocellular function usually is well preserved, and spider nevi, gynecomastia, jaundice, and ascites are uncommon.

In some patients, particularly adolescents in whom irreversible vascular changes have occurred in the lungs, pulmonary hypertension associated with chronic cor pulmonale dominates the clinical picture. Deposition of eggs in the spinal cord may result in transverse myelitis.

DIAGNOSIS AND LABORATORY FINDINGS Diagnosis depends on finding the ova in the stools or the rectal mucosa. By the use of methods such as the formol-ether technique for stool concentration, a greater number of eggs is picked up from a given specimen, and a larger number of cases may be detected. Quantitative egg-counting methods are helpful in estimating the severity of infection and in following response to therapy.

By means of a Jackson's laryngoscopic forceps 35 cm long, a piece of mucosa 2 to 3 mm in diameter can readily be obtained through a proctoscope. When this unstained tissue is compressed between two glass slides, the ova can be recognized easily under the low-powered lens of a microscope. It is believed by many investigators that rectal biopsy is the most reliable method of diagnosis; a very small piece of tissue may contain up to several hundred ova. In many cases in which repeated stool examinations have been negative, rectal biopsy has shown living or dead ova. Occasionally, however, stools contain ova when biopsy is negative.

An intradermal test is available and may be helpful in diagnosis. It is quite sensitive except in children and becomes positive about 2 months after infection. It is not species-specific, however, and 25 percent of patients with a history of "swimmers' itch" also react to the antigen. Because it remains positive despite cure, it is valuable in epidemiologic surveys.

The complement fixation test is the most reliable serologic test available. It becomes positive early in the course of infection, often before eggs can be recovered. Like the intradermal test, it is not species-specific. A cercarial slide flocculation test may provide a simple reliable tool for serologic surveys. Serologic tests do not necessarily reflect active infection and may give false positive as well as false negative results. However, positive serologic or skin tests should lead to a vigorous search for eggs by concentration methods or rectal biopsy, but positive tests are not themselves an indication for treatment.

TREATMENT The principal aim of treatment is the elimination of the parasite. Since the severity of disease is related to the intensity of infection, however, the complete eradication of adult worms is probably unnecessary. Because of the toxicity of available antischistosomal drugs, specific therapy should not be undertaken unless viable eggs are demonstrated in stool or biopsy specimens. Certain trivalent antimony compounds are effective against *S. mansoni.* These are tartar emetic (antimony potassium tartrate), stibophen (Fuadin), and stibocaptate (Astiban). *Tartar emetic* remains the most effective agent available but is also the most toxic. Antimony sodium tartrate is less toxic than the potassium salt and is the form generally used. It is administered intravenously as a freshly prepared 0.5% solution. The drug must be given slowly. Extravasation into surrounding tissue leads to painful necrosis. The initial dose is 0.04 g; subsequent doses are given on alternate days and gradually increased to a maximum of 0.12 g by the fifth dose. A total of 1.8 to 2.2 g should be given. The patient should be hospitalized during treatment and should remain at bed rest for a few hours after each injection. Temporary ECG changes are common during therapy; they consist primarily of repolarization abnormalities which disappear a few days after the drug is discontinued. However, arrhythmias, collapse, and sudden death have been reported. Antimonials also may cause hepatitis, acute nephritis, hemolytic anemia, and thrombocytopenic purpura. Any of these complications calls for immediate discontinuation of therapy. Nausea and joint pains can usually be controlled by decreasing the individual dose or increasing the intervals between doses. Heart, renal, or liver disease constitutes a contraindication to therapy with this group of agents.

Astiban appears to be as effective as tartar emetic but is much less toxic. It is given by intramuscular injection as a 10% solution for five doses for a total of 35 to 50 mg per kg (maximum 2.0 g). Toxic side effects are mitigated if injections are given at weekly intervals.

Fuadin contains 6.3 percent trivalent antimony and is less toxic, but also less effective, than tartar emetic. If the drug can be given intramuscularly, daily injections of 1.5, 3.5, and 5 ml are given for the first 3 days; 5.0 ml is then given every other day until a total of 100 ml of a 6.3% solution has been given. Pain at the site of administration is common.

Ambilhar (niridazole) can be taken orally, 25 mg per kg every day in divided doses for 7 days, and may be as effective as Astiban. Although ECG changes occur with this drug also, they are less common than with antimonial therapy. However, there has been a high incidence of neurologic abnormalities, and as many as 80 percent of patients receiving the drug show electroencephalographic changes. Psychotic episodes or convulsions, which disappear when the drug is discontinued, have also been reported.

Hycanthone is a new preparation that can be administered in a single intramuscular injection. Its hepatotoxicity and mutagenic properties may limit its usefulness. It is not available in the United States.

Success of treatment is judged by the disappearance of eggs from the stool, reduction in eosinophils, and alleviation of symptoms. Patients should be examined monthly for 6 to 12 months to detect relapses. If living eggs in significant numbers are found, retreatment is indicated. In the late stages of the disease, therapeutic measures are palliative, since the patient is suffering from fibrosis of the liver, portal hypertension, or hypersplenism. The indications for surgical procedures are the same as for the other forms of portal hypertension.

PROGNOSIS The prognosis is good. Many patients never develop symptoms, and early states of colonic, hepatic, pulmonary, and central nervous system disease are completely reversible with adequate therapy. In the late fibrotic stage, the prognosis is worse.

SCHISTOSOMIASIS JAPONICA (EASTERN SCHISTOSOMIASIS, KATAYAMA DISEASE)

ETIOLOGY The oval eggs are shorter, wider, and smaller than those of the other two species, measuring about 90 × 70 μm. Mature eggs have a minute hook, or spine, laterally situated and smaller than that of *S. mansoni.* The ova are passed in the feces only. The life cycle is similar to that of *S. mansoni,* but amphibious snails of the genus *Oncomelania* are utilized as intermediate hosts. *Schistosoma japonicum* lives in the superior mesenteric venules but frequently migrates into the venules draining the large intestine and oviposits there. Water buffalo, horses, cattle, pigs, dogs, and cats as well as man may harbor the parasite, and some of these species serve as important reservoirs.

PATHOLOGY *Schistosoma japonicum* resembles the mansoni type, but because of the much greater number of ova deposited by the female worms in the former disease, the manifestations are frequently more severe. Fibrosis of the liver develops earlier, and the duration of the disease is shorter—death often ensuing in 2 to 5 years. In advanced cases the gross postmortem findings are emaciation and pallor; a large or contracted liver with periportal fibrosis; splenomegaly, with fibrosis of pulp; ascites; fibrotic nodules over the colonic peritoneum; fibrous thickening and rigidity of the colon, with small polyps projecting from the mucosa; and thickening and fibrosis of the omentum. Microscopically, the tissue changes are similar to those of schistosomiasis mansoni. Eggs and adult worms are more frequently found in ectopic locations, especially the central nervous system, than is the case with *S. mansoni.*

MANIFESTATIONS Following penetration of cercarias through the skin, allergic manifestations such as urticaria, itching, localized dermatitis, cough, and angioneurotic edema accompanied by fever and diarrhea may appear. From 4 to 6 weeks after exposure, gastrointestinal symptoms are evident, a result of ulcerations produced in the intestinal walls by the large number of eggs. Bloody mucoid stools, or periods of bloody diarrhea accompanied by abdominal pain, may be present. If untreated, symptoms may last for several months. The liver enlarges and becomes tender, and splenomegaly develops.

As the disease progresses, signs of portal obstruction, such as engorgement of superficial abdominal veins, ascites, etc., appear. Some individuals present marked splenomegaly, a small contracted liver, profound anemia, leukopenia, and thrombocytopenia associated with severe malnutrition and hypoproteinemia. The majority of individuals suffering from schistosomiasis japonica die of cirrhosis and cachexia, massive hemorrhage from rupture of esophageal varices, or intercurrent infections.

Central nervous system lesions occur more frequently in the brain than in the spinal cord and appear clinically as an expanding tumor.

DIAGNOSIS AND LABORATORY FINDINGS The characteristic ova must be found in the stools in order to establish the diagnosis. In established cases, ova are more difficult to demonstrate in the stools or in rectal biopsy; positive intradermal and serologic tests in suspected cases should lead to an intensive search for the egg.

TREATMENT In general, *S. japonicum* infections are more difficult to treat, and relapses are more frequent. The drug of choice is sodium antimony tartrate; a total dose of 2.2 g should be given in the manner outlined for *S. mansoni.* If a lesion is present in the brain, prompt treatment may forestall the need for surgical intervention. Astiban may be used as an alternative drug. Portacaval shunt may be necessary to control bleeding from esophageal varices.

PROGNOSIS If the condition is not treated early, prognosis is poor in the majority of cases encountered in endemic communities.

SCHISTOSOMIASIS HAEMATOBIA (GENITOURINARY SCHISTOSOMIASIS, ENDEMIC HEMATURIA)

ETIOLOGY AND LIFE CYCLE The eggs are compact, elongated spindles, dilated in the middle and measuring about 140 by about 50 μm. At one pole they present a short terminal spine. The ova are passed in the urine, and occasionally in the feces. The life cycle is similar to that of *S. mansoni.* The adult worms live in the hemorrhoidal plexus of veins, some going to the rectum for oviposition but most of them passing on to the vesical plexus. The intermediate hosts are snails of the genera *Bulimus, Physopsis,* and *Planorbarius.*

PATHOLOGY In the urinary bladder, large numbers of ova are deposited in the submucosa and give rise to dense infiltration with eosinophils, lymphocytes, and plasma cells. These "pseudoabscesses" apparently represent a delayed hypersensitivity reaction to soluble antigens excreted by the egg. The trigone is involved at first, but soon the entire mucosa is thickened and ulcerated. In chronic infections, the other coats become scarred and the muscularis hypertrophies. Pedunculated papillomas often develop at the trigone and about the urethral orifices. The bladder capacity becomes greatly reduced as the organ loses its contractility. Lesions occur in the distal third of the ureters in many cases, causing obstruction and hydronephrosis. Bacterial pyelonephritis may occur. In about 10 percent of cases, calculi develop in the bladder, renal pelvis, or ureters. Fistulas between the urogenital tract and intestines may develop. The prostate and seminal vesicles may be affected, and lymph blockage may produce an elephantoid condition of the genitalia. The cervix and vagina can be infected by extension from the bladder. Carcinoma of the bladder is a frequent late complication in Egypt but not in other areas. Because the ova are deposited in the vesical plexus, ectopic eggs are carried to the lungs with resulting lesions.

MANIFESTATIONS Painful micturition, frequency, and terminal hematuria are the leading symptoms. Secondary bacterial infection of the urinary tract is frequent, and repeated hemorrhages from the bladder produce severe anemia. Salmonellosis, including the carrier state and bacteremia, is frequently associated with *S. haematobium* infection.

DIAGNOSIS AND LABORATORY FINDINGS As in the other types of schistosomiasis, diagnosis is made by finding the characteristic ova in the urinary sediment, in tissues obtained from vesical mucosa, or, less frequently, in the stools.

TREATMENT Chemotherapy is very effective early in the disease and often results in dramatic reversal of symptoms and obstructive phenomena. The drugs are the same as those recommended for *S. mansoni.* Surgery may be required for abscesses, fistulas, strictures, papillomas, and various other complications involving the bladder. Chemotherapy is indicated for secondary bacterial infections of the urinary tract. The criteria of cure are the absence of ova in the urine and bladder wall and the disappearance of ulcerative granulomatous lesions, as revealed by cystoscopic examination.

PROGNOSIS Provided treatment is started without further delay, prognosis is good in recent infection, fair when damage to the bladder and urinary infection have already occurred. Prognosis is very poor in chronic, late infections. After age forty-five, the mortality rate increases fourfold. The frequent coexistence of infection with *S. mansoni* aggravates prognosis and the clinical picture.

SCHISTOSOME DERMATITIS

DEFINITION AND GEOGRAPHIC DISTRIBUTIONS

Certain nonhuman schistosome cercarias may penetrate the skin of man and cause a dermatitis. This condition is known as *schistosome dermatitis*, or "swimmer's itch," and is common in many parts of the world. The condition apparently does not develop after a single contact with cercarias, but it ensues following multiple exposures. Definitive hosts of some of the schistosomes producing dermatitis are the muskrat and migratory birds. Again, snails are intermediate hosts.

Schistosome dermatitis has been reported from the freshwater areas of North Central and Western United States, Alaska, Canada, Oregon, Central and South America, Western Europe (particularly Switzerland), and the Far East.

A seawater dermatitis believed to be produced by nonhuman schistosome cercarias has been reported in New York, Rhode Island, California, Hawaii, and Florida.

PATHOGENESIS AND CLINICAL MANIFESTATIONS

Because the dermatitis develops only after multiple exposures, the condition is believed to represent an allergic reaction, the nonhuman cercarias being the sensitizing agents. Exposed individuals show positive intradermal reaction when tested with cercarial antigen. The initial symptom is usually a prickling sensation, followed by erythema, urticaria, and ultimately a pruritic papular dermatitis which subsides in 1 to 2 days.

TREATMENT Local application of antipruritic lotions such as calamine with menthol or phenol is used to allay itching and thereby reduce the likelihood of secondary infection. Treatment with antihistaminic drugs will relieve the pruritus.

PREVENTION Immediate drying of the skin after swimming has been recommended as a prophylactic measure. This will not completely prevent lesions, since some penetration occurs during immersion. Dimethylphthalate cream has been reported as an effective cercarial repellent.

In some areas, control has been effected by destruction of snails. Copper sulfate and copper carbonate have been used for this purpose. Treatment of shallow waters where snails are abundant has been moderately effective.

REFERENCES

AMAURY C: Hemodynamic studies of portal hypertension in schistosomiasis. Am J Med 44:547, 1968

CHEEVER AW: A quantitative post-mortem study of schistosomiasis mansoni in man. Am J Trop Med 17:38, 1968

GARCIA-PALMIERI MR, MARCIAL-ROJAS RA: The protean manifestations of schistosomiasis mansoni: A clinical pathologic correlation. Ann Intern Med 57:763, 1962

JORDAN P: Epidemiology and control of schistosomiasis. Br Med Bull 28:55, 1972

KAGAN IG: Serologic diagnosis of schistosomiasis. Bull NY Acad Med 44:262, 1968

LEHMAN JS JR et al: Renal function in urinary schistosomiasis. Am J Trop Med 19:1001, 1970

MAEGRATH BG, GILES HM: *Management and Treatment of Tropical Diseases*, Oxford: Blackwell Scientific Publications, Ltd., 1971

MARCIAL-ROJAS RA, FIAL RE: Neurologic complications of schistosomiasis: Review of the literature and report of two cases of transverse myelitis due to *S. mansoni.* Ann Intern Med 59:215, 1963

ORRIS L, COMBES FC: Clam digger's dermatitis: Schistosome dermatitis from sea water. AMA. Arch Dermatol Syphilol 66:367, 1952

SMITHERS SR: Recent advances in the immunology of schistosomiasis. Br Med Bull 28:49, 1972

WARREN KS: The immunopathogenesis of schistosomiasis: A multidisciplinary approach. Trans R Soc Trop Med Hyg 66:417, 1972

221 OTHER TREMATODES OR FLUKES

JAMES J. PLORDE

INTRODUCTION The trematodes of man, with the exception of schistosomes, are similar in morphology and life cycle. The adult flukes are flat, leaflike hermaphrodites that possess an oral and a ventral sucker. They are generally long-lived and produce progressive damage to the tissues of the host. The operculated eggs, which are passed in the feces (except for *Paragonimus*), hatch in the water to produce a ciliated, free-swimming *miracidium.* The miracidium reaches and penetrates the tissue of an intermediate snail host to undergo a period of development, eventuating in the release of free-living *cercariae* from the snail. These, in turn, must reach a second intermediate host, usually an aquatic animal or vegetation, where they encyst forming *metacercariae.* The definitive host is infected when he ingests the parasitized second intermediate host.

PARAGONIMIASIS Definition Paragonimiasis (endemic hemoptysis) is a chronic infection of the lung caused by trematodes of the genus *Paragonimus.* Geographically, it is probably the most widely distributed disease caused by the hermaphroditic flukes.

Etiology and epidemiology Although *P. westermani,* which is widely distributed in the Far East, is the most common cause of human paragonimiasis, a number of other species, including *P. skigabini, P. heterotremus* (China), *P. africanus* (Cameroons, Nigeria, Zaire), and possibly *P. mexicanus* and *P. caliensis* (Central and South America), may cause the disease. The short, plump adults (7 to 12 mm in length, 4 to 6 mm in width) have a life span of 4 to 5 years which they typically spend encysted in the lung parenchyma of the host. Their golden-brown operculated eggs (50 by 90 μm) reach the bronchioles from where they are coughed up and excreted in the sputum or swallowed and passed in the feces.

The infection is acquired by ingestion of cysts in the second intermediate host, a crab or crayfish. The metacercariae excyst in the duodenum, burrow through the intestinal wall into the peritoneal cavity, and then usually migrate through the diaphragm and into the lung. The worms also may be found in the liver, mesentery, skeletal muscle, subcutaneous tissues, and central nervous system, particularly the brain. The dog, cat, pig, rat, and wild carnivores are definitive hosts for the parasite in addition to man.

Pathogenesis and clinical manifestations An eosinophilic granuloma forms about the adult worm eventually leading to the formation of a fibrous cyst. The pulmonary lesions which measure up to 1 cm in diameter frequently communicate with a bronchiole, resulting in secondary bacterial infection. Small, fibrous nodules representing reaction around deposited eggs also occur. Clinically the picture is one of chronic bronchitis and bronchiectasis with production of brownish sputum and hemoptysis. A poorly resolving pulmonary infiltrate, lung abscess, or pleural effusion may be present in heavy infections.

An abdominal mass, pain, and dysentery characterize intestinal or peritoneal infections. Various types of paralysis and epilepsy occur in cerebral involvement. Homonymous hemianopsia, optic atrophy, and papilledema are common. The cerebrospinal fluid usually shows an eosinophilic leukocytosis and elevated protein. Cerebral calcifications are seen on x-ray in 50 percent of cases. *Paragonimus skijabini* infections are characterized by migratory subcutaneous nodules that contain adult flukes.

Laboratory findings Eosinophilia is a constant finding. Definitive diagnosis depends upon finding the characteristic operculated ova in the sputum, stool, pleural fluid, or subcutaneous nodules. A complement fixation test is available, and the results correlate well with active infection. It usually becomes negative within 6 months of successful therapy. The skin test does not distinguish present and past infections and is used primarily for epidemiologic purposes.

Treatment and prevention Bithionol is the drug of choice. From 30 to 40 mg per kg in divided doses should be given every other day for a total of 10 to 15 treatment days. The symptoms disappear rapidly, and most infiltrates resolve within 3 months. Side effects are minor and consist of nausea, vomiting, and urticaria. Emetine and chloroquine are less satisfactory. Prevention of superinfection by the same parasite is important, because the disease is self-limiting.

The most practical control measure is the adequate cooking of all shellfish before they are eaten.

CLONORCHIASIS Definition Clonorchiasis is caused by *Clonorchis sinensis* and is characterized by hepatic lesions produced by the adult worms in the biliary passages.

Etiology and epidemiology *Clonorchis sinensis,* the most important liver fluke of man, lives in the biliary tree and passes 29 by 16 μm eggs into the intestine. The adult *clonorchis,* which measures 15 by 5 mm, is capable of living as long as 25 years. Infection results from ingestion of the raw, dried, salted, or pickled flesh of freshwater fish containing encysted metacercariae. The larva is released in the duodenum. It enters the common bile duct and migrates to the small bile capillaries, where it develops into the adult form in about 1 month. In addition to man, dogs, cats, pigs, and rats serve as disease reservoirs. The main endemic areas are Korea, Japan, China, and North Vietnam. Infections in the United States are usually due to imported dried, frozen, or pickled fish from the Far East.

Pathogenesis and clinical manifestations During the migration of the larvae, the patient may have fever, chills, tender hepatomegaly, mild jaundice, and eosinophilia. The mature worm causes proliferation of the biliary epithelium, periductal fibrosis, chronic pericholangitis, and atrophy of the parenchyma. Light infections are usually asymptomatic, but heavy worm loads can result in periportal fibrosis with the clinical manifestations of portal hypertension. Attacks of suppurative cholangitis may follow biliary obstruction with dead flukes. These occasionally present as hypoglycemic coma. Cholangiocarcinoma may occur in patients with severe, long-standing infections. The adult worms may infest the pancreatic ducts, where they can cause squamous metaplasia and periductal fibrosis.

Laboratory diagnosis The diagnosis usually depends on the demonstration of the eggs in the feces or the duodenal contents. An antigen extracted from adult worms can be used in a complement fixation test for the detection of the host's antibody response. Skin tests are also useful.

Treatment and prevention No consistently effective treatment is known, but some success has been noted with chloroquine diphosphate. Chloroquine is prescribed in a dose of 0.25 g twice daily for 2 months. Infections which do not respond to this dosage should be treated for an additional 2- to 3-month period. Thorough cooking of freshwater fish will prevent infection.

OPISTHORCHIASIS Opisthorchiasis is caused by *Opisthorchis felineus* or *O. viverini* and is characterized by hepatic lesions produced by adult worms in the larger bile ducts. The life cycle resembles that of *C. sinensis*, with lesions and clinical manifestations like those produced by *C. sinensis*. The geographic distribution differs in that it is endemic in Eastern and Central Europe and in Siberia and occurs in some parts of Asia. The diagnosis usually is based on the finding of the eggs in the feces or duodenal contents. Treatment as recommended for clonorchiasis may be used. Infection can be prevented by eating only well-cooked fish.

FASCIOLIASIS Fascioliasis is caused by *Fasciola hepatica*, which like *Clonorchis*, inhabits the bile ducts of the definitive host. When fully matured, the adult measures about 3 by 1 cm and discharges large operculate eggs 140 by 70 μm.

Fascioliasis produces so-called "liver rot" in sheep, the principal definitive host. The disease is most common in sheep- and cattle-raising countries but has been reported from many parts of the world. In North America it occurs in the Southern and Western United States, Central America, and in the Caribbean Islands.

Infection is contracted by ingestion of the encysted form of the fluke attached to edible aquatic plants such as watercress. The larvae excyst in the duodenum, migrate through the intestinal wall, pass into the peritoneal cavity, penetrate the liver capsule, and finally reach the bile ducts, where they mature. Occasionally larvae may migrate to and mature in ectopic locations including subcutaneous tissue, chest cavity, or brain.

Early clinical manifestations are related to the migration of the larval form to and within the liver. Epigastric pain, fever, diarrhea, jaundice, urticaria, pruritus, arthralgia, and eosinophilia may be observed during this stage. Fibrosis of the liver similar to that found in clonorchiasis appears only after prolonged residence of many adult worms in the bile ducts. Obstruction of the bile duct occurs frequently and may be the presenting manifestation of disease. A pharyngeal form of the disease, called *halzoun*, can result from eating infected raw liver, the young adults attaching themselves to the pharyngeal mucosa, occasionally interfering with respiration.

The diagnosis usually is based on the finding of the eggs in the feces or in the duodenal contents. It is difficult to distinguish the eggs from those of *Fasciolopsis buski*. Complement fixation, hemagglutination, and precipitin tests have been reported to be helpful. A skin test is also available.

Treatment is unsatisfactory. Emetine hydrochloride in dosage of 30 mg per day intramuscularly for 18 days may be helpful and at times curative. The drug should not be given to patients with chronic cardiac or renal disease or to children. Bithionol in an oral dose of 50 mg daily for 20 days has been effective and may be less toxic.

To prevent infection, aquatic plants such as watercress should not be eaten, vegetables grown in fields irrigated with polluted water should be boiled, and safe drinking water should be provided.

FASCIOLOPSIASIS Fasciolopsiasis is caused by the large intestinal fluke *Fasciolopsis buski*, which inhabits the upper part of the intestine of its definitive host. The principal definitive host is the pig. In parts of China, India, and other areas in the Far East, infection of man is contracted following ingestion, or peeling with the teeth, of water chestnuts and other edible aquatic plants. The large adults attach themselves to the intestinal mucosa, and these sites may later ulcerate. Diarrhea and abdominal pain appear early. Later, if heavy infection continues, asthenia with ascites and anasarca occurs. Diagnosis is based upon the history and the finding of eggs in the feces. The eggs resemble those of *Fasciola hepatica*. The prognosis in untreated heavy infections, especially in children, is poor. Either tetrachloroethyline or niclosamide as given for hookworm and tapeworm infections, respectively, is effective. Hexylresorcinol can also be expected to cure or markedly reduce the worm burden in the majority of cases.

REFERENCES

Chan PH, Teoh TB: The pathology of *Clonorchis sinensis* infestation of the pancreas. J Pathol Bacteriol 93:185, 1967

Farcey RV, Marsden PD: Fascioliasis in man: An outbreak in Hampshire. Br Med J 2:619, 1960

Koenigstein RP: Observations on the epidemiology of infections with *Clonorchis sinesis*. Trans R Soc Trop Med Hyg 42:503, 1949

Komiya V: Clonorchis and clonorchiasis, in *Advances in Parasitology*, vol. 4, ed B Dawes, London: Academic, 1966, p. 53

McFadzean AJS, Yeung RTT: Hypoglycemia in suppurative pancholangitis due to Clonorchis sinensis. Trans R Soc Trop Med Hyg 59:179, 1965

Plant AG et al: A clinical study of *Fasciolopsis buski* in Thailand. Trans R Soc Trop Med Hyg 63:470, 1969

Sadun EH, Buck AA: Paragonimiasis in South Korea—Immunodiagnostic, epidemiologic, clinical, roentgenologic and therapeutic studies. Am J Trop Med 9:562, 1960

YOKOGAWA M: *Paragonimus* and paragonimiasis. Exp Parasitol 10:81, 139, 1960
——: *Paragonimus* and paragonimiasis, in *Advances in Parasitology*, vol. 7, ed B Dawes, London: Academic, 1969, p. 375

222 CESTODES OR TAPEWORMS

JAMES J. PLORDE

TAENIASIS SAGINATA Definition *Taenia saginata*, the beef tapeworm, is a hermaphroditic cestode which inhabits the intestinal tract of man, its only definitive host.

Etiology and pathogenesis In its adult stage, *T. saginata* measures 5 to 10 m in length and possesses about 1,000 proglottids. The gravid proglottid measures about 5 × 20 mm and possesses 15 to 20 lateral uterine branches, thus distinguishing it from *Taenia solium*, which has 8 to 12. The head, or scolex, measures 1 to 2 mm in diameter and possesses prominent suckers but no hooks. The eggs are ovid, 30 × 40 μm, and are indistinguishable from those of *T. solium*. When the eggs are ingested by cattle, buffaloes, or llamas, the embryo is released in the intestine, invades the intestinal wall, and is carried by vascular channels to striated muscle in the hind limbs, diaphragm, and tongue, the common sites for formation of the cysticercus stage. The cysticercus measures about 5 × 10 mm and consists of a scolex held in a cystlike structure. After ingestion of the cyst in raw or undercooked beef by man, it requires about 2 months for the adult worm to develop in the intestine.

Epidemiology Taeniasis saginata occurs in all countries in which it is the custom to eat raw or undercooked beef. It is particularly prevalent in Ethiopia, Kenya, the Middle East, Yugoslavia, Mexico, and parts of South America and the U.S.S.R. Beef tapeworm transmission, although uncommon, continues to occur in the United States, particularly in the Northeastern and Western parts of the country.

Clinical manifestations In probably the majority of cases the disease is asymptomatic. Epigastric discomfort, diarrhea, hunger sensations, weight loss, irritability, nausea, and rarely an increase in appetite have been reported in association with *T. saginata* infections.

Movements of the worm are sometimes apparent, and occasionally proglottids may crawl through the anus, appearing in the bed linen or underclothing of the distraught host. Rarely, segments become impacted in the vermiform appendix, with development of appendicitis.

Laboratory findings The diagnosis is usually made by the finding of proglottids in the feces. Eggs may be distributed on the stool or perianal area if a proglottid ruptures during defecation, and should be looked for in the absence of segments. The perianal region may be examined as for pinworm infection, using the Scotch tape swab. By this method 85 to 95 percent of infections may be detected, whereas by stool examination only 50 to 75 percent can be recognized. Since the eggs cannot be distinguished from those of *T. solium*, it is necessary to examine carefully either the proglottids or the scolex to identify the tapeworm species correctly.

Treatment Niclosamide (Yomesan) is a relatively new and highly effective taenicide which kills the scolex and immature segments of the worm on contact. This drug may be given without preparation or purge in a single 2-g dose. Four 0.5-g tablets are thoroughly chewed at one time and swallowed with a small amount of water. Few side effects have been reported. As the worm is digested before it is passed in the stool, no attempt should be made to recover the scolex. The stool should be checked at 3 and 6 months to be certain a cure has been obtained. Alternatively, quinacrine (Atabrine) may be used. This drug, for many years the standard medication for tapeworm, is inconvenient to administer. The evening before treatment, the patient takes 30 g sodium or magnesium sulfate in a glass of water. The following morning, while still fasting, he takes 0.8 g quinacrine as 2 tablets of 0.1 g each at 10-min intervals. Nausea, vomiting, and abdominal pain are common. This may be alleviated somewhat by taking 600 mg sodium bicarbonate with each dose of quinacrine. The entire 0.8-g dose can be mixed in water and given as a single dose through a duodenal tube. Two hours later a second dose of sodium or magnesium sulfate is taken. When successful, such treatment will remove the entire worm, which will be found to be stained yellow. If the scolex has not been removed, the tapeworm will regenerate after 2 or 3 months.

Bithional given in two oral 1-g doses 1 hr apart and followed by a purge 2 to 8 hr later has been found to be highly effective by Japanese workers.

Prevention The only practical means of preventing infection is the thorough cooking of beef. Temperatures as low as 56°C for as little as 5 min will destroy cysticerci. Refrigeration and salting for prolonged periods also destroy the cysticercus. Adequate meat inspection and proper disposal of human excreta will also aid in control.

TAENIASIS SOLIUM Definition *Taenia solium*, the pork tapeworm, inhabits the intestinal lumen of man, its only definitive host. The usual intermediate host is the hog, but in some circumstances, the larval or intermediate stages may also develop in man, resulting in a condition referred to as *cysticercosis*.

Epidemiology Taeniasis solium is worldwide but is most common in the U.S.S.R., Eastern Europe, Asia, Africa, Mexico, and South America. At the present time the disease is practically nonexistent in the United States.

Etiology and pathogenesis The hermaphroditic adult tapeworm measures about 3 m in length and possesses a globular scolex containing a rostellum with about two dozen hooklets. There are seldom more than 1,000 proglottids. The gravid proglottid measures about 6 × 12 mm and contains a uterus with 8 to 12 lateral branchings. The eggs resemble those of *T. saginata* but are infective for both man and hog. Although man may be auto-infected when gravid segments are returned to the stomach by reverse peristalsis, the eggs are more commonly transmitted by the fecal-oral route. When ova are ingested by the intermediate host, the embryo is released from the egg, penetrates the intestinal wall, and is carried by vascular channels to all parts of the body. Localization with development to the encysted larval stage ("bladder worm") occurs predominantly in striated muscle of the tongue, neck, and trunk. The cysticerci are ovoid, gray-white, opalescent structures about 1 cm in diameter. Man becomes infected with the adult stage following ingestion of undercooked pork containing cysticerci. The scolex is freed and attaches itself to the intestinal mucosa; development to the adult stage begins at this time.

Clinical manifestations Clinical manifestations of adult worm infestation resemble those associated with *T. saginata*. The clinical picture is entirely different when man serves as the intermediate host. Cysticerci develop in the subcutaneous tissues, in muscles, in viscera, and—of most significance—in the eye and brain. Only a moderate tissue reaction occurs while the scolex is viable. The dead larva, however, behaves as a foreign body and provokes a marked tissue response. Symptoms are related to active larval encystment only in heavy infections. Muscular pains, weakness, and slight fever may be observed. The involvement in the brain may be in the form of a meningoencephalitis when the cysticerci are widely distributed. However, epilepsy, brain tumor, encephalitis, and other types of neurologic disorder may be simulated. Degenerated cysticerci ultimately calcify.

Infection with the adult worm can be detected by finding eggs in perianal scrapings or in the feces. However, to differentiate *T. solium* from *T. saginata* infection, proglottids or the scolex must be examined. Cysticercosis should be suspected in an individual who has lived in a hyperendemic area and who develops neurologic findings. Biopsy of subcutaneous nodules may lead to the identification of typical encysted larvae. Roentgenograms of the soft tissues also often reveal calcified cysticerci. The cysticercosis hemagglutination test may be of help in the diagnosis. The prognosis is in large part determined by the stage and location of the parasite. Surgery may be necessary in cerebral and ocular cysticercosis.

Treatment For removal of the worm in the adult, quinacrine is given as for taeniasis saginata, above. It is well to administer an antiemetic before giving quinacrine, to prevent reverse peristalsis, with return of the eggs to the stomach and release of the embryos. Niclosamide is also very effective against *T. solium*. However, because it results in the maceration of worms with release of ova, cysticercosis could theoretically occur following the use of this drug.

COENUROSIS This is a rare infection of man by the larval stage, or *coenurus*, of the dog tapeworm *Taenia multiceps*. Over 50 cases have been reported to date from both temperate and tropical countries. Infections have involved the subcutaneous tissue, eye, and central nervous system. Cerebral coenurosis usually presents as a slowly growing tumor which is often fatal. Treatment is surgical.

HYMENOLEPIASIS NANA Definition Hymenolepiasis nana is an intestinal infection of man caused by *Hymenolepis nana*, the dwarf tapeworm.

Etiology The life cycle is unique in that both the larval and adult phases occur in the same host. Man, mice, and rats readily contract infection upon ingestion of the eggs. The adult measures about 2 cm in length and may possess more than 100 proglottids.

Distribution Dwarf tapeworm infection has been reported in temperate and tropical regions around the globe. It is the most common tapeworm found in the United States, most of the infections occurring in the Southern states and involving children.

Clinical manifestations This tapeworm infection is characterized by the presence of many adult worms in the host's intestine. When infection is massive, diarrhea and abdominal pain occur.

Treatment Niclosamide, as prescribed for taeniasis saginata, is given each day for five consecutive doses. Children under eight should receive one-half the adult daily dose and infants one-fourth the adult dose. Cure is obtained in 90 percent of patients.

Prevention This is a difficult problem, similar to that encountered in enterobiasis. Only a single host is involved, and the eggs are immediately infective. Personal hygiene should be stressed. The contamination of food by rats and mice should be prevented.

DIPHYLLOBOTHRIASIS LATUM Definition *Diphyllobothrium latum,* the fish tapeworm or broad tapeworm, produces a disease in its definitive hosts, including man, characterized by the presence of the adult worm in the intestinal lumen.

Etiology and pathogenesis The adult worm may be as long as 5 to 10 m and passes between 3,000 and 4,000 proglottids. Unlike *Taenia*, the gravid segments are retained by the worm and the operculated ova are passed directly in the stool. On reaching water, the egg hatches, releasing a free-swimming embryo. This is eaten by small freshwater crustaceans belonging to the species *Cyclops* or *Diaptornus*, in which it develops into a *procercoid*. When the infected crustacean is swallowed by a fish, the larva migrates into the flesh and grows into a *plerocercoid*, or *sparganum*, larva. Man is infected when he ingests raw infected fish. The tapeworm matures in the intestine and after 3 weeks is an adult capable of discharging eggs. The adults of *D. latum* have been known to survive for 5 to 10 years.

Epidemiology The infection is common in the Baltic and Scandinavian countries, Switzerland, Italy, Russia, Japan, Chile, and Central Africa. It also occurs in the north central United States, south central Canada, and Florida. Women who sample "lüdefisk" or "gefüllte fish" as they prepare these dishes often become infected.

Clinical manifestations Most infections are asymptomatic or produce slight, transient abdominal discomfort. Rarely, there may be severe cramping abdominal pain, vomiting, weakness, and loss of weight.

In a small percentage of infected patients, a tapeworm anemia develops which has many features in common with Addisonian pernicious anemia, including central nervous system involvement. The location of the worm in the intestine is important, anemia occurring only when the tapeworm is in the proximal small intestine. Large amounts of vitamin B_{12} have been demonstrated in the tapeworm, presumably absorbed from the host's intestine. *Taenia saginata*, which does not produce pernicious tapeworm anemia, contains about 2 percent as much vitamin B_{12} as *D. latum*. The appearance of anemia is certainly related to vitamin B_{12} absorption and possibly also to decreased production of intrinsic factor or inadequate extrinsic factor. It is apparent that the tapeworm and the host compete for vitamin B_{12}.

Diagnosis The characteristic operculated eggs are discharged into the stools in large numbers, making the diagnosis quite easy.

Treatment Niclosamide as prescribed for taeniasis saginata will cure most infections. In the presence of severe macrocytic anemia, parenteral vitamin B_{12} should be given.

Prevention The most practical control measure is the thorough cooking of all freshwater fish. Freezing of fish at −10°C for 24 to 48 hr will also prevent transmission.

SPARGANOSIS The *sparganum*, or plerocercoid larva, of *Diphyllobothrium mansoni* will develop in man following ingestion (usually in drinking water) of a *Cyclops* bearing the procercoid larva. Sparganosis also follows ingestion of infected frogs or application of infected fresh frog flesh as a poultice. The frog tissues contain the sparganum, which is capable of invading human tissues. The dog and cat are definitive hosts for *D. mansoni*. The infection often presents as a painful subcutaneous swelling. The periorbital tissues may be involved with marked palpebral edema and destruction of the globe. The location of the larvae determines the prognosis of the infection in man. Surgery and local injection of ethyl alcohol with epinephrine-free procaine to kill the worms is the preferred method of treatment. Novarsenobenzol given intravenously is also said to be effective.

ECHINOCOCCIASIS Definition Echinococciasis may be caused by the larval stage of *Echinococcus granulosus* or *E. multilocularis*. These species of echinococcus are distinct morphologically and biologically. In man, *E. granulosus* produces cystic, expanding lesions, involving the liver and lungs primarily, whereas the lesions of *E. multilocularis* are destructive because of their invasive character.

Etiology The adult *E. granulosus* is found in the intestine of dogs, wolves, and other canines, where it may live for five to 20 months. It is a small worm measuring 5 mm in length. In addition to the scolex and neck, it has three proglottids, one immature, one mature, and one gravid. The eggs, which appear identical to those of *T. saginata*, are passed in the feces. When ingested by an appropriate intermediate host such as sheep, cattle, hogs, deer, or man, the embryos escape from the eggs, penetrate the intestinal mucosa, and enter the portal circulation. Many are filtered out by the liver; the rest lodge in the lung or are carried into the general circulation to involve the brain, kidney, bones, and other tissues. The larvae that are not phagocytosed and destroyed develop into hydatid cysts, reaching the diameter of 1 cm within 5 months. Most cysts are unilocular and consist of an external laminated cuticula and an inner germinal layer. Fluid fills and distends the cyst. Brood capsules and daughter cysts develop from the germinal layer. "Hydatid sand" found in the cyst consists of scolices liberated from ruptured brood capsules. Occasionally, evagination of the cyst wall occurs, with the development of a multilocular or alveolar type of lesion. The cycle is completed when the hydatid cyst is ingested by a carnivore. The enormous number of scolices are released in the intestine and develop into adult worms. The life cycle of *E. multilocularis* is similar except that small rodents serve as the natural intermediate hosts, and the hydatid cyst is always of the multilocular or alveolar type. Most of the cysts develop in the liver, and progressive invasion of that organ usually occurs. The lesions may metastasize when growth extends into blood vessels.

Epidemiology The dog is the principal definitive host of *E. granulosa*, and sheep and cattle are common intermediates. Human echinococciasis has its highest incidence in countries where sheep and cattle raising is carried out with the help of dogs, particularly in northeast and south Africa, the Middle East, Central Europe, South America, Australia, and New Zealand. It has been reported from 15 states in this country, and a new focus was discovered recently among Basque sheep farmers in California. A "sylvatic" focus of *E. granulosa* exists in Alaska and western Canada, where wolves act as the definitive host and caribou and moose as the intermediate host. When man kills these herbivores and feeds their viscera to dogs, a domestic cycle is initiated. A sylvatic cycle involving deer and coyotes also appears to exist in California. In *E. multilocularis* infection, rodents and deer mice are the natural intermediate hosts, while wolves, foxes, and coyotes serve as definitive hosts. A domestic dog and cat may also harbor the adult worms, and an urban cycle involving the cat and common house mouse has been described. Human infections have been reported from Russia, Central Europe, Canada, and Alaska. An extensive sylvatic focus has been described in the North Central United States.

Clinical manifestations Enlarging hydatid cysts usually produce tissue damage by mechanical means. The resulting symptoms depend upon the site, type, and rate of growth of the cystic lesions. The hydatids of *E. granulosa* var. *canadensis*, which occur principally in the lung, are small, grow very slowly, and seldom cause symptoms. The unilocular hydatids produced by other strains of *E. granulosa* also grow slowly but eventually may reach enormous size. Hepatic lesions may remain asyptomatic for 5 to 20 years, finally presenting as a palpable abdominal mass or abdominal pain. Obstruction of the bile duct may result in jaundice. Cough, chest pain, and hemoptysis are the most common presenting symptoms of pulmonary echinococcosis. Asymptomatic cysts are frequently discovered on routine chest x-ray. Bone lesions with pathologic fractures occur, and central nervous system involvement may be manifested by epilepsy or blindness. Unilocular lesions may be secondarily infected, resulting in abscess formation and sterilization of the cyst. Rupture of a hydatid into the bile duct, peritoneal cavity, lung, pleura, or bronchus may produce an anaphylactoid reaction which is occasionally fatal. Release of the numerous scolices leads to dissemination of echinococcal infection. The multilocular or alveolar cyst of *E. multilocularis* usually presents as a slowly growing hepatic tumor, with jaundice and portal hypertension.

Diagnosis and treatment The clinical picture is seldom sufficiently characteristic to suggest the diagnosis. When eosinophilia is present, it is helpful. Pulmonary lesions usually present as round somewhat irregular masses of uniform density. Occasionally hepatic calcifications are seen in plain x-rays of the abdomen. A liver scan with radioactive isotopes is extremely helpful in detecting the presence of hepatic lesions and should always be done in suspected cases. Liver hydatids often show a characteristic rim of opacification on celiac arteriography. The skin test (Casoni's test) is usually positive, but lack of a standard antigen and testing technique limits its usefulness. Moreover, patients with other helminthic diseases, particularly schistosomiasis, may give false positive results. Of the serologic tests, the indirect hemagglutination test seems to be the most sensitive and reliable and gives positive results in up to 90 percent of the patients with hepatic hydatid disease. The results are less encouraging in patients with lung disease. The latex agglutination and bentonite flocculation tests are simpler but not as reliable. Occasionally scolices may be demonstrated in the sputum with the Ziel-Nielsen stain. Because of serious reactions to the leakage of cyst fluid into the tissues and body cavities, diagnostic aspiration should not be attempted.

There is no medical therapy. When the cysts become symptomatic, surgical treatment offers the only hope of cure. The size and location of the lesion will determine whether complete excision or sterilization and drainage should be performed. The contents of the cyst should be sterilized with 10 ml of 10 percent Formalin, 1 percent iodine, or 0.5 percent silver nitrate before an attempt to drain or excise the lesion is made.

Prevention In prevention, (1) contact with infected dogs should be avoided, particularly fecal contamination of the hands and food; (2) infected carcasses and offal should be burned or buried, in order to prevent access of dogs to material containing scolices; and (3) dogs should be treated if found to be infected. The reduction of the incidence of echinococciasis in Iceland is an example of the efficacy of control measures.

REFERENCES

FAUST EC et al: *Craig and Faust's Clinical Parasitology*, 8th ed., Philadelphia: Lea & Febiger, 1970

HERMOS JA et al: Fatal human cerebral coenurosis. JAMA 213:1461, 1970

KAGAN IG et al: Evaluation of intradermal and serologic tests for the diagnosis of hydatid disease. Am J Trop Med 15:172, 1966

KEELING JED: in *Advances in Chemotherapy*, eds A Goldin et al, vol. 3, New York: Academic, 1968, p. 109

MOST H: Drug therapy: Common parasitic infections of man. N Engl J Med 287:495, 1972

NEWMAN CM, ARON BS: Roentgen diagnosis of tapeworm infestation. J Mt Sinai Hosp NY 28:91, 1961

PERERA DR et al: Niclosamide treatment of cestodiasis: Clinical trials in the United States. Am J Trop Med 19:610, 1970

POWELL SJ et al: Cysticercosis and epilepsy in Africans. Ann Trop Med Parasitol 60:152, 1966

RAUSCH, RL: Echinococcosis. Bull WHO 39:1, 1968

SAUDI F, NAZARIAN IJ: Surgical treatment of hydatid cysts by freezing of cyst wall and instillation of 0.5 percent silver nitrate solution. N Engl J Med 284:1346, 1971

SCHULTZ MG et al: Epidemiology of beef tapeworm infection in the United States. Public Health Rep 85:169, 1970

SWARTZWELDER JC et al: Sparganosis in southern United States. Am J Trop Med 13:43, 1964

VON BONSDORFF B et al: Vitamin B_{12} deficiency in carriers of the fish tapeworm, *Diphyllobothrium latum*. Acta Haematol 24:15, 1960

WILLIAMS JF et al: Current prevalence and distribution of hydatidosis with special reference to the Americas. Am J Trop Med 20:224, 1971

WILSON JF et al: Cystic hydatid disease in Alaska. Am Rev Resp Dis 98:1, 1968

section 23 | Diseases of uncertain etiology

223 SARCOIDOSIS

CAROL J. JOHNS

DEFINITION There is no basis for altering the definition adopted by the 1960 International Conference of Sarcoidosis, which states:

Sarcoidosis is a systemic, granulomatous disease of undetermined etiology and pathogenesis. Mediastinal and peripheral lymph nodes, lungs, liver, spleen, skin, eyes, phalangeal bones, and parotid glands are most often involved but other organs or tissues may be affected. The Kveim reaction is frequently positive, and tuberculin type hypersensitivity is frequently depressed. Other important laboratory findings are hypercalcuria and increased serum globulin. The characteristic histologic appearance of epithelioid tubercles with little or no necrosis is not pathognomonic and tuberculosis, fungal infection, beryllium disease and local sarcoid tissue reactions must be excluded. The diagnosis should be regarded as established for clinical purposes in patients who have consistent clinical features together with biopsy evidence of epithelioid tubercles or a positive Kveim test.

ETIOLOGY The cause of sarcoidosis remains unknown. Hypotheses include a special form of tuberculosis (with unusual host reactivity or some alteration in the tubercle bacillus), a single as-yet-unidentified inciting agent, or a tissue reaction induced by differing agents, with factors of genetic susceptibility and unidentified factors of hypersensitivity. The last is supported by familial aggregations of sarcoidosis, observed immunologic abnormalities, and the occurrence in sarcoidosis of manifestations common to hypersensitivity diseases such as erythema nodosum, uveitis, arthritis, and occasionally arteritis, and thyroiditis. A factor related to the tubercle bacillus or a fungus could well serve as an immunologic sensitizer in *some* patients and initiate the widespread granulomatous reaction.

EPIDEMIOLOGY Sarcoidosis has been observed in virtually every country in which it has been sought. Negroes are ten times more commonly affected than Caucasians in the United States, and the incidence in females is usually double that in males. An increased incidence in relation to pregnancy and lactation has been noted, especially in patients with erythema nodosum. The disease is most frequent in the third and fourth decades of life, but the range begins in childhood, particularly around adolescence, and extends to the sixth and seventh decades. Sarcoidosis has been observed in siblings and in parent and child but not in husband and wife. There is no evidence for patient-to-patient transmission.

PATHOLOGY Granulomatous inflammatory changes of sarcoidosis may occur in almost any organ. Disseminated granulomas are probably often present even with clinically localized disease, i.e., hepatic granulomas with only asymptomatic hilar adenopathy. The hard tubercles are generally sharply demarcated from surrounding tissues but may coalesce. Some central fibrinoid necrosis may occur, especially in association with systemic active febrile disease, but caseation is usually absent, and inflammatory reaction is minimal. Giant cells containing laminated calcific Schaumann bodies or stellate "asteroid" bodies are frequent, but neither of these inclusions is found solely in sarcoidosis.

Similar histologic changes may be seen in tuberculosis, fungus infections, leprosy, tertiary syphilis, beryllium disease, "farmer's lung," foreign-body reactions, lymphomas, and lymph nodes draining malignant tumors. The histologic picture in sarcoid is not specific for that disease alone, and the above-mentioned possibilities cannot be excluded in the absence of other data.

Adrenal corticosteroids cause a prompt reduction in the nonspecific cellular inflammatory reaction of an acute or subacute process and hasten involution and resorption of the "sarcoid" tubercles. It is not certain whether these hormones prevent or lessen scarring.

Autopsy material on patients with long-standing sarcoidosis may reveal widespread tubercles in many organs, a few scattered tubercles or focal hyaline scarring, or rarely, no residual changes.

MANIFESTATIONS Clinical manifestations of sarcoidosis generally depend on the activity, degree, and site of tissue involvement and vary from incidental radiographic findings without associated symptoms, to severe incapacity and death. Impaired function is caused both by active granulomatous disease and by secondary fibrosis. Mediastinal and peripheral lymphadenopathy, pulmonary disease, fever, cutaneous lesions, and uveitis are the most frequent presenting manifestations.

Constitutional symptoms Fever, weight loss, and fatigue are often nonspecific presenting complaints, occasionally without other localizing symptoms. Persistent daily spiking fever to 101°F may be observed and necessitates careful exclusion of tuberculosis. This is most commonly observed in association with active granulomatous inflammation in the liver. Fever in association with *erythema nodosum* is another form in which sarcoidosis may become evident. This syndrome includes transient tender erythematous subcutaneous nodules over the pretibial areas, arthralgias, and pulmonary hilar adenopathy on x-ray. Hepatic tubercles and a positive Kveim reaction are frequent. This syndrome has been regarded as an early manifestation of sarcoidosis and noted frequently in young women in Scandinavia and Great Britain. It is also observed in the United States, may be overlooked easily, and has a favorable prognosis.

Lymph nodes Mediastinal and hilar nodes are most frequently involved. Vague substernal discomfort may be present. Readily palpable peripheral nodes which are discrete, firm, and nontender are often prominent. There may be generalized lymphadenopathy, or involvement may be localized to the cervical, axillary, and femoral nodes. Usually, the changes are symmetric, and the epitrochlear nodes are palpable.

Lungs Pulmonary involvement is the most common and, perhaps, the most important manifestation of sarcoidosis. Spontaneous permanent remissions are observed, but significant lung disease represents the most frequent indication for treatment. Serious parenchymal changes, with or without hilar adenopathy, are evident on x-ray in about 50 percent of all patients. Varying and impressive degrees of dyspnea and cough are noted. A discrepancy in which the radiographic changes exceed the symptoms and signs is a diagnostic clue in early sarcoidosis. In some patients, usually Caucasian, striking radiographic changes may be associated with no symptoms and ventilatory and diffusion measurements are normal. In others, often Negroes, pathologic and physiologic abnormalities may be present when the x-ray shows only hilar adenopathy. Dyspnea may be severe and is present in approximately half the patients with parenchymal disease. This results from extensive interstitial changes which impair oxygenation by destruction of effective diffusing surface. Compensatory hyperventilation is often noted. Large rounded intrapulmonary masses which may resemble metastatic tumor are probably a result of primary involvement of lymphoid tissue or localized infiltrates producing minimal physiologic disturbance and minimal symptoms despite their dramatic x-ray appearance. Pleural effusions are unusual and should lead to the suspicion that other disease is present.

Cough may be severe and incapacitating and may occur in paroxysms which can even lead to vomiting. Sputum is scanty; occasional blood streaking results from the strain of coughing or endobronchial granulomas or in association with a picture that resembles bronchiectasis. Wheezing is occasionally produced by localized bronchial lesions with stenosis. Physical findings are variable and nonspecific. Respiratory excursion may be restricted, crackling rales may be heard diffusely or at the lung bases, and the P_2 may be accentuated or split if pulmonary hypertension develops.

Bronchoscopy generally reveals normal mucosa, although in a few cases it shows granulomatous inflammatory changes with endobronchial narrowing. Granuloma may be demonstrated occasionally in grossly normal-appearing mucosa.

In some patients sarcoidosis is a chronic progressive disease, and pulmonary insufficiency and cor pulmonale occur as late features. Bronchiolostenosis, resulting from peribronchial fibrosis and mucosal changes, may result in localized emphysema, giving rise to systic changes, usually in the upper lung fields. With superimposed bacterial infection, a bronchiectasis-like picture results. Large cavitary or bullous lesions are rare but may lead to large and repeated hemoptyses, which are occasionally fatal. Such lesions may also form the locus for an aspergilloma, with which hemoptyses or disseminated *Aspergillus* infection are hazards. However, these "fungous balls" are usually saprophytic and often multiple. They may vary spontaneously in size and number over periods of ten or more years, without invasive disease, even when steroid maintenance treatment is required. Surgical management is rarely feasible because of the diffuse and restrictive nature of the disease. Spontaneous pneumothorax is an occasional complication of lung involvement.

Eyes Acute granulomatous uveitis may be the initial manifestation of sarcoidosis. Ocular disease may progress to severe visual impairment and blindness with corneal and lenticular opacities and secondary glaucoma. A careful slit-lamp examination is worthwhile in all patients with sarcoid to detect early evidence of anterior uveitis. Lacrimal gland enlargement, conjunctival infiltrations, and keratoconjunctivitis sicca of the type seen in Sjögren's syndome (Chap. 363) are common. Exophthalmos has been observed, as have retinal lesions with vasculitis producing papillitis and periphlebitis.

Skin Lesions occur in about 30 percent of patients, most dramatically around the nose, eyes, and mouth, and vary from extensive erythematous, infiltrated, and raised lesions to small nondescript plaques and papules. Mucosal lesions are often associated, extending into the nose, sinuses, and the hard palate. Increased or decreased pigmentation is frequently noted. Sarcoid changes often occur at sites of old scars or recent injury. Subcutaneous nodular infiltrations occur, and in rare instances calcification of such lesions has been observed. Alopecia occurs if the scalp is affected. Skin lesions are associated with chronicity but often with otherwise mild disease. Erythema nodosum in early sarcoidosis usually presents a histologic picture of a nonspecific vasculitis.

Liver Clinical manifestations of hepatic sarcoidosis are present in only about 20 percent of cases. Nevertheless, hepatic tubercles can be found by biopsy in about 75 percent and provide one of the most useful means of obtaining histologic confirmation of the diagnosis. Asymptomatic hepatomegaly is frequent. Severe jaundice is unusual, but mild increase in bilirubin and striking elevation of serum alkaline phosphatase level are observed. Intense pruritus may be the presenting manifestation. The spectrum of hepatic sarcoid includes the incidental tubercle, tubercles with surrounding nonspecific inflammatory reaction, chronic active granulomatous hepatitis, postnecrotic cirrhosis with or without portal hypertension, and portal hypertension without significant cirrhosis. Esophageal varices have been demonstrated in patients with portal hypertension, and shunt procedures occasionally have been required. Response to steroids has been disappointing in severe hepatic sarcoid. In some patients the granulomatous disease is limited to the liver, spleen, and abdominal nodes without other clinical or radiographic evidence of sarcoidosis.

Spleen Mild splenomegaly occurs in 20 to 30 percent of cases and often regresses promptly with administration of corticosteroids. Enlargement may be striking and associated with "hypersplenism," anemia, leukopenia, and thrombocytopenia. It may persist for 10 to 20 years without undue complications, although splenectomy will result in hematologic improvement.

Kidneys Impaired renal function may occur secondary to hypercalcemia and hypercalcuria, secondary to hyperuricemia, and less commonly, because of direct granulomatous involvement. Nephrocalcinosis and renal calculi are observed.

Heart Effects are usually secondary to lung disease, with pulmonary hypertension and cor pulmonale. Primary myocardial sarcoidosis is most commonly manifested by conduction disturbances and paroxysmal arrhythmias.

Salivary glands Asymptomatic enlargement of the parotid, sublingual, and submaxillary glands occurs in about 6 percent of cases. Spontaneous regression commonly occurs. A syndrome of fever, uveitis, and lacrimal and salivary gland enlargement is known as uveoparotid fever, or Heerfordt's syndrome. Facial nerve palsies may be associated with parotid disease.

Muscle Sarcoid granulomas occur in muscles far more frequently than is clinically indicated by pain and weakness. In a few cases symptoms may be severe and incapacitating. Muscle biopsy is likely to be positive in such patients and also in those with polyarthralgias.

Joints Arthralgias may occur independently as an early prominent feature and are common in association with erythema nodosum and fever. Sarcoid tubercles have been observed in biopsies of synovium. Transient knee effusions are occasionally noted. Chronic periarticular swelling and tenderness may be associated with bony changes in the fingers and toes and skin lesions.

Bones Asymptomatic, punched-out lesions in the distal phalanges of the hands and feet are visible in roentgenograms in about 10 percent of cases. Associated overlying skin changes are common. Radiolucent skull lesions have been noted in a few patients. "Routine" hand x-rays are not likely to be abnormal in the absence of overlying skin changes.

Nervous system Neurologic manifestations are variable. Cranial and peripheral nerves may be affected by direct involvement of the nerve sheaths or roots. Facial nerve palsies, which may be bilateral and sequential, are the commonest neurologic finding and may undergo full remission. Swallowing disorders are observed. A granulomatous basilar meningitis can affect the cranial nerves and produce pleocytosis and elevation of the spinal fluid protein level. Pituitary involvement produces diabetes insipidus. Involvement of the choroid plexuses may obstruct the ventricles. Cortical changes may result in convulsive seizures.

Other tissues Involvement of the tonsils and laryngeal, buccal, and nasal mucosa (often with associated sinusitis) has been encountered. Sarcoid lesions have been found in thyroid, parathyroid, and pancreatic tissues, and gastric granulomas have resulted in bleeding and perforation. Sarcoid involving the adrenal, cervix, uterus, epididymis, or testis is very unusual.

LABORATORY FINDINGS Mild anemia, leukopenia, eosinophilia, and elevated sedimentation rate are common in active disease. Thrombocytopenia is unusual but may be severe.

Delayed skin reactions Tuberculin anergy is noted in about two-thirds of patients, but a positive tuberculin reaction occurs if active tuberculosis intervenes. A previously known positive tuberculin reaction may become less reactive with active sarcoidosis. Associated generalized cutaneous anergy to other commonly occurring antigens such as *Candida albicans*, *Trichophyton*, and mumps virus has been noted. This depression of delayed skin reactivity is considered to be an important feature of sarcoidosis, but it varies with the duration and activity of the disease.

Chemical studies Hypergammaglobulinemia and reduction of serum albumin are common. Hypercalcemia and hypercalcuria are infrequent but apparently result from increased intestinal absorption of calcium, which is possibly related to increased sensitivity to vitamin D. Serum uric acid level may be elevated even in the absence of renal insufficiency. Elevation of serum alkaline phosphatase level is attributable to intrahepatic tubercles, rather than to bone lesions, and may reach very high levels.

Roentgenographic studies Approximately 90 percent of patients will eventually show intrathoracic disease on chest x-ray. Bilateral hilar adenopathy, often with associated right paratracheal adenopathy, is a common feature. Unilateral hilar adenopathy is unusual and should initiate a search for other diseases. Patients may be grouped according to apparent severity and chronicity of the radiologic picture as follows: group I—hilar adenopathy with no parenchymal changes; group II—hilar adenopathy and diffuse parenchymal changes; group III—diffuse parenchymal changes without hilar adenopathy; group IV—chronic parenchymal changes of more than 2 years' duration with pulmonary fibrosis. The pulmonary changes are generally symmetric, and may present a diffuse ground-glass appearance, fine reticular or miliary lesions, large nodular lesions, or multiple large confluent infiltrates resembling metastatic tumors. Fine diffuse interstitial fibrosis may be present. Pulmonary fibrosis may produce contraction and distortion, and extensive cystic and bullous lesions are common in the late stages. Bony changes in the phalanges and skull may occur.

Pulmonary function tests These tests commonly demonstrate restriction, decreased compliance, and loss of effective diffusing surface. Vital capacity is reduced. Measurements of oxygen- and carbon monoxide-diffusing capacity are frequently reduced even in the absence of demonstrable radiographic changes or clinical symptoms. Measurements of vital capacity and diffusing capacity may serve as indicators of progression of disease and response to treatment. In diffuse disease, arterial blood studies reveal with exercise a reduced P_{O_2} because of perfusion of poorly ventilated areas of the lung. The arterial P_{CO_2} is commonly below normal because of contemporary hyperventilation. Because ventilatory obstruction occurs only occasionally, and then in severe, late stages of pulmonary fibrosis, carbon dioxide retention with elevation of arterial P_{CO_2} is a late and unusual feature. Significant impairment of pulmonary function frequently remains even after radiographic clearing. Following steroid therapy or a spontaneous remission, the vital capacity tends to return toward normal, but may remain somewhat reduced. The diffusing capacity may improve significantly but usually stabilizes well below normal despite complete remission of all symptoms. Improvement in diffusing capacity is less frequent than is that of the vital capacity. Deterioration of pulmonary function may occur gradually and progressively.

DIAGNOSIS The diagnosis depends on the clinical features along with histologic evidence of epithelioid tubercles from tissue biopsy or from a positive Kveim reaction. It is essential to exclude other recognized causes of granulomatous disease. To exclude local sarcoid tissue reaction, as in nodes draining a malignant tumor, evidence of involvement of more than one site is desirable. Careful search for tubercle bacilli, fungi, and foreign bodies must be made in all histologic sections. A positive Kveim reaction is perhaps the unique feature, and helps to exclude other granulomatous processes, but the specificity of this reaction is uncertain. Tissue biopsy for histologic diagnosis is most readily and easily obtained from superficial or palpable lesions in skin, lymph nodes, conjunctiva, and nasal, buccal, and bronchial mucosa. Almost any palpable lymph node is likely to be positive. Epitrochlear and supraclavicular nodes will verify the diagnosis in a high percentage of cases. Liver biopsies reveal granulomas in 70 to 80 percent of cases even without clinical evidence of impaired hepatic function. Biopsy of the gastrocnemius muscle frequently reveals granulomatous changes in patients with arthralgias and erythema nodosum. In the absence of palpable peripheral lymph nodes, or dermal lesions, biopsy of liver, deeper lymph nodes (as with mediastinoscopy), or muscle is in order. Lung biopsy is generally reserved for patients in whom other diagnostic maneuvers have not been successful or in whom the exclusion of other diseases is urgent. The indicated tissue biopsy is that which combines the least risk with the greatest likelihood of diagnostic yield.

Kveim reaction In 50 to 80 percent of patients with sarcoidosis, the intracutaneous injection of a heat-sterilized suspension of human sarcoid tissues (spleen or lymph nodes) produces a papulonodular lesion with epithelioid tubercles. The nodule must be biopsied in 4 to 6 weeks for routine histologic study. This reveals a spectrum from positive to negative, and includes a middle equivocal group. A positive reaction is limited to those with well-formed *epithelioid tubercles.* Test material must be assayed in patients of known reactivity, and experienced interpretation is essential. The Kveim reaction is very likely to be positive in the presence of sarcoid lymphadenopathy, in association with erythema nodosum, and when sarcoid skin lesions are present. The reaction is less likely to be positive in the absence of lymph node involvement and during steroid therapy. Tests in patients with a variety of granulomatous and collagen vascular diseases have revealed only 2 to 5 percent false positive reactions, but many false negative results are encountered in patients later shown to have sarcoidosis. The nature of the Kveim reaction is not understood, and its relation to other causes of lymphadenopathy must be evaluated.

COURSE Sarcoidosis is frequently no more than an incidental radiographic finding on routine chest x-ray. The course is often one of spontaneous remission over a period of 6 to 24 months, with little or no evidence of residual disease and with normal life expectancy. However, there may be persistent abnormalities with varying disability or progressive deterioration. Death related to sarcoidosis may ensue in 5 to 10 percent of cases and is most frequently related to advanced pulmonary disease. There may be impressive clearing of radiographic lesions, especially when the disease seems limited to the thorax. Following a spontaneous remission, recurrence is most unusual. Remissions are most frequent in the syndrome of erythema nodosum and hilar adenopathy. This "benign" form is more common in Caucasians than in Negroes, where chronic progressive disease is more frequently encountered. Systemic manifestations in skin, bone, eyes, and salivary glands and hepatosplenomegaly herald a less favorable prognosis. Severe uveitis may progress to glaucoma, cataract formation, and blindness.

The influence of steroids on the prognosis is not clear but is probably favorable if there is significant incapacitating disease.

TREATMENT Relatively asymptomatic patients often require no treatment. *Adrenal corticosteroids* dramatically suppress the active inflammatory reaction and provide important symptomatic improvement. Indications for treatment are (1) active ocular disease; (2) persistent or progressive pulmonary involvement; (3) persistent hypercalcemia or hypercalcuria; (4) central nervous system involvement with significant functional impairment; (5) persistent systemic evidence of illness such as fever and weight loss; or (6) significant and progressive involvement of a vital organ. The disease remains in remission in some patients after administration of steroids, but it commonly recurs as the dose is reduced, even when therapy has been continued for two or more years. It is thought that steroids prevent the progression of disease, but healing may occur with hyaline scarring. Steroids clearly cannot reverse a fibrotic process. Early steroid therapy offers more hope than that initiated after 1 to 2 years of disease.

Steroids are most frequently required and beneficial for symptomatic lung disease. Uncertainty as to the value of steroids may stem from attempted evaluation of benefits in patients with asymptomatic minimal disease which probably required no treatment. Even relatively asymptomatic but significant lung disease should be treated if there is no evidence of spontaneous regression in 6 to 12 months, or if there is progression in 3 months. Asymptomatic hilar adenopathy without evidence of pulmonary parenchymal disease does not require therapy.

Prednisone is administered in initial divided daily doses of 40 mg, with 2-week periods on daily doses of 40, 30, and 25 mg, and then in maintenance doses of 20 to 10 mg. Symptomatic improvement occurs in 1 to 2 weeks, and the disease regresses over a period of several months. Therapy probably should be continued for a minimum of 6 months, with periodic attempts thereafter to reduce dosage or eliminate the drug. Objective criteria such as x-rays and measurements of pulmonary function are important. Maintenance therapy for many years has proved necessary in many patients in whom relapses recur at a dose below 10 to 15 mg. Dosage must be tapered slowly, with decrements of 2.5 mg no oftener than at 2- to 4-week intervals if long-term treatment has been used. Lifelong therapy must be required. Careful documentation and observation during tapering are essential in planning treatment. The efficacy of alternate-day dosage is not well established, but this regimen may be used for maintenance therapy. It is probably not advisable for initial management. Endocrine side effects, with weight gain of 20 to 50 lb, have been observed in some women. Diabetes has appeared in some patients, particularly in association with significant hepatic involvement. Local steroid therapy has been effective in ocular sarcoid with anterior uveitis or iritis, although there is the risk of glaucoma. Intradermal steroids have been used with some success for disfiguring cutaneous lesions. Such lesions are not usually considered justification for systemic steroids.

Oxyphenbutasone also has been observed to produce radiographic remission comparable to that of steroids in a small series of relatively asymptomatic patients. There has been less experience with this drug than with steroids.

Chloroquine (Aralen), in doses of 250 to 500 mg daily, has been observed to induce dramatic improvement in skin lesions over periods of several weeks, but relapse is the rule when the drug is withdrawn. With periodic ocular examinations and intermittent treatment periods of 6 months no irreversible retinal damage has been encountered. Remission may be maintained with as little as 125 mg daily. Response to hydroxychloroquine (Plaquenil) has been slower and less satisfactory. Hypercalcemia has also appeared to respond to chloroquine. Other beneficial effects of chloroquine in sarcoidosis have been less certain and slower, although temporary radiographic remissions of lung disease have been noted after 4 months of chloroquine sulfate in 400- to 600-mg daily doses.

Antituberculous therapy is ineffective in sarcoidosis. However, prophylactic isoniazid in association with corticosteroids, is often recommended for Negro patients with extensive pulmonary disease, in areas with high risks of exposure to tuberculosis, and always for patients who are tuberculin-positive. If tuberculosis is really suspected, two drugs should be employed, i.e., isoniazid and ethambutol, especially if corticosteroids are to be administered (Chap. 156).

COMPLICATIONS The complications are related to the effects of severe and progressive disease in various organs, the side effects of therapy, and superimposed infection. An increased incidence (2 to 5 percent) of tuberculosis in association with sarcoidosis has been recognized. Superimposed fungous infections seem to be increasing. Aspergillosis with "fungous balls" developing in cysts has occurred. Candidiasis and cryptococcosis in association with sarcoidosis have also been noted. It is highly probable that long-term steroid and antimicrobial therapy predispose to these fungous infections.

REFERENCES

Emirgil C et al: Long-term study of pulmonary sarcoidosis. The effect of steroid therapy as evaluated by pulmonary function studies. J Chronic Dis 22:69, 1969

Foti PR, Moser KM: Laboratory guides to scalene node or liver biopsy in suspected sarcoidosis. Am Rev Resp Dis 99:610, 1969

Goldstein RA et al: The infrequency of hypercalcemia in sarcoidosis. Am J Med 51:21, 1971

Hirsch JG et al: The Kveim test. N Engl J Med 284:1326, 1971

Israel HL, Goldstein RA: Kveim reaction and lymphadenopathy in sarcoidosis and other diseases. N Engl J Med 284:345, 1971

——, Ostrow A: Sarcoidosis and aspergilloma. Am J Med 47:243, 1969

Longcope WT, Freiman DG: A study of sarcoidosis: Based on a combined investigation of 160 cases including 30 autopsies from The Johns Hopkins Hospital and Massachusetts General Hospital. Medicine 31:1, 1952

Maddrey WC et al: Sarcoidosis and chronic hepatic disease: A clinical and pathologic study of 20 patients. Medicine 49:375, 1970

Mayock RL et al: Manifestations of sarcoidosis: Analysis of 145 patients, with a review of 9 series selected from the literature. Am J Med 35:67, 1963

Reisner D: Observations on the course and prognosis of sarcoidosis, with special consideration of its intrathoracic manifestations. Am Rev Resp Dis 96:361, 1967

La Sarcoidose, Rapports de la IV Conference Internationale Paris, 12-15 Septembre, 1966, eds J Turiaf, J Chabot, Paris: Masson et Cie, 1967

Winnacker JL et al: Endocrine aspects of sarcoidosis. N Engl J Med 278:427, 483, 1968

224
INFECTIOUS MONONUCLEOSIS

JAMES C. NIEDERMAN

DEFINITION Infectious mononucleosis (IM) is an acute and usually benign infectious disease caused by the Epstein-Barr virus (EBV). It occurs most commonly among adolescents and young adults, who have a characteristic clinical picture consisting of fever, pharyngitis, lymphadenopathy, an increase of peripheral lymphocytes with a high proportion of atypical cells, and the development of transient heterophil and persistent EBV antibody responses.

HISTORY Idiopathic lymphadenopathy in children was first reported in the medical literature by Filatov, a Russian pediatrician, in 1885. Pfeiffer described glandular fever (*Drüsenfieber*) as a clinical entity in 1889. It was not until 1920 that the term infectious mononucleosis was employed by Sprunt and Evans; shortly thereafter the condition they described was recognized to be the same disorder as glandular fever.

In 1932, a diagnostic test was introduced by Paul and Bunnell, who demonstrated the development of heterophil antibodies during the course of the disease; the characteristic absorption patterns of this antibody were described by Davidsohn and Walker several years later. Evidence of the etiologic role of EBV was first recognized by Henle et al. early in 1968.

ETIOLOGY EBV, which has the structural and immunologic characteristics of a member of the herpes group, was originally discovered by electron microscopic studies of tumor cells from biopsies of Burkitt's lymphoma grown in tissue culture. EBV antibodies measured by immunofluorescence techniques, complement fixation, and virus neutralization are consistently absent prior to infectious mononucleosis, regularly develop during the course of the disease, and persist with little change for many years thereafter. In addition to IgG, EBV-specific IgM antibody has been demonstrated during acute infectious mononucleosis in serums obtained 7 to 70 days after onset, and in one instance persisted for 6 months in association with protracted clinical symptoms.

Further evidence of a causative relationship is the presence of EBV in leukocytes cultured from acute cases of mononucleosis as well as from subjects with a past history of the disease. The classical heterophil antibody of infectious mononucleosis has been produced experimentally in squirrel monkeys inoculated with EBV-transformed autologous leukocytes. In addition, inadvertent transmission of EBV by transfusion has been reported and in several instances was associated with the development of clinical infectious mononucleosis, including heterophil antibody.

EPIDEMIOLOGY Infectious mononucleosis has been recognized in all parts of the world. Although no yearly or seasonal trends are present in the general population, early fall and spring are periods of high frequency among college students. The most characteristic epidemiologic feature of the disease is its occurrence among young adults, especially in the fifteen- to twenty-five-year age group.

Seroepidemiologic studies have demonstrated that the absence of EBV antibody correlates with susceptibility to infectious mononucleosis and its presence indicates immunity. The age at which infection is acquired is related to socioeconomic factors and hygienic environment. Among disadvantaged groups such as children living in certain tropical countries, antibody is acquired early. In contrast, in middle and upper socioeconomic groups, only 50 to 60 percent have detectable antibody during adolescent years and at the time of entry into college. Among these individuals, infectious mononucleosis is a well-recognized disorder. Studies measuring both apparent and inapparent infections suggest a clinical/subclinical ratio of 1:2 to 1:4 in young adults.

When EBV infection develops in early childhood, a mild and nonspecific or an inapparent illness occurs, both of which are associated with the appearance and persistence of specific antibody. If primary infection is delayed until adolescence or young adulthood, the clinical response is frequently typical infectious mononucleosis with the development of both heterophil and EBV antibodies.

Epidemiologic and laboratory evidence have suggested that transmission of EBV occurs through the oropharyngeal route during close personal contact. Table 224-1 indicates that EBV is present in small amounts in throat washings from 1 week to many months after clinical illness.

This prolonged carrier state following clinical infectious mononucleosis, and perhaps also after inapparent EBV infection, may serve as a principal source of transmission. Investigations utilizing the presence of EBV antibody as an index of immunity have confirmed the low contagiousness of both the infection and the disease among susceptible college roommates; secondary attack rates for EBV infection within family units have also been low.

Pathology Generalized involvement of lymphoid tissue with lymphadenopathy, nasopharyngeal lymphoid hyperplasia, and splenomegaly is the outstanding pathologic feature. Widespread focal and perivascular aggregates of mononuclear cells, including atypical lymphocytes, are found throughout the body. Nonspecific hyperplastic changes in lymph nodes are present without infiltration of the capsule or surrounding tissues. Nonlymphoid organs and tissues, including liver, heart, kidneys, and central nervous system, are also infiltrated, and changes in these organs may be associated with functional disturbances. Bone marrow hyperplasia develops, and occasionally small granulomas are present.

TABLE 224-1
Recovery of EBV in pharyngeal excretions from 25 cases of infectious mononucleosis

Time after onset of symptoms, days	*Virus present in throat*		
	No. specimens tested	*No. specimens positive*	*Percent positive*
0–14	16	13	81.3
15–28	12	10	83.3
29–150	11	11	100.0
>150	3	2	66.7
Total	42	36	85.7

SOURCE: *G Miller et al*

MANIFESTATIONS In young adults an incubation period of 30 to 50 days has been suggested on the basis of contact infection studies. IM associated with the development of heterophil and EBV antibody has occurred in several patients 5 weeks following blood transfusion. Children appear to have shorter incubation periods, in the range of 10 to 14 days, but there is relatively little information on this point.

During a prodromal period of 3 to 5 days, mild symptoms, including headache, malaise, and fatigue, are common. Frank clinical features usually present over the next 7 to 20 days; they are variable in severity, but in over 80 percent of cases include fever, sore throat, and cervical adenopathy. In adults, temperature elevations which peak at 101 to 103°F may persist for 7 to 10 days. In severe cases, a daily rise in temperature to 105°F may continue even longer. On the other hand, children often have little or no fever accompanying the infection.

Sore throat occurs in the first week and is the most common feature of infectious mononucleosis. Hyperplasia of pharyngeal lymphoid tissue with inflammation and edema develops. A grayish-white exudative tonsillitis persisting for 7 to 10 days is present in approximately 50 percent of cases. The uvula and palatal arch frequently have a gelatinous appearance. *Palatine petechiae*, located near the border of the hard and soft palate, are observed in about one-third of patients toward the end of the first week of illness. Although highly suggestive, their presence is not pathognomonic of the disease.

Lymph node enlargement is a hallmark of infectious mononucleosis. The onset is gradual, and anterior and posterior cervical chains are most commonly involved. Generalized adenopathy, including axillary, epitrochlear, and inguinal nodes, may also develop during the course of the disease. The nodes are affected singly or in groups and may be small or grape-sized; they are firm, discrete, and moderately tender on palpation.

Splenomegaly occurs in approximately one-half the patients, and enlargement is greatest during the second and third weeks of illness. Although extremely rare, splenic rupture is one of the few potentially fatal complications of the disease.

Percussion tenderness over the liver and hepatomegaly develop in only about 10 percent of patients, but the majority (90 percent) have abnormal liver function test results which persist for several weeks. Jaundice occurs in no more than 4 to 5 percent of cases and is usually mild and uncomplicated.

During early stages of the disease a transient faint *erythematous maculopapular eruption* on the trunk and extremities is present in about 10 percent of patients. The rash often resembles rubella, but may be urticarial, hemorrhagic, or scarlatiniform in nature. *Bilateral supraorbital edema* may also be a transient finding early in the course.

A wide variety of neurologic manifestations has been described but occurs only rarely. Aseptic meningitis, encephalitis, blurred vision, coma, acute cerebellar syndrome, and the Guillain-Barré syndrome may appear at any time during the illness. Most patients experience complete recovery from central nervous system involvement; however, severe paralysis and/or respiratory incapacity occur in rare instances and are potentially fatal complications.

LABORATORY FINDINGS **Blood picture** Essential to the diagnosis of infectious mononucleosis is an increase in relative and absolute numbers of lymphocytes and monocytes, including 10 to 20 percent atypical forms. The atypical lymphocytes are large cells with oval, horseshoe-shaped, or indented nuclei and basophilic, vacuolated foamy cytoplasm. Nuclear chromatin is usually dense and irregular, and nucleoli are rarely seen. During the first week of illness, the total leukocyte count either is normal or there may be a leukopenia due to granulocytopenia. The total count then rises to between 10,000 and 20,000 leukocytes per mm^3 by the second or third week of illness; rarely, the number of leukocytes may range as high as 50,000 per mm^3. Characteristic leukocyte changes often persist for 4 to 8 weeks or more. Anemia is rare in infectious mononucleosis, but hemolytic anemia has been reported as a complication. Slight to moderate thrombocytopenia, which is usually symptomless, has been recognized during the early weeks of disease. In a few reported cases, the clinical picture has suggested idiopathic thrombocytopenic purpura.

Serologic diagnosis The serum of IM patients characteristically contains heterophil antibodies, i.e., agglutinins against sheep red cells, in high titer. Heterophil antibody is associated with the IgM fraction of serum and usually declines over a period of 3 to 6 months. In general, the higher the titer developed during clinical illness, the longer the antibodies will remain detectable in convalescence. Though a nonspecific serologic response, the heterophil antibody of infectious mononucleosis differs from other antibodies in human serums that also agglutinate sheep red cells. The latter are found at low levels in normal human serums and in high titers in serum sickness. Differentiation is based on absorption techniques utilizing guinea pig kidney and beef erythrocytes. The sheep cell agglutinins of infectious mononucleosis are completely absorbed by beef red cells but not by guinea pig kidney. Serum sickness agglutinins are absorbed by both, whereas nonspecific Forssman agglutinins are absorbed only by guinea pig kidney. A high order of specificity has now been achieved with other qualitative heterophil antibody tests which utilize Formalin-treated horse red cells, ox red cells, and enzyme-treated and -untreated sheep cells.

Usually sheep cell agglutinins are present in the first week of illness but they may be delayed in appearance. During the first 2 weeks after onset of the illness, 60 percent of young adult patients develop a positive heterophil antibody test. This percentage increases to 80 to 90 percent by the end of 1 month. The height of the titer is not related to severity of the disease or to the degree of lymphocytosis. In the presence of clinical and hematologic findings, a sheep cell agglutinin titer of 1:224 or higher before guinea pig kidney absorption and 1:28 after absorption has diagnostic significance. In the beef cell hemolysin test, a titer of 1:480 or higher may be considered significant. A rising titer in early stages of disease is the best criterion.

During acute infectious mononucleosis an increase in

total serum IgM levels up to 100 percent over control values and a 50 percent increase in IgG levels have been observed. Other protein alterations associated with the IgM fraction which may be present in the disorder include cold agglutinating antibody and transiently positive serologic tests for syphilis and rheumatoid factor. In IM, the presence of EBV antibody is a regular feature. Prospective clinical studies have shown that the disease occurs only in individuals who lack antibodies to EBV; patients become seropositive in almost all cases by the time acute symptoms appear. As measured by immunofluorescence techniques, levels of 1:80 to 1:320 are often found during early illness, and in only 15 to 20 percent of cases are significant antibody rises demonstrable. Rarely, the development of both EBV and heterophil antibodies is delayed several weeks following onset of symptoms. The relationships between clinical features and antibody levels in a typical heterophil-positive case are shown in Fig. 224-1.

No direct correlation has been found between the levels of EBV and heterophil antibodies, nor between the anti-EBV titer and severity of clinical symptoms or hematologic findings. Heterophil antibody levels are highest during the first 4 to 6 weeks after onset, and then decline or disappear after several months. EBV antibodies also reach peak titers within 3 to 4 weeks but persist at lower levels for many years thereafter, if not for life. Antibody titers of 1:20 to 1:40 have been demonstrated in serum collected 42 years after laboratory documentation of heterophil-positive infectious mononucleosis.

The appearance of EBV antibody has also been demonstrated in cases which have the clinical and hematologic characteristics of infectious mononucleosis but do not develop heterophil antibody. These EBV-positive, heterophil-negative cases are apparently frequent in infants and children but rare in adults.

Other laboratory abnormalities These consist primarily of abnormal liver function tests and may include an elevation in alkaline phosphatase level, retention of

FIGURE 224-1
Relationships between clinical features, hematologic changes, and antibody levels in a typical case of infectious mononucleosis.

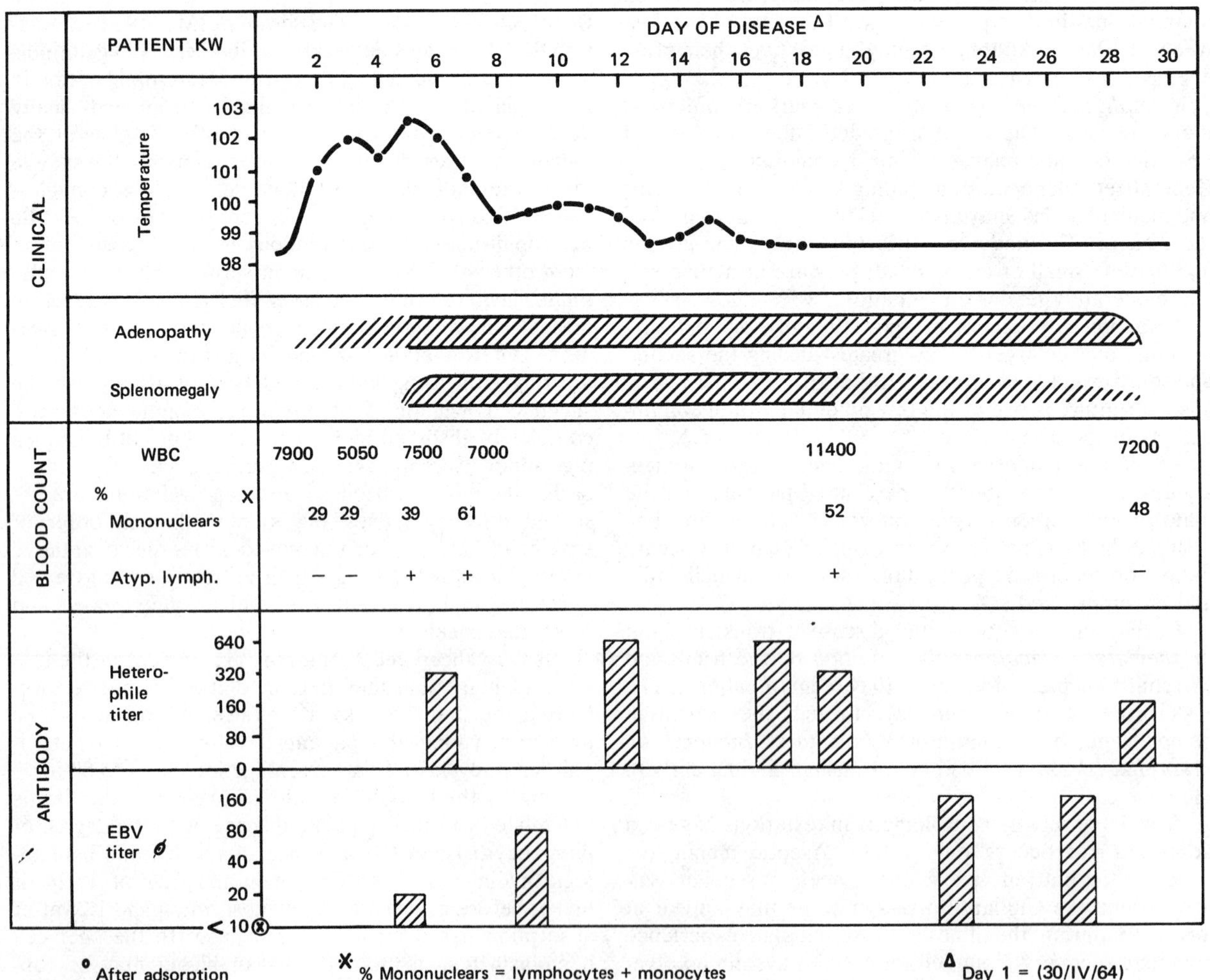

Bromsulphalein, mild abnormalities in serum glutamic oxaloacetic transaminase and serum glutamic pyruvic transaminase, and mild icterus. With recovery, all these values return to normal.

DIAGNOSIS The main diagnostic features of infectious mononucleosis are (1) irregular fever, sore throat, and lymphadenopathy; (2) an absolute increase in lymphocytes and monocytes exceeding 50 percent and including more than 10 percent atypical lymphocytes in the peripheral blood; (3) the transient appearance of sheep cell agglutinins and beef cell hemolysins; (4) the development of persistent antibody against Epstein-Barr virus; and (5) abnormalities of liver function tests.

Since many of these features are also seen in other diseases, IM may resemble a number of febrile disorders, especially those associated with fever, sore throat, adenopathy, and leukocytosis. In early stages of the disease, it is often difficult to distinguish IM from other forms of febrile exudative pharyngotonsillitis such as *streptococcal infections, exudative tonsillitis of viral etiology, Vincent's angina,* and *diphtheria.* Differentiation depends on the results of throat cultures and the development of the hematologic and serologic features characteristic of infectious mononucleosis.

Diseases with some similarities in hematologic abnormalities such as *acute leukemia* and other lymphoproliferative disorders may be mistaken for infectious mononucleosis. Demonstration of very immature leukocytes in blood or bone marrow and the presence of anemia, severe thrombocytopenia, and a negative heterophil antibody test distinguish these disorders from IM.

Cytomegalovirus (CMV) mononucleosis usually involves a slightly older age group, i.e., twenty to thirty years. Splenomegaly, hepatic involvement, and the presence of atypical lymphocytes in blood are common features of this disease, whereas sore throat and cervical adenopathy are usually absent. In transfusion-associated CMV infections, cytomegalovirus is excreted in the urine and a rise in complement-fixing antibody can be demonstrated.

Acute infectious lymphocytosis, a benign disorder of children, should be considered in the differential diagnosis among younger age groups. The majority of these cases are associated with signs of an upper respiratory tract infection; adenopathy is minimal, and splenomegaly is absent. The major feature is leukocytosis consisting of small mature lymphocytes; this abnormal blood picture may persist for 4 to 5 weeks, and occasionally for several months. The heterophil antibody test is negative, and no relationship to EBV antibody has been found.

The prodromal stage of *rubella,* associated with fever, malaise, postauricular and posterior cervical adenopathy, and lymphocytosis, may be indistinguishable from early infectious mononucleosis. A distinguishing feature of the rash of rubella is its invariable presence on the face, while that of IM is prominent on the trunk and usually spares the face; it is rarely as florid as in typical rubella. The appearance of large numbers of atypical lymphocytes in the blood and the development of heterophil and/or EB viral antibodies indicate infectious mononucleosis. Isolation of rubella virus from the throat and demonstration of a rising rubella antibody titer will confirm a diagnosis of rubella.

Acquired *toxoplasmosis* may be associated with fever, generalized adenopathy, splenomegaly, and lymphocytosis. A definitive diagnosis is based on direct isolation of *Toxoplasma gondii* and/or the demonstration of the development of specific serologic responses.

Infectious mononucleosis with jaundice can frequently be confused with *infectious hepatitis.* In hepatitis, fever is often lower and disappears when jaundice develops. Similarly, the presence of atypical lymphocytes is usually transitory during the preicteric phase of hepatitis, and the disease is rarely associated with splenomegaly and leukocytosis.

TREATMENT Therapy is symptomatic. Antibiotics have no effect on uncomplicated cases of infectious mononucleosis. During the febrile period rest in bed is advisable. Salicylates or other analgesics are usually sufficient to control headache and discomfort from sore throat. Gargling and irrigation with saline solutions provide symptomatic relief of pharyngitis and stomatitis. As a rule, most patients recover uneventfully on this regimen in 2 to 4 weeks, with gradual return to normal activities. Patients with splenomegaly should be cautioned against heavy lifting and strenuous athletics until splenic enlargement has disappeared.

In patients with severe toxic exudative pharyngotonsillitis associated with extensive pharyngeal edema, corticosteroids are useful to induce a prompt anti-inflammatory effect. A short course of prednisone may be administered, starting with 40 to 60 mg the first day and decreasing this total dose 5 mg daily over 7 to 10 days. Steroids are not necessary in treatment of the usual patient with infectious mononucleosis. However, full dosages of steroids should be employed in the management of severe complications, including (1) airway obstruction, in which a tracheostomy may also be required, (2) neurologic complications, (3) hemolytic anemia and thrombocytopenic purpura, and (4) myocarditis and pericarditis.

Severe abdominal pain is rare in infectious mononucleosis except in association with splenic rupture. This serious complication requires massive transfusions and immediate splenectomy.

REFERENCES

Carter RL, Penman HG: *Infectious Mononucleosis,* Oxford: Blackwell Scientific Publications, Ltd., 1969

Evans AS et al: Seroepidemiologic studies of infectious mononucleosis with EB virus. N Engl J Med 279:1121, 1968

Henle G et al: Relation of Burkitt's tumor associated herpes-type virus to infectious mononucleosis. Proc Natl Acad Sci USA 59:94, 1968

Hoagland RJ: *Infectious Mononucleosis,* New York: Grune & Stratton, 1967

Miller G et al: Prolonged oropharyngeal excretion of Epstein-Barr virus following infectious mononucleosis. N Engl J Med 288:229, 1973

Niederman JC et al: Prevalence, incidence and persistence of

EB virus antibody in young adults. N Engl J Med 282:361, 1970

——et al: Infectious mononucleosis: Clinical manifestations in relation to EB virus antibodies. JAMA 203:205, 1968

225
FAMILIAL MEDITERRANEAN FEVER (FAMILIAL PAROXYSMAL POLYSEROSITIS)

SHELDON M. WOLFF

DEFINITION Familial Mediterranean fever (FMF) is an inherited disorder of unknown etiology, characterized by recurrent episodes of fever, peritonitis, and/or pleuritis. Arthritis, skin lesions, and amyloidosis are seen in some patients.

HISTORY Although the first report of FMF was by Janeway and Mosenthal in 1908, it was not until the report of five cases by Siegal in 1945 that attention was focused on FMF as a distinct entity. Subsequently, some authors have not applied strict clinical criteria, however, and many patients with other diseases have been reported as having FMF. The detailed and extensive descriptions by Heller and Sohar have clarified many of the clinical aspects of FMF.

TERMINOLOGY The variety of names given to FMF has led to confusion concerning its clinical features. None of the names, including FMF, is completely satisfactory, but FMF has received the widest acceptance. Such terms as *periodic disease, periodic peritonitis, la maladie periodique* are inaccurate because the disease often is not cyclical. *Benign paroxysmal peritonitis* is inappropriate because many of the patients have involvement of serosal surfaces other than the peritoneum, and some die of amyloidosis. *Familial paroxysmal polyserositis* is an acceptable alternative for the term *familial Mediterranean fever.*

ETHNOLOGY AND GENETICS FMF occurs predominantly in patients of non-Ashkenazic (Sephardic) Jewish, Armenian, and Arabic ancestry. However, the disease is not restricted to these groups, and has been seen in patients of Italian, Ashkenazic Jewish, and Irish descent as well as others.

The best studies of the genetics of FMF have been done in Israel, where relatively homogeneous population groups exist. In Israel, the disease appears to be inherited as an autosomal recessive. Nevertheless, approximately 50 percent of patients give no family history of the disease. Consanguinity among the parents of FMF patients is as high as 20 percent, a figure which may be an underestimate because most patients came from very inbred ethnic groups. Approximately 60 percent of patients are male.

ETIOLOGY Although numerous pathogenetic mechanisms have been suggested, the etiology of FMF is unknown. Fever and inflammation are such prominent signs that frequent attempts have been made to implicate infectious agents and/or their products. It has been suggested that FMF is a form of brucellosis or tuberculosis. Suffice it to say that extensive studies utilizing modern microbiologic and serologic techniques have failed to implicate these or any other specific infectious agents.

It has been reported that FMF is due to an allergy or to hypersensitivity, but such hypersensitive states have not been substantiated. There is no firm evidence favoring an autoimmune etiology.

Reimann has suggested that FMF, like many other recurring illnesses (periodic diseases), may be a pathologic exaggeration of normal periodic temperature rhythmicity. However, extensive studies of temperature and other circadian rhythms in FMF patients have failed to demonstrate alterations from normal.

Because many FMF patients note that certain emotional or environmental changes may have profound effects on the frequency with which episodes of their disease occur, a psychosomatic basis has been suggested for the illness. There is no question that most patients eventually have transient or even permanent psychologic alterations, which probably reflect their reaction to a chronic recurring illness that is forever threatening their social, economic, and personal well-being, but there is no evidence for a functional etiology for FMF.

The demonstration that FMF is inherited as an autosomal recessive disorder has led to the thesis that it is another inborn error of metabolism. In view of initial optimistic reports that restriction of dietary fat ameliorates the course of FMF, it was thought that the disorder might be one of altered lipid metabolism. Despite extensive studies, no such error has been found. Reported instances of excessive urinary excretion of porphyrins in FMF are probably examples of true porphyria and not FMF.

It has been reported that blood levels of unconjugated etiocholanolone were elevated during fever in 6 patients with FMF. Subsequent studies, however, showed no correlation between levels of etiocholanolone and fever. The possible role of etiocholanolone and other steroids in FMF is discussed below.

PATHOLOGY Despite the striking clinical manifestations during an acute attack of FMF, no specific pathologic alterations have been found. Most FMF patients undergo at least one laparotomy, and only acute peritoneal inflammation in which the exudate contains a predominance of polymorphonuclear leukocytes is present. A disproportionately large number of male patients develops gallbladder disease with and without cholelithiasis, but extensive histopathologic examination has failed to reveal any specific pathologic changes. Pleural and joint inflammation are also nonspecific.

In the amyloidosis which accompanies FMF, amyloid is deposited in the intima and media of the arterioles, the subendothelial region of venules, the glomeruli, and the spleen. Aside from their vessels, the heart and liver are uninvolved.

MANIFESTATIONS In the majority of patients, the symptoms of FMF begin between the ages of five and fifteen, although attacks sometime commence during infancy, and onset has occurred as late as age thirty-eight. The duration and frequency of attacks vary greatly in the same patient, and there is no set rhythm or periodicity to their occurrence. The usual acute episode lasts 24 to 48 hr, but some may be prolonged for 7 to 10 days. The attacks range in frequency from twice weekly to once a year, but 2 to 4 weeks is the commonest interval. Spontaneous remissions lasting years have been seen. In the majority of cases, pregnancy is associated with an absence of acute episodes, and many patients note less frequent attacks in the summer than in the winter. There tends to be a decrease in the severity and frequency of the attacks with age or with development of amyloidosis.

Fever Fever is a cardinal manifestation of FMF and is present during most but not all attacks. Rarely, fever may be present without serositis. The temperature rise may be preceded by a chill, and will peak in 12 to 24 hr. Defervescence is often accompanied by diaphoresis. The fever ranges from 38.5 to 40°C but is quite variable.

Abdominal pain Abdominal pain occurs in more than 95 percent of patients, and may vary in severity in the same patient. Minor premonitory discomfort may precede an acute episode by 24 to 48 hr. The pain usually starts in one quadrant and then spreads to involve the whole abdomen. The initial site is usually very tender. Tenderness may remain localized with referred pain in other areas, and there may be radiation to the back. There may be splinting of the chest and pain in one or both shoulders, typical of diaphragmatic irritation. Nausea and vomiting sometimes occur. The abdomen is usually distended, and may become rigid with decreased or absent bowel sounds. On x-ray, the wall of the small intestine may appear edematous, transit of barium is slowed, and fluid levels may be seen. Because the manifestations of an acute abdominal attack can simulate those of a perforated viscus so closely, patients should be advised to have an elective appendectomy between attacks so that acute appendicitis will not obfuscate the picture at a later date. An abdominal operation may precipitate an acute attack of FMF which may be confused with other postoperative complications.

Chest pain Most patients with abdominal attacks have referred chest pain at one time or another, and 75 percent also develop acute pleuritic pain with or without abdominal symptoms. In 30 percent, the attacks of pleuritis precede the onset of abdominal attacks by varying periods of time, and a small number of patients never develop abdominal attacks. Chest pain is usually unilateral and is associated with diminished breath sounds, a friction rub, or a transient pleural effusion.

Joint pain In Israel, 75 percent of patients report at least one episode of acute arthritis. Arthritis can be distinct from abdominal or pleural attacks, can be acute or, rarely, chronic, and may involve one or several joints. Effusions are common and the large joints are involved most frequently. Radiologic findings are nonspecific. Despite careful search, frank arthritis rarely has been seen in the United States. Some patients have a history of rheumatic fever-like illness in childhood, but in a large series of patients, including 30 from the Middle East, acute arthritis was not observed. Mild arthralgia is common during acute attacks but is nonspecific and can be seen in many febrile illnesses, including experimentally induced hyperthermia.

Skin manifestations Skin involvement is reported by 25 to 35 percent of patients. These lesions consist of painful, erythematous areas of swelling from 5 to 20 cm in diameter, usually located on the lower legs, the medial malleolus, or the dorsum of the foot. They may occur without abdominal or pleural pain and subside within 24 to 48 hr.

Other signs and symptoms Involvement of other serosal membranes has been reported, but pericarditis is rare, and it is probable that descriptions of recurrent meningitis have been diseases other than FMF. Hematuria, splenomegaly, and small white dots called "colloid bodies" in the ocular fundus are among the findings of questionable significance. Rarely migraine-like headaches accompany acute abdominal attacks, and some patients have become somewhat irrational or show extreme emotional lability during attacks. Whether these are primary manifestations of FMF or secondary effects of pain and fever is not known.

Complications The most serious complication of FMF in the United States is drug addiction or habituation, and obviously efforts should be made to avoid use of narcotics. Depression and lack of motivation are common, and patients with FMF require considerable encouragement and support. A striking number of patients in one American series have developed gallbladder disease.

Another major complication of FMF is *amyloidosis*. Some investigators believe that few patients in Israel escape this complication and that it is an expression of the same gene that is responsible for the other manifestations of FMF. If the attacks occur first, as they do in over 90 percent of the patients, the patients are classified as being of phenotype I. Amyloidosis also occurs in siblings of FMF patients or precedes the abdominal attacks (phenotype II). The infiltration by amyloid involves the kidneys, and death is often attributable to renal failure.

Amyloidosis has been reported in Israel and North Africa, but there have been only two reported instances of amyloidosis complicating FMF in the United States. These findings are even more striking because there are probably as many known FMF patients in the United States as in Israel. These differences are unexplained and suggest that environmental or nutritional, as well as genetic, factors may play a role in the development of amyloidosis in FMF.

LABORATORY FINDINGS There is no specific diagnostic test. Polymorphonuclear leukocytosis ranging from 15,000 to 30,000 is almost invariable during acute attacks. The erythrocyte sedimentation rate is elevated during attacks but returns to normal between attacks. Plasma fibrinogen, serum haptoglobin, ceruloplasmin, and C-reactive protein increase during the episodes. Plasma lipids are normal, and there are no consistent abnormalities of hepatic or renal function. When amyloidosis is present, laboratory findings are typical of a nephrotic syndrome followed by renal insufficiency. Electrocardiographic and electroencephalographic changes are inconstant and nonspecific.

DIAGNOSIS When the typical acute attacks of FMF occur in an individual of appropriate ethnic background who has a family history of FMF, the diagnosis is easy. On the other hand, if the disease has not been present in the family and the patient resides in a community where FMF is rare, the diagnosis can be very difficult.

Most patients with undiagnosed FMF have had one or more abdominal operations with no relief of symptoms. When a patient is seen for the first time, a variety of other febrile illnesses must be excluded by appropriate study or observation. These include acute appendicitis, acute pancreatitis, porphyria, cholecystitis, intestinal obstruction, and other major abdominal catastrophes.

Some of the inherited forms of the hyperlipidemias (Chap. 106) may mimic the clinical picture of FMF, but measurement of serum cholesterol and triglycerides will eliminate them from consideration. The patient with FMF is not immune to the other diseases, and when an attack differs from the usual pattern or is more prolonged, consideration should be given to other diagnostic possibilities. The pleural form of the disease is sometimes difficult to differentiate from acute pulmonary infection or infarction, but the rapid disappearance of signs and symptoms resolves the problem. The joint manifestations may be more prolonged than other forms of FMF, and differentiation from septic arthritis, gout, and acute rheumatoid disease may be necessary. The erythema is sometimes difficult to differentiate from superficial thrombophlebitis or cellulitis.

Whether or not the patient is of the appropriate ethnic group, the most difficult diagnostic problem in FMF is the patient who presents with fever alone. In this situation, an extensive diagnostic work-up for fever of unknown origin may be required. Fortunately, such patients are rare and all eventually develop serosal involvement. Until specific diagnostic tests for FMF are available, patients with recurrent fever but without signs of inflammation of one of the serosal membranes should not be categorized as having FMF.

PROGNOSIS The prognosis of the patient with FMF varies greatly according to the country in which he lives. In the United States, the prognosis for long life is excellent. Despite the severity of the symptoms during some acute attacks, most patients are remarkably free of any debilitation during the intervals between attacks. With encouragement and an understanding of their disease, most FMF patients lead fairly normal lives. The greatest hazard to patients is prolonged periods of hospitalization due to erroneous diagnoses or failure to understand the disease. The liberal and injudicious use of narcotics for analgesia in these patients can lead to major psychologic and health problems. Establishment of a reasonable doctor-patient relation and education of the patient will avoid this hazard. In the United States, the prognosis of patients with FMF does not seem to be different from that of patients with other chronic nonfatal illnesses. Death usually results from causes unrelated to the underlying disease.

The complication of amyloidosis in Israel, parts of North Africa, Turkey, and other parts of the Middle East makes the prognosis quite different from that in America. Approximately 25 percent of FMF patients in Israel are known to have amyloidosis, and this complication usually leads to death. Because a majority of patients under observation in Israel are under forty years of age, it has been suggested that fatal amyloidosis may eventually occur in nearly all patients. This would explain the rarity of older patients in that area.

TREATMENT Many forms of therapy have been tried in FMF, but no specific or uniformly effective therapeutic agent or regimen has been found. Antibiotics, hormones, antipyretic and anti-inflammatory agents, immunotherapy, psychotherapy, elimination diets, and many other agents and programs have been attempted. Chloroquine and phenylbutazone have been reported to be successful in treating FMF, but other investigators have failed to substantiate these findings. Adrenal cortical steroids have been used extensively to suppress some of the signs of inflammation, but attacks recur upon steroid withdrawal. In fact, some patients have noted increased numbers of attacks while taking corticosteroids. Symptomatic therapy and support are all that can be offered to FMF patients. Narcotics should be avoided whenever possible.

ETIOCHOLANOLONE AND THE PYROGENIC STEROIDS

In 1957, Kappas et al. reported that certain 5β-H, C-19 steroids of endogenous human origin would induce inflammation and fever when administered to human volunteers. Etiocholanolone was the prototype of this group of hormone metabolites. Shortly thereafter, Bondy and his colleagues reported high levels of plasma unconjugated etiocholanolone in association with fever in two patients. Since that time, much has been written about the possible role of these steroids in the pathogenesis of certain recurrent fevers of unexplained etiology, including FMF. It is for this reason that special mention should be made of these compounds.

There is no question that many C-19, C-21, C-24 steroids with a 5β-H configuration are potent inducers of fever, inflammation, granulocytosis, and other biologic effects when they are administered to man. Despite these observations, there is considerable doubt that these compounds play a role in human disease. Investigators have been hampered by the lack of a sensitive and reproducible method for detection of minute concentrations in biologic fluids. Nevertheless, the potential importance of compounds such as etiocholanolone in human febrile disease should not be disregarded until such techniques are at hand. When precise methodology is available, some of these endogenous human products may turn out to be important not only in the pathogenesis of FMF but in other conditions of unknown etiology which are characterized by fever and inflammation. In the light of available data, however, none of these steroids has been shown to cause human disease or its symptoms; to assign a pathogenetic role to them at this time leads to confusion and tends to impede the search for the etiology of these diseases.

REFERENCES

Bondy PK et al: Etiocholanolone fever. Medicine 44:249, 1965

Ehrenfeld EN et al: Recurrent polyserositis (familial Mediterranean fever; periodic disease): A report of fifty-five cases. Am J Med 31:107, 1961

George JM et al: Recurrent fever of unknown etiology: Failure to demonstrate association between fever and plasma unconjugated etiocholanolone. J Clin Invest 48:558, 1969

Kappas A, Palmer RH: Thermogenic properties of steroids, in *Methods in Hormone Research*, vol 4, ed RI Dorfman, New York: Academic, 1965

Reimann HA: *Periodic Diseases*, Philadelphia: Davis, 1963

Sohar E et al: Familial Mediterranean fever. Am J Med 43:227, 1967

Wolff SM et al: The biological properties of etiocholanolone. Ann Intern Med 67:1268, 1967

226
MIDLINE GRANULOMA

SHELDON M. WOLFF

DEFINITION Midline granuloma is an uncommon disease characterized by inflammation, destruction, and often mutilation of the tissues of the upper respiratory tract and face. This condition has also been referred to as *lethal midline granuloma*, *malignant granuloma*, and *granuloma gangrenescens*, none of which is an appropriate term. The disease was first described by McBride in 1897.

ETIOLOGY The etiology of midline granuloma is unknown. A variety of microorganisms have been considered as possible causative agents, but detailed microbiologic investigations have failed to detect the consistent presence of pathogenic organisms. In view of the clinical and pathologic features of the illness, some authors have suggested a neoplastic basis for midline granuloma. However, when malignant tissue (usually of a lymphomatous nature) is found in the lesions, the diagnosis of midline granuloma is no longer tenable. Likewise, a localized hypersensitivity reaction has been suggested as the cause of this disease, but no serologic or immunopathologic evidence has been presented to corroborate such a hypothesis.

PATHOLOGY The most characteristic pathologic findings are acute and chronic inflammation with necrosis. Superimposed pyogenic infection of the involved tissues, including the sinuses, may contribute to nonspecific histologic findings. The pathologic hallmark, noncaseating granulomata, with or without giant cells, may be obscured by the inflammatory reaction, but when present is strong evidence in favor of the diagnosis. Primary vasculitis is not seen, and when it occurs, a search for other causes, most notably Wegener's granulomatosis, should be made. The presence of malignant cells makes the diagnosis of midline granuloma unacceptable. Until an etiology is established, the diagnosis of midline granuloma will rest on the characteristic clinical features outlined below.

CLINICAL FEATURES The disease may occur at all ages, but the majority of patients are in the fifth and sixth decades. It is more common in women than men and has been reported in all races. Many patients report recurrent "sinus" problems and some have histories of allergic rhinitis, although the significance of these features is unknown.

The major symptoms are usually related to the nose. Patients frequently complain of nasal stuffiness and occasionally of discharge. The first symptom in a smaller percentage of patients relates to ulceration of the mucosa of the nose, the buccal mucosa, or the gums. This has led to loosening of the teeth, and dentists are often first consulted by these patients. Rarely, patients will present first with eye findings related to conjunctival inflammation or even ulceration. Although the progression of symptoms in some patients may be slow, all too often the disease steadily, and sometimes rapidly, progresses. The characteristic symptoms of nasal discharge, difficulty in breathing through the nose, and pain over the sinuses, nose, or eye become more prominent with time. Once ulceration begins, the disease often progresses rapidly. The ulcers frequently involve the nasal septum and will lead to the characteristic septal perforation and a "saddlenose" deformity. The majority of the patients develop ulceration and eventually perforations of the soft and hard palates. Untreated, the disease can lead to massive destruction and mutilation of the tissues involved, including the skin of the face and the eyes. Frequently, the necrotic tissue becomes infected, and systemic symptoms like fever and anorexia appear. The destructive lesions can become very malodorous. The disease extends to involve local tissues and does not progress below the neck; if this happens, then other diseases should be considered. As the necrotic process progresses and involves vital organs, patients may lose sight in the affected eye, experience dysphagia, and have difficulty in speech. Although spontaneous temporary remissions have been reported, untreated midline granuloma is fatal. The progression of the disease can be rapidly accelerated by surgical procedures in the affected areas. The patient usually dies from secondary infection, although erosion by the process into a major blood vessel or penetration into the central nervous system with superimposed meningitis are also causes of death.

Aside from the granulomatous inflammation, necrosis, and destruction, no other specific clinical or pathologic findings are associated with midline granuloma. Occasionally, with superimposed infection, local lymphadenopathy may be noted, but it is not characteristic of the disease per se.

LABORATORY FINDINGS With progression of the disease, a variety of nonspecific abnormalities may be noted. These changes are characteristic of inflammatory processes in general or of secondary infections. For example, mild anemia, leukocytosis, elevated sedimentation rate, and hyperglobulinemia are common in these patients. Radiographic examination reveals pansinusitis, and as the disease advances, destruction of bone in the involved areas is characteristic.

DIFFERENTIAL DIAGNOSIS The diagnosis of midline granuloma is made by finding the characteristic histologic lesions in biopsies of the affected tissues. When the specimens show only inflammatory tissue, a presumptive diagnosis of midline granuloma can be made only when the characteristic clinical picture is present and other diseases with similar presentation have been excluded. The diagnosis of Wegener's granulomatosis is ruled out by the absence of vasculitis in the biopsy specimens and the localized nature of midline granuloma (i.e., no pulmonary or renal involvement). To differentiate midline granuloma from *granuloma gangrenescens* is difficult. *Granuloma gangrenescens* is clinically similar to midline granuloma but is due to a neoplastic process. The histologic feature of *granuloma gangrenescens* is either a malignant reticulosis or lymphoma, either of which can be associated with granuloma. Other diseases to be excluded by appropriate laboratory techniques are kala azar, rhinoscleroma, syphilis, leprosy, tuberculosis, blastomycosis, coccidiodomycosis, and pseudotumor of the orbit.

TREATMENT The complications of midline granuloma such as superimposed infections can be treated specifically. Although adrenal corticosteroids are often used in the therapy of midline granuloma, they are of no value and probably are contraindicated if infection is present. Sporadic reports on therapy with cytotoxic agents are difficult to interpret, since some of the patients reported clearly had lymphoma or Wegener's granulomatosis, diseases where such agents are of definite value. Surgical removal of the involved tissue has been attempted but is useless and may, in fact, cause rapid progression of the disease.

The treatment of choice is radiotherapy to the local lesion. Although low dosages (1,000 rads and below) have been reported to be effective, many patients relapse after such therapy. Radiotherapy should be given in a dose of 5,000 rads to the involved areas. Where such a regimen is employed, long-lasting (more than 10 years) remissions and possible cures have been achieved. Following irradiation and after an appropriate period to allow for tissue healing (usually 1 year), reconstructive and plastic surgery, which may be of enormous cosmetic and functional value, can be undertaken.

REFERENCES

BLATT IM et al: Fatal granulomatosis of the respiratory tract (lethal midline granuloma—Wegener's granulomatosis). AMA Arch Otolaryngol 70:707, 1959

FECHNER RE, LAMPPIN DW: Midline malignant reticulosis. Arch Otolaryngol 95:467, 1972

STEWART JP: Progressive lethal granulomatous ulceration of the nose. J Laryngol 48:657, 1933

WALTON EW: Reticuloendothelial sarcoma arising in the nose and palate (granuloma gangrenescens). J Clin Pathol 13:279, 1960

PART EIGHT | DISEASES OF THE ORGAN SYSTEMS

section 1 | Disorders of the heart

227
APPROACH TO THE PATIENT WITH HEART DISEASE

EUGENE BRAUNWALD

The initial symptoms of the patient with heart disease result most commonly from myocardial ischemia, from disturbance of the contractile activity of the myocardium, or from an abnormal cardiac rhythm or rate. Coronary insufficiency is manifest most frequently as chest pain, while reduction of the pumping ability of the heart commonly leads to weakness and fatigability or, when severe, produces cyanosis, hypotension, and syncope; elevated intravascular pressures upstream to a failing ventricle often result in abnormal fluid accumulation, which in turn leads to dyspnea, orthopnea, and edema.

A cardinal principle in the evaluation of the patient with suspected heart disease is that myocardial or coronary function which may be totally inadequate during exertion may be quite adequate at rest. Thus, a history of the development of symptoms of chest pain or dyspnea during activity which disappear at rest is characteristic of heart disease, while the opposite pattern, i.e., the appearance of these symptoms at rest and their remission during exertion, is rarely observed in patients with true organic heart disease.

Cardiac arrhythmias often develop suddenly, and the resulting signs and symptoms—palpitations, dyspnea, angina, hypotension, or syncope—generally occur abruptly and may disappear as rapidly as they develop. Patients with cardiocirculatory disease may also be entirely asymptomatic, both at rest and during exertion, but may present an abnormal physical finding, such as a heart murmur, elevated systemic arterial pressure, or an abnormality of the electrocardiogram or of the cardiac silhouette on the chest roentgenogram.

Diseases of the heart and circulation are so common and the laity is so well acquainted with the major symptoms resulting from these disorders, that patients, and occasionally physicians, erroneously attribute many complaints to organic cardiovascular disease. Furthermore, the combination of the widespread fear of heart disease in the Western World with the deep-seated emotional connotations concerning this organ's function results in the frequent development in persons with normal cardiovascular systems of symptoms which mimic those of organic disease. The correct interpretation of symptoms and signs in patients with organic cardiovascular disturbances may be particularly difficult. Such persons, in addition to having symptoms resulting from their disease, may also develop functional complaints referable to the cardiovascular system. The unraveling of symptoms and signs due to organic heart disease from those which are not directly related is an important and challenging task in these patients.

It must be recognized that dyspnea, one of the cardinal manifestations of diminished cardiac reserve, is not limited to diseases of the heart, but is also characteristic of conditions as diverse as pulmonary disease, marked obesity, and anxiety (Chap. 28). Similarly, chest pain (Chap. 7) may result from a variety of causes other than myocardial ischemia. Whether heart disease is responsible for these symptoms can frequently be determined by carrying out a detailed clinical examination. The electrocardiogram and roentgenogram provide additional helpful information; more specialized examinations are often helpful but only occasionally essential.

In every branch of medicine the establishment of the prognosis and development of a rational plan of management are based on a correct diagnostic appraisal. However, in the case of patients with disorders of the cardiocirculatory system, particular care must be taken to establish not only a correct but also a *complete* diagnosis. As outlined by the New York Heart Association, the elements of a complete cardiac diagnosis include consideration of:

1 The underlying etiology. Is the disease congenital, rheumatic, hypertensive, or arteriosclerotic in origin?
2 The structural abnormalities. Which chambers are enlarged? Which valves are affected? Is there pericardial involvement? Has there been a myocardial infarct?
3 The physiologic disturbances. Is an arrhythmia present? Is there evidence of congestive heart failure or of coronary insufficiency?
4 The extent of functional disability. How strenuous is the physical activity required to elicit symptoms?

Two simple examples may serve to illustrate the importance of establishing a complete diagnosis. The identification of exertional chest pain caused by myocardial ischemia is of crucial significance. However, this diagnosis is insufficient, because treatment can be no more than symptomatic until the underlying disease process, e.g., coronary atherosclerosis, aortic stenosis, severe anemia, thyrotoxicosis, or atrial tachycardia, which is responsible for angina pectoris, is identified. Similarly, determining that heart disease is congenital provides an important starting point, but the decision as to whether or not surgical treatment is advisable generally depends upon the specific anatomic defect present and often upon the nature of the physiologic disturbance and the functional impairment.

The establishment of a correct and complete cardiac diagnosis often requires the use of five different methods of examination: (1) history, (2) physical examination (Chap. 228), (3) electrocardiogram (Chap. 229), (4) chest roentgenogram (Chap. 230), and occasionally (5) specialized examinations, such as cardiac catheterization or angiocardiography (Chap. 231). In order to be most effective each of these five techniques should be employed independently of one another as well as with the information derived from the other methods clearly in mind. Only in this way can one avoid overlooking a subtle, though extremely significant, finding. For example, an electrocardiogram should be obtained in every patient suspected of having heart disease. It may provide the critical clue in establishing the correct diagnosis, such as the finding of an atrioventricular conduction disturbance in a patient with unexplained syncope, even when all other methods of examination reveal no abnormal findings. On the other hand, when combined intelligently with the results of other methods of examination, the electrocardiogram may provide essential confirmatory data. Thus, the knowledge that a patient has an apical diastolic rumbling murmur may direct particular attention to the P waves, and the recognition of left atrial enlargement electrocardiographically would support the suggestion that the murmur is caused by mitral stenosis.

In obtaining the history of the patient with known or suspected cardiovascular disease, particular attention should be directed to the family history. Familial clustering is common in many forms of heart disease. Genetic transmission may occur, as in patients with familial hypertrophic subaortic stenosis (Chap. 242) or Marfan's syndrome (Chap. 364). In patients with essential hypertension or coronary atherosclerosis the genetic component may be less obvious but is also of considerable importance. The nature of the response of the myocardium to an increased hemodynamic load, such as hypertension, or a valvular lesion may also be conditioned by hereditary factors. Familial clustering of cardiovascular diseases may not only occur on a genetic basis but may also be related to familial, dietary, or behavior patterns.

When an attempt is made to ascertain the severity of functional impairment in a patient with heart disease, it is essential to determine the precise extent of activity and the rate at which it is performed before symptoms develop. Thus, breathlessness which occurs after running up two long flights of stairs denotes far less functional impairment than similar symptoms occurring after taking a few steps on the level. Similarly, the history must include a detailed consideration of the patient's therapeutic regimen. For example, the persistence or development of edema in a patient whose diet is rigidly restricted in sodium content and who is receiving optimum doses of digitalis and diuretics must be interpreted quite differently from the findings of edema in the absence of these measures.

In addition to a careful examination of the heart, a detailed general physical examination should be carried out in every patient with known or suspected heart disease. Cardiovascular manifestations of systemic illnesses are being recognized with increasing frequency, and often the precise cardiovascular diagnosis can be easily established if the associations are clearly kept in mind. Thus, the occurrence of coarctation of the aorta in patients with Turner's syndrome, of myocardial involvement in the presence of Friedreich's ataxia, of primary pulmonary hypertension in patients with Raynaud's syndrome, and of aortic regurgitation in patients with rheumatoid spondylitis, represent a small sample of a growing list of diseases which affect the cardiovascular and other organ systems. Conversely, identification of the cardiovascular disease should prompt a search for frequently associated noncardiac manifestations of the same underlying disease process.

The phonocardiogram and the graphic indirect recording of pulse tracings, such as the jugular venous pulse, the carotid arterial pulse, and the apex cardiogram (Chap. 230), may in some instances provide information of considerable diagnostic value by amplifying the physical findings. It must be appreciated, however, that these techniques are primarily of aid in the precise timing of specific events, such as heart sounds, murmurs, and pulsations, which are easily elicited on physical examination.

The electrocardiogram (Chap. 229) is an invaluable and essential aspect of every cardiovascular examination. However, with the exception of the identification of arrhythmias, the electrocardiogram rarely permits one to make a specific diagnosis. In the absence of any other abnormal findings, electrocardiographic changes, particularly abnormalities in QRS voltages, S-T segments, and T waves, must not be overinterpreted. The range of normal electrocardiographic findings is wide, and the tracing can be affected significantly by many noncardiac factors, such as age, body habitus, and serum electrolyte concentrations.

Special examinations, such as catheterization of the right and left sides of the heart, selective angiography, and coronary arteriography (Chap. 231), provide precise diagnostic information under many circumstances. For example, they aid in establishing a specific anatomic diagnosis in patients with congenital heart disease, in patients with chest pain of uncertain etiology in whom coronary artery disease is suspected, and in determining the functional significance of valvular abnormalities in patients with rheumatic heart disease being considered for surgical treatment. Although a great deal of attention has been lavished on the newer specialized laboratory examinations, it should be recognized that they serve to *supplement*, not supplant, a careful clinical examination. There is an unfortunate tendency to carry out procedures such as coronary arteriography instead of taking a detailed and thoughtful history; the results often do not provide a definite answer to the question of whether a patient's complaint of chest pain is clearly attributable to coronary arteriosclerosis. Similarly, catheterization of the left side of the heart is all too frequently employed to determine whether operative treatment of valvular disease is indicated, even before the patient has had a trial of medical therapy. Despite their enormous value, it must not be overlooked that these specialized examinations entail some risk to the patient, involve discomfort and cost, and place a strain on existing medical facilities. Therefore, they should be carried out only if there is a specific indication.

REFERENCES

Dressler W: *Clinical Aids in Cardiac Diagnosis*, New York: Grune & Stratton, 1970

Hurst JW (ed): *The Heart*, 3d ed., New York: McGraw-Hill, 1974

New York Heart Association, Inc., Criteria Committee (chairman Rejane Harvey): *Nomenclature and Criteria for Diagnosis of Diseases of the Heart and Great Vessels*, 7th ed., Boston: Little, Brown, 1973

228 PHYSICAL EXAMINATION OF THE HEART

ROBERT A. O'ROURKE
EUGENE BRAUNWALD

The physical examination of the patient with cardiac disease includes careful evaluation of both the arterial pressure pulse and the jugular venous pulse, as well as deliberate precordial palpation and attentive cardiac auscultation.

ARTERIAL PRESSURE PULSE The normal central aortic pulse wave is characterized by a fairly rapid anacrotic rise to a somewhat rounded peak (Fig. 228-1). The anacrotic shoulder, present on the ascending limb, occurs at the time of peak rate of aortic flow just before maximum pressure is reached. The less steep descending limb is interrupted by a high-frequency downward deflection, synchronous with aortic valve closure, called the *incisura*. As the pulse wave is transmitted peripherally, the initial upstroke becomes steeper, the anacrotic shoulder becomes less apparent, and the incisura is replaced by the smoother dicrotic notch. Accordingly, palpation of a peripheral pulse (e.g., the brachial arterial) frequently gives less information than examination of a more central pulse (e.g., the carotid arterial) regarding alterations in left ventricular ejection or aortic valve function. Simultaneous palpation of the radial and femoral arterial pulses, which normally are virtually coincident, is important to rule out aortic coarctation, in which the latter is weaker and delayed (Chap. 237). In order to examine the carotid arteries the sternocleidomastoid muscle should be relaxed and the head rotated slightly toward the examiner. The application of varying amounts of pressure with either the forefinger or the thumb may permit appreciation of the ascending limb, the systolic peak, and the descending limb of the pressure pulse. In most normal persons a dicrotic wave is not palpable.

A small weak pulse is frequently present in conditions with a diminished left ventricular stroke volume, a narrow pulse pressure, and increased peripheral vascular resistance. This may be due to hypovolemia, to left ventricular failure secondary to myocardial disease or myocardial infarction, to restrictive pericardial disease, or to mitral valve stenosis. In aortic valve stenosis, the delayed systolic peak is the result of mechanical obstruction to left ventricular ejection and is often accompanied by the transmission of a coarse systolic thrill. In contrast, a large bounding pulse is usually associated with an increased left ventricular stroke volume, a wide pulse pressure, and a decrease in peripheral vascular resistance. This often occurs in patients with hyperkinetic circulation due to anxiety, anemia, exercise, or fever, or in patients with an abnormally rapid run-off of blood from the arterial system (patent ductus arteriosus, peripheral arteriovenous fistula). Patients with mitral regurgitation or a ventricular septal defect may also have a bounding pulse, since vigorous left ventricular ejection produces a rapid upstroke in the arterial pulse even though the duration of systole and the forward stroke volume may be diminished. In aortic regurgitation the rapidly rising, bounding arterial pulse results from increased left ventricular stroke volume and the associated increased rate of ventricular ejection.

The *bisferiens pulse*, which consists of two systolic peaks, is characteristic of aortic regurgitation (with or without accompanying stenosis) and of idiopathic hypertrophic subaortic stenosis (Chap. 242). In the latter the pulse wave upstroke rises rapidly and forcefully, producing the first systolic peak ("percussion wave"). A brief decline in pressure follows, because of the sudden decrease in the rate of left ventricular ejection as severe obstruction develops during midsystole. This pressure trough is followed by a smaller and more slowly rising positive pulse wave ("tidal wave"), produced by continued ventricular ejection and by reflected waves from the periphery. When the second positive wave is produced by an accentuated and palpable diastolic wave, the pulse is called *dicrotic*. It has been recorded primarily in patients who have very low stroke volume, particularly in those with diffuse myocardial disease.

Pulsus alternans refers to a pattern in which there is a regular alteration of the pressure pulse amplitude, despite a regular rhythm. It is due to alternating left ventricular contractile force; the end-diastolic pressure may or may not vary. It usually denotes severe left ventricular decompensation and usually occurs in patients who also have a loud ventricular filling sound (S_3). Pulsus alternans may also occur during or following paroxysmal tachycardia or for several beats following a premature beat in patients without heart disease. *Pulsus paradoxus* is an accentuation of the decrease in systolic arterial pressure accompanying the reduced amplitude of the arterial pulse which normally occurs during inspiration. In patients with pericardial tamponade, airway obstruction, or superior vena cava obstruction, the decrease in systolic arterial pressure frequently exceeds 10 mm Hg and the peripheral pulse may disappear completely during inspiration.

JUGULAR VENOUS PULSE (JVP) The two main objectives of the bedside examination of the neck veins are inspection of their wave form and estimation of the central venous pressure (CVP). In most patients, the right internal jugular vein is superior for both purposes, but occasionally examination of the left internal jugular vein, the external jugular veins, or the venous pulsations in the supraclavicular fossae may yield more information. In most normal subjects, maximum pulsation of the internal jugular vein is observed when the trunk is inclined by less than 30°. In patients with elevated venous pressure it may be necessary to elevate the trunk further, sometimes to as much as 90°. When the neck muscles are relaxed, a beam of light shone tangentially across the skin overlying the vein exposes the pulsations of the internal jugular vein. Simultaneous palpation of the left carotid artery aids the examiner in deciding which pulsations are venous and in relating the venous pulsations to their timing in the cardiac cycle.

The normal JVP reflects phasic pressure changes in the right atrium and consists of two positive waves and two negative troughs (Fig. 228-1). In considering this pulse, it is useful to refer to the events of the cardiac cycle (Fig. 230-2). The positive presystolic *A* wave is produced by venous distention following right atrial contraction and is the dominant wave in the JVP, particularly during inspiration. Large *A* waves indicate that the right atrium is contracting against an increased resistance, such as occurs with obstruction at the tricuspid valve (tricuspid stenosis or right atrial myxoma) or more commonly with increased resistance to right ventricular filling (pulmonary hypertension or pulmonary stenosis). Large *A* waves also occur during arrhythmias whenever the right atrium contracts while the tricuspid valve is closed by right ventricular systole. Such cannon *A* waves may occur regularly (as during junctional rhythm) or irregularly (as in atrioventricular dissociation or complete heart block). The *A* wave is absent in patients with atrial fibrillation, and there is an increased delay between the *A* wave and the carotid arterial pulse in patients with first degree AV block.

The *C* wave, often observed in the JVP, is a positive wave produced by the bulging of the tricuspid valve into the right atrium during right ventricular isovolumetric systole and by the impact of the carotid artery adjacent to the jugular vein. The *X* descent is due to a combination of atrial relaxation and the downward displacement of the tricuspid valve during ventricular systole. In patients with constrictive pericarditis, there is often increased prominence of the *X* descent wave during systole, but this wave is reduced in dilatation of the right side of the heart and may even be reversed in tricuspid regurgitation. The positive, late systolic *V* wave results from the increasing volume of blood in the venae cavae and right atrium during ventricular systole when the tricuspid valve is closed. After the peak of the *V* wave is reached, the right atrial pressure diminishes because of the decreased bulging of the tricuspid valve into the right atrium as right ventricular pressure declines followed by tricuspid valve opening. With mild tricuspid regurgitation the *V* wave becomes more prominent, and when tricuspid regurgita-

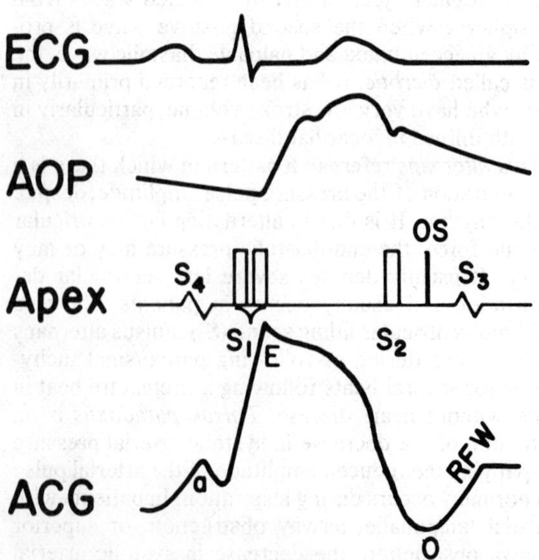

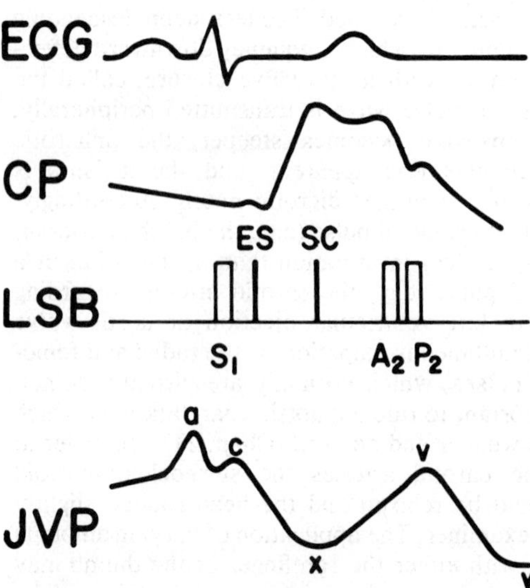

FIGURE 228-1

A *Simultaneous recordings of electrocardiogram, aortic pressure pulse (AOP), phonocardiogram recorded at the apex, and apexcardiogram (ACG). On the phonocardiogram, S_1, S_2, S_3, and S_4 represent the first through fourth heart sounds; OS represents the opening snap of the mitral valve, which occurs coincident with the O point of the apex cardiogram. S_3 occurs coincident with the termination of the rapid-filling wave (RFW) of the ACG, while S_4 occurs coincident with the A wave of the ACG.* B *Simultaneous recording of electrocardiogram, indirect carotid pulse (CP), phonocardiogram along the left sternal border (LSB), and indirect jugular venous pulse (JVP). ES, ejection sound; SC, systolic click.*

tion becomes severe, the prominent *V* wave and the obliteration of the *X* descent result in a single large positive systolic wave ("ventricularization").

Following the summit of the *V* wave there is a negative descending limb, referred to as the *Y* descent or "diastolic collapse," which is produced mainly by tricuspid valve opening and the rapid inflow of blood into the right ventricle. A rapid, deep *Y* descent in early diastole occurs with severe tricuspid regurgitation. A venous pulse characterized by a sharp *Y* descent, a deep *Y* trough, and a rapid ascent to the base line is seen in patients with constrictive pericarditis or with severe failure of the right side of the heart and a high venous pressure. A slow *Y* descent in the JVP suggests an obstruction to right ventricular filling, such as occurs with tricuspid stenosis or right atrial myxoma.

For accurate estimation of the CVP, the right internal jugular vein is best utilized, with the sternal angle as the reference point, since in the average patient, the center of the right atrium lies approximately 5 cm below the sternal angle, regardless of body position. The patient is examined at the optimum degree of trunk elevation for visualization of venous pulsations. The vertical distance between the top of the oscillating venous column and the level of the sternal angle is normally less than 3 cm (3 cm + 5 cm = 8 cm blood). The most common cause of an elevated venous pressure is an elevated right ventricular diastolic pressure. In patients suspected of having right ventricular failure who have a normal CVP at rest, the hepatojugular reflux test may be helpful. The palm of the hand is placed over the right upper quadrant of the abdomen, and firm pressure is applied for 30 to 60 sec. Normally, the jugular venous pressure is not significantly altered, but with impaired function of the right side of the heart the upper level of venous pulsation usually increases. The increased abdominal pressure most likely enhances systemic venous return, and the abnormal right ventricle is unable to accept this additional blood volume, causing pressure in the great veins to rise. Also, abdominal compression may elicit the typical JVP of tricuspid regurgitation when the resting pulse wave is normal.

PRECORDIAL PALPATION The normal left ventricular apex impulse is located at or medial to the left midclavicular line in the fourth or fifth intercostal spaces and is a tapping, early systolic outward thrust localized to a point not more than 2 to 3 cm in diameter. It is due primarily to recoil of the heart as blood is ejected, and it is best evaluated with the patient lying supine. Left ventricular hypertrophy results in an exaggerated amplitude and duration of the normal left ventricular thrust. The impulse may be displaced laterally and into the sixth or seventh interspace, particularly in patients with a left ventricular volume load such as occurs in aortic regurgitation.

Additional abnormal features of the left ventricular apex impulse may become more obvious when the patient is turned on his left side. These include marked presystolic distention of the left ventricle, often accompanying a fourth heart sound in patients with an excessive left ventricular pressure load, and a prominent early diastolic rapid-filling wave, often accompanying a third heart sound in patients with left ventricular failure or mitral valve regurgitation (Fig. 228-1). A double systolic impulse is frequently palpable in patients with idiopathic hypertrophic subaortic stenosis.

Right ventricular hypertrophy results in a sustained systolic lift at the lower left parasternal area which starts in early systole and is synchronous with the left ventricular apical impulse. In patients with chronic obstructive pulmonary disease a right ventricular impulse may often be detected by sliding the fingers up under the rib cage just beneath the sternum. The enlarged right ventricle strikes the ends of the fingertips as an inferiorly directed movement.

Abnormal precordial pulsations occur in patients with motion disorders of the left ventricular wall due to coronary artery disease or to diffuse myocardial disease from some other cause. This is particularly true in patients with a recent transmural myocardial infarction, 70 percent of whom have abnormal left ventricular wall motion which is recordable by graphic methods. These ectopic impulses may occur in early, mid-, or late systole and may be present in some patients only during episodes of anginal pain. They are most commonly felt in the left mid-precordium one or two interspaces above the left ventricular apex. When a systolic bulge occurs in the region of the apex, it is difficult to distinguish it from the impulse of left ventricular hypertrophy.

A left parasternal lift is frequently present in patients with severe mitral regurgitation. This systolic lift occurs distinctly later than the left ventricular apical impulse, is synchronous with the *V* wave in the left atrial pressure curve, and is due to anterior displacement of the right ventricle by the large left atrium. A similar impulse occurring to the right of the sternum has been noted in some patients with severe tricuspid regurgitation and a giant right atrium. A vigorous pulsation of the right sternoclavicular joint may indicate a right-sided aortic arch or aneurysmal dilatation of the ascending aorta. Pulmonary artery pulsation is often visible and palpable in the second left intercostal space and may be normal in children or young adults. However, this pulsation usually denotes pulmonary hypertension, increased pulmonary blood flow, or poststenotic pulmonary artery dilatation.

Thrills are low-frequency vibrations associated with heart murmurs which can be palpated. The diastolic rumble of mitral stenosis and the systolic murmur of mitral regurgitation may be palpated at the cardiac apex. With the palm of the hand placed over the precordium, the thrill of aortic stenosis crosses the palm of the hand toward the right side of the neck, while the thrill of pulmonic stenosis tends to radiate more often to the left side of the neck. The thrill due to a ventricular septal defect is usually located in the third and fourth intercostal spaces near the left sternal border.

Percussion adds little to careful inspection and palpation in the recognition of cardiac enlargement. Occasionally, however, it is useful in detecting an abnormal rightward position of the heart, such as occurs in dextrocardia, dextroversion, right lung atelectasis, and left pneumothorax, as well as in demonstrating an increased area of dullness or flatness to the right of the sternum and at the upper left sternal border in patients with a large pericardial effusion.

CARDIAC AUSCULTATION To obtain maximal information from cardiac auscultation, the observer should keep in mind several principles: (1) In order to hear a faint heart sound or murmur it is necessary to focus attention on that phase of the cardiac cycle during which the auscultatory event may be expected to occur. (2) The accurate timing of a heart sound or murmur necessarily involves ascertaining its relation to other observable events in the cardiac cycle—the carotid arterial pulse, the JVP, or the apical impulse. (3) To determine the significance of a cardiac sound or murmur it is often necessary to observe alterations of it in timing and intensity during various phases of the respiratory cycle, during changes in position, during and following a premature ventricular contraction, and during the administration of vasoactive drugs such as amyl nitrite and phenylephrine.

HEART SOUNDS The major components of heart sounds are vibrations associated with the abrupt acceleration or deceleration of blood within the cardiovascular system, but there is continuing controversy regarding the relative significance of the vibrations of valves, muscles, vessels, and supporting structures in the production of the heart sounds. The intensity of the *first heart sound* (S_1) is influenced by (1) the position of the AV valves at the onset of ventricular systole; (2) the rate of rise of the left ventricular pressure pulse; (3) the presence or absence of structural disease of the mitral valve; and (4) the amount of tissue, air, or fluid between the heart and the stethoscope. The AV valves are wide open at the end of diastole and S_1 is increased in intensity if diastole is shortened because of tachycardia, if flow is increased because of high cardiac output or prolonged because of AV valve stenosis, or if atrial contraction precedes ventricular contractions by a short (P-R) interval. The loud S_1 in mitral stenosis is related not only to the thickening of the cusps but also to a delay in onset of the mitral component of the first heart sound due to the elevated left atrial pressure. A reduction in the intensity of S_1 may be due to a slow rise of the left ventricular pressure pulse, a long P-R interval, or imperfect closure due to reduced valve substance, as in mitral regurgitation. S_1 is also soft when the anterior mitral leaflet is immobile because of rigidity and calcification.

Splitting of the two high-pitched components of S_1 by 10 to 30 msec is a normal phenomenon (Fig. 228-1). For clinical purposes, the first component of S_1 is attributed to mitral valve closure and the second to tricuspid valve closure. A widened split of S_1 is most often due to complete right bundle branch block and the resulting delay in onset of the right ventricular pressure pulse. Reversed splitting of the S_1 with the mitral component following the tricuspid component has occasionally been noted in complete left bundle branch block and is frequently present in patients with severe mitral stenosis or a left atrial myxoma.

The components of the *second heart sound* (S_2) are produced by the sudden deceleration of blood in the aorta and pulmonary artery. Splitting of S_2 into audibly distinct aortic (A_2) and pulmonic (P_2) components occurs normally during inspiration when augmented inflow into the right ventricle prolongs its ejection time. Audible expiratory splitting, heard best at the pulmonic area or left sternal border, is usually abnormal when the patient is in the upright position. Such splitting may be due to delayed activation of the right ventricle (right bundle branch block), to prolongation of right ventricular contraction with an increased right ventricular pressure load (pulmonic stenosis), or to delayed pulmonic valve closure because of an increased right ventricular flow load (atrial septal defect). In pulmonary hypertension, P_2 is increased in intensity and splitting of the second heart sound may be diminished, normal, or accentuated, depending on the cause of the pulmonary hypertension and the presence or absence of right ventricular decompensation. Early aortic valve closure, occurring with mitral regurgitation or a ventricular septal defect, may also produce audible expiratory splitting. In patients with large atrial septal defects the proportion of right atrial filling contributed by the left atrium and the venae cavae varies reciprocally during the respiratory cycle so that right atrial inflow remains relatively constant. Therefore, the volume and duration of the right ventricular ejection are not significantly increased by inspiration, and there is little inspiratory exaggeration of the splitting of S_2. This phenomenon, termed "fixed splitting" of the second heart sound, is of considerable diagnostic value.

A delay in aortic valve closure causing P_2 to precede A_2 results in so-called reversed (paradoxic) splitting of S_2. Splitting is then maximal in expiration, and decreases during inspiration with the normal delay of pulmonary valve closure. The commonest cause of reversed (paradoxic) splitting of S_2 is left bundle branch block. Mechanical prolongation of left ventricular systole, resulting in reversed splitting of S_2, may be caused by severe aortic outflow obstruction, a large aorta-to-pulmonary artery shunt, severe systolic hypertension and ischemic heart disease, or cardiomyopathy with left ventricular failure.

The *third heart sound* (ventricular gallop) is a low-pitched sound produced in the ventricle in early diastole during passive rapid filling. This protodiastolic sound is frequent in normal children and in patients with high cardiac output. However, in patients over forty, an S_3 usually indicates ventricular decompensation, AV valve regurgitation or other conditions which increase the rate or volume of ventricular filling. The left-sided S_3 is best heard with the bell piece of the stethoscope at the left ventricular apex during expiration and with the patient in the left lateral position. The right-sided S_3 is best heard at the left sternal border or just beneath the xiphoid and is increased with inspiration. Often there are physical findings of functional tricuspid regurgitation.

An earlier, higher-pitched third heart sound (pericardial knock) often occurs in patients with constrictive pericarditis; its presence is dependent upon the restrictive effect of the adherent pericardium, which halts diastolic filling abruptly.

The opening snap (OS) is a brief, high-pitched, early diastolic sound which is usually due to stenosis of an AV valve, more commonly the mitral valve. It is usually heard best at the lower left sternal border and radiates well to the base of the heart. The A_2-OS interval during exercise is inversely related to the height of the mean left atrial pressure. At the base an OS is often confused with P_2. However, careful auscultation at the upper left sternal border will reveal both components of the second heart sound, followed by the opening snap during early inspiration. The OS of tricuspid stenosis occurs later in diastole than the mitral OS. Since most patients with tricuspid stenosis also have severe mitral valve disease, the tricuspid OS is often overshadowed by the diastolic rumble and OS originating in the stenotic mitral valve.

The audible *fourth heart sound* (atrial sound) is a low-pitched, presystolic sound produced in the ventricle during ventricular filling, associated with an effective atrial contraction, and is heard best with the bell piece of the stethoscope. The sound is absent in patients with atrial fibrillation. The atrial sound occurs when there is diminished ventricular compliance and is frequently present in patients with systemic hypertension, severe aortic stenosis, cardiomyopathies, coronary artery disease, and acute mitral regurgitation. Most patients with an acute myocardial infarction and sinus rhythm have an audible S_4. The atrial sound is frequently accompanied by visible and palpable presystolic distention of the left ventricle. It is maximal in intensity at the left ventricular apex with the patient in the left lateral position, and is accentuated by mild supine exercise. The right-sided S_4 is present in patients with right ventricular hypertrophy, secondary to either pulmonary stenosis or pulmonary hypertension, and frequently accompanies a prominent presystolic A wave in the JVP.

Audible atrial sounds may be present during increased ventricular filling and normal ventricular compliance such as occurs in patients with severe anemia, thyrotoxicosis, or a peripheral ateriovenous fistula. An S_4 frequently accompanies delayed AV conduction even in the absence of clinically detectable heart disease. The incidence of an audible atrial sound increases with increasing age. Whether an audible S_4 in patients without other evidence of cardiac disease is abnormal remains controversial.

The *systolic ejection sound* is a sharp, high-pitched event occurring in early systole closely following the first heart sound. Ejection sounds occur in the presence of semilunar valve stenosis, i.e., opening snaps of the aortic or pulmonic valves, and in conditions associated with dilatation of the aorta or pulmonary artery. The aortic ejection sound is usually heard best at the left ventricular apex and the second right interspace; the pulmonary ejection sound is of maximal intensity at the upper left sternal border. The latter, unlike most other right-sided acoustical events, is heard better during expiration.

Nonejection systolic clicks, occurring with or without a late systolic murmur, often denote mitral valve regurgitation (Chap. 239). They probably result from functional unequal length of the chordae tendineae of the mitral valve and are heard best along the lower left sternal border and at the left ventricular apex. Systolic clicks may be single or multiple, and they may occur in early, mid-, or late systole. Frequently the midsystolic click is misinterpreted as S_2, and the actual second heart sound is called an OS or S_3.

Heart murmurs Cardiac murmurs result from vibrations set up in the bloodstream and the surrounding heart and great vessels as a result of turbulent blood flow, the formation of eddies, and cavitation (bubble formation as a result of sudden decrease in pressure).

The intensity or loudness of the murmurs may be graded from I to VI. A grade I murmur is so faint that it can be heard only with special effort, and a grade VI murmur is audible with the stethoscope removed from contact with the chest. The configuration of a murmur may be crescendo, decrescendo, crescendo-decrescendo (diamond-shaped), or plateau. The precise time of onset and time of cessation of a murmur depend on the instant in the cardiac cycle at which an adequate pressure difference between two chambers appears and disappears (Fig. 228-2).

Accentuation of a murmur during inspiration with the augmentation of systemic venous return implies that it originates on the right side of the circulation; expiratory exaggeration has less significance. Prolonged expiratory pressure against a closed glottus, the Valsalva maneuver, reduces the intensity of most murmurs by diminishing both right and left ventricular filling. The systolic murmur associated with *idiopathic hypertrophic subaortic stenosis* and the late systolic murmur due to a *billowing mitral valve leaflet* are exceptions and may be accentuated during the Valsalva maneuver. Murmurs due to flow across a normal or obstructed semilunar valve increase in intensity in the beat following a premature ventricular contraction or a long R-R interval in atrial fibrillation. In contrast, murmurs due to AV valve regurgitation or a ventricular septal defect do not change appreciably during the beat following a long cycle length. Standing, which decreases heart size, accentuates the murmur of hypertrophic subaortic stenosis and occasionally the murmur due to a billowing posterior mitral valve leaflet. Squatting, which increases both venous return and systemic arterial resistance, increases most murmurs, except those due to idiopathic subaortic stenosis and mitral regurgitation due to a billowing posterior mitral valve leaflet, which often decrease.

Pansystolic (*holosystolic*) *murmurs* are generated when there is flow between two chambers which have widely different systolic pressures, such as the left ventricle and either the left atrium or the right ventricle. The pressure gradient is established early in contraction and lasts until relaxation is almost complete. Therefore, holosystolic murmurs begin before aortic ejection, and at the area of maximal intensity they begin with S_1 and end after S_2. Pansystolic murmurs accompany mitral or tricuspid regurgitation, ventricular septal defect, and, under certain circumstances, aorta-pulmonary shunts. Although the typical high-pitched murmur of mitral regurgitation continues throughout systole, the shape of the murmur may vary considerably. The pansystolic murmurs of mitral regurgitation and ventricular septal defect are augmented by raising the arterial pressure with intravenous phenylephrine and are diminished by lowering the left ventricular systolic pressure by inhalation of amyl nitrite. The murmur of tricuspid regurgitation associated with pulmonary hypertension is holosystolic and frequently increases during inspiration, a feature of diagnostic importance.

Midsystolic murmurs occur when blood is ejected across the aortic or pulmonary outflow tracts. The murmur starts shortly after S_1 when the ventricular pressure rises sufficiently to open the semilunar valve. Ejection then begins and with it the onset of the murmur; as ejection increases, the murmur is augmented, and as ejection declines, it diminishes. The murmur ends before the ventricular pressure falls enough to permit closure of the aortic or pulmonary leaflets. In the presence of normal semilunar valves an increased flow rate or ejection into a dilated vessel beyond the valve may be responsible for the production of this murmur. Valvular or subvalvular obstruction may also cause such a midsystolic murmur, the intensity being related to the flow. Thus, the murmur of aortic stenosis may become faint or disappear during heart failure and return following the use of digitalis.

The murmur of aortic stenosis is the prototype of the left-sided midsystolic murmur. The location and radiation of this murmur appear to be influenced by the direction of the high-velocity jet within the aortic root. In *valvular aortic stenosis* the murmur is usually maximal in the second right intercostal space, with radiation into the neck. In *supravalvular aortic stenosis*, the murmur is occasionally loudest even higher, with disproportionate radiation into the right carotid artery. In idiopathic hypertrophic subaortic stenosis, the murmur originates within the left ventricular cavity, and is usually maximal at the lower left sternal edge and apex, with relatively little radiation to the carotids. When the aortic valve is immobile (calcified), the closure sound may be soft and inaudible so that the length and configuration of the murmur are difficult to determine.

The patient's age and the area of maximal intensity aid in determining the significance of midsystolic murmurs. Thus, in a young adult with a thin chest and high velocity of blood flow, a faint or moderate ejection murmur heard only in the pulmonary area is usually without significance, while a similar murmur in the aortic area may indicate congenital aortic stenosis. In elderly patients pulmonary flow murmurs are rare, while aortic systolic murmurs are frequent and may be due to aortic dilatation, to a significant degree of valvular aortic stenosis, or to nonstenotic deformity of the aortic valve. Systolic ejection murmurs are intensified by amyl nitrite inhalation and during the cardiac cycle following a premature ventricular contraction. Aortic systolic murmurs are diminished by interventions which increase systemic arterial resistance such as intravenous phenylephrine. Cardiac catheterization may be necessary to separate a prominent and exaggerated functional murmur from one due to congenital semilunar valve stenosis.

Early systolic murmurs begin with the first heart sound and end in midsystole. They may be due to a *ventricular septal defect*, *mitral regurgitation*, or *tricuspid regurgita-*

FIGURE 228-2
Simultaneous recordings of ECG, aortic pressure (AOP), left ventricular pressure (LVP), and left atrial pressure (LAP). HSM is a holosystolic murmur; PSM, a presystolic murmur; MDM, a middiastolic murmur; SEM, a systolic ejection murmur; and EDM, an early diastolic murmur.

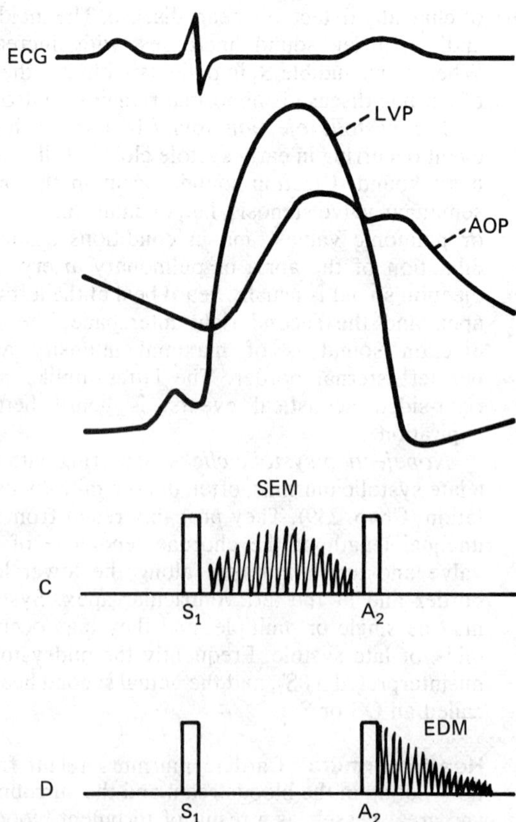

tion. In large ventricular septal defects with pulmonary hypertension the shunting at the end of systole may be small or absent, resulting in an early systolic murmur. A similar murmur may occur with very small muscular ventricular septal defects, the shunt being interrupted in late systole. An early systolic murmur is a feature of tricuspid regurgitation occurring in the absence of pulmonary hypertension. This lesion is common in drug addicts with bacterial endocarditis, in whom a tall regurgitant right atrial *V* wave reaches the level of the normal right ventricular pressure in late systole, confining the murmur to early systole. In patients with acute mitral regurgitation and a large *V* wave in a noncompliant left atrium, a loud early systolic murmur is frequently heard which diminishes as the pressure gradient between left ventricle and left atrium decreases in late systole (Chap. 239).

Late systolic murmurs are faint or moderately loud high-pitched apical murmurs, which start well after ejection and do not mask either heart sound. They may appear only during angina but are common in patients with myocardial infarction or diffuse myocardial disease. They are probably related to papillary muscle dysfunction caused by infarction or ischemia of these muscles or to their distortion by left ventricular dilatation. Late systolic murmurs accompanied by midsystolic clicks are associated with late systolic mitral regurgitation caused by herniation of the posterior and/or anterior leaflet of the mitral valve into the left atrium, which results from inadequate leaflet support due to cusp redundancy and chordae elongation. This abnormality may be congenital, often is familial, occurs frequently in patients with Marfan's syndrome, and may occur in patients with traumatic mitral regurgitation or with coronary artery disease.

Early diastolic murmurs begin with or shortly after the second heart sound as soon as the corresponding ventricular pressure falls sufficiently below that in the aorta or pulmonary artery. The high-pitched murmurs of aortic regurgitation or pulmonary regurgitation due to pulmonary hypertension are generally decrescendo, since there is a progressive decline in the volume or rate of regurgitation during diastole. They may be musical when the regurgitation is associated with a flail, everted semilunar valve cusp. Faint, high-pitched murmurs of aortic regurgitation are difficult to hear unless they are specifically sought by applying firm pressure with the diaphragm over the mid-left-sternal border while the patient sits, leans forward, and holds his breath in full expiration. The diastolic murmur of aortic regurgitation is enhanced by an acute elevation of the arterial pressure and squatting; it diminishes with a decrease in arterial pressure such as occurs during amyl nitrite inhalation. The diastolic murmur of congenital pulmonary regurgitation in the absence of pulmonary hypertension is low to medium pitched. The onset of this murmur is delayed because at the time of pulmonary valve closure the regurgitant flow is minimal, since the diastolic pressure exerted upon the regurgitant valve is negligible. An early diastolic murmur has been occasionally observed in patients with no semilunar valve regurgitation but with partial obstruction of the left anterior descending coronary artery. This murmur is presumably due to diastolic flow through the stenotic segment.

Middiastolic murmurs occur during early ventricular filling and, like ejection murmurs, are due to disproportion between valve orifice size and flow rate. Such murmurs may be loud despite slight AV valve stenosis when there is normal or increased blood flow. Conversely, the murmur may be soft or even absent despite severe obstruction if the cardiac output is significantly reduced. When stenosis is marked, the diastolic murmur is inevitably prolonged and the duration of the murmur is more reliable than its intensity as an index of the degree of valve obstruction.

The low pitched middiastolic murmur of mitral stenosis characteristically follows the opening snap. It should be specifically sought by placing the bell of the stethoscope at the site of the left ventricular impulse, which is best localized with the patient on his left side. Frequently the murmur of mitral stenosis is present only at the left ventricular apex, and it may be increased in intensity by mild supine exercise or by inhalation of amyl nitrite. In tricuspid stenosis the middiastolic murmur is localized to a relatively limited area along the left sternal edge and may increase in loudness during inspiration.

Middiastolic murmurs may be generated across the mitral valve in ventricular septal defect, patent ductus arteriosus, or mitral regurgitation; and across the tricuspid valve in atrial septal defect or tricuspid regurgitation. These murmurs are related to the torrential flow across an AV valve, usually follow a third heart sound, and tend to occur with large left-to-right shunts, or severe AV valve regurgitation. A soft middiastolic murmur may sometimes be heard in patients with acute rheumatic fever (Carey-Coombs murmur). It has been attributed to inflammation of the mitral valve cusps or excessive left atrial blood flow as a consequence of mitral regurgitation.

In acute aortic regurgitation, the left ventricular diastolic pressure may exceed the left atrial pressure, resulting in a middiastolic murmur due to "diastolic mitral regurgitation." In severe chronic aortic regurgitation a murmur is frequently present which may be either middiastolic or presystolic (Austin Flint murmur). This murmur appears to originate at the anterior mitral valve leaflet when blood simultaneously enters the left ventricle from both the aortic root and the left atrium.

Presystolic murmurs begin during the period of ventricular filling that follows atrial contraction and therefore are most prominent during sinus rhythm. They are usually due to mitral stenosis and have the same quality as the middiastolic filling rumble but are usually crescendo, reaching peak intensity at the time of a loud S_1. The presystolic murmur corresponds to the AV valve gradient, which may be minimal until the moment of right or left atrial contraction. A right or left *atrial myxoma* may occasionally cause either middiastolic or presystolic murmurs that resemble the murmurs of mitral or tricuspid stenosis.

Continuous murmurs begin in systole and persist through S_2 into all or part of diastole. These murmurs signify continuous flow due to communication between high- and low-pressure areas without an intervening valve. A *patent ductus arteriosus* causes a continuous murmur as long as the pressure in the pulmonary artery is much below that in the aorta. The murmur is intensified by elevation of the systemic arterial pressure and is reduced by amyl nitrite inhalation. When pulmonary hypertension is present, the diastolic portion may disappear, leaving the murmur confined to systole. A continuous murmur is uncommon in aortopulmonary septal defects, since this malformation is generally associated with severe pulmonary hypertension. Surgically produced aortopulmonary connections, such as subclavian-pulmonary artery anastomosis, result in murmurs similar to that of a patent ductus.

Continuous murmurs may result from congenital or acquired *systemic arteriovenous fistula, coronary arterial fistula,* anomalous origin of the left coronary artery from the pulmonary artery, and communications between the *sinus of Valsalva and the right side of the heart.* Continuous murmurs may also occur when high left atrial pressure results in continuous flow across a small defect in the atrial septum. Murmurs associated with *pulmonary arteriovenous fistulas* may be continuous but are usually only systolic. Continuous murmurs may also be due to disturbances of flow pattern in constricted systemic (e.g., renal) or pulmonary arteries when marked pressure differences between the two sides of the narrow segment persist; a continuous murmur in the back may be present in *coarctation of the aorta*; and *pulmonary embolism* may cause continuous murmurs in partially occluded vessels.

In nonconstricted arteries continuous murmurs may be due to rapid flow through a tortuous bed. Such murmurs typically occur within the bronchial arterial collateral circulation in cyanotic patients with severe pulmonary outflow obstruction. The "mammary souffle," an innocent murmur heard during late pregnancy and early post partum, may be systolic or continuous. The innocent cervical venous hum is a continuous murmur usually heard over the medial aspect of the right supraclavicular fossa with the patient upright. The hum is usually louder during diastole and can be instantaneously abolished by digital compression of the ipsilateral internal jugular vein. Transmission of a loud venous hum to the area below the clavicles may result in a mistaken diagnosis of patent ductus arteriosus.

The *pericardial friction rub,* which may have presystolic, systolic, and early diastolic scratchy components, may be confused with a murmur or extra cardiac sound when heard only in systole. It is best appreciated with the patient upright and leaning forward and may be accentuated during inspiration.

REFERENCES

DOHAN MC, CRISCITELLO MS: Physiological and pharmacologic manipulations of heart sounds and murmurs. Mod Concepts Cardiovasc Dis 39:121, 1970

HURST JW (ed): *The Heart* 3d ed., Part IV: Methods Used to Obtain a Cardiovascular Data Base, Sections A & B (chaps. 11–19), New York: McGraw-Hill, 1974, pp. 138–289

LEATHAM A: *Auscultation of the Heart and Phonocardiography,* London: Churchill, 1970

REDDY PS et al: Cardiac systolic murmurs: pathophysiology and differential diagnosis. Prog Cardiovasc Dis 14:1, 1971

229 ELECTROCARDIOGRAPHY

STANLEY A. BRILLER

INTRODUCTION Electrocardiograms may be interpreted by seeking a match between the observed pattern and one of a large number of patterns previously found to be empirically associated with various conditions, or by using available electrophysiologic knowledge. The latter strategy is not only more satisfying intellectually but can minimize the information which must be committed to memory. In addition, a number of striking advances in understanding the origin of bioelectricity and its alterations by ischemia, ionic changes, and other interventions have made electrocardiographic interpretation by pattern recognition even less appealing. For example, intensive studies on the squid giant axon have led to an understanding of the interrelationships between the generation of both the resting and action potential by this nerve, an understanding which can, in principle, be extended both to skeletal and cardiac muscle.

Studies employing revived human hearts have permitted a precise analysis of the spread of excitation in the normal heart as well as in certain forms of heart disease. Knowledge of conduction defects through the heart has been expanded by studies of the effects of sectioning various tracts below the bundle branches in experimental animals. In sum, much of the mystery and speculation which formerly surrounded electrocardiography has now been exposed, making it possible to account for many, though not all, electrocardiologic observations in health and disease.

THE RESTING POTENTIAL In most excitable animal cells, including the giant axon of the squid and mammalian myocardial cells, a difference in potential of about 90 mV exists between the interior and exterior of the cell in the polarized (resting) state. However, since each myocardial cell is bounded by walls which face equally but oppositely charged walls (Fig. 229-1*A*), no net voltage across the myocardial wall is discernible from the outside. If the cell is pierced by a microelectrode and the voltage of the intracellular potential is compared with that of the extracellular potential, the 90 mV becomes easily measurable. The resting potential is believed to stem largely from a difference in concentration of potassium on either side of the cell membrane; the intracellular

FIGURE 229-1
A *A group of myocardial cells in the resting state.* B *After stimulation by the adjacent electrode.*

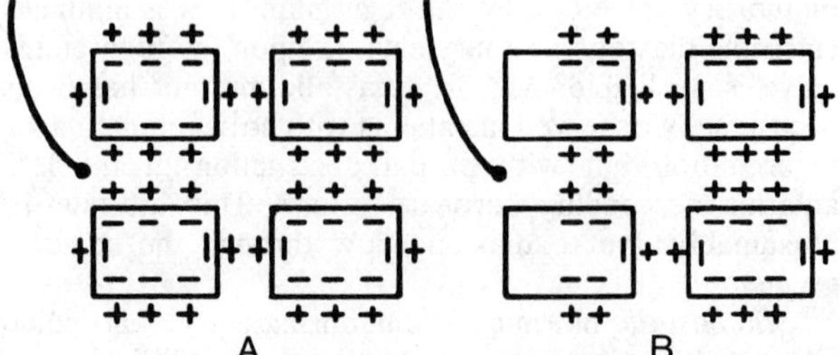

concentration of potassium is approximately twenty times that of the extracellular concentration. This gradient impels a relatively small amount of potassium ion to leave the interior of the cell. In the absence of outward migration of potassium, the interior and exterior cell compartments are electrically neutral, but as the concentration gradient of potassium forces some intracellular ions to the outside, this neutral balance is upset, and the loss of internal positively charged potassium results in a relatively negative internal potential. The outward migration of potassium continues until the mounting potential difference creates a force equal to that resulting from the concentration gradient, at which point equilibrium is achieved during the resting phase.

There is evidence from artificial manipulation of the concentration of various ions during the resting phase that although potassium is by far the most important contributor to the resting potential, other ions such as sodium, conceivably calcium, chloride, and some as-yet-unknown constituents (referred to collectively as "leak") participate. The intracellular potential depends upon whether the specific cationic concentration is richer inside the cell (negative) or outside (positive) and on the resistance offered by the membrane to the passage of each ion. During the resting phase the resistance to the passage of potassium is clearly less than for any other ion.

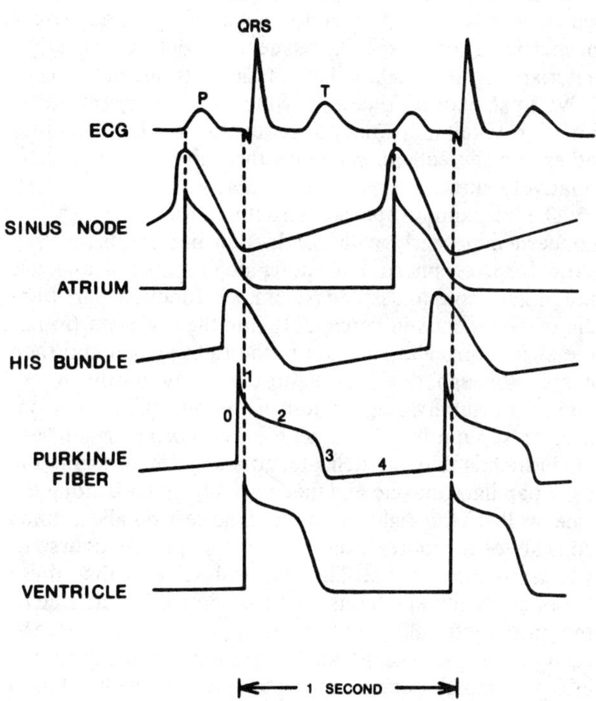

FIGURE 229-2

The relationships among a surface ECG lead and monophasic action potentials in the various cardiac tissues. The dominant pacemaker is the sinoatrial node, which has the fastest rate of rise during phase 4 of any tissue with pacemaker properties. Phase 4 in the sinus node terminated in a smooth curve, indicating its pacemaker function, whereas the acute inflection at the end of diastolic depolarization in the His bundle and Purkinje tissues indicates that they are driven.

THE ACTION POTENTIAL It has long been known that if the resting intracellular potential of a nerve or heart muscle cell is gradually made less negative, a point is reached (threshold) at which cellular mechanisms rapidly make the interior of the cell briefly positive (phase 0). During phase 1 the action potential rapidly declines and then plateaus (phase 2). Phase 3 is a moderately rapid process in which polarization of the membrane and the resting state are restored (Fig. 229-2). These events, which may be triggered by an adjacent active cell, underlie the concept of conduction of a cardiac impulse throughout the heart.

When the cell becomes depolarized the resistance offered by the cell membrane to sodium is less and the resistance to potassium is greater than in the polarized (resting) phase. Since the concentration gradient of sodium across the cell membrane is roughly the reverse of potassium, dominance of sodium movement during the action potential accounts for the positive spike during phase 0. A small amount of calcium accompanies sodium entry, and it participates in generating the positive interior milieu, and plays an extremely important role in excitation-contraction coupling (Chap. 232). The resistance of the cell membrane to potassium then increases, an adjustment which conserves intracellular potassium because the cell interior is now positive and would tend to expel cations.

ELECTRICAL CHARACTERISTICS OF SPECIFIC TISSUES The resting and action potentials described above are characteristic of atrial and ventricular myocardium. The properties of automaticity (the capacity to originate a beat) and facilitated conduction of the impulse through both atria and ventricles are made possible by the presence of specialized conduction tissue.

Normally the property of automaticity is most evident in the sinoatrial node, the dominant pacemaker of the heart which lies in the right atrium. The most distinctive electrophysiologic property of this structure is that the resting potential during diastole is not constant. Following phase 3, i.e., during phase 4, it drifts steadily upward (Fig. 229-2). This phase of diastolic depolarization appears to be due to the gradual loss of intracellular potassium by pacemaker or potential pacemaker tissues. Since the resting potential is largely determined by the concentration gradient of potassium across the cell membrane, a loss of this ion from the cell should produce a loss of potential difference across the membrane. When the potential is reduced to threshold, the sinus node generates an action potential and initiates a chainlike reaction in the right atrium which ultimately pervades the heart. The spread through the atria is probably modulated by three intranodal tracts. All three tracts appear to connect the sinoatrial node with the atrioventricular junction. The most anterior of these (Bachmann) also sends fibers to the left atrium. The middle (Wenckebach) and the posterior internodal tracts (Thorel) all contribute a few fibers, which apparently bypass the atrioventricular junction, connect directly to the bundle of His, and may participate in certain varieties of preexcitation.

The resting potential (phase 4) of the atrioventricular node at the base of the right atrium near the coronary sinus is flat, and it exhibits none of the pacemaker properties of other specific tissues. The outstanding characteristic of atrioventricular junctional tissue is the very slow upstroke of phase 0. Since the atrioventricular junction takes more time to reach its threshold than do other cardiac cells, conduction through this structure is relatively slow.

The remaining specific structures of the heart are concerned primarily with conduction but exhibit a very slow form of phase 4 diastolic depolarization and are potentially able to assume pacemaker function. The bundle of His blends imperceptibly into the lower portion of the atrioventricular junction in the right atrium and then passes through the central fibrous body of the heart, thereafter subdividing on top of the muscular intraventricular septum into the bundle branches. The right bundle branch is thin and delicate, coursing downward to the right papillary muscle and then partially upward along the free wall of the right ventricle. The left bundle branch consists of a proliferation of fibers, the precise course of which is contentious. The classical view is that these fibers gradually spread as they pass down the left side of the intraventricular septum, supplying it with several early fibers and then gradually fanning out to supply the left ventricular endocardium. Another viewpoint, based more upon electrocardiographic than on anatomic findings, is that fibers from the left bundle branch coalesce into anterior and posterior divisions.

The rate of rise of upstroke (phase 0) of the bundle of His, the bundle branches, and the Purkinje system is faster than that of the ventricular myocardium. Normally this results in a rapid and predetermined order of activation of the elements of the ventricles.

THE ORDER OF DEPOLARIZATION (EXCITATION)

Resting, polarized cells produce no *external* potential difference, since, as shown previously, each charged pair is balanced by an equal but oppositely charged pair. Stimulation of a cell (Fig. 229-1*B*) results in abolition of charges adjacent to the point of stimulation, with loss of the potential balance present earlier. The unbalanced charge makes the side adjacent to the point of stimulation negative with respect to the opposite side. Whether conveyed by conductive tissue or by the general myocardium, this current of depolarization causes the transmembrane potential of adjacent resting tissue to exceed threshold, and the process spreads as a chain reaction until the entire myocardium is excited. It is convenient to represent the state of depolarization and the resulting potential by an arrow drawn so that its head points toward the positive charge and its back indicates negativity.

In normal human hearts the depolarization wave originates in the sinoatrial node, which reaches threshold potential more rapidly than any other automatic tissue. The slope of phase 4 is governed by sympathomimetic and parasympathomimetic influences; the former increase the slope of phase 4, allowing threshold to be reached sooner, resulting in an increase in heart rate. In a complementary manner, parasympathomimetic interventions slow heart rate. Having reached threshold, the sinus tissue quickly undergoes complete depolarization and initiates the spread of activation to other constituents of the atrial musculature. Although some spread is undoubtedly directly through the general atrial muscle in a tangential direction, the process is modulated by conduction through the three prominent atrial conduction bands described earlier (Fig. 229-3).

The spread of activity in the atrium is a complex process. After starting at the sinoatrial node, a vast number of pseudopods of activity spread out in every direction, ultimately reaching the atrioventricular junction; the overall spread of atrial activity is from right to left and downward. The spread of activity through the atrioventricular junction is very slow. However, once activity reaches the Purkinje fibers, spread to the ventricular myocardium is extremely rapid, although in an ordered sequence.

The first mass of ventricular myocardium to be activated is the midregion of the septum and a small portion of the anterior wall of the left ventricle. Since the Purkinje system terminates in the endocardium, activity of the ventricle begins internally. Activation then spreads to the lowest portion of the interventricular septum and to the free wall of the right ventricle. Activation of the papillary muscles appears to occur early in the depolarization sequence of the ventricles. Activity spreads quickly through the thin wall of the right ventricle to reach the epicardium. Activation then reaches the apex of the left ventricle. The penultimate areas are the bases of the right and left ventricles, and the final region of heart to be depolarized normally is the crista supraventricularis of the right ventricle.

REPOLARIZATION—THE T WAVE Excitation or depolarization of the myocardium is a passive process arising from ions moving down their concentration gradi-

FIGURE 229-3

A stylized cross section through the heart. SN, sinoatrial node; A, anterior (Bachmann), M, middle (Wenckebach), and Po, posterior (Thorel) internodal tracts; IAS, atrial septum; SVC, superior vena cava; AVN, atrioventricular node; HIS, bundle of His; LBB, left bundle branch; RBB, right bundle branch; P, direction of atrial excitation; 1 to 5, directions and relative magnitudes of forces at successive intervals during depolarization; RT, right ventricle; LT, left ventricle.

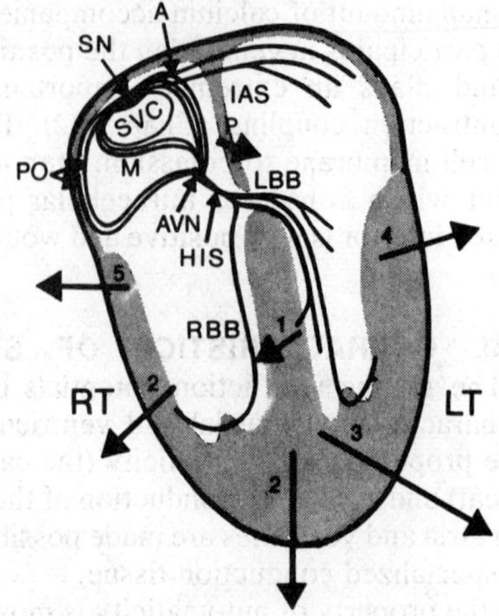

ents. It is an ordered process guided by the conduction system. In contrast, repolarization, or the process underlying the generation of the T wave, is active, since expenditure of metabolic energy is required to restore ionic concentration gradients. Moreover, repolarization is an unguided process in which each area of myocardium repolarizes when it can. T waves may be drastically modified by changes in temperature and by the slightest pressure of a myocardial electrode. Alterations of the T waves accompany a number of conditions, including electrolyte disturbances, ischemia, myocardial hypertrophy, myocardial injury, metabolic disturbance, myocarditis, and cardiomyopathy.

The atria are so thin and the hemodynamic forces acting upon them are so low that pressure, nutritional, and other gradients across their walls are negligible. Consequently those atrial areas excited first recover first. If the four cells in Fig. 229-1*B* are taken to be atrial, the cellular areas free of charge on the left would be the first to be repolarized, making the left side positive with respect to the right during repolarization. This polarity is just the reverse of potential differences accompanying depolarization and accounts for a negative T_a wave ("a" for atria) associated with a positive P wave, or vice versa. T_a waves are only rarely seen in the normal electrocardiogram, since they are usually buried within the much larger forces created by excitation of the ventricles, i.e., the QRS.

Repolarization in the much thicker ventricular walls is more complex. Although excitation spreads generally outward from endocardium to epicardium, the latter repolarizes before the endocardium, presumably because of a better blood supply and less intramyocardial tension. If the right-hand side of Fig. 229-1*B* is now regarded as ventricular epicardium, and the uncharged region as the endocardium, the polarity of charge is identical at corresponding times in excitation and recovery; thus, the normal T wave has the same direction as the QRS.

ELECTROCARDIOGRAPHIC LEADS The earliest practical ECG leads (connections to the body) measure the difference in potential successively between the left arm and right arm (lead 1), the left leg and right arm (lead 2), and the left leg and left arm (lead 3).[1] The polarity of each of these leads was set so that a normal electrocardiogram would usually result in an upright deflection of the major ECG components. A somewhat more complex group of leads is based upon the use of the so-called Wilson terminal, which consists of the junction of two or three resistors of equal value connected to the extremities. Although the Wilson terminal is sometimes described as having a 0 potential, this point of view is at variance with a basic physical principle. However, it does provide a useful commonality for anyone wishing to record leads other than the standard. For example, the Wilson terminal is used paired with each extremity in turn, but the resistor connecting the central terminal to the extremity being measured is dropped by a switch in the electrocardiograph. Such a connection is referred to as an (augmented) extremity lead—aVR, aVL, or aVF, depending upon which limb does not have a resistor connected to it. The full complement of three resistors is used in a Wilson central terminal when measurements are made on the precordium at the standard sites (Table 229-1).

[1] *Connection of the electrocardiographic lead to the right leg is for electronic reference or "grounding."*

TABLE 229-1
Precordial leads

Lead	*Location*
V_1	Fourth intercostal space at the right parasternal line
V_2	Fourth intercostal space at the left parasternal line
V_3	Halfway between V_2 and V_4
V_4	Fifth intercostal space at the left midclavicular line
V_5	On the same horizontal plane as V_4 at the left anterior axillary line
V_6	On the same horizontal plane as V_4 at the left midaxillary line
$(V_{1R} = V_2)$	
$(V_{2R} = V_1)$	
V_{3R}	Halfway between V_1 and V_{4R}
V_{4R}	Fifth intercostal space at the right midclavicular line
V_{5R}	On the same horizontal plane as V_{4R} at the right anterior axillary line
V_{6R}	On the same horizontal plane as V_{4R} at the right midaxillary line
Note:	V_1 to V_6 are the usual leads. V_{1R} to V_{6R}, over the right precordium, are often of use in congenital heart disease.

The most common reference frame for the standard and extremity leads consists of the sides and medians of an equilateral triangle (Fig. 229-4). The utility of this reference system is enhanced by shifting inward the sides of the triangle until they intersect the point where the medians cross. The total result, sometimes called the hexaxial system, appears in Fig. 229-5, including polarity

FIGURE 229-4
The Einthoven triangle. The arrow indicates the direction in which the lead 1 side is transposed to the center (dotted line) in constructing the hexaxial system in Fig. 229-5.

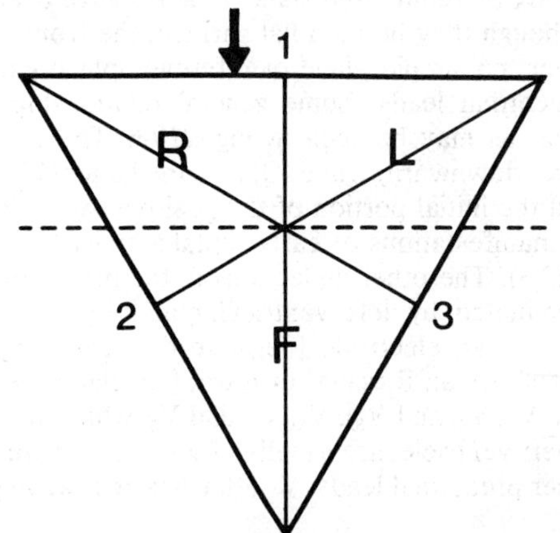

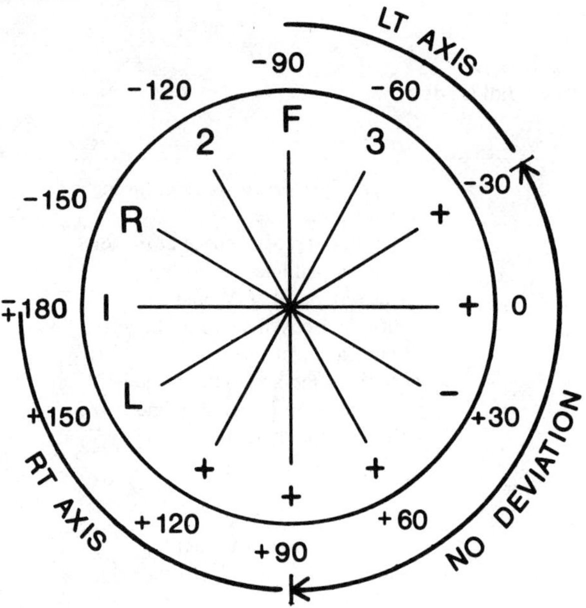

FIGURE 229-5
The hexaxial system.

conventions for each lead. Its use may be illustrated by imagining the largest ventricular excitation force in Fig. 229-3, arrow 3, superimposed on and passing through the center of the hexaxial frame. The head of the arrow is positive. To determine its effect on a particular lead, perpendiculars are erected from the lead to the head and tail of the arrow. The distance between these perpendiculars on the lead axis is proportional to the electrocardiographic deflection. Suppose arrow (or vector) 3 is projected on lead 1. The result would be a force somewhat smaller than vector 3. Since the head (positive potential) of the vector points toward the plus sign on lead 1, the ECG deflection will be upward, or positive.

If vector 3 is projected on lead R, its magnitude would be maximum in this lead, since the vector is parallel to it. However, since the projected head of the vector points to a minus sign, the resultant deflection in R is downward, or negative. In a similar way, all the electrical forces of the heart can be projected on the reference frame, resulting in the amplitude and polarity of the standard and extremity leads shown in the normal example in Fig. 229-6.

The six extremity and standard leads have been treated as though they lie on a flat surface, the frontal plane. However, no simple plane or reference plane exists for the precordial leads. Some general relationships exist, however, as may be seen in Fig. 229-6. The tiny initial negative (downward) wave (Q) in 1, the larger Q in V_5 and V_6, and the initial portion of the positive wave (R) in V_1 are all manifestations of early septal activity (vector 1 in Fig. 229-3). The other deflections in the precordial leads are dominated by left ventricular activity as it points away from an electrode [negative deflection (S) in V_2 which follows an R wave] or toward an electrode site (R wave in V_4, V_5, and V_6). V_3, V_4, and V_5, which are closest to the left ventricle, are usually of greater amplitude than the other precordial leads. V_1 often has an S wave greater than R.

ECG DEFLECTIONS, INTERVALS, AND ESTIMATION OF HEART RATE ECG paper is millimeter graph paper with every fifth millimeter line bold in both directions. Each heavier line along the abscissa is separated from the next one by 200 msec, and the millimeter time intervals are 40 msec. In clinical practice, amplitude (1 mV per cm) and paper speed (25 mm per sec) are standardized. The P wave, due to atrial depolarization, is a gently rounded or slightly peaked deflection, less than 0.3 mV in any lead. Atrial repolarization is usually vastly overshadowed by ventricular activity, but occasionally it appears as a barely perceptible negative displacement following P, the T_a wave. Ventricular excitation gives rise to the Q, R, and S deflections. A deflection is not completed until it crosses the base line, the segment immediately preceding the P wave. The Q wave is the first negative deflection *not* preceded by a positive deflection. The R wave is the first positive deflection; it may or may not be preceded by a Q wave. The S wave is a negative wave following an R wave. Deflections beyond the S wave are designated by prime and double-primed R and S symbols, i.e., S′, R,″ etc. A lead which is entirely negative is referred to as a QS deflection. The S-T segment is a flat segment which begins at the end of the QRS and blends imperceptibly into the T wave. Repolarization of the ventricles begins during the S-T segment and is often in evidence in young people as a slight upward displacement of the S-T segment, e.g., in V_3, V_4, and V_5 of Fig. 229-6. The T wave is a slowly rising and falling wave, upright in all leads except R and V_1 in most adults. The U wave is a very low-amplitude deflection, usually upright, which follows the T (see V_2 and V_3, Fig. 229-6). The origin of the U wave is not proved, but it is believed by many to stem from repolarization of the intraventricular conduction system.

The P-R interval indicates the lapse of time between the onset of atrial and ventricular activation, an *index* of atrioventricular conduction time. This interval is best obtained by measuring the shortest time in any lead between the beginning of P and of the first ventricular deflection—Q, R, or S. The P-R interval normally ranges between 120 and 200 msec. The QRS interval estimates the duration of ventricular electrical activity; the lead with the widest QRS should be chosen for measurement, and it normally does not exceed 100 msec. The Q-T interval estimates the duration of an entire cycle of depolarization and repolarization; this interval is mea-

FIGURE 229-6
A normal electrocardiogram.

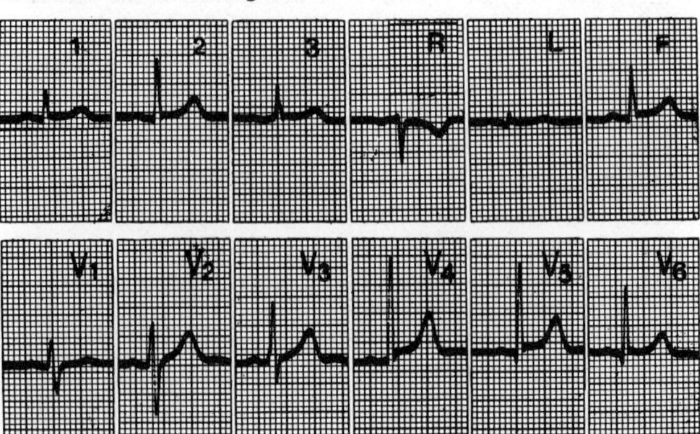

sured from the beginning of QRS to the end of T; it varies with age, sex, and heart rate. Men and children with a heart rate of 100 beats per min can be expected to have a Q-T interval not exceeding 300 msec, whereas women with a heart rate of 50 have a normal Q-T up to 460 msec. Tables giving specific values appear in standard electrocardiographic texts.

When interpreting electrocardiograms, it is convenient to have a simple means for estimating heart rate. What follows is based upon counting the number of complete small boxes (40-msec intervals) between consecutive R waves, P waves, or other identical portions of two electrocardiographic complexes. This number divided into 1,500 provides an estimate which is sufficiently accurate for most clinical purposes.

Electrical axis Some electrocardiographic interpretations depend, at least in part, on the mean or average direction of total electrical activation. The measurement of electrical axis depends on a number of assumptions, including that the body can be represented by a circular disk and that the electrical activity of the heart is adequately represented by a single dipole. Although both these assumptions are invalid, the determination of electrical axis is sufficiently embedded in clinical electrocardiography so that it plays an empirical role in the diagnosis of entities such as ventricular hypertrophy and certain types of conduction defects.

Clinical determination of electrical axis is based on the Einthoven triangle transposed to the hexaxial system shown in Fig. 229-5. This system consists of six intersecting lines pointing in 12 directions. It is therefore possible to determine the axis to within about 30° (360 divided by 12). Lead 1 is used as a reference lead and is assigned the value 0°. The lead containing the smallest QRS is approximately 90° from the direction of the largest or mean electrical axis. For example, if it is ascertained that lead F is the closest of all six leads to 0 area, then the electrical axis must point 90° away, or in a horizontal direction; therefore the axis has a direction of either 0° or ±180°. A decision of which angle is correct is easily obtained by inspecting a second lead. For example, if lead 1 is upright, the axis must be 0°; if lead 1 is inverted, it is ±180°. It is rarely necessary to perform interpolation between intervals of 30°.

FIGURE 229-7
Frontal, right sagittal, and transverse vectorcardiograms (VCGs) and the three orthogonal (X, Y, Z) scalar leads displayed by computer. Only the portion of QRS between cursors 1 and 2 in the right upper corner of the VCG views is displayed. The numbers at the beginning and end of the loops correspond to the cursors. The loop rotates from 1 to 2. Dots on the VCG are separated by 1.25-sec intervals. The vertical bars indicate 0.25 mV.

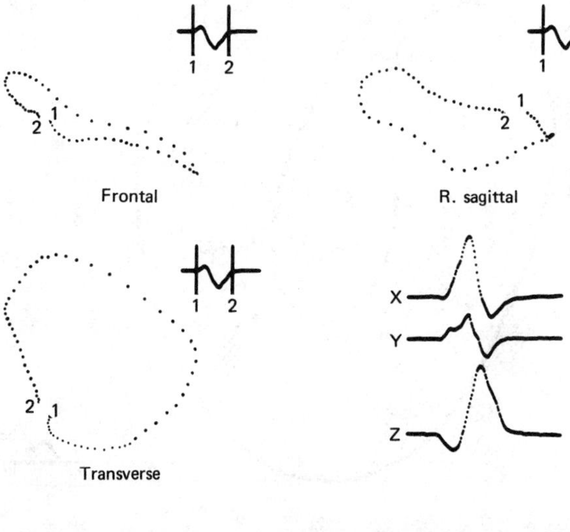

1 2
1 2
Frontal
1 2
1 2
R. sagittal
1 2
2 1
Transverse
X
Y
Z

THE VECTORCARDIOGRAM If the numbered arrows (vectors) in Fig. 229-3 are transposed to a common origin, and the tips of the arrows are connected by a smooth curve interrupted at intervals for timing, the result is a *vectorcardiogram.* The direction and relative size of these vectors depend in part upon the lead system which traditionally had been based on the Einthoven equilateral triangle, shown in Fig. 229-4. This triangle presumes that the heart may be represented electrophysiologically at each instant of its cycle by a pair of charges (a dipole) at the center of a conductive disk or sphere. In order to bring this assumption into accord with the nonspherical shape of a body and the eccentric body location of the heart, a number of corrected vectorcardiologic lead systems have been described. The most popular of these, devised by Frank, consists of seven connections to the body which are interconnected by a resistive weighting network. The outputs of the network are the so-called X, Y, and Z orthogonal (related by right angles) leads, which are displayed and photographed in pairs with a cathode ray oscilloscope. The X-Y pair forms the frontal, the Y-Z the sagittal, and the X-Z the transverse loops or projections, as shown in Fig. 229-7. The P, QRS, and T waves each form a separate loop. Vectorcardiography is of value in the diagnosis of minor intraventricular conduction defects and of unusual varieties of myocardial infarction, in distinguishing myocardial hypertrophy from intraventricular conduction defects, and in confirming the more common electrocardiographic entities.

ISCHEMIA Myocardial ischemia can alter uniformity of polarization, but repolarization, an active process dependent upon a normal blood supply, is more vulnerable. T-wave abnormalities accompany changes in repolarization, whereas alterations in the degree of polarization produce shifts in S-T segments. A most common electrocardiographic pattern accompanying human myocardial ischemia is shown in Fig. 229-8, in which the S-T segment is depressed moderately in leads 1, 2, and V_5, and impressively in V_2, V_3, and V_4. A working hypothesis of these abnormalities is attempted in Fig. 229-9. The arrow in the lower inset indicates that the events in this figure occur before the onset of the QRST deflections, during ventricular electrical diastole. The horizontal line crossing the electrocardiogram is the base-line voltage level which would be present if leads were connected to the recorder. The inset above the diagram of the ventricle shows that during electrical diastole, when most myocardial cells are normally fully polarized, there are cells adjacent to the shaded ischemic zone which are only partially polarized.

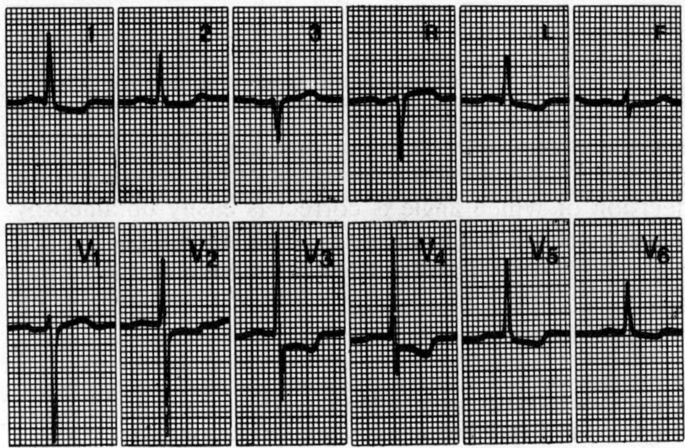

FIGURE 229-8
Subepicardial ischemia.

The result, shown in the large diagram of Fig. 229-9, is the series of double charges oriented with their positive poles facing the anterior electrode and the more distant negative charges facing the central terminal electrode. This charged front causes elevation of the electrocardiographic record during ventricular electrical diastole, which gives the appearance, relatively, of depression of the S-T segments, as in Fig. 229-8. Figure 229-10 presents an explanation of the second abnormality encountered in subepicardial ischemia—inversion of T waves, as in the ECG in Fig. 229-8. The conventions in Fig. 229-10 remain those used in Fig. 229-9. However, the arrow is now located during inscription of the T wave, indicating that the events depicted occur at this time. The upper inset indicates that recovery, or repolarization, commences at the endocardium, because epicardial ischemia delays repolarization in localized areas. As a result, repolarization occurs in a direction the reverse of normal and consists of a negative force directed toward the left and anterior electrodes.

When ischemia is confined to the subendocardial region, the characteristic finding is deeply, symmetrically inverted T waves. The deeply inverted T waves are relatively evanescent unless infarction intervenes. The lower record in Fig. 229-11 was recorded in the same patient 5 days after an episode of chest pain; no enzymatic abnormality or other evidence of myocardial infarction was observed in the interim.

An unusual or variant form of myocardial ischemia causes angina which is often unprovoked by exertion. Attacks of pain often occur at night, awakening the patient from sleep. An electrocardiogram obtained during pain reveals profound S-T segment elevation similar to that present in the early stages of acute myocardial infarction (Fig. 229-12), in which irreversible blockade of a coronary artery occurs. It is believed that variant angina is due to temporarily reversible obstruction, caused perhaps by spasm, of a major coronary artery (Chap. 240). The relatively normal, though thin, layer of epicardium present in subepicardial ischemia (Fig. 229-9) is absent in variant angina, in which malperfusion is more profound. Absence of this normal layer causes an opposite orientation of partially polarized cells (Fig. 229-13) in variant angina compared with subepicardial ischemia, and S-T segment elevation in the former contrasted with S-T depression in the latter.

It must be emphasized that the QRS complex is not directly altered in any of the preceding varieties of myocardial ischemia. Significant distortion of the QRS complex (other than that due to evanescent conduction defects or arrhythmias) is usually consistent with myocardial damage.

MYOCARDIAL INFARCTION Myocardial infarction results when coronary artery thrombosis or other permanent obstruction to coronary artery flow occurs (Chap. 240). The mass of myocardium perfused by the obstructed artery becomes ischemic, and death of the cells followed by replacement of myocardium with fibrous tissue eventually results, if the patient survives. During the acute phase of myocardial infarction, S-T segment changes dominate the electrocardiogram. The most striking change in the upper record of Fig. 229-12 is the presence of greatly elevated S-T segments in all precordial leads except V_6, but especially in V_3, V_4, and V_5. The S-T abnormalities are thought to arise as shown in Fig. 229-13. In this figure the anterior wall of the left ventricle is to the viewer's right, and a detailed section is shown above the ventricle. The shaded zones indicate ischemia, and the dotted area indicates an absence of viable, polarized cells, many of which will ultimately succumb. The inset shows that the ischemic zone contains cells which are partially polarized during electrical diastole, the instant indicated in the schematic ECG in the lower right-hand portion of the figure. Thus, the anteriorly placed precordial electrode will reflect an unvarying negative potential throughout the period of electrical diastole.

FIGURE 229-9
A schematic representation of the origin of S-T depression in subepicardial ischemia. C.T., the central terminal.

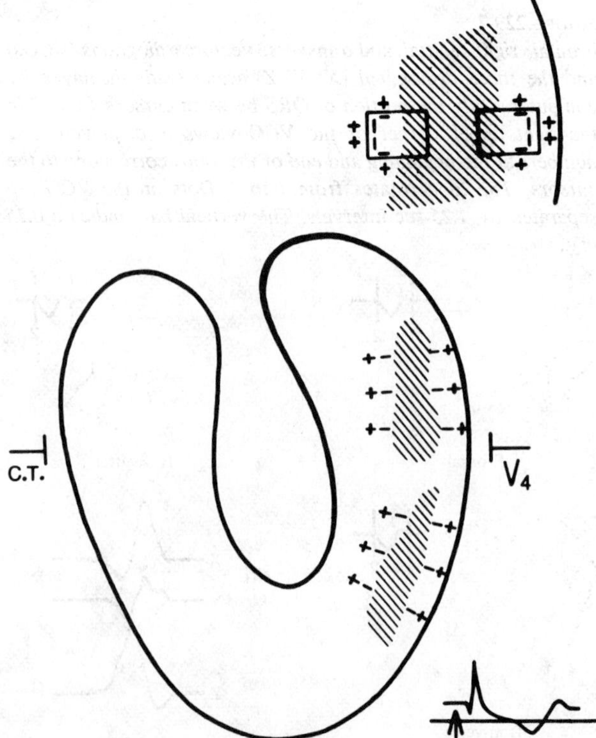

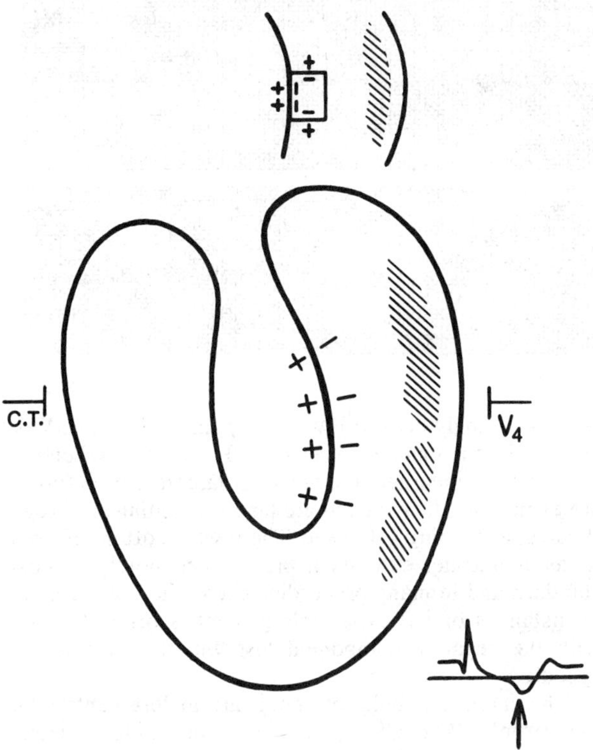

FIGURE 229-10
The origin of T-wave inversion in subepicardial ischemia. Symbols as in Fig. 229-9.

Immediately after depolarization, roughly analogous to phase 2 of the action potential, all charges disappear and the record returns to the base line drawn through it (Fig. 229-13). If the base line is not present, as in the upper record of Fig. 229-12, S-T segments appear to be elevated. Partially polarized cells are in an unstable state; shortly they will either recover or die. Consequently, S-T segment displacements accompanying myocardial infarction can usually be expected to disappear in a few days. The lower record in Fig. 229-12, obtained 2 days after the upper record, shows that S-T segment displacements have been greatly reduced, but several new features are now present. First, the T waves have become inverted in V_3, V_4, and V_5; this is generally believed to be a manifestation of persistent ischemia. Secondly, R waves formerly present in V_2 and V_3 have disappeared and have been replaced by Q-S deflections; the R wave in V_4 is less than half its former size. Q-S and Q waves in myocardial infarction are believed to arise because the nonviable wall of the infarcted ventricle generates insufficient excitation forces to oppose those arising in the opposite wall. If, for example, the wall of the ventricle on the left represents the posterior wall of the left ventricle, activity appearing there is unbalanced by forces in the infarcted anterior wall; negativity is recorded in the anterior precordial lead, as in V_4 of the lower strip in Fig. 229-12. As time passes, the remaining S-T elevations in the lower strip in Fig. 229-12 disappear unless partial depolarization persists because of ventricular aneurysm.

The electrical localization of myocardial infarction is determined by which leads exhibit the most striking findings. In Fig. 229-12 the process is confined to the anterior and left precordium, but careful inspection will reveal that the small septal R wave in V_2 and V_3 disappeared by the time the lower record was obtained. Thus, the records show anteroseptal damage, a further consequence of left coronary artery disease. If the process had involved more lateral regions in the left ventricle, Q waves and ST-T wave abnormalities would be present in leads 1 and aVL.

Figure 229-14 is typical of the electrocardiographic abnormalities encountered after the acute S-T segment changes have subsided in a case of inferior (diaphragmatic) wall infarction. There are deep, slurred Q-S deflections and inverted T waves in leads 3 and aVF (the latter contains a deep notch in the Q-S deflection) and a deep Q and inverted T wave in lead 2. These abnormalities are present in the leads mentioned because the inferior wall of the heart faces the left leg, which is common to leads 2, 3, and aVF. There are also S-T depression in V_5 and T-wave inversion in V_6, suggesting that ischemia of the lateral wall is present. All these abnormalities are due to occlusion of a branch or branches of the right coronary artery.

The chronology of anterior and inferior (transmural) electrocardiographic abnormalities is summarized in Table 229-2. Infarction of the true posterior wall of the left ventricle produces inconstant changes in both the electrocardiogram and the vectorcardiogram. Most com-

FIGURE 229-11
Subendocardial ischemia during pain (top) and 5 days later (bottom).

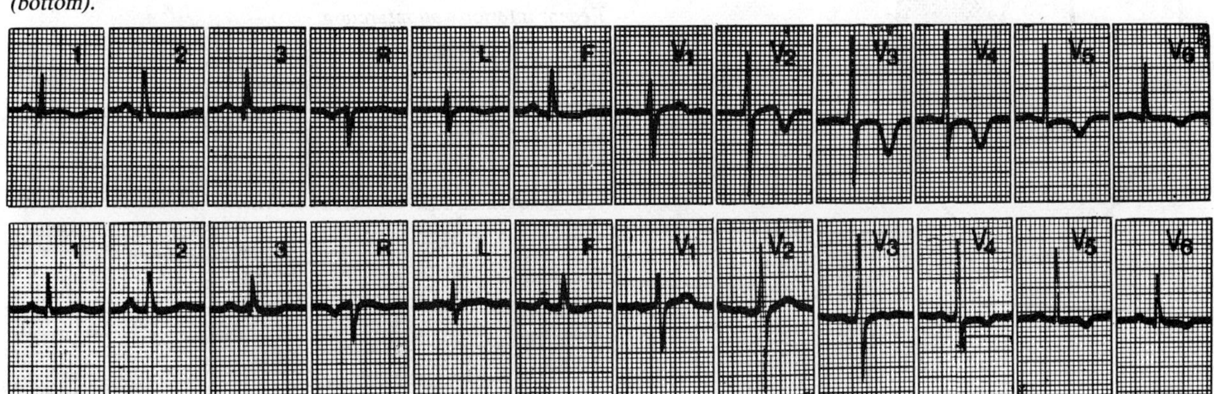

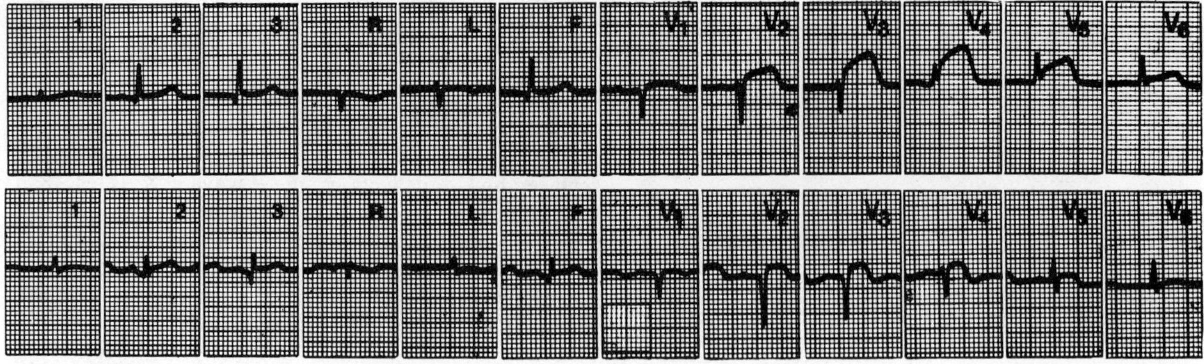

FIGURE 229-12
Acute anteroseptal infarction (top). 48 hr later (bottom).

monly these consist of heightened R and T waves in V_1 and V_2, findings which may be difficult to recognize in the absence of electrocardiograms antedating the illness.

When the arterial blood supply to the subendocardium is sufficiently compromised, infarction of a portion of that zone occurs. The electrocardiographic changes resemble those seen in Fig. 229-11, which represents the changes of subendocardial ischemia. In subendocardial infarction, as in subendocardial ischemia, the abnormalities are confined to the T waves and occasionally to S-T segments; the former are deeply and symmetrically inverted. No abnormalities of QRS are present since a substantial shell of viable, depolarizable epicardium persists.

CHAMBER ENLARGEMENT Depolarization of the right atrium is normally followed by that of the left. When right atrial enlargement occurs, electrical forces that are greater and longer lasting than normal arise from this chamber and summate with normal left atrial forces. The result is a singly peaked P wave (P pulmonale), 0.3 mV or greater, in one or more of leads 2, 3, and aVF. When the left atrium is enlarged, the normally later left atrial forces are even more delayed and are larger, resulting in a broad P wave, exceeding 110 msec. The P wave, often referred to as P mitrale, exhibits a pronounced notch in most standard and in many precordial leads. The P wave in V_1 in instances of left atrial enlargement is often diphasic with the negative component last, but this sign is not specific.

FIGURE 229-13
The origin of S-T elevation in acute anterior wall infarction.

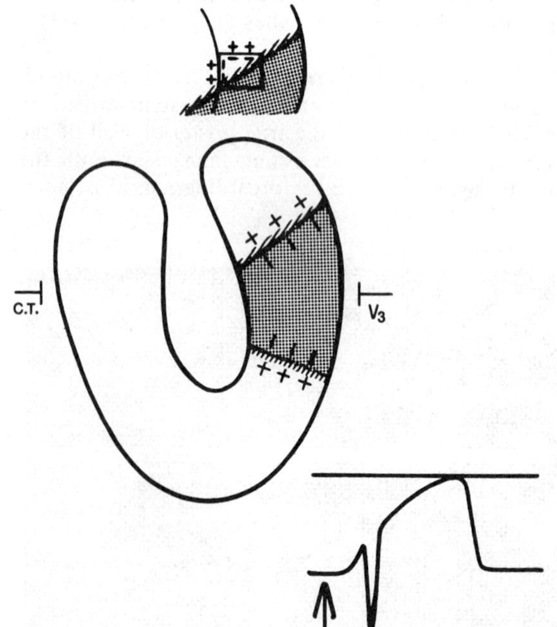

The increased bulk of the heart in left ventricular hypertrophy (Fig. 229-15) might be expected to be detected easily in the electrocardiogram. However, the vast array of indices of left ventricular hypertrophy testify to the difficulty encountered in making this diagnosis. Not a small source of difficulty lies with the internal cancellation of much of the electrical force generated by the hypertrophied left ventricle. Characteristically, the QRS deflections are larger than usual; an R or an S wave in any of the six limb leads exceeding 2 mV, an S wave in V_1, V_2, or V_3 greater than 3 mV, or an R wave exceeding 3 mV in V_4, V_5, or V_6 strongly suggests left ventricular hypertrophy. Although T-wave inversion and sometimes S-T depression accompany these changes, the latter two findings may accompany digitalis administration or ischemia and therefore are nonspecific. Left axis deviation is sometimes present in left ventricular hypertrophy, and the QRS interval may be increased somewhat but not to more than 100 msec.

Interpretation of right ventricular hypertrophy rests upon even fewer observations than in the case of left ventricular hypertrophy. Right axis deviation of more

FIGURE 229-14
Recent inferior wall infarction.

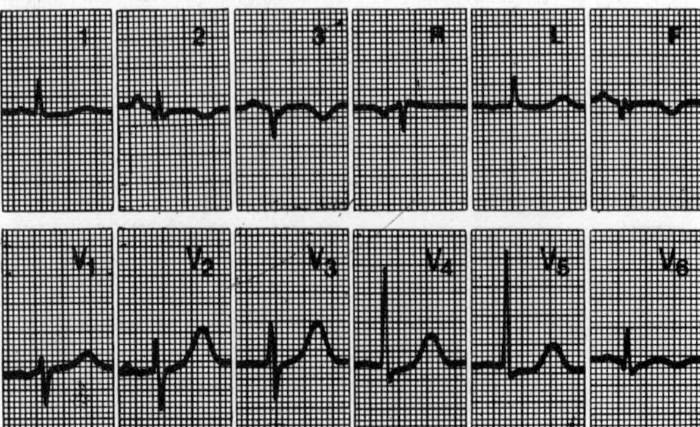

TABLE 229-2
Persistence of ECG findings in uncomplicated transmural infarction

Portion of QRS	*Hours to days*	*Days to weeks*	*Weeks to months*	*Years*
Q	Normal, if present	Broad and deep	Broad and deep	Broad and deep
S-T	Elevated	Less elevated	Normal	Normal
T	Upright; may be concealed in S-T	Inverted	Inverted	Upright, sometimes

than 110° and an R/S ratio in V_1 of 1 or greater with an R wave in V_1 exceeding 0.5 mV are regarded as strong electrocardiographic evidence of right ventricular hypertrophy.

PERICARDITIS In pericarditis, the epicardium is the focus of an inflammatory process and contains a layer of cells temporarily incapable of uniform repolarization (Fig. 229-16; see also Chap. 241). By a mechanism analogous to that present in acute myocardial infarction (Fig. 229-13), S-T segment elevations are seen early in virtually *all* leads, without the reciprocal S-T depression characteristic of acute infarction. The absence of S-T segment depression in most leads during acute pericarditis appears to be due to the ubiquitous nature of the acute inflammation: every electrode (except aVR and sometimes V_1) faces partially polarized cells.

As the acute process heals, S-T segment elevation gradually subsides, only to be replaced by widespread T-wave inversion. T-wave abnormalities, such as those consonant with delayed epicardial recovery, may persist for months.

CONDUCTION DEFECTS Atrioventricular conduction defects are discussed in Chap. 234.

Uncomplicated block of one bundle branch does not result in disturbances of rhythm, since the intact branch remains to transmit the wave of atrial depolarization to the ventricle. Complete right bundle branch block is present when the QRS interval exceeds 110 msec, and an RSR′ pattern is present in V_1 (Fig. 229-15). A broad, prominent S wave in lead 1 is also characteristic of complete right bundle branch block. In V_1 the early R reflects normal depolarization of the interventricular septum by a twig from the left bundle branch, and the S denotes activity arriving normally at the lateral wall of the left ventricle. The R′ in V_1 and the S in lead 1 are due to delayed right ventricular depolarization because of the block.

The sequence of ventricular activation in left bundle

FIGURE 229-15
Electrocardiograms in right ventricular hypertrophy (RVH), left ventricular hypertrophy (LVH), complete left bundle branch block (LBBB), and complete right bundle branch block (RBBB).

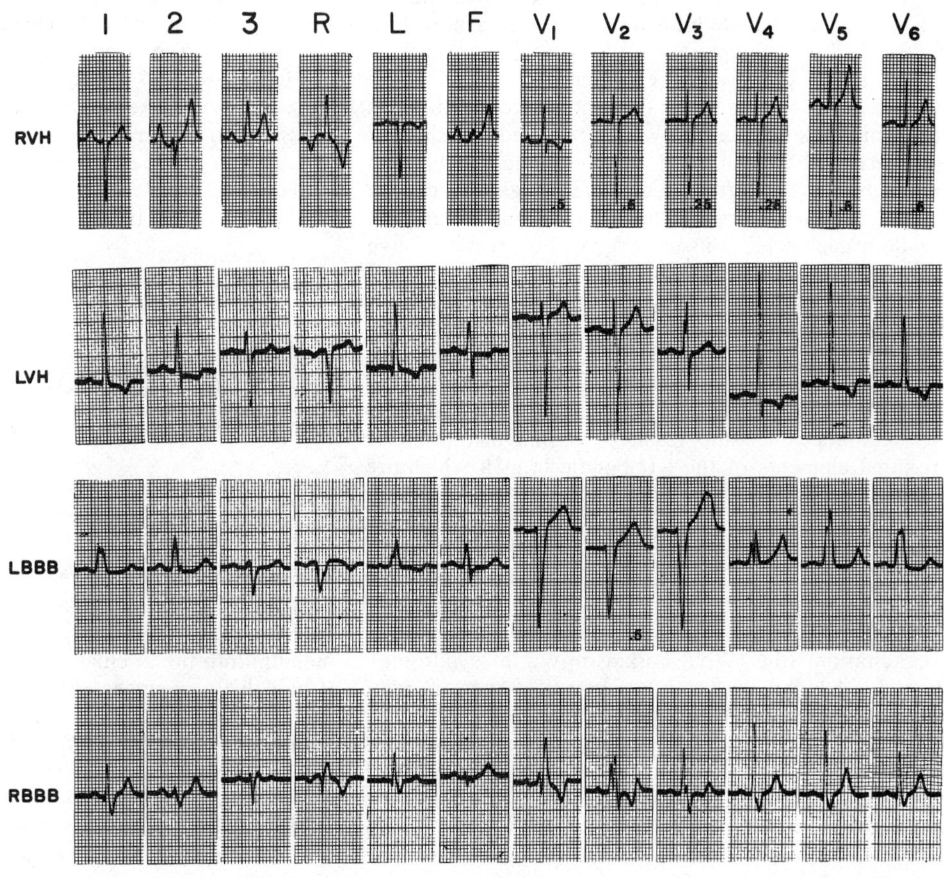

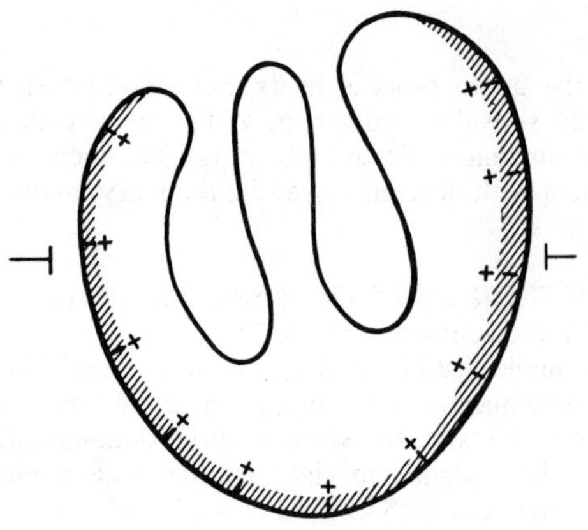

FIGURE 229-16
The source of widespread S-T elevation in acute pericarditis. The electrodes face the right and left ventricles, e.g., V_2 and V_5.

branch block (Fig. 229-15) is initiated by depolarization of the right ventricle via the intact right bundle branch. Thereafter the thick left ventricle is slowly depolarized from right to left and inferiorly. Complete left bundle branch block is typified by QRS complexes in the lateral precordial leads (V_5 and V_6) which are slurred and broad and which almost always consist of only an R wave; there is no RSR′ in V_1, and lead 1 characteristically has no S wave. In complete left, as in right, bundle branch block, the QRS interval exceeds 110 msec. When the morphologic characteristics of right bundle branch block or of left bundle branch block are present but the QRS interval is 110 msec, the bundle branch block, either right or left, is described as incomplete.

For many years electrocardiographers have noted unexplained instances of left (and more rarely, right) axis deviation. Four decades ago Wilson reported situations of this sort in cases of right bundle branch block and deduced that the left axis observed might be due to ". . . a lesion of some of the subdivisions of the left bundle branch. . . ." Wilson's original observations have given birth to the concept of hemiblocks, i.e., conduction disturbances in the anterior and posterior subdividions of the left bundle branch. Although the electrocardiographic findings accompanying hemiblocks are simple and clear, the existence of discrete, cordlike subdivisions within the mane-like left bundle branch is contentious. It is likely that the hemiblocks are the result of partial disruption of proximal elements of the left bundle branch which are destined to supply either the anterior or posterior left ventricular wall.

The dominant feature of anterior hemiblock is a normal QRS interval with left axis deviation in the absence of other causes of left axis deviation such as inferior myocardial infarction, pulmonary emphysema, and preexcitation (the Wolff-Parkinson-White syndrome). Posterior hemiblock may be suspected if there is right axis deviation and the following are not present: extensive lateral wall myocardial infarction, right ventricular hypertrophy, chronic pulmonary disease, and vertical electrical position of the heart. The shift in axis following disruption of some of the left bundle fibers is attributed to unbalanced spread of depolarization in the left ventricle. Immediately beyond the distal end of the bundle of His, the left bundle fibers normally fan out in all directions to embrace the endocardium of that chamber. Those fibers coursing anteriorly are thought to be superior (cephalad) to posterior fibers. Hence, disruption of anterior fibers (anterior hemiblock) is considered to result in unbalanced excitation, starting from the inferior termini of intact posterior fibers. The mean direction of depolarization of the left ventricle will be more or less upward, and left axis deviation is the result. Similar reasoning accounts for right axis deviation in posterior hemiblock.

As *isolated* electrocardiographic entities, left or right axis deviation cannot be practically separated from anterior or posterior hemiblock. In young adults the latter interpretation is unwise. In association with another disorder of the conduction apparatus, the occurrence of left (or right) axis deviation warns that more than a single element is involved. For example, the coexistence of right bundle branch block and left axis deviation (anterior hemiblock) has a very high risk of becoming complete heart block.

REFERENCES

Chou T, Helm RA: *Clinical Vectorcardiography*, New York: Grune & Stratton, 1967

Durrer DD et al: Total excitation of the isolated human heart. Circulation 41:899, 1970

Estes EH: Examination by means of electrocardiography, chap. 21 in *The Heart*, 3d ed., ed JW Hurst, New York: McGraw-Hill, 1974, pp. 297–323

Goldman MJ: *Principles of Clinical Electrocardiography*, 7th ed., Los Altos, Calif.: Lange, 1970

James TN: Anatomy of the conduction system of the heart, chap. 5 in *The Heart*, 3d ed., ed JW Hurst, New York: McGraw-Hill, 1974, pp. 52–62

Langer GA: Ion fluxes in cardiac excitation and contraction and relation to myocardial contractility. Physiol Rev 48:708, 1968

Spach MS et al: The electrical potential distribution surrounding the atria during depolarization and repolarization in the dog. Circ Res 24:857, 1969

230
INDIRECT METHODS OF EXAMINATION OF THE HEART

JOHN ROSS, JR.
ROBERT A. O'ROURKE

The indirect methods for examination of the heart, which encompass special diagnostic approaches other than cardiac catheterization or injection of radiographic contrast medium into the circulation, include electrocardiography (Chap. 229), roentgenography, phonocardiography, external recordings of pulse wave forms, and other special techniques such as echocardiography and the use of radioisotopes.

ROENTGENOGRAPHY Roentgenographic examination of the heart and lungs is one of the most valuable indirect tools available to the physician. Although standard 6-ft posteroanterior and lateral chest roentgenograms may provide adequate information, overpenetrated frontal, lateral, and oblique views obtained when the esophagus is filled with barium paste are essential for visualization of specific regions of the heart.

The cardiac silhouette In the posteroanterior projection (Fig. 230-1*A*), left ventricular enlargement often causes convexity of the left cardiac border, and the cardiac apex is displaced downward, below the level of the diaphragm. Enlargement of the right ventricle, which has no representation in the frontal projection, may result in tipping upward of the cardiac apex. An enlarged left atrium may produce a round "double density" in the center of the cardiac silhouette and upward displacement of the left mainstem bronchus.

In the right anterior oblique (RAO) projection (Fig. 230-1*B*), the barium-filled esophagus courses directly adjacent to the left atrium. This projection is helpful for detecting right ventricular enlargement and is of particular value for recognizing compression or posterior displacement of the esophagus by an enlarged left atrium.

In the left anterior oblique (LAO) projection (Fig. 230-1*C*), the posterior aspect of the left ventricle normally clears the spine with the patient rotated to an angle of 60° or less relative to the plane of the film. When the left ventricle is enlarged, it overlaps the spine when the patient is rotated 60° or more from the posteroanterior position, but it should be appreciated that marked right ventricular enlargement alone can cause posterior displacement of the left ventricle.

The dimensions of the cardiac silhouette relative to the bony thorax can be measured directly from the standard 6-ft chest roentgenogram. The measurement most commonly made is the cardiothoracic ratio, which is obtained by dividing the transverse diameter of the heart (defined as the distance from the outermost point of the right cardiac border to the midsternal line, plus the distance from the outermost point of the left cardiac border to the midsternal line) by the internal diameter of the thorax at its widest point above the diaphragm. Although the cardiothoracic ratio is dependent on the configuration of the chest, generally it is less than 0.5 in normal subjects.

Image-intensification fluoroscopy may be employed to define further the size and the pulsations of the cardiac chambers and great vessels. It also is useful for detecting areas of calcification within the cardiac valves, coronary arteries, or pericardium. The characteristic motion of the cardiac valves observed on fluoroscopy aids considerably in identifying the site of a calcification.

The pulmonary vasculature The size of the central and peripheral pulmonary blood vessels can be evaluated from the standard chest roentgenogram. Estimation of the degree of pulmonary vascularity may be of great diagnostic importance, particularly in patients suspected of having congenital heart disease, and a disproportion between the size of the central and peripheral pulmonary arteries (enlarged main vessels that taper sharply) may suggest an elevated pulmonary vascular resistance.

An unusually prominent pulmonary vascular pattern is observed in lesions associated with left-to-right shunting of blood, and the main pulmonary artery segment often is enlarged. Examination of the heart for specific chamber enlargement often aids in determining the location of the shunt. For example, in patients with atrial septal defect there is right ventricular enlargement, but the left atrium and left ventricle are small because the defect allows decompression of those chambers. In contrast, in patients with ventricular septal defect both the left atrium and left ventricle are enlarged.

A selective increase in the caliber of the upper lobe pulmonary veins can be observed with lesions such as mitral stenosis that produce left atrial hypertension. In addition, the normal pattern in the upright subject, a more prominent vascular pattern at the lung bases than at the apices, may be reversed in patients with an elevated left atrial pressure. Higher levels of pulmonary venous pressure (exceeding 15 to 20 mm Hg) may also be associated with interstitial edema or fibrosis in the interlobular septums, resulting in the Kerley "B" lines, horizontal markings about 1 cm in length appearing above the diaphragm near the rib cage. Pulmonary edema (fluid within the alveoli) may be secondary to acute left atrial hypertension or left ventricular failure and is characterized by bilateral, confluent "butterfly" densities in the central lung fields.

Decreased pulmonary vascularity is observed most commonly with lesions that cause both obstruction to right ventricular outflow and right-to-left shunting of blood. The reduction in pulmonary blood flow results in diminished caliber of the pulmonary arteries and veins, and the left atrium also may be small; such findings are present in patients with tetralogy of Fallot. In patients with pure valvular pulmonic stenosis, since the pulmonary blood flow may be normal, the pulmonary vascularity often is not diminished.

Radioisotopes The intravenous injection of macroaggregated ^{131}I-labeled albumin, with subsequent scanning of the lung fields for underperfused areas, is valuable in the detection of pulmonary emboli (Chap. 256). Another application of this approach is to scan the cardiac silhouette after intravenous injection of the radioisotope; the area of the cardiac silhouette occupied by the labeled intracardiac blood pool is then compared with the cardiac silhouette on the chest roentgenogram for the detection of pericardial effusion. The intravenous injection of a small bolus of a gamma emitter such as ^{99m}Tc pertechnetate permits rapid, sequential visualization of the heart, great vessels, and pulmonary vasculature by use of an Anger scintillation camera. The image usually is recorded, stored on tape, replayed, and photographed. This technique is used in the diagnosis of a variety of congenital and acquired cardiac lesions, as well as for detecting pulmonary emboli and pericardial effusion.

PHONOCARDIOGRAPHY The phonocardiogram provides a graphic display of heart sounds and murmurs, and enhances considerably the assessment of auscultatory events. The modern phonocardiograph is capable of recording sounds in a manner that resembles their detection by the ear. In order to simulate the relative insensi-

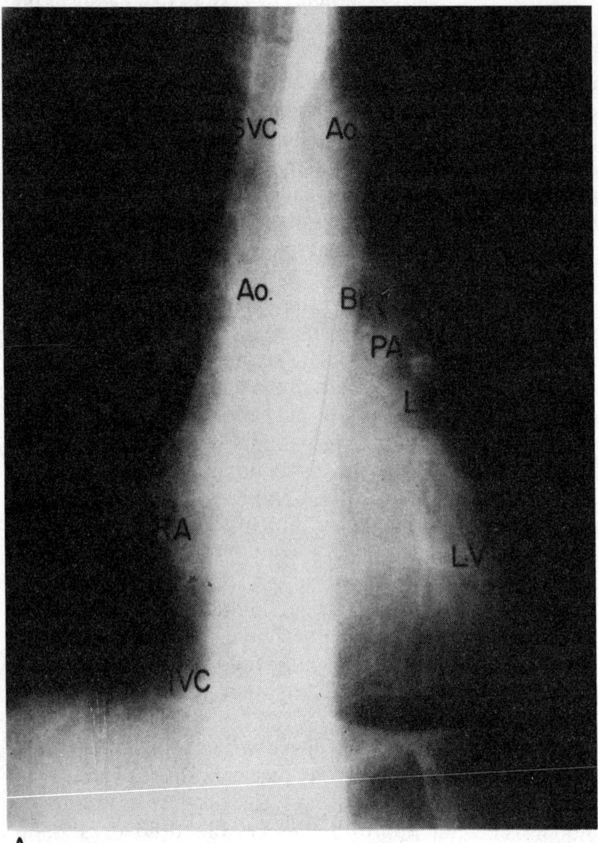

A

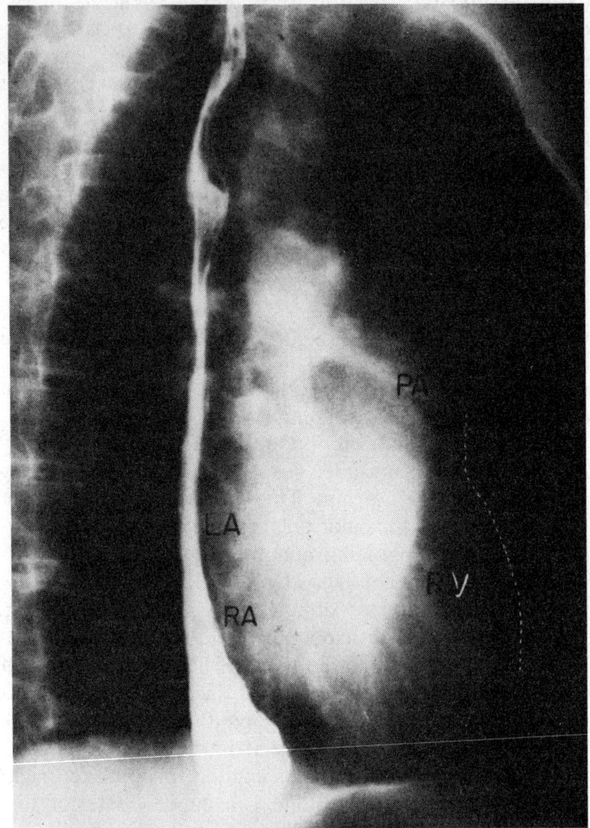

B

FIGURE 230-1
Roentgenograms of a middle-aged woman with coronary heart disease and minimal enlargement of the left ventricle. A *Frontal projection (posteroanterior).* B *Right anterior oblique projection.* C *Left anterior oblique projection. SVC, superior vena cava; AO, aorta; Br, left main-stem bronchus; RA, right atrium; IVC, inferior vena cava; PA, pulmonary artery segment; LA, left atrium; LV, left ventricle; RV, right ventricle; Asc, ascending aorta and Dsc, descending aorta.*

tivity of the human ear to low-frequency vibrations and its great sensitivity to high-frequency signals, so-called logarithmic or high-frequency recordings are used to provide relatively greater amplification of high-frequency components. Filters also are employed to allow selective passage of low- and high-frequency sounds, perhaps the most satisfactory system consisting of a series of band-pass filters which encompass the frequency fields from 15 to 1,000 Hz (cycles per second). The transducer of the phonocardiograph consists of a crystal (piezoelectric) microphone applied directly to the skin, or attached indirectly through an air-coupled diaphragm or bell. The crystals within the microphone alter their electrical properties when stressed by sound pressure waves, and the resulting electrical signal is amplified and recorded on a high-frequency oscillograph.

The phonocardiogram is useful for determining the configuration and frequency composition of individual cardiac murmurs, but perhaps its most important application is in the precise timing of cardiac sounds and

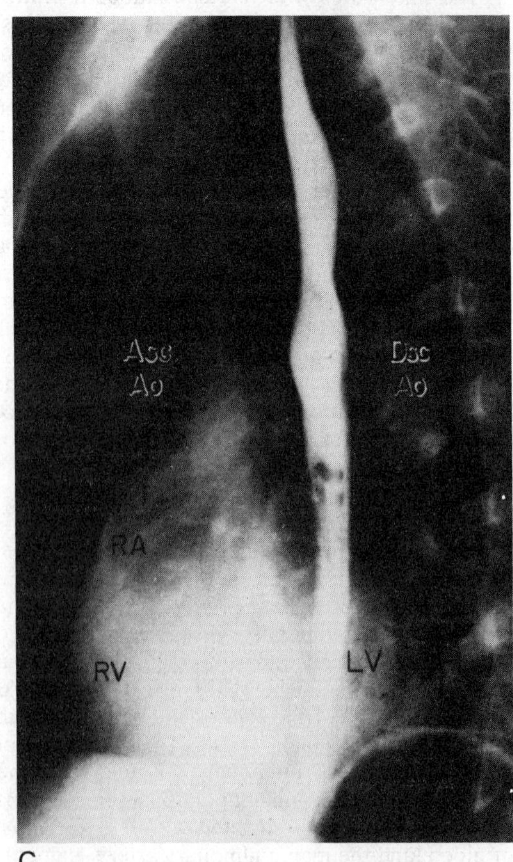

C

murmurs (see Chap. 228). Thus, it allows clear definition of a sequence of events, such as the variation in the splitting of the second heart sound which occurs during respiration, or the differentiation of separate systolic and diastolic murmurs from a continuous murmur which continues throughout late systole and early diastole. The phonocardiogram also may provide quantitative information of significance, such as the precise duration of the interval between the aortic closure sound and the mitral valve opening snap in patients with mitral stenosis, an interval that correlates inversely with the atrioventricular pressure gradient (Chap. 239).

The electrocardiogram is recorded simultaneously with the phonocardiogram to provide a reference signal. Other externally recorded variables that are extremely helpful in timing auscultatory events are the venous pulse tracing (jugular phlebogram), the carotid pulse wave, and the apexcardiogram, each of which is discussed below.

In order to appreciate the significance of alterations in the timing of heart sounds which occur in various disease states and the relation that these sounds bear to external pulse tracings, it is essential to understand the normal temporal relations between the electrical and mechanical events of the cardiac cycle (Fig. 230-2). The normal cycle begins with the P wave of the electrocardiogram, which is followed by right atrial contraction, the initial mechanical event. Left atrial contraction occurs shortly thereafter. The QRS complex ensues, initiating the onset of isovolumetric left ventricular contraction 0.04 to 0.06 sec after the onset of the QRS complex. Right ventricular contraction then starts, and the brief period of isovolumetric right ventricular contraction is then followed by the onset of right ventricular ejection. The onset of left ventricular ejection is the next event, and since the duration of ejection is shorter on the left side than on the right, closure of the aortic valve precedes pulmonic valve closure. Isovolumetric relaxation of the ventricles terminates earlier on the right side than on the left (at the peak of the atrial V wave). A convenient way to remember this normal sequence of mechanical events in the two ventricles (onset of isovolumetric contraction, onset of ejection, end of ejection, end of isovolumetric relaxation) is to recall that isovolumetric phases of left ventricular contraction and relaxation completely encompass those of the right ventricle (Fig. 230-2).

FIGURE 230-2
Diagrammatic representation of pressure tracings recorded within the left and right ventricles correlated with the ECG and the phonocardiogram (Phono). The diagonal cross-hatched areas labeled Isom. represent the isovolumetric phases of left ventricular contraction and relaxation; isovolumetric right ventricular contraction and relaxation is shown in black. M_1 and T_1, sounds produced by closure of the mitral and tricuspid valves, respectively; A_2 and P_2, sounds produced by the closure of the aortic and pulmonic valves; OT and OM, sounds produced by opening of the tricuspid and mitral valves, respectively.

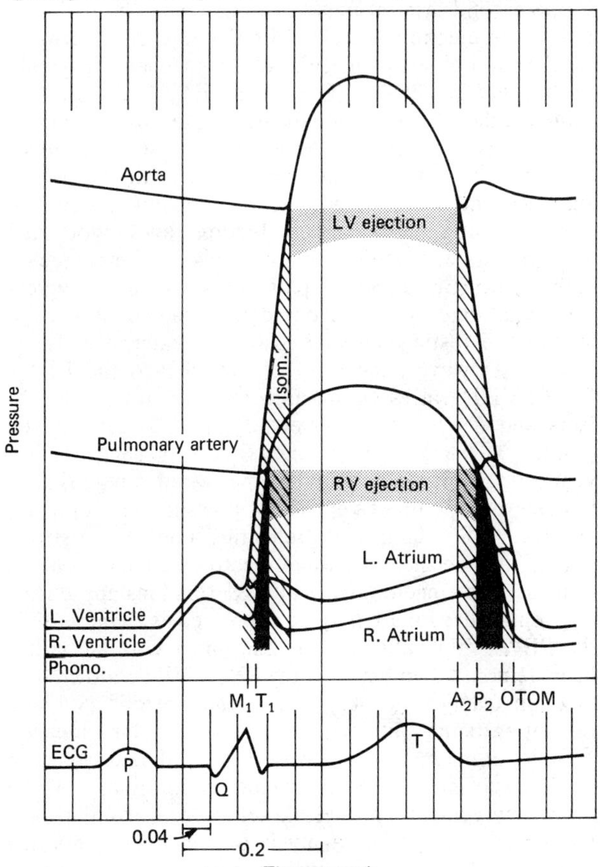

The jugular venous pulse tracing is obtained by applying a cup transducer over the jugular bulb with slight suction; an inner chamber transmits the pressure changes induced by the venous pulsations to a crystal microphone. The nomenclature of the venous waves is the same as that employed in describing intraatrial pressure pulse contours recorded directly (Figs. 228-1 and 231-3). Although some difficulty may be introduced by a variable delay in transmission of the venous waves to the neck (this delay generally averages 0.02 sec), the venous tracing may be extremely helpful in studying the dynamics of the right side of the heart (see Chap. 228).

The indirect carotid arterial pulse wave is recorded with a transducer similar to that employed for obtaining the jugular venous tracing. This signal provides an important means of analyzing the carotid pulse contour and for timing the sounds of aortic and pulmonic valve closure (Figs. 228-1 and 230-3*A*). Alterations in the contour of the carotid arterial pulse are often helpful in the diagnosis of aortic valve disease, idiopathic hypertrophic subaortic stenosis, and left ventricular failure (see Chap. 228). Normally, the ascending limb of the systolic carotid wave is steeper than the descending limb; the upstroke time from onset to peak averages 100 msec (range, 60 to 140 msec),[1] and the normal duration of ejection averages 300 msec (range, 260 to 310 msec).[1]

The aortic component of the second heart sound (A_2), generated at the closure of the aortic valve, can be identified using the incisura of the carotid pulse wave as a reference point (Fig. 230-3*A*). Since there is a slight delay in the transmission of the pulse wave to the neck, the

[1] *Corrected for heart rate by dividing the measured interval by the square root of the cycle length in seconds.*

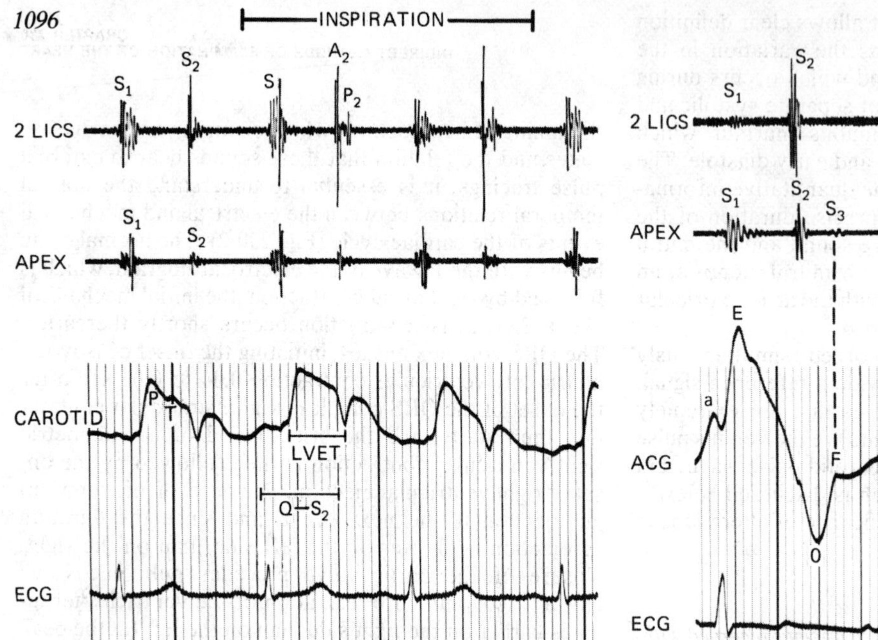

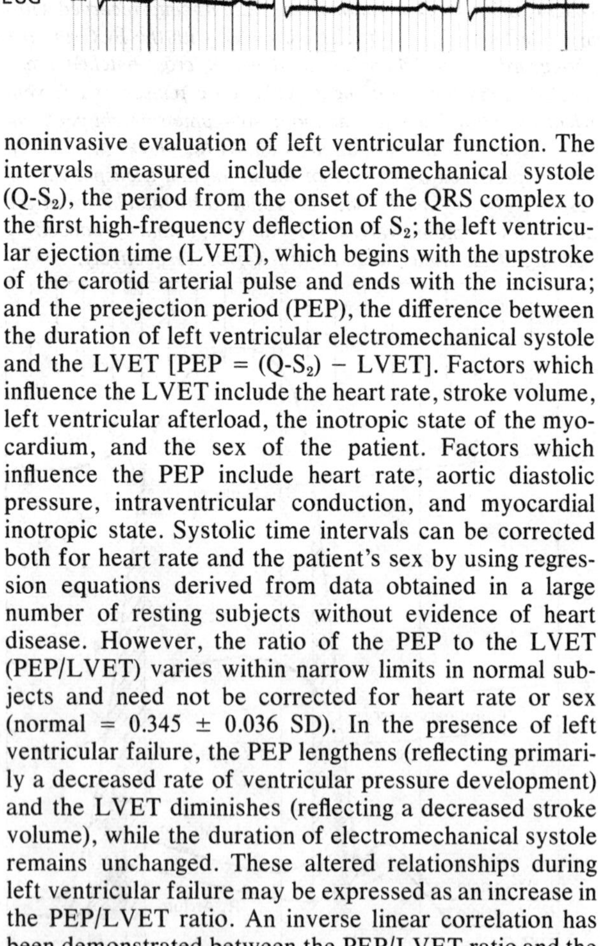

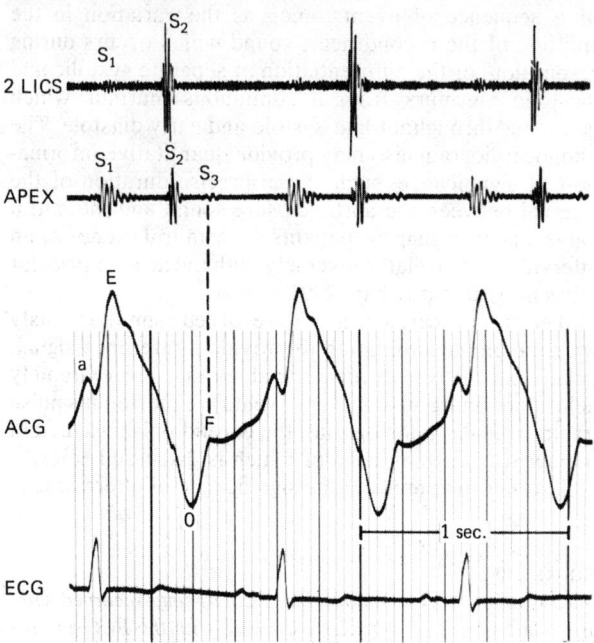

FIGURE 230-3

A *The indirect carotid pulse wave tracing exhibits two normal systolic waves, the initial percussion wave (P) followed by a tidal wave (T). The incisura is then followed by the dicrotic wave. The phonocardiogram is recorded at the second left intercostal space (2 LICS) and the apex, and it demonstrates the normal increase in the interval between the aortic second sound (A_2) and the pulmonic second sound (P_2) which occurs during inspiration. The diminished intensity of P_2 at the apex also may be noted. LVET is the left ventricular ejection time, and the Q-S_2 interval is the duration of electromechanical systole (see text).* B *The apexcardiogram (ACG) in a patient with a third heart sound (S_3). The A wave of the apexcardiogram is coincident with atrial contraction, the E point shortly follows the onset of the first heart sound and coincides approximately with the onset of left ventricular ejection, and the O point corresponds to the time of opening of the mitral valve at the end of isometric ventricular relaxation. The end of the rapid-filling wave in diastole (the F point) is coincident with the third heart sound and is followed by the phase of slow ventricular filling.*

recording of this sound precedes the incisura by approximately 0.02 sec. In the normal person, closure of the pulmonic valve (P_2) always follows A_2 (Fig. 230-2; Chap. 228). Although this interval is narrow during expiration (0.02 sec) and the splitting may be inaudible, it may be recorded on the phonocardiogram (Fig. 230-3*A*).

Lesions that result in prolongation of left ventricular ejection may cause reversal of the normal sequence of aortic and pulmonic valve closure, termed paradoxic splitting of the second heart sound (Chap. 228). That A_2 follows P_2 may be verified on the phonocardiogram using the carotid pulse tracing for timing.

Systolic time intervals are calculated from the simultaneous recording at rapid paper speed of a high-frequency phonocardiogram, the indirect carotid arterial pulse wave, and the electrocardiogram (Fig. 230-3*A*). These measurements frequently are employed in the noninvasive evaluation of left ventricular function. The intervals measured include electromechanical systole (Q-S_2), the period from the onset of the QRS complex to the first high-frequency deflection of S_2; the left ventricular ejection time (LVET), which begins with the upstroke of the carotid arterial pulse and ends with the incisura; and the preejection period (PEP), the difference between the duration of left ventricular electromechanical systole and the LVET [PEP = (Q-S_2) − LVET]. Factors which influence the LVET include the heart rate, stroke volume, left ventricular afterload, the inotropic state of the myocardium, and the sex of the patient. Factors which influence the PEP include heart rate, aortic diastolic pressure, intraventricular conduction, and myocardial inotropic state. Systolic time intervals can be corrected both for heart rate and the patient's sex by using regression equations derived from data obtained in a large number of resting subjects without evidence of heart disease. However, the ratio of the PEP to the LVET (PEP/LVET) varies within narrow limits in normal subjects and need not be corrected for heart rate or sex (normal = 0.345 ± 0.036 SD). In the presence of left ventricular failure, the PEP lengthens (reflecting primarily a decreased rate of ventricular pressure development) and the LVET diminishes (reflecting a decreased stroke volume), while the duration of electromechanical systole remains unchanged. These altered relationships during left ventricular failure may be expressed as an increase in the PEP/LVET ratio. An inverse linear correlation has been demonstrated between the PEP/LVET ratio and the ejection fraction (stroke volume/end-diastolic volume), the latter being obtained by left ventricular cineangiography in patients with a variety of cardiac diseases.

The apexcardiogram, a graphic recording of the precordial movements, provides a reference signal that is of particular value in the analysis of diastolic events and heart sounds. The apexcardiogram is recorded using a bell-type, linear crystal microphone and a filter designed to pass only low frequencies (between 0.1 and 20 Hz). The O point on the apexcardiogram occurs at the end of isovolumetric left ventricular relaxation and at the onset of ventricular filling (Figs. 228-1 and 230-3*B*). Thus, it corresponds closely in time to the opening of the mitral valve and is useful as a reference point for identifying the opening snap in patients with mitral stenosis. Normally, a rapid-filling wave of about 0.08 sec follows the O point. In the presence of mitral stenosis this event is replaced by a slow-filling wave. On the other hand, in patients with myocardial failure, mitral regurgitation, or constrictive pericarditis, an exaggerated rapid-filling wave may terminate in a ventricular diastolic gallop or third heart sound (Chap. 228, Fig. 230-3*B*).

The A wave of the apexcardiogram is absent in patients with atrial fibrillation or mitral stenosis. This wave may be augmented and accompanied by a fourth heart sound in patients with left ventricular failure and in the presence of lesions, such as aortic stenosis, that produce left ventricular hypertrophy. In patients with hypertrophic subaortic stenosis, the apexcardiogram often exhibits a double systolic wave, or even a triple contour if the A wave is prominent as well.

ECHOCARDIOGRAPHY Reflected ultrasound is widely used as a noninvasive technique for evaluating a variety of cardiovascular disorders. With this technique, a ceramic compound such as barium titanate is excited by short, high-frequency (2.5 MHz) electrical signals to provide inaudible ultrasonic pulses. Reflection of the ultrasonic pulses occurs at an interface between two media of different densities, only those interfaces which are relatively perpendicular to the sound beam being sampled. The electromechanical transducer serves as both the emitter and the receiver of ultrasound at a repetition rate of 200 to 1,000 impulses per second. The echoes are amplified and displayed on an oscilloscope. For recording the echoes, a "time-motion" presentation commonly is used which plots distance from chest wall against elapsed time and displays moving structures as undulating lines. Photographs of the echo display can be taken directly from the face of the oscilloscope, or a strip chart recorder may be used. The electrocardiogram and time-distance markers usually are displayed on the oscilloscope as well and used as reference signals on the recorded tracing.

The ultrasound tracing from the normal anterior mitral leaflet exhibits a sharp upstroke representing the anterior movement of the leaflet toward the chest wall as the valve opens. The end of this excursion, the E point, represents the mitral cusp at its most anterior position (Fig. 230-4). This initial opening of the mitral valve in diastole is followed by partial closure of the valve, which is recorded as a downward deflection in the ultrasound tracing. The end-point of partial closure is the F point, and the speed of semiclosure of the mitral valve during diastole can be measured by the slope (ratio of distance to time) of the EF segment (normally 80 to 150 mm per sec). Subsequently, during left atrial contraction the mitral valve again opens further, and this event is recorded as another anterior movement, the A point in the echocardiogram. The valve leaflets then return to their intermediate position, and after the onset of ventricular systole B, the closed valve reaches its most posterior position at point C.

Echocardiographic recordings of the motion of the anterior leaflet of the mitral valve have been particularly valuable in evaluating the status of patients with mitral stenosis, idiopathic hypertrophic subaortic stenosis (Chap. 242), left atrial myxoma, or mitral regurgitation due to a prolapsing mitral leaflet; characteristic movements of the mitral valve leaflet can be observed with each of these lesions (Fig. 230-4). *Mitral stenosis* frequently causes a decrease in the amplitude of anterior leaflet movement (normal = over 20 mm), a reduction of the EF slope (less than 40 mm per sec), and a sustained anterior position during diastole (Fig. 230-4*A*). These phenomena result from the continued pressure gradient and sustained slow forward flow across the stenotic, domed valve, as well as from reduced mitral valve mobility consequent to thickening of the cusps and fusion of the commissures. Ultrasonic evaluation of mitral valve motion is particularly valuable in diagnosing patients with mitral stenosis in whom there is no audible diastolic murmur, despite evidence of severe pulmonary hypertension and a low cardiac output. It also is useful in distinguishing an Austin Flint murmur due to severe aortic regurgitation from the murmur of mitral stenosis.

Abnormal anterior movement of the mitral valve leaflet during systole occurs in patients with *idiopathic hypertrophic subaortic stenosis* (Fig. 230-4*B*). The abnormal systolic movement begins with the onset of ventricular ejection and reaches a peak with the initial peak in the arterial pulse. The characteristic abnormality often can be provoked by maneuvers which increase ventricular contractility or decrease left ventricular volume (e.g., amyl nitrite, Valsalva maneuver). The systolic anterior movement of the mitral valve is probably related to abnormal papillary muscle position and pulling forward of the anterior leaflet into the left ventricular outflow tract as the obstruction to ejection develops. There is also a moderately reduced EF slope, reflecting a reduced rate of left ventricular filling due to diminished ventricular compliance. This phenomenon may be seen in other forms of left ventricular hypertrophy as well.

Ultrasound is a useful technique in detecting left atrial tumors, particularly if the tumor advances partially into the mitral valve orifice at some time during the cardiac cycle. A *left atrial myxoma* may be recognized as an aggregation of multiple echoes behind the anterior leaflet (Fig. 230-4*C*), and there may be a diminished EF slope because of mitral valve obstruction.

Patients with a *prolapsing mitral valve*, in many of whom a midsystolic click and/or late systolic murmur is heard on auscultation, often have a characteristic echocardiogram. Normally, during diastole the posterior mitral valve leaflet echo moves in a direction exactly opposite to that of the anterior leaflet echo (away from the ultrasonic transducer), while during systole the two leaflets come together. In patients with billowing or prolapsing mitral valve leaflets, the echocardiogram may show displacement of the posterior mitral leaflet toward the left atrium during late systole (Fig. 230-4*D*), or

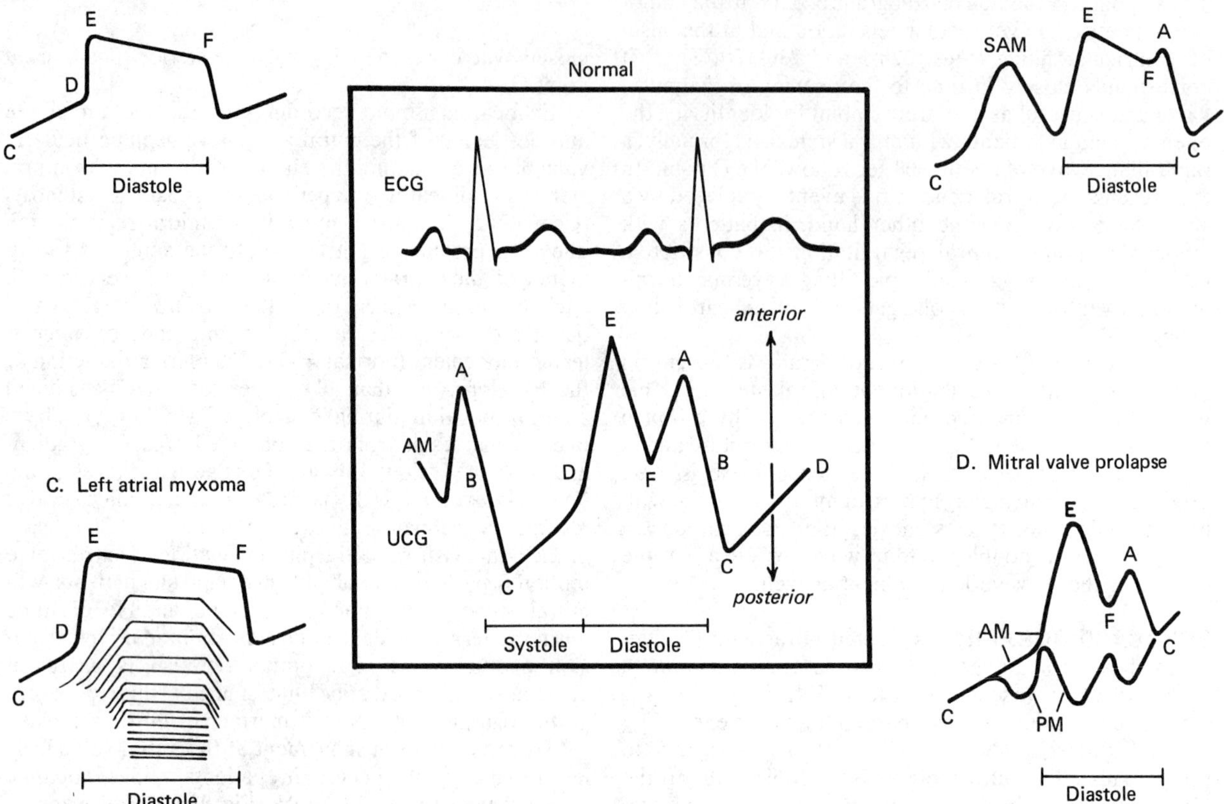

FIGURE 230-4

A schematic presentation of the normal ultrasound recording (UCG) of anterior mitral valve leaflet (AM) motion is shown in the center with the simultaneous ECG. Abnormal mitral echocardiograms which occur in (A) *mitral stenosis,* (B) *idiopathic hypertrophic subaortic stenosis,* (C) *left atrial myxoma, and* (D) *mitral valve prolapse are also depicted. In the UCG, the A point represents the end of anterior movement resulting from left atrial contraction, the C-D segment represents the closed position of AM during ventricular systole, and point E ends the anterior movement as the valve leaflet opens. The slope E-F results from posterior motion of the AM during rapid ventricular filling. In idiopathic hypertrophic subaortic stenosis, SAM represents systolic anterior movement. In the mitral valve prolapse echocardiogram PM is the posterior mitral valve leaflet (see text).*

persistence of the anterior leaflet in a posterior position during late systole.

Echocardiography also provides a simple, noninvasive method of reliably distinguishing *pericardial effusion* from a dilated heart (Chap. 241). In the presence of a pericardial effusion, the prominent posterior echo from the pericardial-pleural surface is stationary, while a second more anterior echo of lower amplitude originating from the posterior left ventricular wall moves with the heartbeat. The echo-free space between the two posterior echoes is roughly proportional to the amount of pericardial fluid present.

In addition to its widespread use for determining anterior mitral valve leaflet motion and for detecting pericardial effusion, reflected ultrasound has been employed to evaluate left atrial size, the presence or absence of left atrial thrombi, the size of the aorta, tricuspid valve motion, prosthetic mitral valve motion, and the pathologic anatomy in various congenital cardiac lesions. Recently, reflected ultrasound has been utilized for the semiquantitative evaluation of left ventricular function from estimates of ventricular end-diastolic volume, end-systolic volume, and the ejection fraction.

REFERENCES

FEIGENBAUM H: Clinical applications of echocardiography. Prog Cardiovasc Dis 14:531, 1972

KERBER RE et al: Echocardiographic patterns in patients with the syndrome of systolic click and late systolic murmur. N Engl J Med 284:691, 1971

KRISS JP et al: Radioisotope angiography. Wide scope of applicability in diagnosis and evaluation of therapy in diseases of the heart and great vessels. Circulation 43:792, 1971

LESTER RG: Radiological concepts in the evaluation of heart disease (I) & (II). Mod Concepts Cardiovasc Dis 37:113; 38:7, 1968

SIEGEL W: Non-invasive graphic methods, chap. 25 in *The Heart*, 3d ed., ed JW Hurst, New York: McGraw-Hill, 1974, pp. 386–402

TAVEL ME: *Clinical Phonocardiography and External Pulse Recording*, 2d ed., Chicago: Year Book, 1972

WEISSLER AM, GARRARD CL JR: Systolic time intervals in

cardiac disease (I) & (II). Mod Concepts Cardiovasc Dis 40:1; 40:5, 1971
WOLF SB et al: Diagnosis of atrial tumors by ultrasound. Circulation 39:615, 1969

231
CARDIAC CATHETERIZATION

JOHN ROSS, JR.

In 1929, Werner Forssman described the insertion of a catheter through his own arm vein into the right atrium and proposed that the procedure might prove useful for physiologic studies. A little more than a decade later, Andre Cournand and his associates introduced the modern era of cardiac catheterization in man by showing that it was possible to advance the catheter with safety further into the right ventricle and pulmonary artery and to perform hemodynamic studies by measuring intracardiac pressures and cardiac output. The technique of angiography also was developed rapidly in the period between 1930 and 1940, as relatively nontoxic opaque organic iodide media were discovered, and their intravascular injection provided definition of a number of congenital and acquired cardiovascular malformations. Since then, the development of techniques for catheterizing the left side of the heart and the coronary arteries, and for selective injection of contrast media into the cardiac chambers combined with exposure of high-speed x-ray motion pictures (cineangiography), has provided understanding of the dynamic anatomy of the heart, cardiac valves, and coronary arteries in the normal state and a variety of cardiac disorders. By permitting accurate anatomic and functional diagnoses of complex cardiac lesions, these procedures now have placed the selection of patients for surgical treatment on a firm, objective basis.

INDICATIONS FOR USE

There are several types of problems for which hemodynamic or angiographic investigations commonly are performed, although other specific indications and contraindications may exist in the individual patient. These broad areas may be summarized as follows:

1 In patients with acquired valvular heart disease, hemodynamic assessment and angiographic studies often are required to determine whether or not the nature and severity of a mechanical valvular defect render it amenable to surgical treatment. In particular, cardiac catheterization studies may be indicated when both the mitral and aortic valves are involved, or when associated tricuspid valve disease is suspected to be of significance.

2 In patients with congenital heart disease, hemodynamic studies and angiography usually are necessary to characterize the primary defect and to determine whether or not associated lesions are present.

3 In patients with chest pain of undetermined cause, angiographic visualization of the coronary arteries may be indicated, and in patients with known coronary heart disease such studies can determine whether or not operative treatment might be feasible.

4 In patients who have undergone cardiac operations, cardiac catheterization studies may be indicated to evaluate the success of the operation, particularly when residual symptoms are present. Such studies may reveal malfunction of a prosthetic valve or residual disease of the ventricular myocardium.

5 In patients with suspected myocardial disease, cardiac catheterization may be undertaken in an effort to exclude lesions potentially amenable to surgical treatment such as mitral regurgitation, coronary heart disease, constrictive pericarditis, and hypertrophic subaortic stenosis.

6 In patients with evidence of pulmonary hypertension, cardiac catheterization should be performed to search for such lesions as mitral stenosis, left-to-right shunts, multiple pulmonary emboli, or peripheral pulmonic stenosis.

COMPLICATIONS The increasingly widespread application of cardiac catheterization procedures has made it imperative to consider carefully the complications that may ensue. Although a retrospective analysis in 1953 of over 500 studies indicated that the mortality rate of catheterization of the right side of the heart was only 0.07 percent, the present tendency to perform more extensive and complex procedures and to study patients who are critically ill called attention to the need for a reappraisal of this risk. In a cooperative prospective study among 16 laboratories on the complications of cardiac catheterization reported in 1968, the incidence of important complications in patients of all ages (including such incidents as cardiac perforation, major arrhythmia, hemorrhage, serious hypotension, infection, vascular thrombosis, as well as death) was about 3 percent. However, when simple right-sided heart catheterization without angiography was performed, this incidence was much less, and lower complication rates also have been reported for coronary arteriography alone. The overall mortality rate, as well as the incidence of major complications, was highly dependent on the patient's age and diagnosis. For example, in critically ill infants studied under the age of 60 days, the mortality rate was 6 percent, whereas it was only 0.05 percent in patients between the ages of five and fourteen years, when most of the procedures were of an elective nature. The mortality rate increased to 0.3 percent in patients aged sixty and over. These figures should be considered whenever a decision concerning the advisability of performing specialized diagnostic procedures is made, and the risks of cardiac catheterization should be weighed carefully in relation to the potential benefits to be derived from an accurate anatomic and functional diagnosis.

GENERAL METHODS OF USE

CATHETERIZATION OF THE RIGHT SIDE OF THE HEART AND ANGIOGRAPHY Catheterization of the right side of the heart is now a well-standardized procedure. An antecubital or saphenous vein is isolated, local anesthesia is used, and a long, flexible radiopaque catheter is introduced. Alternatively, the percutaneous approach is employed, in which a needle is positioned in the vessel, a flexible wire passed through the needle, the needle removed, and a tapered-tip catheter advanced over the guide wire. Using fluoroscopic control, the cardiac catheter is guided into the right ventricle, the pulmonary artery, and the pulmonary arterial wedge position. Blood samples may then be obtained and intracardiac pressures and indicator-dilution curves determined sequentially within the chambers of the right side of the heart in the diagnosis of congenital and acquired lesions, as discussed subsequently in this chapter. The course of the cardiac catheter alone may provide a clue to the diagnosis of certain congenital malformations. The catheter may enter an anomalous pulmonary vein or left superior vena cava; it may directly traverse a patent ductus arteriosus or an atrial septal defect; and inability to cross the tricuspid valve may indicate tricuspid atresia.

Selective injection of radiopaque contrast media at various sites within the right side of the heart also may be performed during cardiac catheterization. Venous injections are particularly useful in detecting the thickened right atrial wall of constrictive pericarditis and for defining certain congenital lesions, such as Ebstein's malformation of the tricuspid valve and tricuspid atresia. Selective right ventriculography commonly is used in the delineation of congenital cardiac lesions such as pulmonic stenosis and tetralogy of Fallot. Injection into the pulmonary artery permits visualization of anomalies affecting the pulmonary venous drainage and may be useful in the detection of thrombi within the left atrium.

CATHETERIZATION OF THE LEFT SIDE OF THE HEART AND ANGIOGRAPHY Various methods for catheterization of the left side of the heart have been devised, and each has found application under certain circumstances. Currently, the retrograde arterial approach is used most widely for catheterization of the aorta and left ventricle. The catheter usually is inserted via the femoral artery using the percutaneous method, or through a small incision directly into the exposed brachial artery. The transseptal approach often is employed to gain access to the left atrium and left ventricle, particularly when disease of the mitral valve is suspected. With this method, a catheter is inserted via the right saphenous or femoral vein, and its tip is positioned in the right atrium. A long, curved needle is introduced through the catheter and employed to puncture the intact interatrial septum in the region of the fossa ovalis. Commonly, the catheter then is advanced over the needle into the left atrium and ventricle. Other methods of catheterization of the left side of the heart are used less commonly; e.g., with the anterior percutaneous approach a needle is introduced directly into the left ventricle in the region of the cardiac apex. This procedure sometimes is useful for measuring the left ventricular pressure in patients with valvular aortic stenosis.

Left ventriculography generally is employed for detecting and estimating the severity of mitral regurgitation and for delineating congenital and acquired lesions affecting the left ventricular outflow tract. Sites of subvalvular, valvular, or supravalvular aortic stenosis may be visualized, and the anatomy of the ventricular septum and mitral valve can be defined in evaluating such lesions as hypertrophic subaortic stenosis or the transposition complexes. In addition, analysis of the left ventricular cavity silhouette from the left ventriculogram is useful for assessing local disorders of left ventricular wall motion in patients with coronary heart disease; regions of absent or reduced contraction (akinesia or dyskinesia), and aneurysm formation resulting from previous myocardial infarction, can thereby be assessed as to severity. Finally, by calibrating the cineangiogram so that the area of the left ventricular cavity can be determined accurately at end diastole and end systole (often with the help of simultaneous biplane exposures), it becomes possible to employ the formula for an ellipse to derive the volume of the chamber. An increased left ventricular end-diastolic volume can be detected (upper limit of normal about 90 ml per m^2 of body surface area) and the total stroke volume of the left ventricle can be calculated; this value, when the forward stroke volume is calculated by an independent method (see below), can then be used to derive the amount of aortic or mitral regurgitation per beat. The ejection fraction, the ratio of end-systolic to end-diastolic volume which normally is approximately 0.66 (lower limit of normal 0.55), when reduced indicates the presence of depressed left ventricular contractility.

Aortography frequently is used for assessing the severity of aortic regurgitation (Fig. 231-1), for determining the size and location of aortic aneurysms, and for the visualization of less-common malformations such as sinus of Valsalva aneurysm. Injection into the left atrium has been used to study the movement of the mitral valve, as well as to detect thrombi within that chamber.

CORONARY ARTERIOGRAPHY Accurate visualization of the coronary vascular bed has assumed practical importance, particularly with the advent of successful surgical procedures for bypassing atherosclerotic lesions within the coronary arteries. In the past, techniques for injecting contrast medium into the ascending aorta or sinuses of Valsalva using retrograde arterial catheterization was partially successful in visualizing the coronary vascular bed, but selective injection of several milliliters of contrast medium directly into each coronary artery has gained general acceptance. Specially designed catheters are used: one type, which has a closed tip and multiple side holes, is inserted via brachial arteriotomy (Sones's technique); another type has a tapered tip and is advanced over a guide wire inserted percutaneously via the femoral artery. The latter catheters are specially curved to allow ready access to the right and left coronary orifices (Judkins's technique). Injections are made into the right and left coronary arteries with the patient placed in several oblique views while cineangiograms or large x-ray films are rapidly exposed, allowing visualization of obstructive lesions within the branches of the coronary vessels (Fig. 231-2), as well as detailed examination of any coronary collateral circulation that may have developed.

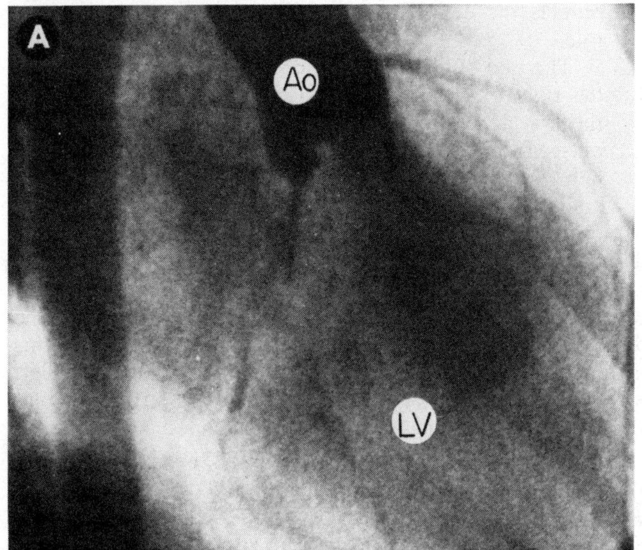

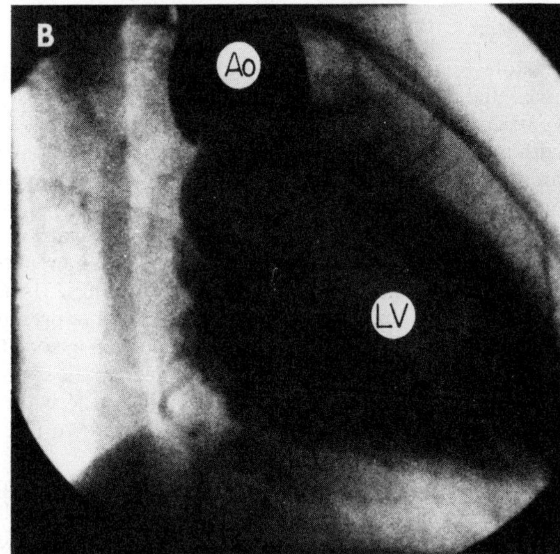

FIGURE 231-1
Cineangiograms with injection of contrast medium into the aortic root. Studies are performed in the right anterior oblique projection in a patient with mild aortic regurgitation in whom the LV is slightly opacified (A), *and in a patient with severe aortic regurgitation in whom the LV is densely opacified* (B). *Ao, aorta; LV, left ventricle.*

MEASUREMENT OF INTRAVASCULAR PRESSURES

The pressures within the great vessels and chambers of the heart ordinarily are measured by means of a catheter-transducer system. The tip of the cardiac catheter is in communication with the transducer by means of the fluid column contained within the catheter lumen. A number of factors, such as movement of the catheter and the presence of air bubbles, can influence the dynamic accuracy of these catheter-transducer systems, and miniature pressure gages attached directly to the tip of the cardiac catheter are finding increasing application. These microtransducers have frequency-response characteristics greatly superior to those of conventional catheter-transducer systems.

INTRACARDIAC PRESSURE PULSES The upper limits of normal for intracardiac pressures and certain other hemodynamic variables are shown in Table 231-1. In understanding the contours of the intracardiac pressure pulses, thorough knowledge of the temporal relations between the electrical and mechanical events of the cardiac cycle is important (see Fig. 231-3, page 1103, and 230-2). Although detailed study of the contours of the atrial pressure pulses has proved less reliable in predicting relative degrees of mitral valve stenosis and regurgitation than once was anticipated, a general understanding of the atrial pressure pulses is useful in the hemodynamic evaluation of a number of cardiac lesions.

The *A* wave in the right atrium normally is larger than the *V* wave, whereas in the left atrium the *V* wave is dominant (Table 231-1). Therefore, when the *V* wave in the right atrial pressure pulse exceeds the *A* wave, abnormal filling of the right atrium during ventricular systole, as occurs in tricuspid regurgitation or atrial septal defect, should be suspected. A characteristic right atrial pressure pulse also may be seen in the presence of tricuspid stenosis, the contour resembling that of mitral stenosis (see below), as well as in constrictive pericarditis, when an early diastolic "dip" and "plateau" elevation of pressure in mid- and late diastole occur. In many patients, the *mean* level of pressure in the left atrium is reflected with reasonable accuracy by the pulmonary artery wedge pressure (also sometimes termed the pulmonary "capillary" pressure), although the excursions of the wedge tracing often do not coincide with those measured directly within the left atrium. The characteristic contours of the left atrial pressure pulse in a normal subject and in patients with several forms of mitral valve disease are shown in Fig. 231-3. In the normal pressure pulse, or in the presence of mitral regurgitation without stenosis, there is a rapid fall in pressure during early diastole (the *Y* descent), and a slow rise in pressure occurs during late

TABLE 231-1
Normal hemodynamic values,* mm Hg

	A wave	*V wave*	*Mean*	*S/D*
Right atrium	7	5	5	
Left atrium	16	20	12	
Right ventricle	. .	. .	. .	30/5
Left ventricle	. .	. .	. .	145/12
Pulmonary artery	. .	. .	20	30/16
Pulmonary artery wedge	7	15	13	

Cardiac index = 2.5–3.6 L/min/m² body surface area.

AV O_2 difference: 4.0–5.2 ml/100 ml.

Pulmonary vascular resistance: 250 dynes/sec/cm^{-5} (3 resistance units).

* *The figures shown indicate the upper limits of pressure (mm Hg) and resistance in normal adult subjects. The values for the pressure waves, the mean pressures, and the systolic and diastolic pressures* (S/D) *are shown; in the ventricles,* D = *end-diastolic pressure. The ranges for cardiac index and arterial-mixed venous O_2 differences are shown.*

diastole (diastasis), reflecting equilibration between the atrial and ventricular pressures during this slow phase of ventricular filling (Fig. 231-3*A*). In contrast, in patients with mitral stenosis the *Y* descent is slow and prolonged; pressure in the left atrium continues to fall throughout diastole, and evidence of diastasis on the left atrial pressure pulse is absent because of the persistent atrioventricular pressure gradient (Fig. 231-3*B*). When mitral stenosis is present with normal sinus rhythm (Fig. 231-3*C*), the *A* wave is abnormally prominent, and a large pressure gradient accompanies atrial contraction (often associated with a loud presystolic murmur in such patients). In patients with pure mitral regurgitation, the *V* wave is prominent and the descending limb of this wave (the *Y* descent) is rapid (Fig. 231-3*D*).

The left ventricular end-diastolic pressure immediately precedes the onset of isometric contraction in the left ventricular pressure pulse. This pressure point therefore follows the *A* wave and precedes the *C* wave, and the coincident pressure point in time in the left atrial tracing is termed the *Z* point (Fig. 231-2*A*). The left ventricular end-diastolic pressure may be elevated in several situations: (1) in the presence of heart failure, (2) when the ventricle bears a high flow load (as in aortic regurgitation), (3) when the ventricle is hypertrophied and relatively noncompliant (restrictive myocardial disease), and (4) in the presence of constrictive pericarditis.

The systolic pressure in the left ventricle is elevated over that in the aorta when any of the various forms of aortic stenosis obstruct outflow. In patients with valvular aortic stenosis, the left ventricular pressure pulse resembles that of an isometric contraction, the contour being more symmetric and the pressure peak more delayed than normal (a similar phenomenon is observed in the right ventricle in patients with pulmonic stenosis). The characteristics of the peripheral arterial pressure tracing also may be distinctive in patients with different types of aortic stenosis. Thus, when valvular stenosis is present, a slow and delayed rise of the peripheral arterial pulse wave is seen, while in hypertrophic subaortic stenosis an initially sharp upstroke is followed first by a rapid decline in pressure and then by a secondary positive wave, which reflects the development of the obstruction during systole.

The rate of change, or slope, of the isometric phase of the right or left ventricular pressure pulse, often called the first derivative, or *dp/dt,* of the ventricular pressure pulse, frequently is used to characterize the contractile behavior of the ventricles. The *dp/dt* may be measured manually by determining the slope of the pressure rise, but more commonly it is recorded by means of an electronic circuit. The peak of this derivative tracing (maximum *dp/dt*) provides an index of the speed of contraction of the ventricle and therefore can help to define the level of the inotropic or contractile state of the heart. This measure tends to be under 1,200 mm Hg per sec in the left ventricles of patients with disease of the left ventricular myocardium, and it may be augmented strikingly by agents which improve the contractility of the heart, such as digitalis or catecholamines.

MEASUREMENT OF CARDIAC OUTPUT

The direct Fick and indicator-dilution methods presently are widely used in man for the determination of volume blood flow, or the cardiac output. In general, the equations used with these techniques are derived from the principle proposed by Adolf Fick which states that the rate at which a substance distributed in a fluid is delivered to an area by the moving fluid stream is equal to the product of the flow rate and the difference between the concentration of the substance at sites proximal and distal to the area. Thus,

$$q = F(C_a - C_v)$$

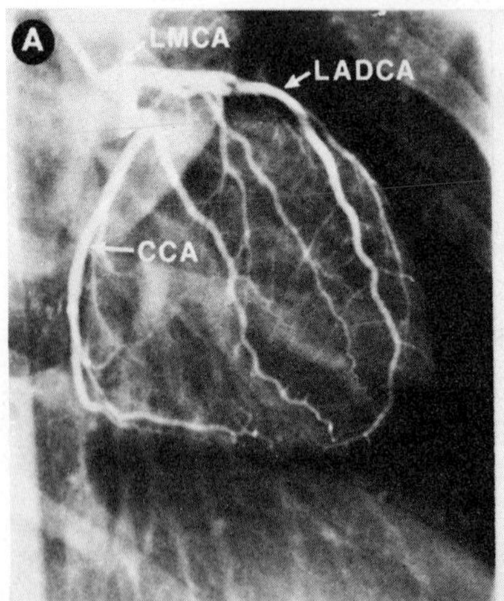

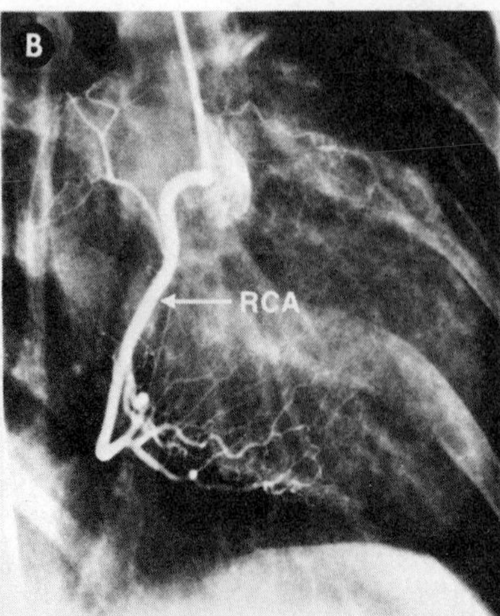

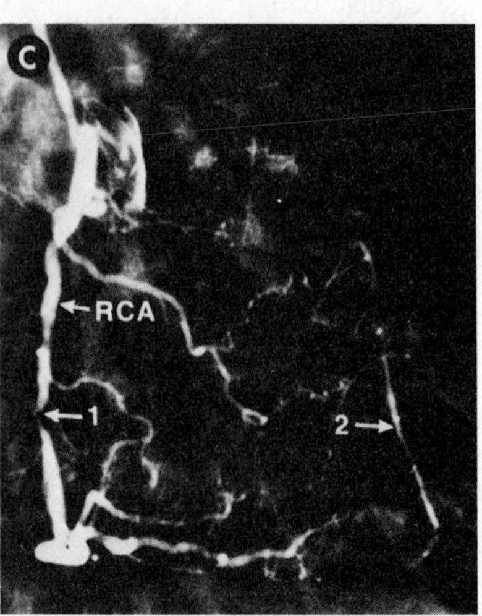

FIGURE 231-2
Selective coronary arteriograms obtained in the right anterior oblique projection. A *and* B *show a normal subject and* C *a patient with severe stenosis of the right coronary artery. LMCA, left main coronary artery; CCA, circumflex coronary artery; LADCA, left anterior descending coronary artery; RCA, right coronary artery. In* C, *arrow 1 indicates the area of narrowing in the right coronary artery, and arrow 2 shows retrograde filling of the anterior descending coronary artery via collateral vessels, indicating that a severe obstruction is present in that vessel as well. (Courtesy of Melvin P. Judkins, Loma Linda University, Loma Linda, Calif.)*

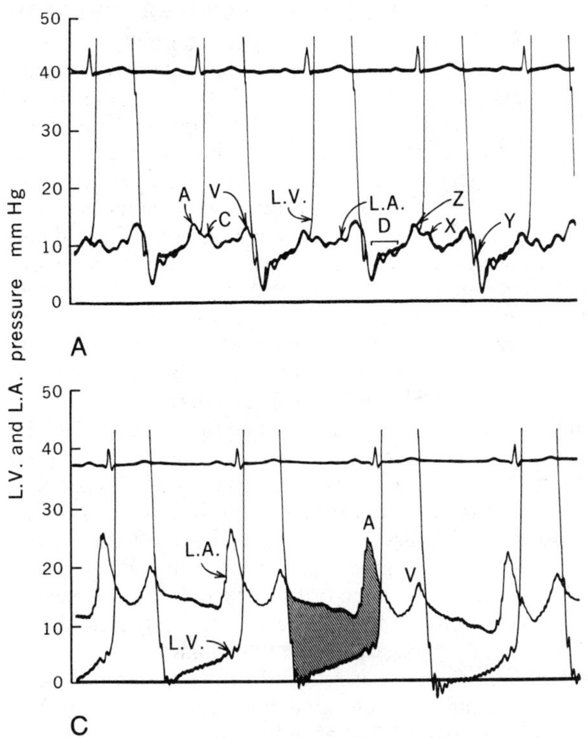

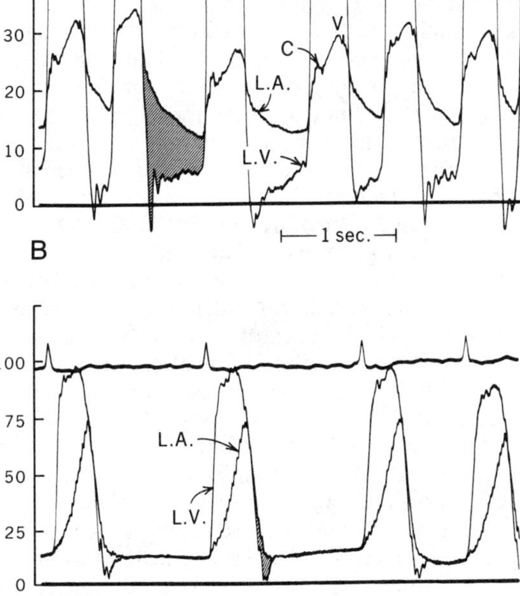

FIGURE 231-3

Simultaneously recorded left ventricular (LV) *and left atrial* (LA) *pressure tracings in a normal subject* (A) *and in patients with various forms of mitral valve disease* (B to D). *The tracings are recorded at high sensitivity (0 to 40 mm Hg), and therefore the top portion of the left ventricular pressure tracing is cut off. The electrocardiogram is recorded in the upper portion of each panel.*

A *In the normal heart, diastole is initiated by a rapid-filling wave, which is followed by a period of slow ventricular filling or diastasis (bracket D), in which atrial and ventricular pressure rise together slowly. This period of diastasis is followed by the atrial contraction wave (A), which precedes the onset of isometric contraction in the ventricle, the end-diastolic pressure, or the Z point in the left atrium. The C wave occurs during the phase of isometric ventricular contraction and is followed by the X descent. The V wave occurs during late systole and the downslope of the V wave, constituting the Y descent, occurs immediately after opening of the mitral valve.*

B *Tracings obtained in a patient with mitral stenosis and atrial fibrillation. The pressure gradient from left atrium to left ventricle during diastole is indicated by the diagonally shaded area. The A wave is absent, and the CV wave is prominent.*

C *Tracings from a patient with mitral stenosis and normal sinus rhythm. The pressure gradient is indicated by the diagonally shaded area. A large pressure gradient occurs at the time of atrial contraction. No pressure rise during the period of diastasis is evident in the left atrial pressure tracings of panels* B *and* C.

D *Tracings from a patient with isolated, severe mitral regurgitation and atrial fibrillation. The C wave is not evident, and the giant V wave in the left atrial pressure pulse is nearly 70 mm Hg. There is small pressure gradient during the phase of rapid ventricular filling, because of the large volume of antegrade flow across the mitral valve.*

where q = the quantity of substance delivered per unit time

F = the flow rate

C_a, C_v = the concentrations of the substance at proximal and distal sampling sites, respectively

(The same equation is applicable to the measurement of the removal rate, or clearance, of a substance.) When flow is the quantity to be derived, the equation is rearranged to

$$F = \frac{q}{C_a - C_v}$$

DIRECT FICK METHOD In this method for measuring the cardiac output it is assumed that at rest the oxygen uptake in the lungs is equal to that used by the tissues, and systemic flow, i.e., left ventricular output, therefore is equated with blood flow through the lungs. It is essential to this method that a sample of mixed venous blood be obtained, because blood samples in the venae cavae and the coronary sinus have widely differing oxygen concentrations, and therefore the venous blood sample generally is withdrawn from the right ventricular outflow tract or the pulmonary artery. In practice, arterial and venous blood samples ($C_a - C_v$) are obtained during the measurement of oxygen consumption, q, over a 3-min period by spirometry and subsequent chemical analysis of the expired gas. Flow F or cardiac output is then calculated. The subject must be in a steady state throughout the period of measurement to avoid transient changes in systemic blood flow or in the rate of ventilation that can negate the assumption that oxygen uptake in the lungs equals that taken up in the tissues.

INDICATOR-DILUTION METHOD This is a special application of Fick's principle. A variety of relatively nondiffusible indicators have been employed, the indicator substance being injected into the circulation and its concentration measured at a downstream sampling site by a suitable detector. For example, the dye indocyanine green is injected intravenously and blood is withdrawn from an artery at a constant rate through a calibrated densitometer, which provides direct measurement of the dye concentration. Generally, a single bolus of the indicator is injected rapidly and is thoroughly mixed in one of the vascular spaces such as a ventricular chamber; the concentration versus time curve then provides a measure of the rate at which indicator was washed out of the mixing site. Prior to recirculation of the indicator, the downslope of this curve is exponential, and therefore extrapolation of the curve using semilog paper permits the elimination of recirculated indicator. The mean concentration $\bar{c}$ of the dye is determined from the area of this corrected curve and its duration. The rate of blood flow F then is directly related to the quantity of indicator injected i and is inversely related to the mean concentration of the indicator $\bar{c}$ and the duration of the curve t (in seconds) by the formula $F = 60i/\bar{c}t$. A simple example will serve to illustrate this principle: if 8 mg of dye is injected and a mean concentration of 2 mg per liter is recorded, and if the indicator takes 60 sec to pass the sampling site, then the flow is 4 liters per min.

MEASUREMENT OF PULMONARY VASCULAR RESISTANCE In calculating the resistance offered by a vascular bed, blood flow is assumed to be laminar and the general resistance formula then can be employed. This formula, in simplified form which omits consideration of vessel length and blood viscosity, states that resistance is directly proportional to the pressure drop or gradient across the bed and inversely proportional to the rate of blood flow. This ratio of mean pressure gradient to volume flow is expressed in dynes per sec per cm^{-5}, the mean pressure gradient across the pulmonary bed being obtained by subtracting the mean left atrial or pulmonary artery wedge pressure from the mean pulmonary artery pressure.[1] The *resistance unit* (i.e., the pressure gradient in millimeters of mercury divided by the cardiac output in liters per minute and expressed in arbitrary units) also is commonly employed as an index of arteriolar resistance (Table 231-1). Estimation of the pulmonary vascular resistance, which normally is about 15 percent of that in the systemic vascular bed, is of importance in patients with congenital heart disease and circulatory shunts, as well as in certain forms of acquired cardiac and pulmonary diseases. Its calculation provides a useful means of interpreting the level of pulmonary arterial pressure relative to pulmonary blood flow, high pressure and high flow obviously bearing a different connotation than high pressure and low flow.

[1]*Resistance* = $\dfrac{\text{PA (mm Hg)} - \text{LA (mm Hg)} \times 1{,}332 \text{ dynes/cm}^2}{\text{cardiac output (ml/sec)}}$

where PA *and* LA *= mean pulmonary artery and left atrial pressures. 1 mm Hg = 1.36 cm water; 1 cm water = 980 dynes per cm² force.*

VALVE ORIFICE SIZE AND VALVULAR REGURGITATION When the cardiac output is normal, the severity of a stenotic valve lesion may be estimated from the magnitude of the pressure gradient across the valve. When the cardiac output is elevated or reduced, however, reliance on the pressure gradient alone may lead to an erroneous estimate of the degree of mechanical obstruction. In addition, it is of importance to consider the heart rate in assessing the significance of a pressure gradient. When the heart rate is rapid, systole occupies a disproportionate amount of time in each cardiac cycle, diastole filling time is limited, and a large pressure gradient across the atrioventricular valve may exist in the face of relatively mild stenosis. The application of the hydraulic formula devised by Gorlin and Gorlin to the calculation of valve orifice size has proved helpful in analyzing the degree of valve stenosis in these situations. In simplest terms, this formula states that the area of a short-bore orifice is directly proportional to the rate of blood flow across the orifice and inversely proportional to the square root of the pressure gradient. For example, if the flow rate across a narrowed valve orifice of fixed size doubles, as may occur when the cardiac output increases during exertion, the pressure gradient will quadruple. Conversely, when the flow rate is reduced, as in patients with heart failure, a small pressure gradient may exist in the presence of a severe degree of valve stenosis. This relationship differs from the general resistance equation discussed above and reflects the fact that the kinetic energy losses across a stenotic valve are high, a large pressure head being expended in developing a rapid flow velocity across the narrowed orifice.

It should be pointed out that use of the orifice formula is not valid when significant valvular regurgitation is present and forward cardiac output alone is measured, since an unknown volume of blood is regurgitated and recrosses the valve during the cardiac cycle. Application of the formula under these circumstances leads to an underestimation of the valve orifice area, since forward flow across the valve is underestimated. The characteristics of the indicator-dilution curve are helpful in the detection of valvular regurgitation, the peak concentration being reduced and the washout slope prolonged (Fig. 231-4*B*), and angiography provides a definitive diagnosis.

DIAGNOSIS OF CIRCULATORY SHUNTS

When a communication exists between the left and the right sides of the heart, and when pulmonary vascular resistance is lower than that in the systemic vascular bed, a left-to-right shunt of oxygenated blood will occur. Conversely, when the resistance in the pulmonary bed is higher than that in the systemic circulation, or an obstruction such as pulmonic stenosis exists distal to an intracardiac communication, a right-to-left shunt of venous blood may occur.

Many types of indicators have been employed in the diagnosis and quantification of circulatory shunts. The indicator may be the oxygen in room air, blood samples being withdrawn and analyzed for oxygen manometrically or by an oximeter. Foreign, inert gases such as hydrogen or krypton 85 may be employed; these, like oxygen, are "injected" into the pulmonary circulation by inhalation and sampled from the right side of the heart. They may be measured by a catheter-tip sensor (hydrogen) or by withdrawal of blood samples for analysis. In obtaining indicator-dilution curves, the substance most commonly injected is indocyanine green dye, detected by withdrawing blood through a densitometer.

The techniques used for localizing and quantifying shunts at cardiac catheterization may be divided into two basic categories: (1) Those methods in which an indicator is delivered distal to the site at which blood is sampled (the so-called upstream sampling method), e.g., indicator is injected into the pulmonary artery or is inhaled to enter the pulmonary veins and left side of the heart. Blood samples are then obtained upstream in the right side of the heart and analyzed for concentration of the indicator. (2) Those methods in which an indicator is delivered proximal to the sampling site (the so-called downstream sampling method), in which most frequently an indicator-dilution curve is obtained by intracardiac dye injection with sampling from a peripheral artery. This approach permits detection of right-to-left as well as left-to-right shunts. Exposure of cineangiograms with selective injections of contrast medium also permits localization of the site of a shunt.

UPSTREAM SAMPLING METHOD Blood samples are withdrawn in serial fashion from the pulmonary artery, right ventricle, right atrium, and venae cavae, the indicator being introduced downstream (in the case of oxygen into the lungs). This approach permits localization of the site of a left-to-right shunt. With the oxygen sampling method, a step-up of 1.5 ml per 100 ml from the venae cavae to the right atrium, or of 1.0 ml per 100 ml from the right atrium to the right ventricle, or from the right ventricle to the pulmonary artery, is considered to be evidence of a left-to-right shunt. The use of a foreign gas improves the sensitivity of this approach, even a small left-to-right shunt being readily detected by appropriate sampling within the right side of the heart using a catheter-tip hydrogen electrode, for example. Upstream sampling has also been applied by injecting an indicator distally into a peripheral pulmonary artery and sampling proximally to detect early recirculation of indicator through a left-to-right shunt.

For determination of the size of a left-to-right shunt, samples of venous blood proximal to the shunt and samples from the pulmonary artery and a systemic artery are obtained in close time sequence. The oxygen uptake at the lungs is measured simultaneously, or estimated, and the pulmonary and systemic blood flow rates (and hence the magnitude of the left-to-right shunt relative to systemic flow) can be calculated using Fick's equations. Generally a pulmonary to systemic flow ratio of 1.5:1 or greater is considered to indicate a left-to-right shunt of substantial magnitude.

DOWNSTREAM SAMPLING METHOD A needle is placed into a systemic artery and a time-concentration curve is recorded following upstream injection of the indicator. This technique is particularly useful for localizing the site of a right-to-left shunt. For example, when a right-to-left shunt exists at the ventricular level, an injec-

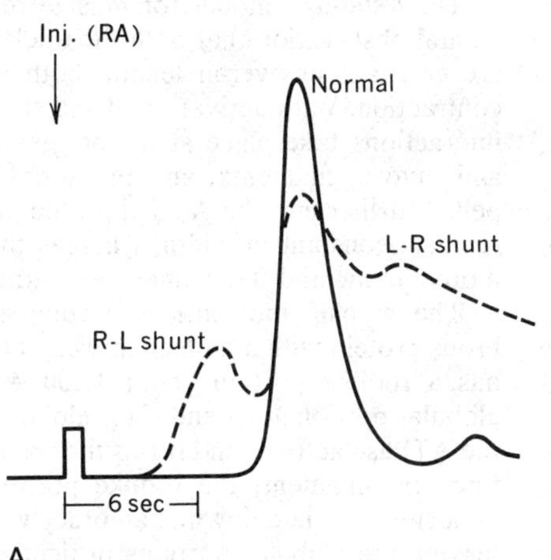

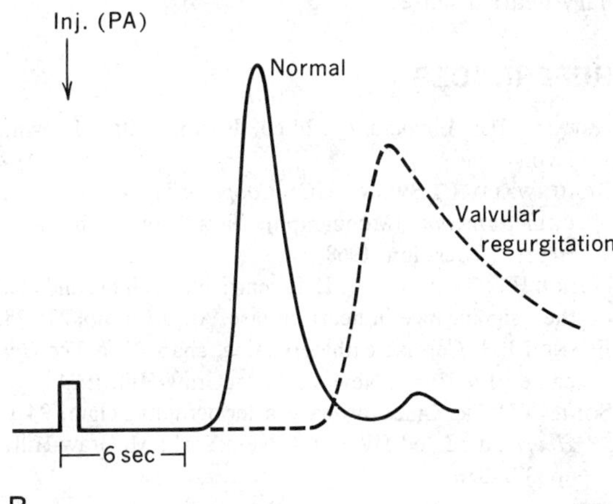

FIGURE 231-4

Diagrammatic representation of indicator-dilution curves in various forms of cardiac disease. The downstream sampling method is employed.

A *The time of injection (Inj.) of an indicator, such as cardiogreen dye, is indicated by the arrow and by the square wave response on the recorded tracing. With right atrial (RA) injection and sampling at a peripheral artery, the normal appearance time is about 8 sec, and the normal contour of the indicator-dilution curve is represented by the solid line. In a patient with a right-to-left (R-L) shunt at the atrial, ventricular, or pulmonary arterial levels, early appearance time of the dye is indicated by the dashed line. In a patient with a left-to-right (L-R) shunt, the appearance time need not be altered, but there is a reduced peak concentration of dye, and a break on the downslope, indicating early recirculation of the indicator.*

B *The indicator-dilution curve in a normal patient with injection into the pulmonary artery (Inj. PA) shows an appearance time of about 6 sec. In a patient with severe regurgitation at the mitral or aortic valves, the appearance time is prolonged and the delayed clearance of the indicator from the left side of the heart results in a prolonged downslope of the indicator-dilution curve (dashed line).*

tion into the right ventricle and at all sites proximal to the right ventricle will result in an early appearance time of dye that has immediately traversed the defect (Fig. 231-4*A*). However, an injection into the pulmonary artery, distal to the right-to-left shunt, shows a normal appearance time. A left-to-right shunt also may be detected, but not localized, by injection of indicator into the right side of the heart using peripheral arterial sampling. The indicator-dilution curve will show a reduced peak concentration of dye and a break on the downslope when compared with a normal indicator-dilution curve (Fig. 231-4*A*). This contour occurs because a portion of the indicator traverses the left-to-right shunt during its initial passage to the left side of the heart, recirculates rapidly through the right side of the heart and lungs, and reappears at the peripheral artery before the downslope of the primary curve has been completely inscribed.

OTHER SPECIAL MEASUREMENT TECHNIQUES A number of technical advances are improving cardiac catheterization methods. For example, special catheters for recording the intracardiac electrocardiogram have made it possible to record potentials from the right atrium, His bundle, and ventricle and are used in the diagnosis of arrhythmias and heart block. Also available are special catheters for measurement of phasic blood flow velocity within the great vessels, catheter-tip pressure transducers, and other special catheters for characterizing and localizing murmurs and heart sounds by intracardiac phonocardiography.

STRESS TESTING Exercise in the supine position, using a bicycle ergometer may be performed during cardiac catheterization and can provide important information concerning the ability of the heart to respond to this mode of stress. For example, certain patients with heart disease may have a normal cardiac output and normal intracardiac pressures at rest but exhibit a markedly impaired response of the cardiac output, or an abnormal elevation of ventricular diastolic pressure, during exercise. Infusion of a pressor agent also has been employed to test the cardiac response to stress, and electrical pacing of the heart to induce mild tachycardia may induce ischemic changes in the electrocardiogram in patients with coronary heart disease.

REFERENCES

Abrams HL: *Angiography*, 2d ed., Boston: Little, Brown, 1971, 2 vols

Braunwald E, Swan HJC: *Cooperative Study on Cardiac Catheterization* (Monograph), New York: The American Heart Association, 1968

Dodge HT, Baxley WA: Left ventricular volume and mass and their significance in heart disease. Am J Cardiol 23:528, 1969

Franch RH: Cardiac catheterization, chap. 23 in *The Heart*, 3d ed., ed JW Hurst, New York: McGraw-Hill, 1974

Sones FM Jr: Cine coronary arteriography, chap. 24 in *The Heart*, 3d ed., ed JW Hurst, New York: McGraw-Hill, 1974, pp. 377–386

232 DISORDERS OF MYOCARDIAL FUNCTION

EUGENE BRAUNWALD
JOHN ROSS, JR.
EDMUND H. SONNENBLICK

CELLULAR BASIS OF CARDIAC CONTRACTION

The myocardium is composed of individual striated muscle cells (fibers), normally 10 to 15 μm in diameter and 30 to 60 μm in length. Under the light microscope, each fiber is seen to contain multiple cross-banded strands (myofibrils), which run the length of the fiber and are composed of a serially repeating structure, the sarcomere. The remainder of the cytoplasm, lying between the myofibrils, contains other cell constituents, such as the single centrally located nucleus, numerous mitochondria, and intracellular membrane systems.

The sarcomere, the fundamental structural and functional unit of contraction, is delimited by two adjacent dark lines, the Z lines (Fig. 232-1). The distance between Z lines varies with the degree of contraction or stretch of the muscle and ranges between 1.5 and 2.2 μm. Within the confines of the sarcomere, alternating light and dark bands are seen, giving the myocardial fibers their striated appearance under the light microscope. At the center of the sarcomere is a broad dark band of constant width (1.5 μm), the A band, which is flanked by two lighter bands, the I bands, which are of variable width. The sarcomere of heart muscle, like that of skeletal muscle, is made up of two sets of myofilaments. Thicker filaments, composed principally of the protein myosin, traverse and are limited to the A band. They are about 100 A in diameter, with tapered ends, and measure 1.5 to 1.6 μm in length. Thinner filaments composed primarily of actin, course from the Z line through the I band into the A band. They are approximately 50 A in diameter and 1.0 μm in length. Thus, there is overlapping of thick and thin filaments only within the A band, while the I band contains only thin filaments (Fig. 232-1). On electromicroscopy, bridges may be seen to extend between the thick and thin filaments within the confines of the A band.

The "sliding" model for muscle rests on the fundamental observation that both the thick and thin filaments are constant in overall length, both at rest and during contraction. With activation of the sarcomere, repetitive interactions take place at the bridges between the actin and myosin filaments, and the actin filaments are propelled further into the A band. In the process, the A band remains constant in width, whereas the I bands become more narrow and the Z lines move toward one another.

The myosin molecule is a complex, asymmetric fibrous protein with a molecular weight of about 500,000; it has a rodlike portion about 1,500 A in length with a globular portion at its end. This globular portion contains the ATPase activity and forms the bridges. In forming the thick myofilament, the rodlike portions of the myosin molecules are laid down in an orderly, polarized manner, leaving the globular portions projecting outward so that they can interact with actin to generate force and shorten-

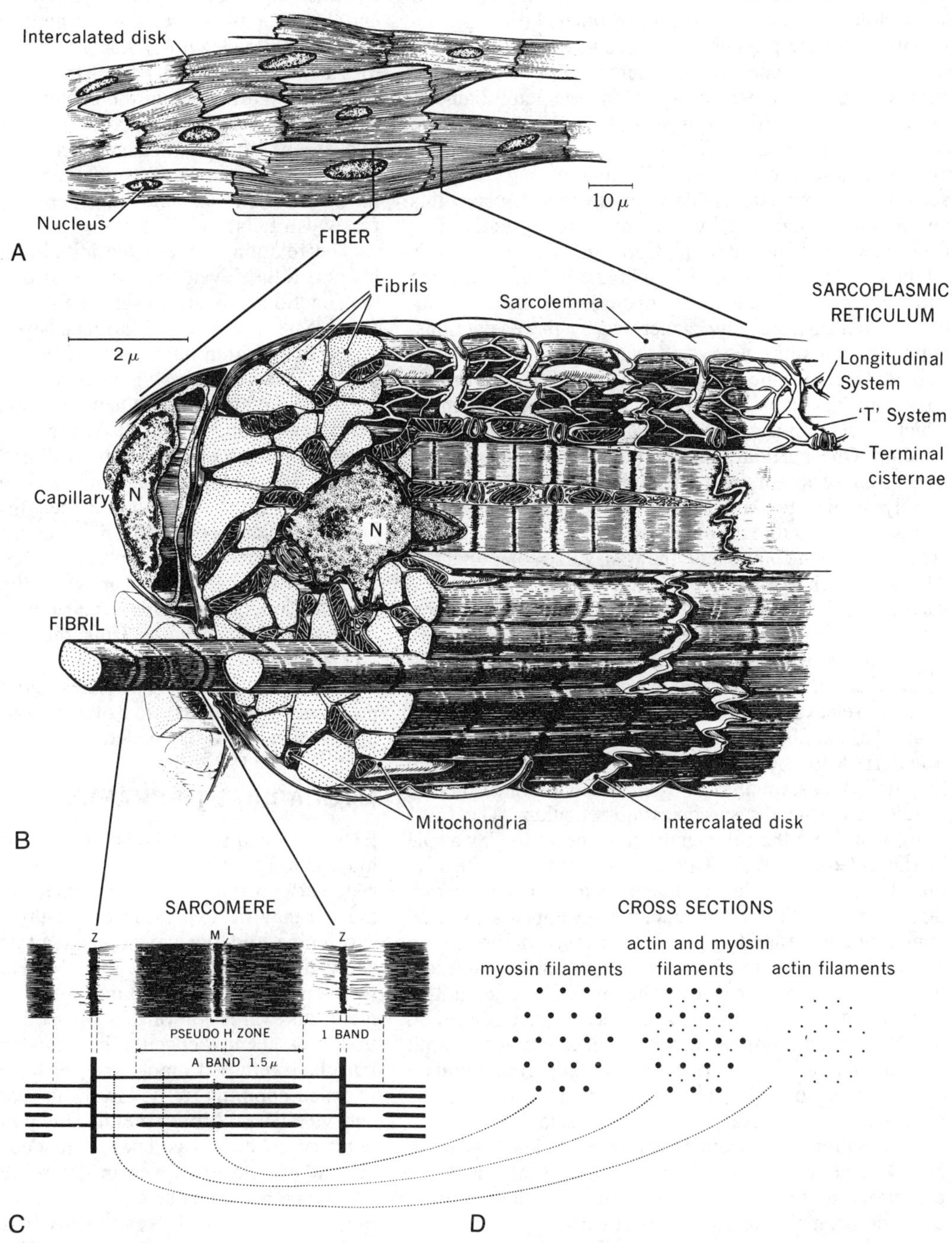

FIGURE 232-1

Microscopic structure of heart muscle. A *Myocardium as seen under the light microscope. Branching of fibers is evident. Each fiber, or cell, contains a centrally located nucleus.*

B *Myocardial cell, reconstructed from electron micrographs. Each cell is composed of multiple parallel fibrils. Each fibril is composed of serially connected sarcomeres (N, nucleus).*

C *Sarcomere from a myofibril, with diagrammatic representation of myofilaments. Thick filaments (1.5 μm long, composed of myosin) form the A band, and thin filaments (1 μm long, composed primarily of actin) extend from the Z line through the I band into the A band. The overlapping of thick and thin filaments is seen only in the A band.*

D *Cross sections of the sarcomere indicate the specific lattice arrangements of the myofilaments. In the center of the sarcomere only the thick, or myosin, filaments arranged in a hexagonal array are seen. In the distal portions of the A band, both thick and thin, or actin, filaments are found, with each thick filament surrounded by six thin filaments. In the I band only thin filaments are present. (From Braunwald et al,* Mechanisms of Contraction of the Normal and Failing Heart, *Boston: Little, Brown, 1968.)*

ing. Actin has a molecular weight of 55,000. The thin filament is composed of a double helix of two chains of actin molecules wound about each other, intimately associated with the protein tropomyosin, which appears to form the central core of this filament. Another protein, *troponin*, is located periodically along the actin filament. In contrast to myosin, actin has no intrinsic enzymatic activity, but it has the ability to combine reversibly with myosin in the presence of ATP and of Mg^{++}, which activates the myosin ATPase. In relaxed muscle this interaction is inhibited by troponin. During activation, Ca^{++} becomes attached to the troponin, and removes this inhibition. As a result, ATP is split and linkages between actin and myosin filaments are made and broken cyclically. Mechanical forces are generated by these reactions, with resultant shortening of the sarcomere.

The sarcoplasmic reticulum, a complex network of anastomosing, membrane-lined intracellular channels, which invests the myofibrils, has two distinct components. One portion, the longitudinal component, consists of a series of interconnecting membrane tubules closely applied to the surfaces of the individual sarcomeres; it has no direct continuity with the outside of the cell. The second component, the transverse component or "T" system, is formed by tubelike invaginations of the sarcolemma, which extend into the myocardial fiber, along the Z lines, i.e., the ends of the sarcomeres.

When an excitatory stimulus results in electrical depolarization of the cell membrane, Ca^{++} bound to the latter is released. When the depolarization reaches the interior of the fiber via the transverse tubular system, it is transferred to the adjacent terminal cisternae of the longitudinal system and Ca^{++} which is contained therein is released from the sarcoplasmic reticulum. The Ca^{++} movement from the cell membrane appears to play a role in this release as well. The Ca^{++} diffuses into the myofibril and activates the myofilaments to produce contraction. The sarcoplasmic reticulum then appears to reaccumulate Ca^{++}, thereby lowering its concentration in the myofibril to a level that inhibits the actin-myosin interaction which is responsible for contraction and in this manner leads to relaxation. Thus, the cell membrane and the sarcoplasmic reticulum, with their ability to transmit an action potential, to release and then reaccumulate Ca^{++}, appear to play a fundamental role in the rhythmic contraction and relaxation of heart muscle.

The ATP formed from substrate oxidation appears to be the source of energy for almost all of the work performed by the myocardial cell. Some of this energy is expended in maintenance chemical work (e.g., in modifying substrates, producing glycogen, synthesizing lipids and proteins, maintaining the integrity of the membranes), although in the normally functioning heart the major fraction of energy is expended in the mechanical work of contraction. The high-energy phosphate stores in ATP are in equilibrium with those in the form of creatine phosphate.

In all forms of striated muscle, including cardiac muscle, the force of contraction depends on initial muscle length. The sarcomere length associated with the most forceful contraction is 2.2 μm. It is at this length that the two sets of myofilaments of the sarcomere are most ideally situated to provide the greatest area for their interaction. In support of the sliding-filament hypothesis, force development diminishes in direct proportion to the decrease in the overlap between thick and thin filaments, and the resultant decrease in the number of reactive sites. At a sarcomere length of 3.65 μm, developed tension falls to zero, and it is at this point that the thin filaments are entirely withdrawn from the A band. Similarly, when the sarcomeres are shorter than 2.0 μm, the thin filaments bypass one another, producing a double overlap of the thin filaments, a less-than-ideal arrangement for interaction between thick and thin filaments (Fig. 232-2), and force also falls.

The relation between the initial length of the muscle fibers and the developed force is of prime importance for the function of heart muscle. This forms the basis of the Frank-Starling relation (Starling's law of the heart), which states that, within limits, an augmentation of initial volume of the ventricle, which is a function of the initial length of the muscle, results in an increase in the force of ventricular contraction. It has been shown for heart muscle that sarcomere length is directly proportional to muscle length along the ascending limb of the length–active tension curve. As muscle length decreases to the point at which developed tension approaches zero and at which sarcomere length approaches 1.5 μm, the I bands at first narrow, then disappear while the A band remains constant in length. At this latter point, the Z line abuts on the edges of the A band. Thus, the sarcomere length–active tension curve forms the ultrastructural basis of Starling's law of the heart. These points concerning the mechanism of contraction of the heart muscle fiber are also applicable to the skeletal muscle fiber.

MYOCARDIAL MECHANICS

Extremely helpful methods for examining the behavior of muscle were provided by the skeletal muscle physiologists early in this century. The mechanical activity of all muscle may be expressed externally in only two ways: shortening and the development of tension. A. V. Hill showed in skeletal muscle that the velocity of shortening is inversely related to the magnitude of tension development, an expression of the so-called force-velocity relation, now acknowledged to be a fundamental property of muscle. Expressed simply, the greater the load the muscle is called upon to lift, the lower the velocity of shortening and vice versa. More recently, the concept of the force-velocity relation has been extended from skeletal to cardiac muscle. However, in this respect there is a basic difference between skeletal and cardiac muscle. Skeletal muscle has a single, essentially fixed, force-velocity curve; i.e., at any given muscle length, force and velocity are always related to each other in the same manner. The contractile activity of skeletal muscle is increased by the recruitment of additional muscle fibers, i.e., motor units, and by increasing the frequency of nerve impulses, while the contractility of each individual fiber remains constant. Although resting length also influences the characteristics of contraction, this variable remains essentially fixed *in vivo*. In contrast, the number of cardiac cells activated remains constant during each contraction. However, the contractile activity of the myocardium may be readily altered under physiologic conditions by changes in resting fiber length and by changes in the inotropic state, i.e., the contractility, both of which shift the myocardial force-velocity curve.

Variations in myocardial contractile activity may be expressed as displacements of the force-velocity curve. However, there are two fundamental ways in which the force-velocity curve can be shifted. Figure 232-3*A* shows a family of force-velocity curves obtained from an isolated cardiac muscle; each curve was obtained at a different preload, i.e., with a different degree of stretch on the muscle. Note that changing the preload alters the intercept of the force-velocity curve on the horizontal axis; i.e., it increases the isometric force developed by the muscle. However, within limits, these alterations in preload do not appear to alter the intrinsic velocity of shortening, since all the curves extrapolate to the same intercept on the vertical axis. Thus, a change in initial length of heart muscle shifts the force-velocity curve primarily by altering the total force which can be developed by the muscle, as illustrated by the isometric length-tension curve, shown in the insert of Fig. 232-3*A*.

This type of shift in the force-velocity curve may be contrasted with that obtained when a positive inotropic agent, such as norepinephrine or digitalis, is added to the muscle while the initial length is held constant (Fig. 232-3, right). These agents not only increase the force which the muscle is capable of lifting, i.e., the intercept of the force-velocity curve on the horizontal axis, therefore shifting the isometric length-tension curve upward, but also increase the velocity of shortening of the unloaded muscle, i.e., the extrapolated intercept on the vertical axis.

It has been postulated that an increase in initial muscle length brings about an increase in the number of force-generating sites operating effectively without any alteration in the qualitative character of the cyclic process at these contractile sites. Such a change would be anticipated from a more advantageous overlap of interdigitating contractile filaments within the sarcomere. On the other hand, a change in the inotropic state, characterized by an increase in the velocity of shortening of the unloaded muscle, could result from an increase in the rate of cyclic force-generating processes at the contractile

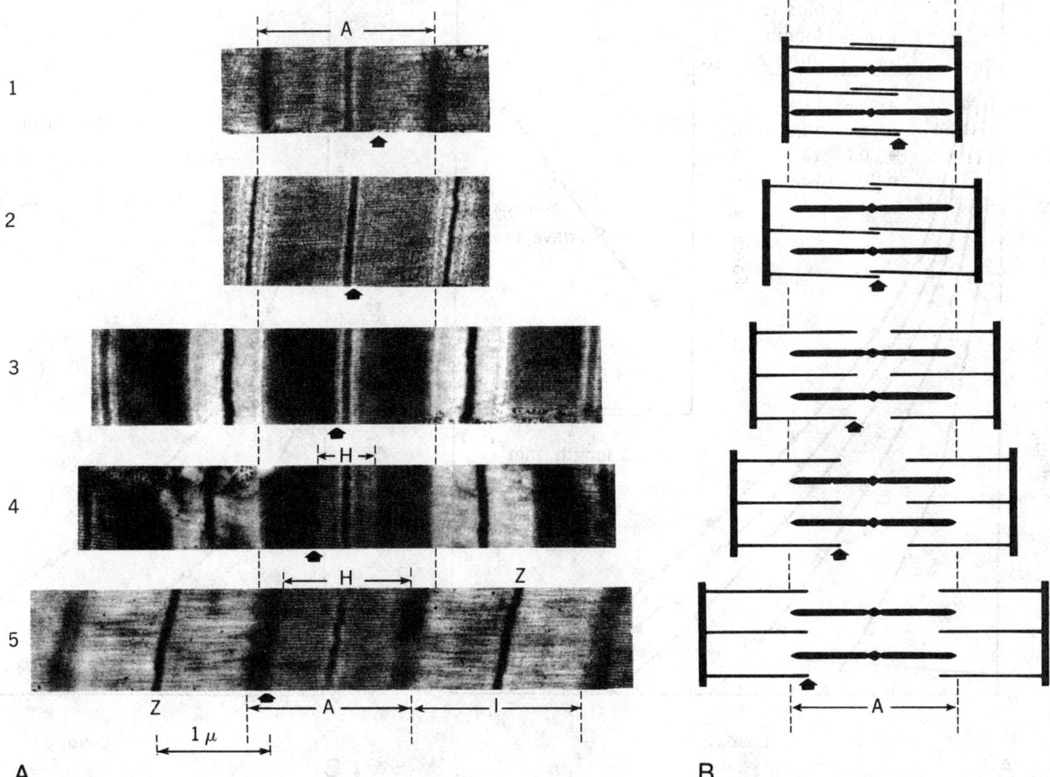

FIGURE 232-2
Relation between sarcomere length and band patterns in skeletal muscle (frog sartorius). A *Band patterns as seen electromicroscopically.* B *Disposition of the thick and thin filaments that create band patterns. The vertical arrows in both panels denote the ends of the thin filaments that insert at the Z line at the left. Line 3 represents the sarcomere at the apex of the length-tension curve, i.e., at L_{max}. In lines 1 and 2, sarcomere length has been progressively decreased, whereas in 4 and 5 it has been progressively elongated. Throughout, the A band remains constant in width. The placement of filaments to provide for maximum overlap is shown in* B*(3). Line 1 shows the sarcomere pattern in the contracted muscle; the I band has disappeared, and a secondary dark band has been formed at the center of the sarcomere, termed the C contraction band, which is due to the passage of thin filaments through this area as in* B*(1). In* A *(4 and 5), an expanding H zone has appeared, owing to the withdrawal of the thin filaments from the A band, as shown diagrammatically in* B (4 and 5). *(From Braunwald et al,* Mechanisms of Contraction of the Normal and Failing Heart, *Boston: Little, Brown 1968)*

sites, without a change in the number of these sites, or alternatively from a greater number of sites that are activated. Increased contractility appears to be related to an increased availability of Ca^{++} within the cell, but whether this alters the quantity or quality of interactions is unsettled.

CONTRACTION OF THE INTACT VENTRICLE

Analysis of the heart as a pump has classically centered upon the relation between the filling pressure, or diastolic volume, of the ventricle (length of the muscle fibers) and its stroke volume (the Frank-Starling relation). It was shown clearly in the heart-lung preparation that the stroke volume is a function of diastolic fiber length, and that the failing heart delivers a smaller-than-normal stroke volume from a normal or elevated end-diastolic volume. Later, the concept of measuring stroke work (the product of stroke volume and mean aortic pressure) over a range of mean atrial or ventricular end-diastolic pressures, using one of these pressures as an index of diastolic volume, was expanded by Sarnoff and his collaborators. They concluded that this relation between the mean atrial or the ventricular end-diastolic pressure and the stroke work of the corresponding ventricle (the ventricular function curve) provided a definition of the level of the contractile, or inotropic, state of the ventricle. Significant increases in the level of ventricular contractility were accompanied by shifts of the ventricular function curve upwards and to the left, while depression of contractility was identified by downward and rightward displacement of this relation (Fig. 232-4).

Considerable effort also has been directed toward a study of the responses of the intact, unanesthetized animal, and it has been observed that during the adrenergic stimulation of the myocardium accompanying a stress such as exercise, relatively little change in ventricular end-diastolic size occurs, while minute cardiac output, aortic flow velocity, and the rate of ventricular pressure development are augmented. Thus, reflex and humorally mediated changes in myocardial contractility, heart rate, venous return, and peripheral vascular resistance may overshadow the effects of the intrinsic Frank-Starling mechanism, i.e., the relation between end-diastolic pressure or volume and stroke work.

The important influence of the neurotransmitter substance norepinephrine on the mechanical and electrical properties of the myocardium has long been recognized. Direct stimulation of the stellate ganglions has been shown to elevate the ventricular function curve, as a consequence of the release of norepinephrine from sym-

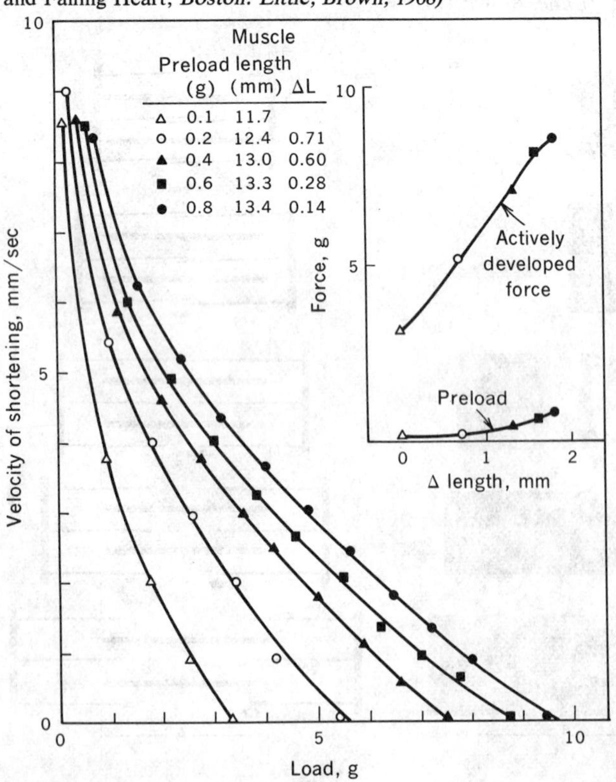

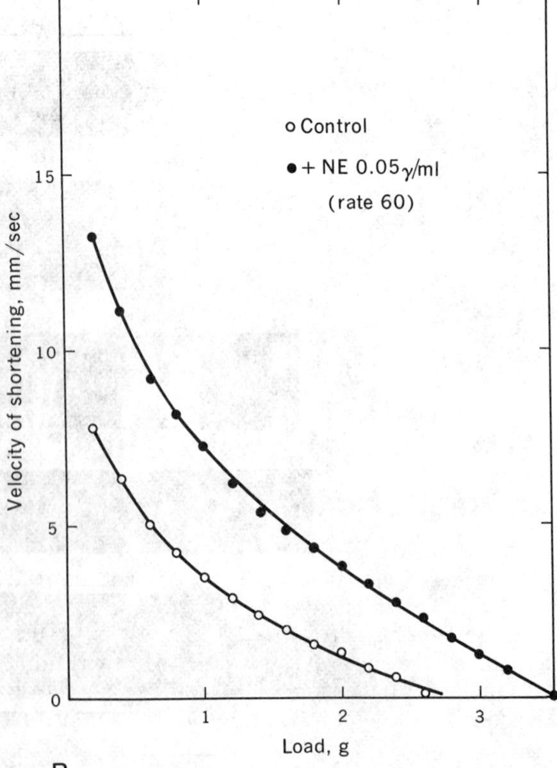

FIGURE 232-3

A *Effects of increasing initial muscle length on the force-velocity relation of the cat papillary muscle. Initial velocity of shortening has been plotted as a function of load for five different muscle lengths. The maximum velocity of shortening (V_{max}) is essentially unchanged, whereas the maximum force of contraction (P_o) is augmented. The insert shows the places along the length-tension curves at which these force-velocity curves were determined.* B *Effects of norepinephrine on the force-velocity relation of the cat papillary muscle. Both V_{max} and P_o have been increased. (From Braunwald et al,* Mechanisms of Contraction of Normal and Failing Heart, *Boston: Little, Brown, 1968)*

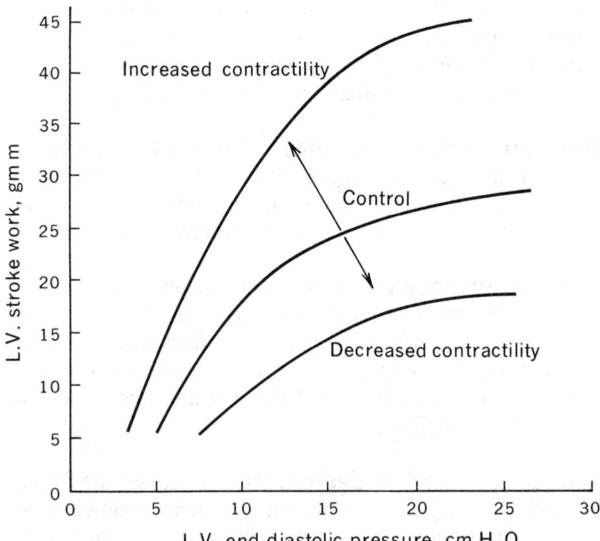

FIGURE 232-4
Diagrammatic representation of ventricular function curves obtained under control conditions, during the administration of a positive inotropic agent (increased contractility), and during a negative inotropic state (decreased contractility). LV, left ventricular. (From Braunwald et al, Mechanisms of Contraction of Normal and Failing Heart, *Boston: Little, Brown, 1968)*

pathetic nerve endings in the heart. In the intact animal, these adrenergic effects are evidenced by tachycardia, a reduction in cardiac dimensions, increased velocity of ejection, and an enhanced rate of tension development. Cerebral ischemia also appears to cause a profound increase in ventricular performance.

Surgically denervated hearts *in situ*, or isolated papillary muscles taken from such hearts, do not exhibit depression of their intrinsic inotropic state despite depletion of the norepinephrine stores within the sympathetic nerve endings of the muscle. The surgically or pharmacologically denervated heart of the intact organism also appears capable of meeting many of the demands of muscular exercise. However, the mechanisms by which the denervated heart increases its output differ from those of the intact animal. Thus, tachycardia is less marked, and the stroke volume and cardiac output rise as a consequence of elevation of ventricular end-diastolic volume. In all these respects the activity of the heart muscle fiber differs from the activity of skeletal muscle fiber, the latter being totally dependent on its nerve supply and unable to contract effectively when denervated.

CONTROL OF CARDIAC PERFORMANCE AND OUTPUT

The extent of shortening of mammalian heart muscle and, therefore, the stroke volume of the intact ventricle are, in the final analysis, determined by four influences: (1) the length of the muscle at the start of contraction, i.e., the preload; (2) the inotropic state of the muscle, i.e., the position of its force-velocity-length relation or function curve; (3) the tension which the muscle is called upon to develop during contraction, i.e., the afterload; and (4) the heart rate, which determines the cardiac output at any stroke volume as long as ventricular filling is maintained.

VENTRICULAR END-DIASTOLIC VOLUME (PRELOAD) At any level of its inotropic state, the performance of the myocardium is influenced profoundly by ventricular end-diastolic fiber length and therefore by diastolic ventricular volume. The following are the major determinants of ventricular end-diastolic volume in the intact organism (see also Fig. 232-5):

1 *Total blood volume.* When it is depleted, as in acute hemorrhage, ventricular performance, as reflected in ventricular stroke work, must decline.
2 *Distribution of blood volume.* At any given total blood volume, the ventricular end-diastolic volume is influenced by the distribution of blood between the intra- and extrathoracic compartments. This distribution in turn is influenced by:
   a *Body position.* Gravitational forces tend to pool blood in dependent portions.
   b *Intrathoracic pressure.* Normally, mean intrathoracic pressure is negative, a factor which acts to increase thoracic blood volume and ventricular end-diastolic volume, particularly during inspiration. Elevation of intrathoracic pressure, as occurs in a tension pneumothorax, during the Valsalva maneuver, or in prolonged bouts of coughing, tends to impede venous return to the heart, diminish intrathoracic blood volume, and ultimately reduce ventricular work.
   c *Intrapericardial pressure.* When elevated, as in pericardial effusion, there is interference with cardiac filling, and the resultant reduction in ventricular diastolic volume lowers ventricular work.
   d *Venous tone.* The veins are not a simple system of passive conduits between the systemic capillary bed and the right atrium. Instead, the smooth muscle in venous walls responds to a variety of neural and humoral stimuli. Venoconstriction occurs during muscular exercise, deep respiration, fright, or marked hypotension, tending to diminish extrathoracic blood volume and to augment intrathoracic blood volume.
   e *The pumping action of skeletal muscle.* During exercise the contracting skeletal muscles tend to squeeze blood out of the veins and, with the aid of the venous valves, to displace it centrally, thereby increasing intrathoracic blood volume, ventricular end-diastolic volume, and ventricular work.
3 *Atrial contraction.* Vigorous, appropriately timed atrial contraction augments ventricular filling and end-diastolic volume. The atrial contribution to ventricular filling is of particular importance in patients with ventricular hypertrophy, in whom the loss of atrial systole (as in atrial fibrillation) tends to reduce ventricular end-diastolic pressure and volume, ultimately lowering myocardial performance.

INOTROPIC STATE (MYOCARDIAL CONTRACTILITY) A number of factors determine the level of ventricular performance at any given ventricular end-diastolic volume, i.e., the position of the ventricular function curve (Fig. 232-6). These influences may be considered to operate by modifying myocardial force-velocity-length relations.

Sympathetic nerve activity The quantity of norepinephrine released by sympathetic nerve endings in the heart is, under ordinary circumstances, dependent on the sympathetic nerve impulse traffic, and variations in the frequency of nerve impulses modify the quantity of norepinephrine released and acting upon the beta-adrenergic receptors in the myocardium. This mechanism is the most important one which acutely modifies the position of the force-velocity and ventricular function curves under physiologic conditions.

Circulating catecholamines The adrenal medulla and other sympathetic ganglions outside the heart, when properly stimulated by sympathetic nerve impulses, release catecholamines, which augment the inotropic state of the myocardium.

The force-frequency relation The position of the myocardial force-velocity curve is influenced by the rate and rhythm of cardiac contraction; e.g., ventricular extrasystoles result in post-extrasystolic potentiation. Sustained improvement in myocardial contractility also can be induced with a bigeminal rhythm or by paired electrical stimulation.

Exogenously administered inotropic agents The cardiac glycosides, isoproterenol and other sympathomimetic agents, calcium, caffeine, theophylline, and their derivatives, all improve the myocardial force-velocity relation (Chap. 235) and therefore may be used therapeutically to augment ventricular performance at any given ventricular end-diastolic volume.

Physiologic depressants Included among these are severe myocardial hypoxia, hypercapnea, and acidosis. Acting either singly or in combination, these influences exert a depressant effect on the myocardial force-velocity curve and lower the level of left ventricular work at any given ventricular end-diastolic volume.

Pharmacologic depressants These include quinidine, procain amide, and other local anesthetics (Chap. 235), barbiturates, as well as many other drugs which exert an effect analogous to that of the physiologic depressants.

Loss of ventricular substance When a portion of ventricular myocardium becomes nonfunctional or necrotic, as occurs in myocardial infarction, total ventricular performance at any given level of end-diastolic volume is depressed, even if the remaining myocardium functions normally.

Intrinsic myocardial depression Although the fundamental mechanisms responsible for depression of myocardial contractility in heart failure still remain to be elucidated, it is now apparent that in this condition the inotropic state of each unit of myocardium is depressed and that the level of ventricular performance at any ventricular end-diastolic volume is thereby lowered.

VENTRICULAR AFTERLOAD The volume of blood ejected by the ventricle during each contraction is ultimately a function of the extent of ventricular fiber shortening during systole. As in isolated cardiac muscle, the velocity and extent of shortening at any given level of diastolic fiber length and myocardial inotropic state is inversely related to the afterload imposed on the muscle. The afterload on the intact heart is dependent on the level of aortic pressure, but it may be defined as the tension or stress developed in the wall of the ventricle during ejection. Therefore, the afterload on the ventricular muscle fibers also is dependent on the size of the heart, according to the Laplace principle, which indicates that the tension of the myocardial fiber is a function of the

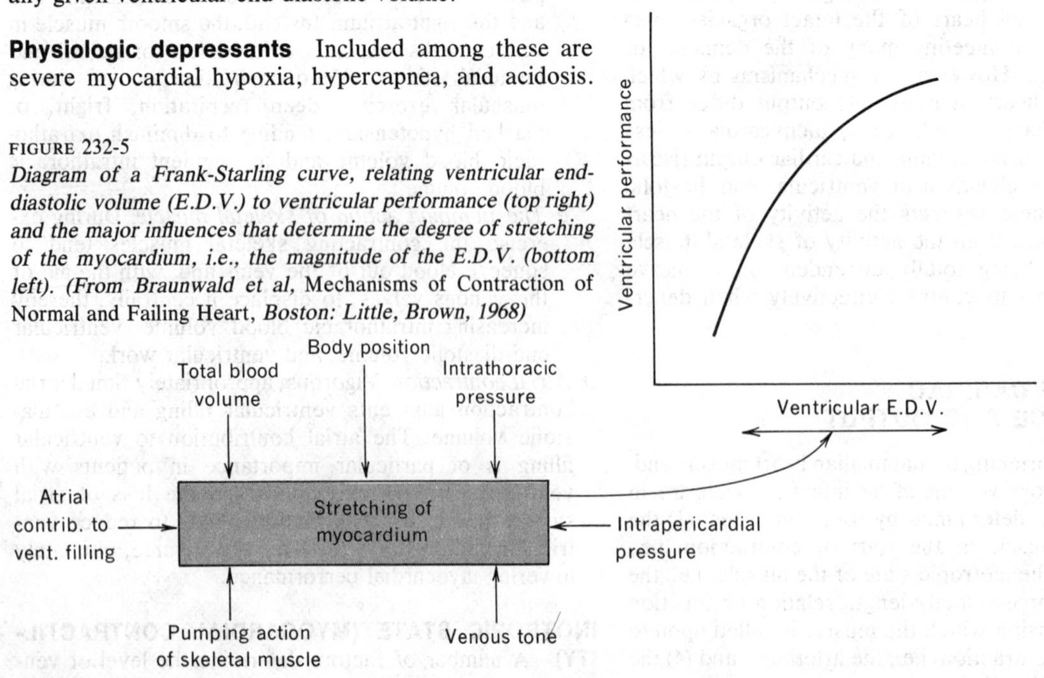

FIGURE 232-5
Diagram of a Frank-Starling curve, relating ventricular end-diastolic volume (E.D.V.) to ventricular performance (top right) and the major influences that determine the degree of stretching of the myocardium, i.e., the magnitude of the E.D.V. (bottom left). (From Braunwald et al, Mechanisms of Contraction of Normal and Failing Heart, *Boston: Little, Brown, 1968)*

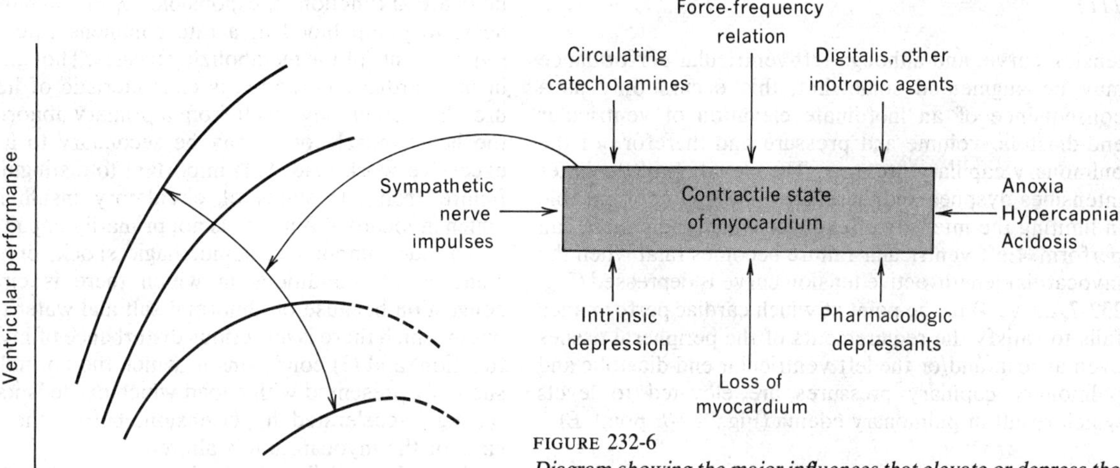

FIGURE 232-6

Diagram showing the major influences that elevate or depress the inotropic state of the myocardium (top right), and the manner in which alterations in the inotropic state of the myocardium affect the level of ventricular performance at any given level of ventricular end-diastolic volume (bottom left). (From Braunwald et al, Mechanisms of Contraction of Normal and Failing Heart, *Boston: Little, Brown, 1968)*

product of intracavitary ventricular pressure and the ventricular radius. Thus, at the same level of aortic pressure, the afterload faced by an enlarged left ventricle is higher than that encountered by a ventricle of normal size. The aortic pressure, in turn, is influenced largely by the peripheral vascular resistance, the physical characteristics of the arterial tree, and the volume of blood it contains at the onset of ejection. At any given ventricular end-diastolic volume and level of the myocardial state, the left ventricular stroke volume is a function of the afterload.

All the influences acting on cardiac performance enumerated above interact in a complex fashion to maintain cardiac output at a level appropriate to the requirements of the metabolizing tissues, and in a normal person interference with one of these mechanisms may not influence the cardiac output. For example, a moderate reduction of blood volume or the loss of the atrial contribution to ventricular contraction can ordinarily be sustained without a reduction in cardiac output. Presumably other factors, such as an increase in the frequency of sympathetic nerve impulses reaching the heart, will, in the normal person, augment contractility and sustain output under these circumstances. Mechanisms are also available which prevent elevation of the cardiac output when there is no physiologic demand for augmented flow. For example, expansion of blood volume or augmentation of myocardial contractility by means of cardiac glycosides does not increase the cardiac output in normal man. Thus, in analyzing the effect of an intervention on cardiac output, it is important to recognize that the inotropic state of the myocardium is not the factor that limits the volume of blood ejected by the heart in the normal individual and that an improvement of myocardial contractility by a drug such as digitalis, should not be expected to elevate the output in a normal subject. On the other hand, in the presence of congestive heart failure, the cardiac output usually is limited by the depressed contractile state of the myocardium, and a positive inotropic influence would be expected to raise cardiac output.

EXERCISE The hemodynamic changes which normally occur during muscular exercise are complex (Fig. 232-7). The hyperventilation of exercise, the pumping action of the exercising muscles, and the venoconstriction which occur, all tend to augment ventricular filling. Simultaneously, the increase in the sympathetic nerve impulses to the myocardium, the increased concentration of circulating catecholamines, and the tachycardia which occur during exercise, all result in an augmentation of the contractile state of the myocardium (Fig. 232-7, curves 1 to 2), and an elevation of stroke volume, with no change or even a decrease of end-diastolic pressure and volume (Fig. 232-7, points *A* to *B*). Vasodilatation occurs in the exercising muscles, thus reducing the impedance to ventricular emptying. This ultimately allows the achievement of a greatly elevated cardiac output during exercise, at an arterial pressure which does not differ greatly from that occurring in the resting state.

In heart failure, the fundamental abnormality resides in depressions of the myocardial force-velocity relationship and of the length-active tension curve, reflecting reductions in the contractile state of the myocardium (Fig. 232-7, curves 1 to 3). In many instances, cardiac output and external ventricular performance at rest are within normal limits but are maintained at these levels only by an elevated end-diastolic fiber length and ventricular end-diastolic volume, i.e., through the operation of the Frank-Starling mechanism (Fig. 232-7, points *A* to *D*). The elevations of left ventricular end-diastolic volume and pressure are associated with similar changes in the pulmonary capillary pressure, contributing to the dyspnea experienced by patients with heart failure. The normal improvement of contractility which is mediated by augmented sympathetic activity during exercise is attenuated or even prevented by norepinephrine depletion which occurs in heart failure (Fig. 232-7, curves 3 and 3′). The factors which tend to augment ventricular filling during exercise in the normal subject push the failing myocardium even farther along its flattened length–active tension curve, and although left ventricular performance may be augmented somewhat, this occurs only as a consequence of an inordinate elevation of ventricular end-diastolic volume and pressure and therefore of the pulmonary capillary pressure. The elevation of the latter intensifies dyspnea and therefore plays an important role in limiting the intensity of exercise which the patient can perform. Left ventricular failure becomes fatal when the myocardial length–active tension curve is depressed (Fig. 232-7, curve 4) to the point at which cardiac performance fails to satisfy the requirements of the peripheral tissues even at rest, and/or the left ventricular end-diastolic and pulmonary capillary pressures are elevated to levels which result in pulmonary edema (Fig. 232-7, point *E*).

THE FAILING HEART

Though heart failure may be readily described as a clinical syndrome, characterized by well-known symptoms and physical signs, a precise physiologic or biochemical definition is far more difficult. However, from the clinical point of view, heart failure may be considered to be the disease state in which an abnormality of myocardial function is responsible for the inability of the heart to pump blood at a rate commensurate with the requirements of the metabolizing tissues. Though a defect in myocardial contraction is characteristic of heart failure, this defect may result from a primary abnormality in the heart muscle or it may be secondary to a chronic excessive work load. It is important to distinguish heart failure from (1) states of circulatory insufficiency in which myocardial function is not primarily impaired, such as cardiac tamponade, hemorrhagic shock, or tricuspid stenosis, (2) conditions in which there is circulatory congestion because of abnormal salt and water retention but in which there is no serious disturbance of myocardial function, and (3) conditions in which the normal heart is suddenly presented with a load which exceeds its capacity, e.g., accelerated hypertension, before the intrinsic state of the myocardium is altered.

FIGURE 232-7
Diagram showing the interrelations between influences on ventricular end-diastolic volume (E.D.V.) through stretching of the myocardium and the contractile state of the myocardium. Levels of ventricular E.D.V. associated with filling pressures that result in dyspnea and pulmonary edema are shown on the abscissa. Levels of ventricular performance required when the subject is at rest, while walking, and during maximal activity are designated on the ordinate. The dotted lines are the descending limbs of the ventricular-performance curves, which are rarely seen during life but which show the level of ventricular performance if end-diastolic volume could be elevated to very high levels. (From Braunwald et al, Mechanisms of Contraction of Normal and Failing Heart, *Boston: Little, Brown, 1968)*

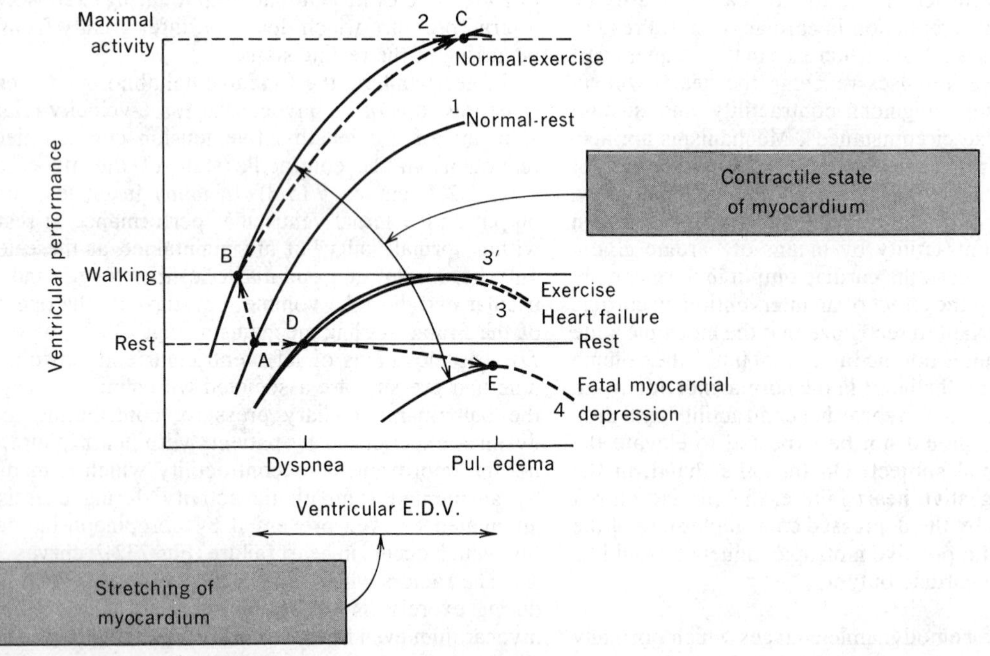

Acute heart failure in the intact canine heart, studied *in situ* or in the heart-lung preparation, is characterized by a depression of ventricular stroke volume or stroke work at any given level of left ventricular end-diastolic volume or filling pressure. Further, as diastolic volume is augmented in the failing heart, an abnormally small increase or no change in stroke volume occurs. Thus, in order to maintain stroke volume at a normal level, the heart dilates and the Frank-Starling mechanism therefore might be considered one of the first lines of defense called upon to maintain cardiac output when myocardial contractility declines. An increase in the end-diastolic volume of the ventricle permits the ejection of a larger stroke volume, even when the extent of shortening of individual muscle fibers remains constant. The fact that in the failing heart the stroke volume is unchanged or is actually diminished when end-diastolic volume is augmented, clearly indicates that a decrease in the relative degree of muscle fiber shortening must have occurred. Thus, an important mechanical defect which can be delineated in acute heart failure is a decrease in the extent of shortening of cardiac muscle fibers.

The intrinsic contractile state of myocardium removed

from normal, hypertrophied, and failing animal hearts has been evaluated, and both ventricular hypertrophy and heart failure were shown to reduce the maximum isometric tension and velocity of shortening to subnormal levels; the changes were more marked in the myocardium of animals in which heart failure had been present than in those with hypertrophy alone. However, ventricular hypertrophy, in the absence of heart failure, also appears to be associated with a depression of the inotropic state per unit of myocardium, although the absolute increase of total muscle mass maintains cardiac compensation. Papillary muscles removed from the left ventricles of patients with heart failure have also shown a depression of the maximum degree of active tension which they can develop. Electronmicroscopic analysis of failing cat papillary muscles fixed at the apices of the length–active tension curves revealed sarcomere lengths averaging 2.2 μm. Thus, the abnormalities of contractility do not appear to be produced by an alteration in the overlap of filaments within the sarcomere.

The failing ventricle may still eject a normal or nearly normal stroke volume despite considerable depression of function, when its end-diastolic volume increases, i.e., through the operation of the Frank-Starling mechanism. As outlined above, an increase in the initial volume of the ventricle is associated with stretching of the sarcomere, a process which augments the number of sites at which the actin and myosin filaments can interact. Furthermore, the development of ventricular hypertrophy may be considered to provide additional contractile units, and thereby constitutes an important compensatory mechanism when the intrinsic myocardial inotropic state is depressed.

Several techniques are available for defining impaired ventricular contractility in intact man. With the patient at rest, the cardiac output and stroke volume may be depressed, but not uncommonly these variables are within normal limits. A more sensitive index is the ejection fraction, i.e., the ratio of stroke volume to end-diastolic volume, which may be estimated by biplane angiography (Chap. 231), and which is frequently depressed in heart failure even when the stroke volume itself is normal. An even more sensitive method for detecting impaired ventricular performance is based on the measurement of the circulatory changes occurring during stresses such as exercise or increased afterload. Thus, left ventricular performance may be estimated accurately by measuring the left ventricular end-diastolic pressure, cardiac output, and total body O_2 consumption at rest and during exercise. In normal persons, the cardiac output rises by more than 500 ml per min for each 100 ml increase in minute O_2 consumption. The left ventricular end-diastolic pressure at rest is less than 12 mm Hg and rises slightly, remains unchanged, or decreases slightly during exercise, while stroke volume usually rises. The failing left ventricle, on the other hand, is characterized by an elevation of end-diastolic pressure during exercise, which reaches a value exceeding 12 mm Hg, accompanied by either no change or a fall in stroke volume. Various degrees of impairment intermediate between the normal response and that of the failing left ventricle during the stress of exercise also have been described.

Another method consists of the measurement of stroke volume, arterial pressure, and ventricular end-diastolic pressure before and after ventricular afterload is increased by means of an infusion of a pressor agent such as angiotensin. Though the normal left ventricle responds to this stress by increasing its stroke work and end-diastolic pressure, in the failing left ventricle the end-diastolic pressure rises markedly, but stroke work either remains constant or actually declines. Thus, as in the acutely failing experimental preparation, the failing human left ventricle appears to exhibit a depression of the relation between end-diastolic pressure and the stroke volume and stroke work which can be achieved. The potential value of stressing the left ventricle in some manner is emphasized by the fact that the basal values for left ventricular end-diastolic pressure, cardiac index, and ventricular stroke work may be in the same range in patients with depressed ventricular function as in normal persons. The response to these stresses may prove useful not only in the detection of the impairment of myocardial function, but also in expressing the severity of this impairment quantitatively.

The performance of the left ventricle in man may also be characterized by examining the instantaneous myocardial force-velocity relations and the extent of shortening during individual cardiac cycles. Angiocardiographic studies and analyses of the rate of change of intraventricular pressure (dp/dt) during isovolumetric contraction have shown that depressions in the velocity of myocardial fiber shortening and of tension development exist in human heart failure. Further evidence for the decreases in the velocity of myocardial fiber shortening is provided by the finding of a reduced mean systolic ejection rate in patients with heart failure and a failure of the mean systolic ejection rate to rise normally during muscular exercise. Noninvasive, graphic techniques are of increasing value in the clinical assessment of myocardial function (Chap. 230).

CARDIAC METABOLISM IN HEART FAILURE

The common forms of low-output heart failure, secondary to arteriosclerosis, hypertension, and certain valvular and congenital lesions, are characterized by an absolute or a relative decrease in the useful external work delivered by the heart. Considerable effort has been directed to the question of whether cardiac failure is due to a defect in the production of energy, its conservation, or its utilization. Only in isolated instances of heart failure, such as those associated with beriberi, are there clear-cut disturbances of myocardial energy production. The major pathway by which pyruvate enters the citric acid cycle and some reactions within the cycle itself are dependent on the presence of adequate concentrations of thiamine (Chap. 78). Thiamine deficiency results in diminished pyruvic acid utilization by heart slices, and in abnormally low pyruvate extraction coefficients in intact dogs and in man.

The myocardial defect in the common forms of low-output heart failure does not appear to reside in an impairment of energy production. In the second phase of cardiac metabolism, energy conservation, the energy of substrate oxidation is converted into the terminal-bond energy of creatine phosphate (CP) and of ATP, the immediate source of chemical energy utilized by heart muscle. This process, known as oxidative phosphorylation, occurs in the mitochondria. The effectiveness of the combined energy production-conservation mechanisms may be studied by measuring the stores of ATP and CP existing in the myocardium, while energy conservation may be evaluated by determining (1) the P:O ratio, i.e., the ratio of high-energy phosphate produced to oxygen consumed in the mitochondria, and (2) the degree of coupling between electron transport and the generation of high-energy phosphate compounds. Although lively controversy exists concerning the status of this phase of metabolism in heart failure, it now appears that severe impairment of myocardial performance may occur without disturbances of mitochondrial function or reduction of high-energy phosphate stores.

In the absence of a definitive abnormality of energy liberation or conservation in the failing myocardium, attention has naturally been directed to the possibility that energy utilization is abnormal. The possibility must be considered that an abnormality of excitation-contraction coupling is an important feature of heart failure. An abnormality of energy liberation could certainly occur if the contractile proteins themselves were altered, and indeed this was once believed to be the basic biochemical abnormality occurring in congestive heart failure, a theory no longer supported. It has been shown that the ATPase activity of myofibrillar preparations is depressed in heart failure, and it is possible that this depression may be responsible for a defect in energy utilization, i.e., in the breakdown of ATP, the process which leads to the shortening and tension development by the contractile filaments.

THE ADRENERGIC NERVOUS SYSTEM IN HEART FAILURE

In view of the importance of the adrenergic nervous system in stimulating the contractility of the normal myocardium, the activity of this system has also been studied intensively in patients with congestive heart failure. An index of the activity of this system, at rest and during exercise, is provided by measurements of the concentration of norepinephrine (NE) in arterial blood. No change or very little increase in the NE concentrations occurs during exercise in normal subjects; much greater increases are seen in patients with congestive heart failure, presumably because of an increased activity of the adrenergic nervous system during exercise in these patients. Marked elevations of 24-hr urinary NE excretion occur in patients with heart failure, indicating that the activity of their adrenergic nervous systems is also augmented at rest.

The importance of the increased activity of the adrenergic nervous system in maintaining ventricular contractility when the function of the myocardium is depressed in congestive heart failure also is shown by the effects of adrenergic blockade in patients with heart failure. Antiadrenergic drugs such as propranolol or guanethidine may cause sodium and water retention, as well as intensify heart failure. The adrenergic nervous system thus plays an important compensatory role in the circulatory adjustments of patients to congestive heart failure, and caution must be exercised in the use of antiadrenergic drugs in the treatment of patients with limited cardiac reserve. (Chap. 233).

The concentration of NE in atrial and ventricular tissue removed at operation in patients with heart failure is less than one-third of that observed in the absence of failure. This is a reduction in NE content in the heart and is not the result of a simple dilution of sympathetic nerve endings in a hypertrophied muscle mass.

The biosynthesis of NE proceeds through a series of steps from tyrosine to dopa to dopamine, the immediate precursor of the neurotransmitter. It is now known that tyrosine hydroxylase, which catalyzes the first reaction (tyrosine to dopa), is the rate-limiting enzyme in the synthesis of NE. Marked reductions in the activity of this enzyme recently have been shown to accompany the NE depletion in the myocardium of dogs with experimental heart failure, and it appears likely that this reduction of enzyme concentration is responsible for the cardiac NE depletion in heart failure.

Although the mechanism ultimately responsible for this reduction of tyrosine hydroxylase in the heart in congestive heart failure remains to be elucidated, some of the consequences of cardiac NE depletion in heart failure are evident. In view of the strongly positive inotropic effect exerted by the NE released from these nerves, the adrenergic nervous system may be considered to provide an important potential source of support to the failing myocardium. However, it has been observed that with supramaximal stimulation of the cardiac sympathetic nerves, the increments of heart rate and contractile force which occurred in animals with experimental heart failure and cardiac NE depletion are abolished or markedly reduced. Thus, it is likely that when congestive heart failure is accompanied by depletion of cardiac NE stores, the quantity of NE released by the sympathetic nerve endings in the heart is deficient relative to the impulse traffic along these nerves.

Cardiac stores of NE are not fundamentally necessary for maintaining the intrinsic contractile state of the myocardium. However, since the reduction of NE stores in heart failure is associated with a diminished release of neurotransmitter, then this depletion of NE may be responsible for loss of the much-needed adrenergic support in the failing heart.

REFERENCES

BRAUNWALD E et al: *Mechanisms of Contraction of the Normal and Failing Heart,* Boston: Little, Brown, 1968

BRAUNWALD E: Mechanics and energetics of the normal and failing heart. Trans Assoc Am Physicians 84:63–94, 1971

GUYTON AC et al: *Circulatory Physiology: Cardiac Output and Its Regulation,* 2nd ed., Philadelphia: W.B. Saunders, 1973

JAMES TN, SHERF L: Ultrastructure of the myocardium, chap. 6 in *The Heart,* 3d ed., ed JW Hurst, New York: McGraw-Hill, 1974, pp. 63–79

KATZ AM, BRADY A J: Mechanical and biochemical correlates of cardiac contraction. Mod Concepts Cardiovasc Dis 40:39–48, 1971

ROSS J JR, SOBEL BE: Regulation of cardiac contraction. Ann Rev Physiol 34:47–90, 1972

Symposium: Neural regulation of the cardiovascular system. Fed Proc 31:1197–1253, 1972

233 HEART FAILURE

EUGENE BRAUNWALD

INTRODUCTION

Heart failure may be defined as the condition in which an abnormality of myocardial function is responsible for the inability of the ventricles to deliver adequate quantities of blood to the metabolizing tissues at rest or during normal activity. Although the fundamental cellular abnormality responsible for heart failure has not been elucidated (Chap. 232), the clinical manifestations resulting from this derangement are usually readily recognized, their pathogenesis is, in general, understood, and means for their alleviation in most patients are available. The underlying cause of heart failure must ultimately be traced to abnormal behavior of the myocardial cell. In many patients heart failure results from anatomic lesions of the heart valves or pericardium which interfere with cardiac filling or emptying, or from severe or prolonged disorders of cardiac rate or rhythm. In most of these instances an abnormality of myocardial function results from, or is associated with, the extramyocardial abnormality. For example, in many patients with rheumatic valvular disease and heart failure, the heart muscle has been damaged as a consequence of the excessive hemodynamic burden imposed by the valvular abnormality, and/or the rheumatic process has impaired myocardial function. In patients with chronic constrictive pericarditis, myocardial damage resulting from infiltration of the heart muscle by the pericardial inflammation and calcification is common (Chap. 241).

In some patients, however, a state which closely resembles heart failure occurs without any detectable abnormality in myocardial function. Such conditions are exemplified by the occurrence in patients with otherwise normal hearts of massive pulmonary embolism, acute hypertensive crisis, and severe valvular regurgitation due to bacterial endocarditis. In such instances, the abnormally elevated hemodynamic load exceeds the ability of even the normal myocardium to pump an adequate quantity of blood to the periphery.

The term *congestive heart failure* is frequently used in clinical medicine because so many of the clinical manifestations of heart failure result from excessive accumulation of fluid. However, effective diuretic therapy is frequently capable of eliminating or markedly reducing these congestive manifestations, while the underlying state of cardiac function may not be altered. Therefore, the simpler term *heart failure* is preferred.

CAUSES OF HEART FAILURE

It is important to identify not only the *underlying cause* of the heart disease but the *precipitating cause* of heart failure as well. The cardiac abnormality produced by a congenital or acquired lesion may exist for many years and produce no or only trivial disability. Frequently, however, serious manifestations of clinical heart failure appear for the first time in the course of some acute disturbance which places an additional load on a myocardium that chronically is excessively burdened, resulting in further deterioration of cardiac function. Identification of such precipitating causes is of critical importance because their prompt alleviation may be lifesaving. However, in the absence of underlying heart disease these acute disturbances do not usually, by themselves, lead to heart failure.

PRECIPITATING CAUSES

1 *Pulmonary embolism.* Patients with low cardiac output, circulatory stasis, and physical inactivity are likely to develop thrombi in the veins of the lower extremities or the pelvis. Pulmonary embolization may result in further acute elevation of pulmonary arterial pressure, which in turn may produce or intensify distention and failure of the right ventricle and may lower the cardiac output further. In the presence of pulmonary vascular congestion, such emboli may lead to infarction of the lung (Chap. 256).

2 *Infection.* Patients with elevated pulmonary venous and capillary pressures are particularly susceptible to pulmonary infections. The fever, tachycardia, hypoxemia, and the increased metabolic demands resulting from pulmonary or other infections may place a further burden on the overloaded, but compensated, myocardium of a patient with chronic heart disease and may thereby precipitate heart failure.

3 *Anemia.* The development of a marked reduction in the oxygen-carrying capacity of the blood may precipitate heart failure because in the presence of severe anemia the oxygen needs of the metabolizing tissues can be satisfied only by an increase in the cardiac output. Though such an increase in the cardiac output might be sustained by a normal heart, a diseased, overloaded, but otherwise compensated heart may be unable to augment the volume of blood which it delivers to the periphery.

4 *Thyrotoxicosis and pregnancy.* Like anemia, these conditions require an increased cardiac output. The development or intensification of heart failure may actually be one of the first clinical manifestations of hyperthyroidism in a patient with underlying heart disease. Similarly, heart failure not infrequently occurs for the first time during pregnancy in women with rheumatic valvular disease; in such women the condition of the heart may remain normally compensated for many years following delivery, after the excessive burden has been eliminated.

5 *Arrhythmias.* Cardiac arrhythmias are among the most frequent precipitating causes of heart failure for a variety of reasons: *(a)* tachyarrhythmias reduce the time period available for ventricular filling; *(b)* the dissociation between atrial and ventricular contractions characteristic of many supraventricular and ventricular arrhythmias results in the loss of the atrial booster pump mechanism, thereby tending to raise atrial pressures; *(c)* in ventricular tachycardia or any arrhythmia associated with abnormal intraventricular conduction, myocardial performance is impaired because of the loss of normal synchronicity of ventricular contraction; *(d)* the marked bradycardia associated with complete atrioventricular block requires a greatly elevated stroke volume if a marked reduction in cardiac output is to be prevented.
6 *Rheumatic and other forms of myocarditis.* The development of acute rheumatic fever and a variety of allergic or infectious processes affecting the myocardium may further impair myocardial function in patients with preexisting heart disease.
7 *Bacterial endocarditis.* The anemia, fever, additional valvular damage, and myocarditis which often occur as a consequence of bacterial endocarditis may, singly or in concert, precipitate heart failure.
8 *Physical, dietary, and emotional excesses.* Sudden augmentation of sodium intake, the discontinuation of diuretics or digitalis glycosides, physical overexertion, excessive environmental heat or humidity, and emotional crises may all precipitate cardiac decompensation.
9 *Systemic hypertension.* Rapid elevation of arterial pressure, as may occur in some instances of hypertension of renal origin or upon discontinuation of antihypertensive medication, may result in cardiac decompensation.

A careful and systematic search for one or more of these precipitating causes should be made in every patient with heart failure, particularly if it is refractory to the usual methods of therapy. If properly recognized, the precipitating cause of heart failure can usually be treated more effectively than the underlying cause. Furthermore, the prognosis in patients with heart failure in whom a precipitating cause can be identified and treated is far more favorable than in patients in whom the underlying disease process has advanced to the point of producing heart failure.

FORMS OF HEART FAILURE

Heart failure may be described as *high-output* or *low-output, acute* or *chronic, right-sided* or *left-sided,* and *forward* or *backward.* Although these terms may be useful in a clinical setting, they are entirely descriptive and do not signify fundamentally different disease states.

HIGH-OUTPUT VERSUS LOW-OUTPUT HEART FAILURE With the development of methods for the measurement of cardiac output, it became useful to classify patients with heart failure into those with a low cardiac output, i.e., *low-output heart failure,* and those with an elevated cardiac output, i.e., *high-output heart failure.* The cardiac output is often depressed in patients with heart failure secondary to coronary artery disease, hypertension, primary myocardial disease, valvular disease, and pericardial disease, but it tends to be elevated in patients with heart failure and hyperthyroidism, anemia, arteriovenous fistulas, beriberi, Paget's disease, and pulmonary emphysema. In clinical practice, however, it may be difficult to distinguish between low-output and high-output heart failure. The normal range of cardiac output is wide (2.6 to 3.6 liters per min per m^2), and in many patients with so-called low-output heart failure the cardiac output may actually be within normal limits at rest, although it may fail to rise normally during exertion. On the other hand, in patients with so-called high-output heart failure the output may not be excessive but rather may be close to the upper limit of normal, particularly when heart failure is severe. Regardless of the absolute level of the cardiac output, however, cardiac failure may be said to be present when the characteristic clinical manifestations described below are accompanied by a depression of the curve relating ventricular end-diastolic volume to cardiac performance (Fig. 232–6).

An integral part of the heart failure syndrome is evidence that the heart does not deliver the quantity of oxygen required by the metabolizing tissues. In the absence of peripheral shunting of blood, such inadequate delivery of oxygen to the metabolizing tissues is reflected in an abnormally widened arterial–mixed venous oxygen difference, relative to the total body oxygen consumption. In mild cases, this abnormality may not be present at rest and may become evident only during exertion. In patients with the high-output cardiac states associated with conditions such as arteriovenous fistula, beriberi, thyrotoxicosis, and Paget's disease, the arterial–mixed venous oxygen difference is often abnormally low, because the mixed venous oxygen saturation is raised by the admixture of blood which has been shunted away from some of the metabolizing tissues, and it may be presumed that even in these patients the delivery of oxygen to the metabolizing tissues is reduced. When heart failure occurs in such patients the arterial–mixed venous oxygen difference may be normal or even reduced, but it still exceeds the level which existed prior to the development of heart failure, and therefore the cardiac output, though normal or elevated, is lower than before heart failure occurred.

The mechanisms responsible for the development of heart failure in patients whose cardiac outputs are initially high are complex and depend on the underlying disease process. In most of these conditions the heart is called upon to pump abnormally large quantities of blood in order to deliver the normal quota of oxygen to the metabolizing tissues. This increased flow load exerts an effect on the myocardium which resembles that produced by regurgitant valvular lesions. In addition, thyrotoxicosis and beriberi may impair myocardial metabolism directly, and severe anemia and chronic pulmonary emphysema may interfere with myocardial function by producing myocardial anoxia.

ACUTE VERSUS CHRONIC HEART FAILURE Frequently there is no fundamental distinction between these two conditions. For example, intensive efforts to prevent expansion of blood volume by means of dietary sodium restriction and the administration of diuretics will frequently delay the development of exertional dyspnea and ankle edema in patients with severe hypertension until an acute episode, such as a small myocardial infarction, an arrhythmia, or further elevation of arterial pressure, results in acute heart failure. Without intensive efforts to restrict blood volume the same patient would have been considered to have been suffering from chronic heart failure, even though his underlying myocardial disease was no further advanced.

RIGHT-SIDED VERSUS LEFT-SIDED HEART FAILURE Many of the clinical manifestations of heart failure result from the accumulation of excess fluid behind one or both ventricles. This fluid may localize upstream to the specific cardiac chamber which is initially affected. For example, patients in whom the abnormal load is placed on the left ventricle develop dyspnea and orthopnea as a result of pulmonary congestion, a condition referred to as *left-sided heart failure.* When heart failure has existed for months or years, such localization behind the failing ventricle may no longer exist. For example, patients with long-standing aortic valve disease or systemic hypertension may have ankle edema, congestive hepatomegaly, and systemic venous distention late in the course of their disease, even though the abnormal hemodynamic burden initially was placed on the left ventricle. In contrast, when the underlying abnormality affects the right ventricle primarily, e.g., valvular pulmonic stenosis or pulmonary hypertension secondary to pulmonary thromboembolism, symptoms resulting from pulmonary congestion such as orthopnea, or paroxysmal nocturnal dyspnea are less common. However, severe exertional dyspnea may be observed in such patients.

Thus, although specific lesions may place an abnormal load on one or the other ventricle, when this load is prolonged, failure of the heart as a whole occurs. Perhaps this is because the muscle bundles composing both ventricles are continuous and both ventricles share a common wall, the interventricular septum. Also, biochemical changes which occur in heart failure and which may contribute to the impairment of myocardial function, such as norepinephrine depletion and alterations in the activity of myofibrillar ATPase, occur in the myocardium of both ventricles, regardless of the specific chamber on which the abnormal hemodynamic burden is placed.

BACKWARD VS. FORWARD HEART FAILURE For many years a controversy has revolved around the mechanism of the clinical manifestations resulting from heart failure. The concept of *backward heart failure,* originated by James Hope in 1832, contends that when heart failure occurs, one or the other ventricle fails to discharge its contents normally, the end-diastolic volume of that ventricle rises, and the pressures and volumes in the atrium and venous system behind the failing ventricle become elevated. According to this concept, retention of sodium and water occurs as a consequence of the elevation of systemic venous and capillary pressures and the resultant transudation of fluid into the interstitial space, as well as from increased renal tubular reabsorption of sodium associated with an elevation of renal venous pressure.

In contrast, the proponents of the *forward heart failure* hypothesis, expounded by MacKenzie in 1913, maintain that the clinical manifestations of heart failure result directly from an inadequate discharge of blood into the arterial system. Salt and water retention, according to this concept, is a consequence of diminished renal perfusion, which not only results in the reduction of glomerular filtration rate but also stimulates sodium reabsorption through activation of the renin-angiotensin-aldosterone system.

The rigid distinction between *backward heart failure* and *forward heart failure* is artificial, since both mechanisms appear to operate to varying extents in most patients with chronic heart failure. However, the rate of onset of heart failure often influences the clinical manifestations. For example, when a large portion of the left ventricle is suddenly destroyed, as in myocardial infarction, acute pulmonary edema may develop rapidly, and although stroke volume is reduced, the patient may die of acute pulmonary edema before the reduced cardiac output can be responsible for the renal retention of salt and water. However, if this same patient survived the acute insult, clinical manifestations resulting from the abnormal retention of fluid within the systemic vascular bed would develop. Similarly, the right ventricle may dilate and the systemic venous pressure may rise to high levels immediately following acute massive pulmonary embolism, but this state may have to be maintained for some days before sodium and water retention sufficient to produce edema occurs.

FLUID RETENTION IN CHRONIC HEART FAILURE

When the volume of blood pumped by the left ventricle into the systemic vascular bed is chronically reduced, and when one or both of the ventricles fails to expel the normal fraction of its end-diastolic volume, a complex sequence of adjustments occurs which ultimately results in the abnormal accumulation of fluid. Though, on the one hand, many of the clinical manifestations of heart failure are secondary to this excessive retention of fluid, on the other hand, this abnormal fluid accumulation constitutes an important compensatory mechanism which tends to maintain cardiac output and therefore perfusion of the vital organs. Except in the terminal stages of heart failure, the myocardium operates on an ascending, albeit depressed, function curve, and the augmented ventricular end-diastolic volume and pressure characteristic of heart failure must be regarded as aiding the maintenance of cardiac output. The expansion of the intravascular blood volume, regardless of the mechanism responsible, tends to elevate ventricular end-diastolic volume and, in accordance with the Frank-Starling principle, tends to augment ventricular performance. On the other hand, the maintenance of right ventricular end-diastolic volume and pressure at elevated levels raises systemic venous and capillary pressures, resulting ultimately in transudation of fluid from the vascular bed and edema formation (Chap. 30).

The redistribution of left ventricular output also serves as an important compensatory mechanism in the presence of severe impairment of cardiac function. This redistribution occurs when cardiac output is limited during the imposition of an additional burden, such as exercise, fever, or anemia in patients with impaired myocardial function, but as heart failure advances, redistribution occurs even in the basal state. Blood flow is redistributed so that the delivery of oxygen to vital organs, such as the brain and myocardium, is maintained at normal or near-normal levels, while blood flow to less critical areas, such as the cutaneous and muscular beds, is reduced. Vasoconstriction mediated by the sympathetic nervous system is primarily responsible for this redistribution of peripheral blood flow.

In the presence of heart failure, effective filing of the systemic arterial tree is reduced, a condition which initiates the complex hemodynamic and hormonal adjustments that interact to promote reduced renal sodium and water excretion by lowering renal cortical blood flow and glomerular filtration rate. The latter falls proportionately less than does the renal plasma flow; hence, the filtration fraction rises. The renin-angiotension system is activated, probably as a consequence of increased renal sympathetic nervous activity and reduced hepatic renin clearance. This, in turn, augments aldosterone secretion by the adrenal cortex. Also, in the presence of hepatic venous congestion, the metabolism of aldosterone by the liver is impaired, and, therefore, in some patients with heart failure, the tubular reabsorption of sodium is increased because of augmented circulating aldosterone. Though this by itself may not be sufficient to produce retention of salt and water, when accompanied by the abnormal renal hemodynamics characteristic of heart failure, the elevated aldosterone levels results in abnormal sodium and hence fluid accumulation. The presence of augmented mineralocorticoid activity in heart failure is reflected in low concentrations of sodium in the urine, sweat, and saliva. There is increasing evidence that factors beside the reduction of glomerular filtration rate and augmented mineralocorticoid activity play a significant role in the sodium retention characteristic of heart failure, but they have not been defined precisely. It appears that the reduction in cardiac output initiates alterations in intrarenal hemodynamics, and raises the concentration of an antinatriuretic substance (hormone) and/or lowers the concentration of a natriuretic substance, resulting in sodium retention. Patients with severe heart failure often exhibit a reduced capacity to excrete a water load, which may result in dilutional hyponatremia. These abnormalities may be caused, in part, by excess antidiuretic hormone activity and/or factors that prevent sodium reabsorption in the distal tubule, such as avid proximal tubular reabsorption of sodium or the action of a diuretic acting on the distal tubule.

The importance of elevated systemic venous pressure and of the aforementioned alterations of renal function vary in their relative importance in the production of edema in different patients with heart failure. In patients with tricuspid valve disease or constrictive pericarditis the elevated venous pressure appears to play the dominant role. On the other hand, severe edema may be present in patients with ischemic or hypertensive heart disease, in whom systemic venous pressure is within normal limits or is only minimally elevated. In such patients, the fluid retention is probably due primarily to a redistribution of cardiac output and a concomitant reduction in renal perfusion. Regardless of the mechanisms involved in fluid retention, patients with congestive heart failure have elevations of total blood volume, interstitial fluid volume, and body sodium. These abnormalities diminish, but may not disappear even after clinical compensation has been achieved by treatment.

CLINICAL MANIFESTATIONS OF HEART FAILURE

DYSPNEA *Dyspnea*, or respiratory distress which occurs as the result of increased effort in breathing, is the most common symptom of heart failure (Chap. 28). It is at first observed only during activity, when it may simply represent an aggravation of the breathlessness which normally occurs under these circumstances. As heart failure advances, however, dyspnea appears with progressively less strenuous activity. Ultimately, breathlessness is present even when the patient is at rest. Thus, the chief difference between exertional dyspnea in normal persons and in cardiac patients is the degree of activity necessary to induce the symptom. Cardiac dyspnea is observed most frequently in patients with elevations of left atrial, pulmonary venous, and pulmonary capillary pressures. Such patients have engorged pulmonary vessels and interstitial pulmonary edema, which reduces the compliance of the lungs and thereby increases the work of the respiratory muscles required to inflate the lungs. The Hering-Breuer reflex, which inhibits inspiration, is enhanced, resulting in the rapid, shallow breathing of cardiac dyspnea. The oxygen cost of breathing is increased because of the excessive work of the respiratory muscles. This is coupled with the diminished delivery of oxygen to these muscles, which occurs as a consequence of the reduced cardiac output and which may contribute to the sensation of shortness of breath.

ORTHOPNEA *Orthopnea*, i.e., dyspnea in the recumbent position, is also characteristic of those forms of heart failure associated with elevations of pulmonary venous and capillary pressures. While orthopnea is usually a symptom of more advanced heart failure than exertional dyspnea, in patients who are physically inactive it may actually precede dyspnea. Orthopnea results from the redistribution of blood from the lower extremities and the splanchic bed to the lungs as the result of the alteration in gravitational forces, when the recumbent position is assumed. This augmentation of intrathoracic blood volume reduces the vital capacity and elevates pulmonary venous and capillary pressures.

The patient with orthopnea generally elevates his head on several pillows at night and frequently awakens short of breath if his head has slipped off the pillows. The sensation of breathlessness usually is relieved by sitting bolt upright, and many patients report that they find relief from sitting in front of an open window. As heart failure advances orthopnea may be so severe that patients cannot lie down at all and must spend the entire night in a sitting position. On the other hand, in other patients with long-standing, severe heart failure, symptoms of pulmonary congestion may actually diminish with time as the function of the right ventricle becomes impaired.

PAROXYSMAL (NOCTURNAL) DYSPNEA Also known as *cardiac asthma*, this term refers to attacks of severe shortness of breath which generally occur at night and usually awaken the patient from sleep. The attack is precipitated by stimuli which aggravate the previously existing pulmonary congestion; frequently the total blood volume is augmented at night because of the reabsorption of edema from dependent portions of the body which occurs with recumbency; the redistribution of blood volume which takes place results in an increase in intrathoracic blood volume and therefore produces pulmonary congestion. When the patient is asleep, he can tolerate relatively severe pulmonary engorgement; he may awaken only when actual pulmonary edema and bronchospasm have developed. The patient awakens with the feeling of suffocation and with wheezing respirations. Though simple orthopnea may be relieved by sitting upright at the side of the bed with legs dependent, in the patient with paroxysmal nocturnal dyspnea coughing and wheezing often persist in this position. The depression of the respiratory center during sleep may reduce ventilation sufficiently to lower arterial oxygen tension, particularly in patients with interstitial lung edema and reduced pulmonary compliance. Also, ventricular function may be further impaired at night because of reduced adrenergic stimulation of myocardial function. Acute pulmonary edema is a severe form of cardiac asthma due to further elevation of pulmonary capillary pressure and associated with extreme shortness of breath, rales over both lung fields, and the transudation and expectoration of blood-tinged fluid. If not treated promptly (page 1126) acute pulmonary edema may be fatal.

CHEYNE-STOKES RESPIRATION Also known as periodic or cyclic respiration, Cheyne-Stokes respiration is characterized by diminished sensitivity of the respiratory center. In this form of respiration there is an apneic phase, during which the arterial P_{O_2} falls and the arterial P_{CO_2} rises. This combination of changes in the arterial blood stimulates the depressed respiratory center, resulting in hyperventilation and hypocapnia, followed in turn by apnea. Cheyne-Stokes respiration occurs most often in patients with cerebral atherosclerosis and other cerebral lesions, but the prolongation of the circulation time from the lung to the brain which occurs in heart failure, particularly in patients with hypertension and coronary artery disease and associated cerebral vascular disease, also appears to precipitate this form of breathing.

FATIGUE AND WEAKNESS These are nonspecific but common symptoms of heart failure and are related to the reduction of cardiac output. Anorexia and nausea associated with abdominal pain and fullness are frequent complaints in patients with severe heart failure; they may be related to the enlarged, congested liver.

CEREBRAL SYMPTOMS In severe heart failure, particularly in elderly patients with accompanying cerebral arteriosclerosis and arterial hypoxemia, there may be alterations in the mental state characterized by confusion, difficulty in concentration, and impairment of memory.

PHYSICAL FINDINGS IN HEART FAILURE

In moderate heart failure the patient appears to be in no distress at rest except that he may become uncomfortable if asked to lie flat for more than a few minutes. In more severe heart failure the pulse pressure may be diminished, reflecting a reduction in stroke volume, and occasionally the diastolic arterial pressure may be elevated as a consequence of generalized vasoconstriction. There may be cyanosis of the lips and nail beds (Chap. 29), as well as peripheral pallor and diaphoresis. Sinus tachycardia is common, as well as evidence of congested neck veins, which fill from below and which become distended with sustained pressure on the liver (positive hepatojugular reflux). *Systemic venous pressure* is often abnormally elevated in heart failure and may be recognized most readily by observing the extent of distention of the jugular veins. In the early stages of heart failure the venous pressure may be normal at rest but may become abnormally elevated during and immediately after exertion.

Early diastolic and presystolic gallop sounds (Chap. 228) are often audible but are not specific for heart failure, and *pulsus alternans,* i.e., a regular rhythm in which there is alternation of strong and weak cardiac contractions and therefore alternation in the strength of the peripheral pulses, may be present. Pulsus alternans may be detected by sphygmomanometry and in more severe instances by palpation; it frequently follows an extrasystole and is observed most commonly in patients with cardiomyopathy or with hypertensive or ischemic heart disease. It is caused by a reduction in the number of contractile units during weak contractions and/or by alternation in the ventricular end-diastolic volume.

BASAL PULMONARY RALES Moist, inspiratory, crepitant rales and dullness to percussion over the posterior lung bases are common in patients with heart failure and elevated pulmonary venous and capillary pressures. In patients with pulmonary edema, rales may be heard widely over both lung fields; they are frequently coarse and sibilant and may be accompanied by expiratory wheezing. Rales may, however, be caused by many other conditions.

CARDIAC EDEMA Cardiac edema is usually dependent, occurring in the legs symmetrically, particularly in the pretibial region and ankles in ambulatory patients, and in the sacral region of individuals at bed rest. Pitting edema of the arms and face occurs rarely and only late in the course of heart failure.

HYDROTHORAX Pleural effusion in congestive heart failure results from the elevation of pleural capillary pressure and transudation of fluid into the pleural cavities. Since the pleural veins drain into both the systemic and pulmonary veins, hydrothorax is observed most commonly in patients with marked elevations of pressure in both venous systems, but may also occur with marked elevation of pressure in either venous bed. It is noted more frequently in the right pleural cavity than the left.

ASCITES This also occurs as a consequence of transudation and results from increased pressure in the hepatic veins and the veins draining the peritoneum (Chap. 43). Ascites occurs most frequently in patients with tricuspid valve disease and with constrictive pericarditis.

CONGESTIVE HEPATOMEGALY An enlarged, tender, pulsating liver also accompanies systemic venous hypertension and is observed not only in the same conditions in which ascites occurs, but also in milder forms of heart failure from any cause. When systemic venous hypertension and hepatomegaly are prolonged and severe, enlargement of the spleen may also occur.

JAUNDICE This is a late finding in congestive heart failure and is associated with elevations of both the direct- and indirect-reacting bilirubin levels; it results from impairment of hepatic function secondary to hepatic congestion and the hepatocellular hypoxia associated with central lobular atrophy. Serum enzyme concentrations, particularly SGOT and SGPT, are frequently elevated.

CARDIAC CACHEXIA With severe, chronic heart failure there may be serious weight loss and cachexia because of (1) elevation of the metabolic rate, which results in part from the extra work performed by the respiratory muscles, the increased oxygen needs of the hypertrophied heart, and the discomfort associated with severe heart failure; (2) anorexia and abdominal fullness, and (3) some impairment of intestinal absorption.

ROENTGENOGRAPHIC FINDINGS IN HEART FAILURE

In addition to the enlargement of the particular chambers characteristic of the lesion responsible for heart failure, vascular changes in the lung fields are common in patients with heart failure and elevated pulmonary vascular pressures. In *acute pulmonary edema* marked mottling usually extends from the hilar regions and may cover both lung fields. With less severe heart failure there may be increased opacity of the hilar regions and dilatation of all central vessels, particularly the veins draining the upper lung fields. Constriction of the arteries and veins to the lower lung zones may occur. The roentgenogram may also present a "ground glass" appearance, with cloudy lung fields due to diffuse interstitial edema. Prolonged elevation of pulmonary venous pressure in excess of 20 mm Hg results in visible, dilated lymphatic vessels (Kerley B Lines), i.e., thin horizontal lines most clearly evident at the bases of the lung fields. Prolonged interstitial edema may also produce nodular deposits because of pulmonary hemosiderosis. Pleural effusions may be present and associated with interlobar effusions. In patients with heart failure associated with systemic venous hypertension, the roentgenogram may show distention of the superior vena cava, hydrothorax, and occasionally evidence of pulmonary infarction.

CLINICAL MANIFESTATIONS OF HIGH CARDIAC OUTPUT STATES ASSOCIATED WITH HEART FAILURE

THYROTOXICOSIS The characteristic clinical features of hyperthyroidism may be so conspicuous even after the development of heart failure that the diagnosis is simple on clinical grounds (Chap. 85). In other cases, when eye phenomena and thyroid enlargement are not striking and other classic manifestations of thyrotoxicosis are obscured and masked by the antagonistic effects of cardiac failure, the overactivity of the thyroid is hardly discernible. Thyrotoxicosis should be suspected as a contributing factor in patients with cardiac disease under the following circumstances: persistent tachycardia that endures after prolonged rest and during sleep; any suggestion of heart failure with a high cardiac output in the absence of other recognizable causes; failure of the usual treatment measures to bring about a satisfactory response; attacks of paroxysmal atrial fibrillation or chronic atrial fibrillation in a person without mitral stenosis, particularly when the ventricular rate is resistant to the slowing effect of full doses of digitalis. The diagnosis is discussed fully in Chap. 85.

After treatment has restored the euthyroid state, remarkable improvement in a previously intractable form of heart disease usually follows. In about one-third of those with atrial fibrillation the rhythm reverts spontaneously to a normal sinus mechanism; angina and congestive failure disappear or become easily controllable.

HEART FAILURE SECONDARY TO ANEMIA The clinical picture is that of high-output failure with anemia. One may find cardiac enlargement, occasionally with hypertrophy; unusually pronounced systolic murmurs because of the combined effects of decreased viscosity, increased flow, and dilatation of the mitral ring; rarely an early diastolic rumbling murmur at the mitral area, due to increased flow, or an aortic diastolic blowing murmur, presumably due to dilatation of the aortic ring. The latter may present a confusing problem of diagnosis. Furthermore, when slight fever is also present, subacute bacterial endocarditis may be mimicked. In patients with sickle-cell anemia with fever and joint pains, acute rheumatic fever may be suspected.

When there is an organic obstruction in a coronary artery, the compensatory increase in coronary flow that would otherwise take place in anemia is prevented and angina may appear; alternatively, anemia may aggravate already existing angina.

HEART FAILURE SECONDARY TO THIAMINE DEFICIENCY (BERIBERI) Thiamine deficiency (Chap. 78) leads to a deficiency of cocarboxylase, resulting in impaired myocardial energy production. The defect in the peripheral tissues causes peripheral vasodilatation, increased venous return and cardiac output, and, consequently, an increased load on a heart already handicapped by the metabolic defect. Cardiac failure is more likely to occur in persons who have the least involvement of the nervous system and a greater capacity for work, i.e., who have a greater opportunity to develop an increased load on the heart.

The usual clinical picture of beriberi heart disease, as seen in the Orient, is characterized by enlargement of the heart, absence of arrhythmia, systemic venous hypertension, bounding arterial pulsations, and the classical phenomena of heart failure with a high cardiac output.

This picture is rarely encountered in the occidental countries; in these areas the more common description is that of a person who has been on a clearly deficient diet over a long period of time, who has had an excessive consumption of alcohol, who has heart disease of uncertain origin, heart failure that does not respond to the usual methods of treatment, signs of mild peripheral neuritis or other manifestations of dietary deficiency, and whose heart failure and cardiac enlargement disappear with the administration of thiamine.

The diagnosis depends mostly on securing a good dietary history and on observing the response to treatment. Beriberi heart disease should be suspected when heart failure with a normal or elevated cardiac output is observed in the absence of thyrotoxicosis or anemia. Furthermore, thiamine deficiency may contribute to the development of heart failure in all alcoholics.

Differential diagnosis

The diagnosis of congestive heart failure may be established by observing some combination of the clinical manifestations of heart failure, enumerated above, together with the findings characteristic of one of the etiologic forms of heart disease. Since heart failure is usually associated with an enlarged heart on physical examination and/or roentgenography, the diagnosis should be suspected when heart size is normal. Heart failure may be particularly difficult to distinguish from pulmonary disease. Patients with dyspnea secondary to pulmonary disease may, like patients with heart failure, be more dyspneic in the supine than in the erect position, but they do not usually have episodes of paroxysmal nocturnal dyspnea. Occasionally, a therapeutic test with dietary salt restriction, digitalis, and diuretics may be helpful in differentiating dyspnea of cardiac from that of pulmonary disease, since the latter is not alleviated by these measures. A prolonged arm-to-tongue circulation time is characteristic of low-output heart failure, while in patients with pulmonary disease the circulation time is normal. An abnormal ventricular impulse on palpation and/or electrocardiographic evidence of left ventricular hypertrophy are helpful in recognizing left ventricular disease in patients with chronic lung disease. Arterial hypercapnia is present in severe pulmonary insufficiency, while hypocapnia is more characteristic of heart failure. Pulmonary function tests, cardiac catheterization, and angiocardiography may be necessary to distinguish these two forms of dyspnea. Pulmonary embolism also presents many of the manifestations of heart failure, but fixed splitting of the second heart sound, a right ventricular left, hemoptysis, pleuritic chest pain, and a perfusion defect on a lung scan should point to this diagnosis (Chap. 256).

Ankle edema may be due to varicose veins, cyclic edema, or gravitational effects, but in these patients there is no generalized systemic venous hypertension at rest, following exertion, or with pressure over the liver. Edema secondary to renal disease can usually be recognized by appropriate renal function tests and urinalysis and is rarely associated with elevation of the venous pressure. Enlargement of the liver and ascites occur in patients with hepatic cirrhosis, but may also be distinguished from heart failure by a normal antecubital venous pressure and absence of a positive hepatojugular reflux.

TREATMENT OF HEART FAILURE

The treatment of heart failure may be divided into three components: (1) removal of the precipitating cause of heart failure; (2) correction of the underlying cause of heart failure; (3) control of the congestive heart failure state. The first two are discussed elsewhere, together with each specific disease entity or complication. The third component of the treatment of heart failure may, in turn, be divided into three categories: (*a*) reduction of the cardiac work load; (*b*) enhancement of myocardial contractility; and (*c*) control of excessive fluid retention. The first two of these forms of therapy should be utilized simultaneously, and if abnormal fluid accumulation persists the third should be applied. The vigor with which each of these measures is pursued in any individual patient should depend upon the severity of the heart failure state. Following effective treatment, recurrence of the clinical manifestations of heart failure may be prevented by continuing those measures that were originally effective.

Reduction of the cardiac work load

A reduction in physical activity in mild cases and rest in bed or in a chair in severe failure remain cornerstones in the treatment of heart failure. Meals should be small in quantity, and every effort should be made to diminish the patient's anxiety. Physical and emotional rest tend to lower arterial pressure, diminish the work of the respiratory muscles, slow heart rate, and reduce the load on the myocardium by diminishing the requirements for cardiac output. These influences act in concert to diminish the need for redistribution of the cardiac output, and in many patients, particularly those with mild heart failure, simple bed rest and mild sedation often result in an effective diuresis.

Rest at home or in the hospital should be maintained for 1 to 2 weeks in patients with overt congestive failure and should be continued for several days after the patient's condition has stabilized. The hazards of phlebothrombosis and pulmonary embolism which occur with bed rest may be reduced with anticoagulants, leg exercises, and elastic stockings. Heavy sedation should be avoided, but small doses of barbiturates or tranquilizers may be helpful in calming the emotionally disturbed patient with heart failure through the first few days of therapy and in allowing essential sleep. In patients with chronic, mild heart failure, bed rest on weekends will frequently allow continuation of gainful employment.

Following recovery from heart failure, the patient's activities must be carefully assessed and in many instances his work load and responsibilities must be reduced. Intermittent rest during the day and the avoidance of strenuous exertion are helpful. Weight reduction by restriction of caloric intake in the obese patient with heart failure also diminishes cardiac work load and is an essential component of the therapeutic program.

Enhancement of myocardial contractility

The improvement of myocardial contractility by means of cardiac glycosides is the second of the three cornerstones in the control of the heart failure state. The pharmacology, indications, contraindications, and methods of administration of glycosides are considered in detail in Chap. 235. Digitalis is most effective in the common forms of heart failure associated with an excessive hemodynamic burden, such as hypertension and valvular heart disease, as well as in ischemic heart disease. It is particularly effective in the treatment of euthyroid patients with atrial fibrillation or atrial flutter and rapid ventricular rates associated with heart failure. In such patients the slowing of the ventricular rate, resulting from prolongation of the refractory period of the atrioventricular node, combined with the improved inotropic state of the myocardium results in striking and rapid clinical improvement. However, even in patients without these arrhythmias digitalis produces considerable clinical improvement as a consequence of its positive inotropic action.

Cardiac glycosides are less effective in diseases primarily affecting the myocardial cell, such as the toxic and infectious myocarditides, the various forms of cardiomyopathy and fibroelastosis, and in those forms of heart failure which are precipitated by infection, fever, anemia, thyrotoxicosis, beriberi, acute rheumatic fever, complete atrioventricular block, and cor pulmonale. Digitalis is contraindicated in patients with second degree or unstable atrioventricular block and in patients with idiopathic hypertrophic subaortic stenosis (Chap. 242).

Three sympathomimetic amines which act largely on beta-adrenergic receptors—epinephrine, isoproterenol, and dopamine—improve myocardial contractility in various forms of heart failure. Dopamine, the immediate precursor of norepinephrine, appears to be most effective, since it also produces renal vasodilatation by a nonadrenergic mechanism and thereby augments sodium excretion. It increases cardiac output substantially but lowers peripheral resistance slightly. It is administered by constant intravenous infusion, in doses ranging from 100 to 1,000 μg per min, and has been found useful in intractable heart failure, particularly in patients with myocardial infarction and shock or pulmonary edema.

Control of excessive fluid retention

Many of the clinical manifestations of heart failure are secondary to hypervolemia and expansion of the interstitial fluid volume. When fluid retention due to heart failure first becomes clinically evident, considerable expansion of the extracellular space has already occurred, and heart failure is already advanced. The quantity of extracellular fluid volume is largely dependent on the extracellular sodium content, and treatment aimed at reducing extracellular fluid volume is dependent primarily on lowering total body sodium stores, while fluid restriction, per se, is of less importance. A negative sodium balance can be achieved by reducing the dietary intake and increasing the urinary excretion of this ion with the aid of diuretics. In severe heart failure mechanical removal of extracellular fluid by means of thoracentesis, paracentesis, hemodialysis, or peritoneal dialysis may also be employed.

DIET In patients with mild heart failure, considerable improvement in symptoms may result from the simple reduction of sodium intake, particularly if this measure is accompanied by bed rest. In patients with more severe failure the sodium intake must be controlled more rigidly, even when other measures such as cardiac glycosides and diuretics are used, and following recovery from a bout of heart failure, at least moderate sodium restriction should be maintained. The normal diet contains approximately 6 to 10 g sodium chloride; this intake can be reduced by half simply by excluding salt-rich foods and salt which is added at the table. Reduction of the ordinary dietary intake to approximately one-fourth of normal may be achieved if, in addition, all salt is omitted from cooking. In patients with severe heart failure, in whom the daily sodium chloride intake is reduced to between 500 and 1,000 mg, milk, cheese, bread, cereals, canned vegetables and soups, some salted cuts of meat and fresh vegetables, including spinach, celery, and beets, must be eliminated. A variety of fresh fruit, green vegetables, specially processed breads and milk, and salt subtitutes are permissible, but such diets are difficult to keep palatable outside the hospital. Water intake may be *ad libitum* in all but the most severe forms of congestive heart failure. However, late in the course of heart failure, dilutional hyponatremia may develop in patients who are unable to excrete a water load, sometimes because of excessive secretion of antidiuretic hormone. In such cases water intake as well as sodium intake must be restricted.

Attention must also be directed to the caloric content of the diet. Substantial improvement can result from caloric restriction in obese patients with heart failure, in whom weight loss will reduce the load placed on the myocardium. On the other hand, in individuals with severe heart failure and cardiac cachexia, an attempt must be made to maintain nutritional intake and to avoid caloric and vitamin deficiencies.

DIURETICS A variety of diuretic agents is available, and in the patient with mild heart failure almost all are effective. The choice of the particular diuretic to be employed depends to some extent on convenience. However, in the more severe forms of heart failure, the selection of diuretics is more difficult, and any existing abnormalities in the serum electrolytes must be taken into account. Hypovolemia must be avoided, since excessive reduction of blood volume may reduce cardiac output, interfere with renal function, and produce profound weakness and lethargy.

Thiazide diuretics These agents are the most widely used diuretics in clinical practice because of their effectiveness when administered orally. In patients with chronic heart failure of mild or moderate severity the continued administration of chlorothiazide or one of its many analogues abolishes or diminishes the need for rigid dietary sodium restriction. Thiazides are well absorbed following oral administration; chlorothiazide and hydrochlorothiazide reach their peak action in 4 hr, and diuresis persists for approximately 12 hr. Thiazide agents reduce the tubular reabsorption of sodium, and chloride and water follow the unreabsorbed sodium into the more distal tubule. Here, potassium-sodium exchange is enhanced, resulting in augmented kaluresis. Thiazides fail to increase free water clearance, and in some instances they reduce it, supporting the hypothesis that these drugs inhibit sodium reabsorption in the cortical diluting segment, at a site where the urine is normally diluted. The carbonic anhydrase-inhibiting properties of the thiazides are of limited importance and need not be invoked to account for most of the diuretic action. Chlorothiazide is administered in doses of up to 500 mg every 6 hr. Many derivatives of this compound are available but offer few, if any, significant advances over the parent compound.

Potassium depletion is the chief adverse effect following prolonged administration of chlorothiazide; it may be prevented by the oral supplementation of potassium chloride solution. However, this is not palatable and may be hazardous in patients with renal failure. Therefore, to control potassium depletion produced by thiazides (as well as by ethacrynic acid and furosemide) intermittent dosage schedules, e.g., omitting the diuretic every third day, and the use of a potassium-retaining diuretic, such as spirolactone or triamterene, may be preferable. The hypokalemia produced by thiazides and other diuretics may seriously enhance the dangers of digitalis intoxication. Other side effects of thiazides include reduction of the excretion of uric acid, which may lead to hyperuricemia, and a hyperglycemic effect, which is particularly troublesome in patients with overt or latent diabetes mellitus. Skin rashes, thrombocytopenia, and granulocytopenia have also been reported.

Mercurial diuretics Presumably these diuretics act by releasing inorganic mercury within the tubule cell, which then combines with sulfhydryl enzymes essential for sodium reabsorption. Mercurial diuretics reduce sodium reabsorption and make a greater quantity of sodium available for exchange with potassium in the distal tubule, thus tending to increase the excretion of potassium. Since these compounds produce a hypotonic diuresis, they may be useful in the treatment of patients with heart failure and dilutional hyponatremia. The most commonly used mercurial diuretic, Mercuhydrin, also contains theophylline.

Mercurial diuretics are not particularly effective when given by mouth and require parenteral administration. They are usually administered intramuscularly in doses of 0.5 or 1.0 ml, but may be given intravenously in patients with severe and refractory heart failure. One commonly available mercurial diuretic, Thiomerin, may be administered subcutaneously. Mercurial diuretics result in a metabolic alkalosis which limits the effectiveness of further administration. Effectiveness may be restored, however, in a patient whose condition is refractory to further mercurial administration, by raising the serum chloride concentration with oral ammonium chloride, 6 to 12 g orally, in divided doses for 3 to 4 days prior to the administration of the mercurial. Rare fatal reactions following intravenous injection have been reported and presumably are due to cardiac arrhythmias. Mercurial diuretics should be administered with caution to patients with renal insufficiency in whom clinical manifestations of mercurialism, i.e., stomatitis, colitis, further renal damage, and salivation, have been reported. Skin rash and fever occur rarely.

Aldosterone antagonists The 17-spironolactones resemble aldosterone structurally and act on the distal renal tubule by competitive inhibition of aldosterone. These agents produce a sodium diuresis, and, in contrast to mercurial diuretics and particularly to chlorothiazide derivatives, they tend to result in potassium retention. Although secondary hyperaldosteronism exists in some patients with congestive heart failure, the spironolactones are effective even in patients in whom the serum aldosterone concentration is within normal limits. Aldactone A may be administered in doses of 25 to 100 mg three to four times daily by mouth. The maximal effect of this regimen is not observed for approximately 4 days. Spironolactones are most effective when administered in combination with thiazide diuretics. The opposing action of these two classes of drugs on urine and serum potassium makes possible a sodium diuresis without either hyper- or hypokalemia when both agents are administered.

Aldactone should not be administered alone to patients with hyperkalemia, renal failure, or hyponatremia. Reported complications include nausea, epigastric distress, mental confusion, drowsiness, gynecomastia, and erythematous eruptions.

Triamterene A pteridine derivative, triamterene exerts a renal effect similar to that of the spironolactones; i.e., it prevents sodium reabsorption and interferes with sodium-potassium exchange in the distal tubules. However, its fundamental mechanism of action differs from that of the spironolactones, since it is active in adrenalectomized animals. The effective dose is 100 mg once or twice daily. Side effects include nausea, vomiting, diarrhea, headache, granulocytopenia, eosinophilia, and skin rash. Although, it resembles Aldactone A in that its diuretic potency is not great, it is extremely effective in preventing the hypokalemia characteristic of thiazide administration.

Ethacrynic acid and furosemide Ethacrynic acid is an unsaturated ketone derivative of aryloxyacetic acid, while furosemide differs from the thiazides in that the thiadiazine ring has been replaced by a furfuryl group on the amino nitrogen of the anthranilic acid.

These are extremely powerful diuretics which inhibit sodium reabsorption throughout the nephron, but especially in the ascending limb of the loop of Henle. These agents produce rates of urine formation which may be as high as one-third of the glomerular filtration rate. While other diuretics lose their effectiveness as blood volume is restored to normal levels, ethacrynic acid and furosemide remain effective despite the elimination of excessive extracellular fluid volume. The major side effects of these agents are due to this marked diuretic potency, which may result in circulatory collapse and in reductions in the renal blood flow and glomerular filtration rate. Alkalosis is produced by a large increase in the urinary excretion of chloride, hydrogen and potassium ions. Hypokalemia and hyponatremia may occur, and hyperuricemia is also observed, as with thiazide diuretics.

Both drugs are readily absorbed orally and are excreted in the bile and urine. They are usually effective by mouth, in doses of 25 to 100 mg two or four times daily, and intravenously in doses ranging from 10 to 100 mg. Weakness, nausea, and dizziness may accompany both diuretics; ethacrynic acid has been associated with skin rash and granulocytopenia, as well as with transient or permanent deafness.

These extremely effective diuretics are useful in all forms of heart failure, particularly in otherwise refractory heart failure and pulmonary edema. Both agents have been shown to be effective in patients with hypoalbuminemia, hyponatremia, hypochloremia, hypokalemia, and reductions in the glomerular filtration rate and to produce a diuresis in patients in whom mercurial and thiazide diuretics are ineffective.

The effectiveness of ethacrynic acid or furosemide may be potentiated by spironolactone, triamterene, a thiazide diuretic, a carbonic anhydrase inhibitor, or an osmotic diuretic, such as mannitol. In turn, when used in combination with mercurials or thiazides, ethacrynic acid or furosemide increases the effectiveness of these agents.

Choice of a diuretic The thiazides, administered orally, are the agents of choice in the treatment of chronic cardiac edema of mild to moderate degree in patients without hyperglycemia or hyperuricemia. Mercurial diuretics are useful when a rapid diuresis is desired, particularly in patients who do not respond adequately to orally administered thiazides, and are also valuable in patients with hyperglycemia or hyperuricemia in whom the administration of thiazide diuretics is not advisable. Spironolactones and triamterene are not potent diuretics when used alone, but they are particularly effective when administered along with other diuretics, particularly the thiazides, ethacrynic acid, and furosemide, which by themselves produce marked potassium loss. However, in patients with heart failure and severe secondary aldosteronism, spironolactone may be extremely effective. Ethacrynic acid or furosemide, given alone or with spironolactone or triamterene, is the agent of choice in patients with severe heart failure refractory to other diuretics.

Refractory heart failure

When the response to treatment is inadequate, heart failure is considered to be refractory. Before assuming that this state simply reflects advanced, perhaps preterminal, myocardial depression, careful consideration must be given to several possibilities: (1) an underlying and overlooked cause of the heart disease that may be amenable to specific surgical or medical therapy, such as silent aortic or mitral stenosis, constrictive pericarditis, bacterial endocarditis, hypertension, or thyrotoxicosis; (2) one or a combination of the precipitating causes of heart failure, such as pulmonary or urinary tract infection, recurrent pulmonary emboli, arterial hypoxemia, anemia, or arrhythmia; (3) complication of too vigorous therapy, such as digitalis intoxication, hypovolemia, or electrolyte imbalance.

Treatment of acute pulmonary edema

Pulmonary edema is life-threatening and must be considered to be a medical emergency. As is the case for the more chronic forms of heart failure, in the treatment of pulmonary edema, attention must be directed to identifying and removing any precipitating causes of decompensation, such as an arrhythmia or infection. However, because of the acute nature of the problem, a number of additional measures are necessary: (1) Morphine is administered by the subcutaneous, intramuscular, or intravenous routes in doses from 10 to 20 mg, depending upon the severity of the problem. This drug reduces anxiety, which tends to perpetuate pulmonary edema, and thereby breaks a vicious cycle. Also, morphine exerts a positive inotropic effect and tends to reduce venous return. Naline should be available in case respiratory depression occurs. (2) High concentration of oxygen must be inhaled because the alveolar fluid interferes with oxygen diffusion, resulting in arterial hypoxemia. Therefore, 100 percent oxygen should be administered, preferably under positive pressure. The latter increases intraalveolar pressure and therefore reduces transudation of fluid from the alveolar capillaries and impedes venous return to the thorax, reducing pulmonary capillary pressure. (3) The patient should be maintained in the sitting position, which also tends to reduce venous return to the heart. (4) Rotating tourniquets should be applied to the extremities and may be followed by a phlebotomy of 500 ml of blood. (5) Aminophylline (theophylline ethylene diamine), 240 to 480 mg intravenously, is effective in diminishing bronchoconstriction, increasing sodium excretion, and augmenting myocardial contractility. (6) If digitalis has not been administered previously, three-fourths of a full dose of a rapidly acting glycoside, such as ouabain, digoxin, or Lanatoside C, should be administered intravenously (Chap. 235). (7) Intravenous diuretics, such as furosemide or ethacrynic acid (25 to 50 mg) or mercuhydrin (1 to 2 ml), will, by rapidly establishing a diuresis, reduce circulating blood volume and thereby hasten the relief of pulmonary edema.

Prognosis

The prognosis in heart failure depends primarily on the nature of the underlying heart disease and on the presence or absence of a precipitating factor which can be treated. When one of the latter can be identified and removed, the outlook for immediate survival is far better than if heart failure occurs without any obvious precipitating cause. The prognosis can also be estimated by observing the response to treatment. When clinical improvement occurs with only modest dietary sodium restriction and/or digitalis without the administration of diuretics, then the outlook is far better than if, in addition to these measures, intensive diuretic therapy is necessary. The long-term prognosis for heart failure is most favorable when the underlying forms of heart disease can be treated.

REFERENCES

Braunwald E et al: *Mechanisms of Contraction of the Normal and Failing Heart,* Boston: Little, Brown, 1968

Cherniack NS, Longobardo GS: Cheyne-Stokes breathing: An instability in physiologic control. N Engl J Med 288:952, 1973

Fowler NO: Congestive heart failure, chap. 11 in *Cardiac Diagnosis,* New York: Harper & Row, 1968

Friedberg CK (ed): Symposium on congestive heart failure. Prog Cardiovas Dis 12:313, 1970

Hurst JW (ed): *The Heart,* 3d ed., Part V, Section A: Heart Failure (chaps. 27–31), New York: McGraw-Hill, 1974, pp. 416–494

Robin ED et al: Pulmonary edema. N Engl J Med 288:239, 292, 1973

Wood P: Heart failure, chap. 7 in *Diseases of the Heart and Circulation,* 3d ed., Philadelphia: Lippincott, 1968

234 CARDIAC DYSRHYTHMIAS

EUGENE BRAUNWALD
BURTON E. SOBEL

The term *dysrhythmia* is not limited to irregularities of the heartbeat but is applied also to disturbances of rate and of conduction. We shall first present certain broad considerations and then deal with specific disorders. The mechanism of action of the most important drugs utilized in the treatment of dysrhythmias is considered in Chap. 235; treatment by electrical methods is the topic of Chap. 236.

GENERAL CONSIDERATIONS

Etiologic factors

Certain dysrhythmias are especially likely to occur in the absence of detectable structural disease of the heart. These include sinus arrhythmia, sinus bradycardia, and sinus tachycardia; atrial and ventricular premature beats; milder forms of first-degree atrioventricular (AV) block (i.e., P-R intervals of 0.21 to 0.25 sec), and paroxysmal atrial tachycardia. Only rarely can a specific agent such as tobacco or coffee be identified as an inciting cause of sinus or atrial tachycardia.

Other dysrhythmias are particularly likely to occur in persons with organic disease of the heart. These include ventricular tachycardia and fibrillation, atrial flutter and fibrillation, and second and third degrees of AV block. Although any type of structural cardiac disease may underlie any dysrhythmia, certain disturbances of rhythm are commonly associated with specific underlying processes. For example, atrial fibrillation in patients with thyrotoxicosis, mitral valve disease, and left atrial enlargement; and ventricular tachycardia in those with ischemic heart disease. Still other disturbances of rhythm should immediately arouse the suspicion that a drug is responsible. Ventricular bigeminy—a disorder in which a ventricular premature beat follows every supraventricular beat—and atrial tachycardia with atrioventricular block are often due to digitalis excess, especially when there is coexistent potassium deficiency induced by diuretics (Chap. 235).

A cardiac dysrhythmia may be a manifestation of a serious circulatory or metabolic disturbance and should result in a careful, deliberate search for the underlying abnormality, which may be (1) a pathologic process in the myocardium, e.g., a myocardial infarction or myocarditis; (2) involvement of the vascular bed, e.g., leakage from an aortic aneurysm, or pulmonary embolization; (3) a sudden drop in blood volume due to hemorrhage such as gastrointestinal bleeding; (4) an endocrine disturbance such as thyrotoxicosis or pheochromocytoma; (5) drug toxicity, especially evoked by cardioactive agents, including digitalis glycosides, catecholamines, and antiarrhythmics (Chap. 235); (6) systemic infections; (7) metastatic disease to the heart, such as carcinoma of the lung, lymphoma, or melanoma; and (8) the rapid development of sudden severe hypoxemia or hypercapnia.

Electrolyte disturbances are of particular importance in the genesis of cardiac dysrhythmias and deserve special consideration. They are rarely isolated but usually multiple; in practice it may therefore be difficult to determine the specific ion abnormality responsible. *Hyperkalemia* leads to AV block, impairment of intraatrial and intraventricular conduction with prolonged P waves and QRS complexes, and rarely sinoventricular conduction. Death may occur from ventricular fibrillation or, less commonly, from ventricular standstill. *Hypokalemia* may produce atrial and ventricular extrasystoles, coupled beats, and tachycardias, as well as mild atrioventricular and intraventricular conduction defects; severe hypokalemia may lead to multifocal premature ventricular contractions deteriorating into ventricular fibrillation. *Hypercalcemia* diminishes conduction velocity and shortens the refractory period, thereby facilitating reentry and the development of coupled ventricular beats, ventricular tachycardia, and ventricular fibrillation.

The treatment of dysrhythmias per se, without identification and management of the underlying abnormality, is often unrewarding. Also, often relatively little may be gained when treatment is directed toward a cardiac dysrhythmia which results from a structural abnormality, e.g., a greatly enlarged left atrium in a patient with mitral valvular disease. Effective control of atrial fibrillation under these circumstances might require surgical relief of the valvular abnormality.

Mechanism of dysrhythmias

Many cardiac dysrhythmias result from abnormalities in the automaticity of cardiac tissue. Increases in automaticity may result from (1) a more rapid rate of diastolic depolarization (Chap. 229); (2) a more negative threshold potential, i.e., a reduction in the potential which must be reached before the cell is excited; (3) a less negative resting potential, which is therefore closer to the threshold potential; or (4) some combination of these abnormalities. Reductions in automaticity are produced by the opposite changes. Certain dysrhythmias, e.g., sinus tachycardia and some ectopic tachycardias, appear to result from increases in automaticity of the sinoatrial node or of pacemaker tissue elsewhere in the heart. Other disturbances, such as atrioventricular junctional rhythm or idioventricular rhythm, usually result from reduction in the automaticity of the sinoatrial node, with control of the cardiac rhythm assumed by a pacemaker which ordinarily exhibits a lower degree of automaticity.

Disturbances in the conduction of the action potential provide another important physiologic basis for cardiac dysrhythmias. Pathologic slowing or failure of propagation of the impulse from the atrium and AV junctional tissue to the ventricles results in various degrees of AV block. However, slowed conduction may also set the stage for the development of tachyarrhythmias. Local ischemia or mechanical stresses may diminish conduction through segments of the myocardium so that when an impulse leaves the area of reduced conduction velocity it finds the adjacent myocardium no longer refractory and restimulates it. This phenomenon is termed *reentry*, and it can result from either focal reexcitation due to the flow of current between adjacent portions of myocardium which are repolarized at different times (asynchronous recovery) or from circus current movement due to local impairment of conductivity. Reentry is frequently responsible for coupled beats, and hence some instances of bigeminal rhythm. Sometimes, conduction is slowed in a diseased area so that unidirectional block is present. When this occurs, reexcitation of normal tissue may be followed by retrograde repetitive excitation of the diseased area and a self-sustaining tachycardia may result. Electrocardiographically, such rhythms appear to be initiated by a rapid ectopic pacemaker. In fact, however, although the dysrhythmia may be initiated by an ectopic impulse, it may be sustained by reentrant mechanisms. Bigeminy due to digitalis, however, is probably due *not* to reentry but rather to increased automaticity associated with instability of Purkinje cells during repolarization.

For a number of years considerable evidence supported the prevailing view that a *circus movement* is responsible for atrial flutter and fibrillation. However, some instances of these rhythms now appear to result from very rapid and irregular stimuli being discharged from a single focus. At the present time conflicting evidence favors and refutes both concepts; it is likely that each applies in different instances.

Concealed conduction is an additional important mechanism involved in complex dysrhythmias. This phenomenon usually affects the AV junction and occurs when an impulse penetrates the junction without traversing it. Thus, it may lead to apparent AV block or augmentation of the severity of block but in reality is due to concealed conduction of ectopic impulses and "resetting" of the refractory period of the junction. Concealed conduction is probably responsible for the nature of the irregularity of the ventricular response in the presence of atrial fibrillation.

Other important physiologic mechanisms which underlie complex dysrhythmias are the *Wedensky effect* (protracted enhancement of excitability after a stimulus of abnormally large amplitude), *Wedensky facilitation* (enhancement of excitability distal to the site of block of propagation of a preceding impulse), and *supernormal conduction* (enhancement of conduction occurring near the end of the relative refractory period of the preceding depolarization). The former probably accounts for appearance of ventricular dysrhythmias after electrical cardioversion (Chap. 236) in the presence of occult digitalis toxicity. Wedensky facilitation probably accounts for the occurrence of enhanced AV conduction immediately after the dropped beat in a Wenckebach period (page 1140). *Supernormal conduction* is recognizable in patients with artificial pacemakers when a subthreshold impulse arising endogenously or initiated by another artificial pacemaker is conducted only when it occurs during the supernormal period of the preceding beat.

Circulatory derangements associated with dysrhythmias

Dysrhythmias alter cardiac function by a variety of mechanisms.

EFFECTS OF CHANGES IN HEART RATE In a resting person with a normal heart, because of compensatory changes in stroke volume, cardiac output remains constant, or almost so, despite variations in heart rate from approximately 40 to 160 contractions per min; output decreases progressively at extremes beyond this range. However, in patients with significant myocardial, valvular, coronary arterial or pericardial disease, the range of heart rates at which the cardiac output is normal is much narrower. Therefore, the sudden development, for example, of a supraventricular tachycardia, with a ventricular rate of 160 beats per min, or of complete AV block with a rate of 40 beats per min, may not alter the resting cardiac output in the absence of serious cardiac impairment. However, such changes may seriously depress cardiac output in patients with heart disease. The effect of bradycardia on cardiac output depends in part on its duration. Thus, in chronic long-standing AV block, cardiac output may be sustained even at rates as low as 35 beats per min. When increased demands are placed on the normal heart, as during exertion, infection, or anemia, the heart rate normally accelerates, and this acceleration contributes importantly to the circulatory adjustment to the stress. However, when third-degree AV block is present with a fixed, slow ventricular rate, the cardiac output fails to rise normally and the patient becomes especially symptomatic during the period of stress.

LOSS OF APPROPRIATELY TIMED, VIGOROUS ATRIAL CONTRACTION The atria are not merely passive conduits for returning blood from the systemic and pulmonary venous beds to the ventricles. Rather, they should be considered as booster pumps which augment ventricular filling. In many dysrhythmias the normal temporal sequence between atrial and ventricular systole is lost. These include all degrees of AV block, AV junctional rhythms, ventricular tachycardia, and many instances of atrial tachycardia and flutter. In atrial fibrillation, effective atrial contraction does not occur.

Loss of atrial booster pump function will not usually lower the cardiac output in persons with otherwise normal cardiac function, since compensatory mechanisms such as augmented sympathetic stimulation of the myocardium help to maintain the output. However, loss of atrial function reduces the maximal cardiac output which can be achieved during marked exertion. On the other hand, in patients with impaired myocardial function (particularly those with overt or incipient chronic heart failure) or with acute myocardial infarction, atrial function is more critical and loss of the atrial booster pump results in a lowering of cardiac output by as much as 40 percent, elevation of atrial pressures or both. In patients with marked ventricular hypertrophy, such as occurs in hypertension, aortic stenosis, idiopathic hypertrophic subaortic stenosis, and the related cardiomyopathies, characterized by ventricular hypertrophy, the atrial contribution to ventricular filling is particularly important, since the thickened ventricular wall impedes the inflow of blood. In patients with these lesions the sudden development of one of the aforementioned dysrhythmias may seriously impair cardiac performance and depress cardiac output and arterial pressure.

EFFECTS ON MYOCARDIAL OXYGEN CONSUMPTION AND CORONARY BLOOD FLOW The frequency of cardiac contraction is one of the major determinants of myocardial oxygen consumption (Chap. 7). Hence, when all other factors are constant, tachycardia increases and bradycardia reduces the need of the heart for oxygen. Coronary blood flow occurs predominantly during diastole, and since the total number of seconds of diastole per minute is reduced during tachycardia, a rapid heart rate may precipitate myocardial ischemia in the presence of coronary arterial narrowing. In turn, the ischemia may result in angina and in impairment of myocardial function. Conversely, the development of AV block and a slow ventricular rate often diminishes the severity of angina in patients with ischemic heart disease.

EFFECTS ON THE VENTRICULAR CONTRACTION SEQUENCE Ventricular function depends on a synchronous, nearly simultaneous ventricular contraction. Though the ventricular myocardium contracts in ventricular fibrillation, the chaotic nature of the contraction prevents the development of sufficient intraventricular pressure to propel blood forward. Lesser degrees of asynchrony occur in dysrhythmias associated with intraventricular conduction abnormalities, such as ventricular tachycardia, ventricular extrasystoles, and supraventricular tachycardias with bundle branch block. Such asynchrony of contraction will not impair the cardiac output in an individual with an otherwise normal heart but may exert a significant depressant effect in patients with serious cardiac disease.

EFFECTS ON MYOCARDIAL FUNCTION Although the responsible mechanism has not been identified, prolonged severe tachycardia can depress myocardial function directly, and this depression may persist even after sinus rhythm has been restored.

Methods of examination

The most precise methods of diagnosis of the various dysrhythmias include electrocardiographic examination and recordings of His bundle electrograms. However, the physician who has regularly correlated his observations by simple physical examination with electrocardiographic tracings can usually recognize many dysrhythmias at the bedside.

The exact ventricular rate should be measured by auscultation for a full minute. Pulse rate may be misleading because of a pulse deficit. The presence or absence of irregularity should be noted. The intensity of the first heart sound and the amplitude of the peripheral pulse should be observed, and it should be especially noted whether they are constant, as in dysrhythmias in which the normal temporal relation between atrial and ventricular contraction is maintained (as in sinus, paroxysmal atrial, or junctional tachycardias), or variable, as in dysrhythmias in which the normal temporal relation between atrial and ventricular contraction is lost (e.g., in complete AV heart block, ventricular tachycardia, or atrial flutter). Atrial sounds independent of the first and second heart sound are frequently audible in patients with third-degree AV block. If the rhythm is irregular, one should distinguish between a basic cadence that is predictable (regular irregularity, e.g., premature beats) and one that is entirely unpredictable (irregular irregularity, e.g., atrial fibrillation). In some instances the effect of mild exercise on the ventricular rate, and likewise on the degree of irregularity, should be observed; whether the deceleration immediately after exercise occurs in the normal gradual fashion (sinus tachycardia) or in one or more abrupt steps (atrial flutter) should also be noted.

Inspection of the jugular venous pulse is helpful, especially when, in a patient with a very slow or rapid rate, an occasional abrupt large venous excursion—"cannon wave"—is seen. This giant A wave occurs when the atria contract simultaneously with or after the ventricles and results from atrial contraction when the tricuspid valve is closed. Occasionally the jugular venous pulse will be of aid in the recognition of atrial flutter, with A waves perceptible at a frequency of 250 to 350 beats per min. Observation of the effect of *carotid sinus massage* on the electrocardiogram may also be valuable. This maneuver elicits vagal efferent impulses which influence automaticity and conduction. After excluding occlusive carotid disease by examination, one may massage for a few seconds on one side. This may cause (1) no change in rate (ventricular tachycardia); (2) an abrupt slowing which persists after discontinuation of massage (atrial tachycardia); (3) a temporary slowing which lasts only during the massage (atrial flutter or sinus tachycardia), the rate then returning to the previous level either gradually (sinus tachycardia), or at once or following a brief period of irregular acceleration (atrial flutter). Carotid massage acts on the atrial mechanism (1) by gradually and temporarily slowing sinus rhythm or by abruptly interrupting a paroxysmal supraventricular tachycardia and/or (2) by increasing AV block.

The *electrocardiogram* should be studied systematically. The first and most important problem is to determine whether the dysrhythmia is ventricular or supraventricular in origin, a decision often made difficult by the presence of intraventricular conduction disturbances. The presence of P waves or flutter waves and their relation to the QRS complex in the tracing is especially important. P waves most often can be seen best in leads II, III, AVF, and/or those leads taken over the right precordium. Occasionally, other types of tracings may be necessary. For example, paroxysmal atrial tachycardia in the presence of a bundle branch block is exceedingly difficult to distinguish from ventricular tachycardia. Similarly, flutter impulses may be superimposed on the QRS complex or upon the T wave and make diagnosis difficult. In these instances, it may be necessary to employ esophageal electrodes or a bipolar anteroposterior lead. The right arm lead is placed over the right ventricle and the left arm lead on the back and the electrocardiograph is set on lead I. Another bipolar chest lead may be used by placing the left arm lead at the cardiac apex and the right arm lead over the right ventricle. Esophageal intraatrial leads or surface electrocardiograms recorded during carotid sinus massage are often helpful in unraveling complex dysrhythmias.

Difficult diagnostic problems may necessitate evaluation with *His bundle electrograms*, recorded with the use of a transvenous electrode catheter positioned with its tip in the right ventricle adjacent to the tricuspid valve. Ordinarily, atrial depolarization (A), His bundle depolarization (H), ventricular depolarization (V), and ventricular repolarization produce well-defined characteristic wave forms on the electrogram (Fig. 234-1). Recognition of each is facilitated by reference to a simultaneously recorded standard surface electrocardiogram and by knowledge of the usual temporal relationships between components of the electrogram. Junctional beats with aberrant ventricular conduction are preceded by an H spike, and the H-V interval is the same as in sinus beats. Ventricular premature beats are not preceded by an H spike, and in fact may be followed by an H depolarization and an A spike indicative of retrograde atrial depolarization. His bundle electrograms are useful in characterizing the nature of AV block. Prolonged A to H intervals are typical of AV junctional disease; prolonged H-V intervals are typical of delayed conduction in more distal portions of the conduction system and hence of trifascicular block. The latter is far more common than the former, and since it is more likely to evolve into sudden third-degree block associated with syncope or sudden death, its recognition is of considerable importance.

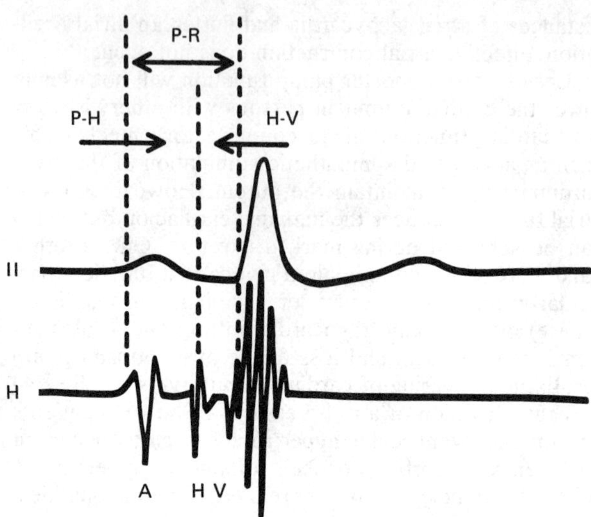

FIGURE 234-1
The relationship between deflections on the conventional electrocardiogram (II) and potentials evident on a simultaneously obtained His bundle recording (H). Three components are readily recognizable on the His bundle recording. The A spike follows the onset of the P wave and represents the atrial electrogram. The H spike represents depolarization of the His bundle. The V potential represents the recording of ventricular depolarization from the catheter electrode. The P-R interval on the simultaneously recorded electrocardiogram is divided conveniently into two components on the basis of the time of occurrence of the H spike. Thus the P-H component represents the time from the onset of atrial depolarization to His bundle depolarization and reflects the duration of conduction through atrial myocardium and the A-V junction. The subsequent component of the P-R interval, namely the H-V component, represents the time required for conduction of the impulse from the common His bundle to the ventricular myocardium. Normally, the P-H interval is between 80 and 140 msec and the H-V interval is between 35 and 55 msec. Prolongation of the PH interval is usually indicative of delay of conduction in the proximal A-V junction and is often associated with Mobitz type I A-V block. Prolongation of the H-V interval is usually indicative of conduction delay in the His bundle, or in both bundle branches or all three fascicles of the distal conduction system, and is frequently associated with Mobitz type II A-V block. Premature supraventricular beats with aberrant conduction are preceded by an H spike at the usual interval prior to the onset of QRS complex on the conventional electrocardiogram. On the other hand, premature ventricular beats are recognized by appearance of a V spike occurring prematurely after an H spike, prior to an H spike or without any association with an H spike.

Treatment

GENERAL MEASURES The success or failure of specific treatment by drugs or by electric shock may be conditioned by appropriate systemic management. A precipitating cause of the dysrhythmia should be sought and treated. Obstruction of the air passages, hypoxia, and disturbances of pH and of electrolyte balance should be corrected. The coexistence of circulatory shock, whether of cardiac or peripheral origin, may render the patient's heartbeat refractory to the usual antiarrhythmic drugs. Thus, it may be necessary first to improve coronary flow by blood or fluid replacement, or by means of inotropic drugs when the heart is primarily at fault. Since pressor amines tend to induce ectopic rhythms at elevated blood pressure levels, the arterial pressure as well as the electrocardiogram should be observed frequently.

Rapidly acting cardiac glycosides such as digoxin, ouabain, or lanatoside C are useful for the treatment of any of the supraventricular tachycardias except, of course, paroxysmal atrial tachycardia with block, which is frequently caused by digitalis intoxication (Chap. 235). The roles of antiarrhythmic drugs and of electric reversion in the treatment of arrhythmias are discussed in Chaps. 235 and 236 and in this chapter in relation to individual arrhythmias. The management of arrhythmias occurring with acute myocardial infarction is discussed in Chap. 240. In general, electrical reversion is most useful in the management of tachyarrhythmias which impair hemodynamics, while the antiarrhythmic drugs are indicated when tachyarrhythmias recur.

Artificial cardiac pacemakers

Two types of electrical pacemakers are commonly employed: the most commonly used is the *direct*, in which the electrode is in contact with the myocardium; the other is the *transthoracic*, in which the electrical pulse is delivered to the chest wall. In the latter, stimuli with a voltage of 25 to 150 volts and a duration of approximately 2 msec are delivered across the precordium by means of a small plate electrode or through subcutaneous needles. The transthoracic pacemaker is rarely used but offers the unique advantage of a rapid, easy start-up; it serves as a useful standby technique until direct pacing can be instituted.

The most common form of *direct* cardiac pacing is the endocardial, in which an electrode catheter is placed, generally in the right ventricle, through the venous route; it is employed with an external power supply for temporary pacing or one that is implanted subcutaneously for permanent pacing. Endocardial pacing of the atrium is more difficult to achieve on a long-term basis, because of electrode instability. Epicardial pacing may be carried out by suturing wire leads to the atrial or ventricular myocardium at the time of thoracotomy and utilizing a totally implanted power supply. Two principal modes of direct myocardial pacing may be employed. In *fixed-rate* pacing, cardiac stimulation is carried out continuously at a preset rate and is independent of the intrinsic electric activity of the heart. Consequently, if AV conduction is reestablished in patients with AV block, competition between the paced beats and the patient's intrinsic rhythm may occur. This competition may result in chaotic rhythms with an attendant, if small, hazard of the development of ventricular fibrillation. Accordingly, this mode of pacing is most appropriate when a return to normal sinus rhythm is unlikely; a distinct advantage is that the simple design of these pacemakers enables them to last longer.

Noncompetitive (demand) pacemakers fire only when the patient's ventricular rate falls below the preset rate of the pacemaker; the output of the pacemaker is inhibited when the frequency of spontaneous ventricular depolarizations is above this level. The advantage of noncompetitive pacing is that if AV conduction returns, the hazards of competitive, fixed-rate pacing are eliminated. It is also useful in patients with paroxysms of symptomatic bradyarrhythmias other than AV block (including sinus bradycardia, SA block, the so-called sick sinus syndrome) and in patients in whom bradycardia alternates with tachycardia. In patients with bradyarrhythmias the implantation of a demand pacemaker permits the administration of antiarrhythmic drugs to suppress the development of ventricular tachyarrhythmias.

SPECIFIC DISORDERS OF RATE AND RHYTHM

Derangements arising in the sinus node

SINUS BRADYCARDIA This is characterized by a slow heart rate (below 60 beats per min) with a normal spread of atrial excitation. It is frequent in athletes and is usually a sign of excellent physical fitness. It occurs also in patients with increased intracerebral pressure, with myxedema, and in hypothermia.

SINOATRIAL ARREST This is due to a sporadic failure of the sinus impulse, and, therefore, there is no sinus node–initiated ventricular excitation. The electrocardiogram shows a prolonged pause between two P waves. Sinoatrial arrest is most frequently due to digitalis or to some other cause of vagal stimulation but may result from myocardial disease. Aside from withholding digitalis and the occasional use of atropine, treatment is usually unnecessary.

SINOATRIAL BLOCK In this dysrhythmia regular sinus impulse formation occurs but there are no atrial or ventricular depolarizations because the impulse is blocked from reaching these structures. The P-P interval is prolonged, usually to some multiple of the regular intervals, but may progressively and periodically shorten, prior to a dropped P wave, when sinoatrial Wenckebach exit block is present. Sinoatrial block is infrequently accompanied by AV block; it may be precipitated by digitalis, quinidine, or hyperkalemia.

SINUS ARRHYTHMIA This dysrhythmia is present in most healthy young persons at rest; it consists of a quickening of the heart rate during inspiration and a slowing during expiration, tends to be intensified by deep breathing, and tends to disappear when the breath is held or when the heart rate is increased by exercise or fever. It has no pathologic significance.

SINUS TACHYCARDIA (Fig. 234-2*B*) Defined as a sinus-initiated heart rate faster than 100 beats per min, this dysrhythmia must be distinguished from the various ectopic tachycardias. The latter group will usually respond to therapy aimed directly at the heart; in sinus tachycardia, the treatment of the rapid rate depends on the management of the underlying condition. A reliable history of abrupt onset and cessation suggests that the attack represents an ectopic tachycardia, rather than sinus tachycardia. However, the patient is often unable to make this differentiation with certainty. When the rate is less than 140 beats per min, the odds favor sinus tachycardia, but a ventricular rate below 140 is also frequent in patients with digitalis-induced atrial tachycardia with AV block and is seen in some persons with atrial flutter or ventricular tachycardia. Rates of 170 or more per minute are almost invariably the result of ectopic rhythms. Difficulty in distinguishing ectopic rhythms from sinus tachycardias occurs chiefly with heart rates between 140 and 170. In sinus tachycardia the rate is less constant than in ectopic tachycardia and is altered somewhat by changes in posture and activity. Anxiety, fever, blood loss, thyrotoxicosis, pregnancy, pheochromocytoma, or some other cause of the tachycardia is usually evident. The response to manual carotid sinus stimulation may help in the differentiation. As described above under Methods of Examination, sinus tachycardia is usually slowed slightly but gradually by such massage.

Extremely rapid sinus tachycardia with heart rates exceeding 130 beats per min is usually due to marked elevation of body temperature, to severe thyrotoxicosis, or to any condition that produces profound circulatory collapse. Frequently, patients with severe advanced chronic airway disease have a sustained tachycardia,

FIGURE 234-2

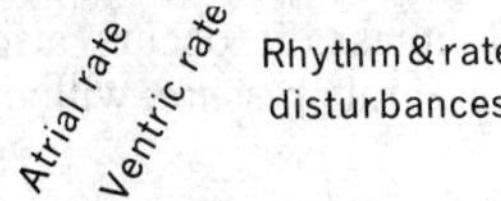

A. Ectopic atrial contraction

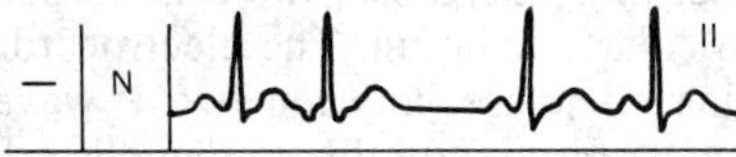

B. Sinus tachycardia

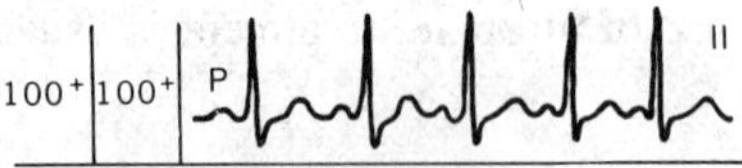

C. Paroxysmal atrial tachycardia

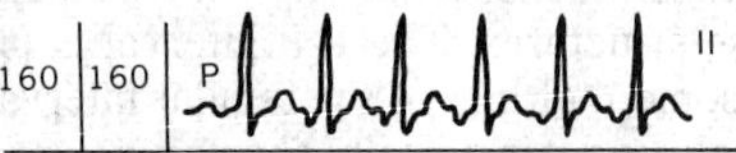

D. Paroxysmal atrial tachycardia with block (2-1)

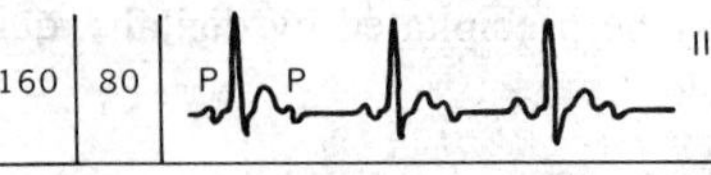

E. Atrial flutter (2:1 block)

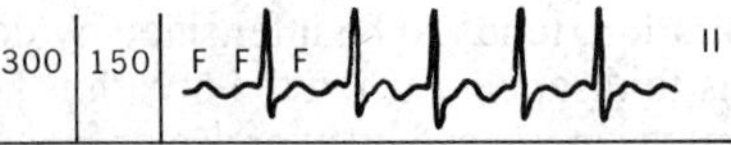

F. Atrial fibrillation

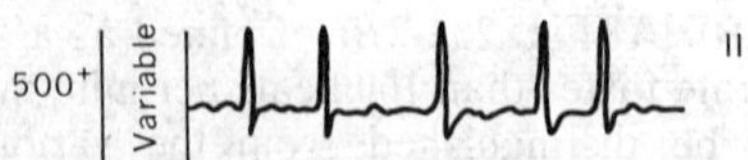

G. Ectopic ventricular contractions

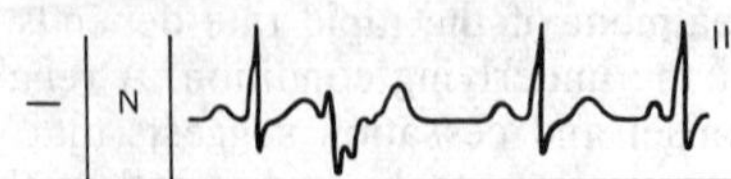

H. Ventricular tachycardia

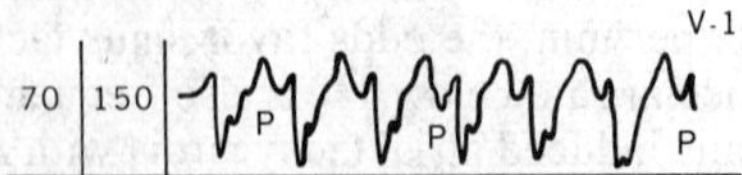

I. Ventricular fibrillation

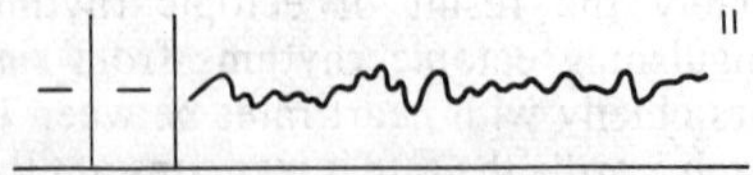

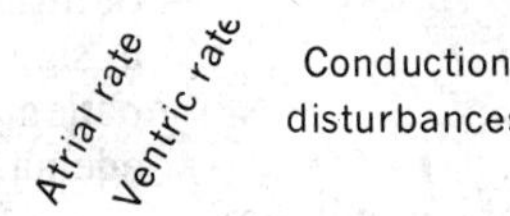

J. First degree heart block

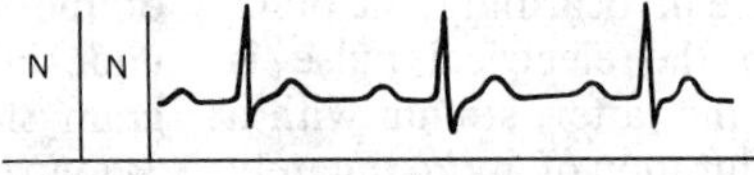

K. Second degree heart block

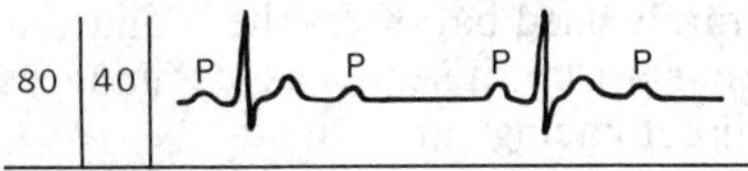

L. Third degree heart block (complete H.B.)

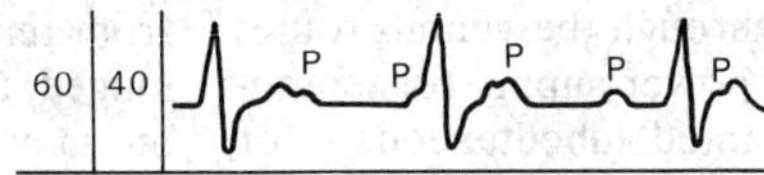

M. Wenckebach

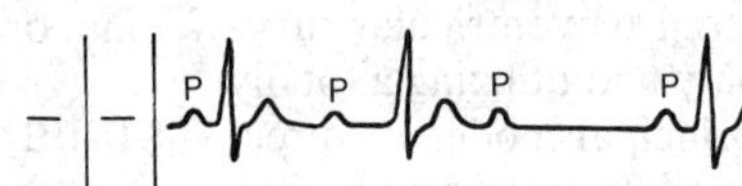

N. Wolff Parkinson White with delta waves

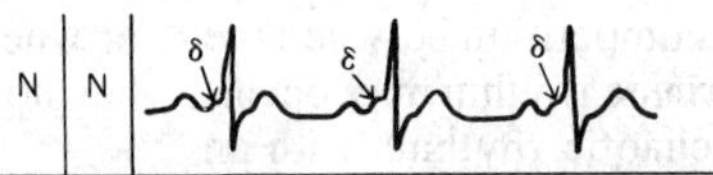

O. Wolff Parkinson White without delta waves

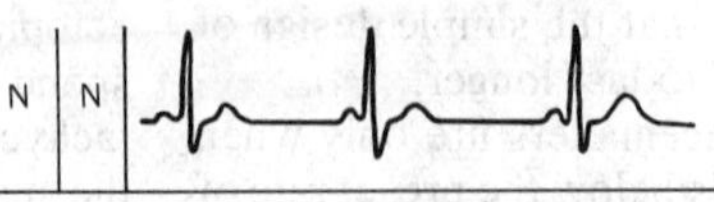

P. Right bundle branch block

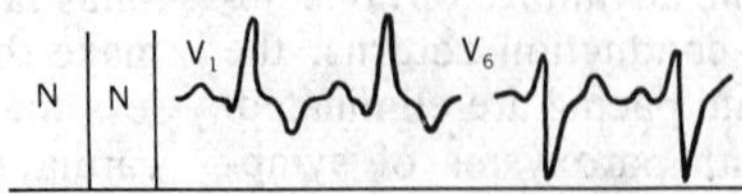

Q. Left bundle branch block

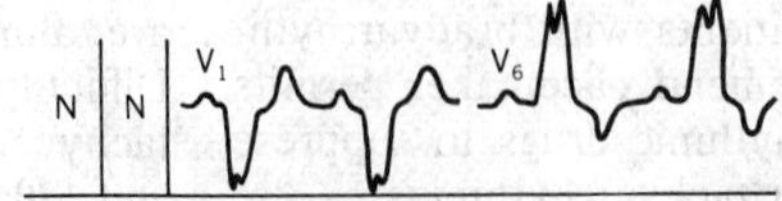

usually not over 120 beats per min; however, during episodes of respiratory decompensation initiated by intercurrent pulmonary infections, heart failure, or obstruction of the airways, the tachycardia may reach 160 beats per min. Consequently, correcting the underlying systemic abnormality is paramount. A similar problem is often present in patients with chronic lung disease following a pneumonectomy or lobectomy. Maintaining airway patency, ventilation, and oxygenation is of great importance. Digitalis or other cardiac therapy is of no therapeutic value in patients with sinus tachycardia unless there are manifestations of congestive heart failure. Effective management of this dysrhythmia requires discovering its basic cause and correcting it.

Derangements arising in the atrium

ECTOPIC ATRIAL BEATS (Fig. 234-2*A*) Also known as premature atrial beats, these originate from an abnormal focus in the atrium rather than the sinus node. Ectopic atrial beats have little clinical significance, but they may precede the onset of sustained atrial dysrhythmias, such as atrial tachycardia, flutter, or fibrillation. Also, their suppression may prevent the onset of these sustained tachyarrhythmias. Recognition of atrial ectopic beats is important, since they may be confused at the bedside with the often more serious ectopic ventricular beats; an electrocardiogram is usually necessary to distinguish between these two disorders. Ectopic atrial beats are easily recognized on the electrocardiogram by the presence of a deformed P wave preceding a QRS complex of normal duration and configuration. They usually occur prematurely after a normal beat and are followed by an incomplete compensatory pause; however, they are not always premature, and therefore the term *ectopic atrial beat* is preferred. Occasionally, there may be aberrant intraventricular conduction in that the QRS complex may be slightly altered in amplitude or configuration and may even resemble the QRS complex of right bundle branch block. In these instances, the presence of the P wave preceding the beat serves as the major distinguishing feature from ectopic ventricular contractions.

PAROXYSMAL ATRIAL TACHYCARDIA (Fig. 234-2*C*) This dysrhythmia has generally been attributed to rapid discharges from an abnormal atrial pacemaker. However, recent evidence suggests that many, if not all, instances of paroxysmal atrial tachycardia are the consequence of sustained reentry and are really manifestations of reciprocating rhythms. This phenomenon will be discussed in connection with the Wolff-Parkinson-White syndrome (page 1142). When reentry occurs as the mechanism of sustained supraventricular tachycardia, it usually involves functional longitudinal stratification in the AV junction, with the reentry pathway encompassing the AV node (Fig. 234-3). Sustained reciprocation may be initiated or terminated by an ectopic beat which precipitates or interrupts the circus current propagating the reentrant pathway. Usually it appears first in youth, and attacks may recur throughout life. The majority of patients with this disorder display no evidence of any other cardiac abnormality, and in the absence of structural disease, atrial tachycardia should be considered benign unless the rate is extremely rapid or the episodes unusually prolonged. Occasionally, the patient presents a history of precipitating events, such as emotional upset, nervousness, fatigue, indigestion, or alcohol ingestion; polyuria may occur after several hours of tachycardia. This arrhythmia may produce great anxiety on the part of the patient and his family. When a patient is seen during an attack, the heart is found to be perfectly regular and the rate ranges from 140 to 250 beats per min. Carotid sinus pressure or other types of vagal stimulation either have no effect or will terminate the attack abruptly. Atrial tachycardia in the presence of intraventricular conduction disturbances may resemble ventricular tachycardia electrocardiographically, and the differentiation may be difficult. In these instances physical signs may be helpful. For example, varying intensity of the first heart sound and irregularly occurring cannon waves in the jugular venous pulse may be sufficient to establish the diagnosis of ventricular rather than atrial tachycardia. Esophageal, intraatrial leads or His bundle recordings may be required to demonstrate the sequence between atrial and ventricular depolarization and thereby differentiate between these two entities.

The causes of atrial tachycardia are not known, since most patients have no signs of organic disease. However, the possibility of underlying causes, such as atrial septal defect, mitral valve disease, and the Wolff-Parkinson-White syndrome, should be considered. Prognosis is excellent unless the attack brings on congestive failure or myocardial ischemia. The keystones of therapy are reassurance, coupled with attempts to prevent recurrences and to terminate the disorder when it occurs. For many patients digitalis is the most effective drug for the prevention of the attacks; in others, quinidine is more useful. Certain patients notice that the attacks are regularly precipitated by specific trigger factors, such as anxiety, digestive disturbances, or hypoglycemic episodes, and avoidance of these factors will have a salutary effect. In many, the attacks occur at such long intervals that the patient himself prefers to treat the disorder only when it transpires rather than to take a drug immediately to prevent the ectopic rhythm.

For the treatment of paroxysmal atrial tachycardia, the patient should assume the recumbent position and be given a sedative, such as sodium pentobarbital or secobarbital 0.2 g intramuscularly. If significant hypotension is present (90 mm Hg systolic or less, slightly higher if the patient has previously been hypertensive), elevation of the arterial pressure by intravenous phenylephrine or methoxamine to not more than 160 mm Hg systolic may suffice to restore a normal rhythm or to make the heart more responsive to other measures. The carotid sinuses should be massaged, each one separately, for about 15 to 20 sec, while the examiner listens to the heart and records the electrocardiogram; the massage is discontinued if the rate slows abruptly. Usually, one of these procedures will be effective; it not, electrical countershock may be employed (Chap. 236). If the ectopic rhythm persists and electrical countershock is not available or is contraindicated, a rapidly acting cardiac glycoside, such as lanatoside C, 0.8 to 1.2 mg may be given slowly intravenously, provided, of course, that the patient has not received digitalis during the preceding 2 weeks. The digitalis acts as a vagal stimulant. If after 1 hr the tachycardia continues, carotid sinus pressure should again be attempted, and if this fails, cholinesterase inhibitors—neostigmine (Prostigmine), 0.5 to 1.0 mg intramuscularly, or Tensilon (edrophonium sulfate), 10 mg intravenously—may be administered, followed again by carotid sinus massage. Some physicians prefer to employ Prostigmine before using digitalis. If all these measures fail, morphine sulfate, 10 to 15 mg subcutaneously, may be given; during the ensuing sleep, the attack will often cease.

Quinidine, propranolol, or procainamide may be given by mouth to prevent recurrences. In patients with recurrent atrial tachycardia resistant to drugs, the insertion of a temporary or permanent pacemaker, which is activated when tachycardia occurs and which stimulates the right atrium or ventricle and thereby interrupts the reentrant pathway, has been found to be effective.

FIGURE 234-3
Diagrammatic representation of possible conduction pathways in a heart exhibiting functional bypass pathways under two conditions: sinus rhythm and reentrant tachycardia. Examples of the electrocardiogram that might be seen in each condition are included below the diagrams. AV, LBB, and RBB represent the AV junction, left bundle branch, and right bundle branch respectively. During sinus rhythm, impulses are initiated at the SA node and propagated simultaneously through the functional bypass pathway and the AV junction. Because of the absence of delay in the bypass tract, the impulse reaches the His bundle first by spread through the ventricular myocardium, accounting for the slurred upstroke in the conventional electrocardiogram as seen in V_6 and leading to both antegrade and retrograde conduction of the impulse in the His bundle. The subsequent portion of the ventricular depolarization occurs conventionally, since impulse transmission through the main branches of the conduction system is more rapid than that resulting from spread of the impulse from the bypass pathway. During reentry tachycardia, perhaps initiated by an appropriately timed supraventricular beat which might find the accessory pathway refractory but the proximal AV junction capable of transmitting the impulse, impulse transmission to the ventricle occurs via the main branches of the conduction system. However, each impulse fragments, with propagation occurring retrograde through the bypass pathway, reentering the atrium, and returning once again to the ventricle through the AV junction, His bundle, and bundle branches. Accordingly, a repetitive reentrant tachycardia results from each QRS complex showing normal morphology and failing to demonstrate the slurred upstroke which was present with sinus rhythm. The horizontal arrows in the conventional electrocardiographic representations indicate that in both sinus rhythm and reentrant tachycardia the "P-J" intervals (from the onset of atrial depolarization to the termination of ventricular depolarization) are identical because in each case the terminal portion of ventricular depolarization results from spread of the impulse through the main branches of the conducting system.

SINUS RHYTHM

AV

Bypass

LBB

RBB

V_6

REENTRANT TACHYCARDIA

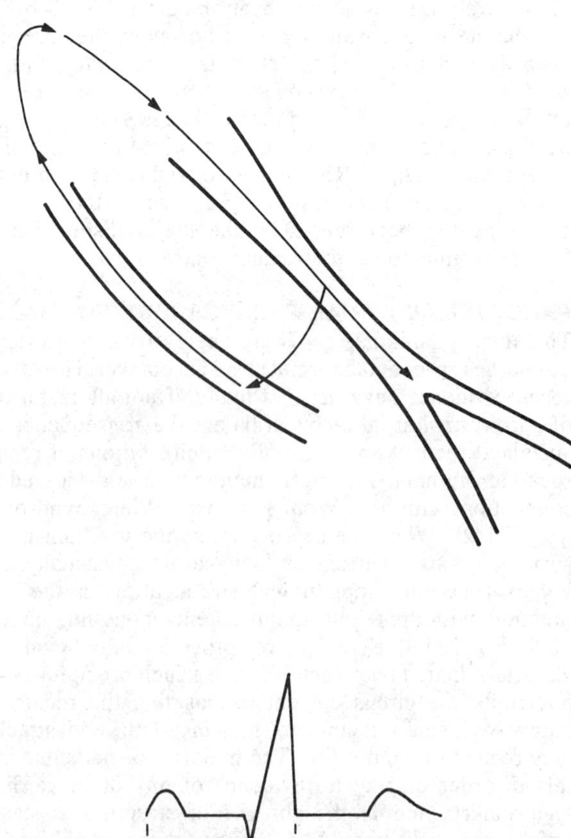

The treatment outlined above refers to the measures taken by the physician. Often, however, the patient has previously learned how to terminate the attack by utilizing carotid sinus pressure, or by inducing gagging and vomiting, or by the Valsalva maneuver (attempting to expire against a closed glottis). Naturally, these simple methods can also be employed by the physician before carotid sinus massage or drug therapy is instituted.

ATRIAL TACHYCARDIA WITH BLOCK (Fig. 234-2*D*) This form of tachyarrhythmia has certain characteristics of flutter in that the responses to vagal stimulation are similar; it resembles atrial tachycardia in that the atrial rate is slower than flutter and usually is between 120 and 250 beats per min. It is generally considered to be a variant of flutter, and the exact mechanism is not known. When atrial tachycardia supervenes in the presence of established AV block, the P waves are usually large, the atrial rate is precisely regular, the onset and offset are sudden, and the response to carotid sinus pressure is typical of ordinary paroxysmal atrial tachycardia.

Digitalis intoxication is a common cause of atrial tachycardia with block (Chap. 235). It usually exhibits gradual onset and offset; small-amplitude P waves, often in a phasic pattern; and an unusual response to carotid sinus stimulation, in which AV block is dramatically accentuated in magnitude and degree and ventricular ectopic beats often become manifest. AV block in this rhythm may be latent and made overt only by carotid massage, which must be employed cautiously. Sensitivity to toxic effects of digitalis increases markedly with potassium depletion, apparently with the severity of heart failure, with hypoxia, and possibly with age. Under these circumstances, serious digitalis intoxication may ensue with doses that would ordinarily be considered therapeutic.

Paroxysmal atrial tachycardia with block should be sought in any digitalized patient who displays other symptoms of intoxication, such as nausea and vomiting, who has received vigorous diuretic treatment, who may otherwise have lost potassium as a result of vomiting or diarrhea, or whose heart rate increases after he has received full doses of digitalis. The electrocardiogram displays an atrial rate of 120 to 250 beats per min, an isoelectric line between P waves of unusual configuration, and some degree of AV block.

The earliest stage is an alteration in the form of the P wave and an increase in the atrial rate, usually with a 1:1 ventricular response. Thus, the ventricular rate may increase to 120 to 140 beats per min and still resemble normal sinus rhythm. At higher atrial rates, 2:1 block usually appears. However, the impaired AV conduction remains inapparent, except when carotid sinus pressure is applied, because every other P wave may be masked by the T deflections of the previous beat. The danger of this abnormal rhythm comes from the fact that although it may be a manifestation of serious digitalis intoxication, it is likely to be confused with sinus tachycardia or atrial flutter and, because of the frequent presence of congestive failure, may be treated with even larger doses of digitalis, or with electrical shock. The proper treatment is prompt cessation of digitalis and of potassium-wasting diuretic drugs and the administration of potassium by mouth or parenterally, depending on the urgency. The serum potassium level must not be relied on as an absolute criterion of diagnosis; most patients with this form of disturbed heart action have little or no diminution in the level of serum potassium. Dilantin or procainamide (Chap. 235) may also be effective.

About one-fourth of patients with atrial tachycardia and block do not suffer from digitalis intoxication and/or potassium depletion. If there is doubt about the role of potassium depletion and there is no evidence of hyperkalemia, potassium therapy may be tried. If this is ineffective, procainamide should be given.

ATRIAL FLUTTER (Fig. 234-2*E*) This dysrhythmia is less common than atrial fibrillation. There is considerable controversy regarding its mechanism. The leading possibility is that it is caused by a rapidly firing ectopic pacemaker. A reciprocating rhythm may be responsible, and a circus movement has not been excluded. The atria contract at a rate of 250 to 350 beats per min. AV block is almost always present, and its ratio is usually even-numbered (e.g., 2:1 or 4:1), with corresponding ventricular rates in the neighborhood of 150 or 75. In a common variation of flutter the ventricular rate is not a constant multiple of atrial rate. This occurs with two sites of block in the AV junction; high junctional 2:1 and low junctional 3:2 Wenckebach block. When the AV block is constant but the ratio is odd (3:1, 5:1, etc.), concealed retrograde conduction of ectopic ventricular beats with antegrade block should be suspected. When the block is constant and of high degree, atrial flutter is usually not suspected without an electrocardiogram. If it is suspected, its presence may be confirmed by the fact that exercise increases the rate suddenly and stepwise rather than gradually, and in the postexercise period slowing occurs suddenly, not gradually. This occurs because exercise has no influence on the rate of the fluttering atrium, but the decrease in vagal tone during exercise reduces the degree of AV block, 4:1 giving way to 2:1 block, for example. Thus, the acceleration of ventricular rate occurs promptly, within one beat; the reverse takes place as vagal tone is restored in the postexercise period. Usually, 2:1 block is present when the ventricular rate is between 140 and 160 beats per min. This fact alone would lead to the suspicion of flutter, because other types of tachycardias are likely to be associated with faster ventricular rates. Carotid sinus pressure slows the ventricular rate in flutter by increasing vagal tone and hence increasing the degree of AV block. The slowing is maintained only for the brief period of pressure, and both the slowing and quickening tend to occur in stepwise fashion rather than gradually, as would be the case with sinus tachycardia if there were any response at all. Occasionally, the block is so variable that the ventricular irregularity is virtually identical to that observed in atrial fibrillation. However, after exercise, the irregularity of flutter tends to disappear, whereas that seen with fibrillation is enhanced.

Careful auscultation frequently reveals an appreciable difference in the intensity of the first heart sound in atrial flutter, because of slight variations in timing of the ventricular contraction in relation to the preceding atrial contraction. The variation in the intensity of the first sound is never present in sinus tachycardia or paroxysmal atrial tachycardia (paroxysmal atrial tachycardia with variable block excepted), but it occurs frequently in ventricular tachycardia and thus serves to help limit the diagnostic possibilities. Atrial flutter is unlike paroxysmal atrial tachycardia without block, but resembles atrial fibrillation and atrial tachycardia with block because it usually occurs in patients with organic heart disease. It occurs most commonly with rheumatic mitral stenosis, but may also be seen with thyrotoxicosis, coronary disease, atrial septal defect, and chronic obstructive pulmonary disease.

The *usual treatment of atrial flutter is the administration of digitalis,* which slows the ventricular rate, by increasing the degree of AV block, and commonly converts flutter to fibrillation. When the drug is withdrawn, atrial flutter will frequently revert spontaneously to normal sinus rhythm; if this does not occur, quinidine may be employed to restore sinus rhythm; if this is unsuccessful, the patient may be maintained in chronic atrial fibrillation and treated appropriately (page 1137). Atrial flutter may be one of the most difficult of all dysrhythmias to revert with drugs, but electrical reversion is often effective (Chap. 236). When flutter persists or recurs, increasing the AV block with digitalis (and when this is ineffective, with propranolol as well) may be necessary for long-term therapy similar to that used to manage atrial fibrillation.

In the presence of atrial flutter, quinidine may slow the atrial rate from about 300 to 200 beats per min. Under these circumstances, the ventricular rate may suddenly increase paradoxically, as the previous 2:1 ratio is replaced by a 1:1 response. Furthermore, vagolytic effects of quinidine may lead to increased ventricular rates, because of enhanced AV conduction, even when the flutter rate remains constant. Accordingly, *quinidine should not be used in patients with flutter without prior or concomitant administration of digitalis.*

ATRIAL FIBRILLATION (Fig. 234-2*F*) This is a dysrhythmia in which the effective contraction of the atria is abolished and the AV node and the ventricles are bombarded with a very rapid and irregular series of stimuli. Many of these impulses are blocked at the AV node, but many are passed through, so that the ventricular contractions in the untreated patient are usually rapid and irregularly irregular.

The untoward effects of atrial fibrillation depend on the rapidity of the ventricular rate and the extent of the pulse deficit (i.e., on the proportion of the ineffective and wasted ventricular beats), on the prior state of the affected heart, on the duration of the dysrhythmia, and on the absence of effective atrial contraction. Cardiac output may be diminished, and heart failure may occur. Stagnation of blood in the atria tends to predispose to the development of thrombi and hence to embolism in both the pulmonary and systemic circulations. Finally, the cardiac irregularity may give an unpleasant consciousness of palpitation (Chap. 31).

When the ventricular rate is rapid, 120 beats or more per minute, the diagnosis is readily made by clinical examination, because atrial fibrillation is the only common condition in which one observes the combination of a marked tachycardia with a gross irregularity. When the rate is normal or only slightly increased, as in digitalized patients, the diagnosis is less apparent on clinical examination alone. The distinction from numerous extrasystoles can be made by noting that it is only in atrial fibrillation that abnormally long pauses occur, in groups of two or more. Moreover, exercise may abolish extrasystoles, whereas it exaggerates the irregularity of atrial fibrillation. More difficult, and frequently impossible, is the differentiation by physical examination of fibrillation from atrial flutter with varying block, and from a shifting pacemaker associated with multifocal atrial ectopic beats. Paroxysmal atrial tachycardia with block is also sometimes confused with atrial fibrillation.

Atrial fibrillation may be paroxysmal or persistent. Occasionally, the paroxysmal form occurs in healthy persons in whom no evidence of structural cardiac disease can be found. These patients (lone fibrillators) may have a variant of the preexcitation syndrome (page 1142), and their dysrhythmia may be due to functional AV junctional reentry pathways. Atrial fibrillation is also encountered in persons who, otherwise normal, develop acute infections such as pneumonia, or in patients with rheumatic heart disease or acute myocardial infarction. Rarely, paroxysmal atrial fibrillation may be the consequence of administration of anesthesia, surgical manipulation within the chest, potassium deficiency, digitalis intoxication, or other forms of poisoning. Most frequently, however, paroxysmal atrial fibrillation is seen in thyrotoxicosis, mitral stenosis, or in elderly persons, many but not all of whom have ischemic heart disease. The paroxysmal attacks frequently occur before the dysrhythmia is permanently established. The bouts may last for a few seconds to a few days, and, as in most types of paroxysmal rapid heart action, the onset and offset are sudden. Unless the patient happens to be observed during an attack, the physician must rely on the patient's observation that the onset was abrupt and that the heart action was highly irregular during the episode.

Permanent atrial fibrillation is confined almost exclusively to patients with myocardial disease, mitral stenosis, constrictive pericarditis, ischemic heart disease, and thyrotoxicosis. In patients with thyrotoxicosis the clinical signs may be absent and the arrhythmia may be the only feature suggesting the possibility of thyroid disease. Rarely, chronic atrial fibrillation may be the sole cause of congestive failure that persists despite full digitalization, and in such instances reversion to normal rhythm improves ventricular performance markedly because of the reestablishment of the atrial transport function. When the ventricular rate fails to slow in the usual fashion after full doses of digitalis, fever may be present, or thyrotoxicosis, a recent silent coronary occlusion, multiple pulmonary infarcts, or acute rheumatic carditis. The onset of this dysrhythmia in a patient who has received therapeutic doses of digitalis and of diuretic drugs may be a manifestation of potassium deficiency and an indication for potassium therapy. Rarely, persistent atrial fibrillation occurs in individuals without other evidence of heart disease.

Treatment In a patient with atrial fibrillation, several choices of therapy are available: (1) allowing the rhythm to remain irregular but attempting to control the ventricular rate with digitalis; (2) abolishing the arrhythmia by quinidine or other antiarrhythmic drugs (Chap. 235); and (3) reverting the arrhythmia by electrical means (Chap. 236). In patients with mitral stenosis, or with marked cardiac enlargement with heart failure, it is rarely possible to restore normal sinus rhythm more than transiently. In other patients with chronic atrial fibrillation, normal sinus rhythm can be restored with large, nearly toxic doses of quinidine. Moreover, it can usually be maintained only with persistent large maintenance doses of quinidine, and even then, for only variable intervals before the dysrhythmia recurs. Quinidine frequently transforms atrial fibrillation into atrial flutter, with the risk of increased ventricular rate. Electrical reversion is usually the treatment of choice for atrial fibrillation (Chap. 236). However, the problem of maintaining sinus rhythm subsequently still remains. In some patients with chronic atrial fibrillation ventricular rate must be controlled with digitalis. Hence, reversion to sinus rhythm with electrical countershock or quinidine is likely to be of value in patients with fibrillation of recent development who are known to have had no evidence of congestive failure prior to the onset of the arrhythmia. Reversion to sinus rhythm should also be considered when the ventricular rate is not well controlled by digitalis, and it may be attempted in patients with intractable heart failure. In patients who cannot be maintained in sinus rhythm and in whom the ventricular rate cannot be slowed sufficiently with digitalis, small doses (5 to 10 mg q.i.d.) of propranolol will often control the ventricular rate. In all cases of atrial fibrillation, therapeutic doses of digitalis should be administered before quinidine is given, but reversion should not be attempted if occult or overt digitalis intoxication is suspected. When atrial fibrillation follows acute myocardial infarction, the first and most important objective is to slow the ventricular rate with digitalis. For the treatment of paroxysmal atrial fibrillation, a rapidly acting digitalis glycoside is preferable; for the control of established atrial fibrillation, one of the slower-acting digitalis preparations should be used.

In many instances of transient atrial fibrillation the administration of digitalis is followed by the disappearance of the dysrhythmia. This probably results from overall hemodynamic improvement, diminished sympathoadrenal myocardial stimulation, and diminution of atrial size, rather than from a direct pharmacologic effect of digitalis on the atria. When atrial fibrillation is of long duration, digitalis rarely abolishes it. Under these circumstances, the ventricular rate slows and becomes less obviously irregular unless complete AV block and a regular idioventricular or AV junctional rhythm develop; but electrocardiographic tracings reveal that the atria continue to fibrillate.

Thromboembolism is one of the dreaded complications in patients with atrial fibrillation (or less commonly with atrial flutter), particularly when the dysrhythmia is chronic and when mitral stenosis is present. Thromboembolism is responsible for about 20 percent of the deaths in patients with mitral stenosis. To prevent such catastrophes, long-term anticoagulant therapy is advocated in patients with atrial fibrillation, and is especially important in patients who have already experienced one or more episodes of embolism. When possible, anticoagulants should be administered for at least 2 weeks prior to attempts to reestablish sinus rhythm in order to minimize thromboembolic episodes associated with pharmacologic or electrical cardioversion.

SINOVENTRICULAR CONDUCTION This unusual dysrhythmia arises in the atria, in which impulses are initiated in the sinoatrial node in a normal fashion and are propagated via internodal pathways to the AV junction. However, spread of the impulse through atrial myocardium fails to occur, and hence no P wave is seen on the electrocardiogram, and atrial contraction is absent. Although the ventricular electrocardiographic complexes may be distorted because of aberrant conduction, ventricular rate varies, as it does in normal sinus rhythm when maneuvers such as carotid sinus stimulation are performed, with exercise, and following drug administration. The major significance of the dysrhythmia is loss of atrial transport function; also, when bizarre QRS complexes are present, there is the possibility of misdiagnosis as ventricular tachycardia.

Derangements arising in the AV junction

ECTOPIC JUNCTIONAL BEATS According to nomenclature popularized in the past, the configuration of the QRS complex on the electrocardiogram depends on whether the junctional beat is thought to originate in the high, mid-, or lower portion of the AV junction (the term junction refers to the AV node and the His bundle). Ectopic beats originating in the atrium near the AV junction exhibit a short P-R interval and P waves of unusual configuration which precede a ventricular complex which is normal in configuration, unless there is aberrant ventricular conduction. In earlier literature these beats were described as high nodal or coronary sinus beats. In fact, the AV node itself has no pacemaking cells. Thus, beats that have been called AV nodal beats actually originate in the atria or His bundle, and probably no junctional beats originate in the AV node itself, which is specialized for decremental conduction and accounts for the normal AV junctional delay of impulse transmission. When the impulse arises in the His bundle, retrograde atrial conduction causes impulse propagation into the atrium at about the same time that the impulse is propagated antegrade into the ventricular conduction system. Consequently, there is no visible electrocardiographic wave of atrial depolarization; again, the QRS complex is usually normal in configuration and duration, resembling a normal supraventricular beat but without a preceding visible P wave. Beats originating at a more distal site in the His-Purkinje system or those associated with delayed retrograde conduction into the atrium exhibit an abnormal P wave that regularly follows the QRS complex.

AV JUNCTIONAL TACHYCARDIAS These are of two types: *idiojunctional tachycardia*, with a ventricular rate usually between 100 and 140 beats per min; and *extrasystolic* (or paroxysmal) *AV junctional tachycardia*, with a ventricular rate generally between 140 and 200 beats per min. In the former there is acceleration of the inherent idiojunctional rhythm, which becomes evident when its rate exceeds that of the SA pacemaker. It may be a manifestation of digitalis toxicity, and has also been noted in patients with acute myocardial infarction and acute rheumatic fever. When idiojunctional tachycardia is due to digitalis toxicity it may be particularly grave, because it may degenerate into ventricular tachycardia and ventricular fibrillation. Reversion may occur after discontinuation of digitalis or administration of intravenous potassium. However, occasionally in critical situations, more vigorous therapy is required; in these instances lidocaine, procainamide, diphenylhydantoin, or propranolol may be effective. Paroxysmal AV junctional tachycardia resembles paroxysmal atrial tachycardia in its clinical significance and management, but is much less common.

AV JUNCTIONAL RHYTHM This is an escape rhythm which occurs when the sinus impulse fails to arrive at the AV junction because of sinoatrial depression, standstill, or block of the sinus impulse proximal to the AV junctional pacemaker. The ventricular rate is 40 to 60 beats per min, and the rhythm is regular. The QRS complex is generally identical to that of the conducted sinus impulses. No treatment is necessary, as the circulation is usually adequate, but atropine or isoproterenol may be helpful to speed the sinus rate if the circulation is compromised by a ventricular rate below 50 beats per min. The presence of AV junctional rhythm is a manifestation of a safety mechanism, rather than a primary derangement affecting the junctional pacemaker.

Derangements arising in the ventricles

ECTOPIC VENTRICULAR BEATS (Fig. 234-2*G*) These are relatively more frequent in patients with structural cardiac disease than ectopic atrial beats, but they are so common in healthy individuals that their presence has no diagnostic significance unless they are invoked or increase in numbers after exercise, originate from the left ventricle, occur during the vulnerable period, or occur in pairs or salvos (Chap. 34). Their prevalence increases markedly with age. In the absence of organic heart disease, premature beats may be due to excessive use of tobacco, coffee, tea, and occasionally alcohol, or to reflexes from the gastrointestinal tract; often they are caused by emotional stress, but in many patients the cause cannot be ascertained.

Ventricular ectopic beats are often easily recognized, as the ventricular depolarization and contraction occur before the next beat would ordinarily occur and are commonly followed by a compensatory pause. The patient may or may not be conscious of the premature beat. When extrasystoles are frequent, they may be confused with atrial fibrillation on clinical examination, an error that may sometimes be avoided by noting that the rhythm becomes regular when the heart rate is accelerated by exercise. There is still uncertainty whether ectopic ventricular beats are produced by an abnormal pacemaker or by reentry; probably each mechanism accounts for some instances of this disorder. In some patients ectopic ventricular beats and even ventricular tachycardia occur during episodes of severe bradycardia. When ectopic ventricular beats arise in an abnormal pacemaker, the latter is probably located in Purkinje cells rather than in myocardial cells per se. Ectopic beats may originate in a *parasystolic focus*, i.e., one "protected" from depolarization initiated elsewhere in the heart. The manifest rate of the parasystolic focus will depend on the degree of exit block from it, the refractoriness of surrounding myocardium, and the interplay between the rate of the focus and other pacemakers which are initiating impulses. Other ectopic beats originate in extrasystolic ventricular pacemakers which are not completely protected from depolarization by impulses arising in other pacemaker cells.

BIGEMINAL RHYTHM This is a state in which every alternate beat is premature; it may be caused by digitalis overdosage and disappears within a few days after the drug has been withheld. It should not be confused with *pulsus alternans* or with *paradoxic pulse*, conditions in which the rhythm remains regular. Bigeminy not due to digitalis is usually, though not always, associated with structural heart disease. Bigeminy probably results from several mechanisms, including electrical instability of the ectopic pacemaker during repolarization, reentry, and enhancement of spontaneous depolarization of the ectopic pacemaker by the preceding beat.

The *treatment of ectopic ventricular beats* depends on the clinical circumstances. When these beats occur occasionally, and evidence of cardiac disease is lacking, no treatment is necessary. If there is reason to believe that tobacco or coffee is a precipitating factor, its use should be discontinued or curtailed. In excitable patients, extrasystoles may disappear following the administration of a mild sedative, barbiturates, reserpine, or other tranquilizers. Ectopic ventricular beats, if caused by digitalis, will disappear if the drug is withdrawn; or if the irregularity occurs after the ingestion of a high-carbohydrate meal, it will be abolished by the administration of potassium. The occurrence of extrasystoles in undigitalized patients does not constitute a contraindication to the use of digitalis if the patient has congestive heart failure. Indeed, with the restoration of myocardial function, the irregularity will often disappear. Lidocaine, procainamide, diphenylhydantoin, and quinidine are all effective in the treatment, and the relative efficacy of each drug varies in different patients. In patients in whom the development of ventricular ectopic beats or ventricular tachycardia is precipitated by bradycardia, increasing the atrial rate with atropine may be helpful.

Although ectopic ventricular beats may ordinarily be considered a benign form of irregularity, the occurrence of numerous such beats may diminish the efficiency of the heart with an impaired cardiac reserve. Moreover, the appearance of ventricular extrasystoles following an acute myocardial infarction should not be viewed with complacency, since they may herald the onset of ventricular tachycardia. An isolated ventricular beat may occur in the "vulnerable" period at the end of the previous systole (the time during ventricular repolarization when recovery is asynchronous, the opportunity for reentry is maximized, and hence the ventricles are especially likely to develop ventricular fibrillation). Such beats are likely to initiate ventricular fibrillation and sudden death. It is for this reason that premature ventricular contractions occurring in patients with acute myocardial infarction should be treated vigorously, with intravenous lidocaine, procainamide, or diphenylhydantoin (Chap. 240). The treatment of premature ventricular contractions in other patients is discussed in Chap. 34.

VENTRICULAR TACHYCARDIA (Fig. 234-2*H*) This dysrhythmia is much less frequent and far more serious than paroxysmal atrial tachycardia. The commonest cause is ischemic heart disease, and ventricular tachycardia frequently occurs within a few days following the development of an acute myocardial infarction (Chap. 240). Less commonly, it is induced by digitalis or quinidine intoxication, and very rarely the arrhythmia appears spontaneously in otherwise healthy persons without any evidence of cardiac disease. The diagnosis should be suspected when the following clinical features are observed: (1) The patient has evidence of coronary disease or has been receiving digitalis or quinidine in large doses. (2) As a rule, there is no history of numerous previous attacks. (3) During the attack, the ventricular rate is usually between 150 and 210 beats per min, and although the rhythm is essentially regular, there are often slight variations in it. (4) Carotid sinus stimulation has no effect on the rate. (5) An intermittent jugular cannon A wave is present. (6) The first heart sound varies in intensity, because the relationship between atrial and ventricular contractions is inconstant. (7) Systolic blood pressure varies because of inconsistent contributions to ventricular filling by fortuitously timed atrial contractions.

Although these clues are useful, the clinical impression should be confirmed by an electrocardiogram, but the interpretation even of the ECG may be rendered difficult because atrial tachycardia may be associated with intraventricular conduction defects (aberrant QRS complexes) which cause the tracing to resemble that of ventricular tachycardia. The diagnosis is supported by evidence that the P-wave rate is independent of the ventricular rate, by evidence that in the intervals between attacks ventricular premature beats occur which are identical in form with the complexes seen during the paroxysm, and by the presence of fusion beats comprising components of depolarization initiated by impulses arising in a supraventricular pacemaker and in the ectopic ventricular site. Nevertheless, the electrocardiographic diagnosis frequently cannot be made with certainty. His bundle recordings may be helpful, since in ventricular tachycardia H spikes may be shown to follow rather than precede the QRS complex.

Since it is but one step removed from the frequently fatal *ventricular fibrillation*, ventricular tachycardia is the most serious of the ectopic tachycardias. If the attack occurs during a bout of acute myocardial infarction, immediate electric countershock is utilized (Chap. 236), but there is a strong possibility that another episode will occur soon after the first. Hence, a maintenance dose of an antiarrhythmic drug (e.g., intravenous lidocaine, procainamide, or diphenylhydantoin, parenteral or oral) should be continued until cardiac electrical activity has become demonstrably stable. When heart failure occurs in an undigitalized patient with ventricular tachycardia, digitalis should be administered despite the dysrhythmia, since the drug is not necessarily more hazardous in such patients than in those without the disturbance.

The cardiac rhythm of patients with ventricular tachycardia who are receiving large doses of quinidine or of procainamide may fail to revert to the normal sinus mechanism, but the ventricular rate may still show marked slowing, to 120 beats per min or less. Under these circumstances the administration of large doses of atropine (up to 2 mg intravenously) may increase the atrial rate to a level above that of the ectopic rhythm, which may permit the sinoatrial node to resume its normal role as pacemaker and restore the normal sinus mechanism; alternatively, atrial overdrive, i.e., electrical stimulation of the atria with an electrode catheter at a rate exceeding that of ventricular tachycardia, may exert a similar effect. The extracardiac toxicities of procainamide and quinidine are not necessarily additive, and therefore it may be desirable to use the drugs simultaneously in patients who are especially liable to such side effects as diarrhea and tinnitus (quinidine) or hypotension, nausea, or a lupus-like syndrome (procainamide).

VENTRICULAR FIBRILLATION (Fig. 234-2*I*) This chaotic rhythm may occur in very brief bursts, last for a few seconds, and then subside spontaneously, following which the rhythm previously present is resumed. These episodes are responsible for some of the Stokes-Adams attacks that occur in patients with prevailing slow rates due to high-grade AV block. Usually, however, unless it is recognized and treated immediately, ventricular fibrillation is synonymous with practically instantaneous death, since effective ventricular contraction and circulation cease (Chap. 34). Aside from AV block, ischemic heart disease is the most common cause of the dysrhythmia, particularly during attacks of acute myocardial infarction. There was no treatment for the calamitous disorder until introduction of externally applied electric shock (Chap. 236). Needless to say, this form of therapy must be applied promptly, because cessation of the circulation beyond 2 to 4 min leads to irreversible damage in the brain and heart. Thus, in individuals particularly susceptible to ventricular fibrillation, such as those with acute myocardial infarction or those with a history of Stokes-Adams attacks, the rhythm must be monitored constantly, and immediate availability and preparedness to apply external electric shock must be assured. Such precautions may be required for weeks, until cardiac electrical stability has been reestablished. In the absence of special equipment for delivering the countershock, closed-chest massage should be employed. This involves manual rhythmic compression of the sternum once per second, plus mouth-to-mouth respiration. Such maneuvers, described in Chap. 34, may be effective in sustaining life during the crucial time required to secure and apply the apparatus needed for countershock.

AV dissociation

As its name implies, in this dysrhythmia the atria and ventricles are controlled by two independent pacemakers. Fundamentally, it may occur in two forms, with antegrade AV block and without it. In the first type, the ventricles are excited by a pacemaker in the AV junction, or the Purkinje system, because impulses arising in the sinoatrial node or atria are blocked in the AV conduction system. In AV dissociation *without* antegrade block the automaticity of the AV junction or ventricle exceeds that of the supraventricular pacemaker, and the impulses from the atrium, while normally conducted to the ventricles, usually find these tissues refractory. Occasionally, the regular ventricular rhythm may be interrupted by a normally conducted impulse which arrives fortuitously, at an instant when the ventricle is not refractory. More precisely, this rhythm should be termed *AV dissociation without antegrade block with capture.* This dysrhythmia must be associated with some degree of retrograde block, or else the atria would be depolarized by the more rapidly firing AV junctional or ventricular pacemaker.

Abnormalities of conduction

Sinoatrial block, which represents a disorder of excitation, has been considered above (page 1137). The term *heart block* as herein employed refers to a condition in which the wave of excitation from the atria is delayed pathologically (or blocked) at the junctional tissues (AV node and His bundle). The P-R interval represents the time required for the impulse to traverse the atrium, the AV node. His bundle, and the bundle branches. The generally accepted upper limit of normal in adults is 0.20 sec; it is somewhat shorter in children. When the P-R interval exceeds the normal duration and all the atrial beats are followed by ventricular beats, *first-degree AV block* exists. A more advanced disturbance in the conduction system, *second-degree block*, is present when from time to time the atrial impulses are incapable of penetrating the conduction system sufficiently to excite the ventricles. *Third-degree* or *complete AV block* describes the condition in which the conduction system is so altered that no atrial impulses reach the ventricles, and the atria and ventricles maintain separate and independent rhythms (atrioventricular dissociation due to third-degree antegrade AV block).

AV block is a general term describing impaired conduction. Despite repeated usage of this term, the actual site(s) of impairment is not necessarily in the AV node itself. Block may exist because of impaired conduction in the atrial myocardium adjacent to the node (AN region); the node itself (N region); or the bundle of His adjacent to the node (NH region). Furthermore, block may exist only in more distal portions of the conduction system, i.e., the His bundle, the right or left bundle branches, or the anterior or posterior fascicles of the latter (Chap. 229). Thus, "AV block" with P-R prolongation on the electrocardiogram may be due in reality to delayed conduction only in distal ramifications of the conduction system, or fascicular block. At each site block may be partial (first or second degree) or complete (third degree), and various sites of block may occur singly or in combination. As discussed below, bundle branch or fascicular block is generally associated with pathologic conditions other than those associated with AV junctional block proper, and it generally indicates a different prognosis. In addition, the electrocardiographic manifestations of these two classes of block are often different. Definitive differentiation between fascicular block and AV junctional block is possible with the aid of His bundle recordings (Fig. 234-1). In third-degree trifascicular block (involving the right bundle and both fascicles of the left bundle branch) ventricular depolarizations occur independently of His bundle depolarizations. However, when block occurs in the AV junction proximal to the His bundle, each ventricular depolarization is preceded by a His bundle depolarization separated from it by the normal interval of approximately 50 msec.

FIRST-DEGREE AV BLOCK (Fig. 234-2*J*) This is usually due to impaired conduction in the AV junction, i.e., proximal to the His bundle. It may be caused by digitalis or by any of the inflammatory, toxic, degenerative, or vascular processes that may affect the heart. Prolongation of the P-R interval, for example as seen in patients with acute rheumatic fever, may be suspected when the intensity of the first heart sound suddenly declines without any other change in the clinical picture and without evidence of fluid in the pericardium, or in patients with mitral stenosis when a presystolic murmur becomes middiastolic in the absence of atrial fibrillation. P-R prolongation may be due to increased vagal tone in a healthy, normal person. In the absence of any other evidence of disease, this one electrocardiographic deviation from an arbitrary norm should not be construed as evidence of organic heart disease, and it requires no treatment.

SECOND-DEGREE, OR PARTIAL AV BLOCK (Fig. 234-2*K*) This form may be divided into two groups. In the *Möbitz type I block*, the P-R interval increases progressively until finally a propagation of an impulse originating in the atrium is completely blocked, the corresponding ventricular beat dropping out (Wenckebach block, Fig. 234-2*M*). The P-R interval after the pause shortens to within the normal range, but each successive one lengthens, and the cycle is repeated periodically. The dropped beat may occur after six to eight conducted beats, or it may take place after every second atrial impulse, thus giving rise to 2:1 AV block and becoming indistinguishable at first glance from the other type of 2:1 block (Möbitz type II), to be described below. With type I block the QRS duration is usually normal. Inhibition of vagal tone, as by intravenous injection of atropine (1 to 2 mg) or exercise, may help to differentiate these two types of block. In type I, the block often diminishes or disappears with such a procedure, whereas with Möbitz type II block it increases or it may temporarily change into a complete AV block. Möbitz type I second-degree block is often due to abnormal conduction in the AV junction proximal to the His bundle; it is frequently accentuated or precipitated by heightened vagal tone, occurring spontaneously or after carotid sinus pressure or following digitalis therapy. It is usually a transitory phenomenon and requires no treatment unless hemodynamic disturbances result or the extent of block increases.

Möbitz type II block is usually a more serious disorder. The P-R interval is either normal or increased but fixed except when beats are dropped; QRS duration is often prolonged. The dysrhythmia exhibits dropped beats, i.e., 2:1, 3:1, or 4:1 block or irregular ratios. This form of block usually results from block in the His bundle or trifascicular block and may be caused acutely by myocardial infarction or by various forms of myocarditis. Although it may be transient, it may progress suddenly to complete block. Idiopathic sclerosis producing damage of the conduction system (Lenegre's disease) and fibrocalcific degeneration of the myocardium involving the conduction system as well (Lev's disease) are perhaps the most common causes of chronic Möbitz type II block. It may also result from coronary narrowing in the absence of an acute episode of infarction; calcification of the mitral annulus; extension of the lesion of calcific aortic stenosis into the septum; any of the diffuse disorders of the myocardium such as cardiac amyloidosis; or congenital heart disease, usually an interventricular septal defect. This type of second-degree block is sometimes characterized by a unique phenomenon, a slowing of the ventricular rate during exercise as 2:1 block suddenly appears when the atrial rate increases.

Syncopal attacks (Stokes-Adams attacks) are common in type II block, and they have the characteristics of all such syncopal attacks that are due to a sudden cessation of the circulation (Chap. 16). The attacks occur suddenly and without warning, with the patient in either the upright or recumbent posture. In contrast, premonitory lightheadedness, faintness, and "blacking out" usually precede simple emotional vasovagal syncope, which develops with the patient in the upright position and is relieved by the recumbent posture. If the heart of a patient with Möbitz type II 2:1 block is monitored during or shortly after the lapse of consciousness, ventricular standstill (or less commonly fibrillation) will be recorded during the syncopal period, often followed by complete block in the early recovery state, 2:1 block being restored after a variable interval. When a person with a slow heart rate or with an electrocardiogram showing second-degree block develops a characteristic syncopal attack, the diagnosis should be simple. However, in a number of patients, syncopal attacks may appear at relatively long intervals over a number of years, during which time the electrocardiogram between episodes remains normal and the P-R interval stays well within the normal range. Intravenous administration of atropine in such persons may unmask concealed block, since the AV conduction system may be unable to follow the accelerated sinus rate. Eventually, most people with type II block, whether overt or concealed, will develop complete block if they do not first succumb in a Stokes-Adams attack.

COMPLETE OR THIRD-DEGREE AV BLOCK (Fig. 234-2*L*) This advanced form of block is caused by any of the disorders responsible for type II second-degree block, as well as by accidental surgical trauma to the AV node or His bundle. Occasionally, one encounters an otherwise normal person with congenital AV block, and rarely a patient with persistent complete block will be found at autopsy to display no demonstrable microscopic lesion in the conduction system. A transitory form, lasting a few seconds, may follow carotid sinus pressure, and it may also be a consequence of digitalis intoxication, disappearing a week or two after the drug is withdrawn. Most cases of chronic and persistent complete heart block are infra-AV nodal, i.e., due to block in the bundle of His or bilateral bundle branch block. The ventricular rate is usually 45 beats per min or less, although in congenital heart block, which is usually due to AV junctional block proximal to the His bundle, the rate may be as rapid as 60 beats per min. In either case the rhythm is regular, and the rate increases only slightly or not at all after exercise. The lesion tends to occur proximal to the bifurcation of the bundle of His in patients with congenital heart block, while acquired third-degree AV block and Möbitz type II second-degree block are usually bilateral bundle branch or trifascicular blocks. When the subsidiary pacemaker is in the AV node or the bundle of His, as is usual in congenital heart block, the QRS complex is usually normal; when it is below the bifurcation of the bundle of His, i.e., within the Purkinje system, as is usual in acquired heart block, the QRS complex is prolonged, notched, and slurred. The intensity of the first heart sound varies from beat to beat, being sometimes almost inaudible and at other times so loud as to merit the term *bruit de canon*; faint atrial contractions can also often be heard, possibly because of diastolic mitral regurgitation caused by atrial relaxation with a momentary reduction of atrial pressure below the ventricular level.

Acute myocardial infarction often precipitates AV block (Chap. 240). Infarcts associated with ischemia in the distribution of the right coronary artery (e.g., inferior or posterior infarctions) commonly cause AV junctional block which is due to impaired conduction proximal to the His bundle bifurcation, is transient, and is usually first or second degree (Möbitz type I block). Even when third-degree block occurs in this setting, recovery of conduction may generally be anticipated. On the other hand, heart block associated with infarcts due to ischemia in the distribution of the left coronary artery is less common and more grave. It usually results from extensive damage of the His bundle and/or all three fascicles of the conduction system, is persistent, and presents as second-degree Möbitz type II or third-degree trifascicular block. The mortality rate associated with infarcts producing this type of block is high, even despite the indicated pacemaker therapy, because of the massive nature of the infarct responsible.

Because myocardial infarction is so common, it is by far the commonest cause of acute AV block. However, coronary artery disease is responsible for only a minority of cases of chronic and persistent complete heart block, which is usually due to primary or secondary degeneration or inflammation of the conduction system.

The prognosis of first- and second-degree, Möbitz type I, AV block is favorable. The outlook for high grades of block (second-degree Möbitz type II or complete AV block) is always uncertain, since the patient is constantly subject to the risk of Stokes-Adams attacks, any of which may be fatal. When such attacks occur frequently in patients with complete block and are uncontrolled, death usually occurs within a year. AV block occurring in the course of acute myocardial infarction is often transient, and if the patient survives with the aid of a pacemaker catheter, sinus rhythm is usually restored after several days. In addition to the hazards of Stokes-Adams attacks, complete AV block may lead to impairment of cardiac reserve or frank heart failure.

TREATMENT OF HEART BLOCK The important problem is the prevention of the Stokes-Adams attacks. Accordingly, in all patients with symptomatic or high-grade block, definitive therapy and the treatment of choice consist of implantation of a permanent transvenous pacemaker. In emergency situations, every effort should be made for prompt institution of pacemaker therapy without undue reliance on drugs. Atropine and isoproterenol or epinephrine are useful adjuncts to accelerate ventricular rate acutely and temporarily. However, since the latter two agents increase myocardial oxygen demand, they may increase ischemic injury or lead to prolonged anginal attacks, if used chronically. Other adjuncts employed in the past include corticotropin and corticosteroids, although the mechanism of their beneficial effect is uncertain. Because potassium depletion accelerates conduction, chlorothiazide, 500 to 1,000 mg, combined with sodium bicarbonate, 10 g, given t.i.d., has been found to exert a favorable effect in some patients with incomplete heart block. In life-threatening situations, external pacemakers may be used for ventricular standstill, external countershock may be applied for ventricular fibrillation, and life may be sustained by these measures and by closed-chest cardiac massage until intracardiac pacing by means of a catheter electrode has been achieved.

When AV block is not complete, digitalis therapy may either improve or worsen its degree. Hence the drug should be withheld unless congestive failure fails to respond to other measures and until a pacemaker has been implanted. Under no circumstances should quinidine, procainamide, or beta-adrenergic blockers be used in the presence of high-grade block unless the ventricular rhythm is first controlled by an artificial electrical pacemaker. However, these agents are useful in patients with complete heart block who manifest frequent ventricular premature contractions despite continued ventricular pacing.

BUNDLE BRANCH BLOCK DISORDERS (Fig. 234-2*P*, *Q*) These are examples of impaired conduction in a specific portion of the conducting system (Chap. 229). When the duration of the QRS complex exceeds 0.12 sec and when the main deflection is positive in leads I and V_6 and negative in leads III and V_1, left bundle branch block is said to be present. Similar prolongation but with opposite directional deflections in the leads mentioned is characteristic of right bundle branch block. Lesser degrees of QRS lengthening are often designated as incomplete left or right bundle branch block. In some instances the ventricular complex may be markedly prolonged without these typical changes; such disturbances are usually considered to be *intraventricular blocks.*

Bundle branch block is related to delayed spread of ventricular excitation. The commonest causes are ischemic heart disease, inflammatory or infiltrative disease of the myocardium, and marked left or right ventricular hypertrophy, with associated delay of impulse propagation via unusual conduction pathways. None of the numerous physical signs which have been attributed to bundle branch block is wholly reliable, although paradoxic splitting of the second heart sound (Chap. 228) may suggest underlying left bundle branch block. The electrocardiogram remains the only consistently accurate method of diagnosis.

These disturbances of conduction are usually encountered in persons with advanced myocardial disease or severe pressure loads, but they may be seen in association with volume loads, incomplete right bundle branch block in atrial septal defect (Chap. 237) being a classic example. It is probable that the abnormal sequence of contraction consequent to the disordered spread of excitation impairs further the effectiveness of ventricular systole. In a patient with heart failure, marked prolongation of the QRS complex adds to the gravity of the prognosis. However, when right bundle branch block is discovered for the first time in an asymptomatic person under the age of forty years who lacks all other objective evidence of cardiac disease, the outlook is excellent, since in this setting, right bundle branch block is probably often of congenital origin and associated with little or no structural heart disease. In asymptomatic patients of any age with left bundle branch block, and in those with right bundle branch block who are older than forty, the prognosis is less certain, because there is always the possibility that the conduction disorder may be the sole manifestation of ischemic heart disease. The treatment of bundle branch block is that of the associated disorder.

THE WOLFF-PARKINSON-WHITE (WPW) SYNDROME (ANOMALOUS ATRIOVENTRICULAR EXCITATION) (Fig. 234-2*N*) This example of a group of *preexcitation syndromes* is a congenital or acquired disorder characterized by the presence of normal P waves, a P-R interval of 0.11 sec or less, increased QRS duration, a slur on the initial phase of the QRS complex (delta wave), and a pronounced tendency for the occurrence of atrial tachyarrhythmias, especially paroxysmal tachycardia, atrial flutter, and atrial fibrillation. Variations include the presence of some but not all of these electrocardiographic features, such as the *Lown-Ganong-Levine syndrome* (LGL syndrome), which is manifested by a short P-R interval but no delta wave or QRS widening. Recent anatomic and electrophysiologic studies have led to a general concept embracing these disorders. The common denominator appears to be the presence of an anatomic and/or functional anomalous conduction pathway which bypasses the AV node (Fig. 234-3). Conduction through the anomalous pathway may be manifest or occult. In the classical Wolff-Parkinson-White syndrome the sinus impulse is conducted concomitantly down the anomalous pathway and the normal pathway. Accordingly, the impulse fragments longitudinally. Ventricular excitation is a composite of early excitation (preexcitation) by the impulse traversing the anomalous pathway and hence not delayed in the AV node, and normal excitation by the impulse conducted normally through the AV node. Thus, "normal" beats are fusion beats containing a delta (preexcitation) wave, accounting for QRS prolongation. The activation from the preexcitation impulse travels more slowly through ventricular myocardium than does the normal impulse through the specialized His-Purkinje system once it has traversed the AV node. Accordingly, a large portion of ventricular depolarization is due to normal conduction, and the preexcitation wave is extinguished by the activation front of the normally conducted impulse.

Surgical interruption of the anomalous pathway (the bundle of Kent) then restores the normal P-R interval and normal QRS duration and obliterates the delta wave. It also eliminates recurrence of atrial tachycardias. Other potential AV node–bypass pathways exist, such as the bypass tract of James and the fibers of Mahaim. However, in many instances the anatomic pathways responsible for anomalous conduction cannot be identified.

Anomalous conduction pathways underlie the genesis of the supraventricular tachyarrhythmias so common in patients with these disorders. Usually these dysrhythmias are initiated by a premature supraventricular beat which finds the anomalous pathway refractory and the normal pathway excitable. Accordingly, impulse transmission proceeds antegrade through the normal pathway; the impulse fragments in the AV node; *antegrade* conduction proceeds within one fragment, leading to ventricular excitation; *retrograde* conduction of the other fragment proceeds through the anomalous pathway, which has become excitable by this time; and the tachyarrhythmia persists because when the impulse reaches the normal pathway again it can be retransmitted antegrade in a persistently reciprocating manner. Thus, during the tachycardia QRS complexes are normal and do not exhibit a delta wave. A fortuitously timed premature beat will terminate the tachycardia by resetting the refractory period of one or both pathways so that the circus movement is interrupted. Termination may occur also by block in one or the other of the pathways, or in both of them, sufficient to interrupt the reciprocating impulse and allow reemergence of sinus pacemaker activity.

A similar mechanism probably underlies many so-called ectopic supraventricular tachyarrhythmias in patients without electrocardiographic evidence of preexcitation. In such cases the anomalous pathway may simply represent longitudinal functional stratification within the AV junction, allowing for fragmentation of impulse propagation because of disparity between recovery times of two or more longitudinal pathways. In many patients with preexcitation syndromes the electrocardiogram shifts between the abnormal preexcitation and the normal intraventricular conduction pattern. The normal pattern may reveal abnormalities masked by the preexcitation form.

Two classical Wolff-Parkinson-White patterns have been recognized. In group A the delta wave is directed anteriorly and there are tall R waves in right precordial leads; in some instances deep Q waves are present in lead aVF. In group B the delta wave is directed to the left and posteriorly, resulting in a Q-S wave over the right precordium and tall R waves in left precordial leads. Therefore, in both types, the tracing may be mistaken for QRS abnormalities indicative of myocardial infarction. The shift to anomalous conduction can sometimes be induced by vagal stimulation, such as that produced by carotid sinus pressure or by digitalis given intravenously. The normal type of conduction may be elicited by vagal inhibition with atropine or exercise, and also by quinidine and procainamide. As noted earlier, during paroxysms of tachycardia, the widened, ventricular complexes usually assume a normal configuration.

The preexcitation syndrome should be suspected in any person subject to paroxysms of tachycardia, particularly when they have occurred from youth. Any patient with a supraventricular tachyarrhythmia in which the ventricular rate exceeds 200 beats per min is a likely candidate, because normal AV nodal delay of conduction usually precludes rates this rapid. Digitalis may terminate a paroxysm of rapid heart action, but it may also paradoxically increase the ventricular rate by facilitating conduction through the AV node–bypass pathway; propranolol is more effective. Procainamide and quinidine control attacks in some patients, perhaps by diminishing the incidence of the precipitating premature beats. Repetitive attacks may be disabling, and rarely sudden death occurs during an attack. If maintenance propranolol or other pharmacologic prophylaxis is ineffective, two procedures merit consideration: implantation of a transvenous atrial, coronary sinus, or ventricular pacemaker which can be activated to interrupt the tachycardia by initiating an appropriately timed beat; and surgical interruption of the anomalous pathway identified by epicardial mapping in carefully selected patients.

REFERENCES

Damato AN et al: Application of His bundle recordings in diagnosing conduction disorders. Prog Cardiovasc Dis 14:601, 1972

Durrer D et al: Pre-excitation revisited. Am J Cardiol 25:690, 1970

Hurst JW et al: Cardiac arrhythmias and conduction disturbances, chap. 32 in *The Heart*, 3d ed., ed JW Hurst, New York: McGraw-Hill, 1974, pp. 495–558

Lown B, Kosowsky BD: Artificial cardiac pacemakers. N Engl J Med 283:907, 971, 1023, 1970

——, Levine SA: The carotid sinus; clinical value of its stimulation. Circulation 23:766, 1961

—— et al: Paroxysmal atrial tachycardia with block. Circulation 21:129, 1960

Papp C: New look at arrhythmias. Br Heart J 31:267, 1969

Rosenbaum MB et al: Intraventricular trifascicular block. Review of the literature and classification. Am Heart J 78:450, 1969

Schamroth L: *The Disorders of Cardiac Rhythm*, Oxford: Blackwell Scientific Publications, Ltd., 1971

Scherlag BJ et al: Catheter technique for recording His bundle activity in man. Circulation 39:13, 1969

Symposium on Cardiac Arrhythmias. Circulation 47:January–June, 1973

Wolff L: Diagnostic clues in the Wolff-Parkinson-White syndrome. N Engl J Med 261:637, 1959

235
PHARMACOLOGIC TREATMENT OF CARDIOVASCULAR DISORDERS

PETER E. POOL
EUGENE BRAUNWALD

The direct cardiac action of drugs may be divided into four major areas: (1) an effect on *contractility* (inotropic effect), reflecting alterations in the myocardial force-velocity relation at any given initial muscle length (Chap. 232); (2) an effect on heart rate, expressed as an alteration in the *rhythmicity*, i.e., the frequency of discharge of normal pacemaker tissue, generally that in the sinoatrial node; (3) an effect on *conductivity*, i.e., on the velocity with which the depolarization wave travels through the myocardium and the atrioventricular conduction system; (4) an effect on *irritability*, referring to the tendency to develop ectopic pacemaker activity, which is dependent on the rate of diastolic depolarization and the threshold potential. In addition to these direct effects, drugs may also alter any or all of these four properties indirectly by altering (1) autonomic influences acting on the heart or (2) the relationship between myocardial oxygen supply (determined largely by coronary blood flow) and oxygen needs.

CARDIAC STIMULANTS **Digitalis glycosides** The basic molecular structure of the digitalis glycosides is a steroid nucleus to which an unsaturated lactone ring is attached at C_{17} (Fig. 235-1*A*). These two elements are called the *aglycone* or *genin*, and it is this portion of the molecule which is responsible for the cardiotonic activity. The addition of a sugar to this basic structure enhances both the potency of the glycoside and the duration of its action, probably as a result of increasing solubility, which allows increased cell penetration. The sugar residue may prevent alterations in the steric structure of the molecule, which would result in a loss of cardiotonic activity.

Although, in the absence of severe malabsorption, digitalis is adequately absorbed from the intestinal tract even in the presence of vascular congestion secondary to heart failure, some glycosides, including ouabain, are poorly absorbed and therefore are effective only when administered parenterally; the intravenous route is preferable to the intramuscular, since absorption is erratic with the latter. When they are administered orally, absorption is close to complete within 2 hr. The fraction of orally administered glycoside which is absorbed varies. Approximately 40 percent of digitalis powder is absorbed, 80 percent of digoxin, and almost 100 percent of digitoxin. Considerable variability of absorption has been found in different commercial preparations of digoxin. Varying degrees of protein binding occur in the bloodstream, and though these differences may account in part for the varying duration of the effect of different glycosides, they are not related to the speed of action of these drugs. The glycosides are directly bound by various tissues, including the heart, but cardiac muscle binds no more glycoside than does kidney or skeletal muscle and actually substantially less than does the liver.

Digitoxin, with a half-life of approximately 7 days, is metabolized chiefly in the liver; digoxin (half-life of 1.5 days) is filtered in the glomeruli and is largely excreted in the urine in unchanged form. Digoxin and the degradation products of digitoxin are chiefly eliminated through the kidneys, and in man biliary excretion is negligible. Serious reductions of the glomerular filtration rate reduce the elimination of tritiated digoxin and therefore may prolong its effect, allowing it to accumulate to toxic levels.

The cardiac effects of all digitalis glycosides are alike; they are listed in Table 235-1. These effects result from augmenting contractility and irritability and from slowing heart rate and atrioventricular conduction. In addition, the cardiac glycosides potentiate the vagal effect on the heart. The most important effect of digitalis on cardiac muscle is to shift its force-velocity relation upward (Chap. 232). This positive inotropic effect is present in normal and nonfailing hypertrophied hearts as well as in failing hearts. In the absence of heart failure, however, when cardiac output is not limited by the contractility of the heart, the drug does not elevate the cardiac output. The finding that digitalis increases the contractility of the nonfailing heart has led to its increasing use prophylactically in patients with heart disease prior to operation or other stressful situations such as serious infections, or in the presence of a chronically increased load, such as hypertension without heart failure. However, definitive evidence of the advantage of its use in these circumstances has not been demonstrated.

Digitalis exerts a negative chronotropic effect, which in part is a vagal effect and in part is due to a direct action on the sinus pacemaker. In heart failure, slowing of the sinus rate following the administration of digitalis results also from withdrawal of sympathetic activity secondary to general improvement in circulatory status due to the positive inotropic effect of the glycoside. In the nonfailing heart the slowing effect is negligible, and digitalis should not be used for the treatment of sinus tachycardia unless heart failure is present. The apparent suppression of pacemaker activity which may take place following high doses of digitalis is probably due not to arrest of the pacemaker but rather to a sinoatrial block related to a depression of conduction.

The slowing of ventricular rate in atrial fibrillation and flutter is due to prolongation of the refractory period of the atrioventricular junction. It also slows conduction through the atrioventricular nodal system. However, conduction velocity is slightly increased in the atrium and ventricle by low doses. Digitalis may increase automaticity sufficiently to initiate pacemaker activity in Purkinje cells and in this manner may lead to the development of ventricular premature beats, bigeminal rhythm, atrial, AV junctional, or ventricular tachycardia, or ventricular fibrillation.

Excitation-contraction coupling is the membrane and intracellular process (p. 1308) most likely involved in producing the positive inotropic effect of digitalis glycosides. The biochemical events probably involve inhibition by digitalis of cell membrane sodium-potassium-activated ATPase and the resulting altered transmembrane distribution of sodium, i.e., an elevation of the intracellular concentration of this ion, which leads to an increased uptake of calcium by the sarcolemma; the latter results in an increment of calcium released to the myofilaments during excitation and therefore a positive inotropic response.

In addition, the digitalis glycosides also have an action on the peripheral vasculature, causing venous and arterial constriction in normal individuals and reflex dilatation in patients with congestive heart failure.

The most important indication for the administration of digitalis is congestive heart failure (Chap. 233). By improving the contractile function of the heart, digitalis aids in restoring normal circulatory function. Another important indication is atrial fibrillation or flutter with a rapid ventricular response (Chap. 234). Digitalis is also indicated both in the prevention and the treatment of recurrent episodes of paroxysmal supraventricular tachycardia. It is of relatively little value in some forms of cardiomyopathy, myocarditis (Chap. 242), beriberi with heart failure, and cor pulmonale when the lung disease is not being treated concurrently. Although digitalis is one of the cornerstones of treatment for heart failure, it is a two-edged sword, because intoxication due to digitalis excess is a common, serious, and potentially fatal complication of its use. The therapeutic to toxic ratio is identical in all cardiac glycosides, and in most patients with heart failure the lethal dose of most glycosides is probably five to ten times the minimal effective dose and only about twice the dose which leads to minor toxic manifestations. In addition, old age, acute myocardial infarction, hypoxemia, magnesium depletion, renal insufficiency, calcium administration, carotid sinus massage, d-c (direct current) cardioversion (Chap. 236), and hypothyroidism all may reduce the tolerance of the patient to the digitalis glycosides or provoke latent digitalis intoxication. The most common precipitating cause of digitalis intoxication, however, is depletion of potassium stores, which often occurs as a result of diuretic therapy and secondary hyperaldosteronism.

Anorexia, nausea, and vomiting, which are among the earliest signs of acute digitalis intoxication, are caused by

FIGURE 235-1
Chemical structure of various cardioactive drugs.

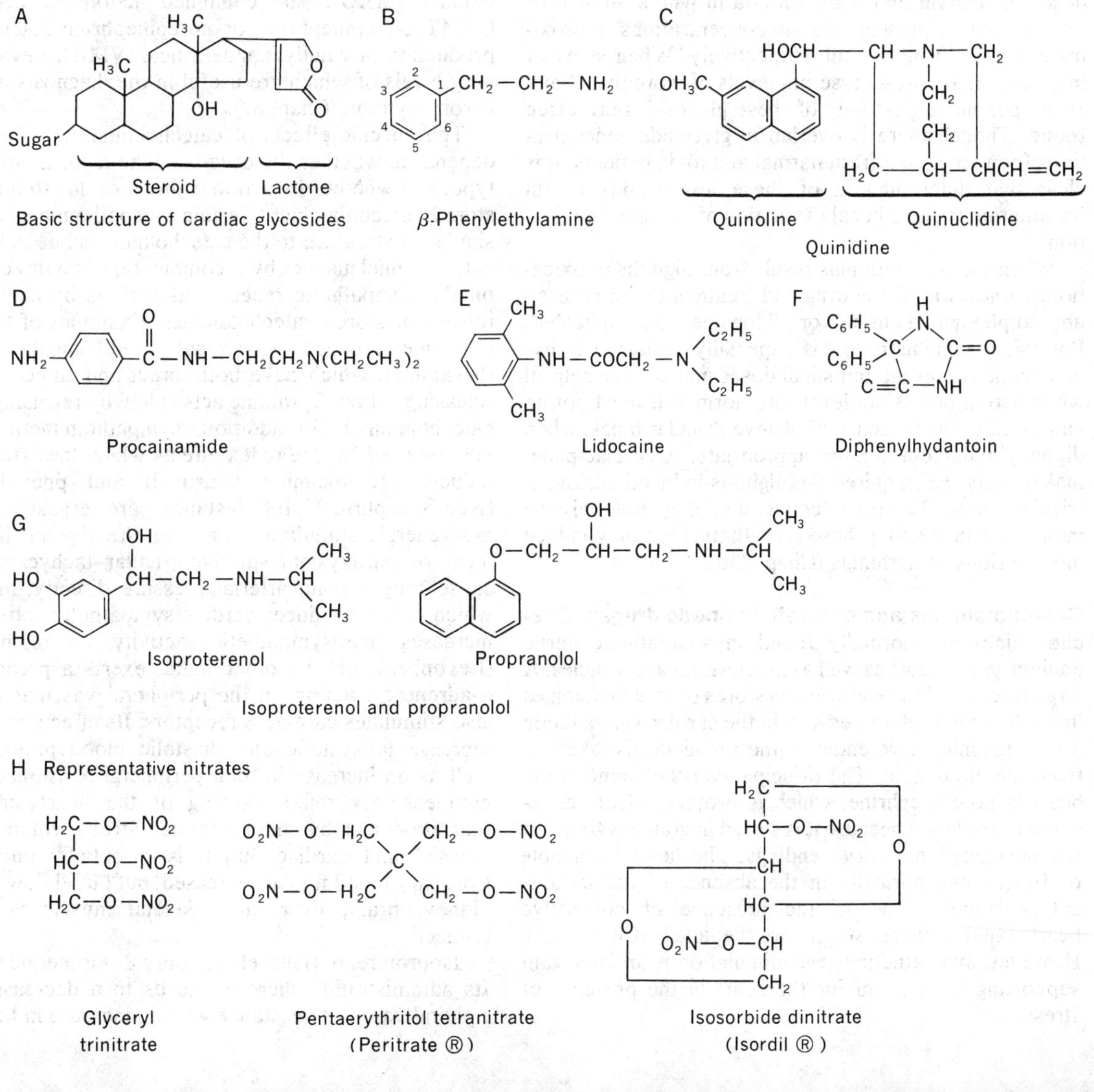

A
H_3C
H_3C
OH
O
O
Sugar
Steroid
Lactone
Basic structure of cardiac glycosides

B
2
3
1
4
6
5
$CH_2-CH_2-NH_2$
β-Phenylethylamine

C
$HOCH-CH-N-CH_2$
OH_3C
CH_2
CH_2
$H_2C-CH-CHCH=CH_2$
Quinoline
Quinuclidine
Quinidine

D
$NH_2-C_6H_4-C(=O)-NH-CH_2CH_2N(CH_2CH_3)_2$
Procainamide

E
CH_3
$NH-COCH_2-N(C_2H_5)_2$
CH_3
Lidocaine

F
H
C_6H_5
C_6H_5
N
C
C=O
C=C—NH
Diphenylhydantoin

G
OH
HO
HO
$CH-CH_2-NH-CH(CH_3)_2$
Isoproterenol

OH
$O-CH_2-CH-CH_2-NH-CH(CH_3)_2$
Propranolol

Isoproterenol and propranolol

H Representative nitrates

$H_2C-O-NO_2$
$HC-O-NO_2$
$H_2C-O-NO_2$
Glyceryl trinitrate

O_2N-O-H_2C CH_2-O-NO_2
C
O_2N-O-H_2C CH_2-O-NO_2
Pentaerythritol tetranitrate (Peritrate ®)

H_2C
$HC-O-NO_2$
O
CH
HC
O
$O_2N-O-CH$
CH_2
Isosorbide dinitrate (Isordil ®)

direct stimulation of centers in the medulla and are not of gastrointestinal origin. The most frequent disturbance of cardiac rhythm caused by digitalis is premature ventricular beats, which may take the form of bigeminy because of increased myocardial irritability or facilitation of reentry. Atrioventricular block of varying degrees of severity may occur. Nonparoxysmal atrial tachycardia with variable atrioventricular block is quite characteristic of digitalis intoxication. Finally, sinus arrhythmia, sinoatrial block, sinus arrest, atrioventricular junctional and multifocal ventricular tachycardia may also occur. Chronic digitalis intoxication, on the other hand, may be insidious in onset and may be characterized by exacerbations of heart failure, weight loss, and cachexia, neuralgias, gynecomastia, yellow vision, and delirium in the elderly.

Digitalis intoxication has been reported to occur in more than 20 percent of hospitalized patients receiving a cardiac glycoside, which emphasizes the importance of the ability to diagnose this condition. The radioimmunoassay for digoxin and digitoxin makes possible the correlation of serum glycoside levels with the presence of toxicity. In patients receiving standard maintenance doses of digoxin and digitoxin and in whom no sign of intoxication is present, serum concentrations approximate 1 and 20 ng per ml, respectively. When signs of intoxication are present, serum levels of more than 2 and 30 ng per ml respectively of these glycosides are often found. Though there is overlap in glycoside concentrations found in serum from normal and toxic patients, it is clear that determination of these levels adds useful information to the clinical evaluation of digitalis intoxication.

When tachyarrhythmias result from digitalis intoxication, withdrawal of the drug and treatment with potassium, diphenylhydantoin, or lidocaine are indicated. Potassium administration is especially indicated if hypokalemia is present, but small doses may also be helpful when serum potassium levels are normal; it must not be employed in the presence of atrioventricular block, when diphenylhydantoin is more appropriate. A cardiac pacemaker may be required in digitalis-induced atrioventricular block. Electrical conversion may not only be ineffective in treating these arrhythmias but may induce more serious arrhythmias (Chap. 236).

Catecholamines and sympathomimetic drugs Catecholamines are normally found in sympathetic nerve endings in the heart as well as in arterioles and venules. A large fraction of the endogenous stores of catecholamines in the heart is synthesized within the cardiac sympathetic postganglionic nerve endings; the remainder is taken up from the circulation. The principal catecholamine in the heart is norepinephrine, which is protected from enzymatic degradation because it is stored in granules found in the postganglionic nerve endings. The heart is capable of functioning normally in the absence of endogenous catecholamines, and in the presence of congestive heart failure, these stores are depleted (Chap. 233). However, sympathetic nerve stimulation is an important supporting mechanism for the heart in the presence of stress.

Catecholamines and other sympathomimetic drugs act upon the circulation by stimulating adrenergic receptors in the effector organs. Activation of α-adrenergic receptors results in vasoconstriction, leading to a pressor response. Stimulation of β-adrenergic receptors results in vascular dilatation and stimulation of cardiac contractility, automaticity, conduction velocity, and irritability (Table 235-1).

The catecholamines are based on the β-phenylethylamine molecule, an aromatic nucleus consisting of a benzene ring and an aliphatic portion, ethylamine (Fig. 235-1*B*). In general, these compounds have a brief duration of action. When administered orally they are rapidly inactivated in the intestinal wall and liver and are therefore ineffective. Epinephrine is rapidly absorbed after intramuscular injection. However, norepinephrine should be administered only intravenously, because it produces necrosis of tissue consequent to intense vasoconstriction when given intramuscularly or subcutaneously. Isoproterenol may be administered parenterally, as an aerosol, or sublingually.

Catecholamines may be inactivated by ortho-methylation by the enzyme catechol ortho-methyl transferase (COMT), or they may be deaminated by monoamine oxidase (MAO). The combined action of MAO and COMT on epinephrine or norepinephrine leads to the production of vanillylmandelic acid (VMA), elevated urinary levels of which are useful in the diagnosis of pheochromocytoma (Chap. 87).

The specific effects of catecholamine administration depend on whether the drug is of the α- or β-adrenergic type, and whether its action is direct or due to release of stored catecholamines. Certain sympathomimetic drugs, similar in structure to the catecholamines but lacking the catechol nucleus, act by a combination of a direct action on the sympathetic receptor as well as by causing the release of stored catecholamines. Examples of this type are metaraminol (Aramine) and mephentermine (Wyamine), which have both direct and catecholamine-releasing action. Tyramine acts solely by releasing stored catecholamines. In addition, sympathomimetic agents may be used for the reflex effects which they frequently induce. Methoxamine (Vasoxyl) and phenylephrine (Neo-Synephrine), for instance, are essentially pure α-adrenergic stimulators, and are effective in the treatment of paroxysmal supraventricular tachycardias because they elevate arterial pressure directly, an effect which reflexly reduces cardiac sympathetic activity and increases parasympathetic activity. Norepinephrine (Levophed), on the other hand, exerts a predominant α-adrenergic action on the peripheral vascular bed but also stimulates cardiac β receptors. Its effects include an increase in systolic and diastolic blood pressures, as well as an increase in total peripheral resistance with a compensatory reflex slowing of the heart similar to that produced by methoxamine. Stroke volume is increased and cardiac output is essentially unchanged. Coronary blood flow is increased, but blood flow through kidney, brain, liver, and skeletal muscle is usually reduced.

Isoproterenol (Isuprel) has pure β-adrenergic activity. Its administration therefore leads to a decrease in peripheral vascular resistance with an increase in heart rate

TABLE 235-1
Classification of drug effects on the heart

Effect on	*Digitalis glycosides*	*β-Adrenergic catecholamines*	*Quinidine and procainamide*	*Nitrites*	*Propranolol*
Contractility	+	+	−	0	−
Rate (automaticity of SA node)	−	+	+(−)	0	−
Conduction	−*	+	−	0	−*
Irritability (automaticity of ectopic pacemakers)	+	+	−	0	−
Vagal tone	+	0	−	0	0

Note: + = positive effect; − = negative effect; 0 = no direct effect. All effects listed represent the overall effect of the drug. Where this differs from the direct effect, the latter is shown in parentheses.
** Predominantly in the atrioventricular junction.*

and contractility and, thus, an increase in cardiac output. Tachycardia and ventricular ectopic rhythms may also occur. The formation of cyclic 3′5′-adenosine monophosphate (cyclic AMP) from ATP (adenosine triphosphate) is an important biochemical consequence of β-receptor stimulation. However, the precise manner in which this relates to the induced alterations in the electrical and mechanical properties of the heart is not clear.

Sympathomimetic amines are useful in the management of a variety of cardiovascular disorders. Isoproterenol is indicated in the treatment of a number of arrhythmias characterized by reduced automaticity and conductivity. It may be administered as a continuous intravenous infusion (1 to 6 μg per min) or sublingually (10 to 20 mg each 2 to 4 hr) in patients with sinus arrest, sinoatrial block, sinus bradycardia, various forms of atrioventricular conduction defects, and Stokes-Adams attacks (Chap. 234). This amine is also indicated in a variety of low cardiac output states, including those following cardiac operations and those associated with septic and hemorrhagic shock, unless the peripheral vascular bed is already dilated; expansion of circulating volume is usually necessary because the vasodilatation produced by the drug may greatly reduce central venous pressure. Methoxamine and phenylephrine, which act almost exclusively by stimulating α receptors, are indicated in hypotensive states secondary to loss of vasoconstrictor tone, in which it is desired to augment peripheral resistance without increasing cardiac contractility or automaticity. These agents are not beneficial in shock due to myocardial infarction and other conditions in which depression of cardiac contractility plays an important role in the genesis of the hypotension. Agents which stimulate both α and β receptors, such as norepinephrine and metaraminol, may be used to elevate arterial pressure when hypotension is secondary to both a depression of myocardial contractility and an inadequate vasoconstrictor response. However, in most hypotensive states peripheral vascular resistance is increased and the α-receptor stimulation provided by norepinephrine may actually be deleterious.

Toxic reactions to the catecholamines include headache, anxiety, severe hypertension, and the production of cardiac arrhythmias. When norepinephrine extravasates from its site of intravenous administration, tissue necrosis and sloughing may occur. Infiltration of the area with an α-adrenergic blocking agent such as phentolamine (Regitine) may prevent necrosis by blocking vasoconstriction. Following prolonged administration of sympathomimetics for the support of arterial pressure, the dose may have to be tapered slowly to prevent vascular collapse. The replacement of endogenous catecholamine stores with nonreleasable congeners such as metaraminol may explain in part the difficulties of weaning patients from these drugs.

ANTIARRHYTHMIC AGENTS Quinidine Quinidine is one of some twenty alkaloids derived from the bark of the cinchona tree, found in certain regions of South America and the Far East. It is composed of a quinoline group attached through a secondary alcohol linkage to a quinuclidine ring (Fig. 235-1*C*). A methoxy side chain is attached to the quinoline ring, and a vinyl to the quinuclidine group.

The electrophysiologic effects of quinidine on ventricular and Purkinje fibers are also shared by procainamide. The duration of the effective refractory period is prolonged more than that of the action potential. Quinidine also reduces the slope of phase 0 of the action potential, and it is this effect which is responsible for slowing conduction velocity. The spontaneous frequency of discharge of ectopic pacemakers is reduced.

Quinidine exerts negative inotropic effects (Table 235-1). In addition, large doses, especially when given parenterally, produce peripheral vasodilatation, which together with a decreased cardiac output may lead to a fall in arterial pressure. The drug also has negative chronotropic effects, depressing both the sinoatrial node and ectopic pacemaker activity. However, this direct negative chronotropic effect of quinidine is often counteracted by its vagal blocking action, which may lead to no change or an actual increase in heart rate and reduce the refractory period of the atrioventricular junction. Quinidine slows conductivity in the atrioventricular junction; therefore, in the presence of depressed atrioventricular conduction, it must be used with great caution. However, in the absence of depressed conduction, its potent vagal blocking action may actually facilitate conduction through this system. Quinidine also increases the threshold of excitability, thereby making atrial, ventricular, and Purkinje tissue less irritable.

There are various interpretations of the means by which quinidine is effective in converting atrial fibrillation to normal sinus rhythm. If atrial fibrillation results from the formation of rapid waves of depolarization in the atrium (Chap. 234), then quinidine, by diminishing the rate of impulse formation of an ectopic pacemaker, may slow this rate below the frequency at which atrial fibrillation occurs. If, on the other hand, atrial fibrillation results from a circus movement of impulses around the atrium, the prolongation of the atrial refractory period by quinidine would interrupt the circus movement, even though the velocity of impulse transmission is also decreased by quinidine.

Diminished intraventricular conduction velocity is reflected in an increase in the duration of the QRS complex, while the delayed repolarization is reflected in the prolongation of the Q-T interval of the electrocardiogram. The anticholinergic action of quinidine may produce sinus tachycardia. The drug may also lead to an increase in ventricular rate when it is used for the treatment of atrial flutter or fibrillation; the slowing of atrial rate produced by quinidine may paradoxically increase the number of impulses conducted to the ventricle.

Though quinidine had been used for years to convert atrial fibrillation to sinus rhythm, electrical countershock is now employed more frequently because of its safety and effectiveness (Chap. 236). Quinidine is now used most frequently for prevention of recurrent atrial fibrillation after sinus rhythm has been restored. Quinidine may also be used in atrial flutter after a trial of digitalis therapy has failed to convert this rhythm to normal sinus rhythm. In the treatment of atrial flutter, however, quinidine frequently leads to a progressive reduction in the degree of block from 4:1 or 2:1 to 1:1, and when this occurs the rapid ventricular response may be hazardous. Quinidine is frequently used to prevent ventricular tachycardia and fibrillation in patients who have had episodes of these serious arrhythmias. However, if atrioventricular block is associated with ventricular tachycardia, quinidine is contraindicated, because suppression of the ventricular focus in the presence of complete heart block may lead to ventricular standstill or fibrillation. Quinidine is also used in the treatment of ectopic premature supraventricular and ventricular beats, but it is not indicated unless the frequency of these ectopic impulses seriously disturbs the patient or unless the onset of a more serious arrhythmia is feared, as in acute myocardial infarction (Chap. 240).

Quinidine may be administered orally or intramuscularly. Following oral administration, maximum effects occur in 1 to 2 hr. If the drug is given at intervals of 2 to 4 hr, effects will be cumulative. Effects are negligible 8 hr following administration. This point may be especially important in the prophylaxis of recurrent supraventricular arrhythmias. If doses are spaced more than 6 hr apart, less than therapeutic serum levels may occur between doses and prophylaxis may fail. More frequent rather than increased doses may avert this problem. Sustained release preparations may also be used. Peak effects occur 30 to 90 min following intramuscular administration. Intravenous administration, however, does not produce instantaneous effects, and therefore, when it is given by this route, the drug should be administered slowly and the dose should not be repeated before peak effect has been achieved.

In therapeutic concentrations approximately 60 percent of quinidine is bound by plasma albumin. Blood concentrations may be measured easily; concentrations of the order of 3 mg per liter are necessary for therapeutic effects; approximately 10 mg per liter usually produces toxicity. Although metabolic degradation of quinidine, mostly to hydroxy derivatives, occurs in most tissues, particularly in the liver, hepatic injury does not appear to influence the rate at which quinidine leaves the plasma. Both the metabolic end product (2-hydroxyquinidine) and the unchanged drug normally are rapidly excreted by the kidneys.

Toxic reactions to quinidine include cinchonism, consisting of ringing in the ears, headache, nausea, and distorted vision. Diarrhea, nausea, and vomiting are common side effects but may be controlled with the phenothiazines. Frequently, in order to convert atrial fibrillation to normal sinus rhythm, it may be necessary to accept moderate levels of toxicity, entailing nausea, vomiting, tinnitus, and minor widening of the QRS complex. Idiosyncratic reactions, thrombocytopenic purpura, and severe hypotension may occur. The myocardial depressant action of quinidine limits its usefulness in the presence of congestive heart failure and hypotensive states. Its use is contraindicated in patients with a history of thrombocytopenic purpura or in individuals with digitalis intoxication who have an atrioventricular conduction disorder. Widening of the QRS complex by 50 percent or greater of control values and reduction of arterial pressure by more than 20 mmHg are serious warning signs and necessitate discontinuation of the drug. The greatest hazard of quinidine is sudden death due to ventricular fibrillation. This may occur even in patients treated with moderate therapeutic doses.

Procainamide In 1936 it was discovered that procaine, applied directly to the heart, elevates the threshold of ventricular muscle to electrical stimulation. Its prominent central nervous system–stimulating effects and rapid enzymatic hydrolysis make it undesirable clinically. Procainamide, which differs from procaine in that an amide structure (—CONH—) is present instead of an ester linkage (—COO—) (Fig. 235-1*D*), has negligible central nervous system effects and is protected from enzymatic hydrolysis by plasma esterases.

Procainamide may be administered by the oral, intramuscular, or intravenous routes. It is rapidly and almost completely absorbed from the gastrointestinal tract and has a peak effect in approximately 1 hr. It is concentrated in most tissues to levels greater than in the plasma. The major metabolites of procainamide are diethylamino-ethanol and para-aminobenzoic acid, which are excreted along with unchanged procainamide in the urine. As a result, the drug may accumulate to toxic levels in patients with renal insufficiency.

The electrophysiologic effects of procainamide on the heart are similar to those of quinidine (Table 235-1). Clinically, procainamide is generally used in the treatment or prevention of ventricular tachyarrhythmias, in which it appears to be slightly more effective than quinidine. Procainamide, especially when given by the intravenous route, may cause hypotension, and α-adrenergic stimulators should be available to counteract this effect.

An initial loading dose of 1 g given intramuscularly will rapidly produce effective blood concentrations (4 to 8 mg), per liter which may be maintained with an average dose of 500 mg orally or intramuscularly every 6 hr. During the chronic administration of procainamide periodic blood counts should be obtained, because this drug has caused fatal agranulocytosis. It is also frequently a cause of drug fever. The commonest problem encountered during chronic administration of procainamide is a lupus erythematosus-like syndrome. After several months of administration, arthralgias are present in about one-third of patients; an even higher proportion have positive antinuclear antibody tests. Cross sensitivity to procaine and other related drugs should also be anticipated. Procainamide is contraindicated in the presence of atrioventricular block and when there is a history of hypersensitivity to local anesthetics.

Lidocaine Although lidocaine is similar to procaine in its antiarrhythmic action, it is not similar to procaine and the other local anesthetics in the aromatic portion of its structure (Fig. 235-1*E*). In addition, lidocaine lacks an ester linkage and may be given to persons sensitive to procaine. Unlike quinidine and procainamide, lidocaine does not prolong the effective refractory period of ventricular myocardium. It diminishes automaticity in the His-Purkinje system and raises the threshold of ventricular fibrillation. Lidocaine enhances conduction at the Purkinje fiber–myocardial junctions, an action that may diminish reentrant arrhythmias (Chap. 234). Lidocaine is ineffective orally; it may be administered intramuscularly, although the intravenous route is preferred. When administered intravenously, it acts almost instantaneously, but its action is quite transient. Because of these properties, it is particularly useful when it may be expected that the inciting cause of the arrhythmia will disappear. Lidocaine, therefore, is widely used during cardiac catheterization and during cardiac operations when the stimuli which produce arrhythmias are short-lived. However, arrhythmias abolished by single injections of lidocaine may reappear in 10 to 20 min.

Lidocaine is the drug of choice for ventricular arrhythmias complicating myocardial infarction. In order to achieve adequate blood levels, administration should be initiated with a bolus intravenous injection of 1 mg per kg body weight, with additional doses every 5 min until the arrhythmia is abolished or 5 mg per kg has been administered, followed by a continuous intravenous infusion of 20 to 40 μg per kg per min. In the presence of congestive heart failure or shock, hepatic metabolism of lidocaine may be impaired and dosage should be reduced by as much as 50 percent to avoid toxicity, which may include myocardial depression and neurologic abnormalities, including convulsions. It is contraindicated in patients with sinoatrial or atrioventricular block. Toxic effects include drowsiness, paresthesias, and convulsions.

Diphenylhydantoin Diphenylhydantoin (Dilantin) was introduced in 1938 as an antiepileptic drug (Fig. 235-1*F*). During the following 20 years a number of studies in animals reported its effectiveness in experimentally produced cardiac arrhythmias, especially those induced by digitalis. Unlike quinidine, diphenylhydantoin does not reduce atrioventricular or intraventricular conduction velocity and does not prolong the ventricular refractory period. However, like quinidine, diphenylhydantoin reduces automaticity in Purkinje fibers and raises the atrial and ventricular fibrillation thresholds.

Soon after intravenous administration, the drug is concentrated in liver, kidney, and salivary glands and to a lesser extent in brain, fat, and muscle. Plasma concentrations decrease rapidly. The liver is the chief site of detoxification, and there is a substantial enterohepatic circulation of metabolites of the drug; urinary excretion of metabolites is also significant. Diphenylhydantoin may be administered orally or intravenously.

To reach antiarrhythmic plasma levels (10 to 18 mg per liter) an oral loading dose of 1,000 mg is given the first day, 500 mg on the next 2 days, and 400 mg per day thereafter. Intravenous doses consist of 100 mg every 5 min until the arrhythmia is abolished or until undesirable effects appear; the total dosage should not exceed 1,000 mg.

Diphenylhydantoin has been frequently used in cardiac arrhythmias resulting from digitalis excess, particularly ventricular arrhythmias. It is particularly useful in these arrhythmias because it does not interfere with atrioventricular conduction, as do several other antiarrhythmic agents. It is also useful in the treatment and prevention of ventricular extrasystoles and tachycardia not caused by digitalis excess, as well as acute ventricular arrhythmias associated with anesthesia, cardioversion, cardiac catheterization, and cardiac surgery. Less success has been reported with diphenylhydantoin in the treatment of supraventricular tachyarrhythmias.

Toxic reactions include transient hypotension and bradycardia; with long-term administration, ataxia, slurring of speech, mild gastric upsets, and skin rashes occur in 2 to 5 percent of patients. During chronic administration, hyperplasia of the gums develops in about 20 percent of patients. Hepatocellular injury and pseudolymphoma are rare complications.

BETA-ADRENERGIC RECEPTOR BLOCKING AGENTS Propranolol (Inderal) is similar in configuration to the pure β-adrenergic stimulant, isoproterenol, except for the addition of a benzene ring (Fig. 235-1*G*). Beta-adrenergic blockage with propranolol is basically of the competitive type and is reversible. Propranolol may be administered both orally and parenterally. It is capable of blocking the effects of catecholamines and sympathetic nerve stimulation on heart rate, cardiac output, and contractility (Table 235-2). It tends to reduce resting heart rate, cardiac index, and arterial blood pressure in normal subjects, but impairment of cardiac performance during muscular exercise is even more pronounced because of blockade of the augmented sympathetic activity which occurs during exercise. In addition, propranolol reduces oxygen uptake by the myocardium and in large doses may cause sodium retention.

Propranolol, alone or in combination with long-acting nitrates, is often effective in patients with angina pectoris in whom nitrates alone have failed to give relief (Chap. 240). Propranolol with isosorbide dinitrate is one such combination which is felt to be effective. The beneficial effects of propranolol in angina pectoris probably are achieved by preventing the increased myocardial oxygen requirements induced by sympathetic nervous discharge during exercise. Because propranolol depresses myocardial contractility, it may intensify heart failure and should be used only with extreme caution in patients with seriously diminished cardiac reserve. Dosage schedules are usually begun with 40 mg per day in divided doses; 120 mg per day is often required for efficacy, and dosage needed has reached 600 mg per day.

A second major use of propranolol is in the treatment of cardiac arrhythmias, particularly ectopic tachycardias. Propranolol is effective in the treatment of tachyarrhythmias resulting from digitalis intoxication, when electric countershock is contraindicated (Chap. 236). It is particularly useful in reducing excessive ventricular rate in patients with atrial fibrillation. Its beneficial effects in this regard result from prolongation of the refractory period in the atrioventricular junction by blocking adrenergic influences on this system. In this regard the effects of propranolol are additive to those of digitalis. Although only the *l*-isomer of propranolol has β-adrenergic blocking activity, *d*-propranolol is also effective against digitalis-induced arrhythmias. Therefore, the antiarrhythmic effects of propranolol may derive both from β-adrenergic blocking action and from direct antiarrhythmic activity, i.e., a "quinidine-like" effect.

Propranolol is also effective in relieving many of the symptoms of idiopathic hypertrophic subaortic stenosis (Chap. 242). Its effects are related to a depression of the contractile state of the heart, leading to lessening of the severity of obstruction. Finally, propranolol has received a trial in the treatment of hypertension, but its efficacy in this condition is limited to patients with labile hypertension, those with high-output states, and those with high levels of circulating renin.

Toxic effects of propranolol, which occur in less than 2 percent of patients, include nausea, fatigue, visual disturbances, diarrhea, cutaneous eruptions, and insomnia. The serious side effects of propranolol include the production of shock and intensification of heart failure. Propranolol is specifically contraindicated in patients with second- or third-degree atrioventricular block, in whom it may produce serious bradycardia or even asystole. The drug is also contraindicated in patients with asthma or pulmonary insufficiency associated with bronchospasm, because β blockade may induce bronchial constriction.

VASODILATORS Glyceryl trinitrate (nitroglycerin) and amyl nitrite have been used for more than a century for their vasodilating properties. In recent years, however, numerous other nitrate compounds have been introduced which have a longer duration of action than nitroglycerin (Fig. 235-1*H*). The nitrite ion is an active vasodilator in both inorganic and organic forms. However, the nitrate ion is active only in organic form. The organic nitrates are absorbed most effectively from the sublingual or buccal mucosa. Many of the longer-acting organic nitrates, however, are also absorbed from the gastrointestinal tract and may be administered orally. However, for optimal absorption, these drugs should be ingested before meals. Once absorbed they disappear rapidly from the bloodstream. Portions of absorbed nitrite ion may be converted to ammonia, and portions are excreted in the urine, but their metabolic fate is largely unknown.

TABLE 235-2
Approximate dosage schedules for cardioactive drugs*

	Initial or loading dose			
Drug	*Orally*	*Intramuscularly*	*Intravenously*	*Usual maintenance dosage*
Ouabain			0.5–1.0 mg in divided doses	
Digoxin	1.0–2.0 mg		0.8–1.6 mg in divided doses	0.25–0.50 mg p.o. daily
Digitoxin	1.0–1.5 mg			0.05–0.15 mg p.o. daily
Digitalis leaf	1.0–2.0 g			0.05–0.15 g p.o. daily
Quinidine	0.2 g q.6h.—increase dose by 0.2 g until arrhythmia is controlled or dose of 0.8 g q.4h. is reached			0.2–0.4 g p.o., q.4h.
Procainamide	0.5–1.0 g	0.5–1.0 g	100 mg q.5 min up to × 10	500 mg p.o. q.6h.
Lidocaine			75 mg (1 mg/kg)	20–40 μg/kg/min
Diphenylhydantoin	250 mg q.i.d.		100 mg q.5 min. up to × 5	100 mg p.o. q.6h.
Glyceryl trinitrate	0.3–0.6 mg sublingually			As needed
Isosorbide dinitrate				10–20 mg p.o., q.i.d. (sublingual)
Propranolol	10–80 mg p.o., q.i.d., or greater for angina 10–40 mg p.o., q.i.d., for arrhythmias		1.0 mg for arrhythmias	Same as initial dose for angina

* *Dosage schedules represent broad ranges and must be modified for individual patients. Initial digitalis doses are total loading doses and should be given in fractional amounts.*

The vasodilators have only one specific therapeutic effect—to relax smooth muscle. The mechanism of this action is not known, and it cannot be blocked by any known inhibitors. For example, nitrite ion can relax smooth muscle even in the presence of the α-adrenergic–stimulating effects of norepinephrine. Administration of organic nitrates leads to generalized arterial and venous dilatation, resulting in a fall in mean systemic arterial pressure and in peripheral pooling of blood. Pulse pressure, stroke volume, and central venous pressure decline, particularly when the patient is in the erect position. The hypotension evokes a compensatory tachycardia. Dilatation of blood vessels in the skin causes marked flushing of the head, neck, and chest, and severe pounding headache may occur because of dilatation of the meningeal vessels.

Though nitroglycerin increases coronary blood flow in normal individuals, there is considerable evidence that it does not always evoke this effect in the presence of diffuse, severe coronary artery disease. Therefore it is difficult to relate the beneficial effects of this drug in angina pectoris to a direct increase in total coronary blood flow. Coronary ischemia, however, may relate not only to the amount of blood which reaches the coronary capillaries, but also to the myocardial demands for oxygen. Since nitroglycerin regularly reduces arterial blood pressure, the work performance and the oxygen requirements of the heart are diminished. The venous dilatation produced by this drug leads to a reduction in heart size, which also tends to reduce myocardial oxygen consumption. Coronary blood flow, however, is not diminished, and therefore the major effect of nitroglycerin may be to improve the relationship between myocardial oxygen delivery and myocardial oxygen requirements. Also, there is some evidence that nitroglycerin dilates collateral vessels, increasing perfusion of ischemic areas.

The nitrates are primarily used for the treatment of angina pectoris; the chest pain is relieved within 1 to 3 min by sublingual nitroglycerin. Because the effects of this drug may persist for 30 min, it may also be used prophylactically to prevent angina pectoris when the patient predicts that it will occur. However, long-term prophylaxis with the longer-acting nitrates has been relatively unsuccessful, perhaps because of the development of tolerance. The most useful of the longer-acting nitrates appears to be sublingual isosorbide dinitrate. When given in adequate doses, nitrates regularly produce cutaneous flushing and headache; if the patient fails to be relieved of angina but also fails to show any side effects, it is possible that the dose of the drug is not adequate.

Toxic effects of the nitrates include headache and hypotension as well as occasional drug rashes. In addition, the nitrate ion readily oxidizes hemoglobin to methemoglobin, which may cause severe hypoxia if large enough doses are ingested.

Other drugs useful in the treatment of patients with disorders of the cardiovascular system are considered in Chap. 233 (diuretics) and in Chap. 245 (antihypertensive agents).

REFERENCES

Bellet S: Drug therapy, sec. 5 in *Clinical Disorders of the Heart Beat*, 3d ed., Philadelphia: Lea & Febiger, 1971, p. 927

Braunwald E, Pool PE: Mechanism of action of digitalis glycosides. Mod Concepts Cardiovasc Dis 37:129, 1968

Butler VP: Assays of digitalis in the blood. Prog Cardiovasc Dis 14:571, 1972

Epstein SE, Braunwald E: Beta-adrenergic receptor blocking drugs: Mechanisms of action and clinical applications. N Engl J Med 275:1106, 1175, 1966

Gettes LS: The electrophysiologic effects of antiarrhythmic drugs. Am J Cardiol 28:526, 1971

Goldberg LI: Pharmacology of cardiovascular drugs, chap. 101 in *The Heart*, 3d ed., ed JW Hurst, New York: McGraw-Hill, 1974

Goodman LS, Gilman A (eds): *The Pharmacological Basis of Therapeutics*, 4th ed., New York: Macmillan, 1970, p. 667

Harrison DC: Beta adrenergic blockade: Pharmacology and clinical uses. Am J Cardiol 29:432, 1972

Krantz JC: Action and nomenclature of nitroglycerine and nitrate esters. Am J Cardiol 29:436, 1972

Langer GA: The mechanism of action of digitalis. Hosp Pract 5:49 (August), 1970

Rosen MR, Hoffman BF: Mechanism of action of antiarrhythmic drugs. Circulation Res. 32:1, 1973

Smith TW: Drug therapy: Digitalis glycosides. N Engl J Med 288:719, 935, 1973

236 ELECTRICAL REVERSION OF CARDIAC ARRHYTHMIAS

BERNARD LOWN

Ectopic arrhythmias of the heart have generally been controlled by means of drugs. Major reliance has been on quinidine, procainamide, and the digitalis glycosides. The use of antiarrhythmic drugs presents a number of problems. To reach an effective dose requires a time-consuming biologic titration involving frequent monitoring of the patient's condition. There is a high incidence of mild as well as serious toxic reactions. Furthermore, a number of rhythm disorders are refractory to drugs. A method is needed that is simple in application, restores sinus rhythm consistently, and is free from untoward side effects. These requirements are satisfied by the use of a specific type of electrical discharge across the intact chest.

THEORETIC BASIS FOR USE OF ELECTRICAL DISCHARGE The use of electrical energy for terminating ectopic arrhythmias is based on three propositions:

1 Chronic ventricular and atrial arrhythmias are initiated by a multiplicity of interacting factors, some of which are transient. Once initiated, the abnormal mechanisms are self-sustaining, perhaps because of a continuing passage of recirculating wave fronts of excitation over fixed or variable pathways (circus movement).

2 When an ectopic disorder is momentarily extinguished,

the sinus node, which has the highest rhythmicity in the heart, resumes as dominant pacemaker.

3 The heart can be depolarized across the intact chest by electrical discharge. When effective, such depolarization abolishes the ectopic mechanism and permits restoration of sinus rhythm.

If electrical discharge were safe it would constitute an ideal form of antiarrhythmic therapy. Ventricular fibrillation has been terminated across the intact chest by 60-cycle alternating current (a-c) shocks. When this type of electrical discharge is administered to normal animals, it may induce cardiac arrest or ventricular fibrillation. The danger of provoking such serious disruptions in cardiac mechanism has deterred adoption of alternating current for the treatment of arrhythmias other than ventricular fibrillation.

CARDIOVERSION Capacitor discharge, or direct current (d-c) shock, may also be employed to defibrillate the heart. A capacitor can be made to yield a great variety of wave forms, depending on the parameters of the discharge circuit. Incorporating an inductance in the circuit reduces the peak voltage released by a capacitor and lengthens the duration of discharge. A single monophasic pulse resulting from the use of an appropriate capacitor and inductor is more effective in depolarizing the heart, induces fewer arrhythmias and less tissue damage than alternating current, and, furthermore, does not provoke cardiac standstill. The one hazard remaining is the sporadic occurrence of ventricular fibrillation.

When the d-c pulse is delivered systematically through the cardiac cycle, ventricular fibrillation occurs only when the discharge is triggered during the final one-third of systole. This vulnerable period appears to be an essential physiologic property of the mammalian heart. It generally has a duration of 30 msec and just precedes the apex of the T wave of the surface electrocardiogram. When a d-c discharge is triggered outside this vulnerable period, ventricular fibrillation does not occur.

Thus by employing a capacitor discharge with a specific underdamped pulse and synchronizing the release of this pulse within a safe part of the cardiac cycle, i.e., 30 msec after the beginning of the QRS complex, the twin dangers of electricity, namely, ventricular standstill and fibrillation, can be avoided. The use of synchronized capacitor shock has been designated *cardioversion* and is employed for terminating a diversity of ectopic arrhythmias.

TECHNIQUE OF CARDIOVERSION The technique employed is essentially the same irrespective of the type of arrhythmia. Cardioversion can be carried out as an outpatient procedure, although brief hospitalization is preferred. No special area is required. In the treatment of atrial fibrillation or atrial flutter, quinidine in a dose of 0.3 g every 6 hr is initiated 24 to 48 hr prior to the procedure. The objective is fourfold:

1 To build up an adequate level of drug in the body so that the arrhythmia will not occur soon after reversion
2 To determine whether quinidine is tolerated
3 To obtain a small dividend of reversion which occurs in about 10 percent of patients with chronic atrial fibrillation who are given this dose of quinidine
4 To decrease the occurrence of postcardioversion arrhythmias

Premedication is limited to a sedative drug given about an hour before the procedure. Amnesia is induced by means of small (10 to 15 mg) intravenous doses of diazepam.

The electrical discharge is applied by means of two insulated electrode paddles. These are covered with thick layers of conductive paste. One electrode is placed below the angle of the left scapula, the other is applied over the right parasternal area of the third intercostal space. The instrument is automatically synchronized to deliver the discharge during inscription of the QRS complex. The initial energy setting is 5 to 10 watt-sec, depending upon the severity of heart disease and uncertainty as to the presence of overdigitalization. If reversion is not accomplished with these low-energy discharges, successive shocks are delivered without delay at increasing energies, proceeding to 25, 50, 100, 200, 300, up to 400 watt-sec. The patient's response consists of a single twitch of thoracic muscle, a slight jerk of the arms, and at times an audible sigh. Normal rhythm is restored instantly; at times a brief episode of nodal rhythm precedes establishment of sinus node dominance.

CLINICAL RESULTS Many thousands of patients have been treated with this method. The good results that have almost always occurred have confirmed theoretic expectations. Cardioversion has been found effective in many ectopic rhythm disorders, whether of ventricular, nodal, or atrial origin.

Ventricular tachycardia In the majority of instances, ventricular tachycardia arises in patients with serious

FIGURE 236-1
Ventricular tachycardia in a forty-two-year-old man with acute myocardial infarction. A single cardioversion discharge restores sinus rhythm.

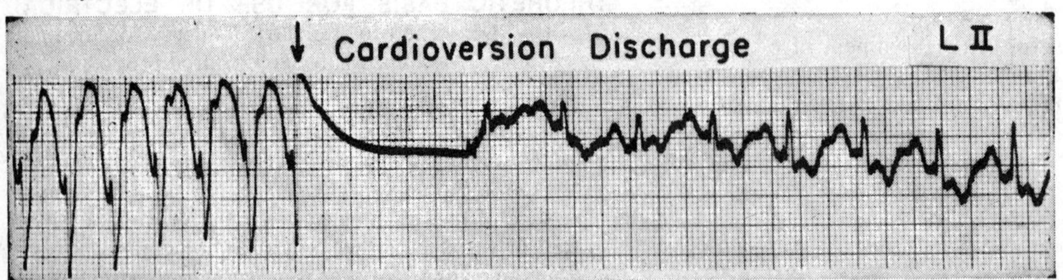

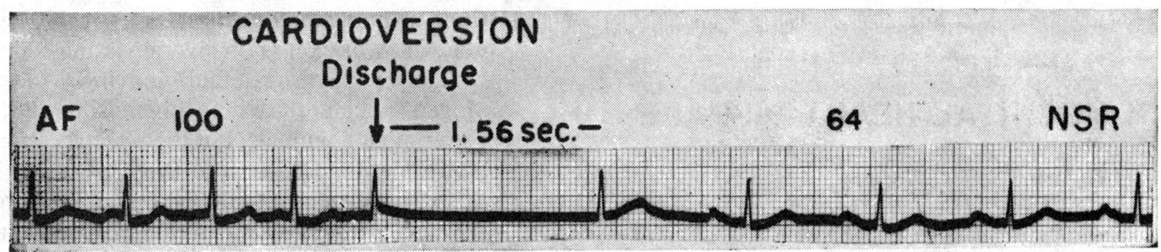

FIGURE 236-2
Restoration of sinus rhythm in a patient with long-standing atrial fibrillation. The isoelectric interval of 1.56 sec represents an artifact due to the massive electrical field across the chest. Note the marked slowing in ventricular rate.

organic heart disease; usually, it occurs in the wake of a myocardial infarction. The rapid heart action and aberrant activation of the myocardium seriously compromise cardiac function. This arrhythmia frequently constitutes a dire emergency. Antiarrhythmic drugs may reduce ventricular contractility and peripheral resistance, and thus further impair cardiac function. Cardioversion is devoid of these adverse actions. Restoration of sinus rhythm is immediate (Fig. 236-1). This method is nearly 100 percent effective and constitutes a treatment of choice for ventricular tachycardia when the disorder does not respond to a 50-mg bolus of lidocaine. In the case of the oft-recurring episodes of ventricular tachycardia which accompany acute myocardial infarction, the use of continuous intravenous infusion of lidocaine is the treatment of choice.

Atrial fibrillation This arrhythmia is the most common chronic disorder of the heartbeat. Until recently treatment has been based on the use of quinidine. Even when it is given to the point of toxicity, the heartbeat of only 50 percent of patients can be restored to sinus rhythm. With cardioversion, atrial fibrillation can be terminated in more than 90 percent of patients. Failures are encountered mainly in patients with mitral valvular disease, with giant left atria, and with continuous arrhythmia for 5 years or longer. A typical example of cardioversion is illustrated in Fig. 236-2. At times, transitional mechanisms are encountered, consisting of nodal rhythm and ectopic atrial beats which generally last for 30 to 60 sec, until the SA node "warms up." Slowing the ventricular rate is one immediate effect of restoration of sinus rhythm. The P-R interval is full, and not infrequently first degree AV block is present. In patients with congestive heart failure, restoration of sinus rhythm results in an increase in the cardiac output. The patient generally feels improved and comments on the newly sensed "calm" in the chest. Compared to the use of quinidine, cardioversion is a more efficient and safer method. Nevertheless, quinidine continues as an invaluable antiarrhythmic drug for maintenance therapy. Without its use a majority of patients would experience recurrence of atrial fibrillation.

Atrial flutter and other arrhythmias Cardioversion has proved nearly 100 percent effective in chronic atrial flutter. Usually, a single low-energy discharge proves adequate. This method is also applicable to other atrial and AV nodal ectopic arrhythmias which have not responded to drug therapy.

Complications Immediate complications have been limited to the development of ventricular ectopic beats, ventricular tachycardia, and, rarely, even ventricular fibrillation. Such disorders can nearly always be avoided if the lowest effective amount of energy for reversion is employed, electrolyte deficits are corrected prior to the cardioversion, and treatment of overdigitalized patients is avoided. Furthermore, the electrical discharge should not be released in the presence of artifacts in the electrocardiogram. Such artifacts may trigger the discharge to occur during the vulnerable period, thereby precipitating ventricular fibrillation. It is probable that most, if not all, of the very rare fatalities which have been reported have been due either to neglect of these precautions or to the excessive and, at times, improper use of such drugs as digitalis and quinidine.

In many patients electrical reversion is only temporarily successful and the arrhythmia soon recurs. It is, therefore, often necessary to continue the use of the drugs mentioned in the previous chapter. Moderate to large doses of quinidine, procainamide, or both, may be needed. Agents such as reserpine or guanethidine, that deplete or antagonize catechols, may be beneficial. In refractory patients antithyroid substances such as propylthiouracil or radioiodine may be necessary as a supplement to the several antiarrhythmic drugs.

Summary Cardioversion is a simple and direct method for terminating various ectopic cardiac arrhythmias by depolarizing the heart transthoracically by means of a synchronized d-c discharge. It is based on physiologic principles and is the most effective and safest means yet devised for restoring a sinus mechanism.

REFERENCES

LOWN B: Electrical reversion of cardiac arrhythmias. Br Heart J 29:469, 1967

RESNEKOV L: Present status of electroversion in management of cardiac dysrhythmias. Circulation 47:1356, 1973

——, MCDONALD L: Electroconversion of lone atrial fibrillation and flutter including haemodynamic studies at rest and on exercise. Br Heart J 33:339, 1971

237 CONGENITAL HEART DISEASE

WILLIAM F. FRIEDMAN
EUGENE BRAUNWALD

GENERAL CONSIDERATIONS

INCIDENCE Approximately 9 births in 1,000 are complicated by a cardiovascular malformation. If the problem is recognized early, these anomalies can now be diagnosed accurately, and most of these babies may be salvaged by aggressive medical and surgical management.

Children with congenital heart disease usually show an overall male preponderance. Moreover, specific defects may show a definite sex preponderance; patent ductus arteriosus and atrial septal defect are more common in females, whereas valvular aortic stenosis, coarctation of the aorta, tetralogy of Fallot, and transposition of the great arteries are more common in males. Table 237-1 demonstrates the frequency of occurrence of specific cardiovascular malformations in clinical and pathologic studies.

ETIOLOGY Congenital cardiovascular malformations are generally the result of aberrant embryonic development of a normal structure or a failure of such a structure to progress beyond an early stage of embryonic development. Malformations appear to result from a complex interaction between multifactorial genetic and environmental systems that does not allow a single specification of etiology; only rarely may a causal factor be implicated in their genesis. Maternal rubella and the ingestion of thalidomide early during gestation are two environmental insults that are known to interfere with normal cardiogenesis in man. The *rubella syndrome* consists of cataracts, deafness, microcephaly, and, either singly or in combination, patent ductus arteriosus, pulmonary valvular and/or arterial stenosis, and ventricular septal defect (see Chap. 196). *Thalidomide* is associated with major limb deformities and occasionally with cardiac malformations without a predilection for a specific lesion. Hypoxia, deficiency or excess of several vitamins, intake of several categories of drugs, and ionizing irradiation are teratogens that are capable of causing cardiac defects in experimental animals, but their precise relation to human malformations requires further definition.

TABLE 237-1
Frequency of occurrence of single cardiac malformations in selected pathologic studies*

Disease	*Percent*
Ventricular septal defect	14.1
Tetralogy of Fallot	9.8
Complete transposition of the great arteries	9.4
Patent ductus arteriosus	8.3
Atrial septal defect	7.1
Coarctation of the aorta	6.2
Single ventricle and biloculare	5.0
"Valvular atresias"	3.3
Pulmonary stenosis	2.4
"Idiopathic hypertrophy of the heart"	2.3
Persistent truncus arteriosus	2.3
Persistent common atrioventricular canal	1.7
Endocardial sclerosis	0.8

* *2,040 studies = 100 percent.*

A single gene mutation may be incriminated in the familial forms of atrial septal defect, ventricular septal defect, congenital heart block, situs inversus, the combination of supravalvular aortic stenosis and peripheral pulmonary arterial stenosis, and idiopathic hypertrophic subaortic stenosis (Chap. 242). Cardiovascular anomalies may also be manifestations of the pleiotropic effects of single genes, as suggested by the large number of syndromes such as the *Holt-Oram* (atrial septal defect and radial defect of the upper extremity), *Ehlers-Danlos* (hyperextensible joints, hyperelastic and friable skin, arterial dilatation or rupture) (Chap. 362), *Marfan's* (Chap. 362), and *Ellis–van Creveld* (chondrodystrophic dwarfism, ectodermal dysplasia, polydactyly, single atrium). Examples of gross chromosomal defects of the cardiovascular system are found in *Turner's syndrome* (Chap. 98), in which coarctation of the aorta and/or pulmonic stenosis may occur; *Down's syndrome* (Chap. 334), which is frequently accompanied by endocardial cushion defects, atrial or ventricular septal defect, and/or pulmonic stenosis; the *trisomy 13–15 (D_1)* and *17–18 (E) syndromes*, which may be associated with ventricular septal defect and more complex cardiovascular anomalies; and the *cri-du-chat* syndrome of partial chromosomal deletion, which may be associated with atrial and ventricular septal defects. Despite this long list, it must be appreciated that recognized chromosomal aberrations and mutations of single genes account for less than 10 percent of all cardiac malformations.

The finding that, with a few exceptions, only one of a pair of monozygotic twins is affected by congenital heart disease indicates that the vast majority of cardiovascular malformations are not inherited in a simple manner. Family studies indicate a two- to fourfold increase in the incidence of congenital heart disease in the siblings of affected patients. The malformations are concordant or partially concordant in at least half of such cases. Nonetheless, the incidence of congenital heart disease in the siblings of an index patient is only 2 to 4 percent. With few exceptions, therefore, patients with isolated heart defects have a negative family history for malformations and a normal chromosome pattern, and it is rarely wise to discourage the parents of one affected child from having additional children. The low recurrence rate and the increasing possibilities for effective therapy for nearly all cardiac lesions usually justify a positive approach to family counseling. If, however, two or more members of a family are affected, the recurrence risk may be quite high, and a pedigree should be obtained prior to further counseling. If a dominant or recessive mendelian pattern is established, the mendelian laws apply, and the risk of recurrence in each pregnancy is equal.

PREVENTION The feasibility of preventive programs will depend upon what is learned about the cause of the 90 percent or more of cardiovascular anomalies for which no cause is now known.

A rubella vaccine has been developed that appears to

be effective, and immunization of children with this vaccine may be anticipated to eradicate maternal rubella and its cardiac consequences. Strict testing in animals of new drugs that may be teratogenic when taken early in pregnancy may be expected to reduce the chances of another thalidomide tragedy. In this regard, no medications should be taken during pregnancy without prior consultation with a physician. Physicians dealing with pregnant women should be aware of known teratogens, as well as of drugs for which inadequate information exists relative to their teratogenic potential. Similarly, appropriate use of radiologic equipment and techniques for reducing gonadal and fetal radiation exposure may be expected to reduce the potential hazards of this likely cause of birth defects.

The presence of a cardiac malformation as one component of the multiple system involvement that may exist in the Down's, Turner's, and trisomy 13–15 (D_1) and 17–18 (E) syndromes may be anticipated in occasional pregnancies by the detection of abnormal chromosomes in fetal cells obtained from amniotic fluid. Similarly, identification in such cells of the enzyme disorders observed in Hurler's syndrome or type II glycogen storage disease may allow one to predict the ultimate presence of cardiac disease.

THE FETAL AND TRANSITIONAL CIRCULATIONS

An understanding of the fetal and neonatal circulations is important to systematic comprehension of congenital heart disease (Fig. 237-1). The fetal circulation is a single circulation in which the pulmonary vasculature exists in parallel with the systemic circulation, not in series with it. Prenatal survival is not endangered by extremely severe cardiac anomalies as long as one side of the heart can drive blood from the great veins to the aorta. Blood can bypass the nonfunctioning lungs both proximally and distad to the heart. Inferior vena caval blood is deflected across the foramen ovale into the left atrium. Most of the blood that reaches the right ventricle bypasses the high-resistance, unexpanded lungs and passes through the patent ductus arteriosus into the descending aorta. In fetal life, pulmonary vessels are surrounded by a fluid medium, have relatively thick walls and small lumens, and resemble comparable vessels in the systemic circulation.

Normally, the fundamental change which occurs at birth is the division of this single circulation into two separate, interdependent circulations. Inflation of the lungs with the first inspiration produces a marked reduction in pulmonary vascular resistance. Fetal pulmonary vessels, heretofore supported by fluid media, are suddenly suspended in air, reducing extravascular pressure. New vessels are opened, and already patent vessels enlarge. Pulmonary arterial pressure falls, and pulmonary blood flow increases greatly. The systemic vascular resistance rises when clamping the umbilical cord removes the low-resistance placental circulation. Increased pulmonary blood flow increases the return of blood to the left atrium and raises left atrial pressure, which in turn closes the foramen ovale. The shift in oxygen dependence from the placenta to the lungs produces a sudden increase in arterial blood oxygen tension, which is one of the

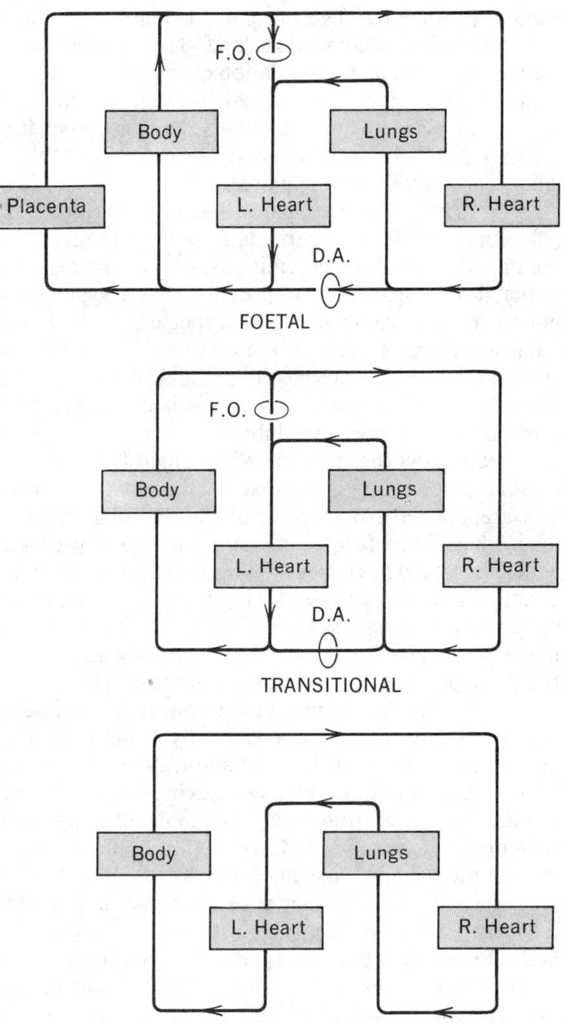

FIGURE 237-1
Diagrams of the fetal, transitional (neonatal), and adult types of circulation. F.O. = foramen ovale; D.A. = ductus arteriosus. (From GS Dawes, Foetal and Neonatal Physiology, *Chicago: YearBook, 1968.)*

factors that initiates constriction of the ductus arteriosus, and total anatomic closure follows within a few days. As yet unclearly defined autonomic and chemical mediators may participate in these events.

Pulmonary hypertension

Pulmonary hypertension frequently complicates congenital heart disease, and the status of the pulmonary vascular bed may determine the clinical picture, its rate of progression, and whether or not corrective surgical treatment is feasible. Elevation of pulmonary blood pressure frequently depends on morphologic alterations in the pulmonary vascular bed. Following the fall in pulmonary arterial pressure, resistance, and vasomotor tone shortly after birth, a gradual reduction of the ratio of pulmonary vessel wall thickness to lumen size occurs for some months postnatally. The muscular media of the pulmonary arterioles become thin, and their lumens widen. Hence, the pulmonary circulation of the normal adult has evolved from a high-pressure, high-resistance, highly reactive vascular bed with relatively small cross-sectional area, to a low-pressure, low-resistance, less-reactive bed with a large cross-sectional area.

As in the other vascular beds, the pressure in the pulmonary artery is determined by the product of the volume of blood flow, per unit of time, and the resistance to that flow. Equalization of pressures in the systemic and pulmonary circulations may be expected if a large communication exists between the two ventricles or the two great arteries in the absence of semilunar valve obstruction. Pulmonary vascular resistance is calculated as the transpulmonary pressure difference per unit of pulmonary blood flow (page 1104). When blood flow increases, existing patent vessels are distended and additional vessels are opened, so that calculated vascular resistance diminishes. Therefore, in a normal pulmonary vascular bed, pressure will rise substantially only if flow is very greatly increased (page 1104). In the vast majority of patients with congenital heart disease and elevated pulmonary vascular resistance, the pulmonary arterioles are the principal locus of this abnormal resistance.

A delay in the normal involution of the pulmonary vascular bed often occurs postnatally in the presence of an intra- or extracardiac communication with a large left-to-right shunt. In patients having high pulmonary arterial pressure from birth, anatomic changes in the pulmonary vessels, in the form of medial thickening and intimal proliferation, usually progress so that in the older child or adult the vascular resistance may ultimately be fixed by obliterative changes in the pulmonary vascular bed. However, if pulmonary arterial hypertension is not present in infancy or childhood, it may never occur or may not develop until the third or fourth decade, or even later.

Because pulmonary vascular obstructive disease may be the factor limiting a decision concerning the advisability of operation, it is important to quantify and compare the ratios of pulmonary to systemic flows and resistances in patients with severe pulmonary hypertension. Furthermore, the lability of the pulmonary vascular resistance should be evaluated; a reduction with the infusion of acetylcholine and tolazoline or the inhalation of oxygen suggests that resistance may fall after successful operation. Some defects between the left and right sides of the heart should be closed in order to eliminate a sizable left-to-right shunt, which, in turn, may result in a significant drop in pulmonary arterial pressure because of reduction of pulmonary blood flow. Conversely, little or no benefit and high mortality rates may be expected from the closure of defects that are associated with bidirectional or predominant right-to-left shunts in patients with high-resistance and obstructive pulmonary hypertension. The designation "Eisenmenger's reaction" is applied to this condition in patients who may have a large communication between the two circulations at the aortopulmonary, ventricular, or atrial levels. The actual mechanism for the persistence, delayed reduction, or late onset of elevated pulmonary vascular resistance is not known.

The clinical manifestations of the hyperkinetic form of pulmonary hypertension, i.e., that associated with a large left-to-right shunt, reflect the specific malformation responsible. When a significant right-to-left shunt exists in patients with pulmonary hypertension, the patient is cyanotic, and polycythemia and clubbing of the digits may be noted (Chap. 29). A dominant A wave in the jugular venous pulse may be seen, reflecting vigorous right atrial contraction; in some instances there are large V waves, which suggest tricuspid regurgitation. A prominent right ventricular parasternal lift and palpable systolic expansion of the pulmonary artery are present. On auscultation, one often hears a soft pulmonary systolic ejection murmur following a loud ejection sound, marked accentuation of the pulmonic component of the second heart sound, and, often, a fourth heart sound produced by right atrial contraction. The decrescendo diastolic murmur of pulmonary valvular regurgitation and/or the holosystolic murmur of tricuspid regurgitation may be heard. The electrocardiogram shows right ventricular hypertrophy (page 1090). Roentgenologic examination reveals enlargement of the right ventricle, a conspicuously enlarged pulmonary artery, prominent hilar pulmonary vascular markings, and attenuated peripheral vessels. The site of the underlying defect may be localized by means of cardiac catheterization and angiocardiography (Chap. 231). Pressures in the right side of the heart are essentially identical to systemic pressures in cyanotic patients if the shunt is at the ventricular or aortopulmonary levels, but they are usually lower than systemic pressure in patients with an interatrial shunt. No specific treatment has proved beneficial for obstructive pulmonary vascular disease.

CIRCULATORY SHUNTS

Although equal quantities of blood flow through the pulmonary and systemic circulations in normal subjects postnatally, the systemic circulation is a relatively high-resistance system usually requiring a systolic pressure in the left ventricle in excess of 100 mm Hg to maintain normal blood flow. The pressure drop across the pulmonary vascular bed, however, is approximately one-sixth that across the systemic bed, indicating that the resistance to flow through the normal pulmonary vascular bed is much lower than that in the systemic bed. Therefore, it may be expected that, ordinarily, if an abnormal communication is present blood will flow from the left to the right side of the heart. The size of the opening and the pressures on either side of it generally determine the direction and magnitude of the shunt flow. A right-to-left shunt usually requires either an obstructive lesion at some point in the right-sided circulation (i.e., tricuspid stenosis or atresia, pulmonary valvular or infundibular stenosis, elevated pulmonary vascular resistance) or an obligatory mixing of systemic venous and arterial blood (i.e., total anomalous pulmonary venous drainage, a single atrium or ventricle, or a persistent truncus arteriosus). The location, direction, and magnitude of the right-to-left shunt may be determined during hemodynamic study by measuring the admixture of venous and arterial blood at various sites in the central circulation, by indicator-dilution curves, and by angiocardiography, as outlined in Chap. 231.

Clinical manifestations of right-to-left shunts

CYANOSIS AND POLYCYTHEMIA These signs are discussed in Chap. 29.

CLUBBING A prominent accompaniment of arterial hypoxemia consists of a widening and thickening of the terminal phalanges of the fingers and toes, accompanied by convex nails. These digits have an increased number of capillaries with increased blood flow through extensive arteriovenous aneurysms, and an increase of connective tissue.

SQUATTING Patients with cyanotic heart disease, especially tetralogy of Fallot, typically assume a squatting posture after exertion to obtain relief from breathlessness. Squatting appears to hasten an increase in the arterial oxygen saturation by increasing systemic vascular resistance and thereby diminishing the right-to-left shunt and by pooling markedly unsaturated blood in the legs. Also, systemic venous return and therefore pulmonary blood flow may rise.

ANOXIC SPELLS A sudden marked increase in cyanosis due to an abrupt reduction in pulmonary blood flow occurs in younger children with certain types of cyanotic heart disease, particularly tetralogy of Fallot. The spells may lead to convulsions and may even be fatal; they may be precipitated by fluctuations in arterial P_{CO_2} and pH, a sudden fall in systemic or increase in pulmonary vascular resistance, or augmented contraction of the hypertrophied muscle in the right ventricular outflow tract. Treatment consists of oxygen administration, placing the child in the knee-chest position, and intravenous administration of sodium bicarbonate to correct the accompanying acidosis. Additional medications that may prove of value include morphine, α-adrenergic receptor stimulants such as phenylephrine or methoxamine, or angiotensin to raise peripheral resistance and to diminish right-to-left shunting, and β-adrenergic blocking agents, which may relieve infundibular spasm by reducing cardiac sympathetic tone.

PARADOXIC EMBOLUS AND BRAIN ABSCESS In patients with cyanotic heart disease, venous blood bypasses the normal filtering action of the lungs, and emboli arising in systemic veins may pass, paradoxically, directly to the systemic circulation. Patients with severe cyanosis or polycythemia have often had previous occlusive microcirculatory damage to the central nervous system. These predisposing factors are primarily responsible for the relatively high incidence (2 to 4 percent) of brain abscess in patients with cyanotic forms of congenital heart disease.

IMPAIRED GROWTH Physical underdevelopment and a delayed onset of adolescence are common features of many types of cyanotic and, to a lesser extent, acyanotic forms of congenital heart disease. Mental development is rarely affected. Various explanations for the mechanisms of growth interference have implicated malnutrition, tissue anoxia, diminished peripheral blood flow, hypermetabolic state, chronic cardiac decompensation, genetic and endocrine factors, and frequency of upper and lower respiratory infections. In many instances, the underdevelopment is influenced little by operative correction of the underlying cardiac anomaly. Thus, it is unwise preoperatively to guarantee to the parents of a child with heart disease that operation will result in accelerated growth and development.

SPECIFIC CARDIAC DEFECTS

Various classifications of congenital cardiovascular lesions have been proposed, depending on hemodynamic, anatomic and radiographic factors. Although there is overlapping between groups, the following arrangement of the more common anomalies is used in this chapter.

1 Communications between the systemic and pulmonary circulation without cyanosis (left-to-right shunts)
2 Obstructing valvular and vascular lesions with or without associated right-to-left shunts
3 Abnormalities in the origins of the great arteries and veins; the transpositions
4 Malpositions of the heart

Communications between systemic and pulmonary circulation without cyanosis (left-to-right shunts)

ATRIAL SEPTAL DEFECT Atrial septal defect, the most common congenital cardiac anomaly in adults, occurs more frequently in females than in males. Defects of the sinus venosus type occur high in the atrial septum, near the entry of the superior vena cava, and are associated frequently with anomalous connection of pulmonary veins from the right lung to the junction of the superior vena cava and right atrium. Most often, an atrial defect involves the fossa ovalis, is midseptal in location, and is of the *ostium secundum* type. This type of defect should not be confused with a patent foramen ovale. Anatomic obliteration of the foramen ovale ordinarily follows its functional closure soon after birth. *Ostium primum* anomalies are a form of endocardial cushion defect that lie immediately adjacent to the atrioventricular valves, either of which may be deformed and incompetent, or which may form together a common atrioventricular canal; this defect may also involve the superior portion of the interventricular septum. Ostium primum defects occur commonly in patients with *Down's syndrome* (mongolism). *Lutembacher's syndrome* is the designation applied to the rare combination of atrial septal defect and mitral stenosis; this component of the malformation almost invariably is the result of acquired rheumatic valvulitis.

The magnitude of the left-to-right shunt through an atrial septal defect depends on the size of the defect, the relative compliance of the ventricles, and the relative resistances in the pulmonary and systemic circulations. In patients with a patent foramen ovale or a small atrial septal defect, the left atrial pressure may exceed the right by several millimeters of mercury, whereas the mean pressure in both atria are identical when the defect is large. The left-to-right shunt causes diastolic overloading of the right ventricle and increased pulmonary blood flow. The pulmonary vascular resistance is usually normal in the child and young adult with atrial septal defect, and the volume load is usually well tolerated even though pulmonary blood flow may be three to six times greater than systemic. Streaming of unsaturated inferior vena caval blood from right to left is not uncommon in patients with ostium secundum defect, even in the absence of pulmonary hypertension.

Patients with atrial septal defect are usually asymptomatic in early life; cardiorespiratory symptoms occur in many of the older patients. Beyond the fourth decade, a significant number of patients develop atrial arrhythmias, pulmonary arterial hypertension, bidirectional and then right-to-left shunting of blood, and cardiac failure. Patients exposed to the chronic environmental hypoxia of high altitude tend to develop pulmonary hypertension at younger ages. Features that suggest that the defect is of the endocardial cushion variety include the onset of disability, pulmonary hypertension, and heart failure in infancy or childhood.

Physical examination usually reveals a prominent right ventricular cardiac impulse and palpable pulmonary artery pulsation. The first heart sound is normal or split, with accentuation of the tricuspid valve closure sound. Increased flow across the pulmonic valve is responsible for a midsystolic pulmonary ejection murmur. The second sound is widely split and is relatively fixed in relation to respiration, because of reciprocal changes in the magnitude of the left-to-right shunt and of the systemic venous inflow into the right ventricle during respiration, so that filling of the right ventricle remains constant throughout the respiratory cycle. A middiastolic rumbling murmur at the fourth intercostal space and along the left sternal border reflects increased flow across the tricuspid valve. In patients with ostium primum defects, an apical thrill and holosystolic murmur indicate associated mitral or tricuspid incompetence or a ventricular septal defect.

The *physical findings* are altered when an increase in the pulmonary vascular resistance results in diminution of the left-to-right shunt. Both the pulmonary and tricuspid murmurs decrease in intensity, the pulmonic component of the second heart sound and a systolic ejection sound are accentuated, the two components of the second heart sound may fuse, and a diastolic murmur of pulmonic incompetence appears. Cyanosis and clubbing accompany the development of a right-to-left shunt.

The *electrocardiogram* in patients with an ostium secundum defect usually shows right axis deviation, right ventricular hypertrophy, and a right intraventricular conduction defect. A coronary sinus pacemaker or first degree heart block is occasionally noted in patients with defects of the sinus venosus type. In patients with an ostium primum defect, the right ventricular conduction defect is characteristically accompanied by left axis deviation and by superior orientation and counterclockwise rotation of the QRS loop in the frontal plane. Varying degrees of right ventricular and right atrial hypertrophy may be seen with each type of defect, depending on the height of the pulmonary artery pressure; prolongation of the P-R interval is most common with defects of the ostium primum variety. Chest roentgenograms reveal enlargement of the right atrium and ventricle, dilatation of the pulmonary artery and its branches, and increased pulmonary vascular markings. Left atrial enlargement is extremely uncommon.

The diagnosis may be confirmed readily at cardiac catheterization by passage of the catheter across the atrial defect. The site at which the catheter crosses, if high in the cardiac silhouette, may suggest a sinus venosus defect, or, if low, a primum defect. Serial determinations of the oxygen saturation, or indicator-dilution curve techniques, may be used to estimate the magnitude of the shunt. In young patients, pressures in the right side of the heart are often normal despite a large shunt; pulmonary arterial hypertension occurs with greater frequency in the older patients. If an endocardial cushion defect is present, a left ventricular angiogram will frequently demonstrate a "gooseneck" deformity of the left ventricular outflow tract caused by an abnormal anterior mitral valve leaflet; it may also show mitral regurgitation. When a high oxygen saturation is found in the superior vena cava, or when the catheter enters pulmonary veins directly from the right atrium, a sinus venosus defect is likely, and indicator-dilution curves and selective angiography will aid in identifying the number and location of the anomalous veins. Partial anomalous pulmonary venous connection, although generally associated with a sinus venosus defect, may occasionally accompany primum and secundum defects.

Patients with atrial septal defect rarely die before the fifth decade. During the fifth and sixth decades, the incidence of progressive symptoms, often leading to severe disability, increases substantially. Medical management should include prompt treatment of respiratory tract infections, antiarrhythmic medications for atrial fibrillation or supraventricular tachycardia, and the usual measures for heart failure (Chap. 233) if these complications occur. Although the risk of subacute bacterial endocarditis is low, antibiotics should be administered prophylactically prior to dental procedures (see Chap. 127).

Operative repair, ideally in patients between five and ten years of age, should be advised for all patients with uncomplicated atrial septal defects in whom there is evidence of significant left-to-right shunting, i.e., with pulmonary-to-systemic flow ratios exceeding approximately 1.5/1.0. Excellent results may be anticipated, at low risk, even in patients beyond forty years of age in the absence of pulmonary hypertension. The defect is closed by suture or with a patch of prosthetic material with the patient on cardiopulmonary bypass. Special attention must be given to the atrioventricular valves in patients with endocardial cushion defects, since suture repair of a cleft in either or both of them, and even replacement with a prosthetic valve, may be necessary to prevent significant regurgitation and failure in the postoperative period. The operative risk and the incidence of such complications as complete heart block and the persistence of significant mitral regurgitation are significantly higher in patients with endocardial cushion defects. Operation should not be carried out in patients with small defects and trivial left-to-right shunts, or in those with severe pulmonary vascular disease without a net left-to-right shunt.

VENTRICULAR SEPTAL DEFECT Isolated defects of the ventricular septum are among the commonest cardiac malformations, and they are encountered as one component of a combination of anomalies more often than any other. Most frequently, the opening is single and situated in the membranous portion of the septum. The functional disturbance caused by a ventricular septal defect is dependent primarily on its age and the status of the pulmonary vascular bed, rather than on the location of the defect. A substantial left-to-right ventricular pressure gradient occurs in the presence of a small defect (*maladie de Roger*), and a small shunt, limited by the size of the defect, occurs throughout systole. The larger the defect, the more likely it is that both ventricles will function as a single pumping chamber with two outlets, equalizing the pressures in the systemic and pulmonary circulations. In such patients, the magnitude of the left-to-right shunt varies inversely with the pulmonary vascular resistance. In patients with large defects and large left-to-right shunts, the left ventricle is overloaded and may fail. Survival through infancy in many of these patients is predicated on delayed regression of the fetal pulmonary vascular pattern, the development of an elevated pulmonary vascular resistance, or the secondary development of infundibular hypertrophy and obstruction to right ventricular outflow. Irreversible obliterative changes in the pulmonary vessels with dominant right-to-left shunts and cyanosis become manifest after the second decade in many patients with large defects. Spontaneous closure of small and even large ventricular defects occurs in a significant number of patients, especially before the age of two years. In some others, the relative size of the interventricular communication may diminish as normal growth of the heart occurs with advancing age.

The clinical picture varies greatly, depending on the patient's age, the size of the defect, and the level of the pulmonary vascular resistance. Patients with small defects are asymptomatic; moderate left-to-right shunts may be associated with effort intolerance and fatigue. Large defects are commonly accompanied by frequent pulmonary infections, growth retardation, and cardiac failure in infancy, but survival past this period is often associated with an amelioration of symptoms until adulthood. In patients with severe pulmonary vascular obstruction, symptoms develop most often in adult life and consist of exertional dyspnea, chest pain, syncope, and hemoptysis. The right-to-left shunt leads to cyanosis, clubbing, and polycythemia.

Patients with moderate-sized defects exhibit cardiomegaly with a forceful left ventricular impulse and a prominent systolic thrill along the lower left sternal border. The second heart sound is normally split, with moderate accentuation of the pulmonic component, and a third heart sound and diastolic rumbling murmur, reflecting increased flow across the mitral valve during rapid ventricular filling, are often audible at the cardiac apex. The characteristic holosystolic murmur results from flow across the defect; it is best heard along the third and fourth interspaces to the left of the sternum, and is widely transmitted over the precordium. A basal midsystolic ejection murmur may also be heard, because of increased flow across the pulmonic valve. In patients with pulmonary vascular obstruction and small left-to-right shunts, both the systolic thrill and murmur decrease in intensity and duration and may disappear entirely, to be replaced by a marked right ventricular precordial lift, pulmonary ejection sound and soft systolic ejection murmur, a closely split second heart sound with accentuation of the pulmonic component, and the diastolic murmur of pulmonic incompetence.

The electrocardiographic pattern, the relative size and contour of the two ventricles roentgenographically, and the appearance of the lung fields serve as indicators of the underlying pathophysiologic condition. The electrocardiogram is generally normal in patients with small defects. Left or combined ventricular hypertrophy is seen with large left-to-right shunts; right ventricular hypertrophy occurs with pulmonary vascular obstruction. The roentgenograms may be normal in patients with small defects; large defects are characterized by an enlarged left atrium, biventricular hypertrophy, a prominent pulmonary artery segment, and increased pulmonary vascular markings. Relative diminution and attenuation of the peripheral pulmonary vasculature occur in patients with obstructive pulmonary vascular disease.

In approximately 90 percent of patients with this malformation, the defect occurs in the membranous septum. A shunt from the left ventricle to the right atrium may occur with a defect in the most superior portion of the ventricular septum, since the tricuspid valve is lower than the mitral valve. The clinical, electrocardiographic, and radiologic findings in these patients do not differ appreciably from those with a simple ventricular septal defect, but the diagnosis can be established by left ventriculography. Prolapse of an aortic valve leaflet through a subpulmonary ventricular defect or the combination of subcristal ventricular septal defect and underdevelopment of an aortic valve commissure may produce aortic regurgitation that is frequently progressive and is the most significant hemodynamic lesion. In these patients complete operative repair may necessitate insertion of a prosthetic aortic valve. The pathophysiology of a single or common ventricle resembles that of a large ventricular septal defect, although the two lesions are dissimilar embryologically. There is an obligatory admixture of systemic and pulmonary venous return in patients with a single ventricle, but there may be little or no cyanosis if selective streaming and increased pulmonary blood flow occur. Severe pulmonary hypertension is invariably present unless pulmonic stenosis coexists. It is imperative to differentiate a large ventricular septal defect from a single ventricle by angiography, because no corrective operation is available for single ventricle.

The risk of bacterial endocarditis is higher in patients with small or moderate-sized defects than in those with large ones, and appropriate prophylaxis is essential. In the small infant with a large left-to-right shunt, congestive failure may be severe and intractable despite intensive medical management; this problem is managed best by surgical constriction of the pulmonary artery, followed, when the patient is older, by a corrective operation.

Closure of the defect of the ventricular septum is indicated in children and adults when there is a moderate or large left-to-right shunt, regardless of the level of pulmonary artery pressure. Operation is contraindicated when the pulmonary vascular resistance is elevated to a level which eliminates the net left-to-right shunt. The recognition of associated cardiac anomalies is imperative if surgical treatment is contemplated. The most common of these are patent ductus arteriosus, ostium secundum atrial defects, pulmonic stenosis, coarctation of the aorta, and corrected transposition of the great arteries.

PATENT DUCTUS ARTERIOSUS The ductus arteriosus is a vessel leading from the bifurcation of the pulmonary artery to the aorta just distad to the left subclavian artery. Normal closure of the ductus immediately after birth may be due to the sudden increase in arterial oxygen tension that accompanies ventilation and/or the release of vasoactive substances. Intimal proliferation and fibrosis proceed more gradually, so that total anatomic obliteration may not occur for several months after birth. Persistent patency of the ductus after birth is a relatively common anomaly, occurring more frequently in females, in the offspring of women whose pregnancies were complicated by first-trimester rubella, in premature infants, and in children born at high altitudes. Although this anomaly occurs most frequently in the isolated form, it may coexist with other malformations, particularly coarctation of the aorta, ventricular septal defect, pulmonic stenosis, and aortic stenosis.

The flow across the ductus is determined by the pressure relationships between the aorta and the pulmonary artery and by the cross-sectional area and length of the ductus itself. Most commonly, pulmonary pressures are normal, and a gradient and shunt from aorta to pulmonary artery persists throughout the cardiac cycle. Physical examination reveals a characteristic thrill and a continuous "machinery" murmur, with a late systolic accentuation at the upper left sternal border. The left atrium and ventricle enlarge to accommodate the increased pulmonary venous return, and flow murmurs across the mitral and aortic valves may be detected. With large or moderate-sized left-to-right shunts, the runoff of blood through the ductus causes a widened systemic pulse pressure and bounding peripheral pulses. The hemodynamic abnormality is reflected by left ventricular and, occasionally, left atrial hypertrophy on the electrocardiogram and by left atrial and ventricular enlargement, a prominent ascending aorta and pulmonary artery, and pulmonary vascular engorgement on the chest roentgenogram.

The clinical recognition of patent ductus arteriosus may be difficult in infancy and in patients with pulmonary hypertension or heart failure. In these circumstances, the pressure gradient between the aorta and pulmonary artery is reduced or absent, as is the typical continuous murmur, and there may be only a systolic ejection murmur at the base, a diastolic blowing murmur of pulmonary regurgitation (Graham Steell), or no murmur audible at all. When severe pulmonary vascular disease results in reversal of flow through the ductus, unoxygenated blood is shunted to the descending aorta, and the toes, rather than the fingers, become cyanotic and clubbed, a finding termed *differential cyanosis*.

Delayed spontaneous closure of the ductus arteriosus has been known to occur in premature babies, even if heart failure was a problem in the neonatal period. Although a large ductus often results in cardiac failure and pulmonary edema in infancy, this anomaly is usually compatible with survival until adult life. The leading causes of death in adults with patent ductus are cardiac failure and bacterial endocarditis. In older patients, severe pulmonary vascular obstruction may cause aneurysmal dilatation, calcification, and rupture of the ductus.

In the absence of severe pulmonary vascular disease with predominant right-to-left shunting of blood, the simple presence of a patent ductus is generally considered a sufficient indication for operation, at least in patients over three years of age. Ligation or division of the ductus is associated with a low risk (under 2 percent) when it is performed electively in an otherwise healthy person. The operative risk is reduced if cardiac failure can be treated successfully before operation. Operation should be deferred for several months in patients treated successfully for bacterial endarteritis, because the ductus may remain somewhat edematous and friable.

AORTOPULMONARY SEPTAL DEFECT Aortopulmonary window, partial truncus arteriosis, and aortic septal defect are other designations applied to this relatively uncommon anomaly, which consists of a communication between the aorta and the pulmonary artery just above the semilunar valves. Such defects are usually large and are accompanied by varying degrees of obstructive pulmonary vascular disease and severe pulmonary arterial hypertension. The anomaly may be difficult to distinguish from patent ductus arteriosus. However, the murmur of aortopulmonary septal defect is rarely continuous, and a basal systolic murmur is most common. Cardiomegaly is present, and pulmonary hypertension is reflected in a loud and palpable sound of pulmonary valve closure. The diagnosis of aortopulmonary septal defect should be suspected whenever a large shunt into the pulmonary artery is demonstrated at catheterization. Distinction from patent ductus and persistent truncus arteriosus is facilitated by selective angiocardiography, with the injection of contrast material into the left ventricle and/or the root of the aorta. Operative correction is usually indicated in children and adults with large left-to-right shunts; total cardiopulmonary bypass is required, and the defect is closed, generally with a prosthetic patch.

AORTIC SINUS ANEURYSM AND FISTULA Congenital aneurysm of an aortic sinus of Valsalva, particularly the right coronary sinus, is an uncommon anomaly with a predilection for males; it consists of a separation, or lack of fusion, between the media of the aorta and the annulus fibrosus of the aortic valve. Progressive aneurysmal dilatation of the weakened area develops but may not be recognized until the third or fourth decade of life, when rupture into a cardiac chamber occurs. The receiving chamber of the aorticocardiac fistula is usually the right ventricle, but occasionally the fistula drains into the right atrium.

The unruptured aneurysm generally does not produce

symptoms or a hemodynamic abnormality, although pressure on the intracardiac conduction system by an unruptured aneurysm occasionally causes atrioventricular block, and myocardial ischemia may be caused by coronary arterial compression. Rupture is often of abrupt onset, causes chest pain, and creates continuous arteriovenous shunting and volume overloading of both right and left heart chambers, with resultant heart failure. Bacterial endocarditis may originate either on the edges of the aneurysm or on those areas in the right side of the heart which are traumatized by the jetlike stream of blood flowing through the fistula. This anomaly should be suspected in a patient with a history of recent onset of chest pain, symptoms of diminished cardiac reserve, bounding pulses, and a loud, superficial, continuous murmur accentuated in diastole when the fistula opens into the right ventricle, as well as a thrill along the right or left lower parasternal area. The electrocardiogram shows biventricular hypertrophy, and the chest roentgenogram demonstrates generalized cardiomegaly. The diagnosis may be established definitively by retrograde thoracic aortography. Operation is indicated in patients with large left-to-right shunts; the aneurysm is closed and amputated, and the aortic wall is reunited with the heart, either by direct suture or with a prosthesis.

CORONARY ARTERIOVENOUS FISTULA Coronary arteriovenous fistula is an unusual anomaly that most often consists of a communication between the right coronary artery and the right atrium or ventricle. The shunt is usually of small magnitude, and myocardial blood flow is not compromised. Potential complications include bacterial endocarditis, thrombus formation with occlusion or distal embolization, rupture of an aneurysmal fistula, and, rarely, pulmonary hypertension and congestive failure when the left-to-right shunt is large. The finding of a loud, superficial, continuous murmur at the lower or midsternal border usually prompts a further evaluation of asymptomatic patients. Retrograde thoracic aortography or coronary arteriography permits identification of the size and anatomic features of the fistulous tract, which may be closed by suture obliteration.

ANOMALOUS PULMONARY ORIGIN OF CORONARY ARTERY In this rare malformation, the left coronary artery originates from the pulmonary artery. Myocardial infarction and fibrosis commonly develop during the first 6 months of life, leading to death within the first year. From 10 to 20 percent of patients survive to childhood or adolescence without surgical correction. As the elevated pulmonary vascular resistance declines immediately after birth, perfusion of the left coronary artery from the pulmonary artery ceases and the direction of flow in the anomalous vessel reverses. Thus, blood flows from the aorta to the right coronary artery, then through collateral channels to the left coronary artery, and finally to the pulmonary artery. Total myocardial perfusion through the right coronary artery increases if adequate collateral channels develop between the two coronary circulations. Occasionally, in older children or adults one may find an example of mitral regurgitation which results from dysfunction of ischemic or infarcted papillary muscles. In some instances the coronary anomaly is unsuspected until a previously well adolescent or adult experiences angina, heart failure, or sudden death.

The diagnosis of anomalous origin of the coronary artery is supported by the electrocardiographic findings of an anterolateral myocardial infarction (Chap. 229). Chest roentgenograms show moderate to severe enlargement of the left atrium and ventricle. Aortic root or coronary angiography demonstrates the retrograde drainage of the coronary vessel into the pulmonary artery and the presence of a single right coronary artery arising from the aorta.

Ideal operative management of these patients consists of anastomosis of the left coronary artery to a systemic artery or to the aorta via a graft. However, the disorder may also be managed by simple ligation of the left coronary artery at its origin, preventing retrograde flow and allowing perfusion of the left ventricle by blood supplied through anastomoses from the right coronary artery. The outcome of operation and ultimate prognosis are influenced significantly by the degree of myocardial damage suffered preoperatively.

PERSISTENT TRUNCUS ARTERIOSUS Persistent truncus arteriosus is a rare but serious anomaly in which a single vessel forms the outlet of both ventricles and gives rise to the systemic, pulmonary, and coronary arteries. It is always accompanied by a ventricular septal defect and frequently by a right-sided aortic arch. The designation "pseudo-truncus arteriosus" refers to the condition in which a single vessel arises from the heart but is accompanied by a remnant of atretic pulmonary artery; this malformation does not differ from tetralogy of Fallot with pulmonary atresia (page 1162). Truncus malformations may be classified embryologically and anatomically according to the mode of origin of the pulmonary vessels from the common trunk, or, from a functional point of view, by the magnitude of flow to the lungs. Pulmonary flow is governed by the size of the pulmonary arteries and the pulmonary vascular resistance. Most often, mild cyanosis coexists with the cardiac findings of a large left-to-right shunt. The most frequent physical findings include cardiomegaly, a systolic ejection sound, a loud, single second heart sound, a harsh systolic murmur accompanied by a thrill, and a low-pitched middiastolic rumbling murmur. Left ventricular hypertrophy, alone or in combination with right ventricular hypertrophy, is present electrocardiographically. Gross cardiomegaly with left or combined ventricular enlargement, left atrial enlargement, and a small or absent main pulmonary artery segment with pulmonary vascular engorgement are the usual radiographic findings. The diagnosis should be suspected at catheterization if the catheter fails to enter the central pulmonary arteries from the right ventricle despite evidence of increased pulmonary blood flow; aortography is the diagnostic procedure of choice.

The early fatal course and, in patients surviving infancy, the development of pulmonary vascular obstructive disease are responsible for the poor prognosis associated with persistent truncus arteriosus. The long-term results of corrective operations employing a homograft of the ascending aorta and aortic valve to construct a pulmonary trunk have yet to be evaluated. In infants and young children, palliative banding of one or both of the pulmonary arteries may be indicated when pulmonary flow is markedly excessive. In patients with inadequate pulmonary blood flow it is usually not possible to enhance pulmonary blood flow with a shunting operation.

VALVULAR AND VASCULAR LESIONS WITH RIGHT-TO-LEFT SHUNT

PULMONARY STENOSIS WITH INTACT VENTRICULAR SEPTUM Obstruction to right ventricular outflow is relatively common; it may be localized to the supravalvular, valvular, or subvalvular levels or to a combination of these sites. Multiple sites of narrowing of the peripheral pulmonary arteries are often a feature of rubella embryopathy and may be associated with both the familial and sporadic forms of supravalvular aortic stenosis. Valvular pulmonic stenosis is the most common form of right ventricular obstruction.

The severity of the obstructing lesion, rather than the site of narrowing, is the most important determinant of the clinical course. In the presence of a normal cardiac output, a peak systolic transvalvular pressure gradient between 50 and 100 mm Hg is considered to be moderate stenosis; levels below and above that range are classified as mild and severe, respectively. Patients with mild pulmonic stenosis are generally asymptomatic and demonstrate little or no progression in the severity of obstruction as they grow older. In patients with more significant stenosis, the severity of the obstruction may increase with time. Progression may be relative and may reflect disproportionate physical growth of the patient, infundibular narrowing due to progressive hypertrophy of the right ventricular outflow tract, or fibrosis of the valve cusps. Atresia of the pulmonary valve is commonly associated with a hypoplastic right ventricle and interatrial communication. Symptoms vary according to the degree of obstruction. Infants with pulmonary atresia often die from hypoxia. Fatigue, dyspnea, and syncope may limit the activity of older patients, in whom moderate or severe obstruction prevents an augmentation of pulmonary blood flow with exercise.

In patients with severe obstruction, the systolic pressure in the right ventricle may exceed that in the left ventricle, since the ventricular septum is intact. Right ventricular ejection is prolonged in patients with moderate or severe stenosis, and the sound of pulmonary valve closure is delayed and soft. Right ventricular hypertrophy reduces the compliance of that chamber, and a forceful right atrial contraction is necessary to augment right ventricular filling. A fourth heart sound, prominent A waves in the jugular venous pulse, and, occasionally, presystolic pulsations of the liver reflect the vigorous atrial contraction. The clinical diagnosis is further supported by the presence of a right parasternal lift and harsh systolic ejection murmur and thrill at the upper left sternal border, often preceded by a systolic ejection sound if the obstruction is valvular. The systolic murmur becomes louder, and its crescendo occurs later in systole, as progressively more severe degrees of valvular obstructions result in increasing prolongation of right ventricular systole. The holosystolic decrescendo murmur of tricuspid regurgitation may accompany severe pulmonic stenosis, especially in the presence of congestive heart failure. Cyanosis usually reflects venoarterial shunting through a patent foramen ovale. In patients with supravalvular or peripheral pulmonary arterial stenosis, the murmur is systolic or continuous and is best heard over the area of narrowing, with radiation to the peripheral lung fields.

The electrocardiogram may be helpful in assessing the degree of obstruction to right ventricular output. In mild cases, the electrocardiogram is often normal, whereas moderate and severe stenoses are associated with right axis deviation and right ventricular hypertrophy. A ventricular strain pattern, as well as high-amplitude P waves in leads II and V_1, indicating right atrial enlargement, is associated with severe stenosis. The chest roentgenogram in patients with mild or moderate pulmonic stenosis often shows a heart of normal size and normal vascularity of the lungs. In the presence of valvular stenosis, poststenotic dilatation of the main pulmonary artery may be evident. In patients with severe obstruction and resultant right ventricular failure, right atrial and right ventricular enlargement are generally evident. The pulmonary vascularity may be reduced in patients with severe stenosis, right ventricular failure, and/or a venoarterial shunt at the atrial level.

Cardiac catheterization and angiocardiography with right ventricular injection are necessary to localize the site of obstruction and evaluate its severity, and to document the coexistence of additional cardiac malformations. The treatment of moderate and severe degrees of pulmonary valvular and subvalvular stenosis is surgical. Direct surgical relief of the obstruction may usually be accomplished at a low risk. Multiple stenoses of the peripheral pulmonary arteries are usually inoperable, but narrowing of a single branch or at the bifurcation of the main pulmonary trunk may be corrected.

TETRALOGY OF FALLOT The four components of this malformation are (1) ventricular septal defect; (2) obstruction to right ventricular outflow; (3) overriding of the aortic orifice above the two ventricular outflow tracts; and (4) right ventricular hypertrophy. Systolic pressures are equal in the right ventricle and aorta as a consequence of the first two components. The overall incidence of tetralogy approaches 10 percent of all forms of congenital heart disease, and it is the most common anomaly responsible for cyanosis after the age of one year. The ventricular septal defect is usually large, approximating the aortic orifice in size, and located high in the septum beneath the crista supraventricularis just below the aortic valve. The aortic root may be displaced anteriorly and straddle or override the septal defect. Infundibular stenosis occurs as the only major site of obstruction to right ventricular outflow in about one-half the patients and coexists with valvular obstruction in another 25 percent. Supravalvular and peripheral pulmonary arterial narrowing may be observed. When the main pulmonary artery, pulmonic valve, or right ventricular infundibulum is atretic, the condition may be called *pseudo-truncus arteriosus* (page 1160. In such cases, the lungs are perfused through enlarged bronchial arteries and/or through the pulmonary arteries via a patent ductus arteriosus. A right-sided aortic knob, arch, and descending aorta occur in approximately 25 percent of patients with tetralogy of Fallot.

The relationship between the resistance to blood flow from the ventricles into the aorta and into the pulmonary vessels plays the major role in determining the hemodynamic and clinical picture. Therefore, it is the severity of obstruction to right ventricular outflow which is of fundamental significance. When right ventricular outflow obstruction is severe, the pulmonary blood flow is markedly reduced and a large volume of unsaturated systemic venous blood is shunted from right to left across the ventricular septal defect, severe cyanosis and polycythemia occur, and symptoms of systemic anoxia are prominent. The term *pink*, or *acyanotic*, *tetralogy of Fallot* is used often to describe an interventricular communication and a milder degree of obstruction to right ventricular outflow with no appreciable venoarterial shunting. In some patients the obstruction to right ventricular outflow is so mild that pulmonary exceeds systemic blood flow and the symptoms resemble those produced by a simple ventricular septal defect.

Most children with tetralogy of Fallot are cyanotic from birth or develop cyanosis before one year of age. Dyspnea with exertion, retarded growth and development, clubbing, and polycythemia are common. When resting after exertion, patients with tetralogy characteristically assume a squatting posture. Spells of severe anoxia and cyanosis (see page 1157) constitute a major threat to survival.

Physical examination reveals variable degrees of underdevelopment and cyanosis. Clubbing of the terminal digits may be prominent after the first year of life. A right ventricular impulse and systolic thrill may be palpable along the left sternal border; there is no generalized cardiomegaly. The second heart sound is single, and the pulmonic component is rarely audible. A systolic ejection murmur is produced by flow across the narrowed right ventricular outflow tract or pulmonic valve. The intensity and duration of the murmur vary inversely with the severity of obstruction, the opposite of the relation existing in patients with an intact ventricular septum and pulmonary stenosis. Polycythemia, decreased systemic vascular resistance, and increased obstruction to right ventricular outflow may all be responsible for a decrease in the intensity of the murmur. A continuous murmur over the paravertebral area may indicate collateral circulation to the lungs through bronchial arteries.

The electrocardiogram ordinarily shows right ventricular and, less often, right atrial hypertrophy. Radiologic examination characteristically reveals a normal-sized, boot-shaped heart (*coeur en sabot*) with prominence of the right ventricle and a concavity in the region of the pulmonary conus. The pulmonary vascular markings are typically diminished, and the aortic arch and knob may be on the right side. Selective angiocardiography with right ventricular injection is necessary to evaluate the architecture of the right ventricular outflow tract, pulmonary valve and annulus, and caliber of the main branches of the pulmonary artery.

Among the factors that may complicate the management of patients with tetralogy are iron-deficiency anemia, subacute bacterial endocarditis, paradoxic embolism, polycythemia, coagulation defects, and cerebral infarction or abscess. The paroxysmal cyanotic spells may respond quickly to oxygen, placing the child in the knee-chest position, and morphine. If the spell persists, metabolic acidosis will develop from prolonged anaerobic metabolism, and infusion of sodium bicarbonate may be necessary to interrupt the attack. Vasopressors, β-adrenergic blockade, or general anesthesia may occasionally be necessary.

Total correction is ultimately advisable for almost all patients with tetralogy of Fallot. However, if cyanosis or symptoms are marked in an infant or young child, the risk of primary repair is high, and a palliative operation designed to increase pulmonary blood flow is recommended. These procedures include aortopulmonary or subclavian-pulmonary arterial anastomosis or transventricular infundibulectomy or valvulotomy. Total correction can then be carried out at a lower risk later in childhood or during adolescence.

EBSTEIN'S ANOMALY In this rare anomaly there is redundancy of tricuspid valve tissue, and the annular attachment of the septal and posterior leaflets of the tricuspid valve is lower than normal; the leaflets originate from the right ventricular wall rather than from the atrioventricular ring. Hence, the portion of the right ventricle that lies between the atrioventricular ring and the origin of the valve is continuous with the right atrial chamber. The tricuspid valve is usually incompetent, the foramen ovale is patent, and the right ventricle exhibits varying degrees of hypoplasia. The clinical manifestations of Ebstein's anomaly are variable, depending on the severity of the anatomic changes. Ultimately, however, progressive cyanosis resulting from the right-to-left shunt across the interatrial communication, symptoms resulting from right ventricular dysfunction, and/or paroxysmal arrhythmias develop.

A prominent systolic pulsation of the liver and a large V wave in the jugular venous pulse accompany the systolic thrill and murmur of tricuspid regurgitation. Wide splitting of the first and second heart sounds and prominent third and fourth heart sounds may produce a characteristically rhythmic auscultatory cadence. The electrocardiogram shows giant P waves, a prolonged P-R interval, and complete or incomplete right bundle branch block. Occasionally, there is a short P-R interval with the Wolff-Parkinson-White (type B) conduction anomaly. Roentgenographic and fluoroscopic studies usually demonstrate an enlarged right atrium, a small right ventricle, and a pulmonary artery with reduced pulsations; the pulmonary vascularity may be reduced if a large right-to-left shunt is present. At cardiac catheterization the intracavitary electrocardiogram recorded just proximal to the tricuspid valve shows a right ventricular type of complex, while the pressure recorded is that of the right atrium.

Ebstein's anomaly may be compatible with a relatively long and active life, most patients surviving to the third decade. In some disabled patients improvement has resulted from anastomosis of the superior vena cava to the right pulmonary artery to divert systemic venous return from the right atrium and to increase pulmonary blood flow. Others have been benefited by prosthetic replacement of the tricuspid valve.

TRICUSPID ATRESIA Atresia of the tricuspid valve, an interatrial communication, and, frequently, hypoplasia of the right ventricle and pulmonary artery, as well as transposition of the great arteries, exist in this malformation. Survival is dependent on a right-to-left shunt at the atrial level. Blood reaches the lungs through a patent ductus arteriosus, bronchial collateral vessels, or the right ventricle and pulmonary artery via a ventricular septal defect. The clinical picture is usually dominated by symptoms resulting from greatly diminished pulmonary blood flow, with anoxic spells and severe cyanosis.

The electrocardiogram showing left axis deviation, right atrial enlargement, and left ventricular hypertrophy in a cyanotic child strongly suggests tricuspid atresia. Many patients die in the first weeks or months of life. Palliative operations, consisting of increasing pulmonary blood flow, often by systemic-arterial or venous-pulmonary artery anastomosis, though capable of producing clinical improvement and/or relieving significant interatrial obstruction, carry a significant risk. Total operative correction of the anomaly has not been successful.

COARCTATION OF THE AORTA Narrowing or constriction of the lumen of the aorta may occur anywhere along its length but is most commonly localized just distad to the origin of the left subclavian artery near the insertion of the ligamentum arteriosum. Coarctation is encountered in approximately 7 percent of patients with congenital heart disease and is twice as common in males as in females, although the lesion occurs frequently in patients with gonadal dysgenesis (Turner's syndrome, Chap. 92). Clinical manifestations depend on the site and extent of obstruction and the presence of associated cardiac anomalies, which occur in about one-third of patients. These include bicuspid aortic valve, patent ductus arteriosus, ventricular septal defect, and congenital aortic stenosis. When the coarctation is located proximal to the ductus arteriosus, right ventricular hypertrophy develops in utero and pulmonary hypertension and congestive heart failure are common in early life. *Differential cyanosis* may result from preferential shunting of unsaturated pulmonary arterial blood through a patent ductus arteriosus to the lower part of the body.

More commonly, the coarctation is postductal and the ductus arteriosus is closed. The majority of children and young adults with isolated postductal coarctation are asymptomatic. Headache, epistaxis, cold extremities, and claudication with exercise may be noted, although attention is usually directed to the cardiovascular system when a heart murmur of hypertension in the upper extremities is detected on routine physical examination. Both mechanical and humoral factors, particularly of renal origin and involving the renin-angiotensin-aldosterone mechanism (Chaps. 86 and 245), play a significant role in the production of hypertension.

Absence, marked diminution, or delayed pulsations in the femoral arteries and a low or unobtainable arterial pressure in the lower extremities with hypertension in the arms are the basic clue to the diagnosis. In adults, enlarged and pulsatile collateral vessels may be palpated in the intercostal spaces anteriorly, in the axillas, or posteriorly in the interscapular area. A midsystolic murmur over the anterior part of the chest, back, and spinous processes is most frequent, becoming continuous if the lumen is narrowed sufficiently to result in a high-velocity jet across the lesion throughout the cardiac cycle. Additional systolic and continuous murmurs over the lateral thoracic wall may reflect increased flow through dilated and tortuous collateral vessels. The *electrocardiogram* reveals left ventricular hypertrophy of varying degree, depending on the height of the arterial pressure proximal to the obstruction and the patient's age; predominant right or combined ventricular hypertrophy may be seen in infants and children, and usually implies a complicated lesion. *Roentgenograms* may show a dilated left subclavian artery high on the left mediastinal border and a dilated ascending aorta. Indentation of the aorta at the site of coarctation and pre- and poststenotic dilatation (the "3" sign) along the left paramediastinal shadow are almost pathognomonic. Notching of the ribs, an important radiographic sign, is due to erosion by dilated collateral vessels, increases with age, and usually becomes apparent between the sixth and twelfth years of life. Cardiac catheterization and aortography may be indicated to localize accurately the site of obstruction, determine the length of the coarctation, and identify associated malformations.

The *treatment* of uncomplicated coarctation of the aorta is surgical; resection and end-to-end anastomosis can be accomplished with excellent results in most patients, although it is occasionally necessary to use a graft in the repair if the narrowed segment is long. Paradoxic hypertension of short duration is often noted in the immediate postoperative period, and occasionally a necrotizing panarteritis of the small vessels of the gastrointestinal tract of uncertain cause complicates the course of recovery. In those who survive the first 2 years of life complications are uncommon before the second or third decade; operation on asymptomatic patients is advised ideally between the ages of five and ten years. The chief hazards to patients with coarctation result from severe hypertension and include the development of cerebral aneurysms and hemorrhage, rupture of the aorta, left ventricular failure, and bacterial endocarditis.

Congenital aortic stenosis

Malformations that cause obstruction to the ejection of blood from the left ventricle include congenital valvular aortic stenosis, the discrete form of congenital subaortic stenosis, congenital narrowing of the supravalvular ascending aorta, and idiopathic hypertrophic subaortic stenosis (Chap. 242).

VALVULAR AORTIC STENOSIS Valvular aortic stenosis occurs in approximately 4 percent of patients with congenital cardiovascular defects and occurs three to four times more often in males than in females. However, the congenital bicuspid aortic valve, which is not necessarily stenotic, may actually be the most common congenital malformation of the heart, although it may go undetected in early life. Because bicuspid valves may become stenotic with time, the lesion may become of clinical significance only in adult life, when it may be difficult to distinguish it anatomically from acquired rheumatic aortic stenosis. Commonly associated anomalies include patent ductus arteriosus and coarctation of the aorta.

One finds thickening and increased rigidity of the valve tissue and varying degrees of commissural fusion. The dynamics of blood flow associated with a congenitally deformed aortic valve commonly lead to thickening of the cusps and, in later life, to calcification. When the obstruction is hemodynamically significant, concentric hypertrophy of the left ventricular wall and dilatation of the ascending aorta occur.

The hemodynamic abnormalities produced by obstruction to left ventricular outflow are discussed in Chap. 239. A peak systolic pressure gradient exceeding 75 mm Hg, in association with a normal cardiac output, or an effective aortic orifice less than 0.5 cm^2 per m^2 body surface area, is considered to represent critical obstruction to left ventricular outflow. The resting cardiac output is generally within normal limits. During exercise, however, the majority of patients with critical stenosis show little elevation, because an increase in blood flow across the stenotic valve can occur only if the transvalvular pressure gradient increases disproportionately.

Most children with congenital aortic stenosis are asymptomatic and grow and develop normally. Usually, a murmur is detected on a routine examination. At least moderately severe obstruction should be suspected if there is a definite history of fatigability and exertional dyspnea. In patients with severe obstruction, the inability of the left ventricle to increase its output and the cerebral flow during exercise may result in exertional syncope, while the disparity between the oxygen supply to the left ventricle and myocardial oxygen requirements may be responsible for anginal pain. The truly symptomatic child with valvular aortic stenosis generally has critical stenosis, although a lack of symptoms does not preclude the presence of moderately severe obstruction. Sudden death, a potential threat to these patients, occurs in from 1 to 7.5 percent. Its precise cause is poorly understood, but ventricular arrhythmias, perhaps initiated by acute myocardial ischemia, may be responsible.

When obstruction is significant, a left ventricular lift is usually palpable and a precordial systolic thrill is felt over the base of the heart, with transmission to the jugular notch and along the carotid arteries. Presystolic expansion is often palpable. A systolic aortic ejection sound, signifying opening of the aortic valves, may be heard at the cardiac apex when the valve is mobile, particularly in patients with mild to moderate stenosis. Delayed closure of the stenotic aortic valve leads to a single or a closely split second heart sound, and paradoxic splitting may be present. A fourth heart sound is generally associated with severe obstruction. The systolic murmur starts after the completion of left ventricular isometric contraction, is rhomboid-shaped, loud, harsh, and best heard at the base of the heart. The murmur, like the thrill, radiates to the jugular notch and carotid vessels, as well as to the apex. In some patients, an early diastolic blowing murmur of aortic regurgitation is present, but unless the valve leaflets have been eroded by bacterial endocarditis, the regurgitation is usually not hemodynamically significant.

Electrocardiographically, left ventricular hypertrophy tends to vary with the severity of obstruction, although a *normal or near-normal electrocardiogram does not exclude severe aortic stenosis.* The left ventricular "strain pattern," which consists of left ventricular hypertrophy combined with S-T segment depressions and T-wave inversion in the left precordial leads, generally, but not always, indicates that severe aortic stenosis is present.

Roentgenographically, the overall heart size is most often normal or slightly enlarged. Left atrial enlargement and concentric left ventricular hypertrophy accompany moderate or severe obstruction. Poststenotic dilatation of the ascending aorta is a common finding. Cardiac catheterization is indicated when the clinical diagnosis of aortic stenosis has been established and when the history, clinical examination, roentgenogram, or electrocardiogram suggests the possibility of severe obstruction. The site and severity of obstruction are established, and associated malformations are identified. In patients with mild obstruction repeat left-sided heart catheterization should be carried out every 5 to 10 years because stenosis may progress.

The medical management of congenital valvular aortic stenosis includes prophylaxis against bacterial endocarditis and, in patients with diminished cardiac reserve, the administration of digitalis and sodium restriction while awaiting operation. If severe aortic stenosis is present, strict avoidance of strenuous physical activity is advised even when the patient is asymptomatic, and participation in competitive sports should probably also be restricted in patients with milder degrees of obstruction. The decision concerning the advisability of operation depends on the severity of obstruction rather than on the symptoms described by the patient. Operation is carried out under direct vision with the aid of total cardiopulmonary bypass, and the fused commissures are opened. Following commissurotomy the valves remain somewhat deformed, and it is possible that further degenerative changes, including calcification, will lead to significant stenosis later.

SUBAORTIC STENOSIS The most common form of subaortic stenosis is the idiopathic hypertrophic variety, which occurs in a congenital form in about one-third of the patients and is discussed in Chap. 242. Both clinically and physiologically, however, it is the discrete form of subaortic stenosis which resembles valvular aortic stenosis. The lesion consists of a membranous diaphragm or fibrous ring encircling the left ventricular outflow tract just beneath the base of the aortic valve. It is less common than isolated valvular obstruction, but it also occurs more frequently in males than in females. There are no clinical criteria which can be relied upon to distinguish the two forms of obstruction, although a systolic ejection sound is rarely heard in patients with discrete subvalvular aortic stenosis and the diastolic murmur of aortic regurgitation is more common than in patients with valvular aortic stenosis. Also, valvular calcification is not observed roentgenographically in patients with subaortic stenosis. Definitive differentiation between valvular and subvalvular obstruction is best accomplished at cardiac catheterization by recording pressure tracings as a cardiac catheter is withdrawn across the outflow tract and valve or by localizing the site of obstruction with selective left ventricular angiocardiography.

There are few differences in the indications for operation in patients with discrete subaortic stenosis and valvular aortic stenosis. Surgical correction consists of excising the membrane or fibrous ridge; it may be expected to improve the hemodynamic state substantially and may be totally curative. However, secondary muscular hypertrophy of the outflow tract and a subaortic pressure gradient may persist following the operative relief of aortic stenosis.

Occasionally, valvular and subvalvular aortic stenosis coexist in the same patient, producing a tunnel-like narrowing of the left ventricular outflow tract. Associated findings are often a small ascending aorta, hypoplasia of the aortic valve ring, and thickened valve leaflets. It may be recognized by angiography. Operative treatment frequently necessitates prosthetic replacement of the aortic valve, as well as enlarging the aortic annulus, proximal aorta, and left ventricular outflow tract.

Several anatomic lesions other than a membrane, ridge, or muscular band that may produce subaortic stenosis are listed in Table 237-2.

SUPRAVALVULAR AORTIC STENOSIS Supravalvular aortic stenosis is a localized or diffuse narrowing of the ascending aorta, originating just above the level of the coronary arteries at the superior margin of the sinuses of Valsalva. In contrast to other forms of aortic stenosis, in the supravalvular variety the coronary arteries are subjected to the elevated pressures that exist within the left ventricle, and are often dilated and tortuous. Adherence of the free edges of the aortic cusps to the site of supravalvular stenosis may interfere with coronary arterial inflow.

The designation *supravalvular aortic stenosis syndrome* has been applied to the distinctive clinical picture produced by coexistence of the cardiovascular lesion and a metabolic disorder, idiopathic infantile hypercalcemia, that is probably related to deranged vitamin D metabolism. Other manifestations of this syndrome include mental retardation, a peculiar "elfin facies," craniosynostosis, strabismus, narrowing of peripheral systemic and pulmonary arteries, inguinal hernias, cryptorchidism in males, premature development of secondary sexual characteristics in females, and abnormalities of dental development. Supravalvular aortic stenosis and peripheral pulmonary arterial stenosis are also seen in familial and sporadic forms unassociated with the other features of the syndrome. Genetic studies suggest that when the anomaly is familial it is transmitted as an autosomal dominant strain with variable expression.

TABLE 237-2
Unusual causes of subaortic stenosis

1 Accessory tissue of the mitral valve
2 Restriction of movement of the anterior mitral valve leaflet
  a Anomalous basal attachment of anterior leaflet
  b Accessory chordae tendineae
  c Abnormal fusion of valvular tissue to the septal wall of the outflow tract
  d Convergence of all mitral chordae into one or two fused papillary muscles ("parachute" deformity)
3 Deficiency of the ventricular septum (endocardial cushion defects)
4 Anomalous subaortic muscle bundle (corrected transposition)
5 Type II glycogen storage disease

The physical findings resemble those in valvular aortic stenosis, except that the sound of aortic valve closure is accentuated, ejection sounds are infrequent, and transmission of the thrill and murmurs into the jugular notch and along the carotid vessels is more prominent; the systolic pressure in the right arm tends to be higher than in the left.

The electrocardiogram reveals left ventricular hypertrophy, but biventricular or even right ventricular hypertrophy may be observed if significant narrowing of peripheral pulmonary arteries coexists. Poststenotic dilatation of the ascending aorta is rarely seen. The diagnosis is confirmed by the demonstration at retrograde aortic catheterization of a pressure gradient just above the aortic valve, and a constriction at this level as revealed by aortography.

Surgical treatment consists of widening the lumen of the aorta by the insertion of an oval or diamond-shaped fabric prosthesis, and operative treatment is indicated if the obstruction is discrete and severe without generalized hypoplasia of the ascending aorta and arch.

HYPOPLASTIC LEFT HEART SYNDROME This designation is used to describe the condition of patients with an obstructive lesion on the left side of the heart associated with hypoplasia of the left ventricle and hypertrophy of the right ventricle. This syndrome, which is a significant cause of neonatal mortality, may be caused by atresia and/or hypoplasia of the aortic and mitral valves and of the aortic arch. The left atrium and ventricle often exhibit endocardial fibroelastosis. The diagnosis should be considered in infants, particularly males, with the sudden onset of cardiac failure, hypotension, and a nonspecific murmur. The electrocardiogram frequently reveals right axis deviation, right atrial and ventricular enlargement, and S-T and T-wave abnormalities in left precordial leads. Chest roentgenograms show moderate to marked cardiac enlargement and increased pulmonary vascular markings in nearly all patients.

Definitive diagnostic studies may be indicated as early as the first 24 hr of life. Presently, the anatomic lesions are inoperable. Results of palliation by means of a systemic arterial–pulmonary arterial anastomosis, banding the pulmonary arteries, and enlarging an interatrial communication have been disappointing.

MALFORMATIONS OBSTRUCTING PULMONARY VENOUS FLOW A number of malformations at or upstream to the mitral valve may cause obstruction to flow of pulmonary venous blood into the left ventricle.

Mitral stenosis Anatomic types of mitral stenosis include the "parachute" deformity of the valve, in which shortened chordae tendineae converge and insert into a single large papillary muscle; an anomalous arcade of obstructing papillary muscles; rudimentary valve commissures and thickened fibrotic leaflets, often associated with endocardial fibroelastosis of the left atrium and ventricle; and a supravalvular circumferential ridge of connective tissue arising at the base of the atrial aspect of the mitral leaflets.

Cor triatriatum In this malformation an abnormal fibromuscular diaphragm divides the left atrium into a posterosuperior chamber, into which the pulmonary veins drain, and an anterointerior chamber, which communicates with the mitral valve and atrial appendage. The diaphragm contains an opening, or occasionally several openings, the size of which determines the degree of obstruction to pulmonary venous return.

Congenital pulmonary vein stenosis This malformation may consist of a localized narrowing at or near the junctions of the pulmonary veins and the left atrium, or individual pulmonary veins may be hypoplastic for variable distances along their intra- or extrapulmonary portions.

The hemodynamic and clinical consequences of each of these lesions result from obstruction to pulmonary venous return. There is severe pulmonary arterial hypertension as a consequence of elevations both of the pulmonary venous pressure and of pulmonary vascular resistance. At cardiac catheterization cor triatriatum and pulmonary vein stenosis may be suspected if the pulmonary arterial wedge pressure is higher than a simultaneous left atrial pressure obtained by transseptal catheterization. A specific diagnosis of each of these anomalies may be established by visualizing the obstructing lesion angiographically. Although these malformations are rare, differential diagnosis is important, since cor triatriatum may be easily corrected at operation.

TRANSPOSITION COMPLEXES

The term *transposition* identifies a complicated group of malformations that have in common abnormal relationships between the cardiac chambers and the great arteries.

COMPLETE TRANSPOSITION OF THE GREAT ARTERIES The aorta arises from the right ventricle to the right of and anterior to the pulmonary artery, which emerges from the left ventricle. This results in two separate and parallel circulations, and some communication between the two circulations must exist after birth in order to sustain life. Almost all patients have an interatrial communication, two-thirds have a patent ductus arteriosus, and about one-half have an associated ventricular septal defect. Transposition occurs more frequently in males than in females. It is a leading cause of death due to congenital heart disease in the first 2 months of life and accounts for approximately 10 percent of all patients with cyanotic heart disease. Without treatment, about 70 percent of the patients with this malformation die by the age of six months. A few survive into childhood, and rarely a patient survives into young adult life. Those who live beyond infancy have, as a general rule, either an isolated large atrial septal defect or a ventricular septal defect and pulmonic stenosis.

The clinical course is determined by the degree of tissue hypoxia, the ability of each ventricle to sustain an increased work load in the presence of reduced coronary arterial oxygenation, the nature of the associated cardiovascular anomalies, and the anatomic and functional status of the pulmonary vascular bed. A bidirectional shunt is always present, because continuous unidirectional shunting would result in a progressive depletion of the circulating volume in either the pulmonary or the systemic vascular bed. The volume of these life-sustaining shunts may be estimated from the effective pulmonary blood flow, since this is a measure of the quantity of systemic venous return that ultimately traverses and is oxygenated in the pulmonary circulation. The magnitude of both the arteriovenous and venoarterial shunts is modified by the number of intercirculatory communications that exist, the presence of associated obstructive intra- and extracardiac anomalies, and the relations between the pulmonary and systemic vascular resistances. Severe morphologic alterations develop in the pulmonary vascular bed by the age of two years in almost all patients with this anomaly with an associated large ventricular septal defect or large patent ductus arteriosus.

The usual clinical manifestations are dyspnea and cyanosis from birth, retardation of growth, and congestive heart failure. Attacks of paroxysmal dyspnea may occur. Murmurs are of little diagnostic significance and are absent or insignificant in approximately 30 percent of these infants.

The usual electrocardiographic findings include right axis deviation, right atrial enlargement, and right ventricular hypertrophy, reflecting that the right ventricle is the systemic pumping chamber. Left ventricular hypertrophy is also present in those patients with large ventricular septal defects or significant obstruction to pulmonary blood flow. The roentgenographic findings are often diagnostic and consist of (1) progressive cardiac enlargement in early infancy; (2) characteristic oval or egg-shaped cardiac configuration in the anteroposterior view and a narrow base of the heart, created by superimposition of the aortic and pulmonary artery segments; and (3) increased pulmonary vascular markings. Cardiac catheterization shows a lower oxygen saturation in the aorta than in the pulmonary artery. Angiocardiography is diagnostic and demonstrates that the anteriorly placed aorta arises from the right ventricle, and the posteriorly placed pulmonary artery from the left ventricle.

Medical treatment is often of limited help but should be vigorous now that total correction of the malformation has become a reality. Conservative measures include use of oxygen, digitalis, diuretics, iron if an associated iron-deficiency anemia is present, and intravenous sodium bicarbonate for severe anoxemic metabolic acidosis. The creation or enlargement of an interatrial communication is the simplest procedure for providing increased intracardiac mixing of systemic and pulmonary venous blood; it may be achieved surgically or by rupturing the valve of the foramen ovale with a balloon catheter during transseptal catheterization of the left side of the heart (Rashkind's procedure). Pulmonary artery banding should be considered as an adjunct in infants with increased pulmonary blood flow and high pulmonary arterial pressure. Systemic-pulmonary artery or superior vena caval–pulmonary artery anastomosis may be indicated in the patient with severe obstruction to left ventricular outflow and diminished pulmonary blood flow. Complete intracardiac repair may be accomplished by rearranging the venous return so that the systemic venous blood is directed to the mitral valve and thence to the left ventricle and pulmonary artery, while the pulmonary venous blood is diverted through the tricuspid valve and right ventricle to the aorta. The risk of this corrective operation is lowest in those patients with an intact ventricular septum and no obstruction to pulmonary flow; it is indicated in patients one year of age or older without associated severe pulmonary vascular disease. A new corrective procedure has been devised for those patients with a ventricular septal defect in whom it is necessary to by-pass completely a severely obstructed left ventricular outflow tract. The operation employs an intracardiac ventricular baffle and extracardiac aortic homograft or prosthesis to replace the pulmonary artery (Rastelli's procedure).

PARTIAL TRANSPOSITION This designation is applied to both the Taussig-Bing malformation (in which the aorta is transposed and arises entirely from the right ventricle, while the pulmonary trunk communicates with both ventricles and overlies a large anterosuperior ventricular septal defect situated above the crista supraventricularis) and to the anomaly referred to as "double-outlet right ventricle" or "origin of both great vessels from the right ventricle." This anomaly consists of transposition of the aorta but not of the pulmonary trunk, and a ventricular septal defect in the posterior portion of the interventricular septum, below the crista supraventricularis, so that the pulmonary trunk does not sit astride the defect. In both lesions, the aortic and pulmonary orifices are situated at about the same vertical level in both the frontal and horizontal planes. Both physiologically and clinically the Taussig-Bing malformation resembles complete transposition with ventricular septal defect and pulmonary vascular obstruction. In double-outlet right ventricle, the ventricular septal defect is the only route of ejection from the left ventricle. Because of the streamlining of blood flow from the left ventricle across the outflow tract of the right ventricle to the aorta, these patients may resemble clinically those with isolated, large ventricular septal defects without cyanosis. However, when there is accompanying pulmonary stenosis, the clinical findings are similar to those of cyanotic tetralogy of Fallot. Diagnosis of these lesions is dependent on careful angiocardiographic analysis, and increased preoperative recognition of the partial transposition anomalies may be expected to result in improved operative results.

CORRECTED TRANSPOSITION The two fundamental anatomic derangements comprising this malformation are transposition, or anteroposterior reversal of the ascending aorta and pulmonary trunk, and inversion, or right-left reversal of the ventricles. This arrangement of the great vessels and ventricles (in contrast to the uncorrected transposition) permits functional correction, so that systemic venous blood passes into the pulmonary trunk while arterialized pulmonary venous blood flows into the aorta. In the heart with corrected transposition, the venae cavae and coronary sinus drain into a right atrium which is normal in position and structure. Venous blood flows from the right atrium, designated as the "venous atrium," across an atrioventricular valve, which has the structure of a normal mitral valve, into the right-sided "venous ventricle." This chamber, however, has the morphologic characteristics of a normal left ventricle, i.e., its interior lining is finely trabeculated, it has no crista supraventricularis, and the bicuspid atrioventricular valve is in continuity with a posteriorly placed semilunar valve. It ejects blood into the pulmonary trunk, which arises posterior to the ascending aorta. Oxygenated blood returns from the lungs to the left atrium, which is normal in position and structure, from which it flows into the left-sided "arterial ventricle" across an atrioventricular valve, which has the structure of a normal tricuspid valve. The interior lining of the arterial ventricle has the morphologic characteristics of a normal right ventricle, i.e., it has coarse trabeculations and a crista supraventricularis; the tricuspid atrioventricular valve is not in continuity with the anteriorly placed semi lunar valve. The arterial ventricle ejects blood into the aorta, which arises anterior to the pulmonary trunk.

In complete, "uncorrected" transposition of the great vessels the maintenance of life is dependent on the presence of associated defects. In contrast, patients in whom corrected transposition exists as an isolated anomaly present no functional alterations and have no symptoms. When a patient with corrected transposition has symptoms and signs of congenital heart disease, it may, therefore, be assumed that one or more associated malformations are present. Ebstein-type anomalies of the left-sided, tricuspid atrioventricular valve, ventricular septal defect, obstruction to outflow from the venous ventricle, and congenital heart block are those malformations most often associated with corrected transposition. Malposition of the heart may further complicate the altered anatomy.

In addition to the manifestations of the associated lesions, patients with corrected transposition frequently have an accentuated, single second heart sound in the second left intercostal space, representing closure of the aortic valve, which lies lateral and anterior to the pulmonic valve. An abnormal direction of initial ventricular depolarization is manifested electrocardiographically by a reversal of the precordial Q-wave pattern (Q waves are present in the right precordial leads and absent on the left). The His bundle is elongated because of the greater distance between the atrioventricular node and the base of the ventricular septum. This arrangement may be a causal factor in a variety of arrhythmias, and atrioventricular conduction disturbances are common. Roentgenographic examination characteristically reveals absence of the normal pulmonary artery segment and a smooth convexity of the left supracardiac border produced by the displaced ascending aorta.

The diagnosis of corrected transposition can usually be established by selective angiocardiography, which allows visualization of the transposed great arteries and morphologic differentiation of the two ventricles. The competence of the left atrioventricular valve may be determined by injection of contrast material into the arterial ventricle.

A high operative mortality rate has attended repair of the lesions associated with corrected transposition; it is related to the elevated pulmonary vascular resistance which may exist in patients with associated ventricular septal defects, which are usually large, and to a high incidence of surgically induced heart block. In addition, the inversion of the coronary arterial system greatly limits and may preclude an incision into the venous ventricle, thereby interfering with exposure of intracardiac defects in the usual manner. The presence of significant regurgitation from the arterial ventricle to the arterial atrium further raises the risk of operation.

TRANSPOSITION OF THE PULMONARY VEINS

When all the pulmonary veins connect either to the right atrium directly or to the systemic veins or their tributaries, the condition is called total anomalous pulmonary venous connection (TAPVC). Because all venous blood returns to the right atrium, an interatrial communication is an integral part of this malformation. Additional major cardiac malformations occur in about one-third of these patients. TAPVC accounts for about 2 percent of the deaths from congenital heart disease in the first year of life. The anomalous connection is usually supradiaphragmatic and to the left brachiocephalic vein, right atrium, coronary sinus, or superior vena cava. The distal site of connection may be below the diaphragm, a condition which is often unrecognized but which is hazardous because it is associated with markedly elevated resistance to pulmonary venous return.

Most infants with the more usual, unobstructed form of supradiaphragmatic TAPVC fail to thrive, are subject to repeated respiratory infections, and have congestive heart failure by the age of six months. At any age the physiologic consequences and, accordingly, the clinical picture depend on the size of the interatrial communication and on the magnitude of the pulmonary vascular resistance. When the interatrial communication is small, systemic blood flow is markedly limited, right atrial and systemic venous pressures are elevated, and hepatic enlargement and peripheral edema are present. On the other hand, the magnitude of the pulmonary blood flow and, therefore, the ratio of the oxygenated to the unoxygenated blood which returns to the right atrium are a function of the pulmonary vascular resistance. Accordingly, the arterial oxygen saturation, which ranges from markedly reduced to normal values, is inversely related to the pulmonary vascular resistance. Therefore, cyanosis is not usually prominent in the absence of congestive failure unless the patient survives long enough to acquire secondary pulmonary vascular changes and a reduction in pulmonary blood flow.

A characteristic physical finding is the presence of multiple heart sounds, consisting of a first sound followed by an ejection click, a fixed, widely split second heart sound with an accentuated pulmonic component, and a third, and often a fourth, heart sound. The electrocardiogram shows right axis deviation, as well as right atrial and ventricular hypertrophy. Roentgenograms of the chest reveal increased pulmonary blood flow; the right atrium and ventricle are dilated and hypertrophied, and the pulmonary artery segment is enlarged. In addition, the specific site of anomalous connection may result in a characteristic appearance of the cardiac silhouette. Thus in patients with TAPVC to the left brachiocephalic vein, the superior vena cava on the right, left brachiocephalic vein superiorly, and left vertical vein on the left produce a cardiac shadow that resembles a "snowman" or figure-of-eight. The upper right cardiac border may be prominent when the anomalous connection is to the right superior vena cava. Selective pulmonary arteriography and indicator-dilution studies at cardiac catheterization are especially helpful in determining the drainage pathways of the pulmonary veins. Indicator injected into the right ventricle or pulmonary artery takes longer to reach the peripheral arterial sampling site than indicator injected into the venae cavae or right atrium. The contour of the dilution curves obtained from a peripheral artery after injection into both the right atrium and a pulmonary vein are identical and show a large right-to-left shunt while the left atrial curve is normal.

Balloon atrial septostomy may provide dramatic palliation for the infant in whom the small size of the interatrial communication limits the amount of blood reaching the left side of the heart and systemic circulation. Unless serious pulmonary vascular disease is present, results of operation for TAPVC in patients more than one year of age are good. The procedure consists of creating an anastomosis between the common pulmonary venous channel and left atrium and closing the atrial defect.

PARTIAL TRANSPOSITION OF THE PULMONARY VEINS In this condition, one of the pulmonary veins (or more than one) is connected to the right atrium or to one or more of its tributaries. An atrial septal defect, particularly one of the sinus venosus type, often accompanies partial transposition of the pulmonary veins, and the usual connection involves the veins of the right upper and middle lobes and the superior vena cava. In the absence of associated anomalies, the physiologic disturbance is determined by the number of anomalous veins and their site of connection, the presence and size of an atrial septal defect, the state of the pulmonary vascular bed, and associated anomalies. In the usual case of isolated partial transposition of the pulmonary veins, the hemodynamic state and physical findings are similar to those in atrial septal defect. Occasionally, drainage is into the inferior vena cava. This condition may be associated with pulmonary parenchymal abnormalities, hypoplasia of the right pulmonary artery and lung, and dextroposition of the heart. This complex has been designated the "scimitar syndrome," because of the characteristic roentgenographic findings of a crescent-like shadow in the right lower lung field which is produced by the anomalous venous channel.

Malposition of the heart

Positional anomalies of the heart refer to conditions in which the cardiac apex is located in the right side of the chest (dextrocardia) or at the midline (mesocardia), or in which there is a normal location of the heart in the left side of the chest but abnormal position of the viscera (isolated levocardia). Knowledge of the position of the abdominal organs is important in diagnosing these malpositions. For example, a mirror-image dextrocardia is usually observed in a patient with complete situs inversus; this condition occurs more frequently in an otherwise normal person than in one with a malformed heart. In contrast, when dextrocardia occurs without situs inversus, associated malformations are the rule. When the heart occupies its normal position but situs inversus of the viscera is present, the heart is almost always seriously malformed. Moreover, when the visceral situs is indeterminate, there is a striking association of asplenia or polysplenia with complex, multiple cardiac anomalies, which usually include a combination of systemic and pulmonary venous abnormalities, defects in the atrial and ventricular septums, and endocardial cushion defects. In addition, pulmonary arterial obstruction and maldevelopment of the great arteries may occur with both asplenia and polysplenia but are more common in the former. It is important to recognize these complex syndromes in order to distinguish them from forms of cyanotic heart disease that may be amenable to corrective surgical therapy. The diagnosis is suggested by a symmetric liver shadow roentgenographically, and by the presence of Howell-Jolly and Heinz bodies in red cells demonstrated by blood smear, and confirmed by a negative or abnormal radioactive spleen scan.

Once the type of visceral situs is defined, it is necessary to describe the basic anatomic structure of the heart and its vascular connection. The atria exhibit a strong tendency to conform to the general orientation of the viscera, so that the right, or venous, atrium lies on the same side of the body as the trilobed lung, liver, and inferior vena cava, while the morphologic left, or arterial, atrium tends to lie on the same side as the stomach, spleen, and bilobed lung. The visceral situs can usually be determined by the location of the stomach bubble and liver on a routine roentgenogram, and the inferior vena cava can be located by the position of a cardiac catheter or by means of a venous or radioisotope angiocardiogram. The location of the ventricles and the relationship between the great arteries may also be demonstrated angiocardiographically. The cardiac chambers should be diagnosed positionally (left- and right-sided), functionally (arterial and venous), and morphologically (in terms of their intrinsic anatomic characteristics). The anatomic right ventricle is equipped with a tricuspid valve, is highly trabeculated, and contains the crista supraventricularis; its infundibulum always lies anteriorly to and superiorly beyond the outlet of the left ventricle. The morphologic right ventricle generally connects with whichever of the two great arteries is the more anterior. The entrance to the anatomic left ventricle is composed of a bicuspid mitral valve with an anterior leaflet which is in continuity with elements of the semilunar valve at its outlet, is smooth-walled, and contains an outlet that lies posterior to the right ventricular infundibulum. Transposition of the great arteries occurs frequently in cardiac malposition.

Once the positional, functional, and morphologic relationships are understood, and the presence of associated anomalies has been established, the principles of medical and surgical treatment apply to these cardiac malpositions as they do to normally located hearts.

REFERENCES

General

HURST JW (ed): *The Heart,* 3d ed., Part VI, Section B: Congenital Heart Disease (chaps. 38-41), New York: McGraw-Hill, 1974

MEYER RA, KAPLAN S: Noninvasive techniques in pediatric cardiovascular disease. Prog Cardiovasc Dis 15:341, 1973

MOSS AM, ADAMS FH: *Heart Disease in Infants, Children and Adolescents,* Baltimore: Williams & Wilkins, 1968

NADAS AS, FYLER DC: *Pediatric Cardiology,* 3d ed., Philadelphia: Saunders, 1972

TATOOLES CJ, MILLER RA: Palliative surgery in infants with congenital heart disease. Prog Cardiovasc Dis 15:331, 1973

Anomalous pulmonary origin of coronary artery

WESSELHOEFT H et al: Anomalous origin of the left coronary artery from the pulmonary trunk. Circulation 38:403, 1969

Aortopulmonary septal defect

SEVERALL PB et al: Aortopulmonary window. J Thorac Cardiovasc Surg 57:479, 1969

Aortic sinus aneurysm and fistula

ONAT A et al: Congenital aortic sinus aneurysms. Am Heart J 72:158, 1966

Atrial septal defect

GAULT JH et al: Atrial septal defect in patients over the age of 40: clinical and hemodynamic studies and effects of operation. Circulation 37:261, 1968

RAHIMTOOLA SH et al: Atrial septal defect. Circulation 37 (suppl. 5):2, 1968

Coarctation of the aorta

CAMPBELL M: Natural history of coarctation of the aorta. Br Heart J 32:633, 1970

Complete transposition of the great arteries

FISHER E, PAUL MH: Transposition of the great arteries: recognition and management. Cardiovasc Clin 2:211, 1970

BONHAM-CARTER RE: Progress in the treatment of transposition of the great arteries. St. Cyres lecture 1972. Br Heart J 35:573, 1973

Congenital valvular aortic stenosis

COHEN LS et al: Natural history of mild congenital heart disease elucidated by serial hemodynamic studies. Am J Cardiol 30:1, 1972

FRIEDMAN WF, BRAUNWALD E: Congenital aortic stenosis, in *Heart Disease in Infants, Children and Adolescents,* eds HJ Moss, FH Adams, Baltimore: Williams & Wilkins, 1968

Coronary arteriovenous fistula

DENEF JJE et al: Congenital coronary artery fistula. Br Heart J 33:857, 1971

Corrected transposition

BERRY WB et al: Corrected transposition of the aorta and pulmonary trunk. Am J Med 36:35, 1964

VAN PRAAGH R, VAN PRAAGH S: Anatomically corrected transposition of the great arteries. Br Heart J 29:112, 1967

Cor triatriatum

BRICKMAN RD et al: Cor triatriatum. J. Thorac Cardiovasc Surg 60:523, 1971

Discrete subaortic stenosis

EDWARDS JE: Pathology of left ventricular outflow tract obstruction. Circulation 31:586, 1965

Ebstein's anomaly

SIMCHA A, BONHAM-CARTER RE: Ebstein's anomaly. Clinical study of 32 patients in childhood. Br Heart J 33:46, 1971

Hypoplastic left-sided heart syndrome

SINHA SN et al: Hypoplastic left ventricle syndrome: Analysis of thirty autopsy cases in infants with surgical considerations. Am J Cardiol 21:166, 1968

Malposition of the heart

STANGER P et al: Diagrammatic portrayal of variations in cardiac structure. Circulation 37(suppl. 4):1, 1968

Partial transposition

GOMES MMR et al: Double-outlet right ventricle without pulmonic stenosis. Circulation 43(suppl. 1):31, 1971

—— et al: Double-outlet right ventricle with pulmonic stenosis. Circulation 43:889, 1971

Patent ductus arteriosus

CAMPBELL M: Natural history of persistent ductus arteriosus. Br Heart J 30:4, 1968

Pulmonary stenosis

JOHNSON LW et al: Pulmonic stenosis in the adult: Long-term follow-up results. N Eng J Med 287:1159, 1972

MOLLER JH, ADAMS P JR.: The natural history of pulmonary valvular stenosis. Am J Cardiol 16:654, 1965

Supravalvular aortic stenosis

BEUREN AJ et al: Syndrome of supravalvular aortic stenosis, peripheral pulmonary stenosis, mental retardation and similar facial appearance. Am J Cardiol 13:471, 1964

FRIEDMAN WF, ROBERTS WC: Vitamin D and the supravalvular aortic stenosis syndrome: The transplacental effects of vitamin D on the aorta of the rabbit. Circulation 34:77, 1966

Tetralogy of Fallot

KIRKLIN JW, KARP RB: *The Tetralogy of Fallot*, Philadelphia: Saunders, 1970

—— et al: Early and late results after intracardiac repair of tetralogy of Fallot. Am Surg 162:578, 1965

Transposition of the pulmonary veins

BONHAM-CARTER RE et al: Total anomalous pulmonary venous drainage. Br Heart J 31:45, 1969

Tricuspid atresia

LEVIN AR et al: Dynamics of interatrial shunting in children with obstruction of the tricuspid and pulmonic valves. Circulation 41:503, 1970

Truncus arteriosus

WALLACE RB et al: Complete repair of truncus arteriosus defects. J Thorac Cardiovasc Surg 57:95, 1969

Ventricular septal defect

CLARKSON PM et al: Prognosis for patients with ventricular septal defect and severe pulmonary vascular obstructive disease. Circulation 38:129, 1968

HOFFMAN JI: Natural history of congenital heart disease: Problems in its assessment with special reference to ventricular septal defects. Circulation 37:97, 1968

238 RHEUMATIC FEVER

ALVAN R. FEINSTEIN

Acute rheumatic fever is an arbitrarily designated portion of the spectrum of inflammatory complications that may follow group A streptococcal infections. As specified in the revised Jones' diagnostic criteria (Table 238-1), rheumatic fever is manifested by the appearance, either alone or in various combinations, of arthritis, carditis, chorea, erythema marginatum, or subcutaneous nodules. A diagnosis of rheumatic fever is usually justified if two of these manifestations are present.

ETIOLOGY The relationship between rheumatic fever and group A streptococcal infection was obscure for many years because the antecedent infection is often clinically asymptomatic or atypical, and because the streptococcus is not always demonstrable in the throat when the rheumatic patient comes to medical attention. With the modern availability of tests for streptococcal antibodies, the organism can now be identified by its "fingerprints" in the serum after it has left the scene of its original "crime" in the throat.

Figure 238-1*A* shows the complex natural spectrum of patients who may have sore throats (a clinical symptom), streptococcal throats (a positive result obtained when material taken from the throat is tested by culture or by fluorescent staining), and streptococcal infections (a positive result in a test of serologic antibodies). This Venn diagram emphasizes that not all sore throats are due to the streptococcus, that not all streptococcal throats are sore, and that streptococcal infections may occur in the absence of both positive cultures and sore throats.

Figure 238-1*B* shows the emergence of rheumatic fever from only a restricted portion of this spectrum: patients whose streptococcal infection produced an antibody rise, with or without sore throats and with or without a positive culture. For this rise to be regularly demonstrated, testing for antibodies may have to be exhaustive, involving the use of multiple antibodies, examination of sequential specimens, demonstration of suitable increments, and concomitant comparisons. Because the antistreptolysin O titer will rise in only about 80 percent of group A infections, more than one type of antibody must be examined; among the most useful of the additional antigens are streptococcal antihyaluronidase and antideoxyribonuclease B. Evidence of a recent infection must be demonstrated by a *change* in the titer of sequential specimens rather than by any single value; the time interval between specimens need not be shorter than 2 weeks, and a significant change can usually be shown even when the specimens are separated by 2 months. Since a difference of one tube dilution may be due to nonspecific variations, a true "change" in titer should not be diagnosed unless the increment spans at least two tubes in the dilutional system used for the test; a knowledge of the laboratory's dilutional system is necessary for meaningful interpretation of the results.

Streptococcal infections that are detected and treated appropriately (Chap. 130) can be prevented from causing rheumatic fever, but when the infection is not treated, the rheumatic attack rate varies according to the clinical type of infection. With symptomatic exudative streptococcal pharyngitis, the rate is about 3 percent; in patients in whom the infection is less severe, the rate may be 0.4 percent or even lower.

In epidemics of exudative streptococcal pharyngitis, rheumatic fever occurs about 2 weeks after the pharyngeal symptoms, but in other clinical circumstances, this latent interval is generally more variable. For chorea, and less often for erythema marginatum, the poststreptococcal latent interval is longer than for other clinical manifestations of rheumatic fever; it may be as long as 6 months. The chorea or the skin rash may appear after other rheumatic manifestations have subsided, and may suggest a spurious posttherapeutic "rebound" or a new rheumatic attack. When chorea is the only clinical manifestation, the long latent interval may preclude successful identification of an antecedent streptococcal infection, because the elevated antibody titers already have returned to normal values. The long-standing belief that "pure chorea" was an isolated disease, unrelated to rheumatic fever, has been refuted by recent examinations of sequential serums obtained in repeated periodic examinations of rheumatic patients. When some of these patients developed a recurrence of "pure chorea," the antibody rise of an earlier asymptomatic streptococcal infection could be demonstrated.

Features that influence susceptibility to a first episode of rheumatic fever are not well defined. Familial clustering has been observed, but clear evidence for genetic transmission has not been found. Acute attacks of the disease seldom occur in patients below the age of four years, are most common in the age group of five to seventeen, and decline in frequency thereafter.

Although poverty and undernutrition are regularly indicted as predisposing factors, their role is difficult to separate from that of the concomitant overcrowding that facilitates transmission of streptococci in this socioeconomic group, and from the statistical bias created when epidemiologic data are based mainly on populations seen in public clinics and wards. Once rheumatic fever has occurred, the patient is more susceptible to recurrences than members of the general population are to first attacks, and the likelihood of recurrences increases with increasing severity of cardiac disease in the preceding attack.

PATHOGENESIS No certainty exists about the pathogenetic pathway by which the streptococcus leads to rheumatic inflammation. Among the proposed mechanisms are a direct invasion of the affected tissues either by the unaltered streptococcus or by "L forms" lacking a cell wall; a direct toxic action by substances produced by the streptococcus, such as streptolysin S; a specific allergic reaction to the organism or its products; or the development of an autoimmune reaction. The theory that supports the last of these mechanisms is currently the most fashionable, although none has been proved unequivocally.

The rheumatic inflammation has relatively few histologic characteristics that are sufficiently distinct to be pathognomonic. For this reason, biopsy of inflamed joints or of subcutaneous nodules is seldom diagnostically rewarding and is generally performed mainly to rule out other diseases. Because of the low fatality rate, the morbid anatomy of chorea is not well defined.

Although the most distinctive histopathologic characteristics of rheumatic fever are found in the heart, not all hearts are involved, and not all of those that are involved show typical lesions. The pericardial inflammation of rheumatic fever does not have a unique histologic appearance but Aschoff bodies in the myocardium are

FIGURE 238-1

A *Spectrum of sore throats, streptococcal throats, and streptococcal infections.* B *Sources of rheumatic fever (shaded area) in the spectrum shown in* A.

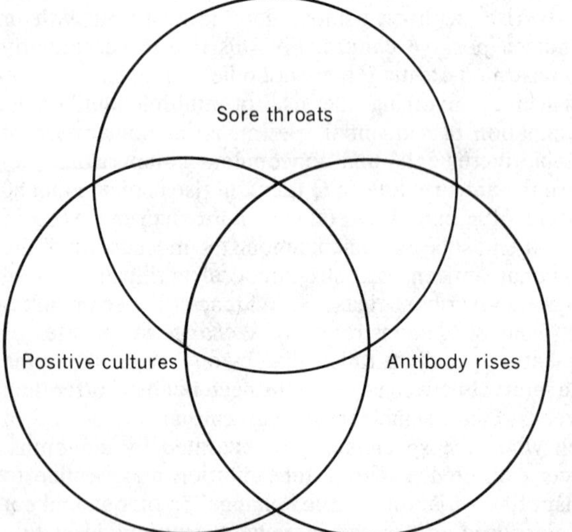

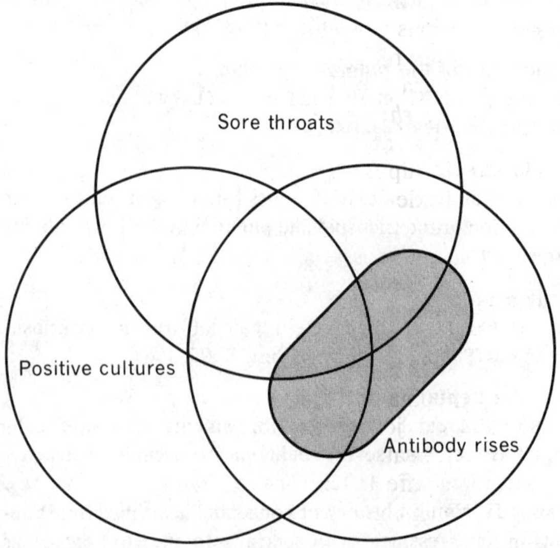

TABLE 238-1
Jones' criteria (revised) for guidance in the diagnosis of rheumatic fever*

Major manifestations	*Minor manifestations*
Carditis	History of previous rheumatic fever or evidence of preexisting rheumatic heart disease
Polyarthritis	Arthralgia
Chorea	Fever
Erythema marginatum	Abnormal erythrocyte sedimentation rate or C-reactive protein test
Subcutaneous nodules	Electrocardiographic changes

**The presence of two major, or of one major and two minor, manifestations, indicates a high probability of the presence of rheumatic fever if supported by evidence of a preceding streptococcal infection.*

pathognomonic of the disease. How often these occur is uncertain, because of the diverse histologic criteria used by different pathologists. Although once believed to represent *acute* rheumatic inflammation, the Aschoff body has been found in many patients with no other clinical or laboratory evidence of inflammation; conversely, Aschoff bodies have been absent from the myocardium despite unequivocal clinical evidence of acute rheumatic inflammation. The most frequent cardiac lesions of rheumatic fever are evident as gross, rather than microscopic, lesions in the valves. Dilatation of valve rings, destruction of valve substance, or contraction of chordae tendineae produces regurgitation; and fusion of cusps or commissures leads to stenosis. The mitral valve is affected most frequently; the aortic next, more commonly in boys than in girls; the tricuspid valve is seldom involved; and the pulmonic, rarely if ever. Although progressive scarring with age can further impair a damaged valve, enough damage may occur to produce significant stenosis or regurgitation even in childhood.

EPIDEMIOLOGY In the United States, rheumatic fever is now diagnosed less frequently than in the past, but because the decline in occurrence began long before the introduction of antibiotics, successful treatment of streptococcal infections cannot be given exclusive credit for the change. Other reasons include more rigorous modern diagnostic criteria to eliminate many minor ailments formerly termed *rheumatic*, and the availability of more precise diagnostic adjuncts that can identify other diseases, such as lupus erythematosus, congenital heart disease, and sickle-cell anemia, that formerly masqueraded as rheumatic fever. In temperate climates, rheumatic fever occurs most frequently during late winter and early spring, when streptococcal infections are more prevalent.

MAJOR CLINICAL MANIFESTATIONS **Arthritis** The pain of rheumatic arthritis usually develops rapidly, and the affected joint may become exquisitely tender before redness, heat, or swelling has appeared. The knees and ankles are affected most frequently, and the next most common are the elbows, wrists, or hips. The shoulders and small joints of the hands or feet are involved uncommonly, and the temporomandibular or vertebral joints, rarely; a disease other than rheumatic fever should be considered when these are the *only* affected joints. Characteristically, the joint pain is migratory and fleeting. No permanent joint deformities occur.

Certain patients develop poststreptococcal arthralgia rather than arthritis. They complain of pain in the joints but have no overt evidence of arthritis, i.e., redness, swelling, or deformity of the joints. Among patients who appear clinically to have *arthralgia*, a more correct diagnosis is often *tendonalgia* or *myalgia*. In such patients, a careful examination will reveal that the pain originates in a neighboring muscle or tendon, not in the joint. With the joint held immobile, isometric tension of the associated muscle or tendon will reproduce or increase the pain, although passive movement of the joint is painless. The common "growing pains" of children and adolescents are an example of this type of musculotendonalgia, and should not be attributed to rheumatic fever.

Chorea Chorea is more common in girls than in boys. Choreic movements are purposeless, nonrepetitive, spasmodic motions that may involve any voluntary muscle, including those of the face and tongue. Although not present during sleep, the movements persist while the patient is awake, and are partially controllable by concentrated voluntary effort, which may, however, also sometimes exacerbate them. With more severe attacks, the extremities and the trunk may be in constant motion, and the patient may need protection from injury. Choreic motions must be distinguished from habit tics or spasms, which are repetitive, and from hyperkinetic movements, which are purposeful and voluntarily controllable. The poststreptococcal episodic type of chorea, often called *Sydenham's chorea,* is also called *chorea minor,* to distinguish it from the hereditary *chorea major* (or *Huntington's chorea,* Chaps. 18 and 333), which usually begins in adult life and is relentlessly progressive.

Carditis Since no specific objective tests are available, the clinical diagnosis of acute carditis may be difficult. Prolongation of the P-R interval on the electrocardiogram cannot be regarded as definitive evidence of carditis, because this finding is nonspecific and present in about one-third of patients with rheumatic fever. It has shown no definite relation to other evidence of cardiac damage or to the long-term cardiac prognosis. The diagnosis of carditis thus becomes dependent on the clinical recognition of four events that may occur alone or in various combinations: abnormal murmur(s), pericardial rub, cardiac enlargement, and congestive heart failure.

The clinical manifestations of congestive heart failure in rheumatic children and adolescents are often similar to those noted in adults (Chap. 233), but certain differences may exist, probably because congestive failure develops more rapidly and is detected more promptly in children than in adults. During acute decompensation due to rheumatic fever, young patients often have dyspnea without rales; an ache in the right upper quadrant or epigastrium due to tenderness of the distended hepatic capsule; and a hacking nonproductive cough, due to pulmonary congestion, that may at first be attributed to a respiratory infection. After antirheumatic treatment has been instituted, congestive heart failure may be diagnosed incorrectly if the tachypnea of salicylate toxicity is mistaken for dyspnea, or if the slight hepatomegaly that may develop with steroid therapy is mistaken for hepatic congestion.

The first heart sound in rheumatic fever is often faint or "muffled," not because of carditis but because prolonged atrioventricular conduction allows the valve leaflets to drift closer together before they close. If heart failure is present, or if a pericardial effusion has occurred, both the first and second sounds may be faint. A third heart sound is a common normal finding in children, and it is frequently audible in patients with acute rheumatic fever. If the sound is long or somewhat roughened, it may be mistaken for a pericardial rub or a middiastolic murmur; if the cardiac rate is rapid, the quick repetition of three sounds will produce a gallop cadence. The short middiastolic noise that is often heard with mitral regurgitation during acute carditis is called a *Carey Coombs murmur*; a phonocardiogram may be required to differentiate it from a third heart sound.

A systolic murmur of mitral regurgitation is the most common auscultatory finding in rheumatic carditis. It is generally at least grade III/VI in intensity, loudest at the apex and transmitted to the anterior axillary line, blowing, high-pitched, and relatively unaltered by respiration and by changes in position. The murmur commonly begins with and masks the first heart sound. Mitral regurgitation is often falsely diagnosed in patients with acute rheumatic fever and a functional systolic murmur, so common in children and young adults, particularly in the presence of fever or tachycardia. This physiologic systolic murmur arises from the pulmonary artery and is generally loudest along the left sternal border; it is an ejection murmur (Chap. 228), rather than holosystolic, as is the murmur of mitral regurgitation, and its intensity is reduced during inspiration. A blowing, high-pitched early diastolic murmur due to aortic regurgitation is most easily audible at the left sternal border, in the third or fourth interspaces, with the patient leaning forward, in expiration, and may also be audible in patients with acute carditis.

The harsh crescendo-decrescendo systolic murmur of aortic stenosis seldom, if ever, occurs alone during rheumatic carditis in young patients. When the aortic valve is involved, the diastolic murmur is almost invariably present, and the associated systolic murmur results either from mild stenosis of the valve or from ejection through the dilated orifice. Aortic stenosis is commonly overdiagnosed when physiologic pulmonary murmurs are audible to the right of the sternum.

The classical acoustic pattern of mitral stenosis—a presystolic rumble merging with an accentuated first sound, as well as the early diastolic sound often regarded as an "opening snap" (Chaps. 228 and 239)—is uncommon during acute carditis. More commonly, the presystolic rumble and accentuated first sound are detected without an "opening snap," or the mitral deformity is manifested by systolic and long diastolic murmurs.

With marked mitral regurgitation, a systolic thrill may be palpable at the apex; as the right ventricle enlarges or is pushed forward by an enlarged left atrium, a left parasternal lift or heave can be felt; with marked aortic valve damage, a systolic thrill may be palpable over the carotid arteries but is seldom felt—in young patients—at the base of the heart. An apical diastolic thrill is uncommon.

A pericardial rub is sometimes the major or sole clinical manifestation of carditis, but more frequently it occurs in patients with cardiac decompensation.

No radiographic findings are characteristic of acute rheumatic carditis, and the cardiac size may remain normal despite unequivocal acoustic evidence of mitral or aortic regurgitation. Certain cardiac chambers may enlarge in accordance with valvular hemodynamic abnormalities; and generalized enlargement of the cardiac silhouette may occur with rheumatic myocarditis, congestive failure, or pericardial effusion.

Erythema marginatum This nonpruritic, flat or slightly raised rash occurs in only about 5 percent of patients with rheumatic fever, and it almost always coexists with arthritis, chorea, or carditis. Serpiginous or circular shapes are formed, usually on the trunk and thighs; the rash is often evanescent.

Subcutaneous nodules These are firm, painless, colorless, seldom larger than 1 to 2 cm; they most commonly develop near tendons or bony prominences of joints, particularly the elbows, are found in about 5 percent of patients with rheumatic fever, and are especially likely to coexist with severe carditis.

Other clinical features The fever of rheumatic fever has no distinguishing pattern. Epistaxis occurs in about 5 to 10 percent of cases, generally along with carditis. Abdominal pain appears in about 10 percent of patients; it may be due to hepatic congestion during cardiac decompensation or to mesenteric lymphadenitis. Pleurisy and pneumonia, previously common manifestations, are now seldom observed. Although pulmonary infarctions and infections regularly occur in association with heart failure, "rheumatic pneumonia" as a clinical or histopathologic entity cannot be defined. Pleurisy, although sometimes found in rheumatoid arthritis and lupus erythematosus, does not occur in rheumatic fever unless heart failure, pneumonia, or pulmonary infarction is present.

PATTERNS OF CLINICAL PRESENTATION Because erythema marginatum and subcutaneous nodules seldom occur alone, the basic clinical spectrum of rheumatic fever may be portrayed (Fig. 238-2*A*) as the overlap of "sets" of patients with arthritis, chorea, or carditis. In Fig. 238-2*B*, the complete clinical spectrum is constructed by further distinguishing a subset of *severe carditis*, and by adding a set of patients with poststreptococcal *arthralgia*. The spectrum shows the wide range of clinical manifestations—some of which are neither "rheumatic" nor "febrile"—that may be diagnosed as rheumatic fever. Arthralgia alone is shown in Fig. 238-2*B* with a dotted outline, because it does not fulfill Jones' diagnostic criteria. This spectrum of diverse clinical constituents shows that rheumatic fever need not have a single pattern of appearance. The presenting features may be as diverse as arthritis alone, "pure" chorea, or congestive heart failure without arthritis or chorea.

In the most common clinical situation, a child or adolescent develops nonspecific symptoms and then develops fever and painful enlargement of a large joint. Joints in other or symmetric contralateral locations then may become affected. Although the term "migratory polyarthritis" is used regularly to describe the articular events of rheumatic fever, the arthritis is often neither "migratory" nor "poly": several joints may begin to hurt simultaneously; and only one joint may remain involved, particularly when bed rest or anti-inflammatory treatment is initiated promptly.

In about 10 percent of cases, the patient seeks medical attention because of fever or arthralgia, and a diagnosis of rheumatic fever may be established only if carditis is found or if chorea develops later. Unless one of these two major manifestations appears, the condition is defined as a poststreptococcal inflammatory state that does not fulfill the Jones diagnostic criteria for rheumatic fever. Somewhat fewer than 10 percent of patients have chorea. Its onset may be so insidious that the patient may have been regarded as behaving peculiarly for weeks before the movements become overt or severe enough to come to medical attention.

Although pericarditis may produce pain, other features of carditis per se are asymptomatic unless congestive failure occurs. Thus, in a first rheumatic episode, carditis often is detected not because of its own manifestations, but because the patient seeks medical attention for arthritis, chorea, or fever. In a patient with only mild carditis without heart failure who does not manifest arthritis, fever, or chorea, rheumatic fever may therefore escape detection during the acute rheumatic episode. In such patients (upper right, Fig. 238-2*B*), the valvular disease develops insidiously, primarily because the patient does not seek medical attention. When the residual evidence of carditis is found in a subsequent examination, the patient is considered to have "rheumatic heart disease without a history of rheumatic fever." Such patients may first reach medical attention in adolescence or adult life as

the result of a recurrence of rheumatic fever, manifested by arthritis.

Definite evidence of carditis occurs in about half the patients having their first attack of rheumatic fever. The percentage of cardiac abnormalities is higher in patients with recurrent rheumatic fever, because patients with previous carditis are particularly likely to develop recurrences.

LABORATORY DATA The erythrocyte sedimentation rate and the level of serum C-reactive protein are always elevated during active rheumatic inflammation, and repeated tests of these acute-phase reactants are useful indexes of the inflammatory activity as the disease progresses. "Pure" chorea, however, may not begin until after the acute-phase reactants have reached normal values. A slight leukocytosis is usually present during the acute inflammatory phase; and in children receiving steroid treatment, the white blood cell count may reach values of 25,000 per mm^3. Because the development of heart failure alone will not return an elevated sedimentation rate to normal, decompensation is probably not due to active carditis when a normal sedimentation rate is found in patients with rheumatic heart disease and heart failure.

Mild degrees of anemia may occur, particularly after a long period of cardiac decompensation. Slight microscopic hematuria, of 2 to 6 red blood cells per high-power field, is sometimes noted during repeated examination of the urine in rheumatic fever, particularly when the patient is febrile, but gross hematuria and overt glomerulonephritis seldom occur, despite their frequent provocation by group A streptococcal infection. Rarely, rheumatic fever may be followed several years later by an episode of

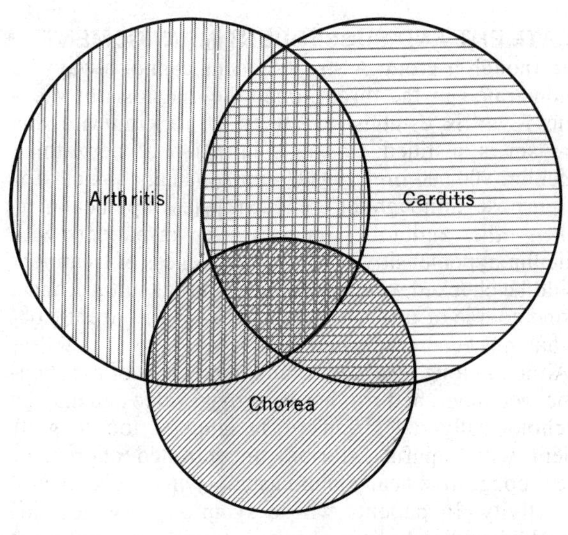

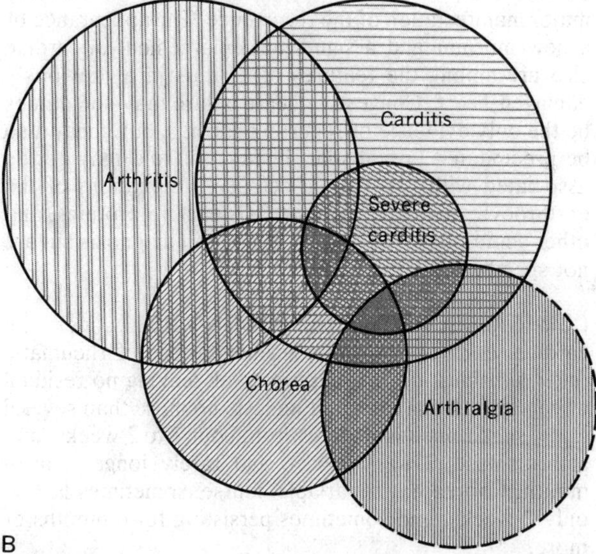

FIGURE 238-2

A *Major constituent sets in rheumatic fever.* B *The clinical spectrum of acute rheumatic fever.*

glomerulonephritis, but the acute simultaneous occurrence of significant renal and articular inflammation suggests an alternative diagnosis, such as lupus erythematosus.

DIFFERENTIAL DIAGNOSIS *Bacterial endocarditis* sometimes makes its appearance with articular symptoms, and the combination of fever, heart murmurs, and arthralgia may suggest rheumatic fever until positive blood cultures are obtained. A suppurative bacterial arthritis can usually be ruled out by the history of trauma or infection elsewhere and by the findings when the joint fluid is examined. The arthritis associated with gout, gonococcal infection, and sickle-cell anemia generally can be excluded by appropriate laboratory tests. Acute leukemia, which may begin with fever and articular symptoms, is identified after the white blood cells are examined. Rheumatic arthritis may be difficult to differentiate from rheumatoid arthritis or lupus erythematosus, because the diagnostic laboratory test results in the latter two diseases often are negative early in the clinical course. A "butterfly" facial rash, pleuritic involvement, and significant renal abnormalities are common in lupus erythematosus and unusual in rheumatic fever, as are the persistence of arthritis and permanent articular deformities, the hallmarks of rheumatoid disease. Furthermore, elevations in streptococcal antibody levels are characteristic of the initial episode or with a recrudescence of the arthritis due to rheumatic fever, but do not occur with systemic lupus erythematosus or rheumatoid arthritis.

Rheumatic carditis must be distinguished from congenital or less-common forms of heart disease, such as tumors or subendocardial fibroelastosis. Cyanosis suggests a congenital origin for the heart disease; otherwise, careful auscultation will often demonstrate that the murmurs are not of rheumatic origin. In doubtful circumstances, cardiac catheterization and angiocardiography are necessary to define the lesion.

A common problem is to identify a recurrence of rheumatic fever in a patient who already has rheumatic heart disease, particularly when such a patient does not develop arthritis or chorea and has carditis as the only major manifestation of the recurrence. The appearance of a new murmur and a significant enlargement in cardiac size are among the features of carditis in a previously damaged heart. Congestive heart failure may sometimes be the only evidence of recurrent carditis, but it may also be precipitated by valvular dysfunction and may not be associated with "rheumatic activity." Elevations of the erythrocyte sedimentation rate, C-reactive proteins, and other acute-phase reactants may help in diagnosis but are not specific.

CLINICAL COURSE AND PROGNOSIS Aside from carditis, each of the major manifestations of rheumatic fever subsides after a finite interval, leaving no residual effects. Erythema marginatum lasts no more than several days; subcutaneous nodules last about 1 to 2 weeks; and arthritis lasts 2 to 3 weeks, and rarely longer than a month. Chorea has a variable course, sometimes lasting only 2 weeks, and sometimes persisting for 6 months or more.

When carditis develops, overt evidence has usually occurred by the time the patient reaches medical attention. Thereafter, the cardiac damage may increase or decrease, but manifestations of carditis will seldom appear *de novo* if not found initially when the patient was carefully examined after the onset of an attack of acute rheumatic fever.

The sedimentation rate returns to normal in about 2 months in the absence of carditis, and in about 3 months in patients with carditis. Occasionally, the sedimentation rate may remain slightly elevated, in the range of 25 to 35 mm per hr, for months or even years after all other clinical evidence of acute inflammation has subsided. In these patients, a normal C-reactive protein test can be taken as evidence that the inflammation has subsided.

The long-term outcome of rheumatic fever depends on the state of the patient during the acute attack. Patients who do not develop carditis almost always remain free of rheumatic heart disease thereafter. Among those with questionably abnormal murmurs, the murmur will become distinctly abnormal in about 10 percent and will disappear in the remainder. In patients with definitely abnormal murmurs but without significant cardiomegaly or congestive heart failure, residual heart disease will be found in about 50 percent. Patients with severe carditis have the worst prognosis: some die during the acute attack; about 20 percent of those who survive will die during the following decade; and residual rheumatic heart disease remains in most of the others.

Susceptibility to recurrences of rheumatic fever increases with increasing severity of cardiac damage but diminishes as the patient grows older and more remote from the preceding rheumatic episode. Though most recurrences take place within a few years after the previous attack, they may occur at any age. As already stated, patients who have had carditis are more susceptible to rheumatic recurrences than those who were free of carditis, and the recurrences often increase the existing cardiac damage.

After cardiac damage is established, the subsequent course of the rheumatic heart disease depends on the hemodynamic effects of the valvular deformity and on the severity of myocardial damage (Chap. 239).

TREATMENT AND SUBSEQUENT MANAGEMENT

Even though a group A streptococcus cannot always be demonstrated in the throat, once the diagnosis of rheumatic fever is established an effort to eradicate this organism is justified. A single injection of benzathine penicillin, 900,000 or 1,200,000 units, usually suffices for this purpose, although different schedules of penicillin, as well as other antibiotics, may be used in patients with penicillin hypersensitivity. The effectiveness of treatment should be checked with a subsequent throat culture, and a second course of treatment is indicated if the streptococcus has not been eradicated.

Although long regarded as an integral part of antirheumatic treatment, bed rest has no proved value and may be psychologically deleterious if maintained too long. A patient with painful arthritis, uncontrolled chorea, or severe congestive heart failure usually will choose to limit his activity. In patients whose symptoms are not sufficiently disabling to limit physical activity, bed rest is not required.

For patients without carditis, treatment with adrenocortical steroids is unnecessary. Acute arthritis can be relieved with codeine or with salicylate, the latter being preferable if fever is also present. When salicylate is used in the therapy of rheumatic fever, the dosage should be increased until the drug produces either a clinical effect, manifested by elimination of fever or joint pains, or systemic toxicity, characterized by tinnitus, headache, or tachypnea. A useful starting daily dose is 15 to 20 mg per kg in children and 6 g in adults, given in four or five portions. Of the various salicylate preparations, ordinary aspirin is both cheapest and most effective. Absorption of enteric-coated preparations is too erratic; buffered preparations seldom contain enough buffer to exert a physiologic effect. Gastric intolerance can usually be avoided by meals or antacids 15 to 30 min following the aspirin.

Chorea should be managed as if it were a self-limited, completely reversible form of cerebral palsy. The most critical aspect of treatment is not the administration of drugs, but the avoidance of intellectual and psychologic trauma. The patient, and all those who deal with him, should be reassured that the peculiar movements are due to a specific neurologic disorder, of finite duration, that does not lead to any impairment of the intellect. Barbiturates or tranquilizers can sometimes be helpful in reducing the intensity of the choreic movements.

Many physicians prefer steroids to salicylates for the treatment of carditis, despite the lack of a demonstrated advantage of adrenal hormones in controlled clinical trials. Although more potent anti-inflammatory agents, steroids are more likely to be followed by a posttherapeutic rebound and have the additional disadvantage of more frequent side effects, particularly acne, hirsutism, and cutaneous striae in young people during prolonged therapy. For this reason, salicylates are the drugs of choice in patients with carditis. However, if these drugs fail to reduce fever and ameliorate heart failure, therapy with steroids should be initiated promptly. Prednisone is administered in dosage of 60 to 120 mg, or higher when necessary, in four divided doses daily. After the inflammation has been brought under control by either salicylate or steroid, treatment should be continued until the sedimentation rate approaches normal values, and should be maintained for several weeks thereafter. Salicylate may then be discontinued abruptly; administration of steroid should be tapered off over a 2-week period. To prevent poststeroid rebounds, an "overlap" course of salicylate therapy should be added when the steroid tapering begins, and this program should be continued for 2 weeks after steroid therapy has been discontinued. Rebounds are usually of short duration and, when mild, are best managed without resuming anti-inflammatory treatment, because a second rebound may occur when it is discontinued.

About 5 percent of rheumatic attacks persist for 8 months or longer, either in the form of spontaneous acute recrudescences or as posttherapeutic rebounds. These "chronic" attacks, which are most likely to occur in patients with cardiac damage and with previous rheumatic episodes, occasionally may be terminated with immunosuppressive agents such as nitrogen mustard or 6-mercaptopurine.

PREVENTION After streptococci are eradicated at the start of treatment, a prophylactic regimen should be initiated to prevent recurrent streptococcal infections that in turn may produce rheumatic recurrences. The most effective regimen is a monthly injection of 1.2 million units of benzathine penicillin. Oral prophylactic therapy avoids the pain and inconvenience of the injections, and a single daily dose of 1.0 g sulfadiazine has been found to be as effective as 250,000 units of oral penicillin twice daily, but is not as good as injected benzathine penicillin. There is no agreement about how long antirheumatic prophylaxis should be maintained. A reasonable policy for all patients is to continue prophylaxis for at least 5 years after the last acute attack and until the patient reaches the age of twenty-five years. Thereafter, prophylaxis may be discontinued in patients who have not had carditis, but should be maintained indefinitely in patients who have had cardiac involvement.

REFERENCES

American Heart Association: Jones criteria (revised) for guidance in the diagnosis of rheumatic fever. Circulation 32:664, 1965

Feinstein AR et al: The prognosis of acute rheumatic fever. Am Heart J 68:817, 1964

——: The natural histories of acute rheumatic fever. Bull Rheum Dis 17:423, 1966

Joint Report of a U.K.-U.S. Co-operative Study: The natural history of rheumatic fever and rheumatic heart disease. Ten-year report of a cooperative clinical trial of ACTH, cortisone, and aspirin. Circulation, 32:457, 1965

Markowitz M, Gordis L: *Rheumatic Fever*, Vol. 2, *Major Problems in Clinical Pediatrics*, 2d ed., Philadelphia: Saunders, 1972

Sellers TF Jr: Etiology of rheumatic fever, chap. 42 in *The Heart*, 3d ed., ed JW Hurst, New York: McGraw-Hill, 1974

Taranta A et al: Prevention of rheumatic fever and rheumatic heart disease. Circulation 41:A-1, 1970

239 VALVULAR HEART DISEASE

EUGENE BRAUNWALD

Specific valve abnormalities are discussed in this chapter. The role of phonocardiography and other indirect graphic techniques in the evaluation of patients with these lesions is considered in Chap. 230, and the role of cardiac catheterization and angiocardiography in Chap. 231.

AORTIC STENOSIS

Aortic stenosis occurs in about one-fourth of all patients with chronic valvular heart disease; approximately 80 percent of adult patients with symptomatic valvular aortic stenosis are male.

PATHOLOGIC PHYSIOLOGY The primary hemodynamic abnormality in aortic stenosis is obstruction to left ventricular outflow which leads to a pressure gradient between the left ventricle and aorta during the systolic ejection period. When severe obstruction is suddenly produced experimentally, the left ventricle responds to this excessive afterload by dilatation and reduction of stroke volume. However, in clinical aortic stenosis, the obstruction may be present at birth or it increases gradually over the course of many years and left ventricular output is maintained by the presence of left ventricular hypertrophy. A large pressure gradient across the aortic valve may exist for many years without a reduction of cardiac output, left ventricular dilatation, or the development of any symptoms. As aortic stenosis progresses in severity, the left ventricular systolic pressure continues to rise but rarely exceeds 300 mm Hg.

As with any stenotic lesion in the cardiovascular system, in order to estimate the severity of obstruction, it is necessary to measure both the transvalvular pressure gradient and the blood flow, preferably simultaneously. A peak systolic pressure gradient exceeding 50 mm Hg in the face of a normal cardiac output or an effective aortic orifice less than 0.7 cm^2 per m^2 body surface area, i.e., less than approximately one-third of the normal orifice, is generally considered to represent critical obstruction to left ventricular outflow. The left ventricular pressure pulse exhibits a rounded summit as the contraction of this chamber becomes progressively more isometric, and pulsus alternans in the left ventricle is a common finding in patients with severe stenosis. The elevated left ventricular end-diastolic pressure observed in many patients with severe aortic stenosis does not necessarily signify the presence of left ventricular failure or dilatation, but may instead reflect diminished compliance of the hypertrophied left ventricular wall.

A large A wave in the left atrial pressure pulse is usually present in patients with severe aortic stenosis, because of unusually forceful atrial contraction and diminished ventricular compliance. Atrial contraction tends to raise left ventricular end-diastolic pressure without producing a concomitant elevation of mean left atrial pressure. This "booster pump" function of the left atrium prevents the pulmonary venous and capillary pressures from rising to levels which would produce pulmonary congestion, while at the same time maintaining left ventricular end-diastolic pressure at the elevated level necessary for effective left ventricular contraction. Loss of an appropriately timed, vigorous atrial contraction, as occurs in atrial fibrillation or atrioventricular dissociation, occasionally results in a rapid aggravation of symptoms or cardiovascular collapse, even when the ventricular response is not particularly rapid.

The cardiac output and stroke volume at rest are within normal limits in the majority of patients with severe aortic stenosis. These variables may fail to rise normally during exercise. Late in the disease the cardiac output, stroke volume, and left ventricular–aortic pressure gradient decline and the mean left atrial, pulmonary artery wedge, pulmonary arterial, and right ventricular pressures become elevated. At this stage, a prominent A wave in the right atrial pressure pulse is also commonly found and hemodynamic evidence of mitral regurgitation, with a tall left atrial V wave and sharp Y descent, may occur in association with marked left ventricular dilatation.

The hypertrophied left ventricular muscle mass and increased myocardial wall tension characteristic of aortic stenosis elevate myocardial oxygen requirements. In addition, there may be interference with coronary blood flow, because the pressure compressing the coronary arteries exceeds the coronary perfusion pressure.

A significant fraction of patients with rheumatic aortic stenosis has associated mitral valve disease. Aortic stenosis intensifies the severity of mitral regurgitation by increasing the pressure driving blood from the left ventricle to the left atrium. The dilatation of the left ventricle which occurs late in the course of the disease in some patients with aortic stenosis further intensifies the magnitude of the mitral regurgitant flow.

ETIOLOGY Aortic stenosis may be congenital in origin, secondary to rheumatic inflammation of the aortic valve, or due to calcification of the aortic cusps of unknown cause. The *congenitally affected valve* may already be stenotic at birth and may gradually become calcified during the first three decades of life, becoming progressively more stenotic. The valve may also be congenitally bicuspid without serious narrowing of the aortic orifice during childhood; its abnormal architecture apparently makes the leaflets susceptible to normal hemodynamic stresses, which ultimately lead to valvular calcification, increased rigidity, and narrowing of the aortic orifice.

Rheumatic endocarditis of the aortic leaflets produces commissural fusion, resulting, at first, in a bicuspid valve. This, in turn, also makes the leaflets more susceptible to trauma, and ultimately leads to calcification and further narrowing. By the time the obstruction to left ventricular outflow causes serious disability, the valve is usually a rigid calcified mass, and even careful examination may make it impossible to determine whether the underlying process was rheumatic or congenital. Rheumatic aortic stenosis is virtually always associated with rheumatic involvement of the mitral valve. A rheumatic etiology is also favored by a history of active rheumatic fever and by associated severe aortic regurgitation. *Idiopathic calcific aortic stenosis* occurs most often in the elderly and is occasionally associated with fibrosis and fusion of the valve cusps; the pathologic process is considered to be a degenerative one—a "wear-and-tear" phenomenon. It may produce many of the characteristic physical signs of aortic stenosis. The valvular obstruction is usually relatively mild and of little if any hemodynamic significance; it may, however, on occasion, produce severe obstruction.

OTHER FORMS OF OBSTRUCTION TO LEFT VENTRICULAR OUTFLOW Besides valvular aortic stenosis, three other lesions may be responsible for obstruction to left ventricular outflow.

1 *Idiopathic hypertrophic subaortic stenosis.* This is the most important of these conditions numerically. It is characterized by marked hypertrophy of the left ven-

tricle, involving in particular the interventricular septum of the left ventricular outflow tract, as described in Chap. 242.

2 *Discrete congenital subvalvular aortic stenosis.* Less common than hypertrophic subaortic stenosis, this condition is produced by either a membranous diaphragm or a fibrous ridge just below the aortic valve (Chap. 237).

3 *Supravalvular aortic stenosis.* This uncommon congenital anomaly is produced by narrowing of the ascending aorta or by a fibrous diaphragm with a small opening just above the aortic valve (Chap. 237).

SYMPTOMS Aortic stenosis is rarely of hemodynamic or clinical importance until the valve orifice has narrowed to approximately one-third of normal. In contrast to mitral stenosis, which results in symptoms as soon as the obstruction becomes severe because the chamber just proximal to the narrowed valve provides little compensation, severe aortic stenosis may exist for many years without producing any clinical disability.

Most patients with pure or predominant aortic stenosis have gradually increasing obstruction for years but do not become symptomatic until the fourth or fifth decade. Exertional dyspnea, angina pectoris, and syncope are the three cardinal symptoms. Dyspnea results primarily from elevation of the left ventricular end-diastolic pressure, which in turn increases the mean left atrial and pulmonary capillary pressures. Angina pectoris usually develops somewhat later and reflects an imbalance between the augmented myocardial oxygen requirements and oxygen availability; the former results from the increased myocardial mass and intraventricular pressure, while the latter may result from the coronary artery disease which is not uncommon in patients with aortic stenosis. Exertional syncope may result from a decline in arterial pressure caused by vasodilatation in the exercising muscles in the face of a fixed cardiac output, or from a sudden fall in cardiac output produced by an arrhythmia. If prolonged, the syncopal episode may be accompanied by convulsions and loss of sphincteric control.

Since the cardiac output is well maintained at rest until the late stage of the disease, marked fatigability, debilitation, peripheral cyanosis, and other clinical manifestations of a low cardiac output are usually not prominent until this stage is reached. Orthopnea, paroxysmal nocturnal dyspnea, and pulmonary edema, i.e., symptoms of left ventricular failure, also occur in the advanced stages of the disease. Severe pulmonary hypertension leading to right ventricular failure and systemic venous hypertension, hepatomegaly, atrial fibrillation, and tricuspid regurgitation are usually preterminal findings.

When aortic stenosis and mitral stenosis coexist, the mitral obstruction masks many of the clinical findings of aortic stenosis. The reduction of cardiac output induced by mitral stenosis lowers the pressure gradient across the aortic valve, diminishes the frequency of anginal episodes, and retards the development of aortic calcification and severe left ventricular hypertrophy. On the other hand, symptoms considered more characteristic of mitral stenosis, such as pulmonary congestion and hemoptysis, occur more frequently in patients with combined stenotic lesions than in those with isolated aortic stenosis. Careful physical, electrocardiographic, and radiologic examinations in patients with aortic and mitral stenosis generally reveal more evidence of left ventricular enlargement than in patients with pure mitral stenosis, and catheterization of the left side of the heart is helpful in defining the relative importance of each valvular abnormality.

PHYSICAL FINDINGS The systemic arterial pressure is usually within normal limits. In the late stages, however, when stroke volume declines, the systolic pressure may fall and the pulse pressure narrows. Systemic hypertension is unusual in patients with marked aortic stenosis, and a basal systolic arterial pressure exceeding 200 mm Hg practically excludes severe narrowing of this valve. The peripheral arterial pulse rises slowly, with a delayed peak. Indirect recordings of the carotid pulse exhibit a gradually ascending limb, often with a prominent anacrotic notch or shoulder on the upstroke, as well as a delayed peak, with coarse systolic vibrations. A palpable double systolic wave, the so-called bisferiens pulse, excludes pure or predominant aortic stenosis, and signifies dominant or pure aortic regurgitation or idiopathic hypertrophic subaortic stenosis (Chap. 242). In the late stages of the disease, when the pulse pressure is reduced, the pulse amplitude is so small that the anacrotic nature of the pulse and the delay in its upstroke may become more difficult to appreciate. The jugular venous pulse may be normal, although in many patients the A wave is accentuated. This results from the diminished distensibility of the right ventricular cavity caused by the bulging, hypertrophied, interventricular septum and/or the presence of pulmonary hypertension.

The apex beat is usually active and displaced inferiorly and laterally, reflecting the presence of left ventricular hypertrophy. A double apical impulse may be appreciated, particularly with the patient in the left lateral recumbent position; the first outward expansion occurs during atrial systole and reflects the important contribution made by atrial contraction to ventricular filling, while the second commences during early ventricular systole and is well sustained during ejection. The right ventricle is usually palpable only when pulmonary hypertension develops in the late stages of the disease. A systolic thrill is generally present at the base of the heart, in the jugular notch, and along the carotid arteries, but occasionally it is palpable only during expiration and with the patient leaning forward. In patients without marked pulmonary emphysema, a thick chest wall, thoracic deformity, or heart failure, *absence of a systolic thrill signifies that the aortic stenosis is relatively mild.*

The rhythm is generally regular; atrial fibrillation should call to mind the possibility of associated mitral valve disease. An early systolic ejection sound, actually the opening snap of the aortic valve, is frequently audible in children and adolescents with noncalcific valvular aortic stenosis. However, this sound usually disappears when the valve becomes calcified and rigid. The sound of aortic valve closure can also be identified most frequently in patients with aortic stenosis with pliable valves, and calcification tends to diminish the intensity of this sound. As aortic stenosis increases in severity, left ventricular systole may become prolonged so that the aortic valve closure sound no longer precedes the pulmonic valve closure sound, and the two components may become synchronous, or aortic valve closure may even follow pulmonic valve closure. This is called paradoxic splitting of the second heart sound (Chap. 228); in patients with aortic stenosis in the absence of a left intraventricular conduction defect this finding usually signifies severe obstruction to left ventricular outflow. An atrial (presystolic) gallop, audible at the apex in many patients with severe aortic stenosis, reflects the presence of left ventricular hypertrophy and an elevated left ventricular end-diastolic pressure; a ventricular (protodiastolic) gallop in adults generally occurs when the left ventricle dilates and fails.

The systolic murmur in aortic stenosis is of the ejection type, i.e., it commences shortly after the first heart sound, increases in intensity to reach a peak toward the middle of the ejection period, and diminishes progressively thereafter to end just before aortic valve closure (Chaps. 228 and 230). The murmur is usually low-pitched, rough, and rasping in character and is loudest at the base of the heart, usually in the second intercostal space just to the right of the sternum. It is transmitted upwards to the jugular notch and along the carotid arteries. In patients with trivial degrees of obstruction or in those with severe stenosis in the late stage of the disease in whom the stroke volume is reduced, the murmur may be relatively soft and brief, and confined to midsystole. However, in almost all patients with significant obstruction, the murmur is at least grade III/VI. Occasionally the murmur is transmitted downward and to the apex and may be confused with the systolic murmur of mitral regurgitation. However, this murmur is usually holosystolic, while that of aortic stenosis is diamond-shaped and of the ejection type (Chap. 228).

ELECTROCARDIOGRAM This reveals left ventricular hypertrophy in the majority of patients with severe aortic stenosis. In advanced cases, S-T segment depression and T-wave inversion in standard leads I, aVL, and in the left precordial leads are evident. However, there is no close correlation between the electrocardiogram and the hemodynamic severity of obstruction, and the absence of electrocardiographic signs of left ventricular hypertrophy does not always exclude severe obstruction. Left bundle branch block or the presence of intraventricular conduction defects with QRS prolongation suggests diffuse fibrotic involvement of the myocardium. The presence of left atrial enlargement should suggest the possibility of associated mitral valve disease.

ROENTGENOGRAPHIC FEATURES The chest roentgenogram may show no or little overall cardiac enlargement for many years, since the development of concentric left ventricular hypertrophy is the initial response to obstruction to left ventricular outflow. Considerable hypertrophy without dilatation may produce some rounding of the cardiac apex in the frontal projection and slight backward displacement in the lateral view; significant aortic stenosis is usually associated with poststenotic dilatation of the ascending aorta. Aortic calcification is usually readily apparent on fluoroscopic examination with an image intensifier; indeed, *the absence of valvular calcification in an adult suggests that severe valvular aortic stenosis is not present.* In later stages of the disease as the left ventricle dilates, there is progressively more evidence of left ventricular enlargement, and there may also be roentgenologic signs of pulmonary congestion, as well as enlargement of the left atrium, pulmonary artery, right ventricle, and right atrium.

CATHETERIZATION AND ANGIOCARDIOGRAPHY Catheterization of the left side of the heart should be carried out in the majority of patients suspected of having severe aortic stenosis, particularly before a final decision concerning operative treatment is made. These investigations are especially indicated in (1) young, asymptomatic patients with noncalcific aortic stenosis, in order to define the severity of their obstruction to left ventricular outflow, since operation may be indicated if severe aortic stenosis is present; (2) patients in whom it is suspected that the obstruction to left ventricular outflow may not be at the aortic valve, but rather in the sub- or supravalvular regions; (3) patients with clinical signs of aortic stenosis and symptoms of myocardial ischemia, in whom associated coronary artery disease is suspected. An effort should be made to determine whether aortic stenosis or coronary atherosclerosis is responsible for the symptoms in this group of patients, and coronary arteriography should be carried out in addition to catheterization of the left side of the heart; and (4) patients with multivalvular disease, in whom the role played by each valvular deformity must be defined before operative treatment is planned.

Angiocardiographic studies with left ventricular injection of contrast material are helpful in defining the size of the left ventricular cavity, the thickness of the wall, the site of obstruction, the degree of deformity and mobility of the aortic valve cusps, the diameter of the ascending aorta, and the presence and degree of accompanying mitral regurgitation. In patients with severe narrowing, a jet of contrast substance passing through the aortic orifice is readily visualized. When contrast substance is injected into the ascending aorta, the aortic valve cusps can also be outlined and associated aortic regurgitation can be detected and its severity assessed.

NATURAL HISTORY The advanced age at death of patients with severe aortic stenosis is a consistent feature of this disease, and averages sixty-three years in males. In several studies, based on analysis of data obtained at postmortem examination, the average duration of various symptoms was as follows: angina pectoris, 3 years; syncope, 3 years; dyspnea, 2 years; and congestive heart failure, 1.5 to 2 years. Moreover, in more than 80 percent of these patients who died with aortic stenosis, symptoms had existed for less than 4 years. Congestive heart failure was considered to be the cause of death in one-half to two-thirds of patients.

Among adults dying with valvular aortic stenosis, sudden death occurred in 10 to 20 percent, and at an average age of sixty years. About one of every six patients dying suddenly has evidence of old or recent myocardial infarction at postmortem examination.

TREATMENT Strenuous physical activity should be avoided even in the asymptomatic stage in patients with *severe* aortic stenosis. Digitalis glycosides, sodium restriction, and diuretics are indicated in the treatment of congestive heart failure, and nitroglycerin is helpful in relieving angina pectoris. The most critical decision in the management of aortic stenosis concerns the advisability of surgical treatment. The indications and results of operation, as well as the techniques, differ considerably, depending on the patient's age and the nature of the valvular deformity.

In children and adolescents with noncalcific aortic stenosis, considerable hemodynamic improvement can be anticipated from simple commissural incision under direct vision. When carried out by an experienced surgeon, this procedure may be expected to enlarge the size of the valvular orifice significantly, without increasing the magnitude of aortic regurgitation, with a mortality rate of less than 5 percent. This operation is recommended not only for symptomatic patients but also for asymptomatic children and adolescents with hemodynamic evidence of severe obstruction to left ventricular outflow, with a peak systolic pressure gradient exceeding 50 mm Hg when the cardiac output is normal, or a calculated effective orifice less than 0.7 cm^2 per m^2 of body surface area. Though this procedure can be expected to result in complete or almost complete relief of obstruction in the majority of patients, the valve cannot be rendered entirely normal anatomically, and it is quite possible that it will become deformed, calcified, and stenotic again in later years, entailing the possibility of reoperation, and perhaps valve replacement at some later date.

In the majority of adults with calcific aortic stenosis, satisfactory valve function cannot be restored, even by deliberate sculpturing procedures carried out under direct vision, and replacement of the aortic valve is necessary. In most instances, it seems prudent to postpone operation in patients with severe calcific aortic stenosis who are asymptomatic, since their future course is difficult to predict and they may continue to do well for many years. However, it is likely that as the results of surgical replacement of the aortic valve improve, many of these patients will become candidates for operation before their disease reaches the symptomatic stage. At this time replacement of the aortic valve should be undertaken in patients with symptoms believed to result primarily from aortic stenosis, and in those who have hemodynamic evidence of severe obstruction.

It is clear that when symptoms of angina pectoris, syncope, or left ventricular decompensation develop in adults with valvular aortic stenosis, the outlook, despite medical treatment, is poor but can be improved significantly by replacement of the aortic valve with a ball valve prosthesis or homograft. Therefore, the risk entailed by operation in this group of patients is considerably lower than the risk involved by nonoperative treatment; moreover, the symptomatic improvement in many survivors of operation has been remarkable. However, the influence of aortic valve replacement on long-term survival and disability has not been established.

Operation should, if possible, be carried out before the development of frank left ventricular failure and failure supervenes; the operative risk is extremely high, and evidence of myocardial disease may persist even when the operation is technically successful. Nonetheless, in view of the very poor prognosis of such patients when they are treated medically, there is usually little choice but to advise surgical treatment. In patients in whom severe aortic stenosis and coronary artery disease coexist, relief of stenosis and revascularization of the myocardium by means of aorto-coronary saphenous vein bypass grafting (Chap. 240) may result in striking clinical and hemodynamic improvement. Since many patients with calcific aortic stenosis are elderly, particular attention must be directed to the adequacy of hepatic, renal, and pulmonary function before valve replacement is recommended. At the present time aortic valve replacement in symptomatic patients with severe obstruction is associated with a higher immediate mortality rate than is aortic commissurotomy in childhood (10 to 20 percent in most centers), and the long-term results and complications associated with the use of available prostheses have still not been defined completely. Accordingly, a more conservative approach to operative treatment is warranted in adults with calcific aortic stenosis than in children with noncalcific stenosis.

AORTIC REGURGITATION

PATHOLOGIC PHYSIOLOGY The total stroke volume expelled by the left ventricle (i.e., the sum of the effective forward stroke volume and the volume of blood which regurgitates back into the left ventricle) is increased in aortic regurgitation. In contrast to mitral regurgitation, in which a fraction of the left ventricular stroke volume is delivered into the low-pressure left atrium, in aortic regurgitation the entire left ventricular stroke volume must be ejected into a high-pressure zone, the aorta. Although the low aortic diastolic pressure facilitates ventricular emptying during early systole, an increase of the left ventricular end-diastolic volume constitutes the major hemodynamic compensation to aortic regurgitation, and the total stroke volume is augmented, primarily through the operation of the Frank-Starling mechanism (Chap. 232). Measurements of aortic regurgitant flow by means of angiocardiographic techniques have revealed that in patients with free aortic regurgitation the volume of regurgitant flow may be of the same order of magnitude as the effective forward stroke volume. The dilatation of the left ventricle allows this chamber to expel a larger stroke volume without requiring any increase in the relative shortening of each myofibril. Therefore, severe aortic regurgitation may occur with a normal effective forward stroke volume and a normal ejection fraction [total (forward plus regurgitant) stroke volume/end-diastolic volume], together with an elevated left ventricular end-diastolic pressure and volume. On the other hand, through the operation of Laplace's law (which indicates that myocardial wall tension is the product of intracavitary pressure and left ventricular radius), left ventricular dilatation increases the left ventricular systolic tension required to develop any given level of systolic pressure. As left ventricular function deteriorates, the end-diastolic volume increases without further elevation of the aortic regurgitant volume; the ejection fraction and forward stroke volume decline. Considerable thickening of the left ventricular wall also occurs with chronic aortic regurgitation, and at autopsy the hearts of these patients may be among the largest encountered, occasionally exceeding 1,000 g in weight.

The reduction of the aortic diastolic pressure in aortic regurgitation shortens the left ventricular isometric contraction period, which is helpful in allowing a longer left ventricular ejection period. The reverse pressure gradient from aorta to left ventricle, which is responsible for the aortic regurgitant flow, falls progressively during diastole, accounting for the decrescendo nature of the diastolic murmur. Equilibration between aortic and left ventricular pressures may occur toward the end of diastole, particularly when the heart rate is slow, and the left ventricular end-diastolic pressure may be elevated, occasionally to extremely high levels (>40 mm Hg). Rarely, the left ventricular pressure exceeds the left atrial pressure toward the end of diastole, and this reversed pressure gradient closes the mitral valve prematurely, or may cause diastolic mitral regurgitation.

In patients with free aortic regurgitation the effective forward cardiac output usually is normal or slightly reduced at rest, but often it fails to rise normally during exertion. In advanced stages there may be considerable elevation of the left atrial, pulmonary artery wedge, pulmonary arterial, and right ventricular pressures, and lowering of the cardiac output at rest. A qualitative index of the severity of aortic regurgitation may be obtained by determining the intensity of left ventricular opacification and the size of the left ventricle during thoracic cineaortography. In addition, this technique allows the detection of associated mitral regurgitation. However, quantitative biplane angiographic techniques are required for accurate estimates of aortic regurgitant flow.

Myocardial ischemia occurs in patients with aortic regurgitation because both left ventricular dilatation and the increased left ventricular systolic pressure tend to elevate the systolic tension developed by the myocardium, and thereby to increase myocardial oxygen requirements. However, the major portion of coronary blood flow occurs during diastole, when arterial pressure is lower than normal; thus, coronary perfusion pressure is reduced.

ETIOLOGY Approximately three-fourths of all patients with pure or predominant regurgitation are males; however, females predominate among patients with aortic regurgitation who have associated mitral valve disease. In approximately 80 percent of patients with aortic regurgitation the disease is rheumatic in origin, resulting in thickening, deformation, and shortening of the individual aortic valve cusps, changes which prevent their proper closure during diastole. Less commonly, bacterial endocarditis may attack a valve previously affected by rheumatic disease, a congenitally deformed valve, or rarely a normal aortic valve, and may result in the perforation or erosion of one or more of the leaflets. Patients with discrete membranous subaortic stenosis may develop thickening of the aortic valve leaflets, which in turn leads to mild or moderate degrees of aortic regurgitation and makes these valves particularly susceptible to bacterial endocarditis. Aortic regurgitation may also occur in patients with congenital bicuspid aortic valves. Prolapse of an aortic cusp, resulting in progressive aortic regurgitation, occurs in approximately 15 percent of patients with ventricular septal defect. Traumatic rupture of the aortic valve is an uncommon cause of aortic regurgitation, but it represents the most frequent serious lesion observed in patients surviving nonpenetrating cardiac injuries. Congenital fenestrations of the aortic valve occasionally produce mild or moderate degrees of aortic regurgitation. In patients with aortic regurgitation due to primary valvular disease, dilatation of the aortic annulus may occur secondarily and intensify the regurgitation.

Aortic regurgitation may be due entirely to marked aortic dilatation, without primary involvement of the valve leaflets; widening of the aortic annulus and separation of the aortic leaflets are responsible for the aortic regurgitation. Syphilis and ankylosing rheumatoid spondylitis may be associated with cellular infiltration and scarring of the media of the thoracic aorta, leading to aortic dilatation, aneurysm formation, and severe regurgitation. In syphilis of the aorta (Chap. 246), the involvement of the intima may narrow the coronary ostia, which narrowing in turn may be responsible for coronary insufficiency. Cystic medionecrosis of the ascending aorta, which may or may not be associated with other manifestations of Marfan's syndrome (Chap. 246), idiopathic dilatation of the aorta, and severe hypertension may also widen the aortic annulus and lead to progressive aortic regurgitation. Occasionally, retrograde dissection of the aorta involving the aortic annulus produces aortic regurgitation.

The coexistence of hemodynamically significant aortic stenosis with aortic regurgitation usually excludes all the rarer forms of aortic regurgitation because it occurs almost entirely in patients whose aortic regurgitation is on a rheumatic or congenital basis.

SYMPTOMS The history is often helpful in determining the cause of aortic regurgitation. A family history may frequently be elicited from patients with Marfan's syndrome, and a history of a heart murmur heard early in life may be obtained from patients with congenital aortic regurgitation. Patients with aortic regurgitation of obscure cause should also be questioned in detail about a positive serologic test for syphilis, and about prior chest trauma; a history compatible with subacute bacterial endocarditis may sometimes be elicited from patients with rheumatic or congenital involvement of the aortic valve, and the infection often precipitates or seriously aggravates preexisting symptoms. Ankylosing spondylitis is usually self-evident.

The interval between the first episode of acute rheumatic fever and the development of hemodynamically significant aortic regurgitation averages approximately 7 years, and this period is followed by an asymptomatic interval of approximately 10 to 20 years, during which the severity of the aortic regurgitation usually increases. Thus, severe aortic regurgitation may exist for many years without producing symptoms.

The first complaint is often an uncomfortable awareness of the heartbeat, especially on lying down. Sinus tachycardia occurring during exertion or with emotion, or premature ventricular contractions may produce particularly uncomfortable palpitations, as well as head pounding. These complaints may persist for many years before the development of exertional dyspnea, usually the first symptom of diminished cardiac reserve. This is followed by orthopnea, paroxysmal nocturnal dyspnea, and excessive diaphoresis. Symptoms of left ventricular failure are more common than symptoms of myocardial ischemia in patients with severe aortic regurgitation. Angina occurs as frequently in younger as in older patients, and it is not necessary to invoke the presence of coronary artery disease to explain this symptom in patients with aortic regurgitation. Anginal pain may develop at rest as well as during exertion. Nocturnal angina may be a particularly troublesome symptom and is frequently accompanied by marked diaphoresis. The anginal episodes may be prolonged and often do not respond satisfactorily to sublingual nitroglycerin. Late in the course of the disease, evidence of systemic fluid accumulation, including congestive hepatomegaly, ankle edema, and ascites, may develop. Patients with severe aortic regurgitation do not tolerate high fevers, infections, or cardiac arrhythmias, and may die in pulmonary edema as a result of one of these complications.

PHYSICAL FINDINGS The general examination should be directed toward the detection of causes predisposing to aortic regurgitation, such as Marfan's syndrome, rheumatoid spondylitis, syphilis, essential hypertension, and ventricular septal defect. Even prior to the examination of the heart of the patient with free aortic regurgitation, the jarring of the entire body and the bobbing motion of the head with each systole can be appreciated and the abrupt distention and collapse of the larger arteries are easily visible. A rapidly rising "water hammer" pulse, which collapses suddenly as arterial pressure falls rapidly during late systole and diastole (Corrigan's pulse), and capillary pulsations (Quincke's pulse), an alternate paling and flushing of the skin at the root of the nail while pressure is applied to the tip of the nail, are characteristic of free aortic regurgitation. A booming, "pistol-shot" sound can be heard over the femoral arteries, and a to-and-fro murmur (Duroziez's sign) is audible if the femoral artery is lightly compressed with a stethoscope.

The arterial pulse pressure is widened, with an elevation of the systolic pressure, sometimes to as high as 300 mm Hg, and a depression of the diastolic arterial pressure. The measurement of arterial diastolic pressure with a sphygmomanometer may be complicated by the fact that systolic sounds are frequently heard with the cuff completely deflated. However, the level of cuff pressure at the time of muffling of the Korotkoff sounds generally corresponds fairly closely to the true intraarterial diastolic pressure. The severity of aortic regurgitation does not always correlate directly with the arterial pulse pressure, and in many instances severe regurgitation exists in patients with arterial pressures in the range of 140/60 mm Hg. As the disease progresses, and the left ventricular end-diastolic pressure becomes markedly elevated, the arterial diastolic pressure may actually rise.

The apex beat is displaced laterally and inferiorly. The left ventricle is hyperdynamic in patients with free regurgitation, and the systolic expansion and subsequent retraction of the apex are prominent and contrast sharply with the sustained systolic thrust characteristic of severe aortic stenosis. A diastolic thrill is often palpable along the left sternal border, and a prominent systolic thrill may be palpable in the jugular notch and transmitted upwards along the carotid arteries. This thrill and the accompanying systolic murmur are due to the markedly increased blood flow across the aortic orifice, and do not necessarily signify the coexistence of aortic stenosis. Palpation, or indirect recording of the carotid arterial pulse, reveals it to be bisferiens, i.e., with two systolic waves separated by a trough, in many patients with pure aortic regurgitation, or with combined stenosis and regurgitation.

In patients with severe regurgitation the aortic valve closure sound is usually diminished or absent, and the indirectly recorded carotid arterial pulse does not usually show a clear-cut incisura. A third heart sound is common, and occasionally a fourth heart sound may also be heard. A loud systolic ejection sound is frequently audible; presumably it results from the sudden dilatation of the aorta by a greatly increased stroke volume.

The murmur of aortic regurgitation is a high-pitched, blowing, decrescendo diastolic murmur which is usually heard best in the third left intercostal space. In patients with mild regurgitation this murmur is brief and usually lasts less than one-third of diastole. However, as the severity increases, the murmur generally becomes louder and longer, and in patients with free aortic regurgitation it is usually holodiastolic. When the murmur is soft, it can be heard best with the diaphragm of the stethoscope and with the patient sitting up, leaning forward, and with the breath held in forced expiration. As it increases in intensity it tends to radiate widely, particularly down the lower sternal edge. In patients in whom the regurgitation is caused by primary valvular disease, the diastolic murmur is usually louder along the left than the right sternal border. However, when the decrescendo diastolic murmur is heard best along the right sternal border, it suggests that the aortic regurgitation is caused by dilatation or an aneurysm of the aortic root.

On a purely statistic basis, a diastolic blowing murmur along the left sternal border is much more commonly caused by aortic than by pulmonic regurgitation. Unless it is trivial in magnitude, the aortic regurgitation can also be recognized by peripheral signs such as a widened pulse pressure or a collapsing pulse. On the other hand, the Graham Steell murmur of pulmonary regurgitation is usually accompanied by clinical evidence of severe pulmonary hypertension, including a loud and palpable pulmonary component of the second heart sound. In addition, the phonocardiogram reveals that the murmur of aortic regurgitation begins with the aortic second sound and therefore commences somewhat before the murmur of pulmonary regurgitation.

A systolic ejection murmur is generally heard best at the base of the heart and is transmitted to the jugular notch and along the carotid vessels. This murmur may be as loud as Grade V/VI without reflecting any organic obstruction; it is often higher pitched and less rasping in quality than the ejection systolic murmur heard in patients with predominant aortic stenosis.

The third murmur which is frequently heard in patients with aortic regurgitation is the Austin Flint murmur, a soft, low-pitched, rumbling diastolic bruit. It is probably produced by the displacement by the aortic regurgitation stream of the anterior leaflet of the mitral valve. However, this displacement of the mitral valve does not appear to be associated with hemodynamically significant obstruction to left ventricular filling. In patients with rheumatic aortic regurgitation it may be difficult to distinguish the Austin Flint murmur from the rumbling diastolic murmur of mitral stenosis. Both are loudest at the apex, but the murmur of mitral stenosis is usually accompanied by a loud first heart sound and immediately follows the opening snap of the mitral valve, while the Austin Flint murmur is often shorter in duration than the murmur of mitral stenosis, and in patients with sinus rhythm the latter more frequently is characterized by presystolic accentuation. A blowing holosystolic murmur at the apex, which is transmitted to the axilla, may also be heard in patients with marked left ventricular dilatation and functional mitral regurgitation.

Electrocardiogram In patients with mild aortic regurgitation there may be no electrocardiographic abnormalities, but as the severity of aortic regurgitation increases, so do the electrocardiographic signs of left ventricular hypertrophy (Chap. 229). In addition to the abnormally tall R waves over the left precordium and deep S waves over the right precordium, patients with severe aortic regurgitation frequently exhibit S-T segment depressions and T-wave inversions in leads I, aVL, V_5, and V_6. Electrocardiographic signs of previous myocardial infarction generally indicate associated coronary artery disease. Left axis deviation and/or QRS prolongation denote diffuse myocardial disease, generally associated with patchy fibrosis; these signs are usually associated with a poor prognosis.

Roentgenogram Moderate or severe degrees of regurgitation are always associated with varying degrees of left ventricular enlargement. The apex is displaced downwards and to the left on the frontal projection, and frequently the cardiac shadow appears to extend below the left diaphragm. Left ventricular enlargement also occurs in the left anterior oblique and lateral projections, in which the left ventricle is displaced posteriorly and encroaches on the spine. In patients in whom primary valvular disease is responsible for the aortic regurgitation, the ascending aorta and aortic knob may be moderately dilated and may extend further to the right than the right atrial shadow in the frontal view. On fluoroscopic examination the aorta and left ventricle pulsate vigorously in opposite directions during systole. When aortic regurgitation is caused by primary disease of the aortic wall, aneurysmal dilatation of the aorta may be seen roentgenographically, and the aorta may fill the retrosternal space in the lateral view.

TREATMENT The left ventricular failure of aortic regurgitation at first usually responds to treatment with digitalis glycosides, salt restriction, and diuretics. Digitalis may also be indicated in patients with severe regurgitation and dilated left ventricles without symptoms of frank left ventricular failure, since it may retard its development (Chap. 235). Cardiac arrhythmias and infections are poorly tolerated in patients with free aortic regurgitation, and must be treated promptly and vigorously. Although nitroglycerin and long-acting nitrites are not as helpful in relieving anginal pain as in patients with coronary artery disease or aortic stenosis, they are worth a trial. Patients with syphilitic aortitis should receive a full course of penicillin therapy (Chap. 159).

As in patients with aortic stenosis, the most critical decision in patients with aortic regurgitation concerns the advisability and proper timing of surgical treatment. Total replacement of the aortic valve with a suitable prosthesis or homograft is generally necessary in patients with rheumatic aortic regurgitation and in many patients with other forms of regurgitation. Rarely, when a leaflet has been perforated during an episode of bacterial endocarditis, or torn from its attachments to the aortic annulus, surgical repair may be possible. When aortic regurgitation is due to aneurysmal dilatation of the annulus and ascending aorta, rather than to primary valvular involvement, it may be possible to reduce the regurgitation by narrowing the annulus or by excising a portion of the aorta without operating on the aortic valve itself. More frequently, however, regurgitation can be eliminated only by replacing the aortic valve, excising the aneurysm responsible for the regurgitation, and replacing the latter with a graft. This formidable procedure probably entails a higher risk than aortic valve replacement alone.

As in patients with aortic stenosis, the risks of aortic valve replacement are largely dependent on the stage of the disease. However, the outlook for symptomatic patients with aortic regurgitation is somewhat better than for patients with aortic stenosis. Surgical treatment should be considered in patients who have free aortic regurgitation and who are symptomatic when engaged in ordinary activity in spite of maximal medical therapy. It is likely, however, that as in the case of aortic stenosis, further reductions of the operative mortality rate and increased confidence in the long-term effects of valvular prostheses and/or homografts will make it possible in the future to recommend operative treatment to minimally symptomatic or even asymptomatic patients with severe regurgitation and cardiomegaly.

MITRAL STENOSIS

PATHOLOGIC PHYSIOLOGY In normal adults the mitral valve orifice is approximately 5 cm^2. In the presence of significant obstruction, i.e., when the orifice is less than one-half of normal, blood can flow from the left atrium to the left ventricle only if propelled by an abnormally elevated left atrioventricular pressure gradient; such a gradient is the hemodynamic hallmark of mitral stenosis. When the mitral valve opening is reduced to 1 cm^2, a left atrial pressure of approximately 25 mm Hg is required to maintain a normal cardiac output. The elevated left atrial pressure in turn raises pulmonary venous and capillary pressures, resulting in exertional dyspnea. The first bouts of dyspnea are usually precipitated by an increased rate of blood flow across the mitral orifice, which results in further elevation of the left atrial pressure. In order to assess the severity of obstruction, it is essential to measure the transvalvular pressure gradient and flow rate. The latter is dependent not only on the cardiac output but on the heart rate as well. An increase in heart rate shortens diastole proportionately more than systole, and diminishes the time available for flow across the mitral valve. Therefore, at any given level of cardiac output tachycardia augments the transvalvular gradient and elevates left atrial pressure.

The left ventricular diastolic pressure is normal in pure mitral stenosis; coexisting mitral regurgitation, aortic valve disease, rheumatic myocarditis, systemic hypertension, or coronary artery disease may be responsible for elevations which reflect impaired left ventricular function and/or reduced left ventricular compliance. In pure mitral stenosis and sinus rhythm, the mean left atrial and pulmonary artery wedge pressures are usually elevated and the pressure pulse shows a prominent atrial contraction (A wave), and a gradual pressure decline after mitral valve opening (Y descent). In patients with mild to moderate mitral stenosis without elevation of the pulmonary vascular resistance, the pulmonary arterial pressure may be normal at rest and may rise only with exercise. However, in severe mitral stenosis and whenever the pulmonary vascular resistance is significantly increased, the pulmonary arterial pressure is elevated even when the patient is at rest and in extreme cases it may exceed the systemic arterial pressure. Further elevations of left atrial, pulmonary capillary, and pulmonary arterial pressures occur during exercise. When the pulmonary arterial systolic pressure exceeds 50 mm Hg, the mean right atrial and right ventricular end-diastolic pressures may also be elevated.

Cardiac output varies considerably in patients with mitral stenosis. Thus, the hemodynamic response to a given degree of mitral obstruction may be characterized by a normal cardiac output and a high left atrioventricular pressure gradient or, at the opposite end of the hemodynamic spectrum, by a greatly reduced cardiac output and low transvalvular pressure gradient. In a small fraction of patients with moderately severe mitral stenosis, the cardiac output is normal at rest and rises normally during exertion; under these circumstances, the high atrioventricular pressure gradient elevates the left atrial and pulmonary capillary pressures, which elevation is responsible for symptoms of pulmonary congestion. In the majority of patients with obstruction of equal severity the cardiac output is normal at rest but rises subnormally during exertion. In patients with severe stenosis, particularly those in whom the pulmonary vascular resistance is strikingly elevated, the cardiac output is subnormal at rest and may fail to rise or may even decline during activity. The depressed cardiac output in patients with mitral stenosis is not only related to the obstruction of the mitral orifice but may also be due to the impairment of left ventricular function which can accompany it.

The clinical and hemodynamic pictures of mitral stenosis are dictated largely by the level of the pulmonary artery pressure. Pulmonary hypertension results from (1) the passive backward transmission of the elevated left atrial pressure, (2) arteriolar constriction, which presumably is triggered by left atrial and pulmonary venous hypertension (reactive pulmonary hypertension), and (3) organic obliterative changes in the pulmonary vascular bed. The elevation of pulmonary vascular resistance may be considered to be a complication of mitral stenosis; in time, the resultant severe pulmonary hypertension results in tricuspid and pulmonary incompetence as well as right-sided heart failure. However, the changes in the pulmonary vascular bed may also be considered to exert a protective effect; the elevated precapillary resistance reduces the likelihood of symptoms of pulmonary congestion by tending to prevent blood from surging into the pulmonary capillary bed and damming up behind the stenotic mitral valve. However, this protection is at the expense of a decreased cardiac output.

ETIOLOGY Mitral stenosis is generally rheumatic in origin. A history of one or more attacks of acute rheumatic fever can be elicited from approximately two-thirds of adult patients with predominant or pure mitral stenosis. The valve leaflets are diffusely thickened by fibrous tissue and/or calcific deposits. The mitral commissures fuse, the chordae tendineae fuse and shorten, the valvular cusps become rigid, and these changes in turn lead to narrowing at the apex of the funnel-shaped valve. While the initial insult to the mitral valve is rheumatic, the later changes may be a nonspecific process resulting from trauma to the valve caused by altered flow patterns. Pure or predominant mitral stenosis is a common valvular abnormality following rheumatic fever, occurring in approximately 40 percent of all patients with rheumatic heart disease. Two-thirds of all patients with mitral stenosis are females. Rarely, mitral stenosis is congenital in origin (Chap. 237), most commonly the so-called "parachute" mitral valve, in which all the chordae insert into a single left ventricular papillary muscle.

SYMPTOMS The asymptomatic or latent period between the initial attack of carditis and the development of symptoms due to mitral stenosis is generally long, on the order of two decades; most patients begin to experience disability in the fourth or fifth decades. In economically deprived areas mitral stenosis tends to progress more rapidly and frequently causes serious symptoms before the age of twenty years.

When valvular obstruction is trivial, all the physical signs of mitral stenosis may be present in the absence of any symptoms. However, even in those patients whose mitral orifices are large enough to accommodate a normal blood flow with only mild elevations of left atrial pressure, extreme exertion, excitement, fever, severe anemia, paroxysmal tachycardia, sexual intercourse, pregnancy, and thyrotoxicosis may precipitate elevations of pulmonary capillary pressure and lead to dyspnea. As stenosis progresses the stresses that precipitate dyspnea become less severe and the patient becomes limited in his daily activities. Redistribution of blood from the dependent portions of the body to the lungs, which occurs when the recumbent position is assumed, leads to orthopnea and paroxysmal nocturnal dyspnea. *Pulmonary edema* develops when there is a sudden increase in flow rate across a markedly narrowed mitral orifice. When moderately severe mitral stenosis has existed for several years, *atrial arrhythmias*—premature contractions, paroxysmal tachycardia, flutter, and fibrillation—tend to occur with increasing frequency. The rapid ventricular rate associated with untreated atrial fibrillation is frequently responsible for acute exacerbations of dyspnea. The development of permanent atrial fibrillation often marks a turning point in the patient's course and is generally associated with acceleration of the rate at which symptoms progress.

Hemoptysis, a complication which is almost never fatal, results from rupture of pulmonary-bronchial venous connections. It tends to occur most frequently in patients who have elevated left atrial pressures without markedly elevated pulmonary vascular resistances. True hemoptysis must be distinguished from the bloody sputum that occurs with pulmonary edema, pulmonary infarction, and bronchitis, three conditions that occur with increased frequency in the presence of mitral stenosis.

When the pulmonary vascular resistance rises or when tricuspid stenosis or regurgitation develops, symptoms secondary to pulmonary congestion may diminish, and the episodes of acute pulmonary edema and hemoptysis become reduced in frequency and severity. Elevation of pulmonary vascular resistance further increases right ventricular systolic pressure, ultimately leading to right ventricular failure, fatigue, weakness, abdominal discomfort due to hepatic congestion, and ankle edema.

Recurrent pulmonary emboli with infarction (Chap. 256) are an important cause of morbidity and mortality late in the course of mitral stenosis, occurring most frequently in patients with right ventricular failure and markedly elevated pulmonary vascular resistance. *Pulmonary infections*, i.e., bronchitis, bronchopneumonia, and lobar pneumonia, commonly complicate untreated mitral stenosis. *Bacterial endocarditis* is rare in pure mitral stenosis but is not uncommon in patients with combined stenosis and regurgitation.

In addition to the aforementioned changes in the pulmonary vascular bed, extensive fibrosis of the alveolar walls and thickening of pulmonary capillary walls occur commonly in mitral stenosis. The vital capacity, total lung capacity, maximal breathing capacity, and oxygen uptake per unit of ventilation are reduced, and in patients with severe stenosis the latter fails to rise normally during exertion. There is uneven distribution of blood flow and ventilation, resulting in physiologic dead space. As in other conditions in which left atrial pressure is elevated, pulmonary blood flow in the erect position is displaced from the basal and the superior segments of the lung (Chap. 249). The diffusing capacity may be lowered, particularly during exertion, as a result of structural changes in the diffusing surface and reduction of the pulmonary capillary blood volume. The reduction of pulmonary compliance that occurs generally correlates directly with the severity of the dyspnea and inversely with the left atrial pressure, and these changes are intensified during exercise. In some patients airway resistance is abnormally increased.

The changes in the lungs are due, in part, to increased transudation of fluid from the pulmonary capillaries into the interstitial and alveolar spaces as a consequence of the elevated pulmonary capillary pressure. A combination of the above-mentioned alterations in pulmonary function, particularly the diminution of pulmonary compliance, contributes to the increase of respiratory work and plays an important role in the genesis of dyspnea in mitral stenosis. However, the thickening of the alveolar and capillary walls tends to impede the transudation of fluid into the alveoli and the development of pulmonary edema at times when the pulmonary capillary pressure exceeds the plasma oncotic pressure. The increased capacity of the pulmonary lymphatic system to drain excess fluid also retards the development of pulmonary edema.

Thrombi may form in the left atria, particularly in the enlarged atrial appendages of patients with mitral stenosis. When they embolize, they do so to the systemic vessels, most commonly the brain, kidneys, spleen, and extremities. This complication occurs much more frequently in patients with atrial fibrillation, in older patients, and in those with a reduced cardiac output. However, it is not particularly more common in patients with extremely severe mitral valve obstruction than in those with only moderate degrees of obstruction; hence systemic embolization may be the presenting complaint in otherwise asymptomatic patients with mild mitral stenosis. At operation, thrombi are not found more frequently in the left atria of patients with past history of embolization than in those without this complication, indicating that it is usually the freshly formed clots that break off. Patients who have had one or more systemic emboli are more likely to have further embolic episodes than are patients with stenosis of comparable severity without previous embolization. Rarely, a large pedunculated thrombus or a free-floating clot may suddenly obstruct the stenotic mitral orifice. Such "ball valve" thrombi produce syncope, angina, and changing auscultatory signs with alterations in position, findings that resemble those produced by a left atrial myxoma (Chap. 243).

PHYSICAL FINDINGS Peripheral and facial *cyanosis* occur commonly in patients with extremely severe mitral stenosis. In advanced cases there is a malar flush and the facies appear pinched and blue. The jugular venous pulse reveals prominent A waves due to vigorous right atrial systole in patients with sinus rhythm who have associated tricuspid stenosis or severe pulmonary hypertension. When atrial fibrillation is present, the jugular pulse reveals only a single expansion during systole (C-V wave). The systemic arterial pressure is usually normal or slightly low. The heart generally presents a right ventricular tap along the left sternal border, signifying an enlarged right ventricle. In patients with associated pulmonary hypertension, the impact of pulmonary valve closure can usually be felt in the second and third left intercostal spaces just to the left of the sternum; the left ventricle is not palpable in severe, pure mitral stenosis. A diastolic thrill may frequently be felt at the cardiac apex, particularly if the patient is turned into the left lateral recumbent position. The apex cardiogram (Chap. 230) reveals a slow rate of left ventricular filling during early diastole; when a rapid left ventricular filling phase is present, either mitral stenosis is very mild or there is associated mitral or aortic regurgitation. The echocardiogram usually shows a decrease in the extent of opening, i.e., the anterior movement of the anterior leaflet of the mitral valve, and a sustained anterior position during diastole (Chap. 230).

On *auscultation*, the first heart sound is generally accentuated and snapping, and since the mitral valve cannot close until the left ventricular pressure reaches the level of the elevated left atrial pressure, it is often slightly delayed, particularly in patients with severe stenosis. In patients with pulmonary hypertension, the pulmonary component of the second heart sound is often accentuated, and the two components of the second heart sound are closely split. A pulmonary systolic ejection click is heard commonly in patients with severe pulmonary hypertension and extensive dilatation of the pulmonary artery. The opening snap of the mitral valve is most readily audible in expiration at, or just medial to, the cardiac apex but may also be easily heard along the left sternal edge or at the base of the heart. This sound generally follows the sound of aortic valve closure by 0.06 to 0.12 sec, i.e., after the pulmonic valve closure sound. Since the opening snap of the mitral valve occurs at the instant at which the left ventricular pressure falls below the left atrial pressure, the time interval between aortic closure and the opening snap will tend to be short, i.e., 0.06 to 0.08 sec, in patients with moderate or severe obstruction.

The opening snap usually ushers in a low-pitched, rumbling, diastolic murmur, heard best at the apex with the patient in the left lateral recumbent position, and often accentuated by exercise carried out just before auscultation. In general, the duration of this murmur correlates with the severity of the stenosis. In patients with sinus rhythm the murmur often reappears or becomes reaccentuated during atrial systole, as atrial contraction reelevates the rate of blood flow across the narrowed orifice. Soft (grade I or II/VI) systolic murmurs are commonly heard at the apex or along the left sternal border in patients with mitral stenosis and do not necessarily signify the presence of mitral regurgitation. Hepatomegaly, ankle edema, ascites, and the physical finding of pleural effusion, particularly in the right pleural cavity, may occur in patients with mitral stenosis and right ventricular failure.

Associated lesions When severe pulmonary hypertension is present in a patient with mitral stenosis, a loud pansystolic murmur produced by functional tricuspid regurgitation may be audible along the left sternal border. This murmur is often accentuated by inspiration, diminishes during forced expiration or during performance of the Valsalva maneuver, may disappear as compensation is restored, and must not be confused with the apical pansystolic murmur of mitral regurgitation, since management is quite different if mitral regurgitation is present.

Once the diagnosis of mitral stenosis is established, the recognition of associated mitral regurgitation is of considerable clinical importance. A presystolic murmur and an accentuated first heart sound may be taken as evidence against the presence of serious associated mitral regurgitation; when the first heart sound and/or the opening snap are soft or absent in a patient with mitral valve disease, it is likely that significant mitral regurgitation and/or serious calcification of the deformed mitral valve leaflets are present. A third heart sound at the apex often signifies that the degree of associated mitral regurgitation is more than trivial. This sound is generally duller and lower pitched and follows the opening snap. Occasionally, in patients with pure mitral stenosis, physical signs may falsely suggest mitral regurgitation. Thus, in the presence of severe pulmonary hypertension and right ventricular failure, a third heart sound may originate from the right ventricle and be audible along the left sternal border. In such patients the enlarged right ventricle may rotate the heart in a clockwise direction and form the cardiac apex, giving the examiner the erroneous impression of left ventricular enlargement. Under these circumstances the rumbling diastolic murmur and the other auscultatory features of mitral stenosis become less prominent or may even disappear. When severe congestive heart failure exists in a patient with calcific mitral stenosis, none of the auscultatory findings typical of severe mitral stenosis may be detectable, but they may become apparent again as compensation is restored. Associated tricuspid stenosis also tends to obscure many of the physical signs of mitral stenosis.

The Graham Steell murmur of pulmonary regurgitation, a high-pitched, diastolic, decrescendo blowing murmur along the left sternal border, results from dilatation of the pulmonary valve ring and occurs in patients with mitral valve disease and serious pulmonary hypertension. This murmur may be indistinguishable from the more common murmur produced by mild aortic regurgitation except that it is rarely audible at the second right intercostal space, and may disappear following successful surgical treatment of the mitral stenosis.

Electrocardiogram The QRS complex may be normal, even in patients with critical mitral stenosis. However, with severe pulmonary hypertension, right axis deviation and right ventricular hypertrophy are usually found. When left ventricular hypertrophy is present in patients with mitral stenosis it generally indicates that an additional lesion that places a burden on the left ventricle, such as mitral regurgitation, aortic valve disease, or hypertension, is present. In mitral stenosis and sinus rhythm the P wave usually suggests left atrial enlargement (Chap. 229). It may become tall and more peaked in lead II and upright in V_1 when severe pulmonary hypertension or tricuspid stenosis complicates mitral stenosis and right atrial enlargement occurs. When atrial fibrillation is present in patients with mitral valve disease, the base line shows coarser undulations than when this arrhythmia occurs as a consequence of coronary artery disease.

Roentgenographic features The earliest changes are straightening of the left border of the cardiac silhouette, prominence of the main pulmonary arteries, dilatation of the upper lobe pulmonary veins, and backward displacement of the esophagus by an enlarged left atrium. In patients with mild or moderate stenosis, the overall cardiac size is not grossly enlarged. In severe mitral stenosis, however, all chambers and vessels upstream to the narrowed valve are prominent, including the pulmonary arteries and veins, right ventricle, right atrium, and superior vena cava. Kerley B lines are fine, dense, opaque, horizontal lines which are most prominent in the lower and mid-lung fields and which result from distention of interlobular septums and lymphatics with edema. These lines usually signify a resting mean left atrial pressure of at least 20 mm Hg. As the pulmonary arterial pressure rises, the smaller pulmonary arteries become attenuated, at first in the lower and then in the mid-lung fields. Deposits of hemosiderin occur in the lungs of patients who have had multiple hemoptyses; the hemosiderin-containing macrophages fill the air spaces, and if they become large enough and confluent result in a fine, diffuse nodulation most prominent in the lower lung fields. Ossified nodules are also more common in this region and are produced by true lamellar bone, which tends to develop in areas of interstitial pulmonary edema.

DIFFERENTIAL DIAGNOSIS Significant mitral regurgitation may be associated with a prominent diastolic murmur at the apex, but this murmur commences slightly later than in patients with stenosis, and there is often clear-cut evidence of left ventricular enlargement on physical examination, roentgenography, and electrocardiography. In addition, a pansystolic murmur of at least grade III/VI intensity as well as a third heart sound should arouse the suspicion of significant associated regurgitation. Similarly, the apical middiastolic murmur associated with aortic regurgitation (Austin Flint murmur) may be mistaken for mitral stenosis. However, in a patient with aortic regurgitation the absence of an opening snap or of presystolic accentuation if sinus rhythm is present points to the absence of mitral stenosis. Tricuspid stenosis, a valvular lesion that rarely occurs in the absence of mitral stenosis, may mask many of the clinical features of mitral stenosis.

Exertional dyspnea and recurrent pulmonary infections may be falsely ascribed to pulmonary emphysema in patients with both *chronic lung disease* and mitral stenosis. Careful auscultation, however, will generally reveal the characteristic opening snap and rumbling diastolic murmur. Similarly, the hemoptysis that occurs in many otherwise asymptomatic patients with mitral stenosis may be improperly attributed to bronchiectasis or tuberculosis. Actually, the latter condition is uncommon in patients with significant mitral obstruction.

Primary pulmonary hypertension (Chap. 259) results in a number of the clinical and laboratory features of mitral stenosis. It is seen most frequently in young women; the opening snap and diastolic rumbling murmur are absent, there is no left atrial enlargement on the electrocardiogram or roentgenogram, and the pulmonary artery wedge and left atrial pressures are normal.

Atrial septal defect (Chap. 237) may also be mistaken for mitral stenosis; in both conditions there is often clinical, electrocardiographic, and roentgenographic evidence of right ventricular enlargement and accentuation of the pulmonary vascularity. The widely split second heart sound of atrial septal defect may be confused with the mitral opening snap, and the diastolic flow murmur across the tricuspid valve considered to be the mitral diastolic murmur. However, the absence of left atrial enlargement on the roentgenogram or electrocardiogram, the absence of Kerley B lines, and demonstration of fixed splitting of the second heart sound all favor atrial septal defect over mitral stenosis.

Cor triatriatum is an unusual congenital malformation that consists of a fibrous ring within the left atrium (Chap. 237). It results in elevation of the pulmonary venous, capillary, and arterial pressures. This lesion can be recognized most readily by means of left atrial angiography.

A *left atrial myxoma* (Chap. 243) may obstruct left atrial emptying, resulting in dyspnea, a diastolic murmur, and hemodynamic changes that resemble those of mitral stenosis. However, patients with left atrial myxoma often demonstrate findings suggestive of a systemic disease, with weight loss, fever, anemia, systemic emboli, elevated erythrocyte sedimentation rate, and increases in the serum gamma-globulin concentration. Usually an opening snap is not audible, there is no clinical evidence of associated aortic valve disease, and the auscultatory findings frequently change with body position. The diagnosis can be established by demonstrating a lobulated filling defect in the left atrium by angiocardiography.

Specialized techniques Left heart catheterization is extremely helpful in deciding whether or not valvulotomy is necessary in patients in whom it is difficult to estimate the severity of obstruction by clinical means alone. When combined with left ventricular angiocardiography, this procedure is particularly valuable in the detection and estimation of associated mitral regurgitation and of coexisting lesions such as aortic stenosis and regurgitation. Left atrial thrombi and tumors may be detected or excluded by angiocardiography, particularly when the contrast medium is injected directly into the left atrium. Catheterization of the left side of the heart is also helpful in the detection of conditions that impair left ventricular function and would thereby contraindicate or reduce the effectiveness of mitral valvulotomy. Detailed physiologic investigations are indicated for most patients who have undergone previous mitral valve operations and who have redeveloped serious symptoms; in such patients clinical assessment is particularly difficult, and the hemodynamic studies allow determination of the severity of the lesion, intelligent planning of the operative procedure when it is indicated, and a more informed estimate of the risk.

TREATMENT In the asymptomatic adolescent with mitral valve disease, penicillin prophylaxis of β-hemolytic streptococcal infections (Chap. 238) and vocational counseling are particularly important; physically strenuous occupations should be avoided so that premature retirement will not be necessary should symptoms develop later. In symptomatic patients considerable improvement can be expected with restriction of sodium intake and maintenance doses of oral diuretics. Digitalis glycosides do not alter the hemodynamics and usually do not benefit patients with pure stenosis and sinus rhythm, but they are necessary for slowing the ventricular rate of patients with atrial fibrillation and for reducing the manifestations of right-sided heart failure in the advanced stages of the disease. Particular attention must be directed to detecting and treating anemia and infections. Hemoptysis is treated by measures designed to diminish pulmonary venous pressure, including bed rest, the sitting position, salt restriction, and diuresis. Anticoagulants are indicated in patients who have had systemic and/or pulmonary embolization.

If atrial fibrillation is of relatively recent origin in a

patient whose mitral stenosis is not severe enough to warrant surgical treatment, reversion to sinus rhythm, by means of either electrical countershock (Chap. 236) or quinidine (Chap. 235), is indicated. Conversion to sinus rhythm is rarely helpful in patients with severe mitral stenosis, particularly those in whom the left atrium is especially enlarged or in whom atrial fibrillation has been present for more than one year, since it is frequently impossible to maintain sinus rhythm, and reversion to atrial fibrillation is common.

Surgical treatment Unless there is a specific contraindication, operative treatment is indicated in the symptomatic patient with pure mitral stenosis whose effective orifice is less than approximately 1.5 cm². Unless recurrent systemic embolization has occurred, valvulotomy is not indicated in patients who are entirely asymptomatic, regardless of hemodynamic findings. In uncomplicated cases, the surgical mortality rate should be less than 3 percent, and a comparison of the natural history of patients with serious symptoms treated by valvulotomy with those who did not receive the benefits of surgical therapy has shown considerable improvement following operation. However, there is no evidence that surgical treatment improves the prognosis of patients with slight or no functional impairment. When there is little symptomatic improvement following valvulotomy, it is likely that the procedure was ineffective, that it induced mitral regurgitation, or that associated valvular or myocardial disease was present. The recurrence of symptoms several years after what appeared to be a satisfactory initial result is usually due to an inadequate valvulotomy, but progression of other valvular lesions, the development of myocardial disease, or restenosis of the mitral valve may also be responsible.

A closed operation is usually preferable for patients with pure mitral stenosis who have not been operated upon previously, in whom no valvular or perivalvular calcification is detected on fluoroscopic examination, and in whom there is no suspicion of left atrial thrombosis. Many surgeons have found that transventricular instrumental dilatation of the mitral valve results in more effective relief of stenosis than transatrial finger fracture, and the importance of loosening any existing subvalvular fusion of papillary muscles and chordae tendineae must be appreciated. In a number of patients with uncomplicated mitral stenosis, closed valvulotomy may be ineffective or may result in severe regurgitation. For these reasons, the ready availability of an extracorporeal system is helpful. Operative treatment of patients with extremely severe obstruction, significant associated mitral regurgitation, valvular calcification, left atrial thrombi, or a mitral valve distorted by previous operative manipulation is usually carried out under direct vision, with open-heart techniques. The valve may have to be replaced with a prosthesis in those patients who were severely symptomatic preoperatively and in whom the surgeon does not find it possible to improve valve function significantly. Since the operative mortality rate of replacement of the mitral valve is still approximately 10 percent in most centers, and since there is some uncertainty concerning the fate of valve replacements, patients in whom preoperative evaluation suggests the possibility that replacement may be required should be operated on only if they are significantly limited and symptomatic on ordinary activity despite optimal medical therapy.

MITRAL REGURGITATION

PATHOLOGIC PHYSIOLOGY The regurgitant mitral orifice may be considered to be in parallel with the aortic orifice, and therefore the resistance to left ventricular emptying is reduced in patients with mitral regurgitation. As a consequence, the left ventricle decompresses itself rapidly into the left atrium early during ejection, and with the marked reduction in left ventricular size there is a rapid decline in left ventricular tension. Therefore, a greater proportion of the contractile activity of the left ventricle is expended in shortening and the cardiac output may be maintained at normal levels for many years even in patients with severe regurgitation. The initial compensation to mitral regurgitation consists of more complete systolic emptying of the left ventricle. However, a progressive increase in left ventricular end-diastolic volume occurs as the severity of the regurgitation increases and the function of the left ventricle deteriorates. The atrial contraction wave in the left atrial pressure pulse (A wave) is usually not as prominent as it is in mitral stenosis, but the V wave is often much taller, since it is inscribed during ventricular systole, when the left atrium fills from the pulmonary veins as well as from the left ventricle. During early diastole, as the distended left atrium suddenly empties, there is a particularly rapid Y descent. The left ventricular end-diastolic pressure is either near the upper limits of normal or somewhat elevated. The effective cardiac output usually declines in seriously symptomatic patients. Although a left atrioventricular pressure gradient persisting throughout diastole signifies the presence of significant associated mitral stenosis, a brief, early diastolic gradient may occur in patients with pure regurgitation as a result of the torrential flow of blood across a normal-sized mitral orifice.

The diagnosis of mitral regurgitation can be established by means of left ventricular angiocardiography and by indicator-dilution curves; the prompt appearance of contrast material indicator in the left atrium following its injection into the left ventricle signifies the presence of mitral regurgitation. The regurgitant volume can be measured by determining the difference between the total left ventricular stroke volume estimated angiocardiographically, while simultaneously measuring the effective forward stroke volume by Fick's method. The results of such studies suggest that the regurgitant volume may be of the same magnitude as the effective forward stroke volume or may even exceed it in patients with severe regurgitation. Qualitative, but clinically useful, estimates of the severity of regurgitation may be made by observation on cineangiograms of the degree of left atrial opacification following the injection of contrast material into the left ventricle.

Patients with severe mitral regurgitation may be divided into several subgroups, depending on the compliance, i.e., the pressure-volume relationship, of the left atrium and pulmonary venous bed, which appears to be capable of affecting the clinical and hemodynamic picture. Among patients with severe mitral regurgitation, three major conditions have been identified: (1) *Normal or reduced compliance.* In this group there is little enlargement of the left atrium, but marked elevation of the mean left atrial pressure, particularly of the V wave. In many patients in this group severe mitral regurgitation develops acutely, as in those in whom it follows rupture of chordae tendineae, infarction of a papillary muscle, or tear of a mitral leaflet. Marked elevation of pulmonary vascular resistance frequently occurs, presumably as a consequence of the left atrial hypertension, and therefore right-sided heart failure is a common clinical manifestation; sinus rhythm is usually present. (2) *Moderate increase in compliance.* By far the most common group consists of patients whose clinical and hemodynamic features are midway between those in the other two groups; i.e., they exhibit variable degrees of enlargement of the left atrium, associated with significant elevation of the left atrial pressure. (3) *Marked increase in compliance.* At the other end of the spectrum from group 1 are those patients with severe chronic mitral regurgitation, massive enlargement of the left atrium, and normal left atrial pressure. The pulmonary artery pressure and pulmonary vascular resistance are normal or only slightly elevated at rest. Clinically, these patients are usually disabled with fatigue and exhaustion, because of a low cardiac output, while symptoms resulting from pulmonary congestion are less prominent. In this group the mitral regurgitation is long-standing and atrial fibrillation is almost invariably present. The association of a normal left atrial pressure with a markedly enlarged, thin-walled left atrium indicates that this chamber must be far more compliant than normal. Thus, long-standing mitral regurgitation may, in some instances, alter the physical properties of the left atrial wall and thereby displace the atrial pressure-volume curve, allowing a normal pressure to exist in a greatly enlarged left atrium.

ETIOLOGY In about half the patients mitral regurgitation is caused by chronic *rheumatic heart disease*, but in contrast to mitral stenosis, pure or predominantly rheumatic mitral regurgitation occurs more frequently in males. The rheumatic process produces rigidity, deformity, and retraction of the valve cusps, commissural fusion, as well as shortening, contraction, and fusion of the chordae tendineae. Mitral regurgitation may also occur as a congenital anomaly (Chap. 237), most commonly as a consequence of (1) a defect of the endocardial cushions; (2) corrected transposition, (3) endocardial fibroelastosis, and (4) the "parachute" mitral valve. It may follow rupture or fibrosis of a papillary muscle or of one of its heads in ischemic heart disease. Myocardial infarction, fibrosis, or a ventricular aneurysm, at the base of the papillary muscle but not necessarily involving it may lead to abnormal anchoring of the latter, also resulting in mitral regurgitation. The latter may also occur during transient periods of ischemia involving a papillary muscle or adjacent myocardium and may accompany bouts of angina pectoris. Mitral regurgitation may occur with marked left ventricular dilatation of any cause in which lateral displacement of the papillary muscle results in coaptation of the valve leaflets. Idiopathic hypertrophic subaortic stenosis also may distort the mitral valve so as to render it regurgitant (Chap. 242). Massive calcification of the mitral annulus of unknown cause which occurs most commonly in elderly women can also be responsible for significant mitral regurgitation.

Abnormal elongation of chordae tendineae and/or redundant posterior cusps of the mitral valve with prolapse of the cusps into the left atrium, the so-called "floppy valve," leading to the syndrome of mid-late systolic click and late systolic murmur is another important cause of mitral regurgitation. The quantity of acid mucopolysaccharide is greatly increased in these valves, which occur most frequently in patients without any of the other stigmata of Marfan's syndrome (Chap. 364), as well as in patients with this syndrome; in the latter the acid mucopolysaccharide is also increased in the ascending aorta and tricuspid valve, leading to regurgitation of these valves as well.

Regardless of etiology, significant mitral regurgitation tends to be gradually progressive since enlargement of the left atrium places tension on the posterior mitral leaflet, pulling it away from the mitral orifice, thereby aggravating the valvular dysfunction. Similarly, the dilatation of the left ventricle increases the regurgitation, which in turn further enlarges the left atrium and ventricle, resulting in a vicious cycle; hence the aphorism, "mitral regurgitation begets mitral regurgitation."

SYMPTOMS Only a small fraction of patients with mitral regurgitation ever experience any reduction of cardiac reserve, but in patients who do become symptomatic, fatigue, exertional dyspnea, orthopnea, and nocturnal dyspnea are prominent complaints. Symptoms resulting from pulmonary congestion tend to be less episodic in nature than in mitral stenosis, since fluctuations of the mean pulmonary capillary pressure are less marked. Indeed, acute paroxysmal pulmonary edema is quite rare in patients with mitral regurgitation. Similarly, hemoptysis and systemic embolism occur far less frequently in mitral regurgitation than in stenosis. On the other hand, fatigability, weakness, exhaustion, weight loss, and even cachexia are more prominent and occur most frequently in patients with marked reduction of cardiac output. Right-sided heart failure, characterized by painful hepatic congestion, ankle edema, distended neck veins, ascites, and evidence of tricuspid regurgitation, is observed commonly in patients with mitral regurgitation who have associated pulmonary vascular disease.

PHYSICAL FINDINGS Although the arterial pressure is usually normal, the arterial pulse is often characterized by a sharp upstroke. The jugular venous pulse shows abnormally prominent A waves in patients with sinus rhythm and marked pulmonary hypertension. A systolic thrill is usually palpable at the cardiac apex, the left ventricle is hyperdynamic, and the apex beat is often displaced laterally. When the left atrium is markedly enlarged, it may extend anteriorly, and its expansion may be palpable along the sternal border late during ventricular systole. The combination of the retraction of the left ventricle and expansion of the left atrium during systole may produce a characteristic rocking motion of the chest with each cardiac cycle. A right ventricular tap and the shock of pulmonary valve closure may be palpable in patients with marked pulmonary hypertension.

The first heart sound at the apex is generally absent, soft, or buried in the systolic heart murmur, and an accentuated mitral closure sound is useful in excluding severe regurgitation. A pulmonary ejection sound is audible in patients with associated pulmonary hypertension. The splitting of the second heart sound is usually normal, although in patients with severe regurgitation, aortic valve closure may occur early, resulting in wide splitting of the second heart sound. An opening snap indicates associated mitral stenosis but does not exclude predominant regurgitation. A low-pitched third heart sound, occurring 0.12 to 0.17 sec after the aortic valve closure sound, at the completion of the rapid-filling phase of the mitral valve, is believed to be caused by the sudden tensing of the papillary muscles, chordae tendineae, and valve leaflets, and is an important auscultatory feature of severe mitral regurgitation. The absence of a third heart sound indicates that if mitral regurgitation exists, it may not be severe. The third heart sound may usher in a short, rumbling, diastolic murmur in the absence of mitral stenosis. A fourth heart sound is heard characteristically in patients with acute severe regurgitation in sinus rhythm. A presystolic murmur is not ordinarily heard in patients with pure regurgitation and sinus rhythm but is present when there is significant associated mitral stenosis.

A systolic murmur, grade III/VI in intensity or louder, is the most characteristic auscultatory finding in patients with severe mitral regurgitation. It is usually holosystolic (Chap. 228). Although the systolic murmur usually radiates into the axilla, in a minority of patients, particularly those with ruptured chordae tendineae or primary involvement of the posterior mitral leaflet, the regurgitant jet strikes the left atrial wall adjacent to the aortic root, and the systolic murmur is referred to the base of the heart and therefore may be confused with the murmur of aortic stenosis. In patients with ruptured chordae tendineae the systolic murmur may have a cooing or "sea gull" quality.

In patients with acute severe mitral regurgitation the systolic murmur may be decrescendo because the tall V wave in the left atrial pressure pulse results in a reduced late systolic left ventricular–atrial pressure gradient. Mid-to-late systolic clicks, single or multiple and introducing a late systolic murmur, are characteristic of prolapse of a cusp of the mitral valve. High-frequency whoops or honks may occur in these patients as well. The clicks are presumably due to sudden tautening of slack elongated chordae tendineae or valve cusps.

Electrocardiogram The electrocardiographic signs of ventricular hypertrophy are variable; in many patients there is no clear-cut electrocardiographic evidence of enlargement of either ventricle. In severe regurgitation the signs of left ventricular hypertrophy are often present, although in many patients associated right ventricular hypertrophy is apparent. Electrocardiographic signs of pure right ventricular hypertrophy occur in patients with severe pulmonary hypertension, and, though unusual in patients with pure mitral regurgitation, they do not exclude this diagnosis. There is electrocardiographic evidence of left atrial enlargement in patients with sinus rhythm, but right atrial hypertrophy may be present when pulmonary hypertension is extreme. Prolonged, severe mitral regurgitation with marked left atrial enlargement is generally associated with atrial fibrillation.

Patients with prolapse of the posterior leaflet of the mitral valve ("floppy valve" syndrome or the syndrome of mid-late systolic click and late systolic murmur) may demonstrate T-wave inversions in diaphragmatic or left chest leads, ectopic rhythms (most frequently ventricular tachycardia), and very rarely sudden death. This syndrome may be familial.

Roentgenographic features The left ventricle and left atrium are the dominant chambers; the latter may be enlarged to aneurysmal proportions and form the right border of the cardiac silhouette. Though both mitral stenosis and regurgitation tend to increase left atrial size, extreme left atrial enlargement usually signifies that regurgitation is the predominant lesion and has existed for many years. On fluoroscopic examination the left ventricle is hyperdynamic and the left atrium exhibits vigorous systolic expansions. Marked calcification of the mitral leaflets occurs commonly in patients with combined severe regurgitation and stenosis but is uncommon in patients with pure regurgitation. Cineangiography commonly reveals late systolic prolapse of a leaflet (usually the posterior) of the mitral valve into the left atrium in patients with the syndrome of mid-late systolic click and late systolic murmur. This abnormal movement of the mitral valve can also be detected by echocardiography.

TREATMENT The nonsurgical management of mitral regurgitation is directed toward restricting those physical activities which regularly produce extreme fatigue and dyspnea, reducing sodium intake, and enhancing sodium excretion with the appropriate use of diuretics (Chap. 233). Digitalis glycosides (Chap. 235) play a more important role in the treatment of mitral regurgitation than in treatment of mitral stenosis, since these drugs augment the output of the overburdened left ventricle even in the presence of sinus rhythm. The same considerations as in patients with mitral stenosis apply to the reversion of atrial fibrillation to sinus rhythm. In the late stages of the disease, anticoagulants and leg binders are used to diminish the likelihood of venous thrombi and pulmonary emboli. Effective surgical treatment of rheumatic mitral regurgitation generally requires total valvular replacement with a suitable prosthesis. The mortality rate of this procedure usually ranges from 5 to 15 percent, depending on the level of compensation, the patient's general condition, and the skill and experience of the operative team. Though most patients who survive operation appear to be greatly improved, some degree of myocardial dysfunction may persist. The development of thrombi around the prosthesis, which may block the valvular orifice or result in systemic embolization, may be a serious hazard, both in the early and the late postoperative periods. The likelihood of this complication may be reduced by some of the newer valves.

When surgical treatment is contemplated, detailed hemodynamic investigations and selective left ventricular angiocardiography are indicated. These studies are helpful in confirming the presence of severe regurgitation, and they aid in the identification of patients with primary myocardial disease and relatively mild, functional mitral regurgitation, who usually do not benefit from operation. Hemodynamic studies are also helpful in detecting and assessing the severity of associated valve lesions, which may have to be dealt with at the time of operation or which might limit the patient's ultimate improvement if they are left untreated.

In the selection of patients for surgical treatment, the chronic, often slowly progressive nature of the disease must be balanced against the immediate risks and long-term uncertainties attendant upon valve replacement. Patients with hemodynamically significant mitral regurgitation who are asymptomatic or who are limited only during severe exertion are not considered to be ideal candidates for surgical treatment, since they may live for many years with relatively little deterioration. However, surgical treatment should be considered seriously in patients who are so disabled that they are no longer able to work full time or carry out normal household activities despite optimal medical management. The risks of valve replacement rise sharply when the patient has developed congestive heart failure which is refractory to medical therapy, or associated severe tricuspid regurgitation. However, conservative management has little to offer these patients, so that operative treatment may be indicated even at these advanced stages of the disease, and occasionally the clinical and hemodynamic improvement following surgical treatment is dramatic. It is likely that both the immediate and long-term results of surgical treatment will improve considerably and will lead to recommendations of operative treatment for selected patients with mitral regurgitation even before they become severely disabled.

TRICUSPID STENOSIS

Tricuspid stenosis, a relatively uncommon valvular lesion, is generally rheumatic in origin. It does not usually occur as an isolated lesion or in patients with pure mitral regurgitation, but most commonly is observed in association with mitral stenosis, and sometimes with combined mitral and aortic stenosis. Hemodynamically significant tricuspid stenosis occurs in 5 to 10 percent of patients with severe mitral valve disease; carcinoid heart disease, fibroelastosis, and endomyocardial fibrosis are rare causes of tricuspid stenosis.

PATHOLOGIC PHYSIOLOGY A diastolic pressure gradient between the right atrium and ventricle is the hemodynamic hallmark of tricuspid stenosis. This gradient can be recorded most accurately and conveniently with a double-lumen cardiac catheter, by placing the distal opening into the right ventricle and the proximal opening into the right atrium. It is augmented when the transvalvular blood flow increases during inspiration, and it is reduced when flow declines during expiration. A mean diastolic pressure gradient exceeding 5 mm Hg is usually sufficient to elevate the mean right atrial pressure to levels which result in systemic venous congestion and, unless sodium intake has been restricted or diuretics have been given, is associated with ascites and edema. In patients with sinus rhythm, the right atrial A wave may be extremely tall and may even approach the level of the right ventricular systolic pressure. The resting cardiac output is usually depressed and fails to rise during exercise. The low cardiac output is responsible for the normal or only slightly elevated left atrial, pulmonary arterial, and right ventricular systolic pressures despite the presence of even moderately severe mitral stenosis.

SYMPTOMS Since mitral stenosis generally precedes the development of tricuspid stenosis, many patients initially have symptoms of pulmonary congestion. Amelioration of the symptoms of pulmonary congestion in a patient with mitral stenosis should raise the possibility that tricuspid stenosis may be developing. Characteristically, patients with hemodynamically significant tricuspid stenosis complain of relatively little dyspnea for the degree of hepatomegaly, ascites, and edema which they present. In some patients tricuspid stenosis may be suspected for the first time when symptoms of right ventricular failure persist after an adequate mitral valvulotomy.

PHYSICAL FINDINGS Severe tricuspid stenosis is associated with marked hepatic congestion, often resulting in cirrhosis, jaundice, serious malnutrition, severe edema, and ascites. The jugular veins are distended, and in patients with sinus rhythm there may be giant A waves. The V waves are less conspicuous, and since the presence of tricuspid obstruction impedes right atrial emptying during diastole, there is a slow, gentle, almost imperceptible Y descent. In patients with sinus rhythm there may be prominent presystolic pulsations of the enlarged liver.

The right ventricle and the shock of pulmonary valve closure are usually not easily palpable. Indeed, a giant A wave in the jugular venous pulse without palpatory evidence of pulmonary hypertension or right ventricular enlargement suggests the possibility of tricuspid stenosis. The pulmonic closure sound is not accentuated on auscultation, and occasionally an opening snap of the tricuspid valve may be heard or recorded phonocardiographically approximately 0.06 sec after pulmonary valve closure. The diastolic rumbling murmur of tricuspid stenosis has many of the qualities of the mitral diastolic murmur, and since tricuspid stenosis almost always occurs in the presence of mitral stenosis, the less-common valvular lesion may be missed on superficial auscultation. However, the tricuspid murmur is generally most readily audible along the left sternal margin and over the xiphoid process. It is augmented during inspiration, when negative intrathoracic pressure increases the velocity of blood flow across the tricuspid orifice, and it is reduced during expiration and particularly during the Valsalva maneuver, when tricuspid blood flow is reduced. The diastolic murmur is reduced in amplitude laterally, only to intensify or reappear as the mitral murmur at the apex. In patients with sinus rhythm the presystolic component is often louder at the tricuspid than at the mitral area; the tricuspid presystolic murmur commences before the mitral, and it often is of the crescendo-decrescendo type. As already indicated, severe tricuspid stenosis may obscure many of the physical signs of accompanying mitral stenosis.

Electrocardiogram and roentgenogram The most striking features are tall, peaked P waves in lead II, as well as prominent, upright P waves in lead V_1. The absence of electrocardiographic evidence of right ventricular hypertrophy in a patient with right-sided heart failure who is believed to have mitral stenosis should suggest the possibility of associated tricuspid valve disease. The chest roentgenograms in patients with combined tricuspid and mitral stenosis show particular prominence of the right atrium and superior vena cava without much enlargement of the pulmonary artery and with less evidence of pulmonary vascular congestion than occurs in patients with pure mitral valve disease.

TREATMENT Patients with tricuspid stenosis generally exhibit marked systemic venous congestion; intensive salt restriction, digitalization, and diuretic therapy are required during the preoperative period. Such a prolonged preparatory period may diminish hepatic congestion and thereby improve hepatic function sufficiently so that the risks of operation are diminished. Surgical treatment of the tricuspid valve is not ordinarily indicated at the time of mitral valve surgery in patients with mild tricuspid stenosis. On the other hand, definitive surgical relief of the tricuspid stenosis should be carried out, preferably at the time of mitral valvulotomy, in patients with moderate or severe tricuspid stenosis who have mean diastolic pressure gradients exceeding 5 mm Hg and tricuspid orifices less than 1.5 to 2.0 cm^2. Tricuspid stenosis is almost always accompanied by significant tricuspid regurgitation; simple finger-fracture valvulotomy often does not result in significant hemodynamic improvement, but may merely substitute severe regurgitation for stenosis. However, open operations utilizing cardiopulmonary bypass may permit substantial improvement of tricuspid valve function. If this cannot be accomplished, the tricuspid valve may have to be replaced with a prosthesis.

TRICUSPID REGURGITATION

Tricuspid regurgitation is usually functional and secondary to marked dilatation of the right ventricle and the tricuspid valve ring. Functional tricuspid regurgitation may complicate right ventricular failure of any cause, and is commonly seen in the late stages of heart failure due to rheumatic or congenital heart disease with severe pulmonary hypertension, as well as ischemic heart disease, cardiomyopathy, and cor pulmonale. Rheumatic fever may also produce organic tricuspid regurgitation, which is associated with tricuspid stenosis in some instances. Less commonly, regurgitation results from congenitally deformed tricuspid valves, and it occurs with defects of the atrioventricular canal, as well as with Ebstein's malformation of the tricuspid valve. Carcinoid heart disease, endomyocardial fibrosis, bacterial endocarditis, trauma and infarction of right ventricular papillary muscles may also produce tricuspid regurgitation.

The clinical features of tricuspid regurgitation result primarily from systemic venous congestion and reduction of the cardiac output. With the onset of tricuspid regurgitation, as cardiac output declines, symptoms of pulmonary congestion diminish, but the clinical manifestations of right-sided heart failure become intensified. The neck veins are generally distended, with prominent V waves, and marked hepatomegaly, ascites, pleural effusions, edema, systolic pulsations of the liver, and positive hepatojugular reflux are common. A prominent right ventricular pulsation along the left parasternal region and a blowing holosystolic murmur along the left sternal margin which is generally intensified during inspiration and reduced during expiration or the Valsalva maneuver are characteristic findings; atrial fibrillation is usually present.

The electrocardiogram is usually characteristic of the lesion responsible for the enlargement of the right ventricle which leads to this form of valvular dysfunction. In the rare instances of isolated tricuspid regurgitation the electrocardiogram often shows incomplete right bundle branch block. Roentgenographic examination usually reveals enlargement of both the right ventricle and right atrium, and the latter chamber expands during systole. The cardiac output is usually markedly reduced, and the right atrial pressure pulse may exhibit no X descent during early systole, but a prominent C-V wave, with a rapid Y descent. The mean right atrial and the right ventricular end-diastolic pressures are often elevated.

Treatment of the underlying cause of heart failure usually reduces the severity of functional tricuspid regurgitation. In patients with mitral valve disease and tricuspid regurgitation due to pulmonary hypertension and massive right ventricular enlargement, effective surgical correction of the mitral valvular abnormality results in lowering of the pulmonary vascular pressures and gradual reduction or disappearance of the tricuspid regurgitation without direct treatment of the tricuspid valve. However, in patients with severe regurgitation secondary to deformity of the tricuspid valve due to rheumatic fever, particularly those without severe pulmonary hypertension, surgical treatment of the tricuspid regurgitation, consisting of either valve replacement or narrowing of the annulus, should be carried out.

REFERENCES

Behrendt DM, Austen WG: Current status of prosthetics for heart valve replacement. Prog Cardiovasc Dis, Valvular Heart Disease 15:369, 1973

Braunwald E: Mitral regurgitation: Physiological, clinical and surgical considerations. N Engl J Med 281:425, 1969

El-Sherif N: Rheumatic tricuspid stenosis: Hemodynamic correlations. Br Heart J 33:16, 1971

Hanning CE, Rowe GC: Tricuspid insufficiency: A study of hemodynamics and pathogenesis. Circulation 45:793, 1972

Harrison DC: Papillary muscle syndromes. DM, January, 1972

Hurst JW (ed): *The Heart*, 3d ed., Part VI, Section C, Rheumatic Heart Disease & Other Acquired Valvular Disease, New York: McGraw-Hill, 1974

Kirklin JW et al: Surgery for acquired valvular heart disease. New Eng J Med 288:133, 194, 1973

Kremkau EL, et al: Acquired, nonrheumatic mitral regurgitation. Clinical management with emphasis on evaluation of myocardial performance, Prog Cardiovasc Dis Valvular Heart Disease 15:403, 1973

Pockeck WA, Barlow JB: Etiology and electrocardiographic features of the billowing posterior mitral leaflet syndrome. Am J Cardiol 51:731, 1971

Rackley CE, Hood WP Jr: Quantitative angiographic evaluation and pathophysiologic mechanisms in valvular heart disease. Prog Cardiovasc Dis (Valvular Heart Disease) 15:427, 1973

Reichek N et al: Clinical aspects of rheumatic valvular disease. Prog Cardiovasc Dis (Valvular Heart Disease) 15:491, 1973

Roberts WC, Perloff JK: Mitral valvular disease. Ann Intern Med 77:939, 1972

Rotman M et al: Aortic valvular disease: Comparison of types and their medical and surgical management. Am J Med 51:241, 1971

Schlant RC, Nutter DO: Heart failure in valvular heart disease. Medicine 50:421, 1971

Selzer A, Cohn KE: Natural history of mitral stenosis: A review. Circulation 45:878, 1972

240 ISCHEMIC HEART DISEASE

RICHARD S. ROSS

INTRODUCTION Ischemic heart disease results from inadequate perfusion of a portion of the myocardium. The designation *ischemic heart disease* is preferred to other widely used terms, such as arteriosclerotic heart disease, coronary heart disease, and coronary artery disease, since it identifies the myocardium as the site of the physiologic and anatomic deficit. By far, the most common cause of ischemic heart disease is atherosclerosis of the coronary arteries, but myocardium can be rendered ischemic by other coronary obstructive lesions, such as arteritis or embolism. Myocardial ischemia also may occur as a consequence of altered hemodynamics in the presence of aortic valve disease or in association with hypotension from any cause. Congenital abnormalities of the coronary circulation occasionally may result in myocardial ischemia and may be important in childhood.

Severe coronary atherosclerosis always produces ischemic heart disease, but lesser degrees of arterial involvement may exist without resulting in disease of the myocardium. The location of the atherosclerotic lesion is important in determining whether or not it will result in significant and, hence, clinically evident ischemia. The state of the collateral circulation is probably another important factor in determining whether or not ischemic heart disease develops as a consequence of coronary atherosclerosis, but the factors responsible for collateral development and their influence on the course of the disease remain uncertain. It seems reasonable to conclude that the potential for the development of collaterals is present in many and possibly all hearts, but that they do not develop sufficiently to be visualized until the stimulus of ischemia is superimposed.

Asymptomatic coronary artery disease develops at an unknown rate and is detected only when death occurs from another cause, such as trauma. The disease begins early in life, as evidenced by the finding of significant lesions in young men killed in war. Middle-aged males become symptomatic in a variety of ways. Myocardial infarction is the most common presentation, but some patients enter the symptomatic phase by developing angina pectoris, and others die suddenly, presumably as a result of an arrhythmia. The problem of sudden death is discussed in more detail in Chap. 335. Angina pectoris and myocardial infarction are at the extremes of the clinical spectrum; another group of presentations is referred to as the intermediate syndromes because they share features with both myocardial infarction and angina pectoris.

Once in the symptomatic phase, the patient may die or recover and return to the asymptomatic stage. Movement from one to another of the symptomatic phases, either directly or after passing through an asymptomatic interval, is also possible. The average expected duration of life following entry into the symptomatic phase of ischemic heart disease is the same whether the initial event be the development of angina pectoris or a myocardial infarction from which the patient recovers. The mortality rate for both groups is 4 percent per year. There are, however, subsets of the angina population with mortality rates that differ by a factor of 4. Angina patients with a normal electrocardiogram and blood pressure have an expected mortality rate of only 2 percent per year, in contrast to those with hypertension and an abnormal electrocardiogram, for whom the expected annual mortality rate is 8 percent per year.

The pathogenesis of myocardial infarction remains a matter of debate. It is clear that the simplistic concept of thrombosis superimposed on an atheroma or hemorrhage into the atheromatous lesion is not adequate. Severe atheromatous disease is usually present, but the role of thrombosis has been questioned, because thrombus material is more likely to be present in patients with myocardial infarction complicated by shock or congestive failure than in patients who die suddenly. These observations raise the possibility that thrombosis may be the result rather than the cause of myocardial infarction in many patients.

PREVENTION By the time the disease has become symptomatic, the process in arteries will be far advanced, and, therefore, prevention must be directed at the asymptomatic disease. A prevention program based upon the control of the "risk factors" which have been found to be associated with the progression of the disease must be initiated in childhood. The three major risk factors are hypercholesterolemia, hypertension, and cigarette smoking; all are subject to control. The mortality rate from arteriosclerotic diseases in men free of these risk factors is one-fifth of that observed in men with all three factors and one-third of that in a group with two of the three. Hypercholesterolemia can be controlled by diet or in certain instances by medication (Chap. 244). Hypertension can and should be controlled by medication; a significant decrease in mortality rate has been observed in association with such control (Chap. 245). Cigarette smoking should be discouraged, especially in young people. Other risk factors, some of which are amenable to control, are diabetes mellitus, obesity, sedentary living, and psychosocial tensions. A family history of premature heart attack is important and should stimulate a search for controllable risk factors such as hypercholesterolemia, diabetes, or hypertension.

PHYSIOLOGIC AND BIOCHEMICAL CONSEQUENCES OF ISCHEMIA

Biochemical, mechanical, and electrical changes result when the blood supply is inadequate relative to the requirements of the myocardium. The biochemical changes which have been noted in the first minute of anoxia are the accumulation of hydrogen ion and the efflux of potassium from the cells. Glycogen stores are reduced as a consequence of the shift to anaerobic metabolism, which also results in an accumulation of lactic acid. Electron microscopy reveals changes in the mitochondria within the first few minutes of anoxia, but these anatomic changes and the biochemical changes do not reach an irreversible stage for a much longer period. The subendocardial region of the left ventricle is particularly susceptible to all the changes of ischemia.

Contractility of the myocardium becomes impaired during the transient ischemia of angina pectoris and also within the first minute following a coronary occlusion. The impaired contractility may be limited to the ischemic portion of the myocardium, in which case there will be an asymmetric and hence inefficient pattern of contraction. The ischemic, or infarcted, portion may bulge outward when the normal portion of the ventricle contracts, thus further reducing the effectiveness of ventricular systole. The compliance of the left ventricle is also reduced by ischemia, and this process impairs the filling of the ventricle. These changes in ventricular function lead to an increase in the left ventricular filling pressure.

The ischemic process also alters the electrophysiology of the heart, the most characteristic early changes in the electrocardiogram being those in repolarization process, as evidenced by inversion of T waves and later by displacement of the S-T segment (Chap. 229). S-T segment shifts are seen clinically in association with angina pectoris and also in the early stages of myocardial infarction. Another important consequence of myocardial ischemia is ventricular irritability, which may result in ventricular premature systoles, ventricular tachycardia, and ventricular fibrillation. Most patients who die suddenly from ischemic heart disease do so from a ventricular arrhythmia.

ANGINA PECTORIS

Angina pectoris is a clinical syndrome characterized by chest pain, which most often is a presenting manifestation of ischemic heart disease but may occur in other situations characterized by myocardial ischemia, such as aortic valve disease and anemia (see Chap. 7).

Diagnosis

Approximately three-fourths of patients with angina are males; the typical patient is in his fifties or early sixties and seeks medical advice because of chest discomfort. The patient commonly declines to apply the word pain to his chest symptom, and has difficulty describing the sensation, but will usually select words such as heaviness, pressure, tightness, choking, or squeezing. The typical discomfort is substernal. The most important feature of angina pectoris is its relation to exertion or emotion. The discomfort comes on during physical activity or emotional disturbance and is relieved by rest. Anger, fright, or merely enthusiastic enjoyment of a sporting event may bring on the syndrome. The threshold for the development of angina varies with the time of day more than from day to day. The typical patient may have to stop at exactly the same spot on his way to work each morning, yet by midday he may be able to cover many times that distance without discomfort. Symptoms which develop soon after arising are common, and the patient may not be able to shave without stopping; yet he may perform moderately heavy manual labor later in the day, after he has "gotten warmed up." Precipitation of angina by coitus is common, and inquiry about this may yield information of value in separating angina pectoris from other syndromes which cause similar chest discomfort but do not interrupt or prevent sexual activity.

Variation in the location and character of the discomfort may occur, so that angina pectoris should not be ruled out just because the location of the pain is atypical, especially if there is a strong relation to exertion. Myocardial ischemia may be characterized by pain in the neck, jaw, throat, shoulder, or arm, with no symptoms in the chest. Radiation to the arms is common in typical angina, and sometimes the only discomfort may be in the arms, where it is often described as a numbness. Sharp pains, especially those of short duration, are rarely due to myocardial ischemia, but the words knifelike and cutting are occasionally utilized to describe ischemia.

The term *angina decubitus* has been applied to the variant of angina pectoris which develops while the patient is in the recumbent position. This form of rest pain represents one of the intermediate syndromes. The patient may report that he is awakened at night by a sensation which is similar to his exertional pain. The syndrome of angina decubitus is similar to that of paroxysmal nocturnal dyspnea, and dyspnea actually often accompanies the chest discomfort. It is postulated but not proved that the pathophysiology is also similar and that angina decubitus is a form of left ventricular failure precipitated by the expansion of the intrathoracic blood volume which occurs with recumbency. Elevation of systemic arterial blood pressure has been demonstrated to precede attacks of pain and may be another precipitating factor. Dreaming has also been implicated in the pathogenesis of this relatively unusual variant of angina.

Physical examination

Physical findings are usually normal in the patient with angina pectoris between episodes, but during an attack of pain certain signs may be present and may be helpful in establishing a diagnosis. The most important of these is the fourth heart sound, which is the auscultatory manifestation of the increased amplitude of the presystolic expansion of the left ventricle. Sometimes this presystolic activity can be felt or even seen. Another manifestation of ischemia is dysfunction of the papillary muscles, which may be manifested as a systolic murmur of mitral regurgitation. For this reason, it is important to inspect, palpate, and auscultate at the apex of the heart if the patient should happen to develop pain during the examination.

Physical examination is also valuable in detecting evidence of a systemic disease or a metabolic state which predisposes to coronary atherosclerosis. For example, systemic hypertension is a finding of great significance because it accelerates the atherosclerotic process and is amenable to treatment. Xanthelasma and xanthoma may indicate an abnormality of lipid metabolism with which an increased incidence of coronary atherosclerosis may be associated (Chaps. 106 and 244).

Laboratory examination

The electrocardiogram, especially, may be very helpful in establishing the diagnosis of ischemic heart disease if characteristic changes are present. The absence of abnormalities is, however, far less specific and does not exclude the diagnosis, because the 12-lead electrocardiogram is normal in approximately 50 percent of patients with typical angina pectoris and demonstrable coronary atherosclerosis. The most definite and diagnostic electrocardiographic changes are those of old myocardial infarction. The characteristic Q-wave changes of a myocardial infarction, especially if they are of the anterior type with changes in leads I, aVL, or the precordial leads, are almost specific for myocardial infarction. The diagnosis can be made with greater certainty when a previously normal electrocardiogram is present and the appearance of the changes of myocardial infarction can be documented (Chap. 229).

T-wave changes are more difficult to interpret as evidence of ischemic heart disease. Inverted T waves may appear as the only manifestation of ischemic heart disease, but they may also occur in other conditions which may be associated with chest pain, such as pericarditis, myocarditis, and abnormalities of vasoregulation.

Great diagnostic significance can be placed upon S-T and T-wave changes which occur during attacks of pain and which disappear thereafter. The most characteristic change is displacement of the S-T segment, with or without T-wave inversion, which is similar in every way to that which is induced during the course of an exercise test. Long-term monitoring with magnetic tape may be useful in documenting the association of ECG changes and chest pain. The S-T segments are usually depressed but rarely may be strikingly elevated, as in the early stages of myocardial infarction.

STRESS TESTING This is a keystone in the evaluation of patients with chest pain which may be due to ischemic heart disease. It has a firm basis because it is designed to reveal the basic physiologic defect, i.e., the inability of myocardial blood flow to increase in proportion to the metabolic demands. The coronary circulation may be adequate to supply blood in sufficient quantity to meet resting demands and, hence, prevent ischemia, but the discrepancy between supply and demand is apparent when demand is increased by exercise or when supply is decreased by hypoxia.

The stress-testing techniques may be divided into three categories on the basis of the system used to determine the exercise load: tests with standardized external work loads, tests which are standardized by heart rate response, and tests designed to reach the maximal possible exercise load. The two-step system of exercise developed by Master is an example of the first variety. The second and third methods employ a treadmill or bicycle and differ only with respect to the method of determining the end point of the exercise. In the "target heart rate" test, exercise is continued until the patient attains 80 to 90 percent of his predicted maximum heart rate. In the maximal exercise test, exercise is progressively increased until maximal work load is attained. Both tests are discontinued at a lower level of work if the patient develops chest pain, signs of cerebral insufficiency, fall in blood pressure, or significant electrocardiographic changes. The percentage of positive tests in a population of patients with angina and arteriographically proved coronary atherosclerosis is greater with the graded exercise methods (85 to 95 percent) than with the tests standardized on the basis of external work load (double two-step test). A physician must be in attendance throughout every graded exercise test to observe the patient, to evaluate the in-exercise ECG, and to decide whether the testing should continue. The risk of an exercise test is small but present, being estimated at approximately one fatality and 2.4 nonfatal complications per 10,000 tests. The test is probably unusually hazardous and hence contraindicated in patients with unstable angina pectoris and patients in the first few weeks of a myocardial infarction.

Approximately 10 percent of patients with positive test results will have changes only during exercise; hence, the sensitivity of the test is improved by monitoring during exercise. Exercise testing is safer with in-exercise monitoring, because S-T segment changes or arrhythmias may develop before pain or other symptoms occur, and the stress can be discontinued before severe ischemia develops. Multiple leads should be recorded, and precordial leads should be included, because one-third of patients with a positive test result will have changes only in one lead; this one lead is most likely to be V_5 or V_6.

A characteristic positive exercise response is seen in the postexercise record in Fig. 240-1. The S-T segment is depressed 1 mm below the base line, and this depression lasts for more than 0.08 sec. The depression is of the "square-wave" or "plateau" type and is flat or slopes downward (unlike the S-T segment depression in the record taken during exercise, which slopes upward, is referred to as a junctional change, and does not constitute a positive test result). T-wave abnormalities, arrhythmias, and conduction disturbances may develop with exercise but do not constitute certain evidence of myocardial ischemia. If 1 mm or more of S-T segment depression is required before the test is considered to be positive, the percentage of false positive results will be small (less than 5 percent) and only about 15 percent of patients with severe coronary atherosclerosis will have negative test results. If the threshold of positivity is set at 0.5 mm, there will be more false positive tests and fewer false negative ones.

Exercise electrocardiography is still the best generally available test for the detection of myocardial ischemia. The negative tests in patients with severe coronary disease and angina can be explained by the experimental observations which show that electrocardiographic changes may not be the earliest manifestation of ischemia. In other patients with severe disease, pain or fatigue causes termination of exercise before ECG changes appear. If collaterals are adequate, severe coronary atherosclerosis, as indicated by arteriography, may coexist with a negative exercise test result.

A particular form of false positive exercise test may be seen in patients who have a disorder of vasomotor control which has been termed vasoregulatory asthenia. These patients frequently develop S-T segment and T-wave changes resembling those of myocardial ischemia when they assume the erect posture prior to the onset of exercise. During the first minute of exercise, typical positive electrocardiographic changes develop, but as exercise continues they are rapidly replaced by junctional S-T segment depressions. The changes can be eliminated by β-adrenergic blockade, and are attributed to an abnormality of autonomic control of the circulation.

Other forms of stress testing have been developed for use in the recumbent subject during the course of cardiac catheterization and angiography. Under these circumstances the heart can be stressed by having the patient perform leg exercise with a bicycle device afixed to the catheterization table or by isometric hand grip exercise produced by having the patient squeeze an ergometer. Probably the most widely used form of stress at catheterization is the pacing stress test, in which the heart rate is increased by electrical pacing of the heart with a pacing catheter in the right atrium. Pacing-induced tachycardia increases the myocardial oxygen demands and hence produces ischemia in the patient with limited ability to increase myocardial blood flow in proportion to oxygen demands. The rate is increased in stages from the resting rate to 160 to 180 beats per minute, or until the patient develops chest pain or an ischemic electrocardiogram. One of the advantages of this form of stress is that it can be conducted on a recumbent subject; and, therefore, hemodynamic measurements can be made during the test. The major disadvantage lies in the fact that pacing-induced tachycardia is not physiologically comparable to exercise in that the cardiac output does not increase, and hence the stroke volume decreases as rate increases.

CORONARY ARTERIOGRAPHY Providing precise and direct information about the atherosclerotic process in the coronary arteries during life, coronary arteriography is of great value in evaluating the status of patients with chest pain of uncertain origin and patients with typical angina pectoris who are being considered for surgical therapy (Chap. 231). Coronary arteriography is clearly indicated in all patients with chest pain of uncertain origin when the uncertainty persists after clinical evaluation and stress testing. The indications are less clear in the group with typical angina and depend upon the attitude of the physician and surgeon concerning surgical therapy. In general, patients with stable angina pectoris of 3 months' duration which is not controlled by medical therapy and which is of sufficient severity to interfere with the patient's life should be subjected to arteriography. The procedure is also indicated for patients with unstable angina and rest angina for whom surgery is being considered.

The best radiographic visualization of the coronary arterial tree is obtained with the selective methods, in which the catheter is introduced directly into the orifice of a coronary artery and radiopaque material is injected (Chap. 231). During the procedure the catheter should be advanced into the left ventricle for pressure measurements and the conduct of left ventriculography to evaluate ventricular function, which is often disordered in ischemic heart disease.

Management of angina pectoris

The term *management* is more appropriate than *treatment* with reference to angina pectoris because far more is required than the prescription of a drug or the recommendation of surgery. The patient must be evaluated with particular reference to the interaction between his disease

FIGURE 240-1
Positive electrocardiographic exercise test. "Square-wave" S-T segment displacement in lead V_4 in postexercise record. Changes during exercise are junctional.

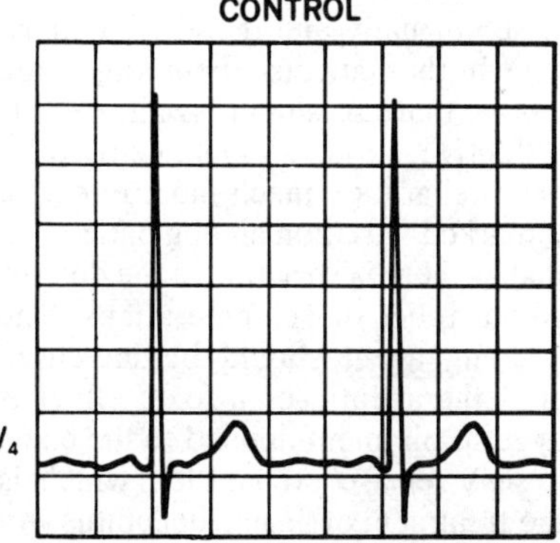

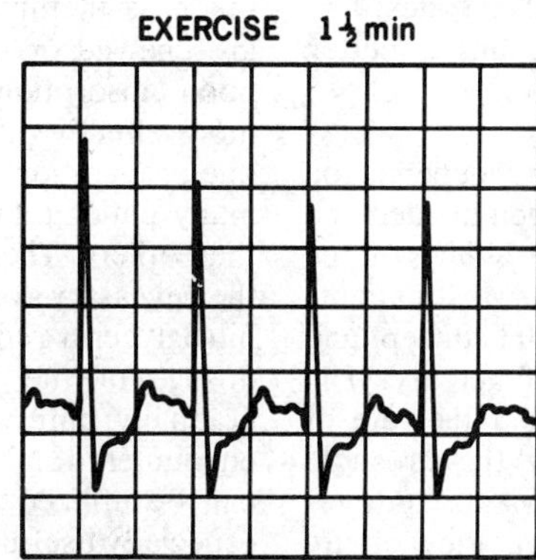

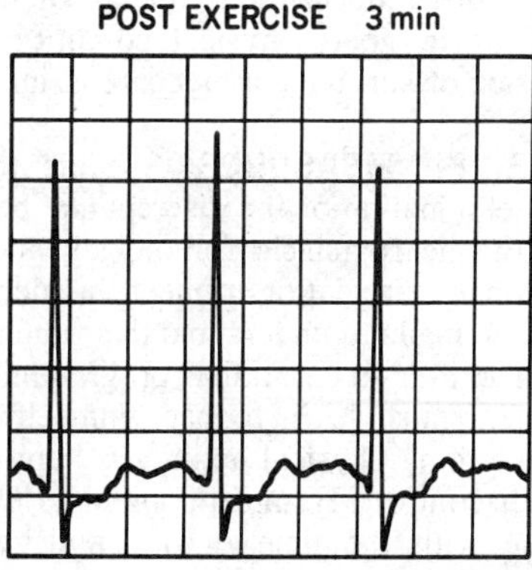

and life pattern. The physical and emotional stresses which precipitate pain and the pleasurable activities prohibited by angina must be identified. The first step in management is reassurance. The patient must be made to realize that long useful life is possible even though he has angina pectoris. It is usually not advisable to quote statistics, but the recital of case histories of persons in public life may be of great value. A realistic explanation of the pathophysiology of the disease is worthwhile for the intelligent patient and can be used as the basis for the life plan which is to be described.

The management plan has two parts: (1) general measures directed toward preventing progression of ischemic heart disease, and (2) measures to prevent or minimize the attacks of ischemia. The general measures also apply to patients in whom the initial presentation of ischemic heart disease is a myocardial infarction or the intermediate syndrome.

GENERAL MEASURES There is no proof that the lesions of atherosclerosis can be made to regress, but it is clear that certain factors accelerate their progression. It seems reasonable, therefore, to make the reduction of these risk factors a keystone of therapy in all patients with coronary artery disease. Ideal weight should be maintained; if the patient is obese he should reduce, but if he is of normal weight when he comes under medical management, his diet should be adjusted to prevent the gain in weight which so often accompanies advancing years, especially if physical activity is restricted because of angina. The caloric content of the diet is most important, but the content of animal and other saturated fats should also be restricted (Chap. 244). Hypertension is associated with an increased incidence of complications of ischemic heart disease; therefore, the blood pressure should be maintained at normal levels. Smoking should be forbidden, unless in the physician's judgment the emotional consequences of abstinence are extreme and greater than the risks of continuing. It has been demonstrated that the mortality rate for people who have stopped smoking is the same as that for those who have never smoked. Thus, the facts do not support the statement often made by patients that it is too late to stop. Diabetes and the hyperlipemias should be treated when they are present (Chap. 244). The patient should be encouraged to engage in regular exercise. The maintenance of good physical condition enables him to perform physical work more efficiently at a lower pulse rate and, therefore, reduces the frequency of anginal episodes. The patient in good physical condition also has a better chance of surviving a myocardial infarction.

SPECIFIC MEASURES Specific therapy depends on the elimination of the discrepancy betweeen the demand of the heart muscle for oxygen and the ability of the coronary circulation to meet this demand. Most patients can be made to understand this fundamental concept and utilize it in the rational programming of activity. The patient must learn to pace himself so that the rate of performing physical activity is kept below the threshold of discomfort. He must appreciate the variation in tolerance with the time of day and see that the activity requirements are reduced in the morning and immediately after meals. It may be necessary to advise a change in job or residence to avoid physical stress, but with the exception of the manual laborer it is usually possible for the patient to continue to function merely by allowing more time for the completion of each task. Emotional tension is often neglected in the planning of a program for the patient with angina. In some patients, anger and frustration may be the most important precipitating factors in daily life.

Nitroglycerin The mechanism of action of nitroglycerin, the most valuable drug in the treatment of angina pectoris, is discussed in Chap. 235. The activity of the agent depends upon its absorption, which is most rapid and complete through the mucous membranes. For this reason nitroglycerin is administered sublingually in tablets of 0.4 or 0.6 mg. Patients with angina should be instructed to take the medication to relieve an attack and also in anticipation of stress which is likely to induce angina. When the patient develops pain on exertion, he should cease activity and place a tablet under his tongue. The discomfort generally disappears more rapidly with nitroglycerin than would be expected if the drug were not administered. A flight of stairs, a walk up a hill, or sexual intercourse may produce pain consistently, but the pain can be prevented by the anticipatory use of nitroglycerin.

The dose of nitroglycerin should be large enough to relieve pain but not large enough to produce a feeling of pulsating fullness in the head or a frank headache, the most common side effect of nitroglycerin, which fortunately only rarely becomes disturbing at doses required to relieve angina. Nitroglycerin deteriorates with exposure to air and sunlight; therefore, if it produces neither relief of pain nor a headache, the preparation may be inactive and a fresh supply should be obtained.

If the patient does not experience relief after the first dose of nitroglycerin, he may take a second but should be instructed not to continue to take the medication if the first few doses prove unsuccessful. If pain continues despite nitroglycerin, the patient should consult his physician, who can evaluate the possibility of his having myocardial infarction or one of the intermediate syndromes (page 1209).

Unfortunately, none of the long-acting nitrates is as effective as nitroglycerin in the relief of angina pectoris. However, several of these preparations are useful in prolonging the time interval between attacks and, hence, in reducing the amount of nitroglycerin which has to be taken as therapy for acute attacks. Preparations which are chewed or taken sublingually and therefore depend upon absorption through the mucous membranes are more effective than those that are simply swallowed. If one preparation is ineffective, another should be tried, as many patients find one preparation much more effective than others. There is marked variation among patients in the necessary dose, just as there is variation in the dose of nitroglycerin required for relief of an acute attack. The dosage of the long-acting agent should be increased gradually until either a therapeutic or a toxic effect is encountered. Nitroglycerin ointment applied to the chest can be utilized as a slow-release preparation which is especially useful in the treatment of angina decubitus. An application of ointment at bedtime may give the patient a night's sleep which had not been possible before.

Cardiac glycosides and diuretics During an attack of angina pectoris, left ventricular function becomes impaired and the left ventricular end-diastolic pressure rises, leading in turn to an elevation in pulmonary vascular pressures. Therefore, agents useful in the treatment of congestive heart failure (Chaps. 233 and 235) also may be valuable in the management of angina pectoris. The cardiac glycosides will be most effective in the patient with an enlarged heart. A decrease in heart size decreases wall tension and hence myocardial oxygen requirements. If the heart is of normal size the cardiac glycosides may aggravate the angina by increasing contractility and hence the oxygen requirements. The addition of an oral diuretic will also prove useful in many patients. These measures are especially valuable in the prevention of attacks of nocturnal angina and of angina at rest, i.e., angina decubitus. When angina pectoris is refractory to the general measures outlined above, digitalis should be tried even though overt congestive failure may be absent.

Beta-adrenergic blockade The β-adrenergic blocking agents such as propranolol represent a useful addition to the pharmacologic treatment of angina pectoris. The effects of β-adrenergic blockade are described best as being the opposite of those of isoproterenol, an agent which stimulates the cardiac beta receptors (Chap. 235). Isoproterenol produces an increase in heart rate, myocardial contractility, cardiac output, and myocardial oxygen consumption, associated with a decrease in total peripheral resistance, while the β-adrenergic blocking agents prevent these changes. The effects of these drugs are most apparent during exercise; there is only a small decrease in cardiac output and heart rate at rest, but beta blockade reduces these variables significantly during exercise. Propranolol is useful in angina pectoris because it reduces the workload associated with exercise, rather than because of any direct effect on the coronary arteries. Propranolol is usually administered in an initial dose of 40 mg per day in four divided doses and is increased as tolerated to doses of 160 to 320 mg per day. Therapy is monitored by observation of the pulse rate and examination for signs of congestive failure.

Surgery During the last quarter-century cardiac surgeons have introduced many procedures as treatment for ischemic heart disease. Symptomatic improvement has followed all of them in a high percentage of patients, but there is no evidence that the natural history of the disease has been favorably altered. The only surgical procedure for coronary artery disease for which there is general enthusiasm is the aorta–coronary vein bypass procedure. A section of vein, usually the saphenous, is used to form a connection between the aorta and the coronary artery distal to the obstructing lesion. The operation is attractive because it represents a simple, direct mechanical attack on the obstructive lesions in the major coronary arteries.

The operative mortality rate is low, being 5 percent or less in patients with good ventricular function. The most impressive result of the operation is the relief of symptoms and hence improvement in the quality of life for the patient with angina pectoris. Although a worthwhile objective, the improvement in symptomatic status in 85 percent of patients does not constitute proof that the operation is changing the disease process. The powerful placebo effect of surgery in patients with angina pectoris makes the evaluation of symptomatic improvement very difficult. Exercise tolerance is also improved after operation, but this may be closely related to the relief of pain. Objective evidence of improved left ventricular function as measured by hemodynamics or angiography has not been consistently present. There is as yet no evidence upon which to base a conclusion about the effect of the operation on the natural history of the disease. Another important unanswered question concerns the long-term fate of the saphenous vein. Available evidence indicates that from 60 to 70 percent of veins remain patent for 2 years. Occlusion of segments of the native circulation with myocardial infarction has also been reported with a frequency of 20 to 30 percent.

The role of this operation in the therapy of ischemic heart disease cannot be defined precisely at this time. It is, therefore, possible to list indications only in terms of current practice. Three factors are usually considered in arriving at a decision to advise vein bypass surgery: (1) symptomatic status; (2) coronary anatomy as shown by coronary arteriography; and (3) ventricular function as determined by angiography and hemodynamics. Most patients advised to have surgery are symptomatic, although the severity of the symptoms in surgical candidates varies widely from one institution to another. The ideal candidate has severe (80 percent or greater) obstructive lesions in the proximal portions of two of the three major coronary arteries. In some centers patients with lesions in a single vessel are also considered to be surgical candidates. Patients with severe lesions in the left main coronary artery are at high risk and should have surgical therapy if there are no contraindications. The best results are obtained in patients with normal ventricular function or at most a single area of impaired myocardial contractility. The mortality rate is high in patients with an ejection fraction of less than 0.45, left ventricular end-diastolic pressure greater than 20, and poor contraction as seen on angiography.

MYOCARDIAL INFARCTION

Austin Flint, Osler, and others were familiar with the pathology of coronary atherosclerosis and coronary occlusion, but the pathologic and clinical features were associated for the first time in 1912 by Herrick.

Clinical presentation

Pain is the most frequent presenting complaint of the patient with myocardial infarction and is usually severe enough to be described as the worst pain the patient has ever experienced (Chap. 7). It is a deep visceral pain, and adjectives commonly applied to it are "heavy," "squeezing," and "crushing." It is similar in character to the pain of angina pectoris but is more severe, lasts longer, and is usually relatively constant. The typical pain involves the central portion of the chest and epigastrium and radiates to the arms in about 25 percent of cases. Less-common sites of radiation are the abdomen, back, jaw, and neck. The location of the pain beneath the xiphoid is responsible for the mistaken diagnosis of acute indigestion. The pain is often accompanied by a feeling of weakness, sweating, nausea, vomiting, and giddiness. It may begin during a period of exertion but does not subside with rest.

Although pain is the most common presenting complaint, it is by no means always present; a minimum of 15 to 20 percent of myocardial infarcts may be painless. The frequency of painless infarcts is probably much higher than this estimate because the patient without pain often does not reach medical attention. The incidence of painless infarcts increases with age, and in the elderly, the presenting complaint of a myocardial infarct may be the sudden onset of breathlessness, which may progress to pulmonary edema. Other less-common presentations in the absence of pain include sudden loss of consciousness, a confusional state, the appearance of an arrhythmia, or merely an unexplained drop in arterial blood pressure.

Physical findings

In most instances, the dominant feature of the patient's presentation is his reaction to the chest pain. He is typically anxious and may be restless, attempting to relieve the pain by moving about in bed, squirming, stretching, belching, or even inducing vomiting. Pallor is common and is often associated with perspiration and coolness of the extremities. The pulse is rapid except in a few patients who exhibit profound bradycardia with heart rates of 40 or 50 beats per min.

The precordium is usually quiet, and the apical impulse may be difficult or impossible to palpate. An abnormal systolic pulsation in the area between the apex and the left sternal border may be noted in a few patients. On auscultation, the heart sounds are usually of diminished intensity, but may be normal. The most common extra sound is the S_4, or atrial gallop sound, which may be detected in the majority of patients with myocardial infarction. An S_3, or ventricular gallop sound, is far less common. Occasionally, the second heart sound is paradoxically split. An apical systolic murmur of mitral regurgitation secondary to papillary muscle dysfunction is present in more than half these patients at some time during their course. A pericardial friction rub will be heard in the majority of patients at some time in their course if they are examined frequently.

Laboratory diagnosis

The laboratory tests of value in confirming myocardial infarction may be divided into three groups: (1) nonspecific indexes of tissue necrosis and inflammation, (2) the electrocardiogram, and (3) the serum enzyme changes.

The nonspecific reaction to myocardial injury is associated with leukocytosis, which often reaches levels of 12,000 to 15,000. The leukocytosis appears within a few hours after the onset of the pain and persists for 3 to 7 days. The magnitude of the leukocytosis yields some information about the size of the infarct, the higher white blood cell counts being associated with larger infarcts. The second nonspecific change is elevation of the erythrocyte sedimentation rate, which rises more slowly than the white blood cell count, peaks during the first week, and remains elevated for several weeks.

ELECTROCARDIOGRAPHIC MANIFESTATIONS The electrophysiologic process within the heart is sensitive to alterations in the perfusion of the myocardium and, hence, the electrocardiogram is of great value in ischemic heart disease (Chap. 229).

If the infarct does not involve the entire thickness of the myocardium it is said to be nontransmural or subendocardial and the characteristic ECG changes described in Chap. 229 will not occur. If the infarct is not transmural, which usually means that only the subendocardial tissue is involved, there will be no Q waves and the characteristic changes will be S-T segment depression, in association with tall, peaked T waves. The amplitude of the R waves in the precordial leads may also be decreased. These changes are nonspecific, and the diagnosis of infarction has to be supported by other clinical and laboratory information. Enzyme studies are especially helpful in this situation.

SERUM ENZYME STUDIES The discovery of increased concentration of serum glutamic oxalacetic transaminase (SGOT) in patients with myocardial infarction ushered in an era of improved accuracy in the diagnosis of the condition. It was learned that certain enzymes present in heart muscle in large quantities are released into the blood when the myocardium is infarcted. The same enzymes are present in tissues other than the heart, and they differ with respect to the rate of liberation following injury. The time course of the serum concentration of the most commonly used enzymes is shown in Fig. 240-2. Levels of two of the enzymes, SGOT and creatinine phosphokinase (CPK), rise and fall rapidly, while that of lactic dehydrogenase (LDH) rises later and stays up longer. SGOT is the most widely used enzyme in the first or rapid group, but it has several disadvantages. In the first place, the levels may have fallen to normal in 3 days and if the first blood sample is not taken until the third day following the infarct, diagnostic changes may not be present. The enzyme is also present in skeletal muscle, liver, and red blood cells and may be liberated from these extracardiac stores. CPK has an advantage over SGOT in that it is not present in significant concentrations in red blood cells, the kidney, liver, or lungs, but only in heart, skeletal muscle, and brain. Therefore, it is more specific and sensitive than SGOT, but its rise is also short-lived and may be missed.

In myocardial infarction, the LDH rises during the first day, with a peak at 3 to 4 days, and returns to the normal range in 14 days. There are five common LDH isoenzymes which may be separated by starch-gel electrophoresis. Tissues differ with respect to the specific isoenzymes which predominate; the rapidly migrating isoenzyme which predominates in the heart is referred to as LDH_1, while the slowly migrating components predominate in liver and skeletal muscle. LDH_1 rises before total LDH in patients with myocardial infarction and may rise

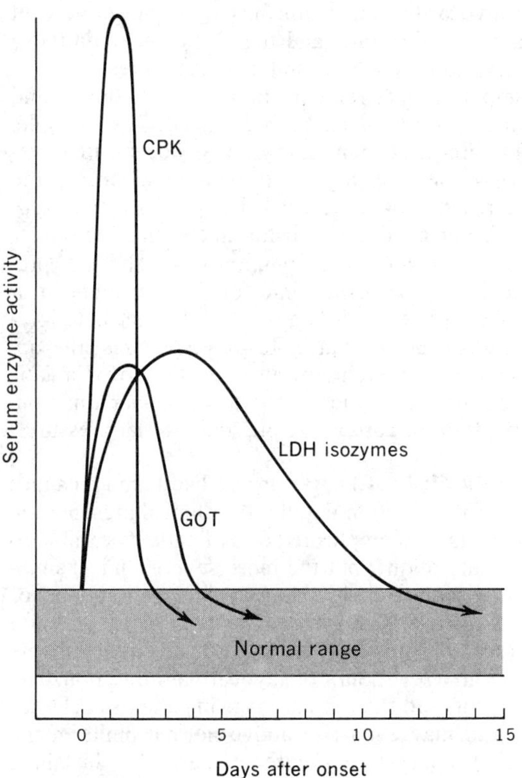

FIGURE 240-2
The time course of serum enzyme concentration changes following a typical myocardial infarction. CPK, creatinine phosphokinase; LDH, lactic dehydrogenase; GOT, glutamic oxaloacetic transaminase.

when there is no change in total LDH. Therefore, increased LDH_1 is a more sensitive indicator of myocardial infarction than total LDH. Its sensitivity exceeds 95 percent.

It is the time course of the change which is important in establishing the diagnosis, and it is appropriate to select an "early riser" like SGOT or CPK and another enzyme with a slower time course such as LDH. The bigger the infarct, the bigger the enzyme response. The mass of heart muscle infarcted can be estimated from analysis of the concentration-time curve of the enzyme and knowledge of the kinetics of the enzyme. The best estimates of the accuracy of enzyme diagnosis are based on the experiences with SGOT. A characteristic rise occurs in more than 95 percent of patients with clinically proved myocardial infarction, and the SGOT generally does not rise in the conditions most often considered as differential diagnostic possibilities in the case of suspected myocardial infarction. Specifically, SGOT does not rise in the intermediate syndromes, rheumatic carditis, or pericarditis. The rise in SGOT which follows pulmonary infarction occurs later and is of a lesser magnitude than that which follows myocardial infarction. The list of conditions other than myocardial infarction which may result in elevated SGOT includes (1) right ventricular failure with hepatic damage due to acute congestion, (2) the administration of salicylates, opiates, or coumarin-type anticoagulants, (3) primary muscle disease, including muscular dystrophy and surgical trauma, (4) cardiac operations, (5) acute pancreatitis, (6) extensive central nervous system damage, (7) toxemia of pregnancy, (8) hemolytic crisis, (9) crush injuries or burns, and (10) infarction of kidney, spleen, or intestine. Of particular importance in the clinical situation is the fact that a two- to threefold elevation of CPK may follow an intramuscular injection even in the absence of local inflammation. This may lead to the erroneous diagnosis of myocardial infarction in a patient who has been given an intramuscular injection of morphine or Demerol for a chest pain of nonspecific origin.

Clinical course

The course and prognosis of the patient with myocardial infarction may be predicted with reasonable accuracy from the original clinical presentation. The system of clinical classification originally proposed by Killip divides patients into four groups as follows: class I—no signs of pulmonary or venous congestion; class II—moderate heart failure as evidenced by rales at lung bases, gallop, tachypnea, or signs of right heart failure including venous and hepatic congestion; class III—severe heart failure, pulmonary edema; class IV—shock with systolic pressure less than 90 mm Hg and evidence of peripheral constriction, diaphoresis, peripheral cyanosis, mental confusion, and decreased urine output. The expected hospital mortality rate of patients in these clinical classes has been established by a number of investigators as follows: class I, 0 to 5 percent; class II, 10 to 20 percent; class III, 35 to 45 percent; and class IV, 85 to 95 percent.

ARRHYTHMIAS It is useful to divide the arrhythmias of myocardial infarction into two groups on the basis of whether the rate is too fast, i.e., tachyarrhythmia, or too slow, i.e., bradyarrhythmia. The tachyarrhythmias may arise in the atrium, the AV node, or the ventricle. *Sinus tachycardia* is the most common tachyarrhythmia to occur in myocardial infarction, but it requires no specific therapy. *Atrial fibrillation* and *flutter* are seen in from 10 to 15 percent of patients and may precipitate congestive failure because of the acceleration of the ventricular rate and the loss of effective atrial systole. The appearance of atrial tachycardia should suggest the possibility of digitalis intoxication.

Coronary care units have had their greatest impact on the mortality rate in myocardial infarction through the detection and control of ventricular arrhythmias. The risk of ventricular fibrillation is highest soon after infarction, being fifteen times greater in the first 4 hr than it is between the fourth and twelfth hours. The ventricular premature beat is generally considered to be a precursor of ventricular fibrillation, and the premature beat which occurs on the T wave of the previous sinus beat is especially likely to initiate a serious ventricular arrhythmia. The highest incidence of fibrillation occurs following beats exhibiting this "R-on-T" phenomenon, but fibrillation may occur following ventricular beats which do not exhibit this relationship or, indeed, in the absence of any premonitory premature ventricular activity of any sort.

Ventricular tachycardia occurs at least once in 10 percent of patients with myocardial infarction, as a self-limited burst of 10 to 25 beats of which the patient may be unaware. It is significant in that it may lead to hemodynamic deterioration or be a precursor of ventricular fibrillation.

It is useful to classify ventricular fibrillation as either primary or secondary. The secondary variety is often a terminal event and associated with shock or congestive failure; and although often contributing to the fatal outcome, it is not the primary cause. Primary ventricular fibrillation is that which develops in the absence of shock or heart failure. It is much more likely to occur in the first few days but may occur at any time, responds well to treatment, but is usually fatal if untreated.

The bradyarrhythmias may be of significance equal to that of the tachyarrhythmias, especially if the prehospital phase of myocardial infarction is considered. *Sinus bradycardia* has been reported in 61 percent of patients with inferior myocardial infarction seen within the first hour of the onset of symptoms. If the degree of slowing is severe, an escape rhythm originating in the AV junctional tissue usually develops.

Failure of the atrial impulse to be propagated to the ventricle is another important cause of bradycardia. The failure to conduct or block may develop at three different levels in the conduction system: the atrioventricular node, the bundle of His, or the more peripheral portions of the conduction system. If the block occurs in the AV node, the QRS complexes will be normal; but when the block occurs distal to the AV node, the QRS structure will be abnormal and it will be prolonged. Rosenbaum has directed attention to disturbances of conduction in the peripheral bundle branches as being of value in predicting the occurrence of AV nodal block. Block of the anterior fascicle is characterized by the appearance of left axis deviation with a mean QRS axis of -45 to $60°$, a small 0.02 sec Q wave in leads I and AVL, and slight prolongation of the QRS complex to between 0.08 and 0.09 sec. This pattern is referred to as left anterior hemiblock or left anterior fascicular block. Block of the posterior division or left posterior fascicular block is recognized by a mean QRS axis of approximately $+120°$ and Q waves of less than 0.02 sec in leads II and III and AVF. Block of the single fascicle to the right ventricle results in the familiar pattern of right bundle branch block with a QRS duration of 0.12 sec and an RSR′ or RR′ wave in lead V_1. When block occurs in any two of the three fascicles, bifascicular block is said to exist; and trifascicular block, or complete heart block, follows in approximately 35 percent of patients. Patients with right bundle branch block and either left anterior or left posterior hemiblock have a particularly high risk of progression to complete heart block.

Conduction disturbances are two to three times more common in patients with inferior infarction. The mortality rate of patients with heart block in association with anterior infarction is, however, three to four times that of patients who develop conduction disturbances with inferior infarction. Atrioventricular block in association with anterior myocardial infarction has an 80 to 90 percent immediate mortality rate, and the risk of death in those who survive to leave the hospital is also increased.

The important interrelations between arrhythmias and hemodynamic states must be recognized. For example, potentially life-threatening arrhythmias occur with a frequency of 45 percent in patients *without* shock, but the incidence reaches 94 percent in a group *with* shock. Both atrioventricular conduction disturbances and ventricular fibrillation are much more common when shock is present. Shock may be responsible for the development of arrhythmias, which may then result in further deterioration of cardiac performance. In other patients, the opposite sequence of events occurs, i.e., the arrhythmia is responsible for impairment of left ventricular function, with depression of cardiac output and arterial pressure.

HEMODYNAMICS Changes in cardiac hemodynamics in myocardial infarction parallel the clinical presentation of the patients. Uncomplicated class I patients exhibit no significant alterations; but the more severe clinical situations are associated with hemodynamic alterations of greater magnitude. The systemic arterial blood pressure may be reduced transiently in up to 80 percent of patients during the first few hours of myocardial infarction. The pressure returns to the normal range in patients in classes I and II and may even rise above normal limits in the presence of congestive failure in class III. Sustained systemic arterial hypotension is present only in class IV.

Left ventricular filling pressure may be measured directly by a retrograde catheter introduced into the left ventricle or indirectly as the pulmonary capillary wedge pressure determined by the Swan-Ganz balloon catheter. The pulmonary artery wedge pressure will be elevated (greater than 12 mm Hg) in approximately 25 percent of patients in class I, 60 to 70 percent of patients in class II, and in 90 percent of patients in classes III and IV. The average wedge pressure in patients in class IV is over 20 mm Hg. The central venous pressure, or right-sided filling pressure, does not accurately reflect the left ventricular filling pressure. It may, however, be useful as a means whereby volume expansion can be monitored. Cardiac output changes are less closely related to clinical status but cardiac output is usually reduced in patients with heart failure and shock (classes III, IV) and is usually normal in class I. There is great variability in the peripheral resistance, but elevation is the rule in class IV. The arterial oxygen tension is reduced in the first week following myocardial infarction in most patients in whom it is measured; this is because of shunting of blood in the lung, i.e., the perfusion of under- or poorly ventilated alveoli. A single set of measurements of hemodynamic variables may provide information useful as a supplement to clinical classification; however, hemodynamic measurements are most useful when made serially over the first few days to predict changes and to monitor the effect of therapy. Rapid change is possible in any patient, even those in class I; therefore, any system which permits early detection of change is of great value.

Management

The objectives of management of the patient with myocardial infarction are to prevent death due to arrhythmia or asystole and to minimize the mass of infarcted tissue. Arrhythmia and asystole can usually be managed successfully if trained personnel and appropriate equipment are available when the complication develops. The importance of rapid action to put the patient in contact with appropriate personnel and equipment can be easily appreciated by consideration of the time of death in myocardial infarction. Sixty-three percent of male subjects under fifty years of age who died of myocardial infarction did so within 1 hour of the onset of symptoms; 85 percent died during the first 24 hr; and only 23 percent lived long enough to be examined by a physician. Experience in coronary care units indicates that the mortality rate is highest during the first few hours; therefore, there is a great urgency in bringing the patient into an environment where complications can be treated. The biggest delay is not in transportation to the hospital but rather between the onset of pain and the patient's decision to call for help. This major and most significant delay can be reduced only by education of the public concerning the significance of chest pain and the importance of early medical attention. The patient can be placed in such a protective environment by admitting him to a coronary care unit in a hospital or by bringing trained personnel and apparatus to him, as in the coronary ambulance unit.

CORONARY CARE UNITS The development of coronary care units has resulted in improved care of patients with myocardial infarction, a reduction in mortality rates, and also a major increase in the body of information about myocardial infarction. The coronary care unit is a specially designed nursing unit, the most important feature of which is a staff of highly trained personnel with authority to take immediate action in emergency situations. The unit should be equipped with systems which permit the continual monitoring of the electrocardiogram of each patient for the first 5 days. Defibrillators, pacemakers, and respirators must also be available, but equipment alone will not make an effective coronary care unit. Of prime importance is the organization of a highly trained team of nurses who can recognize arrhythmias, adjust the dosage of antiarrhythmic drugs, perform cardiac resuscitation, and apply electroshock when necessary. A physician should be available at all times, but many lives have been saved because the nurse treated ventricular tachycardia with electrical shock before the physician arrived.

The policies and procedures for admission to a coronary care unit should assure that patients are being admitted early in their illness when they may expect to derive maximal benefit from the care provided. The threshold for admission must be low, and this is best monitored in terms of the fraction of total admissions with proved myocardial infarcts. If this fraction exceeds 50 percent, the admission policies are too restrictive and not enough patients are admitted because of the suspicion of myocardial infarction which did not develop. Mortality rates for myocardial infarction in coronary care units vary from 12 to 20 percent, and this variation is probably best explained by the delay between the onset of symptoms and the admission to the unit. The earlier patients are brought under observation, the higher will be the incidence of arrhythmias and the higher will be the mortality rate, as a larger fraction of patients subject to the high early mortality characteristic of this disease will be included.

TREATMENT Analgesia Myocardial infarction usually announces itself with severe pain, and therefore, one of the important initial therapeutic objectives is the relief of pain. Morphine, the drug traditionally used for the relief of pain, is still the most effective and remains the drug of choice. It may lower arterial pressure by producing venous pooling and a reduction in cardiac output. This must be recognized but does not necessarily contraindicate its use. The skin may become cool and moist, and the patient may complain of nausea, but these events usually pass and are replaced by a feeling of well-being associated with the relief of pain. It is important to recognize this syndrome as one attributable to morphine, because the hypotension and signs of peripheral constriction may be interpreted as manifestations of the shock syndrome and taken as grounds for the initiation of vasoconstrictor or other therapy which would be inappropriate. The hypotension associated with venous pooling usually responds promptly to elevation of the legs. If associated with bradycardia, this syndrome will often respond to the administration of atropine. Meperidine (Demerol) has similar hemodynamic effects. There is great variability in the analgesic and hemodynamic response of patients to morphine. Because of its potential for producing hypotension, it is advisable to select the minimal effective dose for the relief of pain.

Oxygen The use of oxygen is supported by the observation that the arterial P_{O_2} is reduced in many patients with myocardial infarction, and inhalation of oxygen increases the P_{O_2} of the blood and, hence, increases the concentration gradient responsible for the diffusion of oxygen into the ischemic myocardium from adjacent, better-perfused areas. Certain side effects of oxygen administration may be undesirable under some circumstances. Oxygen elevates peripheral resistance and lowers cardiac output, stroke volume, and heart rate slightly. Although it is possible that these effects may be deleterious, the weight of evidence indicates that oxygen should be administered by tent, face mask, or nasal cannula for the first 4 or 5 days to the majority of patients.

Rest Factors which increase the work of the heart increase the size of the myocardial infarct. Circumstances in which heart rate, arterial blood pressure, cardiac output, or myocardial contractility are increased should be avoided. It has been demonstrated that 6 to 8 weeks are required for the healing which takes place by the replacement of the infarcted myocardium by scar tissue, and the objective of rest is to provide the most favorable possible circumstances for this healing. The development of collateral circulation in and around the area of the infarction is another important and time-consuming part of the healing process. The work of the heart should be maintained at the lowest possible level while this recovery is taking place. It is no longer considered necessary to keep patients at bed rest for 6 weeks, and most cardiologists allow the patient with uncomplicated myocardial infarct to sit in a chair on the second or third day. A schedule should be developed for each patient to provide as much rest as possible with minimal frustration and anxiety. Muscle tone and general body condition are better maintained if the patient is mobilized early in his convalescence, and the incidence of thromboembolic complications is thereby reduced.

All patients with myocardial infarction should be admitted to a coronary care unit and remain there for 3 to 5 days under constant observation by trained personnel utilizing continual electrocardiographic monitoring. A catheter should be introduced into a peripheral vein, advanced into the intrathoracic veins, and kept open by the slow infusion of glucose solution as a route of administration for antiarrhythmic or other drugs which may be necessary. In many units, a flow-directed balloon catheter is utilized to obtain a measurement of pulmonary capillary wedge pressure and hence left ventricular filling pressure. The catheters should be withdrawn in an uncomplicated (class I) case in 24 hr. During the initial period in the coronary care unit the patient should be at bed rest most of the day, with 1 to 2 periods of 15 to 30 min in the bedside chair. He should use the bedpan or a bedside commode, and should be fed and bathed by a nurse. Oxygen will usually be administered continuously during this period. The bed should be equipped with a footboard, and the patient should push his feet against the footboard firmly ten times each hour to prevent venous stasis and thromboembolism, and to maintain the muscle tone in the legs. To help prevent atelectasis, the patient should be instructed to take 10 deep breaths during each hour.

The usual patient whose course has been uncomplicated leaves the coronary care unit on the third day. By this time, he should be spending 30 to 60 min in a chair twice a day and using the bedside commode. It is advisable at this stage to measure the patient's blood pressure when he stands, so as to be aware of the development of postural hypotension, which may be a problem as he begins to ambulate. By the end of the second week, the patient can be allowed to walk to the bathroom; during the third week short walks about the hospital floor are permissible. The patient can usually be discharged at 3 weeks to complete his convalescence at home. Patients in clinical classes II and III usually remain in the hospital for 4 to 6 weeks. It is usual to restrict the patient to one floor until he has completed 6 weeks of convalescence, and then allow only one trip up stairs a day. From 6 to 8 weeks he should be encouraged to increase activity with walking about the house and may be allowed outdoors in good weather. He should still spend 10 hr a day in bed at night and lie down for 1 hr both morning and afternoon.

From 8 weeks onward, the physician must regulate the patient's activity on the basis of his exercise tolerance. It is during this period of increasing activity that the patient may become aware of profound fatigue. Postural hypotension may still be a problem. Most patients will be able to return to work between 12 and 16 weeks.

Diet During the first 5 days, a liquid diet divided into six small feedings is preferred. Cardiac output increases following ingestion of food and, therefore, the quantity of feedings should be kept small. During the second week, solid food may be added. At this time, the importance of restriction of calories and saturated fat may be explained to the patient, and he can be started on an appropriate diet. His willingness to accept dietary restriction will never be greater than it is during this early period of convalesence.

Bowels Bed rest of 3 to 5 days added to the effect of the narcotics utilized for the relief of pain often leads to constipation. The use of the bedside commode after the first day often prevents serious problems with constipation. If a laxative is required, Colace in a dose of 300 mg twice daily is usually effective. Alternate regimens are either mineral oil, 30 ml, or Senokot tablets. It must be remembered that straining at stool is highly undesirable because it serves as a vagal stimulant which may produce bradycardia and provoke arrhythmias. The Valsalva maneuver associated with defecation may also lead to the release of pulmonary emboli. The patient should be reassured that it will not be deleterious to go without a bowel movement for several days, but if he is distressed and uncomfortable, he may be permitted to receive a rectal suppository on the fourth or fifth day.

Sedation Most patients require sedation during the period in the hospital in order to withstand better the period of enforced inactivity. Phenobarbital is utilized most frequently and is usually found to be effective in a dosage of 16 to 32 mg four times a day, but other sedatives and tranquilizers such as diazepam, 5 mg three times a day, may be substituted. The only problem encountered with phenobarbital is related to its use in patients receiving anticoagulants. The destruction of warfarin-type (dicumarol and coumadin) anticoagulant drugs is increased by phenobarbital and many tranquilizing drugs, and therefore a larger dose of the anticoagulant drugs is required if these agents are given simultaneously. In patients in whom the anticoagulant dosage is regulated while they are receiving phenobarbital which is subsequently discontinued, the dosage of anticoagulant drug may be too large. It is advisable, therefore, to discontinue the phenobarbital as the patient's activity is increased and to readjust the anticoagulant dosage before discharging the patient from the hospital. A hypnotic should be given at night to ensure adequate sleep. This is especially important during the first few days in the coronary care unit, where the atmosphere of 24-hr vigilance may interfere with the patient's sleep. Sedation is no substitute for a dark quiet room.

It is not advisable to use morphine or meperidine as sedatives because of their cardiovascular effects. Furthermore, morphine may depress respiration and intensify arterial desaturation. Morphine and meperidine should be reserved for use in the relief of pain.

Anticoagulant and thrombolytic therapy Anticoagulant therapy has been utilized for the treatment of myocardial infarction for more than a quarter century, but unfortunately its efficacy in reducing mortality still remains in doubt because the results of well-designed clinical trials are conflicting. The lack of any statistically clear-cut, valid demonstration of a lower mortality rate in the first few weeks following myocardial infarction suggests that the benefit, if any, of anticoagulant therapy is small. However, there is agreement that anticoagulant therapy decreases the incidence of thromboembolic complications. Evidence also suggests that the mortality in the first year after myocardial infarction may be reduced by anticoagulation.

Anticoagulant therapy is not without hazard and should be avoided in patients with a history of bleeding diathesis, bleeding ulcer, severe hypertension (diastolic pressure > 110 mm Hg), or cerebral hemorrhage. The patient must be willing and able to cooperate and, therefore, inadequate intelligence and an uncooperative attitude also constitute contraindications to anticoagulant therapy.

Despite some uncertainties, anticoagulant therapy is utilized in most patients with myocardial infarction. Thromboembolic complications do not appear in the first few days and, therefore, could be prevented by the use of the slower-acting anticoagulants (coumadin, etc.) alone, but many physicians prefer to administer heparin intravenously during the first 3 days. This practice cannot be supported by statistics but is defended on the theoretic grounds that heparin may prevent the extension of the thrombotic process in the coronary arteries. A case can also be made for the continuation of anticoagulation for 1 to 2 years after infarction, especially in patients with angina pectoris and multiple infarctions.

The potential use of thrombolytic agents in the therapy of acute myocardial infarction is under active investigation. The plasminogen activator, urokinase, present in human urine has been obtained in purified form, utilized in experimental studies, and also tried in patients with pulmonary embolism. The administration of "polarizing solutions" containing potassium, glucose, and insulin has been advocated as a means whereby intracellular potassium is repleted in the cells at the margin of the infarct. The use of agents which reduce left ventricular work by lowering blood pressure or reducing contractility is under active investigation. Although not yet ready for routine clinical use, this approach offers hope of providing a means whereby the size of the infarct may be reduced.

Complications

ARRHYTHMIAS—PREVENTION AND TREATMENT

The improved management of arrhythmias constitutes a most significant advance in the treatment of myocardial infarction. The prevention of the serious and life-threatening arrhythmias depends on the early recognition and aggressive management of their precursors.

Ventricular premature systoles These are the most frequent harbingers of more serious ventricular arrhythmias. Infrequent, sporadic ventricular premature systoles occur in almost all patients and do not require therapy, but prompt treatment is indicated if the premature systoles occur frequently or in certain patterns. In general, more than five isolated ectopic beats per minute is considered an indication for therapy. Similar indications are the occurrence of consecutive or multifocal ventricular extrasystoles. Ectopic beats occurring early in diastole and, hence, superimposed on the previous T wave are also likely to precede ventricular tachycardia and should be treated promptly. Intravenous lidocaine has become the treatment of choice for the precursors of ventricular arrhythmias, because it acts rapidly and its effects disappear soon (15 to 20 min) after its administration is discontinued. Lidocaine is given initially as a single injection of 25 to 50 mg, which usually eliminates the ectopic beats; this initial dose is followed by an intravenous infusion of 20 to 50 μg per kg per min. If the patient is able to take oral medication, he can be maintained on procainamide (500 mg q. 4 h.) or quinidine (300 mg q. 4 h.) (see Chap. 235).

Ventricular tachycardia and ventricular fibrillation
Sustained ventricular tachycardia is treated first with lidocaine, and if it cannot be terminated by a 50- to 100-mg dose, electroconversion should be employed (Chap. 236). Electroshock is used immediately in patients with ventricular fibrillation. If fibrillation has persisted for more than a few seconds, the first shock may be unsuccessful, and in this situation it is advisable to administer closed-chest massage, mouth-to-mouth respiration, and intravenous bicarbonate solution before attempting electroconversion again. The improvement of oxygenation and perfusion and the correction of acidosis increase the likelihood of successful defibrillation.

In considering the efficacy of therapy for ventricular fibrillation, it is useful to divide patients into groups based on the circumstances of origin of the arrhythmia. The long-term survival in patients with primary ventricular fibrillation is good; 87 percent of these patients in one series left the hospital alive. This is in sharp contrast to the prognosis in the patients who develop secondary ventricular fibrillation. A far smaller percentage, 29 percent, of patients in this group was discharged from the hospital alive.

Accelerated idioventricular rhythm Accelerated idioventricular rhythm or slow ventricular tachycardia has been found to occur in 25 percent of patients with myocardial infarction. The rate is usually similar to that of the sinus rhythm which precedes and follows it, and this similarity of rate and the absence of hemodynamic effects make the rhythm impossible to detect other than by electrocardiographic monitoring. The QRS complexes are broad and identical in shape. The rhythm comes and goes spontaneously and is of little prognostic significance. It does not presage the development of fast ventricular tachycardia or ventricular fibrillation and does not require specific treatment.

Supraventricular arrhythmias Although of less potential significance than the ventricular arrhythmias, supraventricular arrhythmias are common and should be treated promptly. The common arrhythmias in this group are nodal rhythm, atrial tachycardia, atrial flutter, and atrial fibrillation. The administration of a short-acting glycoside such as digoxin or ouabain is the treatment of choice. If the abnormal rhythm persists for more than 2 hr with a ventricular rate in excess of 120 beats per min, treatment with electroshock should be utilized. If there is evidence of heart failure or shock, electroshock should be utilized sooner.

Bradycardia Another important precursor of ventricular tachycardia is bradycardia. Lown found the incidence of ventricular tachycardia in patients with sustained bradycardia to be twice that observed in patients with normal heart rates. Atropine is useful in speeding the heart rate and should be given intravenously in doses of 1.0 to 1.5 mg. However, the administration of atropine is not without hazard because tachycardia increases the oxygen consumption of the heart and also has been reported to produce ventricular fibrillation.

Conduction disturbances Electrical pacing provides an effective means of increasing the heart rate of patients with bradycardia due to atrioventricular block, but it is not possible to be sure that such acceleration is always beneficial. For example, patients with anterior infarction and complete heart block usually have large infarcts and severe heart failure, and it is not possible to demonstrate that the uniformly poor prognosis is improved by pacing. Pacing does appear to be beneficial in patients with an inferior infarct who have complete heart block associated with moderate heart failure. Pacing may also be useful in the treatment of syncope or ventricular irritability. Some cardiologists advocate the placement of a pacing catheter prophylactically in patients with conduction disturbances known to be precursors of complete heart block. Unanimity of opinion does not exist on this point.

Asystole The arrhythmia with the poorest results following treatment is asystole. It usually occurs in patients who have heart failure and/or hypotension. Asystole is treated with closed-chest cardiac massage, artificial ventilation, electrical stimulation, and the intravenous administration of bicarbonate, but the salvage rate is low.

Congestive heart failure Some degree of congestive heart failure occurs in over half the patients with myocardial infarction. The most common clinical signs are rales in the lungs and an S_3 gallop rhythm. Elevation of left ventricular filling pressure and pulmonary artery pressure are the characteristic hemodynamic findings. The therapy of congestive failure in association with myocardial infarction is similar to that of congestive failure secondary to other forms of heart disease, with a few exceptions (Chap. 233). The major difference concerns the use of cardiac glycosides, which are of uncertain value early in the course of myocardial infarction. No clear benefit has been demonstrated to follow digitalization. This is not surprising in that the agent would not be expected to improve the function of infarcted tissue, and the function of the noninfarcted tissue is normal. Evidence also suggests that the patient with myocardial infarction may be unusually sensitive to the digitalis glycosides. Diuretic agents are extremely effective in the treatment of congestive failure following myocardial infarction. A fall in left ventricular filling pressure and an improvement in clinical evidence of failure follow the intravenous administration of 40 mg furosemide. This powerful drug should be used with caution, however, as it can result in a massive diuresis with associated decrease in plasma volume, cardiac output, systemic blood pressure, and, hence, coronary perfusion. The patient with pulmonary edema is treated with the usual agents, which include morphine, tourniquets, oxygen, diuretics, and, rarely, phlebotomy (Chap. 233).

THE SHOCK SYNDROME—POWER FAILURE With the development of effective methods for treating arrhythmias, shock or "power failure" has become the most important fatal complication of myocardial infarction. It is useful to consider this syndrome to be a severe form of left ventricular failure. Shock occurs in about 20 percent of patients with myocardial infarction and accounts for at least 50 percent of the deaths now that the mortality rate due to arrhythmias has been reduced. The mortality rate in myocardial infarction with shock (class IV) ranges from 85 to 95 percent.

Hypotension alone is not a basis for the diagnosis of the shock syndrome, because many patients who make an uneventful recovery will have hypotension (systolic pressures of 80 mm Hg) for several days. The shock syndrome is considered to be present when hypotension is accompanied by other clinical signs of circulatory inadequacy. The following criteria for the shock syndrome define a population of patients with a mortality rate of greater than 95 percent: (1) systolic arterial blood pressure of less than 90 mm Hg or 30 mm Hg below the previous level, (2) clinical signs of peripheral circulatory insufficiency; cold, moist skin and cyanosis, (3) dulled sensorium, (4) oliguria with urine flow of less than 20 ml per hr, and (5) failure of improvement following relief of pain and administration of oxygen. Specifically excluded are patients with hypotension secondary to vasovagal reaction, arrhythmia, drug reactions, or hypovolemia.

Pathophysiology The insult to the heart is the cause of the shock syndrome in myocardial infarction, although all organ systems are involved ultimately. The function of the heart is impaired by the initial insult; this results in a decrease in arterial pressure and, hence, in coronary blood flow because of its dependence on aortic perfusion pressure (Fig. 240-3). The reduction in coronary perfusion pressure and myocardial blood flow further impairs myocardial function and may increase the size of the myocardial infarction. Arrhythmias and metabolic acidosis also participate in this deterioration, because they are the result of inadequate perfusion and both tend to perpetu-

FIGURE 240-3
Diagram illustrating the physiologic interrelationships in the shock syndrome following myocardial infarction.

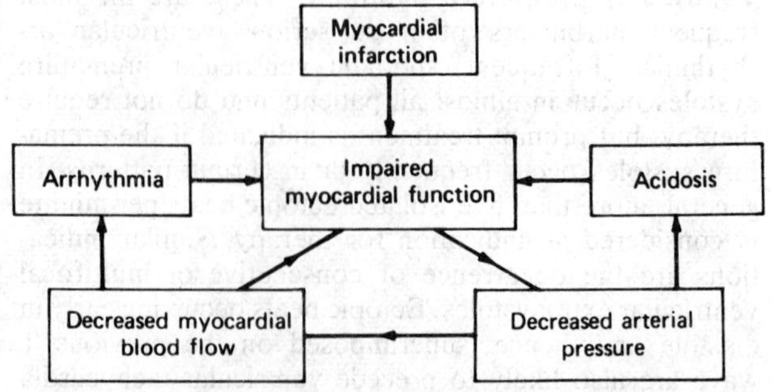

ate the precipitating conditions. It is this positive feedback relationship (impaired cardiac function → arterial hypotension → reduced coronary blood flow → impaired cardiac function) which accounts for the high mortality rate associated with the shock syndrome.

Arterial blood pressure is a function of two factors —the cardiac output (C.O.) and the total peripheral resistance (TPR)—and a decrease in either C.O. or TPR will result in a fall in arterial blood pressure. Cardiac output is lower in a population of patients with shock than in those who do not have the shock syndrome, but this is by no means the whole explanation. Many patients with myocardial infarction without shock have cardiac outputs in the same range as those measured in patients with shock, and therefore it is not possible to characterize these patients on the basis of changes of cardiac output alone.

Total peripheral resistance, the other factor important in determining blood pressure, may be either normal or increased in myocardial infarction. Here again, a similar range of values for total peripheral resistance may be seen in patients in the absence of shock. Normally, a fall in cardiac output is accompanied by a compensatory rise in total peripheral resistance, but in patients with shock due to myocardial infarction the appropriate response in peripheral resistance fails to occur. It appears that the total peripheral resistance is inadequate to support blood pressure at the existing level of cardiac output.

It is necessary to return to the heart itself as the site of the fundamental physiologic alteration in the shock syndrome. It is axiomatic that if the diagnosis of myocardial infarction is correct, there will be a reduction in myocardial contractile function. Direct measurements of left ventricular filling pressure in the form of pulmonary capillary wedge pressure have demonstrated that left ventricular function may be impaired in the absence of the usual clinical manifestations of left-sided heart failure, such as pulmonary edema. A simple schematic diagram depicting the relationship between left ventricular work and filling pressure is seen in Fig. 240-4. The upper curve represents the familiar Frank-Starling relationship in the normal heart; the lower curve shows the relations which might be expected in the patient with shock secondary to myocardial infarction. It is obvious that at all levels of end-diastolic pressure the left ventricular work of the patient with myocardial infarction is depressed. At point *B*, the end-diastolic pressure is elevated; but at point *C*, it may be normal while the myocardial work is well below that expected of the normal heart at this diastolic pressure, as indicated by point *A*.

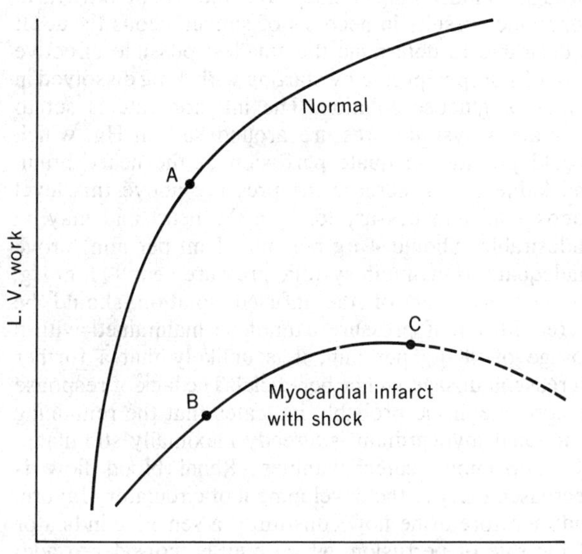

FIGURE 240-4
Schematic representation of the Frank-Starling relationship as applied to patients with the shock syndrome in myocardial infarction.

Treatment The gravity and complex physiology of this condition indicate that all patients with shock should, if possible, have continual monitoring of arterial pressure and pulmonary capillary wedge pressures, and frequent checking of cardiac output. All patients with the shock syndrome should receive 100 percent oxygen continuously. The addition of dissolved oxygen to the plasma helps to combat the hypoxemia which is universally present. The relief of pain is important, as some vasodepressor reflex activity may be a response to severe pain, but narcotics should be used cautiously in view of their propensity to lower arterial pressure.

Treatment is directed at the interruption of the feedback loop (Fig. 240-3), whereby impaired myocardial function leads to a reduction in arterial pressure, decreased coronary blood flow, and a further depression of left ventricular function. This objective is approached by attempting to maintain coronary perfusion by raising the arterial blood pressure without causing the area of ischemia to enlarge. The problem of therapy is complicated by the experimental observation that agents which raise arterial pressure and enhance myocardial contractility may also result in an enlargement of the area of necrosis.

Hypovolemia is an easily corrected condition which may contribute to the hypotension and vascular collapse associated with myocardial infarction in a few patients. Fluid loss may be secondary to reduced intake during the early stages of the illness or to vomiting associated with pain or medications. For this reason it is advisable to be sure that hypovolemia does not exist before embarking upon more vigorous forms of therapy. If the left ventricular filling pressure and/or the central venous pressure are in the normal range, a fluid load should be administered.

VASOPRESSORS The coronary vascular bed distal to an obstructing lesion will be maximally dilated, and therefore myocardial blood flow will be totally dependent on the perfusion pressure. A drop in arterial pressure results in a drop in flow. Norepinephrine (Levophed) is the vasoconstrictor of choice for the treatment of shock in myocardial infarction because it has a positive inotropic effect, as well as having a vasoconstrictor effect on the peripheral circulation. Agents such as methoxamine, Neo-Synephrine, and angiotensin which are pure vasoconstrictors have no place in the treatment of shock due to myocardial infarction, as they increase the work of the heart and hence the myocardial oxygen requirements.

Norepinephrine should be administered intravenously through an indwelling catheter to avoid risk of extravasation, which results in necrosis of subcutaneous tissue. It is desirable to determine the smallest possible effective dose of norepinephrine by starting with 4 mg dissolved in a liter of glucose solution. The infusion rate is set to maintain a systolic pressure around 90 mm Hg, which should provide adequate perfusion of the heart, brain, and kidneys. To increase the pressure above this level imposes an unnecessary load on the heart and may be undesirable. Should 4 μg per min (1 ml per min) prove inadequate to maintain systolic pressure near 90 mm Hg, the concentration of the infused solution should be increased, but if pressure cannot be maintained with a dosage of 48 μg per min, it is unlikely that a further increase in dosage will be beneficial. The lack of response to norepinephrine probably indicates that the remaining functional myocardium is already maximally stimulated by endogenous catecholamines. Renal blood flow is decreased early in the development of circulatory failure, and therefore urine flow constitutes a sensitive indicator of the rate of perfusion, which may be considered adequate if a urine flow of 0.5 ml per min is maintained.

Every effort should be made to use the smallest effective dose of pressor agent for the shortest possible time. Weaning the patient from pressors is often difficult and requires close observation and the exercise of great clinical judgment. The rate of administration must be reduced cautiously. The pressure may fall to 70 mm Hg systolic; but if there are no other clinical signs of circulatory insufficiency, i.e., cyanosis, clouded sensorium, or cold moist extremities, it is wise not to reinstitute therapy. Instead the patient should be observed closely, because the pressure may rise with the passage of time. If, on the other hand, the pressure falls further or clinical signs of circulatory inadequacy appear, therapy must be reinstituted.

Isoproterenol is a synthetic sympathomimetic amine which has enjoyed unjustified popularity in the treatment of shock due to myocardial infarction. It increases the vigor of contraction, increases the heart rate, and, unlike norepinephrine, produces peripheral vasodilatation. The increase in contractility results in an increase in myocardial oxygen consumption, and the increase in wall tension produces a decrease in blood flow to the inner layers of the myocardium. It has also been demonstrated that isoproterenol results in metabolic deterioration, as evidenced by increase in lactate production by the heart. For all these reasons isoproterenol probably does not have a role in the treatment of shock due to myocardial infarction. It may be valuable in other situations when a positive inotropic stimulus is required and the blood pressure is normal.

CARDIAC GLYCOSIDES Consideration of the central role of impaired myocardial function in the shock syndrome leads to the conclusion that cardiac glycosides should be administered to all patients with this condition. The recent experimental work on the extension of infarcts secondary to cardiac glycoside administration suggests that this may not be the case. Obviously, the cardiac glycosides cannot improve the function of necrotic myocardium, but a positive inotropic influence on the noninfarcted myocardium is desirable if it does not result in extension of the infarct. The effect of the cardiac glycosides may be minimal or nonexistent early in the disease at a time when endogenous catecholamines have resulted in maximal stimulation of the myocardium, but the effect may be more evident and beneficial later in the course if congestive failure persists. It has been demonstrated that the incidence of arrhythmia and cardiac rupture is no higher in patients with myocardial infarction treated with digitalis than in a control group.

NEWER FORMS OF THERAPY The basic defect in the shock syndrome is impaired myocardial function; therefore, many mechanical assist devices have been developed to supplement the pumping action of the heart. The largest body of clinical experience has been obtained with the intraaortic balloon system of diastolic augmentation. A balloon is introduced into the aorta on the end of a catheter, and the balloon is inflated at the appropriate time to retard diastolic runoff and enhance coronary flow. It collapses in early systole and therefore reduces the afterload against which left ventricular ejection takes place. Improvement in the hemodynamic status of the patient is associated with balloon pumping in a large number of patients, but long-term survival following balloon pumping alone is still disappointing. The balloon system appears to be of greatest use for the support of patients during angiography and vein bypass surgery.

There is reason to believe that therapy of the shock syndrome secondary to myocardial infarction will continue to be disappointing because a large fraction of patients with the syndrome have severe, diffuse coronary atherosclerosis with large areas of infarcted myocardium.

MITRAL REGURGITATION Apical systolic murmurs of mitral regurgitation appear in more than half the patients during the first 5 days after the onset of a myocardial infarction, but only in a minority of patients is the mitral regurgitation of hemodynamic importance.

In one-third of patients the murmur is present during the acute phase and disappears with recovery. A characteristic and useful clinical sign of the appearance of mitral regurgitation is the development of P-wave changes in the electrocardiogram suggestive of left atrial overload. The most common cause of mitral regurgitation following myocardial infarction is dysfunction of the papillary muscles in the left ventricle, due to ischemia or infarction.

Other pathogenic mechanisms may contribute to or be solely responsible for the development of mitral regurgitation after myocardial infarction. Mitral valve competence depends on the normal spatial relationships between the papillary muscles and the mitral valve; therefore, mitral regurgitation may be the result of alteration in the size or shape of the ventricle due to impaired contractility or to aneurysm formation. Surgical replacement of the mitral valve may be followed by dramatic results in patients in whom heart failure results primarily from mitral regurgitation due to papillary muscle rupture or dysfunction and in whom myocardial function is maintained relatively well.

VENTRICULAR ASYNERGY—VENTRICULAR ANEURYSM Cineradiographic techniques have been responsible for the extension of knowledge of the disorders of ventricular function in ischemic heart disease. Gorlin introduced the term *ventricular asynergy* to describe disorders of ventricular function which occur in 25 to 35 percent of patients with ischemic heart disease. The term ventricular aneurysm is usually used to describe two forms of asynergy: (1) dyskinesis—local expansile paradoxic wall motion: (2) akinesis—local absence of wall motion. Ventricular function is impaired by these disorders because the normally functioning myocardial fibers must increase their degree of shortening if stroke volume and cardiac output are to be maintained.

The clinical manifestations of left ventricular aneurysm are angina pectoris and congestive failure. Apical aneurysms are the most common and the most easily detected by clinical examination. The physical finding of greatest value is a double, diffuse, or displaced apical impulse. The standard roentgenogram frequently reveals an abnormal bulge distorting the contour of the heart, but the roentgenogram may be perfectly normal. The electrocardiographic finding of S-T segment elevation at rest is present in precordial leads in 25 percent of patients with either apical or anterior aneurysms. Ventricular aneurysms may also be responsible for persistent ventricular arrhythmias such as ventricular tachycardia.

THROMBOEMBOLISM Clinical evidence of thromboembolism complicates myocardial infarction in approximately 10 percent of cases, but thrombotic lesions are found in 45 percent of patients in necropsy series, suggesting that thromboembolism is often unrecognized clinically. Thromboembolism is considered to be at least an important contributing cause of death in 25 percent of patients. The left ventricle is the most common locus for mural thrombus, and the rarity of mural thrombi in the right ventricle is consistent with the belief that most pulmonary emboli arise in the leg veins. Thromboembolism most commonly occurs in association with large infarcts and in the presence of congestive failure. The high incidence of thromboembolism constitutes one of the best arguments for the use of anticoagulant therapy in myocardial infarction.

CARDIAC RUPTURE Myocardial rupture is a dramatic complication of myocardial infarction which is most likely to occur during the first week after the onset of symptoms; its frequency increases with the age of the patient. The clinical presentation may often be that of a sudden disappearance of the pulse, blood pressure, and consciousness while the electrocardiogram continues to show sinus rhythm. The electrical activity of the heart continues, and the myocardium continues to contract, but forward flow is not maintained, and blood is pumped into the pericardium instead of into the aorta. Cardiac tamponade ensues, and closed-chest massage is ineffective in producing forward flow. It is conceivable that prompt recognition and surgical intervention might be effective.

SEPTAL PERFORATION The pathogenesis of perforation of the ventricular septum is similar to that of external rupture of the myocardium, but the rate of progression is slower, and, hence, the therapeutic potential is greater. The clinical presentation is one of congestive failure in association with the appearance of a pansystolic murmur typical of a ventricular septal defect. It is often impossible to differentiate this condition from rupture of a papillary muscle. The diagnosis can be established by the demonstration of a left-to-right shunt by limited cardiac catheterization which can be performed at the bedside using a Swan-Ganz flow-directed balloon catheter. Rupture of the ventricular septum is amenable to surgical treatment; but if the clinical condition permits, surgical intervention should be postponed for 6 to 8 weeks, at which time the margins of the defect are composed of firm scar tissue and surgical closure is easier and more likely to be permanently successful.

POST MYOCARDIAL INFARCTION SYNDROME—DRESSLER'S SYNDROME This syndrome, characterized by fever and pleuropericardial chest pain, was first described by Dressler and is thought to be due to an autoimmune pericarditis, pleuritis, and pneumonitis (Chap. 241). It may begin from 1 to 6 weeks after myocardial infarction. The pain often can be distinguished from that of an extending infarction by its characteristic pericardial pattern; it is substernal; it radiates to the neck and shoulders; it is relieved by leaning forward and exacerbated by deep breathing. The syndrome responds promptly to therapy with adrenal cortical steroids.

SHOULDER-HAND SYNDROME A few patients will develop pain and stiffness of the left arm and shoulder following myocardial infarction. The syndrome is probably related to immobility during the early period of therapy and is less frequent in patients who have been mobilized at an early stage in convalescence.

INTERMEDIATE SYNDROMES

The manifestations of ischemic heart disease may be thought of as representing a spectrum ranging from angina pectoris at one end to acute myocardial infarction at the other. In angina pectoris the myocardial blood supply is temporarily inadequate, but there is no death of tissue, as evidenced by the ECG changes of infarction or by elevation of the serum enzyme levels. Myocardial infarction is characterized by death of myocardial tissue associated with the typical changes in the ECG and in serum enzymes. Some patients develop manifestations which logically place them at an intermediate position between these two extremes; hence, the designation "intermediate syndromes." Included under this heading are syndromes known as acute coronary insufficiency, unstable angina, and crescendo angina. These syndromes sometimes represent the prodromal stages of myocardial infarction; hence, the terms preinfarction angina and preinfarction syndrome are sometimes applied. The intermediate syndromes may be superimposed upon a background of stable exertional angina pectoris, or one of the intermediate syndromes may represent the first manifestation of symptomatic ischemic heart disease.

Rest pain—acute coronary insufficiency

The term acute coronary insufficiency has been applied to the condition in which severe ischemic chest pain may come on at rest, but if it begins during exertion, does not disappear with rest. The pain lasts 30 min or more and is of sufficient severity to cause the diagnosis of myocardial infarction to be considered; the patient will often be admitted to a coronary care unit. He may have elevation or depression of the S-T segments of the electrocardiogram in association with the pain, and conduction disturbances may also be present. Myocardial infarction is ruled out by the absence of evolutionary Q-wave changes in the electrocardiogram and the absence of a diagnostic elevation in serum enzyme concentration. Arteriographic study of patients with this clinical presentation has shown that about one-third of the patients will have disease of the proximal portion of a single vessel and hence may be candidates for surgical therapy. A few patients, probably less than 5 percent with this syndrome, will be found to have normal coronary arteries.

In a series of 107 patients presenting with acute coronary insufficiency reported from the Massachusetts General Hospital, there was only one in-hospital death and six patients developed an acute myocardial infarction. The 1-year survival in this group was 86 percent. The results of surgery must be evaluated in the light of these figures for medical treatment.

Crescendo angina

The syndrome of crescendo angina pectoris is usually superimposed upon chronic stable angina pectoris. The patient notes that his pain is precipitated by less severe exertion, comes more frequently, lasts longer, or has changed in pattern. This syndrome may be associated with bouts of rest pain or acute coronary insufficiency.

MANAGEMENT The objective of management of all the intermediate syndromes is to prevent myocardial infarction and death. It is likely that the pathophysiology of all these syndromes is the same and represents a sudden alteration in the balance between myocardial blood supply and demand. The decrease in supply may be due to an occlusion or possibly to spasm of a vessel. The collateral circulation is barely adequate to maintain viability during the critical period. If the collateral circulation is able to increase to meet the new demands, infarction will not occur; but if it fails, tissue will die and myocardial infarction will result. Sometimes the issue may hang in the balance for several days. Reduction in myocardial oxygen demand is the keystone of medical management. Anxiety is reduced by the liberal use of sedatives and tranquilizing agents. Activity should be minimized by placing the patient at bed rest. The myocardial oxygen requirements can be further reduced by the administration of beta-adrenergic blocking agents. Nitroglycerin or long-acting nitrites may be used to relieve pain and further reduce myocardial oxygen demands. Anticoagulation with intravenous heparin is advocated by many on the grounds that it prevents the formation of thrombus in narrowed vessels.

The role of arteriography and vein bypass surgery in this group of patients is poorly defined at the present time, but it appears clear that there is a group who will benefit by early study and operation. The risk of arteriographic study and operation is higher in this group of patients than in a group with stable angina. The mortality rate for operation varies from 5 to 20 percent and depends upon the severity of the arterial disease and the left ventricular dysfunction.

REFERENCES

BLOMQVIST CG: Use of exercise testing and functional evaluation of patients with arteriosclerotic heart disease. Circulation 44:1120, 1971

BONDURANT S: Research on acute myocardial infarction. Introduction. Circulation 40 (IV): 1, 1969

Current problems in acute myocardial infarction and sudden death. I & II. Prog Cardiovas Dis 13:309, 1971

HURST JW (ed): *The Heart*, Part VI, Sect. D, Coronary Artery Disease, 3d ed., New York: McGraw-Hill, 1974

JULIAN DG, OLIVER MF: *Acute Myocardial Infarction*, Proceedings of a Symposium sponsored by the University of Edinburgh, Edinburgh: E&S Livingstone, 1968

STAMLER J et al: Primary prevention of atherosclerotic diseases. Circulation 42 (A): 55, 1970

Symposium. Angina pectoris. A series of articles dealing with all aspects of diagnosis, laboratory evaluation, and management of angina pectoris. Circulation 46: 1035, 1972; republished as AHA Monograph no. 37, American Heart Association, Inc., New York, 1972

Symposium. Myocardial infarction. A series of articles dealing with all aspects of myocardial infarction. Circulation 45:1972; republished as AHA Monograph no. 36, American Heart Association, Inc., New York, 1972

241
PERICARDIAL DISEASE

EUGENE BRAUNWALD

NORMAL FUNCTIONS OF THE PERICARDIUM The visceral pericardium is a serous membrane, separated by a small amount of fluid from a fibrous sac, the parietal pericardium. The pericardium prevents sudden dilatation of the cardiac chambers during exercise and hypervolemia, and facilitates atrial filling during ventricular systole, as the result of the development of a negative intrapericardial pressure during ejection. It holds the heart in a fixed anatomic position, minimizes friction between the heart and surrounding structures, prevents displacement of the heart and kinking of the great vessels, and probably retards the spread of infections from the lungs and pleural cavities to the heart. However, its total absence does not produce obvious clinical disease. In partial left pericardial defects the main pulmonary artery and left atrium bulge through the defect; rarely their herniation may cause sudden death.

It is useful to classify the types of pericarditis both clinically and etiologically (Table 241-1), as it is by far the most common pathologic process involving the pericardium.

ACUTE PERICARDITIS

Pain, a pericardial friction rub, electrocardiographic changes, and pericardial effusion with cardiac tamponade and paradoxic pulse are cardinal manifestations of many forms of acute pericarditis and will be considered prior to a discussion of the most common varieties.

Pain is an important symptom in various forms of acute pericarditis; it is usually present in the acute infectious types and in many of the forms presumed to be related to hypersensitivity or autoimmunity. Pain is often absent in a slowly developing tuberculous, postirradiation, or neoplastic pericarditis. The pain of pericarditis is often severe; its character and location have been described in Chap. 7. It is *usually* pleuritic, but occasionally the steady, constrictive pain, radiating into either arm or both arms and resembling that of myocardial ischemia, may overshadow the pleuritic pain, or it may occur along the arm at the onset of the illness, with the result that confusion with myocardial infarction is not infrequent. This problem becomes even more perplexing when, with acute pericarditis, the serum transaminase level rises to about 80 units. Suffice it to say that a pain felt either in the precordium or in one or both of the shoulders or trapezius ridges, aggravated by coughing, swallowing, inspiration, or rotation of the trunk, and relieved by sitting up and leaning forward should alert one to the possibility of an acute pericarditis.

The *pericardial friction rub* is the most important physical sign; it may have up to three components per cardiac cycle, as described on p. 1082, and may sometimes be elicited only when firm pressure with the stethoscope is applied to the chest wall. It is heard most frequently during forced expiration, with the patient leaning forward or on his hands and knees. The rub is likely to be inconstant and transitory, and a loud to-and-fro leathery sound may disappear within a few hours, possibly to reappear the following day.

The *electrocardiogram* in acute pericarditis without massive effusion usually displays elevation of the S-T segments in two or three standard limb leads and V_2 to V_6, with reciprocal depressions only in aV_R and V_1 and without significant changes in QRS complexes, except occasionally for some diminution in voltage. Several days later, the S-T segments return to normal and the T waves then become inverted. In contrast, in acute myocardial infarction, reciprocal depression of S-T segments is usually more prominent; QRS changes occur, particularly the development of Q waves; and T-wave inversions usually occur before the S-T segments have become isoelectric.

TABLE 241-1
Classification of pericarditis

Clinical classification

- *I* Acute pericarditis (< 6 weeks)
  - *A* Fibrinous
  - *B* Effusive (or bloody)
- *II* Subacute pericarditis (6 weeks to 6 months)
  - *A* Constrictive
  - *B* Effusive-constrictive
- *III* Chronic pericarditis (> 6 months)
  - *A* Constrictive
  - *B* Effusive
  - *C* Adhesive (nonconstrictive)

Etiologic classification

- *I* Infectious pericarditis
  - *A* Viral
  - *B* Pyogenic
  - *C* Tuberculous
  - *D* Mycotic
  - *E* Other infections (syphilitic, parasitic)
- *II* Noninfectious pericarditis
  - *A* Acute myocardial infarction
  - *B* Uremia
  - *C* Neoplasia
    - *1* Primary tumors (benign or malignant)
    - *2* Tumors metastatic to pericardium
  - *D* Myxedema
  - *E* Cholesterol
  - *F* Chylopericardium
  - *G* Trauma
    - *1* Penetrating chest wall
    - *2* Nonpenetrating
  - *H* Aortic aneurysm (with leakage into pericardial sac)
  - *I* Post-x-irradiation
  - *J* Associated with atrial septal defect
  - *K* Associated with severe chronic anemia
  - *L* Infectious mononucleosis
  - *M* Familial Mediterranean fever
  - *N* Acute idiopathic
- *III* Pericarditis presumably related to hypersensitivity or autoimmunity
  - *A* Rheumatic fever
  - *B* Collagen vascular disease
    - *1* Disseminated lupus erythematosus
    - *2* Rheumatoid arthritis
    - *3* Scleroderma
  - *C* Drug-induced
    - *1* Procainamide
    - *2* Hydralazine
    - *3* Other
  - *D* Postcardiac injury
    - *1* Postmyocardial infarction (Dressler's syndrome)
    - *2* Postpericardiotomy

PERICARDIAL EFFUSION Usually associated with an enlargement of the cardiac silhouette, pericardial effusion is especially important when it develops within a relatively short time. There is no definitive contour to the cardiac shadow in effusion, and differentiation from enlargement of the heart may be difficult on physical examination or plain roentgenography. The heart sounds tend to become faint; the friction rub may disappear or remain clearly audible, and the apex impulse may vanish, but sometimes it is felt well within the left border of cardiac dullness. On fluoroscopic examination, the ventricular pulsations may be diminished. When the effusion is large, one often encounters an area of dullness and tubular breath sounds at the angle of the left scapula, probably caused by compression of the lung (Ewart's sign).

A number of laboratory techniques are available for establishing the diagnosis of pericardial effusion. Echocardiography (Chap. 230) has emerged as the most effective, since it is simple, innocuous, and noninvasive and may be performed at the bedside. The presence of pericardial fluid is recorded as a relatively echo-free space between the posterior left ventricular epicardium and the posterior pericardium, and the anterior right ventricle and the parietal pericardium just beneath the anterior chest wall (Fig. 241-1). The diagnosis of pericardial fluid or thickening may be confirmed by: (1) *Cardiac catheterization*: a catheter is introduced into the right atrium and rotated so that its tip makes contact with the lateral right atrial wall. In the presence of an effusion, or pericardial thickening, the tip of the catheter is seen to be separated from the radiolucent lungs by an opaque band. (2) *Angiocardiography*: contrast medium is injected rapidly into the right atrium, and the lateral wall is outlined. (3) *Carbon dioxide angiography*: the intravenous injection of carbon dioxide, with the patient in the left lateral position, also provides contrast between the interior of the right atrium and surrounding structures that makes possible an estimation of the width of the pericardium or the contents of the pericardial sac.

When examination of pericardial fluid is deemed essential, exploration of the pericardium may be required. This should be accomplished with a needle attached to a properly grounded electrocardiographic lead, and intrapericardial pressure should be measured, utilizing the same apparatus employed for measuring cerebrospinal fluid pressure during lumbar puncture. When an effusion develops, the fluid nearly always has the physical characteristics of an exudate. Bloody fluid is commonly due to tuberculosis or tumor, but it may also be found in the effusion of rheumatic fever or in the post-cardiac-injury syndrome (see below). Occasionally, bloody fluid may be found in the effusion of uremic pericarditis and in the hemopericardium following infarction, especially following the administration of anticoagulants.

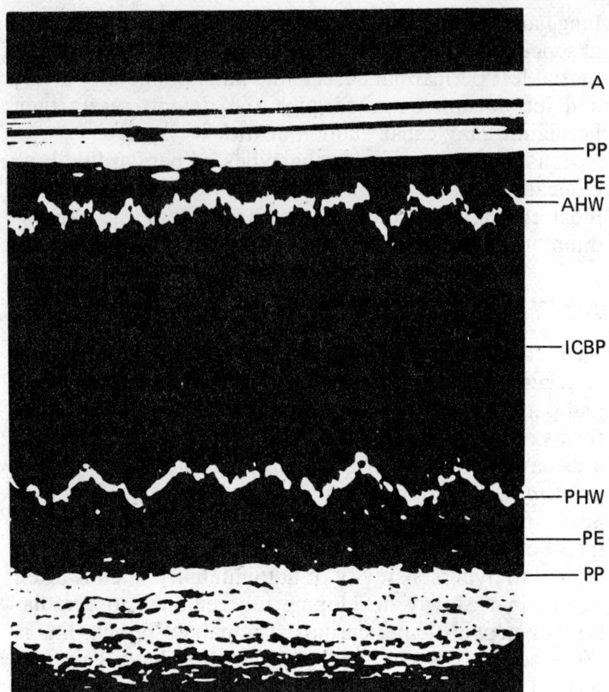

FIGURE 241-1
Echocardiogram in patient with pericardial effusion. A, anterior chest wall. PE, pericardial effusion, i.e., space separating (1) parietal pericardium (PP) and anterior heart wall (AHW); and (2) posterior heart wall (PHW) and parietal pericardium (PP). ICBP, intracardiac blood pool.

CARDIAC TAMPONADE The accumulation of fluid in the pericardium in an amount sufficient to cause serious obstruction to the inflow of blood to the ventricles results in cardiac tamponade. The amount of fluid necessary to produce this critical state may be as small as 250 ml, when the fluid develops rapidly; or it may be over 1,000 ml in slowly developing effusions when the pericardium has had the opportunity to stretch and adapt to the increasing volume of fluid. Tamponade results most often from bleeding into the pericardial space following cardiac operations, trauma (including cardiac perforation during diagnostic procedures), tuberculosis, pyogenic infection, or tumor, but it may occur in acute viral or idiopathic pericarditis, the post-cardiac-injury syndrome, and with hemopericardium associated with anticoagulant therapy of any form of acute pericarditis. The clinical manifestations are due to the fall in cardiac output and to systemic venous congestion. However, the classic findings of arterial hypotension and of a small quiet heart with faint heart sounds usually are seen only with very rapidly developing, severe tamponade, such as occurs with cardiac trauma. More frequently, tamponade develops slowly and the clinical manifestations, resembling those of heart failure, include dyspnea, orthopnea, tachycardia, hepatic engorgement, and a positive hepatojugular reflux. A high index of suspicion is required, since, in many instances, no obvious cause for pericardial disease is apparent. A widening of the area of flatness to percussion across the anterior aspect of the chest wall, a paradoxic pulse (see below), clear lung fields, diminished pulsations of the cardiac silhouette on fluoroscopy, and alteration in the amplitude of the electrocardiographic complexes, i.e., *electrical alternans*, should raise the suspicion of cardiac tamponade. Since immediate treatment may be lifesaving, prompt measures to establish the diagnosis (echocardiography, followed by cardiac catheterization and angiocardiography or CO_2 angiography) should be undertaken.

PARADOXIC PULSE This important clue to the presence of cardiac tamponade consists of *a greater than normal (10 mm Hg) inspiratory decrease in systolic arterial pressure.* When severe, it may be detected by palpating weakness or disappearance of the arterial pulse during inspiration, but usually sphygmomanometric measurement of systolic pressure during slow respiration is required (Fig. 241-2).

The mechanism of paradoxic pulse in cardiac tamponade is complex. Normally, the inspiratory decline in intrathoracic pressure enhances right ventricular filling by virtue of the increased gradient of pressure between the extrathoracic veins and the chambers of the right side of the heart. Right ventricular output increases, but because of the time required for the transmission of this augmented output through the pulmonary vascular bed and left atrium, left ventricular output does not rise until the following expiration. Thus, normally there is a slight inspiratory diminution in systemic arterial pressure. This effect is enhanced by the reduction of cardiac output which occurs in cardiac tamponade, since the respiratory variation then involves a larger fraction of the total output. Also, respiratory distress increases the fluctuations in intrathoracic pressure, which, in addition to exaggerating the mechanism just described, are also transmitted directly to the intrathoracic aorta and hence to the peripheral arterial bed. In addition, the inspiratory increase in venous return distends the right atrium and right ventricle; since these chambers share a tight incompressible covering with the left side of the heart, the volume of the latter declines reciprocally and the fall of left ventricular stroke volume is greater than normal.

Paradoxic pulse is less common in constrictive pericarditis than in tamponade. Furthermore, it is important to bear in mind that paradoxic pulse is not pathognomonic of pericardial disease because it may be observed in various forms of restrictive cardiomyopathies (Chap. 242) and, indeed, in some cases of severe myocardial failure, hemorrhagic shock, chronic obstructive airway disease, and severe bronchial asthma.

TREATMENT All patients with acute pericarditis should be observed frequently and carefully for the possibility of a developing effusion or, if effusion is already present, for signs of tamponade. In the presence of an effusion, arterial and venous pressures and heart rate should be monitored and serial chest roentgenograms obtained. If manifestations of tamponade appear, pericardiocentesis must be carried out at once, since relief of the intrapericardial pressure is often lifesaving.

Viral or idiopathic form of acute pericarditis

This disorder is an important clinical entity because of its frequency and because it may be confused with other more serious illnesses. In some cases a Coxsackie A or B virus or the virus of influenza, echo type 8, mumps herpes simplex, chickenpox, or adenovirus has been isolated from pericardial fluid and/or appropriate elevations in viral antibody titers have been noted; in other instances, acute pericarditis has occurred in association with illnesses of known viral origin and, presumably, was caused by the same agent. In others there is an antecedent infection of the respiratory tract, but in many patients such an association is not evident and viral isolation and serologic studies are negative. Frequently, a viral causation cannot be established nor can it be excluded; the term *acute idiopathic pericarditis* is then appropriate. However, regardless of the specific causative factor, the clinical manifestations are similar. This form of acute pericarditis occurs at all ages but is more frequent in young adults; it is often associated with pleural effusions and pneumonitis. The appearance of fever and precordial pain at about the same time constitutes an important feature in the differentiation of acute pericarditis from myocardial infarction, in which pain precedes fever. The

FIGURE 241-2

Simultaneous recording of electrocardiogram (ECG), blood flow velocity in the superior vena cava (SVC), brachial arterial pressure (BA), and the pneumogram (Pneumo) in a patient with cardiac compression and pulsus paradoxus. A downward deflection of the pneumogram denotes significant inspiration, when SVC blood velocity rises and arterial pressure falls (pulsus paradoxus). Arterial pressure is maintained during prolonged expiratory pause.

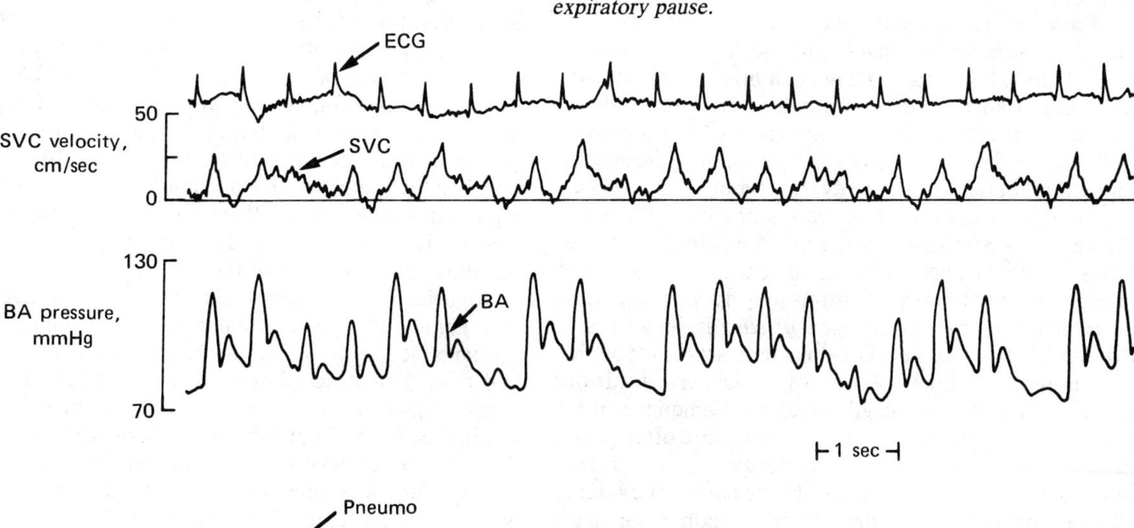

constitutional symptoms are usually mild to moderate, but occasionally the initial symptoms are stormy, the temperature rising to 104 to 105°F. The disease ordinarily runs its course in a few days to 2 weeks, but occasionally after the patient has apparently recovered he may have one or several recurrences, weeks or even months later. Tamponade is unusual, although accumulation of some pericardial fluid is common and constrictive pericarditis develops rarely. A pericardial friction rub is often audible. The ST-T wave alterations in the electrocardiogram are usually transitory, but the abnormal T waves may persist for several years or indefinitely, constituting a subsequent source of confusion in persons without a clear history of pericarditis. Pleuritis and pneumonitis frequently accompany pericarditis. There is no specific therapy, but corticosteroids effectively suppress the clinical manifestations of the acute illness and may be useful in patients who do not respond to supportive nonspecific therapy after the purulent and tuberculous forms of pericarditis have been excluded. Recurrences occur in about one-fourth the patients, and when they are repeated, pericardiectomy may be effective in terminating the illness.

DIFFERENTIAL DIAGNOSIS Differential diagnosis of *acute fibrinous pericarditis* is primarily one of exclusion, as there is no specific test for acute idiopathic pericarditis. Consequently all other disorders that may be associated with acute fibrinous pericarditis must be considered. When associated with *acute myocardial infarction*, acute fibrinous pericarditis may be confused with acute viral or idiopathic pericarditis, and this complication of infarction, described on page 1209, must be differentiated by the time of occurrence of fever and pain and by electrocardiographic abnormalities (such as the appearance of Q waves and earlier T-wave changes in myocardial infarction), the extent of the elevations of myocardial enzymes, and the total clinical picture. More common is the error of assuming that acute viral or idiopathic pericarditis represents acute myocardial infarction.

Acute pericarditis may follow injury to the myocardium. This is the *post-cardiac-injury* syndrome discussed in detail below. Pericarditis from such injury is most likely to be confused with acute idiopathic pericarditis when it follows myocardial infarction or a nonpenetrating bruise to the chest. Such pericarditis is differentiated from acute idiopathic pericarditis chiefly by timing. If it occurs within a few weeks of an infarction or a chest blow, it is justifiable to conclude that the two are probably related. If the infarct has been silent or the chest blow forgotten, the relationship to the pericarditis may not be recognized.

Pericarditis due to collagen disease is important to distinguish from acute idiopathic pericarditis. Most important in the differential diagnosis is the pericarditis due to disseminated lupus erythematosus. Sometimes it appears as an asymptomatic effusion, but more often pain is present, and rarely tamponade develops. Very rarely, when pericarditis occurs in the absence of other evidence of the underlying disorder, differentiation from acute viral and idiopathic pericarditis or tuberculous pericarditis may be made on discovery of LE (lupus erythematosus) cells, a rise in antinuclear antibodies, or by the specific methods for diagnosing tuberculosis. Acute pericarditis is also an occasional complication of *rheumatoid arthritis*, *scleroderma*, and *periarteritis nodosa*, but against other evidence of these diseases is usually obvious. It is important to question every patient with acute pericarditis about the ingestion of *procainamide* and *hydralazine*, both of which can cause this syndrome.

The pericarditis of *acute rheumatic fever* is generally associated with evidence of severe pancarditis and with cardiac murmurs. *Pyogenic pericarditis*, usually secondary to pneumococcal pneumonia and pleuritis or staphylococcal septicemia, is now far less common than before the advent of effective antibiotics. *Uremic pericarditis* is a common finding in patients with uremia. It may be fibrinous or associated with a serous or bloody effusion. A friction rub is common; pain and tamponade are unusual. Pericarditis due to *neoplastic diseases* results from the extension of primary or metastatic tumors (most commonly carcinoma of the lung and breast, malignant melanoma, and lymphomas) to the pericardium or from invasion by a lymphomatous or leukemic process; pain, atrial arrhythmias, and tamponade are complications which occur occasionally. Unusual causes of acute pericarditis include syphilis, fungous infection (actinomycosis, histoplasmosis, coccidioidomycosis), and parasitic infestation (amebiasis, toxoplasmosis, echinococcosis, trichinosis).

Post-cardiac-injury syndrome

During the past few years, it has been recognized that a number of disorders, identical in their clinical manifestations, may appear under a variety of circumstances. They have one common feature: previous injury to the myocardium, with blood in the pericardial cavity. The syndrome has been observed when the injury has been induced in the course of a cardiac operation (postpericardiotomy syndrome or, as it was originally designated, postcommissurotomy syndrome). It may also follow myocardial infarction (Dressler's syndrome) or develop after trauma of the heart (e.g., stab wound, contusions following a nonpenetrating blow to the chest and following perforation of the heart with a pacemaker catheter).

The principal symptom is pain, which usually develops after an interval of 2 to 4 weeks following the cardiac injury but sometimes appears only after a lapse of months. Recurrences are common and may occur up to 2 years or more after the injury. Fever up to 102 to 104°F, pericarditis, pleuritis, and pneumonitis are the outstanding features, the bout of illness usually subsiding in 1 or 2 weeks. The pericarditis, which appears to be the most constant lesion, may be of the fibrinous variety, or it may be a pericardial effusion, which is often serosanguineous and sometimes causes tamponade. Concomitantly, arthralgias, leukocytosis, an increased sedimentation rate, and typical electrocardiographic changes may occur.

The mechanism whereby the clinical manifestations are induced is not certain, but there is a likelihood that they are the result of a hypersensitivity reaction in which the antigen originates from injured myocardial tissue and/or pericardium; the suggested designation *post-cardiac-injury syndrome* for this group of disorders implies that they may have a common pathogenetic mechanism. Circulating autoantibodies to myocardium occur frequently, but their precise role in this syndrome has not been defined.

The clinical picture mimics in practically every detail acute viral or acute idiopathic pericarditis. Moreover, it is possible that the recurrences that occur so frequently in the latter condition are not always caused by an exacerbation of the original (presumably viral) infection, but that the original injury may have initiated the sequence of events that culminates in the post-cardiac-injury syndrome.

TREATMENT Often no treatment is necessary aside from analgesics for pain. The management of pericardial effusion and tamponade has already been discussed. When the illness is severe and is followed by a series of disabling recurrences, therapy with corticosteroids is usually effective.

Tuberculous pericardial effusion

Tuberculous involvement of the pericardium may present as an acute fibrinous pericarditis, but more frequently it presents as a chronic pericardial effusion. With the acute form the history of precordial pain is inconstant and there may be no other evidence of tuberculosis (Chap. 156). The symptoms are those of a chronic, systemic illness in an individual with effusion. It is important to bear this condition in mind when a middle-aged or elderly person with fever has an apparent enlargement of the heart of undetermined origin, with or without congestive failure. Weight loss, fever, and fatigability are sometimes observed. Inasmuch as effective specific methods of therapy have now reduced strikingly the mortality rate from the previous figures of about 70 percent, overlooking a tuberculous pericardial effusion is a serious error. Consequently, no method of examination should be omitted to establish this diagnosis. Included are chest roentgenograms for pulmonary tuberculosis and a search for tuberculosis in other organs; tuberculin skin tests, repeated after several weeks; cultures and smears of gastric washings and of pleural and pericardial fluid. Finally, if the diagnosis is still obscure, a pericardial biopsy, preferably by a limited thoracotomy, should be performed after 1 or 2 weeks of preliminary antituberculous chemotherapy. If definitive evidence is then still lacking, but the specimen shows caseation necrosis, continuous antituberculous chemotherapy for at least 24 months is justified (Chap. 156). Pericardiectomy should be carried out in order to prevent the development of constriction if the biopsy specimen shows a thickened pericardium.

DIFFERENTIAL DIAGNOSIS OF CHRONIC PERICARDIAL EFFUSION *Tuberculosis* is the most common cause of chronic pericardial effusion.

Myxedema may be responsible for a pericardial effusion that is sometimes massive. The other manifestations of myxedema should clarify the diagnosis, but unfortunately, even when they are present the diagnosis is frequently overlooked. It is important, therefore, to carry out appropriate tests for thyroid function (Chap. 85) in patients with an enlarged cardiac outline of undetermined origin.

Neoplasms, disseminated lupus erythematosus, rheumatoid arthritis, mycotic infection, radiation therapy, pyogenic infections, severe chronic anemia, chylopericardium, and cholesterol deposits may also cause chronic pericardial effusion.

Aspiration and analysis of the pericardial fluid may often be helpful in diagnosis. In infections the organism can be identified by smear or on culture. Grossly sanguineous pericardial fluid results most commonly from a neoplasm, tuberculosis, or slow leakage from an aortic aneurysm.

CHRONIC CONSTRICTIVE PERICARDITIS

This disorder results when the healing of an acute fibrinous or serofibrinous pericarditis is followed by obliteration of the pericardial cavity, with the formation of granulation tissue which gradually contracts and forms a firm scar, encasing the heart and interfering with filling. In some reports, a high percentage of all cases has been of tuberculous origin. In other series, tuberculosis has been an infrequent cause. The condition also may follow pyogenic infection, trauma, radiation, histoplasmosis, neoplastic disease, and acute viral or idiopathic pericarditis, rheumatoid arthritis, lupus erythematosus, and chronic renal failure with uremia treated by means of chronic dialysis. In many patients the cause of the pericardial disease is undetermined. Rarely, routine fluoroscopic or radiographic examination may reveal calcification of the pericardium in a person who is free of all symptoms referable to the heart.

The basic physiologic abnormality in symptomatic patients with chronic constrictive pericarditis, as in those with cardiac tamponade, is the inability of the ventricles to fill adequately during diastole because of the limitations imposed by the rigid, thickened pericardium or the tense pericardial fluid. Stroke volume is diminished, and the end-diastolic pressures in both ventricles, as well as the mean pressures in the atria, pulmonic veins, and systemic veins, are elevated to about the same levels. In constrictive pericarditis the central venous and right and left atrial pressure pulses display an M-shaped contour, with sharp A and V waves and X and Y descents; the Y descent is the most prominent deflection and is interrupted by a rapid rise in pressure during early diastole, when ventricular filling is impeded by the constricting pericardium. In cardiac tamponade the pressure contour differs in that the most prominent deflection is the X trough, while the Y descent is usually absent. These characteristic changes are transmitted to the jugular veins, where they may be recorded or recognized by simple inspection. In constrictive pericarditis, but not in cardiac tamponade, both ventricular pressure pulses exhibit characteristic "square root" signs during diastole. These hemodynamic changes, although characteristic, are not pathognomonic of constrictive pericarditis but are also observed in cardiomyopathies characterized by restriction of ventricular filling, as discussed on p. 1220.

CLINICAL FINDINGS IN PERICARDIAL CONSTRICTION Contrary to a widely held impression, dyspnea, though absent or minimal at rest, is present on exertion, and orthopnea is commonly present in chronic constrictive pericarditis, although it is not severe. Attacks of acute left ventricular failure (acute pulmonary edema) practically never occur. The cervical veins are distended and remain so even after intensive diuretic treatment, and in about one-third of the cases a paradoxic pulse may be observed; this may be associated with increased inspiratory venous distention (Kussmaul's sign). Congestive hepatomegaly is pronounced and may impair hepatic function; ascites is common and is more prominent than dependent edema. In about half the patients, the heart is normal in size; if it is enlarged, the enlargement is rarely extreme. The heart sounds may be distant, an early third heart sound, i.e., a pericardial knock, occurring 0.06 to 0.12 sec after aortic valve closure, is often conspicuous, and murmurs are usually absent. The apex beat is poorly defined, and cardiac pulsations under fluoroscopic examination are diminished. Because of the high sustained venous pressure, congestive splenomegaly may be sufficiently pronounced to make the spleen palpable. In the absence of evidence of bacterial endocarditis or tricuspid valve disease, splenomegaly in a patient with congestive heart failure should arouse suspicion of constrictive pericarditis. Protein-losing gastroenteropathy and the nephrotic syndrome sometimes complicate chronic constrictive pericarditis. The electrocardiogram frequently displays low voltage and flattening or inversion of the T waves in most leads; P mitrale is frequently found in patients with sinus rhythm; atrial fibrillation is present in about one-third of these patients.

Systemic and/or pulmonary venous congestion is initially the result of impaired filling of the ventricles caused by the restrictive action of the inelastic pericardium. However, the fibrotic process may extend into the myocardium, and venous congestion may then be due to the combined effects of the myocardial and pericardial lesions. The interference with filling reduces the work of the heart and perhaps this leads to myocardial atrophy. The latter probably accounts for the delayed beneficial effects of operative treatment.

Inasmuch as the usual physical signs of cardiac disease (murmurs, cardiac enlargement) may be inconspicuous or entirely lacking, hepatic enlargement and dysfunction associated with intractable ascites may lead to a mistaken diagnosis of cirrhosis of the liver. This error should be avoided if the neck veins are inspected carefully in all patients with ascites and hepatomegaly. *Given a clinical picture resembling that of cirrhosis, but with the added feature of distended neck veins, careful search for calcification of the pericardium by chest roentgenograms should be carried out and may disclose a curable or remediable form of heart disease.* Since calcification occurs in only about one-half these patients, surgical exploration of the pericardium is justifiable if the clinical picture and cardiac catheterization findings are suggestive enough. Conversely, sometimes a calcified pericardium, clearly visible on the roentgenogram, may cause no symptoms whatsoever and in the absence of clinical manifestations of constriction does not require treatment.

DIFFERENTIAL DIAGNOSIS Like cor pulmonale (Chap. 262), chronic constrictive pericarditis may be associated with severe systemic venous hypertension but with little or no pulmonary congestion; the heart may not appear to be enlarged; and a striking inspiratory fall in arterial pressure may be present. However, in contrast to constrictive pericarditis, in cor pulmonale there is also an inspiratory fall in venous pressure and advanced parenchymal pulmonary disease is evident. *Tricuspid stenosis* may also simulate the picture of chronic constrictive pericarditis; congestive hepatomegaly and ascites may be equally prominent, and the manifestations of left-sided heart failure may be inconspicuous. However, in tricuspid stenosis, the characteristic murmur, the frequent presence of mitral stenosis, the absence of a paradoxic pulse, as well as the absence, in the jugular venous pulse, of the steep, deep Y descent followed by a rapid ascent (manifested by the diastolic shock on palpation and its audible equivalent, the pericardial knock), should make the clinical differentiation possible.

It is of the greatest importance, though often difficult, to distinguish chronic constrictive pericarditis from various forms of heart disease which are characterized by a similar physiologic abnormality, i.e., restriction of ventricular filling, leading to a similar clinical picture. Described in Chap. 242, these include endomyocardial fibrosis, infiltrative cardiomyopathies such as amyloidosis, hemochromatosis, sarcoidosis, scleroderma, and, perhaps most important, *idiopathic myocardial hypertrophy*, in which the marked thickening of the ventricular wall is responsible for the diminished compliance. It has also been shown that diffuse and severe scarring of the endocardium and myocardium caused by *coronary sclerosis*, which, in some instances, has not been associated with the pain of myocardial ischemia, may mimic constrictive pericarditis.

The features favoring the diagnosis of one of the above forms of cardiomyopathy are a well-defined apex beat, conspicuous enlargement of the heart, and pronounced orthopnea with attacks of acute left ventricular failure, left ventricular preponderance, bundle branch block, or significant Q waves in the electrocardiogram. At catheterization, patients with chronic constrictive pericarditis usually are found to have left atrial or pulmonary arterial wedge pressure equaling right atrial pressure, the latter often exceeding 15 mm Hg following intensive medical treatment for heart failure; the pulmonary artery systolic pressure is often less than 50 mm Hg, and the right ventricular end-diastolic pressure often reaches one-third of the systolic pressure; the cardiac output is slightly depressed. In contrast, in patients with restrictive myocardial or endomyocardial disease, the left atrial exceed the right atrial pressures by at least 10 mm Hg, the mean right atrial pressure usually falls to below 15 mm Hg following treatment, the pulmonary artery systolic pressure often exceeds 50 mm Hg, and the right ventricular end-diastolic pressure is usually less than one-third the systolic pressure, while the cardiac output is markedly depressed.

The lesson to be learned is that when a patient has progressive, disabling, and unresponsive congestive failure, and if he displays any of the phenomena of constrictive heart disease, the most careful and detailed clinical and laboratory studies must be carried out in order to detect or exclude constrictive pericarditis. In many instances cardiac catheterization, selective angiocardiography, and coronary arteriography may be required. However, when even these examinations do not yield a definitive diagnosis, the only decisive method of determining whether or not constrictive pericarditis is responsible for the clinical manifestations of heart failure is by surgical exploration of the pericardium.

TREATMENT Surgery is the only definitive treatment of constrictive pericarditis, but diuretic drugs and sodium restriction are useful during preoperative preparation for pericardial resection. Digitalis may be beneficial in the prevention of heart failure when resection of the thickened pericardium permits an increased inflow into the ventricles and hence an enhanced burden on an atrophic myocardium. The benefits derived from cardiac decortication are often striking, and frequently the improvement, though slight at first, is progressive over a period of many months.

Many instances of constrictive pericarditis are of tuberculous origin. Antituberculous therapy during the phase of effusion may prevent the development of constriction, and such therapy should be carried out before and after operation, if a tuberculous origin is suspected or cannot be excluded in a patient with chronic constrictive pericarditis (Chap. 156).

Subacute effusive-constrictive pericarditis

This form of pericardial disease is characterized by tense effusion into a free pericardial space, as well as by constriction of the heart by the visceral pericardium, and thus it shares a number of features both with pericardial effusion producing cardiac compression and with pericardial constriction. It may be caused by tuberculosis, multiple attacks of acute idiopathic pericarditis, radiation, traumatic pericarditis, and uremia. The heart is generally enlarged, there are a paradoxic pulse and a prominent X descent in the atrial pressure pulse, and the atrial pressure remains elevated even after pericardiocentesis. In many patients the condition progresses to the chronic constrictive form of the disease. Surgical removal of both the visceral and parietal pericardium is usually effective.

OTHER DISORDERS OF THE PERICARDIUM

Pericardial cysts appear as rounded or lobulated deformities of the cardiac silhouette, most commonly at the right cardiophrenic angle. They do not cause symptoms, and their major clinical significance lies in the possibility of confusion with a tumor, ventricular aneurysm, or massive cardiomegaly. *Tumors* involving the pericardium are almost always secondary to malignant neoplasms of the mediastinum. Rarely, a tumor, such as a mesothelioma, may originate in the pericardium. The usual clinical picture is that of an insidiously developing, often bloody pericardial effusion.

REFERENCES

CORTES FM (ed): *The Pericardium and Its Disorders*, Springfield, Ill.: Thomas, 1971, 298 pp.

FOWLER NO: Pericardial disease, chap. 76 in *The Heart*, 3d ed., ed JW Hurst, New York: McGraw-Hill, 1974, pp. 1387–1405

HANCOCK EW: Subacute effusive-constrictive pericarditis. Circulation 43:183, 1971

SHABETAI R (ed): Symposium on pericardial disease. Am J Cardiol 26:445, 1970

SPODICK DH: Acoustic phenomena in pericardial disease. Am Heart J 81:114, 1971

WOOD P: Pericarditis, chap. 13 in *Disease of the Heart and Circulation*, 3d ed., Philadelphia: Lippincott, 1968, p. 762

242
THE CARDIOMYOPATHIES AND MYOCARDITIDES

GERALD GLICK
EUGENE BRAUNWALD

CARDIOMYOPATHY

Until recent years, virtually all cases of symptomatic heart disease in adults were classified as ischemic, hypertensive, valvular, or congenital heart disease. When unequivocal evidence for one of these diagnoses was not present in an older patient, the diagnosis of ischemic heart disease was often made, even though a history of a myocardial infarction or angina pectoris could not be elicited. With the development of newer diagnostic techniques, particularly coronary arteriography, it has become clear that ischemic heart disease is not a diagnosis of exclusion, but must meet rigorous and specific criteria (Chap. 240). With this realization, various cardiomyopathies, previously considered uncommon, have emerged as important causes of morbidity and mortality.

The term *cardiomyopathy* is used here to indicate a disease entity in which the presenting signs and symptoms result entirely or predominantly from dysfunction of the myocardium. However, myocardial lesions produced by ischemic heart disease, hypertensive cardiovascular disease, cor pulmonale, valvular heart disease, and congenital heart disease are excluded. The cardiomyopathies may be classified on a pathologic basis as resulting either from primary involvement of the myocardium or from secondary involvement as part of a generalized disease (Table 242-1). From a clinical point of view, however, it is more desirable to classify them on the basis of differences in their pathologic physiology and differences in clinical presentation (Table 242-2).

Congestive cardiomyopathy

The hearts are always dilated and sometimes are also hypertrophied. Mural thrombi are frequently present in the left ventricle, left atrium, and right atrium. On histologic examination the major changes seen are fibrosis and

TABLE 242-1
Pathologic classification of cardiomyopathies

I Primary myocardial involvement
- *A* Idiopathic
- *B* Familial
- *C* Alcoholic
- *D* Post-partum
- *E* Endocardial fibroelastosis
- *F* Endomyocardial fibrosis

II Secondary myocardial involvement
- *A* Amyloidosis
- *B* Hemochromatosis
- *C* Sarcoidosis
- *D* Scleroderma
- *E* Polyarteritis
- *F* Lupus erythematosus
- *G* Leukemia
- *H* Neuromuscular disease
  - *1* Muscular dystrophy
  - *2* Friedreich's ataxia
- *I* Glycogen storage disease (Pompe's disease)
- *J* Hurler's syndrome

myocardial degeneration and hypertrophy. Electron microscopy reveals disorganization, loss of contractile elements, and disorganization of the sarcoplasmic reticulum, both in idiopathic and alcoholic cardiomyopathies. Idiopathic cardiomyopathy most frequently occurs in middle-aged persons, who, when first seen, have the signs and symptoms of congestive heart failure. The failure is both left- and right-sided and is manifested by dyspnea on exertion, fatigue, orthopnea, paroxysmal noctural dyspnea, peripheral edema, and palpitations. In addition, pulmonary and systemic emboli are not uncommon.

PHYSICAL FINDINGS The pulse pressure is small and in the presence of heart failure, the arterial diastolic pressure and the jugular venous pressure may be elevated. Protodiastolic and presystolic gallop sounds (Chap. 228) are present, and the tricuspid and and mitral rings may be dilated, with consequent production of valvular regurgitation and the associated physical signs. However, diastolic murmurs and valvular calcification militate strongly against the diagnosis of cardiomyopathy and point toward a rheumatic origin. As the congestive failure improves with treatment, the abnormal physical findings may return to normal.

Roentgenologic examination commonly reveals the heart to be grossly and diffusely enlarged; pericardial and pleural effusions may be present, and the lung fields may show evidence of venous hypertension and interstitial congestion. The most common abnormalities present in the *electrocardiogram* are left atrial hypertrophy, premature ventricular contractions, nonspecific ST-T wave changes, sinus tachycardia, and atrial fibrillation. Paroxysmal ventricular tachycardia occurs not infrequently and without apparent cause. Left axis deviation is common, and incomplete or complete left bundle branch block or, rarely, right bundle branch block may be present. Frequently, low voltage is noted, but left ventricular hypertrophy may be present.

Hemodynamic study generally reveals a cardiac output which is moderately or severely reduced at rest and which does not increase normally with exertion. The end-diastolic pressures in both ventricles are usually elevated, and consequently the mean atrial pressures are also elevated to abnormally high levels. Angiocardiography characteristically reveals left ventricular dilatation, a reduced ejection fraction, a variably thickened left ventricular wall, and, in some instances, mitral regurgitation.

TREATMENT In its early phases, the congestive heart failure associated with idiopathic cardiomyopathy responds to the usual therapeutic regimen of digitalis, salt restriction, and diuretics, but as the disease enters its more advanced states it frequently becomes refractory to these standard therapeutic measures. Burch and associates believe that prolonged strict bed rest for up to one year or more is important for the optimal management of these patients, but the effectiveness of this form of therapy remains controversial and it is not feasible in most patients; one must usually rely, therefore, on the standard management for congestive heart failure (Chap. 233). Excessive activity, however, is certainly contraindicated. The associated arrhythmias may also be extremely resistant to the usual antiarrhythmic drugs. Anticoagulants are indicated in patients with a history of embolization, atrial fibrillation, or a markedly reduced cardiac output. The usefulness of corticosteroid therapy has not been established.

Until recently, this form of cardiomyopathy characterized by congestive heart failure, has usually been recognized only in its far-advanced stages; as a result, treatment has been difficult and the prognosis poor. As the diagnosis of this disease is established earlier, therapy may prove more effective and the prognosis may be improved.

FAMILIAL CARDIOMYOPATHY In some families a genetic predisposition to cardiomyopathy exists. Aside from the familial occurrence, this type of cardiomyopathy resembles the idiopathic, nonfamilial form just described. Several different types of genetic abnormalities may manifest themselves as familial cardiomyopathy; they appear to be inherited as autosomal dominant traits with incomplete penetrance and variable expressivity.

ALCOHOLIC CARDIOMYOPATHY Animal experiments, as well as studies in man, have demonstrated that ethanol depresses ventricular performance, reduces myocardial uptake of free fatty acids but enhances uptake of triglycerides, and causes myocardial cell injury. These experimental studies have their clinical expression in

TABLE 242-2
Clinical classification of cardiomyopathies

1 Congestive: Characterized by cardiac dilatation, congestive heart failure, arrhythmias, emboli, and murmurs of mitral and tricuspid regurgitation

2 Restrictive: Characterized by restriction to ventricular filling

3 Hypertrophic: With or without obstruction to ventricular outflow

those patients who repeatedly develop congestive heart failure after ingestion of large quantities of alcohol. Because successive insults to the myocardium may lead to increasing irreparable damage, these persons must be instructed to stop all alcoholic intake. Clinically, they resemble patients with idiopathic cardiomyopathy as described above, and should be treated similarly. When the myocardial damage has become widespread and severe, the prognosis is poor. Therefore, ingestion of alcohol must be interdicted as early as possible in the course of the disease. Although thiamine deficiency may be present in many of these patients. alcoholic cardiomyopathy is associated with a low cardiac output and systemic vasoconstriction, in contrast to beriberi heart disease (Chap. 78), in which elevated cardiac output and diminished peripheral vascular resistance occur.

POST-PARTUM CARDIOMYOPATHY When cardiac enlargement and congestive heart failure of unexplained causation develop for the first time in a patient during the first 4 months after delivery, the diagnosis of post-partum cardiomyopathy should be considered. This temporal relation to delivery may not represent a direct consequence of pregnancy itself but may be conditioned by such factors as poor nutrition, familial or hereditary abnormalities, autoimmune mechanisms, unsuspected myocarditis, or some unknown cause. Nevertheless, a clinical picture quite characteristic for this entity has emerged. The patient is usually multiparous, black, over the age of thirty, who has been undernourished, may have a history of hypertension, and may have had a pulmonary embolus. The symptoms and signs are similar to those in patients with idiopathic cardiomyopathy. The prognosis in these patients appears to be closely related to whether or not the heart size returns to normal after the first episode of post-partum congestive heart failure. If the heart returns to a normal size, subsequent pregnancies may sometimes be well tolerated; if the heart remains enlarged, however, further pregnancies frequently produce increasing myocardial damage, ultimately leading to refractory congestive heart failure and death. Therapy is the same as for patients with the idiopathic form of cardiomyopathy, although patients with the post-partum form apparently have an increased sensitivity to digitalis. Patients who recover should be encouraged to improve their nutritional state and to avoid further pregnancies, especially if residual cardiomegaly exists.

NEUROMUSCULAR DISEASE Cardiac involvement is common in many of the muscular dystrophies. In the *Duchenne type of progressive muscular dystrophy,* the myocardial involvement is most often detected electrocardiographically. The most characteristic abnormalities, which do not occur in other forms of muscular dystrophy, are an excessively tall R wave in lead V_1 and a ratio between the amplitude of the R wave and S wave in this lead which exceeds 1.0 but which is not caused by right ventricular hypertrophy. In the terminal stages of the disease, congestive heart failure, arrhythmias, and sudden death may occur. However, cardiomegaly and low cardiac output are not commonly seen. *Myotonic dystrophy* is also marked by electrocardiographic abnormalities, viz., atrioventricular and intraventricular conduction disturbances, left axis deviation, sinus bradycardia, atrial fibrillation, atrial flutter, and frequent ventricular premature contractions. Sudden death may occur, but congestive heart failure is relatively uncommon. The heart is usually of normal size. In *limb girdle dystrophy* cardiomyopathy manifested by congestive heart failure and arrhythmias may appear in middle life. In *fascioscapulohumeral dystrophy* cardiac involvement is absent or exceedingly rare.

The heart is usually involved in *Friedreich's ataxia.* Pathologically, cardiac dilatation, replacement of myocardial fibers with connective tissue, and extensive interstitial fibrosis are seen. The picture is that of a congestive type of cardiomyopathy associated with arrhythmias.

ENDOCARDIAL FIBROELASTOSIS This disease, also of unknown cause, is generally seen in infants and is a relatively common cause of congestive heart failure in this age group. It occurs far less frequently in adults, and is characterized by a thickened endocardium that shows proliferation of elastic tissue. The process generally affects the left ventricle most extensively but may also involve the mitral and aortic valves. Mitral regurgitation is often present, and it may be difficult to determine to what extent the clinical picture results primarily from the endocardial or the valvular lesion. Involvement of the right side of the heart is less common. When first seen, the patient generally has congestive heart failure and shows stigmata of both the congestive and restrictive forms of cardiomyopathy. The electrocardiogram usually shows evidence of left ventricular hypertrophy, and the chest roentgenogram reveals left ventricular and atrial enlargement. Therapy is directed at the congestive failure but is generally unsatisfactory.

ENDOMYOCARDIAL FIBROSIS This is a progressive form of heart disease, seen in the tropics, especially in Africa, occurring most commonly in children and young adults; it is characterized by fibrosis in the inflow tract and the apex of one or both of the ventricles. Fibrosis of the endocardium begins at the apex of either ventricle and extends toward the inflow tract to involve the tricuspid and mitral valves, and also toward the outflow portions of each ventricle. In addition, the disease process extends into the myocardium to produce muscle destruction, fibrosis, and occasionally calcification; tricuspid and/or mitral regurgitation are common.

The clinical picture depends upon which ventricle and atrioventricular valve show dominant involvement. The electrocardiogram generally shows low voltage, and roentgenologically the heart is usually enlarged, primarily as a consequence of atrial enlargement. The most prominent findings at cardiac catheterization are a decreased cardiac output, elevated central venous pressure, and the characteristics of restrictive cardiomyopathy, described below. Thus, endomyocardial fibrosis and endocardial fibroelastosis fall into the category of a cardiomyopathy that has features both of congestive and of restrictive disease.

Restrictive cardiomyopathy

As indicated above, a given disease entity may present certain features of the congestive and restrictive cardiomyopathies simultaneously or sequentially, e.g., as the heart in the congestive form becomes progressively more fibrotic and therefore less distensible, it acquires some of the characteristics of the restrictive form of cardiomyopathy. Infiltrative diseases, such as amyloidosis, may present initially as either congestive or restrictive cardiomyopathies. However, certain of the cardiomyopathies are dominated by the features of restriction to ventricular filling, and the pathologic physiology and clinical presentation are similar even though the causes may be diverse. Thus, patients with restrictive cardiomyopathy resulting from primary amyloidosis, hemochromatosis, sarcoidosis, and Loeffler's fibroplastic endocarditis have similar cardiac findings. As a result of persistently elevated venous pressure, they commonly have dependent edema, ascites, and an enlarged, tender liver. The jugular venous pressure is elevated and does not fall normally or may rise with inspiration (Kussmaul's sign). The heart is usually enlarged, the heart sounds are distant, and third and fourth sounds are common. Murmurs are not distinctive. The electrocardiogram shows low-voltage, nonspecific ST-T wave changes and various arrhythmias. The most important radiologic features are moderate cardiac enlargement and absence of pericardial calcification.

Cardiac catheterization shows a decreased cardiac output, elevation of right and left ventricular end-diastolic pressure, and a dip and plateau configuration of the diastolic portion of the ventricular pressure pulse. This form of cardiomyopathy may be completely indistinguishable from constrictive pericarditis (Chap. 241), both at the bedside and even with the benefit of cardiac catheterization. Certain clues to the differentiation, which are presented on page 1216, may be observed. However, thoracotomy and operative exploration may be necessary to make a definitive differentiation between a restrictive cardiomyopathy and chronic constrictive pericarditis. This distinction is of importance because the latter condition is potentially curable by operation.

DIFFERENTIAL DIAGNOSIS *Amyloidosis* may be diagnosed by biopsy of the rectal mucosa, tongue, gums, or liver. Amyloid deposits may involve the adventitia and media of the intramural coronary arteries, and in these patients angina pectoris and myocardial infarction may occur. *Hemochromatosis* should be suspected if cardiomyopathy occurs in the setting of diabetes mellitus, hepatic cirrhosis, and increased skin pigmentation. *Sarcoid* involvement of the heart is generally associated with other manifestations of generalized disease, such as uveitis, parocortitis, hilar lymphadenopathy, pulmonary infiltrates, and pulmonale (Chap. 223). Although the heart may be involved in *scleroderma,* the major symptoms result from esophageal, pulmonary, and cutaneous involvement. *Loeffler's disease,* or *fibroplastic endocarditis,* is associated with a marked eosinophilia and must be distinguished from cardiac involvement in *polyarteritis, trichinosis, and eosinophilic leukemia.*

Hypertrophic cardiomyopathy

IDIOPATHIC HYPERTROPHIC SUBAORTIC STENOSIS (IHSS) This disease has also been referred to as hypertrophic obstructive cardiomyopathy, muscular subaortic stenosis, and asymmetric ventricular hypertrophy. The various appellations all emphasize the characteristic abnormality, namely, marked hypertrophy of the left ventricle, most striking in the interventricular septum. Obstruction to outflow occurs when the hypertrophied septum abuts on the anterior mitral leaflet during systole (Chap. 230). In contrast to the obstruction to flow seen in patients with valvular aortic stenosis, in whom the size of the narrowed orifice is fixed, in IHSS the obstruction to outflow is dynamic and may change between examinations or even from beat to beat. The severity of obstruction is a function of the width of the outflow tract during systole, which in turn appears to be related to three major factors: (1) the left ventricular end-diastolic volume, (2) the myocardial contractile state, and (3) the pressure that distends the left ventricular outflow tract during systole. Muscular exercise, isoproterenol, and digitalis glycosides, all of which increase the force of myocardial contraction and decrease the size of the ventricle, intensify the obstruction. Similarly, when ventricular volume is decreased by the Valsalva maneuver, nitroglycerin, or tachycardia, the obstruction is once again increased. Conversely, elevation of arterial pressure by phenylephrine, increasing venous return by raising the legs, and expansion of the blood volume, all tend to increase the ventricular volume and to ameliorate the obstruction. Sometimes the hypertrophied septum bulges into the outflow tract of the right ventricle, thereby impeding the ejection of blood from this chamber as well. IHSS occurs in familial form in one-third the cases, whereas in the remainder it occurs sporadically. In some patients it is congenital, but more commonly it is acquired.

Physical findings The most common symptoms are dyspnea, angina, dizziness, syncope, and left ventricular failure. Physical examination usually reveals a prominent A wave in the jugular venous pulse, a double or triple apical impulse, a sharply rising peripheral pulse that is best appreciated in the carotid arteries, and a fourth heart sound. The second heart sound may be paradoxically split, and a third heart sound may be audible. A systolic ejection murmur is heard best along the left sternal border or at the apex, rather than at the aortic area or along the carotid arteries, as in patients with valvular aortic stenosis. Some degree of mitral regurgitation is present in the majority of patients, probably as a result of the displacement of the mitral valve by the grossly hypertrophied left ventricular myocardium. Indeed, IHSS must be distinguished both from isolated mitral regurgitation and from ventricular septal defect, conditions which it resembles superficially. The murmur, itself, probably results both from the obstruction to ventricular outflow and from the mitral regurgitation.

The electrocardiogram commonly shows left ventricular hypertrophy and widespread, abnormally deep, broad Q waves that suggest an old myocardial infarction but probably result from gross septal hypertrophy. Although chest roentgenograms reveal left ventricular hypertrophy, in contrast to valvular aortic stenosis, calcification of the aortic valve is not observed and poststenotic dilatation of the aorta is present only rarely. The indirectly recorded carotid arterial pressure pulse rises unusually rapidly and often displays a double peak during systole. Echocardiography reveals abnormal motion of the anterior leaflet of the mitral valve, with reopening of the valve in midsystole and juxtaposition of the septum and anterior leaflet at the onset of obstruction. Generally a pressure gradient is present between the body of the left ventricle and the area directly below the aortic valve. When a gradient is not present, it frequently can be induced by provocative maneuvers such as infusion of isoproterenol or the Valsalva maneuver. In some patients symptoms may be severe but obstruction to ventricular outflow may be minimal. In these patients the left ventricular end-diastolic pressure is generally elevated, and symptoms probably result from restriction to ventricular filling, a consequence of decreased ventricular compliance. Thus, IHSS may have features of a restrictive cardiomyopathy.

The natural history of IHSS is variable, with some patients improving, some deteriorating, and some remaining stable. Over a long period of time some of these patients lose their murmur as their condition deteriorates and the gradient decreases or disappears, quite likely because the failing heart becomes somewhat dilated and contracts less forcefully. Sudden death occurs in a small fraction of patients but does not seem related to the severity or type of previous symptoms or to the extent of obstruction. Cardiac glycosides or nitroglycerin are ordinarily not helpful, although once congestive failure has developed, digitalis should be tried cautiously. Beta-adrenergic receptor blocking agents reduce the frequency and severity of angina, but if symptoms remain intractable, surgical excision or incision of the hypertrophied portion of the outflow tract may be indicated. Frequently, as a result of operation both the obstruction to ventricular outflow and the mitral regurgitation are significantly improved.

Type II glycogen storage or *Pompe's disease* with cardiac involvement may also show features of obstruction to ventricular ejection. In addition, signs and symptoms of congestion and restriction may also be present.

MYOCARDITIS

Generally, myocarditis is the result of an infectious process, but it may also be present in hypersensitivity states such as acute rheumatic fever (Chap. 238) or be caused by radiation therapy, chemical poisons, or physical agents. The myocarditides may be divided into the acute and chronic forms. In the United States, clinically significant acute myocarditis is caused most commonly by viruses. Thus far, the Coxsackie A and B viral strains, the poliomyelitis, influenza, adeno, echo, rubeola, and rubella viruses have been the best-documented etiologic agents, but as viral studies become more widespread, other viruses probably will be implicated. Generally, when the heart is involved in these diseases, only transient ST-T wave abnormalities are noted and the myocardial involvement does not influence the course of the disease. However, sometimes myocarditis, which may develop either during or several weeks after the respiratory illness, may lead to acute heart failure which may be fatal, more frequently in infants than in adults, or to a variety of cardiac arrhythmias. Myocarditis is frequently associated with acute pericarditis, especially when it is caused by Coxsackie B viruses (Chap. 186).

Physical examination may show the first heart sound to be faint, a ventricular gallop (third heart) sound may be heard, and a soft apical systolic murmur is often present. A pericardial friction rub is usually heard in patients with associated pericarditis.

Measures to combat the congestive failure, such as use of digitalis, diuretics, and salt restriction, may be necessary. Patients with viral myocarditis are sometimes exceedingly sensitive to digitalis; therefore, this drug should be given cautiously and a short-acting preparation should be used. The arrhythmias are occasionally extremely difficult to manage and may be refractory to the usual treatment with drugs such as quinidine, procainamide, diphenylhydantoin, lidocaine, or propranolol. When propranolol is used, care must be taken not to precipitate congestive heart failure. Deaths attributed to heart failure and arrhythmias have been reported. Prolonged bed rest may be helpful, but its efficacy remains to be established. Animal studies suggest that steroids may aggravate the myocardial involvement.

Though viral myocarditis is most often self-limited and without sequelae, active disease may recur, and it is likely that acute viral myocarditis occasionally progresses to a chronic form. In addition, the possibility must be considered that many of the instances of idiopathic cardiomyopathy (page 1218) arise from mild or subclinical episodes of myocarditis. Patients often give the history of a preceding upper respiratory febrile illness, and viral nasopharyngitis or tonsillitis may be evident clinically. The isolation of virus from the stool, pharyngeal washings, or other body fluids and change in specific viral antibody titers are helpful clinically.

ISOLATED MYOCARDITIS Also called *Fiedler's myocarditis,* this is a rare condition in which only the myocardium is involved and the cardiac involvement cannot be related to a previous or concurrent illness. The etiology of this disease is unknown, but a viral causation has been postulated. When first seen by the physician, the patient generally has fulminating congestive heart failure; corticosteroids are occasionally effective, but in general, therapy is unsatisfactory and a fatal outcome follows a brief illness.

Diphtheritic myocarditis is caused by an exotoxin produced by *Corynebacterium diphtheriae* (Chap. 151). Patients may die in acute congestive heart failure or as a result of complete heart block. Widespread immunization against diphtheria has virtually eliminated this disease.

TOXOPLASMOSIS (see also Chap. 214) Toxoplasmosis is a relatively common cause of acute myocarditis in the newborn. The parasite *Toxoplasma gondii* can pass in utero from the mother to the fetus, so that toxoplasmosis may occur in the fetus or in the newborn. Toxoplasma myocarditis may occur in several members of a family. In adults it occurs most often as an opportunistic infection in patients treated with corticosteroids, cytotoxic chemotherapy, or immunosuppressive agents. Myocarditis may be isolated or occur as a feature of miliary toxoplasmosis. This condition should be considered in the differential diagnosis of obscure acute myocarditis or cardiomyopathy. Markedly elevated or rising levels of complement in a complement fixation test or of antibody in the antibody dye test are valuable diagnostic aids. Therapy consists of administration of pyrimethamine and triple sulfonamides, as described in Chap. 214.

CHAGAS' DISEASE (see also Chap. 213) Chagas' disease, caused by *Trypanosoma cruzi,* produces a form of myocarditis that occurs in well-defined acute and chronic forms. It is one of the most common causes of heart disease encountered in Central and South America. The heart is enlarged, the sounds are distant, and a protodiastolic gallop sound may be present. The electrocardiogram may show first degree atrioventricular dissociation and abnormal T waves. The acute myocarditis is usually self-limited, but some patients develop the chronic form which may occur in patients without a history of an acute episode. The chronic form is characterized by dilatation of the cardiac chambers, fibrosis and thinning of the ventricular wall, aneurysm formation in the areas of thinning, especially at the apex, and mural thrombi. At first, the electrocardiogram may show evidence of intraventricular block and frequent premature ventricular contractions. As the patient becomes symptomatic, signs and symptoms of congestive heart failure develop. Premature contractions become more frequent, and serious arrhythmias, such as ventricular tachycardia, may occur. The cause of death is either intractable congestive failure or an arrhythmia. Therapy is directed toward the treatment of the congestive heart failure and arrhythmias.

RADIATION MYOCARDITIS Patients who receive large doses of radiation therapy to the area of the heart (generally in excess of 4,000 rads), most frequently for carcinoma of the lung or breast, may develop acute pericarditis, chronic constrictive pericarditis, and chronic myocarditis.

REFERENCES

Buja LM et al: Clinically significant cardiac amyloidosis. Am J Cardiol, 26:394, 1970

Bulloch RT et al: Myocardial lesions in idiopathic and alcoholic cardiomyopathy. Am J Cardiol 29:15, 1972

Burch GW, Giles TD: The role of viruses in the production of heart disease. Am J Cardiol 29:231, 1972

Burch GE (ed): *Cardiovascular Clinics: Cardiomyopathy*, vol. 4, no. 1, Philadelphia: F.A. Davis, 1972

Demakis JG et al: Natural course of peripartum cardiomyopathy. Circulation 44:1053, 1971

Frank S, Braunwald E: Idiopathic hypertrophic subaortic stenosis: Clinical analysis of 126 patients with emphasis on the natural history. Circulation 37:759, 1968

Friedberg CK: Symposium on cardiomyopathy. Circulation 44:935, 1971

Goodwin JF: Congestive and hypertrophic cardiomyopathies. Lancet 1:731, 1970

Gozo EG Jr et al: Heart in sarcoidosis. Chest 60:379, 1971

Hamby RI: Primary myocardial disease. A prospective clinical and hemodynamic evaluation in 100 patients. Medicine 49:55, 1970

Hurst JW (ed): *The Heart*, 3d ed., Part VI, Section H. Diseases of the Myocardium (chaps. 71–75), New York: McGraw-Hill, 1974, pp. 1311–1386

Perloff JK: Cardiomyopathy associated with heredofamilial neuromyopathic diseases. Mod Conc Cardiovasc Dis 40:23, 1971

Puigbo JJ: Chagas' heart disease, clinical aspects. Cardiologia 52:91, 1968

Theologides A, Kennedy BJ: Toxoplasmic myocarditis and pericarditis. Am J Med 47:169, 1969

Wolstenholme GEW, O'Connor M (eds): *Hypertrophic Obstructive Cardiomyopathy,* Ciba Foundation Study Group No. 37, London: Churchill, 1971

243 CARDIAC TUMORS AND OTHER UNUSUAL FORMS OF HEART DISEASE

GERALD GLICK
EUGENE BRAUNWALD

TUMORS OF THE HEART

MYXOMA Cardiac myxomas, though rare causes of heart disease, are the commonest type of primary tumor of the heart seen in adults. Despite their rarity, myxomas are of clinical importance because they represent a potentially curable form of heart disease; therefore they always present a formidable diagnostic challenge to the clinician. Myxomas, which are histopathologically benign, occur most frequently in the atria, the left atrium being involved three times as often as the right. They are generally pedunculated, with the stem attached to the interatrial septum in the region of the foramen ovale, and they may be either firm and smooth or gelatinous and polypoid. When located in the ventricles, myxomas are generally sessile. The clinical manifestations produced by cardiac myxomas may be divided into three separate groups: (1) symptoms resulting from impediment to blood flow through the heart as a result of mechanical obstruction produced by the tumor itself; (2) symptoms resulting from emboli released from the tumor into the pulmonary or systemic arterial beds; and (3) generalized constitutional abnormalities.

When the myxoma is located in the left atrium, it characteristically mimics mitral stenosis because the pedunculated mass may fall into the mitral orifice, thereby obstructing blood flow into the left ventricle. Less commonly the clinical findings resemble those produced by combined mitral stenosis and regurgitation or pure mitral regurgitation. Presumably the tumor causes regurgitation by interfering with the function of the mitral valve apparatus. The left atrial pressure is elevated, and the increased pressure is transmitted through the pulmonary vascular bed, with consequent pulmonary congestion and pulmonary arterial hypertension. All the symptoms and some of the signs of mitral valve disease therefore may be produced (Chap. 239). In addition, episodes of syncope or sudden relief or exacerbation of symptoms with changes in posture may occur as the myxoma shifts its position in relation to the valve orifice. The pertinent physical findings include splitting of the first heart sound, accentuation of the pulmonic component of the second heart sound, an early diastolic sound attributed to the hitting of the myxoma against the ventricular wall (a tumor "plop"), and both apical pansystolic and middiastolic murmurs. The auscultatory findings may change with alterations in position. Systemic emboli, resulting from the breaking off of pieces of tumor tissue or from the formation of thrombi on the tumor, may involve any organ. In fact, when many organs are involved, attention may be diverted away from the heart. Intracardiac myxomas also produce constitutional symptoms such as weight loss, fever, weakness, anemia, hyperglobulinemia, and an elevated erythrocyte sedimentation rate. These findings may also direct attention away from the heart. Coupled with the finding of changing heart murmurs, they may suggest the diagnosis of subacute bacterial endocarditis.

When the myxoma is located in the right atrium, it may produce the signs and symptoms of tricuspid stenosis. Embolization from these tumors produces pulmonary hypertension as a result of widespread obstruction of the pulmonary vascular bed. Constitutional symptoms are similar to those occurring with left atrial myxomas. Ventricular myxomas are much less common and may obstruct ventricular outflow by involving the semilunar valves or subvalvular regions, as well as by producing emboli.

The diagnosis of intracardiac myxoma can be made by echocardiography and by selective angiocardiography. Surgical removal results in a complete cure, including relief of the constitutional symptoms. Accordingly echocardiography, and if the results are suspicious, angiocardiography should be carried out in patients with valvular heart disease and unusual features or in those with obscure cardiac problems.

Rhabdomyoma This is the most common form of primary cardiac tumor in young children. It is considered to be a hamartoma, i.e., it arises from normal embryonal elements found in the heart, and is therefore benign. It is frequently associated with tuberous sclerosis, a disease in which hamartomas of many organs occur. The left ventricle is the chamber most frequently involved, and multiple nodules are present in the interventricular septum and free wall.

Sarcomas These comprise the malignant primary cardiac tumors. They occur most commonly in the right atrium; as a result they may occlude inflow into the atrium from either vena cava, and produce an inferior or superior vena caval syndrome. Right ventricular outflow may also be obstructed. Metastases to the vertebral column and to parenchymal organs are common. The tumors are named for the dominant cellular element involved, the most common being *fibrosarcomas, rhabdomyosarcomas,* and *angiosarcomas.*

Secondary tumor involvement The heart may be involved in 25 percent of patients with Hodgkin's disease, 37 percent of patients with leukemia, and 60 percent of patients with malignant melanoma. In addition, metastases to the heart occur relatively often in individuals with bronchial carcinoma or carcinoma of the breast. More rarely, metastases may arise secondary to carcinoma of the pancreas, gastrointestinal tract, or kidney. The most common abnormalities produced by secondary involvement of the heart by tumor are the production of arrhythmias and bloody pericardial effusions. Atrial fibrillation is the commonest arrhythmia seen in these circumstances.

OTHER UNUSUAL FORMS OF HEART DISEASE

MALIGNANT CARCINOID In the usual form of carcinoid syndrome with gastrointestinal tumors and hepatic metastases (Chap. 99), the lesions in the heart are mainly on the right side and consist of tricuspid regurgitation and pulmonic stenosis. The clinical manifestations consist of dilated neck veins with prominent V waves, hepatomegaly, ascites, and edema. Predominantly left-sided lesions of mitral stenosis have been reported in patients with bronchial carcinoid tumors and in patients with right-to-left shunts through a patent foramen ovale. It is probable that an as yet unidentified substance released by the tumor is responsible for the development of the valvular lesions, and that this substance is removed or detoxified in the pulmonary circulation.

OBESITY In extremely obese patients, the heart may be markedly enlarged, the left ventricle showing the greatest hypertrophy. This form of heart disease must be distinguished from the Pickwickian syndrome (Chap. 255). The clinical course of obesity heart disease is marked by congestive heart failure, with both pulmonary and systemic venous congestion. Since obesity without cardiac involvement may be responsible for dyspnea and ankle edema, evidence of superimposed congestive failure may be difficult to recognize; measurement of venous pressure and circulation time may be helpful. Also, a therapeutic trial of digitalis, salt restriction, diuretics, and weight loss may be indicated.

MYXEDEMA (see also Chap. 85) The heart is often seemingly enlarged, and electrocardiographic abnormalities such as low voltage, prolonged P-R interval, and T-wave alterations are common. Arrhythmias such as paroxysmal atrial tachycardia and atrial fibrillation and high-grade atrioventricular dissociation may occur. Disappearance of the electrocardiographic abnormalities and arrhythmias is usual after restoration of the euthyroid state, and the marked decrease of the cardiac silhouette makes it likely that the apparent enlargement of the heart is caused by a pericardial effusion. A large amount of fluid, of high protein content, may accumulate in the pericardial space but rarely produces tamponade. On histologic examination myxedema hearts reveal a variety of nonspecific degenerative changes, and lack of thyroid hormone depresses intrinsic myocardial contractility. Nevertheless, early myxedema seldom, if ever, causes actual myocardial failure; when heart failure is present in patients with myxedema, it is likely that some other form of heart disease, such as ischemic heart disease, is associated with the myxedema or that myxedema is of long duration. Thyroid replacement therapy should be carried out with great caution, and the initial dose should be quite small because of the possibility of precipitating anginal attacks or cerebral dysfunction in patients whose arteries have been narrowed by atherosclerotic lesions and in whom, therefore, blood flow may be inadequate to meet the increased oxygen demands of the heart and brain produced by the hormone.

RHEUMATOID ARTHRITIS The heart may be involved in various ways in patients with rheumatoid arthritis. Granulomatous lesions resembling subcutaneous nodules in their histologic characteristics may affect all tissues of the heart. Other lesions that may occur include healed or active pericarditis, focal or diffuse myocarditis, valvular fibrosis, and healed or subacute arteritis. *Ankylosing spondylitis,* an entity probably distinct from rheumatoid arthritis, is associated in about 3 percent of cases with valvular regurgitation, most often of the aortic valve but occasionally of the mitral valve.

TRAUMATIC HEART DISEASE Cardiac damage may be due to both penetrating and nonpenetrating injuries. The most frequent cause of a nonpenetrating injury is impact of the chest against the steering wheel of an automobile. Serious injury of the heart may ensue even though no external sign of thoracic trauma is evident. Although the common type of injury is myocardial contusion, any structure of the heart may be affected by the trauma. If the valve cusps are ruptured, a loud heart murmur may appear, followed by the development of rapidly progressive heart failure. Hemopericardium with fatal tamponade may follow tear of the myocardium, of a pericardial vessel, or of a coronary artery. Myocardial contusion may cause arrhythmias, bundle branch block, or electrocardiographic abnormalities resembling those of infarction. Thus, it is important to bear trauma in mind as a cause of otherwise unexplained electrocardiographic changes. The most serious consequence of nonpenetrating injury is rupture either of the atria or of the ventricles, which is generally fatal; rarely, a patient with a ruptured ventricular or atrial septum may survive. Pericardial effusion may occur weeks or even months after the accident, as a late manifestation of a nonpenetrating injury of the chest wall. In these cases, the pericardial effusion is a manifestation of the post-cardiac-injury syndrome, which resembles the postpericardiotomy syndrome (Chap. 241).

Conservative medical treatment for acute myocardial failure resulting from rupture of a valve, most commonly the aortic, is rarely effective; operative correction is usually necessary. If the electrocardiographic abnormalities are those of myocardial infarction, it may be impossible to distinguish between myocardial contusion and infarction secondary to coronary artery injury; in either case, treatment is the same, namely, that indicated for myocardial infarction due to ischemic heart disease (Chap. 240). Tamponade has been managed successfully by repeated pericardiocentesis. Other authorities recommend open drainage when tamponade recurs rapidly or when bleeding takes place into the thoracic or abdominal cavities. When pericardial hemorrhage leads to constrictive pericarditis, decortication is necessary.

REFERENCES

ABRAMS HL et al: Radiology of tumors of the heart. Radiol Clin North Am 9:299, 1971

GOODWIN JF: Symposium on cardiac tumors. Am J Cardiol 21:307 1968

LEBOWITZ WB: Heart in rheumatoid arthritis. Ann Intern Med 58:102, 1963

SELZER A et al: Protean clinical manifestations of primary tumors of the heart. Am J Med 52:9, 1972

WENGER NK: Cardiac tumors, chap. 78 in *The Heart*, 3d ed., ed JW Hurst, New York: McGraw-Hill, 1974, pp. 1413–1425

section 2 | Disorders of the vascular system

244
ATHEROSCLEROSIS AND OTHER FORMS OF ARTERIOSCLEROSIS

DONALD S. FREDRICKSON

The major cause of death in the United States and most industrialized societies is arterial degeneration. The largest share of this is attributed to *arteriosclerosis*, which is a generic term for thickening and induration of the arterial wall. One type of arteriosclerosis is *atherosclerosis*, the disorder that underlies most *arteriosclerotic heart disease* or *coronary artery disease* (in this chapter referred to as *ischemic heart disease*) and also plays a major role in cerebrovascular disease. Atherosclerosis dwarfs all other single causes of death in the United States (Table 244-1). The major arterial diseases other than arteriosclerosis include *congenital structural defects*, *inflammatory* or granulomatous diseases (e.g., syphilitic aortitis), and *hypersensitivity* or autoimmune diseases. The last tend to affect the smaller vessels; they may include *thromboangiitis obliterans* and possibly the specific capillary lesions of *diabetic angiopathy*, but neither of these disorders has been proved to be an autoimmune disease.

THE NATURE OF ARTERIES

The walls of arteries are conventionally described as having three layers: intima, media, and adventitia.

Intimal layer All blood vessels, with the possible exception of sinusoids, are lined with a single, continuous layer of endothelial cells. The cells are generally oriented parallel to the longitudinal axis of the vessel. The plasma membranes of adjacent cells are closely apposed. There are spaces of as much as 180A in some areas; in others, there are tight junctions in which the outer leaflets of the two membranes are fused. The endothelial cells, at least in smaller vessels, have a clearly defined basement membrane, below which fine elastic fibrils extend to contact the smooth-muscle cells of the media. These fibrils usually appear as a continuous refractile strand, the *internal elastic lamina*. It is particularly prominent in the muscular arteries of medium caliber, and disappears in capillaries. The fibrils of *collagen* and *elastin* are elaborated by mesenchymal cells of fibrocytic or smooth-muscle type and exist in a surrounding amorphous, acid mucopolysaccharide–rich ground substance. The amount of collagen and ground substance generally increases with age.

Medial layer The media consists of smooth-muscle cells and elastic fibers arranged in concentric spirals. In *conducting* or *elastic* vessels like the aorta, the proximal portions of all vessels arising from its arch, and the major pulmonary arteries, elastic lamellas are very prominent. Such arteries expand and increase their elastic tension with the pulse of systole. In diastole, the elastic fibers contract. This propels the blood distally and progressively dampens the pulsatile character of flow toward more terminal vessels. In *distributing* or *muscular* arteries there is a preponderance of smooth-muscle cells and an *external elastic membrane* between the media and adventitia. The muscular arteries (arterioles) regulate peripheral flow by contraction (vasoconstriction) and relaxation (vasodilatation).

Adventitial layer The external coat of the arteries consists mainly of longitudinally directed bundles of collagen fibers. In addition, there are fibroblasts, some elastic fibers, nerve bundles, and small blood vessels (*vasa vasorum*).

An important feature of the anatomy of most arteries is the existence of a "nutritional watershed" located about midway in the media. The vasa vasorum normally do not penetrate beyond this point, and the layers of the arterial wall from there to the endothelium are nourished from the lumen.

METABOLISM AND ADAPTATION Arteries are conduits which must withstand for a lifetime the passage of a viscous and complex suspension under high pressure. Their shape and internal diameter not only vary along the length of the vessel, but are cyclically changing in the

TABLE 244-1
Deaths, by cause, in the United States, 1968

Causes of death	ICDA† Codes, 8th rev.	No. of deaths, thousands: All ages	Under age 65: M	Under age 65: F
All deaths		1,930	474	267
All cardiovascular diseases	390–458, 746,747	1,048	183	83
Ischemic heart disease	410–413	675	133	44
Cerebrovascular disease	430–438	211	21	18
Hypertensive disease*	400–404	27	4	3
Diseases of arteries and veins	440–458	75	9	5
Rheumatic heart disease	390–398	16	5	5
Congenital heart disease	746–747	8	4	3
Other heart disease	420–429	36	8	5

* *A substantial proportion of deaths of hypertensive persons occurs with ischemic heart disease or cerebrovascular disease; such deaths are classified in those categories.*

† *International Classification of Diseases, adapted.*

SOURCE: National Center for Health Statistics, Vital Statistics of the United States, 1968.

same region, especially where flow is pulsatile. The mechanical forces on the arterial wall are complex; tensile stresses imposed mainly by hydraulic force are considerable. Shear or frictional stresses are especially prominent near the orifice and entrance region of branches. The form and manner in which these forces are dissipated depend upon flow, the amount of elastic tension developed, and the tethering or external support provided by surrounding structures. Arteries are also permeable pipes, which constantly exchange fluid and solutes with the blood they carry. They must meet a steady demand for energy production to maintain smooth-muscle tension and to repair and replenish their tissue constituents.

The metabolism of arteries is less well characterized than that of many other tissues, and much of what is known has been deduced from histochemical studies rather than from more precise biochemical analyses. Multiple processes obviously occur, including glycolysis and respiration, the elaboration of proteins (including collagen and elastin, glycosaminoglycans, and other structural elements), as well as many catabolic pathways catalyzed by a variety of enzymes, including fibrinolysins and lysosomal hydrolases. No one biochemical reaction can be singled out as culpable in the production of arteriosclerosis. Because of the prominence of lipids in atheromas, much attention has been directed to lipid metabolism in arteries. They synthesize fatty acids, cholesterol, phospholipids, triglycerides, and other lipids, but it is apparent that many lipids are also taken up from the blood. Large molecules such as ferritin, peroxidase, and albumin pass across the endothelium, both by pinocytosis and by seepage across intercellular junctions. It is not clear which pathway predominates. It also remains to be determined whether the relatively gigantic plasma lipoproteins are taken up intact, as partially degraded remnants, or whether only their lipid moieties may normally enter.

The stresses and demands laid upon arteries change throughout life and sometimes within very short intervals. They have appreciable capacity for adaptation, but the variety of responses is limited. Distinctions between physiologic and pathologic morphologic changes must be assessed in quantitative rather than qualitative terms. An example is change in the amounts of fibrous, muscular, and elastic tissue in the intima and media and in the relative thickness of these layers. The coronary arteries offer an illustration. These are muscular arteries, representing a transition from the elastic aorta. At birth the media is thicker than the intima. During life both layers continue to increase in thickness, but the intima does so more rapidly and often exceeds the width of the media by the thirtieth year. This evolution occurs to about the same degree in men and women and in races which vary greatly in prevalence of arteriosclerosis. This thickening involves the development of smooth muscle and an increase in collagen and elastic tissue within the intima. These changes represent a normal response and enhance intimal resistance to lipid deposition and other signs of deterioration. When such fibromuscular hyperplasia becomes excessive, however, and manifests as discrete raised plaques, it becomes a feature of atherosclerosis. The intimal endothelial cells also are in a constant state of adaptation. Changes in the patterns of flow along the vessel wall alter the orientation of these cells and accelerate their already fairly rapid rate of turnover, processes which seem designed to maintain the integrity of the endothelial barrier.

In considering adaptation of the arterial wall, one cannot forget that the flux of oxygen and substrates and the reverse flow of catabolic products are directed both from the luminal and the adventitial sides of the vessel. Transfer processes across the endothelial wall must be maintained. The success or failure of the arterial wall to assure the nutrition of its inner half throughout a series of adaptive changes is a major determinant of whether arteriosclerosis develops or not.

REACTION TO INJURY The luminal surface of the endothelium is a delicate semipermeable barrier, and doubtless its integrity is maintained by a balance of electrical and chemical forces which can be altered by many kinds of injury. One example, well documented in gross but not molecular terms, is the injury produced by increased shear force or hydraulic pressure, which causes enhanced passage of proteins such as albumin and lipids or lipoproteins into the intima in the injured region. Early in this process vesicles appear within the endothelial cells, and extracellular lipid droplets also appear in the intima, and sometimes in the media. Cells within these layers are then stimulated to several kinds of differentiation. Some become macrophages and seem to phagocytose lipid. Others develop myofilaments and are transformed into smooth-muscle cells. Along with lipid deposition and cell multiplication, there is an increase in collagen, ground substance, and elastic fibrils. Some of these latter responses occur in much the same manner as in "physiologic adaptation," mentioned earlier. The reaction may become more complicated, however, and involve formation of intramural capillaries. If these should hemorrhage, or if necrosis develops, calcification and sclerosis may follow; the wall may become distorted, and the vessel lumen may be narrowed or obliterated. An altered endothelial surface is often attended by thrombus formation, which can compound a reaction that might otherwise have halted at an earlier stage. Some or all of these events can be precipitated by various stimuli such as radiation damage, a jet stream playing on the wall from the orifice of a deformed cardiac valve, or focal endothelial damage due to rheumatic or syphilitic processes. Conversely, abnormal reactions to physiologic stresses may be dictated by molecular defects in components of the arterial wall. A dramatic example is provided by the abnormal collagen elaborated in Marfan's syndrome; perhaps changes induced by diabetes mellitus may some day prove to be another example. There are also reactions to unphysiologic stresses which first occur in the media, as exemplified by massive increases in fibrous and elastic tissue induced in small arteries by severe hypertension. Such medial changes may then act as stimuli to reactive changes in the intima. The forms of arteriosclerosis now to be described all embody one or more of the above reactions to injury. Their classification fails to convey the diversity of the number of prolonged and synergistic insults, or the great variation in responsiveness of the arterial wall, that can determine the causation in a given patient.

FORMS OF ARTERIOSCLEROSIS

Atherosclerosis involves primarily the intimal layer, most commonly in the aorta, coronary, and cerebral arteries. It may accompany or accelerate the other major features of arteriosclerosis, which consist of (1) *involutional* or *senile* changes, (2) *focal calcification*, and (3) *arteriolosclerosis*. They involve primarily the medial layer and usually affect segments of the arterial tree other than those in which atherosclerosis is most prominent.

INVOLUTIONAL CHANGES Some of the age-related adaptive changes which arteries normally undergo are classified as arteriosclerosis only when they occur prematurely, or, perhaps, excessively. After the usual increase in intimal and media thickness has peaked at age twenty-five to thirty-five, rigidity of the vessels gradually increases, despite an increase in the number of elastic fibers. These are the major changes of senescence. Other involutional changes begin in midlife, especially in the abdominal aorta and its iliac, splenic, renal, hepatic, and superior mesenteric branches. The vessels become dilated, elongated, tortuous, and an aneurysm may form, especially if medial degeneration is accelerated by an encroaching intimal plaque. Such "wear-and-tear" lesions are frequently proportional to the vessel diameter and correlated with branching, curvature, and anatomic points of attachment. The amount of external support also determines the ability of vessels, weakened by loss of elasticity, to withstand hydrostatic pressure. The unsupported cerebral arteries may be particularly vulnerable in this regard, although most of the ruptures in the cerebral vessels occur in aneurysms in relatively small vessels. Though senescence is accompanied by the intimal thickening, medial calcification, and elastosis that are features of localized atheromatosis, all in all, there is a lack of direct correlation between many changes of senescence and arteriosclerosis.

FOCAL CALCIFICATION Not to be confused with atherosclerosis is focal calcification of the media of smaller arteries. This includes *Mönckeberg's arteriosclerosis*, common in the lower extremities and thyroidal arteries, and *Fahr's sclerosis*, i.e., calcification of the extramural branches of the cerebral arteries.

ARTERIOLOSCLEROSIS This disorder represents alterations in small arteries that are particularly common in hypertension. Lesser degrees of sustained hypertension characteristically cause *hyaline proliferation* in renal arterioles; more severe or malignant hypertension produces a typical *fibrous and elastic hyperplasia* of the media and intima.

ATHEROSCLEROSIS Although a scourge of modern civilizations, atherosclerosis is an ancient disease which has been detected in Egyptian mummies and described in Greek writings. The term *atheroma* (from the Greek *athere*, gruel) was revived by Albrecht von Haller of Bern (1755) to focus attention on the softening process which often accompanies the sclerosis and the aneurysms that had been emphasized earlier by Da Vinci and then by Vesalius and other anatomists of the sixteenth and seventeenth centuries. For a time in the nineteenth century, it was believed that imbibition of substances from the blood (Virchow) or other events at the endothelial blood interface might cause atheromas (Rokitansky); but by the time the term *atherosclerosis* was coined (Marchand, 1904), the dominant concept was that the lesions were intimal softenings secondary to an increase in subintimal connective tissue that in turn was due to irritative or mechanical forces. The present-day preoccupation with the etiologic importance of lipid infiltration began about 1910 with the demonstration of an increased amount of cholesterol in atheromas (Windhaus, Aschoff) and the experimental production of atherosclerosis by feeding cholesterol (Ignatowski, Anitschkow, and others). Many of the present assumptions about the causes of atherosclerosis are derived from epidemiologic observations based on the occurrence of the complications of the disease.

Morbid anatomy Atherosclerosis is basically a patchy, nodular type of arteriosclerosis. The lesions are commonly classified into two main groups, *fatty streaks* and raised lesions or *plaques*. The latter may be subclassified as *fibrous* or *complicated* plaques. Basically a fatty streak is an area which is stained distinctly by a fat-soluble dye, such as oil-red-O or Sudan IV, and shows no other underlying change. Some fatty streaks are visible without staining as yellow or whitish patches on the intima. At least some fatty streaks are probably precursors of raised lesions, but some additional undefined forces are required for this transformation, and these factors operate very unevenly between the sexes and among different individuals. In all populations that have been carefully studied, the aorta and carotid arteries shows fatty streaks beginning in infancy. The number reaches a peak between twenty and thirty years of age. Fatty streaks begin to appear in the coronary and cerebral arteries during puberty. Between the ages of fifteen and thirty-nine, such lesions are more common in women than in men.

Fibrous plaques are palpably elevated areas of intimal thickening; they sometimes contain lipid in the overlying layer. Raised lesions usually begin to appear after the development of fatty streaks has reached its peak. In populations having the highest incidence of complications of atherosclerosis, fibrous plaques have begun to replace most of the fatty streaks in the coronary arteries in the third decade. There is no correlation between the amount of fatty streaks and raised lesions in the aorta, but there is a rough correlation between them in the coronary arteries, especially in nonblack populations. It is also noteworthy that in populations in which a high incidence of coronary atherosclerosis is preponderant in men, the aorta in men and women tends to have the same degree of involvement by raised plaques. *Complicated plaques* are raised lesions which show some or all of the degenerative changes described earlier, sometimes including calcification.

Localization The raised lesions of atherosclerosis are irregularly distributed. The *aorta* is usually most heavily involved in the arch, about the orifices of its branches, particularly the coronaries and intercostals, in its abdominal portion, and frequently at its bifurcation into the iliacs. There is more atherosclerosis in the lower limbs than in the upper ones. In the legs, the incidence decreases peripherally, as the musculoelastic vessels give way to large muscular arteries and these become smaller vessels, such as the plantar or digital arteries. Plaques and thrombosis are particularly common in the *femoral* artery, in Hunter's canal, and in the *popliteal* artery just above the knee joint. The *anterior* and *posterior tibials* are often occluded together, but in different sites—the posterior where it rounds the internal malleolus, the anterior where it is superficial and becomes the dorsalis pedis artery. The peroneal artery, which is well embedded in muscle, often escapes while other major vessels are occluded, and it may be the main blood supply to the extremity (*peroneal leg*). Atherosclerosis in abdominal branches, except for the renal arteries, causes much less difficulty than in coronary and cerebral vessels.

In the *coronary arteries*, raised lesions are most prominent in the main stems, the highest incidence being a short distance beyond the ostia. Atherosclerosis is nearly always found in the epicardial portions of the vessels, while the intramural coronary arteries are spared. The left coronary artery is usually more affected than the right. Coronary atherosclerosis is nearly always diffuse. The degree to which the lumen is narrowed varies, but once the process is present, all the intima of the extramural portions of the vessel is usually involved. A single tiny plaque occluding an otherwise normal coronary artery is rare. In the cervical and cerebral arteries the distribution of atherosclerosis is patchy, as it may be in other arteries. It first appears in the base of the brain in the carotid, basilar, and vertebral arteries. The proximal portion of the internal carotids in the neck is a site of special predilection. There is a concentration of lesions near bifurcations. Atherosclerosis in the *retinal arteries* may often be secondary to other arteriopathies, such as those due to hypertension or diabetes. Whether atheromas cause the common intrinsic lesions of retinal vessels that lead to decreased choroidal circulation and macular degeneration with aging has not been clarified. Atherosclerosis in the *pulmonary artery* bears no relation to the severity of the disease in the aorta or other systemic arteries. There is some involvement in about half of adults over fifty who have no reason to have pulmonary hypertension. Pulmonary hypertension per se, however, is associated with medial hypertrophy, intimal thickening, and great acceleration of atheroma formation.

Recognition of atherosclerosis There is no blood test for atherosclerosis, nor any satisfactory noninvasive technique for demonstrating its presence. Angiographic visualization of deformity in the lumen of a vessel is the best presumptive test of silent atherosclerosis. Radiographic demonstration of calcification in the location of coronary vessels usually indicates atherosclerosis, but complete luminal obstruction may occur in the absence of any calcification. Calcification, or beading, of peripheral arteries and changes in appearance of retinal vessels are not correlated directly with atherosclerosis. Detection usually waits upon one of the clinical complications attending rupture or a critical decrease of blood flow in an involved vessel, and knowledge of the prevalence and incidence of arteriosclerosis and most of the inferences concerning its causes are derived from tabulations of the appearance of its complications.

Ischemic heart disease (IHD), synonymous with *coronary heart disease* or *arteriosclerotic heart disease*, is the most useful indicator of atherosclerosis available today. Practically all patients with myocardial infarction, as defined by electrocardiographic and enzyme changes, have coronary atherosclerosis. Rare exceptions are due to congenital anomalies of the coronary vessels, emboli, or ostial occlusion due to other types of cardiac or vascular disease. Nontraumatic *sudden death* (Chap. 34) makes up a sizable portion of all deaths eventually certified as due to IHD. At autopsy, evidence of fresh myocardial infarction or of *coronary thrombosis* is usually absent. While ventricular fibrillation may have been due to sudden closure of a partially compromised vessel by a small thrombus or embolus that has subsequently lysed, or from *spasm*, none of these need have preceded a fatal arrhythmia. The majority of victims of sudden death have had a previous diagnosis of IHD; the number who had preexisting diabetes or hypertension is also significant. In epidemiologic studies of IHD, *angina pectoris* and electrocardiographic changes attributable to ischemia without infarction are considered "softer end points" and treated separately.

Cerebrovascular disease (stroke) is a less reliable criterion for the presence of atherosclerosis. It includes *cerebral hemorrhage* and *cerebral thrombosis*. Cerebral thrombosis, including infarction or softening without evidence of embolus, is usually due to atherosclerosis. On the other hand, cerebral hemorrhage is often the result of congenital aneurysms or other vascular defects peculiar to hypertension and diabetes. Dissecting aneurysms, thrombosis of other major vessels, and ischemic renal disease likewise are not used to determine the prevalence of atherosclerosis in a population. For all these reasons, the present discussion of atherosclerosis revolves about IHD. It also concentrates particularly on that which is "premature," arbitrarily defined as IHD appearing before age sixty-five.

ISCHEMIC HEART DISEASE

PREVALENCE According to the National Health Examination Survey, about 5 million Americans have IHD (see Chap. 240), which makes it second to hypertension as the most prevalent cardiovascular disease. It is the leading cause of death in males after age thirty-five and in all persons after age forty-five. Premature deaths from IHD occur preponderantly in men, and a third of all deaths from IHD in males occur before age sixty-five. In fact nearly all of the excess premature mortality rate in American males is due to IHD. Between the ages of thirty-five and fifty-five the death rate is over five times higher in white men than in white women in the United States; this difference narrows after the menopause (Table 244-2). The exceptions are women with hypertension, diabetes, or premature (usually iatrogenic) menopause, who share the risk of the male. A distressing higher mortality rate in nonwhite women (Table 244-2) is probably due mainly to a greater incidence of hypertension in blacks. There is less difference between men and women in the prevalence of angina pectoris than in that of myocardial infarction; after age sixty-five more women than men have angina without a history of infarction.

The death rate from IHD in American men rose appreciably between 1940 and 1960. Now the rate below age sixty-five appears to be at a plateau. There was an appreciable decline in death rates from IHD in white females below age sixty-five between 1940 and 1960, a trend which now may have stopped. The death rate in nonwhite males and females below fifty-five has ceased to increase. There are many other interesting differences in regional death rates from IHD in the United States. The highest rates for both sexes combined are in the Middle Atlantic States. They exceed the lowest, found in the mountain states, by 25 percent. There are even more striking differences within a given locality. In a recent 7-year study in Evans County, Georgia, for example, the age-adjusted incidence of IHD in white males is more than three times that in black males, a discrepancy that appears best related to differences in amount of physical activity.

International comparisons In most well-developed countries, IHD is the major single cause of premature cardiovascular deaths. There are, however, marked differences in premature death rates among them. The six nations leading in death rate in white men, ages forty-five to sixty-four, are South Africa, the United States, Finland, Scotland, Canada, and Australia. Much lower age-adjusted death rates from IHD are found in most Western European countries, Latin America, and Japan. The rates in Japan are about one-fifth of those in the United States. Subsamples obtained in many countries convey the strong impression that upper socioeconomic classes which have adopted the culture of Western industrialized countries have far more IHD than lower socioeconomic classes. Two of the most obvious cultural differences between these groups are fat content of the diet and amount of physical work. In other industrialized nations in the West, mortality rates generally rose much more steeply during the period 1950–1960 than they did in the United States. Especially prominent were 60 and 90 percent increases, respectively, in death rates from IHD in younger men in the Netherlands and Norway in the decade following the war. Paradoxically, in many countries experiencing a rise in male death rates, the rates in females declined.

TABLE 244-2
Death rates in the United States from ischemic heart disease, 1966 (deaths per 100,000)

Sex	*Age*	*White*	*Nonwhite*
Male	25–34	10	22
	35–44	87	115
	45–54	358	346
	55–64	954	880
	65–74	2,115	2,080
	75–84	4,200	2,702
	85–	9,225	4,417
Female	25–34	2	12
	35–44	16	54
	45–54	72	186
	55–64	278	544
	65–74	1,014	1,362
	75–84	2,926	2,123
	85–	8,589	4,083

SOURCE: *Moriyama et al*

Extensive epidemiologic studies have not revealed the reasons for differences between cultures that are superficially similar. Why, for example, do the Scots and North Americans have nearly twice the death rate from premature IHD as Swedes? This difference can be extrapolated to excess of deaths before age sixty-five of about 60,000 males in the United States. Migrants to this country tend to have a higher risk of death from premature IHD than age-matched relatives who remain at home. There are many instances in which different ethnic groups in the same locality have widely differing prevalence of IHD. An example is the difference between whites and Bantus in South Africa. The Indians in Durban also have a peculiarly high propensity for IHD. Nevertheless, there are no epidemiologic data indicating that the great differences between populations in the incidence of IHD are due to genetic variation. Presently it seems that genetic heterogeneity is much more likely to explain some of the striking differences in susceptibility among individuals sharing the same ethnic and cultural setting.

CAUSATION Many of the theories about the origins of accelerated atherosclerosis are derived from relating the prevalence or incidence of premature IHD with other biologic, demographic, and social variables. This is a narrow view, but a practical one, for IHD is overall the most costly and common of the untimely complications of atherosclerosis. Preoccupation with IHD must not blind one, however, to the realization that angina and myocardial infarction are expressions of late-stage atherosclerotic lesions. Factors precipitating these events may be independent of those leading to the initiation of a plaque or its progression to a complicated lesion. Steps taken to prevent recurrence of myocardial infarction or fatal arrhythmia will not necessarily be the same as those taken to delay or prevent formation of atherosclerosis, and the latter should begin earlier in life, long before there is any suspicion of IHD.

It is safe to say that there are many causes of accelerated atherosclerosis. It is somewhat riskier to insist that two of them, *hyperlipidemia* and *hypertension*, are known, since definitive experiments in man have not proved them to be certain causes, but the inferential evidence is overwhelming. Many species of experimental animals develop atherosclerosis when plasma concentrations of low-density or very low-density lipoproteins are elevated; the incidence of premature IHD in both men and women in a given population and in different populations bears a reasonably good correlation with the concentration of cholesterol in plasma. These facts are the main pillars of the *filtration theory*, i.e., that cholesterol in atheromatous lesions comes mainly from the lumen and that flux of lipid into the arterial wall is a function of the plasma cholesterol concentration. As a group, hypertensive men and women have more IHD and a greater involvement of the surface of coronary and other major arteries by atherosclerosis. Presumably lesion development is accelerated by exaggeration of adaptive changes incident to increasing tensile, shear, and other hydraulic forces when diastolic pressure is elevated. Hypertensive animals have more atherosclerosis when also made hyperlipidemic. Perfusion of lipids and protein into experimental arterial preparations is enhanced by increasing the hydrostatic pressure. Hypertension and hyperlipidemia together also give rise to a higher incidence of premature IHD in man than either alone. Thus hypertension and hyperlipidemia appear independently and additively to accelerate atherosclerosis. The facts by no means clarify the etiology of atherosclerosis or, least of all, explain the great variability in susceptibility to complications or in extent of lesions among individuals with one or both of these major "risk factors."

Potentially, there are many other important determinants. These include *initiating* events at the endothelial surface, two of those suggested, but not proved, being fibrin deposition (Duguid) and platelet aggregation, with possible release of factors affecting endothelial permeability. Even these might be secondary to other injury forces changing the chemical or electrical barriers at the endothelial surface. Other possible factors relate to the ability of the wall to respond to increased tensile forces or to greater influx of lipid. It has been considered that altered ground substances may bind lipoproteins with unusual avidity, that enzyme activities catalyzing degradation and removal of lipids might be deficient, or that lipid synthesis *in situ* might be accelerated. Inappropriate excitation of phagocytic activity, structurally abnormal lipoproteins, deficient fibrinolytic activity, excessive platelet adhesiveness, or even sluggish depression of synthesis of collagen or smooth-muscle components needed to withstand a change in hydrodynamics are but some of many other "causes" or aggravations of the atherosclerotic process that have been considered. None has been excluded; none has been established. They remain questions for the experimentalist, and do not yet enter into a rational basis for formulating measures to prevent or decelerate atherogenesis or forestall some of its complications. There are, however, other variables in addition to the hyperlipidemia and hypertension which appear to have some effect on the incidence of IHD, even though their mechanism of action is vague. Because they are amenable to control, they are considered in preventive management of atherosclerosis. The principal ones are listed in Table 244-3 in the rough order of their importance in the population of the United States. Missing from the table is *diet*, which will be discussed under *hyperlipidemia*, even though it is not proved that all dietary factors operate through an effect on plasma lipids.

TABLE 244-3
Factors to consider in prevention of premature atherosclerosis

1 Hyperlipidemia	*5* Physical inactivity
2 Hypertension	*6* Obesity
3 Cigarette smoking	*7* Emotional stress
4 Diabetes mellitus	*8* Positive family history of premature atherosclerosis

PREVENTION No convincing evidence has been obtained in man that atherosclerotic lesions can be made to regress. There is some encouraging evidence in animals, most notably in primates, that relatively uncomplicated plaques induced by hyperlipidemia will regress, and that further progression of atherosclerosis will cease when hyperlipidemia is removed. Prevention, rather than treatment, is the goal and one of the most important tasks facing those responsible for the health of the public and of individual persons. An effective program of prophylaxis has not been established, but enough is known to guide both the identification of some of those with a higher risk and conservative measures that probably will reduce that risk.

Hyperlipidemia

The lipids in plasma of major clinical importance are *cholesterol* and *triglycerides*. They are combined with *phospholipids* and certain proteins (apolipoproteins) in four major classes of plasma *lipoproteins*. *Chylomicrons* are large particles in which glycerides in the diet and cholesterol are transported from the small intestine to the blood via the lymphatics. *Very low-density lipoproteins* (VLDL or pre-beta-lipoproteins) carry endogenously synthesized triglycerides, which are removed by muscle, heart, adipose tissue, and other sites. Major remnants of VLDL metabolism are *low-density lipoproteins* (LDL or beta-lipoproteins), which are probably catabolized in the liver. *High-density lipoproteins* (HDL or alpha-lipoproteins) contain phospholipid and cholesterol complexed with apolipoproteins, the bulk of which differ from those found in VLDL and LDL. HDL are involved in the metabolism of VLDL and the enzymatic reaction by which cholesterol is esterified in plasma.

In the postabsorptive state, a total plasma cholesterol concentration of 200 mg per 100 ml is distributed very roughly as follows: VLDL, 10: LDL, 140; and HDL, 50. Most of the plasma triglycerides above about 50 mg per 100 ml will be found in VLDL. Chylomicrons are present only 2 to 6 hr after ingestion of fat; their presence after an overnight fast is abnormal. A small quantity of fat in the plasma is normally transported by albumin, not by the lipoproteins. These are the *free fatty acids* (FFA), the form in which fat is mainly carried from the adipose tissue stores to meet caloric demand. The normal concentration (0.3 to 0.7 μEq per liter) of FFA is increased when tissue insulin activity is low or glucose utilization is deficient, and by the excessive sympathetic or catecholamine discharge that may arise from such diverse causes as emotional stress, nicotine, and caffeine. The FFA released in excess of those utilized by muscle, liver, or other tissues mainly reappear in plasma as *endogenous glyceride.* FFA play a key role in supplying oxidizable substrate to the heart, are a delicate indicator of the state of carbohydrate metabolism, and have an indirect effect on the concentration of plasma lipoproteins.

PLASMA CONCENTRATIONS There is no absolute definition of hyperlipidemia. For biologic variables, upper limits such as the upper 5 percent of the distribution within the population are often used, but for plasma cholesterol, such statistical limits are probably too high (Table 244-4). Correlations between the cholesterol concentrations in young men in North America and incidence of premature IHD indicate that an increasing risk can be detected when the cholesterol is higher than 220 mg per 100 ml, a value close to the mean for men from forty to forty-nine years of age in this population. Extrapolation of similar data from other populations suggests that a cholesterol concentration of 150 mg per 100 ml would be healthier as far as premature IHD is concerned. The cholesterol level at birth averages 60 mg per 100 ml. Within a month the average has risen to about 120 and by the first year to 175. A second rise begins in the third decade and continues to about age fifty in men and somewhat later in woman. In other populations, such as in southern Italy, this rise in adulthood is far less prominent; it is therefore not to be considered necessarily physiologic. Triglycerides are more variable but also show an age-related increase, in this case possibly correlated with weight gain in early adulthood. The above age-related increases in cholesterol are associated mainly with a rise in LDL concentrations, the increases in triglycerides with a rise in VLDL. HDL concentrations in females average about 20 percent higher than in man. Estrogens and androgens have opposite effects on HDL levels.

CORRELATIONS WITH IHD Hyperlipidemia is associated unequivocally with increased incidence of premature IHD. Hypercholesterolemia has been studied most extensively. It correlates highly with the risk of myocardial infarction in both men and women. In the Framingham study, for both sexes combined, the relative incidence of infarction between ages thirty and forty-nine at starting cholesterol levels >260 mg per 100 ml was three- to fivefold that at cholesterol levels <220. This appears to be a continuous gradient of risk as the cholesterol level ascends. These data are supported by comparisons of prevalence of IHD and cholesterol in many other populations. The concentrations of LDL or LDL + VLDL have roughly the same correlation with IHD as does cholesterol. The relationship of triglycerides and VLDL to IHD is compounded by a rise in cholesterol as VLDL increases. The available data, however, including a prospective study in Swedish men and comparisons of lipoprotein pattern with angiographic data, indicate that increased triglycerides (or VLDL) alone are also correlated with the incidence of premature IHD. A fasting triglyceride >150 mg per 100 ml is therefore considered to be a potential *risk factor* in IHD. All studies indicate that hyperlipidemia is a more meaningful risk factor below age fifty and that it operates independently of hypertension, diabetes, obesity, and other factors. For the population over age fifty-five, there do not exist satisfactory data to suggest that reduction of hyperlipidemia will decrease atherogenesis or its complications.

TABLE 244-4
Plasma lipid concentrations in Americans, mg/100 ml*

Age, yr	*Cholesterol*	*Triglycerides*
1–19	175 (120–230)	70 (10–140)
20–29	180 (120–240)	70 (10–140)
30–39	205 (140–270)	75 (10–150)
40–49	225 (150–310)	85 (10–160)
50–59	245 (160–330)	95 (10–190)

* *The approximate mean and upper and lower 5 percent limits for Americans; significant differences between the sexes in different age groups are ignored.*

CAUSES OF HYPERLIPIDEMIA The relationship of diet to the relative hypercholesterolemia in North Americans is still a subject of debate, particularly with respect to what general public health measures are justified. There is no question but that the plasma cholesterol (and LDL) level is sensitive to the amount of saturated fat and cholesterol in the diet. The "average" adult in the United States eats about 145 g fat per day and 600 mg cholesterol. The mixture of fats ingested usually contains about three times as much saturated fatty acids (mainly myristic, palmitic, and stearic) as polyunsaturated fatty acids (mainly linoleic and linolenic acids). If a healthy young adult switches from this diet to an extremely different one containing the same amount of total fat in which the ratio of polyunsaturates to saturates is reversed and a cholesterol content <300 mg per day, his cholesterol concentration will usually drop by 10 to 30 percent within 2 weeks, and remain depressed on continuation of the diet. Proportionately similar changes are produced in many patients with severe hypercholesterolemia when due to increased LDL (type II hyperlipoproteinemia). These observations in individuals parallel a relationship established in many populations. The average cholesterol level in most populations is more closely related to one variable than to any other: the amount of animal fats (meat, eggs, and milk products, major sources of long- and short-chain saturated fatty acids and cholesterol) in the diet. Increased animal fat consumption also tends to be correlated with greater intake of refined sugars and less of complex carbohydrates, with a lesser proportion of dietary fats that are polyunsaturated, with less physical work, as well as with higher per capita gasoline consumption and many other cultural traits associated with most populations having higher risk of premature IHD. It remains, however, that none of the other variables can be so directly related to an effect on plasma cholesterol. The average triglyceride is more sensitive to total carbohydrate intake, to caloric balance, and to alcohol intake. It is important to note that physical activity, emotional stress, obesity per se (as opposed to positive caloric balance), and smoking are not well correlated with plasma lipid and lipoprotein concentrations. Any relationship these latter factors have to incidence of IHD is probably not operating directly through effects on hyperlipidemia.

For clinical purposes, hyperlipidemia should be considered as either *secondary* to other recognized diseases or *primary*. The latter includes mainly abnormalities induced by diet and other *environmental factors* and by genetically determined errors in lipid or lipoprotein metabolism. *Familial hyperlipoproteinemias* are discussed in Chap. 106. It may be assumed that most of the hyperlipidemia as defined here in the context of prevention is environmental in origin, but much subtle variation in genetic regulation determines the plasma lipid responses of different individuals to the same diet or to other coexisting environmental factors. Present knowledge allows only gross segregation of some of the more obvious types of primary hyperlipoproteinemia.

Diagnosis and management

The screening of individuals for hyperlipidemia now usually occurs during convalescence from a myocardial infarction, a time which may be two or more decades too late. In a program for prevention of premature atherosclerosis based on current incomplete knowledge, arguments may be made for routine cholesterol analysis on cord blood or no later than age two years. A common form of familial hyperbetalipoproteinemia (type II hyperlipoproteinemia) will be easily identifiable by these times in an estimated 1 per 500 or 1 per 1,000 children. Primary hyperlipidemia is *relatively* rare, however, until about the third decade. Screening at this time will be more efficient, both by increasing the yield of abnormal levels and permitting identification of those families in which children will most likely be affected. As more is learned, public health practices will be adjusted. *Today, good health maintenance practice demands a test for detection of hyperlipidemia in all persons between twenty and thirty years of age.*

Hyperlipidemia is detected by two generally available clinical tests, the concentration of cholesterol and triglycerides in serum or plasma. The sample should be obtained before breakfast and during a period when the subject is maintaining weight and taking no medications known to affect lipid concentrations. *In subjects less than fifty-five years of age, a cholesterol concentration (C) greater than 220 mg per 100 ml or triglycerides (TG) greater than 150 mg per 100 ml indicates hyperlipidemia sufficient to require some attention by the physician to the items listed in Table 244-5.* If hyperlipidemia is absent, the tests need not be repeated for 1 to 10 years in an adult who maintains body weight and does not otherwise change in health or life style. Many adults will have a C >220; vigor in pursuing the "causative factors" in Table 244-5 should increase in proportion to the degree of hyperlipidemia. Any adult with C >280 or TG >150 should, however, be checked for *secondary causes* of hyperlipidemia. If all these are absent, it is then useful to convert the presumably primary hyperlipidemia into hyperlipoproteinemia. This may be done by using the plasma C and TG, by observation of the fasting plasma for presence of chylomicrons, and by estimation of the LDL concentration (see Chap. 106). Lipoprotein determinations by electrophoresis or other methods are also helpful. Translation of hyperlipidemia to hyperlipoproteinemia offers better separation of different metabolic bases for hypercholesterolemia or hyperglyceridemia, somewhat sharper identification of genetic disorders, and more rational management.

HYPERLIPOPROTEINEMIA There are three common types of hyperlipoproteinemia as now identified in a recent WHO classification. They are quite frequent in patients with premature IHD and occur in about the same proportions. Type IIa (elevated C; normal TG) is defined by increased LDL and normal VLDL concentrations. In its mild form, this pattern is most commonly due to excessive intake (or abnormal response to a normal intake) of saturated fats and cholesterol. In its more severe form, and nearly always when accompanied by tendon and subcutaneous xanthomas, it is inherited as a mendelian dominant trait. *Familial hyperbetalipoproteinemia* (*familial hypercholesterolemia*) is detected by high cholesterol or LDL levels in childhood, and is associated with an overall five- to tenfold increase in prevalence of premature IHD, and probably increased cerebrovascular disease. Treatment consists of use of a low-cholesterol, low–saturated-fat diet, with or without an increase in polyunsaturated fats. Failure of good diet therapy to bring the cholesterol level below 300 mg per 100 ml warrants a trial of cholestyramine, *d*-thyroxine, or nicotinic acid (see Chap. 106).

Type IV (TG elevated, C normal or increased to a lesser degree) means an increase in VLDL without a rise in LDL. The initial steps in management of primary type IV are reduction to ideal weight, limitation or elimination of alcohol intake, and restriction of carbohydrate intake to 40 percent of calories.

Type IIb (elevated C and TG) means increased LDL and VLDL concentrations. This *mixed hyperlipidemia* is not definitive of any specific disease. It is present in some patients with *familial hypercholesterolemia.* In milder

TABLE 244-5
A check list of factors requiring attention in patients with hyperlipidemia

1 Disorders to which hyperlipidemia is secondary
   a Hypothyroidism
   b Uncontrolled diabetes mellitus
   c Obstructive liver disease
   d Hypoproteinemia (viz., nephrosis)
   e Dysproteinemia (viz., multiple myeloma, lupus erythematosus)
2 Diet
   a Content of saturated fats and cholesterol
   b Unusually high intake of carbohydrate
   c Caloric balance (weight gain)
3 Alcohol intake
4 Xanthomas
5 Hyperglycemia
6 Hyperuricemia
7 History of pancreatitis or recurrent abdominal pain
8 Family history of hyperlipidemia xanthomas or diabetes mellitus

forms, it is often much more responsive than type IIa to weight control and a diet low in saturated fats and cholesterol; the best form of drug therapy for patients with this lipoprotein pattern has not been established. Recent studies of genetic hyperlipidemia in families of patients with myocardial infarction associated with hyperlipidemia have suggested a new and possibly very common form of genetic hyperlipidemia. In this *combined hyperlipidemia*, relatives may have type IIa, IIb, or IV patterns. The genetic defect may be located at sites concerned with VLDL (triglyceride) secretion or disposal, rather than at sites concerned primarily with LDL (cholesterol) metabolism. The heterogeneity disclosed in such families underscores the lack of specificity of any pattern of hyperlipidemia or hyperlipoproteinemia in a given patient. It also implies that screening of all possible first-degree relatives may be necessary to determine phenotypes when the abnormality is shown to be familial.

Type III hyperlipoproteinemia (C and TG elevated to about the same level) is a rare disorder, which is identified by the presence of "abnormal" lipoproteins not seen in significant concentrations in normal persons or in other types of hyperlipoproteinemia (Chap. 106). The ultracentrifuge is required for an absolute diagnosis, a test not generally available. Patients with type III have a marked increase in coronary and peripheral atherosclerosis; sometimes they can be identified by yellow lipid deposits in the palms and reddish-yellow tuberous and eruptive xanthomas on the elbows, buttocks, and knees. Both types III and IV are associated with increased frequency of diabetes and hyperuricemia. Although type III is familial, it is rarely seen in children. The treatment of type III includes maintenance of ideal weight, use of a diet similar to that for type II, and administration of clofibrate; therapy promptly results in a gratifying normalization of plasma lipid concentrations and a disappearance of subcutaneous xanthoma. Two types of hyperlipoproteinemia with very high triglyceride levels (types I and V) are not known to be associated with increased atherosclerosis; they are treated in a different manner, mainly to reduce the danger of pancreatitis (see Chap. 106). It is reemphasized that all the above types of hyperlipidemia or hyperlipoproteinemia may be either secondary or familial. The genetic forms can be recognized only by screening as many relatives as possible.

No proof has yet been obtained that treating hyperlipidemia results in a decrease in the rate of progression of atherosclerosis. The numerous positive correlations of hyperlipidemia with premature atherosclerosis and the success with which blood lipid levels can be lowered, especially in younger patients, indicate the following conservative course to the physician today. He should screen young adults for hyperlipidemia, and if they are abnormal, see that their children are examined. He should recommend, and follow up, appropriate dietary therapy in all patients below age fifty-five. When these measures do not succeed in lowering cholesterol or triglyceride concentrations below 300 mg per 100 ml in the young adult, he should consider a therapeutic trial of an appropriate hypolipidemic drug. If the latter is satisfactory, he should maintain both diet and drug with careful observation. Significant side effects indicate withdrawal of any hypolipidemic agent except under extraordinary circumstances.

The uncertainties still surrounding the treatment of hyperlipidemia also diminish the force of movements to change the dietary patterns of the population as a whole. Nevertheless, several responsible bodies, including the Inter-Society Commission on Heart Disease Resources, have advocated a "prudent diet for everyone, to consist of about 30 percent calories as fat, less than the usual proportion of this as saturated fats, and <300 mg of cholesterol per day." This diet generally means elimination of *whole* milk products, no more than one to two eggs per week, use of lean meats, avoidance of short-chain fats such as coconut oil, and use of predominantly polyunsaturated vegetable oils (corn, soybean, cottonseed, and safflower) for cooking and baking. The elements of such a diet are given in Table 244-6.

Other risk factors

HIGH BLOOD PRESSURE (Chap 245) In the Framingham study, the incidence of IHD in men aged forty-five to sixty-two with blood pressures exceeding a systolic level of 160 or diastolic about 95 was more than five times that in normotensive men (blood pressure 140/90 or less). Hypertension correlates positively with IHD in both men and women, the diastolic pressure perhaps being more important. After the age of forty-five, hypertension has greater weight than hypercholesterolemia as a risk factor. Not only are IHD and cerebrovascular disease increased by hypertension, but also the amount of atherosclerosis found at autopsy in comparisons of many subjects from different countries. A recent intervention study has shown convincingly that reduction of diastolic levels >105 significantly reduces the incidence of strokes and congestive heart failure in men. A decrease in IHD has not yet been demonstrated; studies are underway to test the effect on these complications when patients with diastolic elevations between 90 and 105 are similarly maintained on adequate treatment. Special urgency for relief of hypertension obtains when hyperlipidemia or other risk factors are concomitantly present.

CIGARETTE SMOKING Ample statistical evidence supports a mean increase of about 70 percent in the death rate from IHD in men who smoke one pack of cigarettes per day compared with nonsmokers. The excess morbidity ratio in some instances may be as high as 200 percent. In general, the increase in death rate is proportional to the amount smoked and decreases with age. Excess morbidity from myocardial infarction is also present in women smokers, but the relationship is somewhat less firm than in men. In men, but not in women, smoking is also associated with increased angina pectoris. Smoking involves an excess risk in younger men that is not removed by adustment for hyperlipidemia, hypertension, and other variables. The explanation for the association of smoking and increased IHD is not known. Pipe and cigar smokers have a lesser increase in risk of IHD, presumably because less smoke is inhaled. Smokers dying of causes other than IHD have been found at autopsy to have more coronary atherosclerosis than nonsmokers. The major influence of smoking is upon the incidence of sudden death, however. Those who stop smoking show a prompt decline in risk but may not reach the risk level of nonsmokers until after about 10 years of abstention.

ABNORMAL GLUCOSE TOLERANCE (Chap. 88) There is at least a twofold increase in incidence of myocardial infarction in diabetics compared with nondiabetics. There is an increased tendency toward cerebral thrombosis and infarction but not toward cerebral hemorrhage in diabetes. Gangrene of the lower extremities has been variously estimated to be from 8 to 150 times as frequent in diabetics as in nondiabetics. Diabetes is associated with an increase in atherosclerosis observed at autopsy, but proof is lacking that increased myocardial infarction or gangrene in diabetes can be attributed entirely to either accelerated atherogenesis or an approximately twofold increase in the frequency of hypertension in diabetics. The capillary basement membrane thickening, proliferative lesions, and microaneurysms considered to be pathognomonic of diabetes have not been adequately studied in the hearts of diabetics. They have been demonstrated in peripheral arteries; these lesions may cause small infarcts in vessel walls, interfere with development of collateral circulation, and promote atherogenesis. Studies indicate that insulinopenic diabetics who are well controlled do not have consistent significant elevations in either cholesterol (or LDL) or triglycerides (or VLDL) compared with nondiabetics. It does not seem likely, therefore, that the usual forms of hyperlipidemia are the basis for the increased risk of IHD in diabetics.

PHYSICAL ACTIVITY Data seeking to relate prevalence of IHD to daily (occupational) physical activity are confounded by many variables. Among prospective studies the Framingham data do indicate that the less sedentary an individual is, the less susceptible he is to sudden death. The Evans County Study indicates that physical work may be the major determinant of greatly differing incidences of IHD in Southern males, black or white. How physical activity may operate to decrease death from IHD, or possibly atherogenesis, is not known. Beyond affecting hyperlipidemia as it is related to caloric expenditure, no mechanism has been demonstrated. Moderate exercise, unassociated with weight change, has not yet been proved to have a beneficial effect on blood lipid levels. Advocates of physical activity in primary or secondary prevention of IHD have suggested that exercise improves sympathetic tone or development of collateral circulation. Such arguments are largely intuitive, but steady physical activity is supported as an element of hygiene desirable in a program of preventive maintenance.

TABLE 244-6
Suggested 2400-kcal meal plan*

Food	*Typical portion size of one serving or one "exchange"*	*Portion for* Breakfast	Lunch	Dinner	Snacks	*Remarks*
Milk, nonfat	1 cup (8 oz)	1		1		Skim milk; buttermilk from skim milk
Vegetables:						
Low-carbohydrate			As desired			Raw vegetable salads; leafy vegetables, tomatoes, etc.
Medium-carbohydrate	1/2 cup			1		Carrots, beets, peas, etc.
Fruit	1/2 cup, 1 small apple	1	1	1	2	Fresh, frozen, canned; if sweetened, subtract 2 sugar exchanges per portion
Bread, cereals, starches	1 slice bread, or 1/2 cup cereal, or potato	2	2	2	2	
Lean meat, fish, poultry	1 oz, cooked weight		3	4		11 meals/week—poultry (no skin) veal, fish, uncreamed cottage cheese; 3 meals/week—lean beef, lamb, or pork well trimmed of fat
Eggs						3-4 per week, as substitute for meat (1 egg = 1 oz meat)
Fat	1 tsp		6	9		Vegetable oil (except olive) and salad dressing from these oils
Special margarine	1 tsp	1		1	1	Margarine with 30-40% polyunsaturates; first-named ingredient on label should be "liquid oil"
Sugar, sweets	1 tsp	5	3	2	2	

* *35–40 percent of kilocalories from fat; high in polyunsaturates, low in cholesterol. Total fat, 115.5 g; saturated fat, 30.2 g (11 percent of kilocalories); linoleate, 44.8 g (17 percent of kilocalories); cholesterol 350 mg.*

SOURCE: *Adapted from suggested meal plan included in The Regulation of Dietary Fat, a review prepared by the Council on Foods and Nutrition of the American Medical Association (JAMA 181:411, 1962).*

TABLE 244-7
Sample menu for 2400-kcal meal plan*

Breakfast	*Lunch*	*Dinner*	*Snack*
1/2 grapefruit 2 tsp sugar 1/2 cup cooked cereal 2 tsp sugar 1 slice toast 1 tsp special margarine 1 tsp jelly 1 cup skim milk	Sandwich: 3 oz chicken 1 tbsp mayonnaise 2 slices bread Salad: Lettuce, celery, green pepper 1 tbsp oil, vinegar to taste 1 small apple baked with 1 tbsp sugar	4 oz breaded haddock, fried in 1 tbsp oil (bread crumbs from 1 slice bread) 1/2 cup potatoes, fried in 1 tsp oil 1/2 cup tomato and lettuce salad, 2 tsp oil, vinegar to taste 1/2 cup peas with 1 tsp special margarine 1 tbsp mayonnaise with relish as tartar sauce 1 small pear with 2 tsp sugar (or two sweetened canned pear halves) 1 cup skim milk	2 slices cinnamon toast with 1 tsp special margarine 2 tsp sugar 1/2 cup orange juice 1/2 small banana

* *25–40 percent of kilocalories from fat, high in polyunsaturates, low in cholesterol.*

OBESITY Atherosclerosis of major vessels is not independently associated with either obesity or body habitus; neither is IHD correlated with body weight. An increase in body weight in early adulthood may be correlated with mean triglyceride levels, and weight reduction is important in reduction of both hyperglyceridemia and glucose intolerance. Obesity is also correlated weakly with hypertension. Obesity is an undesirable hazard to cardiovascular function and a poor trait to be tolerated in a population at high risk for premature vascular disease.

PSYCHOLOGIC FACTORS A Western Collaborative Group Study has classified men into two personality types with different incidence of IHD. Type A is compulsive, striving, and deadline-conscious compared with the more sluggish or passive type B. In a prospective study, young type-A men, age thirty to thirty-nine, have had nearly three times the incidence of new IHD as type-B men. This difference is not clearly related to cigarette smoking or other well-established risk factors. The executive and managerial classes tend to include more type-A than type-B men. Yet, in large corporations, it has been observed that premature IHD in men is more common in the laborers. In such comparisons, college-educated men also have lower rates than the non-college-educated. There is a general clinical impression that psychic or other emotional stress and anxiety are associated with sudden death and even with development of IHD. In individual cases this sometimes seems incontrovertible. Except for the above-mentioned study, however, many social and demographic analyses have so far failed to reach any agreement about the etiologic relationships of occupation and similar situational factors and the incidence of IHD.

GENETIC FACTORS Family history is included among the factors to be weighed in prophylaxis. Primarily the family history helps the physician to avoid missing hyperlipidemia, hypertension, and diabetes, all of which tend to be familial. Probably diabetes is the most important known genetic variable in the atherogenesis. The obvious, xanthomatous forms of severe familial hyperlipidemia are relatively uncommon (familial type II is perhaps present in a frequency of 1:200 to 1:1,000 persons), but milder familial forms are likely to account for a sizable proportion of patients with premature IHD. As indicated earlier, genetic influences still appear to be less important than cultural ones in determining overall prevalence of IHD. There are also a few families with excessive premature vascular disease in which none of the known risk factors appears to be operating.

TREATMENT

The above emphasis on prevention of atherosclerosis is based on knowledge that is woefully incomplete, yet adequate enough to begin with, for the emphasis of medical practice must shift away from a preoccupation with the treatment of the complications of atherosclerosis. Programs designed to detect those most susceptible to premature atherosclerosis today emphasize the young adult and children at special hazard for hyperlipidemia or some other increased risk. Tomorrow's programs will undoubtedly begin in early childhood and involve all apparently normal children. We do not yet have enough information to advocate a radical change in the diet in infancy. Indeed, it is difficult to inspire interest in a more "prudent" diet in asymptomatic adults.

Recently, reports have appeared that chronic administration of clofibrate may reduce the incidence of myocardial infarction in patients who have had previous IHD and in previously asymptomatic subjects. This was not correlated with the known hypolipidemic affect of this drug. More evidence is needed of the efficacy of this or similar drugs before their use as preventives might become standard practice. Both the safety and long-term efficacy of any agent used prophylactically must be carefully established. Many other agents, without obvious effect on other risk factors, including vitamins B, C, and E, oral preparations of phospholipids and acid mucopolysaccharides, and enzymes have been advocated. None is backed with necessary proof of efficacy. The ultimate value of any intervention will be based on the degree to which it prevents or retards the underlying damage to the arterial wall as opposed to forestalling the formation of a thrombus or some other terminal event obliterating the lumen of a vessel already in the last stages of function. The former may perhaps be truly prophylactic of atherosclerosis. The latter will still be "treatment" of its complications, a subject dealt with in other chapters. For atherosclerosis, there is no definitive therapy, but there is increasing hope for effective prevention.

REFERENCES

ADAMS CWM: *Vascular Histochemistry*, Chicago: Year Book, 1967

BLUMENTHAL HT (ed): *Cowdry's Arteriosclerosis*, 2d ed., Springfield, Ill.: Charles C Thomas, 1967

DI GIROLANO M, SCHLANT RC: Etiology of coronary atherosclerosis, chap. 48 in *The Heart*, 3d ed., ed JW Hurst, New York: McGraw-Hill, 1974, pp. 987–1003

The Framingham Study, An Epidemiological Investigation of Cardiovascular Disease, sec. 10, Washington: U.S. Government Printing Office, September, 1968

FREDRICKSON DS: A physician's guide to hyperlipidemia, in *Modern Concepts of Cardiovascular Disease*, New York: American Heart Association, 1972

FRY DL: Localizing factors in arteriosclerosis, chap. 7 in *Atherosclerosis and Coronary Heart Disease*, eds W Likoff et al, New York: Grune & Stratton, 1972

GOLDSTEIN JL et al: Genetics of hyperlipidemia in coronary heart disease. Trans Assoc Am Physicians (in press)

INTER-SOCIETY COMMISSION FOR HEART DISEASE RESOURCES: Primary prevention of the atherosclerotic diseases. Circulation 42:A-55, 1970

KEYS A (ed): Coronary heart disease in seven countries. Circulation, 41: I-1, 1970

McGILL HC JR (ed): The geographic pathology of atherosclerosis. Lab Invest 18:463, 1968

MORIYAMA I et al: *Cardiovascular Diseases in the United States*, Cambridge, Mass.: Harvard, 1971

ROSENMAN RH et al: Coronary heart disease in the Western Collaborative Group Study: A follow-up experience of four and one-half years. J Chronic Dis 23:173, 1970

245 HYPERTENSIVE VASCULAR DISEASE

PAUL I. JAGGER
EUGENE BRAUNWALD

When a resting supine adult has an arterial pressure of 160/95 mm Hg or higher, hypertension may be considered to be present. Since, as pointed out in Chap. 32, there is apparently no sharp dividing line between normal and elevated blood pressure, this is an arbitrary definition based on demonstrated deleterious effects and one by which approximately 15 to 20 percent of the adult population of the United States has hypertension.

Diastolic hypertension, a disease complex which is the focus of this chapter, may be *labile* or *sustained.* Though major attention here is directed to sustained diastolic hypertension, most patients with labile hypertension eventually develop sustained hypertension and therefore should be reexamined at regular intervals. Sustained diastolic hypertension may sometimes be further categorized as *accelerated* or *malignant.* The patient with malignant hypertension often has a blood pressure above 200/140 mm Hg, but it is the papilledema, not the level of pressure, that specifically defines malignant hypertension, clinically. Pathologically, in this condition, fibrinoid or necrotizing arteritis involves the kidneys. The term *accelerated* hypertension indicates either a recent significant increase over previous hypertensive levels, or symptoms and signs suggesting malignant hypertension, but without papilledema. Though hypertension that is neither accelerated or malignant has been termed *benign*, hypertension is never truly benign, since even mild elevations of diastolic pressure are associated with increased risks of premature death and of vascular complications involving eyes, brain, heart, and kidneys.

Diastolic hypertension, if severe and/or sustained, results in the development of hypertensive vascular disease, consisting of arteriosclerotic changes in large arteries, thickening of walls, and occlusion of lumens of small arteries and arterioles, and, in the brain, of so-called Charcot-Bouchard aneurysms of the small perforating arteries. In malignant hypertension, there may be necrosis of the walls of small arteries and arterioles. It is, of course, desirable whenever possible to identify patients before they develop hypertensive vascular changes and to institute therapy that will prevent or retard such changes and the attendant illness and death.

SECONDARY HYPERTENSION

To institute the proper therapy for the patient with hypertension, it first must be determined whether hypertension is due to a clearly definable cause, i.e., *secondary* hypertension; if no cause can be identified, *essential* (*primary*) hypertension is present.

RENAL HYPERTENSION The two subdivisions of renal hypertension are *renal arterial hypertension* and *renal parenchymal hypertension.* A simple explanation for renal arterial hypertension is that decreased perfusion of renal tissue, due to stenosis of a main or branch renal artery, activates the renin-angiotensin system, described in Chap. 86. The angiotensin elevates arterial pressure both by direct vasoconstriction and by stimulation of aldosterone secretion, with resultant sodium retention. However, only two-thirds of patients with renal arterial hypertension have elevated circulating levels of plasma renin activity. In animal experiments, partial occlusion of a main renal artery results in early rises in peripheral plasma renin activity sufficient to account for the initial elevations in pressure; however, the hypertension persists while plasma renin activity returns to base-line levels. In spite of these and other observations which indicate that renal hypertension is a complex phenomenon, there is no question as to the usefulness of renin measurements in the clinical evaluation of the patient with a suspected renal arterial lesion. If that lesion is responsible for the hypertension, the circulating renin should come from the involved kidney.

Activation of the renin-angiotensin system also has been offered as an explanation for the hypertension in both acute and chronic renal parenchymal disease. In this formulation, the only difference between renal arterial hypertension and renal parenchymal hypertension is that the decreased perfusion of renal tissue in the latter case results from inflammatory and fibrotic changes involving multiple small intrarenal vessels. However, peripheral plasma renin activity is elevated far less frequently in renal parenchymal hypertension than it is in renal arterial hypertension; also cardiac output usually is slightly elevated in renal arterial hypertension, but normal in renal parenchymal hypertension; circulatory responses to tilting and to the Valsalva maneuver are exaggerated in the former, while blood volumes tend to be low in patients with severe renal arterial hypertension and to be high in patients with severe renal parenchymal hypertension.

Alternate explanations for the hypertension in renal parenchymal disease include the possibilities that the damaged kidneys (1) produce another unidentified vasopressor substance, (2) fail to produce a necessary humoral vasodilator substance (perhaps prostaglandin or bradykinin), (3) fail to inactivate circulating vasopressor substances, and/or (4) are ineffective in disposing of sodium and the retained sodium is responsible for the hypertension. Though all these possible explanations, including participation of the renin-angiotensin system, probably have some validity under certain circumstances, the hypothesis involving sodium retention is the most attractive. It is supported by the observation that those patients with chronic pyelonephritis or polycystic renal disease who are salt wasters do not develop hypertension, and by the observation that removal of salt and water by dialysis or diuretics is effective in controlling blood pressure in the majority of patients with uremia. Sodium retention supposedly leads to sustained hypertension, first by increasing extracellular (including intravascular) fluid volume and, sequentially, venous return to the right side of the heart, and cardiac output; the latter evokes peripheral vasoconstriction to return flow to control levels. Pressure is then maintained at the elevated level by the increased peripheral resistance, even though cardiac output returns toward baseline. It is also postulated that the increased sodium content of arteriolar walls can increase peripheral resistance, either by causing swelling of the walls with narrowing of lumens, or by increasing reactivity of smooth muscles to vasoconstrictor stimuli.

ADRENAL HYPERTENSION Hypertension is a feature of a variety of adrenal cortical abnormalities. In *primary aldosteronism* (Chap. 86) there is a clear relationship between the aldosterone-induced sodium retention and the hypertension. Normal individuals given aldosterone develop hypertension only if they also ingest sodium. Since aldosterone causes sodium retention by stimulating renal tubular exchange of sodium for potassium, hypokalemia is a prominent feature in most patients with primary aldosteronism, and the measurement of serum potassium provides a simple screening test. The effect of sodium retention and volume expansion that is critically important for definitive diagnosis is the chronic suppression of circulating levels of plasma renin activity (Fig. 86-6). In most clinical situations plasma renin activity and plasma or urinary aldosterone levels parallel each other, but in patients with primary aldosteronism, aldosterone levels are high and relatively fixed because of autonomous aldosterone secretion, while plasma renin activity levels are suppressed and respond sluggishly to sodium depletion.

The sodium-retaining effect of large amounts of glucocorticoids also offers an explanation for the hypertension in *Cushing's syndrome* (Chap. 86); however, cortisol itself may be hypertensinogenic. Moreover, increased production of mineralocorticoids also has been documented in some patients with Cushing's syndrome. In the forms of the *adrenogenital syndromes* due to C-11 or C-17 hydroxylase deficiency (Chap. 86), deoxycorticosterone appears to account for the sodium retention and the resultant hypertension, which is accompanied by suppression of plasma renin activity.

Approximately 20 percent of patients who by all other criteria have essential hypertension have suppressed plasma renin activity. Though these patients are not hypokalemic, they have been reported to have expanded extracellular fluid volumes, and it is tempting to implicate sodium retention and renin suppression due to excess production of an unidentified mineralocorticoid. Involvement of the adrenal cortex is supported by the observations that inhibition of steroidogenesis by aminoglutethimide, and large doses of spironolactone, the mineralocorticoid antagonist, can result in sodium loss and lowering of blood pressure in these patients. A search for other mineralocorticoids has revealed increased secretion of 18-hydroxy-11-deoxycorticosterone in a few patients.

In patients with *pheochromocytoma* increased secretion of epinephrine and norepinephrine by the adrenal medullary tumor causes excess stimulation of adrenergic receptors, which results in peripheral vasoconstriction and cardiac stimulation. This diagnosis is confirmed by demonstrating increased urinary excretion of epinephrine and norepinephrine or their metabolites (Chap. 87).

ORAL CONTRACEPTIVES The estrogen component of oral contraceptive agents may be responsible for secondary hypertension in some patients by stimulating the hepatic synthesis of renin substrate, angiotensinogen, which in turn favors the generation of increased amounts of angiotensin and, secondarily, of aldosterone. This form of hypertension is reversible. When a woman taking oral contraceptives presents with hypertension, the contraceptives should be discontinued for at least 6 months so that their contribution to the problem can be assessed.

COARCTATION OF THE AORTA (Chap. 237) The hypertension associated with coarctation may be caused by the constriction itself, or perhaps by the changes in the renal circulation which result in an unusual form of renal arterial hypertension. The diagnosis of coarctation is usually evident from clinical and routine x-ray findings.

HYPERCALCEMIA The hypertension which occurs in up to one-third of patients with hyperparathyroidism ordinarily can be attributed to renal parenchymal damage due to nephrolithiasis and nephrocalcinosis. However, calcium infusions can also have a direct vasoconstrictive effect. In some cases, the hypertension disappears when the hypercalcemia is corrected.

ESSENTIAL HYPERTENSION

After being thoroughly evaluated for secondary hypertension, as described below, approximately 90 percent of patients will remain in the group with essential hypertension. Undoubtedly, this group represents a spectrum of diseases and includes as-yet-undefined forms of secondary hypertension.

Symptoms and signs

Many patients with hypertension are identified in the course of routine examination and have no symptoms referable to the blood pressure elevation. When symptoms do bring the patient to the physician, they fall into three categories. They are related to (1) the elevated pressure itself, (2) the hypertensive vascular disease, and (3) the underlying disease in the case of secondary hypertension. Headache is the most consistent symptom related directly to the pressure elevation; most commonly it is localized to the occipital region, is present when the patient awakens in the morning, and subsides spontaneously after several hours. Other complaints include dizziness, palpitations, and easy fatigability. The earliest complaint referable to vascular disease often is epistaxis or hematuria, but may include blurring of vision due to retinal changes, episodes of weakness or dizziness due to transient cerebral ischemia, pain due to myocardial ischemia, and dyspnea due to cardiac failure. Chest pains due to dissection of the aorta or to a leaking aneurysm are less common presenting symptoms.

Examples of symptoms related to the underlying disease in secondary hypertension are polyuria, polydipsia, and muscle weakness secondary to hypokalemia in patients with *primary aldosteronism*, or weight gain and emotional lability in patients with *Cushing's syndrome*. The patient with a *pheochromocytoma* may present with episodic headaches, palpitations, and diaphoresis.

Clinical evaluation

The evaluation of the patient with hypertension has two principal objectives: (1) to identify secondary forms of hypertension; (2) to determine the presence and extent of hypertensive vascular disease.

HISTORY A strong family history of hypertension, along with the reported finding of labile pressure elevation in the past, favors the diagnosis of essential hypertension. The development of hypertension before the age of thirty-five or after the age of fifty years favors a secondary form. The history of use of *steroids* or *oral contraceptives* has obvious significance. History of repeated urinary tract infections or proteinuria suggests *renal parenchymal disease*; nocturia and polydipsia suggests *renal* or *endocrine disease*, while trauma to either flank or an episode of acute flank pain may be a clue to the presence of *renal injury*. A history of weight gain is compatible with *Cushing's syndrome*, while weight loss suggests *pheochromocytoma*. A number of aspects of the history aid in determining whether vascular disease has progressed to dangerous stages. These include chest pain due to myocardial ischemia, symptoms of cerebrovascular insufficiency, of congestive heart failure, and peripheral vascular insufficiency. Detailed discussions of these symptoms are presented in the chapters dealing with these specific conditions.

PHYSICAL EXAMINATION The physical examination starts with the patient's general appearance. Are the round face and trunkal obesity of Cushing's syndrome present? Are there features of acromegaly or myxedema? Are the purple striae and ecchymoses of Cushing's syndrome or the coarse skin of myxedema evident? Does muscular development in the upper extremities out of proportion to that in the lower extremities suggest coarctation of the aorta? The next step is to compare the blood pressures and pulses in both upper extremities, as well as measurements in the supine position, with measurements taken during standing. A rise in diastolic pressure when the patient goes from the supine to the standing position is most compatible with essential hypertension or renal arterial hypertension; a fall, in the absence of antihypertensive medications, suggests other forms of secondary hypertension. Detailed examination of the ocular fundi is mandatory, since fundoscopic findings provide one of the best indications of the duration of hypertension and of prognosis. The Keith-Wagener-Barker classification of fundoscopic changes (Table 33-2) is useful; the specific changes should be recorded and a grade assigned. Palpation and auscultation of the carotid arteries for evidence of stenosis or occlusion is important, since narrowing of a carotid artery may be a manifestation of hypertensive vascular disease, but it may also be a clue to the presence of a renal arterial lesion, since these two lesions may occur together. In examination of the heart and lungs one should search for evidence of left ventricular hypertrophy and cardiac decompensation. Is there a left ventricular lift? Are third and fourth heart sounds present? Are there pulmonary rales? Are the extracardiac murmurs and palpable collateral vessels that may result from coarctation of the aorta present? Bruits originating in stenotic renal arteries have both systolic and diastolic components and are best heard just to the right or left of the midline above the umbilicus, or in the flanks; they are heard in 80 percent of patients with renal artery stenosis due to fibrous dysplasia and in 40 to 50 percent of those with stenosis due to arteriosclerosis. The abdominal examination should also include palpation for abdominal aneurysm and for the enlarged kidneys of polycystic renal disease. The femoral pulses must be carefully palpated and, if they are decreased and/or delayed, blood pressure in the lower extremities must be measured. Even if it is normal to palpation, arterial pressure in the lower extremities should be recorded at least once in patients in whom hypertension is discovered before the age of thirty years. Finally, the neurologic examination is performed in a search for evidence of a previous cerebrovascular accident or of other intracranial pathologic change.

LABORATORY INVESTIGATION The laboratory tests and special studies that complete the clinical evaluation of the patient with hypertension are listed in Table 245-1. The first group should be performed in all patients with newly documented hypertension. Evaluation of renal status is carried out by urinalysis, a urine culture, determination of the serum creatinine level, and a rapid-sequence intravenous pyelogram. This combination of tests identifies a large majority of patients with renal disease and should give strong indication as to whether a *renal arterial* or a *renal parenchymal lesion* may be present. Findings consistent with renal parenchymal damage will raise the question of whether the damage is the cause or the result of the hypertension. However, the history, severity, and specific pattern of the findings of renal disease and of the hypertension usually are sufficient to answer this question.

Initial tests should also include blood sugar measurements, both because *diabetes mellitus* may be associated with accelerated arteriosclerosis and resultant *renal vascular disease*, and because *primary aldosteronism, Cushing's syndrome,* and *pheochromocytoma* all can cause hyperglycemia. Serum sodium, potassium, chloride, and bicarbonate levels should be obtained to screen for *mineralocorticoid excess*, and the possibility of *hypercalcemia* should be investigated. Serum uric acid should be measured because of the increased incidence of hyperuricemia in patients with *renal* and *essential hypertension*, which may be exaggerated by treatment with thiazide derivatives. Serum cholesterol and triglycerides should be measured to identify these other factors, which, besides hypertension, predispose to the development of *arteriosclerosis*. The electrocardiogram and chest roentgenogram yield information on cardiac status, and the latter also provides the opportunity to look for aortic dilatation or elongation and for the rib notching that occurs in coarctation of the aorta. Finally, the initial studies should include a 24-hr urine collection for measurement of catecholamines or one of their metabolites, metanephrine and vanillylmandelic acid. This test should be included even if the patient does not give a history of episodic attacks suggesting a pheochromocytoma, for this history is obtained in only about two-thirds of cases.

If the results of the above investigations indicate the possible presence of remediable secondary hypertension, the additional studies are needed.

TABLE 245-1
Laboratory tests and special studies for evaluation of hypertension

Always included

1 Urine
- *a* Urinalysis
- *b* Urine culture*
- *c* 24-hr urine catecholamines,* metanephrine, or vanillylmandelic acid

2 Blood
- *a* Na, K, Cl, CO_2
- *b* Creatinine
- *c* Fasting sugar and 2-hr postprandial sugar
- *d* Calcium
- *e* Uric acid
- *f* Cholesterol and triglycerides

3 Other
- *a* ECG
- *b* Posteroanterior chest x-ray
- *c* Rapid-sequence intravenous pyelogram

Sometimes included (on basis of clinical evaluation or results of above)

1 When clinical evaluation suggests Cushing's syndrome:
- *a* A.M. and P.M. plasma cortisol
- *b* 24-hr urine 17-OH or 17-ketogenic steroids
- *c* Fast dexamethasone suppression test

2 When clinical evaluation or intravenous pyelogram suggests renal artery stenosis:
- *a* Radioisotope renogram
- *b* Renal arteriogram
- *c* Renal vein plasma renin activity
- *d* Ureteral catheterization study

3 When hypokalemia suggests primary aldosteronism:
- *a* Plasma renin activity during Na restriction
- *b* Plasma aldosterone or 24-hr urine aldosterone during Na loading
- *c* Adrenal venography
- *d* Adrenal vein aldosterone

* *May be omitted on the basis of clinical evaluation and if patient is over forty years of age.*

Cushing's syndrome A 24-hr urine test for 17-hydroxy- or 17-ketogenic steroids or plasma cortisol levels can be used to screen for the presence of this condition; however, the more definitive text involves the administration of 1 mg dexamethasone at midnight, followed by measurement of plasma cortisol at 8 A.M. Supression of the plasma level to below 5 μg per 100 ml effectively rules out Cushing's syndrome (Chap. 86).

Renovascular hypertension The finding on the intravenous pyelogram of changes compatible with renal artery stenosis will dictate the need for *renal arteriography*. These changes are (1) unilateral delayed appearance and excretion of contrast material, (2) a difference in kidney size of at least 1.5 cm, (3) irregular contour of the renal silhouette, suggesting partial infarction or atrophy, and (4) indentations on the ureter or renal pelvis, possibly due to dilated ureteral arteries (collateral notching). Since these criteria identify only about 85 percent of patients with renal artery stenosis and hypertension, it is also appropriate to proceed to the arteriogram, even when the intravenous pyelogram is normal in certain groups of patients; namely, those who develop hypertension before the age of thirty-five or after the age of fifty years, those with an abdominal bruit, and those with severe or poorly controlled hypertension. The *isotope renogram* which measures differential uptake and excretion by the two kidneys of one of several isotope-labeled substances, can be used as a further screening procedure in these latter groups. Like the intravenous pyelogram, however, it is positive in 85 percent of instances. Because this test has false positives and false negatives and because it provides less substantial information than a pyelogram, suspicion based on the factors outlined above still can dictate proceeding to the arteriogram without performing this test or in the absence of a characteristic abnormality.

The *renal arteriogram* both establishes the presence of a renal arterial lesion and aids in determining whether the lesion is due to atherosclerosis or to one of the fibrous or fibromuscular dysplasias. It does not, however, prove that the lesion is responsible for the hypertension, nor does it permit prediction of the chances of surgical cure; it must be noted (1) that renal artery stenosis is a frequent finding at postmortem in normotensive individuals, and (2) that essential hypertension is a common condition which may occur in combination with renal arterial stenosis, which is not necessarily responsible for the hypertension in the patient with an elevated arterial pressure. Determination of bilateral renal vein *plasma renin activity* is preferred over ureteral catheterization for assessing the functional significance of any lesion. When one kidney is ischemic and the other is normal, all the renin released comes from the involved kidney. In the most straightforward situation, the ischemic kidney has a significantly higher venous plasma renin activity than the normal kidney by a factor of 1.5 or 2.0 to 1.0. Moreover, the uninvolved kidney exhibits levels similar to those in the inferior vena cava below the entrance of renal veins. Significant benefit from operative correction may be anticipated in at least 80 percent of patients with the findings described above in whom the ratio of plasma renin activities from the renal vein on the involved side exceeds 1.5/1.0.

A high sodium intake can mask the differences in renin production between the two kidneys, while sodium depletion accentuates it; therefore, the patient should be placed on a 250- to 500-mg low-sodium diet for 3 to 5 days before the study. Intravenous hydralazine (20 mg) also accentuates the difference. When obstructing lesions in the branches of the renal arteries are demonstrated by arteriography, an attempt to obtain blood samples from the main branches of the renal vein should be made in an effort to identify a localized intrarenal arterial lesion responsible for the hypertension.

Primary aldosteronism The diagnosis of this cause of secondary hypertension is discussed in Chap. 86. Diuretic therapy often complicates the picture when the hypertensive patient with hypokalemia is first seen. To determine if the diuretic is the cause of the hypokalemia, 24-hr urine potassium excretion is measured immediately following discontinuance of therapy, without adding potassium supplements. Excretion of less than 40 mEq ordinarily indicates that potassium conservation is appropriate; excretion of 40 mEq or more, while serum potassium concentration is less than 3.6 mEq per liter is presumptive evidence of inappropriately high aldosterone secretion. The relation between plasma renin activity and the aldosterone level is a key observation in the diagnosis of primary aldosteronism. The aldosterone concentration or excretion is high and plasma renin activity is low in primary aldosteronism, and these levels are relatively unaffected by changes in sodium balance.

A significant number of patients with normal serum potassium levels have suppressed plasma renin activity during sodium restriction. A very small fraction of these have been claimed to have normokalemic primary aldosteronism, but the reason for renin suppression is not clear in most of these patients. Perhaps they have another form of adrenal cortical hypertension. Because of the existence of this group of patients, the argument may be advanced that every patient with hypertension should have a plasma renin measurement during sodium restriction, even though his serum potassium level is normal. Mineralocorticoid measurements would not need to be made unless the plasma renin activity proved to be suppressed. Though the identification of this group of patients with suppressed plasma renin activity may well have therapeutic and prognostic implications (see further on), until further data regarding this important issue become available, the routine measurement of plasma renin activity in hypertensive patients without findings suggestive of renovascular disease or mineralocorticoid excess is better left as an investigative procedure.

Further evaluation of patients with hypertension who prove to have hypercalcemia or whose screening studies suggest a diagnosis of Cushing's syndrome or pheochromocytoma is discussed in the appropriate chapters (Chaps. 86 and 87).

Hypertension is a common condition and affects approximately 20 million Americans. When communities are screened for hypertension, the expense and effort involved may not permit a detailed workup of all hypertensive subjects for secondary hypertension. Under these circumstances it may be possible to limit the rapid-sequence intravenous pyelogram and vanillylmandelic acid to individuals under the age of forty years and to those over the age of forty who present with clinical evidence suggestive of renovascular hypertension or pheochromocytoma and to those who fail to respond to medical treatment. Urine culture might also be deferred unless the need is suggested by the history or by the findings of proteinuria or by white blood cells in the sediment.

Prognosis

When the clinical evaluation has been completed, the next step is to decide upon treatment, which must be considered in the light of current information about the prognosis of hypertension. Abundant statistical evidence indicates that diastolic hypertension results in shortening of life span; studies of large populations have shown an inverse correlation between the height of the arterial pressure and the length of survival. Prognosis for untreated hypertension is worse in males than in females and in blacks than in nonblacks. Obviously, the outlook is poorer if there is evidence of vascular complications when the patient is first seen. Factors affecting prognosis, listed roughly in order of increasing gravity, are shown in Table 245-2. It has been suggested that the level of plasma renin activity may also be of prognostic importance, since patients with low plasma renin activity appear to have a lower incidence of cerebrovascular accident and

TABLE 245-2
Factors indicating an adverse prognosis in hypertension

1 Black race
2 Youth
3 Male
4 Persistent diastolic pressure, >115 mm Hg
5 Marked cardiac enlargement
6 ECG changes of ischemia or left ventricular strain
7 Myocardial infarction
8 Congestive heart failure
9 Cerebrovascular accident
10 Impaired renal function*
11 Retinal hemorrhages and exudates
12 Papilledema

* *When due to hypertensive vascular disease.*

myocardial infarction than patients with normal or elevated renin levels and similar degrees of hypertension.

Prior to the development of effective therapy the mean life span from the time of apparent onset of untreated hypertension was approximately 20 years. This span could be divided into an uncomplicated phase, lasting an average of 15 years and a final phase lasting an average of 5 years, when vascular disease became manifest and led to death. The commonest cause of death was congestive heart failure, but cerebrovascular accident, myocardial infarction, renal failure, and ruptured aortic aneurysm were also observed. Patients with untreated secondary hypertension have factors in addition to the blood pressure elevation which influence prognosis. An example of this is the patient with hypertension due to renal parenchymal disease, whose prognosis depends also upon the nature of renal disease.

Evidence continues to mount in support of the effectiveness of antihypertensive drug therapy in improving prognosis. Impressive validation is supplied by the 5-year prospective study of the Veterans Administration Cooperative Study Group on Antihypertensive Agents. The differences in incidence of severe complicating events between the actively treated and placebo-treated groups with diastolic pressures of 115 to 129 mm Hg became so striking after the first 3 years that the study in these groups was terminated. At the end of 5 years the benefits of therapy also were clear-cut for the groups with diastolic pressures of 90 to 114 mm Hg. In these groups, the estimated risk of developing a morbid event was reduced from 55 to 18 percent by treatment, but the incidence of myocardial infarction was not altered. The study included only male patients, and they were placed in the study on the basis of diastolic pressures determined from the fourth to the sixth day of hospitalization. Since blood pressure usually falls during hospitalization, these patients probably had even higher levels as outpatients. Furthermore, when the patients with the lower diastolic pressures of 90 to 104 mm Hg were considered separately, results showed a beneficial trend, but were not definitive.

The effectiveness of surgical therapy in improving the prognosis in patients with renovascular hypertension is also established, except in the elderly patient with renal artery stenosis due to arteriosclerosis. Such patients are very likely to die within a short period of time from another complication of arteriosclerosis, even though hypertension is successfully treated.

Treatment

STRATEGY Virtually every patient with sustained diastolic hypertension is a candidate for diagnostic studies and for subsequent treatment. This conclusion must be tempered with the arguments that it is difficult to show conclusive benefits in patients with only slight pressure elevations. Since women appear to tolerate elevated arterial pressures better than men do, the conclusions concerning men cannot be directly applied to women, particularly in those with diastolic pressures under 100 mm Hg. Furthermore, it may be argued that it is hard to justify making a patient with mild hypertension who starts with no complaints feel uncomfortable because of the side effects of therapy. On the other hand, it is not difficult to justify side effects in patients with severe hypertension, because they receive the greatest benefit from therapy. Fortunately, the choice of treatment is such that a satisfactory program to control arterial pressure with minimal side effects can be developed for most patients. All men with diastolic pressure above 95 mm Hg on repeated outpatient examinations, and all women with diastolic pressure repeatedly above 100 mm Hg, should be treated unless specific contraindications exist. There is considerable controversy regarding the advisability of treating *isolated systolic hypertension*. Until the results of a well-controlled prospective study provide evidence to the contrary, treatment of isolated systolic hypertension is not recommended. Patients with labile hypertension, isolated systolic hypertension, or borderline levels and who are not treated should have regular follow-up examinations at 6-month intervals, because of the frequent development of progressive increase in the blood pressure.

The identification of an operable form of *secondary hypertension* does not automatically mean that surgical treatment is indicated. The decision depends upon the age and general health of the patient, the natural history of the lesion, and the response of the pressure to drug therapy. In renal artery stenosis the feasibility of vascular repair versus nephrectomy and the degree of overall renal functional impairment must also be considered. Age and general health are particularly important in patients with renal artery stenosis due to arteriosclerosis, because there is no evidence that repair of the stenosis increases life expectancy in the elderly patient. Knowledge of the natural history of the disease is especially important when approaching the decision in the young patient with renal artery stenosis due to fibrous dysplasia. If the arteriographic appearance suggests that the stenosis is due to intimal or subadventitial fibroplasia, the lesion may be expected to progress and operation is required. Medial fibroplasia, on the other hand, often remains stable, and operation may not be necessary if pressure can be controlled by drug therapy. The decision regarding operation should also be considered particularly carefully in the patient with primary aldosteronism when bilateral adrenal venography does not demonstrate a tumor, because this patient may prove to have multinodular hyperplasia. This means that bilateral adrenalectomy would be required to eliminate the aldosterone excess, and even then, hypertension may persist. If hypokalemia can be controlled by spironolactone, then it is reasonable to withhold surgery.

GENERAL MEASURES The general measures employed in the treatment of hypertension are (1) relief of stress, (2) control of diet, and (3) regular exercise. Relief of emotional and environmental stress is one of the reasons for the improvement in hypertension that occurs when the patient is hospitalized and placed at rest. Though it is usually impossible to extricate the hypertensive patient from all his internal and external stresses, he should be advised to avoid any unnecessary tensions. In rare instances, it may be appropriate to recommend a change of job or of life style.

Dietary management has three aspects: (1) Because of the documented efficacy of sodium restriction and volume contraction in lowering blood pressure, patients previously were instructed to curtail sodium intake drastically. Most patients, however, were unwilling or unable to follow a diet low enough in sodium to be of great benefit. The advent of effective oral diuretics provided an additional method of decreasing body sodium stores, and the most practical approach now is to advise mild dietary sodium restriction (up to 4 g salt per day) in conjunction with an oral diuretic. (2) *Caloric restriction* should be urged for the patient who is overweight. Some obese patients will show a significant reduction in pressure simply as a consequence of weight loss. (3) A moderate *restriction in intake of cholesterol and saturated fats* is recommended; this is based on the identification of hypertension as a risk factor in the development of arteriosclerosis and on the suggestive evidence that such a diet may diminish the incidence of arteriosclerotic complications. (4) *Regular exercise* is indicated in every patient within the limits of his cardiovascular status. Not only is exercise helpful in controlling weight, but, in addition, there is evidence that physical conditioning itself lowers arterial pressure.

DRUG THERAPY To make rational use of antihypertensive drugs, the sites and mechanisms of their action must be understood. The only drugs that appear to have a major *central action* are *alpha-methyldopa* and the new investigational agent, *clonidine*. The antihypertensive actions of *rauwolfia alkaloids* and *hydralazine* may also depend, but perhaps to a lesser extent, on a central action. Sedatives and tranquilizers obviously also act on the central nervous system but do not exert a direct effect on blood pressure; however, they may be helpful in particularly anxious patients.

The *ganglionic blocking agents* were the first effective antihypertensive drugs available. These drugs block the action of acetylcholine on the postganglionic neuron and prevent impulse transmission in the autonomic nervous systems. This has little effect when the patient is supine, but prevents reflex vasoconstriction in the upright position. Ganglionic blocking agents interfere with parasympathetic as well as sympathetic function, and this results in such side effects as impairment of visual accommodation, paralytic ileus, retention of urine, and failure of erection and ejaculation. Presently, because of these problems, ganglionic blocking agents are largely reserved for the rapid lowering of arterial pressure in patients with severe hypertension.

Various drugs act at *postganglionic nerve endings*. The *rauwolfia alkaloids* are the oldest members of the group and their long-term effect results from their ability to inhibit the storage of norepinephrine within the vesicles in adrenergic nerve endings and thus lead to depletion of catecholamine stores. When given parenterally they also have a direct effect on vascular smooth muscle. The rauwolfia alkaloids exhibit the undesirable side effects that result from the unopposed activity of the parasympathetic nervous system, including nasal congestion, diarrhea, impairment of sexual function, and increased gastric secretion. Depression is their most serious side effect, and this is most likely to occur in elderly patients. The rauwolfia alkaloids are most helpful in the treatment by the oral route of mild to moderate hypertension in younger patients and in the treatment of malignant hypertension by the parenteral route. The antihypertensive effect of alpha-methyldopa appears to be related mainly to an action on the central nervous system but also to blockade of sympathetic nervous impulses. The commonest side effects are transient drowsiness and a feeling of fatigue; approximately 20 percent of patients develop a positive direct Coombs test result; rarely, this is accompanied by hemolytic anemia. *Guanethidine*, perhaps the most effective antihypertensive agent in general use, blocks the release of norepinephrine from the sympathetic nerve endings. It has a greater postural effect than the other drugs that work at the nerve endings, and orthostatic hypotension is a frequent side effect. The *monoamine oxidase inhibitor*, *pargyline*, acts centrally and peripherally by blocking the degradation of catecholamines. The increased stores of catecholamines that result include amines that are false neurotransmitters, and these may dilute and reduce the quantity of norepinephrine released. The tyramine present in such foods as aged cheese, wine, beer, and pickled herring has the potential for precipitously releasing the increased stores of catecholamines present in patients being treated with monoamine oxidase inhibition and may thus cause a hypertensive crisis.

Phenotolamine and *phenoxybenzamine* block the action of circulating norepinephrine at *alpha-adrenergic receptor sites*. Since high circulating levels of norepinephrine are not present in most patients with hypertension, alpha blockade usually is not effective in lowering pressure. The exception, of course, is the patient with pheochromocytoma. *Propranolol*, an effective *beta-adrenergic receptor* blocking agent, blocks sympathetic effects on the heart (Chap. 235) and should theoretically be effective in reducing cardiac output and in lowering arterial pressure when there is increased sympathetic nerve activity. In practice, however, it is effective more often than that, with about one-third or more of all patients showing some fall in pressure, perhaps resulting primarily from a decrease in cardiac output. However, it has been reported to be particularly effective in patients with essential hypertension and high or normal plasma renin activities. In these cases the antihypertensive action appears to be closely linked to an inhibition of renin secretion. Propranolol can precipitate congestive heart failure and asthma in susceptible individuals, and it is also contraindicated in diabetics receiving hypoglycemic therapy, because it inhibits the usual sympathetic responses to hypoglycemia.

Hydralazine is the most versatile of the drugs that cause direct relaxation of *vascular smooth muscle*; it is effective both orally and parenterally, acting mainly on arterial *resistance*, rather than on venous *capacitance* vessels, as evidenced by lack of postural changes. Unfortunately, the effect of hydralazine on peripheral resistance is partly negated by reflex increases in sympathetic discharges that raise heart rate and cardiac output. These limit the usefulness of hydralazine, especially in patients with severe coronary artery disease. However, the efficacy of hydralazine can be increased if it is given in conjunction with propranolol so that the reflex effects on the heart are blocked. A serious side effect of doses of hydralazine exceeding 200 mg per day has been the production of a lupus erythematosus-like syndrome. A very interesting drug in the same category as hydralazine is the new thiazide derivative, *diazoxide*. It is not a diuretic and, in fact, causes sodium retention. However, like the other thiazides, it reduces carbohydrate tolerance. It must be given rapidly intravenously to guarantee effect, and it begins to act immediately to lower blood pressure. Its effects may last for several hours or more; it appears to be useful for the treatment of hypertensive emergencies.

Drugs active on the *renal tubules* affect arterial pressure primarily by causing sodium diuresis and volume depletion; these agents are discussed in detail in Chap. 233. The thiazides are the most frequently used and most extensively investigated members of this group, and their early effect certainly is related to the diuresis. A reduction in peripheral vascular resistance also has been reported by some workers to be important in the long term. Thiazide diuretics form the cornerstone of most therapeutic programs. Their most frequent side effects are hypokalemia due to renal potassium loss, hyperuricemia due to uric acid retention, and carbohydrate intolerance. The newer and more potent diuretics, *furosemide* and *ethacrynic acid*, also have been shown to be antihypertensive, but the more evanescent actions and great potency do not lend themselves to long-term therapy. It is not yet established whether, like the thiazides, these agents have hypotensive effects beyond sodium diuresis. *Spironolactone* causes renal sodium loss by blocking the effect of endogenous mineralocorticoids, and therefore it is most effective in patients whose mineralocorticoids are present in excess. It provides specific therapy for patients with primary aldosteronism and may also be helpful in hypertensive patients with low plasma renin activity and normal aldosterone levels, as well as in hypertensive patients with signs of secondary aldosteronism. Spironolactone can also be given along with thiazide diuretics to minimize renal potassium loss.

APPROACH TO DRUG THERAPY The aim of drug therapy is to use the agents just described, alone or in combination, to return arterial pressure to normal levels with minimal side effects. When drugs are used in combination, they should have different sites of action. Since many effective antihypertensive agents are available, a number of useful therapeutic regimens have been developed. The following plan of therapy is suggested for patients with essential hypertension without contraindications to specific agents, such as those listed in Table 245-3. The first drug employed is a *thiazide diuretic*. Even if not effective by itself, it potentiates the action of other hypotensive agents. If a second drug is needed, a rauwolfia alkaloid or alpha-methyldopa may be added. Although rauwolfia is less expensive than alpha-methyldopa it is often less well tolerated, particularly by older patients. If the thiazide diuretic and maximally tolerated doses of the rauwolfia alkaloid or alpha-methyldopa are still ineffective in returning pressure to normal levels, *hydralazine* is added. If pressure still is not controlled, the next step is to substitute the more potent sympatholytic drug, *guanethidine* for the rauwolfia alkaloid or for alpha-methyldopa. Patients with diastolic pressures above 120 mm Hg prior to treatment will usually require more than one drug for control, and the combination of a thiazide and rauwolfia or alpha-methyldopa may be started initially in these patients. There are only a few patients in whom blood pressure cannot be adequately controlled with the above approach. In these, use of other drugs discussed in the previous section should be considered. Failure to obtain adequate pressure control may be due to insufficient volume depletion, and more vigorous dietary sodium restriction and diuretic administration may be helpful in resistant cases.

Reduction of arterial pressure in hypertensive patients with impaired renal function is often accompanied by an initial increase in serum creatinine. These changes do not represent further structural renal damage, and they should not deter continuation of therapy, since achievement of blood pressure control may eventually reduce these values toward normal. Therapy in the azotemic patient, however, should emphasize the use of those drugs that have the least propensity to lower renal blood flow, namely, hydralazine, clonidine, and alpha-methyldopa. However, the latter drug may accumulate in the presence of renal failure, and the dosage might have to be reduced.

The patient with severe hypertension who becomes unresponsive to a previously effective antihypertensive regimen presents a special problem. An approach that has proved effective in some patients involves the use of intravenous injections of diazoxide for 7 to 10 days. This program may result in sustained lowering of blood pressure and, for the reasons that are not clear, may restore responsiveness to other antihypertensive agents. It is postulated that this program resets pressoreceptors downward toward "normal."

It must be emphasized that a very small fraction (probably less than one-fifth) of hypertensive patients in the United States is being treated effectively. Only a small number of these failures is related to drug unresponsiveness. The majority are related to (1) failure of detection of hypertension; (2) failure of institution of effective treatment of the asymptomatic hypertensive subject; and (3) failure of the asymptomatic hypertensive subject to adhere to therapy. In order to improve this deficiency, widespread screening for hypertension is necessary, and patients must be educated to continue treatment once an effective regimen required for a particular patient has been identified. Side effects of treatment must be minimized or counteracted in order to obtain the patients' continued cooperation.

MALIGNANT HYPERTENSION

In addition to marked blood pressure elevation in association with papilledema, the full-blown picture of malignant hypertension usually includes manifestations of *hyper-*

TABLE 245-3
Drugs used in treatment of hypertension—listed according to site of action

Site of action	*Drug*	*Dosage*	*Indications*	*Contraindications*	*Frequent or peculiar side effects*
Central	Clonidine	Oral: 0.2–0.6 mg q.i.d.	Mild to moderate hypertension, renal disease with hypertension		Postural hypotension, drowsiness, dry mouth
	Alpha-methyldopa (also acts by blocking sympathetic nerves)	Oral: 250–750 mg t.i.d–q.i.d. IV: 500–1000 mg q.4–6 h. (tolerance may develop)	Mild to moderate hypertension (oral), malignant hypertension (IV), in patients who cannot take oral treatment, renal disease with hypertension	Pheochromocytoma, active hepatic disease (IV), during MAO inhibitor administration	Postural hypotension, sedation, fatigue, diarrhea, impaired ejaculation, fever, gynecomastia, lactation, positive Coombs tests (occasionally associated with hemolysis)
	Sedatives and tranquilizers		Tense or anxious patient with hypertension		Drowsiness, fatigue
	Phenobarbital	Oral: 15–30 mg t.i.d.–q.i.d.			
	Diazepam	Oral: 2–10 mg q.i.d.			
Ganglions			Severe or malignant hypertension	Severe coronary artery disease, cerebrovascular insufficiency, diabetes mellitus (on hypoglycemic therapy), glaucoma, prostatism	Postural hypotension, visual symptoms, dry mouth, constipation, urinary retention, impotence
	Trimethaphan	IV: 1–10 mg/min			
	Pentolinium	IV: 1–5 mg/min IM: 2–5 mg q.2–6 h.			
	Mecamylamine	Oral: 2.5–10 mg q. 8–12 h. (most completely absorbed of oral blocking agents)			Tremors, confusion
Nerve endings	Rauwolfia alkaloids		Mild to moderate hypertension in young patient	Pheochromocytoma, peptic ulcer, depression, during MAO inhibitor administration	Depression, nightmares, nasal congestion, dyspepsia, diarrhea, impotence
	Reserpine	Oral: 0.1–0.5 mg q.d.			
	Guanethidine	Oral: 10–300 mg q.d.	Severe hypertension	Pheochromocytoma, severe coronary artery disease, cerebrovascular insufficiency, during MAO inhibitor administration	Postural hypotension, bradycardia, dry mouth, diarrhea, impaired ejaculation, fluid retention
	Pargyline	Oral: 10–100 mg q.d.	Depressed patient with moderate to severe hypertension	Pheochromocytoma, severe coronary artery disease, cerebrovascular insufficiency, hyperthyroidism, paranoid schizophrenia, during administration of other drugs that act at same site	Postural hypotension, insomnia, nightmares, diarrhea, muscle twitching, acute hypertension (induced by tyramine-containing foods and certain drugs)

tensive encephalopathy, such as severe headache, vomiting, visual disturbances (including transient blindness), transient paralyses, convulsions, stupor, and coma. These have been attributed to spasms of cerebral vessels and to cerebral edema. In some of these patients who have died, multiple small thrombi have been found in the cerebral vessels. Cardiac decompensation and rapidly declining renal function are other critical features of malignant hypertension. Oliguria may, in fact, be the presenting feature. The vascular lesion characteristic of malignant hypertension is fibrinoid necrosis of the walls of small arteries and arterioles, which may be reversed by effective antihypertensive therapy.

The pathogenesis of malignant hypertension is unknown. Many patients show evidence of a microangiopathic hemolytic anemia; this appears to be a secondary phenomenon, which could, however, contribute to the deterioration of renal function. Most patients also have elevated levels of peripheral plasma renin activity and increased aldosterone production which may be critically involved in causing severe vascular damage.

About 5 percent of hypertensive patients develop the malignant phase, which occurs in the course of both essential and secondary hypertension and occasionally is the first manifestation of the blood pressure problem. The average age at diagnosis is forty, and men are more often affected than women. Prior to the availability of effective therapy, life expectancy after the diagnosis of malignant hypertension was less than 2 years, with most deaths being due to uremia, cerebral hemorrhage, or congestive heart failure. With the advent of effective antihypertensive therapy, at least a third of patients survive for more than 5 years.

Malignant hypertension requires immediate therapy. A

TABLE 245-3 (*continued*)

Site of action	*Drug*	*Dosage*	*Indications*	*Contraindications*	*Frequent or peculiar side effects*
Alpha receptors	Phentolamine	IV: 1–5 mg	Suspected or proved pheochromocytoma	Severe coronary artery disease	Tachycardia, weakness, dizziness, flushing
	Phenoxybenzamine	Oral: 10–50 mg q.d.–b.i.d., (tolerance may develop)	Proved pheochromocytoma		Postural hypotension, tachycardia, miosis, nasal congestion, dry mouth
Beta receptors	Propranolol	Oral: 10–40 mg q.i.d.	Mild hypertension (especially with evidence for hyperdynamic circulation), adjunct to hydralazine therapy, pheochromocytoma	Congestive heart failure, asthma, diabetes mellitus (on hypoglycemic therapy), during MAO inhibitor administration	Dizziness, depression bronchospasm, nausea, vomiting, diarrhea, constipation, heart failure
Vascular smooth muscle	Hydralazine	Oral: 10–50 mg q.i.d. IV or IM: 10–50 mg q.6h. (tolerance may develop)	As adjunct in treatment of moderate to severe hypertension (oral), malignant hypertension (IV or IM), renal disease with hypertension	Lupus erythematosus, severe coronary artery disease, mitral valvular rheumatic heart disease	Headache, tachycardia, angina pectoris, anorexia, nausea, vomiting, diarrhea, lupus syndrome
	Diazoxide	IV: 300 mg rapidly	Severe or malignant hypertension	Diabetes mellitus, hyperuricemia, congestive heart failure	Hyperglycemia, hyperuricemia, sodium retention
	Rauwolfia alkaloids Reserpine	IM: 2.5–5 mg q.6 h.	Malignant hypertension	Pheochromocytoma, during MAO inhibitor administration	Lethargy, nasal congestion, facial flushing, extrapyramidal signs
Renal tubule	Thiazides		Mild hypertension, as adjunct in treatment of moderate to severe hypertension	Diabetes mellitus, hyperuricemia, primary aldosteronism	Potassium depletion, hyperglycemia, hyperuricemia, dermatitis, purpura
	Hydrochlorothiazide	Oral: 25–50 mg q.d.–b.i.d.			
	Furosemide	Oral: 20–40 mg q.d.–b.i.d.	Mild hypertension	Hyperuricemia, primary aldosteronism	Potassium depletion, hyperuricemia, nausea, vomiting, diarrhea
	Ethacrynic acid	Oral: 25–50 mg q.d.–b.i.d.	Mild hypertension	Hyperuricemia, primary aldosteronism	Potassium depletion, hyperuricemia, diarrhea
	Spironolactone	Oral: 25–100 mg t.i.d.–q.i.d.	Hypertension due to hypermineralocorticoidism, adjunct to thiazide therapy	Renal failure	Hyperuricemia, diarrhea, gynecomastia, menstrual irregularities
	Triamterine	Oral: 100 mg q.d.–t.i.d.	Hypertension due to hypermineralocorticoidism, adjunct to thiazide therapy	Renal failure	Hyperkalemia, nausea, vomiting, leg cramps

useful preliminary step is to perform a phentolamine test or check urinary catecholamine levels to screen for the presence of a pheochromocytoma. Unless previous evaluations have excluded the diagnosis, it is imperative that this be done. Though a positive phentolamine test is not absolutely diagnostic for pheochromocytoma, it alerts the physician to avoid using drugs that have the potential for releasing the increased catecholamine stores (e.g., rauwolfia alkaloids, alpha-methyldopa, and guanethidine). The initial aim of therapy should be to reduce diastolic pressure toward, but not below, 90 mm Hg. Preliminary reports suggest that diazoxide may be the ideal drug for initial control of malignant hypertension. If a delay of approximately 2 hr in attainment of the full effect is acceptable, intravenous *alpha-methyldopa* is an effective drug with which to begin therapy. A dose of 500 mg alpha-methyldopa in 100 to 200 ml of 5 percent dextrose in water is given intravenously over 30 min; if the effect is inadequate in 2 to 4 hr, a second dose of 500 to 1,000 mg is given. Additional intravenous doses may then be given every 6 hr until the pressure has stabilized. If alpha-methyldopa is ineffective, or if a more rapid response is desired, intravenous *hydralazine* can be used. It usually begins to work within 10 min; an effective protocol involves giving 10-mg doses intravenously every 10 to 15 min until the desired effect has been obtained or until a total of 50 mg has been administered. The total dose required for response may then be repeated intramuscularly or intravenously every 6 hr. Hydralazine should be used with caution in patients with significant coronary artery disease. Intramuscular reserpine in doses of 1 to 2.5 mg also is an effective agent, and has an onset of action in 2 to 4 hr. Unfortunately, some patients demonstrate unexpected sensitivity, and the resulting hypotension may persist for several hours. Also, marked central nervous system depression often occurs, especially in elderly patients.

If the above measures fail, if the patient is having convulsions, or if arterial pressure must be reduced rapidly, it may be necessary to use a ganglionic blocking agent. *Trimethaphen* or the longer-acting *pentolinium* is diluted in 5% dextrose in water and infused at a rate to maintain the desired pressure level. The patient should be in the sitting position and the pressure monitored closely, preferably in an intensive care unit. After the pressure has been controlled for 8 to 24 hr it should be possible to switch to intramuscular pentolinium on a 3-to 6-hr schedule, and then to the more conventional oral agents. Guanethidine almost certainly should be one of the oral agents in patients who need an intravenous ganglionic blocking agent for initial control. As an alternative to ganglionic agents, intravenous *nitroprusside* may be employed. This is perhaps the most potent of all antihypertensive agents. The drug acts similarly to diazoxide, but its onset and offset are almost immediate. It should be made up fresh, 100 mg in 500 ml dextrose, and given by pump, under carefully supervised conditions, to achieve desired response.

The potent diuretics, furosemide and ethacrynic acid, are important adjuncts to the therapy just discussed. Given either orally or intravenously they serve to maintain sodium diuresis in the face of a falling blood pressure and thus will speed recovery from encephalopathy and congestive heart failure. If hypokalemia is a problem, *spironolactone* may be given. *Digitalis* (Chap. 235) also is indicated if there is evidence of cardiac decompensation.

There is some hope even for patients who fail to respond sufficiently to any of the forms of therapy and who show progressive deterioration in renal function. In some, a period of peritoneal dialysis or hemodialysis to deplete extracellular fluid has resulted in better blood pressure control and eventual improvement in renal function. In other patients with refractory hypertension and renal failure who do not respond to volume depletion, particularly those with marked elevation of plasma renin activity, bilateral nephrectomy has resulted in amelioration of hypertension; subsequently these patients have been maintained on chronic dialysis or have received renal homografts.

REFERENCES

Biglieri EG: Evaluation of renal vascular hypertension and primary hyperaldosteronism. Calif Med 115:40, 1971

—— et al: Adrenal mineralocorticoids causing hypertension. Am J Med 52:623, 1972

Bourne HR, Melmon KL: Guides to the pharmacologic management of essential hypertension. Ration Drug Ther 5:1, 1971

Brown JJ et al: Comparison of surgery and prolonged spironolactone therapy in patients with hypertension, aldosterone excess, and low plasma renin. Brit Med J 2:729, 1972

Crane MG et al: Hyporeninemic hypertension. Am J Med 52:457, 1972

Dustan HP et al: Differential diagnosis of etiologic types of hypertension. Prog Cardiovasc Dis 14:210, 1971

Freis ED: The treatment of hypertension. Why, when, and how. Am J Med 52:664, 1972

Freis ED et al: Guidelines for the detection, diagnosis and management of hypertensive populations. Circulation 44:A-263, 1971

Hurst JW: *The Heart*, 3d ed., Part VI, Section E, Systemic Hypertension (chaps. 56–65) New York: McGraw-Hill, 1974, pp. 1162–1247

Hunt JC (ed): Hypertension in man and the experimental animal. Supplement to Circulation Research Vol. 21, 1973

Kaufman JJ et al: Hypertension—primary and secondary. Ann Intern Med 75:761, 1971

Laragh JH et al: Renin, angiotensin, and aldosterone system in pathogenesis and management of hypertensive vascular disease. Am J Med 52:633, 1972

Ledingham JM: Mechanisms in renal hypertension. Proc Roy Soc Med 64:409, 1971

Melby JD et al: 18-Hydroxy-deoxycorticosterone in human hypertension. Circ Res 28-29 (suppl. 2):143, 1971

Perera GA: Hypertensive vascular disease; description and natural history. J Chron Dis 1:33, 1955

Veterans Administration Cooperative Study Group on Antihypertensive Agents: Effects of treatment on morbidity in hypertension. JAMA 202:116, 1967; 213:1143, 1970

246 DISEASES OF THE AORTA

VICTOR A. McKUSICK

DISSECTING ANEURYSM OF THE AORTA

Dissecting aneurysm occurs more commonly in men. Under the age of forty years, approximately half the instances of dissecting aneurysm in women occur in relation to pregnancy. Hormonal changes associated with pregnancy seem to be responsible for effects on connective tissues, including those of the aorta.

Usually from an intimal rent in the ascending aorta, dissection extends proximally to the aortic ring and distally for a variable distance. (Occasionally an intimal rent is absent. Bleeding into the media from the vasa vasorum is obviously important in such cases and probably is important in the initiation of most cases; hence the synonyms for dissecting aneurysm: medial hematoma and dissecting hematoma of the aorta.) "Reentry" may take place at some site such as just beyond the left subclavian orifice or in the abdominal aorta, with creation of a "double-barrel aorta." Prognosis is better in such cases. The dissection may extend for a considerable distance into one or several of the branches of the aorta, from the coronary arteries to the iliac arteries. The proximal dissection may distort the aortic ring and result in aortic regurgitation. (Cystic medial necrosis antedating the dissection may have resulted in dilatation of the sinuses of Valsalva and aortic regurgitation.) Rupture of the aorta into the pericardial or pleural cavity occurs in a majority of cases, although other sites of rupture such as the transverse portion of the duodenum are occasionally observed. Rupture into the pericardial sac is not surprising since the pericardial deflections extend high on the ascending aorta in many persons.

DeBakey proposed the following useful anatomic classification of dissecting aneurysm: type I, those starting in the ascending aorta and extending for a variable distance beyond the arch, often the entire length of the aorta; type II, those limited to the ascending aorta, a finding particularly in the Marfan syndrome; type III, those limited to the aorta beyond the mouth of the left subclavian artery.

The clinical manifestations of dissecting aneurysm may be classified as follows: (1) pain, (2) aortic regurgitation, (3) interference with the blood supply through branches of the aorta, (4) x-ray evidence of progressive widening of the aorta, (5) rupture of the aorta.

In addition, tissue destruction may be of sufficient proportions to produce mild fever, leukocytosis, and elevation of sedimentation rate.

The pain of dissecting aneurysm is sometimes described as tearing in quality. It is questionable that its quality is truly different from that of myocardial infarction. Characteristically it attains peak intensity very shortly after onset. It may involve the anterior part of the chest, back, lumbar area, or abdomen, sometimes in a progression. Dissecting aneurysm may occur, however, with little or nothing the patient describes as pain. The blood pressure may drop precipitously during the dissection, but maintenance of hypertension or increased blood pressure in response to the pain is often the finding.

The most frequently observed evidence of disturbance at the orifices of the branches is discrepancy in the pulses and blood pressure readings in the arms. Asymmetric diminution in these signs may occur. The same observations may be made in the carotid and femoral vessels. Myocardial infarction or changes of myocardial ischemia, neurologic signs from interference with cerebral and/or spinal blood flow, intestinal symptoms, and hematuria may occur.

Rupture of the aorta is, of course, usually fatal. However, in rare instances leakage into the pericardial cavity may be interrupted and the patient may survive for months or even years. The chest pain, together with a pericardial friction rub, may indicate the presence of leaking dissecting aneurysm hours before the leak proceeds to the point of producing cardiac tamponade.

In the differential diagnosis of dissecting aneurysm, myocardial infarction and pulmonary embolus present the greatest problems. Pain reaching a rapid peak of intensity, especially if followed within minutes or hours by signs of arterial occlusion, favors the diagnosis of dissecting aneurysm. Unconsciousness may result from involvement of the cephalic trunks in the dissection and is unusual in myocardial infarction in the absence of severe hypotension or arrhythmia. The maintenance of arterial hypertension favors the diagnosis of dissecting aneurysm, although profound hypotension may occur in both dissection and myocardial infarction.

Only a few patients survive more than a few days after an acute dissection. Most of the survivors succumb to rupture of the aorta or other complications within a year. Pharmacologic hypotension in those cases with maintained hypertension during the acute dissection has a rational place in treatment of the early stages. In normotensive patients, reserpine or propranolol in subhypotensive doses, by changing the shape of the ventricular ejection curve and reducing the abruptness of ejection, may be beneficial. (Reserpine has been effective in reducing the incidence of aortic rupture in strains of turkeys predisposed to this accident.) Significant aortic regurgitation, evidence of encroachment on the ostiums of branch arteries, especially the renals, inability to maintain a normal blood pressure, evidence of progressive dissection or of adventitial rupture are all indications that surgical intervention should be considered.

CYSTIC MEDIAL NECROSIS This is the most frequent morphologic substrate of dissecting aneuryms. It is not the only structural change which can lead to dissection, and conversely it can produce clinical manifestations (e.g., aortic regurgitation) in the absence of dissection. Cystic medial necrosis appears to be a nonspecific change in the aorta in response to hemodynamic stresses. The frequency with which it is found at autopsy increases with age of the group studied. (The age distribution of cases of dissecting aneurysm is similar.) Its anatomic distribution is also characteristic, being most marked in the ascending aorta and decreasing progressively as one passes farther from the aortic valve, especially beyond the vessels which branch at the aortic arch. Hypertension accelerates the development of cystic medial necrosis. Furthermore, cystic medial necrosis and dissecting aneurysm are occasional complications of coarctation of the aorta. The hemodynamic changes produced by aortic stenosis and regurgitation accelerate the development of cystic medial necrosis in the ascending aorta. In the genetically defective aorta—that of Marfan's syndrome (Chap. 364) is the clearest example one can cite—the ordinary hemodynamic stresses lead to early development of cystic medial necrosis, especially in the ascending aorta, with progressive dilatation and/or dissecting aneurysm. (In all dissecting aneurysm, the intimal rent occurs most often in the ascending aorta.) All these features suggest that cystic medial necrosis is a relatively nonspecific morphologic expression of "wearing-out" of the aorta in response to hemodynamic stress. The stress to which the ascending aorta is particularly subject is repetitive expansile pulsation. With each heartbeat the ascending aorta is subjected to greater expansile pulsation than any other part of the aorta, especially more than that beyond the aortic arch.

Cystic medial necrosis sometimes results in aneurysm, usually of the ascending aorta, without dissection. The clinical behavior resembles that of syphilitic aneurysm in many respects. In other cases, aortic regurgitation is the main and presenting problem. Surgical treatment has been successful in some of these instances.

Syphilitic aortitis does not lead to dissection, nor does atherosclerosis per se.

SYPHILITIC AORTITIS

Syphilitic involvement is limited largely to the thoracic aorta, particularly the ascending aorta. Syphilitic cardiovascular disease rarely occurs in persons who have had syphilis for less than 10 years or in those who received even a moderate amount of antisyphilitic treatment in the early stage of the infection. On the other hand, so great is the predilection of *Treponema pallidum* for the aorta that a majority of patients with untreated cases have involvement of that vessel. Fortunately, the frequency of syphilitic cardiovascular disease has decreased markedly in the last decade.

The predominant localization of syphilitic change to the ascending aorta may be the result of the combination of the particular hemodynamic stress (see Cystic Medial Necrosis, above) with the medial damage by the treponemal infection. Other explanations are probably less satisfactory.

Aortic regurgitation, fusiform aneurysm, or saccular aneurysm may result. Syphilitic aortitis uncomplicated by any of these three may betray its presence by a change in the quality of the aortic second sound usually referred to as "tambouric" (scarcely a pathognomonic sign, however) and by the presence of intimal, shell-like calcification in the first part of the ascending aorta. In some cases this calcification even extends proximally to outline the sinuses of Valsalva. Atherosclerosis alone usually does not produce calcification in the first part of the ascending aorta. The primary lesion of syphilitic aortitis is medial, but intimal atherosclerosis is accelerated by the damage to the media. Occlusive change in the ostiums of branch arteries, such as the coronaries with production of angina pectoris or the aortic arch vessels with production of the aortic arch syndrome, occurs through a similar mechanism.

Syphilitic aneurysms occur with diminishing frequency from the ascending aorta distally toward the abdominal aorta. They may be single or multiple, diffuse or sharply localized, fusiform or saccular, smooth-walled or thrombus-filled. Symptoms are likely to be due to compression (e.g., of trachea, pulmonary artery, or superior vena cana) or erosion (e.g., of the sternum or vertebral column). Rupture into the superior vena cava or pulmonary artery may occur and the patient may survive for some time, with dramatic physical findings. Sudden death may result from external rupture or rupture into the tracheobronchial tree, pericardium, esophagus, etc. Happily, with improved public health control of syphilis and with better treatment, syphilitic aneurysm may soon become a matter of no particular concern to the clinician.

There has never been convincing evidence that specific treatment given after the development of clinical signs of cardiovascular syphilis prolongs life. There is evidence that aortic regurgitation is more frequent in syphilitic aortitis than previously thought; however, the prognosis in these patients is better than previously realized.

Herxheimer reactions following closely after the administration of penicillin have been observed in early syphilis, in which fever may occur, and in central nervous system syphilis, in which fever and aggravation of mental disturbances may be seen. Although the occurrence (after penicillin treatment) of Herxheimer reactions involving the coronary ostiums remains to be established, it is probably wise in a patient with cardiovascular syphilis and angina pectoris or electrocardiographic signs of myocardial ischemia to improve the myocardial status as much as possible before antisyphilitic therapy and to institute such therapy only under conditions of optimal rest and observation.

Surgical therapy for syphilitic aneurysms has made outstanding advances. With cardiopulmonary bypass, aneurysms of the ascending aorta can be resected. Operation is indicated for all except small aneurysms, for which observation is warranted.

ARTERIOSCLEROTIC ANEURYSMS

Arteriosclerotic aneurysms occur most frequently, although not exclusively, in the abdominal aorta, especially in that portion between the ostiums of the renal arteries and the bifurcation. The patients are usually men in the sixth or seventh decade of life or older. Both dilatation and buckling of the aorta are usually involved, and the buckling is usually predominantly to the left.

Manifestations include primarily pain in the back or anterior part of the abdomen and a pulsatile abdominal mass which usually presents in the epigastrium. (As projected on the anterior abdominal wall, the bifurcation lies at approximately the level of the umbilicus.) The patient may discover that the knee-elbow position relieves the pain. The diagnosis may be obvious from ordinary roentgenograms of the abdomen if an eggshell-like or other calcification outlines the aneurysm. Aortograms permit the definitive anatomic diagnosis. About two-thirds of cases are asymptomatic, and almost one-fifth are discovered on roentgenograms taken for other purposes. Discovery of aneurysm is important because death can be averted by timely operation.

Rupture of arteriosclerotic aneurysms is frequently the mechanism of death. Rupture is likely to begin in the ulceration of an atheromatous plaque. There is usually no more than short medial dissection. Rupture may result in the rapid development of a mass in the left flank. The hematoma may dissect retroperitoneally into the groin and produce manifestations simulating incarcerated inguinal hernia. Rupture into the duodenum, another indication of the high location of these aneurysms, may occur.

Embolization may occur in the legs from a clot in the aneurysm, or from an associated atherosclerotic ulcer, and give rise to manifestations of large- or small-vessel occlusion.

Arteriosclerotic aneurysm of the abdominal aorta has been treated surgically with good results. Resection of the affected portion and replacement with a synthetic prosthesis have been performed successfully in literally thousands of patients. If the general condition of the patient permits, all except small aneurysms should be resected. In the minority of cases in which the renal arteries and higher branches of the aorta are involved in the wall of the aneurysm, modifications of the basic procedure are necessary.

AORTIC ARCH SYNDROMES

(Pulseless disease, young female arteritis, Takayasu syndrome, reverse coarctation)

Slowly progressive change may lead to partial or total obliteration of the major branches of the aortic arch. Intimal atherosclerosis alone can produce at least a partial aortic arch syndrome, and it often collaborates with other factors such as syphilis and trauma in producing obliteration. Severe trauma to the upper part of the chest, especially if the neck is extended, may rupture elements of the media in the region of the ostiums of the arch branches and thus lay the groundwork for progressive intimal atherosclerosis at these sites. An inadequately understood progressive disorder occurs especially in young females, for which reason the designation *young female arteritis* has been used. Histopathologically these cases have been characterized by collections of chronic inflammatory cells, including giant cells. In this disorder the obliteration of major branches is especially likely to be complete, and the designation *pulseless disease* is particularly appropriate. Because of the absence of pulses in the upper part of the body with normal femoral pulses and hypertension in the legs, the term *reverse coarctation* has also been applied to this group of conditions.

In addition to the loss of palpable pulses, clinical manifestations include easy fatigability of the arms, atrophy of the muscles and other soft tissues of the face, necrosis of the cartilaginous nasal septum, and cataract. Systolic murmurs may be heard just above and below the clavicles if the occlusion is partial. If the pressure proximal to the obstruction is higher than that distad to the obstruction at all times in the cardiac cycle, a continuous murmur simulating that of patent ductus arteriosus may be heard in the same area. Syncopal attacks, especially with quiet standing after exercise, also occur.

Surgical replacement of the aortic arch has been formed in a few cases and will undoubtedly become increasingly feasible in the future.

THROMBOTIC OBLITERATION OF THE BIFURCATION OF THE AORTA (LERICHE SYNDROME)

The bifurcation of the aorta is, like the bifurcation of the common carotid artery and the coronary arteries, an Achilles heel of the arterial tree as far as the development of atherosclerosis is concerned. Slowly progressive thrombosis at the bifurcation can result in complete obliteration of the aorta. The patients are usually men and may be as young as in the fourth decade. Some of the patients have hypercholesterolemia. The same clinical picture may result from saddle embolism of the bifurcation, as in mitral valve disease or myocardial infarction, if the patient survives the acute episode and is not operated on early.

The clinical manifestations of Leriche's syndrome are (1) intermittent claudication, with pain in the low part of the back or *gluteal area* which may be mistaken for "sciatica"; (2) loss of the ability to maintain a stable erection, because of the poor blood supply to the penis; (3) globose, i.e., symmetric, atrophy of the legs, which may be difficult to appreciate because of its symmetry; and (4) absence of both femoral pulses. Most of the patients have manifestations of atherosclerosis elsewhere—cerebral, coronary, aortic arch ostia—and hypertension is frequent. Differentiation from coarctation of the aorta is afforded by feeling an aortic pulse in the epigastrium and by the absence of certain other signs of coarctation such as notching of the ribs and dilated collateral vessels over the thorax. Lateral roentgenograms of the lumbar spine may reveal basket-like or other calcification in the region of the bifurcation. Aortograms can make the diagnosis definite.

Surgical replacement of the aortic bifurcation with a synthetic prosthesis has been performed in a large number of patients, with great success.

TRAUMA OF THE AORTA

Penetrating wounds of the chest may be rapidly fatal because of puncture of the aorta. Nonpenetrating trauma to the chest, most commonly the steering wheel injuries in automobile accidents, may lead to rupture of the aorta. In over one-third of cases such rupture is just beyond the mouth of the left subclavian artery. If the victim survives the acute tear, a false aneurysm may result at this site. Such aneurysms are susceptible to surgical resection. As mentioned above, progressive obliteration of ostia at the aortic arch with production of the aortic arch syndrome may be a late complication of trauma of a particular type.

AORTIC SINUS ANEURYSM

Aneurysms may occur in the sinuses of Valsalva from syphilis or idiopathic cystic medial necrosis, or on a presumably congenital (ill-understood) basis. Rupture into the right atrium or right ventricle may occur. Successful surgical closure has been effected in such cases. Aneurysm of the aortic sinuses, usually with symmetric involvement of all three sinuses, occurs as a characteristic feature of the Marfan syndrome. Such aneurysms rarely if ever rupture into the right side of the heart.

UNUSUAL FORMS OF AORTITIS

Unusual forms of aortitis include mycotic aneurysm, such as that produced by aortic tuberculosis, temporal arteritis with aortic involvement, and granulomatous aortitis of the proximal few centimeters in ankylosing spondylitis.

Coarctation and other congenital anomalies of the aorta are discussed elsewhere (Chap. 237).

REFERENCES

DEBAKEY ME et al: Surgical management of dissecting aneurysms of the aorta. J Thorac Cardiovasc Surg 49:130, 1965

——, BEALL AC JR: Surgical treatment of diseases of the aorta and major arteries, chap. 99 in *The Heart*, ed JW Hurst, 3d ed., New York: McGraw-Hill, 1974

DOMINGO RT et al: Acquired aorto-arteritis. A worldwide vascular entity. Arch Surg 95:780, 1967

LINDSAY J JR: Diseases of the aorta and venae cavae, chap. 95 in *The Heart*, 3d ed., ed JW Hurst, New York: McGraw-Hill, 1974, pp. 1586–1598

——, HURST JW: Clinical features and prognosis in dissecting aneurysm of the aorta. A re-appraisal. Circulation 35:880, 1967

MCFARLAND J et al: Medical treatment of dissecting aortic aneurysms. N Engl J Med 286:115, 1972

WHEAT, MW JR, PALMER RF: Dissecting aneurysms of the aorta. Curr Probl Surg July:1-43, 1971

247 VASCULAR DISEASES OF THE EXTREMITIES

D. EUGENE STRANDNESS, JR.

In approaching the patient with a suspected peripheral vascular disorder, the physician must seek answers to the following questions: (1) Is the disease arterial, venous, or lymphatic in origin? (2) Is the process primary or secondary to some underlying disorder? (3) What segment(s) of the vascular system is involved? (4) How useful and specific are the symptoms and signs in establishing the diagnosis? (5) Under what circumstances are special tests necessary to make a correct diagnosis and to plan therapy? (6) What are the complications associated with the disorder? and (7) What is the prognosis with and without therapy? The following discussion will present the pertinent, available information that permits at least a partial answer to some of these questions.

ARTERIAL DISORDERS

Acute arterial occlusion

Sudden interruption of the blood supply to all or a portion of an extremity results in a spectrum of symptoms and signs which are dependent upon the location and extent of the occlusion and the immediately available collateral circulation. The major causes of acute arterial occlusion are *embolism, thrombosis,* and *injury*. In the upper extremity the heart is the source of the emboli in 95 percent of the patients with this problem. Less common causes include emboli from ulcerated plaques in the subclavian artery and aorta (especially aneurysms), as well as paradoxic emboli via an interatrial septal defect.

In the lower extremity somewhat over half of emboli will lodge in either the superficial femoral or the popliteal artery. The abdominal aorta is occluded in about one-sixth of cases, with the iliac arteries involved in approximately one-fifth. The remaining emboli will lodge in the three major vessels distal to the popliteal artery. The heart is the most common source of emboli to the leg arteries, but they may also originate from ulcerated plaques and aneurysms in the thoracic and abdominal aorta.

A variety of diseases involving the heart must be considered when a patient has acute arterial occlusion. Diseases of the aortic or mitral valve secondary to rheumatic endocarditis, particularly when associated with left atrial enlargement, atrial fibrillation, or atrial flutter, are common sources of emboli. Mural thrombi on the wall of the left ventricle which form secondary to a myocardial infarction may also be a source of the problem. A prosthetic aortic or mitral valve should also be considered a possible source of arterial emboli.

Arterial thrombosis occurs secondary to a number of causes, which include injury to the arterial wall, arteriosclerosis obliterans, collagen vascular disorders, myeloproliferative disorders, disseminated intravascular coagulation, and the dysproteinemias. Determining the exact cause of acute sudden arterial thrombosis is not always easy.

SYMPTOMS AND SIGNS Acute arterial occlusion produces an immediate fall in both the mean and pulse pressures in the distal arteries. Tissue P_{O_2} decreases markedly during the initial period after the insult. If collateral artery function is adequate to sustain viability, both the distal arterial pressure and tissue P_{O_2} gradually increase. The rapidity with which perfusion improves depends largely upon the resistance offered by the collateral arteries.

If acute arterial occlusion involves a critical segment of the arterial system where the collateral potential is poor, the clinical picture is dramatic. The initial complaint is pain in the most distal part of the limb; this is rapidly accompanied by pallor, coldness, and a sensation of numbness. Cutaneous sensation is usually lost within the first hour. After about 6 hr ischemic muscular contracture develops. Subcutaneous hemorrhage, focal gangrene, and fixed staining of the skin also develop after about 6 hr. Fixed staining of the skin is a certain index of loss of viability.

When the arterial inflow is marginal, ischemic rest pain involving the distal foot and toes may be present. The foot is nearly always cool, with very reduced capillary filling, particularly of the toes.

Though the diagnosis is rarely difficult when the extent of the ischemia is as outlined above, there are important variations in the clinical picture. If the immediately available collateral circulation is sufficient to maintain viability, the patient may complain only of a sensation of numbness, usually accompanied by a decrease in the temperature of the part. Under these circumstances, the circulation will nearly always improve, with these minor symptoms disappearing over the course of several hours.

DIAGNOSIS The physical examination is helpful in establishing the most proximal level of the occlusion and the extent of the peripheral ischemia. The combination of pain, pallor, and paralysis clearly indicates that limb viability will be lost unless the proximal occlusion can be immediately corrected. If limb viability is not in question, the major physical findings include loss of pulses distal to the site of occlusion and a decrease in skin temperature. Light touch sensation is usually intact, even though the patient may complain of numbness. Detection of a bruit from the subclavian artery is common when an arterial plaque or aneurysm is the source of emboli to the hand.

When the leg is affected, it is important to determine whether a previous history of arterial insufficiency existed. If there is a history of intermittent claudication, it is likely that the basis for the acute change is thrombosis on a preexisting plaque. With *cholesterol emboli* from the aorta, the clinical picture may be confusing. If the emboli arise from the thoracic aorta it is common for the patient to present with hematuria, abdominal pain, and ischemic rest pain in both feet. When the emboli arise from the abdominal aorta (including aneurysms), the ischemic rest pain in the feet is often the only complaint. The ischemic pain is accompanied by prominent livedo reticularis of both feet, as well as petechiae. The final diagnosis can be established with certainty only by histologic examination of the occluded digital arteries where the cholesterol clefts can be seen.

TREATMENT In any situation where the collateral circulation is clearly inadequate, immediate operation is required, if feasible. Time is of the essence, since tissue death is progressive, often reaching an irreversible stage in about 6 hr. If limb viability is not in question, the indications for operation are not as clear. In the arm, occlusions of the radial, ulnar, or brachial artery can often be treated nonoperatively with good results. However, patients with brachial artery occlusions may later complain of arm claudication, particularly if their occupation requires heavy physical labor. In the leg, acute occlusions distal to the popliteal artery rarely require operative intervention. If the obstruction is in or proximal to the popliteal artery, embolectomy should be carried out (with few exceptions), because of the high incidence of limb loss and subsequent disability if nonoperative treatment is employed.

Operative extraction of emboli can now be successfully managed with a balloon catheter. Since this can be accomplished if necessary under local anesthesia, regardless of the site of occlusion, the operation should rarely be withheld, even in the critically ill patient.

Anticoagulants (with heparin) for the short term and oral coumadin for the long term are used to treat the underlying cause of the emboli and prevent extension of the peripheral thromboembolism (Chap. 256). If a cardiac lesion is the source of the embolus, serious consideration must be given to operative correction of the underlying problem. If that is not feasible, the patient should be given anticoagulants for an indefinite period. Patients with cholesterol emboli from aortic atherosclerosis are treated expectantly, with the prognosis depending entirely upon the extent of occlusion. In some cases, amputation is required to control the ischemic rest pain and tissue loss which may occur.

Immediately after acute arterial occlusion, the head of the bed is elevated so that the legs are in the dependent position. The patient must be kept warm, but heat should not be applied to the ischemic limb; vasodilator drugs have not been shown to be helpful.

Arteriosclerosis obliterans

The primary lesion of arteriosclerosis is the intimal plaque, which progressively narrows and, in many instances, leads to complete occlusion of large and medium-sized arteries. In the abdomen the disease has its highest incidence in the aorta and common iliac arteries. The external iliac arteries are often spared. Distal to the inguinal ligament occlusions are most common in the adductor canal, with the popliteal artery itself down to the level of its three major branches having a much lower incidence of involvement. In the lower leg, the posterior tibial artery at the ankle and the anterior tibial at its origin are most commonly diseased. Arteriosclerosis obliterans is usually a segmental disease, with marked variation from patient to patient in its extent.

CLINICAL FEATURES Unless complicated by thrombosis, the symptoms and signs that develop secondary to arteriosclerosis obliterans rarely have an abrupt onset, since the process is a gradual, progressive one. The most common symptom occurs with exercise and is termed *intermittent claudication,* i.e., the pain that occurs in a muscle(s) with an inadequate blood supply that is stressed by exercise. The patient often describes the discomfort as a cramp which disappears within 1 or 2 min after stopping the exercise. Occasionally, profound weakness will be noted as exercise progresses. The walking distance required to produce the claudication is usually quite constant from day to day. The pain is more severe and the walking distance is always shortened when the patient walks upstairs and up a hill.

A point not often appreciated is that with arteriosclerosis obliterans claudication does not occur with occlusions in the anterior tibial, posterior tibial, or peroneal arteries. The location of the involved muscle group(s) is useful in predicting the most proximal level of occlusion.

For example, calf and thigh claudication suggests that the primary involvement is proximal to the origin of the thigh muscles, i.e., the profunda femoris artery. The combination of hip, thigh, and buttock claudication with impotence in the male indicates terminal aortic occlusion, *the Leriche syndrome.*

The second important group of symptoms are those which occur at rest and are the result of either multiple levels of occlusion or involvement of a critical arterial segment where the major collaterals are also obstructed. Paresthesias and indeed numbness may occur but are less common than continuous pain in the toes or foot, which may be partially or completely relieved by dependency. Ulceration and gangrene of the toes and distal foot are a common occurrence when the disease reaches this advanced stage.

The patient with diabetes mellitus often presents variations in the clinical picture. Approximately 30 percent of patients with diabetes have a peripheral neuropathy which results in loss of deep pain sensation and sympathetic tone. When diabetics with a neuropathy develop ulcers with or without arterial occlusion, the lesions are typically painless. The combination of chronic arterial occlusion, peripheral neuropathy, and a nonhealing ulcer is a difficult therapeutic problem.

The physical examination is useful in substantiating the diagnosis and localizing the levels of disease. Patients with single occlusions in the aortoiliac or superficial femoral artery often have limbs which are normal in appearance. Patients with far-advanced disease secondary to multiple levels of disease often have ulcers, gangrene, loss of hair, trophic nail changes, and dependent rubor. Chronic arterial narrowing and occlusion lead to loss of pulses distal to the most proximal level of disease. The pulses should be examined in the groin in the popliteal fossa, and at the level of the ankle. If the involvement results in narrowing only, bruits are commonly heard which are transmitted to varying degrees downstream from the stenosis. Auscultation should be performed from the level of the midabdomen to the popliteal artery; one should listen for the characteristic sound which is diagnostic of arterial narrowing.

SPECIAL DIAGNOSTIC TESTS The magnitude of the physiologic derangement can be assessed simply by measuring the ankle systolic blood pressure at rest and following exercise to the point of claudication. Since arterial occlusion forces the blood to follow alternate pathways (collaterals) which have a greater-than-normal resistance to flow, an abnormal pressure gradient develops which lowers the pressure recorded at the ankle. The pressure may be measured by a variety of plethysmographs or the ultrasonic velocity detector. In general, if the systolic pressure at the ankle is greater than one-half that recorded from the arm, occlusion of one segment is most likely. Ankle pressures less than one-half arm systolic pressure are most often observed with multiple levels of disease.

When the patient with intermittent claudication exercises to the point of pain, the postexercise ankle blood pressure falls, often to unrecordable levels, requiring several minutes to return to the prewalking level. With exercise there is a marked fall in arterial resistance in the muscle. The amount of inflow available through the collateral arteries is inadequate, because of their high resistance to flow. As a consequence, distal arterial pressure falls and blood is shunted away from the foot. These changes explain the pallor in the foot which is so commonly observed during and immediately following exercise to the point of claudication. This test is most useful in following the progress of disease with and without therapy and is the most sensitive index of change available. Its great utility lies in the fact that each patient can serve as his own control.

Arteriography is essential prior to operation to localize precisely the disease and the extent of the involvement. However, it is rarely required to establish the diagnosis of arterial narrowing or occlusion secondary to arteriosclerosis obliterans.

DIFFERENTIAL DIAGNOSIS It is rarely difficult to make the diagnosis of chronic arterial narrowing or occlusion if the clinical picture is combined with measurements of ankle blood pressure. There is a recently recognized entity, referred to as "pseudoclaudication," which may be secondary to neurospinal disease. The features of the symptom-complex which are useful in distinguishing it from true intermittent claudication include the following: (1) the exercise-pain-rest cycle is not constant; (2) the symptoms may include numbness, tingling, weakness, incoordination, and clumsiness; (3) patients with pseudoclaudication may have to sit down or even lie down for relief; and (4) the time required for the pain to disappear often exceeds the few minutes observed in claudication due to arterial occlusion.

THERAPY Patients with mild or moderate intermittent claudication may benefit from a rigorous, daily-exercise training program. The essential features of this program include (1) repetitive daily walks to 75 percent of the claudication distance with interspersed periods of rest (1 to 2 min); (2) weekly retesting of maximum walking time with readjustment of walking distance; and (3) continuation of the exercise program—this is essential, since evidence suggests that cessation of the daily walking periods will result in loss of the improvement that often results. Vasodilator drugs have been advocated and used for the treatment of intermittent claudication, but evidence supporting their efficacy is lacking.

Weight reduction can be useful in patients with intermittent claudication by simply reducing the workload involved. It is also important that *smoking be stopped* entirely. All patients with arteriosclerosis should have their serum lipid levels determined, since they may be found to have a treatable disorder (Chap. 244). Direct arterial surgery may be effective in bypassing or removing areas of occlusion but should be reserved for those patients with disabling claudication.

Most patients with ischemic rest pain, ulcers, or gangrene present serious problems which can be helped only by direct arterial surgery. Lumbar sympathectomy may be useful but should be used *only* in patients with mild rest pain. If the rest pain is controlled by nonnarcotic analgesics and transient dependency, about 50 percent of these patients can obtain permanent pain relief by lumbar sympathectomy.

The majority of patients with arteriosclerosis obliterans will never require surgical therapy even though they do suffer some disability. The nondiabetic will have a limb loss rate of about 2 percent per year, which increases to 7 percent per year if the patient has diabetes mellitus. Meticulous foot care, which includes properly fitting shoes, and immediate attention to cuts and blisters are critical in proper management. This is particularly true in patients with diabetes and a peripheral neuropathy who are unable to appreciate deep pain.

Thromboangiitis obliterans (Buerger's disease)

In 1908 Buerger described a nonatheromatous lesion involving arteries, veins, and nerves occurring in young males which frequently led to nonhealing ulcers and gangrene. Though there has been some controversy concerning the existence of this disease as a specific entity, sufficient evidence is available to recommend its continued recognition. The exact pathogenesis is obscure, but there appears to be a definite relationship with tobacco smoking or chewing.

The disease typically occurs in young males and has a characteristic location and set of clinical manifestations. Whereas arteriosclerosis obliterans is a segmental disease of large- and medium-sized arteries, Buerger's disease starts in the smaller arteries of the hands and feet. There is usually an intense inflammatory component, which in later stages results in arterial and venous occlusion as well as fibrous encasement of the entire neurovascular bundle.

CLINICAL FEATURES The diagnosis of Buerger's disease should be suspected when male patients in the twenty- to forty-year age range give the following history. A superficial, migratory nodular phlebitis may occur early in the disease. These nodules are well localized, associated with cutaneous erythema, and tender to touch. Cold sensitivity of the Raynaud's type occurs in about one-half the patients and is frequently confined to the hands. The fingers turn white when exposed to cold, then blue, and finally red—the so-called triphasic color response.

One of the most characteristic and typical symptoms of Buerger's disease is instep claudication. Exercise results in pain in the instep, promptly relieved by rest. Calf claudication may occur but is unusual, since the disease does not commonly progress proximally to involve and occlude either the popliteal or superficial femoral artery. When there is hand involvement, the occlusions may be bilateral, are often symmetric, and may lead to the development of hand claudication and fingertip ulcers which are exquisitely painful and difficult to heal.

The following findings during *physical examination* should lead one to suspect Buerger's disease: (1) intense rubor of the feet even in the supine position; (2) absent foot pulses in the presence of a normal femoral and popliteal pulse; and (3) reduction or absence of the radial and/or ulnar pulses.

THERAPY There is only one effective treatment, and that is permanent, complete abstinence from tobacco. However, for some unknown reason, patients with Buerger's disease rarely quit smoking even though amputation is usually the inevitable consequence and only method available of controlling the severe rest pain and ulceration which ultimately develop.

Arteriovenous fistulas

ACQUIRED Most acquired arteriovenous fistulas occur secondary to penetrating injuries; however, they may in certain circumstances occur secondary to blunt trauma. Malignancy, infection, and arterial aneurysms have also been responsible for the development of arteriovenous communications.

Clinical picture Patients with penetrating injuries of an extremity should all be suspected of having an arteriovenous fistula. Initially there are no distinguishing symptoms which alert the physician to the presence of the fistula. The diagnosis is made by noting a continuous murmur and palpable thrill over the abnormal communication. Compression of the feeding artery will obliterate the murmur and thrill. With large fistulas compression of the feeding artery results in an abrupt slowing of the heart rate (Branham's sign). In rare instances distal arterial perfusion may be so severely impaired that gangrene develops.

With chronic fistulas the clinical manifestations may mimic those of venous disease, with varicose veins, stasis pigmentation, and cutaneous ulcers. Cardiac enlargement with or without failure may be seen in long-standing fistulas. Infection (bacterial endarteritis) may complicate large fistulas.

Therapy The proper treatment of arteriovenous fistulas is division of the communication with maintenance of arterial continuity. Immediate operation may be indicated with large fistulas between such vessels as the abdominal aorta and inferior vena cava where cardiac failure may develop very quickly.

CONGENITAL The development of anomalous communications between arteries and veins can pose both diagnostic and therapeutic difficulties. When there is an arrest in the development of the circulation during the stage of an undifferentiated capillary network, a *cavernous hemangioma* results. There is at this period an interlacing system of blood spaces which contain mixed blood and it is impossible to distinguish the arterial and venous components.

When the development is arrested at the stage of differentiation, intercommunicating arteriovenous channels may persist. If the fistulas are large enough to be visualized arteriographically, the term used is congenital *macrofistulous arteriovenous* aneurysm. When the fistulas are too small to be visualized by arteriography, the term *microfistulous communication* should be used. This classification, based upon the size of the communications, is useful from a therapeutic standpoint.

Clinical manifestations The clinical manifestations are extremely variable and largely depend upon the location and extent of the abnormal communications. The most common symptoms are (1) cosmetic changes due to the presence of the fistulas in the subcutaneous tissue and skin; (2) limb swelling and hypertrophy; (3) visible pulsations in some cases with macrofistulous communications; and (4) varicose veins in atypical locations. In long-standing cases stasis pigmentation and cutaneous ulcers may develop in response to the continued venous hypertension.

Diagnosis The presence of arteriovenous fistulas should be suspected when the following findings are presented: (1) unilateral leg or arm swelling; (2) cutaneous hemangioma of the "port-wine" variety; (3) varicose veins in atypical locations; and (4) an increase in temperature of the part. An important syndrome which may be confused with congenital arteriovenous fistulas is the *Klippel-Trénaunay* syndrome. The triad of this syndrome consists of varicose veins, "port-wine" hemangioma of the skin, and bone and soft-tissue hypertrophy. Arteriovenous fistulas are usually not demonstrable on arteriographic studies, but there is either agenesis or obstruction of the deep venous system.

Therapy The management of congenital arteriovenous fistulas depends entirely upon location, extent, and clinical manifestations. Treatment is largely conservative, with support stockings used to control the venous hypertension and valvular incompetence which often produce symptoms identical with those of the postphlebitic syndrome. If the fistulas are limited in extent, it may be possible to excise the lesion in its entirety, but this is usually not feasible.

Thoracic outlet syndromes

The neurovascular bundle, by virtue of its course from the neck and thorax, is subject to compression by both muscular and skeletal structures.

SCALENUS ANTICUS SYNDROME The subclavian artery and brachial plexus normally pass through the interscalene triangle in their course to the arm. These structures may be compressed by an accessory cervical rib or by variations in the insertion of the scalenus anterior muscle. In some instances, the subclavian artery may pass through the muscle itself.

CERVICAL RIB When a cervical rib is present, the subclavian artery may be angulated in passing over the rib. If the rib is incomplete there is apt to be compression of the brachial plexus.

COSTOCLAVICULAR SYNDROME Symptoms of neurovascular compression may be observed when the shoulders are moved backward and downward. Several anatomic defects have been noted as possible causes of this syndrome, including (1) old clavicular fractures; (2) cervicodorsal scoliosis; (3) failure of the anterior curvature of the clavicle to develop; (4) abnormalities of the first rib; (5) hypertrophy of the subclavius muscle; and (6) abnormalities of the costocoracoid ligament.

HYPERABDUCTION SYNDROME When symptoms appear with the arms in the hyperabducted position, there are two possible sites of compression: (1) the point where the neurovascular bundle passes beneath the tendon of the pectoralis minor; and (2) the retroclavicular space between the clavicle and the first rib.

Clinical manifestations The symptoms that may occur secondary to the thoracic outlet syndromes include pain, paresthesias, numbness, weakness, and swelling involving the arm and hand. In rare instances digit ulceration and gangrene may develop. Raynaud's phenomenon has also been reported. The symptoms themselves are usually not helpful in distinguishing the underlying anatomic defect.

Diagnosis The diagnosis of the underlying defect rests upon (1) reproduction of the symptoms by the appropriate position; (2) disappearance of the radial pulse which coincides with the appearance of symptoms (it must be remembered that disappearance of the radial pulse is not in itself sufficient to make the diagnosis); (3) x-ray examination of the cervical spine, clavicles, and shoulder girdle, which must always be carried out when the diagnosis of thoracic outlet compression is entertained.

Specific maneuvers that have been recommended to establish the site of compression include (1) disappearance of the radial pulse with deep inspiration, extension of the neck, and turning the chin toward the side being examined (a positive test is indicative of compression of the subclavian artery in the scalene triangle with or without a cervical rib); (2) if the symptoms are produced with the shoulders moved backward and downward (the exaggerated military position), the costoclavicular syndrome is likely. In the *hyperabduction syndrome*, the position responsible for the symptoms is with the arms brought together above the head with the elbows flexed.

When a *cervical rib* is present with compromise of the interscalene triangle, bruits are commonly heard and exaggerated in the position that produces symptoms.

A *herniated nucleus pulposus* and *cervical osteoarthritis* can produce symptoms which are often confused with the thoracic outlet syndromes. Cervical spine films must be obtained in all cases of suspected thoracic outlet compression. In some cases a cervical myelogram may be indicated.

Therapy The costoclavicular and hyperabduction syndromes rarely produce symptoms sufficient to warrant operative correction. Physical therapy to strengthen the muscles of the neck and shoulder girdle may be helpful. The scalenus anticus syndrome may be treated by division of the anterior scalene muscle. When a cervical rib is responsible for the compression, the rib should be resected. Thrombosis of the subclavian artery or embolization to the arteries of the arm is most apt to occur when a cervical rib is present.

Vasospastic disorders

Those diseases which are properly classified as arteriospastic disorders include acrocyanosis, livedo reticularis, and cold sensitivity of the Raynaud type. The challenge with these entities is not in making the correct clinical diagnosis but rather in differentiating between the primary and secondary forms of the diseases. The primary forms are benign, rarely lead to digit ulcers, and never terminate fatally. The secondary causes of the arteriospastic disorders are frequently serious and may have a fatal outcome.

COLD SENSITIVITY OF THE RAYNAUD TYPE In evaluating and determining whether a patient has a true sensitivity to cold or emotional stimuli it is necessary to establish whether or not the "triphasic" color response occurs, i.e., pallor, cyanosis, and rubor, in sequence. The most important element from a diagnostic standpoint is the pallor, during which the digits turn absolutely white.

LIVEDO RETICULARIS Livedo reticularis presents with a persistent cyanotic mottling of the skin which has a typical "fishnet" appearance. In contrast to Raynaud's disease, a phenomenon which is confined to the digits, livedo reticularis may involve all parts of the extremities and trunk. This cutaneous pattern is often accentuated by exposure to cold.

ACROCYANOSIS The most uncommon of the vasospastic disorders is acrocyanosis, which is characterized by a persistent diffuse cyanosis of the fingers, hands, toes, and feet. This disease is benign and not associated with an underlying disorder. The involved parts are nearly always cold, with excessive perspiration being a common accompanying feature.

Diagnosis *Raynaud's disease* is more common in women, often starting in the late teens, is usually bilateral and symmetric, and uncommonly leads to fingertip ulceration or gangrene. The hands are much more commonly involved than are the feet. The factors in the clinical presentation which should lead the clinician to suspect that the Raynaud's phenomenon is secondary to some underlying disorder include (1) abrupt onset with rapid progression to tissue necrosis; (2) late onset in life (> fifty years), particularly in men; (3) unilateral involvement, especially when only one or two digits are affected; and (4) associated symptoms compatible with a systemic disease.

Sorting out the underlying causes is often difficult because of the wide variety of diseases which may have Raynaud's phenomenon as a part of their clinical picture. The following diseases must be kept in mind: (1) chronic arterial disease, most particularly thromboangiitis obliterans; (2) the collagen vascular disorders, with scleroderma being the most common; (3) occupational and industrial exposure to vibrating instruments; (4) poisoning with lead and arsenic; (5) ingestion of drugs, namely, the ergotamine preparations, methysergide, and propranolol; (6) hematologic disorders, namely, cryoglobulins, cold agglutinins, and dysproteinemias; (7) bilateral thoracic outlet syndromes; (8) late sequelae of bilateral cold injury; (9) primary pulmonary hypertension; and (10) occult carcinoma.

The secondary causes of livedo reticularis include (1) collagen diseases, in particular periarteritis nodosa and disseminated lupus erythematosus; (2) hematologic disorders, i.e., hyperviscosity syndrome, macroglobulinemia, and cryoglobulinemia; (3) cholesterol emboli arising from ulcerated plaques in the thoracic and abdominal aorta; (4) Cushing's syndrome (5) drug ingestion, i.e., adrenal corticosteroids; (6) prolonged dependency or immobilization; (7) late result of cold injury; and (8) prolonged exposure to or the local application of heat.

Therapy The primary forms of cold sensitivity, i.e., livedo reticularis and acrocyanosis, rarely require treatment other than assurance and instruction relative to the dangers of prolonged exposure to cold. Sympathectomy has been widely applied, with inconsistent results, in the treatment of Raynaud's disease. Lumbar sympathectomy, probably due to the higher incidence of permanent denervation, is more likely to give good results than cervicodorsal sympathectomy. Sympathectomy, particularly in the upper extremity, should be performed only when conservative measures fail to control the symptoms. Reserpine and methyldopa have been reported to reduce the frequency and severity of the attacks.

When there are secondary causes for the vasospastic disorders, treatment is directed at the cause of the problem. It is important to remember that drugs and sympathectomy are rarely effective with the secondary forms of the disease.

Erythromelalgia

This rare disorder of unknown etiology expresses itself as burning, tingling, and often itching of the foot and lower leg which appears as the ambient temperature increases. There is usually a critical temperature for each patient above which the symptoms appear (usually in the range of 89 to 97°F). During the attack the patient's feet and lower legs become bright red. The patient quickly finds that his symptoms are related to temperature and will assiduously avoid those circumstances which bring out the symptoms. Characteristically, patients wear sandals, avoid stockings, sleep with their feet outside the bedcovers, and use fans to reduce the skin temperature.

The *diagnosis* is established by the history and the examination of the extremities during an attack. The pedal pulses are intact, and the skin is warm and bright red. The disease is usually primary but has, in rare instances, been associated with myeloproliferative disorders.

Therapy is usually unsuccessful, but some patients have reported relief with aspirin or methysergide maleate.

VENOUS DISORDERS

Varicose veins

Varicose veins are dilated, tortuous superficial veins whose valves are incompetent. The greater and lesser saphenous systems are most commonly involved, but it is not unusual for secondary branches of the superficial system of veins also to become dilated. They most often appear after the age of twenty, but in females often develop in relation to puberty, during pregnancy, and with commencement of the menopause. In men there is a fairly even distribution in the onset of symptoms by decades up to age seventy.

The etiology remains largely obscure, but varicose veins are known to be aggravated by hormonal factors in the female, increased intraabdominal pressure, and, in rare instances, arteriovenous fistulas. Hereditary factors are important but have been poorly studied.

CLASSIFICATION It is important to classify varicose veins as either primary or secondary. Primary varicose veins occur in the absence of deep venous disease and generally have a benign course. Varicosities which occur secondary to obstruction and valvular incompetence of the deep venous system are much more serious.

CLINICAL FEATURES Primary varicose veins are brought to the attention of the patient first by the cosmetic deformity and secondly by the symptoms which develop with prolonged standing. The patient complains of a feeling of heaviness in the leg, combined with fatigue, that gets progressively worse toward the end of the day. Elevation of the legs will result in rapid and impressive relief from the symptoms. When the varicose veins are secondary to deep venous obstruction, loss of valves, and incompetent perforating veins, the symptoms are more severe and accompanied by swelling (see postphlebitic syndrome).

DIAGNOSIS The diagnosis of primary varicose veins is made largely by inspection of the legs in the upright position. The varicosities appear as dilated, often tortuous channels which are most commonly observed in the greater and lesser saphenous systems. When isolated clusters are observed in atypical locations, the possibility of an underlying incompetent perforating vein or arteriovenous fistula should be considered. To assess whether or not incompetent perforating veins are contributing factors, the Trendelenburg test may be employed. With the legs elevated and the superficial veins empty, a tourniquet is applied about the thigh close to the groin. The patient then quickly stands, and the pattern of filling is noted. If the superficial veins do not fill in 30 sec, it is unlikely that incompetent perforating veins are contributing to the etiology of the varicose veins.

THERAPY The majority of patients with symptomatic primary varicose veins should be treated initially with compression stockings. If the deep veins and perforating channels are patent and competent, it is very unusual for primary varicose veins to lead to stasis pigmentation and ulceration. In those rare instances in which treatment with compression stockings is inadequate, high ligation and stripping of the long and/or short saphenous veins may be required.

Thrombophlebitis

Thrombophlebitis encompasses a spectrum of symptoms and signs of acute venous disease which has as its end point thrombosis of the involved segment(s). It is important in approaching this problem to classify the disease by the anatomic area(s) involved—superficial, deep, or both.

ETIOLOGY The known precipitating factors responsible for thrombosis of the venous system of the extremities include trauma, infection, and chemical irritation. Each of these processes injures the vein wall, leading to thrombosis at the site of the insult. There is, however, a much larger group of patients who develop superficial and/or deep venous thrombosis for which no definite cause can be found. Though it is not possible at the present time to identify a specific etiologic factor, the conditions under which thrombosis is most apt to occur are well recognized. These common risk factors include (1) prolonged bed rest; (2) severe illness; (3) immobilization; (4) malignancy, particularly of the pancreas, lung, and gastrointestinal system; (5) administration of estrogens, including oral contraceptives; (6) polycythemia vera; (7) disseminated intravascular coagulation; (8) congestive heart failure; (9) the post-partum period; (10) orthopedic injuries; and (11) the postoperative state.

The exact factors responsible for venous thrombosis remain obscure. However, it is known that the earliest lesions are observed in the sinus of the venous valve, where stasis would be expected. Attachment of the thrombus to the vein wall rapidly occurs, but as the process advances there is propagation beyond the margin of the valve cusp into the lumen of the vein. At this stage, venous outflow may be completely obstructed, with secondary venous thrombosis. The most dangerous sequel is the release of all or a portion of the thrombus, resulting in pulmonary embolism. It is important to recognize that inflammation of the vein wall is not a prominent part of this sequence, particularly in the earlier stages.

LOCATION OF DISEASE In superficial thrombophlebitis, the greater saphenous vein is the most common site of involvement. When the deep venous system is occluded, it is important to consider the following three areas: (1) illofemoral area; (2) femoropopliteal segment; and (3) the small veins of the calf. When the calf veins alone are involved, propagation proximally is not a common occurrence and the likelihood of developing a large pulmonary embolus is remote. The most dangerous and potentially lethal emboli arise from the iliac and femoral veins.

CLINICAL FEATURES Superficial thrombophlebitis results in pain, tenderness, and erythema at the site of inflammation in the involved vein. Local swelling may be prominent, and as the process advances, the vessel becomes thrombosed.

Thrombophlebitis of the deep venous system results in a clinical picture which varies greatly, depending upon the location and extent of the occlusion. It is critically important to remember that deep venous thrombosis often develops *without any* symptoms or signs apparent either to the patient or the physician. Though edema, increased calf girth, and local deep tenderness are the most reliable physical findings, it is important to remember that deep venous thrombosis can and does occur without the presence of these physical findings. The first symptoms and signs which might lead the physician to suspect deep venous thrombosis are often those observed with pulmonary embolism.

DIAGNOSIS The involved vein is reddened, tender, swollen, and associated with local edema. It rapidly becomes firm as the thrombus begins to organize. The diagnosis of deep venous thrombosis should be suspected when the patient complains of local deep tenderness and swelling. Occlusions of the iliofemoral and femoropopliteal segments may be determined at the bedside by using the ultrasonic velocity detector. Calf vein thrombosis is usually not detectable with the velocity detector. The ^{125}I-labeled fibrinogen test is the best method available to detect calf vein thrombosis, but it is severely limited in its application. The isotope must be given prior to the development of the thrombosis in order reliably to permit incorporation of the tagged material into the forming clot. Since pulmonary embolism is always a potential danger with deep thrombophlebitis, it is important in questionable cases to verify the diagnosis by venography.

DIFFERENTIAL DIAGNOSIS Bacterial cellulitis and lymphangitis are the most common causes of leg pain, tenderness, and swelling which may be confused with thrombophlebitis. In these cases the cutaneous erythema and tenderness are usually more pronounced, as in the systemic response to the process. Myositis, muscle cramps, and arthritis may also be confused with phlebitis; meticulous physical examination and venography may be required for differential diagnosis.

Though uncommon, a ruptured Baker's cyst can produce marked, acute swelling of the calf, ankle, and foot. The rapidity of the onset, initial location of the pain (popliteal fossa and posterior calf), and absence of superficial venous collaterals should lead the examiner to suspect this diagnosis. The diagnosis is simply made by an arthrogram, which demonstrates extravasation of the contrast material in the posterior compartment of the lower leg.

THERAPY The treatment of thrombophlebitis is directed at control of the thrombotic process already initiated. With superficial phlebitis, heat and elevation are the cornerstones of therapy. Anticoagulation is not necessary unless the deep system is also involved by the process.

When deep venous thrombosis is present, heparin is the most potent and effective drug available. It should be administered intravenously (5,000 to 10,000 units) every 4 to 6 hr. Clotting times may be assessed prior to each dose to assure that cumulative effects are not occurring. This type of therapy gives the so-called "picket fence" response, in which it is the objective to elevate the Lee-White clotting time (Chap. 59) to two or three times the normal control. If hemorrhagic complications occur, the heparin effect can be reversed immediately by giving an equivalent dose of protamine sulfate intravenously.

The duration of anticoagulant therapy is also unsettled, but probably should be continued for at least 10 to 14 days in cases of extensive deep venous thrombosis with or without pulmonary embolism. One of the coumarin preparations may be begun and heparin discontinued when a satisfactory level of anticoagulation with the oral anticoagulant has been reached. Warfarin, 40 to 60 mg, is ordinarily given by mouth on the first day; none is given on the second day; the dosage on the third day and thereafter ranges from 2 to 15 mg daily as an effort is made to maintain the one-stage prothrombin time approximately two to two and one-half times the control.

The question of long-term anticoagulation will depend upon the individual patient. For single episodes of thrombophlebitis associated with severe illness or operation, there would appear to be little need for continued anticoagulation. However, when repeated episodes of thrombophlebitis have occurred, particularly when associated with pulmonary embolism, one should recommend anticoagulation for a minimum of 6 months with one of the coumarin drugs, at a dose necessary to maintain the prothrombin time approximately twice the control.

Operative therapy for acute deep venous thrombosis may be considered under the categories of thrombectomy and venous interruption. Thrombectomy should be considered in those patients with iliofemoral thrombosis who appear within 24 to 48 hr after the onset of symptoms. However, it must be recognized that thrombectomy is still a controversial procedure. Venous plication or ligation, usually at the level of the inferior vena cava, or the insertion of an "umbrella" to prevent upward passage of thrombi is reserved for those patients who sustain pulmonary emboli while receiving adequate doses of heparin or who are not candidates for anticoagulant therapy.

Postphlebitic syndrome

Patients who have single or multiple episodes of deep venous thrombosis will frequently have irreversible changes in the veins which lead to further morbidity. The acute venous thrombosis often leads to residual chronic occlusion and destruction of the venous valves.

The loss of the valvular mechanism in the deep venous system forces the blood to follow abnormal pathways, particularly during exercise. In the standing position or during walking the muscle pump pushes the blood proximally, distally, and out through the perforating veins into the superficial system. By increasing venous and capillary pressures, this sequence of events, over a period of many years, leads to edema, and to rupture of small superficial veins in the vicinity of the perforating veins. The subcutaneous hemorrhage leads to deposition of hemosiderin pigment (stasis pigmentation), subcutaneous fibrosis, cutaneous atrophy, and lymphatic obstruction. These chronic changes lead to the development of stasis ulcers, which are difficult to manage.

CLINICAL FEATURES AND DIAGNOSIS The important features of this disorder consist of swelling which is always worse at the end of the day, pain, cutaneous pigmentation, (usually in the region of the medial malleolus), and nonhealing ulcers which develop secondary to minor trauma. Repeated trauma, subcutaneous hemorrhage, and cellulitis can produce changes in the skin and subcutaneous tissues that are indistinguishable from those of the postphlebitic state. In questionable cases venography is useful in establishing the cause of the problem.

THERAPY The most important factor in the treatment of the postphlebitic syndrome is to reduce the hydrostatic pressure and to prevent "high-pressure leaks" through the perforating veins when the patient is erect. This can best be accomplished by a tailored pressure-gradient stocking, which must be worn at all times that the patient is ambulatory, and by elevating legs when possible.

When an ulcer is present, healing may be accomplished by bed rest and elevation of the legs with or without concomitant skin grafting. In selected cases, removal of the incompetent superficial veins with ligation of the perforating veins may be necessary. Support stockings must be worn regardless of the therapy directed at the ulcer, because the deep venous system remains incompetent and edema will continue to develop without adequate external support.

LYMPHATIC DISORDERS

Lymphedema

Lymphedema, an abnormal accumulation of lymph in the extremities, occurs from multiple causes, which include (1) lymphedema from organisms such as *Wuchereria bancrofti*; (2) infectious lymphedema resulting in thrombosis of lymphatics; (3) congenital lymphedema with arrest in lymph growth, which is apparent at birth or shortly thereafter; (4) traumatic lymphedema secondary to direct injury, burns, operations, and radiation; (5) essential lymphedema—so-called Milroy's disease which appears at puberty and is most commonly observed in females; (6) allergic lymphedema occurring secondary to exposure to drugs and pollens; (7) postthrombotic lymphedema, which represents combined venous and lymphatic obstruction; and (8) malignant lymphedema, which occurs secondary to either direct invasion or obstruction of the lymphatics by tumor cells.

CLINICAL FEATURES Painless swelling of the involved extremity is the earliest and most common symptom and sign with most types of lymphedema. The swelling usually starts in the foot and ankles and then progresses proximally. Initially the swelling tends to subside somewhat at night, but as the process progresses, the swelling becomes permanent secondary to fibrosis of both the skin and subcutaneous tissues. Skin color and texture are normal until the late stages, when the skin becomes thickened and brown and has multiple papillary projections—so-called lymphostatic verrucosis.

DIAGNOSIS The location and nature of the edema readily separate lymphedema from that due to other causes. In the legs, the dorsum of the toes and foot are nearly always involved, which is uncommon in other causes of swelling. The edema is often brawny in character and pits only with difficulty. Though the other forms of edema often improve with bed rest, elevation, and diuretics, lymphedema, even in early stages, responds poorly to these measures. In later stages when fibrosis develops in the skin and subcutaneous tissues, these conservative measures are of little, if any, value. Lymphangiography in selected cases may be of value in localizing and elucidating the cause of the lymphedema.

THERAPY Therapy must be directed at removing the cause of the obstruction, but this is rarely possible. Most often attention is directed at minimizing the swelling by wearing pressure-gradient stockings and the use of intermittent-pressure devices at night. Patients with lymphedema are subject to recurrent attacks of cellulitis, most commonly due to the beta-hemolytic streptococcus and less commonly the staphylococcus. In late stages with marked swelling, disfigurement, and recurrent ulcers, excision of the edematous tissue with skin graft replacement may be required.

ANTERIOR TIBIAL COMPARTMENT SYNDROME

Acute swelling of the anterior tibial compartment may occur secondary to intensive exercise, increased capillary permeability, and hematomas within the enclosed space. It may follow aneurysmectomy or placement of iliofemoral grafts. It is associated with sudden, severe pain in the compartment. The overlying skin is warm, red, and tight, reflecting the increased pressure in the muscle. The muscles and nerves in the compartment will undergo ischemic degeneration unless the overlying fascia is divided. Once the diagnosis is established, *immediate* fasciotomy is indicated, since delays of only a few hours may lead to permanent neuromuscular damage and a foot drop.

REFERENCES

DEBAKEY ME, BEALL AC JR: Surgical treatment of diseases of the aorta and major arteries, chap. 99 in *The Heart*, 3d ed., ed JW Hurst, New York: McGraw-Hill, 1974, pp. 1666–1683

FAIRBAIRN JF et al: *Peripheral Vascular diseases*, 4th ed., Philadelphia: Saunders, 1972

GIFFORD RW JR et al: Diseases of the peripheral arteries and veins, chap. 96 in *The Heart*, 3d ed., ed JW Hurst, New York: McGraw-Hill, 1974, pp. 1599–1635

HAEGER K: *Venous and Lymphatic Disorders of the Leg*, Philadelphia: Lippincott, 1966

HUME M et al: *Venous Thrombosis and Pulmonary Embolism*, Cambridge, Mass.: Harvard, 1970

MITCHELL JRA, SCHWARTZ CJ: *Arterial Disease*, Philadelphia: Davis, 1965

ROSATI LM, LORD JW: *Neurovascular Compression Syndromes of the Shoulder Girdle*, New York: Grune & Stratton, 1961

STRANDNESS DE JR: *Peripheral Arterial Disease: A Physiologic Approach*, Boston: Little, Brown, 1969

SUMNER DS: Arteriovenous fistula, chaps. 2 to 4 in *Collateral Circulation in Clinical Surgery*, ed DE Strandness, Jr., Philadelphia: Saunders, 1969

section 3 Disorders of the respiratory system

248
APPROACH TO THE PATIENT WITH DISEASE OF THE RESPIRATORY SYSTEM

EUGENE BRAUNWALD

As in other branches of medicine, a careful and detailed history and physical examination are essential in establishing an accurate diagnosis in patients with disorders of the respiratory system. In addition, the roentgenographic examination occupies a particularly important role in the evaluation of patients with lung disease. Since abnormalities of the respiratory system are frequently a manifestation of a systemic process, not only must attention be focused on the chest, but a comprehensive evaluation of the patient's entire health status is essential. For example, the presence of a pulmonary lesion may be due to metastatic disease, and hemoptysis may be due to a disorder of hemostasis. Systemic scleroderma may result in diffuse pulmonary infiltrative disease (Chaps. 254, 362), and multiple pulmonary cavities associated with rhinitis, sinusitis, and renal insufficiency may be a manifestation of Wegener's granulomatosis (Chap. 71). Carcinoma of the lung (Chap. 260) may be accompanied by prominent extrathoracic manifestations, which may overshadow the pulmonary lesion. These include myopathy, peripheral neuropathy, hypertrophic pulmonary osteoarthropathy, and a variety of endocrine and metabolic manifestations, including Cushing's syndrome, the carcinoid syndrome, a hyperparathyroid-like picture, inappropriate secretion of antidiuretic hormone, gonadotropin, and increased frequency of pulmonary infections. Contact with both wild and domestic animals may result in pulmonary symptoms such as bronchospasm in the subject allergic to a pet, or acute pneumonitis in the patient with ornithosis (Chap. 189), tularemia (Chap. 141), or Q fever (Chap. 182).

In eliciting the history of patients with pulmonary disease, it must be appreciated that an increasing fraction of the population is exposed to materials which are potentially toxic to the lung (Chap. 258). The history must therefore contain a detailed *occupational history* with a description of exposure to industrial hazards such as coal, silica, asbestos, beryllium, bagasse, iron oxide, tin oxide, cotton dust, titanium oxide, silver, and nitrogen dioxide. A history of tobacco consumption must also be sought. A record of the patient's *previous residence* is of considerable importance in the diagnosis of histoplasmosis, coccidioidomycosis, or tropical eosinophilia. For example, pulmonary mass lesions in patients in the Mediterranean Basin may be due to hydatid cysts; hemoptysis in patients from Central China may be caused by paragonimiasis (Chap. 221), and cor pulmonale in Egypt frequently results from schistosomiasis (Chap. 220).

The *family history* should consider pulmonary diseases which may be on a genetic basis, such as cystic disease of the lung, cystic fibrosis, asthma, hereditary telangiectasia, Kartagener's syndrome, and alveolar microlithiasis, as well as infections due to the tubercle bacilli where exposure to involved family members is important.

Dyspnea is a cardinal manifestation of diseases involving the respiratory and cardiovascular systems (Chap. 28). A detailed physical examination of both organ systems is therefore mandatory in every patient with this symptom. Dyspnea secondary to cardiac disease is often recognized by the presence of other evidence of heart failure, of cardiac enlargement, gallop sounds, and of cardiac murmurs. It may be difficult to differentiate paroxysmal nocturnal dyspnea due to pulmonary edema of cardiac origin from nocturnal attacks of bronchial asthma, but a detailed description of the circumstances in which this symptom occurs is most useful. Dyspnea is a common functional complaint, and an important clue in the identification of this form is the observation that shortness of breath often occurs at rest and is relieved during exertion; the opposite is the case in patients in whom this symptom is secondary to cardiac or pulmonary disease. Equally important in the differential diagnosis is a careful elucidation of the relationship of dyspnea to other symptoms such as cough or angina pectoris.

Patients with diseases involving the respiratory system may also present with *chest pain* which is frequently caused by inflammation of the pleura, occurring in pneumonia, pulmonary thromboembolism, tuberculosis, and malignancy (Chap. 7). Pleuritic pain is usually localized to one side of the chest and is related to movements of the thorax and to respiration. Lesions confined to the pulmonary parenchyma do not produce pain, while diseases involving the organs in the mediastinum (Chap. 261) may cause local discomfort with radiation characteristic of the specific organ. Pain may also originate in or be referred to the chest wall; it may be due to intercostal neuritis, as in herpes zoster, or to compression of the intercostal nerves as they leave the spinal cord. Such pain is often superficial in character and may be related to coughing and straining. Thoracic pain may also be due to myositis, costochondral disturbances, myocardial ischemia, pericarditis, esophageal disease, and aortic dissection and aneurysm (Chap. 7).

Cough and *expectoration* are also cardinal features of pulmonary disease (Chap. 35). Few patients can describe the severity of cough or quantity of expectoration reliably, and it is therefore extremely desirable for the physician to inspect a 24-hr collection of sputum. Cough is often precipitated by foreign materials irritating nerve endings in airways and is frequently caused by inflammation of the bronchi; the latter may be persistent (as in patients with a cigarette cough and chronic bronchitis) or acute (as in a variety of viral and bacterial infections). The time of occurrence of the cough and the character and quantity of expectorated material may point to the diagnosis. For example, bronchiectasis and lung abscess produce purulent sputum which may have an offensive odor or be streaked with blood (Chap. 253). Paroxysmal cough may also be the presenting feature in patients with bronchial asthma, in whom physical examination reveals wheezing respirations and squeaking musical sounds (Chap. 67), as well as in patients with left ventricular failure, in whom it generally occurs at night and in the recumbent position (Chap. 233). Pulmonary tuberculosis (Chap. 156), though less common than previously, remains a common cause of chronic cough, as do neoplasms of the lung (Chap. 260). A change in the character of a chronic cough, unaccompanied by an acute infection, should alert the physician sufficiently to carry out a detailed examination.

In addition to a detailed examination of the thorax, a meticulous *general physical examination* is mandatory in patients with disorders of the respiratory system. A careful search for infection in the teeth, gums, tonsils, or sinuses is recommended in patients known or suspected of having bronchiectasis or lung abscess. Neurologic findings including headache, drowsiness, papilledema, and other evidence of increased intracranial pressure may occur in patients with pulmonary disease who have hypoxia and hypercapnia. Vascular collapse is a late complication of carbon dioxide intoxication and is characterized by hypotension, flushed skin, sweating, and tachycardia.

Hemoptysis is often a frightening symptom (Chap. 35). Faint streaking of the sputum with blood may be observed in acute infections of the respiratory tract. However, many patients with bloody sputum have serious disease, such as pulmonary thromboembolism, tuberculosis, mitral stenosis, neoplasm of the lung, or bronchiectasis. In all instances it is necessary to exclude sources of blood in the nasopharynx and bleeding of gastric or esophageal origin. The character of the bloody expectorate should be defined, since it may be helpful in establishing the underlying disease process. Sputum which is frankly bloody without mucus or pus may be due to pulmonary thromboembolism (Chap. 256). When pus is present, pneumonia, bronchiectasis, or lung abscess should be considered. Dilute, pink, frothy sputum should suggest acute pulmonary edema (Chap. 233).

The *roentgenographic examination* of the chest represents the cornerstone of the diagnostic workup of the patient with suspected pulmonary disease, and it is the integration of the information obtained from the clinical examination and the roentgenogram which often provides the key to diagnosis. Unfortunately, in recent years, physical examination of the chest has been deemphasized, largely because of the recognition of the enormous value of radiographic techniques. However, abnormalities such as small or moderate amounts of fluid in the alveoli or in the mediastinum, bronchospasm, and pleural effusions can often be detected more accurately by physical examination than by chest roentgenography. It must also be appreciated that a number of other abnormalities may be associated with normal roentgenograms. These include solitary lesions less than 6 mm in diameter, acute pulmonary thromboembolism without infarction, early interstitial pneumonia, diffuse granulomatous disease such as miliary tuberculosis, interstitial disease such as scleroderma and systemic lupus erythematosus, bronchiectasis, acute chronic bronchitis, mild to moderate emphysema, endobronchial masses only partially obstructing the airways, and the majority of instances of hypoventriculation due to disorders of the central nervous system or neuromuscular disease. On the other hand, gross abnormalities of thoracic structure; pulmonary, mediastinal, and pleural masses; parenchymal consolidation, cysts, cavities, and abnormalities of the pulmonary vascular bed are all detected more reliably by roentgenographic than by physical examination.

An abnormal chest roentgenogram may be the presenting feature in an otherwise symptomless patient. In such circumstances the physician must make every effort to obtain earlier films in order to determine whether the lesion is new or old. Laminography, angiocardiography, and pulmonary photoscanning are additional procedures which may be helpful in establishing a diagnosis in a patient with an abnormality on the plain chest roentgenogram.

A variety of other diagnostic procedures are helpful in the workup of the patient with known or suspected pulmonary disease. These are are presented in Chap. 250 and include skin tests for tuberculosis, histoplasmosis, coccidioidomycosis, etc., as well as appropriate serum complement fixation tests, culture of the sputum, pleural fluid, bronchial washings, and gastric aspirate, as well as cytologic examination of the sputum and of bronchial washings. Bronchoscopy and bronchoscopic biopsy have been greatly facilitated by the development of the fiberoptic bronchoscope. Mediastinoscopy, scalene node and mediastinal node biopsy, pleural and lung biopsy may also be instrumental in establishing a diagnosis in an otherwise asymptomatic patient. Particularly important points which must be investigated in the history of the asymptomatic patient with a lesion discovered on a routine chest roentgenogram include exposure to individuals with tuberculosis, previous tuberculin and fungus skin tests, residence in or visits to areas of the country where fungal disease is endemic, a history of smoking and of exposure to dusts, and symptoms of systemic disease such as fever, sweat, fatigue, and weight loss.

In establishing the diagnosis in a patient suspected of having pulmonary disease, consideration must be given to the observation that substantial changes in the relative incidence of disease affecting the respiratory system have taken place in the United States during the past three decades. Chronic infectious disorders such as tuberculosis, lung abscess, and bronchiectasis have decreased. On the other hand, patients with chronic bronchitis and with emphysema now survive longer and form an increasing fraction of patients with chronic respiratory disease, as do patients with environmental lung disease. Modern intercontinental travel has increased the appearance in the lung of parasitic infestations in the Western world. Also, the reduction of immunologic competence which occurs in the treatment of patients with a variety of malignancies (Chap. 320) and following organ transplantation (Chap. 66) has led to an increasing incidence of opportunistic infections of the lungs with a variety of microorganisms rarely pathogenic in the past.

249 DISTURBANCES OF RESPIRATORY FUNCTION

JOHN B. WEST

The prime function of the lung is to exchange gas between the inspired air and the venous blood. A convenient starting point, therefore, for a discussion of disturbances of respiratory function is the alveolar membrane across which gas exchange occurs (Fig. 249-1). This blood-gas barrier is less than 1 μm thick and has a surface area of some 100 m^2. It is therefore ideally suited to its gas exchange function.

Air is pumped to one side of this membrane and blood to the other. The air flows through conducting tubes, the bronchi; these are not lined with blood capillaries, with the result that no gas exchange can occur within them. These conducting airways, therefore, comprise a *dead space.* Beyond these airways is the *alveolar gas,* which makes up most of the volume of the lung. This gas is in a constant state of agitation because of molecular diffusion, and thus all the alveolar gas has access to the capillary blood via the alveolar membrane.

On the other side of the membrane, blood is pumped from the right side of the heart to the pulmonary capillaries. These delicate vessels have diameters of only about 10 μm, so that the blood is spread out in a thin film, one or two red blood cells thick, around the air sacs.

It is worth emphasizing two features of the basic lung unit shown in Fig. 249-1: (1) its symmetry, i.e., air and blood are equally important in the central process of gas exchange (this simple fact is sometimes forgotten in clinical medicine, where the patient's difficulties in moving air in and out of the lung often dominate the picture); (2) the simplicity of the lung unit compared with, say, the nephron. The structure of the lung is simple because its main role is simple, i.e., bringing together air and blood so that gas exchange can occur by passive diffusion. By contrast, the kidney carries out many functions involving active transport, and its structure is correspondingly complicated.

VENTILATION

This is the process of moving inspired air into the alveolar gas compartment, where the gas exchange with the blood occurs. It is worth attaching some typical values for ventilation to the lung shown in Fig. 249-1. A normal breath is about 500 ml, so that with a breathing frequency of 15 per min, some 7 to 8 liters of air enters the lung each minute. However, because the volume of the conducting airways (dead space) is about 150 ml, only 350 of the 500 ml of air inhaled with each breath reaches the alveolar gas compartment. The rest remains behind in the airways and is subsequently exhaled. Thus, the volume of fresh gas entering the alveoli each minute is about 350 ml × 15, or some 5 liters. This is known as the *alveolar ventilation* and is of key importance to gas exchange. Of the 5 liters of air entering the alveoli, some 300 ml of oxygen moves across into the blood each minute to be replaced by about 250 ml of carbon dioxide. Thus less than 5 percent of the gas volume inhaled is exchanged with the gas in the blood.

The above figures apply to resting conditions. On exercise, the oxygen uptake may rise as high as 4 to 6 liters per min and the minute volume of air inspired may increase twentyfold. This is accomplished by an increase in both tidal volume and the frequency of breathing.

It should be noted that inspired air passes only a limited distance down the airways by ordinary bulk flow. Before it gets to the alveoli, its forward velocity is reduced to something like a millimeter per second, because of the enormous combined cross-sectional area of the small bronchi. In addition, the volume of gas in the small bronchi is so large that the alveoli and their ducts have completed their expansion before the fresh inspired air reaches them. The last few millimeters of its travel are therefore accomplished by molecular diffusion within the small airways. This process is very rapid for gas molecules but exceedingly slow for dust particles if they are over 1/2 μm in size. For this reason most inhaled dusts and aerosols never reach the alveoli, and many are deposited in the region of the terminal bronchioles.

MEASUREMENT OF VENTILATION The minute volume of air passing the lips is easily measured by connecting to the patient a large bag or spirometer via a mouthpiece and one-way valve. The resting and exercise ventilations are increased when disease impairs the efficiency of pulmonary gas exchange, but the measurement of ventilation by itself is not often useful because it is partly under voluntary control and is often changed by the stress of the measurement.

The maximum ventilation, or maximum breathing capacity, can be measured by asking the patient to breathe as fast and deep as he can for 15 sec. This measurement gives information about the mechanical properties of the

FIGURE 249-1
The functional lung unit. The alveolar membrane across which gas exchange takes place has alveolar gas on one side and pulmonary capillary blood on the other.

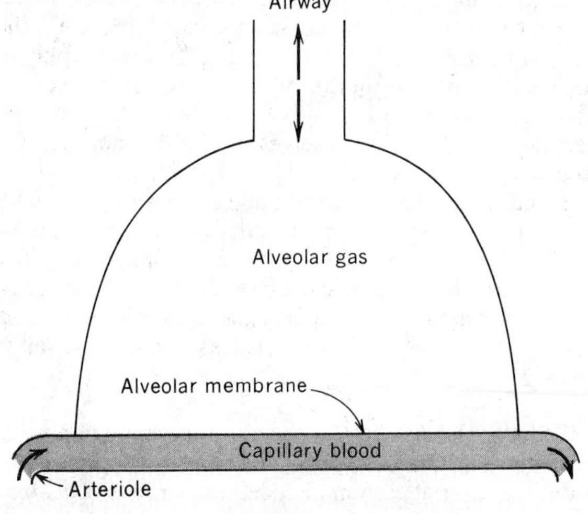

lungs, but it has largely been replaced by a less demanding measurement, the forced expiratory volume (see below).

CONTROL OF VENTILATION The rhythmic act of breathing is initiated in the respiratory centers of the pons and medulla. The level of ventilation is closely controlled from minute to minute by the medullary chemoreceptors which respond to changes in the carbon dioxide tension of arterial blood. There is evidence that these chemoreceptors are exquisitely sensitive to a fall in pH of the cerebrospinal fluid bathing them, which occurs when carbon dioxide diffuses across the blood-brain barrier.

Arterial hypoxemia also increases the ventilation through its action on the peripheral chemoreceptors in the carotid bodies. This hypoxic stimulus is normally relatively weak and variable but may dominate during chronic hypoxia, for example, following ascent to high altitude. This is also often the situation in patients with chronic respiratory failure, with the result that the administration of oxygen may cause hypoventilation and severe carbon dioxide retention.

The pH of the arterial blood has an effect on ventilation which is independent of the carbon dioxide tension. This is why ventilation may be altered during metabolic acidosis and alkalosis, thus displacing the arterial carbon dioxide tension away from its normal range.

HYPOVENTILATION When inspired air reaches the alveoli, oxygen is removed from it and carbon dioxide is added. The concentrations, or partial pressures, of these two gases in the alveoli depend on a balance between two processes. On the one hand, the removal of oxygen from (or addition of carbon dioxide to) the alveolar gas is determined by the metabolic demands of the body. On the other hand, the addition of oxygen to (or removal of carbon dioxide from) the alveolar gas depends on the amount of alveolar ventilation. Thus, if the alveolar ventilation is low in relation to oxygen uptake and carbon dioxide output, the partial pressure of oxygen in alveolar gas and arterial blood falls, and the level of carbon dioxide rises. This is hypoventilation.

Hypoventilation is commonly caused by disease outside the respiratory system and may exist in the presence of normal lungs. Causes include depression of the respiratory center by drugs or anesthesia, damage to the medulla by disease, diseases affecting the nerve supply to the muscles of the thorax or the muscles themselves, injury to the chest wall, and obstruction to the airways. Because the lungs themselves are often normal, the prognosis may be excellent if the precipitating cause is removed. Note that hypoventilation always causes both hypoxemia and hypercapnia, although the first can be abolished by adding oxygen to the inspired air. The carbon dioxide retention can be relieved only by increasing the ventilation, e.g., by using a ventilator. Disorders leading to hypoventilation are discussed in more detail in Chap. 255.

HYPERVENTILATION If the alveolar ventilation is abnormally high for the carbon dioxide production of the body, the arterial carbon dioxide tension falls. This may occur in metabolic acidosis, e.g., uremia, in which the chemoreceptors respond to the low blood pH. Hysterical hyperventilation is also not uncommon. The sensation of respiratory distress, or *dyspnea,* which should be clearly distinguished from *hyperpnea*, is considered in detail in Chap. 28.

DIFFUSION ACROSS THE ALVEOLAR MEMBRANE

Oxygen and carbon dioxide move across the blood-gas barrier by a process of simple physical diffusion from a region of high partial pressure to one of low, just as water runs downhill. Consider a red blood cell as it enters a pulmonary capillary. The oxygen tension in mixed venous blood (in the pulmonary artery) is typically about 40 mm Hg, and as the cell enters the capillary, it encounters an oxygen tension in alveolar gas of some 100 mm Hg, less than a micrometer away. Oxygen therefore moves rapidly across the barrier into the cell to combine with hemoglobin, and the oxygen tension rises. As a consequence, the oxygen pressure difference between the cell and the alveolar gas falls, and the rate of inflow of oxygen is reduced. However, under normal conditions, the diffusion properties of the alveolar membrane are so good and the rate of combination of oxygen with hemoglobin so rapid that before the cell has spent more than about a third of its time in the capillary, its oxygen tension has virtually reached that of the alveolar gas. This transfer of oxygen is helped by the shape of the oxygen dissociation curve, which ensures that the driving pressure difference is maintained until almost all the oxygen is moved across. Thus, under ordinary circumstances, there is no measurable difference between the oxygen tension of alveolar gas and that of the blood at the end of the pulmonary capillary. Indeed, the normal lung has plenty of reserve diffusion in hand.

Two factors which stress the diffusion ability of the lung are exercise and the inhalation of a low oxygen mixture. During strenuous exercise, the time spent by the red blood cells in the capillaries is greatly reduced, perhaps to a third of that at rest, so that the time available for the diffusion process is curtailed. Even so, the oxygen tension in the capillary blood almost reaches that of the alveolar gas, except possibly during the most exhausting work. Additional stress occurs if the lung inspires a low oxygen mixture, thus reducing the alveolar oxygen tension. Because the pressure difference between the oxygen in the gas and that in the red blood cells as they enter the capillary is lowered, the rate of movement of oxygen across the membrane is slowed. There is evidence that heavy work when the inspired oxygen tension is very low (e.g., at high altitude) causes lowering of the arterial oxygen tension because of inadequate diffusion into the pulmonary capillary. It is generally believed that carbon dioxide transfer is never limited by diffusion across the alveolar membrane, because of the much higher diffusion rate of this gas.

MEASUREMENT OF DIFFUSING CAPACITY This can be done using carbon monoxide. The subject inspires a low concentration (approximately 0.1 percent), and the rate of uptake of the gas by the blood is calculated from the difference between the inspired and expired concentrations. The measurement can be made during the course of a single 10-sec breath-holding period, or over a minute or so of steady breathing. In both cases, the diffusing capacity is expressed as the milliliters per minute of carbon monoxide taken up by the lung per millimeter of mercury of partial pressure of carbon monoxide in the alveolar gas. Normal values are in the region of 20 ml per min per mm Hg at rest, rising to 60 or more on exercise.

The reason why the uptake of carbon monoxide measures the diffusing capacity is the remarkable avidity of the blood for this gas. This means that appreciable amounts of carbon monoxide can be combined with hemoglobin in the blood at an exceedingly low partial pressure. As a result, the rise in tension of carbon monoxide in the red blood cells as they pass along the pulmonary capillaries is negligible and the amount of the gas which is transferred into the blood is determined only by the diffusion properties of the alveolar membrane and the rate of combination of carbon monoxide with hemoglobin. The latter depends on the oxygen tension in the alveoli; by measuring the carbon monoxide uptake at various inspired oxygen tensions, it is possible to determine separately the diffusing capacity of the alveolar membrane itself and the volume of blood in pulmonary capillaries.

The measurement of carbon monoxide uptake is a relatively simple procedure, and there is no problem in following changes of diffusing capacity in the normal lung under a variety of conditions. Unfortunately, however, it is very difficult to say how far the carbon monoxide uptake reflects the true diffusion characteristics of the alveolar membrane and the capillary blood in the presence of appreciable lung disease. The reason for this is that gross inequality of ventilation and blood flow in the lung reduce the carbon monoxide uptake, even in the absence of impaired diffusion. For this reason, the test when used in the clinic is sometimes said to measure the *transfer factor* of the lung for carbon monoxide and should be looked upon as a general index of the efficiency of gas exchange in the lung, rather than as a specific test of diffusion.

A method of measuring diffusing capacity using oxygen has also been described, but its validity is uncertain and the test is now rarely done.

IMPAIRMENT OF DIFFUSION There are generalized lung diseases, such as diffuse interstitial fibrosis (Chap. 254), sarcoidosis (Chap. 223), asbestosis (Chap. 258), and alveolar carcinomatosis (Chap. 260), in which microscopically the alveolar wall is thickened, and it is tempting to attribute any hypoxemia to defective diffusion. The term "alveolar-capillary block" was coined for this situation, and it is certainly an easy one to remember. However, the importance of impaired diffusion as a cause of the hypoxemia in these diseases has been questioned. The chief reason for this is that it is impossible to imagine normal ventilation and blood flow in an alveolus which has a thickened wall, and indeed several studies have shown marked inequality of ventilation and blood flow in the lung in these conditions. Since it is now recognized that uneven ventilation-perfusion ratios constitute a potent cause of hypoxemia (see below), the role of impaired diffusion is not clear. Furthermore, because the uptake of carbon monoxide in these diseases is undoubtedly reduced by the presence of uneven ventilation and blood flow, it is difficult to see how the question can be resolved. It is safer, therefore, to attribute the bulk of the hypoxemia in these generalized lung diseases to ventilation-perfusion inequality and leave the question of the importance of diffusion impairment open.

BLOOD FLOW

Mixed venous blood is pumped to the pulmonary capillaries directly from the right side of the heart so that the total *pulmonary blood flow* is equal to the cardiac output, say 5 or 6 liters per min in a normal adult. We saw earlier that the volume of fresh inspired air entering the alveoli each minute, the *alveolar ventilation,* is some 5 liters. Thus, the overall ratio of ventilation to blood flow, or *ventilation-perfusion ratio,* is about 1.

Even though the volumes of fresh gas and blood reaching the alveoli each minute are about the same, the volumes involved in exchanging gas at any instant are very different. Thus, while the alveolar gas volume is 2 to 3 liters at the end of a normal expiration, the capillary blood volume is only some 70 ml. This is why the lung microscopist sees chiefly air.

The pressures in the pulmonary circulation have long been considered the domain of the cardiologist, but they have an important bearing on gas exchange in the lung. The normal pulmonary arterial pressure is only just sufficient to raise blood to the top of the upright lung; if the pressure is reduced, as in hemorrhagic shock, the upper part of the lung is unperfused and gas exchange is impaired. Alterations in the pulmonary venous pressure, too, affect the distribution of blood flow in the lung.

VENTILATION-PERFUSION RELATIONSHIPS

Up to this point, we have been assuming that all lung units behave identically. Thus, Fig. 249-1 has been taken to refer to an alveolus, a group of alveoli with their duct, a lobe, or even the whole lung. In fact, however, the lung is not homogeneous, and the differences in behavior between the millions of units are responsible for the great bulk of the hypoxemia and hypercarbia seen in clinical practice. We shall see that even in the normal lung, there are marked regional differences in blood flow and ventilation which affect gas exchange, while in diseased states, the inhomogeneity becomes so severe that respiratory failure may ultimately develop.

NORMAL DISTRIBUTION OF BLOOD FLOW It is possible to measure the regional distribution of blood flow and ventilation in the lung by using radioactive gases. In one technique, the inert gas ^{133}xenon is employed. To measure blood flow, the xenon is dissolved in saline solution and injected into a peripheral vein. On reaching the lung, it is evolved into alveolar gas because of its poor solubility; there it remains during breath holding and can be detected by external counters. To measure ventilation, the patient inhales a single breath of the radioactive gas and again its regional distribution is measured. In both instances, a further measurement after a period of rebreathing of xenon allows a correction for lung volume to be made.

In the normal upright lung, blood flow per unit volume decreases rapidly from bottom to top, reaching very low values at the apex (Fig. 249-2). This pattern is affected by change of posture and exercise. When the subject lies supine, the apical and basal blood flows become the same, but the posterior (dependent) part of the lung has a higher blood flow than the anterior region. In the lateral position, the dependent regions are best perfused. On exercise in the upright position, both apical and basal blood flows increase, so that the proportion of the total flow going to the apex rises.

The cause of this uneven distribution of blood flow lies in the hydrostatic pressure differences within the lung. The pulmonary circulation is unique in that air and blood are separated by a very delicate membrane over a vertical distance of some 30 cm, and consequently, the hydrostatic effect of this large column of blood determines the caliber of the small vessels. It has been shown that the distribution of blood flow depends on the relative magnitudes of the pulmonary arterial, venous, and alveolar pressures. In particular, if pulmonary arterial pressure falls (as in hemorrhage, shock, and anesthesia) or alveolar pressure is raised (as in positive-pressure ventilation), the distribution of blood flow becomes more uneven. The normal pattern is also commonly affected by both heart and lung disease.

NORMAL DISTRIBUTION OF VENTILATION Ventilation also increases down the upright lung, though the changes are less marked than for blood flow (Fig. 249-2). This distribution of ventilation which is seen under normal resting conditions is altered at low lung volumes. It has been shown that when a normal subject exhales as far as he can (to residual volume) and then gradually inhales in small steps, initially very little air goes into the lower zones, but the upper zones are well ventilated. However, before he reaches his normal resting lung volume (functional residual capacity), this distribution is reversed and the lower zones are better ventilated than the upper. This pattern is then maintained right up to maximal volumes. The poor ventilation of the dependent regions of the lung at low lung volumes is seen in the erect, supine, and lateral positions, and it has important implications in clinical situations where the lung volume is low, e.g.. in obesity or following abdominal surgery. Since the dependent regions are the best perfused, the impairment of gas exchange may then be severe.

The cause of the uneven distribution of ventilation has to do with the way the lung is supported inside the chest. It is known that the expanding pressure on the lung is less in the dependent zones, presumably because these regions help to support the lung above them. Thus, the intrapleural pressure is less negative at the bottom of the lung than at the top. The reason for the greater ventilation of the dependent regions at normal volumes is twofold: (1) these alveoli have a smaller resting volume, and (2) their increase in volume is relatively large because they are so distensible. By contrast, these dependent regions are poorly ventilated at low lung volumes, because the expanding forces on them are then too weak to inflate them. Indeed, under these conditions, the airways to these alveoli may close and the alveoli become unventilated.

The volume at which the lower-zone airways close (the *closing volume)* is considerably less than the resting lung volume in normal young subjects. However, as the lung ages, and especially in the presence of chronic obstructive lung disease, the closing volume increases until it encroaches on the normal breathing range. Thus elderly normal subjects and patients with chronic bronchitis and emphysema frequently close their lower-zone airways during resting breathing; this results in a poorly ventilated region which impairs gas exchange.

VENTILATION-PERFUSION RATIO We have seen that while blood flow increases greatly down the upright lung, the change in ventilation is less. As a result, the ventilation-perfusion ratio varies from a high value at the top of the lung to a low value at the bottom (Fig. 249-2). The ventilation-perfusion ratio is of key importance because it determines the gas exchange which occurs in any part of the lung.

Consider a lung unit as shown in Fig. 249-1. It can

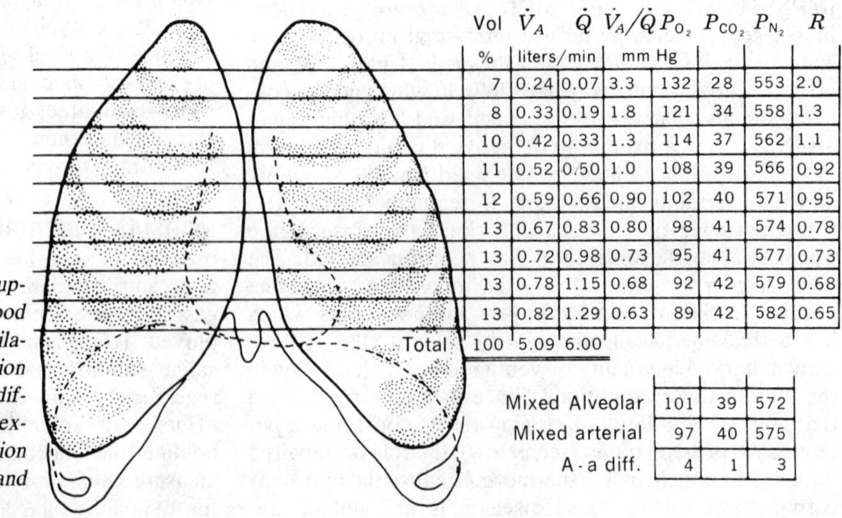

Vol	$\dot{V}_A$	$\dot{Q}$	$\dot{V}_A/\dot{Q}$	P_{O_2}	P_{CO_2}	P_{N_2}	R
%	liters/min			mm Hg			
7	0.24	0.07	3.3	132	28	553	2.0
8	0.33	0.19	1.8	121	34	558	1.3
10	0.42	0.33	1.3	114	37	562	1.1
11	0.52	0.50	1.0	108	39	566	0.92
12	0.59	0.66	0.90	102	40	571	0.95
13	0.67	0.83	0.80	98	41	574	0.78
13	0.72	0.98	0.73	95	41	577	0.73
13	0.78	1.15	0.68	92	42	579	0.68
13	0.82	1.29	0.63	89	42	582	0.65
Total 100	5.09	6.00					

	P_{O_2}	P_{CO_2}	P_{N_2}
Mixed Alveolar	101	39	572
Mixed arterial	97	40	575
A-a diff.	4	1	3

FIGURE 249-2
Regional differences within the normal upright lung. Note the large inequality of blood flow Q and the smaller inequality of ventilation V_A. The resulting ventilation-perfusion ratio (V_A/Q) inequality causes regional differences in gas exchange. Overall gas exchange is impaired, as shown by the tension differences between mixed alveolar gas and arterial blood.

readily be seen that the partial pressure of oxygen in the alveolar gas (and therefore in the end-capillary blood) will be set by a balance between the rate of its removal by the blood flow on the one hand, and the rate of its replenishment by the ventilation on the other. Thus, if the ventilation is gradually reduced but the blood flow is maintained, the oxygen partial pressure will gradually fall. The limit is reached when the unit is not ventilated and the oxygen tension becomes that of venous blood. This is a ventilation-perfusion ratio of zero. By contrast, if perfusion is gradually reduced, the oxygen tension will rise. The limit now occurs when the unit is unperfused and the oxygen tension in the alveolus is the same as that of inspired air. This is a ventilation-perfusion ratio of infinity.

Thus, the crucial factor determining the oxygen partial pressure is the ventilation-perfusion ratio; this is true also for the partial pressure of carbon dioxide, and indeed of any other gas that might be present. Figure 249-2 shows some of the regional differences in gas exchange which are calculated to occur in the normal upright lung as a consequence of the uneven ventilation-perfusion ratios.

OVERALL GAS EXCHANGE Though these regional differences in gas exchange are of interest, more important is the effect of uneven ventilation-perfusion ratios on overall gas exchange, i.e., the ability of the lung to take up oxygen and put out carbon dioxide. The reason why gas transfer is impaired by uneven ventilation and blood flow is made clearer by referring to Fig. 249-2. It can be seen that the base of the lung is much more important than the apex in determining the arterial blood composition, because it contributes most of the blood. However, the base has a low oxygen tension (because of its low ventilation-perfusion ratio). Thus, inevitably the arterial oxygen tension is depressed because it is loaded with less-well-oxygenated blood. For the same reason, the carbon dioxide tension in the blood is elevated. It is as if uneven ventilation-perfusion ratios set up a barrier between the gas and the blood, with the result that the arterial oxygen tension is depressed and the carbon dioxide tension is raised.

There is an additional reason why the arterial oxygen tension is reduced by ventilation-perfusion ratio inequality. Though the oxygen content of blood draining from alveoli with a low ventilation-perfusion ratio is always abnormally low, alveoli with a high ventilation-perfusion ratio are not able to oxygenate their blood much more than normal alveoli. This is because the blood is normally almost fully saturated with oxygen owing to the shape of the oxygen dissociation curve. This additional reason does not apply to carbon dioxide.

In the normal lung (Fig. 249-2), the effects of uneven ventilation-perfusion ratios on overall gas exchange are trivial; the arterial oxygen tension is reduced by a few millimeters of mercury and the carbon dioxide tension is raised by less than 1 mm Hg. Both these liabilities can be met if the total ventilation of the lung and thus its overall ventilation-perfusion ratio are increased. Indeed, the level of overall ventilation is normally set by the respiratory center via the arterial carbon dioxide tension. Thus, if uneven ventilation-perfusion ratios elevate the arterial carbon dioxide tension, this is brought back by the increased respiratory drive and the consequently higher overall ventilation.

In the diseased lung, the effects of ventilation-perfusion ratio inequality on gas transfer may be very severe because the degree of uneven ventilation and blood flow is far greater than in the normal lung. The arterial oxygen tension may be depressed by 50 or more millimeters of mercury, and in practice no amount of increased ventilation can return it to its normal level. The carbon dioxide tension, however, is often brought down by an increase in total ventilation. The reason why an increase in ventilation to diseased lungs can reduce the carbon dioxide tension but not increase the oxygen tension to normal levels lies in the different shapes of the two dissociation curves. If the ventilation is not increased, the carbon dioxide tension remains elevated. Ventilation-perfusion ratio inequality is much the commonest cause of hypoxemia and hypercarbia in generalized lung disease.

MEASUREMENT OF VENTILATION-PERFUSION INEQUALITY Unfortunately, it is difficult to derive much information about the pattern of uneven ventilation and blood flow in the diseased lung. Because much of the inequality is at the microscopic level, radioactive gas detectors which "see" relatively large regions of lung give little indication of the extent of the unevenness. The best method as yet is by the analysis of expired gas and arterial blood.

We saw in Fig. 249-2 that the arterial oxygen tension is depressed in the presence of ventilation-perfusion ratio inequality because it is loaded with less-well-oxygenated blood from the well-perfused lung base. By contrast, the expired alveolar gas receives a disproportionately high contribution from the apex, where the oxygen tension is high. An alveolar-arterial oxygen difference therefore develops, and the magnitude of this difference is a measure of the amount of ventilation-perfusion ratio inequality.

Though arterial blood can be collected by puncture, a representative sample of mixed alveolar gas is often impossible to obtain in the diseased lung because of its disturbed pattern of emptying. An alternative is to collect all the expired gas (including the dead space from the bronchi), using a valve box and a large bag or spirometer, and to calculate what is called the *ideal alveolar oxygen tension.* This is the value which the alveolar gas would have in the absence of ventilation-perfusion ratio inequality. This calculation is made using the arterial carbon dioxide tension and the alveolar gas equation.

The oxygen tension difference between ideal alveolar gas and arterial blood chiefly reflects those alveoli with an abnormally *low* ventilation-perfusion ratio, i.e., the alveoli which are overperfused in relation to their ventilation. These alveoli cause the hypoxemia, and their presence has the same effect as the admixture of some venous blood with arterial blood. Indeed, it is possible to express their contribution *as if* a certain proportion of the venous blood bypassed the lung altogether and was then added to the arterial blood. This is called *venous admixture,* or wasted blood flow, and is calculated from the oxygen tension difference between ideal alveolar gas and arterial blood. Normally, calculated venous admixture is only about 2 percent of the pulmonary blood flow, but it may rise to 30 percent or higher in the presence of severe ventilation-perfusion ratio inequality.

The alveoli with an abnormally *high* ventilation-perfusion ratio, i.e., those which are overventilated in relation to their perfusion, mainly affect carbon dioxide elimination. They behave as if a certain proportion of the inspired gas bypassed the alveoli altogether, i.e., as if the dead space were increased in size, thus resulting in wasted ventilation. Their contribution can be calculated from the carbon dioxide tension of arterial blood and mixed expired gas, using Bohr's equation. This gives a value for the *physiologic dead space,* which includes not only the volume of the bronchi but also the so-called alveolar dead space attributable to the overventilated alveoli. Normally the physiologic dead space is less than 30 percent of the tidal volume at rest, but it may rise to 50 percent or more in the presence of severe disease. Both venous admixture and physiologic dead space are typically increased in chronic obstructive pulmonary disease (Chap. 252) and infiltrative diseases of the lung (Chap. 254); in pulmonary thromboembolism (Chap. 256), an increase in dead space predominates.

MEASUREMENT OF VENTILATION INEQUALITY
Because the measurement of ventilation-perfusion ratio inequality is a relatively difficult procedure, the simpler measurement of uneven ventilation is often made. Although theoretically it would be possible for a patient to have ventilatory inequality but no mismatch of ventilation and blood flow, this is not seen in practice.

Two methods of measuring uneven ventilation are in use. In the single-breath test, the patient takes a single inspiration of pure oxygen and then exhales fully. A rapid nitrogen meter analysis of the expired nitrogen concentration at the lips and analysis of the expired volume are recorded simultaneously. After 750 ml has been expired (sufficient to clear the dead space), the rise in nitrogen concentration over the next 500 ml is measured. This is less than 1.5 percent in normal subjects. However, in patients with uneven ventilation, the nitrogen concentration rises more rapidly because the degree of dilution of the nitrogen by the inhaled oxygen varies throughout the lung, and also because the poorly ventilated regions (which received little oxygen and therefore have the most nitrogen) always empty last. This is a simple, quick, and useful test.

Uneven ventilation can also be detected by the multibreath washout method. Pure oxygen is breathed via a one-way valve, and again expired nitrogen concentration at the lips is measured. When the nitrogen concentration is plotted against the number of breaths on semilogarithmic paper, an almost straight line is found in normal subjects. This is because the successive dilution of the nitrogen in the lung by each breath of pure oxygen causes an exponential decay in nitrogen concentration. However in the presence of uneven ventilation, the line becomes successively flatter, because different regions of the lung lose their nitrogen at different rates, until finally only the nitrogen in the worst-ventilated spaces is being washed out. An additional check can be made after 7 min of washout. A forced expiration will show a nitrogen concentration of less than 2.5 percent in normal subjects but a higher value in patients with uneven ventilation because of delayed washout of the poorly ventilated spaces.

VENTILATION-PERFUSION RATIO INEQUALITY IN DISEASE Virtually all generalized diseases of the lung, such as emphysema, chronic bronchitis, diffuse interstitial fibrosis, and the pneumoconioses, result in mismatch of ventilation and blood flow. Very little is known about the pattern of unevenness in these conditions, though it is not difficult to imagine that an area of fibrosis or a bulla, for example, must interfere with both ventilation and blood flow.

There is evidence that in general, areas of the lung which are poorly ventilated are also poorly perfused. One reason for this is that local pathologic change tends to disturb both processes by its mechanical effects. However, there are other physiologic mechanisms which reduce the mismatch of uneven ventilation and perfusion. One is the reduction in blood flow to a poorly ventilated, hypoxic region of the lung, which has now been demonstrated on many occasions. The precise mechanism is unknown, but it appears to be a local response to alveolar hypoxia, since it occurs in the isolated denervated lung. Another mechanism is the reduction of ventilation which has been shown to follow obstruction to a branch of the pulmonary artery. This is apparently due to an increase in resistance of the small airways caused by a fall in carbon dioxide tension in the region.

How far these two mechanisms operate in practice is unknown, but it has been shown that the administration of various bronchodilator and vasodilator drugs to patients with generalized lung disease can exaggerate their hypoxemia. For example, isoproterenol (by aerosol) and epinephrine and aminophylline (by injection) have been shown to reduce the arterial oxygen tension of some patients with chronic obstructive lung disease. It is likely that one of the actions of these drugs is to interfere with these active mechanisms which reduce ventilation-perfusion ratio inequality.

MECHANICS OF BREATHING

This section deals with the forces involved in supporting and moving the lung and chest wall so that ventilation can be accomplished. The bellows function of the lung is one of the easiest to measure and also one of the most informative measurements in practice. Serious malfunction of the lung is almost always accompanied by a reduced ventilatory capacity.

LUNG AND CHEST WALL The lung is elastic and collapses if it is not held expanded. The pressure *inside* the lung (alveolar pressure) is the same as atmospheric pressure at the end of inspiration or expiration if the glottis is open. The pressure *outside* the lung (intrapleural pressure) is less than atmospheric pressure, or "negative." This pressure keeps the lung inflated and is developed by the chest wall, which is also elastic and tends to bow outwards. If air is introduced into this space and a pneumothorax is produced, the lung collapses inwards and the chest wall moves outwards.

During quiet breathing, inspiration is produced by the action of the diaphragm and intercostal muscles, and expiration results from the passive elastic recoil of the lungs. During deep breathing, the accessory muscles such as the sternomastoids and scaleni are called upon, and patients with diseased lungs may use these even at rest. Under these conditions, expiration is often assisted by the abdominal muscles.

COMPLIANCE This is the term used to describe the elastic properties of the lung and chest wall. The normal lungs expand by about 200 ml when the expanding pressure (intrapleural pressure) changes by 1 cm of water. Thus the compliance (or distensibility) of the lungs is said to be 200 ml per cm of water. In fact, this figure only applies at normal resting lung volumes; at high lung volumes, the lungs are less easy to expand and their compliance falls. The compliance of the normal chest wall is about the same as that of the lungs, and the compliance of both lung and chest wall together is therefore about half this value, i.e., 100 ml per cm of water.

The compliance of lung depends very much on how much tissue is present. A single lobe, for example, will clearly not change its volume by as much as a whole lung for the same change in expanding pressure. Compliance is therefore sometimes corrected for lung volume and called *specific compliance.*

The normal elastic behavior of the lungs is only partly caused by the elastic tissue within it. An important component is the surface tension of the fluid lining the alveoli. The lungs may be regarded as composed of 300 million tiny bubbles which tend to collapse for the same reason that a soap bubble on the end of a bubble pipe does. During the last few years it has been found that the cells lining the alveoli produce a phospholipid which lowers the surface tension of the lining fluid to extremely low values. The substance is known as a *surfactant.* This lowering of the surface tension has great physiologic importance, because it helps to maintain the stability of the alveoli and discourage atelectasis. About half the normal compliance of the lung is due to these surface forces.

The normal elastic behavior of the lung is disturbed by many diseases. Diffuse pulmonary fibrosis, pleural thickening, healed tuberculosis with scarring, and atelectasis all reduce the compliance of the lung. Heart disease, such as mitral stenosis and left ventricular failure, also commonly lowers compliance, although it is often difficult to be certain whether the volume of ventilating lung is reduced by edema in the airways, for example, or whether the elastic behavior of lung tissue itself is altered. An absence of surfactant is thought to be responsible for the alveolar collapse and the stiff lungs seen in hyaline membrane disease of the newborn. In emphysema and old age, the lungs become more compliant and have an abnormally large volume at normal expanding pressures.

AIRWAYS RESISTANCE So far we have been looking at the static forces involved in maintaining the expansion of the lung. However, during ventilation, additional forces are required to move air along the airways, because of the resistance offered to flow. This is expressed as the pressure difference between the alveoli and the mouth per unit of airflow rate. The normal value is in the vicinity of 1 to 2 cm water per liter per sec of flow at normal flow rates. The resistance rises at higher flow rates.

The airways resistance is higher during expiration than inspiration, and it is greater at small lung volumes because the airways are then not held open so much. A single deep inspiration often reduces the resistance, but the inhalation of cigarette smoke or other irritants increases it. During a forced expiration, airways resistance rises greatly, because of collapse of parts of the bronchial tree, and the expiratory resistance increases with respiratory effort. The reason for this is that the expiratory pressure is applied not only to the alveoli in an effort to empty them, but also to the outside walls of the airways which lie within the chest. As a result, the expiratory flow rate is independent of respiratory effort over a large range. In normal subjects, this is true only for forced expirations, but it often occurs much more readily in patients with emphysema, because the diseased airways collapse easily.

Diseases which increase airways resistance include bronchial asthma, chronic bronchitis, and pulmonary emphysema. The resistance may rise to many times its normal value and even during clinical remissions of the disease can be shown to be abnormally high. Lung volume increases in these conditions, and this has two helpful consequences: the airways are pulled open more, thus limiting the increase in resistance, and the higher passive recoil pressure of the lung assists expiration.

WORK OF BREATHING In order to move the lungs and chest wall and force air along the airways, work is required and the respiratory muscles must consume oxygen. In normal subjects, the work of breathing is very small except during the large ventilation of heavy exercise. In patients with obstructive lung disease, however, the frictional resistance to airflow is high even at rest and the work of breathing is much increased, perhaps to five or ten times its normal value. Under these conditions, the oxygen cost of breathing may become an appreciable fraction of the total oxygen consumption.

Patients with a reduced compliance of the lungs or chest wall have a higher work of breathing, because the stiffer structures are more difficult to move. These patients tend to use rapid shallow breaths, which reduces their oxygen cost of ventilation. However, if breathing becomes too shallow, the volume of air merely moved in and out of the bronchial dead space becomes disproportionately high, and gas exchange is consequently impaired. A compromise is therefore reached.

MEASUREMENTS OF MECHANICS One of the most useful tests in the armamentarium of the pulmonary function laboratory is the analysis of a single forced expiration. The patient makes a full inspiration and then exhales as hard and as fast as he can into a lightweight spirometer. Typical records are shown in Fig. 249-3. It can be seen that for a normal subject the total volume exhaled, the *vital capacity* or VC, is large, and also that about 80 percent of this volume is exhaled in 1 sec. This is called the *forced expiratory volume* or FEV_1. In *obstructive lung disease,* e.g., emphysema, the vital capacity is reduced because the airways close and limit expiration before the patient has breathed out fully. In addition, the FEV_1 is grossly reduced, as is the FEV/VC percentage. This is because of the high airways resistance, which slows down the rate of expiration. In *restrictive lung disease,* e.g., ankylosing spondylitis, the VC is low because of the limited expansion of the lung or chest wall. However, the FEV_1 is often not reduced proportionately, because airway resistance is normal. Thus the FEV/VC percentage is normal or high.

The FEV_1 is closely related to the maximum breathing capacity, and since it is a much simpler test to perform, it has largely replaced it. Impaired lung function is almost always associated with a reduced FEV_1, and the test is therefore a valuable screening procedure. It is also useful in assessing the efficacy of bronchodilator therapy and in following the progress of patients.

Other lung volumes can also be measured at the same time. The *inspiratory capacity* is the maximum volume which can be inspired from the resting volume of the lungs, which is called the *functional residual capacity.* The maximum volume which can be expired from the resting level is the *expiratory reserve volume.* This leaves the *residual volume* still in the lungs, and this can be measured only indirectly. One technique is to connect the patient to a spirometer circuit containing helium and measure the degree of dilution of this gas which occurs after several minutes of rebreathing. Another is to use a body plethysmograph (see below).

The measurement of compliance and airways resistance is more difficult. In order to determine lung compliance, i.e., volume change per unit of pressure change, the pressure expanding the lungs must be known. In practice this can be found by passing a small rubber balloon connected to a manometer down into the esophagus. Esophageal pressure is then taken as a measure of intrapleural pressure. To measure airways resistance, i.e., the pressure drop along the airways per unit of airflow, alveolar pressure must be known. This can be found by seating the patient in a large airtight box, or plethysmograph. First, he is asked to try to breathe against a complete obstruction, and from the change in box pressure, lung volume can be calculated. Next, he is asked to pant in and out, and again box pressure is recorded. Alveolar pressure can then be derived and airway resistance calculated. This equipment is available only in specialized centers.

ACID-BASE DISTURBANCES If pulmonary gas exchange is impaired, carbon dioxide tension in the arterial blood may rise, thus tending to depress the pH and causing *respiratory acidosis.* The compensatory mechanisms which are then brought into play are discussed in Chap. 265.

MEASUREMENT OF BLOOD GASES Blood gas measurements play a vital role in the management of respiratory failure. Arterial blood can be obtained by direct puncture, and the oxygen and carbon dioxide tensions and the pH measured by electrodes. Oxygen saturation can be derived from the oxygen content of the blood using van Slyke's method before and after complete oxygenation, or the saturation can be calculated from an oxygen dissociation curve.

HYPOXEMIA

The four main causes of a low arterial oxygen tension are ventilation-perfusion ratio inequality, right-to-left shunt, hypoventilation, and impaired diffusion. In addition, living at high altitude or deliberately inspiring a low oxygen mixture causes hypoxemia. Ventilation-perfusion ratio inequality is the commonest cause and is responsible for

FIGURE 249-3
Measurement of the forced expiratory volume, FEV_1, and vital capacity, VC. The patient makes a full inspiration and then exhales as hard and as fast as he can. As he exhales, the pen moves down. The FEV_1 is the volume exhaled in 1 sec; the VC is the total volume exhaled. Note the differences between the normal, obstructive, and restrictive patterns.

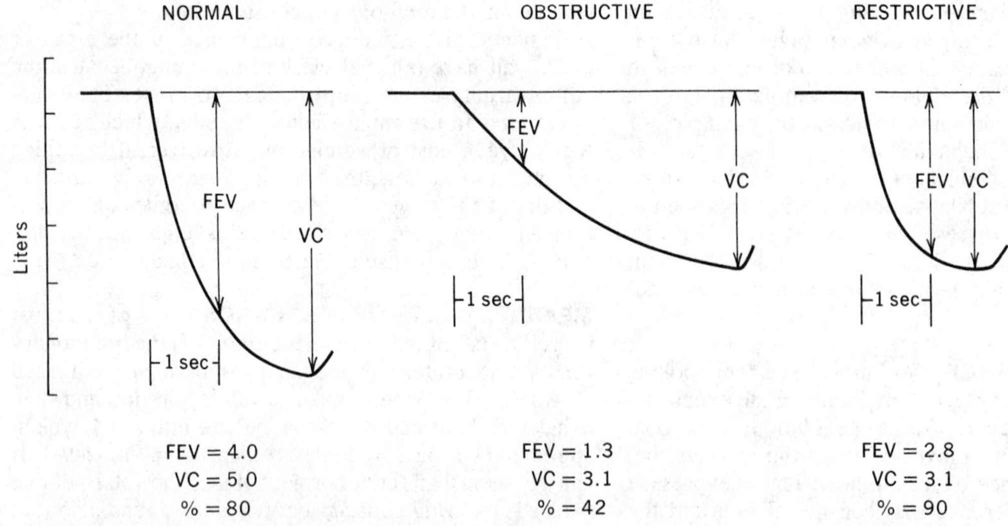

almost all the hypoxemia seen in chronic lung disease. Specific tests of ventilation-perfusion inequality are not available; it is generally deduced by exclusion. The demonstration of ventilatory inequality (see above) is a useful pointer. Mild degrees of ventilation-perfusion ratio inequality may be present without hypoxemia, and considerable inequality may exist without hypercapnia if overall ventilation is increased. However, carbon dioxide retention almost always develops eventually. The hypoxemia is abolished by the administration of 100 percent oxygen, though with severe inequality, the arterial oxygen tension may take many minutes to rise to normal values, because of very poorly ventilated areas. Exercise may or may not aggravate the hypoxemia and hypercapnia (see Table 249-1).

Shunted blood, i.e., blood which has not circulated through ventilated areas of the lung, causes hypoxemia. Patients with right-to-left shunts through congenital heart defects belong to this group. Patients with ventilation-perfusion ratio inequality often have some parts of the lung completely unventilated, and the contribution of these regions is indistinguishable from that of a shunt. The hypoxemia due to shunt is not abolished (though it is reduced) by administering 100 percent oxygen, and this test will distinguish it from the other causes of hypoxemia. The level of the arterial oxygen tension under these conditions allows the percentage of shunted blood to be measured. The arterial tension rises to some extent because of the addition of dissolved oxygen to the pulmonary blood, and a measurement of arterial saturation may not permit detection of the hypoxemia. It is therefore important to measure oxygen tension. The hypoxemia of shunt may be exaggerated by exercise. Hypercapnia does not occur unless the shunt is very gross, because the respiratory center increases the ventilation, thus holding the arterial carbon dioxide tension down.

Hypoventilation always causes both hypoxemia and hypercapnia. Because of the shape of the oxygen dissociation curve, considerable carbon dioxide retention may be present without recognizable cyanosis. If the patient is inhaling an enriched oxygen mixture, e.g., in the anesthetic recovery room, hypoxemia is not present but the hypercapnia may be severe.

Impaired diffusion causes hypoxemia but not hypercapnia. The hypoxemia is accentuated by exercise but abolished if an enriched oxygen mixture is administered. As we have seen, diffusion impairment may occur in normal subjects during work at very high altitude, but its importance as a cause of hypoxemia in disease is disputed.

TABLE 249-1
Features helpful in distinguishing the various causes of hypoxemia and hypercapnia

	Hypoxemia	*Hypercapnia*	*Hypoxemia on exercise*	*Hypercapnia on exercise*	*Hypoxemia on 100% O_2*
Ventilation-perfusion ratio inequality	Yes	Yes or no	Yes	Yes or no	No
Shunt	Yes	No	Yes	Possible	Yes
Hypoventilation	Yes	Yes	Often severe	Often severe	No
Impaired diffusion	Yes	No	Often severe	No	No

HYPERCAPNIA

The two chief causes of carbon dioxide retention are ventilation-perfusion ratio inequality and hypoventilation. Ventilation-perfusion ratio inequality is the commonest cause, although many patients have some degree of uneven ventilation and blood flow without hypercapnia. A combination of the two causes is common.

Why does a patient with chronic lung disease develop hypercapnia? Progressive lung disease (perhaps aggravated by an acute infection) causes increasing mismatch of blood flow and ventilation and greater impairment of carbon dioxide transfer. For a time, the respiratory center is able to hold the arterial carbon dioxide tension down by increasing the ventilation, but the work of breathing is usually high because of airways obstruction, so that eventually a compromise is reached and the arterial and alveolar tensions are allowed to rise. This has the advantage that more carbon dioxide tension is put out for the same ventilation, so that it may be looked upon as a compensatory mechanism, albeit a hazardous one. As the ventilation-perfusion ratio inequality becomes worse, the tendency is for the arterial carbon dioxide tension to rise further.

A particularly dangerous situation may arise if the patient is given oxygen to breathe. The chief stimulus to ventilation in these patients is often hypoxia, and when this is suddenly relieved, the ventilation may drop precipitously and the arterial carbon dioxide tension climb rapidly. The carbon dioxide retention and acidosis may then cause unconsciousness, muscular twitching, and a raised intracranial pressure. This is known as *carbon dioxide narcosis.* Drugs which depress the respiratory center may produce a similar effect. Thus while oxygen administration is generally indicated in these patients because of their severe hypoxemia, it should be given with caution.

Another hazardous situation often arises when these patients are taken off oxygen because they are retaining too much carbon dioxide. Since the body stores of carbon dioxide are so large, many minutes elapse before the alveolar carbon dioxide tension returns to reasonable levels. During this recovery period, this high alveolar carbon dixoide dilutes the alveolar oxygen and may cause profound hypoxemia.

REFERENCES

BASS H: Pulmonary function studies: Aid to diagnosis for dyspnea. Prog Cardiovasc Dis 14:621, 1972

BATES DV et al: *Respiratory Function in Disease,* 2d ed., Philadelphia: Saunders, 1971

CHERNIACK RM et al: *Respiration in Health and Disease,* 2d ed., Philadelphia: Saunders, 1972

COMROE JH et al: *The Lung: Clinical Physiology and Pulmonary Function Tests,* 2d ed., Chicago: Year Book, 1962

WEST JB: *Ventilation/Blood Flow and Gas Exchange,* 2d ed., Oxford: Blackwell Scientific Publications, Ltd.; Philadelphia: Davis, 1970

250 DIAGNOSTIC PROCEDURES IN THE PATIENT WITH RESPIRATORY DISEASE

KENNETH M. MOSER

In seeking a definitive diagnosis in the patient with respiratory disease, a wide choice of diagnostic procedures is available. These procedures vary considerably, not only in diagnostic reliability and specificity, but also in terms of the discomfort and hazard to the patient. Hence, an orderly sequence of test selection is mandatory. This sequence should begin with procedures involving little risk and move on to those which entail higher morbidity and mortality rates only if necessary.

RADIOGRAPHIC PROCEDURES The *chest roentgenogram* serves two major roles in the search for a diagnosis in the patient with respiratory disease: *detector* and *guide.* Often, in its role as a detector, the routine chest roentgenogram initiates the diagnostic search by disclosing an abnormality in an asymptomatic individual. More commonly, it permits detection of pulmonary involvement in someone already ill. Rarely, detection may coincide with diagnosis; e.g., in spontaneous pneumothorax or when a radiopaque foreign body has been aspirated.

Far more frequently, however, the roentgenogram, having detected potential disease, provides a guide to the selection of subsequent diagnostic procedures. Many radiographic findings are quite characteristic of certain diseases. A number of radiographic patterns are sufficiently repetitive to warrant descriptive names, such as bilateral hilar adenopathy, solitary pulmonary nodule, diffuse interstitial infiltrate, alveolar filling pattern, multinodular lesion, honeycomb lung. Thus, a particular radiographic finding, combined with other pertinent data, often permits establishment of a reasonable list of possible diagnoses. For example, the roentgenographic detection of bilateral hilar adenopathy in an asymptomatic, twenty-six-year-old Negro male immediately places sarcoidosis at the top of the list. A chest roentgenogram disclosing upper lobe cavities in a febrile male whose brother recently was admitted to a tuberculosis sanitarium would make tuberculosis the most likely entity. Or a "diffuse interstitial" infiltrate—for which more than 100 etiologies exist—may yield a prompt diagnosis of varicella pneumonia when combined with the classical skin lesions.

In some instances, special radiographic technique may provide valuable diagnostic insights.

Fluoroscopy allows visualization of the thoracic contents in a dynamic rather than static manner and also permits a wide range of special views. It also indicates whether a lesion is pulsatile, what its precise location in the thorax is, whether the hemidiaphragms move normally, i.e., whether they are fixed or more paradoxically, and how various zones of the lung behave during inspiration and expiration.

Tomography (laminography, planography) is a radiographic technique by which a sequence of roentgenograms, each representing a "slice of the lung" at a different depth, is obtained. Ordinarily, "cuts" at 0.5-to-1.0-cm distances through the area of interest are made. Tomograms can identify a number of features which were not appreciated on the "routine" roentgenogram, including the presence of calcium or cavity in a lesion; the presence of hilar adenopathy; abnormalities in configuration of the trachea and major bronchi; and the contours of masses in the mediastinal area.

SKIN TESTS Having arrived at a tentative list of diagnostic possibilities based on the history, physical examination, and the radiographic appearance, the physician should move to other procedures. One of the simplest and most commonly overlooked is the application of *skin tests* with specific antigens. Antigens are now available to assist in the diagnosis of tuberculosis, histoplasmosis, coccidioidomycosis, blastomycosis, trichinosis, and toxoplasmosis. A negative battery of skin tests may provide a diagnostic clue by suggesting a disorder associated with skin anergy, such as sarcoidosis.

SEROLOGIC TESTS These tests also may be useful in the diagnosis of histoplasmosis, blastomycosis, coccidioidomycosis, toxoplasmosis, mycoplasma pneumonia, and a variety of other infectious diseases involving the lungs. Often, more extensive diagnostic procedures can be avoided if appropriate serologic tests are obtained.

SPUTUM EXAMINATION Another rapid, innocuous diagnostic procedure is *sputum examination.* It is important that the specimen contain sputum, not saliva. The gross nature of the sputum—color, odor and the presence of blood—may provide valuable clues. Carefully stained smears of the sputum should be examined next, for these will disclose the causative organism in many bacterial pneumonias, in tuberculosis, and in some fungus infections. Often valuable time is lost because the sputum smear is not examined and results of culture are awaited instead.

Culture of the sputum is not a substitute for careful microscopic examination of stained sputum specimens. Proper results from sputum culture require attention to detail. Specimens for culture should be collected and delivered to the laboratory promptly. If unusual organisms are anticipated, the laboratory should be alerted so that implantation on all appropriate media will be assured.

Exfoliative cytology of the sputum is helpful in the diagnosis of carcinoma of the lung. Again, proper handling of such specimens is essential. Sputum samples often can be obtained in a patient who is not coughing by having him inhale a heated mixture of a mildly irritative solution which induces cough.

EXAMINATION OF PLEURAL FLUID Like sputum, pleural fluid can supply definitive information and should be examined for specific gravity, white blood cell count and differential count, hematocrit and/or red blood cell count, protein and glucose concentrations, amylase, appropriate cultures, and exfoliative cytology. The gross appearance of the fluid, the quantity obtained, and the precise location of the thoracentesis should be recorded. Specific diagnostic findings in pleural fluid may include the opalescent, pearly fluid characteristic of chylothorax; cytologic evidence of cancer; positive cultures for tuberculosis or other infections; a marked elevation of amylase, indicative of effusion secondary to pancreatitis; and the very low glucose value often seen in effusions associated with rheumatoid arthritis.

PULMONARY FUNCTION TESTS These tests may serve as diagnostic guides. Certain "patterns" of derangement in spirometric tests, arterial blood gases, diffusing capacity, and other functional parameters are particularly suggestive of certain pulmonary diseases. For example, diffuse interstitial fibrotic diseases of the lungs produce a "restrictive" spirometric defect, reduced pulmonary compliance, and an alveoloarterial oxygen tension gradient which is widened at rest and widens further with exercise. Emphysema characteristically causes expiratory obstruction, lung hyperinflation, decreased static elastic recoil (increased compliance), and a reduced diffusing capacity (Chap. 249).

PULMONARY SCINTIPHOTOGRAPHY This technique can provide a visual image of the distribution of both blood flow and ventilation in the lungs, as well as quantitative data on such distribution. Scintiphotos ("scans") are obtained by a variety of "scanning" devices which record the pattern of pulmonary radioactivity after intravenous injection or inhalation of gamma-emitting radionuclides. Injection (perfusion) photoscans have proved especially valuable in detecting zones of absent or decreased blood flow compatible with embolism (Chap. 256). When ventilation scans, obtained with radioactive gases, are combined with perfusion studies, ventilation/perfusion patterns are provided which permit recognition of parenchymal lung diseases and vascular disorders including embolism.

All the above procedures involve minimal risks and discomfort to the patient. These approaches should be exhausted before the techniques discussed below are considered, unless the condition of the patient demands immediate diagnosis.

BRONCHOSCOPY Bronchoscopy is employed to visualize directly the trachea and its major subdivisions. A lighted mirror-lens system is introduced into the anesthetized tracheobronchial tree. In addition to permitting observation of abnormalities such as tumors or granulomatous lesions, it enables one to obtain biopsy material from suggestive or obvious lesions, as well as bronchial washings for culture and cytologic examination. The standard rigid bronchoscope permits visualization only of lobar bronchi and the orifices of some segmental bronchi. The flexible fiberoptic bronchoscope extends the range of view and biopsy to segmental and subsegmental bronchi, and reduces the discomfort of the patient associated with the use of the larger rigid instrument.

BRONCHOGRAPHY In this method, radiopaque material is instilled into the tracheobronchial tree via a catheter. Positioning the patient and catheter permits the material to coat all portions of the tracheobronchial tree for a sufficient period so that their outline can be recorded on chest roentgenograms. Bronchography is required for the diagnosis of bronchiectasis, for the identification of obstruction in distal bronchi, and for the detection of other types of congenital and acquired forms of tracheobronchial distortion or malformation.

PULMONARY ANGIOGRAPHY Just as bronchography outlines the tracheobronchial anatomy, pulmonary angiography permits visualization of the pulmonary vasculature. Radiopaque materials are injected rapidly by vein or via a catheter into the systemic veins, right chambers, or the pulmonary artery. The distribution of this material in the pulmonary vasculature is recorded on film (angiography), by a high-speed camera (cineangiography), or on videotape (Chap. 231). Angiography is frequently used to detect pulmonary emboli and a variety of congenital and acquired lesions of the pulmonary vessels.

Often, despite the application of the procedures discussed above, a definitive diagnosis is still lacking, and biopsy of tissue is indicated. If a pleural effusion exists, *pleural biopsy* is often worthwile. This can be carried out with either a "closed" or "open" technique. In the former, a needle specially constructed for biopsy is inserted at the time of thoracentesis. All available needles have a cutting edge and some mechanism for retaining the biopsy specimen. The needle is introduced into the effusion and seated on the parietal pleura, from which a biopsy is then obtained with the cutting edge. The procedure is sufficiently safe and productive to warrant its performance in every thoracentesis done when there is an effusion of obscure cause. Pleural fluid should be obtained prior to biopsy because bleeding after parietal pleural biopsy may obscure the true character of the fluid. Usually, three biopsies are taken from differing sites at the same session. Care should be exercised to place the needle in a position least likely to impinge upon the intercostal vessels.

The absence of pleural fluid increases the hazard of "closed" biopsy, because the needle cannot be placed into the pleural space with assurance. Bleeding, pneumothorax, and bronchopleural fistula induced by cutting through visceral pleura are more likely, and a satisfactory biopsy specimen is less likely to be obtained. Therefore, in the absence of effusion—or when "closed" biopsy has not provided a diagnosis—"open" biopsy is indicated. This involves a limited thoracotomy, requiring anesthesia. A small intercostal incision is made, and the parietal pleura is biopsied under direct visualization. The incision is then closed, often without an intercostal tube. "Open" biopsy has several advantages because a larger specimen is obtained and the pleura and underlying lung can be seen and palpated. When pleural involvement is "spotty," open biopsy increases the possibility of establishing a diagnosis.

Another favored site for biopsy is the *scalene fat pad.* Because the lymph nodes invariably present in this fat pad receive lymphatic drainage from the lungs, they often disclose intrathoracic diseases such as carcinoma, granulomatous infections, and sarcoidosis. Scalene biopsy can be performed under local anesthesia. In some clinics, scalene node biopsy has been combined with, or replaced by, *mediastinoscopy.*

Mediastinoscopy This involves insertion of a lighted mirror-lens system, much like a bronchoscope, through an incision at the base of the neck anteriorly. The instrument is advanced under visual control into the mediastinum, where inspection and biopsy can be carried out.

Lung biopsy Finally, if the diagnosis still remains unclear, biopsy of the lung may be required. Again, "closed" and "open" approaches are available. Closed needle biopsies of the lung are a subject of some debate because pneumothorax and bleeding are encountered in a substantial number of patients. In addition, the pulmonary architecture leads to difficulty in cutting and retaining the specimen. Finally, because of its small size, the specimen of tissue obtained may be inadequate for diagnosis. Advocates of closed lung biopsy emphasize that, in experienced hands, pneumothorax and bleeding are rare, mild, and easily controlled; and that a substantial number of diagnoses can be established without resort to open biopsy.

Those who prefer open (surgical) biopsy feel that the risk and morbidity of a limited thoracotomy are not substantially greater than those encountered in closed biopsy and are counterbalanced by the fact that an adequate, representative lung biopsy will provide a reliable answer to the diagnostic problem. The decision in favor of closed lung biopsy usually depends upon local expertise. However, there is general agreement on three points: (1) closed biopsy is particularly hazardous in patients with pulmonary hypertension; (2) prior to needle biopsy, provision should be made for prompt treatment of pneumothorax and bleeding; and (3) large solid lesions abutting, or attached to, the thoracic wall are the most favorable for closed biopsy. Needle biopsy of such lesions is safer and more likely to provide a diagnosis than is needle biopsy of lesions located deeply in the pulmonary parenchyma.

All specimens obtained by biopsy should be both cultured and processed for pathologic examination.

REFERENCES

BATES DV et al: *Respiratory Function in Disease,* Philadelphia: Saunders, 1971

BAUM GL: *Textbook of Pulmonary Diseases,* Boston: Little, Brown, 1973

FRASER RG, PARÉ JAP: *Diagnosis of Diseases of the Chest,* Philadelphia: Saunders, 1970

LILLINGTON GA, JAMPLIS RW: *A Diagnostic Approach to Chest Diseases,* Baltimore: Williams & Wilkins, 1965

251 DISEASES OF THE UPPER RESPIRATORY TRACT

JOSEPH W. WALIKE
IVAN L. BENNETT, JR.
ROBERT G. PETERSDORF

This chapter summarizes some of the diseases that are manifested in whole or in part by structural alterations or dysfunction of the nose, nasopharynx, paranasal sinuses, and larynx. In the course of their normal function of warming, humidifying, and preliminary cleansing (by impingement of inhaled particles upon the mucosa) of inspired air, these passages are exposed to a multitude of irritants and infectious agents. Their lining membranes contain many mucous glands and deposits of lymphoid tissue; the vascular bed of the nasal mucosa is capable of such rapid and extensive alterations in response to local or systemic stimuli that it is often classified as erectile tissue. Engorgement, hypersecretion of mucus, and hyperplasia of the adenoids and other lymphatic foci in response to irritation or infection can produce acute or chronic obstruction of the passages draining the sinuses, conjunctivas, and middle ears. This leads to initiation or aggravation of bacterial infection in these areas.

The annoying and distracting discomfort occasioned by interference with inspiration and speech, coupled with the frequency of viral and allergic disorders of this region, makes upper respiratory disease a most important transient disability.

DISEASES OF THE NOSE AND NASOPHARYNX

Anosmia, total loss of olfactory sense, is common during acute infections of the nose. It may occur if the olfactory fissure is blocked by swollen mucosa, polyps, or tumors. Anosmia following head trauma is often permanent. Idiopathic cases may respond to 200,000 units of vitamin A twice daily.

Hay fever, vasomotor rhinitis, and complicating nasal polyposis are discussed in Chap. 67. Acute coryza and other forms of viral rhinitis are discussed in Chap. 186. The upper respiratory prodrome of measles is discussed in Chap. 195.

Among *bacterial infections,* the persistent rhinitis ("snuffles") of congenital syphilis, nasal diphtheria, and furunculosis of the nares (which occasionally may be complicated by cavernous sinus thrombosis) are the more important.

Clear, watery discharge characterizes *cerebrospinal rhinorrhea.* The instillation of a small amount of methylene blue into the cerebrospinal fluid may provide the diagnosis, although radioactive tracers are preferred for locating the leakage. Testing the cerebrospinal fluid for sugar content does not provide accurate diagnostic information because in most children nasal discharge contains glucose. Chronic mucoid discharge is frequent in children with enlarged adenoids. Unilateral purulent or sanguineous discharge suggests a foreign body, diphtheria, or tumor.

Perforation of the nasal septum This condition may result from habitual nose picking, but syphilis, occupational exposure to chromate, complications of cautery for epistaxis, and sequelae of nasal septal surgery are other causes. Septal perforation has also been documented in patients with rheumatoid arthritis, disseminated lupus erythematosus, scleroderma, and psoriatic arthritis. Many diseases are characterized by extensive destructive and deforming lesions of the nose and adjacent structures. These include leprosy (Chap. 157), the gangosa and goundou lesions of yaws (Chap. 160), the espundia type of American leishmaniasis (Chap. 212), South American blastomycosis (Chap. 167), midline granuloma (Chap. 226), Wegener's granulomatosis (Chap. 363), and phycomycosis (Chap. 172).

Rhinosporidiosis Caused by a yeast-like organism, *Rhinosporidium seeberi*, this disease is common in India and Ceylon; sporadic cases occur in many other areas. Soft, pinkish, sessile or pedunculated polyps appear on the nasal mucosa; sometimes the conjunctivas and, rarely, other mucosal surfaces are involved. Treatment is simple excision (see Chap. 174).

Rhinophyma Also called Pfundnase, this progressive, deforming, nodular enlargement of the alae nasi is due to hypertrophy of sebaceous follicles in patients with chronic, severe acne rosacea. There is no specific treatment; dramatic improvement can be achieved by plastic surgery.

Ozena This is a severe chronic rhinitis of unknown cause characterized by thick, greenish discharge, mucosal crusts, turbinate atrophy, and an offensive odor. Patients eventually become anosmic. Even when the nasal passages are widened and resistance to airflow is decreased, obstruction is a constant complaint. Cultures grow gram-negative bacilli (*Klebsiella, Pseudomonas*, etc.). Treatment, aimed at reducing the odor, includes use of local or systemic antibiotics and large doses of vasodilators (Priscoline, nicotinic acid). Local cleansing by means of repeated saline irrigation is extremely important to get rid of the foul-smelling crusts. Surgical treatment of the nasal airway affords relief in many cases.

Mycosis leptothrica So called because infection by *Leptothrix* was thought to be its cause, this is a focal hyperkeratosis of the tonsils, pharynx, and larynx that occurs in young adults. The many small, white, raised patches over the mucosa are striking and are often mistaken for exudate; removal causes no bleeding. Patients are sometimes asymptomatic but may complain of a "scratchy" throat. There is no treatment; the lesions regress after months or years.

Epistaxis Recurrent, profuse epistaxes occur with hypertensive vascular disease, familial telangiectasia, coagulation defects, and tumors.

Carcinoma of the nares Both basal-cell and squamous-cell carcinoma are common about the nasal skin and vestibule. These lesions respond well to either surgical excision or radiotherapy; choice of therapy depends on size and location of the tumor. Carcinomas of the nasal mucosa are unusual; they occur in elderly individuals and invade or metastasize late.

Carcinoma of the nasopharynx Also called *lymphoepithelioma*, this condition occurs in young and middle-aged adults and is especially common among Chinese. These tumors metastasize early. Large, cancerous cervical lymph nodes often result from a primary lesion so small that it is found with great difficulty. These tumors tend to occur near the orifice of a eustachian tube, and the combination of *cervical adenopathy and ipsilateral ear pain or deafness* is a signal for careful examination of the nasopharynx. These tumors are radiosensitive, and survival for several years with repeated courses of therapy is usual; complete cures are effected less than 30 percent of the time.

Lymphoma Lymphoma and reticulum-cell sarcoma are often first detected as nasopharyngeal masses. Isolated plasmacytomas of the nasopharynx are found predominantly in elderly males, some of whom develop multiple myeloma. Two tumors of children deserve mention. A highly malignant and rapidly fatal lesion which tends to arise in the nasopharynx or soft palate is the sarcoma botryoides or embryonal rhabdomyosarcoma. Nasopharyngeal angiofibromas are benign tumors that occur almost exclusively in adolescent boys. They usually arise from the base of the sphenoid, may extend into the pterygomaxillary space, nose, cheek, and sinuses, and on rare instances may spread intracranially. These highly vascular tumors may cause spontaneous life-threatening epistaxis. Biopsies are advised only in an operating room, with adequate help and instrumentation. Radiation therapy is not recommended. Stilbestrol (5 mg per day for 30 days) matures the collagen and vascular components. Surgical excision should be planned and carried out immediately following the course of stilbestrol. Spontaneous regression after puberty has been thought to occur in some cases; however, it has not been adequately documented. Watchful waiting is not recommended.

DISEASES OF THE PARANASAL SINUSES The mucosa of the ethmoid and maxillary sinuses may become involved by the polyposis that occurs in patients with allergic rhinitis (Chap. 67). Although primary tumors of the sinus mucosa are rare, encroachment by neoplasms arising in contiguous structures is common and easily visualized by x-ray. Osteoma of the frontal sinus is the most frequent lesion of this type; neoplasms of the maxilla and mixed tumors of the salivary gland type arising in the palate invade the antrum.

Sinusitis In the vast majority of cases, acute sinusitis is a bacterial infection brought on by impairment of drainage by the boggy, engorged nasal mucosa of allergic or viral rhinitis. Occasionally, pressure changes of air travel may result in an "aerosinusitis" similar to "aerotitis media"; deviations of the nasal septum are contributory.

The manifestations are local pain and tenderness, sometimes with edema of the overlying facial skin, headache, and fever. The headache is worse in the morning, when exudate has accumulated overnight, and tends to improve with upright posture and drainage during the day. If fluid has filled the frontal or maxillary sinuses, they cannot be transilluminated. Treatment consists of administration of analgesics and appropriate antibiotics, and, most important, the establishment of adequate drainage. In the acute stage, drainage is achieved most effectively by reduction of nasal swelling by astringents such as Neo-Synephrine, ephedrine, or antihistaminics in patients with allergy. Aspiration or irrigation of the infected cavity by an otorhinolaryngologist should be avoided during the acute stage but frequently is indicated after acute symptoms subside, particularly in maxillary sinusitis. Often, however, acute sinusitis clears up promptly when acute coryza or allergic rhinitis has subsided.

About 10 percent of antral infections are secondary to dental sepsis or result from fractures of the bony floor during dental extractions.

Complications of acute sinusitis are statistically rare but may be serious. Frank suppuration and abscess may lead to osteomyelitis and spread of infection to the orbit (retrobulbar abscess, cavernous sinus thrombosis), the meninges (see pneumococcal meningitis, Chaps. 128 and 329), and brain (via the diploic veins). Surgical drainage of frontal and ethmoid abscesses is sometimes an emergency procedure. About 10 percent of brain abscesses originate from frontal sinusitis, and infection of the frontal or sphenoid sinus precedes almost every case of subdural empyema. A serious complication of frontal suppuration is osteomyelitis of the skull, recognized by doughy edema of the forehead ("Pott's puffy tumor") and rapid destruction of bone.

With repeated episodes of acute infection, there may be thickening of the sinus mucosa, continual partial obstruction, and chronic inflammation that flares up with even slight obstruction such as may follow smoking, ingestion of spicy foods, the use of alcohol, or chilly, damp weather. Each acute episode becomes more difficult to control, and the patient may be continuously miserable. Rigid control of exposure to allergens and extremes of temperature, correction of structural defects such as deviated septum, and intensive treatment of acute exacerbations will sometimes bring relief, but radical surgery to ensure free drainage is eventually necessary in many instances. Chronic sinusitis is present in 50 percent of patients with bronchiectasis (Chap. 253). *Kartagener's syndrome* is the association of bronchiectasis, chronic sinusitis, and dextrocardia.

Cerebral phycomycosis in patients with diabetic acidosis (Chap. 172) usually originates as a sinusitis and invades the orbit and cranium secondarily.

When a diagnosis of "sinusitis" has been made radiologically, distinctions among acute, chronic, and inactive disease may be impossible and the diagnosis must depend on the patient's symptoms as well as on accurate bacteriologic identification of the causative organism. Nasal swab cultures are never sterile, and the choice of an antibiotic should be based on the predominating pathogenic organism in cultures of exudate from the sinus; usually these are group A streptococci, pneumococci, and staphylococci, and may be treated with a penicillin, erythromycin, or lincomycin. Gram-negative pathogens are common in patients who have received antibiotics, and it is fruitless to change antimicrobial drugs in these patients.

DISEASES OF THE LARYNX The two most important manifestations of laryngeal diseases are hoarseness and respiratory obstruction. Hoarseness that persists for more than 3 weeks in an adult calls for intensive investigation; tumor, chronic infection (tuberculosis, mycosis), and vocal cord paralysis are the important possibilities. Respiratory obstruction by edema, exudate, foreign body, or bilateral cord paralysis is an acute emergency.

Among infectious agents, the diphtheria bacillus, *Hemophilus influenzae*, the viral agents of croup and laryngotracheitis, *Treponema pallidum*, the tubercle bacillus, and fungi, especially monilia, are the ones most likely to attack the larynx. Laryngitis and hoarseness are not complications of streptococcal pharyngitis; their appearance in a patient with sore throat indicates a viral etiology or diphtheria.

Laryngeal papillomatosis is believed by many to be a viral disease. The lesions are multiple pedunculated growths on the cords, which are easily excised but recur. They are seen most commonly, but not invariably, in children and are rare after puberty.

Laryngeal acanthosis or hyperkeratosis (pachydermia laryngis) causing hoarseness may be a result of misuse of the voice, smoking, and probably of alcoholism; it is not a precancerous lesion. Leukoplakia of the larynx has the same significance in terms of later development of cancer that it has elsewhere and calls for local excision. It is important not to confuse acanthosis and leukoplakia.

The so-called *singers' nodule* is a lesion of the vocal cord that appears in individuals who have strained or misused their voices. If discovered early, the lesions may regress as proper voice modulation is practiced. Once the nodule becomes firm, treatment is excision; the lesion does not recur.

Systemic diseases affecting the larynx These include cystic fibrosis, lipoid proteinosis, myxedema, acromegaly, hypogonadism, hypoparathyroidism, diabetes mellitus, amyloidosis, and the collagen diseases. Significantly, rheumatoid arthritis may involve the cricoarytenoid joint in 25 percent of cases; rarely an arytenoidectomy may be required to provide an adequate airway.

Carcinoma of the larynx This tumor is ten to twelve times more common in men than in women; it appears at an average age of sixty. Tumors arising on the vocal cords are classified as "intrinsic" and constitute about 70 percent of the lesions; those extending beyond the cords are "extrinsic." Hoarseness is an early symptom of intrinsic cancer; it is often delayed in the extrinsic type. Treatment varies, but radiation alone is recommended only for small lesions of the middle third of the cord. Total or partial laryngectomy is the treatment of choice for many cancers; preoperative radiation and extensive removal of lymph nodes are used in many clinics. Partial supraglottic laryngectomy is preferable in some patients with cancer of the epiglottis and/or false cords because it permits patients to retain normal speech without jeopardizing their chances for cure. The overall cure rate for cancer of the larynx is excellent particularly for early lesions (around 90 percent).

Paralysis of the vocal cords Among the many causes of partial or complete paralysis of the vocal cords are pressure by aortic aneurysm; mediastinal tumors; metastatic cancer; neuritis (sometimes following meningitis); cervical and mediastinal infections; viral infections by poliomyelitis, mumps, measles, and Coxsackie viruses; polyneuritis (Guillain-Barré syndrome); infectious mononucleosis; sarcoidosis; tuberculosis; leprosy; diphtheria; neuropathy of diabetes mellitus, rheumatoid arthritis, alcoholism, poisons, and toxins; trauma, including surgical trauma (especially thyroidectomy). If a nerve is cut at operation, there will be sudden stridor; if stretching and edema are affecting the nerve, the onset of stridor and hoarseness will be gradual. Bilateral injury may cause sudden obstruction, necessitating tracheostomy.

REFERENCES

BERNSTEIN L: Surgery of the nasal sinuses, in *The Otolaryngology Clinics of North America*, ed L Bernstein, Philadelphia: Saunders, 1971

SISSON GA: Problems of the larynx, in *The Otolaryngology Clinics of North America*, ed L Bernstein, Philadelphia: Saunders, 1970

252 CHRONIC AIRWAY OBSTRUCTION DUE TO ASTHMA, BRONCHITIS, AND EMPHYSEMA

NORMAN L. JONES
E. J. MORAN CAMPBELL

For a century, three diagnoses have been applied to diseases in which there is breathlessness due to airway obstruction: *asthma*, *chronic bronchitis*, and *emphysema*. These have usually been treated as discrete disease entities or differential diagnoses, and because of lack of agreement on the precise meaning of these terms there has been much confusion regarding many aspects of the conditions—the structural abnormalities, pathophysiologic effects, incidence, and prognosis. Recently efforts have been made to define them more precisely in order to establish criteria for their diagnosis based on the following definitions.

Chronic bronchitis is characterized by excessive mucus production in the bronchial tree, sufficient to cause excessive expectoration of sputum.

Emphysema is characterized by distention of the air spaces distal to the terminal bronchiole, with destruction of their walls.

Asthma is characterized by widespread narrowing of the airways, which varies considerably from time to time, either spontaneously or as the result of treatment.

As defined above, these conditions are not mutually exclusive and there is little doubt that these definitions will be improved over the next few years. It is likely that asthma will come to be defined in terms of an increased reactivity of the airways to a variety of stimuli; that bronchitis will be defined in terms of changes in the structure and function of mucous glands in the smaller bronchi; and that emphysema will be more quantitatively defined in morphometric terms. It is important where possible that criteria be established to aid in categorizing these conditions. To diagnose asthma we need evidence of variable airway obstruction at some stage of the clinical course; for chronic bronchitis, a measure of sputum production; and for emphysema, evidence that destructive changes are present in the lung. Even when such criteria are developed, the diagnoses will not be mutually exclusive; it is common to see patients with chronic cough and sputum production who have an element of reversibility in their airway obstruction and who may also show some evidence of emphysema. The application of a diagnostic label to a patient's condition should not be taken as any more than a convenient first approximation.

It has been suggested that all patients with airway obstruction be classified as suffering from *chronic nonspecific lung disease*. This usage has *not* been widely adopted and is not to be encouraged; even more insidious is the term *chronic obstructive pulmonary disease*, because this also implies that the patients are suffering from a single disease. It is preferable to recognize multiple causes and to describe the clinical, structural, and functional changes in individual patients separately. An assessment of the extent to which each of the factors contributes to the total clinical picture will carry therapeutic and prognostic implications.

PATHOPHYSIOLOGY

The airway narrowing which is common to all patients with these conditions is produced by various mechanisms; although there is considerable overlap among the three conditions defined above, it is possible to recognize certain pathologic features characteristic of each.

CHRONIC BRONCHITIS The airway narrowing in this condition is due mainly to an increase in the mucous glands in the large bronchi (Fig. 252-1) and to chronic inflammatory changes in the smaller airways. The mucous gland hypertrophy may be expressed as a gland/wall ratio (the Reid index, Fig. 252-1); normally this is less than 0.4, but in bronchitis, because of the considerable hypertrophy of the glands, this ratio may reach 0.7. In addition, there is some increase in the amount of bronchial muscle; and in active infection, edema and inflammatory infiltration of the bronchial wall are present. These changes increase airway resistance, but in the early stages of the condition the smaller airways (less than 2 mm in diameter) may be mainly affected, and the symptoms and physiologic disturbances are then minimal (page 1279). As larger airways become involved, airway obstruction becomes more severe. Regional variations in airway resis-

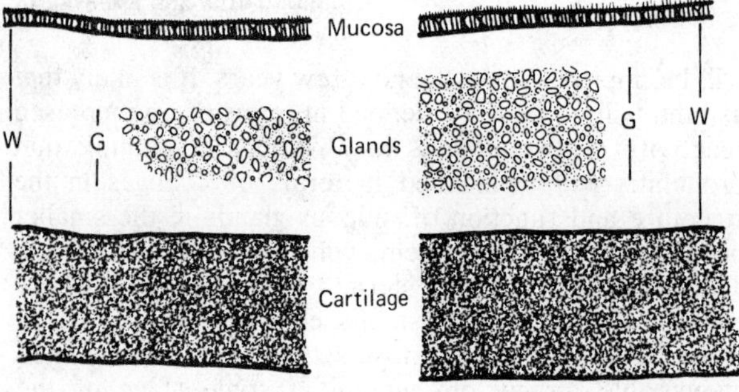

FIGURE 252-1
Diagram of bronchi in cross section to show the Reid index (gland/wall ratio) in a normal person (left) and in a patient with bronchitis (right). W = wall; G = gland.

tance lead to areas which are underventilated, resulting in a lowering of the arterial P_{O_2}; other areas become overventilated in relation to their perfusion, leading to an increase in the physiologic dead space (Chap.249). The disturbance of ventilation, increased work of breathing, and a low central responsiveness to carbon dioxide often lead to chronic hypercapnia.

In many patients with moderate or early airway obstruction, the hypoxia in poorly ventilated areas of the lung leads to localized active pulmonary vasoconstriction and a reversible increase in pulmonary vascular resistance. These "pulmonary vascular responders" to hypoxia are more likely eventually to develop pulmonary hypertension and right-sided heart failure (Chap. 262). On the other hand, in patients whose pulmonary vessels constrict less in response to hypoxia, the development of pulmonary hypertension is less likely, but their P_{O_2} is lower because of the relative overperfusion of poorly ventilated areas. In patients with long-standing pulmonary hypertension, muscular hypertrophy in the small pulmonary vessels and right ventricular hypertrophy occur.

EMPHYSEMA Two main categories of emphysema are recognized, *panlobular* and *centrilobular* (Fig. 252-2). Some argument exists as to whether these two types have different physiologic effects and produce different clinical features. In the panlobular type the alveolar distention and destruction are peripheral and involve the whole primary lung lobule; the changes usually affect all regions of the lung, although it has been noted that the lung bases are most affected in patients with antitrypsin deficiency. In centrilobular emphysema the distention is mainly limited to the respiratory bronchiole and alveolar ducts, with relatively less change peripherally, and the abnormalities tend to be more severe at the lung apices. Minor degrees of centrilobular emphysema are very common; it is considered by some to be almost a normal variant. When emphysema is severe, it is difficult to distinguish the two types, which often coexist in the same lung. Both types lead to a loss of alveolar surface area and a loss in the support of small airways by the lung parenchyma, causing expiratory airway narrowing and increases in the total lung capacity and, in particular, the residual volume. A major abnormality in centrilobular emphysema is the impairment of gaseous diffusion within the primary lobule; in panlobular emphysema the major abnormality is the reduction in the alveolar capillary interface. The overall effect is to impair pulmonary gas exchange, which is recognized by a reduction in the carbon monoxide–diffusing capacity and a fall in arterial P_{O_2} (Chap. 249).

ASTHMA The characteristic finding in asthma is hypertrophy of the bronchial muscle. It seems likely that muscle contraction is the main mechanism through which bronchial hyperreactivity is expressed; mucosal edema, infiltration with mononuclear cells and eosinophils, and changes in the basement membrane are also found. In severe exacerbations of asthma, excessive mucus is produced and there may be widespread blockage of airways by mucous plugs containing eosinophils. When these changes become chronic, features of chronic bronchitis will also occur. All these factors lead to an increase in airway resistance with a fall in expiratory flow rates; an improvement is usually obtained in flow rates by a nebulized bronchodilator. When airway obstruction is severe, hyperinflation of the lungs occurs, and reduction in regional ventilation/perfusion ratios leads to a fall in the arterial P_{O_2}. Airway obstruction is usually extremely severe before hypercapnia develops, and the development of CO_2 retention is far less common than a normal or even low P_{CO_2}, despite marked reduction of the FEV_1 (forced expired volume in 1 sec).

THE CLINICAL SYNDROMES

The clinical features of chronic airway obstruction due to asthma, chronic bronchitis, or emphysema show considerable overlap, and many patients exhibit a mixed picture. However, there are characteristic features which can be used to separate them.

Until recently it was widely accepted that chronic breathlessness in patients with chronic respiratory symptoms and without other disease signified destruction of the lungs by emphysema; when this was accompanied by a history of cough and sputum production, the patient was said to have chronic bronchitis *and* emphysema.

TYPE A (EMPHYSEMATOUS TYPE) These patients generally present a history of effort intolerance due to shortness of breath; cough may be absent or productive of only small amounts of sputum; the frequent infective exacerbations of chronic bronchitis do not occur. On examination they are usually found to be asthenic in build, with evidence of weight loss. Signs of chronic airway obstruction (see below) are found, but there are no clinical signs which are diagnostic of emphysema. Hyperresonance to percussion, poorly heard breath sounds, reduced cardiac and lowered hepatic dullness, and a barrel-shaped chest are usually present but are of little help in assessing the severity of airway obstruction or the degree of emphysema. Radiologic signs may also be misleading; a low, flattened diaphragm with a long, narrow heart shadow and increased retrosternal translucency on the lateral x-ray are all signs of overinflation and may not relate closely to structural changes of emphysema. However, attenuation and narrowing of the peripheral pulmonary vessels correlate well with severe changes of emphysema in the underlying lung. Pulmonary function tests show airway obstruction, increased residual volume and total lung capacity, and reduced elastic recoil and diffusing capacity; blood gases generally show normal P_{CO_2} and P_{O_2} which is normal or only slightly low at rest but which falls during exercise. Patients with this clinical syndrome generally maintain normal resting arterial blood gases for many years in spite of severe airway obstruction and, presumably because of this, avoid the recurrent episodes of fluid retention and right-sided heart failure which are found in type B patients. Because resting hypoxemia is absent and ventilation is high, maintaining normal P_{CO_2} in spite of abnormal gas exchange function, these patients are described as "pink and puffing" (Table 252-1). Postmortem, widespread panlobular emphysema is the characteristic finding.

TYPE B (BRONCHITIC TYPE) Typically, the patient comes to the physician after the age of forty with an already established history of chronic cough and sputum production; almost invariably the patient has been a cigarette smoker for many years. At first the cough is present only in the winter months, but it then becomes constant, with infective exacerbations becoming more prolonged and disabling. By the time the patient seeks the advice of the physician he is usually found to have a severe degree of airway obstruction with a fall in ventilatory capacity as assessed by FEV_1, or maximal voluntary ventilation, to 50 percent or less.

These patients are typically short and fat, with a plethoric complexion and wet cough. There are signs of chronic airway obstruction; variable wheezes and basal rales are usually present. Pulmonary function tests show severe reduction in expiratory flow rates and in the FEV_1; residual volume is usually increased, but the total lung capacity is frequently within normal limits; diffusing capacity measured by carbon monoxide transfer is not severely impaired; arterial blood gases usually show a low resting P_{O_2}, and if the obstruction is severe, an increase in P_{CO_2}. During exercise the P_{CO_2} rises, but, perhaps surprisingly, the P_{O_2} may also rise, because of an improvement in ventilation/perfusion relationships. After blood gas abnormalities determined with the patient at rest have been present for some time, *polycythemia* develops, and signs of fluid retention appear, with dependent edema and elevated jugular venous pressure. Such patients are likely to be admitted to hospital repeatedly in episodes of respiratory failure and cor pulmonale (Chap. 262). Radiologic examination generally shows an enlarged heart, evidence of pulmonary congestion, and frequently changes due to recent or past infection. This type of patient, because of the polycythemia, frequent hypoxia, and cor pulmonale, has been termed "blue and bloated" (Table 252-1). Postmortem, chronic inflammatory changes in the bronchi are found; although most of these patients are found to have a moderate degree of centrilobular emphysema, some of them have no emphysema.

ASTHMA The pathogenesis and clinical picture are dealt with in detail in Chap. 67.

In any patient with airway obstruction, it is important to establish whether there is variation in airway obstruction, either at present or at the onset of the illness. However, it is not uncommon for long-established asthma to lead to severe chronic airway obstruction, and at this stage there is little spontaneous variability or response to acutely administered bronchodilator. An occupational history should be taken to exclude exposure to such agents as isocyanates, enzyme detergents, red cedar dust, hemp dust, organic gums, and soldering fluxes containing ethyl ethanolamine. Seasonal variations may indicate environmental causes, such as pollens, molds, and fungi. Sometimes it may be difficult to recognize a specific cause because of delayed reactions, which may not be produced until several hours following exposure.

There is frequently an infective element to episodes of asthma, but this factor has been overrated in the past. It should be proved, rather than treated on suspicion; eosinophilic sputum appears purulent but does not require treatment with an antibiotic. The central problem in asthma is an increase in airway reactivity; asthmatics frequently develop symptoms on exposure to cigarette smoke and in highly polluted or dusty atmospheres. Symptoms may also follow strenuous exercise. The history should be supplemented by skin tests. Positive reactions should be interpreted with respect to the history when deciding whether an offending allergen is of clinical importance. Blood and sputum should be examined for excessive number of eosinophils, which may be the only indication of asthma in patients with chronic intrinsic asthma, which might otherwise be diagnosed as severe chronic bronchitis. Allergic bronchopulmonary aspergil-

FIGURE 252-2
The lung parenchyma in health, in centrilobular emphysema, and in panlobular emphysema, showing the changes distal to the terminal bronchiole (TB), in respiratory bronchioles and ducts (RB), and in alveoli (A).

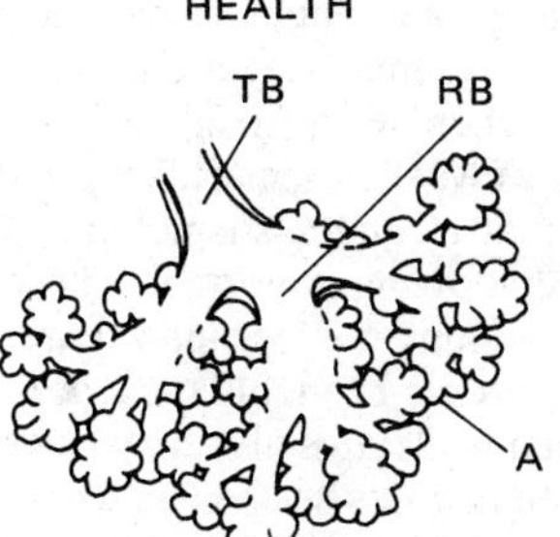

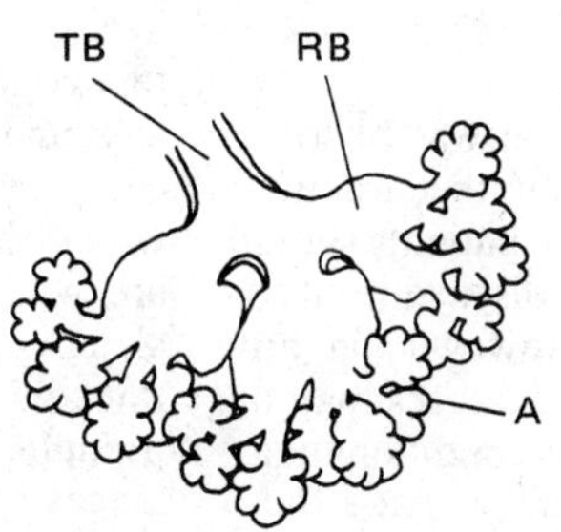

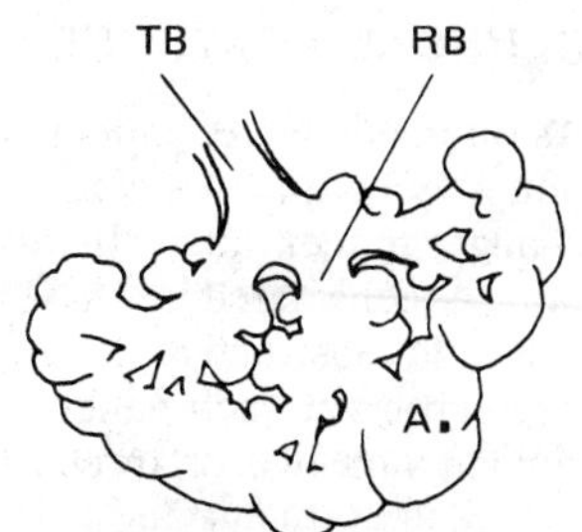

losis, characterized by episodes of asthma, has become increasingly recognized over the last few years (Chap. 67); variable airway obstruction may occur in carcinoid tumor (Chap. 99) and in polyarteritis nodosa (Chap. 71).

CRITERIA FOR DIAGNOSIS **Airway obstruction** The most widely used criterion has been slowing of the respiratory air flow, as shown by one of several indices based on forced expiratory spirograms—the FEV_1, the FEV_1/VC ratio, and the maximum midexpiratory flow rate (MMFR) (see further on, under Physiology). Other techniques are mentioned below. In the last few years it has become recognized that these indices are influenced to a large extent by the caliber of larger bronchi and that widespread obstruction of small airways may be present without much impairment of results in these tests. This is because the small airways contribute only a small proportion of the total airway resistance. As chronic bronchitis may first develop in smaller airways, newer tests—those of closing volume and frequency dependence of compliance—have been introduced to identify these early changes.

Chronic bronchitis, at least for purposes of classification and epidemiology, is diagnosed in any patient with chronic or recurrent cough productive of sputum which has been present for at least 3 months of the year for three consecutive years. Chronic obstructive bronchitis is diagnosed in a patient with airway obstruction in addition (an FEV_1 of less than 70 percent of the predicted normal values). The absence of radiologic or functional evidence of emphysema (normal total lung capacity, CO-diffusing capacity, and elastic recoil pressure) and the presence of elevated arterial P_{CO_2}, polycythemia, or cor pulmonale constitute supportive evidence for the type B patient.

Emphysema is diagnosed in a patient with chronic airway obstruction in whom the characteristic changes of emphysema are found in the chest x-ray (see below). Increased total lung capacity, low CO-diffusing capacity, and reduced elastic recoil pressure support the diagnosis, but the values which should be used as criteria are debatable.

Asthma is diagnosed in the presence of airway obstruction in three situations: (1) the airway obstruction may be seen to change spontaneously or as the result of bronchodilator therapy; (2) an increase in airway reactivity may be identified symptomatically or by the use of a nonspecific provocative agent such as methacholine; (3) a specific provocative agent which causes a change in airway obstruction may be recognized. The finding of blood or sputum eosinophilia supports the diagnosis.

CLINICAL FEATURES

As outlined above, patients with chronic airway obstruction may be *quite dissimilar* with regard to the structural changes in their lungs. In this sense, these patients should *not* be considered as having a single disease entity—"chronic obstructive lung disease." However, in any large group of such patients the clinical features may be similar, and two or three of the causal conditions may coexist, making separation of the causal conditions difficult or even impossible.

HISTORY At first patients with chronic bronchitis produce sputum only in the early morning and mainly in the winter. Sputum is mucoid and may be accepted by the patient as "normal phlegm" or a "smoker's cough." Usually the patient gives a history of cigarette smoking or less commonly of occupational exposure or childhood infection. In the absence of any of these causative factors, one should take particular care to exclude other causes of cough and sputum production. Later the cough becomes persistent throughout the year and throughout the 24 hr, and exacerbations, in which the sputum becomes purulent, become increasingly frequent. Shortness of breath occurs after many years of cough; severe dyspnea in a patient with little or no cough or asthma suggests the presence of panlobular emphysema.

PHYSICAL EXAMINATION The most reliable sign of airway obstruction is a prolongation of the time taken to perform a forced expiration. This may be measured as the forced expired time (FET): the patient is asked to inhale fully and then expire forcibly and completely through the wide open mouth; the time to completion of airflow is measured. Normally the vital capacity can be expired within 3 sec; prolongation of the FET to over 6 sec indicates a significant degree of airway obstruction. In long-standing airway obstruction, particularly in older patients, signs are found related to hyperinflation of the chest—poor expansion of the chest with paradoxic or biphasic movement of the lower ribs, hyperresonant percussion note, reduced cardiac and lowered hepatic dullness to percussion, and an inspiratory tracheal tug. On auscultation, harsh breath sounds and rhonchi are heard in both phases of respiration, generally of higher pitch on expiration than on inspiration; inspiratory crepitations may be heard when there are retained secretions or in an area of bronchiectasis. These sounds may be altered by coughing if they are due to secretion, but otherwise their character and loudness have little functional significance. Other signs which may be present are plethora due to polycythemia; cyanosis due to arterial hypoxemia; and edema with or without elevated jugular venous pressure. Clinical signs of hypercapnia are usually absent unless there has been a rapid increase in carbon dioxide pressure, but edema almost invariably signifies CO_2 retention.

RADIOLOGY Chest x-rays may appear normal even in patients with severe symptoms. Flattening and depression of the diaphragm to below the level of the seventh rib anteriorly, widening of the rib spaces, and an increase in the retrosternal air space to 4 cm or more all indicate overinflation of the lungs. Although these changes are not necessarily due to emphysema, they are usually found in this condition, which when severe leads also to a patchy loss and attenuation of vascular markings, detected by comparing an area that is under suspicion with one in which the vascular shadowing is normal. These changes are well seen in whole-lung tomographs. Parallel linear shadows are seen in chronic bronchitis and are related to thickening of bronchial walls; this also may be detected in perihilar bronchi, seen in cross section as rings. Irregular and poorly defined linear markings are frequently seen; the underlying structural abnormality is uncertain, but it is generally thought that they are due to subsegmental atelectasis. Characteristic bronchographic features of chronic bronchitis are the presence of diverticula in the larger bronchi, because of the dilated mucous gland ducts, and also truncation of the peripheral airways and localized variations in airway caliber. In patients with chronic respiratory failure, cardiac enlargement and prominent central pulmonary vessels are usually seen.

PHYSIOLOGY *Airway obstruction* may be assessed in several ways. The simplest technique is *dynamic spirometry*; airway obstruction leads to a reduction in expiratory flow rates, which is generally detected by changes in three main indices: (1) the forced expired volume in 1 sec (FEV_1) is reduced; although the total expired vital capacity (VC) may also be reduced, the FEV_1/VC ratio is always low, allowing the reduction to be distinguished from that occurring in a restrictive lung disorder; (2) the maximum midexpiratory flow rate (MMFR) is reduced; (3) the peak expiratory flow rate is also low. Body plethysmography may be used to study the mechanical factors influencing airflow; the two main factors are the resistance of airways and the alveolar driving pressure. Airway resistance, the measurement of interest in these conditions, is determined by relating the airflow to the intrathoracic pressure change. The alveolar driving pressure is a function of the lung volume and the elastic recoil properties of the lung (Chap. 249). Conventionally, the reciprocal of the resistance, the airway conductance, is divided by the lung volume to obtain the specific conductance. All these measurements may fail to show changes in patients in whom abnormalities are limited to the smallest airways, i.e., those of less than 2 mm in diameter; in order to detect an increase in resistance in this "silent zone," the techniques of "closing volume" and of frequency dependence of compliance have been introduced. The closing-volume technique uses the measurement of the expired concentration of an inert gas; during inspiration this gas will be distributed unequally to the upper and lower parts of the lung. During expiration a constant alveolar "plateau" will be seen as alveoli empty synchronously, but when basal airways begin to close, a change in the expired gas concentration is detected. The volume at which this occurs is related to an increase in resistance of small airways. The measurement of dynamic compliance at varying frequencies of breathing in the body plethysmograph will detect reduction of the volume response to a change in intrathoracic pressure, where small changes in airway caliber are present; the detection of frequency-dependent compliance is a sensitive indicator of increased flow resistance in small airways. Reduction in flow rates due to an increase in airway resistance leads to a reduction in the maximal voluntary ventilation, which may be measured directly as the maximum breathing capacity (MBC) or estimated indirectly from the FEV_1.

Changes in the lung volume occur because of the increase in airway resistance and reduced lung elastic recoil. Thus, the most marked increases in total lung capacity occur particularly when these two factors are combined, as in emphysema. The total lung capacity and the residual volume may be measured by an inert gas technique using a closed-circuit helium technique or an open-circuit nitrogen washout technique. The lung volumes can also be measured by body plethysmography; this technique measures the total thoracic gas volume and

TABLE 252-1
Clinical types of patients with severe chronic airway obstruction

	Type of patient	
	A	*B*
Pathology	Severe emphysema, both panlobular and centrilobular.	Severe bronchitis: little emphysema, usually centrilobular
Radiology	Sparse and narrow peripheral vessels, overinflation	Normal or congested lung fields: minor changes (infection, bronchiectasis)
Clinical features	Dyspnea	Cough, sputum
		Cyanosis
		Polycythemia
	Cor pulmonale a late feature	Fluid retention, cor pulmonale
	"Pink, puffing"	"Blue, bloated"
Physiology	FEV_1 low	FEV_1 low
	TLC high	TLC often normal but may be increased
	Elastic recoil low	Elastic recoil normal
	CO transfer low	CO transfer normal
	P_{CO_2} normal	P_{CO_2} high
	Resting P_{O_2} often > 70	Resting P_{O_2} usually < 70
	P_{O_2} falls on exercise	P_{O_2} does not fall on exercise
Clinical course	Unrelenting, but often slow increase in obstruction and gas exchange abnormality	Recurrent infection, respiratory failure and heart failure

Note: FEV, forced expiratory volume; TLC, total lung capacity

thus permits detection of very poorly ventilated or nonventilated areas in the lung. A large discrepancy between the total lung capacity measured by an inert gas technique and the thoracic gas volume yields an estimate of the size of lung bullae.

The mechanical properties of the lung may be analyzed in terms of the airway resistance by measuring dynamic pressure-flow relationships and of compliance by the measurement of static pressure-volume relationships. The measurement of airway resistance has already been mentioned. The change in volume for a given change in intrathoracic pressure yields an index of compliance of the lung (Chap. 249); in emphysema the maximal elastic recoil pressure is low and compliance increased. In chronic bronchitis and asthma the static pressure volume relationships are usually normal; a transient reduction in lung elastic recoil has been noted in episodes of acute asthma.

The distribution of ventilation may be assessed by the "wash-in" of an inert gas such as helium or by the "wash-out" of lung nitrogen by oxygen breathing. The wash-in and wash-out curves yield an index of the rate at which inspired gas is distributed to various areas of the lungs. The rate may be analyzed in terms of two compartments—a "fast space," indicating areas which are relatively well ventilated, and a "slow space," in which gas equilibration takes place extremely slowly and which often comprises the majority of the lung volume and receives the majority of the pulmonary blood flow, leading to an extremely low ventilation/perfusion (V/Q) ratio (Chap. 249).

Regional ventilation/perfusion ratios may be measured using radioactive gas techniques (Chap. 249). Gross changes in these ratios may be found in all three conditions, (asthma, bronchitis, and emphysema), although a greatly reduced regional flow is characteristically found in an area affected by severe emphysema or in one that is the site of bullous disease.

Overall lung gas exchange is assessed using carbon monoxide–diffusing capacity and by analysis of arterial blood gases. In asthma and chronic bronchitis normal values for diffusing capacity, are usually found; in emphysema a gross reduction is the rule.

Measurement of arterial blood gases combined with expired gas analysis allows measurement of alveolar ventilation, the physiologic dead space, and the alveolar to arterial P_{O_2} difference. More information regarding the reserve capacity of the lungs is obtained by performing these measurements during exercise. Frequently, ventilation is adequate at rest but during exercise the arterial P_{CO2} may rise, indicating an inadequate increase in effective alveolar ventilation. The physiologic dead space—made up of airway dead space and a contribution from areas with high V/Q ratios—is increased particularly in emphysema, when values as high as 60 percent of the tidal volume may be found during exercise. The alveolar to arterial P_{O_2} difference (A-a gradient) yields an index of oxygen uptake in the lung, being increased by the presence of low V/Q areas and poor diffusion; marked widening of the gradient is seen both in chronic bronchitis and in emphysema; characteristically there is little change or a reduction during exercise in chronic bronchitis, but in patients with emphysema an increase in the difference usually occurs, because of the gross disturbance in gas exchange function in this condition.

CLINICAL-FUNCTIONAL CORRELATIONS

1 *Dyspnea.* Although the degree of dyspnea correlates with the degree of airway obstruction, there is considerable variation among patients. Patients with emphysema tend to be more dyspneic than bronchitic patients with a similar degree of airway obstruction.
2 *Physical work capacity.* Reduced ventilatory capacity, arterial hypoxemia, and physical unfitness due to a chronically reduced activity in everyday life lead to severe effort intolerance, which again is most severe in emphysema. It is important to recognize that the relationship between the pulmonary function abnormality and effort intolerance is nonlinear; the loss of pulmonary function may be considerable before any limitation occurs (Fig. 252-3). Conversely, considerable symptomatic improvement may follow relatively minor improvement in pulmonary function.
3 *Carbon dioxide retention.* The worse the airway obstruction, the more frequently will carbon dioxide retention be found, but considerable variation is present. There is a well-established relationship between the arterial P_{CO_2} and the FEV_1 (Fig. 252-4), but generally, for a given degree of airway obstruction patients with emphysema have a lower P_{CO_2} than do patients with chronic bronchitis. The condition of patients with an FEV_1 of less than 1 liter and those who have had CO_2 retention in the past should in practice be followed closely with measurements of arterial P_{CO_2}.

PREVALENCE

Information regarding the prevalence of chronic bronchitis and of emphysema has been difficult to obtain because of variation in diagnostic habits and the lack of internationally accepted criteria for diagnosis. These fac-

FIGURE 252-3
Work performance related to severity of airway obstruction in patients with chronic airway obstruction.

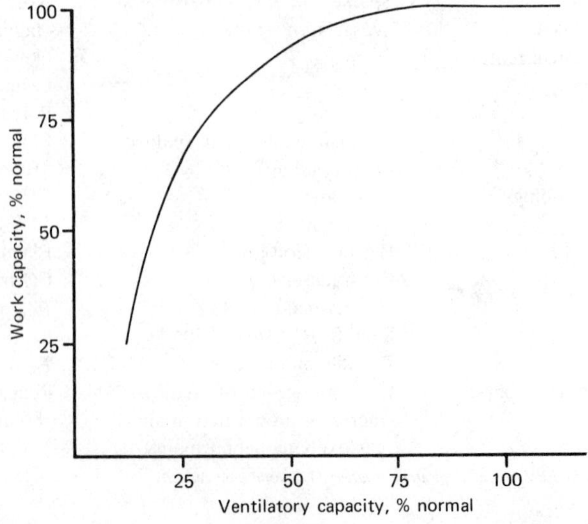

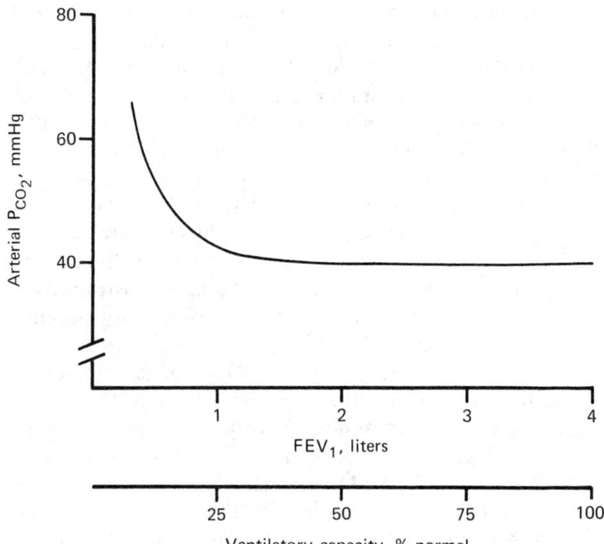

FIGURE 252-4
Arterial P_{CO_2} in patients with chronic airway obstruction. Values in type A patients tend to lie below the curve, and in type B patients, above.

tors particularly affect statistics obtained from mortality rates; a comparison made by the World Health Organization in 1964 showed that mortality from bronchitis in men varied from a high of 90 deaths per 100,000 in England and Wales to a low of 4 deaths per 100,000 in the United States. More recent epidemiologic studies have suggested that these wide differences are largely related to diagnostic criteria, although true differences may exist which may be due to variations in air pollution, smoking habits, climate, and other factors. Studies of chronic bronchitis in the general population have shown a prevalence varying between 8 percent and 17 percent in men and 3 percent and 8 percent in women. The prevalence has been shown to be higher in urban areas and among the smoking population. Estimates of the prevalence of asthma have also shown wide variations: according to the more conservative estimates, its prevalence is between 1 percent and 2 percent of children and 0.5 percent and 1 percent of adults; epidemiologic studies using more sensitive indications of airway obstruction have suggested an incidence as high as 20 percent of children.

ETIOLOGY

SMOKING There is a clear relation between smoking habits and bronchitis death rates; the mortality risk increases with increasing cigarette consumption to over twenty times that of nonsmokers; the risk in exsmokers is similar to that in persons smoking small numbers of cigarettes, but is five times higher than in nonsmokers. Epidemiologic surveys have shown that chronic bronchitis is almost confined to smokers; the incidence ranges from 20 percent in heavy smokers to 5 percent in exsmokers. Experimental work has also supported the impression that it is the major cause of bronchitis. Cigarette smoke inhibits ciliary movement and macrophage activity in the lung and produces hypertrophy of the mucous glands. Smoking a cigarette leads to a rise in the resistance of small airways, which can be abolished by atropine, suggesting that a vagal reflex is involved. The incidence of emphysematous changes in lungs studied postmortem is related to cigarette smoking, and emphysema has been produced experimentally in dogs by smoking.

AIR POLLUTION The mortality rate from both chronic bronchitis and emphysema is higher in urban areas and is correlated with air pollution. Exacerbations of bronchitis are associated with periods of high pollution, particularly by sulfur dioxide and smoke particles. When variations due to air pollution have been taken into account, smoking still exerts a major effect, suggesting that it is the more important factor etiologically.

OCCUPATION The incidence of chronic bronchitis is higher in men working in industrial occupations, such as coal miners, steel workers, and workers in the flax industry, but again even in these men smoking appears to be more important. The part played by occupational factors in the etiology of emphysema is also unclear. Coal miners are likely to develop centrilobular emphysema.

INFECTION There is some evidence that viral respiratory infections early in life may lead to persistently increased airway resistance. Exacerbations of chronic bronchitis have been shown to be related to viral infections and also to infection by *Hemophilus influenzae* and *Diplococcus pneumoniae*. Although information regarding the earliest phases is lacking, it appears unlikely that infections play as important an initiating role as cigarette smoking.

GENETIC FACTORS Studies in twins have suggested some genetic predisposition to bronchitis which cannot be explained by smoking habits, but the mechanism by which this is expressed is uncertain.

A notable advance in the etiology of emphysema has been the discovery of a deficiency in α_1-antitrypsin in many patients with emphysema. The techniques of acid starch gel and immunofixation electrophoresis have led to genetic typing of the protease inhibitory (Pi) system. Most normal persons have two M genes and a normal amount of α_1-antitrypsin in the serum (>250 mg per 100 ml). The Z gene is responsible for a low production of α_1-antitrypsin; individuals who are homozygous ZZ have a level of less than 50 mg per 100 ml. Heterozygotes having MZ genes are found to have levels of around 150 mg per 100 ml. Other phenotypes have been identified but are less common and not as important in relation to emphysema. The clinical picture of emphysema is seen in ZZ homozygotes; it consists of the early onset of dyspnea—sometimes even in childhood—without much cough. Severe panlobular emphysema is found in almost all these subjects by the age of fifty; the process usually affects the lung bases predominantly. There is an equal incidence between males and females. Both parents are found to be MZ heterozygotes. At the present time there is argument regarding the incidence of heterozygotes in the general population, but it may be as high as 5 percent.

It is also not clear how many will develop emphysema. The finding of poor vascular perfusion of the lung bases may indicate early changes in such individuals, particularly if they are smokers. Alpha$_1$-antitrypsin has been shown to inhibit trypsin, elastase, and collagenase, as well as a variety of other enzymes, and the serum level normally rises in response to several inflammatory reactions. It is tempting to believe that the structural integrity of lung elastin and collagen depends on the presence of this antienzyme to protect it from proteases released from leukocytes and platelets as a result of various injuries. Recent experimental observations have provided some support for this concept. Emphysema can be produced in animals by the injection of papain, a potent protease, and by penicillamine, which breaks down elastin and collagen.

The α_1-antitrypsin level should be measured in all patients with emphysema. The finding of low levels should lead to screening of relatives, with counseling regarding cigarette smoking and early chemotherapy of infections.

CHRONIC BRONCHITIS AND ASTHMA AS CAUSES OF EMPHYSEMA Chronic bronchitis, airway obstruction, recurrent cough, and infection have often been implicated as causes of emphysema. Chronic asthma has also been thought to cause emphysema; gross overinflation and some loss of elastic recoil are common during a severe attack of asthma and many patients in remission have evidence of small-airway obstruction. There is, however, little evidence that asthma causes the permanent alveolar damage of emphysema. Although it seems likely that many of these factors may predispose to centrilobular emphysema, there is a high incidence of this condition in postmortem studies of people without respiratory complaints, making cause and effect difficult to establish.

NATURAL HISTORY

Most studies have been carried out in patients who exhibit the late features of these conditions, and there is less information regarding the earlier stages. The condition of men with established bronchitis has been followed over a number of years to enable some of the factors influencing outcome to be identified. The general pattern is one of steady deterioration, which is, however, extremely variable. This progression is punctuated by respiratory infections of increasing severity, increasing dyspnea and incapacity, and finally edema and cor pulmonale. The progression of airway obstruction is strongly influenced by cigarette smoking, being most marked in heavy smokers; the rate of decline is only slightly greater in ex-smokers than in nonsmokers. Although there is an argument for getting smokers with bronchitis to give up their habit, by the time severe airway obstruction is present the response is usually disappointing. Recurrent respiratory infection has long been held responsible for the deterioration of persons with bronchitis, but recent evidence suggests that it is unlikely to account for the decline in ventilatory capacity in most patients. However, there are well-documented instances of sudden and persistent deterioration following an acute infection.

The wide variation in individual response to such factors as cigarette smoking has led to the hypothesis that variations in bronchial reactivity within the population may influence the onset and outcome of bronchitis, patients with the most reactive airways being likely to develop the most severe bronchitis.

Once chronic bronchitis and emphysema are well established, a number of factors have been shown to be related to outcome. The severity of airway obstruction is a major factor; in a recent study, 80 percent of patients presenting with an FEV_1 of more than 1.25 liters survived 5 years, but in patients with an FEV_1 of less than 0.75 liters, the survival fell to 25 percent. The mortality rate is influenced by the presence of respiratory failure; of patients having an increase in P_{CO_2}, 85 percent were dead within 5 years. Elevated arterial P_{CO_2} and low P_{O_2} are major factors influencing the onset of pulmonary hypertension and cor pulmonale. In spite of these general rules, the wide variation in clinical course allows one to take a less gloomy outlook in individual patients. Some patients develop rapidly progressive airway obstruction and run a tragically short course over 2 or 3 years, whereas other patients may survive for many years with a stable severe degree of airway obstruction. In view of this it is important to use simple measurements in order to follow the course of an individual patient over a number of years; this information is more reliable from a prognostic point of view than measurements made at any one time.

ACUTE RESPIRATORY FAILURE IN CHRONIC AIRWAY OBSTRUCTION Patients with established chronic airway obstruction are liable to episodes of respiratory failure, which are usually triggered by an increase in airway resistance, due often to a respiratory infection. The loss of ventilatory capacity and the effects of poorly ventilated and atelectatic areas on gas exchange lead to worsening hypoxemia and CO_2 retention. Patients with impaired central ventilatory control mechanisms are more likely to develop respiratory failure during an infective or asthmatic exacerbation.

The clinical features are not pathognomonic, nor need they be dramatic. The patient is often afebrile, but usually the sputum becomes more purulent; breathlessness usually increases; cyanosis appears or becomes more intense; edema and other signs of heart failure may appear; the patient becomes confused and develops neuromuscular twitching; sleep is disturbed, and hypoxemia may lead to nocturnal disorientation and agitation, which may lead to ill-advised administration of a sedative. Cough eventually becomes depressed and less effective, and this leads to sputum retention, with further deterioration of respiratory function, severe hypoxemia, and CO_2 retention. Although mental deterioration occurs with increasing hypoxemia, unconsciousness is unusual unless the patient is given uncontrolled oxygen therapy or a sedative. Clinical signs of carbon dioxide retention are unreliable. Such classical signs as flapping tremor, bounding pulse, and engorgement of fundal veins are highly variable and are related more to the rate at which respiratory failure is developing than to absolute levels of arterial P_{CO_2}, P_{O_2}, or pH.

When such patients are admitted to the hospital, typical values for arterial blood gases show an arterial P_{O_2} of 20 to 40 mm Hg (oxygen saturation of 40 to 70 percent), P_{CO_2} of 60 to 80 mm Hg, and a pH of 7.30 to 7.20. The main danger is that of hypoxia due to hypoxemia, rather than of CO_2 retention or acidosis; a P_{CO_2} of more than 90 mm Hg is almost never found unless oxygen has been administered. The relief of hypoxemia is a cornerstone of treatment; however, the administration of oxygen may lead to deterioration of respiratory function, probably in two ways; (1) by removing chemoreflex hypoxic stimuli to breathing, and (2) by reducing pulmonary vasoconstriction, which to some extent regulates the blood flow to poorly ventilated parts of the lung. These two factors may, when O_2 is given without control, lead to a rise of P_{CO_2} to narcotic levels (over 90 mm Hg), with further depression of consciousness and cough. These considerations influence the choice of treatment, as outlined in Chap. 263.

Respiratory failure may develop very insidiously following operations, particularly emergency abdominal operations. Patients may be judged to have primary cardiac disease, and may be given sedation; this is of particular importance in patients whose condition is diagnosed as pulmonary edema and who may be given large doses of morphia.

PRINCIPLES OF TREATMENT

CHRONIC AIRWAY OBSTRUCTION The only measure shown to influence the progress of chronic bronchitis, and that only in its early stages, is the cessation of smoking. No other measure has been shown by controlled trial unequivocally to cure or reverse the condition. On the other hand most individual patients improve symptomatically and functionally with adequate treatment. Management is guided by the following principles.

1 A full initial assessment of the patient will give much information on which to base logical treatment. This should include a careful history, with particular enquiry into causal factors, and a physical examination, together with some measurements to assess ventilatory and gas exchange function and working capacity. The requirements from this point of view are spirometry, CO-diffusing capacity, and a simple standardized exercise test to assess work capacity and the cardiac and ventilatory responses to exercise. Ventilation during exercise gives a measure of the patient's true ventilatory capacity, which may not be adequately reflected by spirometry. Exercise assesses the reserve present in the respiratory system by imposing the stress of an added load of O_2 and CO_2. Arterial blood gas studies at rest and, if possible, during exercise should be made in any patient in whom the ventilatory capacity or gas exchange function is severely reduced; a large rise in arterial P_{CO_2} during exercise is an indication that the patient will be likely to develop respiratory failure when airway obstruction becomes severe. In relating the physiologic assessment to the patient's symptoms, particularly if the symptoms are disproportionate to the functional state, it is important to assess the patient's personality. In addition to explaining unexpectedly severe symptoms, personality may be one of the factors influencing the response of respiratory control mechanisms to airway obstruction.

2 The patient should be given as detailed an explanation of his condition as he is capable of following.

3 *The patient must stop smoking.* This advice should be strongly given, particularly to patients in the early stages of their illness; in patients with very severe obstructive bronchitis it is less easy to show that cessation of smoking improves the outlook, but even they should stop.

4 The patient's status should be reassessed two or three times a year; this allows the rate of progression to be established and will also allow observation of the physical findings and functional status at the patient's best, thus setting the goal for the therapeutic measures during relapses.

5 Excess weight should be reduced, and the patient should take regular exercise.

6 Simple bronchodilators often ease the patient's symptoms and may be given in aerosol or tablet form. Some patients, particularly those with chronic asthma, will respond to steroids, but these should not be used except in a strictly controlled situation with measurements of ventilatory capacity.

7 Chemotherapy should be used during infective exacerbations. Long-term chemotherapy reduces the severity but not the frequency of episodes and is not to be recommended in most patients. Antibiotics are best used at the first sign of an increase in sputum purulence. As the commonest organisms found are *Hemophilus influenzae* and *Diplococcus pneumoniae, tetracycline* and *ampicillin* are the most useful agents.

8 Portable oxygen may sometimes be of help in patients who are extremely disabled because of hypoxemia; in view of the dangers of uncontrolled oxygen therapy, however, it should be used only when there is good evidence of symptomatic and objective improvement with it.

9 Surgery has sometimes been advocated for the removal of areas in the lung particularly affected by emphysema. Occasionally a large bulla may interfere with the function of the rest of the lung, and when this can be established, good results may be expected from its removal. However, the coexistence of severe changes in the rest of the lungs often leads to disappointment in these measures, particularly in the long term.

CONDITIONS WHICH OVERLAP CLINICALLY AND PATHOLOGICALLY

BRONCHIECTASIS (Chap. 253) Minor degrees of bronchial deformity and dilatation are seen in chronic bronchitis, together with the dilatation of mucous gland ducts, which may be seen in bronchograms. Conversely, a localized bronchiectasis is usually accompanied by a more widespread chronic bronchitis. The bronchial changes lead to retention of secretions and infection and are a source of hemorrhage. Localized bronchiectasis is usually not important functionally, although the disturbed ventilation-perfusion relationships in the area may lead to a reduced arterial P_{O_2}.

DISEASE OF SMALL AIRWAYS Airways of less than 2 mm in diameter, consisting of the smallest bronchi and bronchioles, have been termed by Macklem the "quiet zone." They earn this description for two reasons: (1) they form only a small part of the total resistance to airflow and thus have to be widely obstructed or narrowed before they increase total airway resistance sufficiently to affect spirometric measurements; (2) if they become obstructed, air spaces distal to them continue to receive ventilation through collateral channels. Disease at this level appears to be a feature of many conditions, from the effects of cigarette smoking and acute lower respiratory infections to chronic bronchitis and asthma. At present the lesion is difficult to detect because it does not cause an obstructive pattern in the spirogram, and the techniques of frequency dependence of compliance and of the closing volume (see above) are required to detect it.

Disease of small airways may have little effect on lung function in adults, but in infants serious effects may ensue, because of the smaller caliber of airways and less collateral ventilation. In adults it may eventually be found to be related to the development of chronic bronchitis.

VARIANTS OF EMPHYSEMA In addition to the two main forms of emphysema described above, other types are recognized pathologically but are less important functionally. Air space distention and destruction are often found around areas of fibrosis ("scar emphysema") and along the borders of lobes ("paraseptal emphysema"). They may occur rarely in infants, probably as a result of valvular obstruction of a lobar bronchus ("infantile lobar emphysema"). *Unilateral emphysema* may be detected radiologically by finding unilateral hypertransradiancy (McLeod's syndrome, Swyer-James syndrome). The finding of a normal complement of airways with a reduced number of alveoli in affected lungs has been interpreted as an indication of disease occurring in early life, before the age of eight years. This is a period of development in which bronchi have reached adult numbers but alveoli are still being formed. In most cases the pulmonary artery on the affected side is hypoplastic, but it is not known whether this is a primary developmental abnormality or is secondary to an initiating illness. Usually the condition is detected coincidentally, but sometimes a severe unilateral abnormality is found which may on rare occasions lead to functional impairment sufficient to warrant surgical removal of the lung.

EMPHYSEMATOUS BULLAE OR CYSTS Air spaces greater than 1 cm in diameter may be congenital but are often found complicating generalized emphysema, chronic bronchitis, and many fibrotic pulmonary conditions. They may sometimes increase in size progressively, compressing surrounding lung. Because considerable structural abnormality usually exists in other parts of the lungs, complex techniques (radioactive gas studies, lobar gas sampling) are required to measure the regional effects of bullae. When it can be shown that the regional effects are of greater importance on overall lung function than any coexisting generalized abnormalities, removal of the bulla usually leads to functional improvement. In general, such improvement is more likely if the bulla is large, is subject to valvular airway obstruction (i.e., is seen on fluoroscopy to cause air trapping on the affected side), and is compressing potentially functional lung. Usually improvement is short-lived because of the existence of other bullous areas which become larger after surgery.

PNEUMOCONIOSIS (Chap. 258) Chronic bronchitis commonly occurs in occupational dust diseases, and the incidence of centrilobular emphysema is also increased in such cases. As the patient is usually a smoker as well, it becomes difficult to decide whether the chronic bronchitis is occupational or unrelated to the pneumoconiosis. Although the reliance usually placed on radiographic features for compensation purposes is understandable, functional effects due to occupation may be severe in their absence.

CYSTIC FIBROSIS (Chap. 302) This condition has many of the clinical and pathologic features of chronic bronchitis and bronchiectasis, and an abnormality of mucus secretion has long been suspected as a cause of chronic bronchitis. The finding of abnormal sweat electrolytes and upper intestinal enzyme deficiencies in some patients was taken as evidence in support of this hypothesis, but lack of confirmation of these findings makes it doubtful that there is a strong direct relationship.

REFERENCES

General review

Bates DV: Medical progress: Chronic bronchitis and emphysema. N Engl J Med 278:546, 1968

Etiology and prevalence

Auerbach O et al: Relation of smoking and age to emphysema. Whole lung section study. N Engl J Med 286:853, 1972

Lambert PM, Reid DD: Smoking, air pollution and bronchitis in Britain. Lancet 1:853, 1970

Reid DD et al: An Anglo-American comparison of the prevalence of bronchitis. Br Med J 2:1487, 1964

Talamo RC: The α_1-antitrypsin in man. J Allergy Clin Immunol 40:240, 1971

Pathology and definitions

Ciba Guest Symposium. Terminology, definitions and classification of chronic pulmonary emphysema and related conditions. Thorax 14:286, 1959

Reid L McA: *The Pathology of Emphysema.* Chicago: Year Book, 1967

Thurlbeck WM et al: A comparison of three methods of measuring emphysema. Hum Pathol 1:215, 1970

Pathophysiology and clinical types

Bates DV et al: *Respiratory Function in Disease*, 2d ed., Philadelphia: Saunders, 1971

Burrows B et al: The emphysematous and bronchial types of chronic airways obstruction. Lancet 1:830, 1966

Macklem PT et al: Chronic obstructive disease of small airways. Ann Intern Med 74:167, 1971

Pain MC et al: Changes of arterial carbon dioxide tension in patients with chronic lung disease breathing oxygen. Australas Ann Med 14:195, 1965

Prognosis

BURROWS B, EARLE RG: Course and prognosis of chronic obstructive lung disease. N Engl J Med 280:397, 1969

Treatment

CAMPBELL EJM: The management of acute respiratory failure in chronic bronchitis and emphysema. (The J. Burns Amberson Lecture). Am Rev Resp Dis 105:626, 1967

MEDICAL RESEARCH COUNCIL: Value of chemoprophylaxis and chemotherapy in early chronic bronchitis. Br Med J 1:1317, 1966

REBUCK AS, READ J: Assessment and management of severe asthma. Am J Med 51:789, 1971

SYKES MK et al: *Respiratory Failure*, Oxford: Blackwell Scientific Publications, Ltd., 1969

253 BRONCHIECTASIS, LUNG ABSCESS, AND BRONCHOLITHIASIS

JOHN F. MURRAY

This chapter considers three principal disease entities: bronchiectasis, lung abscess, and broncholithiasis. These disorders have certain features in common. Each can be defined on the basis of abnormal morphology, and each has numerous, rather than single, underlying causes. It was formerly believed that bronchial obstruction was a sine qua non in all three, contributing to the pathogenesis of bronchiectasis and lung abscess and arising as a consequence of broncholithiasis. This is no longer thought to be true.

The widespread availability and extensive use of antibiotic drugs has dramatically altered the course and prognosis of most bacterial diseases and their sequelae. Like other chronic infectious diseases, bronchiectasis and lung abscess, though still important medical problems, have been transformed during the antibiotic era so that their pathogenesis, clinical manifestations, treatment, and prognosis are strikingly different from what they were 20 years ago.

BRONCHIECTASIS

DEFINITION Bronchiectasis can be defined as a permanent abnormal dilatation of one or more large (greater than 2 mm in diameter) bronchi due to destruction of the elastic and muscular components of the bronchial wall. Since the disorder is defined in morphologic terms, its diagnosis depends on the demonstration, usually through the use of bronchography, of widened bronchi. But the appearance of the bronchi and the extent of involvement differ markedly between patients and even in the same patient.

Classification is therefore difficult and is not useful in indicating the severity of the disease; however, certain descriptive terms are in common use, and understanding them is important. The simplest classification is one in which the abnormal bronchi show either saccular or cylindrical changes. *Saccular (cystic) bronchiectasis,* occurs mainly in the proximal large bronchi; affected airways show marked dilatation ending in large sacs at about the fourth bronchial division. *Cylindrical (fusiform) bronchiectasis* involves airways from the sixth to the tenth generation; the bronchographic appearance shows mild to moderate uneven widening, without a great increase in diameter, of bronchi that often look beaded and end squarely and abruptly. Saccular and cylindrical bronchiectasis are different degrees of the same process; they frequently coexist, along with intermediate stages ("varicose" bronchiectasis), in the same patient.

Although "true" bronchiectasis is not reversible, the concept of reversibility is an important one, because abnormalities displayed by bronchography in some patients with reversible lung diseases (atelectasis, tracheobronchitis) may simulate bronchiectasis. Atelectasis causes shortening and tortuosity of airways in the involved region, producing an accordion-like appearance on bronchography. Similarly, ulcerations of the bronchial mucosa, which are common in viral infections of the lower respiratory tract, appear as an irregular pattern on bronchography. Both conditions resemble cylindrical bronchiectasis. Reexpansion of the collapsed lung and/or regeneration of the epithelium results in reversibility of the "pseudobronchiectasis."

PATHOGENESIS Since bronchiectasis is defined by the presence of morphologic changes in the caliber of large bronchi, its pathogenesis depends on antecedent factors that either cause or lead to necrosis of the bronchial wall and supporting tissues. The origin of the destructive process is nearly always a bacterial infection, but usually other factors—hereditary, congenital, or mechanical—are also present and predispose to the development of the infection. The infection may be a primary event, such as suppurative necrotizing pneumonia, or it may be secondary to local or systemic abnormalities that impair defense mechanisms (i.e., cellular, humoral, and clearance) and promote bacterial growth. The use of antibiotic drugs has resulted in a marked decline of primary pneumonia, while improvements in medical care may actually have resulted in an increase in the incidence of secondary infections, such as those that arise as a consequence of diminished host resistance.

Hereditary and congenital factors Several hereditary and congenital disorders have been identified in which there is a high incidence of secondary bronchiectasis. *Congenital bronchiectasis* occurs at the site of a pre- or postnatal developmental defect of the bronchial system. The formation of cysts, cul-de-sacs, or bronchomalacia leads to pooling of secretions and bacterial infection. The generalized disorder of exocrine gland secretions in patients with *cystic fibrosis* affects the physical properties of tracheobronchial mucus; this causes retention of secretions, with partial or complete plugging of airways, that provides a nidus for implantation and growth of bacteria. Most deaths of patients with cystic fibrosis are now caused by the consequences of chronic bronchopulmonary suppuration. The diffuse bronchiectasis occasionally encountered in patients with *atopic bronchial asthma,* in whom there is often a strong familial association (Chap. 67), presumably is related to diffuse obstruction, as described below.

A variety of hereditary *immune-deficiency diseases,* secondary to either cellular or humoral defects, is associated with a high incidence of bacterial infections. Involvement of the sinuses and airways is particularly common, and the tendency for infections to recur in the lower airways often leads to bronchiectasis in patients with impaired immunologic mechanisms.

Bronchiectasis may be associated with dextrocardia and sinusitis *(Kartagener's syndrome),* but its pathogenesis in this disorder has never been elucidated satisfactorily. Similarly, a high incidence of unexplained bronchiectasis has been observed in Eskimo families and in the Maoris of New Zealand.

Obstruction Postobstructive bronchiectasis was much commoner in preantibiotic years than it is today. The availability of antimicrobial therapy and corrective surgical procedures accounts for the decreased incidence in this form of the disease. It is now recognized that obstruction per se does *not cause* bronchiectasis but *favors its development* by impairing clearance mechanisms, which enhances bacterial infection. Any process that leads to bronchial obstruction, therefore, may be associated with bronchiectasis distal to the site of involvement. Since the disorders causing obstruction are usually confined to one part of the bronchial system, postobstructive bronchiectasis is of the localized rather than the diffuse variety found in most forms of congenital-hereditary bronchiectasis. An exception is the bronchiectasis associated with diffuse obstruction of airways in patients with chronic bronchitis, atopic asthma, and cystic fibrosis.

Endobronchial tumors or foreign bodies, compression of airways from enlarged hilar lymph nodes or tumor masses, and bronchostenosis from endobronchial inflammatory disease (especially tuberculosis) all cause bronchial obstruction and may favor the development of postobstructive bronchiectasis.

Necrotizing inflammation Virtually all forms of bronchiectasis are associated with bacterial infections. Usually other causative factors are present, such as hereditary disorders and bronchial obstruction, that predispose the patient to secondary bacterial involvement, but bronchiectasis may also occur as the result of necrotizing infections in a previously healthy individual. This presumably is the mechanism underlying the bronchiectasis that follows the staphylococcal, some gram-negative, and the suppurative pneumonias that occasionally complicate measles, pertussis, and influenza.

In rare instances, bronchiectasis may follow the introduction of corrosive chemical substances, commonly hydrocarbons, into the tracheobronchial tree. Similarly, the repeated aspiration of gastric fluid into the lungs may cause bronchiectasis. Since ulceration from chemical causes is invariably associated with secondary bacterial infection, it is difficult to dissociate the contributions of these two factors.

CLINICAL MANIFESTATIONS The signs and symptoms of bronchiectasis depend on the extent, severity, location, and presence of complications of the disease, but the hallmarks of the disease are chronic cough with sputum production, hemoptysis, and recurrent pneumonia. Even these vary greatly in frequency and severity, and may be absent if the disease is mild or involves only the upper lobes of the lung.

The most frequent symptom is a *chronic cough* that produces sputum. The amount of sputum varies considerably but may be voluminous and is apt to be purulent during bouts of intercurrent infections. Streaks of blood in the sputum are common, and frank hemoptysis of large amounts of blood may develop if epithelial and parenchymal necrosis is severe. Exacerbation of chronic bronchial infection is frequent and may progress to pneumonia with or without lung abscess and empyema formation. Associated systemic features of bronchiectasis are fever, weight loss, and weakness; these usually indicate the presence of active sepsis from severe disease or untreated intercurrent bacterial infection.

In what was once the typical patient with bronchiectasis, symptoms develop during infancy or early childhood; the onset is usually acute and follows suppurative pneumonia or pulmonary infection complicating measles or pertussis. However, because of the success of antimicrobials and vaccines in treating or preventing these disorders, acute onset of bronchiectasis at an early age is becoming infrequent, except in those areas of the United States and other countries where, owing to isolation or poverty, good medical care is not available.

Although chronic childhood bronchiectasis is decreasing, another group of patients with a different form of the disease is increasing: These patients have recurrent lower respiratory tract infections that initially respond to treatment, with symptom-free intervals between episodes. The infections usually begin during childhood or young adulthood. As the number of recurrent bouts increases, the time between them tends to shorten and the response to treatment becomes less complete. Finally, chronic symptoms of cough and sputum develop. Patients in this category are likely to have cystic fibrosis, immune-deficiency diseases, or atopic asthma. The number of patients with late-onset bronchiectasis is increasing, because, owing to the availability of potent antimicrobial agents, patients now survive the acute episodes of bacterial infection that complicate their underlying disease, only to develop chronic suppurative sequelae.

Sinusitis is a common accompaniment of diffuse bronchiectasis and may be an expression of the vulnerability of the entire respiratory tract in these patients. Development of digital clubbing, metastatic abscesses (often brain), and amyloidosis were common complications in the past but are less frequent now. If the disease is widespread, it may resemble other forms of chronic obstructive lung disease, with generalized wheezing and ultimate progression to cor pulmonale; this constellation is occurring more often, owing to the increased longevity of patients with bronchiectasis and to the frequency with which it is found in patients with underlying systemic abnormalities that lead to diffuse pulmonary involvement.

DIAGNOSIS Bronchiectasis is defined as a morphologic disorder; hence its diagnosis depends on demonstrating the abnormal anatomy of the bronchial system. Ordinarily this is accomplished by roentgenographic techniques, usually *bronchography.* The diagnosis should be *suspected* in any patient with chronic productive cough, especially if his sputum intermittently becomes more purulent and streaked with blood. Physical examination seldom reveals the severity and extent of distribution of the disease. Inspiratory rales are often the only evidence of pulmonary involvement. Occasionally, advanced cases of saccular bronchiectasis can be diagnosed by routine (plain) chest roentgenography; in such cases multiple 1- to 2-cm cystic lesions or fluid levels in poorly delineated sacs can be seen. More often, however, plain chest roentgenograms show only streaky infiltrations and loss of volume in involved areas; at times the chest films may appear completely normal.

Bronchography is performed under topical anesthesia by instilling radiopaque material through a catheter, positioned under fluoroscopic guidance, in the tracheobronchial tree. Liquid iodine compounds are conventionally used, but tantalum powder, which may be insufflated into the airways, appears to be a promising contrast material and will probably find more widespread use in the future. Bronchography should not be performed in patients during exacerbations of their cough and sputum production, but only after the manifestations have been thoroughly treated (see next section) and the volume of secretions is minimal. Postural drainage and vigorous tracheobronchial toilet help to prepare patients with copious secretions for bronchography. If liquid contrast material is used, it is much safer to study one lung at a time, owing to alterations in pulmonary function and to occasional inflammatory reactions induced by the procedure. Bronchograms in patients with bronchiectasis show combinations of the cylindrical, varicose, and saccular changes in the caliber of the diseased bronchi, but filling must be adequate and all segments must be visualized if the study is to be considered satisfactory for diagnostic purposes.

Bronchography should be performed in all patients whose symptoms are severe or disabling. It is crucial in the evaluation of patients for possible surgery, and it documents sites of involvement so that effective postural drainage can be prescribed. Since the information from bronchography contributes little to the management of patients in whom surgery is contraindicated, such as those with generalized involvement or with obstructive airways disease, the procedure should be avoided in these patients because of its hazards.

Bronchoscopy does not establish the diagnosis of bronchiectasis but may be useful in identifying the source of secretions in patients with cough and sputum and in determining the site of bleeding in patients with hemoptysis.

All patients with multiple episodes of sinopulmonary infections should have an immunologic survey to detect immune-deficiency diseases. Similarly, patients with suspected cystic fibrosis and allergic disorders should have appropriate diagnostic studies to establish the presence of these important predisposing causes of bronchiectasis.

The sputum volume, color, cellular content, and bacterial inhabitants are useful guides to the presence of active infection. During exacerbations of the disease, the sputum increases in volume, becomes more purulent, and contains large numbers of polymorphonuclear leukocytes and bacteria that can be identified by Gram's stain. Culture of the sputum often reveals normal nasopharyngeal flora and, less commonly, *Diplococcus pneumoniae* or *Hemophilus influenzae.* Fetid sputum signifies the presence of anaerobic microorganisms, and appropriate cultures often yield *Bacteroides* species or anaerobic *Streptococcus* species. Sputum from patients receiving prolonged or frequent treatment with broad-spectrum antibiotic drugs may grow *Staphylococcus* species or *Pseudomonas aeruginosa;* this finding is especially common in children with cystic fibrosis. It is of significance only in patients who have active infections and is of little importance in asymptomatic individuals.

The blood count is apt to be within the normal range but may reveal anemia, reflecting chronic infection, or leukocytosis, signifying active suppuration. The urinalysis is normal except in the rare instances of *amyloidosis* when proteinuria occurs. The electrocardiogram is normal until the late stages, when *cor pulmonale* may supervene. Owing to the wide variations in the extent and severity of the disease, only broad generalizations about pulmonary function abnormalities are possible, although a correlation exists between the overall impairment of lung function and the number of involved segments. Vital capacity and expiratory flow rates tend to be reduced but may be within normal limits if the disease is mild. In the late stages of diffuse bronchiectasis, functional abnormalities similar to those of emphysema are found, except that the total lung capacity is usually reduced. A mild to moderate reduction in arterial oxygen tension (P_{O_2}) reflects regional abnormalities in the distribution of ventilation with respect to perfusion. Mismatching of ventilation and perfusion is the physiologic hallmark of bronchiectasis and can now be examined in regions of the lung by the use of radioactive gases, e.g., xenon 133 (Chap. 249). Pulmonary function studies are helpful in defining the extent and severity of abnormalities, in assessing the effects of therapy, and in evaluating patients for surgery.

TREATMENT Since bacterial infections are associated with most forms of bronchiectasis initially and are responsible for its exacerbation, antibiotics are the major weapons for its prevention and treatment. The choice of antimicrobial agents should be guided by the results of sputum culture; however, as indicated, these may reveal "normal flora" and no valid pathogen. Patients with this finding nearly always respond to either ampicillin or one of the tetracyclines. When pneumococci are present, it is best to avoid the tetracycline drugs, as some of these organisms are resistant to these agents. Antibiotics should be given until sputum production becomes minimal and purulence disappears; this desirable therapeutic result is usually achieved swiftly (5 to 7 days) if antibiotics are started early in the course of an exacerbation—as soon as the patient's cough increases and becomes productive of sputum in greater quantity and purulence than customary—but much longer periods are required if the infection is well established. Antibiotics should be administered either orally or by injection, *not* by nebulization (owing to failure of delivery and inactivation of the antibiotic).

Adjuvant medical measures are of great benefit in diminishing the consequences of bronchiectasis. Postural drainage and physical therapy facilitate removal of secretions. The treatment regimen depends on the location of the disease segments and is best administered under the supervision of a skilled respiratory physical therapist. Bronchodilators, expectorants, and humidifiers are of questionable value in many patients but are useful in those with bronchospasm or thick tenacious sputum. The need for expectorants can be reduced if the patient maintains a good fluid intake and stays well hydrated. Bronchoscopy is useful in identifying sites of endobronchial disease and sources of secretions and permits removal of secretions by aspiration under direct vision. The development of fiberoptic bronchoscopy, which is simpler than conventional bronchoscopy and provides access to subsegmental bronchi, should prove useful in the management of the unusual patient with problems of sputum retention. Similarly, bronchial lavage has been tried as a "last resort" in patients with large volumes of inspissated secretions. Oxygen should be given to patients with hypoxia during acute exacerbations; it can be administered outside the hospital to patients who are severely and chronically hypoxic. Inflammation from any cause will aggravate the effects of chronic bronchiectasis; therefore, smoking should be prohibited, exposure to air which is excessively polluted should be avoided, and influenza vaccine should be administered yearly.

Resectional surgery, once the mainstay of treatment, is used far less often now than previously for two reasons: (1) medical management is very effective in controlling bronchiectasis and preventing disability from it; (2) many patients with bronchiectasis have a generalized disorder that makes their entire tracheobronchial system vulnerable; although their bronchiectasis may appear well localized when evaluated initially, new sites of involvement may appear later. Operation should be considered in patients with localized (i.e., resectable) disease who do not respond to medical management or who are sufficiently disabled by complications that either their livelihood or their emotional life is impaired. Bouts of hemoptysis, especially if massive, and intercurrent pneumonias are the usual complications that require hospitalization, cause recurrent disability, and indicate the need for surgery.

PREVENTION The best approach to bronchiectasis is preventive. Patients with heritable diseases that predispose to bronchiectasis and their families should obtain genetic counseling to minimize the incidence of these disorders. Prompt diagnosis and effective antimicrobial treatment of bacterial infections of the lower respiratory tract is the best way of avoiding their potential chronic sequelae. The eradication of measles and pertussis by vaccines should eliminate these diseases as harbingers of bronchiectasis.

Prompt removal of foreign bodies, tumors, and other causes of bronchial obstruction should diminish postobstructive bronchiectasis.

LUNG ABSCESS

DEFINITION Lung abscess can be defined as a lesion of the lung parenchyma that contains purulent material. A classification of causes of necrosis and liquefaction of lung tissue with formation of an abscess cavity is presented in Table 253-1.

Many of the specific causes of lung abscesses are considered elsewhere in the text, and this discussion will mainly be concerned with what has been improperly called either "primary" or "nonspecific" lung abscess. Obviously a lung abscess must have a cause, and both expressions reflect the previous inability to identify the etiologic agents; improved collection and microbiologic techniques now permit isolation of pathogenic microorganisms from most patients with lung abscess; therefore the terms should be abandoned.

PATHOGENESIS The lower respiratory tract is normally sterile, even though it has been shown that oro- and nasopharyngeal contents are aspirated into dependent airways during sleep. This implies that local defense mechanisms are capable of controlling bacteria introduced under *most* circumstances and that development of infection requires additional predisposing conditions. Defense mechanisms may be overwhelmed by large numbers of microorganisms and/or unusually virulent bacteria, or they may be suppressed or modified by alcohol, smoke, drugs, or disease. Local factors such as obstruction by food particles or necrosis from gastric fluid also enhance the development of bacterial infection.

TABLE 253-1
Classification of lung abscesses according to cause

I Necrotizing infections
- *A* Pyogenic bacteria (*Staphylococcus aureus, Klebsiella,* group A streptococcus, *Bacteroides, Fusobacterium,* anaerobic and microaerophilic cocci and streptococci, other anaerobes, *Nocardia*)
- *B* Mycobacteria (*Mycobacterium tuberculosis, M. kansasii, M. intracellularis*)
- *C* Fungi (*Histoplasma, Coccidioides*)
- *D* Parasites (amebas, lung flukes)

II Cavitary infarction
- *A* Bland embolism
- *B* Septic embolism (various anaerobes, *Staphylococcus, Candida*)
- *C* Vasculitis (Wegener's granulomatosis, periarteritis)

III Cavitary malignancy
- *A* Primary bronchogenic carcinoma
- *B* Metastatic malignancies (very uncommon)

IV Other
- *A* Infected cysts
- *B* Necrotic conglomerate lesions (silicosis, coal miner's pneumoconiosis)

Any event or underlying disorder that is associated with aspiration may lead to lung abscess. Improved techniques of anesthesia and surgery have virtually eliminated the problem of lung abscesses associated with general anesthesia and tonsillectomy. But alcoholic stupor, drug overdosage, unconsciousnesness during seizures or strokes, defective swallowing, and prolonged debility impair protective reflexes and allow excess material from the oro- and nasopharynx and stomach to enter the tracheobronchial system.

Once introduced, liquid material flows down the airways until it reaches the most dependent region. Where material will localize in the lungs varies with body position at the time of aspiration; if aspiration occurs in a supine person, the anatomy of the airways favors movement into the right lung and then into either the posterior segment of the upper lobe or the superior segment of the lower lobe, providing an explanation for the frequent location of aspiration lung abscesses in these two segments.

The microorganisms that reach the lungs during aspiration will be the resident flora of the oro- and nasopharynx. In this context, the almost invariable association between lung abscess and poor dental and oral hygiene becomes obvious. Anaerobic organisms, especially *Bacteroides, Fusobacterium,* and streptococci and other cocci, are the principal inhabitants of diseased mouths and are likely to produce an abscess when carried into the lungs. A condition favoring aspiration and/or oral sepsis can be found in nearly 80 percent of patients with lung abscesses caused by anaerobic microorganisms. The fastidious growth characteristics of these organisms probably explains why they were not until recently considered responsible for most "aspiration" lung abscesses. When the normal flora has been modified by antimicrobial agents and/or hospitalization (with exposure to nosocomial organisms), other bacteria such as *S. aureus* and *Klebsiella* may be involved.

Although anaerobic organisms and the pathogenic sequence described above are responsible for most lung abscesses, they do not cause all of them. Staphylococcal and *Klebsiella* pneumonias and the less common pneumonias caused by other microorganisms with necrotizing potential are frequently associated with lung abscesses. Staphylococcal and *Klebsiella* pneumonias usually develop in patients with alcoholism, diabetes, or other causes of impaired host defenses; the organisms presumably are introduced into the lungs by aspiration—hence the frequency of upper lobe involvement—and cause swiftly progressive disease. Necrosis from liquefaction of lung tissue rapidly ensues and leads to the early formation of small ("micro") abscesses that coalesce and increase in size as further lung destruction occurs.

Tubercle bacilli are more likely to reach the upper lobes by bloodstream dissemination than through the airways, but they also cause necrosis of lung tissue and abscesses; these lesions conventionally are called "cavities," but pathogenetically they are really abscesses. Although the clinical course differs in acute necrotizing pneumonia on the one hand and pulmonary tuberculosis on the other, both may resemble anaerobic lung abscess and should, therefore, be considered in the differential diagnosis. Other organisms, notably the staphylococci, may also reach the lung by dissemination through the bloodstream and cause single or multiple lung abscesses.

CLINICAL MANIFESTATIONS Lung abscesses occur about three times more often in men than in women, presumably because conditions causing aspiration are more common in men. The spectrum of illness varies greatly, ranging from mild chronic productive cough to acute disease with severe systemic manifestations. The most common feature is cough productive of moderate to large amounts of purulent sputum that is often fetid and bloody. Fever and pleuritic or dull chest pain, are present in most patients. Symptoms gradually increase in severity during the next several weeks. Associated findings are anorexia and weakness (extremely common in children), dyspnea, and weight loss.

Physical examination reveals malodorous breath and evidence of dental caries, gingivitis, and periodontal infection. Pulmonary findings consist of signs of consolidation, rales, and (occasionally) amphoric or cavernous breath sounds over the involved area. Clubbing of the fingers may occur but is uncommon. Polymorphonuclear leukocytosis with an increased percentage of immature forms is usually present, and if the infection persists for more than a few weeks, anemia and hypoalbuminemia may be found. The diagnosis may be suspected from the medical history and physical findings, but these are obviously nonspecific. However, foul-smelling sputum clearly indicates an anaerobic pulmonary (rarely, bronchial) infection, often with abscess formation. Definitive diagnosis rests on the demonstration of an abscess cavity by chest roentgenography and the identification of the causative organism in the microbiology laboratory.

The chest roentgenogram reveals an area of consolidation containing a radiolucency. Not all radiolucent areas are abscesses, however, and either a wall or a border completely around the lucent area, or a fluid level within it must be delineated if an abscess cavity is to be diagnosed. Even these criteria are not certain, since infected cysts or bullae or an empyema with a bronchopleural fistula may resemble lung abscesses.

Examination of the sputum by both microscopy and culture is essential. Gram's stain reveals numerous polymorphonuclear leukocytes and abundant gram-positive cocci and/or pleomorphic gram-negative bacilli, fusiform rods, or coccobacilli. Sputum culture for anaerobic organisms yields one or more species of *Streptococcus* or gram-negative bacilli. Since anaerobic organisms are universal inhabitants of the mouth, caution must be exercised in attributing pathogenic significance to an organism isolated from an expectorated specimen. For this reason, either sputum obtained by transtracheal aspiration or transthoracic lung puncture or empyema fluid is preferred for cultural identification. Material for anaerobic culture should be placed immediately in an oxygen-free atmosphere in a tube or bottle for transport to the laboratory. Sputum obtained by nasotracheal suction or by bronchoscopy is distinctly less reliable. Blood cultures, which are often sterile, should be obtained before treatment is instituted.

TREATMENT Because of the difficulties encountered in the past in isolating the causative organism(s), the treatment of lung abscess has been largely empirical. In the initial evaluation of patients with a lung abscess it is vital to identify (or exclude) the presence of aerobic pyogenic organisms (especially *Staphyloccus* and *Klebsiella),* mycobacteria, etc., that cause necrotizing pneumonias; this can usually be accomplished by consideration of the history, the physical abnormalities, the chest x-ray findings, and, most importantly, the results of careful examination of Gram's stain of the sputum. Where a predominant organism is found, treatment with an antimicrobial agent appropriate for it is instituted. However, if the clinical evidence suggests aspiration and if Gram's stain suggests probable anaerobic microorganisms (often two or three types or more), a treatment regimen should be chosen that is effective against anaerobic bacteria. Penicillin is usually the drug of choice and should be given in high doses (e.g., aqueous penicillin, 5 to 10 million units daily, intravenously). However, *Bacteroides fragilis*, which is resistant *in vitro* to penicillin, may be found in up to 25 percent of patients; therefore, if the patient is seriously ill or fails to respond to penicillin, chloramphenicol, which is active against almost all anaerobes, is the preferred drug. In addition to chloramphenicol, alternate drugs for the penicillin-sensitive patient include tetracycline and lincomycin. Clindamycin and metronidazole, both still experimental for the treatment of lung abscess, are very active against most anaerobes, including *B. fragilis.*

The duration of antibiotic therapy is determined empirically. In view of the partial resistance of anaerobic organisms and the tendency for signs and symptoms to recur if antimicrobial agents are discontinued prematurely, prolonged treatment for 4 to 6 weeks is necessary. The antibiotic regimen should be changed only when there is definite clinical or radiographic evidence of relapse, and *not* simply on the basis of changing flora in serial sputum cultures. Penicillin can be given intramuscularly or orally instead of intravenously *after* all signs of systemic toxicity (i.e., fever, leukocyte count) have subsided and when serial roentgenograms show appreciable clearing of the contiguous pneumonia, reduction in the size of the cavity, and absence of a fluid level within the cavity. The antibiotic drug may be stopped when the surrounding infiltration has disappeared, even though a thin-walled abscess cavity persists. Serial roentgenograms of the chest should show gradual diminution of the cavity in subsequent months. Delayed closure is common, and as long as resolution progresses, no further therapy is indicated.

Ancillary measures to loosen secretions and facilitate their removal are helpful. Hydration and postural drainage with physical therapy are important adjuncts that should be used in the initial management of most patients with lung abscesses.

The role of bronchoscopy is somewhat controversial. Some clinicians believe that every patient with a lung abscess deserves bronchoscopy soon after admission to the hospital; others believe it should be used in special circumstances, e.g., in the patient who fails to respond as anticipated after beginning antibiotic therapy, when tumor or foreign body is suspected, to promote drainage from a poorly communicating cavity, and to obtain specimens for cultural and cytologic examination. Fiberoptic bronchoscopy should be used increasingly because of its ease and convenience and its high yield of positive reliable bacteriologic results when combined with aspiration and bronchial brushing.

Medical management is successful in the majority of cases of lung abscess, so that surgical intervention is seldom necessary. Tube thoracostomy or some other form of surgical drainage may be needed to manage uncontrolled sepsis and systemic manifestations in patients with poorly draining acute lung abscesses; although only rarely indicated, such treatment may be lifesaving. Another uncommon complication of acute lung abscess that requires emergency surgery (i.e., thoracotomy and resection) is massive hemoptysis.

Incomplete resolution of a chronic lung abscess is not sufficient reason for resectional surgery, since delayed closure is common. Resection is indicated for severe or recurrent hemoptysis, recurrence of infection, associated symptomatic bronchiectasis, and suspicion of malignancy.

PROGNOSIS Antibiotic drugs have had a dramatic effect on the prognosis of patients with pyogenic lung abscesses. Instead of a disease with a high mortality rate (35 percent) and prolonged morbidity from numerous complications, the disease can be readily treated by medical measures in most cases. The prognosis is now influenced mainly by associated disorders—alcoholism, drug addiction, central nervous system disease—that affect the patient's ability to tolerate severe infection.

PREVENTION Lung abscess from anaerobic microorganisms should be preventable. Since two phenomena underlie its pathogenesis—aspiration and oral sepsis—efforts should be directed toward prevention of aspiration and treatment of dental and periodontal disease. Dental care will substantially reduce the reservoir of anaerobic bacteria that may reach the lungs should aspiration occur; therefore, patients with high risk of aspiration (those with epilepsy or swallowing difficulties or those receiving electroshock therapy) should maintain good oral hygiene. If a known bout of aspiration takes place, the patient should be carefully observed and followed with chest roentgenograms. At the earliest sign of pulmonary infection, cough, sputum, fever, leukocytosis, or radiographic infiltration, a sputum culture should be obtained, and appropriate antibiotic therapy should be begun promptly.

BRONCHOLITHIASIS

Broncholiths, or bronchial stones, occur when calcified particles in a lymph node or the lung parenchyma erode into a contiguous bronchus. Broncholithiasis, therefore, is a secondary complication of an antecedent disease that has resulted in residual intrathoracic calcifications. Numerous disorders leave calcified deposits which can be detected by chest roentgenography, but clinically significant broncholithiasis is rare. It is usually a late complication of one of the three common granulomatous infections: tuberculosis, histoplasmosis, and coccidioidomycosis. Of these, histoplasmosis has the greatest tendency to heal with multiple residual calcifications and coccidioidomycosis is the least; hence brocholithiasis in the United States, especially in the Central and Eastern regions, is most likely related to previous infection with *Histoplasma capsulatum.*

The clinical consequences of broncholithiasis are related to the movement of stones through the airway wall and their release into the lumen. The process of erosion is often accompanied by paroxysms of cough, intermittent hemoptysis, and bronchopulmonary infection. The overlying inflammatory reaction impairs bronchial clearance and narrows the lumen; these conditions may lead to distal recurrent infections or, if the obstruction is complete, atelectasis. The hallmark of broncholithiasis is the coughing and expectoration of chalky sediment, sandy (gritty) particles, or stones. Such episodes are usually single but may be multiple.

Broncholithiasis should be suspected in any patient with recurrent cough and hemoptysis who has multiple calcifications in the lung and/or mediastinal lymph nodes on the chest roentgenograms. The diagnosis can be established by recovering stones in the sputum, by visualizing broncholiths penetrating the bronchial wall at the time of bronchoscopy, or by establishing that calcified particles have disappeared on serial chest x-ray films. Tomography may be helpful in determining with greater precision than routine roentgenograms the presence and location of calcifications in and around bronchi.

Treatment depends on the magnitude of the symptoms. The disorder is self-limiting once the stone has eroded into the lumen and is coughed up; however, ulceration of the particle may be slow and attended by significant symptomatology. Antimicrobial agents are useful in the treatment of associated bacterial infection. Bronchoscopy should be performed and the stone removed if possible. At times, thoracotomy and lung resection are necessary, usually for obstructive complications or massive hemoptysis.

REFERENCES

Bronchiectasis

BASS H et al: Regional structure and function in bronchiectasis: A correlative study using bronchography and ^{133}Xe. Am Rev Resp Dis 97:598, 1968

CROFTON J: Diagnosis and treatment of bronchiectasis: I. Diagnosis. II. Treatment and prevention. Br Med J 1:721, 783, 1966

FIELD CE: Bronchiectasis: Third report on a follow-up study of medical and surgical cases from childhood. Arch Dis Child 44:551, 1969

ROSENZWEIG DY, STEAD WW: The role of tuberculosis and other forms of bronchopulmonary necrosis in the pathogenesis of bronchiectasis. Am Rev Resp Dis 93:769, 1966

Broncholithiasis

ARRIGONI MG et al: Broncholithiasis. J Thorac Cardiovasc Surg 62:231, 1971

WEED LA, ANDERSEN HA: Etiology of broncholithiasis. Dis Chest 37:270, 1960

Lung abscess

BARNETT TB, HERRING CL: Lung abscess: Initial and late results of medical therapy. Arch Intern Med 127:217, 1971

FELNER JM, DOWELL VR JR: *"Bacteroides"* bacteremia. Am J Med 50:787, 1971

SCHWEPPE HI et al: Lung abscess: An analysis of the Massachusetts General Hospital cases from 1943 through 1956. N Engl J Med 265:1039, 1961

254 DIFFUSE INFILTRATIVE DISEASES OF THE LUNG

JOHN F. MURRAY

Infiltration means the diffusion into or accumulation in a tissue of substances not normal to it. Infiltrates of the lung are usually either cellular (e.g., inflammatory or neoplastic infiltration) or noncellular (e.g., infiltration by edema fluid, amyloid, or other substances). Numerous clinicopathological entities, therefore, are associated with diffuse infiltration of the lung. Although the pathogenesis of the lung lesion in these disorders differs considerably —and is obscure in many instances—they commonly produce widespread structural involvement and cause characteristic alterations in pulmonary function. Because of these similarities, they are often accompanied by identical signs, symptoms, and roentgenographic changes.

The lung, like other organs, has a limited capacity to react to injury; accordingly, the interstitial pneumonias, the most common cause of diffuse pulmonary infiltration, are regarded as a spectrum of pathologic changes that represent a common response to diverse stimuli. In contrast to the acute polymorphonuclear *intra*alveolar exudative process that characterizes most bacterial pneumonias, the reaction in the infiltrative diseases is primarily *inter*alveolar. In the latter the acute cellular infiltrate is usually composed of round cells (histiocytes, lymphocytes, and plasma cells) and is accompanied by interstitial edema and a proteinaceous exudate, containing some cells or cellular debris, that accumulates in alveolar spaces and bronchioles; organization of this material leads to hyaline membrane formation. A later phase consists of abundant hyperplasia and/or metaplasia of bronchial and alveolar epithelium. Following necrosis of the interalveolar septa, scarring and reepithelialization occur progressively incorporating the intraalveolar inflammatory exudate (fibrosing alveolitis); this eventually causes extensive fibrosis with gross lung destruction and "honeycombing." When the changes become advanced ("end-stage lung"), any specific histologic or identifying hallmarks that were present are usually lost. Although the cellular population causing the infiltrate differs considerably depending on whether infiltration is by neoplastic or inflammatory cells, the resulting functional alterations and clinical consequences are similar.

It follows from these considerations that the number of diffuse infiltrative diseases of the lung is large. Table

254-1 lists the most important causes but is by no means inclusive.

PATHOGENESIS

INFECTIONS Several members of each of the major classes of infectious agents are known to cause diffuse infiltration of the lung parenchyma. Viruses that affect the lower respiratory tract cause an acute interstitial inflammatory infiltration of lymphocytes, histiocytes, and plasma cells that may be accompanied by occasional hyaline membranes. Although most viral interstitial pneumonias resolve without significant residual lesions, experimental and clinical evidence has linked viruses with chronic, progressive diffuse interstitial disease. Necrotizing pyogenic bacteria and infections causing widespread granuloma formation, especially tuberculosis and fungus disorders, are likely to heal with fibrous tissue (scar) formation and hence cause infiltrative disease that may be permanent. The migration of parasites through the lungs causes pulmonary infiltrations, presumably on an immunologic basis, as shown by positive immediate skin test reactions, presence of precipitating or complement-fixing antibodies, systemic eosinophilia, and (at times) asthma. Infections of the lung are chiefly focal rather than diffuse processes, because they are acquired through the tracheobronchial tree. Hematogenous dissemination of organisms, however, may result in widespread, fairly uniform distribution of lesions throughout the lung parenchyma. Infections are not a common cause of *diffuse* infiltration

TABLE 254-1
Causes of diffuse infiltrative diseases of the lungs

I Infections*
- *A* Viruses: influenza, chickenpox, measles
- *B* Bedsonia: psittacosis (ornithosis), lymphopathia venereum
- *C* Rickettsia: Q fever, Rocky Mountain spotted fever
- *D* Bacteria: miliary tuberculosis, staphylococcal infection, streptococcal infection, *Klebsiella* infection, mycoplasma infection, brucellosis, salmonellosis, shigellosis, tularemia, glanders, pneumonic plague, pertussis
- *E* Fungi: histoplasmosis, coccidioidomycosis, blastomycosis, cryptococcosis, candidiasis, aspergillosis, actinomycosis, nocardiosis, geotrichosis, sporotrichosis
- *F* Parasites: schistosomiasis, *Pneumocystis carinii* infection, filariasis, toxoplasmosis, paragonimiasis, ascariasis, trichinosis, hookworm infestation, strongyloides, visceral larva migrans, amebiasis, echinococcosis

II Occupational causes
- *A* Mineral dusts: silicosis, asbestosis, berylliosis, coal miner's pneumoconiosis, Shaver's disease (bauxite), diatomaceous earth disease, talc pneumoconiosis, siderosis (arc welder's disease), pneumoconiosis from barium, silver, tin, vanadium, manganese
- *B* Chemical fumes: nitrogen dioxide (silo-filler's disease), chlorine, ammonia, sulfur dioxide, phosgenes, acetylene, kerosene, carbon tetrachloride, bromine, hydrogen fluoride, hydrochloric acid, nitric acid, picric acid

III Neoplastic causes: bronchioloalveolar carcinoma, hematogenous metastases, lymphangitic carcinomatosis, leukemia, lymphoma, polycythemia vera

IV Congenital or familial causes: cystic fibrosis, Niemann-Pick disease, Gaucher's disease, neurofibromatosis, tuberous sclerosis, familial dysautonomia (Riley-Day syndrome), pulmonary alveolar microlithiasis, familial idiopathic pulmonary fibrosis (congenital cystic disease with pulmonary fibrosis and familial fibrocystic pulmonary dysplasia)

V Metabolic causes: uremic pneumonitis

VI Physical agents: postirradiation fibrosis, thermal injury, oxygen toxicity, blast injury

VII Circulatory causes
- *A* Thromboembolic: multiple pulmonary emboli, fat embolism, lymphangiography, sickle-cell anemia, foreign body vasculitis (drug addicts, schistosomiasis)
- *B* Hemodynamic: pulmonary edema, chronic passive congestion with fibrosis (possibly with hemosiderosis and/or bone deposition)

VIII Immunologic causes
- *A* Hypersensitivity pneumonia
  - *1* Inhaled antigens: farmer's lung, bagassosis, byssinosis, bird fancier's disease, maple bark disease, sequoiosis, mushroom grower's disease, pneumonitis from pituitary snuff, exposure to *Bacillus subtilis* enzymes (detergent manufacturing), or smallpox vaccine
  - *2* Drug reactions: sensitivity to hydralazine, busulfan, nitrofurantoin, hexamethonium, mecamylamine, methysergid(e), and bleiomycin
- *B* Collagen diseases: scleroderma, rheumatoid arthritis, lupus erythematosus, periarteritis nodosa, Wegener's granulomatosis, dermatomyositis, Sjögren's syndrome
- *C* Goodpasture's syndrome

IX Unknown origin
- *A* Sarcoidosis
- *B* Histiocytosis X: Letterer-Siwe disease, Hand-Schüller-Christian disease, eosinophilic granuloma
- *C* Idiopathic hemosiderosis
- *D* Pulmonary alveolar proteinosis
- *E* Desquamative interstitial pneumonia
- *F* (Idiopathic) organizing interstitial pneumonia (synonyms: usual interstitial pneumonia, chronic interstitial pneumonitis, diffuse idiopathic pulmonary fibrosis, idiopathic interstitial pulmonary fibrosis, acute diffuse interstitial fibrosis of the lungs, diffuse fibrosing alveolitis, chronic diffuse sclerosis, alveolitis, chronic Hamman-Rich syndrome, bronchiolar emphysema, and muscular cirrhosis of the lung)

* *Infections are not a common cause of diffuse infiltrative disease of the lungs. More commonly they cause focal processes.*

of the lung, but they are important to recognize because most are treatable.

NEOPLASTIC DISEASE Widespread pulmonary neoplasms (Chap. 260) are an important cause of diffuse pulmonary infiltrations and may occur in three different locations: (1) the surface epithelium. (2) the blood vessels and lymph channels and their surrounding spaces, and (3) the interstitial tissues. Bronchioloalveolar carcinoma is a primary lung cancer that may cause either focal tumor deposits or extensive epithelial infiltration (pulmonary adenomatosis). Some varieties grow slowly and are not invasive; others spread rapidly and are highly malignant. The lung parenchyma may become diffusely infiltrated by hematogenous or lymphatic metastases from a primary tumor anywhere in the body. Similarly, widespread interstitial pulmonary involvement may occur during the course of any of the lymphomas (Hodgkin's disease, lymphosarcoma, reticulum cell sarcoma), in mycosis fungoides, and in Kaposi's sarcoma.

Infiltration of the lung with leukemic cells can be identified microscopically in a high proportion of patients with leukemia, but the involvement, in most cases, is not associated either with radiographically recognizable lesions or with clinically significant symptoms. Acute and chronic lymphatic leukemias are much more likely than myelogenous leukemias to cause pulmonary infiltrations. The presence of fever and detectable pulmonary infiltrations in a patient with leukemia usually indicates the presence of an infection, often by an "opportunistic" organism, and these conditions should not be regarded as leukemic until a thorough search has been made for potential pathogens. Untreated polycythemia vera is often associated with congestion of the pulmonary circulation and occasionally has been reported to cause interstitial pulmonary fibrosis.

CONGENITAL OR FAMILIAL DISEASES Several unrelated congenital or familial diseases are associated with diffuse pulmonary infiltration; most are systemic disorders, and the pulmonary component may be a relatively infrequent manifestation that can be overshadowed by involvement of other organs that are more important sources of morbidity and mortality. Extensive parenchymal scarring with overinflation of distal airspaces occurs in *cystic fibrosis* as a result of the frequent and troublesome lower respiratory tract infections that accompany and worsen the pulmonary component of the disease. Recurrent infections are due to the presence of viscous tracheobronchial secretions. *Familial dysautonomia* may be associated with pulmonary scarring secondary to pneumonitis resulting from frequent aspiration caused by autonomic nervous system dysfunction. Diffuse pulmonary fibrosis has been found in 10 to 20 percent of patients with *tuberous sclerosis* or *neurofibromatosis* (von Recklinghausen's disease). In *Niemann-Pick disease* and *Gaucher's disease* (usually the infantile form), chest roentgenograms may reveal fine reticulonodular shadows that reflect the presence of diffuse infiltration by cells containing the abnormal lipids that characterize the diseases.

Pulmonary microlithiasis is a sporadic or familial disease in which there are innumerable intraalveolar calcified particles. The disorder presumably begins at an early age and is often recognized accidentally by chest roentgenography in an asymptomatic patient. There are no identifiable alterations in calcium and phosphorus metabolism, but local physicochemical abnormalities in lung tissue may account for the deposition of calcium salts. *Familial idiopathic pulmonary fibrosis* is identical to organizing interstitial pneumonia (described in more detail later) but has, in addition, a definite familial incidence and a tendency to afflict younger persons. The pathogenesis in both sporadic and familial cases remains obscure.

METABOLIC DISORDERS Two relatively common clinical disorders, uremia and hypercalcemia, are associated with diffuse pulmonary infiltration. The pathologic findings in *uremic pneumonitis* consist of a fibrinous exudate in the alveoli (most marked in the hilar regions of the lung), often organized into dense hyaline membranes, and an interstitial pneumonia with varying degrees of organization. Similar changes have been observed in chronic left ventricular failure in the absence of uremia; a controversy exists whether the lung lesions are caused by uremia since congestive heart failure often accompanies uremia or are related to the associated heart disease. Available data indicate that, in patients with uremia, a dialyzable substance may accumulate that affects capillary permeability generally and contributes to the development of lung lesions.

Hypercalcemia from virtually any cause, e.g., hyperparathyroidism, extensive bone malignancy, and hypervitaminosis D, may be associated with multiple deposits of calcium salts in the lungs. The lung, like the gastric mucosa and renal tubules, is a preferred site of involvement, presumably owing to local changes in pH which favor calcification. Although metastatic calcification of the lung parenchyma may be extensive when examined microscopically, it is often undetectable by chest roentgenography and seldom produces symptoms.

PHYSICAL AGENTS *Radiation pneumonitis* results from the acute effects of irradiation of the lung. The areas of involvement are usually sharply confined to the target sites, but if either the area irradiated or the secondary scatter is extensive, most of the lung parenchyma may be involved. The pathologic process consists of varying degrees of capillary congestion, interstitial edema, cellular infiltration, lymphangiectasis, and hyaline membrane formation. In the chronic phase, dense interstitial fibrosis develops, and blood vessels become narrowed or obliterated. Virtually every patient who acquires radiation pneumonitis also develops radiation fibrosis; however, fibrosis may occur in the absence of a clinically significant acute phase, presumably through the organization of a subacute and more indolent reaction. There is wide variation in the response of patients to a given dose of irradiation, suggesting that "host factors" may substantially modify the response. *Thermal and blast injuries* initiate a similar series of pathogenetic events: diffuse parenchymal injury, followed by organization and repair. There is also abundant experimental and clinical evidence that *oxygen,* given in high concentrations for several days, also injures the lung; moreover, its acute effects and subsequent evolution are similar to those of irradiation but proceed more rapidly. Exposure to 100 percent oxygen damages pulmonary capillary endothelium and initiates an acute infiltrative-edematous phase, often with hyaline membrane formation, followed by a proliferative phase leading to fibrosis and collagen deposition.

CIRCULATORY DISORDERS Numerous thromboembolic conditions and a variety of hemodynamic complications of disorders of the left side of the heart and the pulmonary venous system may cause obliteration of or leakage from small pulmonary blood vessels. Diffuse pulmonary infiltrations ensue if *thromboemboli* elicit a perivascular inflammatory response or, if abnormal hydrostatic forces are sufficiently imbalanced, promote accumulation of fluid in the interstitium; when excessive fluid is retained in the lung parenchyma for prolonged periods, as in *mitral stenosis* and *chronic left ventricular failure,* hemosiderin is deposited, and possibly it or other factors cause slowly progressive interstitial fibrosis. At times, focal organization may progress to bone deposition.

IMMUNOLOGIC DISORDERS The disorders in this category are presumed to originate through aberrant immunologic mechanisms; this assumption remains unproven because antigen, antibody, and (at times) complement have not been consistently demonstrated at the sites of the pulmonary lesions and in other involved organs. Three major subgroups can be differentiated on the basis of their clinical manifestations and immunologic characteristics:

Hypersensitivity pneumonia A good example of how numerous apparently varied disorders express themselves through a common pathogenetic mechanism can be found in hypersensitivity pneumonia [also called allergic interstitial pneumonitis (Chap. 257)]. The factors that determine the pathogenesis of pulmonary infiltration following inhalation of dust include the immunologic reactivity of the host, the nature and size of the inhaled organic dust, and the degree and duration of exposure. The onset may be acute if exposure is great or if the patient is exquisitely sensitive to the antigen; conversely, the onset may be insidious in the nonsusceptible, weakly sensitized subject or when exposure is limited.

Hypersensitivity to a suspected (specific) antigen can be established by demonstrating precipitating antibodies in the patient's serum, and by the presence of a positive intermediate skin reaction (Arthus type) 4 to 8 hr after intradermal testing. Evidence for an etiologic role for the antigen is obtained by reproducing an acute attack, with attendant pulmonary function abnormalities, following inhalation of an aerosol containing the antigen. If the patient is also atopic, he may show a positive immediate skin reaction. Allergic bronchopulmonary aspergillosis (Chap. 174) is an example of an infiltrative disease in which both immediate and intermediate hypersensitivity mechanisms contribute to the pathogenesis.

The pathogenesis of pulmonary lesions following the long-term ingestion of certain drugs is unclear. The acute interstitial pulmonary inflammatory reaction they provoke is similar to that found following the inhalation of sensitizing antigens, but direct evidence of an allergic mechanism is lacking and their classification is inferential. Specific examples of immunologic disorders involving the lung are detailed in Chap. 257.

"Collagen diseases" This group of diseases share such common features as multisystem involvement, considerable overlap in organ dysfunction (e.g., arthritis, nephritis), and the presence of excessive quantities of immunoglobulins and circulating non-organ-specific "autoantibodies." Although antigen-antibody complexes have been implicated in the pathogenesis of the nephritis of lupus erythematosus, there is no direct evidence that they cause the associated pulmonary infiltrates, nor have immune complexes been identified in the other "collagen diseases." Pathologically, the prototype lesion is vascular, and pulmonary vasculitis is found in periarteritis nodosa (and related disorders like Churg-Strauss allergic granulomatosis) and Wegener's granulomatosis. Vasculitis may also be present in scleroderma, rheumatoid arthritis, lupus erythematosus, dermatomyositis, and Sjögren's syndrome, but a more common pulmonary lesion is organizing interstitial pneumonia (diffuse interstitial fibrosis). The pathogenesis of the interstitial pneumonia is unknown but may pertain to the unique vulnerability of the lung. The lung receives more blood flow, and hence more circulating antigens, antibodies, or immune complexes, than other organs and offers a much greater surface area than the skin for contact with environmental antigens. Procaineamide–induced lupus erythematosus, for example, is associated with a higher incidence of pulmonary infiltration than the naturally occurring disease.

Goodpasture's syndrome This syndrome is differentiated from the collagen diseases on the basis of clinical and experimental evidence that it is mediated by a cytotoxic tissue-specific antibody rather than by immune complexes. There appear to be antigenic similarities between alveolar and glomerular basement membranes, and antibodies to them have been identified in the serum and on the basement membranes of the respective organs. However, how the presence of the specific antibodies induces injury after combination with tissue antigens is poorly understood.

OCCUPATIONAL CAUSES A wide variety of mineral dusts and chemical fumes may be inhaled (Chap. 258). Whether or not disease is produced depends on a number of factors, including the duration of exposure and concentration of the agent, its chemical properties (e.g., whether or not it is inert, fibrogenic, granuloma-inducing), and the susceptibility (including immunologic responsiveness) of the host.

Diffuse parenchymal infiltration results from the tissue

injury produced by the toxic substances and from the subsequent organization and evolution of the pathology. Once exposure ceases, the process may remain stable, as in early ("simple") silicosis, or it may progress slowly and become clinically apparent only many years later, as in asbestosis. The growth and conglomeration of the early small infiltrates of either coal miner's pneumoconiosis or silicosis into progressive massive fibrosis may occur spontaneously (as in Caplan's syndrome or rheumatoid pneumoconiosis), but it often signifies coexisting tuberculosis.

UNKNOWN ORIGIN Although the basic pathogenesis of many of the diseases just discussed (e.g., drug reactions, congenital disorders, immunologic diseases) is not known, they can be classified according to major subject headings that allow inferences to be made concerning their etiology. There remain several important diffuse infiltrative diseases of the lung that cannot be conveniently grouped and so are listed separately under disorders of unknown origin.

Sarcoidosis Sarcoidosis (Chap. 223) is a multisystem disease with characteristic, but *not* pathognomonic, noncaseating granulomas commonly involving the lungs, lymph nodes, and liver. Interalveolar and interstitial granulomas may be undetectable roentgenographically but can be recognized by sensitive tests of pulmonary function. The natural history of sarcoidosis is variable and capricious. Spontaneously, the pulmonary lesions may either resolve completely or organize by extensive scarring and disruption of alveoli (honeycombing) with devastating loss of pulmonary function.

Histiocytosis X Histiocytosis X (Chap. 317) is a generic term that includes *Letterer-Siwe disease, Hand-Schüller-Christian disease, eosinophilic granuloma,* and their variants. The disorder is characterized by proliferation of and infiltration by histiocytes into various tissues. The stimulus for the histiocytic proliferation is unknown, and inflammatory, immunologic, and neoplastic causes have been considered. Tissue eosinophilia may occur, and the presence of foam cells, collagenization, and fibrosis indicates older organizing lesions. The major variations of histiocytosis X depend on the age of the patient, the extent of involvement, and the duration of the disease. The pulmonary complications vary, therefore, in a manner analogous to the progression in sarcoidosis, from acute cellular infiltration to chronic extensive scarring of the lung parenchyma.

Idiopathic pulmonary hemosiderosis This rare disease is encountered much more commonly in children than adults, and its chief manifestations are diffuse pulmonary infiltration, anemia, and hemoptysis. Bleeding into the lung interstitium accounts for the anemia and, when brisk, for the hemoptysis. Hemosiderin-filled macrophages, the clinical hallmark of the disease, can be found in the sputum during exacerbations and are abundant in the lung at all times. The presence of blood or blood products appears to initiate a fibrogenic response that leads to an increase in reticulum, collagen, and, ultimately, fibrous tissue. The prognosis is poor, and death usually occurs during an acute episode of bleeding; however, if the patient survives for several years, extensive interstitial fibrosis may result. Theories about etiology have included immunologic mechanisms, vascular defects, and abnormal iron storage, but none is proved.

Pulmonary alveolar proteinosis In 1958 Rosen, Castleman, and Liebow described 27 cases of a new entity they called pulmonary alveolar proteinosis. The disorder is characterized by diffuse pulmonary infiltrations which, in contrast to the disorders described earlier, are confined to alveolar spaces; alveoli in involved areas are filled with a dense granular material that stains vividly with the periodic acid–Schiff technique. The material has been identified as a lipoprotein with many chemical similarities to pulmonary surfactant, but with different physical properties. Although hyperplasia of alveolar epithelium is usually present, inflammation and fibrous thickening of the interalveolar septa are conspicuously absent, and, in the absence of infection, fibrous tissue organization to the stage of honeycombing has never been reported. In contrast to the relatively uniform roentgenographic and pathologic appearance of the lungs in pulmonary alveolar proteinosis, the clinical manifestations are extremely varied; they range from asymptomatic involvement to total disability or death from hypoxia, cor pulmonale, or secondary infection (often with "opportunistic" microorganisms, notably *Nocardia).* The etiology is unknown, and the natural history is poorly defined and appears to be variable: both spontaneous resolution and worsening have been reported.

Desquamative interstitial pneumonia (DIP) There are pathologic similarities between pulmonary alveolar proteinosis and DIP and between organizing interstitial pneumonia (see below) and DIP; however, DIP appears sufficiently distinct to justify its separate classification. In DIP there is striking hyperplasia of the alveolar epithelium with large cells (probably type II granular pneumocytes or possibly macrophages) that slough into and fill the alveolar spaces. DIP is unlike alveolar proteinosis and is similar to the usual interstitial pneumonias in that there is an impressive interstitial cellular infiltrate and, at times, an interstitial fibrotic reaction of varying severity. The tendency to severe fibrosis is less in DIP than in organizing interstitial pneumonia, but it may occur, and progression to honeycombing has been observed. The cause of DIP is unknown, but the disease may arise from multiple factors that initiate similar pathogenetic responses.

(Idiopathic) organizing interstitial pneumonia (OIP) The lack of specificity of the pulmonary pathologic reaction in the large number of diffuse pulmonary infiltrative disorders is best illustrated by the many known causes of or associations with organizing interstitial pneumonia. *Identical* pathologic findings have been documented in cases caused by infections, occupational exposure, hypersensitivity reactions, a variety of familial disorders, irradiation or oxygen inhalation, prolonged circulatory failure, "collagen disease," and desquamative interstitial pneumonia. The term *"usual* organizing interstitial pneumonia" (UIP) has been recommended for all these disorders, because it correctly describes the similar pulmonary pathology in all of them, but, being descriptive, it ignores what is known about etiology and pathogenesis. In most large series of cases of UIP, the etiology or pathogenesis can be identified in about half, and the remaining half are labeled "idiopathic." Those that are idiopathic *must* have a specific origin, and unquestionably many entities will be sorted out and properly classified in the future. The confusion about nomenclature is reflected in the number of synonyms listed in Table 254-1 that are mainly descriptive, each having some advantages and some disadvantages over the others. Idiopathic organizing interstitial pneumonia is used because it recognizes the etiologic heterogeneity of this (presumed) group of diseases rather than their pathologic homogeneity.

Idiopathic organizing pneumonia presumably begins with an alveolar wall injury leading to interstitial and alveolar exudate and to hyaline membranes. The next phase consists of cellular infiltration and regeneration of alveolar epithelium around the material in the alveolar spaces; during this phase fibroblasts appear and progressive fibrosis occurs, with obliteration of gas exchange units and marked alteration of parenchymal architecture. The sequence from injury to fibrosis may evolve in weeks (acute organizing pneumonitis or Hamman-Rich disease), or much more slowly over a period of years, which is the typical course of idiopathic organizing pneumonia.

CLINICAL MANIFESTATIONS

The symptoms, signs, and results of laboratory tests obviously vary, depending on the extent of the pulmonary process and its rate of progress. Moreover, if diffuse pulmonary infiltration is but one component of a systemic disorder (e.g., in collagen diseases), the clinical manifestations may pertain to other organ system disease. In addition, pulmonary involvement is substantially augmented by the presence of secondary complications —infection, cor pulmonale, and pneumothorax.

The predominant complaint caused by pulmonary infiltration is dyspnea, which is usually insidious in development, related primarily to exercise at its onset, and progressive. Weakness and fatigue often occur and are difficult to dissociate from breathlessness. Cough is present much less commonly than in most pulmonary diseases and, if productive, especially if associated with fever, signifies the coexistence of bronchopulmonary infection. A variety of uncharacteristic and variable pleuritic and substernal chest pains may develop during the evolution of the disorder. Physical examination may be unremarkable, especially in the early stages. The most characteristic findings are increased transmission of breath sounds and showers of superficial crackling rales at the lung bases. Clubbing of the digits and cyanosis indicate more severe involvement; signs of cor pulmonale (loud pulmonary second sound, parasternal heave, venous distention, hepatomegaly, and peripheral edema) imply marked lung dysfunction with hypoxia and obliteration of the pulmonary vascular bed.

Chest roentgenograms characteristically reveal diffuse reticular or reticulonodular densities that are most marked in the lung bases. At times roentgenograms may not show any abnormalities, even in the presence of significant symptoms and pulmonary function abnormalities, or the lungs may have a homogeneous "ground-glass" haziness. With progression of the process, the linear densities become coarser; small cystic lesions appear (honeycombing); marked loss of lung volume occurs (shown primarily by elevation of the diaphragm); and central pulmonary arterial dilatation and right ventricular enlargement may become apparent. Pleural involvement (thickening, effusions, plaques, and calcification) is uncommon except in asbestosis and collagen diseases.

Routine laboratory studies are not very helpful. Anemia may be present in chronic infection, hemosiderosis, or collagen diseases. Polycythemia may be present if hypoxia has been severe and prolonged. Pulmonary function studies, however, provide valuable documentation of the severity of impairment that is useful in deciding whether treatment is indicated or not and in defining prognosis; they are also useful in following the course of the disease and objectively determining its response to treatment. However, pulmonary function studies do *not* delineate etiology or pathogenesis because, as might be anticipated from the similar pathologic involvement of the lungs in the various disorders, the functional impairment is also similar.

The earliest detectable physiologic abnormality is a reduction in resting arterial oxygen tension or, more precisely, an increase in the alveolar-arterial oxygen tension difference. Unwarranted emphasis has been placed on the contribution of impaired diffusion of oxygen (the so-called "alveolar-capillary block syndrome") to the alveolar-arterial oxygen tension difference, which is now recognized as being caused by mismatching of the distribution of inspired air and blood flow (ventilation-perfusion imbalance) (Chap. 249). Infiltrative diseases of the lung are the classic cause of a restrictive ventilatory defect, manifested by a loss of both vital capacity and residual volume, the former proportionately more than the latter. Associated with the reduction in lung volumes is a reduction in lung compliance (Chap. 249).

A corollary finding is alveolar hyperventilation (presumably owing to stimuli from hypoxia and stretch reflexes) that occurs despite an increased physiologic deadspace. Arterial carbon dioxide tension is thereby reduced, while the disease process progresses through most of its course; carbon dioxide tension becomes normal and finally elevated only in the terminal stages of the illness.

DIAGNOSIS

Careful historical examination is essential to the diagnosis of occupational lung diseases and hypersensitivity pneumonias. Chills, fever, weight loss, fatigue, and other nonspecific symptoms suggest that either an infectious process or a systemic disorder underlies the diffuse pulmonary infiltration. Physical examination is not likely to contribute to the differential diagnosis of those disorders confined to the lungs but may reveal important evidence of multisystem involvement in infectious, neoplastic, familial, metabolic, immunologic, and circulatory diseases as well as in sarcoidosis and histiocytosis X.

The results of routine blood counts, urinalysis, and blood chemistries are not likely to reveal important abnormalities or provide clues to the etiology of the underlying pulmonary disorder. Infections may be identified by appropriate cultural or serologic studies; hypersensitivity and immunologic diseases may be established by finding circulating antibodies or immune complexes; and neoplasms may be diagnosed by cytologic examination of the sputum. However, specific diagnosis of most diffuse infiltrative diseases, if it can be made at all, requires examination of tissue.

Biopsy is often the only method of documenting the type and cause of pulmonary disorder. The source of biopsy material is determined by the likelihood of obtaining diagnostic tissue and by the risks inherent in the procedure. Skin, lymph nodes, and liver are useful biopsy sites in disseminated infections, neoplasms, and at times sarcoidosis. But finding noncaseating granulomas is by no means pathognomonic of sarcoidosis, and a biopsy from within the thorax is more likely than one from a more peripheral organ to discriminate among the multiple causes of granulomas. If cervical or supraclavicular lymph nodes are palpable, they should be examined histologically and culturally. If nodes are not palpable, but hilar or mediastinal nodes are evident roentgenographically, scalene node biopsy or mediastinoscopy is indicated; this latter procedure is preferable, since it entails virtually no additional risk and has a substantially higher yield of positive diagnoses.

The majority of diffuse pulmonary infiltrative diseases are not associated with significant lymphadenopathy; if a diagnosis cannot be documented by other means, lung biopsy is indicated. Open lung biopsy by thoracotomy is more desirable than a percutaneous needle biopsy, because it has a higher yield and fewer complications in the patient whose general condition and pulmonary function permit general anesthesia. Open biopsy allows removal of a suitable piece of selected lung tissue that can be cultured and examined histologically by light and electron microscopy; in addition, a portion can be frozen for special studies at a later date (virus cultures, chemical or spectroscopic analysis). It is useful in the diagnosis of *diffuse* pulmonary infiltrative disease. Percutaneous needle biopsy of the lung should be reserved for the seriously ill patient in whom diagnostic information is imperative and the risks of thoracotomy are grave, unless a large solitary nodule near the periphery is present.

TREATMENT

The majority of diffuse pulmonary infiltrations do not respond well to therapy, but some are eminently treatable, and the value of making an etiologic diagnosis lies in determining which, of the many available therapeutic agents, should be used. Specific chemotherapy is available for most infectious agents. Removal from exposure diminishes the risk of occupational pulmonary diseases and may allow clearing of hypersensitivity pneumonias.

Corticosteroids are useful in the treatment of many of the causes of organizing interstitial pneumonia, especially when administered early. They are helpful in patients with hypersensitivity pneumonias, chemical injuries of the lungs, sarcoidosis, histiocytosis X, and desquamative interstitial pneumonia; their role in idiopathic hemosiderosis and acute idiopathic interstitial pneumonia (Hamman-Rich disease) is questionable. They are seldom of benefit in the treatment of collagen diseases, diseases due to occupational dusts, and chronic organizing interstitial pneumonia.

When corticosteroids are used, they should be given in sufficient doses to ensure that a response will occur if one can be elicited. Patients with disorders that usually improve (sarcoidosis, etc.) customarily do so when given prednisone, 40 to 60 mg per day (or its equivalent); the dosage is reduced 5 to 10 mg per day each week until maintenance levels are reached—usually 5 to 15 mg per day or 10 to 30 mg every other day. The patient's response must be followed objectively by serial chest roentgenograms and, more importantly, by appropriate tests of pulmonary function (arterial blood gases, lung volumes, diffusing capacity), since subjective responses to corticosteroids are notoriously unreliable. Patients with infiltrative disorders in which improvement is less predictable (organizing interstitial pneumonia, collagen diseases) should be started on even higher doses (60 to 100 mg prednisone per day) in an attempt to achieve a response; if pulmonary function studies document that no improvement has occurred, the drug should be rapidly discontinued.

Immunosuppressive therapy has produced striking long-term remissions of severe forms of Wegener's granulomatosis, usually a progressive and fatal disease. Rheumatoid arthritis and lupus erythematosus have responded to cytotoxic drugs in short-term controlled trials, but whether the fibrotic pulmonary infiltrations associated with these diseases will resolve remains to be determined.

PROGNOSIS

It follows from the information presented in previous sections that the course and prognosis of diffuse infiltrative diseases of the lung is extremely variable. The outlook is determined by the natural history of the underlying cause of the disorder, how far advanced it is when diagnosed, its response to therapy, and the presence of complicatons. The prognosis is favorable in those diseases with a reversible component, either spontaneous or induced by easily tolerated therapy (infections, chemical injuries, hypersensitivity pneumonias, and sarcoidosis). The prognosis is poor in most collagen diseases, progressive occupational dust diseases, idiopathic organizing interstitial pneumonia, and in any condition that has advanced to severe lung fibrosis and honeycombing; these disorders are associated with slow but relentless lung destruction, with progressive hypoxia and finally death from cor pulmonale or secondary bronchopulmonary infection.

REFERENCES

HERBERT FA et al: Pathophysiology of interstitial pulmonary fibrosis. Report of 19 cases and follow-up with corticosteroids. Arch Intern Med 110:628, 1962

HINSON KFW: Diffuse pulmonary fibrosis. Hum Pathol 1:275, 1970

LEWIS JG: Eosinophilic granuloma and its variants with special reference to lung involvement. Q J Med 33:337, 1964

LIEBOW AA et al: Desquamative interstitial pneumonia. Am J Med 39:369, 1965

LIVINGSTON JL et al: Diffuse interstitial pulmonary fibrosis: A clinical, radiological, and pathological study based on 45 patients. Q J Med 33:71, 1964

MCCOMBS RP: Diseases due to immunologic reactions in the lungs. N Engl J Med 286:1186, 1245, 1972

ROSEN SH et al: Pulmonary alveolar proteinosis. N Engl J Med 258:1123, 1958

SCADDING JG, HINSON KFW: Diffuse fibrosing alveolitis (diffuse interstitial fibrosis of the lungs): Correlation of histology at biopsy with prognosis. Thorax 22:291, 1967

STEINBERG AD et al: Cytotoxic drugs in treatment of nonmalignant diseases. Ann Intern Med 76:619, 1972

255 DISORDERS OF REGULATION OF RESPIRATION

JOHN B. WEST

The principles governing pulmonary ventilation and its regulation are discussed in Chap. 249. The fine control of ventilation is normally carried out by the central chemoreceptors near the central surface of the medulla which respond to changes in pH of the cerebrospinal fluid bathing them. For example, a fall in pH caused by diffusion of carbon dioxide across the blood-brain barrier increases respiratory drive, thus holding the arterial P_{CO_2}* within close limits (Fig. 255-1). The extreme sensitivity of this feedback control is seen when a normal subject inhales air containing carbon dioxide. Typically the ventilation may double for a rise in P_{CO_2} of only 2-3 mm Hg.

Arterial hypoxemia constitutes a coarse control through its action on the peripheral chemoreceptors in the carotid and aortic bodies. Although this control is minor under normal conditions, it becomes very important during chronic hypoxia, as in people living at high altitude, or in patients with chronic lung disease. Under these conditions the increased ventilation lowers the P_{CO_2} of the arterial blood and cerebrospinal fluid, but the pH of the cerebrospinal fluid is reset to its normal level of about 7.32, possibly by active transport of bicarbonate. Additional control is afforded by changes in pH of the arterial blood irrespective of its P_{CO_2}. This relatively weak regulation apparently occurs through stimulation of the peripheral chemoreceptors, and although it is seldom seen under normal conditions, it may dominate in the control of ventilation in metabolic acidosis and alkalosis.

Disorders of the regulation of respiration include hypoventilation, hyperventilation, and abnormal patterns of breathing. A cardinal feature of hypoventilation is carbon dioxide retention, and indeed these terms are often used virtually interchangeably. This can be misleading, but, following common usage, the various types of carbon dioxide retention are grouped here under the heading of hypoventilation.

HYPOVENTILATION

CARBON DIOXIDE RETENTION CAUSED BY PURE HYPOVENTILATION (NORMAL LUNGS) In this group of diseases, the amount of air going into the lungs each minute is reduced. Strictly it is the volume of air entering the alveoli, or *alveolar ventilation,* which is crucial (Chap. 249). However, in practice, the volume of

FIGURE 255-1
Scheme to illustrate the various causes of carbon dioxide retention. These include: 1, disorders of the respiratory center or, 2, of the supplying nerves or, 3, of muscles of ventilation or, 4, some mechanical problem in lung or chest wall including obstruction to the upper airways. All these conditions result in hypoventilation. However, chronic obstructive pulmonary disease, 5, in effect diverts blood from the ventilated regions, so that carbon dioxide retention occurs in spite of a normal (or high) ventilation. In addition, the ventilatory response is inappropriate for the level of carbon dioxide in these patients because of the increased work of breathing.

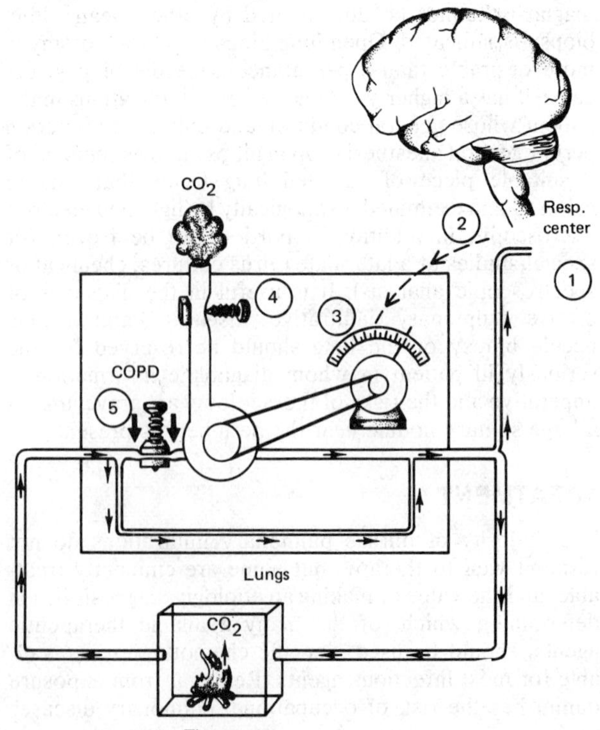

* *Unless otherwise stated, the partial pressures refer to arterial blood.*

the conducting airways remains fairly constant so that, if the amount of air passing the lips is abnormally low, hypoventilation is said to be present.

The alveolar ventilation and alveolar P_{CO_2} are related by the following equation:

$$P_{CO_2} = \frac{CO_2 \text{ output}}{\text{alveolar ventilation}}$$

In normal lungs, the P_{CO_2} of arterial blood is virtually the same as that in alveolar gas, and the carbon dioxide output at rest remains fairly constant. Thus the expression implies that, if the alveolar ventilation is halved, the arterial P_{CO_2} is doubled.

The level of alveolar ventilation also influences the P_{O_2}. As the ventilation falls and the P_{CO_2} rises, the P_{O_2} falls, though the change is slightly smaller. An important practical point is that, if the P_{CO_2} is considerably increased by pure hypoventilation, say 70 mm Hg, the P_{O_2} may still be well above the level at which cyanosis can be detected clinically. Thus a patient may have serious carbon dioxide retention and yet appear a "healthy" pink color. Note also that, if a patient is given an oxygen-enriched mixture to breathe, the hypoxemia will be abolished, but the hypercapnia remains (Chap. 263).

Conditions affecting the respiratory center During normal *sleep,* the P_{CO_2} rises by 3 or 4 mm Hg. Patients with idiopathic hypoventilation or with the "Pickwickian syndrome" (see below) are particularly likely to develop depressed breathing when they are asleep. One of the commonest causes of hypoventilation is depression of the respiratory center by *drugs.* These include many anesthetics, the barbiturates, and morphine and its derivatives. Respiratory center depression is often seen in the postoperative recovery room, before the effects of anesthetic and preoperative sedatives have worn off, and also in the emergency room in patients who have taken an overdose of barbiturate (Chap. 113). In these circumstances, the P_{CO_2} should be monitored, and assisted ventilation following endotracheal intubation or tracheostomy may be lifesaving. Depression of the respiratory center is often accompanied by impairment of the cough reflex and difficulties with swallowing, so that aspiration of fluid into the lungs may occur and lead to pneumonia. An additional advantage of intubation is that it allows the airways to be sucked free of secretions and inhaled material (Chap. 263).

Central nervous system abnormalities which may cause hypoventilation include inflammation, hemorrhage, trauma, and rarely neoplasms. Encephalitis and acute bulbar poliomyelitis (in the absence of weakness of the respiratory muscles) may cause slowing and shallowness of respiration. Irregularities of rhythm and periods of apnea may develop. The first signs of these abnormalities often appear during sleep. The ventilatory response to inhaled CO_2 mixtures is depressed. These patients can return their blood gases to normal by voluntarily increasing their ventilation, and indeed they can sometimes be managed by being reminded to breathe when periods of apnea develop. However, they may die because of apnea during sleep. Respiratory depression may be associated with loss of the cough and swallowing reflexes and consequent accumulation of secretions.

Neuromuscular disorders Neuromuscular disorders affecting the respiratory muscles are important causes of hypoventilation. These include the Guillain-Barré syndrome, amyotrophic lateral sclerosis, poliomyelitis, myasthenia gravis, and muscular dystrophies. The most important muscle of respiration is the diaphragm, and patients with progressive disease often do not complain of dyspnea until the diaphragm is involved. By then their ventilatory reserve is severely compromised, and they must be carefully observed. The progress of the disease can be monitored by measuring the vital capacity and the arterial blood gases. Again, the treatment of hypoventilation in these conditions is assisted ventilation either by oropharyngeal intubation in acute states, or with a tracheostomy for long-term management (Chap. 263). Patients with chronic paresis of their respiratory muscles are prone to develop chest infections because of their difficulty in getting rid of secretions.

Metabolic alkalosis This may also be associated with hypoventilation, although it causes no symptoms and is difficult to detect clinically. The commonest causes include severe vomiting and potassium loss such as that caused by diuretics or steroid therapy. Blood gas analysis shows an increased P_{CO_2} associated with an elevated base excess, and typically an increased pH, which indicates that the metabolic alkalosis has been only partly compensated for by the hypoventilation.

Thoracic cage abnormalities CRUSHED CHEST An increasingly common cause of hypoventilation is trauma to the thoracic cage resulting from automobile accidents. Frequently this is caused by impact of the steering wheel with the sternum, or the chest is crushed when a wheel of a car runs over it. Usually there are multiple injuries. There may be dissociation of movement of the chest wall, so that one region is sucked in while the remainder of the chest wall moves out during inspiration ("flail chest"). Prompt intubation and assisted ventilation is often required, and careful monitoring of the arterial blood gases is mandatory.

KYPHOSCOLIOSIS Bony deformity of the chest can lead to respiratory failure with a raised P_{CO_2}. Kyphosis refers to posterior curvature of the spine, and scoliosis to lateral curvature. The effects of scoliosis on cardiopulmonary function are the most serious, especially if the angulation is situated high in the vertebral column. Scoliosis is frequently associated with rotation of the spine giving the appearance of an added kyphosis. Some 80 percent of cases of kyphoscoliosis are idiopathic in origin. The rest are caused by neuromuscular disorders such as poliomyelitis or by bone tuberculosis or are congenital in origin.

The initial complaint is dyspnea on exertion. Later hypoxemia develops; eventually carbon dioxide retention and signs of failure of the right side of the heart may supervene. Sometimes bronchitis may complicate the picture, especially in smokers. The chief cause of the CO_2 retention is the deformity of the chest wall, which leads to an inefficient action of the respiratory muscles and a great increase in the work of breathing. The compliance of the chest wall is reduced (it is stiffer), especially in older patients, and this results in rapid shallow breathing, so that an increasingly large fraction of the tidal volume is wasted in the dead space of the bronchi. The hypoventilation causes not only hypercapnia but also hypoxemia. Pulmonary vasoconstriction results, pulmonary artery pressure rises, and the work of the right heart is also raised by the polycythemia which develops (Chap. 262).

It should be noted, however, that these patients also have abnormal lungs. These tend to be remarkably small, and the restricted pulmonary vascular bed probably also plays a role in the development of pulmonary hypertension. Areas of atelectasis are common, presumably because the volume of the thoracic cage is greatly reduced. Uneven ventilation of the lungs has been demonstrated in many cases, so that ventilation-perfusion inequality contributes to the hypoxemia.

Pulmonary function tests show a reduction in all lung volumes; indeed the total lung capacity may be reduced to half of the predicted normal value. Some of the inequality of ventilation can be explained by airway closure in dependent regions of the lung as a result of the gross reduction of lung volume. Airways resistance in relation to lung volume is approximately normal, but the maximum breathing capacity is reduced because of the restricted vital capacity. The diffusing capacity of the lung for carbon monoxide is not markedly abnormal when related to lung volume. When CO_2 retention develops, a reduced ventilatory response to inhaled carbon dioxide can be demonstrated. This is probably related to the large increase in work of breathing caused by the deformity of the chest wall.

Little specific therapy is available. Just as the cause of most cases of the disease is unknown, so the factors determining its progression are poorly understood. Some help can be obtained from orthopedic braces in the early stages of the disease. Any pulmonary infection should be promptly and vigorously treated with appropriate antibiotics. If hypoxia is severe and O_2 therapy is required (Chap. 263), the patient should be carefully watched for evidence of increasing hypoventilation. Cor pulmonale and right heart failure should be treated with diuretics, digitalis, and perhaps venesection if the polycythemia is severe.

Other conditions associated with an abnormal chest wall include ankylosing spondylitis and pectus excavatum. In *ankylosing spondylitis* there is immobility of the vertebral joints and fixation of the ribs, so that movement of the chest wall may be grossly reduced. There is a reduction of vital capacity and total lung capacity, but good movement of the diaphragm is preserved so that the ventilatory capacity is unimpaired. Some fall in the compliance of the chest wall has been reported and also some uneven ventilation, the latter possibly caused by the reduced lung volume. In general, however, the lungs are virtually normal and do not show the pathological changes seen in kyphoscoliosis. Hypoventilation is not a feature, and secondary heart failure does not occur.

Pectus excavatum is a congenital abnormality in which the lower part of the sternum is depressed towards the spine. In spite of the bizarre appearance of the chest, little interference with pulmonary function is the rule. There may be a slight reduction in vital capacity, total lung capacity, and maximum breathing capacity, but gas exchange is virtually normal, and hypoventilation does not occur. Surgical correction for cosmetic reasons may be considered.

Obstruction to the upper airways Tracheal stenosis can be caused by neoplasms such as thymoma in structures adjacent to the trachea, by scarring following injury, by aortic aneurysm, or by a congenital abnormality. Tumors originating in the upper airways and foreign bodies may also be responsible for airways obstruction. Hypoventilation with CO_2 retention may occur, and this may be of long standing. It is possible to distinguish tracheal obstruction from the airways obstruction of chronic obstructive lung disease by the stridor and from the flow patterns of maximal inspiration and expiration. In addition, pulmonary function tests show no inequality of ventilation.

Idiopathic hypoventilation Idiopathic, or primary, hypoventilation is a rare disease of unknown etiology occurring in patients whose lungs and chest wall are normal. Most of the reported cases have been between twenty and sixty years of age, with a preponderance of males. Typical symptoms include lack of energy, somnolence, headache, and some breathlessness on exertion. Cyanosis, especially when the patient is asleep, is a common observation, this being caused by a combination of the hypoxemia and polycythemia. Periodic breathing is often noted at night. Occasionally unusual sensitivity to sedatives or hypnotic drugs given preoperatively has been a feature. In some cases, an acute respiratory infection has prompted awareness of the condition. Several patients have had a past history of encephalitis, neurosyphilis, or schizophrenia. Signs of heart failure including engorged neck veins, enlarged heart, palpable liver, and peripheral edema have been described in severe cases.

The P_{CO_2} is elevated, generally in the range of 55 to 80 mm Hg, and the P_{O_2} is depressed, and these can rapidly be restored to near normal by asking the patient to increase his ventilation voluntarily. Indeed some observers have found considerable variability in the P_{CO_2}, because, when the patients are tested and become aware of their breathing, they tend to breathe more. For this reason the finding of a raised plasma bicarbonate may be a useful diagnostic pointer. The hematocrit is typically between 50 and 70 percent. The ventilatory response to inhaled CO_2 is greatly impaired, though the work of breathing is not increased. Tests of pulmonary function are generally normal with no indication of airways obstruction. The pulmonary arterial pressure is typically increased because of the alveolar hypoxia.

No specific pathological changes have been found in the central nervous system of these patients. Congestive heart failure and respiratory infections should be treated vigorously.

Hypoventilation associated with obesity ("Pickwickian syndrome") Some extremely obese patients hypoventilate, and the association of obesity, somnolence, polycythemia, and excessive appetite has been dubbed the *Pickwickian syndrome,* after the fat boy, Joe, in Charles Dickens's "Pickwick Papers." Apart from the obesity, the clinical features are similar to those patients with idiopathic hypoventilation and in the fully developed form include marked obesity (body weight typically over 300 lb), somnolence, twitching, cyanosis, periodic respiration, secondary polycythemia, right ventricular hypertrophy, and right heart failure.

The obesity may have been present for years, but in some cases a recent rapid gain in weight has been described. The somnolence may be a striking feature, the patient sometimes dozing off halfway through a sentence. The cyanosis and periodic breathing are particularly marked during sleep. Ankle edema is a common symptom, and an enlarged liver and engorged neck veins are seen.

Blood gas measurements show an elevated P_{CO_2} and depressed P_{O_2}; the former may be as high as 70 mm Hg. Lung function tests show a reduction in lung volumes, particularly in the expiratory reserve volume (the volume which can be forcibly exhaled from normal end-expiration). The vital capacity is also reduced, as is the compliance of the chest cage. The abdominal pressure is raised, especially when the patient is supine, thus forcing the diaphragm into the chest. There is no indication of airways obstruction and little inequality of ventilation, but the energy cost of moving the chest wall is abnormally high. The ventilatory response to inhaled CO_2 is generally greatly decreased. In these respects the syndrome is similar to kyphoscoliosis. The reduction of lung volume causes airway closure in the dependent regions of the lung, and this contributes to the hypoxemia. There is an increase in the resting oxygen consumption of these patients which aggravates the effects of their impaired ventilation.

A striking feature of this syndrome is the dramatic improvement that takes place in all symptoms when the patient loses weight. Objective indices of improvement include a fall in P_{CO_2}, rise in P_{O_2}, increases in vital capacity, total lung capacity, and minute ventilation, and an enhanced ventilatory response to inhaled CO_2. In addition, signs of heart failure often disappear. Even a loss of 30 to 40 lb is often sufficient to bring about a remarkable improvement in well-being. Treatment by caloric restriction is indicated.

It is important to note that not all extremely obese patients develop hypoventilation. Some investigators have suggested that the Pickwickian individual is simply a patient with idiopathic hypoventilation who happens to be obese. The term "Pickwickian syndrome" is often used rather loosely. It should be reserved for very obese patients who have an increased P_{CO_2} without evidence of lung disease. The cause of the hypoventilation is not clear but presumably is related to the high energy cost of moving the chest wall. In addition the reduction in lung volumes caused by elevation of the diaphragm causes shallow inefficient breathing. However the association of marked somnolence and voracious appetite suggests that, in some patients at least, there is an abnormality in the central nervous system.

CARBON DIOXIDE RETENTION ASSOCIATED WITH CHRONIC LUNG DISEASE The commonest clinical situation in which CO_2 retention is seen is the patient with chronic lung disease. Such patients are often said to be "hypoventilating," but the cause of their hypercapnia is clearly very different from that in the patients with normal lungs whom we have considered so far. Historically it is easy to see how the term hypoventilation came to be applied so indiscriminately. When in the late 1950s it became possible to measure the P_{CO_2} of arterial blood in the clinical setting, CO_2 retention was found to be a common and serious complication of chronic lung disease which could always be abolished by artificially increasing the ventilation. Thus it was natural to say that these patients had a reduced ventilation, and this term had the advantage of keeping an important therapeutic option in the forefront.

It is important to understand the factors leading to CO_2 retention in these patients if they are to be managed most effectively. Figure 255-1 shows a scheme of the factors determining CO_2 elimination in patients with lung disease. CO_2 is produced in the tissues at a rate which depends on the level of metabolic activity; at rest there is little variation. It is transported to the lungs in the venous blood and pumped out by the ventilation. The speed of the pump is normally set by the level of the P_{CO_2} via the medullary chemoreceptors. In the presence of lung disease, the efficiency of the pump is impaired. Thus, for the same level of ventilation, less CO_2 is eliminated. This is principally because ventilation and blood flow are unevenly matched within the lung (see Chap. 249) and possibly because of limited diffusion. In any event the result is that, for a normal level of ventilation, inadequate amounts of CO_2 are excreted, and CO_2 retention occurs.

When the increased arterial P_{CO_2} is sensed by the medullary chemoreceptors, the ventilation is increased. This usually returns the P_{CO_2} to normal, because fortunately even lungs with grossly mismatched ventilation and blood flow can greatly increase their elimination of CO_2 when their ventilation is raised. (Contrast this with the behavior of O_2, where uneven ventilation and blood flow invariably result in a low P_{O_2}; this follows from the shape of the O_2 dissociation curve.) Thus a common end result is a normal P_{CO_2}, but at the expense of increased ventilation. However in the presence of severe disease, the ventilation may not be increased enough to restore the P_{CO_2} to normal, and CO_2 retention therefore occurs.

One of the factors affecting the regulation of ventilation (servoloop of Fig. 255-1) is the work of breathing. It has been shown that, if normal subjects breathe through a resistance, their ventilatory response to inhaled CO_2 is depressed. Indeed the relationship between increase in ventilation and inspired CO_2 concentration may become indistinguishable from that observed in patients with chronic airways obstruction. In most cases of chronic obstructive lung disease, the resistance to airflow is high, so that the increase in ventilation for a given rise in P_{CO_2} is depressed. This is one of the chief reasons for the inappropriate ventilatory response in these patients.

When CO_2 retention becomes established, the respiratory center becomes reset at a higher arterial P_{CO_2}. This can be explained by an increase in bicarbonate concentration in the cerebrospinal fluid, which probably occurs through the active transport of bicarbonate across the blood-gas barrier. As a result the pH of the cerebrospinal fluid is returned to its normal value of 7.32 in spite of its increased P_{CO_2}. Since this pH apparently determines the response of the medullary chemoreceptors, respiratory drive may then not be increased despite the raised P_{CO_2}.

Further CO_2 retention occurs in some patients with chronic lung disease, especially following the administration of oxygen. These patients have chronic hypercapnia and hypoxemia but normal pH in arterial blood (compensated respiratory acidosis) and in their cerebrospinal fluid. Their main stimulus to ventilation may be the arterial hypoxemia via the peripheral chemoreceptors so that, when this is relieved, ventilation almost ceases. The ensuing rise in P_{CO_2} may further depress ventilation because of the narcotic effect of high levels of carbon dioxide. This extremely dangerous situation should be avoided by giving carefully controlled O_2 concentrations, for example, 24 to 28 percent, and assiduously watching the patient. CO_2 retention in chronic obstructive lung disease is considered in Chap. 252 and the treatment of acute and chronic respiratory failure in Chap. 263.

HYPERVENTILATION

Hyperventilation can be caused by lesions of the central nervous system, metabolic acidosis, and anxiety states. A patient with severe cerebral hemorrhage causing coma may exhibit deep, regular respirations of a mechanical nature. This causes a reduced P_{CO_2} in the arterial blood, which initially shows a high pH and normal base excess. Irregularities of breathing such as Cheyne-Stokes respiration may also occur. In metabolic acidosis caused, for example, by uncontrolled diabetes mellitus or by chronic renal insufficiency, deep regular respiration known as *Kussmaul breathing* is frequently seen. Active rather than passive expiratory movements are a feature of this pattern. Here the low P_{CO_2} is accompanied by reduction in base excess and a low pH (see Chap. 265).

In the hyperventilation of anxiety states, the patient may be very apprehensive and complain of shortness of breath, difficulty in taking a deep breath, a feeling of chest tightness, or a sense of suffocation. The patient is often a nervous, anxious woman who has other functional disturbances due to tension. There are often accompanying symptoms such as numbness in the limbs, palpitations, and epigastric discomfort. The fall in P_{CO_2} and the consequent alkalosis may be severe and cause tetany with carpopedal spasm. The reduced plasma bicarbonate level and relatively normal arterial pH (compensated respiratory alkalosis) distinguish chronic hyperventilation from the acute hyperventilation with fall in P_{CO_2} which frequently accompanies an arterial puncture. The patient may complain of fainting spells and blurring of vision; these are probably related to the reduction in cerebral blood flow caused by low P_{CO_2}. The finding of slow waves of high voltage in the EEG suggests that these changes may be the result of hypoxia. The changes can be reversed by hyperbaric oxygenation. The serum calcium remains normal. It is likely that some of the cardiovascular symptoms are related to the release of epinephrine.

The patient is usually not aware of the overbreathing, although he may admit to periods of sighing. It is often possible to reproduce many of the symptoms of an attack by encouraging him to overbreathe spontaneously. It is also useful to demonstrate to the patient that he can hold his breath for a considerable period even during an attack. An attack can sometimes be terminated by having him breathe in and out of a plastic bag, or inhale a 5 percent CO_2 mixture. However attention to the underlying anxiety state is indicated.

ABNORMAL PATTERNS OF VENTILATION

CHEYNE-STOKES BREATHING This is a form of periodic breathing characterized by alternating periods of apnea and hyperpnea. The patient often lies motionless for 15 to 20 sec and then begins to breathe shallowly at first, then with increasing amplitude, and finally shallowly again. The respirations during this period of breathing are regular in time.

The cause of this disturbance presumably lies in some delay in the control process which results in "hunting" for the equilibrium condition. Periodic breathing can be produced in experimental animals by lengthening the distance over which blood travels from the thorax to the brain. As a result, the response of the medullary chemoreceptors lags behind the blood gas changes produced by the lungs, and a cyclical chain of events is created. Conditions in which Cheyne-Stokes breathing is seen include congestive heart failure when the circulation time is prolonged (Chap. 233), brain damage caused by trauma or cerebral hemorrhage, and chronic hypoxia. It occurs in normal subjects living at high altitude, especially during sleep.

BIOT'S BREATHING This is another form of periodic breathing in which periods of apnea are punctuated by a few deep breaths which may be irregular and which do not have the waxing and waning pattern of Cheyne-Stokes respiration. It is most frequently associated with brain damage.

REFERENCES

BERGOFSKY EH et al: Cardiorespiratory failure in kyphoscoliosis. Medicine (Baltimore) 38:263, 1959

BURWELL CS et al: Extreme obesity associated with alveolar hypoventilation—A Pickwickian syndrome. Am J Med 21:811, 1956

FISHMAN AP et al: General alveolar hypoventilation: A syndrome of respiratory and cardiac failure in patients with normal lungs. Q J Med 35:261, 1966

PLUM F: Breathlessness in neurological disease: The effects of neurological disease on the act of breathing, in *Breathlessness,* ed EJM Campbell, JBL Howell, Oxford: Blackwell Scientific Publishers. Philadelphia: Davis, 1966

SYKES MK et al: *Respiratory Failure,* Oxford: Blackwell Scientific Publications. Philadelphia: Davis, 1969

WEST JB: Causes of carbon dioxide retention in lung disease. N Engl J Med 284:1232, 1971

256 PULMONARY THROMBOEMBOLISM

KENNETH M. MOSER

Pulmonary thromboembolism (PTE) is a leading cause of morbidity and mortality, and can appear in many clinical contexts. Epidemiologic surveys indicate that PTE is responsible for more than 8,000 deaths in the United States annually. Autopsy statistics further emphasize the magnitude of the problem. Routine autopsies disclose evidence of recent or remote pulmonary embolism in 25 to 30 percent of all patients. When special techniques are applied at autopsy, the frequency of discovery exceeds 60 percent. Even these data underestimate incidence, since many emboli present at the time of death resolve without trace and are not found at postmortem examination. The high incidence of PTE at autopsy contrasts sharply with the incidence of antemortem diagnosis. Available information suggests that an antemortem diagnosis is made in only 10 to 30 percent of all cases.

The three factors involved in thrombogenesis are stasis, abnormalities in the vessel wall, and alterations in the blood coagulation system. Coagulation alterations have been studied extensively, but as yet, there is no reliable test for a state of "hypercoagulability" in a given patient. Conditions which are associated with a high risk of venous thromboembolism include the postoperative period; pregnancy, particularly the postpartum period; in the opinion of many, the use of anovulatory drugs; congestive heart failure; chronic pulmonary disease; fractures or other injuries of the lower extremities; chronic deep venous insufficiency of the legs; prolonged bed rest; and carcinoma.

Although there is increasing awareness of the conditions which predispose to PTE, detection of embolism in the majority of patients remains poor. One reason is inadequate understanding of the natural history of pulmonary embolism.

NATURAL HISTORY OF EMBOLISM

THE ACUTE EVENTS The immediate result of thromboembolism is complete or partial obstruction of the pulmonary arterial blood flow to the distal lung. This obstruction leads to a series of pathophysiologic events which can be categorized as the "respiratory" and "hemodynamic" consequences of PTE.

Respiratory consequences Embolic obstruction produces a zone of the lung which is ventilated but not perfused—an intrapulmonary "dead space" (Chap. 249). Because it cannot participate in the process of gas exchange, ventilation of this nonperfused area is "wasted," in the functional sense. Another consequence of embolic obstruction is a constriction of the airspaces and airways in the affected lung zone. This "pneumoconstriction" appears to be due to the bronchoalveolar hypocapnia that results from cessation of pulmonary capillary blood flow, because experimentally it can be abolished by inhalation of carbon dioxide—enriched air. This constrictive response may be viewed as beneficial since it decreases the amount of "wasted" ventilation.

Another disturbance caused by embolic obstruction —loss of alveolar surfactant—does not occur immediately. This surface-active lipoprotein is required to maintain alveolar stability. In its absence, alveolar collapse occurs. Cessation of pulmonary capillary blood flow leads to reduction in surfactant within 2 or 3 hr, which becomes severe at 12 to 15 hr. Frank atelectasis—the morphologic expression of alveolar instability—can be detected at 24 to 48 hr after interruption of blood flow.

Hemodynamic consequences The primary hemodynamic consequence of thromboembolic obstruction is a reduction in the available cross-sectional area of the pulmonary arterial bed. This loss of vascular capacity increases the resistance to pulmonary blood flow; this resistance, if marked, leads to pulmonary hypertension and acute failure of the right ventricle. Tachycardia, and often a decline in cardiac output, also occur.

The factors which determine the severity of these hemodynamic changes have been a subject of continued debate. There is agreement that the *extent of embolic obstruction* is a key factor. However, the reserve capacity of the pulmonary arteriocapillary bed is so extensive that more than 50 percent of the vascular area must be obstructed before significant elevation in pulmonary arterial pressure results. Because pulmonary hypertension occurs in some patients with occlusion of lesser extent, investigators have searched for reflex or humoral vasoconstrictor mechanisms associated with embolism. Despite long and careful search for such mechanisms, their extent and frequency in human PTE remains unknown. Hence, some workers maintain that the degree of embolic obstruction itself is the only determinant of hemodynamic impairment. They suggest that instances of apparent disparity between the extent of embolism and clinical response reflect only clinical underestimation of the magnitude of the embolism. Other investigators, however, have presented compelling evidence to support the occurrence of vasoconstriction with embolism. Some have demonstrated that constriction is associated with obstruction of the smaller, but not the larger, pulmonary arterial vessels. Another thesis holds that serotonin, a known pulmonary vasoconstrictive-bronchoconstrictive substance, is released from platelets coating fresh emboli as they lodge in the pulmonary tree. This thesis introduces the attractive concept that an embolus should be regarded as a packet with pharmacologic, as well as obstructive, potential. A consensus view, then, suggests that, while the extent of embolism is a key factor, humoral and/or reflex influences probably are operative in certain patients and compromise the pulmonary circulation to a greater extent than might be expected on an anatomic basis alone.

The cardiopulmonary status of the patient prior to embolism is also critical in determining the clinical severity of embolism. A small embolus may have limited impact upon an otherwise healthy individual but may have serious consequences in someone with advanced cardiac or pulmonary disease.

Both experimental and clinical studies have established that infarction—death of lung tissue—rarely accompanies embolic occlusion. It is likely that less than 10 percent of emboli in man lead to infarction. That infarction rarely follows embolism should occasion little surprise. The lung has three avenues for obtaining its oxygen requirements: the pulmonary arterial circulation; the bronchial arterial circulation; and the airways. Thus, infarction occurs infrequently, and its appearance usually requires simultaneous compromise of bronchial arterial flow and/or airways to the involved area.

BEYOND THE ACUTE STATE The vast majority of pulmonary emboli resolve, and resolve rather quickly. Resolution of fresh emboli begins within the first few days and is well advanced in 10 to 14 days. Two powerful mechanisms promote restoration of vascular patency: the fibrinolytic system and the process of organization. The fibrinolytic system seems specifically designed to dissolve fibrin thrombi wherever they occur in the body and is responsible for the rapid phase of thromboembolic resolution. Organization is a slower process, requiring some days. As it proceeds, the thrombus is gradually transformed into a small scar attached to the vascular wall.

The availability of these two efficient mechanisms raises the question as to why all emboli do not resolve. There may be some impairment of the intrinsic fibrinolytic system. The emboli may have been well organized prior to their lodgment in the lung so that they are subject to neither fibrinolytic attack nor further organization. Alternatively, some emboli may be recurrent, so that their failure to resolve is more apparent than real.

Another important element of the natural history of thromboembolism is the development of bronchial arterial collateral circulation. If pulmonary arterial obstruction persists, bronchial arterial flow increases substantially over a period of several weeks, restoring flow to the capillary bed. With the return of flow, surfactant production is restored, so that alveolar stability is regained, atelectasis resolves, and alveolar hypocapnia and its resultant pneumoconstriction also subside.

Finally, it should be recognized that many emboli are not totally occlusive. Some distal pulmonary arterial flow often persists and modifies the cardiopulmonary events described above.

DIAGNOSTIC FEATURES

Sudden onset of unexplained dyspnea should suggest the diagnosis of embolism. This symptom, related to the sudden addition of alveolar "dead space," is usually the only one which occurs. *Pleuritic chest pain and hemoptysis are present only when infarction has occurred* and, because bland embolism rarely leads to infarction, are usually absent. With extensive embolism, severe substernal oppressive discomfort may be present. Patients also may present with syncope, suggesting a neurologic disorder. The most reliable symptom, however, is breathlessness. Severe, persistent dyspnea is an ominous sign, for it usually indicates extensive embolic occlusion.

PHYSICAL EXAMINATION The *physical examination,* like the history, may be deceptively normal. Examination of the lungs may disclose a few atelectatic rales, and localized wheezes may be heard. A pleural friction rub or evidence of pleural effusion will not be present unless infarction has occurred.

On cardiac examination, the single consistent finding is tachycardia. Only in the rare cases of massive embolism will such signs as a right ventricular gallop, a palpable "lift" over the right ventricle, a loud pulmonary closure sound, or prominent A waves in the jugular venous pulse be found. A scratchy systolic ejection-type murmur may be heard in the pulmonic area. Also, a systolic or continuous murmur accentuated by inspiration may be audible over the lung fields. These murmurs appear to be generated by turbulence of flow in vessels partially obstructed by emboli since they disappear after resection or resolution of emboli. They should be carefully sought in any patient suspected of PTE. Wide, often fixed, splitting of the second heart sound may be present. This indicates extensive embolic obstruction and implies both severe pulmonary hypertension and right ventricular failure. As embolic resolution occurs, this finding disappears. Absence of an accentuated pulmonic closure sound is not a reliable guide to the severity of PTE, since, when embolism is sufficiently massive to reduce cardiac output, pulmonary closure may be normal or diminished.

The detection of *deep venous thrombosis* qualifies as an excellent clue to the diagnosis of embolism, but its absence should by no means rule out the diagnosis. Even when sought with diligence, thrombophlebitis is found in less than half of patients with PTE. Not only may emboli arise from sites other than the veins of the extremities, but even when deep venous thrombosis is present, it may not be detectable. Often, the entire venous thrombus may have detached as an embolus. *Fever* in patients with pulmonary embolism is uncommon without complicating infection or infarction. With infarction, fever of 100 to 101°F (oral) is the rule; but temperature elevations to 103°F or above may occur, making difficult the differentiation between pulmonary infarction and infection.

On clinical grounds alone, then, a firm diagnosis of embolism is rarely possible, and the clinical suspicion of embolism requires confirmation by laboratory studies.

LABORATORY STUDIES Routine laboratory studies contribute little toward the diagnosis. Leukocytosis and elevation of the sedimentation rate are rarely present in the absence of infarction. A diagnostic "triad" of elevation of serum lactic dehydrogenase (LDH) and bilirubin with a normal serum glutamic oxalacetic transaminase (SGOT) has been proposed but is of limited value.

Aside from tachycardia, the *electrocardiogram* is normal in most patients. With extensive embolization, there may be evidence of acute pulmonary hypertension; rightward shift of the QRS axis; a tall, peaked P wave; and ST-T changes indicative of right ventricular "strain" and "ischemia." These changes are often transient, lasting minutes to hours, but when persistent, suggest severe pulmonary vascular obstruction.

The *chest roentgenogram* may show a parenchymal infiltrate and evidence of a pleural effusion if *infarction* has occurred. Characteristically, the infiltrates caused by infarction abut against the pleura. However, their shape varies, and they do not usually appear until 12 to 36 hr after the infarction has occurred. The effusion, which often precedes the infiltrate, is characteristically small. Thoracentesis usually yields hemorrhagic fluid, with the characteristics of an exudate.

The radiographic findings with embolism alone are more subtle. *Differences in diameter between vessels which should be of equivalent size* should raise the suspicion of embolism. For example, embolic obstruction of the right main pulmonary artery can lead to dilation of the left main pulmonary artery because that vessel must accept the entire pulmonary flow. There may be *abrupt "cutoff"* of a vessel; i.e., as the vessel is traced distally, it suddenly disappears. Clot has the same radiodensity as blood, accounting for the proximal shadow; the absence of flow beyond the clot explains the sudden radiographic "disappearance" of the vessel.

Organization of a clot within a pulmonary artery may lead to retraction of the vessel's walls and a so-called *"rattail configuration,"* in which the vessel is relatively normal proximally and suddenly tapers to a sharp point. Finally, there may be *abnormal radiolucency* in some lung zones due to absent or decreased flow. Such abnormally lucent areas, indicative of proximal arterial obstruction, are best appreciated by examining comparable areas in the two lung fields.

Even in embolization without infarction, the roentgenogram may show small infiltrates, which appear in about 24 hr and reflect atelectasis secondary to surfactant depletion. They are not associated with effusion, may fail to touch a pleural surface, and disappear without the linear scarring characteristic of infarction. It should be emphasized that a *normal chest roentgenogram does not exclude the diagnosis of PTE.*

Fluoroscopy While clot and blood have the same radiodensity, a vessel containing clot will exhibit reduced or absent pulsations. Fluoroscopic discovery of a nonpulsatile vessel is a good clue to PTE.

Analysis of arterial blood gases This may be of diagnostic value, since massive embolism is commonly associated with arterial hypoxemia, hypocapnia, and respiratory alkalosis. In addition, the difference between alveolar P_{CO_2} and arterial P_{CO_2} ("A-a" P_{CO_2} gradient) is widened owing to the increase in alveolar dead space (Chap. 249).

The laboratory tests discussed thus far are often negative in PTE and are relatively nonspecific. Therefore, it is usually necessary to proceed to two more definitive techniques: the pulmonary-perfusion radiophotoscan and the pulmonary angiogram.

Pulmonary perfusion scintiphotography Scintiphotographs (photoscans) are obtained by intravenous injection of gamma-emitting radionuclides. The most commonly used material is macroaggregated albumin (MAA), labeled with iodine 131 or technetium 99m. The radioactive particles, 50 to 100 μm in size, are trapped in the pulmonary capillary bed because the pulmonary capillaries approximate 10 μm in diameter. Alternatively, xenon 133 gas, dissolved in saline, may be used, but the patient must hold his breath. The distribution of MAA particles entrapped in capillaries, or of xenon 133 evolved from them, accurately depicts the distribution of pulmonary blood flow.

After injection, a gamma-detecting device records the pattern of radioactivity within the lungs. This radioactive image can be recorded on radiographic film, on special photographic film, as a television image, or on videotape. Normal scans exhibit homogeneous distribution of radioactivity, smooth margins, and a configuration which corresponds to the normal anatomy of the lungs. Any deviation from these characteristics requires explanation because it represents an abnormality in blood flow distribution.

The lung photoscan has been most valuable in the diagnosis of embolism. Zones of absent or sharply decreased radioactivity in the patient whose other findings are compatible with PTE provide substantial diagnostic support. Scanning is simple, safe, and rapid. It can be repeated to define the resolution, or recurrence, of obstructive vascular phenomena. Like any laboratory test, however, the photoscan must be applied and interpreted with care. It is important, for example, to obtain multiple scan views, because lesions not apparent in one view may be easily detected in another. Furthermore, the lung photoscan demonstrates only abnormalities of the *distribution of blood flow.* It does not provide anatomic information. Many disorders other than PTE are associated with abnormalities in the distribution of pulmonary blood flow. Any disease process, such as pneumonia, atelectasis, or pneumothorax, which reduces the ventilation of a lung zone will decrease its perfusion. Parenchymal diseases, such as emphysema, sarcoidosis, bronchogenic carcinoma, and tuberculosis, can all produce scan defects. Therefore a perfusion defect lacks specificity. Specificity is enhanced by also assessing the distribution of ventilation in the region(s) of abnormal blood flow. This is accomplished by performing a ventilation scan following inhalation of a radioactive gas such as ^{133}Xe. If a perfusion defect is due to vascular disease (e.g., embolism, vasculitis), ventilation in that lung zone is preserved (the "alveolar dead space" is visualized). If parenchymal disease causes the perfusion abnormality, a defect in ventilation also is present.

Occasionally, emboli may not produce obvious perfusion scan defects, either because they only partially obstruct the vascular lumen or because the obstructed zones are too small to be detected by current techniques. Despite these limitations, the perfusion photoscan has been invaluable in the diagnosis of embolism when interpreted properly.

Pulmonary angiography This is the only means for providing anatomic information about the pulmonary vasculature. Injection of radiopaque material, preferably through a cardiac catheter advanced into the pulmonary artery, provides a visual image of the pulmonary vessels. Cardiac catheterization and angiography require specialized personnel, a reasonable period for preparation and performance, and do entail more risk than the procedures discussed above. However, the procedure has the advantage of providing valuable hemodynamic data which may be necessary for therapeutic decisions. Interpretive limitations of angiography are of three types: (1) *Injection artifacts* may occur which suggest absence of flow to a vessel. Injection should be repeated whenever the question of such artifacts exists. (2) The inability to evaluate the patency of small vessels is another limitation. Emboli in vessels below the resolving capability of the method cannot be detected with certainty. (3) Interpretive errors may also be a consequence of *not looking for the proper type of defect.* Classically, the angiogram shows an *abrupt "cutoff"* of a vessel at the point of embolic impaction. However, complete embolic obstruction is uncommon. Therefore, *filling defects* are the most frequent finding; i.e., the embolus creates a "negative" shadow as the radiopaque material flows around it. Also, a *decrease in filling* of a lung zone suggests embolic obstruction.

How far one should proceed down the diagnostic pathway outlined above depends on many factors, the major ones being the severity of the patient's symptoms and, therefore, the urgency of the need for prompt and precise diagnosis. There should be no complacency in dealing with this potentially lethal disease. Photoscanning should be employed in any suspected case. Furthermore, there should be no hesitancy in proceeding to catheterization and angiography when a correct therapeutic decision is at stake.

TREATMENT

Once a diagnosis of PTE has been established, management is determined by two considerations: (1) the degree to which the circulation has been compromised; and (2) the natural history of the disease. In time, most emboli will resolve. Therefore, the goals of therapy should be to sustain life until resolution can occur and to prevent embolic recurrence. In most instances, *medical therapy* with anticoagulant drugs is adequate. Heparin is the drug of choice for several reasons: immediate onset of action; potent inhibition of the coagulation system; enhancement of fibrinolytic dissolution of fresh thrombi; inhibition of platelet breakdown (and therefore serotonin release); and prompt reversibility of anticoagulant action.

There are some differences of opinion regarding the specific techniques by which the drug should be given. A consensus would suggest that therapy should be initiated with an intravenous injection of 15,000 units, followed by intravenous administration of 5,000 to 7,500 units every 4 hr. If intravenous therapy cannot be maintained reliably, heparin should be given subcutaneously in doses of 7,500 units every 6 hr or 10,000 units every 8 hr. Intramuscular injection should be avoided because hematomas result. The need for, and utility of, clotting times to guide therapy is debated. If done improperly, this test is worthless, and may be misleading. If used appropriately, the usual objective is to keep the clotting time, measured *just prior to the next dose* of drug, two to three times the base-line clotting time (or 20 to 30 min, assuming a normal clotting time of 8 to 10 min). Heparin therapy should be maintained until the patient's cardiopulmonary status has stabilized and any evidence of venous thrombosis has resolved. Because thrombi become firmly attached to vessel wall and are well along the road toward organization within 5 to 7 days, patients should be maintained at bed rest for at least that period. If possible, ambulation is begun on heparin therapy, with elastic supports applied to the legs. If symptoms do not recur, the heparin may be tapered over the next 36 to 48 hr and then discontinued.

Prothrombinopenic drugs are not suitable for initial therapy in embolism. Their only role is in maintaining anticoagulant protection for prolonged periods. This is advisable if conditions exist which suggest that venous thrombosis and embolism are likely to recur, such as congestive heart failure, chronic venous insufficiency of the lower extremities, or the need for prolonged bed rest. In the absence of such indications, heparin alone suffices.

Thrombolytic (fibrinolytic) agents such as plasmin and urokinase have the potential of actually dissolving fresh thromboemboli. Despite extensive study, their efficacy and safety for routine clinical use remains to be established. Thrombolytic drugs should have their greatest utility in patients with massive embolism in whom surgical intervention would otherwise be contemplated.

Surgical therapy should be reserved for those patients in whom heparin therapy is deemed inadequate or impractical. Anticoagulant therapy may be contraindicated by the presence of a bleeding diathesis, or the patient may be in such critical condition that it is felt unwise to await a response to medical therapy. In such instances *venous ligation* and *pulmonary embolectomy* must be considered.

The objective of venous ligation is to prevent immediate recurrence of embolism. Ligation of the superficial femoral vein offers no protection against embolization from the deep femoral venous system, and ligation of the common femoral vein is unacceptable because of severe obstruction to venous drainage. Furthermore, these procedures must be bilateral to grant protection from a suspected embolic focus in the legs. For these reasons, interruption of the inferior vena cava has replaced more distal ligation procedures. A number of surgical procedures have been applied to the inferior vena cava: simple ligation; plication, in which fine channels are preserved; and the application of totally or partially occlusive "clips." Nonsurgical interruption also can be accomplished by introducing "umbrella" or balloon devices, attached to catheters, into the inferior vena cava via neck or upper-extremity veins. Each procedure has advantages and disadvantages. For example, total interruption leads to variable degrees of edema of the legs; successful plication does not prevent small emboli from reaching the lungs; devices introduced into the cava may migrate upward or be badly placed. Unfortunately, no form of inferior vena caval interruption precludes embolic recurrence. There are several reasons for this: sizable collateral channels develop weeks to months after interruption of the cava, through which embolization may recur; thromboembolism may originate at the site of caval manipulation; caval blockade does not prevent embolization from foci within the right cardiac chambers. Therefore, because most pulmonary emboli do resolve, caval interruption should be regarded as a *lifesaving procedure* to be restricted to patients who could not tolerate an *immediate* embolic recurrence. To elect this procedure, definite evidence of cardiopulmonary compromise by embolism is required, and there should be reasonable assurance that the embolic source is in the caval drainage area.

Caval interruption is not a formidable surgical procedure but may be associated with substantial morbidity. It should be used therefore only when required, and with recognition that it does not necessarily provide long-term protection. There is one instance, however, in which prompt caval ligation is the therapy of choice: septic thrombophlebitis of pelvic origin with multiple septic pulmonary emboli. If these patients do not respond promptly to a heparin-antibiotic regimen, they may die unless caval (and left ovarian vein) ligation is carried out promptly.

The decision to carry out emergency *pulmonary embolectomy* has many features in common with the decision to interrupt the inferior vena cava. In addition, however, since embolectomy is a major, complex operation which has been associated with a 50 percent mortality, the decision to carry out this procedure is a difficult one. However, there is agreement that two criteria should be met before embolectomy is performed: (1) there must be evidence of severe hemodynamic compromise due to embolism which is not responsive to supportive measures; and (2) the personnel and equipment required for embolectomy must be available.

These criteria require angiographic confirmation of the extent and location of the embolus except under the most unusual circumstances when a scan might suffice. Hemodynamic measurements are extremely helpful. Facilities for cardiopulmonary bypass should be available. Unless these requirements are met, the opportunity for error is great and the chances of a successful outcome are limited—indeed, less than with medical therapy.

SPECIAL CONSIDERATIONS Total resolution of emboli does not always occur. If residual vascular obstruction is substantial, the patient may present, months or years after the actual embolic events, with dyspnea and pulmonary hypertension of uncertain etiology. Multiple undetected recurrent small emboli may produce the same picture. These patients may masquerade with the diagnosis of "chronic lung disease" or "primary" pulmonary hypertension (Chap. 259).

Such patients should be studied by appropriate techniques, since larger emboli are potentially resectable, even after having been present for months to years. These patients represent potentially curable forms of otherwise fatal pulmonary hypertensive disease.

Embolism should also be suspected in other clinical contexts: as a precipitating cause for cardiac arrhythmia; as a reason for sudden or progressive worsening of congestive heart failure (Chap. 233); as an explanation for sudden deterioration in the patient with chronic obstructive pulmonary disease; and as a possible alternative to the diagnosis of "psychic" hyperventilation.

PROPHYLAXIS The ultimate goal in thromboembolism is its prevention, and certain measures can be invoked to limit the occurrence of venous thrombosis and pulmonary embolism. Elastic stockings or bandages should be used in any patient requiring a prolonged period of bed rest, particularly when venous stasis is present. Early ambulation should be encouraged in the postpartum and postoperative periods. Prophylactic use of anticoagulant drugs is indicated in patients over the age of forty years with fractures of the pelvis or lower extremities for whom a period of 10 days of immobilization is anticipated, and in patients with severe congestive heart failure. The potential risk of anovulatory therapy should be recognized. Truly effective prophylaxis, however, must await a better understanding of the pathogenesis of thrombosis, and techniques which can identify individuals with thrombotic tendencies or subclinical venous thrombosis. Several techniques—the use of radiolabeled fibrinogen, assay of fibrin split products, impedance plethysmography, and ultrasonic (Doppler) devices—offer promise in such early detection of venous thrombosis.

REFERENCES

DEXTER L, DALEN JE: Pulmonary embolism and acute cor pulmonale, chap. 67 in *The Heart*, 3rd ed., ed JW Hurst, New York: McGraw-Hill, 1974

MOSER KM, STEIN MS (eds): *Advances in Cardiopulmonary Diseases—Pulmonary Thromboembolism,* Chicago: Year Book, 1973

MOSER KM et al: Assessment of pulmonary photoscanning and angiography in experimental pulmonary embolism. Circulation 39:663, 1969

PARASKOS JA et al: Late prognosis of acute pulmonary embolism. N Engl J Med 289:55, 1973

POLLAK EW et al: Pulmonary embolism: An appraisal of therapy in 516 cases. Arch Surg 107:66, 1973

257 HYPERSENSITIVITY REACTIONS OF THE LUNG

PHILIP S. NORMAN

THE EOSINOPHILIC PNEUMONIAS

A series of syndromes of undoubtedly diverse but often unknown etiology are grouped together under the terms *pulmonary eosinophilia,* or *eosinophilic pneumonia*. The consistent anatomical feature is the filling of alveoli with a mixture of large mononuclear cells and eosinophils along with edema and infiltration of the connective tissue of the lung with large numbers of eosinophils accompanied by varying numbers of large and small mononuclear cells and plasma cells. Fibrinous exudates are common, granulomas can occur, and there may be eventual organization. Mucous plugging of the bronchi occurs frequently and can cause atelectasis.

Clinically, these syndromes are commonly divided into 5 groups:

1 *Loeffler's syndrome:* This consists of transitory and migratory pulmonary infiltrations, fever, and peripheral blood eosinophilia with minimal or no pulmonary symptoms. Recovery usually occurs within a month.
2 *Prolonged pulmonary eosinophilia:* When eosinophilic infiltrations of the lung are prolonged beyond a month,

they may be accompanied by high fever, malaise, productive cough, and chest pain. Although by definition "Loeffler's syndrome" is not chronic, there are all gradations between the transient and chronic infiltration; hence the distinction may well be artificial.

3 *Pulmonary eosinophilia with asthma:* Asthma (Chap. 67) is occasionally accompanied by transient infiltrations. When eosinophilic infiltrations are prolonged as a late complication of chronic asthma, the term eosinophilic pneumonia may be used. At times, some degree of bronchial obstruction may be a part of the course of a typical eosinophilic pneumonia.

4 *Tropical eosinophilia:* This condition simply is eosinophilic pneumonia occurring in the tropics. As usually described, fever, dyspnea (or asthmatic attacks), and weight loss are more prominent than in the nontropical form. About 35 percent of patients respond to arsenical therapy, and this has been considered a diagnostic feature, but it may merely reflect a different therapeutic practice in the tropics, since asthma in the temperate zone has been shown to respond to arsenic also.

5 *Polyarteritis nodosa:* This disorder (Chap. 71) may occasionally present as asthma or pulmonary infiltrates with eosinophilia.

The etiology remains obscure in many if not most cases of pulmonary eosinophilia; yet evidence of parasitic infestations and exposure to chemicals and drugs seems to provide an etiology in a number of cases. The following intestinal parasites with a phase of migration through the lung have been associated with the syndrome: *Ascaris lumbricoides, Necator americanus, Ancylostoma brasiliense, Trichinella spiralis, Fasciola hepatica,* and *Strongyloides stercoralis.* In the more severe tropical eosinophilia, complement fixation tests with filarial antigens (usually the dog heartworm, *Dirofilaria immitis)* are regularly positive, and the antiparasitic drug diethylcarbamazine usually produces a gratifying response. Microfilariae are not usually found in the peripheral blood.

Inhalation of *nickel carbonyl vapors* has resulted in asthma, dermatitis, infiltration of the lungs, and eosinophilia. The most frequent chemicals to be associated with the syndrome are, however, drugs and include penicillin, para-aminosalicylic acid, hydralazine, nitrofurantoin, chlorpropamide, and sulfonamides. Allergic aspergillosis, occurring in asthmatics, is often accompanied by pulmonary infiltrations and eosinophilia (Chap. 174). Presumably, in all these instances the disease arises as a hypersensitivity reaction to a foreign antigen which finds its way into the lung.

The *diagnosis* of the eosinophilic pneumonias is made on the basis of migrating nodular or patchy pulmonary infiltrates accompanied by sputum or blood eosinophilia. Ventilatory ability is often normal unless there is asthma, but diffusing capacity may be reduced when the pulmonary infiltrates are at their peak. In prolonged cases a lung biopsy may be necessary because of the possibility of more serious conditions, such as Hamman-Rich syndrome, sarcoidosis, polyarteritis, nodosa, or specific granulomatous infections. The tropical form is commonly accompanied by a false positive serologic test for syphilis and a high titer of cold agglutinins.

TABLE 257-1
Agents which cause allergic interstitial pneumonitis

Form of hypersensitivity	*Agent*
Farmer's lung	*Micropolyspora faeni*
Moldy-hay disease	*M. faeni; A. fumigatus*
Bagassosis	*Thermoactinomyces vulgaris*
Mushroom-worker's disease	*M. faeni and T. vulgaris*
Suberosis (oak-bark)	*M. faeni and T. vulgaris*
Malt-worker's lung	*A. fumigatus and A. clavatus*
Maple-bark stripper's lung	*Cryptostroma corticale*
Sequoiosis	*Graphium and Auerobasidium*
Cheese-worker's lung	*Penicillium*
Insect-antigen's lung (wheat weevil)	*Sitophilus ghonvirus*
Pituitary-snuff-taker's lung	Pituitary snuff
Pigeon breeder's disease	Pigeons and budgerigars (avian antigen)
Enzyme lung	*Bacillus subtilis*
Sisal-worker's disease	?
Coffee-worker's disease	?
Wood-dust pneumonitis	Oak and mahogany dust
Humidifiers and air-conditioner pneumonitis	Thermophilic actinomycetes

SOURCE: Adapted from RM Katz, and WT Kniker, N Engl J Med 288:233, 1973

In most instances there is no therapy unless a specific parasite can be uncovered by examination of the stool. Persons residing in, or recently removed from, the tropics deserve a trial of diethylcarbamazine, 2 mg per kg three times a day for 3 or 4 weeks. In cases with severe bronchospasm or prolongation of the syndrome with no trend toward improvement, corticosteroids are indicated and will often cause a dramatic response. Relapse when the drug is withdrawn occasionally occurs.

PNEUMONIAS FROM SPECIFIC EXPOSURES

Inhalation of a variety of organic dusts produces a series of hypersensitivity syndromes characterized by interstitial granulomatous reaction of the lung *without* eosinophiles. The period of exposure required to establish specific sensitization accompanied by precipitating antibodies is unknown, but a new inhalation of the antigen commonly leads to an acute illness in hours.

FARMER'S LUNG Agricultural workers may develop chills, fever, cough, and dyspnea rapidly, a few hours after exposure to moldy organic dusts (hay, grain, corn, tobacco, etc.). In nearly half the patients with farmer's lung, however, dyspnea, cough, and weight loss develop insidiously over several weeks or months. Whether the initial onset is acute or insidious, subsequent attacks may vary; acute attacks may develop in patients whose previous attacks were characterized by a gradual onset, while in patients with an acute initial episode, slow inexorable deterioration may occur as long as exposure to the antigen continues. Dyspnea often is accompanied by tightness or pain in the chest. There are occasionally small hemoptyses, but cough is usually nonproductive. There are usually loud crackling rales at the lung bases, and early in the disease, the chest roentgenogram shows diffuse interstitial or nodular infiltrates. Although the disease improves in a few days or weeks when exposure stops, recurrence upon reexposure is usual. Furthermore, prolonged or recurrent exposure may result in pulmonary fibrosis which may not be entirely reversible.

Moldy hay is rich in the thermophilic actinomycetes, *Micropolyspora faeni* (formerly, *Thermopolyspora polyspora)* and *Micromonospora vulgaris*, as well as a number of fungal species *(Aspergillus, Cladosporium, Mucor, Penicillium,* and *Humicola)*. Growth of the actinomycetes is favored by spontaneous heating during mold growth. The serum of patients with farmer's lung contains precipitating antibodies against extracts of moldy hay dust but none to clean hay dust. Furthermore, when inhaled by aerosol, extracts of moldy hay of cultures of the actinomycetes will produce typical attacks in patients with farmer's lung while extracts of clean hay will not. Precipitins against thermophilic actinomycetes and molds repeatedly have been demonstrated in the serum.

The *physiologic derangement* is a direct result of the interstitial infiltrate. Compliance is reduced and pulmonary gas diffusion is defective, but airway resistance is normal or nearly so.

Diagnosis depends on a history of exposure to moldy agricultural products, a finely granular reticular pattern on chest roentgenogram, pulmonary function tests showing reduced compliance and diffusion of gases, and improvement when exposure is discontinued. Eosinophilia is not part of the syndrome. A lung biopsy is not ordinarily necessary but may be required in cases which do not resolve quickly. The demonstration of precipitating antibodies to moldy hay extracts or to thermophilic actinomycetes may also be helpful. Although skin tests to mold or hay extracts are often positive, they are not useful in diagnosis because they are frequently positive not only in exposed individuals who do not have symptoms but also in some normal individuals, possibly because of endotoxin in the extract. Coworkers of patients with farmer's lung who are exposed to similar substances do not develop the illness, indicating that this is truly a disease of hypersensitivity.

If exposure is continued, the physiologic derangements, particularly the diffusion defect, may lead to right-sided heart failure, with a fatal outcome in some instances. When exposure is stopped, symptoms, pulmonary infiltrates, and physiologic derangements all tend to abate. Eventually, complete recovery occurs, although some patients, particularly those with prolonged exposure, have residual interstitial pulmonary fibrosis.

DISEASE FROM HUMIDIFIERS AND AIR CONDITIONERS Typical allergic interstitial pneumonitis has been reported in several instances from contamination of either home or office central heating or air conditioning systems where the installation permits the growth of microorganisms in a location where they might be spread by the flow of forced air through the system. Leaking water pipes in a central heating system may be located near the heating element and provide the heated moist environment favorable to growth of thermophilic actinomycetes. Susceptible individuals are particularly apt to suffer attacks when returning after a weekend away from the contaminated environment. In other instances, home humidifiers installed near the hot-air plenum provided a reservoir of heated water for the growth of these organisms. The humidifier then atomized the contaminated water into the airstream, resulting in typical inhalation disease. The usual history is that a housewife notes respiratory disease in the winter which remits during the summer when the heat is off or when she is away on vacation. The findings are typical of other forms of interstitial pneumonitis and resolve when exposure ceases. Much detective work may be required to find the source of contamination. When home humidifiers are installed in forced-air systems, they should be placed away from the source of heat and should be of a type that provides direct evolution of water vapor from a piped source of water rather than from a reservoir which may grow mold or bacteria.

MAPLE BARK DISEASE Sawmill or logging workers may develop typical attacks of interstitial pneumonitis after shaving or peeling bark from maple logs that have been stored for some time after cutting. Examination of the logs reveals heavy growth of the sporulating mold *Cryptostroma corticale*, just beneath the outer bark. Lung biopsies may show a number of inhaled spores; these spores have not germinated or grown mycelium, but by their presence, they initiate a strong hypersensitivity reaction. Skin tests with extract of *C. corticale* give both immediate (wheal and erythema) as well as delayed reactions. Serum precipitins to *C. corticale* also appear. Improved ventilation in sawmills and methods for storing logs to prevent continued dampness will usually eradicate the problem in a logging operation. Similar syndromes occur after exposure to redwood or elm sawdust and may be due to sensitivity to fungi of the genus *Graphium*. As in other conditions in this group, cessation of exposure usually results in complete recovery.

MUSHROOM-WORKER'S LUNG Mushrooms are cultivated commercially on beds of aged horse manure. The manure, admixed with straw, is aged under conditions of warm temperature and high humidity which encourage the growth of the same thermophilic actinomycetes implicated in farmer's lung. When the aged manure is spread in beds to be sown with the spawn of the mushrooms or when the spent manure is removed after harvest of the mushrooms, workers may develop attacks of allergic interstitial pneumonitis. These individuals have serum precipitins against *T. polyspora* and *M. vulgaris*. A change of job usually results in complete relief.

BAGASSOSIS Bagasse is the dried fiber of sugarcane after the sugar-bearing juice is pressed out. It is used as a source of cellulose for a variety of manufactured goods. Bagassosis results from the inhalation of the dust of bagasse when the bales are eventually opened or the fibers shredded. Fresh bagasse is not a problem, and the condition is not observed in sugarcane workers or at sugar mills. The baled bagasse is often stored, usually outdoors, without protection against moisture before being used, and there is often evident mold growth.

Attacks of chills, fever, and dyspnea accompanied by granulomatous pneumonia have been described in bagasse workers in many parts of the world.

Precipitins to moldy bagasse can be demonstrated in the serum of 80 to 100 percent of patients with bagassosis but are also found frequently in bagasse workers without pulmonary disease and occasionally in individuals with no known contact with bagasse. Cultures of moldy bagasse show a variety of thermophilic actinomycetes, with *M. vulgaris* being the most frequent. Precipitins to this organism are found in a majority of bagassosis patients, but there are rarely precipitins to the other microorganisms in bagasse. Precipitins to *M. vulgaris* are rare in bagasse workers without the disease and appear to be in low titer. Immediate hypersensitivity to moldy bagasse with wheal and erythema skin reactions is clearly not diagnostic because it is as common in workers without disease as in those with disease.

The clinical picture and the physical and laboratory findings are quite similar to those of farmer's lung, and prolonged exposure may lead to pulmonary fibrosis and chronic restrictive disease. The presence of the typical clinical syndrome and of serum precipitins to *M. vulgaris* is strong presumptive evidence for bagassosis. Ordinarily the disease improves when jobs are changed. If the bagasse is moistened before handling, the exposure can be considerably reduced, and when exposure to moldy bagasse is curtailed, precipitins to *M. vulgaris* tend to disappear over several years.

PIGEON BREEDER'S DISEASE Acute attacks of chills, fever, cough, and breathlessness recently have been observed in individuals who breed and race pigeons or keep parakeets. The attacks occur a few hours after handling the birds and are accompanied by rales at the lung bases and by a fine diffuse interstitial pneumonia which appears with each episode. As with farmer's lung, some patients have insidious onset of exertional dyspnea without dramatic episodes of chills and fever. Weight loss may be striking. Exposure to aerosols of pigeon droppings reproduces the acute attacks and is accompanied by a drop in pulmonary diffusing capacity within 24 hr. The patient's serum contains precipitins against pigeon serum or pigeon egg white, and immunoglobulin levels are almost always elevated. Challenge with 3 ml of aerosolized pigeon serum also reproduces the disease so that it appears that molds or actinomycetes do not play a role. The relation of serum precipitins to the disease is not clear as some pigeon breeders have serum precipitins to pigeon antigens but do not develop the illness after handling the birds. Symptoms disappear and precipitin levels decline when exposure is stopped. Similar conditions occur after inhalation of pituitary snuff and grain weevil dust. In these cases the antigens are also proteins not derived from microorganisms.

TREATMENT In this group of diseases, cessation of exposure is usually the only treatment required. Acute episodes may dictate bed rest and supportive measures such as oxygen and antipyretics for fever. It is possible to hasten resolution of the process with corticosteroids, but this is not always necessary. When cor pulmonale and right-sided heart failure occur, they should be treated as described in Chap. 262.

REFERENCES

LIEBOW AA, CARRINGTON CB: The eosinophilic pneumonias. Medicine (Baltimore) 48:251, 1969

PEPYS J: Farmer's lung. Br Med J 2:359, 1965

REED CE et al: Pigeon breeder's lung, a newly observed interstitial pulmonary disease. JAMA 193:261, 1965

WEILL H et al: Bagassosis: A study of pulmonary function. Ann. Intern Med 64:737, 1966

258 ENVIRONMENTAL LUNG DISEASE

AREND BOUHUYS
J. BERNARD L. GEE

Ample opportunity exists for interactions in the lungs between the host and inhaled materials, including allergens, viruses, bacteria, air pollutants, and dusts. Both the environmental factors and their interactions with the host are acknowledged to be complex, while the frequency and clinical importance of environmental lung disease are increasingly recognized. An understanding of the pathogenesis and control of these diseases leans heavily on other disciplines, including environmental hygiene, chemistry, engineering, meteorology, epidemiology, and statistics. These disciplines are required for an accurate description of the environment, and for a definition of the effects of common environmental exposures on individuals of different age, sex, and genetic background. At present, attempts to influence the environment constitute the main tool in prevention of environmental lung disease. It is to be hoped that in the future, the identification of host factors will permit the selection of workers at minimum risk of developing disease despite industrial exposure.

The Federal Occupational Safety and Health Act of 1970 charges employers in the United States with the provision of a workplace "free from recognized hazards" to all employees. The Secretary of Labor is in charge of implementing the act, with the Occupational Safety and Health Administration serving as a resource for prevention, control, and the setting of adequate standards, and with the National Institute for Occupational Safety and Health serving as a research resource. Adequate implementation of the act could greatly decrease the incidence of occupational lung diseases but will require the understanding and cooperation of the medical professions.

Exposures to industrial agents that may cause lung disease are undoubtedly widespread. In a survey of some 800 establishments with 260,000 employees in the Chicago area, dust hazards were found in 20 percent of the plants visited. Exposure to gaseous inhalants may be even more prevalent. Before considering such specific exposures, classified according to pathologic and physiologic criteria, some general principles of pulmonary transport require discussion.

TRANSPORT OF MATTER

VAPORS AND GASES A volatile substance can be absorbed from inspired air at a maximum rate equal to the product of its concentration and the alveolar ventilation. The quantity actually absorbed depends on its solubility in body tissues and fluids; the toxic effects depend, in addition, on its rates of excretion and metabolism. Effects of irritant gases on upper airways are common with highly soluble gases such as NH_3 and SO_2, which dissolve immediately in the mucus of the nose and throat, while only minimal amounts reach lower airways. Less soluble gases, such as Cl_2 and phosgene, are not as readily removed by the scrubbing action in the upper airways and can therefore elicit violent responses in the peripheral airways and pulmonary parenchyma.

AEROSOLS An aerosol is a suspension of liquid or solid particles in air. When inhaled, some particles are deposited in the airways and lungs, depending on their size, weight, shape, and especially their settling velocity. Large particles (>10 μm in diameter) tend to impact or settle in the nose and upper airways, while very small particles (<0.1 μm in diameter) may behave like very large molecules; if retained at all, they are deposited in small airways and alveoli. Particles of intermediate size tend to settle by gravity (sedimentation). Many aerosols of medical interest consist of particles in this intermediate size range (0.1 to 10 μm in diameter), for which it is difficult to define a precise pattern of deposition.

Theoretical models of particle deposition are usually based on particles of uniform size and shape, which occur only within the laboratory. Actually most "natural" aerosols contain particles with a wide range of sizes; with liquid aerosols, a relatively small number of large particles contain more than 90 percent of the toxic or therapeutic substance. Thus, the effects depend primarily upon the site of deposition of the large particles, not on that of the much more numerous small particles, which account for only a small fraction of the total aerosol mass. For instance, bronchodilator aerosols with a few large droplets may deposit most of the drug in upper airways, where they have no useful action, while systemic absorption from this site may cause undesirable side effects. Predominant deposition in smaller airways is obtained with aerosols of a more restricted size range, e.g., 0.5 to 5 μm in diameter. The deposition pattern of aerosols of solid particles (dusts) is more complex than that of liquid droplets, because it depends not only on their size but also on their shape and specific gravity; e.g., long, thin, straight fibers may penetrate to much smaller airways than round particles of equivalent mass.

ASPIRATION Solid food or fluids, including saliva, may be aspirated into the lungs in states of disturbed consciousness, in debilitating diseases, disorders of deglutition, obstructing lesions of the esophagus, after local anesthesia of the pharynx, and in drowning. Emulsions and oils may be aspirated even in the absence of overt disturbances of deglutition, particularly following their intranasal instillation, or in older persons who frequently ingest laxative mineral oils. Small amounts of such materials may coat the pharyngeal mucosa and may be aspirated without evoking a cough reflex.

MUCOCILIARY CLEARANCE Normally, small particles entering the bronchial tree are engulfed in a layer of mucus produced by bronchial glands and goblet cells. The respiratory cilia move this layer toward the pharynx, where it is swallowed. Mucociliary clearance is probably not effective beyond the first generation of bronchioles, at which point phagocytic cells appear to take over; these cells probably reach "the first rung of the mucociliary ladder" by their own motility.

The amount and regulation of normal mucus production are unknown, but it has been established in experiments with animals that vagal stimulation increases mucus production in the tracheobronchial tree, while atropine decreases it. Mucus is not homogeneous and has elastic, plastic, and viscous properties. Two layers of mucus cover the airways—a watery layer, the sol phase, in which the cilia beat, and, superficial to that, a more viscous layer, the gel phase, which moves toward the pharynx. The frequency of the ciliary beat is probably regulated by the quantity of mucus to be transported. In addition to its important role in the removal of particulate matter from the lungs, mucus also has an antibacterial function, provided by secretory antibodies and lysozyme.

PHAGOCYTOSIS The two principal phagocytes in the lung are the leukocyte and the alveolar macrophage, both of which are mobilized in response to inhaled particles and vapors. Leukocytes respond vigorously to acute, high-intensity challenges and to the chemotaxis of inflammatory responses. Alveolar macrophages are mobilized in response to the more chronic application of less intense stimuli and to agents which evoke little acute inflammation, such as fibrogenic dusts and carbon, as well as in delayed hypersensitivity responses. Once ingested, particles are subjected to biochemical events within the cell. Lysosomal hydrolases may degrade inhaled organic materials and, together with peroxidative metabolism, exert antimicrobial action. Other ingested materials injure the phagocytes and may kill them. Silica and asbestos injure lysosomal membranes, and the release of lysosomal enzymes within the cell then initiates autodigestion. Yet other agents, including oxides of nitrogen and ozone, impair the ingestion of particles and modify the actions of lysosomal hydrolases. A similar effect is exerted by cigarette smoke, which impairs the ingestion of particles by alveolar macrophages in vitro. Alveolar macrophages obtained from the lungs of cigarette smokers show increases in glucose oxidation and in the activity of lysosomal hydrolases, but the phagocytic competence of such cells does not seem to be impaired. Cell surface and membrane events may be of critical importance in determining particle ingestion. The lysosomal enzymes of the phagocytic cells usually exert important defensive actions, but the release of these enzymes may also lead to lung injury and inflammation.

Following ingestion of the particles, some phagocytes remain viable, migrate to lymphatics, and are trapped in regional lymph nodes, where they deposit the ingested material. Cells that die soon after particle ingestion, on the other hand, may either disintegrate locally or be removed via the mucociliary ladder.

COUGH Cough is primarily a protective reflex and a mechanism for the removal of mucus in the tracheobronchial tree. Its mechanism is discussed elsewhere (Chap. 35).

GENERAL RESPONSES TO INHALED MATERIALS

PROTECTIVE REFLEXES Irritant gases cause subjective sensations such as unpleasant odor or throat irritation, which in turn elicit behavioral responses designed to avoid further exposure. In addition, reflex responses may lead to sneezing, glottal closure, apnea, or rapid shallow breathing, cough, and constriction of lower airways. Some of these responses can help to limit absorption or to remove inhaled matter. The reflex responses also serve as warning signals to the patient to minimize exposure; noxious gases, such as phosgene, that do not elicit these reflexes can cause grave lung injury.

MUCUS PRODUCTION This is increased acutely by SO_2 and other irritant gases in high concentration, and chronically by cigarette smoke. An increase in mucus production occurs in the early years of smoking and results in hypertrophy of bronchial glands and an increase in goblet cells. Since mucus production often decreases when cigarette smoking is discontinued, it appears that the changes in the mucous glands are at least partially reversible.

PULMONARY EDEMA This is a prominent feature of the response to "deep-lung irritants" such as phosgene. The predominant symptom is dyspnea, followed by cyanosis and other signs of asphyxia.

AIRWAY CONSTRICTION Airway caliber may decrease because of mucosal swelling, mucus accumulation, deposition of foreign matter, or contraction of smooth muscle. The latter occurs in response to allergens in asthma and to some toxic dusts. This response is mediated by histamine and possibly by other locally released substances. Reflex airway constriction can be induced by stimulation of the upper airway, larynx, or trachea with mechanical stimuli or irritant gases. This is usually a short-lived response, while release of chemical mediators is often effective for several hours.

EMPHYSEMA Epidemiologic data have shown an association of emphysema with cigarette smoking and certain occupational exposures. Loss of elastic recoil in the lung may occur in workers with enzyme detergents and textiles, suggesting structural damage of the kind found in emphysema (Chap. 252).

PARENCHYMAL RESPONSES The cellular reactions in environmental lung diseases include (1) acute necrotizing and inflammatory responses induced by chemicals; (2) edema and inflammatory responses with leukocyte mobilization induced by organic antigens (extrinsic allergic alveolitis, see Chap. 257); (3) formation of granulomas, as in beryllium exposure; (4) mobilization of macrophages after exposure to dusts; (5) pleomorphic cellular responses following exposure to asbestos and hard metals; and (6) fibrosis, a late reaction to many of the above.

Three forms of fibrosis occur: (1) diffuse interstitial; (2) focal or nodular; and (3) progressive massive fibrosis (PMF). Diffuse and focal fibrosis are progressively disabling conditions which restrict lung volumes and decrease gas transport. Their early stages may include destruction of the alveolar basement membrane and release of lysosomal enzymes from macrophages. Indestructible particles, such as asbestos and silica, may recycle through macrophages and cause sustained low-grade inflammation. Collagen formation may depend on reactions to such inflammation or to products of autolyzed macrophages. Some particles, such as asbestos, may transform macrophages directly into fibroblasts. These mechanisms do not explain the distribution of fibrous tissue, which, for example, is diffuse in asbestosis and nodular in silicosis. Instead, this distribution may result from different patterns of deposition, which in turn are a function of the size and shape of particles.

The fibrogenic properties of dusts vary. In some instances (e.g., siderosis) they depend on the varying silica contents of the inhaled material. The cause of PMF in patients with silicosis and coal workers' pneumoconiosis is unknown; it is manifested by confluent opacities on the chest roentgenogram of patients who usually have severe dyspnea. Tuberculous infection is not a prerequisite for its development. PMF lesions may develop cavities, perhaps from ischemic necrosis, and these lesions account for about 25 percent of all fatal cases of coal workers' pneumoconiosis.

COMBINED EXPOSURES Exposures to more than one agent may result in independent or additive effects, or interactions between multiple agents may occur. The high risk of lung cancer in asbestos workers who smoke is one example of interaction. Since many workers exposed to occupational inhalants also smoke, assessing the relative risk of each agent requires that nonsmokers as well as smokers be studied.

Smoking and occupational exposure to irritant gases or dusts are common features of the history of patients with chronic bronchitis, emphysema, and other chronic obstructive lung diseases (Chap. 252). The terminal stages of these diseases include widespread obstruction of the small airways and ventilatory failure, but their early stages and natural history may differ considerably. For instance, patients with chronic airway obstruction may have cystic fibrosis, α_1-antitrypsin deficiency, or an occupational disease such as byssinosis. Since the majority of patients with chronic airway obstruction probably have some environmental injury to the lungs and airways, prevention will require more precise delineation of the environmental and genetic factors involved.

HOST VARIABILITY Some individuals respond to environmental toxic agents that do not harm others. Such individual differences may result from atopy (Chap. 67), acquired sensitization, a normal distribution of sensitivities, or a bimodal distribution, with distinct groups of "reactors" and "nonreactors" in the population at risk.

Among textile workers there are reactors who develop byssinosis and nonreactors who do not, a difference which is not acquired by sensitization. The autonomic innervation of airways may play a role in determining reactor status. Thus, a nonreactor to textile dust can temporarily be converted to a reactor by the blockade of beta-adrenergic receptors with propranolol (Chap. 235), while parasympathetic blockade with atropine renders a reactor temporarily insensitive. Interaction between neural and humoral endogenous stimuli with environmental factors in airway smooth muscle may be an important determinant of individual sensitivity. Temporal variations in sensitivity include those induced by drugs (e.g., atropine, adrenergic agonists and antagonists, antihistamines), tachyphylaxis (temporary desensitization after exposure), the efficacy of the various protective mechanisms, and the state of the effector organ (e.g., normal versus constricted airways).

DIAGNOSTIC METHODS

HISTORY AND PHYSICAL EXAMINATION A detailed environmental and occupational history is usually the key to the diagnosis of environmental lung diseases. It should include details on cough, sputum, and dyspnea, and factors influencing the severity of these symptoms, as well as a complete, quantitative record of past and present smoking habits, residences since birth, and all jobs held since leaving school.

Respiratory symptoms may be analyzed by using a standard questionnaire in epidemiologic studies as well as in clinical settings. Inquiries must be made about exposures to irritant gases, fumes, dusts, and vapors at work or in hobbies. The nature of the work, characteristics of the workplace, and type of materials handled are more important than the title of the position. For example, an electrician may be exposed to silica in a foundry, to asbestos in construction work, or to cotton dust in a textile mill. A mesothelioma in an executive, diagnosed in 1970, may be due to exposure to asbestos during 2 years of work in a shipyard in World War II.

Exposures at home may include dust, smoke, paints, and solvents. Exposure to noxious agents occurs not only in modern industry but also in primitive societies. For example, the grinding of corn between siliceous stones indoors is a cause of silicosis in Africa, while the batting and hackling of flax or soft hemp fibers may cause disabling byssinosis. In industry, technical procedures are more complex, and specific information on exposures may be difficult to obtain.

IDENTIFICATION OF INHALED MATERIAL This may be less crucial for diagnosis than may appear at first sight. For instance, the presence of asbestos bodies in the sputum merely confirms that exposure has taken place, not that asbestos-induced disease is present. Similarly, the finding of free silica in tissue obtained by means of lung biopsy confirms that exposure has occurred but does not indicate the extent of the disease. Environmental monitoring of the workplace provides a simpler confirmation of exposure, without risk to the worker. Lung biopsy is rarely required to diagnose environmental lung disease.

CHEST ROENTGENOGRAPHY Together with a history of exposure, the chest roentgenogram provides important diagnostic information. A classification scheme has been developed under the auspices of the International Labor Office which allows interpretation of films in a standardized and semiquantitative form. The "UICC/Cincinnati Classification" should be used to classify the roentgenograms of all cases of mineral-dust diseases of the lungs. In large groups of miners there are positive correlations between roentgenographic changes and lung dust content. Thus, on the basis of autopsy data, the chest roentgenogram has been found to be a semiquantitative guide to dust exposure in mineral-dust diseases, in which the dust deposits or the tissue lesions, or both, are radiopaque. This is of great diagnostic importance, especially when the composition of the inhaled dust is known. However, roentgenographic findings bear little relation to the degree of disability, in particular in coal workers' pneumoconiosis. This discrepancy is related to the variable presence of additional lesions, such as airway obstruction, which are not visible on the roentgenogram.

LUNG FUNCTION AND DISABILITY Spirometric and other lung function tests are discussed in Chapter 249. Sensitive tests are needed to detect early stages of lung disease; maximum expiratory flow/volume (MEFV) curves are useful for this purpose (Fig. 258-1). They offer several advantages: (1) VC (vital capacity) and FEV_1 (forced expiratory volume in 1 sec) data are available; (2) specific curve patterns are of diagnostic value; (3) performance of the patient is easily monitored, and thus reproducibility of data is assured; (4) the portion of the MEFV curve which is independent of the patient's effort can be used to measure flow rates at small lung volumes. The latter are often reduced when other indices of obstruction (e.g., FEV_1/VC) are still normal, for instance in patients with asymptomatic asthma or in young cigarette smokers.

Restrictive function loss (Chaps. 249 and 254) occurs in a variety of diffuse interstitial diseases, including environmental lung diseases. The airways are not obstructed, and elastic recoil may be increased because of diffuse fibrosis. Hence, expiratory flow rates are high, with an FEV_1/VC ratio approaching 1. The reduced VC and the high flow rates produce a typical MEFV curve pattern (Fig. 258-1*A*). With *obstructive function loss*, forced expiratory flow rates are reduced, but VC may be normal. Flow reduction is usually most pronounced at low lung volumes, since the caliber of airways decreases with lung volume. This results in another typical configuration of the MEFV curve, with a curvature opposite in direction from that in restrictive function loss (Fig. 258-1*A*). The sensitivity of flow measurements on MEFV curves, at small volumes, is illustrated by an example taken from a study on teenage smokers (Fig. 258-1*B*). In that instance, maximum flows at 50 percent VC discriminated much better between smokers and nonsmokers than did the FEV_1. Among tests of gas exchange, the single-breath diffusing capacity for carbon monoxide (Chap. 249) is suitable for epidemiologic work on interstitial lung disease of occupational origin.

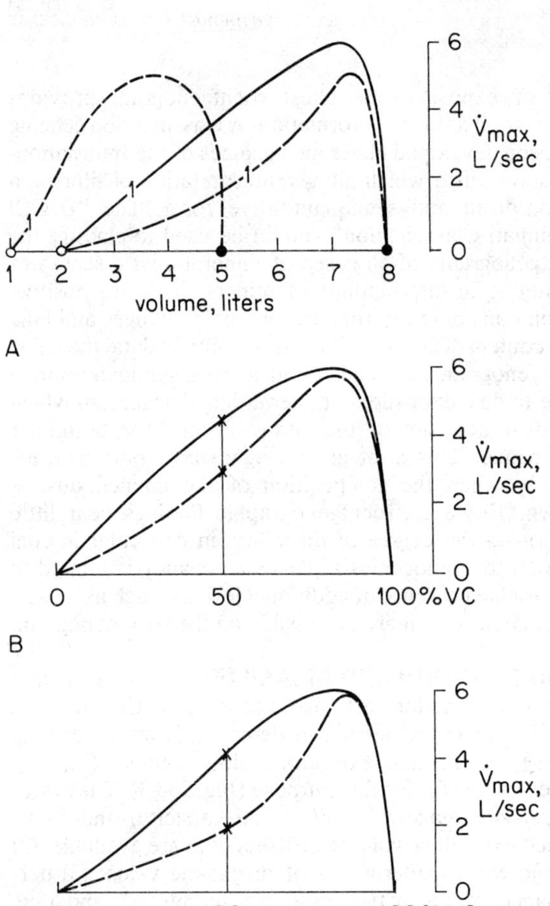

FIGURE 258-1

Maximum expiratory flow volume (MEFV) curves. Ordinate shows flow in liters per second. Curves indicate maximum expiratory flow produced during forced expiration from total lung capacity. Abscissa shows lung volume in absolute values (thoracic gas volume). 1 = volume expired in 1 sec (FEV_1). A *Solid line = normal. Long dashes = obstructive. Short dashes = restrictive. On the abscissa, total lung capacity is indicated by the dots at 5 and 8, residual volume by the circles at 1 and 2. The abscissa in* B *and* C *shows lung volume as percent of vital capacity (VC). X= V_{max} at 50 percent VC.* B *Solid line = nonsmoking teenager. Dashed line = smoking teenager.* C *Textile worker before (solid line) and after (dashed line) 4 hr of dust exposure.*

Airway obstruction and restrictive function loss are relatively simple to detect when overt clinical disease is present. In epidemiologic studies, however, it is important to detect functional loss related to environmental exposure in asymptomatic subjects. This can be accomplished by comparing the groups at risk with suitably matched control groups. If these groups are sufficiently large, even small differences in lung function may be statistically significant and indicative of environmental risks.

The clinician must often decide whether a certain degree of lung function loss provides a basis for disability. The Social Security Administration assumes total disability when the FEV_1 is less than 1.1 to 1.5 liters, depending on body height. Such patients are usually short of breath during minimal exertion and can perform only desk work or similar activities. Persons who are more active physically in their jobs may be disabled from working, even though their FEV_1 is above these limits. Objective criteria for decreased work performance in lung disease are as yet unsatisfactory. Many persons with restrictive disease or airways obstruction reach the limit of their exercise tolerance because of their limited ventilatory capacity. This can be shown by comparing ventilation during exercise with maximum ventilatory performance (Fig. 258-2). In severe lung disease, an abnormally low arterial O_2 tension, if it occurs at rest or during light exercise, is an indicator of clinical disability.

ACUTE SPECIFIC EXPOSURES

CHEMICAL INFLAMMATION Many agents listed in Table 258-1 produce acute inflammation of mucous membranes (conjunctiva, nose, pharynx, larynx, and lower airways) and pulmonary edema. The more irritant chemicals (acid mists and ammonia) produce severe, immediate reactions, with intense lacrimation, sore throat, and reflex

FIGURE 258-2

Expiratory flow volume curves. Dotted line = tidal expiration (V_T) at rest. Dashed line = V_T during moderate exercise. Solid line = V_T during heavy exercise. All expiratory flow volume loops are drawn within contours of MEFV curves in a healthy person (A) *and in two patients with moderate* (B) *and severe* (C) *obstructive disease. Limits of expiratory performance are reached at rest in* C, *during moderate exercise in* B, *and during heavy work in* A. *Patient represented by* C *is dyspneic at rest, and the patient represented by* B *is dyspneic during moderate exercise.*

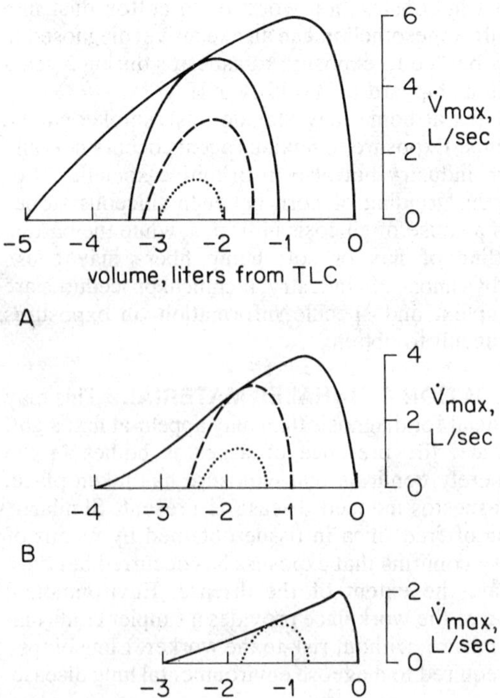

cough. Other chemicals (oxides of nitrogen, chlorine, phosgene, and cadmium fumes) provoke less noxious effects immediately and prolonged exposure may occur; since inflammation of lower airways and pulmonary edema may take several hours to develop, 24-hr observation is indicated after exposure to these fumes. Clinical features following such exposure include cough, expectoration, chest tightness, cyanosis, and dyspnea, with rhonchi, diffuse rales, or both. Roentgenographic change may be minimal despite the presence of severe arterial desaturation; usually, however, pulmonary edema or bronchopneumonia is obvious on the roentgenogram. Arterial oxygen saturation is often low, because of intrapulmonary shunting of blood. Treatment includes administration of steroids to diminish the inflammatory response, of oxygen to combat arterial desaturation, and of antibiotics to prevent infection.

Similar but less acute responses occur in workers in polymerization processes such as the production of rubber and plastic, including polyurethanes. The specific chemicals involved have not been precisely identified, but di-isocyanates, aromatic amines, and aldehydes may be involved. Continued exposure leads to chronic cough, mucus expectoration, and minor hemoptysis, sometimes with low-grade fever and malaise, initially worse at the beginning of the work week but more persistent later. FEV_1 and pulmonary diffusing capacity are reduced, and moderate arterial desaturation may be present; partially reversible airway obstruction also occurs. The chest roentgenograms may show minor patchy and soft opacities. Most patients recover in a few weeks after termination of exposure, but residual disability and permanent lung damage may occur.

Exposure to oxides of nitrogen, as may occur in silo-fillers, may lead to progressive *bronchiolitis obliterans*, with disabling dyspnea due to closure of peripheral airways and restrictive function loss. However, febrile reactions some weeks after silage exposure are probably cases of *farmer's lung* (Chap. 257), rather than of silo-filler's disease.

Metal fumes (Table 258-1) and products of combustion of polymers, notably Teflon, cause *metal-fumes fever*, characterized by febrile reactions, shaking chills, diaphoresis, malaise, and leukocytosis. Pulmonary symptoms and signs may be sparse. Chest roentgenograms are usually normal, and the conditions appear to be benign, may pass for a viral syndrome, and usually last for 24 to 48 hr. Some metals, in particular cadmium, cause severe chemical inflammation as well as fever. Acute *cadmium pneumonitis* is easily misdiagnosed as acute infection; since steroid therapy may be lifesaving in these cases, recognition of the exposure is imperative. A similar syndrome has been observed after severe acute exposures to *beryllium* and its salts.

TABLE 258-1
Acute chemical reactions

Agents	*Industries*
Ammonia	Chemical, refrigeration, coal distillation, fertilizers, explosives
Nitrogen dioxide	Silage, metal etching, explosives, rocket fuels, welding
Acid fumes, HF, HCl, H_2SO_4, HNO_3	Chemical, steel, metal, bleaching, glass and metal etching
Halides (Cl, Br, F)	Chemical, bleaching
Metal fumes, As_2O_3, Cd Oxide, Hg, Ni, Zn, Mn, Cu, Co, Be, V, Al_2O_3	Metal industry, brass and zinc foundries, galvanizing, chrome plating, welding, metal grinding
Phosgene	Munitions, welding (chlorinated solvent)
Osmic acid	Electron microscopy
Polymerizing chemicals, amine accelerator and hardeners, epoxy resins, isocyanates	Rubber, plastics, resins, electron microscopy, polyurethane foam rubber
Plastics, polymers, Teflon, polyethylene	Machining and manufacture of plastics

ASPIRATION PNEUMONIA Aspiration of gastric contents produces an acute inflammation resulting from hydrochloric acid and obstructive atelectasis from inhaled solid materials. The pneumonia frequently progresses to necrosis and suppuration. In addition to the administration of antibiotics, steroids, and oxygen, bronchoscopic aspiration is required when solid materials have been inhaled. A recurrent subacute or chronic lower lobe aspiration pneumonitis occurs in the presence of obstructive esophageal disease, e.g., achalasia, with recurrent aspiration.

ALLERGIC ALVEOLITIS See Chap. 257.

REVERSIBLE AIRWAY OBSTRUCTION Environmental exposures always need to be explored in detail in patients with bronchial asthma (Chap. 67). Sensitization to organic materials occurs in many industries (Table 258-2), but not all these instances are related to IgE-mediated reaginic allergy. Other inhaled agents causing asthma act via direct release of histamine, e.g., textile dusts, platinum salts.

Byssinosis This disease occurs among cotton textile workers (carders and others) and among preparers of flax and soft hemp fibers. Its symptoms include chest tightness, cough, and wheezing, initially on first workdays after a temporary absence from work ("Monday dyspnea"). Chronic respiratory symptoms and permanent dyspnea follow in many cases after 10 to 20 years of exposure. The acute symptoms may occur in up to 70 to 80 percent of all workers exposed to dust in a cotton cardroom.

"Monday dyspnea" in byssinosis goes with decreases of FEV_1 and of flow rates on MEFV curves, and with impairment of intrapulmonary mixing (Fig. 258-1 *C*). Since isoproterenol reverses symptoms and function loss, the airway obstruction in byssinosis is probably caused by contraction of smooth muscle. It is of interest that

TABLE 258-2
Chronic occupational lung diseases

Disease	Agent	Industries	Effects
Mineral dusts			
Aluminosis, bauxite lung	Aluminum and aluminum oxide dusts	Corundum smelting, explosives, paints, fireworks	Fibrosis, bullae, pneumothorax
Asbestosis	Asbestos: Chrysotile Amosite Crocidolite	Insulation, lagging, construction, shipyards, and textiles	Fibrosis, pleural plaques, lung cancer, mesothelioma
Baritosis	$BaSO_4$	Mining	Dust deposits
Beryllium disease	Be compounds	Aircraft manufacturing, metallurgy, rocket fuels	Pneumonitis, granuloma, interstitial fibrosis
Coal workers' pneumoconiosis	Coal dust	Mining, coal trimming, graphite	Dust deposits, fibrosis, bronchitis
Hard-metal pneumoconiosis	Cobalt, tungsten carbide, titanium, tantalum carbide	Cutting tool industry	Interstitial disease
Kaolinosis	Hydrated Al silicates	China clay	Dust deposits, fibrosis
Platinum asthma	Platinum salts	Electronics, chemical	Reversible airway obstruction
Siderosis	Iron oxide	Welding, iron ore mining	Dust deposits
Silicosis	Silica (SiO_2)	Mining (gold, tin, copper, graphite, coal), pottery, sand blasting, foundries, quarries and masonry (granite, slate, sandstone)	Dust deposits, fibrosis
Stannosis	Tin oxide	Smelting	Dust deposits
Talcosis	Hydrated Mg silicates	Rubber industry	Perivascular fibrosis
Organic dusts			
Asthma (see Chap. 67)	Castor bean	Castor oil manufacturing	Reversible airway obstruction
	Flour	Bakeries	
	Tamarind seed	Yarn finishing	
	Gum acacia	Printing industry	
	Grain weevil	Grain handlers	
	Guinea pig hair	Laboratory workers	
	Grass pollen	Gardeners, grounds keepers	
Allergic alveolitis (see Chap. 257)	Various fungi; vegetable dusts and animal matter	Farming, sugar cane (bagasse), mushrooms, malt workers, bird fanciers	Acute and chronic interstitial pneumonitis, fibrosis
		Lumber, sawmills	
Byssinosis	Cotton, flax, and hemp dust	Textiles	Airway obstruction, loss of elastic recoil

textile dusts contain agents that release histamine from nonsensitized human lung in vitro; one of these is derived from the bracts of the cotton boll which contaminate raw cotton. Healthy, nonallergic laboratory subjects have chest tightness and airway obstruction after 10 to 20 min of inhalation of aerosols of tyrode extracts of cotton dust or bracts, the same effects as occur in textile workers after dust exposure. Thus, the acute stage of byssinosis can be adequately explained by chemical agents in textile dusts.

The chronic stage of byssinosis develops most frequently in workers who have suffered from the acute effects of the dust for years. Disabled persons with chronic byssinosis usually have severe airway obstruction and diminished elastic recoil. Varying degrees of chronic bronchitis and emphysema have been found at autopsy to provide a structural basis for these irreversible changes in lung function. Byssinosis was recognized as a compensable disease in Great Britain in 1940.

Di-isocyanates These compounds, including toluene di-isocyanate (TDI), which are used in the manufacture of polyurethane, can cause acute reversible airway obstruction, often more severe at the beginning of the work week. Responses vary from subclinical decreases in FEV_1 to overt wheezing and dyspnea. Chronic exposure causes persistent reductions in FEV_1.

Enzyme detergents The "enzymes" in laundry detergents are concentrated autolysates from *Bacillus subtilis*. In workers exposed to dust of the concentrate, wheezing, chest tightness, dyspnea, and cough develop within a few hours after leaving work. Responses to skin testing do not correspond to the time sequence of the respiratory symptoms. Some enzyme workers have a progressive decrease of lung elastic recoil, which suggests permanent damage of the type found in emphysema. The enzyme material may have a proteolytic action similar to that of papain.

CHRONIC SPECIFIC RESPONSES

The two main forms of chronic parenchymal response to mineral dusts are (1) diffuse interstitial responses, with pleomorphic cellular reactions and diffuse fibrosis, e.g., asbestosis and aluminosis; and (2) focal responses, which occur in silicosis and coal workers' pneumoconiosis. The former present functionally as purely restrictive disease; the latter may combine features of obstructive and restrictive disease.

DIFFUSE INTERSTITIAL RESPONSES These feature progressive dyspnea, dry cough, clubbing of the fingers, increased risk of spontaneous pneumothorax, and diffuse roentgenographic changes (Chap. 254).

Asbestosis Asbestos includes several fibrous minerals, consisting of hydrated silicates. Asbestos fibers are extremely resistant to heat and acid, and have high tensile strength and low electrical conductivity. These properties make asbestos a unique mineral with multiple uses. It is virtually indestructible and persists indefinitely after uptake in the lungs. Autopsies have shown asbestos or ferruginous bodies in the lungs of city dwellers, similar to those in the sputum and lungs of asbestos workers. The origin of the inhaled asbestos is not clear, but there is concern about asbestos-induced disease associated with urban air pollution. The widespread distribution of asbestos fibers and the associated risks have led to a search for safe asbestos substitutes. However, caution should be exercised with the use of any substitute material that is as persistent and indestructible as asbestos.

Asbestosis is an interstitial process which slowly develops into diffuse pulmonary fibrosis after a long latent period. There are instances of massive exposure with a rapid course, but the disease is usually recognized after ten or more years of exposure and then continues to progress even after cessation of exposure. Its incidence has been as high as 15 percent of the population at risk in shipyard and insulation workers.

Aluminosis (bauxite lung) This condition results from exposure to aluminum dust, which may cause a syndrome similar to that found in smelters of metallic corundum in the abrasives industry, in which Al_2O_3 is employed. Acute chemical inflammation may occur, but the usual course is a subacute interstitial pneumonitis with subsequent fibrosis. In addition, metallic aluminum causes a febrile response.

Hard-metal disease The process of hardening metals employs various alloys and metallic carbides, including cobalt, tungsten, manganese, and cadmium. Machining, grinding, and polishing of such metals may cause interstitial pneumonitis and fibrosis. Chronic airway disease with cough and sputum has been described in these workers. In one series of workers exposed to tungsten carbide and cobalt for periods varying from 1 month to over 20 years, 8 of 12 died.

Silicatoses Acute and chronic interstitial disease may occur after exposure to mica, kaolin, or talc dusts; the latter may contain free silica as well as asbestos fibers, which may account for its fibrogenic properties. Fatal cases of kaolin pneumoconiosis with massive fibrosis have been described. Talc has occasionally caused acute lethal disease in infants who were heavily exposed at home.

Berylliosis Acute pneumonitis occurs after heavy exposures, but more commonly there is formation of focal, noncaseating granulomas which are difficult to distinguish from sarcoidosis (Chap. 223). There is, however, no lymph node or ocular involvement or hypercalcemia.

Lipoid pneumonitis Aspiration of oils is rarely an occupational hazard. However, aspiration produces chronic low-grade inflammatory and granulomatous responses which sometimes evoke localized fibrotic reactions; symptoms are few and nonspecific. The chest roentgenogram may show patchy or nodular lesions, particularly at the lung bases. Occasionally, a larger or circumscribed lesion simulating a tumor, the so-called paraffinoma, is produced. The diagnosis of lipoid pneumonitis is suggested by a long history of using oily nasal drops or mineral oil laxatives; it may be confirmed by demonstrating fat-filled macrophages in fresh sputum with Sudan III or IV.

FOCAL RESPONSES **Silicosis** A major component of the earth's crust is free crystalline silica (SiO_2) which occurs in several crystal forms, such as quartz. Mines and other industries with exposure risks to silica dust are listed in Table 258-2. Acute forms of silicosis are now rare. Chronic silicosis, which still occurs in primitive as well as modern industries, usually has a latent period of ten or more years, with gradual worsening of dyspnea on exertion, cough, expectoration, and eventual disability. Advanced cases may develop cor pulmonale, and there is an unexplained high incidence of scleroderma in silicosis. Tuberculosis is still a common complication, though less so than in the past and requires adequate chemotherapy.

The radiologic patterns include diffuse nodular fibrosis, notably in the upper lobes and "calcified rings" or "egg shells," which affect hilar and bronchopulmonary nodes. Lung-function changes are variable and do not correlate well with roentgenographic changes. There may be a combination of restrictive and obstructive defects, the former predominating in advanced cases. The early changes have been inadequately described, but it has been reported that arterial desaturation may occur during exercise at a time that lung volumes are near normal.

There is no specific therapy. In the early stages of the disease one must decide whether or not to advise the patient to stop work. Although there are no adequate data on postexposure progression, we believe that termination of exposure is advisable. Silicosis is still a significant hazard, especially when organized industrial medical surveillance is lacking.

Coal workers' pneumoconiosis (CWP) Lung disease among coal miners was recognized as a compensable occupational disease in Great Britain in 1936 and in some states in the United States in the 1960s. A "Black Lung" Act has provided compensation to all eligible coal miners in the United States since 1969. The prevalence of CWP varies with the type of coal mined, its silica content, and perhaps its content of aluminum and iron oxide. Silica increases the risk, while aluminum and iron oxide may render CWP more benign. Mechanization may increase dust production; construction of shafts and tunnels poses high risks. The prevalence of CWP is high; in one United States study which included retired miners, roentgenograms revealed pneumoconiosis in 46 percent.

Although inhaled dust contains carbon and varying amounts of silica, there is no longer any doubt that CWP can occur in the absence of silica exposure; typical lesions occur in lungs without silica deposits, and pure carbon dust (graphite) can cause CWP. The lesions include deposits of carbon dust along respiratory bronchioles, with development of a reticulin fiber network and bronchiolar widening due to loss of wall structure. Thus, early lesions in CWP include dilatation of respiratory bronchioles and centrilobular emphysema. At this stage ventilatory function may be normal, but gas distribution and ventilation/perfusion relations may already be disturbed. At a later stage, nodular lesions appear, with a radial type of fibrosis and a preponderance of reticulin rather than collagen fibers. Silicotic nodules may be found if there is concomitant SiO_2 exposure; progressive massive fibrosis is discussed on page 1296. Caplan has described an association between seropositive rheumatoid arthritis and CWP.

Other dust deposits Several mineral dusts are inhaled and deposited in the lungs and elicit only minimal tissue responses. These include iron oxide (siderosis), tin oxide (stannosis), and barium sulfate (baritosis). In mining iron oxide there may be associated SiO_2 exposure and thus silicosis.

CIGARETTE SMOKING Cigarette smoking accounts for a large excess in mortality and morbidity due to lung cancer and chronic airway obstruction, as well as in cardiovascular and peripheral vascular disease. Cigarette smoke contains a complex mixture of particulates and volatile substances, several of which have biologic actions. For instance, "tar" contains several chemical substances which can induce cancerous lesions experimentally. Nicotine in smoke may be responsible for pharmacologic dependence on cigarettes; other constituents of smoke release histamine from lung tissue, stop the ciliary beat, delay particle clearance from lungs, cause reflex bronchoconstriction, induce changes in alveolar macrophage cells and their function, and cause cytotoxic effects in lung explants. Carbon monoxide is an important constituent of the smoke (see page 1319).

Long-term smokers often have chronic cough, sputum production, and increased dyspnea on exertion, as well as a greatly increased risk of lung cancer. Function studies show airway obstruction, loss of diffusing capacity, and decreased arterial oxygen tension, especially in the supine position. After only 3 to 5 years of smoking, teenagers have an excess of respiratory symptoms and decreased flow rates on MEFV curves (Fig. 258-1*B*). The anatomic substrate for these functional changes is unknown, and in young people the changes are probably partially reversible. Progression of airway obstruction in people who continue to smoke is inferred from the severe disease found in older smokers. Abolition of cigarette smoking would probably be the single most important measure for decreasing the prevalence, morbidity, and mortality rates of lung disease. Such programs are particularly needed in industries where there may be interaction between cigarette smoke and industrial dust, such as the asbestos industry.

PLEURAL DISEASE (see also Chap. 261) Asbestos exposure is frequently associated with pleural lesions, including symptomless calcified plaques which occur on the visceral pleura and in interlobar fissures, with frequent involvement of diaphragmatic and pericardial surfaces. Asbestos may also produce mesotheliomas of the pleura and the peritoneum. The asbestos exposure has always occurred at least 20 years previously and may have been of relatively short duration (1 to 3 years). Clinically, these malignant tumors are often silent until local invasion has occurred, and they are generally inoperable once diagnosed. Asbestos fibers, which are long and thin, probably cause pleural disease by inhalation and penetration of the pleura. The risk is greater with the straight fibers of amphibole asbestos (crocidolite, amosite) than with the curled chrysotile fibers, but both cause pleural disease when injected into the pleural cavity of animals.

LUNG CANCER (see also Chap. 260) An increased risk of developing bronchogenic carcinoma has been documented for workers exposed to asbestos, chromates, nickel, arsenic, radioactive dusts, and possibly for those exposed to beryllium. The association between occupation and lung cancer is best documented for asbestos, where there is also evidence for positive interaction between cigarette smoke and asbestos as etiologic agents. Cigarette smoking remains the major cause of lung cancer, in terms of the total number of persons affected.

AIR POLLUTION

In the past few decades, acute air pollution disasters occurring in Donora, Pennsylvania; in the Meuse Valley, Belgium; and in London have demonstrated that large masses of air severely contaminated with smoke and other industrial and domestic wastes can cause large increases in morbidity and mortality rates from lung disease.

At present there is increasing concern about the long-term health hazards of levels of air pollution commonly present in urban air. Though there is no doubt that some air pollutants can have acute effects on the respiratory tract, their contribution to the prevalence of chronic respiratory diseases is not well established, although evidence is mounting that they may aggravate preexisting lung diseases. Statistical studies based on mortality data, hospital admissions, and similar indices point to an association between urban residence and the prevalence of chronic bronchitis and emphysema, but the "urban factors" have not been precisely defined and need not be identical with air pollution.

Children living in high-pollution areas in the United Kingdom have a higher prevalence of lower respiratory tract infections than do controls in low-pollution areas. The prevalence of chronic cough and sputum in nonsmoking, not occupationally exposed women over sixty-five years of age has been found to correlate significantly with residence in low- or high-pollution areas. In North American studies, more respiratory symptoms and lower values for various lung functions have been found in a random sample of an industrialized area than in a rural community; correction for smoking habits did not abolish this difference. These and similar studies suggest deleterious chronic effects of polluted air on respiratory symptoms, although proof for this is not yet at hand. Physicians should probably advise patients with serious chronic lung disease who live in high-pollution areas to move to a clean-air area. The matter should, however, be put in the proper perspective; such a move makes sense only if the patient has stopped smoking and is not exposed to occupational or other specific pollutants.

The two main types of polluted air masses are oxidant smog and reducing smog.

OXIDANT SMOG The "Los Angeles-type" smog arises by photochemical oxidation of products of automobile exhaust in atmospheric air. Since oxidant smog is linked with sunlight and traffic patterns, it shows striking diurnal variations, with peak levels a few hours after the morning rush hour. Its main components are oxides of nitrogen (an unstable mixture of several oxides), ozone, nitroolefins, and peroxyacetyl nitrate. Oxidant smog clearly needs to be controlled, since its components have important biologic actions. Ozone concentrations similar to those in oxidant smog cause significant changes in lung function in acute experiments. NO_2 and O_3 impair pulmonary bacterial clearance, but whether this promotes lung infections is unclear. NO_2 [1 part per million (ppm)] for several hours causes lipid peroxidation of unsaturated fatty acids, and O_3 impairs bronchial mucus lysozyme activity and decreases the number of sulfhydryl groups in lung tissue.

SULFUR DIOXIDE This is an irritant gas, a major component of reducing smog, that is largely absorbed in upper airways. It causes changes in lung function in concentrations of about 1 ppm, higher than those in urban air. SO_2 may, however, dissolve in water and form ionic SO_3; it is also possible that SO_2 and its derivatives can be adsorbed on particles and thus reach the airways in concentrated form. In any case, measurement of SO_2 levels indicates the amount of air pollution produced by burning of fossil fuels, as occurs in industry, home heating, and power plants.

PARTICULATES Particles are responsible for lack of visibility, soiling, and similar undesirable effects of air pollution. Even relatively inert particles can affect the airways, although large amounts are required to reproduce such effects in the laboratory. The size and shape of particles and their chemical constituents are more important than their absolute quantities. Specific particles with demonstrated health hazards that may be associated with community exposures are asbestos, coal dust, and cotton dust.

CARBON MONOXIDE (CO) This pollutant, contained in cigarette smoke and automobile exhaust, is one cause of toxic effects from smoke inhalation during fires or from improperly vented domestic water heaters. It combines avidly with hemoglobin; low levels of CO (in the order of 10 ppm) produce significant defects in O_2 transport by excluding hemoglobin from combination with O_2 and also by impairment of O_2 unloading at the periphery, with a shift to the left of the hemoglobin-O_2 dissociation curve (Chap. 29). Low levels of inspired CO may be associated with subtle decrements in performance. Severe exposures lead to frequently fatal anoxia (when CO in the hemoglobin exceeds 50 percent of the total hemoglobin), to acute myocardial infarction, or to anoxic brain damage. Recovery from the latter may be incomplete; parkinsonism may be a late complication. The symptoms of chronic CO intoxication, resulting from repeated or continuous low-level exposures, include those of anemia and disturbances of mental function. Occupational CO exposures occur in traffic policemen, vehicular tunnel personnel, and blast furnace workmen. Such persons may be exposed to levels of 30 to 50 ppm CO for several hours; the long-term effects of such exposures are not well documented but may be significant. Protective devices should be recommended in these situations.

OTHER HEALTH EFFECTS OF AIR POLLUTION There is no conclusive evidence that community air pollution is a causal factor in lung cancer, although asthma may be precipitated by pollutants. Widespread low-grade exposure results from the presence of lead in automobile exhaust, but has so far not been demonstrated to be a significant health hazard.

PREVENTION AND CONTROL

SMOKING By abandoning smoking, many physicians have set an example that will help to decrease the prevalence of lung disease. The motives involved in smoking are complex, but individual counseling and mass media propaganda against smoking have made limited inroads on the problem. Rational programs, directed at youth in particular, must be developed to reduce the prevalence of smoking. A "safe cigarette" does not exist, since any type of smoked organic material exposes the smoker, at a minimum, to inhalation of CO.

AIR POLLUTION Current pollution levels usually cause subtle and even equivocal health effects, but deterioration of the prevailing air quality in cities must be prevented. Stringent control of sources of air pollution (automobile exhaust, fossil fuel burning, and other industrial effluents) is required to prevent pollution levels from increasing beyond their current range.

OCCUPATIONAL ENVIRONMENT Here, the physician can have a direct impact on prevention and control programs, since the absence of disease should be the final criterion for their success. Until recently, the emphasis has been on control of industrial exposures by technical methods to limit exposure to established "safe" levels, termed "threshold limit values." In recent years, medical and environmental studies have shown that for several substances, such as asbestos, cotton dust, and radioactive materials, no unequivocal "safe limits" can be set. As exposure decreases, the risk becomes less but does not disappear. Thus, a radical change in the approach toward prevention and control of certain occupational diseases is in order. Engineering controls alone are no longer sufficient, since even with modern controls some persons will probably continue to have health effects resulting from minimal exposure. The addition of medical surveillance is required to detect and protect individuals at risk.

Technical control of exposure may include substitution of nonhazardous materials, prevention of accidents with irritants, or changes in industrial procedures. Dust sources must be enclosed and provided with exhaust and dust collection systems, whose effectiveness should be assessed by measuring the actual dust levels existing in workrooms. Masks are needed during short hazardous exposures, or as emergency measures until technical controls can be implemented.

Medical surveillance includes preemployment and periodic medical examinations. Persons with preexisting lung disease should usually not be assigned to dusty work areas. Periodic examinations should include a full-sized chest roentgenogram and pulmonary function tests, including vital capacity and FEV_1, in all industries in which occupational lung diseases occur. Transfer to other work should be advised only after full consideration of medical as well as financial, social, and legal implications for the worker. For instance, the risk of progression of silicosis must be weighed against financial and social factors (decreased wage, loss of seniority) involved in a transfer. Such arbitrary judgments can largely be avoided if adequate environmental control is practiced in industry.

REFERENCES

AYRES SM, BUEHLER ME: The effects of urban air pollution on health. Clin Pharmacol Ther 11:337, 1970

BOHLIG H et al: UICC/Cincinnati classification of the radiographic appearances of pneumoconioses. Chest 58(1):57, 1970

BOUHUYS A: *Breathing—Physiology, Environment and Lung Disease,* New York, Grune and Stratton, 1974.

The Health Consequences of Smoking: A Report of the Surgeon General, 1972, U. S. Dept. of Health, Education, and Welfare Publ. 72-7516

LOURENCO RV (guest ed): Inhaled aerosol symposium. Arch Int Med 131(1), 1973

PATTY FA (ed): *Industrial Hygiene and Toxicology,* 2d ed., 2 vols., New York: Interscience, 1958 and 1963

SPENCER H.: *Pathology of the Lung,* 2d ed., Oxford: Pergamon, 1968

Task Force on Research Planning in Environmental Health Science: *Man's Health and the Environment,* Washington: U.S. Government Printing Office, 1970

259 PRIMARY PULMONARY HYPERTENSION

JOHN ROSS, JR.

Primary (or idiopathic) pulmonary hypertension is an uncommon disease, the diagnosis of which can be established only after a thorough search for the usual causes of pulmonary hypertension. The patient with primary pulmonary hypertension typically is a young female between the ages of twenty and forty, although older and younger patients of either sex have been described. The clinical and laboratory features of severe pulmonary hypertension are present, but there is no evidence of parenchymal pulmonary disease or organic cardiac disease, nor is there cause to suspect the occurrence of pulmonary emboli. In the past, anatomic verification often has been necessary to distinguish clearly the primary form of pulmonary hypertension from that due to multiple pulmonary emboli, although angiography and radioisotope scanning methods have facilitated this differentiation considerably.

PATHOLOGY The findings on pathologic examination of patients with primary pulmonary hypertension usually are confined to the right side of the heart and lungs. The right atrium often is enlarged and the right ventricle is hypertrophied. Frequently, the large pulmonary arteries exhibit atherosclerotic plaques. The disease process involves the small pulmonary arteries (between 40 and 300 μm in diameter), which exhibit muscular hypertrophy and intimal hyperplasia, sometimes with fibrosis. Abnormal vascular structures or plexiform lesions also have been described and are attributed by some investigators to recanalization of thrombi, by others to abnormal vascular anastomoses. On occasion, a necrotizing arteritis may be encountered. Fowler and his associates have contrasted these pathologic findings with those in thromboembolic pulmonary hypertension, in which similar disease of the small pulmonary vessels may be observed, but in addition thrombotic material is present in the larger pulmonary vessels (300 μm to 1.5 mm in diameter). Rarely, disease of the systemic arterial vascular bed resembling that found in the pulmonary blood vessels has been described. The syncope and sudden death which may occur in this disease has been attributed to involvement of the coronary arterial branch supplying the sinoatrial node.

ETIOLOGY The cause of primary pulmonary hypertension is unknown, but a number of possible etiologic factors have been suggested. A few patients with primary pulmonary hypertension have been reported in whom minimal changes were found in the pulmonary vessels on pathologic examination, and this observation has raised the possibility that a neurohumoral vasoconstrictor mechanism is involved. Support for this view has been provided by the observation that the pulmonary vascular resistance can be acutely reduced in some patients with this disease by the intrapulmonary injection of vasodilators, or by breathing oxygen. A febrile illness may precede the onset of the disease by a variable period and has been implicated in the etiology. The occurrence of the disease in young females has prompted the suggestion that unrecognized thromboemboli or amniotic fluid emboli during pregnancy may play a role. In other patients, it seems quite possible that the disease may represent an end stage of earlier, unrecognized emboli originating from the legs or pelvic veins.

Raynaud's disease has preceded the onset of primary pulmonary hypertensive disease by a number of years in an appreciable number of patients. This association and the occurrence of Raynaud's disease in scleroderma, disseminated lupus erythematosus, rheumatoid arthritis, and dermatomyositis have led to the speculation that primary pulmonary hypertension may represent a form of collagen vascular disease. It also has been suggested that the disease may be congenital and present from birth; however, the closely packed, parallel elastic fibers in the main pulmonary arteries in patients having Eisenmenger's syndrome from birth, described by Heath and Edwards, usually have not been observed in patients with primary pulmonary hypertension. Finally, primary pulmonary hypertension has been reported in a number of families; sometimes more than two members and up to three generations have been affected.

PATHOPHYSIOLOGY Some studies have suggested that the response of the pulmonary vascular bed is labile early in the course of this disease, as evidenced by a response to vasodilating agents and oxygen. It also has been proposed that the disease tends to progress. Thus, serial cardiac catheterizations have shown a tendency for the pulmonary vascular resistance to increase and to become fixed. With the development of severe pulmonary vascular disease, abnormal elevation of the pulmonary arterial pressure occurs, often to a striking degree, and the pulmonary arterial pressure may be equal to that in the systemic arterial bed. The pulmonary arterial wedge pressure is normal in patients with primary pulmonary hypertension, the cardiac output is normal or reduced, and no intracardiac shunts are detected. In many patients the mean right atrial pressure is elevated, and the A wave in the right atrium may be markedly elevated, an indication of the forceful atrial contraction necessary to fill the hypertrophied right ventricle. With the long-standing overload on the right side of the heart, right ventricular failure finally develops. In some patients, peripheral cyanosis occurs secondary to reduced cardiac output, and occasionally central cyanosis becomes evident at the end stage of the disease due to right to left shunting through a patent foramen ovale. Mild systemic arterial desaturation is quite common, even in the absence of heart failure, and may be due to shunting within the lungs. Pulmonary function in patients with primary pulmonary hypertension generally is normal, although hyperventilation often is present, resulting in hypocapnia and a decreased serum bicarbonate concentration.

CLINICAL PICTURE

The patient, usually a young female, gives a history of relatively recent onset of symptoms. Ordinarily, the natural course of the disease encompasses less than 5 years. Not uncommonly, patients with primary pulmonary hypertension are classified as neurotic early in the course of their disease because of the hyperventilation, chest discomfort, and the relative paucity of objective findings. Precordial pain on exertion occurs in from 25 to 50 percent of patients, and occasionally severe chest pain has been associated with a dissection of the main pulmonary artery. Other common symptoms are weakness, fatigue, exertional dyspnea, and effort syncope. Hoarseness may be noted because of compression of the left recurrent laryngeal nerve by the enlarged pulmonary artery. Unexplained, sudden death occurs relatively often. Sudden death also has occurred during cardiac catheterization or surgical procedures and after the administration of barbiturates or anesthetic agents. The terminal course usually is characterized by right-sided heart failure.

On physical examination, the jugular venous pulse usually shows a prominent A wave, there is a right ventricular heave, and an impulse may be felt over the region of the main pulmonary artery. An ejection click may be audible at the pulmonic area, the second heart sound is narrowly split, and the pulmonic closure sound is markedly accentuated. Often, an atrial gallop sound is heard at the lower left sternal border, and in some patients there is an ejection murmur at the pulmonic area, or the early diastolic murmur of pulmonic regurgitation. The chest roentgenogram may show cardiac enlargement with right ventricular and right atrial prominence, and there is marked dilatation of the pulmonary artery segment. Peripherally, the pulmonary arteries taper sharply, and the lung fields appear oligemic. The electrocardiogram almost always shows some evidence of right ventricular enlargement, with right axis deviation, right ventricular hypertrophy in the precordial leads, and sometimes inverted T waves over the right precordium. Right atrial enlargement also may be evident on the electrocardiogram.

DIFFERENTIAL DIAGNOSIS It is imperative that the diagnosis of primary pulmonary hypertension not be made until potentially treatable causes of elevated pulmonary arterial pressure have been excluded. The presence of pulmonary hypertension and cor pulmonale caused by chronic pulmonary disease can be established readily by finding abnormalities in pulmonary function. Cardiac catheterization studies are necessary to search for a primary cardiac defect, and angiography or radioactive lung-scanning studies also may be indicated to detect pulmonary emboli (Chap. 256). Patients having chronic emboli to the lungs are difficult to distinguish from those with primary pulmonary hypertension, but the distinction is important because anticoagulants, inferior vena caval or common femoral vein ligation, and pulmonary embolectomy sometimes have been effective in patients with embolic disease. Often a site of origin for emboli cannot be identified in the leg veins, and other possible sources should be considered, such as right atrial thrombus, or ovarian and pelvic vein thromboses.

Several congenital cardiac conditions must be considered and excluded by appropriate cardiac catheterization studies. Valvular pulmonic stenosis usually can be distinguished from pulmonary hypertension by identification of the delayed, soft pulmonic closure sound, but peripheral stenoses of the pulmonary arteries may be associated with an increased second heart sound. A left-to-right shunt at the pulmonary arterial, ventricular, or atrial levels should be sought. The wide, fixed splitting of the second heart sound should be helpful in identifying patients with atrial septal defect. Eisenmenger's syndrome in a patient with ventricular septal defect or patent ductus arteriosus (Chap. 237) may be confused with primary pulmonary hypertension, but usually in Eisenmenger's syndrome cyanosis, polycythemia, and clubbing are present, and at cardiac catheterization a large right-to-left shunt at the ventricular or pulmonary arterial level can be demonstrated.

The murmurs of tricuspid or pulmonic regurgitation, and the atrial gallop sounds heard in patients with primary pulmonary hypertension may be mistaken for the murmurs of rheumatic mitral and aortic valve disease, or vice versa. Before making the diagnosis of primary pulmonary hypertension, the presence of left atrial hypertension due to undetected mitral stenosis, or to a more unusual lesion such as left atrial myxoma, should be specifically sought and excluded. This can be done by obtaining a pulmonary arterial wedge pressure tracing or by catheterization of the left side of the heart, with angiography if necessary.

THERAPY Presently, no definitive treatment is available for patients with primary pulmonary hypertension, and therapy during their progressive downhill course therefore must be palliative. The use of anticoagulants is of doubtful value, provided chronic pulmonary embolic phenomena can be excluded. Right-sided heart failure should be treated with a cardiotonic and diuretic regimen (Chap. 233). Since there is no hypercapnia in these patients, the hypoxia which may accompany heart failure can be treated safely with oxygen therapy.

Pharmacologic approaches to therapy have proved disappointing, and though transient reductions in pulmonary vascular resistance may be observed with intrapulmonary arterial injection of acetylcholine or tolazoline, the chronic oral use of these agents has not been effective. The possibility of performing total lung transplantation has, of course, been under consideration for many years, and much experimental work is directed toward this goal.

REFERENCES

BLOUNT SG JR, GROVER RF: Pulmonary hypertension, chap. 66 in *The Heart*, 3d ed., ed JW Hurst, New York: McGraw-Hill, 1974

FOWLER NO et al: Idiopathic and thromboembolic pulmonary hypertension. Am J Med 40:331, 1966

MELMON KL, BRAUNWALD E: Familial pulmonary hypertension. N Engl J Med 269:770, 1963

WALCOTT G et al: Primary pulmonary hypertension Am J Med 49:70, 1970

WINTERS WL JR et al: Pulmonary hypertension and Raynaud's phenomenon. Arch Intern Med 114:821, 1964

260 NEOPLASMS OF THE LUNG

GENNARO M. TISI

At the turn of the century Adler, in his classical monograph, was able to collect only 374 cases of cancer of the lung from the world's literature. During the past 50 years, there has been a slow but steady increase in the incidence of cancer of the lung. Currently, lung cancer is the most common form of malignancy in the male, reaching a peak between the fifth and seventh decades and accounting for 1 in 4 male cancer deaths. The sex incidence is at least 5 to 1, male to female.

EPIDEMIOLOGY

It has been approximately 30 years since Müller first drew attention to the relationship between lung cancer and heavy cigarette smoking. Extensive statistical analysis has confirmed this relationship. It has been demonstrated that the more cigarettes a person smokes, the greater is his risk of developing cancer of the lung. Hammond and Horn report the death rate in cancer of the lung per hundred thousand is 3.4 in the male nonsmoker; 59.3 for ten to twenty cigarettes daily; and 217.3 for forty or more cigarettes daily. If a person stops smoking, he is less likely to develop lung cancer than his counterpart who continues to smoke. Although smoking has attracted the principal interest in the epidemiology of lung cancer, other factors also have been implicated. Considerable attention has been directed to the potential role of air pollution, exposure to ionizing radiation, and numerous occupational hazards, including exposure to chromates, metallic iron and iron oxides, arsenic, nickel, beryllium, and asbestos. In many tissues, chronic inflammatory changes are known to precede cancer. In the lung, fibrosis may follow focal destructive and proliferative lesions. Numerous studies report an increased incidence of peripheral adenocarcinomas in such areas of chronic scarring (so-called "scar carcinoma").

PATHOLOGY

Primary cancer of the lung can be classified, in terms of its anatomic location, into *central* or *peripheral* categories. Central lesions involve the tracheobronchial tree from the primary to the distal bronchi, while peripheral lesions involve the distal bronchi and bronchioles. The relative frequency of cancer of the lung, when divided into these broad anatomic categories, is approximately equal. This simple classification helps in understanding many of the vagaries of the clinical presentation, the pattern of growth, the avenues of metastasis, and the preferential diagnostic approach.

There is not universal agreement on the histologic classification of primary pulmonary carcinoma. The classification offered here has been selected because it stresses the correlation between a histologic pattern and particular mode of clinical-pathologic behavior. Four basic histologic patterns of primary lung cancer and their approximate relative incidences are recognized: (1) *Squamous cell* carcinoma (epidermoid carcinoma)—60 percent; (2) *adenocarcinoma*—15 percent; (3) *undifferentiated* or anaplastic carcinoma including the round-cell, large-cell, and oat cell types—20 percent; and (4) *bronchioloalveolar* cell carcinoma (alveolar cell carcinoma)—2 percent. In some instances it is difficult to discern a uniform histologic pattern, and this leads to the diagnosis of mixed patterns.

With reference to this histologic classification, the following observations should be considered: (1) Squamous cell or epidermoid carcinoma is virtually always associated with cigarette smoking, usually occurs in central locations, produces earlier symptoms due to the potential for bronchial obstruction, spreads generally by continuity, and may undergo cavitation; (2) adenocarcinoma has been associated with focal lung scars and chronic interstitial fibrosis, occurs primarily in peripheral locations, may spread by all routes but particularly by the bloodstream, and often remains clinically silent until distant hematogenous metastases occur; (3) undifferentiated carcinoma is found in a relatively younger age group than the other types, occurs predominantly in the male (as does squamous cell carcinoma), occurs with equal frequency in central and peripheral areas, and metastasizes early; and (4) bronchioloalveolar cell carcinoma classically presents with a diffuse or multinodular type of lesion, significant bronchorrhea, progressive dyspnea, and increasing hypoxemia usually associated with hyperventilation. This combination of hypoxemia and hypocapnia is classical of diffuse interstitial processes. Considerable controversy centers on whether alveolar cell carcinoma has a multicentric or unicentric origin. The principal evidence favors a unicentric origin, providing philosophically a brighter approach to therapy.

Primary carcinoma of the lung may spread by any of four routes: (1) direct local extension; (2) hematogenous dissemination; (3) lymphatic spread; and uncommonly (4) transbronchial spread. The preferential sites of extrapulmonary metastasis include the prescalene lymph nodes, liver, brain, adrenal glands, and bones.

CLINICAL PRESENTATION

PRIMARY TUMORS The clinical presentation of carcinoma of the lung depends upon many variables including cell type; site of origin; the concept of biologic predetermination of cancer behavior; and immunologic mechanisms, at present poorly understood. The resulting symptom complexes should be viewed as constituting two modes of presentation: early and late.

The *early* mode of presentation has special clinical significance because a reasonable expectation of cure can be anticipated. In this stage of the disease, a patient may present with symptoms attributable to an intrabronchial lesion, such as a mild cough or a change in the pattern of a chronic cigarette cough. He may instead have symptoms secondary to local bronchial obstruction and/or surrounding inflammation including fever, chills, sputum production, a localized wheeze, or hemoptysis. The latter is alarming but a presenting symptom in only 7 to 10 percent of patients. In many instances a patient may be entirely asymptomatic, the sole reason for referral to medical attention being an abnormal chest roentgenogram. Unfortunately, in the early cases, the physical examination may be entirely negative. A localized wheeze over a segmental bronchus brought out by a forced expiratory or panting maneuver may be an early sign. As the lesion progresses, the classical physical signs due to obstruction may develop, including those of atelectasis, pneumonitis, abscess formation, and loss of lung volume.

The *late* mode of presentation indicates that a lesion has extended beyond the stage of resectional or curative surgery. In this stage of his disease, depending upon the degree or direction of spread, a patient may present with one or a combination of the following: (1) nonspecific systemic symptoms; (2) signs and symptoms of intrathoracic spread; (3) signs and symptoms of extrathoracic extension; and (4) classical systemic syndromes.

A patient with advanced disease may present with *nonspecific systemic* symptoms such as weight loss, anorexia, nausea and vomiting, and weakness. The longer the duration of such symptoms, the more likely the lesion is nonresectable.

When the patient is first seen, evidence for *intrathoracic spread* already may be present. Evidence for such spread includes hoarseness, due to involvement of the recurrent laryngeal nerve; pleuritis with or without effusion, due to pleural extension; a unilaterally paralyzed diaphragm with paradoxical motion, due to involvement of the phrenic nerve; dysphagia due to esophageal involvement; Horner's syndrome, due to involvement of the cervical thoracic sympathetic nerves; and superior vena caval obstruction due to entrapment of the superior vena cava.

Symptoms of *extrathoracic spread* or distant metastasis may also be present. The symptoms in any given patient depend upon the sites of metastasis. Commonly involved are one or more of the following: prescalene lymph nodes, brain, liver, adrenal glands, and bone.

The fourth symptom complex includes numerous *systemic syndromes.* These syndromes are of diagnostic value in that, in some instances, they may antedate the roentgenographic appearance of a pulmonary lesion. The list of syndromes associated with cancer of the lung (particularly the oat cell variety) continues to grow. This intriguing array of classical systemic syndromes can be divided into five categories: (1) *metabolic* including hypercalcemia, the syndrome of inappropriate ADH secretion, Cushing's syndrome, gynecomastia, and carcinoid syndrome (the latter is usually associated with bronchial adenoma); (2) *neuromuscular* including peripheral neuropathy, corticocerebellar degeneration, and nonspecific myopathy; (3) *connective tissue* abnormalities including hypertrophic pulmonary osteoarthropathy, clubbing, and nonspecific arthralgias; (4) *dermatologic* abnormalities including acanthosis nigricans and dermatomyositis; (5) *vascular* abnormalities including thrombocytopenic purpura, leukemoid reaction, myelophthisic anemia, and nonbacterial thrombotic endocarditis.

Two modes of presentation deserve separate mention: the patient with a solitary pulmonary nodule (coin lesion) and the patient with a bronchial adenoma.

A *solitary pulmonary nodule* is one with minimal satellite lesions in the pulmonary parenchyma and normally aerated lung around it. Its shape may be round or oval; lobulations, if present, must be minimal. Its margins are circumscribed and its contour smooth, and there must be minimal, if any, associated pneumonitis, atelectasis, or regional adenopathy. Most patients with such a lesion have no symptoms on initial questioning, but upon closer interrogation, a number may admit to a slight cough. Several roentgenographic features should be stressed. The presence of indentation or umbilication of the nodule's border has been referred to as a potential sign of malignancy ("notch sign"). Review of old roentgenograms is of particular importance in the evaluation of a patient with a solitary pulmonary nodule, since a demonstrable increase in size suggests that the lesion is neoplastic. The pattern of calcification within a lesion is of paramount importance. The presence of a calcific fleck or of peripheral calcification does not exclude the presence of a malignant lesion. However, centrally located or "core" calcification, lamination, and dense generalized calcification are often associated with benign lesions. In reviewing series of resected solitary pulmonary nodules, one must bear in mind that preoperative evaluation excludes the obviously benign lesions, and therefore these surgical series are weighted to favor a higher incidence of malignant lesions. In 1956, Davis collected 1,203 cases of resected solitary pulmonary nodules from the literature. Of resected lesions, 36.7 percent were malignant, with bronchogenic carcinoma comprising the major subgroup. The remaining 63.3 percent were benign, with granulomas accounting for approximately two-thirds of the benign group. In the individual patient surgical excision remains the only absolute assurance of benignity.

Bronchial adenomas (carcinoid bronchial adenoma) comprise 3 to 10 percent of all surgically excised pulmonary neoplasms. They are primarily central in location with approximately 90 percent visible at bronchoscopy. The characteristics of central location, slow growth, and marked vascularity account for the common types of clinical presentation: (1) recurrent hemoptysis; (2) localized wheezing; (3) infection distal to bronchial obstruction; and (4) history often antedating diagnosis by 5 or more years. Distant blood-borne metastases are rare. Bronchial adenoma, like oat cell carcinoma, has been associated with multiple endocrinopathies.

METASTATIC TUMORS The pulmonary capillaries, with a mean cross-sectional diameter of 12 μm, are ideally suited to the entrapment of tumor emboli. This feature and the rich lymphatic supply of the lung account, in large part, for the high incidence of metastatic (secondary) carcinoma in the lung. The great majority of pulmonary metastatic lesions are adenocarcinomas from the gastrointestinal tract, genitourinary tract, and glandular tissues. Metastases to the lung are usually spherical in shape, variable in size, multiple, and bilateral. These roentgenographic features combined with symptoms suggesting an extrapulmonary source help in the differential diagnosis of primary from metastatic carcinoma.

Early diagnosis and improved therapy have produced an increase in the number of long-term survivors of nonpulmonary, primary malignancies. If such a surviving patient presents with a new pulmonary lesion in the course of his long-term follow-up, what are the etiologic possibilities? The problem of distinguishing among late metastasis to the lung, a new primary in the lung, or a benign pulmonary lesion has been reviewed by Adkins. The majority of such patients will present with ancillary evidence of metastatic spread from the original primary tumor. The pattern of spread will depend upon the sites of predilection of the original primary. However, if the patient is asymptomatic and if diagnostic evaluation fails to provide evidence for other distant metastases, a substantial percentage of such lesions will prove to be either a new primary or a benign lesion.

DIAGNOSTIC EVALUATION

There are three principal aims in the diagnostic evaluation of a patient with carcinoma of the lung: (1) identification of the lesion as a carcinoma; (2) determination whether the pulmonary lesion has extended *(a)* beyond the pulmonary parenchyma and *(b)* beyond the thoracic cavity; and (3) preoperative cardiopulmonary evaluation to determine whether the patient with an operable lesion will be able to tolerate the degree of resection anticipated.

In most instances, the initial diagnostic approach is *roentgenographic*. Many times the x-ray may display the only abnormality in an asymptomatic patient. In all cases, inquiries about past roentgenograms should be made, and every attempt should be made to obtain these films promptly. The initial x-ray lesion may be of any size, shape, or location. Early roentgenographic signs include the solitary pulmonary nodule, areas of localized overinflation due to intrabronchial obstruction, atelectasis with unilateral loss of volume, and the appearance of localized inflammatory changes. All patients over the age of forty with pneumonia should be followed with serial chest films to the point of complete resolution. Such an approach may lead to the diagnosis of a slowly resolving pneumonia and be the first indication of carcinoma of the lung. Roentgenographic signs of intrathoracic spread include pleural thickening and/or effusion (providing an inflammatory basis is excluded), elevation of a diaphragm, rib erosion, hilar metastasis, and lymphatic obstruction with Kerly B lines. Multiple roentgenographic views, including lateral and oblique projections, and tomography may be invaluable in defining the features described above, particularly the presence of calcification within solitary pulmonary nodules. Fluoroscopy may help in determining the mobility of a diaphragm and in differentiation of neoplastic processes from vascular lesions, granulomatous diseases, inflammatory lesions, thromboemboli, and artifacts. Common artifacts include chest wall lesions such as warts and hemangiomas, nipple shadows, and technical artifacts due to film processing.

The triad of bronchoscopy, scalene lymph node biopsy, and cytologic smear will provide information on both the tissue diagnosis and the extension of lung cancer. *Bronchoscopy* and bronchoscopic biopsy are of principal value in central epidermoid carcinomas. Lower-lobe tumors, which less commonly metastasize to the anterior scalene nodes, are usually accessible to bronchoscopy and bronchoscopic biopsy. It has been reported that a positive diagnosis of epidermoid carcinoma can be established in 26 to 60 percent of patients by means of bronchoscopy and bronchoscopic biopsy. Bronchoscopy is obviously of less value in peripheral adenocarcinomas. However, it is significant that *scalene node biopsy* is most successful in the diagnosis of those lung cancers which are inaccessible to bronchoscopy. The yield in scalene node biopsy is greater when the lesion involves the upper rather than the lower lobes, and greater when the lesion is a peripheral adeno- or undifferentiated carcinoma than when it is a central squamous cell carcinoma. The side selected for a scalene node biopsy should preferentially include the side of parenchymal involvement and all palpable nodes. Reports of *cytologic smears* illustrate considerable lack of uniformity and success in the detection of lung cancer. The primary variables here are the training of the cytologist and the method of sputum collection. The range of positive cytologic smears has been reported anywhere from 44 to 95 percent. Most observers have noted a decreased yield in the cytodiagnosis of peripherally situated lung carcinomas compared to more centrally located lesions.

If a pleural effusion is observed as an isolated presentation or related to a parenchymal lesion, *thoracentesis* and *needle biopsy* of the *pleura* should be performed. The fluid should be sent for cytologic analysis. The character of the pleural fluid in malignancy is usually exudative (specific gravity greater than 1.015 and protein greater than 3.5 g per 100 ml) with an increased red blood cell count (greater than 10,000 red blood cells per ml).

When the initial clinical presentation, physical examination, or initial laboratory examination suggests one of the classical patterns of metastatic spread to liver, brain, or bone, further evaluation should include, in the instance of suspected brain metastasis, skull films, echoencephalogram, brain scan, and lumbar puncture; in the instance of suspected liver metastasis, liver function tests and liver scan and biopsy; and in the instance of bone metastases, a skeletal x-ray survey, radioisotopic bone scan, and biopsy where possible.

The efficacy of closed-chest *needle biopsy* of the lung in establishing a diagnosis of pulmonary carcinoma has been stressed by many centers. The primary use of this procedure is reserved for those patients who have probable inoperable or nonresectable lesions and in whom a tissue diagnosis should be obtained prior to institution of second-line therapy such as radiation and/or chemotherapy.

In patients with carcinoma of the lung, *pulmonary scintiphotoscans* with radioisotope-labeled macroaggregated albumin may provide nonspecific information on the status of arteriocapillary pulmonary perfusion. The combination of ventilation and perfusion scintiphotoscans should allow differentiation of primary perfusion defects from those which are secondary to decreased or absent ventilation (Chap. 250). It is hoped that pulmonary scintiphotoscans and pulmonary angiograms in selected patients may provide potentially valuable and reliable information on resectability and operability.

Several centers have reported their experience with *interosseous azygography*. This procedure allows roentgenographic evaluation of the mediastinal venous pattern. A definite deformity or a complete blockade may provide evidence of the mediastinal extension of an intrathoracic lesion and thus offer evidence of nonresectability. *Mediastinoscopy* with acquisition of biopsy material may provide similar evidence of extension and for nonresectability. Recent experience with *fiberoptic bronchoscopy* indicates that the tracheobronchial tree will be more accessible to diagnosis than previously. This technique provides the means for visual inspection, localized biopsy, and regional lung washings and brushings for cytologic examination.

Although a patient may have a pulmonary lesion, which by all criteria is operable, with potential for a curative resection, a decisive problem remains. Will the patient's cardiopulmonary reserve allow him to tolerate the degree of pulmonary resection anticipated? If there are no clinical signs of cardiopulmonary disability, simple determination of static lung volumes, dynamic flow rates, and resting arterial blood gas tensions and pH is sufficient, but if these studies are abnormal, further evaluation is indicated. The patient with obvious pulmonary disability presents a more complex physiologic problem. In this group of patients the determination of the type and degree of disability is essential. The more extensive the patient's clinical disability, the more extensive and sophisticated should be his preoperative evaluation.

Indications of nonoperability include laboratory evidence of (1) a *severe* restrictive and/or obstructive defect (determined by static lung volumes, dynamic flow rates, and measurement of pulmonary compliance and total pulmonary resistance by body plethysmography (Chap. 249); (2) a *markedly reduced* functional pulmonary arteriocapillary bed (determined by a decreased diffusion capacity for carbon monoxide, an increase in calculated wasted ventilation, i.e., ventilation of nonperfused areas, and resting hypoxemia with a widening of the alveolar-arterial oxygen gradient under conditions of exercise); (3) *grossly abnormal* ventilation-perfusion relationships (determined by pulmonary scintiphotoscans with radioisotope-labeled macroaggregated albumin, xenon (^{133}Xe) ventilation-perfusion scans, and pulmonary angiography); (4) *marked alveolar hypoventilation* (determined by a level of alveolar ventilation inadequate to maintain a normal arterial carbon dioxide tension); (5) *serious* pulmonary hypertension and cor pulmonale (determined by right-sided heart catheterization with measurement of cardiac output, pulmonary artery pressure, and total pulmonary vascular resistance).

TREATMENT

If a patient has had adequate diagnostic evaluation, the therapeutic approach will follow naturally. The currently preferred therapeutic approach is surgical resection of the primary pulmonary carcinoma. In most instances, in an attempt to conserve pulmonary function, lobectomy rather than pneumonectomy is the operation of choice, provided the lesion can be excised completely by lobectomy.

An operative candidate is an individual who has no demonstrable evidence of intra- or extrathoracic spread of his malignancy and whose cardiopulmonary status does not preclude resectional surgery. Accepted contraindications to thoracotomy and pulmonary resection for primary carcinoma include (1) evidence of metastatic lymph node involvement; (2) superior vena caval obstruction; (3) recurrent laryngeal or phrenic nerve paralysis; (4) pleural thickening and/or effusion, with histologic evidence of carcinomatous involvement of the pleura, and/or the presence of malignant cells in the pleural fluid; (5) distant metastasis to liver, brain, adrenal glands, or bones; (6) multicentric or multilobar distribution of the lesion; and finally (7) a *serious* cardiopulmonary functional defect.

The *classical systemic syndromes,* with which a patient may present, by themselves do not constitute contraindications to resection. To the contrary, since they may contribute significantly to the patient's discomfort and demise, resection of the pulmonary parenchymal lesion may offer significant palliation. As a rule, many of these syndromes abate with resection and recur with metastasis.

The management of a patient with inoperable pulmonary carcinoma includes *supervoltage radiotherapy* and *chemotherapy.* Radiotherapy alone is seldom curative, while chemotherapy alone is generally ineffective. However, both modalities have a definite role in the palliative treatment of some patients with distressing manifestations of pain, superior vena caval obstruction, bleeding, and bronchial obstruction. The physiologic evaluation of the candidate for radiotherapy is as critical as that of the operative candidate, for the patient with severe cardiopulmonary disability may be converted to a cardiopulmonary cripple by extensive radiation therapy as well as by resection.

There is renewed enthusiasm for the use of preoperative supervoltage radiation in an attempt to obtain sterilization of local lymph nodes and reduction in size of the primary parenchymal lesion. Both of these goals, especially with regard to superior sulcus tumors, may increase the percentage of resectable lesions and improve the survival statistics.

PROGNOSIS

The prognosis of primary carcinoma is a direct function of the cell type and the extent of the malignant process at the time of diagnosis. The statistics of survival for the patient with inoperable carcinoma are universally poor; the average survival time from diagnosis to demise has been variously reported as between 5 and 14 months. Of all patients with carcinoma of the lung, one-third are inoperable at the time of diagnosis. Of the remaining patients only 30 to 50 percent of those subjected to exploratory thoracotomy prove to be resectable. The 5-year survival of this selected resectable group is approximately 20 percent. This results in an overall 5-year survival of all patients with primary pulmonary carcinoma of approximately 5 percent. It is apparent that any major therapeutic gains and improved prognoses, at this time, hinge upon the early diagnosis of the early lesion. Jackman and associates support this tenet by reporting a resectability rate of 98 percent and a 5-year survival of 45 percent for bronchogenic carcinoma presenting as a solitary nodule (less than 4 cm in diameter).

REFERENCES

Adkins PC et al: Thoracotomy on the patient with previous malignancy: Metastasis or new primary. J Thorac Cardiovasc Surg 56:351, 1968

Feinstein AR: Symptomatic patterns, biologic behavior, and prognosis in cancer of the lung. Ann Intern Med 61:27, 1964

Hajek M, Homan Van Der Heide JN: Early detection of mediastinal spread of pulmonary carcinoma by mediastinoscopy. Thorax 25:720, 1970

Jackman RJ et al: Survival rates in peripheral bronchogenic carcinoma up to four centimeters in diameter presenting as solitary pulmonary nodules. J Thorac Cardiovasc Surg 57:1, 1969

261 DISEASES OF THE PLEURA, MEDIASTINUM, AND DIAPHRAGM

DAVID C. SABISTON, JR.

THE PLEURA

The pleura and pleural cavities are the sites of a variety of medical and surgical disorders. An understanding of their development is important in consideration of the diseases related to these structures. During embryogenesis the two pleural cavities become separated from the central pericardial cavity by the pleuropericardial membranes. Although initially they are continuous with the peritoneal cavity, further development of the pleuroperitoneal membrane ultimately separates these serous cavities. However, defects may remain and may be the site of a hernia connecting the pleural and peritoneal cavities. The parietal pleura covers the inner surface of the chest wall, the diaphragm, and the mediastinum, and is reflected at the pulmonary hilum to cover the entire lung. The pleura is composed of a very thin layer of connective tissue with a mesothelial surface. Both smooth-muscle and elastic fibers are present, and numerous lymphatics and small vessels form a diffuse network in the pleural wall. In addition, the pleura is supplied with many nerve fibers, a factor of considerable importance in the presence of inflammation or stretching of the pleura, either of which is apt to produce a highly *painful* response.

Several important physiologic principles affect the pleura. Normally, the intrapleural pressure is negative and varies between −4 to −8 cm H_2O at the end of inspiration and −2 to −4 cm at the end of expiration. In patients with severe pulmonary emphysema, the intrapleural pressure is apt to be less negative than normal; in pneumothorax the pressure is usually elevated, frequently to a high level. Air or gas in the pleural cavity produces a partial collapse of the underlying lung. The disappearance of the gas in the pleural cavity is related to the partial pressure of the specific gas in the blood, among other factors. For example, oxygen is more rapidly absorbed than nitrogen, and with the passage of time, air in the pleural cavity has a higher concentration of nitrogen. Since carbon dioxide is present in the blood, equilibrium is established between this gas and the blood, yielding a higher concentration of carbon dioxide than is present in normal air.

In the normal pleural cavity the surfaces of the pleural membranes are moist, no appreciable fluid being present. In various disease processes, fluid may accumulate in the pleural cavities; such fluid has been arbitrarily divided into two groups: (1) transudates and (2) exudates. The transudates have a specific gravity less than 1.015 with a protein content under 2 or 3 g per 100 ml. Transudates are usually clear, although they may have a tinge of color and at times may contain blood. Few cells are present. Examples of transudates are the fluid accumulations in congestive heart failure, cirrhosis of the liver, and nephritis. Exudates are generally thicker and may be either clear or cloudy. They may contain a considerable number of cellular elements as well as bacteria. Such fluid is found in inflammation and infection of the pleura.

HYDROTHORAX The accumulation of significant amounts of fluid in the pleural cavity may be the result of a variety of causative factors. The diagnosis may be established by abnormal physical findings which include prominence of the interspaces on the affected side, increased dullness on percussion, impaired transmission of breath sounds, and deviation of the trachea to the opposite side. The chest roentgenogram confirms the diagnosis with evidence of marked radiopacity of the involved pleural cavity. Perhaps the most common cause of noninflammatory fluid collection in the pleural cavity is congestive heart failure. Other causes include nephrosis with hypoproteinemia, trauma, and cirrhosis of the liver. Primary or metastatic neoplastic involvement of the pleura may produce a transudate or an exudate. Some females with an ovarian fibroma may also have an associated pleural effusion (Meigs's syndrome), a poorly understood transudate which disappears following removal of the ovarian neoplasm. The "phantom tumor" is an interesting form of pleural effusion which can present a diagnostic problem. This lesion is usually found on a chest roentgenogram and is actually an interlobar effusion occurring with congestive heart failure or following pleural inflammation.

Another cause of pleural effusion is that which has been termed "sympathetic effusion." An inflammatory process beneath the diaphragm, such as a subphrenic abscess or acute pancreatitis, can stimulate the accumulation of fluid in the pleural cavities as a response to injury. In the early stages such fluid is usually a transudate and sterile, although later it may become thicker and infected.

CHYLOTHORAX Chyle may accumulate in the pleural cavity as a result of several causes. As the thoracic duct passes through the posterior mediastinum, it may be ruptured by trauma, invaded by tumor, or injured in a thoracic surgical procedure. Chyle has a milky appearance, a specific gravity between 1.020 and 1.030, a protein content of 3 to 4 g per 100 ml, and fat content from 1 to 4 g per 100 ml. In most instances, chylothorax can be managed by aspiration or continuous catheter drainage. In refractory cases, thoracotomy with direct closure of the lymph fistula is indicated.

PLEURITIS Inflammation of the pleura is apt to produce severe pain, which is often sharp and stabbing in quality, aggravated by deep inspiration, and augmented by coughing and sneezing. The cause of acute pleurisy may be pneumonia, viral infections, tuberculosis, and pulmonary embolism or abscess. The inflammation usually resolves with subsidence of the primary disease. *Fibrinous pleurisy* may be a sequel and may be associated with a friction rub. The treatment of pleuritis and fibrinous pleurisy is generally directed toward the primary disease. The use of analgesics, strapping, and intercostal block may at times be symptomatically helpful. Failure of the process to resolve completely may produce chronic *adhesive pleuritis*. In this condition, marked pleural thickening may be sufficient to interfere with pulmonary function. It may be the final result of an empyema, tuberculous effusion, or unresolved hemothorax. If pleuritis is chronic, and especially when it is productive of symptoms, surgical removal of the thickened pleura (decortication) may be indicated.

EMPYEMA Empyema is defined as the presence of purulent fluid in the pleural cavity. It is the result of extension of infection from a contiguous structure, and may be a complication of pneumonia, pulmonary abscess, subdiaphragmatic abscess, perforation of a carcinoma into the pleural cavity, perforation of the esophagus, or penetration from an acute mediastinitis. In most instances, acute empyema is a serious infection and produces prominent clinical manifestations. Malaise, fever, and tachycardia are generally present and are accompanied by appropriate physical signs of fluid accumulation within the chest. The chest roentgenogram also usually shows evidence of fluid, although the definitive diagnosis rests upon thoracentesis with aspiration of purulent material and subsequent culture for the specific organism. Some of the more frequently encountered organisms responsible for empyema include *Staphylococcus aureus,* anaerobic *Streptococcus, Escherichia coli, Pseudomonas aeruginosa,* and *Klebsiella pneumoniae.*

The therapy of empyema is directed both at the control of the specific organism by appropriate use of antimicrobial drugs and at drainage of the pleural cavity. Needle aspiration of the pleural cavity is rarely effective in the management of empyema, and surgical drainage is most often required in adults. Moreover, surgical drainage is apt to be followed by rapid amelioration of symptoms and marked improvement in the clinical course of the patient. In selected patients *closed* drainage employing a trocar for introduction of a tube is satisfactory, but in the majority open drainage with resection of a small portion of rib is the treatment of choice. The empyema cavity gradually becomes obliterated with expansion of the underlying lung. Occasionally, decortication for removal of a fibrous peel surrounding the lung may be necessary in order to produce expansion and obliteration and healing of the empyema cavity. In rare instances, when treatment is delayed, the empyema presents beneath the skin and drains spontaneously (*empyema necessitatis*). Treatment of empyema is more difficult in the presence of a bronchopleural fistula and requires suction under negative pressure in order to expand the lung. If the fistula is the result of a benign inflammatory process, it is likely to close spontaneously, but if due to neoplastic disease, spontaneous closure is very unlikely.

Chronic empyema If the acute process is not treated adequately, chronic empyema may result. Continuous drainage of purulent material from the chest may lead to chronic debilitation, including anemia, malnutrition, and, occasionally, secondary amyloidosis. Treatment should be directed toward the surgical closure of the empyema cavity by decortication or rib resection. In postpneumonectomy empyema, cure may result from antibiotic instillation and closure of the drainage tract.

SPONTANEOUS PNEUMOTHORAX The term *spontaneous pneumothorax* is applied to a condition frequently encountered in otherwise healthy patients who suddenly exhibit symptoms of pneumothorax. Formerly, it was thought that the onset of this condition was truly *spontaneous,* but subsequent evidence has shown that it is nearly always produced by rupture of an emphysematous bleb on the pleural surface. The severity of the clinical manifestations varies in proportion to the magnitude of the pneumothorax. At times the amount of air may be minimal, producing only slight pleural pain. In some patients the amount of air in the pleural cavity is great, collapsing the lung, with resultant shift in the mediastinum, heart, and trachea to the opposite side, and producing severe dyspnea and cyanosis. Spontaneous pneumothorax is characterized by a sudden onset of unilateral chest pain associated with dyspnea. The pain is often sharp and agonizing and produces considerable apprehension in the patient, especially during the first attack. The chest roentgenogram establishes the extent of the pulmonary collapse and, together with the gravity of the symptoms, dictates the choice of therapy. Though the majority of spontaneous pneumothoraxes result from rupture of emphysematous blebs, the condition is known to follow other pulmonary diseases such as sarcoidosis, silicosis, infection, and neoplasms in rare instances. If the amount of air is minimal, with only slight collapse of the lung, observation alone may suffice. More commonly, it is necessary to perform a thoracentesis, removing the air, and preferably inserting an indwelling chest catheter for continuous drainage of the pleural cavity.

One of the characteristics of spontaneous pneumothorax is its *tendency to recur.* Following the first attack, a second one occurs in half the patients; there is an even higher likelihood of a third attack after a second one. Though the first and second attacks are most often treated only by removal of the air, either by thoracentesis or the use of an intercostal catheter, the third and subsequent attacks are generally best treated by open thoracotomy. The surgical procedure is designed to produce an adherence of the parietal pleura to the visceral pleura so that a pneumothorax cannot recur. This can be accomplished by pleurectomy or by the application of irritants to the pleural surfaces (*poudrage*). When pleural blebs are present, these can also be resected at the time of operation.

THE MEDIASTINUM

The mediastinum is an anatomic division of the thorax which may be the site of numerous disorders, including neoplasms, cysts, inflammation, emphysema, and aneurysms (Fig. 261-1). Anatomically, the mediastinum extends from the superior aperture of the thorax to the diaphragm; it is bounded laterally by the mediastinal pleura and posteriorly by the vertebral column. For descriptive purposes, the mediastinum is customarily divided into three major compartments: the superior, anterior (or middle), and posterior divisions. The clinical manifestations of the various disorders of the mediastinum are due in part to pressure or invasion of the multiple structures present within the mediastinum. In the

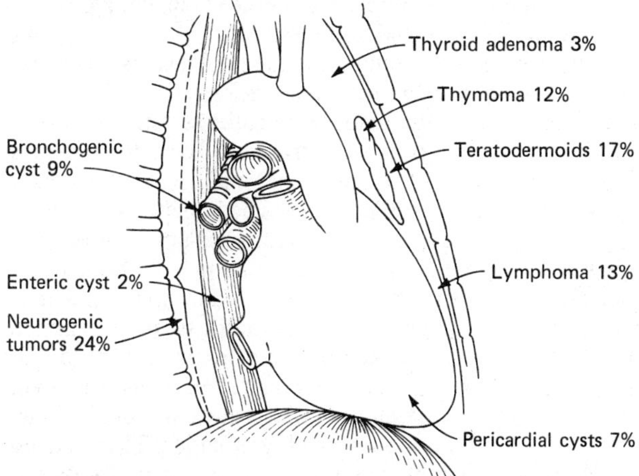

FIGURE 261-1
Diagrammatic illustration of usual anatomic sites of primary cysts and neoplasms of the mediastinum. The figures given refer to those shown in the series presented in Table 261-1.

superior division are the thymus gland, trachea, esophagus, thoracic duct, aortic arch, innominate vein, and the phrenic, vagal, and recurrent nerves. The *anterior* mediastinum contains the heart, pericardium, lymph nodes, and substernal fibroareolar tissue. In the *posterior* division are the esophagus, thoracic duct, descending thoracic aorta, and the intercostal and the vagus nerves.

TUMORS AND CYSTS OF THE MEDIASTINUM The mediastinum is the site of a variety of primary and metastatic neoplasms. In addition, a number of specific cysts originate in the mediastinum, including those arising from the pericardium, thymus, bronchi, and esophagus. Lymphomas are particularly common in the mediastinum because of the significant amount of lymphoid tissue present. The large variety of neoplasms and cysts which may occur in the mediastinum is demonstrated by a collection of 1,000 patients (Table 261-1). The remarkable number of specific histologic diagnoses responsible for mediastinal lesions emphasizes the problems involved in diagnosis and management.

Diagnosis One of the more interesting aspects of the clinical manifestations of mediastinal lesions is that these disorders may be asymptomatic, even when massive. However, in about two-thirds of patients symptoms are present. In the remainder, the diagnosis is first suggested as a result of a routine chest roentgenogram. The most frequent symptoms include chest pain, cough, and dyspnea. Symptoms are most apt to be associated with a malignant lesion. In most patients with malignant neoplasms, the most common symptoms are chest pain and cough. In one series, these were present in 94 percent of the patients, whereas only 6 percent of malignant lesions were asymptomatic and found on routine chest roentgenogram. A variety of syndromes with characteristic symptoms may be associated with lesions in the mediastinum. Several examples include von Recklinghausen's disease in association with neurofibroma, hypertrophic osteoarthropathy with neurogenic tumors, red blood cell aplasia with thymomas, hypertension and diarrheal syndromes with pheochromocytomas and ganglioneuromas, and hypoglycemia with mesotheliomas and teratomas. Pressure symptoms are also common, resulting from encroachment on or invasion of the trachea, esophagus, heart, various nerves, or great veins.

The diagnostic evaluation begins with a careful history to determine the site and extent of the lesion, with especial emphasis on manifestations which suggest a specific lesion. Roentgenographic studies are essential, and the chest roentgenograms in the anteroposterior, oblique, and lateral positions usually outline the size and extent of the lesion. The use of fluoroscopy (to establish the presence of intrinsic pulsations), esophagram, and tomography are helpful. Angiocardiography plays an important role in the differentiation of vascular lesions involving the great veins, pulmonary vessels, and aorta. Radioisotope scanning is helpful in the diagnosis of substernal thyroids. Parathyroid lesions within the mediastinum may be localized by selective venous catheteriza-

TABLE 261-1
Incidence of neoplasms and cysts of the mediastinum, in a collected series of 1,000 patients*

Type of tumor or cyst	*Herlitzka and Gale, 1958*	*Morrison, 1958*	*Key, 1954*	*Harrington, 1949*	*Oldham and Sabiston, 1967*	*Total*	*%*
Neurogenic tumors	35	101	10	51	43	240	24
Cysts							
Pericardial	17	13	4	7	33	74	7
Bronchogenic	24	23	3	10	27	87	9
Enteric	2	6		4	10	22	2
Nonspecific	4	6		8	13	31	3
Teratodermoids	26	36	31	40	36	169	17
Thymomas	14	47	4	8	52	125	12
Lymphomas	12	33	43		38	126	13
Other	20	26	6	30	44	126	13
Total	154	291	101	158	296	1,000	100

* *Excluding primary carcinoma of the mediastinum and substernal extension of cervical goiter. From HN Oldham Jr and DC Sabiston Jr, in* Davis-Christopher Textbook of Surgery, *10th ed., ed DC Sabiston Jr, Philadelphia: Saunders, 1972*

tion with radioimmunoassay for parathyroid hormone levels. Mediastinoscopy and bronchoscopy may also be useful, especially in establishing the histologic diagnosis. The differentiation between vascular lesions and primary mediastinal tumors and cysts is of considerable importance. In a recent study a distinct group of patients (8 percent) was initially thought to have primary cardiovascular abnormalities. The original diagnosis was made on the basis of chest roentgenograms and the associated clinical findings. Angiocardiography showed the mediastinal mass to be nonvascular in each case. Similarly, it is important to employ angiocardiography in the diagnosis of those lesions which indeeed are vascular, in order to be prepared properly at the time of surgical exploration. For example, extracorporeal circulation may be necessary in the treatment of aneurysms and other vascular abnormalities.

The anatomic site of the lesion is often of diagnostic significance. Characteristically, the superior mediastinum is the location in which substernal goiters and thymic tumors occur. The anterior (and middle) mediastinum is the most common site of teratomas, dermoid cysts, and lymphomas. Pericardial and bronchogenic cysts are also found in this location. The posterior mediastinum is the well-recognized site of nearly all neurogenic tumors. It is thus possible to evaluate mediastinal lesions statistically in a meaningful manner according to their location.

Neurogenic tumors are the most common mediastinal lesions found in most series. They occur in all age groups, but the malignant variants are most often present in childhood. Nearly all neurogenic tumors arise in the posterior mediastinum near the paravertebral gutter. These lesions arise from the intercostal nerves, the sympathetic chain, and embryonal neurogenic rests. Though many are asymptomatic, pain and/or cough are present in approximately two-thirds of neurogenic tumors. Hormonal activity may be present in ganglioneuromas and neuroblastomas, and diarrhea, hypertension, flushing, and sweating may occur in these patients. The urine may show excretion of vanillylmandelic acid (VMA). *Neurofibromas* may occur either singly or in association with von Recklinghausen's disease. Neurilemmomas arise from the sheath of Schwann. *Ganglioneuromas* originate from the sympathetic chain and have a stronger potential to become malignant, especially in children. Neuroblastomas may also occur in the mediastinum, usually in children, and are especially responsive to x-ray therapy. Pheochromocytomas may arise from sympathetic tissue along the vertebral column and are capable of secreting epinephrine and norepinephrine with corresponding symptoms. Other chromaffin tumors are also present and may be hormonally inactive.

Teratodermoid tumors characteristically occur in the anterior mediastinum. In its simplest form, the lesion is an isolated cyst with ectodermal components alone. However, the majority of these lesions, even in the cystic form, contain cells from each of the three primary germ layers and are therefore more properly called teratodermoids. The lesions often contain teeth, which may be seen in the chest roentgenogram. Most of the lesions become apparent in adult life and may become quite large. Unless removed, they have a tendency to become malignant. Approximately 10 percent undergo malignant change, usually in the epithelial component.

Thymomas are common mediastinal lesions, especially in association with myasthenia gravis (Chap. 347). The incidence of the latter disorder in patients with thymomas has been reported to range from 10 to 50 percent, whereas the presence of thymomas in patients with myasthenia gravis is lower (8 to 10 percent). The beneficial effects of thymectomy in patients with myasthenia gravis have been greatest in the young female without a thymoma, especially if the disease is of short duration. Similarly, patients with myasthenia gravis and a thymoma have a poorer prognosis. Thymomas are often malignant (about 25 percent), but they rarely metastasize. Their malignant potential is demonstrated by direct invasion of the lung, pericardium, blood vessels, and lymphatics. Thus, a diagnosis of a malignant thymoma is made primarily on the basis of its invasiveness, rather than on the basis of the histologic cell type. Fortunately, the malignant lesions are usually sensitive to x-ray therapy.

Lymphomas are especially common in the mediastinum, and involvement of lymph nodes with leukemia, lymphosarcoma, Hodgkin's disease, and the various types of reticulum sarcoma are well recognized. Though most of these tumors are widespread, solitary lesions also occur. The chest roentgenogram usually demonstrates multiple lesions, and the supraclavicular nodes are frequently involved as well. If the lesions are localized, surgical extirpation may be performed. Additional treatment with irradiation and chemotherapy is also indicated.

Mediastinal *thyroid* lesions usually occur in the superior mediastinum and receive their blood supply from the thyroid vessels. Totally intrathoracic thyroid (or ectopic) mediastinal lesions are rare.

Parathyroid adenoma in the mediastinum has been recognized for many years. Among 400 patients with hyperparathyroidism in one series, 84 (21 percent) had a mediastinal adenoma. Of these, three-fourths were removed by a cervical incision, and the remainder required mediastinotomy.

Primary *cysts* are among the most common mediastinal lesions. The vast majority of these cysts occur in the *anterior* mediastinum. In the collected series shown in Table 261-1, these lesions comprise 21 percent of the total. Approximately two-thirds of the lesions are asymptomatic, and the diagnosis is made on routine chest roentgenogram. Pericardial cysts are attached to the pericardium and most often occur at the inferior cardiophrenic angles. Since they contain clear fluid, they have also been termed *spring-water cysts*. These lesions rarely communicate directly with the pericardium. Bronchogenic cysts are also common and occur in close approximation to the main bronchi usually near the carina. The cyst wall is characteristically comprised of ciliated respiratory epithelium with cartilage, smooth muscle, and mucous glands. Rarely, communication with the bronchus or trachea is present. These lesions are benign but may produce troublesome pressure symptoms, especially if the contents become infected. *Enteric* cysts occur along the esophagus and usually contain a mucosal lining more akin to gastric or intestinal epithelium. Although they rarely communicate with the esophagus, infection and abscess formation may occur. The presence of hydrochloric acid in some of these cysts may lead to ulceration, perforation, and bleeding. Mediastinal cysts are encountered which have only a fibrous wall and no specific histologic lining. These lesions have been termed *nonspecific* cysts for lack of a more appropriate designation. Their exact nature is poorly understood; they may actually represent lesions in which the original lining has disappeared.

Other types of neoplasms and cysts are rare. Among them are fibromas, leiomyomas, mesotheliomas, hemangiomas, liposarcomas, and lymphangiomas. Also of importance are metastatic lesions in mediastinal lymph nodes. These occur especially as a result of primary tumors of the lungs and bronchi. Sometimes the enlarged hilar lymph nodes may be more prominent than the primary lesions. Carcinoma of the breast, lymphomas, and tumors of the intestinal tract may also metastasize to the mediastinum. Moreover, the mediastinal metastases may occur before the primary lesion appears. Therefore, in every patient with a mediastinal lesion attention should be directed toward the elimination of a distant primary site as the responsible factor.

THE SUPERIOR VENA CAVAL SYNDROME Superior mediastinal lesions characterized by a dense infiltration and obstruction of the superior vena cava produce a characteristic clinical syndrome. These manifestations usually include marked cyanosis, swelling of the head, neck, and upper extremities, and the development of numerous superficial venous collateral vessels. Primary mediastinal tumors—especially lymphomas—aneurysms, and carcinoma of the lung are the most common causes of this condition. Occasionally, mediastinal *fibrosis* may be responsible for this syndrome. This condition may occur at any age but is most common in middle or late life. Initial symptoms in mediastinal fibrosis include facial edema with spread to the arms, conjunctival suffusion, headache, tinnitus, and dyspnea. Nonpitting edema involving the upper thorax and arms becomes progressively more severe. A helpful roentgenographic finding associated with mediastinal fibrosis is the absence of positive changes on the chest roentgenogram. Pathologically, dense fibrosis is present in the mediastinum, involving the superior vena cava and occasionally the pulmonary veins. If the latter are involved, pulmonary hypertension may ensue. In some patients, histoplasmosis has been shown to be the cause and has been demonstrated in microscopic sections. Fortunately, in many instances spontaneous amelioration occurs because an adequate venous collateral circulation develops.

MEDIASTINITIS Although uncommon, acute infection in the mediastinum is usually serious. Acute suppurative mediastinitis accompanies esophageal perforation, which may be due to external trauma, esophageal erosion, or perforation, or may develop as a result of endoscopy. Symptoms usually appear promptly and consist of substernal pain, subcutaneous emphysema, fever, tachycardia, and leukocytosis. If untreated, overwhelming sepsis follows, producing prostration and collapse. Though acute mediastinitis may respond to antimicrobial therapy alone, prompt surgical drainage is also indicated in most patients.

MEDIASTINAL EMPHYSEMA Air within the planes of the mediastinum may produce few clinical manifestations, but in the presence of an increased pressure it can produce severe pain, which may spread to the surrounding tissues. Mediastinal emphysema may result from traumatic perforation of the trachea or esophagus, from rupture of pulmonary alveoli in interstitial emphysema of the lung, from spread along the fascial planes of the neck or pharynx, or from dissection from the retroperitoneal space. Traumatic rupture of the bronchial tree in association with pneumothorax following puncture wounds or associated with endotracheal anesthesia may be the antecedent cause.

The escape of air from ruptured alveoli producing *spontaneous mediastinal emphysema* was first described by Hamman. Air dissects along the vascular structures of the lung to the hilum and thence into the various planes of the mediastinum. From the mediastinum it may spread to the subcutaneous tissues of the neck or through the diaphragm to retroperitoneal structures. If a large amount of air is involved, and especially if it is under pressure, it may produce collapse of the veins in the mediastinum, with impaired venous return to the heart.

Though small amounts of air in the mediastinum are generally without clinical consequence, severe substernal pain may result, and a characteristic crunching noise synchronous with the heartbeat is often heard over the precordium. Dyspnea, cyanosis, and distention of the cervical veins may follow. The chest roentgenogram demonstrates air shadows in the mediastinum, usually along specific planes. Moreover, air shadows are seen in the soft tissues of the neck and over the chest wall. In most instances, sedation and oxygen suffice as treatment. Rarely, surgical relief of the increased mediastinal pressure is indicated.

DISORDERS OF THE DIAPHRAGM

The most common abnormality of the diaphragm is *displacement.* The diaphragm may be displaced upward or downward by a variety of abdominal and thoracic disorders. Normally, the right side of the diaphragm is approximately 4 cm higher than the left, because of the right lobe of the liver. Upward displacement of the diaphragm may be associated with intraabdominal masses, ascites, marked obesity, or pregnancy. Disorders within the thorax can also produce displacement. The diaphragm may be depressed because of pleural effusion or pneumothorax. Phrenic nerve paralysis will produce upward displacement and paradoxic motion of the diaphragm with respiration. Phrenic paralysis is most commonly caused by direct invasion of metastatic tumor, but it may be the result of infection and trauma.

Diaphragmatic hernia may occur in several specific sites. The most common location is the esophageal hiatus through which the stomach can pass into the posterior mediastinum. The diagnosis and management of hiatus hernia are discussed in Chap. 281. In addition, congenital defects occur on either side of the sternum (foramen of Morgagni) and posterolaterally (foramen of Bochdalek). In addition, blunt trauma to the abdomen or chest may rupture the diaphragm, usually in its central portion. Direct trauma, such as incised wounds and missile wounds, may produce an opening which is followed by herniation of abdominal contents into the thorax. Traumatic diaphragmatic hernias may produce symptoms of intestinal obstruction and should be corrected surgically as soon as the diagnosis is established.

Eventration of the diaphragm is a condition in which the diaphragm is quite thin and membranous. The muscular portion of the diaphragm is usually confined to the posterior third, with a thin membrane constituting the remainder of the diaphragm. This causes marked upward displacement of the diaphragm and results in the presence of abdominal contents in the thoracic cage. Though often asymptomatic, eventration may produce pulmonary insufficiency. The chest roentgenogram, particularly following ingestion of barium, is diagnostic, and in most instances no therapy is required. However, in patients in whom symptoms are present, surgical correction is indicated.

Neoplasms in the diaphragm occur but are uncommon. Direct spread or lymphatic involvement may occur from primary neoplasms within the abdomen, e.g., in the stomach or colon. Also, direct involvement may occur from primary carcinoma of the lung. Primary tumors of the diaphragm are rare and include lipomas, fibromas, mesotheliomas, and neurogenic tumors. Approximately half are benign and the remainder malignant. Surgical removal is indicated.

REFERENCES

DOCTOR AH: Mediastinoscopy: A critical evaluation of 220 cases. Ann Surg 174:965, 1971

HAMMAN L: Spontaneous mediastinal emphysema. Bull Johns Hopkins Hosp 64:1, 1939

NATHANIELS EK et al: Mediastinal parathyroid tumors: A clinical and pathological study of 84 cases. Ann Surg 171:165, 1970

OLDHAM HN JR, SABISTON DC JR: The mediastinum, in *Davis-Christopher Textbook of Surgery*, 10th ed., ed DC Sabiston Jr, Philadelphia: Saunders, 1972

SAMSON PC: Empyema thoracis: Essentials of present-day management. Ann Thorac Surg 11:210, 1971

262 COR PULMONALE

ALFRED P. FISHMAN

Cor pulmonale denotes enlargement of the right ventricle secondary to malfunctioning lungs. The malfunction may be a consequence of either intrinsic pulmonary disease or an abnormal chest bellows or a depressed ventilatory drive from the respiratory centers (Table 262-1). Invariably, if the cause is in the lungs, the disease will be diffuse, bilateral, and extensive, in most cases affecting airways as well as parenchyma.

Pulmonary arterial hypertension ("pulmonary hypertension") systematically precedes cor pulmonale. Indeed, cor pulmonale is synonymous with pulmonary hypertensive heart disease. But the discriminating proviso for the diagnosis of cor pulmonale is that *neither disease of the left side of the heart nor congenital heart disease be responsible for its pathogenesis.* Cor pulmonale need not be associated with, or terminate in, failure of the right side of the heart.

Enlargement of the right ventricle is usually much more difficult to detect and to quantify clinically and at autopsy, than is left ventricular hypertrophy. Moreover, dilatation may predominate if pulmonary hypertension is recent in onset and too brief in duration for considerable hypertrophy to have occurred. Consequently, it is difficult to assess the nature of right ventricular enlargement during life without a clear understanding of the etiology and natural history of the antecedent pulmonary disorder.

These qualifications have several practical implications. By identifying the pulmonary disorder as the critical element in the pathogenesis of cor pulmonale, they underscore the fact that prognosis and treatment of cor pulmonale *depend more on the lungs and their response to treatment than on the heart.* Moreover, by stressing *enlargement* of the right ventricle as the hallmark of cor pulmonale, they indicate that pulmonary hypertension may exist without straining the right ventricle to the stage of enlargement and that right ventricular failure is a complication, rather than an essential feature, of cor pulmonale.

TYPES OF COR PULMONALE By tradition, the designation "acute" is generally reserved for the dilatation of the right side of the heart which follows acute embolization of the lungs. The designation "chronic" is less specific. Usually chronicity is judged by the type and duration of the pulmonary disorder that led to the cardiac enlargement (Table 262-1). Just how long, and how much, the heart remains enlarged depends on fluctuations in the level of pulmonary arterial pressure.

INCIDENCE Reliable estimates of the prevalence of chronic cor pulmonale are sparse. However, because predisposing chronic obstructive lung disease (COLD) and chronic bronchitis and/or emphysema[1] are so prevalent (Chap. 252), cor pulmonale is a common type of heart disease. Indeed, in parts of the world where cigarette smoking is popular, air pollution severe, and COLD rampant, cor pulmonale may comprise up to one-quarter of all types of heart failure. By virtue of exposure rather than predisposition, men are more often affected than women. Chronic cor pulmonale is also the rule in other bronchitic disorders, such as adult cystic fibrosis of the pancreas. In contrast, it is an unusual complication of allergic asthma.

Most diffuse pulmonary diseases are either too limited in extent or too circumscribed in their effects on alveolar-capillary gas exchange to set in motion the train of events leading to cor pulmonale. Thus, the bulk of patients with silicosis, emphysema, or diffuse fibrosis

[1] *Definitions of chronic bronchitis, emphysema, and chronic airway obstruction are dealt with in Chap. 252. All these disease entities are included in the designation "chronic obstructive lung disease" (COLD) as used in this chapter.*

TABLE 262-1
Pulmonary disorders predisposing to chronic cor pulmonale

Intrinsic disease of the lungs and airways
- Chronic obstructive lung disease (COLD)
- Diffuse pulmonary interstitial disease
- Pulmonary vascular disease

Malfunctioning chest bellows
- Kyphoscoliosis
- Neuromuscular incompetence
- Marked obesity ("Pickwickian syndrome")

Inadequate ventilatory drive from the respiratory centers
- Primary or idiopathic alveolar hypoventilation ("Ondine's curse")
- Chronic mountain sickness

suffer from breathlessness for years but fail to develop pulmonary hypertension or cardiomegaly.

PATHOGENESIS

Pulmonary hypertension is a prerequisite for cor pulmonale. Although a large cardiac output, tachycardia, an expanded blood volume, or myocardial damage from hypoxia and acidosis may contribute to the pulmonary hypertension, the crux in the pathogenetic sequence is an increase in pulmonary vascular resistance to blood flow through small muscular arteries and arterioles. The increase in vascular resistance may be anatomical or vasomotor in origin; often both mechanisms are involved (Table 262-2).

ANATOMIC INCREASE IN PULMONARY VASCULAR RESISTANCE In the normal resting individual, the pulmonary circulation is a highly distensible, low-resistance circuit, accommodating the same blood flow as the systemic circulation at approximately one-fourth the mean blood pressure; during moderate exercise, tripling the blood flow elicits only slight increments in pulmonary arterial pressure. Even after pneumonectomy, the residual pulmonary vascular bed accepts considerable increments in pulmonary blood flow with only slight increase in pulmonary artery pressure as long as the lung is free of fibrosis, emphysema, or pulmonary vascular change. Similarly, disappearance of a large portion of the pulmonary capillary bed in emphysema generally fails to elicit pulmonary hypertension.

However, when pulmonary vascular reserve has been exhausted by progressive reduction in the extent and distensibility of the pulmonary vascular tree, even the increments in blood flow associated with daily living may suffice to elicit marked pulmonary hypertension. The essential component of this vulnerability is a decrease in the cross-sectional area of the pulmonary resistance vessels. The restricted vascular bed stems from widespread narrowing and obstruction of small pulmonary arteries and arterioles, usually accompanied by a decrease in the distensibility not only of the vessels but also of the adjacent lung.

VASOMOTOR INCREASE IN PULMONARY VASCULAR RESISTANCE (HYPOXIA AND ACIDOSIS) The most potent stimulus for pulmonary vasoconstriction is alveolar hypoxia which acts directly on adjacent small pulmonary arteries and arterioles; systemic arterial hypoxemia supplements the local effects of alveolar hypoxia indirectly by way of the sympathetic nerves to the pulmonary circulation. In chronic hypoxia, these effects

TABLE 262-2
Pathogenetic mechanisms in chronic pulmonary hypertension and cor pulmonale

Pathogenetic mechanism	*Intermediaries*	*Examples*
Primary mechanisms		
Anatomical increase in pulmonary vascular resistance	Obliteration, obstruction, reduction, and stiffening of pulmonary vascular tree	*Vascular disease:* Primary pulmonary hypertension; recurrent pulmonary emboli *Extravascular disease:* Diffuse interstitial disease; fibrosing alveolitis; pneumoconiosis
Vasomotor increase in pulmonary vascular resistance	Pulmonary vasoconstriction by hypoxia and acidosis	*General alveolar hypoventilation with normal lungs:* *1* Disorders of chest bellows: neuromuscular; extreme obesity; kyphoscoliosis *2* Diminished ventilatory drive: primary alveolar hypoventilation; sleep; hypercapnia
Combined anatomical restriction and vasomotor	Combination of above	*Net alveolar hypoventilation with abnormal lungs:* Chronic obstructive lung disease: "blue bloater"; cystic fibrosis of pancreas
Secondary mechanisms		
Increase in cardiac output	Increase in metabolic rate; acute hypoxia	Daily activities; acute respiratory infection
Increase in blood viscosity	Secondary polycythemia	Chronic hypoxia
Tachycardia	Aggravation of hypoxia	Heart failure

may be intensified by increased viscosity of the blood arising from secondary polycythemia. Experiments in dogs indicate that severe acidosis (pH <7.2) also elicits pulmonary vasoconstriction. In man, acidosis acts synergistically with hypoxia, whereas alkalosis diminishes the pressor response to hypoxia. The biological basis for this interplay remains unclear.

HYPERCAPNIA In contrast to the effects of hypoxia and acidosis, the effects of CO_2 on the pulmonary circulation appear to be by way of the acidosis that it generates rather than by a direct action on pulmonary vessels. However, because heart failure in cor pulmonale is often associated with respiratory insufficiency and because management of the respiratory insufficiency generally determines the prognosis, the noncardiac effects of hypercapnia merit consideration.

Hypercapnia affects mainly the central nervous system, producing cerebral vasodilatation, increased cerebrospinal fluid pressure, and neurologic derangements ranging from weakness, irritability, lassitude, and cloudy sensorium to somnolence, confusion, and coma. These derangements are most apt to occur if hypercapnia is acute in onset and severe, or if chronic hypercapnia is acutely aggravated. In contrast, during chronic hypercapnia, the patient may be virtually free of central nervous system disturbances if respiratory acidosis is fully compensated. When severe hypoxemia and hypercapnia coexist, it may be impossible to distinguish between their neurologic effects because severe hypoxia causes anatomic damage to nervous tissues.

Carbon dioxide retention, with elevated CO_2 tensions in the blood and tissues, is self-perpetuating. On the one hand, hypercapnia from any cause blunts the responsiveness of the respiratory center to the CO_2 stimulus; on the other, hypercapnia promotes retention of bicarbonate by the kidney. Not only the hypercapnia originating in disorders of the lungs or ventilation, but also the hypercapnia of metabolic alkalosis causes ventilatory depression. This is the reason that patients with chronic hypercapnia are particularly vulnerable to the effects of sedatives or oxygen breathing, both of which may cause calamitous increments in the degree of hypercapnia: sedatives do so by depressing further the respiratory centers in the brain; oxygen by abolishing the hypoxic peripheral drive to ventilation. It is usually in the severely hypoxic, hypercapneic patient that right-sided heart failure occurs.

ALVEOLAR HYPOVENTILATION A large disparity between the degree of pulmonary hypertension recorded during life and the anatomic changes in the lungs and pulmonary vessels at autopsy is common and is particularly marked in patients with COLD, in whom the anatomic changes in the gas-exchanging parts of the lungs consistently appear to be inadequate to explain either the blood-gas abnormalities or the pulmonary arterial pressor response. Similarly, the most extensive emphysema may be associated with normal levels of blood gases and normal pulmonary arterial pressures. Much of this discrepancy disappears when account is taken of alveolar hypoventilation, an important functional disorder which cannot be quantified at autopsy. Recognizing that alveolar hypoventilation is an essential component in the pathogenesis of cor pulmonale is critical for two reasons: (1) elimination of the initiating mechanism (e.g., acute respiratory infection) usually reverses the alveolar hypoventilation, and (2) unless alveolar ventilation is improved, other therapeutic measures are apt to be ineffective.

PULMONARY HYPERTENSION

Two distinct patterns characterize the natural history of cor pulmonale at sea level: (1) *episodic* pulmonary hypertension and cor pulmonale which may, but need not, be succeeded by sustained pulmonary hypertension, cor pulmonale, and right-sided heart failure; this sequence is characteristic of COLD with periodic exacerbations that elicit episodic alveolar hypoventilation (see below and Chap. 252), and (2) *progressive*, unremitting pulmonary hypertension and cor pulmonale leading inexorably to right-sided heart failure; this pattern is generally a consequence either of progressive pulmonary vascular or interstitial disease or of unremitting hypoxia (as in continuing alveolar hypoventilation). Distinction between the two sequences tends to become blurred if intercurrent respiratory infections decrease the intervals between bouts of hypoxia and pulmonary hypertension. Also, each bout of pulmonary hypertension may predispose to a subsequent bout of cor pulmonale because of residual hypertrophy of the muscular pulmonary arteries or further curtailment of the extent and distensibility of the pulmonary vascular tree. Consequently, although relief of hypoxia may restore the pulmonary arterial pressure to normal or near-normal levels, with each attack the pulmonary vascular tree seems to lose some of its adaptability and the patient moves a little closer to the verge of persistent cor pulmonale.

FROM PULMONARY HYPERTENSION TO COR PULMONALE In patients destined to develop cor pulmonale, pulmonary hypertension first appears either when blood flow is increased (exercise; fever) or during a bout of acute hypoxia (bronchopulmonary infection). In time, pulmonary hypertension is present even at rest. The highest pulmonary artery pressures occur in pulmonary vascular and interstitial disease; they are much less impressive and fixed in chronic obstructive lung disease, even during an acute exacerbation. At first, the pulmonary hypertension during exercise or hypoxia is associated with normal end-diastolic pressure in the right ventricle. But as pulmonary hypertension is prolonged or becomes more severe, abnormally high filling pressure (end-diastolic) develops in the right ventricle, a reflection of right ventricular dilatation and/or of diminished ventricular compliance associated with hypertrophy; cardiac output is still normal at rest and increases normally during exercise (cor pulmonale without heart failure). Finally, the onset of right-sided heart failure is identified by abnormally high end-diastolic pressures in the right ventricle; the cardiac output, which may still be normal at rest, fails to increase normally during exercise; the systemic veins are engorged, reflecting the inability of the right ventricle to empty normally.

THE LEFT VENTRICLE IN COR PULMONALE Except for those few altitude dwellers who develop mountain sickness, the left ventricle does not share in the cardiomegaly of high altitude. Consequently, tolerable levels of hypoxia do not exert serious noxious effects on the myocardium nor are they associated with an inordinate hemodynamic load on the left ventricle. Conversely, severe, high intolerable levels of hypoxia and arterial hypoxemia at altitude may impair myocardial function of both ventricles as well as produce right ventricular overload. The left ventricle then enlarges and fails, primarily because of inadequate oxygen delivery to the myocardium.

At sea level, cor pulmonale is not associated with left ventricular enlargement as long as arterial hypoxemia is modest in degree. But, in pulmonary disorders associated with severe hypoxemia, left ventricular enlargement and malfunction may occur. In the latter group, a complicated interplay seems to be involved in the pathogenesis of abnormal left ventricular performance: independent disease of the left ventricle, particularly arteriosclerotic heart disease, aggravated by the direct effects of inadequate oxygen delivery to the myocardium plus the noxious effects of severe hypoxemia and acidosis on the myocardium. In turn, the respiratory insufficiency which initiated the impaired myocardial performance by causing abnormal levels of arterial blood gases is intensified if left ventricular failure causes interstitial and alveolar pulmonary edema.

CLINICAL MANIFESTATIONS OF COR PULMONALE

The ease of diagnosing cor pulmonale depends on recognition of the fact that the underlying pulmonary disorder can culminate in pulmonary hypertension. The diagnosis is generally straightforward in obliterative vascular disease. It is much more elusive in COLD; chronic bronchitis and bronchiolitis are not always self-evident, and clinical indices of pulmonary hypertension are not always reliable. Therefore, the cor pulmonale that follows COLD may be appreciated only retrospectively, i.e., after an episode of overt right ventricular failure. Detection may be particularly difficult if the systemic venous congestion and peripheral edema develop insidiously, over days to weeks, rather than appearing suddenly in the course of an acute bronchopulmonary infection.

DIFFERENTIAL DIAGNOSIS This is particularly troublesome and important in the elderly patient who is of the proper age for arteriosclerotic heart disease, has had cough and sputum for many years ("chronic bronchitis"), and clearly manifests right ventricular failure. Analyses of arterial blood gases are then most helpful in deciding whether the primary cardiac disorder is in the right or left ventricle, since appreciable arterial hypoxemia, hypercapnia, and acidosis are unusual in left-sided heart failure unless frank pulmonary edema is also present.

Support for the diagnosis of cor pulmonale may be adduced from roentgenographic and electrocardiographic evidence of right ventricular enlargement. Rarely is catheterization of the right side of the heart needed to settle the question, once suspicion of cor pulmonale is aroused. But, if necessary, cardiac catheterization will typically show pulmonary arterial hypertension, normal left atrial ("pulmonary wedge") pressures, and the classical hemodynamics of right ventricular failure.

The conventional signs of right ventricular enlargement include a cardiac thrust along the left sternal border or immediately below the sternum and a fourth heart sound arising in the hypertrophied ventricle. Concomitant pulmonary hypertension is suggested by a cardiac thrust in the second left interspace adjacent to the sternum, an unusually loud second component of the second heart sound in the same area, and occasionally the murmur of pulmonary valvular insufficiency. If the right ventricle fails, tricuspid insufficiency and a right ventricular gallop sound are often added. Hydrothorax is uncommon, even after the advent of overt right ventricular failure. Permanent arrhythmias, such as atrial flutter or fibrillation, are unusual, but transitory arrhythmias are common during severe hypoxia or when respiratory alkalosis has been induced by mechanical hyperventilation.

The diagnostic value of the *electrocardiogram* in cor pulmonale depends on the underlying pulmonary or ventilatory disorder (Table 262-3). It is most valuable in pulmonary vascular or interstitial disease, particularly if COLD is absent, or in alveolar hypoventilation with normal lungs. Conversely, because of the hyperinflated lungs and the episodic nature of the pulmonary hypertension and right ventricular overload, patterns diagnostic of right ventricular hypertrophy are uncommon in cor pulmonale secondary to COLD. Consequently, even if right ventricular enlargement in the course of COLD is marked, as during a bout of acute upper respiratory infection, electrocardiographic evidence may be inconclusive because of rotation and displacement of the heart, widened distances between electrodes and the cardiac surface, and the predominance of dilatation over hypertrophy in the cardiac enlargement. Thus a reliable diagnosis of right ventricular enlargement can be made in only one-quarter of patients with COLD whose hearts show right ventricular hypertrophy at autopsy, whereas the diagnosis is easily and reliably made in the great majority of patients with cor pulmonale originating in pulmonary disorders other than COLD.

Roentgenography has more diagnostic value in arousing suspicion of or confirming than in detecting enlargement of the right ventricle. Suspicion is aroused by evidences of an antecedent predisposing pulmonary disorder coupled with large central pulmonary arteries and a pruned peripheral arterial tree, i.e., evidence of pulmonary hypertension. Serial x-rays are generally more useful than a single examination for heart size, particularly in COLD, where dramatic changes in heart size may occur between a bout of acute respiratory insufficiency and recovery.

CLINICAL FORMS OF COR PULMONALE AND THEIR TREATMENT

No matter how initiated—anatomic, vasomotor, or both—chronic pulmonary hypertension tends to be self-perpetuating because of continuing narrowing and obliteration of the pulmonary vascular bed by muscular hypertrophy of small arteries and arterioles, arteriosclerosis, thrombosis, and devious malformations in the course of small arteries and arterioles (*glomus formations*).

ANATOMICAL INCREASE IN PULMONARY VASCULAR RESISTANCE These abnormalities may be sorted into two general categories (Table 262-2):

Vascular disease; occlusive disease of the small pulmonary arteries In these disorders, widespread occlusion of the small pulmonary vessels takes place over months to years. Most often, the cause is multiple pulmonary emboli (Chap. 256); less common are multiple thromboses such as those which complicate sickle-cell anemia. A rare cause is "primary pulmonary hypertension" (Chap. 259).

Tachypnea, persisting during sleep, is an outstanding feature of multiple pulmonary emboli. This increase in respiratory frequency is associated with alveolar hyperventilation as indicated by characteristically low values for alveolar and arterial P_{CO_2} and for serum bicarbonate. Incapacitating breathlessness occurs on mild exertion. Precordial or thoracic pain is not uncommon: occasionally the pain mimics angina; at other times it is clearly pleuritic, intensifying during inspiration. Clinical criteria, roentgenography, and electrocardiography are classical for right ventricular enlargement. Cyanosis, which is rarely impressive before heart failure, usually becomes striking after the right ventricle fails. Objective evidence for pulmonary emboli is conventionally sought by photoscanning and pulmonary angiography (Chaps. 250 and 256).

Of all patients who develop cor pulmonale, those with multiple pulmonary emboli have the highest pulmonary arterial pressures; these may equal or even exceed systemic arterial pressures. The cardiac output tends to be low. Mild arterial hypoxemia is the rule and seems to arise from shunting within the lungs. Whether the shunts represent blood flow through recanalized vessels (e.g., glomus formations) that are no longer in contact with alveoli, or too-rapid passage of the entire cardiac output through unoccluded and dilated portions of the pulmonary vascular tree, or blood flow through anatomic pulmonary arteriovenous channels that are ordinarily inoperative, is conjectural. During right-sided heart failure, these shunts cause profound arterial hypoxemia because the shunted (mixed venous) blood has an extremely low O_2 content.

Once pulmonary hypertension is fixed, treatment directed at the process in the lungs is rarely effective, since organization of emboli has led to irreversible occlusions of innumerable small arteries. Continuous administration of O_2 enriched mixtures is standard. Caution must be exercised to avoid oxygen toxicity by administering as little additional oxygen as possible. Unfortunately, compromises are often required, because the arterial blood is not easily restored towards normal levels of oxygenation because of the magnitude of the venous shunts.

The grim outlook for treating the cor pulmonale of multiple pulmonary emboli, as well as the ever-present prospect of catastrophic pulmonary embolization, has emphasized the need for prophylactic measures in patients judged to be candidates for pulmonary emboli (Chap. 256). Heart failure is treated by the usual cardiotonic measures in conjunction with measures directed at improving arterial oxygenation. Rarely does it respond dramatically as long as the hemodynamic overload persists.

TABLE 262-3
ECG patterns in chronic cor pulmonale

*Chronic obstructive lung disease (suggestive, but not diagnostic, of right ventricular enlargement)**
- "P-pulmonale" (in leads II, III, AVF)
- Right axis deviation (>90°)
- R:S ratio in $V_1 > 1$; in $V_6 < 1$
- rSR′ in right chest leads
- Right bundle branch block (partial or complete)

Pulmonary vascular or interstitial disease; general alveolar hypoventilation (diagnostic of right ventricular enlargement)
- Classic pattern in V_1 or V_3R (dominant R or R′ with inverted T waves in right chest leads)
- Often associated with "suggestive" criteria above

* *Among the "suggestive" criteria, it is difficult to distinguish right ventricular enlargement (hypertrophy and enlargement) from changes in the anatomic and electrical positions of the heart produced by the hyperinflated lungs. Consequently, the "suggestive" criteria are more useful as confirmatory, than as diagnostic, evidence.*

Diffuse interstitial fibrosis and granuloma Among the diverse entities included in this category are (1) sarcoidosis, berylliosis, and the "nonspecific" granulomatoses (Chap. 258); (2) scleroderma of the lung (Chap. 254); (3) the various interstitial or alveolar-septal fibroses such as "fibrosing alveolitis," radiation fibrosis, or pulmonary asbestosis, and the special progressive form of interstitial disease known as the Hamman-Rich syndrome (Chap. 254); (4) immunopathologic disease of the lungs, exemplified by "farmer's lung" (Chap. 257); and (5) diffuse carcinomatous infiltration of the lung, such as "alveolar-cell" or lymphangitic carcinoma (Chap. 260).

Clinically, the respiratory difficulty often begins with an acute respiratory illness that fails to resolve. Tachypnea persists. The roentgenogram shows fine nodular or fibrotic lesions widely disseminated throughout both lung fields. In the resting subject, the arterial P_{O_2} is sustained at near-normal levels by chronic hyperventilation; during exercise, it drops precipitously. The arterial P_{CO_2} is normal or slightly low, reflecting the balance between the augmented ventilation, the oxygen consumption, which is often increased, and the partition of the augmented ventilation between the alveoli and the dead space.

As long as hypoxemia is mild, pulmonary hypertension is modest. But as the disease progresses and as hypoxemia increases—in part because of ventilation-perfusion abnormalities—the level of pulmonary hypertension also increases, and cor pulmonale begins to evolve. Right ventricular failure generally occurs late in the course of the disease. At first, it responds well to oxygen mixtures and a cardiotonic program (Chap. 233). Oxygen therapy is quite useful since it affords relief of dyspnea and improves oxygenation without threat of carbon dioxide retention. However, oxygen dependence may become marked, and the hazards of oxygen toxicity increase *pari passu* with the increasing concentrations of inspired oxygen and the duration of exposure.

Relief of heart failure is usually transient unless the initiating mechanism is controlled. Rarely is the underlying lesion in the lung reversible, even though steroids occasionally have been associated with dramatic benefit, especially in some of the granulomatoses and "fibrosing alveolitis." More apt to be rewarding is the successful treatment of a superimposed respiratory infection which has toppled a stable patient into heart failure.

VASOMOTOR INCREASE IN PULMONARY VASCULAR RESISTANCE For convenience, alveolar hypoventilation, a prime cause of elevated pulmonary vascular resistance, can be identified by a value for arterial P_{CO_2} greater than 45 mm Hg; the disorder may be regarded as either "general" or "net."

Alveolar hypoventilation: general The critical importance of abnormal values for blood gases in the pathogenesis of cor pulmonale is illustrated by the syndrome of alveolar hypoventilation coexistent with normal lungs ("general alveolar hypoventilation"). In these patients, some abnormality, either in the regulation of ventilation or in the neuromuscular apparatus, rather than intrinsic pulmonary disease, is responsible for the hypoxia and hypercapnia. The syndrome may have diverse etiologies (Chap. 255).

Alveolar hypoventilation: net The common denominator in this group of disorders is the imbalance between alveolar ventilation, blood flow, and diffusion, resulting in hypercapnia and hypoxemia. In contrast to *general* alveolar hypoventilation, in which the same abnormalities of arterial blood gas levels occur despite normal lungs, intrinsic lung disease is the basis for the abnormal values for blood gases in *net* alveolar hypoventilation.

The assortment of obstructive airway diseases predisposing to cor pulmonale has been pictured as a spectrum of bronchopulmonary disorders, ranging from pure obstruction of the airways at one end to pure emphysema at the other; between the two ends are the mixtures which are most prevalent (Chap. 252). Most pertinent to cor pulmonale is the patient with bronchitis and bronchiolitis, usually with some emphysema, in whom obstructive disease of the airways has so deranged the balance between alveolar ventilation, blood flow, and diffusion as to cause the characteristic syndrome of cyanosis (hypoxemia), somnolence (hypercapnia), and right ventricular failure; these are the "blue bloaters." In contrast, the "pink puffers," with comparable degrees of airway obstruction by conventional tests, do not develop hypoxia in the course of their breathless existence; only during an intercurrent respiratory infection, as hypoxia is superimposed, do they become candidates for cor pulmonale. Emphysema without bronchitis is rarely associated with cor pulmonale since alveolar ventilation and capillary blood flow seem to be commensurately curtailed, as after pulmonary resection, so that neither hypoxia nor pulmonary hypertension become appreciable.

Successful treatment of the "blue bloater" with cor pulmonale depends on relieving the bronchitis and bronchiolitis (Chap. 263). Cardiotonic agents are useless unless oxygenation is improved. If the patient succeeds in maintaining good oxygenation, digitalis and diuretics can usually be discontinued. Relief of airway obstruction is more readily accomplished in some disorders than in others. For example, it is generally easier in chronic bronchitis than in cystic fibrosis of the pancreas, in which most of the airways remain plugged with abnormal, thick, tenacious sputum despite heroic therapeutic efforts.

Cor pulmonale is uncommon in uncomplicated silicosis or tuberculosis. On the other hand, it is not uncommon when silicosis, anthrosilicosis, or long-standing fibrotic tuberculosis is complicated by extensive, conglomerate, massive fibrosis, distorted adjacent parenchyma, shrunken lobes, and bronchitis. The likelihood of cor pulmonale is increased further by chronic pleurisy, fibrothorax, or excisional surgery. In such cases, a combination of anatomic restriction of the vascular bed and disturbances in gas exchange is involved in the pathogenesis of the pulmonary hypertension. Indeed, the disturbances in gas exchange, often brought to clinical levels by an acute respiratory infection, are the most reversible element of this disorder.

Although it is convenient to separate "net" from "general" alveolar hypoventilation on pathogenetic grounds, the therapeutic principles are basically the same for both and are described in Chap. 263. The present section will deal only with the circulatory abnormalities.

Since the pulmonary hypertension in the most prevalent pulmonary disorders is rarely anatomically fixed but arises mainly from hypoxia and acidosis, relief of alveolar hypoventilation is usually remarkably successful in restoring the circulation to normal. Measures to improve alveolar ventilation vary considerably. In mild cases, simple measures, such as hydration, antibiotics, and bronchodilators, often suffice; in more severe degrees of hypoxemia and hypercapnia, in which heart failure is associated with respiratory insufficiency, mechanical aids to respiration are usually needed.

It has been noted above that treatment of right-sided heart failure is less important than restoring the blood gas values to tolerable levels. The usual therapeutic measures for heart failure (Chap. 233) apply: low salt regimen, digitalis, diuretics. However, measures to decrease the circulating blood volume (and hematocrit) are of greater importance. Several phlebotomies, each draining 300 to 400 ml, may be needed within a period of 2 to 3 weeks to bring hematocrit and blood volume back to normal; repeated phlebotomies at monthly or bimonthly intervals may have to be instituted to prevent return of the hypervolemia. Diuretics have to be given with more care than usual because the metabolic alkalosis, which may complicate the use of potent diuretics such as ethacrynic acid, aggravates ventilatory insufficiency by depressing the effectiveness of the CO_2 stimulus on the respiratory centers.

The effects of vigorous therapy, directed mainly to the pulmonary disorder, are often dramatic in improving the blood gas abnormalities and heart failure. Other manifestations usually clear more slowly. Indeed, several weeks to a month may elapse before the arterial blood gases, the hematocrit, cardiac output, and pulmonary arterial pressures return to optimal levels. But therapy throughout is guided by the fact that the final outcome in cor pulmonale usually depends on the ability to cope with the underlying pulmonary disorder rather than with the changes in the heart and circulation.

REFERENCES

FISHMAN AP: Dynamics of the pulmonary circulation, in *Handbook of Physiology*, eds WF Hamilton, P Dow, vol. 2, *Circulation*, Washington: American Physiological Society, 1963

——: The left ventricle in "chronic bronchitis and emphysema," N Engl J Med 285:402, 1971

——, HECHT H: *The Pulmonary Circulation and Interstitial Space*, Chicago: University of Chicago Press, 1969

—— et al: General alveolar hypoventilation. A syndrome of respiratory and cardiac failure in patients with normal lungs, Q J Med 35:261, 1966

HEATH D et al: *Cor Pulmonale in Emphysema*, Springfield: Charles C Thomas, 1968

INGRAM RH JR, GROSSMAN GD: Chronic cor pulmonale, chap. 68 in *The Heart*, 3d ed., ed JW Hurst, New York: McGraw-Hill, 1974

PEÑALOZA D, SIME F: Chronic cor pulmonale due to loss of altitude acclimatization (chronic mountain sickness), Am J Med 50:728, 1971

263 MANAGEMENT OF ACUTE RESPIRATORY FAILURE

KENNETH M. MOSER

The management of acute respiratory failure is simple in terms of the concepts which guide therapy but complex with respect to the specific means applied. Furthermore, the fundamental concepts of therapy are well established while the specifics are continuously evolving. This chapter focuses upon the principles, rather than the details of the management of acute respiratory failure, a condition which is said to exist when, as a consequence of impaired respiratory function, arterial hypoxemia and/or hypercapnia are present; at sea level and with the patient at rest, an arterial $P_{O_2} < 60$ mm Hg and a $P_{CO_2} > 49$ mm Hg are useful guidelines in establishing the diagnosis. Clearly, substantial mechanical, biochemical, hemodynamic, and structural abnormalities may long antedate significant impairment of pulmonary gas exchange.

Therefore, respiratory failure is a laboratory diagnosis. Its detection requires (1) arterial puncture, a simple, safe procedure which should be familiar to any physician responsible for the diagnosis and treatment of patients with acute respiratory failure; and (2) determination of the P_{O_2},[1] P_{CO_2}, and pH; the development of instrumentation which can analyze the P_{O_2}, P_{CO_2}, and pH precisely and within minutes has helped to shape the modern management of acute respiratory failure.

In clinical practice, two forms of acute respiratory failure are encountered: the hypercapneic type, in which the P_{CO_2} is elevated and the P_{O_2} is lowered, and the hypoxemic type, in which the P_{CO_2} is normal or even depressed. These two forms differ with respect to pathogenesis, clinical presentation, pathophysiology, and therapy.

HYPERCAPNEIC RESPIRATORY FAILURE Patients with acute hypercapneic respiratory failure are categorized into two major groups: those with essentially normal lungs and those with intrinsic lung disease. Carbon dioxide retention in the first group is due to an absolute reduction in alveolar ventilation because of abnormalities in respiratory control, in the neuromuscular events required to maintain ventilation, or in the behavior of the chest wall (Chap. 255). Acute respiratory failure is often overlooked in these patients, who do not have pulmonary disease. The second type of patient with acute hypercapneic respiratory failure has intrinsic lung disease—most often emphysema, bronchitis, and/or asthma (Chap. 252). In these patients, alterations in the mechanical and gas exchange characteristics of the lungs lead to inadequate CO_2 elimination (alveolar hypoventilation), even though minute ventilation may be normal to increased (Chap. 255). Occasionally, mixed forms occur. A common example is the patient with chronic obstructive lung disease who receives sedatives or narcotics because of anxiety or because of a misdiagnosis of left ventricular failure. Such therapy, by depressing ventilation, may make the patient appear to be more comfortable. However, since a high level of ventilation is required to maintain adequate elimination of CO_2, the decreased ventilation may lead to acute respiratory failure and, often, to hypercapneic coma.

Consequences of hypercapnia Regardless of the events responsible for hypercapnia, all forms are complicated by hypoxemia, by respiratory acidosis if hypercapnia develops acutely, by an increase in pulmonary arteriolar resistance, and by dilatation of the cerebral vessels. This plays an important role in the increase in intracranial pressure which is sometimes seen in acute respiratory failure, including the development of papilledema, and perhaps the asterixis, seen in some patients. This increase in intracranial pressure, combined with the direct effects of hypercapnia and hypoxemia on cerebral function, also explains the disorientation, personality changes, and coma that may appear in the course of respiratory insufficiency.

HYPOXEMIC RESPIRATORY FAILURE In this form of acute respiratory insufficiency, the central problem is failure of the lungs to deliver sufficient O_2 to the pulmonary capillary blood, resulting in arterial hypoxemia. Carbon dioxide elimination is normal or even increased in these patients, so that the P_{CO_2} is normal to reduced. This form of respiratory failure occurs in a variety of circumstances (Table 263-1), including a group of disorders which may be grouped under the label "adult respiratory distress syndrome"; these disorders are characterized by

[1] *Unless otherwise stated in this chapter, P_{O_2} and P_{CO_2} refer to the partial pressures of these gases in arterial blood.*

TABLE 263-1
Pathogenetic factors in hypoxemic acute respiratory failure

1 Diffuse pulmonary infections (viral, bacterial, fungal, pneumocystis)
2 Aspiration pneumonia
3 Interstitial pneumonias of unknown cause
4 Inhalation of irritating gases, e.g., smoke, NO_2, chlorine
5 Oxygen toxicity
6 Fat embolism
7 Post-trauma, postcardiopulmonary bypass, post-shock ("wet lung," "shock lung," "perfusion lung")
8 Immunologic disorders (systemic lupus erythematosus, rheumatoid arthritis, Goodpasture's syndrome, drug-induced disorder, inhaled allergens)
9 Alveolar-filling diseases (lipoid pneumonia; alveolar proteinosis)
10 Pulmonary burns

injury of the alveolar-capillary membrane, which permits leakage of fluid and cellular components from the blood into the interstitial spaces of the lung and, as the process advances, into the alveoli themselves. The injurious agents differ, and include a variety of infectious and chemical agents (Chap. 258), as well as immunologically mediated forms of pulmonary injury (Chap. 257). Whatever the cause, the clinical sequence observed is characteristic. At the time of the initial injury, and for some hours thereafter, the patient may be without respiratory symptoms. Tachypnea then appears, and the patient may complain of dyspnea. Measurements of P_{O_2} at this time will disclose significant hypoxemia despite a normal P_{CO_2}; therefore, a widened alveolar-arterial O_2 tension difference is present. Lung compliance is reduced (Chap. 249). Findings on physical examination are usually unremarkable at this juncture; a few fine rales may be present.

The hypoxemia is due to severe ventilation/perfusion imbalance (Chap. 249). In multiple zones of the lung there is diminished to absent ventilation, while perfusion continues. Where alveoli are filled with exudate, a true intrapulmonary shunt exists. Reduced lung compliance is due to the extensive accumulation of fluid, first of interstitial and later of intraalveolar fluid. Some degree of pulmonary hypertension is usually present because of arteriolar constriction from focal alveolar hypoxia and arteriolar compression by fluid in the perivascular space. Ventilation is markedly increased because of the hypoxemia and the stimuli arising from the stiff pulmonary parenchyma.

MANAGEMENT OF THE PATIENT WITH ACUTE RESPIRATORY FAILURE

The most dangerous feature of respiratory failure, the abnormality which threatens the patient's life, is the impairment of gas exchange. Therefore, the first goal of therapy is to assure that hypoxemia, hypercapnia, and acidosis do not reach hazardous levels, which are defined rather arbitrarily, since coexisting conditions modify such definitions. For example, a degree of hypoxemia which may be tolerated by a young adult with barbiturate overdosage may be dangerous in an elderly person who has recently sustained a myocardial infarction. However, there is reasonable agreement that P_{O_2} levels below 40 mm Hg are poorly tolerated by adults. Such levels are commonly associated with cardiac arrhythmias, impaired cardiac and cerebral function, and functional or anatomic damage to other organs, such as the liver and kidney. The danger level of pH is more difficult to establish, but strenuous efforts should be made to avoid or correct values below 7.2. Patients have survived brief episodes of pH 6.9 and below, but the mortality rate increases with each decrement below 7.2. The deleterious effects of severe acidosis potentiate the actions of hypoxemia and include the induction of pulmonary hypertension, depression of myocardial contractility, and compromise of cellular function throughout the body. There is no generally accepted "danger" level of P_{CO_2}, because the injurious effects of P_{CO_2} relate importantly to the degree of associated acidosis. Thus, chronic hypercapnia of 60 mm Hg with a nearly normal pH is not dangerous, while a sudden rise to 60 mm Hg sharply elevates hydrogen ion concentration and has much greater functional impact. However, when the P_{CO_2} exceeds 70 mm Hg, even when this level has been reached slowly, many patients become confused or comatose.

MAINTENANCE OF ADEQUATE OXYGENATION

The principle guiding oxygenation is to use the simplest method and the lowest inspired oxygen tension which will achieve the desired result. Reference to the oxyhemoglobin dissociation curve (Fig. 29-1) provides general guidance in defining the latter. At a P_{O_2} of approximately 50 to 60 mm Hg, the curve reaches its flat portion. Above this level, substantial increments in P_{O_2} lead to only modest increments in hemoglobin saturation and total O_2 content of the arterial blood. Therefore, a reasonable objective of O_2 therapy is to achieve a P_{O_2} of 50 to 60 mm Hg. It is not necessary to attempt to achieve a *normal* or even supernormal P_{O_2}, because there is little gain in O_2 content of the blood, as noted above. Also, any increase in arterial P_{O_2} carries significant risk of causing respiratory depression and direct lung injury.

The hazard of respiratory depression with O_2 is confined to patients with the hypercapneic form of respiratory failure in whom the normal stimuli to ventilation are compromised. The major central drives to respiration are reviewed in Chap. 255. Acute CO_2 retention provides potent drives to respiration through a decline in the pH of cerebrospinal fluid, a fall in arterial pH, and a decrease in the P_{O_2}. However, with chronic hypercapnia, cerebrospinal fluid pH readjusts to normal within 24 hr and arterial pH returns toward normal within 3 to 5 days by rises in cerebrospinal fluid and blood bicarbonate levels respectively. Thus, after several days, hypercapnia itself no longer provides a major stimulus to ventilation. Only hypoxemia and cortical factors remain. If the patient is sedated or obtunded, little cortical "drive" is provided. If O_2 is now given to the patient, the last major drive to respiration, i.e., hypoxemia, is severely blunted. The patient therefore ventilates less, and the P_{CO_2} climbs. Often, hypercapneic coma and death ensue.

It is critical, then, to avoid both sedatives and excessive

O_2 delivery in patients with chronic hypercapnia. Such patients *need* O_2 and, while fears of respiratory depression should not prevent adequate relief of hypoxemia, use of O_2 should be judicious, with frequent monitoring of P_{O_2} and P_{CO_2}, i.e., the administration of a concentration of O_2 in the inspired gas (FIO_2) which restores the P_{O_2} to acceptable levels of 50 to 60 mm Hg, without raising P_{CO_2}.

The second toxic risk of a high FIO_2 is direct injury to the lung. The mechanisms underlying this injury are debated, but its nature and gravity are well established. High concentrations of inspired O_2 injure some component(s) of the alveolar-capillary membrane, presumably the endothelium of the pulmonary capillary, with consequent increase in permeability and the leak of blood components into the interstitial and alveolar spaces. Some alveoli are flooded with proteinaceous fluid and red blood cells; in others, hyaline membranes form. In their advanced form, the lesions induced are lethal, because of progressive hypoxemia. In its end stage the lung damage by O_2 resembles that of the infant dying with hyaline membrane disease or the adult dying with devastating viral pneumonia or "shock lung."

The risks of O_2 toxicity are related to at least two factors; the FIO_2 and the duration of O_2 administration. For example, hyperbaric O_2 at several atmospheres of pressure can induce the lesion of O_2 toxicity within hours. As the FIO_2 is lowered, the period of safe exposure lengthens. Thus an FIO_2 of 100 percent at ambient partial pressure may take several days to produce lung injury. Whether an inspired FIO_2 below 50 percent is safe when given for many days is debatable. All available data indicate that the best rule is to use the lowest FIO_2 possible to maintain adequate oxygenation and for the shortest time necessary.

Means for delivering O_2 These are multiple; soft nasal prongs through which O_2 is delivered at the required flow rate are used most commonly. The net FIO_2 entering the trachea will be determined by the minute ventilation of the patient, and the flow rate of O_2. The best procedure is to start at very low flow rates (0.5 to 1.0 liter per min) and measure the response of the P_{O_2}, P_{CO_2}, and pH, gradually increasing the flow rate until the desired response has been achieved. Such "titration" by monitoring the arterial blood gases provides a safe way to guide O_2 administration.

An alternative method of O_2 delivery involves the use of masks which have been designed to deliver known, fixed concentrations of O_2. Such masks achieve a fixed concentration (regardless of the oxygen flow rate to the mask) by the *Venturi* principle. These "Venturi" masks can be obtained in rated concentration (FIO_2 = 24 percent, 28 percent, etc.). They are "high-flow" masks, fitting lightly over nose and mouth, thus providing the patient with a microenvironment of fixed FIO_2. The major advantage of masks over nasal prongs is that, regardless of the total ventilation, FIO_2 remains constant. With prongs delivering a fixed flow, the FIO_2 varies inversely with total ventilation. The disadvantage of masks is that dyspneic patients often cannot tolerate devices over their nose and mouth.

These simple means of O_2 delivery suffice in the great majority of patients with hypoxemia. However, in some patients with hypercapneic respiratory failure, masks and prongs may be unable to achieve adequate P_{O_2} without inducing marked hypercapnia, and in some patients with hypoxemic respiratory failure, it may not be possible to achieve the desired P_{O_2}. The next step is to provide the patient with a mechanical device, i.e., a ventilator, to assist respiration, and simultaneously to raise P_{O_2} and lower P_{CO_2}. This is a major decision, since it requires tracheal intubation and attachment of the patient to a mechanical device. Thus, the patient is in a "closed system" over which he can exert only limited control, and he becomes heavily dependent, or if obtunded, totally dependent, on those attending him. Furthermore, intubation and ventilation expose the patient to the additional risks described below. Therefore, it is a decision which should not be undertaken until it is clear that simpler measures will not suffice.

If assisted ventilation is required, basically two kinds of ventilator are available; the pressure-cycled and volume-cycled devices. The inspiratory phase of a pressure-cycled ventilator can be initiated by the negative-pressure inspiratory effort of the patient or by an automatic timer. Inspiration is terminated when the pressure in the device reaches a preset value of positive pressure. Thus, the volume delivered is determined by the respiratory flow rate and the time required to reach the preset pressure limit. In a volume-cycled device, the operator sets the desired volume and either the inspiratory time or the inspiratory flow rate. The machine generates whatever pressure is required to achieve the volume selected.

Each type of ventilator has its advantages and disadvantages. The major limitation of pressure-cycled devices is their inability to attain the high inspiratory pressure which may be required in patients with poorly compliant lungs. The major hazard of volume-cycled respirators is the very high pressures which they can achieve, with potential deleterious effects on venous return and cardiac output and an increased risk of pneumothorax. Patients with hypoxemic respiratory failure usually have poorly compliant lungs and require a volume ventilator. Most patients with hypercapneic respiratory failure, who have normal or highly compliant lungs, can be managed with pressure-cycled devices which are less costly.

In *hypercapneic respiratory failure*, ventilatory assistance provides several potential gains: (1) concern about respiratory depression of ventilatory drive due to increased FIO_2 is reduced, since the respirator will continue to ventilate the patient even if respiratory drive ceases, as long as the device is set to cycle automatically; (2) ventilation can be augmented at will, thus decreasing the P_{CO_2} and leading to a rise in P_{O_2} (often allowing the use of an FIO_2 approaching room air); (3) the patient's own ventilatory effort may be reduced, making him more comfortable and decreasing both O_2 needs and CO_2 production.

In *hypoxemic respiratory failure*, the ventilator is used to achieve improvement of oxygenation, by assuring adequate lung inflation and restoring a better match between ventilation and perfusion. Even areas of the lung with marked disturbances in airway resistance and compliance can be ventilated. An additional dividend is that

O_2 requirements may diminish as the respirator assumes a portion of the patient's ventilatory workload.

In some patients assisted ventilation does not suffice. They "fight" the respirator and are unable to cycle with it effectively; their ventilation must therefore be controlled. This usually can be accomplished by sedation and setting the respirator to cycle automatically. If sedation does not achieve this goal, the patient can be paralyzed with curare-like drugs.

The condition of almost all patients with hypercapneic respiratory failure can be managed by the maneuvers described above. However, some patients with severe hypoxemic failure remain dangerously hypoxemic—even with controlled volume ventilation at 100 percent O_2. Clearly, in this situation, there is the risk of inducing O_2 toxicity in an effort to maintain the patient's life. Two additional maneuvers may be considered at this point. One is the use of positive end-expiratory pressure (5 to 15 cm H_2O), or maintenance of a continuous positive pressure. This practice has been shown to increase arterial P_{O_2} in many such patients and to allow a reduction in FIO_2. However, it may also induce a decrease in venous return and cardiac output. If the increase of positive end-expiratory pressure required to elevate P_{O_2} is large, it may be necessary to measure cardiac output to determine whether oxygen delivery has actually been increased, since the P_{O_2} alone may be misleading—if it rises at the expense of a sharp decline in cardiac output and mixed venous P_{O_2}.

The second and final resort in severely hypoxemic patients is the application of cardiopulmonary bypass. Membrane oxygenators capable of maintaining adequate gas exchange for many days are now becoming available. They appear capable of sustaining patients who cannot be saved with respirators or who are placed at hazard by the need for prolonged administration of 100 percent O_2 at high pressures via respirators.

How rapidly these escalating maneuvers to assure adequate oxygenation must be employed depends on the clinical situation. Patients who have severe hypoventilatory respiratory failure because they have inadvertently received excess sedation or O_2 may require immediate intubation and ventilation, as do many patients with a fulminant form of the acute respiratory distress syndrome. Guided by the condition of the arterial blood gases, the physician can make these decisions rapidly and evaluate the patient's response.

TREATMENT OF THE PRIMARY PROBLEM Once the life-threatening derangements of gas exchange have been controlled, attention can be focused on the treatment of the problem which induced respiratory failure. In patients with absolute hypoventilation, the primary problem usually can be identified rapidly and appropriate treatment initiated. In patients with drug overdosage, treatment with dialysis or other methods to enhance drug excretion should be considered. Similar specific measures are available for patients with myasthenia gravis (Chap. 347) or myxedema (Chap. 85). In other patients, such as those with the Guillain-Barré syndrome (Chap. 323), long-term ventilatory support is required until the process runs its course.

In patients with relative hypoventilation due to obstructive lung disease, therapy is directed toward removing the problems which caused acute deterioration in the effectiveness of gas exchange. The most frequent problems are accumulation of secretions, bronchospasm, and infection. Treatment of these abnormalities will improve the mechanical dysfunction of the lungs, restore ventilation/perfusion relationships toward normal, and thereby reduce the disturbances in gas exchange.

If bronchospasm is present, therapy usually begins with administration of xanthine drugs such as aminophylline, parenterally, by mouth, or rectally; or by administration of beta-adrenergic stimulating drugs (e.g., isoproterenol) by aerosol. The usual adult dose of intravenous aminophylline is 250 to 500 mg dissolved in 10 to 20 ml diluent and delivered over a 5- to 10-min period every 2 to 6 hr. Rectal and oral doses are comparable. Isoproterenol is usually delivered by nebulizer as a 1:200 solution for 5 to 10 deep inhalations; it may be repeated hourly if necessary. If severe bronchospasm persists, adrenocortical steroids should be administered promptly by mouth or parenterally. A starting dose of 100 to 200 mg hydrocortisone is appropriate and may be repeated at hourly intervals until bronchospasm is controlled, at which point both dose size and frequency are reduced. Again, only blood gas analysis can determine how rapidly therapy should be escalated and tapered.

The attack upon secretions is two-pronged and should include measures to liquefy and to remove them. Liquefaction is best achieved by adequately hydrating the patient. Drugs which may assist in liquefaction of sputum include inorganic iodide preparations (10 drops saturated solution of potassium iodide in a glass of liquid every 6 hr or equivalent intravenous potassium iodide), glyceryl guaiacolate (15 to 30 ml by mouth every 4 to 6 hr), and acetylcysteine (5 ml of a 10% solution delivered by aerosol every 2 to 6 hr). However, by far the most effective technique for liquefying sputum is fluid administration, and adequate hydration is the keystone to sputum mobilization. If adequate hydration cannot be accomplished by mouth, oral delivery can be supplemented intravenously or by aerosol delivery of water. Furthermore, all inspired gases (oxygen or compressed air delivered from wall sources or via ventilators) should be well humidified to avoid dehydration and the accompanying thickening of nasotracheobronchial secretions.

Secretions are best removed by encouraging the patient to cough. The likelihood that coughing will be productive is greatly enhanced if a skilled respiratory or physical therapist is available to encourage the patient, assure that proper postural drainage positions are used, and supplement the patient's efforts with percussion and vibration. When spontaneous cough is either depressed or inadequate, nasotracheal or transtracheal insertion of a catheter will assist in inducing cough and removal of secretions. Transtracheal catheters, which must be kept scrupulously clean, can also be used for installation of water and other agents and for obtaining reliable sputum for culture. Finally, bronchoscopy, which is no longer a formidable procedure since introduction of the flexible fiberoptic bronchoscope, can be performed even in patients receiving continuous ventilator support. This procedure has special value in assessing the extent and distribution of secretions and in assuring that they have been removed.

Respiratory infection This is both a frequent cause and a common complication of respiratory failure in patients with obstructive lung disease. Indeed, it is so common that therapy is usually initiated with broad-spectrum antibiotics (ampicillin, tetracycline) on the presumption that infection is present. The antibiotic regimen is altered, if necessary, on the basis of the results of sputum culture. Finally, there should be a thorough search for other factors which may have induced respiratory failure, particularly left ventricular failure and pulmonary embolism.

In the hypoxemic type of acute respiratory failure, treatment of the primary problem is usually not feasible, since injury to the alveolar-capillary membrane is involved and no effective method is available for restoring its integrity. Therefore, treatment usually consists of maintenance of adequate gas exchange while awaiting resolution of the initial injury. If the latter has been caused by an infectious agent, identification and appropriate treatment are important. Occasionally, lung biopsy may be required for the rapid identification or exclusion of infectious agents, particularly in the case of viral and *Pneumocystis carinii* infections, although specimens obtained by fiberoptic bronchoscopy should be examined first.

Corticosteroids often are useful in those forms of the acute respiratory distress syndrome which are mediated through the immune system or are responses to injurious inhalants (e.g., irritant gases, chemical substances, or thermal injuries). High doses of these agents should be used in an effort to halt inflammation and restore the integrity of cell membranes (e.g., 100 to 200 mg hydrocortisone or its equivalent every 2 to 4 hr). If a response is to occur, it should be apparent within a few days and the dose of corticosteroids should then be tapered. The value of corticosteroids remains controversial in many of the forms of the adult respiratory distress syndrome, such as aspiration pneumonia and fat embolism. Nevertheless, their use is warranted when the lung injury is severe. It is also essential that the presence of left ventricular failure, masquerading as or complicating the adult respiratory distress syndrome, be ruled out.

Tracheostomy There are three major indications for tracheostomy in patients with acute respiratory failure: (1) to facilitate removal of secretions; (2) to provide a port for long-term ventilator attachment; (3) to bypass upper airway obstruction (e.g., croup, allergic edema). These indications are relative, since an endotracheal or nasotracheal tube can be used for attaching ventilators and other means for removal of secretions are available. However, when copious secretions are a major problem, tracheostomy often is of great value in reversing respiratory failure. Tracheostomy is preferable to an endo- or nasotracheal tube in patients who require ventilatory assistance for more than a few days, particularly alert patients.

THE RESPIRATORY INTENSIVE CARE UNIT The patient with acute respiratory insufficiency requires expert care in terms of both monitoring and therapy. These special requirements are intensified if the patient requires ventilatory support. Such requirements are best satisfied in a unit specifically devoted to the care of such patients; i.e., a respiratory intensive care unit. The central elements of such a unit include: (1) a staff of physicians and nurses highly trained in the diagnosis and therapy of respiratory failure, supported by respiratory and chest physical therapists; (2) immediate and continuous availability of special equipment for ventilation, resuscitation, aspiration, and of monitoring equipment, including instruments for arterial blood gas analysis; and (3) a geographic area designed for these purposes. Such a pooling of personnel and resources available 24 hr a day, 7 days a week, is an expensive undertaking, but this cost appears to be justified by the more favorable results of therapy. Though not every hospital needs to develop a respiratory intensive care unit, one such unit should be available within a reasonable transport time for patients in any given geographic region. Indeed, many respiratory intensive care units now offer transport teams which move patients to the unit from his home or from other medical facilities.

Complications of respiratory intensive care Certain complications occur frequently in patients being treated for acute respiratory failure; when sudden deterioration of the patient with acute respiratory failure occurs, the reasons will usually be among those listed below:

1 *Cardiac arrhythmias* of all types are very common. Potential causes of arrhythmias in respiratory failure are multiple: hypoxemia, wide swings in pH, electrolyte disturbances, and the action or interaction of pharmacologic agents such as aminophylline and isoproterenol employed in the treatment of acute respiratory failure. Digitalis toxicity, for example, is potentiated by hypoxemia, and the arrhythmic potential of isoproterenol is well recognized. For these reasons, continuous monitoring of cardiac rhythm is essential.
2 *Gastrointestinal hemorrhage* is also frequently seen in these patients. In part, this reflects the high incidence of peptic ulcer in patients with obstructive lung disease, but it also is related to other factors such as stress, the possible effects of severe blood gas derangements and of alterations in cardiac output upon the gastrointestinal circulation, and the use of adrenocortical steroids, aminophylline, aspirin, and other drugs. Bleeding occurs almost exclusively from the stomach and duodenum and may be both massive and sudden.
3 *Pulmonary infection* already has been mentioned. Scrupulous cleansing of respiratory equipment is essential, lest these devices populate the patient's lungs with pathogenic bacteria. All personnel caring for such patients must observe strict aseptic techniques in all manipulations of the patient (e.g., nasotracheal suction, cleaning tracheostomy tubes).
4 *Pneumothorax* occurs with more than chance frequency in patients with acute respiratory failure, especially in those requiring ventilator support. Volume ventilators and end-expiratory positive pressure in

particular predispose to this complication. Sudden respirator malfunction or respiratory distress should promote a prompt search for a pneumothorax, since its persistence may be lethal and its correction can be accomplished simply and rapidly.

5 *Bronchial obstruction by endotracheal or tracheostomy tubes* often occurs. These tubes, when too long or poorly anchored, slide into one mainstem bronchus, usually the right one because of its less angulated origin from the trachea. The tube then blocks ventilation of the other mainstem bronchus, and atelectasis may ensue. Such an event usually causes abrupt deterioration in the patient with respiratory failure. It is detected readily by physical examination, which reveals the absence of breath sounds over the occluded lung. The tube should immediately be pulled back slowly if this complication is suspected.

Other common complications during acute respiratory failure include (1) acute right ventricular failure, due to pulmonary hypertension and hypoxia (Chap. 262); (2) left ventricular failure, detectable by means of right-sided heart catheterization carried out at the bedside with flow-guided catheters; (3) pulmonary interstitial and alveolar edema from overhydration and increased pulmonary capillary permeability. Diuretics and oncotic substances, such as salt-poor albumin, may be helpful in the treatment of this complication; (4) pulmonary oxygen toxicity, reviewed previously; (5) convulsions due to hypoxia or to sudden induction of alkalosis with ventilators; and (6) tracheal injury due to excessive pressure in the occluding cuffs of endotracheal-tracheostomy tubes or pressure exerted by the tubes themselves.

Those caring for patients with acute respiratory failure must be alert to all these complications. Their prevention—or prompt detection and reversal—often spell the difference between survival and death. The ability of all personnel in the respiratory intensive care unit to deal with these problems is another factor which enhances the likelihood of survival of the patient in the respiratory intensive care unit environment.

MANAGEMENT OF CHRONIC RESPIRATORY FAILURE See Chap. 252.

REFERENCES

Campbell EJM: The management of acute respiratory failure in chronic bronchitis and emphysema. Am Rev Resp Dis 96:626, 1967

Hedley-Whyte J: Causes of pulmonary oxygen toxicity. N Engl J Med 283:1518, 1970

Inter-Society Commission for Heart Disease Resources, Study Group on Pulmonary Heart Disease: Resources for the optimal care of acute respiratory failure. Circulation 43:A-185, 1971

Petty TL, Ashbaugh DG: The adult respiratory distress syndrome. Chest 60:233, 1971

Symposium on Management of Chronic Obstructive Lung Disease and Acute Respiratory Failure. Chest 58(suppl 2):407, 1970

section 4 | Disorders of the kidneys and urinary tract

264
DISORDERS OF FLUIDS AND ELECTROLYTES

LOUIS G. WELT

PHYSIOLOGIC CONSIDERATIONS

VOLUMES OF BODY FLUID The total volume of body fluid is equivalent to 50 to 70 percent of the body weight. Since adipose tissue is relatively free of water, the figure is closer to 50 percent in the obese and approximates 70 percent in lean individuals. This fluid is compartmented into two major phases, the *intracellular* and the *extracellular,* and several subdivisions thereof. Approximately two-thirds of the total water is within the cells. The extracellular fluid (one-third of the total, approximately equivalent to 16 to 20 percent of the body weight) is further partitioned between the plasma and interstitial fluid. The smallest component represents about 2.5 percent of the total volume of water and is referred to as *transcellular.* It includes the fluid within the gastrointestinal tract, the tracheobronchial tree, the excretory system of the kidneys and glands, the cerebrospinal fluid, and the aqueous humor of the eye.

The volume of several of these major compartments can be estimated. The technique entails administration of some material whose distribution is considered to be uniform throughout the compartment in question. If a known amount of the test material is administered, and if the amount lost from the body during the time necessary for complete mixing can be determined and the concentration per liter at the time of equilibration can be estimated, the volume of distribution of the test substance can be calculated. The volume of total body water can be estimated by using water labeled with deuterium or tritium. A variety of substances, such as inulin, sucrose, and sulfate, have been used to define the volume of the extracellular fluid. The volume of the intracellular fluid cannot be estimated directly but may be inferred from the difference between the total volume of body water and the volume of the extracellular fluid. Plasma volume (approximately 4 percent of the body weight) has been calculated from the volume of distribution of protein-bound dyes, such as T-1824, and of albumin tagged with ^{131}I. However, since the proteins, particularly albumin, are not wholly confined to the vascular compartment and gain access to the interstitial spaces and the lymph, the volume of distribution of tagged albumin is likely to be in excess of the plasma volume itself. The volume of the red blood cell mass is considered to be more reliable and may be estimated utilizing erythrocytes tagged with an isotope of iron, phosphorus, or chromium. From the red blood cell mass and the hematocrit one can readily calculate the plasma volume.

Each of these measurements has been of value in investigating both normal and pathologic exchanges of water and electrolytes. There is no doubt that such measurements would provide considerable aid in managing patients whose illness is complicated by a disorder of hydration and of electrolyte imbalance.

COMPOSITION OF BODY FLUIDS There are major differences in the composition of the intra- and extracellular fluids, and minor differences among the several components of the latter. The composition of the extracellular fluid is better understood and more precisely defined, both because it is a simpler fluid and because it is available for analysis in the form of serum and transudates into the serous cavities. The only cells that can be obtained in relatively pure form in any bulk are the erythrocytes. Generalizations from the characteristics of this unique and highly specialized cell to all cells would, of course, be most hazardous.

The *interstitial fluid* of the extracellular compartment is an ultrafiltrate of serum and differs from the latter in that it contains very low concentrations of large-molecular species such as proteins and lipids. The usually accepted normal range of values for the concentrations of electrolytes in serum is as follows:

Cations, mEq/liter	
Sodium	132–142
Potassium	3.5–5.0
Calcium	4.5–5.5
Magnesium	1.5–2.0
Anions, mEq/liter	
Chloride	98–106
Total CO_2	26–30 (mmol/liter)
Phosphate and sulfate	2–5
Organic anions	3–6
Proteins	15–25

The average total cation concentration approximates 150 mEq per liter, and this is considered to be identical with the total anion concentration. Although these concentrations are conventionally expressed in relation to a unit volume of serum, it is understood that these ions are for all intents and purposes distributed in the aqueous phase of the serum. The average water content of serum is about 93 percent, and hence to express these concentrations in terms of serum water, they should each be divided by 0.93. The concentrations in the water of serum can then be translated to the concentrations in the interstitial fluid by applying a correction factor to account for the asymmetric distribution of ions across the capillary membrane. This latter is related to the presence in the serum of nondiffusible ions, the proteins. The Donnan ratio that describes the relative concentrations between serum and an ultrafiltrate thereof is approximately 1.05 for the univalent cations and 0.95 for the univalent anions. For example, the calculations of the concentrations of sodium or chloride in the interstitial fluid are performed as follows:

$$Na_{IF} = \frac{Na_s}{SW} \times 1.05$$

and

$$Cl_{IF} = \frac{Cl_s}{SW} \times 0.95$$

where IF = interstitial fluid, SW = fraction of serum that is water.

The compositions of joint fluid, aqueous humor of the eye, and cerebrospinal fluid are all similar to an ultrafiltrate of serum, but there are enough differences in the aqueous humor and spinal fluid to suggest that these are not pure dialysates but are, in part at least, formed by active transport processes.

The composition of the intracellular fluids cannot be examined directly, and hence the characteristics of cell fluid are inferred from analyses of whole tissue and the use of certain "reasonable" calculations. The total tissue water can be readily estimated from the difference in weight between the fresh wet tissue and the weight after it has been dried. The volume of this water that is to be ascribed to the extracellular phase is calculated from knowledge of the concentration of some substance in the tissue and serum, with the assumption that that particular substance is confined to an extracellular position. In the past, most of these calculations were made on the assumption that chloride was confined to the extracellular phase. This is obviously not true, and for more precise data one must employ other agents, such as inulin. The values for the volume of the extracellular fluid and the concentrations of sodium and potassium in this fluid (as derived from their values in serum) are used to calculate the quantity of these two ions in the noncellular phase. The difference between the total tissue sodium and potassium and the quantity in the extracellular phase represents the amount in cells. The difference between the total water and the extracellular volume is the intracellular water. The concentration of sodium and potassium in the intracellular fluid can then be calculated. These details have been recited to emphasize the indirectness with which cell composition is defined.

The average data, derived largely from muscle analyses, obtained in this inferential manner are as follows:

Cations, mEq/liter	
Sodium	10
Potassium	150
Magnesium	40
Anions, mEq/liter	
Bicarbonate	10 (mmol/liter)
Phosphate and sulfate	150
Proteins	40

Granting the calculations are valid, much is still unknown about the physiochemical state of these materials. For example, the characteristics of the phosphate, sulfate, and proteins in terms of valence are unknown. It is not certain that all the potassium and magnesium is in a free and ionized state. Furthermore, it is probably unrealistic to speak of intracellular fluid as an entity, since diverse tissue cells have major differences in composition. Lastly, the intracellular fluid of a single cell type is probably not an entity, since it, in turn, is compartmented into extra- and intramitochondrial fluid, nuclear fluid, etc.

Another important technique to evaluate the composition of body tissues employs radioactive isotopes. These are used to calculate a value that is referred to as the *total exchangeable quantity* of a given ion. This method involves administration of a known quantity of the particular radioactive material. After a sufficient period of time, allowing the isotope to equilibrate with as much of the stable element as it will readily exchange with (approximately 24 hr), one then determines the specific activity in serum; with this datum plus knowledge of the quantity that has been lost by decay as well as that which has been excreted in the urine, one can calculate the total quantity of the ion that is readily exchangeable. This figure is usually expressed as a unit of body mass. The data collected by Moore and his colleagues provide the following average figures:

	mEq/kg body weight	
	Male	*Female*
Sodium	39.5	38.3
Potassium	48	39.4
Chloride	29.3	28.6

It must be cautioned that these figures do not represent the *total* quantity of these ions in the body, since the total is not readily exchangeable. For example, approximately 75 percent of the total body sodium and 85 percent of the total body potassium are exchangeable.

The most complicated characteristics of cell composition and the marked differences between it and the environment of the cells serve to emphasize the highly specialized functions of cells, the complex mechanisms that must be available to maintain these compositional differences, and the possibilities for alterations in metabolic pathways that may result from even subtle alterations in composition.

In contrast to the marked differences in the composition of these two major phases, it is believed that the total solute concentration in these fluids is identical. This, in turn, is due to the presumed free permeability of most of the cell membranes to water. This concept has been challenged in recent years. Although a categorical statement is not appropriate, the preponderance of evidence continues to support the concept that the cellular fluids are, in fact, isotonic with respect to their environmental fluid. This may not apply for those cells which secrete a hypotonic fluid, such as the sweat and salivary glands, and for the renal tubular cells that tolerate fluids of markedly different osmolalities on each surface.

Internal exchanges of water

When two aqueous solutions are separated by a membrane that is freely permeable to water, molecules of water will move from one compartment to the other. There will be an equilibrium with respect to water when the same number of water molecules pass in each direction per unit of time. At such a time there is no *net* alteration in volume in either of the compartments separated by the membrane. The tendency for the molecules of water to pass from one compartment to the other is spoken of as an "escaping tendency" and is referred to as the *chemical potential* of the water. Whenever the chemical potentials of the water of two contiguous solutions differ, there will be a net movement of water from the phase with the higher chemical potential to that with the lower, until equilibrium is reached. The chemical potential of water is reduced when solutes are added, and the reduction is proportional to the concentration of solutes. In contrast, the chemical potential of water molecules is enhanced by increases in hydrostatic pressure and temperature.

Thus, the addition of a solute that can traverse a membrane with freedom will result in its uniform distribution throughout the volumes of fluid separated by that membrane. The addition of this solute will diminish the chemical potential of the water molecules, but since the water in both compartments is influenced to the same degree, there is no *net* change in the volume of water on either side of the membrane. The only effect is that fewer molecules of water, but an equal number of them, move in each direction per unit of time. In contrast, if the added solute were unable to permeate the membrane in question, it would be confined to the side to which it was added and would diminish the chemical potential of the molecules of water on that side alone. Under this circumstance molecules of water would continue to *enter* this phase at the rate which obtained prior to the addition of the solute, but water molecules would *escape from* this compartment at a slower rate and there would be a net change in volume, such that water would accumulate in the compartment to which the solute had been added. The redistribution of water would continue until a new state of equilibrium was established.

This problem may be looked at a little more carefully in terms of the pore theory of membranes. In the context of the discussion just presented, imagine a membrane separating two aqueous solutions and visualize a pore that permeates the membrane. Assume that the solutions in the two phases are pure water and that exchange (with no *net* movement) occurs owing to the random movement of molecules of water. Now if one adds to side I a solute that cannot permeate the membrane, it is clear that more molecules of water will move from the pore at its interface with solution I than will move from solution I into the pore. This loss of water molecules at the interface must promote a pressure drop across the pore and be responsible for the net movement of water into solution I. This is emphasized by pointing out that there is only pure water within the pore and, hence, no tendency for the molecules of water to move more in one direction than another. The situation that conditions the movement must, in fact, be the pressure gradient across the pore. Ordinarily these problems are discussed in terms of osmotic pressure. In this context, the addition of a solute that can permeate membranes freely, such as urea, contributes to the total osmotic pressure, but it is not effective in promoting a redistribution of water. Glucose, which is not free to enter cells by passive diffusion, not only contributes to the total osmotic pressure of a solution to which it is added, but contributes what is referred to as an *effective osmotic pressure* (as opposed to *total* osmotic pressure) and does condition a redistribution of water.

With respect to biologic fluids and membranes, it may be said that an increase in the concentration of those solutes that permeate membranes freely augments the total osmotic pressure (decreases the chemical potential of the water molecules) in all compartments of the body fluids. However, an increase in the concentration of a solute that cannot penetrate a membrane freely will increase the *effective* osmotic pressure as well as the total (diminish the chemical potential of the molecules of water) in the fluid in which the concentration has been altered. If this fluid is separated by a membrane freely permeable to water, there will be a net alteration in volume in favor of the compartment to which the solute has been added. Despite long usage and familiarity, the terms *total* and *effective osmotic pressure* will be replaced in the rest of this discussion with the terms *total* and *effective osmolality*. This should serve to recall that it is the activity of molecules of water that is under discussion, not the technique (utilizing hydrostatic pressure) used to estimate these activities. However, since hydrostatic pressure increases the chemical potential of molecules of water, a change in hydrostatic pressure may counterbalance the influence of solutes so that a *difference* in total solute concentration across a membrane may be unassociated with net transfers of water.

Sodium salts represent almost all the solutes that usually contribute to the effective osmolality of the extracellular fluid. Hence, in most instances an increase or a decrease in the concentration of sodium in the serum may be equated with an increase or decrease in the effective osmolality of the extracellular fluid and, in turn, will promote movement of water from or into the cellular compartment.

There are two circumstances when depressed concentration of sodium in serum may not necessarily represent diminished effective osmolality of the serum water. It will be recalled that it would be more precise to speak of the concentration of an ion such as sodium in terms of its concentration in the water of serum. Since the determination is actually performed on a diluted aliquot of serum, and since the percentage of serum that is water is so commonly between 90 and 93 percent, the convention is to refer the concentration to a unit (usually a liter) of serum. In circumstances characterized by hyperlipemia, the lipids may occupy a significant volume of the serum, and the percentage of serum that is water may be drastically reduced, to as low as 70 to 80 percent. An average concentration of sodium of 138 mEq per liter in a serum of which the water content was 93 percent would represent a concentration of 148.3 mEq per *liter* of serum *water* (138/0.93). If this same concentration obtained in the water of a *lipemic serum* where the water content was only 75 percent, the concentration per liter of *serum* would be 111.2 mEq (148.3 × 0.75). Thus, a striking hyponatremia in this instance would not mean a diminished effective osmolality of the water of the serum. This may also obtain with unusual hyperproteinemias.

Although glucose contributes to the effective osmolality of the extracellular fluid, the magnitude is usually small. At a concentration of 100 mg per 100 ml (1,000 mg per liter) this would amount to 5.5 mOsm per liter. However, if hyperglycemia supervenes, the corresponding increase in the effective osmolality will promote a movement of water from the cells. This will dilute the concentration of sodium and may depress the level to the point of frank hyponatremia. In this instance the interpretation that the hyponatremia signifies a decrease in effective osmolality would be in error. For these reasons the concentration of sodium in a patient with diabetes mellitus should be interpreted with knowledge of the simultaneous concentration of glucose in the serum.

Significance of hyponatremia

Hyponatremia is observed frequently in hospital practice. Not all instances of hyponatremia have the same pathogenesis; many are poorly understood, and a decision about management may be difficult. This discussion excludes those instances in which hyponatremia is not equivalent to a decrease in the effective osmolality of the body fluid, such as those cited in relation to hyperlipemia and hyperglycemia.

The commonest situations in which hyponatremia is observed are those cases of dehydration or edema in which salt has been lost in excess of water or water has been retained in excess of salt. A modest deficit of sodium is frequently accompanied by an equivalent loss of water. The sequence of events may be something as follows: (1) the loss of sodium induces a mild reduction of the concentration of this cation in the extracellular fluids; (2) this, in turn, suppresses the secretion of the antidiuretic hormone (ADH) (and furthermore the loss of salt impairs the ability to elaborate an appropriately concentrated urine); (3) the excretion of water is increased until the concentration of sodium has been restored. This is frequently referred to as a "sacrifice of volume in the interests of tonicity of the body fluids." However, as the volume deficit assumes more significant proportions, equivalent losses of water no longer follow further deficits of sodium salts and hyponatremia is established. It may be that the deficit in volume, or some expression thereof, is a stimulus for the secretion of ADH despite hyponatremia, and the volume deficit may influence renal function, in some fashion independent of ADH, to conserve water. It is clear from this sequence that one very important implication of a state of dehydration accompanied by hyponatremia is that the intensity of the dehydration is not trivial. In addition, the decrease in effective osmolality of the extracellular water will have promoted movement of water into the cellular compartment. Thus, the deficit in volume of the extracellular phase is greater than the total external loss. Lastly, the dilution of the intracellular fluid may be expected to have untoward consequences with respect to cell functions. These latter are most clearly expressed on a clinical level by a clouded sensorium, which may progress to frank coma and may be accompanied by seizures. In addition, there are data that hyponatremia (with or without cellular dilution) promotes an increased rate of production of urea nitrogen and induces a rise in the serum level of potassium.

Hyponatremia may occur in the absence of dehydration. In fact, there are some indications that it may develop in patients with no apparent alteration in the volume or disposition of body water; and it may certainly occur in patients with edema. There is some value in a tentative effort to characterize the several pathogeneses of hyponatremia other than that already discussed with regard to dehydration.

ESSENTIAL HYPONATREMIA There is a group of patients who have hyponatremia but no other obvious disturbances in body fluid physiology. These patients have advanced and debilitating diseases and are frequently in preterminal status. They excrete in the urine the approximate quantity of salt ingested. They are able to conserve sodium when this ion is removed from their regimen, and they are able to excrete an appropriately dilute urine when a water load is administered. No aspect of their symptom complex is apparently favorably modified by attempts to restore the concentration of sodium in serum to the normal range. If this is attempted, the patient becomes thirsty, ingests water, and then excretes salt and water until the volume and tonicity of the body fluids have been restored to the level from which they began.

It is clear that the basic defect of this syndrome is mysterious, but it may be suggested that a generalized cellular disorder promotes a new "setting" of the osmolality of the body fluids. Some have referred to this as the "sick cell syndrome." It is not difficult to discriminate between this syndrome and the condition in patients with hyponatremia and dehydration or in those whose condition is deteriorating as a consequence of adrenal cortical insufficiency. The physical examination and collateral laboratory data such as a normal level of serum urea nitrogen and potassium are important clues. The disorder from which it must be differentiated is inappropriate secretion of antidiuretic hormone.

INAPPROPRIATE SECRETION OF ADH More and more examples of this condition have been noted. Many of these patients have intrathoracic lesions, both benign and malignant. Some of the latter have been found to secrete a material that cannot be differentiated from lysine vasopressin. Other intrathoracic lesions may interfere with neural pathways that normally translate the message of increased volume to promote suppression of secretion of the antidiuretic hormone by the neurohypophyseal system. Many other instances are associated with intracranial lesions, including trauma, infection, and tumor. These lesions may promote the secretion of antidiuretic hormone by partial destruction of the posterior lobe of the pituitary gland, with escape of hormone; or by virtue of an irritative focus that promotes the secretion of the hormone (Chap. 84). In addition, the syndrome is noted in an odd variety of circumstances which defies a unifying concept.

The problem is that the patient is secreting antidiuretic hormone (or an antidiuretic substance of other origin) under inappropriate circumstances. This implies that ADH is secreted in abundance in the absence of an osmometric or volumetric stimulus. The consequence is that the continued ingestion of water is not followed by its excretion and the patient develops a positive balance of water and dilutional hyponatremia. This hypotonic expansion of the body fluids usually promotes an increased glomerular filtration rate and an augmented excretion of salt. At this point, the urine osmolality may not be as high as it was initially, owing to the solute diuresis and perhaps in part to some suppressive influence on the secretion of ADH by the severe hypoosmolality of the body fluids. In any event, the urine osmolality is still inappropriately high for the degree of dilution consequent to the positive balance of water.

Since there is frequently an increased rate of glomerular filtration, it is not uncommon to find that these patients have serum urea nitrogen at the lowest levels of normal. Although these patients have an expanded volume of total body water, it is distributed throughout both the cellular and the extracellular compartments, and one usually finds only the most subtle signs of edema.

The treatment of these patients is clearly aimed at dissipating the positive balance of water. This is usually accomplished by drastic restriction in the volume of water ingested until a normal concentration of sodium in serum has been achieved. Then one must find, in an empirical fashion, what food and fluid regimen will be comfortable for the patient and yet not permit a positive balance of water to be achieved once again.

There are occasional circumstances when the level of hyponatremia is so extreme as to produce clouding of consciousness, coma, or seizures. These instances demand more rapid correction, and there are two courses available. One may administer solutions of mannitol, hypertonic glucose, or urea to induce a solute diuresis that will dissipate part of the positive balance of water via the urine and restore the concentration of sodium in serum to a more nearly normal level quickly. Alternatively, one may administer a volume of hypertonic saline solution sufficient to increase the concentration of sodium to a level where the hazards attendant on hyponatremia no longer obtain. This should be employed as the last resort, since, in fact, the patient already has an expanded body fluid volume.

It is almost certain that what was formerly referred to as "cerebral salt wasting" was, in fact, misinterpreted and represented instances of inappropriate secretion of ADH.

HYPONATREMIA WITH EDEMA There are many instances of patients who have hyponatremia associated with lesser or massive degrees of edema. These conditions are usually classified in two general categories: *chronic dilutional* and *acute dilutional hyponatremia.*

Chronic dilutional hyponatremia (1) It seems reasonable that some of these patients may well have what is called *essential hyponatremia*. In that circumstance there would obviously be no value to restoring the concentration of sodium in serum to "normal." In fact, the patient would then have the discomfort of thirst added to his other problems. (2) Some of these patients may well have *inappropriate secretion of* ADH. The best management is to dissipate the relative positive balance of water by restricting intake. As in the instances of this syndrome without edema, there may be occasions when more aggressive measures are required, such as administration of a solution to provoke a solute diuresis. There may be *rare* occasions when the administration of small volumes of hypertonic saline solution is justified if the hyponatremia per se is truly hazardous. However, since these patients are already markedly expanded with fluids and may already have congestive heart failure, it is obvious that the treatment itself is dangerous and should be employed only under the most dire circumstances. (3) Lastly, it is quite probable that in many states of edema the rate of glomerular filtration is markedly reduced. Under these circumstances the quantity of water that escapes reabsorption in the more proximal portions of the nephron may be so small that very little gains access to the more distal segments where it might escape into the bladder. Why patients in such circumstances do not lose their thirst and thereby automatically prohibit a positive balance of water is certainly not clear. Nevertheless, drinking and eating patterns in man are such that a positive balance of water can be readily achieved under these circumstances. Once again, the treatment is dissipation of the positive balance of water.

Acute dilutional hyponatremia (1) One example of this disorder is simply the consequence of administering water or urging a patient with edema to ingest quantities of water in excess of his ability to excrete the load. This is possible in any circumstance including health but is much more easily achieved in patients with edema who have altered renal hemodynamic and other parameters. In any event, the first point to emphasize is that this is preventable. Secondly, should it occur, the treatment again demands restriction of water to rid the body of this relative excess. Lastly, under duress the use of hypertonic solutions may be employed to encourage a solute diuresis. (2) A second example is observed in patients who develop considerable thirst after a successful therapeutic measure aimed at ridding the edematous patient of a volume of fluid. This may be noted after a brisk diuretic response and more commonly after a large abdominal paracentesis. The reasons for the intense thirst are not clear but may relate to a sudden loss of volume in some crucial segment of the vascular system. These complications are preventable. Patients should be warned that they may develop thirst, and their ingestion of water should be limited by themselves and carefully monitored and restricted when indicated by those responsible for their care.

The point of emphasis in managing patients with hyponatremia and edema is that if the concentration of sodium in serum is to be restored, it should be accomplished by dissipating the relative positive balance of water by restricting intake or by hastening excretion through the use of an osmotic load. Some patients, reflecting a state referred to as essential hyponatremia, may, in fact, be more comfortable with hyponatremia than with "normal" concentrations of sodium in serum. The indications for administration of hypertonic saline solutions are *exceedingly rare*, and the measure is only to control what are considered hazardous symptoms from the hyponatremia per se. Even under these circumstances saline solution should be administered in a small quantity sufficient only to restore the sodium concentration to levels that no longer represent a hazardous state.

Another way that hyponatremia might develop is by movement of sodium from the extracellular compartment to cells or to bone. There is some evidence that such an intercompartmental shift of sodium may occur in adrenal cortical insufficiency. Sodium may accumulate in cells deficient in potassium, and some investigators have considered that certain instances of hyponatremia are related to this transfer from the extracellular compartment.

An assessment of the pathogenesis of hyponatremia can usually be made on the basis of the above discussion, and hence the therapeutic implications can usually be arrived at according to the above criteria.

Significance of hypernatremia

In contrast to hyponatremia, an increase in the concentration of sodium in the serum reflects loss of water in excess of salt or administration (or ingestion) of salt in excess of water. The hypernatremia, which is the chemical expression of a water deficit, in turn, incites the following responses, which result in the acquisition of more water, the most efficient conservation of same, and the most desirable distribution of the available water:

1 Thirst
2 Secretion of ADH, which promotes excretion of a concentrated urine
3 Movement of water from the cells to the extracellular space, thus mitigating the deficit of volume in this latter compartment
4 Diminution in the loss of insensible perspiration
5 Decrease in the rate of secretion of sweat

At least one report leaves little doubt that there may well be circumstances in which there is hypernatremia with no other disorder in body fluid physiology and the patient appears to operate with a new "setting" of body fluid osmolality. This may be the counterpart of essential hyponatremia and perhaps should be referred to as *essential hypernatremia*.

Comments on correction of hypo- and hypernatremia

One other implication of the free permeability of cell membranes to water and a uniform osmolality throughout the body fluids concerns the manner in which the concentration of sodium in the serum is restored to normal from both hypo- and hypernatremic levels.

If hyponatremia complicates an illness and it is considered advisable to correct this abnormality by administering a hypertonic solution of sodium salts, the amount of sodium required is equivalent to the deficit in concentration per liter multiplied by the estimated number of liters of *total body water.* If there is to be osmotic equality throughout the body fluids, it is implicit that the concentration of sodium in the extracellular phase cannot be increased without an equivalent increase in solute concentration in the cellular fluid. The administered sodium will increase the osmotic activity of intracellular fluid, not by entering the cells, but by promoting movement of water from the cells to the extracellular compartment as the osmolality of the latter is increased. If it is desired to restore the concentration of sodium reasonably promptly, or if it is to be accomplished with a small volume of fluid, the sodium salts must be administered in hypertonic solution. The amount of sodium that must be administered to restore the concentration to normal is equal to the normal concentration of Na_s (138 mEq per liter) minus the current concentration of N_s multiplied by the total volume of body water. For example, in a 70-kg adult with an assumed body water content of 60 percent (42 liters) and a concentration of sodium in the serum of 128 mEq per liter,

$$(138 - 128) \times 42 = 420 \text{ mmol deficit of sodium chloride}$$

Since there are 17.1 mmol per g NaCl, 420/17.1 or 24.56 g NaCl would be necessary to restore the sodium to 138 mEq per liter. This could be supplied in 500 ml 5% NaCl solution.

The same principles apply to estimating the volume of water that may be necessary to reduce the concentration of sodium in the serum from hypernatremic to normal levels. Since the intensity of the hypernatremia (due to the loss of water in excess of or without salt) is proportionate to the deficit of total body water, the following relationship obtains:

$$\frac{\text{Normal concentration } Na_s}{\text{Elevated concentration } Na_s} = \frac{\text{current vol total body } H_2O}{\text{assumed normal vol total body } H_2O}$$

The value for the current volume of total body water can be calculated, and the difference between it and the assumed normal volume for total body water represents the deficit of water. For example, in the same adult mentioned above but with a concentration of sodium in the serum of 160 mEq per liter:

$$\text{Current vol total body } H_2O = \frac{138}{160} \times 42 = 36.2 \text{ liters}$$

The deficit would be 42 — 36.2 = 5.8 liters of water.

Although these calculations are of value, it should be cautioned that there may be some danger in the too-rapid correction of the elevated or depressed concentration of sodium in extracellular fluid. This, in turn, may be related to adaptive alterations that have obtained. The important feature to be kept in mind in the management of a patient with dehydration and an abnormal concentration of serum sodium is that, in the net, the hyponatremic subject should receive salt in excess of water, and the hypernatremic patient should receive water in excess of salt.

Exchanges between plasma and interstitial fluid

The net exchange of fluid between the plasma and interstitial space is conditioned by a series of forces. Some of these forces favor transudation from the vascular system, such as the hydrostatic pressure within the vessels and the colloid osmotic pressure of the tissue fluids. The tissue tension and the colloid osmotic pressure of the plasma favor the reabsorption of fluid from the interstitium (see Chap. 30). It should be emphasized that, unlike the cell membranes, the capillary endothelial membrane is freely permeable not only to water but to all the solutes of the plasma except the large molecular species such as the proteins and the lipids. Thus, the concentration of sodium and its salts does not influence the distribution of water between these two major components of the extracellular compartment. Although the proteins do not contribute a large osmolality, they alone contribute to the effective osmolality since they are unable to permeate the endothelial membrane except in very small quantity. Thus, hypoalbuminemia may promote expansion of the interstitial fluid, with diminution in plasma volume and hemoconcentration, with normal values for the concentration of sodium.

A change in the forces governing the net exchange between the plasma and the interstitial fluid need not necessarily condition a redistribution of volume between these two compartments. A net increase in transudation could be largely compensated by the return of this increment of fluid to the vascular system by way of the lymphatic vessels. Lymphatic flow is frequently increased when the interstitial fluid volume is expanded, and this influence must be carefully considered when analyzing the forces that govern the disposition of fluid within the extracellular compartment.

Internal exchanges of electrolytes

Although it is apparent that ions such as sodium, potassium, and magnesium move in and out of cells, it is equally apparent that their net movements are not a consequence of free passive diffusion. The measurements of the electric potential differences across the membranes as well as the determination of the concentration gradients make it clear that these ions are not in a state of equilibrium but exist in what is referred to as a *steady state away from equilibrium.* This demands a series of operations dependent on sources of energy and referred to in general terms as *active transport.* The special permeability or "leakiness" characteristics of the plasma membranes of cells with regard to the several ionic species as well as the specific active transport mechanisms and the factors that regulate their rates are ultimately the determinants of the steady state composition of the several cell types. Any change in the permeability characteristics or rates of transport could readily influence the cell composition. It is presumed that metabolic reactions are necessary to maintain cell membrane structure, which, in turn, establishes the permeabilities to passive diffusion as well as the mechanisms involved in the active phases of transport. There are data which establish adenosine triphosphate (ATP) as the ultimate source of energy for active transport, and, lastly, there is an enzyme within the membrane structure itself, ATPase, which may play an important role in making the energy available for the work of transport.

In some instances there appear to be elements of active transport in which the movement of two ionic species in opposite directions may be linked. Although hypothetical, an illustration of the manner in which muscle cells become laden with sodium in the face of potassium deficits can be offered. For example, assume that the level of potassium outside the cell is one of the factors which regulate the rate at which sodium is actively extruded from within the cell. Assume, further, that the rate of extrusion of sodium from the cells controls the inward movement of potassium from the extracellular fluid to the intracellular space. When potassium is lost from the extracellular fluid owing to augmented urinary excretion, or losses from the gastrointestinal tract, etc., the level in the extracellular fluid tends to diminish. This creates initially a larger gradient for potassium from inside to outside the cell, and perhaps more potassium leaks out by passive diffusion. However, this is still inadequate to raise the extracellular fluid concentration of potassium to normal levels. At the same time sodium is constantly diffusing into the cells only to be actively extruded. However, if the diminished level of potassium in the extracellular fluid imposes a rate-limiting influence on the extrusion of sodium from the cells, the latter should accumulate within the cells. The advantage of this is that with the higher intracellular concentration of sodium more of this ion can now be extruded (despite the lower external concentration of potassium), and restoration toward normal of the rate of sodium extrusion at the expense of the higher intracellular concentration of this ion promotes the ability to implement the movement of potassium back into the cell. All these alterations induce a net change characterized by a loss of cell potassium, an increase of cell sodium, and the achievement of new steady state away from equilibrium. This may very well be fanciful in detail, but it provides an overall context in which one may view some of the problems.

The most prominent hypothesis relating to a mechanism of active transport is referred to as the *carrier hypothesis*. In an oversimplified fashion this may be described as suggesting that a compound resides at one side of the cell membrane and has a particular affinity for the sodium ion. Because of this characteristic it becomes linked with this ion; it is now a new species of compound with a higher concentration at one side of the membrane than the other. As a result, it diffuses passively to the other side of the membrane, where a reaction splits the sodium ion from the carrier. This reaction again modifies the compound, and it can be postulated that it now has an affinity for potassium. The latter ion articulates with the carrier and, again, owing to the establishment of a diffusion gradient in this fashion, it moves back to the original side of the membrane, where the potassium ion is split off and the carrier is returned to its original state with a great affinity for sodium; the process is repeated over and over again.

This discussion of active transport has been too simple and succinct to provide more than a vague conceptual framework. The interested reader is referred to Ussing and other sources for detailed discussions of this fascinating and fundamental property. It should be emphasized that the active transport of ions is responsible at the least for the maintenance of cell volume and tissue excitability as well as what must be a vast array of phenomena that are dependent on the details of intra- and extracellular fluid composition.

Bone as a reservoir of ions other than calcium has attracted increased attention. Approximately one-third of the total body sodium is in bone, and only 15 percent of this can be ascribed to the extracellular phase. About one-half of the total body content of magnesium is in bone. Potassium is present in much smaller amounts. Deficits of sodium, potassium and magnesium are shared by bone, and this tissue participates in exchanges that articulate with alterations in acid-base relationships. (See also Chap. 265, Acidosis and Alkalosis.)

External exchanges of electrolytes and water

THIRST In considering the net exchange of water between the individual and his environment, it seems reasonable to begin with thirst. This is the sensory impression that motivates the ingestion of water. Several stimuli may give rise to the sensation of thirst, and the most important of these is an increase in the effective osmolality of the body fluids. This appears to hold true whether the hypertonicity is promoted by loss of water in excess of salt or by administration of salt in excess of water. These two circumstances differ in that in the first instance the volume of the extracellular fluid is decreased, and in the second this volume is expanded. However, in each circumstance the volume of the cells is diminished by virtue of a shift of water to the extracellular phase. A secondary stimulus is related somehow to a deficit of volume (or some expression of such a deficit) in some key portion of the extracellular space. Other factors that condition and modify the sensation of thirst include exposure of the oropharyngeal and esophageal tissues to water, the fullness of the stomach, and emotional as well as social factors. The central nervous system is responsible for the appreciation of and the response to thirst in both a specific and a nonspecific manner. There is now abundant evidence that lesions in key portions of the central nervous system—predominantly in the hypothalamus—may induce hypodipsia or polydipsia. The latter need not be accompanied by diabetes insipidus. The polydipsic center can be stimulated by exposing it to tiny volumes of hypertonic, but not isotonic, saline solutions. It can also be aroused by electrical stimulation.

In a less specific sense the nervous system conditions the reception and response to stimuli provoking thirst in relation to the level of the state of consciousness. The frequency with which patients with a clouded sensorium or coma are allowed to develop significant deficits of water is sufficient justification for emphasizing the obvious fact that such patients can neither appreciate nor respond to their own thirst mechanism.

Potassium depletion may be accompanied by thirst and polydipsia. This may reflect, in part, the inability of the kidneys to conserve water appropriately in this condition. However, it is also possible that there may be a primary influence on some aspect of the stimulus-response pathways concerned with thirst.

INSENSIBLE PERSPIRATION Water is continuously lost from the body in the expired air and from the skin. The sum of these losses is spoken of as "insensible loss" of water and is equivalent to about 600 to 1,000 ml per day in the average adult. This loss is augmented with increase in metabolic activity (fever, exercise, hyperthyroidism) and respiratory exchange. The catabolism of tissues produces 200 to 300 ml water per day; hence the *net* loss of insensible water may be considered at 400 to 700 ml per day. Since this loss is water without solutes, it should be replaced as water without salt (e.g., 5 percent glucose in water when fluid balance is being maintained by parenteral techniques).

SWEAT The production of sweat is primarily responsive to heat. The latter presumably excites afferent impulses to centers that regulate motor activities promoting the loss of heat. The important centers in the central nervous system are in the anterolateral portions of the hypothalamus. Sweat is not a simple fluid, and the details of its secretion are not well understood. It is always a hypotonic solution except in adrenal cortical insufficiency and in patients with fibrocystic disease (mucoviscidosis) of the pancreas. Among other influences, the rate of sweating is diminished by an increase in the effective osmolality of the body fluids. An average composition for sweat, in millimoles per liter, is as follows: sodium 48.0, potassium 5.9, chloride 40.0, ammonia 3.5, and urea 8.6. The characteristics of this fluid dictate the replacement of losses incurred as sweat by a solution that is one-third to one-half isotonic saline. This is readily satisfied for intravenous administration with 1 part isotonic saline to 1 or 2 parts of 5 percent glucose in water.

GASTROINTESTINAL TRACT The exchange of water and solutes between the body fluids and the lumen of the gastrointestinal tract is large. It is contributed to by saliva and the secretions of the stomach, liver, pancreas, and intestinal mucosa. The volume of these secretions may exceed 8 liters per day under ordinary circumstances, but the net loss from the body is negligible. However, when there are losses through vomitus, diarrhea, or drainage from enterostomies, colostomies, or fistulas, the deficits of water and electrolytes may be prodigious. Loss of fluid through these routes probably represents the commonest pathogenesis of significant dyhydration in clinical practice.

Aside from saliva, which is a hypotonic solution, the secretions mentioned are close to isotonicity with the extracellular fluids. However, they differ from the latter in composition. For example, the gastric secretion, if it contains free HCl, has a much lower pH, less sodium and bicarbonate, and more chloride than the extracellular fluids. In contrast, the pancreatic secretion has a higher pH and more bicarbonate. Most gastrointestinal secretions have more potassium than the extracellular fluid. Thus, although losses of gastrointestinal secretions per se represent isotonic deficits, the derangements that accompany the dehydration will be conditioned by the particular portion of the gastrointestinal tract from which the lost fluid derived. In many instances, however, these losses can be successfully replaced by equal volumes of isotonic saline solution. The potassium lost with these secretions and the consequences thereof must also be adequately managed.

RENAL EXCHANGES OF ELECTROLYTES AND WATER The kidneys represent the major organs of conservation as well as of excretion in the net balance of water and electrolytes. The kidneys can excrete large volumes of excess water and large quantities of unwanted ions and other solutes. In addition, they respond to the need to conserve water by excreting small volumes of highly concentrated urine. Their response to a sodium deficit is to excrete a urine virtually free of salt. The conservation of magnesium is also good, and subjects subsisting on a diet deficient in magnesium may excrete as little as 1 mEq of this ion per day. Although the excretion of potassium is very much diminished when there is a deficit of this cation, the efficiency with which the kidneys conserve potassium is not quite so great as it is with sodium, chloride, or magnesium.

The excretion of sodium is markedly reduced when there is primarily a deficit of water, even though this is accompanied by hypernatremia. This has the advantage of eliminating a major solute from the urine and, by reducing urine flow, furthers the conservation of water.

The kidneys display other exquisitely sensitive responses to most of the alterations in the composition, volume, tonicity, and pH of the body fluids. Details of these responses and the mechanisms involved therein are discussed in Chap. 47.

CLINICAL CONSIDERATIONS

An understanding of the pathogenesis and management of disorders of fluid and electrolyte balance depends on an appreciation of the approximate net exchanges of water and the several ions that have occurred during the course of a patient's illness. In essence, many of the problems concerning clinical disorders of hydration are resolved by the simple expediency of setting up a balance sheet in which the total estimated losses are accumulated, the total intake is summated, and the net differences are calculated. Although not quantitatively precise, this practice usually defines the qualitative nature of the alterations and provides an approximation of the quantitative characteristics. Many of these data can be obtained from the carefully taken history or the well-documented hospital chart. In addition, the physical examination, the chemical analyses of serum and urine, and other laboratory data provide additional insights. The management of the problem then becomes largely one of providing those materials which will restore the normal state of hydration. It is not an oversimplification to state that the majority of these problems are easily resolved with simple arithmetic.

In many instances a disordered state of hydration could have been avoided by provision of adequate replacement of certain predictable and mandatory losses. It is desirable, therefore, to define the characteristics of the basal requirements for water and electrolytes, and to describe how they are modified by a variety of conditioning circumstances.

BASAL REQUIREMENTS For the purposes of this discussion it will be assumed that the patient must receive the necessary water, electrolytes, and other materials by parenteral routes, that he has accumulated no antecedent deficits, that he is not sustaining any unusual losses, and that he has normal renal function. One other qualification is that the problem is one of short duration and that the need for calories and protein is not a major consideration. The task then is to prescribe a regimen which will maintain a normal state of hydration, avoid depletion of the major essential minerals, and minimize the most immediate threats of starvation.

The volume of water recommended per day is the sum of (1) the probable net insensible loss, 400 ml; (2) a reasonable volume for urine, 1,000 ml; and (3) perhaps a small additional volume, 400 ml, which is provided to anticipate other losses such as sweat but which, if not lost by extrarenal routes, can be readily excreted in the urine. These total 1,800 ml.

If a patient has been previously ingesting an average diet, he has probably been receiving about 8 to 10 g (135 to 170 mmol) NaCl per day. If the intake of salt is suddenly eliminated, the patient will probably be able to excrete a urine essentially free of sodium in about 5 days. During this interval of 5 days a negative balance of sodium is allowed to develop. This is likely to be accompanied by an equivalent loss of water in the interests of maintaining a normal concentration of sodium in the extracellular fluid. This deficit in volume is probably not harmful in itself, but it prejudices the patient's ability to withstand subsequent losses. Therefore, unless there is some specific contraindication, it is recommended that the patient receive 4 to 5 g (70 to 85 mmol) NaCl each day.

As noted earlier, the conservation of potassium is not quite so efficient as that of salt, and unless the urinary excretion of this cation is replaced, a deficit of potassium will be ultimately achieved. From 40 to 60 mmol potassium per day should be adequate to avoid a negative balance of this cation.

Although the mechanisms of conservation for magnesium are quite good, one of the settings in which depletion of this cation is observed is prolonged parenteral fluid management. The administration of as little as 2 to 4 mmol magnesium per day ought to suffice under most circumstances.

It has been stated that approximately 100 g carbohydrate is necessary for the operation of the Krebs cycle. Unless this is made available from preformed endogenous or exogenous carbohydrate, the catabolism of protein and fat will be accelerated and 4-carbon ketones will be formed faster than they can be utilized. The acid products of protein catabolism and the excess ketones must be excreted to avoid a metabolic acidosis; they are excreted in part as sodium salts, which adds another drain to the body's store of sodium. Each of these complications can be avoided by the provision of an adequate quantity, 150 to 200 g of glucose per day.

The total basal requirements are the following:

Water	1,800 ml
NaCl	70–85 mmol/ (4–5 g)
KC1	40–60 mmol/ (3–4.5g)
$MgSO_4$	2–4 mmol (1–2 ml 50% $MgSO_4 \cdot 7H_2O$)
Glucose	150–200 g

An appropriate fluid prescription to meet these requirements is the following:

1,300 ml 10% glucose in water
500 ml 5% glucose in isotonic saline solution
4 g KCl (added to the total water to be administered)
2 ml 50% $MgSO_4 \cdot 7H_2O$ (added to the total water to be administered)

It should be reemphasized that this prescription is appropriate for the patient with qualifications set forth in the initial paragraph of this discussion on basal requirements.

ADDITIONAL REQUIREMENTS There are many circumstances which would require revision of the above prescription. Fever, restlessness, and increased respiratory activity will augment the loss of water as insensible perspiration. A hot environment and fever will promote sweating. Water loss in urine will be accelerated during an osmotic diuresis due to glycosuria or unusual amounts of urea. The latter situation is observed when unnecessarily large amounts of protein are administered to patients who are experiencing a reaction to injury and hence are limited in the ability to store nitrogen. Additional amounts of salt may be lost with glycosuria. Impaired renal function will demand an increased volume of urine, and the conservation of sodium may be less efficient than in patients with normal kidneys.

FLUIDS AVAILABLE FOR PARENTERAL ADMINISTRATION There are available a number of specially prepared solutions, such as "gastric replacement fluid" and "intestinal replacement fluid," aimed at meeting the requirements of particular types of loss. Their use should be discouraged. The basic tenet of the individualization of therapy applies here, as it does elsewhere in clinical practice. The proper management of disorders in fluid and electrolyte balance demands an analysis of the specific characteristics of the distortion in the particular patient at hand. The routine use of a special solution tends to diminish the diligence with which this analysis is made through the false sense of security provided by the claims of the value of the particular solution. This is not to imply that solutions other than glucose in water and isotonic saline are not frequently needed. However, when the need arises, the appropriate fluid should be designed for the particular patient and his problem. A great variety of special problems can be met by preparation of a special solution from the following list of raw materials:

5%, 10%, 50% glucose in water
0.9% NaCl (154 mmol/liter)

5.0% NaCl (855 mmol/liter)
7.5% $NaHCO_3$ (900 mmol/liter)
14.9% KC[1] (2,000 mmol/liter or 2 mmol/ml)
50%[1] $MgSO_4 \cdot 7H_2O$ (2 mmol/ml)

Lastly, it should be emphasized that the most appropriate replacement fluid for lost blood is whole blood; and where the particular need is to expand plasma volume, the use of whole blood, single units of plasma, or, preferably, 25 percent salt-poor albumin or some other plasma expander, is recommended.

TECHNIQUES OF ADMINISTRATION OF FLUIDS

Fluids may be given by vein, by hypodermoclysis, or by gavage into the stomach. The latter method has many advantages, especially when the problem is likely to last for some time and when considerations of calories, proteins, and other essential foodstuffs merit attention. The intravenous route is convenient, and the use of plastic tubing threaded into larger veins has eliminated some of the technical problems.[2] The rate of administration of fluid deserves some attention, and in cases of cardiovascular disease the patient should be observed carefully and frequently to ensure the earliest recognition of an untoward response. The potential hazard of cardiovascular complication may serve to modify the fluid prescription and the speed with which the fluids are administered. However, it should certainly not interfere with the proper management of dehydration.

The subcutaneous route may have some advantages in patients with heart disease. The access of fluid from the subcutaneous tissue to the bloodstream is obviously slower than when fluid is introduced directly into the vein, but, in addition, its absorption may be even further delayed if there is a rise in venous pressure. In this fashion there is an added factor of safety. If fluids are administered by hypodermoclysis, two precautions must be borne in mind:

1 The fluid should be isotonic with the plasma. If it is hypertonic, there will be a tendency initially for water to leave the plasma and enter the clysis pool. This will cause an initial decrease in plasma volume, which is undesirable, especially if the patient is already dehydrated. Moreover, a hypertonic solution may be irritating to the subcutaneous tissue and result in a bad slough of tissue.
2 A solution of 5% glucose in water should not be administered by clysis if the patient is dehydrated. When glucose is administered in this fashion, concentration gradients are established for the diffusion of glucose from clysis pool to plasma and for diffusion of sodium from plasma to clysis pool. Sodium diffuses more rapidly than glucose; the fluid in the pool, therefore, becomes hypertonic, and this, in turn, promotes movement of water from the plasma. This reduction in plasma volume superimposed on the antecedent deficit may be sufficient to induce a state of peripheral vascular collapse.

[1] *These solutions are highly concentrated and should never be administered unless they are diluted.*
[2] *The site of the plastic intravenous catheter should be changed every 48 hr if at all possible. Significant incidence of infection and phlebitis usually appears after 2 days.*

DEHYDRATION

The term *dehydration* continues to mislead, since it implies to many physicians the loss of water alone. Clinical dehydration is rarely a pure deficit of water. Dehydration is usually associated with losses of both salt and water (in proportionate or disproportionate quantities), with deficits of other ions such as potassium, and with the frequent complication of a disturbance in acid-base equilibrium. All these factors must be considered in planning appropriate management. For purposes of orientation and discussion, clinical dehydration may be classified into three major groups as follows:

1 Loss of water in excess of sodium
2 Loss of sodium in excess of water
3 Isotonic losses of sodium and water

LOSS OF WATER IN EXCESS OF SODIUM The failure to drink is the commonest cause of a water deficit. This is observed most frequently in severely debilitated patients with clouding of consciousness or coma. Not only are these patients too weak and ill to respond to thirst, but they are even unable to communicate the fact that they are thirsty to their families or to their physicians. The size of the water deficit, though it may increase each day, may be small and hence easily overlooked. However, this deficit can achieve significant proportions and contribute greatly to the severity of the patient's illness.

Solute diureses due to glycosuria are usually characterized by a loss of water in excess of salt. This is the situation, for example, in almost all patients with significant degrees of diabetic acidosis.

Another type of solute diuresis may be responsible for a deficit of water. Many physicians have become impressed with the therapeutic value of feeding large quantities of protein. There are many situations in which this is desirable. However, in the early stages of reaction to injury, the ability to store nitrogen may be very seriously impaired, and large amounts of protein (usually administered by gavage) will find their way to urea, demanding excretion in the urine. If the patient is able, he may complain of thirst if the urine flow is large enough to induce a deficit of water. The unconscious patient cannot provide this help. Delay in recognition is due, in great measure, to misinterpretation of the significance of a large flow of urine, especially when the latter is not concentrated. This is equated with an appropriate state of hydration, whereas, in fact, the large volume of unconcentrated urine may be causing the deficit of water (see Chap. 84).

Diabetes insipidus may be responsible for large deficits of water. Unfortunately, acute diabetes insipidus is commonly associated with trauma or infection in the central nervous system, and hence a clouded or comatose state is not unusual. Major deficits of water may occur in a matter of hours. A large volume of very dilute urine should alert the clinician to this possibility. The defect in the tubular reabsorption of water is easily corrected by the administration of pitressin (see Chap. 84).

The loss of sweat contributes to a deficit of water in excess of salt loss. To the extent that water alone is ingested and retained to replace the volume of lost sweat, a dehydration characterized by a loss of water in excess of salt loss is readily converted to one characterized by a loss of salt in excess of water loss. This serves to emphasize the point that the characteristics of the net deficit are conditioned not only by the quantity and quality of the fluid lost but also by the characteristics of the replacement fluid.

The hallmark of dehydration characterized by a loss of water in excess of salt loss is an increase in the effective osmolality of the extracellular fluids. In most instances this is reflected in an increase in the concentration of sodium in the serum, and the intensity of the hypernatremia may be used as a gage to calculate the relative deficit of water (see above).

DEFICIT OF SALT IN EXCESS OF WATER DEFICIT *Adrenal cortical insufficiency* is probably the classic example of this type of dehydration (see Chap. 86). Although the loss of sodium may be the primary event in the pathogenesis of the dehydration in this disorder, it does not necessarily follow that the concentration of sodium will be depressed in the early phase (see Significance of Hyponatremia, earlier in this chapter). However, as the contraction of volume becomes more significant, further deficits of sodium salts are not accompanied by equivalent deficits of water, and hyponatremia supervenes. The dehydration is severe, the cells are overhydrated, and the contracted volume of the plasma may compromise the renal blood flow and glomerular filtration rate, leading to azotemia and some degree of acidosis. The excretion of potassium is diminished. This is owing to the failure to reabsorb sodium at a site in the renal tubule where potassium secretion is coupled with sodium reabsorption. Hyperkalemia out of proportion to the azotemia and hyponatremia is characteristic of this disorder. Peripheral vascular collapse is common, as are hypoglycemia, restlessness, and an altered sensorium.

Patients with *chronic renal insufficiency* may exhibit an inability to conserve salt properly. This may be of striking proportions and has been known to mimic and be misdiagnosed as adrenal cortical insufficiency. More commonly, the defect is much less intense and may be unmasked only when such patients are advised to restrict the use of dietary salt. The loss of salt each day may not be great, but in the course of time a significant deficit may develop, accompanied by hyponatremia. The dehydration is associated with alterations in renal hemodynamics, and further reduction of an already deficient renal function is a common and dangerous complication. The hazard of a salt-poor regimen in patients with chronic renal disease should be recognized, and it is the responsibility of the physician to make certain that the patient can tolerate the treatment. Careful evaluation of daily weights, observations with respect to changes in concentration of blood urea nitrogen and the concentration of sodium in serum, and an estimation of the total 24-hr excretion of salt in the urine are helpful in evaluating the response.

ISOTONIC DEFICITS OF SALT AND WATER In general, these deficits are primarily incurred by losses of fluid from the gastrointestinal tract. The ultimate character of the net deficit will be determined in part by the quality and quantity of fluids that the patient may receive. If the patient refrains from taking fluid and none has been administered by a parenteral route, the continued loss of insensible perspiration, sweat, and urine will determine a net deficit characterized by the loss of water in excess of salt loss. If the patient drinks water and vomits, the net deficit will be a loss of salt in excess of water loss.

ANALYSIS OF THE CHARACTERISTICS OF DEHYDRATION The discussion presented above concerns the pathogenesis of dehydration in rather isolated terms, and in the hope of achieving clarity the price of oversimplification has been paid. Most patients have experienced a variety of physiologic insults of different magnitudes and for shorter or longer periods of time. The essence of the analysis of the characteristics of the dehydration is an assessment of all the data, in both quantitative and qualitative terms. These data are derived from the history, the physical examination, and the laboratory.

History A careful review of the sequence of events during the course of the illness provides most important information concerning the quality and magnitude of the deficits of electrolytes and water. These data should actually be tabulated, and it is most desirable to develop the habit of preparing a balance sheet to use in the analysis. A sheet with the simple headings indicated below will usually suffice:

Intake:	*Output:*
Date/time	Diarrhea
Weight	Vomitus
Character of fluid	Urine
Volume	Insensible loss
	Sweat
	Blood

The systematic analysis of these data should provide a fair estimate of deficits in terms of volume, salt, potassium balance, and acid-base equilibrium. In an illness of short duration, information relating to the patient's usual and current weight may be helpful in estimating the volume of fluid that has been lost. The presence or absence of fever and sweating is relevant, as are data concerning the possibility of renal insufficiency or diabetes mellitus. Information concerning the usual level of blood pressure is helpful, since a "normal" blood pressure may be hypotensive for a patient whose blood pressure is usually in the hypertensive range. The symptom of thirst is most significant and can be most helpful in calling the physician's attention to a disorder of hydration which might otherwise be neglected. Thirst is most often due to a primary deficit of water, although it may also reflect a contracted volume, even when salt has been lost in excess of water.

A disorder of hydration may develop during the course of hospitalization. The data referred to above should certainly be available in a precise fashion in the hospital chart. The administration of parenteral fluids should be recorded with as much attention to detail as in the record of drug therapy.

Physical examination The physical signs may provide important information for the analysis of the deficits of electrolytes and water. The appearance of the skin, its elasticity, texture, temperature, and color, the appearance of the mucous membranes, the tension of the eyeballs, the blood pressure, and the pulse rate all contribute to an estimation of the magnitude of the deficit. The state of consciousness may be related to the magnitude of the deficit. Muscle weakness and diminished-to-absent deep-tendon reflexes may suggest potassium depletion.

The character of respiratory activity may suggest a disequilibrium in acid-base relationships. The respirations in metabolic acidosis, with dehydration as an almost invariable concomitant feature, are deep and eventually accelerated, and one can usually detect an effort toward the end of expiration. A systemic alkalosis is suggested by a positive Chvostek reflex; this may also be present if the patient has hypocalcemia despite a concurrent acidosis. Clinically detectable changes in respiration in alkalosis can rarely if ever be appreciated. The odor of acetone on the breath implies a ketonemia.

Laboratory data The value of the *packed cell volume* (hematocrit), the concentration of *hemoglobin*, and the concentration of *total proteins* in the serum can help in evaluating the degree of contraction (or expansion) of the plasma volume. Since this inference is dependent on *changes* in the concentrations, these data are of help primarily in evaluating those disorders that develop while the patient is under observation and in following the progress of a patient whose dehydration is undergoing correction.

It is worthwhile to reemphasize that the concentration of sodium per se cannot possibly be equated with the presence or absence of a state of dehydration. The *concentration* of sodium is merely a statement of the amount of sodium in a liter (or any other unit of volume) of extracellular fluid. The patient with a normal concentration of sodium in the serum may have no disorder of hydration, he may have gained many liters of fluid, or he may have lost a large volume of fluid.

The excretion of urea is related to the amount filtered less the amount reabsorbed through the renal tubules. This latter process is considered to be primarily passive. There are data suggesting that some component of urea reabsorption may be active. However, to the extent that it is passive it is favored by high concentration gradients between renal tubular and interstitial fluid. Therefore, it is clear that a diminished rate of filtration at the glomerulus, or a highly concentrated urine, or both will favor a diminished rate of excretion and an increase in urea concentration in the body fluids. To the extent that dehydration is responsible for these alterations in renal function, the concentration of urea in blood may serve as a gross index of the severity of the dehydration.

The urinalysis contributes considerable information. In the first place it provides information concerning the probability of renal disease. A urine of high specific gravity, in the absence of glucose or protein, suggests good renal function and an antidiuretic response. This, in turn, carries certain implications with respect to alterations in the internal environment. The excretion of salt despite hyponatremia may indicate one of the salt-wasting disorders or the syndrome of inappropriate secretion of antidiuretic hormone.

The concentrations of potassium and total CO_2 content of the serum may be altered, and these deviations are frequently accompanied by disturbances in acid-base equilibrium. These matters are discussed in more detail in Chap. 265. Hypo- or hypermagnesemia may be present. The former is not uncommon in the same situations that are characterized by deficits of potassium such as diabetic acidosis, gastrointestinal disturbances including the malabsorption syndrome, and the postoperative period.

PRINCIPLES OF MANAGEMENT OF DEHYDRATION The initial goals of the management of a state of dehydration are simple and include the restoration of the body fluids to normal volume, effective osmolality, composition, and acid-base relations. The quality and quantity of fluids required to satisfy these goals depend on the analysis of the characteristics of the dehydration. On the basis of this analysis it should be possible to outline a course of action. Since the analysis cannot be expected to be precise, it is wise to include in the outline a plan to interrupt therapy at an appropriate point to allow a reevaluation of the status of the patient. This reevaluation should employ all the available clinical and laboratory data relevant to the problem. The initial plan of management may then be modified in accord with this second analysis. Like the management of many other clinical problems, management of dehydration requires a combination of information, logic, and empiricism. In many instances the restoration of normal volume and tonicity of the body fluids, and the repair of a deficit of potassium, if present, will be accompanied by the coincidental correction of a complicating disturbance in acid-base balance. The administration of insulin and, at an appropriate time, of glucose and potassium is obviously necessary in a patient with diabetic acidosis. Since the alleviation of the acid-base disturbance is dependent on normal renal and respiratory function, these problems are more complex in patients with renal and pulmonary disease. The basic principles of the management of adrenal cortical insufficiency do not differ from those presented above; however, cortisone or hydrocortisone and 9α-fluorohydrocortisone are added to the regimen. The management of the water deficit in diabetes insipidus differs from that of other deficits of water only insofar as the patient with diabetes insipidus should be given a preparation of the posterior pituitary gland to replace the deficiency of the ADH.

When these first goals have been realized, plans must be made to maintain the normal state of hydration. The fluid prescription must be developed in relation to the usual basal requirements and their possible alterations in this particular patient and to the need to replace losses other than those included in the former category.

DEFICIT OF POTASSIUM
(See Chap. 265)

DEFICIT OF MAGNESIUM
(See also Chap. 81)

There are approximately 2,000 mEq magnesium in the average 70-kg adult, and of this approximately one-half resides in bone. The concentration in serum is between 1.5 and 2.0 mEq per liter and is remarkably constant; approximately one-third of this is bound to protein. The residual magnesium is in the skeleton, muscles, and parenchymal tissues.

Magnesium deficiency in man is frequently accompanied by hypocalemia. There are data to suggest both a lack of responsiveness to parathormone as well as deficient secretion of this peptide in magnesium deficiency. Very little more is known about the chemical and anatomic correlates of magnesium deficiency in man. Hypomagnesemia can ensue when the negative balance of this ion is as small as 10 to 20 mEq. On the other hand, large deficits of this ion do not occur easily in adults unless malabsorption and inadequate intake coincide. Thus, the clinical circumstances in which magnesium deficiency is likely to be observed include the malabsorption syndromes, chronic alcoholism, prolonged and severe losses of body fluids, diabetic acidosis, cirrhosis of the liver, and primary aldosteronism. It may be seen in patients who must be treated for long periods of time by the parenteral route when no magnesium salt is added to the administered fluid. It is also noted following removal of a parathyroid adenoma, and this is more likely when there is evidence of bone demineralization.

The symptoms consist primarily of neuromuscular disorders and others related to the central nervous system. In the former area the prominent features include weakness, muscle fasciculation, tremors and occasionally a positive Chvostek's sign, and tetany. With reference to the central nervous system there may be personality changes, agitation, delirium, frank psychoses, and coma. Choreiform and athetoid movements have been noted.

The presence of hypomagnesemia does not *necessarily* imply a significant deficit of this cation. If normal subjects are provided with a diet which contains less than 1 mEq magnesium per day, the urinary excretion will diminish to this level in 4 to 5 days. The negative balance by way of the urine will be no more than 10 to 20 mEq. Despite this, the serum level of magnesium will be depressed by more than three standard deviations from the mean. Hence, a patient who has been on an alcoholic binge for 4 to 5 days with the ingestion of little or no food may have hypomagnesemia but a trivial magnesium deficit.

It is difficult to evaluate the specific characteristics of the response to magnesium therapy. This is because magnesium in pharmacologic doses may readily improve some of the signs and symptoms noted above when their origins are not necessarily ascribable to magnesium deficit. Nevertheless, in the presence of these symptoms with evidence of magnesium deficiency, these patients should be treated with appropriate amounts of magnesium, since such treatment can be performed safely.

Since one cannot define antecedently the quantitative nature of the deficit, the repletion program must be empirical. The use of the intramuscular route for the injection of magnesium sulfate is appropriate, and if modest doses, such as 5 mM magnesium (2.5 ml 50 percent $MgSO_4 \cdot 7H_2O$), are given at intervals and the serum levels checked, it is unlikely that one will promote hazardous hypermagnesemia. In general, levels as high as 3 to 4 mEq per liter in the serum are unassociated with untoward effects.

REFERENCES

Edelman IS, Leibman J: Anatomy of body water and electrolytes. Am J Med 27:256, 1959

Tosteson D: Active transport, genetics, and cellular evolution. Fed Proc 22:19, 1963

Ussing HH et al: The alkali metal ions in biology, in *Handbuch der Experimentellen Pharmakologie*, eds O Eichler, A Farah, Berlin: Springer 1960

Wacker WEC, Parisi AF: Magnesium metabolism. N Engl J Med 278:658, 712, 772, 1968

Welt LG: Agents affecting volume and composition of body fluids, chap. 36 in *The Pharmacologic Basis of Therapeutics*, 3d ed., eds LS Goodman, A Gilman, New York: Macmillan, 1970, p. 773

265
ACIDOSIS AND ALKALOSIS

LOUIS G. WELT

Physiologic considerations

Understanding the physiologic regulation and the clinical disorders of acid-base balance is often needlessly difficult because of the multiple uses and misuses of the terms *acid* and *base*. In the past these terms have been applied to anions and cations. This is not now acceptable, although the respectability of long usage has tended to perpetuate the error. Moreover, this is not a semantic quibble, since the use of these inadequate and misleading definitions creates a major handicap in the efforts to appreciate the very nature of the problem. In this discussion the term *acid* refers to any substance that can donate a hydrogen ion (H^+), and *base* means any substance that can accept a hydrogen ion. This statement may be rewritten as follows:

$$\text{Acid} \rightleftharpoons \text{base} + H^+$$

Some substances may serve as an acid *or* a base. For example, $H_2PO_4^-$ can dissociate to H^+ and HPO_4^{--}, or it can accept a hydrogen ion to form H_3PO_4. In the first instance it serves as an acid, and in the second as a base. These definitions serve to focus attention on the hydrogen ion as the significant item in acid-base balance. The manner in which the concentration of hydrogen ions may be expressed and the inferences drawn from this expression therefore become highly relevant.

The dissociation of an acid, HA, may be expressed in the following manner:

$$HA \rightleftharpoons H^+ + A^- \quad (1)$$

The rate at which this reaction proceeds to the right is proportional to the molar concentration of the acid and may be said to be equivalent to $k_1[HA]$. Likewise, the rate at which the reaction proceeds to the left is proportional to the product of the molar concentrations of H^+ and A^- and may be described as equivalent to $k_2[H^+]\,[A^-]$. At equilibrium the two rates are equal, and therefore

$$k_1\,[HA] = k_2\,[H^+]\,[A^-] \quad (2)$$

This equation can be rearranged to

$$\frac{k_1}{k_2} = \frac{[H^+]\,[A^-]}{[HA]} \quad (3)$$

The ratio of the two constants can be included in one new constant, K, and the statement can be rearranged to function as an expression of the concentration of hydrogen ions:

$$[H^+] = K\,\frac{[HA]}{[A^-]} \quad (4)$$

Sörenson introduced the alternative method of expressing the concentration of hydrogen ions as the negative logarithm. The latter is denoted as pH, and the following statement emerges:

$$pH = pK + \log\frac{[A^-]}{[HA]} \quad (5)$$

This may be stated in the more general form:

$$pH = pK + \log\frac{[base]}{[acid]} \quad (6)$$

which is referred to as the *Henderson-Hasselbalch equation.* The logarithm of 1 is zero, and therefore when the concentrations of the base (the hydrogen ion acceptor) and the acid (the hydrogen ion donor) are equal to each other, the pH is equal to pK.

BUFFERS A buffered solution is able to minimize the deviation of pH owing to the addition to that solution of a strong acid or a strong base. A buffer pair is composed of a weakly dissociated acid or base and a highly dissociated salt. Such a pair might be designated as HA and NaA. The addition of a strong acid, such as HCl, to this solution would promote the following reaction:

$$HA + NaA + HCl \rightarrow 2HA + NaCl$$

In this fashion a weak acid is substituted for the strong acid. The concentration of hydrogen ions will be increased to the extent that the increment of weak acid dissociates. This increase is clearly considerably less than that which would have occurred had the HCl been added to pure water.

The pH of a buffered solution will be defined by the ratio of the molar concentrations of the members of the buffer pair:

$$pH = pK + \log\frac{[NaA]}{[HA]}$$

Several characteristics of buffer activity are implicit in this equation. The deviation in pH consequent to the addition of an acid stronger than HA will be equated with a decrease in the concentration of A^- (represented by the numerator of the ratio) and an increase in the concentration of HA. This implies that, for a given increment of acid, the least change in pH will occur when the buffer ratio has a value of 1. Another implication is that at *any* specific ratio of the concentrations of the pair, the addition of a given quantity of acid will alter the ratio less if the concentrations of the members of the pair are high rather than low. Finally, it is apparent that the capacity to buffer is lost when there is no hydrogen ion acceptor (base) left.

A solution may contain several buffers. The ratio of the concentrations of the components of each buffer pair is determined by the pH and, in turn, determines the pH. The ratios of each pair will be different at a specific pH in accordance with the individual dissociation constant for the system. Therefore, in a solution with several buffers a change in one component of any pair will dictate a change in the ratio for every other pair.

As mentioned in the preceding chapter, the body fluid most accessible for analysis is the plasma, and the pH of the extracellular fluid can be defined by the relationship between $NaHCO_3$ and H_2CO_3, or, more precisely, the tension of CO_2 (P_{CO_2}).[1] This is expressed by the equation

$$pH = 6.1 + \log\frac{NaHCO_3}{H_2CO_3 + \text{dissolved } CO_2}$$
$$\downarrow\!\uparrow$$
$$CO_2 + H_2O$$

The ratio of the concentrations of sodium bicarbonate and the carbonic acid plus dissolved CO_2 is 20:1 at the pH of serum 7.40. This is far removed from the more efficient ratio of 1:1, and in a closed system this would be a poor buffer pair at that pH. However, the buffer is unique in that its acid component is a gas whose excretion can be rapidly accelerated or diminished by variations in respiratory exchange, and it is ubiquitous in that it is constantly being formed as a metabolic end product.

Although much of the buffer activity within the body is reflected and mirrored in the bicarbonate–carbonic acid system, this is by no means the only important buffer system in the body's fluids. The proteins of the plasma, the hemoglobin of the red blood cells, and the bicarbonate, phosphate, and proteins of the intracellular fluids all play a significant role in buffer activity. The sum total of the anions of the buffer salts capable of accepting hydrogen ions (i.e., the sum total of *base*) represents the first line of defense in absorbing the insult of the accession of an acid load in the body. The total of all body buffers (including those contributed by cations from cells and bones) cannot be estimated readily; some indication of their magnitude and a reflection of changes therein may be obtained from a consideration, as developed by Singer and Hastings, of the buffers present in whole blood alone.

[1] *The term* P_{CO_2} *refers to the partial pressure of carbon dioxide and is usually close to 40 mm Hg.*

The buffers in whole blood include the bicarbonate, proteins, and phosphate of the plasma and the hemoglobin, bicarbonate, and phosphate salts in the red blood cells. In addition, since the anionic properties of hemoglobin vary between the reduced and oxygenated state, the degree of saturation of hemoglobin with oxygen must be stipulated. The sum of these buffers has been referred to as *buffer base.* Initially this term was used to mean the cation equivalents of the buffer anion. It is now more proper to use the term interchangeably with *buffer anion* itself. The range of normal values for the sum of the buffer base is 46 to 52 mmol per liter. The values for buffer base and P_{CO_2} can be read from a nomogram prepared by Singer and Hastings if the pH of the blood, the hematocrit, the oxygen saturation of the hemoglobin, and the total CO_2 content of whole blood or plasma are known. Since the anionic properties of the proteins vary directly with pH, the primary retention or loss of carbon dioxide and bicarbonate, as in respiratory disturbances, is accompanied by reciprocal changes in the buffer base value for the proteins. Hence, the characteristic of respiratory acidosis and alkalosis will be the lack of deviation from normal in the value for buffer base. In contrast, the value for buffer base will be diminished in metabolic acidosis and increased in metabolic alkalosis.

Astrup and Siggaard-Andersen have emphasized the concept of *standard bicarbonate,* from which one can calculate a base excess or a base deficit. In a sense this represents a somewhat more refined and sophisticated method of determining what was alluded to above as the buffer base of Singer and Hastings. The essence of the concept is to remove from consideration the contribution made by the respiratory regulatory defenses. In this technique the pH of the blood is determined as drawn. Following this the pH is again measured at two different levels of P_{CO_2}, and the hemoglobin is rendered fully oxygenated. From a nomogram one can then determine the standard bicarbonate. The normal values range between 21 and 25 mEq per liter. If the determined value is greater, there is a base excess, and if lower, a base deficit. Thus, if the pH of the blood as originally drawn is depressed or elevated and there is neither a base excess nor deficit, the disturbance is respiratory in origin. Those who champion this system consider an additional advantage to be the quantitative nature of the determination and stress its usefulness in management of the clinical problem. In contrast, others have indicated that this technique offers little that is not readily available through less elaborate methods; and they point out in addition that the specific datum of base excess or deficit can be misleading.

There is a difference between the concentration of sodium and the sum of the concentrations of total carbon dioxide and chloride in serum. The magnitude of this difference is normally 5 to 15 mmol per liter and is referred to as the "anion gap." This quantity of anion is composed of phosphate, citrate, lactate, and other known and unknown negatively charged species. If this anion gap is absent, the implication is that one or more of the chemical determinations is incorrect. In a metabolic acidosis due to the accession of acids other than hydrochloric or carbonic acid, the anion gap will be enhanced.

ACID-BASE RELATIONSHIP

It should be clear from the above that the status of the acid-base relationship cannot be evaluated solely from knowledge of the total CO_2 content of the serum. This latter represents the sum of the members of the buffer pair and includes bicarbonate as well as carbonic acid and CO_2 gas. The total provides no information with respect to the relative proportions of the components of the buffer pair. In fact, a high or low concentration of total CO_2 is compatible with either acidosis or alkalosis. The pH of arterial blood (or blood obtained from a limb vein after warming the part at 45°C for about 10 min) is ultimately necessary to define the acid-base relationship. The pH, however, may be found to be disturbed more or less than the deviation in total CO_2 content of the serum. This depends, in part, on the sequence of events, the speed with which the distortion has supervened, and the success or failure of the compensatory mechanisms. Furthermore, in more complicated circumstances, the estimation of both P_{CO_2} and whole-blood buffer base may be necessary to unravel the nature of the disturbance in acid-base relationships.

CALCULATION OF P_{CO_2} AND PARTITION OF TOTAL CO_2 CONTENT The quantity of carbon dioxide dissolved in a liquid is proportional to the P_{CO_2} and may be expressed in millimoles per liter as equal to alpha P_{CO_2}. The term *alpha* is equal to 0.0301 (mmol/liter/mm Hg) for plasma at a temperature of 38°C. At different body temperatures an appropriate correction must be made. In turn, dissolved CO_2 is in equilibrium with H_2CO_3, and therefore the sum of dissolved CO_2 and carbonic acid may be said to be proportional to P_{CO_2}. Since the quantity of dissolved CO_2 is so much greater than the concentration of carbonic acid, this value will be used as the denominator in the Henderson-Hasselbalch equation.

In the sample calculation to follow, it will be assumed that the pH is 7.40, the total CO_2 content is 26 mmol per liter, and the pK for the bicarbonate-CO_2 system is 6.10. The Henderson-Hasselbalch equation may be written as follows:

$$\text{pH} = 6.10 + \log \frac{(\text{HCO}_3^-)}{(\alpha P_{CO_2})}$$

Since the concentration of bicarbonate in plasma is equal to the difference between the total CO_2 content and P_{CO_2}, the equation may be rewritten:

$$\text{pH} = 6.10 + \log \frac{(\text{total CO}_2) - (\alpha P_{CO_2})}{(\alpha P_{CO_2})}$$

$$7.40 = 6.10 + \log \frac{(26) - (0.0301 P_{CO_2})}{(0.0301 P_{CO_2})}$$

$$7.40 - 6.10 = 1.3 = \log \frac{(26) - (0.0301 P_{CO_2})}{(0.0301 P_{CO_2})}$$

$$\text{antilog } 1.3 = \frac{(26) - (0.0301 P_{CO_2})}{(0.0301 P_{CO_2})}$$

$$\text{antilog } 1.3 = 19.95$$

therefore,

$$19.95(0.0301 P_{CO_2}) = (26) - (0.0301 P_{CO_2})$$

$$19.95(0.0301 P_{CO_2}) + (0.0301 P_{CO_2}) = 26$$

$$0.6306 P_{CO_2} = 26$$

$$P_{CO_2} = \frac{26}{0.6306}$$

$$P_{CO_2} = 41.2 \text{ mm Hg}$$

The sum of the concentrations of dissolved CO_2 and H_2CO_3 is equal to

$$0.0301 P_{CO_2} = 0.0301 \times 41.2 = 1.24 \text{ mmol/liter}$$

Since the concentration of bicarbonate ion is the difference between total CO_2 content and the value for dissolved CO_2 and H_2CO_3,

$$(HCO_3^-) = 26 - 1.24 = 24.76 \text{ mmol/liter}$$

REGULATION OF ACID-BASE EQUILIBRIUM In general, the problem of regulating acid-base balance in health is to protect the pH from alterations induced by the continuous formation of acid end products of metabolism. In health the pH of the extracellular fluids is maintained at a level between 7.35 and 7.45. This is accomplished by buffer activity (discussed earlier), by exchange of ions between the two major fluid compartments, and by adaptations of respiratory and renal function.

Regulation by ion exchange The exchange of *anions* across membranes appears to be most free in the red blood cells and, probably, the renal tubular cells. Chloride and bicarbonate ions can diffuse across the erythrocyte membrane, and their distribution between the red blood cell and plasma water is responsive to changes in their concentrations and pH. For example, an increase in the P_{CO_2} of the plasma due to the addition of carbon dioxide is followed by diffusion of the gas into the red blood cell, where part of it is hydrated to H_2CO_3. The dissociation of this acid increases the concentration of bicarbonate ions, and these diffuse from the cell. This, in turn, is accompanied by a movement of chloride into the red blood cells. The net effect of this redistribution of anions in terms of the acid-base relationships of the extracellular fluid is to increase the concentration of bicarbonate in this compartment. This increase in the concentration of HCO_3^- tends to offset the effect of the initial increase in P_{CO_2} on the buffer ratio of the Henderson-Hasselbalch equation.

The exchange of *cations* such as sodium, potassium, and perhaps calcium as well from muscle cells and bone for hydrogen ions in the extracellular fluid (and vice versa) plays a significant role in modifying the alterations in pH of the extracellular fluids. It has been estimated, for example, that approximately 50 percent of an acid load administered to dogs was neutralized by such an exchange of sodium and potassium for hydrogen ions. In another study it was suggested that 25 percent of the "neutralization" of an infusion of $NaHCO_3$ had been achieved by the exchange of extracellular sodium for intracellular hydrogen ions. Similar exchanges are reported in studies of both respiratory acidosis and respiratory alkalosis.

Respiratory regulation The lungs play a major role in the excretion of acid as carbon dioxide. Moreover, the centers that regulate the rate and depth of ventilation are exquisitely sensitive to subtle changes in the composition of the blood and extravascular fluids. The central chemoreceptors located in the medullary respiratory centers are responsive to the P_{CO_2} and pH of their environment in such a way that an increase in P_{CO_2} or hydrogen ion concentration promotes an increase in pulmonary ventilation. In contrast, a decrease in CO_2 tension or increase in pH tends to inhibit ventilation. In either case it is clear that the alteration in respiratory activity tends to correct the primary deviation in P_{CO_2} or pH. The P_{CO_2} appears to be the more potent stimulus of the two. In addition, there are peripheral chemoreceptors located in the carotid and aortic bodies. These are relatively insensitive to pH and P_{CO_2} but are responsive to the arterial oxygen tension (P_{O_2}).

An interesting aspect of the chemoregulation of pulmonary ventilation concerns the phenomenon of a change in the "sensitivity" of the central respiratory centers to a specific P_{CO_2}. It appears as though a period of hypercapnia diminishes "sensitivity," and hypocapnia enhances the intensity of the response to a given tension of CO_2. The precise nature of this altered response is not clear. An appreciation of this adaptation is helpful in understanding certain complications of acid-base disorders, which will be discussed in more detail later (see Chap. 29 for a more complete discussion of respiratory regulation).

Renal regulation The kidneys contribute to the regulation of acid-base balance by varying the net rate of excretion of hydrogen ions and by processes of selective reabsorption and rejection of cations and anions. These two processes are interdependent to the extent that the reabsorption of sodium is closely related to the secretion of hydrogen ions and potassium. The total rate of *secretion* of hydrogen ions by the tubular cells may be calculated from the sum of the titratable acid, ammonium ion, and a fraction equivalent to the difference between the filtered and excreted bicarbonate.

The rate of *excretion* of acid is calculated from the sum of the titratable acid plus ammonium ion *minus* the bicarbonate.

The titratable acid is equivalent to the quantity of NaOH that must be added to the urine to change its pH to that of the plasma. It represents the hydrogen ions present in free acid compounds and incorporated in the buffer components of the urine. Caution must be exercised to avoid the error of necessarily equating a low urinary pH with a high rate of excretion of acid. A small quantity of dissociated acid in a poorly buffered urine will lower the pH considerably. This same quantity of titratable acid in a buffered solution might be accommodated with very little depression of pH.

Pitts and his collaborators demonstrated that the urinary excretion of acid may be in excess of what can be accounted for by filtration and preferential reabsorption. They developed the hypothesis that hydrogen ions are secreted into the tubular fluid in exchange for sodium. The source of the hydrogen ions for this secretory process is not known for certain, although it is usually represented as having been derived from carbonic acid.

The latter, in turn, is believed to be formed from the hydration of carbon dioxide:

$$\left.\begin{array}{c} H_2O + CO_2 \\ \rightleftharpoons \\ H_2CO_3 \end{array}\right\} \text{This reaction accelerated by the enzyme carbonic anhydrase}$$

$$\rightleftharpoons$$

$$H^+ + HCO_3^-$$

The rate of tubular *secretion* of hydrogen ions is probably conditioned by many factors, some of which include the pH of the renal tubular cell fluid, the P_{CO_2} (rather than the pH) of the extracellular fluid, the availability of buffers in the tubular fluid, the intensity of the stimuli primarily responsible for the reabsorption of sodium, and the status of the stores of potassium in the tubular cells. A decreased pH in the cell fluid, hypercapnia, and a diminished content of potassium in the renal tubular cells tend to favor the secretion of hydrogen ions. These ions cannot be secreted against a concentration gradient in excess of approximately 800:1. A diminished tubular content of buffer will therefore impose a restriction on the rate of secretion of hydrogen ions by failing to resist the decrease in pH consequent to this secretion.

In essence one may view the major role of the kidney in combating acidosis as reabsorbing all the filtered bicarbonate and, in addition, regenerating the bicarbonate that is continuously dissipated by the buffer action of strong acids with the bicarbonate–carbonic acid system. These operations may be portrayed as follows:

1 The reabsorption of filtered bicarbonate.

Interstitial fluid — Tubular cell — Tubular fluid

H^+ HCO_3^- Na^+ HCO_3^-

$NaHCO_3 \longleftarrow NaHCO_3$ H_2CO_3

$CO_2 \longleftarrow CO_2 + H_2O$

It will be noted that the reabsorption of the filtered bicarbonate is somewhat indirect. The sodium which is reabsorbed by exchange with hydrogen ion is then transported from the cell to the interstitial fluid of the kidney along with the bicarbonate remnant of the carbonic acid that donated the hydrogen ion. The carbonic acid left behind in the tubular fluid is then dehydrated to CO_2 and H_2O, and the carbon dioxide diffuses back to the body fluids.

2 The reabsorption of bicarbonate that is *not* filtered.

Interstitial fluid — Tubular cell — Tubular fluid

H^+ HCO_3^- Na^+ $NaHPO_4^-$

$NaHCO_3 \longleftarrow NaHCO_3$ NaH_2PO_4

In this way sodium of a salt other than bicarbonate is reabsorbed in exchange for a hydrogen ion that becomes incorporated in a buffer. In a somewhat similar fashion the following reaction may obtain when the anion accompanying sodium is relatively unable to permeate the tubular cell membrane:

Interstitial fluid — Tubular cell — Tubular fluid

H^+ HCO_3^- Na^+ X^-

$NaHCO_3 \longleftarrow NaHCO_3$ HX

In addition to excretion as titratable acid, as illustrated above, hydrogen ions are excreted as ammonium, NH_4^+, as well. The sequence of events leading to enhanced excretion of ammonium depends in part on the reaction just described. The active transport of sodium produces a potential difference across the tubular membranes such that the lumen is negative. This creates a driving force which can be accommodated either by reabsorption of an anion with a negative charge along the established electrochemical gradient or by secretion of a positively charged cation. If the anion cannot permeate, the second alternative must obtain. Hydrogen ions can be secreted until the luminal fluid pH falls to a level against which no more hydrogen ions can be transported. Ammonia is considered to be in diffusion equilibrium between tubular cells and lumen and can move freely in either direction, but NH_4^+ cannot. Thus, if hydrogen ions are secreted and all filtered buffers are exhausted, the NH_3 in the luminal fluid can buffer the hydrogen ion. The NH_4^+ which is formed cannot diffuse back and hence is excreted into the urine. This sets the direction of the reaction pathway for ammonia, the hydrogen ion gradient is reduced, and now more hydrogen ions can be secreted. This may be illustrated in the following fashion:

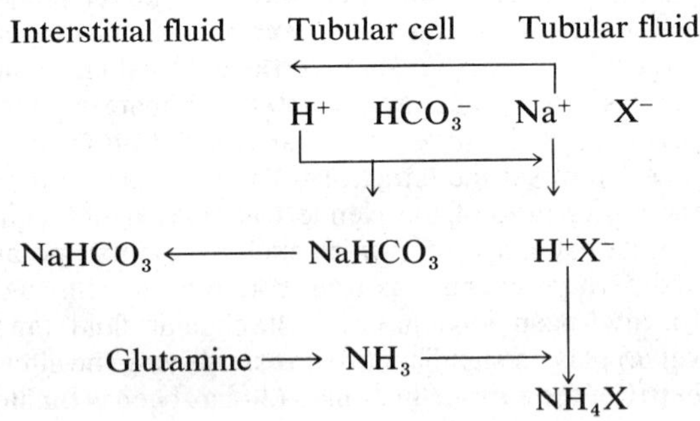

The rate of excretion of ammonia does not change as acutely as is the case with titratable acid, but in appropriate circumstances it may make a greater contribution in quantitative terms. Ammonia is formed in the tubular cells, and the largest fraction is derived from glutamine. The manner in which ammonia derives from glutamine, alanine, and other precursors is still unclear, as is the nature of the delay of full activation of these mechanisms.

In these several ways the renal tubules regenerate the bicarbonate that is dissipated (and excreted as CO_2) by the buffer activity consequent to the accession of an acid load in the body fluids.

The reabsorption of sodium may be associated with an exchange for potassium in lieu of hydrogen ion. These alternatives are frequently pictured as competing one with the other. These interrelationships may explain, in part, the aciduria which may accompany potassium depletion despite an extracellular alkalosis; and this may also explain why the administration of $NaHCO_3$ is accompanied by an augmented excretion of potassium.

The administration of a carbonic anhydrase inhibitor suppresses all these reactions that depend on a readily available source of hydrogen ions. Such an agent promotes increased excretion of sodium, bicarbonate, and potassium and decreases the rate of excretion of titratable acid and ammonia. Some of these alterations are observed in patients with renal disease characterized by tubular dysfunction. The defect in some instances is due to inability to transport hydrogen ions against a concentration gradient.

The role of the kidneys in acid-base regulation will be discussed further later in this chapter. The nature of the specific responses in each type of acid-base disturbance will serve to illustrate the particular contributions of the kidneys.

A comment is in order concerning the significance of *compensation.* The responses just described are initiated by a distortion of one or more of the physicochemical characteristics of the body fluids. If the response were such as to efface the distortion, the stimulus for the response would be removed and the distortion would reappear. Thus, it is unlikely that compensation can ever be perfect since it would automatically be self-destructive so long as the initial basis for the disturbance persisted. Hence, if a patient with an obvious acid-base disturbance has a normal value for pH, or P_{CO_2}, or total CO_2 content, the implication is that this is almost certainly an instance of a *mixed* acid-base disturbance.

CLINICAL CONSIDERATIONS

There are four major disturbances in acid-base equilibrium, and it is convenient to discuss them individually and as separate entities. Nevertheless it should be remembered that mixed disturbances occur fairly frequently. In this discussion the aim is to analyze each disorder in terms of the primary alteration, the impact of this insult and the compensatory respiratory and renal responses on the Henderson-Hasselbalch equation, the nature of the compositional changes, and the approach to the management of the disorder. The Henderson-Hasselbalch equation is re-presented here with respect to the bicarbonate–carbonic acid buffer system. Reference to this equation, which defines the pH, is most helpful in visualizing the sequence and consequence of primary and secondary events in the pathogenesis of acidosis and alkalosis:

$$pH = 6.1 + \log \frac{NaHCO_3}{\underset{\substack{\downarrow\uparrow \\ CO_2 + H_2O}}{H_2CO_3} + \text{dissolved } CO_2}$$

The ratio of the concentrations of the buffer pair is 20:1.

RESPIRATORY ACIDOSIS Respiratory acidosis is due to inadequate elimination of CO_2 by the lungs because of hypoventilation or because of uneven ventilation in relation to blood flow. It is unlikely to be associated solely with impaired diffusion across the alveolar capillary membranes, since the diffusion of CO_2 is so rapid. Respiratory acidosis is found commonly in patients with conditions such as emphysema, pulmonary fibrosis, and cardiopulmonary disease.

The retention of CO_2 will increase the P_{CO_2} and the concentration of carbonic acid. The increase in the value for the denominator of the buffer ratio will change this to something less than 20:1 and will define a decrease in the pH. The CO_2 can penetrate cell membranes freely, and in this fashion a considerable quantity of acid can be buffered in the intracellular fluids. In addition, there is evidence that hydrogen ions from the extracellular fluids exchange for potassium and sodium from cells and bone.

The increase in P_{CO_2} and the decrease in pH both serve to stimulate ventilation, and further accumulation of CO_2 may be prevented or at least retarded thereby. The renal response is characterized by increased excretion of titratable acid, ammonium, and chloride and diminished excretion of bicarbonate. The above-mentioned response clearly implies a net increase in the total rate of *secretion* of hydrogen ions by the renal tubule, which is not necessarily the case in metabolic acidosis (see below). In this manner the kidneys help eliminate acid, but, in addition, they alter electrolyte composition so that the concentration of bicarbonate in the extracellular fluid increases at the expense of chloride. To the extent that this increase in the concentration of bicarbonate restores the buffer ratio toward 20:1, the deviation of the pH is minimized. The ability to tolerate a high P_{CO_2} has an additional advantage in that a greater quantity of CO_2 is excreted per unit of ventilation. This increment may be sufficiently large to allow the excretion of CO_2 to equal its production. In this circumstance no further increase in P_{CO_2} will occur unless the primary disease worsens.

It was stated earlier that the increase in CO_2 tension stimulated respiratory activity, but as the hypercapnia is maintained the respiratory centers appear to develop decreased sensitivity to this stimulus. A diminution in the respiratory response to the next increment of P_{CO_2} will promote a more intense hypercapnia. This new level of P_{CO_2} serves to maintain some increase in ventilation until a new level of desensitization develops, and the vicious cycle is repeated. Ultimately the hypercapnia becomes extreme, and the increased P_{CO_2} no longer serves as an appropriate stimulus to increase ventilation. At this time the most important stimulus for respiratory activity is the accompanying hypoxia. It has been said that if patients with respiratory acidosis were left to their own devices, they would probably succumb to hypoxia rather than to hypercapnia or acidosis. The slower diffusion of oxygen would be expected to promote incapacitating hypoxia before the development of CO_2 narcosis or a pH incompatible with life. However, if such patients are treated by exposure to a breathing mixture with a high content of oxygen in an effort to relieve the hypoxemia, they may quickly become confused, lapse into coma, and die. The improvement in the hypoxia may remove the last effective stimulus for respiratory activity. As a result of the diminished ventilation, there is a further decline in the excretion of CO_2, leading to the grave consequences of extreme hypercapnia. This should not be interpreted to suggest that such patients should never be treated with oxygen; it emphasizes the need for close observation when oxygen therapy is used to detect the earliest evidences of this complication. If morphine is given these patients, it should be administered with caution, since this drug may affect the respiratory center in such a manner as to induce hypoventilation. This, in turn, will promote a sharp increase in the P_{CO_2}, the intensity of the acidosis, and the degree of hypoxia.

The management of these patients includes all those measures which may be expected to improve the basic disease condition responsible for pulmonary insufficiency, as discussed in Chap. 263. However, these measures may fail, and the extreme hypoxia and hypercapnia may require immediate attention. In this situation artificial respiration (by mechanical respirator) may offer a valuable therapeutic approach. The increase in ventilatory exchange induced by the respirator improves the hypoxia and promotes an increased excretion of CO_2. In the course of a few days this may be successful in reducing the P_{CO_2} to more nearly normal levels. This, in turn, may restore the sensitivity of the respiratory center to lower levels of CO_2, and a rising P_{CO_2} may again serve as a proper stimulus to respiratory activity.

The compositional changes in the serum have been mentioned; a fairly typical pattern of concentrations of electrolytes in a patient with respiratory acidosis is

Na	137 mEq/l
K	4.5 mEq/l
Total CO_2	40 mmol/l
Cl	90 mEq/l
pH	7.31
P_{CO_2}	79 mm Hg

The pattern, neglecting pH and P_{CO_2}, would also be compatible with metabolic alkalosis. The gross characteristics of the underlying clinical problem will usually dictate the appropriate selection between these two alternatives. The normal concentration of potassium suggests that this is not metabolic alkalosis. The arterial pH clearly resolves the problem in the above instance.

METABOLIC ACIDOSIS Metabolic acidosis is due to either an accumulation of acids or a primary loss of bicarbonate. An accumulation of acids is observed classically in diabetic acidosis and in renal insufficiency, and a primary loss of bicarbonate may be observed in renal disease as well. In diabetes the offenders are the 4-carbon ketones, and if these may be represented by the expression HK, the consequences of their accession to the extracellular fluid may be visualized as follows:

$$HK + NaHCO_3 \rightleftharpoons NaK + H_2CO_3$$

If this buffering of the ketone acid is related to the effect on the Henderson-Hasselbalch equation, it is readily observed that the reduction in bicarbonate and increase in carbonic acid will decrease the ratio to something less than 20:1 and will define a decrease in the pH. The latter as well as the presumed initial increase in P_{CO_2} both serve as stimuli to increase pulmonary ventilation, the excretion of CO_2 will be accelerated, P_{CO_2} will fall, the buffer ratio will be restored toward 20:1, and the deviation in pH is minimized. The violent respiratory response to acidosis characterized by an increase first in depth and later in frequency of respirations is referred to as *Kussmaul breathing*. If one observes the characteristics of this respiratory activity closely, it is usually noted that the effort appears to be on the expiratory phase in contrast to the inspiratory effort noted in patients with oxygen lack.

Since the P_{CO_2} is depressed along with the decrease in pH, the inference is either that the latter is now solely responsible for the increased respiratory activity or CO_2. The latter appears quite likely, and it has been pointed out that during the recovery phase of several types of metabolic acidosis, the pH reaches normal values while the P_{CO_2} is still depressed. This would be an unlikely event unless the respiratory center was responsive to these lower levels of P_{CO_2}.

The renal response to this metabolic acidosis includes virtual total reabsorption of filtered bicarbonate and an increase in the net *urinary excretion* of acid as titratable acid and ammonia. The increase in net excretion of acid does not necessarily imply an increase in the net *secretion* of hydrogen ions. This will be apparent if it is recalled that the secretion of hydrogen ions to effect total reabsorption of a small filtered load of bicarbonate may be considerably less than that needed for incomplete reabsorption of bicarbonate when there is a much higher filtered load, as is the case normally or in respiratory acidosis. The net rates of excretion of acid may be similar in respiratory and metabolic acidosis, although presumably more hydrogen ion is secreted in the former to effect the larger bicarbonate reabsorption. Thus, although higher levels of P_{CO_2} favor the secretion of hydrogen ions, the renal response, in terms of the *net excretion* of acid, is not jeopardized by the hypocapnia of metabolic acidosis.

A fairly typical pattern of the concentrations of electrolytes in the serum in diabetic acidosis is

Na	125 mEq/l
K	3.5 mEq/l
Total CO_2	5 mmol/l
Cl	90 mEq/l
Glucose	800 mg/100ml
pH	7.01
P_{CO_2}	19 mm Hg

It will be noted that the sum of the concentrations of CO_2 and chloride is 95 mEq per liter. The difference between this sum and the concentration of sodium is 30 mEq per liter, so that the anion gap is significantly higher than the usual value of 5 to 15 mEq per liter and implies an unusual concentration of some anion other than bicarbonate and chloride. In diabetic acidosis this is likely to be almost all represented by ketones. (Although the concentration of sodium is depressed, the effective osmolality of the extracellular fluids will be found to be increased if one calculates the osmolar contribution of the elevated concentration of glucose.)[2]

[2] *The osmolar contribution of glucose is calculated as follows: mg/100 ml glucose × 10 = mg/l; mg/l divided by 180 (molecular weight of glucose) = the number of milliosmols of glucose. Thus: 800 × 10 = 8,000; 8,000 divided by 180 = 44.4 mOsm/l.*

The management of the acid-base disturbance in diabetic patients is not usually a primary concern. The administration of adequate amounts of insulin can be expected to promote the utilization of glucose and to decrease the production of ketones. Under these circumstances the ketonemia is soon dissipated by utilization and excretion, and as the ketonemia subsides, the concentration of bicarbonate increases and the pH is soon restored to more nearly normal levels.

Metabolic acidosis due to the loss of bicarbonate in the urine is not uncommon in chronic renal insufficiency. It is due, presumably, to inadequate reabsorption of bicarbonate by the renal tubular cells. This may, in turn, be due to one of several steps that must precede the actual secretion of hydrogen ions in the process of exchange with sodium. Since this is primarily a reflection of tubular dysfunction, it has been stated that it is seen more commonly in chronic pyelonephritis than in glomerulonephritis or other forms of chronic Bright's disease; it may occur, however, in all types of chronic renal failure. In one rather rare form of renal disease there is relatively little functional evidence of glomerular disease. In some of these disorders, the tubular defect may be congenital in origin. In this last instance the defect appears to be concerned not with the formation of hydrogen ions but with the inability to secrete these ions against the concentration gradient. The net effect of the defect is reduced concentration of bicarbonate in the extracellular fluids, accompanied by reciprocally increased concentration of chloride. The diminution in concentration of bicarbonate defines a decrease in the pH of the extracellular fluid. This latter serves as a stimulus to respiratory activity, increased excretion of CO_2 promotes a decrease in P_{CO_2}, and pH approaches a normal value as the ratio of the buffer pair approaches a value of 20:1. Since the ability to secrete hydrogen ions is not totally defunct, the excretion of bicarbonate diminishes only to the point where the filtered load of bicarbonate reaches a value no longer in excess of the residual capacity to secrete hydrogen ions. This disorder may also be associated with increased excretion of calcium and potassium. The latter is not unexpected by virtue of the competitive relationship between hydrogen ions and potassium for exchange with sodium. The reason for the augmented excretion of calcium is less clear. It may be due, in part, to the effect of systemic acidosis in mobilizing calcium from bone. It may also represent some specific renal response of an adaptive nature.

A characteristic set of concentrations of electrolytes in the serum is

Na	134 mEq/l
K	3.5 mEq/l
Total CO_2	12 mmol/l
Cl	115 mEq/l
PO_4	2 mEq/l
pH	7.25
P_{CO_2}	26 mm Hg

It should be noted that the sum of the concentrations of CO_2 and chloride, 127 mEq per liter, differs only by 7 mEq per liter from the concentration of sodium and that the phosphate concentration is normal. This makes it clear that the depression of CO_2 cannot be ascribed to the accumulation of anions other than chloride. This same pattern might be observed in a patient who had received large doses of NH_4Cl or Diamox or who had respiratory alkalosis. The determination of the pH readily resolves the directional deviation in this instance. In clinical situations the history alone should reveal whether this pattern resulted from a renal lesion or from the administration of ammonium chloride or a drug.

In instances of renal insufficiency accompanied by a significant decrease in filtration rate and renal mass, there is an inability to regenerate bicarbonate. This may be due in part to the filtration of lesser quantities of sodium salts, diminished buffer capacity in the tubules, and failure to excrete ammonia properly owing to the loss of the tissue responsible for this function. The diminished filtration rate is presumably responsible for the retention of phosphate, sulfate, and other anions of fixed acids as well. This constellation of defects is characterized by a diminution in the total CO_2 content as well as an increase in what is commonly referred to as the ***undetermined anions*** or anion gap. Hence, the sum of the concentrations of total CO_2 and chloride subtracted from the concentration of sodium in the serum will usually equal a value in excess of 5 to 15 mEq per liter. This type of acidosis is the one most commonly encountered in chronic renal failure. A characteristic set of concentrations is

Na	130 mEq/l
K	5 mEq/l
Total CO_2	12 mmol/l
Cl	93 mEq/l
PO_4	7 mEq/l
pH	7.25
P_{CO_2}	26 mm Hg

Note that the total CO_2 plus chloride subtracted from the sodium equals 25 mEq per liter. The hyperphosphatemia accounts for part of this excess, and sulfates would, if measured, probably be equally increased. Note also the slight hyperkalemia.

Metabolic acidosis due to renal insufficiency can be corrected by administering sodium bicarbonate. In this fashion the concentration of bicarbonate can be increased and the buffer ratio restored to a normal value. Correction can be made effectively in many instances simply by prescribing the ingestion of sodium bicarbonate either in addition to or in lieu of table salt. The reduction in the intake of NaCl is particularly desirable where there is some reason to avoid an excessive intake of sodium or where the substitution of sodium bicarbonate for sodium chloride is indicated because acidosis is due to a primary loss of bicarbonate and the concentration of chloride is already high. The amount of sodium bicarbonate necessary as a daily supplement must be gaged in an empirical manner by correlating the dosage with the response. The use of 2 to 4 g $NaHCO_3$ per day is safe to start with. Two complications may mar the success of this treatment. Since the kidneys of these patients have lost the capacity to discriminate properly, it is possible to overcorrect the acidosis. The possibility of overcorrection may be increased by the maintenance of a low P_{CO_2} due to increased sensitivity of the respiratory center to CO_2 as a stimulus. The second complication deals with the possible development of tetany. Many of these patients have hyperphosphatemia and hypocalcemia. The acidosis may protect against tetany from hypocalcemia, and this protection may be lost as the pH is corrected with $NaHCO_3$. The ingestion of several grams of calcium gluconate or lactate may prevent this complication. The obvious advantages of the correction of the metabolic acidosis include elimination of the hyperpnea which may be a troublesome symptom, in most cases some relief from subjective discomfort, and maintenance of an internal environment better able to buffer sudden increments of acid. The increase in excretion of calcium and potassium that may accompany the acidosis may be diminished as well. However, it is unnecessary to raise the level of bicarbonate in excess of 20 mmol per liter.

So far this discussion has concerned management in a noncritical chronic phase of the disease. When patients with renal insufficiency experience an episode of dehydration with further decompensation in renal function, they may develop acute and more intense disturbances in acid-base balance. However, it is frequently in these very circumstances that the physician may be most effective in correcting a disabling acidosis. The efficient correction of acidosis depends on increasing the concentration of bicarbonate in the extracellular fluid. This can be accomplished most dramatically when hyponatremia accompanies the disorder, since the concentration of sodium can be raised together with the bicarbonate by administering a hypertonic solution of $NaHCO_3$. The quantity of sodium to administer is calculated as discussed in Chap. 264. This could represent too much bicarbonate, and blood should be sampled during the course of therapy to ensure that the treatment is not excessive. The second most dramatic correction may be accomplished when the patient with acidosis has a normal concentration of sodium but is dehydrated. The administration of an isotonic solution of a sodium salt will expand the volume of the extracellular fluid and repair the dehydration. If the salt is the bicarbonate, the concentration of this anion will be increased.

The possibility of provoking hypocalcemic tetany must always be considered when sodium bicarbonate is administered in these circumstances. It is recommended that prior to the infusion of $NaHCO_3$ the patient should receive at least 10 ml 10 percent solution of calcium gluconate intravenously. In addition, the presence of Chvostek's reflex should be checked during the administration of the bicarbonate and more calcium administered if the reflex is elicited. The solution of calcium should not be mixed with bicarbonate, since calcium carbonate will precipitate.

RESPIRATORY ALKALOSIS Respiratory alkalosis is due to hyperventilation and results from the excretion of carbon dioxide in excess of its production. This reduces the tension of CO_2, increases the value for the ratio of the buffer pair, and defines an increase in pH. This disorder may be observed in the early phases of pulmonary and cardiopulmonary disease when hyperventilation is induced by hypoxia. It is more commonly observed as a manifestation of anxiety and tension, and it may be due to a lesion in the area of the central nervous system responsible for respiratory regulatory regulation. This last is the least common variety, but it is the circumstance in which one may see the most significant deviations from normal.

The anxious and tense patient, usually a woman, who hyperventilates in response to emotional stimuli may develop acute, although transient, alkalosis accompanied by a variety of symptoms, which include giddiness and light-headedness, circumoral and peripheral paresthesias, muscle tremors, and frank carpopedal spasm. Since these episodes are short-lived, there is insufficient time for a significant renal response in the nature of a compensatory effort. For the same reasons the only compositional changes are the increase in pH and decrease in P_{CO_2}.

In those instances of relatively sustained hyperventilation, as with an irritative lesion in the reticular formation of the medulla, compensatory responses and compositional changes may be prominent. The renal responses are characterized by increased excretion of bicarbonate, decreased excretion of chloride, and augmented excretion of potassium and sodium. The diminution in renal tubular reabsorption of bicarbonate is due, presumably, to decreased secretion of hydrogen ions for the exchange with sodium. This may be due to hypocapnia. The lessened secretion of hydrogen ions may be responsible for an increase in the secretion and excretion of potassium. The most significant consequence of these renal responses is decreased concentration of bicarbonate in the extracellular fluids. This alteration tends to reduce the value for the ratio of the buffer pair toward 20:1 and hence minimizes the deviation in pH. The other alterations in composition include an increase in the concentration of chloride in the serum, along with a tendency to a lowered concentration of sodium and potassium.

These alterations in the electrolyte pattern may mimic those of metabolic acidosis. It is important to recognize respiratory alkalosis as distinct from metabolic acidosis, since the administration of bicarbonate, which may be desirable for acidosis, may be detrimental to the patient who is already alkalotic.

The management of patients with hyperventilation as a manifestation of anxiety and tension is primarily directed toward helping the patient to understand the pathogenesis of the disorder. It is frequently helpful to have the patient induce an episode by voluntary hyperventilation and then to demonstrate how this may be modified by rebreathing into a paper bag or by holding the nose and covering the mouth. This demonstration is usually quite convincing and helps to furnish the motivation for the patient to train herself to discontinue this habit. In those instances where hyperventilation has provoked carpopedal spasm, the immediate need is to use some technique to increase the P_{CO_2} of the body fluids. This is most easily accomplished by having the patient rebreathe into a paper bag.

METABOLIC ALKALOSIS Metabolic alkalosis is characterized by increased concentration of bicarbonate unattended by an equivalent increase in the P_{CO_2}, so that the ratio of the concentrations of the buffer pair is in excess of 20:1 and the pH is elevated. This condition may arise as a consequence of (1) the administration of sodium bicarbonate (or sodium salts of organic acids such as citrate or lactate); (2) the loss of chloride as HCl, as in vomiting or gastric suction; (3) the loss of chloride with sodium in a ratio in excess of that which characterizes their relative concentrations in the extracellular fluid; (4) excessive excretion of acid in the urine; (5) the movement of hydrogen ions from the extracellular fluid to the cells in consequence of a deficit of potassium. The interrelationships among these possible primary events are intimate, and each of them provokes responses of an interdependent character, so it is rare to find metabolic alkalosis that is not multicausal. The interplay of primary events and subsequent responses can be illustrated by examining the sequence that may follow each of the major initiating events.

Throughout the discussion it will be well to visualize the effects of compensatory mechanisms that tend to mitigate the deviation in pH as these may be surmised from the Henderson-Hasselbalch equation. These include an increase in the CO_2 tension, which may be induced by hypoventilation, and a reduction in the concentration of bicarbonate in the extracellular fluid. Hypoventilation would, presumably, be favored by the increase in pH. However, this path of compensation is not usually of great quantitative significance. There are limiting influences on hypoventilation, which include the development of hypoxia and hypercapnia. These are both stimuli to increased respiratory activity. Reduction in the high concentration of bicarbonate may be achieved to some extent by the accelerated excretion of $NaHCO_3$ in the urine. To the extent that an increase in P_{CO_2} tends to enhance the reabsorption of bicarbonate, it may be said that a more successful hypoventilatory response would impose serious limitations on the efficiency of the renal response. Other limitations imposed on the compensating mechanisms will be illustrated in the discussions to follow. Furthermore, there may be specific deleterious effects on renal function and anatomic integrity as a consequence of certain features of metabolic alkalosis. One of these effects is potassium depletion.

Alkalosis induced with sodium bicarbonate The administration of $NaHCO_3$ will induce metabolic alkalosis, which depends, in part, on the magnitude and rapidity with which a particular load of this salt is administered. However, the ability to accelerate the excretion of $NaHCO_3$ in the urine is so great that it is difficult to maintain any serious degree of alkalosis in this fashion in the absence of other conditioning influences. The ingestion or administration of $NaHCO_3$ is accompanied by an augmented excretion of potassium. If the ingestion or administration of potassium is inadequate to match the accelerated urinary loss, a deficit of potassium develops. The depletion of potassium has several consequences that tend to intensify rather than mitigate alkalosis:

1 A potassium deficit tends to diminish the secretion of potassium and enhance the exchange of hydrogen ions for sodium in the renal tubular reabsorptive mechanism. The augmented secretion of hydrogen ions promotes increased reabsorption of sodium as bicarbonate, which imposes a limit on the efficiency with which bicarbonate may be excreted.

2 A large experimental literature dealing with the production of potassium depletion utilizing diets essentially free of this cation and administering $NaHCO_3$ describes an increase in the quantity of sodium in tissue cells. However, in most instances the quantitative relationship is such as to suggest that some other cation has gained access to the cell along with sodium. In some instances, at least, this appears to be hydrogen ion. To the extent that this transfer of hydrogen ions from the extracellular fluids to cells operates, the intensity of the extracellular alkalosis will be augmented.

As long as potassium depletion is avoided, large amounts of administered bicarbonate may fail to induce significant alkalosis.

Metabolic alkalosis due to loss of gastric secretion by vomiting or suction The primary cause of alkalosis in this instance is the loss of HCl with the consequent increase in the bicarbonate concentration and decrease in the chloride concentration in the extracellular fluids. The renal response to this alkalosis is similar to that just described and is characterized by accelerated excretion of sodium and potassium bicarbonate in the urine. The loss of potassium in the urine added to the loss of this ion in the gastric fluid represents an early potassium deficit. The nature of the primary event precludes retention of ingested food or fluid, and if potassium is not administered parenterally and the gastric losses continue, the intensity of the potassium depletion increases. Furthermore, the loss of sodium in the gastric fluid and in the urine, if unreplaced, induces a deficit of this ion as well. The deficits of potassium and sodium both impose limitations on the mechanisms that tend to compensate for alkalosis. Those related to potassium depletion have just been described. The limits imposed by sodium depletion may operate as follows: As the deficit of sodium develops, there is a loss of fluid. If no water is ingested or administered, the net deficit tends toward a loss of water in excess of sodium loss. If water is ingested and promptly vomited, or if water without salt (e.g., glucose in water) is administered by vein, the net deficit will be of sodium in excess of water. In either event, there will be a contraction of the extracellular volume. This, in turn, will promote a decreased rate of sodium excretion. To the extent that renal tubular reabsorption of sodium is increased (owing to the sodium depletion and the consequent hypovolemia) and the concentration of chloride in plasma is diminished, a set of circumstances is created that dictates an increase in acid secretion and excretion. As alluded to earlier, the reabsorption of sodium from the tubular urine will be associated with the reabsorption of the accompanying anion or the secretion of a positively charged ion such as potassium or hydrogen. One of the determinants of these options relates to the ease with which the anion can permeate the renal tubular cells. This varies, and chloride may be the most permeant, bicarbonate the least, with the others in intermediate positions. Hence, if there is hypochloremia, virtually all the chloride may be reabsorbed along with sodium before the luminal fluid reaches more distal sites. Under these circumstances, the nonchloride salts of sodium predominate, and since their permeability is limited, the option for reabsorption of the anion may be likewise limited. The alternative of the secretion of a positively charged ion is then likely to play a more important role. If there is accompanying potassium depletion, hydrogen ion will be secreted in response to the reabsorption of sodium; and the reabsorbed sodium will then relate to bicarbonate in the cell and enter the interstitial fluid as sodium bicarbonate. These conditioning factors are, presumably, the genesis of the *paradoxic aciduria* that may be noted in clinical disorders associated with metabolic alkalosis. The paradoxic aciduria in the context of an alkalosis is presumptive evidence of sodium depletion and, probably, of potassium depletion as well. In most instances the urine will become alkaline if the sodium deficit is repaired with saline solution, since in the absence of volume depletion the demands for sodium reabsorption are diminished and sodium bicarbonate can then escape into the urine.

These considerations have very important therapeutic implications and serve to emphasize the need for an overall evaluation of the problem in management. For example, administration of ammonium chloride to such a patient could correct the state of alkalosis but add the complications of metabolic acidosis; it would probably enhance the loss of potassium and sodium and serve very poorly to improve the patient's status. In contrast, the clearly indicated therapeutic measures include the following:

1 Dehydration should be corrected by administration of salt and water. The proportion in which they should be administered depends on the net character of the deficits. If there is hypernatremia, the patient needs more water than salt; if he is hyponatremic, the need is for more salt than water. If one is in doubt, isotonic saline solution will usually be adequate. The amount to administer must be judged by an evaluation of the quantity of the deficit, made on the basis of history, physical examination, laboratory data, and the observed response to therapy (see Chap. 264).
2 The deficit of potassium must be corrected. The manner in which this may safely be accomplished will be discussed below under Deficit of Potassium.
3 Sufficient carbohydrate should be administered to minimize protein catabolism and ketonemia.

Once the antecedent deficits are restored, care must be taken to ensure appropriate replacement of current losses so that a new state of depletion will not obtain.

Altered urinary composition due to diuretic and steroid therapy The administration of many diuretic agents promotes potassium loss and alkalosis. The precise manner in which this occurs is not clear. However, it is most probably a consequence of the delivery of greater quantities of sodium to sites where its reabsorption articulates with secretion of hydrogen ions or potassium. In the first instance this would tend to induce alkalosis with its attendant consequences; and in the second instance it induces a loss of potassium, which, in turn, tends to provoke a state of alkalosis.

The naturally existing adrenal cortical hormones tend to enhance the excretion of potassium. This appears to be a secondary rather than a primary event, since it does not occur when the dietary regimen is free of sodium. The suggestion is that the steroids enhance reabsorption of sodium and to the extent that this promotes the secretion of potassium, more of this latter ion is excreted in the urine. The synthetic steroids, employed for reasons other than replacement therapy, have a considerably diminished activity in this regard.

Deficit of potassium (see also Chap. 81) The manner in which a deficit of potassium interrelates with a state of metabolic alkalosis has already been described. There are many causes of a deficit of this ion, including prolonged periods of parenteral alimentation without addition of potassium, excessive losses in gastrointestinal fluid, diarrhea due to disease or induced with cathartics, excessive losses in the urine as with the use of organic mercurial diuretics, chlorothiazide, and steroid hormones, potassium-losing renal disease, Cushing's syndrome, and primary aldosteronism.

Potassium is the major intracellular cation, and depletion is accompanied by disorders of structure and function in various tissues. These tissues include skeletal muscle, smooth muscle of the gastrointestinal tract, myocardium, cartilage, kidneys, and gastric mucosa. Weakness of the muscles and hyporeflexia are common, alterations in the electrocardiogram are well established, and abnormalities in the motor and secretory activity of the gastrointestinal tract are well documented. Inability to concentrate the urine appropriately, decreased rate of filtration at the glomerulus, and defective transport of para-aminohippurate have all been reported.

Although a potassium deficit may have serious consequences, judgment must be exercised in the technique of repletion to avoid the complications of therapy. The most significant hazard is the possibility of administering a potassium salt in too great a quantity or too rapidly so that cardiotoxic levels are reached in the serum.

In the course of the development of a potassium deficit, the patient may become sufficiently dehydrated or acidotic that the depletion is not mirrored in hypokalemia. This is seen quite often, for example, in diabetic acidosis. It would appear to be safer under these circumstances to refrain from administering potassium until partial correction of the dehydration and utilization of the carbohydrate have induced a decrease in the concentration of potassium in the serum and there is clear evidence of satisfactory flows of urine. Potassium salts may be administered more safely by mouth than parenterally. There is sufficient delay in absorption from the gastrointestinal tract to provide some assurance that a sudden increase in the concentration of potassium in the serum will not obtain.

These precautionary comments should not be interpreted to mean that potassium salts cannot be safely administered intravenously. There are many circumstances where for obvious reasons the salt cannot be administered orally and potassium repletion is clearly indicated. However, some control should be exercised with respect to the rate of administration. It is reasonably safe to administer potassium at a rate of about 20 mEq per hr, but it would be desirable to limit the first replacement to 50 to 100 mEq. After this first phase of replacement has been completed, the level of potassium in the serum should be determined. A change in the pattern of the electrocardiogram may also be used as a guide. The change in concentration will provide some indication as to the safe dosage for the next phase of therapy. Unfortunately, there is no way to estimate the magnitude of the deficit with any precision from knowledge of the concentration of potassium in the serum. There is, of course, a gross correlation, but this is an inadequate premise on which to base a safe prediction.

Since the rate of infusion may vary with change of position of the needle, it is always possible that the plan of administration may fail. An additional safeguard is provided by limiting the concentration of potassium in the infusate to approximately 50 mEq per liter. Under this circumstance an accidental increase in the rate of administration of the infusion will have less effect on the rate of administration of potassium.

The particular salt of potassium that is used may be very important. If there is no source of chloride in the diet (as might well be the case with hypertensive or edematous patients who have become potassium-depleted), the potassium should be given as potassium chloride. Other salts of potassium such as acetate, bicarbonate, or citrate may make it difficult to retain potassium under these circumstances. The reasons for this relate to some of the earlier discussion of renal regulation of acid-base equilibrium. Chloride is quite able to permeate the renal tubular epithelium, so when sodium is reabsorbed and an electric gradient established, the reabsorption of sodium will usually be accompanied by chloride if it is present. However, when there is a deficit and no dietary source of chloride, more sodium may be reabsorbed at sites where chloride is no longer present. Since the other anions are less able to permeate, there will be a tendency for the reabsorption of sodium to articulate with the secretion of hydrogen ions or potassium. If it is the former, alkalosis will be established that promotes potassium excretion; if it is potassium, it is obvious that its excretion will be enhanced. In either event the retention of potassium is not as efficient. This has several important consequences. First, the ill effects of potassium depletion are not reversed appropriately. Secondly, if the patient has hypertension and is potassium-depleted and it appears difficult to effect repletion, the clinical state may be misinterpreted as primary aldosteronism.

Once again it must be emphasized that, although this discussion has presented the disturbances of acid-base equilibrium as four distinct and separate entities, mixed clinical pictures are common. However, these should not be too difficult to analyze if the principles described are recalled. In addition, it must be remembered that a disturbance in acid-base equilibrium may be only one aspect (and not necessarily the most important) of the patient's total disease picture. In fact, in some instances attention to the primary disorder may improve the disturbance in acid-base equilibrium so that no therapy for the disequilibrium per se is necessary. Moreover, there are circumstances in which a correction of abnormal chemical values may be undesirable in that it may destroy an adequate compensation.

REFERENCES

BERLINER RW: Outline of renal physiology, in *Diseases of the Kidney*, 2d ed., eds MB Strauss, LG Welt, Boston: Little, Brown, 1971, p. 31

DAVENPORT HS: *The ABC of Acid-Base Chemistry*, 4th ed., Chicago: The University of Chicago Press, 1958

KASSIRER JP et al: The critical role of chloride in the correction of hypokalemic alkalosis in man. Am J Med 38:172, 1965

SIGGAARD-ANDERSEN O: *The Acid-Base Status of the Blood*, 2d ed., Copenhagen: Munksgaard, 1964

266 APPROACH TO THE PATIENT WITH RENAL DISEASE

FRANKLIN H. EPSTEIN

INTRODUCTION The patient with renal disease may have any one of a wide variety of problems. He may complain of symptoms easily recognized as originating in the urinary tract, such as dysuria, frequency, and polyuria (Chaps. 46 and 47), or of those generally (and sometimes wrongly) attributed to the kidneys, such as back pain. He or his doctor may have noticed blood in the urine. Proteinuria may have appeared on a routine examination. Often, however, the presenting complaints and signs are less overt and specific, more general, and hence more confusing. The kidneys must be suspected in cases of unexplained fever, lassitude, anorexia, nausea, weakness, and anemia. Hypertension, heart failure, or edema may dominate the clinical picture. Neurologic disturbances such as headache, tremor, coma, or convulsions often monopolize attention when the patient is first seen. Stunted growth may be the chief concern of the child or adolescent with chronic renal disease. Abnormalities in bone metabolism caused by renal insufficiency may masquerade as arthritis, gout, or rickets.

Certain curable but rare disorders may produce clinical pictures almost identical with those caused by more common but less treatable diseases. These include the possibility that hypertension may be due to unilateral renal disease and the fact that drug sensitivity and syphilis are rare but curable causes of the nephrotic syndrome. In a patient with renal insufficiency, the diagnosis of chronic uremia should not be accepted until all reversible disorders which depress renal function have been considered and excluded. The most important of these are acute glomerulonephritis, acute tubular necrosis, obstructive nephropathy, circulatory insufficiency (including shock or congestive heart failure), and depletion of water and salt. Proper management of renal insufficiency requires above all an expert appreciation of the physiology of body fluids. Treatment should be individualized and animated by a concern with the specific problems of a particular patient rather than with general formulas which fit only an average.

APPROACH TO THE DIAGNOSIS OF PROTEINURIA AND RENAL DISEASE Some points in the study of the patient with abnormal urinary findings deserve special emphasis. *Postural proteinuria* should be ruled out, as well as the proteinuria which is normally associated with exercise or which follows certain febrile diseases. A careful history should inquire into the possibility of recent respiratory or skin infections, recurrent pyelitis, edema or hypertension during pregnancy, arthritis, rash, and drug sensitivity. The patient should be asked specifically about the intake of analgesics, phenacetin-containing compounds, and methysergide. A history of enuresis past the age of six may suggest congenital structural or neurologic anomalies of the urinary tract or chronic childhood pyelitis. The results of prior examinations for employment, insurance, or military service should be ascertained. The family history may be positive for renal and vascular diseases; inquiry should also be made about gout and diabetes. Blood pressure should be checked in the erect as well as the supine position, and retinal as well as peripheral vessels should be examined. Amyloidosis may be suggested by an enlarged liver or spleen; palpable masses in both upper quadrants should also raise the question of polycystic kidneys. Physical examination should not overlook the possibility of a cystocele or an enlarged prostate.

A fresh urine sample should be examined by the physician and the urine should be cultured. Clinical tests of renal function should include a measure of blood urea and serum creatinine. A 24-hour urine collection should be made and the amount of protein excreted per day measured quantitatively. The same urine sample may serve for the measurement of creatinine output, so that the creatinine clearance can be calculated. Occasionally, a disproportionate elevation of blood uric acid level will suggest underlying gouty nephropathy. Examination of the blood for lupus erythematosus cells or of the serum for antinuclear antibodies may permit detection of early lupus erythematosus. Electrophoresis of the serum may reveal globulins characteristic of multiple myeloma. The serum complement level may be depressed in certain forms of active nephritis; e.g., acute streptococcal nephritis, membranoproliferative glomerulonephritis, and lupus nephritis.

The size and shape of the kidneys as well as the structure of calyces and ureters may be ascertained from an *intravenous pyelogram.* High-dose infusion pyelography can provide useful information even when the glomerular filtration rate is depressed, down to a level of about 7 ml per min, but care must be taken not to dehydrate the patient in preparation for x-ray. At the conclusion of this examination, a postvoiding film of the bladder gives information about residual urine without the necessity for catheterization. The size of the kidneys can be estimated in relation to the vertebral shadows on the plain x-ray of the abdomen; normal kidneys are approximately as long as three to three and one-half lumbar vertebral bodies. When one kidney is shrunken and the other has failed to hypertrophy, disease is usually bilateral. Very large kidneys suggest obstruction or polycystic disease. Renal failure with kidneys of normal size suggests an acute rather than a chronic process. Irregular scarring of the renal outlines and clubbed calyces suggest chronic pyelonephritis or analgesic nephropathy.

Renal biopsy is invaluable in distinguishing among the various causes of the nephrotic syndrome, in making the diagnosis of amyloidosis, periarteritis, or interstitial nephritis, or in assessing the nature, severity, and course of glomerular diseases. Biopsy is clearly indicated in patients with heavy proteinuria in whom treatment with steroids is contemplated, since it enables the physician to distinguish forms of the nephrotic syndrome that are likely or unlikely to respond to treatment. It is most useful in diffuse glomerular diseases of the kidney, rather than in those with focal pathologic change. The hazards of percutaneous biopsy (serious bleeding into the capsule or the urine, intrarenal arteriovenous fistula) are uncommon and can be minimized by expert technique and fluoroscopic control, and by avoiding the procedure in patients with bleeding tendencies, uremia, or severe hypertension. The extent to which percutaneous biopsy of the kidney is employed in diagnosis and management is best governed by the expertise available—not only in performing the biopsy but also in preparing the specimen and interpreting the results. Thin sections (less than 3 μm) are essential to proper interpretation by light microscopy. Immunofluorescent staining and electron microscopy are necessary adjuncts to full exploitation of the diagnostic power of the procedure.

Finally, in addition to being innocuous, the diagnostic maneuver of following the course of the patient's condition has a great deal to recommend it. Acute or self-limited processes, even when the histologic picture is clear, can sometimes be diagnosed only in retrospect.

APPROACH TO THE TREATMENT OF RENAL INSUFFICIENCY The approach to the patient with chronic renal failure is shaped by the relationship between renal function and the signs and symptoms of renal insufficiency. Figure 266-1 illustrates the hyperbolic relation between the plasma level of urea or creatinine and the rate of glomerular filtration. When clearance is low, small fluctuations in glomerular filtration produce large changes in concentration of plasma urea or creatinine. The relationship between functioning renal tissue and the clinical signs of renal failure may be visualized in the same fashion, as in Fig. 266-2. This curve, illustrating the nature of the physiologic reserve of the kidneys, also clarifies certain aspects of the course of many chronic progressive renal diseases characterized by a long "latent" period and rapid terminal progression. One can visualize a slowly progressive process, relentlessly destroying renal substance, which is relatively asymptomatic for many years. When the limits of renal reserve are reached, symptoms appear in swift succession and the condition of the patient deteriorates rapidly, though there may be little actual acceleration of the rate of parenchymal destruction of the kidneys.

Figure 266-2 provides a rationale for the treatment of patients with renal disease. The less kidney tissue there is

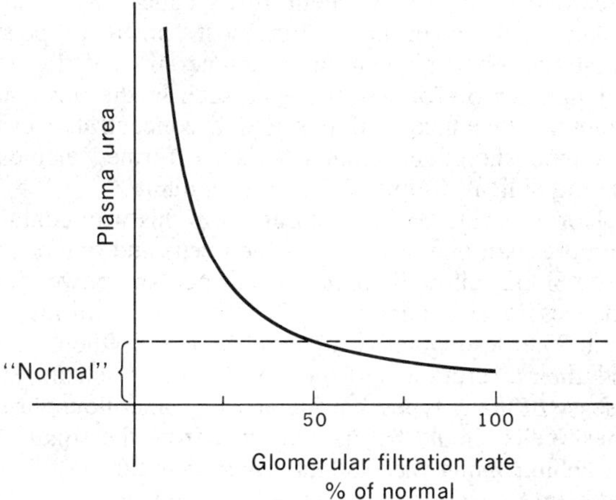

FIGURE 266-1
Relation between plasma level of urea or creatinine and rate of glomerular filtration.

remaining, the more difference an increment in function makes to the patient. The fragility of patients with little remaining renal function is apparent. Prolonged dehydration, the depressant effects of anesthesia, or the septic shock of septicemia may be tolerated easily by a person with normal or slightly impaired renal reserve but may be disastrous to a patient balanced on the knife-edge of renal decompensation. In treating a patient with advanced renal disease, the extent of damage that is reversible is obviously tremendously important. The goal must be the discovery and treatment of reversible disorders, no matter how insignificant they may appear. For a patient on the steeply ascending portion of the curve, a small improvement in function may mean the difference between life and death. Treatable causes of renal failure include obstruction of the urethra or ureters, congestive heart failure, infection, dehydration, salt depletion, potassium deficiency (Chap. 264), and hypercalcemia. Renal failure may seem worse than it is because urea production is increased by bleeding into the intestine, excessive intake of protein, infection, surgery, trauma, diabetes mellitus, or administration of adrenal steroids or tetracycline. Finally, chronic renal disease is sometimes complicated by self-limited disorders of the kidney which will eventually resolve if the patient does not die in the meantime. These include acute glomerulonephritis, acute exacerbations of chronic glomerulonephritis, and acute tubular necrosis. These reversible aggravating factors must be sought and corrected if possible in every patient with renal insufficiency. When doubt as to their presence exists, peritoneal dialysis or hemodialysis will provide time for investigation and treatment of reversible complications.

REACTIONS OF THE KIDNEY TO DRUGS The kidney is a target organ for a variety of allergic and toxic reactions to drugs. *Hypersensitivity angiitis* occurring in the course of a serum sickness reaction (e.g., to penicillin) frequently produces microscopic hematuria and protein in the urine. Renal biopsy may show a mild focal nephritis, but it is uncommon for this to produce renal insufficiency.

The *nephrotic syndrome*, usually without other systemic allergic symptoms, has been reported as a reaction to drug antigens such as tridione, mercurials, probenecid, and penicillamine. Immune complexes visible by electron microscopy are deposited in the glomerular basement membrane. The condition usually remits when the offending drug is discontinued, but improvement may take several weeks or months. Recovery may be speeded by administration of prednisone, but this is not clearly established.

Acute tubulo-interstitial nephritis is a hypersensitive reaction involving the tubules and interstitial tissue rather than the glomeruli. Most reports have implicated sulfonamides, methicillin, or large doses of other penicillin-related antibiotics. The lesions are characterized by irregular interstitial accumulation of leukocytes containing many mononuclear cells, plasma cells, and eosinophils, and by tubular damage. Arteritis is not a feature. The clinical picture is often characterized by fever, eosinophilia, and occasionally a morbilliform rash, all suggesting hypersensitivity. Hematuria and mild to moderate proteinuria are present. Renal insufficiency may develop very rapidly, occasionally with oliguria, so that the picture resembles acute tubular necrosis or acute glomerulonephritis. There is usually slow improvement when the antibiotic is withdrawn; prednisone is said to produce rapid remission.

Tetracycline antibiotics have an antianabolic action and may therefore increase azotemia in patients who accumulate high concentrations of the drug because of renal insufficiency. In addition, certain outdated lots of tetracycline have been shown to damage the proximal tubule, producing Fanconi's syndrome.

Amphotericin B, in toxic dosage, decreases filtration rate and renal blood flow, selectively damages the distal tubule, produces tubular acidosis and potassium wasting, and leaves distal tubular calcification in its wake. Although improvement occurs after cessation of therapy, renal function is usually permanently impaired to some degree.

Streptomycin, gentamicin, vancomycin, kanomycin,

FIGURE 266-2
Relation between functioning renal tissue and clinical signs of renal failure.

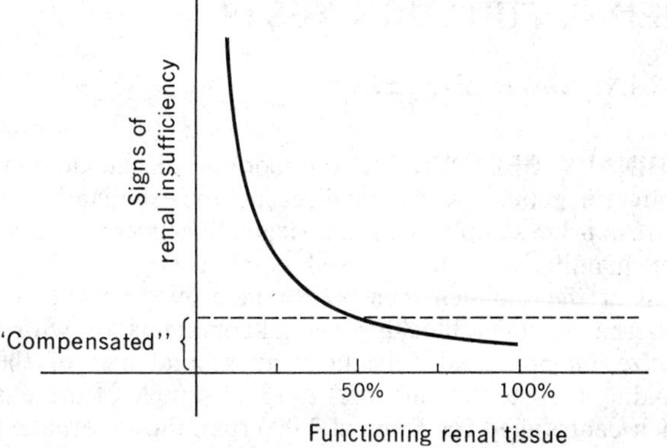

and *neomycin* are toxic to the eighth cranial nerve as well as to the kidneys. Renal toxicity consists of proximal tubular necrosis (heralded by proteinuria and abnormalities in the urinary sediment) and azotemia, which is reversible (though sometimes only after weeks) when the antibiotic is stopped. *Colistin* and *polymixin* are also sometimes toxic to the kidneys in amounts given therapeutically. Renal failure occurring in the wake of a gram-negative septicemia thus poses a diagnostic problem: the cause may be ischemic tubular necrosis secondary to shock, or a toxic nephritis due to drugs employed to treat the infection, or a combination of both.

Analgesic nephropathy Certain patients who habitually consume large amounts of analgesic preparations containing phenacetin develop a chronic interstitial nephritis. The characteristic feature is papillary necrosis, often with superimposed bacterial infection. Calyceal clubbing is frequent, and pyuria is common even when the urine culture is sterile. Renal colic may be caused by ureteral obstruction with a necrotic papilla. Progressive renal failure is associated with inability to concentrate the urine and a tendency to salt wasting. When analgesics are stopped, there is often initial improvement, much of which can be ascribed to the treatment of dehydration and infection. Some patients show further slow improvement, probably related to removal of the noxious agent combined with the natural tendency of the kidney to compensatory growth. In others, however, especially those in whom hypertension and vascular disease have appeared, uremia continues to progress slowly.

REFERENCES

BALDWIN DS et al: Renal failure and interstitial nephritis due to penicillin and methicillin. N Engl J Med 279:1245, 1968

BELL D et al: Analgesic nephropathy: Clinical course after withdrawal of phenacetin. Br Med J 3:378, 1969

BLACK DAK: *Renal Disease*, 3d ed., Philadelphia: Davis, 1972

FRIMPTER GW et al: Reversible Fanconi syndrome caused by degraded tetracycline. JAMA 184:111, 1963

STRAUSS MB, WELT LG: *Diseases of the Kidney*, 2d ed., Boston: Little, Brown, 1971

267
RENAL FUNCTION TESTS

FRANKLIN H. EPSTEIN

URINARY SEDIMENT An important diagnostic maneuver in patients with renal disease is the examination of a fresh urine sample by the physician. Specimens suitable for quantitative culture as well as microscopic examination of the sediment can be obtained by cleansing the external genitalia, blocking vaginal contamination with a gauze tampon, and collecting the second half of the voiding in a sterile container. A 15-ml sample of urine is then centrifuged for 5 min at 3,000 rpm, the supernatant discarded, and the sediment resuspended in the few remaining drops of urine. For most clinical purposes, qualitative or semiquantitative enumeration of the type and number of formed elements seen in the unstained sediment is sufficient. If possible, a concentrated urine specimen should be examined, since formed elements may be difficult to find if the urine is dilute.

Normal urine collected carefully in this way contains no more than one or two red blood cells and one or two white blood cells and epithelial cells per high-power field. An occasional hyaline cast per low-power field may be seen. The desquamation of renal tubular epithelial cells and their excretion into the urine is increased in renal disease of many types, particularly in glomerulonephritis. These cells should be distinguished from the squamous epithelium lining the bladder which may fill the urinary sediment in cystitis. Tubular cells choked with fat, called "oval fat bodies," as well as fatty casts, are characteristically found in the urine of patients with heavy proteinuria.

The composition of casts is particularly significant, since the entrapment of red blood cells or leukocytes in casts establishes their origin in the renal parenchyma. Casts are formed by the agglutination of protein, cells, or cellular debris in the lumen of renal tubules.

Hyaline casts are clear, colorless cylinders barely seen against the usual background. They result from the precipitation in the renal tubules of Tamm-Horsfall protein, a high molecular weight mucoprotein originating in the cells lining the renal tubules distal to the loop of Henle. Its solubility is decreased in the presence of albumin. When the urine contains bile pigment or hemoglobin, the protein making up hyaline casts will be stained this color. They are seen in concentrated acid urines in which much protein is excreted. *Broad casts*, sometimes referred to as *renal failure casts*, are characteristically found in advanced renal disease where there is hypertrophy of some remaining renal tubules together with stasis of urine in lower reaches of the collecting duct system. *Leukocyte casts* and clumps of leukocytes suggest pyelonephritis or sterile interstitial inflammation of the kidneys. White blood cell casts are also found in the exudative stage of acute glomerulonephritis. *Epithelial cells entrapped in casts*, together with red blood cells, and casts containing lipid droplets, should suggest glomerulonephritis without permitting distinction among its various causes. *Granular casts* are said to represent a further stage in the degeneration of cellular casts. *Red blood cell casts* often are orange or rusty brown in color, even when the cell outlines have deteriorated, but when only a few erythrocytes are present they may appear colorless. Their presence in association with hematuria almost invariably signifies a destructive lesion of the glomerulus, such as an active glomerulonephritis, lupus, arteritis, or malignant hypertension. The absence of formed elements does not rule out either chronic glomerulonephritis or pyelonephritis.

When urinary infection is suspected, a Gram stain of the urinary sediment in a freshly voided specimen may permit prompt diagnosis and early initiation of therapy.

PROTEINURIA Some protein is filtered by normal glomeruli, and there is a small amount of protein in normal urine, but protein excretion in excess of 150 mg per day or

20 mg per 100 ml urine is abnormal. Proteinuria may be induced in normal subjects by injections of epinephrine, by exercise, or by renal ischemia resulting from dehydration, surgery, hemorrhage, or salt depletion. Continuous proteinuria implies disease of the kidneys.

The bulk of urinary protein in most renal diseases is albumin, which passes into the urine through damaged glomeruli. If the increase in glomerular permeability is extremely selective, as in lipoid nephrosis, little other protein is present. With more disruptive glomerular disease, as in proliferative or membranous glomerulonephritis, the proportion of other proteins rises. In myeloma, macroglobulinemia, and primary amyloidosis, the excretion of globulin may exceed that of albumin, because of the presence of abnormal nonalbumin proteins in the serum, which are filtered and excreted.

Circulating proteins of low molecular weight pass the glomerular filter but are normally reabsorbed from the proximal tubules and do not appear in the urine. Lysozyme is an example of these. When proximal tubules are damaged, reabsorption is incomplete and "tubular proteinuria" can be detected, in which lysozyme and other nonalbumin proteins are prominent.

Heavy proteinuria, in excess of 4 g daily, signifies a gross increase in glomerular permeability, usually the result of a generalized glomerular disease. Venous congestion of the kidneys and malignant hypertension may also cause proteinuria of this degree. When such large amounts of protein are excreted into the urine, the degree of proteinuria is influenced by both the glomerular filtration rate and the level of serum albumin. For example, when a dose of prednisone is given which increases filtration rate, protein excretion rises.

Renal diseases that may be present without proteinuria include polycystic disease, pyelonephritis, disease of the large or small blood vessels, hypercalcemic or hypokalemic nephropathy, obstruction, stone, congenital malformations, and tumor. Proteinuria is usually absent or scant in renal insufficiency because of dehydration or "prerenal azotemia."

Orthostatic and functional proteinuria In perhaps three-quarters of adolescents and young adults, proteinuria may be induced by prolonged standing in the erect position or by strenuous exercise. The effect is more pronounced when a lordotic posture is assumed. Changes in the renal circulation secondary to peripheral sequestration of blood are probably involved, since proteinuria can be produced in susceptible individuals by applying tourniquets in the supine position, prevented by having the subject stand upright in water, and aggravated by the peripheral vasodilatation induced by heat. In patients with orthostatic proteinuria, urine passed early in the morning, before arising, is free of protein, although of high specific gravity. Care must be taken to have the patient empty his bladder at midnight, without getting up, so that urine formed in the erect position during the previous evening is discarded. Urine produced after the patient has been up may contain as much as 1 to 3 g protein per liter, although usually less than 1 g protein is excreted per day. The excretion of casts and other formed elements may also increase with the appearance of protein. Often a history of easy flushing, fainting, or other evidence of autonomic instability is obtained.

In most young individuals with intermittent orthostatic proteinuria, the condition is entirely benign and unassociated with other evidence of renal disease. The fact that proteinuria is intermittent does not, however, rule out organic disease. A small percentage of apparently healthy patients with intermittent orthostatic proteinuria are found on renal biopsy to have some form of nephritis, and some of them eventually develop signs of chronic renal diseases.

CLINICAL MEASUREMENTS OF GLOMERULAR FILTRATION RATE In a healthy adult, blood flow to both kidneys accounts for approximately one-quarter of the cardiac output, or about 1,250 ml per min. Renal plasma flow is about 600 ml per min, and glomerular filtration rate is 100 to 150 ml per min. The rate of glomerular filtration can be estimated by measuring the plasma clearance of a substance such as inuline or mannitol, which appears in the glomerular filtrate in the same concentration as in plasma but which is neither reabsorbed nor secreted by renal tubules.

The clearance of a substance is given by the equation,

$$\text{Clearance} = \frac{\text{excretion rate}}{\text{plasma concentration}} = \frac{\text{mg/ml urine} \times \text{ml urine/min}}{\text{mg/ml plasma}}$$

The clearances of urea and creatinine or their plasma levels, although determined in part by tubular processes, are related closely enough to glomerular filtration rate to make them convenient clinical indices of glomerular function. Urea is filtered at the glomerulus and variably reabsorbed, presumably as a passive consequence of the concentration gradient established by water reabsorption, so that its clearance is 40 to 70 percent of the true glomerular filtration rate. The back diffusion of urea is diminished when urine flow is increased; hence urea clearance approaches a maximum when daily urine volume exceeds 3 liters, but it decreases out of proportion to glomerular filtration when urinary output is low. Furthermore, for the same rate of urine flow and of inulin clearance, urea clearance is higher during solute diuresis than during water diuresis.

The clearance of endogenous creatinine in general approximates inulin clearance. Creatinine excretion is independent of urine flow, and its level in plasma is relatively stable. Creatinine clearance may therefore be determined over 24 hr by collecting all the urine formed during this time and drawing one sample of blood within this period. Normal values for men are 140 to 200 liters per day (97 to 140 ml per min); for women, 120 to 180 liters per day (85 to 125 ml per min). The quantity of creatinine formed and excreted per day is related to muscle mass and does not change appreciably with changes in diet or protein breakdown. Serum creatinine is therefore more reliable than blood urea as an index to serial changes in glomerular filtration when renal function is compromised. At low serum levels the usual analytic methods for creatinine in serum are less accurate, and a variable portion of the result can be ascribed to noncreatinine chromogens of plasma, unless special precautions are taken by the laboratory.

The creatinine clearance provides a convenient index against which to evaluate the excretion of other substances (e.g., phosphorus) whose excretion is influenced by changes in glomerular filtration. For any substance, that fraction of the amount filtered at the glomerulus which is excreted in the urine (E/F) is given by dividing its urine/plasma concentration ratio by that of creatinine.

$$\frac{\text{Clearance substance}}{\text{Clearance creatinine}} = \frac{U \text{ substance } V}{P \text{ substance}}$$

$$\div \frac{U \text{ creatinine } V}{P \text{ creatinine}} = \frac{(U\,/\,P) \text{ substance}}{(U\,/\,P) \text{ creatinine}}$$

where U = urine concentration
P = plasma concentration
V = urinary volume (ml/min)

MEASUREMENT OF TUBULAR FUNCTION Phenolsulfonphthalein excretion Phenolsulfonphthalein (PSP), like Diodrast, para-aminohippurate, and penicillin, is secreted into the urine by the proximal tubules. Only 4 percent of the PSP reaching the bladder is filtered through the glomeruli. With the usual 6-mg intravenous dose, the plasma level of PSP is no more than one-fifth of that normally needed to saturate tubular capacity to secrete the dye. Its excretory rate is therefore usually limited by renal plasma flow, and with severely impaired kidneys by proximal tubular function. Errors in interpretation of the test may arise from incomplete emptying of the bladder; hence the patient should be loaded with water before the test is begun. Inadequate urine volumes (< 150 ml) in the 15-min sample may be avoided by injecting the dye only after the patient feels the urge to void. Normal values are given in Table 267-1. The 15-min period is the most significant.

Urinary concentration When dehydrated, normal adults can concentrate the urine to 750 to 1,400 mOsm per liter (specific gravity 1.020 to 1.032). Withdrawal of fluids for 12 to 18 hr overnight is often not a satisfactory stimulus to the kidneys to reabsorb water maximally in patients with edema who are diuresing, or in those whose diurnal pattern of urine flow is reversed. In such cases and in other states (e.g., renal insufficiency) where dehydration may be dangerous, concentrating ability may be tested by measuring urinary specific gravity or osmolarity after an injection of 5 units of vasopressin in oil. Slightly lower values are achieved when the kidneys are induced to concentrate by an injection of vasopressin rather than by prolonged dehydration. For practical purposes, if the specific gravity of a casual urine sample or one obtained after a short period of dehydration or an injection of vasopressin reaches 1.022 or more, concentrating ability may be considered intact. The measure of specific gravity may be misleading when heavy solutes, such as glucose, protein, or contrast dyes, are excreted abundantly in the urine. Freezing-point measurements of urinary osmolarity avoid this difficulty.

TABLE 267-1
Excretion of PSP by normal subjects

	Excretion of PSP, percentage	
Time, min	*Minimum*	*Average*
15	28	35
30	13	17
60	9	12
120	3	6
Total for 2 hr	53	70

The production of a concentrated urine depends on the development of a high concentration of sodium and urea in the interstitial fluids of the renal medulla as a consequence of the active transport of sodium out of the thin medullary loops and of the countercurrent pattern of flow through loops of Henle and medullary capillaries. Disease processes which disturb the function or structure of the medulla should therefore be expected to produce early, marked, and disproportionate impairment of concentrating ability. This occurs in patients with acute tubular necrosis, pyelonephritis, papillary necrosis, obstructive uropathy, potassium depletion, hypercalcemic nephropathy, medullary cysts, and sickle-cell disease. Maximum urinary concentration is reduced in normal persons by starvation, by a low-protein diet, and by excessive water drinking and overhydration.

Urinary dilution Normal persons can excrete 70 percent of a load of water equal to 2 percent of the body weight within 5 hr of drinking it, and can reduce urinary solute concentration to 50 mOsm per liter. Water diuresis and urinary dilution are impaired in states characterized by inappropriate liberation of antidiuretic hormone (such as severe infections, cerebral injuries, and lung carcinoma), circulatory disturbances (heart failure, hepatic cirrhosis), and adrenal insufficiency, as well as in renal insufficiency of whatever cause. Tests of urinary dilution are therefore not specific nor especially sensitive in the detection and the follow-up of patients with renal disease.

Other tests of tubular function All the *glucose* normally present in glomerular filtrate is completely reabsorbed by the proximal tubules. The appearance of glucose in the urine when the blood glucose level is below 180 mg per 100 ml may therefore signify proximal tubular damage. In certain patients, renal glycosuria is present as a heritable, isolated tubular defect, without other signs of renal disease; the condition has no serious consequences. *Renal glycosuria* may be present, without implying tubular dysfunction, when the load of glucose presented to the tubules is greatly increased because of an increase in the glomerular filtration rate (GFR), as in *pregnancy*.

A useful test of *urinary acidification* is to give 0.1 g ammonium chloride per kilogram body weight, in a non-enteric-coated capsule by mouth, and to collect hourly urine samples from 2 to 8 hr after giving the drug. Normally the urine pH falls promptly to 5.3 or below. Inability to lower urinary pH to this degree is abnormal and characteristic of renal tubular acidosis. The test should not be done if a random urine pH is found to be 5.3 or less, or if the patient is already acidotic.

Importance of serial tests Early in chronic disease of the kidneys, any of the clinical tests of function may be impaired while others are normal. Serial measurements of any or all functions may therefore be helpful in evaluating progress. When azotemia supervenes, PSP and concentration tests usually change in rough proportion to filtration rate. In severe renal insufficiency, urinary specific gravity becomes fixed near 1.010 and no longer reflects changes in GFR and PSP excretion. The blood urea is influenced by the intake and breakdown of protein, and the urea clearance by water and solute diuresis, as well as by GFR. *Serial measurements of filtration rate by creatinine clearance or serum creatinine level therefore remain the most suitable way of following the course of chronic azotemic renal disease.*

REFERENCES

Lippman RW: *Urine and the Urinary Sediment: A Practical Manual and Atlas,* Springfield, Ill.: Charles C Thomas, 1957

Pitts RF: *Physiology of the Kidney and Body Fluids,* 2d ed., Chicago: Year Book, 1968

268
CHRONIC RENAL FAILURE:
PATHOPHYSIOLOGY, CLINICAL MANIFESTATIONS, AND TREATMENT

FRANKLIN H. EPSTEIN
JOHN P. MERRILL

PATHOPHYSIOLOGY A great deal of the disturbed physiology of renal disease can be understood by considering what happens when kidney tissue is progressively ablated in experimental animals, so that fewer and fewer nephrons must do more and more work. As total glomerular filtration rate (GFR) falls, the blood urea level rises along the hyperbolic curve illustrated in Fig. 266-1. Remaining nephrons become hypertrophied. An increase in the load of solutes traversing each remaining nephron therefore occurs, contributed to by the rise in plasma concentration of urea and also by an increase in filtration rate per glomerulus. Among the consequences of this are an impairment of the concentrating ability of intact nephrons and interference with the ability of the kidneys to excrete a salt-free urine. The initial result is polyuria. Urine flow declines, however, as severe renal insufficiency approaches. When the GFR is reduced to 5 or 10 percent of normal and urinary output is correspondingly limited, the normal dietary intake of salt and water can no longer be excreted. Hypertension, edema, and congestive heart failure then ensue unless intake of salt and water is restricted.

Water Because they are unable to excrete a concentrated urine, patients with renal insufficiency must drink and excrete more water than normal in order to handle the usual load of urinary solutes. Polyuria and polydipsia are therefore among the first signs of advancing impairment of renal function. Reversal of the normal diurnal excretory pattern contributes to nocturia, since water and solute ingested during the day are now excreted at night.

The *decrease* in *renal concentrating ability* which characterizes patients with renal insufficiency has been ascribed to a solute diuresis provoked by the concentration of urea in the glomerular filtrate and the resulting increase in solute load per individual intact nephron. This is not the only explanation in patients with far-advanced disease, for when the load of urea per nephron is reduced in advanced renal failure by hemodialysis, the urinary osmolarity usually fails to rise. Most patients with renal disease are able to excrete a urine as concentrated in solutes as is the glomerular filtrate, but hypotonic urine is often excreted by patients with selective destruction of the renal medulla. Urine persistently hypotonic to plasma and unresponsive to vasopressin (nephrogenic diabetes insipidus) may be encountered in obstructive uropathy, chronic pyelonephritis, medullary cystic disease, amyloidosis, nephrocalcinosis, and familial nephrogenic diabetes insipidus.

Because polyuria is obligatory, dehydration is readily produced by relatively brief abstention from fluids. Thirsting and purgation in preparation for x-ray studies may prove fatal in the patient with renal decompensation who has achieved a delicately balanced status. In such patients it is usually unnecessary and unwise to withhold fluids before blood is drawn for chemical determinations in the morning. Even minor surgical procedures should be undertaken against a background of adequate hydration, by the intravenous route if necessary. Overnight polyuria in many patients results in early-morning thirst and a feeling of hunger on awakening, which quickly turns to nausea and vomiting, thereby perpetuating the vicious circle of dehydration. This can sometimes be prevented by a drink of water taken after urinating at night or a small preliminary feeding immediately on awakening.

Although restriction of fluid intake is seldom indicated, there is no reason to push fluids to the point of discomfort. The efficiency of the kidney in excreting urea and other solutes appears to reach a maximum at a urine volume of about 3,000 ml; even the diseased kidney is not much more effective at higher volumes. Moreover, the ability to excrete large loads of water rapidly is impaired in most patients with azotemia. Excessive administration of water, especially when salt is limited, is therefore likely to result in hyponatremia, with its attendant symptoms of nausea, muscle cramps, and mental disturbances.

Sodium Normal man reduces his urinary output of sodium to negligible levels within 2 or 3 days after taking a salt-free diet. Patients with renal insufficiency are unable to restrict renal losses of sodium this efficiently, and continue to leak variable amounts of sodium into the urine when salt is restricted. At first, losses of water may occur in parallel with sodium so that the serum sodium concentration is normal even though extracellular fluid is contracted. Later hyponatremia develops as water is no longer lost proportionately. The degree of hyponatremia, then, is not a reliable guide to the magnitude of sodium deficit, but must be supplemented by a clinical estimate of extracellular fluid depletion. One mechanism contributing to the salt-wasting tendency in renal disease is the increased solute load excreted by each intact nephron, since osmotic diuresis in normal kidneys results in obligatory salt losses. Specific damage to salt-resorbing portions of the renal tubule is also responsible in many cases. Salt wasting is particularly common in patients with chronic pyelonephritis, interstitial nephritis, polycystic disease, medullary cystic disease and obstruction, rather than in chronic glomerulonephritis, though it should be suspected in renal insufficiency from any cause, when polyuria is prominent. In such cases the triad of asthenia, dehydration, and hyponatremia may suggest the diagnosis of Addison's disease. From 50 to 100 mEq sodium daily is often required to prevent sodium depletion, and as much as 200 mEq sodium may be necessary. The diagnosis of salt wasting may be established by measuring the urinary sodium. In the presence of obvious volume depletion or of hyponatremia, an output of more than 10 mEq sodium per day or per liter of urine is suggestive. In the terminal stages of renal failure salt losing disappears or becomes less marked as glomerular filtration becomes progressively compromised and oliguria supervenes. With marked constriction of blood volume, or in heart failure, a fall in glomerular filtration rate may enable a sodium-free urine to be excreted, even when underlying renal disease is severe.

In addition to urinary losses, vomiting and diarrhea commonly produce sodium depletion in uremic patients. Anorexia may defeat attempts to replace deficits by oral feeding, and since hyponatremia commonly causes nausea, a vicious circle ensues. Where anorexia is a limiting factor, the use of intravenous fluid or peritoneal dialysis may reverse the cycle in a matter of 1 or 2 days, thus enabling the patient to ingest adequate fluid, electrolytes, and calories, and saving days and sometimes weeks of hospital time. Depletion of extracellular volume, with or without hyponatremia, compromises renal failure by reducing renal blood flow and glomerular filtration, even when the degree of volume depletion is not readily detected by physical examination. Although a fall in blood pressure, a dry mouth, and some loss of skin turgor are often present, listlessness, fatigue, nausea, and mental clouding may dominate the picture. As sodium depletion progresses, muscle cramps and generalized muscle twitches or convulsions may appear, and the patient becomes confused, somnolent, and comatose. It is important not to mistake these signs of sodium deficit for an inevitable progression of uremia.

In azotemic patients without edema, hypertension, congestive heart failure, or oliguria, restriction of salt is unwise and unnecessary. The intake of sodium should be encouraged, preferably in the form of salty foods and drinks, rather than by use of pills of sodium chloride, which irritate the stomach. Ingestion of bouillion which contains 2.5 g of NaCl per cube is a palatable and useful way of increasing sodium chloride intake. If acidosis is present, part of the sodium requirement should be taken as sodium bicarbonate or citrate. The slight expansion of extracellular fluid induced by a diet high in sodium is often reflected in improved renal blood flow and glomerular filtration. Excretion of urea, sulfates, and phosphates is augmented, and the secretion of acid and potassium is promoted. Because salt stimulates thirst, the intake of water, in a natural fashion, is encouraged, and urinary flow is improved. The appearance of ankle edema at the end of the day or a decrease in vital capacity which may be measured with a portable apparatus which the patient can be easily trained to use at home gives warning of impending overhydration and possible congestive heart failure.

Because of the beneficial effects of salt on renal function, an attempt should be made to control early congestive heart failure in patients with chronic renal disease with digitalis, rather than by rigid limitation of dietary sodium.

While many patients with renal failure require or tolerate liberal quantities of salt, many others do not. Additional sodium in them merely exaggerates hypertension and the signs of heart failure. This tendency becomes more pronounced as GFR and daily urinary volume progressively decline. The hypertension can usually be controlled by the restriction of salt or its removal by dialysis. Control of hypertension by salt removal is usually accompanied by a decline in kidney function, but this is unimportant if the patient is being dialyzed regularly, or if the additional renal insufficiency can be tolerated without symptoms. If this is not the case, the patient and his physician may have to choose between hypertension with somewhat better renal function, and normotension with uremia.

Potassium Although the kidneys are the main route for excretion of the 50 to 80 mEq potassium in a normal diet, hyperkalemia does not commonly complicate chronic renal insufficiency so long as urinary output is well maintained. The enormous capacity of the distal tubules to secrete potassium into the urine is usually adequate to maintain the level of potassium in the serum close to normal even though glomerular filtration is greatly restricted. An increased secretion of aldosterone, observed in some patients with renal failure, may be one mechanism for increasing potassium secretion in the presence of a decreased filtration rate. The increased flow through intact distal tubules of urine containing high concentrations of the impermeant anions, sulfate and phosphate, also encourages the secretion of potassium by remaining nephrons of diseased kidneys. Tubular secretion of potassium is enhanced by a high-sodium diet and depressed when sodium excretion is reduced. Serum potassium level may therefore rise in patients with chronic azotemia when they are placed on salt-free diets, especially when juices and fruits, high in potassium content, are simultaneously given in large amounts to "force fluids." If the supply of potassium from diet or breakdown of tissue is not excessive and urinary output is adequate, the cause of an elevated serum potassium level is usually found to be acidosis. Hydrogen ions are buffered by intracellular proteins, which release potassium to the extracellular fluid. Restoration of serum bicarbonate to normal usually reduces the serum potassium concentration. Persistent hyperkalemia in the absence of excessive potassium intake, salt restriction, oliguria, or acidosis should raise the suspicion of adrenal insufficiency. Patients with adequate urine volume may maintain some degree of elevated serum potassium concentration (5 to 6 mEq per liter) without hazard, and strenuous efforts to treat this are not warranted.

When oliguria supervenes, and urinary output falls below 500 to 1,000 ml daily in patients with renal decompensation, serum potassium may rise to dangerous levels. Clinical manifestations and management of hyperkalemia are discussed in Chap. 269.

Inability to conserve potassium is not a feature of most primary diseases of the kidney, though hypokalemia with potassium wasting may complicate renal tubular acidosis, nephrocalcinosis, and Fanconi's syndrome, and may sometimes occur during the diuretic phase of recovery from tubular necrosis. Renal potassium losing, with urinary potassium in excess of 15 to 20 mEq per day or per liter in the presence of hypokalemia, is characteristic of primary aldosteronism but may also be seen in malignant hypertension, presumably because of the high level of circulating aldosterone in this condition. When patients with azotemia are depleted of potassium by vomiting or diarrhea, additional renal damage may result; repair of the deficit, with care taken not to cause hyperkalemia, is therefore indicated.

Acidosis About 40 to 60 mEq acid (H^+) is excreted daily by the kidneys of a normal man eating 70 g protein per day. Most of this is produced in the body by the oxidation of sulfur-containing amino acids to sulfuric acid and of phosphorus to phosphoric acid. About half the load of H^+ appears in the urine as NH_4^+; the rest is buffered by phosphate. In most patients with renal insufficiency the capacity to produce NH_4^+ is reduced; hence the excretion of acid is impaired. Interestingly, the ability to reduce urinary pH below 5 often remains, but it requires a greater degree of systemic acidosis. Bicarbonate wasting, or inability to reabsorb all the filtered bicarbonate at normal levels of serum bicarbonate, also contributes to the retention of H^+ in body fluids and the production and maintenance of systemic acidosis.

The excess of acid produced over that excreted is neutralized by body buffers, including bone. Acidosis therefore contributes to osteoporosis and negative calcium balance in renal disease. When renal tubular secretion of H^+ is specifically and disproportionately impaired, and glomerular filtration rate is well maintained, *renal tubular acidosis* results, characterized by a high serum chloride and low serum bicarbonate, without azotemia. There is no rise in "undetermined anions" (mostly sulfate and phosphate) in the serum, as in ordinary uremic acidosis, since these substances can be excreted by glomerular filtration. Since serum sodium is maintained at a normal level, serum chloride level must rise. When distal tubular function is predominantly at fault, urinary pH is consistently above 5.5, even during severe systemic acidosis. In "proximal tubular acidosis," on the other hand, urine pH may drop below 5 when the serum bicarbonate level has been lowered, but bicarbonate is wasted in the urine in huge amounts when the serum bicarbonate level is brought near normal by the administration of alkali. "Distal tubular acidosis" is a familial, inherited disorder associated with calcification of the kidney. It can also be produced by calcium nephropathy and amphotericin toxicity, and is seen in some patients with pyelonephritis. "Proximal tubular acidosis" may be observed in any of the disorders which cause Fanconi's syndrome.

Systemic acidosis is often responsible for nausea, fatigue, malaise, and breathlessness on exertion, long before Kussmaul's respiration is clinically apparent. Acidosis may be avoided by prescribing an amount of alkali equal to the daily production of acid, or 40 to 60 mEq per day. This is contained in 1 to 2 tsp baking soda, or 2 to 4 tbsp 10% sodium citrate in syrup of wild cherry. Taken in divided doses after meals, this usually suffices to maintain the serum bicarbonate level at 18 to 22 mEq per liter, thereby avoiding the unpleasant side effects of acidosis. Excessive administration of alkali must be avoided, especially in the presence of hypocalcemia, when correction of acidosis without the simultaneous administration of calcium may precipitate tetany and convulsions. Large amounts of sodium bicarbonate or lactate are also contraindicated in congestive heart failure.

Calcium, phosphate, and bone (see Chap. 349) Calcium and phosphate ions are normally present in extracellular fluid at concentrations close to the limit of solubility of calcium phosphate salts. When the concentration of phosphate is increased, therefore, calcium phosphate tends to be deposited in soft tissue and bone, and the calcium level in serum tends to fall. Phosphate is excreted by glomerular filtration, and 80 percent or more of filtered phosphate is usually reabsorbed, chiefly in the proximal tubule. As glomerular filtration rate diminishes, phosphate is retained, depressing the serum calcium level slightly and thus stimulating the parathyroids to secrete hormone. The action of parathyroid hormone reduces renal tubular reabsorption of phosphate and tends to restore serum calcium and phosphate levels to normal. In the course of progressive renal disease, therefore, the fraction of filtered phosphate reabsorbed by the tubules decreases, so as to keep phosphate clearance constant and maintain a normal level of inorganic phosphorus in the plasma. When GFR decreases to about 20 ml per min, however, phosphate excretion can no longer be maintained by this method of compensation, since the kidneys cannot secrete phosphate into the urine in excess of the amount filtered. The serum phosphate level then begins to rise. In an attempt to keep the serum calcium level normal the secretion of parathyroid hormone increases further, and its circulating level reaches heights far in excess of those seen in patients with primary parathyroid adenoma. With advanced renal failure the effect of this excess of parathyroid hormone, is, paradoxically, to increase serum phosphorus further, since dissolution of bone induced by hormone adds phosphate as well as calcium to the extracellular fluid. Parathyroid secretion can be diminished, at least in the early stages of renal failure, by limiting the intake of phosphate or retarding its absorption from the intestine with aluminum gels.

Serum calcium level is thus characteristically depressed in renal decompensation. A portion of the decrement is a result of decrease in the protein-bound fraction, since the serum albumin level is often low, but the ultrafiltrable portion of serum calcium is also regularly reduced. The level of ionized calcium is further decreased by the tendency of calcium to form undissociated but soluble complexes with sulfate, phosphate, and citrate ions. Though hyperphosphatemia contributes to hypocalcemia, the serum calcium level may not return to normal when serum phosphorus levels are reduced by oral aluminum hydroxide gel. Other factors must therefore be partly responsible for the low serum calcium level of renal insufficiency. One of these is impaired absorption of calcium from the gastrointestinal tract. Increased fecal excretion of calcium and decreased urinary calcium can in fact be detected quite early in azotemic renal disease. Calcium absorption improves in uremic patients only after very large doses of vitamin D (from 50,000 to 200,000 daily), which commonly produce hypercalcemia in normal patients.

Resistance to vitamin D in uremia has a physiologic basis in the sequence of chemical transformations necessary to transform calciferol into the active form of vitamin. This is normally accomplished by a series of hydroxylation steps that take place in the liver and the kidney. Vitamin D_3 is transformed to 25-hydroxy-cholecalciferol in the liver. This compound is in turn hydroxylated by the kidney to 1-25-hydroxy-cholecalciferol, which is more potent than any of the other calciferol derivatives in stimulating intestinal transport of calcium. With extensive destruction of renal tissue, formation of the active metabolite is presumably impaired (see Chap. 349).

When chronic renal failure associated with secondary parathyroid hypertrophy has been present for a long time, parathyroid adenomas may develop in the overgrown glands. This complication is marked by a rise in serum calcium above normal. Whether or not there is an autonomous adenoma, pronounced secondary hyperparathyroidism may produce extensive osteitis fibrosa, bone pain, and extraskeletal depositon of calcium, especially around the joints, in the skin (suggested by severe itching), in the conjunctivas (producing the "red eyes of renal failure"), and in the walls of blood vessels (producing gangrene). Parathyroidectomy sometimes relieves symptoms dramatically, while lowering both serum calcium and phosphate levels.

When the serum phosphorus level is rapidly lowered by dialysis or transplantation, the serum calcium level may rise above normal because of persistent parathyroid secretion by very large parathyroids. The hypercalcemia can be modified by giving supplements of inorganic phosphate in the diet, but it usually disappears spontaneously over a period of weeks or months, as the hypertrophied glands regress.

Bone disease in renal failure thus has several contributory causes: parathyroid overactivity, disturbance in vitamin D metabolism, fecal losses of calcium, and acidosis. The development of osteodystrophy appears to be conditioned by the rate of skeletal growth and the chronicity of the renal failure. Renal osteodystrophy is consequently more common in children and in patients with congenital anomalies of the kidney and with slowly progressive renal disease such as chronic pyelonephritis with normal blood pressure. Radiographic changes in bone are of three general types: (1) widening of osteoid seams at the growing ends of bones, as in rickets (hence the term "renal rickets"); (2) erosive and cystic changes of osteitis fibrosa, as in hyperparathyroidism, in which the earliest signs are of subperiosteal resorption in the phalanges and long bones; and (3) hyperostosis or osteosclerosis, most marked at the upper and lower margins of the vertebras, producing the radiologic appearance of "rugger jersey spine." The serum alkaline phosphatase level is usually high but may be normal. Growth is retarded. Bones and joints are often tender. Painful, swollen joints, often with deposits of calcium in the bursae, may mimic classical gout. Proximal muscular weakness, producing a waddling gait, may be mistaken for myopathy or neuritis but improves dramatically with administration of vitamin D.

Aseptic necrosis of the hip occurs with distressing frequency in patients with renal failure, particularly when they are kept alive for long periods by dialysis or transplantation. The use of steroids contributes to it, but a number of patients with this lesion have never had steroids.

Azotemic osteodystrophy may be treated with vitamin D, 50,000 to 200,000 units daily. Elevation of the serum calcium level above 10 mg per 100 ml, the development of lassitude, anorexia, and nausea, or a rising blood urea level not attributable to other causes, warn of vitamin D intoxication and should signal the complete withdrawal of medication, since the action of vitamin D persists for about 2 weeks. Calcium carbonate, lactate or citrate, in amounts of 10 to 20 g daily, may be given to supplement dietary calcium. Aluminum hydroxide gel, 30 to 60 ml with each meal, will reduce phosphate absorption, and if given early in the course of renal failure, may prevent secondary parathyroid oversecretion. One of the hazards of treatment is that these medications sometimes interfere with the patient's already poor appetite.

During chronic hemodialysis, signs of secondary hyperparathyroidism slowly regress, though histologic evidence of bone disease usually persists. Successful renal transplantation produces complete recovery of renal osteodystrophy.

Magnesium The serum magnesium level does not usually rise until the GFR falls below 30 ml per min. It may be lowered by starvation or diarrhea and by diuretics. Even in severe renal insufficiency, the serum magnesium level does not generally rise high enough to cause symptoms (4 mEq per liter) unless magnesium salts have been given as laxatives or antacids, or parenterally to control convulsions. Under these circumstances, bladder retention, drowsiness, muscle weakness, and coma may ensue.

Uric acid The blood uric acid level may be slightly increased early in renal insufficiency but does not usually rise above 10 mg per 100 ml, even in severe renal failure, because of increased uricolysis in the gut. Secondary gout is rare, though "calcium gout" caused by calcium phosphate crystals may be mistaken for it. Repeated episodes of classical gout in a patient with uremia suggest a gouty family background or primary uric acid nephropathy.

Urea Urea diffuses readily across most cell membranes

and into all body secretions. The hydrolysis of urea to ammonia in the mouth is responsible for the uremic odor and bad taste of advanced uremia. The formation of ammonia by urease-producing bacteria in the stomach and intestines may contribute to gastrointestinal irritation and "uremic ulcerations." Ammonia formation in the intestines in uremia permits the recycling of some nitrogen through the amination of the carbon skeletons of amino acids that may be manufactured by the body or introduced in the diet.

The contribution of elevated blood levels of urea per se to the symptoms of uremia is not at all clear. Uremic symptoms are correlated in only a rough way with the concentration of urea in blood. Hemodialysis against a bath containing high concentrations of urea has been reported to produce subjective improvement in "uremic" symptoms. Anorexia, nausea, and vomiting are perhaps easier to correlate with blood urea than are other symptoms, and they respond more consistently to artificial manipulation of the urea level by diet or dialysis.

Carbohydrate metabolism Mild carbohydrate intolerance, manifested by a diabetic glucose tolerance curve, is present in more than half of patients with chronic uremia. The fasting blood sugar level is not usually elevated, and the condition does not give rise to any important clinical problems. The defect appears to be due to resistance to insulin, since insulin levels are normal. It disappears several weeks after adequate dialysis.

Other chemical abnormalities Indoles, phenols, certain amino acids, various organic acids, and derivatives of guanidine appear in increased concentration in the blood in renal decompensation, but their contribution to the clinical syndrome of uremia is not firmly established. Guanidinosuccinic acid, which accumulates in the blood in renal failure, has been implicated as a cause of the qualitative defect in platelet function of uremia.

PHARMACOLOGY OF RENAL FAILURE Drugs predominately excreted by the kidneys rapidly accumulate when they are given to patients with renal insufficiency, and their dosage must be modified to avoid toxic side effects. A useful rule is to give the standard initial or loading dose, since this serves to establish the therapeutic level in body fluids. The maintenance dose may be roughly calculated by dividing the usual dose by the serum creatinine concentration in milligrams per 100 ml. Renal clearance of the drug will be reduced in approximately inverse proportion to the elevation of serum creatinine, since this roughly parallels the fall in the GFR. Alternatively, the interval between doses may be lengthened in proportion to the height of the serum creatinine level. Regulation of dosage and determination of the plasma level of drug are particularly important in the case of ototoxic antibiotics.

Antimicrobials chiefly excreted by the kidney include cephalothin, cephaloridine, colistin, polymyxin B, gentamicin, kanamycin, streptomycin, penicillin, vancomycin, nitrofurantoin, and sulfonamides. Tetracycline is partially excreted into the urine. Phenobarbital is excreted entirely by the kidneys. Other barbiturates and most other sedatives are not, though toxic hepatic metabolites of the phenothiazines may accumulate to cause excessive sedation, rigidity, and hypotension in renal failure. Ethacrynic acid, mercurials, and thiazides are cleared by the kidneys; furosemide is not. The dose of azothiaprine must be reduced in renal insufficiency, an important consideration in the treatment of patients after kidney transplantation.

The choice and dose of *cardiac glycosides* are also conditioned by their mode of elimination and the presence and degree of renal failure. Digoxin is normally completely excreted by the kidneys; its advantage of rapid excretion is therefore lost in renal insufficiency, and it becomes a "long-acting" digitalis glycoside. Digitoxin is metabolized chiefly in the liver; the standard dose need therefore be reduced by only one-quarter to one-third even in severe renal failure.

PROXIMAL TUBULAR SYNDROMES Reabsorption of glucose, phosphate, amino acids, urate, and bicarbonate is a normal function of the proximal tubule. When proximal tubular reabsorption is interfered with, therefore, these substances appear in the urine in excessive amounts. This occurs when there is selective damage to the proximal tubules, as in cystinosis (de Toni-Fanconi disease of children), heavy-metal poisoning, hepatolenticular degeneration (in which copper deposition is responsible for tubular injury), galactosemia, and some cases of myeloma (because of injury by abnormal low molecular weight proteins filtered and absorbed by proximal tubules). The generic term, *Fanconi's syndrome*, is used to denote the cluster of chemical derangements, including hypophosphatemia, glycosuria, aminoaciduria, and hypouricemia, and sometimes including acidosis and hypokalemia, that results from dysfunction of the proximal tubules.

Proximal tubular function in intact residual nephrons is altered in uremia even though no anatomic damage is specifically localized to this segment of the tubule. The high levels of parathyroid hormone not only reduce tubular reabsorption of phosphate; reabsorption of other constituents of proximal tubular urine is also retarded. Hence a slight degree of "bicarbonate wasting," and aminoaciduria as well as minimal glycosuria, may accompany severe chronic renal insufficiency from any cause. For the same reason, hypophosphatemia and bicarbonate-wasting hyperchloremic renal tubular acidosis are sometimes seen during the first several weeks after a healthy kidney is transplanted into a chronically uremic patient.

Clinical manifestations The onset of chronic renal failure is insidious. Polyuria and nocturia may be the only signs at first. Later the patient complains of feeling weak and unwell, of easy fatigue, insomnia, and slight breathlessness. Appetite is lost, and there is a bad taste in the mouth. Intractable nausea, especially in the morning, frequently brings the patient to the physician. He looks pale and may be referred to the hematologist because of anemia. When acidosis and azotemia become more severe, the patient takes to bed, becomes increasingly lethargic, and may be troubled by hiccups and uncontrollable twitching of the limbs. If renal failure is untreated, heart failure, progressive anemia, and bleeding into the skin, mucous membranes, and gastrointestinal tract herald the final illness. The skin becomes dry, with a sallow tint, the breath uriniferous. Exophthalmos may be present. Vision is impaired as hemorrhages and exudates appear in the fundi. The urinary output becomes progressively reduced. Fibrinous pericarditis or pleurisy, usually but not always painless, may appear within a few weeks of death. Disorientation and coma mercifully precede the end.

Cardiovascular manifestations Although chronic renal insufficiency per se does not produce congestive heart failure, hypertension and hypertensive heart disease are so often associated with renal disease that heart failure is one of the most common complications of uremia. In addition to hypertension, anemia may aggravate heart failure. Finally, when renal failure is so severe that oliguria is present, continued intake of salt and water will expand the circulatory volume and produce circulatory congestion with pulmonary edema that is not relieved by digitalis.

When *edema* is present in patients with renal disease, heart failure or hypoproteinemia is usually the cause. The edema of acute glomerulonephritis and toxemia of pregnancy are exceptions to this rule. Edema without heart failure or hypoproteinemia may also be seen during oliguria in acute tubular necrosis or terminal renal insufficiency, when the intake of fluid has been excessive.

The contribution of *heart failure* to renal insufficiency can sometimes be assessed only by a therapeutic trial of digitalis. Diuretics are generally ineffective when glomerular filtration rate is greatly restricted, i.e., when the blood urea nitrogen level is over 100 mg per 100 ml. Large intravenous doses of furosemide or ethacrynic acid may cause transient increases in urine flow in patients with this degree of renal impairment, but the toxicity of these two drugs in patients with chronic renal failure should be appreciated.

In many patients with renal insufficiency, *pulmonary edema* tends to be central, producing a "butterfly pattern" on the chest roentgenogram; this condition is sometimes miscalled "uremic pneumonia." Because congestion without alveolar edema is common, rales may be absent. Increasing agitation and restlessness, coupled with accentuation of the second pulmonic heart sound, are often the first warning to the physician of an impending explosion of paroxysmal dyspnea, which may be warded off with digitalis.

Pericarditis, although usually painless, may sometimes produce excruciating pain and bloody effusion. A coarse rub and characteristic electrocardiographic signs are commonly found. In untreated patients it is unusual for uremic pericarditis to be present when the blood urea nitrogen level is below 80 mg per 100 ml; however, this occurs with some frequency in patients who have been on the Giordano-Giovanetti low-protein diet. Although it is not clear what causes uremic pericarditis or uremic pleuritis, signs of pericardial inflammation or pleurisy usually disappear soon after hemodialysis, though they may return later when the blood urea and serum creatinine levels rise. Chronic pericardial effusion may exist for many weeks in patients on dialysis, producing an enlarged cardiac shadow but none of the classical signs of tamponade. Occasionally tamponade develops, sometimes as a result of pericardial bleeding secondary to heparinization in the course of dialysis, and pericardiocentesis must be performed.

Hypertension is almost always present at some stage of chronic renal failure; with worsening renal insufficiency salt retention is a major contributing cause. Plasma renin levels are very high in only a few patients, who have malignant hypertension. Continued secretion of renin in the presence of salt overload may play a part in sustaining hypertension in the remainder. Unfortunately, salt depletion and drug-induced postural hypotension tend to reduce renal function, so that vigorous treatment of high blood pressure may be hazardous when the blood urea nitrogen level is more than 80 mg per 100 ml. Under these circumstances a small reduction in perfusion pressure and blood flow through the kidneys may precipitate renal decompensation, treatable only by dialysis, or by abandoning salt restriction and drugs. Treatment of hypertension becomes a pressing necessity, however, when headache, retinopathy, or hypertensive heart failure produces symptoms. The long-range prospect of further vascular and renal deterioration caused by severe high blood pressure provides an additional rationale for its treatment in patients with renal disease.

Methyldopa, 750 mg to 3 g per day, is a useful drug. It can be combined with propranolol, 10 to 40 mg three times daily, or with hydralazine, 25 to 75 mg three times daily. Small doses of dibenzyline (10 mg three times daily) may occasionally produce striking improvement without deterioration of renal function. Guanethidine, 10 to 25 mg daily, may be required. Diuretics lose their effectiveness as antihypertensive agents with advancing renal decompensation, since they no longer increase the excretion of sodium. Hypertensive headaches may be treated with analgesics and by elevating the head of the bed (see Chap. 245).

Gastrointestinal manifestations The *mouth ulcers* and *parotitis* which complicate advanced uremia are related to bacterial breakdown to ammonia of the urea present in high concentration in saliva, to mouth breathing in acidosis, and to dehydration. Careful attention to cleansing of the mouth and removal of tartar from teeth helps to prevent these complications.

Anorexia, hiccups, nausea, and *vomiting* are common symptoms of uremia. In about half the patients with severe uremia, the vomitus contains no free acid and therefore does not result in alkalosis. Bleeding from small ulcers may occur from anywhere in the gastrointestinal tract. Bloody diarrhea is a distressing complication. Abdominal pain occurs with severe vomiting and diarrhea but may also be due to pericarditis or pancreatitis. The latter diagnosis is sometimes difficult to establish because serum amylase levels are often high in advanced renal insufficiency, even without pancreatitis.

The treatment of nausea should include close attention to proper hydration, correction of acidosis, and treatment of sodium depletion. Anorexia is one of the first signs of a low serum sodium concentration, and nausea often improves dramatically when hyponatremia is corrected.

Sometimes, however, nausea and vomiting persist despite full correction of serum electrolyte levels. In such cases, small doses of phenothiazine or of diphenhydramine HCl several times daily coupled with small frequent feedings may prove helpful. The pattern of meals should be adjusted flexibly to take advantage of the sometimes unpredictable periods of hunger and well-being, and the meals offered should be small. When vomiting is persistent, all feedings should be stopped and fluids should be given intravenously for a few days. Nausea and vomiting usually subside after peritoneal dialysis or hemodialysis. If they persist, the possibility of hiatus hernia should be considered, especially in patients with polycystic kidneys.

Neuromuscular disturbances *Mental clouding, inability to concentrate, drowsiness*, and *lethargy* are the rule in advanced uremia. The EEG is frequently abnormal. Psychotic disturbances may be troublesome. The patient may alternate between periods of torpor and uncontrollable restlessness. Hyponatremia, acidosis, and dehydration may cause coma, which often disappears when these are corrected. Accumulation of sedative drugs normally excreted by the kidney may cause hypotension and unconsciousness, which should not be mistaken for the terminal coma of uremia. Chloral hydrate (1 to 2 g nightly) and diphenhydramine HCl (100 mg) are useful sedatives.

Although *hypocalcemia* in renal failure is frequent, tetany is rare. The reasons for this are not completely clear. Acidosis may protect against tetany by increasing the dissociation of calcium from protein complexes as well as by a direct action on neuromuscular irritability. The high levels of serum magnesium in uremia also counteract the tendency to tetany.

Frank tetany is often brought out by alkali therapy in the presence of hypocalcemia and can be relieved by intravenous administration of calcium salts (1 g Ca^{++} intravenously as the gluconate or chloride). Hypocalcemia or alkalosis may trigger convulsions, however, without the warning signs of tetany. The gross tremors, twitchings, and jactitations of uremia are usually not caused by hypocalcemia and are not improved by the administration of calcium. Occasionally they disappear or improve when hyponatremia is corrected. They are usually relieved by dialysis, suggesting that they have a metabolic, rather than a vascular, origin. A flapping tremor may mimic that seen in liver disease. Rigidity, tremor, and even convulsive episodes sometimes follow overdoses of the phenothiazine drugs in azotemic patients. Grand mal seizures are more common when hypertension is present and are usually thought to have a vascular basis. They are best controlled by sodium phenobarbital or diazepam given intravenously or intramuscularly, and diphenylhydantoin sodium may help to prevent a recurrence. Convulsions may also be caused by hyponatremia, which is most commonly due to water intoxication.

Rapid reduction of the blood urea level by hemodialysis sometimes is associated with drowsiness, headache, and convulsions, attributed to cerebral edema caused by rapid reduction of the osmotic pressure of extracellular fluid (the "disequilibrium syndrome"). An alternative explanation of the propensity to convulsions of uremic patients who are dialyzed is the rapid removal of cerebral depressants that accumulate in the uremic state, presenting an analogy with the withdrawal of alcohol or barbiturates.

Nocturnal muscle cramps may be a sign of dehydration or salt depletion. They often accompany strenuous therapy of hypertension and then suggest vascular insufficiency. They may be the first signal of peripheral neuritis.

Peripheral demyelinating neuropathy, most marked in the legs, appears in patients who have lived many months with severe uremia, or in patients who have been inadequately dialyzed. Nerve conduction time is prolonged. The patient may complain of numbness, tingling, and burning. Once muscular weakness has appeared, wasting and paralysis often progress rapidly. Pyridoxine, thiamine, and other vitamins do not seem to help. Progress of the disease can be prevented by intensive hemodialysis, and slow improvement can sometimes be detected on this regimen. The neuropathy is usually cured by successful kidney transplantation.

Hematologic disturbances *Normocytic, normochromic anemia* is the rule, and though it is usually proportionate to the degree of azotemia, there are many exceptions. The mechanism of anemia in renal failure is complex. Hemolysis and bone marrow depression both contribute. Marrow function is reduced, with a consequent decrease in erythrocyte iron turnover, but the extent to which this is seen depends on erythropoietin levels, iron stores, and the presence of hemolysis. Reticuloendothelial metabolism is also abnormal, so that there is impaired release of iron derived from hemoglobin catabolism and a consequent fall in serum iron with reduction in supply to the marrow. Lack of folate and ascorbate as well as low plasma concentrations of erythropoietin may also contribute to depression of erythropoiesis in uremia. Although the degree of tolerance to anemia varies greatly, weakness, shortness of breath, and poor appetite are likely to be improved by transfusions when the hemoglobin is below 7 g per 100 ml. Strenuous efforts to maintain normal or near-normal hemoglobin levels by transfusion are, however, unwise and unnecessary. Unless serum proteins are depleted, or hemostatic defects are present (in which case whole blood should be given), transfusions should consist of plasma-free packed red blood cells derived from fresh blood. Transfusion should be given cautiously in the presence of congestive heart failure, but treatment of severe anemia should not be neglected because the heart is failing; in such circumstances, transfusions should be of packed red blood cells given slowly in small amounts, with the patient in a sitting position.

Though anemia may produce symptoms, there are important reasons to avoid unnecessary transfusion in patients who are on chronic dialysis or who anticipate eventual kidney transplantation. Repeated transfusions greatly increase the risk of viral hepatitis and may sensitize a prospective donor to leukocyte antigens that might be present in a transplanted kidney. Most patients on chronic dialysis tolerate a hematocrit as low as 15 to 20 percent reasonably well. The anemia can sometimes be partly ameliorated by replacing iron lost as blood in the dialysis apparatus, and by giving androgens.

In a few patients with polycystic disease and uremia, anemia is absent or very mild; this has been ascribed to the overproduction of erythropoietin.

The *bleeding tendency of uremic patients* often makes venipuncture and the therapeutic use of tubes in the nose, esophagus, and bladder distressingly complicated. Ecchymoses, nosebleeds, and oozing from mucous membranes are prominent. Bleeding and clotting times are usually normal, though capillary fragility may be increased. The platelet count is often low. Abnormal prothrombin consumption and thromboplastin generation are sometimes present, suggesting a qualitative defect in platelets. Where the platelet defect is associated with bleeding tendency, ADP-mediated platelet aggregation is characteristically disturbed. Platelet adhesiveness is reduced and is not restored by a low-protein diet. The only treatment is symptomatic, consisting of transfusions of fresh whole blood or platelet-rich plasma. Regular hemodialysis reduces the bleeding tendency and restores platelet function to normal.

Skin Accumulation of carotene-like pigments in renal insufficiency combines with anemia to give the skin a sallow, yellow cast. The high concentration of urea in sweat gives rise to uremic frost when the sweat dries. Itching is an inconstant symptom, not closely correlated with the level of blood urea and aggravated by dryness and superficial irritation of the skin. Severe itching has been ascribed to calcium deposition in the skin, since it is seen in some cases of severe secondary hyperparathyroidism and sometimes responds dramatically to parathyroidectomy. Itching may sometimes be controlled by daily baths, bland lubricating ointments, and the use of diphenhydramine HCl. Topical adrenal cortical steroids occasionally give relief. Meticulous daily cleansing with antibacterial soaps helps to reduce the tendency to superficial skin infections.

Infection Although mildly azotemic patients do not seem to be unusually susceptible to infection, with advanced renal insufficiency septic complications are common. The leukocyte count is not depressed by uremia, but the ability of white blood cells to phagocytize and kill bacteria is impaired. Cellular immunity is also interfered with, as evidenced by impairment of delayed hypersensitivity and improved tolerance of skin and kidney grafts. Poor nutrition, pulmonary congestion and edema, inanition and coma, vascular insufficiency, and the use of indwelling catheters, tubes, and cannulas undoubtedly predispose to sepsis. The necrotizing cystitis and subsequent bacteremia triggered by an indwelling bladder catheter may prove fatal. In a uremic patient, an unexplained fall in blood pressure or any sudden lapse into disorientation or coma should spur a search for infection and bleeding.

TREATMENT OF END-STAGE RENAL DISEASE

Role of dietary protein When oliguria is present at any stage of renal disease, it is clear that the dietary intake of protein should be restricted, if not eliminated. Similarly, there is general agreement that protein intake should be increased in the nephrotic syndrome. Controversy still surrounds the proper prescription of protein in the diet of the large number of patients with chronic renal disease and azotemia who have an undiminished or increased urinary output. Restriction of dietary protein will reduce the blood urea nitrogen and the rate of accumulation of metabolic acids, without, however, improving renal function. Derivatives of testosterone may induce a positive nitrogen balance and a slight fall in blood urea for a few weeks in some patients with renal insufficiency, but this action is self-limited and is not generally useful in the chronic treatment of renal disease.

A low-protein diet is most efficacious in reducing blood urea when the protein eaten is of high biologic value (eggs and milk) and the intake of carbohydrate and calories is sufficient to prevent ketosis and loss of weight. Protein restriction is useless if caloric intake is inadequate, since endogenous protein will be broken down to supply energy. If these conditions are met, and protein is restricted to 18 to 20 g daily, the blood urea may be expected to fall to 50 to 60 percent of the level present at a daily intake of 40 to 60 g protein. Nausea, vomiting, and lethargy often respond temporarily to this form of dietary treatment. It is most useful in the symptomatic treatment of patients with a creatinine clearance between 10 and 3 to 4 ml per min, but it need not be used if symptoms are not present or can be controlled in other ways.

The treatment of advanced renal insufficiency has been transformed by the development of techniques for dialysis and kidney transplantation. Transplantation is discussed in detail in Chap. 66.

Role of dialysis in the treatment of renal failure It is now clear that intermittent dialysis of blood may rehabilitate a majority of uremic patients, although not all of them. With adequate sodium restriction or depletion, hypertension and hypertensive disease may be markedly improved. In most instances peritoneal dialysis and hemodialysis with the artificial kidney are the two techniques used.

Peritoneal dialysis Physiologic fluid (dialysate) is introduced into the peritoneal cavity via an indwelling plastic catheter placed by paracentesis. The dialysate is left in place for 20 min to 1 hr, during which time solute (urea, phosphate, uric acid, etc.) diffuses from the blood across the peritoneal membrane into the dialysate. The dialysate is then removed. This process is repeated for the desired number of times, usually 30 to 40. Disposable equipment and solutions are now available commercially. There are four indications for peritoneal dialysis in the treatment of chronic renal failure: (1) As an adjunct to the conservative regimens described above. Patients critically ill with uremia but whose disease has a reversible element may be dramatically improved by 2 or 3 days of peritoneal dialysis, which enables them to take adequate amounts of fluid and electrolyte and a low-protein diet. (2) As a "holding action." Peritoneal dialysis in conjunction with a diet of 20 g protein and adequate caloric content may be used until the patient can enter a program of chronic dialysis with the artificial kidney (hemodialysis) or receive a renal allograft. (3) Peritoneal dialysis may be used to introduce the severely uremic patient to a program of long-term chronic dialysis. The slower amelioration in abnormalities of body composition which occur with this technique may prevent the "disequilibrium syndrome." This syndrome, characterized by psychoses and convulsions, may occur with the more efficient artificial kidney during the first treatment of a chronically ill patient. Alternatively, the disequilibrium syndrome may be avoided by deliberately making the first hemodialysis less efficient or by treating the patient with hemodialysis before he becomes severely decompensated. (4) Patients who cannot be trained at home for hemodialysis.

Chronic peritoneal dialysis In general, because the use of most permanently indwelling plastic prostheses providing access to the peritoneal cavity has not been successful for more than a few months at a time, long-term peritoneal dialysis has not been popular. In addition, the complications of such therapy are infection, protein loss into the peritoneal cavity, pain, and occasional bleeding. However, although it has not received widespread acceptance, a program of long-term peritoneal dialysis in the home has now been successfully accomplished in at least one series. Dialysis may be carried out by the patient himself or by a family member utilizing sterile solutions prepared in the home and taking advantage of the fact that a permanent means of access to the peritoneal cavity has now been devised which eliminates the necessity for puncture of the peritoneal cavity three times a week. This study reports no difficulty with protein loss, a common complication of long-term dialysis. Infection occasionally occurs around the site of insertion of the cannula but usually can be handled by intraperitoneal use of antimicrobials. Although this technique is cheaper than hemodialysis, most patients prefer the use of the artificial kidney.

Hemodialysis Hemodialysis with the artificial kidney is now a well-established method for treatment of chronic renal failure. The development of permanent inlying plastic arteriovenous "shunts" has made the technique a painless and relatively simple one. Cannulas placed surgically in an artery and a vein of the leg or the arm are connected by a bypass. The bypass may be removed at will so that the cannula in the artery can be connected to the inflow end of an artificial kidney and that in the vein to the outflow end to receive the blood returning from the artificial kidney after it has been dialyzed. A surgically established subcutaneous arteriovenous fistula has been used as another method of establishing portals for the connection to the artificial kidney. This requires percutaneous puncture of the proximal portion of the venous limb of the fistula for the outflow of blood from the patient and the distal portion for the inflow. This technique has the advantage of eliminating the externalized "shunt" with the hazard of infection in the exit sites, but it has the disadvantage of requiring a percutaneous puncture on each occasion.

Two types of apparatus are in general use for hemodialysis, one in which the cellophane tubing is spirally wound between a polypropylene screen (twin-coil artificial kidney), and the other in which sheets of cellophane are compressed between plastic plates (Kiil type). The twin coil is immersed in a tank through which dialysate is pumped, whereas in the Kiil type, dialysate fluid flows in a countercurrent fashion between the cellophane and the plastic plates. Smaller, equally effective types of artificial kidney (the capillary kidney) which do not require priming with blood prior to the onset of dialysis are now under active clinical trial. A number of centers for the treatment of patients with chronic renal failure by hemodialysis have been established throughout this county and in Europe. The centers vary in size from 4 to 30 beds. Usually patients report for treatment two or three times a week and are treated for 4 to 6 hr if the twin coil is used and for 10 to 12 hr if a Kiil type of artificial kidney is employed.

Where *home dialysis* is not possible, self-dialysis in a satellite unit staffed largely by paramedical personnel can be successfully accomplished and is considerably cheaper than hospital dialysis. Such units have been successfully established in trailers, providing unusual mobility for rural areas.

Since the object of chronic hemodialysis is the rehabilitation of patients with debilitating chronic disease, the successful institution of self-dialysis at home has been a major advance in this field. Patients with arm shunts may be treated by spouses or nurses who have been trained in the technique of hemodialysis. Ideally, the shunts are placed in the leg so that with arms free of shunts the patients are able to use their hands to treat themselves. One of the advantages of home dialysis lies in the fact that a patient may arrange his schedule to suit himself; e.g., dialysis may be done in the evening after work.

Although theoretically the ideal form of treatment, many patients are unwilling or unable to undertake home dialysis. Factors involved are motivation, intelligence, and environment. The chances are poor, for example, of mounting a successful home dialysis effort in a tenement apartment in an urban slum area.

The major criterion for the initiation of chronic hemodialysis is the inability of the patient to maintain useful comfortable existence without it. The major criterion for selection of patients is that the disability be due to primary renal failure without any underlying disease. A rare exception is the removal of localized cancer in a single kidney. Physiologic rather than chronologic age is the limiting factor for selection of patients. In general children do not adjust well to the strict routine of dialysis, although there are many exceptions. Patients with severe diabetes usually do not thrive on chronic dialysis, but this fact seems related to the degree of coronary and cerebrovascular disease rather than to glucose intolerance. The patient and/or his assistant must be intelligent, adequately motivated, willing, and able to learn. Psychiatric problems may arise during long-term dialysis, particularly in the home. It is important, however, to remember that psychiatric findings in the patient while he is terminally ill with uremia may be quite different from those in the same person after he has been adequately dialyzed for a period of weeks. Another problem of chronic hemodialysis is its cost, which at present is estimated at $25,000 (range $20,000 to $30,000) per patient per year in hospital centers. "Satellite-center" dialysis costs range from

$10,000 to $20,000 per year. The cost of home dialysis is considerably less, averaging approximately $5,000 per year after the initial investment in equipment.

Management of the patient on chronic dialysis

Where adequate facilities exist, the patient should be begun on hemodialysis early rather than late to prevent some of the irreversible complications of renal failure such as the bone disease and peripheral neuropathy. With adequate dialysis, dietary protein need not be restricted, but in most patients some degree of sodium and water restriction is necessary. Although it is possible to remove sodium and water by ultrafiltration during hemodialysis, large swings in the state of hydration make the patient uncomfortable. Moreover, hypertension, edema, and congestive heart failure may ensue if proper sodium and fluid restriction is not practiced. Since a major cause of death in the chronic-dialysis patient is vascular disease, blood pressure control is of paramount importance. Prior to beginning the dialysis program, the procedure should be carefully explained to the patient and his family in a factual, not a threatening, fashion. He must be indoctrinated in the fact that he will be responsible for at least part of his well-being, but this idea should be presented to him not so that he feels isolated from physician or paramedical personnel but so that he feels part of a team endeavor. This rapport and reassurance must be continued throughout the procedure, even in patients on home dialysis. Recent trends in hemodialysis quite correctly stress self-care and the use of paramedical personnel in satellite units. It must be always emphasized, however, that a physician is available for any emergency. Finally, it is important that each unit retain an individual whose major function is to assist the patient in seeking sources for adequate and continuing financial support.

Complications of chronic dialysis *Peripheral neuropathy* may be prevented and to some extent reversed by adequate dialysis, but once firmly established, it is not often markedly improved. *Anemia* usually is not corrected and may require transfusion of packed red blood cells during the first year. There is increasing evidence, however, that if the patient is not transfused, erythropoiesis may be improved over a period of months or years and that he may be able to maintain an adequate hematocrit without transfusion. Patients who have undergone bilateral nephrectomy become considerably more anemic than those with kidneys, even though these are badly diseased. This is particularly true for patients with polycystic disease. The problem of transfusion is highlighted by the occasional occurrence of hepatitis both in patients and in staff. Patients should be carefully screened for the presence of Australia antigen, and persons found to have this antigen should be handled with particular care. If icteric or anicteric *hepatitis* occurs, the patient must be isolated, no other patient should use his artificial kidney, the staff should observe glove-gown precautions, needles and stools must be carefully handled, and eating must not be allowed in the area. Most of these cases are serum hepatitis, and the prophylactic use of gamma-globulin for staff and other patients is not effective. Extreme care in detecting patients with serum hepatitis early and in isolating them represents the proper course.

Blood transfusion containing even small amounts of platelets and white cells may sensitize the recipient to human transplantation antigens, markedly decreasing the chances for prolonged survival of a renal allograft. The use of frozen plasma-free red cells, though expensive, seems to minimize both these risks. *Pruritus* may occasionally persist even in adequately dialyzed patients; occasionally such pruritus may respond dramatically to parathyroidectomy. Pericarditis, with or without hemorrhagic effusion, may occur even in patients on adequate dialysis. Although this complication may be treated with conservative measures, pericardiotomy is required in occasional cases.

Osteoporosis and *metastatic calcification* are complications that are becoming less frequent as more careful attention is given to calcium intake and to levels of calcium in the dialyzing fluid. It has been shown that *parathyroid activity* may be supernormal even in adequately dialyzed patients. To some extent parathormone levels can be reduced by elevating the level of magnesium in the bath fluid. Since metastatic calcification depends upon an elevated (calcium X phosphate) product, the use of aluminum hydroxide gels to reduce serum phosphate concentrations may be helpful. An alarming increase in the incidence of one form of bone disease, aseptic necrosis of the hip, has been reported from several centers in patients who have been on chronic dialysis for 2 years or more.

Infection and clotting of external shunts represent a continuing problem. These can be minimized by careful asepsis and care, particularly by the patient himself. The "declotting" of a shunt may be undertaken with streptokinase. Care should be taken in attempting to dislodge the clot that retrograde arterial emboli are not produced. It has been demonstrated that as little as 4 ml saline solution injected in a retrograde fashion into the arterial limb of a shunt may produce cerebral emboli. Experience and skill in the insertion of the needle so that the vascular intima is not damaged are important in preventing clotting in the arteriovenous fistula. Although such fistulas have been shown to increase the cardiac output by 400 to 600 ml per min, this does not usually represent a major hazard.

The *contamination of tap water* used in making up the dialysate by copper, fluoride, or excess amounts of magnesium or calcium has been reported to impair the beneficial results of dialysis.

Hypertension occurs frequently in individuals whose salt and water intake is excessive. In general, this condition can be controlled in most patients by a combination of restricting intake and removing sodium and water by ultrafiltration. Although hypertension is largely related to sodium excess, uremic patients appear to have a resetting of the pressoreceptors which regulate the level of blood pressure, and are peculiarly sensitive to both volume excess and volume depletion. Even modest sodium depletion by hemodialysis may cause extreme orthostatic hypotension for 24 hr after the procedure. Occasionally hypertension does not respond to drastic sodium depletion. Under such circumstances bilateral nephrectomy may be necessary for the control of blood pressure. Such patients may be identified by extremely high peripheral venous renin concentrations.

Prognosis in chronic dialysis In most centers, from 4 to 15 percent of patients per year are lost to the program, exclusive of those who receive kidney allografts. With adequate dialysis in centers, satellite units, or at home, restoration to full productive activity may be expected in 50 to 75 percent of the patients treated for more than 1 year. The causes of death in dialysis patients are usually infection or vascular disease. Psychologically, the necessity to "tie my life to a machine," as well as the financial problems entailed, is a constant source of anxiety in some 20 percent of patients. The use of hemodialysis in conjunction with a vigorous transplantation program is the optimum treatment for end-stage renal failure, and offers patients on hemodialysis a chance at release from their bonds, while the patient with an allografted kidney may have his fears of graft rejection somewhat assuaged by the fact that he can always resume hemodialysis. It must be remembered, however, that even the well-dialyzed patient is not normal, and careful studies can detect continuing evidence of peripheral neuropathy, inability to perform certain psychologic tests normally, and evidence of chronic malnutrition, such as consistently low serum levels of essential amino acids. Some 10 to 15 percent of patients "fail to thrive" even on adequate dialysis. This may be due to a combination of "residual uremia" plus age and vascular disease. Recently it has been suggested that the removal of so-called middle molecules, i.e., those with molecular weights greater than 5,000, may be important in the treatment of uremia by dialysis. With this in mind, dialyses using membranes with greater permeability, larger surface area, and slower blood flows have been utilized.

REFERENCES

HAMPERS CL, SCHUPAK E: *Long-term Hemodialysis: The Management of the Patient with Chronic Renal Failure*, New York: Grune & Stratton, 1967

MERRILL JP, HAMPERS CL: *Uremia: Progress in Pathophysiology and Treatment*, New York: Grune & Stratton, 1971

269 ACUTE RENAL FAILURE

FRANKLIN H. EPSTEIN

The term *acute renal failure* has been used loosely to include all forms of acute urinary suppression, generally secondary to acute parenchymal damage. *Acute tubular necrosis* (or lower nephron nephrosis) indicates the clinical and pathologic syndrome which results when renal excretory function is temporarily lost because of renal tubular degeneration caused by renal ischemia or toxic agents.

PATHOLOGY Microdissection studies of kidneys with acute tubular necrosis reveal two types of lesions. When renal toxins (bichloride of mercury, carbon tetrachloride, diethylene glycol) have been administered, there is diffuse necrosis of the proximal tubular cells, while the basement membrane of the proximal tubules, from which a new lining may regenerate, is spared. The lesion caused by ischemia, on the other hand, occurs at random among nephrons and in any part of a nephron. It consists of complete destruction of limited stretches of tubular lining scattered along the course of an otherwise well-preserved nephron. The basement membrane is frequently disrupted. During recovery from both types of lesions mitotic cells may be seen. Except when extremely severe and prolonged ischemia has produced renal cortical necrosis, the glomeruli are intact. Casts packed with degenerating epithelial cells and hemoglobin are seen in the straight tubules of the medulla. The most important inference to be drawn from the nature of the pathologic process is that should the patient survive his other injuries, the renal lesions will be repaired.

ETIOLOGY AND PATHOGENESIS *Acute tubular necrosis* typically occurs in a setting of sudden injury or illness usually associated with shock or with intense renal vasoconstriction. Even those cases which follow the administration of known tubular poisons are generally aggravated by vascular collapse and renal ischemia. Nevertheless, perhaps because of difficulty in recognizing and quantifying the ischemic state, the cause goes undiagnosed in as many as 25 percent of patients. Common causes include hemolysis and hypotension following extensive burns, rapid hemorrhage or hypotension on the operating table, bacteremic shock, crushing injuries in which the toxic effects on the kidney of myoglobin are added to those of vasoconstriction and shock, and intravascular hemolysis from transfusion of mismatched blood or rapid infusions of distilled water (e.g., during transurethral prostatectomy). Following operations on the heart, aorta, or great vessels, during which renal circulation is interrupted, some degree of acute tubular necrosis is almost invariable. Pregnancy appears in some way to predispose to ischemic renal insults; in a large proportion of most published series, acute renal failure followed placenta previa, septic abortion, post-partum hemorrhage, or eclampsia. Other conditions which have triggered tubular necrosis include sudden defervescence following salicylate administration and status epilepticus. Acute renal failure is the most important cause of death in epidemic hemorrhagic fever.

Tubular necrosis resulting from many poisons is enhanced by prior dehydration and tends to be prevented by infusions of saline solution or mannitol if these are given before the noxious agent is presented to the kidneys. Paradoxically, healthy renal tubules are more susceptible to certain types of injury than are poorly functioning ones. A dose of uranium nitrate that induces acute tubular necrosis in a healthy dog may not interrupt the urine flow when given again to the same animal during the diuretic phase of early recovery from renal insufficiency. The role of free pigments derived from blood and muscle in the pathogenesis of tubular necrosis is not clear. Infusions of purified hemoglobin decrease renal blood flow and may be toxic to tubular cells. In addition, intravascular hemolysis may liberate other vasoconstrictor substances which promote renal ischemia.

PATHOPHYSIOLOGY OF ANURIA The formation of casts which occlude the renal tubular lumens may play some part in the pathogenesis of oliguria. In most patients, however, casts appear to be a result of diminished urinary flow, rather than its cause. An exception is the renal failure which follows dehydration in *multiple myeloma* and which is characterized by extensive gel formation by abnormal proteins in renal tubules.

Following the acute renal ischemia which usually initiates tubular necrosis, renal blood flow is decreased to approximately one-third to one-half normal during the first days of oliguria. The reduction in blood flow is more marked in the outer cortex than in the inner cortex and medulla. There is some evidence that the reduction in glomerular filtration is a vasoconstrictive response mediated through the macula densa and the juxtaglomerular apparatus. Increased interstitial pressure secondary to edema probably reduces renal blood flow and filtration rate and collapses tubules. The presence of interstitial edema may be inferred from the increase in the weight of the kidneys during acute tubular necrosis. Experimental measurements of wedged renal vein pressure and of pressures at the end of a fine needle inserted directly into the kidneys have not shown elevation. The pressures may nevertheless be sufficient to collapse renal tubules which are distended with less than normal pressure derived from glomerular filtration and urine flow. In any case, much of the fluid which is filtered at the glomerulus must leak back into the substance of the kidney through the widely scattered disruptions in the denuded tubular basement membranes. As tubular repair proceeds and these leaks are mended, urinary flow improves.

CLINICAL FEATURES In the majority of cases, acute tubular necrosis is characterized by a period of oliguria and increasing clinical and chemical evidence of renal failure, lasting from a few days to as long as 3 weeks, and averaging about 10 to 14 days. This is succeeded by a period of relatively rapid return of urine flow and improvement in renal function, while water and metabolites accumulated during the oliguric phase are excreted.

During the first few days of *oliguria*, the clinical picture is dominated by the underlying illness. The urine is scanty and usually bloody. Although the specific gravity may be high owing to the presence of red blood cells and protein, its freezing point is close to that of plasma, and the sodium concentration is usually over 50 mEq per liter. Traces of glucose may appear in the urine. Complete anuria for more than 24 hr is infrequently encountered, though it is common to see less than 30 to 40 ml urine for several days. If the condition is not recognized early, edema and/or hyponatremia may develop as a result of the unrestricted intake of fluids. If this pitfall is avoided and shock is successfully treated, the only symptoms during the first week may be lethargy and nausea. The latter is related partially to the development of metabolic acidosis. Fever is uncommon after the first day or two. Leukocytosis, on the other hand, is the rule with or without infection. It should be emphasized that severe systemic symptoms during the first several days are usually a result *not* of renal failure but of associated conditions.

Serum amylase and lipase concentrations may be elevated as a result of renal failure per se, without implying active pancreatitis. The blood urea nitrogen level rises at a rate influenced by the degree of tissue necrosis and endogenous protein catabolism. In a chronically ill patient who has had a mismatched transfusion, a daily rise of 20 mg per 100 ml might be expected; increments of 50 mg per 100 ml per day in blood urea nitrogen are not uncommon in previously healthy persons who have undergone severe crushing injuries of overwhelming infections. Disproportionate elevations in serum phosphate or serum creatine levels have been proposed as diagnostic aids in the detection of devitalized tissue.

During the second week of oliguria, nausea, weakness, and somnolence become more prominent as azotemia mounts, acidosis increases, and the serum potassium level becomes elevated. Thirst is commonly present and may be severe, although the serum sodium level is frequently depressed, extracellular fluid volume is expanded, and there are no clear signs of shock or heart failure.

Cardiovascular complications arise in most patients during the oliguric phase of acute renal failure. Although overhydration is the most important cause of pulmonary edema, signs of pulmonary congestion and cardiac failure may appear even in patients who have not gained weight, probably because water has been added to the extracellular fluid from the dissolution of tissue. Pulmonary edema may develop in the absence of hypertension and without peripheral edema. Diastolic hypertension becomes evident in about 25 percent of patients during the second week of oliguria. The fundi, however, remain normal. In exceptional instances in which the tension is very high, arteriolar necrosis develops. Arrhythmias are frequent and are not necessarily associated with potassium intoxication or removal. Pericarditis may develop but does not have the grave prognosis attached to its appearance in chronic renal disease. It may be extremely painful and simulate intraabdominal disease. Occasional patients die of acute cardiorespiratory failure characterized by apprehension, tachypnea, inconstant respiratory wheezing, progressive cyanosis, and hypotension. At postmortem examination no evidence is found of pulmonary emboli, and the lungs show mild to moderate terminal congestion.

Potassium intoxication may arise because of the liberation of large amounts of potassium from injured or infected muscle, intravascular hemolysis, or hematomas. It rarely occurs in the course of renal failure following a postoperative hemorrhage or transfusion reaction in which the rate of tissue catabolism is not increased and in which proper attention has been paid to hydration and caloric needs from the inception of the disease. The rate of rise of the serum potassium level reflects the catabolic response of the patient to injury. In addition, anoxia, acidosis, and dehydration are important determinants of the rate of loss of potassium from cells. The dangers are cardiac arrhythmias and standstill. Serious electrocardiographic abnormalities rarely occur when the serum potassium level is below 7 mEq per liter but are almost always present about 9 mEq per liter. As serum potassium concentration rises, the T waves become high and peaked. The P wave disappears, the QRS complex becomes broad and slurred, bradycardia and arrhythmias ensue, and the ventricular complexes finally resemble those of ventricular tachycardia. These changes may be modified by digitalis and by correction of acidosis and hyponatremia. Susceptibility of the heart to vagal standstill is enhanced, and sudden death may occur, even in the absence of characteristic electrocardiographic changes of potassium intoxication. The electrocardiogram, though a necessary adjunct, is not a satisfactory replacement for the flame photometer in evaluating such situations.

Infection is the most frequent complication of acute tubular necrosis and the most common cause of death. Sepsis may often be overlooked because of confusion with uremic symptoms. Pulmonary and bloodstream infections with "hospital" organisms, particularly the staphylococcus, are frequent in exhausted, semicomatose patients. Common predisposing factors are loss of ability to cough or change position, drying of the pharyngeal mucosa from constant mouth breathing, and the aspiration of inspissated mucous plugs or vomitus. Healing of surgical wounds seems to be impaired, and infection or dehiscence of incisions is common. Infection of the urinary tract, sometimes silent but often with fever, flank pain, and gram-negative septicemia, may result from the use of inlying catheters or repeated instrumentation of the bladder.

Neurologic manifestations are common, the two most important being coma and convulsions. Hyponatremia may be responsible for somnolence or seizures early in the course of acute renal failure and may be corrected by hypertonic saline solution, with proper regard for the complications of overhydration and heart failure. Hypocalcemia may also predispose to convulsions, as may too-vigorous administration of alkali without accompanying calcium in the treatment of acidosis. Seizures may be focal in nature or generalized; some presumably have a vascular basis. They sometimes appear to be triggered by vomiting, heart failure, or the rapid changes in body volume and composition which may accompany the onset of profuse diuresis.

Anemia usually appears in the second week, even without bleeding, presumably as a result of a mild increase in erythrocyte destruction and a deficiency in red cell production. Defects in hemostasis are commonly encountered and include thrombocytopenia, abnormal prothrombin consumption time, and other less well-defined coagulation deficiencies.

In some patients tubular necrosis is not associated with oliguria, or the period of diminished urine flow is so short as to pass unrecognized. The urine volume in such cases is, however, not flexible or responsive to body needs and may be fixed at perhaps 800 to 1,200 ml per day. The diagnosis is appreciated only when the blood urea nitrogen level is seen to rise at the rate of 15 to 20 mg per 100 ml per day and when the patient becomes edematous owing to retention of fluids in excess of the excretory capacity of the kidneys. The urine, unlike that in most other edema-forming states, contains sodium in a concentration higher than 20 to 30 mEq per liter, and the concentration of total solutes does not differ significantly from that of plasma.

After the first few days of oliguria the urine loses its grossly bloody character and becomes clear, increasing slightly in amount every day. The onset of tubular recovery is usually heralded by an increase in daily urinary output to 400 ml. At this point the urine usually contains very little protein, although the sediment may still contain red blood cells and many large dark hematin casts. Further increases in flow are sometimes dramatic, the urine volume increasing by 50 to 100 percent each day until polyuria exceeds 3,000 ml daily. In other patients daily urine volume only gradually approaches a liter over the course of a week or two. If brisk diuresis is not achieved, the blood urea concentration falls only slowly or not at all, and the urine contains more than 3 to 4 g protein per liter, cortical necrosis must be suspected. The blood urea *usually continues to rise* for several days after urinary output exceeds 1 liter per day, until the excretion of urea exceeds its production. In addition, during the early diuretic phase of recovery, hyperkalemia, congestive heart failure, and convulsions may complicate the clinical picture. Pyelonephritis sometimes makes its appearance at this time, and death from infection, when it occurs, is commonly during diuresis. The onset of the diuretic phase, therefore, should not cause the physician to relax his vigilance.

Diuresis is usually associated with a striking weight loss, representing loss of fluid accumulated during the period of oliguria. The urinary concentration of sodium usually varies from 50 to 75 mEq per liter. Some of the excreted sodium is derived from edema fluid, but if the remainder is not replaced, hyponatremia and dehydration may ensue. Elevated levels of serum sodium and chloride are observed during the diuretic phase when water replacement is inadequate and the patient is allowed to dehydrate himself through the obligatory excretion of a large volume of urine containing sodium at a lower concentration than plasma. Occasionally, urinary losses of potassium so greatly exceed intake that the serum potassium level falls below normal. Once established, diuresis proceeds smoothly unless interrupted by urinary obstruction or shock, and azotemia regresses over the course of 1 to 3 weeks. *If diuresis is interrupted by a second period of oliguria and rising blood urea concentration, obstruction to bladder or ureters must be seriously considered.*

After the patient has been discharged from the hospital, anemia sometimes persists for weeks or months, gradually disappearing without benefit of hematinics. Muscle weakness and joint stiffness slowly improve. Although azotemia generally disappears and renal function may be restored, renal blood flow and glomerular filtration rate usually do not return completely to normal. Hypertension is not a sequel in those who recover from acute tubular necrosis, though it may complicate the unusual case of cortical necrosis in a patient who survives anuria.

DIFFERENTIAL DIAGNOSIS The physician is frequently faced with an oliguric patient who has just passed through an episode which might have produced tubular necrosis, but in whom this diagnosis is not yet established. Vigorous treatment of shock, congestive heart failure, dehydration, or hyponatremia frequently resolves the question by promoting diuresis. Urinary osmolarity is not appreciably higher than that of plasma after the first few hours of acute tubular necrosis, whereas it may be elevated in simple dehydration and other prerenal causes of oliguria. The sodium concentration of the urine in acute tubular necrosis is usually over 30 mEq per liter; in oliguria secondary to acute glomerulonephritis or renal arterial occlusion it is usually much less than this. Low urinary sodium concentrations may, however, be observed in tubular necrosis associated with terminal hepatic or cardiac failure, and in the presence of shock. Failure of the blood urea level to rise in a stepwise fashion makes the diagnosis of tubular necrosis unlikely, even though oliguria is present. If doubt persists, a liter of 10 percent mannitol may be infused rapidly to determine the effect on urine flow.

Lower urinary tract *obstruction* must always be kept in mind. A plain roentgenogram of the abdomen should be obtained in all patients with acute renal failure to delineate the size of the kidneys and detect radiopaque stones. If the possibility of ureteral obstruction exists, gentle investigation of the patency of one ureter is indicated.

Complete anuria for more than 48 hr should suggest obstruction, bilateral renal arterial emboli or thrombosis, cortical necrosis, or acute glomerulonephritis. Atheromatous emboli to the small renal arteries sometimes produce irreversible anuria following attempts at aortic resection. Carcinomatous obstruction to the ureters and idiopathic retroperitoneal periureteral fibrosis are frequently associated with intermittent oliguria, alternating with periods of polyuria and diuresis. Occasionally, acute papillary necrosis is attended by oliguria. Uric acid crystals may obstruct both ureters temporarily in patients with leukemia or lymphoma who have received antineoplastic therapy. Similar obstruction may be caused by certain sulfonamides given to dehydrated individuals. The prolonged anuria which occasionally follows bilateral retrograde pyelography is probably a result of obstruction to the lower ureteral orifices by inflammatory edema.

Oliguria attending the terminal stage of chronic kidney disease can usually be distinguished by the history, presence of hypertension, abnormal fundi, and smallness of the kidneys. During the terminal stages of hepatic failure, especially in cases complicated by dehydration, hemorrhage, or low blood pressure, a syndrome of oliguria and progressive azotemia appears which is associated with the lesions of tubular necrosis at postmortem examination but differs in some respects from the course of acute tubular necrosis outlined above. The oliguria is not severe, urine flow usually exceeding 150 ml per day. Urinary osmolarity may in some instances be distinctly elevated above that of plasma, and urinary sodium concentration is low. Vigorous transfusion and the use of vasopressor agents improve urinary flow only inconstantly and transiently. Although progression of the syndrome may in rare instances be halted, a typical diuretic phase does not ensue.

TREATMENT Perhaps more than in any other renal disease, the course of acute renal failure is determined by the therapy the patient receives. Treatment during the initial stages of the disease must be directed toward reversing circulatory failure, which may have initiated the ischemic episode. Although overhydration predisposes to later pulmonary edema if renal failure is established, too timid replacement of blood or saline solution in shocked or dehydrated patients may perpetuate oliguria and permit tubular necrosis to develop. If vasoconstrictor agents are substituted for blood in hypovolemic shock, further renal damage with ischemic coagulative necrosis of cortical tubules may result.

Once circulatory efficiency has been restored, only current losses should be replaced. The patient should receive enough water and salt to provide for obvious extrarenal (e.g., gastrointestinal) and urinary losses and, in addition, enough water to compensate for insensible perspiration and water in expired air. Under average conditions of environmental and body temperatures, normal hydration in an adult patient can be maintained by the daily administration of about 600 ml water in addition to other measured losses (since some water is provided from oxidized foodstuffs and tissue breakdown). Accurate daily weights provide a reliable index of fluid balance; ideally the patient should lose $^1/_4$ to $^1/_2$ lb daily as a result of consuming his own fat calories.

At least 100 to 150 g carbohydrate should be given daily, to minimize protein breakdown and prevent ketosis. Its effect in this direction is enhanced if it is administered throughout the day rather than over a short period of time. There is no evidence that high-calorie mixtures containing more carbohydrate and much fat are appreciably more efficacious in reducing protein catabolism *when the intake of protein is interdicted*, as it must be in acute renal failure. When nausea is not present, 50 g lactose, 25 g sucrose, and 25 g glucose may be dissolved in the daily water requirement, flavored with a little lemon and served cold, to be sipped throughout the day. Ordinary food, especially juices, should not be given, since potassium intake is undesirable. *Oral feedings should not be attempted in the presence of nausea or vomiting.* Sodium lactate, accompanied by calcium, may be given in amounts of 40 to 80 mEq per day to avoid further acidosis, when the plasma CO_2 has fallen to 16 mEq per liter. Larger amounts may be indicated, especially when overhydration is not apparent and congestive heart failure is not present.

Potassium intoxication is prevented in many cases by proper attention to requirements for water and glucose, as well as by the prophylactic oral administration of a teaspoon of potassium-exchange sulfonic resin, sodium polystyrene sulfonate (Kayexalate, Winthrop), three times daily. Larger amounts of the latter may be used if necessary. One tablespoon four times daily by mouth or enema usually serves to reduce an elevated serum potassium level by 1 or 2 mEq every 24 to 48 hr. If hyperkalemia is associated with acidosis, it is frequently brought under control by infusions of sodium bicarbonate or sodium lactate. Infusions of hypertonic glucose solution with insulin have a similar but more transient effect. The deleterious action of potassium on the heart may be counteracted to some extent by infusions of calcium or by the administration of digitalis. If hyperkalemia cannot be controlled by these measures, artificial dialysis is indicated.

Heart failure should be treated with digitalis in the usual doses (Chap. 235). Artificial dialysis, with the removal of several kilograms of edema fluid by ultrafiltration, may be dramatically effective in relieving pulmonary edema. Testosterone propionate or norethandrolone, 25 to 50 mg daily, may be given during the first 2 weeks in an attempt to reduce nitrogen breakdown. Its action is frequently overwhelmed by the intense catabolic reaction to acute injury.

Scrupulous care should be taken to avoid *infection*. After the diagnosis is established, an accurate estimate of the daily output may be obtained by catheterizing the patient, using sterile precautions, only once in 24 to 48 hr, thus dispensing with an inlying bladder catheter. As the urinary volume reaches a significant level, most patients will be able to void spontaneously. In alert patients, deep breathing and forced coughing should be stressed to avoid atelectasis. Tracheotomy should be considered early if there is difficulty in handling bronchial secretions. Careful mouth care, with prevention of crusting and ulceration, is important in avoiding parotitis and aspiration of infected material. Prophylactic administration of antibiotics should be avoided.

The prime indication for *artificial dialysis* in acute renal failure is uncontrollable hyperkalemia. (It should be remembered that suddenly lowering the serum potassium level by dialysis may induce dangerous arrhythmias in digitalized patients.) Acidosis cannot be successfully treated by measures short of dialysis without giving sodium; mounting acidosis in the presence of congestive heart failure is therefore another clear indication for dialysis. Dialysis is especially helpful in temporarily inducing a return of appetite and clearheadedness in azotemic patients. Repeated dialyses may make management during oliguria simpler by permitting patients to continue to eat and drink and by preventing clinical deterioration due to uremia. Peritoneal dialysis has the advantage that if necessary large amounts of fluid can be easily removed from the body by the use of concentrated glucose in the irrigating solution. Artificial dialysis may also be used to remove exogenous toxins such as barbiturates, bromide, and salicylates. Indeed, a portion of the clinical improvement following dialysis in some patients with uremia may be related to removal of sedatives. Although the majority of patients in civilian practice can recover without dialysis if proper care is instituted from the onset of anuria, extensive wounds, severe infection, or prolonged oliguria are likely to necessitate its use.

During the *early diuretic phase*, every effort should be made to avoid salt depletion and dehydration and to sustain diuresis by replacing the previous day's urinary losses. Daily weights and determinations of serum and urinary electrolytes serve as guides; a useful approximation for replacement is to give one-quarter of the urine volume as 0.9% saline solution, one-quarter as $^1/_6$ M sodium lactate, and one-half as 5% glucose in water, in addition to replacing other losses. Equivalent quantities of sodium and water may be provided by mouth if oral feedings are tolerated. As azotemia recedes, tubular ability to reabsorb salt and water improves, and the daily provision of large volumes of fluids becomes unnecessary. In a patient who is alert, spontaneous intake of food and water may usually be trusted to prevent depletion after the blood urea nitrogen level has fallen below 80 mg per 100 ml. At this time protein may be allowed in the diet and will generally be well utilized in repleting tissue stores.

PREVENTION The development of toxic or ischemic tubular necrosis in experimental and clinical situations is conditioned by the state of hydration and the concentration of the urine. Renal vasoconstriction is potentiated in dehydrated animals. Hemorrhagic shock is enhanced by dehydration and modified by prior infusions of saline solution. It would seem wise to give enough saline and glucose solution before and during surgical operations to compensate for antecedent losses as well as those anticipated during the operative procedure. Since dehydration contributes to the production of shock, it is likely that these simple measures will reduce the necessity for transfusions and therefore the likelihood of transfusion reactions.

Mannitol diuresis, initiated before operation, appears to reduce the incidence of acute renal failure in the course of aortic and open-heart surgery. The effect is partly related to expansion of extracellular fluid volume, but in part also to an additional protective action of osmotic diuresis, the mechanism of which is not understood. After acute tubular necrosis has been established, there is no evidence that mannitol or other diuretics can reverse the process, though they may cause a slight transient increase in urine flow.

PROGNOSIS Even though in most cases the damage to tubular epithelium is theoretically reparable, acute tubular necrosis carries a serious prognosis. The mortality rate in many large series is about 50 percent, in spite of the most careful attention to details of fluid and electrolyte balance and with the aid of the artificial kidney. The outcome depends to a large extent on the background of associated illness leading up to the acute episode and the course of infections or cardiorespiratory failure acquired during its course. A number of patients regain normal function only to die of their underlying disease.

When renal ischemia is extremely intense or prolonged, *acute cortical necrosis*, with destruction of glomeruli, may occur. Such lesions are not reversible, and most patients die without emerging from anuria. Most instances of acute cortical necrosis have followed complications of pregnancy, particularly premature separation of the placenta, eclampsia, and septic abortion, although the disease is also encountered following severe shock in nonpregnant patients with preexisting vascular disease. Anuria for several days is common, followed by prolonged oliguria. The protein content of the urine is elevated. In the few patients who survive, renal calcification and contraction of the kidneys may be observed and death may occur within 12 to 18 months from malignant hypertension.

REFERENCES

FRANKLIN SS, MERRILL JP: Acute renal failure. N Engl J Med 262:711, 1960

HALL JW et al: Immediate and long-term prognosis in acute renal failure. Ann Intern Med 73:515, 1970

VERTEL RM, KNOCHEL JP: Nonoliguric acute renal failure. JAMA 200:118, 1967

270 GLOMERULONEPHRITIS

FRANKLIN H. EPSTEIN

Glomerular disease accounts for about half of all patients with severe renal disease treated in the hospital and for two-thirds of patients requiring transplantation. Glomerular inflammation, exudation, cellular proliferation, and membrane thickening and scarring occur in the course of many diseases. The terms acute glomerulonephritis and chronic glomerulonephritis should therefore be regarded as general descriptions of a pattern of reaction of the kidneys, rather than as individual diseases with a single specific cause or course.

In the past several years rapid advances have been made in elucidating the natural history and clinical course of different forms of nephritis by renal biopsy. Several entities with distinctive clinical features and responses to therapy are now distinguishable, and their immunopathogenesis is discussed in Chap. 69.

ACUTE GLOMERULONEPHRITIS

Acute glomerulonephritis is an acute diffuse inflammation of the glomeruli of the kidneys. It represents about 0.5 percent of all admissions to general hospitals in the United States and is found at autopsy in 0.1 to 0.2 percent of deaths. The disease is twice as frequent in males as in females. Although it is more common in children than in adults, it is found in adults of every age.

ETIOLOGY *Preceding infection with the group A, beta-hemolytic streptococcus is the most common cause.* The infection usually arises in the upper part of the respiratory tract, and its severity is not necessarily related to the incidence or severity of the ensuing nephritis. Streptococcal infection of the skin or of wounds may also be followed by glomerulonephritis. There is considerable evidence that only certain strains of group A streptococci are nephritogenic; these include types 12, 4, 25, and Red Lake.

The latent period between streptococcal infection and the first symptoms of nephritis, which may be as long as 1 to 4 weeks but averages 10 to 14 days, represents the time necessary for the development of circulating antibodies to the streptococcal antigens. The fall in serum complement level characteristic of an attack of acute nephritis is a result of combination with antigen-antibody complexes in the kidney. All components of complement are lowered. The concentration of β_{1C}-globulin (the third component of complement) is usually depressed for about 6 weeks. The anti-streptolysin-O titer is elevated in 80 percent of patients with streptococcal nephritis within the first few weeks. However, a raised antibody titer in renal disease is not a rigid demonstration of streptococcal etiology, since streptococcal infections are not rare and may have occurred without relationship to the bout of nephritis.

Acute nephritis has been reported as a complication of an epidemic of acute pharyngitis, presumably of viral origin, in which streptococcal infection was excluded by bacteriologic and immunologic evidence. Bacterial endocarditis is frequently complicated by acute glomerulonephritis. Glomerulonephritis has occasionally been reported to follow other infections, such as malaria, typhoid fever, and secondary syphilis, as well as many virus infections, including mumps, measles, hepatitis, mononucleosis, chickenpox, echo virus, and adenovirus.

Acute nephritis superficially resembling the poststreptococcal variety may occur in the course of lupus erythematosus, periarteritis, or erythema nodosum. It is commonly seen as a complication of the allergic purpuras, associated with joint or abdominal pain. Finally, it may be a manifestation of hypersensitivity to drugs or other foreign agents.

PATHOLOGY The kidneys are normal in size or swollen. The surfaces are smooth and spotted with fine punctate hemorrhages; the pyramids are markedly congested. All or almost all glomeruli are generally involved; yet the degree of inflammation may vary from one to another and be focal in distribution inside the glomerular tuft. In poststreptococcal nephritis, the glomeruli are usually swollen and hypercellular, with thickened glomerular loops, infiltrating polymorphonuclear leukocytes, and proliferation of endothelial and epithelial cells. Occasionally, however, especially when function is completely recovered but while the urine sediment is still abnormal, renal biopsy will reveal glomeruli which appear normal except for occasional focal thickening of basement membranes. Red blood cells and red blood cell casts are present in the tubular lumens. Tubular cells may appear flattened or vacuolated, but pathologic changes in tubules are minimal compared with those in the glomeruli. Afferent arterioles sometimes show focal medial necrosis with perivascular cellular infiltrates, and there may be similar lesions of the interlobular vessels.

As the disease process subsides, there may be complete resolution of the inflammatory process, with restoration of normal architecture. More frequently, hyalinized glomeruli, glomerular adhesions, and vascular changes persist, with wedge-shaped areas of atrophy and fibrosis separated by areas of relatively well-preserved tissue in which the remaining tubules are dilated. Even after the urine has completely cleared, focal hypercellularity and thickening of the stalks of glomerular lobules may persist. Widespread proliferation of the capsular epithelium, producing glomerular "crescents," is a characteristic finding when the condition deteriorates rapidly; the patient dies with hypertension and oliguria within 1 to 12 months of the onset of the disease.

CLINICAL FEATURES AND PATHOLOGIC PHYSIOLOGY The typical patient with streptococcal nephritis develops a pharyngitis with fever and malaise. Microscopic hematuria may be found during the first few days of the respiratory illness when fever is present, but it then disappears. One or two weeks after the onset of the infection, when the initial symptoms have completely subsided, weakness and anorexia return. The patient awakens with puffiness of the eyes and notices shortness of breath or swelling of the ankles during the day. The urine is scanty and looks like Coca-Cola or diluted coffee. Abdominal pain, nausea, and vomiting may be prominent. High blood pressure, usually asymptomatic, may be heralded by headache or an unexpected convulsion. The clinical picture is often dominated by one or more manifestations which overshadow the rest and which initially mislead the physician who anticipates a "classical" pattern.

Fatigue and *anorexia* are almost universal; it is unusual for a patient with acute glomerulonephritis to feel as well as before the illness or to have a good appetite.

Pain in the loins or abdomen may be colicky or steady and, in exceptional instances, may be so severe as to simulate a surgical condition. Fever generally does not exceed 101°F and usually subsides within a few days. Persistent fever may be caused by residual streptococcal or other infection, by a reaction to antibiotics, or by vasculitis.

Although facial *edema* is extremely common, edema of the legs without any swelling of the face is frequent, especially in older persons. Edema may be generally distributed and hence unapparent; and the only clue to its presence may be a 5- or 8-lb weight loss after the patient is put to bed and given a low-salt diet. Localization of edema about the eyes is best explained by the low tissue turgor in this region. The absence of orthopnea, at least during the early stages of the disease, further favors accumulation of fluid in the upper half of the body during the hours of sleep.

Whether salt and water retention in acute nephritis is primarily due to renal disease per se or is secondary to other circulatory disturbances which provoke even normal kidneys to retain sodium is not entirely clear. Considerable evidence suggests that disproportionate reduction in glomerular filtration rate is responsible for the initial oliguria and subsequent retention of sodium which result in excessive accumulation of extracellular fluid. Edema formation is generally associated with some decrease in the inulin clearance and with diuresis which produces a fall in blood urea nitrogen level. Nevertheless, diuresis may be initiated in acute nephritis without any measurable improvement in a depressed filtration rate; the relationship between impaired inulin clearance and sodium retention is therefore not simple or clear-cut. Generalized capillary damage is probably *not* a cause of edema in nephritis, since the edema fluid does not contain increased amounts of protein. Although hypoalbuminemia resulting from extensive losses of plasma protein into the urine may contribute to edema in some cases, this factor cannot be the most important one in the many instances where plasma volume, by direct measurement, is increased or normal. Urinary excretion of aldosterone is low in acute glomerulonephritis in the presence of edema, even when the patient is on a salt-free diet. As might be expected in such a situation, spironolactone does not provoke diuresis. Renal retention of sodium under these circumstances is probably a result of altered renal hemodynamics, rather than of excessive secretion of salt-retaining hormone by the adrenal cortex.

Together with edema, signs and symptoms of *congestive heart failure* are often prominent, whether or not arterial hypertension is present. The sudden onset of heart failure in a previously well person may be the manifestation which brings the patient with acute nephritis to the doctor. Fatal pulmonary edema may be precipitated by convulsions. The heart is usually somewhat enlarged, and the venous pressure may be elevated. Nonspecific alterations in the electrocardiogram are common. Unlike the pattern of "low-output" cardiac failure, the circulation time is typically normal or short, and cardiac output is normal even when edema is present or increasing. Under such circumstances cardiac output does not rise further when digitalis is administered. It seems probable that, in most cases, circulatory congestion is a result of fluid retention rather than its cause. However, heart failure responsive to digitalis (and associated with a prolonged circulation time) may at times complicate acute nephritis. When orthopnea is present, especially if accompanied by rales or gallop rhythm, digitalis should be prescribed. In other instances of edema and elevated venous pressure, a careful therapeutic trial of digitalis should be undertaken, with the knowledge that in many instances it will be found ineffective.

Hypertension is observed in approximately 50 percent of adults with nephritis admitted to a general hospital. The incidence is lower in mild cases detected in the course of a streptococcal epidemic. The onset is usually coincident with the first abnormal urinary findings, although in certain cases it may even precede and in others follow them.

The reason for the high blood pressure is not established. It is probably contributed to both by pressor substances (renin) liberated by the kidney, and by overfilling of the circulation due to retention of salt and water.

The optic fundi are generally normal but may show arteriolar narrowing, a glossy sheen, and, in exceptional circumstances, papilledema, hemorrhages, and fluffy exudates.

When the blood pressure rises rapidly, headache, somnolence, and convulsions may develop (hypertensive encephalopathy), simulating the clinical picture of brain tumor. The differential diagnosis in such instances is not made easier by the fact that proteinuria and microscopic hematuria are often detected immediately following generalized seizures of any origin. Vomiting, dehydration, and heart failure appear to predispose to convulsions. They are not dependent on nitrogen retention but are probably the result of cerebral ischemia or tiny hemorrhages secondary to changes in the cerebral vasculature.

Mild anemia occurs frequently in acute glomerulonephritis, especially with edema. Total red blood cell mass has been found to be normal in many such patients, in whom the low hematocrit reflects dilution. In addition, depression of the bone marrow and increased destruction of red blood cells contribute to anemia in certain azotemic patients. Serum albumin level may be low as a result of urinary losses and of the excessive catabolism of protein observed in many acute diseases or injuries. Serum cholesterol level is sometimes elevated even when serum albumin is not greatly decreased. The presence of anemia and hypercholesterolemia, then, does not necessarily mean that nephritis is chronic or progressive.

Changes in renal function which occur in acute nephritis are characteristic. Glomerular filtration rate is usually depressed, and to a greater degree than renal blood flow. The latter may, indeed, be elevated, though in severe cases it falls as well. Filtration fraction is therefore reduced. Blood urea nitrogen level is elevated in perhaps half the patients with glomerulonephritis. Acid urine of high specific gravity may be excreted early in the course of the illness, despite pronounced azotemia. *The combination of azotemia with well-maintained phenolsulfonphthalein excretion and high urinary specific gravity is seen in few diseases of the kidney other than acute glomerulonephritis.*

The *urine* may be grossly bloody or coffee-colored; on the other hand hematuria may be apparent only on careful inspection of the spun sediment. The identification of red blood cells embedded in casts establishes the glomerular origin of the bleeding. Granular and epithelial cell casts, especially the latter, are characteristically present. Lipid droplets and fatty casts are usually not seen at the very onset of the disease, but may appear within the first few weeks, regardless of the presence or absence of hyperlipemia in the serum. Leukocytes and white blood cell casts reflect the essentially inflammatory character of the glomerular lesion. Proteinuria may reach impressive levels, over 6 to 8 g daily, but is more often below 2 g per day. Especially during recovery, protein may disappear from the urine while red blood cells and red blood cell casts continue to be excreted.

The disease is sometimes ushered in by a period of *oliguria* which may progress to complete anuria. Usually this lasts only a few days, but an occasional case has been reported of acute glomerulonephritis with anuria lasting more than 20 days, followed by complete recovery. The oliguria which occurs at the onset of acute nephritis has a much better prognosis than that which may supervene when the disease has been active for several weeks. In contrast to the condition in patients with acute tubular necrosis and oliguria, urinary sodium concentration is very low (less than 15 mEq per liter) and urinary osmolarity is usually above that of plasma.

Extrarenal vasculitis may be an important concomitant of nephritis. Its myocardial and cerebral manifestations have already been mentioned. Purpuric rashes, subungual hemorrhages, and even acute arthritis may rarely be seen in the course of severe poststreptococcal nephritis. At postmortem examination, necrotizing and organizing lesions of periarteritis may be found in the kidneys and elsewhere.

Pulmonary infiltration and hemoptysis occur most frequently in acute nephritis as a result of circulatory congestion and do not necessarily imply a bad prognosis. In most patients with nephritis, hemoptysis is associated with foamy sputum and is the result of left ventricular failure with pulmonary hypertension and edema. Lung involvement together with nephritis should, however, call to mind the possibility of Wegener's granulomatosis or Goodpasture's syndrome.

Finally, patients may develop acute nephritis with no symptoms and no abnormal physical or laboratory findings other than mild proteinuria and an abnormal urinary sediment. Several cases have been documented in which the renal biopsy showed typical changes of acute glomerulonephritis although the urine was normal.

DIFFERENTIAL DIAGNOSIS Periorbital edema, occurring as an initial symptom of urticaria, trichinosis, infectious mononucleosis, or insect bites about the face may suggest acute nephritis until the urine is examined. The finding of red blood cell casts and the coincidence of an elevated blood urea nitrogen level with normal phenolsulfonphthalein excretion serve to exclude many other diseases of the urinary tract, in which glomeruli are not primarily affected. The nephritis associated with lupus erythematosus, polyarteritis nodosa, and subacute bacterial endocarditis will often be recognized as a complication of the primary disease, but sometimes may be its only manifestation. The characteristic elevation and subsequent fall of antistreptolysin titer is excellent evidence of preceding streptococcal infection, but it may not be present, especially when the infection has been treated with penicillin. Gross hematuria with lower urinary symptoms is much more likely to be due to hemorrhagic cystitis or prostatitis. In middle-aged or elderly men, azotemia and hematuria may be mistakenly ascribed to the prostate until the daily excretion of protein is found to be greater than 2 g, suggesting the correct diagnosis of glomerulonephritis. The presence of small kidneys or of severe anemia (less than 8 g hemoglobin) suggests chronic renal disease, as does prolonged hypertension in heart or fundi. In the elderly, acute nephritis is often misdiagnosed as heart failure, until disproportionate oliguria and the abnormal urinary sediment call attention to the kidneys.

Idiopathic malignant hypertension accompanied by hematuria and azotemia may present diagnostic difficulties, though such patients often have a previous history of high blood pressure and the degree of hypertension is greater than in the usual case of nephritis. Spontaneous improvement in blood pressure and renal function is unlikely in malignant hypertension and favors a diagnosis of glomerulonephritis. *The appearance of acute nephritis immediately following a respiratory infection, without a latent period, suggests an acute exacerbation of chronic nephritis.* Persistent fever, cardiac murmurs, or a palpable spleen should spur a search for subacute bacterial endocarditis.

COURSE AND PROGNOSIS The course and outlook

of acute glomerulonephritis vary widely. In children or young adults who develop nephritis following streptococcal infection, the entire disease may be over within 2 to 4 weeks. Most children recover completely, although a small number (less than 10 percent) go rapidly downhill and die within the first few months. On the other hand, in the adult population of a general hospital the likelihood of chronicity is much greater. It has been estimated that 50 percent of adult patients hospitalized with acute glomerulonephritis either succumb to the acute episode or develop chronic disease. The latter may be quiescent for long periods and manifested only by proteinuria and an abnormal urinary sediment. The ultimate outcome bears a rough relation to the initial severity of the illness, though there are many exceptions to this rule. The most frequent duration of the disease in hospitalized adults is probably about 2 to 3 months. Blood pressure usually returns to normal before the urine clears. Heavy proteinuria lasting longer than 3 to 4 months suggests a poor prognosis, though nephritis may heal completely even after proteinuria has been present for as long as 2 years. Microscopic hematuria commonly persists for some months after proteinuria has disappeared or diminished to a faint trace. Postural dizziness, easy flushing, and other signs of autonomic instability, as well as postural proteinuria, are not infrequent during convalescence. After the urine has become completely normal on several examinations, a second attack of nephritis is unlikely, probably because of the persistence of type-specific antibodies to the hemolytic streptococcus.

TREATMENT *Penicillin* should be given to eradicate residual streptococcal infection even when this is not proved but only suspected. It has been suggested that early treatment of streptococcal infections with penicillin may prevent nephritis, but in the only study performed to test this hypothesis the number of patients observed was too small to permit statistically valid conclusions to be drawn.

During the acute stages *bed rest* is indicated, at least until the systemic manifestations of the disease have disappeared. There is no critical evidence to establish that further rest in bed appreciably modifies the course, although most studies concerned with this problem have been carried out in children with mild nephritis in whom complete recovery is the rule. If proteinuria or microscopic hematuria is the only remaining sign after 6 weeks to 2 months of rest in bed, the patient may be allowed up.

In the presence of edema or signs of *heart failure* intake of salt should be restricted. Treatment for congestive heart failure is discussed above. During the initial stages of the disease, when urinary output is restricted, it may be wise to limit the intake of protein as outlined in Chap. 269. There is no reason, however, to restrict intake of protein during convalescence.

Hypertensive crises may be treated with 0.5 to 2.5 mg reserpine intramuscularly two to four times a day, by alpha-methyldopa, or by an infusion of magnesium sulfate (Chap. 245), by parenteral hydralazine, guanethidine, or ganglionic blocking agents.

Adrenal steroids have no clear-cut beneficial effect in acute nephritis. When massive doses of steroids or azathioprine have been used in occasional instances of rapidly progressive glomerulonephritis with oliguria, they have failed to modify the course.

CHRONIC GLOMERULONEPHRITIS

Chronic glomerulonephritis is not a single entity but a melange of different diseases which predominantly affect the glomerular tufts, causing inflammatory changes and subsequent scarring.

Though it affects all ages it is more frequent before forty. It is more common in men than in women. Only a few patients give a clear-cut history of acute nephritis following infection, and although some cases of chronic nephritis probably originate in an inapparent infection with streptococcus, following which edema or bloody urine was not noticed, it seems likely that most instances represent some disease other than poststreptococcal glomerulonephritis.

CLINICAL COURSE Since "chronic glomerulonephritis" is a collection of diseases, its clinical pattern varies widely. Many patients progress into the terminal stage without ever having experienced edema. An occasional patient develops clear-cut acute glomerulonephritis following respiratory infection, succeeded by a "nephrotic stage," which yields over a period of years to slowly progressive renal insufficiency and mounting hypertension, but it is not usual to observe this full sequence of events in one individual. More characteristic patterns are considered below.

Explosive course The entire illness lasts only a few months, usually less than a year. Sometimes it originates in acute nephritis following an infection. In other instances evidence for an infectious origin is absent and the beginning of the disease can be dated only by the last normal examination. In any case, fatigue, anemia, and breathlessness quickly appear, hypertension is prominent even though the heart may initially not be enlarged, and the urine contains large quantities of protein and red blood cells and may be grossly bloody. Oliguria and rapidly advancing uremia, complicated by pulmonary edema, characterize the terminal weeks. The kidneys are usually normal in size, and the glomeruli are swollen, with intense proliferation of the capsular epithelium, resulting in widespread crescent formation.

Slowly progressive course *Abnormal urinary findings* may be detected in a completely asymptomatic patient in the course of a routine physical examination. *Renal biopsy* shows a patchy glomerulitis, with focal thickening of glomerular loops, occasional capsular adhesions, and some completely hyalinized glomeruli. Other glomeruli may appear completely normal. Alterations in arterioles of the kidney can sometimes be detected even though blood pressure is normal.

Hypertension is often absent. The fundi are normal.

Results of the usual tests of renal function may be completely within normal limits, and serial studies over many years show no or very slow progression of functional impairment. The character of the *urinary sediment* is a poor guide to prognosis; moderate proteinuria, red blood cells, and red blood cell casts may be present intermittently or continuously for years, with a normal or only slightly elevated serum creatinine level. The pathologic process is continuously active at a low level, though counterbalanced by forces of repair and renal hypertrophy. Some patients live normal lives for decades without any change, and some are cured; others eventually develop severely impaired renal function and hypertension.

Nephrotic syndrome Glomerulonephritis in some patients begins insidiously with nightly swelling of the ankles and early-morning puffiness of the eyes. Proteinuria is in excess of 5 g daily, and the serum albumin level is low. Hypertension may or may not be present initially but eventually makes its appearance. In many cases, edema remits as the glomerular filtering area is progressively restricted and the excretion of protein falls; in others, hypoalbuminemia and edema persist to the end (see Chap. 271).

Hypertension Many patients with chronic glomerulonephritis seek medical attention because of complaints associated with hypertension. Sometimes high blood pressure will be found to have developed without significant impairment of renal function. Such cases may be indistinguishable in their clinical manifestations and course from benign essential hypertension, except that proteinuria, dating in occasional instances from a clear-cut attack of acute nephritis, has antedated the hypertension. In some instances "malignant hypertension," with papilledema and extremely high diastolic blood pressure, may develop and dominate the picture. In patients in whom azotemia has not become pronounced, judicious use of hypotensive agents may produce a remission in the pattern of malignant hypertension without seriously damaging renal function.

By the time azotemia has appeared, hypertension is present in most patients with glomerulonephritis, and as the disease approaches its terminus, blood pressure is elevated in all. When progression is very slow, both azotemia and mild hypertension may be borne without symptoms for years.

Exacerbations of chronic nephritis Respiratory infections, especially with the streptococcus, sometimes cause an increase in proteinuria, hematuria, and hypertension as well as a decrease in renal function in patients with chronic nephritis. These exacerbations may be distinguished from attacks of acute nephritis, which they resemble, by the short latent period between the onset of the infection and the exacerbation. There is little evidence that the tendency to progression seen in most patients with chronic glomerulonephritis is related to infection. In some patients, reversible exacerbations of vascular disease characterized by rising blood pressure, hematuria, and retinitis occur without evidence of preceding infection and subside spontaneously.

PROGNOSIS It is almost impossible, except in the most advanced cases, to offer an accurate prognosis from a single set of clinical observations and tests of renal function. Serial observations of the level of blood urea nitrogen or serum creatinine, phenolsulfonphthalein excretion, the degree of proteinuria and anemia, and the blood pressure level afford an estimate of the velocity and character of the process. Anemia eventually develops in most patients by the time renal insufficiency makes its appearance. In patients in whom renal failure has developed only slowly, fatigue associated with anemia may be the presenting symptom. Severe anemia, recurrent after transfusions, implies a poor prognosis. *Probably because of the intensity of the associated vascular disease, the prognosis is much worse in glomerulonephritis with renal insufficiency than in pyelonephritis with azotemia of comparable severity.*

Regardless of the character of the glomerular involvement in the early stages of the disease, it is usually difficult to discern its nature at postmortem examination, since the kidneys are shrunken and fibrotic. Many glomeruli are completely hyalinized; in others there is only partial eccentric fibrosis, with varying degrees of adhesion of capillary loops to one another and to Bowman's capsule. The few glomeruli which are not injured are enlarged, as if stimulated to compensatory hypertrophy.

DIFFERENTIAL DIAGNOSIS In patients with renal insufficiency, the possibility of other diseases of the kidney must be kept in mind. A history of acute nephritis with edema is helpful if present, but a detailed account of the illness should be obtained because what the patient refers to as nephritis may have been a urinary infection. Multiple myeloma and amyloid disease mimic chronic nephritis in the middle-aged and elderly. Hypercalcemia may produce polyuria, azotemia, and anemia, all of which are potentially reversible.

Heavy proteinuria (over 2 to 3 g daily) is present in most patients with chronic glomerulonephritis (and the various other disorders which cause the nephrotic syndrome) but in few other renal diseases unless heart failure or malignant hypertension is present. Epithelial cell casts, red blood cell casts, and lipid droplets in the urinary sediment are useful in distinguishing the disease from pyelonephritis or primary nephrosclerosis. The kidneys are of equal size, usually without evidence of distortion of the calyxes on pyelography, and if small, are contracted symmetrically. The possibilities of lupus erythematosus, periarteritis, and bacterial endocarditis should be kept in mind. Elderly patients with endocarditis, without fever or audible murmurs, may come to the physician with what appears to be nephritis and may die of progressive renal insufficiency without a correct diagnosis having been made.

TREATMENT Restriction of activity is indicated in patients with heart failure, acute exacerbations of nephritis with hematuria, or intercurrent infections. Patients who feel well enough should be permitted to be up and about and should be encouraged to lead normal lives. Diet should not be restricted except for the clear indications mentioned in Chap. 269. Strenuous exertion leading to fatigue is probably best avoided. Pregnancy may be safely undertaken by patients in whom hypertension has not appeared and whose blood urea nitrogen level is normal. In others the risk of preeclampsia or exacerbation of nephritis is greatly increased. Moving to a warm climate has been recommended to patients with nephritis; there is no evidence that it influences the natural history of the disease. Prophylactic administration of penicillin has not been shown to alter the course of the disease. Treatment of the nephrotic syndrome is dealt with in Chap. 271, and management of renal insufficiency, in Chap. 269.

RAPIDLY PROGRESSIVE ("SUBACUTE," "CRESCENTIC") GLOMERULONEPHRITIS

The anatomic hallmark of this syndrome is a diffuse proliferative glomerular inflammation involving the capsular epithelium with widespread crescent formation. The kidneys are normal in size. Abrupt onset and rapid progression are the rule, with bloody urine, anemia, oliguria, and azotemia. Most patients die within 6 to 12 months.

Glomerular crescents may be stimulated by a variety of injuries; hence rapidly progressive nephritis is associated with several different disorders. Some can be distinguished by electron microscopy and immunofluorescence studies. Causes include poststreptococcal glomerulonephritis, bacterial endocarditis, Goodpasture's syndrome, lupus erythematosus, anaphylactoid purpura, and periarteritis. There is also a group of patients who do not have any sign of extrarenal vasculitis but do not have poststreptococcal disease.

The prominence of fibrin thrombi in the glomeruli has suggested the use of heparin and other anticoagulants in treatment. In some cases these agents have resulted in improved renal function, though extrarenal hemorrhage is a distressing complication.

Successful renal transplantation has been carried out in occasional patients with rapidly progressive nephritis. When transplantation is considered, bilateral nephrectomy should be done, followed by several months of dialysis, in order to permit concentrations of circulating immune complexes and anti-kidney antibodies to fall.

FOCAL NEPHRITIS WITH RECURRENT HEMATURIA

This is a common condition affecting children and young adults, usually male, in whom episodes of frankly bloody urine or microscopic hematuria occur within days of a respiratory infection or following exercise. Proteinuria is usually slight (less than 0.5 g per day) or absent. There is no hypertension. Red blood cell casts in the urinary sediment often provide the critical clue that enables one to avoid unnecessary instrumentation of the urinary tract. Renal biopsy shows focal increases in the mesangial matrix and clumping of mesangial cell nuclei without endothelial or epithelial proliferation or glomerular scarring. A number of patients, but not all, have glomerular deposits of IgA immunoglobulins, demonstrable by immunofluorescent techniques.

Though the manifestations are alarming, the prognosis is benign and renal insufficiency does not appear to develop, though red blood cells are seen from time to time in the urinary sediment. The condition may be distinguished from Alport's syndrome (hereditary deafness with nephritis), membranoproliferative nephritis, and mild diffuse glomerulonephritis by the negative family history, the normal serum complement, and the renal biopsy. In a minority of patients with recurrent hematuria, diffuse glomerular changes consistent with chronic glomerulonephritis are seen. Usually, but not invariably, these may be clinically distinguished by their higher excretion of protein (more than 0.5 to 1.0 g per day).

No special treatment is required. Adrenal steroids are said to prevent attacks of hematuria, but their side effects are worse than the disease. Renal biopsy is often useful in reassuring the patient that his outlook is good and in putting an end to investigative procedures unnecessarily repeated with each episode of hematuria.

CHRONIC LOBULAR, MEMBRANOPROLIFERATIVE, HYPOCOMPLEMENTEMIC GLOMERULONEPHRITIS

This distinctive disease occurs in both sexes and at all ages but particularly in children and young adults. The onset resembles that of streptococcal nephritis, with the sudden appearance of edema, hypertension, and hematuria, often following a respiratory infection. Streptococcal antibody levels, however, are not elevated. Proteinuria is frequently massive, so that the picture is that of the nephrotic syndrome associated with hematuria. Renal biopsy shows enlarged glomeruli with marked accentuation of the lobular pattern, caused by proliferation of mesangial cells in the center of the lobule with encroachment on the peripheral capillary space. Splitting and reduplication of the glomerular basement membrane is apparent on electron microscopy. Complex trapping may occasionally be present, usually in the mesangium, but it does not have the characteristic subepithelial location and bumpy appearance seen in poststreptococcal nephritis. Immunofluorescent studies show deposition of $\beta_{1\text{-c}}$-globulin and other immunoglobulins in the mesangium. The distinctive laboratory feature is a profound, prolonged depression of $\beta_{1\text{-c}}$-globulin, ascribed to anticomplementary factors circulating in the blood.

Though partial, temporary, spontaneous improvement may occur, the typical course is that of gradual progression of the renal disease, with eventual death from renal failure. Glucosteroids and immunosuppressive agents do not appear to help the condition.

HEMOLYTIC-UREMIC SYNDROME

This disease occurs chiefly in infants and young children and is characterized by severe hemolytic anemia, thrombocytopenia, and renal failure. The onset, typically a few days to 2 weeks after a respiratory illness or gastroenteritis, is marked by weakness, pallor, purpura, jaundice, and oliguria. Coma or convulsions are observed in almost half the patients. Hypertension may or may not be present. The prodrome and the occurrence of the disease in epidemics suggest an infectious cause, but no single causative agent has yet been identified.

Hematologic studies support the diagnosis of a hemolytic anemia, with reticulocytosis and absent serum haptoglobin. The platelet count is depressed, though bone marrow aspiration shows plentiful megakaryocytes. The white blood cell count is moderately elevated. The peripheral blood smear shows large numbers of fragmented erythrocytes and "Burr cells," typical of microangiopathic hemolysis.

The urine resembles that seen in acute nephritis. Oliguria is the rule, and total anuria is not infrequent. Serum complement level is normal.

Renal biopsy shows focal occlusion of glomerular capillaries and renal arterioles by fibrin thrombi. Some crescent formation and glomerular cell proliferation may also be seen. In fatal cases renal cortical necrosis is common. The changes resemble those seen in the generalized Shwartzman reaction.

The course of the disease is variable, the mortality rate in some series being 40 percent. Recovery, when it occurs, takes place within 2 to 4 weeks. Some children who recover from the acute disease have persistent renal disease or chronic hypertension.

Heparin has been advocated for treatment of the acute episode, but there is no evidence that the results are better than those obtained without anticoagulation. The urgent requirement is to tide patients over the often prolonged period of renal failure and oliguria, if necessary by dialysis.

A similar hematologic picture is seen in adults with *thrombotic thrombocytopenic purpura* (see Chap. 313), which, however, rarely leads to renal failure.

ANAPHYLACTOID (SCHÖNLEIN-HENOCH) PURPURA

Renal complications of this generalized vasculitis associated with purpuric skin lesions, gastrointestinal symptoms, and arthralgia occur in about 40 percent of patients. The glomeruli are involved by a spectrum of changes varying from focal and segmental hypercellularity with focal fibrin capillary thrombi to widespread and diffuse crescentic glomerulonephritis. Electron microscopy reveals subendothelial electron-dense deposits but no subepithelial bumps. Deposits of fibrin and immunoglobulins are apparent in the mesangium when immunofluorescent techniques are used. Arteritic lesions are usually not observed in the kidney.

Although symptoms often follow a respiratory infection, the incidence of positive anti-streptolysin-O titers is only slightly higher than that expected in patients with nonstreptococcal illness. In contrast to what occurs in acute poststreptococcal nephritis, the serum complement is normal.

Microscopic hematuria and albuminuria signal renal involvement by the vascular process, but this may not become evident until several months after onset of the characteristic syndrome. The proteinuria may be so heavy as to produce the nephrotic syndrome. With mild focal glomerulopathy, about half the patients improve rapidly and are well in 3 months. When glomerular involvement is diffuse, with much crescent formation, the prognosis is poor and renal failure is progressive. Prednisone does not improve matters consistently or dramatically, and the role of immunosuppressive agents is still not determined.

NEPHRITIS IN LUPUS ERYTHEMATOSUS

INCIDENCE (see Chap. 70) In about two-thirds of all patients with lupus erythematosus the kidneys are involved. Renal failure is a frequent cause of death. Lupus erythematosus is more frequent in women than in men, and is a common cause of the nephrotic syndrome in young women.

PATHOLOGY The fundamental lesion is the deposition of electron-dense antigen (DNA)-antibody complexes in the mesangium and the basement membrane, where they evoke a variable inflammatory response. The deposits are characteristically subendothelial or intramembranous in location but occasionally extend to the subepithelial region. The earliest change seen by light microscopy is a focal glomerulitis with small areas of endothelial proliferation in the periphery of the glomerular tuft. As the disease advances, the glomerular process becomes more generalized, with diffuse thickening of the basement membrane, resulting in "wire-loop" formation and intense focal cellular proliferation, with capsular adhesions and epithelial crescent formation, progressing to hyalinization. Lesions are frequently seen in various stages of development, and they overlap morphologically with those observed in other forms of chronic glomerulonephritis. Some of the morphologic differences may be expressions of the relatively rapid rate of progression of the disease. Thus, contracted kidneys with many fibrotic and hyalinized glomeruli are uncommon, while focal zones of necrosis in the glomeruli, with nuclear fragmentation, are frequent. Hematoxylin bodies, consisting of depolymerized ribonucleic acid, are occasionally observed in the glomeruli.

A special pattern of "membranous lupus nephropathy" is seen when numerous intramembranous electron-dense complexes cause diffuse thickening of glomerular basement membranes without much inflammation or necrosis; this is associated with a distinctive clinical course.

CLINICAL FEATURES Lupus nephritis may present as acute glomerulonephritis, "latent" nephritis with asymptomatic albuminuria, nephrosis, or chronic glomerulonephritis with renal insufficiency. The urinary sediment is characteristic of active glomerulonephritis, with leukocytes, red blood cell casts, doubly refractile lipid granules, and broad granular casts. Renal involvement is usually signaled by these urinary abnormalities, but as in acute glomerulonephritis, the renal biopsy may occasionally show lupus nephritis even when the urine shows no involvement. The serum complement is usually low when the disease is active, but there are too many exceptions to rule out lupus nephritis with confidence merely because the complement level is found to be normal. The course may be fulminating, with death in uremia after only a few weeks of onset, or the patient may live for years, with proteinuria and microscopic hematuria regarded as merely subsidiary to the other vicissitudes of the disease. In its early phases, and when the distribution of the lesions is "focal," i.e., when less than half the glomeruli in the renal biopsy appear involved, signs of renal disease may remit spontaneously. When glomerular involvement is diffuse, on the other hand, and especially when massive proteinuria or azotemia has appeared, the course of untreated patients is generally rapidly downhill within 1 to 3 years. Hypertension is rare unless azotemia is present or the patient is being treated with steroids. Other systemic signs of lupus erythematosus, such as rash and arthritis, as well as a positive reaction to the LE test, may disappear while the nephritis is active; this is especially likely with the development of the nephrotic syndrome or signs of uremia. In the membranous form of the disease, the course is more indolent and the prognosis more favorable. Proteinuria is mild to moderate, often in the nephrotic range, but with spontaneous fluctuations. Hypertension appears late, as a consequence of progressive renal scarring. Late in the disease, when signs of active lupus are long gone, high blood pressure, heart failure, or renal insufficiency may become the main problem, as in any patient with chronic glomerulonephritis.

TREATMENT Treatment with relatively small doses of adrenal steroids (e.g., 20 mg prednisone daily), which may be enough to suppress fever and arthritis, rarely improves diffuse advanced lupus nephritis and does not prevent its development, though mild proteinuria and hematuria associated with focal disease may show improvement. The nephrotic syndrome responds to steroid treatment in a minority of cases, often requiring more than 6 weeks of treatment. Even large doses of prednisone (e.g., 60 to 80 mg daily) are frequently ineffective in producing a sustained remission of diffuse proliferative lupus nephritis. On the other hand, azathioprine or cyclophosphamide, 2 to 3 mg per kg per day, produces clinical remission and improvement in the renal biopsy in a majority of instances. The drugs are given for several months, usually in combination with a low dose (15 to 20 mg) of prednisone. After azotemia and hypertension have appeared, however, many cases progress regardless of treatment.

SCLERODERMA

About one-third of patients with scleroderma die of renal failure, and in two-thirds renal changes are present at death. The characteristic lesions consist of extensive intimal thickening of the interlobular arteries, fibrinoid necrosis of the cortical arterioles, thickening of glomerular loops, and spotty ischemic cortical necrosis. These changes are indistinguishable from those seen in malignant hypertension. Proteinuria does not generally exceed 2 g per day. The blood pressure is usually elevated, especially terminally. In exceptional instances, however, it may be normal, even in patients with widespread arterial and arteriolar lesions at postmortem examination. Minimal proteinuria may be the only sign for long periods. Once renal involvement is moderately advanced, the course is rapid, leading to death from renal insufficiency within a few weeks or months after azotemia has appeared. Terminal oliguria or anuria is common. The rapid progression of renal insufficiency frequently appears to be precipitated by the use of hypotensive agents. Adrenal steroids do not prevent or ameliorate the renal disease; it has been suggested that they accelerate it, but the evidence for this is not convincing.

PERIARTERITIS NODOSA—HYPERSENSITIVITY ANGIITIS

The kidney is said to be involved in approximately 80 percent of all patients with periarteritis nodosa. Precise nosology in this area is complicated by the fact that arteritic lesions nearly always occur in the course of malignant hypertension and occasionally appear in the course of glomerulonephritis.

PATHOLOGY Renal lesions in periarteritis are of two types. The first is characterized by segmental fibrinoid necrosis of part or all of an arterial wall, with an inflammatory perivascular infiltrate. Usually, arteries of medium size are involved (arcuate arteries or larger), but arterioles and even capillaries may be attacked. Signs of organization are evident, with fibrous replacement of the damaged media and the formation of aneurysms at weakened spots in the larger muscular arteries. Multiple infarctions and gross cortical scars are apparent in the renal parenchyma. There is scattered focal glomerulitis of varying age and activity. Necrotic or scarifying lesions may involve only a portion of a glomerulus while the remainder appears untouched. The second type of involvement is characterized by an active, rapidly progressive glomerulonephritis, with widespread fibrinoid necrosis of glomeruli and epithelial crescent formation. Combinations of these types of lesions may occur.

CLINICAL FEATURES With lesions of the larger renal arteries, hypertension is usual and may dominate the clinical picture. Albuminuria is almost always present, and the urinary sediment frequently contains red blood cell casts and fat bodies. Episodes in which the urine is grossly bloody are common. Uremia may be noted terminally, but azotemia frequently is absent or mild and only slowly progressive. Remissions and relapses often mark the clinical course. Persistent hypertension may be a serious sequel when the disease is no longer active.

When the clinical and pathologic features of acute glomerulonephritis are present, hypertension is more often absent, even in the presence of marked azotemia. Although death from renal insufficiency usually takes place within 6 months to a year of onset, in milder cases permanent spontaneous remissions have been observed.

Periarteritis should be suspected in patients with renal failure or hypertension, especially when features suggesting glomerulonephritis are present, when other organ systems are involved, or in the presence of obscure fever or unexplained leukocytosis or eosinophilia.

Large doses of adrenal steroids (60 to 80 mg prednisone daily) usually control systemic manifestations and produce improvement in renal function in some patients. In a few of these cases, the manifestations of renal involvement completely disappear and the remission persists after steroids are withdrawn. In others, maintenance on steroids and azathioprine is necessary to sustain the remission, and in many patients the renal lesion appears to progress in spite of treatment. The response to steroids appears to be related to the extent and stage of the lesions when therapy is begun. Early diagnosis and treatment are therefore important. Other immunosuppressive agents such as azathioprine and cyclophosphamide probably improve the effectiveness of the regimen.

WEGENER'S GRANULOMATOSIS

(See also Chap. 71)

Renal lesions indistinguishable from those found in other varieties of periarteritis are also seen in Wegener's granulomatosis. Without treatment they progress inexorably. Remission in kidney disease has been reported, however, when azathioprine or cyclophosphamide has been given, usually in conjunction with prednisone. Prednisone alone has no effect once renal insufficiency has appeared.

GOODPASTURE'S SYNDROME

(See also Chap. 69)

This term has been used to identify a group of patients with hemoptysis and glomerulonephritis. Since hemoptysis may complicate many forms of nephritis, it seems best to restrict the definition to those patients without polyarteritis in whom frank lung hemorrhage is associated with a proliferative glomerulonephritis caused by antibody to glomerular basement membrane.

The initial event is usually severe hemoptysis in patients who have normal renal function and occasionally even an initially normal urinalysis. In a short time this is followed by signs of severe nephritis, including hematuria and progressive renal failure. Hypertension is seldom seen early in the disease, although it may appear as the nephritis progresses. The histologic picture in the lung resembles that of pulmonary hemosiderosis.

The earliest change seen in the kidney is a focal and local glomerulonephritis resembling the nephropathy of anaphylactoid purpura. In later stages there is a severe diffuse glomerulonephritis with necrosis of glomerular tufts and crescent formation. The hallmark of the disease is the linear deposition of IgG globulin along the basement membrane, visible by immunofluorescence. The observation that glomerular basement membrane has antigens in common with lung alveoli may explain the pathogenesis of the disorder.

A group of patients has been identified in whom heavy chronic exposure to hydrocarbon fumes preceded the development of Goodpasture's syndrome; it may be significant that prolonged exposure to gasoline fumes has also been shown to produce nephritis in rats.

Though the majority of patients die within a few months, a few have survived for prolonged periods when treated with large doses of steroid or immunosuppressive drugs early in the course of the disease. Several cases have also been reported in which pulmonary hemorrhage ceased after the kidneys were removed and the patient placed on chronic hemodialysis. A few patients have had renal transplants without recurrence of hemoptysis.

LIPOID NEPHROSIS

(See also Chap. 271)

This term was first used to describe the nephrotic syndrome but is now used to designate a distinctive pathologic lesion which is usually associated with a characteristic clinical course. In early stages of the disorder the glomeruli appear normal by light microscopy. By electron microscopy the glomerular capillary basement membranes are normal but glomerular epithelial foot processes are coalesced. In advanced stages the glomeruli may show sclerosis but never more than slight mesangial cell proliferation by light microscopy. By electron microscopy, thickening of the basement membranes and mesangial thickening may be seen. Electron-dense deposits consistent with antigen-antibody complexes are, however, never found. Unlike other forms of glomerulonephritis, no glomerular localization of immune globulin IgG, $\beta_{1\text{-c}}$, or fibrin is demonstrable by immunofluorescent techniques. The "atopic antibody," IgE, has been identified within the glomeruli in a few instances.

This is the most common cause of the nephrotic syndrome in children. It also affects adults of all ages, accounting for perhaps one-fourth of adults with the nephrotic syndrome. It is more common in males than in females. Rapid onset of heavy proteinuria is the rule, with selective excretion of proteins of small molecular size. The majority of patients do not have hypertension, microscopic hematuria, or azotemia, but any of these findings may be present in individuals with the specific lesion of lipoid nephrosis. Care must be taken not to misinterpret prerenal azotemia due to contraction of blood volume and increased breakdown of protein, which is reversible. This is sometimes wrongly ascribed to glomerular sclerosis. Fever and leukocytosis are not part of the clinical picture. Slight eosinophilia is sometimes present, and there is said to be a high incidence of atopic allergy in children with the disease. Serum complement level is not depressed.

The *characteristic features of the course* of lipoid nephrosis, in adults as well as children, are its good prognosis, the tendency to spontaneous remission, the excellent response to treatment with steroids, and the tendency to relapse.

Spontaneous remission occurred in 30 to 50 percent of patients in the era before steroid treatment. With prednisone, 75 percent of children and adults eventually recover completely. The remainder have persistent or recurrent proteinuria. Some of these patients, unresponsive to steroids, develop a focal glomerular sclerosis that may progress to cause renal insufficiency over a period varying from 1 to 2 years to much longer.

Treatment is usually started with 60 to 80 mg prednisone daily. If double the dose of steroid is given every other day, the incidence of remission is the same but side effects are said to be less troublesome (see page 523). Remission generally requires the development of Cushing's syndrome. Improvement is usually apparent after 10 to 20 days of steroid therapy and is signaled by a fall in protein excretion, diuresis, and a rise in serum albumin. The earliest sign of a therapeutic effect is a diminution in the number of grams of protein excreted daily. High doses of prednisone tend to increase glomerular filtration rate, so that the serum creatinine often falls during treatment. The blood urea nitrogen level, however, often rises because the catabolism of protein is increased by steroids. If no improvement in protein excretion can be detected after 4 to 6 weeks of treatment with large amounts of prednisone, it is unlikely that further treatment with steroids alone will be beneficial, though spontaneous remission will occur in approximately 25 percent of these cases.

In the majority of patients, proteinuria disappears completely or diminishes to a constant low level. After no further improvement can be detected, the dose of steroid is gradually reduced over 4 to 6 weeks. If administration of the drug is interrupted at this time, some patients continue in remission indefinitely, but many relapse at varying intervals following cessation of treatment. At least one relapse after a remission induced by prednisone is the rule in 70 to 80 percent of children with the disease, though relapses are less frequent in adults. Most relapses occur within the first 2 to 3 years after the initial episode, though in rare instances they may also occur after an asymptomatic interval of 15 to 20 years. If the initial episode of nephrosis has responded to steroid treatment, subsequent ones usually do so as well.

In a few patients, proteinuria reappears promptly when the dose of steroid is lowered (steroid-dependent) or else recurs repeatedly when steroids are discontinued (chronic relapsers). There is some evidence that the addition of cyclophosphamide or azathioprine to the regimen may permit sustained remission in some such cases at the same time that the dose of prednisone is lowered to escape the evil effects of Cushing's syndrome.

Complications of steroid treatment include hypertension, muscular weakness and cramps, peptic ulcer, potassium depletion, diabetes, and osteoporosis (Chap. 86).

MEMBRANOUS NEPHROPATHY

This distinctive entity may be separated from lipoid nephrosis by its pathologic appearance and clinical behavior. The single most significant morphologic change is a uniform thickening of the glomerular capillary wall unaccompanied by any significant increase in mesangial, endothelial, or epithelial cells. With PAS (periodic acid–Schiff) or silver methenamine stains the basement membrane shows numerous small silver or PAS-positive projections protruding outward from the basement membrane to form a characteristic "spike-and-dome" pattern. Under the electron microscope this pattern is seen to be formed by large intramembranous and epimembranous electron-opaque deposits interspersed with spikelike projections of a basement membrane–like substance.

The clinical picture varies from asymptomatic proteinuria to full-blown nephrotic syndrome. The disease is more common in adults than in children. Hypertension and microscopic hematuria are each seen in about one-third of the patients. The proteinuria is less "selective" than in lipoid nephrosis. There is usually no history of preceding infection, and the serum complement level and antistreptolysin titer are normal.

The outstanding feature of the natural history is the indolent and benign course found in most patients. Though there is no good evidence that prednisone or immunosuppressive drugs help the disease, complete or partial spontaneous remissions occur in 40 to 50 percent of cases. Though proteinuria diminishes in such patients, the renal biopsy may remain abnormal. A few patients show remarkable spontaneous variations in protein excretion, suggesting an intermittent or polycyclic course. In others there is a slow but steady progression of glomerular scarring, with gradual reduction in glomerular filtration rate leading to uremia after many years.

Because of the poor response to steroids and the high incidence of spontaneous clinical remission, membranous nephropathy should not be treated with prednisone. Supportive measures designed to relieve the edema (see Chap. 271) during several months of watchful waiting will frequently be rewarded by spontaneous improvement.

REFERENCES

COMERFORD FR, COHEN AS: The nephropathy of systemic lupus erythematosus. Medicine 46:425, 1967

HENDLER ED et al: Clinicopathological correlations of primary hematuria. Lancet 1:458, 1972

HERDMAN RC et al: Chronic glomerulonephritis associated with low serum complement activity (chronic hypocomplementemic glomerulonephritis). Medicine 49:207, 1970

HOPPER J JR et al: Lipoid nephrosis in 31 adult patients: Renal biopsy study by light, electron, and fluorescence microscopy with experience in treatment. Medicine 49:321, 1970

MCCLUSKEY RT, BALDWIN DS: Natural history of acute glomerulonephritis. Am J Med 35:213, 1963

POLLAK UE, MENDOZA N: Rapidly progressive glomerulonephritis. Med Clin North Am 55:1397, 1971

271 NEPHROTIC SYNDROME

FRANKLIN H. EPSTEIN

The nephrotic syndrome is a clinical constellation characterized by (1) massive proteinuria, (2) hypoalbuminemia, and (3) edema. Hyperlipemia is frequently but not invariably present. The term "nephrosis" is sometimes used by pathologists to indicate degenerative changes in renal tubular epithelium, but this definition should not be confused with the clinical syndrome under discussion.

ETIOLOGY The nephrotic syndrome is the result of diffuse injury to the glomerulus. The injury may therefore occur in the course of any of the forms of glomerulonephritis discussed in the preceding chapter. It can be caused by amyloid infiltration of the glomeruli and by diabetic intercapillary glomerulosclerosis. It is occasionally observed in allergic reactions to plant pollens, poison ivy, poison oak, or insect stings, or as a manifestation of sensitivity to trimethadione or paramethadione. It may occur as a complication of secondary syphilis or malaria and has sometimes appeared in the course of treatment with mercurial diuretics and salts of gold and bismuth. Massive proteinuria may result from the marked elevation in glomerular capillary pressure which follows thrombosis of the renal veins or constrictive pericarditis. Nephrosis has also been reported in association with a variety of malignant lesions, especially lymphoma. Uncomplicated pyelonephritis or nephrosclerosis does not cause the nephrotic syndrome.

CLINICAL FEATURES The patient usually comes to the physician because of the insidious onset of *edema.* This is often particularly noticeable in the face because of the absence of orthopnea. The edema is characteristically soft and pits easily. Ascites and pleural effusions are frequently present, but pulmonary edema does not occur without heart failure. Though edema may be the only manifestation, other symptoms are often present, vaguely suggesting the extensive depletion of body proteins that hypoalbuminemia betokens. Loss of appetite is frequent, although not so common as in poststreptococcal glomerulonephritis. A previously active child may feel tired and run-down. Amenorrhea or some irregularity in menses is the rule in women. The course is sometimes punctuated by unexplained episodes of abdominal pain, vomiting, and diarrhea.

The blood pressure is often normal, and in the absence of hypertension the heart is not enlarged. The fundi are normal except when diabetic glomerulosclerosis is the cause of the disorder. The skin looks puffy and pale; there may be a mild normocytic anemia, but the hematocrit is usually higher than the pasty appearance of the patient suggests. Mild generalized osteoporosis is frequently observed, especially in children.

The daily urine usually contains more than 4 to 5 g protein, *chiefly albumin,* but significant quantities of α_1-, β-, and *γ-globulins* are found as well. Some nephrotic patients excrete as much as 20 to 30 g protein each day. The serum proteins are grossly reduced in concentration, especially the albumin and, less predictably, the γ-globulin fraction. Serum γ-globulins are said to be normal in the nephrosis caused by lupus erythematosus or amyloid disease; they may also be within normal limits in the nephrosis associated with membranous glomerulonephritis. Alpha-2-globulin levels are generally elevated, but this occurs in many chronic diseases. Serum albumin concentration is usually below 2.0 to 2.5 g per 100 ml when edema is present, and with massive edema it is frequently below 1 g per 100 ml. The overall increase in the lipid-carrying globulins conceals a reduction in the concentration of the smaller metal-carrying proteins, transferrin (iron) and ceruloplasmin (copper). The serum calcium level is low, entirely as a result of a decrease in the fraction bound to albumin. The plasma fibrinogen level is often elevated, and the sedimentation rate is greatly accelerated. The cholesterol, phospholipid, and triglyceride levels in the serum are usually elevated, and the serum is often lactescent. The low-density β-lipoproteins, to which these molecules are attached, increase in concentration. When caloric intake has been low and nutrition poor, however, serum cholesterol and triglyceride levels may be normal. This is frequently the case in instances of the nephrotic syndrome caused by lupus erythematosus and Kimmelstiel-Wilson disease.

The *basal metabolic rate* is usually low, perhaps as a result of malnutrition and, in some cases, failure to correct for edema fluid in estimating weight. The impression of hypothyroidism may be strengthened by a puffy face and pasty appearance, by an elevated serum cholesterol level, and by the decrease in serum precipitable iodine, which, however, is a consequence of the low concentration of thyroxine-binding proteins in the serum, rather than of impaired thyroid function. Treatment with thyroid produces no improvement.

The *urinary sediment* is filled with granular and epithelial cell casts and casts in which highly refractile lipid droplets are embedded. Fat bodies may be seen in the urine even when the serum cholesterol level is normal. Red blood cells are often absent, but many patients show some degree of continuous or intermittent microscopic hematuria.

The *glomerular filtration rate* is frequently normal or above normal early in the course of the nephrotic syndrome, and the blood urea level is not elevated. In patients with progressive nephritis azotemia gradually develops, together with a fall in filtration rate and filtration fraction. In others renal function may remain normal, despite edema, for years, or may be depressed transiently, particularly during or immediately following infections. With severe hypoalbuminemia and consequent reduction in plasma volume, prerenal azotemia may be present, glomerular filtration rate falling because of hypovolemia. This reversible depression of renal function must not be taken for progressive renal insufficiency due to destruction of renal tissue. Tubular functions such as concentrating ability and phenolsulfonphthalein excretion are generally normal. Occasionally aminoaciduria or renal glycosuria is observed, presumably as a result of interference with proximal tubular reabsorption.

PATHOLOGIC PHYSIOLOGY The *glomerular basement membrane* is abnormally permeable to proteins. Those of low molecular weight and small size, such as albumin, are lost into the urine in greatest quantity. Although it is conceivable that failure of the renal tubular epithelium to reabsorb protein might contribute to proteinuria, the massive amounts of protein excreted by some nephrotic patients and the striking increase in protein excretion observed following infusions of concentrated serum albumin suggest that increased glomerular permeability is the major determinant of the nephrotic syndrome. Indeed, there is good reason to believe that tubular reabsorption of protein is increased. There is no evidence (except in nephrosis associated with multiple myeloma) that abnormal proteins appear in plasma or urine. Hypoalbuminemia is chiefly a result of the extensive urinary losses of this protein; its synthesis is normal or even increased. In addition, in some patients the rate of catabolism of albumin is accelerated in a manner similar to that observed in a variety of acute injuries or infections. Associated with the reduction in amount of serum albumin there is usually marked wasting of tissues, which may be clinically evident only after the edema disappears. Balance studies carried out in nephrotic patients during refeeding with high-protein, high-calorie diets suggest that for every gram of protein added to the plasma, 20 to 100 g tissue protein must be incorporated in tissue.

The *decrease in plasma albumin* and consequent fall in the oncotic pressure of plasma results in an increased transudation of fluid from the bloodstream to extravascular spaces. Plasma volume falls. The reaction of the kidneys to these events is to diminish the excretion of sodium and of water, as in many other situations where the integrity of the effective circulating blood volume is threatened. Secretion of aldosterone by the adrenal cortex is augmented.

The primary role of sodium in the production of nephrotic edema is demonstrated by the fact that, when administered without salt, water may be excreted normally. When the intake of sodium is continued, it is retained by the kidneys and sequestered with water in an expanded interstitial fluid. Despite edema, plasma volume remains normal or low. If albumin is added to the bloodstream in increased amounts, or its rate of loss is diminished, the sequence of events will be reversed and diuresis will ensue.

When the quantity of circulating albumin is increased in a nephrotic patient, plasma volume is expanded by dilution with extravascular edema fluid, thereby minimizing the expected rise in albumin *concentration.* For this and other reasons, diuresis and edema formation need not be correlated with the exact concentration of albumin in the serum.

Serum cholesterol, phospholipids, and triglycerides usually are all increased in nephrotic patients. The rise in level of triglycerides may be so marked that the serum is milky. At least one reason for the elevation in serum cholesterol level is its increased solubility in fatty serum, though increases in amount of serum cholesterol may also be observed in the absence of lactescent serum and even when serum triglyceride levels are normal. Decreases of cholesterol and lipid phosphorus frequently coincide with periods of especially severe anorexia or vomiting; increases, with periods in which appetite is good. Nevertheless, the most intense lipemia may be observed in wasted patients with extreme hypoproteinemia and the most massive edema. Though hyperlipemia usually disappears when elimination of edema marks regression of or recovery from the disease, it may persist in rapidly progressive cases despite advanced azotemia and hypertension.

The cause of *hyperlipemia* is not clear. It is not secondary to increased synthesis of fat or to difficulty in disposing of fat in the diet. Infusions of albumin produce an immediate fall in serum lipid level, often, but not always, to normal. In general, elevation of serum lipid level tends to be inversely proportional to the level of serum albumin. Infusions of dextran which store the colloid osmotic pressure of serum also result in a fall in serum lipid level in patients with nephrosis. Overproduction of β-lipoproteins may be responsible for hyperlipemia. Since albumin binds and transports unesterified fatty acids, a deficiency of binding sites for free fatty acids, with consequent "trapping" of neutral fat in the plasma, has also been suggested.

There seems to be an increased tendency to *vascular thrombosis* in the nephrotic syndrome. This is probably contributed to by contraction of plasma volume in severe hypoalbuminemia, and by the production of Cushing's syndrome in patients treated with adrenal steroids.

TREATMENT Although a few days in bed help to mobilize edema, there is no indication for prolonged bed rest. Hospitalization is indicated at the onset of the disease to confirm the diagnosis and to obtain base-line studies but need not be prolonged.

The *diet* should be low in sodium and high in protein. Except in the presence of hyponatremia, water should not be restricted. Very low-sodium diets (200 mg) are unpalatable, although the development of "sodium-free" milk and milk powders has made a satisfactory high-protein, low-salt diet more feasible. Sodium restriction should, however, be considered an emergency measure to control edema; it is not indicated during convalescence from the nephrotic syndrome or when edema is minimal. A high consumption of protein (120 to 150 g daily for an adult), together with adequate calories, leads to steady replenishment of wasted tissues. Since the goal is to restore body proteins, not simply to prevent further wastage, additional intake of protein above the normal requirement of 1 g per kg per day, plus urinary losses, is of importance. If the additional protein is to be utilized, sufficient calories must be given. The proportion of fat and carbohydrates is determined, as a practical matter, by the composition of the supplements of milk or milk powder. There seems to be no great advantage to restriction of fat. With such liberal intake of protein and calories, there is usually some subjective increase in feeling of well-being, as well as, over many months, a slow rise in plasma albumin concentration. The increase in blood urea level which invariably occurs on a high-protein diet reflects the additional amount of urea presented to the kidney for excretion, rather than deterioration of renal function. Proteinuria may also increase when serum albumin level rises.

Diuretics may be used, in conjunction with sodium restriction, to control edema. Agents (such as spironolactone) that block the action of aldosterone are useful, in conjunction with stronger diuretics (ethacrynic acid, furosemide) in resistant cases. The action of diuretics is enhanced by infusions of albumin, plasma, or dextran. These agents raise the oncotic pressure of plasma and expand plasma volume temporarily but are rapidly lost into the urine through the leaky glomerular filter. The diuretic effect of recumbency can be utilized by giving, for example, 40 to 80 mg furosemide before an afternoon nap, or before bedtime, and by elevating the feet whenever possible, when the patient sits down. Diuresis is not an end in itself; a little edema is often to be preferred to the complications of too-vigorous diuretic therapy.

Adrenal steroids should not be given indiscriminately in nephrosis. Their use should depend on a diagnosis established as specifically as possible by renal biopsy, as suggested in Table 271-1.

TABLE 271-1
Nephrotic syndrome: causes and response to prednisone treatment

Renal biopsy finding	*Therapeutic response*
Lipoid nephrosis	Yes
Membraneous glomerulonephritis	No
Acute diffuse proliferative glomerulonephritis	No
Mild proliferative glomerulonephritis	Sometimes
Lupus erythematosus	Sometimes
Lobular (membranoproliferative) glomerulonephritis	No
Amyloid	No
Diabetic nephropathy	No
Preeclampsia	No
Renal vein thrombosis	No
Henoch-Schönlein purpura	Probably not

REFERENCES

EARLY LE et al: Nephrotic syndrome. Calif Med 115:23, 1971

MILLER RB et al: Long-term results of steroid therapy in adults with idiopathic nephrotic syndrome. Am J Med 46:919, 1969

272
VASCULAR DISEASE OF THE KIDNEY. TOXEMIA OF PREGNANCY

FRANKLIN H. EPSTEIN

NEPHROSCLEROSIS (see also Chap. 245) **Definition and pathology** Although early in the course of "essential" hypertension there may be no morphologic changes in the kidney at all, structural alterations in the small arteries and the arterioles are almost always present in the kidneys of patients who die in the course of hypertensive disease. In about 10 percent of such patients the changes are severe enough to produce marked renal insufficiency. Large and medium-sized arteries show intimal thickening. This change is more ubiquitous and more severe in the small arteries and arterioles. In addition, an eosinophilic hyaline thickening frequently involves the entire wall of arterioles and prearterioles. These changes lead to mild generalized atrophy of the cortex with focal scars. Hyalinized glomeruli are a conspicuous microscopic feature.

In patients who die with rapidly progressive, "malignant" hypertension, especially after renal insufficiency has appeared, there is often intense intimal hyperplasia of the medium-sized and small arteries, so that the lumen is substantially reduced. Necrosis of the preglomerular arterioles is present, which frequently extends into the glomerular tufts. There are hemorrhages into Bowman's space and occasional crescent formation.

It is not generally realized that similar but less intense changes may be found at postmortem examination in patients without systemic hypertension. Arteriolosclerosis is observed in the renal biopsies of a few patients with normal blood pressure and mild asymptomatic proteinuria. Definite arteriolosclerosis was described by Bell in 10.6 percent of normotensive patients fifty to sixty years of age, and it increased in intensity and frequency in older age groups. It seems clear that renal arteriolosclerosis may occur in the absence of systemic hypertension, though it rarely produces symptoms or signs. Such vascular changes may account for the moderate decrease in renal reserve often observed in elderly patients.

Clinical features Hypertension antedates proteinuria by many years in most patients with "essential" hypertension. When proteinuria does appear it is usually minimal. The urinary sediment is usually not remarkable, although microscopic hematuria and occasionally gross urinary bleeding may occur in the accelerated phase, when the excretion of protein may also increase to more than 4 g daily, reflecting widespread necrosis of glomerular capillaries. The anemia associated with advanced renal insufficiency occurs in some patients with nephrosclerosis as in other renal diseases, although the appearance of hypertensive neuroretinopathy with azotemia *in the absence of anemia* should suggest primary vascular disease. The patient with hypertension and uremia whose optic fundi are normal usually has glomerulonephritis or pyelonephritis. At the inception of the hypertensive process, renal blood flow is usually depressed more than glomerular filtration rate. The opposite is true in glomerulonephritis, but the difference has no important clinical significance.

The course of nephrosclerosis is extremely variable and cannot be reliably predicted from the height of the blood pressure. Proteinuria and even mild azotemia may not be symptomatic for many years. The abrupt change in course which marks the onset of the malignant phase is characterized by an increase in proteinuria and hematuria. Extremely high blood pressure, retinal hemorrhages and papilledema, heart failure, and hypertensive encephalopathy complicate the rapidly progressive uremia, which is fatal. Most patients in whom this syndrome occurs have been known to have hypertension for less than 8 years.

The term "malignant hypertension" has been used variously to indicate (1) hypertension with papilledema, (2) hypertension with rapidly progressive renal insufficiency, or (3) hypertension with necrotizing arteriolitis. These arbitrary definitions should not be confused or allowed to obscure the facts in individual cases. Papilledema, hematuria, weight loss, advancing uremia, and necrotizing arteriolitis usually coexist in hypertensive patients, but it is not unusual for any of these features to be absent in the presence of the others. Thus, 23 percent of 68 cases studied by Goldring and Chasis with excessively high diastolic pressure and rapidly advancing uremia did not have papilledema. In some, the fundi showed only arteriolar narrowing without hemorrhage. Contrariwise, papilledema may be present in occasional patients at intervals for many months or even years without advanced renal involvement or necrotizing arteriolitis. In some patients the uremic syndrome appears over the course of a year to two but hematuria and proteinuria remain minimal, and neuroretinopathy may never be present. Such patients are likely to have massive cellular intimal hyperplasia of the interlobular arteries with little necrotizing glomerulitis.

In addition to "primary" nephrosclerosis, the clinical syndrome of malignant hypertension may occur in the course of chronic pyelonephritis, glomerulonephritis, periarteritis nodosa, scleroderma, pheochromocytoma, and unilateral renal arterial occlusion.

RENAL ARTERIAL OCCLUSION *Arterial infarction* of the kidney is usually attended by sudden sharp unremitting pain in the upper part of the abdomen or flank. The most common cause is embolic occlusion. Fever and moderate leukocytosis are common, especially when a major branch of the renal artery has been occluded. Gross hematuria is not unusual, and microscopic hematuria is present in more than half the cases. The blood urea nitrogen usually is not abnormal unless there is contralateral disease. Shortly after a renal infarct, the kidney may not function on intravenous pyelography, although it appears normal in size and retrograde pyelograms are normal. During the ensuing days or weeks, function is slowly regained.

When occlusion of the renal artery is *incomplete* as a result of atherosclerotic narrowing, or if a branch of the main renal artery is occluded and viability of kidney tissue is preserved by collateral circulation, hypertension may ensue which is often of the rapidly progressive type, though reversible by nephrectomy. In such patients, intravenous pyelograms carried out at 1 and 2 min characteristically show differences in filling times between the affected kidney and the uninvolved one. In a significant minority of cases, albuminuria is absent and the urinary sediment may be completely normal. The diagnosis may be made by studies of the volume and composition of urine obtained on bilateral ureteral catheterization, by aortography, and by measurement of renal venous renin. Often the affected kidney is contracted. (See Chap. 245.)

RENAL VEIN THROMBOSIS **Etiology** One or both of the kidneys may be involved by renal vein thrombosis. Occlusion of both renal veins usually implies thrombosis of the inferior vena cava as well. A common cause is invasion of the veins by *hypernephroma* or compression by *malignant metastases* to retroperitoneal lymph nodes at the level of the celiac axis. *Thrombophlebitis* of the legs with extension upward, *periarteritis, congestive heart failure*, or severe *dehydration*, especially in children, may be etiologic factors. The venous occlusion may follow an *abdominal injury* or *operation*. In adults, renal vein thrombosis may occur as a secondary and often terminal complication of renal disease which has previously caused perinephric inflammation or reduction of renal blood flow. It is particularly likely to occur in *papillary necrosis* and in renal *amyloidosis*.

Clinical features Sudden complete thrombosis of a renal vein causes severe lumbar pain, enlargement of the affected kidney, hematuria, and proteinuria. If the condition is bilateral, oliguria and death from uremia usually ensue. If the occlusion is more gradual, renal function may be partially preserved by the development of collateral venous channels. These can be diagnosed on the intravenous pyelogram by the ureteral notching which they cause. In a few such cases, massive proteinuria results in a full-blown *nephrotic syndrome*; in other instances, proteinuria is not prominent and is overshadowed by hematuria. The blood pressure is usually normal, and when hypertension occurs it is not severe. The presence of collateral abdominal veins with upward blood flow, unexplained edema of the legs and lower part of the trunk, or recurrent pulmonary emboli may suggest the diagnosis, which can be established by venography of the inferior vena cava.

PREECLAMPSIA AND ECLAMPSIA—TOXEMIAS OF PREGNANCY The term *toxemia of pregnancy* includes those disorders encountered during gestation or shortly after delivery which are characterized by the appearance of hypertension, edema, and proteinuria (preeclampsia) and, in severe cases, convulsions and coma (eclampsia). There is no reason to believe that patients with convulsions suffer from a disease essentially different from that of patients with preeclampsia. Such a clinical classification usually includes many patients with diverse diseases of the kidneys and blood vessels which begin or are exacerbated during pregnancy. The following discussion will be concerned with a specific disease affecting the kidneys and the vascular system, usually commencing in the last trimester of pregnancy, which in most cases is improved dramatically when the pregnancy is terminated.

Pathology The most common histologic finding in the kidneys in toxemia of pregnancy is marked swelling of the endothelial and epithelial cells of the glomeruli. In severe or prolonged cases, thickening of afferent arterioles may be apparent. Generalized and focal thickening of the glomerular basement membrane and fibrinoid necrosis of glomerular tufts have been described at postmortem examination, but these changes are rarer in renal biopsies obtained from patients who recover. Tubular necrosis is present in almost all patients who die of acute toxemia of pregnancy. Necrosis of liver cells and hemorrhages in the periportal areas are present in some but not all fatal cases; it has been suggested that these as well as the necrotic lesions of the kidneys are secondary to vascular spasm and shock.

A characteristic lesion in toxemia of pregnancy is the deposition of fibrin in glomeruli. Fibrin deposits can be demonstrated by immunofluorescent techniques even when they are not apparent with the usual stains. Unlike acute glomerulonephritis, antigen-antibody complexes and complement do not seem to be involved in the pathogenesis of the disease, and the serum complement is normal. In its severe forms, when *cortical necrosis* appears, the condition bears a tantalizing resemblance to the generalized Shwartzman phenomenon, because of widespread fibrin deposits in small blood vessels.

Clinical features Toxemia occurs more often in women pregnant for the first time and in those over thirty-five. It is more common with twins than in single pregnancies. Its incidence is especially high in mothers bearing hydatidiform moles, in which albuminuria and hypertension characteristically appear early rather than late in pregnancy, suggesting that the disorder is associated with the placenta, rather than the fetus. As with most vascular disorders, its manifestations are more frequent and pronounced in the obese, though paradoxically its incidence is higher in economically underprivileged segments of the population. Toxemia of pregnancy is especially frequent in patients with prior renal and vascular disease. A significant percentage of pregnant women with preexisting hypertension can expect to have their pregnancy complicated by a toxemic episode. The incidence increases in general with the height of the diastolic blood pressure and is especially high if in previous pregnancies preeclampsia was superimposed upon chronic hypertensive vascular disease. Preceding toxemia of pregnancy appears to predispose to recurrence in 30 to 60 percent of patients even if blood pressure and urine have been normal between pregnancies. Evidence of pyelonephritis is encountered clinically in about one-fifth of patients with preeclampsia. Patients with diabetes are not especially susceptible to the disorder unless vascular or renal disease is present.

The *onset* may be either insidious or shockingly abrupt. Although toxemia commonly appears after the twenty-fourth week of gestation and frequently only a day or two before delivery, it may begin earlier, particularly in patients with underlying renal disease. *Hypertension* is usually an early sign. Because of the normal decline in blood pressure during the latter two-thirds of pregnancy, the physician should not disregard the significance of a *rising blood pressure*, even though it may not exceed 140/90. With hypertension, *headaches* and visual disturbances are frequent but not universal complaints. The *fundi* often show narrowing and spasm of the retinal arterioles. The retina may appear glistening or wet, but this sign is not specific. Exudates and hemorrhage are late occurrences in severe cases.

The appearance of *proteinuria* is usually coincident with hypertension, although it may follow (less often, precede) the rise in blood pressure by a week or so. The amounts may vary from a trace of protein to 8 or 10 g in 24 hr. Granular and hyaline casts are found in the urinary sediment. Unlike acute glomerulonephritis, toxemia does not usually cause red blood cells and cellular casts in large numbers in the urinary sediment. Renal concentrating ability is generally unimpaired except in severe cases and in patients with previously decreased renal function. The blood urea nitrogen level does not often rise above 20 mg per 100 ml. Nevertheless, glomerular filtration rate is diminished by the disease in most cases. Even slight nitrogen retention must be interpreted with due regard to the physiologic increase in glomerular filtration rate and fall in blood urea which characterize the normal pregnancy. Blood *uric acid* level is commonly though not invariably elevated, reflecting a decrease in the renal clearance of urate. In fulminant cases, oliguria may be prominent and may presage the acute renal failure of tubular necrosis.

The *edema* which characterizes preeclampsia resembles that of acute glomerulonephritis in its distribution and its pathogenesis. Edema may be absent when the toxemia has been explosive in its onset, as with convulsions. In other cases excessive weight gain with puffiness of the face, fingers, and ankles is the earliest symptom, antedating hypertension or proteinuria. Edema is usually contributed to by hypoalbuminemia; yet the serum albumin, though diminished, is not often below 2 g per 100 ml, and the edema of toxemia is not so dramatically relieved by injecting serum albumin as is the edema of nephrosis.

Signs of *cardiac failure* are present in a significant proportion of cases. With the appearance of edema, orthopnea and exertional dyspnea are often exaggerated. These symptoms frequently subside with bed rest, administration of digitalis, and diuresis. As in glomerulonephritis, the circulation time may be normal while the venous pressure is elevated.

Certain patients with severe toxemia, with or without eclamptic convulsions, may develop multiple clotting deficiencies or intravascular hemolysis, often following delivery, in a syndrome of *consumptive coagulopathy*.

Convulsions are often preceded by the development of hyperactive tendon reflexes and occasionally by epigastric pain. Though convulsions are often associated with marked hypertension, their appearance is not necessarily correlated with the height of the blood pressure. They may occur within the first day or two following delivery, as well as before or during labor. Petechial hemorrhages are observed in the brain in most patients who die of eclampsia.

Termination of the pregnancy is usually followed by prompt improvement of the mother. Proteinuria and hypertension usually disappear by the end of 1 or 2 weeks, though occasionally they persist longer. Nevertheless, in perhaps 35 percent of patients with preeclampsia, hypertensive vascular disease indistinguishable from essential hypertension develops later. The incidence of irreversible renal changes and of late hypertension increases significantly with the duration of the toxemia.

Treatment The most effective treatment is prompt emptying of the uterus. *Ganglionic blocking agents should not be used* to treat the hypertension, since they cross the placental barrier and may injure the fetus. Abrupt and severe hypotension induced by drugs may result in fetal distress and cause acute renal failure in the mother. In mild cases, hypertension may be treated with vasodilating agents such as reserpine, hydralazine, alpha-methyldopa, or magnesium sulfate. Edema can be eliminated with diuretics, bed rest, and a low salt diet. Simple sedatives, such as phenobarbital, help prevent convulsions, and parenteral barbiturates are useful in controlling seizures. When proteinuria and hypertension persist, however, it is doubtful that such symptomatic treatment prevents further vascular injury to the placenta and the kidneys. In such instances attempts to prolong the pregnancy for several weeks are associated with a high fetal mortality rate and the risk for the mother of permanent vascular disease.

POST-PARTUM RENAL FAILURE This is a rare condition, not clearly related to preeclampsia. Within several weeks after delivery of a normal child after a normal pregnancy, progressive azotemia develops, associated with microangiopathic hemolytic anemia. The blood pressure may be normal or elevated. The renal lesion resembles that of rapidly progressive malignant hypertension, even when hypertension is absent. Biopsy shows thrombosis in glomerular capillaries and necrotic foci in glomerular loops. The lumen of arterioles is greatly narrowed by intimal thickening of a loose, cellular type. Progression to oliguric renal failure is usually unrelenting, though early treatment with heparin has occasionally reversed the process.

REFERENCES

HARRISON CU et al: Clinical aspects of renal vein thrombosis. Quart J Med 25:285, 1956

KINCAID-SMITH P et al: The clinical course and pathology of hypertension with papilledema (malignant hypertension). Quart J Med 27:117, 1958

POLLACK VE, NETTLES JB: The kidney in toxemia of pregnancy: A clinical and pathological study based on renal biopsies. Medicine 19:469, 1960

ROBSON JS et al: Irreversible postpartum renal failure. Quart J Med 37:423, 1968

VASALLI P et al: The pathogenic role of fibrin deposition in the glomerular lesions of toxemia of pregnancy. J Exp Med 118:467, 1963

273 PYELONEPHRITIS AND OTHER INFECTIONS OF THE URINARY TRACT, INCLUDING PROSTATITIS

LAWRENCE R. FREEDMAN
FRANKLIN H. EPSTEIN

INTRODUCTION Bacterial infections of the urinary tract constitute one of the major medical problems encompassing all fields of practice. They are extremely common and some are notoriously resistant to treatment and are likely to recur. In most instances they do not produce serious renal disease (pyelonephritis) or serve as a source of bloodstream infection.

It is important to define *urinary tract infection* and pyelonephritis, since these terms do not have the same meanings for all physicians. Urinary tract infection is taken to exist when significant numbers of bacteria are detected in the urine. Pyelonephritis is considered to be disease resulting from the immediate or late effects of bacterial infection of the kidney. A person with pyelonephritis might or might not have a urinary tract infection at a given point in time. Similarly, a patient with a urinary tract infection might or might not have pyelonephritis, and might or might not develop it in the future.

The majority of persons with a urinary infection are unaware of its presence. Careful questioning and follow-up, however, reveal that symptoms have often occurred but are either intermittent or not recognized by the patient as arising from the urinary tract. These patients are sometimes referred to as having asymptomatic bacteriuria.

In many instances infections take the form of acute infectious disease; occasionally they are first recognized because of growth retardation in children, anemia, hypertension, or uremia—consequences of severe renal damage.

INFECTIONS OF THE URINARY TRACT

Etiology Many different microorganisms can infect the tissues and fluids of the urinary organs, but by far the commonest belong to the coli-aerogenes group of gram-negative bacilli. Other microorganisms which may be found include enterococci, *Proteus, Pseudomonas*, achromobacteria, staphylococci, and certain yeasts. Infection by other than the coli-aerogenes organisms is generally related to previous instrumentation of the urinary tract, with or without the use of chemotherapeutic agents. *Proteus* and *Pseudomonas* urinary infections, for example, are rarely seen except in patients who have had catheters or other instruments passed through the urethra. Staphylococci play a minor role in the total problem of urinary tract infection. Their detection has been overemphasized in the past because of the use of qualitative cultural techniques which did not permit their identification as contaminants. Viruses have been shown to be able to produce pyelonephritis in animals and may increase the susceptibility of the kidney to infection with coliform bacteria. In man, viruses are commonly recovered from the urine in subjects without evidence of urinary tract disease, but recently they have been implicated as a cause of hemorrhagic cystitis.

PATHOGENESIS Sources of infection The common urinary pathogens are usual inhabitants of the large intestine. In the majority of instances these bacteria gain access to the bladder cavity via the urethra. Under normal circumstances bladder urine is sterile and large numbers of bacteria placed in the bladder cavity are cleared rapidly in man and animals. However, the balance between bacterial multiplication rates and host defense mechanisms is a delicate one. In animals as many as 10,000,000 *Escherichia coli* may be cleared rapidly from the bladder cavity, whereas slight physiologic alterations may permit the survival of as few as 10 microorganisms which multiply rapidly and persist for prolonged periods.

The entire urinary tract must be looked upon as a single anatomic unit with a minute column of urine constantly maintaining a channel of communication between bladder and kidney. The ascent of bacteria within this channel from the bladder is the usual pathway for the majority of renal parenchymal infections. *Most patients with bacteria in the bladder urine do not, however, have evidence of renal parenchymal infection,* and the factors which determine whether the kidney will become infected are as a rule not clinically apparent.

Hematogenous pyelonephritis occurs most often in the late stages of terminal illness when there is general lowering of resistance to infection, either because of the primary illness or because of the use of potent agents which interfere with host antibacterial defenses. Staphylococcal pyelonephritis, however, may be seen following dissemination of bacteria from distant septic foci such as a carbuncle or osteomyelitis. Tuberculous pyelonephritis also results from bloodstream dissemination.

Associated conditions AGE AND SEX Urinary infections are found in about 1 to 4 percent of females from childhood to the childbearing age. The prevalence of infection then rises, with the greatest increment occurring at about age sixty, beyond which age infections are detected in 5 to 10 percent of women. In men, on the other hand, urinary infections are rare below age fifty, and even in older age groups are considerably less common than in women. There is evidence that race and socioeconomic status also influence the rates of infection.

PREGNANCY Depending on the socioeconomic status of the persons studied, urinary infections are detected in perhaps 4 to 8 percent of pregnant women. Another increment of infections occurs if bladder catheterization is performed at the time of or following delivery. The majority of infections during pregnancy are established before the time when dilation of the ureters occurs.

It has been suspected that urinary infections and pyelonephritis are more common in toxemia of pregnancy. However, data utilizing modern bacteriologic techniques do not support such a relation. There are, in addition, conflicting data concerning possible increased rates of prematurity and of newborn mortality in the offspring of women with urinary infections.

DIABETES MELLITUS Despite reports that pyelonephritis at autopsy is very common in diabetics, clinical surveys of hospital and nonhospital populations have failed to document any convincing difference in the prevalence of urinary tract infections in diabetic and nondiabetic persons of the same age. This suggests either that diabetics with urinary infections are more likely to develop pyelonephritis or that in the presence of severe vascular and glomerular lesions in diabetic kidneys, morphologic changes result which are similar to those of bacterial infection. The problem requires further study. Irritation of the vulva in women with heavy uncontrolled glucosuria probably increases the rate of false positive voided cultures and may predispose to bladder infection. When diabetic neuropathy has interfered with normal bladder function, persistent infections of the urine are frequent.

Urinary infection may produce difficulties in the regulation of carbohydrate metabolism and may precipitate diabetic acidosis. The risk of additional renal disease caused by infection in persons already subject to severe vascular and glomerular disease is, of course, to be avoided whenever possible. Diabetics are also likely to develop necrotizing papillitis, a fulminating form of renal disease usually associated with infection. It is likely that more slowly developing forms of papillary sclerosis also occur in diabetics.

OBSTRUCTIVE UROPATHY Any impediment to the free flow of urine—tumor, stricture, or stone—results in hydronephrosis and a greatly increased frequency of urinary tract infection. Infection superimposed on urinary tract obstruction may lead to the rapid destruction of renal tissue. It is of utmost importance, therefore, when infection is present, to repair obstructive lesions. On the other hand, when minor degrees of obstruction are present and not progressive and when this obstruction is not associated with infection, great caution must be exercised in attempting surgical correction. The introduction of infection in such patients may be more damaging than uncorrected minor obstructions which do not significantly impair renal function.

INSTRUMENTATION Infection of the lower urinary passages is sometimes initiated by bacteria carried on catheters or other instruments being passed through the urethra into the bladder. Although the risk is small in normal people, it undoubtedly rises considerably in patients in hospital. Indwelling catheterization for 24 to 48 hr is usually accompanied by the initiation of a urinary infection, unless careful attention is directed to the proper use of closed drainage systems or the use of antibacterial lavage of the bladder and drainage system. These special techniques considerably lessen the risk of short-term catheterization (up to 1 week), but even with these precautions, infection rates steadily increase thereafter.

RENAL DISEASE AND HYPERTENSION Experimental and clinical evidence indicates that various renal diseases increase the susceptibility of the kidney to infection. In addition, persons with abnormal urinalyses or hypertension are likely to have had some diagnostic procedures involving urinary tract instrumentation and thereby providing access of bacteria to the urinary tract. A careful medical history is essential but often not sufficient to distinguish cause from effect.

In surveys of nonhospital populations it has been found that mean blood pressure levels are likely to be slightly higher in women with urinary infections than in those without infections. The significance of this relation remains to be determined, and the data are not sufficient to ascertain whether rising blood pressure or urinary infection is primary. Too few infections have been found in men in these surveys to study the problem in that sex.

NEUROGENIC BLADDER DYSFUNCTION Interference with the nerve supply to the bladder, as in spinal cord injury, tabes dorsalis, multiple sclerosis, etc., is likely to be associated with urinary tract infection. The infection may be initiated by the use of catheters for bladder drainage and is favored by the prolonged standing of urine in the bladder. Additional factors which often operate in these patients are bone demineralization due to immobilization, causing hypercalciuria, calculus formation, and obstructive uropathy.

EXPERIMENTAL EVIDENCE Urinary tract infections can

be produced in experimental animals by several methods, including inoculation of bacteria into the pelvis or substance of the kidney, or into the bladder urine. Certain organisms such as *Pseudomonas*, enterococci, staphylococci, and monilias are capable of causing infection in the normal kidney when they are injected by the intravenous route. Coliform organisms will not do this as a rule, unless intrarenal hydronephrosis or acute obstruction of the ureter is present. It has also been shown that the renal damage resulting from a virus or staphylococcal infection can render the kidney susceptible to infection by colon bacilli injected intravenously.

The frequent association of urinary tract infection with an obstructive lesion has led to the widespread view that stasis of urinary flow is a prime factor in the development of infection. In support of this is the fact that urine is a good medium for growth of bacteria; hence, prolonged opportunity for multiplication during slow passage along the tract would provide a heavier inoculum to which the kidneys and other tissues of the tract are exposed. The effect of increased hydrostatic pressure may be an additional factor to explain the association between obstruction and urinary infection. To assess the relative importance of stasis and increased pressure is difficult, since slowing of flow is an inevitable accompaniment of obstruction and dilatation of the passages above the level of obstruction. Even when a profuse diuresis is obtained in a patient with a partially obstructed urinary tract, this seldom if ever achieves cure of infection, whereas relief of the obstruction, with or without diuresis, may be followed by subsidence of infection. Even if the urinary infection is not cured, relief of obstruction materially reduces the risk of renal damage.

The pathogenesis of urinary tract infection is mediated by the interaction between the tissues and the urine itself, and it seems clear that infection beginning in one can spread to the other. The pathogenesis of chronic nonobstructive pyelonephritis is not well understood. Chronic pyelonephritis may be an indolent process consisting of many isolated microabscesses, some of them within single tubules. Here bacterial growth may be slow, phagocytosis inefficient, and antibacterial drugs incapable of acting optimally. Yet such areas may, from time to time, discharge their contents into the urinary passages, affording opportunity for rapid bacterial multiplication and spread to other parts of the system. In the urine phagocytosis is probably less effective than it is in tissues, and elimination of bacteria may call for more than simple bacteriostasis. This line of reasoning leads to the conclusion that optimal results in drug treatment require the use of an agent or a combination of agents capable of killing the infecting bacteria both in tissues and in the urine. However, there is no clinical or experimental proof to support this contention.

Clinical and experimental evidence has shown that the papillae and medulla of the kidney are particularly susceptible to bacterial infection. This is where bacterial multiplication begins in animals with pyelonephritis, and in this normally hypertonic environment host defense mechanisms such as leukocyte migration, phagocytosis, and complement activity are likely to be impaired. In addition, forms of bacteria with defective cell walls such as spheroplasts or protoplasts (a consequence of the action of antibiotics or complement and antibody) can survive in the hypertonic environment of the renal medulla, whereas they would be expected to die in tissues isotonic to plasma. Thus, in patients without urinary obstruction, decreasing the osmolarity of the papillae by drinking large quantities of water would be expected to increase the resistance of the kidney to infection. However, experiments testing the effect of water diuresis on urinary infections vary in outcome, depending on animal species, test organism, means by which bacteria gain access to the urinary tract, and presence of underlying renal disease. In man, water diuresis may temporarily lower the concentration of bacteria in the urine, but the long-term consequences of water diuresis on the natural history of urinary infections or on the outcome of antibiotic treatment is unknown.

CYSTITIS

This is the name used by many physicians to refer to urinary tract infection with pathognomonic local symptoms: frequency and urgency of micturition, and burning pain felt in the urethra during and immediately following the act. Prominent systemic manifestations of infection, such as fever above 101°F, muscular pain, nausea, vomiting, and prostration, should cause the physician to suspect concomitant infection in the kidney, prostate, or some other part of the body. Even in the absence of systemic manifestations of infection, it is usually not possible to be certain that infection is limited to the bladder area in patients with cystitis.

ACUTE PYELONEPHRITIS

The symptoms of acute pyelonephritis generally develop rapidly over a period of a few hours or a day or two. The characteristics are aching pain in the lumbar region, and fever which may be high (103 to 105°F), often with shaking chills. There may be nausea, vomiting, and diarrhea or, occasionally, constipation. Dysuria and frequency are also common.

On physical examination, in addition to fever and some generalized tenderness of the muscles, the key finding is tenderness on deep pressure in one or both of the costovertebral areas or on bimanual palpation of the kidney region. Occasionally, this sign is absent.

Except in individuals with papillary necrosis or urinary obstruction, the manifestations of acute pyelonephritis usually subside within days, even without specific antibacterial therapy. The patient becomes symptom-free although laboratory tests may show that bacteriuria with or without pyuria is still present. When pyelonephritis is severe, fever subsides more slowly and may not disappear for several days, even after appropriate antibiotic treatment has been started.

Most persons recover completely and permanently after an attack of acute pyelonephritis, but in a considerable proportion of cases there are repeated attacks, at irregular intervals, sometimes over a period of many years; between these attacks the patient may be symptom-free. Bacteriuria and pyuria are often demonstrable during these symptom-free intervals. Infection in any part of the urinary tract is capable of subclinical continuation for months or years, during which a patient may have no symptoms and may live an apparently normal life, even though urine cultures provide continuing evidence of active infection.

LABORATORY FINDINGS In acute pyelonephritis there is a *polymorphonuclear leukocytosis*, whereas in patients with localized or few symptoms the white blood cell picture is normal. The urine sediment usually reveals numerous leukocytes occurring singly, in clumps, and in casts, and occasionally some red blood cells. Sometimes in cystitis there is gross hematuria. The persistence of hematuria after localized or generalized symptoms of infection have subsided is unusual and should alert one to the possibility of a stone, a tumor, or tuberculosis within the genitourinary tract. In chronic infections of low-grade activity, diagnosis may be very difficult on the basis of urine sediment. There may be a few pus cells, or they may be found only intermittently during repeated urinalyses.

Enumeration of the numbers of bacteria in the urine is the most important diagnostic procedure. In symptomatic infections of the urinary tract, bacteria are virtually always easily demonstrable in the urine in large numbers. The absence of easily demonstrable bacteria in uncentrifuged bladder urine indicates that urinary infection is not likely to explain the patient's symptoms. Quantitative estimation of the number of bacteria in the urine, as a rule, makes it possible to distinguish contaminants (from the anterior urethra or elsewhere) from bacteria multiplying in the bladder urine and is, therefore, essential for the interpretation of urine cultures.

A rough quantitative estimate of the situation can be made by means of Gram's stain or microscopic examination of uncentrifuged, freshly voided urine. If bacteria can be found by this method, it may be assumed that the number present is approximately 100,000 per milliliter. Since bacteria multiply in urine, when bacterial infection is present they usually achieve concentrations in excess of 100,000 viable units per milliliter. In culturing voided urine specimens contamination is common. It is essential, therefore, to examine two or three urine specimens bacteriologically before starting treatment in patients with few or no symptoms. In patients who are sufficiently ill to require prompt antibiotic therapy, a single quantitative estimate of the number of bacteria in the urine combined with symptoms typical of infection is sufficient to make the diagnosis of urinary infection. If fewer than 10,000 viable bacterial units per milliliter are cultured from a voided urine specimen, they are likely to be of no significance. If 10,000 to 100,000 are present, no positive conclusion can be drawn. Since the large numbers of bacteria in the bladder urine are due in part to bacterial multiplication during residence in the bladder cavity, samples of urine from the ureters or renal pelves might contain considerably fewer bacteria and yet indicate infection. If the urine contains antibacterial substances or if the pH is low (about 5), inhibition of bacterial multiplication will also result in lower numbers of bacteria in the presence of the infection. For this reason, antiseptic solutions should not be used in washing the periurethral area prior to collection of the urine specimen.

Intravenous pyelograms may be of value in the diagnosis of pyelonephritis and may show asymmetry between the kidneys, as judged by their size and the density of the renal shadows. This is a reflection of the patchy distribution of the pyelonephritis lesion. Careful radiographic studies will show hypotony of the calyxes, pelvis, and ureters in a high proportion of these cases. Particular attention should be paid to papillary deformities and corresponding cortical scars. Needle biopsy of the kidney is of limited value for demonstrating pyelonephritis because of the spotty distribution of the lesions.

TREATMENT Treatment is based on the concept of the urinary tract as a complex system in which infection introduced into any one part may spread. An essential principle in management is to consider what factors may be contributing to the infection, such as obstruction, faulty bladder innervation, etc. Relief of obstruction may be an essential factor in eradicating the infection (see Chap. 274).

The best results from antibacterial agents are obtained when treatment is individualized. In view of the varying conditions under which bacteria grow in urine and in urinary tract tissues, it seems probable that the ideal chemotherapeutic attack is one which is capable of bactericidal, not simply bacteriostatic, action. The synthetic penicillins meet this requirement. The sulfonamides are splendid for lower urinary tract infections. Determination of possible synergistic or antagonistic effects of combinations of agents on the bacteria to be attacked is occasionally necessary. Enterococcus infections may be treated with ampicillin. For *Proteus* infections, the antibiotics most likely to be beneficial are gentamicin, kanamycin, ampicillin, cephalothin, and penicillin in massive doses. For *Pseudomonas* infections, gentamicin, carbenicillin, polymyxin, or colistin may be required (see Chap. 125).

There is now good evidence that lower urinary tract infections can be treated with short courses of antibiotics but that upper tract infections do better following long courses. There is a clear-cut difference in the results of the treatment of both these types of infection.

Whatever the *length of treatment*, it is essential to obtain follow-up urine cultures after discontinuing treatment, to avoid overlooking smoldering asymptomatic infection, with its potentialities for eventual development of serious disease. The minimum number of follow-up cultures should be carried out approximately 1 to 3 weeks, 2 to 3 months, and 1 year after stopping treatment. Any recurrence of symptoms should serve as an indication for urinalysis and culture. It is wise to avoid catheter specimens for urine examinations, since catheterization may actually cause reinfection of the urinary tract. With proper care it is possible to obtain suitable "clean-voided" specimens of urine from females as well as males. Since bacteria multiply rapidly in urine, a specimen should be cultured or refrigerated immediately. Specimens kept at about 4°C for as long as 1 to 4 weeks are still suitable for bacteriologic culture.

It has now been established that many cases of

recurrent urinary infection can be managed effectively with very low dosages of several antibacterial agents given over a prolonged period of time. As little as 50 to 100 mg nitrofurantoin or 0.5 to 1.0 g nalidixic acid or 0.5 to 1.0 g of a soluble short-acting sulfonamide given at bedtime, with perhaps another dose upon arising, may keep the urine sterile in patients who up to the time of treatment had been subject to recurrent symptomatic infections at monthly intervals. Even patients with nonprogressive urinary obstruction, neurogenic bladder, or staghorn calculi may respond dramatically to such treatment. In most instances discontinuing antibiotics is associated with prompt reappearance of bacteriuria or recurrence of infection. These antibacterial agents interfere with bacterial multiplication sufficiently to permit host defenses to be effective.

PROGNOSIS It is usually possible to obtain a dramatic cessation of symptoms in the treatment of acute urinary infection not complicated by other diseases. The potentially dangerous feature is persistence of relatively asymptomatic infection. It is not possible to state which patients with urinary infections will eventually suffer renal damage and which patients may have persistent infection without significant damage to the kidney. There is little doubt that patients with underlying urinary abnormalities such as obstruction and stone and patients with conditions capable of producing primary papillary injury (sickle-cell disease, excessive ingestion of phenacetin-containing analgesic mixtures, diabetes mellitus, hypertensive or occlusive vascular disease) are at greater risk. In the absence of these underlying conditions, however, the evidence currently available indicates that renal damage is only rarely attributable to urinary infections in patients followed for as long as 5 to 10 years. One must exercise considerable caution, therefore, in recommending diagnostic or therapeutic procedures without proved benefit and with some degree of risk in this category of patients.

In patients with some of the complicating diseases mentioned above (particularly neurogenic bladder, irremediable obstruction, or multiple stones), eradication of urinary tract infection is exceedingly difficult, if not impossible. Even here, however, the extent of the process can be minimized by comprehensive care, including surgical measures, prevention of stone formation, and appropriate chemotherapy guided by reliable laboratory procedures.

CHRONIC PYELONEPHRITIS

Chronic pyelonephritis is that variety of chronic interstitial nephritis resulting from bacterial infection of the kidney. The recognition of the nonspecificity of traditional morphologic diagnostic criteria has led to a serious reevaluation of the generally accepted concepts of this disorder. In contrast to the state of affairs pertaining to urinary tract infections, for which simple diagnostic criteria are available, the diagnosis of chronic pyelonephritis is reached only after careful consideration of various nonpathognomonic clinical and pathologic findings. Reliable data are difficult to obtain and are too often available for only a fraction of the patient's illness. As a consequence there are no reliable data concerning the prevalence of chronic nonobstructive pyelonephritis.

ETIOLOGY Urinary obstruction is a common accompaniment of chronic pyelonephritis, but in a large proportion of cases obstruction cannot be demonstrated anatomically. Most patients with renal lesions which fulfill criteria for chronic pyelonephritis at autopsy have sterile kidney cultures and were not known to have had clinical episodes of bacterial urinary infection. These observations have stimulated investigations into factors other than obstruction which make the kidney susceptible to infection and into other injuries which may result in morphologic changes in the kidney resembling those produced by bacterial infection.

PATHOLOGY The kidneys are frequently asymmetric in size. The parenchyma is scarred, and the surface is coarsely and irregularly pitted. In many areas glomeruli and tubules are completely replaced by connective tissue, which may contain lymphocytes and plasma cells. Foci of active interstitial inflammation may be seen throughout the medulla and cortex, and leukocyte casts are found in some tubules. Other tubules are dilated and contain large amounts of homogeneous eosinophilic material (colloid casts). Most glomeruli appear relatively normal in comparison with the nearby atrophic tubular and inflammatory interstitial changes. The capsule of many glomeruli is disproportionately thickened and fibrotic in contrast to the relative integrity of the Malpighian tufts. Some glomerular loops may be thickened or hyalinized, probably as a result of vascular changes proximally; in the cortex there are clusters of fibrotic glomeruli, especially within the wedges of atrophic areas. Often, distinctive inflammatory changes in the pelvic mucosa are lacking. A proliferative endarteritis is usually present, most marked in areas of chronic inflammation. More generalized and severe vascular changes develop with the onset of hypertension.

Even at autopsy, the diagnosis of chronic pyelonephritis is often not clear-cut. None of the foregoing changes is pathognomonic of chronic infection of the kidneys, though when taken together they are useful in suggesting the diagnosis. Similar morphologic features may be encountered as a result of many diseases, including the nephropathy of chronic potassium depletion, nephrocalcinosis, chronic poisoning with analgesic mixtures, primary vascular disease of the kidneys, obstruction, diabetes mellitus, and tubular necrosis. The kidney responds similarly to a variety of insults. When the damage is principally interstitial, the reaction will take the form of what is called acute or chronic interstitial nephritis. Chronic pyelonephritis is chronic interstitial nephritis resulting from bacterial infections. Since urinary infections are common and frequently initiated by instrumentation of the urinary tract in attempting to diagnose renal disease, the determination of the contribution of infection in any particular patient with renal disease may not be possible.

CLINICAL FEATURES The original description of Longcope[1] is worth quoting:

Starting with a pyelitis in childhood, an infection of the urinary tract during pregnancy, or, in rare instances, an acute pyelonephritis, there may be from time to time attacks of unexplained fever, with or without slight or fairly severe pain in the lumbar regions. These attacks are often accompanied by the passage of cloudy urine. Occasionally there is a history of albuminuria of many years' duration. Often there is a story of malnutrition or sometimes of retarded growth in children, leading occasionally to rickety deformities. In some instances, the progress of the disease is, for years, symptomless.

Early symptoms are particularly infrequent in the group with bilaterally atrophic, nonobstructed kidneys. A history of acute pyelitis in childhood may be especially difficult to obtain because the symptoms are mainly gastrointestinal, the physical signs are scanty, and pyuria is difficult to demonstrate; a history of persistent enuresis is sometimes the only helpful clue.

Patients often, therefore, come to the attention of the physician only when renal failure or hypertension has made its appearance, or because of the accidental discovery of proteinuria. However, proteinuria is characteristically absent or minimal in pyelonephritis. Fatigue and lassitude associated with anemia may be the presenting complaints. If renal failure is severe, nausea and vomiting or breathlessness may be present. Edema is rare, and when it occurs it is a result of heart failure.

Many patients with chronic pyelonephritis develop hypertension at some time in the course of their illness. It has been suggested that this is related to the contraction of scar tissue and to endarteritis obliterans with focal renal ischemia, rather than to diffuse renal damage. Occasionally, the blood pressure may become elevated long before there is measurable impairment of renal function, and only a persistently positive urine culture or characteristic changes in the intravenous pyelogram may distinguish the clinical picture from that of "essential" or "malignant" hypertension.

In general, glomerular filtration and renal blood flow decline together and proportionally as the disease progresses. As might be expected, there is usually more disparity between the function of the right and left kidneys than is generally the case in diffuse diseases of the kidney such as glomerulonephritis or nephrosclerosis. Maximum concentrating ability tends to become impaired earlier in the course of the disease than in patients with chronic glomerulonephritis. Occasional patients with advanced azotemia may excrete a urine hypotonic to plasma, even when they are dehydrated. Many patients are unable to conserve sodium on a low-salt diet, even when only mild azotemia is present. Polyuria and nocturia are prominent in such cases. Hyperchloremic acidosis as a result of impaired renal excretion of acid and reabsorption of bicarbonate is more often a feature of chronic pyelonephritis than of glomerulonephritis. Proteinuria is usually less than 2 g (rarely as much as 4 to 6 g) daily, except when congestive heart failure supervenes.

[1] *Longcope WT, Winkenwerder WL: Clinical features of the contracted kidney due to pyelonephritis. Bull Johns Hopkins Hosp 53:255, 1933*

Careful examination of the *urinary sediment* may be the key to diagnosis. Leukocytes may be numerous or infrequent, but the appearance of white blood cell casts should alert the physician to the possibility of chronic pyelonephritis. Bacteria and pus cells may be present on the fresh stained smear but often appear intermittently or not at all in the chronic stage of the disease. In fact the urine sediment may be normal, and, especially with a dilute urine of fixed specific gravity, albuminuria may not be detected. On intravenous or retrograde pyelography, distortion, flattening, and reduction in size of the renal pelves can be seen. The renal cortices may be narrowed unevenly and the underlying pyramid distorted or destroyed, producing "blunting" of the calyces. The absence of roentgenographic changes does not, however, rule out chronic pyelonephritis.

When pyelonephritis is not accompanied by hypertension, the course may be prolonged and compatible with comfortable and useful life even after considerable encroachment upon renal function. In perhaps no other disease of the kidneys can fluctuations in renal function be so marked or so frequent. During acute infections or episodes of dehydration, renal decompensation may progress to the stage of advanced uremia; yet the patient may be able to recover and carry on with adequate though impaired renal function for years. Nonspecific complaints of fatigue, anorexia, and weakness often remit remarkably when the urine is sterilized by an appropriate course of antibiotics and when acidosis, dehydration, and salt depletion are adequately treated.

The problem of *recurrent infections*, sometimes with resistant bacteria, is important and unsolved. An effort should be made to treat urinary tract obstruction and to improve bladder emptying, when residual urine is present. Reducing the bacterial population of bladder urine by the prolonged administration of urinary antiseptics may offer some hope for halting the indolent progression of the disease.

Even when one kidney appears small and the other normal in size, pyelonephritis is in most instances bilateral. Nephrectomy which is undertaken in the hope of eradicating infection is generally doomed to failure. Excision of a hydronephrotic, pus-filled renal shell will, however, sometimes permit a successful therapeutic attack on infection in the opposite kidney.

This general view of the frequency of asymptomatic destruction of the kidney in pyelonephritis may be incorrect, since some of the patients may have had some other form of chronic interstitial nephritis, rather than pyelonephritis. Proper understanding of the problem requires continued careful study with clear recognition of the possible error of traditional concepts.

PAPILLARY NECROSIS

When severe infection of the renal pyramids is present in association with vascular diseases of the kidney or urinary tract obstruction, renal papillary necrosis is likely to result. Patients with diabetes, sickle-cell hemoglobin, chronic alcoholism, and vascular disease seem peculiarly susceptible to this complication. Hematuria, pain in the flank or abdomen, chills, and fever are the most common presenting symptoms. Acute renal failure with oliguria or anuria sometimes occurs. Rarely, sloughing of a pyramid may take place without symptoms in a patient with chronic urinary infection, and the diagnosis is made when the necrotic tissue is passed in the urine or identified as a "ring shadow" on pyelography. If renal function deteriorates suddenly in a diabetic patient or one with chronic obstruction, this diagnosis should be entertained, even in the absence of fever or pain.

The chronic overuse of drug mixtures containing phenacetin and perhaps other analgesics predisposes to necrotizing papillitis which may be unassociated with renal infection or obstruction and which may present the picture of slowly progressive renal insufficiency. This problem is much more common than generally recognized, and diagnosis requires careful attention to historical information obtained from the patient.

RENAL ABSCESS AND PERINEPHRIC ABSCESS
(See Chap. 126)

PROSTATITIS

This term is loosely used to designate various inflammatory conditions affecting the prostate. These include acute and chronic infections with specific bacteria and, more commonly, instances where signs and symptoms of prostatic inflammation are present but no specific organisms can be detected. Patients in this category usually have low-back pain and perineal or testicular discomfort. They may have microscopic pyuria or hematuria without any other evidence of genitourinary disease. Such patients are generally treated symptomatically by prostatic massage and warm sitz baths, but many of them are given antibiotics, with variable results. In some cases infection may be secondary to the T strain of *Mycoplasma* which has been incriminated in the pathogenesis of urethritis.

ACUTE BACTERIAL PROSTATITIS This disease generally affects young male adults when it occurs spontaneously, but it may be associated with an indwelling urethral catheter. It is characterized by fever, chills, dysuria, and a tense or boggy, extremely tender prostate. Palpation of the prostate is the key to diagnosis. The infection is generally due to one of the common urinary tract pathogens or *Staphylococcus aureus*, and the response to antibiotics is usually prompt. The long-term prognosis is good, although in some instances, acute infection may result in abscess formation and a residual chronic bacterial prostatitis. Since the advent of antibiotics, the frequency of acute bacterial prostatitis has diminished markedly, and it is now an uncommon cause of acute urinary tract infection. Many so-called cases of "acute prostatitis" are probably posterior urethritis. Antibiotics penetrate poorly into prostatic fluid.

CHRONIC BACTERIAL PROSTATITIS This entity is less well defined. Symptoms are usually absent, the prostate feels normal on palpation, and although many white blood cells may be seen in the urinary sediment, results of conventional bacteriologic studies are negative. Chronic bacterial prostatitis is characterized by the presence of small numbers of bacteria which may be cultured from the expressed prostatic secretion. The presence of these bacteria can be determined only by careful quantitative bacteriologic techniques when the bladder urine is sterile. The usual symptoms of frequency and dysuria occur when infection spreads to the bladder urine, but infection confined to the prostate is asymptomatic. Antibiotics are of limited value in eradicating the foci of chronic infection in the prostate, even though they may relieve the symptoms of the acute exacerbations promptly. The relative ineffectiveness of antimicrobials is due in part to the poor penetration of most antibiotics into the prostate because the low pH which prevails in this organ precludes solubility of most drugs. The macrolide group of drugs (erythromycin, oleandomycin) do enter the prostatic secretions, but these agents are generally ineffective against gram-negative organisms. These patients should be treated with prolonged courses of antimicrobials with a view toward suppressing symptoms and keeping the bladder urine sterile.

Urinary infections are much less common in men than in women, perhaps because of the antibacterial properties of prostatic fluid. The pattern of recurrent bladder infection in the male with chronic bacterial prostatitis is clinically not very different from that seen in the recurrent cystourethritis of the female. It has been suggested that this pattern of infection in women is due to chronic bacterial infection of the paraurethral glands and ducts, which are in fact vestigial remnants of the prostate.

REFERENCES

FREEDMAN LR: Urinary tract infection, pyelonephritis and other forms of chronic interstitial nephritis, in *Diseases of the Kidney*, 2d ed., eds MB Strauss, LG Welt, Boston: Little, Brown, 1971

KINCAID-SMITH P, FAIRLEY, KF: *Renal Infection and Renal Scarring*, Melbourne: Mercedes Publishing Services, 1970

MEARES EM, STAMEY TA: Bacteriologic localization patterns in bacterial prostatitis and urethritis. Invest Urol 5:492, 1968

NORDEN CW, KASS EH: Bacteriuria of pregnancy: A critical appraisal. Ann Rev Med 19:431, 1968

O'GRADY F, BRUMFITT W: *Urinary Tract Infection*, London: Oxford, 1968

274 OBSTRUCTIVE UROPATHY

BERNARD LYTTON
FRANKLIN H. EPSTEIN

OBSTRUCTION OF THE BLADDER OUTLET The importance of obstruction as a cause of renal failure is indicated by the fact that a considerable percentage of deaths from uremia may be attributed wholly or in part to obstructive disease. Obstruction of urinary flow occurs most frequently at or below the bladder outlet. The principal causes are meatal stenosis, congenital or acquired urethral strictures, urethral valves, bladder neck contracture, prostatic and urethral carcinoma, and, most commonly, benign overgrowth of the prostate.

Prostatic obstruction may cause frequency, slowing of the stream, hesitancy, urgency, terminal dribbling, pain, and hematuria. Sometimes, however, progressive obstruction occurs with few or no urinary symptoms and the patient comes to the physician with signs of uremia or a palpable mass in the lower part of the abdomen due to a distended bladder which may be mistaken for some other abdominal tumor. It is estimated that some 30 to 50 percent of men will develop symptoms of prostatism after the age of fifty, but only 1 in 10 will require surgical relief of obstruction before reaching the age of eighty.

Obstruction of the bladder neck is a late symptom in *carcinoma* of the *prostate,* since this usually arises in the posterior part of the gland. The disease often goes unrecognized until distant metastases or obstruction of the ureters develop.

An obstructive lesion of the bladder outlet may be closely mimicked by neurogenic vesical dysfunction, as in tabes, multiple sclerosis, or diabetic neuropathy. The effect of minor degrees of obstruction of the vesical neck is commonly magnified by neurogenic vesical dysfunction (see Chap. 46).

Although bladder neck obstruction is usually signaled by dysuria, frequency, or incontinence, it is important to remember that nausea and vomiting may be the only outward signs of a distended bladder in a bedridden patient.

Chronic obstruction of the bladder outlet in children is frequently associated with *vesicoureteral reflux.* Reflux of urine from bladder to ureters in association with infection leads to progressive dilatation of the upper part of the urinary tract and chronic pyelonephritis. Some patients who have vesicoureteral reflux without any bacteriologic or histologic evidence of infection have kidneys with the radiologic and pathologic appearances associated with chronic pyelonephritis. The renal parenchymal disease in these cases is often progressive and does not appear to be improved by ureteral reimplantation. It is unclear whether the reflux is responsible for the parenchymal damage or whether it is merely an associated condition, since reflux may occur in normal individuals, particularly children, without infection. In adults with obstruction of the bladder outlet, on the other hand, reflux occurs less commonly and is detectable in only about 10 percent of cases. Ureteral reflux may also be caused by anatomic abnormalities of the ureterovesical junction. Acute cystitis can cause reflux which resolves completely after control of the infection. Reflux can therefore be caused by infection of the bladder even when obstruction is not present, and in that case perhaps contributes to the development of parenchymal renal damage.

URETERAL OBSTRUCTION *Obstruction of the ureters* can be caused by calculi, cancer, injury, congenital anomalies, or retroperitoneal fibrosis. Obstruction of a single ureter may pass unrecognized unless colic or bleeding occurs, as with a calculus (see Chap. 275). Anomalies of the ureteropelvic junction, often associated with aberrant vessels or congenital bands, produce hydronephrosis through the mechanism of partial obstruction. Sometimes this is intermittent, especially when the kidney is excessively mobile. Intermittent obstruction of the pelvicalyceal system can also be produced by calculi. Pain in the flank is the usual complaint, but the discomfort may be more vague, referred to the upper part of the abdomen, and confused with gastrointestinal disease. The pains of intermittent hydronephrosis may be precipitated by exercise or drinking large amounts of fluid, and relieved by recumbency. Pyelographic x-rays taken in the erect position and during forced diuresis are helpful in diagnosis.

Congenital neuromuscular abnormalities of the lower part of the ureter, producing functional obstruction, may give rise to massive dilatation of the ureter, which can be corrected by excision of the lower segment, with ureteral revision and reimplantation. This sometimes occurs bilaterally in infants, resulting in hydroureteronephrosis, and may cause chronic uremia and failure to thrive.

Retrocaval ureter, a developmental anomaly, presents a typical J-shaped deformity of the upper part of the ureter on pyelographic examination and is often associated with obstruction. Hypertrophy and dilatation of the ovarian vein, usually the right, may cause partial obstruction of the ureter at the pelvic brim. Temporary ureteral dilatation is associated with pregnancy and may persist for many months post partum.

After *pelvic surgery,* vascular or mechanical injury to a ureter may cause stenosis. Obstruction developing several months after treatment of a pelvic tumor may be the first indication of a recurrence of the growth.

Bilateral ureteral obstruction is most commonly due to malignant disease, either from local extension of tumors of the pelvic organs or from metastases in the retroperitoneal lymphatics. Occlusion of both ureters may also be caused by calculi.

Retroperitoneal fibrosis is a chronic inflammation of unknown cause which involves the cellular tissue surrounding the great vessels in the lower lumbar area. It has been related in some instances to the taking of methysergide derivatives (Sansert) for the relief of migraine. The resulting fibrous constriction may obstruct the vena cava and occasionally the aorta. Rarely the process spreads to the upper part of the abdomen and mediastinum, leading to obstruction of the duodenum, bile ducts, and superior vena cava. It frequently involves the midportion of the ureters, which become drawn medially. Ureteral compression leads to hydronephrosis and finally to azotemia. Patients, usually males of middle age, complain of abdominal and low-back pain, anorexia, weakness, weight loss, and fever. Urinary symptoms include frequency, hematuria, and, depending on the degree of obstruction, either polyuria or anuria. Ureterolysis with lateral transposition or intraperitoneal placement of the ureters is the most effective treatment for the urinary obstruction. Occasional spontaneous remissions have been recorded. The condition must be distinguished from lymphomas and metastatic malignant diseases which involve the retroperitoneal tissues.

PATHOLOGIC PHYSIOLOGY Complete obstruction of a ureter causes eventual atrophy of its kidney while the opposite kidney undergoes a compensatory increase in growth and function. Failure of these compensatory changes to occur indicates severe disease in the contralateral kidney, although some degree of functional improvement may occur in the presence of a moderate degree of parenchymal damage.

Increases in ureteral pressure produce a fall in glomerular filtration rate and renal blood flow and impairment of renal concentrating capacity. Partial obstruction of the urethra or of both ureters may therefore result in progressive azotemia associated with an apparently adequate or even excessive urinary output. Polyuria is the result of loss of renal concentrating power from tubular damage by the obstruction. When the urinary passage is greatly narrowed, small changes in the size of the lumen produce large alterations in flow and in pressure proximal to the obstruction. *Unexplained wide fluctuations in blood urea or urinary output in patients with azotemia should always raise the question of partial urinary obstruction.*

When obstruction is relieved, a profuse obligatory diuresis may follow. The urine is dilute and alkaline, and contains much sodium. This is caused in part by an osmotic diuresis, resulting from excretion of the large amounts of urea which have accumulated during obstruction. In addition, the capacity of the renal tubules to reabsorb water and salt and to excrete acid is impaired as a result of increased back leak of sodium from the interstitial fluid into the dilated tubules. There may also be an increase in secretion of potassium consequent to the dehydration. Adequate amounts of both water and salt must be provided to avoid dehydration during the early postobstructive period. *Rapid dehydration is probably responsible for some cases of shock following sudden decompression of an obstructed bladder.*

In an occasional patient with chronic obstruction, concentrating power may be so severely impaired that urine more dilute than plasma is excreted, even after vasopressin is given. The state of nephrogenic diabetes insipidus is often reversible when obstruction is relieved. The special susceptibility of the obstructed kidney to infection is discussed in the previous chapter on pyelonephritis (Chap. 273).

CLINICAL FEATURES The distended bladder is often felt as a cystic swelling arising out of the pelvis, in the lower part of the abdomen. It may be displaced to one side, either from an asymmetric enlargement or by a large diverticulum. The bladder may be difficult to detect in obese individuals or when the abdominal muscles are poorly relaxed, and the passage of a urethral catheter to establish the diagnosis may be a lifesaving procedure. Even though on rectal palpation the prostate appears normal or only slightly enlarged, it may still be causing obstruction. Conversely, a considerable degree of prostatic hypertrophy may be present without any obstruction. The important factor is the degree of distortion of the bladder neck and intraurethral anatomy. The diagnosis of partial obstruction of the urinary tract may be suggested by the pattern of excretion of dye, following an intravenous pyelogram with a "bladder holdup."

Urinary obstruction may mimic or complicate uremia due to chronic parenchymal renal disease. In the bedridden patient with obtunded senses, unrecognized functional difficulty in bladder emptying (often precipitated by sedatives, but treatable with bethanechol chloride or Prostigmine) may cause rapid and otherwise inexplicable deterioration. If an obstruction is suspected, delineation of the upper part of the urinary tract is necessary to establish the diagnosis. This can be achieved in some cases by injecting large doses of contrast material for excretory urography and tomography; if this fails, retrograde pyelography is required. The absence of residual urine in the bladder after spontaneous voiding, or of any evidence of hydronephrosis, makes it unlikely that obstruction contributes to azotemia. Catheterization to obtain a single urine specimen for culture and measurement of residual urine is important.

Obstruction of the bladder or ureters does not usually cause hypertension unless it is complicated by renal scarring and atrophy. Simple relief of obstruction, therefore, cannot be expected to cure chronic high blood pressure when this is present in cases of hydronephrosis, although improvement has been reported in some instances.

Patients with obstructive uropathy usually improve remarkably with drainage. The greater part of the recovery of renal function occurs within 2 to 3 weeks, but some improvement may continue slowly for several months after this. During the period of drainage, recurrent infections of the kidneys and the bloodstream remain as potential hazards. After occlusion of one ureter lasting four or more months, recovery of function is unlikely, especially if the opposite kidney has undergone compensatory growth. It may, however, retain its potential for recovery for a long time, but this would become apparent only after loss of or injury to the normal kidney.

REFERENCES

Bricker NS, Klahr S: Obstructive Uropathy, in *Diseases of the Kidney,* eds MB Strauss, LW Welt, Boston: Little Brown, 1971, p. 997

Brunschwig A et al: Return of renal function after varying periods of ureteral occlusion. JAMA 118:125, 1964

Massry SG et al: Studies on the mechanism of diuresis after relief of urinary tract obstruction. Ann Intern Med 66:149, 1967

275 NEPHROLITHIASIS

FRANKLIN H. EPSTEIN

Renal stones vary in size from tiny particles to large staghorn calculi which fill the entire renal pelvis. They may be asymptomatic or continue to be formed and passed for years with no deleterious effect on renal function and no discomfort except occasional renal colic. Even a large staghorn calculus may produce no symptoms save perhaps for occasional nagging abdominal or flank pain. Often, however, renal calculi are associated with infection and progressive encroachment on renal function. Stones passed from above are rarely retained in the bladder unless obstruction and residual urine are present.

CLINICAL MANIFESTATIONS The typical attack of renal colic is exquisitely painful, causing the patient to double up in agony. The crampy pain begins in the side or back, radiating to the lower part of the abdomen, genitals, and inner thigh. The attack usually persists for several hours, although it may be over in a matter of minutes. Dysuria is frequently present, and even after the attack has subsided, tenderness along the course of the ureter often persists. Fever and leukocytosis signal associated infection. Hematuria and proteinuria are almost always present. Sometimes the pain is not referred in the usual manner and may simulate gallbladder disease, appendicitis, peptic ulcer, or disease of the spine. Renal colic may also be produced by blood clots or pus obstructing the ureter.

PATHOGENESIS *Chronic dehydration* is an important cause of stone formation, probably responsible for the high incidence in tropical climates, or in patients with chronic diarrhea. *Urinary obstruction* is another predisposing factor, perhaps because of the association with infection. A *family history* of stone is often obtained. The mucoprotein found in stone matrices may be excreted in excessive amounts by some patients who form stones.

Hypercalcuria In approximately one-half of all patients with renal calculi, some predisposing metabolic cause can be found. The chief causes include disorders that increase the excretion of calcium in the urine as in hyperparathyroidism, excessive ingestion of milk, alkali, and vitamin D, bone disease producing hypercalcuria, sarcoid, and renal tubular acidosis. Idiopathic hypercalcuria is found in a large proportion of patients with recurrent calcium stones. In such cases urinary calcium excretion exceeds 250 to 300 mg daily in patients on a normal diet who seem otherwise healthy. These patients may be examples of one "tail" of the distribution of calcium excretion in the general population. In many of them, the intestinal absorption and urinary excretion of calcium are unusually responsive to changes in the calcium content of the diet.

Cystinuria (see Chap. 98) This congenital disorder is characterized by decreased tubular reabsorption of cystine, arginine, ornithine, and lysine. Owing to its relative insolubility, cystine tends to precipitate in the urinary tract to form stones, which are radiopaque on account of their high content of sulfur. The condition may be diagnosed from the hexagonal appearance of cystine crystals in the urine and their characteristic reaction with nitroprusside. Cystine stones may be dissolved or prevented from forming if the reaction of the urine is kept alkaline and the urine volume high.

Glycinuria Hereditary glycinuria is a rare familial disorder associated with nephrolithiasis and excessive urinary excretion of glycine unaccompanied by other amino acids.

Uric acid stones Uric acid stones are radiolucent, form most readily in acid urine, and may be prevented if the urine is kept persistently alkaline (Chap. 100). They frequently complicate gout and may appear in a variety of hematologic diseases, notably polycythemia. More than half of all patients with urate calculi have neither hyperuricemia nor increased urinary excretion of uric acid. In this group of patients an unexplained tendency to excrete urine of pH below 5.5 may predispose to uric acid stones.

Hyperoxaluria Although most patients with calcium oxalate stones do not excrete excessive amounts of oxalate, the rare condition of primary hyperoxaluria is characterized by progressive calcium oxalate urolithiasis and nephrocalcinosis beginning in early childhood (see Chap. 97). Patients with an *ileostomy* may form calcium oxalate stones because of the excretion in the urine of excessive oxalate, derived from glycine conjugates of bile salts.

Renal infection Finally, primary renal infection, especially with urea-splitting organisms and in the presence of hydronephrosis, may promote the formation of renal calculi.

TREATMENT Every effort should be made to obtain stones for analysis, since this often provides the key to an underlying disorder. A stone consisting predominantly of calcium oxalate can have a small central nucleus of uric acid or cystine, and magnesium ammonium phosphate may be deposited in layers around a central calcium phosphate core.

Treatment must be individualized and governed by the patient's symptoms and the signs of associated renal disease. A small asymptomatic calculus entrapped in a renal calyx and unassociated with infection may be best left alone. Many stones pass spontaneously, but in the majority of instances special urologic and surgical procedures are eventually required. Daily urine volume should be kept over 2,500 ml. Special emphasis should be placed on drinking before retiring and once more during the night. Infection should be vigorously treated. Unless hypercalcuria is clearly present, calcium excretion is rarely changed much by reducing the dairy content of the diet. A much easier way to decrease the tendency to crystallization is to increase water intake. Urinary calcium can be reduced by feeding phosphate. In addition, certain complex phosphates interfere with crystal formation and are excreted into the urine when phosphate is supplied in the diet. Perhaps for this reason, a mixture of sodium and potassium neutral phosphates, made isotonic to reduce the cathartic effect, and given in three divided doses totaling 1.5 g *phosphorus* per day, is efficacious in preventing the growth of new calculi in patients with recurrent calcium stones.

REFERENCES

Maurice PF, Henneman PH: Medical aspects of renal stones. Medicine 40:315, 1961

Smith LH Jr.: Symposium on stones. Am J Med 45:649, 1968

276 CYSTIC DISEASES OF THE KIDNEYS

FRANKLIN H. EPSTEIN

POLYCYSTIC KIDNEYS In this disorder normal renal tissue is gradually replaced and encroached upon by multiple cysts of the renal parenchyma of varying size. The disease is congenital and in one-half to two-thirds of adult cases appears to be familial. The condition is bilateral, though one kidney may be involved to a greater extent than the other.

Pathology The kidneys are enlarged to several times normal size and are filled with grapelike clusters of cysts containing clear or hemorrhagic fluid. Between the cysts islands of normal or partially fibrotic renal parenchyma persist. In infants the cysts are said to be closed and do not communicate with the renal pelvis; in adults there is evidence that the cysts are functional. In patients with polycystic kidneys, cysts of the liver may be present and, more rarely, cysts of the pancreas and spleen. These are usually asymptomatic. There is a high associated incidence of intracranial aneurysms, and death from cerebral hemorrhage occurs in about 10 percent of cases.

Clinical features The infantile familial form of polycystic kidney disease with enlarged kidneys and a very high perinatal mortality rate is often associated with other malformations, particularly cystic disease of the liver, and appears to be inherited as an autosomal recessive trait. In contrast, the adult familial disease is an autosomal dominant trait, with virtually complete penetrance if the bearers of the gene survive to the ninth decade. The two diseases appear to be distinct, since families have not been reported in which both the infantile and the adult forms have appeared. Multiple cysts observed in adult kidneys in the absence of symptoms and of a family history may represent the asymptomatic stage of the familial disease, or an unrelated and nonprogressive disorder. The condition in the adult is commonly discovered in the fourth, fifth, or sixth decade, frequently in the course of a routine physical examination or as part of an investigation of asymptomatic hematuria, proteinuria, or hypertension. Both kidneys are usually palpable; in one-fifth of the cases, only one can be felt, and occasionally no mass can be palpated. In all instances, however, intravenous or retrograde pyelography demonstrates enlarged kidneys with elongation of the pelvis, flattening of the calyxes, and indentations due to the cysts. Lumbar and abdominal ache is a frequent complaint, owing to the weight of the kidney which produces tension on the pedicle, to intracystic hemorrhages, or to pressure on other organs. The pain is often increased by exertion and relieved by lying down. Pain may also be colicky and associated with hematuria and the passage of clots or with concomitant renal calculi. Massive and prolonged bleeding into the urine is a distressing complication; it sometimes responds to a tight abdominal binder. Hypertension appears in the third or fourth decade, when symptoms referable to high blood pressure may predominate. After the age of forty or forty-five, the more common presenting complaints are those associated with renal insufficiency. When a patient comes to the physician with uremia and a palpable "liver" and "spleen," the diagnosis of polycystic kidneys must be considered. Polyuria is common and oliguria is rare, even terminally. The average age at death is between fifty and sixty years; several patients have lived past seventy. Although the rate of progression may be extremely slow, patients generally do not live longer than 5 years after the blood urea nitrogen level rises above 50 mg per 100 ml. Superimposed pyelonephritis occurs frequently and may induce renal decompensations, which can be reversed by appropriate treatment.

Treatment In some patients polycystic kidney disease is compatible with a normal life span. Puncture or marsupialization of the cysts has not been demonstrated to prolong life and may introduce a disastrous infection. Because of the high incidence of bilateral disease, excision of one polycystic kidney is practically never indicated unless it is irretrievably infected or causing alarming hemorrhage, and then only after the other kidney has been shown to have fair function and to be only moderately involved in the cystic process. Hematuria usually responds to bed rest but should be disregarded if it is microscopic and asymptomatic. Pregnancy may be undertaken before hypertension and azotemia have appeared. Uremia and infection require treatment similar to that of other types of renal disease.

MEDULLARY CYSTIC DISEASE This is a rare disorder in which the kidneys are not large and may be contracted. Cysts varying in size from a few microns to a centimeter in diameter occupy what once was the corticomedullary junction and are lined with a single layer of epithelium. Completely normal as well as hyalinized glomeruli are found in the thinned cortex, together with chronic interstitial inflammation and fibrosis. Few abnormalities are seen in the urine, other than an inability to concentrate it. The blood pressure is usually normal until late in the course of the disease. Anemia, polyuria, and salt wasting are prominent. Bone disease is common. Death of renal insufficiency before the age of thirty is the rule, but patients have been reported in their fifth decade. There appears to be a familial incidence in some cases, especially those described in Europe as "familial juvenile nephronophthisis," but in others there is absolutely no evidence for familial inheritance.

MEDULLARY SPONGE KIDNEY Medullary sponge kidney, an entirely separate condition, has been recognized primarily as a radiologic abnormality; it is usually asymptomatic and nonprogressive, with a good prognosis. The cysts, which often appear as tiny clusters of radiopaque material adjacent to the calyxes on intravenous and, less commonly, on retrograde pyelography, often contain small calculi. Occasionally these calculi erode to produce bleeding, colic, obstruction, or infection. No familial incidence has been noted. The chief importance of the accidentally discovered sponge kidney is that it may be mistaken for renal tuberculosis or diffuse nephrocalcinosis.

OTHER CYSTS OF THE KIDNEY *Solitary cysts* usually occur at the lower pole, projecting from the surface of the kidney. They contain a serous fluid which is not urine. They may be associated with a dull, dragging pain in the side but are most often asymptomatic unless complicated by hemorrhage or infection. Occasionally one kidney is completely replaced by *multiple congenital cysts,* while the other is uninvolved. *Multiple small retention cysts,* secondary to obstruction of tubules, are common in nephrosclerosis and pyelonephritis.

REFERENCES

LAGERGREN C, LINDVALL N: Medullary sponge kidney and polycystic disease of the kidney: Distinct entities. Am J Roentgenol Radium Ther Nucl Med 88:153, 1962

MONGEAU JG, WORTHEN HG: Nephronophthisis and medullary cystic disease. Am J Med 43:345, 1967

OSATHANONDH V, POTTER EL: Pathogenesis of polycystic kidneys: Survey of results of microdissection. Arch Pathol 77:510, 1964

STRAUSS MB: Clinical and pathological aspects of cystic disease of the renal medulla. An analysis of eighteen cases. Ann Intern Med 57:373, 1962

277 OTHER CONGENITAL AND HEREDITARY DISORDERS OF THE KIDNEY AND URINARY TRACT

FRANKLIN H. EPSTEIN

HEREDITARY NEPHRITIS The most widely recognized form of familial nephritis is associated with nerve deafness and sometimes with cataracts or other defects of the lens. Although it is transmitted as an autosomal dominant trait, males are affected more severely than females and usually die before the age of forty of renal failure; hence the disease is more often transmitted by the mother. Gross microscopic hematuria is common and is often worse after nonspecific infections. In childhood, while renal function is normal, renal biopsy may show nothing but blood in the tubules. At autopsy, on the other hand, the picture may resemble either chronic glomerulonephritis or advanced interstitial nephritis ("pyelonephritis"). Foam cells containing anisotropic lipid are frequently found in the interstitial tissue. Families are also found with a high incidence among the members of glomerulonephritis, toxemia of pregnancy, and asymptomatic albuminuria, but without deafness or lenticular abnormalities. It is not clear whether or not these cases all represent variants of the same inherited affection of the kidneys.

ANGIOKERATOMA CORPORIS DIFFUSUM This is a familial disorder characterized by deposition of an abnormal glycolipid in vascular smooth muscle, myocardium, cells of sympathetic ganglions and the central nervous system, and epithelial cells of the renal glomeruli. The disease is recognized by characteristic punctate skin lesions (most profuse around the genitals and buttocks), acroparesthesias, dependent edema, defective sweating, and unexplained attacks of fever and pain. Proteinuria develops in the majority of cases in the second decade. Lipid globules and foam cells may be seen in the urine. Uremia and hypertension usually supervene in the fourth or fifth decade.

NAIL-PATELLA SYNDROME (OSTEOONYCHODYSPLASIA) Transmitted as an autosomal dominant trait, this condition involves arthrodysplasia of the elbows (webbed elbows), rudimentary patellas, split deformed nails, and iliac horns. The kidneys are the site of a mild chronic glomerulonephritis that is usually asymptomatic but may progress slowly to renal insufficiency.

NEPHROGENIC DIABETES INSIPIDUS This hereditary defect in tubular function occurs more often in males than in females. Like pituitary diabetes insipidus, it is characterized by the excretion of large volumes of dilute urine, with osmolality well below that of plasma, but is distinguished by the failure of the kidneys to respond to vasopressin. Polyuria and polydipsia are apparent early in life ("water babies"). There are no associated genetic abnormalities of tubular function, but atonic bladder and hydronephrosis often result from the high rates of urine flow with prolonged voluntary retention of urine. Treatment consists of adequate water intake combined with chlorothiazide (Chap. 84), which probably acts by producing mild salt depletion, resulting in increased reabsorption of fluid in the proximal segment of the renal tubule.

OTHER MALFORMATIONS Congenital malformations of the kidney are sometimes associated with malformations of the external ear. Complete *absence of one kidney* occurs about once in 500 births. *Unilateral hypoplasia* is a rarer congenital anomaly. *Horseshoe kidney* results from fusion of the renal blastemas, generally at their lower poles, at the eighth to tenth fetal week. The common location is close to the region of the aortic bifurcation. The anomaly is found once in every 500 to 1,000 autopsies and in most instances is asymptomatic and compatible with long life. It may, however, be complicated by renal calculi, recurrent pyelonephritis, hematuria, and abdominal pain. A few patients have nausea and vomiting associated with abdominal pain which is accentuated by hyperextension and relieved by leaning forward (Rovsing's syndrome). In some, a mass may be palpated in the lower part of the abdomen. In *crossed ectopia* the renal blastema becomes deviated to the opposite side, where it usually lies caudad to the normal kidney, with which it may fuse. Its ureter usually crosses the midline to terminate in the normal position. Such kidneys, as well as *unilateral fused kidneys,* are predisposed to hydronephrosis and pyelonephritis but not to other renal lesions. Pain is the most common symptom; many patients are entirely asymptomatic.

Anomalies of the ureter include bifurcation, complete reduplication, and abnormal implantation in the bladder, as well as stricture at the ureteropelvic or ureterovesical junction. Anomalies of the vesical neck may underlie enuresis in children, which is sometimes treated as a behavior problem, while the kidneys are irretrievably damaged.

REFERENCE

PERKOFF GT: The hereditary renal diseases. N Engl J Med 277:79, 1967

278 TUMORS OF THE URINARY TRACT

BERNARD LYTTON
FRANKLIN H. EPSTEIN

Benign renal tumors rarely present a clinical problem as they are usually small and asymptomatic. The majority are adenomas, but a variety of fibrolipomyomas also occurs. When they enlarge they may be difficult to differentiate clinically from malignant growth of the kidney or suprarenal gland. They have a potential for malignant change.

Malignant tumors of the kidney occur chiefly in childhood and after forty. The incidence in adults is considerably higher in men.

NEPHROBLASTOMA The common malignant tumor of children is nephroblastoma (Wilms's tumor), which probably arises from embryonic nephrogenic tissue and may contain both epithelial and connective tissue elements. It constitutes 20 to 25 percent of all malignant neoplasms of childhood and is observed before the age of seven in 90 percent of cases. The tumor usually presents as a palpable abdominal mass and may grow to enormous size. It is associated in a high proportion of cases with hypertension which is relieved by nephrectomy. It has to be differentiated from multicystic kidney, neuroblastoma, hydronephrosis, and renal cyst. The tumor is present bilaterally in 1 to 2 percent of cases. Treatment consists of a combination of surgery, chemotherapy, and irradiation, which has resulted in a dramatic improvement in the prognosis. Dactinomycin (Actinomycin D) administered during the first week after operation and subsequently at intervals during the next year, together with postoperative radiation of the tumor bed, has achieved a 5-year survival of 60 to 70 percent. The most favorable prognosis is in those children in whom the diagnosis is made before the age of two years. Preoperative irradiation may be employed to render a large tumor operable.

CARCINOMA OF THE KIDNEY (HYPERNEPHROMA, GRAWITZ'S TUMOR) This is the commonest neoplasm of the kidney in adults. One or more of the classic triad of hematuria, flank pain, and abdominal mass is present in about half the cases, but not infrequently the first symptoms arise from metastases to lung, bone, liver, or brain. Obscure fever together with a moderate leukocytosis, without infection, is a fairly common presenting symptom. Occasionally gastrointestinal symptoms are prominent. Serum alkaline phosphatase level is sometimes elevated even in the absence of bony metastases. Calcification within the tumor mass is occasionally seen on the plain x-ray of the abdomen. The diagnosis of a renal mass has been greatly improved with the advent of renal angiography. This is probably best performed by the transfemoral route, which allows selective injections to be made into individual renal vessels if required. Solid renal tumors are generally opacified on nephrotomography, as compared to the lucency and sharply defined margins seen when a cyst is present. The arteriogram shows the characteristic pooling of the contrast material in the venous sinusoids which occurs in these tumors and is a result of the small arteriovenous communications which develop. The hypervascularity of the tumor is responsible for the "tumor blush." Epinephrine injection into the renal artery during arteriography may accentuate visualization of tumor vessels. A small number of renal carcinomas do not exhibit the typical neovascularity; these are usually papillary adenocarcinomas rather than the usual clear-cell tumors. Nephrotomography may be helpful in these cases in establishing the presence of a solid lesion. Rarely, the wall of a renal cyst will be found to contain a small focus of tumor. Needle aspiration of cystic lesions with examination of the fluid for cells and fat content, together with radiographic visualization of the wall, provides an additional method for diagnosis in patients who are a poor surgical risk. Abnormal tumor vessels are generally not seen in transitional-cell carcinomas of the renal pelvis invading the parenchyma. Renal arteriography, nephrotomography, and cyst puncture have markedly improved the accuracy in diagnosis of renal mass lesions, but the distinction between cyst and tumor still cannot always be made with certainty.

Lactic dehydrogenase activity in the urine has been shown to be elevated in the presence of carcinoma of the urinary tract, but is of no value as a diagnostic test. There are a significant number of false negative results, and a high proportion of patients with pyuria from a variety of causes have an elevated level.

In rare instances *polycythemia* may be observed, unaccompanied by leukocytosis, thrombocytosis, or splenomegaly. It is thought to be due to an erythropoietic factor produced by the tumor. A similar factor has also been detected in the fluid of some renal cysts. In such cases the polycythemia may be cured by removal of the tumor. *Polyneuritis* and *myopathy* found in association with other forms of malignant disease are occasionally seen in carcinoma of the kidney and bladder. Abnormalities in liver function tests may occur, in the absence of metastases, which resolve after extirpation of the tumor. An elevated serum calcium and a low phosphorus level, suggesting hyperparathyroidism, may be caused in occasional cases by a parathormone-like substance elaborated by the tumor. Hypertension, if present, is usually coincidental and is not improved by nephrectomy. Renin-secreting tumors of the juxtaglomerular cells producing severe hypertension, which is relieved by nephrectomy, have been reported. Extension of carcinoma into the renal veins may cause acute varicocele or produce venous thrombosis. A few cases have been reported in which there has been evidence of spontaneous regression of lung metastases following nephrectomy; unfortunately, progression of the lesions is more common. Long-term survival after the excision of solitary pulmonary and cerebral metastases has also been recorded. About one-quarter of the patients with renal carcinoma survive more than 10 years after nephrectomy. The value of preoperative irradiation is undetermined. The tumors are relatively radioresistant, but some improvement in survival has been ascribed to irradiation. Administration of progestational agents and androgens to control metastatic disease has been successful in isolated cases, but the results in general have been disappointing. Vinblastine has produced significant regression of metastatic lesions in a few patients.

Papillary transitional-cell neoplasms of the renal pelvis These growths are often associated with similar tumors of the ureter and bladder. Hematuria is the outstanding symptom. An association with calculi and infection is frequent in the less common squamous-cell carcinoma, which has a poor prognosis. Nephroureterectomy is the treatment of choice. Carcinoma of the renal pelvis may appear deceptively benign, and failure to find infiltration at operation does not ensure prolonged survival. The prognosis is worse than with parenchymal carcinoma.

Carcinoma of the bladder This condition is seen in two main forms, papillary and solid. Where possible, surgical extirpation by partial or total cystectomy is the treatment of choice and has the advantage that radiotherapy can be used subsequently in the event of recurrence. Supervoltage irradiation offers results approaching those of surgery and is the preferred treatment in patients who are poor surgical risks, or for palliation. There may be considerable morbidity from radiation cystitis and proctitis.

Papillary tumors These growths are often relatively benign and may be single or multiple. Those which show no evidence of invasion of the bladder wall are usually well controlled by endoscopic resection and fulguration, but as the entire bladder mucosa appears susceptible to the neoplastic change, the appearance of further tumors is likely and careful follow-up by cystoscopy is essential. Repeated local instillation of triethylenethiophosphoramide is sometimes effective in the treatment of multiple lesions and in the prevention of recurrences. A small group of these tumors become invasive after a variable period of time and behave like the solid lesions. Prognosis depends on the depth of penetration and the degree of anaplasia. A tumor which has penetrated to the perivesical tissues and is poorly differentiated is associated with a very small chance of cure after any form of treatment. The most frequent symptom is *painless hematuria.* Dysuria and frequency are also common even in the absence of infection. Ureteral obstruction seen on the pyelogram indicates invasion of the bladder wall. A cystogram may be helpful in the localization of the lesion. Individuals exposed to xenylamine and to intermediate products in the manufacture of aniline dyes (1- and 2-naphthylamines, benzidine, and 4-aminodiphenyl) have been noted to have a high incidence of bladder tumor. These tumors usually develop after a long latent period of between 3 to 40 years. A threefold increase in the incidence of bladder cancer has been noted in heavy cigarette smokers.

Benign overgrowth of the prostate A result of an irregular, multifocal hyperplasia of the fibromuscular stroma, with a varying amount of secondary invasion by glandular elements, this condition affects principally the lateral and middle lobes. The degree of enlargement may be up to ten times normal. The enlarging hyperplastic nodules compress the normal prostatic tissue into a thin shell, the surgical capsule, from which they may readily be enucleated or resected transurethrally, as in subtotal prostatectomy. The enlargement produces varying degrees of urethral obstruction as a result of compression, elongation, or ball valve action of the middle lobe. The cause remains obscure, but the condition is associated with senescence and is thought to be due to hormonal imbalance, the exact nature of which is undetermined. About 50 percent of men over fifty develop clinical symptoms of prostatic hypertrophy, but only about 10 percent require surgical relief of obstruction. It has been thought by some that benign hypertrophy is a precancerous lesion, but there is little evidence to support this view.

Adenocarcinoma of the prostate One of the most common tumors in men, adenocarcinoma of the prostate accounts for 10 percent of deaths from malignant disease in males in the United States. The *incidence* rises rapidly with advancing age, and microscopic lesions have been found at autopsy in 15 to 20 percent of men in the fifth decade, increasing to as high as 60 percent in the eighth decade. Less than one-sixth however, become clinically apparent prior to death, the remainder being latent carcinomas. Three-fourths of the tumors arise in the posterior lobe, and urinary symptoms therefore tend to occur late in the disease. Frequent *routine rectal examinations* are the best means of demonstrating the early and operable tumors. A solitary indurated nodule confined to one part of the prostate should be investigated by open perineal biopsy in patients who are suitable for radical surgery, as this is the most reliable procedure for a definitive diagnosis. About one-half these nodules subsequently prove to be malignant. The more advanced carcinoma is indicated by a hard irregular nodularity, generalized induration, loss of the normal contour of the prostate, and infiltration extending upwards and laterally over the vesicles with fixation of the gland. One-fifth of the patients present symptoms due to distant metastases. *Needle biopsy* is a useful method of obtaining histologic diagnosis, particularly in the more advanced cases, but failure to demonstrate the presence of cancer in such a specimen does not exclude the diagnosis. The "prostatic" fraction of the serum acid phosphatase, though a more sensitive estimation than that of the total enzyme, is not elevated with tumor confined to the prostate but is elevated in a high proportion of cases when local or distant dissemination has occurred. Elevation of the prostatic acid phosphatase level may occur for 24 hr after palpation of the normal prostate, and is found in a small number of cases without evidence of carcinoma. The serum alkaline phosphatase level is frequently elevated in prostatic carcinoma, but this occurs in a wide variety of conditions so that it is of little aid in diagnosis. Biopsy of the marrow from the sternum or ilium in patients with unexplained anemia will sometimes reveal metastatic prostatic cancer in the absence of radiologic changes in the bones or elevation of the acid phosphatase level. Radioactive strontium scanning of the skeleton has proved to be helpful in the detection of metastases in the absence of radiologic changes. Bony metastases are usually osteoblastic, and prostatic cancer is by far the commonest cause for such lesions.

Radical prostatectomy remains the treatment of choice for tumors confined to the gland but is applicable to only 5 percent of cases. About 40 percent live for 10 years postoperatively without evidence of recurrence. An intravascular coagulopathy, probably due to release of thromboplastic materials from the tumor, has been observed occasionally in association with prostatic carcinoma and has resulted in severe and uncontrollable hemorrhage postoperatively. Fibrinolysins which were previously thought to be responsible for this condition are probably produced in excess as a secondary phenomenon. Treatment with heparin is helpful in controlling the bleeding, but aminocaproic acid is of doubtful value. *Orchiectomy* and *estrogen therapy* appear to provide the most effective palliation in patients with symptomatic cancer of the prostate and are also used as adjuncts to surgery. *Diethylstilbestrol 1 mg*, or the equivalent dose of other estrogenic products, is administered daily. There is evidence that the mortality from cardiovascular disease may be significantly increased in patients receiving hormonal therapy for carcinoma of the prostate. *Caution should therefore be exercised in the administration of estrogens to patients with asymptomatic prostatic cancer.* Obstruction may be relieved by transurethral resection. A 2-year remission may be expected in 70 to 80 percent of patients. If dissemination is not present at the outset of treatment, 44 percent survive for 5 years, but in the presence of metastases only 20 percent survive. However, only 5 to 10 percent of all patients may be expected to live 5 years without treatment. When relapse occurs following estrogen therapy, further remissions may sometimes be obtained by adrenal suppression with corticosteroids, adrenalectomy, or transsphenoidal hypophysectomy; such remissions are thought to be due to suppression of extragonadal sources of androgen.

Supervoltage irradiation and direct injection of *radioactive gold* have been used, with variable results, in the treatment of tumors confined to the pelvis. Local irradiation of skeletal metastases may effectively relieve bone pain when hormone therapy fails.

Penile warts or papillomas These growths occur usually in the coronal sulcus and are often associated with poor hygiene. Occasionally they may involve the external meatus. Treatment is by fulguration or application of 25 percent podophyllum in mineral oil. The surrounding normal skin must be protected with petrolatum when the latter irritant is used.

Carcinoma of the penis This rare condition affects elderly uncircumcised men. The disease may reach a fairly advanced stage before diagnosis if phimosis is present. Small superficial tumors may be adequately treated by irradiation, but partial or complete amputation in conjunction with excision of the regional lymph nodes is usually required.

Carcinoma of the scrotum Primarily an occupational disease, this carcinoma occurs as a result of contact with petroleum and its products which may soil the workman's clothes. The classic example is the mule spinners' cancer. Arsenical medicines may give rise to epitheliomatous changes in the scrotal skin and elsewhere.

REFERENCES

Bennington JL, Kradjian RM: *Renal Carcinoma*, Philadelphia: Saunders, 1967

Jewett HJ: Tumors of the bladder, in *Urology*, 3d ed., eds MF Campbell, JH Harrison, Philadelphia: Saunders, 1970

Scott WW, Schirmer HKA: Carcinoma of the prostate, in *Urology*, 3d ed., eds MF Campbell, JH Harrison, Philadelphia: Saunders, 1970

279
OTHER DISEASES AFFECTING THE KIDNEYS

FRANKLIN H. EPSTEIN

DIABETIC NEPHROPATHY—INTERCAPILLARY GLOMERULOSCLEROSIS (KIMMELSTIEL-WILSON DISEASE) Pathology In about 25 percent of patients with diabetes mellitus a distinctive nodular glomerular lesion is evident at autopsy, which was first described by Kimmelstiel and Wilson as *intercapillary glomerulosclerosis.* The typical, ball-like, hyaline, acidophilic masses are situated at the periphery of the glomerular tuft, often with an apparently intact capillary running over the surface. The mass often contains cell nuclei, but they are usually distributed around its periphery. The wall of the afferent arteriole is usually hyalinized, and hyaline change in the efferent arteriole is frequently present as well. (The latter change is said to be so characteristic of diabetes as to be almost specific.) The nodules may be sparse or frequent; they rarely involve every glomerulus but completely obliterate some. In addition, a more diffuse hyaline thickening of the glomerular basement membrane is apparent in many cases of diabetes, even when the nodules are absent, although this change is more difficult to distinguish from similar "axial thickenings" in such diseases as benign nephrosclerosis and membranous glomerulonephritis. Examination of renal biopsies from patients with diabetes by the electron microscope usually demonstrates some thickening of the glomerular basement membrane, even though the diabetes is of short duration, proteinuria and hypertension are absent, and conventional histologic sections appear normal. In patients with long-standing diabetes, three renal diseases are likely to be present: intercapillary glomerulosclerosis, arteriolar nephrosclerosis, and pyelonephritis.

Clinical features and pathophysiology The usual textbook description is of a patient with 10 years or more of diabetes who develops proteinuria and hypertension. Though the patient is asymptomatic at first, massive urinary losses of protein produce hypoproteinemia, and edema and anasarca follow. The blood urea level slowly rises, and vision is impaired by retinopathy. Within 5 years after proteinuria is first noted, death occurs from uremia complicated by infections, anemia, and heart failure (Chap. 88).

Departures from the classic picture are legion. Although both *hypertension* and *proteinuria* are present in 80 percent of diabetic patients with eosinophilic glomerular nodules, one-fifth have normal blood pressure, and occasional patients have no detectable proteinuria. Both hypertension and proteinuria can, of course, be caused in diabetic patients primarily by pyelonephritis or nephrosclerosis rather than Kimmelstiel-Wilson disease, and if this is true, the prognosis is probably better. In some cases, slight proteinuria, with fluctuating retinopathy, may persist for years with little or no impairment of renal function. In other instances, the interval from onset of proteinuria to death is as short as 2 years, and the intensity and rapidity of the deterioration in renal function reminds one of a subacute glomerulonephritis, though at postmortem there is only widespread nodular intercapillary glomerulosclerosis.

The appearance of *heavy proteinuria* (over 4 to 5 g daily) usually signifies extensive involvement of the glomeruli by the diffuse or the nodular type of diabetic lesion. Heavy losses of albumin into the urine produce hypoalbuminemia, which in turn predisposes to edema and pleural effusions. Poor appetite and inadequate intake of protein and calories often contribute to the low concentration of albumin in serum. The serum cholesterol level, unlike that in childhood nephrosis, is often normal in the nephrosis of diabetes. When much protein is excreted, the urine also contains many granular and fatty casts and epithelial cells choked with doubly refractile lipid, called *fat bodies*. Hematuria is unusual except with malignant hypertension.

As renal reserve declines, glomerular and tubular functions deteriorate in parallel, so that *blood urea nitrogen rises* while creatinine clearance, phenolsulfonphthalein excretion, and concentrating capacity fall. The kidneys are scarred and contracted somewhat in size, but very small kidneys are not characteristic of Kimmelstiel-Wilson disease, in contrast to chronic end-stage glomerulonephritis. It is not uncommon to see kidney outlines normal or only slightly reduced and a creatinine clearance one-tenth normal.

With advanced renal insufficiency, *glycosuria may not be an accurate guide to levels of blood sugar*. There is no consistent change in insulin requirements with progression of renal disease, though many patients require less insulin as their appetite wanes and they lose weight.

Retinopathy precedes proteinuria in practically all cases of diabetic glomerulosclerosis. Thus, although diabetic retinopathy may be present without clinical manifestations of glomerulosclerosis, marked proteinuria or azotemia in Kimmelstiel-Wilson disease without retinopathy is rare. *When the retinas are absolutely normal in a diabetic with nephrosis, the cause of the difficulty is not likely to be the diabetes.*

Because of the generalized vascular disease that is always present, *myocardial infarcts*, *congestive cardiac failure*, and *cerebral vascular accidents* punctuate the course of diabetic nephropathy. They are responsible for more deaths in such patients than is uremia. When edema is present, heart failure is usually a contributing cause. A sudden deterioration in renal function may be the only reflection of a critical weakening of myocardial function or a silent myocardial infarct.

Sclerosis of the intrarenal arteries, infection, and in some cases, ureteral dilatation and reflux secondary to neurogenic bladder may combine to produce *papillary necrosis*. This is usually asymptomatic, though it may be attended by pain, colic, hematuria, and the passage of bits of tissue in the urine. Occasionally, papillary necrosis is the cause of rapid progression of renal insufficiency or acute oliguric renal failure.

Factors predisposing to *urinary infection* in diabetes include incomplete emptying of the bladder because of *diabetic neuropathy*, and repeated instrumentation of the bladder during hospitalization. *Uncontrolled glycosuria* with associated vaginal itching and irritation probably contributes to the incidence of urinary infections in women.

Retention of urine in the bladder because of difficulty in emptying commonly causes nausea and accentuates azotemia in bedridden diabetics. In patients with neurogenic bladders, proper emptying, using suprapubic pressure and full doses of urecholine, may permit infection to be controlled. In a few patients, residual urine may be eliminated by resection of the bladder neck.

Prevention and treatment The development of intercapillary glomerulosclerosis does not seem to be avoided by rigid control of the blood sugar, and there are several well-documented cases in which the fasting blood sugar level was normal. It seems likely, on the other hand, that prevention of urinary infection (e.g., by avoiding unnecessary catheterization of the bladder) and proper treatment and follow-up of those infections which do occur may be important in preventing ultimate renal scarring from pyelonephritis in at least some diabetic patients.

Adrenal steroids do not alter the proteinuria of diabetic glomerulosclerosis. Hypoalbuminemia may, however, sometimes be improved by a more generous intake of protein and calories. Edema can usually be eliminated by salt restriction and diuretics if renal insufficiency is not severe and heart failure is not present. Because heart failure occurs at some time in almost every patient with Kimmelstiel-Wilson disease, digitalis should be given a therapeutic trial in every patient with edema or uremia in whom the heart is enlarged. Heart failure should be controlled by digitalis if possible rather than by restricting the intake of fluid and salt or by sole dependence on diuretics. When the latter become necessary, they should not be pushed to the point of dehydration. Modest edema is often to be preferred to progressive azotemia with its attendant weakness and nausea. Dehydrating procedures in the hospital such as fluid restriction and castor oil before intravenous pyelography should be carefully avoided in azotemic patients.

Alpha-methyldopa and reserpine are useful in moderating the blood pressure in situations where hypertension is clearly responsible for symptoms (e.g., intractable vascular headaches) or menaces vision (severe diastolic hypertension with hemorrhagic retinitis). The tendency to postural hypotension induced by drugs used to lower high blood pressure is greatly accentuated by diabetic neuropathy. See the discussion of treatment in Chap. 245, Hypertension.

Normocytic, normochromic anemia usually appears in diabetic nephropathy when the blood urea level is elevated, and contributes to fatigue and weakness. It is due to renal insufficiency and responds only to transfusions. When anemia is severe and recurrent, an attempt should be made to give blood before the critical level is reached at which the patient complains of symptoms.

Frequent feedings with adequate quantities of carbohydrate and insulin to prevent ketosis and to avoid excessive breakdown of protein are especially important in treating patients with diabetic nephropathy, since sudden increases in the load of urea and acid presented to the kidneys, which are excreted with ease in patients with normal renal function, are retained in renal insufficiency and augment azotemia and acidosis.

Peritoneal dialysis is often useful in tiding a uremic diabetic patient over a reversible episode which temporarily decreases renal function, such as, for example, systemic or renal infection, decreased cardiac output secondary to myocardial infarction; or salt depletion from vomiting or diarrhea.

AMYLOID KIDNEY (see Chap. 107) Renal amyloidosis, a relatively rare condition, is most commonly encountered as a complication of chronic suppurative diseases, such as osteomyelitis, tuberculosis, tertiary syphilis, and leprosy, as well as Hodgkin's disease, ulcerative colitis, regional enteritis, and rheumatoid arthritis. As the incidence of chronic infection has declined owing to the introduction of antibiotics, the amyloid kidney of "primary amyloidosis" and amyloidosis secondary to multiple myeloma (Chap. 65) and rheumatoid arthritis have become relatively more prominent. Amyloid involvement of the kidneys, as well as of other organs, commonly occurs in the course of familial Mediterranean fever, in which renal insufficiency secondary to amyloidosis is usually the cause of death. The clinical and pathologic features of the renal disease produced by "primary" and "secondary" amyloidosis are similar.

Amyloid deposition in the kidney may be most prominent in the walls of blood vessels (especially the small arteries), or in the glomeruli, or surrounding the collecting tubules and small blood vessels of the medulla. In all these locations its distribution tends to be patchy rather than diffuse and uniform.

The clinical picture is influenced by the location and degree of involvement. When amyloid deposits are limited to blood vessels and to occasional focal deposits in glomeruli, mild proteinuria, sometimes with hematuria, is the only sign. On the other hand, when glomeruli are massively infiltrated, heavy proteinuria is the rule, associated with the nephrotic syndrome. In such cases, glomerular filtration may be surprisingly well maintained despite extensive deposits of amyloid in the Malpighian tufts. The rare instance of amyloidosis confined chiefly to the medulla is marked by polyuria resistant to vasopressin. Hypertension is unusual unless the disorder has progressed to the stage of azotemia and contracted kidneys. Heart failure, purpura, generalized muscular weakness, difficulty in swallowing, and postural hypotension are frequent accompaniments of primary amyloidosis. Biopsy of the kidney, liver, or rectal mucosa is useful in establishing the diagnosis. The course of the disease is generally prolonged, but in some cases secondary to advanced tuberculosis, only 6 months may elapse from the first appearance of albuminuria to the development of advanced uremia. Death occurs from the primary disease, amyloid involvement of the myocardium, intercurrent infection, or renal insufficiency. *Renal vein thrombosis* causing anuria is a special complication of amyloidosis. The disease does not respond to steroid treatment. In those instances in which a chronic suppurative disease can be eradicated, a complete remission has occasionally been observed.

THE KIDNEY IN MULTIPLE MYELOMA (see Chap. 65) Impairment of renal function occurs in over 50 percent of patients with multiple myeloma. Proteinuria is even more common. Renal damage can be related in many cases to the excretion of abnormal proteins of low molecular weight and the injurious effect of these substances on the renal tubules and ultimately on the entire nephron. Impairment of renal function is not necessarily correlated, however, with the *degree* of albuminuria or Bence Jones proteinuria. Hypercalcemia may produce transient or irreversible renal damage. In some cases the kidney is infiltrated by amyloid. Rarely, deposits of myeloma cells diffusely infiltrate the kidneys.

The major early change produced by the Bence Jones proteins is in the tubules. Proximal tubular cells are swollen and have droplets or rodlike inclusions. Large obstructing casts form along the entire length of the renal tubule, most prominently in the straight tubules of the medulla. These are often laminated and surrounded by multinucleated giant cells possibly derived from degenerating tubular epithelium. In addition, there is usually distinct thickening of the glomerular basement membrane, without cellular proliferation or crescent formation. Vascular sclerosis is not common; when it occurs it is probably coincidental.

Alteration in renal function is most frequently characterized by nitrogen retention and loss of concentrating power, without hypertension, retinitis, or edema. Proteinuria is usually present, consisting of albumin as well as certain globulins and Bence Jones proteins which may be excreted only intermittently. Anemia may seem out of proportion to the degree of azotemia. The disease may superficially resemble the chronic forms of glomerulonephritis or pyelonephritis. The nephrotic syndrome probably does not occur in multiple myeloma unless the disease is complicated by amyloidosis. In unusual instances before azotemia has become prominent, disturbances in renal tubular function dominate the picture, with renal glycosuria, aminoaciduria, low levels of serum uric acid, and renal potassium wasting. Loss of concentrating power is common, and nephrogenic diabetes insipidus has been reported. Renal loss of phosphate with consequent hypophosphatemia and elevation of the serum alkaline phosphatase level may, in rare cases, cause confusion with hyperparathyroidism. Because of the exceptional tendency to formation of obstructive casts, procedures which cause dehydration must be carefully avoided in the patient with multiple myeloma. Acute anuria has been observed in several instances following intravenous pyelography, probably as a result of the dehydration which is often induced in preparing for this procedure. Acute renal failure with anuria or oliguria which follows an episode of dehydration in an elderly person should suggest the possibility of myeloma kidney.

SICKLE-CELL NEPHROPATHY (see Chap. 307) Patients with sickle-cell anemia often develop progressive changes in renal function as a result of multiple small ischemic and hemorrhagic infarcts in the kidney. In children the principal anatomic finding is congestion of blood vessels, with sickled erythrocytes most prominent in the medulla. The glomeruli appear engorged and stuffed with red cells. In adults interstitial fibrosis and areas of cortical necrosis and hyalinization may be seen, resembling those of chronic glomerulonephritis or chronic pyelonephritis. Papillary necrosis may occur in patients with the homozygous disease or the trait. There is early impairment of renal concentrating ability, even when blood urea nitrogen, glomerular filtration rate, and renal plasma flow are normal. This selective disturbance in renal function may be present in patients with sickle-cell trait as well as in the full-blown disease. It is said to be temporarily reversed in children by transfusion of normal blood, but this is not the case in adults. Gross and microscopic hematuria occur frequently; bleeding may come from lesions in the papillae and pelvic mucosa as well as miliary infarctions in the cortex. Renal insufficiency may eventually develop in adults with sickle-cell anemia as a result of renal scarring. Despite the high incidence of at least minimal renal changes, the sickle-cell trait does not appear to predispose to toxemia of pregnancy.

CHYLURIA The chief cause of chyluria is filariasis (Chap. 219) with obstruction between the abdominal lymphatics and the thoracic duct, producing lymph varices in the kidney which rupture into the renal tubules. The urine is milky and on standing settles into a top layer of fatty material, a middle pinkish layer, often containing a clot, and a bottom layer containing blood and debris. Hematuria is common, and pyelonephritis is almost universal. Microfilarias are usually found in the urine for about 6 weeks after an acute infection but not thereafter unless the patient is in an endemic area. The lymph and blood may coalesce into ureteral casts, causing flank pain and renal colic. Chyluria may disappear with recumbency and be aggravated by exertion. The condition is entirely suppressed in some cases by wearing a tight abdominal corset.

RADIATION NEPHRITIS (see Chap. 119) Following the administration of large doses of x-ray (2,300 R during 5 weeks) to the kidneys in the course of therapy for abdominal carcinoma or lymph node metastases from testicular tumors, a characteristic syndrome develops. The clinical disease may mimic either benign or malignant hypertension or chronic glomerulonephritis. The latent period between irradiation and the appearance of symptoms is usually at least 6 months but may be much longer. Hypertension invariably appears and may lead to congestive heart failure, retinopathy, and encephalopathy. Refractory anemia is often prominent. Uremia is usually progressive, but in some cases renal insufficiency may be reversible, improvement commencing about 6 months after the onset of symptoms. Proteinuria is present but slight; hematuria is characteristically absent. Oliguria is never observed except with heart failure. Histologic features include widespread fibrosis between atropic tubules, damage to almost all the glomeruli, and fibrinoid necrotic lesions of arterioles.

HYPERCALCEMIC NEPHROPATHY (see Chap. 350) Acute elevations of serum calcium level are associated with marked polyuria, succeeded by dehydration, oliguria, and rapidly advancing azotemia. Prolonged hypercalcemia and/or hypercalcuria, as in hyperparathyroidism, vitamin D intoxication, sarcoid, multiple myeloma, or carcinomatosis, may result in diffuse nephrocalcinosis and present as renal insufficiency, insidious in onset and only slowly progressive. In such cases, severe disturbances in renal function need not be associated with stones or with radiologic evidence of calcification in the kidneys. Patients who have drunk several quarts of milk daily and ingested large amounts of absorbable alkali for prolonged periods of time to assuage symptoms of peptic ulcer sometimes develop azotemia, hypercalcemia without elevation of the serum alkaline phosphatase level, and calcinosis manifested by band keratopathy (milk-alkali syndrome).

Impairment of urinary concentrating capacity is an early sign of chronic calcium nephropathy, and polyuria and polydipsia are frequent, although not invariable. In more severe cases, filtration rate and renal blood flow are depressed, with retention of nitrogen. The urinary sediment may contain red blood cells, as well as leukocytes and white blood cell casts; in many patients, however, it is remarkably free of formed elements. Unless congestive heart failure is present, proteinuria is slight. Hypertension is common when nephrocalcinosis is established and does not disappear when the serum calcium level has returned to normal, even though renal function improves. Renal insufficiency may sometimes be completely or partially reversed when hypercalcemia is eliminated. In other cases, uremia and hypertensive vascular disease progress to a fatal termination despite the disappearance of hypercalcemia. The degree of reversibility of renal impairment is related to the extent of scar formation and permanent medullary obstruction by calcium precipitates, as well as to the presence of vascular disease and infection.

THE KIDNEY IN GOUT (see Chap. 100) From 30 to 50 percent of gouty patients die of renal disease. The kidneys of most patients with gout contain characteristic fan-shaped clefts containing deposits of urate in the interstices of the medulla. Pyelonephritis is a frequent finding, and arteriolar sclerosis is almost always present.

Urate calculi occur in approximately 15 percent of patients with gout and are particularly common during uricosuric therapy if a high fluid intake is not maintained. Both uric acid stones and interstitial deposits of urate crystals in the kidney may occur in patients with hyperuricemia who have never had gouty arthritis.

The most common indications of early renal damage are mild proteinuria, decreased excretion of phenolsulfonphthalein, and a reduction in concentrating ability. Slowly progressive azotemia with minimal albuminuria and little or no abnormality in the urinary sediment characterizes the course of this disease in some patients. Though hypertension may be absent, the blood pressure is commonly elevated; in fact, it has been suggested that hypertension and vascular sclerosis, especially nephrosclerosis, occur as part of a constitutional diathesis of which gout or hyperuricemia is a component part. Hyperuricemia and evidence on renal biopsy of arteriolar sclerosis may occasionally be the only positive findings in patients with asymptomatic proteinuria.

In rare instances of gouty kidney, renal function has been reported to improve slowly and urate stones to dissolve following the long-term maintenance of a high fluid intake and use of alkali in association with uricosuric agents. Administration of allopurinol, which blocks the formation of uric acid, is a rational treatment to use in the hope of preventing progression in gouty nephropathy.

REFERENCES

Berkman J, Rifkin H: Newer aspects of diabetic microangiopathy. Ann Rev Med 17:83, 1966

Epstein FH: Calcium and the kidney. Am J Med 45:700, 1968

Gellman DD et al: Diabetic nephropathy: A clinical and pathological study based on renal biopsies. Medicine 38:321, 1959

Luxton RW: Radiation nephritis. Quart J Med 22:215, 1953

Perillie PE, Epstein FH: Sickling phenomenon produced by hypertonic solutions. A possible explanation for the hyposthenuria of sicklemia. J Clin Invest 42:570, 1963

Sanchez LM, Domzy CA: Renal patterns in myeloma. Ann Intern Med 52:44, 1960

Schlitt LE, Keitel HG: Renal manifestations of sickle-cell disease: A review. Am J Med Sci 239:773, 1960

section 5 | Disorders of the alimentary tract

280
APPROACH TO THE PATIENT WITH GASTROINTESTINAL DISEASE

KURT J. ISSELBACHER

GENERAL CONSIDERATIONS Gastrointestinal symptoms occur not only with primary gastrointestinal tract disease but frequently as manifestations of other systemic diseases. Thus anorexia, nausea, and vomiting may be seen in congestive failure and uremia, and diarrhea or constipation may be seen as a consequence of metabolic derangements such as electrolyte changes or alterations in thyroid function. With today's technical advances one finds too often that the physician is willing to diagnose (or misdiagnose) gastrointestinal disease simply by relying on routine x-ray studies of the upper and lower parts of the gastrointestinal tract. Such an overwhelming dependence on technical procedures often leads to great pitfalls. In order to define the most probable and profitable area to study, the proper approach requires careful attention to the history and physical examination before ordering the appropriate diagnostic tests.

IMPORTANCE OF THE HISTORY To evaluate gastrointestinal symptoms, a careful history is crucial. Pain or indigestion is the most common intestinal complaint. Correlation between pain and gastrointestinal function must of necessity be chronologic. There should be a meticulous inquiry as to the frequency and specificity of the complaint. The questioning should include the location of the pain and whether it is circumscribed or diffuse. It is important to determine what factors aggravate or relieve the discomfort. *Does eating produce the symptom?* If so, determine whether the discomfort occurs *while eating* (as in esophageal disorders and abdominal angina), shortly *after the meal* (as often occurs in biliary tract disease), or *30 to 90 min later* (as typically seen with peptic ulcer). *Does eating relieve the symptom,* and if so, for how long? Temporary relief of epigastric pain is characteristic of gastritis and peptic ulceration. Many patients have tried or taken antacids by the time they come to the physician, and a history indicating relief of epigastric pain by antacids is suggestive of peptic disease of the upper part of the intestine. *What is the relation of pain to bowel movements?* The patient with ulcerative colitis often obtains temporary relief from his lower abdominal cramps by defecation.

Attention should be paid to *anorexia* and weight *loss;* their combined occurrence should make one suspicious of an underlying malignancy. If weight loss is accompanied by an increased appetite, one must consider the diagnosis of malabsorption or maldigestion as well as a hypermetabolic state, such as thyrotoxicosis. If *diarrhea* is present, one should determine the average number of the stools and their consistency. To some patients, diarrhea means an increased number of stools, even though they are relatively normal in consistency; to others, diarrhea means watery stools. In a patient with diarrhea one should ask about stool *odor* (malodorous stools being typical of pancreatic insufficiency and sprue), change in stool *color* (light-colored stools are seen with steatorrhea or cholestasis), and whether blood or mucus has been noted. (Blood is characteristic of ulcerative colitis but is hardly ever noted in mucous colitis.)

Finally, careful attention must be given to a "drug history." We are living in a "medicated society." Unless asked, the patient may forget to mention that he takes aspirin almost daily for headache, and this may indeed account for the occult blood in his stool. Many patients take daily laxatives, which may explain chronic diarrhea and colonic changes on x-ray. It was through a careful analysis of drug therapy that the syndrome of intestinal ulceration due to the ingestion of enteric-coated KCl was recognized.

PHYSICAL EXAMINATION AND ENDOSCOPY A vague history of abdominal distress may be brought into focus by a thorough physical examination. Upper abdominal distress together with tenderness in the right upper quadrant suggests that cholecystitis or hepatitis may be present. The history of intermittent abdominal pain together with a palpable mass or tender loop of bowel in the right lower quadrant should make one suspicious of regional enteritis. All too often, however, in gastrointestinal diseases the routine physical examination is negative and other techniques for examining the intestine are needed. Among the techniques which should almost be routine as an extension of the physical examination is *sigmoidoscopy.* This technique is important in the diagnosis of colonic cancer because (1) approximately 50 percent of large-intestine malignancies are within the reach of the sigmoidoscope; and (2) small rectosigmoid tumors may be missed on examination after a barium enema because of the tortuosity and redundancy of the intestine in this area. Sigmoidoscopy also permits inspection of the mucosa for edema, erythema, friability, or ulceration. In a patient with diarrhea due to nonspecific causes, the mucosa may be normal; with dysentery due to agents such as *Shigella,* the mucosa may become friable, edematous, and hyperemic; if the latter findings are combined with extensive ulcerations, ulcerative or amebic colitis may be present.

With the advent of *fiberoptic instruments,* it has become much easier and less hazardous to perform endoscopic procedures. Gastroscopy is valuable in helping to determine whether a gastric ulcer is benign or malignant. Endoscopy has become an increasingly routine technique in the approach to selected patients with upper gastrointestinal bleeding. Colonoscopy with fiberoptic equipment permits direct examination of mucosa beyond the customary 25 cm of the rigid sigmoidoscope.

RADIOLOGIC EXAMINATION Perhaps in no other organ system is the use of x-ray examination as important to diagnosis as in disorders of the intestinal tract. In fact, with few exceptions investigation of the patient with gastrointestinal symptoms is not complete without appropriate x-ray examination. However, all too often x-ray examination is ordered by the physician without attention to a number of important factors.

Initial considerations by the internist To obtain the best and most effective use of gastrointestinal x-rays, the physician must decide (1) which *organ system* is most likely to be involved, (2) in what *sequence* to perform the x-rays, and (3) whether there are any *contraindications* to the proposed radiologic study.

If the physician orders an upper gastrointestinal series and the results are negative, he may decide to order a barium enema only to find that it must be delayed because of the presence of barium from the prior study. Therefore, if a thorough study of the intestinal tract is contemplated, the sequence should be (1) oral cholecystogram, (2) barium enema, and (3) upper gastrointestinal series. Preparation or prior cleansing of the intestinal tract is important for a proper barium enema examination, but the physician must keep in mind that with obstructing lesions of the colon or small intestine or in the presence of active ulcerative colitis, the use of strong cathartics may be hazardous and even life-threatening. *No x-ray preparation should be considered routine.* In fact, the barium examination itself may aggravate an acute ulcerative colitis or precipitate colonic perforation or the onset of toxic megacolon. Similarly, if partial obstruction of the intestine is detected by plain x-ray of the abdomen, the physician must be wary of introducing barium from above for fear of producing further or complete intestinal obstruction.

Consultation with the radiologist One cannot overemphasize the importance of providing the radiologist with as much information as possible about the nature of the disease process under investigation. Though this can be done in writing (on the x-ray requisition), it is often preferable to do it verbally. In fact, in difficult cases it is advantageous for the physician to join the radiologist during the study. In addition, the radiologist may suggest, for example, that instead of barium an iodinated radiopaque dye may be preferable; that the study should be supplemented with angiography, especially in the patient with gastrointestinal bleeding or portal hypertension; or that the examination be repeated with more adequate preparation of the patient.

Interpretation All too often the busy physician allows a negative x-ray report to be the decisive factor in his diagnosis. If the patient has had weight loss and a change in bowel habits and the physician suspects a colonic neoplasm, inspection of the x-rays (by himself or preferably with the radiologist) may in fact reveal that the patient had too much retained fecal material in his colon or that the area of concern was never well visualized. Similarly, if the patient has typical ulcer symptoms or a classic history of biliary colic, the physician should not discard his diagnosis merely because of a negative x-ray report.

On the other hand the physician must be able to determine whether the abnormal finding is causally related to the symptoms. This is especially true in older patients where the presence of a hiatus hernia, gallstones, or diverticulosis is not unusual and hence may be coincidental.

DIAGNOSTIC APPROACHES **Problems of swallowing** The approach should be as follows:

1 Careful visual and *neurologic examination* of the pharynx, with tests for myasthenia gravis if indicated.
2 *Routine esophageal x-rays* in the upright and lateral or Trendelenburg position. The horizontal views are essential for demonstration of the swallowing mechanism, unaided by gravity, and of the esophagogastric junction. For details of the pharyngoesophageal area cineradiography is necessary because of the rapidity with which the contrast media passes through. Hiatus hernia is extremely common (in 15 to 35 percent of persons over fifty) and often asymptomatic unless reflux of gastric contents can be demonstrated to occur repeatedly.
3 *Esophagoscopy* is desirable to describe lesions suggested by x-ray, or if the lesion is unsuspected, to obtain biopsies from masses or abnormal mucosa, and to obtain washings for exfoliative cytologic study. The diagnosis of peptic esophagitis is best made endoscopically. Esophageal varices can be identified by this approach when they are too small to be seen radiologically, although the latter technique will pick up 70 percent of large varices.
4 *Manometric studies* of the pharyngoesophageal area, particularly in conjunction with cineradiography, at present offer the best differential between disorders primary in the central nervous system, primary pharyngeal muscular disease, and cricopharyngeal dystonia. Manometry of the esophagus is useful in the diagnosis of diffuse esophageal spasm, achalasia, and infiltrative diseases which can alter esophageal motility.

Peptic or digestive disorders The approaches to these disorders include:

1 *Insertion of a nasogastric tube.* This is used to establish whether significant gastric retention (more than 75 ml) exists, and whether there is acid, bile, blood, or other material in these contents. If pyloric obstruction or gastric atony is present, the tube is used to maintain suction while the patient's electrolyte and fluid balance is restored to normal; the stomach is kept as clean as possible so that reliable radiologic investigation may be carried out.
2 *Radiologic examination* of stomach, duodenum, and the upper part of the jejunum is the most important single procedure in this area. The single examination of the stomach carries an overall accuracy of about 80 percent if the lumen is carefully cleaned out beforehand; duodenal lesions are more precisely identified (90 percent). However, gastritis and superficial ulcers of the duodenum may be missed with routine barium studies.
3 When lesions are noted radiographically in the stomach, *gastroscopy* may be very helpful in identifying the diffuseness of the mucosal response in gastritis or, together with biopsy and brushings for cytology, in differentiating between peptic and neoplastic ulcerating lesions. Gastroscopy may permit the diagnosis of superficial erosive gastritis and Mallory-Weiss syndrome as a cause of bleeding when the x-ray examination is negative. Gastroscopy is particularly helpful in inspecting the postoperative stomach, especially when stomal ulceration is expected. It is useful in detecting bile reflux.
4 *Exfoliative cytologic study* of gastric contents, in the hands of experts, is capable of an accuracy of 85 to 95 percent in diagnosing mucosal abnormalities such as malignancies and the gastric changes of pernicious anemia. The method is of value in follow-up studies of patients with high probability of developing gastric neoplasms.
5 *Gastric acid–secretory studies* are useful in the diagnosis of the Zollinger-Ellison syndrome and suspected carcinoma or atrophic gastritis, and for determination of completeness of vagotomy. They should not be obtained for the routine diagnosis of uncomplicated duodenal ulcer. There is no convincing evidence that acid studies are useful in determining the type of surgery for duodenal ulcer.

The only reliable technique for measuring rates of gastric acid production employs an indwelling tube and requires careful attention to details of tube placement, handling of samples, and analysis. Presently this method is used in one of two ways: (1) "Basal secretion" is that obtained in the morning after an overnight fast in an unstimulated stomach; it measures vagal plus hormonal factors acting on the gastric mucosa. After discarding the first aspirate, four samples are taken over a period of an hour, while the patient expectorates any saliva. The absence of hydrochloric acid in any of the four samples is considered incompatible with the presence of an active duodenal ulcer. (2) "Maximum acid output" is assessed by collecting samples every 15 min for an hour in a patient who has previously received a parenteral antihistaminic drug and then an amount of parenteral histamine equal to 0.04 mg histamine acid phosphate per kilogram body weight; if the safer analogue, betazole, is used, 2 mg per kg body weight is administered. One may also give pentagastrin (6 μg per kg) intramuscularly. With these drugs one attempts to obtain maximal stimulation of parietal cells. The maximum output is proportional to the total "parietal cell mass." Achlorhydria is defined as the failure of the stomach so stimulated to produce a juice with a pH less than 6. The normal basal fasting secretion is 30 to 70 ml per hr, with acid production being 1 to 2.5 mEq per hr. Maximal acid output is 20 to 25 mEq per hr. In the Zollinger-Ellison syndrome basal acid secretion is usually greater than 10 mEq per hr and exceeds 60 percent of the maximal acid output. An increased serum gastrin level may confirm the diagnosis.

Obstructive and vascular disorders of the small intestine When intestinal problems present as obstructive syndromes, the plain x-ray of the abdomen is the most important diagnostic adjunct to careful physical examination. Patterns of dilatation of individual loops of intestine may be characteristic, as in volvulus or acute pancreatitis; erect and decubitus views will often show fluid levels in the affected segments. Air under the diaphragm is diagnostic of a perforated viscus; air in the portal vein usually results from intestinal necrosis secondary to mesenteric vascular occlusion. The diagnostic accuracy of the plain x-ray in all types of intestinal obstruction is about 75 percent. Celiac artery angiography is of particular value in the diagnosis of mesenteric vascular disease.

Inflammatory and neoplastic diseases of small and large intestine Patients with these conditions are usually identified by history, physical examination, and careful examination of the stools for exudate and blood. Sigmoidoscopy is valuable in identifying mucosal and neoplastic lesions of the lower 25 cm of the colon; anal lesions commonly accompany inflammatory disease of the ileum and colon. The radiologic examination of the small intestine is highly reliable in identifying the prestenotic and stenotic lesions of Crohn's disease. In the colon a single examination in a well-prepared patient has a diagnostic accuracy of 80 to 85 percent; the addition of air-contrast technique brings the accuracy up over 90 percent, but none of these figures is meaningful if the patient is poorly prepared for the examination. In the demonstration of small polyps the degree of accuracy is understandably not so high, but for polyps larger than 1 cm, which are of greater clinical importance, it is satisfactory. The cecal area is the hardest to examine adequately because of its anatomy; flat plaquelike lesions on the posterior wall are particularly hard to demonstrate. The rectal area is usually better visualized proctoscopically than radiologically. It is hoped that immunologic tests, such as those for the *carcinoembryonic antigen* will be increasingly useful in the diagnosis of colonic cancer.

Peroral biopsy of the small intestine and forceps biopsy of the rectosigmoid are of considerable importance in revealing mucosal disease. Rectal biopsy is an excellent means of demonstrating amyloidosis, schistosomiasis, and amebiasis. Submucosal disease is not seen in these superficial biopsies. Hirschsprung's disease is histologically diagnosed by a deep surgical biopsy of the lower part of the rectum.

Malabsorption syndromes Malabsorption may be suspected on the basis of history and physical examination and is confirmed by examination of the stools. Radiologic examination is of general help in ruling out local lesions and suggesting motor and secretory dysfunction, but it is rarely diagnostic unless calcifications in the pancreas or short circuits between intestine and stomach are demonstrated.

The tests useful in the diagnosis of malabsorption are discussed in Chap. 284. Analyses of 3-day stool collections for volume, fat, and nitrogen content on a standard diet are used to establish the diagnosis of malabsorption. The D-xylose absorption test is about 90 percent accurate in separating mucosal disease from pancreatic insufficiency. Peroral biopsy of the small intestine is of value in the diagnosis of celiac disease, and may show the less common infiltrations of the mucosa by amyloid or bacterial mucoproteins (Whipple's disease). Leakage of protein into the intestinal lumen may cause hypoproteinemia and can be demonstrated by the recovery in stools of intravenously administered markers such as albumin labeled with iodine or chromium isotopes.

Biliary tract Cholecystography and intravenous cholangiography cannot be performed in the jaundiced patient because the liver is unable to secrete the contrast material. *Percutaneous cholangiography* or cannulation of the *papilla of Vater* via the fiberoptic endoscope may give diagnostic information when biliary tract obstruction is suspected. When air is seen in the biliary tree, it may coexist with gallstone ileus, representing the fistula formed between the gallbladder and duodenum by the passed stone.

Barium studies of the duodenum for the changes produced by pancreatic masses, pancreatitis, and retroperitoneal nodes have been markedly improved in recent years, especially by the use of *hypotonic duodenography*, but the accuracy of such examinations is still not over 80 percent. *Exfoliative cytologic studies* of the second and third portions of the duodenum are reliable in expert hands, particularly when they are used after "flushing" the pancreatic ducts with secretin. The accuracy of this technique for cancer of the pancreas in the best hands approaches 80 percent; negative results thus may not have important significance. The same kind of intubation technique can be used to demonstrate cholesterol crystals and microspheroliths in aspirated bile for the positive diagnosis of gallstones, and with the addition of an indwelling gastric tube for suction, to carry out tests of pancreatic secretion as stimulated by secretin and cholinergics (see Chaps. 301, 302, and 334).

REFERENCES

BLENDIS LM: Carcinoma of stomach: Evaluation of individual and combined diagnostic accuracy of radiology, cytology and gastrophotography. Br Med J 1:656, 1967

COOLEY RN: The diagnostic accuracy of radiologic studies of biliary tract, small intestine, and colon. Am J Med Sci 246:610, 1963

COTTON PB et al: Cannulation of papilla of Vater via fiberduodenoscope: Assessment of retrograde cholangiopancreatography in 60 patients. Lancet 1:53, 1972

POLLARD JJ, NEBESAR RA: Abdominal angiography. N Engl J Med 279:1035, 1093, 1148, 1968

281 DISEASES OF THE ESOPHAGUS

THOMAS R. HENDRIX

Although the exact correlation of anatomic, radiologic, and functional features of the esophagus and the cardioesophageal junction in particular continues to be debated, it is useful to consider disorders of the esophagus in functional terms. In normal swallowing the activities of the striated muscle of the pharynx and upper esophagus and the smooth muscle of the lower esophagus are so closely integrated that they function as a single tissue. The esophagus proper is separated from adjacent segments of the alimentary tract by two sphincters. (A sphincter is a segment that has a resting tone greater than the adjacent segments and that relaxes in response to the appropriate stimulus—swallowing in the case of the esophagus.) The upper esophageal sphincter (cricopharyngeus) separates the pharynx from the esophagus and prevents air from filling the esophagus during inspiration. The lower esophageal sphincter is the barrier to reflux of gastric juice into the esophagus. It relaxes during swallowing, regurgitation, belching, and vomiting.

Other structures illustrated diagrammatically in Fig. 281-1 have been assigned varying roles in preventing reflux. These include the infradiaphragmatic segment of the lower esophageal sphincter, the possible flap valve mechanism provided by the angle of His, and the diaphragm itself. The first phase of swallowing, the movement of the bolus from the mouth to the pharynx, is voluntary, but subsequent events are involuntary. As the upper sphincter relaxes, the bolus is propelled into the esophagus. The lower esophageal sphincter relaxes prior to the arrival of the bolus in the lower esophagus. Finally, the esophagus is swept clean by a peristaltic wave proceeding from pharynx to lower esophageal sphincter.

SYMPTOMATOLOGY Dysphagia (see Chap. 37) Difficulty in swallowing can be produced by the derangement or incoordination of any part of the swallowing act as well as by the narrowing of the lumen by tumor or an inflammatory stricture. Dysphagia of oropharyngeal origin is characterized by failure to move a bolus out of the mouth, regurgitation into the nose, or aspiration into the trachea. Esophageal dysphagia is characterized by the complaint that food is sticking somewhere behind the sternum. Dysphagia occurs only with swallowing and must be differentiated from globus hystericus, a persistent sensation of a lump or tightness in the throat.

Dysphagia is usually localized to the level of the lower sternum corresponding to the most frequent site of esophageal disease. In other instances dysphagia is localized higher in the chest or at the base of the neck, either because the responsible lesion is situated higher in the esophagus or because in some patients sensations from the distal esophagus are referred to the level of the sternal notch.

Dysphagia may be painless, but more often it is distressing and sometimes causes pain of alarming proportions. It commonly appears gradually or in intermittent attacks, although on occasion the onset is abrupt and reaches maximum intensity rapidly. Certain foods, notably beef and soft breads, are often the first offenders, probably because these elastic solids are wedged by peristalsis into the segment narrowed by esophageal disease. The impacted bolus may be forced through the narrowed area by drinking liquids, or forceful retching may be required to dislodge the food, and on occasion it must be removed through the esophagoscope.

Pain Heartburn, or pyrosis, is the most common type of esophageal pain. Heartburn, a burning, tight, or searing sensation, appears intermittently beneath the lower sternum and spreads upward in a wavelike fashion to the throat or even into the angles of the jaw. It is often associated with increased salivation. Heartburn is most likely to occur 10 to 60 min after eating, especially after overindulging, and is accentuated by bending over or lying down. Heartburn is the consequence of reflux of irritant material into the esophagus, usually acid gastric juice, but intestinal juice containing bile and pancreatic enzymes is equally irritating and is more difficult to inactivate.

Esophageal pain frequently accompanies dysphagia and may be severe if the bolus is unable to pass the constricted segment. In addition, esophageal pain may occur in the absence of dysphagia or obvious heartburn. At times its onset is so abrupt and severe that myocardial infarction is the initial diagnosis. Esophageal pain may mimic ischemic heart pain even to the radiation of pain down the ulnar aspect of the arms. Referral of esophageal pain to the epigastrium is common, and referral to the back is encountered on occasion.

Belching A belch is caused by the forceful regurgitation of air from the stomach or esophagus. Although belching is an esophageal phenomenon, it is not a common manifestation of esophageal disease. More often it is a functional disorder or is indicative of peptic, cardiac, or biliary tract disease.

Regurgitation Regurgitation, as contrasted to vomiting, is the effortless appearance of esophageal or gastric contents in the mouth. A functional disorder of esophageal motility, a retrograde flow of material forced by normal peristalsis against an obstructed segment, or a gravitational effect, as in the case of the dilated esophagus of cardiospasm, may be responsible for regurgitation.

GASTROESOPHAGEAL REFLUX AND ESOPHAGITIS

Reflux of small amounts of gastric juice into the lower part of the esophagus is a common event. Its frequency is increased by overindulgence. Whether or not reflux occurs and whether it produces symptoms are determined by three factors: (1) the competency of the lower esophageal sphincter, the primary barrier to reflux; (2) the irritant nature of the refluxed material; and (3) the sensitivity of the esophageal mucosa to the refluxed material. Although the symptoms of reflux were attributed in the past to inflammation of the esophagus, i.e., esophagitis, it is clear that esophagitis is a complication of severe reflux rather than being the cause of the symptoms associated with reflux. On the other hand, the competency of the lower esophageal sphincter correlates well with the presence or absence of reflux. Refluxed acid gastric juice is the most common cause of reflux symptoms; the reflux of alkaline intestinal juice, which may occur after gastric resection, also causes reflux symptoms which are particularly difficult to manage.

SYMPTOMS Heartburn, the typical symptom of reflux, is characterized by burning epigastric or retrosternal pain which spreads upward. Typically, heartburn appears after meals, especially large meals, and is aggravated by bending over, lying down, or straining. It is relieved by standing up or drinking something, especially antacids. In severe episodes, the pain may radiate to the base of the neck, the angles of the jaw, or down one or both arms, simulating angina pectoris. Although heartburn is often a trivial complaint without serious consequences, it must be differentiated from other causes of chest pain and may be the manifestation of esophagitis. In some cases, when the patient is asleep, there is a reflux of material into the hypopharynx and this material is aspirated. The patient awakens coughing and strangling on the refluxed material. If this process is severe or recurrent, pneumonitis or pulmonary fibrosis may ensue.

DIAGNOSIS To establish that a patient's chest pain is caused by reflux, it must be shown that reflux occurs and that the esophagus is sensitive to the refluxed fluid. The most sensitive test of reflux is to measure intraesophageal pH after instilling a volume (300 ml) of 0.1 *N* HC1 into the stomach. If the sphincter is competent, intraesophageal pH will remain above 5 or 6. In patients with reflux the pH falls intermittently to pH 1.5 or 2, and in those with free reflux the pH never rises above intragastric levels as the pH electrode is withdrawn from the stomach into the esophagus. Radiographic studies can demonstrate reflux in no more than 40 percent of symptomatic patients. To determine if reflux causes the patient's symptom, reflux may be mimicked by perfusing the esophagus alternately with saline solution and 0.1 *N* HC1 at 120 drops per minute. In patients with symptoms due to reflux, pain is produced by acid perfusion but not with saline, whereas the asymptomatic individual or a patient with chest pain of different origin is unable to distinguish between saline and acid perfusion.

TREATMENT Medical management aims to protect the esophagus by decreasing reflux of gastric juice and by decreasing the irritant effect of the refluxed juice. The first aim may be achieved by decreasing the volume of gastric contents available for reflux, by positioning the patient so that gravity acts to impede reflux, and by improving the function of the lower esophageal sphincter. In practical terms, the patient is advised to take small meals and not to eat in the 2 to 3 hr before retiring. Patients should avoid those foods which they may have found to be associated with dyspepsia and heartburn. Four to six-inch blocks elevating the head of the bed lessen nocturnal gastroesophageal regurgitation.

Although anticholinergic drugs decrease the volume of gastric secretion, they are not indicated in the treatment of peptic esophagitis because in effective doses that decrease tone in the lower esophageal sphincter they decrease the volume of alkaline saliva, and they decrease frequency of secondary peristalsis, which functions to return refluxed gastric juice to the stomach. To aid in decreasing the irritant effect of refluxed gastric juice, 15 to 30 ml of a liquid, viscous antacid preparation, such as aluminum hydroxide gel, should be taken at hourly intervals while the patient is awake. The medication should be taken "straight" and should not be followed by other material. After 2 weeks the frequency usually can be decreased because the esophageal mucosa has become less sensitive to the refluxed material.

Finally, in stocky or obese patients, weight loss is beneficial.

Chronic reflux esophagitis

Reflux esophagitis is inflammation of the esophageal mucosa caused by reflux of acid gastric or alkaline intestinal juice. One-fourth of patients with symptoms severe enough to be considered indicative of reflux esophagitis have normal esophageal biopsies, and less than 20 percent have acute inflammatory changes. On the other hand, reflux may lead to severe damage or loss of the squamous epithelium of the lower part of the esophagus. When such severe esophagitis heals, the squamous epithelium may be replaced by columnar epithelium. If esophagitis is persistent or severe, an inflammatory stricture will develop.

SYMPTOMS The symptoms of esophagitis are symptoms of reflux. In some patients heartburn worsens, cold and hot foods and slightly acid foods are increasingly painful to swallow, and eventually dysphagia appears. Dysphagia is most frequently due to acid-induced esophageal spasm. In some patients, not necessarily those with the most impressive reflux symptoms, an inflammatory stricture develops, causing progressive dysphagia. With advancing disease, malnutrition is inevitable, and occasionally slow blood loss occurs.

DIAGNOSIS The diagnosis of esophagitis may be suspected on clinical, radiographic, and esophagoscopic findings but is established by demonstrating inflammatory changes in an esophageal biopsy. Esophagitis is not necessarily a primary process but may be the manifestation of a variety of diseases such as peptic ulcer, cancer, and scleroderma.

TREATMENT The treatment of esophagitis is the treatment of reflux, but the end point in addition to relief of symptoms is healing of the inflammatory process so that strictures do not develop. If healing does not occur, symptoms are not controlled, or bleeding or stricture develops during 3 to 6 months of carefully controlled medical therapy, surgical therapy should be offered. The fundoplication operations of Belsey, Hill, or Nissen have given the best results. If a severe stricture has developed, it may be necessary to resect the involved segment and interpose a segment of colon.

Hiatal hernia

Hiatal hernia is defined as a herniation of a portion of the stomach into the chest through the esophageal hiatus of the diaphragm. Clinically it is useful to classify hernias as rolling, or paraesophageal, and sliding, or direct. In the first, the gastric cardia rolls through the hiatus beside a gastroesophageal junction that is normally situated with respect to the diaphragmatic hiatus (Fig. 281-1*B*). In the second, the sliding, or direct, hernia, both the stomach and the gastroesophageal junction slip up into the chest, thereby placing the gastroesophageal junction above the diaphragmatic hiatus (Fig. 281-1*C*). This position of the junction may make the esophagus appear shortened, but actual shortening occurs rarely. Many hernias are mixed and present features of both types.

Sliding hernia is three to ten times as common as the rolling and mixed hernias combined. Paraesophageal hernias are primarily a disorder of women, being ten times as frequent in women as in men.

SYMPTOMS The major symptoms that can be attributed to a sliding hernia are those initiated by reflux into the esophagus.

Symptoms due to the herniated pouch of the stomach are almost exclusively limited to the rolling, or mixed, type of hernia. On rare occasions a patient with a paraesophageal hernia comes to the physician with acute prostration due to strangulation of the hernia. Although chronic and acute bleeding commonly are attributed to hernias, bleeding most often originates in mucosal erosion, peptic ulcers, and esophagitis, all of which may be associated with diaphragmatic hernia. It is uncommon, however, for gastrointestinal bleeding to be *proved* to be originating from the hernia itself or from the esophagus.

The principal complications of sliding hiatal hernias are due to gastroesophageal reflux and peptic esophagitis.

DIAGNOSIS The diagnosis of diaphragmatic hernia is often suspected on the basis of reflux symptoms. The definitive diagnosis, however, must rest on radiographic evidence. Superficially it would seem a simple matter to determine whether or not the stomach is in its rightful place in the abdomen, because the commonly accepted criteria seem precise. The application of these criteria apparently presents great difficulty, and the incidence of diaphragmatic hernia has been reported to be as low as 10 percent and as high as 70 percent in routine barium meal studies performed for the investigation of dyspepsia. There is also no agreement as to the frequency with which diaphragmatic hernias produce symptoms, and it has been claimed that the incidence of symptoms varies from 30 to 97 percent. Symptoms ascribed to diaphragmatic hernia are diverse and may resemble those of coronary insufficiency, biliary colic, pancreatitis, gastric and duodenal ulcers, esophageal disorders, and functional digestive disorders. Association, however, does not establish a cause-and-effect relation. The important clinical question is not whether the patient has a hernia but whether significant reflux is present.

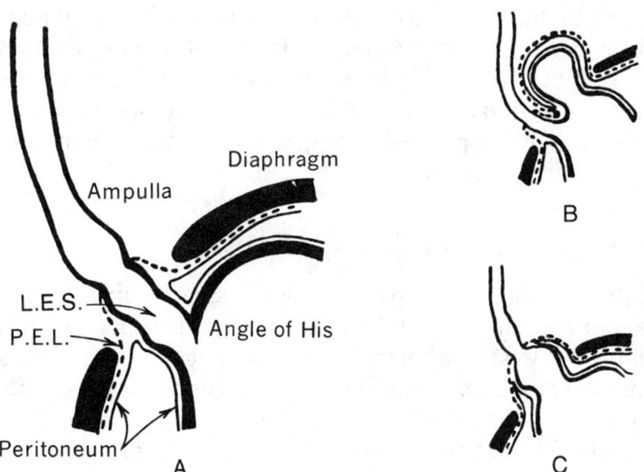

FIGURE 281-1
Diagrammatic representation of the structure and relations of the lower esophagus. A *Normal esophagus.* B *Parahiatal hernia.* C *Sliding hernia. In this type of hernia the distinction between the lower esophageal sphincter and the herniated cardia is lost, and the angle of His has become obtuse. L.E.S. = lower esophageal sphincter. P.E.L. = phrenoesophageal ligament. The location of the gastroesophageal junction is a matter of opinion. It may be defined as located at the level where the tube of the esophagus widens into the sac of the stomach, but sometimes the transition from one shape to the other is gradual rather than abrupt. Alternatively, the junction is placed at the serrated line where squamous esophageal and glandular gastric mucosas meet, but this epithelial boundary is located somewhat above the level of the angle of His and thus does not coincide with a division of stomach and esophagus based on gross shape and muscular function.*

TREATMENT The aim of treatment is to decrease gastroesophageal reflux. Operative repair of paraesophageal hernias is indicated if they have been identified as causing esophageal obstruction, respiratory symptoms, perforation, strangulation, repeated or chronic bleeding, or severe distress not affected by intensive use of medical measures.

Acute esophagitis

Mild acute esophagitis, with substernal pain aggravated by swallowing, may complicate infections of the upper part of the respiratory tract. Severe esophageal inflammation with variable necrosis may occur in moribund states, in diseases of the central nervous system, after extensive burns or trauma, after operations, especially if vomiting is pronounced or gastric intubation prolonged, with herpetic oral lesions that extend into the esophagus, and with monilial esophagitis that may appear in those weakened by chronic disease, especially if antibiotics or adrenocortical hormones have been used. In many of these conditions debility, ischemia, the trauma of vomiting, or exposure of the esophageal mucosa to acid gastric contents must be important pathogenic factors.

The ingestion of alkaline corrosive agents produces a

form of acute esophagitis which, if not immediately fatal, may terminate in extensive esophageal stenosis. Immediate treatment consists of administration of parenteral analgesics for pain and avoidance of oral intake for 3 to 7 days. The use of adrenocorticosteroids to contain the tissue reaction responsible for the stricture, intubation to maintain an esophageal lumen, and antibiotics to prevent mediastinitis are controversial.

DIFFUSE ESOPHAGEAL SPASM

Diffuse esophageal spasm is not a specific disease but rather a common disorder of esophageal motility which is caused by several unrelated conditions. It may be a manifestation of aging (presbyesophagus), ganglion degeneration (as seen in early stages of some patients with achalasia), mucosal irritation (most commonly encountered in gastroesophageal reflux), obstruction at the cardia, neuromuscular disorders such as diabetic neuropathy and amyotrophic lateral sclerosis, or if none of these features is present it may be labeled idiopathic. Diffuse spasm in severe form produces retrosternal pain or dysphagia or both. Many patients may, however, have radiographic or manometric evidence of the disorder without symptoms. In patients with this disorder, peristalsis is initiated normally by swallowing, but as the wave approaches the distal third of the esophagus, the progressive contraction is supplanted by "spastic" or simultaneous contractions. Contrary to what happens in achalasia, relaxation of the lower esophageal sphincter is usually normal in diffuse esophageal spasm.

SYMPTOMS Dysphagia or substernal distress occurs episodically. Symptoms frequently, although not necessarily, are triggered by ingestion of elastic boluses (such as meat) or cold or carbonated beverages, and by eating when tense or upset. On occasion a bolus becomes so firmly lodged in the "spastic" segment that relief is achieved only by retching and regurgitating the offending bolus. Often following such an episode the patient can return to the table and finish his meal without incident. Weight loss and aspiration pneumonia are rarely features of diffuse spasm. Substernal pain of esophageal origin may be acute and severe, and may be confused with angina pectoris, especially if symptoms are not associated with eating.

DIAGNOSIS The diagnosis is suggested by the history of intermittent dysphagia and chest pain. X-ray findings (with barium swallow) confirm the existence of disordered esophageal motility. The mildest abnormality is tertiary or segmental contractions without a peristaltic wave in the distal esophagus. The contour of the lower esophagus may take a variety of bizarre shapes described as curling, pseudodiverticulosis, corkscrew, or rosary-bead esophagus. Symptoms, however, do not clearly correlate with the extent of the abnormality seen on barium swallow. Indeed, only a minority of patients with this disturbed motor pattern have significant symptoms. The motility abnormalities of diffuse esophageal spasm may be recorded by esophageal manometry.

TREATMENT The first step in the treatment of diffuse spasm is to reassure the patient as to the benign nature of the disorder. The second step is to minimize the contribution of gastroesophageal reflux by giving antacids and small meals and by elevating the head of the bed as already described under Gastroesophageal Reflux and Esophagitis.

An occasional patient obtains gratifying control of symptoms with the use of sublingual nitroglycerin at mealtime. Anticholinergic drugs, however, have not provided symptomatic relief. In patients with severe, poorly controlled symptoms forceful distention of the lower esophagus and sphincter by a pneumostatic dilator may be employed. As a last resort, a longitudinal myotomy of the entire distal esophagus has been successful in providing relief. This is, however, an extensive operation for a benign disorder.

ACHALASIA

The terms *achalasia* and *cardiospasm* are used interchangeably for a disease usually presenting as slowly progressive dysphagia. Neither describes the nature of the disease completely. Actually, achalasia is a motor disorder involving the entire distal two-thirds of the esophagus. The pressure within the lower esophageal sphincter is twice normal, and relaxation of the sphincter in response to a swallow is incomplete. In addition, there is no peristaltic response to swallowing in the esophagus above the sphincter. For this reason, the name *aperistalsis* is used in Brazil. Finally, the massive dilatation seen in some patients has, in turn, given rise to the name *megaesophagus*.

The motor disorder of achalasia appears to reflect impaired cholinergic innervation of the esophagus. Although the greatest attention has been given to the damage and loss of postganglionic parasympathetic neurons of the myenteric plexuses, pathologic lesions have also been described in the brainstem and extrinsic vagal fibers. Pharmacologic studies have shown that the administration of a cholinergic agent produces violent, segmental contractions of the affected esophagus. This response, when interpreted in the light of Cannon's finding that denervated structures respond maximally to neurohumoral stimulation, provides additional evidence that in achalasia the cholinergic innervation of the esophagus is deficient. Recently, the response of the lower esophageal sphincter to gastrin, which is medicated through the postganglionic parasympathetic fibers, has been shown to be hyperactive in achalasia. Since the normal neuromuscular interactions and the pathology of achalasia are incompletely understood, it is not possible to define the mechanisms responsible for the loss of peristalsis and normal sphincter function in achalasia. In Brazil, the remarkable prevalence of achalasia in areas where Chagas' disease is prevalent has fostered the conviction that the intrinsic esophageal denervation is a late result of esophageal infestation by *Trypanosoma cruzi*. This agent cannot be implicated in achalasia in the United States.

SYMPTOMS Cardiospasm affects patients of all ages and of both sexes. Its course is usually chronic, with dysphagia gradually worsening over months to years, leading to progressive weight loss. In some patients, the process is painless; in others spasms of substernal pain may follow eating. Occasionally the initial episode of dysphagia appears with dramatic suddenness, either after bolting food or after an emotional upset. In either case, however, the condition has probably been present in latent form before the acute episode. As the disease progresses, extreme and tortuous dilatation of the esophagus may develop. When the patient lies down, the copious amount of food residue and saliva contained in the spacious esophageal sac runs freely back into the pharynx and mouth. If the regurgitated material is aspirated, recurrent aspiration pneumonia is a potential complication. Although stagnation of food in the esophagus may be striking, esophagitis rarely if ever occurs in untreated cardiospasm.

DIAGNOSIS Diagnosis is usually made without difficulty on the basis of the history and the characteristic radiologic findings of abnormal esophageal motor function with smooth, beaklike narrowing of the distal esophageal segment. An occasional case presents as diffuse esophageal spasm and over many years evolves into a completely typical example of achalasia. In some cases, cancer originating in the gastric cardia and infiltrating the esophagus may present a somewhat similar x-ray appearance. This possibility is best excluded by esophagoscopic examination of the distal esophagus and cardia. These problems in differential diagnosis should be less frequent if it is remembered that the radiologic abnormalities of achalasia consist of deranged peristalsis as well as narrowing in the area of the sphincter.

TREATMENT Symptomatic medical treatment consisting of sedatives, semisoft foods, nitrites, and anticholinergic drugs is not effective. The best available therapy is forceful dilatation of the narrowed sphincter with the specific purpose of tearing some of the muscle fibers in this area. Passing graduated mercury-tipped bougies does not accomplish this and therefore relieves dysphagia only briefly. It is necessary to use bags that can be inflated under pressure or a mechanical (Starck) dilator. In experienced hands, these instruments, when positioned under fluoroscopic control, rarely cause esophageal rupture, and dysphagia is relieved successfully for years, or even permanently, in over 75 percent of cases. Forceful dilatation does not restore normal esophageal motility, but it impairs the contractile power of the sphincter and thus permits the esophagus to empty under the influence of hydrostatics and transmitted oropharyngeal pressures. Improved esophageal emptying, in turn, prevents further distention of the lumen and aspiration of esophageal contents.

When the esophagus is extremely dilated and sufficiently tortuous to warrant the adjective sigmoid, mechanical dilation of the narrowed area is often not feasible and surgical intervention becomes necessary. Unfortunately any procedure that removes the sphincter between the dilated esophagus and the stomach permits, when the patient lies down, reflux of gastric contents into an already damaged esophagus which cannot muster the peristaltic force necessary to return the gastric contents to the stomach. As a consequence severe esophagitis, which is often more distressing than the achalasia, occurs and also may be a major source of blood loss. If technically feasible, the surgical procedure favored at present is the Heller myotomy, which is based on the same principle as forceful dilatation: the contractile power of the sphincter is reduced by placing a longitudinal cut through the muscle, but not the mucosa, of the narrowed segment. Myotomy is, however, not invariably successful in alleviating dysphagia or preventing reflux esophagitis. In advanced cases, with unsuccessful previous operative procedures, colonic interposition may have to be used to replace the hopelessly malfunctioning gastroesophageal segment.

CANCER

SYMPTOMS The importance of dysphagia as a symptom and the urgent necessity of determining its cause are no better exemplified than by the patient with esophageal cancer. Difficulty in swallowing solids is the patient's first, and usually his only complaint as the tumor encroaches upon the lumen. Although initially intermittent, the dysphagia is inexorably progressive over a course of rarely more than 6 months. Pain under the sternum, the back, or in the neck, is common and may merely be caused by associated esophagitis, but it usually indicates spread of the tumor through the wall of the esophagus. In some cases an early symptom not to be ignored is substernal burning on swallowing hot liquids. Slow oozing of blood is a frequent complication, but brisk bleeding is rare. When esophageal stenosis is severe, regurgitation of esophageal contents, which are sometimes blood-flecked, is common.

Approximately 25 percent of squamous esophageal cancers are in the upper third, 50 percent in the middle, and 25 percent in the lower third of the organ. The lesions in the upper two-thirds are derived squamous esophageal mucosa. In the distal esophagus over half the cases prove to be adenocarcinomas, indicating that many cancers in this area are gastric in origin. Origin in the stomach is, in fact, often evident at operation in cases which radiologically appear to be purely esophageal.

COURSE Physical examination is usually negative, and even those patients with advanced disease may present no more than the signs of malnutrition. Although metastases to lymph nodes occur in three-fourths of the cases, only 5 percent have palpable nodes in the supraclavicular or other accessible areas. Because the liver and lung each are involved eventually in 20 to 25 percent of the cases, hepatomegaly or pulmonary lesions may be evident. Other organs subject to metastatic foci are bone, kidneys, and adrenal glands. Sometimes direct invasion of adjoining structures leads to dramatic complications: (1) mediastinitis with subcutaneous emphysema in the neck, (2) tracheoesophageal or bronchoesophageal fistula, with an apoplectic cough induced by swallowing liquids, or (3) aortic perforation with precipitous exsanguination.

DIAGNOSIS Esophageal cancer occurs in the usual cancer age groups, and predominantly in males, in a ratio of 4:1. In the United States and Europe it accounts for only 7 percent of all cancers in males, whereas in some parts of Asia it is one of the most common cancers. X-ray often reveals the irregular and sometimes surprisingly long luminal defect caused by esophageal cancer, but supplemental diagnostic information must usually be sought by esophagoscopy and biopsy. The initial examination with either procedure is not, however, invariably adequate in differentiating cancer from inflammatory stricture. In these cases, cytologic examination of material obtained by esophageal lavage is indicated. This procedure, depending upon the interest and experience of the cytologic laboratory, yields 75 to 95 percent positive results in patients with esophageal cancer.

TREATMENT Lesions that appear to be resectable are usually treated surgically. Calculated on the basis of all esophageal cancer patients who enter a hospital, the 5-year cure rate is still a disappointing 0 to 7 percent. In some hands, however, 5-year cure rates in patients who at operation have no gross evidence of extension are over 15 percent for cancers in the lower third of the esophagus. Somewhat better results have been obtained by combining resection with preoperative irradiation. Successful resection of middle and upper-third lesions is more difficult or impossible, and such lesions are usually treated with radiotherapy. In the case of inoperable tumors of the fungating variety, a remarkable degree of palliation may sometimes be achieved by deep radiotherapy.

OTHER ESOPHAGEAL DISORDERS

DIVERTICULA Diverticula are found in the esophagus in about 5 percent of older patients who are given a swallow of barium. Most of these pouches occur in the midesophagus and distal esophagus, but they are usually small (1 to 4 cm in diameter) and do not cause symptoms. Extremely rarely an esophageal diverticulum is subject to ulceration or becomes large enough to cause dysphagia. A diverticulum of great clinical importance, however, is Zenker's diverticulum, a pouch which actually arises in the posterior aspect of the hypopharynx above the upper esophageal sphincter but which extends downward between the spine and the esophagus. Patients with this condition—elderly men for the most part—suffer dysphagia because swallowed material tends to fill the diverticular sac, which then compresses the esophagus. Regurgitation of stagnant food and nocturnal fits of coughing may complicate the picture. The diagnosis can usually be made by x-ray provided the pharynx is adequately studied as the patient swallows barium. Surgical treatment is necessary to relieve the symptoms of Zenker's diverticulum. Myotomy of the upper sphincter has improved the results of surgical treatment.

LOWER ESOPHAGEAL RING This is the name given to a thin, symmetric, diaphragm-like structure located 1 to 4 cm above the diaphragmatic hiatus. Ten to twenty percent of adults have asymptomatic rings, but if the residual lumen is less than 12 mm in diameter, the ring may cause a highly characteristic syndrome consisting of intermittent attacks of dysphagia, recurring over years, unassociated with any other esophageal abnormality and precipitated only when the patient swallows meat or other elastic chunks without proper chewing. Treatment usually consists of avoiding hasty swallowing. Dilatation is inconstantly successful. In a few, unusually severe cases, surgical treatment with cutting or fracture of the diaphragm is indicated.

SCLERODERMA (PROGRESSIVE SYSTEMIC SCLEROSIS) Scleroderma is associated with loss of esophageal peristalsis and sphincter tone in 80 percent of the cases. Although gastroesophageal reflux and esophagitis are common, heartburn is not a prominent feature, and dysphagia, which is much less striking than that encountered with achalasia, does not become prominent until esophagitis has led to stricture of the esophagus. Chronic blood loss may be an important complication. Esophageal aperistalsis is not limited to scleroderma but may be seen occasionally in other disorders, particularly those associated with Raynaud's phenomenon.

DERMATOMYOSITIS Oropharyngeal dysphagia (see Chap. 37) complicates the course of patients with dermatomyositis because of involvement of the striated muscle of the pharynx. Difficulty in propelling the bolus from the mouth into the esophagus, regurgitation into the nose, and aspiration are the consequences of pharyngeal muscle weakness. Aperistalsis of the esophagus is seen occasionally in patients with polymyositis. It is sometimes difficult to categorize these patients, because they may have features of both scleroderma and dermatomyositis.

PEPTIC ULCER A solitary peptic ulcer is occasionally found in the distal esophagus. This lesion differs from peptic esophagitis in that the ulcer is sharply localized, penetrates deeply, and may perforate or cause massive bleeding. The solitary peptic ulcer in the distal esophagus resembles a benign gastric ulcer in many respects. Indeed many ulcers at the lower end of the gullet actually involve either a herniated portion of stomach or a section of the esophagus that is lined with gastric mucosa.

PERFORATION AND RUPTURE Perforation of the esophagus may complicate esophagitis, peptic ulcer, or neoplasm. Rupture may be induced by external trauma or, more commonly, during instrumentation of the esophagus. Sometimes it develops spontaneously in a previously healthy organ. The consequences are a syndrome comprising (1) severe pain, usually substernal but occasionally epigastric or precordial, intensified by swallowing, (2) free air in the mediastinum, producing a mediastinal crunch and subcutaneous emphysema palpable within 1 to 12 hr, (3) digestion of mediastinal pleura by pressure and gastric juice with resultant hydropneumothorax or hemopneumothorax and respiratory embarrassment, (4) shock, and (5) secondary infection.

Spontaneous rupture is a specific entity that develops suddenly during vomiting or coughing, or occasionally merely after injudicious gluttony. The tear, 1 to 8 cm in length, almost invariably is in the posterolateral portion of the esophagus immediately proximal to the diaphragmatic hiatus. The diagnosis should be suspected in elderly men (80 percent of cases) who suddenly have pain while vomiting or coughing; it is established by x-ray (air in the mediastinum or neck, demonstration of laceration by having the patient swallow radiopaque material, pleuropulmonary abnormalities), detection of methylene blue in the pleural fluid after a swallow of the dye, and exclusion of myocardial infarction, pancreatitis, and ruptured abdominal viscus. Air under the diaphragm is never found in spontaneous esophageal rupture.

Perforation of the esophagus is fatal if not treated vigorously. In early cases, constant esophageal suction and parenteral administration of antibiotics, which are active against both enteric gram-negative organisms and enterococci, should be given. Surgical drainage and repair of the laceration are indicated as soon as possible.

A disorder closely allied to spontaneous esophageal rupture is vertical laceration of the gastroesophageal junction producing severe and occasionally exsanguinating hemorrhage. This so-called "Mallory-Weiss syndrome" usually develops when vomiting follows an alcoholic bout.

PATTERSON-KELLY (PLUMMER-VINSON) SYNDROME This syndrome, also known as *sideropenic dysphagia*, is a cause of dysphagia in women with hypochromic anemia. A crescentic fold indenting the anterior aspect of the cricopharyngeal area and mucosal atrophy and inflammation of the hypopharynx are features of this disorder. A good diet and iron are usually therapeutically effective, but sometimes supplemental instrumental dilatation is required. This lesion predisposes to pharyngeal carcinoma.

FOREIGN BODIES Foreign bodies may cause dysphagia, pain, or perforation of the esophagus. Rigid bodies usually are arrested above the aortic arch, and elastic material usually is held up in the distal esophagus. Not infrequently a structural abnormality or disease of the esophagus is responsible for stopping the foreign body.

VARICES Esophageal varices are discussed in Chaps. 41 and 296. They do not cause dysphagia or other esophageal symptoms. Radiologically, however, they may be confused with cancer or esophagitis.

BENIGN INTRAMURAL TUMORS OF THE ESOPHAGUS Tumors such as cyst (usually of respiratory tract origin), leiomyoma, fibroma, and neurofibroma may cause intermittent dysphagia and sharply defined radiologic defects with smooth margins. Some benign tumors, especially adenomas, may produce intraluminal polyps.

The esophagus may be affected by leukoplakia, acanthosis nigricans, sarcoma, Hodgkin's disease, and leukemia.

EXTRINSIC DISEASE Diseases of the aorta, heart, respiratory tract, or mediastinal lymph nodes often displace the esophagus and may appear to narrow the lumen. Aneurysms of the aortic arch and an aberrant right subclavian artery may compress the esophageal lumen; however, dysphagia is rarely produced by extrinsic esophageal masses. Invasion of the esophagus by bronchogenic carcinoma occurs rarely.

REFERENCES

Adams CWM et al: Achalasia of the cardia. Guy's Hosp Rep 110:191, 1961

Atkinson M: Mechanisms protecting against gastro-oesophageal reflux: A review. Gut 3:1, 1962

Bayless TM: Management of esophageal disease. Mod Treat 7:1081, 1970

Bennett JR, Hendrix TR: Diffuse esophageal spasm: A disorder with more than one cause. Gastroenterology 59:273, 1970

Benz L et al: A comparison of clinical measurements of gastroesophageal reflux. Gastroenterology 62:1, 1972

Cohen S, Harris LD: Does hiatus hernia affect competence of the gastroesophageal sphincter? N Engl J Med 284:1053, 1971

——, Lipshutz W: Lower esophageal sphincter function in achalasia. Gastroenterology 61:814, 1971

Ismail-Beigi F et al: Histological consequences of gastroesophageal reflux in man. Gastroenterology 58:163, 1970

Kramer P: Does a sliding hiatus hernia constitute a distinct clinical entity? Gastroenterology 57:442, 1969

Skinner DB et al: *Gastroesophageal Reflux and Hiatal Hernia*, Boston: Little, Brown, 1972

282
PEPTIC ULCER

WILLIAM SILEN

A rational understanding of the pathophysiology of gastric secretion and peptic ulcer requires a sound knowledge of the normal mechanisms which control the function of the stomach.

PHYSIOLOGY OF THE STOMACH

Gastric secretion

MECHANISMS It is generally accepted that gastric juice is the result of two types of secretion: a component actively produced by the parietal cells and consisting of a slightly hyperosmotic secretion of hydrochloric acid and potassium chloride; and a nonparietal component, possibly of extracellular origin and virtually identical in composition to interstitial fluid. An alternative theory suggests that the final composition of gastric juice is derived from primary gastric secretion after back diffusion of hydrogen ion and some exchange of hydrogen for sodium has taken place. The rate of gastric secretion is virtually linearly related to mucosal blood flow, although agents such as histamine and gastrin may exert a stimulatory effect on gastric secretion in vitro without producing alterations in the circulation. The role of endogenous histamine as a final common pathway by which other stimuli act remains controversial.

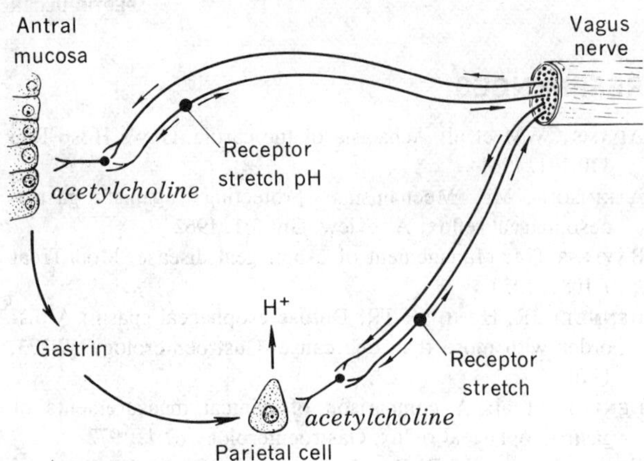

FIGURE 282-1
Diagrammatic representation of neurohumoral control of gastric secretion. The two cholinergic end effects, cholinergic stimulation of parietal cells and release of gastrin, are identical for the cephalic and gastric phases. (Modified after MI Grossman, Physiologist 6:349, 1963)

THE CONTROL OF GASTRIC ACID SECRETION *The cephalic phase* of gastric secretion consists of (1) a direct vagal stimulation of the parietal cell mediated over long vagal tracts and causing elaboration of acid gastric juice rich in pepsin, and (2) an indirect component, also carried over long tracts of the vagus, which results in the release of antral gastrin. The *gastric phase* of gastric secretion also consists of two components: (1) a direct component in which activation of local cholinergic reflexes by *fundic* distention is by itself a rather weak stimulus, although potentiation of other stimuli such as gastrin or histamine is marked, and (2) an indirect component which consists of secretion of antral gastrin in response to local antral stimuli such as distention or the presence of an alkaline solution in the lumen. The indirect component of the gastric phase is mediated by local antral cholinergic reflexes. Since all four components are thus cholinergically influenced, neurohumoral relationships are the key to the control of gastric secretion. A variety of stimuli may thus ultimately produce the same two cholinergic end effects, namely the direct stimulation of parietal cells or the release of antral gastrin (Fig. 282-1).

Gregory has succeeded in establishing the structure of gastrin and in purifying and synthesizing it (Fig. 282-2). Gastrin is a polypeptide composed of 17 amino acids. The active moiety of the molecule is contained in the terminal tetrapeptide, and all the actions of the entire molecule can be produced by a peptide consisting of the terminal four amino acids arranged in the proper sequence. The terminal tetrapeptide is the same in the gastrin of all species identified to date. Immunoassay studies have shown that there exists a "big" circulating gastrin with a molecular weight of about 6,000, but the functional and physiologic significance of this gastrin remain unknown. On a molar weight basis gastrin is about 500 times as potent as histamine in its capacity to stimulate gastric secretion. The actions of pure gastrin are (1) stimulation of gastric acid and pepsin secretion, (2) stimulation of gastric and intestinal motility, (3) increase of volume and enzyme output by the pancreas, (4) increase of flow of hepatic bile, (5) increase in tone of the lower esophageal sphincter, (6) increase in output of intrinsic factor. Since pancreozymin and cholecystokinin are similar to each other structurally and possess the same terminal tetrapeptide as gastrin, some of the extragastric effects of gastrin are more easily understood. The length and composition of the remainder of the molecule may thus modify the intensity of the various effects of the hormones. Several investigators have been successful in producing antibodies to gastrin or one of its analogues after coupling them with other protein moieties, so that routine determination of levels of serum gastrin are now available.

FIGURE 282-2
Amino acid sequence of human gastrin I. The amino acids in positions 14 through 17 comprise the active tetrapeptide. Gastrin II possesses a tyrosyl o-sulfate in position 12. The leucine at position 5 is replaced by methionine in hog gastrin and by valine in sheep gastrin.

1 2 3 4 5 6 7 8 9 10 11 12 13 14 15 16 17
Glu-Gly-Pro-Try-Leu-Glu-Glu-Glu-Glu-Glu-Ala-Tyr-Gly-Try-Met-Asp-PheAla-NH_2

The *intestinal phase* of gastric secretion consists of a small stimulatory effect when various foodstuffs, especially peptones, are introduced into the small intestine; it is likely that this effect is mediated by a humoral substance. Of greater importance is the role of the small intestine as an inhibitor of gastric secretion. Resection of long segments of small intestine is often followed by the development of gastric hypersecretion, probably because of loss of the inhibitory influences of the small intestine. Perfusion of all portions of the small intestine with stable fat emulsions causes inhibition of gastrin-stimulated gastric secretion. It is possible but not yet proved that this inhibition is caused by the release of enterogastrone, a hormone whose structure has not been defined. Bathing the duodenum in an acid medium (pH of 2.5) similarly inhibits gastric secretion. It is likely that such inhibition is produced by secretin and perhaps cholecystokinin released from the duodenum, especially because the administration of exogenous secretion or cholecystokinin also inhibits gastric secretion.

RESISTANCE OF THE MUCOSA TO INJURY The gastric mucosa is remarkably resistant to injury. Two factors normally protect the stomach from autodigestion: (1) gastric mucus and (2) the epithelial barrier.

The application of an irritant to the gastric mucosa is followed by the outpouring of large quantities of mucus, the protective capacity of which is largely attributable to its physical characteristics. These properties are more beneficial in protecting the mucosa from thermal or mechanical trauma than from chemical injury, because acid and other chemical substances readily penetrate the mucus barrier. Only about 1 percent of fasting acid secretion can actually be neutralized by the gastric mucus. An additional protective effect of mucus is its ability to adsorb pepsin. Cortisone and acetylsalicylic acid produce qualitative changes in the gastric mucus that may facilitate its degradation by pepsin, and in addition they decrease the total output of mucus.

Mucus-producing cells are generously distributed throughout the gastric mucosa. This epithelial lining has remarkable properties of repair and is able to reproduce itself within 36 to 48 hr. Aspirin, alcohol, bile salts, and other substances injurious to the gastric mucosa alter the permeability of the epithelial barrier, allowing back diffusion of hydrochloric acid, with resultant injury to underlying tissues, especially blood vessels. Pepsin is released in large quantities when the barrier is injured and may contribute to destruction of the mucosa. It is possible that the gastric mucosal barrier to ionic diffusion may also be disrupted in a variety of disease states, especially in gastritis and benign gastric ulcer.

The resistance of the small intestine to trauma or peptic ulceration deserves comment. The thick layer of Brunner's glands in the duodenum produces a highly alkaline (pH of 8), viscid mucoid secretion which has a high buffering capacity and which appears to have an important protective action. Possible loss of, or a defect in, these secretions requires greater attention, since the intraduodenal pH differs little between normal individuals and those with duodenal ulcers. Except for the duodenal Brunner glands, there is little if any inherent difference in susceptibility to acid peptic digestion from jejunum to ileum.

Gastric motility and gastric emptying

The musculature of the upper half of the stomach produces weak peristaltic waves which scarcely disturb its contents. The function of this portion of the stomach is mainly an adaptive one enabling great changes in volume with insignificant alterations in pressure. Thus, after a distal gastrectomy, gastric emptying must occur mainly by gravity. Studies of electrical activity indicate the presence of a "pacemaker" in the cardia from which an impulse is propagated to the remainder of the stomach.

The "gastric pump" resides in the antrum and pylorus, which should be regarded as a unit, because the pylorus is not truly a sphincter but is rather an integral part of the pumping mechanism, contracting at the culmination of a peristaltic wave and relaxing the remainder of the time. In fact, the pylorus does not act in opposition to the antrum, and because it is usually relaxed, the term "sphincter" is misleading. During its contraction at the end of a peristaltic wave, the pylorus serves to prevent reflux into the stomach when the pressure in the duodenum is raised and also turns back larger solid particles which need further gastric trituration. The action of the pyloroantrum may thus be likened to the squeezing of the gastric contents toward a pointed funnel which narrows as the squeezing proceeds.

The regulation of gastric emptying is complex. The extrinsic nerve supply in the stomach seems important, since vagotomy produces marked gastric retention, resulting not as has been commonly suggested from pylorospasm but rather from a disturbance of normal antral peristalsis. The duodenum contains osmoreceptors which when exposed to hypertonic solutions inhibit gastric emptying. The instillation of fat or acid chyme into the small intestine similarly causes gastric motor inhibition, perhaps by a humoral mechanism. Although gastrin increases the frequency of antral contractions, this hormone actually decreases the rate of gastric emptying. Secretin and cholecystokinin inhibit antral peristalsis and gastric emptying.

DUODENAL ULCER

INCIDENCE AND PATHOLOGY Duodenal ulcer comprises about 80 percent of all peptic ulcers. At one time during their lives, approximately 10 percent of the population probably suffer from duodenal ulcers, many of which may be asymptomatic. Mainly because of hemorrhage or perforation, as many as 10,000 lives are lost yearly in the United States as a result of this disease. Duodenal ulcer is most common in men between the ages of twenty and fifty years. The preponderance of males varies from 3:1 to 10:1, but no significant differences in occurrence between the sexes is evident before puberty or after the menopause. While gastric ulcer is relatively more common in females, the absolute incidence of duodenal ulcer in females is greater than the occurrence of gastric ulcer.

Duodenal ulcers are usually found within 3 cm of the pylorus and occur with about equal frequency on the anterior and posterior walls. The depth of the ulcer varies from a shallow erosion confined to the mucosa to a full-thickness destruction of the wall of the duodenum. Juxtaposition to adjacent organs and rapidity of destruction of the wall are the two factors which determine whether a lesion *perforates* into the free peritoneal cavity or *penetrates* into an adjacent organ. *Perforation* indicates a free communication between the gut and the peritoneal cavity and usually occurs during a period of extremely active ulceration. *Penetration* signifies that a free perforation has not occurred but that an adjacent organ, usually the pancreas, has become adherent to a slowly progressive but chronic ulcer which ultimately erodes that structure. In the process, a posterior penetrating ulcer may erode the gastroduodenal artery or one of its branches and cause sudden massive hemorrhage.

Grossly, duodenal ulcers are generally round with a slightly irregular outline. The base is white, gray, or yellow, and the surrounding mucosa is soft, pliable, and of normal color although occasionally somewhat edematous and hyperemic. Microscopically the base of the ulcer consists of mucus and necrotic debris surmounting a bed of granulation tissue and scar containing variable amounts of inflammatory reaction. Ulcers arising from exposure to gastric juice have a similar appearance whether they occur in the duodenum, stomach, jejunum, or the base of a Meckel diverticulum which contains gastric mucosa. Hence the term *acid-peptic ulceration*, or *acid-peptic disease*, can be applied correctly to all these ulcerations.

Occasionally, anterior and posterior duodenal ulcers coexist. The simultaneous occurrence of gastric and duodenal ulcers is common and may be noted in as many as one-third of patients with duodenal ulcers. It is unusual for a gastric ulcer to precede a duodenal ulcer, and it is safest from a therapeutic standpoint to assume that a patient with both has primarily a duodenal ulcer diathesis. A chronic duodenal ulcer which causes delay in gastric emptying and consequent gastric stasis stimulates the production of gastrin and thus the development of a gastric ulcer.

PATHOPHYSIOLOGY In the development of duodenal ulcer in a given patient, it is likely that a multiplicity of causative and contributing factors is involved.

Hypersecretion of gastric juice Duodenal ulcer *never* occurs in the absence of acid. No single test of gastric secretion shows abnormal hypersecretion in much more than half of duodenal ulcer patients, with the unexplained exception of the caffeine-stimulated test. An explanation for the absence of excessive acid secretion in some patients with duodenal ulcer is lacking. Dragstedt has proposed that duodenal ulcer arises from hypersecretion caused by excessive vagal stimulation. This thesis is based upon the fact that the nocturnal or basal hypersecretion in most patients with duodenal ulcer is abolished by complete division of the vagus nerves. Absolute proof for this theory is not available. The amount of gastrin or gastrin-like substance in the antrums of patients with duodenal ulcer appears to be greater than that found in those with benign gastric ulcer or in normal persons. Whether this results from excessive vagotonia or is by itself a primary etiologic factor is unknown.

There is a linear correlation between the parietal cell mass, or the total number of parietal cells secreting acid, and the secretion achieved by maximal gastric stimulation with histamine and pentagastrin. The factors which control the population of parietal cells are not well understood.

Tissue resistance and disturbances in motility It has been suggested that the resistance of the duodenal mucosa is diminished in patients with duodenal ulcers, but substantiation is lacking. There is no clear evidence that disturbances in gastric motility have a *pathogenetic* role in the development of duodenal ulcer.

Genetic factor A family history of duodenal or gastric ulcer may be striking in some patients, and endocrine factors should be sought in such families. However, familial tendency to ulcer is often absent, and the importance of genetic factors in the development of most duodenal ulcers is not clear. The blood group substances are mucopolysaccharides with antigenic properties present in the red blood cell which in certain individuals are secreted into the gastrointestinal tract (secretors) and which may protect against the development of ulceration. Duodenal and stomal ulcers are more common in patients with the O blood grouping and in nonsecretors.

Neuropsychiatric factors Emotional factors may alter gastric function profoundly. However, studies of patients with gastric fistulas have shown that different types of stimuli affect the stomach in varying ways which differ from one individual to another. Patients with duodenal ulcers can often clearly point to an emotional upset which may have triggered the onset or exacerbation of their ulcer. Although it is true that many patients with duodenal ulcer are hard-driving, ambitious executives, many exceptions are found. Psychiatric factors may play a role in the pathogenesis of duodenal ulceration but are in all likelihood not the sole causative factor.

Endocrine factors Because peptic ulceration is more common in males, it has been suggested that estrogenic hormones may protect against the development of ulcer. Gastric secretion is not altered by pregnancy, however, and a lesser gastric secretion in normal females than in males may indicate only a genetically determined smaller parietal cell mass rather than a primary effect of estrogens.

The role of adrenal steroids has received much attention. In the absence of the adrenal glands, in patients with Addison's disease, or in hypopituitarism, gastric hyposecretion occurs and ulcer is virtually nonexistent. Responsiveness of the parietal cells has been restored after total adrenalectomy by treatment with glucocorticoids but not with mineralocorticoids. It is likely therefore that adrenal steroids play a permissive role in the regulation of gastric secretion. The acute administration of glucocorticoids or ACTH exerts no effect on gastric secretion in normal man or animals. Chronic glucocorticoid administration to dogs with intact adrenals increases acid and pepsin secretions, but evidence for this is inconclusive in man. No abnormalities in adrenal function have been detected in patients with duodenal ulcer. In patients who receive large doses of steroids for prolonged periods ulcer-like symptoms often develop, and peptic ulcers develop in some. Whether the true incidence of duodenal or gastric ulcers among patients receiving long-term steroid therapy is greater than the incidence occurring in the disease for which the treatment is being administered is debatable. In the presence of sepsis or burns, which of themselves are probably ulcerogenic, steroids may be dangerous. It is likely that steroids not only affect gastric secretion but also may cause serious injury to the mucosal epithelial barrier.

A high incidence of peptic ulceration has been reported in patients with hyperparathyroidism, and in certain cases, gastric acid hypersecretion has reverted to normal after surgical cure of the hyperparathyroidism, but this has by no means been uniform. Calcium must be present in adequate amounts for the normal gastric secretory process to occur. In addition, an increase in serum calcium causes a rise in serum gastrin level.

Other predisposing diseases An increased incidence of peptic ulceration is found in cirrhosis of the liver, chronic pancreatitis or cystic fibrosis, chronic pulmonary emphysema, and rheumatoid arthritis. While gastric hypersecretion is present in some of the patients with these diseases, it is often absent, possibly because of a preexistent abnormality of the stomach. In cirrhosis, failure of the liver to inactivate a gastric secretagogue (histamine?) normally present in portal blood, either because of functional deterioration or because of portacaval shunting, is the probable mechanism of hypersecretion. In chronic pancreatitis or cystic fibrosis, the loss of the buffering capacity of pancreatic juice in the duodenum and of the inhibitory effect of normally digested fat upon gastric secretion may contribute to the development of ulcer. Patients with chronic pulmonary disease are subjected to stress, hypoxia, and hypercapnia, all of which may play a role in enhancing the development of peptic ulcer. The cause of the increased incidence of ulcers in rheumatoid arthritis is unknown.

CLINICAL FEATURES Duodenal ulcer is a chronic disease characterized by exacerbations and remissions. Although many individuals have only one encounter with active duodenal ulceration, the diathesis seems to recur or persist in most patients. Characteristically symptoms last for a few days, weeks, or months and disappear for varying periods of time, only to reappear with or without therapy or frequently without identifiable precipitating cause. Classically exacerbations appear to occur more frequently in spring and fall. Eighty to ninety percent of patients with duodenal ulcer have a relatively benign course interrupted occasionally by the inconvenience of necessity for therapy. In the remaining 10 to 20 percent intractability or other complications develop, and these patients become candidates for operation. Many patients have ulcers sufficiently asymptomatic to evade detection, and in about 20 to 30 percent of cases of perforation or hemorrhage no antecedent symptoms can be elicited.

The symptoms have a remarkably uniform pattern. The development of pain followed by the relief of discomfort after ingestion of food or alkali is such a characteristic sequence that the absence of this periodicity should raise serious question as to the correctness of the diagnosis. The pain is a steady, gnawing, burning, aching, or hungerlike discomfort high in the midepigastrium or slightly to either side of the midline, especially on the right. It is located over a limited area and does not radiate unless penetration of the pancreas has occurred, in which case spread of pain to the back is common. The pain usually begins about 2 or 2 $^{1}/_{2}$ hr after meals and usually is relieved immediately by the ingestion of alkali or food. The pain may awaken the patient between midnight and 3 A.M., but for unknown reasons, it is almost never present upon awakening before breakfast. The mechanism of the pain is disputed, but most observers believe that the acid bathing the ulcer causes the discomfort especially because buffering of acid within the stomach produces relief. Some patients have no pain even prior to a major and serious complication.

A variety of other gastrointestinal symptoms may be present, many of which are often found in the general population. Heartburn, a sensation of retrosternal burning, is very common, as is *water brash*, the regurgitation of sour fluid into the mouth, and both may be especially severe in patients who have an incompetent lower esophageal sphincter (see Chaps. 37 and 281). Alterations in bowel habits, including both constipation and diarrhea, often related to medications, are not infrequently observed. The appetite is unusually good, and gain in weight is common, because these patients eat so frequently to relieve discomfort. Weight loss is uncommon unless chronic duodenal obstruction has been present. Physical examination of patients with active duodenal ulcers may be negative or show only mild tenderness in the epigastrium or to the right of the midline.

Atypical symptoms occur in certain types of duodenal ulcer and may herald subacute perforation or pyloric obstruction. In childhood the pain is frequently bizarre in type and location and may even be accentuated by the ingestion of food. Bleeding or perforation is often the initial manifestation in children. Ulcers in the second portion of the duodenum or in the pyloric canal may have unusual pain patterns, and the pain-food-relief sequence is less common. Interference with the normal antropyloric pump by ulcers of the pyloric canal often causes nausea, vomiting, anorexia, weight loss, and cramping pain shortly after ingestion.

Ulcers in this region respond poorly to medical therapy.

DIAGNOSIS The most important criterion in the diagnosis is the elicitation of the typical sequence of *pain-food-relief*. A variety of nonspecific symptoms such as heartburn, belching, intolerance to certain foods, and vague diffuse abdominal discomfort are frequent symptoms in the general population. Although they are often equated with duodenal ulcer, more frequently other diseases or no specific underlying diseases are found. The typical periodicity of relief of discomfort by the ingestion of food or alkali is usually helpful in excluding these other diseases. The presence of pain at night and its absence in the early morning are also important diagnostic features. The response of the discomfort to medical treatment is important but must be interpreted carefully, because some patients with nonspecific symptoms or other diseases also may improve. If the history is atypical and the radiologic findings do not substantiate the presence of a duodenal ulcer, further diagnostic steps including barium examination of the colon and small intestine and cholecytography should be taken lest serious lesions in other portions of the gastrointestinal tract be missed.

X-ray examination with barium is the most definitive diagnostic step. The demonstration of a crater persistent on several films is the only means by which the presence of an active duodenal ulcer can be clearly established (Fig. 282-3). Giant craters in the duodenal bulb may be missed because of their enormous size. The presence of a persistent deformity of the duodenal bulb does not necessarily indicate that *active* duodenal ulceration is present but signifies only that at one time ulceration was present which in the process of healing produced the deformity (Fig. 282-4). Not infrequently active ulcers are present in these deformed bulbs, but they may be difficult to demonstrate. Only a history compatible with active disease together with the presence of a deformed bulb can define active duodenal ulceration when a crater is not demonstrable.

Gastric analysis is generally unnecessary in patients with typical duodenal ulcer. In certain instances of fulminating or atypical disease or when the possibility of marginal ulceration exists and cannot be confirmed radiologically, examination of gastric secretion may be useful. Near-maximal output of acid in the basal state combined with a minimal increment to maximal histamine stimulation strongly suggests that the parietal cell mass is already maximally stimulated under basal conditions and that the

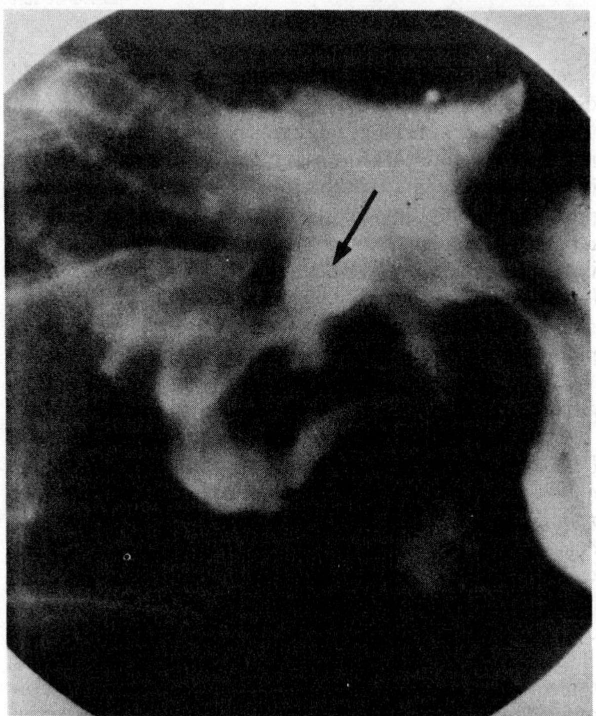

FIGURE 282-3
Duodenal bulb showing a persistent fleck of barium, representing a true crater with radiating folds of mucosa.

Zollinger-Ellison (Z-E) syndrome may be present. A 12-hr nocturnal test of gastric secretion is uncomfortable and unnecessary, and careful determination of the 1-hr basal acid output coupled with the maximal histamine stimulation provides as much information. True achlorhydria excludes a benign peptic ulcer.

TREATMENT Medical treatment Virtually every conceivable dietary regimen and drug has been advocated at one time or another. Yet, in controlled studies, the rate of healing of ulcers has been significantly altered by few things. Certain recommendations can be made, however, which will provide greater comfort and relief of symptoms. Rather than uniformly imposing an extremely restrictive dietary and pharmacologic regimen, each patient can be treated in a manner most suitable for him without significantly altering the incidence of recurrence or complications.

Antacids Antacids are the mainstay of therapy. The rationale of antacid therapy is to elevate the pH of the gastric contents to at least 5, where the proteolytic capacity of pepsin is virtually abolished and the damaging effect due to acidity is minimal. Some antacids also inactivate pepsin by an adsorbent effect. When given to the *fasting* patient with duodenal ulcer most antacids have an effect lasting for only 20 to 30 min. This evanescent effect is related not to the inadequacy of the buffering capacity of the antacid but rather to rapid gastric emptying. The effect of antacid therapy can be prolonged markedly if the agent is taken 1 hr after eating, the gastric acidity decreasing to 30 to 40 percent of its control values as long as 4 hr after the meal.

The choice of antacid is important, but the ideal antacid probably does not exist. Absorbable antacids such as sodium bicarbonate should not be used, because they induce systemic alkalosis. Especially if combined with the prolonged ingestion of milk, absorbable antacids and occasionally even nonabsorbable agents may produce the milk-alkali syndrome, consisting of hypercalcemia, alkalosis, azotemia, and nephrocalcinosis. Nonabsorbable antacids, either singly or in combination, are the most frequently employed agents. Calcium carbonate is probably the most effective antacid, because its neutralizing action is prolonged and it reduces peptic activity, although "acid rebound" of gastric contents after this agent may be caused by gastrin stimulation. It should not be used for patients with a history of renal calculi or for those with dehydration and electrolyte imbalance because of its tendency to cause hypercalcemia and hypercalcuria. Magnesium oxide is eight to ten times more potent than magnesium trisilicate or magnesium carbonate, and the aluminum hydroxide gels have little neutralizing capacity. Calcium carbonate and aluminum hydroxide have the disadvantage of producing severe constipation and fecal impaction, especially in the aged. These side effects may be countered by the replacement of one or two of the daily doses with 4 g magnesium oxide. The high sodium content of many alumina preparations may be disadvantageous in patients who require a

FIGURE 282-4
Markedly deformed duodenal bulb with "cloverleaf" deformity.

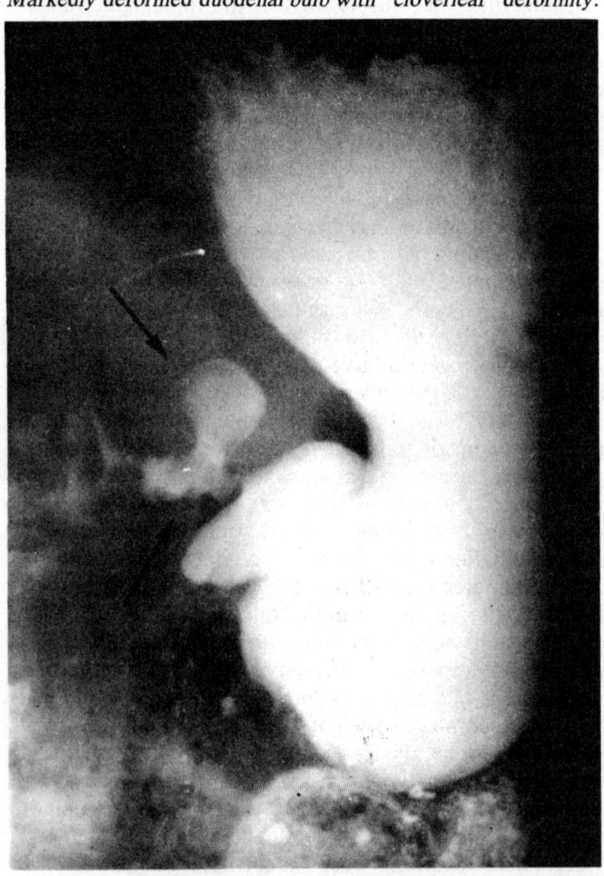

low sodium intake. The binding of phosphate in the intestine by alumina preparations is usually not a severe problem, because the diet ingested by these patients is generally high in phosphorus.

Liquid antacids are dispersed more readily within the stomach and are hence somewhat more effective than tablets. The usual dose of calcium carbonate, magnesium oxide, or alumina tablets is 4 g, and the dose of alumina gels is 15 to 30 ml, enough to neutralize 50 mEq acid in 1 hr. The usual ambulatory regimen consists of administration of the antacid 1 hr after meals, at bedtime, and on any other occasion when discomfort arises. Should adequate relief not be obtained, a more stringent regimen may be required. In intensive therapy for active acute ulceration, antacids may be given every hour in the usual dose without serious side effects if constipation is avoided. The presence of nocturnal discomfort should dictate the use of antacid at night until complete relief of pain is obtained.

In certain instances of severe ulceration with unrelenting pain, continuous neutralization of gastric acidity must be accomplished. This can be achieved by continuous gastric aspiration, by the constant intragastric installation of one of the liquid alumina hydroxide or magnesium preparations, or by the continuous administration of a milk and cream drip. These instances are not common but are more often encountered in patients with pyloric channel ulcers.

Anticholinergic drugs Anticholinergic drugs theoretically not only inhibit the direct effect of the vagus nerve upon the parietal cells but also decrease the vagal release of gastrin and excessive gastric motility. These agents reduce the *output* of gastric acid but do not decrease the concentration of acid or the output of pepsin. Consequently anticholinergic drugs do *not* reduce the peptic digestive capacity of gastric juice but facilitate the neutralization of gastric juice by food and antacids. Prolonged use of anticholinergic agents probably diminishes the incidence of exacerbations of duodenal ulcer disease. However, the doses necessary to produce the desired gastric action also have undesirable systemic effects. These symptoms include *dryness of the mouth, blurring of vision, atony of the bladder* (often producing urinary retention or slowing of the urinary stream in older men), *constipation, drowsiness,* and *mental confusion.* Anticholinergics should not be used in patients with glaucoma or prostatic hypertrophy or when pyloric obstruction is present or imminent. Atropine (0.3 to 0.4 mg) and tincture of belladonna (12 to 15 drops) are often prescribed and given to tolerance by increasing the dose until side effects such as blurred vision and dryness of the mouth appear. The dose is then reduced until symptoms become tolerable. *They are usually given 30 min before meals and at bedtime.* Many agents with similar antisecretory actions are available, such as propantheline (Pro-Banthine) 15 mg, glycopyrrolate (Robinul) 1 mg, isopropamide (Darbid) 1 mg, oxyphencyclimine (Daricon) 5 mg. These drugs are also generally given at least four times daily (before meals and at bedtime). No single anticholinergic drug excels, although often the patient may tolerate one drug better than another. They are generally prescribed continuously during the treatment of an active peptic ulcer. However, there is no good evidence that these agents actually accelerate the healing of a duodenal ulcer.

Dietary management Controlled observations indicate that there is no clear-cut therapeutic effect of diet therapy. From a practical standpoint, frequent small bland feedings are likely to be tolerated more readily than a routine diet, because nonspecific food intolerances are common and large meals may cause discomfort to some patients, especially in the acute phases of duodenal ulcer. This is begun with six small feedings consisting of skim milk or protein snacks which have a high buffering capacity and avoidance of highly seasoned foods, roughage, and greasy or fried foods. As soon as pain is diminished or has completely disappeared, the diet is gradually liberalized.

Sole reliance upon dietary therapy for buffering the excess acid is not physiologically sound, since considerable stimulation of acid secretion occurs after the initial buffering effect of the meal has worn off. Antacid therapy 1 hr after eating should also be employed. The traditional administration of large quantities of cream and milk has been implicated in causing a higher incidence of atherosclerosis in ulcer patients. The high fat content of such a diet may tend to accentuate the symptoms of biliary tract disease.

Rest, sedatives, and tranquilizers Rest and adequate sleep are strongly advised, and patients are urged to curtail their business and social responsibilities. Controlled investigations have revealed that rest in the form of hospitalization has proved beneficial in patients with gastric ulcer, but data are not available for an assessment of its effect in duodenal ulcer patients. Should symptoms from a duodenal ulcer persist despite active therapy on an outpatient basis for 5 or 6 days, the more rigid therapy and enforced rest produced by hospitalization will frequently become effective. Though sedatives and tranquilizers have not been shown to affect the course of duodenal ulcer materially, they may be helpful in the anxious and tense patient. There is no need to administer these agents routinely.

Psychotherapy Psychotherapy has no proved beneficial effect on the healing or recurrence of duodenal ulcer. In fact, intensive psychotherapy during phases of acute activity of a duodenal ulcer is probably contraindicated, because it may result in exacerbations. However, a warm and sympathetic attitude on the part of the physician, reassurance, and support are important aspects of the care of the ulcer patient. If specific indications for psychotherapy exist, it is better carried out during quiescent phases of ulcer activity.

Interdictions Ingestion of alcohol is strictly contraindicated. Alcohol not only produces direct stimulation of the parietal cell but may also cause the release of gastrin. In addition, it probably injures the gastric mucosal epithelial barrier. Coffee, tea, and cola drinks stimulate gastric secretion because of their caffeine content and are also interdicted. Cigarette smoking has been documented to be a definite cause of delayed healing of gastric ulcers. Nicotine is known to decrease the output of water and bicarbonate by the pancreas and hence, cessation of smoking is similarly recommended for duodenal ulcer patients. In most patients the habit of cigarette smoking is so firmly ingrained, however, that absolute abstinence may be extremely disturbing. Consequently, the ideal therapeutic regimen must be tempered by the judgment of the physician.

Drugs which may contribute to peptic ulceration such as the xanthine alkaloids, anti-inflammatory drugs, reserpine, adrenal steroids, and salicylates should be discontinued if not absolutely necessary.

Irradiation of the stomach Irradiation of the stomach has a definite though small role in the treatment of duodenal ulcer. The administration of approximately 1,500 R in 10 divided doses with conventional therapy or 2,000 R with cobalt teletherapy generally produces marked depression of gastric secretion. True achlorhydria is rare after irradiation, and the usually resultant hypochlorhydria is frequently transient. Within 6 to 12 months, the acid secretion returns to normal in at least half the patients. For reasons which are incompletely understood, however, rates of recurrence remain reasonably low. This mode of therapy is useful in a limited number of patients who have not responded adequately to medical therapy but who are extremely poor risks for surgical procedures.

Other forms of therapy Claims of therapeutic success have been made for an enormous variety of additional therapeutic modalities, but none has survived the test of time. The remarkable tendency for spontaneous remission makes the evaluation of any form of therapy difficult at best, and only carefully controlled clinical trials can confirm the efficacy of any therapeutic regimen. A perfect example is the wave of enthusiasm which followed the introduction of gastric freezing. Only after an "excessive" period did it become clear that improvement was transient and complications frequent. Gastric freezing may be regarded as a transient curiosity with no place in our therapeutic armamentarium.

Therapy between recurrences Since a duodenal ulcer may take from several weeks to months to heal depending upon its size and depth, active therapy should be continued for 2 to 3 months in all patients with an acute exacerbation. Spontaneous recurrence is frequent despite continued therapy, and because most patients who are feeling well do not tolerate severe restrictions, the physician must outline an acceptable interim regimen.

That recurrent symptoms are likely should be explained to the patient, since 50 to 95 percent of duodenal ulcers will recur within 5 years. Therapy may not prevent such recurrences; hence dietary and antacid management should be liberalized after the initial 2 to 3 months of active therapy. Indeed, medications may be discarded in many patients with the admonition that gastric stimulants be avoided and that moderation be used in smoking and other aggravating factors. At the first inkling of recurrent symptoms, active therapy should be reinstituted immediately and should be continued for 2 to 3 weeks, or longer if relief is not immediate. Even in the absence of symptoms prophylactic therapy for a short period should be advised if the patient is about to enter a period of emotional stress or a potentially ulcerogenic situation.

The long-term use of anticholinergic drugs has been shown in a few controlled studies to reduce the recurrence rate below 10 percent. Because of the side effects of these drugs, the routine use of anticholinergic drugs is not warranted.

Surgical treatment INDICATIONS The indications for operation in patients with duodenal ulcer are the complications of the disease: (1) perforation, (2) organic obstruction, (3) intractable bleeding, and (4) refractoriness to medical therapy. Surgical therapy is indicated in the minority of patients. The indications are usually clear, with the possible exception of those patients with intractability to medical management. The decision to advise operation in a patient with duodenal ulcer must balance the risks of the disease with those of operation. The repeated discomfort, cost of frequent hospitalization, time lost from work, possible mortality, the threat of complications are the factors which influence the decision against continued medical treatment. These must be compared with operative and anesthetic risks, the incidence of recurrent ulcers, and some of the symptoms which occur following operations for duodenal ulcer. The risks on the surgical side must be evaluated in light of the experience of the surgeons with whom the internist works closely and not solely from results reported in the literature. In many instances the results are either markedly better or worse than those which are published, a consideration generally given insufficient attention.

ACCEPTABLE SURGICAL PROCEDURES The goals of surgical therapy are identical with those of nonoperative therapy, namely, profound and lasting decrease of the secretion of hydrochloric acid and pepsin. There is probably no single operation which is suitable for all patients with duodenal ulcer, and contemplated procedures should be tailored to fit the individual patient.

Vagotomy and drainage operation are designed to ablate any direct effects of vagal stimulation upon the parietal cell as well as the vagal release of gastrin. Stimulation of the antrum by chemical means or by distention remains operative in the presence of a vagotomy. From a physiologic standpoint, pyloroplasty has theoretical advantages over gastroenterostomy for drainage purposes, because pyloroplasty maintains duodenal continuity, is less frequently associated with the dumping syndrome, and should preserve any acid-inhibitory influence of the duodenum. Interestingly, however, the recurrence rate of ulceration following either of these procedures is about the same (5 to 8 percent), and the incidence of postoperative digestive symptoms is virtually identical. The operative mortality rate for elective vagotomy and drainage throughout the country is approximately 1 percent, the lowest figure for any operative procedure. Recent controlled studies indicate not only that selective gastric denervation ("selective vagotomy") accomplishes complete vagotomy more frequently than the truncal technique, but also that the incidence of postoperative diarrhea has been significantly reduced.

Subtotal distal gastric resection is the time-honored procedure for duodenal ulcer, preferably with reconstruction by gastroduodenostomy because of nutritional advantages derived from the establishment of normal gastrointestinal continuity and because of the preservation of inhibitory influences of the duodenum. The operation removes approximately 75 percent of the stomach, including the antrum and a generous portion of the parietal cell mass. In all probability, if mobilization of the stomach is extensive, nondeliberate vagal denervation may also be produced. The operative mortality rate for elective operation by well-trained surgeons is approximately 3 percent, and the recurrence rate of ulceration is also approximately 3 percent. Subtotal gastrectomy has a higher incidence of dumping than does vagotomy with an emptying operation.

Vagotomy and antrectomy have become extremely popular procedures. The overall mortality rate is about 3 percent, although in selected series it has been as low as $^1/_2$ to 2 percent. Removal of the antrum and denervation of the remaining parietal cell mass entail the lowest rate of recurrence, less than 1 percent. The nutritional consequences are about the same as those for vagotomy and drainage operation and for subtotal distal gastrectomy.

GASTRIC ULCER

It is useful clinically to separate the approach to gastric and duodenal ulcers, because the implications of the two are very different, even though the ulcers are similar pathologically.

INCIDENCE AND LOCATION Clinically gastric ulcers are less common than duodenal ulcers in the ratio of about 1:4, but autopsy studies show a roughly equal incidence of duodenal and gastric ulcer. This indicates that many gastric ulcers may be asymptomatic and also that terminal acute gastric ulcers are probably included in the autopsy studies. Males usually predominate by a ratio of 3.5:1, somewhat less than the predominance noted in duodenal ulcers. Although gastric ulcers may appear at any age, they tend to occur between forty-five and fifty-five years of age, whereas the maximal incidence for duodenal ulcer is about 10 years earlier.

Gastric ulcers occur most often in the antrum or at the junction of the antral and fundic tissue. They are usually single and often located on the lesser curvature or in the prepyloric area. About 20 percent of gastric ulcers occur in patients who have had past or present duodenal ulceration, but it is very unusual for duodenal ulcer to follow the onset of pure gastric ulceration.

PATHOPHYSIOLOGY With the exception of those patients having concomitant duodenal and gastric ulceration, the average basal gastric secretion and maximally stimulated gastric secretion and, hence, parietal cell mass are either decreased or normal. True achlorhydria following maximal stimulation is so exceptional that its demonstration should virtually exclude the presence of a benign gastric ulcer.

Several theories have been proposed to explain the development of benign peptic ulceration in the stomach. Dragstedt suggested that gastric ulcers are due to hypersecretion of gastric juice of hormonal origin dependent upon *prolonged or excessive secretion of gastrin.* Although this theory may explain the ulceration which occurs secondary to gastric stasis produced by vagotomy without a drainage operation, or duodenal stenosis resulting from a duodenal ulcer, it is by no means a satisfactory explanation for the vast majority of spontaneously occurring gastric ulcers. No proof has been provided that gastric hypomotility or stasis is more prevalent in patients with gastric ulcer than in the normal population.

Other hypotheses which have been proposed include a decreased resistance of the stomach to ulceration by injury of the epithelium or by *a decrease in gastric mucus.* It has been suggested that *regurgitation of bile* into the proximal parts of the stomach is more common in patients with gastric ulcer and that such regurgitation injures the mucosa so that acid-peptic ulceration may occur. This is consonant with the findings of Davenport that injury to the gastric mucosa by various substances enhances the back diffusion of hydrogen ion, causing destruction of blood vessels and possible ulceration. Patients with gastric ulcer may therefore actually have hypersecretion of acid which cannot be detected because of the back diffusion of hydrogen ion, accounting for the usual clinical finding of normal or low acid secretion. Although qualitative and quantitative changes in gastric mucus have been described following the administration of salicylates or steroids, there is no evidence for the exhaustion of the mucus-secreting cell or the excessive destruction of mucus in patients with gastric ulcer.

CLINICAL FEATURES Asymptomatic gastric ulcers are common, so that some are found by chance and others are heralded only by severe complications such as perforation or bleeding. Symptomatic ulcers produce a picture more variable than that associated with duodenal ulcer. Atypical symptoms such as vague bloating or nausea after eating are common. Although the rhythmicity of the pain-food-relief sequence may occur, it is not as frequent or as clear-cut as it is in duodenal ulcer. In fact, food often aggravates the pain. The discomfort may be burning or cramping in nature and is usually less localized and more diffuse than that found in patients with duodenal ulcers. Pain occurring at night is uncommon. Nausea, anorexia, and vomiting are not infrequent and may occur in the absence of obstruction. Weight loss is frequent. The symptoms of gastric ulcer tend to be chronic, sometimes respond poorly to medical management, and frequently recur.

DIAGNOSIS The history is not as informative or diagnostic as it is in duodenal ulcer. Only a high index of suspicion will result in the proper diagnosis in patients who so frequently have vague symptoms. The diagnosis is almost completely dependent upon radiologic and gastroscopic examinations. Roentgenologic examination with barium will detect a gastric ulcer in the majority of cases. The radiologic features which allow this distinction include the smooth oval nature of the defect extending beyond the projected wall of the stomach, the absence of a mass lesion, ready passage of peristalsis through the area, and the presence of normal or slightly edematous mucosal folds to the very edge of the lesion (Fig. 282-5). Gastroscopic examination is almost as accurate as roentgenologic demonstration of the ulcer in differentiating benign from malignant lesions if the lesion can be visualized, and when taken together, diagnostic accuracy is about 93 percent. Gastroscopic biopsy may be useful; however, if benign tissue is obtained, it must be emphasized that the specimen represents but a very small superficial segment of the lesion in question. The major concern in the diagnosis lies in the ability to distinguish between benign and malignant ulcers.

DIFFERENTIATION OF BENIGN AND MALIGNANT GASTRIC ULCER Although the vast majority of gastric ulcers are benign, about 7 percent of ulcerating gastric lesions in which a clear-cut diagnosis was not evident originally will prove to be carcinoma of the stomach. The diagnostic accuracy of approximately 90 percent can be improved by the rigid application of criteria to be mentioned. In case of doubt, the ulcer should be considered malignant until proved otherwise. The 5-year survival rate in patients with initially indeterminate gastric ulcers which proved to be carcinomas at operation is approximately 50 percent, roughly five times the overall survival rate in gastric cancer. It is not uncommon to see patients with operable and potentially curable lesions who have been treated nonoperatively for as long as 2 or 3 years and who later appear with either inoperable, unresectable lesions or with distant metastases. Furthermore, an error in making a diagnosis of gastric cancer when such does not exist may also be forgiven in view of the high recurrence rate of medically treated gastric ulcer. Within a 5-year period, 75 to 80 percent of patients with benign gastric ulcer will have recurrent morbidity, and 3 to 4 percent will die from complications of the ulcer, a figure comparable to the mortality rate of gastric resection for benign ulcer. Since the surgical therapy of gastric ulcer is usually successful, it cannot be emphasized too strongly that procrastination is to be clearly avoided. These statements should not be misconstrued to indicate that the majority of gastric ulcer patients should be subjected to operation. On the contrary a sober and rational approach may be achieved by utilizing the following criteria:

FIGURE 282-5
Typical benign lesser curvature gastric ulcer. Note ulceration beyond projected margins of the stomach and collar of edema.

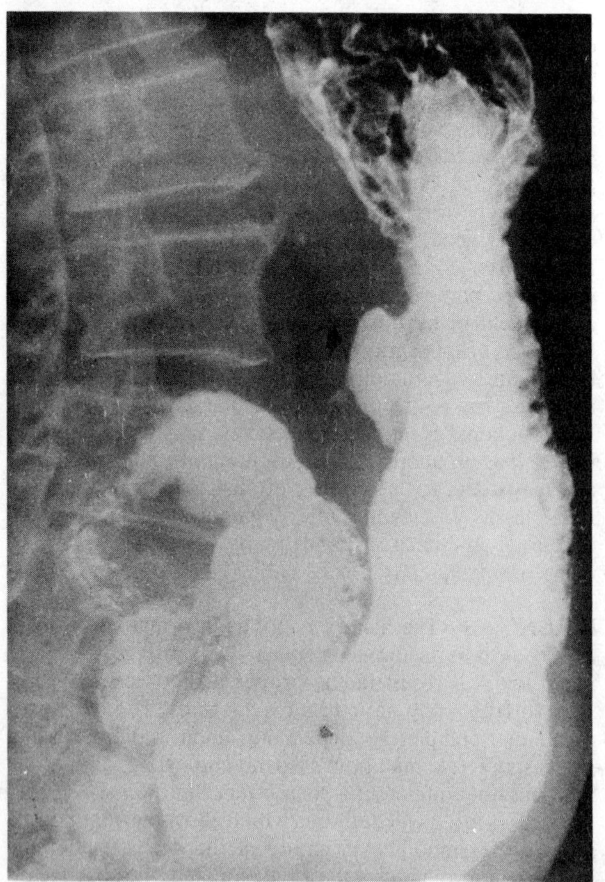

1 *Roentgenologic examination of the stomach.* This is probably the most important diagnostic aid. In the hands of an expert roentgenologist, the correct differentiation between a benign and malignant lesion can be made in 80 to 85 percent of the cases.
2 *Gastroscopy.* As available instrumentation improves so that virtually all of the interior of the stomach can be visualized and biopsied, this tool is now almost indispensable. It should be used if any question of the benignancy of a gastric lesion exists.
3 *Cytologic examination of the gastric juice.* When properly performed, this yields a diagnostic accuracy as high as 80 to 90 percent. The errors usually encountered are in the direction of false negatives. False positive results are uncommon.
4 *Examination of the gastric acid.* This may be of some value. If true histamine-fast achlorhydria is present, the diagnosis of carcinoma cannot be excluded no matter what other criteria are present. On the other hand, should acid be present, gastric carcinoma cannot be ruled out, because gastric secretion persists in many patients with carcinoma.
5 *Response to medical therapy.* Should one of the four criteria outlined above provide evidence of the presence of malignancy or should there be suggestive findings in two of these, operation is clearly indicated. However, if all these studies suggest that the lesion is benign, then a trial of medical therapy should be instituted, a test at least equal in importance to the other criteria. Strict rules for this test must be applied so that serious errors will not be made. The patient should be placed on an intensive medical regimen similar to the one described for duodenal ulcer. Roentgenologic examination should be repeated between 2 and 3 weeks after medical therapy has begun. By this time the benign ulcer should be approximately half its original size, and a small ulcer may show virtually complete healing. If less or no improvement has occurred, operation should be undertaken. If healing is progressing well, the medical regimen is continued for another 2 to 3 weeks, and a second gastrointestinal

series is then obtained, at which time healing should be complete. If it is not, then operation must be recommended.

If one adheres rigidly to these criteria, diagnostic errors will be kept to an absolute minimum. Undue procrastination may allow patients with carcinoma of the stomach to go untreated for inordinate periods. It should be recognized that patients with carcinoma of the stomach improve symptomatically on a medical regimen and that some healing or diminution in the size of the malignant ulcer may occur.

There is no conclusive pathologic demonstration of the transition of a benign gastric ulcer to a malignant one. Malignant degeneration is probably a rare event. Nevertheless the diagnostic criteria outlined above must be followed to be certain that an early malignant lesion is not missed.

TREATMENT The *medical therapy* of gastric ulcer is identical to that for duodenal ulcer except that anticholinergic agents should not be used. Anticholinergic drugs prolong gastric emptying and may contribute to ulcerogenesis by stimulating elaboration of gastrin. Randomized controlled prospectives studies have shown that hospitalization of the patient with gastric ulcer has a beneficial effect. Consequently, hospitalization for a 2- to 3-week period will not only provide the opportunity for adequate work-up but will also permit supervision of the medical therapy. The follow-up roentgenologic examination can be obtained at the end of the second or third week of therapy, and the patient may be discharged if 50 percent healing has occurred. The rationale for antacid therapy in benign gastric ulcer lies in the protection of the diseased gastric mucosa from destruction by normal or even subnormal quantities of acid and pepsin. Carbenoxolone sodium, a hydrolytic product of glycyrrhizinic acid derived from licorice, has been shown in randomized studies to have a salutary effect in patients with gastric ulcer, but it has sodium-retaining properties and may produce fluid retention. This drug has not been widely used in this country, although it has received extensive trial elsewhere. Its mechanism of action is unknown.

Surgical therapy is indicated for perforation, bleeding, obstruction, and intractability, the same indications used in the operative treatment of duodenal ulcer. Failure to heal completely in a period of 6 weeks is an important addition to this list. The surgical therapy of gastric ulcer generally consists of subtotal, distal gastrectomy which encompasses mainly the gastric antrum. Wide resection of the parietal cell-bearing areas is unnecessary, because gastric hypersecretion is uncommon and a less radical resection almost invariably is associated with an extremely satisfactory result. The recurrence rate of benign gastric ulcer after antrectomy is less than 1 percent. Reconstruction should be by gastroduodenostomy. Lesser procedures such as pyloroplasty and vagotomy have been advocated for benign gastric ulcer, but controlled randomized trials indicate that the incidence of recurrence is higher than after distal gastrectomy while the frequency of postoperative digestive symptoms is no less. A small but significant number of carcinomas will be missed even if operative biopsy is performed, and therefore resection is preferred.

STRESS-INDUCED ULCERS AND DRUG-INDUCED ULCERATIONS

Stress-induced ulcers and ulcerations caused by various drugs are similar in many respects. These ulcers are usually acute, tend to be superficial, and frequently occur without symptoms. When symptomatic, bleeding and perforation are the most common manifestations. *Stress ulcers* are far more common in the stomach than in the duodenum. They are encountered commonly in diseases of the central nervous system, especially after trauma, operation, or vascular accidents, and under these circumstances are known as *Cushing's ulcers.* They may also appear in patients with burns (Curling's ulcer), severe sepsis, or injury. The mechanism whereby stress ulceration develops is not readily apparent. However, hypersecretion of acid gastric juice is not the sole causative factor, and vascular alterations produced by changes in splanchnic blood flow or by stimulation or irritation of the hypothalamic areas may be important. Stimulation of the anterior hypothalamic nuclei is known to increase gastric secretion and blood flow, whereas the opposite effect is seen after stimulation of the posterior hypothalamus.

Drug-induced ulcerations or erosions may be caused by a variety of therapeutic agents. In many instances the exact mechanism by which these agents produce ulceration is unknown. Perhaps the most common substance known to cause ulceration or erosion is *acetylsalicylic acid.* Salicylates damage the mucosal epithelial barrier, allowing the back diffusion of hydrogen ion, with subsequent injury to the underlying tissue. Other anti-inflammatory agents such as phenylbutazone, indomethacin, cinophen, acetophenetidin, and colchicine may produce similar types of injury. Reserpine in large oral doses or given parenterally augments gastric secretion by accentuating the vagal release of gastrin. The role of adrenal steroids in the production of peptic ulceration has already been discussed. Although any of these agents may induce ulceration, they may, in addition, reactivate a preexisting duodenal or gastric ulcer.

Because stress- and drug-induced ulcerations are often asymptomatic prior to a major complication, attempts to prevent them with antacids should be made in high-risk situations, such as burns in children, or where large doses of corticosteroids are used. Drugs known to induce ulceration should be avoided in such situations.

STOMAL OR GASTROJEJUNAL ULCERATION

The incidence of stomal or gastrojejunal ulceration is reasonably low in acceptable operations for duodenal ulceration, but these types of ulceration develop in approximately 20 to 30 percent of patients with simple gastrojejunostomy without vagotomy.

The *causation of stomal ulcers* usually is related to a defect in the original therapy, although an underlying Z-E syndrome may be present (see below). Stomal ulceration following simple gastroenterostomy is due to the direct effect of the vagus nerve upon the parietal cell and the persistent vagal release of gastrin. The regurgitation of alkaline juices into the antrum of the stomach also enhances the chemical release of gastrin. If marginal or stomal ulceration occurs following distal gastrectomy, the possibility that not all of the distal antrum was resected should be considered. This occurs if a difficult duodenum was encountered in the first operative procedure, so that closure of the duodenal stump occurred proximal to the pylorus. The constant bathing of the excluded antrum in alkaline juice produces profound hypersecretion, which may reach proportions resembling those of the Z-E syndrome.

The *symptoms* are often extremely vague. A poorly localized burning sensation associated with a mild degree of cramping abdominal pain is common. This discomfort is often but not always relieved by antacid therapy. Massive hemorrhage alone is sometimes the sole presenting manifestation. Free perforation into the peritoneal cavity or penetration into adjacent organs producing a gastrojejunocolic fistula are also less frequent complications of stomal ulceration. The diagnosis may be extremely difficult, because approximately two-thirds to three-fourths of stomal ulcers are not visible roentgenologically because of their superficial nature. Under these circumstances gastroscopy is valuable because the stoma usually can be visualized. An occasional marginal ulcer may occur as a result of a granuloma around a nonabsorbable suture in the gastrojejunal or gastroduodenal suture line.

Medical therapy of marginal ulceration is generally unsatisfactory, and this diagnosis is usually an indication for reoperation. All attempts should be made prior to reoperation to ascertain the possible physiologic causes for the recurrent ulcer, so that inappropriate therapy can be avoided. When the Z-E syndrome can be ruled out, vagotomy is the most successful treatment if it has not previously been carried out or if it has been shown to be incomplete in the presence of an adequate distal gastric resection. In cases of retained antrum, removal of the stump of distal gastric antrum may be all that is necessary. Occasionally resection and vagotomy are required if a gastroenterostomy alone has been previously carried out or if the resection is inadequate.

ULCEROGENIC TUMOR OF PANCREAS (ZOLLINGER-ELLISON SYNDROME)

PATHOGENESIS The Zollinger-Ellison (Z-E) syndrome is the clinical entity of fulminant peptic ulceration associated with a non-beta cell islet tumor of the pancreas. Although most of these tumors occur in the pancreas, approximately 10 percent are aberrant and are located in the region of the duodenum or within the duodenal wall itself. Microscopically, the tumors either resemble islet cells or often have a striking resemblance to carcinoid tumors. In 50 percent of the cases, metastases have already occurred at the time of operation and are located in the regional lymph nodes which drain the pancreas, as well as in the liver. However, these patients rarely die from malignant spread but rather succumb to the adverse effects of the excessive release of gastrin from the tumor or its metastases. In 20 percent of cases more than one tumor is present. In approximately 10 to 20 percent multiple endocrine adenomas have occurred, particularly in the parathyroid, pituitary, adrenal, and thyroid glands. In these instances of polyendocrine adenomatosis, familial incidence is very common. Gastrin has been isolated from these tumors, and immunoassays of plasma gastrin show markedly elevated levels, found otherwise only in patients with pernicious anemia and certain types of gastritis. Plasma calcitonin levels are elevated in many patients; it has been suggested that this is due to the stimulation of calcitonin release from the thyroid by gastrin.

CLINICAL FEATURES The symptoms of the Z-E syndrome are in many cases similar to those of the usual duodenal ulcer. On the other hand, the tendency toward fulminant ulceration with severe complications is great. Rapidly recurrent ulceration after previously adequate surgical therapy should raise the possibility of the Z-E syndrome, particularly if ulceration occurs in the jejunum. Profound gastric hypersecretion is present, and basal rates of secretion between 10 and 30 mEq per hr are almost invariable. Since the stomach is almost maximally stimulated at all times, further stimulation by histamine produces only a small or no increment in secretion over the basal state. *A ratio of basal to maximally stimulated secretion of 0.6 or greater is considered highly suggestive* but not diagnostic.

Diarrhea and *malabsorption* may be the only presenting manifestations of the Z-E syndrome, or they may occur in conjunction with symptoms of peptic ulceration. The highly acid environment of the lower regions of the small intestine in patients with Z-E syndrome causes inactivation of pancreatic lipase and tends to precipitate bile salts; as a consequence malabsorption occurs. Injury to the intestinal mucosa by acid also contributes to malabsorption. The enormous volume of highly acid gastric juice also accentuates the diarrhea. The diarrhea of the Z-E syndrome must be clearly distinguished from that produced by another non-beta, non-insulin-producing islet cell tumor of the pancreas. These tumors have not been associated with ulcerogenesis and do not cause gastric hypersecretion. The cause of the diarrhea in these instances is not known, although it has been suggested that these tumors elaborate a substance (polypeptide) which alters the intestinal transport of water and electrolytes.

TREATMENT The *ulceration* present in patients with Z-E syndrome is notably resistant to both medical and ordinarily satisfactory surgical therapy. It is tempting to postulate that removal of the tumor without operation upon the stomach will cure the patient. However, the extremely high incidence of multiple lesions, particularly of a metastatic nature, usually causes this form of therapy to fail. After radical therapy these patients often do not die of malignant disease, and the weight of evidence is overwhelming that nothing short of total gastrectomy will suffice. Leaving only a tiny remnant of the stomach is fraught with hazard and will only result in recurrent ulceration and possibly death. The mortality rate in cases without total gastrectomy is as high as 90 percent, whereas when total gastrectomy is carried out, the mortality is about 10 to 15 percent. Several instances of spontaneous regression of metastases and return of serum gastrin levels to normal after total gastrectomy have been recorded.

COMPLICATIONS OF PEPTIC ULCERS

The complications of benign peptic ulceration include perforation, obstruction, and hemorrhage.

HEMORRHAGE Hemorrhage is the most common complication. Any discussion of hemorrhage from peptic ulceration must include other major causes of gastrointestinal hemorrhage, since the latter account for almost half the instances of massive gastrointestinal hemorrhage.

Diagnostic approach (see also Chap. 41) A vigorous diagnostic approach must be taken in all instances. For example, it is dangerous to assume that a patient with cirrhosis of the liver is bleeding from esophageal varices, since peptic ulcer is more common among patients with cirrhosis than in the general population. Similarly, a malignant lesion of the colon may be overlooked in a patient with a chronic duodenal ulcer if the assumption is made that the long-standing ulcer is the cause of the bleeding.

An initial assessment of the level of the bleeding is of the utmost importance. Hematemesis almost invariably means that the bleeding point is proximal to the ligament of Treitz, although in rare instances the lesion is in the upper jejunum. Intubation of the stomach should be carried out in every patient with gastrointestinal bleeding in the absence of hematemesis, because blood in the aspirate has the same significance as does hematemesis. The intubation should be carried out *while the patient is bleeding* to increase the opportunity of localizing the site of hemorrhage. The character of the stool is helpful in determining the location of the bleeding. A massive hemorrhage from esophageal varices may be associated with passage of bright-red blood by rectum if bleeding has been sufficiently rapid and the transit time short. Conversely, if hypomotility is present, a lesion in the cecum may produce a rather dark, tarry stool. If transit time is slow or normal, bright-red or dark-red liquid stools usually point to lesions of the terminal ileum or colon. Tarry stools in the presence of a normal transit time usually indicate bleeding from the upper part of the tract. Tarry black stools are not to be confused with the dark, blackish-green stools of patients receiving iron or bismuth therapy.

In general, these simple measures are adequate to define the level of bleeding. *Under very special circumstances,* other methods may be employed. *Intubation of the small intestine* with a long intestinal tube can be carried out. During the passage of the tube gentle aspiration should be done every 20 to 30 min. If bloody aspirate is obtained, a small amount of barium is given under fluoroscopic control, and careful study of the area in question is carried out. It may be necessary to withdraw the tube 6 to 8 in. prior to the x-ray examination, so that the tube does not migrate distal to the lesion. This method is generally applicable only to patients with slow and intermittent bleeding when there is adequate time for the necessary manipulations. If the site of bleeding is identified and the findings on roentgenologic examination are normal, the tube should remain in place, so that the surgeon may more readily identify a possibly otherwise undetectable lesion at operation. Selective visceral angiography has become increasingly useful and is indicated *before* barium examination when no cause for the hemorrhage has been found by conventional techniques during a prior episode of bleeding, or in those cases of initial hemorrhage in which the history, physical examination, and endoscopy provide no clue to the source (see Chap. 41).

Specific diagnostic tests may reveal the exact nature of the lesion once the level of bleeding has been determined. The most important of these is the roentgenologic examination which can be done in a leisurely fashion if the patient is not bleeding rapidly. If upper gastrointestinal tract bleeding is massive, the stomach should be emptied of clots with a large gastric tube using iced saline solution for irrigation. When the bleeding is under reasonable control, an emergency gastrointestinal series can be carried out and is rewarding in a surprisingly large number of patients. Since bleeding usually stops after irrigation of the stomach, useful information can be obtained if gastroscopy and esophagoscopy are carried out immediately before the x-rays are taken. A thorough discussion of the diagnostic approach to gastrointestinal bleeding will be found on pages 220–221.

Complete evaluation of the patient is extremely important, since a variety of systemic diseases may be associated with hemorrhage. A bleeding diathesis must always be ruled out. Investigation of hepatic function should be included, because cirrhosis of the liver is so often associated with bleeding esophageal varices, gastritis, or peptic ulceration.

Clinical features Syncope or other symptoms of acute blood loss usually signify a blood loss of at least 1,000 to 1,500 ml. Melena alone in the absence of any other symptoms is surprisingly common. Bleeding from duodenal or gastric ulcers occurs without prior symptoms in 20 percent of patients. In individuals who have had prior symptoms of ulcer, these complaints often disappear at the onset of bleeding, because blood in the stomach and duodenum buffers the highly acid gastric juice. Hyperperistalsis and frequent bowel movements are common, because blood within the gastrointestinal tract is irritating.

Treatment The treatment of gastrointestinal hemorrhage from peptic ulcer will depend upon the magnitude of the hemorrhage. In the majority of patients the therapy is nonoperative, and if the general condition permits, all patients should undergo the diagnostic tests outlined above. *Surgical consultation should always be obtained from the outset.* The decision to operate or not to operate should be made jointly by internists and surgeons. Occasionally, operation may be necessary as a diagnostic as well as therapeutic maneuver.

Sedation is important, because apprehension is common and may contribute to hypersecretion of acid. Replacement with blood should be early and adequate, and frequent monitoring of the physical findings and vital signs are mandatory. Careful records of the frequency, character, and output of stools must be made. Continuous gastric aspiration for the first 6 to 12 hr may be helpful, not only in determining whether bleeding is continuing, but also in removing acid from the ulcerated area. This may be supplanted by a drip of milk or alkali or by the stringent antiacid regimen described above. Thorough ice-water lavage may be useful. In poor-risk patients, infusion of vasopressin or norepinephrine by selective catheterization of a visceral artery as a means of controlling hemorrhage has been employed with benefit, but its true place is not yet known (see Chap. 41).

There is fairly universal agreement on the indication for operation in most cases. Operation should be considered *urgent* when exsanguinating hemorrhage is present, and such a patient may need to be taken to the operating room under less than optimal circumstances. In patients with esophageal varices, a Sengstaken-Blakemore tube may be used when hepatic function is so poor as to preclude operative therapy. A second group of patients requiring *emergency operation* are those who have continued to bleed sufficiently briskly to require as much as 500 ml blood every 8 hr after initial replacement of blood loss. Those patients who *rebleed* in the hospital after the initial episode constitute a third group about whom there is unanimity in favor of emergency operation. Such patients frequently have a large crater in either the stomach or duodenum. Even if bleeding stops, a previous history of multiple hemorrhage or other indications for operation should suggest that an opportune time for operation has arrived.

Factors which adversely affect the outcome of a gastrointestinal hemorrhage include age over sixty, previous massive hemorrhage, long-standing ulcer, or previous perforation. Bleeding from a gastric ulcer is much less likely to cease than is bleeding from a duodenal ulcer. Any of these factors might dictate operative therapy when other indications are equivocal.

Patients who bleed intermittently from an undetermined site following extensive evaluation should be operated on only when bleeding, because the chance of finding a lesion at operation in such an individual when he is not bleeding is very small.

PERFORATION Perforated ulcers are usually located on the anterior wall of the duodenum but may occur either on the anterior or posterior wall of the stomach.

Clinical features The onset of pain is usually sudden and severe. The pain begins in the epigastrium or right upper quadrant, is of a constant, steady nature, and may radiate to the superclavicular area if soiling of the subdiaphragmatic surfaces has occurred. The pain is accentuated by movement, coughing, or straining. Hence, the patient usually lies quietly in bed, often with flexed thighs. Vomiting of gastric content may occur once or twice, but persistent profuse vomiting is rare. On occasion, patients give a history suggesting preexisting symptoms of ulcer, but at least 10 to 20 percent of patients with perforation do not have such a history. Examination shows a quiet abdomen usually with marked direct and rebound tenderness, and severe rigidity, although these findings are greatly attenuated in the elderly. Liver dullness may be absent, and there may be tenderness on rectal examination if the irritating gastric juice has migrated to the cul-de-sac. Shock is rare until late in the course of the disease and is caused by the extravasation of large quantities of fluid into the peritoneal cavity, the extent of which may be assessed by the rise in hematocrit if no significant bleeding has occurred.

Diagnosis The diagnosis rests mainly upon the clinical findings. The shift of pain from the epigastrium to the right lower quadrant may be confused with acute appendicitis, but the findings of peritoneal irritation are usually more striking in patients with perforated ulcer, and a carefully taken history is usually adequate to distinguish between these diseases. Confusion is particularly likely to occur in patients who are examined 6 to 10 hr after perforation and in whom sealing of the perforation has occurred by adherence of the liver or other adjacent structures to the lesion. Rapidly progressive clinical improvement serves to differentiate this special group from patients with acute appendicitis.

Roentgenologic examination of the abdomen in the flat and upright position is often extremely helpful to detect free air under the diaphragm though approximately 15 percent of patients with perforated ulcers do *not* show this sign. The absence of free air must not be misconstrued to indicate that perforated ulcer is not present. The white blood cell count is usually increased, with a concomitant increase in the number of immature cells. An *elevated serum amylase level* is not infrequent and should not be a contraindication to operation if the clinical diagnosis suggests perforated ulcer. Intravenous cholangiography may be useful to exclude acute cholecystitis. Examination of the stomach and duodenum with water-soluble contrast material (gastrografin) may identify the perforation in equivocal cases, but false negative results occur.

Treatment Operation is the mainstay in the treatment of perforated ulcer. Nonoperative therapy should probably be reserved for those patients in whom sealing of the perforation has already taken place and in whom marked and progressive clinical improvement has occurred when they are first seen. Nonoperative treatment consists mainly of careful continuous gastric suction to ensure complete emptying of the stomach. In addition, antibiotics and adequate fluid therapy are given. The major objections to nonoperative therapy are that intraabdominal and subphrenic abscesses are more common than after surgical treatment.

Preparation of the patient for operation should include intubation of the stomach and replacement of fluid losses. The magnitude of the "third space" losses in these patients is often underestimated, but even 3 or 4 hr after a perforation, as much as 3,000 ml fluid may be required if contamination of the peritoneal cavity has been massive. For the majority of patients simple closure of the ulcer is the safest therapy associated with the lowest mortality rate. If the patient is seen within 6 to 8 hr of the perforation and should other indications for surgical therapy of the peptic ulcer disease already exist, definitive surgical therapy of the ulcer may be undertaken, especially if peritoneal soiling is minimal. The results of definitive treatment have been gratifying in these carefully selected cases. Biopsies should always be taken of perforated gastric ulcers, but if carcinoma is likely, gastric resection is indicated.

GASTRIC OUTLET OBSTRUCTION Obstruction to the outlet of the stomach is most commonly associated with duodenal ulceration, but in a significant minority of cases, a distally located antral ulcer may produce the same clinical picture. Carcinoma of the stomach, congenital anomalies, and a variety of other lesions may also cause gastric outlet obstruction.

Pathophysiology Obstruction is usually the result of edema associated with active ulceration or fibrous stenosis or both. The severity of the symptoms is related to the degree and rapidity of onset of the obstruction and depends upon the competence of the antral musculature, the so-called "antral pump." An effectively compensated antral pump may overcome a high-grade stenosis for prolonged periods and may be associated with mild or no symptoms. On the other hand, less severe degrees of obstruction may produce severe symptoms if the antral pump decompensates, a more common finding when the obstruction is sudden rather than slowly progressive.

Clinical features Anorexia, nausea, and fullness after eating are the most frequent symptoms. Surprisingly, vomiting may not occur until late when decompensation of the antral pump has occurred. A vague aching pain after eating associated with hyperperistalsis may also be present and is usually relieved by vomiting. Spontaneous vomiting without pain may occur only once a day, and generally the vomitus consists of the food ingested during the previous 24-hr period. Vomiting rarely occurs more than two or three times daily despite severe obstruction. Weight loss and constipation are frequent. As the obstruction progresses, severe extracellular fluid deficits and hypokalemic and/or hypochloremic alkalosis often supervene. Roentgenologic examination of the abdomen usually shows an enormously dilated stomach, often occupying as much as two-thirds of the abdomen. Definitive examination of the upper part of the gastrointestinal tract with barium before adequate decompression and cleansing of the stomach is unrewarding, because accurate assessment of the cause of the obstruction is difficult or impossible. Such studies are best delayed for a few days, since they often exhaust an already seriously ill patient.

Differential diagnosis In addition to gastric and duodenal ulcer, tumors of the stomach and foreshortening secondary to antral gastritis may produce gastric outlet obstruction. Occasionally, corrosive gastritis from the ingestion of alkali, postoperative stenosis of gastroduodenal anastomoses or pyloroplasties, congenital anomalies, and inflammatory disease of adjacent organs also produce outlet obstruction.

Neuromuscular defects must also be considered. Diabetic autonomic neuropathy, vagotomy without a drainage operation, anticholinergic drugs, severe postoperative ileus, potassium deficiency, hypothyroidism, and acute and chronic disease of the central nervous system may all be associated with gastric dilatation because of failure of the antral pump. Sometimes a single lesion cannot be identified, and the dilatation is attributed to severe debility, aging, and protein deficiency.

Treatment The response to therapy is of great value in determining whether organic irreversible stricture or edema is the predominant cause of the obstruction. Fluid and electrolyte deficits can usually be within the first 24 hr, particularly if azotemia is not present. *Continuous* gastric aspiration for 72 hr is the most important part of the therapeutic regimen and will almost always allow differentiation between organic stricture and edema. Resolution of the obstruction after 72 hr of continuous aspiration is generally excellent when edema is the predominating feature, whereas large gastric residuals of over 500 ml persist in organic strictures.

Repeated attempts to produce resolution of the obstruction beyond 72 to 92 hr cause undue delay and further deterioration of the patient. If the obstruction is so marked that 5 to 6 days of aspiration is required, operation is undoubtedly indicated anyway. Following the original period of gastric suction, a stringent antacid regimen and clear-liquid diet are begun. Anticholinergic drugs are contraindicated, because gastric emptying is delayed. The gastric residual volume is determined 24 hr after the institution of such a regimen and occasionally 48 hr later. Should gastric obstruction be evident by the indication of large residual volumes, then operation is immediately indicated.

SYNDROMES AFTER GASTRECTOMY OR VAGOTOMY

The immediate postoperative complications are those which may follow any abdominal operation in addition to a small group of special complications peculiar to gastric operations. A full discussion of these is not within the purview of this chapter, and it is the late complications to which attention will be directed.

Anatomic and functional derangements

FAILURE OF GASTRIC EMPTYING After vagotomy there is failure of the normal antral pump mechanism. Since the advent of the combination of an emptying procedure (pyloroplasty or gastroenterostomy) with vagotomy, this complication is not common. In rare instances of long-standing preoperative obstruction where decompensation of the antral pump has occurred, pyloroplasty in the presence of an elongated J-shaped stomach may fail to provide adequate gastric emptying after vagotomy. Gastroenterostomy or resection may be necessary to overcome this problem. Obstruction of a gastroduodenal or gastrojejunal anastomosis may be a delayed occurrence and usually results from faulty surgical technique, although rarely the development of recurrent ulcer or carcinoma of the stomach may be a causative factor. Obstruction of the efferent loop of a gastrojejunostomy more commonly results from adhesions or kinking, however, and may require operative intervention.

OBSTRUCTION OF THE AFFERENT LOOP This complication occurs only in the presence of a gastrojejunostomy and is slightly more frequent when the afferent loop is anastomosed to the greater curvature of the stomach. The usual symptoms are a marked feeling of fullness, bloating, and nausea after meals. These symptoms are dramatically relieved 20 to 60 min after the ingestion of the food by the vomiting of clear bilious material not containing the ingested food. Food is absent because the efferent loop is patent, while the bilious vomiting is caused by the sudden release of the secretions from the afferent loop. Usually the symptoms are chronic, although occasionally acute severe complete obstruction may develop. The latter condition resembles acute pancreatitis clinically, and elevation of the serum amylase level is common. The diagnosis is usually difficult, since lack of filling of the afferent loop on radiologic examination is not infrequently observed in the absence of afferent loop obstruction. Treatment consists of surgical revision of the anastomosis. Afferent loop obstruction may be associated with the blind loop syndrome (see Chap. 284) due to bacterial overgrowth in the obstructed afferent loop.

JEJUNOGASTRIC INTUSSUSCEPTION AND RETROANASTOMATIC HERNIATION Retrograde intussusception of the jejunum into the gastric pouch may cause acute obstruction of either the afferent or the efferent loop of the gastrojejunal anastomosis and may occur early or many years after operation. Herniation of the afferent loop or the efferent loop behind the gastrojejunal stoma or herniation of the jejunum through the mesocolon if a posterior gastrojejunal anastomosis has been carried out may also be the cause of acute obstructive symptoms. These complications are associated with repeated vomiting and require immediate surgical intervention.

GASTRITIS In addition to the usual factors which may cause irritation of the gastric mucosa, the loss of the pylorus allows almost continuous regurgitation of alkaline juices into the stomach. Bile salts and phospholipase A are known to disrupt the gastric mucosal barrier. Consequently, microscopic gastritis is present in a high percentage of patients following gastric operations, although overt gastroscopic gastritis is somewhat less frequent. So-called "bile gastritis" may be much more common than previously suspected and might be a more frequent cause of bilious vomiting than afferent loop obstruction. In certain patients, surgical diversion of bile and pancreatic juice from the anastomosis is curative.

Metabolic and other derangements

EARLY AND LATE POSTPRANDIAL POSTGASTRECTOMY SYNDROMES The *early syndrome*, often referred to in the literature as the *dumping syndrome*, is characterized by the development of weakness, nausea, a feeling of warmth, palpitation, pallor, borborygmi, diarrhea, and distention, 20 to 30 min after a meal. There is often a strong urge to assume the recumbent position, and recumbency usually relieves the symptoms. The syndrome is most violently and frequently produced by a high-carbohydrate intake. The *late syndrome*, not truly dumping, consists of profound weakness, tremulousness, palpitation, and sweating without hyperperistalsis and diarrhea, usually occurring approximately 2 to 3 hr after the meal.

The causes of the symptoms of the early and late syndromes are different. Loss of the pylorus, by whatever surgical operation, allows the introduction of hyperosmolar substances into the small intestine, with a resultant outpouring of fluid from the plasma, to produce an isosmotic intestinal content. However, the lack of correlation of decreases in plasma volume with the severity of the symptoms has led to a search for other causes of the early postprandial dumping syndrome. The release of serotonin from the small intestine, and rapid and prolonged alimentary hyperglycemia have also been implicated, but their role is uncertain. Elevations of circulating kinin levels have been found to correlate with the vasomotor symptoms in these patients, but further studies are required to assess the importance of these findings. Enteric glucagon released in response to glucose may contribute to the diarrhea, since glucagon inhibits sodium absorption by the small intestine. The late postprandial symptoms clearly result from a functional hypoglycemia which may be caused by excessive production of insulin or an insulin hypersensitivity. The diagnosis of the early postprandial syndrome is relatively easy if a careful history is taken. The late hypoglycemic syndrome can be diagnosed by the finding of hypoglycemia late in the course of a 6-hr oral glucose tolerance test.

Attempts at prevention of the early postprandial dumping syndrome by surgical narrowing of the original gastroenteric stoma have not been uniformly successful and may be associated with early or late stomal obstruction. Treatment consists of frequent small meals low in sugar and starch in order to decrease the osmolarity of the meal. Fluids are permitted between meals only, because the concomitant administration of food and fluids permits the production of a hypertonic solution. Anticholinergic drugs may retard the hyperperistalsis and are often helpful. Serotonin antagonists have been disappointing and probably are of little value. In those patients with prolonged alimentary *hyperglycemia*, excellent results have been obtained by the administration of tolbutamide. The usual dose is 0.5 to 1 g tolbutamide 10 to 30 min before meals. The late prandial *hypoglycemic* symptoms are best treated with a high-protein–low-carbohydrate diet.

Although any patient may develop the dumping syndrome after loss of normal pyloric function, significant symptoms occur in only about 5 to 10 percent of patients. In only 1 percent are the symptoms sufficiently severe that operative reconstruction is contemplated. In selected instances the introduction of an antiperistaltic loop of intestine has been helpful.

Anemia Anemia is probably the most common complication of partial gastrectomy. If patients are carefully studied after gastrectomy, 20 to 50 percent will show some anemia. Anemia is more common after gastrojejunostomy than after gastroduodenostomy and is more prevalent after resection than after simple vagotomy with emptying operation. It often represents a combination of iron deficiency and vitamin B_{12} deficiency. The iron deficiency results not only from decreased oral intake but also from impaired iron absorption caused by hypochlorhydria, rapid gastric emptying, and bypass of the duodenum, especially after gastrojejunostomy. Chronic blood loss from stomal gastritis may contribute to the iron deficiency. The treatment of iron-deficiency anemia is discussed in Chap. 304. Vitamin B_{12} deficiency may result not only from extensive removal of the source of intrinsic factor but also from the ensuing gastritis in the gastric remnant. The afferent loop syndrome described above may be contributory. Vagotomy also reduces the amount of intrinsic factor in gastric juice. Folic acid deficiency after gastrectomy is rare. Every patient who undergoes gastrectomy should be carefully surveyed for anemia at least once yearly for the remainder of his life and appropriate therapeutic measures undertaken if anemia appears.

Malabsorption and weight loss Weight loss following gastric operations is common if the patient is overweight at the time of operation. On the other hand, when patients have lost a great deal of weight prior to operation, they will often gain after the procedure but do not usually reach their previous level. Weight loss is caused by poor eating habits, fear of eating because of the dumping syndrome or mechanical abnormalities, and malabsorption. The cause of the malabsorption is not completely understood, but causative factors include poor mixing of bile and pancreatic secretions with food, rapid intestinal transit, and the effects of bacterial overgrowth in the afferent loop if afferent loop obstruction is present. When truncal vagotomy is performed, decreased release of secretin and cholecystokinin from the duodenum may contribute to the malabsorption. Osteomalacia may occur as a result of poor absorption of vitamin D and calcium. Careful demonstration of the etiologic factors is important, and treatment includes an adequate diet occasionally supplemented by pancreatic extracts and bile salts. Courses of broad-spectrum antibiotics may be dramatic in reversing the malabsorption if afferent loop obstruction accompanied by overgrowth of bacteria is an important factor. Surgical revision may be considered should these nonoperative methods fail.

POSTVAGOTOMY EFFECTS An increasing number of instances of development of gallstones after total abdominal vagotomy is being recognized. This is probably caused by poor emptying of the gallbladder, not only because of loss of its nerve supply, but also because of inadequate stimulation of bile flow by secretin and cholecystokinin and lack of contraction of the gallbladder by cholecystokinin, especially if the duodenum has been bypassed. Consequently, this complication may also occur after high subtotal gastric resection with gastrojejunostomy.

Postvagotomy diarrhea has been reported in as many as 50 to 60 percent of individuals undergoing vagal resection. However, as a troublesome symptom it occurs in only 4 to 5 percent of patients. It consists of intermittent pale, greasy stools, associated with sudden, explosive, loose bowel movements, seemingly occurring without any predisposing factor. This occurs once every week or two, lasts 1 or 2 days, and then subsides as rapidly as it commenced. The cause of the diarrhea is unknown, but selective denervation of the stomach alone has been successful in preventing this complication.

REFERENCES

FORTRAN JS, WALSH JA: Gastric acid secretion rate and buffer content of the stomach after eating. Results in normal subjects and in patients with duodenal ulcer. J Clin Invest 52:645, 1973

GEAR MLW et al: Gastric ulcer and gastritis. Gut 12:639, 1971

GOLIGHER JC et al: Five- to eight-year results of truncal vagotomy and pyloroplasty for duodenal ulcer. Br Med J 1:7, 1972

HARVEY RF, LANGMAN MJS: The late results of medical and surgical treatment for bleeding duodenal ulcer. Quart J Med 39:539, 1970

KAY AW: Memorial lecture: An evaluation of gastric acid secretion tests. Gastroenterology 53:834, 1967

LITTMAN A (ed): The Veterans Administration cooperative study on gastric ulcer. Gastroenterology 61:567, 1971

MCGUIGAN JE, TRUDEAU WL: Differences in rates of gastrin release in normal persons and patients with duodenal ulcer. N Engl J Med 288:64, 1973

RHODES J et al: Increased reflux of bile into the stomach in patients with gastric ulcer. Gastroenterology 57:241, 1969

SAKITA T et al: Observations on the healing of ulcerations in early gastric cancer. The life cycle of the malignant ulcer. Gastroenterology 60:835, 1971

SCHILLER KFR: Haematemesis and melaena, with special reference to factors influencing the outcome. Br Med J 2:7, 1970

SIZEMORE GW et al: Calcitonin and gastrin in Zollinger-Ellison syndrome and medullary carcinoma of thyroid. N Engl J Med 288:641, 1973

283
CANCER, GASTRITIS, AND OTHER DISEASES OF THE STOMACH

EDWIN ENGLERT, JR.

GASTRIC CARCINOMA Carcinoma of the stomach is asymptomatic during early growth. Later, local and systemic symptoms appear through necrosis, bleeding, ulceration, obstruction, disturbed motility, invasion of adjacent structures, metastasis to distant organs, and the effects of advanced malignancy. Resultant clinical patterns range widely, and diagnosis may be easy or extremely difficult. Unfortunately, clinical descriptions of gastric carcinoma relate almost exclusively to late manifestations and are not of much help to the physician who wishes to make the diagnosis early enough to effect a cure by complete excision.

Incidence There has been a striking, continuous, but unexplained decline in the reported death rate of gastric carcinoma in the United States from 34 per 100,000 population in 1930 to 8 per 100,000 currently, but world figures indicate that cancer of the stomach remains a major health problem. Men are affected twice as often as women. The disease afflicts all races, but as in other gastroduodenal diseases, there appear to be unexplained geographic and cultural differences in incidence. It attacks all ages, although rarely before the third decade, and the risk rises progressively thereafter. The antrum is the leading site of gastric carcinoma, followed by the lesser curvature, cardia, and body of the stomach.

Predisposing factors *Genetic* predisposition is evident from the familial occurrence of carcinoma of the stomach as well as the increased incidence of blood group A among its victims. *Alteration of the gastric mucosa* requires special mention, because it defines patients at high risk. The cancer rate increases progressively in patients with hypochlorhydria, achlorhydria, gastric atrophy, gastric polyps, and pernicious anemia, reaching 6 to 12 percent in the last group. Mucosal changes may also explain the increased risk of cancer in the gastric remnant which occurs many years after gastrectomy performed for any reason, since gastritis is virtually universal in these pouches.

Polyps are not found frequently in cancer-bearing stomachs, but some polyps in fact are malignant, particularly those over 2 cm in diameter. There is no convincing evidence that malignant change occurs in the benign adematous polyp.

The adult form of *acanthosis nigricans*, a pigmented papillomatous skin disease of intertriginous areas, face, and flexor surfaces, is frequently associated with visceral carcinoma, often of the stomach. The mechanism is unknown (see Chap. 367).

Environment may also play a role. Factors such as rural residence, ingestion of very hot foods, smoked fish, soya bean paste, and aflatoxins have been implicated.

Clinical features The early carcinoma may be frustratingly silent, and the late manifestations extremely variable. The course may be fulminating or insidious, short or prolonged. Anorexia is a remarkably constant feature, and patients with advanced cases exhibit abdominal discomfort, weight loss, anemia, weakness, and rapid filling on eating. Discomfort varies from mild intermittent epigastric pain to constant severe pain often boring into the back. Pain may be poorly localized and may reflect a sensation of fullness, aching, or bloating initiated or aggravated by meals. In ulcerated carcinoma, the pain may mimic ulcer pain.

Gastric carcinoma *invades* locally and *metastasizes* by way of the lymphatics, by way of the bloodstream, and by free passage across the peritoneum. Commonly it extends into the lower esophagus, proximal duodenum, omentum, colon, peritoneum, or pancreas. Pulmonary metastases may be lymphangitic and diffuse, or hematogenous and nodular. Local and distant spread also produces symptoms in liver, pleura, bone, nervous system, and skin. There may be gastric retention or obstruction, diarrhea, thrombophlebitis, nausea, vomiting, backache, cough, hiccup, pleurisy, fever, and melena. Perforation and massive bleeding are unusual.

Physical examination Physical findings are entirely normal during the early course, but in late cases there is evidence of local and metastatic tumor. Commonly there are signs of anemia and weight loss, mass or tenderness in the epigastrium, low-grade fever, and a nodular enlarged liver. There are numerous eponymic metastases of gastric carcinoma, such as Virchow's left supraclavicular lymph node, the Irish left pectoral node, Blumer's shelf on rectal examination, and Krukenberg's tumor in the ovary, but these occur in only 10 percent of cases, or less. There may be bone tenderness, ascites, pleural effusion, succussion splash, peripheral or central neurologic signs, jaundice, pericardial rub, skin rash, or an umbilical mass. The wasted cachetic look of terminal malignancy is rare.

Roentgenographic and gastroscopic examination Rarely employed in early, unsuspected carcinoma in this country, these techniques have been revolutionized by the advent of photographic fiberoptic endoscopy and careful innovative investigations from Japan, where the accuracy of visualizing early cancer less than 1 cm in diameter is about 60 percent. For all carcinomas, accuracy is over 90 percent and virtually reaches 100 percent when both x-ray and endoscopy are combined with direct biopsy and cytology. Both methods reveal features of one of several types of growth: (1) polypoid mass, (2) tumor with punched-out ulceration, (3) ulcerative mass blending into adjacent stomach wall, (4) diffusely infiltrating intramural tumor, or (5) superficial spreading mucosal plaque. X-ray features of the mass and ulceration were described in Chap. 282, but it may be reemphasized that differentiation of benign from malignant ulcers is clear-cut in over 80 percent of cases. In the small remaining group, the radiologist is less certain. It is for this reason that gastric ulcers which are not obviously malignant and destined for early surgical therapy should be evaluated thoroughly by the combined use of x-ray, gastroscopy, cytology, examination of gastric acidity, and trial of medical management as outlined in Chap. 282.

Diffuse infiltrating carcinomas may not produce roentgenographic evidence of a mass. Instead, they cause concentric narrowing of the lumen or areas of flattening, beading, rigidity, and absent peristalsis (Fig. 283-1). This variety is responsible for the "leather bottle stomach" deformity and the term *linitis plastica*, referring to a network of dense fibrous tissue interspersed with isolated carcinoma cells.

Biopsy and cytology Though "blind" biopsy is of no value, *direct-vision biopsy* through the gastroscope is diagnostic in 90 percent of cases. Japanese investigators, who pioneered this method, emphasize the importance of *multiple* biopsies of each lesion and of biopsying *inside* the crater in cases of malignant ulcer. *Cytology* yields the highest accuracy, but unfortunately this is achieved only in centers which make a major commitment to painstaking technique and interpretation. "Blind" lavage with

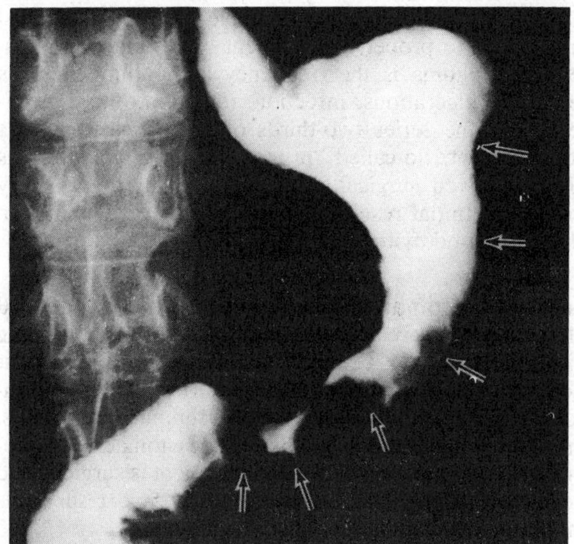

FIGURE 283-1
Diffusely infiltrating gastric carcinoma (linitis plastica). The stomach is rigidly contracted to a narrow channel throughout most of its length. Note fine irregularities in the wall, absence of peristaltic contractions, and nodular tumorous masses in the distal third.

chymotrypsin solutions may detect over 90 percent of adenocarcinoma with less than 1 percent false positives; over 95 percent accuracy has been attained in Japan with lavage or with brushing of the lesion through the gastroscope.

Laboratory findings In late or symptomatic cancers laboratory findings include *anemia*, usually of chronic-blood-loss type, and *occult blood* in the stools in most patients. True *achlorhydria* with maximum pentagastrin, betazole, or histamine testing is found in half the patients, and *hypochlorhydria* in another quarter. Since many patients therefore have normal secretion, the presence of acid is of no value in differential diagnosis. Moreover, true hypersecretion, although rare, does not rule out carcinoma. *Hypoalbuminemia* due to leakage of serum albumin into the stomach is found occasionally. Gastric secretions contain elevated levels of *lactic acid* (>100 μg per ml) in 50 percent of patients with carcinoma but in only 2 percent with gastric ulcer. Gastric contents also reveal increased β-*glucuronidase* (>1 unit per mg protein) in 90 percent of subjects with cancer or atrophic gastritis. As in other malignant conditions, there may be elevated levels of serum haptoglobin and abnormal spikes in the serum protein electrophoretogram, usually due to an IgG globulin. Although carcinoembryonic antigen (CEA) appears in the serum of some patients with stomach cancer, it is not specific and occurs with greater frequency in colonic cancers (see Chap. 288).

Diagnosis Diagnosis of advanced carcinoma may be easy when the clinical and roentgenographic findings are clear-cut. In other cases, the condition defies analysis completely or mimics other diseases. It is wise to *insist* on histologic diagnosis before concluding that the patient has inoperable gastric cancer. This may be obtained by endoscopic biopsy; cytology, lymph node biopsy, blind needle biopsy of the liver; needle biopsy of metastatic nodules in liver, pleura, or bone marrow; or limited surgical exploration.

Early cases are regrettably silent, but sudden changes in upper gastrointestinal function, particularly the appearance of anorexia in men over forty years of age, should arouse suspicion. Clinical judgment must be exercised in deciding how far to proceed, but the minimum is an x-ray study of the stomach and repeated tests of the stool for occult bleeding. If any doubt exists, cytology, gastroscopy, secretory studies, repeated x-ray, and gastroscopy with biopsy of any suspicious area and exploration are the next steps to be taken in sequence.

Cancer screening programs Roentgenographic surveys of the normal population have been made to detect silent carcinomas of the stomach, but the yield of curable lesions did not justify their routine use in the United States. Mass surveys in Japan by x-ray or endoscopy found a 0.25 to 0.5 percent incidence of cancer with one-half still in the early stage. In high-risk patients, such as those with pernicious anemia, gastric polyps, and gastric atrophy, it is desirable to carry out semiannual examinations with alternating gastric cytology, gastroscopy, and roentgenography. In past surveys of these groups, unsuspected tumors were detected five times more often and had spread beyond the possibility of surgical cure less often than in surveys of the normal population. Periodic testing of the stool for occult bleeding also is indicated in these patients.

Treatment *Surgical treatment* to attempt *complete excision* of the tumor is indicated in every patient in whom careful clinical investigation fails to reveal evidence of spread beyond the stomach. Moreover, *palliative operation* is necessary to relieve obstruction in some patients and rarely for emergencies induced by perforation or massive bleeding.

The natural history of the disease too often places the surgeon at the disadvantage of being able to do too little too late. Surgical statistics, on the other hand, are nonrandom, uncontrolled, and confusing. Consequently, it is difficult if not impossible to be certain of the real effectiveness of surgical treatment or even to compare one surgical series with another. It is believed that the overall *5-year survival rate* in all patients undergoing operation for carcinoma of the stomach is *10 to 20 percent.* In one study of patients who were *not* operated on it was 2 percent.

In comparison, high survival rates may be expected with tumors of low invasiveness and slow growth characteristics, such as small ulcerating and superficial spreading carcinomas. The same appears to be true for occasional patients with augmented host resistance to the tumor, although such cases are poorly understood and therapeutically unexplored. Sporadic reports of prolonged survival without surgical treatment and of true recurrence (rather than an independent primary cancer)

10 or more years postoperatively also reflect these factors. This suggests that a long history of the disease may mean slow growth and a favorable prognosis. Other factors which determine the outcome of surgical therapy are location and extent of tumor, condition of the patient, and the presence of metastases at exploration. When no metastases are found in regional lymph nodes, 5-year survival may occur in as many as half the patients of this group. An experience unique to Japan is the frequent occurrence of cancer confined to mucosa and submucosa (roughly 20 percent of cases); in this group 5-year survival after surgery may reach 90 percent!

Formerly, attempts at curative operation employed total gastrectomy, but comparable results have attended the use of radical subtotal resection for all but high gastric cancers near the cardia. The latter procedure is more extensive than in ulcer operations, since local and lymphatic pathways of extension are included in the resection. Surgical mortality rate is 8 to 43 percent after total gastrectomy and 5 to 13 percent after subtotal gastrectomy, figures considerably higher than those for noncancer gastric surgery. The incidence and types of postgastrectomy syndromes depend on the extent of resection (see Chap. 282).

Cancer chemotherapy has been tried in inoperable carcinoma of the stomach, but the lack of well-controlled clinical trials makes it difficult to assess its possible effectiveness. 5-Fluorouracil in schedules of 15 mg per kg for 2 or 3 days, then 7.5 mg per kg on alternate days until toxicity, and weekly maintenance with 500 to 1,000 mg is said to induce some tumor regression for an average of 5 months in 10 to 20 percent of patients. However, such agents may actually shorten the patient's life through toxic effect on other tissues, such as bone marrow.

OTHER MALIGNANT TUMORS OF THE STOMACH

Carcinoma of the stomach comprises 90 percent of gastric malignant tumors, and lymphoma accounts for most of the remainder. A rare group of sarcomas, the most common of which is leiomyosarcoma, includes fibrosarcoma, neurogenic sarcoma, neurofibrosarcoma, and myxosarcoma. They usually are misdiagnosed as carcinoma or found by chance.

Lymphoma of the stomach Lymphoma of the stomach generally is a lymphosarcoma or reticulum-cell sarcoma. It appears in about one-fifth of patients with systemic lymphomatous involvement and also occurs as a "primary" lymphoma without obvious disease elsewhere. There are no distinctive gastric symptoms, and indeed there often are no gastric symptoms in patients with widespread disease. Epigastric pain or mass and weight loss are frequent in the "primary" variety. Lymphomas are often indistinguishable from carcinoma by acid studies, gastroscopy, and even by their appearance at operation. Biopsy via the gastroscope or at laparotomy is thus essential for diagnosis.

Characteristically, the patient's general condition is good when first seen. Lymphoma of the stomach bleeds massively or perforates more often than carcinoma but usually presents a similar roentgenographic and gastroscopic appearance. However, large stiff folds or a submucosal mass may be the sole finding. Of special importance to proper management of patients with systemic lymphoma is the frequency of nontumor lesions (erosions, ulcerations, infection, radiation, and drug effects); in one series two-thirds of gastric bleeding was nonmalignant. So-called "primary" gastric lymphoma is often removed surgically and the patient subsequently irradiated. Initial results of such therapy or of radiation alone are good, with 5-year survival in half the patients.

Leiomyosarcomas These tumors often ulcerate and bleed, but there are no distinctive clinical features. A long history is common. On x-ray and gastroscopic examination, these tumors appear as exogastric masses, circumscribed globular filling defects, or submucosal tumors, most often toward the fundus of the stomach and frequently with central ulceration. Treatment is surgical, and because of slow growth characteristics 5-year survivals may be expected in one-half these patients.

Benign tumors of the stomach The benign gastric tumors are adenomas, leiomyomas, fibromas, lipomas, and neurofibromas. Except for adenomas, these are rare. Usually they do not produce symptoms, but those derived from mesenchyme and ectoderm may ulcerate and bleed. Although features of benignancy are generally evident on x-ray and gastroscopy, these tumors often are removed, because malignancy cannot be excluded with certainty.

Adenomatous polyps These tumors occur in the distal two-thirds of the stomach and often are multiple. They appear in about 2 percent of achlorhydric patients and in 5 percent of patients with pernicious anemia. Conversely, 85 percent of patients with polyps will be found to be achlorhydric. Roentgenographically they produce smooth, oval filling defects within the gastric lumen, and gastroscopy reveals a berrylike mass with an intact mucosa.

Polyps over 2 cm in diameter are actually polypoid carcinomas 50 percent of the time, while those under 2 cm are cancerous in only 1 percent. Since the weight of evidence indicates that adenomas do not themselves become cancers, small polyps should receive no treatment but follow-up (see Cancer Screening Programs, above). Polyps over 2 cm, those which grow and bleed, and those which appear suggestive on x-ray, gastroscopy, or biopsy should be removed surgically.

Leiomyomas Leiomyomas occur in the antrum, body, and fundus of the stomach, and they commonly bleed. By x-ray, gastroscopy, and even histology they may be difficult to distinguish from leiomyosarcomas. When diagnosed, they should be removed surgically. Although rare clinically, careful search reveals small ones in 16 to 50 percent of autopsies; there is no evidence that they undergo malignant change.

Pseudotumors *Benign lymphoid or reactive lymphoreticular hyperplasia*, or pseudolymphoma, may occur in the stomach as well as in other organs and cause a long history of vague dyspepsia. Such lesions may ulcerate and bleed and produce a variety of appearances on x-ray and gastroscopic examination, simulating carcinoma or peptic ulcer. Simple surgical excision is curative. *Eosinophilic granuloma*, or inflammatory fibroid polyp, may be related to diffuse eosinophilic gastroenteritis, an alleged hypersensitivity state. Such granulomas may be found throughout the gastrointestinal tract but especially in the gastric antrum, where they produce episodic cramps and vomiting or ulceration and bleeding. X-ray and gastroscopic appearances mimic adenoma, carcinoma, or antral narrowing, and there may be peripheral eosinophilia. Some cases respond to corticosteroid therapy. *Fundoplication* of the lower esophagus (in Belsey Mark IV and Nissen operations) for repair of hiatus hernia routinely produces a pseudotumor at the upper medial aspect of the stomach, which projects into the gastric air bubble. In patients with portal hypertension, *gastric varices* may appear, predominantly in the fundus as lobulated, smooth masses and in the antrum as coarse, turgid folds. Thickened rugae occur also in *uremia* and in patients undergoing chronic hemodialysis. Intramural *hematoma* may follow trauma or occur spontaneously in disorders of coagulation and vascular disease and be mistaken for carcinoma. Numerous *inflammatory conditions* may also simulate tumor. (See Other Forms of Gastritis, below.)

Functional dyspepsia Symptoms caused by *disturbances of physiologic functions* are termed functional disorders. They are the *commonest illnesses* in the United States, and the gastrointestinal tract is the organ system most often involved. The two leading functional gastrointestinal syndromes are functional dyspepsia and the irritable colon (Chap. 288). Because it is ubiquitous, functional dyspepsia may coexist with one or more organic lesions, be mistaken for a normal, physiologic event, or be confused with other diseases of the upper part of the gastrointestinal tract.

Clinical features *Symptoms* include dry mouth, a lump in the throat, difficulty in initiating swallowing, anorexia, belching, flatus, abdominal distention or rumbling, nausea, vomiting, sourness, "water brash," and epigastric or midabdominal discomfort. The latter ranges from vague epigastric fullness to cramps and "burning." The patient may complain of persistent but poorly defined pain. In contrast to peptic ulcer disease, pain or discomfort generally occurs before breakfast, is usually quite diffuse, and is frequently aggravated or initiated by eating. Characteristically it is difficult for the patient to provide specific details of his discomfort, its timing, and its relationship to bodily functions or associated symptoms. Extremely common is *flatulent indigestion* after eating fatty foods.

The *course* of functional symptoms is chronic, with tendencies to wax and wane. Despite great concern, the patient sleeps well and appears healthy. Typically there is no weight loss, even when the patient has a fear of eating or when vomiting prevents adequate nutrition. Often there are *neurasthenic* symptoms in addition to gastrointestinal complaints, and many patients have *headaches*, chronic *fatigue*, and acute or chronic *anxiety* or *depression*.

Findings on *examination* may be normal, but usually evidence is disclosed of coincident unrelated disease, visceral dysfunction, and the associated functional disturbances. There may be epigastric tenderness, distention, hypo- or hyperactive bowel sounds, hyperresonance, clammy palms, postural hypotension, depression, and other functional symptoms.

Laboratory confirmation is rarely necessary, but when there is doubt, visceral dysfunction can be documented by appropriate testing, e.g., motility studies or cinefluoroscopy *during* a period of active symptoms. Results also serve as excellent visual aids with which to explain symptoms to the patient. In addition, every patient with functional dyspepsia should have a thorough upper gastrointestinal workup (Chap. 38), to permit diagnosis of coincident symptomatic and "silent" diseases. The physician must be extremely cautious not to make the common error of blaming every symptom on any and all organic aberrations found.

Diagnosis If the history is taken carefully, with the timing and relationship of symptoms to body functions and patient activities, and if the functional and psychomotor findings on examination are not passed off as normal variants, the symptom patterns and associations outlined permit clear-cut diagnosis. It is, therefore, a *serious error* to diagnose functional disease only when organic lesions cannot be demonstrated. It is also important not to jump to the conclusion, once the diagnosis of functional disease is clear, that the condition is psychogenic. It most often is, but the physician must remember to rule out the many other causes of functional symptoms [see Gastric Retention (Atonia and Dilatation), below].

Treatment This consists of thorough *examination* to identify and treat accompanying organic disease, sympathetic but firm *explanation* of symptoms, strong *reassurance*, and *symptomatic measures*. Since symptoms do have a physiologic basis, temporary relief often follows judicious use of agents known to influence the physiologic abnormalities demonstrated in any given patient, e.g., anticholinergic agents for cramps and hypermotility (Chap. 282), antacids for pain and sourness (Chap. 282), or thiopropazate hydrochloride 10 mg 20 min a.c. for nausea and vomiting. Metoclopramide, a gastric motor stimulant not approved for use in the United States, in doses of 10 mg t.i.d. (30 min before usual timing of symptoms in relation to meals) has been shown to be effective in treating the whole flatulent dyspepsia syndrome. Other measures are discussed under Treatment below.

Symptomatic relief is temporary, but reexamination often reveals changing physiologic events which justify changing the symptomatic agent. It is helpful to agree with the patient and proscribe foods believed by him to cause distress. *Sedatives and tranquilizers* usually are recommended. Two controlled trials of a tranquilizer plus an anticholinergic agent demonstrated effectiveness against anxiety symptoms (diazepam 2.5 mg and propantheline bromide 15 mg q.i.d.) and against visceral symptoms (chlordiazepoxide 5 mg and clidinium bromide 2.5 mg q.i.d.). In some patients, there is a marked psychopathologic condition with gross psychiatric symptoms over and above the functional gastrointestinal complaints. Such patients require psychiatric treatment.

One of the physician's prime responsibilities to these patients is to remain alert for the development of new symptoms, which are difficult to separate from the numerous functional complaints but which may herald the onset of serious organic disease.

NONSPECIFIC GASTRITIS Gastritis is *common*, the reported incidence of the chronic variety starting at 28 percent in childhood and rising to 96 percent of the population past age sixty! It is usually asymptomatic, and its clinical significance therefore lies largely in its complications: bleeding, neoplasia, impaired digestion and nutrition (loss of acid, pepsin, and intrinsic factor). The cause seems evident in some patients but is as yet unproved in most. The disease is confined to the gastric mucosa and cannot be detected by standard x-ray techniques. *Multiple biopsy* is the only reliable diagnostic method although *gastroscopy alone* is also accurate in the acute and advanced atrophic varieties.

Acute gastritis Acute alcoholism, food poisoning, shock, certain drugs, acute illnesses, uremia, and heavy metal poisoning may be associated with acute gastritis. *Symptoms* include anorexia, nausea, vomiting, diffuse epigastric discomfort, fever, and in severe cases, the systemic fluid and electrolyte consequences of persistent vomiting. Brisk hemorrhage is common and in alcoholic patients often occurs suddenly, without prior gastric symptoms. Physical examination may reveal tenderness in the epigastrium or left upper part of the abdomen, the area often corresponding to the subcostal projection of the gastric silhouette. *Pathologically* there are inflammation and bleeding in the lamina propria, and surface denudation and exudation. The process lasts for hours to days but heals rapidly. Therefore, the diagnosis is missed if gastroscopy and biopsy are delayed until symptoms abate. *Treatment* of acute gastritis is supportive, since the process heals spontaneously. Bleeding, when present, generally is self-limited. Since increased back diffusion of hydrogen ions into the mucosa is believed to play a causative role, massive bleeders require acid neutralization. This may be achieved via intragastric drip of 1 mEq per ml sodium bicarbonate solution at a rate of 1,000 mEq per day (with care to avoid systemic alkalosis) or of milk, cream, and liquid nonabsorbable antacids. Often emergency operation is required, which is followed by recurrence in one-third or more patients unless vagotomy is added to the surgical procedure. The vagal effect is thought to lead to reduction in both acid secretion and mucosal blood flow.

Chronic gastritis The *cause* of chronic gastritis is unknown, but it occurs in association with carcinoma of the stomach, pernicious anemia, gastric polyps, gastric ulcer, duodenogastric reflux, all types of thyroid disease, sprue, chronic wasting diseases, pituitary or adrenal insufficiency, diabetes mellitus, Sjögren's syndrome, chronic iron deficiency, x-ray and surgical treatment of the stomach, chronic use of acetylsalicylic acid, and normal aging. Antibodies to the microsomal fraction of gastric parietal cells are found in 60 percent of patients with atrophic gastritis, 90 percent with pernicious anemia, 30 percent with thyroid disease, and 2 to 16 percent of the general population. Blocking or binding antibodies to gastric intrinsic factor in serum or gastric juice are not found in atrophic gastritis, but occur in virtually all patients with pernicious anemia (Chap. 305). These observations, limited experimental results in animals, and the clinical association of atrophic gastritis with so-called "autoimmune" diseases, such as thyroiditis, have led to the suggestion of an immunologic cause for atrophic gastritis. Alternatively, the antibody responses have been considered nonspecific reactions to mucosal damage of a variety of causes.

The pathology of chronic gastritis may be described in three categories: chronic superficial gastritis, chronic atrophic gastritis, and gastric atrophy. These may represent stages of progression of the same process. *Histologically*, one finds necrobiosis in the generative layer of the mucosa (the neck cells between the gastric pits and gastric tubules), chronic inflammatory cell infiltration, erosion of surface epithelium, loss of parietal and chief cells, epithelial cell abnormalities, proliferation of enterochromaffin cells, and metaplasia ("intestinalization"). These cellular changes convert the gastric mucosa from a secretory to an absorptive type, with concomitant changes in mucosal enzymes and gastric function. As atrophy progresses, mucosal lymphoid follicles and patchy areas of irregular hyperplasia develop. There may be two types of gastric atrophy. In one, there is antral sparing, increased "G"-cell mass of gastrin-producing cells, hypergastrinemia, and the presence of parietal cell antibodies; most patients with pernicious anemia belong to this group. The other has antral involvement, small "G"-cell mass, normogastrinemia, and rarely parietal cell antibodies or pernicious anemia. There may be other differences in the atrophy accompanying pernicious anemia, including differences in mucosal immunoglobulin types, delayed hypersensitivity, and perhaps in the incidence of cancer, blood group A, and response to steroid therapy (Chap. 305). *Gastroscopically* the mucosa appears normal or is reddened, granular, mammillated, and thinned, with patches of erosions and surface exudate. As atrophy advances, the mucosa becomes dull gray-blue and transparent and permits visualization of submucosal veins. Hyperplastic zones appear as excrescences of polyps. Follow-up of patients with atrophic gastritis for a decade or more revealed no change in two-thirds and regression or progression in the rest; adenocarcinoma developed in 10 percent.

Chronic gastritis is *asymptomatic*, but there may be intermittent or persistent vague complaints. These include constant mild nausea; anorexia; nausea on seeing or smelling food; sense of distention or pain on eating, which is related to the size of the meal; easy satiety; bad taste in the mouth, particularly before breakfast; vomiting after eating; and diffuse dull epigastric discomfort or burning. At times pain may be severe and radiate into the back; despite hypochlorhydria, it is often relieved by alkali. These symptoms are difficult to differentiate from those of functional dyspepsia and indeed may be caused by secondary alterations of gastric motor function. Findings on *physical examination* are negative, or there may be mild epigastric tenderness. Hemorrhage is uncommon, but occult bleeding may occur, leading to hypochromic microcytic anemia.

Laboratory features Since gastritis may be patchy, diagnosis depends on multiple "blind" *biopsies* or biopsy directed through the gastroscope. Gastroscopy alone is often misleading, except in the acute and advanced atrophic varieties. The laboratory findings include *anemia* from brisk or chronic blood loss, *occult blood* in the stool, and *impaired gastric secretion*, which is transient in acute gastritis but persistent and related to the stage of histologic change in chronic gastritis. *Hypochlorhydria* is the rule in early cases; true *achlorhydria* upon maximum pentagastrin, betazole, or histamine stimulation is found in complete gastric atrophy. Serum *gastrin* levels depend on the histopathologic changes in the antrum (see above). *Hypoalbuminemia* may follow leakage of proteins from the bloodstream into the stomach. Elevated levels of β-*glucuronidase* in gastric juice (see Gastric Carcinoma, above) and the appearance of certain *enzymes*, particularly alkaline phosphatase and leucine aminopeptidase, in biopsies or in abraded cytologic samples are diagnostic of metaplasia. In atrophy without pernicious anemia, small amounts of intrinsic factor continue to be secreted; vitamin B_{12} deficiency is therefore unusual.

Treatment Restoration of a normal histologic picture has been reported in atrophic gastritis treated with dexamethasone, 10 to 30 mg per day for 5 months, but atrophy may recur on cessation. Pain frequently responds to antacid gels and powders. In contrast, sipping of dilute (0.1*N*) hydrochloric acid with meals (1 to 2 tsp in a glass of fruit juice) may aggravate it severely! Other measures are those outlined above under Functional Dyspepsia, as well as frequent small feedings in place of large meals; correction of anemia, chronic sinusitis, and pyorrhea; and the use of mucosal "coating" agents such as bismuth subnitrate and bismuth subcarbonate powder and aluminum hydroxide gels. The dose of powder is 1 tsp with sufficient water to make a thick paste, and of gel, 1/2 oz. For demulcent usage these are prescribed every 2 to 4 hr and after every drink or snack which could remove them from the mucosa.

A mixture of a topical anesthetic agent with an alumina preparation (oxethazaine, 10 mg in 5 ml alumina, in dose of 1 to 2 tsp) may provide good symptomatic relief; the potential toxicity of the anesthetic limits the use of such mixtures to four daily doses. Finally, in view of the necrobiotic, atrophic, and inflammatory nature of the disease, cigarettes and irritants are often prohibited, or permitted only with simultaneous doses of alumina gels (Chap. 282).

BENIGN GIANT HYPERTROPHIC GASTRITIS This rare condition, also known as Ménétrier's disease, is characterized by marked hypertrophy of the gastric mucosa. It should not be confused with a cobblestone appearance of the mucosa occasionally found in normal or diseased stomachs and known by the obsolete gastroscopic term "hypertrophic gastritis," or with large gastric rugae, which occur normally and can be effaced by air insufflation during gastroscopy or by the examiner's finger during fluoroscopy.

Etiology, symptomatology, and pathophysiology are unclear. Mucosal hypertrophy, inflammation, metaplasia, thickening of the muscularis mucosa, and edema produce huge convoluted and interconnecting gastric rugae, pseudopolyps, and cystic dilatations extending into the submucosa. The condition may be diffuse or localized to the greater curvature. There may be ulcer-like symptoms or excessive mucus secretion and achlorhydria. Bleeding occurs in 40 percent. Some patients have *hypoproteinemia*, with edema and ascites secondary to massive leakage of serum proteins into the stomach, which occurs in over 70 percent of these cases (Chap. 284). Others have vomiting, diarrhea, and weight loss. Roentgenographically, the gastric hypertrophy may be confused with gastric neoplasms, particularly lymphoma. Diagnosis can be made only by full-thickness biopsy of the stomach. Treatment includes supportive measures, including replacement of albumin. Gastric resection is indicated for intractable symptoms, bleeding, or severe protein-losing gastropathy.

OTHER FORMS OF GASTRITIS Specific gastritis resulting from known physical, microbiologic, and infiltrative processes is rare.

Corrosive gastritis This follows ingestion of strong acids and, less often, strong alkalies or iron poisoning. It usually affects the cardia or pylorus but occasionally other parts of the stomach as well as the oropharynx and esophagus (Chap. 281). It may cause perforation or it may heal with scarring and obstruction. Such complications depend upon the concentration, duration of exposure, volume and type of dilution and neutralization, rapidity of vomiting, and delay before therapy. Treatment is expectant, with the stomach kept empty during the acute episode. Operation may be necessary for perforation or obstruction.

Phlegmonous and emphysematous gastritis These acute infections of the gastric wall are very rare in the United States. Bacteria gain entry through infarction, surgical manipulation, ulcerative disease, or through the bloodstream. These diseases constitute a serious threat to life and must be treated with parenteral fluid administration, vigorous specific antibiotic therapy based on the results of blood and gastric cultures, and good surgical principles of drainage and resection of focal abscesses. *Nonbacterial interstitial gastric emphysema*, following rupture of a pulmonary emphysematous bleb, pyloric obstruction with vomiting, instrumentation, or pneumatosis cystoides intestinalis (Chap. 289), causes similar radiologic findings but is a benign, self-limited condition.

Granulomas and infiltrations Under this heading are included sarcoidosis, eosinophilic granuloma (see Benign Tumors of the Stomach, above), berylliosis, pseudoxanthoma elasticum, and xanthomatosis. They rarely produce symptoms. When extensive, these lesions may ulcerate, interfere with gastric motor function, or be detected on x-ray examination, in which event the uncertainty in distinguishing them from cancer often leads to surgical resection.

Antral gastritis Antral gastritis, or periantritis, is a confusing condition. It produces antral deformity, often a lengthy segment of persistent concentric narrowing, which leads to a roentgenographic diagnosis of carcinoma (Fig. 283-2). Gastroscopy may show no abnormality or only partial restriction of motility and some pitting and reddening of the mucosa. Fibrosis or chronic inflammation of the antral wall is common, but mucosal gastritis is variable. The patient may be asymptomatic or exhibit atypical ulcer pain.

The process follows repeated ulceration in some cases. Obstruction is uncommon. Therefore each case requires careful investigation to avoid unnecessary surgery. Most helpful in differential diagnosis are the absence of consistency in the deformity on sequential spot films during radiography and the gastroscopic evidence of normal expansibility and nontumorous mucosa. When intramural neoplasm cannot be excluded, exploration is necessary.

MISCELLANEOUS CONDITIONS OF THE STOMACH

Hypertrophic pyloric stenosis A condition similar to congenital hypertrophic pyloric stenosis of infancy occurs in adults, but is rare. Uncritical interpretation of radiographs and surgical pathologic changes often inflate the statistics on incidence, however, and it is necessary to employ strict roentgenographic and pathologic criteria for this diagnosis, lest common lesions (e.g., antral gastritis and neuromuscular causes of gastric retention) be missed and inappropriate therapy be instituted.

Symptoms date from birth or appear at any age. Pathologically, there is true pyloric muscle hypertrophy and scarring. The clinical features are those of slowly progressive obstruction and gastric retention (Chap. 282).

FIGURE 283-2

Antral gastritis. Smooth, asymmetric, conical, narrowed deformity of the distal antrum. Modest variation in size and shape on other films argued against a diagnosis of infiltrating carcinoma. Gastroscopy demonstrated normal expansibility and hemorrhagic erosive gastritis. The roentgenographic appearance returned to normal over a 2-year period following treatment.

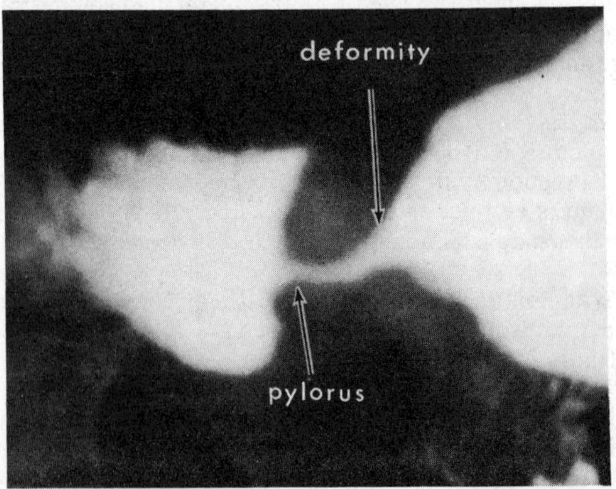

The characteristic olive-sized mass in neonatal patients is rare in adults. X-ray demonstrates persistent flexible elongation and narrowing of the pyloric segment and establishes the diagnosis. The Fredet-Ramstedt operation of pyloromyotomy is said to be less effective in adults than in infants, and limited gastric resection or pyloroplasty is the procedure of choice in the former. Rare *congenital pyloric* or *antral diaphragms* or *band* are also silent or lead to gastric retention; treatment is simple excision if gastric motility is normal.

Gastric retention (atonia and dilatation) The term *gastric retention* is preferable to pyloric obstruction, because failure of gastric motor function may be neuromuscular as well as secondary to relative obstruction or organic stenosis (Chap. 282) at the gastric outlet. There are numerous *neuromuscular* causes, many of which are uncommon, which produce only mild retention. These include anticholinergic drugs, vagotomy, diabetic autonomic neuropathy (Fig. 283-3), migraine, acute and chronic diseases of the central nervous system, spinal injury, the postoperative state, fluid and electrolyte disturbances, hypocalcemia, hypothyroidism, and poorly understood effects of acute illness, abdominal trauma, protein deficiency, debilitating diseases, extreme aging, body casts, overloading of starved stomach, and psychiatric disease.

Symptoms vary with the degree and rate of development of motor failure. If the diagnosis of retention is in doubt, it can be confirmed by the saline loading test: retention of more than 400 ml 30 min after instilling 750 ml isotonic saline solution into the fasting stomach is diagnostic. The clinical features and early treatment of hypotonia are similar to those of pyloric stenosis (Chap. 282) except that operation rarely is necessary. Most patients respond to gastric decompression for 3 to 5 days followed by a clear-fluid diet, which is gradually augmented every few days as tolerated to full fluids, soft foods, and finally solids. Motor stimulants such as methacholine in gradually increasing doses to tolerance, starting at 10 mg before meals, or metoclopramide (see Functional Dyspepsia, above) plus the noted modifications of diet consistency may suffice for initial therapy of mild retention in ambulatory patients.

Gastric torsion and volvulus Torsion, i.e., rotation of the stomach on its long axis (organoaxial) with the greater curvature rising anteriorly and superiorly to lie cephalad to the lesser curvature, is present on 0.5 percent of gastric x-ray examinations. Usually, it is asymptomatic. Rarely it causes twists at the cardia and pylorus or one twist in the midfundic region, which may be incomplete and recurrent or complete and disastrous. When complete it constitutes true volvulus, which produces acute obstruction and is a surgical emergency. Mesenterioaxial volvulus, or a combination of the two, may also occur. The cause is uncertain, but associated hernias, adhesions, lax ligaments, and anomalous spaces and mobility of stomach or duodenum frequently are blamed.

The recurrent variety frequently defies diagnostic analysis, since symptoms may be vague, variable, or intermittent. Retching which cannot yield vomitus, and relationships to eating, size of meal, and posture are

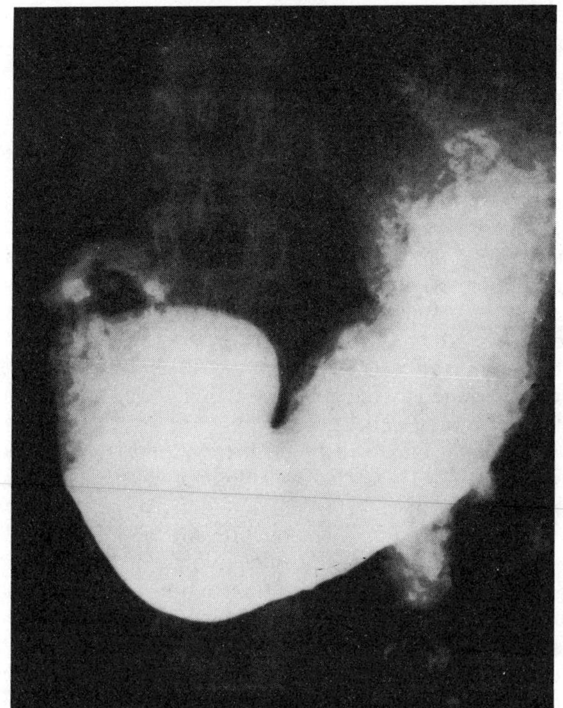

FIGURE 283-3
Gastric retention due to gastric hypotonia in a patient with diabetic autonomic neuropathy. The stomach is dilated moderately, peristaltic contractions are weak, and little barium has entered the duodenum. The mottled appearance is caused by dilution and flocculation of barium by retained gastric secretions.

significant clues. Inability to pass a gastric tube beyond the cardia during an attack is the crucial physical finding. Other features are those of gastric retention (Chap. 282). Patients learn to empty the sac with the aid of position and movement or the use of a nasogastric tube. Only when symptomatic cause and effect are demonstrable is surgical correction indicated in chronic volvulus.

Cardioesophageal laceration Exsanguination from laceration at the junction of esophagus and stomach is known as the Mallory-Weiss syndrome, and perforation with mediastinitis or peritonitis as the Boerhaave syndrome. Nonfatal lacerations occur and indeed are relatively common causes of gastrointestinal bleeding, accounting for 5 to 15 percent of massive gastrointestinal hemorrhage in modern series. A clue to the diagnosis is the time lag between severe retching without bleeding (presumably the cause of the laceration) and subsequent hematemesis. Rarer reported causes have been coughing, childbirth, straining at stool, chest trauma, convulsions, and accidental insufflation with compressed air. Most patients are alcoholics, and many have hiatus hernia. Diagnosis may be suspected by history, chest x-ray, extension of swallowed dye. Confirmation of the diagnosis can be made by selective arterial angiography, esophagogastroscopy, or laparotomy. Treatment of bleeding by gastroesophageal cooling or selective celiac arterial perfusion of epinephrine 10 to 20 μg per min for 20 min is highly effective. Reported use of gastric tamponade with the Sengstaken-Blakemore tube is sparse and ineffective. All patients with esophageal perforation urgently require operation.

Gastric diverticula These are uncommon, almost always congenital, and situated posteromedially near the cardia. Very rarely, acquired traction or pulsion diverticula may be found anywhere in the stomach. Virtually all diverticula are asymptomatic and require no treatment, but small ones may be mistaken for ulcers on x-ray examination. Some, such as those in paraesophageal hiatus hernia, produce mild complaints and may be relieved by postural maneuvers. Only when a symptomatic cause-and-effect relationship is objectively demonstrable can a rational case be made for surgical removal. In rare instances hemorrhage and perforation may occur.

Hourglass deformity Midgastric narrowing may appear to be rigid on roentgenographic examination, the general outline of the stomach vaguely resembling the shape of an hourglass. The most common cause is disordered gastric motor function adjacent to a gastric ulcer with a segment of tonic contraction forming an incisura on the contralateral curvature, which seems to point at the ulcer. Occasionally, this persists after the ulcer heals. Rarely, disease in the stomach wall, e.g., infiltrating carcinoma, scarring after corrosive gastritis, or gastric syphilis, produces a similar configuration.

Foreign bodies and bezoars A wide variety of foreign objects may be found in the stomach, but all are rare except in certain groups with specific predilections—psychotics, pregnant women with *pica, clay and laundry starch eaters* in the southern and western United States, and malingering prison inmates. Some occur *occupationally* without the patient's knowledge, e.g., the upholsterer who swallows a tack. Others follow *gastric hypotonia* or *gastric surgery* after which gastric mucus, ingested food, medicines, or diagnostic agents such as barium sulfate are not passed. *Gastroconiosis*, i.e., foreign-body granulomas in the mucosa, follows long-continued ingestion of particulate matter, e.g., chalk, kaolin, or silica. Clay and starch, taken as cultural habit or folklore medicine, bind iron, prevent its absorption, and produce iron-deficiency anemia. *Dirt* and *asphalt* may be eaten, and alcoholics who take to drinking alcoholic solutions of *resins* may retain resinous masses. Anyone may accidentally swallow a fragment of bone in a bolus of meat, and children ingest a variety of small objects such as coins and marbles.

An interesting group of foreign bodies are the *bezoars*, balls of hair (trichobezoar), plant fibers (phytobezoar), or mixtures of hair and fiber. In the United States, human hair ingestion and unripe persimmon eating (diospyrobezoar) are the leading causes of bezoar formation. Only the unripe fruit contains the phlobatannin, shibuol, which is converted by gastric acid to an insoluble coagulum.

Most foreign bodies are asymptomatic or pass through the intestinal tract without incident, but complications may occur. Sharp objects may perforate, produce localized abscesses, or migrate through the peritoneum, abdominal viscera, or parietal structures. Bezoars and blunt objects may lie freely in the lumen for long periods or become embedded and cause gastric retention, erosion, ulcerations, and bleeding. Some cause intestinal obstruction and perforation after leaving the stomach.

Diagnosis begins with a history of ingestion or the detection of a mass on roentgenographic examination. Gastroscopy usually establishes the nature of the mass. Once an object has reached the stomach, there is 90 percent likelihood that it will pass through the gastrointestinal tract; *treatment* is therefore expectant. If the mass fails to leave the stomach, or progression ceases after the pylorus is passed, or complications of bleeding, obstruction, or penetration occur, surgical intervention is indicated. With gelatinous and plastic masses, cessation of oral intake of the material, lavage, and restoration of gastric motility (see Atonia, above) often lead to breakup and passage. Bezoars can be torn apart by gastroscopic biopsy forceps. Phytobezoars have disappeared after administration of cellulase, 225 mg per day, and diospyrobezoars have responded to 0.5 g papain with 1 g sodium bicarbonate in 120 ml water, q.i.d., orally or by lavage.

REFERENCES

AVERY JF, GUMMER JWP: *Clinical Gastroenterology*, 2d ed., Oxford: Blackwell Scientific Publications, Ltd., 1968

EDWARDS FC, COGHILL NF: Clinical manifestations in patients with chronic atrophic gastritis, gastric ulcer and duodenal ulcer. Quart J Med 37:337, 1968

GOLDBERG LS, FUDENBERG HH: The autoimmune aspects of pernicious anemia. Am J Med 46:489, 1969

JARNUM S, BIRGER JK: Plasma protein turnover in Ménétrier's disease (giant hypertrophic gastritis): Evidence of non-selective protein loss. Gut 13:128, 1972

KAUFMAN S: Current concepts: 5-Fluorouracil in the treatment of gastrointestinal neoplasia. N Engl J Med 288:199, 1973

MILLER NE: Learning of visceral and glandular responses. Science 163:434, 1969

MORRISSEY JF: Gastrointestinal endoscopy (includes biopsy and cytology). Gastroenterology 62:1241, 1972

SHERLOCK P et al: Treatment of gastrointestinal cancer: Current status and recent progress. Gastroenterology 53:630, 1967

TANNER NC: Chronic and recurrent volvulus of the stomach: with late results of "colonic displacement." Am J Surg 115:505, 1968

WELLS RF: A common cause of upper gastrointestinal bleeding: The Mallory-Weiss syndrome. South Med J 60:1197, 1967

284
DISORDERS OF ABSORPTION

NORTON J. GREENBERGER
KURT J. ISSELBACHER

MECHANISMS OF ABSORPTION

Diseases of the small intestine are frequently accompanied by alterations in intestinal function, and clinically this impaired function is seen as the malabsorption syndrome. In order to obtain a better appreciation of the derangements which occur in the many disorders of intestinal function the processes of normal absorption will first be reviewed.

It is important to distinguish between digestion and absorption, since an increased loss of nutrients in the stool may be a reflection of a derangement of either process. Digestion involves the breakdown or hydrolysis of nutrients to smaller molecules in order to prepare the ingested substances for absorption, or transport across the intestinal cell. It will be recalled that most of the digestive process is initiated in the stomach by acid and pepsin and is continued in the upper small intestine primarily by the action of pancreatic enzymes such as lipase, amylase, and trypsin. As a result of these digestive actions carbohydrates are broken down to monosaccharides and disaccharides, proteins to peptides and amino acids, and fats to monoglycerides and fatty acids. In the adult it is in this form that nutrients are, to a large extent, transported across the epithelial surface of the intestinal cell.

Anatomic and physiologic factors

The intestine has an enormous surface area. This can be attributed in large part to its length, which in the adult is more than 12 ft, and to the foldings of the surface plicae. At the light microscopic level, the villi of the small intestine provide additional surface area, which is further augmented by the presence of microvilli (approximately 2×10^8 per cm^2) on the outer, or brush border, region of epithelial cells. Thus the total absorptive area of the small intestine is enormous.

Motility (contractility) of the bowel is an important process which permits nutrients to remain in intimate contact with the intestinal cells and possibly influences the continued movement of the nutrients *into* and along the absorbing channels, such as the lymphatics. Two types of motility aid in this process: the gross motility of the intestine itself and the motility of individual villi. Entrance of the nutrients into the general circulation is achieved via the capillaries into the portal system or via the lacteals into the intestinal lymphatics.

Types of absorption

Four mechanisms have been considered to be important in the transport of substances across the intestinal cell membrane, namely, active transport, passive diffusion, facilitated diffusion, and pinocytosis (Table 284-1).

Active transport involves the transport of a substance across the cell against an electric or chemical gradient; this process requires energy, is carrier-mediated, and is

TABLE 284-1
Mechanisms of transport across the intestinal cell

Types of transport	Properties: Energy-dependent	Carrier-mediated	Competitive inhibition	Electric or chemical gradient
Active	+	+	+	+
Diffusion:				
Passive	0	0	0	0
Facilitated	0	+	+/0	0
Pinocytosis	0	0	0	0

subject to competitive inhibition. *Passive diffusion* is the opposite of this process; energy is not required, transport is with (rather than against) the electric or chemical gradient, the process is not carrier-mediated, and it does not show properties of competitive inhibition. Thus active transport may be viewed as "uphill" transport, whereas passive diffusion is equivalent to "downhill" transport. *Facilitated diffusion* is similar to passive diffusion except that such a process shows evidence of being carrier-mediated and frequently subject to competitive inhibition.

Pinocytosis, which literally means "cells drinking," is a process akin to phagocytosis. By this mechanism nutrients (soluble or particulate) upon entering the cell are surrounded by the components of the outer plasma cell membrane. In the intestinal tract pinocytosis has been definitely demonstrated only in the neonatal period, and the quantitative significance of this process in the adult organism seems to be limited.

It should also be emphasized that not every substance presented to the intestinal surface is subject to transport or absorption, because the normal epithelial cell is able to exclude many substances. Generally water-soluble compounds with a high molecular weight (above 300) or with pK less than 4 or greater than 9, especially polyvalent ions, tend not to be absorbed. When the mucosa is damaged, as for example by mesenteric vascular disease, the ability to exclude substances may be lost, and compounds of high molecular weight may be absorbed.

Sites of absorption

While many substances are absorbed throughout the length of the small intestine, certain nutrients tend to be absorbed in one region more than the others. The proximal intestine is a major area for the absorption of iron, calcium, water-soluble vitamins, and fat (monoglycerides and fatty acids). Sugars are absorbed in the proximal small intestine and also in midintestine. While the major absorption of amino acids appears to occur in the middle of the small intestine or jejunum, some absorption also occurs in the upper and lower areas. The distal small intestine appears to be the *major* absorptive area for bile salts and vitamin B_{12}. As is emphasized below, this factor is of clinical significance in circumstances where there has been removal or disease of the ileum.

The colon is important for the absorption of water and electrolytes, a process which occurs predominantly in the cecum. Although the rectum is not a usual site for absorption of ingested foodstuffs, drugs introduced by rectum may be absorbed there. Thus drugs introduced by this route, such as salicylates or steroids, may be absorbed systemically.

Absorption of specific nutrients

CARBOHYDRATE ABSORPTION Much of the carbohydrate we ingest is in the form of starch, a complex polysaccharide consisting of many hexose units (attached either in a 1,4 or 1,6 linkage). By the action of salivary and pancreatic amylase, starch is hydrolyzed to oligosaccharides, then to dissacharides (mostly maltose), and a small amount to monosaccharides. While monosaccharides such as glucose are readily absorbed, disaccharides are not. Disaccharides are split enzymatically into their component sugars by enzymes located on or within the microvilli of the intestinal epithelial cells. By the action of these *disaccharidases*, lactose is split into glucose and galactose, sucrose into glucose and fructose, and maltose into two molecules of glucose. The resultant monosaccharides are then transported through the cell into the portal circulation.

Sugars such as glucose and galactose are absorbed by an active transport mechanism. Most actively transported sugars possess a hydroxyl group at the C-2 position. Fructose, a hexose lacking a hydroxyl group at the C-2 position, is absorbed by passive diffusion, and after its entry there is also some conversion of fructose to glucose and lactic acid within the mucosal cell. The transport of xylose, a pentose frequently used in absorption studies, is complex. At low concentrations xylose transport is active; at higher concentrations some is by facilitated diffusion.

The exact mechanism for the active transport of sugars such as glucose and galactose has not been elucidated. However, *sodium* ions appear necessary for the *entry* of the sugar into the cell, and *energy* is required for the *accumulation* of the sugars within the cell. Glucose and galactose presumably are transported by a carrier-mediated mechanism, but the nature of this carrier remains to be determined.

PROTEIN AND AMINO ACID ABSORPTION Dietary proteins are initially subject to degradation in the stomach by pepsin. However, complete hydrolysis is largely achieved by the action of the pancreatic enzymes trypsin, chymotrypsin, and carboxypeptidase. By these enzymatic processes polypeptides, dipeptides, and amino acids are formed. Just as there are disaccharidases in mucosal cells to digest disaccharides, there are also dipeptidases to split dipeptides. Dipeptidases are located in the cytoplasm as well as on the microvilli. Dipeptides are absorbed more rapidly than amino acids and presumably their uptake involves a separate mechanism. Contrary to earlier beliefs proteins can also be absorbed by the adult intestine. Although quantitatively limited, protein absorption probably is immunologically significant.

Most naturally occurring amino acids are L-amino acids, and these are subject to a number of different transport processes. *Neutral* amino acids seem to share a common "pump," or pathway; thus amino acids such as tryptophan and alanine show competitive inhibition. Among the *basic* amino acids which appear to have a distinct transport mechanism are arginine, ornithine, lysine, and cystine. There is also a separate transport system for the *imino* acids proline and hydroxyproline. Therefore, in genetic disorders, such as cystinuria, one will find impaired absorption not only of cystine but also of arginine, ornithine, and lysine. Similarly in Hartnup disease, a defect in the transport of neutral amino acids (especially of tryptophan, phenylalanine, histidine) is found. In these genetic disorders uptake and absorption of dipeptides is normal.

The actual mechanism of the absorption of amino acids by the intestine has not been elucidated. As in the case of carbohydrates, sodium ions appear to be required for entry, and energy for concentration within the cell. Since pyridoxine deficiency interferes with the transport of amino acids, pyridoxine may be involved in amino acid transport, but its exact role is not understood.

FAT ABSORPTION (Fig. 284-1) Most of the ingested dietary fats are in the form of long-chain triglycerides. These triglycerides contain both saturated fatty acids (such as palmitic and stearic) and unsaturated fatty acids (such as oleic and linoleic). The particle size of the fat is decreased largely by the churning action of the stomach. The entry of fat into the duodenum plus the presence of acid causes release of secretin and pancreozymin-cholecystokinin, which in turn leads to a stimulation of the flow of bile and pancreatic juice.

Role of pancreatic lipase For the hydrolysis of triglycerides by pancreatic lipase, the fats must be emulsified. The detergent properties of the bile salts permit the enzyme to gain access to the water-insoluble lipids. The enzymatic action of lipase results in the stepwise hydrolysis to diglycerides, monoglycerides, and fatty acids with the concomitant liberation of glycerol. Normally only 25 to 30 percent of the triglyceride is completely hydrolyzed to fatty acids. Monoglycerides constitute the major end product of hydrolysis (i.e., 70 to 75 percent of the ingested fat). Usually less than 5 percent of the fat remains in the form of diglycerides or triglycerides.

Role of bile salts (Fig. 284-2) Bile salts play an important role in the digestion and absorption of fat. They are synthesized in the liver (approximately 200 to 600 mg daily) from cholesterol and excreted in the bile in the form of their glycine or taurine conjugates. In man the principal bile acids excreted are the conjugates of cholic and chenodeoxycholic acid. Bile salts are good detergents, because they have both polar (hydrophilic) and nonpolar (hydrophobic) groups. During digestion the concentration of conjugated bile salts in the lumen is in the range of 5 to 15 micromoles per ml, and at these concentrations the bile salts aggregate to form *micelles*. Fatty acids and monoglycerides enter these micelles, forming mixed micelles. An emulsion of triglyceride is turbid; mixed micelles containing bile salts, fatty acids, and monoglycerides are clear solutions. The formation of *mixed micelles* and hence the solubilization of fatty acids and monoglycerides is much more effectively achieved with *conjugated bile salts* at the pH which normally exists in the intestinal lumen (Fig. 284-2).

There are additional properties of bile salts important in fat absorption and digestion. Bile salts shift the pH optimum of pancreatic lipase from 8.5 to 6.5. This is important because the pH in the upper small intestine is normally 6 to 6.5. Most conjugated bile salts are absorbed in the ileum and after entering the portal vein are subject to an enterohepatic circulation. By this process about 90 percent of the conjugated bile salts reaching the ileum are reabsorbed. As a consequence only about 200 to 600 mg bile salts is excreted in the feces per day, while, as part of the enterohepatic circulation, as much as 20 to 30 g bile salts recirculates daily between the liver and intestine. If the ileum is diseased or removed, absorption of bile salts is impaired, and a significant fecal loss of bile salts will occur. As a consequence of this bile salt depletion, the concentration of bile salts in the intestinal lumen will also

FIGURE 284-1
Scheme of intestinal digestion, absorption, esterification, and transport of dietary triglycerides. TG, triglycerides; FA, fatty acids; MG, monoglyceride; BS, bile salts.

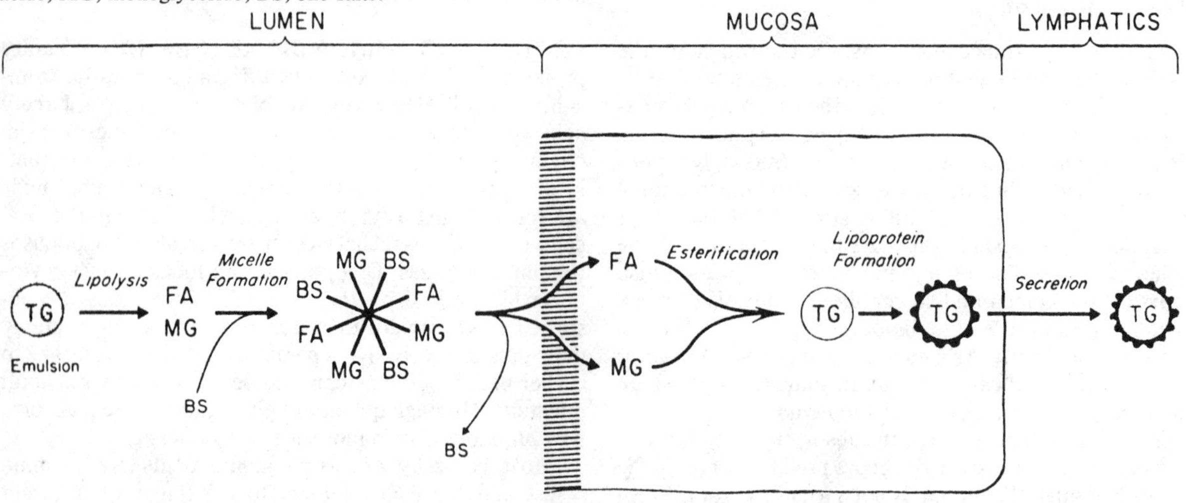

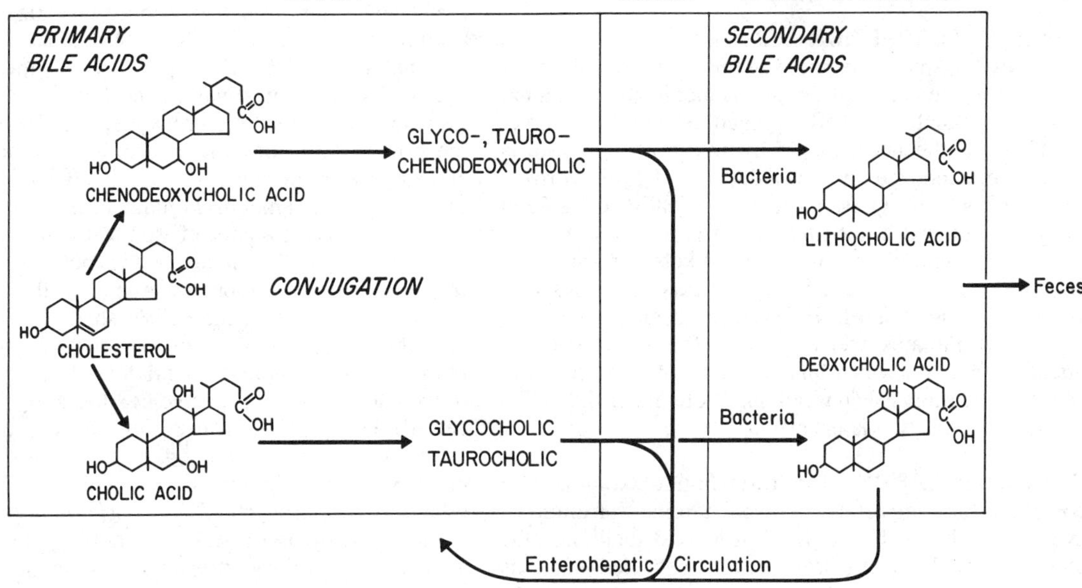

FIGURE 284-2

Scheme of hepatic and intestinal metabolism of bile salts and the enterohepatic circulation (from ileum to liver). Note that bacteria lead to the formation of secondary bile acids; of the latter, only deoxycholic acid is absorbed to any appreciable extent.

decrease, leading to further impairment of fat absorption. A similar result will occur if bile salt reabsorption is prevented by chelating agents, such as cholestyramine (see below).

Intramucosal aspects of fat absorption (Fig. 284-1) After the hydrolysis of fatty acids to monoglycerides and their interaction with bile salts to form mixed micelles, the lipids pass through an "unstirred" water layer covering the cell surface. The mixed micelles apparently do not enter the cell, but instead the component fatty acids and monoglycerides are released from the micellar phase and then enter the cell by diffusion. Upon entry fatty acids may interact with specific binding proteins. The subsequent fate of the intracellular lipid is strongly influenced by the fatty acid chain length. Fatty acids and monoglycerides derived from long-chain triglycerides (i.e., containing C-16 to C-18 fatty acids) are promptly *reesterified to triglycerides* by enzymes of the endoplasmic reticulum. These triglycerides then interact with specific apolipoproteins plus cholesterol and phospholipid leading to the formation of chylomicrons and very low density lipoproteins. These initially accumulate in the Golgi region of the cell and then are secreted into the lacteals and the intestinal lymph. There are thus four major steps in the absorption of long-chain fatty acids and monoglycerides: (1) mucosal uptake and interaction with binding proteins, (2) reesterification to triglycerides, (3) lipoprotein formation, and (4) secretion into lymph.

By contrast, fatty acids derived from medium-chain triglycerides (i.e., containing C-8 and C-10 fatty acids) are *not reesterified* to any significant extent within the cell and are not incorporated into lipoproteins. Instead, they rapidly enter the portal venous system, where they are transported as fatty acids bound to albumin. The major aspects of fat absorption are summarized in Fig. 284-1.

ABSORPTION OF CHOLESTEROL AND FAT-SOLUBLE VITAMINS (A, D, E, K) In addition to contributing significantly to the total body synthesis of cholesterol, the intestine also plays an active role in the absorption of cholesterol and its esters. Within the lumen, cholesterol esters from the bile and diet are hydrolyzed by a pancreatic esterase. There is also a separate cholesterol esterase in the intestinal microvilli, which completes this hydrolysis. As a result only free cholesterol appears to enter the intestinal cell. However, just as in the case of long-chain fatty acids, much of the cholesterol is reesterified and is then secreted primarily into lymph.

The absorption mechanisms of the fat-soluble vitamins A, D, E, and K are not well understood. The intestine is able to convert beta-carotene into vitamin A. The vitamin A thus formed or absorbed from the lumen is esterified in the mucosa primarily with palmitic acid, transported in the chylomicrons of the lymph, and stored as retinyl palmitate in the liver. The other lipid-soluble vitamins also appear in lymph chylomicrons, but esterification with fatty acids does not appear to be necessary for their transport.

WATER AND SODIUM ABSORPTION In spite of extensive investigations the main mechanisms of water and electrolyte transport are not well understood. To explain water movement across the lipid membrane of the mucosa, it is believed that this surface has aqueous-filled channels or pores. These allow diffusion of water as well as bulk flow; the latter refers to water movement in response to osmotic pressure differences. The largest fraction of net water movement appears to be the result of bulk flow.

Sodium ions are absorbed largely by active transport and are linked in some manner to the brush border ATPase. Sodium movement is also linked to the transport or metabolism of glucose; sodium transport usually ceases in the absence of glucose. Some sodium transport accompanies the movement of water (i.e., solvent drag).

CALCIUM ABSORPTION Calcium is actively transported by the small intestine, and this process is intimately linked to the action of vitamin D metabolites. Vitamin D_3 or cholecalciferol is hydroxylated to 25-hydroxycholecalciferol in the liver; the 25-hydroxycholecalciferol is further metabolized in the kidney to 1,25-dihydroxycalciferol, which represents the biologically active form of cholecalciferol in the intestine. The impaired absorption of calcium found in renal rickets, uremia, and anephric man may be due to decreased synthesis of vitamin D metabolites. It has also been shown that vitamin D initiates the synthesis of a protein in the intestinal mucosa which binds calcium, but the relationship between this calcium-binding protein and the active transport of calcium is uncertain.

IRON ABSORPTION The formation of soluble iron complexes is important for maintaining intraluminal iron in an absorbable form. Gastric acid facilitates the chelation of inorganic iron with substances such as ascorbic acid, sugars, amino acids, and bile; these macromolecular complexes then remain soluble in the more alkaline duodenum and jejunum. A regulatory mechanism for the absorption of inorganic iron appears to exist within the small-intestinal mucosal cells. Iron is actively transported by the small intestine, and the duodenum is the principal site of iron absorption. The absorption of elemental iron in man and animals involves at least two distinct steps: (1) mucosal uptake of iron from the lumen and (2) mucosal transfer of iron to the plasma. Much of the iron entering the mucosal cell is not transferred to the plasma but remains trapped within the cell and is excreted into the lumen when the cell is shed. Iron lost by this mechanism seems to vary inversely with body iron stores. However, this mucosal regulatory mechanism can be overcome when pharmacologic doses of iron are ingested. Hemoglobin iron is also absorbed by human subjects depending upon body requirements for iron; the heme is split from globin in the lumen and absorbed as an intact metalloporphyrin. The absorption of inorganic iron is increased by ascorbic acid. Similarly, the presence of anemia, liver injury, pregnancy, idiopathic hemochro-

TABLE 284-2
Tests useful in the diagnosis of malabsorptive disorders

		Typical findings in		
Test	*Normal values*	*Malabsorption (nontropical sprue)*	*Maldigestion (pancreatic insufficiency)*	*Comment*
Quantitative determination of stool fat	< 6 g/24 hr; > 95% coefficient of fat absorption	> 6 g/24 hr	> 6 g/24 hr	Best test for establishing presence of steatorrhea
D-Xylose absorption (25-g oral dose)	5-hr urinary excretion > 4.5 g; peak blood level > 30 mg/100 ml	↓	Normal	A good screening test for carbohydrate absorption
Small-intestinal x-rays		Malabsorption pattern	Normal or minimal malabsorption pattern; occasionally pancreatic calcification	Moulage sign and other abnormalities may be present in several disorders (see text)
Small-intestinal mucosal biopsy		Abnormal	Normal	A specific diagnosis can be established in a small number of disorders (see text)
Schilling test for vitamin B_{12} absorption	> 8% urinary excretion in 48 hr	Frequently ↓	Usually normal	Useful in determining whether vitamin B_{12} malabsorption is due to gastric or small-intestinal disorders
Secretin test	Volume: > 1.8 ml/kg/hr—bicarbonate concentration: > 80 mEq/l	Normal	Abnormal	See discussion of pancreatic insufficiency in Chap. 301
Serum calcium	9–11 mg/100 ml	Frequently ↓	Usually normal	
Serum albumin	3.5–5.5 g/100 ml	Frequently ↓	Usually normal	Decreased levels of both serum albumin and globulins should raise the question of protein-losing enteropathy
Serum cholesterol	150–250 mg/100 ml	↓	Frequently ↓	Usually decreased in disorders associated with significant steatorrhea
Serum iron	80–150 μg/100 ml	Frequently ↓	Normal	Low values may reflect decreased body iron stores
Serum carotenes	> 100 IU/100 ml	↓	Usually ↓	Fairly satisfactory screening tests for malabsorption
Serum vitamin A	> 100 IU/100 ml	↓		

matosis, or a portacaval shunt may result in increased iron absorption. Conversely, the prior ingestion of large doses of iron and the presence in the lumen of phosphates, carbonates, and phytates may lead to decreased absorption of inorganic iron. Impaired absorption of iron is frequent in disorders (such as nontropical sprue) which involve the duodenal mucosa.

WATER-SOLUBLE VITAMINS The absorption of *vitamin B_{12}* is discussed in Chap. 305. In the case of *folic acid absorption*, it must be emphasized that folates exist in food conjugated with glutamyl peptides. These *polyglutamates* must be deconjugated (by folic deconjugase) to monoglutamates for absorption to occur. Certain drugs such as diphenylhydantoin inhibit this conjugase, decrease the absorption of dietary polyglutamates, and hence can cause folate deficiency. Thiamine and riboflavin appear to be absorbed by passive diffusion.

Tests useful in the diagnosis of malabsorption

Most of the tests useful in the diagnosis of malabsorption indicate the presence of abnormal absorptive or digestive function, and only a few tests may suggest a specific diagnosis. Accordingly, it is frequently necessary to employ a combination of tests to establish a diagnosis. To illustrate the use of various tests, the characteristic findings in nontropical sprue, an example of a primary malabsorptive disorder, and pancreatic insufficiency, an example of impaired digestion, are compared in Table 284-2.

STOOL FAT The qualitative examination of the stool for undigested muscle fibers, neutral fat, and split fat is a simple and reliable screening test for steatorrhea. The finding of an increased number of muscle fibers indicates impaired intraluminal digestion. Properly performed, the qualitative microscopic examination of a stool specimen with the Sudan III stain is of value and correlates well with the quantitative determination of fecal fat by the Van de Kamer method. The latter remains the most reliable measurement of steatorrhea. A normal fecal fat

TABLE 284-2 (*continued*)

		Typical findings in		
Test	*Normal values*	*Malabsorption (nontropical sprue)*	*Maldigestion (pancreatic insufficiency)*	*Comment*
Prothrombin time	70–100%; 12–15 sec	Frequently	Frequently ↓	
Urine 5-hydroxyindoleacetic acid (5-HIAA)	2–9 mg/24 hr	↑	Normal	Slightly increased level (12–16 mg/24 hr) characteristically found in nontropical sprue
Urine indican	< 100 mg /24 hr	↑	Normal or ↑	Increased values found in several malabsorptive disorders as well as in bacterial overgrowth syndromes
Duodenal fluid analysis				
a Conjugated bile salts	> 2mmol/ml	Normal	Normal	May be decreased with bacterial overgrowth, ileal resection or ileal inflammatory disease
b Unconjugated bile salts	Not present	Normal	Normal	Increased with bacterial overgrowth
c Micellar lipid	> 50% ingested lipid in micellar phase	Normal or decreased	Decreased	Decreased with a deficiency of conjugated bile salts or pancreatic lipase
d Bacteria (culture)	< 10^3 organisms/ml	Normal	Normal	> 10^5 organisms/ml indicate bacterial overgrowth
Glycocholic acid metabolism (oral glycine-1-^{14}C glycocholate)*	< 1% of dose excreted as $^{14}CO_2$ in 4 hr	Normal	Normal	Increased $^{14}CO_2$ excretion with bacterial overgrowth or bile acid malabsorption (due to ileal resection or inflammatory disease)
	< 4% of dose excreted in stools			Increased fecal excretion of ^{14}C in bile acid malabsorption

* *For details of procedure, see H Fromm and AF Hofmann,* Lancet, *2:621, 1971.*

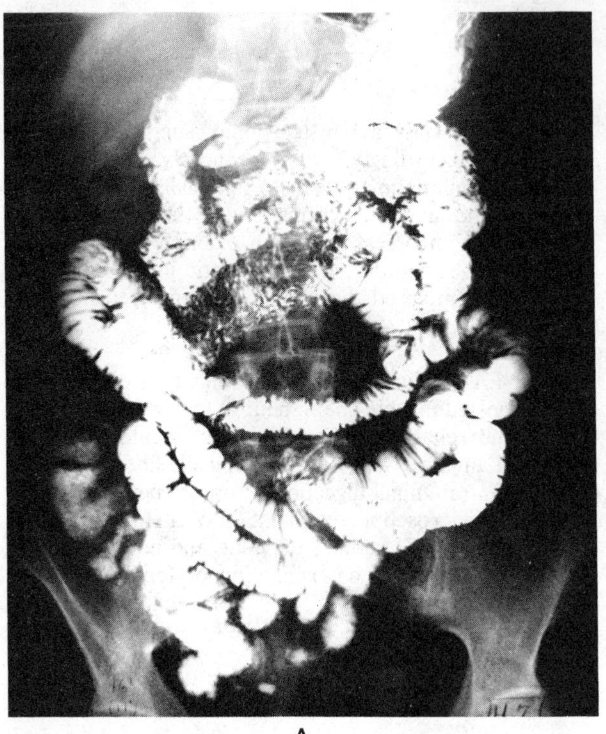

A

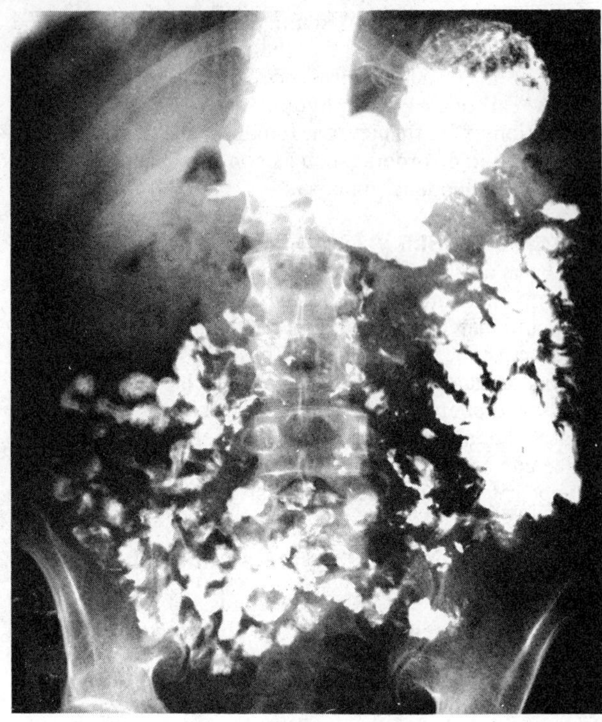

B

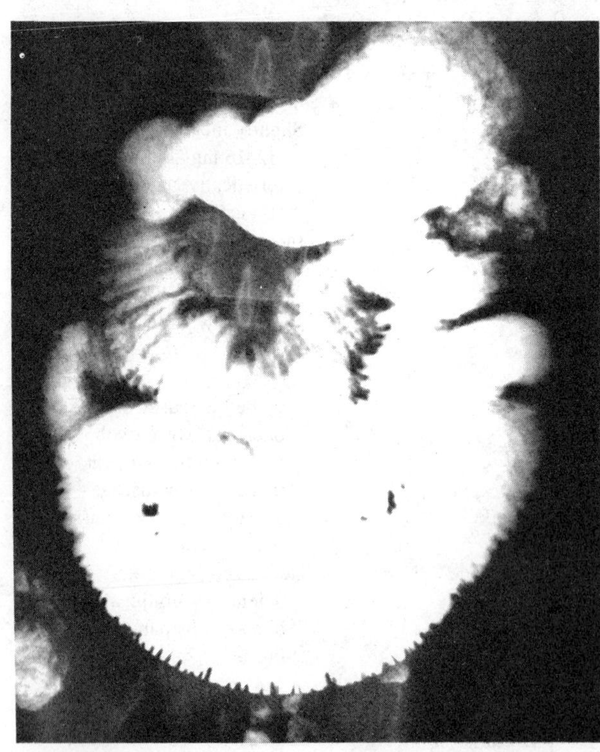

C

FIGURE 284-3
A *X-ray of a normal small intestine showing good mucosal pattern.* B *Intestinal x-ray of a patient with nontropical sprue. Note dilatation of small bowel, lack of mucosal markings, and segmentation and clumping of barium.* C *Intestinal x-rays of patient with obstructed lymphatics due to Kohlmeier-Degos disease. Note "accordion-pleated" pattern at lower edge of film.*

excretion is less than 6 g for 24 hr, or less than 5 percent of ingested fat.

XYLOSE ABSORPTION In the most commonly employed form of the xylose absorption test, the patient ingests 25 g D-xylose. A 5-hr urine xylose excretion of 4.5 g or greater is considered normal. There is some decreased renal excretion with age, and over age sixty-five 3.5 g is the normal value. Falsely low values may be obtained in patients with ascites, intestinal bacterial overgrowth, or renal insufficiency, after administration of certain drugs (e.g., acetylsalicylic acid, indomethacin), and most commonly if the urine collection is incomplete. To obviate difficulties in interpreting the test, it is advisable to determine the blood xylose level 2 hr after ingestion of xylose. A blood xylose level of 30 mg per 100 ml or greater indicates normal absorption of D-xylose. An abnormal D-xylose absorption test is found most frequently in disorders affecting the mucosa of the proximal small intestine, such as nontropical and tropical sprue.

GASTROINTESTINAL X-RAY STUDIES All patients with malabsorption should have radiographic examinations of the small intestine and, in many cases, of the esophagus, stomach, and colon as well. Occasionally, the latter two examinations may provide important clues to the presence of such disorders as gastroileostomy, scleroderma, Zollinger-Ellison syndrome, ulcerative colitis, and intestinal fistulas. The typical small-bowel radiographic abnormalities in patients with a malabsorption syndrome are a breaking up of the barium column with segmentation, clumping, and coarsening of the mucosal folds. Segmentation or clumping of the barium in a small-bowel loop is often termed a *moulage sign.* Less frequently there is dilatation of the proximal small bowel and loss of a normal mucosal pattern. Collectively, these changes have been referred to as a *malabsorption pattern.* These findings are nonspecific and may be found in several of the disorders listed in Table 284-3. Some representative examples of abnormal small-bowel radiographs are shown in Fig. 284-3.

SMALL-INTESTINAL BIOPSY The most commonly used instruments for obtaining peroral biopsy specimens from the small intestine include the Rubin and Shiner tubes, and the Crosby, Carey, and Ross-Moore capsules. Examination of small-bowel biopsy specimens has proved to be of considerable value in the differential diagnosis of malabsorptive disorders. Table 284-3 lists disorders associated with abnormalities in intestinal biopsies and Fig. 284-4 depicts some illustrative lesions.

SCHILLING TEST FOR VITAMIN B_{12} ABSORPTION The Schilling test is valuable in the differential diagnosis of malabsorption and is frequently carried out in three stages: (1) without intrinsic factor, (2) with intrinsic factor, and (3) after a course of treatment with antibiotics. Since vitamin B_{12} is absorbed primarily in the distal ileum, an abnormal Schilling test may indicate a pathologic condition of the distal small bowel. In disorders affecting the terminal ileum such as regional enteritis and lymphomas, the first-stage Schilling test is frequently abnormal. The ileal receptor site appears to be damaged in these disorders, and the impaired absorption of B_{12} is not corrected by the addition of intrinsic factor or the use of antibiotics. The Schilling test may also be useful in establishing a diagnosis of abnormal bacterial overgrowth of the small bowel which may be present in disorders such as blind loop syndrome, scleroderma, and multiple small bowel diverticula (Table 284-3). In the blind loop syndrome, for example, the bacteria can actually take up vitamin B_{12} with resultant impaired absorption of B_{12}. Under these conditions the first-stage Schilling test is frequently abnormal. After appropriate antibiotic treatment the Schilling test usually returns to normal.

TABLE 284-3
Disorders associated with abnormalities in small-bowel biopsy specimens

A Disorders in which biopsy is of diagnostic value
- *1* Celiac sprue: shortened or absent villi; hypertrophied crypts; damaged surface epithelium; mononuclear infiltrate
- *2* Whipple's disease: lamina propria infiltrated with macrophages containing PAS-positive glycoproteins
- *3* Abetalipoproteinemia: villus structure normal; epithelial cells vacuolated due to excess fat
- *4* Agammaglobulinemia: flattened or absent villi; increased lymphocyte infiltration; absence of plasma cells

B Disorders in which biopsy may be of diagnostic value
- *1* Intestinal lymphoma: infiltration of lamina propria and submucosa with malignant cells
- *2* Intestinal lymphangiectasia: dilated lacteals and lymphatics in lamina propria; clubbed villi
- *3* Eosinophilic enteritis: diffuse or patchy eosinophilic infiltration in lamina propria and mucosa
- *4* Amyloidosis: presence of amyloid confirmed by special stains
- *5* Regional enteritis: noncaseating granulomas
- *6* Parasitic infestations: parasitic invasion of mucosa; adherence of trophozoites to mucosal surface
- *7* Systemic mastocytosis: mast cell infiltration of lamina propria

C Disorders in which biopsy may be abnormal but not diagnostic
- *1* Tropical sprue: lesion similar to celiac sprue with shortened or absent villi; lymphocyte infiltration
- *2* Folate deficiency: shortened villi; megalocytosis; decreased mitoses in crypts
- *3* Vitamin B_{12} deficiency: similar to folate deficiency
- *4* Acute radiation enteritis: similar to folate deficiency
- *5* Systemic scleroderma: fibrosis around Brunner's glands
- *6* Bacterial overgrowth syndromes: patchy damage to villi and increased lymphocyte infiltration

SOURCE: *Modified from JS Trier, N Engl J Med 285:1470, 1971*

SECRETIN TEST The secretin test and the secretin pancreozymin test, which may be useful in establishing a diagnosis of pancreatic insufficiency, are discussed in detail in Chap. 302.

SERUM CALCIUM, ALBUMIN, CHOLESTEROL, MAGNESIUM, AND IRON Abnormal serum calcium, albumin, cholesterol, magnesium, and iron values may be found in several malabsorptive disorders. The primary value of such tests is to suggest that abnormal intestinal absorptive function may be present. These tests are usually of limited value in the *differential diagnosis* of malabsorption but if abnormal may be helpful in supporting this diagnosis.

SERUM CAROTENES, VITAMIN A, AND PROTHROMBIN TIME Absorption of the fat-soluble vitamins A, D, K, and E is frequently impaired in patients with steatorrhea. Measurements of serum carotene and vitamin A levels are useful as screening tests for malabsorption. However, other tests not only are more sensitive but often give more specific information than the serum carotene and vitamin A levels. The blood prothrombin time is an important test, since patients with malabsorption may present with abnormal bleeding due to vitamin K deficiency. If the decreased prothrombin activity is due to malabsorption, it should be readily correctable with parenteral vitamin K.

5-HYDROXYINDOLEACETIC ACID (5-HIAA) AND URINE INDICAN Patients with malabsorption frequently have abnormalities in tryptophan metabolism which are reflected by an increased urinary excretion of tryptophan metabolites. Such patients frequently have a deficiency of vitamin B_6 (pyridoxine) which results in decreased conversion of tryptophan to xanthurenic acid, kynurenic acid, and nicotinamide. Consequently, increased amounts of tryptophan are converted to other metabolites such as 5-hydroxyindoleacetic acid (5-HIAA) and indole-3-acetic acid.

In untreated nontropical sprue in relapse there is characteristically a modest increase in the urinary excretion of 5-HIAA, usually in the range of 10 to 20 mg per 24 hr. This reverts to normal after institution of a gluten-free

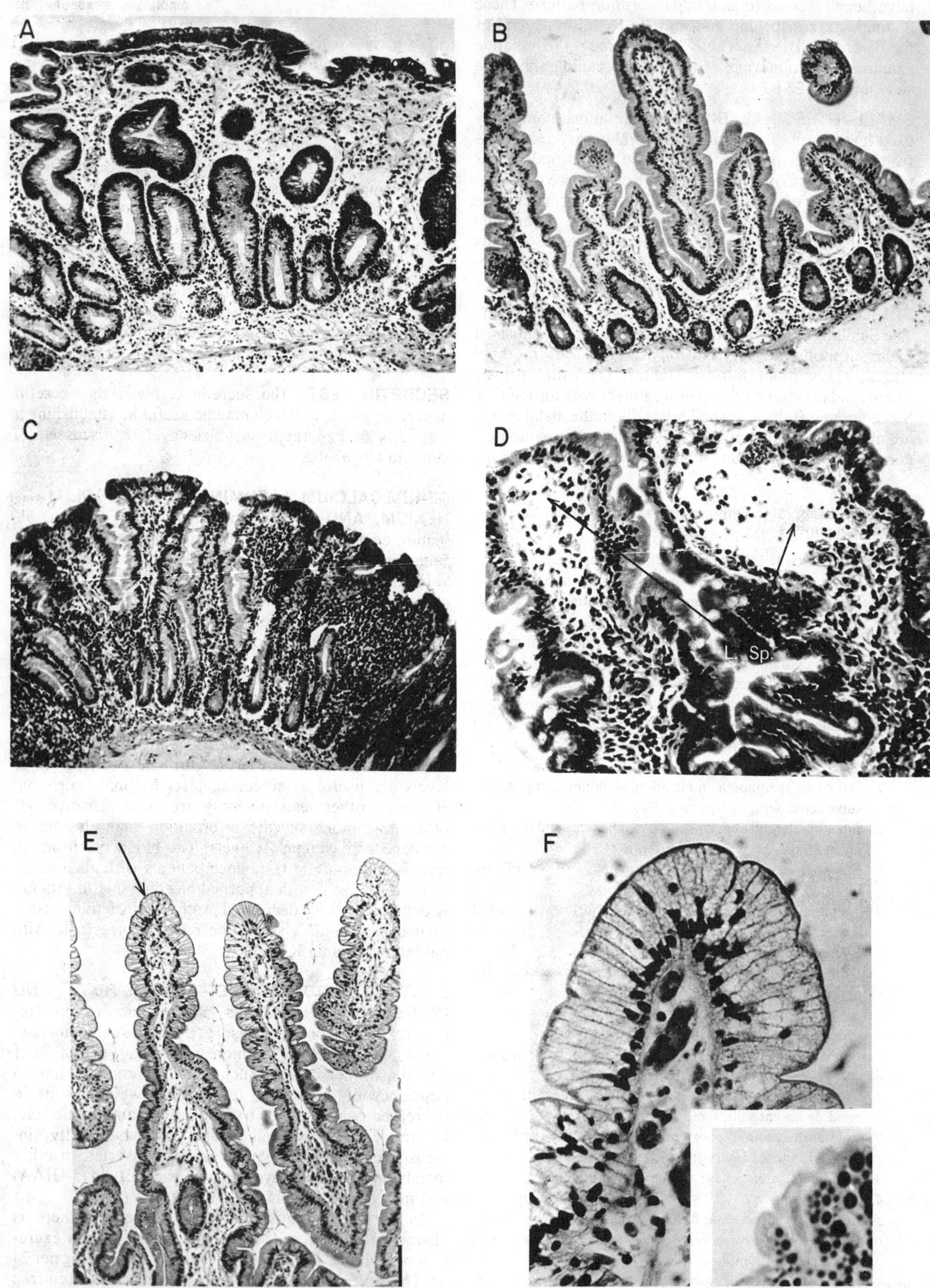
A
B
C
D
L
Sp
E
F

diet. Indican (indoxylsulfate) is another metabolite of tryptophan. Bacteria within the gut lumen cleave the side chain of tryptophan to form indole, which is absorbed, hydroxylated, and esterified with sulfate in the liver. Urine indican excretion greater than 100 mg per 24 hr is abnormal. The urine indican excretion is useful as a screening test for bacterial overgrowth in the gastrointestinal tract. Abnormal values are frequently found in the blind loop syndrome and scleroderma. An increased urine indican excretion is not specific for such disorders, and elevated values have also been found in patients with nontropical sprue, tropical sprue, and regional enteritis.

Pathophysiologic basis for symptoms and signs in malabsorptive disorders

The common symptoms and signs found in malabsorptive disorders are listed in Table 284-4. The most frequent symptoms are those of malnutrition, weight loss, and diarrhea. However, in each of the clinical settings listed in Table 284-4, it is important to consider the cause of the malabsorption.

TABLE 284-4
Pathophysiologic basis for symptoms and signs in malabsorptive disorders

Symptom or sign	*Pathophysiology*
Generalized malnutrition and weight loss	Malabsorption of fat, carbohydrate, and protein → loss of calories
Diarrhea	Impaired absorption of sodium and water; effect of unabsorbed fatty acids and bile acids
Nocturia	Delayed absorption of water
Anemia	Impaired absorption of iron, vitamin B_{12}, and folic acid
Glossitis, cheilosis	Deficiency of iron, vitamin B_{12}, folate, and other vitamins
Peripheral neuritis	Deficiency of vitamin B_{12}
Edema	Impaired absorption of amino acids → protein depletion → hypoproteinemia
Amenorrhea	Protein depletion and "caloric starvation" → secondary hypopituitarism
Bone pain	Protein depletion → impaired bone formation → osteoporosis Calcium malabsorption → demineralization of bone → osteomalacia
Tetany, paresthesias	Calcium malabsorption → hypocalcemia; magnesium malabsorption → hypomagnesemia
Hemorrhagic phenomena	Vitamin K malabsorption → hypoprothrombinemia
Weakness	Anemia; electrolyte depletion (hypokalemia)

DISORDERS ASSOCIATED WITH MALABSORPTION

Inadequate digestion

LIVER AND BILIARY TRACT DISEASE It is not generally appreciated that patients with acute or chronic liver disease may develop malabsorption due to impaired intraluminal digestion. Steatorrhea has been described in acute viral hepatitis, chronic extrahepatic biliary tract obstruction, primary biliary cirrhosis, and postnecrotic and nutritional cirrhosis. Absorption of D-xylose and vitamin B_{12} are usually normal, and small-intestinal mucosal biopsy specimens are generally unremarkable. The steatorrhea associated with liver and biliary tract disease is thought to be due to impaired hepatic synthesis or excretion of conjugated bile salts resulting in impaired formation of micellar lipid. In addition to steatorrhea, patients with liver disease may have impaired absorption of vitamin D and calcium resulting in severe metabolic bone disease. This is particularly common in patients with primary biliary cirrhosis. Skeletal roentgenograms may show increased porosity of bone, cortical thinning, vertebral compression, and spontaneous pathologic fractures. Patients with alcohol-induced liver disease may also have exocrine pancreatic insufficiency. Accordingly, pancreatic function should be evaluated in patients with liver disease and malabsorption.

FIGURE 284-4
(On facing page.) Typical peroral intestinal biopsies.
A *Jejunal mucosa of patient with nontropical sprue. Note virtual absence of villi, elongated crypts (some are cut in cross section), mononuclear infiltrate, cuboidal instead of columnar epithelium on top of villi (X300).*
B *Biopsy from the same patient as in* (A), *after 9 months on a gluten-free diet. Note the reappearance of villi with normal-appearing columnar cells, and reduction in infiltrate and crypt height (X300).*
C *Biopsy from patient with agammaglobulinemia. The features bear a striking resemblance to those of nontropical sprue. There is a marked mononuclear infiltration, some of it in aggregates (X200).*
D *Close-up of villi of patient with protein-losing enteropathy. Tips of villi are broadened and dilated. Lymphatic spaces are present (arrows) (X450).*
E *Intestinal biopsy from patient with abetalipoproteinemia. The villus tips have a "lacy" appearance (arrow) due to retained fat (X300).* [*This is more apparent at the higher magnification shown in F.*]
F *High-power micrograph of villus from patient with abetalipoproteinemia. The vacuoles are filled with lipid (X750). Insert shows dark-staining (osmium) lipid droplets in mucosal cells (osmium counterstained with Giemsa; X800).*

POSTGASTRECTOMY MALABSORPTION The presence of a malabsorption syndrome has been documented frequently in patients after subtotal gastrectomy. Steatorrhea is more common with a Billroth II than a Billroth I type of anastomosis. Usually the fat loss is minimal, ranging from 7 to 10 g per 24 hr. Patients with gross steatorrhea usually have impaired intraluminal fat digestion due to several factors: First, with a Billroth II anastomosis the duodenum is bypassed, and there is a decreased entry of stomach contents into the proximal duodenum (i.e., afferent loop). This leads to a decreased stimulus for the release of *secretin* and *pancreozymin* from the pancreas and in essence is a form of functional pancreatic insufficiency. Second, there may be *inadequate mixing* of the pancreatic enzymes and bile salts secreted into the proximal duodenum with the gastric contents entering the jejunum. Third, there may be *stasis* of intestinal contents in the afferent loop resulting in abnormal bacterial proliferation in the proximal small bowel. This in turn may lead to abnormalities in bile salt metabolism (see Pathophysiology, below). Fourth, the presence of maldigestion may lead to *protein depletion*, which in turn may produce further impairment in pancreatic function. Fifth, the *loss of the reservoir function of the stomach* may result in decreased intestinal transit time. In some patients treatment with pancreatic enzymes may lead to significant improvement. Specimens of duodenal or jejunal fluid should be obtained for culture of both aerobic and anaerobic organisms and appropriate antibiotic therapy instituted if there is evidence of abnormal bacterial overgrowth (colony count of greater than 10^5 per ml jejunal fluid). Because the duodenum is the principal site of absorption of iron and calcium, in patients with a Billroth II anastomosis impaired absorption of calcium and iron may also develop.

Inadequate absorptive surface
(See Regional Enteritis, Chap. 285)

Malabsorption due to bacterial overgrowth of the small bowel

The proximal small intestine is often bacteriologically sterile. When bacteria are isolated from the upper small bowel, they are frequently contaminants transported from the mouth and upper respiratory tract, and the colony count rarely exceeds 10^4 per ml jejunal fluid. The major mechanism limiting the growth of bacteria in the small intestine is normal peristalsis. Any disorder leading to impaired intestinal motility may result in abnormal stasis of intestinal contents with ineffective mechanical cleansing of bacteria. This in turn may lead to abnormal bacterial proliferation and malabsorption. Several malabsorptive disorders have been associated with bacterial overgrowth of the small bowel, and these are listed in Table 284-5.

PATHOPHYSIOLOGY Bacterial overgrowth may result in changes in bile salt metabolism, and these are believed directly and indirectly to account for the steatorrhea. First, bacteria (especially anaerobic gram-positive bacteria) may lead to the intraluminal deconjugation of bile salts with a consequent production of free bile acids. In contrast to conjugated bile salts, unconjugated bile salts may be absorbed in the proximal small bowel by nonionic diffusion resulting in decreased intraluminal concentrations of bile salts in the jejunum. Second, the decreased bile salt concentrations, the increase of unconjugated bile salts, and the decrease of the conjugated salts all serve to contribute to impaired intraluminal micelle formation and hence fat malabsorption. There is little evidence that decreased lipolysis of triglycerides by pancreatic lipase or increased fecal excretion of endogenous lipid are important factors in the pathogenesis of steatorrhea in the blind loop syndrome. The impaired absorption of vitamin B_{12} is not related to the disturbed bile salt metabolism but appears to be due to uptake of vitamin B_{12} by microorganisms.

Many of the above abnormalities in bile salt metabolism may be reversed by appropriate antibiotic therapy. When such treatment is instituted, unconjugated bile salts in the jejunal fluid decrease, an increase in the micellar lipid phase will occur, and steatorrhea diminishes or disappears. In addition, significant improvement in the absorption of vitamin B_{12} will occur with broad-spectrum antibiotics such as tetracycline.

CLINICAL MANIFESTATIONS The diagnosis of a malabsorption syndrome due to abnormal bacterial overgrowth of the small intestine is usually established on the basis of the following findings: (1) steatorrhea of a moderate degree, usually in the range of 15 to 30 g fecal fat per 24 hr; (2) macrocytic anemia with a megaloblastic bone marrow; (3) impaired absorption of vitamin B_{12} which is not corrected by intrinsic factor; (4) large numbers of microorganisms (greater than 10^5 per ml) in cultures of duodenal or jejunal fluid; (5) correction of steatorrhea and impaired vitamin B_{12} absorption by antibiotic therapy, together with a decrease in the number of microorganisms in the small-intestinal fluid; and (6) increased urinary indican excretion which reverts to normal with antibiotic therapy. Absorption of D-xylose, peroral small-intestinal biopsy specimens, and other tests of absorptive function (Table 284-2) may be normal in these patients.

SCLERODERMA Although there are numerous reports of small-intestinal involvement in scleroderma, frank malabsorption has been reported infrequently. It has been suggested that malabsorption may be due to several factors: (1) lymphatic obstruction; (2) reduced arterial blood supply to the gut; (3) impaired intestinal motility leading to relative stasis of intestinal contents and hence bacterial overgrowth; and (4) involvement of the intestinal wall by the disease. At present there is little data to support the first two postulated mechanisms. In some cases abnormal bacterial proliferation in the upper small bowel has been documented, and in these patients antibiotic therapy has resulted in decrease in steatorrhea, gain in weight, and increased absorption of vitamin B_{12}. In the intestinal wall there may also be extensive deposition of collagen, especially in the muscular mucosa, submucosa, and muscularis externa, with significant muscle atrophy. Electron microscopic studies have revealed a paucity of nexuses (cell junctions) between adjacent muscle cells in the small intestine of these patients. Since nexuses are important in the propagation of electric impulses, the loss of contact between muscle cells may result in impairment of muscular contraction. This may be an important factor in the dilatation, atony, and stasis of intestinal contents in scleroderma.

Disorders associated with lymphatic obstruction

WHIPPLE'S DISEASE This is a rare disorder characterized clinically by arthralgia, abdominal pain, diarrhea, progressive weight loss, and impaired intestinal absorption. The disease is unusual in women and occurs predominantly in men of middle age. Wasting, low-grade fever, increased skin pigmentation, and peripheral lymphadenopathy are frequently present. In addition, there may be enlargement of mesenteric, periaortic, and celiac lymph nodes. Laboratory examination usually reveals the presence of steatorrhea, impaired xylose absorption, abnormal small-bowel x-rays, hypoalbuminemia, and anemia. Hypoalbuminemia is due to excessive loss of serum albumin into the gastrointestinal tract as well as impaired synthesis of albumin. Serum calcium, cholesterol, and iron levels are usually low and often inversely correlated with the degree of malabsorption.

The diagnosis is established by demonstrating the presence in the mucosa of macrophages containing large cytoplasmic granules which give a brilliant magenta stain with periodic acid–Schiff reagent (PAS). Such macrophages may also be seen in other tissues such as lymph nodes, spleen, or liver. The PAS-positive reaction is due to the presence of glycoproteins. The finding of PAS-positive macrophages in the lamina propria is not specific for Whipple's disease, but virtual replacement of most cellular elements in the lamina propria by these macrophages has been seen only in this disorder. In addition to the PAS-positive macrophages, jejunal biopsies frequently show dilated lymphatics and some degree of blunting of the intestinal mucosal villi.

Electron microscopic studies have revealed the presence of rod-shaped structures (or bacilliform bodies) 0.3 by 1.5 to 2.5 μm within and adjacent to the macrophages in the lamina propria as well as within epithelial cells, and polymorphonuclear leukocytes. The ultrastruc-

TABLE 284-5
Classification of the malabsorption syndromes

A Inadequate digestion
- *1* Post-gastrectomy steatorrhea*
- *2* Deficiency or inactivation of pancreatic lipase
  - *a* Exocrine pancreatic insufficiency
    - *1* Chronic pancreatitis
    - *2* Pancreatic carcinoma
    - *3* Cystic fibrosis
    - *4* Pancreatic resection
  - *b* Ulcerogenic tumor of the pancreas (Zollinger-Ellison syndrome)*

B Reduced intestinal bile salt concentration (with impaired micelle formation)
- *1* Liver disease
  - *a* Parenchymal liver disease
  - *b* Cholestasis (intrahepatic or extrahepatic)
- *2* Abnormal bacterial proliferation in the small bowel
  - *a* Afferent loop stasis
  - *b* Strictures
  - *c* Fistulas
  - *d* Blind loops
  - *e* Multiple diverticula of the small bowel
  - *f* Hypomotility states (diabetes, scleroderma)
- *3* Interrupted enterohepatic circulation of bile salts
  - *a* Ileal resection
  - *b* Ileal inflammatory disease (regional ileitis)
- *4* Drug-induced (by sequestration or precipitation of bile salts)
  - *a* Neomycin
  - *b* Calcium carbonate
  - *c* Cholestyramine

C Inadequate absorptive surface
- *1* Intestinal resection or bypass
- *2* Gastroileostomy

D Lymphatic obstruction
- *1* Intestinal lymphangiectasia
- *2* Whipple's disease*
- *3* Lymphoma
- *4* Köhlmeier-Degos disease (primary progressive arterial occlusive disease)*

E Cardiovascular disorders
- *1* Constrictive pericarditis
- *2* Congestive heart failure
- *3* Mesenteric vascular insufficiency
- *4* Vasculitis

F Primary mucosal absorptive defects
- *1* Inflammatory or infiltrative disorders
  - *a* Regional enteritis*
  - *b* Amyloidosis
  - *c* Scleroderma*
  - *d* Lymphoma*
  - *e* Radiation enteritis
  - *f* Eosinophilic enteritis
  - *g* Tropical sprue
  - *h* Infectious enteritis (e.g., salmonellosis)
  - *i* Collagenous sprue
  - *j* Nonspecific ulcerative jejunitis
  - *k* Mastocytosis
  - *l* Dermatologic disorders (e.g., dermatitis herpetiformis)
- *2* Biochemical or genetic abnormalities
  - *a* Nontropical sprue (gluten-induced enteropathy); celiac sprue
  - *b* Disaccharidase deficiency
  - *c* Hypogammaglobulinemia
  - *d* Abetalipoproteinemia
  - *e* Hartnup disease
  - *f* Cystinuria
  - *g* Monosaccharide malabsorption

G Endocrine and metabolic disorders
- *1* Diabetes mellitus
- *2* Hypoparathyroidism
- *3* Adrenal insufficiency
- *4* Hyperthyroidism
- *5* Ulcerogenic tumor of the pancreas (Zollinger-Ellison syndrome)*
- *6* Carcinoid syndrome

* *Malabsorption caused by multiple defects.*

tural features of these bacilliform bodies suggest that they are microorganisms. It is of particular interest that after treatment with antibiotics the bacilliform bodies decrease or disappear together with a decrease in the number of PAS-positive macrophages. In addition, the reappearance of the bacteria often heralds the onset of a clinical relapse after antibiotics have been withdrawn. Despite the fact that the presence of bacilliform bodies is usually associated with active disease, the exact role of the bacilli in the pathogenesis of Whipple's disease is unclear. The microorganism has not been identified with certainty, and the disease has not been reproduced in animals.

Whipple's disease at one time was thought to be invariably fatal. However, it is now clear that therapy with antibiotics, with or without corticosteroids, will usually induce a clinical remission. In a few cases there has been complete reversal of the histologic abnormalities in the jejunal mucosa, and some of these cases have been followed for 10 years. It is recommended that patients with Whipple's disease be treated with antibiotics such as tetracycline for at least 1 year and then followed closely with serial small-bowel biopsies. The most important parameter for following the disease and predicting its course is the presence or absence of bacilli in sections of small-bowel biopsies.

INTESTINAL LYMPHOMA Steatorrhea is an uncommon manifestation of intestinal lymphoma. The disease occurs predominantly in men, and the mean age of onset of symptoms is about fifty years. The diagnosis should be suspected in patients with malabsorption with the following findings: (1) a malabsorption syndrome in which clinical and biopsy features resemble those of nontropical sprue but in which there is an incomplete response to a gluten-free diet, (2) the presence of abdominal pain and fever, and (3) signs and symptoms of intestinal obstruction. It should be emphasized that the usual stigmas of generalized lymphoma are frequently absent. Hepatomegaly, splenomegaly, palpable abdominal masses, and peripheral adenopathy are usually not found. Lymphangiography may reveal abnormal intraabdominal nodes. The diagnosis can be established by laparotomy and often may be made by thorough examination of multiple mucosal biopsy specimens obtained perorally. There may be a total absence of villi or lesser degrees of blunting and shortening of the villi. In contrast to nontropical sprue, the lamina propria is usually massively infiltrated with lymphoid cells. Malignancy may be diagnosed by demonstrating lymphoid cells with the cytologic features of malignancy, the presence of reticulum cells outside of germinal centers, and infiltration and destruction of crypts by pleomorphic lymphoid cells. Some patients elaborate or secrete a fragment of the heavy chain of IgA immunoglobulins (*alpha chain disease*). The latter is probably a variant of intestinal lymphoma.

The mechanism of malabsorption in intestinal lymphoma may be related to several factors: (1) diffuse involvement of the small-intestinal mucosa; (2) involvement of the bowel wall with lymphatic obstruction; and (3) localized stenosis with stasis of intestinal contents and bacterial overgrowth. It should be emphasized that it is often difficult, by clinical and morphologic features alone, to distinguish nontropical sprue from intestinal lymphoma. Indeed, there is evidence to suggest that lymphoma may develop as a late complication of nontropical sprue.

The course of intestinal lymphoma has ranged from 4 months to 4 years from the onset of symptoms. Perforation, bleeding, and intestinal obstruction are common terminal complications. There is insufficient data to determine whether radiation therapy, chemotherapy, or localized surgical resection modify the natural course of the disease.

Cardiovascular disorders

Steatorrhea has been described in patients with chronic congestive heart failure, superior mesenteric artery insufficiency, and constrictive pericarditis. Abnormal dilated mucosal lymphatics and excessive enteric loss of protein have been demonstrated in patients with constrictive pericarditis. The mechanism of steatorrhea in patients with chronic heart failure remains uncertain. It might be due to congestion and edema of the mucosa, mucosal hypoxia, or abnormalities in pancreatic function. Although pronounced steatorrhea is uncommon in congestive heart failure, these patients are frequently anorectic, and a low fat intake could mask a latent steatorrhea. Steatorrhea is quite infrequent in patients with vasculitis and is thought to be due to segmental infarction of the small bowel in addition to intestinal ischemia.

DEFECTS IN MUCOSAL FUNCTION

Inflammatory or infiltrative disorders

REGIONAL ENTERITIS The clinical features of regional enteritis are described in Chap. 285. Malabsorption in regional enteritis may result from several factors: (1) inadequate absorbing surface due to intestinal resection; (2) changes in mucosal cell structure and function; (3) inflammatory cell infiltration of the lamina propria; (4) strictures and fistulas with secondary stasis of intestinal contents and bacterial overgrowth; and (5) impaired absorption of bile salts due either to ileal resection or to the presence of active inflammatory disease in the ileum. After intestinal resection, the functional capacity of the remaining small bowel will depend on the site and extent of resection as well as the presence of residual inflammatory disease. Massive intestinal resection usually results in impaired absorption of all food constituents. Such patients should be treated with a low fat diet, and substitution of medium-chain for long-chain triglycerides may be beneficial. When the malabsorption is due to strictures and blind loops as a result of previous surgical therapy, antibiotic therapy may be helpful, but surgical removal of these areas is usually necessary for long-term improvement. With diffuse inflammatory disease a florid malabsorption syndrome may occur with steatorrhea, hypocalcemia, impaired vitamin B_{12} absorption, and hypoalbuminemia due to increased enteric protein loss. Treatment with salicylazosulfapyridine and corticosteroid drugs may be beneficial.

After *ileal resection,* patients frequently have bothersome diarrhea. This appears to be due to *interruption of the enterohepatic circulation* whereby increased amounts of bile salts reach the colon, where they interfere with water and electrolyte absorption and thus have a cathartic effect. The *bile salt–induced diarrhea* after ileal resection may respond to treatment with cholestyramine, an exchange resin which binds bile salts and causes them to lose their biochemical effect on the bowel. Patients with ileal resection of less than 100 cm and fecal fat excretion less than 20 g per day show the best symptomatic response to cholestyramine.

AMYLOIDOSIS This disorder is discussed in detail in Chap. 107. The intestinal tract is involved infrequently in amyloidosis. Diarrhea and steatorrhea are thought to be due to (1) infiltration of the intestinal wall with amyloid and (2) involvement of the autonomic nervous system. Metachromatic and congophilic amyloid has been demonstrated in small and medium-sized blood vessels in the intestine, in nerve bundles in Meissner's sub-mucosal and Auerbach's myenteric plexus, and in the thoracolumbar and celiac sympathetic ganglions. With involvement of the autonomic nervous system, patients may show uncontrollable diarrhea, orthostatic hypotension, trophic ulcers, anhydrosis of the distal extremities, and impotence. The clinical features closely resemble those found in "diabetic diarrhea." The diagnosis can be established by demonstrating amyloid deposits in rectal and small-intestinal biopsy specimens. In addition to malabsorption, rare manifestations include intestinal perforation, colonic infarction, and excessive enteric loss of protein. There is no effective treatment for the disease.

RADIATION INJURY TO THE SMALL BOWEL Extensive morphologic damage of the small-intestinal mucosa often follows after normal or excessive abdominal irradiation. These changes include a decrease in crypt mitoses, marked shortening of the villi, megalocytosis of epithelial cells, and inflammatory cell infiltration of the lamina propria. This may be associated with transient diarrhea and impaired intestinal absorption. However, restoration of normal intestinal architecture is usually complete within 2 weeks after cessation of therapy. Persistent diarrhea and malabsorption may develop shortly after x-ray therapy, or there may be a latent period of several years before the onset of diarrhea. Steatorrhea, ranging from 10 to 70 g per day, has been frequently observed, but impaired absorption of calcium, iron, D-xylose, or vitamin B_{12} is less common. In some patients intestinal strictures may develop following irradiation, and thus stasis of intestinal contents and abnormal bacterial proliferation may occur. In others, intestinal lymphangiectasia, presumably due to lymphatic obstruction, has been documented. Diarrhea and malabsorption may be refractory to all methods of management. Treatment with antibiotics, pancreatic enzymes, gluten-free diet, adrenal corticosteroids, anticholinergic drugs, and opiates has met with but limited success.

EOSINOPHILIC ENTERITIS Eosinophilic gastroenteritis is a disorder of the stomach and small bowel of unknown etiology characterized by peripheral blood eosinophilia and eosinophilic infiltration of the gut wall but without evidence of vasculitis. The clinical manifestations, usually recurrent, are protean and relate to the site of gastrointestinal tract involvement. Three main patterns have been identified. First, predominant mucosal disease manifested by iron-deficiency anemia, hypoalbuminemia due to protein-losing enteropathy, and mild steatorrhea. Second, predominant muscle layer disease characterized by marked thickening and rigidity of the stomach and proximal small bowel with obstructive symptoms and radiologic features of pyloric narrowing and obstruction. Third, predominant subserosal disease in which the cardinal manifestation is ascites with marked eosinophilia in the ascitic fluid. Small-bowel thickening and subserosal infiltration of eosinophils may also be present. Patients in the first group often present with a malabsorption syndrome and a history of intolerance to specific foods. However, specific elimination diets are frequently only transiently effective, and many patients require prolonged corticosteroid therapy to remain well. Thus eosinophilic gastroenteritis does not appear to be a simple reversible allergic reaction to specific foods.

DERMATITIS AND MALABSORPTION A malabsorption syndrome, usually mild, has been reported in patients with a variety of dermatological disorders including psoriasis, eczematoid dermatitis, and dermatitis herpetiformis. Proximal intestinal mucosal abnormalities are almost invariably found in patients with dermatitis herpetiformis. In one study 21 of 22 patients had lesions ranging in severity from a completely "flat" to an almost normal intestinal mucosa. The mucosal lesions were often patchy in distribution. Clinical and laboratory evidence of significant malabsorption was infrequent, possibly due to the limited length of small intestine involved in this skin disorder. In some patients with dermatitis herpetiformis, blunted and flattened intestinal mucosal lesions and steatorrhea, there may be a striking improvement in villous architecture and regression of steatorrhea after withdrawal of gluten from the diet. This raises the interesting question as to whether certain patients with dermatitis herpetiformis and a malabsorption syndrome have nontropical sprue.

Biochemical or genetic abnormalities

NONTROPICAL SPRUE Definition Nontropical sprue is a disorder characterized by malabsorption, abnormal small-bowel structure, and intolerance to gluten, a protein found in wheat and wheat products. It has been appropriately referred to as *gluten-induced enteropathy*. Celiac disease in children and nontropical sprue of the adult are probably one and the same disorder with the same pathogenesis.

There are insufficient data to provide an accurate estimation of the incidence of nontropical sprue in any population. This is largely because the severity of the disease varies greatly and individuals may have typical mucosal change and yet have no overt symptoms. The incidence in siblings appears to be many times higher than that in the general population, and it has been suggested that sprue may be inherited through a dominant gene of incomplete penetrance. Seventy percent of the cases in most reported series are in women.

Pathophysiology Gluten and the related substance gliadin are high molecular weight proteins found especially in wheat. These proteins are unique in that glutamine accounts for about 40 percent of the component amino acids. These proteins as well as the larger peptide hydrolysis products (containing glutamine) are toxic when administered to patients with sprue in remission. The exact mechanism for this effect is not clear, but two theories have been proposed: One possible mechanism is that patients with sprue lack a specific mucosal peptidase, such that gluten or its larger glutamine-containing peptides are not effectively hydrolyzed to smaller peptides (i.e., dipeptides or amino acids). As a consequence "toxic" peptides might accumulate in the mucosa. It has been demonstrated that patients with sprue in remission will develop steatorrhea and typical mucosal changes when they are given gluten. Similar results will occur with the administration of peptide hydrolyzates containing at least eight amino acids with a terminal glutamine residue. It has been shown that when gluten is instilled into the *ileum* of sprue patients, histologic changes begin to occur within hours, but not in the upper jejunum, suggesting that the effect is immediate and local rather than systemic. After noxious gluten fractions damage surface absorptive cells, the damaged cells are sloughed rapidly from the mucosal surface into the gut lumen. To compensate for this, cell proliferation increases, crypts hypertrophy, and cell migration is accelerated to replace the damaged and sloughed epithelial cells. This more rapid than normal epithelial cell renewal can be reversed by a gluten-free diet. The intestinal mucosa of patients with sprue shows many enzyme alterations including decreased levels of disaccharidases, alkaline phosphatase, and peptide hydrolases as well as impaired ability to digest gluten peptides. However, these abnormalities usually revert toward normal after successful treatment with a gluten-free diet. No persistent, specific, or selective peptidase deficiency has been demonstrated.

It has also been suggested that gluten or gluten metabolites may initiate a hypersensitivity reaction in the intestinal mucosa. The presence of a mononuclear inflammatory cell infiltrate in the lamina propria of the mucosa, the beneficial response to corticosteroid drugs, and the finding of abnormal antibodies to gliadin in the serum of sprue patients have all been cited as evidence in support of this hypothesis. There are no firm data indicating that an abnormal (immune) mechanism is important in initiating or perpetuating this disease process.

Jejunal biopsy specimens from patients with nontropical sprue usually show a characteristic lesion. There is blunting and flattening of the mucosal surface, with villi either absent or broad and short. The crypts are elongated, and there is generally a dense infiltration of inflammatory cells in the lamina propria. The surface epithelium is altered with a sparse brush border, cuboidal rather than the normal columnar cells, and infiltration of inflammatory cells in the epithelial layer. These changes are usually most severe in the proximal small bowel, presumably because this area of the bowel is exposed to the highest gluten concentration. The typical morphologic changes are illustrated in Fig. 284-4. It should be emphasized that these changes are characteristic of nontropical sprue but are not specific. Similar changes have been described in other conditions including lymphoma, tropical sprue, and hypogammaglobulinemia associated with malabsorption. Many biochemical abnormalities have been demonstrated in mucosal biopsy specimens from nontropical sprue patients. Impaired esterification of fatty acids to triglycerides, decreased uptake of amino acids, and decreased activity of intestinal disaccharidases (especially lactase) have been well documented. The latter observation may account for the high incidence of milk intolerance in untreated sprue patients or those in relapse.

Since the mucosa is severely damaged in patients with nontropical sprue, there is *decreased release of pancreatic tropic hormones* (secretin and cholecystokinin-pancreozymin). This results in decreased stimulation of the pancreas with lower than normal intraluminal levels of pancreatic enzymes in response to a meal. In addition, impaired release of cholecystokinin may result in absent or minimal contractions of the gallbladder leading to sequestration of bile salts in an inert gallbladder. These two defects may result in impaired intraluminal digestion of fat and protein which will be superimposed on the defect in intestinal transport caused by a damaged mucosa.

Clinical features Most patients with nontropical sprue will have a typical malabsorption syndrome characterized by weight loss, abdominal distention and bloating, diarrhea, steatorrhea, and abnormal tests of absorptive function. The characteristic alterations in tests of intestinal absorption are outlined in Table 284-2. It should be emphasized, however, that some sprue patients may present with isolated abnormalities which initially do not suggest the diagnosis of nontropical sprue. Thus, a patient may be admitted for investigation of iron deficiency anemia without apparent blood loss or of abnormal bleeding due to hypoprothrombinemia, but not have diarrhea or overt steatorrhea. Likewise, sprue patients may present with puzzling metabolic bone disease without diarrhea or steatorrhea. Such patients usually complain of bone pain and tenderness and frequently are found to have extensive demineralization of bone, compression deformities, kyphoscoliosis, and Milkman's fractures. Emotional disturbances are common in these patients, and many individuals with a diagnosis of weight loss initially considered related to severe anxiety and depression are subsequently found to have nontropical sprue. In each of the above clinical settings, the diagnosis of sprue should be considered in the differential diagnosis.

Since there is no specific diagnostic test, three criteria should be met in order to establish a definite diagnosis of nontropical sprue: (1) evidence of malabsorption, (2) an abnormal small-bowel (jejunal) biopsy showing blunting and flattening of the villi along with changes in the surface epithelium (i.e., subtotal villous atrophy), (3) clinical, biochemical, and histologic improvement after institution of a gluten-free diet. In equivocal cases, the patient can be challenged with 30 to 50 g gluten orally, and if this promptly results in increased diarrhea and steatorrhea, the diagnosis of gluten-induced enteropathy is established. It should be emphasized that tests of intestinal absorption may reveal abnormalities which range from very minimal alterations to severe changes. Abnormalities in absorption tests have been shown to correlate reasonably well with the length of small-bowel involvement and to a lesser extent with the severity of the proximal lesion. A possible variant of nontropical sprue is "collagenous sprue," which is characterized by refractory malabsorption and small-bowel biopsy alterations showing a blunted and flattened mucosa and large masses of eosinophilic hyaline material in the lamina propria. Its relation to nontropical sprue is unclear.

Treatment Despite the uncertainties concerned with the diagnosis of nontropical sprue, approximately 80 percent of the patients improve after institution of a *gluten-free diet*. Symptomatic improvement usually occurs within a few weeks, but improvement in tests of absorptive function and small-bowel histologic characteristics may not occur for months. It has been repeatedly demonstrated that strict adherence to a gluten-free diet more consistently results in improvement than suboptimal gluten restriction. Nevertheless, even with strict diet adherence some cases show little improvement in intestinal histologic features. Patients with nontropical sprue treated with corticosteroids but continuing a normal gluten-containing diet have shown symptomatic improvement as well as improvement in intestinal histology and tests of intestinal absorptive function. The mechanism by which prednisolone protects the mucosa from the effects of gluten is not clear.

If a patient with nontropical sprue does not respond to a gluten-free diet, other possibilities or complicative factors must be considered: (1) the diagnosis is incorrect, (2) the patient is not adhering strictly to the diet, (3) there may be another concurrent disease, such as pancreatic insufficiency, (4) the patient may have ulceration of the jejunum or ileum, (5) lactase deficiency may be present with resultant milk intolerance, (6) the patient may have "collagenous sprue," or (7) he may have developed intestinal lymphoma, a disease which appears to occur more frequently in sprue than in the general population. Finally, it should be emphasized that a small number of patients show a markedly delayed response to a gluten-free diet, with significant improvement occurring only after 24 to 36 months of therapy.

DISACCHARIDASE DEFICIENCY SYNDROMES As indicated above, the hydrolysis of disaccharides occurs on or within the brush border (microvilli) of intestinal epithelial cells by specific disaccharidases located there. As would be anticipated, both primary (genetic or familial) and secondary (acquired) deficiencies of these disaccharidases have been observed.

Lactase deficiency in the adult Instances of isolated deficiency of mucosal lactase occur which are associated with symptoms of lactose intolerance. Since lactose is the principal carbohydrate of milk, such individuals show milk intolerance with symptoms of abdominal cramps, bloating, or distention, and diarrhea. Similar symptoms will occur following the ingestion of lactose. The symptoms are due to the fact that lactose, when not hydrolyzed, is not absorbed and its osmotic effect in the lumen leads to shifts of fluid into the intestinal tract. The pH of the stool will also decrease because of the production of lactic acid and short-chain fatty acids from the fermentation of lactose by colonic bacteria. Although primary intestinal lactase deficiency seems to be hereditary, lactose or milk intolerance may not become clinically evident until puberty or late adolescence. There are significant racial differences in the incidence of this entity. It would appear that about 5 percent of the adult white population show intestinal lactase deficiency, but in American Negroes, Bantus, and Orientals, the incidence has been reported as high as 60 to 90 percent.

The diagnosis may be suspected by obtaining a history of gastrointestinal symptoms following milk ingestion. That these symptoms are not due to allergic reactions to the proteins in milk (i.e., milk allergy or hypersensitivity) can be demonstrated by performing a lactose tolerance test. This test consists of administering an oral dose of lactose (usually from 0.75 to 1.5 g per kg body weight) and obtaining serial blood samples for measurements of blood glucose. In a positive test, intestinal symptoms occur, and the blood glucose increases less than 25 mg per 100 ml above the fasting level. Because false positive tests occur in about 20 percent of normal subjects, a positive test should be confirmed by direct enzymatic measurements of lactase on peroral mucosal biopsy specimens. In primary lactase deficiency the intestinal mucosa is normal histologically.

Acquired lactase deficiency is often seen in association with a variety of gastrointestinal diseases, in many of which there is histologic evidence of mucosal damage. The disorders in which lactose intolerance and lactase deficiency may occur include nontropical and tropical sprue, regional enteritis, bacterial infections of the intestinal tract, giardiasis, abetalipoproteinemia, cystic fibrosis, and ulcerative colitis.

Deficiency of other disaccharidases Damage to the intestinal mucosa may produce decreased levels of other disaccharidases such as invertase (sucrase), but usually these are not as depressed as lactase, and symptoms of specific intolerance, such as sucrose intolerance, are uncommon. There are instances of primary and apparently hereditary invertase intolerance, but these always occur in association with isomaltase deficiency. There have been no reports of maltose intolerance, perhaps reflecting the fact that there are at least four mucosal enzymes capable of hydrolyzing maltose.

HYPOGAMMAGLOBULINEMIA There are several reports documenting the association of malabsorption in hypogammaglobulinemia or agammaglobulinemia. The hypogammaglobulinemia may be of the congenital or the acquired type with the onset either in childhood or adulthood. When malabsorption has been noted, it has included impaired absorption of fat, D-xylose, and vitamin B_{12}. Peroral intestinal biopsy may reveal changes comparable to those seen in nontropical sprue, but often one finds a more striking mononuclear infiltrate giving a nodular appearance to the mucosa both microscopically and macroscopically. Diarrhea and steatorrhea may precede or follow the development of hypogammaglobulinemia, and these may worsen during infections and subside after the infection is controlled with antibiotics. Arthritis, resembling rheumatoid arthritis, and thymoma have also been described in patients with this syndrome. In some patients improvement in diarrhea and malabsorption may occur spontaneously, whereas in others improvement may follow treatment with a gluten-free diet, corticosteroids, antibiotics, injections of γ-globulin, and cholestyramine. These forms of therapy have not been uniformly successful. Although transient improvement is common, complete cessation of symptoms is distinctly unusual.

The relationship between hypogammaglobulinemia and malabsorption remains obscure. There is no evidence to date indicating that excessive enteric loss of γ-globulin or alteration of the intestinal microflora occurs, but abnormalities in IgA metabolism may be important in this syndrome. This immunoglobulin is the predominant one in the intestinal mucosa and is found in many exocrine secretions including tears, saliva, gastric juice, and intestinal juice. A few patients have been described with malabsorption and selective deficiency of IgA.

ABETALIPOPROTEINEMIA See Chap. 106.

HARTNUP DISEASE See Chap. 97.

CYSTINURIA See Chap. 97.

Endocrine and metabolic disorders

DIABETES MELLITUS The occurrence of diarrhea and steatorrhea in patients with diabetes mellitus has been well documented. When steatorrhea accompanies diabetes, it may be due to the presence of (1) exocrine pancreatic insufficiency, (2) coexistent nontropical sprue, (3) abnormal bacterial proliferation in the proximal small bowel, and (4) severe and uncontrolled diabetes per se (e.g., so-called "diabetic diarrhea"). Patients falling into the first three categories will usually respond in a satisfactory manner to treatment with pancreatic extracts, a gluten-free diet, and antibiotics, respectively. The pathogenesis of diarrhea and steatorrhea in patients in the fourth category remains poorly understood, and the response to various forms of therapy has been quite variable. It has been demonstrated that patients with "diabetic diarrhea" and steatorrhea may have involvement of the autonomic nervous system with degenerative changes in the sympathetic and parasympathetic nerves and ganglions. In some patients bacterial overgrowth in the stomach and proximal small bowel may occur and contribute to the diarrhea and steatorrhea.

The clinical features in patients with diarrhea and steatorrhea due to diabetes per se seem to be fairly uniform. Diabetes usually develops at a young age and is often severe and difficult to control. There is a distinct predominance of males. Several signs of autonomic neuropathy are usually present including postural hypotension, anhydrosis, impotence, and bladder irregularities. Peripheral vascular disease and peripheral neuropathy are also common. Gastrointestinal x-rays may show delayed gastric emptying and disordered transit through the small bowel. Peroral small-bowel biopsy specimens are normal. Tests of intestinal absorptive function are normal except for steatorrhea and azotorrhea. There has been no consistent response to therapy with pancreatic extracts, gluten-free diet, corticosteroids, and cholinergic drugs such as Urecholine. When bacterial overgrowth is present, broad-spectrum antibiotics may be helpful. In a few patients improvement in steatorrhea and diarrhea occurs after satisfactory control of diabetes.

HYPOPARATHYROIDISM Steatorrhea has been documented in several patients with idiopathic hypoparathyroidism. In addition to hypocalcemia, impaired absorption of D-xylose and vitamin B_{12}, decreased serum iron values, and abnormal small-intestinal roentgenograms have been demonstrated in some cases. In such patients the serum phosphorus level is elevated (due to the hypoparathyroidism) rather than low (as in primary malabsorption). The cause of malabsorption in this disorder is unclear. It is possible that hypocalcemia causes impaired neuromuscular function, which in turn may lead to hypomotility, stasis of intestinal contents, and abnormal bacterial proliferation in the small bowel. The latter abnormality could account for the development of steatorrhea and malabsorption of vitamin B_{12}.

ADRENAL INSUFFICIENCY Although there are few studies on fat excretion in adrenal insufficiency in man, malabsorption, especially of fat, would appear to occur more frequently than has been generally appreciated. Patients with adrenal insufficiency have been found to have steatorrhea which was corrected by therapy with adrenal corticosteroids. Jejunal biopsies in a small number of these patients were normal. It is possible that the diarrhea and weight loss seen in adrenal insufficiency may be due in part to malabsorption.

HYPERTHYROIDISM There are few detailed studies on intestinal absorptive function in patients with hyperthyroidism. Mild to moderate steatorrhea, impaired absorption of D-xylose and vitamin B_{12}, and hypoalbuminemia have been reported. These abnormalities usually revert to normal after successful treatment of hyperthyroidism. Experimental studies suggest that steatorrhea in hyperthyroidism is not due to any defect of pancreatic, biliary, or small-intestinal mucosal function but is a result of a disturbance in the intraluminal phase of fat absorption caused by rapid gastric emptying and intestinal transit.

ULCEROGENIC TUMOR OF THE PANCREAS (ZOLLINGER-ELLISON SYNDROME) The clinical features of ulcerogenic tumor of the pancreas are described in Chapter 282. Malabsorption is frequently found in this disease. The acidification and dilution of intestinal contents caused by gastric acid hypersecretion leads to major disturbances in fat digestion and absorption. Impaired formation of micellar lipid due to inactivation of pancreatic lipase is probably the major factor in the production of steatorrhea. Other factors contributing to fat malabsorption in this disorder include (1) precipitation of glycine conjugated bile salts due to low intraluminal pH, (2) alteration of the intestinal mucosa with ulceration and metaplasia, and (3) impaired fatty acid esterification and chylomicron formation.

CARCINOID SYNDROME (see Chap. 99) Although diarrhea is common in the carcinoid syndrome, malabsorption with significant steatorrhea is unusual. In many of the cases of carcinoid syndrome with steatorrhea there has been a prior intestinal resection (usually ileal), and in these cases the resection is the important factor in the causation of steatorrhea. However, direct involvement of the bowel wall and mesentery by the carcinoid tumor have been well documented. That abnormalities in serotonin metabolism may also be important is suggested from the decrease in the steatorrhea observed in some of these patients when treated with the antiserotonin drug methysergide. Although side effects may occur, for control of diarrhea and steatorrhea, patients may be given a trial of 8 to 12 mg methysergide per day.

Protein-losing enteropathy

The gastrointestinal tract has been shown to play a significant role in the metabolism and physiologic degradation of plasma proteins. The exact magnitude of the normal gastrointestinal protein loss in man has remained unclear, but studies with ^{131}I- or ^{125}I-labeled albumin and ^{51}Cr-labeled albumin have suggested that between 10 and 20 percent of the normal turnover of albumin may be accounted for by enteric protein loss. However, under certain pathologic conditions, excessive gastrointestinal protein loss may develop. An extensive number of disorders have been found to be associated with intestinal protein loss. Some of these are listed in Table 284-6.

PATHOPHYSIOLOGY Several mechanisms have been proposed for the passage of plasma proteins across the gastrointestinal mucosa both normally and in certain disease states: First, plasma proteins may pass into the gastrointestinal tract through an inflamed or ulcerated mucosa and account for the protein loss occasionally seen in regional enteritis and ulcerative colitis. Second, plasma protein loss may occur as a result of disordered mucosal cell structure. For example, patients with nontropical sprue have abnormal villous structure and surface epithelium, and these changes could facilitate the diffusion of plasma protein between the cells. Third, in the presence of increased lymphatic pressure, there may be increased passage of plasma proteins into the lumen via the intercellular spaces of the mucosal epithelium. This might be expected to occur in disorders in which there is granulomatous or neoplastic involvement of lymphatics. Fourth, dilated lymph vessels in the mucosa may rupture through the surface epithelium, discharging their contents into the intestinal lumen. This is thought to be important in the pathogenesis of steatorrhea and hypoproteinemia in patients with idiopathic intestinal lymphangiectasia (see Intestinal Lymphangiectasia, below).

Several techniques have been developed for the detection and quantitation of gastrointestinal protein loss. Most of these involve the use of intravenously administered radioactive-labeled macromolecules such as ^{131}I- and ^{125}I-labeled serum albumin, $^{51}CrCl_3$, ^{51}Cr-labeled albumin, and ceruloplasmin. ^{51}Chromium-labeled albumin and $^{51}CrCl_3$ (both of which rapidly become attached to circulating transferrin) are the compounds used most frequently. After the intravenous administration of 25 to 30 microcuries of the labeled compound to normal subjects, between 0.1 and 0.7 percent of the administered radioactivity is recovered in the stool over a 4-day period. Patients with excessive enteric protein loss may excrete from 2 to 40 percent of the injected radioactive label. False positive results may be obtained if the stool specimen is contaminated with urine.

TABLE 284-6
Disorders associated with protein-losing enteropathy

A Stomach
- *1* Gastric carcinoma
- *2* Giant hypertrophy of the gastric mucosa
- *3* Atrophic gastritis
- *4* Postgastrectomy syndrome

B Small intestine
- *1* Nontropic sprue
- *2* Tropical sprue
- *3* Regional enteritis
- *4* Whipple's disease
- *5* Lymphoma
- *6* Intestinal lymphangiectasia
- *7* Intestinal tuberculosis
- *8* Acute infectious enteritis
- *9* Scleroderma
- *10* Jejunal diverticulosis
- *11* Allergic gastroenteropathy

C Colon
- *1* Colonic neoplasm
- *2* Ulcerative colitis
- *3* Granulomatous colitis
- *4* Megacolon

D Cardiac
- *1* Congestive heart failure
- *2* Constrictive pericarditis
- *3* Interatrial septal defect
- *4* Primary cardiomyopathy

E Miscellaneous
- *1* Esophageal carcinoma
- *2* Gastrocolic fistula
- *3* Agammaglobulinemia
- *4* Nephrosis

SOURCE: *Modified from Waldman, Gastroenterology. 50:422, 1966.*

Using intravenously administered radioiodinated albumin, the decline in radioactivity in the serum and whole body can be followed and the rate of albumin synthesis and degradation determined. Such studies carried out in patients with protein-losing enteropathies have demonstrated a reduced circulating (intravascular) and total body pool of albumin, a normal or increased rate of albumin synthesis, markedly shortened albumin survival, and increased fecal protein loss. Whereas normal subjects catabolize 5 to 10 percent of their intravascular albumin pool each day (the fractional catabolic rate), patients with excessive enteric protein loss may have fractional catabolic rates of 50 to 60 percent.

Studies utilizing radioiodinated immunoglobulins have

demonstrated a decreased intravascular globulin pool and increased fractional catabolic rate. However, the synthesis of IgG is usually normal, suggesting that a decreased level of IgG and increased enteric protein loss is not a potent stimulus for IgG synthesis. The increase in fractional catabolic rate is comparable for albumin, IgG, and IgM immunoglobulins, further suggesting that there is bulk loss of plasma proteins into the intestinal tract and not a selective loss of certain proteins. The finding of decreased globulins often is an ancillary aid in excluding renal, cardiac, and hepatic causes of hypoalbuminemia.

Several studies have demonstrated that abnormalities in albumin and globulin metabolism in patients with a protein-losing enteropathy may be reversed or diminished within a few months after the institution of appropriate therapy. It is obviously important that a specific etiologic diagnosis should be established in all patients with treatable disorders, who may be expected to have a remission induced by the appropriate therapy for the underlying disease. The intestinal protein loss in patients with nontropical sprue, Whipple's disease, constrictive pericarditis, regional enteritis, ulcerative colitis, and Menetrier's disease has been ameliorated by therapy appropriate for the underlying disorder.

INTESTINAL LYMPHANGIECTASIA Pathophysiology Intestinal lymphangiectasia is a disorder characterized by increased enteric loss of protein, hypoproteinemia, edema, lymphocytopenia, malabsorption, and abnormal dilated lymphatic channels in the small intestine. The high incidence of chylous effusions and abnormal peripheral, retroperitoneal, and thoracic lymphatics indicates that intestinal lymphangiectasia is part of a generalized congenital disorder of the lymphatic system. It has been suggested that the hypoplastic visceral lymphatic channels result in obstruction to lymph flow with the subsequent development of increased intestinal lymphatic pressure. This in turn may lead to dilated lymphatic vessels throughout the small-bowel wall and mesentery. Hypoproteinemia and steatorrhea are thought to be due to rupture of the dilated lymphatic vessels with discharge of lymph into the bowel lumen. In adults approximately 1,500 ml lymph, containing 70 g fat and 50 g albumin, passes through the thoracic duct each day. The leakage of a small amount of this lymph might be expected to result in considerable loss of protein and fat into the intestinal lumen. In addition, absorption of dietary long-chain triglycerides stimulates lymph flow, and this may increase further the retrograde leakage of intestinal lymph into the lumen. Three lines of evidence support the concept of intestinal leakage of lymph in intestinal lymphangiectasia: (1) chylous fluid has been recovered from the duodenum in these patients; (2) retrograde passage of contrast material from retroperitoneal lymphatics into the duodenum and jejunum has been documented; and (3) significant steatorrhea may persist in patients after institution of a completely fat-free diet, suggesting an increased enteric loss of endogenous fat present in lymph.

Clinical features The disease affects primarily children and young adults. All patients have edema, which may be asymmetrical because of hypoplastic peripheral lymphatics. Chylous effusions and diarrhea are common symptoms. The primary laboratory finding is hypoproteinemia with decreased serum levels of albumin, immunoglobulins IgG, IgA, and IgM, transferrin, and ceruloplasmin. Despite moderate to severe hypogammaglobulinemia there does not appear to be an increased incidence of pyogenic bacterial infections. In addition, circulating antibody response to challenge with *Brucella* and typhoid antigens is normal. Steatorrhea is usually mild, although in some instances fat loss may be as much as 40 g per day. Some patients have hypocalcemia and impaired absorption of vitamin B_{12}. Lymphocytopenia (due to the loss of lymphocytes in lymph) is common, with lymphocyte counts ranging from 400 to 1,000 per ml (normal: 1,500 to 4,000 per ml). This is associated with abnormal delayed hypersensitivity as evidenced by prolonged homograft survival and impaired cutaneous responsiveness to antigens such as mumps and monilia.

Small-bowel roentgenograms are frequently abnormal, showing changes of mucosal edema and a malabsorption pattern. Lymphangiograms may demonstrate hypoplastic peripheral and visceral lymphatics with the absence of groups of retroperitoneal lymph nodes. Specimens of jejunal mucosa characteristically reveal dilated and telangiectatic lymphatic vessels in the lamina propria and submucosa. The villi may be club-shaped because of distortion from grossly dilated lymphatics (Fig. 284-4). Such changes in the intestinal mucosa may be reversed after appropriate therapy. The diagnosis of intestinal lymphangiectasia is, therefore, established by (1) small-intestinal biopsy and (2) demonstration of increased enteric protein loss using radioactive macromolecules.

Treatment A low fat diet, by decreasing lymph flow, usually results in significant improvement with decreased fecal fat excretion, decreased enteric protein loss, increased serum calcium and albumin levels, and an increased half-life of injected ^{131}I-labeled albumin. Similar results may be obtained by the substitution of medium-chain triglycerides (MCT) for dietary long-chain triglycerides, since MCT are transported as medium-chain fatty acids by the portal vein rather than via the lymph.

REFERENCES

Ament ME et al: Structure and function of the gastrointestinal tract in primary immunodeficiency syndromes. Medicine 52:227, 1973

Benson GD et al: Adult celiac disease with emphasis upon response to the gluten-free diet. Medicine 43:1, 1964

Falchuk ZM, Strober W: Increased jejunal immunoglobulin synthesis in patients with non-tropical sprue as measured by a solid-phase immunoadsorption technique. J Lab Clin Med 79:1004, 1972

Hellier MD et al: Dipeptide absorption in man. Gut 13:965, 1972

Hofmann AF: The syndrome of ileal disease and the broken enterohepatic circulation: Cholerheic enteropathy. Gastroenterology 52:752, 1967

Klipstein FA: Tropical sprue in New York City. Gastroenterology 47:457, 1964

Krone CL et al: Studies on the pathogenesis of malabsorption:

Lipid hydrolysis and micelle formation in the intestinal lumen. Medicine 47:89, 1968

SAVILAHTI E: Intestinal immunoglobulins in children with coeliac disease. Gut 13:958, 1972

TABAQCHALI S: The pathophysiological role of small intestinal bacterial flora. Scand J Gastroenterol (Supp) 6:139, 1970

TRIER JS et al: Whipple's disease: Light and electron microscopic correlation of jejunal mucosal histology with antibiotic treatment and clinical status. Gastroenterology 48:684, 1965

WALDMANN TA: Protein-losing enteropathy. Gastroenterology 50:422, 1966

WEINSTEIN WM et al: Collagenous sprue: Unrecognized type of malabsorption. N Engl J Med 283:1297, 1970

WELCH JD: Isolated lactase deficiency in humans: Report on 100 patients. Medicine 49:257, 1970

WHALEN GE et al: Diabetic diarrhea: A clinical and pathophysiological study. Gastroenterology 56:1021, 1969

WILSON FA, DIETSCHY JM: Differential diagnostic approach to malabsorption. Gastroenterology 61:911, 1971

285 DISEASES OF THE SMALL INTESTINE

ALBERT I. MENDELOFF

DIVERTICULOSIS

It is usually impossible on clinical grounds to decide whether diverticula of the intestinal tract are congenital or acquired. The rarer congenital diverticula contain the entire thickness of the intestinal wall, whereas acquired diverticula consist of mucosa and serosa alone. Probably the defect in the muscular wall through which the mucosa herniates is always potentially present, usually at the points where the nutrient arteries perforate the serosal and muscular layers. As with other forms of herniations, these potential tunnels are widened as life proceeds, so that all forms of diverticulosis are more common among persons in the later decades of life. Some individuals display great numbers of diverticula of the gastrointestinal tract, from esophagus to anus, but more often diverticula of the stomach and small intestine are solitary; they are more common in the duodenum (in possibly 5 percent of all persons having barium studies of this area), next most frequent in the jejunum, and rare in the ileum, except for Meckel's diverticulum.

Diverticula of the duodenum are most commonly found on the medial surface of the second portion of the duodenum, in close proximity to the entrance of the pancreatic and common ducts. They are usually wide-necked, about 1 cm in diameter, and appear to fill with and expel intestinal contents with ease.

The location of duodenal diverticula constitutes the main reason for suspecting their pathogenicity. Although statistically few patients harboring these common outpouchings suffer any misfortune from their presence, there are documented cases in which obstruction to the neck of the diverticulum has led to acute diverticulitis, hemorrhage, and necrosis of the wall; pressure exerted by obstructed diverticula on pancreatic ducts has definitely resulted in acute pancreatitis, pressure on the common duct in obstructive jaundice. When diverticula occur along the third portion of the duodenum they have occasionally been the site of acute inflammation and free perforation, with consequent peritonitis.

Diverticula of the jejunum, while less common, seem to be more subject to the development of acute inflammation and necrosis of the wall, with severe upper abdominal pain and occasionally massive intestinal hemorrhage ensuing. The acute process may go on to suppurate; a definite mass and localized peritonitis are the accompanying physical findings. Another way in which multiple diverticula of the jejunum may result in disease is the effective replacement of normal absorbing jejunal surface by multiple bacteria-filled sacs (Fig. 285-1), resulting in a loss of surface and bacterial action which deconjugates bile salts and actively competes for such nutrients as vitamin B_{12} (see Chap. 284).

Meckel's diverticulum, resulting from persistence of the omphalomesenteric duct, is reasonably common, occurring in about 3 percent of all laparotomized children in whom a definite search is made and in about 2 percent of autopsied adults. Even though only a small percentage of these diverticula cause trouble, the possibility must be thought of in every case of gastrointestinal hemorrhage and obstruction. The diverticula are usually found on the antimesenteric border within the last 90 cm of the ileum, and most frequently within 50 cm of the ileocecal valve. They may be wide-mouthed or narrow, short or long, sometimes a nubbin hard to find on the smooth surface of the ileum, occasionally a long 10- to 20-cm funnel attached like a stout pipe to the umbilicus. Diverticula lying within the mesentery are rare and do not arise from the

FIGURE 285-1
Multiple diverticula of jejunum in a 55-year-old man with macrocytic anemia.

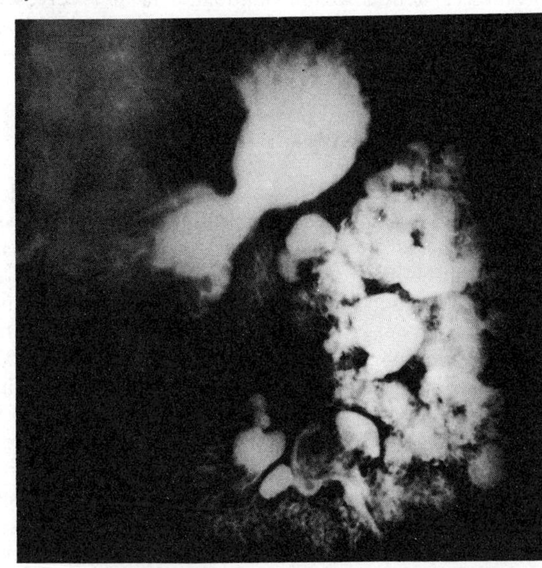

omphalomesenteric duct. The diverticulum may be lined with normal ileal mucosa, or it may contain varying amounts of ectopic gastric, pancreatic, duodenal, or colonic epithelium. Symptoms are more common in males by at least 3:1. Coincident malformations are infrequently met. There is no hereditary pattern. In children and adolescents, bleeding from this epithelium is the striking clinical feature, with or without the presence of a palpable mass. The source of bleeding is almost invariably an ulceration, and this is generally of peptic origin. The gastric mucosa in Meckel's diverticulum has been shown to secrete acid peptic juice, which acts on bordering ileal epithelium to produce the ulcer. Pathologically the ulcer is always near the junction of gastric and ileal mucosa, on the ileal side; it thus resembles the usual anastomotic ulcer occurring after gastrojejunostomy. In the young adult the clinical picture begins to change, inflammatory processes becoming more prominent, and varying degrees of intestinal obstruction, either of the ileum proximal to the diverticulum or of neighboring loops of bowel trapped behind the inflammatory mass, constitute the most serious presenting symptoms. Free perforation of Meckel's diverticulum is relatively uncommon, but sealed-off localized perforations are very common once the initial inflammatory process has distorted the bowel enough to set up the pathologic requisites for cyclic bouts of inflammation. A number of these patients have repeated bouts of low-grade abdominal cramps referred to the infraumbilical area, usually aggravated by eating. The diagnosis is rarely made by x-ray studies of the small or large intestine, but these are necessary in order to eliminate other possible lesions. The treatment is entirely surgical.

BRUNNER'S GLAND HYPERTROPHY

Occasionally one notes on radiologic examination a cobblestone appearance of the duodenal bulb caused by hypertrophy of Brunner's glands, submucosal structures secreting an alkaline mucoid material of unknown function, highly viscid, and apparently affording a mechanical protective action to the duodenum as it receives acid chyme. Most patients showing this hypertrophy have no evidence of disordered duodenal function, but occasionally they have peptic symptoms.

MOTOR DISTURBANCES

OBSTRUCTIVE SYNDROMES The natural tendency of smooth muscle when operating against a pressure gradient is to stretch and contract forcibly. This increased distention is pain-producing (see Chap. 8). Thus all syndromes in which normal small bowel is trying to force luminal contents past nonrelaxing segments of more distal bowel, whether occasioned by a tumor, a stricture, an occluding gallstone, or a constricting band, are primarily characterized by *painful cramps at the onset*, progressing to loss of pain sensation as the bowel loses its viability. Associated with the progress of events are many others which may assume prominent roles in coloring the symptoms evoked. Intermittent jejunal or ileal obstruction, with poor maintenance of oil-water interfaces, will lead to malabsorption (see Chaps. 8 and 286).

Motor abnormalities of the duodenum associated with many psychic disturbances (e.g., anorexia nervosa) or with generalized disorders like lupus erythematosus may result in severe bouts of nausea and vomiting. The radiologist may get the impression of an organic obstruction of the third portion of the duodenum at the point at which the superior mesenteric vessels cross anterior to the gut. Such impressions have given rise to many diagnoses of "mesenteric root compression syndrome" which fail to be borne out on surgical exploration to remove the source of the obstruction. An atonic or sluggish duodenum proximal to this "compressed" area will of itself produce the apparent obstructive picture, just as gastric atony may make a normal pyloric area appear to be "obstructing." Only if the peristaltic activity of the first and second portions of the duodenum is normal or hyperactive can one suspect an organic obstruction of the third portion of the duodenum. If this is identified, exploration is indicated and a bypassing operation justified.

STASIS Complete stasis of the duodenum occurs rarely, usually in association with mesenteric vascular catastrophes. On x-ray examination, dilatation of the duodenum with a peculiar churning of the barium meal is characteristically noted in the patient with anorexia nervosa and, occasionally, in those suffering from severe ulcerative colitis. Elsewhere in the small intestine, stasis is the result of loss of vascular integrity, and exhaustion following mechanical or paralytic ileus (Chap. 286).

SPASM Spasm of the duodenum occurs in peptic disorders, acute pancreatitis, or in various conditions associated with severe nausea. Experimental nausea, as, for example, that produced by vestibular stimulation, gives characteristically a tetanic spasm of the duodenum.

PAIN Migratory or steady pain around the umbilicus may result from *insufficiency of the mesenteric vessels*, usually as a result of degenerative aortic disease encroaching on the lumina of the vessels. The celiac axis can be compressed by fibrous portions of the diaphragm, eliciting attacks of high epigastric pain. Angiography is necessary to identify such pathologic processes.

REGIONAL ENTERITIS (CROHN'S DISEASE)

The most disabling and discouraging affliction of the small intestine known to the internist is regional enteritis, an unpredictable granulomatous response of the submucosa to an unknown agent or agents, in which damage is done by encroachment upon the lumen, scarring of the muscle, ulceration of the mucosa, and necrotic breakdown with fistula formation between loops of bowel, bowel and skin, and bowel and perirectal spaces. Any, all, or none of these sequelae may follow the initial bout of the disease, and single attacks are well documented. Much more common, however, is recurrence and slow spread of the lesion to involve contiguous areas of the intestine, including occasionally the duodenum. Involvement of the antrum of the stomach by a similar process has been described.

Since the original description by Crohn, Ginzburg, and Oppenheimer in 1932, in which this disorder was localized to the terminal ileum, a number of different clinical syndromes have been distinguished from the classic forms, but our knowledge is far from satisfactory as to causes, course, and proper management.

EPIDEMIOLOGY The disorder is worldwide in distribution and occurs among all races. In the United States its exact incidence is unknown, but it appears to be about one-third as common as chronic ulcerative colitis. In the United States, the annual incidence is about 2 to 3 per 100,000. It has been reported as having its onset in every decade of life, the peak incidence being between the ages of fifteen and thirty-five. Both sexes are equally affected; Negroes are less commonly affected than whites.

The patients are often of Jewish origin; in some series Jews are affected three times more often than their distribution in the population would suggest. The patients show urban backgrounds more commonly than rural and reach higher levels of schooling than usual and slightly higher economic status than ordinarily encountered. Despite some evidence to the contrary, severely disturbed personalities are not routinely met with in these patients, particularly early in the course of the disease or antedating the onset of the disease. Many such patients show remarkable fortitude in meeting the innumerable difficulties wrought by progressive destruction of the intestine; a number have distinguished themselves in the arts, sciences, professions, and business despite prolonged and progressive disease.

Familial occurrence of the disease has been recognized from the onset. In various series the percentage of cases occurring in siblings ranges from 2 to 10; father-daughter, mother-son, and father-son patterns are recorded in all large series of cases. No genetic markers have as yet been identified.

ETIOLOGY AND PATHOGENESIS No specific cause of this disease has been identified. Investigations have been carried out on the possible etiologic relationship of bacterial and viral organisms identified no more frequently in the gastrointestinal tract of these patients than in normal subjects, but all such studies have been fruitless. Certain disorders of the mesenteric arteries seen in the aging population have occasionally given rise to a submucosal inflammatory and cicatricial reaction producing a picture similar to that of regional enteritis, but in the majority of cases of regional enteritis no such arterial lesions can be found. The enlarged and succulent lymph nodes of the mesentery seem to result from the submucosal inflammation rather than cause it; remarkable alterations in the autonomic ganglions of the bowel wall, frequently seen in excised specimens, are rarely present early in the course of the disease. Histochemical studies are remarkably normal, particularly with respect to the columnar epithelium of the bowel luminal surface. Noncaseating tubercles are found in about half the cases in the bowel submucosa and in the serosa; these show giant cells but no evidence of fungi or inclusion bodies. The fistulous tracts usually show only granulation tissue and a purulent response.

The earliest lesions, as seen in the terminal ileum, are rarely minute and more usually involve appreciable (6 to 20 cm) lengths of gut in a swollen beefy glistening mass, occasionally rather purplish, but more often intensely red. The serosa is often injected and the mesenteric fat edematous. Large lymph nodes in the mesentery nearby are commonly noted. The luminal surface of the bowel is thrown up into injected folds stretched over the heaped-up submucosal hypertrophy (Fig. 285-2). Ulceration of this mucosa, although common, is usually superficial in the early stages of the disease, when microscopically the nonulcerated areas of mucosa appear healthy.

There is usually gradual demarcation between the diseased and healthy bowel; the appendix may be involved by a similar process or may merely show lymphoid hyperplasia and venous congestion as a result of the adjacent inflammatory reaction. The initial process may disappear rather quickly, may remain indolent only to flare up months or years later, or may slowly progress to involve ileal segments more cephalad. "Skips" are well documented in which an initial ileal lesion subsides and a midjejunal lesion of similar character develops later, the intervening area remaining uninvolved. Adjacent or contiguous small or large intestine may be involved, if not invaded, by this inflammatory process; cicatrization, local perforations, abscesses, and fistulas commonly characterize the development of such a process. The fistulas may go from intestine to colon, from intestine to skin, or from one loop of intestine to another. Loops low in the pelvis or involving sigmoid colon may fistulize into the adnexae or vagina and produce perirectal or ischiorectal abscesses, perirectal nodular masses seen on proctoscopy, or a patchy proctitis.

A number of changes—endothelial cell proliferation in lymphatics, giant-cell aggregations in the edematous submucosa, ischemic contraction of smaller arterioles, and increased numbers of ganglion cells and neurofibrillar accumulations—occur characteristically in surgical and autopsy material and in such profusion as to render the pathologic diagnosis of the disease easy to make. However, the primacy of any one of these changes, or even the proper sequence of lesions, is not clear.

The endothelial reaction in lymphatics and the presence of granulomas have suggested to many that the disease must be a reaction to some irritant absorbed in the lymphatics; the absence of foreign bodies in the giant cells would lead one not to suspect particulate foreign matter as the offending agent; attempts have been made to produce the disease experimentally by abnormal fatty substances, but so far these studies have been fruitless. Sarcoidosis, tuberculosis, and reaction to abdominal trauma seem unrelated to the characteristic forms of this disease, even though some of the granulomas may be indistinguishable from the characteristic lesions of these processes. There is a peculiarly indolent reaction of lymphocytes in these patients, both of those cells surrounding the submucosal lymphatics and of those in the peripheral blood. Some have postulated an immunological deficit in the response to the unknown inciting agent in the bowel analogous to the sluggishness of the blastic transformation of peripheral lymphocytes to phytohemagglutinin.

SYMPTOMS These depend on the location of the inflammatory lesion, its extent, its acuteness, the amount of obstruction it produces, the peritoneal reaction, if any, and its relationship to contiguous structures. A certain number of such patients may present only with the systemic features of a febrile illness without localizing symptoms or signs. Even in these cases, a careful history will often document abdominal discomfort, loose stools, rectal urgency, and mild anorexia made worse by the feeling that abdominal discomfort increases after eating. Spondylitis occurs in a small percentage.

Acute ileitis presents as the sudden development of right lower quadrant pain and tenderness, with fever, localized guarding, and some disturbance of bowel motility—either diarrhea or constipation. It thus presents the clinical picture of appendicitis, and the differential diagnosis can be made only at laparotomy, when the characteristic beefy red terminal ileum, boggy mesenteric fat, and succulent lymph nodes of the mesentery tell the surgeon that appendicitis alone could not produce the picture. The appendix also may be involved in the primary lesion, or it may be obstructed secondarily by the acute submucosal edema of the adjacent ileitis.

In one large series, diarrhea, colicky pain, and weight loss were encountered as presenting symptoms in over two-thirds of 600 patients. Fever occurred in one-third, and a history of bright red rectal bleeding or melena in less than one-sixth. Symptoms related to rectal and anal complications predominated in about 10 percent.

Approximately half the patients have initial involvement of the terminal ileum, another 15 percent have both ileum and cecum affected at the onset, and less than 4 percent present initial symptoms due exclusively to jejunal or duodenal involvement. Various other combinations of jejunal, ileal, and colonic lesions may be seen at the time the patient first consults the physician.

Variants of this picture include (1) a full-blown *malabsorption syndrome* (Chap. 284) with any one or many malnutritive derangements capturing the spotlight, (2) *acute perforation and generalized peritonitis* (less than 1 percent), or (3) *massive melena*, seen in less than 2 percent of cases. The advanced case, with cutaneous fistulas, easily appreciable masses throughout the abdomen, increased pigmentation, and severe proctitis, presents little difficulty in diagnosis. Amyloidosis due to regional enteritis is becoming a more frequent complication and may be responsible for the patient's death in renal failure.

As experience with the disease as a whole has expanded, a small number of patients have been encountered who present a diffuse involvement of jejunum and ileum when first seen. These patients have been described by Crohn as having a subtype of regional enteritis in which the lesions are more superficial but much more extensive, less prone to suppurative complications and fistula formations, but likely to lead to

FIGURE 285-2
Regional enteritis: resected specimen of ileocecal area demonstrating the hypertrophy of ileal submucosa (right), *with nodular encroachment on the lumen and minute areas of mucosal hemorrhage.*

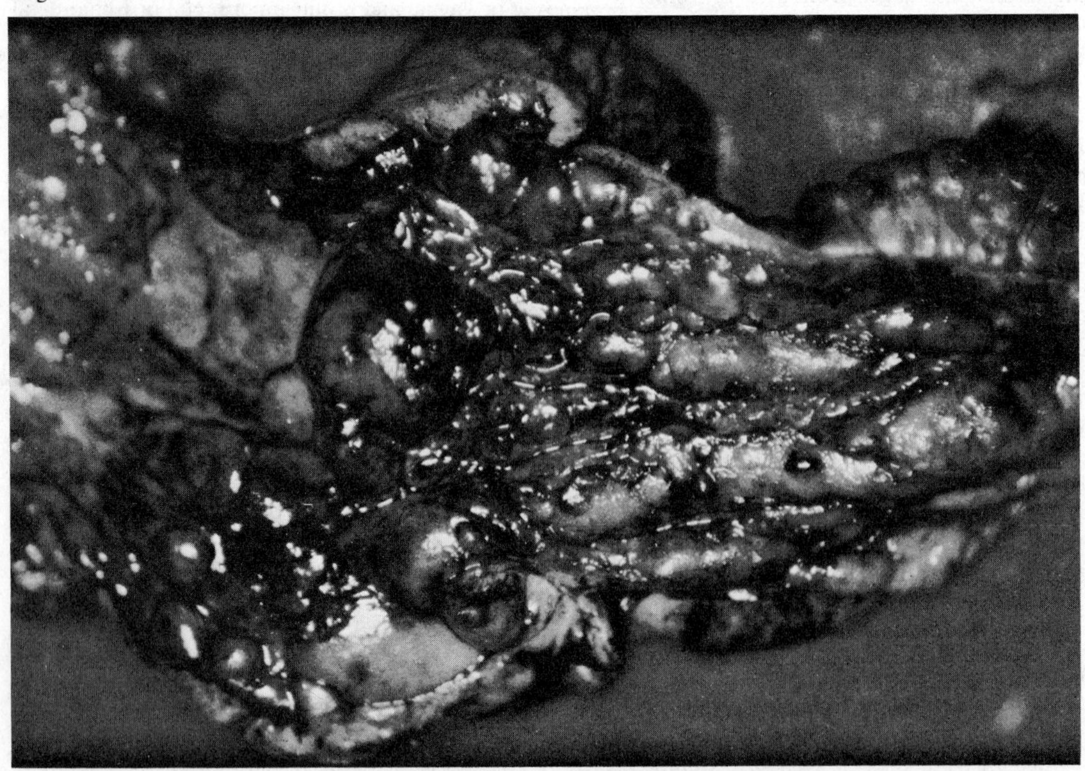

malabsorptive symptoms, fever, splenomegaly, and clubbing of the fingers, the reasons for which are not understood.

On physical examination patients with enteritis characteristically show evidence of undernutrition and malnutrition if the symptoms are of long standing. Clubbing of the fingers and acrocyanosis are common. Special attention to the abdominal examination is necessary, since a definite mass or doughy aggregations of bowel loops can be felt in one-third of the patients. Fistulous tracts between the involved bowel and the abdominal skin are classic complications of the disease and are easily appreciated. More readily overlooked are the perirectal and ischiorectal fistulas found in nearly 10 percent of chronic cases; rectal digital examination will disclose an anorectal stricture in half of these cases and in 3 to 4 percent of those without fistulas. Proctoscopic examination is abnormal in 10 to 15 percent; the abnormalities may include nodular submucosal masses, acute proctitis, ulceration, or stricture in the rectosigmoid junction. Rectovaginal fistulas are noted in a small percentage of cases.

DIAGNOSIS Regional enteritis should be suspected on clinical grounds in most instances when a patient presents with a history of intermittent chronic diarrhea, fever, weight loss, crampy abdominal pain, or joint symptoms, and on physical examination shows abdominal masses, perianal suppuration, and anal strictures. It should be part of the differential diagnosis of all types of malabsorption (Chap. 284), fever of unexplained origin, intermittent small-bowel obstruction, polyarthritis, and amyloidosis.

Laboratory features of regional enteritis parallel the severity of the (1) inflammatory reaction: leukocytosis, elevated sedimentation rate; (2) blood loss by ulceration: iron deficiency anemia; (3) undernutrition and malabsorption: hypoalbuminemia, hypocalcemia, hypokalemia, elevated serum alkaline phosphatase level, hypoprothrombinemia, and macrocytic anemia; (4) possibly more specific changes related to disturbed protein metabolism: increased seromucoids in the serum and hypergammaglobulinemia. The inflammatory lesion may cause a continual leak of albumin from the blood, leading to hypoalbuminemia. None of these laboratory tests is diagnostic.

The most helpful adjunct to the clinician suspicious of regional enteritis is the radiologist, who generally establishes the diagnosis short of histologic confirmation. Marshak and Wolf have tried to separate the nonstenotic phase of regional enteritis from the stenotic phase on radiologic grounds, despite the fact that occasionally both phases may be encountered in the same patient. In the nonstenotic phase the principal changes are loss of detail in the mucosa, stiffening of the submucosa to form a tubular pattern on the radiograph, and separation of the tubular loops by inflammation in the mesentery. The stenotic phase is characterized by narrowing of the lumen, with dilatation of normal bowel proximally. In the dilated area poor oil-water interfaces and retained mucus secretions produce abnormal puddling of the barium. Fistulous tracts are often seen, particularly in the ileocecal area, and are virtually diagnostic, the only other disease likely to produce a similar picture being actinomycosis. When the duodenum or upper jejunum is involved by regional enteritis, the stenotic phase predominates from the onset, whereas ileal involvement characteristically is nonstenotic and ulcerative early in its course (Fig. 285-3). The unoperated case usually demonstrates little radiologic change after the first studies are completed, except for fistula formation.

Definitive diagnosis on histologic grounds is established under the microscope, although most surgeons can make an accurate diagnosis by inspection at the operating table of the beefy reddish-to-bluish serosa, edematous mesentery, and large lymph nodes. Differential diagnosis in the operating room includes tuberculosis, various lymphomas, sarcoidosis, and fungus diseases. Biopsies of the bowel and lymph nodes provide adequate bases for histologic diagnosis.

COURSE AND PROGNOSIS Acute regional ileitis apparently is self-limited in over two-thirds of the cases; the remaining one-third go on to develop chronic enteritis. Since many patients first operated upon for seemingly acute symptoms present to the surgeon the picture of *chronic* disease with acute exacerbation, reported differences in the course of patients so operated upon must reflect differences in the criteria for making the diagnosis of "acute" disease.

Accurate prognostication in this disease is at present impossible. Those who develop symptoms before age 20 generally have a more severe illness, require surgery earlier, and have more recurrences. Almost every large series of cases consists of a heterogeneous population

FIGURE 285-3
Regional enteritis. Several involved loops of ileum communicate via multiple fistulous tracts. Small bowel proximal to involved areas is dilated (upper).

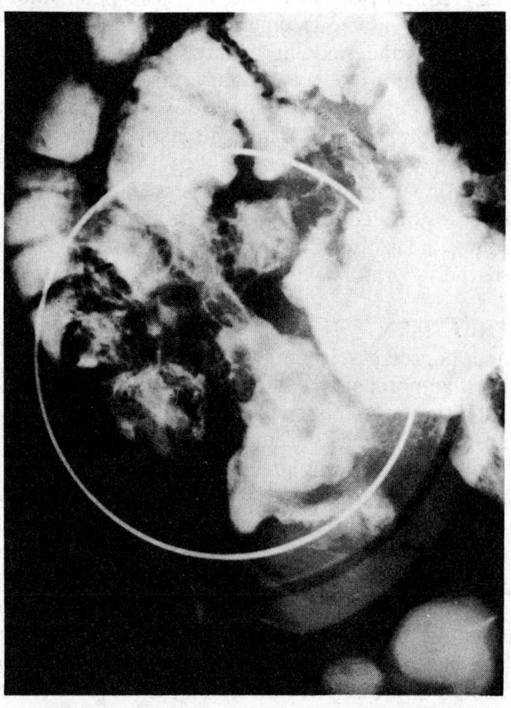

with enteritis of different longevity and severity, the majority of whom require surgery for some complication of the original disease. The extent of the intestinal lesions in an unoperated case tends to remain at the level present when the patient was first seen, except for the development of fistulas. If operation is carried out to remove the entire diseased bowel, as was the custom soon after the disease was first identified, approximately half the cases have a recurrence of the disease within a few years of the operation. Whether this is due to failure at operation to recognize "skip" areas of enteritis proximal to the resected area or whether new foci of enteritis develop in hitherto normal bowel is not clear. In any case, the physician should expect a patient with regional enteritis to have exacerbations and remissions over a period of many years; these exacerbations usually involve the same areas of bowel established as diseased in the first attack, but ulceration, fistulas, and stenosis may supervene at any time. Extension of these suppurative and necrotic lesions to neighboring loops of small bowel, colon, bladder, and perirectal tissues may be constantly suspected and looked for by the physician. Gallstones are more commonly encountered in these patients than expected, no doubt due to disturbance of the enterohepatic circulation of bile salts. Right hydronephrosis is an important sequel of inflammatory spread deep to the ileocecal region, involving the right ureter. The incidence of cancer of the small intestine is probably increased in patients with chronic regional enteritis.

Involvement of the colon by a granulomatous inflammatory process is reported by some workers in half their cases of enteritis, and there is no question that primary Crohn's disease of the colon is a definite entity (see Chap. 288).

Involvement of more distant organs and organ systems unrelated to the intestine has been reported with increasing frequency as these patients have been studied more closely over a long time span. Liver abnormalities are common, and nodular pancreatitis has been reported; their relation to the primary disease is probably important, despite the transfusions, injections, and drugs these patients receive and the many nutritional deficiencies they incur. More significant is the incidence of arthritic symptoms which also are noted in a proportion of cases of ulcerative colitis. The arthritis involves larger joints and is often of the spondylitis type, unaccompanied by the laboratory data suggestive of rheumatoid disease.

TREATMENT In a chronic disease of unknown cause and unpredictable course, medical management of the most comprehensive type is mandatory. Regardless of the validity of the theory that psychiatric disorder underlies or determines the onset and progression of this disease, it is clear that careful attention to personality factors must proceed *pari passu* with meticulous attempts to meet the nutritional requirements of these patients. These must be combined to assure physical and mental rest as part of the program for combating the discouraging periods during which all efforts of physician and patient seem unable to slow the progress of the process. Psychiatric assistance will be needed in evaluating a number of these cases and should form the principal management in a small percentage. Supportive care consists first of all in explaining to the patient the problem which faces him, the relatively limited areas in which pharmacologic and surgical maneuvers can aid him, and yet at the same time repeatedly pointing out that adequate hyperalimentation, rest, and the more specific measures can enable him to "ride out" the disease; it is generally true that the activity of the disease does slow down after a number of years, at which time the patient will have residua demonstrable on x-ray and physical examination but will be able to lead a reasonably normal life. For women it should be made clear that pregnancy is not something to avoid; many women with severe ileitis but with a genuine wish to have children have produced normal offspring without undue hazard to themselves. Even menstrual function seems preserved better in women with ileitis than in those with ulcerative colitis.

Specific measures Chemotherapeutic and antibiotic drugs are of assistance in managing the purulent complications of enteritis but have little or no effect on the primary disease process. Nonabsorbable sulfonamides have been the most beneficial of these agents.

Medical therapy is directed at suppressing inflammation. For this purpose one has available the adrenal steroids and ACTH, salicylazosulfapyridine, and immunosuppressive drugs. Of the latter, azathioprine has been most extensively employed, but at doses much lower than those used for pronounced immunosuppression.

The results of successful inflammatory inhibition would be expected to reduce the number of inflammatory cells and to allow edema to subside, the intestinal lumen to regain its normal caliber, and the pseudo-obstructive syndrome to disappear. For such results, the *corticosteroids and ACTH* are most effective in producing dramatic immediate improvement. Doses employed should be high—equivalent to 40 to 60 mg prednisone daily for a 2- to 3-week period. After the patient has improved acutely, the dose should be decreased to a maintenance level of 10 to 20 mg prednisone daily; at this point many authorities add salicylazosulfapyridine in doses of 2 to 3 g daily, and then maintain the patient for many months on this dual regimen. Alternate-day steroid therapy is often possible, and offers advantages in reducing the side reactions of hypercorticism.

When such measures fail, and particularly when recurrences are associated with increasing evidence of obstruction or of multiple foci of disease, *azathioprine* may be added to the regimen, at doses of 1.5 to 3.0 mg per kg. Results of this additional therapy are unpredictable, but dramatic improvement has resulted in a small percentage of patients of every series so treated. In patients with diffuse jejunoileitis without obstructive features the use of this combined program probably is the only effective regimen other than purely supportive measures.

Surgical therapy, originally used solely for the complications of a then little-understood process, has gone through a number of stages only to return full circle to its original status. In the 15 years from 1932 to 1947, surgical therapy was thought to effect a cure of the disease; radical resection of the involved ileocecal area in the original group of patients with disease localized there was advocated as curative. The disease recurred in half these patients, usually at the anastomotic site. More conservative by-pass surgery was then advocated; although the operative mortality was probably reduced, recurrence rates were not. Most surgeons now prefer to excise diseased bowel if this can be carried out safely. Overall recurrence rates are about 35 percent, but many of the recurrences are not severe, and respond to medical therapy. Patients who develop their disease in the first two decades of life have more early surgery and are more prone to serious recurrences. Overall, reoperation is necessary in about 25 percent of all those who require one resection; the operative mortality is about 5 percent for each major procedure. Experiments with diverting ileostomies and irrigated loops are of unproven value. About 70 percent of large series of patients who have recurred more than once still maintain reasonably good health, and there is reason to hope that this record can be improved. Whether these recurrences result from outward spread of disease foci not seen at the time of operation or from activation of the disease process by newly contiguous bowel is not clear.

Since surgical measures are not curative, they have now returned to their original place in the therapy of enteritis, as a means of eliminating complications of the disease which are producing serious symptoms on their own. Among these are intermittent intestinal obstruction, blind loops leading to macrocytic anemia, ulcerating lesions in fixed stenotic bowel, and fistulas between the bowel and adjacent hollow viscera.

The case fatality rate for all patients with regional enteritis, regardless of therapy, probably ranges from 5 to 10 percent. Primary cancer of the intestine is a small but definite risk; amyloidosis and renal failure account for a few deaths. Most deaths are due to peritonitis and sepsis.

The sequelae of resections of the small intestine have been of considerable interest in throwing light on the mechanisms of nutrient absorption. The physician caring for a patient with unoperated enteritis must have a good understanding of the nutritional derangements produced by the disease; when that patient has lost, in addition, a sizable segment of his small intestine by resection, the physician must be much more alert in detecting and correcting the multitude of nutritional defects which inevitably result (see Chap. 284).

UNUSUAL DISORDERS OF THE SMALL INTESTINE

MESENTERIC ARTERIAL INSUFFICIENCY The splanchnic area is supplied with arterial blood by the celiac axis, superior mesenteric, and inferior mesenteric arteries. In recent years, as the population of older persons has increased, a growing number of patients presenting ischemic symptoms referred to the periumbilical and general abdominal area has been observed. Gradual luminal encroachment by atherosclerotic or other degenerative changes in the aorta or in any two of these three arteries can produce these painful syndromes, initially brought on 1 or 2 hr after eating, but with further progression resulting in pain that is not only steady but often agonizing. The relationship of pain to food discourages the sufferer from eating; weight loss is therefore prominent. In addition, chronic arterial insufficiency may produce mucosal and mural deterioration, leading to malabsorption, which aggravates the weight loss. When the symptoms are intermittent, the term *abdominal angina* is often used, but this rarely remains static for long, going on either to the development of adequate collateral circulation or to the production of mesenteric infarction. The diagnosis may be confirmed by mesenteric angiography, which is not without serious risk in these patients, of course, but the disease is life-threatening. The only definitive treatment is surgical removal of the obstruction or the construction of bypass arterial grafts to the ischemic bowel.

STENOSING ULCERS OF THE SMALL INTESTINE
Although the existence of rare solitary and unexplained ulcers of the small intestine has been recognized for many years, a recent sharp increase in their incidence has led to studies which appear to implicate a vascular factor producing ischemic necrosis of the mucosa in one or more areas of the small bowel. Most of these newly recognized ulcers occur in patients receiving enteric-coated tablets of materials recognized to be highly caustic to mucosa; the most commonly identified material has been potassium chloride, given routinely to patients receiving chronic diuretic therapy. The symptoms are those of abdominal pain and obstruction, rarely with peritonitis and perforation. The treatment is discontinuance of the medication and surgical excision of the damaged segment if symptoms warrant. Sometimes severe atherosclerotic disease of the mesenteric vessels is the underlying cause.

PROTEIN-LOSING ENTEROPATHY See Chap. 284.

TUMORS OF THE SMALL INTESTINE

Generally, this is an infrequently occurring group of lesions, but because of the variety of symptoms they produce, they may be very difficult to diagnose. It is perhaps best to describe them according to their pathology, since any or all of them may produce identical symptoms.

BENIGN TUMORS *Leiomyomas* of clinical significance are rare in the small intestine, but they may produce intussusception with obstruction, ulceration and hemorrhage, with fatal outcome, or varying degrees of intestinal obstruction alone. The mucosa becomes stretched tightly over these solid tumors and frequently ulcerates to produce gastrointestinal hemorrhage of mild to fatal severity. Malignant change may occur at any time.

Hemangiomas of the small intestine, although rare, are very difficult to identify by clinical methods or radiologic examination. When they bleed suddenly into the bowel wall, they often collapse, so that they do not present to radiologic study any space-occupying defect in the barium-filled bowel. Here mesenteric angiography may be very successful in demonstrating the tumor and its leakage of contrast material into the lumen. The occurrence of these various syndromes as hereditary disorders is well documented, and a hint as to the existence of an intestinal hemangioma may well be gleaned from identification of hemangiomas of the skin or mucous membrane.

Lipomas are more common than leiomyomas or hemangiomas in the small intestine and, like them, may be involved in developmental anomalies of supporting tissues in the bowel and elsewhere. Although a number of these could be considered to be hamartomas, they do exhibit the neoplastic ability to grow and expand. Characteristically, they are found in middle adult life, although they may have been growing slowly for many years before making clinical mischief. Sex incidence is probably equal. It is probable that they arise from adipose tissue anywhere in the body. Since the mesentery of the small intestine contains a large amount of such tissue, a variety of lipomas involving the wall of the bowel to produce obstruction have been documented.

Polypoid tumors of the small intestine usually turn out to be hamartomas. These have been thoroughly studied as part of the Peutz-Jeghers syndrome (see Chap. 55). Such tumors are rarely malignant but may cause intussusception and hemorrhage.

MALIGNANT TUMORS Malignant tumors of the small intestine are not common in the United States, accounting for less than 1 percent of all digestive tract cancers. In Africa, on the other hand, primary tumors of the small intestine have been described among some races as more common than carcinoma of the stomach.

Adenocarcinoma of the duodenum is more frequent as an independent lesion than is carcinoma of the jejunum or ileum. However, in recent years diffuse carcinomas of the small bowel have been described in patients with long-standing regional enteritis. The most frequently involved area of duodenum is the second, near the papilla of Vater. The tumor usually causes ulceration with hemorrhage or high obstruction and may be easily confused radiologically with chronic peptic ulcer in the same area. Carcinoma of the jejunoileum may present as diffuse foci of intestinal obstruction due to early metastases to the peritoneum, as ascites, or as a malabsorption syndrome.

Argentaffine tumors are found in 0.5 percent of all surgically removed appendixes, as a yellowish indurated area. They are the most common epithelial tumors of the small intestine and may appear anywhere from the duodenum to the colon. They arise from argentaffin cells in the crypts of Lieberkühn and grow as clumps or strands of small closely packed polyhedral cells. The degree to which these tumors are regarded as malignant varies among pathologists, but there is increasing recognition of their invasive tendencies. They are often multiple, but when solitary some 60 percent arise in the ileum, enlarging to form plaques projecting into the muscularis and serosa. Adenofibrosis of the surrounding tissues accompanies this spread so that ulceration from the luminal spread and compromise of the lumen by pressure of the inflammatory reaction may produce the symptoms. They are tumors of middle age, more common in males. Remote spread is infrequent and late. For some reason, lesions of the duodenum tend less to invade surrounding tissues. When metastases invade the liver, the characteristic *carcinoid syndrome* results (see Chap. 99).

Lymphosarcoma, which may develop in any region where lymphoid tissue is present, is an important invader of the small intestine. Reticulum cell sarcoma usually develops in retroperitoneal lymph nodes, secondarily involving the bowel; localized lymphosarcoma usually involves the ileum as a solid bulky tumor which may cause ileal obstruction. It may remain stationary for a long time and can produce an x-ray picture simulating that of localized ileitis. When it spreads, it does so slowly, to regional lymph nodes. Hodgkin's granuloma and sarcoma may invade any organ in the body, but they rarely cause localized lesions in the small intestine. Enlarged retroperitoneal nodes may distort the x-ray picture of the upper small intestine, but localized infiltrations are uncommon. *Alpha-chain disease*, a variant of Mediterranean lymphoma, affects young people of Mediterranean origin, producing severe abdominal pain and diarrhea, with malabsorption and often hypoproteinemia.

Both *liposarcomas and leiomyosarcomas* are infrequently encountered in the small intestine. The symptoms may be the same as those of the benign tumors or of any malignant lesion.

DIAGNOSIS Tumors of the small intestine should be thought of in the differential diagnosis of obstructive syndromes of any type, of gastrointestinal bleeding, and of malabsorptive states. They are less likely to cause fever than is regional enteritis or tuberculosis, but in all other respects benign inflammatory disease, benign tumors, and malignant tumors of this organ can produce identical clinical syndromes. The reason for this is not hard to find, since most symptoms are due to (1) ulceration of mucosa with bleeding, (2) obstruction of the lumen behind which mucosal bowel wall contracts forcibly, giving rise to crampy pain, (3) necrosis and inflammation of the wall, giving rise to persistent pain and tender masses, (4) interference with intraluminal, mucosal, and lymphatic aspects of digestion and absorption of nutrients, producing abnormal stools, weight loss, anorexia, vomiting, and occasionally intestinal obstruction.

Radiologic techniques designed to differentiate localized from generalized lesions, pressure of enlarged nodes or inflammatory abscesses on the intestines, "deficiency patterns" and flocculation of barium in the bowel lumen, distortion of outlines of the bowel by stiffened mesentery—all these may be of the greatest diagnostic assistance or may indicate in only a general way the nature of the underlying disease.

Localization of a specific bleeding point may be achieved either by use of a long plastic tube through which intraluminal contents are aspirated and tested for blood or, especially if bleeding is brisk, by mesenteric angiography of the celiac axis or superior mesenteric artery.

Careful microscopic and chemical testing of the stools may confirm the presence or absence of an inflammatory exudate, cancer cells, and malabsorbed or maldigested foodstuffs, as well as blood, abnormal concretions, or parasites.

If a diagnosis of tumor is made presumptively or if symptoms persist and no diagnosis can be arrived at, laparotomy is indicated. Therapy for most of the tumors described is entirely surgical. In the case of lymphomas and lymphosarcomas, local removal and general irradiation or chemotherapy are employed.

REFERENCES

ALEXANDER-WILLIAMS J et al: A comparison of results of excision and bypass for ileal Crohn's disease. Gut 13:973, 1972

BOCKUS HL (ed): Regional enteritis, chap. 50 in *Gastroenterology*, 2d ed., vol. 2, Philadelphia: Saunders, 1964

BOLEY SJ et al: Experimental evaluation of thiazides and potassium as a cause of small-bowel ulcer. JAMA 192:93, 1965

CROHN BB, YARNIS H: *Regional Ileitis*, 2d ed., New York: Grune & Stratton, 1958

DOE WF et al: Five cases of alpha chain disease. Gut 13:947, 1972

FRY WJ, KRAFT RO: Visceral angina. Surg Gynecol Obstet 117:417, 1963

THAYER WR JR: Crohn's disease (regional enteritis). Scand J Gastroenterol 5:(suppl. 6)165, 1970

286
ACUTE INTESTINAL OBSTRUCTION

ALBERT I. MENDELOFF
ARNOLD M. SELIGMAN

DEFINITION Acute intestinal obstruction may be defined as a failure of progression of intestinal contents, whether due to mechanical causes or to inadequacy of intestinal muscular activity.

ETIOLOGY The most useful classification is based on the immediate need for surgical or medical therapy. The *mechanical* type of intestinal obstruction usually requires surgical intervention for its correction. This type is due either to intraluminal obstruction by foreign bodies, gallstones, meconium, bezoars, enteroliths, and worms or to mural obstruction due to encroachment by compression of the intestinal wall, as in adhesions, stenosis, hernia, volvulus, intussusception, tumors, and atresia. *Nonmechanical obstruction* is referred to as *ileus.* Ileus is either adynamic (paralytic) or dynamic (spastic).

Adynamic ileus occurs (1) reflexly after certain surgical manipulations, diagnostic studies such as retrograde pyelography, or trauma; (2) secondary to peritoneal insult by chemical agents (hydrochloric acid or blood), pancreatic enzymes, or bacterial agents; (3) as the result of metabolic changes secondary to generalized dislocation of electrolyte equilibrium, especially abnormally low serum potassium levels, interference with the enzymes and coenzymes involved in acetylcholine synthesis (pantothenic acid), or drug effects (especially ganglionic blocking agents); (4) following mechanical *hypoactivity* in which the musculature of the intestinal wall loses its functional integrity on the basis of localized hypoxia secondary to compromised blood supply. This can happen suddenly as a result of arterial spasm secondary to venous or arterial thrombosis or embolism of intestinal vasculature, or more slowly when obstructing factors progress to a degree that embarrasses the arterial or venous blood flow through localized portions of the bowel.

Spastic ileus is an uncommon form of mechanical *hyperactivity* of the normal bowel behind a spastic segment or segments of the gut. It is seen in toxic conditions such as uremia, heavy metal poisoning, porphyria, infections, and extensive ulcerations.

Untreated ileus with progressive distension enhances mechanical obstruction as well as circulatory embarrassment in the wall of the involved segment. In this way partial mechanical occlusion may progress to complete obstruction and eventually strangulation.

SYMPTOMS Acute mechanical intestinal obstruction is characterized by colicky pain, nausea, vomiting, distention, and constipation or obstipation. Obstruction high in the intestinal tract produces earlier and more severe vomiting, whereas obstruction low in the intestinal tract produces earlier obstipation, more distention, and later vomiting. When obstruction is accompanied by strangulation, the pain is more severe and constant, and evidence of sepsis soon develops. Diagnosis of the strangulation is relatively easy when a large segment of bowel is involved, but the diagnosis of devitalized bowel, although equally important, is difficult when only a few centimeters of bowel is involved. When the obstruction is primarily due to adynamic ileus, pain is absent, obstipation is present, and discomfort results when distention is severe enough to cause a tight abdomen, at which time tachypnea, tachycardia, and oliguria are the result of pooling of fluids in the intestinal lumen and interference with diaphragmatic respiration.

Pain in acute mechanical obstruction of the small bowel is referred to the midabdomen and occurs in severe paroxysms that reach a crescendo and cease abruptly. In acute mechanical obstruction of the large bowel, colicky pain is less severe and is referred to the lower part of the abdomen. When the ileocecal valve is competent, distention is confined to the colon, and vomiting occurs late if at all. As distention progresses, the intensity of the pain decreases, and the paroxysms become less frequent. When strangulation supervenes, the discomfort becomes constant, and pain becomes more localized to the quadrant of the abdomen in which the strangulated loop of bowel resides.

Vomiting occurs earlier and is more severe, the higher the obstruction in the intestinal tract. High obstructions result in earlier dehydration and alkalosis due to loss of hydrochloric acid, whereas lower obstructions result in slower dehydration and loss of alkaline fluid, and they produce acidosis. Vomitus at first contains bile and mucus but later becomes brown and fecal in odor because of putrefaction of protein in the small bowel. When the ileocecal valve is competent, little or no vomiting occurs in colonic obstruction.

Obstipation results in all cases of complete obstruction after the intestinal tract distal to the obstruction is emptied. In high obstruction, the lower bowel may function quite well for a time, e.g., expelling an enema readily, whereas in low intestinal obstruction and colonic obstruction obstipation occurs early. Blood in the scanty stool suggests strangulation in low lesions. Diarrhea is not encountered, except in those rare situations where mechanical obstruction is precipitated by gastroenteritis in already mechanically embarrassed loops of intestine. When the onset of constipation is gradual but steadily increasing in severity, chronic intestinal obstruction due to encroachment on the lumen of bowel by the growth of neoplasm should be suspected. The progression of symptoms may be marked by bouts of obstipation, distention, and cramps, only to be relieved by purgation with the passage of fecal impaction. Eventually these measures fail to give relief, and complete obstruction supervenes, with the added hazard of perforation into the peritoneal cavity of bowel proximal to the obstruction.

PHYSICAL FINDINGS The physical findings vary from very few at the onset, to severe dehydration and alkalosis or acidosis from continued vomiting, to localized or generalized distention with abdominal tenderness after several hours of obstruction. Severe sepsis and shock revealed by pallor, sweating, cold and clammy extremities, rapid pulse, hypotension, and stupor supervene when strangulation and perforation occur. Disorientation may be one of the earliest evidences of peritonitis, especially in older persons, occurring before shock becomes manifest. Clinical evidences of shock indicate extensive fluid and blood loss into bowel lumen, bowel wall, and peritoneal cavity as well as loss of fluid by vomiting. The shock state is also produced by endotoxemia from colonic organisms in the peritoneal cavity. Shock is seen early when the intestine is infarcted, whether because of vascular occlusion or strangulation of bowel wall. Involuntary spasm of the abdominal muscles is noted only when strangulation with local peritonitis occurs and is not a prominent feature of acute obstruction. During paroxysmal painful contractions of small intestine, proximal to the point of obstruction, there is noted voluntary rigidity of the abdominal wall, but this subsides when the contraction subsides. These paroxysms of bowel contraction are accompanied by auscultatory sounds that are exaggerated, gurgle more than normal because of the abnormal amounts of fluid in the bowel, and become more high-pitched as gaseous distention increases. Sometimes one can locate the noisy proximal bowel in one quadrant of the abdomen by auscultation with a stethoscope. The sounds become more tinkling in character as the ileus progresses and distention increases. The abdomen is silent when ileus becomes adynamic, which occurs when peritonitis is superimposed or when large segments of bowels are infarcted.

Distention in high obstruction may be limited to the upper part of the abdomen and in low colonic obstruction may outline the colon. Most of the gas in the distention that accompanies acute intestinal obstruction is from swallowed air. In those who tend to swallow air readily and unconsciously, gaseous distention may develop very rapidly indeed and to a degree not only to aggravate mechanical obstruction but to endanger life by respiratory embarrassment, cardiac arrhythmias, and the precipitation of vascular insufficiency of the gut with perforation. When perforation results, it usually occurs on the antimesenteric surface.

Detection of a large heart with irregular rhythm or the definitive finding of mitral stenosis may suggest that an embolus to the superior mesenteric artery has occurred. Embolism to that artery is also suggested by a history of recent myocardial infarction, subacute bacterial endocarditis, or other embolic phenomena. In an older patient, palpation of an abdominal aortic aneurysm, evidence of defective arterial circulation to the legs, or history of diffuse abdominal pain exacerbated by eating all suggest diffuse aortic arteriosclerosis with encroachment on the lumina of vessels supplying the intestine. Rarely, periarteritis nodosa will cause thrombosis of the superior mesenteric artery or one of its branches. When portal hypertension is present, thrombosis of the portal venous bed may occur, with resultant mesenteric venous thrombosis. Polycythemia vera, postsplenectomy states, and disorders of the coagulating mechanism such as thrombotic thrombocytopenic purpura are rare but documented causes of venous mesenteric thrombosis.

ROENTGENOGRAPHIC FINDINGS An x-ray is a very valuable adjunct to the physical examination in demonstrating whether gas is present in loops of small bowel with or without fluid levels, whether gas is in the upper part of the small bowel or the entire small bowel, or in single loops of intestine, or primarily in the colon. A clue to the point of obstruction may be obtained often by a flat film together with a film of the patient sitting up or lying on his side. Classic radiologic evidence of obstruction of the small intestine is seen in Fig 286-1, the stepladder distribution of distended small-bowel loops being readily identified. Distention of the large bowel is usually recognized on the flat films from the distribution of the air-filled colon, the haustral markings extending not entirely across the lumen. Volvulus of the sigmoid colon presents a very characteristic radiologic picture, and various forms of internal or sliding hernias give characteristic radiologic patterns. The diagnosis may be much more difficult when low-grade or early obstruction is present or when large fecal masses obscure the picture. In low acute obstructions it is not wise to give barium by mouth, although in chronic situations contrast media can sometimes be injected through a tube in the intestinal tract to visualize the point of obstruction. If evidence points to colonic obstruction, a carefully administered barium enema will often demonstrate the point of obstruction and reveal its cause.

LABORATORY FINDINGS Laboratory findings are usually related to the amount of necrosis, the presence of peritonitis, and other chronic diseases which may underlie the catastrophe. Leukocytosis is usually of moderate degree, the hematocrit may be high, and electrolytes are disturbed to various degrees. Lactic dehydrogenase levels in the serum are often very high in intestinal infarction. The stool may be grossly bloody if a large area of small bowel has been strangulated.

TREATMENT Therapy consists of (1) correcting fluid and electrolyte imbalance, (2) alleviating vomiting and distention by intubation and decompression, (3) control

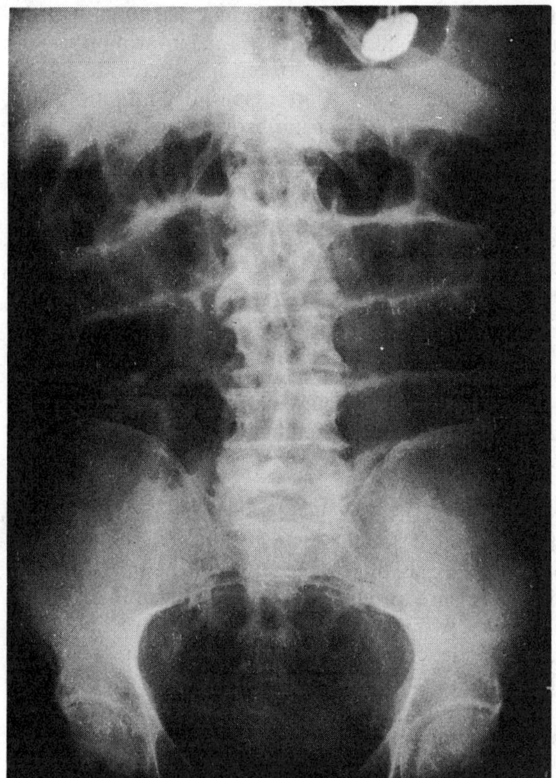

FIGURE 286-1
Paralytic ileus due to thrombosis of the superior mesenteric artery.

of peritonitis, if present, and blood transfusion for shock, if present, and (4) removal of the obstruction and restoration of bowel continuity and function.

Since the efflux of fluid into the dilated gut and peritoneal cavity results in dehydration and often in hemoconcentration and since chloride is lost in high obstructions and both sodium chloride and potassium chloride are lost in lower obstructions, the administration of saline solution and potassium chloride is indicated. Extra water should also be given in the form of 5% glucose. Because these patients have not taken anything by mouth and will not do so for several days, caloric requirements (2,000 per day) must be met by continuous infusion of glucose, and parenteral vitamin preparations should be given. Adequate hydration can be gauged by measuring urinary excretion, which should be kept near a liter per day. The hematocrit is also useful in determining the results of combating hemoconcentration. Determination of sodium, chloride, potassium, and bicarbonate ionic levels in the serum twice a day in very sick patients serves as a useful guide to electrolyte therapy and control of acidosis or alkalosis. No attempt to maintain nitrogen equilibrium other than by blood and plasma infusion is indicated in short periods of disability.

Decompression is best achieved by intubation with one of the long, weighted intestinal tubes attached to gentle continuous suction. Single-lumen tubes drain more effectively than double-lumen tubes. This method of decompression is useful in adynamic ileus. However, there is great danger in relying solely on intubation for relieving mechanical obstruction whenever there is any question of strangulation of bowel or when large-bowel obstruction occurs in the presence of a competent ileocecal valve. Early operative intervention is required in all such cases.

In the majority of cases, surgical intervention is necessary to remove the obstructing agent and restore normal bowel continuity and function. In some cases due to adhesions and hernia, relief by decompression suffices, and in some cases of intussusception or volvulus a barium enema under fluoroscopy restores normal continuity. Many cases of adynamic ileus are cured by tube decompression alone. However, if the patient does not improve rapidly on such conservative measures, operation within 24 hr is indicated to establish an accurate evaluation of the cause of obstruction and to effect a cure. When *severe* distention is not relieved *promptly* by intubation or when there is x-ray evidence of a closed-loop type of obstruction (due to obstruction of both inlet and outlet of a segment of herniated bowel), surgical intervention is required for immediate decompression by means of enterostomy, colostomy, or resection. However, treatment of shock metabolic acidosis and of dehydration should be instituted before surgical therapy is undertaken in order to lessen the operative risk. In very poor risk patients, total parenteral hyperalimentation is now possible, providing time to restore the patient to better status and lessen his operative risk.

PROGNOSIS The prognosis is always guarded, depending upon the level of obstruction, being poorer in high obstruction than in low intestinal obstruction, and upon the viability of the bowel wall, the length of time the bowel has been obstructed and strangulated, and the amount of bowel involved in the strangulation. Patients with complicating peritonitis from perforation have a poorer prognosis, and this is especially true in very young infants or in elderly patients with complicating cardiovascular or renal disease.

REFERENCES

DEMUTH WE et al: Mesenteric vascular occlusion. Surg Gynecol Obstet 108:209, 1959

NOER RJ: Intestinal obstruction, chap. 33 in *Textbook of Surgery*, eds WH Cole, RM Zollinger, New York: Appleton-Century-Crofts, 1970

287 ACUTE APPENDICITIS

ALBERT I. MENDELOFF
ARNOLD M. SELIGMAN

Inflammation of the vermiform appendix constitutes one of the most common and most important acute disease processes. Although descriptions of isolated cases of the disease had been written in the seventeenth and eighteenth centuries, and appendiceal abscesses had been described at autopsy, it was Reginald Fitz in 1886 who first collected a series of cases in which clinicopathologic correlations were established.

EPIDEMIOLOGY The disease occurs in all age groups but appears to be productive of higher mortality rates in the group aged five to fourteen and after age fifty-five. It is estimated that in 1946, in England and Wales, one case occurred every year for every 700 of the population. The incidence of the disease is somewhat higher in males, and the death rates for the period prior to 1946 were 40 percent higher in males. A consistent feature of the disease has been its greater incidence and mortality in the upper socioeconomic stratum and its tendency to decline in frequency during periods of food shortages. In Western Europe and in the United States, the death rates for the disease have shown a steady decline, ranging from 8.1 per 100,000 of the population in 1941 to less than 1.0 per 100,000 in 1970. There is also definite evidence that the incidence of the disease has recently decreased; despite great increases in the number of admissions of surgical patients to American hospitals since World War II, the absolute number of acutely inflamed appendixes removed has steadily declined by 30 to 60 percent, and approximately at the same rates in urban and rural institutions. It is difficult to explain this decrease by single causation. Possible factors are the greater use of effective antibiotics and chemotherapeutic agents to treat upper respiratory infections, some of which undoubtedly have been associated with appendicitis, and a lessened infestation with helminths. Changes in diet have also occurred, changes which many feel have increased the incidence of degenerative disease but may have sharply reduced the incidence and the mortality from appendicitis. Surgeons are also probably more careful about removing nearly normal appendixes now than heretofore. None of these explanations is adequate to clarify in its totality what appears to be a progressive and definite decrease in the incidence of one of our most important acute inflammatory diseases.

PATHOGENESIS Appendicitis is an inflammation of the vermiform appendix involving all layers of the organ, beginning either as a focal ulceration or as a diffuse phlegmon. Evidence of a focal point of obstruction due to fecalith or stricture is sometimes found. The appendiceal artery is an end artery, and its tributaries are susceptible to occlusion from the increased pressure within the lumen of the obstructed appendix or direct pressure of a fecalith. Inflammation and edema, therefore, may also lead to obstruction of venous return, with resulting congestion and final impairment of arterial flow. Infections lead to vascular thrombosis, local necrosis, and infarction resulting in perforation. Streptococcal involvement, which rises in frequency when acute respiratory infections are prevalent, adds to the necrotic process and to the virulence of the disease. The process either subsides early or progresses to gangrene or perforation with abscess or peritonitis. Chronic inflammation occurs only with the granulomatous infections such as tuberculosis, amebas, or actinomycosis. Recurring appendicitis due to spontaneous subsidence of acute attacks should not be considered chronic appendicitis. Recognition of the disease as an entity was first made by Fitz, and treatment by appendectomy was introduced thereafter by Morton, Ochsner, Murphy, McBurney, and Deaver. Since then to the present time, acute appendicitis is the most common major surgical disease.

CLINICAL PICTURE The history of onset should be carefully obtained, for the history may be the *only* clue to a correct diagnosis of retrocecal appendicitis, when abdominal signs are absent. The first symptom in an otherwise well individual is acute periumbilical or epigastric pain. In young children the abdominal pain cannot be localized and is usually generalized. Pain varies from mild or vague to quite severe and is followed by anorexia, nausea, or vomiting. The sequence of these symptoms is very important. When the illness is initiated by nausea and vomiting, which is then followed by abdominal pain, one should suspect an infection capable of producing extensive toxic absorption such as is noted in cases of gastroenteritis, tonsillitis, scarlet fever, and pneumonia, rather than the early stage of appendiceal inflammation. Pain is the first symptom of appendicitis and is due to distention of the appendiceal serosa by edema. Stretching of the serosa stimulates sympathetic nerve endings in the wall of the appendix, producing pain first and, because of continued stimuli, anorexia, nausea, and vomiting afterward. For this reason it is important to determine whether abdominal pain preceded the nausea and vomiting. The only other mechanism for producing pain is by the acute contractions of the appendiceal musculature which occurs in appendiceal colic, when the lumen is obstructed by stricture, fecalith, worms, or foreign bodies. Since the sensory innervation of the appendix corresponds to the tenth spinal segment, the pain is referred to the periumbilical region like sensory impulses originating anywhere in the entire small bowel.

At the time of the initial symptoms, inflammation is confined to the appendix. Fever and abdominal signs are not prominent at the onset. High fever, like vomiting, as an initial symptom is suggestive of some other diagnosis. Within a few hours, when the inflammatory process has begun to involve peritoneal surfaces of neighboring loops of bowel, omentum, and finally the anterior parietal peritoneum, pain shifts to the right lower quadrant of the abdomen, and tenderness, spasm, and rebound tenderness become increasingly prominent. In a sixth of the patients, diarrhea may appear owing to irritation of the bowel. Contralateral rebound tenderness, like pain in the right lower quadrant on sneezing, is a particularly reliable sign of parietal peritoneal inflammation. Although direct pressure of the examining hand produces pain, it may do so in the distended gut of gastroenteritis as well.

However, release of tension by the examining hand, as in demonstrating rebound tenderness, can produce pain only when peritoneal surfaces are inflamed. Sudden cessation of abdominal pain some hours after onset signifies perforation of a distended appendix, infarction of the appendix, or the accumulation of enough peritoneal fluid to lubricate the moving inflamed surfaces.

In the absence of anterior abdominal signs and a history of onset consistent with appendicitis, one must suspect that the appendix is in the retrocecal position. Evidence for inflammation in this area may be obtained by stretching the iliopsoas muscle either by passive hyperextension of the legs on the torso or by actively flexing the iliopsoas by straight-leg raising. When the appendix lies over the brim of the pelvis, evidence of inflammation is more striking on rectal examination than on abdominal examination. After 24 hr, progressive appendicitis results in localized peritonitis and abscess formation, when the signs remain confined to the right lower quadrant with the appearance of a tender mass. Diffuse peritonitis develops as a result of perforation before adequate adhesions by omentum and neighboring loops of bowel have been able to form. This is more common in children than in adults. Tenderness and spasm are generalized, ileus becomes evident, and progressively severe toxicity develops, with high fever, severe leukocytosis, vomiting, dehydration, rapid pulse, and shock. When a history of illness for 2 to 3 days is obtained, one should expect to find evidence of appendiceal abscess with mass or more generalized peritonitis with ileus, rather than signs of appendicitis alone.

Atypical clinical pictures of appendicitis are distressingly common and difficult to identify. If one remembers that appendicitis is the most common acute intraabdominal focal inflammation, the onset of unexplained weakness, anorexia, and tachycardia in the elderly may lead the physician to suspect the appendix; similarly, in patients obtunded by cerebral disease or whose pain pathways are disturbed by neurologic degeneration or whose appreciation of pain is blunted by sedatives or ganglionic blocking agents, the objective signs of early peritonitis may be the only clue that an acute appendicitis has occurred. Retrocecal appendicitis can easily be confused with disease of the right kidney or ureter or with colonic disease, as noted below. In the elderly, abdominal distention may be the only objective sign of appendicitis, and is often mistaken for an obstructing carcinoma.

DIFFERENTIAL DIAGNOSIS *Gastroenteritis* may produce vomiting, abdominal pain, and fever that are difficult to distinguish from those of acute appendicitis. However, vomiting is often the first and predominating symptom in the former and is later followed by diarrhea. Sometimes diarrhea ushers in the illness. Although tenderness is sometimes present, especially after considerable retching has occurred, spasm and rebound tenderness are absent. Systemic muscle aching and prostration are common, and bowel sounds are loud and "whooshing." The illness may occur in epidemics or affect several members of a family, making diagnosis somewhat easier.

Referred pain from diaphragmatic irritation in *pneumonia* may simulate appendicitis, especially in children. This is especially the case when the signs of appendicitis are found to be higher in the abdomen than usual and are attributed to malrotation of the colon. However, fever and vomiting are more prominent at the onset of abdominal symptoms and respiration is more rapid in pneumonia. Abdominal spasm and rebound tenderness should be absent in pneumonia, unless pneumococcal peritonitis has occurred.

Abdominal pain from mesenteric *lymphadenitis* is very difficult to distinguish from acute appendicitis and is frequently a cause of illness in children. Less spasm and rebound tenderness, lower leukocytosis, and more gradual onset of symptoms help distinguish it from appendicitis.

Since free blood in the peritoneal cavity produces the symptoms and signs of peritoneal irritation, a *ruptured graafian follicle* or a *ruptured tubal pregnancy* will simulate the acute abdominal condition of appendicitis, although the onset is marked by more localized lower abdominal pain rather than by generalized pain and nausea. The signs are less localized, however. Other acute processes accompanied by a mass are torsion of an ovarian cyst and acute salpingitis. These conditions are usually readily distinguished on vaginal examination by noting tenderness mainly on movement of the cervix. The local signs are usually more pronounced than the general illness of the patient would warrant.

Other acute processes such as *acute cholecystitis*, *diverticulitis* of the *colon*, and *perforation* of *carcinoma* of the *colon* are often difficult to distinguish, especially in older patients. The history is the most helpful means of making a correct diagnosis. Urologic conditions such as *stone* and *pyelonephritis* of the right kidney may give symptoms referred to the right lower quadrant. The urine is usually abnormal, and pain begins in the costovertebral angle and radiates to the groin or pubic area. However, a retrocecal appendicitis may also cause the appearance of blood cells in the urine.

In all these conditions, with the exception of pneumonia, it is usually safer to operate in the suspected case of acute appendicitis than to wait until the signs and symptoms of peritonitis make diagnosis relatively easy. The more patients who are operated upon after peritonitis has occurred, the higher the mortality will be.

TREATMENT If appendicitis is a possible diagnosis, cathartics are absolutely contraindicated.

Once the diagnosis of acute appendicitis is made, the patient is prepared for operation by initiating parenteral administration of fluid and electrolytes, and the appendix is removed as soon as possible, at any hour of the day or night. Uncomplicated appendicitis results in prompt recovery; with early ambulation, the patient may be able to eat within 2 days and be discharged within a few days thereafter. The complications of appendicitis such as local abscess, peritonitis with ileus, and intestinal obstruction require surgical intervention such as drainage or lysis of adhesions, prolonged hospitalization, energetic treatment with gastrointestinal intubation, antibiotics, and careful control of fluid, glucose, and electrolyte balance by parenteral means.

REFERENCES

Condon RE: Appendicitis, chap. 32 in *Textbook of Surgery*, ed DC Sabiston, Philadelphia: Saunders, 1972.

Cope Z: *The Early Diagnosis of the Acute Abdomen*, 13th ed., London: Oxford University Press, 1968, chap. 5

288 DISEASES OF THE COLON AND RECTUM

ALBERT I. MENDELOFF
J. THOMAS LAMONT
KURT J. ISSELBACHER

SYMPTOMS OF COLONIC AND RECTAL DISEASE

Man can exist without a colon and rectum, although with some difficulty. This basic fact has allowed important observations regarding the function of the large bowel and the adjustments which result when it is no longer present. The increasing frequency with which resections of the organ, bypassing operations, and colostomies have been carried out has led to significant advances in our understanding of normal functions of the colon, although our comprehension of many of its diseased states is still rudimentary.

PAIN REFERENCE (see also Chap. 8) Pain of colonic origin is lateralized to the right or left sides of the abdomen, as opposed to pain of small intestinal origin which is usually periumbilical. Pain fibers from the cecum and ascending colon accompany sympathetic fibers to the lower ganglions of the celiac plexus; fibers from the transverse colon, sigmoid, and rectum accompany fibers passing into the inferior mesenteric ganglions. Interconnections of these fibers with somatic nerves permit a considerable amount of localization of pain, roughly corresponding to the distribution of the colon in the peritoneal cavity. Pain from the rectum is projected to the sacral nerve distribution; the lower it arises, the more accurate the localization. Anal pain, which arises from the skin near the mucocutaneous junction, is very accurately localized.

Colonic pain may arise from distention, spasm, or inflammation of that organ. In the noninflamed colon, stretching of the muscularis layer causes pain. Thus, a large-bowel obstruction is accompanied by pain arising from the greatly dilated segment proximal to the obstructing lesion. Pain may also result when the wall of the large intestine is inflamed or infiltrated. In the presence of peritoneal inflammation secondary to colonic disease, pain becomes much more sharply localized and may be accompanied by spasm of the abdominal muscles and rebound tenderness.

MOTOR DISORDERS The colon is a rather sluggish organ, contracting desultorily at rates not exceeding 1 per min, compared with regular contraction frequencies in the small intestine ranging from 10 to 12 per min in the duodenum to 3 to 4 per min in the ileum. The transition between the innervation of the ascending colon and that of the transverse colon occurs just distal to the hepatic flexure, where radiologists often note irregular propulsion of barium (Cannon's ring). The colon husbands its motor activity for the processing of ileal contents, waiting until a certain volume has accumulated in the cecum. Any gas entering the cecum from the small intestine, which is intolerant of air and passes it rapidly downward, diffuses into the colon and distributes itself along the length of that organ. About 100 ml gas is contained in the large intestine, obeying the law of gravity, rising to the most superior portion of the colon—the flexures—when the subject is erect, the transverse colon when he is supine, the rectum when he is in the knee-chest position. Symptomatic disturbances of motor activity tend to be related to the infrequent mass propulsive waves which deliver the fecal bolus to an adjacent and more distal colonic region. The same types of disturbance which cause motor difficulties in the small intestine are also seen in the colon—intraluminal obstruction, destruction or paralysis of muscle, compromise of vascular integrity, pressure from neighboring masses, or infectious processes. The colon differs from the small intestine, however, in its more successful accommodation of these processes, distending to much greater degrees without serious symptoms than the small bowel can. In particular, obstructive lesions of the left colon characteristically produce gradual enlargement of the right colon, occasionally to the point of cecal perforation.

DEFECATION PATTERNS These have been described in Chap. 40. It is still not common knowledge among physicians how varied are the defecatory habits of their fellow citizens, how fanciful their interpretation of deviations from those habits. It is well to ask the patient to describe in some detail what he regards as his normal defecatory pattern, with particular attention to time of day or night, relation to meals, sensation during actual expulsion of stool, and aftersensations. Symptoms of rectal disease include alteration of the pattern of defecation, change in the caliber of the stool, and blood or pus in the stool.

BLEEDING Bleeding from the colon may be occult, massive, or of any grade between. Most often it is occult, an important early sign of malignancy, often of the right colon. Melena or tarry stools rarely result from colonic bleeding. Bright-red blood, either by itself or coating the stools, may originate from any portion of the lower ileum as well as from the colon. Bleeding may result from localized lesions such as polyps, hemorrhoids, or tumors or more generalized disturbances such as colitis or hereditary telangiectasia. Hemorrhoids are so common that their presence can never allow the physician to abandon the search for other bleeding lesions.

DIAGNOSTIC PROCEDURES

EXAMINATION OF THE ABDOMEN Careful examination will often disclose masses or palpable colonic contents strongly suggesting more distal narrowing. Colonic outlines distended by gas have similar significance in leading one to the diagnosis of a more distal obstructing lesion. Spasm and guarding in the left lower quadrant are characteristic of an acute diverticulitis; a distended loop of sigmoid percussed in the midline at the level of the umbilicus may represent a sigmoid volvulus. Generalized hypogastric tenderness is associated with acute inflammations of the colon, such as the dysenteries and ulcerative colitis, both of which may also be accompanied by abdominal distention out of proportion to the habitus of the patient.

DIGITAL EXAMINATION This is a simple and highly efficient procedure provided that the finger's education is maintained by steady use. A digital rectal examination should permit recognition of perianal, sphincteric, and ampullary lesions, gross deformities of prostate and cervix, and perception of even small neoplastic masses in the rectum. About half of all rectal carcinomas lie within reach of the index finger. When one considers that these cancers not only account for 10 percent of all gastrointestinal cancers but have a favorable prognosis if removed early, the importance of digital rectal examination is easily appreciated. Examination of the material coating the gloved finger on its withdrawal from the rectum is often of diagnostic importance, and physicians should form the routine habit of testing the finger specimen for occult blood.

PROCTOSIGMOIDOSCOPY A proctosigmoidoscope is an inexpensive instrument of extraordinary importance in the detection of colonic disease. Contrary to the general impression, it is not difficult to master, and it can be introduced into the rectum as the examining finger is removed without discomfort to the patient.

The physician should learn to evaluate friability of the mucosa, one of the earliest signs of proctitis and colitis, abnormal vascular patterns, edema, ulcerations, and polyps. Ninety percent of tumors of the rectum and rectosigmoid can be directly visualized with this instrument; 60 percent of all tumors of the large intestine lie within the terminal 25 cm of the colon which it can bring into view. This area is particularly difficult to visualize radiographically, so that the *proctosigmoidoscope is the most important diagnostic instrument in this region.* In addition, radiography in the pelvis carries a radiation hazard to the gonads which can frequently be minimized or avoided by making the diagnosis endoscopically.

In addition to the visual inspection of the area, bacteriologic, parasitologic, and cytologic studies can be made on washings obtained through the instrument, and biopsy of a suspicious lesion is easy to perform. The newly available fiberoptic colonoscope permits direct visualization and biopsy of lesions of the transverse and descending colon, a major advance in handling the problem of colonic polyps.

STOOL EXAMINATION Stools constitute important objective evidence of disease processes; some of the difficulties in obtaining them and describing them are discussed in Chap. 40. One must distinguish blood streaking on otherwise normal stools from dark stools containing blood, tarry stools from the gray-black formed stools passed by patients ingesting iron, and, most importantly, the inflammatory mucopurulent exudate passed by patients with inflammatory rectal and sigmoid disease from true diarrheal stools. Microscopic examination of the freshly passed stool or rectal swab is useful not only for parasitologic study but for demonstration of the characteristic exudate of ulcerative colitis and bacillary dysentery and the presence of malignant cells (Papanicolaou technique). Small-bowel diseases and viral invasion of the gut almost never produce purulent exudate in the stools. Stools should be tested for occult blood (Chap. 41).

To summarize, the digital examination should be a routine feature of the general physical examination of all adults. Finger specimens obtained during the examination should be inspected and tested for blood. Whenever abdominal complaints, stool abnormalities, unexplained weight loss, changes in defecation patterns, or a strong family history of colonic disease are features of the history, proctosigmoidoscopy should be carried out. Any patient with anorectal disease should have routine proctosigmoidoscopy prior to surgical treatment.

When these procedures have been carried out, it is usually necessary to visualize the colon proximal to the rectosigmoid by radiologic techniques. The routine barium enema is a very accurate diagnostic tool for the identification of structural abnormalities of the colon. For detection of mucosal abnormalities such as small polyps or early ulcerative colitis, it is often necessary to follow it with an air-contrast enema. The combined use of the digital examination, proctosigmoidoscope, and radiologic investigation of the colon will identify 95 percent of inflammatory, neoplastic, congenital, and vascular diseases of this organ. Negative results of these procedures constitute strong evidence that disorders of a functional type are producing symptoms.

DEVELOPMENTAL DISORDERS

MEGACOLON Aganglionic megacolon, or Hirschsprung's disease, is a congenital disorder manifesting symptoms in early infancy, occurring more often in boys, often in familial clusters. There is abdominal distention, occasionally reaching massive proportions; the sigmoid colon is the earliest segment to be distended, and visible peristalsis is common. The stools consist of characteristically very small pellets or ribbons of pasty consistency. On rectal examination the ampulla is empty of feces, and the anal sphincter feels normal. X-ray examination shows a narrowed lumen in the rectosigmoid area, with a distended sigmoid colon above the constricted area. The anorectal ring always, the rectum often, and the sigmoid less frequently have no ganglion cells in Auerbach's plexus. This area is thus unable to relax in advance of the normal peristaltic activity of the colon proximal to it (Fig. 288-1). Diagnosis is made by deep surgical biopsy under anesthesia or by special rectal balloon motility patterns in the unanesthetized patient.

The condition may also be acquired. In Brazil a large number of acquired megacolon cases have been reported in the aged; pathologic specimens show all degrees of

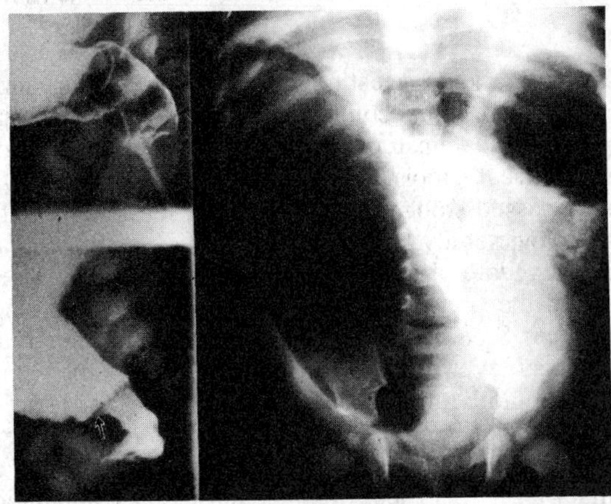

FIGURE 288-1
Aganglionic megacolon. The contracted rectal segment is seen on the left, the dilated colon on the right.

degeneration of the ganglion cells of Auerbach's plexus, and in some cases a relation to infection with *Trypanosoma cruzi* (Chagas' disease) has been demonstrated. In a small number of patients generalized aganglionosis of the esophagus, ureters, and colon has been described, and thiamine deficiency has been incriminated as the etiologic agent.

Treatment of this condition is largely surgical, although a number of borderline cases may be carried along on measures designed to empty the colon. Definitive diagnosis is made by a rectal biopsy deep enough to include the muscularis layer of the rectum; failure to find adequate numbers of ganglion cells indicates that the most effective treatment is resection of the aganglionic segment and a "pull-through" anastomosis to the intact anal sphincter.

CHRONIC IDIOPATHIC MEGACOLON This condition has its onset later in childhood, usually at the time toilet training begins; it is characterized more by constipation than by distention, and the rectal ampulla is invariably found distended with feces. X-ray examination shows the entire colon to be distended from the anal sphincter cephalad; no narrowed segment is seen, and rectal biopsy discloses the normal complement of ganglion cells in Auerbach's plexus. The treatment is based on education in normal bowel habits, but a long course of enemas may have to be carried out concomitantly. It should be pointed out that water intoxication may occur in small children whose enormously dilated colons are vigorously irrigated with tap water; saline enemas are probably safe.

DISORDERS ASSOCIATED WITH COLONIC DIVERTICULA Diverticula of the colon are more common than those of the small intestine; in Western populations they can be found in more than 20 percent of all persons over fifty years of age. The frequency of colonic diverticula increases with age. The outpouchings are nearly always composed of mucosa and serosa following the course of a nutrient artery perforating the muscularis of the bowel wall. The mechanism of diverticular formation may be increased intraluminal pressure, which is thought to account for the fact that they are much more common in the muscular, smaller-lumened sigmoid colon than in the larger and less heavily muscled ascending colon. When diverticula occur solely in the ascending colon, they may be associated with diverticula in the stomach or small intestine, and may represent a special kind of weakening of the muscularis at points where different muscle groups merge. Diverticulosis in itself is usually asymptomatic, but the peculiarities of diverticular structure and origin provide the basis for two serious complications, *diverticulitis* and *hemorrhage*.

Acute diverticulitis Acute inflammation can occur in or around the diverticular sac. The causes of this diverticulitis are probably mechanical, related to poor emptying from these outpouchings of undigested food residues and bacteria. It is believed that such conditions compromise the blood supply to the thin-walled sac (made up solely of mucosa and serosa) and render it susceptible to invasion by colonic bacteria. Mild attacks of this type are thought to be frequent in the elderly, the process resolving uneventfully. Some believe that all acute diverticulitis represents perforation of the sacs, due to increases in intraluminal pressure, and that the resulting inflammation is thus a peridiverticular abscess with localized peritonitis. The published literature on this subject lends itself to either interpretation and suggests therefore that a spectrum of inflammatory complications of diverticulosis exists, most of which heal with minimal clinical symptoms, leaving residual scars that may then complicate future attacks. Diverticulitis occurs more often in men than women, and three times as often in the descending than in the right colon. This suggests that diverticulitis may be related to the higher intraluminal pressures in the sigmoid and the more solid fecal composition in this area.

Acute diverticulitis may present clinically as a mild illness with lower abdominal pain and tenderness. In more serious cases there may be abscess formation, pelvic peritonitis secondary to perforation, or obstruction from a pericolonic inflammatory mass. The clinical features of acute diverticulitis are lower abdominal pain, made worse by defecation, and the signs of peritoneal irritation—muscle spasm, guarding, fever, and leucocytosis. Although constipation may not have been noted by the patient prior to the onset of this illness, the inflammation around the colon usually results in some degree of constipation; the stools may be fluid or pasty, but are almost always small in caliber. Rectal bleeding, usually microscopic, is noted in 25 percent of these patients; it is rarely massive. As the process develops, it may produce a tender abdominal mass. Behind such a mass partial colonic obstruction may occur, and in low grade or recurrent diverticulitis the picture may resemble an obstructing carcinoma. Occasionally, and especially in the elderly, the acute process ruptures freely into the peritoneal cavity. These patients may present with generalized peritonitis, ileus, and shock.

In the less acute situation, the differential diagnosis is principally that of a neoplasm in the area of known or suspected diverticulosis. Proctoscopy may show an acutely inflamed mucosa over what seems to be an extrinsic mass; it is usually impossible to pass the instrument through the contracted lumen. Radiologic findings on barium enema may be diagnostic (see Fig. 288-2), but

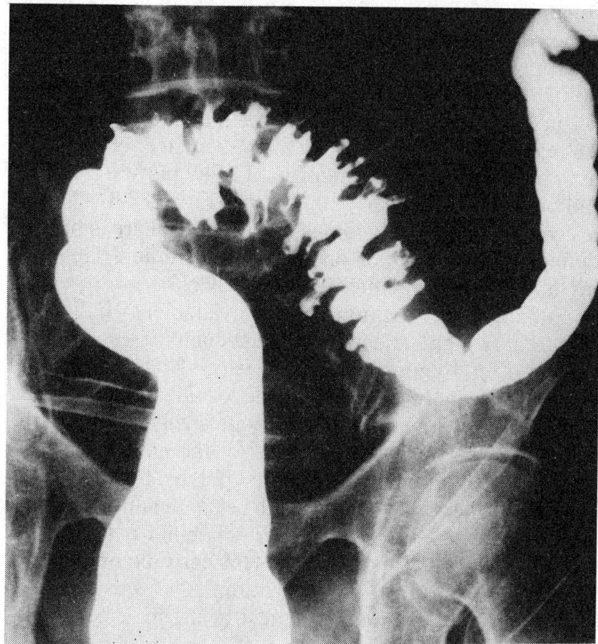

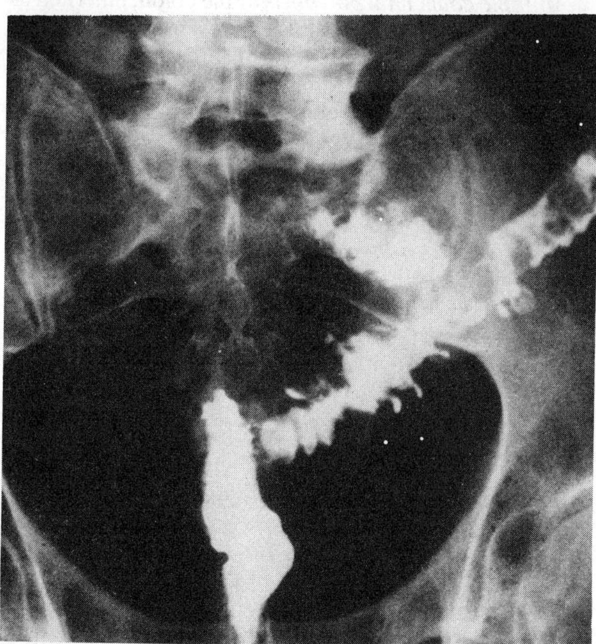

FIGURE 288-2
A *Diverticulosis with marked spasm of the sigmoid colon.* B *Rupture of acutely inflamed diverticula with extravasation of barium into the peritoneal cavity.*

often the distortion caused by inflammation prevents a clear distinction between cancer and diverticulitis. Such a distribution may even be difficult for the surgeon to make when inspecting the bowel at laparotomy.

Treatment in the mild case without signs of perforation consists of bed rest, stool softeners, a liquid diet, and a wide-spectrum antibiotic such as tetracycline or ampicillin. Hospitalized patients with suspected abscess or perforation require intravenous antibiotics directed against gram-negative anaerobic bacteria. Surgical intervention is frequently necessary to drain abscesses or resect an obstructing inflammatory mass. The usual procedure is a diverting colostomy with resection of the involved colon; reanastomosis can be performed at a second operation.

Repeated attacks may result in the development of fistulous tracts between the diverticular perforation and neighboring structures, especially the bladder and vagina. These are particularly difficult to manage surgically, and there is considerable difference of opinion as to the proper surgical approach. There is general agreement, however, that after medical management has been carefully followed, repeated attacks of diverticulitis in the same area of the left colon require surgical resection of the involved segments.

Hemorrhage into the colon This complication usually occurs in the absence of evidence of acute inflammation. The basis for the hemorrhage seems to consist of the glomus-like capillary and arteriolar vascular network left exposed in the colonic lumen when the diverticular sac pushes out along the nutrient artery. In older patients these vessels, often rendered stiff by arteriosclerosis, are presumably damaged by contact with hard fecal aggregates and may rupture and bleed violently. In patients with diverticulosis presenting with massive colonic bleeding, nearly a fourth are found to be bleeding from the right rather than the left colon. Attempts to identify the exact bleeding site may be difficult, but air-contrast enemas, colonoscopy, and mesenteric angiography have been utilized to demonstrate its location and permit surgical correction if the bleeding cannot be controlled.

Diverticular disease associated with irritable colon In some persons with symptoms of the irritable colon syndrome (see below), a peculiar thickening of the circular smooth muscle of the rectosigmoid and sigmoid can be identified. On barium enema, one finds a sawtooth pattern representing the lumen narrowed by the thickened musculature. Intraluminal manometric studies have shown this colonic segment to produce very high pressures after eating and particularly after the administration of morphine. Apparently the muscle fails to relax after stimulation, and with time becomes grossly hypertrophic and hyperreactive to the normal stimuli which provoke its contractions. In the majority of such patients these repeated bouts of high intraluminal pressure push mucosa out through the nutrient artery tunnels, and the sawtooth pattern on barium enema then demonstrates multiple diverticula as well. On a worldwide basis, this disorder is exceedingly rare in populations consuming diets with a high fiber content, and has thus far been recognized only in Western populations. Treatment consists of increasing the bulk (hemicellulose) in the diet, mild sedation during the more acute phase of the disorder, and the regimen outlined for irritable colon. Surgical excision of the most involved segments has been followed by recurrence of the disease process in the remaining colon and hence is of little value.

POLYPOSIS A polyp is a structure which arises from a mucosal surface and projects into the lumen. Polyps of the colon may be classified as *solitary* or *multiple*, and in either category may be described as *neoplastic* (adenoma, papillary adenoma, or villous papilloma), *hamartomatous* (juvenile, Peutz-Jeghers), *inflammatory* (benign lymphoid, inflammatory, or pseudopolypoid), or *unclassifiable* (metaplastic).

In adults, single polyps of the adenomatous type are identified in 2 to 8 percent of the population. Small mucosal tags are very common and have no particular significance. True adenomatous polyps are more common in men than in women and are found more commonly with increasing age. The lobulated surface of adenomatous polyps is in contrast to the smooth vascular surface of childhood retention polyps or to the frondlike, soft appearance of papillary or villous adenomas. All such adenomatous polyps are rare in patients under thirty; when one is discovered, more should be sought, since familial polyposis does occur in this age group and almost always bespeaks prospective malignancy. In children polyps are frequently large, vascular, and on long pedicles, and may produce intussusception or massive hemorrhage. In adults the polyps are more frequently sessile, arise from the glandular epithelium of the crypts, and bleed less frequently. Less often, polyps arising from the surface epithelium may form villous masses which secrete watery discharges rich in potassium. Such villous adenomas, although infrequent, can lead to watery diarrhea of remarkable magnitude, but the primary danger they pose is their high capacity for malignant transformation. Probably 50 percent of these polypoid tumors will become cancers if not totally removed; fulguration is usually followed by prompt recurrence.

The relation of adenomatous polyps, whether sessile or pedunculated, to the development of cancer of the colon is at present a subject of hot debate among pathologists. There is dispute as to whether the distribution of such polyps in the colon is parallel to or totally unlike that of the distribution of rectal and colonic cancers, the evidence favoring the latter idea. Colonic specimens resected for cancer frequently show adenomatous polyps in close proximity to the malignant tissue; polyps removed from noncancerous patients have been observed to show all grades of differentiation known to occur in the progression from benignancy to frank malignancy.

Clinically, polyps are usually silent. When they do give rise to symptoms, these usually consist of recurrent episodes of either bleeding, overt or occult, or intermittent obstruction. The latter occurs when a large sessile polypoid mass weakens the wall to which it is attached or a pedunculated polyp flips caudal, causing the wall from which it arises to buckle. In either case a partial intussusception may result, with the production of crampy pain, occasionally an abdominal mass, and often a bloody exudate.

Treatment of polyps in adults is influenced by the debate as to their possible malignant transformation. Unfortunately, there is no certain way of determining whether a given polyp is benign or malignant when first identified until it has been studied microscopically. Exfoliative cytologic examination of colonic contents obtained by repeated enemas may be of help. However, fiberoptic colonoscopy is more valuable since it permits both visualization and biopsy of lesions in the entire colon. Small polyps may be resected by means of biopsy forceps. Polyps less than 1 cm in diameter, or those on long pedicles, are rarely malignant; they may be followed radiologically at yearly intervals (Fig. 288-3). Larger lesions, all villous adenomas, and polyps in areas hard to define radiologically or endoscopically require laparotomy and resection of the involved bowel.

Sufficient information is now available to indicate a remarkably high incidence of recurrence of adenomatous polyps after fulguration and excision. In approximately 40 to 50 percent of patients who have had polyps removed from the colon and rectum, new polyps will develop in the following decade. Although most of the new polyps will be of the same type as the original polyps, about 15 to 20 percent of the new polyps will be malignant when the original polyps were benign. The reliability of the serum carcinoembryonic antigen to detect early colonic malignancy is still under investigation. The possible importance of this immunologic test in the management of patients with polyps is obvious.

Multiple congenital polyposis of the colon, inherited as a simple dominant gene and thus present in many members of the families affected, is a disorder in which many adenomatous polyps are found from the ileocecal valve to the anus. The polyps are not present at birth but appear in childhood and adolescence. These may give rise to some symptoms, usually diarrhea or bleeding, but once such a disorder has been identified in a patient, it is imperative

FIGURE 288-3
Two adenomatous polyps in the sigmoid.

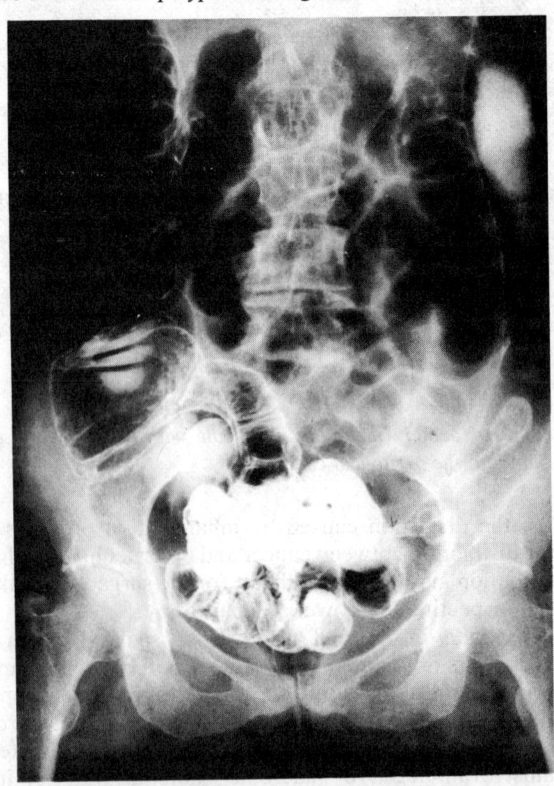

that the entire family be examined sigmoidoscopically and radiologically to detect the characteristic polyps. *The probability of malignancy occurring in these polypoid colons approaches 100 percent by age forty.* Hence, prophylactic colectomy is recommended when full adult growth is attained. Some authorities prefer total colectomy and ileostomy; others leave the rectum which allows the patient to have normal bowel movements. If the rectum is retained, frequent follow-up proctoscopy is necessary to detect malignant degeneration of polyps in the rectal stump.

Gardner's syndrome refers to the coexistence of multiple adenomatous polyps of the colon with various benign tumors elsewhere such as lipomas, fibromas, epidermoid and sebaceous cysts, and osteomas, particularly of the mandible. The colonic polyps develop at a somewhat later age than in multiple congenital polyposis; however, the predisposition to malignancy is the same and hence colectomy is also recommended.

FUNCTIONAL DISTURBANCES

IRRITABLE COLON SYNDROME This name is applied to a triad of symptoms—abdominal distress following the colonic distribution of pain, defecation habits varying from constipation to diarrhea, and the passage of small-caliber stools at the time when abdominal distress is at its worst. The stools may be hard and pelletlike or soft and pasty, but they are characteristically of smaller size than when the patient is asymptomatic. The physiologic basis for most of these symptoms is described in Chap. 40. In the past, many different terms have been applied to this syndrome: some, such as *unstable colon* or *colonic neurosis*, stress the anxiety which characterizes these patients; others, like *spastic colitis*, emphasize the symptoms of pain and distress; still others, such as *mucous colitis*, describe the increased mucus content of the stools and the pain which is usually relieved by defecation.

In its milder forms the syndrome is extremely common. It is more frequently seen in women between ages fifteen and forty-five but may be observed in both sexes under conditions of emotional tension. Constipation and pain in the left lower quadrant relieved by defecation are the most common symptoms when the disorder is mild. Extremely severe pain, diarrheal stools accompanied by much mucus, and various degrees of generalized disability are much less common and carry a rather serious prognosis; patients with such complaints are often severely psychoneurotic. Vasomotor instability and disabling headaches frequently occur in many patients even when the colonic symptoms are minimal. Aerophagia is a frequent accompaniment of the attacks, the swallowed air producing further difficulties when irregularly handled by the "irritable" colon. Bloating, borborygmi, explosive flatulence, and low backache are often described during the days or weeks when the symptoms are at their worst.

On *physical examination* these patients are anxious, often sweaty, but otherwise normal. During intense pain the abdomen may be distended, but no visible peristalsis is noted, the abdominal musculature is relaxed, and in the left lower quadrant a tender sigmoid full of feces may be palpated. Characteristically, the rectal ampulla is empty of feces. Proctoscopic examination usually is entirely normal or may show prominent vascular patterns in an otherwise unremarkable mucosa. Large amounts of clear mucus are frequently encountered during the examination, and there is often difficulty in negotiating the rectosigmoid curve at 13 to 15 cm from the anus because of violent spasm of the rectosigmoid.

The *diagnosis* of the irritable colon syndrome is suggested by the length of the history without obvious signs of physical deterioration, the intermittent character of the disability, and the relation of distress to periods of environmental or emotional stress. Nevertheless, each patient presenting such symptoms deserves not only a careful history but also a complete physical examination including proctosigmoidoscopy, stool examinations for blood, parasites, and pathogenic bacteria; a barium enema is also indicated. The radiographic study serves to rule out other lesions, since there are no findings diagnostic for this syndrome, although spasticity of the sigmoid, accentuated haustra, and tubular descending colon may be observed if the patient is having symptoms at the time of the examination.

The *differential diagnosis* includes all disorders of the colon, female genital tract diseases, regional enteritis, malignant tumors of stomach or pancreas, and those common disorders which are often associated with the irritable colon—gastric and duodenal ulcer and cholelithiasis.

Treatment of the irritable colon syndrome is that of any chronic anxiety neurosis, with more specific symptomatic medication. The relation between patient and physician can be established on the firm grounds of reassurance that the syndrome does not lead to the development either of ulcerative colitis or colonic malignancy, although it should be stated that it confers no protection against these eventualities. From this point the patient should receive a sympathetic ear from the physician as he talks over the circumstances surrounding the onset of his symptoms and those characterizing his present difficulties. Attempts should be made to discover in what way situational and emotional stresses differ when symptoms are present and when they are absent. The emphasis is placed on the patient and his relation to others in his environment rather than on the symptoms and long discussions of what is "normal" bowel physiology. Repeated x-ray examinations are avoided insofar as possible, but general physical examinations, hemograms, and stool examinations are carried out at regular intervals.

Lactose deficiency may masquerade as irritable colon. In any recurrent attack of abdominal pain it is wise to limit the intake of fluid milk, to add hydrophilic colloids at night, to reduce the intake of alcoholic beverages and tobacco, to avoid laxatives, and to employ sedatives and reassurance. Most patients who have experienced many such attacks have learned what is helpful in minimizing discomfort.

Warm saline enemas may be helpful; often viscous lidocaine instillations may overcome severe rectosigmoid spasm. Of all analgesics, codeine is probably the most useful; morphine is best avoided, especially in those patients with diverticular disease.

Follow-up studies reported by many workers in this field show that patients rarely lose their symptoms, but tolerate them much better as the years go by. No specific therapeutic measures seem as important in this respect as general support by physicians; an occasional patient is remarkably helped by cyproheptadine, and some patients believe that diphenoxylate is much more beneficial than anticholinergic or other spasmolytic agents. An important part of the therapeutic program is an increase in the bulk of the diet, either by fibrous foods or by hydrophilic colloids.

CONSTIPATION AND URGENCY OF RECTAL ORIGIN In Chap. 40 the mechanism of defecation is discussed. Disorders involving the sensory or motor components of this mechanism may arise from destruction of the nerves subserving these functions, from invasion or inflammation of the rectosigmoid itself, or from central nervous system dysfunction based on conditioning abnormalities or structural disorganization. If the afferent stimulus from the rectal wall cannot reach the brain or if, upon reaching it, no efferent action occurs, defecation is not initiated. If defecation is initiated but muscular power is lessened or lost, the act is not carried to completion. If all anatomic pathways are intact but habitual neglect of the afferent impulses is established, defecation is not initiated. The result of all these disorders, regardless of cause, is failure of the rectum to empty its contents. Accordingly, physical examination of such patients reveals the rectal ampulla to be full of stool, often to the astonishment of the patient.

Aside from degenerative disease of the central nervous system, severe psychoses, the use of ganglionic blocking drugs, and morphine addiction, the most common cause of this type of rectal or "simple" constipation is voluntary suppression of the defecation reflex. Such inhibitory activity is essential in the daily routines of civilized society; disordered bowel habits are therefore very common in civilized life. Toilet training in infancy leads to a powerful development of these inhibitory actions; repeated experiences in suppressing defecation because of social impropriety, unaccustomed surroundings, uncomfortable commodes, or intercurrent factors lead to a habit pattern in which suppression of defecation becomes simpler than its achievement. When constant distention of the rectum with feces becomes habitual, anorectal disorders, in particular hemorrhoidal itching and bleeding and anal fissures, make defecation painful, thus reinforcing the inhibitory impulses. The next step for the patient is the use of laxatives, which soon becomes as much a constant feature of the regimen as is the voluntary suppression of defecation.

TREATMENT The principal bulwark of therapy for rectal constipation is education. The chain of events leading up to the ineffective rectum is evaluated by careful physical examination of the status of the abdominal musculature, neurologic defects, drug effects, postural abnormalities, and accompanying local lesions of the anus and rectum. Such lesions as can be treated are taken care of, but the therapy may take a long time and usually must be carried out concomitantly with efforts to modify anal sphincteric spasm when it is present. Attention to regular habits of diet and time of defecation is most important; although defecation for most persons is best accomplished following meals, particularly breakfast, in these patients it is more important to select for evacuation whatever time is as free as possible from the pressure of daily events. Habit patterns of many years' standing may have to be altered, one may need to force the patient to get up earlier in the morning, to take some form of physical exercise—for older patients walking briskly outdoors is often helpful—to abandon the usual laxatives and cathartics, to pay more attention to defecatory urges (without becoming excessively bowel-conscious), and to space out the workday in such a way as to honor these urges when they arise.

The elderly patient may be feebly motivated to make such sweeping changes; under such circumstances one must proceed cautiously, making sure impactions are broken up by the physician's finger, that oil retention enemas at night are utilized, that sigmoidoscopy above the impaction reveals no tumor or diverticulitic encroachment on the lumen. The use of hydrophilic colloid laxatives or enemas of tap water may be required for the remainder of the patient's life, if motivation for more drastic alteration of living, eating, and defecatory habits cannot be stimulated or if poor muscle tone, difficulties in ambulation and in achieving a comfortable posture at stool, or cerebral arteriosclerosis are major factors.

As described in Chap. 40, the presence of unaccustomed fecal masses in the rectosigmoid may produce rectal urgency in the patient who has always had normal defecatory responses to such masses. Sudden onset of rectal urgency in a previously healthy person demands immediate investigation. Usually it is seen in young adults required by emergency surgical indications to lie very still in bed (classically, in ophthalmologic, orthopedic, or neurosurgical disorders); intolerable urgency accompanied by the passage of watery exudate of small quantity suggests that an impaction has occurred. Severe urgency accompanied by the frequent passage of an exudate rich in blood, pus, or mucus usually signifies the presence of an acute proctitis (see below).

ACUTE INFLAMMATION OF THE COLON

Acute inflammation of the colon is most often due to the sudden invasion by parasites, bacteria, or viruses. It is characterized by the passage of an inflammatory exudate when there is infection with bacteria and viruses, and by the passage of blood without pus in most parasitic infestations. There is also an important group of nonspecific inflammatory disorders which may have their onset as an acute inflammation, or may first come to attention as a mildly acute exacerbation of what is obviously a chronic disease. In the following discussion emphasis will be placed on the methods by which such distinctions can be effected, and on the inferences as to etiology and course which such distinctions permit.

Patients suffering from acute diarrheal states with fever, cramps, and the passage of bloody stools are

and small intestinal mucosa, while leukocytes from normal individuals and from patients with Crohn's disease are not inhibited. Lymphocyte transformation by various antigens has not revealed any specific changes; likewise, secretory IgA concentration of colonic epithelium has not shown any diagnostic features.

Psychologic features of patients with ulcerative colitis were first stressed by Sullivan in 1932. Since then there have been many suggestions of a relation between the onset of the disorder and certain striking abnormalities in the personality structure of the patients and with their ways of coping with life stresses. Emphasis has been placed on the juvenile appearance of such patients, as well as their frequent feelings of "helplessness or hopelessness" in meeting routine life stresses. They often display an underlying hostility and have poorly developed interpersonal relations. On the other hand, about half the patients with ulcerative colitis appear to be normal in their psychologic behavior; these subjects have a resilient personal and work history, are successful in their educational pursuits, trade, or profession, and have maintained strong interpersonal relations. However, the other half present many of the features noted above.

A small number of patients have been studied prior to and subsequent to total colectomy; of these, about half have shown dramatic improvement of their depressive and despondent reactions, whereas underlying personality disorders persist in the remainder. The disease itself, with its relapses and remissions, its cost in time, money, and damaged career hopes, is usually associated with some degree of depression and anxiety in all patients. These reactions are important factors in modifying both the course of the disease and the response to therapy. There is little doubt that in a significant proportion of patients with ulcerative colitis deep-seated personality changes exist. However, it is not at all clear whether or how such psychopathology is related to the colonic inflammatory process.

CLINICAL FEATURES The major symptoms of chronic ulcerative colitis are *bloody diarrhea, abdominal pain, fever,* and *weight loss.* The extent of bleeding and diarrhea is quite variable, ranging from several semiformed stools per day to frequent passage, up to 20 times daily, of liquid stools with blood and pus. It should be emphasized that in as many as 25 percent of patients, specific colitic symptoms may be almost absent and only such nonspecific complaints as fatigue, malaise, or failure to thrive (in children) can be elicited. Rarely, a patient with ulcerative colitis may present with constipation alternating with bouts of diarrhea.

In most patients, very little will be found on routine physical examination, except that the abdomen may be rather prominent. In some patients one finds signs of extracolonic manifestations such as jaundice, ocular inflammation, or arthritis. The laboratory findings in ulcerative colitis are quite nonspecific. Anemia, due to a combination of iron deficiency and chronic inflammation, is common. Leukocytosis with a shift to the left is frequent, especially during acute febrile exacerbations. Hypoalbuminemia, electrolyte disturbances, and elevations of the sedimentation rate are often found.

Whether the disease is localized to the rectum or involves varying lengths of descending colon, about 50 percent of patients give a history of *an insidious, often cyclic or recurrent, course,* punctuated by more acute episodes. These latter are often misdiagnosed as acute infectious dysentery for which antibiotics or antidiarrheal drugs have been prescribed. About 40 percent of patients, regardless of the anatomic distribution of their disease, have an acute onset, with blood in the stools, diarrhea, and abdominal cramps or pain. The remaining 10 percent of patients present with an *acute, fulminant colitis* (toxic megacolon) in which the entire colon is involved. The hallmarks of this form of fulminant colitis are tachycardia, weakness, abdominal distention, fever, and the passage of large volumes of fluid stools, suggesting that the absorbing function of the colon has been almost totally lost. The distention of the transverse colon may be easily confirmed by plain films of the abdomen. While normally the diameter of the transverse colon usually does not exceed 8 cm, in these patients not only is the diameter greater than 8 cm, but often islands of necrotic tissue or gas in the bowel wall itself may be seen on the abdominal x-ray.

DIAGNOSIS In addition to having a high index of suspicion when patients present with any of the clinical features noted above, the physician must think of ulcerative colitis when patients present with obscure fever, anemia, arthritis, weight loss, and evidence of unexplained liver disease. The single most important procedure for the diagnosis is sigmoidoscopy. X-ray studies of the colon aid in determining the extent of more proximal changes. Further information may be obtained by the use of the colonoscope, but the friable, thinned bowel of the patient with ulcerative colitis presents a major hazard to the introduction of any instrument above the peritoneal floor, as does the preparation needed for this procedure.

The typical sigmoidoscopic appearance of the rectum and colon involved by ulcerative colitis consists of (1) loss of the normal mucosal vascular pattern, (2) friability of the mucosa to swabbing, (3) edema, (4) ulceration, (5) purulent mucosal exudate, which, when swabbed, exposes a bare and bleeding mucosa, (6) inflammatory polyps, and (7) strictures, most commonly noted just inside the anal canal or about 8 to 9 cm above this area. The most subtle but important early change is mucosal friability; later manifestations are inflammatory polyps and strictures. It is important to determine the volume of the rectum by digital examination and by sigmoidoscopy. Characteristically, the rectal capacity is markedly reduced by muscular contraction and eventually by some degree of fibrosis. Confirmation of the inflammatory process may be obtained by rectal biopsy, which in the rectum can be safely carried out with biopsy forceps, but when applied to the mucosa about the peritoneal reflection, requires special suction biopsy techniques.

The radiologic examination of the colon is an important part of the diagnostic work-up, but the *preparation of very ill patients for barium enema is hazardous.* For the patient not presenting with acute or fulminant manifestations, the standard x-ray preparation can be safely followed. The barium study may reveal shortening and straightening of the rectosigmoid and sigmoid, together with a very symmetric mural involvement with small ulcerations, loss of normal haustral patterns, and a pipelike appearance of the descending colon. The important diagnostic features are the *continuous* involvement of the process, the symmetry of the abnormal appearance of the bowel wall, and the demonstration of inflammatory polyps when they exist (see Fig. 288-5). Later changes include strictures and complications such as localized perforations and carcinoma. *In the acutely ill patient barium studies are not indicated*; plain films of the abdomen will permit the physician to diagnose and follow the course of colonic distention.

Stool cultures for pathogenic bacteria, and stool examination, rectal swabbings, or rectal biopsy for the presence of amebas are also important diagnostic tests. If significant anal abnormalities are noted on physical examination, a Frei test for lymphopathia venereum may be carried out.

DIFFERENTIAL DIAGNOSIS In distinguishing ulcerative colitis from other disorders, one must consider primarily the clinical symptoms, together with the sigmoidoscopic and radiologic features. When the primary complaint is rectal bleeding, *hemorrhoids* are commonly found and considered to be the cause. However, since hemorrhoids are very common, they should never be considered the sole cause of rectal bleeding until sigmoidoscopy and barium enema have ruled out other lesions. The next most important cause of rectal bleeding is *carcinoma of the colon*; here the combination of sigmoidoscopic and radiologic studies, plus cytology or colonoscopy, will serve to differentiate most cases. However, it must be remembered that ulcerative colitis and carcinoma may coexist. *Crohn's disease of the colon* may present with rectal bleeding; the differential diagnostic features are found in Table 288-1. *Amebiasis* may present initially as rectal bleeding, and such bleeding is commonly found even when other features are more prominent. Sigmoidoscopic demonstration of discrete ulcers, microscopic studies of the fecal swabbings showing hemorrhage without purulent exudate, isolation of amebas from colonic mucus, and demonstration of trophozoites in rectal biopsies are the most important differential findings. *Radiation proctitis* shows localized telangiectasia, submucosal atrophy, and friability in the midrectum; such a patient usually has a history of prior pelvic irradiation. Large rectal ulcers, aphthous oral ulcers, uveitis, and genital ulcers occur in *Behçet's syndrome.* The proctoscopic picture is not that of ulcerative colitis but more suggestive of amebic disease; the other manifestations may, in combination with rectal bleeding and ulceration, be more difficult to separate from ulcerative colitis.

FIGURE 288-5
Inflammatory disease of the colon. A *Chronic ulcerative colitis showing continuous involvement of descending colon and rectum.* B *Crohn's disease, showing discontinuous lesions at ileocecal valve and in descending colon.*

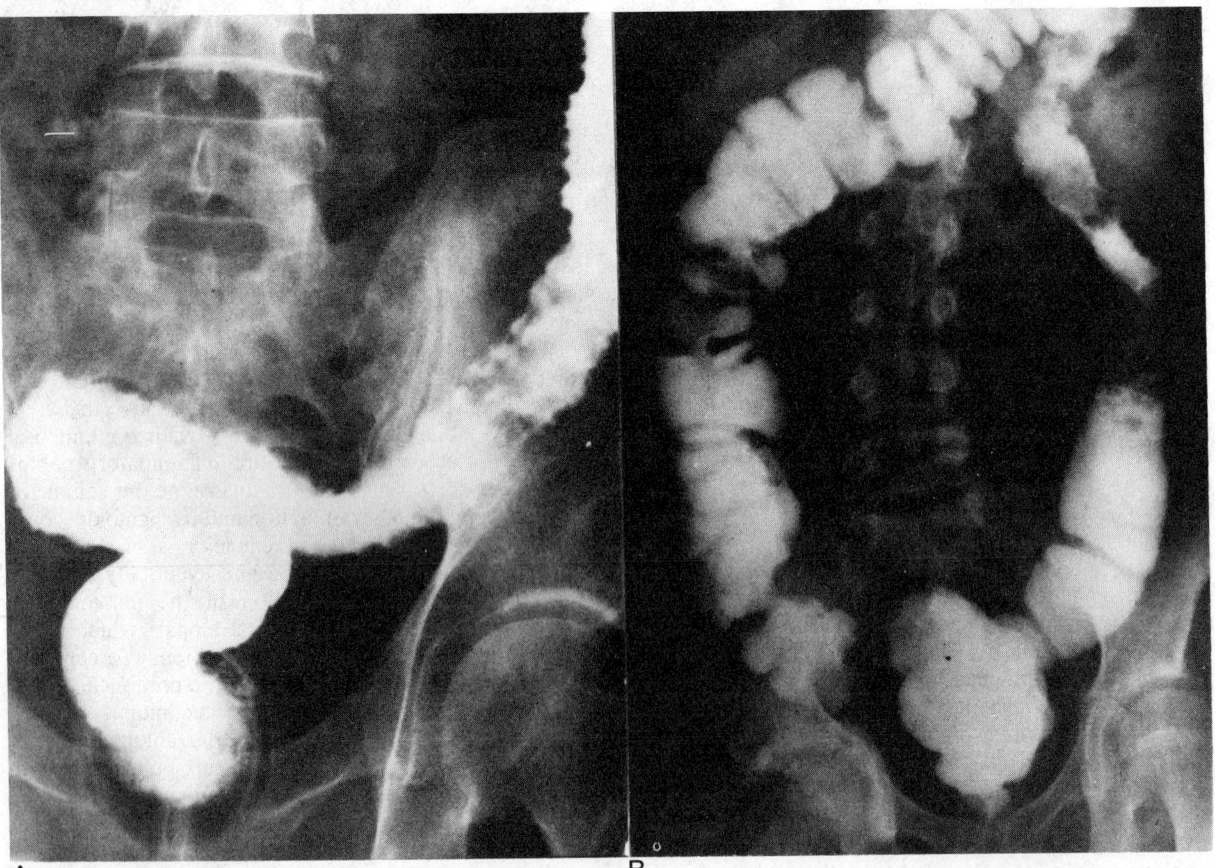

When diarrhea is the presenting symptom, the most important entities to be differentiated are the specific infections. *Acute* bacillary dysentery, especially shigellosis, produces hemorrhagic and purulent involvement of mucosa which may be proctoscopically indistinguishable from ulcerative colitis. The diagnosis therefore must be made by stool culture or serologic studies since the mucosal biopsy is not diagnostic. *Tuberculosis* of the intestine characteristically involves the terminal ileum and adjacent cecum. Pulmonary lesions may be absent. The lesion in tuberculosis is usually a hyperplastic process so that x-ray findings tend to resemble Crohn's disease or carcinoma of the ileocecal area rather than ulcerative colitis. Ulcerative tuberculosis of the colon is rare except in patients with far-advanced pulmonary tuberculosis. *Other causes of diarrhea which produce large bulky stools and other evidence of malabsorption* must be differentiated by their lack of inflammatory components, and by more specific tests such as intestinal biopsy, pancreatic function tests, and x-ray evidence of "blind loops" or diverticular disease of the small intestine.

Abdominal pain in association with rectal bleeding and sudden disturbance of bowel habits may be due to *ischemic colitis*, usually seen in older patients, especially those with generalized vascular disease. The proctoscopic examination is usually normal, unless the ischemic area involves the rectum. If the affected area is visible, one may observe edema, hyperemia, bleeding, and occasionally ulceration which can be confused with ulcerative colitis. The radiologic features of segmental bowel infarction have been well described, and should serve to provide adequate evidence for making this diagnosis.

Disturbance in bowel function, particularly constipation with rectal urgency (i.e., tenesmus with inability to expel stool) but with passage of mucus, blood, or pus is a feature of *ulcerative proctitis*. This diagnosis is totally dependent on proper interpretation of sigmoidoscopic findings, and x-ray studies are usually negative. Stinging rectal pain with creamy pus in the rectum suggests *gonorrheal proctitis*. In such patients, the discharge should be cultured for gonococci, and a history of anal intercourse should be sought. The *irritable bowel syndrome* (see above) usually first manifests itself in persons of the same age and sex as those at greatest risk of developing ulcerative colitis, but they do not have abnormal proctoscopic findings, fever, leucocytosis, or blood and pus in the stools. The barium enema is normal. Patients with chronic laxative abuse give a history of diarrhea which may be associated with hypokalemia and evidence of right-sided colonic dysfunction—very voluminous watery stools, but without the proctoscopic features of inflammation. The radiologic picture is quite characteristic, showing slowly changing muscular contractions, dilated ascending colon, and loss of haustrations of the left colon. The history of laxative taking, although often concealed, will confirm this diagnosis.

COURSE OF THE DISEASE When patients with ulcerative colitis are studied during their first clinical attack of the disease, and one eliminates from consideration all patients with histories longer than 1 year when first seen by a physician, certain facts with regard to their course and ultimate outcome may be established. In one study from England about 70 percent of such patients showed a remission with medical treatment—that is, the disease became totally asymptomatic. Another 16 percent showed marked symptomatic improvement; nearly 12 percent required surgical removal of the colon. About 4 percent died from the disease or its treatment. If one establishes criteria for assessing the severity of the initial and subsequent attacks of colitis, it can be shown that the worst outlook for the patient occurs when the initial attack is very severe, the entire colon is involved, and the patient is under fifteen or over fifty years of age.

Follow-up studies of these patients indicated that about 50 percent of patients became symptom-free after the first year of illness; in the other half, one or more attacks of the disease occurred annually. There was little indication that this proportion changed appreciably with the passage of time; in other words, the findings do not support the concept that the disease "burns itself out." However, for many the disease becomes such a lowgrade inflammation as to provoke little disability; patients become accustomed to minor diarrhea and tenesmus and will often deny that they are ill.

When the first attack of colitis occurs in children before age twelve years, there may be a number of special features. Many of these children pass normally formed stools coated with blood; radiologic findings are often equivocal, but sigmoidoscopic examinations show marked friability. Growth failure may be a feature of the illness, particularly if the entire colon is involved. As these children mature, they show a very high incidence of malignancy of the colon, which may be as high as 20 percent by age forty. These patients develop malignancy after having had their colitis for up to 25 years, and the unusual duration of the colitis must play some role in this alarming cancer incidence.

Patients who develop ulcerative colitis after age fifty also show distinctive features. Perhaps as a result of underlying aging of connective tissue or of vascular changes, local complications of the disease can be very severe even when the extent of the colitis is not great. The overall annual mortality resulting from such complications in elderly patients is about 11 percent when the entire colon is involved and about 5 percent for all cases of colitis. Cancer occurs in about 1 to 3 percent of such patients when followed for about 20 years; however, spontaneously occurring colonic cancer not related to colitis is also an important disease in this age group.

Patients with *ulcerative proctitis* show the same lesions in the rectal mucosa as are seen more proximal in ulcerative colitis; on rectal biopsy the lesions are identical. It is generally agreed that the course of the disease is milder, extra colonic manifestations are rare, and response to therapeutic measures more immediate than in those with more extensive disease. About 10 percent of these patients will show a gradual extension of the inflammatory process into the rectosigmoid. Patients presenting with ulcerative proctitis appear to have the same age-sex distribution and personality and ethnic characteristics as are found in the total spectrum of patients with inflammatory bowel disease.

It should be emphasized that an acute proctitis may be due to other factors such as antibiotic therapy, radiation, or other illness. It is unwise to label any patient with proctitis as having chronic ulcerative colitis when he is suffering a first attack of proctitis. Such patients should be carefully followed; if they do not have another bout within several years, their prognosis is good and recurrences are unlikely.

COMPLICATIONS OF ULCERATIVE COLITIS These are listed in Table 288-2. The percentages are based on a large series of patients followed in Leeds, England. Since the bowel is thinned out by the disease, it is subject to perforation as the inflammatory process advances. *Acute perforation* occurs most often with the first severe attack and is more likely to occur with extensive colonic involvement. Perforation most often involved the sigmoid colon, but can occur at any colonic site. The typical features are those of peritonitis, with evidence of systemic toxicity; diagnosis is made by abdominal x-rays showing air under the diaphragms. In patients with chronic disease, perforation may not be "free," but may manifest itself by increasing abdominal pain or the presence of a newly demonstrated stricture on the barium enema. Conservative management of patients with perforation carries a high mortality; most authorities believe that a demonstrated perforation is an indication for colectomy.

Acute dilatation or toxic megacolon can occur with any inflammatory disease of the colon, but is most often seen in ulcerative colitis. It is usually a manifestation and reflection of the severity of the underlying process. The patient typically has high fever, tachycardia, electrolyte imbalance, hypoalbuminemia, and pronounced diarrhea. Sometimes acute dilatation or toxic megacolon occurs suddenly in a patient with pancolitis in remission, with the onset of distention, abdominal pain, cessation of stools, and anorexia. Events which often precede this complication are excessive use of antimotility drugs (such as diphenoxylate, anticholinergics, or morphine) or vigorous use of cathartics and enemas in preparation for barium studies. This process probably goes unrecognized in many patients with chronic colitis, and may be spontaneously reversible. Generally, it can be described as a paralysis of the motor function of the transverse colon, with rapid dilatation of that segment of the bowel, best diagnosed by the plain film of the abdomen. The diameter of the colon exceeds 8 cm, and the wall may be noted to contain gas. Often the borders on the luminal side are shaggy; sometimes islands of necrotic mucosa can be seen to alternate with preserved mucosa. The predilection of the dilatation for the transverse colon suggests a functional obstruction at the splenic flexure, which is almost always severely diseased in these patients.

TABLE 288-2
Local complications of ulcerative colitis

		Patients, %
I Anorectal		17.6
A Abscess	6.0	
B Fistula in ano	5.4	
C Rectovaginal fistula	2.2	
D Fissure in ano	12.3	
II Pseudopolyposis		12.5
III Stricture		11.2
IV Perforation		2.8
V Carcinoma		1.7
VI Dilatation, all types		3.4
VII Massive hemorrhage		1.5
Total		50.7

SOURCE: *JC Goligher et al*, Ulcerative Colitis, *Baltimore: Williams & Wilkins, 1968*

This complication, occurring usually in patients with severe pancolitis, is associated with a high mortality. The overall mortality in reported cases is about 30 percent. Death may be the result of localized perforation and excessive fluid loss into the lumen, leading to hypovolemic shock and infection. Some of these patients respond to massive fluid replacement and very high doses of corticosteroids. However, if such therapy does not result in marked improvement within a few days, most patients require emergency surgical intervention, the extent of the surgery depending on the patient's ability to tolerate a total colectomy. Staged procedures have also been used with success.

Anorectal complications such as fissures, fistulas, and abscesses may be the presenting symptoms in about 10 percent of patients. Many of the anal complaints occur secondary to the diarrhea itself. For the patient, the discomfort and anxiety produced by anorectal complications are often of more concern than the other symptoms of colitis; the discomfort may discourage attempts by the physician to examine the patient with the sigmoidoscope or to carry out necessary diagnostic studies. Local anesthetics may be helpful under such circumstances; short-acting general anesthesia is warranted if it is impossible otherwise to carry out such studies because of pain. The management of such complications consists of the local measures, as noted below, and treatment of the colitis itself. In some patients the entire function of the anorectal segment is lost; this is an indication for colectomy and ileostomy.

Rectovaginal fistulas may occur as a result of the breakdown of the wall between the rectum and vagina. The development of colonic *strictures* may be caused by muscular hypertrophy, fibrosis, or malignancy. Inflammation and hypertrophy of the muscularis may cause narrowing which varies over the course of time. Hence, "strictures" of this sort may be reversible. True fibrosis is unusual in ulcerative colitis, but when present may mimic a constricting carcinoma. For this reason, when a narrowed segment or stricture is found, it is important to exclude the presence of carcinoma; if the narrowed area can be seen and reached directly, biopsy and brush cytology may be diagnostic. The radiologic differentiation of benign from malignant stricture is not simple; colonoscopic examination may be helpful.

Inflammatory polyps or "pseudopolyps" may appear within a few months of a first attack of severe colitis; more commonly, however, they are noted within the first or second year after the onset of the colitis. They are a response to mucosal ulceration, and thus define to some extent the severity of the mucosal damage. They are not of themselves precancerous, but they occur in the patients with severe disease who are more likely to develop colon cancer. They produce no symptoms and require no specific treatment. When present they may make it difficult for the endoscopist to note early carcinoma developing in mucosa adjacent to the polypoid changes.

Carcinoma of the colon is a significant complication, although the overall incidence is difficult to define unless one subgroups the colitic population. Patients with localized ulcerative proctitis are *not* subject to increased risk of carcinoma of either rectum or colon. In patients whose colitis begins before age fifteen, the risk of colon cancer is about 20 percent in those who have the disease for 20 years. This risk continues and increases with age. Adult patients with recent onset of colitis have a cancer risk of 2 to 3 percent. Factors increasing the risk are (1) disease duration greater than 10 years, (2) pancolitis, and (3) family history of colonic cancer. In general, patients with ulcerative colitis (other than proctitis) have an incidence of colonic cancer which is at least ten times greater than that of a matched control population.

Carcinoma of the colon in patients with colitis tends to be difficult to diagnose for many reasons. Symptoms are often those of colitis. The tumors often arise multicentrically, have a poorly defined outline radiologically, and even grossly have spreading, indurated margins which blend into the abnormal colitic mucosa. Since the diagnosis is so difficult, other means of suspecting carcinomatous changes have been proposed. Morson and Pang believe that a generalized precancerous stage can be identified in rectal or rectosigmoid biopsies of patients who either have or will soon develop cancer of the colon. In their view, suspicious microscopic changes consist of epithelial tubules penetrating the muscularis, and atypical epithelial cells, with stratification of enlarged nuclei and increased mitotic activity. It is hoped that refinements and increasing specificity of the carcinoembryonic antigen (CEA) test will permit serologic identification of patients who are in danger of developing colonic carcinoma. Without such help, one must depend on radiologic criteria, cytologic studies, and possibly colonoscopic biopsy for determining early malignancy. Because all such methods are uncertain and the disease carries such a high fatality rate, some authorities advocate prophylactic proctocolectomy for children with colitis of more than 10 years' duration, and for all adults with pancolitis of more than 20 years' duration. There is, however, no general agreement on this approach.

Systemic complications (see Table 288-3) *Nutritional and metabolic complications* result from deficient colonic intake as well as from increased nutritional requirements and losses. Most patients with moderately severe ulcerative colitis have some anorexia; severely ill patients have in addition nausea and often vomiting. Weight loss and loss of muscle mass are to be expected under such circumstances. The negative nitrogen balance seen in all febrile inflammatory states is enhanced by increased corticosteroid production and increased levels of circulating catecholamines; these serve to mobilize fat from adipose tissue and stimulate gluconeogenesis. Muscle breakdown releases potassium from cells, and potassium deficits are common in these ill patients. Many such patients are initially unable to take oral feedings and are fed parenterally with fluids which are usually deficient in calcium and magnesium. Magnesium deficiency is an important complication and may account for some of the irritability seen

in the severely ill patient. The large surface area of mucosal ulceration also permits losses of albumin, red blood cells, and potassium in the stools. Anemia may be due to iron deficiency or secondary to chronic inflammation. Drug-induced hemolytic anemia may develop in patients with deficiency of glucose 6-phosphate dehydrogenase receiving salicylazosulfapyridine or other sulfonamides; such a process may be suspected by the presence of Heinz bodies in the peripheral blood smear. Defects in blood coagulation may also occur; most often this is due to increased coagulability, with the production of thromboembolic phenomena. In both ulcerative colitis and Crohn's disease there may be an increase in the number of circulating platelets when the disease is active.

A major systemic complication of chronic ulcerative colitis is liver disease. The incidence of liver biopsy abnormalities in patients with colitis ranges from 50 to 90 percent; however, the incidence of significant clinical liver disease is approximately 1 to 3 percent. A common histologic abnormality, especially in autopsy material, is fatty *infiltration.* This lesion has been related to nutritional deficiencies and chronic inflammation. *Pericholangitis* is characterized pathologically by inflammation of the portal tract, bile duct proliferation, and fibrosis around the bile ductules. These changes may be related to portal bacteremia which occurs intermittently in some patients with colitis. Patients with pericholangitis may have normal or only mildly abnormal liver function tests. Others present with jaundice and elevation of the alkaline phosphatase which mimic extrahepatic obstruction. Post necrotic and biliary *cirrhosis* are also seen in some patients with colitis, although the etiology is not clear. Finally, *chronic active hepatitis* may complicate colitis. Although colectomy may arrest the progress of pericholangitis in some patients, this benefit must be weighed against the increased surgical morbidity and mortality in colitis patients with concomitant liver disease.

A variety of *skin lesions* may occur in up to 5 percent of patients. Erythema nodosum appears most often in females with colitis. Pyoderma gangrenosum is a suppurative ulcerating lesion found on the legs and ankles,

TABLE 288-3
Systemic complications of ulcerative colitis

I Nutritional and metabolic changes
- *A* Loss of muscle mass
- *B* Electrolyte losses (K^+, Ca^{++}, Mg^{++})
- *C* Hypoalbuminemia
- *D* Iron-deficiency anemia
- *E* Vitamin deficiencies
- *F* Hypocholesterolemia
- *G* Disturbed growth and maturation

II Arthritis
III Hepatic inflammation, fatty infiltration
IV Skin disorders
V Uveitis
VI Stomatitis
VII Venous thrombosis and thromboembolism
VIII Renal stones

usually in patients with very active colitis. These lesions often improve as the colitis is brought under control, either by medical or surgical treatment. However, some patients have persistent pyoderma in the face of inactive colitis, and occasionally after removal of the colon. *Uveitis* has been reported in about 3 to 10 percent of patients. Although the uveitis may respond well to local or systemic corticosteroid therapy, dramatic disappearance of the lesion may be noted when colectomy is done for other indications.

Joint manifestations may be found in 10 to 20 percent of patients. In ulcerative colitis and Crohn's disease, an acute arthritis may occur, especially in knees, hips, and ankles. The bouts of synovitis correlate with the activity of the colitis, although occasionally the arthritis may precede the colitis. Rheumatoid factor is not present in the serum, and no specific organisms can be found in synovial fluid. This type of arthritis is usually self-limited and does not lead to permanent joint deformity. Spondylitis, especially of the sacroiliac joints, occurs in both ulcerative colitis and Crohn's disease. The course of the spondylitis is not well correlated with activity of the intestinal disease, and it may persist during remissions or following colectomy. Since ankylosing spondylitis is ordinarily a disease of men, the occurrence of sacroileitis in a woman should suggest the possibility of an underlying inflammatory bowel disease.

TREATMENT Medical management Except for those patients with disease limited to the rectum, an acute attack of ulcerative colitis requires hospitalization for proper treatment. The disease can be explosive, and it is often impossible to anticipate its course from the initial presentation. The aims of therapy are to replace nutritional losses and to control the inflammatory process as quickly as possible. It is often best to recommend bed rest and to prohibit any oral intake of foods for several days. Fluid and electrolyte losses are replaced by intravenous fluids, and anemia is corrected by blood transfusions. Sedatives and tranquilizers are best withheld; instead, support and judicious psychotherapy are both important and preferable. Particular attention must be paid to poor prognostic signs such as persistent tachycardia, abdominal distention, and continuous diarrhea without oral intake of food or fluids.

Attention must be directed at replacement of calories, electrolytes, and vitamins. These can be supplied initially by the parenteral route. Parenteral hyperalimentation may be resorted to if the nutritional status is poor or if oral feedings aggravate the colitis. Oral intake can usually be resumed within a few days of admission, as the inflammatory process is being treated and contained.

Specific *anti-inflammatory measures* generally do not include the use of antibiotics unless a specific infection complication is suspected or operation is planned. The two drugs which have been proved most useful in controlling the inflammatory reaction are (1) adrenal corticosteroids, most particularly prednisone (or prednisolone) and ACTH, and (2) salicylazosulfapyridine (Azulfidine). The latter drug is a poor antimicrobial agent but seems to exert an anti-inflammatory effect while bound to the intestinal wall.

For the acutely ill patient the administration of corticosteroids or ACTH is the logical anti-inflammatory therapy. The advantages of ACTH over corticosteroids have not been conclusively established except possibly for treatment of the most severely ill patients; for the usual patient it is impossible to demonstrate any superiority. The usual practice is to give the patient 40 to 80 units ACTH in a slow drip of 500 ml glucose and saline over an 8-hr period, supplemented with 20 to 40 mEq potassium. (Some authorities give as much as 120 units ACTH.) As the patient improves, usually by the fourth or fifth day, the ACTH dosage is reduced by half. After about 10 days oral prednisone may be substituted, usually starting at a level of 30 to 40 mg daily. If prednisone (or prednisolone) rather than ACTH is given initially, it should be administered in daily doses of 40 to 60 mg. After the acute phase begins to subside, the total daily dosage is reduced by 5 mg every 3 or 4 days or by 10 mg at weekly intervals. It is important to give large doses of corticosteroids immediately in order to gain quick control of the inflammation rather than using lower doses in the hope of avoiding the complications of corticosteroid therapy.

After initial improvement has occurred, oral food intake may be started, and the dosage of prednisone reduced. Many physicians add Azulfidine to the regimen, at a level of about 3 g daily in divided doses. During the first week of Azulfidine therapy headache and nausea may occur; hence, the drug is not given initially to patients who already have nausea and anorexia. The combined therapy permits a more rapid reduction in steroid dosage, so that the patient may be maintained on daily doses of Azulfidine, 2 to 3 g daily, and prednisone, 15 to 20 mg daily. Some physicians find alternate-day prednisone therapy effective (i.e., 30 to 40 mg every other day), but there is no uniform agreement on the effectiveness of alternate-day therapy in ulcerative colitis.

The above regimen results in satisfactory control of nearly 90 percent of patients presenting with first attacks. Since the main thrust of medical therapy is to control the inflammatory process as quickly as possible, the use of antimotility drugs, antianxiety or antidepressive preparations, and anabolic steroids during this initial period may make the physician's task more rather than less difficult. *Identifying the patient who will not respond and who needs emergency surgery is most important.* Careful and frequent observations of the patient, including abdominal x-rays, are necessary. *Barium enemas should not be performed during the acute phase of the illness.* Repeated proctoscopies may be needed to evaluate mucosal responses, but these may bear little relation to the general condition of the patient, and are better deferred during the first 10 days of hospitalization. The patient should be seen by both the surgeon and the internist during this initial period.

In patients with ulcerative proctitis or mild attacks of known ulcerative colitis, a different approach may be taken. These patients do not require hospitalization and may respond to therapy with Azulfidine, since this agent is particularly effective in reducing friability and bleeding. The usual initial dosage is 1 to 2 g four times daily with meals. If tenesmus continues, such patients often are markedly relieved by the intrarectal instillation of topical steroids, of which there are many available preparations.

In general, 20 mg prednisone (or 100 mg hydrocortisone) in 60 to 100 ml saline administered in the knee-chest position at bedtime provides good control without producing appreciable steroid side effects. The newer disposable retention enema units or foams containing hydrocortisone are a practical approach to the problem. If large doses of rectal steroids are needed to control symptoms, it is preferable to put the patient instead on oral prednisone at doses of about 20 mg per day. Such patients may do well on alternate-day prednisone, at levels of 20 to 40 mg per dose.

The side effects of corticosteroid therapy (described in Chap. 86) may be difficult to interpret in the treatment of patients with acute ulcerative colitis, who are frequently undernourished, anemic, febrile, and emotionally disturbed on admission. Gastrointestinal bleeding and sepsis are particularly difficult to assess in patients with colitis taking corticosteroids. Azulfidine toxicity, as manifested by rash, leucopenia, or hemolytic anemia, may occur within 3 to 4 weeks after start of the drug.

Psychotherapy Psychiatric approaches to patients with ulcerative colitis are in some dispute. Most psychiatrists agree that the acutely ill patient is approachable only with the most superficial forms of supportive psychotherapy. This is supplied by the physician managing the case, who needs to establish a strong physician-patient relation. The physician should search the patient's history and behavior for indications of inner resources and motivations which can be converted to therapeutic use. Attempts to manipulate the immediate home and work environment of the patient are necessary, but may require professional psychiatric assistance. This is particularly true in children and pregnant women. Ulcerative colitis beginning during pregnancy is often very severe and often creates profound psychologic disturbances. The attending physician should create an attitude of optimism, warm concern, and orderly management; frequent visits and examinations are the cornerstone of good medical management.

In the chronically ill patient, in particular children or adolescents, psychiatric help is often crucial in assessing and strengthening adaptive responses, and in preparing patients for colectomy. When ulcerative colitis occurs in elderly patients, it is often in a setting of despondency which may require emergency psychiatric care. Suicide accounts for a small but appreciable number of deaths from this disease.

Surgical therapy Colectomy should be considered in chronic ulcerative colitis under the following circumstances: (1) in acute fulminant disease with persistent dilatation of the colon, fever, tachycardia, and diarrhea despite vigorous therapy; (2) severe life-threatening hemorrhage; (3) perforation; (4) for control of systemic complications such as pericholangitis or pyoderma gangrenosum; (5) in patients with chronic debilitating disease poorly controlled by medical management; (6) for stricture or suspected malignancy; and (7) as prophylaxis for carcinoma in colitis of greater than 10 years' duration. These indications for surgery are not absolute, and the decision to operate must be weighed carefully in each case. Many patients are extremely reluctant to have surgery and require much support prior to operation. It is very helpful for the patient to speak with someone with an ileostomy who is of his own age and sex. This can be very helpful in reducing anxiety and allowing the patient to face and accept permanent ileostomy.

Colitis and pregnancy *Colitis and pregnancy* pose a special problem. The pregnancy itself is not adversely affected by the existence of the colitis (i.e., of women with colitis who become pregnant, 85 percent will have normal offspring). Ulcerative colitis developing during pregnancy may be more severe than usual. It was previously believed that such patients did poorly, perhaps because of the severe psychologic stresses associated with the pregnancy. Recent data indicate that the incidence of a relapse of colitis in women of childbearing age is similar (i.e., about 45 percent) with or without pregnancy. However, attacks occur more frequently in the first trimester and in the early puerperium.

SUMMARY Ulcerative colitis is a chronic inflammatory disease of the colon, encountered in all age groups, always involving the rectum, and any area of colon more proximal, always in continuity. About 75 percent of patients will be able to cope with it medically, despite the remissions and exacerbations which characterize its course. The disease is more severe when its onset is in childhood or in those over fifty. Ulcerative proctitis carries no threat to life, and patients with proctitis alone are rarely hospitalized. Among those with more extensive disease who are hospitalized, approximately 10 percent die of their disease or its complications, including carcinoma of the colon. Surgical intervention is necessary in about 20 percent of patients with colitis, and as patients survive longer on medical therapy it is likely that more local and neoplastic complications will be encountered and require further surgical treatment.

Crohn's disease of the colon (granulomatous colitis)

In the last decade numerous studies have confirmed the existence of a chronic inflammatory colitis with features similar to Crohn's disease of the small intestine, and separate from chronic ulcerative colitis. This entity is called *Crohn's disease of the colon* or *granulomatous colitis.* (The latter term is less accurate since not all cases have granulomas.) Although the pathologic and clinical features overlap with those of ulcerative colitis, there are sufficient differences to allow Crohn's disease of the colon to exist as a separate diagnostic entity (see Table 288-1). However, a significant number of patients cannot be categorized as having Crohn's disease or ulcerative colitis because features of both entities coexist.

PATHOLOGY The major findings are similar to those seen in the intestine in regional enteritis (see Chap. 285). The presence of sinus tracts and granulomas in the colon help to distinguish it from ulcerative colitis. This is a *transmural* disease, affecting all layers of the colon, but the mucosa least severely. The bowel becomes thickened and may become attached to adjacent tissues or viscera leading ultimately to enteroenteric fistulas. Perianal fistulas and abscesses are common, and in females rectovaginal fistulas are found. The principal feature of the inflammation is its patchy distribution. The rectum is often spared; the disease may involve only the right colon segments of the transverse or descending colon, or the entire colon including the rectum. However, the involvement is not of the continuous and symmetric character as in ulcerative colitis. Crohn's disease of the colon alone is believed to occur in about 10 percent of all cases of Crohn's disease; the colon and small bowel are both involved in about 30 percent of cases. It is estimated that Crohn's disease of the colon composes up to 50 percent of all cases of chronic inflammatory bowel disease.

EPIDEMIOLOGY AND ETIOLOGY The features are generally those of ulcerative colitis. The sex ratio is more nearly equal compared with ulcerative colitis. The disorder probably begins somewhat earlier in life; approximately 20 to 30 percent of cases occur before the age of twenty. However, it is not uncommon to find the first evidence of the disease over the age of fifty. Epidemiologic studies suffer from the insidious onset of this disorder, associated lesions such as diverticulosis, and inadequacy of initial studies for generally vague complaints. Extensive Crohn's disease has been found at autopsy in patients with no prior history of gastrointestinal symptoms. At present the views as to possible etiology are similar to those of Crohn's disease of the small bowel (Chap. 285).

CLINICAL FEATURES Fever, abdominal pain, diarrhea often without urgency, and generalized fatigability are the principal complaints as in ulcerative colitis. The presence of severe anorectal complications such as fistula and abscess formation are important clinical clues in the diagnosis of Crohn's disease of the colon. The radiographic features of this disease are cobblestoning, skip areas, internal fistulas, and asymmetric involvement of the bowel wall. Arthritis, uveitis, aphthous ulcerations of the oral or genital mucosa, hepatic functional derangements (including pericholangitis), and fistulous involvement of the anal and pudendal areas constitute the main complications. As with the small-intestinal form, colonic Crohn's disease is a recurrent, often low-grade inflammatory process which fluctuates in intensity from inactivity to the production of a toxic megacolon indistinguishable clinically from that seen in ulcerative colitis. Colonic malignancy is significantly more common in these patients than in the general population, but the incidence is not as great as in ulcerative colitis.

DIFFERENTIAL DIAGNOSIS The principal features of ulcerative colitis versus Crohn's colitis are outlined in Table 288-1. The other diseases from which the disease must be distinguished are tuberculosis, lymphoma, ischemic colitis, diverticulitis, and cancer.

TREATMENT The approaches to medical management are similar to those used for ulcerative colitis, but Azulfidine and corticosteroids are not as effective in Crohn's disease. Results are usually satisfactory with respect to control of fever, diarrhea, and systemic manifestations. Temporary remissions as well as recurrences are common. The disease tends to be less explosive than ulcerative colitis; free perforations or general peritonitis are not frequent. Of importance is the fact that the disease tends to progress despite apparent clinical well-being.

The principal problem in management relates to the results of surgery. Whereas total proctocolectomy in ulcerative colitis may be regarded as curative, this is not the case in Crohn's colitis, especially when the small intestine is also involved. A recurrence rate ranging from 35 to 50 percent after 10 years has been found in patients subject to proctocolectomy for Crohn's disease of the colon. This recurrence rate is even higher for those with disease of both the large and small intestine. The operative mortality for each operation is at least 4 to 5 percent. Healing of the perineal wound site is often delayed for months, in marked contrast to the patient with ulcerative colitis following colectomy. In spite of this rather gloomy outlook, some studies have shown 80 percent of all patients to be reasonably well some 12 to 15 years after surgery; they may have occasional symptoms but generally are able to work and lead satisfactory lives.

ISCHEMIC COLONIC DISEASE (SEGMENTAL INFARCTION, ISCHEMIC COLITIS)

Ischemia of the colon is a disease most often affecting the elderly population, owing to the greater frequency of vascular disease in that group. Although some cases of large-bowel infarction are caused by embolus or thrombosis of the mesenteric artery, the majority of cases do not have a demonstrable arterial occlusion. In these patients, the ischemia is probably secondary to spasm of mucosal vessels or shunting of blood flow away from the end arterioles. The exact pathogenesis of nonocclusive ischemic colitis is currently unknown.

Clinically, ischemia of the colon can present as acute fulminant colitis, subacute colitis, or as postischemic stricture. In the acute fulminant variety there is severe lower abdominal pain and massive rectal bleeding, often accompanied by shock. Since perforation of the colon is common, barium enema should not be performed. Arteriography may reveal an obstruction of the inferior mesenteric artery or severe spasm of mucosal vessels. Irreversible necrosis and gangrene of the colon are frequently found; hence, surgical resection is usually required.

The commonest clinical variant of ischemic colonic disease is subacute ischemic colitis. These patients have lesser degrees of pain and bleeding, often occurring over several days or weeks. The left colon is usually involved, and if the process extends low enough, sigmoidoscopy will reveal edema, hemorrhage, and ulceration of the mucosa which is difficult to distinguish from ulcerative colitis. Arteriography may reveal tapering or spasm of the colonic vessels, but occlusion is not observed. Barium enema shows irregularity and cobblestoning of the mucosa caused by submucosal hemorrhage and edema. Occasionally stricture formation may follow a bout of ischemic colitis, or may present *de novo* without a history of antecedent pain and bloody diarrhea. Most cases of nonocclusive ischemic colitis resolve in 2 to 4 weeks and do not recur. Surgery is usually not required except for obstruction secondary to postischemic stricture.

TUMORS OF THE COLON AND RECTUM

Neoplasms of the large intestine and rectum account, in the United States, for about 20 percent of all deaths due to malignant disease. These lesions represent 45 percent of all deaths due to neoplasms of the digestive tract, being twice as frequent as the number of deaths due to cancer of the stomach. They occur equally among males and females and in all age groups but are most frequently encountered in persons over age forty-five.

ETIOLOGY Although the causes of colonic malignancy are not established, there appears to be an intimate relation between the adenomatous polyp and the development of carcinoma. All stages of carcinomatous change have been recognized in polyps, and there appears to be a definite risk of malignant polypoid growth and of malignancy in the colons of patients who have polyps, whether or not the tumor originates in or near the polyps. Congenital multiple polyposis of the colon has an astonishingly high malignant potential; chronic inflammatory disease of the colon, as seen in ulcerative colitis, also seems to potentiate or stimulate the development of carcinoma in the diseased bowel. Other lesions of the large intestine seem to bear no causal relation to cancer. As with malignant disease generally, familial aggregates of the disease are well documented, and multiple malignant lesions have been shown to occur in certain members of such families.

PATHOLOGY The majority of tumors originating in the colon and rectum are of epithelial origin. Those which are not are usually benign; they include lipomas, endometriosis, benign lymphomas, leiomyomas, and hemangiomas. Nonepithelial malignant lesions are infrequent but should be mentioned because of the necessity for recognizing them in a treatable stage of their development. *Carcinoids* of the rectosigmoid and rectum ordinarily form yellowish elevations between the muscularis mucosae and mucosa. They are usually discovered by chance sigmoidoscopy, although a few have been indicted as causing bleeding. If the muscularis is invaded, the tumor is malignant and will require wide excision. It is estimated that 10 percent of rectal carcinoids will metastasize. Those beginning in the ileocecal valve or in the cecum, although not ulcerating deeply, metastasize early to regional nodes and the liver; radiologically they may present as a rounded filling defect. *Leiomyosarcomas* of the colon are usually found in the sigmoid or rectum, where they may grow to large size and produce mucosal ulceration with bleeding. *Lymphosarcomas* of the colon and rectum may present as do carcinomas, but there is less fixation of the wall as the tumor grows, so that intussusception is occasionally the presenting syndrome. Colon carcinomas affect women more often than men; rectal carcinomas are seen more commonly in men. They have been recorded at all ages, but their peak incidence is in the fifth, sixth, and seventh decades. The cecum and ascending colon are involved in 15 percent of all carcinomas of the large bowel and rectum, the transverse colon in 10 percent, and the descending colon, rectosigmoid, and rectum in 75 percent. Thus, nearly 60 percent of all cancers of the large intestine are within reach of the sigmoidoscope. In most series of cases, multiple primary colonic cancers are found in about 3 percent of patients operated on or autopsied. Lesions of the colon which seem statistically to favor the development of carcinoma are multiple polyposis, adenomatous polyposis, and chronic ulcerative colitis of over 10 years' duration. In addition to the statistical "precancerous" nature of these lesions, definite observations have been made of the malignant transformation of villous adenomas, single adenomatous polyps, multiple adenomatous polyps, and multicentric foci in ulcerative colitis.

In the colon above the rectum, adenocarcinoma is the common cell type. Classifications of the tumors according to their microscopic appearance—papillary, medullary, scirrhous, or colloid—are not of great assistance to the physician. Obviously, scirrhous carcinomas tend to constrict the lumen of the bowel, thereby producing obstructive syndromes, especially in the sigmoid area. Colloid tumors, most common in the right colon, can grow to enormous bulky mucinous masses, often forming mucous fistulas to the overlying skin. The common medullary tumor grows as a solid mass, the bulk of which may produce intermittent obstructive symptoms. Papillary tumors of the distal colon usually bleed early. All tumors invade the regional lymph nodes and spread through the lymphatics and portal veins to the liver; direct spread into the paravertebral venous plexus is occasionally seen.

Symptoms of colon carcinoma are usually vague and nonspecific at the outset. Weight loss and malaise are common, often disregarded by the patient. It is convenient to divide cancers of the colon into those affecting the right and left sides. Cancers of the cecum and ascending colon are usually flat or polypoid, while those in the rectosigmoid are frequently annular and constrict the lumen. A large tumor in the cecum is often "silent" clinically because it does not obstruct the lumen or cause visible bleeding in the stool. Cancer of the rectosigmoid may obstruct the lumen or bleed and hence cause the patient to seek medical advice. The following symptoms are important clues to the presence of colonic carcinoma.

1 *Changes in bowel habits* are most frequent when carcinoma affects the left colon. These changes are often minimal but progressive alterations in the frequency or time of evacuation, in the size of the stool, and most significantly, in a sensation that evacuation has been incomplete.
2 *Bleeding* occurs in left-sided lesions in about 70 percent of cases and is usually noticed by the patient. When the lesion is in the ascending colon or cecum, fewer than 25 percent of patients notice any blood in or with the stools, no doubt because the blood is thoroughly admixed with the fecal slurry in the right colon. It is important that the physician *not* attribute to hemorrhoids or anal fissures bleeding that is dark, associated with clots, well-mixed with mucus, or adherent to the stool.
3 *Pain* in the lower part of the abdomen is occasionally a symptom of lesions of the cecum or ascending colon.

The pain is characteristically severe on climbing stairs or on bending forward. Pain in left colonic lesions may be related to varying degrees of bowel obstruction above a constricting carcinoma. Occasionally a sigmoid carcinoma may present as an acute bowel obstruction.

4 Symptoms of *anemia* are frequent in right-sided colonic cancer. Cardiac insufficiency and angina may be striking manifestations of the anemia, which reaches a remarkably severe degree in the absence of symptoms calling attention to the diseased bowel.

5 *Anorexia, weight loss,* and *malaise* may occur at any time.

PHYSICAL EXAMINATION As with most malignant tumors early signs are not found. Aside from the pallor due to anemia and the wasting suggestive of chronic disease, the signs are principally those due to masses, partial obstruction of the bowel, fistulas, and invasion of abdominal wall, bladder, uterus, and liver. Fecal masses are often felt behind partially obstructing neoplasms or inflammatory aggregates which have surrounded a perforation due to tumor. Rectal examination with the patient in the lithotomy or right decubitus position will often detect an intussuscepting lesion of the rectosigmoid. Marked distention in the right lower quadrant may represent an accommodation of bowel contents to incomplete obstruction by carcinoma of the left colon. Caution should be exercised in palpating the cecal area under such circumstances, as perforation, always imminent, may be precipitated by digital manipulation from either the abdominal or the intrarectal areas.

LABORATORY FINDINGS There are no diagnostic laboratory procedures. Detection of occult blood or gross blood in the stools is the most important laboratory technique for early identification of the possibility that malignancy of the colon exists. Iron-deficiency anemia is also an important laboratory finding. In the presence of liver metastases there is elevation of the serum alkaline phosphatase and increased Bromsulphalein retention. The role of CEA as an effective diagnostic test for colonic malignancy remains to be determined. The anemia is usually hypochromic and is present in over half the patients with right-sided lesions, even when occasional stool specimens do not contain occult blood. Patients with left-sided lesions may also be anemic, but to a much less severe degree and not so frequently, since their blood loss is more easily appreciated in the appearance of the stools.

DIAGNOSIS Carcinoma of the colon is one of the most common malignant tumors and therefore must be thought of whenever a patient complains of changes in bowel habits, regardless of the kind of change. The finding of gross or occult blood in the stools, a mass or distended colon on routine physical examination, definite abnormalities on rectal examination, or evidences of weight loss and chronic illness should make one consider the diagnosis very seriously. Vague dyspeptic symptoms, especially when hypochromic anemia is present, also should lead the physician to investigate the right colon in particular.

The combination of digital and proctosigmoidoscopic examination should bring 60 percent of all cancers of the colon and rectum into direct view. The lesion may present itself directly as a polypoid or solid mass, frequently ulcerated, as a large ulcer with a rolled margin, or as a deformity of the colonic wall producing obstruction to the passage of the instrument. Instillation of Ringer's solution through the sigmoidoscope and centrifugation of the returning fluid will yield exfoliative cytologic smears of diagnostic value in many cases. Biopsy of suspicious lesions should be carried out whenever possible.

Radiologic diagnosis of lesions above the peritoneal reflection is highly accurate, but not infallible. In the presence of rectal bleeding it is important to follow a barium enema which has been reported as normal with an air-contrast study; such air-contrast enemas may reveal small lesions (greater than 5 mm in diameter) as well as nondistensible portions of the bowel wall. A cecal area which does not respond satisfactorily to preparative enemas and laxatives and shows poor radiologic detail should be particularly suspected of harboring a tumor.

The radiologist looks for structural and physiologic abnormalities reflecting the various ways these tumors may present, as described above under Pathology. (1) Tumors may project into the bowel, giving rise to a filling defect in the barium column (Fig. 288-6). (2) They may partially or completely encircle the bowel, producing a narrowing of the barium column proximal to which the bowel is often dilated (Fig. 288-7). (3) They may, by contiguous infiltration, distort the position of the colon, so that it is not free to follow gravity during the radiologist's maneuvering of the patient. (4) After the patient has expelled the barium, films of the mucosal relief may show defects due to tumor which has not penetrated the muscular coat. (5) Some tumors give rise to no defects as such but interfere with peristalsis, so that irritability, fluid retention, and spasticity may be noted. It is worth emphasizing that the accuracy of barium enema in the diagnosis of rectal cancer is not high. It is imperative, therefore, that a careful sigmoidoscopic examination precede the barium enema.

Differential diagnosis of carcinoma of the ascending

FIGURE 288-6

Filling defect in the cecum produced by a carcinoma.

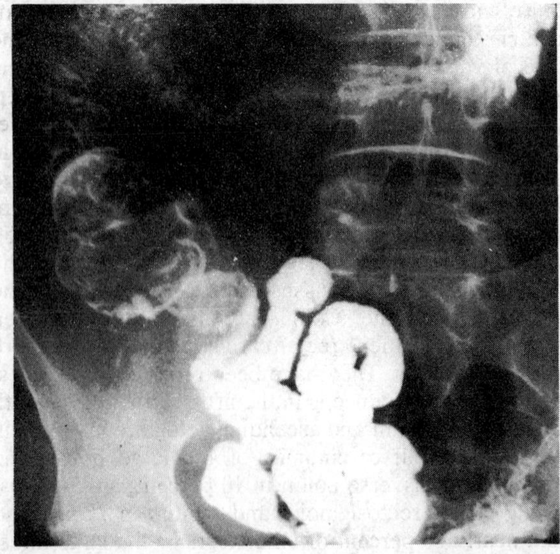

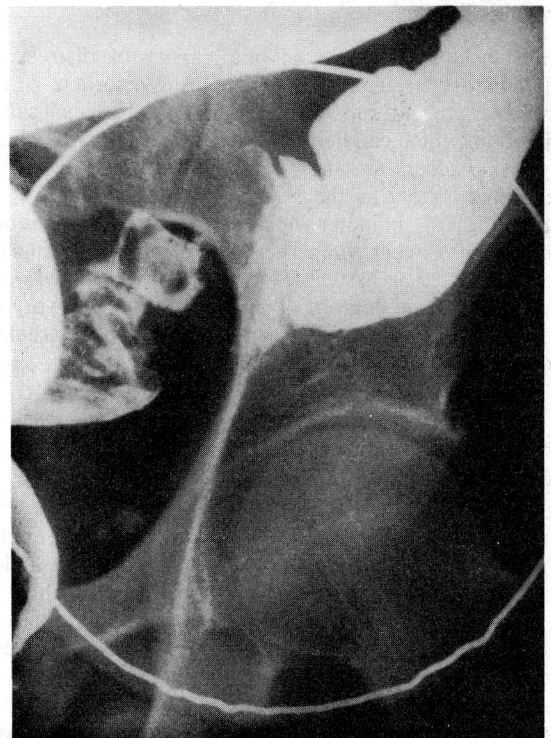

FIGURE 288-7
Obstructing carcinoma of the sigmoid.

colon includes (1) benign lesions: gastric and duodenal ulcer, cholecystitis and cholelithiasis, liver disease; (2) inflammatory processes: appendiceal abscess, amebiasis, regional enteritis, segmental colitis, tuberculosis; (3) other tumors, such as carcinoids, lymphomas, lipomas, gastric cancer, renal cancer; (4) blood dyscrasias and uremia. In the descending colon carcinomas must be distinguished from diverticulitis, endometriosis, ulcerative colitis, lymphogranuloma venereum, and benign tumors. Strictures secondary to chronic diverticulitis or ischemic colitis may be difficult to differentiate from a cancer.

Carcinoma of the rectum and anus presents more specific early symptoms than do the lesions discussed above. Bleeding, intolerable rectal urgency, pain, and soiling are the most frequent symptoms. The principal difficulty occurs when preexisting abnormalities have been present for so long a time that the patient and his physician do not detect subtle changes in them. Most frequently such problems arise when the patient has had an irritable colon syndrome, ulcerative colitis, simple constipation, or a variety of anorectal disorders, often complicated by surgical procedures.

These carcinomas are more frequent in men than in women (5:4) and comprise both adenocarcinoma in the rectum and squamous carcinoma in the anal skin, as well as mixed tumors in the anal canal. Malignant melanoma and basal cell carcinoma may arise in the anal skin; lymphoma, carcinoids, tumors arising from neighboring structures—prostate, cervix, ovary—as well as the seeding of upper abdominal carcinoma into the pelvic peritoneum may present as though they were primary lesions of the rectum.

Diagnosis is made by inspection, digital examination, anoscopy, proctoscopy, biopsy, and exfoliative cytology. Fiberoptic colonoscopy is of much promise in visualizing and performing a biopsy of suspicious areas of the left colon.

COMPLICATIONS Since it is characteristic for tumors to invade, many tumors of the colon may first be diagnosed because of a complication of the original lesion. The tumor may perforate the bowel wall, giving rise to acute peritonitis, may perforate slowly and wall itself off, giving rise to local inflammatory mass and localized peritonitis, or may invade blood vessels to produce an episode of brisk rectal bleeding. More often, the tumor partially obstructs the bowel lumen for a long period of time, during which the colon proximal to the tumor dilates slowly without dramatic change in symptoms until frank obstruction occurs. This occurs most often when the tumor is in the sigmoid, where the stool is driest. Tumors also weaken the colonic wall in such a way that an intussusception may occur, the tumor leading the intussusception. Similarly, fixation of the bowel wall by a tumor may produce a volvulus, which is most frequently seen in the sigmoid colon. Very large and slowly growing tumors may produce symptoms by pressure on neighboring organs such as uterus, bladder, or ureters. Inguinal hernias may become apparent as the first sign of such increased pressure. Fistulas between the colon and pelvic organs suggest a thorough search for an underlying neoplastic infiltration. Abscesses inside the peritoneal cavity and cellulitis of the abdominal wall secondary to tumor infiltration are not infrequent.

TREATMENT Although the only readily available therapeutic techniques are surgical, there are indications that radiotherapy combined with surgical therapy and some new chemotherapeutic means may significantly improve the outlook for patients with colonic and rectal cancer. Surgeons generally prefer abdominoperitoneal resection and colostomy for tumors located below the peritoneal reflections; above this area there is considerably more freedom of choice, depending primarily on the size and the extent of the lesions. It is important to realize that good preoperative management and operative skill will ensure that 75 to 90 percent of all cases can receive either extirpative or palliative surgical therapy with an operative mortality under 10 percent. The operative mortality is somewhat higher for lesions in the left colon. On the other hand, the survival rate for tumors of the left colon which can be resected is slightly higher than for right colon cancer, perhaps because they are discovered earlier.

The overall 5-year survival rate for all patients undergoing resection for colonic malignancy is approximately 50 percent. The 5-year survival rate after resection for patients free of local or distant spread is 75 to 80 percent. When nodal metastases are found at the time of resection, only 25 percent of these patients will be alive at 5 years. It is important that palliative surgical attempts not be discouraged, as the symptomatic relief they bring may allow the patient to live in comfort the remaining months of his life.

Discussion of the complications of surgical therapy and the management of colostomies can be found in surgical texts.

OBSTRUCTION OF THE COLON AND RECTUM

Chronic colonic obstruction has been discussed above in the sections dealing with its principal causes—tumors, diverticulitis, and megacolon. Additional disorders which may present as chronic large-bowel obstruction are strictures resulting from inflammatory processes (ulcerative colitis, lymphogranuloma venereum, perirectal abscess), from ischemic colitis, from pelvic disease (endometriosis, tumors), from traumatic scarring (either postoperative or crushing), or from radiation fibrosis secondary to treatment of pelvic cancer.

The presenting symptoms in all cases are similar, the diagnosis is made clinically and radiologically, and the treatment is surgical.

ANORECTAL PROBLEMS

Complaints centered in this area are among the most common and most troublesome encountered by the physician. Because of failure to understand the anatomy and function of perianal skin, anal sphincters, lower rectal mucosa, and levator muscles, many misdiagnoses are made, and therapy based on these misconceptions prolongs or even aggravates the difficulties. There is no way in which the physician can move with assurance in evaluating these complaints unless he learns the anatomy and constantly performs careful and thorough physical examinations directed to an appreciation of the disturbed physiology.

Fistulas and abscesses

These septic disorders may be the first signs of chronic inflammatory bowel disease, enteritis, or diverticulitis, as previously discussed, or may be complications of surgical procedures employed for these or other conditions. *Fistula in ano*, a tract leading from the rectal lumen to the perianal skin, usually results from local crypt abscesses; fewer than 5 percent of such lesions found in medical practice in the United States are due to tuberculosis or cancer. The fistula is a chronically inflamed tube made up of fibrous tissue surrounding granulation tissue, the lumen of which may be difficult to demonstrate. *Perirectal abscesses* often represent the tracking down into the anal area of purulent material escaping from the rectosigmoid; diverticulitis, enteritis, or colitis may be the source. Previous anal or rectal surgical therapy may be causal. *Fistulas* between the rectum and vagina and between the rectum and bladder represent serious complications of granulomatous, septic, or malignant disorders and require that the patient be hospitalized for definitive diagnostic and therapeutic procedures.

Anal lesions

These lesions comprise a wide variety of distressing inflammatory, traumatic, and neoplastic disorders. *Anal fissures* represent superficial erosions of the anal canal epithelium which can heal rapidly with conservative therapy. *Anal ulcers* are more chronic and deep and give symptoms largely as the result of painful spasm of the external anal sphincter during and after defecation. Bleeding may occur with either fissure or ulcer; healing of the ulcer often is associated with a hypertrophied anal papilla and some degrees of anal contracture. Crypt abscesses may produce pain early and should be treated promptly.

Hemorrhoids

The internal hemorrhoidal plexus of veins is located in the submucosal space above the valves of Morgagni. The anal canal separates it from the external hemorrhoidal venous plexus, but the two spaces communicate under the anal canal, the submucosa of which is attached to underlying tissue to form the interhemorrhoidal depression. Whenever the internal hemorrhoidal plexus is enlarged, there is associated increase in supporting tissue mass, and the resultant venous swelling is called an *internal hemorrhoid.* When veins in the external hemorrhoidal plexus become enlarged or thrombosed, the resultant bluish mass is called an *external hemorrhoid.*

Both types of hemorrhoids are very common and are associated with increased hydrostatic pressure in the portal venous system, characteristically noted during pregnancy, straining at stool, chronic liver disease, and sudden increases of intraabdominal pressure, or with local factors associated with diarrhea, tumors, or incomplete evacuation of feces. When internal hemorrhoids enlarge, pain is not a usual feature until the situation is complicated by thrombosis, infection, or erosion of the overlying mucosal surface. Most persons complain of bright-red blood on the toilet tissue or coating the stool, with a feeling of vague disquiet about the state of their anus. The discomfort is increased when the hemorrhoidal enlargement becomes great or prolapses through the anus; prolapse is often accompanied by edema and sphincteric spasm. Prolapse, if not treated, usually becomes chronic as the muscularis stays stretched, and the patient complains of constant soiling of underclothing with very little pain. Prolapsed hemorrhoids may become infected or thrombosed; the overlying mucous membrane may bleed profusely as the result of the trauma of defecation.

External hemorrhoids, lying as they do under the skin, are quite often painful, particularly if there is a sudden increase in their mass. These episodes result in a tender blue swelling at the anal verge due to thrombosis of a vein in the external plexus and need not be associated with enlargement of the internal veins. Since the thrombus usually lies at the level of the sphincteric muscles, anal spasm often occurs.

The diagnosis of internal and external hemorrhoids is made by inspection, digital examination, and direct vision through the anoscope and proctoscope. Since such lesions are very common, they must not be regarded as the cause of rectal bleeding or chronic hypochromic anemia until a thorough investigation has been made of the more proximal gastrointestinal tract. Acute blood loss can occasionally be attributed to internal hemorrhoids. Chronic anemia in the presence of large but not definitely bleeding hemorrhoids should provoke a search for a polyp, cancer, or ulcer.

Most hemorrhoids respond to conservative therapy, employment of sitz baths or other forms of moist heat, compresses, suppositories, medications to soften the stool, and bed rest. Internal hemorrhoids which remain permanently prolapsed are best treated by surgical means; milder degrees of prolapse or enlargement with pruritus ani or intermittent bleeding can be successfully handled by the injection of sclerosing solutions. External hemorrhoids which become acutely thrombosed are treated by incision, extraction of the clot, and compression of the incised area following clot removal. No surgical procedure should be carried out in the presence of acute inflammation of the anus, ulcerative proctitis, or ulcerative colitis. Both proctoscopy and barium enema should always be performed before a patient is subjected to hemorrhoidectomy.

REFERENCES

BUNTAIN WL et al: Collective review: Premalignancy of polyps of the colon. Surg Gynecol Obstet 134:499, 1972

BURKITT DP: Epidemiology of cancer of the colon and rectum. Cancer 28:3, 1971

DEDOMBAL FB, GOLIGHER JC: Early and late results of surgical treatment for Crohn's disease. Br J Surg 58:805, 1971

DYKES PW, KING J: Carcinoembryonic antigen. Gut 13:1000, 1972

FLEISCHNER F: Diverticular disease of the colon; Gastroenterology 60:316, 1971

GOLIGHER JC et al: *Ulcerative Colitis*, Baltimore: William & Wilkins, 1968

HARVEY RF, READ AE: Effect of cholecystokinin on colonic motility and symptoms in patients with the irritable bowel syndrome. Lancet 1:1, 1973

KIRSNER JB et al: Polyps of the colon and rectum. Gastroenterology 39:178, 1960

LENNARD-JONES JE et al: Clinical and pathological differentiation of Crohn's disease and proctocolitis. Gastroenterology 54:1162, 1968

LOCKHART-MUMMERY HE, MORSON BC: Crohn's disease of the large intestine. Gut 5:493, 1964

MARSTON AM et al: Ischemic colitis. Gut 7:1, 1966

MENDELOFF AI, DUNN JP: *Digestive diseases*, Cambridge: Harvard, 1971

NIXON HH: Megacolon and other congenital anomalies of the colon, in *Surgery of the Anus, Rectum, and Colon*, ed JC Goligher, Springfield, Ill.: Charles C Thomas, 1961

WALLER SL, MISIEWICZ JJ: Prognosis in the irritable bowel syndrome. Lancet 753, 11 October, 1969

WOLFE WI, SHINYA H: Polypectomy via the fiberoptic colonoscope. N Engl J Med 288:329, 1973

289 DISEASES OF THE PERITONEUM AND MESENTERY

KURT J. ISSELBACHER
J. THOMAS LAMONT

ACUTE PERITONITIS Peritonitis is a localized or generalized inflammatory process of the peritoneum that may appear in both acute and chronic forms. In the acute form the motor activity of the intestine is decreased, and the intestinal lumen becomes distended with gas and fluid. Fluid accumulates as a result of failure to reabsorb the 7 or 8 liters normally excreted daily into the lumen and absorbed from the distal small bowel and colon. While acute peritonitis is usually of bacterial origin, it may also result from entry into the abdominal cavity of blood, urine, bile, or pancreatic juice.

Etiology Peritonitis may be due to entry of bacteria into the peritoneal cavity from a perforation in the gastrointestinal tract or from an external penetrating wound. It may be secondary to severe chemical reactions from the release of pancreatic enzymes, the digestive juices of the upper gastrointestinal tract, or bile as a result of injury or perforation of the intestine or biliary tract.

The most common causes of bacterial peritonitis are appendicitis, perforations associated with diverticulitis, peptic ulcer, gangrenous gallbladder, and gangrenous obstruction of the small bowel from adhesive bands, incarcerated hernia, or volvulus. Any lesion leading to the escape of intestinal bacteria may be a source, including a perforating carcinoma, foreign body, and ulcerative colitis. The peritoneal cavity is remarkably resistant to contamination, and unless continuing contamination occurs, the disease process becomes localized. Patients with alcoholic cirrhosis and ascites have an increased susceptibility to spontaneous bacterial peritonitis, usually from enteric pathogens. This complication occurs in the absence of recognizable perforation of a viscus, and may be due to leakage of bacteria through the intestinal wall.

Clinical features These usually consist of increasing abdominal pain, distention, nausea and vomiting, inability to pass feces or flatus, fever, hypotension, tachycardia, thirst, and oliguria. On physical examination the patient appears acutely ill, febrile, and with a variable degree of abdominal distention. The abdomen is usually acutely tender and tympanitic, often with rebound tenderness. The location of the pain and tenderness depends on the underlying cause, and whether the inflammation is localized or generalized. In *localized* peritonitis, as seen in uncomplicated appendicitis or diverticulitis, the physical findings are limited to the area of inflammation. With widespread peritoneal inflammation there is *generalized* peritonitis with diffuse abdominal tenderness and rebound.

Peristalsis may be present initially but usually disappears as the illness progresses. Hypotension is common, as is leukocytosis, which often is greater than 20,000 cells per mm^3. X-ray examination of the abdomen shows dilatation of the large and small bowel with edema of the small-bowel wall as evidenced by the distance between adjacent loops of gas-filled small intestine. Diagnostic paracentesis is valuable in determining the nature of the exudate as well as whether bacteria can be demonstrated or cultured. Lead, colic, gastric crises, and acute porphyria may cause severe abdominal symptoms that resemble the picture of acute peritonitis.

Systemic effects Spreading and progressive peritonitis usually results in an increased demand on the circulatory system, because the exudation of fluid leads to a reduction in the effective circulating blood volume. Some of the fluid is lost into the peritoneal cavity and the rest into the intestinal lumen.

With severe peritonitis, respiratory demands are increased, and elevation of the diaphragm reduces ventilatory capacity and respiratory exchange. There is usually an increase in adrenal activity with increased production of glucocorticoids and aldosterone resulting in potassium loss and sodium retention. Catecholamines may be liberated in increased amounts, and the resulting peripheral vasoconstriction with increased peripheral resistance results in decreased organ perfusion, usually affecting renal and cardiac function.

GONOCOCCAL PERITONITIS This usually involves an extension of gonococcal infection from a primary focus in the female reproductive tract. The signs of inflammation usually are limited to the pelvis, but there may be findings of a mild generalized peritonitis. Occasionally the patient has right upper quadrant pain and tenderness caused by gonococcal perihepatitis involving the liver capsule and adjacent peritoneum (Fitzhugh-Curtis syndrome) (see also Chap. 132).

PSEUDOMYXOMA PERITONEI This is a rare condition resulting from rupture of a mucocele of the appendix or of a mucinous ovarian cyst. The abdomen becomes filled with masses of jellylike material. Occasionally, with removal of the mucocele or the ovarian cyst and most of the myxomatous material, a cure may ensue. In other cases, however, the mucoid material recurs, leading to progressive wasting and eventual death. Colloid carcinoma arising from the stomach or colon with peritoneal implants may resemble pseudomyxoma at laparotomy. The course of this type of highly malignant tumor is one of rapid cachexia and early death. The diagnosis can usually be made by the appearance of many highly malignant cells in the peritoneal implants.

CANCER OF THE PERITONEUM Aside from mesothelioma, which appears uniquely associated with asbestosis but is otherwise very rare, cancer of the peritoneum is usually secondary to a neoplasm within the abdomen, most commonly of the stomach and ovary. Invariably this type of metastatic malignancy is associated with progressive ascites with a high specific gravity and high protein content, often with large numbers of red cells or even gross blood. The diagnosis is established by demonstrating malignant cells in the fluid. The clinical progress of this malignant spread can sometimes be arrested by installations of radioactive gold, nitrogen mustard, or chloroquine.

BENIGN PAROXYSMAL PERITONITIS See Chap. 255.

PNEUMATOSIS CYSTOIDES INTESTINALIS This is a condition in which multiple gas-filled blebs or cysts accumulate in the intestinal wall beneath the serosal surface of the bowel. The exact source of the gas has not been explained satisfactorily. In some instances, this disease is associated with specific ulceration of the intestinal mucosa, in particular peptic ulcer with outlet obstruction. Cysts in the wall of the small bowel are seen as an occasional complication of mesenteric vascular occlusion. In the large bowel, these cysts are usually benign, may be seen with a variety of other disorders, and usually disappear in time.

There are no specific physical findings secondary to the pneumatosis, and the diagnosis is made either by x-ray or at laparotomy. Occasionally the subserosal cysts may rupture, resulting in pneumoperitoneum.

CHYLOUS ASCITES This term refers to the accumulation of chyle (intestinal lymph) in the peritoneal cavity. The condition is sometimes associated with chylothorax. The fluid in the peritoneal cavity appears milky or creamy because of the presence of fat. This fat may be demonstrated microscopically by staining with Sudan III and may be removed by acidification of the fluid followed by extraction with ether. The chyle (lipid) will then go into the ether phase. Many conditions may be associated with the cloudy or milky-appearing peritoneal fluid, so-called "pseudochylous ascites." The milky or turbid appearance is usually due to the presence of protein and desquamated cells. The turbidity of this fluid will not be removed with the ether but will clear with addition of alkali.

The causes of chylous ascites include (1) penetrating or nonpenetrating trauma that damages the main duct in the lymphatic system within the abdomen, (2) intestinal obstruction if it is associated with rupture of a major lymphatic channel, (3) congenital lymphangiectasia, (4) malignant disease or tuberculous infection that obstructs the intestinal lymphatics, or (5) filariasis.

The sudden accumulation of chyle in the peritoneal cavity often results in abdominal pain, signs of peritoneal irritation, and leukocytosis. These symptoms gradually subside, leaving the patient with a distended but nontender, fluid-filled abdomen. The roentgenographic technique of lymphangiography is of value in determining the location of the leak or site of obstruction to the lymphatic channels. The course depends upon the underlying etiologic factors.

MESENTERIC PANNICULITIS This is a rare disorder usually affecting middle-aged women and characterized pathologically by thickening of the mesentery with foci of fat necrosis similar to that seen in the skin of patients with Weber-Christian disease (see Chap. 363). These patients present with ill-defined abdominal pain and occasionally an abdominal mass. The diagnosis is made at laparotomy by demonstration of thick fibrous masses at the root of the mesentery with retraction and distortion of the bowel loops.

REFERENCES

Conn HO, Fessel JM: Spontaneous bacterial peritonitis in cirrhosis. Medicine 50:161, 1971.

Ogden WW et al: Mesenteric panniculitis: Review of 27 cases. Ann Surg 161:864, 1965.

Rhoads JE et al: *Surgery: Principles and Practice*, Philadelphia: Lippincott, 1970.

section 6 | Disorders of the hepatobiliary system

290 APPROACH TO THE PATIENT WITH LIVER DISEASE

KURT J. ISSELBACHER

GENERAL CONSIDERATIONS While disease of the liver or biliary tract may be directly responsible for the symptoms that bring the patient to the physician, examination for nonhepatic complaints may occasionally provide the clues to otherwise asymptomatic or occult hepatobiliary disease. Liver function studies and other diagnostic procedures such as biopsy (as discussed in Chap. 292) are crucial, but much valuable information as to the possible nature and extent of liver disease can be obtained by a carefully elicited history and thorough physical examination.

Importance of clinical history Since laboratory tests often do not establish the specific cause of liver disease, the history is of the greatest significance. *Family history* is important with respect to jaundice, anemia, splenectomy, or cholecystectomy; a positive history may be helpful in diagnosing hemolytic anemia, congenital or familial hyperbilirubinemia, or gallstones. In Wilson's disease (hepatolenticular degeneration), there may be a family history of tremor or neurologic abnormalities. *Occupation* should be reviewed in detail, and *environmental factors* need to be examined. Note should be made of any contact with rats or other animals possibly carrying Weil's disease and of exposure to toxins such as carbon tetrachloride or beryllium. The patient should be asked about travel to other countries, especially to areas where hepatitis may be endemic. Careful questioning regarding alcohol intake is important in most cases. Since the alcoholic often denies or understates the amounts consumed, it is desirable to check the validity of the history with close friends or relatives of the patient.

Contact with jaundiced patients should be noted, especially in hospitals, schools, or the military where viral hepatitis is frequent. If the patient has had any *injections* in the previous 6 months, hepatitis B (long-incubation hepatitis) may be the underlying disease. Injections include blood tests, blood or plasma transfusions, tatooing, and dental treatment. The patient should be asked about narcotics, hallucinogens, or stimulant *drugs* taken parenterally, as well as about agents taken orally, such as chlorpromazine or contraceptive drugs known to affect liver function.

A previous history of indigestion, fat intolerance, and right upper quadrant pain suggests cholelithiasis or choledocholithiasis. Jaundice following shortly after operation on the biliary tract suggests residual stone, that which occurs within 6 months suggests hepatitis B, and that occurring after 1 or more years may be due to stricture of the common bile duct. Postoperative jaundice may be due to the anesthetic, especially multiple uses of halothane, or to the impaired hepatic excretory function resulting from relative hypoxia of liver cells during the operative or postoperative period.

The *onset of the illness* should be noted. The relatively abrupt onset of nausea, anorexia, and aversion to smoking followed by progressive jaundice suggests infection with hepatitis A virus. A gradual development of jaundice associated with pruritus suggests cholestasis. Jaundice associated with fever and chills makes cholangitis and extrahepatic biliary obstruction likely possibilities.

The patient with hepatitis generally feels ill, and dark urine and light stools occur before the appearance of scleral or skin icterus. In cholestatic hepatitis, the patient may feel relatively well and complain only of symptoms due to the obstruction, such as pruritus.

Physical examination Pallor indicative of anemia may be a reflection of hemolysis, cirrhosis, or neoplasm. Significant cachexia, especially of the extremities, may be associated with cancer or active cirrhosis. If the patient is jaundiced, the color of the jaundice should be observed; with hemolysis the jaundice is a mild *yellow*, with parenchymal disease, more *orange*, and with prolonged biliary obstruction, a more *greenish* hue may at times be observed. In the alcoholic one should look for stigmas of cirrhosis such as parotid gland enlargement, Dupuytren's contracture, gynecomastia, testicular atrophy, and diminished axillary or pubic hair.

The *skin examination* may reveal ecchymoses due to prothrombin deficiency, or purpura due to thrombocytopenia. *Palmar erythema* or *spider angiomas* may reflect acute or chronic liver disease. Spider angiomas are usually found above the umbilicus and especially on the face, neck, shoulders, forearms, and dorsum of the hands. The presence of a few spider angiomas is not abnormal in women, especially during pregnancy. However their appearance in males is always abnormal and should be carefully searched for. In chronic cholestasis, *scratch marks*, *finger clubbing*, and *xanthoma* of the eyelids and extensor surfaces of the tendons of the wrists and ankles may be found. A *slate color* to the skin due to increased melanin should suggest the presence of hemochromatosis.

Evaluation of the *mental state* and *neurologic function* is important. Slight deterioration of the intellect and minimal personality changes may suggest hepatocellular disease or the presence of portal-systemic venous shunts, but care must be taken to exclude other causes such as primary or metastatic brain tumors. The presence of flapping tremor of the hands (asterixis) may be found in association with portal-systemic encephalopathy or impending hepatic coma.

Abdominal examination may reveal ascites, which together with dilated periumbilical veins, suggests cirrhosis and extensive portal collateral circulation. A very large nodular and rock-hard liver suggests the presence of hepatoma or hepatic metastases. Careful percussion is necessary to evaluate the size of a nonpalpable liver. A small liver may indicate cirrhosis (especially postnecrotic); a small liver which diminishes in size suggests severe hepatitis or massive hepatic necrosis. In the alcoholic, fatty infiltration and cirrhosis often produces a uniform enlargement of the liver. The liver edge is tender in hepatitis, in congestive heart failure, and occasionally in malignant disease and with alcoholism (especially "alcoholic hepatitis").

A palpable and sometimes visibly enlarged gallbladder (Courvoisier's sign) suggests extrahepatic biliary obstruction often due to pancreatic cancer. A tender gallbladder and positive Murphy's sign suggests cholelithiasis or choledocholithiasis. A palpable spleen may indicate hepatitis; significant splenomegaly may be a reflection of portal hypertension.

Abdominal auscultation may reveal the presence of a venous hum over dilated collateral veins radiating from the umbilicus, the so-called "caput medusae." In advanced cirrhosis this venous hum is virtually diagnostic of significant portal hypertension. A bruit may sometimes be heard over large regenerating nodules in cirrhosis, and occasionally over hepatomas and metastatic nodules in the liver. The presence of a friction rub strongly suggests neoplastic disease or a hepatic abscess. A friction rub may occasionally be heard over hepatomas and metastatic liver nodules.

Diagnostic procedures These are reviewed in Chap. 292. For the proper evaluation of liver and biliary tract diseases chemical and biochemical tests of blood, urine, and stool are essential, and liver biopsy is often needed to help determine the nature of the liver disease. In addition, peritoneoscopy and special radiologic techniques such as cholangiography, angiography, and scintiscans of the liver may be employed. In the problem case, laparotomy should be performed. The exploration should be thorough, and if the diagnosis remains in doubt, should include operative liver biopsy and direct operative cholangiography or angiography.

CLASSIFICATION OF LIVER DISEASE The classification of the various types of liver disease has been

TABLE 290-1
Classification of liver disease

I Parenchymal
- *A* Hepatitis (viral, drug-induced, toxic)
  - *1* Acute
  - *2* Chronic [persistent or "active" (aggressive)]
- *B* Cirrhosis
  - *1* Laennec's (portal, nutritional, "alcoholic")
  - *2* Postnecrotic
  - *3* Biliary
  - *4* Hemochromatosis
  - *5* Rare types (e.g., Wilson's disease, galactosemia, cystic fibrosis of pancreas)
- *C* Infiltrations
  - *1* Glycogen
  - *2* Fat (neutral fat, cholesterol, gangliosides, cerebrosides)
  - *3* Amyloid
  - *4* Lymphoma, leukemia
  - *5* Granuloma (e.g., sarcoidosis, tuberculosis)
- *D* Space-occupying lesions
  - *1* Hepatoma, metastatic tumor
  - *2* Abscess (pyogenic, amebic)
  - *3* Cysts (polycystic disease, *Echinococcus*)
  - *4* Gummas
- *E* Functional disorders associated with jaundice
  - *1* Gilbert's syndrome
  - *2* Crigler-Najjar syndrome
  - *3* Dubin-Johnson and Rotor syndromes
  - *4* Cholestasis of pregnancy and benign recurrent cholestasis

II Hepatobiliary
- *A* Extrahepatic biliary obstruction (by stone, stricture, or tumor)
- *B* Cholangitis

III Vascular
- *A* Chronic passive congestion and cardiac cirrhosis
- *B* Hepatic vein thrombosis (Budd-Chiari syndrome)
- *C* Portal vein thrombosis
- *D* Pylephlebitis
- *E* Arteriovenous malformations

difficult because in many instances the etiology and pathogenetic mechanism are obscure. As a consequence, one finds an abundance of labels and names applied to hepatic disorders. Some individuals use the term *hepatitis* to imply viral infection, others simply to connote evidence of hepatic inflammation. One finds ambiguity in the use of the words acute, subacute, and chronic. *Chronicity* should refer to continuing or recurrent disease (i.e., duration). *Activity* should refer to evidence of the presence of perpetuation of liver cell injury; this is most readily identified on biopsy by the degree of hepatocellular necrosis and by serum transaminase elevations.

Because of the difficulties involved in defining the etiology of many types of liver disease, in most instances the process is best defined and described by an examination of the morphologic character of the lesion. Therefore, a *morphologic classification* of liver disease, as outlined in Table 290-1, appears at present more practical than one based on etiology.

REFERENCES

SCHIFF L: *Diseases of the Liver*, 3d ed., Philadelphia: Lippincott, 1969

SHERLOCK S: *Diseases of the Liver and Biliary System*, 4th ed., Philadelphia: Davis, 1968.

291 DERANGEMENTS OF HEPATIC METABOLISM

DAVID H. ALPERS
KURT J. ISSELBACHER

The liver is an organ with a variety of metabolic functions, both synthetic and degradative. Although there are three major cell types which make up the liver—the hepatocyte, biliary epithelial cell, and Kupffer cell—most metabolic functions are carried out by the hepatocyte. Several observations are pertinent to derangements in liver function when the liver is damaged: (1) in view of its large reserve capacity, mild to sometimes moderate injury often may not be accurately reflected by changes of its synthetic or degradative activity; (2) some functions of the liver are much more sensitive to injury than others, and hence derangements may be found in some liver functions (and function tests) and not in others; (3) there is *no one single test* or procedure which effectively measures the total function of the liver. Therefore proper understanding of the metabolic responses of the liver to injury depends on a comprehension of the many known functions of the liver. Some of these are discussed below.

PROTEIN SYNTHESIS The liver actively synthesizes many proteins, but of these *albumin* is quantitatively the most important. The body contains about 5 g albumin per kg body weight, and in the normal adult the daily albumin production by the hepatic endoplasmic reticulum is about 120 to 200 mg per kg. The half-life of serum albumin is 17 to 20 days. The liver is the only organ which synthesizes albumin. The rate of synthesis is limited and can be doubled only under conditions of excessive albumin loss or destruction. Once albumin is synthesized, it is transported from the rough endoplasmic reticulum to the smooth endoplasmic reticulum and the Golgi apparatus and from there to the hepatic sinusoids. During liver injury changes may occur in the actual synthesis of albumin or in its intracellular transport and release. When the liver is damaged, synthesis of albumin is usually affected more than catabolism, but in view of its half-life, several weeks may elapse before a pronounced decrease in serum albumin levels occurs. In general, albumin catabolism tends to continue at a relatively constant rate, even in the presence of liver injury, and this rate is proportional to its plasma concentration.

Other proteins produced by the liver include many of the bloodclotting factors: fibrinogen, prothrombin, and factors V, VII, and X. All of them have a half-life shorter than that of albumin, varying from 6 hr (factor VII) to 20 hr (prothrombin). For some proteins (e.g., fibrinogen) the degradation is constant irrespective of their plasma concentrations. Therefore when fresh blood is administered, the prothrombin level will be elevated only transiently, while more significant increases in serum albumin will result. Unlike albumin, not all globulins are synthesized by the hepatocytes; much of the α- and β-globulins are produced by liver cells, but normally most γ-globulins are synthesized by reticuloendothelial cells lining the sinusoids and in the spleen and bone marrow. In addition, infiltrating plasma cells and lymphocytes may be of importance in some forms of liver disease associated with hyperglobulinemia (such as chronic active hepatitis and primary biliary cirrhosis). The production and localization of γ-globulins in the liver in these conditions can be detected by immunofluorescence techniques but probably account for only a portion of the γ-globulin production.

Clinically, *hypoalbuminemia* can result from inadequate amino acid supply as in protein caloric malnutrition or malabsorption, or from decreased synthesis, as in cirrhosis. Corticosteroids can increase hepatic synthesis of albumin, but do not affect the plasma concentration very much, demonstrating the complex relationship between synthesis and degradation of plasma proteins.

ENZYMES In view of the many chemical reactions carried out by the liver, this organ contains thousands of protein catalysts or enzymes. Some are unique to the liver, while many others also are found in nonhepatic tissues. The leakage of enzymes out of liver cells into the bloodstream occurs with liver injury, and measurements of these serum enzymes are useful tests of abnormal liver function. When increased serum levels of enzymes such as the transaminases are found, several points must be kept in mind: (1) leakage of enzymes out of the liver cell occurs not only with *necrosis* but also with changes in *cell permeability* which may be produced by ischemia or hypoxia; (2) there is *no direct quantitative correlation* between the amount of liver cell injury and the height of serum enzyme levels, although in general, higher levels are found with more severe injury; (3) if the serum enzymes are measured sometime *after* the acute insult or injury, the initial rise may have been missed, and thus normal or *low* serum enzyme levels may be found as a consequence of a decreased functioning liver cell mass.

In liver disease some enzymes may increase in the blood not because of changes in cell permeability but as a result of *increased enzyme synthesis.* Thus the increased serum alkaline phosphatase with cholestatic liver disease has been shown to be due to increased synthesis of the enzyme. Alkaline phosphatase is also present in tissues such as bone, intestine, kidney, and placenta, and a variety of techniques are available to distinguish these various alkaline phosphatase *isoenzymes.* For example, electrophoresis may be used to separate some of these isoenzymes; heat treatment tends to inactivate the bone alkaline phosphatase; L-phenylalanine selectively inhibits the intestinal enzyme. Another useful approach to determine whether an elevated alkaline phosphatase level reflects hepatic disease is to measure a related enzyme, *5′-nucleotidase*, which is elaborated by hepatic canalicular microvilli but is not found in bone.

AMINO ACID METABOLISM The liver is the major site of amino acid metabolism in the body. Amino acids are derived either from the diet, from tissue protein catabolism, or from direct synthesis, and reach the liver via the bloodstream. In the liver they are subject to anabolic (i.e., protein synthesis) or degradative processes. Catabolism or degradation of amino acids in the liver involves two major reactions. One of these is *oxidative deamination*, resulting in the formation of a keto acid and ammonia. This reaction is catalyzed by L-amino acid oxidases, with but two exceptions: glycine oxidation is catalyzed by glycine oxidase and glutamic acid oxidation by glutamic dehydrogenase.

Transamination, the process by which the amino group of an amino acid is transferred to a keto acid, is a more important mechanism. The two major enzymes are the glutamic-oxalacetic acid and the glutamic-pyruvic transaminases. As a result, amino acids are able to enter the citric acid cycle to function in the intermediary metabolism of carbohydrates and lipids (see Chap. 72). Conversely, by transamination amino acids may be synthesized from keto acids. When the liver is acutely and severely damaged (e.g., in massive hepatic necrosis), utilization of amino acids by the liver is impaired, free amino acid levels in the blood increase, and an "overflow" type of aminoaciduria occurs.

Urea synthesis occurs primarily in the liver and involves the participation of four amino acids: ornithine, citrulline, arginine, and aspartic acid. By this process ammonia is rapidly removed and detoxified. The steps of the urea (Krebs-Henseleit) cycle are shown in Fig. 291-1. Because all the enzymes of the urea cycle reside in the liver, in the presence of severe liver damage urea synthesis may be depressed, and blood urea nitrogen (BUN) levels may fall significantly. In the absence of severe liver damage most of the free NH_3 is formed in the intestinal tract, primarily in the colon. Normally, approximately 25 percent of blood urea is excreted into the intestine, and NH_3 is produced by the action of bacterial ureases or

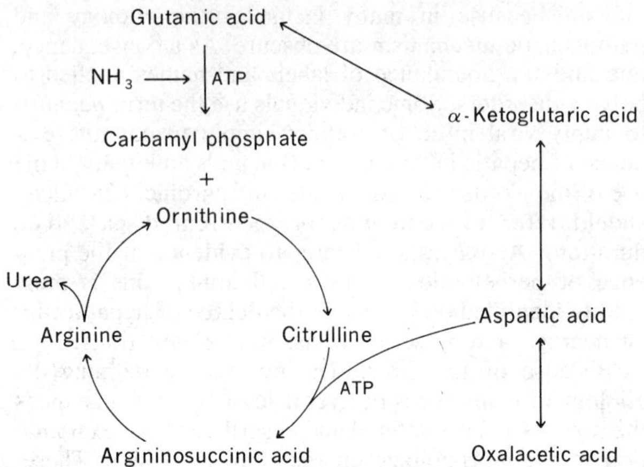

FIGURE 291-1
The chemical steps of the urea (Krebs-Henseleit) cycle.

from bleeding into the intestinal tract. Protein from the diet serves as a major source of ammonia because of the normal digestion of protein to amino acids and the subsequent deamination by bacterial enzymes. The ammonia formed in this manner enters the portal vein and is then detoxified in the liver by being converted to urea.

The four principal mechanisms leading to an increased blood NH_3 level in chronic liver disease are illustrated in Fig. 291-2. (1) If hepatic function is significantly depressed, *decreased urea synthesis* may occur with reduced removal of NH_3. (2) If portal hypertension accompanies cirrhosis, venous anastomoses will develop between the portal vein and systemic venous channels, and these *portal-systemic shunts* will allow NH_3 to escape hepatic detoxification, leading to elevated blood ammonia levels. (3) If there is *excessive nitrogenous material* in the intestine (from bleeding or dietary protein), excessive amounts of NH_3 will be formed by bacterial deamination of amino acids. (4) If metabolic alkalosis and hypokalemia accompany hepatic decompensation, there may be increased *renal* NH_3 *production* from glutamine by the action of glutaminase, leading to increased peripheral blood levels, because the NH_3 concentration in the renal veins is inversely proportional to the amount excreted in the urine.

Two additional factors are probably of importance in determining whether or not a given NH_3 level in the blood will be injurious to the tissues. First, NH_3 is removed from the blood by a variety of tissues, including brain, lungs, and muscle, and the degree of utilization is affected by the presence of AV shunts, which often occur in chronic liver disease. Second, the more alkaline the blood pH, the more toxic a given level of NH_3 is likely to be. At 37°C the pK of NH_3 is 8.9—i.e., close enough to the pH of blood so that small changes of blood pH might affect the NH_4+/NH_3 ratio. Because *un-ionized* NH_3 *crosses membranes more readily than ionized* NH_4+ *ions*, alkalosis favors the entry of ammonia into the brain by shifting the equilibrium of the following reaction to the right:

$$NH_4^+ + OH \rightleftharpoons NH_3 + HOH$$

Alkalosis then not only increases the peripheral blood levels of NH_3 by renal mechanisms but also increases tissue levels by its effect on the diffusion of NH_3 ions.

LIPID METABOLISM Approximately 5 percent of the normal liver weight is due to fat, including phospholipids, triglycerides, fatty acids, cholesterol, and cholesterol esters. The liver is active in the synthesis of lipids, especially triglycerides. While some remain in the liver, most triglycerides are excreted into the bloodstream in the form of lipoproteins. The major steps in hepatic fatty acid and triglyceride metabolism are shown in Fig. 291-3.

Under normal conditions, most of the *fatty acids* taken up by the liver and *esterified to triglyceride* are derived from adipose tissue or the diet. Some fatty acids (especially saturated ones) are synthesized in the liver from acetate. The fatty acids may then be converted enzymatically to triglyceride, esterified with cholesterol, incorporated into phospholipids, or oxidized to CO_2 or ketone bodies. Most of the triglyceride is produced for export and in order to be secreted must be converted to *lipoproteins* by combining with relatively specific apoprotein moieties. Thus, protein synthesis is important for the release and secretion of triglyceride from the liver.

Studies on the production of a fatty liver have shown that singly or in combination one or more of these steps depicted numerically in Fig. 291-3 may lead to excessive hepatic triglyceride accumulation and hence a fatty liver. *Increased influx* of fatty acids (1) such as may occur with drugs producing lipid mobilization from adipose tissue or in diabetic ketosis may lead to a fatty liver. Similarly *increased levels of fatty acids in the liver*, either from enhanced fatty acid synthesis (2) or from decreased oxidation (3), may lead to increased triglyceride formation. In some instances there may also be *increases* in the specific *enzymes* involved in fatty acid esterification to triglyceride (4). Since release of triglyceride involves the formation of lipoproteins, lipid accumulation may occur because of *decreased apoprotein synthesis* (5). In the case of fatty livers produced by toxins such as carbon tetrachloride, phosphorus, and ethionine, and by antibiotics like tetracycline, the major mechanism for lipid accumulation appears to be impaired apoprotein synthesis. Finally, impaired lipoprotein synthesis (i.e., coupling of lipid with *apoprotein*) (6), or lipoprotein secretion from the liver (7). Alcohol is perhaps the most common agent leading to a fatty liver, but the mechanism whereby alcohol leads to increased liver triglyceride is less clear. Alcohol administration, depending on dose or duration, may affect any of the seven steps shown in Fig. 291-3, and the primary factor for the production of the alcohol-induced fatty liver still remains to be determined.

Cholesterol synthesis is also carried out by the liver and to some extent by the intestine. In the plasma cholesterol exists either *free* or combined with fatty acids in the form of *cholesterol esters*; both are found primarily in association with beta-lipoproteins. The plasma and liver also contain cholesterol acyl transferase, an enzyme involved in the conversion of free cholesterol to its esterified form. Free cholesterol exchanges readily between tissues, and thus changes in plasma cholesterol levels reflect changes in total body cholesterol. However, decreases in plasma cholesterol esters may reflect hepatic damage.

FIGURE 291-2
Major factors (steps 1 to 4) influencing the level of blood ammonia. In cirrhosis with portal hypertension, venous collaterals allow ammonia to bypass the liver (5), allowing for the entry of ammonia into the systemic circulation (portal-systemic shunting).

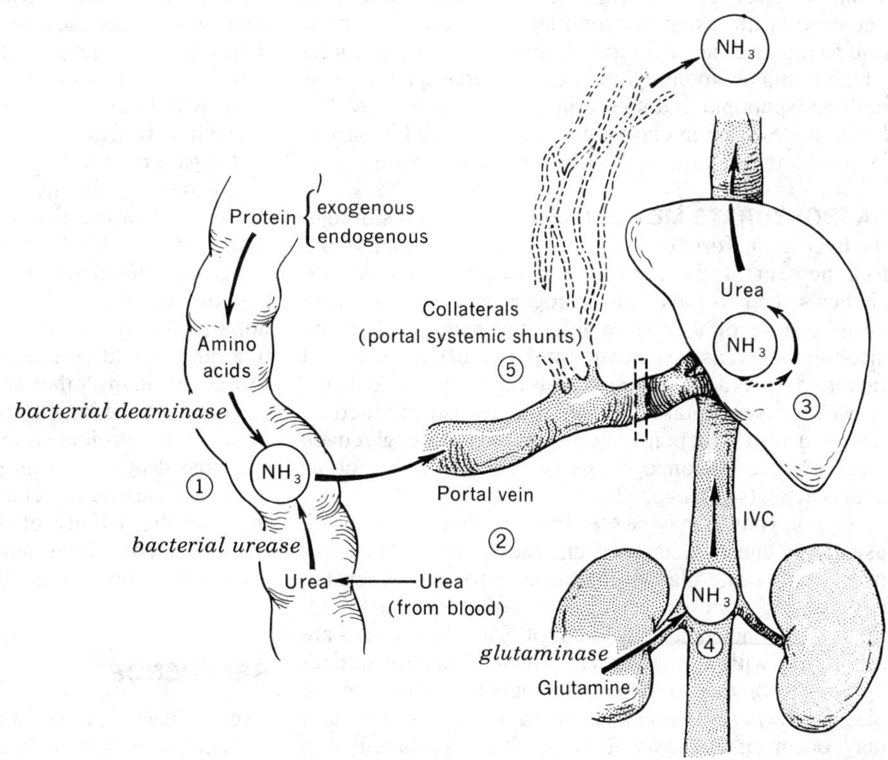

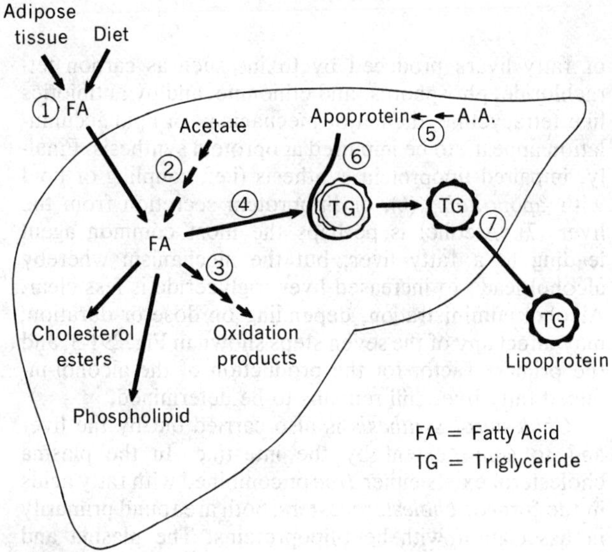

FIGURE 291-3
Factors in the uptake and esterification of fatty acids to triglyceride by the liver including the formation and release of triglyceride as lipoprotein. The numbers refer to steps, which, if altered, may result in increased liver triglyceride (i.e., fatty liver).

Severe liver injury often leads to a decrease in total serum cholesterol levels, including both free and esterified fractions. This may be due to decreased cholesterol and cholesterol ester synthesis, decreased apolipoprotein synthesis, or both. In cholestasis (intra- or extrahepatic) *total serum cholesterol often increases* strikingly. On the other hand, the serum cholesterol ester level increases to a much lesser extent, with the result that there is a *decrease* in the *ester fraction* (i.e., ester/total). There is also found an abnormal serum lipoprotein (lipoprotein X) which contains apolipoprotein C, and large quantities of both phospholipid and unesterified cholesterol. The cholestered elevation in cholestasis may be related in part to increased production of this abnormal lipoprotein.

CARBOHYDRATE METABOLISM Glucose is stored in the liver in the form of glycogen; the latter accounts for 5 to 7 percent of the normal liver weight. Persons with cirrhosis tend to have less glycogen than normal, probably because of a reduced liver cell mass, and in the alcoholic decreased glucose intake is often an added factor. The blood glucose level represents a balance between tissue uptake and hepatic glucose production, which in turn is dependent on dietary glucose, glycogen reserves, and gluconeogenesis from precursors such as amino acids (see Chap. 72).

Hypoglycemia may be seen in severe liver damage and usually is due to decreased gluconeogenesis. This may occur with acute alcohol ingestion, especially when hepatic glycogen stores are depleted, because of the inhibition of gluconeogenesis by alcohol. Some hepatomas are associated with hypoglycemia, which in some instances appears to be due to increased insulinlike activity in the plasma. *Hyperglycemia* and *impaired glucose tolerance* may occur in cirrhosis. This is often associated with normal or increased plasma insulin levels, suggesting that the diabetes associated with liver disease is due to insulin resistance. Galactose is metabolized primarily by the liver, and *impaired galactose tolerance* occurs in liver disease. The galactose tolerance test was once used to evaluate liver function but is now employed rarely.

DETOXIFICATION MECHANISMS The liver plays a key role in the detoxification of many substances, both exogenous (e.g., drugs) and endogenous (e.g., hormones). This is accomplished by two mechanisms: First, there is *conjugation* which converts *water-insoluble substances to water-soluble derivatives,* so that they can be excreted into the bile or urine and eliminated. This is accomplished by *conjugation* with glucuronic acid, sulfate, etc. The second process involves *inactivation* of drugs by reduction, oxidation, or hydroxylation.

Hormones, such as corticosteroids and aldosterone, are first inactivated by reduction to their tetrahydro derivatives and then conjugated mostly with glucuronic acid, so that they may be excreted in bile and urine. Estrogens, such as estradiol, may be converted to estriol and estrone and then conjugated with glucuronic acid or sulfate. Abnormalities in estrogen metabolism have often been considered the cause of spider angiomas, gynecomastia, loss of axillary or pubic hair, and testicular atrophy. However, there is no direct correlation between plasma or urine estrogen levels and these clinical features.

Estrogens also act directly on the liver by impairing hepatic secretory activity. Estradiol and related estrogens, such as those present in contraceptive pills, interfere with Bromsulphalein (BSP) excretion and may also elevate the plasma alkaline phosphatase level (see Chap. 293). Related steroids such as etiocholanolone and pregnanediol have also been shown to stimulate δ-aminolevulinic acid (ALA) synthetase activity leading to porphyrinuria. Since these steroids exert these effects only in their free (i.e., nonglucuronide) form, the increased hepatic levels of δ-aminolevulinic acid synthetase in patients with Laennec's cirrhosis may be due to the effect of gonadal steroids.

Drugs are another important class of compounds inactivated by the liver. The impairment of morphine conjugation or inactivation of barbiturates (by side-chain oxidation) in the liver is an important factor in the increased effectiveness or toxicity of these drugs in hepatic disease. All the barbiturates, except phenobarbital and barbital, are primarily metabolized in the liver and should be used with caution in hepatic disease. Moreover, many other sedatives (Librium, paraldehyde) are metabolized largely by the liver, and their effect may be markedly prolonged in a patient with hepatic failure.

Some drugs, such as phenobarbital and ethanol, can stimulate the smooth endoplasmic reticulum and thereby increase the activity of detoxifying enzymes. Thus, the effect of some drugs may be decreased when taken in combination with other drugs.

REFERENCES

ISSELBACHER KJ, GREENBERGER NJ: Metabolic effects of alcohol on the liver. N Engl J Med 270:351, 1964

KAPLAN MM: Alkaline phosphatase. Gastroenterology 62:452, 1972

KAPPAS A: Biologic actions of some natural steroids on the liver. N Engl J Med 278:378, 1968.

ROTHSCHILD MA et al: Albumin synthesis. N Engl J Med 286:748, 1972

SEIDEL D: Plasma lipids and lipoproteins in patients with liver disease. Scand J Gastroenterol 7:105, 1972

TAVILL AS: The synthesis and degradation of liver produced proteins. *Gut* 13:225, 1972

ZIEVE L: Pathogenesis of hepatic coma. Arch Intern Med 118:211, 1966

292 DIAGNOSTIC PROCEDURES IN LIVER DISEASE

KURT J. ISSELBACHER
J. THOMAS LaMONT

Prompt recognition of liver disease and determination of its nature and extent require an understanding of the physiologic bases of a wide variety of techniques that assess liver function. Since no "battery" of tests is universally applicable, those most appropriate to a given clinical problem must be selected, their potential value and risk considered, and the results interpreted in relation to the clinical findings.

LIVER FUNCTION TESTS

Many liver function tests are based on a wide variety of biochemical reactions, such that the clinician can select combinations of tests that often measure different aspects of hepatic function. Many tests, however, are still empiric and semiquantitative, and no single test is universally helpful in diagnosis. Some methods are too sensitive and lack diagnostic specificity, others are affected by nonhepatic factors, and many simply do not measure any true physiologic function of the liver.

The physician concerned with clinical liver disease should be guided by several practical principles: (1) The tests selected should assess different parameters of liver function. (2) Liver function tests should be used *serially* in order to evaluate the evolution or course of the disease. (3) All such tests should be interpreted within the total clinical context with the recognition that any laboratory test may be fallible. The discussion that follows deals with representative and commonly used tests and should be read in conjunction with Chaps. 42 and 291.

SERUM BILIRUBIN (see Chaps. 42 and 293) Spectrophotometric determinations of serum bilirubin in the clinical laboratory measure two pigment fractions: (1) the water-soluble conjugated fraction that gives a *direct reaction* with the diazo reagent and consists largely of bilirubin diglucuronide, and (2) the lipid-soluble *indirect-reaction* fraction that represents primarily unconjugated bilirubin. The serum of normal adults contains less than 0.25 mg direct-reacting bilirubin per 100 ml and 1 mg or less total bilirubin per 100 ml serum. As noted in Chap. 42, in classifying the type of jaundice it is initially helpful to measure both the direct and total serum bilirubin in order to determine whether the patient has predominantly unconjugated or conjugated hyperbilirubinemia.

URINE BILIRUBIN Clinically significant concentrations of urine bilirubin are measured by the foam test, Harrison spot test or the Ictotest tablet method (see Chap. 42). Bilirubinuria only occurs when there is an increase of the ultrafilterable portion of the serum conjugated bilirubin. The demonstration of bilirubinuria indicates an elevation of conjugated serum pigment levels above a "threshold" of about 0.4 mg per 100 ml. The presence of bilirubinuria suggests underlying hepatocellular or obstructive biliary tract disease. Bilirubinuria may often be detected before the patient appears clinically jaundiced.

URINE UROBILINOGEN Although of limited usefulness as a test of liver function, semiquantitative measurements of urobilinogen can be made on a freshly collected 2-hr urine specimen by the Watson method (normal values 0.2 to 1.2 units). Interpretation of results is often difficult when both liver cell damage and cholestasis are present. With liver injury there is decreased removal of urobilinogen from the portal blood and increased urine urobilinogen excretion. With cholestasis there is decreased enteric production of urobilinogen and reduced urinary excretion. Administration of broad spectrum antibiotics reduces the intestinal flora and decreases urobilinogen production. A portacaval shunt will lead to decreased hepatic removal of urobilinogen and an increased urinary excretion of urobilinogen.

BROMSULPHALEIN (BSP) EXCRETION Several dyes, including BSP (a phenolphthalein derivative), indocyanine green, and radioactive rose bengal, have been used to assess hepatic excretory function. Of these, the BSP test is the most widely used. BSP is taken up rapidly by liver cells, concentrated and stored within the cytoplasm, and conjugated enzymatically with glutathione. Both free BSP and BSP-glutathione are secreted into the bile, since conjugation is *not* obligatory for biliary secretion. In diseases that produce hepatic cell dysfunction or impaired bile secretion, significant quantities of conjugated BSP may escape excretion and reenter the bloodstream. Although it was once considered to be a simple index of liver blood flow and excretory competence, the clearance of BSP from the blood depends also on the rate of hepatic uptake, storage capacity, conjugating activity, and an overall blood-to-bile transfer maximum. However, the techniques that measure these different parameters of BSP metabolism are not routine diagnostic tools.

The BSP test is simple, quantitative, and sensitive but notably *nonspecific*. A standard amount (5 mg per kg body weight) of BSP dye is injected carefully into a vein, a blood sample is withdrawn 45 min later from another venous site and analyzed for total BSP concentration.

The result is expressed as the percentage of injected dye retained in the circulation. Normally, less than 5 percent of the test dose remains in the serum at 45 min.

Despite its simplicity and sensitivity, the BSP test is often difficult to interpret. Abnormal retention may reflect the *presence* of liver cell damage or loss, as in hepatitis or cirrhosis, and may not be a direct measure of the *extent* of parenchymal disease. Many diverse processes such as partial bile duct obstruction, focal intrahepatic duct obstruction by tumor, and cholestasis may produce BSP retention. Decreased hepatic blood flow as in shock or congestive heart failure results in marked BSP retention. The BSP test is therefore a sensitive index of overall liver cell function.

A few practical aspects of the BSP test should be noted: (1) The dye is a local tissue irritant, and extravasation during injection produces painful inflammation and necrosis. (2) Rare *anaphylactic reactions* have been described and hence the test must be used with caution. (3) Gross obesity and fluid retention make calculation of an appropriate dose difficult, and under these circumstances results may be falsely high because of abnormal dye distribution. (4) Fever and certain drugs (notably the gallbladder dye iopanoic acid and the synthetic androgen norethandrolone) may produce BSP retention without apparent liver cell damage. (5) The test is of no value in the presence of jaundice since retention will occur regardless of the nature of the underlying disease.

FLOCCULATION AND TURBIDITY TESTS A number of empirical flocculation and turbidity tests have been used in the past to detect quantitative changes in the serum proteins of patients with hepatobiliary disease. In general, increased levels of γ-globulins and decreased albumin concentrations alter the stability of the colloidal solutions and produce positive reactions. These tests, which are nonspecific and affected by many nonhepatic factors, have been replaced in large part by chemical determinations of albumin and globulin concentrations, protein electrophoretic methods, and serum enzyme measurements.

SERUM ENZYME ASSAYS Measurements of many serum enzymes have been used to quantify liver damage or to distinguish between hepatocellular (i.e., functional) and mechanical cholestasis. No specific or truly diagnostic test has been devised to solve either problem, but the enzymatic liver function tests described below have proved helpful in the clinical study of many hepatobiliary diseases.

Alkaline phosphatase Serum contains alkaline phosphatase, an enzyme which hydrolyzes synthetic phosphate esters at pH 9. As indicated in Chap. 291, this enzyme is produced by many tissues, especially bone, intestine, liver, and placenta, and is excreted in bile. Most of the enzyme present in normal serum is derived from bone. In hepatobiliary disease, there is an increased release of the hepatic enzyme into the bloodstream apparently due to increased enzyme synthesis. In the absence of bone disease and pregnancy, an elevated serum alkaline phosphatase level generally reflects impaired hepatic excretory function.

Several methods of comparable accuracy and sensitivity are available to measure alkaline phosphatase activity. The most widely used are the Bodansky (normal: 1.5 to 4.5 units) and the King-Armstrong methods (normal: 4 to 13 units). Growing children and women in late pregnancy have serum levels that may be twice normal.

Slight to moderate increases in alkaline phosphatase (6 to 10 Bodansky units) occur in many patients with parenchymal liver disorders such as hepatitis and cirrhosis, and transient increases may occur in all types of liver disease. The most striking and persistent increases in activity, however, occur in association with cholestasis. Over 80 percent of patients with malignant biliary obstruction have phosphatase values in the range of 15 to 30 Bodansky units; about 60 percent of those with benign obstruction have levels above 15 Bodansky units, and most with intrahepatic cholestasis have values above 12 Bodansky units. Extremely high values may be associated with biliary obstruction complicated by cholangitis or tumor invasion of the liver. Two features of this test make it especially useful in cases of obscure liver disease: (1) increases in serum alkaline phosphatase may precede elevations of the serum bilirubin level in obstructive biliary disease; (2) focal hepatic lesions (for example, granulomas, inflammatory infiltrates, and tumor metastases) may produce elevation of alkaline phosphatase level with little other evidence of liver dysfunction. Since bone is a source of the enzyme, extensive Paget's disease, bony metastases and other diseases associated with increased osteoblastic activity may produce high levels of alkaline phosphatase in the absence of liver disease.

5′-Nucleotidase This enzyme which is elevated in obstructive biliary disease is sometimes measured because it is *not affected by bone disease*. However, elevations may be found with various hepatocellular diseases, and in general alkaline phosphatase is a more sensitive measure of impaired bile excretion.

Transaminases Assays of many serum enzymes have been proposed as measures of hepatocellular damage. Of these, the serum glutamicoxaloacetic (SGOT) and glutamic-pyruvic (SGPT) transaminases have proved to be the most practical. GOT occurs in all body tissues, expecially in heart, liver, and skeletal muscle. GPT is present primarily in the liver and to a lesser extent in kidney and skeletal muscle. Although many studies have shown that the height and duration of serum enzyme elevations parallel the extent of liver cell damage (i.e., necrosis or altered cell permeability), precise quantitative correlations cannot be made in most clinical conditions (Chap. 291). Normal serum contains less than 40 Karmen units of GOT and less than 40 Karmen units of GPT.

In the absence of acute necrosis or ischemia of other organs such as the myocardium, high SGOT and SGPT levels suggest liver cell damage. With extensive acute hepatic necrosis, as in severe viral hepatitis, serum enzyme levels of 1,000 to 3,000 units may be found. Less severe necrosis produces transient levels of 500 to 1,000 units. Mild chronic or focal liver diseases (e.g., subclinical or anicteric viral hepatitis, Laennec's cirrhosis, granulomatous infiltrations, and tumor invasion) may be associated with transaminase levels of 50 to 200 units. With intrahepatic or extrahepatic cholestasis (in the absence of hepatic cell necrosis) SGOT and SGPT levels usually are not significantly elevated and rarely exceed 300 units.

Serial determinations of SGOT and SGPT are helpful in following the course of a patient with liver disease, especially with acute or chronic hepatitis. Caution is needed in the interpretation of abnormal levels. Serum transaminases may actually *decrease* in some patients with fulminant hepatitis, because of the previous excessive release of enzymes from the liver. Laennec's cirrhosis and postnecrotic cirrhosis may be associated with only slight transaminase elevations.

Lactic dehydrogenase (LDH) Measurement of serum LDH is usually not helpful diagnostically because it is present in all organs and released into the serum from a variety of tissue injuries. Fractionation of LDH into its five tissue specific isoenzymes may give useful information about the site of origin of the LDH elevation. Moderate elevations of LDH levels are common in acute viral hepatitis and in cirrhosis; biliary tract disease may produce slight elevations. High serum levels may be found in metastatic carcinoma of the liver.

SERUM PROTEINS Albumin, prothrombin, fibrinogen, and several other serum proteins are synthesized exclusively by liver cells, and extensive liver damage may lead to decreased blood levels of these proteins. The level of serum immunoglobulins, produced by lymphocytes and plasma cells, varies widely in hepatobiliary disease and reflects inflammatory or immune responses rather than liver cell dysfunction. Thus, analyses of the various serum proteins may provide helpful insights into the nature and extent of liver disease. However, as noted in Chap. 291, many nonhepatic factors also affect the metabolism of these proteins.

Albumin and globulins Total concentrations of serum albumin (normally 3.5 to 5 g per 100 ml) and globulin (normally 2 to 3.5 g per 100 ml) may be determined chemically. The level of each should be evaluated separately, because the *albumin/globulin, or A/G, ratio* has no physiologic significance. The concentrations of α_1-, α_2-, β-, and γ-globulins are usually measured by electrophoretic methods.

Hypoalbuminemia may occur in subacute and massive hepatic necrosis, chronic active hepatitis, cirrhosis, and other disorders with significant destruction or replacement of liver cells. The serum albumin level also serves as a useful guide to prognosis and therapy in these diseases. *Hyperglobulinemia* suggests the presence of chronic inflammatory disorders such as cirrhosis and chronic active hepatitis. Neoplastic and inflammatory diseases of the liver may produce increased levels of α_2-globulins, and some patients with bile duct obstruction have high β-globulin levels (see Chap. 106).

Immunoglobulins Nonspecific immunoglobulin abnormalities occur in a variety of acute and chronic liver diseases. The major immunoglobulin fractions may be increased slightly in the course of acute viral hepatitis. Increased concentrations of IgA and IgG are common in Laennec's cirrhosis, striking elevations of IgG levels are characteristic of chronic active hepatitis, and high levels of IgM may be seen in primary biliary cirrhosis. None of these changes, however, are specific or diagnostic.

Clotting factors The serum activities of most clotting factors may be estimated by special tests, but direct determinations of fibrinogen and of the one-stage prothrombin time (which reflects activities of prothrombin, fibrinogen, and factors V, VII, and IX) are the most useful.

Prolongation of the one-stage prothrombin time may occur in severe hepatitis or cirrhosis and in patients with chronic bile duct obstruction. A single abnormal prothrombin determination should not be interpreted as a sign of liver cell failure, because intestinal malabsorption of vitamin K may produce reductions in prothrombin levels. However, the persistence of an abnormal prothrombin time 24 and 48 hr after parenteral injections of vitamin K_1 (10 mg per day) suggests liver cell dysfunction.

BLOOD LIPIDS Measurements of serum total cholesterol (normal: 130 to 230 mg per 100 ml) and cholesterol esters (normal: 50 to 70 percent of total cholesterol) are frequently made in patients with liver disease. Acute or chronic diffuse liver disease often results in decreased total values and a decrease in the ester fraction; cholestasis, whether functional or mechanical, characteristically produces moderate to extreme elevations of the total cholesterol level but with a decrease in the percent esterified. In cholestasis one also finds variable elevations of serum triglycerides and of an abnormal lipoprotein (lipoprotein X) (see Chap. 293).

IMMUNOLOGIC TESTS Immunologic derangements occur in a variety of liver diseases. Antimitochondrial antibodies are frequently found in primary biliary cirrhosis (85 percent of cases) although they may also be positive in some patients with chronic active hepatitis and drug hepatitis. In chronic active hepatitis the LE cell test may be positive and antinuclear as well as antismooth muscle antibodies may be present in the blood. Immunologic methods are the key to the detection of the hepatitis B antigen (HBAg) in long-incubation or serum hepatitis. Alpha-fetoprotein is of value in the diagnosis of hepatoma. Measurements of alpha-1-antitrypsin may be performed in infants with cirrhosis since they may have an hereditary deficiency of this enzyme.

RADIOLOGIC PROCEDURES

ABDOMINAL ROENTGENOGRAM Films of the upper abdomen and lower thorax rarely provide accurate estimates of liver size and shape, but gross hepatomegaly and hepatic masses that elevate or distort the diaphragm may be detected. However, the abdominal film is more accurate in determining the presence of splenomegaly and is often helpful in detecting minimal degrees of splenic enlargement. Plain films of the abdomen may reveal calcific densities in the gallbladder, biliary tree, pancreas, or liver (as echinococcal cysts, hemangioma, or, rarely, a metastatic tumor mass).

BARIUM STUDIES OF THE GASTROINTESTINAL TRACT An upper gastrointestinal series should be performed in suspected cases of portal hypertension, because esophagogastric varices can be demonstrated with about 70 to 90 percent accuracy when they are present. Enlargement of the left lobe of the liver (as with tumor, abscess, or cirrhosis) may displace the barium-filled stomach laterally and posteriorly. Tumors of the head of the pancreas often produce displacement or irregularity of the second portion of the duodenum.

CHOLECYSTOGRAPHY AND CHOLANGIOGRAPHY The *oral cholecystogram* provides limited information in most patients with overt hepatobiliary disease, because parenchymal dysfunction and impaired bile excretion lead to decreased excretion of the contrast material and hence nonvisualization of the gallbladder. An *intravenous cholangiogram* may permit demonstration of the intrahepatic and extrahepatic bile ducts and the localization of obstructing lesions of the major ducts. Even faint visualization of a normal-sized biliary tree may be helpful in the differential diagnosis of obstructive jaundice. However, as with the oral cholecystography, liver dysfunction and moderate cholestasis may prevent adequate secretion of dye to permit visualization on x-ray. In general, intravenous cholangiography will not be successful if the serum bilirubin is greater than 3 mg per 100 ml.

Percutaneous transhepatic cholangiography is sometimes used to distinguish between mechanical biliary obstruction and intrahepatic cholestasis. This approach may be useful when decreased liver function precludes the use of intravenous cholangiography. With experience and proper precautions, dilated major ducts proximal to an obstructing lesion can be cannulated and visualized in 75 to 90 percent of cases; the normal or small ducts associated with intrahepatic cholestasis are rarely demonstrated. This procedure should be carried out together with a surgeon, because when a dilated duct is punctured and visualized, exploration of the biliary system should be carried out within several hours to avoid bile peritonitis. *Operative cholangiography* should be performed at the time of laparotomy in all cases of obscure obstructive jaundice.

Endoscopic pancreatocholangiography with the fiberoptic duodenoscope has recently been developed and may provide a reasonable alternative to exploratory laparotomy in certain patients with obscure jaundice. The papilla of Vater is cannulated under direct vision and contrast material is injected into the biliary and pancreatic ducts. Additional information can be obtained by biopsy, such as of lesions of the ampulla.

ANGIOGRAPHY An increasingly useful and effective approach for visualizing the hepatic and portal circulation involves *selective angiography* of the celiac, superior mesenteric, and hepatic arteries. In most centers it has replaced splenoportography since by injection of these arteries one can visualize both the arterial (hepatic) and venous (hepatic and portal) systems. Selective arteriography is quite safe. It is useful (1) in demonstrating the hepatic arterial circulation which will be deranged in cirrhosis and in the diagnosis of primary and secondary liver tumor masses; (2) in visualizing the portal circulation for evidence of a collateral circulation, venous obstruction, anomalous vessels, etc. In major medical centers, next to liver biopsy this angiographic method is increasingly used as a diagnostic tool for the study of chronic liver disease and portal hypertension.

RADIOISOTOPE LIVER SCANS (SCINTISCANS) Hepatic scintiscans are performed by the intravenous injection of gamma-emitting isotopes that are extracted selectively by the liver, followed by external radiation scanning of the upper abdomen. There are basically two types of liver scans: the *colloidal scan*, which depends on uptake of a labeled colloid by Kupffer cells, and the *rose bengal scan*, in which the dye is taken up and executed by hepatocytes. The colloidal scan (with ^{198}Au colloidal gold, ^{99m}Tc sulfur colloid or ^{67}Ga citrate) is useful in detecting splenomegaly and intrahepatic masses such as tumors, abscesses, or cysts. The ^{131}I–rose bengal scan may indicate extrahepatic biliary obstruction if no isotope is detected in the intestine in 24 hr. In the presence of cirrhosis, liver scans are seldom used to diagnose liver tumors because the patchy uptake produced by the lobular architecture is difficult to differentiate from the abnormalities produced by multiple or diffuse neoplastic lesions.

Hepatic scanning should be regarded as a supplement to other methods of evaluating liver function, and its indications and limitations must be emphasized. Although tumor nodules larger than 3 cm in diameter can be demonstrated in about 80 percent of cases, false negative scans occur in about 20 percent of most series of metastatic cancer of the liver, because many hepatic metastases are too small to be detected by this method. Abscesses and cysts may be outlined with accuracy, but nonopaque areas may result from parenchymal disorders such as cirrhosis.

OTHER DIAGNOSTIC PROCEDURES

PORTAL AND HEPATIC VEIN MANOMETRY Measurement of the splenic pulp pressure (a reliable reflection of the actual portal venous pressure) by *percutaneous portal manometry* and estimation of the wedged hepatic venous pressure (WHVP—an approximation of the postsinusoidal intrahepatic venous pressure) by *hepatic vein catheterization* are useful in the study of patients with known or presumed portal hypertension. While determination of the WHVP is not a routine procedure, the demonstration of a normal or slightly elevated WHVP in a patient with proved portal hypertension serves to localize the obstruction to the extrahepatic portion of the portal vein, the portal inflow system (as in schistosomiasis), or the presinusoidal vessels (as in some cases of fatty liver or portal fibrosis). Splenic pulp pressure greater than 25 to 30 cm saline solution indicates significant portal hypertension.

PERCUTANEOUS NEEDLE BIOPSY OF THE LIVER

Percutaneous needle biopsy is a safe, simple, and valuable method of diagnosing liver disease. Although the needle biopsy sample is small, *diffuse parenchymal disorders* such as cirrhosis, hepatitis, and drug reactions may be diagnosed with remarkable accuracy. In *disseminated focal diseases* (such as granulomas or tumor infiltrates) serial sections may demonstrate the lesion.

The biopsy is performed under local anesthesia usually with the Menghini (aspiration) or Vim-Silverman (cutting) needle using either the transpleural or subcostal approach. If the operator is skillful and the patient is carefully selected, morbidity should be low and limited to occasional postbiopsy pain or vasovagal reactions.

Some of the major indications for needle biopsy are (1) unexplained hepatomegaly or hepatosplenomegaly, (2) cholestasis of uncertain cause, (3) persistently abnormal liver function tests, (4) suspected systemic or infiltrative diseases such as sarcoidosis or miliary tuberculosis, and (5) suspected primary or metastatic liver tumor.

Needle biopsy should not be performed if (1) the patient is not able to cooperate, (2) clinical or laboratory evidence indicates impaired hemostasis (for example, the one-stage prothrombin time is greater than 50 percent of control, thrombocytopenia or purpura are present, or the partial thromboplastin time is prolonged), (3) there is infection of the right pleural space or septic cholangitis, (4) profound anemia or (5) tense ascites are present, or (6) compatible blood is not available for transfusion in case of hemorrhage. Amyloidosis and carcinoma of the liver may increase the hazard of postbiopsy hemorrhage. Although biopsy in mechanical biliary obstruction may lead occasionally to the escape of bile and localized bile peritonitis, this complication is uncommon.

PERITONEOSCOPY With this technique the serosal lining, liver, gallbladder, spleen, and other abdominal organs can be visualized with minimum discomfort and hazard. Diagnosis may be made by inspection or directed needle biopsy. Peritoneoscopy is useful in the study of debilitated patients and in those with hepatomegaly, unexplained ascites, or abdominal masses.

LAPAROTOMY When the most thorough clinical, laboratory, and biopsy studies fail to define the precise nature of hepatobiliary disease, exploratory laparotomy may be necessary. However, it must be reemphasized that when there is evidence of significant hepatocellular necrosis (e.g., markedly elevated SGOT levels) laparotomy will often be accompanied by an increased morbidity and mortality. When laparotomy is performed, the medicosurgical team should be prepared to obtain full benefit from this direct approach, using biopsy, culture, cholangiography, and angiography as required.

REFERENCES

Liver function

BRADLEY SE: The circulation and the liver. Gastroenterology 44:403, 1963

FEIZI T: Immunoglobulins in chronic liver disease. Gut 9:193, 1968

KAPLAN M: Alkaline phosphatase. N Engl J Med 286:200, 1972

SCHOENFELD LJ: Sulfobromophthalein transport and metabolism. Gastroenterology 48:530, 1965

WALKER G, DONIACH D: Antibodies and immunoglobulins in liver disease. Gut 9:266, 1968

Radiologic and other diagnostic procedures

BAGGENSTOSS AH: Morphologic and etiologic diagnosis from hepatic biopsies without clinical data. Medicine 45:435, 1966

CONN HO et al: Comparison of radiologic and esophagoscopic diagnosis of esophageal varices. N Engl J Med 265:160, 1961

COTTON PB et al: Cannulation of papilla of Vater via fiberduodenoscope. Lancet 1:53, 1972

GOTTSCHALK A: Liver scanning, in *Principles of Diagnostic Radiology*, eds EJ Potchen et al, New York: McGraw-Hill, 1971

LOMAS F et al: Increased specificity of liver scanning with the use of ^{67}gallium citrate. N Engl J Med 286:1323, 1972

293 DISTURBANCES OF BILIRUBIN METABOLISM

KURT J. ISSELBACHER

The normal metabolism of bilirubin and the approach to the patient with jaundice have been presented in Chap. 42. With a consideration of these pathways, the disorders of bilirubin metabolism can be divided into four major categories, namely, those due to (1) increased pigment production, (2) reduced hepatic uptake of bilirubin, (3) impaired hepatic conjugation, and (4) decreased excretion of the conjugated pigment from the liver into bile. The first three of these disorders are associated with predominantly unconjugated hyperbilirubinemia (i.e., more than 80 percent of serum bilirubin is unconjugated, or indirect-reacting). The fourth group, defective excretion, is associated with predominantly conjugated hyperbilirubinemia (i.e., more than 50 percent of serum bilirubin is conjugated, or direct-reacting) and with bilirubinuria.

DISORDERS CAUSING PREDOMINANTLY UNCONJUGATED HYPERBILIRUBINEMIA

Overproduction of bilirubin

INCREASED DESTRUCTION OF CIRCULATING ERYTHROCYTES (INTRAVASCULAR AND EXTRAVASCULAR HEMOLYSIS) In disorders associated with hemolysis, most commonly the hemolytic anemias, the rate of bilirubin production is increased and may even exceed the amount that can be removed by a normal liver. The resulting jaundice is primarily an unconjugated hyperbilirubinemia. There is often also a small but definite increase in the serum conjugated bilirubin, when the amount of bilirubin glucuronide formed exceeds the amount that the liver can excrete (see Chap. 42). If there is significant anemia or if other adverse factors are present (e.g., fever, sepsis, hypoxemia, or vascular collapse), the ability of the liver to handle the pigment load will be compromised, and the degree of jaundice will be greater.

The clinical and diagnostic features of the various hemolytic anemias are described in Chap. 306. The presence of reticulocytosis, shortened red cell survival and increased fecal urobilinogen, in the absence of clinical and laboratory evidence of liver disease, strongly suggest hemolysis and overproduction of bilirubin as the cause of the jaundice. It is obvious, however, that in some cases (e.g., cirrhosis, tumors, and sepsis), hemolysis *plus* deranged liver function may be present. In most cases of uncomplicated hemolytic states, the mean serum bilirubin level will be in the range of 3 to 5 mg per 100 ml; rarely, levels up to 10 mg may be seen.

Jaundice due to increased pigment production may also be seen as a consequence of *tissue infarction* (e.g., pulmonary infarcts) and large *collections of blood in tissues* (e.g., leakage from blood vessels after catheterization studies, rupture of an aortic aneurysm). If hypotension and hypoxia also supervene, jaundice is usually more pronounced, and the resulting impairment of liver function may also lead to a significant increase in the serum conjugated bilirubin level (see Postoperative Jaundice, later in this chapter).

With the exception of early infancy, elevations of serum unconjugated bilirubin levels are not generally harmful per se, and the prognosis is that of the hemolytic process itself. However, in the neonatal state and infancy, unconjugated bilirubin levels above 20 mg per 100 ml may lead to *kernicterus* due to bilirubin deposition in the lipid-rich basal ganglions (see Chap. 332). Chronic overproduction of bilirubin may result in the formation of gallstones composed predominantly of bilirubin ("pigment stones"). In this situation, all the potential complications of calculus disease of the biliary tract (Chap. 300) may be superimposed on the chronic hemolytic state which produced it.

INCREASED PRODUCTION OF BILIRUBIN FROM SOURCES OTHER THAN CIRCULATING ERYTHROCYTES As indicated in Chap. 42, about 15 to 20 percent of the circulating bilirubin is normally derived from sources other than the destruction of circulating red cells. This represents the so-called "early-labeled fraction"; it includes the synthesis of bilirubin from nonhemoglobin heme in the liver and from hemoglobin heme in the marrow.

In some conditions, jaundice results from an increased destruction of red cells or red cell precursors in the marrow—a process referred to as *ineffective erythropoiesis* (see Chaps. 42 and 58). In patients with thalassemia, pernicious anemia, and congenital erythropoietic porphyria, such an increased rate of formation of the early-labeled bilirubin fraction has been demonstrated. It is possible that some cases of unexplained unconjugated hyperbilirubinemia may be caused by an increased hepatic production of bilirubin from nonhemoglobin heme, but this phenomenon has not yet been demonstrated clinically.

Impaired hepatic uptake of bilirubin

DRUGS While numerous drugs may theoretically interfere with uptake of bilirubin by the liver, only one agent has been definitely shown to influence this process. Flavaspidic acid, an active ingredient of male fern extract used in the treatment of tapeworm infestation, may cause unconjugated hyperbilirubinemia, as well as impairment of Bromsulphalein (BSP) clearance, during its administration. The jaundice readily subsides following treatment. Flavaspidic acid competes with bilirubin for intrahepatic binding sites (presumably the Y and Z cytoplasmic binding proteins), leading thereby to unconjugated hyperbilirubinemia. The jaundice which may occur with novobiocin and the iodinated agent bunamiodyl is also apparently due to an interference in bilirubin uptake.

GILBERT'S SYNDROME (CONSTITUTIONAL HEPATIC DYSFUNCTION; FAMILIAL NONHEMOLYTIC JAUNDICE) Since the original report by Gilbert in 1907, there have been increasing reports of patients with this disorder characterized by unexplained mild, chronic elevations of the indirect-reacting bilirubin level in the serum. The patient with Gilbert's syndrome may show jaundice in the neonatal period, but more often it is first detected after the second decade. The patient often is unaware of jaundice until physical or laboratory examination reveals a mild or low-grade hyperbilirubinemia, usually ranging from 1.2 to 3 mg per 100 ml and rarely higher than 5 mg per 100 ml. The jaundice is chronic, and the degree of icterus fluctuates. It is often noted after stress or trauma. It may be first noticed following prolonged fasting, surgery, infection, excessive exertion, or alcohol ingestion. While there may be a history of fatigue or asthenia, one can frequently ascribe these symptoms to the associated disorder which brings the patient to the physician. Liver function tests are normal (except for occasional slight increases in BSP retention), and liver histology shows no specific changes.

This disorder often goes unrecognized. At least one study suggests a prevalence of up to 5 percent of the male population. There are no specific tests for this disease, and *the diagnosis is one of exclusion* in a patient with unconjugated hyperbilirubinemia in whom occult or compensated hemolysis has been eliminated. The underlying defect is considered to be due to *impaired bilirubin uptake*. However, some studies have also shown a *decrease in liver glucuronyl transferase*. Thus the exact mechanism (i.e., impaired uptake, decreased conjugation or both) is not yet clear.

Often cases of unconjugated hyperbilirubinemia are initially called Gilbert's syndrome because *overt* hemolysis has not been detected. However, in many instances, subsequent studies with more sensitive techniques (e.g., bilirubin clearance, ^{51}Cr red cell labeling) do reveal *occult* hemolysis or ineffective erythropoiesis. Thus, many cases labeled "Gilbert's syndrome" may in fact be patients with mild or compensated hemolytic states. In view of these factors and since there is no specific diagnostic test, Gilbert's syndrome may not be a single disease entity.

POSTHEPATITIS HYPERBILIRUBINEMIA Some patients, after recovering from an attack of acute viral hepatitis, are found several months or years later to have a mild unconjugated hyperbilirubinemia. The histologic features of the liver are normal, and the bilirubin increase is of the same order of magnitude as Gilbert's syndrome. Except for a history compatible with a prior attack of viral hepatitis, *these patients have no unique features to distinguish them from patients with Gilbert's syndrome*; in fact, they probably belong to this same broad disease group. It is important to reassure the patient that the mild unconjugated hyperbilirubinemia is of no clinical consequence and is not an indication that chronic liver disease has supervened.

Impaired bilirubin conjugation (decreased activity of bilirubin glucuronyl transferase)

NEONATAL JAUNDICE (PHYSIOLOGIC JAUNDICE OF THE NEWBORN) Almost every infant exhibits some transient unconjugated hyperbilirubinemia between the second and fifth days of life. While during gestation the placenta serves to clear bilirubin from the fetus, after birth the infant must detoxify the pigments himself. However, at this stage the hepatic enzyme system is still "immature" and inadequate for the task. As a result, unconjugated bilirubinemia develops, usually not exceeding 5 mg per 100 ml serum. The activity of glucuronyl transferase increases within several days to 2 weeks after birth, and concomitantly the serum bilirubin returns to normal. In the premature infant the glucuronyl transferase activity is less, and the neonatal jaundice may be more pronounced. The "maturation" of the fetal and neonatal liver may be enhanced by treatment of the pregnant mother or the newborn infant with phenobarbital or related drugs. This results in a clear-cut reduction of the degree and duration of unconjugated hyperbilirubinemia in the newborn. In infants with a superimposed hemolytic process (e.g., erythroblastosis), the excessive pigment load leads to more pronounced jaundice, and bilirubin levels may exceed 20 mg per 100 ml serum. It should be emphasized that neonatal jaundice is not present at the time of delivery; if jaundice is present at birth, other causes must be considered.

Two soluble, low-molecular-weight cytoplasmic liver cell proteins (Y and Z) have been described. These appear to be involved in the normal binding of bilirubin and drugs by the liver (Chap. 42). In experimental animals the Y protein which appears to bind bilirubin is low in the neonatal state and increases with age. It has been proposed that deficiency of this protein may contribute to neonatal jaundice.

An additional facet of the "immature" liver is a concomitant defect in the excretion of *conjugated* bilirubin. Rarely this defect persists beyond the time needed for the development of adequate glucuronide conjugation and may explain the occasional presence of conjugated hyperbilirubinemia in infants with erythroblastosis (*inspissated-bile syndrome*).

When in the neonatal state unconjugated bilirubin levels approach levels of 20 mg per 100 ml, the infants may develop and die of *kernicterus*. The latter condition results from unconjugated bilirubin deposition in the lipid-rich basal ganglia. Treatment consists of exchange transfusions. Albumin infusions may be given to increase binding of bilirubin in the circulation and diminish its entry into the brain. An alternate approach is phototherapy; intense illumination of these patients with strong white or blue light leads to photooxidation of bilirubin to water-soluble derivatives (probably dipyrroles) that are rapidly excreted in the bile and urine without the need of conjugation.

CONGENITAL NONHEMOLYTIC JAUNDICE (GLUCURONYL TRANSFERASE DEFICIENCY) This disorder is now known to exist in two forms. Type I is the clinically *severe* form (known as the Crigler-Najjar syndrome) due to *absence of glucuronyl transferase.* Type II has more *moderate* clinical findings due to *partial deficiency of glucuronyl transferase.* The major differences between the two variants are summarized in Table 293-1.

Type I (Crigler-Najjar) is a rare disorder. Infants develop high unconjugated bilirubin levels in the serum (20 to 45 mg per 100 ml). Absence of the enzyme can be demonstrated in the liver. Indirect measurements of the defect include evidence of impaired urinary excretion of glucuronides following the oral administration of drugs such as menthol. Routine liver function tests are normal, as is the liver histology. Because of the absence of glucuronyl transferase no conjugated bilirubin is formed by the liver; hence no bilirubin is secreted by the liver and the bile is colorless.

Albumin and exchange transfusions, as well as phototherapy, may temporarily and transiently reduce the unconjugated bilirubin level. Phenobarbital has no effect since the enzyme defect is complete and no drug "induction" is therefore possible. Affected infants usually die

TABLE 293-1
Comparison of two types of congenital nonhemolytic jaundice

Features	*Type I (severe)*	*Type II (moderate)*
Eponym	Crigler-Najjar syndrome	
Inheritance	Autosomal recessive	Autosomal dominant
Glucuronyl transferase	Absent	Partial deficiency; induced with phenobarbital
Bile		
a Appearance	Colorless	Yellow
b Bilirubin content	0	+
Serum bilirubin	20 mg/100 ml	6–18 mg/100 ml
Kernicterus	Common	Unusual
Treatment	Albumin infusions; phototherapy	Phenobarbital
Prognosis	Poor	Good

within the first year of life, although some patients have survived to the second and third decade of life. Death is usually from kernicterus.

A strain of rats (Gunn rat) with the type I defect exists and is widely used as an animal model of the Crigler-Najjar syndrome.

Type II patients have a partial deficiency of glucuronyl transferase, and their disorder is less severe. Serum unconjugated bilirubin levels are lower (6 to 18 mg per 100 ml), jaundice may not appear until adolescence, and neurologic complications are uncommon. The bile contains variable amounts of conjugated bilirubin, although none is detectable in the plasma. Phenobarbital, a microsomal enzyme inducer, is effective in lowering the serum bilirubin level in type II patients. However, the disorder is relatively benign. Its relationship to the type I defect remains to be determined.

ACQUIRED DEFICIENCY OF GLUCURONYL TRANSFERASE As with any enzyme, glucuronyl transferase is susceptible to inhibition by a variety of agents, and because of the decreased activity of the enzyme in neonatal state, such inhibition may be more evident at that time. Neonatal jaundice may be aggravated or prolonged in infants treated with *drugs* such as chloramphenicol or novobiocin, or with *vitamin K.* In some breast-fed infants jaundice has been ascribed to the presence in *breast milk* of pregnane-3β,20α-diol, a good inhibitor of glucuronyl transferase. When the infant is removed from the breast, the "breast-milk jaundice" subsides.

Hypothyroidism delays the normal "maturation" of glucuronyl transferase. In cretins, neonatal jaundice may be prolonged for weeks or months. In fact, the presence of prolonged unconjugated hyperbilirubinemia after birth may be a clue to an underlying hypothyroidism.

In the infant, as well as in the adult, *liver cell damage* leads to impairment in glucuronide conjugation as a result of decreased transfer-activity. However, since excretion is probably the rate-limiting step in bilirubin metabolism and since this step is always interfered with to a greater extent than conjugation in parenchymal liver disease, the pigment which accumulates in the blood is predominantly conjugated bilirubin.

DISORDERS CAUSING PREDOMINANTLY CONJUGATED HYPERBILIRUBINEMIA

In jaundice due to primary liver disease, the plasma usually exhibits elevated levels of both conjugated and unconjugated bilirubin, and *urine contains bilirubin.* The relative proportions of the two pigments are highly variable. In many familial hepatic abnormalities (described below) and in some forms of drug-induced liver injury, the jaundice is almost entirely due to conjugated hyperbilirubinemia, 60 to 80 percent of the serum bilirubin giving a direct van den Bergh reaction. Such a pigment pattern is also seen with extrahepatic biliary obstruction.

In jaundice associated with diffuse liver cell damage as in hepatitis and cirrhosis, the conjugated bilirubin levels may be somewhat less than in the above cholestatic syndromes, with the direct-reacting values ranging from 50 to 70 percent of the total serum bilirubin. However, the pattern is quite variable, and in all the above hepatic disorders, once the serum bilirubin components have been measured, repeated fractionation during the course of the disease is of little diagnostic or prognostic value. One cannot differentiate intrahepatic and extrahepatic causes of jaundice from either the levels or proportions of the two pigment types (i.e., unconjugated and conjugated bilirubin) in plasma. Thus the main purpose of the initial fractionation of the plasma bilirubin is to distinguish hepatic parenchymal and biliary obstructive disease from the disorders associated with predominantly unconjugated hyperbilirubinemia.

Familial defects in hepatic excretory function

DUBIN-JOHNSON SYNDROME (CHRONIC IDIOPATHIC JAUNDICE) This disorder is characterized by a mild, chronic hyperbilirubinemia and the frequent presence of a *dark pigment in the liver cells.* It is an autosomal inherited disease of hepatic excretory function. The hyperbilirubinemia, which may begin at any age, is predominantly of the conjugated type, with total serum levels usually ranging from 3 to 10 mg per 100 ml. The patient may be asymptomatic or have vague constitutional or gastrointestinal symptoms. Not infrequently the liver is slightly enlarged; in about one-fourth of the cases there is mild hepatic tenderness. Oral and intravenous cholangiography usually fails to visualize the biliary tract. Liver function tests are variably affected, but BSP excretion is consistently diminished. In performing the BSP test, the serum level falls at 30 and 45 min, but then the BSP *may increase again* at 90 and 120 min. The increase is primarily in conjugated BSP; this temporal pattern, while not specific, is characteristic of this disorder. In the liver the striking feature is the presence of a brown or black pigment in the hepatocytes. This nonbilirubin pigment, initially considered a lipofucin, appears to be a melanin polymer.

These patients also show an abnormality in coproporphyrin excretion. Normal urine contains mostly coproporphyrin III and small amounts of coproporphyrin I; Dubin-Johnson patients show a reversal of this pattern, i.e., a predominant excretion of coproporphyrin I. Heterozygotes show an intermediate excretory pattern.

There is impaired excretion of many metabolites, including conjugated bilirubin, BSP, and iodinated dyes. Oral contraceptive agents may accentuate hyperbilirubinemia or may produce jaundice for the first time. Features of cholestasis such as pruritus or steatorrhea are usually lacking, and serum alkaline phosphatase levels are *not* elevated. Impairment in the excretion of epinephrine metabolites may account for the accumulation of the melanin pigments. The overall prognosis of the disorder is excellent.

Rotor syndrome is similar in most respects to the Dubin-Johnson syndrome. However, *there is no pigment in the liver cells*, and the gallbladder is usually visualized on cholecystography. The BSP excretion pattern is similar to that seen in the Dubin-Johnson syndrome. The fact that in members of a family with chronic idiopathic jaundice one may find some with hepatic pigment and others without strongly suggests that the Rotor and Dubin-Johnson syndromes are genetically related variants.

BENIGN FAMILIAL RECURRENT CHOLESTASIS This is a relatively rare syndrome characterized by recurrent attacks of pruritus and jaundice. During an attack the serum alkaline phosphatase level is markedly elevated, and liver biopsy shows the morphologic features of cholestasis. However, at laparotomy, biliary obstruction is not found, and operative cholangiography reveals a patent and apparently normal biliary tree. Remissions are the rule, and at such times hepatic function tests and liver morphologic features are usually normal. The cause of the disorder is unknown; cirrhosis does not develop, and disorder is benign. A congenital origin has been postulated based on the early age of onset and familial incidence.

RECURRENT JAUNDICE OF PREGNANCY (INTRAHEPATIC CHOLESTASIS OF PREGNANCY) During a normal pregnancy some changes in liver function occur, especially during the last trimester. Usually these consist of slight increases in BSP retention and of serum alkaline phosphatase. This mild increase in alkaline phosphatase during pregnancy is normally of placental rather than hepatic origin. Bilirubin increases never exceed 2 mg per 100 ml serum and usually are hardly detectable.

In a small number of pregnant patients an intrahepatic cholestasis may appear. This usually occurs in the third trimester but may develop any time after the seventh week of gestation. The clinical features consist primarily of pruritus and jaundice. Serum bilirubin levels are usually less than 6 mg and rarely higher than 8 mg per 100 ml. The serum alkaline phosphatase and cholesterol levels are elevated significantly, while other liver function tests are only mildly deranged. Histologically the liver shows varying degrees of cholestasis but only a few parenchymal cell changes. The clinical and laboratory abnormalities subside promptly after delivery and are usually completely normal with 7 to 14 days.

This condition has been seen more frequently in Scandinavia and Europe than in the United States. Since steroid hormones and specifically estrogens can induce changes in hepatic excretory function in normal individuals (see Chap 291), these patients probably have an increased susceptibility or sensitivity to the hepatic effects of estrogenic and progestational hormones. The intrahepatic cholestasis is usually termed *recurrent*, since the syndrome often (but not always) reappears in subsequent pregnancies. The process is benign and self-limited, and treatment is usually not needed, but cholestyramine administration will diminish the pruritus. This disorder must be distinguished from the the many other causes of jaundice not unique to pregnancy, such as viral hepatitis. It must also be distinguished from the idiopathic *acute fatty liver of pregnancy* and the *tetracycline-induced* fatty liver. The latter two conditions are rare, occur in the last trimester, and have a high fatality rate; however, in these disorders there is evidence of diffuse parenchymal damage and not just cholestasis.

Acquired defects of hepatic excretory function

DRUG-INDUCED CHOLESTASIS A condition entirely analogous to the intrahepatic cholestasis of pregnancy may occur in some women following the use of oral contraceptive agents. A significant number of individuals using these drugs show mild increases in BSP retention, and even more have decreased BSP excretory capacity as measured by infusion tests. In some mild cholestatic jaundice may occur, liver function returns to normal when the drugs are withdrawn, and chronic liver disease does not appear to result. It is relevant that one-third of the reported patients with jaundice due to oral contraceptives also have a history of recurrent intrahepatic cholestasis of pregnancy.

The nature of these changes produced by the natural and synthetic female sex hormones is very similar to those resulting from the administration of certain testosterone analogues, esepcially those with α-substitutions at the 17 position of the steroid nucleus. These agents (such as methyltestosterone and norethandrolone) commonly cause BSP retention and less commonly cause jaundice or significant changes in other liver functions. However, unlike the female hormones, these agents have been implicated as a cause of chronic liver disease, especially biliary cirrhosis.

Because of these phenomena, synthetic steroid sex hormones should not be used in patients with liver disease. Conversely, in individuals using these agents the appearance of jaundice or abnormalities in transaminase or alkaline phosphatase contraindicates their further use. However, mild to moderate increases in BSP retention alone are probably not of clinical significance, although liver function tests should be carried out periodically.

As is discussed in detail in Chap. 294, there are many drugs which may produce not simply cholestasis but liver injury resembling acute hepatitis or cholestatic hepatitis. In contrast to the jaundice produced by the steroid hormones the clinical features are those of fever, rash, arthralgia, and eosinophilia, with the liver showing a pronounced inflammatory reaction. These features suggest that such reactions are *allergic* or *toxic* in nature and therefore differ from the effects caused by the steroid

TABLE 293-2
Conditions causing or contributing to postoperative jaundice

I Increased pigment load
- *A* Hemolytic anemia
- *B* Transfusions (especially of stored blood)
- *C* Resorption of hematomas, blood in extravascular spaces

II Impaired hepatocellular function
- *A* Hepatitis-like picture
  - *1* Halothane anesthesia
  - *2* Drugs
  - *3* Shock
  - *4* Infection with hepatitis virus A or B
- *B* Cholestatic picture
  - *1* Hypotension, hypoxemia
  - *2* Drugs
  - *3* Sepsis

III Extrahepatic obstruction
- *A* Bile duct injury
- *B* Choledocholithiasis

hormones, which probably represent an exaggerated response by the liver to the normal action of these hormones.

POSTOPERATIVE JAUNDICE The occurrence of postoperative jaundice is a problem of increasing importance. It is perhaps seen more frequently now than in earlier years, because patients are able to undergo major surgical procedures (i.e., cardiac surgery, repair of ruptured aneurysms) and survive. In approaching this problem the possible pathogenic mechanisms listed in Table 293-2 need to be considered. The patient may have *pigment overload*, especially from blood transfusions (due to hemolysis of stored blood), from resorption of blood in extravascular spaces, and less commonly from hemolytic anemia. *Hepatocellular damage* and decreased liver cell function may occur due to concurrent use of hepatotoxic drugs (Chap. 294) or anesthetics such as halothane. Hepatocellular necrosis may follow profound shock; with lesser degrees of hypotension or hypoxemia, morphologic damage may be slight, but significant impairment of function may occur. Hence prior shock or

TABLE 293-3
Laboratory features in icteric states

Bilirubin disorder	*Bilirubin* *Serum* *Unconjugated*	*Conjugated*	*Urine*	*Urobilinogen* *Urine*	*Stool*	*Comments*
Overproduction:						
Hemolysis (intra- and extravascular)	↑	N	0	↑	↑↑	
Ineffective erythropoiesis	↑	N	0	↑	↑↑	Splenomegaly; normal RBC survival; normoblasts in marrow
Defective uptake:	↑	N	0	N-↓	N-↓	Normal liver biopsy; normal RBC survival; direct/total bilirubin <20%. Some have ↓ transferase
Gilbert's syndrome						
Posthepatitic hyperbilirubinemia						
Some drugs (e.g., flavaspidic acid)						
Defective conjugation:	↑	Low	0	↓	↓	
Congenital nonhemolytic jaundice (Types I and II)						Genetic absence or deficiency of glucuronyl transferase
Neonatal jaundice						Delay in enzyme development; ? ↓ Y protein
Drug inhibition (pregnanediol, chloramphenicol, vitamin K)						Of importance in neonatal period
Defective excretion:						
Intrahepatic obstruction:						
Familial syndromes	↑	↑↑	+	Variable	↓	
Dubin-Johnson						Abnormal BSP curve, hepatic lipochrome pigment (melanin); ↑ urinary coproporphyrin I
Rotor syndrome						Same, but no liver pigment
Drugs (e.g., chlorpromazine, methyltestosterone)	↑	↑↑	+	↓	↓	↑ Alkaline phosphatase but other usually normal
Benign recurrent cholestasis	↑	↑↑	+	↓	↓	↑ Alkaline phosphatase
Recurrent jaundice of pregnancy (3d trimester)	↑	↑↑	+	↓	↓	↑ Alkaline phosphatase in afflicted subjects may be reproduced or exacerbated by estrogens or progesterone
Hepatitis (see below)						
Extrahepatic obstruction (tumors, stone, stricture of bile duct):						↑↑ Alkaline phosphatase (often > 15 Bodansky units)
Partial	↑	↑↑	+	N-↓	↓	
Complete	↑	↑↑	+	0	0	
Hepatocellular disease:*						
Hepatitis	↑	↑↑	+	↑	↓	Direct/total bilirubin > 20%; liver biopsy important for diagnosis
During obstructive phase	↑	↑↑	+	↓-0	↓	
Cirrhosis: same as hepatitis						

* *Note that in hepatic cellular disease there is generally an interference in all pathways of bilirubin metabolism (i.e., impaired uptake, conjugation, and excretion).*

hypotension plus pigment overload may produce significant jaundice. Extensive sepsis can also produce jaundice, often of a cholestatic type. Concurrent renal impairment due to hypotension and hypoxemia may enhance the degree of jaundice because the renal excretion of conjugated bilirubin is decreased. *Extrahepatic obstruction* due to surgical damage or stones needs to be considered, but may be difficult to exclude.

A form of jaundice referred to as *benign postoperative intrahepatic cholestasis* may be seen. In the typical case the patient has had major and prolonged surgery for a catastrophic event such as a ruptured aortic aneurysm complicated by hypotension and hypoxemia, extensive blood loss into tissues, and massive blood replacement. Jaundice may be noted on the second or third postoperative day and the serum bilirubin, predominantly conjugated, may reach 20 to 40 mg per 100 ml by the eighth to tenth day. Alkaline phosphatase levels range from 15 to 40 Bodansky units. Typically the SGOT is only mildly elevated. The liver morphology is striking in that necrosis is not seen but only cholestasis and erythrophagocytosis.

The cause of this type of postoperative cholestatic jaundice is uncertain. However, in all likelihood it reflects (1) increased pigment load, (2) decreased liver function due to hypoxemia and hypotension, and (3) decreased renal bilirubin excretion due to varying degrees of tubular necrosis as a result of shock. This diagnostic possibility must be considered in the postoperative patient with marked cholestatic jaundice. The course of the jaundice is self-limited and will subside if the other systemic complications do not predominate and lead to death.

HEPATITIS AND CIRRHOSIS These disorders, discussed in detail in Chaps. 294 to 296, constitute the *most common disorders associated with jaundice.* As has been stated previously, when the liver cell is damaged, as in viral hepatitis, there is often impairment in all three major hepatic phases of bilirubin metabolism, namely, uptake, conjugation, and excretion. Since the excretory step is one which is rate-limiting and most readily affected by injury, significant amounts of conjugated bilirubin reenter the systemic circulation. There are also usually lesser increases in the serum unconjugated bilirubin. The latter is probably a reflection of the impaired uptake and conjugation, and in part due to the shortened red cell life span often found in liver disease. In most patients with hepatitis and cirrhosis, the total serum bilirubin levels tend not to exceed 50 mg per 100 ml, but on rare occasions levels of up to 90 or 95 mg per 100 ml have been described.

Extrahepatic biliary obstruction

Anatomic or mechanical obstruction of the bile ducts is most commonly due to stones, tumors, or strictures. The clinical picture is quite similar to that of intrahepatic cholestasis with pronounced elevation of the alkaline phosphatase level. Usually, but not always, fever, pain, and chills may be present. While the amount of direct-reacting (conjugated) bilirubin predominates in the serum, the amount of the total serum bilirubin which is direct-reacting is variable (60 to 80 percent) and of no real diagnostic or prognostic significance. In contrast to hepatitis and cirrhosis, the serum bilirubin level often tends to plateau and rarely exceeds levels of 35 mg per 100 ml. The reason for this plateau is not clear but may be related to renal excretion of conjugated bilirubin or alternative pathways of bilirubin catabolism in obstructive jaundice.

REFERENCES

Benign familial recurrent cholestasis

Lesser PB: Benign familial recurrent intrahepatic cholestasis. Am J Digest Dis 18:259, 1973

Schapiro RH, Isselbacher KJ: Benign recurrent intrahepatic cholestasis. N Engl J Med 268:708, 1963

Dubin-Johnson and Rotor syndromes

Butt RH et al: Studies of chronic idiopathic jaundice (Dubin-Johnson syndrome): II. Evaluation of a large family with the trait. Gastroenterology 51:619, 1966

Wolkoff AW et al: The inheritance of the Dubin-Johnson syndrome. N Engl J Med 288:113, 1973

Gilbert's disease; glucuronyl transferase deficiency

Arias IM et al: Chronic non-hemolytic unconjugated hyperbilirubinemia with glucuronyl transferase deficiency: Clinical, biochemical, pharmacological and genetic evidence for heterogeneity. Am J Med 47:395, 1969

Berk PD et al: Constitutional hepatic dysfunction (Gilbert's syndrome). Am J Med 49:296, 1970

——, Blaschke TF: Detection of Gilbert's syndrome in patients with hemolysis. Ann Intern Med 77:527, 1972

Hunter JO et al: Inheritance of type 2 Crigler-Najjar hyperbilirubinaemia. Gut 14:46, 1973

Neonatal jaundice

Arias IM et al: Prolonged neonatal unconjugated hyperbilirubinemia with breast feeding and a steroid pregnane-3(alpha),20(beta)diol, in maternal milk that inhibits glucuronide formation in vitro. J Clin Invest 42:913, 1963

Levi AJ et al: Deficiency of hepatic organic anion-binding protein as a possible cause of non-haemolytic unconjugated hyperbilirubinaemia in the newborn. Lancet 2:139, 1969

Postoperative jaundice

Kantrowitz PA et al: Severe postoperative hyperbilirubinemia simulating obstructive jaundice. N Engl J Med 276:591, 1967

La Mont JT, Isselbacher KJ: Postoperative jaundice. N Engl J Med 288:305, 1973

Recurrent jaundice of pregnancy

Boake WC et al: Intrahepatic cholestatic jaundice of pregnancy followed by Enovid-induced cholestatic jaundice. Ann Intern Med 63:302, 1965

Haemmerli UP: Jaundice during pregnancy, with special emphasis on recurrent jaundice during pregnancy and its differential diagnosis. Acta Med Scand (suppl 444), 1966

294
ACUTE HEPATITIS

RAYMOND S. KOFF
KURT J. ISSELBACHER

ACUTE VIRAL HEPATITIS

Acute viral hepatitis is a systemic infectious disease affecting predominantly the liver. It occurs in two immunologically distinct but clinically similar forms—hepatitis A and hepatitis B. This nomenclature is preferred to the formerly used terms, infectious hepatitis and serum hepatitis, which are no longer satisfactory since both diseases may be transmitted by either the oral or the parenteral route. Synonyms for hepatitis A include infectious hepatitis, short-incubation hepatitis, and MS-1 hepatitis. Hepatitis B is also known as serum hepatitis, long-incubation hepatitis, MS-2 hepatitis, and hepatitis B antigen (HBAg) or hepatitis-associated (Australia) antigen positive hepatitis.

Both hepatitis A and hepatitis B are characterized pathologically by hepatic cell necrosis and inflammation. The usual clinical picture consists of an anicteric prodromal period followed by jaundice and subsequent recovery. However, many cases are mild with no overt symptoms and are recognized or suspected only by the presence of abnormal liver function tests.

PROPERTIES OF THE HEPATITIS VIRUSES Transmission studies in human volunteers have indicated that the infectious agents of hepatitis are viruses, but neither agent has yet been isolated. Although the precise size of virus A is unknown, virus B has been postulated to be less than 26 nm in diameter on the basis of filtration studies. Both agents resist freezing and are not destroyed by heating at 56°C for ½ hr. Virus B is inactivated by heating at 60°C for 10 hr; virus A is probably also inactivated by such treatment. Both viruses are resistant to ether. Virus A remains infective after exposure to chlorine (1 part per million).

In the majority of patients with hepatitis B, serologic and electron microscopic studies have revealed the presence of a circulating antigen referred to as hepatitis B antigen (HBAg). HBAg can be transiently detected during the incubation period or early acute phase of the illness and usually disappears within 3 to 12 weeks. HBAg is a specific marker of hepatitis B and is not found in epidemiologically documented virus A infections. HBAg is infrequent (0.1 percent) in normal populations in the United States and Western Europe. However, it has been found to have a prevalence of 3 to 25 percent in some tropical countries, as well as in Down's syndrome, in lepromatous leprosy, in patients with chronic renal disease receiving hemodialysis, and in needle-using drug addicts. It is not clear whether persons with persistent circulating HBAg are carriers of virus B, are affected with chronic anicteric hepatitis, or both. In liver cells HBAg has been localized to the nuclei, and less commonly the cytoplasm, by direct immunofluorescence and electron microscopy.

Three types of HBAg-carrying particles have been observed in serum. These include small spherical particles approximately 20 nm in diameter, rod-shaped (sometimes tubular) particles approximately 20 by 230 nm, and larger (Dane) particles approximately 42 nm in diameter with an outer coat and an inner core. Purified HBAg has a molecular weight of 2.4×10^6 and consists of approximately 75 percent protein, 20 percent lipid, and 2 to 5 percent nucleic acid. Heating of diluted serum containing HBAg for 1 min at 98°C destroys the infectivity but not the antigenicity of the serum.

Antibodies to HBAg (anti-HBAg) have been detected after primary and secondary hepatitis B infection, and may persist in serum for long periods. Anti-HBAg can be detected when HBAg is present in serum, and in some instances immune complexes of HBAg and anti-HBAg have been identified in serum. It has been suggested that HBAg is an antigenic subunit of hepatitis B or an incomplete hepatitis B virus. A number of HBAg subtypes differing in antigenic specificities exist and may prove useful in epidemiologic studies and in vaccine development. However, it is not clear whether antigenemia can be equated with either viremia or infectivity of serum.

EPIDEMIOLOGY The incubation period of hepatitis A varies between 15 and 50 days, irrespective of route of inoculation, and in most epidemics averages about 30 days. The incubation period of hepatitis B is longer, with a range of 50 to 180 days. Oral inoculation of virus B results in a longer incubation period than does parenteral transmission. As shown in Table 294-1, viremia occurs during the incubation period and the early phase of the illness of both hepatitis A and B; namely, 2 to 3 weeks before the onset of jaundice in hepatitis A and as early as 3 months before jaundice in hepatitis B. The duration of viremia is less clear. Viremia was not demonstrated 1 month after the onset of hepatits A or during convalescence from hepatitis B in volunteer studies. In recent studies persistence of circulating HBAg has been observed in 5 to 10 percent of previously healthy adults following virus B infection. Some of these individuals with persistent antigenemia have no evidence of continuing liver disease, but may act as inapparent carriers, while others may have chronic hepatitis (chronic active or chronic persistent hepatitis). Excretion of virus into the urine or nasopharyngeal secretions has not been conclusively demonstrated in hepatitis A or B. Fecal excretion of virus in hepatitis A has been shown during the last 2 weeks of the incubation period and during the first few days of the acute phase of illness, regardless of the route of inoculation. Fecal shedding of virus after the disappearance of jaundice is extremely rare in hepatitis A.

Fecal excretion of hepatitis B virus and HBAg-like material has been suggested in recent studies, and it is now clear that transmission of hepatitis B by the oral route may occur. The frequency of such transmission is not definitely known, although it is not uncommon in closed institutions with extremely poor sanitary standards. The detection of HBAg in more than 50 percent of urban adults with "sporadic" hepatitis suggests that nonparenteral transmission of hepatitis B is more common than previously suspected.

Homologous immunity has been shown for both hepatitis A and B under experimental conditions, more convincingly for hepatitis A than B. It is not clear whether immunity is complete or lifelong, since reinfections have been well documented. However, second attacks may be due to different antigenic strains of virus. Heterologous immunity has not been demonstrated. Whether a humoral or cell-mediated mechanism is responsible for immunity in hepatitis is not yet clear.

Hepatitis A is a disease primarily of children and young adults; hepatitis B has no specific age preponderance and only about 15 percent of healthy adults have circulating antibody to HBAg, indicating previous exposure to virus B. While no seasonal variation in the incidence of hepatitis B has been noted, in temperate climates the incidence of hepatitis A rises in late autumn, peaks in the winter, and drops in late spring and through the summer. Both hepatitis A and hepatitis B are worldwide in distribution.

Fecal-oral transmission, primarily by person-to-person contact, is the most common mode of spread of hepatitis A. A gradual buildup of cases, peak distribution in young children, familial aggregations, and geographic proximity of cases are typical of person-to-person transmission. History of recent contact with jaundiced persons or known hepatitis cases is found in at least 20 to 30 percent of patients in whom person-to-person transmission occurs. In addition, exposure to children and adults with anicteric infections or to asymtomatic carriers probably represents a significant source of infection. Estimates of the ratio of icteric to anicteric cases of hepatitis A have ranged from 1:1 in adults to 1:10 in children.

A respiratory route of infection and a role for arthropods as mechanical vectors of hepatitis has been suggested, but not proved. Careful epidemiologic studies have shown that a significant risk of hepatitis exists for animal handlers in contact with newly imported nonhuman primates and have suggested that these species may act occasionally as carriers of virus A or B and may, in fact, be susceptible to human hepatitis virus infection.

Extensive outbreaks of hepatitis A but not hepatitis B have been traced to contaminated water or milk, and to the ingestion of other foods, including uncooked clams and oysters. Such common-source epidemics more frequently affect adults than children, and the occurrence of a large number of cases in adults during an epidemic (especially in the summer) is suggestive of common-source rather than person-to-person spread.

Parenteral transmission would seem to be a major mode of spread of hepatitis B and an important source of hepatitis A. Virus has been transmitted in as little as 0.00004 ml blood. Contamination of needles, syringes, lancets, and tattooing instruments has been associated with outbreaks of hepatitis B. Epidemics of either hepatitis A or hepatitis B have been associated with multidose syringe practices and traced to the use of contaminated hypodermic or infusion equipment. The sharing of needles among drug addicts has been responsible for sporadic cases as well as for epidemics of hepatitis.

Transfusion-associated hepatitis may be either hepatitis A or hepatitis B, and the two are clearly differentiated at present only by the presence of circulating HBAg in hepatitis B. Hepatitis A is probably as frequent a complication of transfusion as hepatitis B. The risk of posttransfusion hepatitis increases almost linearly with the number of units of blood transfused and is closely related to standards of donor selection. The incidence of clinically apparent hepatitis following transfusion has been variably reported between 0.3 and 9 cases per 1,000 units transfused, or between 0.5 and 13 cases per 100 patients transfused. The risk of *anicteric hepatitis* following transfusion may be 3 to 10 times greater than that of *clinical hepatitis* with jaundice. The risk of viral hepatitis after transfusion of blood derivatives is dependent upon the methods by which these products are processed (Table 294-2).

Transfusion of frozen-stored red blood cells has been associated with a reduced incidence of hepatitis, probably as a result of elution of virus during the multiple washings required in the preparation of this material. Unfortunately, no effective method has been found for the inactivation of the viruses in whole blood.

TABLE 294-1
Comparison of epidemiologic features of hepatitis A and B

Feature	*Hepatitis A*	*Hepatitis B*
	Infectious Hepatitis (IH), MS-1, short incubation hepatitis	*Serum Hepatitis (SH), MS-2, long incubation hepatitis*
Incubation period	15–50 days	50–180 days
Presence of hepatitis B antigen	0	+
Route of infection:		
Oral	+	+ (< hep.A)
Parenteral	+	
Presence of viremia:		
Incubation period and acute phase	+	+
Convalescence	Rare	5–10%*
Presence of virus in feces:		
Incubation period and acute phase	+	Rare†
Convalescence	Rare	?
Asymptomatic carriers	Rare	0.1%
Epidemiologic patterns:		
Sporadic cases	+	+
Posttransfusion and needle-associated	+	+
Common-source outbreaks	+	0‡

* *Persistent circulating hepatitis B antigen*
† *Probably rare; only limited data available.*
‡ *Except for outbreaks in hemodialysis centers and among contacts of parenteral drug abusers.*

PATHOLOGY The characteristic morphologic lesions of hepatitis A and B are identical and consist of a combination of hepatic cell necrosis and regenerative activity, a diffuse mononuclear inflammatory reaction,

TABLE 294-2
Hazard of hepatitis from blood products

Average risk—single donor products
- Whole blood
- Packed red cells
- Single donor plasma, fresh-frozen or aged
- Single donor platelet or antihemophilic factor concentrates

High risk—multiple donor products
- Pooled plasma, ultraviolet-irradiated or stored at 31.6°C or room temperature for 6 months
- Fibrinogen
- Antihemophilic factor concentrates

No risk—multiple donor products, adequately treated*
- Human albumin
- Plasma protein fraction
- Immune serum globulin
- Hyperimmune serum globulin

* *Treatment refers to heating at 60°C for 10 hr or cold ethanol fractionation (method of Cohn).*

hyperplasia of Kupffer cells, and variable bile stasis. During the late incubation and acute prodromal phase of the disease, liver cell plates are disrupted, although the reticulin framework of the hepatic lobule is preserved. Liver cell damage is evident in the form of diffuse areas of hepatic cell degeneration and necrosis, with hepatic cell dropout, ballooning of cells, and acidophilic (Councilman-like) bodies. Nuclear size and staining are variable, and inclusion bodies are not seen. Liver cell regeneration is suggested by numerous mitotic figures, multinucleated cells, thickened parenchymal plates, and cytoplasmic basophilia. So-called "rosette" or "pseudoglandular" hepatic cell formation may be seen occasionally. Mononuclear cell infiltrates are present in the portal zones and in areas of lobular necrosis. Polymorphonuclear cells and eosinophils comprise only a minor fraction of the inflammatory reaction. Kupffer cells appear prominent and often contain abundant yellow-brown (lipofuscin) pigment. Ductular proliferation is common. Bile stasis, in the form of bile plugs or thrombi in dilated bile canaliculi and bile droplets within parenchymal and Kupffer cells, is variable in extent, occasionally resembling that produced by mechanical bile-duct obstruction. Fatty infiltration is not a feature of viral hepatitis, but rarely may be present in mild form during the late convalescent phase. The morphologic lesions of anicteric viral hepatitis are qualitatively identical to those described above, but quantitatively are usually more subtle. Electron microscopic studies of biopsy material from patients with acute viral hepatitis have shown disruption and dilatation of the endoplasmic reticulum, enlarged mitochondria, and prominent, vacuolated lysosomes. Focal dilatation of the bile canaliculi may be seen with loss of microvillous configuration. Intranuclear and cytoplasmic viruslike particles have been identified in some patients with HBAg-positive hepatitis.

Features of typical acute viral hepatitis

PRODROMAL PHASE In most patients with acute viral hepatitis, the onset of jaundice is preceded by nonspecific constitutional and gastrointestinal symptoms. From 2 to 14 days before the appearance of jaundice, the patient abruptly develops anorexia, fatigue, malaise, and lassitude. This may be followed or accompanied by nausea, vomiting, diarrhea, and occasionally arthralgia.

Abnormalities of olfaction and taste may be associated with a striking loss of appetite which often includes a positive aversion for food. Distaste for cigarettes is another common and curious symptom. Right upper quadrant or epigastric discomfort, described as either a sense of fullness or pain, is common. Fever between 100 and 104°F and symptoms of a "flulike" illness, with cough, coryza, pharyngitis, myalgias, and photophobia are frequent with hepatitis A and less common with hepatitis B, which usually begins insidiously. However, when parenterally transmitted, hepatitis A may begin insidiously and usually without fever. Occasionally urticaria, skin rashes, angioneurotic edema, and polyarthritis may be noted during the prodromal phase of hepatitis B and less frequently of hepatitis A. In hepatitis B this serum sickness-like syndrome may be related to the formation and deposition of circulating immune complexes of HBAg and anti-HBAg with complement.

In 1 to 4 days before the onset of jaundice, the urine darkens because of bilirubinuria, and often the stool color lightens. Pruritus may be a prominent symptom at this stage, but is usually transient. The clinical disease may be very mild in some patients, and overt jaundice may not be present at any time (anicteric cases). Physical findings may be minimal in the early prodromal phase, but hepatic enlargement and tenderness are present in most patients.

ICTERIC PHASE Once jaundice appears, the clinical features of hepatitis A and hepatitis B are identical. The prodromal gastrointestinal symptoms usually decrease in severity within a few days, and fever subsides promptly. The jaundice usually reaches a maximum between the first and second weeks and decreases steadily thereafter. The duration of jaundice is variable but lasts less than 6 to 8 weeks in typical cases. Weight loss of 5 to 10 lb during the prodromal and early icteric phase is common. The stools, which may have been clay-colored with the development of icterus, become darker again as the jaundice subsides.

Physical findings in the icteric phase include hepatic enlargement and tenderness. The liver begins to decrease in size and tenderness 1 to 2 weeks after the onset of jaundice and returns to normal size over a number of weeks. Posterior cervical lymphadenopathy and splenomegaly are present in about 20 percent of cases. Rarely, a few spider angiomas appear during the icteric phase and then disappear during convalescence.

RECOVERY PHASE Immediately following the subsidence of jaundice, the patient usually feels well, but recovery is seldom complete at this stage. The liver may still be enlarged and mildly tender, and abnormalities of hepatic function are still evident. Fatigue is often a prominent symptom. The duration of this posticteric phase varies from 2 to 6 weeks but may be longer in some instances. Full clinical and biochemical recovery is to be expected within 3 to 4 months in most cases.

MORTALITY The mortality of acute viral hepatitis appears to depend in part on the mode of transmission. Patients with hepatitis A contracted via the fecal-oral route have a case fatality rate of 0.1 to 0.4 percent. Patients with parenterally transmitted hepatitis A or B have a case fatality rate of about 1 percent. *However, posttransfusion hepatitis A or B with icterus has a case fatality rate of 10 to 12 percent.* Increasing age, debility, the presence of malignancy, and possibly pregnancy have adverse effects on survival. Anicteric disease is rarely fatal.

LABORATORY FINDINGS The presence of circulating HBAg in hepatitis B is the only distinction which can be made between hepatitis A and B by laboratory tests. During the preicteric phase, the leukocyte count is usually within the normal range, but mild leukopenia may be seen. Neutropenia and lymphopenia are transient, followed by a relative lymphocytosis. Atypical lymphocytosis varying between 2 and 20 percent is common during the acute phase; these so-called "virocytes" are indistinguishable from the atypical lymphocytes of infectious mononucleosis. The heterophil agglutination test may be positive, but guinea pig kidney cell adsorption removes the antibody from hepatitis sera. Although unusual, mild reticulocytosis and slight hemolysis have been reported. As a rule, anemia is not a feature of viral hepatitis.

During the initial prodromal phase of illness the first detectable abnormality may be either the presence of HBAg (in hepatitis B only) or a *progressive elevation of the serum transaminase* levels. Both serum glutamic oxaloacetic transaminase (SGOT) and serum glutamic pyruvic transaminase (SGPT) may be elevated 7 to 14 days prior to the onset of jaundice, reflecting altered hepatic cell permeability with enzyme leakage into the blood. In general, the SGPT levels are higher than SGOT values at all stages of the disease. The actual serum transaminase levels are variable, but peak SGPT values between 400 and 3,000 units are typical of acute viral hepatitis. The laboratory diagnosis of anicteric hepatitis is often based solely on transaminase elevations, although the serum conjugated bilirubin may be mildly elevated despite the absence of clinical jaundice. Bromsulphalein (BSP) retention can be observed commonly before the onset of scleral icterus and in anicteric cases. When jaundice appears, the serum bilirubin is usually above 3 mg per 100 ml and typically reaches 5 to 20 mg per 100 ml. Higher levels or a progressive, erratic rise later in the course may indicate more severe disease. However, patients with glucose-6-phosphate dehydrogenase deficiency or sickle-cell anemia (SS hemoglobin) may develop severe hemolysis and profound hyperbilirubinemia during the course of viral hepatitis.

Serum alkaline phosphatase may be normal or only mildly elevated to levels of 5 to 15 Bodansky units. Urine urobilinogen may increase in the preicteric phase and then decline with the appearance of acholic stools, with a secondary rise when normal stool color returns later in the course of the illness. The total serum protein levels may remain near normal, but in some patients a slight decrease in the serum albumin occurs. Serum globulin levels may be mildly elevated due to an increase in the gamma-globulin fraction. Protein immunoelectrophoresis reveals that IgG and IgM levels are elevated, while IgA is slightly increased or normal.

During the icteric phase serum cholesterol may be normal or slightly low, with a decrease in the cholesterol ester fraction. The prothrombin activity may be moderately decreased during the period of jaundice, but rarely produces clinical bleeding problems.

In a few patients mild and transient steatorrhea has been noted as well as slight microscopic hematuria and minimal proteinuria.

Other clinical forms of acute viral hepatitis (Fig. 294-1)

ANICTERIC HEPATITIS Although the above description of acute viral hepatitis with jaundice serves as a prototype of the clinical expression of hepatitis virus infection, *many patients with acute viral hepatitis do not show clinical jaundice* (i.e., they have anicteric hepatitis). In children anicteric infection is the rule rather than the exception, and unexplained fever and symptoms of an upper respiratory infection or gastroenteritis may be the initial or only feature of viral hepatitis. In adults with anicteric acute viral hepatitis a prodrome may or may not be present, but it is usually less prominent than in hepatitis with jaundice. Fever, gastrointestinal symptoms, and anorexia and malaise, if present, are usually quite mild and short-lived. Hepatomegaly and mild hepatic tenderness are the only signs of liver disease in these patients, but may be absent in some cases. Helpful laboratory studies include the presence of circulating HBAg in hepatitis B and of elevated serum transaminase levels, BSP retention, and minimal conjugated hyperbilirubinemia. The course of the disease is frequently short, and rapid subsidence of symptoms with early improvement of liver function abnormalities is common. In the absence of a local epidemic, *the diagnosis of anicteric viral hepatitis may be very difficult* unless there is a high index of suspicion.

FIGURE 294-1
Scheme showing variants and sequelae of acute viral hepatitis.

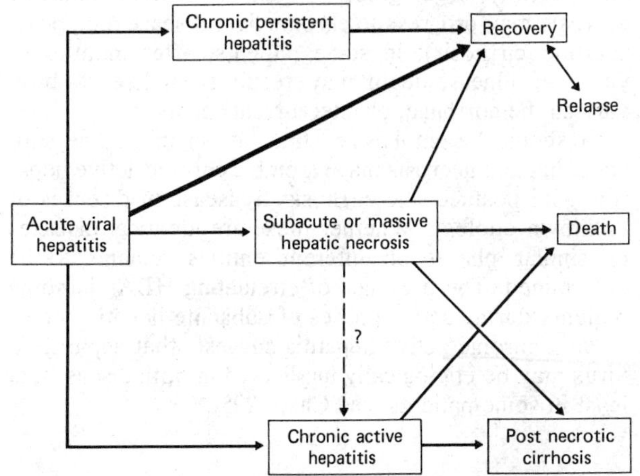

CHOLESTATIC HEPATITIS Less than 5 percent of patients with either hepatitis A or B may have a clinical course resembling that of bile duct obstruction, with severe pruritus and prolonged jaundice with acholic stools. Despite the pruritus and deep jaundice, these patients generally feel well and improve in time, although a number of weeks may be necessary for the jaundice to clear. Liver function studies, in these instances, reveal hyperbilirubinemia in the range of 20 to 30 mg per 100 ml, and the alkaline phosphatase may be 10 to 30 Bodansky units. Serum transaminase values are elevated, often exceeding 300 units. Liver biopsy reveals a striking degree of bile stasis, hepatic cell necrosis of variable severity, and an unusual number of polymorphonuclear leukocytes in the portal zone infiltrates.

SUBACUTE HEPATIC NECROSIS (BRIDGING) This appears to be an extremely uncommon variant of acute viral hepatitis, particularly hepatitis B. The prodromal and early acute phase may be quite similar to that of typical acute viral hepatitis, but the preicteric phase usually begins insidiously and is often longer than 2 weeks. Once jaundice is present, *the course of the illness is clearly different from that of typical acute viral hepatitis.* The patient continues to feel ill, and weakness and vomiting may persist. The serum bilirubin level may still be increasing after 2 weeks, and although it may fluctuate, the bilirubin tends gradually to plateau at levels greater than 20 mg per 100 ml. In contrast to typical viral hepatitis, transaminase levels remain elevated for many weeks. Hepatosplenomegaly persists, and spider angiomas and palmar erythema may be prominent. Hypoalbuminemia, hyperglobulinemia, and hypoprothrombinemia are often striking, and signs of fluid retention, portal hypertension, and hepatic encephalopathy may develop.

Liver tissue from patients with subacute hepatic necrosis reveals extensive zones of confluent liver cell necrosis with an inflammatory infiltrate of variable extent. *The distinguishing morphologic feature is the presence of bands of cell dropout with reticulin collapse bridging adjacent portal triads and central veins.* This "bridging" necrosis is felt to be of prognostic value. After many weeks or months of illness, some patients experience complete clinical recovery with either minimal fibrosis or no residual abnormality on liver biopsy. Another and possibly larger group of patients with submassive necrosis may progress to chronic liver disease (i.e., postnecrotic cirrhosis); in some patients, after months or years of illness, death may result from liver failure, variceal hemorrhage, or intercurrent sepsis.

It should be emphasized that late in its course subacute hepatic necrosis may resemble chronic active hepatitis with postnecrotic cirrhosis, a disease or diseases of unknown etiology. Whether these are identical diseases or similar phases of different entities remains to be determined. The presence of circulating HBAg in some patients during active phases of subacute hepatic necrosis and chronic active hepatitis suggests that hepatitis B virus may be etiologically implicated in both diseases, at least in some patients (see Chap. 295).

MASSIVE HEPATIC NECROSIS (FULMINANT HEPATITIS, ACUTE YELLOW ATROPHY) Sudden shrinking of the liver, as determined by palpation and percussion, over a period of hours or days is an ominous sign of fulminant and often fatal hepatitis. The development of hepatic coma and a rapid decrease in liver size is associated with a case fatality rate of 60 to 90 percent. The interval between the onset of illness and death is usually less than 2 weeks. Profound depression of the serum prothrombin activity with overt bleeding is common prior to death. Transaminase levels, while previously high, may be only moderately elevated or near normal at the time of death. Severe hypoglycemia is an occasional feature. Hypotension and renal failure are common.

The striking feature at postmortem examination is the finding of a small, soft liver. Histologic examination reveals massive necrosis and dropout of liver cells of most lobules. The reticulin framework of the liver may be preserved, but characteristically there is collapse and condensation wherever necrosis has occurred. In patients who recover, hepatic fibrosis may be found subsequently on liver biopsy, although rarely liver biopsy may be completely normal.

EXTRAHEPATIC COMPLICATIONS Acute pancreatitis, myocarditis, and atypical pneumonia have been reported infrequently in viral hepatitis, and the association with hepatitis may be merely fortuitous. However, viral invasion of these organs during the period of viremia is possible. Similarly, neurologic abnormalities other than hepatic encephalopathy, such as acute myelitis, aseptic meningitis, and peripheral neuropathy, have been reported very rarely. In a small number of patients, aplastic anemia may occur during the convalescent phase. This complication is usually fatal.

Differential diagnosis

In the preicteric phase (or in anicteric cases) viral hepatitis may closely resemble other viral acute infectious diseases. Gastroenteritis and influenza may be considered, but hepatitis can usually be distinguished by the presence of liver enlargement and tenderness, transaminase elevations, circulating HBAg in hepatitis B, and the subsequent course. Infectious mononucleosis with hepatitis may be clinically indistinguishable from viral hepatitis. However, large, tender lymph nodes, pharyngitis, and splenomegaly are much more common in infectious mononucleosis. Eventually the differential heterophil agglutination or EB virus antibody test will provide the answer.

During the icteric phase, other infectious diseases to be considered include dengue fever, Q fever, and yellow fever, and these may be excluded by geographic and epidemiologic considerations. Leptospiral liver involvement is usually accompanied by severe myalgia, conjunctivitis, evidence of renal damage, and often leukocytosis. Drug and toxic injury may result in jaundice, and abnormalities of liver function and histology in drug-induced hepatitis may closely resemble those of viral hepatitis. The presence of fatty change and zonal necrosis on liver biopsy suggests toxic injury, and a careful documentation of all exogenous drugs and occupational toxin exposures is necessary. Similarly "alcoholic hepatitis" must be considered, but usually the serum transaminases are not as markedly elevated, other stigmas of alcoholism may be present, and the finding of fatty infiltration, a neutrophilic inflammatory reaction, and alcoholic hyalin on liver biopsy would be consistent with alcohol-induced disease rather than viral injury. Chronic liver disease may present with jaundice; however, the physical findings of cirrhosis may be present and helpful in excluding viral hepatitis. The absence of recurrent fever, chills, and right upper quadrant pain is helpful in excluding acute cholangitis or cholecystitis. Extrahepatic bile duct obstruction due to choledocholithiasis or pancreatic carcinoma may resemble cholestatic hepatitis. Radiologic studies including duodenograms and intravenous cholangiography and percutaneous or retrograde cholangiography through the fiberoptic duodenoscope will aid in diagnosis.

The patient with viral hepatitis does not tolerate major surgery well during the acute phase. Therefore, a number of procedures, including percutaneous liver biopsy, may be necessary to exclude the possibility of viral hepatitis prior to exploratory laparotomy in the diagnosis of surgical jaundice.

Management

TYPICAL ACUTE VIRAL HEPATITIS There is no specific treatment. Hospitalization may be required for diagnosis, for clinically severe illness, atypical variants, and for those with posttransfusion hepatitis because of the high mortality. Although acute viral hepatitis tends to be self-limited, the extreme variability in the severity and course of viral hepatitis has resulted in a clinical impression that enforced and prolonged bed rest is essential to rapid recovery without residual chronic hepatic disease. It has been clearly shown, however, in young, previously healthy men, that strict bed rest has no advantage over a program with 1 hr of absolute rest after each meal. Furthermore, the incidence of cirrhosis was not increased 10 years later in patients treated with this rest program. However, regardless of age, most patients with severe symptoms will feel better with restricted physical activity and will desire bed or chair rest. A high-caloric balanced diet should be encouraged.

Intravenous feeding is necessary in the acute stage if the patient has persistent vomiting and cannot maintain oral intake. In previously well-nourished patients there is no evidence that dietary supplements are needed. If hepatic precoma develops, protein intake should be reduced and an oral, nonabsorbable antibiotic, such as neomycin, should be prescribed.

Drugs capable of producing adverse hepatic reactions or those metabolized primarily by the liver should be used with caution. There is no indication for systemic antibiotics. In an occasional patient pruritus may be severe, and the use of the bile-salt-sequestering resin, cholestyramine, will usually alleviate this symptom. Although administration of prednisone or other corticosteroids undoubtedly increases the appetite and sense of well-being in some patients with viral hepatitis and may also lower serum bilirubin levels, there is no evidence that these agents shorten significantly the convalescent phase or alter significantly the morphologic features of hepatitis. These drugs are usually reserved for patients with subacute hepatic necrosis or fulminant hepatitis.

Rigid isolation of the patient with hepatitis is not warranted. However, both patient and hospital staff must be reminded of proper hygienic practices, including careful washing of one's hands after examining the patient. A private room and bathroom to minimize inadvertent fecal spread is desirable.

Patients may be discharged from the hospital after the serum bilirubin has fallen below 2.0 mg per 100 ml and when other signs or symptoms indicate that the illness is waning. Mild elevation of SGOT or SGPT should not be considered contraindications to the gradual resumption of normal activity. Mild SGPT elevation may persist for 24 months or longer in some patients and has no prognostic significance.

SUBACUTE AND MASSIVE HEPATIC NECROSIS While corticosteroids are not indicated in the treatment of typical viral hepatitis, they are occasionally prescribed in patients with subacute hepatic necrosis and fulminant hepatitis. Massive doses of corticosteroids often are given when liver function deteriorates progressively, when the course is prolonged with deepening jaundice, or when hepatic encephalopathy develops during the course of illness. The effectiveness of steroids in reversing serious hepatitis has not yet been established. Similarly the role of immunosuppressive agents in the treatment of these diseases is not clear. The goal of treatment of fulminant hepatitis is to support the patient by maintenance of fluid balance and an open airway, support of the circulation, control of bleeding, and correction of hypoglycemia until liver cell regeneration and repair occur. Protein intake is usually restricted, and oral neomycin is administered. In some cases administration of L-dopa, exchange transfusion of whole blood, human cross-circulation, and porcine liver cross-perfusion have resulted in lightening of hepatic coma, but only rarely in survival. Human liver transplantation has been suggested, but technical difficulties have precluded its widespread use.

Prevention

HEPATITIS A Because virus is excreted for as long as 2 weeks before the onset of jaundice and usually before the diagnosis of hepatitis is suspected, the benefit of isolation or quarantine measures is limited. Spread of disease by the anicteric or subclinical case further compounds this difficulty.

It is generally agreed that 0.01 ml immune serum globulin per lb body weight given intramuscularly early in the incubation period will prevent symptoms and jaundice in exposed contacts. Instead, these individuals probably develop subclinical infection with serum transaminase elevations, followed by immunity. Immune serum globulin administration is indicated for intimate contacts (adults and children who are household members). Pregnant women and elderly or debilitated patients, in whom the disease may be more severe, should receive immune serum globulin prophylaxis even if exposure is casual. While larger doses of immune serum globulin (0.05 to 0.06 ml per lb) may provide a modifying effect for longer periods (perhaps up to 6 months), they are not more effective than the lower dosage in acute epidemic situations. The larger dose is recommended for individuals who are traveling in areas in which hepatitis is endemic and who require protection for more than 2 to 3 months.

PARENTERALLY TRANSMITTED HEPATITIS A AND B The use of disposable hypodermic equipment is essential, and multidose syringe techniques must be avoided. Sterile blood products should be substituted for whole blood when possible, and blood transfusions should be given only when essential. The cornerstone of establishing minimal hepatitis levels rests upon careful blood procurement programs that avoid drug addicts, patients with a past history of transfusion or hepatitis, and donors of questionable reliability. The screening of donors with liver function tests has proved to be of limited value because of a high frequency of both false positive and false negative results. Exclusion of donor blood containing HBAg may reduce the incidence of posttransfusion hepatitis by approximately 25 percent.

Standard immune serum globulin, containing low titers of antibody to HBAg, given intramuscularly, in both small and large (10 ml) doses during the first and fourth weeks following transfusion is ineffective in reducing the total incidence of hepatitis. In one trial the severity of the disease appeared to be modified by globulin administration. Similarly a preparation of globulin modified for intravenous administration has been reported to reduce the incidence of posttransfusion hepatitis with jaundice but not anicteric transfusion-associated hepatitis.

The role of hyperimmune serum globulin, containing high titers of antibody to HBAg in the prevention of posttransfusion hepatitis and parenterally transmitted hepatitis B still remains to be determined. In one recent study immune serum globulin with a high titer of hepatitis B antibody was shown to decrease the incidence of both HBAg positive and negative nonparenterally transmitted hepatitis in U.S. soldiers stationed in Korea.

Relapses or recurrence and sequelae

Approximately 5 percent of patients with viral hepatitis have an exacerbation of the disease within 6 months of the onset. This is manifested by a recurrence of the initial symptoms, elevated transaminase levels, and in some patients, jaundice. In certain patients HBAg reappears in the serum. Characteristically the recurrence is clinically milder than the initial episode. No distinction, however, between relapse and recurrent infection can be made. Only in special circumstances such as the addict who is reexposed and in whom two or more recurrences may follow is there a suggestion of repeated infection. These recurrences or relapses do not alter the prognosis, and residual liver disease has not occurred. Treatment is similar to that of the original episode.

POSTHEPATITIS SYNDROME Postviral infection asthenia, malaise, and other vague symptoms may occur for 6 to 12 months following hepatitis in some patients. These symptoms have no functional significance and require no treatment other than reassurance. Liver function tests are completely normal, and liver biopsy usually shows no evidence of active hepatic disease. In a small number of patients, mild unconjugated hyperbilirubinemia may persist for weeks, months, and occasionally years. No evidence of chronic liver disease or abnormal histology is evident on liver biopsy (see Chap. 293).

CHRONIC PERSISTENT HEPATITIS (DELAYED CONVALESCENCE) In approximately 5 to 10 percent of patients with viral hepatitis the disease may run a mild and prolonged course, lasting 4 to 8 months in about two-thirds of cases. In the remainder hepatomegaly and intermittently abnormal liver function tests may persist for several years. Elevation of the serum transaminase levels may be the only laboratory finding indicating continuing disease activity. Although some cases of chronic persistent hepatitis begin insidiously, approximately 70 percent begin as typical acute viral hepatitis. One or two exacerbations are not uncommon during the course of the illness. Liver biopsy discloses portal mononuclear infiltration, minimal hepatocyte degeneration without lobular disarray, and slight portal fibrosis. Nodular regeneration, zonal collapse and cirrhosis are not seen. Despite the delayed convalescence of patients with chronic persistent hepatitis, *full recovery is the rule.*

CHRONIC ACTIVE HEPATITIS The presence of circulating HBAg in some patients with chronic active hepatitis, a progressive destructive disorder leading to postnecrotic cirrhosis, suggests that hepatitis B may be etiologically implicated in this disease. Although about one-third of patients with chronic active hepatitis have an onset of illness resembling acute hepatitis, the development of chronic active hepatitis in patients with acute viral hepatitis is uncommon. A full discussion of this disease is found in Chap. 295.

POSTNECROTIC CIRRHOSIS There is still considerable debate as to whether typical acute viral hepatitis may lead to postnecrotic cirrhosis. Although an occasional patient with postnecrotic cirrhosis gives a history of an episode of antecedent jaundice, the identity or nature of such an episode will remain obscure until serologic tests for hepatitis viruses are available in these patients. Prospective follow-up of a large number of patients with acute viral hepatitis has not revealed an increased incidence of cirrhosis. However, as stated above, if patients with subacute or fulminant hepatic necrosis survive, a scarred and cirrhotic liver may be found.

OTHER SEQUELAE Rarely glomerulonephritis with the nephrotic syndrome or hematuria has followed recovery from hepatitis B. Glomerular deposition of immune complexes of HBAg and antibody to HBAg has been demonstrated in a few patients. A polyarteritis-like syndrome, resembling if not identical to polyarteritis nodosa, has also been noted in occasional patients with circulating immune complexes following hepatitis B. The demonstration of circulating HBAg in some patients with primary hepatic cancer (hepatoma) has raised the question of an etiologic relationship which requires further investigation.

TOXIC AND DRUG-INDUCED HEPATITIS

Liver injury may follow the inhalation, ingestion, or parenteral administration of a number of chemical agents. These include industrial toxins (e.g., carbon tetrachloride, yellow phosphorus), the toxic cyclic peptides of *Amanita phalloides* (mushroom poisoning), or more commonly, pharmacologic agents used in medical therapy. It is essential that any patient presenting with jaundice or impaired liver function be carefully questioned about exposure to chemicals used in work or at home and drugs taken by prescription or home remedies bought "over the counter." In general, two major types of chemical hepatitis have been recognized: (1) "*direct toxic*" and (2) "*hypersensitivity*."

As shown in Table 294-3, *toxic hepatitis* is one which *occurs with predictable regularity* in individuals exposed to the offending agent and is dose-dependent. The latent period between exposure and liver injury is usually short (often several hours), although clinical manifestations may be delayed for 24 to 48 hr. Agents producing toxic hepatitis are generally systemic poisons, and liver injury is only one facet of the toxicity. In certain instances, particularly when the toxin is ingested, gastrointestinal symptoms may be more prominent, and liver injury may go unrecognized until jaundice appears. The direct hepatotoxins result in morphologic abnormalities which are reasonably characteristic and reproducible for each toxin. For example, carbon tetrachloride and chloroform characteristically produce a centrilobular zonal necrosis, whereas yellow phosphorus poisoning typically results in periportal injury. *Amanita phalloides* toxin usually produces massive hepatic necrosis.

Drug *hypersensitivity* reactions lead to a morphologic pattern that is more *variable*; a single agent is often capable of inciting a variety of lesions, although certain patterns tend to predominate. In contrast to toxic hepatitis, the occurrence of hypersensitivity hepatitis in those exposed to the agent is *unpredictable*, the response is *not dose-dependent*, and *may occur at any time* during or after exposure to the drug. Immunologic evidence of classic hypersensitivity mechanisms (i.e., the demonstration of specific circulating or tissue-fixing antibodies) is not available. A role for lymphocyte-mediated immune mechanisms in drug-induced hepatotoxicity has also been postulated but has not been proved. However, extrahepatic clinical manifestations of hypersensitivity are common and include arthralgias, rashes, fever, leukocytosis, and eosinophilia. Depending on the agent involved, hypersensitivity hepatitis may result in a clinical picture indistinguishable from viral hepatitis (e.g., halothane) or may simulate extrahepatic bile duct obstruction (e.g., chlorpromazine). In some cases there may be features of both cholestasis and hepatocellular damage.

These major differences between toxic and hypersensitivity hepatitis do not permit a classification of all adverse hepatic drug reactions. For example, oral contraceptive agents, combining estrogenic and progestational compounds, regularly result in impairment of hepatic function and occasionally in jaundice, but they do not produce necrosis or fatty change in lower species and differ from the agents producing hypersensitivity hepatitis because manifestations of hypersensitivity are absent.

Because viral hepatitis is necessarily a presumptive diagnosis, and many adverse drug reactions produce a clinicopathologic picture resembling it, the establishment of an etiologic relationship between the use of a drug and subsequent liver injury may be most difficult. The relation is most convincing when the frequency of hepatic impairment following administration of the specific agent is high, when the latent period between the start of therapy and impaired function is short, and when rechallenge, after an asymptomatic period, results in a recurrence of signs, symptoms, and morphologic and biochemical abnormalities. Rechallenge is often ethically unfeasible, and documentation of adverse hepatic reactions must often await the collection of other clinical cases.

Treatment of toxic and drug-induced hepatic disease is largely supportive and does not differ from that for acute viral hepatitis. Withdrawal of the suspected agent is indicated at the first sign of an adverse reaction. In the

TABLE 294-3
Some features of toxic and drug-induced hepatic injury

	Type of hepatic reaction			
		Hypersensitivity		*Other*
Features	*Direct toxic effect (e.g., carbon tetrachloride)*	*(e.g., halothane)*	*(e.g., chlorpromazine)*	*(e.g., oral contraceptive agents)*
Predictable and dose-related toxicity	+	0	0	+
Latent period	Short	variable	variable	variable
Arthralgia, fever, rash, eosinophilia	0	+	+	0
Liver morphology	Necrosis, fatty infiltration	Similar to viral hepatitis	Cholestasis *with* portal inflammation	Cholestasis without portal inflammation

TABLE 294-4
Principal alterations of hepatic morphology produced by some commonly used drugs and chemicals

Principal morphologic change	*Class of agent*	*Example*
Cholestasis	Anabolic	Methyl testosterone
	Antithyroid	Methimazole
	Chemotherapeutic	Para-aminosalicylic acid*
	Oral contraceptive	Norethynodrel with mestranol (Enovid)
	Oral hypoglycemic	Chlorpropamide
	Tranquilizer	Chlorpromazine
Hepatitis	Anesthetic	Halothane
	Anticonvulsant	Diphenyl-hydantoin
	Antihypertensive	Alpha-methyl dopa
	Chemotherapeutic	Sulfonamides†
	Diuretic	Chlorothiazide
	Laxative	Oxyphenisatin
Toxic	Hydrocarbon	Carbon tetrachloride
	Metal	Phosphorus
	Mushroom	*Amanita phalloides*

* *Occasionally associated with hepatitis.*
† *Occasionally associated with cholestasis.*

case of the direct toxins, liver involvement should not divert attention from renal or other organ involvement which may prove a greater threat to survival than the liver disease. In Table 294-4, several classes of chemical agents are listed together with examples of the pattern of liver injury produced by them.

The following are the patterns of adverse hepatic reactions for some prototypic agents:

CARBON TETRACHLORIDE HEPATOTOXICITY (DIRECT TOXIN) Poisoning may result from inhalation, accidental or purposeful ingestion, or possibly by skin absorption. Initial clinical manifestations include headache, dizziness, drowsiness, nausea, vomiting, and vasomotor collapse. Liver injury may be evident 1 to 4 days following intoxication, with jaundice and hepatomegaly, and serum transaminase levels may be markedly elevated. The striking pathologic features are centrilobular hepatic necrosis and diffuse fatty infiltration. Renal injury may be evident concomitantly or shortly thereafter, with azotemia, albuminuria, and oliguria progressing to anuria. Fatalities during the first week are usually due to liver injury, while deaths later in the course are usually the result of renal damage. When recovery occurs, it is complete by 4 to 6 weeks. Residual liver or renal disease has not been clearly demonstrated following a single acute exposure.

HALOTHANE HEPATOTOXICITY (HYPERSENSITIVITY REACTION) Halothane, a nonexplosive fluorinated hydrocarbon anesthetic agent, structurally similar to chloroform, has been reported to result in severe hepatic necrosis in a small number of individuals, many of whom have previously been exposed to this agent. The failure to produce similar hepatic lesions in animals, the rarity of the hepatic impairment in humans, and the delayed appearance of hepatic injury suggests that halothane is not a direct hepatotoxin, but may be a sensitizing agent. Fever, moderate leukocytosis, and eosinophilia may occur in the first week following halothane administration. Jaundice usually is noted 7 to 10 days after exposure, but occasionally may be seen as long as 30 days later. Nausea and vomiting may precede the onset of jaundice. Hepatomegaly is often mild, but liver tenderness is common. Liver function tests are consistent with parenchymal cell damage, with elevated levels of SGOT. The pathologic changes seen at autopsy have been indistinguishable from massive hepatic necrosis due to viral hepatitis. The case fatality rate of halothane hepatitis is not known, but may be close to 40 percent in cases with severe liver involvement. In a single instance, involving an anesthesiologist, cirrhosis has been observed following repeated bouts of halothane hepatitis. It is strongly suggested that patients in whom unexplained spiking fever or jaundice develops after halothane anesthesia not receive this agent again. Because cross-reactions between halothane and methoxyflurane have been reported, the latter anesthetic should probably not be used after halothane reactions.

CHLORPROMAZINE HEPATOTOXICITY (CHOLESTATIC HYPERSENSITIVITY REACTION) About 1 percent of patients receiving chlorpromazine develop intrahepatic cholestasis with jaundice after 1 to 4 weeks of treatment. In rare instances, jaundice has been reported after a single exposure. Anicteric reactions are probably quite frequent. The onset may be abrupt with fever, rash, arthralgias, lymphadenopathy, nausea, vomiting, and epigastric or right upper quadrant pain. Pruritus may precede the appearance of jaundice, dark urine, and light stools. Eosinophilia with or without mild leukocytosis may be present, and conjugated hyperbilirubinemia, moderately elevated serum alkaline phosphatase, and mildly elevated serum transaminase levels of 100 to 200 are noted. Liver biopsy reveals bile stasis, bile plugs in dilated bile canaliculi, and a dense portal infiltrate of polymorphonuclear, eosinophilic, and mononuclear leukocytes. Occasionally, scattered foci of hepatic parenchymal necrosis may be evident. Jaundice and pruritus usually subside within a few weeks following cessation of therapy, without sequelae, and fatalities are extremely rare. Cholestyramine may be of value in relieving severe pruritus. In a small number of patients, jaundice is prolonged for several months to years, and a picture of primary biliary cirrhosis may develop.

ORAL CONTRACEPTIVE HEPATOTOXICITY (CHOLESTATIC REACTIONS) The administration of oral contraceptive combinations of estrogenic and progestational steroids results in significant BSP retention in a high proportion of patients, and, to a far lesser extent, elevation of serum alkaline phosphatase. Weeks to months after taking these agents, intrahepatic cholestasis manifest by pruritus, jaundice and dark urine, is noted in a small number of patients. Patients who have had recurrent idiopathic jaundice of pregnancy or severe pruritus of pregnancy seem to be especially susceptible. Laboratory studies, with the exception of liver function tests, are negative, and extrahepatic manifestations of hypersensitivity are absent. On liver biopsy, cholestasis is present with bile plugs in dilated canaliculi, and striking bile staining of liver cells. In contrast to chlorpromazine-induced cholestasis, portal inflammation is absent. The lesion is reversible on withdrawal of the agent, and sequelae have not been reported. The two steroid components appear to act synergistically on hepatic function, although the estrogen may be primarily responsible. The use of oral contraceptives in patients with a history of recurrent jaundice of pregnancy is contraindicated.

REFERENCES

Acute viral hepatitis

BARKER LF et al: Antibody responses in viral hepatitis, type B. JAMA 223:1005, 1973

BEEBE GW, SIMON AH: Cirrhosis of the liver following viral hepatitis: A twenty-year mortality follow-up. Am J Epidemiol 92:279, 1970

BOYER JL, KLATSKIN G: Pattern of necrosis in acute viral hepatitis: Prognostic value of bridging (subacute hepatic necrosis). N Engl J Med 283:1063, 1970

GINSBERG AL et al: Prevention of endemic HAA-positive hepatitis with gamma globulin: Use of a simple radio-immune assay to detect HAA. N Engl J Med 286:562, 1972

LE BOUVIER GL: Subspecificities of the Australia antigen complex. Am J Dis Child 123:420, 1972

NIELSEN JO et al: Differential distribution of Australia-antigen-associated particles in patients with liver diseases and normal carriers. N Engl J Med 288:484, 1973

PRINCE AM et al: Immunologic distinction between infectious and serum hepatitis. N Engl J Med 282:987, 1970

RITT DJ et al: Acute hepatic necrosis, an analysis of thirty-one patients. Medicine (Baltimore) 48:151, 1969

SHERLOCK S: Long-incubation (virus B, HAA-associated) hepatitis. Gut 13:297, 1972

ZUCKERMAN AJ: Laboratory investigation into the aetiology of human viral hepatitis. Br Med Bull 28:134, 1972

Toxic and drug-induced liver disease

ISHAK KG, IREY NS: Hepatic injury associated with the phenothiazines: Clinicopathologic and follow-up study of 36 patients. Arch Path 93:283, 1972

KLATSKIN G: Toxic and drug-induced hepatitis, in *Diseases of the Liver*, 3d ed., ed L Schiff, Philadelphia: Lippincott, 1969, pp. 498-601

ZIMMERMAN, HJ: Clinical and laboratory manifestations of hepatotoxicity. Ann NY Acad Sci 104:954, 1963

295 CHRONIC ACTIVE HEPATITIS

RAYMOND S. KOFF
KURT J. ISSELBACHER

DEFINITION Chronic active hepatitis (active chronic hepatitis) is a progressive, destructive liver disease characterized by a prolonged course with continuing or episodic hepatic necrosis, inflammation, and fibrosis leading to cirrhosis. In many patients extrahepatic manifestations and sero-immunologic abnormalities are found and as a result a variety of terms have been used to describe this disorder. Thus *autoimmune hepatitis, lupoid hepatitis, acute juvenile cirrhosis, plasma cell hepatitis, subacute hepatitis,* and *chronic liver disease in young women* have been used in the past and are synonymous with chronic active hepatitis. Although these terms suggest a spectrum of disorders, the pathologic process appears to be relatively homogeneous. *Chronic active hepatitis* would seem the most appropriate designation for this clinicopathologic entity, regardless of the etiology and the clinical variations.

ETIOLOGY The cause of most cases of chronic active hepatitis is unknown, but probably more than one factor can initiate this disorder. In about one-third of patients the disease begins abruptly following an illness typical of acute viral hepatitis, most often hepatitis B. Persistence of the hepatitis B antigen (HBAg) (see Chap. 294) in the serum has been found in 10 to 25 percent of patients with chronic active hepatitis. These HBAg-positive patients usually do not have antinuclear antibodies and the lupus erythematosus (LE) factor in the blood. Other patients with chronic active hepatitis are HBAg-negative but may have antinuclear antibodies and the LE factor in their serum. A third group appears to be neither HBAg-positive or have antinuclear antibodies or the LE factor. These data suggest that in some but not all patients *persistent hepatitis B virus infection may be related to the development of chronic active hepatitis.* The transition of viral hepatitis induced subacute hepatic necrosis (see Chap. 294) to chronic active hepatitis has been observed in a few instances. It is possible that the chronicity or activity of the hepatitis may be related to cell-mediated or humoral immunologic reactions to viral antigens or to virus-altered host tissues. The relative importance of host and viral factors (e.g., viral subtypes) in the persistence of viral infection and in initiating the immune responses is not well understood.

Drugs may also be involved in the pathogenesis of this disorder. Thus, for example, clinical, biochemical, and histologic features of chronic active hepatitis have been found in some patients in association with the ingestion of laxative preparations containing oxyphenisatin. In these patients challenge with oxyphenisatin led to increased activity of the disease; discontinuance of the drug resulted in clinical and biochemical improvement. Although none of these patients had circulating HBAg, several had positive LE cell tests, plus antinuclear or smooth-muscle antibodies. These observations suggest that chemical agents may also play a role in the production of chronic active hepatitis. However, since only a small number of patients ingesting oxyphenisatin develop liver disease, immune mechanisms may still be involved in the production of chronic active hepatitis in those patients.

The role and importance of deranged immune mechanisms or autoimmunity in the pathogenesis of chronic active hepatitis is a matter of considerable debate. *Abnormal immunologic reactions* are found in a significant number of patients; these reactions include false-positive serologic reactions for syphilis, positive latex agglutination tests, the LE cell phenomenon, the presence of antinuclear, smooth muscle and antimitochondrial antibodies, and antibodies to gastric mucosal, thyroid and other epithelial cells. Additional circumstantial evidence for autoimmunity includes the presence of hypergammaglobulinemia (IgG is often strikingly elevated), the occurrence of polyarthritis, pleurisy, nephritis, etc., and the occasional coexistence of other diseases suspected of having an autoimmune basis (e.g., ulcerative colitis, Hashimoto's thyroiditis). It must be emphasized that the tissue-antibody and organelle-antibody reactions observed in chronic active hepatitis are neither species nor organ specific; chronic active hepatitis has in fact occurred in patients with congenital agammaglobulinemia, in whom circulating antibodies are absent. Thus, no direct pathogenetic significance can as yet be attributed to these immunologic phenomena, and the role of autoimmune mechanisms in the development of chronic active hepatitis is inconclusive. It has also been suggested that cell-mediated immune responses, directed against liver cell antigens altered by viruses, drugs, or other agents, may play a central role in the pathogenesis of chronic active hepatitis. However, this latter concept also remains unproved.

PATHOLOGY The characteristic histopathologic features in the liver include: (1) a dense mononuclear and plasma cell infiltration of the portal zones with extension of this inflammatory process into the adjacent parenchyma, (2) necrosis or degeneration of the hepatocytes at the periphery of the liver lobule ("piecemeal necrosis"), and (3) connective-tissue septa (fibrosis) extending from the portal zones into the lobule, isolating parenchymal cells into clusters and enveloping bile ductules. This process may be patchy and individual liver lobules may remain uninvolved. Degeneration of single liver cells and Councilman-like bodies may be seen in the periportal parenchyma. In some patients the "bridging" lesion of subacute hepatic necrosis has also been present.

The above combination of morphologic alterations has been termed "chronic aggressive hepatitis." However, on liver biopsy cirrhosis can be demonstrated in 30 to 50 percent of patients with chronic active hepatitis even early in the course of the disease. Serial biopsies suggest that progression of fibrosis to cirrhosis is common, and at autopsy, postnecrotic cirrhosis is usually found. Although the inflammation and necrosis may subside during remissions or inactive phases of the disease, remnants of periportal hepatocellular necrosis and inflammation may still be identified in many of these cirrhotic livers.

In a few patients with chronic active hepatitis some of the histologic features of primary biliary cirrhosis have been observed.

CLINICAL FEATURES Characteristically, chronic active hepatitis is a disease of adolescent and young women, although all age groups may be affected and men comprise about 25 per cent of the cases. In approximately two-thirds of patients the disease has an *insidious onset* over a period of weeks to months. In the remainder an abrupt onset similar to acute viral hepatitis is seen, but features of chronic active hepatitis develop during the ensuing 6 months. *Fatigue* is the predominant symptom. Persistent or recurrent *jaundice* is noted in about 80 percent of cases. In some patients liver disease may be unsuspected since presenting symptoms may consist of fever, abdominal pain, joint complaints, pleurisy, acne, amenorrhea, or chronic diarrhea. Intermittent deepening of jaundice and recurrent symptoms of malaise, anorexia and fever, suggestive of a superimposed acute hepatitis, are common throughout the course of the illness.

Physical findings include hepatomegaly (80 percent), splenomegaly (50 percent), and spider angiomas. Ascites, abdominal venous collaterals, and other signs of underlying cirrhosis may be present on initial examination or may develop as the disease progresses. Extrahepatic manifestations are often found. Recurrent polyarthralgia and acute migratory polyarthritis of the large joints or fingers may dominate the clinical picture. Pleurisy and pericarditis are observed in less than 10 percent of patients. Skin lesions are more common and include acne vulgaris of the face, transient maculopapular eruptions, erythema nodosum, urticaria, purpura, striae, and ulcerating nodules. The sicca syndrome of keratoconjunctivitis and xerostomia is frequently found. Ulcerative colitis or nonspecific chronic diarrhea may be noted years before or following the diagnosis of chronic active hepatitis. In a few patients renal disease is manifest by the nephrotic syndrome or recurrent hematuria. Kidney biopsies in such instances have revealed membranous or proliferative glomerulonephritis. Renal failure is unusual. In a small number of patients renal tubular acidosis, polyneuropathy, seizures, myocarditis, thyroiditis, generalized lymphadenopathy, and fibrosing alveolitis have been observed.

The *course* of chronic active hepatitis is variable and the disease may persist for long periods without overt clinical manifestations of liver disease. In as many as a third of patients the disease may remit clinically into an inactive phase, although cirrhosis is present in the majority of such patients. Rarely, the histologic lesion may reverse itself completely before the establishment of cirrhosis. During the first few years of the illness the case fatality rate is high (25 to 50 percent) when death occurs as a result of liver failure with jaundice and hepatic coma. Later in the course of the disease, death is often due to the complications of cirrhosis—variceal hemorrhage or intercurrent infection. Primary hepatic cancer (hepatoma) is an uncommon complication. In a small number of patients clinical and histologic features of primary biliary cirrhosis may be noted during the course of typical chronic active hepatitis.

LABORATORY FINDINGS Normochromic anemia, leukopenia, and thrombocytopenia are often found, especially when hypersplenism is present. Infrequently a Coombs-positive hemolytic anemia or thrombocytopenic purpura occur. Liver function tests are invariably abnormal but may not correlate with the clinical severity or histopathologic findings in the individual case. The serum bilirubin is usually moderately elevated (3 to 10 mg per 100 ml) but rarely exceeds 20 mg per 100 ml. Serum glutamic oxaloacetic transaminase levels are elevated and fluctuate in the range of 100 to 1,000 units in most cases, although values as high as 4,000 units have been reported.

Hypergammaglobulinemia (>2.0 g per 100 ml) is common, particularly in patients with abundant plasma cell infiltration of the liver. Mild hypoalbuminemia occurs in patients with active disease or in those with advanced cirrhosis. Serum alkaline phosphatase levels are either moderately elevated (twofold) or near normal. The prothrombin time is often prolonged, but is usually within the range that permits liver biopsy. BSP retention is noted even during inactive phases of the disease.

The LE cell phenomenon is found in 10 to 35 percent of patients, and antinuclear antibodies are common (20 to 60 percent). Smooth-muscle antibodies are demonstrable in a high percentage of cases, and like the LE cell and antinuclear factors, may be more common in those patients with chronic active hepatitis who are HBAg-negative. Antimitochondrial antibodies, detected by immunofluorescence, are found in 10 to 20 percent of patients, usually those without HBAg. Abnormal serologic reactivity may be persistent or transient, and limited studies indicate that serum complement activity is either normal or mildly depressed.

DIFFERENTIAL DIAGNOSIS Early in the course of chronic active hepatitis the disease may resemble typical *acute viral hepatitis.* The fluctuating and progressive character of the illness over the ensuing months indicate, however, that a chronic disorder is present. The major entity which may be confused with chronic active hepatitis is *chronic persistent hepatitis* (delayed convalescence) (Chap. 294). As indicated in Table 295-1, the onset of illness resembling acute viral hepatitis is more common in chronic persistent hepatitis, while recurrent episodes of acute illness and progression to cirrhosis are more frequent in chronic active hepatitis. The presence of extrahepatic manifestations, hypergammaglobulinemia, and signs of cirrhosis point to chronic active rather than chronic persistent hepatitis; definitive differentiation cannot be made without liver biopsy.

The presence of "rheumatic" features in the early phase of chronic active hepatitis may cause confusion with connective tissue diseases such as rheumatoid arthritis and systemic lupus erythematosus. The existence of progressive liver disease clearly distinguishes chronic active hepatitis from these disorders. In young patients Wilson's disease may be excluded. Late in the course of chronic active hepatitis some patients may present with postnecrotic cirrhosis without evidence of active hepatitis. This lesion, termed cryptogenic cirrhosis, may represent an end stage of other destructive liver diseases (e.g., primary biliary cirrhosis) as well as chronic active hepatitis (see Chap. 296 for differential diagnosis of postnecrotic cirrhosis).

TABLE 295-1
Distinguishing features of chronic active and chronic persistent hepatitis

Features	*Chronic active hepatitis*	*Chronic persistent hepatitis*
Clinical:		
Onset like acute viral hepatitis	30%	70%
Recurrent acute episodes	Common	Infrequent
Extrahepatic involvement (e.g., arthralgias, pleuritis, colitis)	Common	Rare
Prognosis	Poor	Good
Liver histology:		
Piecemeal necrosis	Characteristic	Inconstant
Site of inflammation	Portal extending into lobule	Portal
Lobular architecture	Distorted	Preserved
Fibrosis	Common	Slight
Progression to cirrhosis	Common	Rare

MANAGEMENT Ideal treatment of chronic active hepatitis should produce prompt remission of the clinical and biochemical features of active disease, decrease the high early mortality, and reverse or halt the progression to postnecrotic cirrhosis. Unfortunately a regimen capable of achieving all these goals is not yet available.

During episodes of active disease the patient should be managed as in acute viral hepatitis with general supportive care. Hospitalization may be required to define the severity and extent of disease and the presence of extrahepatic involvement, and to confirm the diagnosis by percutaneous liver biopsy. Bed rest is indicated during active phases, but prolonged bed rest following remission is probably unnecessary. With no specific drug therapy as many as 25 percent of patients will remit and lose the clinical features of chronic active hepatitis. However, *corticosteroid therapy* (prednisone 15 to 20 mg per day) has been shown to be effective in prolonging survival during the first few years of illness when the mortality rate is high. Relief of fatigue and anorexia is noted within days to several weeks, and over a period of months the serum bilirubin and globulin levels fall, while serum albumin levels rise. Decreases in serum transaminase levels alone do not appear to be a useful marker of recovery or an adequate guide to the dose of corticosteroids to be employed. Reduction of suppressive doses of corticosteroids should be performed cautiously, since even small decrements in therapy may be associated with clinical worsening, and increasing dosage may be needed for control of spontaneous exacerbations. Unless complications of corticosteroid therapy require discontinuation of this agent, treatment should be continued for several months, or perhaps longer, after clinical and biochemical improvement. Whether corticosteroid therapy will prevent or interrupt the development of cirrhosis is uncertain.

Other immunosuppressive agents have also been tried. Azathioprine in a dose of 100 mg daily has been used but by itself is generally less effective than steroids in increasing survival. In some patients the combination of azathioprine and corticosteroids may be as effective as, or in some instances more effective than, steroids alone.

REFERENCES

BULKLEY BH et al: Distinction in chronic active hepatitis based on circulating hepatitis-associated antigen. Lancet 2:1323, 1970

COOK GC et al: Controlled prospective trial of corticosteroid therapy in active chronic hepatitis. Q J Med 40:159, 1971

DONIACH D et al: "Autoallergic" hepatitis. N Engl J Med 282:86, 1970

DUDLEY FJ et al: Natural history of hepatitis associated antigen positive chronic liver disease. Lancet 2:1388, 1972

GOLDSTEIN G B et al: Drug-induced active chronic hepatitis. Am J Dig Dis 18:177, 1973

MISTILIS SP, BLACKBURN CRB: Active chronic hepatitis. Am J Med 48:484, 1970

MURRAY-LYON IM et al: Controlled trial of prednisone and azathioprine in active chronic hepatitis. Lancet 1:735, 1973

NIELSEN JO et al: Incidence and meaning of persistence of Australia antigen in patients with acute viral hepatitis: Development of chronic hepatitis. N Engl J Med 285:1157, 1971

SOLOWAY RD et al: Clinical, biochemical and histological remission of severe chronic active liver disease: a controlled study of treatments and early prognosis. Gastroenterology 63:820, 1972

296 CIRRHOSIS

WILLIAM A. TISDALE
J. THOMAS LAMONT
KURT J. ISSELBACHER

DEFINITION Morphologic Cirrhosis is a generic term that includes all forms of chronic diffuse liver disease characterized by significant loss of liver cells, collapse and fibrosis of the supporting reticulin network with distortion of the vascular bed, and nodular regeneration of the remaining liver cell masses. The basic causative element of this complex lesion is diffuse liver cell death; the network of scars, the regenerating cell masses, and the changes in hepatic circulation develop secondarily. Less constant pathologic features of most types of cirrhosis include intralobular or portal inflammation, focal or widespread bile stasis, and proliferation of ductular cells.

Clinical and functional The morphologic elements of cirrhosis often have dramatic clinical counterparts. Progressive loss of liver cells may produce jaundice, ascites and edema, central nervous system dysfunction, cachexia, and death—the syndrome of hepatic insufficiency. The advancing fibrosis leads to distortion of the intrahepatic vasculature, which in turn contributes to the development of portal venous hypertension with resultant esophageal and gastric varices and splenomegaly. Nodular regeneration often leads to distortion of liver shape and compression of intrahepatic venous and lymphatic radicles, which may result in ascites and portal hypertension. No clinical, etiologic, or morphologic classification of cirrhosis is satisfactory at present. Clinical signs and symptoms may not reflect accurately the extent and precise nature of the cirrhotic process; the etiology of types of cirrhosis remains uncertain or unknown; pathologic patterns may represent nonspecific hepatic responses to many different forms of liver cell injury. However, in spite of these limitations, it is possible to categorize most cases of cirrhosis clinically, adding qualifying morphologic or etiologic terms when possible. Most types of cirrhosis can be classified as follows: (1) Laennec's, (2) postnecrotic, (3) biliary (either primary or secondary), (4) hemochromatosis, (5) cardiac or congestive, or (6) rare and nonspecific cirrhosis.

LAENNEC'S CIRRHOSIS

DEFINITION This form of cirrhosis, the most common variety encountered in North America and many parts of Western Europe, is characterized by diffuse fine scarring, a fairly uniform loss of liver cells associated with fatty infiltration or active necrosis, and small (often less than lobule-sized) islands of preserved or regenerating parenchyma. The terms *alcoholic*, *portal*, and *fatty cirrhosis* have also been used to describe this type of chronic liver disease. However, each of these terms has misleading implications: alcoholism is usually but not always a factor in the pathogenesis of Laennec's cirrhosis; the fibrosis and scarring may not be centered about the portal triads; and cirrhosis may develop in the absence of significant fatty infiltration of liver cells.

ETIOLOGY Many epidemiologic studies have implicated *chronic alcoholism* as a major cause of Laennec's cirrhosis: between 10 and 20 percent of chronic alcoholic patients in the United States have clinical or morphologic evidence of cirrhosis. About 75 percent of patients with Laennec's cirrhosis admit to heavy drinking; the Prohibition era led to a temporary but distinct decline in deaths due to cirrhosis. Experimental studies of both normal and alcoholic subjects have shown that ethanol (in moderate to large doses) produces liver dysfunction and fatty infiltration (Chap. 291) despite the ingestion of a well-balanced diet. However, some individuals develop an inflammatory reaction with polymorphonuclear infiltration and liver cell necrosis in addition to fatty changes. This lesion of *alcoholic hepatitis* may be the forerunner of Laennec's cirrhosis, since during healing there is fibrosis which distorts the normal lobular architecture.

Most chronic alcoholics consume protein- and vitamin-poor diets, many develop other clinical syndromes clearly related to faulty nutrition (exemplified by folate deficiency or Wernicke's syndrome), and treatment of cirrhotic patients with protein-rich diets often produces clinical and morphologic improvement. For these and other reasons, absolute or relative *malnutrition* is regarded as a contributing factor to the evolution of cirrhosis. Although malnutrition per se does not lead to Laennec's cirrhosis, a reasonable concept, based on much circumstantial evidence, is that a combination of *chronic alcohol ingestion plus impaired nutrition* leads to liver cell damage and Laennec's cirrhosis.

Intercurrent bacterial *infections* are common in cirrhotic patients and seem, on occasion, to accelerate the course of the disease. There are, however, no firm data to implicate overt or latent infection in the pathogenesis of Laennec's cirrhosis. Icteric or anicteric subacute hepatitis, presumably of viral origin, may lead to the development of a finely nodular cirrhosis resembling Laennec's cirrhosis in its general morphology, perhaps explaining the frequent reports of portal cirrhosis in nonalcoholic patients in England. Serial biopsies in these cases do not show many of the characteristic histologic features of progressive alcoholic cirrhosis (see below), and such cases may represent variants of postnecrotic cirrhosis.

No *metabolic defect* has been identified in cirrhotic patients or their families that would suggest a unique "susceptibility" to ethanol or its toxic effects. It is clear, nonetheless, that individual tolerance to ethanol and its capacity to induce cirrhosis vary widely and that a true biological predisposition to ethanol-induced liver diseases may exist.

PATHOLOGY AND PATHOGENESIS In the early stages of Laennec's cirrhosis the liver is enlarged, yellow, greasy, and firm. The parenchymal cells are usually diffusely abnormal, and many are distended by cytoplasmic fat vacuoles, which disappear with therapy and recur promptly after resumption of alcohol ingestion. A characteristic cytologic feature of active Laennec's cirrhosis is the *Mallory body* or *alcoholic hyalin*. These beadlike clumps of perinuclear eosinophilic material are found in damaged cells and consist of swollen and fragmented cell organelles. An abundance of Mallory bodies usually indicates significant hepatic damage in association with alcohol ingestion. Except for childhood cirrhosis of India, the Mallory body is not often found in other nonalcoholic varieties of finely nodular cirrhosis. As the liver disease advances and hepatocytes are destroyed, weblike *septums of connective tissue appear in periportal zones* and in other areas of active cell degeneration. These fibrous septums become denser and more confluent, connecting portal triads and central veins. The fine connective tissue network contains small vessels, lymphatics, and other remnants of portal triads and surrounds small masses of liver cells. These lobular remnants undergo regeneration and form nodules. Inflammation is usually mononuclear, inconspicuous, and concentrated within portal triads and areas of active liver cell damage. Bile stasis is usually minimal and transient, but may be a prominent morphologic feature during acute exacerbations of the disease. As the fatty infiltration subsides and the liver cell mass diminishes, the liver shrinks in size, acquires a finely nodular (hobnail) appearance, and becomes hard.

Laennec's cirrhosis is basically a progressive disease, but appropriate therapy and strict avoidance of alcohol may arrest the disease at most stages and permit repair and functional improvement. Continued loss of liver cells by focal necrosis, however, results in progressive stromal collapse, fibrosis, and vascular distortion. Although regeneration occurs within the small remnants of parenchyma, cell loss eventually exceeds replacement, the liver cell mass dwindles, and a phase of irreversible, or end-stage, cirrhosis is reached.

CLINICAL FEATURES Signs and symptoms Men are affected more frequently than women, but this sex difference has decreased steadily in recent years as drinking habits have changed in many Western countries. Although the average age of onset of symptoms is about fifty years, Laennec's cirrhosis may be found in alcoholic patients in the third or fourth decade of life.

Advanced Laennec's cirrhosis may be clinically silent, and about 10 percent of cases are discovered incidentally at laparotomy or autopsy. Typically, however, after 5 to 15 years of alcoholic excess, evidence of progressive liver dysfunction, fluid retention, and portal hypertension appears. Over a period of weeks or months, the patient notes gradually increasing weakness and fatigability, anorexia, slight weight loss, jaundice, intermittent ankle edema, and increasing abdominal girth due to ascites. A firm and enlarged liver may be the only sign of disease, but additional typical findings include muscle wasting, jaundice, arterial "spider" angiomas, gynecomastia and testicular atrophy (in the male), palmar erythema, splenomegaly, and ascites. Loss of body hair, parotid gland enlargement, purpura, clubbing of the fingers, Dupuytren's contractures, and diffuse hyperpigmentation of the skin are common but less important clinical signs. Low-grade fever without shaking chills is frequent in patients with active disease.

Jaundice and other signs of hepatic dysfunction may subside with therapy, but continued alcoholic excess and poor dietary habits lead to further episodes of hepatic decompensation. Acute acceleration of alcoholic liver damage may follow protracted drinking bouts. Fever, nausea and vomiting, deepening jaundice, hepatic precoma, and ascites may occur rapidly in association with widespread liver cell loss and inflammation. Although some patients die during the acute exacerbations, most recover after several weeks. A few patients experience one or more transient episodes of cholestatic jaundice during the course of alcoholic liver disease. Clinical and laboratory studies may suggest the diagnosis of mechanical biliary obstruction, but liver biopsy and the response to conservative therapy usually support the diagnosis of intrahepatic cholestasis. Over a period of 3 to 5 years, the cirrhotic patient becomes emaciated, weak, and chronically jaundiced, and ascites and signs of portal hypertension become increasingly prominent. Most patients with advanced cirrhosis die in hepatic coma, often precipitated by hemorrhage from esophageal varices or intercurrent infection. Acute and chronic pancreatitis and peptic ulceration occur with greater frequency in cirrhotic patients than in normal subjects. Gram-negative bacteremia, acute bacterial peritonitis, and hepatoma are uncommon complications.

Laboratory findings Anemia is common. The etiology is almost always complex, and acute and chronic gastrointestinal blood loss, folic acid deficiency, hypersplenism, and a direct toxic effect of alcohol on the bone marrow are contributing causes. Hemolytic anemia accompanied by hypercholesterolemia and unusual spurlike projections of the erythrocyte membrane (acanthocytosis) have been described in some alcoholics with cirrhosis. Leukopenia and thrombocytopenia may result from hypersplenism, a direct effect of alcohol on the bone marrow, or folate deficiency, Liver function tests reveal hyperbilirubinemia, BSP retention, and variable elevations of serum alkaline phosphatase and transaminase. The serum albumin is usually depressed, while globulins are increased. Quantitative immunoglobulin determination reveals elevations of all classes, especially IgG. In severe cirrhosis clotting factor deficiencies are common, as manifested by prolongation of the prothrombin and partial thromboplastin times. Elevated serum ammonia levels reflect a combination of impaired liver function and shunting of portal blood around the liver into the systemic circulation.

A diabetic type of glucose tolerance may occur in cirrhosis and is a reflection of endogenous insulin resistance; however, clinical diabetes is uncommon. Low or low normal levels of blood urea nitrogen are seen in some patients with severe cirrhosis; hence the serum creatinine is a more accurate index of renal function. Hyponatremia and hypokalemia are frequent in patients with ascites and edema.

DIAGNOSIS Laennec's cirrhosis should be strongly suspected in patients with a history of prolonged or excessive alcohol intake, hepatomegaly and other signs of chronic liver disease, plus laboratory evidence of hepatic dysfunction. If there are no contraindications, most patients should have a needle biopsy of the liver to confirm the diagnosis as well as to determine the stage of the disease process. When the course of an otherwise stable cirrhotic patient changes without obvious explanation, complicating conditions such as occult bleeding, hepatoma, and portal vein thrombosis should be sought.

Alcoholic hepatitis should be considered in an alcoholic with recent heavy drinking who presents with an enlarged, tender liver, jaundice, fever, and ascites. Morphologically this condition is characterized by alcoholic hyalin, polymorphonuclear infiltration, evidence of hepatocellular necrosis, and varying degrees of fatty metamorphosis. This variant of alcoholic liver disease has a high mortality rate, and variceal bleeding, infection, and hepatic encephalopathy are common. Although corticosteroids may cause a decrease in serum transaminase and bilirubin levels, their role in altering the prognosis of alcoholic hepatitis is debatable.

PROGNOSIS Both retrospective and prospective studies of the natural history of Laennec's cirrhosis show that early, vigorous, and meticulous medical care will prolong life, decrease morbidity, and delay or prevent the appearance of certain complications. Patients who abstain from alcohol and consume nutritious diets have a 5-year survival rate of about 60 percent, whereas those who continue to drink have a 40 percent 5-year survival rate. This generalization must be qualified by the fact that mortality rates are higher for those who develop one of the major complications of cirrhosis, and the 5-year survival after onset of either ascites or jaundice is reduced to about 50 percent. Massive variceal hemorrhage is a major direct or contributing cause of death in many patients. Although surgical shunts are effective in reducing portal hypertension, the overall prognosis often remains poor in patients with advanced, irreversible liver disease.

TREATMENT Laennec's cirrhosis is a serious chronic illness that usually requires prolonged medical supervision and management. In most instances it is desirable to hospitalize the patient for initial study and assessment of his response to therapy as well as for dietary and medical instruction.

In the absence of signs of impending hepatic coma, a *diet* containing at least 1 g protein per kg body weight and 2000 to 3000 kcal per day should be prescribed. Because the patient with active cirrhosis is often anorectic or nauseated, these dietary aims may be achieved by offering the patient three or four small meals with supplemental feedings of eggnog or ice cream. Vitamin supplements, in the form of multivitamin capsules, may be given, but there is no rationale for the clinical use of lipotropic agents. The patient should understand clearly that neither nutritious diet nor added vitamins will protect his liver against the effects of further alcohol. *Alcohol should be absolutely forbidden.*

Minimal ascites and edema may disappear with bed rest alone, but more persistent fluid retention should be treated with a combination of *salt restriction*, utilizing diets that contain 200 to 500 mg of sodium, and *water restriction*, limiting fluid intake to volumes that equal the measured fluid loss of the prior day. Diuretics should be used with great caution in order to prevent electrolyte depletion, hypovolemia, and hepatic encephalopathy (see Ascites, later in this chapter).

Confusion, drowsiness, or other signs of impending *hepatic coma* should be treated by prompt decrease in protein intake to levels of 20 to 30 g daily or less. A careful search for gastrointestinal hemorrhage should be made, including the aspiration of gastric contents, and appropriate therapy to control bleeding should be instituted. Possible offending drugs, especially diuretics and sedatives, should be omitted and any electrolyte imbalance corrected promptly (see Hepatic Coma, later in this chapter).

Anemia should be characterized and corrected by appropriate means. *Fever*, especially when low-grade and unaccompanied by chills or other signs of infection, may be a manifestation of active cirrhosis. However, the presence of hectic or persistent fever or shaking chills requires a vigorous search for septic processes, especially urinary tract infection, pneumonia, and gram-negative bacteremia.

Progressive *renal failure* ("hepatorenal syndrome") is a serious complication of cirrhosis characterized by advancing azotemia, oliguria, and intractable ascites. This may follow a bout of severe gastrointestinal bleeding, sepsis, or too rapid attempts at diuresis or paracentesis. The urine output falls to 200 to 400 ml per day, with gradual elevation of the serum creatinine and marked sodium retention. Death may occur with uremia, gastrointestinal bleeding, or hepatic coma. The cause of this complication is unknown, but it appears to involve a decrease in renal perfusion. Other factors include marked hyperaldosteronism, decreased effective circulating plasma volume, and increased intraabdominal pressure from tense ascites. The kidneys are structurally intact; urinalysis, pyelography, and renal biopsy are usually normal. Treatment is usually unsuccessful, although some patients with hypotension and decreased plasma volume may respond to infusions of salt-poor albumin with increasing urine output and gradual loss of ascites. Salt and water restriction and diuretic therapy are also usually employed, but recovery seems to be most closely correlated with improvement in liver function. In a few cases, recovery has followed a portacaval shunt; however, most patients are not candidates for surgery because of severe liver disease.

POSTNECROTIC CIRRHOSIS

DEFINITION This form of chronic liver disease, the most common type of cirrhosis on a worldwide basis, is characterized morphologically by (1) confluent, often massive loss of liver cells, (2) stromal collapse and fibrosis that produce broad bands of connective tissue containing the remains of many triads, and (3) irregular, often large nodules of intact or regenerating parenchyma. This pattern, which may vary considerably in extent and severity, results from an overall but unequal injury to the liver. As with other forms of cirrhosis, the appearance of advanced postnecrotic disease offers little insight into the original or potentiating causes of the liver cell damage.

The terms *toxic cirrhosis*, *coarsely nodular cirrhosis*, *posthepatic cirrhosis*, *cryptogenic cirrhosis*, *multilobular cirrhosis*, and *healed yellow atrophy* are synonymous with postnecrotic cirrhosis.

ETIOLOGY The cause of postnecrotic cirrhosis is still unknown, but epidemiological and serological evidence suggests that *viral hepatitis* is an antecedent factor in many instances. In this country about 25 percent of patients with postnecrotic cirrhosis have a history compatible with recent or remote attacks of acute viral hepatitis. A few patients with persistent hepatitis and with positive blood tests for the antigen for long-incubation (virus B) hepatitis develop postnecrotic cirrhosis; and 5 to 20 percent of patients with established postnecrotic disease have positive serological tests for hepatitis B antigen (HBAg).

A small percentage of cases stems from documented *intoxications* with industrial chemicals (e.g., phosphorus), poisons (e.g., *Amanita phalloides* toxins), or drugs (chloroform, iproniazid). Finally, certain *infections* (e.g., brucellosis), *parasitic infestations* (clonorchiasis), *metabolic disorders* (hepatolenticular degeneration), and *advanced alcoholic liver disease* may produce confluent cell loss and result in postnecrotic cirrhosis.

PATHOLOGY AND PATHOGENESIS Typically, the postnecrotic liver is small, grossly distorted in shape, and composed of nodules of liver cells separated by dense, wide, sunken scars. Microscopically, the established lesion includes (1) large islands of parenchymal cells with rounded (inactive) or ragged (active) margins; (2) interdigitating broad to thin fibrous septums containing distorted vessels, lymphatics, and bile ducts derived from many portal areas; and (3) prominent mononuclear inflammatory infiltrates, often in the form of follicles or clusters.

Current evidence suggests that infectious, toxic, metabolic, or nutritional factors initiate the postnecrotic process. The destruction appears to progress as the result of similar repeated or persistent insults or possibly on the basis of "autoimmune" liver cell injury.

CLINICAL FEATURES Postnecrotic cirrhosis should be suspected in nonalcoholic patients with evidence of chronic liver disease, especially in those in the younger age group.

Signs and symptoms Like those with Laennec's cirrhosis, a few patients with postnecrotic disease may have little clinical evidence of advanced cirrhosis, the diagnosis being made at operation or postmortem examination or by a needle biopsy performed to investigate asymptomatic hepatosplenomegaly. About 25 percent of patients present with signs and symptoms suggesting active hepatitis, but often with atypical features such as prolonged illness, intense and protracted jaundice, ascites, or manifestations of portal hypertension. Still others have bouts of upper abdominal pain, the sudden onset of unexplained ascites, episodes of hepatic precoma, or massive variceal hemorrhage as the major or initial clinical feature. The signs and symptoms of postnecrotic cirrhosis resemble those of Laennec's cirrhosis and reflect the loss of liver cell reserve, advancing portal hypertension, and disorders of salt and water metabolism. In general, however, patients with postnecrotic cirrhosis show less wasting and more persistent jaundice early in their clinical illness than do patients with Laennec's cirrhosis. A few patients experience migratory polyarthritis or protracted itching. About 15 percent of cases develop hepatoma.

Laboratory findings The results of hematologic and liver function tests resemble those of Laennec's cirrhosis, but protracted and pronounced hyperbilirubinemia, persistent moderate elevations of serum transaminases, and hypergammaglobulinemia (3 to 4 g per 100 ml serum) are often present.

DIAGNOSIS AND PROGNOSIS Postnecrotic cirrhosis should be suspected in young persons and nonalcoholic adults with signs and symptoms of cirrhosis. Most laboratory and radiologic studies are nondiagnostic, and needle or operative liver biopsies are the definitive diagnostic procedures. About 75 percent of cases tend to progress despite supportive therapy and terminate in death after 1 to 5 years from exsanguinating variceal hemorrhage, hepatic coma, or superimposed hepatoma.

TREATMENT Because the primary cause of this disease is rarely detectable or treatable, long-term care must include appropriate rest, control of ascites (see later), avoidance of drugs or excessive protein intake that may induce hepatic coma (see later), prompt treatment of infections, and surgical treatment of portal hypertension (see later) if variceal hemorrhage occurs.

BILIARY CIRRHOSIS

DEFINITION *Biliary cirrhosis* refers to a disorder in patients with clinical and chemical signs of chronic impairment of bile excretion and morphologic evidence of progressive liver destruction centered about the intrahepatic bile ducts. Major clinical concomitants of impaired bile excretion include protracted itching; progressive and prolonged jaundice; steatorrhea; the development of cutaneous xanthelasmas and xanthomas; hepatomegaly; laboratory findings of marked elevations of serum alkaline phosphatase, cholesterol, and other lipid fractions; and slowly progressive decline of health. Morphologically, most forms of biliary cirrhosis evolve from chronic inflammatory lesions of the periportal liver cells, ductules, and interlobular ducts, and true cirrhosis represents a late and often nonspecific phase.

ETIOLOGY Biliary cirrhosis can be classified either as *primary*, in which case the process is related to chronic intrahepatic cholestasis, or as *secondary* to obstruction of the common bile duct or its large branches.

The etiology of *primary biliary cirrhosis* is still unknown. The nearly exclusive (over 90 percent) occurrence of this disorder in adult, often middle-aged, women strongly suggests an endocrine contribution. The occasional onset of primary biliary cirrhosis following a bout of atypical (so-called "cholangiolitic") hepatitis has led to speculation that viral destruction of liver and duct cells initiates the disease process. Although no drug has produced a picture of *typical* progressive biliary cirrhosis, the occasional appearance of many elements of the syndrome in patients treated with phenothiazines suggests that drug hypersensitivity may be one etiologic factor. Hepatic copper levels have been found to be elevated, but the relationship of this abnormality to the disease process is unknown. The occasional association of this form of cirrhosis with calcinosis, Raynaud's phenomenon, sclerodactylia, and telangiectasia (so-called "CRST syndrome") suggests that in some cases abnormalities of connective tissue may be related to primary biliary cirrhosis.

Primary biliary cirrhosis is associated with a number of specific and nonspecific immunologic features:

1 Elevated serum levels of IgM (gamma-M-globulin) are seen in about 80 percent of patients with primary biliary cirrhosis, but this abnormality is nonspecific and occurs occasionally in patients with mechanical bile duct obstruction.
2 Immunofluorescent studies have demonstrated a circulating antibody that reacts with the cytoplasm of bile ductular cells in 75 percent of patients with primary biliary cirrhosis. However, similar antibody changes occur in many patients with viral hepatitis.
3 Periductal lymphocytes in liver biopsy specimens from patients with primary biliary cirrhosis have been shown to form IgM immunoglobulins, again raising the possibility of a self-perpetuating immune process.
4 Impaired lymphocyte transformation has been documented in some patients, suggesting derangement of delayed immune responses.
5 A circulating antibody (IgG) is present in the serum of patients with primary biliary cirrhosis that reacts with mitochondria-rich cells (mitochondrial antibody). These antibodies have been detected in over 80 percent of patients with primary biliary cirrhosis but only rarely in other forms of liver disease. These observations suggest strongly that disordered immune responses play a major role in the initiation or progression of the chronic hepatic lesion of biliary cirrhosis, but the exact mechanisms involved are unclear.

Most instances of *secondary biliary cirrhosis* result from long-standing partial or total obstruction of the common bile duct or its major branches. In adults, chronic bile duct obstruction by postoperative strictures or by gallstones, usually with superimposed infectious cholangitis, is the most common cause of this type of biliary cirrhosis. Tumors of the pancreas, biliary tree, or gallbladder that produce obstruction of the common bile duct occasionally induce cirrhosis but only rarely permit survival to this stage. A few patients with the peculiar pericholangitis of ulcerative colitis or with idiopathic sclerosing cholangitis develop secondary biliary cirrhosis. Congenital atresia of the intra- or extrahepatic bile duct system, a relatively common anomaly, induces rapidly advancing periportal fibrosis in infants; most cases are inoperable and eventually fatal. In neither acquired nor congenital biliary obstruction is the exact pathogenesis of the cirrhotic process understood. Simple pressure effects, local toxicity of bile constituents, and secondary infection alone do not explain the morphologic events satisfactorily.

PATHOLOGY AND PATHOGENESIS The earliest recognizable lesion of *primary biliary cirrhosis* might be termed "chronic nonsuppurative destructive cholangitis," a diffuse necrotizing and inflammatory process centered about the portal triads. This is characterized by destruction of ductular and portal duct cells, infiltration with acute and chronic inflammatory cells, local fibroblastic reaction, and variable bile stasis. At times, periductal granuloma and lymph follicles may be seen. Progression of this process over a period of months to years (usually 3 to 5 years) leads to loss of liver cells, the formation of pseudolobules, expansion of periportal fibrosis into a network of connective tissue scars, with apparent loss of interlobular ducts and the development of true cirrhosis. End-stage primary biliary cirrhosis may be indistinguishable from postnecrotic cirrhosis in its gross and microscopic appearance.

Unrelieved obstruction of the extrahepatic bile ducts leads to (1) centrilobular bile stasis, cell degeneration, and focal areas of necrosis; (2) proliferation and dilatation of the portal ducts and ductules; (3) sterile or infected cholangitis with accumulation of polymorphonuclear infiltrates around bile ducts; and (4) progressive expansion of portal tracts by edema and fibrosis. Bile may collect in the peripheral areas of necrosis to form "bile lakes." While patients may tolerate biliary obstruction for several years without the appearance of irreversible secondary biliary cirrhosis, eventually a finely nodular cirrhosis develops with isolated bile-stained pseudolobules surrounded by dense connective tissue septums. In both primary and secondary biliary cirrhosis, the liver is initially enlarged and greenish-yellow in appearance, but evolves to a smaller, firmer, more coarsely nodular organ as the disease progresses.

CLINICAL FEATURES Signs and symptoms Although not diagnostic, the early clinical course of *primary* *biliary cirrhosis* is quite characteristic. Typically, the patient is a middle-aged woman who develops persistent generalized itching (the earliest symptom in about 50 percent of cases), dark urine, pale stools and jaundice, with some darkening (melanosis) of the exposed areas of the skin. In contrast to many other forms of cirrhosis, there are few early signs of liver cell failure and hepatic fibrosis, and most of the features reflect impaired bile excretion. Steatorrhea with associated malabsorption of lipid-soluble vitamins often produces purpura, diarrhea, and osteomalacia; the latter may be manifested by backache and bone pain. Protracted elevation of serum lipids, especially cholesterol, leads to the deposit of yellowish plaques or nodules in the subcutaneous tissues in the form of periorbital xanthelasmas and xanthomas over joints, in skin folds, and at sites of trauma. Over a period of months to years, the itching, jaundice, and hyperpigmentation slowly increase. At that time the pruritus and skin lipid deposits may decrease, ascites and edema usually appear, and signs of liver cell failure and portal hypertension supervene. Most patients die within 5 to 10 years from the first signs of the illness. Death usually is due to hepatic insufficiency that is often precipitated by variceal bleeding, intercurrent infection, or surgical procedures.

Physical examination may be entirely normal in the early phase of the disease when pruritus is the sole complaint. In addition, however, there may be jaundice of varying intensity, hyperpigmentation of exposed skin areas, xanthelasmas and xanthomas, moderate to striking hepatomegaly, splenomegaly, and clubbing of the fingers. Fever and chills are rare and usually indicate mechanical biliary obstruction or other associated diseases. Muscle wasting, spider angiomas, palmar erythema, ascites and edema, and the bony tenderness of osteomalacia appear in advanced stages of the disease.

Patients who develop *secondary biliary cirrhosis* usually have a long-standing history and evidence of previous biliary tract disease. Pain varies in type. There may be right upper quadrant pain due to stretching of the liver capsule or due to disease in the gallbladder or bile duct. Signs and symptoms of true cirrhosis appear slowly; ascites and massive upper gastrointestinal hemorrhage usually occur terminally.

Laboratory findings The major chemical abnormalities of evolving biliary cirrhosis result from impaired bile excretion. Late in the course of the illness, evidence of failing liver cell function develops. There is usually conjugated hyperbilirubinemia, and total bilirubin concentrations range from 3 to 20 mg per 100 ml serum or higher. In the final stages, bilirubin levels may exceed 50 mg per 100 ml. Serum alkaline phosphatase levels are usually dramatically elevated, and transaminase levels rarely exceed 150 to 200 units. Nonspecific increases in α_2- and γ-globulin, and IgM are noted. Hyperlipidemia is common in early biliary cirrhosis, with the most striking elevations being in unesterified cholesterol. An abnormal, unique lipoprotein (lipoprotein X) found in the plasma of patients with cholestasis is also present in this disorder. Serum bile salts (especially trihydroxy) are increased, and the elevations correlate reasonably well with the intensity of itching. Hypoprothrombinemia and mild to moderate steatorrhea are common. The mitochondrial antibody test is positive in most cases of primary but usually not in secondary biliary cirrhosis.

DIAGNOSIS Biliary cirrhosis should be considered in any patient with signs, symptoms, and laboratory evidence of protracted obstruction to bile flow. The major diagnostic challenge, regardless of the duration of symptoms, is to exclude remediable causes of mechanical bile duct obstruction before permanent liver damage has occurred. Although patients with transient drug reactions and hepatitis may require only careful observation, those with chronic unexplained obstruction after study by liver biopsy and cholangiography (intravenous or percutaneous) will in most instances require laparotomy with thorough exploration and direct visualization of the biliary system. A positive mitochondrial antibody test suggests the presence of primary biliary cirrhosis. However, since false positive results occur, this test should not be used by itself to make the diagnosis but rather be combined with liver biopsy, cholangiography, or laparotomy.

TREATMENT Complete correction of any mechanical obstruction to bile flow is the most important step in the prevention and therapy of *secondary biliary cirrhosis*. The patient with well-documented *primary biliary cirrhosis*, a chronic and incurable disease, requires prolonged medical therapy with careful attention to the many complications of itching, malabsorption, fluid retention, portal hypertension, and late-stage hepatic insufficiency. A reasonably balanced high-caloric *diet* is usually adequate, but some patients report relief of bothersome diarrhea when fat intake is decreased below 30 to 40 g per day. *Itching* is often extremely distressing to the patient. Topical menthol lotions, sedation, and antihistamine therapy may provide some relief. Systemic corticosteroids and various synthetic androgen compounds may decrease itching without altering the course of the disease. The bile salt–sequestering resin *cholestyramine* usually relieves itching in doses of 8 to 12 g daily. Prompt relief of itching, without obvious effects on other aspects of the disease process, has been reported in a few patients treated with azathioprine. The *fat-soluble vitamins* D, A, and K should be given by parenteral injection at regular intervals to help prevent or correct osteomalacia and hypoprothrombinemia. Salt restriction and judicious use of oral diuretic agents usually prevent disabling ascites and edema (see Ascites, later in this chapter). The occurrence of esophagogastric variceal hemorrhage may require a portacaval shunt.

HEMOCHROMATOSIS
(See Chap. 101)

CARDIAC CIRRHOSIS

DEFINITION Cardiac cirrhosis is a relatively rare form of chronic liver disease associated with severe right-sided congestive heart failure such as may be found with protracted and pronounced tricuspid valve disease and constrictive pericarditis. However, heart failure itself rarely leads to cirrhosis. Thus, cardiac cirrhosis must be carefully distinguished from passive congestion of the liver resulting from acute right-sided heart failure. With acute hepatic congestion there is no hepatic fibrosis, and the changes are reversible if the heart failure can be corrected.

ETIOLOGY Excluding primary diseases of the hepatic venules (veno-occlusive disease) and major hepatic veins (Budd-Chiari syndrome), only cardiovascular disorders that produce prolonged or recurrent hypertension of the cavae and right atrium can be listed as causes of cardiac cirrhosis; these include mitral or tricuspid valvular disease, prolonged constrictive pericarditis, and decompensated cor pulmonale.

PATHOLOGY AND PATHOGENESIS The acutely congested liver is swollen, tense with blood and edema fluid, and dark-colored. Chronic congestion leads to thickening of the capsule and increasing fine trabeculation, occasionally with prominent centrilobular stellate or bandlike scars. Many patients with known chronic hepatic congestion have both a finely and coarsely nodular cirrhosis at autopsy, suggesting that factors other than simple passive congestion have contributed to the process.

CLINICAL FEATURES The demonstration of slight jaundice, a firm and somewhat enlarged liver, and ascites in a patient with valvular heart disease, constrictive pericarditis, or cor pulmonale *of long duration* (usually more than 10 years) should suggest cardiac cirrhosis. In cases of marked tricuspid insufficiency, the liver often is pulsatile, but this feature disappears as cirrhosis develops. Variceal bleeding and coma are uncommon and are usually overshadowed by cachexia, fluid retention, and circulatory derangements. In acute congestion the liver is enlarged and tender, and there may be severe right upper quadrant pain due to stretching of the liver capsule. Splenomegaly may result from simple passive congestion and does not necessarily indicate cirrhosis.

Liver function tests are usually abnormal. Conjugated hyperbilirubinemia, BSP retention, hypoalbuminemia, increased transaminase levels, and mild elevations of serum alkaline phosphatase are the most common abnormalities.

DIAGNOSIS The enlarged and chronically congested liver is readily diagnosed clinically, but the recognition of a definite cardiac cirrhosis is difficult. However, it is rarely necessary to establish the diagnosis of cardiac cirrhosis with certainty, although needle biopsy can be safely used.

TREATMENT Prevention or treatment of cardiac cirrhosis depends on proper diagnosis and therapy of the underlying cardiovascular disorder. If constrictive pericarditis is present and pericardectomy is possible, liver function may improve within 6 to 12 months and fibrous bands will become narrower and avascular.

RARE AND NONSPECIFIC TYPES OF CIRRHOSIS

Clinical, etiologic, and morphologic classifications of cirrhosis do not encompass all cases. The efficiency of detection and study of patients with cirrhosis varies widely throughout the world, but unexpected and unexplained cirrhosis accounts for about 10 percent of cases of this chronic liver disease seen at autopsy. Equally important, many patients with cirrhosis are "classified" improperly during life. A small and unrepresentative biopsy specimen from a patient with a poor history often accounts for the errors in diagnosis.

Cirrhosis may be found in association with the following diseases:

1 *Metabolic disorders*: galactosemia, diabetes mellitus, glycogen storage diseases, hereditary tyrosinemia, alpha-1 antitrypsin deficiency, and the Fanconi syndrome
2 *Infectious diseases*: brucellosis, schistosomiasis, clonorchiasis, neonatal cytomegalovirus, and *Toxoplasma* infections
3 *Infiltrative diseases*: sarcoidosis
4 *Gastrointestinal disorders*: ulcerative colitis and cystic fibrosis of the pancreas
5 *Chemical intoxications*: pyrrolidizine alkaloids (veno-occlusive disease)

NONCIRRHOTIC FIBROSIS OF THE LIVER

Several diseases, either congenital or acquired, may be associated with localized or generalized hepatic fibrosis. The clinical manifestations in such cases may suggest on occasion the diagnosis of true cirrhosis, but the absence of clinical and functional evidence of hepatocellular damage, the lack of nodular regenerative activity, and the localized nature of the scarring usually serve to distinguish these conditions from true cirrhosis.

IDIOPATHIC PORTAL HYPERTENSION (NONCIRRHOTIC PORTAL FIBROSIS, HEPATIC PHLEBOSCLEROSIS, HEPATOPORTAL SCLEROSIS) Not infrequently patients with so-called *portal hypertension* and *splenomegaly* have no clinical or morphologic evidence of cirrhosis. Instead of cirrhosis, careful inspection of the liver often shows some fibrosis in the portal areas and variable thickening of the walls of the portal vein branches in the liver. There appear to be three variants of the process. Some patients have only *intrahepatic phlebosclerosis* and *fibrosis*. Others have in addition segmental thickening or *sclerosis of the portal and splenic veins*, and a third group may show actual *thrombosis* of these vessels. Such cases have been reported from many parts of the world, some of them under the term "Banti's syndrome."

SCHISTOSOMIASIS (see also Chap. 220) The ova of *Schistosoma mansoni* elicit granulomatous and fibrotic reactions along the portal tracts, the result of a delayed hypersensitivity reaction or of a nonspecific foreign-body host response. The characteristic hepatic lesion of schistosomiasis is, therefore, noncirrhotic portal ("pipestem") fibrosis, which produces progressive occlusion of the portal venules with resultant presinusoidal portal hypertension. True cirrhosis may be present in some cases, but nutritional deficiencies and other factors contribute to this process. Clinically, the signs of portal hypertension predominate. The liver and spleen are moderately enlarged. Hepatocellular function is usually normal, but BSP retention and elevation of serum alkaline phosphatase may be noted. Jaundice is uncommon.

CONGENITAL HEPATIC FIBROSIS This disorder is a variant of polycystic disease of the liver, which is congenital and, in some instances, familial. Typically, the patient is young, has no history or signs of hepatocellular disease, and presents with unexplained hepatosplenomegaly or hemorrhage from esophagogastric varices due to portal hypertension. Surgical correction of the portal hypertension may permit long-term survival because progressive liver failure is rare. The biopsy findings are distinctive: normal masses of liver parenchyma are separated by mature fibrous bands containing networks of bile ducts. The cellular damage, inflammation, and nodular regeneration of cirrhosis are notably absent.

MAJOR SEQUELAE OF CIRRHOSIS

Patients with any form of cirrhosis, with its progressive loss of liver cell function and advancing distortion of intrahepatic vasculature, are threatened by three major complications: *portal hypertension* and its associated complications of variceal hemorrhage and splenomegaly, disabling *fluid retention* in the form of ascites and edema, and *hepatic coma.* One-third of deaths in patients with Laennec's cirrhosis are related to variceal hemorrhage; ascites occurs in 60 to 85 percent of cases of advanced cirrhosis; and about 50 percent of patients with cirrhosis die in hepatic coma. Other complications include portal vein thrombosis and hepatoma (especially in postnecrotic cirrhosis and hemochromatosis).

Portal hypertension

DEFINITION The normal adult liver is perfused by about 1,500 ml of blood per min, 60 to 75 percent by way of the portal vein. A balance among portal vein and hepatic artery inflows, hepatic vein outflow, and vascular resistance maintains a fairly constant low pressure within the portal system. Constriction of any major portion of the portal-hepatic venous bed with consequent increase in resistance to blood flow may lead to rising portal venous pressures despite the development of extensive but inefficient collateral channels. Portal hypertension may be defined as persistent portal pressure in excess of 25 to 30 cm of saline, with sluggish flow in major venous trunks, evolution of numerous portal-systemic venous collaterals, and passive congestion of the spleen and other viscera.

PATHOGENESIS As summarized in Table 296-1, portal hypertension results from a combination of *increased resistance to flow, sustained high splanchnic inflow*, and *inadequate collateral decompression.* With few exceptions, however, the primary factor in the development of portal hypertension is *obstruction* of the portal vein, the intrahepatic venous bed, or rarely the hepatic veins.

TABLE 296-1
Factors in the pathogenesis of portal hypertension

I Increased vascular resistance
- *A* Intrahepatic
  - *1* Cirrhosis
  - *2* Infiltrations (e.g., tumors, sarcoidosis)
  - *3* Polycystic disease
  - *4* Schistosomiasis
  - *5* Noncirrhotic portal fibrosis (hepatic phlebosclerosis)
- *B* Portal vein
  - *1* Thrombosis
  - *2* Tumor
  - *3* Infection (pylephlebitis)
- *C* Hepatic veins
  - *1* Thrombosis (Budd-Chiari syndrome)
  - *2* Veno-occlusive disease

II Sustained high splanchnic inflow
- *A* Splenomegaly
- *B* Diffuse AV shunts(?)
- *C* Major AV fistulae

III Inadequate decompression via venous collaterals
- *A* Esophageal
- *B* Retroperitoneal
- *C* Periumbilical
- *D* Hemorrhoidal

Most cases of portal hypertension in the United States are caused by *cirrhosis*, which produces mechanical obstruction of blood flow through the liver by fibrosis, thrombosis, and nodular regeneration. About 30 to 60 percent of patients with cirrhosis have significant portal hypertension. The second most common cause of portal hypertension is *mechanical obstruction* of the extrahepatic portal vein, usually the result of thrombosis or tumor invasion. *Occlusion of the major hepatic veins* (Budd-Chiari syndrome) or their small intrahepatic branches (as in veno-occlusive disease) may lead to portal hypertension. About 5 to 10 percent of patients with cirrhosis and portal hypertension have associated *portal vein thrombosis.* As mentioned above, a small but significant number of patients with sustained portal hypertension have no evidence of cirrhosis but show variable degrees of fibrosis and sclerosis of the intrahepatic portal veins (noncirrhotic portal fibrosis).

CLINICAL FEATURES Many patients with portal hypertension of intra- or extrahepatic origin have symptoms or signs related only to the primary disease, and portal hypertension is tolerated without incident for years. Three major clinical consequences of portal hypertension may, however, lead to its recognition: (1) The development of extensive *portal-systemic venous collaterals*, with gastrointestinal hemorrhage; (2) the appearance of *congestive splenomegaly* with hypersplenism; and (3) the onset of episodic stupor or *portal-systemic encephalopathy.*

The *development of collateral channels* between the portal and systemic venous beds is the most characteristic consequence of portal hypertension. Major sites of collateral flow involve dilated veins around the rectum (hemorrhoids), cardioesophageal junction (esophagogastric varices), and retroperitoneal space and the falciform ligament of the liver (periumbilical or abdominal wall collaterals). Although hemorrhoids bleed frequently and varices of the bowel rupture occasionally, massive hemorrhage from thin-walled varices in the upper stomach and lower esophagus is the major complication of portal hypertension. Variceal bleeding occurs without obvious precipitating cause and presents usually as painless massive hematemesis or melena. Abdominal wall collaterals are helpful clinical signs of portal hypertension and appear as slightly tortuous epigastric vessels that radiate from the umbilicus towards the xiphoid and rib margins. Extreme prominence of these collaterals (*caput Medusae*) is rare. Vascular bruits may be heard over the upper abdomen, the *Cruveilhier-Baumgarten syndrome. Splenomegaly*, the result of passive congestion, fibrosis and siderosis, is present in most patients with significant and long-standing portal hypertension. The absence of splenomegaly is not, however, convincing evidence against portal hypertension because splenic size correlates poorly with the level of portal pressure. As noted in Chap. 317, splenic enlargement may be accompanied by abnormal sequestration and destruction of the circulating blood cells (hypersplenism). Patients with portal hypertension and extensive portal-systemic venous shunting may experience bouts of *portal-systemic encephalopathy* or *hepatic coma*. These episodes are often precipitated by gastrointestinal hemorrhage and a moderate to high protein diet.

DIAGNOSIS Portal hypertension should be suspected in all patients with cirrhosis or other chronic hepatic diseases, in those with unexplained splenomegaly, and in all patients with massive upper gastrointestinal hemorrhage not clearly due to peptic ulcer or intestinal neoplasm. Three diagnostic questions should be answered in these cases. (1) Is portal hypertension present? (2) Is the underlying cause hepatic or extrahepatic? (3) If gastrointestinal hemorrhage has occurred, is a ruptured esophageal varix the source? The combination of prominent abdominal collateral veins, an enlarged spleen with pancytopenia, and ancillary signs of cirrhosis suggests portal hypertension. Direct measurement of the portal venous pressure may also be obtained by splenic puncture, although in a small percentage of patients this may be followed by severe hemorrhage. The portal system may be visualized by splenoportography or abdominal angiography (Chap. 292). If no occlusion of the splenoportal trunk is demonstrated by x-ray examination and if clinical or laboratory evidence suggests associated liver disease, needle biopsy of the liver should be carried out to define the precise nature of the hepatic lesion. A careful barium swallow with cinefluoroscopy of the esophagus and stomach may demonstrate varices with reasonable certainty (60 to 80 percent) and serves to exclude other lesions as possible sources of bleeding. If possible, esophagoscopy should be carried out promptly during or after a bout of hematemesis.

TREATMENT General Vigorous treatment of patients with early Laennec's cirrhosis, chronic active hepatitis, and other liver diseases may lead to a fall in portal pressure and to the disappearance of varices. As a rule, however, portal hypertension caused by established cirrhosis or portal vein occlusion persists, and variceal hemorrhage remains a grave threat. No precise prognosis can be made in individual cases, but over 30 percent of patients with cirrhosis and varices experience a major hemorrhage within 5 years and have an overall mortality of 60 to 80 percent. In contrast, patients with normal liver function and variceal hemorrhage secondary to portal vein block tolerate episodes of hemorrhage relatively well. Despite technical improvements in surgical methods of portal vein decompression, shunts should be reserved for patients who bleed from varices. Controlled studies have shown little justification for prophylactic portacaval anastomosis. Several methods of portacaval and splenorenal anastomosis are used. Most produce satisfactory decreases in portal pressure, and recurrent variceal hemorrhage is rare. However, long-term survival ultimately depends on the extent of the underlying liver disease.

Acute variceal hemorrhage Prompt and effective care of the patient with massive hematemasis or melena from a ruptured varix requires coordinated medical-surgical efforts. The basic elements of management include the following:

Quantitative replacement of blood loss is essential to prevent further deterioration of liver function. It is often advisable to use fresh blood if massive replacement therapy is required (one unit of freshly drawn blood for each four units of stored blood). *Demonstration of esophageal varices, location of the actual bleeding site,* and *exclusion of other causes of gastrointestinal hemorrhage* by endoscopy or radiography are critical. It should not be assumed that cirrhotics with proved or probable varices are bleeding from the varices, because at least one-third have other potential bleeding sites in the upper gastrointestinal tract.

Temporary control of variceal bleeding may be achieved by vasopressin infusions, gastric cooling, or balloon tamponade. Infusion of 20 units of vasopressin over a 15- to 30-min period may lead to temporary decrease in variceal hemorrhage by lowering splanchnic blood flow and portal pressure. Transient decreases in cardiac output and effects of this agent on smooth muscles may make the use of vasopressin hazardous to patients with ischemic heart disease. Although the infusions may be repeated every 2 to 4 hr, the effects diminish with time. Insertion and inflation of a gastric cooling balloon has been used but demands special apparatus and careful monitoring to detect rebleeding or aspiration of esophageal contents. The Sengstaken tube or a modified single-balloon tube may be inserted into the stomach, inflated, and attached to traction to provide local compression of the submucosal veins. Although often effective in producing temporary control of massive hemorrhage, this device is difficult to place accurately and uncomfortable for the patient, and its use is often complicated by rebleeding, esophageal erosions, airway obstruction, or aspiration. Both cooling balloons and Sengstaken tube must be regarded as temporizing measures that should, in most instances, be used to prepare the patient for definitive surgery. Active steps must be taken to *prevent or treat impending hepatic coma* (see Hepatic Coma, later in this chapter).

Evaluation of liver function and *assessment of operative risk* are important but difficult. No single clinical test of liver function can predict accurately the immediate postoperative morbidity and mortality. In general, however, patients with compensated or stable cirrhosis have a much more favorable outlook than those with deepening jaundice, ascites, or signs of precoma. Careful medical management for 2 or 3 weeks may permit considerable recovery of liver function in patients with active Laennec's cirrhosis.

Emergency portacaval shunts to arrest bleeding may be performed within a few days. The mortality is understandably high, but the operation does prevent exsanguination, usually prevents future variceal bleeding, and may permit considerable recovery of liver function.

In many patients, *elective shunt surgery* may be advisable. The results of many large clinical series indicate that the immediate and long-term mortality depends largely on the hepatic reserve, because variceal bleeding rarely recurs if a satisfactory portacaval shunt has been established. The type of surgical shunt procedure (i.e., portacaval or splenorenal) often depends on the experience and judgment of the surgeon. Portal decompression does not usually correct the pancytopenia of hypersplenism. In infants and in other patients with extensive portal vein disease, effective portal-systemic shunts may be constructed, using other branches of the portal vein and the trunk of the inferior cava. Late complications in patients with functioning portacaval shunts include hepatic coma (15 to 20 percent), peptic ulceration (10 to 15 percent), slight unconjugated hyperbilirubinemia, and, rarely, accumulation of iron within the cirrhotic liver.

Ascites
(See also Chap. 43)

DEFINITION Ascites, the accumulation of abnormal volumes of fluid within the peritoneal cavity, is a frequent manifestation of cirrhosis and other types of diffuse parenchymal liver disease. The development of ascites is often accompanied by hemodilution, edema, and oliguria. These and other clinical findings reflect the complex abnormalities of electrolyte, water, and protein metabolism that may complicate severe liver disease and other disturbances of the hepatic circulation.

PATHOGENESIS Ascites is usually demonstrable clinically when 500 ml or more of fluid has accumulated in the peritoneal cavity. It results from disturbances of both local and systemic mechanisms that regulate the passage of fluid and solutes across vascular and serosal membranes. The *local or intraabdominal factors* favoring ascites formation in cirrhosis include the following:

1 *Portal hypertension.* Uncomplicated chronic portal hypertension of the extrahepatic type usually is *not* associated with ascites. However, portal hypertension plays an important "permissive" role in ascites formation when combined with salt retention or hypoalbuminemia.
2 *Obstruction to hepatic vein radicles.* Postsinusoidal block or diffuse block of the hepatic venous system (by cirrhosis, infiltrative disease, or thrombi) leads to ascites.
3 *Elevated intrahepatic pressure.* This alteration is typically present in most forms of cirrhosis.
4 *Increased flow of hepatic lymph.* This may substantially contribute to ascites in some patients with severe hepatic inflammation. An elevated protein concentration in ascitic fluid greater than 3 g per 100 ml (in the absence of infection) often reflects ascites formation on this basis.

The most important *systemic factors* include the following:

1 *Increased sodium retention.* Although the exact mechanism by which hepatic disease initiates increased production of aldosterone is unclear, patients with cirrhosis and ascites have striking secondary aldosteronism and consequently marked sodium retention.
2 *Impaired water excretion.* Patients with ascites have decreased renal free water clearance and delayed excretion of a water load, a factor which may contribute to ascites.
3 *Decreased plasma colloid osmotic pressure.* Impaired synthesis of albumin, the serum protein that determines the colloid osmotic pressure, is at times a major consequence of hepatocellular damage and poor nutrition. In some patients with cirrhosis, low serum albumin levels may reflect increased albumin catabolism or loss of protein into the intestinal lumen or ascitic fluid.

DIAGNOSIS When clinical examination suggests the presence of ascites, careful aspiration of 50 to 100 ml of fluid from a flank or low midline site should be attempted. Even in the most typical cases of cirrhosis, a sample of ascitic fluid should be examined for its appearance, color, cell count, presence of microorganisms, protein content, and the presence of malignant cells.

TREATMENT With rare exceptions, ascites produced by diffuse liver disease disappears as the underlying process resolves. Therefore, the *major therapeutic objective is to improve liver function.* In addition, dietary and drug therapy designed to control the local and systemic factors involved in ascites production may be required to produce the desired daily weight loss of 0.5 to 1.0 kg. Sodium retention may be minimized by the use of a *low sodium diet* (250 to 500 mg sodium per day), and fluid intake should be restricted to 1,000 to 1,500 ml daily or to a volume equal to the urine output of the preceding day. If this regimen fails to induce a spontaneous diuresis in 5 to 7 days, *combined diuretic therapy* with an aldosterone antagonist such as spironolactone (Aldactone, 100 mg two or three times daily) and an agent like ethacrynic acid (50 mg once or twice daily) or furosemide (Lasix, 40 or 80 mg daily) is indicated. These measures require careful monitoring for the complications of hypokalemia, azotemia, and hepatic precoma. Hypovolemia can be avoided if negative fluid balance is limited to 300 ml per day in patients without peripheral edema and 1,000 ml per day in the presence of edema.

Infusions of *mannitol* may induce transient osmotic diuresis, and the administration of *salt-poor albumin* may produce temporary elevations of the plasma colloid osmotic pressure, but neither method is especially effective or practical. Both agents are distributed rapidly within the vascular and ascitic fluid spaces, and the effective increase in water transport from the abdomen into the plasma and then to the kidney is short-lived. In addition, repeated infusions of osmotically active substances may lead to significant elevations of portal venous pressure and therefore increase the hazard of variceal hemorrhage.

"*Therapeutic*" *paracentesis* should be avoided because major hemodynamic changes, altered renal function, and significant protein loss are likely to occur. The intravenous infusion of ascitic fluid removed by paracentesis, while theoretically avoiding some of these complications, has limited usefulness in clinical practice. *Surgical procedures* designed to overcome intractable ascites are rarely required. However, since the creation of a portacaval shunt for treatment of variceal hemorrhage often leads to loss of ascites, such surgery has been carried out in the rare case with "intractable ascites."

Hepatic coma

DEFINITION Hepatic coma (hepatocerebral intoxication, portal-systemic encephalopathy) is a complex syndrome characterized by disturbances in consciousness, fluctuating neurologic signs, asterixis or "flapping tremor," and distinctive electroencephalographic changes. This metabolic disorder of the nervous system may appear in the course of acute or chronic hepatocellular disease or as a complication of portal-systemic venous shunting. It may be *acute* and self-limiting or *chronic* and progressive.

DIAGNOSIS The recognition of hepatic coma depends on four major elements. (1) The patient should have evidence of advanced hepatocellular disease, extensive portal-systemic collateral shunts, or both. The liver disease may be acute and massive, as in toxic or fulminant viral hepatitis, or chronic and advanced, as in cirrhosis. The portal-systemic venous shunts, which must permit a significant portion of the portal blood to bypass the liver, may be either *spontaneous* (e.g., naturally developing collaterals) or *surgical* (e.g., large portacaval anastomoses). Most patients who develop hepatic coma have, in fact, elements of both liver disease and portal-systemic shunting. (2) Disturbances of awareness and mentation are characteristic, and forgetfulness and confusion progress to stupor and finally to deep coma. (3) Mental changes are accompanied by shifting combinations of neurologic signs, which include rigidity, hyperreflexia, extensor plantor signs, and rarely seizures. A peculiar "flapping tremor" (asterixis), a nonrhythmic lapse in voluntary sustained posture of extremities, head, and trunk, is often seen in precoma and in advancing hepatic coma but cannot be elicited in the presence of coma. This neurologic picture is nonspecific and is encountered also in patients with uremia, ventilatory failure, and other forms of metabolic brain disease. (4) Most patients with the clinical features of hepatic coma have characteristic symmetrical, high-voltage, slow-wave (2 to 5 per sec) patterns on the electroencephalogram. *Fetor hepaticus*, a unique musty odor of the breath and urine, may be noted in patients with hepatic coma and also in those with an extensive collateral circulation. Several clinical variants of the "classic" syndrome of hepatic coma have been recognized. *Chronic progressive hepatocerebral degeneration*, which may develop in patients with stable liver disease or with portacaval anastamoses, is characterized by a slow decline in intellectual function, cerebellar ataxia, tremor, and choreoathetosis. Isolated signs of *myelopathy*, including spasticity and hyperreflexia of the legs, may antedate the other elements of hepatic coma by several months. Both of these conditions must be distinguished from other nonhepatic causes of deranged nervous system function, as well as from Wilson's disease.

PATHOGENESIS No single biochemical or physiologic defect has been shown to be the actual cause of hepatic coma. Most studies have shown that hepatic coma and its associated disorders of cerebral function result from (1) the shunting of portal blood directly into the systemic circulation, so that the blood largely bypasses the liver, and (2) severe hepatocellular damage and dysfunction. Both circumstances have a common result: nitrogenous substances absorbed from the intestines are not metabolized by the liver before reaching the cerebral circulation. Ammonia is one such compound, and many patients with hepatic coma have elevated systemic arterial and venous blood levels of ammonia, so-called *ammonia intoxication*. Hyperammonemia is most often found in patients with portal-systemic venous shunting and in hepatic cell failure.

Undoubtedly, "toxic" substances other than ammonia are involved in the genesis of hepatic coma. The administration of methionine to patients with portal-systemic shunts has been shown to precipitate stupor or coma in the absence of hyperammonemia. The liver is believed to produce substances that are essential for normal brain metabolism, and in liver failure these may be reduced. Decreased cerebral oxygen uptake and impaired intermediary metabolism of glucose in the brain are common but nonspecific features of hepatic coma.

Most patients with recurrent or progressive forms of hepatic coma have distinctive enlargement and proliferation of protoplasmic astrocytes in many areas of the brain, and a few develop bandlike cerebral cortical necrosis. These findings suggest that the syndrome may progress from a functional to a structural or irreversible phase.

TREATMENT Early recognition and prompt treatment of hepatic coma are essential, because patients in profound coma respond poorly to all forms of therapy and are vulnerable to the added hazards of coma itself. Slight confusion, deterioration in self-care and handwriting, unusual somnolence, and asterixis should be sought for. It may be desirable to grade or classify the stages of hepatic coma, since this is often helpful in charting the course of the illness and gauging the effects of therapy. One useful classification is based on the severity of mental and neurologic signs, and ranges from grade I (slight apathy or euphoria with or without objective neurologic signs) to grade V (true coma).

Basic steps in therapy include: (1) *Specific and supportive therapy of the associated liver disease.* This includes treatment of conditions like fatty liver and fulminating viral hepatitis and more general measures such as providing nitrogen-sparing calories (e.g., 2000 kcal per day as 20 to 25% glucose solutions through a nasogastric tube or intravenously into a large vein). (2) Steps to *reduce blood levels of ammonia and other "toxic" nitrogenous substances.* Protein is excluded from the diet for 2 to 3 days, and it is reintroduced in 10- to 20-g increments every 2 to 4 days as the patient improves. Laxatives such as magnesium citrate, 30 to 50 ml orally, and Fleet enemas may be used to evacuate colonic contents. Persistent or progressive hepatic precoma should prompt the administration of neomycin, a poorly absorbed antibiotic, in doses of 6 to 12 g orally each day to decrease the intestinal production and absorption of ammonia. Bleeding into the gastrointestinal tract should be sought for and controlled by appropriate means. (3) *Factors that potentiate or compound coma should be corrected.* These include respiratory alkalosis, hyponatremia, hypokalemia, anemia, infections, and hypoglycemia. Special efforts should be made to exclude temporarily all drugs, such as opiates, sedatives, and diuretics. (4) *Heroic measures* may be tried in patients with potentially reversible liver disease. Exchange blood transfusions, hemodialysis, plasma exchanges, extracorporeal pig-liver perfusion and liver homotransplantation are experimental therapies that have limited practical application. L-dopa therapy may produce temporary improvement of mental and neurological function in some cases.

Chronic encephalopathy, or episodic coma, may respond to combinations of prolonged protein restriction (30 to 40 g per day) and small (2 to 4 g) daily doses of neomycin. The synthetic disaccharide lactulose, given as 25 to 30 ml of syrup three times daily, often produces clinical improvement and a lessened requirement for protein restruction and neomycin, presumably by altering colonic flora, diminishing fecal pH, and decreasing ammonia absorption. Rarely, patients who are incapacitated by chronic neuropsychiatric symptoms may benefit from surgical procedures that are designed to "isolate" the colon and thereby reduce ammonia production. Ileosigmoidostomy and colonic exclusion have been partially effective in some cases.

REFERENCES

Biliary and other types of cirrhosis

DATTA DV, SHERLOCK S: Cholestyramine for long-term relief of pruritus complicating intrahepatic cholestasis. Gastroenterology 50:323, 1966

KLATSKIN G, KANTOR FS: Mitochondrial antibody in primary biliary cirrhosis and other diseases. Ann Int Med 77:533, 1972

PARONETTO F et al: Immunocytochemical and serologic observations in primary biliary cirrhosis. N Engl J Med 271:1123, 1964

Hepatic coma

GABUZDA GH: Ammonium metabolism and hepatic coma. Gastroenterology 53:806, 1967

KERSH ES, RIFKIN H: Lactulose enemas. Ann Int Med 78:81, 1973

VICTOR M et al: The acquired (non-Wilsonian) type of chronic hepatocerebral degeneration. Medicine (Baltimore) 44:345, 1965

ZIEVE L: Pathogenesis of hepatic coma. Arch Intern Med 118:211, 1966

Laennec's and postnecrotic cirrhosis

EPSTEIN M et al: Renal failure in the patient with cirrhosis. Am J Med 49:175, 1970

LEEVY CM: Clinical diagnosis, evaluation and treatment of liver disease in alcoholics. Fed Proc 26:1474, 1967

POWELL WJ, KLATSKIN G: Duration of survival in patients with Laennec's cirrhosis. Am J Med 44:406, 1967

STONE WD et al: The natural history of cirrhosis. Q J Med 37:119, 1968

Portal hypertension and ascites

CONN HO et al: Prophylactic portacaval anastomosis. Medicine (Baltimore) 51:27, 1972

GABUZDA GH: Cirrhosis, ascites and edema. Gastroenterology 58:546, 1970

WITTE MH et al: Physiological factors involved in the causation of cirrhotic ascites. Gastroenterology 61:742, 1971

297 TUMORS OF THE LIVER

ELLIOT ALPERT
KURT J. ISSELBACHER

PRIMARY CARCINOMA Carcinomas arising within the liver may be of liver cell (hepatoma), duct cell (cholangioma), or mixed origin. In most series hepatomas account for 80 to 90 percent of liver carcinomas. There is, however, little purpose in distinguishing between the two types, since both may be found in different parts of the same tumor and the clinical course is similar.

Incidence and epidemiology Primary liver cancers account for only 1 to 2 percent of malignant tumors found at autopsy in North and South America and Europe. However, in parts of Africa and Asia they comprise 20 to 30 percent of all malignant conditions. Liver carcinoma is two to four times more frequent in men than women, the peak incidence occurring in the fifth and sixth decades of life in the United States and two decades earlier in areas with a high incidence.

The actual cause of hepatic cancer is unknown, but three observations are noteworthy: (1) About 75 percent of hepatomas and 20 to 50 percent of cholangiomas are found in association with cirrhosis; (2) hepatomas occur in 10 to 15 percent of cases of postnecrotic cirrhosis and hemochromatosis but are less common in patients with Laennec's cirrhosis; (3) certain known hepatic carcinogens, such as aflatoxins, are ingested in foodstuffs in some parts of the world, such as Africa and Asia, where one also finds a very high incidence of hepatoma.

Clinical features Hepatic cancers often may escape clinical recognition during life because they often occur in patients with underlying cirrhosis, and the symptoms and signs may initially suggest simply a progression of the underlying liver disease. There are other clinical features often associated with hepatic carcinoma which should alert the clinician to the diagnosis: (1) Pain, usually moderate in degree and localized to the upper abdomen or the right side of the chest, is a major complaint in more than half the cases; (2) blood-tinged ascites or hemoperitoneum which occurs in about 20 percent of cases; (3) a mass in the liver, particularly if tender; (4) the presence of a friction rub or bruit over the liver; (5) the presence of rare metabolic features such as polycythemia, hypoglycemia, endocrine changes (such as precocious puberty), acquired porphyria, hypercalcemia, and dysglobulinemia. Jaundice is characteristic of cholangiomas but is relatively uncommon in hepatomas.

Anemia, leukocytosis, moderate Bromsulphalein (BSP) retention, and elevated alkaline phosphatase levels are common laboratory findings. A disproportionately high alkaline phosphatase in relation to other abnormal liver function tests in a patient with cirrhosis is often a clue to an infiltrating or partially obstructing liver carcinoma.

Diagnosis The clinical features outlined above should suggest the possibility of primary carcinoma of the liver. Liver scintiscans may document the presence of one or more hepatic masses but unfortunately may not distinguish between primary and metastatic liver tumors and cannot prove the existence of a solitary and possibly resectable lesion. Celiac axis angiography may show distortion of vessels or "tumor blushes," but this technique does not distinguish primary cancer from metastatic disease.

A unique "fetal" alpha-1-globulin (alpha fetoprotein) is found in the serum of a high percentage of cases with hepatoma (as well as in embryonal teratoblastoma of the gonads). It occurs only rarely in patients with gastrointestinal tumors metastatic to liver and only transiently in an occasional patient with acute hepatitis. Alpha fetoprotein is detectable in 75 to 95 percent of hepatoma patients in Africa, but only 50 percent of white patients have shown a positive test. The detection and persistence of alpha fetoprotein in a patient with chronic liver disease strongly suggests primary carcinoma of the liver.

Needle biopsy of the liver is helpful, especially if the biopsy is taken in the area of a palpable nodule. False negatives may occur if the liver biopsy is simply performed in a routine manner using the intercostal approach. Cytologic examination of ascitic fluid is usually negative for tumor cells. For these reasons peritoneoscopy or laparotomy with open liver biopsy is often required. This direct approach has the additional advantage of selecting the rare patients who are suitable for partial hepatectomy.

The course of the disease is usually rapid. Most patients die within 6 months from gastrointestinal hemorrhage, progressive cachexia, or hepatic failure.

Management If the patient is young, in good general health, and has no obvious extrahepatic involvement, solitary hepatic lesions may be excised or partial hepatectomy carried out. Persistence or appearance of alpha fetoprotein after excision is indicative of residual tumor. Chemotherapy, particularly by regional perfusion of the hepatic artery, may be considered for relief of pain. To a limited extent liver transplantation has been used in the treatment of hepatic cancer. Frequent recurrence of tumor or appearance of metastases after liver transplantation, however, has limited the value of this procedure. It is possible that in the future liver transplantation may prove to be of value.

BENIGN TUMORS OF THE LIVER These tumors are very rare. Single or multiple hemangiomas are the most common of the benign tumors. They are usually single and small but occasionally may be multiple or large. A vascular hum may be heard over the liver tumor. Needle liver biopsy is contraindicated if the diagnosis is suspected because of the likelihood of hemorrhage. Scintillation scanning using radioactive technetium shows a *defect* in the liver. In contrast, a scan using labeled albumin will show an initial *localization* of isotope in the vascular tumors. The diagnosis can frequently be made by celiac angiography. Treatment is usually not indicated, and attempts at surgical removal are often associated with excessive bleeding.

Other benign tumors include hamartomas, adenomas, and benign cholangiomas.

METASTATIC TUMORS OF THE LIVER Metastatic malignant tumors of the liver are common in clinical practice, probably ranking second only to cirrhosis as a cause of fatal liver disease. In the United States the incidence of metastatic carcinoma is at least twenty times greater than that of primary carcinoma. Hepatic metastases have been reported at autopsies in 30 to 50 percent of patients dying from malignant disease.

Pathogenesis The liver is uniquely vulnerable to invasion by tumor cells: its size, high rate of blood flow, and double perfusion by hepatic artery and portal vein combine to make it the most common site of metastases except for the lymph nodes. In addition, local tissue factors appear to support the growth of metastatic implants. Virtually all types of neoplasms except those primary in the brain may metastasize to the liver. The most common primary tumors are those of the gastrointestinal tract, lung, or breast, melanomas, and lymphoma. Less common are metastases from tumors of the thyroid, prostate, and skin.

Clinical features Most patients with metastatic malignancy of the liver present with (1) symptoms referable only to the primary tumor, asymptomatic hepatic involvement being discovered in the course of clinical evaluation; (2) nonspecific symptoms of weakness, weight loss, fever, sweats, and loss of appetite; or (3) features indicating active hepatic disease, especially abdominal pain, ascites, or jaundice.

Most patients with significant metastatic liver involvement have suggestive clinical signs: about two-thirds have hepatic enlargement; many have localized induration or tenderness of the liver; signs of portal hypertension may be present; a friction rub may be found, usually over tender areas of the liver; when present, it usually means either diffuse hepatic metastases or nodes around the porta hepatis.

Abnormal liver function tests are frequent but often nonspecific. They reflect the effects of fever and wasting, as well as the neoplastic process itself. *Increases in serum alkaline phosphatase*, moderate to marked BSP retention, and mild elevation of transaminase levels are most common. *Two of these three tests are abnormal in about 80 percent of cases.*

Diagnosis Evidence of metastatic invasion of the liver should be sought actively in any patient with a primary malignancy, especially of the lung, gastrointestinal tract, or breast, before therapy is undertaken. Serial studies of liver function and hepatic scintiscans may provide presumptive answers. Needle biopsy of the liver is usually indicated, affording positive diagnoses in 60 to 80 percent of cases with established metastases. Serial sectioning of specimens, repeat biopsies, or cytologic examination of biopsy fragments may increase the diagnostic yield by 10 to 15 percent. Liver biopsy may, on occasion, be the first and only proof of widespread malignancy when the primary tumor is occult.

Treatment Most metastatic carcinomas respond poorly to all forms of treatment, which is usually palliative. Surgical removal of a large metastasis is occasionally feasible. Systemic chemotherapy with methotrexate and 5-fluorouracil may in some cases appear to prolong life by a matter of several months. Metastases from the primary colonic tumors seem more responsive to such chemotherapy than do those from other tumors.

REFERENCES

ALPERT E et al: α-Fetoprotein in human hepatoma. Gastroenterology 61:137, 1971

———, DAVIDSON CS: Mycotoxins: A possible cause of primary carcinoma of the liver. Am J Med 46:325, 1969

FENSTER LF, KLATSKIN G: Manifestations of metastatic tumors of the liver: A study of 81 patients subjected to needle biopsy. Am J Med 31:238, 1961

MARGOLIS S, HOMCY C: Systemic manifestations of hepatoma. Medicine 51:381, 1972

SHERLOCK S: Hepatic tumors, in *Diseases of the Liver*, 4th ed., Philadelphia: Davis, 1968

298 SUPPURATIVE DISEASES OF THE LIVER

WILLIAM A. TISDALE

Suppurative diseases of the liver include isolated or disseminated microabscesses or macroabscesses of bacterial, fungal, or amebic origin. The infecting agents, single or multiple, usually reach the liver by way of the portal vein, hepatic artery, or bile ducts. Less often, the infection results from direct trauma or by extension from adjacent structures. Hepatic suppuration is actually quite rare in view of the frequent occurrence of transient bacteremias, biliary obstruction, and abdominal infections. This resistance to sepsis reflects the capacity of the liver to trap and destroy organisms.

PYOGENIC (NONAMEBIC) LIVER ABSCESS Many septic processes may be complicated by self-limited and undiagnosed microabscesses of the liver. Necropsy examination of livers from patients dying with bacteremic states often show multiple tiny foci of bacteria, cell loss, and inflammation. Rarely, focal lesions progress to gross liver abscesses and produce dramatic clinical features.

Etiology Infected obstruction of the biliary tract (usually nonmalignant in nature) accounts for about 30 percent of abscesses, sepsis in organs drained by the portal vein (especially perforated viscera, infected surgical wounds, and colonic disease) for another 40 percent, and systemic septicemia for 10 to 15 percent. A few abscesses arise from penetrating or blunt trauma with secondary infection, or by extension from contiguous abscesses. A significant number of liver abscesses (40 percent in some series) have no obvious associated or primary lesion, most of these probably resulting from cryptic bowel infections. Abscesses are usually multiple, especially in association with cholangitis. The infecting agents are also usually multiple with coliform bacteria, *Bacteroides*, and other gram-negative organisms, staphylococci and streptococci being the most common organisms.

Clinical features Signs of the associated septic or traumatic process may obscure those of acute liver abscess. However, persistent or hectic fever, sweats and chills, pronounced weight loss, nausea and vomiting, a tender and enlarged liver, and, on occasion, slight jaundice are characteristic of evolving abscesses. Leukocytosis in the range of 16,000 to 25,000 cells per mm^3 is the rule; leukopenia may occur and indicates a poor prognosis. Nonspecific changes in liver function are common. The development of hypoalbuminemia usually signifies an unfavorable prognosis.

Elevation and decreased movement of the diaphragm, occasionally associated with lower lobe atelectasis and pleural effusion, are usually noted on radiologic examination. Liver scans or gamma camera studies using ^{99m}Tc are valuable in localizing abscesses greater than 2 to 3 cm in diameter. Ultrasonic scans may distinguish solid from fluid-filled lesions. In all such patients a careful search should be made for metastatic abscesses in the lungs and brain.

Management Pyogenic liver abscesses should be treated vigorously by medical and surgical means. Blood, wound exudates, or T-tube drainage fluids should be cultured aerobically and anaerobically in an attempt to identify the infecting organisms and to determine their antibiotic sensitivity. Empiric treatment with antibiotics effective against both gram-positive and gram-negative organisms should be instituted until specific pathogenic organisms have been isolated. In most cases, the combination of intravenous gentamicin (5 mg per kg per day) and lincomycin (2 to 4 g per day) will provide adequate initial control. However, the use of antibiotics alone is not sufficient, and well-established abscesses, after they are localized, must be drained surgically since simple aspiration is not sufficient. In fact, multiple drainage is often necessary.

AMEBIC ABSCESS Although less common in North America than pyogenic liver abscess, "hepatitis" (cellulitis) and abscesses due to *Entamoeba histolytica* occur throughout the world, complicating symptomatic intestinal amebiasis in 10 percent of cases. More often clinical evidence of an evolving amebic abscess appears without antecedent intestinal symptoms. Most abscesses are single and occur in the right lobe of the liver.

The clinical presentation tends to be more gradual and less dramatic than that of pyogenic abscess, but the signs, symptoms, and laboratory features are similar. Amebic abscesses often produce anterior and medial elevations of the right diaphragm by x-ray. Hepatic scintiscans, "gamma snaps," and ultrasonic scans are helpful in detecting and following the evolution of amebic abscesses. The most reliable and helpful serologic aid in the detection of extraintestinal amebiasis is the indirect hemagglutination test.

The trophozoites of *E. histolytica* are rarely demonstrated by stool examination and sigmoidoscopy in patients with amebic liver abscesses. Therefore, if the diagnosis is suggested by the clinical features and a positive indirect hemagglutination test, antiamebic therapy should be instituted. A regimen of chloroquine phosphate (Aralen), 0.5 g twice daily for 2 days, followed by 0.250 g twice daily for 4 weeks, usually produces remission and obviates the need for surgical drainage of most abscesses. Metronidazole (Flagyl), 750 mg three times daily for 10 days, is considered to be equally potent and has the added advantage of being effective against the intestinal phase of the infection (see Chap. 209).

REFERENCES

BUTLER TJ, MCCARTHY CF: Pyogenic liver abscess. Gut 10:389, 1969

LAMONT NM, POOLER NR: Hepatic amoebiasis. Q J Med 27:389, 1958

MILGRAM EA et al: Studies on the use of the indirect hemagglutination test in the diagnosis of amebiasis. Gastroenterology 50:645, 1966

REYNOLDS TB: Amoebic abscess of the liver. Gastroenterology 60:952, 1971

299 INFILTRATIVE AND METABOLIC DISEASES AFFECTING THE LIVER

KURT J. ISSELBACHER
J. THOMAS LAMONT

Many disseminated, systemic, or metabolic diseases involve the liver in a diffuse manner by the infiltration of abnormal cells or the accumulation of chemical substances or metabolites. Although infiltrative diseases may vary widely in their etiology and extrahepatic manifestations, the findings in the liver may be quite similar. Generalized enlargement and firmness of the liver, gradual and nonspecific deterioration of liver function, and, less often, signs of portal hypertension or ascites are typical features of this group of diseases. Differential diagnosis by clinical means may be difficult on occasion, but the diffusely infiltrated liver provides an excellent source of tissue for diagnostic purposes.

The infiltrative process may involve one or more of the structural components of the liver: the hepatocytes, the Kupffer cells and other elements of the reticuloendothelial system, the interstitial tissue, or the blood vessels.

LIPID INFILTRATIONS

FATTY LIVER Slight to moderate enlargement of the liver due to diffuse infiltration of liver cells by neutral fat (triglyceride) is a common clinical and pathologic finding. Although minimal fatty changes are often transient and have no clinical significance, persistent or extensive fatty infiltration may produce dysfunction and symptoms that require careful evaluation.

Etiology The major causes of fatty liver encountered in clinical practice depend on the age, geographic location, and metabolic-nutritional status of the patient population. *Chronic alcoholism* is the most common cause of fatty liver in this country and in other countries with a high alcohol intake. Over three-quarters of patients in most series are heavy drinkers, and the severity of fatty involvement is roughly proportional to the duration and degree of alcoholic excess. *Protein malnutrition*, especially in infancy and early childhood, accounts for most cases of severe fatty liver in the tropical zones of Africa, South America, and Asia. The hepatic changes may be associated with other clinical and pathologic features of kwashiorkor. Patients with adult-onset diabetes mellitus, especially those who are overweight and have poorly controlled disease, may have fatty livers. *Obesity* is commonly associated with fatty infiltration of the liver, which recedes as weight reduction occurs. In patients with Cushing's syndrome and in those receiving large doses of corticosteroids, fatty infiltration of the liver may occur. In many *chronic illnesses*, especially those complicated by impaired nutrition or malabsorption, increased fat is found in liver cells. For example, patients with ulcerative colitis, chronic pancreatitis, or protracted heart failure frequently have moderately fatty livers at the time of death. Patients maintained on prolonged *intravenous hyperalimentation* may also develop a fatty liver.

Acute fatty changes, often associated with clinical symptoms and overt liver cell necrosis, may be produced by a number of *hepatotoxins*. Carbon tetrachloride intoxication, DDT poisoning, and ingestion of substances containing yellow phosphorus result in severe fatty liver. Acute and prolonged alcohol ingestion may also be considered in this category and may be associated with a rapidly enlarging and fat-laden liver. Minor degrees of fatty infiltration are seen following acute alcoholic intoxication, but this is rarely of clinical significance. Two types of acute fatty liver deserve special comment: *Acute fatty liver of pregnancy*, a rare but often fatal condition seen during the third trimester of pregnancy, is characterized by nausea, vomiting, and abdominal pain, renal failure, and coma. *Massive tetracycline therapy*, in amounts of 3 to 12 g administered intravenously, has resulted in acute fatty liver and fatal hepatic coma in some pregnant patients.

Pathogenesis The hepatic lipid deposits, which consist largely of triglycerides and lesser amounts of phospholipid and cholesterol, appear as vacuoles of varying size within the cytoplasm of liver cells. In extreme cases, every liver cell is involved, and lipids comprise up to 30 to 40 percent of the total liver weight.

The biochemical mechanisms leading to hepatic triglyceride accumulation have been described in Chap. 291. Fatty infiltration has been produced in experimental animals by a variety of toxic agents and drugs, such as alcohol, carbon tetrachloride, and orotic acid. Dietary deficiencies, such as choline deficiency, readily lead to increased fat in the liver in the rat. However, with few exceptions these experimental studies cannot be used directly to explain the pathogenesis of fatty liver in clinical disease. Moderate doses of ethanol may produce both acute and chronic fatty changes in human subjects, probably by its direct effects on hepatic triglyceride and fatty acid metabolism (Chap. 291). Protein deficiency seems to account for the fatty liver of kwashiorkor and impaired protein synthesis for the fat accumulation following tetracycline and carbon tetrachloride administration. In diabetes mellitus and in starvation, increased mobilization of fatty acids from adipose tissue may be involved.

Clinical features A majority of patients with moderate to severe fatty livers have no symptoms. Massive fatty infiltration, especially if it is rapid in onset, may be associated with abdominal pain and anorexia. A firm and generally enlarged liver is present in most cases. Jaundice with features of cholestasis occurs in some alcoholic patients after bouts of heavy drinking.

Bromsulphalein (BSP) retention, hyperbilirubinemia, and elevated levels of serum alkaline phosphatase are characteristic of the acute "obstructive," or cholestatic, phase of alcoholic fatty liver disease. These changes may be recurrent, and hence causes of extrahepatic biliary obstruction have to be excluded.

Correction of the underlying nutritional or metabolic disorders leads in most instances to mobilization of the excess liver fat and to complete clinical recovery. Signs of cirrhosis may develop in patients with persistently fatty livers and chronic alcoholism. *There is, however, no evidence that a fatty liver per se leads to cirrhosis.* Sudden death from intercurrent infection or fat embolization to the lungs has been reported.

Diagnosis The findings of a firm, nontender, and generally enlarged liver with minimal hepatic dysfunction in a patient with chronic alcoholism, malnutrition, poorly controlled diabetes mellitus, or obesity should suggest a fatty liver. Needle biopsy of the liver will demonstrate the increased fatty content and possibly the underlying primary disorder. In acute fatty liver of pregnancy, especially when associated with tetracycline therapy, and in most cases of Reye's syndrome (see below), fat accumulates in small vacuoles rather than in large cytoplasmic droplets.

Treatment Attention to nutritional factors, removal of alcohol or offending toxins, and correction of any associated metabolic disorders usually result in recovery. There is no clinical rationale for the use of lipotropic agents such as choline. When indicated, attention should be directed to abstinence from alcohol, careful control of diabetes, weight loss, or correction of intestinal absorptive defects. In the alcoholic fatty liver there is gradual disappearance of fat from the liver after 4 to 8 weeks of adequate diet and abstinence from alcohol.

REYE'S SYNDROME (FATTY LIVER WITH ENCEPHALOPATHY) This acute illness has been described in children up to twelve to fifteen years of age. It is characterized by vomiting, progressive central nervous system damage, signs of hepatic injury, and hypoglycemia, and morphologically by extensive fatty vacuolization of the liver and renal tubules. The cause is unknown, although viral and toxic agents have been implicated. Cases have been reported from several countries; infants and children of either sex are affected; and familial occurrences have been described. In fatal cases, the liver is enlarged and yellow, with striking diffuse fatty microvacuolization of cells. Peripheral zonal hepatic necrosis has also been present in some cases. Fatty changes of the renal tubular cells and marked edema and neuronal degeneration of the brain are the major extrahepatic changes.

The onset often follows an upper respiratory tract infection in a previously healthy child. Within 1 to 3 days persistent vomiting occurs together with stupor, which usually progresses rapidly to generalized convulsions and coma. The liver is enlarged, but *jaundice and clinical signs of hepatic failure are characteristically absent or minimal.* Marked increase in serum transaminases, hypoglycemia, metabolic acidosis, and elevated serum ammonia levels are the major laboratory findings. Death from cerebral damage occurs in most patients after 3 or 4 days. However, a few children have recovered following the administration of large quantities of glucose and the use of general supportive therapy. Other patients have survived following exchange transfusions.

Since the disease appears typically to follow apparent upper respiratory tract infections or chicken pox or influenza, virologic studies have been carried out. Isolations from stool and tissues have included Coxsackie virus, influenza viruses, echo virus 11, and adenovirus type 3. The role of these viral agents in the pathogenesis of the disease is still unclear.

The condition bears some resemblance to the "vomiting sickness" of Jamaica, in which hypoglycemia and vomiting follow the ingestion of unripe akee fruit containing a hypoglycemic agent (hypoglycin). In this disease the liver also contains increased fat but also shows periportal hepatic necrosis.

NIEMANN-PICK DISEASE (see Chap. 317) This rare heritable disorder, found mainly in Jewish infants, is characterized by the accumulation of sphingomyelin and cholesterol in reticuloendothelial cells of the liver, spleen, bone marrow, and brain. Hepatomegaly and splenomegaly are present, but jaundice and other evidence of hepatic dysfunction are rare. The liver shows clusters of lipid-filled foamy Kupffer cells. Diagnosis is made by lipid analysis of the tissue.

GAUCHER'S DISEASE (see Chap. 317) Accumulations of large reticuloendothelial cells containing glucocerebrosides (Gaucher's cells) in the liver and spleen account for the characteristic moderate to massive hepatosplenomegaly. Rarely, ascites or portal hypertension is produced by compression of the intrahepatic vasculature. The diagnosis may be made readily by liver biopsy and demonstration of the Gaucher's cells.

WOLMAN'S AND CHOLESTEROL ESTER STORAGE DISEASES Wolman's disease is a rare and fatal familial lipidosis of infancy producing hepatosplenomegaly and stippled calcification of the adrenal glands. Liver biopsy shows clusters of foam cells (reticuloendothelial cells filled with cholesterol ester and triglycerides), hepatocytes containing fat, and patchy fibrosis. A related but less severe genetic disorder is cholesterol ester storage disease. In this condition there is hypercholesterolemia and accumulation of both cholesterol esters and triglycerides in hepatic lysosomes. Both these storage disorders are associated with hepatic deficiencies of cholesterol ester hydrolase and triglyceride lipase.

Other rare lipid disorders associated with hepatomegaly and increased fat in the liver include abetalipoproteinemia (Chap. 106), Tangier disease (Chap. 106), Fabry's disease (Chap. 106) and type I and V hyperlipoproteinemia (Chap. 106).

HEPATIC GLYCOGEN ACCUMULATION

DIABETIC GLYCOGENOSIS Hepatic enlargement caused by distension of liver cells with glycogen is present in some poorly controlled and often juvenile diabetic patients. Ketoacidosis and vigorous insulin therapy may further enhance hepatic enlargement and glycogen deposition. In the absence of cirrhosis, the hepatomegaly usually decreases with careful control of the diabetes.

GLYCOGEN STORAGE DISEASE (see Chap. 104) The normal liver contains 1 to 5 percent glycogen (by weight). In types I, II, and VI hereditary glycogen storage disease, increased amounts of glycogen (and fat) are found. Types III and IV are associated with derangements of glycogen structure, and cirrhosis may be present. Enzymatic and chemical analysis of liver tissue is usually needed for diagnosis.

GALACTOSEMIA (See Chap. 105)

Hepatic changes are common in patients with unrecognized or untreated galactosemia. In early weeks of life fatty infiltration and cholestasis may be noted in acutely ill infants. If the disease goes unrecognized for months or years, cirrhosis may develop.

OTHER INFILTRATIVE DISEASES

HURLER'S SYNDROME (see Chap. 362) This is an uncommon hereditary disease characterized by the widespread tissue deposition of mucopolysaccharide (chondroitin sulfate B and heparin sulfate) in many tissues. The liver is frequently enlarged and firm. Microscopically, Kupffer cells and other macrophages are enlarged and filled with metachromatic granular material. Cirrhosis may be a late complication.

ALPHA$_1$ ANTITRYPSIN DEFICIENCY Patients with the genetic deficiency of serum alpha$_1$ antitrypsin are prone to develop emphysema. Hepatocytes of such patients contain PAS (periodic acid–Schiff)-positive material although liver function may be normal. However, some infants with the homozygous defect have been described in whom jaundice and progressive cirrhosis develop; these patients die from liver failure in the first few years of life.

RETICULOENDOTHELIAL DISORDERS (See Chaps. 317 and 318)

Moderate to massive hepatomegaly and splenomegaly occur frequently in the various types of leukemia and lymphoma. Jaundice, when present, is usually slight and results from hemolysis. Deep and protracted jaundice is distinctly rare and is caused by obstruction of the intrahepatic or extrahepatic bile ducts by tumor. Liver biopsy specimens reveal portal and sinusoidal infiltrates in most cases of leukemia, but the cellular pattern may be mixed and nonspecific. Liver biopsy may provide a tissue diagnosis in patients with lymphoma or Hodgkin's disease; however, if the biopsy needle misses the tumor nodules, the cellular infiltrates may show a nondiagnostic pattern.

Myeloid metaplasia and other myeloproliferative disorders associated with extramedullary hematopoiesis produce hepatomegaly which may reach huge proportions, especially following splenectomy. BSP retention and alkaline phosphatase elevations are often found. Ascites and portal hypertension, apparently caused by diffuse involvement of portal venules and lymphatics, are rare complications.

GRANULOMATOUS INFILTRATIONS

Systemic granulomatous diseases, including sarcoidosis, miliary tuberculosis, histoplasmosis, brucellosis, schistosomiasis, berylliosis, and drug reactions, produce focal infiltrative hepatic lesions with great regularity. In addition, isolated granulomas of no diagnostic importance may be found occasionally in patients with various forms of cirrhosis and hepatitis. The liver infiltrated by granulomas may be slightly enlarged and firm, but hepatic dysfunction is usually limited to BSP retention and increased serum alkaline phosphatase levels. In a few patients with sarcoidosis or brucellosis portal hypertension may develop, and extensive postnecrotic scarring or postnecrotic cirrhosis may follow healing of the granulomatous lesions.

Needle biopsy of the liver reveals granulomas and often provides the first definite evidence of a systemic or disseminated granulomatous disease. In patients with sarcoidosis who have neither clinical nor laboratory evidence of hepatic involvement, needle biopsy is positive in about 80 percent of cases. Portions of the biopsy specimen should be cultured if infections such as brucellosis or tuberculosis are suspected, but special stains rarely demonstrate the infecting organism. Serial sections of the biopsy specimen should be examined if granulomas are not apparent. Individual granulomas are rarely specific in their microscopic appearance, and final diagnosis usually requires other clinical, laboratory, or histologic data.

AMYLOIDOSIS
(See Chap. 107)

Systemic amyloidosis, whether primary and idiopathic, familial, or secondary to chronic inflammatory or neoplastic diseases, often involves the liver. Grossly, the liver infiltrated with amyloid is enlarged and pale and rubbery in consistency. Microscopically, the birefringent amyloid deposits appear as homogeneous waxy material within the space of Disse, often being concentrated in the periportal areas with atrophy of adjacent liver cell plates. Selective involvement of the walls of blood vessels, especially of the hepatic arterioles, may be a striking feature of primary amyloidosis. With this possible exception, however, the hepatic lesions are the same in all forms of amyloidosis and are present in 60 to 90 percent of cases.

An enlarged and firm liver is found in about 60 percent of patients, and ascites occurs in advanced stages of the disease in about 20 percent. Jaundice, portal hypertension, and other signs of chronic liver disease are usually absent. Liver function changes, although frequent, correlate poorly with the extent of liver infiltration. Hypoalbuminemia, BSP retention, and elevated serum alkaline phosphatase levels are common.

The presumptive diagnosis of hepatic amyloidosis is often made after examination of biopsy material obtained from other organs. The frequency and diffuse nature of liver involvement by the amyloid infiltrate make needle biopsy a valuable diagnostic procedure. However, bleeding may occur after liver biopsy, and the procedure must therefore be used with caution.

REFERENCES

ALPERS DH, ISSELBACHER KJ: Fatty liver: clinical and biochemical aspects, in *Diseases of the Liver*, 4th ed., ed L Schiff, Philadelphia: Lippincott (in press)

GUCKIAN JC, PARRY JE: Granulomatous hepatitis. Ann Intern Med 65:1081, 1966

ISHAK KG et al: Cirrhosis of the liver associated with α_1-antitrypsin deficiency. Arch Path 94:445, 1972

RILEY HD JR: Reye's syndrome. J Infect Dis 125:77, 1972

300
DISEASES OF THE GALLBLADDER AND BILE DUCTS

PHILIP J. SNODGRASS
AMERICO ABBRUZZESE

PHYSIOLOGY OF THE BILIARY SYSTEM AND CHEMISTRY OF BILE Bile formation begins at the microvilli of the bile capillaries which are formed from the cell membranes of two opposing liver cells. These membranes contain at least three active transport systems, one secreting conjugated *bile salts*, another secreting various organic anions, such as conjugated *bilirubin*, and a third secreting sodium ions. Phospholipids (greater than 90 percent lecithin) and cholesterol enter bile by a mechanism as yet unexplained, but closely related to bile salt secretion. Water follows the osmotic gradient produced by these solutes, and potassium diffuses passively into bile.

Bile is secreted continuously and flows either directly into the duodenum or, in the fasting state, into a relaxed gallbladder. Within the gallbladder, hepatic bile is modified by the active mucosal absorption of sodium, chloride, and bicarbonate, with water following passively. This process results in an increase of solids from 3 to 11 percent and a reduction in pH from 7.6 to 6. The total volume of bile secreted averages 15 ml per kg per day.

The rate of bile secretion is variable, responding to nervous, hormonal, and chemical stimulation. The cephalic phase of digestion increases bile flow directly via the vagus nerve and indirectly via vagally induced gastrin release. Gastric chyme entering the duodenum stimulates the mucosal release of the hormones secretin and cholecystokinin-pancreozymin (CCK). Secretin stimulates the biliary ductal cells to secrete sodium bicarbonate, while CCK contracts the gallbladder and relaxes the sphincter of Oddi. Most of the bile salts entering the intestine are actively reabsorbed in the distal ileum, returned to the liver via the portal vein (enterohepatic circulation), and resecreted into the bile (Chap. 284). The mass of circulating bile acids is the *bile acid pool*, normally about 3 g. This entire pool circulates three times through the small bowel lumen during each meal, a total daily secretion of 27 g. The daily fecal loss of bile acids is 0.5 g, and this is the amount of primary bile acids synthesized each day.

Primary bile acids, cholic acid (the 3,7,12α-hydroxy form) and chenodeoxycholic acid (the 3,7α-hydroxy form), are synthesized from cholesterol in hepatic cells and are conjugated with either glycine or taurine to form bile *salts*. Glycine ($pK = 4$) and taurine conjugates ($pK = 2$) are stronger acids than are free bile acids ($pK = 6$) and therefore remain completely ionized (water soluble) at the pH of the gallbladder and small intestine. Although bile *acids* are reabsorbed by the intestinal mucosa (Chap. 284), the ionized *salts* are *not* absorbed in the duodenum or jejunum and thus maintain a critical micellar concentration (see below) in the intestinal lumen. The *secondary bile acids*, deoxycholic acid and lithocholic acid, are formed in the colon by bacterial dehydroxylation of the cholic acid and chenodeoxycholic acids which escaped ileal absorption. Deoxycholic acid is readily absorbed from the colon, returned to the liver, and conjugated with taurine or glycine; it accounts for about 13 percent of the bile acid pool. Lithocholic acid is insoluble at body temperature and is poorly absorbed from the normal colon (Chap. 284). Thus normal hepatic bile contains cholic, chenodeoxycholic, deoxycholic, and lithocholic acids in concentration ratios of about 10:10:5:1.

FIGURE 300-1
The three major components of bile solids (bile salts, lecithin, and cholesterol) are plotted on triangular coordinates. Synthetic mixtures of the three components were made up so the solids totaled 10 percent and water 90 percent. The molar ratios of the three components were then varied, and the presence or absence of cholesterol crystals noted at each point. Point P represents bile consisting of 80 mol percent bile salt, 5 percent cholesterol, and 15 percent lecithin. Line ABC represents the maximal solubility of cholesterol in varying mixtures of bile salt and lecithin. Because point P falls below line ABC and within the zone of a single phase of micellar liquid, this bile is less than saturated with cholesterol. Bile with a composition that would place it above line ABC could contain excess cholesterol in supersaturated or precipitated form. (From DM Small, N Engl J Med 279:588, 1968)

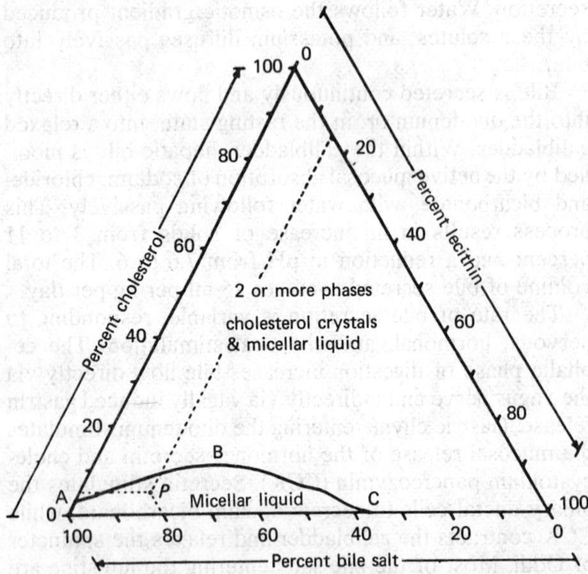

Bile salts are water-soluble, detergentlike molecules which in aqueous solutions, above a critical concentration and temperature, form aggregates called *micelles*. Mixed micelles are complexes of bile salts and phospholipids. They are able to solubilize a nonpolar lipid like cholesterol, forming a water-clear solution. These mixed micelles are thought to resemble bimolecular disks with the bile salts at the perimeter, the polar groups of lecithin projecting into the water phase at the top and bottom, and the nonpolar fatty acid chains in the center. Cholesterol molecules interdigitate between the fatty acids of the phospholipids. The amount of cholesterol which can be solubilized by these mixed micelles is limited and depends on the relative concentration of bile salts and lecithin. The phase diagram (Fig. 300-1) graphically illustrates this relation. Bile obtained from either gallbladders or duodenal drainage has been similarly analyzed and the physical state of cholesterol predicted. Bile with a composition outside the micellar zone (lithogenic bile) is associated with a high incidence of cholesterol gallstones (see below).

The formation of micelles explains why gallbladder bile is isosmolar with plasma yet contains very high concentrations of bile salts and sodium. The aggregation of bile salts in micelles reduces their osmotic effectiveness, and, in addition, micelles bind sodium and potassium, removing them from the ionic, osmotically active state. The sodium ion activity in gallbladder bile, measured with a sodium-sensitive electrode, is 148 to 186 mmol per liter, whereas the sodium content is 220 to 340 mmol per liter. The other ionic consitituents of bile are listed in Table 300-1.

CLINICAL FEATURES OF BILIARY TRACT DISEASE

The primary symptoms of extrahepatic biliary tract disease, pain and jaundice, are caused by obstruction and inflammation. Fever and chills can occur with biliary disorders, even in the absence of pain and jaundice. Nausea and vomiting are reflex phenomena which occasionally dominate the clinical picture. Dyspepsia, flatulence, bloating, and fatty food intolerance have long been considered "the inaugural symptoms of gallbladder disease" (Moynihan, 1908), but controlled studies have dispelled these symptoms as being hallmarks of gallstones. Dyspeptic symptoms are encountered more frequently in patients with normal cholecystograms than in those with abnormal cholecystograms, and patients with histories of fatty food intolerance experience no symptoms when fed meals high in concealed fat. Thus the association of dyspepsia and gallstones seems fortuitous, while fatty food intolerance appears to be a subjective bias rather than a characteristic symptom of biliary tract disease.

Pain The alimentary canal develops from midline endodermal cells, and pain emanating from its derivative

TABLE 300-1
The ionic constituents of bile

Constituent	*Hepatic bile, mmol/liter*	*Gallbladder bile, mmol/liter*
Na^+	174	220–340
K^+	6.6	6–10
Cl^-	55–107	1–10
HCO^-_3	34–65	0–17
Bile salts	28–42	290–340
Ca^{++}	6	25–32
Mg^{++}	0.5	
Osmolality, mOsm/liter	299	299

organs is felt at various levels of the midline. One cause of visceral pain is a tonic response to the sudden distention of a hollow viscus, the pain fibers being conveyed to the spinal cord along with sympathetic afferents (see Chaps. 5 and 8). In the conscious patient gradual elevation of pressure within the common bile duct evokes only vague discomfort, but abrupt elevation of pressure, to identical levels, causes severe epigastric pain. This pain has been traditionally called biliary "colic" and is caused by sudden obstruction of the biliary outflow system by stone or spasm. The pattern of biliary colic differs from the paroxysms of pain caused by violent peristalsis of the gut. Intestinal colic waxes to an agonizing peak and then wanes only to recur at intervals of 5 to 10 min. In contrast, biliary colic is abrupt in onset and reaches a level of maximal intensity which may last for several hours. The attack abates as suddenly as it begins, leaving a residual soreness. The pain is not intensified by moving about; most patients are restless and may pace the floor.

The most common cause of biliary colic is a gallstone suddenly wedged into the cystic duct. The pain is felt predominantly in the epigastrium but often radiates along the costal margin to the right hypochondrium and inferior angle of the right scapula. Less usual sites of referral are the right shoulder or neck and the left upper quadrant of the abdomen. Tenderness or rigidity, localized to an area overlying the gallbladder, is caused by inflammation of the contiguous parietal peritoneum. In approximately 5 percent of cases with gallbladder disease, inflammation is, as far as can be determined, the sole cause of pain (acalculous cholecystitis).

Sudden and brief occlusion of the distal common bile duct produces acute epigastric pain. However, abrupt and protracted obstruction (calculus) may produce a more complex pain response. As the entire biliary tree distends proximal to the obstruction, additional visceral and somatic sensory receptors are stimulated, causing, in addition to epigastric pain, pain in the right upper quadrant, the right shoulder and neck, or the inferior angle of the right scapula. Gradual stenosis of the common duct is painless: the early pain of carcinoma of the head of the pancreas is due to perineural tumor infiltration and is not caused by the raised intraductal biliary pressure.

Jaundice Mechanical blockage of the common bile duct is followed by jaundice, although there may be a variable lag period before both conjugated and unconjugated bilirubin increase in the blood and tissues. The variability of the interval between obstruction and jaundice depends on the state of the gallbladder mucosa and the distensibility of the gallbladder and bile ducts. Normal gallbladder mucosa can concentrate bile tenfold by absorbing water and electrolytes. When an otherwise normal biliary system is obstructed, these factors stabilize ductal pressure for hours despite the steady flow of hepatic bile into a closed system. Eventually the rate of absorption falls behind that of secretion, the biliary tree becomes maximally distended, and intraductal pressure rises. At a pressure of 23 mm Hg hepatic bile flow is suppressed, and conjugated bilirubin regurgitates into the blood. The rise in the unconjugated serum bilirubin level probably represents impaired uptake into the liver cells. Jaundice may not occur until several days after the block. However, when the gallbladder is absent or diseased, obstruction precipitates these events sooner, and scleral icterus appears within 24 hr.

Common duct stones (choledocholithiasis) occasionally cause persistent jaundice. More commonly, a stone acts as a ball valve, creating intermittent obstruction and a fluctuating bilirubin. An unexplained hyperbilirubinemia (rarely over 5 mg per 100 ml) accompanies some cases of acute cholecystitis without common duct calculi or pancreatitis.

Obstructive jaundice may produce secondary effects such as pruritus, steatorrhea, and bleeding tendencies. Although a definite correlation has not been established between the serum level of bile salts and pruritus, bile salts do accumulate in the skin during biliary obstruction and are thought to cause the itching. Steatorrhea and poor hemostasis are due to the exclusion of bile salts from the small bowel. Since conjugated bile salts are essential for the normal digestion and absorption of lipids, their absence causes excessive loss of fat and the fat-soluble vitamins A, D, E, and K in feces. The loss of vitamins A, D, and E are of little clinical consequence unless the obstruction is of long duration (biliary cirrhosis). However, vitamin K deficiency develops rapidly, within 1 to 3 weeks, depressing the synthesis of prothrombin (factor II), proconvertin (factor VII), Christmas factor (factor IX), and Stuart factor (factor X).

Fever and chills Fever is a common symptom of acute cholecystitis but is uncommon in the chronic form. The presence of fever may be due to sterile, obstructive inflammation in some patients, but infection may play a major role in most cases of acute cholecystitis, as bacteria are cultured from 75 percent of the gallbladder specimens or bile. Cultures are positive in less than 50 percent of patients with chronic cholecystitis. Chills and fever signal bacteremia and are usually associated with complications of biliary tract disease such as choledocholithiasis, strictures, and fistulas. When accompanied by pain in the right hypochrondrium, with or without hyperbilirubinemia, fever and chills suggest cholangitis. A combination of infection plus incomplete biliary stasis results in cholangitis.

Cancers which obstruct the common bile duct rarely lead to clinical cholangitis, and bile cultures from such patients are usually negative. The reasons for this useful differential fact are unclear, because all cancers for some time will produce only partial ductal obstruction. Partial (stones) or remitting obstruction (some cases of ampullary carcinoma) is occasionally complicated by cholangitis.

Bleeding Hemorrhage into the biliary passages (hemobilia) is rare, dramatic, and sometimes lethal. The diagnostic triad is right upper quadrant pain, obstructive jaundice (secondary to clots in the biliary tree), and gastrointestinal bleeding. This typical presentation may be altered by massive bleeding or by slow, intermittent blood loss. The biliary system is such an unusual source of gastrointestinal hemorrhage that a diagnosis of hemobilia is seldom made preoperatively; it should be suspected when other causes of bleeding have been eliminated by investigation and exploration. A wide variety of diseases produce hemobilia, most commonly ruptured aneurysms of the hepatic artery or its branches, tumors and inflammatory diseases of the biliary system, trauma (including T-tube pressure necrosis or liver biopsy), choledocholithiasis, and rarely cholecystitis, with or without stones.

BILIARY TRACT RADIOLOGY In 1923 the gallbladder was opacified for the first time by Graham and Cole using an intravenous iodinated phthalein dye. Prior to this, the diagnosis of gallbladder disease depended entirely upon the demonstration of radiopaque calculi, calcium deposits in the gallbladder wall, and milk of calcium bile or gas within the biliary ducts. Although only one in five gallstones contains enough calcium to be visible on plain abdominal films, oral cholecystography identifies 70 percent of all gallstones. In an additional 20 to 28 percent, nonvisualization of the gallbladder is presumptive evidence of disease. Nonvisualization is defined as failure of the gallbladder to opacify following a second dose of contrast medium. The overall accuracy of oral cholecystography, proved in the operating room, is 90 to 98 percent. Only 3 percent of nonfunctioning gallbladders are normal at operation, and less than 2 percent of gallbladders, normal by cholecystogram, contain stones.

This high level of accuracy requires that certain conditions be satisfied: intestinal motility and absorption must be normal, hepatocellular function must be adequate to excrete the dye, and the serum bilirubin must not be increasing or greater than 3 mg per 100 ml. Thirty percent of the nonvisualizing and 64 percent of the poorly concentrating gallbladders will opacify normally following the second dose. Small stones may be obscured if the gallbladder still concentrates the dye normally; upright or lateral spot films should be done to avoid this error (Fig. 300-2). A fatty meal, given if stones are not obvious, stimulates gallbladder evacuation and enhances the detection of low-density stones obscured by a heavy concentration of dye. "Failure to contract" or poor concentration of dye has little diagnostic significance.

Despite its value in detecting gallbladder disease, oral cholecystography yields little information about the hepatic ductal system. Common or hepatic duct stones are present in 15 percent of all patients with cholelithiasis but are identified in 2 percent by oral cholecystography. In 1953, the availability of sodium iodipamide made possible *intravenous cholangiography*. The larger biliary channels opacify in 10 to 30 min, reaching maximal concentrations at 30 to 40 min, provided liver function is normal. A maximally opacified common duct, with an unimpeded flow of dye into the duodenum, decreases in radiodensity within 60 min. Partial obstruction of the common duct prevents normal emptying and prolongs maximum opacification up to 2 hr. The normal common duct diameter is variable; values greater than 9 to 10 mm are considered abnormal, yet one out of four patients with stones has a common duct less than 10 mm in diameter. The common duct dilates very little (approximately 1 mm) after cholecystectomy, but a more accurate correlation between duct size and pathologic changes can be obtained if the preoperative dimensions of the common duct are available for comparison. Adverse reactions to intravenous cholangiography include nausea, vomiting, hypotension, and rare anaphylactic reactions. The procedure should be reserved for patients with previous cholecystectomies, nonvisualizing oral cholecystograms, and acute conditions of the upper abdomen.

A third method for exploring the biliary system is *operative cholangiography*. The procedure involves the introduction of contrast substance into the gallbladder, cystic duct, or common duct at operation, followed by radiography. Properly utilized, operative cholangiography is a valuable adjunct to cholecystectomy. In one large series, the procedure decreased the need for choledochotomy by nearly 50 percent while doubling the number of positive explorations. This was achieved at no increase in morbidity or mortality.

Percutaneous transhepatic cholangiography helps to distinguish extrahepatic from intrahepatic obstruction. A needle is inserted into the liver, and when it enters a dilated intrahepatic duct, bile is drained through a flexible polyethylene catheter, and radiopaque dye is injected to define the biliary anatomy (Fig. 300-2). If, after several hepatic punctures, a dilated duct is not entered, the jaundice is assumed to be of hepatocellular origin and a possibly harmful exploration deferred. Percutaneous cholangiography should be performed only on good surgical candidates, because bleeding or bile peritonitis necessitates immediate intervention in 5 percent of patients.

Finally, fiberoptic duodenoscopy is becoming a more frequently used procedure and, in experienced hands, is a relatively simple and noninvasive method of visualizing the biliary-pancreatic ductal systems. Intubation of the papilla of Vater followed by injection of contrast material under fluoroscopic control has produced excellent diagnostic cholangiograms (and pancreatograms).

BILIARY TRACT MANOMETRY Biliary radiomanometry is a diagnostic technique combining simultaneous pressure readings and contrast roentgenographic studies of the gallbladder and bile ducts, and is commonly done during biliary surgical procedures in many European and Latin American countries. Its proponents point out that although cholangiography provides excellent anatomic detail, it does not reveal motor dysfunction of the ducts or sphincter. Because operative fluoroscopy is impractical, intraluminal manometric pressure curves are substituted. The fact that these pressures are recorded during anesthesia and surgical manipulation of the ducts raises doubt as to their physiologic significance.

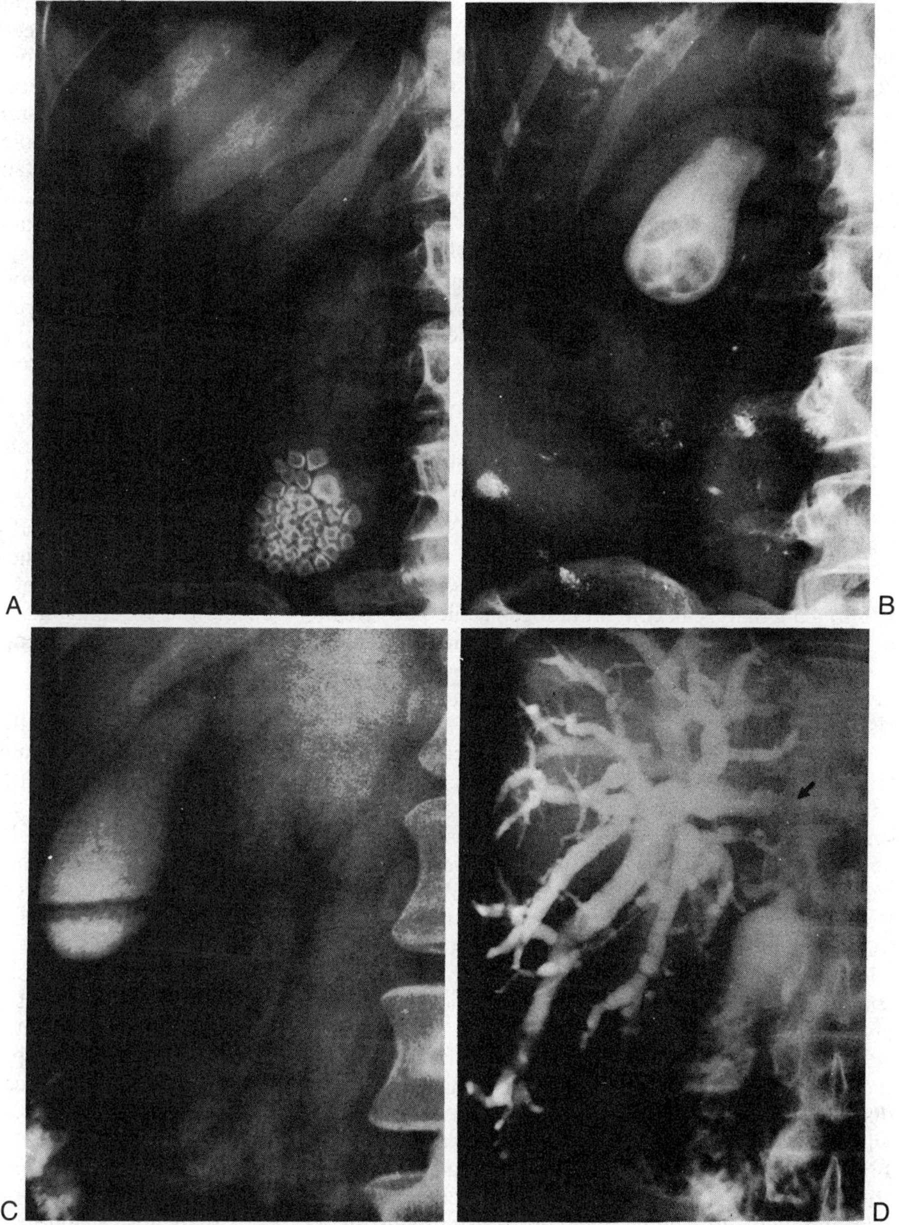

FIGURE 300-2

Contrast studies of the biliary tract. A *Cholelithiasis. Multiple radiopaque stones in a gallbladder with impaired concentrating ability.* B *Cholelithiasis. Nonopaque stones of varying sizes are shown as negative shadows within a gallbladder outlined by concentrated dye.* C *Cholelithiasis. Numerous small stones are grouped in a layer near the bottom of the gallbladder. This picture was taken with the patient standing. Small stones such as these are dispersed when the patient is in a horizontal position and may be difficult to see.* D *Percutaneous transhepatic cholangiogram. The needle, seen in the center of the figure, has punctured a dilated bile duct, and the injected contrast medium shows marked distention of the bile ducts in the right lobe of the liver but no filling of the left lobe. This was due to a bile duct carcinoma which completely blocked the left main hepatic duct and partially occluded the right main duct (*black arrow*), allowing a small amount of dye to enter the duodenum (*lower right*) and the gallbladder, which overlies the duodenal bulb.*

GALLSTONES Etiology Although many questions concerning the pathogenesis of different types of gallstones remain unanswered, recent work has advanced the hypothesis that the cholesterol gallstone, the common gallstone of the United States and westernized countries, is a result of hepatic dysfunction and not a disease of the gallbladder. The evidence suggests that the primary abnormality is the secretion by the liver of an abnormal (lithogenic) bile that is supersaturated with cholesterol. This "pre-stone" state is endemic among young American Indians of various tribes. The true age-specific prevalence of gallstones in Indian men increased only gradually between the ages of fifteen and sixty-five years but increased from less than 1 percent at age eighteen to greater than 75 percent at age thirty-one in women. In those with gallstones when hepatic bile was analyzed for biliary lipids and plotted on triangular coordinates, as in Fig. 300-1, the composition fell outside the micellar zone, and cholesterol microcrystals were visible by microscopy. Gallbladder bile composition fell on the line of saturation. Similar findings are also present in Caucasian patients with gallstones.

Patients with cholesterol stones have a decreased bile salt pool, reduced hepatic secretion of bile salts and phospholipids, and a cholesterol secretion which is not proportionately diminished. The defect in the control of bile acid synthesis which leads to and maintains the low pool size is unclear.

The formation of cholesterol gallstones occurs in stages:

1 *Chemical stage:* secretion of lithogenic hepatic bile supersaturated with cholesterol.
2 *Crystallization stage:* the excess cholesterol precipitates as monohydrate microcrystals in the gallbladder.
3 *Growth stage:* coalescence of cholesterol crystals to form macroscopic stones.

It has been shown that feeding chenodeoxycholic acid, 0.75 to 4.5 g daily, can convert lithogenic bile into bile of normal composition and cause the dissolution of cholesterol gallstones *in situ*. Such therapy, if proved safe, may also *prevent* gallstone formation among persons in high risk groups.

An increased fecal loss of bile salts occurs whenever the enterohepatic circulation is interrupted. The liver can compensate for this loss by increasing the rate of bile salt synthesis. However, when the fecal loss exceeds 30 percent of the bile salts secreted, the liver's synthetic capacity is insufficient to maintain a normal bile salt pool. Depletion of the bile salt pool may result in the secondary formation of lithogenic bile. It is this alteration in hepatic bile which is presumably responsible for the high prevalence of gallstones in patients with regional enteritis involving the distal ileum.

Infection is considered to play a role in lithogenesis by the following theories. (1) The proteinaceous debris produced by inflammatory injury is a potential focus upon which various salts precipitate and stone growth begins. Injury alters normal mucosal function, causing a reabsorption of bile salts and lecithin. (2) Deconjugation of bilirubin diglucuronide by β-glucuronidase-producing organisms (*Escherichia coli*); the free bilirubin seeds bile as insoluble calcium bilirubinate crystals. (3) Deconjugation of bile salts (e.g., by *Streptococcus fecalis*) leads to precipitation or absorption of bile acids, and hence to reduced solubility of cholesterol in bile.

Stasis was regarded by Aschoff as "the essential and common cause of gallstone formation." Factors which change the normal physiochemical composition of bile can produce cholesterol monohydrate or calcium bilirubinate crystals. To form gallstones, the net rate of formation of these substances must exceed the net rate of crystal dissolution or passage out of the gallbladder. Stasis would influence this equilibrium, favoring stone growth. A common cause of gallbladder stasis is total vagotomy. Acute animal studies suggest that bile obtained from vagotomized animals has lithogenic potential. Thus, patients with lithogenic bile who undergo pyloroplasty and total vagotomy have an increased risk of developing gallstones.

Nucleation of lithogenic bile is poorly understood. Possible candidates as seeding agents for cholesterol are bile pigments, bacteria, precipitated bile salts, and calcium carbonate. Modern analytic techniques do not disclose one dominant substance in the center of gallstones but a mixed core of cholesterol, bilirubin, and protein. Once the nucleus is established, small stones must be trapped within the gallbladder, perhaps by mucus. For the stones to enlarge, a constant supply of crystals containing abnormal bile is necessary.

The principal stone-forming constituents of bile are cholesterol, calcium bilirubinate, and calcium carbonate. Traditionally, gallstones have been classified as pure (10 percent), mixed (80 percent), and combined (10 percent), with the implication that "pure" gallstones are a product of a metabolic derangement or of excessive bilirubin excretion, while mixed stones are caused by infection. Modern analytic techniques do not disclose one dominant substance in the center of gallstones but a mixed core of cholesterol, bilirubin, and protein, suggesting a common cause. However, once the nucleus has been established, gallstones grow by accretion, and their final composition reflects the predominant bile constituents at the time of crystallization. For example, in chronic hemolytic anemias, the stones contain mainly calcium bilirubinate.

Prevalence Although the true prevalence of gallstones in the United States is unknown, it is estimated that 12 million women and 4 million men have gallstones, with an additional 800,000 new cases appearing annually. Each year 500,000 people are hospitalized for gallstones, and more than half have a cholecystectomy. Considering the magnitude of the problem, the associated mortality is relatively low (about 6,000 annually).

The aphorism "forty, female, fertile, and fat" may describe certain patients, but it does not characterize a typical gallstone patient. Above twenty years of age, stones are more frequent in women than in men, but the sex difference becomes progressively less after age fifty. There is no clear evidence that pregnancy predisposes to the formation of gallstones, but in patients with gallstones symptoms are more likely to develop during pregnancy. When obese, normal-weight, and thin patients are compared, the frequency of gallstones does not differ. However diabetics, at autopsy, have a greater incidence of stones (2:1) than nondiabetics.

Symptoms and signs Gallstones may be silent (50 percent) or give rise to excruciating pain, chills, and fever. Between these extremes are a multitude of nonspecific abdominal disturbances which may represent coexisting disease rather than symptomatic gallstones. Right upper quadrant pain or tenderness and jaundice are the most clinically useful expressions of cholelithiasis.

Diagnosis The characteristic manifestation of gallstones is biliary colic. The simplest and most rewarding test of gallbladder function is an oral cholecystogram, provided the necessary criteria are fulfilled. If this and other roentgenologic techniques do not elucidate the diagnosis, some clinicians find duodenal drainage useful. The recovery of cholesterol crystals or, to a lesser degree, bilirubinate granules is important supportive evidence of cholecystic disease in the symptomatic, nonjaundiced patient with a normal Bromsulphalin (BSP) excretion.

Course and indications for surgical treatment The most important complications of gallstones are acute and chronic cholecystitis, choledocholithiasis, and pancreatitis. Less common complications are cholangitis, hepatic abscesses, biliary cirrhosis, empyema, fistulous communication to adjacent viscera, and gallstone ileus.

Biliary colic, with or without associated complications, is an indication for cholecystectomy, the cure rate approaching 90 percent. Patients can live a normal life and eat a normal diet without a gallbladder. Medical management of symptomatic gallstones is unsatisfactory because low-fat diets and anticholinergic drugs do not prevent recurrent attacks. However, therapeutic recommendations for patients with chronic, intermittent "digestive symptoms" who are found to harbor gallstones require deliberation. In many, symptoms will not respond to cholecystectomy despite the presence of stones. Therefore, a search for coexisting disease which might be responsible for "digestive symptoms" is mandatory before proceeding to cholecystectomy.

The management of the "silent" gallstone has been debated for years. Statistics pointing out the various complications of surgically untreated gallstones are compiled from symptomatic patients who have refused surgical treatment. Unfortunately, there are no prospective studies of patients with truly silent and surgically untreated stones. Until such information becomes available, silent stones in patients over sixty years of age should be treated conservatively, since the risks of elective surgical treatment beyond this age exceed the risks of developing complications of the gallstones. If and when biliary colic develops, cholecystectomy is indicated. Diabetics with silent stones are an exception to this policy: diabetics and nondiabetics tolerate elective cholecystectomy equally well, but the morbidity and mortality of emergency cholecystectomy is greater in diabetics. Sixty to 80 percent of primary gallbladder cancers have associated gallstones. Despite this high correlation, the evidence is against a direct causal relation. Nevertheless, there is statistic evidence suggesting that prophylactic removal of asymptomatic stones in patients under forty five years may prevent cancer. Above age sixty five, the surgical mortality exceeds the risk of succumbing to cancer.

As mentioned above, the prolonged oral bile acid administration (chenodeoxycholic and cholic) appears to be moderately effective in the dissolution of gallstones. Bile acid administration favors stone dissolution by increasing the total bile acid pool. Except for diarrhea, no toxic side effects have been noted, but the overall role of oral bile acid feeding in the dissolution of stones, especially silent gallstones, remains to be determined.

ACUTE CHOLECYSTITIS Acute cholecystitis is associated with a gallstone impacted in the cystic duct in 90 to 95 percent of cases. Sudden distention of the gallbladder compromises its blood supply and lymphatic drainage, and commensal bacteria which normally inhabit calculous gallbladders proliferate. Approximately five percent of all cases of acute cholecystitis have no associated gallstones (acalculous cholecystitis). Trauma and surgery, unrelated to the biliary system, appear to be the most common antecedent cause of acalculous cholecystitis.

Symptoms and signs Severe right upper quadrant pain, nausea, vomiting, fever, and minimal icterus suggest the diagnosis. However, the pain can be mild, sensed only as an epigastric distress, often relieved by vomiting. If pain radiates to the shoulder or subscapular region, the diagnosis is strengthened. Severe epigastric pain with overt jaundice suggests the complication of choledocholithiasis. Fever is found in over two-thirds of the patients. Local signs include muscle guarding or tenderness in the gallbladder area with discomfort on fist percussion over the liver. A tender mass comprising the swollen gallbladder and adherent omentum is palpable in approximately 50 percent of cases.

Laboratory findings and x-rays The leukocyte count is elevated over a wide range of values, depending on the inflammatory reaction. Low-grade hyperbilirubinemia, increased serum alkaline phosphatase activity, and retention of BSP are often found. Serum glutamic transaminase and lactic dehydrogenase activities are occasionally increased; marked, transient increases in both enzymes suggest common duct stones. Oral cholecystography is of little diagnostic value during the acute attack.

Diagnosis Pain and tenderness in the right upper quadrant are the most frequent and important diagnostic clues to acute cholecystitis, and a past history of similar disturbances makes the diagnosis nearly certain. The differential diagnosis should include, in decreasing order of the frequency with which they simulate cholecystitis, myocardial infarction, perforated or penetrating ulcer, pancreatitis, right lower lobe pneumonia, intestinal obstruction, and acute right kidney disease. X-rays of the chest and abdomen, electrocardiograms, serum amylase or lipase determinations, and urinalysis will exclude, in the majority of patients, many of the diseases mentioned. Intravenous cholangiography has been used to differentiate between acute cholecystitis and pancreatitis. Opacification of the common duct without gallbladder filling favors cholecystitis, whereas opacification of the biliary ducts and gallbladder excludes cholecystitis. However, impaired excretion of the dye and no visualization is common in both diseases. Cancers of the gallbladder and bile ducts have no clinical features which distinguish them from benign gallbladder diseases.

Course Approximately 75 percent of patients with acute cholecystitis have complete remission of symptoms within 1 to 4 days on conservative management. Patients with *only* local evidence of cholecystitis can be treated at home with bed rest and appropriate analgesics in anticipation of radiologic examination of the biliary and gastrointestinal tracts. Those with signs of systemic toxicity will require hospitalization and intensive fluid and antibiotic treatment. In 25 percent toxemia is progressive and urgent surgical intervention is necessary to prevent lethal complications (gangrene, perforation, empyema, pancreatitis, and cholangitis). In the aged patient cholecystitis is a particularly dangerous disease, because fever and leukocytosis may occur with minimal clinical or chemical evidence of gallbladder disease.

CHRONIC CHOLECYSTITIS Repeated attacks of mild to severe acute cholecystitis merit the clinical diagnosis of chronic cholecystitis. Pathologically, the gallbladder mucosa and smooth muscle are partly replaced by fibrous tissue, and biochemically the ability to concentrate bile is impaired. The symptoms are similar to the acute form and range from biliary colic to indolent right upper quadrant and epigastric distress. Low-grade fever and hyperbilirubinemia are common. The diagnosis is confirmed by failure of the gallbladder to opacify after two doses of contrast medium. At operation, 95 percent of these gallbladders are sclerotic and contain stones. Cholecystectomy will cure 9 of 10 patients with this clinical presentation. Patients with chronic, vague abdominal discomfort and dyspeptic symptoms are often thought to have chronic cholecystitis despite roentgenographic evidence of a normally functioning gallbladder. Their surgical specimens may show minor mucosal abnormalities, but the patients usually obtain no relief from their symptoms.

CHOLEDOCHOLITHIASIS Calculi usually reach the bile ducts by expulsion from the gallbladder. This organ can generate an impressive force even in the presence of disease. Thus stones, demonstrated radiographically to be filling the gallbladder and the cystic and common ducts, have been shown to be completely dislodged from the biliary tree following a typical attack of biliary colic. The incidence of unsuspected common duct stones during routine cholecystectomy is 6 to 26 percent, the figure increasing with age. Common duct stones may be found without concomitant stones in the gallbladder or may occur years after cholecystectomy. These stones appear because of stasis or infection and may also form in the hepatic ducts.

Symptoms and signs The symptoms of choledocholithiasis are pain, jaundice, fever, and chills. The pain is steady, is localized to the epigastrium, often radiates to the back and right hypochondrium, and is associated with vomiting. Common duct stones rarely cause persistent obstruction; the jaundice is usually transient and mild, and frequently is missed entirely. Twenty percent of patients with choledocholithiasis have no pain and 25 percent no evidence of jaundice. Spiking fevers indicate cholangitis. The most frequently identified organisms are of enteric origin (*E. coli* and *S. fecalis*). Intermittent fever with chills and sweats but without pain or clinical jaundice has been referred to as *Charcot's hepatic fever*.

Physical signs of common duct stones include jaundice and upper abdominal tenderness. A history of cholecystectomy and common duct exploration does not exclude common duct stones; the frequency of residual calculi is an alarming 10 percent. While most gallbladders associated with choledochal stones are fibrotic and unable to dilate, a distended (but not always palpable) gallbladder occurs with 20 percent of obstructing common duct stones. Intravenous cholangiography will directly identify common duct stones in 50 to 60 percent of cases. When delayed emptying and dilatation of the common duct are included as indirect signs of stones, cholangiography detects 90 percent of cases.

Laboratory findings and x-rays The laboratory features of choledocholithiasis may include leukocytosis, elevated levels of serum bilirubin, alkaline phosphatase, glutamic transaminase, and amylase, and BSP retention. The true incidence with which these biochemical alterations accompany common duct stones is uncertain, since the changes may be fleeting. The transaminases usually do not exceed 300 units. Bromsulphalein retention is the most sensitive indicator of choledochal calculi but is not as specific for obstruction as the alkaline phosphatase. Striking increases in alkaline phosphatase can occur with minimal increases in bilirubin. One of four patients will present with an elevated amylase level, presumably due to passage, or impaction of, a stone in the ampulla of Vater, causing pancreatic edema and occasional hemorrhagic necrosis.

Diagnosis Common duct stones may be present without clinical, chemical, or radiologic clues to their existence. These asymptomatic cases may develop suppurative cholangitis, which is often lethal in older patients. A painless common duct stone with jaundice must be differentiated from malignant disease and various forms of hepatitis. Intravenous cholangiography is of little value when the serum bilirubin is rising. If the disease is hepatitis, exploration increases its mortality. Percutaneous transhepatic cholangiography is useful in this situation; failure to enter a dilated duct after five hepatic punctures is presumptive evidence of hepatocellular disease. Liver biopsy may be attempted later.

GALLSTONE ILEUS

Intestinal obstruction secondary to a gallstone is an unusual complication of cholelithiasis and accounts for 2 percent of all small-bowel obstructions. The stone usually lodges at the terminal ileum, the narrowest portion of the normal gut, but stones can become impacted in the pylorus, duodenum, jejunum, or colon. The pathophysiology involves repeated episodes of acute cholecystitis, adhesions to adjacent hollow viscera, and the opening of a cholecystoenteric fistula. Most fistulas develop between the gallbladder and duodenum, but communications into the stomach and colon can occur. Stones less than 3 cm in diameter usually pass through the gut spontaneously.

Gallstone ileus is a disease of the elderly. Early symptoms may be vague and transient, because of intermittent obstruction. Even when the classic symptoms of intestinal obstruction are present, there is often delay before the urgency of the situation is appreciated. The average mortality is 30 percent. Helpful in the diagnosis of gallstone ileus is a history of cholecystitis, abdominal films showing intestinal obstruction with a radiopaque density in the lower abdomen, or x-ray evidence of a changing level of obstruction. Air outlining the biliary tree, in the absence of previous biliary surgical treatment, is virtually pathognomonic of a cholecystoenteric fistula.

Meticulous surgical exploration is necessary to exclude additional stones; the recurrence rate of gallstone ileus is 10 to 15 percent.

HYDROPS, EMPYEMA, AND ABSCESS A gallstone wedged into the cystic duct will cause hydrops or empyema in some 15 percent of cases. In both conditions, the gallbladder becomes distended to several times its normal volume. The trapped bile is sterile in the case of hydrops and infected in empyema. A curious and rare sequela of cystic duct obstruction is the deposition of milk of calcium bile within the gallbladder. It is of clinical importance, because the homogenous distribution of calcium salts produces a shadow compatible with a normal dye-filled gallbladder. Frank perforation of the gallbladder causing generalized peritonitis occurs in less than 1 percent of patients with acute cholecystitis. The omentum and serosa of contiguous viscera localize the perforation early, often producing a palpable mass and a friction rub. Cholecystostomy or cholecystectomy is indicated, depending on the clinical situation.

TREATMENT OF GALLSTONES AND THEIR COMPLICATIONS Symptomatic cholelithiasis is a surgical disease. The internist's role is to alleviate symptoms and prepare the patient for surgical treatment. Morphine is commonly used to relieve biliary colic despite the fact that it increases intrabiliary pressure. The spasmogenic effect of morphine on the sphincter of Oddi is nullified by combination with atropine. Meperidine, contrary to earlier opinion, shares with morphine the capacity to produce sphincter spasm. Less acutely ill patients respond to analgesics, sedation, and bed rest. Cholangitis should be treated with antibiotics effective in gram-negative infections.

Although intolerance to fats is not related to a specific disease, fat restriction in patients with documented gallstones is rational because it diminishes cholecystokinin response and lessens the chances of precipitating biliary colic. Gastric acid or peptones also liberate cholecystokinin, but together with fat cause the most prolonged release of the hormone.

The following general rules apply to the surgical management of biliary tract diseases:

1 Acute cholecystitis is ideally treated by cholecystectomy, but the timing of the operation is controversial. Many physicians favor intervention within the first 48 hr. Others, citing the predisposition to traumatic bile duct injury in edematous cholecystitis, prefer to wait 1 to 3 weeks unless the patient deteriorates.

   It is prudent not to attempt cholecystectomy with impending perforation or necrosis of the gallbladder. In this situation, as in the debilitated patient with acute cholecystitis, simple gallbladder drainage (cholecystostomy) may be lifesaving. Cholecystostomy is also indicated when, at surgical dissection, inflammation obscures vital structures. Fifty percent of these patients who survive over 2 years will eventually need cholecystectomy.

2 If jaundice is the presenting symptom, diagnosis is more difficult, and clinical observation for 1 to 3 weeks may be necessary. Jaundice per se seldom requires immediate exploration unless cholangitis is suspected. The liver will tolerate uninfected obstruction for 6 weeks before fibrosis develops.

3 The decision to explore the common duct is based on the following criteria: a history of jaundice or pancreatitis, palpable ductal stones, gallbladder gravel or calculi smaller than the diameter of the cystic duct, and a dilated common duct. The frequency with which choledochostomy is performed varies from 7 to 42 percent, reflecting individual interpretation of these criteria. Stones are found in approximately half of the common ducts explored. Theoretically, with a combination of history, laboratory data, preoperative cholangiography, and the surgeon's evaluation at operation, exploration will be positive in 93 percent of cases, will miss stones in 2 percent, and will be unnecessary in only 5 percent. Following choledochostomy, a T tube is left in the common duct draining bile to the exterior of the body. The tube also serves for postoperative cholangiography and is pulled out after 12 days.

POSTCHOLECYSTECTOMY SYNDROME

The postcholecystectomy syndrome describes a group of symptoms of variable severity and cause which follow removal of the gallbladder. Much confusion is associated with this entity, because it is used loosely to cover symptoms unrelated to gallbladder disease. It is a misnomer in many patients who complain of the same symptoms they had prior to cholecystectomy. Analysis of these patients reveals that, in the majority, the indications for cholecystectomy were not clear. Symptoms in this group are commonly due to extrabiliary causes: hiatus hernia, ulcer diathesis, chronic pancreatitis, or functional colonic disorders. However, there are patients with bona fide indications for cholecystectomy whose symptoms continue postoperatively as well as some who develop new symptoms referable to the biliary tract. This group is most representative of the postcholecystectomy syndrome. Symptoms are usually due to incomplete surgical measures (residual choledocholithiasis, cystic duct and gallbladder remnants, overlooked malignancy, biliary fistula) or surgical trauma (bile duct strictures, stenosis of the sphincter of Oddi). The postcholecystectomy syndrome is "often disregarded by the surgeon, recognized by the physician, battled with by the general practitioner and must prove such a bitter disappointment to the patient" (Mallet-Guy, 1956).

STRICTURE

Stricture is the most common complication of operative damage to the extrahepatic ducts. In a series of 1,600 biliary strictures, 96 percent were related to trauma during biliary surgical procedures. One out of 300 to 500 cholecystectomies results in a stricture, with fatal sequelae in about 30 percent of cases. Factors which predispose to these injuries are anatomic abnormalities and surgical treatment during the edematous or late fibrotic phase of cholecystitis. The repair of a stricture often entails a series of difficult reconstructive operations, and some patients remain permanently disabled by secondary liver damage.

Postoperative jaundice or a biliary fistula suggests bile duct injury. Jaundice is the most common finding, evident within the first postoperative week. An external fistula should be suspected if the wound continues to discharge bile after 7 days. Spontaneous internal choledochoduodenal fistulas may leave the patient entirely asymptomatic, but few function adequately. Fever, chills, and varying degrees of jaundice soon appear. Early recognition and repair offer a good prognosis.

BILIARY CIRRHOSIS

(See also Chap. 296)

Biliary cirrhosis, secondary to chronic choledocholithiasis or bile duct stricture, is a disastrous complication of gallstones, usually resulting from lack of recognition or failure of therapy by the physician, or neglect by the patient. While hepatic fibrosis develops as early as 2 months after complete obstruction, even in the absence of significant infection, its progression can generally be stopped and reversed by relief of the obstruction at this early stage. With continuing obstruction and particularly with infection, pruritus, jaundice, steatorrhea, and portal hypertension progressively afflict the patient. Treatment of pruritus is difficult: local applications are of little value; antihistamines help some patients; methyltestosterone or norethandrolone suppress itching but may aggravate the hyperbilirubinemia; cholestyramine, an anion exchange resin, interrupts the enterohepatic circulation of bile salts and improves pruritus but aggravates steatorrhea by further reducing the bile salt concentration in the gut lumen. Calcium supplements and intramuscular vitamin D and K may be necessary.

OTHER DISEASES

BILIARY DYSKINESIA Under normal circumstances, food entering the duodenum stimulates smoothly integrated evacuation of bile from the biliary tree. The concept that pain may arise from a purely motor derangement has been postulated since 1887, when Oddi stated that interference with the coordination of biliary kinetics, i.e., contraction of a gallbladder against a tonic sphincter, could result in pain, jaundice, or both. Since then a vast literature has accumulated concerning "biliary distress" without demonstrable organic lesions in the extrahepatic system. Biliary dyskinesia includes three different kinds of motor dysfunction: disturbances in evacuation (dyskinesia), disorders of tone (dystonia), and disturbances of coordination (dyssynergia).

Biliary dyskinesia can be compared with the spastic colon syndrome, as both conditions share a negative clinical and laboratory evaluation. However, they differ in that many patients with biliary dyskinesia undergo surgical procedures based on operative biliary dynamics, including sphincterotomy, choledochoduodenostomy, vagotomy, or splanchnicectomy. Few patients benefit from these procedures, and a lack of correlation among symptoms, pressure studies, and surgical results has evoked skepticism in the United States and Great Britain regarding biliary dyskinesia as a disease entity.

Symptoms, signs, and diagnosis The clinical manifestations of biliary dyskinesia may run the gamut of traditional symptoms of acute or chronic cholecystitis with the exception that fever, chills, and leukocytosis are rarely noted. The patients are usually anxious females whose symptoms correlate well with emotional tension, situational stress, and fatigue. Their past histories often include investigations for nausea, headaches, giddiness, diarrhea, or constipation. Comprehensive evaluation of liver and pancreatic function together with conventional roentgenographic studies of the biliary system reveal no abnormalities. The following are used by enthusiasts to evaluate these patients: (1) pain, indistinguishable from biliary colic, precipitated by morphine, is taken as evidence of sphincter dysfunction; (2) timed duodenal drainage compares the appearance, volume, and duration of flow of various bile fractions (gallbladder versus hepatic bile); (3) cinecholecystography is used to compare structure and function of the biliary tree; (4) operative radiomanometry is considered in many areas of the world as a definitive investigation.

Treatment The management of patients suspected of biliary dyskinesia requires careful assessment of the symptoms in relation to food, alcohol, chronic intake of medications, and tensions. Reassurance, phenothiazines, sedation, analgesics, and anticholinergics, alone or in combination, should be tried on an empiric basis.

PRIMARY SCLEROSING CHOLANGITIS This is a rare entity involving the extrahepatic biliary ducts, producing progressive biliary cirrhosis. It may appear alone or associated with ulcerative colitis, regional enteritis, gallstones, or other primary fibrotic processes such as periureteral or pulmonary fibrosis. The presenting symptoms are those of biliary obstruction. A definitive diagnosis is possible only at exploration. Attempts at both medical and surgical treatment have provided, at best, only temporary relief. However, some patients have done well with high steroids every other day, depending on changes in bilirubin levels. Antibiotics such as tetracycline may be given 5 to 7 days of each month.

CANCER OF THE GALLBLADDER Primary cancer of the gallbladder is predominantly a disease of older women. In gallbladder operations it has been recorded with a frequency of 0.2 to 5 percent, the higher figure occurring in patients over sixty-five years of age. A causal relation between gallstones and cancer of the gallbladder is not established. Carcinoma of the gallbladder is insidious; persistent right upper quadrant pain with weight loss and anorexia should alert the clinician. A common physical finding is a hard mass associated with the liver. Jaundice is usually a terminal event, due to obstruction of the common duct or metastasis to the liver. Five-year survival is less than 3 percent, regardless of treatment.

CANCER OF THE BILE DUCTS Carcinoma of the bile ducts is also a disease of old age but is more prevalent in males. It is encountered in 1 of every 1,000 biliary tract operations, the common duct most often being involved. Although the jaundice of ampullary carcinoma sometimes fluctuates because necrotic tumor sloughs into the duodenum, the jaundice of bile duct carcinoma is unremitting. Contrary to the poor results of radical surgical treatment with other biliary tract carcinomas, ampullary carcinoma has a 5-year survival rate of 40 percent. Approximately one-third of the patients with ampullary or bile duct cancer have a palpable gallbladder and two-thirds an enlarged liver. Percutaneous cholangiography is the most useful procedure available, often localizing the lesion for operation.

CONGENITAL ABNORMALITIES Congenital abnormalities of the gallbladder include complete absence of the viscus, anomalous structure such as double gallbladder, and unusual position within the liver. The bile ducts are also subject to numerous congenital defects, among which atresia and cystic dilatation are the most prominent. Surgeons must be wary of many normal variations of the biliary tree and blood vessels.

UNUSUAL INFECTIONS *Cholecystitis* due to *Salmonella typhosa* still accounts for some typhoid carriers. Patients with salmonellosis and gallstones should undergo cholecystectomy after antibiotic treatment of the *Salmonella* infection. Tuberculosis, syphilis, actinomycosis, and septic emboli are very infrequent causes of biliary tract infection. The characteristic lesions of periarteritis nodosa are sometimes prominent in the walls of the gallbladder, which may not fill on cholecystography.

Ascaris worms, liver flukes, and *echinococcus cysts* may cause biliary obstruction with cholangitis and jaundice.

Small *polypoid masses* are occasionally found in the gallbladder, but their clinical significance is controversial. Many of these polyps are merely mucosal prominences containing localized cholesterol deposits; some are hamartomas, and rarely true adenomatous growths occur. The lesions cannot be held responsible for symptoms. That the adenomatous polyps progress to cancer is an unproved assertion used by those who insist on cholecystectomy whenever a polyp is discovered radiologically in the gallbladder. Adenomyomatosis is the solitary, segmental, or diffuse proliferation of surface gallbladder epithelium with the formation of either ducts, crypts, or diverticula (Rokitansky-Aschoff sinuses). It is a congenital lesion and is without clinical significance.

REFERENCES

Bouchier IAD: Gallstone formation. Lancet 1:711, 1971

Blumgart LH et al: Endoscopy and retrograde choledochopancreatography in the diagnosis of the jaundiced patient. Lancet 2:1269, 1972

Danzinger RG et al: Dissolution of cholesterol gallstones by chenodeoxycholic acid. N Engl J Med 286:1, 1972

Donaldson RM: Diet and gastrointestinal disorders. Gastroenterology 52:897, 1967

Flemma RJ et al: Bacteriologic studies of biliary tract infection. Ann Surg 166:563, 1967

Hofmann AF, Small DM: Detergent properties of bile salts: Correlation with physiological function. Annu Rev Med 18:333, 1967

Northfield TC, Hoffmann AF: Biliary lipid secretion in gallstone patients. Lancet 1:747, 1973

Shaffer EA et al: Bile composition at and after surgery in normal persons and patients with gallstones. Influence of cholecystectomy. N Engl J Med 287:1317, 1972

Small DM: Gallstones. N Engl J Med 279:588, 1968

section 7 | Disorders of the pancreas

301 APPROACH TO THE DIAGNOSIS OF PANCREATIC DISEASE

PHILIP J. SNODGRASS

The discussion in Chap. 302 indicates that diseases of the pancreas are characterized by a wide spectrum of possible symptoms and signs and a lack of sterotyped clinical patterns. Thus a so-called "classic case" is the exception rather than the rule for acute or chronic pancreatitis or pancreatic carcinoma. Diagnosis is difficult, because pancreatic pain is usually nonspecific in character and radiation, and the retroperitoneal position of the gland makes it inaccessible to physical examination. Roentgenographic studies offer less diagnostic aid than they do in diseases of other abdominal organs, so that laboratory tests must be relied upon to a greater extent than in other abdominal diseases in order to detect or confirm the presence of pancreatic pathologic changes. Based on the considerations discussed in Chap. 302, an operational approach to the differential diagnosis of acute and chronic pancreatitis and pancreatic cancer will be described. This brief summary should serve as a practical guide to the evaluation of these patients.

Acute pancreatitis should be considered in the differential diagnosis of any acute abdominal emergency or any obscure hypotensive state. Unless another diagnosis is obvious, determination of serum amylase activity pays excellent dividends as a screening test in the patient with acute abdominal or back pain. An activity greater than

180 Somogyi units per 100 ml serum raises the question of pancreatic involvement, and a value over 500 units makes pancreatitis highly likely. Other major abdominal emergencies that may also be associated with an elevated serum amylase level are perforated peptic ulcer, acute cholecystitis, and obstruction or infarction of bowel. Although the serum amylase level rarely exceeds 500 units in these diseases, the separation of such entities from pancreatitis occasionally can be very difficult. Prompt abdominal x-rays are necessary to look for free peritoneal air, pancreatic calcifications, or opaque gallstones. A peritoneal tap with a short-bevel intravenous needle plus a flexible plastic catheter in the midlateral quadrants will often yield a cloudy yellow to "prune juice" type of fluid with an amylase level higher than the serum activity. In acute pancreatitis, bile is not detected in the fluid as in a perforated duodenal ulcer, and bacteria are not seen on direct Gram's stain of the fluid as in bowel infarction, although both these entities can be associated with peritoneal fluid very high in amylase.

If the history and physical examination suggest another diagnosis, prompt treatment for pancreatitis should be instituted. The appropriate measures consist of nasogastric suction, plasma and electrolyte replacement, and meperidine for pain. Surgical intervention should be avoided unless perforation, strangulation, or necrosis of gut cannot be ruled out.

Confirmation of the diagnosis of *chronic pancreatitis* during painful episodes requires increases in serum or urinary amylase or serum lipase activities. During quiescent periods, stimulation with secretin and pancreozymin will result in increases in the serum amylase or lipase activities in 50 percent or more of patients whose acinar tissue is not destroyed. When exocrine insufficiency is suspected, the simplest screening procedure is macroscopic inspection of the stool for gross fat and microscopic examination of a stool emulsion, looking for undigested meat fibers and for increased numbers of fat globules after Sudan IV staining. Quantitative proof of steatorrhea should be obtained by chemical fat analysis of a 3-day stool collection on a known fat intake. Pancreatic insufficiency as the cause of steatorrhea is implied by a normal D-xylose absorption test or a normal small-bowel pattern after a barium meal.

A secretin test is the most precise and accurate method of measuring exocrine functional capacity. The greatest experience has been gathered using the method of Dreiling: a double lumen tube is passed into the stomach and duodenum under fluoroscopic control, and duodenal contents are collected uncontaminated by gastric juice. Secretin is given as a single intravenous dose of 1 to 2 clinicals units per kg body weight. Then four 20-min collections are obtained by intermittent suction, and the volumes and bicarbonate concentrations are measured. The usual response in chronic pancreatitis is a decreased bicarbonate concentration in a normal volume of pancreatic juice. The maximum bicarbonate concentration discriminates best between normal subjects and patients with proved chronic pancreatitis, can be measured accurately in any laboratory, and does not require complete volume recovery.

A logical sequence of diagnostic procedures when *pancreatic carcinoma* is suspected would be (1) serum and urinary amylase measurements, (2) an upper gastrointestinal barium study, (3) a glucose tolerance test if the patient is not already diabetic, and (4) if icterus is present, liver function tests designed to separate obstructive from hepatocellular jaundice. If these studies are consistent with the diagnosis of pancreatic tumor, it may be visualized by a selective celiac arteriogram or by a selenomethionine scan. The diagnosis of pancreatic cancer can be confirmed only by surgical exploration.

302 DISEASES OF THE PANCREAS

PHILIP J. SNODGRASS

BIOCHEMISTRY AND PHYSIOLOGY OF THE EXOCRINE PANCREAS Enzyme synthesis and secretion The human exocrine pancreas synthesizes and secretes more protein per gram of tissue than any other organ. Pancreatic juice contains 6 to 12 g digestive enzymes in an average daily volume of 2,500 ml. The proteolytic enzymes are secreted as the inactive precursors (zymogens) trypsinogen, chymotrypsinogen, proelastase, and procarboxypeptidases A and B. When trypsinogen enters the duodenum, it is activated by enterokinase, an enzyme from duodenal mucosa which cleaves one unique lysine-isoleucine bond of trypsinogen. This limited proteolysis releases an N-terminal hexapeptide and allows the molecule to refold, forming the active site of trypsin. Trypsin is critical to the activation process, because autocatalytically it activates other trypsinogen molecules and in addition activates the other zymogens to produce chymotrypsin, elastase, and carboxypeptidases A and B. These five proteases, along with a less well-characterized prolinase, hydrolyze the dietary proteins to di- and tripeptides and amino acids by the time the proteins reach the upper jejunum.

The reserve capacity of the pancreas is tremendous; 90 percent of a dog's pancreas must be removed before protein digestion is impaired. The zymogens are synthesized in the acinar cells of the pancreas, where the proteins are assembled on ribosomes attached to the membranes of the rough-surfaced endoplasmic reticulum. The enzyme proteins are secreted into the tubules of the endoplasmic reticulum and travel through this tubular system to the Golgi apparatus, where the proteins are enclosed in lipoprotein membranes and are condensed into zymogen granules which accumulate at the apex of the cells. The zymogen granules are secreted into the ductal lumen by fusion of their lipoprotein membranes with the membrane of the cell, and their release is initiated by the peptide hormone pancreozymin or by vagal stimulation. The protective mechanisms which prevent autodigestion of the pancreas by these proteases are the synthesis of the enzymes as inactive zymogens; investment in lipoprotein membranes within the cell; the synthesis of two trypsin inhibitors, one being present in the gland and the other secreted into pancreatic juice; and the presence of trypsin and other protease inhibitors in the α_1- and α_2-globulin fractions of plasma. The trypsin inhibitor in human pancreatic juice acts reversibly, allowing free trypsin to be released in the intestinal lumen.

Pancreatic juice contains a ribonuclease and a deoxyribonuclease, but they are not secreted as zymogens. α-Amylase splits starch to limit dextrins and disaccharides, principally maltose. The fat-splitting enzymes are lipase, phospholipases A and B, and cholesterol esterase. Phospholipase A exists as a zymogen and requires trypsin activation. Pancreatic juice also contains a nonspecific esterase which cleaves water-soluble esters of fatty acids. Conjugated bile salts are important in digestion of lipids; when bile is excluded from the gut, 60 percent of ingested triglycerides are lost in the stool, whereas only 40 percent are lost when bile is present but pancreatic juice is diverted. Bile salts emulsify triglycerides and thereby stimulate lipase which functions at water-lipid interfaces, and they also shift the pH optimum of lipase to 6.5, the pH of the jejunal contents. Bile salts function as direct activators of the phospholipases, cholesterol esterases, and the nonspecific esterase.

Water and bicarbonate secretion Water, bicarbonate, and electrolytes are secreted into pancreatic juice by the centroacinar and the ductal cells of the pancreas. Water and bicarbonate output is stimulated by *secretin*, a peptide hormone whose 27 amino acid sequence has been established by Jorpes and Mutt and is closely homologous to glucagon. Secretin, like glucagon, can release insulin from the beta cells of the islets of Langerhans. In addition, secretin stimulates the biliary epithelium to add water and bicarbonate to bile. The human pancreas produces 1,500 to 4,000 ml juice a day which is iso-osmotic with plasma and contains the following electrolytes: Na^+, 140 mEq per liter; K^+, 6 mEq per liter; Ca^{++}, 1.7 mEq per liter; Mg^{++}, 0.7 mEq per liter, and HCO_3^-, which varies from 27 mEq per liter in the resting state to a maximum of 140 mEq per liter during maximum secretin stimulation.

The pH varies directly with the bicarbonate concentration, ranging from 7.5 to 8.5, and chloride concentration varies inversely with bicarbonate. The bicarbonate output of 7 to 18 g per day is sufficient to neutralize gastric acid production, resulting in a pH in the distal duodenum near 7, which is close to the optimal pH for the function of the various pancreatic enzymes. Secretin is released from undefined mucosal cells when acid enters the duodenum; it acts in a feedback manner to inhibit gastrin-stimulated acid production and gastric motility. *Pancreozymin* (also called *cholecystokinin*) is released by entry of fat, amino acids and acid (pH 1 to 2) into the duodenum. This hormone contracts the gallbladder and relaxes the sphincter of Oddi in addition to releasing pancreatic enzymes. Its five C-terminal amino acids are identical to those of gastrin; thus by itself it can weakly stimulate gastric acid production. Pancreozymin usually competes with gastrin for binding to parietal cells and therefore inhibits gastric acid secretion and motility. *Gastrin* stimulates pancreatic zymogen release and gallbladder contraction because of its structural similarity to pancreozymin.

Vagotomy reduces pancreatic secretion in response to endogenous stimuli. Gastrin and pancreozymin release are lessened, so pancreatic enzyme output decreases. Gastric acid output, release of secretin, and potentiation of secretin by pancreozymin are all reduced, so bicarbonate output falls. These findings illustrate the importance of cholinergic stimulation on the hormonal phase of pancreatic secretion. However, vagotomy in man does not result in clinically recognized impairment in digestion.

PANCREATIC FUNCTION TESTS These tests are based on the biochemistry and physiology of the pancreas and depend upon analyzing the blood, the intestinal contents, or both for pancreatic secretory products. Normally there is an exocrine-endocrine partition of pancreatic enzyme secretion wherein a small fraction of the secretory enzymes enters the lymphatics and plasma. When functioning acinar cells secrete into a ductal system which is blocked by edema, stricture, stone, or tumor, an increased regurgitation of the enzymes occurs. In the serum of normal adults amylase activity varies from 60 to 180 Somogyi units per 100 ml serum and lipase activity from 0 to 1.5 Cherry-Crandall units per ml serum. Isoenzymes of α-amylase are detected in the γ-globulin fraction of human serum by use of electrophoretic methods; one isoenzyme is derived from pancreas and one from salivary glands. Rarely amylases derived from fallopian tube or ovary appear in serum.

Thus elevated *total serum amylase* activities are not specific for pancreatitis, but can occur with mumps or salpingitis. In diseases where pancreatic amylase can diffuse from the gut lumen into the peritoneum, such as with a perforated or infarcted small bowel, amylase is absorbed and elevates the serum level. Acute cholecystitis can also elevate serum amylase levels without affecting the pancreas directly. In renal failure, because of impaired urinary excretion of amylase, elevated serum amylase activities may occur. In rare instances one may find patients without pancreatic disease who have persistently elevated serum amylase levels but low urinary amylases. In these patients the serum amylase is either bound to γ-globulins or circulates as an amylase polymer. These large *macroamylases* cannot be filtered by the glomerulus, and result in the benign condition of macroamylasemia.

The assay of any *trypsin* or other pancreatic proteases is interfered with by trypsin inhibitors in the plasma. The α_1-trypsin inhibitor can bind 0.8 mg crystalline trypsin and the α_2-macroglobulin 0.1 mg trypsin, chymotrypsin, elastase, or plasmin. If trypsin is assayed by use of synthetic ester substrates, a low level of activity is detected in normal plasma because trypsin bound to α_2-macroglobulins has esterase activity but cannot hydrolyze protein substrates. Serum *lipase*, when measured earlier by methods which require 12 to 24 hr of incubation, was thought to be less sensitive than amylase in detecting pancreatitis; however with improved methods the serum amylase and lipase activities appear to parallel each other during pancreatitis.

Latent pancreatic disease causing a partial secretory block may sometimes be brought to light by "evocative" tests. When the normal pancreas is stimulated by intravenous secretin and pancreozymin, serum levels of amylase and lipase change little; but in early cases of pancreatic cancer or chronic inflammation where functioning acini secrete against an obstruction, pancreatic stimulation may produce serum enzyme activities which exceed resting levels by 100 percent or more. If the gland is extensively destroyed, stimulation of pancreatic secretion is incapable of causing increased serum enzyme activities; in such cases extensive pancreatic damage is revealed by a diabetic glucose tolerance test and abnormal secretory responses on duodenal intubation.

Pancreatic and salivary amylases have molecular weights of about 55,000 and are filtered by the renal glomerulus. The normal renal amylase clearance is 1 to 4 ml per min; the 24-hr output varies from 800 to 6,000 Somogyi units. A 2-hr collection of urine allows this test to be used in the emergency diagnosis of acute or relapsing pancreatitis; an excretion of more than 300 units per hr is abnormal, and more than 1,000 units per hr is usual in acute pancreatitis. If renal failure is not present and circumstances permit an accurate urine collection, the 2-hr urine amylase test is abnormal more often and for a longer time than the serum amylase or lipase activities. Although the serum amylase activity is often increased in acute renal failure and in some cases of chronic renal failure, the situation can be differentiated from acute pancreatitis by measuring the urinary amylase. In acute pancreatitis both serum and urine amylase activities are increased, while in renal failure only the serum amylase level is above normal. A convenient method of resolving these problems consists of measuring the amylase (units per milliliter) and creatinine (milligrams per milliliter) in serum and in a simultaneously voided urine specimen. The clearance (UV/P) of amylase expressed as percentage of creatinine clearance is calculated as (U/P) of amylase/(U/P) creatinine × 100. (For details of renal clearance calculations, see Chap. 267.) Normally this ratio is 2.3 ± 0.1 percent (SEM). In renal failure the ratio remains at 2.1 ± 0.2 percent because both clearances decrease in parallel fashion. In macroamylasemia the ratio falls to 0.34 ± 0.13 percent, and in acute pancreatitis it rises to 6.6 ± 0.3 percent. Studies in primates indicate that the increased ratio in pancreatitis is due to an increased urinary clearance of pancreatic amylase over that of salivary amylase.

Direct measurement of pancreatic secretion is accomplished by quantitative collection of duodenal contents after stimulation with secretin alone or in combination with pancreozymin. A double-lumen tube is passed into the duodenum, and the proximal part is used to remove gastric contents which interfere with bicarbonate and enzyme measurements. Results vary with the secretin preparations used and with the various doses employed. Using an augmented dose of highly purified secretin (2 clinical units per kg body weight intravenously), Hartley and his associates found the lower limits of normal to be 1.8 ml juice per kg body weight per hr, maximum bicarbonate concentration at least 82 mEq per liter, and bicarbonate output 6.2 mEq per hr. *The most reproducible measurement* with the highest level of discrimination between normal persons and patients with chronic pancreatitis *appears to be the maximum bicarbonate concentration after secretin.* Secretin also stimulates flow of water and bicarbonate in bile, reaching levels of 60 mEq per liter. When the gallbladder has been surgically removed, pancreatic juice is constantly diluted by bile, and as a result higher volumes and lower bicarbonate concentrations are to be expected. In this situation the output of trypsin or amylase after pancreozymin is a more reliable test of pancreatic function. When pancreozymin is given in addition to secretin, the output of amylase, lipase, or trypsin in the subsequent 10 to 20 min is occasionally reduced in chronic pancreatitis even when the maximum bicarbonate concentration is still normal. Pancreozymin tests present problems because the pancreatic enzymes are more difficult to measure, quantitative collections of duodenal juice are necessary, and severe protein malabsorption can result in secondary deficiencies of pancreatic enzymes.

Pancreatic function can also be tested by instilling a test meal containing carbohydrate, protein, and fat into the duodenum and relying on the endogenous release of secretin and pancreozymin (the Lundh test). The peak concentrations or hourly outputs of trypsin, amylase, or lipase are measured. This method tests whether the duodenum contains and releases pancreozymin and whether the pancreas responds; therefore the Lundh test can be abnormal in mucosal diseases such as gluten-induced enteropathy even though the pancreas responds normally to exogenous pancreozymin and secretin.

Early in the course of pancreatic disease exocrine function may be retained to the extent that duodenal intubation studies are within normal limits. At this point in the spectrum of disease the serum evocative tests offer the greatest chance of detecting pancreatic disease. However, as the pancreatic reserve is progressively impaired, more patients will show an abnormal result with duodenal intubation studies, and fewer will show a response to the evocative test. The accuracy of these tests is a function of the type of patient studied as well as the stimuli and collection methods employed.

When pancreatic insufficiency is advanced, microscopic examination of the stool shows *neutral fat droplets* when the stool is emulsified with saline and stained with Sudan IV. Split fats (fatty acid globules and crystals) may also be seen after heating an emulsion of stool with Sudan IV and 33% acetic acid because bacterial lipases in the colon can hydrolyze significant amounts of triglycerides. Neutral fat is usually not seen with intestinal causes of steatorrhea. The presence of *undigested meat fibers* with sharp edges indicates deficient pancreatic protease activity. Intestinal biopsies are usually normal, and D-xylose absorption is relatively unaffected by pancreatic insufficiency. Although abnormal glucose metabolism is a frequent manifestation of chronic pancreatic disease, evidence of impaired glucose tolerance is not specific for pancreatic disease because of the high incidence of genetic diabetes in the population. A practical and simple method of suspecting pancreatic enzymes is to institute a therapeutic trial with pancreatic enzymes (e.g., Cotazym or Viokase). Improvement in symptoms with weight gain and reduction in steatorrhea is strong circumstantial evidence for exocrine pancreatic insufficiency. However, *when exocrine pancreatic insufficiency is suspected, the only way to settle the issue definitively is to demonstrate impaired output of bicarbonate or enzymes into the duodenum after stimulation with hormones or test meals.*

ACUTE PANCREATITIS The pathologic spectrum of acute pancreatitis varies from pancreatic edema, to edema with fat necrosis, to necrosis with variable degrees of hemorrhage. The mortality rate is proportional to the severity of the pathologic process; it is 5 to 10 percent with pancreatic edema, 20 to 30 percent with partial necrosis, and 50 to 80 percent with total hemorrhagic necrosis of the gland. The clinical manifestations vary widely, reflecting the severity of the pathologic process.

Etiology Acute pancreatitis occurs most commonly in association with *alcoholism* or *biliary tract disease.* Occasionally it occurs as a complication of peptic ulcer, mumps, viral hepatitis or following the use of drugs such as glucocorticoids or chlorothiazide. Metabolic disorders associated with acute pancreatitis include *hyperlipidemia* (types 1 and 5) and *hyperparathyroidism.* The mechanism for the increased incidence of acute pancreatitis in patients with hyperparathyroidism is unknown. The common denominator seems to be hypercalcemia, because pancreatitis has been observed in other hypercalcemic states such as multiple myeloma and sarcoidosis. Genetic disorders associated with pancreatitis include a rare hereditary pancreatitis with onset in childhood which is associated with calcifications and an increased incidence of pancreatic carcinoma. Trauma is a relatively frequent cause of pancreatitis; it may result from a severe blow to the abdomen, a penetrating injury from a bullet or knife wound, inadvertent trauma from surgical procedures in the upper abdomen, or rarely electric shock. *Approximately 20 percent of patients with acute pancreatitis have no apparent underlying or predisposing cause.*

The pathogenesis of pancreatitis presumably depends on intrapancreatic activation of proteolytic and lipolytic enzymes with consequent digestion of pancreatic tissue and blood vessels. How pancreatic autodigestion is initiated is unclear. Considering the key role of trypsin in the activation of the proteolytic zymogens and of prophospholipase, some explanation for the initial conversion of trypsinogen to trypsin must be found. When a major pancreatic duct is blocked in animals and secretion is stimulated, pancreatic edema results; necrosis supervenes only if the blood supply to the gland is also impaired. Only localized pancreatitis tends to occur with direct injury such as from arterial ischemia, trauma, or a penetrating peptic ulcer.

Reflux of bile into the pancreatic ducts is believed to be involved in the production of acute pancreatitis. A common channel, 5 mm or more in length, exists at the end of the bile and pancreatic ducts in 60 to 70 percent of normal individuals, allowing for mixing of bile and pancreatic juice and their potential reflux into either ductal system. However, the secretory pressure in the pancreatic duct normally exceeds that in the bile duct except during gallbladder contraction. Injection of bile or of trypsin separately into the main pancreatic duct causes pathologic lesions unlike human pancreatic necrosis while elastase injections produce vascular lesions and hemorrhage. However, when a mixture of bile and pancreatic juice is preincubated and injected into the pancreatic duct under low pressure, a pancreatitis results which closely resembles the human disease. The critical components of the two secretions seem to be the lecithin of bile and the phospholipase A of pancreatic juice. The latter enzyme converts lecithin to lysolecithin which damages cell membranes and can by itself produce pancreatic necrosis when injected into the pancreatic duct. The missing link in this pathogenetic scheme is how trypsinogen is converted to trypsin which then activates prophospholipase.

Opie proposed that reflux into the pancreatic duct could occur when a "common channel" was present and a gallstone became impacted in the ampulla of Vater. Such a situation is actually quite rare, but the presence of common duct stones is often associated with acute pancreatitis, implying that reflux into the pancreatic duct does occur. When stones are not present, reflux is postulated to result from inflammation and fibrosis of the papilla of Vater. Such lesions are detected by biopsy of the papilla, but similar lesions are also found at autopsy in patients without pancreatic disease. Morphine can lead to spasm of the sphincter of Oddi and may elevate the serum amylase but does not produce pancreatitis. Fatal cases of pancreatitis have been seen in patients whose pancreatic duct enters the duodenum separately from the common duct. Reflux of duodenal contents into the pancreatic ducts is postulated as the etiologic factor in these cases. All these phenomena indicate that *the reflux mechanism for acute pancreatitis is a plausible but unproved etiologic theory.*

There is an increased incidence of acute pancreatitis in patients with gallstones, even without evidence of common duct calculi. Removal of the gallstones usually cures this type of recurrent acute pancreatitis, but the mechanism for the relation remains obscure.

How chronic alcoholism produces pancreatitis is also uncertain. An occasional bout of heavy ethanol ingestion in healthy individuals rarely causes an acute attack. Acute pancreatitis in alcoholics is usually superimposed on chronic pancreatitis (see below), where many small ducts are blocked by protein plugs, fibrosis, and stones. Alcohol stimulates pancreatic secretion indirectly by increasing gastric acid output and secretin release. The combination of pancreatic stimulation by alcohol and ductal obstruction appears to cause bouts of pancreatic edema, but the mechanism for the production of pancreatic necrosis in chronic alcoholism is unexplained.

Incidence Pancreatitis is rare in children, except in individuals with hereditary pancreatitis or hyperlipidemia. Acute pancreatitis affects adults of any age, both sexes equally. In one autopsy series the incidence was about 4 percent, but in only 0.46 percent was pancreatitis considered the cause of death. As might be anticipated from the prevalence of predisposing disorder, pancreatitis associated with alcoholism, duodenal ulcer, or trauma is more frequent in men than women, while that associated with gallstones is more common in women.

The percentage of cases of acute pancreatitis associated with alcoholism or gallbladder disease varies greatly; thus, the rate due to alcoholism is high in the United States and France, while gallbladder disease accounts for most of the pancreatitis seen in England.

Symptoms Severe upper abdominal pain is the outstanding symptom of pancreatitis. The location of the pain is determined by the retroperitoneal position of the pancreas and corresponds roughly in location to the position of the lesion; lesions of the tail of the pancreas cause pain in the left upper quadrant, those in the body are perceived in the epigastrium, and diseases of the head in the epigastrium or right upper quadrant. A high percentage of pancreatic lesions cause pain referred to the back at the level of the tenth thoracic to second lumbar vertebras. Patients with pancreatic pain occasionally obtain relief by sitting with the trunk flexed, knees drawn up, and forearms folded across the abdomen to exert pressure upon it. The degree of pain varies with the severity of the pancreatic injury, but in most cases it is intense and the patient requires analgesics. Centered initially in the upper midabdomen, the steady, boring pain usually diffuses to the back, chest, or lower abdomen. Nausea and vomiting, abdominal distention, and constipation are frequent complaints.

Physical examination The patient is distressed, anxious, and restless. Mottled skin, cold sweaty extremities, tachycardia, and shock are hallmarks of severe pancreatitis. Fever is not usually present initially but rises to 100 to 102°F within the first few days. Tenderness, voluntary resistance, and spasm in the upper abdomen are present to a variable degree, but in contrast to the intense pain these signs may be unimpressive. A boardlike abdomen as is seen in a perforated peptic ulcer is unusual. Various degrees of ileus occur, but some patients continue to have bowel sounds in spite of severe pain. Ten percent of patients have gastrointestinal bleeding, usually from ulcerations of the stomach, duodenum, or colon. Acute pancreatitis can produce rales in the lower lobes of the lung; pleuritis and pleural effusion, especially on the left side, also occur.

Laboratory data Urinary output is depressed if there is hypotension and a decrease in circulating plasma volume; acute tubular necrosis is not uncommon when shock is severe. The white cell count ranges from 8,000 to 20,000 with an increased percentage of polymorphonuclear leukocytes; occasionally there are leukemoid reactions with the white cell count as high as 50,000. The more severe cases show hemoconcentration with hematocrit values sometimes exceeding 60 percent. Plasma loss is due to tremendous subcapsular and peripancreatic edema and later to the diffuse "peritoneal burn" that results from intraabdominal enzymatic digestion. Transient hyperglycemia is common and is attributed to islet cell damage and the patient's marked adrenal response to stress. Mild jaundice may occur within 1 to 3 days of onset in 25 percent of the cases due to edema of the head of the pancreas producing compression of the common bile duct. This jaundice in association with acute pancreatitis does not necessarily indicate the presence of a stone in the common duct.

Serum pancreatic enzymes provide the most helpful laboratory information. Within 8 hr of onset, serum amylase values rise in 90 percent of cases, the values usually exceeding 250 Somogyi units. Levels above 500 units are strongly suggestive of acute pancreatitis. After 48 hr, even with clinical evidence of continuing pancreatitis, amylase values tend to return to normal. When massive hemorrhagic necrosis of the pancreas occurs, the amylase level may not rise at all. Serum lipase activity increases in parallel with the amylase but tends to subside more slowly. In patients with fat necrosis, blood calcium levels fall and remain depressed for 1 to 9 days. The initial fall is due in part to precipitation of calcium soaps, from fatty acids liberated by lipolytic destruction of the mesenteric and retroperitioneal fat. The persistent depession of serum calcium is unexplained. Frank or latent tetany may be seen in such patients; tetany that persists after restoration of calcium to a normal level may be associated with a low serum magnesium concentration. In patients with clinical evidence of pancreatic necrosis, a normal serum calcium level may be a clue to underlying hyperparathyroidism.

Occasionally lipemic serum is seen in association with acute pancreatitis and is due predominantly to an increase in chylomicrons or very low density lipoproteins. Most patients with hyperlipidemia and pancreatitis, when subsequently examined, show evidence of an underlying hyperlipidemia which probably antedated the pancreatitis. Electrocardiograms can be abnormal in acute pancreatitis with transient S-T segment depressions and T-wave changes due either to hypotension and myocardial ischemia or rarely to inflammatory changes in the pericardium. If shock is persistent in older patients, myocardial infarction may result.

X-ray Abdominal films may reveal moderately distended gas-filled loops of intestine; paralytic ileus particularly affects the duodenum, the jejunum near the pancreas ("sentinel loops"), and occasionally the transverse colon. Calcifications in the region of the pancreas are diagnostic of previous pancreatitis. Later, abdominal films may show a generalized haziness due to ascites and a loss of psoas shadows due to retroperitoneal edema and hemorrhage. Chest films often reveal elevation of the left side of the diaphragm and fluid in the left side of the chest which, if tapped, has an amylase activity higher than that in serum. Though rarely necessary, a barium meal usually demonstrates delayed gastric emptying and enlargement of the duodenal loop due to edema of the head of the pancreas. Intravenous cholangiography is of little help in differential diagnosis, because a nonvisualizing gallbladder often occurs with pancreatitis, as it does with cholecystitis, and the common duct may be dilated because of edema of the head of the pancreas.

Course Pancreatic edema usually subsides in 2 or 3 days, and patients feel well and eat normally in 1 week. Acute necrotizing pancreatitis causes a prolonged illness in which hyperglycemia, hypocalcemia, persistent ileus, and collections of necrotic debris in and around the pancreas develop. Suppurative pancreatitis usually occurs in the second or third week, when bacteria invade the necrotic collections, and is associated with a secondary rise in temperature and white cell count. In cases where massive necrosis occurs, the patient may die suddenly. The major cause of death in the first few days is refractory hypotension. One reason for this may be massive hemorrhage, due to digestion of the walls of major blood vessels, but in addition to losses of blood and plasma, hypotension may be aggravated by the release of kinins from the pancreas into the lymphatics and plasma. Kallikrein, an enzyme plentiful in the pancreas, catalyses the release from a plasma α_2-globulin of the vasoactive peptides kallidin and bradykinin. These are potent vasodilators and mediate an inflammatory response, causing migration of leukocytes, increased capillary permeability, pain, and smooth muscle stimulation. Trypsin also can produce bradykinin directly from the α_2-globulin substrate (kallidinogen). These vasoactive peptides have been demonstrated in plasma, lymph, and in peritoneal fluid both in experimental and in human pancreatitis.

Fat necrosis is commonly seen in the pancreas and the peripancreatic tissues, often involves the amentum and mesenteric fat, and occasionally extends to the perinephric and retroperitoneal fat. Rarely fat necrosis involves the pleura, pericardium, mediastinum, bone marrow, skin, and even the brain. The mechanism for disseminated fat necrosis is not certain; it has been attributed to the action of lipolytic enzymes circulating in lymphatics or blood. Peritoneal fluid often accumulates in acute pancreatitis; in milder cases it is a "beef broth" type of fluid, high in amylase activity, often containing gross or microscopic fat globules. In hemorrhagic necrosis, the fluid is turbid and bloody and accumulates in volumes ranging from 500 to 2,000 ml. The fluid contains many polymorphonuclear leukocytes but shows no bacteria on Gram stain and usually contains no bile.

Hemorrhagic phenomena may become obvious 3 to 6 days after onset by a blue-green-brown discoloration in the flanks (Grey Turner's sign) due to the seeping of blood to the abdominal wall by retroperitoneal routes. Rarely blood dissects beneath the anterior abdominal muscles, resulting in a bluish discoloration around the umbilicus (Cullen's sign). Abnormalities in the blood-clotting system occasionally occur in severe pancreatitis; these changes are postulated to result from a local release of trypsin in excess of its inhibitors, because free trypsin is able to convert prothrombin to thrombin, fibrinogen to fibrin, and plasminogen to plasmin. In rare cases there is evidence of diffuse intravascular coagulation (consumption coagulopathy).

By the second or third week, abscesses or pseudocysts may complicate pancreatitis. Abscesses occur as collections within the pancreas and pseudocysts as collections outside the pancreas, but both contain pancreatic secretions, necrotic debris, and inflammatory cells. These collections may become infected by staphylococci, coliform organisms, or even by gas-forming anaerobes, and surgical intervention to drain the collections is necessary.

Differential diagnosis Any severe pain in the abdomen or back should suggest pancreatitis. A history of previous attacks of pain is often obtained but is not specific for pancreatitis. If pancreatitis is suspected, the diagnosis can be established by the measurement of serum pancreatic enzymes, by exclusion of conditions most likely to simulate pancreatitis, and by the course of the disease. In considering the differential diagnoses (Table 302-1), it should be remembered that coronary occlusion and biliary colic are twenty times as common as acute pancreatitis, perforated ulcer is three times as common, mesenteric vascular occlusion is less common, and dissecting aneurysm is rare. One of the most difficult problems of differential diagnosis occurs in the patient who has either perforation of a peptic ulcer or obstruction or infarction of gut with leakage of intestinal contents into the peritoneal cavity. In these situations the pancreatic enzymes are absorbed via lymphatics into the blood, resulting in increased serum amylase activities and a picture that closely mimics acute pancreatitis. Peritoneal fluid containing more than 7,000 Somogyi units amylase is characteristic of acute pancreatitis, but other acute intestinal emergencies such as perforated peptic ulcer may give ascitic fluid amylases as high as 4,800 units. When bowel is perforated, the peritoneal fluid usually contains bile or bacteria, and abdominal films often show air under the diaphragm on upright films. Acute cholecystitis may be accompanied by increases in amylase activity and can be confused with acute pancreatitis. Because a perforated, obstructed, or infarcted viscus requires early operative intervention, a laparotomy should be done whenever these diagnoses cannot be clearly differentiated from acute pancreatitis. In contrast to previous beliefs, mortality from pancreatitis is not increased greatly by a diagnostic laparotomy.

Treatment The rationale of therapy is (1) to maintain an adequate circulating blood volume, (2) to keep pancreatic secretory activity at a minimum, and (3) to prevent potential and to treat actual complications.

Direct surgical attack with drainage of the necrotic areas of the pancreas has been generally abandoned as ineffective and incurs the risk of external pancreatic fistula. Shock and hemoconcentration are treated with plasma or human serum albumin and electrolyte solutions, using the hematocrit, central venous pressure, and urine output as indexes of adequate volume replacement. Whole blood usually is required in hemorrhagic pancreatitis. Meperidine or pentazocine is recommended for pain rather than opiates because either causes less spasm of the sphincter of Oddi, but these often prove inadequate. In some patients, morphine or its derivatives may have to be used. Nothing is given by mouth, and constant gastric suction is employed to reduce intestinal distention and stimulation of pancreatic secretion by acid entering the duodenum. Placing of the nasogastric tube with radiologic monitoring is necessary in order to achieve complete collection of gastric juice, and nasogastric suction is continued until intestinal activity returns to normal. When shock is controlled, water, electrolytes, and glucose are given intravenously to meet daily nutritional needs. Because secondary infection of necrotic tissue, of partially obstructed biliary passages, and of atelectatic lung accounts for much of the late mortality, appropriate antibiotic therapy of *established* infection is crucial. Prophylactic antibiotic therapy is often employed, but adequately controlled studies showing that it reduces mortality are lacking.

Other, less well-established, measures may be used. Anticholinergics in full parenteral doses (e.g., 30 mg propantheline bromide) can be given every 6 to 8 hr to inhibit the vagal stimuli of pancreatic secretion, but these obscure interpretation of the pulse rate and tend to dry secretions, leading to further pulmonary problems. Their value in the successful management of pancreatitis is questionable. Paravertebral, splanchnic, or epidural procaine blocks sometimes relieve pain dramatically, but these are rarely necessary. Hypocalcemia should be treated by slow intravenous injections of calcium gluconate, 10 ml of a 10% solution every 4 hr. The amounts needed are determined by the patient's clinical response and the serum calcium level. Peritoneal dialysis with rapid exchanges of slightly hypertonic fluid may sometimes reverse the downhill course of patients unresponsive to all other measures. A polypeptide (Trasylol), a potent kallikrein and trypsin inhibitor which is extracted from beef parotid gland, has been employed extensively in Europe to treat acute pancreatitis. Experimental pancreatitis responds to this inhibitor, but the agent must be given before or at the onset of the pancreatitis. This time factor may account for the lack of significant objective improvement in mortality and morbidity observed in controlled clinical trails.

As the patient improves, food may be given gradually. Usually one begins with carbohydrate, which stimulates the pancreas least; protein and minimal amounts of fat can then be added. Recrudescence of symptoms may occur with food and signals the need for drainage of obstructing pancreatic collections or pseudocysts.

PSEUDOCYSTS When collections of pancreatic juice and cellular debris break through the capsule of the pancreas, pseudocysts may form which are lined by fibroblasts and the serosal surfaces of adjacent organ structures. Usually located in the middle or left upper abdomen, the cysts occur in the lesser peritoneal sac, between the stomach and colon, the stomach and liver, or between the leaves of the transverse mesocolon. Pseudocysts may fluctuate in size or form tremendous masses that create symptoms by pushing the duodenum to the right, the stomach forward (Fig. 302-1), the left diaphragm upward, and the transverse colon downward. Aching distress rather than acute pain is the usual presenting complaint, and the pseudocysts are tender and usually readily palpable. The most common time for these to form is 3 to 4 weeks after a bout of acute pancreatitis.

TABLE 302-1
Differential diagnosis of acute pancreatitis*

Disease	*History*	*Physical examination*	*Laboratory findings*
Acute pancreatitis	Sudden onset, often with immediate maximal development of pain Past or recent history of gallstones, alcoholism, peptic ulcer, trauma, or upper abdominal surgical procedures	Abdominal findings moderate as compared violence of pain Tenderness extends to left of epigastrium Abdominal distention moderate or absent Peristaltic noises diminished or absent Shock and cyanosis may be striking Patient may be restless	Elevation of amylase in serum and urine Hypocalcemia in severe cases Paracentesis: evidence of fat necrosis, sometimes sanguineous fluid, high amylase levels X-ray may show fluid at base of left pleural cavity
Perforated viscus, especially peptic ulcer	History of ulcer	Boardlike spasm and tenderness in epigastrium Patient fears movement and jarring; shock rare	X-ray usually shows free intraperitoneal air
Mesenteric vascular occlusion	Elderly patient with cardiovascular disease or recent operation Development of pain may be gradual		WBC over 20,000 per mm^3 Paracentesis: sanguineous fluid; stool may contain blood; angiography often shows vascular defect
Acute intestinal obstruction	Intermittent colic with relative comfort between pains Past history of abdominal operation or of inguinal or femoral hernia	Abdominal distention with loud peristalsis Shock rare Patient moves around with colic	X-ray of abdomen shows characteristics of mechanical obstruction
Biliary colic	Pain more right-sided, more gradual in onset, and less prostrating than that of pancreatitis	Tenderness maximal on right side of abdomen	
Coronary occlusion	Pain usually maximal in chest, neck, or arms	Relatively few abdominal findings Shock and restlessness often present	Electrocardiographic abnormalities
Dissecting aneurysm of aorta		Impaired femoral pulsations Shock and restlessness often present	Hematuria

* *The points listed are, if present, important guides toward the correct diagnosis, but they are not invariable features of the diseases under which they are grouped.*

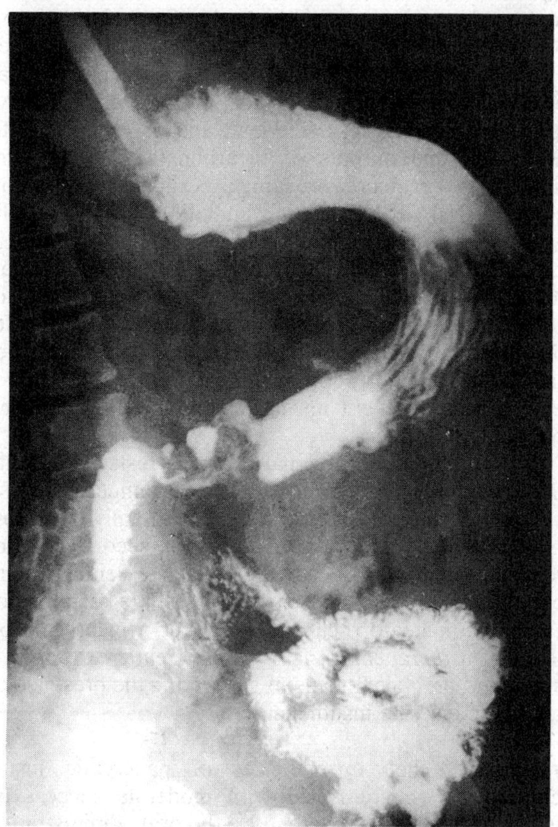

FIGURE 302-1
Pancreatic pseudocyst. In this lateral view the body of the stomach appears to be pushed forward by a large mass between it and the spine. The cause of the pseudocyst is well shown—a large penetrating duodenal ulcer.

Signs of fluid or atelectasis at the left lung base are common. Barium contrast studies establish the location of the mass and exclude lesions of the gastrointestinal tract and kidneys. Jaundice occurs in 10 percent of cases, and occasionally a persistently increased serum amylase activity is a clue to the diagnosis. Pseudocysts should be differentiated from retention cysts, which are cystic dilatations of the ductal system within the substance of the gland.

The principal differential diagnosis is upper abdominal neoplasm, particularly of the pancreas. If an attack consistent with pancreatitis has occurred within weeks or months, the history is helpful, but in approximately one out of three pseudocysts the initiating bout of pancreatitis is atypical and goes unrecognized. In these instances the existence of conditions predisposing to pancreatitis such as gallstones, alcoholism, duodenal ulcer, or trauma provides a basis for suspecting a pseudocyst. Pseudocysts endanger life by rupturing into the peritoneal or pleural cavities, or by dissecting into the mediastinum, the retroperitoneum, or even into the neck. A rare complication of a ruptured pseudocyst is chronic pancreatic ascites, detected by the high amylase, lipase, and protein contents of the peritoneal fluids. Therapy consists of external or internal drainage of the cyst; the lowest mortality and morbidity accompanies anastostomosis of the cyst wall to the stomach or to a loop of small bowel.

CHRONIC PANCREATITIS Chronic pancreatitis is manifested by as broad a spectrum of clinical symptoms as acute pancreatitis. The chronic relapsing form of the disease may be initiated by a severe attack of acute pancreatitis, but in the majority of patients it begins insidiously with mild recurrent bouts of abdominal pain. The most typical pattern resembles recurrent acute edematous pancreatitis. A persistent form of chronic pancreatitis without acute exacerbations is characterized by almost constant abdominal and back pain, and contrasts sharply with the pattern in a small number of patients in whom exocrine insufficiency and diabetes develop without any episodes of pain. In half the cases, calcific deposits form in the ducts or the parenchyma (Fig. 302-2); calcareous pancreatitis is particularly common when the cause is chronic alcoholism.

The same histopathologic changes occur in all clinical types but vary in extent and severity and consist of the following: replacement of acinar cells by fibrous tissue; focal inflammation, edema, and necrosis; deposits of proteinaceous material in the ductal lumens, with metaplasia and dilatation of the ductal system; development of calcium carbonate calculi in the ducts; and relative preservation of the islets of Langerhans. In some patients the

FIGURE 302-2
Chronic relapsing pancreatitis. In this film of the upper abdomen the entire pancreas is shown outlined by extensive calcific deposits.

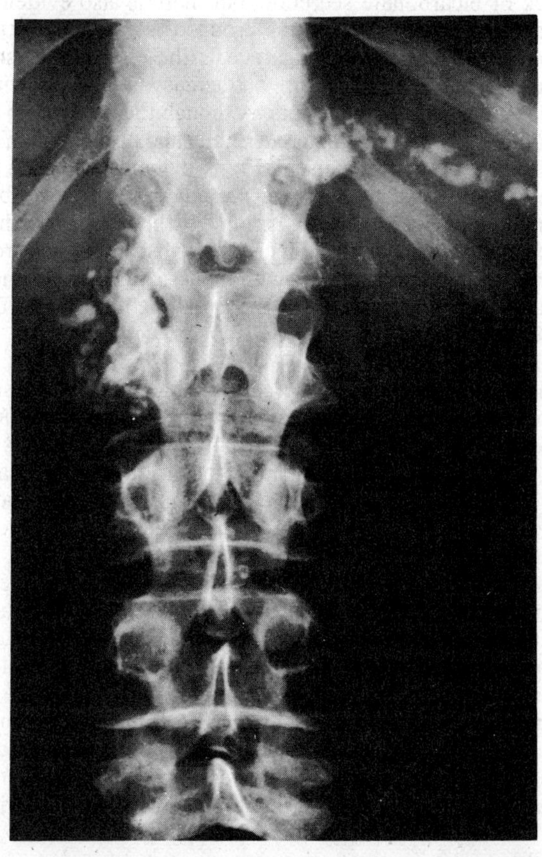

pathologic process is limited to the head of the pancreas, in others it is a patchy process throughout the gland, and in its most extensive state the pancreas is reduced to a fibrous mass with multiple areas of stricture and duct dilatation. The formation of pseudocysts or intrapancreatic retention cysts is an occasional complication. Chronic pancreatitis is associated primarily with alcoholism, occasionally with hyperparathyroidism or hyperlipemia, and occurs infrequently as a result of gallstones, trauma, or peptic ulcer. Hereditary pancreatitis is usually chronic. Atheromatous embolization may involve the pancreas and leads to a fibrotic gland without much inflammation. Twelve to forty percent of cases have no recognizable predisposing factors. Diffuse fibrosis without inflammation or clinical symptoms occurs in hemochromatosis.

Chronic alcoholism usually exists 5 to 10 years before the onset of clinically recognizable pancreatitis. Sarles has been able to produce a form of chronic pancreatitis in rats by feeding an adequate diet containing ethanol for 2 years. The inspissated ductal material, fibrosis, and chronic inflammation resemble human alcoholic disease. These findings suggest that alcoholism can cause a "cirrhosis" of the pancreas as well as of the liver.

Early in the disease there is minimal impairment of exocrine function. As inflammation and resulting fibrosis continue, pancreatic insufficiency gradually develops. When enzymatic secretion becomes inadequate, digestion is impaired, large amounts of fat and protein are lost in the stool, and weight loss is severe. An increased incidence of duodenal ulceration has been attributed to the lack of bicarbonate secretion, but there is also evidence that the obstructed pancreas produces a gastric secretagogue. Careful questioning reveals the presence of steatorrhea with bulky, light, and greasy stools showing occasional gross oil droplets. Although the absorption of vitamins D and K is impaired, tetany and purpura such as occur in spruce are unusual. Frank diabetes occurs in 10 percent of cases and is a sign of advanced disease, but impaired glucose tolerance is found earlier and in a higher percentage of patients. Increased absorption of iron occurs in some patients with pancreatic insufficiency leading to hemosiderosis of the liver; the mechanism for the increased iron absorption is unknown.

Diagnosis Chronic pancreatitis is a good diagnostic possibility in all patients having recurrent upper abdominal pain especially if (1) the pain or tenderness extends to the left of the midline, (2) alcoholism or gallstones are present, and (3) more common abdominal disorders have been excluded. The disease may explain mild recurrent jaundice, diabetes mellitus without a family history, or vague symptoms of indigestion, particularly if these phenomena are accompanied by recurrent low-grade fever and a persistently elevated sedimentation rate. If pancreatic calcification is seen on abdominal films, the diagnosis is obvious, but especially positioned oblique or lateral views may be necessary to demonstrate small calcareous deposits in the region of the pancreas. Before the acinar cells are greatly reduced in number, the diagnosis may be confirmed by repeated serum or urine amylase determinations taken within 8 to 12 hr of episodes of pain or by serum amylase and lipase responses to secretin and pancreozymin stimulation. As more acinar cells are destroyed, elevations of serum or urinary amylase levels become less frequent, and patients begin to show abnormal outputs of bicarbonate after secretin stimulation, or decreased amylase, lipase, or trypsin secretion after pancreozymin stimulation. The abnormality in response to secretin or pancreozymin stimulation is *qualitative*. The volume output usually remains normal, while the concentrations of bicarbonate and enzymes in the pancreatic juice are reduced. This pattern contrasts with the *quantitative* defect seen when tumors obstruct ducts in the head or body of the pancreas, resulting in a decreased volume but normal bicarbonate and enzyme concentrations.

Interpretation of duodenal drainage tests in patients with severe malabsorption syndromes is difficult, because in these patients protein deficiency eventually develops, and they may then show evidence of secondary pancreatic insufficiency due to the lack of essential amino acids. As mentioned previously, a positive response of reduction of steatorrhea and improved weight gain by means of a *therapeutic trial with pancreatic extracts* is a simple and practical means of suspecting the presence of pancreatic enzyme insufficiency.

Treatment The consequences of pancreatic insufficiency can be controlled with moderate success by dietary restriction of fats and by the oral administration of 5 to 10 g potent pancreatic extracts daily (Viokase or Cotazym), divided into doses of 1.5 g with each meal and 0.6 g with between-meal snacks. Supplements containing medium-chain triglycerides are useful, because this form of fat is well absorbed without lipolysis. Control of pain in chronic pancreatitis is often unsatisfactory, and many patients become addicted to narcotics. Low-fat diets, anticholinergics, and antacids given in the hope of controlling gastric acidity and lessening the stimuli for pancreatic secretion are inconsistently effective.

Surgical treatment is most successful if a biliary tract abnormality can be corrected. Direct attack on obstructions within the pancreatic ducts is also possible. The sites of obstruction may be visualized by cannulation of the papilla of Vater during fiberoptic duodenoscopy, followed by injection of contrast medium. Such pancreatograms can also be done at surgery by cannulating the pancreatic duct. When strictures or stones involve primarily the head of the pancreas and the ductal system has become dilated distally, reverse drainage can be established by resecting the pancreatic tail and anastomosing the duct to a loop of jejunum. If the entire ductal system is involved with strictures and stones, it is sometimes necessary to split the gland longitudinally, open the main pancreatic duct, and sew a Roux-en-Y loop of jejunum over the pancreas. Once the gland has been destroyed functionally and the patient has developed intractable pain, the best symptomatic results have been obtained by a 95 percent resection of the pancreas, leaving a small cuff of gland along the duodenal loop; this maneuver avoids the more major procedure of a pancreaticoduodenectomy. Vagotomy, subtotal gastrectomy to reduce gastric secretion, or cutting of a normal sphincter of Oddi have produced variable results. Bilateral sympathectomy and splanchnicectomy may be used to relieve pain, but relief is often temporary.

CYSTIC FIBROSIS Many organ systems are affected by this disorder of infancy and childhood, which is transmitted as an autosomal recessive trait: (1) The pancreatic acini are replaced by fibrotic tissue, multiple cysts, inspissated mucus, and eventually fat. The clinical manifestations of the consequent pancreatic insufficiency are malnutrition and steatorrhea. (2) In the newborn infant a thick meconium, due to viscous intestinal mucous secretions, may cause meconium ileus. Later the child may develop fecal impaction, rectal prolapse, and intussusception. (3) The mucous glands of the entire gastrointestinal tract may show this inspissation, so that the diagnosis can be made by rectal biopsy. (4) In a few cases the smaller hepatic biliary channels are plugged, with the consequent development of cirrhosis and portal hypertension. The gallbladder often contains gelatinous material and is hypoplastic. (5) The sweat contains high concentrations of sodium and chloride; in hot weather this abnormality may cause acute salt depletion and at times death. (6) The most disabling obstructive pathologic changes affect the lungs with chronic bronchitis, emphysema, and bouts of bronchopneumonia.

The cause is obscure. One hypothesis holds that the abnormally viscid mucus blocks small tubular structures in the various organs involved. This concept of "mucoviscidosis," however, does not explain the abnormal composition of sweat, because sweat glands secrete no mucus. The diagnosis is made on the basis of the clinical picture, deficiency of pancreatic enzymes, and high levels of sweat electrolytes. Various methods of inducing sweating allow the sodium or chloride concentration to be measured; 95 percent of affected children will have sweat sodium and chloride concentrations of 60 mEq per liter or greater, while normal children will have values below 60. Eighty percent of patients have severe pancreatic exocrine insufficiency, 10 percent mild deficiency, and 10 percent normal pancreatic function.

Treatment consists of pancreatic substitution therapy; a high-calorie, high-protein, low-fat diet; water-soluble forms of vitamins A, D, and K; liberal use of salt; appropriate antibiotics for acute pulmonary injections and prophylactic broad-spectrum antibiotics; and postural drainage, mist tents, and expectorants.

Because of an increasingly long survival of moderately severe cases and because of failure to recognize mild cases in childhood, adult fibrocystic disease may be more prevalent than heretofore appreciated. Some young adults regarded as having "idiopathic" pancreatitis, chronic bronchitis and emphysema, or cirrhosis may in fact have cystic fibrosis. Sweat sodium and chloride levels increase in adult life to values as high as 92 and 75 mEq per liter, respectively; as a result, there is some overlap between cystic fibrotic patients and normal persons. Heterozygotes have normal sweat electrolytes. Diagnosis in adults rests upon the presence of three or more of the following: suggestive clinical features, positive family history, sweat chlorides greater than 80 mEq per liter, pancreatic insufficiency, and characteristic changes in mucous glands on biopsy.

CANCER OF THE PANCREAS **Incidence** Cancer of the pancreas predominantly affects patients over forty, attacks men twice as frequently as women, and accounts for about 1 in 20 deaths due to cancer. It now occurs more frequently than gastric cancer and one-third as often as colonic and rectal cancer in men and women. Diabetic patients are believed to have an increased incidence.

Symptoms Weight loss, pain, and unremitting jaundice are the outstanding symptoms. Digestive disorders, including anorexia, nausea, loose stools, or, more commonly, constipation, are prevalent. The site of the lesion, however, to a great extent influences the character of the symptoms and their time of onset. Considering the total course of all types of pancreatic cancer, jaundice occurs less frequently than weight loss or pain, but diagnostically it is the most important symptom. Jaundice points specifically to the biliary passages, and lesions near the ampulla of Vater give early warning before extensive growth or metastases have taken place. The course and intensity of the jaundice depend on the degree of biliary obstruction (Table 302-2). Itching is an associated symptom in three-fourths of the patients with jaundice, and may antedate clinical icterus.

Literally painless jaundice characterizes cancer in the head of the pancreas in only a few cases. More frequently, the patient has vague abdominal distress and fullness, which may be made either worse or better be eating. The severe pain of cancer in the body or tail may, however, be diagnostic; it bores through to the midback when the patient lies supine, and he obtains relief only by standing or by sitting haunched up with arms clasped about the knees. A number of patients with cancer of the pancreas complain of depression and a sense of impending doom before the onset of abdominal pain; this occurs in cancer of the pancreas to a much greater degree than in other abdominal neoplasms.

Physical examination Physical examination may reveal nothing except evidence of weight loss, jaundice, and the excoriations of scratching. In spite of biliary obstruction, hepatic enlargement is not striking unless the liver is involved by metastases. The gallbladder is enlarged in nearly all malignant obstructions of the common duct but can be palpated in only half the cases. The finding of an enlarged, nontender gallbladder in a jaundiced patient without biliary colic may, therefore, be taken as a reliable sign of malignant choledochal obstruction (Courvoisier's law). No diagnostic inference is warranted if the gallbladder is not palpable. Unfortunately, by the time the diagnosis is suspected, the liver is often involved by metastases, or positive nodes are present in the left supraclavicular area. The spleen may be enlarged secondary to malignant invasion and thrombosis of the splenic vein.

Laboratory data The urine, blood, and feces of nonicteric patients are often normal. Those with icterus have persistent and progressive bilirubinemia and choluria.

The stools may be greasy, "abundant, of a pultaceous consistence, very deficient in bile, and most dreadfully foetid" (Richard Bright, 1838). In at least half the cases, however, the clay-colored stools are not grossly fatty and are more like putty than butter. Because bile salts are important for the absorption of vitamin K, hypoprothrombinemia develops with prolonged biliary obstruction.

Pancreatic tumors lead to ductal obstruction and occasionally to local areas of pancreatitis. The serum amylase and lipase activities are abnormal in only 10 percent of cases, but the 1-hr urine amylase excretion is increased in as many as 30 percent. Lesions in the head of the pancreas, blocking the larger ducts, result in a diminished volume of pancreatic juice after secretin stimulation, although the bicarbonate concentration is often normal. Glucose tolerance tests or intravenous tolbutamide tests are abnormal in 50 to 70 percent cases, but the patient's age or antecedent diabetes partly accounts for this finding. Because ampullary cancers tend to ulcerate and form fistulas between the biliary and alimentary tracts, the serum bilirubin may fluctuate, occult blood is often found in the stools, and bouts of cholangitis may occur (Table 302-2). All these findings are less common in carcinoma of the head of the pancreas.

Course Pancreatic cancer leads to death by inanition, biliary obstruction, local extension, or distant metastases. By direct extension, the cancer may invade the liver, spleen, stomach, duodenum, colon, portal venous system, or peritoneum. Invasion of the gut or development of varices following malignant occlusion of the portal vein can cause moderate to severe gastrointestinal blood loss. Peritoneal seeding or, very rarely, portal obstruction is responsible for ascites. Metastatic lesions develop in the regional lymph nodes, liver, lungs, mediastinal and cervical lymph nodes, and bone.

Diagnosis In jaundiced patients, cancer of the head of the pancreas must be differentiated from liver disease, common duct stones, and ampullary or bile duct carcinomas. Liver function tests tend to show conjugated hyperbilirubinemia and an elevated serum alkaline phosphatase. Favoring pancreatic cancer is a gradual onset of symptoms in elderly patients without antecedent acute malaise, intermittent colicky pains, or chills and fever. If itching is noticed before the onset of jaundice, mechanical obstruction of the biliary passages is likely. In early cases, before the diagnosis is made obvious by massive or metastatic growth, cancer is suggested by finding an enlarged gallbladder, a slightly enlarged, nontender liver, and by the absence of stigmas of liver disease such as spider angiomas, dilated abdominal veins, and splenomegaly.

Common duct stones rarely cause complete and unremitting biliary obstruction; light-colored stools which contain urobilin or urobilinogen are unusual in pancreatic tumors and suggest stones or ampullary carcinoma. Radiologic procedures may show the encroachment of the pancreatic lesion on other organs. Changes in the mucosa or configuration of the duodenal loop or stomach rarely appear early, but are usually signs of advanced disease. Greater detail of the duodenal loop and its mucosa can be brought out by administering 60 mg propantheline bro-

TABLE 302-2
Clinical features and laboratory findings in cancer of the bile ducts and pancreas*

Clinical feature	*Cancer of ampulla of Vater*	*Cancer of bile ducts*	*Cancer of head of pancreas*	*Cancer of body and tail of pancreas*
Pain	Absent—60% Moderate—40%	Absent—40% Moderate to severe—60%	Absent to mild—15% Moderate to severe—85%	Almost invariably present. Agonizing and boring. Often worse in back and accentuated when patient is supine
Jaundice:				
Onset	Early	Early	Variable	Late to terminal
Character	Progressive and marked—80% Fluctuating—20%	Progressive and marked—90% Fluctuating—10%	Progressive and marked	Mild to moderate
Weight loss before onset of jaundice†	None to mild	None to moderate	Occasionally none, but often 10 to 20 lb	Marked, 10 to 60 lb
Fever and chills	20%	10%	None	May have low-grade fever. No chills
Hepatomegaly	None to slight	Slight in some cases, but may be extreme	Moderate. Marked only if metastases present	None to marked. Size depends on degree of metastatic involvement
Enlarged gallbladder palpable or visible	50%	20%	50%	0%
Splenomegaly	None	None	None	Occasional
Bile in stools and urobilinogen in urine	Absent—80% Fluctuating—20%	Absent—90% Fluctuating—10%	Absent	Present
Occult blood in stools	82%	15%		Rare

* *Because of their anatomic proximity, advanced cancers of the ampulla of Vater, the bile ducts, and the pancreatic head at times cannot be distinguished clinically.*
† *All these cancers cause impressive weight loss sooner or later.*

mide intramuscularly to induce atony of the duodenum, followed by infusion of barium through a duodenal tube (hypotonic duodenography). Selective celiac and superior mesenteric arteriography occasionally identifies a tumor but more commonly demonstrates narrowing of pancreatic vessels due to encroachment by tumor or displacement of vessels by a mass. Percutaneous cholangiography can confirm that there is an obstruction of the common duct in the region of the head of the pancreas, but the distinction between stone and tumor still requires surgical exploration. Pancreatography via a fiberoptic duodenoscope can also demonstrate a block in the ductal system.

Because the pancreas avidly takes up circulating amino acids and transforms them into secretory proteins, it is possible to scan the pancreas for nonfunctioning areas involved by tumor. Radioactine selenium (^{75}Se), a gamma-emitting isotope, can be used to label methionine, which, following intravenous injection, allows external scanning of the gland. Uptake of selenomethionine by the liver often obscures the pancreatic outline, but the liver radioactivity can be subtracted if prior scanning of the liver with radioactive colloidal gold is done. The visualization of the pancreas is poor compared with liver or kidney scanning techniques, and false positive results average 20 to 30 percent. Ductal carcinomas do not take up the isotope. Diffuse defects in uptake occur in chronic pancreatitis as well as in the atrophic gland behind a tumor in the head of the pancreas. However, since false negative scans occur in only 5 to 10 percent, a normal scan is a reliable means for excluding tumor or chronic pancreatitis.

When the patient is not jaundiced, early diagnosis is difficult. Persistent pain and progressive weight loss with negative radiologic studies of the alimentary, renal, and biliary passages should raise the suspicion of pancreatic cancer. In patients with ascites, the character of the fluid and its cellular content often permit the diagnosis of cancer, but differentiation from ovarian, gastric, or primary hepatic cancer is usually not possible. In expert hands, duodenal drainage after secretion stimulation will yield malignant cells in 40 percent of patients with cancer of the pancreas or bile ducts.

Treatment Resection of cancers of the pancreas is usually undertaken only for those involving the head of the gland, because tumors of the body and tail are rarely detected before metastases have occurred. Of every 100 patients presenting to a physician with cancer of the head of the pancreas, only about 15 to 20 are suitable for resection at the time of exploration. Resection of the head of the pancreas and duodenum and anastomosis of the bile duct and pancreatic duct to the jejunum, combined with a subtotal gastrectomy (Whipple procedure), entail a 15 to 20 percent mortality. Eventually only 1 to 2 patients of the original 100 patients survive 5 years, an indication of the tendency for early lymphatic and blood vessel invasion. In jaundiced patients palliative anastomosis of the gallbladder to the intestinal tract affords relief from intolerable itching but does not prolong life. Radiotherapy and chemotherapy are usually ineffective.

OTHER CONDITIONS The islets of Langerhans are also a source of benign and malignant tumors, some of which have the remarkable propensity of producing hormonally mediated clinical syndromes. *Insulin-secreting beta-cell tumors* are discussed in Chap. 90. *Non-beta-cell tumors* or islet cell hyperplasia may be associated with gastric hypersecretion and unusually placed and intractable peptic ulcer disease (Zollinger-Ellison syndrome). Gastrin secreted by these tumors accounts for the gastric secretory stimulation. Other patients with non-beta-cell tumors present a syndrome of severe diarrhea and hypokalemia not associated with gastric hypersecretion. This has led to the postulate of another pancreatic hormone derived from the non-beta cells. Adenomatous involvement of other endocrine glands, in particular parathyroid, adrenal, and pituitary, is seen in a fourth of these patients; usually the disorder is familial (Chap. 282).

Ectopically placed pancreatic tissue may be found in the gastrointestinal tract, Meckel's diverticulum, and various other areas. Nearly all pancreatic rests discovered in adults, however, occur in the distal stomach and duodenum. Unusual pancreatic neoplasms are cystadenomas, cystadenocarcinomas, or hemangiomas.

REFERENCES

BECK IT, SINCLAIR DG (eds): *The Exocrine Pancreas*, London: J & A Churchill, 1971

CREUTZFELDT W, SCHMIDT H: Aetiology and pathogenesis of pancreatitis (current concepts). Scand J Gastroenterol (Suppl) 6:47, 1970

DEREUCK AVS, CAMERON MP (eds): *The Exocrine Pancreas, Normal and Abnormal Functions: Ciba Foundation Symposium*, London: J & A Churchill, 1962

DI SANT'AGNESE PA, TALAMO RC: Pathogenesis and physiopathology of cystic fibrosis of the pancreas. N Engl J Med 277:1287, 1967

FERRUCCI JJ JR, EATON SB: Radiology of the pancreas. N Engl J Med 288:506, 1973

HARTLEY RC et al: Pancreatic exocrine function: Comparison of responses to augmented secretin stimulus, augmented pancrozymin stimulus, and test meal in health and disease. Am J Dig Dis 11:27, 1966

HOWAT HT (ed): Clinics in Gastroenterology, vol. 1. *The Exocrine Pancreas*, Philadelphia: Saunders, 1972

LEVITT MD et al: The renal clearance of amylase in renal insufficiency, acute pancreatitis, and macroamylasemia. Ann Intern Med 71:919, 1969

section 8 | Disorders of the hematopoietic system

INTRODUCTION

M. M. WINTROBE

The hematopoietic system includes the circulating blood, the bone marrow, the spleen, and the lymph nodes, supplemented by the reticuloendothelial cells scattered about the body. The liver, through the presence in it of reticuloendothelial cells as well as by reason of other functions, is also intimately concerned in blood formation and destruction.

Since the blood and its constituents are so intimately related to the body as a whole, much will be found concerning the blood in various chapters in this book. In regard to the red blood corpuscles, attention is called especially to Chap. 58, Pallor and Anemia, where the synthesis and the destruction of hemoglobin and the classification, pathogenesis, and management of anemia are considered, as well as the symptoms and methods of study of a patient with anemia. The platelets, the phenomenon of coagulation, and the various ways in which bleeding is produced receive attention in Chap. 59, Bleeding. Alterations in leukocytes in various circumstances and the functions and kinetics of the white blood cells are discussed in Chap. 61. The significance of enlargement of the lymph nodes and of the spleen is described in Chap. 60.

In the present section, disorders of the hematopoietic system are considered. It is evident that such disorders make themselves known in a variety of ways. They may be such that discovering their cause may tax the acumen of even the most discerning physician. In the main, however, they are characterized in part or whole by symptoms and signs such as pallor, cyanosis, jaundice, bleeding, or enlargement of the lymph nodes or spleen. A thorough understanding of these manifestations of disease is a prerequisite to the correct differentiation as well as the effective treatment of the disorders of the hematopoietic system.

The *approach* to the patient suspected of having a hematopoietic disorder is discussed, therefore, in Part Two under headings such as Pallor and Anemia, Bleeding, and Enlargement of Lymph Nodes and Spleen. Although in the following pages, descriptions of the various recognized disorders of the hematopoietic system are found and their treatment discussed, it is urged that the reader confronted with a problem, for example, of anemia, first study Chap. 58; he will find there a discussion of anemias in general and will thereby be able to make his way more readily through the pages that follow or, for that matter, through other sections in this volume. The same is true, in principle, if the problem is one of bleeding, lymph node enlargement, or splenomegaly.

303
POSTHEMORRHAGIC ANEMIA

M. M. WINTROBE

Anemia resulting from blood loss may have developed acutely because of the rapid loss of a large quantity of blood, or it may have come about very gradually over a period of many months or even years. Obviously there are also many possible variations between these two extremes. The causes of posthemorrhagic anemia are numerous, and the manifestations differ widely, the latter depending in part on the nature of the underlying disorder and in part on the quantity and speed of the blood loss. It is convenient to consider acute and chronic posthemorrhagic anemias separately, because their manifestations and, in certain respects, their treatment differ so greatly. It should be realized, however, that these two syndromes represent two extremes which depend, in the main, on the same underlying defect.

ACUTE POSTHEMORRHAGIC ANEMIA

Etiology Trauma, the bleeding of a peptic ulcer, the rupture of an ectopic pregnancy, and hemorrhage in connection with hemophilia or thrombocytopenic purpura are examples of the widely varied possible causes of acute blood loss. They indicate that the blood loss may be external and recognizable at once, or internal and, consequently, sometimes not readily discovered.

Symptomatology The rapid loss of blood leads to reduction in blood volume, and the clinical manifestations are mainly circulatory. If the blood loss is great, "acute posthemorrhagic shock" develops (see Chap. 32). If the hemorrhage is visible to the patient, whether the amount of blood lost is great or small, symptoms may arise from the psychic effect of such bleeding. Generally speaking, symptoms are likely to appear sooner and are more pronounced in relation to the amount of blood lost when the bleeding is external than when it is not recognizable by the patient. The manifestations of anemia in general have been discussed already (Chap. 58). In addition, the symptoms of the underlying disorder may be present as well.

Blood picture Polymorphonuclear leukocytosis, with the leukocyte count rising even to 20,000 per μl and an increase in the number of platelets are the first discernible changes. A few metamyelocytes and an occasional myelocyte may be seen in the differential count. Because the blood vessels of the skin and muscles constrict in response to the need to maintain the blood supply of the vital organs, because plasma is lost as well as red cells, and because restoration of plasma is slow, the volume of packed red cells or hemoglobin level will not adequately reflect the true degree of blood loss. In the course of the succeeding 24 to 48 hr, however, fluid passes into the bloodstream and anemia becomes apparent. At the same time, the bone marrow is stimulated and reticulocytes begin to increase in 1 or 2 days, reach a peak of 5 to 15 percent in 4 to 7 days, and, in the absence of continued bleeding, return to normal levels in about 10 days. At the same time as reticulocytosis occurs, polychromatophilia develops and even nucleated red cells may be seen. Since immature red cells are larger than older ones, the anemia may become macrocytic temporarily. The leukocyte count should return to normal in 3 or 4 days. A persistent reticulocytosis, forming a plateaulike curve, suggests that bleeding is continuing, for cessation of hemorrhage is marked by quick restoration of physiologic balance, with rapid regression of the signs of stimulated hematopoiesis. If the iron stores of the body are good and the blood loss has not been extreme, iron deficiency does not occur and hypochromia is slight or absent. When the drain on iron is greater than can be readily replenished, iron deficiency begins.

Very severe blood loss, of a degree which requires replacement with 5,000 ml or more of blood per 24 hr, is associated with thrombocytopenia.

When the acute hemorrhage is internal, destruction of the blood and absorption of the products may lead to an increased excretion of urobilinogen in the urine and stools, and, rarely, even slight bilirubinemia may be found. Bowel hemorrhage is often associated with an increase in the blood urea nitrogen level; this increase is due both to temporary impairment of renal function (prerenal azotemia, Chap. 269) and to absorption of large amounts of protein.

Diagnosis When acute hemorrhage is not evident, such signs as pallor, faintness, restlessness, sweating, and palpitation should lead to a search for hemorrhage. If the subject is recumbent, much blood may be lost before these signs appear. They can be brought out by tilting the patient to the erect position. Late signs of acute blood loss are air hunger, thirst, and a falling blood pressure.

Prognosis The amount and rapidity of the blood loss, the acuteness of the physician in discovering it, the availability of blood for transfusion, and the accessibility of the site of bleeding are the important considerations.

Treatment Stopping of the hemorrhage, combating shock, and restoring the blood volume to normal are the essentials. Transfusions of whole blood are best, but a plasma expander such as dextran, 0.9 percent sodium chloride in water, or 5 percent glucose in 0.9 percent sodium chloride, may be used, in that order of preference, while blood is being matched. In civilian practice it is now rarely necessary or justifiable to resort to unmatched universal donor blood. Speed in restoration of blood volume is more important than whether plasma or whole blood is used.

Other medical or surgical procedures depend on the cause of the hemorrhage. Rest and quiet, induced by morphine if necessary and not otherwise contraindicated, are important. Following the acute phase, a high protein diet should be provided. Whether iron is given depends on the extent to which the iron stores are thought to have been drained and the degree to which this loss has been counteracted by blood transfusion. Other supplements are not necessary.

CHRONIC POSTHEMORRHAGIC ANEMIA This refers to that state in which blood loss has produced a chronic anemia and a deficiency of substances necessary for blood formation has developed. Although the factors essential for erythropoiesis are many, the chief deficiency resulting from chronic blood loss is that of iron. The manifestations of chronic posthemorrhagic anemia can therefore be discussed in the chapter which follows.

304 IRON-DEFICIENCY ANEMIA AND OTHER HYPOCHROMIC MICROCYTIC ANEMIAS

M. M. WINTROBE
G. R. LEE

IRON-DEFICIENCY ANEMIA

INCIDENCE In most developed countries iron deficiency is by far the most common cause of anemia. Between 8 and 64 percent of infants, about 20 percent of adult women, 50 percent of pregnant women, and 3 percent of adult males are iron-deficient. In Asia, the Middle East, and in some parts of Africa and of Central and South America this anemia not only is very prevalent but may be very severe. An understanding of iron metabolism provides the explanation for these facts.

IRON METABOLISM Iron is normally obtained by digestion of food. The newborn infant starts with a supply derived from the mother, but as growth occurs, dietary sources are necessary to meet the demands of the ever-expanding vascular space. In the female, with the onset of menarche, iron is needed to make up for the loss of blood; later, the demands of pregnancy exceed the saving due to amenorrhea.

The body of a normal adult male contains approximately 50 mg iron per kilogram of body weight; that of females contains 35 mg per kg. About two-thirds of this amount is found in hemoglobin, and only about 3 mg circulates in the plasma as transferrin. A very small proportion of the total body iron is present in myoglobin and the heme enzymes (0.15 g). The remainder (about 1 g in men, 200 to 400 mg in women) represents a reserve which can be called upon for hemoglobin production and is stored in the liver, spleen, and bone marrow as ferritin and hemosiderin.

The average adult diet in the United States provides about 6 mg iron per 1000 kcal, or about 10 to 20 mg per day. However, only 5 to 10 percent of this amount is absorbed. When there is increased need for iron, absorption may be more efficient (10 to 20 percent). Iron derived from hemoglobin and other heme proteins of animal origin is absorbed as the intact heme molecule. Most other forms of iron must be converted to ferrous iron in the stomach and duodenum in order to be absorbed. Absorption is most efficient in the duodenum and upper part of the small intestine. Iron is transported through the mucosal cell, but the exact mechanism is still uncertain. The absorbed iron is then bound by plasma transferrin, a β_1-globulin, and transported to the bone marrow for hemoglobin synthesis. The normal plasma iron level is 60 to 190 μg per 100 ml, but the turnover is rapid, so that 25 to 40 mg iron is transported in the plasma per day.

Conservation is the characteristic feature of iron metabolism. The iron derived from the breakdown of hemoglobin joins the body pool and is used again and again. Loss of iron from the body is minimal: probably about 1 mg per day in men and an average of 2 mg per day in menstruating women. Most of this amount is contained in cells desquamated from mucosal surfaces or the skin. In women, menstrual iron loss is highly variable but undoubtedly is the greatest normal cause of iron loss. A normal woman loses an average of 17 mg iron during a normal period. The net loss of iron during a normal pregnancy is about 700 mg, i.e., an average of about 2.5 mg per day.

It follows that, in a temperate climate, the requirement for iron in a normal man or postmenopausal woman is 0.5 to 1 mg per day. For menstruating women it is 1 to 2 mg per day. During pregnancy at least 2.5 mg per day is required. The iron requirement for growth during infancy and childhood varies with the rapidity of growth at different periods. During the first year of life the need may be as high as 1 mg per day but averages 0.6 mg; during childhood the average is about 1.0 to 1.5 mg per day. However, for the adolescent girl another 0.5 to 1.0 mg must be added to allow for menstrual loss.

CAUSES OF IRON DEFICIENCY From this review of the iron economy of the body, it follows that children, female adolescents, and women in their reproductive years, are most in danger of developing iron deficiency. However, any circumstance which leads to a greater demand on the iron stores of the body than can be met results in iron deficiency. The possible factors leading to iron deficiency are (1) insufficient iron in the diet, (2) impaired absorption, (3) increased requirements, and (4) loss of blood. In many instances, more than one of these factors is responsible for the resulting deficiency.

Except in infants and in rapidly growing children, *chronic loss of blood* by hemorrhage is by far the most common factor in the development of iron deficiency. Excessive menstruation and occult bleeding from the gastrointestinal tract (peptic ulcer, hookworm infection, esophageal varices, etc.) are the most common types of bleeding which may result in iron deficiency. A woman may lose as much as 200 ml blood during each menstrual period and not be aware that the loss is excessive. In an adult male, the discovery of iron-deficiency anemia should cause a diligent search for a source of bleeding, and this is most likely to be found in the gastrointestinal tract.

On the other hand, *decreased assimilation* of iron, whether from dietary deficiency of iron or from impaired absorption, or both, is rarely an important cause of iron deficiency unless the iron stores are already poor, demands for iron (as by rapid growth or frequent pregnancies) are great, or blood loss has occurred. Diets high in cereal content and low in animal protein are relatively poor sources of iron. Furthermore, the nature of the diet itself, other than its iron content, influences the assimilation of iron. Thus, both phosphates in the diet and phytates in cereals complex with iron and reduce its absorption. Ascorbic acid favors iron assimilation, probably by promoting the reduction of ferric iron in food to the ferrous form. Some protection against dietary iron deficiency is being provided in the United States and elsewhere by fortifying flour, bread, and infant cereals with iron, but the influence of long-established cultural practices, food faddism, and generally poor dietary habits is hard to overcome.

The gastric hydrochloric acid favors ionization and thus absorption; yet many persons are found in whom achlorhydria has existed for years without iron deficiency developing. Nevertheless, iron deficiency develops ultimately after total or partial gastrectomy in the absence of evidence of bleeding. Postsurgically, increased motility also reduces iron absorption. Likewise, chronic diarrhea prevents efficient absorption, and in steatorrhea iron absorption has been shown to be impaired. Not only is the absorption of dietary iron inefficient in these situations, but increased absorption in response to need, which occurs normally, does not take place.

Nevertheless, since the normal loss of iron from the body is relatively small, none of these circumstances of impaired iron assimilation is likely to be an important cause of iron deficiency unless blood loss or increased needs have developed. The high requirements for iron in infants, children, adolescents, and premenopausal women, have been outlined above.

The syndrome of *chlorosis*, the "green sickness" of the last century and before, may have been no more than iron deficiency in adolescent girls in whom dietary iron was insufficient to meet the needs for growth and menstruation. Likewise the chronic hypochromic anemia of women thirty to forty-five years of age represents the ultimate combined effect of chronic loss of blood, frequent pregnancies, and poor diet in a person whose iron deficiency may have had its beginning in adolescence. It is of interest that in many of these patients certain constitutional features similar to those encountered in pernicious anemia have been observed, such as early graying of the hair and achlorhydria.

SYMPTOMATOLOGY Iron deficiency develops insidiously, and mild to moderate anemia is usually asymptomatic. With more severe anemia, depending on the constitution of the patient and the cause of the deficiency, the accompanying clinical manifestations are those common to all chronic anemias, such as increasing fatigability, headache, anorexia or capricious appetite, heartburn, palpitation, dyspnea, edema about the ankles, neuralgic pains, vasomotor disturbances, or numbness and tingling.

It is evident that such symptoms also are found in the absence of anemia. Attempts to relate some of these manifestations to deficiencies of cellular iron metalloenzymes have not been successful.

Abnormalities in epithelial tissues, including sore tongue, sore mouth, angular stomatitis, thinning or spooning of the nails (*koilonychia*), or dysphagia, may occur in an occasional patient who is iron-deficient. The Plummer-Vinson syndrome (sideropenic dysphagia) is characterized by the feeling of food sticking in the throat, and a stricture at the mouth of the esophagus may be found, or the opening may be partially closed by a thin, mucous web which has been demonstrated roentgenographically and is easily ruptured by the passage of an endoscope.

Menstrual disturbances are common—menorrhagia, irregularity of flow, or even amenorrhea.

In the fully developed state, the clinical picture is striking: a tired, lifeless appearance; pallor; inelastic and often dry and wrinkled skin, sometimes with a brownish hue; dry and often scanty hair; and pearly white scleras are found. In many cases, some degree of papillary atrophy of the tongue, slight cardiac enlargement, functional systolic murmurs, a slightly enlarged liver, and a palpable spleen are discernible. When the deficiency is severe, the nails may be flattened, longitudinally ridged, or even concave (koilonychia) and may break easily. Findings on neurologic examination are nearly always normal.

BLOOD PICTURE When significant anemia is present, a good blood smear will reveal thin, pale red corpuscles poorly filled with hemoglobin. In severe cases these may be mere rings. Tiny microcytes, "target-like" cells, elliptic cells, and bizarre poikilocytes also are found, as well as a certain proportion of normally filled corpuscles. The red corpuscle count may be normal or nearly so, or even greater than normal, while the hemoglobin and volume of packed red corpuscles are greatly reduced. The anemia is hypochromic and microcytic. The hypochromia is more significant than the microcytosis, although the latter may be extreme (mean corpuscular volume even 55 to 70 femtoliters). Reticulocytes are usually normal in number but may increase temporarily following an acute episode of blood loss. The leukocyte count is normal or slightly reduced, and slight thrombocytopenia may exist.

The *bone marrow* is hyperplastic and contains relatively increased numbers of normoblasts.

The augmented histamine test has shown true achlorhydria in 16 percent. Superficial gastritis or moderate atrophy has been demonstrated by gastric mucosal biopsy in many instances. Iron therapy may be associated with return of free hydrochloric acid secretion, especially in younger persons, but in many patients neither the secretory nor the morphologic changes are relieved.

DIAGNOSIS Before significant anemia will occur, the iron stores must be depleted. Consequently, in equivocal instances, when the blood picture is not clear-cut or the anemia is not sufficiently severe to produce the classical picture, it is useful to measure the serum iron and the quantity of iron-binding protein. Although the serum iron is reduced both in iron deficiency and in association with chronic disorders (Chap. 308), in the latter the iron-binding capacity falls below normal while in the former it is often increased (greater than 400 to 450 μg per 100 ml).

An additional useful procedure is the examination of the bone marrow after staining for iron. In iron-deficient subjects, no stainable iron will be visible, whereas marrow iron is normal or increased in the anemia of chronic disorders. If neither serum iron determinations nor bone marrow iron stains are available, a therapeutic trial of iron may aid in establishing the diagnosis. The clearest results from therapeutic trials are obtained when the anemia is severe and when there are no complicating illnesses to prevent an adequate response. If such a trial is to be made, it is helpful if serial observations of the reticulocyte count are made during the first 10 days of therapy. A significant reticulocytosis occurring 7 to 10 days after the onset of iron administration indicates a response. In a therapeutic trial period of 3 to 4 weeks, under such circumstances hemoglobin should increase an average of 0.2 gm or more per day.

Iron deficiency is not the only cause of hypochromic microcytic anemia, even though it is the most common one. Other microcytic hypochromic anemias will be discussed in the next section.

TREATMENT True iron deficiency can be relieved by the administration of iron, but this alone does not constitute adequate therapy; it is imperative to seek and, if possible, to correct the cause. Here the onus rests heavily with the physician, since effective iron therapy alone will satisfy the patient temporarily, but the opportunity to cure a malignant neoplasm (e.g., carcinoma of the cecum) or some other treatable condition may be lost if the cause is not discovered.

Contrary to the blandishments of the pharmaceutical manufacturers and their agents, nothing better has been devised for the correction of iron deficiency than ferrous sulfate. The addition of other minerals such as cobalt or copper, combination with vitamins, or the introduction of devices to improve absorption has accomplished nothing other than to increase the cost of therapy to the patient. Ferrous sulfate (300 mg hydrated ferrous sulfate or 200 mg of the exsiccated salt), 3 or 4 tablets per day, is the optimal amount, but the dose should be increased gradually (1 tablet the first day, 2 the second, etc.) because tolerance for iron is thereby built up and fewer gastrointestinal side effects develop. It is easier to take iron when the stomach contains food, but if it can be tolerated when the stomach contains little food, absorption is better.

The administration of ferrous sulfate is followed by a reticulocyte response, and hemoglobin regeneration ensues. Three tablets of $FeSO_4$ per day will provide about 35 mg iron if about 20 percent is absorbed. Treatment for at least 6 months is needed in most cases if the body stores are to be replenished.

It is rare that parenteral therapy is required. When iron is absorbed poorly, as in *some* cases of steatorrhea, or when a condition such as regional ileitis, ulcerative colitis, iliostomy, or colostomy prevents its use, iron-dextran may be given intramuscularly. The first dose should be limited to 50 mg, because reactions, sometimes severe, occur. By repeated injections, a total of 1.5 to 2.0 gm may be given in this way. Intravenous administration also is possible in patients who cannot tolerate intramuscular injections. One or two drops should be given intravenously and then, if no untoward symptoms develop in the next 5 min, 500 mg is injected slowly over the next 10 min.

Transfusion of blood is rarely if ever needed, and free hydrochloric acid is not required, even if achlorhydria is present, because an excess of ferrous iron is prescribed and it is mainly the absorption of ferric rather than ferrous iron which is enchanced by the presence of acid.

OTHER HYPOCHROMIC MICROCYTIC ANEMIAS

Although iron deficiency is by far the most common cause of hypochromic, microcytic anemia, other causes (Table 58-2, II) should be considered. *Thalassemia* (Chap. 307) results in hypochromia and microcytosis with little or no anemia in the heterozygous, or "minor," form and causes severe hypochromic, microcytic anemia with features of hemolysis in the homozygous, or "major," form.

The *anemia of chronic disorders* (Chap. 308) usually is normocytic and normochromic. Occasionally, when the condition is of long standing, modest hypochromia and even microcytosis are observed. An incorrect diagnosis of iron deficiency may be made, not only because of the morphologic changes, but because the serum iron concentration may be reduced. In contrast to iron deficiency, however, the iron-binding capacity is normal or reduced, and iron is found in appropriately stained bone marrow specimens.

SIDEROBLASTIC ANEMIAS. These anemias (Table 304-1) are a group of heterogeneous disorders in which a population of circulating hypochromic, microcytic erythrocytes is found in association with "ringed" sideroblasts in the bone marrow. Sideroblasts are red cell precursors containing granules which take the Prussian blue stain for nonheme iron. In normal subjects, one to three small, blue granules may be seen in 30 to 50 percent of normoblasts. In patients with sideroblastic anemias, both the size and number of these iron-containing granules are increased and the granules tend to form a ring around the nucleus. By electron microscopy, these "ringed" sideroblasts are characterized by extensive mitochondrial iron deposits. In contrast, visible nonheme iron in normal erythroblasts is found in the cytoplasm in the form of ferritin.

Sideroblastic anemias are characterized further by increased total body iron. This is manifested by increased serum iron concentration with complete or nearly complete saturation of the iron-binding protein, and by markedly increased reticuloendothelial iron stores and deposition of iron in parenchymatous organs. The last may be severe enough to cause hyperpigmentation of the skin and impaired function of the liver, pancreas, and heart. Hepatosplenomegaly may be found on examination. The leukocyte and platelet counts are usually normal but may be slightly reduced.

TABLE 304-1
The sideroblastic anemias

- *I* Hereditary or congenital sideroblastic anemias (usually pyridoxine-responsive)
  - *A* X-linked
  - *B* Autosomal recessive
- *II* Acquired sideroblastic anemias
  - *A* Idiopathic refractory sideroblastic anemia
  - *B* Complicating other diseases
    - *1* Neoplastic (e.g., myelomas, lymphoma)
    - *2* Inflammatory (e.g., rheumatoid arthritis)
    - *3* Hematologic disorders (e.g., myelofibrosis, hemolytic anemia)
    - *4* Metabolic (e.g., myxedema, uremia)
  - *C* Associated with drugs or toxins
    - *1* Ethanol
    - *2* Lead
    - *3* Antituberculosis agents (isoniazid, cycloserine)
    - *4* Chloramphenicol
    - *5* Antineoplastic agents

Kinetic studies often reveal "ineffective erythropoiesis": plasma iron turnover is increased, but red cell iron utilization is impaired. Red cell survival is normal or only slightly reduced, and there is erythroblastic hyperplasia in the marrow, but the reticulocyte count is normal. There may be modest "indirect" hyperbilirubinemia and increased fecal urobilinogen excretion.

Sideroblastic anemias may be divided into two categories, hereditary or congenital and acquired (Table 304-1). Most patients with hereditary sideroblastic anemia respond to pyridoxine (vitamin B_6) therapy with reticulocytosis and an increase in blood hemoglobin concentration. However, it is unlikely that correction of a pyridoxine-deficient state accounts for the improvement since (1) the amount of pyridoxine required greatly exceeds the estimated daily nutritional requirement; (2) the response is usually incomplete—the anemia is not completely relieved, and morphologic abnormalities in the erythrocytes persist; (3) prompt relapse occurs when therapy is discontinued; and (4) no neurologic signs of vitamin B_6 deficiency are found.

Most of the patients with hereditary or congenital sideroblastic anemia have been males. An X-linked hereditary pattern has been demonstrated in several families. In one family the affected patients were females. In them there was a striking difference in the appearance of the normal and abnormal red cell populations, possibly on the basis of X-chromosome inactivation (Chap. 62). In some of the reported patients, the free erythrocyte proptoporphyrin content was reduced prior to institution of pyridoxine therapy and became normal or increased with treatment. Since pyridoxal phosphate is a cofactor for the enzymatic synthesis of delta-aminolevulinic acid (Chap. 58), it has been suggested that the genetic defect lies in this enzyme system.

A congenital form of sideroblastic anemia which does not respond to pyridoxine also appears to be inherited as an X-linked trait. In patients with this disorder, the free erythrocyte coproporphyrin is markedly increased and the free erythrocyte protoporphyrin is reduced. This finding suggests a deficiency in the enzyme coproporphyrinogen oxidase (Chap. 58).

Idiopathic refractory sideroblastic anemia usually is found in middle-aged or elderly subjects. In this condition, the proportion of hypochromic erythrocytes is small, as a rule, so that the mean corpuscular hemoglobin concentration (MCHC) is not abnormal; however, a careful examination of the blood smear will detect the abnormal erythrocytes ("partial hypochromia"). In some of these cells, basophilic stippling is present. The pathogenesis is not known. In a few of these patients, the anemia is partially relieved by the administration of pyridoxine, but in the majority this does not occur. About half the patients do not require therapy. In the remainder, the anemia is so severe that periodic transfusions are necessary. High-dose androgen therapy is sometimes useful in the latter group. The prognosis generally is fairly good; median survival is about 10 years. However, a proportion of the patients (7.5 percent) develop acute myeloblastic leukemia.

Symptomatic or secondary sideroblastic anemia has been observed in association with certain underlying illnesses. These include malignancies, such as Hodgkin's disease, multiple myeloma, and carcinoma of the prostate, and chronic inflammatory diseases, e.g., rheumatoid arthritis. Certain drugs (isoniazid, cycloserine, pyrazinamide) have been reported to induce sideroblastic anemia, apparently by interfering with vitamin B_6 metabolism. The drug-induced syndromes may be corrected by administering pyridoxine or by withdrawing the offending agent.

Sideroblastic anemia occurs in about 30 percent of *alcoholics* who are ill enough to require hospitalization. In them, in addition to the usual findings of sideroblastic anemia, vacuolization of erythrocyte precursors is prominent. The anemia is corrected by withdrawal of alcohol or by administration of coenzyme B_6 (pyridoxal phosphate) but not by pyridoxine itself. For this reason, alcohol is thought to act by inhibiting conversion of pyridoxine to the coenzyme form.

Lead inhibits several of the enzymes of heme synthesis, and lead poisoning often is accompanied by sideroblastic anemia. This type of anemia is also found as a less common side effect of several other drugs (Table 304-1).

TREATMENT Management of patients with sideroblastic anemia requires that all possible offending drugs be withdrawn and underlying diseases searched for and treated. If these steps are ineffective, the patients should be given pyridoxine in a dose of 50 to 200 mg per day for about 2 months. If no response occurs, further pyridoxine therapy is of no value. Some patients who do not respond to pyridoxine will improve when given androgens in a regimen similar to that used in aplastic anemia (Chap. 309). Since the ultimate prognosis often is related to the degree of iron loading, it follows that iron-containing medications are contraindicated, and blood transfusions should be kept to a minimum. It is rarely necessary to maintain the volume of packed red cells at more than about 25 ml per 100 ml.

REFERENCES

Bainton DF, Finch CA: The diagnosis of iron deficiency anemia. Am J Med 37:62, 1964

Bothwell TH, Finch CA: *Iron Metabolism*, Boston: Little, Brown, 1962

Harris JW, Horrigan DL: Pyridoxine responsive anemia—prototype and variations on the theme, in *Vitamins and Hormones*, vol. 22, eds RS Harris et al, New York: Academic 1964, p 721

Hines JD, Grasso JA: The sideroblastic anemias. Semin Hematol 7:86, 1970

Kushner J et al: Idiopathic refractory sideroblastic anemia. Medicine 50:139, 1971

Lee GR et al: Hereditary X-linked sideroblastic anemia. Blood 32:59, 1968

Wintrobe MM et al: *Clinical Hematology*, 7th ed, Philadelphia: Lea & Febiger, 1974

305 PERNICIOUS ANEMIA AND OTHER MEGALOBLASTIC ANEMIAS

M. M. WINTROBE
G. R. LEE

It was pointed out earlier (Chap. 58) that anemia characterized by an increase above normal in the mean corpuscular volume may be due (1) to the presence of large numbers of immature red corpuscles, i.e., "nonmegaloblastic macrocytic anemias" (see Table 305-1); or (2) to a qualitative alteration in erythropoiesis which results in the formation of an abnormal erythrocyte precursor, the megaloblast, from which are derived abnormally large red blood cells. The clinical differentiation of these two types of anemia is easy. The treatment of one differs greatly from the treatment of the other. The megaloblastic anemias are the subject of the present discussion. Macrocytic anemia in hypothyroidism and in liver disease is discussed on page 1592.

Pernicious anemia may be considered to be the prototype of this group of anemias. Not only is it of great historic importance, but it remains the most common cause of megaloblastic anemia in temperate zones. Moreover, many aspects of the symptomatology, laboratory picture, and pathologic physiology of pernicious anemia apply as well to other types of megaloblastic anemia. A thorough understanding of pernicious anemia, therefore, forms a logical foundation upon which understanding of other disorders within this group can be built. For these reasons, pernicious anemia will be discussed initially. This will be followed by a discussion of the etiology, pathologic physiology, diagnosis, and therapy of the entire group of megaloblastic anemias.

PERNICIOUS ANEMIA

Pernicious anemia is characterized by megaloblastic anemia, achylia gastrica, and neurologic damage. It may be classed as a "conditioned" deficiency, in that it arises as the result of failure of the gastric fundus to secrete amounts of "intrinsic factor" sufficient to ensure intestinal absorption of vitamin B_{12}.

INCIDENCE This disorder is the most prevalent form of vitamin B_{12} deficiency in North America and Europe. In persons of Scandinavian, English, or Irish extraction the prevalence of pernicious anemia is about 0.13 percent and 9 new cases are detected per 100,000 population per year. In developing and tropical countries, pernicious anemia is uncommon, but certain other forms of megaloblastic anemia are abundant.

Adult pernicious anemia is much less common in Southern Europeans, Orientals, and Negroes. Perhaps because of this racial distribution, a typical somatotype is said to characterize the patient with pernicious anemia: many of the patients are found to be of "large and bulky frame," with prematurely gray hair and blue, widely set eyes. However, there are many exceptions to this generalization.

Both sexes are affected equally. The average age of onset of pernicious anemia is sixty years. It is rare in persons under the age of thirty, and its incidence increases with age. An exception is congenital pernicious anemia, a very rare form observed in children, which differs from that seen in adults in that gastric atrophy and achylia gastrica are not observed.

TABLE 305-1
Classification of macrocytic anemia

Disorder or condition	*Pathogenesis*
Nonmegaloblastic macrocytic anemia	
Acute posthemorrhagic anemia	Accelerated erythropoiesis
Hemolytic anemias	Accelerated erythropoiesis
Hypothyroidism	Unknown
Liver disease	Unknown
Aplastic anemia	Unknown

Disorder or condition	*Main abnormality*	*Probable pathogenesis*
Megaloblastic macrocytic anemia		
Pernicious anemia	Vitamin B_{12} deficiency	Lack of intrinsic factor
Gastrectomy, especially total	Vitamin B_{12} deficiency	Lack of intrinsic factor
Fish tapeworm infestation	Vitamin B_{12} deficiency	Competition for vitamin
Blind loops, strictures, diverticuli	Vitamin B_{12} deficiency*	Small-intestine bacterial overgrowth; competition for vitamin
Nutritional macrocytic anemia	Folate deficiency†	Poor diet—regional (e.g., tropics) or individual (alcoholism, senility, etc.)
Sprue and other malabsorption syndromes	Folate deficiency†	Defective intestinal absorption
Pregnancy, infancy	Folate deficiency	Increased needs, poor diet
Hemolytic anemias, thalassemia, etc	Folate deficiency	Increased needs, poor diet
Congenital folate malabsorption‡	Folate deficiency	Folate malabsorption
Imerslund's syndrome‡	Vitamin B_{12} deficiency	Selective vitamin B_{12} malabsorption
Other hereditary disorders (orotic aciduria, Lesch-Nyhan syndrome, etc.)‡	Disorders of DNA synthesis	Hereditary enzyme deficiency
Chemotherapeutic agents	Inhibition of folate metabolism	Administration of methotrexate
	Inhibition of purine metabolism	Administration of 6-mercaptopurine
	Inhibition of pyrimidine metabolism	Administration of cytosine arabinoside
Other therapeutic agents:		
Anticonvulsants, contraceptives	Folate deficiency	Inhibition of intestinal conjugase, impairment of folate absorption
Para-aminosalicylic acid	Vitamin B_{12} deficiency	Impairment of vitamin B_{12} absorption

Note: In practice, the most common cause of what appears to be macrocytic anemia is laboratory error.
* *Folate deficiency sometimes associated.*
† *Vitamin B_{12} deficiency sometimes associated.*
‡ *Rare inherited disorders.*

HISTORY Although pernicious anemia was described at least as early as 1823 by Combe, it was the descriptions given by Thomas Addison in 1855 and by Biermer in 1872 which drew attention to what was then an ultimately fatal (therefore "pernicious") anemia. Subsequent developments completely changed the prognosis. In 1926, stimulated by the pioneering investigations by Whipple and his associates of the effects of various foods on experimental anemia in animals, Minot and Murphy showed that large amounts (1/2 lb per day) of fresh liver consistently produced remissions in pernicious anemia.

Castle, in 1929, elucidated the role of the stomach in the pathogenesis of the disease. It had been observed previously that pernicious anemia is almost invariably accompanied by a greatly reduced total volume of gastric secretions (achylia) and by the absence of hydrochloric acid in these secretions. Castle demonstrated a more significant abnormality of gastric secretion; namely, the lack of an "intrinsic factor" which normally acts on an "extrinsic factor," present in beef muscle and other foods. The two factors were regarded as combining to form an "anti-pernicious anemia principle" which was stored in the liver.

The subsequent isolation of vitamin B_{12} and the demonstration of its therapeutic efficacy in pernicious anemia clarified some of the puzzling aspects of the pathogenesis of the disease. It is now apparent that the effect of liver observed by Minot and Murphy is accounted for by the high vitamin B_{12} content of liver, and that vitamin B_{12} is identical both with extrinsic factor and the "anti-pernicious anemia principle." Intrinsic factor, a thermolabile glycoprotein, is required for absorption of the vitamin.

CLINICAL DESCRIPTION The onset of the disease generally is insidious. In many instances at least two of the diagnostic triad of symptoms are encountered; namely, weakness, sore tongue, and numbness and tingling in the extremities. However, other complaints may overshadow these, and the presenting clinical picture may suggest some disorder of the digestive tract because of anorexia, diarrhea, and various other gastrointestinal symptoms; it may simulate cardiac dysfunction of the anginal or the congestive failure type; or one may be led to search for some malignant neoplasm or an obscure infection. In some instances the neural involvement is so pronounced that a primary neurologic disease is considered. Even renal or genitourinary disease or a mental disorder may be simulated.

The degree of soreness of the tongue varies greatly, and the involvement may be complete or patchy. The tongue may be "beefy" red when the symptoms are pronounced and is less red and smooth when they subside. The gastrointestinal symptoms also vary greatly. However, one consistent finding in relapse is anorexia. This may be accompanied by a moderate degree of weight loss (average 15 lb). Symptoms referable to the circulatory system include dyspnea, palpitation, sensations of extra heartbeats, weakness, vertigo, tinnitus, and precordial pain. Since pernicious anemia often appears for the first time in the older age groups, it may be difficult to determine to what extent anemia or the degenerative changes of old age have contributed to the development of heart failure.

Pallor; a flabby rather than wasted appearance; a slight or pronounced yellowish color of the skin together with faint icterus of the sclera; a tongue which is often glazed in appearance and sometimes is red and sore; a rapid pulse with slight cardiac enlargement and often precordial hemic murmurs; in many, a spleen which is just palpable; and often a slightly enlarged liver are the chief findings outside the nervous system. In the nervous system, loss of vibratory sense in the lower extremities (not necessarily symmetric), incoordination of the lower extremities, loss of finer coordination of the fingers, signs suggestive of lateral as well as posterior spinal cord involvement, and evidence of peripheral nerve degeneration are the most common findings and may be present in all degrees from slight or none to extensive involvement. Positive Babinski response, positive Romberg's sign, disturbed position sense, spasticity, increased or diminished reflexes and sphincter disturbances may be encountered. Minor mental disturbances (irritability, memory disturbances, mild depression) or more serious mental symptoms may develop.

LABORATORY FINDINGS **Blood** The anemia is usually more severe than the complaints and physical examination would lead one to suspect. In the blood smear, macrocytes, often oval in shape, are characteristically seen (Fig. 305-1), but there is actually a great range in the size of the cells, and in addition, many bizarre-shaped corpuscles are found (poikilocytosis). Since the abnormally large cells predominate, the mean corpuscular volume is found to be greater than normal and ranges between 100 and 160 femtoliters (fl). There is a corresponding increase in the hemoglobin content of the red corpuscles (mean corpuscular hemoglobin), so that the concentration of hemoglobin in the corpuscles (mean corpuscular hemoglobin concentration) is normal. The red corpuscles in pernicious anemia and in other macrocytic anemias are not "hyperchromic," but, being thicker as well as larger in diameter than normal corpuscles, they appear to be supersaturated with hemoglobin, as one looks at them through a microscope. Some degree of diffuse polychromatophilia as well as basophilic stippling is found, and occasional nucleated red corpuscles may be encountered. The most striking changes, described in classic cases, are observed only when the anemia is very severe. Since the anemia is macrocytic, the red corpuscle count is reduced more than proportionately as compared with the hemoglobin or the volume of packed red corpuscles. Reticulocytes are usually within normal limits in untreated patients or, at most, are not greater than 3 or 4 percent.

Hypersegmentation of the nuclei of neutrophilic leukocytes is one of the earliest and most consistent blood findings in patients with pernicious anemia (Fig. 305-1*C*). If more than three cells with five lobes or even a single cell with six or more lobes are seen, a presumptive diagnosis of hypersegmentation may be made. Other

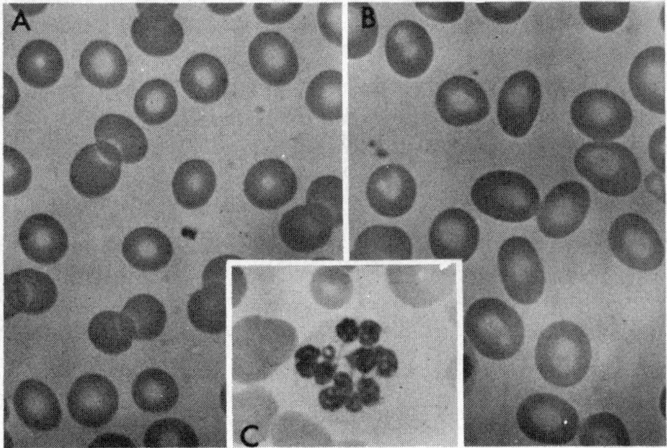

FIGURE 305-1
The blood smear in megaloblastic anemia. A *Normal blood smear for comparison.* B *Pernicious anemia. Most of the erythrocytes are large, oval, and well filled with hemoglobin.* C *Pernicious anemia. Striking hypersegmentation of a neutrophilic leukocyte.*

leukocyte abnormalities also are common in pernicious anemia in relapse. The neutrophils may be exceptionally large, there usually is mild to moderate neutropenia, and an occasional myelocyte may be seen on the blood smear.

Platelets generally are reduced in number and may be large and bizarre in appearance. In exceptional cases, purpura is observed.

Bone marrow The bone marrow is red and is found to be crowded with cells. Cells of the red series make up 30 to 50 percent, rather than about 20 percent, of the cells of the marrow. The degree of hyperplasia and the degree of immaturity of the cells are roughly proportional to the severity of the anemia. The nucleated red corpuscles ("megaloblasts") differ from those found in other types of anemia in several respects. They are exceptionally large, and, more significantly, the nuclear chromatin is fine and sievelike, unlike the relatively coarse and "lumpy" material seen in normoblasts. The cytoplasm of these cells may be polychromatophilic or orthochromatic, and in a few is basophilic. Many abnormal mitotic figures may be present. At the same time, extraordinarily large leukocytes may be found in the marrow; in particular, large ("giant") metamyelocytes may be seen with bizarrely shaped nuclei and peculiarly staining or vacuolated cytoplasm. Megakaryocytes may be reduced in number and may be morphologically abnormal.

Other laboratory findings With very rare exceptions, histamine-fast achlorhydria is found in patients with pernicious anemia. In addition, the total volume of the gastric secretion and its enzyme content are markedly reduced. Mild hyperbilirubinemia due to an increase in the unconjugated or "indirect" fraction is not uncommon. Furthermore, the urobilinogen content of urine and feces is greater than normal. The urinary excretion of methylmalonic acid is markedly increased when vitamin B_{12} is deficient, because this vitamin is required for the enzymatic conversion of methylmalonyl coenzme A to succinyl CoA, a step in the catabolism of proprionic acid.

PATHOLOGY The significant findings are in the alimentary tract, the bone marrow, and the nervous system. The tongue usually appears smooth, and the papillae may be absent. Atrophy of the gastric mucosa may be striking, particularly in the fundus, where the parietal and chief cells are usually absent. The findings in the bone marrow have been described above.

In the nervous system, degenerative changes are found in the dorsal and lateral columns and, in more advanced cases, in the peripheral nerves. The earliest abnormality is loss of the myelin sheath, followed by degeneration of the axon and, finally, by death of the neuron. With appropriate therapy, all but the last are reversible.

Appropriate staining reveals the liver, spleen, and kidneys to be abnormally laden with iron. In the liver, this is found in the periphery of the lobules and in the Kupffer cells. There also may be fatty degeneration in the central cells of the lobules of the liver. The heavy deposit of iron is the consequence of the fault in red blood cell formation which leads to the development of anemia; when active blood regeneration follows therapy, the iron is used in blood formation.

PATHOLOGIC PHYSIOLOGY OF MEGALOBLASTIC ANEMIA

The megaloblast is a morphologic expression of a metabolic defect, namely, disordered synthesis of deoxyribonucleic acid (DNA). Both vitamin B_{12} and folic acid are essential to DNA synthesis. A deficiency of one or both vitamins is the underlying abnormality in the overwhelming majority of patients with megaloblastic anemia.

Vitamin B_{12}, a reddish compound possessing a cobalt-containing tetrapyrrolic ring, is synthesized by certain microorganisms and is principally available to man in the flesh of animals having access to bacterial products. Efficient absorption of dietary vitamin B_{12} ("extrinsic factor") requires its interaction with a thermolabile glycoprotein with a molecular weight of about 50,000 to 60,000 ("intrinsic factor"), secreted in the gastric fundus. This substance has an unusually strong binding affinity for vitamin B_{12}. By attaching to specific receptors in the wall of the distal ileum, intrinsic factor facilitates absorption of vitamin B_{12}. In the presence of intrinsic factor, about 70 percent of ingested vitamin B_{12} is absorbed; less than 2 percent is absorbed in its absence.

Normally, after a delay of several hours in the intestinal wall, the vitamin B_{12} brought there through the intermediation of intrinsic factor is carried through the bloodstream by a specific protein carrier, transcobalamin II. A second protein, transcobalamin I, probably serves a storage rather than a transport function. The serum concentration of vitamin B_{12} in normal subjects is 200 to 900 pg per ml, most of which is bound to transcobalamin I. The total body vitamin B_{12} content is the normal adult is about 5,000 μg (range, 2,000 to 10,000 μg), of which 1,700 μg is stored in the liver. Since biochemical evidence of deficiency is not seen until the total body content drops to less than 500 μg, the surplus of 4,500 μg constitutes a large storage pool. The average daily requirement for vitamin B_{12} in the normal adult is approximately 2.5 μg, but the requirement no doubt is increased during periods of rapid growth and in pregnancy. It has been postulated that the requirement is also increased in hemolytic anemias, in thyrotoxicosis, and even in infection.

The exact role of vitamin B_{12} in DNA synthesis is not certain, but it is clear that it is related to certain functions of folic acid. It is probable that in deficient subjects the vitamin B_{12}–dependent synthesis of methionine is blocked. As a result, folate tends to accumulate in the form of N^5-methyltetrahydrofolate. The latter normally is converted to tetrahydrofolate during methionine synthesis. By this mechanism a relative deficiency of other folate coenzymes develops, including N^5,N^{10}-methenyltetrahydrofolate, a cofactor essential for the synthesis of the DNA precursor, thymidylic acid.

The term *folic acid* has been used to denote either a single chemical substance (pteroylglutamic acid, PGA) or a whole group of unconjugated, conjugated, or formylated compounds owing their activity to the PGA radical; but the term *folate* or *folacin* (Chap. 73) is preferable for the latter, the term folic acid being used to refer to PGA only. Folates are synthesized by higher plants as well as by microorganisms, and are found in many vegetables, as well as in liver. About 90 percent of natural folic acid is conjugated with two to seven glutamate residues. These must be converted to the monoglutamate by intestinal conjugases for absorption to occur. A normal balanced diet may contain 1 to 2 mg folic acid, but little is known about the efficiency of absorption of natural folates. The daily requirement in normal adults is about 50 μg per day but may be as high as 300 μg per day in certain stressful situations, such as pregnancy. Destruction by cooking or loss by aqueous extraction may greatly reduce the amount of folate derived from the diet. Synthetic PGA is absorbed readily and rapidly throughout the small intestine. The serum contains 5 to 20 ng of folate per milliliter in normal subjects. Body stores of folic acid and its derivatives are less substantial than those of vitamin B_{12}. The estimated storage pool of 5 to 10 mg may be depleted after only several months of dietary deprivation.

After absorption, folates are reduced through specific liver enzymes to tetrahydrofolic acid, which is capable of accepting single-carbon fragments such as formyl, methyl, and formimino radicals. N^5-formyltetraphydrofolate (folinic acid, "citrovorum factor"), N^5-methyltetrahydrofolate, and N^5,N^{10}-methenyltetrahydrofolate are among the metabolites that are produced. In these forms folic acid acts as a carbon-transfer agent and as a coenzyme in the synthesis of nucleoprotein. It is essential for the synthesis of carbons 2 and 8 in purines, as well as for the synthesis of thymidylic acid from deoxyuridylic acid.

The alteration in DNA synthesis induced by deficiency of vitamin B_{12} or folate affects many of the tissues of the body, but is especially evident in the hematopoietic system. Before a cell can divide, it must precisely double its DNA content. When DNA synthesis is impaired, cell division is retarded. This is manifest morphologically in an alteration in the nuclear pattern of the red blood cell and an increase in its total size. The abnormal nuclear pattern in the megaloblast presumably results from the prolonged time between cell divisions, allowing for a greater degree of dispersion of nuclear material. Cytoplasmic processes are unaffected; consequently, hemoglobin formation proceeds normally and cell size increases. The maturation of granulocytes and megakaryocytes also is altered, accounting for the presence of giant metamyelocytes in the bone marrow and hypersegmented polymorphonuclear leukocytes in the blood. Cell division in nonerythropoietic tissues also is affected; in the mouth, stomach, and vagina, giant epithelial cells have been demonstrated.

The disordered metabolism of the erythrocytes which characterizes the megaloblastic macrocytic anemias is also manifested by erythroid hyperplasia in the bone marrow. This many be attributed, in part, to the fact that erythropoiesis is ineffective; i.e., many of the red corpuscle precursors, being imperfect, probably are destroyed in the marrow or very shortly after they have been released into the circulation. When red blood cell survival is measured it is found to be mildly shortened; however, the usual techniques for labeling red blood cells do not detect cells which are destroyed in the marrow and, therefore, do not appraise accurately the magnitude of the ineffective erythropoiesis. Ineffective erythropoiesis also accounts for the increased serum bilirubin and increased urobilinogen excretion that so often are found in these disorders. When radioactive glycine is fed to patients with megaloblastic anemia, a disproportionate amount appears in the so-called "early-labeled" bile pigments, indicating that much of the pigment is derived from a very short-lived population of erythrocytes.

The *neurologic damage* seen in some forms of megaloblastic anemia appears to be related specifically to deficiency of vitamin B_{12} rather than of folic acid, and therefore probably is not related to the disordered synthesis of DNA. The biochemical basis for the neurologic changes is unknown.

In pernicious anemia, vitamin B_{12} deficiency is conditioned by lack of intrinsic factor. In other forms of megaloblastic anemia, deficiency is produced in other ways, as will be discussed in the next section. The relatively high familial incidence of pernicious anemia suggests that the defect in intrinsic factor secretion may be genetically determined. In *family studies,* about 13 percent of patients with pernicious anemia have been found to have relatives with this disease. There also is an increased incidence of gastric autoantibodies (see below) in relatives of pernicious anemia patients. Still more impressive is the evidence for an hereditary basis for *congenital pernicious anemia.* A number of pairs of siblings have been reported with this illness, including at least one set of monozygotic twins. The congenital and adult forms of pernicious anemia, however, do not appear to be related genetically.

Several observations suggest that pernicious anemia is produced by autoantibodies directed against the gastric mucosa and that the tendency to form such antibodies may be genetically determined. Antibodies directed against gastric parietal cells are found in 84 percent of patients with pernicious anemia. Similar antibodies are detected in about 50 percent of patients with atrophic gastritis without pernicious anemia, but are uncommon in normal subjects. A second type of antibody, one which reacts directly with intrinsic factor, is found in 56 percent of patients with pernicious anemia but not in other patients with gastric atrophy. The incidence of both types of antibody is greater in relatives of patients with pernicious anemia than in the general population. Still other observations have been made which have been cited as reasons for considering pernicious anemia as representing an autoimmune disorder. Thus, pernicious anemia has been observed to be associated more frequently than would be expected on the basis of chance alone with autoimmune disorders of the thyroid and with certain other conditions of possibly autoimmune nature, such as vitiligo, Addisonian adrenal atrophy, and hypoparathyroidism. In addition, the chronic inflammatory lesions of the stomach in patients with pernicious anemia have been said to resemble those in the thyroid in patients with Hashimoto's thyroiditis. Furthermore, administration of adrenocorticosteroids may improve vitamin B_{12} absorption and induce hematologic improvement in pernicious anemia. Nevertheless, despite the above observations, a cause and effect relationship between the autoimmune phenomena and the gastric lesions in pernicious anemia remains to be demonstrated. It is possible that the antibodies are the consequence of a genetically determined defect in the gastric mucosa, rather than its cause.

MEGALOBLASTIC MACROCYTIC ANEMIAS OTHER THAN PERNICIOUS ANEMIA

Dietary deficiency of folate, of vitamin B_{12}, or of both; impaired absorption of these vitamins; increased requirements; or faulty metabolism may singly or in combination produce this type of anemia. Probably because of its less-efficient storage, folate deficiency is relatively common among the malnourished. In contrast, even in the strictest vegetarians ("vegans") vitamin B_{12} deficiency of a degree sufficient to produce megaloblastic anemia is very rare. Pure folate deficiency with macrocytic anemia has been produced experimentally in swine, but dietary deficiency of vitamin B_{12} alone has not resulted in macrocytic anemia.

The various forms of megaloblastic anemia are listed in Table 305-1, where those due to vitamin B_{12} deficiency and to folic acid deficiency are listed separately. However, a number of conditions are found under both categories. This may be accounted for, in part, by the intimate relationship of these two vitamins in metabolism, as discussed earlier. This explains why, in a disorder such as pernicious anemia, when the specific fault is inability to absorb vitamin B_{12} efficiently from the diet, a hematologic response, albeit temporary or incomplete, follows administration of folic acid. Actually the propensity of an individual to develop a deficiency of these vitamins depends on many factors. Thus, in a person with imperfect means for absorption of vitamin B_{12}, the development of deficiency will depend on the degree and duration of intrinsic factor deficiency (e.g., lifetime or only since the performance of a gastrectomy), on intestinal factors influencing its absorption or permitting its utilization or destruction, or on altered metabolic requirements. Furthermore, other factors being equal, folic acid deficiency is likely to develop more readily than lack of vitamin B_{12} because storage of folic acid is less efficient than that of vitamin B_{12}.

The hematologic manifestations of *folic acid deficiency* are the same as those of vitamin B_{12} deficiency. The gastrointestinal manifestations are similar but may be more widespread and more severe than those of pernicious anemia. Thus diarrhea is often present and may be accompanied by distention, flatulence, and the roentgenographic picture of sprue. Cheilosis and glossitis are common, and ulcerative stomatitis, pharyngitis, esophagitis with dysphagia, and perirectal and peroneal weeping and ulcerations may appear. However, neurologic abnormalities like those seen in pernicious anemia do not occur.

Certain syndromes may now be discussed separately.

FOLLOWING SURGERY Following *total gastrectomy* or extensive damage to gastric mucosa as, for example, by ingestion of corrosive agents, megaloblastic anemia may develop because the source of intrinsic factor has been removed. In such patients the absorption of orally administered vitamin B_{12} is impaired. Megaloblastic anemia may also follow partial gastrectomy, but the incidence is very much lower than after total gastrectomy, although iron-deficiency anemia is relatively common. The macrocytic anemia seen in association with intestinal strictures, diverticula, anastomoses, and "blind loops" may be attributed to colonization of the small intestine by large masses of bacteria which divert vitamin B_{12} from the host. Hematologic responses have been observed when tetracyclines were given.

IN FISH TAPEWORM INFESTATION True megaloblastic macrocytic anemia is seen, in Finland especially, in persons harboring the tapeworm, *Diphyllobothrium latum*. The anemia is attributable to competition between the worm and the intrinsic factor of the host for vitamin B_{12}.

NUTRITIONAL MACROCYTIC ANEMIA This term refers to macrocytic anemia arising from dietary folate deficiency, as distinguished from deficiency resulting from lack of intrinsic factor or from faulty absorption. The condition is particularly common in pregnant women, infants, and the aged. Weakness, shortness of breath, sore mouth, sore tongue, diarrhea, and edema are common complaints. In contrast to pernicious anemia, achlorhydria is no more common than in the population in general, and degenerative changes in the nervous system are practically never found. The blood picture and bone marrow are indistinguishable from those of pernicious anemia.

Since nutritional macrocytic anemia has been seen most often in the tropics, *tropical macrocytic anemia* is sometimes used as a synonym. However, tropical sprue is another common cause of megaloblastic anemia in certain tropical regions. Tropical macrocytic anemia thus is not a single clinical entity. In many patients the anemia has been relieved by the administration of yeast, Marmite (autolyzed yeast), or liver. In some cases a good hematopoietic response has followed the administration of folic acid, and in a few patients (probably those with tropical sprue) a good response to vitamin B_{12} and even to oral penicillin has been reported. That some form of dietary deficiency is the cause of this disorder is indicated by the observation that it does not recur if the diet is satisfactory.

Nutritional macroctyic anemia is less common in the temperate zones. However, it has been found in as many as 40 percent of alcoholics who become ill enough to be hospitalized. In such patients the VPRC averages 30 ml per 100 ml, but the degree of macrocytosis (average MCV 105 fl) tends to be less than that found in pernicious anemia, possibly because the condition often is complicated by sideroblastic anemia. In addition to nutritional deficiency, effects of alcohol on folate absorption and on hepatic folate metabolism may contribute to the development of megaloblastic anemia. Some of the instances of macrocytic anemia seen in pellagra may be accounted for by a lack of vitamin B_{12} in the diet.

MALABSORPTION SYNDROMES In other instances faulty absorption is important, and in many patients both mechanisms play a role. In malabsorption syndromes, as described elsewhere (Chap. 284), inadequate absorption is the main cause for the development of macrocytic anemia. In Great Britain, in particular, occult idiopathic steatorrhea with insignificant alimentary symptoms but accompanied by megaloblastic macrocytic anemia is not uncommon. The latter usually responds much better to the administration of folic acid than to vitamin B_{12}. A specific, selective vitamin B_{12} malabsorption disease beginning in infancy and childhood, familial in occurrence, and characterized by relapsing megaloblastic anemia and proteinuria has been described in Norway.

IN PREGNANCY Megaloblastic anemia may be observed during the third trimester of pregnancy. In most cases it appears to be due to folate deficiency occurring as the result of a marginal diet and the demands of the developing fetus. The syndrome is most common in geographic areas where nutritional macrocytic anemia is observed. Occasionally, however, it is encountered in temperate zones, and historical evidence of dietary inadequacy may be difficult to elicit. Even in such cases, the serum folate level is reduced and a response to the administration of folate may be expected. Exceptional cases have been reported in which vitamin B_{12} appeared to be the deficient nutrient.

IN INFANCY Megaloblastic anemia was observed in infants fed on unsupplemented, heat-treated dried milk formulas. The anemia was frequently accompanied by signs of scurvy. Addition of folate and ascorbate to infant-feeding formulas has largely eliminated this form of anemia, especially in better-developed countries.

IN PRESENCE OF EXCESSIVE DEMANDS In rare instances of very active hematopoiesis, especially in hemolytic anemias, the hemoglobinopathies, myelofibrosis, sideroblastic anemia, and multiple myeloma, megaloblastic anemia has been observed, presumably because of excessively great demands for building materials in persons whose stores of these substances were marginal.

HEREDITARY DISORDERS ASSOCIATED WITH MEGALOBLASTIC ANEMIA *Selective vitamin B_{12} malabsorption* has been described as a rare familial disorder, inherited as an autosomal recessive trait, which appears in the first 2 years of life and is associated with proteinuria (*Imerslund's syndrome*). The defect may be due to impairment of a stage of vitamin B_{12} absorption that follows ileal attachment of the intrinsic factor–vitamin B_{12} complex and can be circumvented by the parenteral administration of vitamin B_{12}.

Congenital folate malabsorption also has been described as a rare disorder associated with mental retardation and ataxia.

An inherited autosomal recessive disorder of pyrimidine metabolism (*orotic aciduria*) is characterized by megaloblastic anemia, excessive excretion of orotic acid, and impairment of growth and development. This condition does not respond to folate or vitamin B_{12} but is corrected by the administration of uridine.

The *Lesch-Nyhan syndrome*, which results from lack of the enzyme hypoxanthine-guanine phosphoribosyltransferase, has been reported in one instance to be associated with megaloblastic anemia which responded to the administration of adenine. Other extremely rare instances of megaloblastic anemia due to metabolic abnormalities, congenital or inherited, include *N^5-methyltetrahydrofolate transferase deficiency, formimino transferase deficiency, dihydrofolate reductase deficiency, and transcobalamin II deficiency.*

DRUG-INDUCED MEGALOBLASTIC ANEMIA There are two main forms of megaloblastic anemia in this category.

1. Megaloblastic anemia is one of the predictable toxic effects of certain drugs used in the chemotherapy of leukemia, lymphomas, and solid tumors. These include methotrexate, 6-mercaptopurine, cytosine arabinoside, cyclophosphamide, and 5-fluorouracil. These drugs are used because they *interfere with DNA synthesis* and thereby impair the growth of rapidly dividing tissues. The folate antagonists act chiefly by competitive inhibition of dihydrofolate reductase. A similar although less pronounced effect is one of the side effects of certain drugs used for other purposes, such as pyrimethamine, triamterine, pentamidine, and trimethoprine.
2. The use of certain *anticonvulsant drugs,* such as diphenylhydantoin (Dilantin), primidone (Mysoline), and phenobarbital, has been claimed to be associated with evidence of folate deficiency and mild hematologic changes resulting from inhibition of intestinal conjugase, with consequent failure to absorb either folic polyglutamates or perhaps free folate. A similar defect in folate absorption has been reported in women taking oral contraceptive medications, but requires confirmation.

The intake of a folate-deficient diet and poor folate stores increase the likelihood that megaloblastic anemia will occur in the various situations mentioned above.

Megaloblastic anemia has also been reported as a rare effect of para-aminosalicylic acid (PAS) therapy. This drug *impairs vitamin B_{12} absorption.* Similar reversible malabsorption has been observed in patients taking colchicine, neomycin, or ethanol.

MISCELLANEOUS DISORDERS In patients such as those described at one time as having achrestic anemia and refractory megaloblastic anemia, because they failed to respond to liver therapy, there may be impaired metabolism of folic acid or complex deficiencies of folic acid, ascorbic acid, choline, or perhaps other substances essential for the metabolic steps which result in normal erythropoiesis.

In hypothyroidism Macrocytic anemia is sometimes seen in hypothyroidism, but the bone marrow is usually hypoplastic and normoblastic, and desiccated thyroid, not vitamin B_{12} or pteroylglutamic acid, is effective in relieving the anemia. Defective intestinal absorption of vitamin B_{12}, uninfluenced by intrinsic factor, has been demonstrated in some cases.

In liver disease Macrocytic anemia occurs in a variable number of patients with chronic liver disease, and in a few it is megaloblastic. Because of the detergent effects of retained bile salts, erythrocyte membrane lipids may become altered, and an increase in membrane area results. This phenomenon may account for nonmegaloblastic macrocytosis in certain patients with liver disease. No wholly satisfactory explanation for the occasional case of megaloblastic anemia has been found. It is conceivable that the requirements for folic acid and vitamin B_{12} may be increased or that their absorption, storage, or utilization is impaired.

DIAGNOSIS

Optimum therapy in macrocytic anemia is completely dependent on accurate diagnosis. In nonmegaloblastic anemias, therapy with folic acid or vitamin B_{12} is valueless. In megaloblastic anemias, correction of the underlying fault, if possible, and in any event selection of the proper vitamin are of critical importance. For example, if folic acid is given to a patient with pernicious anemia, transient hematolotic improvement may be observed but neurologic lesions may appear and progress.

THE CLINICAL SETTING When megaloblastic anemia is found together with neurologic symptoms in an elderly subject with a history of an adequate diet, pernicious anemia is the most likely diagnosis. The detection of neurologic disease is of great diagnostic help, since it occurs only in vitamin B_{12} deficiency; however, only a small proportion of patients exhibit such findings. The demonstration of achylia gastrica supports a diagnosis of pernicious anemia. This impression may be further confirmed by means of a Schilling test. Megaloblastic anemia in an infant, a pregnant woman, or an alcoholic suggests folate deficiency, and confirmation may be sought by the determination of serum vitamin content. A careful history should reveal exposure to the drugs associated with megaloblastic anemia, or uncover symptoms of malabsorption.

LABORATORY EVIDENCE OF SPECIFIC VITAMIN DEFICIENCY When the clinical setting is complex, it is helpful to determine whether there is a deficiency of vitamin B_{12} or of folate. Two indirect tests are available for this purpose. Excessive *urinary excretion of methylmalonic acid* is a sensitive and relatively specific test for vitamin B_{12} deficiency. The *histidine loading test,* which consists of measurement of urinary formiminoglutamic acid (FIGlu) after the oral administration of histidine is a sensitive test for folate deficiency; however, abnormal values also have been observed in some patients with severe vitamin B_{12} deficiency.

More direct evidence for specific vitamin deficiency consists of the determination of serum vitamin levels. Serum vitamin B_{12} concentration may be determined by means of a *microbiologic bioassay* system employing *Euglena gracilis* or by a simpler technique based on radioisotope dilution. The normal range is 200 to 900 pg per ml, and values less than 100 pg per ml may be considered diagnostic of vitamin B_{12} deficiency. A microbiologic assay for folate is available which employs *Lactobacillus casei* as the test organism. The normal serum concentration ranges from 6 to 21 ng per ml; values of 4 ng per ml or less are diagnostic of folate deficiency.

Because of the technical problems associated with microbiologic assays, they are not generally available. The indirect tests are somewhat simpler, but they, too, are not available in most routine clinical laboratories. For this reason, clinicians often must depend on *therapeutic trials* to establish the diagnosis. In performing a therapeutic trial, it is important to employ minimal effective doses, since larger doses may induce nonspecific responses. The minimal effective dose of vitamin B_{12} is 1 μg per day; in the case of folate, it is 200 μg per day. During a trial, after a 5- to 10-day period of observation, one of these vitamins is administered parenterally. Reticulocyte counts should be performed daily during the control and trial periods, and the volume of packed red blood cells and hemoglobin should be determined at 5-day intervals. A response is detected when a significant reticulocytosis occurs 5 to 10 days after the onset of therapy, and reduction in the degree of anemia should follow. A typical response to minimal doses of vitamin B_{12} is illustrated in Fig. 305-2.

The Schilling test The discovery of vitamin B_{12} and the fact that the cobalt contained therein can be labeled radioactively have provided methods whereby the absorption of this vitamin can be measured. They offer a means by which defective absorption of the vitamin from the gastrointestinal tract can be demonstrated even in the absence of anemia. This is useful in treated cases of pernicious anemia, and to some extent is helpful in distinguishing pernicious anemia from other disorders of vitamin B_{12} absorption. Several different techniques are available, but the most commonly used one, the Schilling test, depends on measurement of the excretion of the administered radioactive material in the urine. When radioactive vitamin B_{12} is given by mouth to persons who can absorb it, radioactivity will appear in the urine if the person is simultaneously given a very large amount (1,000 μg) of nonradioactive vitamin B_{12} intramuscularly. Normal individuals have been found to excrete 5 to 40 percent of the orally administered radioactivity in the urine in the next 48 hr if an oral dose of 2 μg is used. Patients with pernicious anemia excrete less than 5 percent under these conditions. In them, the simultaneous oral administration of intrinsic factor and radioactive vitamin results in increased excretion. In contrast, although excretion is also reduced in patients with one of the malabsorption syndromes (Chap. 284), no improvement occurs when intrinsic factor is added.

MANAGEMENT AND PROGNOSIS

PERNICIOUS ANEMIA AND OTHER VITAMIN B_{12} DEFICIENCY STATES With appropriate therapy it is now possible to restore the blood to normal and to promote a return of the general nutrition to normal. If changes are present in the nervous system, their advance can at least be halted, and in those cases in which death of nerve cells has not occurred, the neurologic lesions are reversible. The danger in pernicious anemia arises from failure to continue therapy and from complications and intercurrent conditions. In a chronic ailment like pernicious anemia, other diseases develop in the course of time. Among these, carcinoma of the stomach is particularly noteworthy, since the incidence of this disease in patients with pernicious anemia is more than three times as great as in other persons. When changes in the nervous system exist, particularly if they involve the urinary sphincter, infection may occur. The existence of infection at the time of relapse may seriously interfere with the response to therapy.

Treatment, insofar as the blood changes are concerned, is extremely simple. The administration of an adequate amount of vitamin B_{12} is followed by a reticulocyte response which reaches its maximum 5 to 7 or 8 days following initiation of therapy (Fig. 305-2). This is succeeded, as the reticulocyte count falls to normal, by a rapid disappearance of anemia and by the production of cells of normal size and shape. The leukocyte and the platelet counts likewise return to normal, bilirubinemia disappears, and the increased quantities of urobilinogen in the urine and stools are reduced to the normal range. The gastric achlorhydria persists.

Effective treatment may produce subjective improvement within 48 hr, and evidence of a change is often noted by the patient before the reticulocytes increase in number. He will experience a gain in appetite and a sense of well-being. Tongue symptoms, if present, disappear promptly. On the other hand, neural symptoms do not change quickly. Although the blood usually becomes normal in the course of 2 months from the beginning of

FIGURE 305-2
The response to a minimal effective dose of vitamin B_{12} (cyanocobalamin, 1 μg per day) in a patient with pernicious anemia. The earliest change is an increase in the reticulocyte count, which usually reaches a peak 5 to 7 days after therapy is begun. (Courtesy of Dr. Victor Herbert, N Engl J Med 268:368, 1963)

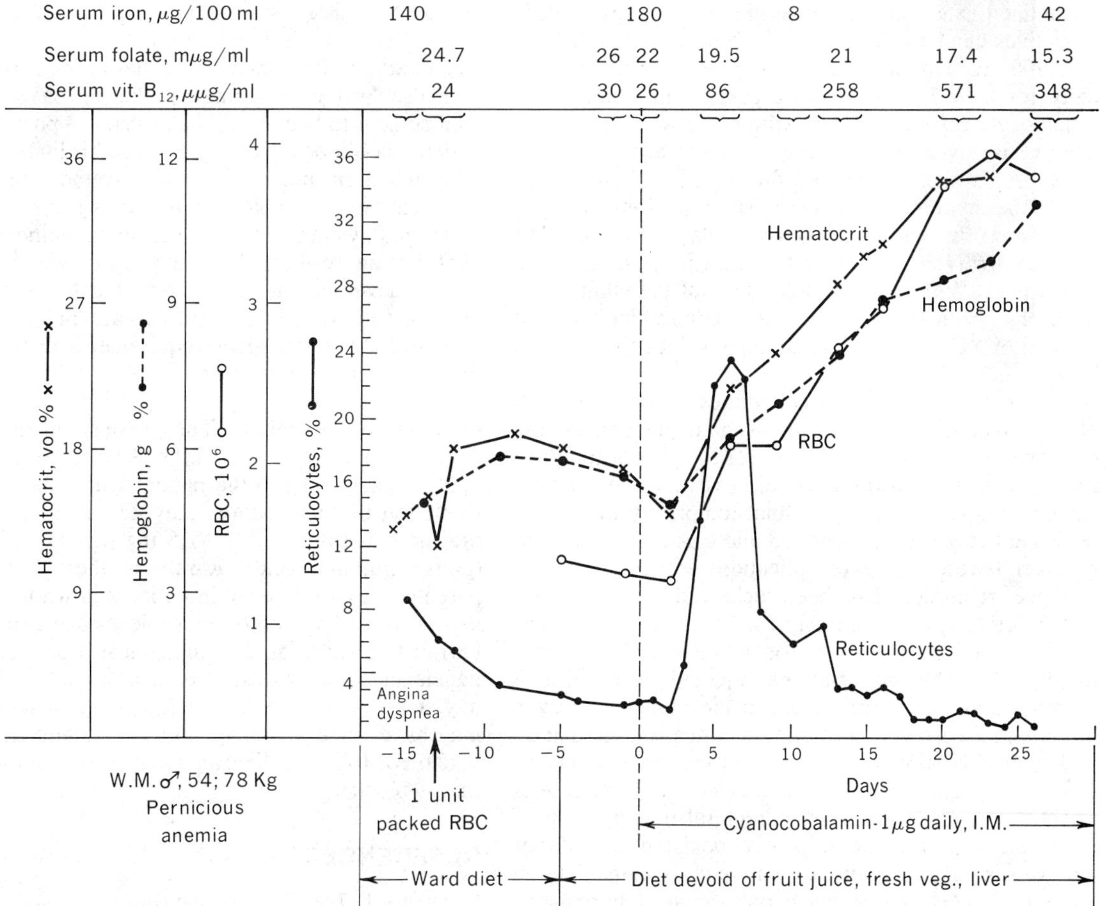

treatment, the neurologic symptoms may still be present. However, those of milder intensity are likely to decrease or disappear.

The most efficient means of treatment is by the intramuscular injection of vitamin B_{12}. Intravenous therapy is effective but unnecessary. The effects of vitamin B_{12} in pernicious anemia are very much more pronounced when the vitamin is given parenterally than when it is taken orally (60 to 100 times). Two forms of vitamin B_{12} are available for therapeutic use, namely, cyanocobalamin and hydroxocobalamin. The two preparations differ in degree of retention in the body and excretion in the urine, but both are capable of inducing and maintaining remission and both are nontoxic, except for very rare allergic reactions. On the average, hydroxocobalamin provides higher serum concentrations of vitamin B_{12} for a longer period than does cyanocobalamin, but there is considerable individual variation, and from the practical standpoint it is not important whether one or the other preparation is used. The minimal effective intramuscular dose of vitamin B_{12} is 1 μg daily. Larger amounts, up to 80 μg or more daily, produce greater effects, the mean response being roughly proportional to the logarithm of the dose. As larger doses are given, however, a greater proportion is promptly excreted.

In a patient with pernicious anemia in relapse, vitamin B_{12} must be given to induce a remission and to reestablish body stores of the vitamin. Then these stores need to be maintained, and this requires lifelong therapy. These objectives can be achieved by the following schedule: at first 100 μg cyanocobalamin is given intramuscularly daily for 6 to 7 days. If the characteristic clinical and reticulocyte response occurs within the week, the same amount is given on alternate days for another seven doses. A distinct increase in the VPRC or hemoglobin should be evident by this time. The injections are continued now only every third or fourth day for another 2 to 3 weeks, to give a total of 1.8 to 2.0 mg in the course of 5 or 6 weeks. With this schedule much of the vitamin B_{12} which has been given should have been retained and, at the end of 5 or 6 weeks, hematologic values should have become normal.

Alternatively, only five weekly injections of 1 mg each of hydroxocobalamin can be given, depending on the desirability in the individual case for the patient to return for medical supervision. Early discovery of the patient's failure to respond promptly and completely allows interfering factors to be identified and corrective action to be taken before further complications ensue.

Once remission has been achieved, 100 μg cyanocobalamin is given monthly for life. If circumstances preclude monthly injections for maintenance therapy, 1 mg hydroxocobalamin may be injected every 2 to 4 months, and examinations are made at least every 4 months to ascertain that remission status is maintained.

Under exceptional circumstances vitamin B_{12} may be given orally, e.g., to those patients who refuse parenteral injections or those in whom parenteral therapy may be hazardous (e.g., those who have a coexistent disorder of hemostasis or sensitivity to parenterally administered vitamin B_{12}). However, since only about 1 percent of orally administered vitamin B_{12} is absorbed, doses that are very large in relation to the body's requirement must be given, usually 300 to 1,000 μg per day. This is preferable to the use of vitamin B_{12}–porcine intrinsic factor combinations. Although this combination facilitates vitamin B_{12} at the outset, patients eventually become refractory to the action of such heterologous intrinsic factor because of the development of antibodies. Patients maintained with oral vitamin B_{12} require much closer supervision than those to whom the vitamin is given parenterally, because the risk of hematologic or neurologic relapse due to forgotten or otherwise omitted treatment is ever present.

Folic acid, in doses which greatly exceed the normal daily requirement, induces a hematopoietic response in pernicious anemia. However, while the administration of vitamin B_{12} relieves or prevents the advancement of the neurologic manifestations of pernicious anemia, these may appear and progress when only folic acid is given.

The diet should be such as to restore the patient to a state of normal nutrition and to maintain this state, but it need not contain any unusual foods.

Transfusion is rarely, if ever, required in pernicious anemia, since a physiologic response can be achieved in 48 to 72 hr if vitamin B_{12} is given parenterally. Since the patient's anemia has developed gradually, he has become adjusted to it. When the cardiovascular system is imperfect, transfusion, by producing a sudden increase in blood volume, may sometimes be harmful and may precipitate acute cardiac failure with pulmonary edema. Iron is not needed as an adjunct except when iron deficiency exists as well. Supplementary therapy with various vitamins is likewise unnecessary. These can be and should be furnished in the diet in the form of food.

Particularly when changes in the nervous system exist, confinement to bed should be as brief as possible and the patient should be encouraged to use his limbs even when lying in bed. In addition, passive movement, massage, and dry heat are valuable for improving the tone of the muscles. Physiotherapy may permit adjustment to permanent damage resulting from the neurologic changes.

The development of an intercurrent disease, particularly infection, calls for an increase in the amount of vitamin B_{12} therapy, since requirements under such conditions seem to be increased.

FOLATE DEFICIENCY The above comments regarding general supportive care and the use of blood transfusions apply equally well to the patient with folate deficiency. Repletion of folate stores may be accomplished by the oral administration of 1 to 5 mg per day of folic acid (pteroylglutamic acid). Rarely is there any need for parenteral therapy, even in patients in whom absorption is defective. Apparently, these doses can circumvent the barrier to absorption. For antagonist-produced folic acid deficiencies, larger doses, as much as 100 to 200 mg per day, may be required. Folinic acid (citrovorum factor) may have some advantage in such situations, since conversion of folic to folinic acid may be one of the reactions that is blocked.

REFERENCES

Chanarin I: *The Megaloblastic Anemias,* Philadelphia: Davis, 1969

DONALDSON RM: Small bowel bacterial overgrowth. Adv Intern Med 16:191, 1970

DONIACH D, ROITT IM: An evaluation of gastric and thyroid autoimmunity in relation to hematologic disorders. Semin Hematol 1:313, 1964

EICHNER ER, HILLMAN RS: The evolution of anemia in alcoholic patients. Am J Med 50:218, 1971

GOUGH KR et al: Megaloblastic anemia due to nutritional deficiency of folic acid. Q J Med 32:243, 1963

LINDENBAUM J, KLIPSTEIN FA: Folic acid deficiency in sickle cell anemia. N Engl J Med 269:875, 1963

Symposium on vitamin B_{12} and folate. Am J Med 48:539, 1970

WINTROBE MM et al: *Clinical Hematology*, 7th ed., Philadelphia: Lea & Febiger, 1974

306 HEMOLYTIC ANEMIAS

ARTHUR HAUT
M. M. WINTROBE

Definition Shortening of the "life span" of the red corpuscles is the essential feature of a hemolytic anemia. As outlined in an earlier chapter (Chap. 58), however, shortened erythrocytic life span characterizes a large variety of anemias. Therefore, to this criterion of hemolytic anemia must be added that of greatly accelerated destruction of mature red corpuscles.

PATHOGENESIS

The formation and destruction of hemoglobin were discussed earlier (Chap. 58), as were the pathogenesis and manifestations of various types of anemia. The causes of increased red blood cell destruction may be separated into three main groups: (1) Those which depend mainly on an intrinsic defect of the red corpuscle, (2) those which are extracorpuscular in origin, and (3) those in which both an intrinsic corpuscular defect *plus* an extracorpuscular factor bring about hemolysis (see the accompanying classification).

Phagocytosis, agglutinins and hemolysins, osmotic lysis, mechanical factors, and sequestration with erythrostasis condition or cause the destruction of red corpuscles. Intrinsic defects of erythrocyte metabolism predispose to the three last-named pathways of erythrocytic destruction. The importance of *phagocytosis* in the pathogenesis of hemolysis is not clear. However, contact between IgG-coated erythrocytes and phagocytic mononuclear cells spheres the erythrocytes even if they are not phagocytosed. Red cells thus altered are susceptible to splenic entrapment (see below). Various types of *hemagglutinins* and *hemolysins* have been described (see Serologic tests below). Immune hemolysins are not found free in the serum except in disorders which require special conditions for their maximum effect. Thus in paroxysmal cold hemoglobinuria (see below), a fall in temperature is required for maximum activity of the hemolytic system. In most instances immune hemagglutinins remain attached to the red corpuscle. The *Coombs test* serves to demonstrate such factors (see below).

The importance of *mechanical factors* is indicated by the fact that the osmotic and mechanical fragilities of the red corpuscles increase when the corpuscles are placed in natural or artificial immune serums in which hemolysins and agglutinins are present. Similar changes in fragility have been observed in association with hemolytic agents, such as saponin, or physical factors, such as heat. It is a plausible hypothesis that mechanical trauma is the ultimate mechanism whereby cell destruction occurs under normal circumstances and in many varieties of hemolytic anemia. In march hemoglobinuria, in certain distance runners, and in karate practitioners, very intense physical stress applied to red cells in the tissue capillaries results in hemolysis. These are examples of "pure" physical-mechanical forces producing hemolytic disease or anemia. The hemolytic anemia associated with defective aortic valve prostheses is an intravascular counterpart of the same phenomenon. *Osmotic lysis*, usually determined by the familiar hypotonic saline fragility test, probably does not operate in vivo except perhaps in the spleen under certain conditions. It has been shown that nearly spheric cells, strongly agglutinated cells, and those with weakened cell membranes are abnormally susceptible to mechanical destruction. In certain cases of acquired hemolytic anemia, increased mechanical fragility has been observed when osmotic fragility was normal. The increased mechanical fragility of sickled masses of erythrocytes may contribute to the increased red corpuscle destruction in sickle-cell anemia (Chap. 307).

Sequestration, by the *spleen*, plays an important part in hemolytic anemias when spherocytes are in the circulation. The spleen appears to have the property of selectively detaining and removing spheroidal cells, as distinguished from normal erythrocytes. This is equally true for the spleen of a patient with hereditary spherocytosis and for a normal spleen or one from a patient with another hematologic disorder but free of a hemolytic process. The spleen also entraps red cells which are not deformable or resilient, e.g., the rigid red cells which are sickled or contain hemoglobin C crystals, or those with acquired membrane defects.

In sequestering sensitized red corpuscles from the circulation, the spleen behaves as a highly proficient, passive filter. Thus, when sensitized red corpuscles are injected into the circulation of normal subjects, they are agglutinated by the plasma globulins, following which they are sequestered in the spleen and are hemolyzed within a few minutes. The speed of the hemolysis is such as to suggest the presence of a preformed lysin; leukocytes may be involved in this lytic process. In reactions involving "complete" antibodies (as when red corpuscles are injected into normal subjects hyperimmunized against them), sequestration and destruction occur in the liver to a greater extent than in the spleen. This is in contrast to the fate of sensitized corpuscles coated with "incomplete" antibodies described above.

Once spherocytes are mechanically trapped by the spleen, other mechanisms may bring about their destruction. The term *erythrostasis* has been applied to the processes to which red corpuscles are subjected when denied free access to fresh plasma. Erythrostasis in the sinusoids of the spleen may lead to depletion of glucose and other energy-yielding substrates. In the absence of these substrates, ATP accumulation ceases and the ATP-dependent sodium pump fails. This results in a lag of sodium efflux from red corpuscles and a net gain of sodium and water, which, in turn, could result in hemolysis not unlike the "osmotic hemolysis" of in vitro tests.

Following tagging of red corpuscles with ^{51}Cr, the relative importance of the spleen and liver in the hemolytic process can be estimated by comparing the radioactivity over the spleen with that over the heart and liver.

CLINICAL MANIFESTATIONS

Whether anemia develops and what the clinical manifestations may be depend on (1) the rate at which the increased breakdown of red corpuscles is occurring; (2) the ability of the bone marrow to make up for the shortened survival of the red corpuscles by increasing red blood cell production; (3) the capacity of the liver to extract from the plasma the increased quantity of bilirubin resulting from the breakdown of the red blood cells; (4) the quantity of haptoglobin available to bind the free

TABLE 306-1
Classification of hemolytic disorders

I Intrinsic erythrocytic defects
- *A* Congenital
  - *1* Membrane defects
    - *a* Hereditary spherocytosis
    - *b* Hereditary elliptocytosis
    - *c* Stomatocytosis
    - *d* Acanthocytosis
  - *2* Hereditary deficiency of enzymes of the Embden-Meyerhof pathway (anaerobic glycolysis)
    - *a* Pyruvate kinase
    - *b* Hexokinase
    - *c* Glucosephosphate isomerase
    - *d* Phosphofructokinase
    - *e* Triosephosphate isomerase
    - *f* Glyceraldehyde 3-phosphate dehydrogenase
    - *g* Phosphoglycerate kinase
    - *h* 2,3-Diphosphoglycerate mutase
  - *3* Abnormalities of the phosphogluconate oxidative pathway ("hexosemonophosphate shunt")
    - *a* Glucose 6-phosphate dehydrogenase deficiency
      - (*1*) Negro-type, "primaquine-sensitive"
      - (*2*) Chronic hemolytic anemia
    - *b* Glutathione reductase deficiency
    - *c* Deficiency of reduced glutathione
    - *d* Glutathione peroxidase deficiency
  - *4* Unknown mechanisms, associated with erythropoietic porphyria
  - *5* Qualitative abnormalities of globin peptides (hemoglobinopathies S, C, etc.)
  - *6* Quantitative abnormality in globin peptide synthesis (thalassemia syndromes)
- *B* Acquired
  - *1* Vitamin B_{12} deficiency*
  - *2* Folic acid deficiency*
  - *3* Paroxysmal nocturnal hemoglobinuria

II Extraerythrocytic Factors
- *A* Due to factors extraneous to the patient
  - *1* Isoantibodies due to, or reacting with:
    - *a* transfused incompatible erythrocytes
    - *b* fetomaternal incompatibility: Rh, ABO
  - *2* Chemical agents and drugs
    - *a* Related to size of dose: (1) phenylhydrazine, (2) toluene, (3) trinitrotoluene, (4) benzene, (5) acetanilid, (6) phenacetin, (7) aniline, (8) methyl chloride, (9) arsine, (10) lead
    - *b* Secondary immunohemolytic anemia, due to (1) haptene type: penicillin; (2) "innocent bystander" reaction: stibophen, quinidine, quinine, phenacetin, etc.; (3) alpha-methyldopa type
  - *3* Infectious agents
    - *a* Malaria (blackwater fever)
    - *b* *Bartonella* (Oroya fever)
    - *c* Septicemia: *Clostridium welchii, Vibrio comma* (cholera), rarely others
    - *d* Viruses (atypical pneumonia, infectious mononucleosis)
  - *4* Physical agents
    - *a* Heat: severe thermal burns
    - *b* Intravascular trauma
      - (*1*) Aortic valve disease
      - (*2*) Valve prostheses
      - (*3*) Microangiopathic [malignant hypertension, cancer, dissecting intravascular coagulation (DIC), lupus erythematosus, etc.]
    - *c* Gamma irradiation
    - *d* March hemoglobinuria
  - *5* Vegetable poison: castor bean (ricin)
  - *6* Animal poisons
    - *a* Snake venoms (lecithinase)
    - *b* Brown-spider venom (*Loxoceles reclusa*)
- *B* Conditions developing within the body, with and without demonstrable autoantibodies
  - *1* Idiopathic acquired hemolytic anemias (Coombs-positive)
    - *a* Antibodies reactive at or near 37°C ("warm" antibodies)
    - *b* Antibodies most reactive at or near 4°C ("cold" antibodies)
  - *2* Secondary or "symptomatic" hemolytic anemias, associated with:
    - *a* Hodgkin's disease
    - *b* Chronic lymphocytic leukemia, lymphosarcoma
    - *c* Disseminated lupus erythematosus
    - *d* Metastatic carcinomatosis
    - *e* Sarcoidosis; myelofibrosis, myeloid metaplasia
    - *f* Liver disease; ovarian tumors
    - *g* Thrombotic thrombocytopenic purpura
    - *h* Renal cortical necrosis (hemolytic-uremic syndrome); sometimes chronic renal disease
  - *3* Paroxysmal cold hemoglobinuria

** Also characterized by defective DNA synthesis.*

hemoglobin and to prevent its escape through the kidneys; (5) the nature and manifestations of the disorder responsible for the reduced corpuscular life span; and (6) the occurrence of certain complications, such as gallstones or cholestasis, resulting from the increased formation of bilirubin. In certain instances, sudden depression of erythropoiesis takes place and a relatively stable state of balance between production and destruction may be upset. In this event, severe anemia develops suddenly (*hyporegenerative crisis*).

Jaundice is a sign common to all forms of hemolytic anemia, but its degree may be such that it is barely perceptible (when it is often overlooked, especially in yellowish incandescent illumination) or striking. Other symptoms may be entirely absent. Thus patients with hereditary spherocytosis are "more yellow than sick" except when a hyporegenerative crisis occurs.

In chronic hemolytic anemia of any cause, *splenomegaly* is common and the liver also may be enlarged. Complications such as cholelithiasis, due to bilirubin stones, or chronic leg ulcers may develop.

In some instances, there may be slowly progressive *anemia* and gradually increasing jaundice. The anemia may become profound, but if there has been time for cardiovascular adjustment (Chap. 58), there may be few manifestations. The age of the patient and underlying cardiopulmonary disease will affect the degree of this adjustment.

On the other hand, the onset of hemolytic anemia may be heralded by a severe, shaking chill followed by high fever, malaise, headache, and pain in the back, abdomen, or limbs. The abdominal pain may be so severe and may be accompanied by such marked muscular rigidity and spasm as to simulate an acute condition requiring surgery. Hemoglobin and methemoglobin in the urine may render it a dark color. If the hemolysis is rapid and severe enough, profound prostration and shock, accompanied by anuria and oliguria, may ensue. Jaundice develops rapidly. Weakness, palpitation, dyspnea, tachycardia, cyanosis, cardiac enlargement, hemic murmurs, vertigo, faintness, and other manifestations of rapidly developing anemia (Chap. 303) then appear. In certain types of acute hemolytic reactions, urticaria, vascular disturbances suggesting Raynaud's phenomenon, and thrombosis and gangrene may be present (Chap. 247).

All grades of hemolytic anemia, from such acute fulminating disorders of several days' duration to extremely benign conditions of many years' standing, may be encountered. A chronic, congenital acquired anemia may be interrupted by acute exacerbations.

It is possible for the survival of red corpuscles to be reduced to 20 days or a little less without development of anemia, provided there is compensatory acceleration of effective erythropoiesis of equivalent magnitude. Such a compensated state may be maintained for long periods of time. On the other hand, especially in association with an acute infection, sudden depression of erythropoiesis may take place. In such hyporegenerative crises the reticulocyte count falls, anemia develops rapidly, and the bone marrow may show hypoplasia. In other instances of reticulocytopenia, the maturation of the red blood cells may seem to be arrested, and megaloblasts have been demonstrated in some cases. In these instances, it is assumed that a relative deficiency of folic acid has developed, in which the demands of accelerated erythropoiesis are not met from the available dietary sources. Supplementary amounts of folic acid (0.5 mg daily) then allow restoration of erythropoiesis.

HEMATOLOGIC MANIFESTATIONS

The hematologic manifestations which accompany acute blood destruction consist of an initial phase of rapid destruction of red corpuscles and a second phase of rapid blood regeneration. These two phases usually overlap, especially when the hemolytic stimulus acts over a prolonged period of time.

The *anemia* may be mild or severe, depending on the intensity and duration of the hemolytic process. It is usually normocytic but may be macrocytic, especially during the stage of rapid regeneration when many relatively immature cells and reticulocytes, which are larger than mature erythrocytes, are present. It is not uncommon to find 10 to 25 percent reticulocytes in chronic cases, and as many as 60 percent or even more in acute cases. Polychromatophilia, stippling, nucleated red blood corpuscles, and Howell-Jolly bodies are usually present. There generally is marked variation in the size of the cells (anisocytosis), but there may be little variation in their shape (poikilocytosis). *Spherocytes* may be numerous, or *schistocytes* (irregularly shaped, "fractured red blood cells") may be found. In sickle-cell anemia and in elliptocytosis the characteristically shaped cells are present.

A crude quantitative assessment of erythropoiesis can be made by calculating from the percentage of reticulocytes and the red cell count the total output of reticulocytes per microliter of blood. This can be somewhat refined by calculating the "*reticulocyte index*." This involves "correcting" the reticulocyte percentage by multiplying it by that fraction (or multiple) by which the hemoglobin or volume of packed red cells (VPRC) differs from the normal; for example, if the VPRC in an adult male is 24 ml per 100 ml and the percentage of reticulocytes is 10, the corrected figures would be $10 \times 24/47$ or approximately 5 percent, the normal VPRC being taken to be 47. Since normally only 1 percent of the red cells are reticulated, this would imply that erythropoiesis has been accelerated fivefold. Such a conclusion must be made with some reservation, however, since the calculation assumes that other conditions, such as rate of release of reticulocytes into the circulation, are the same in disease as in normal persons and that their stage of maturation when released also is the same. These assumptions are not necessarily correct nor are the responses the same in all types of anemia.

Stimulation of the *leukopoietic tissues*, in proportion to the severity of the hemolytic process, is the rule. Leukocytosis and a "shift to the left," with metamyelocytes, myelocytes, and even, rarely, myeloblasts in the circulation, accompany the accelerated erythropoiesis. *Platelets* may also increase in number, and large, bizarre forms may appear. In a minority of cases, however, such as certain cases of acquired hemolytic anemias with demonstrable "autoantibodies," in disseminated lupus erythematosus, and especially in paroxysmal nocturnal hemoglobinuria, leukopenia and thrombocytopenia may be present.

The *bone marrow* is hyperplastic. There is a great increase in the number of normoblasts and a consequent reduction in the myeloid-leukocyte/erythrocyte ratio from the normal 4:1 or 5:1 to about 1:1 or even less. The normoblasts are chiefly polychromatophilic and orthochromatic forms; as a rule there are proportionately not many pronormoblasts or basophilic normoblasts, although they may appear prominent because of the quantitative increase in erythroblastic elements. Megaloblasts, so characteristic of pernicious anemia and related macrocytic anemias, are not present unless a relative folic acid deficiency supervenes, as mentioned earlier.

PIGMENT METABOLISM

When the degree and rate of blood destruction are very great, hemoglobin is liberated into the plasma and, if the hemoglobin-binding capacity of the plasma (haptoglobin, hemopexin, Chap. 58) is exceeded, free hemoglobin is excreted by the kidneys and hemoglobinuria results. However, *red urine* must not be assumed to be necessarily indicative of hemoglobinuria. It may also be produced by intact red corpuscles (hematuria) or by myoglobinuria (both of which also give a positive guaiac or benzidine reaction), or by uroporphyrinuria. Microscopic and spectroscopic examination of the urine will usually suffice to reveal the cause of the abnormal color. Under certain circumstances, hematin (Chap. 58) may be released. Porphyrinuria can be recognized by the salmon-pink fluorescence in ultraviolet light of the porphyrins extracted into dilute hydrochloric acid or into organic solvents. More often, blood destruction is less rapid. Then hemoglobinemia and hemoglobinuria are not found and there is only an increase in the plasma icterus index, serum bilirubin, and urobilinogen excretion in the urine and feces.

The *stools* assume a dark color, and increased quantities of urobilinogen may be found in the stool and urine (Chap. 58). The fecal urobilinogen may be increased when the urine urobilinogen and the bilirubin in the blood are not significantly greater than normal. Fecal urobilinogen determinations are of limited value, however, because (1) the bowel is incompletely evacuated, (2) urobilinogen is partially reabsorbed from the gut, (3) the heme of red corpuscles is not the only source of urobilinogen, and (4) the measurement of urobilinogen does not include all oxidation products of heme degradation. Nevertheless, a threefold or greater increase in the daily fecal urobilinogen excretion, as estimated from analysis of random 10-g stool collections on two successive days, compared with that anticipated from an individual with the same degree of anemia but having a normal red blood cell survival, provides helpful evidence of excessive destruction of red corpuscles. Although the quantity of urobilinogen in the urine is related to the rate of blood destruction, it is so readily affected by liver function and by renal function, that this seemingly simple and aesthetically more acceptable approach to estimating urobilinogen production is not recommended.

The quantity of bilirubin in the plasma may rise as high as 10 mg per 100 ml. The reaction is indirect, but some increase in direct or "1-min" bilirubin (bilirubin glucuronide) may also occur. The intensity of the bilirubinemia depends not only on the extent of the blood destruction but also on the capacity of the liver to remove the pigment from the bloodstream and excrete it in the bile. A normally functioning liver is capable of excreting large quantities of bilirubin, but in some cases of extraordinarily severe hemolysis conjugated bilirubin accumulates in the bloodstream.

CLASSIFICATION

As stated above, hemolytic anemias are conveniently classified as due to intrinsic defects of the red corpuscles or to extracorpuscular influences acting alone or in concert (see Table 306-1). In the main, those associated with intrinsic erythrocytic defects are familial and hereditary.

This classification is useful in considering therapy. When the disorder is attributed to a *congenital* intrinsic erythrocytic defect, usually little can be done to alter the rate of red blood cell destruction; when the lesion is *acquired*, it may be reversed. When there is a significant extracorpuscular factor as well as an intrinsic defect (Table 306-2), even though the inherited intrinsic defect may be unalterable, eliminating the extracorpuscular cofactor will allow partial or even complete relief of hemolysis; conversely, addition of the cofactor will aggravate hemolysis in a previously stable situation. Patients with only intrinsic erythrocytic defects will not destroy transfused, compatible normal erythrocytes at an excessive rate. The second principal category identifies patients who will hemolyze transfused red blood cells as readily as their own. Treatment for this group requires alteration or eradication of the extracorpuscular factors.

The category *hereditary nonspherocytic hemolytic anemia* is now used only as a provisional description when evaluating a patient. The term encompasses all but hereditary spherocytosis among the hereditary disorders listed in the classification. Present-day knowledge of precise defects of the Embden-Meyerhof and phosphogluconic oxidative pathways provides a better basis for identifying cases of hemolytic anemia which previously could be classed only by the terms *hereditary* and *nonspherocytic.*

DIAGNOSIS

The first step is to *suspect* that a hemolytic process may be present. The most common clues are (1) reticulocytosis, sustained for weeks or longer without relief of anemia; (2) persistent reticulocytosis in the absence of anemia; (3) rapid aggravation of anemia, with or without accompanying reticulocytosis; (4) acholuric jaundice; and (5) unexplained splenomegaly in the presence of anemia.

In all the situations just named, both *overt and covert blood loss must be excluded* before hemolysis can be said to be present. Reticulocytosis per se is not evidence of hemolysis, but rather of accelerated erythropoiesis. When it persists, it may be deduced that abnormal blood destruction (or blood loss) is occurring only *if* the expected result of accelerated production, i.e., a rise in the volume of packed red blood cells, does not occur. The

TABLE 306-2
Hemolytic anemias due to intrinsic red cell defects which are significantly affected by extracorpuscular factors

Disease	*Factor*
Hereditary spherocytosis	Spleen
Glucose 6-phosphate dehydrogenase deficiency ("primaquine-sensitive" type)	Certain drugs: (1) primaquine, pamaquine, (2) nitrofurantoin, (3) vitamin K substitutes, (4) sulfonamides, (5) paraaminosalicylic acid, (6) naphthalene, (7) sulfones, (8) phenacetin, acetanilid, acetylsalicylic acid, (9) probenecid
	Plant poison: fava bean (*Vicia fava*)
Paroxysmal nocturnal hemoglobinuria	Normal serum factors (complement)

absence of reticulocytosis does not weigh against the occurrence of excessively rapid red blood cell destruction, but merely indicates that erythropoiesis is not accelerated.

The rate of red blood cell destruction can be estimated, when the degree of anemia is not changing, by measuring the survival time of the patient's red blood cells after tagging them with radioactive chromium (^{51}Cr), or diisopropylfluorophosphate (^{32}DFP), as discussed below. If compatible *normal donor cells* are tagged in a similar fashion and disappear from the patient's circulation at a rapid rate, a hemolytic disorder has been demonstrated; in addition, this fact proves that the cause of the excessive destruction must reside outside the patient's own red blood cells; i.e., an extracorpuscular factor is operating to produce hemolysis.

Tagging of the red corpuscles is most useful when the volume of packed red blood cells is constant and when a series of reticulocyte counts does not indicate whether erythropoiesis is accelerated or not. If sustained reticulocytosis of 7 percent or more is found and persistent blood loss has been excluded, the radioisotope test is not necessary to determine the presence of hemolysis. If the volume of packed red blood cells is rising or falling at the time the test is to be conducted, the results of red blood cell tagging may be erroneous and misleading.

If objective evidence of hemolysis has been found, the second step in diagnosis is to identify the particular cause of the hemolytic disease.

Certain additional tests have been devised which help in determining the nature of the underlying disorder and point to the precise diagnostic classification. These are discussed below. The several *screening tests and specific diagnostic tests* that are used to identify the individual hemolytic disorders are without value in the diagnosis of anemias other than hemolytic anemias, and they *should not be carried out unless it has been clearly established that a hemolytic disorder is present.* To do otherwise may subject the patient to needless discomfort, inconvenience, delay in diagnosis, and expense.

Osmotic fragility test Spherocytes will characteristically hemolyze in solutions of higher tonicity than will normal red corpuscles. Usually, defibrinated blood and solutions of sodium chloride are used, the latter buffered to pH 7.4 with sodium (or potassium) phosphate. The test generally is positive in hereditary spherocytosis, and is sometimes positive in autoimmune hemolytic anemia provided "acquired" spherocytes are present. It is usually negative in other forms of hemolytic anemia. If the test is negative but spherocytosis is suspected, the sensitivity of the test can be increased by incubating the defibrinated blood under aseptic conditions at 37°C for 24 hr before adding it to the saline solutions. Under such conditions the fragility of normal corpuscles is increased slightly while that of corpuscles from patients with hereditary spherocytosis is increased markedly. The plotted curves of increased hemolysis are symmetric. In contrast, in hemolytic anemias without spherocytes, an asymmetric increase in osmotic fragility is more likely to be observed after incubation. In thalassemia, in which leptocytes are present, and less consistently in some of the hemoglobinopathies, osmotic fragility is decreased (Chap. 307).

A *simple screening test* to detect spherocytes and leptocytes by their abnormal osmotic fragility in solutions osmotically equivalent to 0.50% and 0.21% sodium chloride (about 170 and 70 mOsm, respectively) can be performed by adding 0.02 ml capillary or anticoagulated venous blood to three centrifuge tubes. The first tube should also contain 4.0 ml isotonic (0.85%) sodium chloride; the second, 2.3 ml isotonic sodium chloride and 1.7 ml distilled water; and the third tube, 1.0 ml isotonic sodium chloride and 3.0 ml distilled water. After mixing by inversion and then centrifuging the tubes, there should be no hemolysis in the first tube, which serves as a control; hemolysis occurs in the second tube only if spherocytes are present; complete hemolysis occurs in the third tube except when leptocytes are present, in which case erythrocytes containing hemoglobin will be seen at the bottom of the tube.

AUTOHEMOLYSIS This test measures the amount of hemolysis which occurs spontaneously in sterile defibrinated blood incubated for 24 and 48 hr at 37°C. The test is useful in differentiating hereditary spherocytosis from congenital *nonspherocytic* hemolytic anemias due to deficiency of enzymes of the Embden-Meyerhof pathway or the phosphogluconate oxidation pathway and helps to some extent in distinguishing among these when specific enzyme assays are not available. It is based on the effects of the addition of glucose and of adenosine triphosphate (ATP) on the degree of autohemolysis (Table 306-3). Normally, 0.05 to 0.5 percent hemolysis occurs at 24 hr and 0.4 to 4.5 percent at 48 hr, as indicated in Table 306-3. If glucose is added to give a final concentration of about 5 mg per ml, then hemolysis of normal red corpuscles is not more than 0.4 percent at both 24 and 48 hr.

In hereditary spherocytosis, autohemolysis is considerably increased, but it is kept at normal levels, or nearly so, by the prior addition of glucose, or of ATP in a final concentration of about 12 mg per ml. In glucose

6-phosphate dehydrogenase (G-6-PD) deficiency, there is a moderate increase in autohemolysis above normal, and this is only partially prevented by the addition of glucose (type I autohemolysis of Selwyn and Dacie). In pyruvate kinase (PK) deficiency, autohemolysis is greatly increased; the addition of glucose is not protective, but ATP is protective (type II autohemolysis). In triosephosphate isomerase (TPI) deficiency, as in hereditary spherocytosis, both glucose and ATP are protective.

In autoimmune hemolytic anemias with spherocytosis, the autohemolysis may be increased but the effect of adding glucose is variable. In hereditary elliptocytosis, there may be type I autohemolysis.

Erythrocyte enzyme assays For the specific identification of hemolytic anemias due to enzyme deficiencies, quantitative assays are necessary. Simple screening tests are available, however, for the two most common forms, namely, G-6-PD and PK deficiency. These "spot tests" depend on noting whether, after activation with long-wave ultraviolet light, pyridine nucleotide has been reduced (in the case of G-6-PD screening) or oxidized (in the case of PK screening).

Serologic tests If presumptive tests are negative for *warm hemolysins* and *cold hemolysins*, and for hemolysis in *acidified serum*, the latter being characteristic of erythrocytes from patients with paroxysmal nocturnal hemoglobinuria, the diagnoses associated with these types of hemolysis may be excluded with little further laboratory investigation. When one of these tests is positive, the appropriate complete test must be carried out with suitable controls, in order to identify correctly the basis for the observed hemolysis. For example, if the presumptive test for a cold hemolysin is positive, the complete Donath-Landsteiner test should be carried out.

A *simple presumptive test* is performed by placing 0.05 ml washed red corpuscles from freshly defibrinated blood in each of three test tubes containing 0.5 ml serum. The first is incubated for 1 to 2 hr at body temperature and then centrifuged. If hemoglobin is present in the supernatant serum, the presence of a *warm hemolysin* is suggested. The second tube is chilled for 20 min in cracked ice, then incubated for 1 hr and centrifuged. If the result is positive, a *cold hemolysin* is probably present. The test tube should be examined before it has been warmed. If only cold agglutinins are present and no hemolysins, the red corpuscles agglutinate in the cold but fail to hemolyze when the tube is warmed, the clumps disappearing instead. When cold agglutinins are present, care must be taken not to shake the cells too much while they are agglutinated in the cold, since they may hemolyze and give a false reaction to the cold hemolysin test. The blood placed in the third tube is acidified with 0.05 ml 0.2 *N* HCl. If hemolysis is apparent after incubation for 1 hr and subsequent centrifugation, the complete acidified-serum test for paroxysmal nocturnal hemoglobinuria (Ham's test) should be performed.

The *"direct" Coombs antiglobulin test* is carried out by mixing the patient's washed red blood cells with serum from rabbits immunized to human gamma-globulin, and examining the mixture for agglutination. It serves to demonstrate the presence of "incomplete" antibodies, i.e., those which are attached at some points on the surface of the red corpuscles and require a completing substance, such as antihuman globulin, to cause agglutination. A positive result is found in cases of acquired hemolytic anemia due to antibodies; in the type of paroxysmal cold hemoglobinuria associated with syphilis (see Paroxysmal Cold Hemoglobinuria below); and sometimes in hemolytic anemia associated with various physical or chemical agents, and also when isoimmunization has occurred, as in hemolytic disease of the newborn and in patients with hemolytic anemia due to intrinsic erythrocytic lesions who have received many transfusions. The test is negative in hereditary spherocytosis and in other forms of hemolytic anemia due to intrinsic erythrocytic lesions, including paroxysmal nocturnal hemoglobinuria.

The *"indirect" Coombs test* permits detection of antibodies in the patient's serum. In the indirect test, antihuman globulin serum is mixed with normal group O, Rh-positive, and Rh-negative red corpuscles which have been incubated in the patient's serum. If agglutination occurs with both Rh-positive and Rh-negative cells, Rh (anti-D) antibodies may be excluded and the conclusion drawn that other circulating antibodies are present.

In performing the Coombs test it is important that potent antiserum be used and adequate controls carried out. False negative results may occur if the red corpuscles have not been washed sufficiently or as a result of a prozone reaction due to inadequate dilution of the serum. Cold hemagglutinins may cause a false positive reaction.

The detailed elucidation of a case of hemolytic anemia

TABLE 306-3
Diagnostic patterns of autohemolysis tests

	Hemolysis after 24- and 48-hr incubation at 37°C		
Disorder	*No additive*	*Glucose added**	*ATP added**
Normal	(0.05-0.5%/ 0.4-4.5%)	(0.4%)	(0.4%)
	0/0 to +	0	0
Hereditary spherocytosis; Triosephosphate isomerase deficiency	++	0	0
Glucose 6-phosphate dehydrogenase deficiency; Hexokinase deficiency; Glucose phosphate isomerase deficiency; Phosphoglycerate kinase deficiency; Hereditary elliptocytosis	++ or +++	+	+
Pyruvate kinase deficiency	++++	++++	+

* *See text for quantities of additives.*
Note: Zero and plus signs refer to degree of increase of hemolysis after 24 and 48 hr as compared with the tabulated normal values.

of the antibody type will often require the use of still other procedures, but these, in the main, are quite simple. They include (1) the setting up of agglutination tests at various temperatures and in several media, such as isotonic sodium chloride solution, bovine albumin solution, or polyvinylpyrrolidone (PVP), which are helpful in demonstrating and characterizing the agglutinin, and (2) the treatment of the red corpuscles with proteolytic enzymes, such as papain and trypsin, which renders them more susceptible to the demonstration of antibodies. For the antibody tests it is necessary in some instances to use the patient's own red corpuscles rather than any available group O red corpuscles, as is often the practice.

Heinz bodies These are found in certain hemolytic anemias. They are intracorpuscular structures which probably represent denatured globin derived from hemoglobin in the course of an irreversible reaction with a toxic substance. They appear under phase-contrast microscopy as refractile, irregularly shaped bodies often lying at or close to the periphery of the red blood cell, and sometimes are attached to the outer surface of the cell. They range in size from minute particles to bodies up to 3 μm in size. Several bodies may be present in the same cell, but the largest ones usually appear singly. They are not visible in blood films stained with Wright's stain, since the bodies and the surrounding hemoglobin stain the same pink color, but they can be stained supravitally with crystal violet. Some Heinz bodies can be produced in normal blood by mixing it with acetylphenylhydrazine, but a great many more develop in "primaquine-sensitive" (see below) red blood cells. They also are observed in hemolytic anemias unrelated to exposure to recognized toxic agents ("inclusion body" anemia, "hereditary Heinz-body anemia," anemia associated with a chemically unstable hemoglobin, Chap. 307).

Sucrose test This three-tube screening test depends on the enhanced hemolysis of complement-dependent systems in isotonic solutions of low ionic strength. One-half milliliter oxalated or citrated (but not EDTA-anticoagulated) blood is added to 4.5 ml isotonic (10 percent) sucrose. As controls, in place of sucrose, tube 2 contains isotonic NaCl or NaCl–sodium phosphate buffer (pH 7.4), and tube 3 contains distilled water. These controls are designed to measure hemolysis unrelated to the low ionic strength of the sucrose test solution, and to measure complete hemolysis, respectively. After inversion, the tubes must stand at room temperature for about 30 min for hemolysis to occur; they are then centrifuged. Hemolysis in the supernatant solution of tube 1 is presumptive evidence of paroxysmal nocturnal hemoglobinuria (PNH). In PNH there should be little or no hemolysis in tube 2. Quantitation of hemolysis can be achieved by measuring the absorbance at 540 nm (nanometers) of the supernatant from tube 1 (sucrose solution) and dividing this by the absorbance of the supernatant from tube 3, both values having been first reduced by the absorbance of the supernatant from tube 2. Disorders other than PNH may give a positive result and then other procedures pertaining to PNH should be performed (see Chronic Hemolytic Anemia with Paroxysmal Nocturnal Hemoglobinuria below); a negative test is acceptable evidence against the diagnosis of PNH.

Red blood cell survival tests The principles and limitations of these widely used tests should be borne in mind whenever their use is contemplated. Radioactive chromium (^{51}Cr), as sodium chromate, and radioactive diisopropylfluorophosphate (^{32}DFP) are used to tag red corpuscles and to measure their survival in vivo. The techniques are equally applicable to the patient's red corpuscles and to those of a healthy donor and therefore can distinguish between intrinsic erythrocytic defects and extraerythrocytic causes for hemolysis.

Radioactive chromium is not an ideal cell label because it elutes from normal red corpuscles at a rate which approximates 1 percent daily. Hence, loss of the isotope from the circulation does not necessarily mean loss of the red blood cell with which it had been associated. It has been assumed that the same elution rate also applies to abnormal erythrocytes, but this may not be the case. Normally, half the isotope leaves the circulation ($T^1/_2$) in about 29 days. This contrasts with the actual survival time of normal red corpuscles of 120 days; i.e., an actual $T^1/_2$ of 60 days. The gamma radiation of ^{51}Cr is sufficiently penetrating to allow body-surface counting over the liver and spleen to measure isotope localization.

^{32}DFP binds irreversibly to the erythrocytic cholinesterase and, because it is not eluted from the red corpuscle, is a better label. However, the beta radiation of ^{32}P does not allow body-surface counting.

In the most commonly employed autotransfusion techniques, these procedures actually measure the rate of replacement of tagged red corpuscles by unlabeled, new corpuscles, rather than the "survival time" of the tagged corpuscles. Thus they indirectly measure red corpuscle production, rather than destruction. The amount of isotope present is measured as the "specific activity," which is isotope concentration per unit volume of blood. This may be recorded as a certain number of counts per minute (cpm) or disintegrations per second (dps) *per* milliliter packed red corpuscles or per unit volume of whole blood.

The effect of varying red corpuscle replacement rates on the apparent change in isotope "specific activity" warrants special consideration by all who order this test. Only when the patient is in hematologic equilibrium will the rate of fall of red cell specific activity be interpretable with reference to the normal situation. When the rate of red corpuscle production is *less than* the rate of red corpuscle destruction, the recorded rate of change of isotope specific activity will be less than that anticipated from the rate of red blood cell destruction alone. If red corpuscle production were zero, were it not for the rate of elution of the isotope from the red corpuscles, the specific activity would be unchanged with time, and the apparent $T^1/_2$ would be indefinitely long. On the other hand, when the rate of red corpuscle production *exceeds* the rate of corpuscle destruction, the specific activity will fall faster than that attributable to the rate of red corpuscle destruction and equivalent replacement, and the $T^1/_2$ *will be shortened. Abnormally short values for the* $T^1/_2$ *could be obtained when red blood cell survival is in fact normal but the volume of packed red blood cells is rising because of transfusion or any one of a number of causes unrelated to active hemolysis.* It is because the $T^{1/2}$ is altered in an inverse relation to changes from the normal balance of red corpuscle production and destruction that red blood cell survival tests become difficult to interpret if performed in patients in whom there is a significant rise or fall in the volume of packed red blood cells during the period that the test is carried out.

In cross-transfusion experiments, when a small volume of labeled red corpuscles with an *intrinsic defect* is given to a *normal recipient* (differing from the usual procedure of labeling and autotransfusing the patient's own cells), the survival of the red corpuscles is measured directly by the disappearance of the radioisotope.

PROGNOSIS AND TREATMENT

Useful therapy of hemolytic anemia requires either (1) decreasing the rate of corpuscular destruction, or (2) increasing the rate of manufacture and release of new red corpuscles, or both. The bone marrow in adult man is capable of increasing red blood cell production at least six- to eightfold, and a healthy *bone marrow* approaches compensation for the decreased survival of the circulating red blood cells. If erythropoiesis already is accelerated maximally, effective therapy depends on reducing the rate of destruction.

Prognosis and treatment depend on the nature and cause of the hemolytic disorder. If the causative agent is a parasite or chemical, it must be removed. In such cases, no other therapy may be needed. An acute attack of hemolysis requires rest, maintenance of fluid balance, and relief of pain. Blood transfusion may be dangerous if the cause of the hemolysis is extracorpuscular and has not been removed, because the introduced blood may also be destroyed. Yet, when blood destruction is so acute that hemoglobinemia and hemoglobinuria are present, the possibility of death from circulatory collapse is so great that frequent and sometimes massive blood transfusions must be given. However, the utmost caution is necessary in typing and matching both the patient's and the donor's blood and in its administration.

In the acquired hemolytic anemias, both in the "symptomatic" and in the idiopathic varieties (see Idiopathic Autoimmune Hemolytic Anemia below) and especially in cases associated with antibodies, *corticosteroids* provide an effective and rapid means for controlling the hemolytic process. Furthermore, where the anemia is so severe that transfusion is necessary, blood can be given with much less chance of a reaction if steroids have been given. The oral administration of 40 mg prednisone daily, or of its equivalent in related compounds, often suffices, but in some cases twice this amount, or even more, may need to be given at first. Methyl prednisolone or dexamethasone may be given by the intravenous route as the sodium succinate derivative when the patient is unable to take oral medication. It is preferred over hydrocortisone, which may also be given intravenously, because of the potentially dangerous salt-retaining effect of hydrocortisone when large doses are used. The most alarming manifestations of the hemolytic process usually subside within a few days, and then intravenous therapy may be replaced by oral administration of corticosteroids, and the dose may be reduced gradually. Patients vary widely in the amount of these hormones required to control the hemolysis and for maintenance therapy. In some, therapy may be discontinued entirely after several months, but in others it must be continued for years. When corticosteroids are employed for prolonged periods, careful consideration should be given to minimizing the undesirable side effects and the potential complications such as peptic ulcer, diabetes mellitus, osteoporosis, tuberculosis, and other infections (Chap. 86).

In cases of "symptomatic" hemolytic anemia of known cause, treatment of the underlying disorder may relieve the hemolytic anemia as well. When this does not occur, a trial of steroid therapy is justified. In certain instances splenectomy may be helpful, especially if leukopenia and thrombocytopenia are also present and the picture is that of "hypersplenism."

Splenectomy is almost invariably beneficial in hereditary spherocytosis, but it is much less successful in the other hereditary forms of hemolytic anemia. Furthermore, if splenectomy is carried out in an acute hemolytic phase, the operative mortality rate is high. In idiopathic acquired hemolytic anemia, therefore, corticosteroid hormones should be used first, at least in preparation for operation.

Corticosteroid therapy is less likely to be effective in cases of acquired hemolytic anemia without demonstrable antibodies than in those in which antibodies are present. In any event, splenectomy is advisable whenever steroid therapy has not caused the hemolysis to disappear. Even if splenectomy is not successful in completely eliminating the hemolytic process, corticosteroid therapy is at least likely to be more effective than before operation, and smaller doses may suffice. At the time of operation, evidence of underlying disease which may be responsible for the hemolytic anemia should be searched for and treated appropriately if found.

Splenectomy is of no value in sickle-cell anemia, thalassemia, or paroxysmal nocturnal hemoglobinuria except when immune isoantibodies have developed as a result of multiple transfusions.

HEREDITARY DEFICIENCIES OF ENZYMES OF THE EMBDEN-MEYERHOF PATHWAY

Hemolytic anemias in this category are congenital and are due to "inborn errors" in the main glycolytic, energy-yielding pathway of erythrocytes. They have the following additional features in common: (1) They are inherited as autosomal recessive traits. (2) Hemolytic anemia occurs in homozygotes, who are necessarily deficient in the particular enzyme, whereas heterozygotes possess intermediate quantities of the specifically affected enzymes but are free of hemolytic disease. (3) In homozygotes, slight or even moderate macrocytosis occurs and some irregularly crenated erythrocytes and spicule forms are present. (4) Spherocytes are absent. (5) Hemolysis and anemia persist after splenectomy, although some benefit may result from the operation. (6) During in vitro incubation, the erythrocytes tend to lose potassium rather than, as in the case of hereditary spherocytosis, gain sodium.

The degree of anemia and of the hemolytic process itself varies not only among the different enzyme lesions represented in the group, but even among patients with the same enzyme deficiency. In these disorders glycolysis in mature erythrocytes is abnormal and red corpuscle survival may be extremely brief. However, reticulocytes are produced in large numbers in response to the anemia, and these immature corpuscles, in contrast to mature erythrocytes, contain mitochondria. These organelles provide an alternate pathway from which to derive energy: oxidative phosphorylation. As long as the young erythrocyte in the circulation retains this metabolic capability, it can survive despite its inborn error in the Embden-Meyerhof pathway. However, as it matures, it is destined to an early death, the timing of which depends on the site and severity of the enzymatic lesion in the glycolytic pathway. In turn, the location and severity of the lesion determine the severity of the hemolytic process and the resultant clinical syndrome.

Pyruvate kinase deficiency This disorder, first described by Valentine et al. in 1961, is the most common cause of hemolytic anemia among the identifiable enzyme lesions of the Embden-Meyerhof pathway (Fig. 306-1). At

FIGURE 306-1
Pathways for the metabolic breakdown of glucose in the red corpuscle and some of the enzymes involved. The various reactions are numbered in sequence: Embden-Meyerhof pathway, 1–11; phosphogluconate oxidative pathway (pentose phosphate shunt), 12–15.

Interrupted lines indicate that some steps have been omitted. HK, hexokinase; PGI, phosphoglucose isomerase; PFK, phosphofructokinase; ALD, aldolase; TPI, triosephosphate isomerase; PGD, phosphoglyceraldehyde dehydrogenase (glyceraldehyde phosphate dehydrogenase): PGK, phosphoglyceric acid kinase; PGM, phosphoglyceromutase; DPGM, diphosphoglyceratemutase; DPGP, diphosphoglycerate phosphatase; PK, pyruvate kinase; LDH, lactic dehydrogenase; G-6-PD, glucose 6-phosphate dehydrogenase 6PGD, 6-phosphogluconic dehydrogenase; PRI, phosphoribose isomerase; Ep, epimerase; TRK, transketolase; TRA, transaldolase; AD, adenosine deaminase; NP, nucleoside phosphorylase; PRM, phosphoribomutase. (From MM Wintrobe et al., Clinical Hematology, *6th ed., Philadelphia: Lea & Febiger, 1967)*

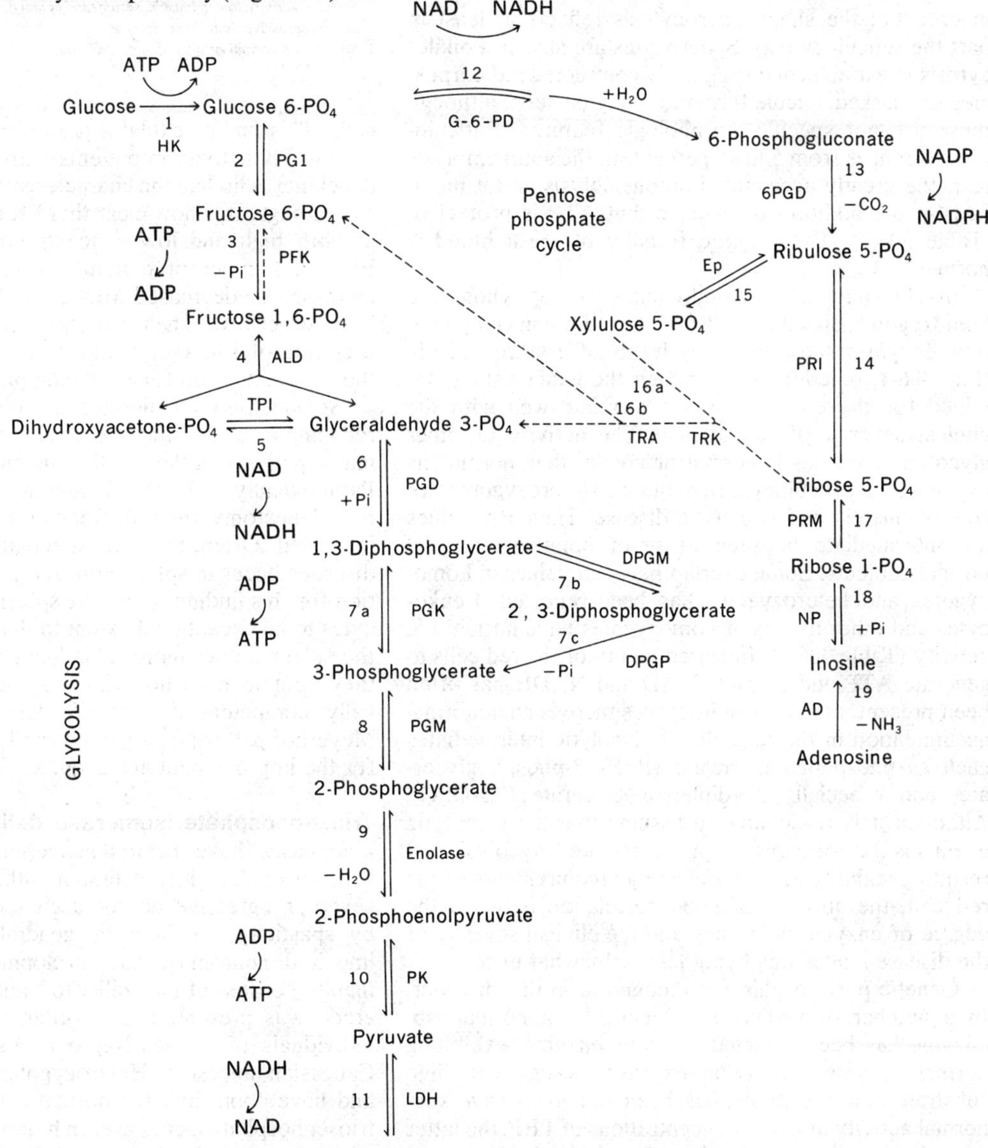

least 136 proved cases have been reported. It may be considered the prototype of the inherited erythrocytic enzyme deficiency disorders.

The disease has most frequently been reported in people of Northern European extraction, but the geographic distribution of the mutant gene is virtually worldwide. Most cases are discovered in infancy or early childhood. In some patients, marked anemia is found in the newborn period. In rare instances, in a seemingly healthy adult relative of a patient, the disorder is mild and fully compensated. Most patients, however, have the characteristic symptoms and signs of chronic hemolytic disorders (see above under Clinical Manifestations). Despite the severity of the hemolytic process, survival to adult life is common. Pregnancy has been tolerated without unusual complications, although blood transfusions have been required.

The anemia is moderately severe, and the volume of packed red corpuscles may be between 15 and 35 ml per 100 ml. The red corpuscles are normochromic and slightly macrocytic; the slight macrocytosis reflects at least in part the reticulocytosis. Spherocytes are absent. Poikilocytosis is variable, and irregularly contracted red corpuscles or marked spicule formation may be seen, although these are not specific morphologic features. Reticulocytosis ranges from 5 to 45 percent. In the autohemolysis test, the greatly accelerated autohemolysis is not modified by the addition of glucose, but ATP is protective (Table 306-3). The osmotic fragility of fresh blood is normal.

In clinically affected individuals, all of whom are homozygotes, specific assays of the red blood cell glycolytic enzymes show very low levels of erythrocyte PK (Fig. 306-1, reaction 10), although the exact values obtained for the enzyme do not correlate well with the clinical severity of the disease. The activity of other glycolytic enzymes is normal or greater than normal, as expected of reticulocyte-rich blood. Heterozygotes are free of anemia and hemolytic disease. Their PK values are intermediate between those of homozygotes and normal subjects. Some overlap between values in homozygotes and heterozygotes has been reported. Leukocytes and other tissues of homozygotes have normal PK activity (Table 306-4). Impaired ability of the red cells to generate ATP and to cycle NAD and NADH has often been present, and in most instances there is an abnormal accumulation in the red cells of glycolytic intermediates such as phosphoenolpyruvate (PEP), 3-phosphoglycerate, and especially 2,3-diphosphoglycerate (2,3-DPG). Although it is reasonable to assume that the hemolytic anemia is the consequence of the impaired glycolysis and resulting inability to meet the energy requirements of the red cell, the absence of good correlation between the degree of enzyme deficiency and the clinical severity of the disease makes this hypothesis somewhat uncertain.

Genetic polymorphism is recognized in this disorder. In a number of pedigrees a kinetically abnormal isoenzyme has been detected. Such an enzyme, exhibiting normal enzyme activity in ex vivo assays with high substrate concentrations, has been shown to have subnormal activity at lower concentrations of PEP, the latter more likely reflecting the situation within the intact red

TABLE 306-4
Some features of inherited red blood cell enzyme disorders

RBC enzyme deficiency	*WBC enzyme concentration*	*Other tissues*	*Mode of transmission*
Pyruvate kinase	Normal	Normal	Autosomal recessive
Hexokinase	Normal	Normal	Autosomal recessive
Glucose 6-phosphate dehydrogenase	Variable*	Low†	X-linked; variable expression in females
Triosephosphate isomerase	Low	Low‡	Autosomal recessive
Glucosephosphate isomerase	Low§	Low in plasma	Autosomal recessive
Phosphoglycerate kinase	Low§	Low	X-chromosome linked

** Sometimes low in affected Caucasians; normal in Negroes.*
† Enzyme activity also low in ocular lenses and in platelets, liver, and other organs.
‡ Enzyme activity low in muscle, serum, and spinal fluid; this disorder is accompanied by a progressive neurologic disease.
§ Sometimes normal or only slightly reduced.

cells. This finding explains prior reports of normal erythrocytic PK activity in patients with clinically typical PK deficiency who had the characteristic collateral biochemical findings. It is now clear that PK assays must be made at both high and low concentrations of the substrate, PEP. A number of mutant isoenzymes with either an increased or decreased Michaelis-Menten constant have been described. Their existence complicates the interpretation of PK assays and especially interpretation of the spot tests used for screening purposes.

Splenectomy ameliorates the disease in most cases, reducing or eliminating the need for blood transfusion in many patients, although the anemia generally persists. Paradoxically, although anemia may be partially relieved by splenectomy, the reticulocytosis has been found to be increased. Often, the highest reticulocyte counts in this disorder occur in splenectomized patients. One explanation for this finding is that the spleen sequesters reticulocytes to an exceptional extent in this disease. Removal of the spleen allows more reticulocytes to circulate, and as they contain mitochondrial enzymes and are metabolically competent despite the lesion of the Embden-Meyerhof pathway, they temporarily survive and account for the improvement achieved.

Triosephosphate isomerase deficiency Since 1965, nine cases have been discovered. Hemolytic anemia became evident in the first month of life. In addition, severe, progressive, neuromuscular disease characterized by spasticity and later by generalized flaccidity, with impaired neuromuscular development resulting in the inability or loss of the ability to stand, sit or hold the head erect, was present. The disorder has been observed in individuals of French-Negro ancestry and of English-Caucasian ancestry. Heterozygotes are clinically well, and have about half the normal activity of erythrocytic triosephosphate isomerase. In homozygotes, erythrocytic triosephosphate isomerase activity (Fig 306-1, reaction 5) is about 10 percent (or less) of the values found in normal persons; in addition, leukocytes, muscle, cerebrospinal fluid, and serum are deficient in the enzyme (Table 306-4). Elevated activity of several of the other erythrocytic enzymes is attributed to the presence of reticulocytes.

The usual features of chronic hemolytic anemia are present. The hemoglobin concentration may be from 5.5 to 10.5 g per 100 ml, and reticulocytes number about 15 percent. The autohemolysis test is abnormal (Table 306-2), but the osmotic fragility of fresh blood is normal.

Five of seven patients died prior to the age of five years; two were alive with severe generalized disease at four and one-half and five years of age. Deaths were attributable to the chronic hemolytic anemia, neuromuscular disorder, and infections, and possibly to cardiac involvement. The effect of splenectomy has not been reported.

Triosephosphate isomerase represents the only known means whereby dihydroxyacetone phosphate formed from 6-carbon compounds may be further metabolized by the Embden-Meyerhof pathway. A block at this step had been anticipated to result in an accumulation of dihydroxyacetone phosphate and a loss of that half of the three carbon moieties, this resulting in a decline in the rate of ATP synthesis (Fig 306-1, reactions 7a and 10). However, measurements have revealed an increase in the rate of glucose utilization even greater than that generally observed in patients with similar elevations of the reticulocyte count, and only small decreases in ATP levels. The amount of lactate formed from glucose has not been deficient. Thus, a compensatory pathway, most likely the phosphogluconate oxidative pathway, appears to be activated in affected red corpuscles. Dihydroxyacetone phosphate does indeed accumulate in affected red corpuscles, but the paucity of other metabolic abnormalities leaves the biochemical mechanism for ths striking clinical abnormalities unexplained.

Hexokinase deficiency Congenital hemolytic anemia in an eleven-year-old girl was attributed to erythrocytic hexokinase deficiency. Hepatomegaly, jaundice, and anemia were present from birth. Osmotic fragility was markedly increased after incubation for 24 hr at 37°C, and the autohemolysis test was abnormal (Table 306-2). The anemia was partially relieved by splenectomy, and the osmotic fragility became normal. Postsplenectomy blood smears showed darkly staining red corpuscles, some bearing spicules, rare target cells, and rare spherocytes.

The patient had less than normal erythrocytic hexokinase (HK) (Fig. 306-1, reaction 1), despite persistent reticulocytosis, which ordinarily results in high HK values. In her brother, free of hemolytic disease, the levels of HK were even lower, whereas both parents had intermediate values. From a study of the family members it appeared likely that the patient is homozygous for a defective gene, the disorder being transmitted, like the other enzymopathies in this group, as an autosomal recessive trait. The significance of the strikingly reduced HK value in the hematologically and clinically normal sibling is not clear. In sharp contrast to the low HK values in the proposita, all other erythrocytic enzyme activities were normal or increased, conforming with the experience in other specific enzymopathies.

Hexokinase is strategically located at the first step in glycolysis, and in vitro it has the lowest activity of any of the glycolytic enzymes of the erythrocytes. Many consider HK as rate-limiting in glycolysis, and since there is no known substitute for its activity, it represents a critical step in energy production for the mature erythrocyte. The patient's red corpuscles utilized fructose and glucose at rates below those of normal cell populations and far below those of samples with comparable numbers of reticulocytes. The leukocytes were unaffected (Table 306-1). Other cases, differing somewhat in clinical features and enzyme kinetics, are indicative of genetic polymorphism.

Glucosephosphate isomerase deficiency Four patients, in two unrelated Caucasian families, have been described in whom erythrocytic glucosephosphate isomerase (GPI) activity averaged about one-fifth of mean normal values. Leukocyte GPI was similarly affected. Other erythrocytic glycolytic enzymes were normal or increased in value, probably because of concomitant reticulocytosis. There were severe congenital hemolytic anemia and splenomegaly. Spherocytes were absent, the osmotic fragility of fresh blood was normal, and only slight abnormality was found after incubation at 37°C for 24 hr. The autohemolysis test was abnormal (Table 306-3). Splenectomy reduced the need for blood transfusions, but anemia persisted. Normal or only slightly reduced leukocyte GPI activity was found in other patients, indicating that this, too, is marked by genetic polymorphism.

Parents of the affected patients and their unaffected siblings lacked clinical evidence of hemolytic disease. Their erythrocytic GPI activity was about one-half of normal values. The disorder was deduced to be transmitted as an autosomal recessive trait (Table 306-4). Several additional cases have been reported.

Erythrocytic GPI reversibly catalizes the interconversion of glucose 6-phosphate and fructose 6-phosphate, the second step in the Embden-Meyerhof pathway of anaerobic glycolysis (Fig. 306-1, reaction 2). In the reticulocyte-rich blood of affected patients, total metabolism of glucose to lactate is greater than normal, and partial compensation for the inborn error is accomplished through bypassing the deficient enzyme step via the phosphogluconate oxidative pathway. How the enzymatic lesion results in premature hemolysis of erythrocytes is unknown. The erythrocytic GPI patterns were electrophoretically dissimilar among affected pedigrees, suggesting that in some cases two abnormal genes may interact to produce the lesion.

Other causes Still other red cell enzyme deficiencies have been reported, all quite rare. Thus, chronic hemolytic anemia associated with neurologic disease and behavioral disturbances has been reported in two young boys of a single pedigree. The red corpuscles and leukocytes of both patients were found to be severely deficient in *phosphoglycerate kinase* (PGK) (reaction 7a, Fig. 306-1). The characteristic clinical and hematologic findings of chronic hemolytic anemia were present. Spherocytes were absent. Osmotic fragility was normal, but the autohemolysis test was not. It seems probable that the disorder is transmitted as an X-chromosome–linked disease. Severely affected males have been tentatively designated as hemizygotes. Females with hemolytic anemia and females who clearly transmitted the disorder were designated as heterozygotes in the pedigree studied. The propositus, an eleven-year-old Chinese boy, was partially improved by splenectomy, but moderate anemia and hemolysis persisted. Female heterozygotes were less severely affected. In another family, leukocyte PGK in a female patient was normal. Again genetic polymorphism must be present, and variations in this clinical syndrome should be anticipated. The enzyme PGK catalyzes the interconversion of 1,3-diphosphoglycerate and 3-phosphoglycerate (3-PG). ATP is generated in the forward reaction, in which 3-PG is the product; in the backward reaction, ADP is formed from ATP. The generation of ATP in the forward reaction may be bypassed if triose is metabolized via 2,3-DPG through the Rapoport-Luebering shunt. Interference in the Embden-Meyerhof anaerobic pathway, with reduction in the synthesis of erythrocytic ATP, is presumed to be the mechanism resulting in hemolysis.

Chronic hemolytic anemia associated with deficiency of *2,3-DPG mutase* (Fig. 306-1, reaction 7b) has been recorded in several pedigrees, illustrating different clinical manifestations and different patterns of inheritance. In one, autosomal recessive inheritance was indicated. The enzyme deficiency was associated with low 2,3-DPG content of red corpuscles but a normal glycolytic rate. It has been postulated that the profound decrease in 2,3-DPG was rate-limiting for the monophosphoglycerate mutase reaction, wherein 2,3-DPG serves as a catalyst in the conversion of 3-PG to 2-phosphoglycerate in the main line of the Embden-Meyerhof pathway.

Congenital hemolytic anemia in a 24-year-old man was associated with half-normal activity of erythrocytic *phosphofructokinase* in the propositus and in two preceding generations.

Other hereditary hemolytic syndromes possibly associated with *nonglycolytic enzyme deficiencies* include adenosine triphosphatase (ATPase) deficiency and the "*high ATP*" *syndromes*; in some instances severe hemolytic anemia was associated. In addition, an erythrocyte disorder in which intracellular erythrocyte sodium was increased and potassium diminished (*high Na, low K syndrome*) has been reported to lead to hemolytic anemia. Thus a great variety of erythrocyte abnormalities have been discovered. The great variability of associated clinical manifestations raises questions concerning the ways in which these abnormalities lead to shortened red cell survival.

ABNORMALITIES OF THE PHOSPHOGLUCONATE OXIDATIVE PATHWAY Although only 10 percent of the glucose in mature red blood cells is metabolized via the phosphogluconate oxidative (hexose monophosphate, HMP) pathway, enzymatic abnormalities in this "shunt" may result in chronic hemolytic anemia or, alternatively, in acute hemolytic anemia following administration of certain drugs or chemicals. The exact biochemical mechanism which results in hemolysis in these disorders is not clear, although failure to defend normal concentrations of soluble intraerythrocytic and membrane-bound reduced thiol compounds appears to be a critical factor common to the several lesions discussed below.

Glucose 6-phosphate dehydrogenase deficiency A deficiency of G-6-PD (Fig. 306-1, reaction 12) is due to the inheritance of any one of a large number of abnormalities in the structural gene which codes the amino acid sequence of this enzyme. More than 100 G-6-PD variants have been described. The most prevalent G-6-PD enzyme of Caucasians and of Negroes is termed B or B+. A common G-6-PD isoenzyme with normal activity found in some other American Negroes is known as A or A+. It has a greater electrophoretic mobility at pH 8.6 than does the B type isoenzyme and differs from B by a single amino acid; asparagine is replaced by aspartic acid. The A− mutation, the most common clinically significant type of abnormal G-6-PD among American Negroes, is synthesized in normal quantity, but intraerythrocytic decay of enzyme activity is accelerated as the erythrocyte ages. This instability of the enzyme in vivo accounts for the diminished G-6-PD activity found in the mixed-age populations of red cells obtained from affected Negro men, whereas when there is reticulocytosis and young erythrocytes predominate in the circulation, normal G-6-PD activity may be found.

G-6-PD Mediterranean, the variant most common among Caucasians, results in the formation of decreased numbers of enzyme molecules, each with approximately normal enzyme activity but with unusual properties. G-6-PD Oklahoma and Milwaukee are associated with the production of enzymes which exhibit abnormal kinetics and hence are functionally deficient.

It has been estimated that 100 million or more persons of all races throughout the world are affected by G-6-PD deficiency. The frequency of the disorder varies from 0.1 to 50 percent among different Caucasian populations and from 10 to 14 percent among male Negroes in the United States. It is especially common among Caucasians of Mediterranean background, Sephardic and especially Kurdish Jews, and Sardinians, and is common in Iranians. A deficiency of G-6-PD also is found commonly among certain Chinese populations and in Southeast Asia. One of these variants is G-6-PD Canton.

The gene determining the structure of G-6-PD is carried on the X chromosome. Being sex-linked, the defect is fully expressed in affected males (hemizygotes) and is transmitted from mother to son. In heterozygous females penetrance may vary from virtually undetectable to fully expressed enzyme deficiency, a phenomenon explained at least in part by the X-chromosome mosaicism resulting from random X inactivation (Chap. 62).

The clinical manifestations of G-6-PD deficiency range from none whatsoever unless exposure to an oxidant drug takes place, as is characteristic of the primaquine-sensitive type, first described in Negroes in the United States (see below), to a variety of manifestations which are usually referred to as the *Caucasian type*. In these, not only is hemolytic anemia precipitated by ingestion of various drugs, but chronic hemolysis (nonspherocytic congenital hemolytic anemia) may be present from infancy or childhood, and may be first manifested as neonatal jaundice which, if untreated, may result in kernicterus. The disorder in Caucasians and Orientals in general is more severe than in Negroes; not only may hemolytic anemia be present in occasional individuals in the absence of drugs (see below) or other extracorpuscular factors which induce anemia (including infections), but these individuals may have more sensitivity than A− type individuals to primaquine and other compounds and even to aspirin. In particular, exposure to *fava beans* may induce even within a few hours a severe hemolytic episode.

Except as noted above, the features of the Caucasian type of G-6-PD deficiency are similar to the more thoroughly studied examples of this disorder in Negroes (Table 306-2) discussed later in this chapter.

Glutathione reductase This enzyme enables reduction of oxidized glutathione (GSSG) to reduced glutathione, using NADPH as hydrogen donor. It is strategically located for recycling NADPH-NADP for enablement of the G-6-PD reaction.

Deficiency of *glutathione reductase* (GSSG-R) has been reported in some patients with hemolytic anemia and in a number of other, diverse conditions. The significance of the deficiency and its relation to the hemolytic disease is unclear, because in most of the reports, the assay evaluated only the active form of the enzyme [with bound flavin adenine dinucleotide (FAD)] and the amount of apoenzyme which could have been activated had there been prior incubation with FAD, or had riboflavin been administered to the patient, was unknown. In at least one family, the latter approach confirmed genetically determined GSSG-R deficiency. There is also good evidence that mutant GSSG-R does occur. However, drug-induced hemolytic anemia due to true GSSG-R deficiency is probably much more rare than had previously been considered.

A well-compensated hemolytic anemia without spherocytosis but with susceptibility to hemolysis induced by primaquine or fava beans has been described in individuals with virtually complete red cell *glutathione (GSH) deficiency*. The disorder is transmitted as an autosomal recessive trait. The defect in most of these cases is due to deficiency of glutathione synthetase, the second of the two enzymes concerned with GSH synthesis in red cells. It mediates the attachment of glycine to glutamyl cysteine in the enzymatic synthesis of glutathione. Deficiency of γ-glutamyl-cysteine synthetase, the first enzyme concerned with glutathione synthesis, was established in two other cases of a well-compensated chronic hemolytic anemia in adults, brother and sister. This lesion, too, is transmitted as an autosomal recessive. The small amounts of radioactive chromate which are perfectly acceptable for red blood cell survival studies in other disorders (1 mmol per liter red corpuscles) have a markedly adverse effect on the in vivo viability of glutathione-deficient red corpuscles.

A compensated hemolytic disorder in newborn infants, associated with hyperbilirubinemia and increased susceptibility of red corpuscles to Heinz body formation in vitro, has been ascribed to *erythrocytic glutathione peroxidase (GSH-Px) deficiency*. The syndrome was self-limited, and evidence of hemolysis disappeared by three months of age. The significance of these observations is unclear, although for some time it has been suspected that deficiency of glutathione peroxidase might result in increased susceptibility to Heinz body formation and drug-induced hemolytic anemia.

Chronic hemolytic anemia or drug-induced hemolytic disease in four adults has been ascribed to partial deficiency of glutathione peroxidase. Drugs and agents resulting in hemolysis in G-6-PD deficiency would be expected to act similarly in GSH and GSH-Px–deficient subjects. It is important to remember that the Heinz body test with acetylphenylhydrazine and the ascorbate-cyanide test are nonspecific and would be expected to be positive with any of the lesions discussed in this section. Measurement of red cell GSH and specific enzyme assays are required to make the precise diagnosis.

OTHER INTRINSIC ERYTHROCYTIC DEFECTS

Hemolytic anemia may be associated with *congenital erythropoietic uroporphyria* (Chap. 102) and *protoporphyria*. Considerable improvement may follow splenectomy.

Elliptic red corpuscles may be present in small numbers in the blood of some individuals. In about 0.04 percent of the population, as many as 50 to 90 percent of the red corpuscles may be elliptic or oval in shape. This condition, known as *hereditary elliptocytosis*, is inherited as an autosomal dominant trait, but there is wide variation in gene penetrance or expression. In many instances the disorder is harmless; in others a mild compensated hemolytic state is present or the hemoglobin is maintained at slightly below normal, reticulocytes are slightly increased, and haptoglobin levels are depressed. In possibly as many as 10 to 15 percent of cases, however, frank hemolytic anemia occurs, splenomegaly is found, and the accelerated blood destruction is usually terminated by splenectomy. The gene for elliptocytosis has been found to be linked with the Rh blood type in most instances, but the severe hemolytic anemias have been observed as a rule in those families in which such a linkage was not present or, in a few instances, where homozygosity for the trait was found. A membrane permeability defect necessitating an increased rate of ATP utilization similar to that present in hereditary spherocytosis is postulated to be present, but the underlying difference between asymptomatic and hemolytic cases is unknown.

Abetalipoproteinemia is accompanied by a hereditary hemolytic anemia (*acanthocytosis*) with altered phospholipid content of the red cells, which is secondary to the altered plasma phospholipids. Another type of hereditary hemolytic anemia, associated with an increased red cell content of lecithin but without alteration of plasma lipids, is transmitted as an autosomal dominant.

Often grouped together are those congenital hemolytic anemias associated with qualitative or quantitative abnormalities in the synthesis of the globin peptide moieties. These result in the *hemoglobinopathies* and *thalassemia* syndromes, respectively (Chap. 307).

The anemia of vitamin B_{12} deficiency exhibits features

of a hemolytic disorder, apparently because of an acquired, intrinsic erythrocytic defect (Chap. 305).

HEMOLYTIC ANEMIAS FROM COMBINED EFFECTS OF INTRINSIC ERYTHROCYTIC DEFECT AND EXTRAERYTHROCYTIC FACTOR

Recognition of the role of an extraerythrocytic factor in sustaining the hemolytic process in these disorders provides an approach to treatment which is not possible in those congenital hemolytic anemias due to an intrinsic erythrocytic defect *alone*. In the present group, removal or addition of the extraerythrocytic factor may result in relief or aggravation, respectively, of the hemolytic process.

HEREDITARY SPHEROCYTOSIS (HS) (CONGENITAL HEMOLYTIC JAUNDICE) This disorder, long considered the prototype of hemolytic anemias due to intrinsic erythrocytic defects, actually differs from most of that group by virtue of the crucial role played by the spleen in the pathogenesis of the anemia. In this disorder, removal of the spleen—the extraerythrocytic factor—relieves the anemia even though the intrinsic erythrocytic defect persists.

Definition This is a familial and hereditary disorder characterized by a variable degree of hemolytic anemia and "acholuric" jaundice, spherocytosis, and increased osmotic fragility of the red corpuscles.

History During the early part of the present century, this familial disorder was clearly defined, becoming known as the type of Chauffard and Minkowski, and was distinguished from the acquired form described by Hayem and Widal.

Etiology Transmitted as an autosomal dominant trait and especially common in people of Northern European stock, this disorder is due to an inherited defect of the red corpuscles, which tend to be more spheric than normal as they age in the circulation. Spherocytes are more rigid than normal red cells and are especially subject to entrapment and destruction by the spleen (see Pathogenesis above). The corpuscular abnormality is related to excessive permeability of the red blood cell membrane to the ingress of sodium ion. As increased amounts of sodium gain access to the interior of the cell, the ATPase mechanism is stimulated, increasing the outward pumping rate of sodium ion and at the same time requiring an increased rate of glycolysis for replenishment of ATP. The abnormality is aggravated by *erythrostasis* in the spleen (see Pathogenesis above). Fragmentation of spherocyte membranes occurs in the circulation, and minute portions can be recovered by ultracentrifugation of the plasma. It is now believed that the total and relative amounts of the various membrane lipids are normal. The nature of the membrane protein components in erythrocytes is an unresolved question. Electrophoretic studies of urea-treated, denatured, or hydrolyzed extracts of erythrocytic membrane proteins have suggested an abnormality characteristic of HS. An abnormality of aggregation of membrane protein subunits in HS has also been suggested. Further study is required to relate these observations to the pathogenesis of spherocytes and to explain why the erythrocytes in this disorder may appear normally biconcave when they are reticulocytes, and spherocytic later.

Pathology The spleen is always enlarged, often weighing 1,000 to 1,500 g. The pulp and, to a lesser extent, the sinuses are greatly congested. Depending on the degree of anemia and the extent of blood destruction, hyperplasia and even metaplasia of the bone marrow occur, and deposits of iron pigment are found in the liver, kidneys, and even lymph nodes.

Symptoms Jaundice and splenomegaly are the most common manifestations; they may pass unnoticed for many years. A persistent sallow appearance, rather than obvious jaundice, may be present. Symptoms of anemia may be absent or mild. At any time from birth to late adult life attention may be drawn to the disorder by the *crise de déglobulization*, which is characterized by fever, lassitude, palpitation, and shortness of breath or even by violent abdominal pain, vomiting, and anorexia. Rather than being merely episodes of increased blood destruction, as had long been assumed, these crises have been found to be associated with sudden, temporary reduction, or even cessation of blood formation (see Clinical Manifestations above). Such "aplastic" or more correctly hypoplastic crises, characterized by relative or absolute reticulocytopenia, are especially likely to be associated with infections, even commonplace ones. Since the life span of the red corpuscles in this hemolytic disease is very brief, anemia develops rapidly under these circumstances.

The liver may or may not be enlarged. Other developmental anomalies are often present. Chronic leg ulcers may be found, and striation and thickening of the frontal and parietal bones of the skull may be seen on roentgenographic examination. Cholelithiasis is a frequent complication, and symptoms of this complication may first bring the patient to the physician.

The anemia is usually moderate in degree but may be very mild or severe. It is normocytic or microcytic in type, but not hypochromic. When severe and associated with marked reticulocytosis, it may be macrocytic. There is little poikilocytosis, but very many small, deeply staining red corpuscles without central pallor (spherocytes) are seen, scattered among the cells of normal size. Polychromatophilia and sometimes even normoblasts may be seen in the blood smear. The leukocytes may be normal in number, or increased, and the same is true of the platelets. Reticulocytes are characteristically increased in number, most often accounting for 5 to 20 percent of the erythrocytes.

Increased osmotic fragility of the red corpuscles is characteristic (see Osmotic Fragility Test above). Hemolysis, beginning at 220 mOsm, equivalent to about 0.64 percent saline solution, is not unusual. It may be complete at the point where hemolysis of healthy erythrocytes normally begins; i.e., about 150 mOsm, equivalent to about 0.44 percent saline.

Hyperbilirubinemia of the "indirect" type, consisting

almost entirely of nonconjugated bilirubin, produces "acholuric jaundice," i.e., jaundice without bilirubin in the urine. There is an increased quantity of urobilinogen in the stools and in the urine, as is characteristic of hemolytic disorders.

Diagnosis Splenomegaly, acholuric jaundice, spherocytosis, reticulocytosis, and an increase of osmotic fragility and of autohemolysis, the latter prevented by the prior addition of glucose (Table 306-3), are characteristic findings in affected patients. Examination of other, even asymptomatic family members for the very same features is most valuable in establishing the diagnosis of *hereditary* spherocytosis in the patient at hand. The failure to find historical evidence of anemia or jaundice in other family members is an unreliable criterion for excluding relatives who may potentially be involved, and should not be a deterrent in seeking further evidence by physical and laboratory examination. Moreover, the absence of evidence of the disease in both parents of a patient does not necessarily exclude the diagnosis of hereditary spherocytosis. About 20 to 25 percent of cases are sporadic, probably the result of incomplete penetrance in the parent or of the occurrence of new cases through genetic mutation.

The Coombs test is negative except in occasional cases. In these it is likely that a superimposed acquired immunohemolytic process has developed. When the picture is not entirely typical, a careful study must be made to rule out other types of hemolytic anemia.

Treatment During a "crisis," many blood transfusions may be needed to avoid a very serious degree of anemia. As the lesion is intrinsic to the patient's erythrocytes, transfused red corpuscles survive normally in the patient's circulation, and the beneficial effects of the transfusions should persist until the patient recovers his usual degree of accelerated erythropoiesis and hematologic equilibrium. In the longer view, splenectomy remains the best treatment.

This is the one disorder in which *splenectomy* is associated with consistently satisfactory results. Although remissions may develop without splenectomy and latent periods of many years' duration may occur, as illustrated by the occasional first recognition of the disease after the age of forty or fifty years, permanent spontaneous recovery does not take place. The risk of hyporegenerative crises and serious anemia, progressive cholelithiasis, and the consequent risk of carcinoma of the gall bladder is always present. Splenectomy is usually deferred in infancy because of possible lowered resistance to infection when splenectomy is performed prior to two years of age. It is best performed as an elective procedure when the patient is otherwise in good health. At operation, a careful search should be made for accessory spleens, and those which are found should be removed. After splenectomy, anemia, jaundice, and reticulocytosis disappear. The spherocytosis as well as the increased osmotic fragility of the red blood cells persists, because the abnormal cells remain in the circulation as they are no longer subject to removal by the spleen. Should such red blood cells be transfused into a recipient with an intact spleen, they would be promptly removed from the circulation.

GLUCOSE 6-PHOSPHATE DEHYDROGENASE DEFICIENCY (PRIMAQUINE-SENSITIVE TYPE) About 11 percent of male Negroes and a variable percentage of individuals of other races, who are otherwise free of hemolytic disease and anemia, respond to the administration of amounts of primaquine and certain other compounds (see Table 306-2) which are innocuous to other individuals, with an abrupt hemolytic episode characterized by dark urine, marked anemia, jaundice, and reticulocytosis. The acute hemolytic phase ends spontaneously in about a week even if the drug is continued, and the anemia is gradually relieved, though reticulocytosis may persist for a while. Glucose 6-phosphate dehydrogenase is concerned with the regeneration of NADPH, which, in turn, is required in the regeneration of reduced GSH from oxidized glutathione (GSSG). Primaquine and other redox compounds oxidize GSH and stimulate the phosphogluconate oxidative pathway (Fig. 306-1, reactions 12 to 15). When these compounds act in the case of G-6-PD deficiency, there is a rapid fall in erythrocytic GSH concentration and Heinz bodies form in red corpuscles. Hemolysis follows, but the exact biochemical mechanism by which this is brought about remains obscure.

Because of the prevalence of the condition among certain population groups, it is worthwhile testing for G-6-PD deficiency in individuals at high risk before prescribing drugs capable of inducing the hemolytic reaction. Simple screening tests are available, including the spot test (see Erythrocyte Enzyme Assays above), the methemoglobin reduction test and the brilliant cresyl blue reduction test. These will detect the fully expressed cases in males and females and many of but not all the intermediate cases occurring in heterozygous females. *Heinz bodies* (see Heinz Bodies above) are readily formed when the blood of G-6-PD-deficient patients is incubated with acetylphenylhydrazine. Accurate diagnosis depends on specific enzyme assay.

Individuals deficient in G-6-PD will usually escape without a hemolytic episode even though the intrinsic erythrocytic defect is present if they are not given the compounds listed in Table 306-2. The abnormality usually has no significant deleterious effect on the individual or on the red corpuscle life span in the absence of the offending chemical agent. In some cases, acute illnesses, such as infectious hepatitis, diabetic acidosis, and pneumonia, may be accompanied by a hemolytic episode even in the absence of known offending drugs.

CHRONIC HEMOLYTIC ANEMIA WITH PAROXYSMAL NOCTURNAL HEMOGLOBINURIA AND PERPETUAL HEMOSIDERINURIA (MARCHIAFAVA-MICHELI SYNDROME) This is a rare disorder usually referred to as *paroxysmal nocturnal hemoglobinura*, or *PNH*. In this disorder, an intrinsic erythrocytic defect renders these cells uniquely susceptible to the hemolytic action of serum complement.

Clinical features This disease occurs most commonly during the third or fourth decade but no age and neither sex is exempt. It is characterized by hemolytic anemia and intravascular hemolysis. The hemoglobinemia and consequent hemoglobinuria, originally regarded as occurring mainly during sleep, fluctuate throughout the 24 hr of a day and from day to day; the classic nocturnal hemoglobinuria is seen in only about 25 percent of cases. The urine may be brown or reddish brown. The symptoms are those of long-standing anemia, but there may be abdominal, lumbar, or substernal pain, which often ushers in an attack of hemoglobinuria. The findings, similar to those in other hemolytic anemias, include splenomegaly and well-marked anemia. The osmotic fragility of the red corpuscles is normal, and spherocytosis is not characteristic. There may be hemoglobinemia even when there is no hemoglobinuria. The urine contains increased amounts of urobilinogen as well as hemoglobin and hemosiderin. The urinary iron loss may amount to 10 mg daily, and iron-deficiency anemia may develop. Hemosiderin can often be demonstrated in leukocytes or epithelial cells of the urine. Leukopenia is usual and may be marked, and there may be thrombocytopenia as well. Indeed, this is one of the few types of severe hemolytic anemia which is accompanied by pancytopenia, and may lead to an erroneous diagnosis of aplastic anemia because of failure to consider the possibility of PNH. Thrombotic episodes involving abdominal, peripheral, or even cerebral veins are a serious complication.

Pathogenesis The red cells from patients with PNH consist of at least two populations, one very sensitive to the lytic action of the third component of complement (C3), the other less sensitive but still usually somewhat more sensitive than normal. The proportion of these two populations varies from patient to patient but in most instances is stable for a given patient for long periods of time. The exact site and cause of complement lysis in PNH have not been defined. Abnormalities on the surface of PNH cells demonstrable by electron microscopy, once considered to be related to their susceptibility to hemolysis, probably do not represent lesions specific for PNH. The first steps of the C′ sequence seem to be the same for normal and PNH cells, and presumably it is the later stages which are involved. Initiation of activation of the C′ sequence in bringing about lysis of PNH cells does not depend on specific antibody; a specific protein, properdin, can do the same. The increase in susceptibility to immune lysis of the complement-sensitive cells of PNH, especially at an acid pH and in isotonic media of low ionic strength, is exploited in the acidified-serum test (Ham's) and the sucrose test for PNH (see Sucrose test above).

A second definable abnormality of PNH red cells is an abnormally low acetylcholinesterase content. The severity of the disease is paralleled by the degree of decrease in this enzyme activity, and the latter, in turn, reflects the number of complement-sensitive cells; such cells contain no detectable acetylcholinesterase. It is postulated that the enzyme deficiency is due to the same membrane defect as the complement-sensitivity, but its nature is obscure. An abnormality of the protein of the membrane is thought to be more likely than a defect in the lipid components.

In contradistinction to the majority of hemolytic diseases due to intrinsic erythrocytic defects, the PNH lesion appears to be acquired rather than hereditary or congenital, perhaps the result of a somatic mutation.

It has been demonstrated that a much greater proportion than normal of complement-sensitive cells is delivered each day by the bone marrow. This would explain the increase in hemoglobinemia which has been observed when erythropoiesis is stimulated in these patients as, for example, by iron therapy. The *hypercoagulable state* (see below) has been attributed to the intravascular release of thromboplastin which is contained within red cells or of some other substance which accelerates coagulation. The mechanism by which the hemolytic system is activated during sleep is obscure.

Diagnosis In addition to the findings of intermittent hemoglobinemia and hemoglobinuria, perpetual hemosiderinuria, and other findings characteristic of hemolytic anemia, there is pancytopenia, a positive acidified-serum test, a positive sucrose screening test, a low leukocyte alkaline phosphatase score, and abnormally low erythrocyte acetylcholinesterase. In some instances, patients with negative tests for PNH and a seemingly established diagnosis of aplastic anemia have been found to have positive tests for PNH months or years later.

Treatment This is purely symptomatic. Splenectomy is of no value, and serious and even fatal thrombotic episodes may follow surgery. The intensity of the hemolytic process varies; crises of severe anemia may occur. Transfusion of whole blood, packed red blood cells, or plasma usually precipitates hemolytic crises, perhaps because of the additional complement which is provided. Another explanation is that the reaction of antileukocyte antibody with transfused leukocytes initiates the complement sequence. Saline-washed leukocyte and platelet-poor blood can usually be given with impunity, and only these should be administered if transfusion is required. Iron deficiency may complicate the picture, but iron salts or iron-dextran complex for parenteral administration should be given with caution because the hemolytic process may be aggravated, perhaps due to accelerated production of red cells, including the complement-sensitive population. The starting dose of iron should be reduced to one-tenth or one-twentieth of the usual daily dose and the dose may be increased gradually if a ferrous sulfate solution is given. The potent androgens, fluoxymesterone and oxymetholone, given in daily doses of 0.5 to 1.0 and 0.5 to 1.5 mg per kg body weight, respectively, have brought about reduction in hemoglobinuria and partial or complete relief of anemia in a number of cases. Relapses have occurred if the androgen was abruptly withdrawn. A trial of one of these drugs for 3 months or longer seems warranted, especially for the more severely affected patients. Although thrombocytopenia is common, purpuric or hemorrhagic manifestations are unusual; in fact, thrombotic complications are not infrequent. It has been reported that the anticoagulant dicoumarin (Dicumarol) impedes hemolytic activity in this disease; it has also been employed to prevent thrombotic complications. Coumarin compounds are best reserved for the latter indication e.g., post-partum or after surgery. Heparin should be avoided, since it is thought to accelerate hemolysis. Infections are frequent in these patients, partly, perhaps, because of the associated leukopenia.

Great care must be taken to differentiate the abdominal pain which may accompany an acute hemolytic crisis from a true surgical emergency, because needless abdominal operations may only further aggravate the hemolysis and lead to serious deterioration in the patient's condition. The prognosis varies greatly. Although a fatal termination may ensue in several years, in some cases the disorder has been compatible with life for many years and has even been known to disappear.

HEMOLYTIC ANEMIA DUE TO EXTRAERYTHROCYTIC FACTORS

AGENTS EXTRANEOUS TO THE PATIENT The naturally occurring isoagglutinis α and β cause hemolysis when incompatible blood is given by transfusion. Proper cross-matching technique and identification of the blood type of donors and of recipients of transfusions will avoid such disasters. When hemolytic transfusion reactions take place in spite of A, B, and O blood group compatibility, they are attributable in most instances to the development of anti-RH (D) agglutinins. Next in frequency are the Kell antigen and antibody. Other blood groups are only rarely involved (Chap. 310).

Erythroblastosis fetalis (*hemolytic disease of the newborn*) is due to the action of immune isoantibodies which enter the fetal circulation from the mother, via the placenta. The mother becomes immunized by an antigen which is lacking in her own red blood cells but is present in fetal red blood cells (which escape into her circulation) carrying a "foreign" antigen inherited from the father; or she may have been immunized by transfusion with blood containing erythrocyte antigens dissimilar to hers but similar to those of the fetus; or immunization may have been brought about by heterogenetic stimuli such as tetanus toxoid or vaccine containing group A substance. Spherocytosis and hyperbilirubinemia are prominent; the direct Coombs test is strongly positive when the condition is due to Rh, Kell, Kidd, and Duffy blood group systems; the test is weakly positive or even negative when erythroblastosis is due to anti-A.

ABO incompatibility is the most common cause of hemolytic disease of the newborn, the mother usually being of blood group O, and the iso-antibody anti-A_2. Rh incompatibility is, nowadays, a less-frequent cause of erythroblastosis, especially among Negroes, in whom the Rh-negative characteristic occurs only half as frequently as in Caucasians. The lower incidence is explained also by the fact that the Rh erythroblastotic child is more likely the result of the second or later pregnancy, whereas in the case of ABO incompatibility about half of the cases occur in the first pregnancy. Passive immunization of Rh-negative mothers with anti-Rh antibodies has proved to be an effective means of protecting infants against Rh hemolytic disease.

Certain chemical agents and drugs may produce hemolysis as a consequence of their usual pharmacologic activity, and in these instances (see Table 306-1, group *II, A, 2*), the effect is related to the size of the dose.

Three types of *immunohemolytic anemia* secondary to drug administration have been identified. The *haptene type* is exemplified by the development of hemolytic anemia with an anti-γG type of positive direct Coombs reaction (and a negative anti-C′ Coombs reaction) following the administration of penicillin in the range of 20 million units daily. The drug is firmly bound to the red corpuscle, perhaps through covalent linkage of a degradation product, benzylpenicilloyl. Anti-penicillin antibodies responsible for the hemolytic anemia and the positive Coombs test are present in the serum and red blood cell eluate. The antibodies react only with penicillin-coated red corpuscles, not with normal uncoated corpuscles, thereby distinguishing this condition from the autoimmune type of hemolytic anemia (see Idiopathic Autoimmune Hemolytic Anemia below).

In the "*innocent bystander*" *type* of drug-induced hemolytic anemia, produced by quinine and stibophen, the red corpuscle is injured by the binding to its membrane of a drug-antibody complex formed in the plasma. The complex activates the complement mechanism at the cell membrane, heavily coating the cell with complement and producing a positive anti-C′ Coombs reaction. These red corpuscles may lyse or may be removed from the circulation by the reticuloendothelial system. Meanwhile, the drug-antibody complex dissociates from the damaged red corpuscle to injure others. The relatively small number of complexes present accounts for the negative anti-γG Coombs reaction in this type of immunohemolytic anemia.

The *alpha-methyldopa type* of immunohemolytic anemia differs from the two preceding types in that the Coombs reactions is of the anti-γG type but the antibodies react not with the drug or drug-coated corpuscles, but with antigens, usually of the Rh system, of the patient's own red corpuscles, or other normal red corpuscles. The phenomenon appears to be that of a cross-reaction in which an exogenous agent may induce the production of an antibody that reacts with the host's own erythrocytic antigens. From 10 to 20 percent of patients treated with alpha-methyldopa develop a positive Coombs test, but hemolytic anemia follows in only about 1 percent of these patients. Withdrawal of the drug results in a gradual reversal of this process. The antibody induced by alpha-methyldopa possesses all the characteristics of typical "warm antibody," the kind seen in Rh sensitization and in patients with severe "auto-immune" hemolytic anemia. The latter should always be considered as possible examples of drug-induced disease and should be studied carefully for an etiologic agent which can be eliminated, thereby permitting reversal of the process.

Infectious agents (Table 306-1, group *II, A, 3*) may produce hemolytic anemia by direct attack or infestation of the red corpuscles, through the production of toxin, or, as in the case of mycoplasma infection, by a type of cross-reaction similar to the response to alpha-methyldopa described above. In the case of mycoplasma, a cold antibody, usually reactive with the I antigen of the red corpuscles, results.

A number of *physical agents* produce hemolytic anemia (Table 306-1, group *II, A, 4*). Among them is the mechanical trauma produced by the impact of red corpuscles on prosthetic heart valves. This results in random destruction of red corpuscles of all ages, appearance of fragmented and so-called "helmet" cells in the circulation, and, because of intravascular hemolysis, a significant loss of iron in the form of hemosiderin in the urine, leading to iron deficiency anemia.

In addition to the exogenous agents discussed above, there are *endogenous causes* for extraerythrocytic mechanisms which produce hemolytic anemia.

SECONDARY ("SYMPTOMATIC") HEMOLYTIC ANEMIAS These types of anemia may be associated with a variety of disorders. The most common ones are listed in Table 306-1, group *II, B, 2.* In addition to the manifestations of hemolytic anemia, which may or may not be associated with autoantibodies of the type described above, there will be symptoms and signs of the underlying disorder, which are often not readily apparent and must be sought out carefully. In younger women, the possibility of disseminated lupus erythematosus should be considered, while in older patients, chronic lymphocytic leukemia or lymphosarcoma is a frequent cause of an immune type of hemolytic anemia. In many cases, the course of the hemolytic disease may be chronic and mild. In others, e.g., lupus erythematosus or chronic lymphocytic leukemia, the hemolytic anemia may be the predominating clinical feature. In such cases, treatment must be directed toward both the underlying disorder and the hemolytic process. Particularly in the case of lymphomas, where therapy might entail the use of agents which suppress erythropoiesis, control of the hemolytic process should be achieved early because reduction in the rate of red corpuscle regeneration might be expected to result in aggravation of the anemia if the hemolytic disorder is severe.

A great proportion of hemolytic anemias due to endogenous causes, including the secondary or so-called "symptomatic" hemolytic anemias already mentioned, are due to the production of "autoantibodies." Frequently, the Coombs test is positive (anti-γG reagent), indicating the presence of erythrocyte-bound antibodies, but no associated disease or causative agent is found. Such instances, diagnosed as "idiopathic" Coombs-positive hemolytic anemia, or idiopathic autoimmune hemolytic anemia, are diagnoses by exclusion.

IDIOPATHIC AUTOIMMUNE HEMOLYTIC ANEMIA The term *autoimmune* as used here signifies the presence of immunologic processes with specificity for antigens found on the tissues of the individual making the response. Explanations offered for the production of antierythrocyte antibodies include (1) alterations in the patient's erythrocytes which make surface antigens no longer recognizable as self; (2) disturbances of immune responsiveness, including the emergence of forbidden clones; and (3) genetically determined peculiarities of immune responsiveness which lead to cross-reactivity of normal immune responsiveness with the patient's own tissue antigens.

It is likely that in the variety of circumstances under which "autoimmune" hemolytic anemia develops, any one of the above mechanisms may play a role. In addition, as mentioned above in the discussion of immunohemolytic anemia secondary to drug administration, autoimmunity may be the result of a normal immune response toward a foreign antigenic determinant which cross-reacts with an autologous tissue constituent. The fact that in a number of instances other abnormalities of globulin synthesis are observed, such as hypergammaglobulinemia, anticomplementary substances, cryoglobulinemia, and antibodies against lipid antigens such as those which give rise to false positive biologic reactions for syphilis, suggests that a generalized disturbance of immune systems is present. Also noteworthy is the fact that many of the red cell autoantibodies interact with normal antigenic determinants, particularly those belonging to the Rh group of antigens.

Both specific and nonspecific antibodies may be found in the same patient. Furthermore, there is considerable variation from one patient to the next, in the temperature requirements, specificity, chemical nature, and in vitro reactions of the antibodies. "Warm" antibodies react well at 37°C and are not potentiated at lower temperatures. They usually are IgG globulins, but nongamma G globulins or mixtures of both types have been found in some cases. Most commonly, these are "incomplete antibodies," i.e., they coat normal erythrocytes and may be detected by antiglobulin serum but do not cause agglutination in a saline medium, nor do they cause hemolysis. The fixation of these antibodies to red corpuscles is not inhibited by previous heat inactivation of the patient's serum at 56°C, to destroy complement, and it is only slightly increased by acidification of the serum to pH 7 or 6.5. "Cold" antibodies are markedly potentiated by reducing the temperature of the in vitro test system below 37°C and especially below 22°C. These antibodies are usually of the 19S, IgM type. They may act as agglutinating antibodies and under certain circumstances may fix complement and also bring about hemolysis.

The mechanism whereby hemolysis is initiated in vivo is not entirely clear because most of the autoantibodies encountered are not hemolytic in vitro. In a small proportion of cases, following the antigen-antibody reaction on the red blood cell membrane, the complement fixation sequence (C 1,4,2,3) ensues and defects appear in the membrane surface, representing holes of about 103 A diameter, which may be visualized by electron microscopy. The nature of the reaction by which complement produces the holes in the lipid layer of the cell membrane is unknown. Lysis need not be by direct loss of hemoglobin through the hole, since excess water or ion transfer can cause the red corpuscle to reach the critical hemolytic volume at which the membrane becomes permeable to hemoglobin. In many cases, complement is not bound to the cell membrane, and in these cases another explanation has been offered. Red corpuscles coated with IgG antibody may become adherent to receptor sites of monocytes and macrophages in vivo, and then sphere. This may well be the first step of the fixed tissue macrophages of the reticuloendothelial system in trapping and destroying red corpuscles coated with "incomplete" antibodies.

The *clinical manifestations* range from insidious and chronic anemia to an acute, severe, and fulminating illness. Remissions and exacerbations may occur spontaneously. The hematologic and clinical features are similar to those of other hemolytic anemias (see Clinical Manifestations above). In cold agglutinin disease, acrocyanosis may be a major complaint and a significant clue to the diagnosis. Spherocytosis may not be prominent, but, may be marked during periods of brisk hemolysis, and at such times the osmotic fragility and mechanical fragility of the red corpuscles are increased. Because the hemolytic system is dependent on extraerythrocytic factors, even normal transfused red blood cells will be hemolyzed, at a rate equivalent to that of the patient's red blood cells, and may also become spherocytes with abnormal osmotic fragility. If reticulocytosis is great, the anemia is likely to be macrocytic. In some cases when a thin film of anticoagulated blood is examined with the unaided eye, or under low-power magnification, a granular appearance is seen, attributable to the agglutination of the red corpuscles in the plasma. Sometimes, this may be detected when blood is first drawn from the patient by venipuncture; it can be observed along the inside of the glass container after mixing the blood with the dry anticoagulant, thus providing an early clue to the diagnosis. The direct Coombs test and the indirect Coombs test detect the globulin attached to the cell surface and the "autoantibodies" in the patient's serum, respectively. It is useful to determine the specificity of the serologic reaction, i.e., whether anti-γG, anticomplement, or anti-γA or -γM. Occasionally anti-red cell antibodies cannot be demonstrated by routine techniques, and in such cases of hemolytic anemia the more sensitive complement-fixing antibody consumption technique is helpful. Tests for warm and cold hemolysins and cold agglutinins should be performed (see Serologic Tests above). Serums of patients with the idiopathic cold hemagglutin syndrome usually belong to the γM class of immunoglobulins, fix complement, and have anti-I specificity.

Treatment was described earlier.

PAROXYSMAL COLD HEMOGLOBINURIA This is an uncommon disorder characterized by the sudden passage of hemoglobin in the urine, following local or general exposure to cold. Aching and pain in the back, legs, or abdomen, and other symptoms of acute hemolysis, such as a chill, fever, and malaise, are associated with the passage of dark brownish urine. Other findings are those characteristic of acute hemolytic anemia. Symptoms may appear at any time from a few minutes to 7 or 8 hr following exposure.

Donath and Landsteiner showed that the hemoglobinuria is due to the sudden intravascular hemolysis of blood as the result of the action of an autohemolysin contained in the patient's blood. The D-L hemolysin unites with the red corpuscles only at a low temperature, but destruction of the cells occurs only after the temperature of the blood has returned to normal body temperature. Appropriate screening and detailed tests have been devised to demonstrate this cold hemolysin (see Serologic Tests above), which has been found to be a complement-fixing 7S, gamma-G-globulin. A the time of hemolytic attacks produced by chilling, strongly positive direct antiglobulin (Coombs) reactions have been observed, but these become negative after the attacks.

Classically described in patients with congenital or tertiary syphilis, paroxysmal cold hemoglobinuria is seen also in the absence of this disease. Now it is seen more often following viral infections. About a third of all patients with this antibody have a positive Wassermann test, but the D-L hemolysin has been shown to be separate from the antibodies which give rise to the various biologic tests for syphilis.

The acute attack is treated symptomatically. Acute postinfectious forms usually terminate spontaneously. Only temporary protection from cold exposure is needed as a rule. Syphilis, if present, is treated.

March hemoglobinuria is not likely to be confused with any of the conditions described above if the characteristic history is elicited. The symptoms usually are trivial, though alarming to the patient: dark urine (hemoglobinuria) is noted following prolonged walking or running. The amount of blood which is hemolyzed probably is small, and the condition is benign. Jaundice is unusual and anemia does not develop. Traumatic destruction of red cells as they circulate through the capillaries in the soles of the feet produces the syndrome. The type of footgear worn and the hardness of the surface walked on play roles in inducing this condition.

REFERENCES

Allgood JW, Chaplin H Jr: Idiopathic acquired autoimmune hemolytic anemia. Am J Med 43:254, 1967

Brain MC: Microangiopathic hemolytic anemia. Annu Rev Med 21:133, 1970

Dacie JV, Worlledge SM: Autoimmune hemolytic anemias. Progr Hematol 6:82, 1969

Harris JW, Kellenmeyer RW: *The Red Cell: Production, Metabolism, Destruction; Normal and Abnormal*, Cambridge, Mass.: Harvard, 1970

Hartmann RC et al: Paroxysmal nocturnal hemoglobinuria: Clinical and laboratory studies relating to iron metabolism and therapy with androgen and iron. Medicine 45:331, 1966

Lieberman E: Hemolytic uremic syndrome. J Pediatr 80:1, 1972

Mollison PL: The role of complement in antibody-mediated red-cell destruction. Br J Haematol 18:249, 1970

Tanaka KR, Paglia DE: Pyruvate kinase deficiency. Semin Hematol 8:367, 1971; Br J Haematol 22:651, 1972

Valentine WN: Deficiencies associated with Embden-Meyerhof pathway and other metabolic pathways. Semin Hematol 8:348, 1971

Wintrobe MM et al: *Clinical Hematology*, 7th ed., Philadelphia: Lea & Febiger, 1974

Worlledge SM: Immune drug induced hemolytic anemias. Semin Hematol 6:181, 1969

307 THE HEMOGLOBINOPATHIES AND THALASSEMIAS

ARTHUR HAUT
M. M. WINTROBE

NORMAL AND ABNORMAL HEMOGLOBINS

The fact that a molecular abnormality in a single protein may produce serious ill effects and can be identified by simple, readily applicable procedures was discovered as the result of investigations concerning the nature of a hereditary, hemolytic anemia which causes serious illness in the Negro and is characterized by sickling of the red cells in vitro when they are deprived of oxygen. The elaboration of electrophoretic methods and the application of more complex techniques led to the discovery that hemoglobin is not a single homogeneous protein and that quantitative and qualitative differences in the various hemoglobins are inherited abnormalities which may produce few or no clinical changes or may cause serious ill health. These investigations have enriched our understanding not only of the pathogenesis of human disease but also of genetics and anthropology (Chap. 62). One of the abnormal hemoglobins, the sickle-cell anomaly, is believed to have conferred on its carriers increased ability to resist malarial infections.

About 97 percent of the hemoglobin in the red corpuscles of normal human adults is termed *hemoglobin A* (Hb A) and consists of two pairs of coiled polypeptide chains: two α chains, each formed of 141 amino acids, and two β chains, each made up of 146 amino acids. Hence, the designation, Hb $\alpha_2^A\beta_2^A$ or, more simply, Hb $\alpha_2\beta_2$. The minor fraction of the hemoglobin of normal adult erythrocytes is Hb A_2 and comprises 2.54 ± 0.35 percent of the total hemoglobin present. It possesses a different second set of polypeptide chains, δ chains in place of β chains, and is designated $\alpha_2^A\delta_2^{A_2}$. In fetal life, a different hemoglobin is present and progressively decreases in amount during infancy. Like Hb A_2, fetal hemoglobin (Hb F) possesses a pair of the same α chains as in Hb A, but the second set is different. Hb F is therefore designated $\alpha_2^A\gamma_2^F$. Amino acid substitutions, occurring in the α, β, γ, and δ polypeptide chains, are transmitted as hereditable traits. The genetic control of production of α, β, γ, and δ chains is mediated via autosomal alleles. It is thought that α and β chain production is controlled by genes located on separate chromosomes. Those for the control of synthesis of β, γ, and δ chains are thought to be located in close proximity to one another on the same chromosome. Each parent contributes one member of an allelic pair of genes (Fig. 307-1). Thus a normal genotype would be α/α, β/β. Mutant genes may appear in the heterozygous or homozygous state, depending on the genotypes of the parents. However, only one allele can be inherited from each parent.

With the exception of Hb C_{Harlem}, only a single amino acid substitution has been found in each of the abnormal hemoglobins studied. In most instances, the exact location and nature of the amino acid substitution has been identified. If an α chain abnormality occurs, both the major hemoglobin component and the minor components (A_2, F) will be affected because they all incorporate α chains. Both α and β chain abnormalities may be present in the same individual, and each is inherited and transmitted separately. In addition to these qualitative differences in hemoglobin peptides, in certain hematologic disorders quantitative alterations in the percentages of the normal hemoglobin peptides have been found. Furthermore, complete deletion of a pair of chains may occur. Thus, Hb H is made up of four β chains (β_4), and Hb Bart's consists of four γ chains (γ_4).

NOMENCLATURE The abnormal hemoglobins at first were identified serially by alphabetic letters because they were discovered by their individual electrophoretic mobility at alkaline pH. As the list grew longer and abnormal hemoglobins with the same electrophoretic mobility but certain other different characteristics were found, the geographic area where the abnormal hemoglobin was discovered was indicated as well; thus, Hb $G_{San\ Jose}$ and Hb $G_{Philadelphia}$. When the exact amino acid sequence structure of the normal hemoglobins was determined, and as the nature and position of the amino acid difference in the abnormal hemoglobin was identified, it became possible to indicate the nature of the abnormality in a simple way. Thus Hb S (sickle-cell hemoglobin) is Hb $\alpha_2^A\beta_2^{6\ val}$. This means that the α chains in Hb S are normal, as in A hemoglobin, but in the β chains the sixth amino acid, which a diagram of the normal amino acid constitution of the β chain indicates is glutamic acid, has been replaced by valine. The genotype of the heterozygous state would indicate that this abnormality is present in only one of the chromosomes governing β chains, whereas in the homozygous state, both chromosomes would code for this abnormality (Fig. 307-1).

The hemoglobin disorders are referred to as *hemoglobinopathies* when they are related to qualitative differences in hemoglobin. These have been called *traits* when heterozygous, and *diseases* when homozygous, because as a rule the trait is harmless, whereas the homozygous state may have deleterious effects. Thalassemia, on the other hand, is thought to be due to the inheritance of a subnormal rate of synthesis of one or the other of the normal hemoglobin peptides and consequently is designated separately. Mixtures of abnormal hemoglobins and combinations of abnormal hemoglobins and thalassemia, due to double heterozygosity for different genes for controlling hemoglobin synthesis, also have been identi-

FIGURE 307-1
Schematic model for synthesis of the globin portion of hemoglobin. Only the abnormal polypeptide chain is labeled (β^s).

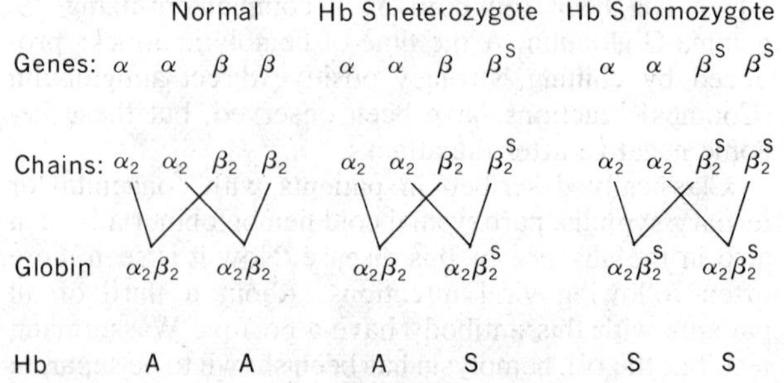

fied. Hemoglobinopathies may also occur in combination with other anomalies of the red cell which are inherited independently, viz., hereditary spherocytosis (Chap. 306).

STRUCTURE OF HEMOGLOBIN By means of x-ray crystallography and model building it has been possible to gain insight regarding the normal functioning of hemoglobin and the ways in which genetic abnormalities have altered function. The *primary* structure of hemoglobin, as mentioned above, consists of the two pairs of polypeptide chains, α and β. These chains are in part straight and in part helical arrays (*secondary* structure). There are eight helical arrays of amino acids, identified by consecutive letters from A to H. The straight-chain sections occur at the amino and carboxy terminals and also between the helices, thus allowing bending. This structure is stabilized by hydrogen ion bonds between the carboxy and amino groups of adjacent coils. The nonpolar amino acids are directed toward the inner core of the molecule, rendering it stable, and the polar amino acids are presented to the molecular surface where they interact with water, rendering the molecule soluble (*tertiary* structure). Heme, one molecule to each chain, is situated in the nonpolar environment, thereby making it possible for Fe^{++} to form reversible bonds with oxygen without being oxidized to the ferric form. It is suspended between the E and F helices, forming covalent bonds with the proximal histidine at F8. When oxygen is bound, it forms covalent bonds with heme and the distal histidine (E8). The contacts between the four chains (*quaternary* structure) also are important because they are located close enough to the heme group to suggest that the heme environment can be significantly altered by their movement when hemoglobin is oxygenated. The affinity for oxygen thereby changes as each of the four oxygen binding sites becomes occupied ("heme-heme interaction"). Such movement can also prevent attachment of 2,3-DPG.

Because the position of an amino acid substitution is now recognized as being of importance in determining whether it will interfere with the function of hemoglobin, in addition to stating the chain and the location on that chain where a substitution has taken place, the helix and the location on that helix also are often indicated.

A classification based on the functional consequence of the different hemoglobin abnormalities is presented in Table 307-1.

HEMOGLOBINS WITH AMINO ACID SUBSTITUTIONS OR DELETIONS The location of many amino acid substitutions is not such that it alters their function, and therefore there are no clinical sequelae. These hemoglobinopathies are of great interest from the points of view of genetics and anthropology. Other alterations, however, alter oxygen affinity, decreasing or increasing it. Such hemoglobin molecules may be stable or unstable. When oxygen affinity is decreased, there is enhanced tissue oxygen supply and reduced bone marrow response. If the variant molecule is stable, the hemoglobin concentration is reduced but there is no true, corresponding deficit in tissue oxygen. If the variant is unstable, hemo-

TABLE 307-1
Classification of the disorders of globin synthesis

I Qualitative abnormalities of the globin peptides (amino acid substitutions or deletions)
- *A* With clinical sequelae
  - *1* Abnormal heme-oxygen interaction
    - *a* Diminished oxygen binding
      - (*1*) Fe^{++} heme: Hemoglobins Kansas, Yoshizuka, Seattle[1]
      - (*2*) Fe^{+++} heme-methemoglobins: Hemoglobins M: Boston (Osaka), Hyde Park (Akita), Iwate (Kankakee) Milwaukee-1, Saskatoon (Chicago)
    - *b* Increased oxygen affinity: Hemoglobins Bethesda, Brigham, Chesapeake, Hiroshe, Hiroshima, $J_{Capetown}$, Kempsey, Little Rock, Malmö, Rainier, Tacoma[2], Yakima, Ypsi, H[3], Bart's[4]
  - *2* Normal heme-oxygen interaction
    - *a* Readily precipitating (forms Heinz bodies): Hemoglobins Bibba, Borås, Bristol, Bucaresti, Christchurch, Columbia, Etiobicoke, Freiburg[5], Genova, Gun Hill[6], H[3], Hammersmith, Köln (Ube I), Olmsted, Peterborough, Philly, Riverdale-Bronx, Sabine, Santa Ana, Savannah, Seattle[1], Shepherds Bush[8], Sinai (Sealy, Hashiron), St. Mary's, Sydney, Tacoma[2], Tochigi[7], Torino[8], Wien, Zürich[8]
    - *b* Aggregating and interacting: Hemoglobins S[9], C, I[9], D_{Punjab}, C_{Harlem}[9]
- *B* Not accompanied by clinical or physiologic sequelae: Hemoglobins J, K, L, N, O, P, Q, and others

II Quantitative abnormality of globin peptide synthesis
- *A* Inherited
  - *1* α chain: α thalassemias (silent, mild, severe): Includes Hb Bart's hydrops fetalis syndrome, Hb H disease
  - *2* β chain: β thalassemias
    - *a* High $A_2\beta$ thalassemia (severe, mild, silent)
    - *b* δβ (F) thalassemia
    - *c* Other forms: A_2F thalassemia, etc.
    - *d* Hemoglobin Lepore syndromes
    - *e* Hereditary persistence of fetal hemoglobin
  - *3* δ chain: δ thalassemia
- *B* Acquired, in association with various hematologic disorders
  - *1* Fetal hemoglobin
  - *2* Hemoglobin H, Hb Bart's

Note: Some of the other names applied to the same amino acid substitution are given in parenthesis.
[1] Has decreased oxygen affinity and is unstable.
[2] Has both increased oxygen affinity and is unstable.
[3] Has both increased oxygen affinity and is unstable. Is composed of four normal β chains; α chains absent. Forms inclusion bodies in addition to Heinz bodies.
[4] Composed of four normal γ chains; α chains absent.
[5] Also a methemoglobin.
[6] Beta chain lacks a heme group, and five amino acids are deleted.
[7] Four amino acids are deleted.
[8] These hemoglobins are sensitive to sulfonamides.
[9] These hemoglobins "sickle."

globin levels are found to be reduced below those expected from the degree of hemolysis. If oxygen affinity is increased and the hemoglobin is stable, polycythemia results. When the molecule is unstable, the patient's hemoglobin concentration is higher than expected from the severity of the hemolytic process.

DECREASED OXYGEN AFFINITY A reduction in the percent saturation of hemoglobin occurring at various values for P_{O_2}, or decreased oxygen-binding capacity (diminished capacity of hemoglobin to reversibly combine with O_2 at any value of P_{O_2}), or both, result when certain amino acid substitutions occur (Table 307-2) in the α or β chain peptides about the critical regions of the crevice (E, F helices) where the heme prosthetic group is located (Table 307-1, *A, 1, a*). Affected individuals are *cyanotic*, but they generally are asymptomatic. Their hemoglobin has a *decreased oxygen saturation* at normal levels of arterial blood P_{O_2} if considered with reference to the total number of heme groups present per mole hemoglobin. Erythrocytosis is usually absent. Only heterozygotes have been discovered. It is thought that the homozygous condition would be lethal in utero for want of oxygen delivery to fetal tissues. Distinctive absorption spectra and characteristic electrophoretic mobility of the oxidized hemolysates allow the presumptive diagnosis of these hemoglobins. Other features of the syndrome and its differential diagnosis are described in Chap. 312.

Hemoglobin *Kansas* maintains all its iron atoms in the ferrous (Fe^{++}) state. It has a distinctive spectral absorption pattern and is chromatographically and electrophoretically distinguishable from normal Hb A even though it has a neutral amino acid substitution. In the "methemoglobin M" disorders, the iron atoms in the hemes of the abnormal chains are stable in the ferric (Fe^{+++}) state, and the affected half of the molecule is incapable of the normal reversible association with oxygen. In four types of methemoglobin M, the altered function of the hemoglobin is attributed to substitution of *tyrosine* for one of the *histidines* of the globin peptides. In Hb $M_{Milwaukee-1}$, the substitution is different but it also occurs in the E helix. The profound changes in the physiologic function of these hemoglobins are the result of a single amino acid substitution and in turn reflect single mutations in the triplet base codon of the gene. Thus, the amino acid substitution *His* → *Tyr* would be the result of the codon change CAC → UAC.

Search for these abnormal hemoglobins is important in the evaluation of cyanotic patients who have normal arterial blood P_{O_2}. Treatment is not ordinarily required. Measures designed to reverse methemoglobinemia of other causes would not be helpful here. As in other hemoglobinopathies, transfusions may be employed as a temporary measure in the face of acute complicating illnesses.

INCREASED OXYGEN AFFINITY The converse of the lesion just described results from other amino acid substitutions in the regions near the F and G helices. These abnormal hemoglobins fail to release oxygen in the normal manner despite the low oxygen tension in the tissue capillaries. Their oxygen dissociation curve is hyperbolic rather than sigmoidal.

Eight of the abnormal hemoglobins which are associated with increased oxygen affinity (Chesapeake, $J_{Capetown}$, Malmö, Yakima, Kempsey, Ypsilanti, Hiroshe, Brigham) involve the contact area between the α_1 and β_2 chains. It has been shown that normally on oxygenation the contact area at the $\alpha_1\beta_2$ interface shifts from one dovetailed position to another. It is postulated that the amino acid substitution interferes with this action. Four of the abnormal hemoglobins (Rainier, Bethesda, Hiroshima, Little Rock) involve the carboxy terminal. Interference with heme-heme interaction, or impairment of the binding of 2,3-DPG have been suggested as the functional alterations which lead to the development of erythrocytosis. Of the above abnormal hemoglobins, erythrocytosis has been observed in association with all but Hb $J_{Capetown}$.

It is likely that some of the individuals carrying these abnormal hemoglobins in the past have been considered to be examples of familial polycythemia or of benign erythrocytosis. White blood cell and platelet counts have been normal. Venesection is unnecessary and inadvisable. Most of these abnormal hemoglobins have been demonstrable by starch-gel electrophoresis.

UNSTABLE HEMOGLOBINS Readily susceptible to precipitation Certain amino acid substitutions, mainly in the β chain and sometimes involving the same sites as those already mentioned, produce unstable hemoglobins which are denatured prematurely in vivo or in vitro and result in *hemolytic disease, erythrocytic inclusion bodies*, and sometimes pigmenturia. In this group (Table 307-1, *1A, 2a*), hemolytic anemia may occur in heterozygotes even though less than half of the hemoglobin in each corpuscle is abnormal. In contrast, as described below, in conditions such as Hb S and Hb C, heterozygotes are usually asymptomatic, and only the homozygous state results in hemolytic anemia.

Many of the cases of hemolytic anemia with red cell inclusion bodies (Table 306-1) are included in this category. In some cases, Heinz bodies (Chap. 306) occur only after exposure to certain chemicals or after splenectomy; in others, they are found at all times. Some patients are free of anemia because the hemolytic disorder is fully compensated unless certain drugs are administered; others have a chronic hemolytic anemia.

Heterozygotes for Hb *Zürich* develop overt hemolysis, anemia, and Heinz bodies in their erythrocytes after administration of sulfonamides or primaquine and related oxyquinolones. This is also true of Hb Shepherds Bush and Hb Torino. In Hb Zürich, the same amino acid residue is affected as in methemoglobin $M_{Saskatoon}$ (β 63), but a different amino acid has been substituted (Table 307-2). Hb *Sydney* is another unstable hemoglobin associated with chronic hemolysis. The same residue that is abnormal in methemoglobin $M_{Milwaukee-1}$ is affected here (β 67) but, again, with a different substitution. Hb *Freiburg* has the properties of both an unstable hemoglobin and a methemoglobin: affected individuals are cyanotic and have hemolytic anemia. Hemoglobin *Gun Hill* is unique because five amino acids are deleted from the β chain and this peptide lacks heme groups—necessarily reducing its oxygen-carrying capacity. A compensated hemolytic anemia and splenomegaly have been described in these cases. Hb *Hammersmith* results in a severe chronic hemolytic anemia, and Hb *Köln* results in chronic hemolysis with anemia provoked by minor infections and thrombocytopenia may be present. These examples point out the value of examining for an abnormal hemoglobin by electrophoresis and testing for hemoglobin stability at 50 to 60°C when an otherwise unexplained hemolytic anemia is encountered. This is especially important if red cell inclusions are demonstrated or pigmenturia is present, or if the anemia appears to be drug-related and a red cell enzymopathy is not found. Treatment is not fully satisfactory, except in the case of Hb Zürich and Hb Shepherds Bush where, if the inciting drugs are not given, anemia may be avoided. In other diseases with chronic hemolysis, some benefit has resulted from splenectomy. Knowledge of the correct diagnosis avoids inappropriate treatment, such as corticosteroid hormones, which might be harmful and offer no potential benefit.

AGGREGATING AND INTERACTING HEMOGLOBINS Sickle hemoglobin (Hb S) was the first of the abnormal hemoglobins to be recognized. It was electrophoretically separated from Hb A, and was shown to be the product of a single, identifiable, amino acid substitution. The studies of Pauling, Itano, and later, Ingram opened a whole new field of investigation: that of molecular biology. Sickle hemoglobin gained its name from the sicklelike shape assumed by some of the red cells containing it when the oxygen tension was lowered (Fig. 307-2). The sickling phenomenon is explained by physical events in solutions of Hb S as the oxygen tension is reduced. At a concentration of approximately 20 g per 100 ml, molecular aggregation of Hb S occurs, as evidenced by increasing viscosity and gelling. At higher concentratures: birefringent tactoids with parallel alignment of long chains of the molecules. These tactoids are responsible for the peculiar shape of the sickled red cell. The phenomenon is reversible upon reoxygenation, but repeated cycles within the intact red corpuscle result in loss of some of the substance of the sickled cell and, eventually, hemolysis. At the molecular level, the tactoids are attributed to an interlocking between the α chains of one molecule and the abnormal β chains of the next. In Hb S, the substitution of the hydrophobic *valyl* for the hydrophilic *glutamyl* at β 6 allows that part of the β chain to stabilize in a ring formation through hydrophobic bonding between the normal N terminal valyl and the anomalous valyl at position number 6. The ring thus formed in the β chain fits into the complementary region in an α chain. Deoxygenation increases the distance between the β chains, and this is thought to facilitate the fit between the complementary sites of adjacent molecules; reoxygenation diminishes the distance between β chains and disrupts the interlock, dissolving the tactoid and reversing the sickling. Tactoid formation is also disrupted by cool-

FIGURE 307-2
A *Sickled red corpuscles from a patient with sickle-cell anemia (formalin-fixed after sickling, X 1050). (MM Wintrobe et al:* Clinical Hematology, *1967. 6th ed., Philadelphia: Lea & Febiger)*
B *Sickled erythrocyte, seen by the scanning electron microscope. (Courtesy of Dr. Fernando Padilla)*

A

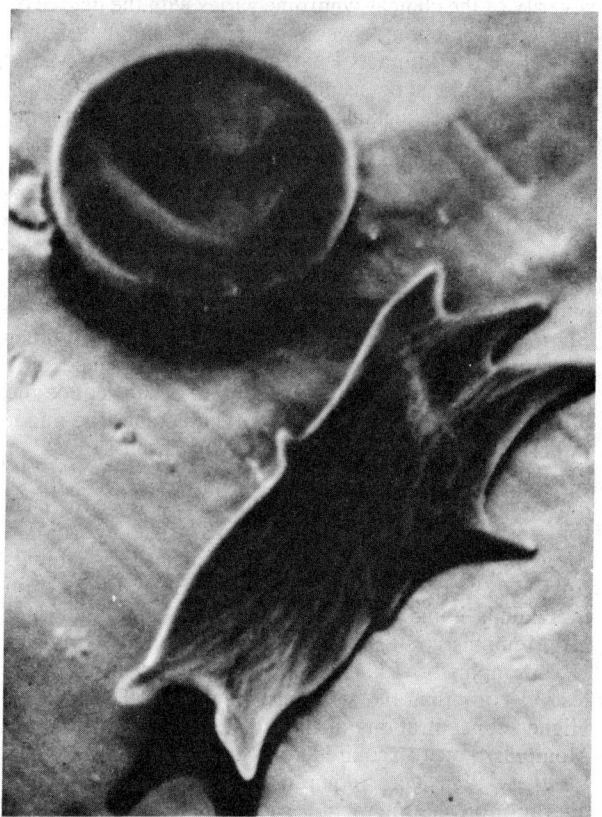

B

ing to low temperature, which decreases ring formation; the same effect results from reaction with propane gas, which forms stronger hydrophobic bonds with the critical valyls than the latter do to each other. These observations and the electron micrographs of "microtubules" formed by the longitudinal array of Hb S molecules support the hypothesis. Perutz and Lehman have proposed a different scheme for the linear aggregation of Hb S based on the presence of two valines in Hb S and two adjoining sites related by a symmetric axis in each molecule which permits a chain linkage to take place.

The extent to which sickling occurs depends upon the oxygen tension, the concentration of Hb S within the red corpuscle, the amount of Hb F, and the type and amount of any other hemoglobin present in the same cells which contain the Hb S. The proportion of Hb S in the blood of heterozygous individuals (sickle-cell trait) has been found to vary from 20 to 45 percent, whereas the amount in the blood of homozygotes (sickle-cell anemia) has ranged from 76 to 100 percent. These variations have been explained on the ground that the expression of the Hb S gene may be under the modifying influence of other genetic factors; the lower and higher proportions of Hb S are a familial characteristic. In the homozygous condition, the amount of sickling which occurs at moderate oxygen tensions and the associated clinical syndrome are far greater than in the case of the simple heterozygote. In the individual who is doubly heterozygous for two abnormal hemoglobins, the relation between the concentration of Hb S within the cell, oxygen tension, sickling, and the severity of the clinical syndrome varies with the degree of physical interaction between the hemoglobin types within the cell. Hb F interacts least, and patients heterozygous for both Hb S and persistence of fetal hemoglobin (high F gene) have less sickling and relatively few symptoms despite the high proportion (70 percent) of Hb S in their red corpuscles. The combination of Hb C and Hb S results in greater interaction than between Hb A and Hb S, and the syndrome associated with the former (*Hb SC disease*) is intermediate in severity between sickle trait (Hb AS) and sickle-cell anemia (Hb SS). Hb D_{Punjab} interacts most with Hb S, and its clinical syndrome (*Hb SD disease*) is also more severe than that of the other doubly heterozygous conditions. The coexistence of a gene for β thalassemia and one for Hb S can reduce the proportion of Hb A present so that it becomes the minor rather than the major component. The result is a higher concentration of Hb S within the red corpuscles and a more severe syndrome than would otherwise be the case for a simple heterozygote (Hb AS). The hybrid Hb *Memphis/S* is composed of the α chains of Hb Memphis ($\alpha_2^{23\ Glu \rightarrow Gln}\ \beta_2^{A}$) and the β chains of Hb S. Blood from individuals homozygous for Hb S but heterozygous for Hb Memphis contained 50 percent Hb S and 50 percent Hb Memphis/S. When deoxygenated, it was markedly less viscous than blood from patients with Hb S alone. Higher concentrations of the isolated, deoxygenated Hb Memphis/S were required for comparable increases in viscosity than were required for isolated Hb S. Thus, alteration in the interaction between the α and β chains seems to affect the sickling process. The clinical syndrome of patients with Hb Memphis/S is less severe than that of patients homozygous for Hb S without the additional abnormality. On the other hand, in a similar situation with simultaneous homozygosity for Hb S and heterozygosity for Hb $G_{Philadelphia}$, an α-chain variant, a moderately severe syndrome characteristic of sickle-cell anemia is found; 63 percent of the hemoglobin is Hb S and 36 percent is of a hybrid type—Hb $G_{Philadelphia}$/S ($\alpha_2^{68\ Asn \rightarrow Lys}\ \beta_2^{Glu \rightarrow Val}$).

An unusual variant of the Hb S structure is Hb C_{Harlem}. This hemoglobin was first identified by the letter "C" to indicate that it had the same electrophoretic mobility at pH 8.6 as did Hb C (and therefore probably two fewer negative charges at that pH than does Hb A). It has since been shown to have the same substitution at β 6 as does Hb S (accounting for one unit charge difference) and, in addition, it has a second amino acid substitution—being unique in this regard—further along the same β chain (Table 307-2). The first substitution accounts for the ability of this Hb C to sickle, while the second accounts for the additional charge difference and hence the "Hb C-like" mobility of this sickling hemoglobin. Compared with Hb S, the Hb C_{Harlem} requires a higher concentration for equivalent change in viscosity upon deoxygenation. The molecular basis for the aggregation of Hb I, which sickles erythrocytes exposed to 4% sodium metabisulfite, when it is present in 70% concentration, is not evident. The disorder is benign. In some individuals with only Hb C, crystallike structures may be seen within the red cells; these are more evident after mixing the blood with 3 percent sodium chloride. Intraerythrocytic crystals are prominent in individuals with both *hemoglobins S and C* coexisting in the same red corpuscles (*Hb SC disease*).

CLINICAL SYNDROMES

In most instances no illness is associated with the inheritance of an abnormal hemoglobin from only one parent. This applies to hemoglobins B_2, J, K, L, N, O, P, and Q, among others. Consequently, the *heterozygous* forms in many cases are of interest and value chiefly for genetic and anthropologic reasons. They can be recognized by simple paper electrophoresis or other similar techniques. The abnormal hemoglobins may manifest anodal mobility on electrophoresis at pH 8.6 which is slower or faster than that of Hb A. Some of these are represented in Fig. 307-3. Hemoglobins having the same electrophoretic mobility at pH 8.6 may actually have distinct primary structures. Thus there are four hemoglobins D, one due to an α-chain mutation and three resulting from β-chain mutations, named for 10 different geographic areas, and 10 hemoglobins G, four due to α-chain mutations and six to β-chain mutations, named for a total of 20 geographic areas.

Those abnormal hemoglobins with altered heme-oxygen reactivity and the readily precipitating (unstable) hemoglobins produce recognizable clinical syndromes even though they constituted less than half of the hemoglobin and the patients are only heterozygous for the abnormal gene.

Other abnormal hemoglobins which produce anemia and serious disease in patients who are homozygous for the responsible gene may be innocuous in the heterozygous state. *Hemoglobin C trait* and *sickle-cell trait* are examples. The phenotype *Hb AS* is rarely the cause of

TABLE 307-2
Characteristics of some hemoglobinopathies

Manifestations				*Hemoglobin*			
					Peptide chains[1]		
Condition	*Syndrome*	*Anemia*	*RBC morphology*	*Helix*	α	β	*Pathologic physiology*
Heterozygous							
Hb Yakima	Erythrocytosis	No	Normal	G1	Normal	99 Asp → His	
Hb Kempsey	Erythrocytosis	No	Normal	G1	Normal	99 Asp → Asn	Increased oxygen affinity
Hb Ypsi	Erythrocytosis	No	Normal	G1	Normal	99 Asp → Tyr	
Hb Chesapeake	Erythrocytosis	No	Normal	FG4	92 Arg → Leu	Normal	
Hb $J_{Capetown}$	None	No	Normal	FG4	92 Arg → Glu	Normal	
Hb Ranier	Erythrocytosis	No	Normal	HC3	Normal	145 Tyr → Cys	
Hb Hiroshima	Erythrocytosis	No	Normal	HC2	Normal	146 His → Asp	
Hb Kansas	Cyanosis	No	Normal	G4	Normal	102 Asn → Thr	Decreased oxygen affinity[3]
Hb M_{Boston}	Cyanosis	No	Normal	E7	58 His → Tyr	Normal	
Hb M_{Iwate}	Cyanosis	No	Normal	F8	87 His → Tyr	Normal	
Hb $M_{Saskatoon}$	Cyanosis	No	Normal	E7	Normal	63 His → Tyr	Methemoglobin
Hb $M_{Hyde\ Park}$	Cyanosis	No	Normal	F8	Normal	92 His → Tyr	Methemoglobin
Hb $M_{Milwaukee\text{-}1}$	Cyanosis	No	Normal	E11	Normal	67 Val → Glu	Methemoglobin
Hb Freiburg	Cyanosis	Hemolytic	Inclusion bodies	B5	Normal	12 Val → 0	Unstable Hb
Hb Zürich	Sensitive to sulfonamide	Hemolytic	Inclusion bodies	E7	Normal	63 His → Arg	Unstable Hb
Hb Köln	Chronic hemolysis	Severe	Inclusion bodies	FG5	Normal	98 Val → Met	Unstable Hb
Hb Genova	Chronic hemolysis	Severe	Inclusion bodies	B10	Normal	28 Leu → Pro	Unstable Hb
Hb Hammersmith	Chronic hemolysis	Severe	Inclusion bodies	CD1	Normal	42 Phe → Ser	Unstable Hb
Hb H		Mild	Inclusion bodies[5]		None	β_4 Tetramer	Unstable Hb[5]
Hb Gun Hill	Chronic hemolysis	No	Normochromic[6] inclusions[4]		Normal	91-97 → 0	β Chains lack heme[6]
Hb Santa Ana	Chronic hemolysis	Severe		F4	Normal	88 Leu → Pro	Unstable Hb
Hb Sydney	Chronic hemolysis	Slight	Normochromic inclusions[8]	E11	Normal	67 Val → Ala	Unstable Hb
Hb Sabine	Chronic hemolysis	Severe	Inclusions	F7	Normal	91 Leu → Pro	Unstable Hb[9]
Hb Bibba	Chronic hemolysis	Severe	Heinz bodies	H19	136 Leu → Pro	Normal	Unstable Hb[10]
Hb Sinai	Hemolysis, thrombocytopenia, splenomegaly	Variable	Normal	CD5	47 Asp → His	Normal	Unstable Hb[11]
Hb S	Asymptomatic	No		A3	Normal	6 Glu → Val	Sickles
Hb C	Asymptomatic	No	Target cells	A3	Normal	6 Glu → Lys	
Hb C_{Harlem}[7]	Asymptomatic	No	Occasional target cells		Normal	6 Glu → Val also 73 Asp → Asn	Sickles
Hb D_{Punjab}	Asymptomatic	No	Normal	GH4	Normal	121 Glu → Gln	
Hb I	Asymptomatic	No	Normal	A14	16 Lys → Glu	Normal	Sickles[12]
Doubly heterozygous							
Hb SC	Hemolysis, pain, infarction	Marked	Many target cells		Normal Normal	6 Glu → Val and[13] 6 Glu → Lys	Sickles
Hb SD	Hemolysis, pain, infarction	Marked	Target cells		Normal Normal	6 Glu → Val and[13] 121 Glu → Gln	Sickles
Hb Memphis/S	Hemolysis, pain, infarction	Marked	Target cells		23 Glu → Gln Normal	6 Glu → Val and[13] 6 Glu → Val	Sickles
Hb $G_{Philadelphia}$/S	Hemolysis, pain, infarction	Marked	Target cells		68 Asn → Lys Normal	6 Glu → Val and[13] 6 Glu → Val	Sickles
Hb S thalassemia	Chronic hemolysis	Severe	Target cells		Normal	6 Glu → Val	Sickles
Homozygous							
Hb SS	Hemolysis, pain, infarction	Marked	Target cells		Normal	6 Glu → Val	Sickles
Hb CC	Arthralgia, splenomegaly, hemolysis	Mild	Many target cells		Normal	6 Glu → Lys	Crystals[14]
Hb EE	Slight	Mild	Target cells; microcytosis		Normal	26 Glu → Lys	

[1] *The number and name of the replaced residue is followed (→) by its replacement. Abbreviations for amino acid residues:* Ala, *alanyl;* Arg, *arginyl;* Asn, *asparaginyl;* Asp, *aspartyl;* Gln, *glutaminyl;* Glu, *glutamyl;* Gly, *glycyl;* His, *histadyl;* Leu, *leucyl;* Lys, *lysyl;* Phe, *phenylalanyl;* Tyr, *tyrosyl;* Val, *valyl;* Met, *methionyl.*

[2] *Some cases of methemoglobinemia have been accompanied by mild erythrocytosis.*

[3] *Also, methemoglobinemia with decreased oxygen binding capacity.*

[4] *After incubation with brilliant cresyl blue.*

[5] *Also, high oxygen affinity.*

[6] *MCHC low because β chains lack heme; normochromic appearance on stained smear indicates normal concentration of protein component of hemoglobin in the red cells.*

[7] *Probably the same as Hb $C_{Georgetown}$.*

[8] *After 50°C or 48 hr at 37°C.*

[9] *Also deficient in heme groups.*

[10] *12% methemoglobin also present.*

[11] *Precipitated at 60°C.*

[12] *In 4% metabisulfite, rather than 2% as with Hb S.*

[13] *There are two types of abnormal hemoglobin molecules present in these conditions; single molecules do not contain two different kinds of β (or α) chains.*

[14] *Intraerythrocytic hemoglobin crystals have been seen.*

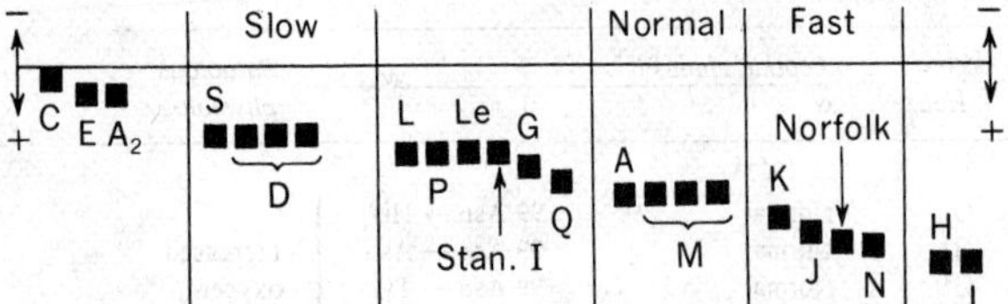

FIGURE 307-3
Relative mobilities of normal and abnormal hemoglobins on paper electrophoresis at pH 8.6. The mobility of hemoglobin M (Chap. 312) is similar to that of normal hemoglobin (hemoglobin A). Other hemoglobins can be classified as slow (e.g., hemoglobin S; this group includes the D hemoglobins and Stanleyville II), very slow (e.g., hemoglobin C; this group includes the normal hemoglobin A_2 as well as the abnormal hemoglobins E and O), or moderately slow [e.g., the G hemoglobins; this includes L, P, Q, Lepore(Le), and Stanleyville I]. In addition, there are fast hemoglobins with electrophoretic mobilities faster than that of hemoglobin A. These include H, I, J, K, N, Norfolk, and Hopkins-1 and Hopkins-2.

clinical problems. When a person with the sickle-cell trait is exposed to extremely low oxygen tension, as in high-altitude flying in unpressurized aircraft, or inadvertently under general anesthesia, intravascular sickling may occur in the spleen, cerebral vessels, or lungs, and thrombotic phenomena or infarction may result. Hyposthenuria and idiopathic hematuria, probably the result of hemorrhage from the renal papillae, have also been noted in *sickle-cell trait.* Though usually brief, the hematuria may last many weeks and may be recurrent often enough to result in a significant loss of iron. It must be differentiated from other, more serious causes of hematuria. Awareness of this complication may avoid premature surgical intervention for some patients.

The phenotype *Hb AC* is asymptomatic and free of anemia. Target cells are found on the blood smears. It occurs in about 2.5 percent of American Negroes. Its incidence is highest in the Gold Coast of Africa.

Hemoglobin E is frequent among the peoples of Southeast Asia (13 to 35 percent), and *Hb H* is frequent among the Chinese and also other racial groups. Hb H (β_4) is an unstable hemoglobin and has a high oxygen affinity (Table 307-2). Hb H is abnormal only in the sense that it is composed only of normal β chains and lacks α chains entirely. Patients with Hb H disease are thought to be doubly heterozygous for two types of α-thalassemia genes. One of these genes (alpha-1) severely, or moderately, depresses α-chain synthesis as in the usual α-thalassemia heterozygote; the other (alpha-2) may be so mild in its effect that when present alone, as in one of the patient's parents, its expression may escape detection. Less than half of the hemoglobin in affected red corpuscles is Hb H. There is slight or moderate hemolytic anemia with hypochromic red corpuscles, and the clinical manifestations suggest thalassemia. The spontaneous denaturation of Hb H within intact erythrocytes is accelerated in vitro by redox compounds, and spheric-inclusion bodies are formed, which stain with vital dyes. *Bart's hemoglobin,* a γ_4 tetramer, is the fetal hemoglobin analogue of Hb H. It occurs in the newborn affected with Hb H.

SICKLE-CELL ANEMIA, OTHER HOMOZYGOUS ABNORMAL HEMOGLOBIN STATES, AND COMBINATIONS THEREOF

DEFINITION Sickle-cell anemia is a chronic, hereditary, hemolytic disease which is due to the inheritance from each parent of a gene for Hb S. The red corpuscles lack Hb A; when they are deprived of oxygen, they assume sickle and other bizarre, but mainly crescentic, shapes.

PATHOGENESIS The sickled cell is a hemoglobin tactoid, thinly veiled and somewhat distorted by the cell membrane. In the homozygous individual the erythrocytes contain sufficient Hb S to sickle even when within the physiologic range of oxygen tensions. When sickled red corpuscles become trapped in the smaller vessels, erythrostasis occurs. Deoxygenation and reduced pH favor further sickling and further increase in blood viscosity. Plugs or masses of sickled erythrocytes become solid enough to occlude vessels, and thrombosis and infarction readily follow. A vicious cycle leading to more sickling develops. Among the clinical consequences are the painful "crises" which characterize this disorder, impaired circulation ultimately resulting in the formation of chronic leg ulcers, infarction, and later, marked shrinkage of the spleen (*autosplenectomy*), hepatomegaly, aseptic necrosis of bone, hematuria, priapism, pulmonary infarction, and central nervous system and other complications. The picture of shock may develop in patients with the abdominal crisis of sickle-cell anemia because capillary hypoxemia may result in plasma loss, hemoconcentration, and further stagnation. Shock may also be cardiogenic, and the clinical picture then resembles myocardial infarction or acute myocarditis. Bone pain may be due to distention of the intramedullary cavity by the vascular engorgement. In some cases there may be focal infarction of bone and of marrow. It is possible that the irregular sclerosis visible in roentgenograms of the long bones is due to healing of such infarcted areas with scarring and subsequent osteoid deposition. Other changes in the bones may perhaps be the result of marrow hyperplasia compensatory to the increased blood destruction.

After stasis, when red cells are released into free circulation, a certain proportion, having been fixed in irreversible sickled form, have also become more fragile in terms of mechanical trauma. Consequently, they are more than normally susceptible to destruction by the trauma associated with circulation. Even when sickling is reversed by reoxygenation, there may be loss of part of the filamentous portions of the cell substance as the cell resumes its discoid shape. This process also leads toward hemolysis.

CLINICAL MANIFESTATIONS This disorder is almost entirely confined to Negroes. The normal fetal hemoglobin which is present at birth lacks the abnormal β chain characteristic of Hb S. In infancy, as β chain synthesis replaces γ chain synthesis, Hb F is replaced by Hb S. The clinical manifestations develop as the proportion of Hb S within the red corpuscles rises. For reasons not fully understood, the time of onset of symptoms may vary widely. The course is that of a chronic, hemolytic anemia which is interrupted by periods of increased weakness, episodes of aching pain in the joints or elsewhere in the extremities, especially in the hands and feet (dactylitis), chest pain with accompanying electrocardiographic changes; or sudden attacks of severe abdominal pain which have often been mistaken for perforated peptic ulcer, intestinal obstruction, or some other abdominal emergency.

The victims of sickle-cell anemia may be poorly developed, and there may be some degree of retardation of secondary sex characteristics. There may be bony deformities of various types. The scleras are icteric. Short, dark-red, comma-shaped or corkscrewlike vascular segments, seemingly isolated from other vessels, may be seen if the lower bulbar conjunctivas are examined with the +40 diopter lens of the ophthalmoscope. These are found in most patients with sickle-cell anemia, rarely in patients with Hb SC disease, and not at all in individuals with the sickle trait or in normal persons. Tortuous, irregularly dilated vessels frequently can be seen in the ocular fundi. There may be slight general lymph node enlargement, but splenomegaly is rare in the adult. The heart may be enlarged, and the cardiac signs may closely simulate those of mitral stenosis or mitral regurgitation while the peripheral findings resemble those of aortic insufficiency.

Impaired ability to concentrate urine is common in both sickle-cell anemia and the sickle trait. Limitation in free water reabsorption has been ascribed to a failure to maintain a high solute concentration in the medullary interstitium. Indirect evidence attributes the latter to an increased renal medullary blood flow and to dilated and tortuous medullary blood vessels which distort spatial relations and thereby decrease the efficiency of the countercurrent exchange system. The low oxygen tension and hyperosmolality of the renal medulla, which could result in sickling of erythrocytes passing through that area, may also play a role. The relative importance of these explanations is unclear, for the sodium pump in the ascending loop is anaerobic and there is no direct measure of medullary blood flow.

In many instances chronic leg ulcers are found over the internal or external malleoli. Roentgenograms may reveal radial striation in the skull, osteoporosis in the vertebral bodies, or areas of increased density or of aseptic necrosis resulting from infarction.

The anemia is usually severe and may be normocytic or macrocytic. The volume of packed red corpuscles is commonly 20 ml per 100 ml or less. Oval, cigar-shaped, sickled, or other bizarre forms of red corpuscles may be seen in the stained blood smear. The sickling is brought out clearly in wet films of blood which are examined under a cover glass sealed with petrolatum. In patients with sickle-cell anemia the typical sickled and oat-shaped forms with elongated, pointed filaments appear within a few hours. When only the sickle-cell trait exists, 24 hr is often required to produce this change, and only a proportion of the cells, rather than practically all, are affected. If reducing agents, such as 2% sodium metabisulfite, are used, the characteristic forms appear promptly.

In sickle-cell anemia, reticulocytosis, polychromatophilia, normoblasts, leukocytosis with "shift to the left" in the myeloid series, and an increase in platelets are found on the blood smear. Hyperbilirubinemia and increased urobilinogen in the urine and stools also occur. Osmotic fragility is decreased. The bone marrow shows striking normoblastic hyperplasia. Occasionally, megaloblasts may be found. These are due to a superimposed deficiency of folic acid. The gap between the increased demands of the hyperplastic marrow and the relatively limited supply of that vitamin in the diet of the often impoverished Negro with sickle-cell anemia is increased by the custom of boiling "greens" for many hours, further lowering the folic acid content of the food.

Hyporegenerative crises with reticulocytopenia may develop, especially following infections, as in other hemolytic anemias (Chap. 306). Infections of the respiratory tract are frequent, as are osteomyelitis and bacteremia, particularly with *Salmonella.* Cerebral vascular accidents occur, and severe renal insufficiency is frequent in the third decade and later. Pregnancy is not associated with excessive hazard, but there is increased morbidity and fetal loss.

DIAGNOSIS Sickle-cell anemia is often mistaken for some other disease. Rheumatic fever, myocarditis, peptic ulcer, renal or biliary calculus, osteomyelitis, and various neurologic disorders may be simulated. Suspicion is raised by the finding of a hemolytic anemia and the demonstration of sickling. Ultimately, the diagnosis rests upon the finding of only Hb S in the patient's erythrocytes. The Hb SS phenotype is indistinguishable from Hb SD disease if the hemoglobin electrophoresis is carried out at only pH 8.6. It may also be simulated by the simultaneous presence of heterozygosity for Hb βS and also for β thalassemia. However, Hb SD may be distinguished from Hb SS by electrophoresis at pH 6.2, and both conditions may be identified by appropriate studies of family members. Hb D does not sickle red corpuscles. Performance of both the sickle test and Hb electrophoresis, on the parents of the patient, will permit the correct identification of the AS and AD phenotypes.

In distinguishing persons with the sickle-cell trait who may also have another disorder accompanied by anemia from those who have sickle-cell anemia, it must be kept in mind that individuals with sickle-cell trait may develop any type of anemia (e.g., iron deficiency anemia), while sickle-cell anemia is always hemolytic. The proportions of target cells present, the finding of intraerythrocytic crystals, or the demonstration of inclusion bodies in the red corpuscles gives clues concerning disorders resulting from combinations of the gene for Hb S with the genes for other abnormal hemoglobins or with the thalassemia gene. Study of the blood smears, electrophoresis of hemoglobin, and the alkali denaturation method for the demonstration of Hb F are simple and essential procedures which should be employed.

Homozygous *Hb C disease* is relatively rare. The hemolytic anemia is usually mild, and patients are rarely disabled. Mild icterus and moderate splenomegaly may be found. The blood contains as many as 80 percent *target cells.*

The *combination of hemoglobin C with S hemoglobin* is accompanied by sickling of the red corpuscles as well as by a hemolytic syndrome similar to sickle-cell anemia.

It differs in that the hemolytic anemia is milder, target cells are more plentiful in the blood, and there is slowly progressive splenomegaly. It is very probable that most of the cases formerly reported as forms of sickle-cell anemia intermediate between the asymptomatic carrier state and the homozygous classic disease actually were cases simultaneously heterozygous for S and C hemoglobin. The correct diagnosis may be made by electrophoresis of the patient's hemoglobin. Hb S and Hb C are found; Hb A is absent. In individuals with *Hb SC* disease, mortality in pregnancy has been relatively high as the result of hemorrhagic and thrombotic complications. Aseptic necrosis of bone, particularly of the head of the femur, is common.

Hemoglobin SD disease is another combination found in the United States. The manifestations are less severe than in most cases of sickle-cell anemia, but differentiation may be difficult unless electrophoretic and family studies are carried out. Cases have been reported in Caucasians who have no evidence of Negro lineage. This may have been the disorder in some of the cases previously considered to have been sickle-cell anemia in Caucasians. In addition to Hb S, one of the Hb D's is present in all the red corpuscles. Hb A is lacking because the gene to produce β^A chains has been replaced in both chromosomes. The volume of packed red corpuscles is often in the range of 20 to 30 ml per 100 ml blood, and reticulocytes number 10 to 40 percent. The spleen is not enlarged.

Hemoglobin E disease, the homozygous condition for Hb E, is characterized as a rule by mild microcytosis, normochromic anemia, and minimal signs of hemolytic anemia. Target cells are plentiful. The spleen is normal in size or only slightly enlarged.

TREATMENT AND PROGNOSIS Because these abnormal hemoglobin syndromes represent inherited anomalies, no treatment other than symptomatic therapy can be provided; no means has been devised whereby the abnormal state might be altered. A number of the conditions are asymptomatic. Sickle-cell anemia, however, is ultimately fatal, often before the age of thirty. Death may result from intercurrent infection, renal or cardiac failure, thrombosis or hemorrhage involving vital tissues, or it may follow one of the abdominal crises. Blood transfusions may be of value in abdominal crises with shock or in aplastic crises which accompany serious infections. In the interim between acute crises, the patient usually is adjusted to the chronic, severe, hemolytic anemia, and transfusions in that situation will only create the additional risks of homologous serum jaundice, transfusion reactions (Chap. 310) and, ultimately, hemosiderosis. Folic acid is useful only if megaloblastic transformation of the marrow has occurred (Chap. 306). Iron, vitamin B_{12}, and other antianemia agents are of no value. Splenectomy also has no place in therapy. In acute crises, it is important to maintain adequate hydration and electrolyte balance, correcting acidosis if it occurs. The claim that urea is helpful in the treatment of sickle-cell crises when given by either the oral or parenteral route has yet to be substantiated. When given intravenously in the doses advocated for the treatment of sickle-cell crises, it may cause a dangerous degree of dehydration. Pain may be relieved through anodynes. One should search for infections which would respond to antibiotic therapy. There are no "specific" agents to reverse sickling in vivo or infarction.

QUANTITATIVE ABNORMALITY IN GLOBIN PEPTIDE SYNTHESIS

Thalassemia and thalassemia syndromes

DEFINITION The term *thalassemia* refers to a group of genetically determined diseases which are caused by partial or complete interference in the synthesis of one of the normal hemoglobin peptide chains. They are characterized by the presence of unusually thin red corpuscles (leptocytes), microcytosis, hypochromia, various degrees of anemia, and, when the anemia is severe, numerous nucleated red corpuscles in the blood.

HISTORY Cooley and Lee (1925) described a chronic progressive anemia commencing early in life that was associated with a characteristic mongoloid facies, splenomegaly, and a familial and racial incidence (*Cooley's anemia*). Later it became clear that this severe and fatal disease was the *homozygous* form of a disorder which is also seen in milder form at all ages as the *heterozygous* state (*thalassemia minor*). In the *homozygous* condition (*thalassemia major; Cooley's anemia*), there is a drastic abnormality in the synthesis of normal hemoglobin. The conditions have also been known as *erythroblastic anemia* and *hereditary leptocytosis.*

Those first discovered to be affected were chiefly of Italian, Greek, Syrian, or Armenian parentage; that is, individuals whose ancestors lived in countries bordering the Mediterranean. In certain communities of Italians, the anomaly has been observed in as many as 20 percent of those examined. Once called *Mediterranean anemia*, this disorder is now known to occur throughout the world and in all racial groups. A high incidence occurs in Thailand and elsewhere in the Far East. The range of severity is now recognized to be much broader than defined by the two categories, thalassemia minor and thalassemia major. Furthermore, a number of distinct, though related, biochemical lesions have been described for the different types of the disorder.

TYPES OF THALASSEMIA AND PATHOGENESIS Although there is a disturbance in iron metabolism and heme synthesis in thalassemia, the primary defect is in the *rate of hemoglobin synthesis.* The selective deficiency in the rate of amino acid incorporation was first demonstrated in β chains during their synthesis on polyribosomes obtained from reticulocytes of patients with the common clinical forms of thalassemia major and minor. Synthesis of α, δ, and γ chains was not reduced. The gene products, the affected peptides, are *qualitatively normal* and therein are distinct from the hemoglobinopathies; they only are quantitatively deficient (Table 307-1).

When the genetic anomaly depresses only β chain synthesis, the disorder is termed β *thalassemia.* This type has been thought to comprise the majority of cases and is expressed in both heterozygous and homozygous forms. Corresponding lesions, selectively depressing synthesis of α chains or δ chains, result in α thalassemia and δ thalassemia, respectively.

In the most common form of β *thalassemia,* in *heterozygotes,* the production of δ chains is increased to 0.26 picogram (pg) from a normal of 0.18 pg of δ chains, per δ gene per red corpuscle. This, together with the reduced production of Hb A resulting from deficient synthesis of β chains, produces a characteristic *increase in the proportion of Hb* $A_2(\alpha_2\delta_2)$ (5.11 ± 1.36 percent, as compared with the normal of 2.54 ± 0.35 percent). For this reason, this form is also known as *A_2 thalassemia.* Hb F is usually normal or only slightly elevated. In the *homozygous* state, there may be nearly complete absence of Hb A, for want of β chains, and the hemoglobin which is present in the hypochromic red corpuscles is mainly Hb F. The Hb F is distributed in an irregular fashion, from cell to cell, in contrast to the situation in hereditary persistence of Hb F (see below), when its distribution is quite uniform. Hb A_2 is normal in most patients but is elevated in some.

Another type of β thalassemia, which is less common than the form of β thalassemia associated with high levels of Hb A_2, is termed $\delta\beta$ *(or F) thalassemia* because both δ and β chain syntheses are suppressed but α and δ chain syntheses are not; as a consequence Hb F concentrations are usually considerably elevated while Hb A_2 is not increased. There are also other, and rare, variants, such as *A_2F thalassemia,* so-named because there is a marked elevation of the Hb A_2 level (5.3 to 7.6 percent), and Hb F levels (5.1 to 14.4 percent) are also significantly increased.

Also included among the β thalassemias are two additional varieties of thalassemia-like syndromes, those associated with the *Lepore hemoglobins* and hereditary persistence of fetal hemoglobin. Lepore hemoglobin is the product of abnormal crossover and fusion of the δ and β genes (Fig. 62-15). It has an abnormal electrical mobility similar to that of Hb S. Hb A_2 is normal or decreased. In the homozygous state and in individuals doubly heterozygous for both Lepore hemoglobin and β thalassemias, the effect on hemoglobin synthesis and the clinical result are the same as in thalassemia major, or somewhat less severe. In these cases Hb F is the principal hemoglobin component, and Hb_{Lepore} makes up only a small proportion of the total pigment. Hb_{Lepore} seems to be inherited as a single gene, resulting in the synthesis of an abnormal hemoglobin and depression of normal β-chain synthesis. Several varieties of Hb_{Lepore} have been recognized, and the study of this abnormal hemoglobin has provided some important clues regarding the genetics of thalassemia.

Hereditary persistence of fetal hemoglobin is characterized by the persistence of elevated levels of Hb F into adult life and the absence of associated red cell changes.

Differing from the β thalassemias mentioned above and quite rare is δ *thalassemia,* characterized by the complete absence of Hb A_2. In contrast, α *thalassemia,* in which α chain synthesis is suppressed, affects a significant number of persons carrying the thalassemia trait, especially in Southeast Asia. Alpha chains are common to Hbs A, A_2, and F; consequently, synthesis of all these hemoglobins is affected. Hb A_2 and F levels are not increased, and suspicion that one is dealing with α thalassemia may arise only because of the presence of very mild thalassemic red cell changes and some decrease in red cell fragility.

Alpha thalassemia is most easily diagnosed in newborn infants because the decrease or absence of α chains results in the formation of *Bart's hemoglobin* (γ_4). The homozygous form of α thalassemia results in intrauterine fetal death, with severe hydrops fetalis. Complete absence of α chains has been demonstrated in such cases; essentially only γ_4 tetramers were present as the hemoglobin. Hemoglobin H is a tetramer of β chains (β_4). *Hemoglobin H disease* is thought to be the result of interaction of at least two α thalassemia genes, one of these being so mild in heterozygotes as to be completely "silent" clinically, or to be caused by the inheritance of the mild α thalassemia gene from each parent.

The thalassemia disorders are the result of autosomal gene mutations. These are not strictly dominant or recessive, for in some heterozygotes there are clinical manifestations, whereas in others there are none. It seems that there are "mild" and even "silent" genes as well as clearly expressed ones. Many theories have been proposed concerning the genetic basis of thalassemia. Best supported is the view that in β thalassemia there is defective transcription of messenger RNA, perhaps because of a reduced amount of β-mRNA, with reduced β-chain synthesis resulting. Possibilities which have not been entirely excluded include deletion of the β gene in that form of β thalassemia in which no β chains are synthesized, mutations resulting in the formation of codons which dictate chain termination, or the development of a mutation which would call for a different or less available transfer RNA to read a given codon. The genetic mechanism of α thalassemia is even more uncertain.

In δ thalassemia no red cell changes are seen, presumably because this is a minor hemoglobin. Also in hereditary persistence of fetal hemoglobin few or no clinical manifestations occur. On the other hand, in other forms of thalassemia there is accelerated intramarrow destruction of erythroid cells, and the life span of the erythrocytes in the blood is shortened. In β thalassemia, free α chains accumulate, and these free chains are thought to exert deleterious effects on the red cell membrane and its permeability. These changes are associated with shortened red cell survival. Why defective peptide chain synthesis results in leptocytes and target cells, rather than simple microcytosis and hypochromia, is not understood.

The excessive destruction of red cells stimulates erythropoiesis, and this causes pronounced medullary and extramedullary hyperplasia. Since these effects are produced in the earliest period of life when growth is taking place, the diploë of the bones expands. Simultaneously iron-containing pigment derived from the breakdown of red cells is deposited in the enlarged spleen, liver, pancreas, and other tissues.

CLINICAL SYNDROMES The clinical manifestations of thalassemia as now defined range from none whatsoever to the very serious disorder described by Cooley, or the severe hydrops fetalis and intrauterine death of the homozygous form of α thalassemia. Silent, mild, and severe forms of β and α thalassemia have been described, and the following descriptions fit only the majority of cases and describe the classic ones.

Thalassemia major Homozygous β thalassemia major develops insidiously within the first year or two of life, perhaps starting at birth. There is marked pallor and great enlargement of the spleen and even of the liver. The child often has a mongoloid appearance. Roentgenograms reveal great thickening of the diploë of the skull, with perpendicular striation, increase in the medullary portion of the long bones and thinning of the cortex, and other changes attributable to the extreme hyperplasia of the bone marrow. Anemia is severe, hypochromic, and microcytic; the red corpuscles are very thin and contain very little hemoglobin pigment. The peculiar distribution of hemoglobin in the cells gives them the "bull's-eye" appearance of targets. Hence the name *target-cell anemia.* The red corpuscles are unusually resistant to hemolysis in hypotonic saline solutions. Normoblasts in the circulation, as well as polychromatophilia, basophilic stippling, Howell-Jolly bodies, and moderate reticulocytosis (19,000 to 25,000 per μl) with a "shift to the left," reflect the myeloid hyperactivity of the bone marrow. There is usually slight or moderate hyperbilirubinemia, with a corresponding increase in the urobilinogen content of the urine and stool. Serum iron levels are high. Hemoglobin F values may be elevated, even to a level of 90 percent or more. The concentration of hemoglobin A_2, relative to the total hemoglobin pigment, is within normal limits.

Thalassemia minor Thalassemia minor is usually asymptomatic and may pass entirely unnoticed; painstaking examination may be necessary to reveal any abnormality. Slight anemia or splenic enlargement, microcytosis and hypochromia, target cells, poikilocytosis out of proportion to the existent anemia, basophilic stippling of the red corpuscles, decreased fragility in hypotonic saline, and hyperbilirubinemia are some of the signs which, singly or in various combinations, mark this disorder. In other patients, pallor, fatigue, or routine examination of the blood, as during pregnancy, may lead to the discovery of moderate anemia. The volume of packed red corpuscles may be 30 to 35 ml per 100 ml in women and 35 to 40 ml per 100 ml in men. Serum iron levels are normal. In a number of patients, a history may be obtained of protracted, ineffectual treatment with iron, even parenteral iron, because the hypochromic appearance of the red corpuscles has suggested iron deficiency. Roentgenographic changes in the bones similar to those found in thalassemia major, though less pronounced, may be observed.

This description, however, applies only to the most commonly recognized condition which results from the inheritance of the β thalassemia gene from one parent. The heterozygous form of β thalassemia is now thought to occur in at least three genetic forms. In the *silent* form there are no clinical or hematologic abnormalities. The silent form is detected only when it occurs in combination with another thalassemia gene or by sensitive radioactive labeling techniques. In the *mild* and the *severe* forms of β thalassemia, hematologic manifestations such as those described above are discoverable, but these two forms are distinguishable from one another mainly when they are associated with a β chain hemoglobinopathy, such as Hb S. Then, in the mild form, some Hb A can be found, whereas in the severe form no Hb A can be demonstrated.

Terms such as *thalassemia intermedia* and *thalassemia minima* have been used, and even additional clinical subdivisions have been proposed, but the last are not very useful. *Thalassemia minima* refers to instances in which clinical manifestations are very slight. *Thalassemia intermedia* refers to cases in which the clinical manifestations are more severe than in thalassemia minor, yet less serious than in thalassemia major. The term has been applied to less serious forms of homozygous disease or, more often, to cases of double heterozygosity for two different types of retardation of β-chain synthesis, such as heterozygosity for β and δβ thalassemia, β thalassemia and a structural hemoglobin variant, or β thalassemia and Hb_{Lepore}.

Microdrepanocytic disease is the name given to the simultaneous heterozygosity for sickle-cell and thalassemia genes which results in a chronic hemolytic anemia with some of the characteristics of both sickle-cell disease and thalassemia. It is more commonly called *sickle-thalassemia disease.*

DIAGNOSIS The morphologic features of the red corpuscles are most important. The finding of hypochromic red corpuscles and only a slight reduction of the mean corpuscular hemoglobin concentration (MCHC), together with a greater reduction in the mean corpuscular volume (MCV) than would be estimated by judging from the corpuscular diameters on the blood smear, should suggest the possibility of leptocytosis and, hence, *thalassemia minor.* The other characteristic morphologic features were mentioned above. The serum iron and marrow iron stores are normal or increased, and the total serum iron-binding capacity is normal. These are important points in differentiating this condition from iron deficiency anemia. If the Hb A_2 concentration is increased, as determined by electrophoresis on starch block or starch gel or, less commonly, by chromatography on ion exchange cellulose, there is strong evidence to support the diagnosis of β thalassemia. If the Hb A_2 is not increased, one may be dealing with α, δ, or (δβ) thalassemia, or a nonthalassemic disorder. Examination of family members often resolves uncertain cases by demonstrating the hereditary nature of the disorder.

Inclusion bodies are seen characteristically in Hb H disease and can also be demonstrated in β thalassemia when the excess of α chains results in their precipitation. They may be seen by phase contrast microscopy or after methyl violet vital staining of red corpuscles or normoblasts.

The various forms of congenital hemolytic anemia, as well as plumbism, pyridoxine-responsive anemia, and various acquired forms of "refractory" anemia, must be distinguished from thalassemia. The hemoglobinopathies which may be associated with thalassemia, and the Lepore hemoglobin which may mimic thalassemia, are inherited independently of one another. These may be distinguished from "pure" thalassemia by hemoglobin electrophoresis. The Hb F content should be measured by the alkali denaturation technique or electrophoresis on agar gel. Thalassemia minor and minima have occasionally been confused with polycythemia vera because the erythrocyte count may be greater than normal. However, in thalassemia the hemoglobin concentration and volume of packed red cells are usually slightly below the average normal values because the red corpuscles are microcytic and hypochromic. In polycythemia, if the red corpuscles are hypochromic, the serum iron would be low rather than normal or high as is the case of thalassemia.

The *homozygous* forms of thalassemia rarely present a problem in diagnosis because the physical signs and the blood examination are usually quite characteristic. Both parents of the affected child usually show clear evidence of β thalassemia minor if that is the nature of the abnormality. However, as mentioned earlier, it may be difficult or impossible to diagnose the α thalassemia heterozygote.

PROGNOSIS This depends on the nature and severity of the inherited disorder. Classic Cooley's anemia was usually fatal, and those affected often did not reach adulthood. With present-day management the outlook is better. The prognosis is more grave the earlier the disease becomes manifest. Less severe forms are compatible with longer life. The heterozygous form may have no influence whatever on life span.

TREATMENT This is the most common form of hypochromic microcytic anemia in man which does not respond to iron therapy. In fact, iron stores are often excessive and severe hemosiderosis may develop, especially if blood transfusions are given repeatedly. Treatment with iron, either by the oral or parenteral route, is contraindicated unless iron deficiency, the result of a separate disease process, is specifically shown to be present (see Chap. 304). Multiagent "anti-anemia preparations," even those sold as "ethical drugs" and available only by prescription, are of no value. In rare instances, when megaloblastic changes occur in the bone marrow as a result of relative folic acid deficiency, 0.1 to 1 mg folic acid orally, daily, for 1 month, will overcome that component of the anemia and replenish the liver stores of the vitamin. Repeated transfusions have been advocated in thalassemia major in amounts to maintain the hemoglobin at about 10 g with the hope of minimizing bone changes and improving the patient's health and activity. Transfusions, however, must be repeated, often at intervals of 3 to 4 weeks, and consequently represent an enormous burden on the patient and the family and subject the patient to many risks, especially hepatitis and iron overload. While the use of iron-chelating agents counteracts the latter to some degree, the risks remain great. Which is the best choice, "hypertransfusion" as this form of therapy has been called, less frequent transfusions, or none at all, must be decided according to many individual factors. Considered from the standpoint of the patient's comfort and convenience as measured in years as such a treatment program must be, unless the anemia is very severe (< 6 g per 100 ml), it is better in many instances to permit him to adjust to the chronic state of anemia which is his lot without encumberment with constant medical attention. It is remarkable how the human organism can adjust itself to handicaps when there is a need. Splenectomy is of no value except where the spleen is cumbersome because of its size or when a superimposed acquired hemolytic anemia develops as the result of repeated transfusions.

REFERENCES

CARRELL RW, LEHMANN H: The unstable haemoglobin haemolytic anaemias. Semin Hematol 6:116, 1969

COMINGS DE: The hemoglobinopathies and thalassemias, in *Genetic Disorders in Man*, ed RM Goodman, Boston: Little, Brown, 1969

FINK HAROLD (ed): Second conference on the problems of Cooley's anemia. Ann NY Acad Sci 165:1, 1969

JAFFÉ ER: Hereditary hemolytic disorders and enzymatic deficiencies of human erythrocytes. Blood 35:116, 1970

MORIMOTO H, LEHMANN H: Molecular pathology of human haemoglobin: Stereochemical interpretation of abnormal oxygen affinities. Nature 232:408, 1971

STAMATOYANNOPOULOS G et al: A study of 31 families with simple heterozygotes and combinations of F-thalassemia with A_2 thalassemia. Am J Med 47:194, 1969

—— et al: Abnormal hemoglobins with high and low oxygen affinity. Annu Rev Med 1971, p. 221

WEATHERALL DJ, CLEGG JB: *The Thalassemia Syndromes*, 2d ed., Oxford: Blackwell, 1972

WINTROBE MM et al: *Clinical Hematology*, 7th ed., Philadelphia: Lea & Febiger, 1974

ZUCKERKANDL E: The evolution of hemaglobin. Sci Am 212:110, 1965

308 ANEMIA ASSOCIATED WITH CHRONIC SYSTEMIC DISEASE

G. R. LEE
M. M. WINTROBE

Anemia is found commonly in association with a wide variety of chronic diseases. These include long-standing infections; noninfectious inflammatory diseases, such as rheumatoid arthritis; malignancies; renal insufficiency; hepatic disease; and certain endocrine-deficiency states. The anemias of infection, rheumatoid arthritis, and cancer appear to be related in that they are accompanied by a characteristic disturbance of iron metabolism manifested by hypoferremia and reticuloendothelial siderosis.

In this chapter, the use of the term *anemia of chronic disorders* will be confined to those situations in which this disturbance of iron metabolism occurs regularly. While it is recognized that this terminology is not entirely satisfactory, as yet no alternative has found general acceptance. The anemias of renal insufficiency, hepatic disease, and endocrine deficiency are not characteristically accompanied by hypoferremia. The anemia of renal disease will be discussed below. The anemias of hepatic disease and endocrine deficiency were considered in Chap. 58.

ANEMIA OF CHRONIC DISORDERS **Clinical description** Anemia associated with hypoferremia and reticuloendothelial siderosis has been found in almost any inflammatory illness which lasts several months or longer. Examples are subacute bacterial endocarditis, tuberculosis, empyema, chronic fungal infections, lung abscess, pyelonephritis, rheumatoid arthritis, rheumatic fever, and other collagen diseases. This type of anemia may also occur in malignant disorders, including Hodgkin's disease, leukemia, and carcinoma of the lung, but it must be distinguished from the "myelophthisic" type of anemia that occurs with extensive bone marrow invasion (see below).

In most clinical circumstances, the anemia of chronic disorders becomes established during the first 2 months of illness and thereafter does not progress unless the underlying disease becomes worse. The anemia tends to be mild to moderate in severity; rarely is the blood hemoglobin concentration found to be less than 9 g per 100 ml. There is a rough correlation between the degree of anemia and the severity of the underlying disease. For example, in one study of patients with rheumatoid arthritis the mean blood hemoglobin concentration was 13.2 g per 100 ml in females with "slightly active" disease and 11.3 and 9.6 g per 100 ml in males and females, respectively, with "very active" disease. This moderate degree of slowly developing anemia rarely produces significant symptoms.

The erythrocytes are usually normocytic and normochromic; occasionally they are hypochromic, and only rarely are they both hypochromic and microcytic. In other respects, the red cells are morphologically normal, with little variation in size and shape and with no polychromatophilia or stippling.

Kinetic studies indicate that the anemia results from an inability of the bone marrow to compensate for a mild to moderate decrease in erythrocyte life span. These kinetic alterations are subtle, and significant deviations from normal in the reticulocyte count, serum bilirubin, or stool or urine urobilinogen are uncommon.

When studies of iron metabolism are performed, the serum iron is found to be reduced and the total serum iron-binding capacity is normal or reduced. Reticuloendothelial iron stores are increased and sideroblast iron is decreased. The free erythrocyte protoporphyrin is increased.

Pathogenesis Cross-transfusion studies indicate that the shortened erythrocyte life span is due to an extracorpuscular mechanism rather than to a defect in the red cell itself. The nature of the extracorpuscular disturbance is unknown, but it may be related to a nonspecific increase in the phagocytic activity of the reticuloendothelial system. In view of the fact that the cellularity of the bone marrow is normal or increased and that it can respond to erythropoietin, the failure of the bone marrow to increase red cell production to a level sufficient to compensate for the shortened red cell life span is puzzling. The erythropoietin-secreting mechanism is intact, and yet the amount of erythropoietin produced is not as great as would normally be expected for the given degree of anemia. It is therefore postulated that chronic systemic disease in some manner induces an alteration in the mechanisms controlling erythropoietin production which causes the erythropoietic "thermostat" to be set at a somewhat reduced level.

The designation *thesauric hypoferremic anemia* epitomizes the paradoxic association of hypoferremia with increased iron stores, phenomena which suggest that a barrier exists to the normal flow of iron from reticuloendothelial cells to plasma. Studies of hemoglobin or red cell iron "reutilization" with labeled iron have supported this suggestion. Neither the nature of the barrier nor the way in which it is produced is known.

Treatment Therapeutic measures should be directed at the underlying chronic illness. The anemia will subside spontaneously if such measures are successful. None of the usual forms of antianemia therapy, such as vitamin B_{12} or iron, is effective. Cobalt chloride has been shown to stimulate red cell production in this type of anemia and to cause the volume of packed cells to increase. However, cobalt therapy is not recommended, since no particular benefits accrue to the patient from the increased number of red cells, and also because the gastrointestinal toxicity of cobalt may be significant. Sometimes, if anemia becomes severe (hemoglobin less than 7 g per 100 ml), blood transfusions may be necessary, but these should be used sparingly.

ANEMIA IN MALIGNANT DISEASE Malignant disease is not necessarily accompanied by anemia. When it is, a number of etiologic factors must be considered. In carcinoma involving the gastrointestinal tract, *blood loss* is the most common cause of anemia. Depending on the amount lost and the duration of the process, the anemia may be that of acute blood loss (Chap. 303) or of iron deficiency (Chap. 304). In other malignancies, including the lymphomas, leukemias, and metastatic carcinomas, the *anemia of chronic disorders* (see above) may be observed.

Carcinoma of the kidney, breast, prostate, thyroid, and lungs, in particular, Hodgkin's disease rarely, and other lymphomas may invade the bone marrow, and in such an event, *myelophthisic anemia* may develop. This type of anemia usually is accompanied by alterations in leukocytes and platelets. Thus, there may be pancytopenia (Chap. 309), or a leukemoid picture, marked by leukocytosis and myeloid immaturity, may result. Sometimes these changes are accompanied by the appearance of nucleated red cells in the circulation; the term *leukoerythroblastic anemia* appropriately describes such an association. Morphologic alterations in the erythrocytes may be extreme, and wide variations in shape and size are common; teardrop-shaped erythrocytes are particularly characteristic of marrow invasion. In addition, polychromatophilia, coarse stippling, and a modest reticulocytosis may be observed. The last is thought to result from the premature release of reticulocytes from marrow (*"shift" reticulocytosis)* rather than from an increase in production of red cells.

Therapeutic measures should be directed at the underlying disease. When palliative therapy with radiation or chemotherapeutic agents is effective, partial relief of the anemia may be observed. On the other hand, adverse effects of such therapy may lead to an increase in the degree of anemia. Thus, serial determinations of the volume of packed red cells, in conjunction with other hematologic measures and evidence of tumor activity, serve as useful guides to management.

ANEMIA OF RENAL INSUFFICIENCY Anemia is as typical of the uremic state as azotemia. The nature of the underlying renal disease has little influence on the development of anemia, except that its degree may be less in patients whose kidneys fail as the result of polycystic disease than in those with other types of renal disease. The patient's presenting complaints in some cases are those due to anemia rather than renal disease. There is a crude correlation between the degree of anemia and the degree of renal insufficiency as estimated by the magnitude of the azotemia or the impairment in glomerular filtration rate. Ultimately the hematocrit level in most patients stabilizes between 15 and 30 ml per 100 ml and thereafter does not progress unless complications occur.

Like the anemia of chronic disorders, the anemia of renal insufficiency is characterized kinetically by a shortened red cell survival and a subnormal marrow response. Two kinetic patterns have been described that differ from one another according to which of these abnormalities predominates. The more common pattern is that found in the *hypoproliferative anemia* of renal disease in which reduced red cell production predominates. The less common *hemolytic anemia* of renal disease is more severe and is characterized by a markedly shortened red cell life span.

The hypoproliferative anemia of renal disease is classified morphologically as normocytic and normochromic. The production defect is attributable to impairment of the erythropoietin-producing function of the kidney. Morphologic changes in erythrocytes on blood smear are minor, at most only crenated ("burr") cells being seen. The reticulocyte count is normal. On the other hand, in the hemolytic anemia of renal disease there may be macrocytosis, reticulocytosis, polychromatophilia, stippling, anisocytosis, poikilocytosis, and normoblasts in the peripheral blood. Burr cells should be distinguished from schistocytes, the distorted or fragmented red cells with peripheral sharp projections characteristically found in association with disease of the small blood vessels *(microangiopathic hemolytic anemia)* and in thrombotic thrombocytopenic purpura (Chap. 313). In addition to microangiopathy, shortened red cell survival in such cases may result from toxic impairment of the erythrocyte membrane cation transport as well as of the red cell phosphogluconate oxidative pathway (Chap. 306).

As in the anemia of chronic disorders, cobalt administration may induce reticulocytosis, but the disadvantages of such therapy outweigh the benefits. Therapy should be directed at the underlying renal disease, and in those few situations in which adequate renal function can be reestablished the anemia will be relieved. In patients treated with long-term dialysis there may be a modest decrease of anemia, making it possible to avoid blood transfusions. In those in whom the renal transplant has been successful, the hematologic response may be dramatic. Normal and even supranormal values may be achieved if the response is not delayed by the immunosuppressive measures that are employed.

REFERENCES

ADAMSON JW et al: The kidney and erythropoiesis. Am J Med 44:725, 1968

BRAIN MC: The hemolytic-uremic syndrome. Semin Hematol 6:162, 1969

CARTWRIGHT GE, LEE GR: The anemia of chronic disorders. Semin Hematol 3:351, 1966; Br J Haematol 21:147, 1971

ERSLEV AJ: Anemia of chronic renal disease. Arch Intern Med 126:774, 1970

WEST CD et al: Myelophthisic anemia in cancer of the breast. Am J Med 18:923, 1955

309 BONE MARROW FAILURE

M. M. WINTROBE
T. C. BITHELL

Some degree of bone marrow insufficiency or failure is present in many varieties of anemia, not only in those which result from infection and chronic systemic disease (Chap. 308) or disseminated cancer, but also in those which are associated with deficiency of essential substance (vitamin B_{12}, folic acid) (Chaps. 304 and 305), abnormalities of heme or globin synthesis (the sideroblastic anemias, Chap. 304, the hemoglobinopathies, Chap. 307), and even accelerated destruction of erythrocytes (the hemolytic disorders, Chap. 306). However, the term is generally used more specifically to refer to those disorders, to be discussed in this chapter (Table 309-1), in which marrow failure is the primary pathogenetic feature and is not the result of the aforementioned processes. In these disorders, the marrow is unable to produce sufficient cells to replace those normally utilized, and usually there is a reduction in the number of erythrocytes, platelets, and leukocytes (*pancytopenia*). In most cases, the precursor cells in the marrow also are reduced in number (*marrow hypoplasia* or *aplasia*), fat having replaced the blood-forming tissue. However, the morphologic appearance of the marrow may not correlate well with its functional capacity, and pancytopenia may sometimes be associated with a normally cellular or even a hypercellular marrow. For such cases, the term *refractory anemia* is more appropriate than *aplastic anemia.* The last is best used in the traditional sense as applying to disorders characterized by hypoplastic bone marrow and pancytopenia. The term *pure red cell aplasia* refers to cases in which only the red corpuscles and their precursors are affected, the white cells, platelets, and their marrow precursors being normal.

APLASTIC ANEMIA Etiology and pathogenesis In approximately half of the cases of aplastic anemia, no etiologic agent is apparent. Such "idiopathic cases" are most common in adolescents or young adults, and their pathogenesis is obscure. The rare Fanconi syndrome appears in young children and is associated with chromosomal aberrations, being inherited as an autosomal recessive trait in many cases.

Another large category comprises cases associated with exposure to various *chemical agents* or to *ionizing irradiation.* These agents may be divided into two groups (Table 309-1): (1) Those which regularly produce marrow hypoplasia or aplasia if a sufficient dose is given (*the myelosuppressive agents*), and (2) those which are only occasionally associated with such a change, i.e., which presumably depend on *idiosyncracy.* Agents in the first category have been or are used in the chemotherapy of leukemia, the lymphomas, and other tumors. Aplasia or hypoplasia of the marrow represents a predictable pharmacologic effect which generally depends on the dose of such agents administered. However, the bone marrow findings and the extent to which the three blood elements are affected vary considerably, and the pancytopenia and acellular marrow of classic aplastic anemia in some instances may be only the ultimate result of a series of stepwise changes. Benzene, for example, not only may produce aplastic anemia but also can be associated with a "regenerative" blood picture including even a leukemoid reaction, and the bone marrow may be hyperplastic rather than acellular. Likewise, internal irradiation produced by the ingestion of radium by radium-dial painters was associated with macrocytic anemia, nucleated red cells in the peripheral blood, and marrow hyperplasia. Both irradiation and benzene may produce chromosomal abnormalities, and both have been implicated in the production of leukemia.

Even less clearly understood are cases of aplastic anemia which are associated with the administration of usually innocuous drugs. The evidence that these drugs are etiologic is only circumstantial, since aplastic anemia has been observed only in a small proportion of those exposed, e.g., 1 of 25,000 individuals given quinacrin (Atabrine). However, in the case of those drugs with definite toxic potentiality (Table 309-1), a sufficient number of cases has been reported to make it seem very likely that the development of aplastic anemia was caused by exposure to the drug. Of particular note is *chloramphenicol.* Although the incidence of aplastic anemia in association with this antibiotic is very low in terms of its widespread use, this drug has so frequently been associated with this dyscrasia that there is little doubt of its etiologic role. Aplastic anemia associated with those drugs listed as probably toxic is even less common. However, even the most widely used and innocuous of drugs, such as aspirin, or streptomycin and tripelennamine, may be associated with serious bone marrow failure in rare susceptible individuals.

The mechanism by which these drugs produce aplastic anemia is obscure. Marrow aplasia is unrelated to a pharmacologic effect of the drug and is usually not dose-related, often developing after prolonged or intermittent administration of small doses and even long after the drug has been stopped. Reticulocytopenia, vacuolization of bone marrow normoblasts, and mild pancytopenia have been demonstrated in many patients receiving chloramphenicol. However, aplastic anemia has not developed in such individuals, and these findings may represent reversible suppression of bone marrow function unrelated to the pathogenesis of aplastic anemia. Most of the evidence favors the hypothesis that drug-induced aplastic anemia represents an idiosyncratic reaction in susceptible individuals, but attempts to demonstrate hypersensitivity in the sense of an antigen-antibody reaction have not been successful. It has been suggested that this idiosyncracy may reside in an intrinsic, possibly hereditary abnormality in the precursor cells of the marrow, such as an enzyme deficiency, analogous to that which conditions certain drug-induced hemolytic anemias (Chap. 306). As yet there is little experimental evidence to support this concept.

In most cases, *pure red cell aplasia* appears to be idiopathic. A congenital form has been described in infants (the *Blackfan-Diamond syndrome*), and drugs such as chloramphenicol and diphenylhydantoin may produce a similar picture. Erythroid hypoplasia also may develop transiently during the course of various infections and hemolytic disorders (*aregenerative "crisis," acute erythroblastopenia*) and for a longer time in association with benign thymoma. There is indirect evidence to

TABLE 309-1
Aplastic or hypoplastic anemias: Disorders characterized by primary bone marrow failure

I Aplastic anemia
- *A* "Idiopathic"
- *B* Fanconi syndrome, pancreatic deficiency syndrome in children
- *C* In association with chemical or physical agents
  - *1* Agents which predictably produce marrow hypoplasia
    - *a* Ionizing irradiation (x-rays, radioactive isotopes)
    - *b* Benzene and derivatives (TNT)
    - *c* Cytostatic agents (alkylating and antimitotic agents, antimetabolites)
    - *d* Other toxic agents (inorganic arsenic, estrogens)
  - *2* Drugs which occasionally produce marrow hypoplasia as an idiosyncratic effect
    - *a* Of "definite" toxic potentiality; chloramphenicol, phenylbutazone, mephenytoin (Mesantoin), gold compounds, quinacrin (Atabrine), organic arsenicals, potassium perchlorate
    - *b* Of "probable" toxic potentiality; trimethadione, tolbutamide, carbutamide, diphenylhydantoin (Dilantin), sulfamethoxypyridizine (Kynex), acetazolamide (Diamox), sulfisoxazole (Gantrisin), insecticides [Parathion chlordane, chlorphenothane (DDT)]
- *D* Miscellaneous: with viral infections, Simmonds' disease, etc.

II "Pure" red cell hypoplasia
- *A* "Idiopathic"
- *B* Congenital (the Blackfan-Diamond syndrome)
- *C* In association with tumors of the thymus
- *D* Drugs
- *E* Transient "aregenerative crises" in infections and hemolytic disorders

suggest that pure red cell aplasia is the result of an autoimmune process in some cases, but in the majority the pathogenesis is obscure.

Clinical manifestations As a rule, the onset of aplastic anemia is insidious. The symptoms are attributable to anemia, or the effects of thrombocytopenia or of neutropenia may dominate the clinical picture. Progressive weakness, fatigability, and a "waxy" pallor are commonly seen. Mild purpura is usually the first bleeding manifestation and frequently is an early sign, but hemorrhage from the nose, gums, vagina, gastrointestinal tract, or into the retina may occur. Infection is common later in the course of the disorder. Indolent ulcerations in the mouth or pharynx, around the nose, rectum, or vagina are common, as are recurrent systemic infections.

Patients with aplastic anemia may carry on without serious trouble for months with very low leukocyte and platelet counts, but complications eventually develop, and in some cases serious bleeding or fulminant infection may appear suddenly, e.g., subarachnoid hemorrhage or septicemia. Such complications may suggest an explosive onset of the disease. Weight loss is unusual, and there is no sternal tenderness, hepatomegaly, or splenomegaly. Fever and lymphadenopathy, if present, are usually the result of infection.

After many transfusions, hemosiderosis (Chap. 310) develops, and then the spleen may become just palpable and the liver moderately enlarged. Bronzing of the skin may produce a misleading "healthy" picture, but examination of the nail beds and mucous membranes will reveal the true picture.

Fanconi's syndrome usually develops in the first decade of life, but in contrast to congenital pure red cell aplasia, is uncommon in neonates. This disorder is associated with a variety of congenital defects (bone abnormalities, particularly of the forearms and thumbs, microcephaly, hypogenitalism, genitourinary tract abnormalities) and a generalized olive-brown pigmentation of the skin.

Laboratory diagnosis The *peripheral blood* usually reveals pancytopenia with absolute neutropenia, the majority of the leukocytes being normal lymphocytes. The anemia usually is normocytic, sometimes macrocytic; the red cells vary little in size and shape, and polychromatophilia, basophilic stippling, and other evidences of accelerated red cell production are absent. The reticulocyte count is very low or zero. In pure red cell aplasia, however, these signs of red cell production sometimes may be seen.

Bone marrow examination is essential and can be done safely in spite of the thrombocytopenia and neutropenia if careful aseptic technique is used and if gentle pressure is maintained over the puncture site. In classic aplastic anemia, the marrow aspirate is composed mainly of erythrocytes and lymphocytes. In cases in which the marrow is only hypoplastic, various abnormalities have been described, including the presence of erythroid precursors and a picture suggesting "arrest of maturation" of the granulocyte precursors. Stainable iron is abundant, but "ringed" sideroblasts are not seen.

A dry tap should not lead to the assumption that the marrow is aplastic. Puncture at another site may yield marrow, and it is well to obtain an adequate specimen by means of biopsy with the Jensen or other appropriate needle.

Tests of *blood coagulation* usually are normal, but the bleeding time is prolonged, the tourniquet test positive, and clot retraction impaired as a result of thrombocytopenia. Although moderate shortening of the red cell life span may be demonstrated by *isotopic techniques*, this is of little significance, and other evidence of accelerated red cell destruction, such as indirect bilirubinemia or elevated fecal urobilinogen, is lacking. Ferrokinetic studies will reveal slow plasma iron turnover and poor tracer iron utilization for hemoglobin synthesis, but such measurements may be difficult to interpret and are not needed to establish a diagnosis. The *serum iron* usually is elevated, and the total *iron binding capacity* is moderately reduced. The *fetal hemoglobin* may be elevated.

Differential diagnosis The diagnosis of aplastic anemia should be one of exclusion, for pancytopenia alone is not indicative of bone marrow failure. The causes of pancytopenia are many (Table 309-2), and appropriate steps must be taken to rule them out. Early acute myeloblastic leukemia (Chap. 316), disseminated tuberculosis (Chap. 156), and paroxysmal nocturnal hemoglobinuria (PNH) (Chap. 306), in particular, may simulate bone marrow failure, and the last may actually represent a stage of or be a sequel to aplastic anemia. The presence of nucleated red cells or polychromatophilia in the blood smear, immature leukocytes, or large morphologically abnormal platelets suggest "myeloproliferative" or myelophthisic disease (Chap. 308) rather than aplastic anemia.

TABLE 309-2
Causes of pancytopenia

I The hypoplastic or aplastic anemias (Table 309-1)
II "Aleukemic," leukopenic, or subleukemic leukemia (Chap. 316)
III Myelophthisic "anemias" (Chap. 308)
- *A* Metastatic carcinoma in bone marrow
- *B* Multiple myeloma, other dysproteinemias (Chap. 65)
- *C* Myelofibrosis
- *D* Osteopetrosis (Marble bone disease)

IV Disorders involving the spleen—"hypersplenism"
- *A* Lymphomas (Chap. 318)
- *B* Congestive splenomegaly (Chap. 317)
- *C* Infiltrative (Gaucher's disease, Niemann-Pick disease, Letterer-Siwe disease, Chap. 317)
- *D* Infections (kala azar, military tuberculosis, syphilis)
- *E* Of unknown etiology [Sarcoidosis (Chap. 223), "primary" hypersplenism (Chap. 317)]

V Disorders due to deficiency of essential substances (pernicious anemia and other megaloblastic macrocytic anemias, Chap. 305)
VI Paroxysmal nocturnal hemoglobinuria (rarely) (Chap. 306)
VII Miscellaneous conditions (rarely): disseminated lupus erythematosus, sarcoid, some refractory anemias, etc.

SOURCE: *Adapted from MM Wintrobe et al,* Clinical Hematology, *7th ed., Philadelphia: Lea & Febiger, 1974*

The presence of splenomegaly, sternal tenderness, hyperglobulinemia, or lymphadenopathy should arouse suspicion that one is not dealing with aplastic anemia. In multiple myeloma and the other dysproteinemias, metastatic carcinoma, Gaucher's disease, and acute leukemia, the diagnosis may often be made by a careful examination of the bone marrow. If an enlarged lymph node is accessible, it may be advisable to examine it microscopically. Numerous other studies may be required in the search for the underlying disorder, e.g., roentgenograms of the bones and chest, serum protein electrophoresis, and PNH test.

The diagnosis of idiopathic aplastic anemia requires that exposure to chemicals be excluded. This is difficult, because of the prevalence of potentially toxic substances in the environment, and the physician must maintain an unusually high "index of suspicion" regarding chemical exposure, e.g., benzene in industry; solvents, insecticides, and hair dyes in the home; and various medications, including presumed innocuous drugs.

When there is pure red cell aplasia, one must avoid overlooking a causative chronic infection, systemic disease, or drug. Thymomas are rare, usually asymptomatic, and may be demonstrable radiologically. In some cases of the Blackfan-Diamond syndrome, splenic and hepatic enlargement and even generalized lymphadenopathy have been described.

Treatment The mainstays in the treatment of aplastic anemia are good general supportive care, the judicious use of transfusions, steroid therapy, and in certain circumstances, splenectomy.

Supportive care is aimed at the removal of possible etiologic factors and the prevention and treatment of the complications of pancytopenia. Exposure to potentially toxic agents should be absolutely eliminated, even if the evidence is only circumstantial, which is usually the case. Antibiotics should not be used prophylactically when there is neutropenia, since this will favor the emergence of resistant bacteria and fungi and more will be lost than gained. It is better to be alert to the development of an infection and to identify the causative organisms, thus permitting specific therapy. Intramuscular and subcutaneous injections should be avoided if possible, and when performed, should be carried out with careful antisepsis. Mouth hygiene is very important, and wounds and abrasions of the mucous membranes and skin should be guarded against. "Reverse isolation" should be employed when patients with severe neutropenia are hospitalized.

Blood transfusions should be held to a minimum, since they may be required for many years. Hemosiderosis will develop ultimately, and sensitization to minor blood groups, leukocytes, and platelets may occur. These patients tolerate hemoglobin levels of 9 g per 100 ml and even lower levels quite satisfactorily. Blood selected for transfusion should be as type-specific and as fresh as possible. Platelet concentrates are valuable in the treatment of life-threatening hemorrhage.

Among the numerous agents which have been used to stimulate marrow function, only adrenocorticosteroids and androgenic hormones deserve mention. Hematinics such as vitamin B_{12}, folic acid, iron, and crude liver extract are valueless in the treatment of aplastic anemia. Cobalt is usually ineffective, and bone marrow transplantation still is in the experimental stage. Success has been reported in cases in which an identical twin was available as a donor. Anabolic steroids (methyltestosterone, testosterone proprionate, oxymetholone), 1 to 2 mg per kg per day, may be given orally and are preferred to parenteral preparations. Moderate relief of anemia and sometimes considerable improvement have been observed in about 50 percent of patients, but the response is slow and treatment must be continued for months. Neutrophils reappear less often and still more slowly, and platelets may increase little or not at all. Adrenal corticosteroids are less useful than the anabolic steroids but occasionally seem to have been helpful. In children, however, they may help to counteract androgen-induced bone maturation. Corticosteroids have been most helpful in the Fanconi syndrome and in congenital red cell aplasia, but treatment usually must be maintained indefinitely.

Splenectomy may be of significant benefit in a few carefully selected patients with aplastic anemia. These include patients in whom there is evidence of accelerated destruction of red cells by the spleen, decreased survival of ^{51}Cr-labeled erythrocytes with splenic "sequestration" of labeled cells, patients with unusually high transfusion requirements, and those with long-standing aplastic anemia and evidence of some persisting marrow function. Splenectomy is seldom of value in the Fanconi syndrome or in congenital red cell aplasia and is rarely curative in the other forms, but it may decrease transfusion requirements, and may reduce the dose of anabolic steroids or corticosteroids required to maintain the patient. In red cell aplasia associated with thymomas, removal of the tumor is indicated but is without effect in many cases.

Prognosis Death usually results from infection or hemorrhage. Spontaneous remission may occur in about 20 percent of patients with congenital red cell aplasia and in a few cases due to toxic agents where the cause has been recognized and further exposure eliminated. About 50 percent of patients live a year or more, and approximately 40 percent live 3 years or more.

REFERENCES

Bithell TC, Wintrobe MM: Drug-induced aplastic anemia. Semin Hematol 194, 1967

Diamond LK, Shahidi NT: Treatment of aplastic anemia in children. Semin Hematol 278, 1967

Scott JL et al: Acquired aplastic anemia: An analysis of thirty-nine cases and review of the pertinent literature. Medicine, 38:119, 1959

Wintrobe MM et al: *Clinical Hematology*, 7th ed., Philadelphia: Lea & Febiger, 1974

310 BLOOD GROUPS AND BLOOD TRANSFUSION

J. FOERSTER
M. M. WINTROBE

BLOOD GROUPS

Blood groups represent systems of antigenic determinants found on the surface of red cells. These antigens are inherited according to simple mendelian laws, and the major systems (for example, ABO and Rh-Hr) are inherited independently of each other.

Blood groups are most readily identified by means of specific antibodies occurring in serum, either "naturally" or after immunization with foreign red cells or soluble blood group substances. Unfortunately, the chemical characterization of blood group antigens has lagged far behind serologic and genetic studies and so far only the ABO, Lewis, and, to a lesser extent, the Ii and MN systems have lent themselves to extensive biochemical analysis. The study of the ABO and Lewis systems has been greatly facilitated by the discovery that the antigens in question occur not only as surface components of cells, but are also found in water-soluble form in the tissue fluids and secretions of most people.

ABO AND LEWIS SYSTEMS The *A and B antigens* are inherited as simple mendelian characters, the blood group of an individual depending on the presence of one or both of two allelic genes (A and B) or their absence (O). The possible genotypic and corresponding phenotypic combinations are listed in Table 310-1. Antibodies reacting with A or B antigens are regularly found in the serum when the corresponding antigen is absent from the red cells. These antibodies were originally thought to occur "naturally" but are now known to arise early in life as a result of exposure to ABO-like polysaccharides occurring ubiquitously in food and other exogenous sources.

In addition to antibodies against A and B antigens, reagents are known which react preferentially with O cells. The antigen defined by these reagents is known as *H-substance*, and its synthesis is under the control of an allelic pair of genes, Hh, which is inherited independently of the ABO system. Indeed, since there is no true O antigen, group O individuals are most correctly identified as group H individuals, and the group O designation is retained solely for historical reasons.

The *H* gene in single or double dose gives rise to the H character, and the rare h allele, when present in double dose, results in its absence. The H-active material is a precursor substance which, under the influence of A and B genes, is converted into A- and B-active substances, respectively, thereby accounting for the presence of large quantities of H-substance in O individuals. It also follows that the rare hh individuals, who are said to have the *Bombay phenotype*, lack A, B, or H antigen on their erythrocytes and in their secretions (Table 310-2). Nevertheless they appear to have normal A and B genes which can be expressed in the next generation if the children acquire an H gene from the other parent.

Approximately 80 percent of Northern Europeans with A, B, or H antigen on their red cells also have the corresponding antigen in various tissue fluids and secretions. While the A, B, and H antigens on red cells are predominantly glycolipids (see below), their soluble counterparts in secretions are glycoproteins. The capacity to secrete these substances is under the control of a pair of allelic genes, Sese. Se is considered dominant over se, and only homozygous sese individuals are therefore "nonsecretors" of A-, B-, or H-substance.

TABLE 310-1
ABO blood groups

Phenotype (group)	*Genotype*	*Antigens on red cells*	*Antibodies in serum*
O	*OO*	None	Anti-A Anti-B
A	*AA* *AO*	A	Anti-B
B	*BB* *BO*	B	Anti-A
AB	*AB*	A and B	None

SOURCE: *MM Wintrobe et al,* Clinical Hematology, *7th ed, Philadelphia: Lea & Febiger, 1974*

The Lewis system is closely related to the ABO system, although the two allelic genes, Le and le, which define this system, are inherited independently of the ABO, Hh, and Sese genes. In single or double dose Le gives rise to Le^a specific structures; le in double dose results in their absence. Le^b specificity, once thought to arise from the activity of an allele of the Le gene, is now considered to be an interaction product between the *H* and *Le* genes. Thus three Lewis phenotypes are possible which are designated Le (a+b−) or Le^a, Le (a−b−), and Le (a−b+) or Le^b.

The Le^a and Le^b antigens, unlike their ABH counterparts, are not integral parts of the red cell membrane, but are acquired from the plasma. Since the secretion of Le^a substance is *not* under the control of the *Sese* gene, nonsecretors have Le^a antigens on their red cells and in their secretions as long as the *Le* gene is present. However, since the secretion of *H* gene products is under the control of the *Sese* genes, the Le^b antigen, which is an interaction product between the *H* gene *and* the *Le* gene, is found only in the secretions and on the red cells of secretors (Table 310-2).

The *chemical composition of secreted ABH and Lewis substances* is remarkably similar. They are composed of a carbohydrate moiety which constitutes about 85 percent of the molecule and an amino acid moiety which makes up the remaining 15 percent. They are heterodisperse, with an average molecular weight of 300,000, but the molecules of different sizes have similar composition and molecular properties. The peptide residues are always composed of the same 15 amino acids, and 4 of these, threonine, serine, proline, and alanine, make up two-thirds of all the amino acids present. The peptides appear to have structural functions only and are thought to form a firm, spiny backbone to which a large number of relatively short oligosaccharide chains, constituting the

TABLE 310-2
Relation between genotype, erythrocyte phenotype, and antigenic specificities detectable in secretions

Probable gene combination	Antigens detectable on red cells: ABH	Le^a	Le^b	Specificities detectable in secretions: ABH	Le^a	Le^b
1 ABO, H, Se, Le	+++	−	++	+++	+	++
2 ABO, H, sese, Le	+++	+++	−	−	+++	−
3 ABO, H, Se, lele	+++	−	−	+++	−	−
4 ABO, H, sese, lele	+++	−	−	−	−	−
*5** ABO, hh, Le (se or sese)	−	+++	−	−	+++	−
*6** ABO, hh, lele (Se or sese)	−	−	−	−	−	−

** Groups 5 and 6 correspond to very rare individuals of the Bombay phenotype (B1) who lack ABH antigens on their red cells and secretions.*

blood group substances, are attached at intervals. The carbohydrate moiety of all the ABH and Lewis substances is qualitatively similar in composition. Each contains a methylpentose, L-fucose; a hexose, D-galactose; two amino sugars, *N*-acetyl-D-glucosamine and *N*-acetyl-D-galactosamine; and a 9-carbon sugar, *N*-acetylneuraminic acid. One of these sugars appears to be immunodominant in each of the blood group substances studied.

Cellular blood group substances are much more difficult to isolate, but both A- and B-active materials have been obtained in water-soluble form. In contrast to the blood group substances found in secretions, most of the cell-derived extracts are glycolipids, although some glycoprotein residues have been found as well. Nevertheless it appears that the oligosaccharide chains which confer blood group specificity on the glycolipid blood group substances of red cells as well as the glycoprotein substances found in secretions are identical, thereby accounting for the similarities in the specificity of antigenic determinants on red cells and in secretions.

The complicated interrelation between A, B, H, and Lewis substances was clarified considerably when it was recognized that the gene systems controlling these four expressions appear to act sequentially on a common glycoprotein precursor substance. Genetic control presumably comes about through the formation of specific glycosyl transferase enzymes or through some mechanism controlling their function. A simplified version of such a proposed scheme is illustrated in Fig. 310-1.

Two precursor chains are recognized on the basis of a 1→3 (type 1) or 1→4 (type 2) linkage of the terminal galactosyl unit to the subterminal *N*-acetylglucosamine residue. The latter precursor chain has cross-reactivity with antiserums to type XIV pneumococcal polysaccharide.

The transferase controlled by the *H* gene is thought to add L-fucose in α-linkage to the carbon 2 position of either chain to form an H-active structure. The enzyme controlled by the *Le* gene, also a fucosyl transferase, adds L-fucose in α-linkage to the 4 position of the subterminal *N*-acetylglucosamine unit in chains of type I only, as chains of type 2 already are substituted at this position. The resultant structure has Le^a specificity. Nevertheless a type 2 oligosaccharide containing fucose linked to C-3 of *N*-acetylglucosamine may also have very weak Le^a activity. When both *H* and *Le* genes are present, two fucosyl units are added to adjacent sugars on chains of type 1, resulting in a structure which, on the basis of inhibition experiments, is thought to be that of the Le^b determinant. Type 2 difucosyl chains have weak Le^b activity.

The presence of the fucosyl unit conferring H specificity to the precursor substance is considered to be essential for the functioning of the transferases controlled by the *A* and *B* genes. Thus *N*-acetyl-D-galactosamine added in α-linkage to carbon 3 of the terminal galactosyl unit confers A specificity to the H-active precursor substance, whereas addition of D-galactose in identical linkage results in B specificity. The addition of these terminal nonreducing sugars effectively masks the serologic reactivity of the H-active groupings, and the Le^a active determinants are similarly masked by the substitutions controlled by the H gene. It would appear, however, that Le^b-substance does not serve as substrate for the *A* and *B* genes, since it is usually found in good concentration on the red cells and in the secretions of A, B, and AB subjects.

Among individuals who possess the *A antigen, two main subclasses* have been identified. Subgroup A_1 includes about 80 percent of Europeans whereas the remainder belong to subgroup A_2. Similarly, 80 percent of AB samples are A_1B, whereas 20 percent are A_2B. A_1 and A_1B individuals do not form anti-A_2 antibodies, but a small proportion of A_2 individuals (1 percent) and a larger proportion of A_2B individuals (25 percent) form anti-A_1 antibodies.

The basis for the difference between A_1 and A_2 specificity has been in dispute from the moment of its discovery. One view holds that the A_1 and A_2 antigenic determinants are chemically identical, but that A_1 individuals simply have many more determinants on their red cells than do A_2 individuals. The other view contends that there is a qualitative difference between the antigenic determinants of A_1 and A_2 individuals, and it has been suggested on the basis of immunochemical studies that A_2 substances lack type 1 A determinants (see Fig. 310-1), whereas A_1 substances contain both type 1 and type 2 A determinants. This would also account for the observed higher H and Le^b activity in A_2 substances, since the addition of the terminal sugar conferring A reactivity ordinarily masks the H or Le^b active determinants on the precursor chain. Definite proof of molecular differences between A_1 and A_2 determinants will have to await the isolation and structural analysis of A_2 substances.

Numerous variants of A_2 have been described which can be characterized by a variety of serologic techniques. A_3, for instance, is thought to be a "weaker" form of A_2, and even "weaker" forms (A_x, A_4, A_5, A_o, A_m) have been reported. These variants are very rare, but may on occasion cause difficulty during typing or cross-matching procedures. The structural basis for these lesser variants, if indeed this is the cause of their poor performance as A antigens, is completely unknown.

THE Ii SYSTEM The red cells of almost all healthy adults carry an antigen I and smaller amounts of a related antigen, i. Very rare individuals, perhaps 1 in 10,000, have little or no I antigen, and have anti-I in their serum. All newborns appear to have the phenotype i since they react strongly with anti-i and weakly with anti-I. During the first 18 months of life the cells gradually change to the I phenotype, and in healthy individuals this reaction pattern appears to be retained throughout life.

In patients with a variety of hematologic disorders, i activity of the red cells may increase again, usually without a demonstrable decrease in I activity. This is particularly true in situations of marrow stress, such as occur in thalassemia major or chronic hemolytic anemia, but it may also be seen in hypoplastic anemia and leukemia. In the last instance the i reactivity of red cells may disappear when the patient goes into remission.

A relation between the ABO and Ii systems has been suspected for many years because the red cells of some Oi individuals were found to react very weakly with anti-H serums and because cells of the Bombay phenotype (see above) usually give a higher score with anti-I than do ordinary OI cells. Immunochemical studies suggest that I specificity appears at intermediate stages in the biosynthesis of A, B, H, Le^a, and Le^b substances and that the enzyme produced by the *I* gene acts on a common precursor just prior to the steps controlled by the *A*, *B*, *H*, and *Le^a* genes.

THE Rh SYSTEM In 1939 Levine and Stetson reported that the mother of a stillborn baby had a severe hemolytic reaction to her husband's blood and her serum agglutinated not only her husband's red cells but also those of 80 out of 104 ABO-compatible individuals. They correctly suggested that the mother had become sensitized to a "new" antigen, which she lacked herself, but which her stillborn baby had inherited from the father. One year later Landsteiner and Wiener made the discovery that the serums of rabbits and guinea pigs immunized with the red cells of rhesus monkeys agglutinated not only the donor erythrocytes, but also those of most Caucasian New Yorkers. Individuals whose red cells were agglutinated by these serums were termed *Rh-positive*, the others, *Rh-negative*. It was subsequently discovered that heterologous antirhesus antibodies do not actually react with red cell antigens presently known to be part of the Rh system, but rather with another antigen, now called LW, which is shared by rhesus and human cells. The original observation did, however, stimulate immediate inquiry into the nature of unexplained intragroup transfusion reactions, and the incompatibilities between mother and child which cause erythroblastosis fetalis (Chap. 306). It was soon discovered that most of these reactions could be accounted for by antibodies resembling those described by Landsteiner and Wiener.

From this modest but auspicious beginning has evolved the most complex of human blood group systems, currently characterized by over 30 antigens and antibodies and an almost unlimited number of apparently complex alleles. Unfortunately much confusion has

FIGURE 310-1
Proposed composite structure of A, B, H, Le^a, and Le^b specific blood group substances linked to serine or threonine spines of the polypeptide backbone. Gal refers to galactose; Fuc to fucose; GNAc to N-acetylglucosamine; GalNAc to N-acetylgalactosamine. The numeric notations (e.g., 1→4) refer to the respective carbon positions at which linkage occurs. The precursor substance is identified by bold type; the determinants characteristic of a given blood group substance are in light type and are identified by their appropriate symbols, namely A, B, H, Le^a, and Le^b. The structure shown is a composite which includes all determinants. In individual blood group substances certain residues will be missing; e.g., H, Le^a, and Le^b specific blood group substances lack A and B specific determinants, and Le^a substance also lacks the H specific determinant. See text and references for details. (After KO Lloyd et al, Biochemistry 7:2976, 1968)

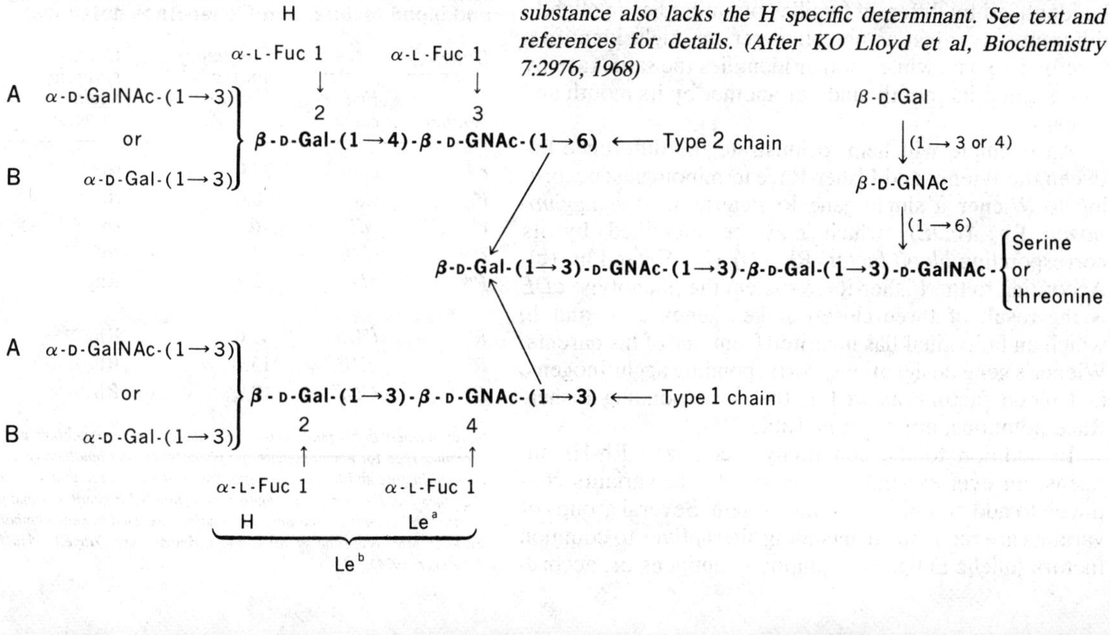

H
α-L-Fuc 1 ↓ 2
α-L-Fuc 1 ↓ 3
A α-D-GalNAc-(1→3) or B α-D-Gal-(1→3) } **β-D-Gal-(1→4)-β-D-GNAc-(1→6)** ⟵ Type 2 chain

β-D-Gal
↓ (1→3 or 4)
β-D-GNAc
↓ (1→6)
β-D-Gal-(1→3)-D-GNAc-(1→3)-β-D-Gal-(1→3)-D-GalNAc- { Serine or threonine

A α-D-GalNAc-(1→3) or B α-D-Gal-(1→3) } **β-D-Gal-(1→3)-β-D-GNAc-(1→3)** ⟵ Type 1 chain
2 ↑ α-L-Fuc 1 (H)
4 ↑ α-L-Fuc 1 (Le^a)
Le^b

arisen over nomenclature and genetic mechanisms, and in the ensuing battle between opposing camps, acrimony and dogma have frequently replaced sweetness and light. It is hoped that biochemical characterization of antigenic structures will eventually resolve all outstanding issues.

Two systems of nomenclature are still in common use, and therefore both need to be considered. According to Fisher the inheritance of Rh antigens is determined by three pairs of closely linked allelic genes, *Cc*, *Dd*, and *Ee*. Each parent contributes three genes, *C* or *c*, *D* or *d*, *E* or *e*, each defining a single antigen. Since every person carries a chromosome from each parent, various combinations of genotypes are found. A person might therefore inherit CDe from one partner and cde from another (*CDe/cde*); or he may be *CDe/CDe*, *cde/cde*, *cDe/cde*, or *CDe/cDe*, to mention only the most common types. So far the postulated anti-d has not been found.

Fisher's theory also assumes that crossover of linked genes can take place, thereby accounting for the maintenance of the rarer combinations by occasional crossing over from common heterozygotes. Some workers doubt that this occurs. Moreover, intermediate forms and other variants are being discovered which do not fit neatly into Fisher's scheme.

The second system of nomenclature is that of Wiener, which is based on a different genetic theory. According to Wiener, the inheritance of Rh antigens is determined by a series of allelic genes at one locus. Thus, according to Wiener, the inheritance of Rh antigens is determined by a single gene, rather than three separable ones, as had been postulated by Fisher. This assertion may well be correct.

In order to understand Wiener's nomenclature, two terms need to be explained. The term *agglutinogen* is used to describe the whole antigen complex determined by a given gene. Unfortunately its structure and physicochemical properties are not yet known, but it can nevertheless be identified by its *blood factors*, the serologic specificities defined by antibodies directed against various facets of its structure. According to Wiener, the terms *blood factors* and *antigenic determinant* are *not* synonymous, since the same antigenic determinants may be identified by different families of antibodies in slightly different ways, just as one blind person might identify a face by its nose, while another identifies the same face by its nose and its mouth, and yet another by its mouth and its ears.

An example will help to illustrate the difference between the Wiener and Fisher-Race terminologies: according to Wiener a single gene R^2 determines the *agglutinogen* Rh_2 (*cDE*), which may be identified by its corresponding *blood factors* Rh_0 (*D*), rh″ (*E*), and hr′ (*c*). According to the Fisher-Race system the phenotype *cDE* is the result of three closely linked genes *c*, *D*, and *E*, which an individual has inherited from *one* of his parents. Wiener's gene designations, corresponding agglutinogens, and blood factors, as well as the corresponding Fisher-Race notations, are given in Table 310-3.

In addition to the commonly recognized Rh-Hr antigens, an ever-expanding number of rare variants continues to add complexity to the system. Several groups of variants are recognized, including alternatives to common factors (allelic antigens); compound antigens or, according to the Fisher-Race interpretation, joint products of theoretically separable genes; and deletions or suppression of some Rh antigens. A discussion of these variants is found in textbooks dealing specifically with blood groups.

MN, Ss, U SYSTEM, AND MN VARIANTS The inheritance of M, N, and MN blood groups appears to be controlled by two allelic genes, L^m and L^n. The corresponding M and N antigens are identified by specific antibodies evoked in rabbits since they are poorly immunogenic in man; naturally occurring anti-M is rare and anti-N even rarer.

It has been suggested that the synthesis of MN antigen is similar to that of the ABH antigens, being the result of sequential gene-controlled changes in a common precursor substance. This is suggested by the association of both M and N activities with the same macromolecule, by the presence of N activity in M preparations derived from cells of the genotype *MN*, and the exposure of common specificities in M and N preparations by the removal of *N*-acetylneuraminic acid. The chemical nature of M and N substances has been investigated extensively, and it appears that carbohydrate units with terminal nonreducing *N*-acetylneuraminic acid residues are important constituents of the determinant structures of both.

The Ss antigens are closely related to M and N. Approximately 55 percent of human red cells react with anti-S antiserums irrespective of the MN type, and about 90 percent of human red cells react with anti-s. The antigens defined by these serums appear to be the products of allelic genes, and although the Ss antigens cut across the M, N distribution, a close statistical linkage with the MN system can be demonstrated, with a bias towards MS/MS and Ns/Ns.

The red cell antigen U is found in all Caucasians and most Negroes. The allele *u* is at least relatively common in Negroes (1 percent) but is not seen in Caucasians. Individuals lacking the U antigen are designated S^u S^u. Uu is closely linked to the Ss system, since no S or s antigens

TABLE 310-3
Wiener's gene designations, corresponding agglutinogens and blood factors, and Fisher-Race notations

Genes		*Frequency among Caucasoids, %*	*Corresponding agglutinogens*	*Blood factors present*
Wiener	*Fisher-Race*			
r	*cde*	38.0	rh	hr′, hr″, hr
r′	*Cde*	0.6	rh′	rh′, hr″
r″	*cdE*	*0.5*	rh″	rh″, hr′
r^y	*CdE*	0.01	rh^y	rh′, rh″
R^0	*cDe*	2.7	Rh_0	Rh_0hr′ hr″hr
R^1	*CDe*	41.0	Rh_1	Rh_0rh′hr″
R^2	*cDE*	15.0	Rh_2	Rh_0rh″hr′
R^z	*CDE*	0.2	Rh_z	Rh_0rh′rh″

Note: Wiener, in his publications, uses italics for gene symbols and for genotypes, regular type for agglutinogens and phenotypes, and boldface type for symbols for blood factors and for the corresponding antibodies used to detect the blood factors in question. Further, to distinguish the symbols for genotypes and phenotypes, the letter "h" is omitted and only superscripts are used in gene symbols.

SOURCE: *MM Wintrobe et al:* Clinical Hematology, *7th ed, Philadelphia: Lea & Febiger, 1974*

have so far been detected in u individuals, suggesting that U may perhaps be a precursor substance for Ss antigens. A large number of MNSs variants has been described.

THE P SYSTEM The P blood group system is now thought to be determined by three alleles, P^1, P^2, and the very rare gene p, which in double dose results in the absence of P_1 and P_2 antigens (Table 310-4). Recognition of the complexity within this system was largely due to the discovery of a rare antiserum, anti-Tj^a, which was soon shown to react with red cells of P_1 and P_2 phenotypes and was later also shown to contain anti-P^k antibodies. The P^k determinant also seems to be associated with the P system, but is genetically independent of the P^1, P^2 genes (K7). It has been postulated that the P^k determinant, like the Bombay phenotype of the ABO system, results from the absence of a very frequent gene dominant in character. The potential clinical importance of the P blood group system derives from the fact that antibodies regularly occur in the serum of individuals who lack the corresponding antigen (Table 310-4). Thus anti-P_1 serums are found in P_2 donors and react specifically with P_1 cells. Anti-P serums react with P_1 or P_2 cells, but when these serums are absorbed with P_2 cells, only anti-P_1 activity remains. Anti-P antibodies are found in pp and P^k subjects. Anti-P+P_1+P^k serums, previously called anti-Tj^a, react with P_1, P_2, and P^k determinants and are found in individuals of the *pp* phenotype. Clinically significant transfusion reactions due to anti-P_1 must be exceedingly rare, although rapid destruction of isotopically labeled cells has been demonstrated. Anti-P+P_1, found in *pp* and P^k individuals and as the Donath-Landsteiner antibody in paroxysmal cold hemoglobinuria (see Chap. 306), is very rare; it occurs predominantly in offsprings from consanguinous marriages and in isolated geographic areas. P_1 antigen activity is thought to be associated with a carbohydrate structure, and D-galactose in α-linkage appears to be the immunodominant sugar.

Many other blood group systems have been described (Table 310-5), some of which possess clinical or anthropologic significance because of their high incidence in the population (for example, k, Vel), difficulties associated with their detection in the laboratory (Kidd), or peculiarities in ethnic distribution (Diego). So-called "private antigens" (for example By, Sw^a, Levay) are of little or no clinical significance, except in the families in which they exist.

TABLE 310-4
The frequency of P phenotypes and their antibodies

Phenotype of cells	*Frequency of phenotype*	*Antibody in serum*	*Frequency of antibody*
P_1	75%		
P_2	25%	Anti-P_1	90%
P^k	Very rare	Anti-P + P_1	?
p	Very rare	Anti-P + P_1 +P^k (anti-Tj^a)	100%

BIOLOGIC SIGNIFICANCE OF BLOOD GROUPS

Blood transfusion reactions are of great variety. Those related to blood group incompatibility are among the most serious. The blood groups A, B, and Rh_0 are involved in by far the greatest majority, perhaps 95 percent, of all cases. This is because anti-A and anti-B antibodies occur "naturally," and Rh_0 is, like A and B, a good antigen to which antibodies are produced readily. The first encounter with ABO-incompatible blood may result in a hemolytic transfusion reaction; the first exposure of an Rh-negative person to Rh-positive blood will not, because of the lack of natural (or preformed) antibodies. Such a transfusion may, however, sensitize the individual to the Rh antigens in question, and the resultant antibodies may then lead to a hemolytic transfusion reaction on subsequent exposure to similarly incompatible cells. The Kell system (Kk) also is important because many K-negative persons can be sensitized to K by transfusion. The same holds true for rh″ and hr′, but the danger is smaller. The remaining blood groups are of comparatively minor clinical importance, although most transfusions are potentially sensitizing. Scarcity of serums and the labor involved make it impractical to type routinely for all the known antigens, but the use of a sensitive cross-match test together with the Coombs test for "incomplete" antibodies is a helpful and essential safeguard.

Blood group incompatibility is responsible for at least one disease, *erythroblastosis fetalis* (Chap. 306). In addition, the anti-red cell antibodies of some other acquired hemolytic anemias have specificity for blood group antigens, most commonly those belonging to the Rh system. This includes many cases of idiopathic autoimmune hemolytic anemia and certain instances of drug-induced hemolytic anemia, most notably those seen in association with alpha-methyldopa therapy.

ABO antigens are also known to act as potent *transplantation antigens* in man. It has been found, for instance, that hyperimmunization with incompatible ABO antigens will result in accelerated skin graft rejection when the donor is incompatible for the same ABO antigen, whereas skin grafts from ABO-compatible individuals are accorded survival times characteristic of first grafts in nonsensitized individuals. It has also been found inadvisable to use donor kidneys containing A or B antigens lacking in the recipient. In one study, 46 percent of kidney transplants with ABO incompatibility failed to show initial function, as compared with only 9 percent in ABO-compatible pairs.

For several decades the ABO groups have been suspected of contributing to *infertility and fetal loss*, but the reports have been conflicting and often speculative. Cumulative evidence now indicates that ABO incompatibility between mother and fetus results in a small but significant decrease in fertility, which may be due to prezygotic selection, prevention of fertilization, or fetal death.

Alterations in red cell phenotypes have been observed in a variety of malignant conditions. Loss or suppression of the A_1 antigen has been seen in leukemia. The change is usually confined to red cells and is accompanied by increased H activity. Acquisition of B-like antigens by patients with malignant disease or infections is also described.

TABLE 310-5
Blood groups

Name of system	Antigens of major clinical importance	Other identified antigens
ABO, Hh, Lewis	A, B, Le^a	H, Le^b
Rh	D	D^u
	C, c	C^u, C^w, C^x
	E, e	E^u, E^w
MNSs	S	M, N, s, M_1, M_2, M^g, Mi^a, Vw, Hu, He, U
P		P_1, P_2, P^k, Tj^a
Kell	K	k, Kp^a, Kp^b, Js^a, Js^b, K^u, K^w
Duffy	Fy^a	Fy^b
Kidd	Jk^a	Jk^b
Lutheran		Lu^a, Lu^b
Ii		I, i
Diego		Di^a, Di^b

Association of blood groups with disease Significant departures from expected ABO frequencies have been observed in patients with disorders involving the gastrointestinal tract: group A individuals have been reported to be more susceptible to gallstones, cirrhosis of the liver, and tumors of the salivary glands, stomach, and pancreas, as well as the ovary. In addition, duodenal ulceration was found to be more common in nonsecretors than secretors of blood group antigens and especially in group O individuals. An increased incidence of myocardial infarction and diabetes mellitus has been reported in group A individuals. The reasons underlying these correlations are not understood.

Medicolegal and anthropologic importance The usefulness of serologic examinations in medicolegal and anthropologic work is readily apparent. It has been calculated that, with the ABO system and the two subgroups of A, the MNSs blood groups, P, the Rh system, Lutheran, Lewis, and Kell, the total number of possible different combinations of serologic recognizable phenotypes is over 20,000, and the number of genotypes is nearly a million. Because of technical and other difficulties, the P, Lewis, Kell, Duffy, and Kidd systems are not recommended for use in problems of parentage or identity, but even without them, when blood of the mother, the child, and the alleged father is available, it is possible to exonerate a majority of men who are wrongfully accused of paternity.

Of additional medicolegal importance is the fact that the antigens A, B, and H are present in the secretions of most individuals and can readily be extracted with aqueous solutions from tissues and organs, especially salivary glands and gastric mucosa. High concentrations of blood group substances can also be found in secretions such as saliva, gastric juice, and semen. As a consequence it is possible to apply blood grouping to the examination of dried stains of these secretions as well as to saline extracts of muscle tissue.

In human genetics and anthropology the blood groups are of the utmost value for a number of reasons. The first is that they are sharply distinguishable "all-or-none" characteristics which do not grade into each other. Then again, they are simple, genetically speaking, and are inherited in a known way according to mendelian principles. Furthermore, they owe nothing to environment in their inheritance, nor are they subject to variations because of natural selection, as is the case, for example, with skin color. Hence, the blood groups are especially fitted to throw light on the moderately remote as well as the recent origins of mankind. Wide differences in frequency in different races have been observed. Consequently the blood groups provide valuable anthropometric measurements.

Considerable and interesting data are being accumulated concerning the ethnologic distribution of the blood groups. Thus the incidence of B has been found highest in certain parts of Asia and declines in all directions from central Asia except for a subsidiary high center in Africa. In the Old World the lowest figures have been found in the Scandinavian countries, and in Australia the gene seems to have been absent until very recent times. A similar complete absence has been found in the living aborigines of North America as well as in the Basques. Group O reaches levels of practically 100 percent among certain Indian tribes in the United States. In the aborigines of North America the gene for N is relatively rare, while in those of Australia it is very common. The factor P is much commoner in the blood of American Negroes than in that of American whites. The Rh-negative gene (cde) has been found in 13 to 17 percent of modern inhabitants of Europe and in white inhabitants of America. In the Basques it reaches very high levels (28.8 percent); in contrast, in a study of Eskimos only 1 out of 2,522 was found to be Rh-negative.

BLOOD TRANSFUSION

BLOOD AND BLOOD COMPONENTS AND INDICATIONS FOR THEIR USE Blood transfusions must be regarded as a form of therapy which carries a significant risk and is potentially lethal; clear indications for their use must therefore exist. The physician must consciously and deliberately weigh the potential benefits against the known risks. When transfusion seems indicated, the physician must also decide whether the patient needs whole blood or blood components and how much needs to be given.

Whole blood By far the most important use of whole blood is for the restoration of an adequate circulating volume after hemorrhage or trauma. In such situations the restoration of an adequate volume is usually more important than an adequate red cell mass, and for this purpose whole blood transfusion has no equal. Saline, plasma, and plasma expanders such as low molecular weight dextran may be useful stopgap measures until the typing and matching have been done. It should be noted, however, that the use of dextran may give rise to difficulties in blood matching, and an adequate blood sample should therefore be removed for these purposes *before* dextran is given.

Accurate assessment of the amount of blood loss is difficult, although an estimate can often be made from the blood pressure, pulse rate, and the patient's general appearance. The signs and symptoms of severe blood loss include pallor, vasoconstriction, sweating, thirst, air hunger, and restlessness. When such manifestations of oxygen want are present, transfusion is of course always mandatory. When there is evidence of acute ongoing hemorrhage, however, it is unwise to wait for the development of these extreme signs and symptoms, as many adults may lose as much as 1,500 ml blood without showing any of them, so long as they remain in the horizontal position. Under such circumstances the blood pressure and other clinical parameters should be observed in the horizontal and the tilted position. Acute blood loss in excess of 1,500 ml produces clinical shock in most patients.

If the blood pressure is less than 100 mm Hg, the blood volume is probably less than 70 percent of normal, but it is dangerous to rely on this sign alone when the patient's prehemorrhage pressure is not known. Thus a systolic pressure of 150 mm Hg may be very significant in a hypertensive patient whose usual systolic pressure is 200 mm Hg. Similarly, the pulse rate is by itself an unreliable guide, although in an actively bleeding patient a persistent pulse rate of 100 or more probably indicates blood loss in excess of 20 percent. Estimation of the hemoglobin or hematocrit may be misleading shortly after an acute hemorrhage, since compensatory vasoconstriction will keep these values at normal levels until the intravascular volume has been reexpanded with fluids from extravascular sources. This usually occurs between 3 and 6 hr after hemorrhage, and rapidly falling hemoglobin levels during this period of time indicate blood loss of serious proportions. The skillful physician will of course not allow these signs of major blood loss to develop.

The loss of blood during surgical procedures is largely a reflection of the skill and care of the operator and to a lesser extent, the type of surgery. The common practice of replacing all blood losses by transfusion is of course totally unjustified. Obviously the loss of 500 ml blood is well tolerated by most patients. Indeed, even patients undergoing open heart surgery and other major surgical procedures in which blood loss exceeds 1,000 ml can be managed without blood transfusions, so long as intravascular volume is maintained with crystalloid solutions or even with simple saline infusions. When noncolloid solutions such as buffered saline are used, the volume administered needs to be two to three times the volume of blood lost.

Whole blood is indispensable for exchange transfusions such as those used in the treatment of hemolytic disease of the newborn (see Chap. 315). It is also most commonly used to prime the equipment for extracorporeal shunts, including renal hemodialysis units and heart-lung machines. It has been suggested by some, however, that packed red cells suspended in suitable balanced salt solutions are preferable for these purposes, while others have recommended priming extracorporeal circuits with blood substitutes such as crystalloid or colloid solutions.

Packed red cells Except as outlined in the previous section, most transfusions are given in order to improve the oxygen-carrying capacity of the blood. The only component of donor blood which can accomplish this is the red cell, and under such circumstances all other components are wasteful or dangerous (see below). In addition, the plasma can be used for the preparation of various plasma fractions such as albumin, cryoprecipitate, or gamma-globulin, as well as platelets.

Indications for packed cell transfusions include the following.

1 *Hemolytic anemia*, especially in aplastic crisis. These patients are frequently very ill and may be found to have hemoglobin values as low as 2 to 3 g per 100 ml. The cardiovascular system of such patients is often on the verge of collapse, and even a small transfusion may precipitate cardiac failure and death. These patients can be managed safely only by constant monitoring of the central venous pressure and by exchanging packed cells cautiously for the patient's blood. A careful balance sheet must be kept, and initially it is well to remove perhaps 10 percent more volume than is replaced. Packed cells should be as fresh as possible. Under no circumstances must a patient with an elevated central venous pressure be subjected to a transfusion without continuous central venous pressure monitoring and the concomitant removal of blood, if necessary, because otherwise cardiac failure will almost inevitably get worse. Digoxin and diuretics may on occasion be useful ancillary measures but are not sufficiently reliable to make an exchange of packed red cells for whole blood unnecessary.

   In acute acquired forms of hemolytic anemia the transfused cells may be destroyed as rapidly as those of the recipient. When hemolysis is due to antibody-mediated mechanisms, it may be possible to identify the specificity of the antibody in order to allow for the proper selection of donor blood.

   In the more chronic forms of hemolytic anemia a state of equilibrium is frequently reached, and when this is so blood transfusions have little to offer.

2 When the severity of the anemia and clinical manifestations require it, packed red cells are the treatment of choice for the support of patients with *chronic hypoplastic anemias* for which no other forms of therapy are available, including the various aplastic anemias, the anemia accompanying chronic renal disease, and others.

3 Patients suffering from acute and chronic leukemia, lymphomas, or other malignancies may need packed-cell transfusions, especially while undergoing therapy. Both chemotherapy and radiotherapy will seriously affect marrow function, which may already be compromised because of disease.

4 Transfusions have been used to *suppress endogenous erythropoiesis* in patients with sickle-cell anemia or thalassemia, but the dangers of transfusion hemosiderosis limit the usefulness of this method.

5 Patients suffering from chronic anemias due to lack of vitamin B_{12} or iron usually respond well to specific therapy and do not require transfusions. Occasionally, however, a patient will be first seen critically ill with cardiac failure, angina pectoris, cerebral insufficiency

or infection, sometimes complicated by leukopenia and thrombocytopenia, and under such circumstances transfusion therapy may be lifesaving. This should be done under close supervision with constant monitoring of central venous pressure and, if necessary, by exchange transfusion.

Platelets Platelet transfusions are given to stop or prevent bleeding due to thrombocytopenia or thrombocytopathia. If the function of individual platelets is adequate, bleeding does not usually occur until the platelet count is 20,000 per μl or less, and many patients, especially those with thrombocytopenia due to immune destruction, may have no bleeding episodes for long periods of time, even though the platelet count is as low as 5,000 per μl. For patients with other illnesses such as leukemia, however, the threat of serious hemorrhage has been estimated to be in excess of 1 percent per day for counts of 20,000 per μl, with a rise of 20 percent per day when the count drops to 1,000 per μl. The risk of hemorrhage is particularly great in the presence of fever and infection, or when thrombocytopenic patients are inadvertently treated with drugs which interfere with platelet function. All these situations require immediate support with platelet transfusions.

In addition, platelet transfusions are indicated in patients with severe thrombocytopenia due to other forms of marrow failure; in patients with thrombocytopenia due to disseminated intravascular coagulation (Chap. 315), but only if they are being treated with heparin; in patients whose platelets have been depleted by massive transfusions or the use of extracorporeal circuits; and in patients who are bleeding because of qualitative platelet defects, whether these are congenital or acquired. However, in the case of acquired platelet defects it is usually necessary to eliminate the underlying defect such as drug therapy or uremia, in addition to giving platelet transfusions, as the transfused platelets will otherwise quickly acquire the same defect. Platelet therapy is not helpful in patients with thrombocytopenia due to immune destruction, since the transfused platelets usually are promptly eliminated.

Platelets are usually supplied as concentrates and are best given as fresh as possible. One unit contains about 10^{11} platelets and can therefore be expected to yield an increment of 10 to 12,000 platelets per μl per m^2 body surface, unless destruction of the transfused platelets is unduly rapid. The frequency of transfusions will depend on the half-life of the transfused platelets; this, in most patients without antibodies, is between 1 and 2 days.

From a clinical standpoint HL-A (transplantation) antigens constitute the most important system of antigens on platelets, and sensitization readily follows repeated transfusions. Unfortunately it is impossible to prevent this complication of transfusion therapy in most instances, since the estimated 20,000 possible HLA phenotypes make matching for HLA antigens impractical. If the recipient has siblings, however, they should always be HL-A typed, since the mode of inheritance of HL-A antigens is such that 25 percent of all siblings have a statistical chance of being HL-A identical. When HL-A-identical siblings are available, they are the donors of choice and may be used as donors repeatedly.

White blood cell transfusions The routine use of platelet transfusions has made infection the leading cause of death in patients with hematologic malignancies. The most common indication for leukocyte transfusions therefore is bacterial sepsis, unresponsive to appropriate antibiotic therapy and occurring in association with severe leukopenia due to malignant disease of the marrow or myelosuppression due to cytotoxic drugs. In addition, patients with granulocytopenia due to a variety of drug reactions and patients with aplastic anemia may benefit from granulocyte transfusions when they develop severe infections. The value of prophylactic granulocytic transfusions, in the absence of infection associated with granulocytopenia, remains to be proved.

The modern techniques of continuous flow centrifugation or filtration leukopheresis permit the collection of large numbers of granulocytes from single normal donors. Histocompatible siblings are preferred (see under Platelets above). When these more sophisticated methods are not available, leukocytes may be obtained from chronic myelogenous leukemia donors by standard leukopheresis techniques using plastic collecting bags and ACD anticoagulant. In either case the percent recovery of transfused leukocytes is closely linked to the goodness of the HL-A match and the presence of preformed anti HL-A antibodies. If granulocyte transfusions are used, they should be repeated daily until the infection is under control, since a progressive improvement in patient survival is seen with increasing numbers of transfusions.

Plasma component therapy Fresh frozen plasma and plasma fractions such as cryoprecipitate can provide clotting factors for the treatment of patients suffering from specific defects. These are discussed in Chaps. 59 and 314. Plasma is also used as an expander of intravascular volume, and human serum albumin is sometimes valuable in certain patients with hepatic cirrhosis, the nephrotic syndrome, idiopathic hypoproteinemia, and the edema of malnutrition.

COMPLICATIONS OF BLOOD TRANSFUSION

Transfusion reactions are of several types but are conveniently classified under the headings of immune and nonimmune mechanisms. The former include (1) reactions due to red cell incompatibility and (2) reactions due to leukocyte and platelet incompatibilities, as well as other forms of allergic reactions. Nonimmune transfusion reactions include (1) those caused by overloading of the circulation, (2) those related in particular to massive transfusions, (3) transmission of infections, and (4) miscellaneous ill effects such as thrombophlebitis, air and fat embolism, and transfusion siderosis.

Immunologically mediated transfusion reactions Hemolytic transfusion reactions may be due to rapid intravascular breakdown of transfused cells or to extravascular destruction of antibody-sensitized erythrocytes, predominantly in the reticuloendothelial system. *Intravascular hemolysis* of red cells is most commonly associated with an incompatibility in the ABO system, since anti-A and anti-B antibodies are usually IgM and capable of binding complement, leading to almost instantaneous lysis of transfused cells in a sensitized individual. Fortunately the administration of incompatible blood is usually associated with the onset of symptoms before much blood has been introduced, and, if the transfusion is stopped, no serious harm may result. The symptoms observed include restlessness, anxiety, flushing of the face, precordial oppression and pain, an increase in pulse and respiratory rate, generalized tingling sensations, and pain in the back and thighs. Nausea and vomiting may follow, and cyanosis, shock with cold, clammy skin, coma, and a failing pulse may develop. A chill, followed by a rise of temperature to 105°F or higher, and possibly delirium may ensue. Leukopenia is followed by leukocytosis.

Not infrequently a hemorrhagic tendency develops immediately after the transfusion of incompatible blood, and blood may ooze from the site of transfusion, from mucous membranes, or from the operative site, if such exists. Fibrinogen and other labile clotting factors are usually found to be depleted, probably as the result of fibrin formation after liberation of thromboplastic substances from red cells hemolyzed intravascularly. Thrombocytopenia may be present as well.

Massive intravascular hemolysis frequently leads to oliguria or anuria, probably as a result of circulatory failure and, subsequently, the precipitation of hemoglobin in functionally impaired nephrons.

Rh incompatibility is by far the most common cause of *extravascular hemolysis;* others include incompatibilities involving Lewis, Kell, and Duffy systems. Of the various components of the Rh-Hr system, anti-Rh_0 (anti-D) is by far the most common, and anti-Rh_1 (anti-D plus anti-C) is another common cause. Anti-hr′ (anti-c), anti-rh″ (anti-E), anti-Rh_2 (anti-D plus anti-E) are not rare, but other antibodies involving this system are found in less than 1 percent of cases.

The clinical manifestations of extravascular hemolysis are less spectacular than those of intravascular red cell destruction. Fever and chills develop frequently and may be delayed in onset for an hour or so. It has been suggested that these febrile reactions are somehow related to splenic sequestration. Acute renal failure is not characteristic of extravascular hemolysis.

Delayed transfusion reactions are most commonly due to isoantibodies such as those directed against Rh-Hr antigens and may not appear until 2 to 14 days after the transfusion of blood. Occasionally hemolytic transfusion reactions occur in the *absence* of *demonstrable* incompatibility.

The laboratory investigation of hemolytic transfusion reactions (Table 310-6) includes (1) the demonstration of red cell destruction, (2) serologic tests to determine the cause of the transfusion reaction, and (3) laboratory tests for the presence of disseminated intravascular coagulation (Chap. 315). The appropriate investigations have been listed in Table 310-6.

Tests demonstrating hemolysis include indirect hyperbilirubinemia and, in cases of intravascular hemolysis, elevated plasma hemoglobin levels and hemoglobinuria. Reduced haptoglobin levels also indicate intravascular hemolysis and are particularly useful in mild reactions. With severe intravascular transfusion reactions, plasma hemopexin levels also decrease and methemalbuminemia may appear. When transfusion reactions are mild, comparison with pretransfusion pigment values are valuable but are not always possible. It is important to draw blood carefully since artifactually induced hemolysis may make interpretation of data difficult.

TABLE 310-6
Tests to be done in suspected hemolytic transfusion reactions

- Demonstrating red cell destruction
  - Increased plasma hemoglobin
  - Hemoglobinuria
  - Reduced haptoglobin levels
  - Methemalbuminemia
  - Hyperbilirubinemia
- Tests for intravascular coagulation
- Serologic studies
  - Complete retyping of patient and donor blood
  - Direct Coombs test on recipient's cells
  - Indirect Coombs
    - Recipient's cells and donor serum
    - Donor cells and recipient's serum
- Others
  - Aerobic and anaerobic culture of donor blood
  - Tests of renal function

Serologic tests include a complete retyping of the patient's and the donor's blood in an effort to identify the responsible blood group incompatibility. The cross match should be reconfirmed. In addition the patient's red cells should be tested for surface immunoglobulin and complement by the direct Coombs test; the patient's serum should be tested for antibodies against donor cells, and the donor's serum should be tested for antibodies which may react with recipient cells.

It is also wise to examine the administered blood for aerobic and anaerobic bacterial contamination. The urine output should be monitored carefully, and the blood should be watched for the development of azotemia.

Treatment The prevention of renal complications is most important and depends on appropriate therapy of intravascular coagulation, when present; establishing and maintaining urine flow with osmotic diuretics such as mannitol, except where acute tubular necrosis has already occurred; increasing renal blood flow with α-adrenergic blocking agents such as phenoxybenzamine; and treating shock with *compatible* transfusions or fluids. If renal shutdown has already occurred, treatment should follow that outlined in Chap. 259.

Nonhemolytic febrile transfusion reactions occur in 1 to 20 percent of cases, but an incidence of 3 to 4 percent would be a reasonable figure for most transfusion centers. These reactions may be due to immune sensitivity to leukocytes, platelets, and various plasma constituents, or they may be due to bacterial and other pyrogens. With the advent of modern transfusion technology the latter have become quite infrequent. Often no cause whatsoever may be discovered.

Sensitization to white cell or platelet antigens is one of the most common causes of nonhemolytic febrile reactions, especially in patients who have received large numbers of transfusions. Occasionally the reaction may be severe and even life-threatening. Accurate diagnosis depends on the demonstration of antileukocyte antibodies in the recipient, but this information is usually not available when the physician is called upon to differentiate between hemolytic and nonhemolytic transfusion reactions. While hemolytic transfusion reactions call for the immediate cessation of the transfusion, nonhemolytic febrile responses are often well tolerated with minimal supportive care, usually consisting of antipyretics (where these are not contraindicated, as in thrombocytopenia) or antihistamine therapy. Antihistamines are most effective if given before the transfusion. A peculiar manifestation of leukoagglutinin transfusion reactions is the appearance of pulmonary infiltrates.

Nonimmune transfusion reactions CIRCULATORY OVERLOAD The administration of excessively large quantities of blood, or smaller amounts given too rapidly ("speed reaction"), can cause circulatory failure, especially when there is myocardial weakness. This is often heralded by the onset of a series of short, sharp coughs, precordial and back pain, dyspnea, cyanosis, and finally a productive cough. The symptoms may develop at any time from 1 to 24 hr after transfusion, and death may result from pulmonary edema. Overloading of the cardiovascular system can be prevented by transfusing blood from which most of the plasma has been removed, and by giving the blood slowly by the gravity-drip method, with the patient in a propped-up position if there is any question of cardiac failure. The rate of administration should not exceed 1 ml per lb body weight per hr and often may well be slower than this. Only when there has been acute and severe hemorrhage does blood need to be given quickly. Measurement of the patient's venous pressure before transfusion provides a useful guide to the probability of inducing cardiac failure: Worsening of failure is likely if the pretransfusion venous pressure is above normal. When there is any doubt about the patient's cardiovascular status, continuous central venous pressure monitoring can be used to signal a dangerous increase in venous pressure. When the central venous pressure is decidedly elevated before the transfusion or rises during the transfusion, blood can be given safely only by exchange.

Other complications of massive transfusion include hypercalcemia, citrate toxicity, and hemorrhage. The potassium is derived from red cells during storage and may reach concentrations of 15 to 20 mEq per liter after 10 to 14 days. Citrate usually is metabolized rapidly, but when large quantities of ACD solution are transfused, ionized calcium concentrations decrease, and skeletal muscle tremors, prolongation of the QT internal, and cardiac arrest may develop. Calcium gluconate usually eliminates these manifestations of citrate toxicity.

Bleeding may result from the dilution of labile clotting factors by stored blood, and this complication can be avoided by the use of fresh blood. If an incompatible transfusion is given, intravascular coagulation may also contribute to the bleeding tendency.

Infections such as hepatitis, cytomegalovirus, syphilis, malaria, toxoplasmosis, and brucellosis are sometimes transmitted by transfusion. In addition the blood may become infected during handling and storage.

Of all the transfusion-transmitted infections, *hepatitis* is the most common and the most serious. The viruses causing hepatitis are hardy and highly infectious (Chap. 294): As little as $^{1}/_{10,000}$ ml icterogenic plasma may cause clinically obvious hepatitis, and as little as $^{1}/_{10,000,000}$ ml may lead to serologically detectable evidence of infection. This is why pooled blood products are so dangerous, since virus from one donor, though diluted, is widely distributed. While both Australian antigen–positive (long incubation) hepatitis and Australian antigen–negative (short incubation) hepatitis may be transmitted by transfusion, only carriers of Australian antigen–positive hepatitis can currently be identified by specific serologic techniques (Chap. 294). Australian antigen–associated virus appears to be implicated in approximately 25 to 30 percent of patients with posttransfusion hepatitis.

The reported incidence of viral hepatitis following transfusion of blood and blood products varies widely and is influenced by several factors. When the diagnosis is based on clinical evidence such as icterus, the risk is considerably less than 1 percent per unit of blood administered, but may be in excess of 50 percent when Australian antigen–positive blood is given. However, when the diagnosis is based on elevated enzyme levels, the incidence is much higher and may reach 3 percent per unit of Australian antigen–negative blood and 50 to near 100 percent for recipients of Australian antigen–positive blood. When blood is derived from commercial sources, rather than from volunteer donors, the risks of hepatitis are particularly high. In one study the number of Australian antigen–positive units was thirteenfold greater in commercial donor blood than in volunteer blood, and similar differences probably exist for the infectious hepatitis virus for which no specific test is yet available.

Other *miscellaneous ill effects* include thrombophlebitis, air embolism, and hemosiderosis.

REFERENCES

MOLLISON PL: *Blood Transfusion in Clinical Medicine*, 5th ed., Philadelphia: Davis, 1972

RACE RR, SANGER R: *Blood Groups in Man*, 5th ed., Philadelphia: Davis, 1968

WINTROBE MM et al: *Clinical Hematology*, 7th ed., Philadelphia: Lea & Febiger, 1974

311 POLYCYTHEMIA RUBRA VERA

M. M. WINTROBE
ARTHUR HAUT

DEFINITION Polycythemia vera ("erythremia"), so-called to distinguish it from polycythemia which develops in response to some known stimulus (secondary polycythemia, "erythrocytosis") and from false ("spurious") or relative polycythemia, is a disease of unknown cause, insidious onset, and chronic course. It is characterized by a striking absolute increase in the quantity of circulating red corpuscles and usually also by evidence of increased production of myeloid leukocytes and platelets. Splenomegaly and a red "cyanosis" of the skin, as well as increase in the viscosity of the blood and in the total volume of the blood, are additional features of this disorder.

HISTORY Vaquez in 1892 described a case of polycythemia which he had originally attributed to congenital heart disease. Osler gave a more complete description in 1903.

ETIOLOGY AND PATHOGENESIS In an earlier chapter (Chap. 29) various forms of polycythemia were discussed. In polycythemia vera none of the circumstances or disorders known to be associated regularly, or even occasionally, with polycythemia can be found; significant oxygen unsaturation of the blood is lacking, whereas splenomegaly, leukocytosis due to an increased number of granulocytes, and other signs suggesting myeloid hyperplasia, including thrombocytosis, are present. These features suggest a close relation to the various so-called "myeloproliferative" disorders, especially chronic myelocytic leukemia. In polycythemia vera, as distinguished from hypoxic polycythemias, absent or significantly reduced serum and urinary erythropoietin have been found in most instances. These rise to normal values when the volume of packed red cells is reduced to normal limits by venesections.

Most commonly, polycythemia vera appears in middle or later life. In very rare instances, polycythemia of unknown cause has been seen in children; equally rarely, it appears as a familial disorder. Such cases have not been characterized by signs of generalized myeloid hyperplasia and are probably unrelated to the classic disorder described by Vaquez and by Osler. Contrary to the view once held, there probably is no preponderance of the disease in any particular racial group. Men are somewhat more often affected than women.

PATHOLOGY AND PATHOLOGIC PHYSIOLOGY The striking pathologic changes are those related to the increase in total blood volume. All the organs are engorged with blood, the veins stand out like "bunches of thick worms," and there may be thromboses or anemic infarcts. The bone marrow is dark red and very cellular. Microscopically, this is found in most instances to be due to hyperplasia of all the marrow elements. In some patients the percentage of normoblasts is increased, in others the proportions of myelocytes and myeloblasts or of basophilic and eosinophilic cells may be greater than normal.

The spleen is enlarged, chiefly from hyperplasia of the pulp and distention with blood. Infarcts are common. There may be foci of extramedullary blood formation in the spleen, the liver, and occasionally elsewhere as well.

The relative quantity of red cells per unit of blood causes a great increase in blood viscosity, and this, probably, is responsible for many of the clinical manifestations. Although cardiac output and work, pulmonary functions, and the arterial oxygen saturation of the blood and the oxygen dissociation curve are normal, the circulatory minute volume is reduced, and the velocity of blood flow is greatly lowered. The resulting visceral stasis, together with the thrombocytosis, may explain the high incidence of intravascular thrombosis seen in this disorder. The existence of a hemostatic defect has been postulated mainly because of the excessive bleeding which may be associated with minor injuries or at operations. This can be explained in part by the physical distention of the vascular bed. Decreased platelet factor 3 activity and excessive friability of the blood clot have been reported, as well as defects in platelet adenosine diphosphate (ADP) release and aggregation and in platelet adhesiveness.

SYMPTOMATOLOGY The onset is insidious and the progress gradual. Headache, dizziness, ringing in the ears, or visual disturbances; dyspnea, lassitude, or weakness; skin or mucous membrane hemorrhages; pruritis, especially after a hot shower or bath; a sense of weight in the abdomen because of the enlarged spleen; or irritability, depression, forgetfulness, or vague symptoms suggesting neurasthenia are complaints which may be encountered in many patients. Various gastrointestinal symptoms, such as fullness, belching, or constipation, may be present, or symptoms of peptic ulcer may be found. Sometimes the symptoms are those attributable to increased metabolism: lassitude, increased sweating, and loss of weight. Swelling and pain in the extremities may be very troublesome. However, in still other patients the symptoms are so insignificant that the polycythemia is discovered only accidentally.

The face is a deep red rather than truly cyanotic. The color is most noticeable in the lips, cheeks, tip of the nose, ears, and neck. The distal portions of the extremities may be more truly cyanotic, since the highly viscous blood circulates more sluggishly there than is normal. Ecchymoses are common, and epistaxis and bleeding of the gums are frequently encountered. Cardiac abnormality is unusual, but vascular disturbances, including venous thromboses, coronary thrombosis, and cerebrovascular accidents, are common. The blood pressure is more often normal than elevated. Enlargement of the liver is frequent, and splenomegaly is found in at least 75 percent of cases. The spleen may be just palpable, or it may extend even to the pelvic brim.

Blood The volume of packed red cells may be 55 to 83 ml per 100 ml whole blood. Unless hemorrhage has occurred or venesections have been performed, there is a corresponding increase in hemoglobin concentration. The number of erythrocytes, which may reach 7 to 10 million cells per μl may be increased out of proportion to the hemoglobin and the volume of packed red corpuscles if iron reserves are limited or frank iron deficiency is present. The volume of packed white cells and platelets, i.e., the buffy coat which is seen on carefully examining the hematocrit, is also increased and may be from 1.5 to several ml per 100 ml blood, signifying the presence of leukocytosis, thrombocytosis, or both. On the blood smear, the individual red corpuscles appear normal, although occasional polychromatophilia or basophilic stippling may be noted. The finding of nucleated red corpuscles and the appearance of small numbers of myelocytes and even earlier forms in the blood give a clue to the hyperplastic state of the bone marrow; leukocytosis, occasionally of marked degree (60,000 leukocytes per μl), due to an increase of the granulocytes, and high platelet counts give further evidence of overactivity. Basophilic and eosinophilic leukocytes are more numerous than normal. The percentage of reticulocytes is not increased unless there has been recent bleeding. Leukocyte alkaline phosphatase generally is high, therein distinguishing polycythemia vera from secondary polycythemia and chronic myelocytic leukemia, but it may be normal, and only rarely has it been found to be low. The red cell life span usually is normal, and the osmotic fragility of the red corpuscles is not significantly altered. Rarely is there evidence of increased blood destruction in the form of slight bilirubinemia and increased excretion of urobilinogen. The viscosity of the blood is greatly increased, even five- to tenfold. The thick, sticky blood may be slow to coagulate, and the clot may not retract. However, conventional coagulation tests usually are normal.

The total blood volume is substantially increased (150 to 300 percent of normal). This may be attributed to the increase in red corpuscle mass, but it does not entirely reflect the full magnitude of the latter, since the plasma volume is most often decreased, particularly in cases with the greater volume of packed red cells.

Other laboratory findings Hyperuricemia and hyperuricosuria, reflecting the increased synthesis and degradation of nucleoprotein associated with the excessive cellular proliferation in this disease, are found in about 30 percent of patients at the time of diagnosis. The serum vitamin B_{12} content and the capacity of the serum to bind additional B_{12} added in vitro are both increased. In untreated polycythemia vera, the plasma iron turnover often is greater than normal due to a shortening of the half time for plasma iron disappearance. This ferrokinetic feature can be attributed to depleted iron stores and can be changed toward normal by iron repletion. A regularly occurring chromosomal anomaly has not been seen in this disease, although aneuploidy, translocations, and deletions have been found; the last, in some cases, perhaps are the result of antecedent treatment with radioactive phosphorus.

DIAGNOSIS The symptoms may suggest a variety of disorders, but once the blood has been examined, the problem is to differentiate secondary forms of polycythemia from the "primary" disorder (polycythemia vera). The discovery of an increased volume of packed white corpuscles and platelets in the hematocrit tube, in addition to the increased volume of packed red corpuscles, and the absence of a bluish cyanosis and hypoxemia immediately favor the diagnosis of polycythemia vera. Splenomegaly is very unusual in secondary polycythemia, even when the hemoglobin or hematocrit is very much increased. Furthermore, one rarely finds persistent neutrophilic leukocytosis, immature granulocytes, basophilia, eosinophilia, thrombocytosis, or an increase in the neutrophil alkaline phosphatase. Normoblasts are much more common in the blood in polycythemia vera than in the secondary forms although, in the latter, hypoxemia may lead to their appearance in the circulation.

Finding an increase in the volume of packed red corpuscles, the hemoglobin concentration, or the erythrocyte count, does not of itself allow one to conclude that there is an increase in the total quantity of red corpuscles in the body. Those findings could also result from a decrease in plasma volume without alteration in the red corpuscle mass, a situation termed *relative polycythemia*. Such instances are most often recognized by the associated clinical circumstances which have resulted in a reduction in plasma volume, e.g., fulminant diarrhea, protracted vomiting, extensive burns of the body surface, and other situations resulting in extraordinary fluid losses and dehydration.

Contrasting with these straightforward examples of hemoconcentration with resulting polycythemia are patients in whom such complaints are lacking. In these, usually middle-aged, often heavily built males, in addition to persistent abnormally high hemoglobin and hematocrit levels, hypertension (Gaisböck's syndrome), elevation of serum cholesterol and uric acid, and a high incidence of thromboembolic disease are common. Because these individuals often are unusually active and tense, the term *stress erythrocytosis* has been applied. First attributed to reduced plasma volume alone, further studies have indicated that the total red cell volume is in the high normal and plasma volume in the low normal range. The total body hematocrit normally is less than (0.9) that of the large vessels ("venous hematocrit"). In persons with this form of spurious polycythemia the difference is thought to be even greater than is found normally. What causes the shift of red cells into the large-vessel pool is obscure.

The total red cell volume may be readily determined by using, for example, the dilution principle and injecting a measured small volume of the patient's own red corpuscles tagged with radioactive chromium (^{51}Cr). Total blood volume may be calculated from the total red cell volume and the ratio of plasma to packed red cells in the venous hematocrit, but it is more accurate to measure plasma volume directly, adding this to the determined total red cell volume. Predicted values for healthy persons, based on studies of 201 men and 101 women, are given in the Appendix. Height, weight, and body surface area are recognized as having bearing on predicted values. The influence of age, lean body mass, and muscularity, though important, is less well understood. For some patients, especially those with the less common body proportions, the base of reference is important in evaluating the measured red corpuscle mass and total blood volume. Calculation per unit of body weight, per unit of body surface area, or per unit of lean body mass, sometimes results in different interpretations regarding the normality or abnormality of the value obtained. One should be aware of this possibility and not place too much reliance on the measurements alone, but rather give consideration to all the clinical and laboratory findings. In equivocal cases, it is better to make additional observations at a later date in order to establish a sounder foundation before making a diagnosis.

Measurements of blood volume differentiate relative from absolute polycythemia but do not distinguish the absolute forms from one another. *Measurement of arteri-*

al oxygen saturation is useful in differentiating erythrocytosis due to cardiac or pulmonary disease, for in the latter, oxygen saturation is altered more or less in inverse proportion to the degree of polycythemia, whereas in polycythemia vera it is normal or nearly normal. Other clinical features and laboratory procedures helpful in differentiating various forms of cyanosis and polycythemia are discussed elsewhere (Chaps. 29, 307, and 312). Attention should also be given to other possible causes of secondary polycythemia: renal carcinoma, adenoma, cysts, hydronephrosis; cerebellar hemangioblastoma; adrenocortical carcinoma, or hyperplasia, pheochromocytoma; ovarian carcinoma, uterine fibroids; hepatoma; familial erythrocytosis; or increased oxygen affinity. Not to be overlooked are patients with polycythemia vera who present with anemia due to evident or occult blood loss. Careful attention to leukocyte, platelet, and erythrocyte morphology on the blood smear, measurement of the neutrophil alkaline phosphatase, and sometimes even resort to bone marrow biopsy will avoid confusion between "anemic polycythemia" and myelofibrosis or chronic myelocytic leukemia. A normal serum vitamin B_{12} concentration and absence of the Ph^1 chromosome further diminishes the likelihood of leukemia.

Unfortunately, some patients do not present all the classic features of polycythemia vera, and since many are advanced in years, cardiac or pulmonary disease may be present as well. In approximately 20 percent of cases leukocyte and platelet counts are within normal limits, and in about 25 percent of patients the spleen is not palpable. The finding of papilledema or of an abdominal mass other than the spleen may be helpful, but even the demonstration of a renal lesion does not in itself prove that it is the cause of the polycythemia. In some cases great judgment is needed in making the differentiation. One must be patient in equivocal cases, for example, those without leukocyte or platelet increases and without apparent cause. Additional observations after there has been some opportunity for evolution of the disease may resolve the question.

COURSE AND COMPLICATIONS The course of polycythemia vera depends on the degree to which each cell type is involved in the proliferative process and on the success of the therapeutic measures which are taken. Myeloid metaplasia, splenomegaly, and myelofibrosis gradually increase in degree. As extramedullary hematopoiesis increases, marked anisocytosis and poikilocytosis may develop, increased numbers of nucleated red cells may be found in the blood, and red cell life span may become shorter, perhaps because of increasing splenic sequestration and ineffective erythropoiesis. Barring the development of serious complications, however, the course of polycythemia vera, if appropriately treated, is often compatible with many years of life. The median survival has been found to be as long as 16 years, although this varies widely; a standard deviation of more than 6 years has been recorded. The most dangerous complications are vascular: thrombosis or hemorrhage. Therapy, by keeping the red corpuscle mass at a nearly normal level, can effectively reduce blood viscosity and thus serves to reduce the likelihood of such vascular accidents. Intercurrent infections, especially of the respiratory tract, may be troublesome, and bronchitis and emphysema may develop. Peptic ulcer and gout are frequent complications. Thrombotic and other complications are influenced by modifying factors, such as advancing age and the presence and degree of atherosclerosis and hypertension. Myelofibrosis may develop and polycythemia may be replaced by anemia. Acute leukemia has been reported in 10 to 15 percent of patients treated with radioactive phosphorus (^{32}P), but the relative importance of the cumulative dose of the radioisotope, the duration of the disease in a given case, and other factors in these retrospective observations are uncertain. Acute leukemia has occurred in nonirradiated patients also, albeit in a much smaller percentage.

TREATMENT Treatment is symptomatic, since the cause is unknown. When the diagnosis is not clear, it is best not to embark on treatment with radioisotopes or chemotherapy, although these are appropriate for the overt cases, as detailed below. *Venesections* may be prescribed if these make the patient feel better, even in the absence of a firm diagnosis, and in established cases symptomatic relief is most quickly accomplished by venesection. Approximately a pint of blood is removed twice a week or even more often, care being taken to ensure normal hydration so that the plasma volume may be expanded promptly. The procedure is repeated until the volume of packed red corpuscles approaches normal. Then venesection may need to be repeated only once a month or less often. In emergency situations, multiple phlebotomies can be performed in a shorter time by returning the patient's own plasma to him after each venesection, thus rapidly reducing blood viscosity without the hazards of reduced systemic blood flow which result from acute, substantial reductions in blood volume.

Once the volume of packed red corpuscles has been reduced to normal values by venesections, recurrence of polycythemia can eventually be prevented by induction of iron deficiency if repeated phlebotomies become necessary. Usually it is preferable to inhibit erythropoiesis by irradiation or by chemotherapy. The effects of irradiation are slow to appear, however. The intravenous injection of ^{32}P is more satisfactory than roentgen therapy. Although ^{32}P may be incorporated in bone, placing this agent in a strategic position, its biologic effect probably results from its incorporation into DNA and ATP, where the effect of radiation at close range and the conversion of radioactive ^{32}P into stable radioactive sulfur (^{32}S) by radioactive decay may critically affect molecular reactions. Three to five mCi (millicuries) ^{32}P is given at first. After 10 to 12 weeks, if symptomatic and hematologic improvement are inadequate, a second, usually smaller dose is administered. Sometimes another venesection or two may be needed. Subsequent therapy is "titrated" according to need, but intervals between injections should not be shorter than 10 weeks, and leukocyte and platelet counts should be included in the blood examinations as guides in avoiding marrow hypoplasia from overdosage. Remissions of 6 to 15 months are common, but much longer ones are not unusual. In spite of its probable leukemogenic effect, ^{32}P therapy has greatly reduced the morbidity associated with polycythemia vera and lengthened survival. By combining the use of venesections and the conservative use of ^{32}P, the danger of the patient's developing leukemia may be minimized.

Agents such as chlorambucil and busulfan also have been shown to be effective in the treatment of erythremia. However, they require more frequent examinations of the patient's blood than is the case with radioactive phosphorus. Furthermore, alkylating agents are mutagenic and can produce chromosomal derangement. It remains to be seen whether their long-term use will result in a lower rate of occurrence of acute leukemia than is now the case, or whether survival will be equivalent to that achieved with radioactive phosphorus.

REFERENCES

LAWRENCE JH: The nature and treatment of polycythemia. Medicine 32:323, 1953; Am J Med Sci 233:268, 1957; Ann Intern Med 70:763, 1969

MODAN B, LILIENFELD AM: Polycythemia vera and leukemia—The role of radiation treatment. Medicine 44:305, 1965

——, MODAN M: Benign erythrocytosis. Br J Haematol 14:375, 1968

OSGOOD EE: Polycythemia vera: Age relationships and survival. Blood 26:243, 1965

WINTROBE MM et al: *Clinical Hematology*, 7th ed., Philadelphia: Lea & Febiger, 1974

312 METHEMOGLOBINEMIA AND SULFHEMOGLOBINEMIA

GEORGE E. CARTWRIGHT

METHEMOGLOBINEMIA

The iron in the hemoglobin molecule is normally in the reduced or ferrous state (Fe^{++}), whether bound to oxygen or carbon dioxide or unbound. When reduced hemoglobin is oxidized, the iron is converted to the ferric state (Fe^{3+}) and methemoglobin is formed.

$$HbFe^{++} + H_2O_2 \rightleftharpoons 2HbFe^{3+}\ OH$$

Methemoglobin is formed continuously in the erythrocyte and exists in equilibrium with reduced hemoglobin. Normally about 99 percent of the hemoglobin is in the reduced state and only 1 percent is oxidized. Since methemoglobin is incapable of binding oxygen or carbon dioxide, erythrocytes must of necessity possess mechanisms for maintaining hemoglobin in the reduced state. These mechanisms require energy and, therefore, are dependent on the metabolism of glucose.

The first and most important mechanism employs reduced nicotinamide adenine dinucleotide ($NADH_2$) ("DPNH"), formed from the oxidation of glucose, as the electron donor. Methemoglobin is reduced by $NADH_2$ in the presence of the $NADH_2$-dependent enzyme, methemoglobin reductase (diaphorase enzyme) (MR-E).

$$1/2 \text{ glucose} + NAD \rightarrow \text{pyruvate} + NADH_2$$

$$NADH_2 + HbFe^{3+} \xrightarrow{\text{MR-E}} NAD + HbFe^{++}$$

A second mechanism for reducing hemoglobin is provided by the generation of reduced nicotinamide adenine dinucleotide phosphate ($NADPH_2$) ("TPNH"). When glucose 6-phosphate (G-6-P) is metabolized to 6-phosphogluconate (6-PG) by glucose 6-phosphate dehydrogenase (G-6-PD) in the first step in the pentose-phosphate pathway, $NADPH_2$ is produced. Methemoglobin is then reduced by the $NADPH_2$-dependent enzyme methemoglobin reductase (MR-E) in the presence of a cofactor (CoF). Methylene blue can substitute for the cofactor in the electron transfer system, and the activity of this pathway is enhanced greatly by the addition of methylene blue (MB).

$$\text{G-6-P} + NADP \xrightarrow{\text{G-6-PD}} \text{6-PG} + NADPH_2$$

$$NADPH_2 + HbFe^{3+} \xrightarrow[\text{COF or MB}]{\text{MR-E}} NADP + HbFe^{++}$$

A third mechanism for maintaining hemoglobin in the reduced state is through the glutathione pathway. $NADPH_2$ in the presence of glutathione reductase (GR) reduces oxidized glutathione (GSSG) to reduced glutathione (GSH). Reduced glutathione, in the presence of glutathione peroxidase (GP), is capable of destroying oxidant compounds such as hydrogen peroxide (H_2O_2) which have the capability of oxidizing hemoglobin.

$$NADPH + GSSG \xrightarrow{\text{GR}} NADP + GSH$$

$$GSH + H_2O_2 \xrightarrow{\text{GR}} GSSG + H_2O$$

Under physiologic conditions, it is the $NADH_2$-dependent pathway which plays the major part in methemoglobin reduction. When the cells are exposed to excess oxidant compounds, the $NADPH_2$-dependent pathway, the glutathione pathway, and catalase, in addition to the $NADH_2$-dependent pathway, all may play a significant part in regulating the levels of methemoglobin in erythrocytes.

ETIOLOGY The known causes of methemoglobinemia are listed in Table 312-1. Methemoglobinemia may be either inherited or acquired.

Hereditary methemoglobinemia due to a deficiency of the $NADH_2$-dependent methemoglobin reductase enzyme (*diaphorase*) is transmitted as an autosomal recessive trait. The disorder may be due to a deficiency of the enzyme or to the synthesis of an abnormal enzymic protein with reduced activity. A number of electrophoretic variants have been described, some with and some without functional abnormalities.

Individuals homozygous for the trait are completely lacking in the enzymic activity, and in them 5 to 60 percent of the hemoglobin is present as methemoglobin. The rate at which hemoglobin is reduced is greatly impaired. The cyanosis is manifest at birth; life expectancy is probably not affected adversely in most cases. The patients are "more blue than sick." Mental retardation and other manifestations of central nervous system involvement have been observed in some patients. Whether this is coincidental or related to the disease has not been established.

Individuals heterozygous for the trait have about half the normal activity of the enzyme and 98 to 99 percent of the hemoglobin is in the reduced state. Such persons have an increased susceptibility to methemoglobin-producing drugs and chemicals and when given these substances may develop cyanosis. Methemoglobinemia provoked by malarial chemoprophylaxis has been described in heterozygotes.

Patients with a hereditary deficiency of erythrocyte $NADPH_2$-dependent methemoglobin reductase and with a deficiency of erythrocyte glutathione have been described, but in neither of these conditions has methemoglobinemia been found.

Hereditary methemoglobinemia associated with an abnormal hemoglobin (HbM) is transmitted as an autosomal dominant trait. At least 12 different M hemoglobins have been described. Those which have been fully characterized are listed in Table 312-1. In these diseases, the formation of methemoglobin is due to decreased oxygen affinity or binding capacity, as discussed earlier (Chap. 307), not to a slow rate of methemoglobin reduction. The hemoglobin Ms with an α chain anomaly are associated with cyanosis, which is present at birth. The patients are otherwise asymptomatic, and life expectancy is not impaired. In patients with a β chain anomaly, cyanosis is absent at birth; it does not appear until HbF disappears; and it is frequently accompanied by a mild hemolytic anemia and splenomegaly.

Acquired (secondary) methemoglobinemia is more common than hereditary methemoglobinemia and is caused by contact with certain drugs and chemicals (Table 312-1). These agents preferentially oxidize hemoglobin and, in sufficient amounts, overcome the normal reducing mechanism of the *erythrocytes*. When exposure to the offending drug ceases, the methemoglobin is rapidly converted to the reduced compound and the cyanosis disappears.

TABLE 312-1
Causes of methemoglobinemia

I Hereditary
- *A* Enzymatic
  - *1* $NADH_2$-methemoglobin reductase deficiency (recessive)
  - *2* Others (?)
- *B* Hemoglobin M disease (dominant)*
  - *1* HbM_{Boston} ($\alpha_2^{58\ tyr}\beta_2$)
  - *2* HbM_{Iwate} ($\alpha_2^{87\ tyr}\beta_2$)
  - *3* $HbM_{Milwaukee\text{-}1}$ ($\alpha_2\beta_2^{67\ glu}$)
  - *4* $HbM_{Hyde\ Park}$ ($\alpha_2\beta_2^{92\ tyr}$)
  - *5* $HbM_{Saskatoon}$ ($\alpha_2\beta_2^{63\ tyr}$)
  - *6* $HbM_{Freiburg}$ ($\alpha_2\beta_2^{23\ val\rightarrow 0}$)
  - *7* HbM_{Sidney} ($\alpha_2\beta_2^{67\ ala}$)

II Acquired
- *A* Nitrites
- *B* Nitrates
- *C* Chlorates
- *D* Quinones
- *E* Aminobenzenes
- *F* Nitrobenzenes
- *G* Nitrotoluenes

* *Boston = Gothenburg, Osaka, Kishunhalas; Iwate = Kankakee, Oldenburg; Hyde Park = Akita; Saskatoon = Emory, Kurume, Chicago, Radom.*

Nitrates after ingestion may be converted to nitrites by intestinal bacteria, and after absorption from the intestine they produce methemoglobin. Cases of methemoglobinemia due to nitrates or nitrites have been reported following the use of bismuth subnitrates or of ammonia or potassium nitrate, from the therapeutic use of amyl nitrite or nitroglycerin, from food high in nitrates, in infants drinking well water high in nitrates, from the inhalation of nitrous gases by arc welders, and from corning syrup. Aniline dyes may produce methemoglobinemia by penetration of the intact skin. Contact with dyed blankets, laundry marks on diapers, and freshly dyed shoes has produced methemoglobinemia. The ingestion by children of certain red wax crayons containing *p*-nitroaniline has resulted in methemoglobinemia. Certain sulfonamides, such as sulfanilamide, Prontosil, sulfathiazole, and sulfapyridine, but not sulfadiazine or sulfamerazine, produce the condition.

The commonly used analgesic and antipyretic drugs, acetanilid and phenacetin, are aniline derivatives and frequently the cause of methemoglobinemia and sulfhemoglobinemia. Drug abuse with these compounds is not uncommon. Patients ingesting these compounds daily are not infrequently neurotic and complain of headaches, constipation, abdominal pain, or a multitude of other symptoms. Drug use may be denied, and in such cases it is necessary to examine the urine for drug metabolites. The older concept of "enterogenous cyanosis," implying that methemoglobinemia and sulfhemoglobinemia can be produced by intestinal dysfunction alone, can best be explained by analgesic drug ingestion.

CLINICAL MANIFESTATIONS When as little as 1.5 g methemoglobin is present in 100 ml blood, recognizable cyanosis results. In contrast, as discussed earlier (Chap. 29), about 5 g reduced hemoglobin must be present before a comparable degree of cyanosis occurs. Since methemoglobin is incapable of combining with oxygen, the symptoms of methemoglobinemia are attributable to the hypoxia produced by the lowered oxygen capacity of the blood. The severity of the symptoms is related to the quantity of methemoglobin present, the rapidity with which the methemoglobinemia develops, and the capacity of the patient's cardiorespiratory and hematopoietic systems to adjust to the hypoxia. In general, levels of less than 20 percent methemoglobin are usually not associated with symptoms. At levels of 20 to 50 percent, fatigue, weakness, dyspnea, tachycardia, headaches, and dizziness may occur. Only rarely is enough methemoglobin present to cause coma and death.

DIAGNOSIS Methemoglobinemia should be suspected in any patient with cyanosis, particularly if physical examination fails to reveal evidence of cardiovascular or pulmonary disease and if the cyanosis is not promptly relieved by oxygen therapy. If blood withdrawn from the vein shows the characteristic chocolate-brown coloration, the diagnosis of an abnormal pigment is almost certain, especially if the color remains after shaking the blood in air.

A family history of cyanosis suggests the hereditary form of the disease; a recent history of exposure to drugs or chemicals suggests the acquired form. The inherited forms which are due to enzymic causes can be differentiated by specific techniques. The diagnosis of the hemoglobin M disorders can be established by starch block electrophoresis (pH 7.0 to 7.2) of hemolysates and by spectrophotometric absorption analysis.

Methemoglobin (other than M hemoglobins) may be differentiated from sulfhemoglobin by examining a 1:10 or 1:100 aqueous dilution of blood in a hand spectroscope. The absorption band of methemoglobin (630 nm) may be confused with that of sulfhemoglobin (618 nm), but on the addition of 2 or 3 drops of 5% potassium cyanide the band due to methemoglobin disappears, whereas the sulfhemoglobin band is unchanged. The addition of hydrogen peroxide causes dissolution of the sulfhemoglobin band, but not of the methemoglobin band.

TREATMENT It is not necessary to treat most patients with *hereditary* methemoglobinemia. However, therapy may be required in the severe cases or in the milder cases for the relief of minor symptoms or for cosmetic purposes. The reducing agent ascorbic acid may be given daily by mouth in an amount of 100 to 500 mg. Methylene blue accelerates the reduction of methemoglobin and is effective in a daily dose of 100 to 300 mg by mouth. These agents are of no value in alleviating the cyanosis due to hemoglobin M.

In most patients with mild *drug-induced* methemoglobinemia no therapy is necessary other than removal of the offending agent, since the methemoglobin is reduced rapidly as a result of the intact normal reconversion mechanism. In those patients in whom therapy is necessary, methylene blue, 1 to 2 mg per kg body weight given intravenously over a 5-min period in a 1 percent solution, is the agent of choice. If cyanosis has not disappeared within an hour, a second dose of 2 mg per kg body weight should be given. The total dose should not exceed 7 mg per kg, since toxic effects such as dyspnea, precordial pain, restlessness, apprehension, a sense of oppression, and fibrillar tremors may occur.

SULFHEMOGLOBINEMIA

Sulfhemoglobin is a hemoglobin derivative of unknown composition which is not found in erythrocytes under normal circumstances. Once it has formed it cannot be converted to hemoglobin. The abnormal derivative remains in the erythrocytes until they are destroyed.

Sulfhemoglobinemia may result when one of the oxidizing drugs listed in Table 312-1 has been taken. Phenacetin (A.P.C., Empirin Compound, Stanback) and acetanilid (Bromo Seltzer) are the drugs found most frequently to be the causative agents.

Sulfhemoglobin is inert as an oxygen carrier, and when it is present intense cyanosis results. Somewhat less than 0.5 g sulfhemoglobin per 100 ml blood causes a degree of cyanosis equal to that of 1.5 g methemoglobin or 5 g reduced hemoglobin. Although the concentration of sulfhemoglobin may be found to be as high as 10 g per 100 ml, the life of the patient is not endangered and symptoms which can be attributed to the sulfhemoglobinemia are rarely present. Since many of the patients in whom sulfhemoglobinemia develops are neurotic or are taking drugs for a chronic headache or constipation, the symptoms which can be elicited are probably not attributable to the sulfhemoglobinemia. Symptoms of bromide intoxication frequently complicate the clinical picture in those ingesting Bromo Seltzer. Once formed, there is no way of removing the sulfhemoglobin except by phlebotomy. In time the affected red corpuscles wear out and are destroyed. Treatment requires interdiction of the offending drug.

Rare cases of acquired hemolytic anemia with paroxysmal sulfhemoglobinemia and methemoglobinemia have been reported, and there is one reported instance of congenital sulfhemoglobinemia.

REFERENCES

AZEN EA et al: Obscure hemolytic anemia due to analgesic abuse. Does enterogenous cyanosis exist? Am J Med 48:724, 1970

FINCH CA: Methemoglobinemia and sulfhemoglobinemia. N Engl J Med 239:470, 1948

JAFFE ET, HSIEH H-S: DPNH-methemoglobin reductase deficiency and hereditary methemoglobinemia. Semin Hematol 8:417, 1971

SHIBATA S et al: Hemoblogin M's of the Japanese. Bull Yamaguchi Med Sch 14:141, 1967

313
DISORDERS OF PLATELETS

T. C. BITHELL
M. M. WINTROBE

Disorders of platelets may be conveniently divided into *quantitative forms*, i.e., those characterized by a reduced or an excessive number of platelets (the thrombocytopenias and thrombocytoses), and the *qualitative forms*, in which the platelets are normal in number but functionally inadequate. All these disorders are manifested clinically by purpura (Chap. 59), and are frequently referred to by the terms *thrombocytopenic* and *nonthrombocytopenic purpuras*. The latter term includes platelet dysfunction, to be discussed below, and disorders due to vascular abnormalities (Chap. 314).

THROMBOCYTOPENIA

Thrombocytopenia is the most common cause of abnormal bleeding, and may result from three pathophysiologic mechanisms: (1) accelerated platelet destruction, (2) deficient platelet production, and (3) abnormal pooling or distribution of platelets within the body. The numerous etiologic factors which may produce thrombocytopenia by each of these mechanisms are summarized in Table 313-1.

ACCELERATED PLATELET DESTRUCTION

IDIOPATHIC THROMBOCYTOPENIC PURPURA

Idiopathic thrombocytopenic purpura (ITP, purpura hemorrhagica) refers to instances of thrombocytopenia in which no etiologic factor is apparent. This disorder is most common in females and in children and young adults, and often develops following an acute infection.

Etiology and pathogenesis There is accumulating evidence that in most cases ITP is due to accelerated platelet destruction as the result of an immunologic process. Evidence for this hypothesis is provided by the following observations: (1) Platelets disappear from the circulation of patients with ITP with extraordinary rapidity. (2) This is the result of a process extrinsic to the platelet since normal isologous platelets survive no longer than those of the patient. (3) Platelet destruction is caused by a humoral substance, because the plasma of patients with this disease produces thrombocytopenia when injected into normal recipients, and the placental transfer of this humoral factor produces thrombocytopenia in infants born of affected mothers. These effects closely resemble those produced by the infusion of plasma containing clearly defined platelet antibodies. (4) In most cases, the "thrombocytopenic factor" in plasma is identifiable as an IgG immunoglobulin.

The nature of the "immunizing event" leading to ITP remains obscure, and the demonstration of platelet antibodies by serologic methods has proved difficult. The most sensitive techniques have yielded positive results in approximately 70 percent of cases, but they are of limited diagnostic value because of the frequency of falsely positive and falsely negative reactions. These difficulties may reflect the exquisite sensitivity of the platelet to immunologic injury. Thus, minute amounts of drug-induced autoantibodies, discussed below, which are undetectable in vitro by the most sensitive serologic tests, may lead to platelet sensitization and sequestration in vivo. Alternatively, it is possible that incomplete or blocking antibodies, similar to those found in isoimmune thrombocytopenia, or antigen-antibody complexes, are involved in the pathogenesis of ITP.

The bone marrow findings and the therapeutic effectiveness of splenectomy in ITP also are consistent with the autoimmune hypothesis. Thus, the spleen is responsible for the removal of damaged platelets, and also may be important in ITP as a site of antibody synthesis. Platelet antibodies also may damage the megakaryocyte and thereby lead to deficient platelet production, but this

TABLE 313-1
Pathophysiologic classification of thrombocytopenia

I Accelerated platelet destruction
- *A* Due to immunologic processes
  - *1* Autoantibodies
    - *a* ITP and related syndromes
    - *b* Drugs:
      - Acetazolamide (Diamox)
      - Allylisopropylcarbamide (Sedormid) and congeners
      - Antazoline
      - Carbamazepine
      - Chlorothiazides
      - Chlorpropamide (Diabenese)
      - Desipramine
      - Digitoxin
      - Diphenylhydantoin (Dilantin)
      - Gold salts
      - Hydroxychloroquin
      - Methyldopa
      - Novobiocin
      - Organic arsenicals
      - *p*-Aminosalicylic acid (PAS)
      - Quinidine
      - Quinine
      - Rifamycin
      - Stibophen (Fuadin)
      - Sulfamethazine
      - Sulfathiazole
    - *c* Miscellaneous (hemolytic anemias; systemic lupus erythematosus, lymphoreticular disorders, hyperthyroidism)
  - *2* Isoantibodies (fetal-maternal incompatibility; following transfusions)
  - *3* Other immunologic processes (allergies, erythroblastosis fetalis, anaphylactic reactions, some infections)
- *B* Due to nonimmunologic processes
  - *1* Diffuse intravascular coagulation (Table 315-1) [Kasabach-Merritt syndrome (giant hemangioendotheliomas); many infections]
  - *2* Microangiopathic processes (thrombotic thrombocytopenic purpura; prosthetic cardiac valves; many others)
  - *3* Miscellaneous (massive transfusions and exchange transfusions, extracorporeal circulatory devices, fibrinogenolysis, ristocetin, some infections)

II Deficient platelet production
- *A* Hypoplasia or suppression of megakaryocytes
  - *1* Chemical and physical agents
    - *a* Those which produce generalized bone marrow suppression (Table 309-1)
    - *b* Those which selectively suppress the megakaryocyte (chlorothiazides, tolbutamide, ethanol)
  - *2* Bone marrow failure (idiopathic aplastic anemia and related disorders, congenital amegakaryocytic thrombocytopenia, Fanconi syndrome, others)
  - *3* Myelophthisic processes, some viral infections
- *B* Ineffective thrombopoiesis (disorders due to deficiency of vitamin B_{12} or folic acid; paroxysmal nocturnal hemoglobinuria; some hereditary forms; others)
- *C* Disordered control mechanisms (deficiency of thrombopoietin, tidal platelet dysgenesis, cyclic thrombocytopenia)
- *D* Miscellaneous (many hereditary forms)

III Abnormal platelet distribution or pooling
- *A* Splenomegaly (neoplastic, congestive, infiltrative, infectious, of unknown etiology)
- *B* Hypothermic anesthesia

appears to be of minor importance in the production of thrombocytopenia. The morphologic changes observed in the megakaryocytes in this syndrome, previously attributed to a suppressive or injurious effect of the spleen, appear to be the result of compensatory acceleration of platelet production, since similar changes are found in the marrow of normal human beings and animals rendered thrombocytopenic by plasmapheresis.

It is possible that in some cases autoantibodies may damage the vascular endothelium as well, but direct evidence for this hypothesis is lacking.

There is much to suggest that ITP is a syndrome which may arise in a number of different ways. Although platelet antibodies are probably present in many cases, it is possible that mechanisms still unrecognized are operative in others.

Clinical manifestations ITP provides the prototype of purpuric bleeding. The lesions may range from the size of a pinpoint or slightly larger (petechiae) to much bigger areas (ecchymoses). Mucosal hemorrhage is common and sometimes severe. Menorrhagia may be the chief complaint and the only prominent clinical sign. Epistaxis is particularly common. Bleeding may occur into any tissue and from any orifice, and slow, continuous oozing is frequently noted following surgical procedures or injuries. This is in contrast with the rapid and voluminous posttraumatic bleeding which is characteristic of the disorders resulting from abnormalities in the process of coagulation (Chap. 315).

Fever of mild degree may be present in acute cases. The spleen may extend a fingerbreadth below the costal margin but usually is not palpable. There is no lymphadenopathy, hepatomegaly, or sternal tenderness.

ITP may begin abruptly and disappear just as suddenly; alternatively its manifestations may seem to have been present a long time. The bleeding may be mild with only a few inconspicuous petechiae; or it may be severe and lead to serious blood loss or to hemorrhage into vital areas, such as the brain or the diaphragm. All variations between these extremes may be encountered.

The clinical features of acute postinfectious ITP in children are distinctive in several respects; namely, there is no sex predilection, and spontaneous remissions may be expected in over 80 percent of cases. In contrast, the disorder in adults seldom develops following an infection, and is much more common in women than in men. In adult cases, a chronic fluctuating clinical course is characteristic, and spontaneous remissions are uncommon.

Laboratory diagnosis Examination of the blood may reveal anemia, which is proportional to the amount of blood lost. If there has been significant acute bleeding, signs of accelerated erythropoiesis (reticulocytosis, polychromatophilia, even occasional nucleated red blood cells) and a moderate leukocytosis with slight "shift to the left" will be found. In some chronic cases, lymphocytosis has been observed. The few platelets which may be seen in the blood smear often are large and morphologically abnormal.

In the bone marrow, the number of megakaryocytes is normal or increased. Immature and morphologically abnormal forms may be seen, and in contrast to the normal picture, a few or no platelets are found about their margins. However, these findings are not diagnostic of ITP, and the primary value of bone marrow examination in this disorder is to exclude the common causes of secondary thrombocytopenia, e.g., acute leukemia, myelophthisic processes.

The bleeding time is prolonged, whereas the coagulation time, prothrombin time, partial thromboplastin time, and other tests of blood coagulation are normal. Thrombocytopenia may be confirmed by a positive tourniquet test, impaired clot retraction, and an abnormal prothrombin consumption test, but these tests are not required and are rarely helpful.

Differential diagnosis The diagnosis of ITP is one of exclusion, and the numerous other causes of thrombocytopenia must be considered (Table 313-1). The history, physical examination, and bone marrow aspirate will serve to rule out many of these conditions. Lymphadenopathy, hepatosplenomegaly, and sternal tenderness, as well as anemia out of proportion to the blood loss, even in the absence of striking changes in the leukocytes, should suggest leukemia. Persistent leukopenia suggests leukemia, aplastic anemia, sequestration in the spleen, or disseminated lupus erythematosus. The last-named disorder may be characterized by persistent thrombocytopenia for months or years before other characteristic manifestations appear. Purpuric lesions must be differentiated from telangiectases and small angiomas (Table 314-1).

A prolonged bleeding time may rarely be found in various coagulation disorders, including hemophilia (Chap. 315), but is characteristic of von Willebrand's disease and various disorders of platelet function. The platelet count is normal in all these disorders, which may be further distinguished from ITP by various ancillary tests (Chaps. 59 and 315).

Treatment An initial period of *expectant management* is usually recommended because spontaneous remissions are common. Such remissions may be complete and permanent, and are especially likely to occur in children, if the onset of the disorder was acute and followed an infection. Unfortunately the danger of bleeding into a vital organ such as the brain makes the waiting period a trying one. Recurrences are twice as common in females as in males. Splenectomy is indicated in cases in which spontaneous remission has not occurred after 6 or more months observation, and the clinical manifestations are moderate or severe.

Administration of *corticosteroids* often produces a significant increase in the platelet count, and a decrease in the severity of the bleeding phenomena. These effects are likely to be transitory; these hormones alone produce complete remissions in only 30 percent of patients. Corticosteroids are nevertheless widely used as the initial therapeutic measure in ITP. They also are valuable in the preoperative preparation of patients for splenectomy, and in the treatment of patients in whom splenectomy has proved ineffective. Those which can be given orally are preferred, e.g., 20 to 60 mg prednisone per day, in divided doses.

Splenectomy results in "cure" in at least two-thirds of patients, and remains the ultimate therapeutic procedure of choice in ITP. Even when splenectomy is not followed by complete recovery, some increase in platelet numbers may be expected. Bleeding often diminishes even though the platelet count may not have increased greatly.

The operation is not indicated early in the first episode of ITP, especially in children, since spontaneous recovery is common, and, according to some authorities, not in acute fulminating cases, in which surgical mortality is high. However, others consider this to be an indication for emergency splenectomy, and the question must be considered unsettled. Although the evidence is not conclusive, the hazards of infection following splenectomy favor postponement of this operation in infants and in young children.

The hazards of splenectomy outweigh the adverse effects of corticosteroids in pregnant women, and these hormones should be used and splenectomy avoided if at all possible in the management of ITP in the pregnant patient. Claims that splenectomy causes "dissemination" of unrecognized lupus erythematosus have not been substantiated.

In chronic cases of ITP, if neither corticosteroid therapy nor splenectomy has been helpful, and if bleeding manifestations are sufficiently troublesome, a cautious trial of an immunosuppressive agent may be justified.

Supportive therapy, in addition to appropriate nursing care, includes transfusions if blood loss has been severe, and iron if indicated. Platelet transfusions are of limited therapeutic value in ITP because of the short platelet life span in this disorder. Nevertheless, the administration of platelet concentrates may be valuable in the preparation of the patient for surgery if bleeding is severe, and in the treatment of life-threatening hemorrhage, e.g., subarachnoid bleeding.

DRUG-INDUCED PLATELET ANTIBODIES Thrombocytopenia due to drug-induced platelet autoantibodies is rare, and like many other drug-induced blood dyscrasias, appears to be a manifestation of individual idiosyncrasy. Among the drugs which may induce the formation of such antibodies (Table 313-1), quinidine and quinine are by far the most frequently involved. Many other drugs not listed in Table 313-1 have been associated with thrombocytopenia, but in the reported cases serologic evidence for the presence of platelet antibodies was not convincing. It is nevertheless probable that many of these drugs produce thrombocytopenia by means of an immunologic mechanism.

The antibodies may be demonstrated by various serologic techniques, including platelet agglutination, complement fixation, and antiglobulin tests. The mechanisms by which these drugs provoke platelet antibodies are as yet unclear. Most evidence suggests that the drug acts as a hapten, and that the antibody is not directed against an intrinsic platelet antigen. These observations have led to the hypothesis (the "innocent bystander" hypothesis) that the platelet suffers immunologic injury as the result of its "spongelike" tendency to absorb drug-antibody complexes.

In thrombocytopenia due to drug-induced platelet antibodies, fulminant bleeding may develop rapidly when a sensitized person has been given the offending drug, but the platelet count will usually rise promptly when the drug is stopped. Splenectomy is contraindicated, and therapeutic measures are limited to the prohibition of potentially toxic agents and to supportive care.

MISCELLANEOUS IMMUNOLOGIC THROMBOCYTOPENIAS Thrombocytopenia in the newborn may result from the placental transfer of platelet antibodies. Such *congenital immunologic thrombocytopenia* may arise from the active immunization of the mother by fetal platelet isoantigens, or from the passive transfer of autoantibodies present in the maternal circulation as the result of various disorders, for example, ITP. In affected neonates, bleeding is seldom severe and thrombocytopenia usually is self-limited.

Isoantibodies may also form following repeated transfusions of incompatible platelets. Many of these antibodies are of the incomplete or blocking type. They may lead to the destruction of transfused platelets at an abnormally rapid rate, a process which eventually limits the therapeutic usefulness of platelet transfusions (Chap. 310). Rarely, isoantibodies formed following transfusion may act as autoantibodies and produce severe thrombocytopenia. The explanation of this curious phenomenon remains obscure.

Thrombocytopenia in association with *systemic lupus erythematosus*, various autoimmune hemolytic anemias, chronic lymphocytic leukemia, and other lymphoreticular disorders may be caused by autoantibodies, and resembles ITP in most respects.

NONIMMUNOLOGIC PLATELET DESTRUCTION

Intravascular coagulation (Table 315-1) is a common cause of thrombocytopenia. Thrombocytopenia in association with *giant hemangioendotheliomas* (Kasabach-Merritt syndrome) is relatively uncommon but is of unusual interest in that these vascular tumors appear to act as abnormal sequestering sites for platelets, and frequently produce either localized or disseminated intravascular coagulation. In the bleeding which may be associated with heat stroke, massive burns, and snake bites, thrombocytopenia appears to be but one facet of a more generalized bleeding diathesis, which may also involve intravascular coagulation.

Thrombotic thrombocytopenic purpura usually is a fulminating disorder with fever, hemolytic anemia of the microangiopathic type, migratory neurologic signs and symptoms, and renal involvement. The basic lesion is a vasculitis which leads to mechanical damage to erythrocytes and the utilization of platelets in diffuse microthrombi. Occlusions are found in terminal arterioles and capillaries of all organs of the body. On the basis of limited experiences, splenectomy and the administration of adrenocorticosteroids and of heparin intravenously have been advocated, but there is as yet no treatment of proved effectiveness. Various other forms of microangiopathic hemolytic anemia also may be associated with thrombocytopenia, e.g., the hemolytic uremic syndrome, prosthetic cardiac devices (Chap. 306).

Thrombocytopenia due to mechanical platelet damage is a predictable result of surgical procedures which employ extracorporeal circulatory devices. The transfusion of massive amounts of stored blood containing no viable platelets also produces thrombocytopenia, presumably as the result of a "washout" phenomenon. In both cases, thrombocytopenia is seldom severe, and rarely is associated with bleeding.

DEFICIENT PLATELET PRODUCTION

Many *drugs and chemicals* produce thrombocytopenia by suppressing platelet production. Those which are commonly associated with generalized bone marrow suppression are summarized in Table 309-1 and discussed in Chap. 309. Others may be associated with isolated thrombocytopenia, in the absence of platelet antibodies or other evidence of generalized bone marrow suppression. Evidence implicating many of these drugs is circumstantial. In the case of ethanol and some chlorothiazides, thrombocytopenia appears to result from selective suppression of the megakaryocytes.

Thrombocytopenia due to deficient platelet production is common in disorders characterized by bone marrow failure and in the *myelophthisic processes.* These disorders, together with others which are characterized by pancytopenia, are discussed in Chap. 309.

Thrombocytopenia is common in the megaloblastic anemias, e.g., pernicious anemia. In this, and in related disorders, platelet production is deficient despite a marked increase in the number of megakaryocytes. This abnormality, termed *ineffective thrombopoiesis*, is similar to that which impairs erythropoiesis in these disorders (Chap. 305).

Rarely, abnormalities in the processes which normally regulate thrombopoiesis may give rise to deficient platelet production, e.g., cyclic thrombocytopenia, tidal platelet dysgenesis, deficiency of "thrombopoietin."

MISCELLANEOUS THROMBOCYTOPENIAS Numerous disorders, which span the entire field of medicine, may be associated with thrombocytopenia ("symptomatic" thrombocytopenias). The pathophysiology of thrombocytopenia in many of these diseases is poorly understood, and a detailed discussion of each is beyond the scope of the present chapter.

Infectious diseases, ranging from mild viral exanthems to serious rickettsial infections, are common causes of thrombocytopenia. Viruses may infest the precursor megakaryocyte and impair platelet production, or may damage the circulating platelet leading to its sequestration. Antigen-antibody complexes of either bacterial or viral origin, as well as various bacterial toxins, also may damage platelets. In serious bleeding (purpura fulminans) associated with fulminant bacterial infections such as meningococcemia (Chap. 131) and gram-negative septicemia (Chap. 124), thrombocytopenia apparently is the result of intravascular coagulation (Chap. 315).

The *hereditary and congenital thrombocytopenias* are relatively rare. Both shortened platelet survival and deficient platelet production are present in many of these, and additional, qualitative abnormalities of platelet function also are commonly associated. In the Wiskott-Aldrich syndrome (Chap. 64), thrombocytopenia is associated with recurrent infections and a fatal termination in early life. Congenital *amegakaryocytic thrombocytopenia* is characterized by hypoplasia of the bone marrow precursors as well as by various congenital abnormalities such as agenesis of the radii. Thrombocytopenia is one feature of the May-Hegglin anomaly (Chap. 61). Other varieties of hereditary thrombocytopenia are characterized by strikingly large and morphologically abnormal platelets.

In disorders characterized by *splenomegaly*, moderate thrombocytopenia may result from platelet pooling within the abnormally enlarged spleen, although the total platelet mass may be normal. Splenic sequestration may also explain thrombocytopenia associated with *hypothermic anesthesia.*

THROMBOCYTOSIS

Like thrombocytopenia, thrombocytosis may result from various inflammatory, neoplastic, and hematopoietic disorders. In such disorders ("secondary" or reactive thrombocytosis), the elevated platelet count is significant mainly because of its diagnostic implications. Thus, in rheumatoid arthritis and ulcerative colitis, the platelet count may provide a good index of the activity of the underlying disease. In other cases, thrombocytosis may provide a valuable clue to the presence of an occult disease, e.g., various carcinomas, Hodgkin's disease. Thrombocytosis may persist for several weeks following splenectomy.

Thrombocythemia (primary, essential, or hemorrhagic thrombocythemia) is an uncommon disorder, characterized by hyperplasia of the megakaryocytes, accelerated platelet production, and very high platelet counts. In this condition, platelet production apparently is unresponsive to normal control mechanisms, and is thus said to be *autonomous*. The disorder may be related to the myeloproliferative syndromes (Chap. 317), and is difficult to distinguish from cases of polycythemia vera with markedly elevated platelet counts. Thrombocythemia is manifested clinically by the paradox of thromboembolic complications and recurrent bleeding. Platelet dysfunction appears to be the major cause of hemorrhage. Splenomegaly and neutrophilic leukocytosis are commonly present. Therapy with ^{32}P-phosphate or antimitotic drugs is usually effective in lowering the platelet count. Anticoagulants and thrombocytophoresis may be valuable therapeutic adjuncts in some cases.

DISORDERS OF PLATELET FUNCTION

The disorders of platelet function are characterized by a prolonged bleeding time and frequently by morphologically abnormal platelets. The platelet count and the results of various tests of blood coagulation are normal. Numerous varieties have been reported, but only a few have been adequately characterized.

THROMBOASTHENIA (GLANZMANN'S DISEASE)

This term refers to a disorder of platelet function which is inherited as an autosomal recessive trait and is characterized by diminished clot retraction and deficient platelet aggregation. Platelets of affected patients do not aggregate in the presence of ADP. As a consequence, platelet aggregation induced by agents which trigger the release of platelet-contained ADP also is deficient. This "total" failure of aggregation results in deficient platelet adhesion to glass, and may explain the associated deficiencies in platelet factor 3 activity as well as the absence of clot retraction. The major pathophysiologic defect in this syndrome appears to reside in the platelet membrane, possibly in the content or reactivity of its contractile proteins (thrombosthenin).

In contrast to most disorders of platelet function, bleeding in thromboasthenia may be incapacitating. Petechiae are uncommon, but spontaneous bruising may be marked. Postoperative hemorrhage also is a significant hazard. Transfusion of normal isologous platelets may be therapeutic; otherwise treatment is supportive.

DEFICIENT RELEASE REACTION (THROMBOPATHIA, "PORTSMOUTH" SYNDROME) This term refers to a group of disorders of platelet function characterized by a deficiency of platelet nucleotides, or a metabolic abnormality which impairs the mechanisms by which such nucleotides are extruded from the platelet during the release reaction (Chap. 59). In vitro, platelet aggregation is normal in the presence of ADP, but it is deficient when induction of aggregation is attempted by the use of agents which normally release platelet-contained nucleotides, e.g., epinephrine, collagen fibers. Clot retraction is normal, but platelet factor 3 activity is variably deficient. Hereditary forms have been described, but the disorder is more commonly acquired, e.g., in association with uremia, certain myeloproliferative disorders, various dysproteinemias. It is manifested clinically by a mild hemorrhagic diathesis. Easy bruising and menorrhagia are common. There is no specific therapy.

Many *drugs*, including aspirin, produce marked impairment of the release reaction. Although it may lead to serious diagnostic confusion, the hemostatic consequences of this effect usually are minimal. However, serious bleeding may result when such drugs are administered to patients with other abnormalities of hemostasis or coagulation, e.g., hemophiliacs, patients receiving anticoagulants.

The *thrombocytopathies* are a poorly characterized group of disorders in which deficient coagulant activity of platelet phospholipids (platelet factor 3) is thought to be the major abnormality. This may be manifested by abnormal prothrombin consumption or by defective "thromboplastic" function of the platelets as measured in the thromboplastin generation test. The status of thrombocytopathy as a specific entity remains uncertain, and it is probable that in many cases the basic abnormality is a deficient release reaction.

REFERENCES

Amorosi EL, Ultmann JE: Thrombotic thrombocytopenic purpura. Medicine 45:139, 1966

Hirsh J, Doery JCG: Platelet function in health and disease. Prog Hematol 7:185, 1972

Horowitz HI, Nachman RL: Drug purpura. Semin Hematol 2:287, 1965

Oski FA, Naiman JL: *Hematologic Problems in the Newborn*, Philadelphia: Saunders, 1972

Ratnoff OD: *Bleeding Syndromes*, Springfield, Ill.: Charles C Thomas, 1960

Shulman NR et al: Similarities between known antiplatelet antibodies and the factor responsible for thrombocytopenia in idiopathic purpura. Ann NY Acad Sci 124:499, 1965

Wintrobe MM et al: *Clinical Hematology*, 7th ed., Philadelphia: Lea & Febiger, 1974

Zucker MB, Lundberg A: Platelet transfusions. Anesthesiology 27:385, 1966

314 BLEEDING DISORDERS CAUSED BY VASCULAR ABNORMALITIES

T. C. BITHELL
M. M. WINTROBE

THE VASCULAR PURPURAS

These disorders are poorly understood, and in general seldom lead to serious blood loss. Results of laboratory tests of hemostasis and blood coagulation usually are normal, and the diagnosis must usually be made from the appearance of the skin lesions and the associated clinical findings, which often are characteristic (Table 314-1).

ALLERGIC PURPURA This disorder, also called Henoch-Schönlein purpura, is characterized by serosanguinous effusions into the subcutaneous, submucous, and subserous tissues. These effusions and the resulting perivascular inflammation produce, in addition to purpura, various localized and constitutional symptoms. The pathogenesis of this disorder is obscure, although there is much indirect evidence to suggest an allergic basis. However, only in a minority of cases has an allergen been demonstrated. In some instances this appears to have been bacterial (streptococci, typhoid vaccine), while in other cases an article of food (milk, eggs, pork, strawberries, etc.) appears to have been the responsible allergen. Rarely hypersensitivity to cold has been implicated. There is considerable epidemiologic evidence which suggests a close relation between allergic purpura and acute glomerulonephritis.

Clinical manifestations This disorder is more common in children and young adults than in older persons. The *skin lesions* are variable in appearance, but purpura is usually associated with one or more of the common manifestations of allergy, such as erythema or urticaria. The lesions are usually located on the extremities, and may appear in crops. In contrast to most other purpuric lesions, they may be accompanied by itching or paresthesias. Necrotic areas, bullae, or ulcers may develop, and submucosal lesions may lead to external hemorrhage such as epistaxis or melena but serious blood loss is uncommon.

Effusions into the joints or viscera may produce

TABLE 314-1
Bleeding disorders caused by vascular abnormalities

I Autoimmune vascular purpuras
 A The allergic purpuras
 B Drug-induced vascular purpura (iodides, belladonna, atropine, quinine, procaine penicillin, phenacetin, aspirin, merbaphen, chloral hydrate and other sedatives, various sulfonamides, coumarins, others)
 C Purpura fulminans (Chap. 313 and *IIA*, below)
II Infections
 A *Bacterial* (meningococcemia and septicemia due to other organisms, typhoid fever, scarlet fever, diphtheria, tuberculosis, endocarditis, bacterial products, others)
 B *Viral* (smallpox, influenza, measles, others)
 C *Rickettsial* (Rocky Mountain spotted fever, typhus, others)
 D *Protozoal* (malaria)
III Structural malformations
 A Hereditary hemorrhagic telangiectasia
 B Hereditary disorders of connective tissue (Ehlers-Danlos syndrome, osteogenesis imperfecta, pseudoxanthoma elasticum)
 C Acquired disorders of connective tissues (scurvy, corticosteroid purpura, Cushing's disease, purpura senilis, and "cachetica")
IV Miscellaneous
 A Autoerythrocyte sensitization and related syndromes (DNA hypersensitivity, cutaneous hyperactivity to hemoglobin, psychogenic purpura, vicarious bleeding, stigmata)
 B Paraproteinemias (Chap. 65) (hyperglobulinemic purpura, cryoglobulinemic purpura, Waldenström's macroglobulinemia)
 C Purpura simplex and related disorders ("orthostatic" and "mechanical" purpura, factitious purpura)
 D Purpura in association with certain skin diseases (annular telangiectatic purpura, angioma serpiginosum, Schamberg's disease, pigmented purpuric lichenoid dermatitis)
 E Others (bloodborne tumor emboli, snake venoms, hemochromatosis, amyloidosis, other chronic diseases)

SOURCE: *MM Wintrobe et al,* Clinical Hematology, *7th ed, Philadelphia: Lea & Febiger, 1974, by permission*

various *localized symptoms.* Thus, there may be concomitant joint pain and swelling (*Schönlein's purpura*) or crises of abdominal pain (*Henoch's purpura*). In the latter form, serohemorrhagic effusion into the intestinal wall may lead to intussusception. The renal lesion consists of a glomerulitis and may result in hematuria, proteinuria, and profound though usually temporary disturbances of renal function. *Constitutional symptoms* such as fever and malaise are present in many cases.

Diagnosis The skin lesions of allergic purpura often are characteristic, and this disorder should be suspected whenever erythematous or urticarial lesions are associated with purpura. When accessible lesions are present, the diagnosis may be confirmed by skin biopsy. Serious diagnostic difficulties may arise when purpura is not obvious or is absent altogether. For example, bouts of abdominal pain accompanied by fever, leukocytosis, or melena cannot be readily distinguished from acute abdominal conditions which call for surgical intervention. Hematuria may be a prominent symptom when the kidney is involved, and is readily mistaken for acute post-streptococcal glomerulonephritis. Similarly, when joint symptoms predominate, it is easy to confuse the disease with rheumatic fever.

Examination of the *blood* may reveal modest neutrophilia or eosinophilia. Tests of hemostasis and blood coagulation are normal.

Treatment and prognosis The results of corticosteroid therapy have been equivocal or disappointing, and treatment is purely symptomatic. If an etiologic agent is discovered or suspected, further exposure should be eliminated.

Allergic purpura usually is self-limited. Individual attacks last from 1 to 6 weeks, during which the clinical manifestations may wax and wane in intensity, extent, or nature. Recurrences at intervals of months or years are not unusual, however, and in a significant proportion of patients, renal involvement may become chronic.

MISCELLANEOUS VASCULAR PURPURA A multiplicity of *drugs* may lead to striking, generalized purpuric eruptions, which subside when administration of the drug is discontinued. The pathogenesis of drug-induced vascular purpura is unclear, but the disorder is thought to be the result of an allergic reaction. *Infectious processes* too numerous to list may produce vascular purpura. This may result from direct endothelial injury by the infectious agent (e.g., some viruses, meningococci, rickettsia). In other cases, bacterial products or toxins, or autoimmune processes, may be responsible. Various hemostatic abnormalities other than vascular injury may be present in many of these cases. The purpuric manifestations of vascular injury should be distinguished from the embolic phenomena that also occur in some of these disorders, such as subacute bacterial endocarditis.

Mild purpura occasionally results from atrophy of the subcutaneous tissue (purpura cachectica and purpura senilis), skin fragility (Cushing's syndrome), hyperlaxity of the skin (Ehlers-Danlos syndrome), or degeneration of elastic tissue or collagen (pseudoxanthoma elasticum). Various *dermatologic conditions* may be associated with cutaneous hemorrhagic manifestations. These include annular telangiectatic purpura (Majocchi's disease), angioma serpiginosum, Shamberg's disease, and pigmented purpuric lichenoid dermatitis. Hemorrhagic manifestations have also been noted in cases of hemochromatosis and primary amyloidosis.

Scurvy (Chap. 79) may be associated with serious bleeding manifestations, including gingival bleeding and hemorrhage into the subcutaneous tissues, muscles, and skin, where the distribution of petechiae around hair follicles is characteristic. Subperiosteal hemorrhages may occur in children. The bleeding in scurvy is attributed to a defect in the intercellular cement and perivascular collagen of small blood vessels, and promptly ceases after the administration of ascorbic acid.

Autoerythrocyte sensitization is an uncommon disorder characterized by spontaneous painful ecchymoses surrounded by erythema and edema. Often heralded by prodromal stinging or burning, the lesions may enlarge progressively and are commonly associated with headache, nausea, and vomiting. These ecchymoses can often be produced by the intradermal injection of a small volume of autologous red blood cells or their stroma. This condition is frequently associated with striking psychoneurotic symptoms, and it has been thought that the bleeding may be psychosomatic in origin. *Hypersensitivity to DNA* and cutaneous hyperreactivity to hemoglobin are closely related disorders.

Purpura simplex is a term generally applied to instances of mild purpuric skin manifestations in otherwise healthy persons. This appears to be particularly common in women ("Devil's pinches"); a hereditary form also has been described.

HEREDITARY HEMORRHAGIC TELANGIECTASIA

This disorder is a hereditary vascular abnormality characterized by widespread telangiectases in the skin and mucous membranes. *Histologically*, there is diffuse involvement of small veins and capillaries, which are dilated, tortuous, and extremely thin, often consisting only of an endothelial layer. As a consequence, vascular support is poor and the contractility of the affected vessels is diminished. The disorder is inherited as an autosomal dominant trait of high penetrance.

Clinical manifestations The *lesions* range from pinpoint to about 3 mm in diameter, are round and bright red or violaceous in color, and characteristically blanch on pressure. They are most commonly found on the lips, tongue, and ears, and on the palmar and plantar surfaces of the fingers and toes. Although the lesions may be found in childhood, they usually increase in number and size as age advances, and in elderly patients some may become spiderlike.

The symptoms are a result of bleeding and the consequent anemia and usually become progressively more severe as age advances. Severe iron-deficiency anemia (Chap. 304) may develop. In general, telangiectases of the skin are less likely to bleed than are those of the mucous membranes. Trivial trauma may nevertheless produce profuse bleeding from superficial lesions, but significant postoperative bleeding is uncommon. Epistaxis is especially common, but bleeding may originate from telangiectases wherever they are: the face, tongue, lips, respiratory, or urinary tracts. Gastrointestinal bleeding is one of the most serious manifestations and is common after middle age. Involvement of various visceral vessels may produce symptoms. Pulmonary arteriovenous fistulas have been reported in a number of cases and may lead to hemoptyses, recurrent pulmonary infections, or significant cardiovascular symptoms (Chap. 232).

Diagnosis In the presence of the characteristic lesions and a typical family history, the diagnosis of hereditary hemorrhagic telangiectasia is not difficult. In cases in which externally visible lesions are lacking or are overlooked, perplexing diagnostic problems may result. This disorder should always be remembered in recurrent or intractable gastrointestinal bleeding of obscure cause. In such cases, visceral angiography may be helpful in diagnosis. *Laboratory* tests of blood coagulation and hemostasis are usually entirely normal.

The lesions must be differentiated from purpuric lesions (Chap. 313), spider telangiectases of liver disease, senile cherry hemangiomas, and the rare *angiokeratoma corporis diffusum universale* (CDU) or Fabry's disease (Chap. 106) (Table 314-2).

Treatment There is no effective treatment for this disorder. Blood tranfusions and the administration of iron may be indicated for the relief of anemia. Local measures

TABLE 314-2
Differentiation of hereditary hemorrhagic telangiectases from other telangiectases and small angiomas

Lesion	*Appearance*	*Distribution*	*Duration; effect of pressure*	*Associated findings*
Hereditary hemorrhagic telangiectases	Usually flat and round; red to purple, pinpoint to 3 mm in size	Centrifugal (face, lips, tongue, ears, nasal mucosa, palmar and plantar surfaces)	Permanent; blanch	Gastrointestinal bleeding, epistaxis common; pulmonary AV fistulas
Cherry angiomas	Elevated, nodular, bright red, 1–3 mm in diameter	Chest and abdomen	Permanent; do not blanch	None
Spider telangiectases	Flat or slightly raised with characteristic spider "legs"; bright red, 2–5 mm in size	Chest, clavicles, face, upper extremities	Permanent; blanch; "legs" fill from center	Liver disease, pregnancy
Angiokeratomas (Fabry's disease)	Flat to slightly raised; dark red to blue-black; pinpoint to pinhead in size; associated with cornlike lesions and subcutaneous nodules	Centripetal (mainly chest and abdomen, umbilicus); in groups	Permanent; few blanch	CNS, renal, pulmonary and myocardial disease; pain in limbs and fever in children

SOURCE: *MM Wintrobe et al,* Clinical Hematology, *7th ed, Philadelphia: Lea & Febiger, 1974, by permission*

to control the bleeding include nasal packs and the use of topical hemostatic agents and styptics, e.g., Gelfoam, thrombin. Electrocoagulation may be of temporary value in the case of accessible lesions of the skin or mucosa, but satellite lesions usually reappear nearby.

REFERENCES

RATNOFF OD: *Bleeding Syndromes*, Springfield, Ill.: Charles C Thomas, 1960

WINTROBE MM et al: *Clinical Hematology*, 7th ed., Philadelphia: Lea & Febiger, 1974

315
DISORDERS OF BLOOD COAGULATION

T. C. BITHELL
M. M. WINTROBE

A classification of the disorders of blood coagulation is presented in Table 315-1. The *hereditary disorders* are rare and usually are the result of deficiency or qualitative abnormality of a single coagulation factor. The clinical picture is dominated by profuse and often life-threatening hemorrhage from trivial injuries and by certain characteristic hemorrhagic manifestations which begin in childhood and persist throughout life. In contrast, *the acquired coagulation disorders* are common, but usually are the result of deficiencies of several coagulation factors; platelet and vascular abnormalities often are present as well and the clinical picture frequently is dominated by signs and symptoms of an underlying disease. The bleeding, with few exceptions, is seldom as severe as that encountered in the hereditary forms.

THE HEREDITARY COAGULATION DISORDERS

ETIOLOGY AND PATHOGENESIS The hereditary nature of hemophilia was recognized in antiquity. Most evidence suggests that the genetic abnormality alters the biosynthesis of a single protein which is essential in the coagulation phase of hemostasis. Because conventional methods for the study of most coagulation factors measure only their biologic activity, they do not distinguish between a deficiency of the requisite protein, i.e., a quantitative disorder, and qualitative aberrations in its structure which alter its function. In the case of fibrinogen, which can be studied directly by biochemical methods, quantitative deficiency (afibrinogenemia) and at least 10 different qualitative abnormalities of this protein (dysfibrinogenemias) have now been recognized. As with abnormal hemoglobins, qualitatively abnormal fibrinogens are designated by the name of the city in which they were discovered, e.g., fibrinogen$_{\text{Baltimore}}$, fibrinogen$_{\text{Zurich}}$. In the case of fibrinogen$_{\text{Detroit}}$, the molecular abnormality has been shown to be due to a single amino acid substitution.

Qualitative and quantitative forms of other hereditary coagulation disorders have now been demonstrated indirectly by immunologic techniques. Thus, classic hemophilia and factor XIII "deficiency" are now known to be the result of qualitative abnormalities, whereas the diminished factor VIII activity found in most patients with von Willebrand's disease is the result of a true deficiency of this protein. Both qualitative and quantitative abnormalities have been shown to be responsible for "deficiencies" of prothrombin, and factors VII, IX, and X. As yet, qualitatively abnormal forms of factors XII, XI, and V have not been demonstrated.

Since the clinical manifestations of the qualitative and quantitative forms of the hereditary coagulation disorders are the same, the term "deficiency" will be used with reference to both forms in the discussion to follow.

TABLE 315-1
A classification of disorders of blood coagulation

I Inherited disorders
- *A* Sex-linked recessive traits
  - *1* Factor VIII deficiency (classic hemophilia)
  - *2* Factor IX deficiency (Christmas disease)
- *B* Autosomal recessive traits
  - *1* Factor XI deficiency (PTA deficiency)
  - *2* Prothrombin deficiency
  - *3* Factor V deficiency (parahemophilia)
  - *4* Factor VII deficiency
  - *5* Factor X deficiency
  - *6* Fibrinogen deficiency (hereditary afibrinogenemia)
  - *7* Factor XII deficiency (Hageman trait)
  - *8* Factor XIII deficiency
- *C* Autosomal dominant traits
  - *1* Von Willebrand's disease (pseudohemophilia, vascular hemophilia)
  - *2* Congenital dysfibrinogenemias

II Acquired disorders
- *A* Deficiencies of vitamin K–dependent coagulation factors
  - *1* Liver disease
  - *2* Drugs (coumarins, indanediones; rarely salicylates, broad spectrum antibiotics)
  - *3* Hemorrhagic disease of the newborn
  - *4* Biliary tract obstruction
  - *5* Malabsorption syndromes (sprue, celiac disease)
  - *6* Dietary deficiency (rare)
- *B* Accelerated destruction of coagulation factors
  - *1* Disseminated intravascular coagulation
  - *2* Pathologic proteolysis
- *C* Abnormal inhibitors of coagulation
  - *1* Inhibitors of specific coagulation factors
  - *2* Nonspecific inhibitors (antithrombins, antithromboplastins, others)
- *D* Miscellaneous coagulation disorders
  - *1* Liver disease
  - *2* Disorders of the hematopoietic system
    - *a* Leukemia, acute and chronic
    - *b* Polycythemia vera
  - *3* The dysproteinemias (multiple myeloma, hyperglobulinemia, macroglobulinemia)
  - *4* Amyloidosis

INCIDENCE The hereditary coagulation disorders are relatively rare, the *absolute incidence* averaging only 1 in 20,000 persons. However, for the patients and their families the economic and psychosocial consequences of these disorders are very great.

The *relative incidence* of the various forms varies, depending on the particular population studied. In most large series, factor VIII deficiency (classic hemophilia) comprises approximately 80 percent, factor IX deficiency (Christmas disease) approximately 13 percent, factor XI deficiency (PTA deficiency) approximately 6 percent, and the remainder, which are exceedingly rare, total 1 percent. There is evidence for the existence of several additional hereditary coagulation disorders due to deficiencies of factors which have not yet been recognized in the international nomenclature.

GENETICS The mode of inheritance of the various hereditary coagulation disorders is seen in Table 315-1, and the details of the various genetic mechanisms involved are discussed at length elsewhere (Chap. 62). The genetics of factor VIII deficiency and factor IX deficiency are virtually identical, and provide a classic example of *sex-linked recessive inheritance* (Chap. 62, Fig. 62-11). In such disorders, the defective gene is located on the X chromosome and produces only an asymptomatic carrier state in females because of the presence of a normal allele. Since males lack a normal allele, the defect is manifested as clinical hemophilia. The Y chromosome is normal, and as a result, the affected male will not transmit the disorder to his sons, but all his daughters will be carriers of the trait. Such female carriers will transmit the disorder to one-half of their sons and the carrier state to one-half of their daughters. The carrier state cannot exist in normal males.

Thus, for practical purposes, the genetic abnormality in factor VIII and in factor IX deficiency is carried by both sexes but affects only males. The exception to this generalization, *hemophilia in the female*, is very rare, but may occur as the result of a mating between a carrier female and an affected male, a mating between a carrier female and an unaffected male who introduces a newly mutant gene, or from an abnormal complement of chromosomes.

The regularity with which the abnormal gene is suppressed by the normal allele in female carriers is somewhat variable due to the *phenomenon of X chromosome inactivation* (Chap. 62). As a result, many carrier females will have slightly lower blood levels of the deficient factor than the normal population. The detection of such carriers in the laboratory is of great practical importance, but in the case of factor VIII, the deficiency is slight and is difficult to detect except by immunologic methods which are not readily available. Female carriers of factor IX deficiency have more clear-cut deficiencies and can be more readily detected. A mild bleeding diathesis may be present in an occasional carrier female.

Approximately 30 percent of patients with hereditary coagulation disorders give a negative family history, an observation which has been ascribed to an unusually high mutation rate for the responsible gene. Consequently, although the occurrence of abnormal bleeding in family members may be of great help in diagnosis, particularly if it occurs in a characteristic pattern, *a negative family history does not exclude a hereditary coagulation disorder.*

The mode of inheritance of the disorders listed in Table 315-1 as autosomal recessive traits is not firmly established because of their extreme rarity and because of the inherent difficulty in distinguishing between a dominant trait with variable penetrance and a recessive or "intermediate" trait. In the case of the only common variety, i.e., factor XI deficiency, the study of several large kindreds has led to conflicting conclusions, the results suggesting an incompletely recessive trait in some, an autosomal dominant trait in others.

CLINICAL PICTURE The hereditary coagulation disorders produce quite similar signs and symptoms regardless of the particular factor which is deficient. Consequently, their clinical picture can conveniently by described in terms of that encountered in the commonest forms, i.e., in factor VIII and IX deficiencies and by citing at the same time important differences between this prototype and less common forms.

Undoubtedly the most dramatic manifestation of the hereditary coagulation disorders is exsanguinating hemorrhage from a *traumatic injury*. However, the most characteristic bleeding manifestations, such as hemarthrosis, often develop without significant trauma, and their frequency and severity are generally proportional to the blood levels of the deficient factor. For example, in the case of factor VIII, *severe deficiency* (factor VIII levels 0 to 1 percent of normal) is clinically manifested by repeated and severe hemarthroses which almost invariably eventuate in crippling. Hemarthrosis is uncommon, however, *in mild factor VIII deficiency* (factor VIII levels 4 to 25 percent of normal), although serious bleeding may follow surgery or traumatic injuries. A comparable correlation between the clinical picture and blood levels of the deficient factor can be made in the other hereditary coagulation disorders, although information is more limited. Most are associated with less severe bleeding manifestations than is the case in either factor VIII or IX deficiency. This is particularly true of factor XI deficiency, in which the bleeding is considerably milder, and serious hemorrhage usually occurs only after trauma or surgery.

Factor XII deficiency (Hageman trait) is not associated with a significant hemorrhagic diathesis, despite gross abnormalities in the various tests of blood coagulation. This apparent paradox is of great theoretic interest, but for practical purposes factor XII deficiency remains a laboratory curiosity.

Hemarthrosis Hemarthrosis is the most common, the most painful, and the most physically, economically, and psychiatrically debilitating feature of the hereditary coagulation disorders. The knee joint is most commonly affected, the elbow and the ankle are next in frequency, and the shoulder, wrist, and hip joints are less commonly involved. The earliest symptom is pain, which results from the distention of the joint with blood. If untreated, this may progress until the subchondral and synovial vessels become ischemic. Physical examination reveals muscle spasm and limitation of motion of the affected joint, which is usually held in a position of flexion. The affected joint may be warm and grossly distended and discolored, but in chronically damaged joints external evidence of bleeding may be minimal or absent. Hemorrhage into the periarticular structures is a common complicating feature.

The joint may regain normal function following the first episodes of hemarthrosis, but with each recurrence the synovia becomes progressively more thickened and vascular. Together with the weakening and imbalance of the periarticular supporting structures, this predisposes the joint to recurrent episodes of bleeding. Repeated bouts of subchondral and synovial ischemia produce a progressive loss of hyaline cartilage, subchondral bone necrosis, cyst and osteophyte formation, and ultimately, ankylosis of the joint. Hemarthrosis has been described in all hereditary coagulation disorders where sufficient data are available, but is very rare in factor V deficiency.

Patients with coagulation disorders may not bleed abnormally from small cuts, e.g., razor nicks, and the onset of bleeding is frequently delayed for several hours following significant trauma (*delayed bleeding*). These phenomena probably reflect the hemostatic efficacy of the platelet thrombus in small wounds and its temporary value in larger injuries. *Petechiae*, characteristic of disorders of vessels and platelets, are rare in the coagulation disorders, but ecchymoses and *subcutaneous hematomas* are common. The latter often are large, and characteristically dissect deeper structures. Such dissecting hematomas may spread to involve an entire limb and produce serious consequences from the compression of vital structures, e.g., ischemic contracture of the forearm, femoral nerve palsy as a result of bleeding into the psoas sheath. Bleeding into the tongue, throat, or neck is especially dangerous, and may compromise the airway with surprising rapidity.

Internal soft tissue hemorrhages may create serious diagnostic problems. Bleeding into the retroperitoneal space or the psoas sheath may mimic acute appendicitis, and hemorrhage into the intestinal wall may be confused with bowel obstruction.

Gastrointestinal bleeding is not uncommon in the hereditary coagulation disorders. The source of bleeding is usually in the upper gastrointestinal tract, and in the majority of cases when bleeding is persistent or recurrent, is found to originate from some organic lesion, e.g., peptic ulcer, gastritis. To the contrary, *hematuria* often develops in the absence of demonstrable pathology in the genitourinary tract. *Menorrhagia* is common in the autosomal traits. Bleeding into the *central nervous system* is relatively rare, unless it is the result of significant trauma. Bleeding from the *umbilical cord* is uncommon in all the hereditary coagulation disorders, with the exception of afibrinogenemia, the dysfibrinogenemias, and factor XIII deficiency, disorders which may also be associated with defective *wound healing*. Intraocular hemorrhage is uncommon, but the orbit is frequently involved.

LABORATORY DIAGNOSIS In a previous chapter (Chap. 59) it was emphasized that most hemorrhagic disorders can be detected and categorized by four "primary" screening tests (Table 59-4). In addition, the results of the partial thromboplastin (PTT) and the prothrombin time identify the abnormality as being in either the intrinsic, extrinsic, or common pathways of coagulation (Fig. 59-3), and together with the bleeding time separate the hereditary coagulation disorders into five categories (Table 315-2*A-E*). When interpreted in terms of the relative incidence of the various disorders (column 4), and when supplemented by simple ancillary tests such as the clotting time and the thrombin time (column 5), a reasonably accurate "presumptive" diagnosis can usually be made without special equipment or reagents. More elaborate confirmatory tests are usually required for a definitive diagnosis (column 6).

A *prolonged PTT and a normal prothrombin time* (Table 315-2*A*) suggests a defect in the *intrinsic* pathway of coagulation (Chap. 59, Fig. 59-3), i.e., a deficiency of factor VIII, IX, XI, or XII. Together, these disorders comprise over 95 percent of all hereditary coagulation disorders. Factor XII deficiency can be readily excluded, since it is not associated with significant bleeding.

Among the ancillary tests, the results of the clotting time vary, depending on the severity of the deficiency. Neither the clotting time nor the prothrombin consumption test (Chap. 59) should be relied upon to exclude a coagulation disorder, since both will usually be normal in mildly affected persons. This point deserves emphasis both because the diagnosis of hemophilia is often erroneously equated with a prolonged clotting time and also because the most serious diagnostic errors are usually made in the case of the mildly affected patient. Such patients may have an equivocal bleeding history and a normal clotting time but nonetheless may develop serious and unexpected bleeding following traumatic injuries or surgery.

Among the confirmatory tests which serve to distinguish between deficiencies of factors VIII, IX, and XI (Table 315-2, column 6), the *thromboplastin generation test* is the most reliable.

A *prolonged PTT and a prolonged prothrombin time* (Table 315-2*B*) suggest the presence of a defect in the *common* pathway of coagulation which may result from an isolated deficiency of factor V, X, prothrombin, or fibrinogen, or from abnormalities in multiple pathways. Deficiencies of these factors are present in many of the most common acquired coagulation disorders, but hereditary forms are exceedingly rare. Consequently, *the presence of a prolonged prothrombin time strongly suggests the presence of an acquired coagulation disorder.* Hereditary afibrinogenemia can be excluded by a fibrinogen determination and the thrombin time; the erythrocyte sedimentation rate is markedly reduced in this disorder. The thrombin time usually is prolonged in the congenital dysfibrinogenemias. Deficiencies of factors V, X, and prothrombin can be distinguished from one another by simple correction tests and by the thromboplastin generation test.

Factor VII deficiency is very rare and is the only disorder characterized by a *prolonged prothrombin time and a normal PTT* (Table 315-2*C*). Since factor VII is essential only in the tissue-activated *extrinsic* pathway of coagulation, this diagnosis can be confirmed by the presence of a normal clotting time, prothrombin consumption test, Stypven time, and thromboplastin generation test.

The coagulation tests listed in Table 315-2 may be normal in the case of the mild or partial forms of von Willebrand's disease (see below) and in mild factor XI deficiency. Specialized techniques are required for the laboratory diagnosis of these disorders.

All coagulation tests will be normal in factor XIII deficiency (Table 315-2*E*). In this disorder, the fibrin polymers are not cross-linked by stable covalent bonds, and the clot will dissolve in solvents such as urea (the clot solubility test).

THERAPY Various styptics, drugs, and hormones have periodically been advocated for the treatment of the hereditary coagulation disorders. These include vitamin K, rutin, corticosteroids, and extracts of peanuts. None of these remedies is of proved value. Topical hemostatics (thrombin, fibrin-foam) may be of temporary value in small injuries. However, *replacement therapy*, i.e., the intravenous infusion of the deficient coagulation factor in the form of normal blood or blood products, remains the only reliable method of treatment.

Concentrated preparations of fibrinogen, factor VIII, and a concentrate containing the four vitamin K–dependent factors (prothrombin, and factors VII, IX, and X) are now commercially available. Concentrated factor VIII may be prepared by several fractionation methods, e.g., glycine precipitation or by the technique of cryoprecipitation. Concentrates avoid the problem of circulatory overload which may be encountered with plasma and produce fewer adverse effects in some patients, e.g., urticarial or febrile reactions (Chap. 310). They are the preparations of choice in the treatment of major hemorrhage due to deficiencies of factors VIII and IX, because adequate blood levels can seldom be attained with plasma. High cost and contamination with the virus of serum hepatitis are relative drawbacks to their use.

Plasma remains the only preparation available for the treatment of deficiencies of factors V and XI, and is still widely used in the treatment of factor IX deficiency. Fresh or fresh frozen plasma is preferred for the treatment of factor V deficiency, but with this exception stored plasma is usually adequate. Plasma is now seldom used in the treatment of factor VIII deficiency. Plasma is

TABLE 315-2
Laboratory diagnosis of the hereditary coagulation disorders

[1] "Primary" screening tests			[2]	[3]	[4]	[5] Ancillary tests		[6]
Partial thromboplastin time	*Prothrombin time*	*Bleeding time*	*"Presumptive" diagnosis*	*Probable deficiency*	*Relative incidence, %*	*Clotting time*	*Thrombin time*	*Confirmatory tests*
A Prolonged	Normal	Normal[1]	Defect in *intrinsic* pathway	VIII	80	Prolonged[2]	Normal	Presumptive correction tests
				IX	13	Prolonged[2]		
				XI	6	Prolonged[2]	Normal	Thromboplastin generation test; Specific assays
				XII	?	Prolonged[2]	Normal	Significant bleeding absent
B Prolonged	Prolonged	Normal	Defect in *common* or *multiple* pathways	Fibrinogen[4]	<1	Prolonged[2]	Abnormal	Qualitative tests; specific assay
				Prothrombin	<1	Prolonged[2]	Normal	Presumptive correction tests
				V	<1	Prolonged[2]	Normal	Thromboplastin generation test
				X	<1	Prolonged[2]	Normal	Specific assays; Stypven time
C Normal	Prolonged	Normal	Defect in *extrinsic* pathway	VII	<1	Normal	Normal	Specific assay; Stypven time
D Prolonged	Normal	Prolonged	"Hybrid" defect	VW disease	Common ?	Normal[3]	Normal	Factor VIII assay; "new" factor VIII synthesis following plasma infusion; platelet adhesion to glass
E Normal	Normal	Normal		XIII, others	<1	Normal	Normal	Clot solubility test for factor XIII

Note: The platelet count, clot retraction, whole blood clot lysis time, and euglobulin lysis time are normal in all uncomplicated hereditary coagulation disorders.

[1] *In severe deficiencies, a prolonged bleeding time and a positive tourniquet test are occasionally found.*

[2] *The coagulation time is abnormal only in severe deficiencies.*

[3] *The coagulation time is usually normal unless the factor VIII deficiency is severe.*

[4] *In hereditary afibrinogenemia, the bleeding time is prolonged, presumably because of platelet dysfunction (Chap. 313).*

probably preferable to purified fibrinogen for the treatment of hereditary afibrinogenemia.

Regimen Replacement therapy should be individualized. Most instances of *minor bleeding* (hemarthrosis, small hematomas) due to factor VIII deficiency will respond to a regimen of 15 to 20 units factor VIII per kg body weight as a loading dose, followed by 10 units per kg every 12 hr. In many patients, a single large daily dose of therapeutic material will suffice. In *major bleeding* (traumatic injuries, surgery, multiple tooth extractions, soft-tissue bleeding in vital areas) larger doses and more frequent administration are required, the exact regimen depending on whether the patient is mildly or severely affected, the site of the bleeding, the in vivo survival time of the deficient factor, and the presence of complicating factors, e.g., external blood loss. As a general rule, replacement therapy, even if for minor bleeding, should be continued for at least 72 hr; in major surgery or following traumatic injuries, therapy for 10 to 14 days or even longer may be required. Experience has taught that the two commonest mistakes in replacement therapy of the coagulation disorders are starting too late and stopping too soon.

The administration of therapeutic material on a maintenance schedule may diminish the frequency and severity of spontaneous bleeding manifestations, particularly hemarthrosis. The use of such prophylactic therapy is restricted because of expense and limitations in availability of the therapeutic material.

Supportive therapy All patients with *hemarthrosis* should receive prompt and adequate replacement therapy, since only in this manner can the permanent disability which results from repeated joint bleeding be minimized. Replacement therapy is particularly effective if given at the first sign of joint bleeding. This provides the rationale for various early home care programs. Supportive therapy includes immobilization and the administration of analgesics. Addicting narcotics should be avoided, and aspirin is contraindicated, since this drug may impair platelet function and provoke or aggravate hemorrhagic episodes as a consequence. *Arthrocentesis* is usually unnecessary, but may be of significant benefit when the joint is severely distended or when resolution of the hemarthrosis is delayed despite adequate replacement therapy. Early ambulation and careful *physiotherapy* aimed at restoring full range of motion to the joint should be instituted as soon as the acute stage of hemarthrosis has resolved.

Special attention should be given to the preventive *dental care* of patients with hereditary coagulation disorders, so as to minimize the hazards, complications, and expense of operative dental procedures. Although deciduous teeth may be shed without significant difficulty, the extraction of even a single permanent tooth requires adequate replacement therapy. Multiple extractions save time and expense but create a major bleeding hazard, and should be carried out only in a hospital. Hypnosis and fibrinolytic enzyme inhibitors such as epsilonaminocaproic acid (EACA) or tranexamic acid may help in minimizing postextraction bleeding.

Von Willebrand's disease

Von Willebrand's disease (pseudohemophilia, vascular hemophilia) occupies a unique position among the hereditary coagulation disorders in that it is characterized by a "dual" or "hybrid" hemostatic defect, i.e., a deficiency of factor VIII and a prolonged bleeding time, the latter suggesting an additional abnormality in the vascular or platelet phases of hemostasis.

Accurate figures concerning the incidence of this disorder are lacking, but it appears to be second only to factor VIII deficiency in frequency, and may be even more common. Von Willebrand's disease is inherited as an autosomal dominant trait.

The *pathophysiology* of von Willebrand's disease is poorly understood. In patients with this disorder, the infusion of normal plasma produces a gradual and sustained rise in the factor VIII level over a 12- to 24-hr period. This cannot be attributed to the factor VIII present in the infused plasma, since comparable results are obtained with factor VIII–deficient plasma. This phenomenon, termed *new factor VIII synthesis*, is presumably the effect of a factor present in the administered plasma which stimulates previously deficient factor VIII biosynthesis for a time and is a specific although cumbersome confirmatory test for von Willebrand's disease.

The transfusion of plasma or cryoprecipitates may also produce a transient shortening of the bleeding time in patients with this disorder. The responsible plasma factor has not been identified, but it appears to differ from that which induces "new factor VIII" synthesis. Platelets of patients with this disorder do not adhere normally to glass beads in vitro, but other tests of platelet function are normal. The bleeding time and the PTT usually are prolonged (Table 315-2*D*), the latter reflecting a slight to moderate reduction in factor VIII.

These findings are compatible with the hypothesis that factor VIII deficiency in von Willebrand's disease is due to lack of a plasma factor which is essential for factor VIII biosynthesis. The cause of the abnormal bleeding time, and its relation to the deficiency of factor VIII, remain obscure.

The bleeding manifestations of von Willebrand's disease also are consistent with the hybrid nature of the disorder. Thus, although the clinical picture is usually dominated by cutaneous and mucosal bleeding characteristic of a "purpuric" disorder, symptoms suggesting a superimposed coagulation defect, e.g., dissecting intramuscular hematomas, serious posttraumatic hemorrhage, and rarely hemarthrosis, occur in severely affected patients.

Perplexing features of this disorder are the tendency of the laboratory abnormalities to vary from time to time and the frequency with which mild or partial forms of the disorder occur. It has been suggested, not unreasonably, that von Willebrand's disease is a syndrome rather than a specific entity.

TREATMENT Von Willebrand's disease should be treated in essentially the same manner as factor VIII

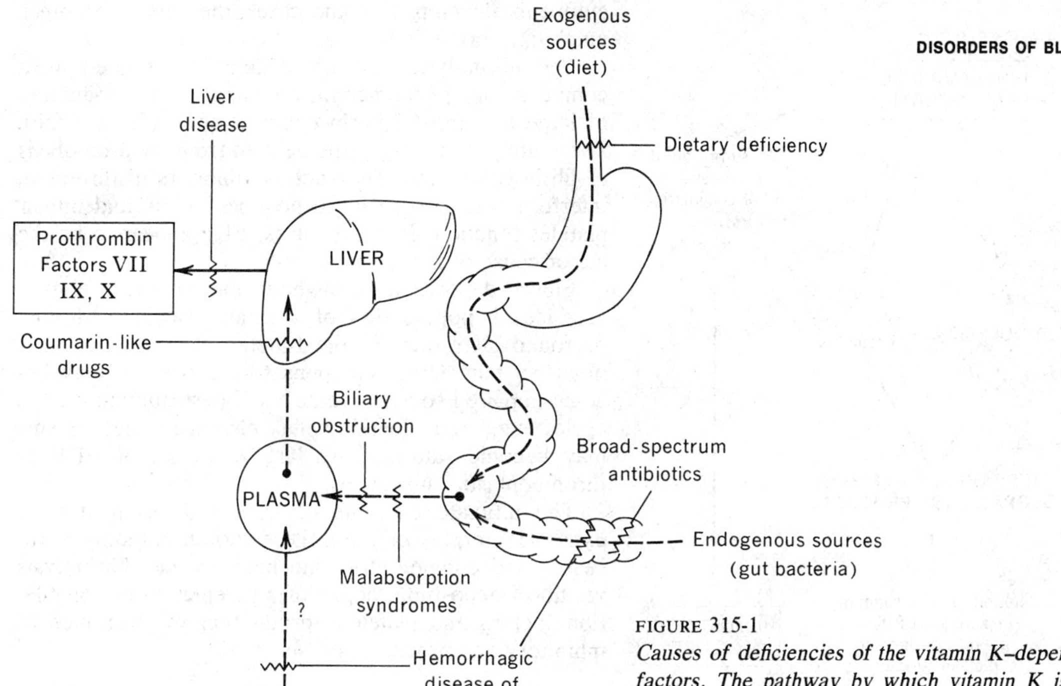

FIGURE 315-1
Causes of deficiencies of the vitamin K–dependent coagulation factors. The pathway by which vitamin K is normally transported is illustrated by dashed lines.

deficiency. Unfortunately the bleeding time seldom is shortened and the clinical response, particularly in the case of mucosal bleeding, such as gastrointestinal hemorrhage and menorrhagia, is unpredictable and often transient. Cryoprecipitates or fresh plasma may be preferable to commercial factor VIII concentrates in the treatment of mucosal bleeding. Since the factor VIII levels attained by replacement therapy may be supplemented by "new" factor VIII synthesized by the recipient, prophylactic therapy should be initiated 24 hr. before surgery.

THE ACQUIRED COAGULATION DISORDERS

DEFICIENCIES OF THE VITAMIN K–DEPENDENT COAGULATION FACTORS Four coagulation factors, i.e., factors VII, IX, X, and prothrombin, are synthesized in the liver by a process which requires vitamin K (Chap. 80). A combined deficiency of these *vitamin K–dependent coagulation factors* develops in diverse clinical situations and is probably the most common of all coagulation disorders (Fig. 315-1).

Liver disease is the most frequent cause of this complex coagulation defect. Here, the hepatic cells cannot synthesize the required coagulation factors despite the presence of adequate amounts of vitamin K. Various additional hemostatic abnormalities are frequently present in severe liver disease. These abnormalities commonly include a deficiency of factor V and, rarely, a deficiency of fibrinogen, both of which are synthesized in the liver but are not vitamin K–dependent. Thrombocytopenia may be present in as many as 50 percent of patients with severe liver disease. In many patients this may be due to sequestration of platelets in the spleen in association with portal hypertension (Chap. 317). Pathologic proteolysis and intravascular coagulation, discussed below also may develop in some cases. The bleeding manifestations in liver disease are usually chronic and include bleeding into the skin and mucosa, recurrent epistaxis, gastrointestinal bleeding, and protracted hemorrhage following minor surgical procedures, e.g., liver biopsy.

Bleeding is a common complication of therapy with *coumarin-like drugs.* Hematuria and epistaxis are particularly common, and may develop while the prothrombin time is within the "therapeutic range." Self-intoxication with these drugs is not uncommon in psychotic and neurotic individuals. Salicylates may antagonize the hepatic biosynthesis of the vitamin K–dependent coagulation factors, but these drugs alone rarely produce abnormal bleeding.

Hemorrhagic disease of the newborn is the result of vitamin K deficiency in the neonate (Chap. 80) and is no longer commonly seen in this country. The pathogenesis of the disorder is complex, but the most important factors appear to be a sterile gut, prematurity, maternal deficiency of vitamin K, and blood loss or other obstetric complications at birth. Petechiae are rare, but ecchymoses and mucosal bleeding, hematomas of the scalp, melena, and bleeding from the umbilical cord are commonly seen. The last named symptom is rare in the commoner hereditary coagulation disorders.

Vitamin K (Chap. 80) is a fat-soluble substance and is absorbed only in the presence of bile salts. Consequently, deficiencies of the vitamin K–dependent coagulation factors may develop in *biliary tract obstruction.* Sprue, celiac disease, and other *malabsorption syndromes* also produce this abnormality, as does the sterilization of the gut by the prolonged administration of *broad-spectrum antibiotics.*

The *laboratory findings* in deficiencies of the vitamin

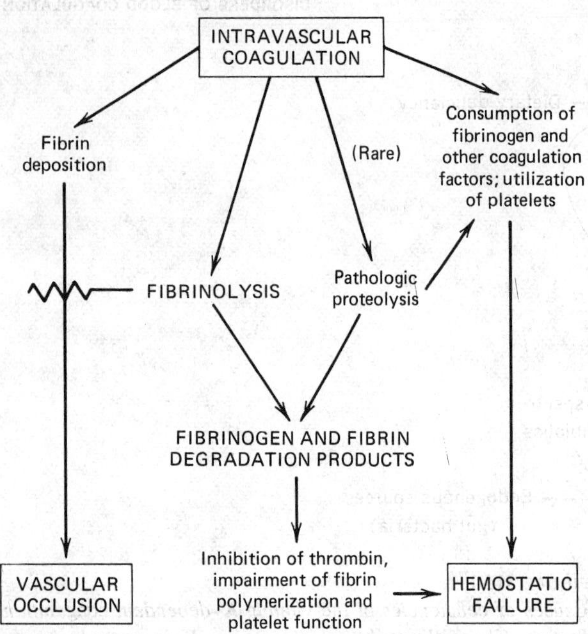

FIGURE 315-2
The pathophysiology of intravascular coagulation.

K–dependent coagulation factors are basically the same, regardless of the etiology, and are reflected in the screening tests by a prolongation of both the prothrombin time and the partial thromboplastin time. Except in the case of liver disease, the coagulation abnormalities will respond specifically and rapidly to the parenteral administration of vitamin K_1 in doses of 10 to 20 mg in adults, and 0.5 to 1.0 mg in neonates with hemorrhagic disease.

INTRAVASCULAR COAGULATION Diffuse intravascular coagulation (DIC, defibrination syndrome, consumption coagulopathy) is one of the most serious of the acquired coagulation disorders. It arises in diverse clinical situations, and is characterized by an exceedingly complex hemostatic defect (Fig. 315-2).

Pathophysiology Diffuse intravascular coagulation is initiated by many pathologic processes. These have in common the capacity to activate the coagulation mechanism to a degree that normal homeostatic mechanisms (Chap. 59) are overwhelmed. The entry of large amounts of thromboplastic substances into the general circulation appears to be the initiating cause in some disorders, e.g., abruptio placentae, various neoplasms. In others, such as gram-negative septicemia, DIC may result from several initiating factors, e.g., activation of factor XII, damage to endothelium and platelets. In many forms of DIC, the pathophysiology is obscure.

Once DIC begins, thrombin is persistently or recurrently elaborated within the circulation. This leads to the utilization of fibrinogen, various other coagulation factors (particularly prothrombin and factors V and VIII), and platelets, in much the same manner as occurs during in vitro coagulation. If utilization proceeds more rapidly than repletion, deficiencies of these factors and thrombocytopenia develop; in some cases, the plasma becomes much like serum.

The fibrinolytic enzyme system is activated as a compensatory phenomenon, resulting in the production of large amounts of fibrin degradation products (FDP). These are protein fragments derived from the proteolysis of fibrin (Chap. 59). They act as inhibitors of thrombin, interfere with normal fibrin polymerization, and impair platelet function. In many cases, FDP appear to be the major cause of hemorrhage.

Fibrin deposition throughout the microvasculature produces hypoperfusion of various vascular beds and profound alterations in the function of virtually every organ system. Other compensatory processes may become impaired so as to create a self-perpetuating vicious cycle; e.g., reticuloendothelial clearance mechanisms may become saturated by large amounts of FDP or thromboplastic substances.

The ultimate outcome of DIC is determined by a dynamic interplay between these various pathologic processes and compensatory mechanisms, i.e., fibrinolysis vs. fibrin deposition, depletion vs. repletion of coagulation factors and platelets, production vs. clearance of inhibitory and procoagulant substances.

Diagnosis The clinical picture of DIC usually is characterized by the sudden onset of hemorrhage, which is often of serious proportions and is frequently associated with profound circulatory collapse. The predominant bleeding manifestations relate to the underlying disorder. Thus, in obstetric accidents, profuse vaginal bleeding is seen, and in postsurgical defibrination syndromes uncontrollable bleeding from the incision is usually the first sign. In severe cases there is bleeding from all bodily orifices, venipuncture sites, and into the skin and mucosa. In others, e.g., disseminated carcinoma, bleeding into the skin and mucosa may be chronic and persistent, and in such patients a premonitory stage of "hypercoagulability" clinically manifested as a thromboembolic diathesis may be seen.

The laboratory diagnosis of full-blown DIC is relatively easy. All the screening tests of coagulation are grossly abnormal, the fibrinogen level is low, and reductions in other coagulation factors of variable degree are usually found. The thrombin time is a valuable ancillary screening test in these disorders, since it is sensitive not only to the level of fibrinogen but also to the inhibitory effects of FDP. Thrombocytopenia is a consistent finding, and schistocytes are seen in peripheral blood smears. The euglobulin lysis time and whole clot lysis time usually are normal, but may reveal evidence of systemic fibrinolysis. Fibrinogen degradation products usually are present. In the subacute or chronic forms of DIC, many of the above-mentioned laboratory findings may be lacking, and such an incomplete or fluctuating laboratory picture may lead to confusion.

Therapy The underlying disorder and existing complications such as shock should be treated promptly and energetically. Despite the seeming paradox of treating a bleeding disorder with an anticoagulant, heparin has been effective in many cases of DIC, particularly the subacute or chronic forms of the disorder. It is of uncertain value in acute DIC, particularly that associated with sepsis.

Replacement therapy usually is disappointing unless the basic pathophysiologic process has been arrested, but platelet transfusions may be of some value in selected cases. In DIC due to abruptio placentae, no treatment other than evacuation of the uterus is ordinarily required. Fibrinolytic enzyme inhibitors must be used with great care, if at all, in DIC, since they may favor the development of disseminated thrombosis.

PATHOLOGIC PROTEOLYSIS The activation of the fibrinolytic enzyme, plasmin, in amounts which exceed the capacity of the antiplasmins (Chap. 59, Fig. 59-2) leads in the general circulation to pathologic proteolysis of fibrinogen (*fibrinogenolysis*) and of other coagulation factors (particularly factors V and VIII). Even when insufficient to deplete coagulation factors, the persistent or recurrent activation of plasmin may cause bleeding as the result of the production of large amounts of FDP, and the dissolution of hemostatically important fibrin plugs.

Pathologic proteolysis is much less common than was previously supposed. It has been described most commonly in liver disease, following surgery employing extracorporeal circulatory devices, and in association with carcinoma of the lung, pancreas, or prostate. These disorders are also commonly associated with DIC and secondary fibrinolysis. Enzyme inhibitors such as EACA are therapeutically effective in the treatment of pathologic proteolysis, but usually are contraindicated in DIC. The differentiation between the two processes is thus of practical importance. It can usually be accomplished in the laboratory. The most reliable criteria are the platelet count, which usually is normal in pathologic proteolysis, and the severity of the coagulation defect, which is often relatively mild in pathologic proteolysis in contrast to intravascular coagulation, where the blood often is incoagulable. Rapid clot lysis and a shortened euglobulin lysis time may be present in either case, but these two abnormalities are rarely as markedly or persistently abnormal in intravascular coagulation as in pathologic proteolysis.

ACQUIRED INHIBITORS OF COAGULATION (THE "CIRCULATING ANTICOAGULANTS") The acquired inhibitors of coagulation factors are uncommon and poorly understood, but may produce serious bleeding. One variety impairs coagulation by inactivating various individual coagulation factors. Such *specific inhibitors* appear to be antibodies to coagulation factors and are most commonly directed against factor VIII. They may develop in patients with factor VIII deficiency, where they produce a marked resistance to replacement therapy, or may arise as a complication of pregnancy, in association with various collagen vascular diseases, and in elderly persons without obvious underlying disease. The clinical picture and laboratory findings resemble those of a specific deficiency of the factor against which the inhibitor is directed. Where inhibitors of factor VIII are involved, the severe case is indistinguishable from severe classic hemophilia (Table 315-2). Specific inhibitors which inactivate fibrinogen, factors V, IX, and XIII, also have been described.

Other inhibitors apparently antagonize various active intermediates in coagulation rather than specific coagulation factors. Among these *nonspecific inhibitors,* those which arise in association with collagen vascular diseases, particularly systemic lupus erythematosus, appear to be the most common. They act by inhibiting an intermediate in prothrombinase formation. The clinical and laboratory picture resembles hemophilia, but in contrast to hemophilia and the aforementioned disorders due to specific inhibitors of factor VIII, the prothrombin time usually is prolonged.

Increased amounts of antithrombins may be found in the plasma in many disorders, and may be contributory factors in various complex hemostatic defects, e.g., liver disease. Antithrombins alone seldom produce significant bleeding, and in many cases may be merely the result of circulating FDP. Of uncertain validity are reports of heparin-like anticoagulants.

Specialized tests are required for the demonstration of inhibitors of coagulation. They are all based on the principle that, in contrast to disorders due to deficiency of an essential factor, the addition of control plasma to inhibitor-containing plasma fails to correct the coagulation abnormalities.

Therapy of bleeding caused by acquired inhibitors of coagulation is difficult. In some cases, corticosteroids, immunosuppressive therapy, and exchange transfusion have been effective. In patients with specific inhibitors of factor VIII, bleeding can usually be stopped by the administration of factor VIII concentrates, but heroic doses often are required.

MISCELLANEOUS ACQUIRED COAGULATION DISORDERS Coagulation abnormalities may be encountered in virtually any serious chronic disease, e.g., amyloidosis, the nephrotic syndrome, various hematologic disorders (leukemia, polycythemia vera, myelofibrosis), and the dysproteinemias. These are discussed elsewhere (Chap. 313), since purpura is often the predominating bleeding manifestation, and the platelet and vascular abnormalities usually overshadow the coagulation defects. Although calcium is essential for normal blood coagulation, hypocalcemia per se, even if severe, does not produce abnormal bleeding.

REFERENCES

BIGGS R: *Human Blood Coagulation, Haemostasis and Thrombosis,* Oxford: Blackwell, 1972

DEYKIN D: The clinical challenge of disseminated intravascular coagulation. N Engl J Med 283:636, 1970

RATNOFF O: *The Treatment of Hemorrhagic Disorders,* New York: Hoeber, 1968

SHULMAN NR et al: The physiologic basis for therapy of classic hemophilia (factor VIII deficiency) and related disorders. Ann Intern Med 57:856, 1967

WINTROBE MM et al: *Clinical Hematology,* 7th ed., Philadelphia: Lea & Febiger, 1974

316 THE LEUKEMIAS

DANE R. BOGGS
M. M. WINTROBE

DEFINITION Leukemia is a disease characterized by an abnormally large number of a specific type of leukocyte within the body in the absence of a demonstrable cause. Types of leukemia are differentiated according to the leukocytic system involved and on the basis of cell maturity. Depending on the type of leukemia and the efficacy of the therapy employed, patients may die within a few days of diagnosis or live for decades. With rare exceptions, all types of leukemia are eventually fatal.

HISTORY Knowledge of leukemia can be traced to the period from 1839 to 1845 when Donné made the first microscopic observations, and Craigie, Bennett, and Virchow distinguished the clinical entity. Virchow recognized that the cells involved were leukocytes and distinguished a lymphatic and a splenic form. After Ehrlich's blood-staining methods were developed, Neumann, in 1891, identified the splenic form as myelocytic. Acute leukemia was described by von Friedreich in 1857, and Naegeli distinguished between lymphoblastic and myeloblastic leukemia in 1900.

Useful, palliative therapy for the chronic leukemias came with development of therapeutic x-ray equipment in the 1920s. However, until folic acid antagonists and adrenal glucocorticosteroid therapy became available in 1948 and 1949, no therapy was of appreciable benefit in the acute leukemias. In the search for a cure there is encouragement in the fact that at the present time a few patients with acute leukemia are alive who have been in remission for from 10 to 20 years. However, for practical purposes, leukemia still is incurable and, while research into its etiology holds promise, the pace of progress toward prevention or cure remains slower than one would wish.

CLASSIFICATION The leukemias usually are classified as acute or chronic and are further categorized according to the predominant cell involved. Actually, the terms *acute* and *chronic* have lost some of their prognostic implications because of present therapeutic regimens. Patients with acute lymphoblastic leukemia may live longer than some patients with chronic myelocytic leukemia. Nonetheless, the terms acute and chronic are still applicable, since in the former the illness often is acute in onset, while in chronic leukemia the onset usually is insidious. A variety of clinical features help to distinguish the various forms of leukemia, but final diagnosis is based on microscopic examination of the blood and/or bone marrow.

Two common forms of leukemia arise from the lymphocytic system of cells: *acute lymphoblastic leukemia* and *chronic lymphocytic leukemia.* The lymphoblast, a large cell with homogeneous and rather granular chromatin, is the most common cell in acute lymphoblastic leukemia, while the small lymphocyte, with its nucleus of densely clumped chromatin, is the common cell in the chronic form. Plasma cells may be closely related to the lymphocytic system and when multiple myeloma is complicated by the release of large numbers of myeloma or plasma cells into the blood, the patient is considered to have *plasma cell leukemia* (see Chap. 65). Patients with lymphosarcoma may develop marked lymphocytosis or lymphoblastosis in the blood (*lymphosarcoma cell leukemia*), and when this occurs, the disease may be indistinguishable from that of patients with lymphocytic or lymphoblastic leukemia.

There are two common forms of leukemia involving the granulocytic cell system: *acute myeloblastic leukemia* and *chronic myelocytic leukemia,* as well as a wide variety of variants and/or subtypes of the granulocytic leukemias. In chronic myelocytic leukemia the entire spectrum of the neutrophilic series from myeloblast to segmented neutrophil is present in abnormally large numbers, and eosinophils and basophils usually are increased as well. Acute myeloblastic leukemia is characterized by an increase in myeloblasts, but with a hiatus of maturation beyond this point. Many patients who otherwise are virtually indistinguishable from patients with acute myeloblastic leukemia have cells with some morphologic features suggesting monocytes (*myelomonoblastic leukemia*); still others show a predominance of promyelocytes (*promyelocytic leukemia*). For purposes of clinical management patients with acute myeloblastic, myelomonoblastic, and promyelocytic leukemia can be considered as the same.

Other rare forms of leukemia include *eosinophilic leukemia*, which takes two forms. One mimics chronic myelocytic leukemia in clinical manifestations, whereas the other is more acute and cardiac manifestations are a cardinal feature. *Basophilic leukemia* has been described. Some patients with myeloblastic leukemia form prominent solid tumors composed of myeloblastic tissue. When their cut surface is exposed to air, these tumors turn green because of their content of myeloperoxidase; they have been termed *chloromas.* In the bone marrow of patients with myeloblastic leukemia, bizarre erythroblasts which bear some resemblance to megaloblasts may be found. In a few patients, such changes in red cells may precede and/or overshadow the myeloblastic hyperplasia. Occasionally, such a patient with anemia and a hyperplastic "megaloblastoid" marrow has died without myeloblastosis. Patients with the above type of erythroid changes have been classified as having the *di Guglielmo* syndrome (*erythroleukemia,* erythremic myelosis). *Monocytic leukemia,* in which the cells are without appreciable myeloblastic features, is occasionally observed. In a clinically acute form the cells are usually very large and bizarre (Schilling type leukemia). In another form which follows a more chronic course, the monocytes are more or less normal in appearance.

Still other rare forms of leukemia do not easily fit into variant patterns of the lymphocytic and granulocytic cell systems. In patients with congenital or acquired urticaria pigmentosa (Chap. 367) increased numbers of mast cells are found in various tissues and organs. Such patients occasionally develop blood mastocytosis (*mast cell leukemia*). Patients with idiopathic thrombocytosis and megakaryocytic hyperplasia of the bone marrow sometimes have been referred to as having *megakaryocytic leukemia.* These patients eventually develop a clinical picture compatible with myeloid metaplasia or myelofibrosis.

INCIDENCE, AGE, AND SEX DISTRIBUTION The incidence of leukemia in the United States is approximately 6 per 100,000. Leukemia incidence was reported to be increasing steadily until approximately 1955 but has since stabilized.

The incidence of the various types of leukemia differs according to age. Acute myeloblastic leukemia and chronic myelocytic leukemia may occur at any age, although they are found most commonly in young adults. Chronic lymphocytic leukemia does not occur in children and is uncommon under the age of forty. Acute lymphoblastic leukemia is primarily a disease of children, but it occurs with decreasing frequency throughout life. Most series suggest that acute lymphoblastic leukemia is the most common of these diseases, followed in order of decreasing frequency by acute myeloblastic leukemia, chronic myelocytic leukemia, and chronic lymphocytic leukemia. Leukemia is the most common form of cancer in children but constitutes only 3.6 percent of deaths due to cancer in the general population.

In all types of leukemia, a slight predominance of male patients is found (approximately 3:2), and in chronic lymphocytic leukemia males predominate 2:1.

ETIOLOGY The etiology of leukemia is unknown, although certain contributing factors have been recognized.

Ionizing irradiation in relatively large doses is a predisposing factor in the development of acute myeloblastic and chronic myelocytic leukemia, but there is little evidence to suggest that it plays a role in lymphoid leukemias. Survivors of Hiroshima and Nagasaki, pioneering radiologists, and patients given therapeutic irradiation have all developed granulocytic leukemia with uncommon frequency. Whether there is a "threshold" of irradiation dose below which there is no attendant increase in risk of developing leukemia or whether any exposure carries a slightly increased risk is uncertain.

Chemical leukemogens are recognized, and they are typified by benzol. Certain drugs, such as phenylbutazone, also are suspected as contributing factors in the development of leukemia. Acute myeloblastic and chronic myelocytic leukemia have been the usual types of leukemia following such exposure or therapy.

Genetic influences are suggested by certain observations. Patients with Down's syndrome, characterized by trisomy of chromosome 21, develop acute myeloblastic leukemia at least three times as frequently as do normal children. Instances of familial leukemia are rare but have been reported frequently enough in chronic lymphocytic leukemia to arouse suspicion of a genetic factor in this disease. Concordance of acute leukemia is significantly more frequent in monozygotic than in fraternal twins. Chronic myelocytic leukemia is characterized by deletion of the long arms of chromosome 22 (Philadelphia chromosome, Ph-) in myelocytic, erythrocytic, and megakaryocytic cells, but since this abnormality is not present in lymphocytes or buccal mucosal cells it would appear to be an acquired rather than an inherited abnormality. Chronic lymphocytic leukemia is rare in the Orient, but whether this represents a racial or environmental factor is not clear.

Many other factors, such as trauma, bacterial infections, and psychologic influences, have been suggested as contributing factors in the development of leukemia, but the evidence supporting these suggestions is questionable.

Murine leukemia and that of a number of other mammals as well as of fowls have been demonstrated to be etiologically related to a *virus*. In certain instances the virus has been shown to be inherited and may be passed in mothers' milk as well. The incidence of leukemia in mice known to carry the virus varies from one strain to another, and the incidence can be increased or the age at which leukemia develops can be influenced by irradiation and by a variety of other leukemogenic agents. These observations suggest that the presence of a virus is essential to the development of leukemia, but that environmental and genetic factors may modify the frequency with which leukemia develops in its presence. There is suggestive but not definitive evidence that human leukemia may be caused by a virus. The presence of RNA-dependent DNA polymerase as well as leukemia-specific antigens in leukemic cells may reflect the presence of an RNA-type tumor virus. Normal marrow cells, transplanted into leukemic patients, have acquired leukemia, suggesting that the disease may be due to a transmissible agent.

CELLULAR PROLIFERATION PATTERNS In the acute leukemias and in chronic myelocytic leukemia, studies with radioactive cell labels and of uric acid excretion suggest that an abnormally large number of leukocytes are produced and destroyed each day. An excessive rate of total cell production appears to be an essential part of these diseases. However, such evidence presently is lacking in chronic lymphocytic leukemia. In none of the leukemias has a shortened cellular generation time been demonstrated, and indeed, the percentage of potentially proliferating cells which are engaged in active DNA synthesis may be decreased. Thus, the overproduction of cells reflects a marked expansion of a potentially proliferating compartment of cells. However, the rate of self-replication of individual cells within this compartment is normal or even subnormal. The life span of leukemic cells may be abnormally long, and this may contribute significantly to cellular accumulation in the disease.

The failure of cells in acute leukemia to mature normally is generally assumed to represent a cellular defect rather than a defect in extracellular factors regulating growth. In chronic myelocytic leukemia, the presence of the Philadelphia chromosome in myelocytic and erythrocytic precursors as well as in megakaryocytes suggests that the primary cellular defect in this disease lies in a stem cell which is pluripotential for these three systems of cells.

The mechanism which prevents the release of large numbers of immature cells to the blood in normal subjects apparently is intact in certain patients with acute leukemia and in a few patients observed very early in the course of chronic myelocytic leukemia. *Aleukemic leukemia* refers to those cases of acute leukemia in which no "blasts" are found in the blood although they are increased over normal in the bone marrow. Leukopenia is seen in such cases as a rule, since the number of normal leukocytes usually is decreased. Patients with acute leukemia with blasts in the blood, but with a normal total leukocyte count, have been termed *subleukemic*.

CLINICAL MANIFESTATIONS

The various types of leukemia are characterized by different signs, symptoms, and complications, but have certain features in common. Clinical manifestations can usually be related to one or more of the following factors: (1) formation of masses composed largely of leukemic cells (splenomegaly, lymphadenopathy, meningeal infiltration, bone pain, etc.); (2) reduced numbers of normal blood cells (thrombocytopenia with resultant hemorrhage, anemia with resultant fatigue, and neutropenia with resultant bacterial infection); (3) other specific problems (excess uric acid production with gout and/or uric acid nephropathy, failure to produce circulating antibodies in chronic lymphocytic leukemia with attendant bacterial infection); or (4) poorly understood manifestations, such as fever and weight loss.

CHRONIC MYELOCYTIC LEUKEMIA The onset is insidious, and the first symptom usually is mild fatigue, bone pain, or a mass in the left side of the abdomen. At the time of diagnosis, physical abnormalities usually are limited to a palpable spleen and a small area of tenderness over the body of the sternum. Fever may be present occasionally, and some weight loss may have been noted. In a few patients with less than 50,000 neutrophils per μl there may be few or no immature neutrophilic leukocytes in the blood, but in most cases the entire spectrum of neutrophils from myeloblasts to segmented neutrophils is represented in the blood. Most patients have more than 100,000 neutrophilic cells per μl in the blood at the time of diagnosis, and the count may exceed 1 million. Morphologic examination of the marrow is of no diagnostic help. It usually discloses that the barrier to release of immature cells is not completely destroyed, since the proportion of immature cells is higher in the marrow than in the blood. Until blastic crisis supervenes, it is the well-differentiated neutrophilic myelocytes and later forms which are found in the blood, and segmented neutrophils predominate. Basophils and eosinophils usually are increased in proportion or even out of proportion to the increase in neutrophilic cells. Monocytes may be normal or increased while lymphocytes usually are normal in absolute number. The severity of the disease is usually reflected by the height of the leukocyte count, and the count tends to increase as the disease progresses. Most patients are mildly anemic at the time of diagnosis, and anemia becomes severe in the terminal phase. Platelets often are increased at the time of diagnosis, and thrombocytopenia rarely develops spontaneously in the absence of a blastic crisis.

The most common cause of death in chronic myelocytic leukemia is the development of a phase which is heralded by an increasing percentage of myeloblasts in blood and marrow (*blastic crisis*). When this develops, the clinical picture approximates that of patients with acute myeloblastic leukemia.

ACUTE MYELOBLASTIC LEUKEMIA Rapidly developing fatigue and a general sense of poor health, often accompanied by hemorrhagic manifestations and fever with or without bacterial infection, bring the patient to a physician. Physical examination usualy discloses pallor, hepatosplenomegaly, sternal tenderness, petechiae and less often ecchymoses. An occasional patient has no demonstrable physical findings. The number of blasts in the blood ranges from none to more than a million. In approximately 40 percent of cases the total leukocyte count is not increased at the time of diagnosis. Normal blood leukocytes are almost always decreased, although an occasional patient has basophilia or eosinophilia. Anemia is present in more than 90 percent of patients at diagnosis and rapidly becomes more severe as the disease advances. Thrombocytopenia is present in most patients and bleeding from the nose or elsewhere is common. Death is usually due to bacterial infection or to hemorrhage.

The course of patients with myelomonocytic or promyelocytic leukemia is similar to that of patients with myeloblastic leukemia, except that in myelomonocytic leukemia, gum infiltration is more commonly present, while in promyelocytic leukemia, hemorrhage due to disseminated intravascular coagulation may occur.

ACUTE LYMPHOBLASTIC LEUKEMIA The above description of the "typical" patient with acute myeloblastic leukemia also is valid for many patients with acute lymphoblastic leukemia. However, patients with this disease do differ from the former in certain clinical manifestations. Presentation with bone and joint pain is much more common in lymphoblastic leukemia. Whether this reflects the youth of the population affected, as compared with the older age of most of those with myeloblastic leukemia, or is due to a difference in the diseases, is uncertain. Infiltration of the meninges causing symptoms of increased intracranial pressure is a common manifestation of lymphoblastic leukemia. Lymph node enlargement may be present in myeloblastic leukemia, but lymph nodes are more commonly palpable and may be larger in lymphoblastic leukemia. Splenomegaly and hepatomegaly tend to be more prominent in lymphoblastic leukemia. The number of blasts in the blood and the severity of anemia, thrombocytopenia, and neutropenia are similar in the two diseases.

As will be discussed later, the most dramatic difference between the two diseases is the frequency of therapeutically induced remissions in lymphoblastic leukemia, as compared with the distressing resistance to therapy in myeloblastic leukemia. Bleeding and infection are the common modes of death in lymphoblastic leukemia.

CHRONIC LYMPHOCYTIC LEUKEMIA This disease is so insidious in onset that in approximately one-fourth of patients it is discovered in an asymptomatic stage during a routine examination or during examination for unrelated disease. A vague sense of not feeling well, often accompanied by a specific complaint of fatigue is the most common presenting symptom, although presentation with a bacterial infection or because of an enlarged node is not uncommon. On physical examination, most patients have enlarged lymph nodes. A palpable spleen is the next most common physical sign (three-fourths of patients), and one-fourth have hepatomegaly. Sternal tenderness is less common than in other forms of leukemia. An increase in blood lymphocytes is a necessary diagnostic feature, and patients with bone marrow infiltration without increased blood lymphocytes are classified as having lymphosarcoma (Chap. 318). Leukocyte counts generally are not as high as in patients with chronic myelocytic leukemia, being less than 100,000 lymphocytes per μl in two-thirds of cases. Although a cursory look at a blood smear of a patient with chronic lymphocytic leukemia may suggest that he has no blood leukocytes except small lymphocytes, careful differential counts reveal that normal absolute numbers of neutrophils, eosinophils, monocytes, and basophils are usually present in untreated patients. Mild anemia is common, as is mild thrombocytopenia. However, except when hemolytic anemia supervenes or complications of cytotoxic therapy are induced, most patients do not develop severe anemia or thrombocytopenia for some years.

Since chronic lymphocytic leukemia is primarily a disease of old age, many patients die of causes apparently unrelated to leukemia. The most common complication and the usual cause of leukemia-related death is bacterial infection.

MANIFESTATIONS OF INFILTRATION WITH LEUKEMIC CELLS

The presence of excessive numbers of leukocytes is assumed to be directly or indirectly responsible for the manifestations of leukemia.

Splenomegaly is the most common physical manifestation of the leukemias. At diagnosis a palpable spleen is present in almost all patients with chronic myelocytic leukemia, in about 85 percent of patients with acute lymphoblastic leukemia, and 60 percent of those with acute myeloblastic leukemia. The relative size of the spleen in the different forms of leukemia tends to parallel this frequency. *Hepatomegaly* is detectable in approximately half of all patients at diagnosis. Enlarged *lymph nodes* are common at the time of diagnosis in chronic lymphocytic leukemia (80 percent) and acute lymphoblastic leukemia (75 percent). While enlarged nodes may be found in myeloblastic and myelocytic leukemia, they generally are smaller. Cervical nodes are most commonly involved, although nodes in any area may be enlarged. Unless the patient notices the mass, none of these infiltrations leads to symptoms or organ failure. Splenic infarcts may produce pain, and splenic rupture is reported very occasionally, but neither of these events has any apparent relation to the size of the spleen. Liver function tests are likely to be normal even in patients with markedly enlarged, infiltrated livers. These observations suggest that the leukemic cells are not "invasive" in the sense that the cells of many carcinomas are invasive, since in general, they tend not to destroy the function of the organs that they infiltrate.

Almost any organ or area of the body has been reported as being infiltrated by leukemic cells, but infiltrations other than those noted above which are most likely to produce symptoms and signs are those of the central nervous system, kidneys, lungs, bones, and skin.

Serious problems with *central nervous system infiltration* can occur with any of the leukemias but are common only in the acute leukemias. In as many as 80 percent of patients with lymphoblastic leukemia, the leptomeninges are infiltrated to a degree that a symptomatic increase in intracranial pressure is produced. This complication is less frequent in myeloblastic leukemia and rare in other varieties. Headache, nausea and vomiting, stiff neck, seizures, blurred vision, and cranial nerve palsy are the attendant symptoms. Papilledema is a common finding. Examination of the spinal fluid usually reveals increased pressure and increased cell content (identifiable as blasts with proper methods), and protein often is elevated and sugar decreased. If the patient still is responsive to corticosteroids, this therapy will often reverse the process, but intrathecal methotrexate, 0.2 mg per kg body weight, repeated at twice-weekly intervals until the spinal fluid is normal, is the treatment of choice. Irradiation of the entire brain area is efficacious but induces alopecia. Most of the commonly employed antileukemia drugs do not enter the spinal fluid, and presumably for this reason, this complication may develop in patients who otherwise are in complete remission.

Intracerebral infiltration is a cause of death in perhaps 10 percent of patients with myeloblastic leukemia and in an occasional patient with lymphoblastic leukemia. In such patients there appears to be a sudden spurt of growth of leukemic cells. The number of blasts in the blood begins to increase exponentially, and "leukostatic" lesions of rapidly growing cells occlude cerebral vessels. Cerebral hemorrhage accompanies rupture of these vessels as the leukemic mass expands, and large intracerebral hemorrhages with grossly visible solid leukemic tumors in their center are found at autopsy.

Infiltration of spinal meninges, compression of the spinal cord by leukemic tumors, and involvement of peripheral nerves are observed occasionally.

Renal enlargement is found with some frequency in the acute leukemias if routine radiographic studies are made, but this rarely results in renal failure. Most renal problems in all types of leukemia are referable to uric acid excess, hemorrhage, infection, or unrelated processes. Parenchymal *pulmonary* lung infiltration of serious degree is uncommon in any of the leukemias and almost never occurs in chronic lymphocytic leukemia. When parenchymal pulmonary infiltration arises in the acute leukemias, it is usually diffuse in nature and can be distinguished from pulmonary infection only by its failure to disappear after appropriate antibiotic therapy. Mediastinal or hilar lymph node enlargement and/or pleural effusions are the usual intrathoracic manifestations of leukemic infiltration. A variety of radiologically demonstrable *bone lesions* are described in all forms of leukemia, but only patients with lymphoblastic leukemia commonly develop pain from such lesions. Pathologic fractures are extremely rare. Bone lesions which may produce excruciating pain are bone infarcts (which may not be demonstrable radiographically), infiltration raising the periosteum, and discrete circumscribed radiolucent lesions.

Skin infiltration with leukemic cells is rarely a serious symptomatic problem but is observed in a small percentage of patients with any type of leukemia. Such infiltrates usually are circumscribed, raised tumors which may be red or purplish in color. They rarely ulcerate or cause pain, but they may itch. An occasional patient with chronic lymphocytic leukemia may develop a very pruritic generalized infiltration of the skin, and at times, this may precede blood lymphocytosis. Such patients have been said to have lymphocytes which contain more PAS-staining material than lymphocytes of other patients with chronic lymphocytic leukemia (*Sézary syndrome*). Skin lesions in patients with leukemia not due to infiltration by leukemic cells have been termed leukemids.

The treatment of choice for localized, troublesome infiltration with leukemic cells, if accessible, is x-ray therapy. A relatively small dose of x-ray will usually eradicate a local infiltrate.

MANIFESTATIONS DUE TO A REDUCTION IN NORMAL HEMATOPOIETIC CELLS Reduced numbers of normal cells are responsible for many of the symptoms and signs and constitute the usual cause of death. It has been assumed that thrombocytopenia, neutropenia, and anemia are due to decreased cell production, although other kinetic changes in these cell systems may play a role as well. The reason for the reduced production of normal cells is not clear. The obvious explanations, crowding out by leukemic cells or competition for nutrients, appear unlikely for a variety of reasons. It now seems clear that erythrocytes, neutrophils, megakaryocytes, and perhaps even lymphocytes share common pluripotential stem cells. An attractive hypothesis is that the primary defect in leukemia is in a stem cell and that the regulatory function for differentiating into various normal cells is disturbed, leukemic cells being produced instead.

Anemia Decreased erythrocyte production is accompanied by a reduction in reticulocytes, and the erythrocytes usually are normocytic and normochromic. An occasional nucleated erythrocyte is not uncommon in patients with acute myeloblastic or chronic myelocytic leukemia, and may be seen in acute lymphoblastic and even chronic lymphocytic leukemia if anemia is severe. In myeloblastic leukemias with "megaloblastoid" marrows, large macrocytes may predominate and large numbers of erythroblasts may be observed in the blood. A modest reduction in red cell survival often is detectable in isotope-labeling studies, but frank hemolytic anemia with hyperbilirubinemia is rare in all types of leukemia except chronic lymphocytic leukemia. In that disease approximately 20 percent of patients may develop severe hemolysis. This complication occurs suddenly at any time during the course of the disease. The Coombs test usually becomes positive, and consequently, the accelerated red cell destruction is assumed to be an autoimmune phenomenon. This anemia usually responds to corticosteroid therapy, although an occasional patient requires splenectomy.

Anemia other than the rare hemolytic anemia is relieved by appropriate treatment of the leukemic process. The indications for transfusion are those which apply to any anemic patient and are discussed in Chap. 310.

Hemorrhage usually is related to thrombocytopenia. In an occasional patient, generally with acute promyelocytic leukemia, hemorrhage is due to disseminated intravascular coagulation or other nonthrombocytopenic causes. Life-threatening hemorrhage rarely develops unless the platelet count is less than 20,000 per μl, but in patients with fewer than 50,000 platelets, ecchymoses and petechiae usually are present. Bleeding from almost any site or organ may be observed, but the most common forms of fatal or life-threatening hemorrhage are intracranial and intraintestinal. Fatal gastrointestinal hemorrhage is more common in lymphoblastic than in myeloblastic leukemia. Intracranial hemorrhage due to thrombocytopenia is usually subarachnoid. Most instances of intracerebral hemorrhage are related to leukemic infiltration.

Decreased production is the probable cause of thrombocytopenia in most patients with leukemia, but an occasional patient with chronic lymphocytic leukemia develops severe thrombocytopenia in the presence of large numbers of megakaryocytes in the bone marrow. In this circumstance, steroid therapy and/or splenectomy usually is effective. In most thrombocytopenic patients there is no effective means of inducing increased platelet production except by inducing a remission in the leukemia by specific therapy.

Thrombocytopenic hemorrhage can be interrupted or prevented by administration of enough platelet transfusions. Fresh whole blood or platelet concentrates properly prepared from fresh whole blood must be used. The number of platelets which must be transfused to raise the platelet count above the danger level depends upon the size of the patient. Platelets from as much as 5 liters of blood may be required to stop hemorrhage in an adult. Since the life span of platelets in the blood is only about 10 days and that of transfused platelets usually shorter, the effect of platelet transfusion is quickly dissipated. However, in treatment centers where platelets are regularly administered prophylactically to thrombocytopenic patients, hemorrhage has become a less frequent cause of death in leukemia than it once was. The repeated use of a single platelet donor, coupled with in vitro tests for platelet compatibility, can reduce the frequency of formation of significant levels of antiplatelet antibodies by the patient.

Fever and infection are common problems in all types of leukemia, although bacterial infection is not particularly common in chronic myelocytic leukemia until blastic crisis supervenes. Fever in chronic lymphocytic leukemia is almost always due to infection, but in other forms of leukemia fever often occurs in the absence of infection as an intrinsic part of the disease. However, in any febrile leukemic patient an intensive search for infection, including blood and urine cultures, should be carried out before concluding that the fever is noninfectious. A "therapeutic trial" of antibiotics is not advisable in the absence of overt infection. Antibiotic-induced changes in the bacterial flora of the patient permit growth of antibiotic-resistant types of infection. Prophylactic antibiotic therapy should not be considered for routine use in these diseases for the same reason. However, the frequency of infection can be reduced by the use of prophylactic antibiotics in conjunction with a sterile environment such as is provided by laminar flow rooms at certain treatment centers.

The frequent bacterial infections which develop in leukemia are explainable on the basis of neutropenia or of failure to form circulating antibodies in response to an antigenic challenge. Failure to form antibodies generally is limited to chronic lymphocytic leukemia and is often reflected by hypogammaglobulinemia. Cytotoxic drug therapy may impair antibody response in any of the leukemias. Neutropenia is present in most patients with active acute leukemia and is a frequent complication of cytotoxic therapy in any of the leukemias.

The impaired resistance of the leukemic patient leads not only to frequent infections but also to infections of unusual severity. Bacterial infections spread with startling rapidity, and bacteremia is frequent. In patients who have not recently received antibiotics, the organisms responsible for infection usually are pneumococci, streptococci, staphylococci, or *Escherichia coli.* However, when a second infection follows closely on the heels of the first (superinfection), unusual organisms such as *Pseudomonas, Candida,* or *Aspergillus* are more frequently encountered. Most infections in patients with leukemia appear to arise from the patients' microbial flora, so that the alteration of the flora induced by antibiotics dictates to some degree the type of infection which is encountered. Almost all the rare organisms have been reported as causes of infection in leukemia, and organisms which are ordinarily nonpathogenic may assume a pathogenic role in such patients.

Therapy of infection in patients with leukemia must be swiftly and aggressively applied, and antibiotics should be as specific as possible for the offending organism. Prompt surgical drainage of abscesses is advisable, as is scrupulous local care of skin infections. Anti-infectious therapy is, at best, a delaying action unless specific antileukemic therapy leads to general improvement in the disease. As long as the defects in host defense persist, antibiotic control of one infection is usually followed with distressing rapidity by infection with another organism. Unfortunately, therapy of chronic lymphocytic leukemia fails to lead to improvement in antibody production.

Excessive production of uric acid reflects the rate of cell turnover in the leukemias. Elevated serum and urine urate levels are common in all leukemias except chronic lymphocytic leukemia. Therapy with cytotoxic agents increases the rate of urate production. Gout may develop, but the most distressing complication of excess urate production is precipitation of urate crystals in renal collecting tubules. Anuria may develop in this circumstance.

If anuria follows institution of cytotoxic therapy, spontaneous recovery is the rule if proper fluid management is followed, although an occasional patient requires dialysis. If oliguria or anuria develops without relation to cytotoxic therapy, more vigorous management is indicated. The xanthine oxidase inhibitor, allopurinol, blocks the conversion of hypoxanthine to uric acid, thereby reducing the excessive urate load. Its prophylactic use will prevent uric acid nephropathy. Alkalinization of the urine increases urate solubility and should be used in oliguric patients. Antigout drugs such as Benemid (*p*-di-*n*-propylsulfamylbenzoic acid) are contraindicated because they increase the concentration of urates in the collecting tubules.

DIFFERENTIAL DIAGNOSIS

The symptoms and signs of the leukemias are found in many other diseases, but diagnostic difficulty should occur only in relation to those diseases in which the leukocytic changes observed in the leukemias are approximated (*leukemoid reactions*). Other instances of diagnostic confusion are due to inadequate attention to examination of the blood.

In the presence of certain infections (e.g., pneumococcal, meningococcal, tuberculosis), in a few patients with malignancy, especially if metastasizing, and following the use of certain toxic drugs, a *picture mimicking that of chronic myelocytic leukemia* may be observed. In most such patients, although leukocytosis is present, there are far fewer myelocytes and more older neutrophils in the blood than in chronic myelocytic leukemia. More reliable differentiating points are the absence of increased basophils and eosinophils in leukemoid reactions, the normal or high, rather than low, leukocyte alkaline phosphatase, and the absence of the Philadelphia chromosome. Neutrophils from more than 90 percent of patients with chronic myelocytic leukemia show an abnormally reduced staining reaction for alkaline phosphatase. The presence of the Philadelphia chromosome in neutrophil precursors is for all practical purposes pathognomonic for chronic myelocytic leukemia, although its absence does not rule out the disease, since a few patients with seemingly typical chronic myelocytic leukemia do not show this finding.

Certain findings suggesting *myelofibrosis* or *polycythemia vera* may cause confusion and make it impossible to clearly categorize the patient. In cases of absence of a low alkaline phosphatase score and the Philadelphia chromosome, one should hesitate to make a diagnosis of chronic myelocytic leukemia.

Infectious mononucleosis may be mistaken for acute leukemia, but this diagnostic confusion reflects lack of experience in examining blood smears. Antibody studies also will be helpful (Chap. 224). Certain infections (e.g., pertussis, infectious lymphocytosis) may be associated with transient increases in numbers of small lymphocytes in the blood, but there are no causes of a marked and sustained increase in small lymphocytes in the blood other than chronic lymphocytic leukemia. Certain types of tumor cells in the bone marrow, such as those from neuroblastoma, may be confused with lymphoblasts. There are reports of patients with tuberculosis in whom a "leukemoid reaction" mimicking acute myeloblastic leukemia was observed. It is not certain whether these represented a leukemoid reaction or the association of myeloblastic leukemia and tuberculosis. As the neutrophil system recovers from drug-induced hypoplasia, the immaturity of bone marrow cells may temporarily suggest myeloblastic or myelocytic leukemia.

There is real difficulty in distinguishing between *lymphoblastic leukemia* and *myeloblastic leukemia* in patients in whom the blasts are very immature. The clinical differences between the diseases which were outlined previously may be of some help in this distinction. The most reliable method for distinguishing lymphoblasts from myeloblasts is a difference in nuclear chromatin discernible on properly prepared and stained thin smears of blood or bone marrow. The nuclear chromatin of myeloblasts is very fine or reticular and the nuclear membrane is thin and of uniform thickness, while some clumping of chromatin and irregularities of thickness of nuclear membrane are found in lymphoblasts. Special stains may be of some value, but no single stain provides infallible differentiation between lymphoblasts and myeloblasts. Myeloblasts stain with the peroxidase stain if they contain specific granules, but when enough cells stain with peroxidase to be of great diagnostic benefit, the myeloid character of the leukemia usually should be discernible on Wright's stained smears. Sudan black stain is of the same significance as peroxidase stain. Mature neutrophils in myeloblastic leukemia are likely to take up less alkaline phosphatase stain than normal neutrophils, while these cells take up more than normal amounts of the dye in many lymphoblastic leukemias. Lymphoblasts are more likely to stain with PAS than are myeloblasts.

Preleukemia represents a form of leukemia which can be distinguished from aplastic anemia or normocytic normochromic anemia of nonleukemic cause only by observation. When first seen, these patients are anemic, granulocytopenia may be present, platelets may be abnormally high or low, and bone marrow examination is nondiagnostic. After weeks, months, or even in an occasional patient, years, myeloblastic leukemia develops. Whether such patients represent a very early stage of the leukemic process or whether their initial syndrome is a different disease which predisposes to the development of leukemia is unknown.

TREATMENT

While the cure of leukemia is an objective which has not been assuredly attained in any patient to date, it is well established that its treatment reduces morbidity and prolongs life in the acute leukemias. Appropriate management also is very important in the chronic leukemias. To provide the patient a maximum of comfort and happiness, whether or not cure will ever be possible, should be the physician's aim. To do this a sound understanding of medicine as a whole is necessary, in addition to familiarity with the various forms of leukemia and the pros and cons of the available therapeutic agents. He must be able to give wise counsel and should be prepared to discuss the many questions which arise as the result of the advice of well-intentioned but usually poorly informed friends and neighbors or the false hopes engendered by premature statements appearing in the various news media. The desperate desire to secure help and the wish for a miracle drug must be treated sympathetically. Kindness, thoughtfulness, and wisdom are as important in therapy as the therapeutic agents themselves. Reassurance, if founded on understanding and good care, is a most valuable therapeutic agent.

Hospitalization, visits to the physician or hospital, and needle punctures should be held to the minimum consistent with care. The patient should be encouraged to maintain normal activities, whether these be play, going to school, housework, or breadwinning. The therapy which is chosen should be the simplest as well as the cheapest that is consistent with effective management.

The goals of therapy are accomplished through the use of antileukemia therapy which attempts to reduce and control the growth of the total mass of leukemic cells, and the employment of adjunctive therapy which is aimed at controlling complications such as infection, hemorrhage, the formation of troublesome localized leukemic tumors, hemolytic anemia, or uric acid nephropathy. Adjunctive therapy was discussed earlier in relation to the common complications and forms as important a part of the management of the patient as does antileukemic therapy. The principles of adjunctive therapy which were outlined previously are applicable to all types of leukemia, but more specific antileukemic therapy differs for the four common leukemias and will be discussed separately for each type.

CHRONIC MYELOCYTIC LEUKEMIA *Busulfan* is the treatment of choice, although radioactive phosphorus and x-ray to the spleen are effective modes of therapy also. Although it is unclear whether therapy prolongs the life of patients with chronic myelocytic leukemia, there is no question that therapy provides excellent and often prolonged symptomatic relief. The severity of this disease is reflected in the height of the leukocyte count, and patients with more than 50,000 leukocytes per μl blood usually are symptomatic. This figure can be used as a rough guide to the need to begin antileukemia therapy in chronic myelocytic leukemia.

Busulfan (Myleran) is given in oral doses of 4 mg daily and is continued until the leukocyte count is reduced to 10,000 per μl. Most patients with active chronic myelocytic leukemia are mildly anemic, and as the leukocyte count decreases, the anemia usually is corrected. Sternal tenderness usually disappears, and the spleen shrinks in response to therapy. However, some evidence of disease persists in most patients, such as a small but palpable spleen, persistent basophilic leukocytosis or an occasional immature myeloid cell in the blood. The duration of therapy required to bring the leukocyte count to normal depends primarily upon the height of the leukocyte count when therapy was begun. The curve of leukocyte decrease is an exponential function, so that the leukocyte count is reduced by one-half at fairly predictable intervals. In most patients approximately 2 months of continuous therapy will be required to accomplish these objectives.

Toxic reactions to busulfan that require interruption of the above type of therapeutic course are unusual. A few patients develop gastric discomfort, but the most serious complications are thrombocytopenia and leukopenia. If either develops, therapy with the drug should be discontinued. After many courses of busulfan or after prolonged maintenance therapy, patients commonly develop hyperpigmentation of the skin and a few develop interstitial pulmonary fibrosis, amenorrhea, testicular atrophy, gynecomastia, or a syndrome mimicking adrenal insufficiency.

If therapy is interrupted when the leukocyte count reaches normal levels, months and occasionally a year or more elapse before the patient again becomes symptomatic. When the leukocyte count increases to 50,000 or more cells per μl, busulfan therapy is resumed. Repeated remissions can be induced in this way. The duration of remission tends to become shorter with each successive course of the drug, but this is not always the case.

An alternative to repetitive, interrupted courses of busulfan is to reduce the dosage of the drug when the leukocyte count reaches normal levels with the hope of maintaining the leukocyte count within normal limits. Nothing is gained by this, however. Such maintenance therapy should be reserved for patients in whom the duration of unmaintained remissions has become distressingly short. Interrupted therapy requires fewer visits to the physician during remission than does maintenance therapy, and the incidence of the various toxic complications of the drug probably is lower with intermittent than with continuous busulfan administration.

The development of a progressive increase in the proportion of myeloblasts in blood and bone marrow (blastic crisis) signals the end of busulfan responsiveness, and at this point treatment is similar to that for acute myeloblastic leukemia.

CHRONIC LYMPHOCYTIC LEUKEMIA The indications for therapy and the beneficial effects of antileukemic therapy are not clear in this disease. Corticosteroid therapy and a variety of alkylating agents, such as cyclophosphamide or chlorambucil, administration of radioactive phosphorus, or irradiation of the spleen will reduce the mass of lymphoid tissue, but the overall benefit is unclear. The most common serious complication and the major cause of death in chronic lymphocytic leukemia is bacterial infection. As outlined previously, this is usually due to inability to form circulating antibodies and often is reflected in hypogammaglobulinemia. There is no evidence that any of the above modes of therapy benefit the antibody-forming mechanism, whereas the likelihood of serious infection may be enhanced by superimposing or accentuating neutropenia by the use of one of these agents. However, some patients report that they feel better after a course of therapy, and at present, hematologic opinion ranges from recommending no therapy except when specific indications, such as anemia, develop to the recommendation that the leukocyte count should be kept within normal limits as much of the time as possible.

If severe anemia (usually but not invariably an overtly hemolytic anemia) or severe thrombocytopenia develops in chronic lymphocytic leukemia, *corticosteroid therapy* is indicated. In most such patients, prompt improvement is induced by administration of 20 to 40 mg prednisone per day, or more. As soon as the anemia and/or the thrombocytopenia is corrected, the drug dosage should be gradually tapered and stopped as soon as possible. If large doses of prednisone are required to maintain the improvement, splenectomy should be considered. The risk of long-term prednisone therapy may outweigh the risk of splenectomy, and in many patients splenectomy will relieve the hemolytic anemia or thrombocytopenia sufficiently to make prednisone therapy unnecessary.

In addition to its salutary effect upon anemia and thrombocytopenia, corticosteroid therapy is markedly lymphocytolytic. The blood lymphocyte count rises initially, but then it decreases and a rapid reduction in the size of enlarged lymph nodes, spleen, and liver takes place. However, these advantages are outweighed by the frequency of bacterial infections which often are associated with long-continued corticosteroid therapy. Consequently, such treatment cannot be recommended for the routine management of this disease.

Therapy with an *alkylating agent* such as chlorambucil will lead to a reduction in blood lymphocyte levels and in the size of enlarged organs and lymph nodes. In some patients anemia is improved. However, anemia, thrombocytopenia, and neutropenia may become more severe during therapy and often fail to return to pretreatment levels when therapy is stopped. Hence, chlorambucil, if used, should be employed in modest dosage (0.1 mg per kg per day) and packed red cell volume, leukocytes, and platelets should be checked at frequent intervals.

ACUTE LYMPHOBLASTIC LEUKEMIA In the last 25 years a true revolution in therapy has occurred in this disease, leading to a marked prolongation in survival. With proper management at least one complete remission can be induced in almost all patients and as many as three successive complete remissions are not unusual. The drugs which are of proved benefit in this disease are listed in Table 316-1 and are divided into drugs which are useful in inducing a remission and those which are useful both in inducing and maintaining a remission. Corticosteroids and vincristine will induce remission, but the duration of the induced remission is not prolonged by continuing these drugs once a complete remission has been induced. Methotrexate (a folic acid antagonist) and 6-mercaptopurine prolong the duration of remission if administered on a continuous basis during remission. Whether cyclophosphamide will maintain, as well as induce, remissions is not entirely clear.

In inducing remissions with a single drug, *prednisone,* 40 mg per day, is probably the drug of choice because of the frequency of remission and its lower toxicity in comparison with the other drugs. Maximum improvement is achieved within 6 weeks after the start of therapy. At this point the drug should be tapered rapidly and then discontinued. Half of the patients who achieve a complete remission with the first course of prednisone will respond to a second course, but a steady reduction in number of responders is seen with subsequent courses. *Vincristine,* 0.1 mg per kg, given intravenously at weekly intervals, is effective in inducing remission but has very serious toxic effects. After three or four doses, deep tendon reflexes disappear in many patients, and unless the drug is discontinued, neurologic toxicity may progress until the patient is paralyzed. However, some patients can be brought into remission before neurologic toxicity supervenes. Asparaginase, 1,000 units intravenously each day, is effective in approximately 50 percent of patients.

Methotrexate and 6-*mercaptopurine* can be used singly as remission-inducing drugs but are more commonly used to induce remission in combination with other drugs or are used to maintain remissions induced with prednisone or vincristine.

If more than one of the remission-inducing drugs is given, the frequency of remission increases (80 percent with prednisone and 6-mercaptopurine, 90 percent with prednisone and vincristine), but so does the toxicity. If *combined therapy* is used, prednisone in combination with one of the other drugs is preferred because the toxic effects of the two drugs used will be qualitatively different. Small groups of patients treated experimentally with prednisone, vincristine, methotrexate, and 6-mercaptopurine (VAMP) administered in combination to induce remission, and patients treated by several other combinations of drugs, have remained in remission, unmaintained by drug therapy during remission, for much longer than have patients treated by any of the drugs administered alone. However, toxicity is severe and necessitates hospitalization and intensive supportive care. Hence, the role of such regimen in the general management of this disease remains to be determined.

For maintenance therapy after remission has been induced, methotrexate, 6-mercaptopurine, and, perhaps, cyclophosphamide are useful. Methotrexate may be administered daily by mouth, but the duration of remission is longer if it is given orally in a dose of from 15 to 30 mg per square meter of body surface twice each week. A daily dose of 6-mercaptopurine is given orally in the amount of 2.5 mg per kg. Therapy is continued at full dosage until relapse occurs or until toxicity supervenes. If hematologic toxicity, gastrointestinal side effects, or oral ulceration develop, the drug should be discontinued until toxicity disappears and then should be cautiously restarted, often at a somewhat reduced dose. Liver disease is an occasional side effect of both methotrexate and 6-mercaptopurine therapy. This is an indication for permanent discontinuation of the offending drug. If relapse occurs while the patient is receiving 6-mercaptopurine or methotrexate, the usefulness of this drug is ended, but if relapse occurs after the drug has been discontinued, a later trial with that agent is warranted. Attempts to delay the onset of drug resistance by alternating maintenance drugs during remission appear to be unsuccessful. Multiagent remission maintenance, used as repeated short, intensive courses of therapy, leads to longer remissions than single-agent regimens, but toxicity may be severe.

TABLE 316-1
Chemotherapeutic agents of proved effectiveness in the treatment of acute lymphoblastic leukemia

Agent	Useful in: Inducing remission	Maintaining remission	Rate of remission induction, %	Duration of remission, av.
Prednisone	Yes	No	60	
Vincristine	Yes	No	50	
Asparaginase	Yes	No	50	
Daunomycin	Yes	?Yes	40	
Cytosine arabinoside	Yes	?	30	
6-Mercaptopurine	Yes	Yes	40	6 months
Methotrexate	Yes	Yes	20	12 months*
Cyclophosphamide	Yes	?Yes	20	3 months

* *When administered as a twice-weekly dose; if given daily, duration is only about three months.*

The exact method of therapy that one adopts for a patient with lymphoblastic leukemia is probably not too important. One should attempt to induce successive remissions and maintain each for as long as possible. Intensive multiagent therapy leads to a higher percentage of 5-year survivors than does less aggressive therapy. However, periods of morbidity associated with drug toxicity reduce the quality of the remissions induced and maintained by intensive therapy. If a significant number of patients are cured, intensive therapy should be used, but it is not yet clear that this is so. While there are now many patients who have been in remission for more than 5 years, relapse has been noted after as long as 16 years in remission.

ACUTE MYELOBLASTIC LEUKEMIA This disease and its common variants, myelomonoblastic leukemia and promyelocytic leukemia, are very resistant to therapy. Of the agents listed in Table 316-1, only cytosine arabinoside, 6-mercaptopurine, and daunomycin are of proved effectiveness in acute myeloblastic leukemia. Whether the other agents have no salutary effect whatever or whether they are of some slight benefit, particularly if combined with an effective agent, is an open question.

The optimal regimen for cytosine arabinoside has not been determined but when given intravenously, every 8 hr, in a daily dose of 100 mg per m- body surface, approximately 30 percent of patients will achieve remission. This dose is given for 5 days followed by 7 days of rest, and then it is repeated. If remission has not been achieved by the third course, it is unlikely to occur.

6-Mercaptopurine is given in doses of 2.5 mg per kg daily by mouth. If remission occurs, some improvement will be evident within 8 weeks of beginning therapy. If improvement takes place, the drug should be continued until the patient relapses. Only 15 percent of patients achieve a complete remission with 6-mercaptopurine alone, and some 10 percent achieve partial remission. Daunomycin, an antibiotic, has severe and somewhat unpredictable hematologic toxicity and is usually used in combination with other drugs.

The low remission rate observed when single agents are employed has led to attempts to improve the rate by combining drugs. Combining 6-mercaptopurine or thioguanine and cytosine arabinoside failed to increase the remission rate above 40 percent in most studies. Short, intensive courses of cytosine arabinoside combined with daunomycin and other less effective drugs may be somewhat more efficacious.

The development of new drugs in the treatment of leukemia is discussed in Chap. 320.

DURATION OF SURVIVAL AND FACTORS INFLUENCING SURVIVAL A statistically demonstrable prolongation of life has attended therapy in acute lymphoblastic and acute myeloblastic leukemia, but such a lengthening of survival is not certain in chronic myelocytic and chronic lymphocytic leukemia. The natural history of chronic lymphocytic leukemia is much longer than that of the other forms of leukemia. Patients in whom the diagnosis was made before symptoms developed have lived an average of 10 years, and survival for two and three decades has been reported. Analysis of a series of patients presenting with all degrees of severity at the time of diagnosis showed that more than half such patients with chronic lymphocytic leukemia lived more than 5 years from diagnosis. Patients with chronic myelocytic leukemia rarely live as long as 10 years, most commonly 3 or 4 years, and blastic crisis usually signals the end of the disease.

The survival of patients with the acute leukemias averaged but 3 months from diagnosis before the present drugs became available, and survival for more than a year was exceptional. Now the average duration of life is steadily increasing in acute lymphoblastic leukemia, being more than 3 years in recent reports. A slight but significant prolongation of life has been observed in acute myeloblastic leukemia, attributable primarily to the few patients who respond favorably to therapy.

The duration of survival in acute lymphoblastic and acute myeloblastic leukemia depends primarily upon the number and duration of remissions. However, there are other prognostic factors in these diseases which help in predicting the duration of remissions and the duration of life. Patients in whom the total leukocyte count is low, few blasts are present in the blood, and sternal tenderness is absent, and who do not have serious hemorrhagic problems at the time of diagnosis tend to live longer than patients who do not present these findings. In patients with chronic lymphocytic leukemia the duration of life from diagnosis is shortened by the presence of any of the parameters of active disease and is inversely related to their severity.

REFERENCES

Boggs DR et al: The acute leukemias. Medicine 41:163, 1962

—— et al: Factors influencing the duration of survival of patients with chronic lymphocytic leukemia. Am J Med 40:243, 1966

——, Frei III E: Clinical studies of fever and infection in cancer. Cancer 13:1240, 1960

Burchenal JH et al: Treatment of acute lymphoblastic leukemia. Annu Rev Med 23:77, 1972

Crowther D et al: Combination chemotherapy using L-asparaginase, daunomycin and cytosine arabinoside in adults with acute myelogenous leukemia. Br Med J 4:513, 1970

Freireich EJ et al: The effect of 6-mercaptopurine on the duration of steroid-induced remissions in acute leukemia: A model for evaluation of other potentially useful therapy, Blood 21:699, 1963

Gallo RC et al: RNA-dependent DNA polymerase of human acute leukemic cells. Nature 2:228, 1970

Haut A et al: Busulfan in the treatment of chronic myelocytic leukemia: The effect of long term intermittent therapy. Blood 17:1, 1961

Rosenthal DS, Moloney WC: The treatment of acute granulocytic leukemia in adults. N Engl J Med 286:1176, 1972

Thomas ED et al: Leukaemic transformation of engrafted human marrow cells in vivo. Lancet 1:1310, 1972

Wintrobe MM et al: *Clinical Hematology,* 7th ed., Philadelphia: Lea & Febiger, 1974

317 DISEASES OF THE SPLEEN AND RETICULOENDOTHELIAL SYSTEM

D. R. BOGGS
M. M. WINTROBE

The functions of the spleen were outlined in an earlier chapter (Chap. 60). Disorders of the spleen most frequently produce enlargement of this organ. The significance of splenic enlargement and the differential diagnosis of splenomegaly were discussed in Chap. 60. Here several disorders which involve the spleen, but which have not been discussed before, will be described.

Congenital anomalies of the spleen may take various forms.

The spleen may be *absent.* This may be suspected when Howell-Jolly bodies, occasional nucleated red cells, target cells, decreased osmotic fragility, siderocytosis, leukocytosis, and a variable degree of thrombocytosis are found in the absence of a discoverable cause and particularly when there is associated congenital heart or intestinal malformation.

Functional asplenia has been suggested in children with sickle-cell anemia and in patients with lymphomatous enlargement of the spleen. In this circumstance the splenic reticuloendothelial system fails to engulf normal quantities of radiopaque dyes.

Instead of being a single organ, the spleen may be subdivided into numerous small spleens, or a spleen of normal size and shape may be accompanied by an accessory spleen, or more than one. Rarely, the spleen assumes a retroperitoneal position and may force the left kidney downward. A movable spleen may be found in any part of the abdomen. If its pedicle becomes twisted, there may be sudden pain, enlargement, and signs of shock, as well as fever and vomiting if the torsion has developed acutely. Less severe symptoms occur if the process is more gradual.

Rupture of the spleen may occur following trauma, particularly if the spleen is diseased. Malaria, typhoid fever, leukemia, and infectious mononucleosis are among the diseases in which this has been observed. Agonizing abdominal pain or pain in the left scapular region, together with signs of internal hemorrhage, characterizes this catastrophe. When subcapsular hemorrhage develops with the original trauma, rupture may be delayed for a few hours. Anemia develops rapidly, and leukocytosis occurs. Prompt surgical treatment is imperative. After traumatic rupture autotransplantation of splenic tissue throughout the peritoneal cavity (*splenosis*) sometimes occurs.

Infarction of the spleen may be sterile, in which event it is followed eventually by fibrosis and shrinkage. This has been observed as a complication of leukemia, as well as in sickle-cell anemia and the sickle-cell trait, and in sickle-cell-hemoglobin-C disease. A septic infarct may terminate with the formation of an abscess. The most common symptom of infarction is pain. Careful examination will reveal a friction rub if the infarcted splenic surface abuts the peritoneum. Unless an abscess forms, necessitating surgical intervention, sedation and abdominal support to impair movement of the spleen suffice.

Aneurysms of the splenic artery are rare but may cause vague, crampy pain in the left upper part of the abdomen and even splenic enlargement. Occasionally the aneurysm is palpable and a bruit may be heard. Found predominantly in women and most frequently after middle age, rupture has been reported during pregnancy.

CHRONIC CONGESTIVE SPLENOMEGALY Definition This syndrome (Banti's syndrome) is characterized by splenic enlargement, leukopenia, anemia and often thrombocytopenia, a tendency to gastric hemorrhage, and, in many cases, cirrhotic changes in the liver.

History The term *splenic anemia* was originally used (1866) to refer to cases of anemia with splenomegaly which were not frank leukemia. Banti, in 1882 and subsequently, described a form of splenomegaly of unknown cause associated in its earliest stages with leukopenia, asthenia, and occasional hemorrhagic episodes. In the intermediate stage, hepatic enlargement occurred, as well as urobilinuria and a dirty-brownish discoloration of the skin. The final stage consisted of liver atrophy and ascites.

Etiology Banti considered the spleen to be the primary seat of the disease. However, later work indicated that the pathologic changes in the spleen are not specific and can be encountered particularly when there is increased venous pressure in the portal bed. That there is portal hypertension has been demonstrated by measurement (225 to 500 or more mm H_2O), and now most students of this syndrome consider the portal hypertension to be due to intrahepatic causes such as Laennec's cirrhosis or schistosomiasis, or to extrahepatic factors. Thus the designation *chronic congestive splenomegaly* has arisen. Cirrhosis of the liver, cavernous transformation of the portal vein, portal vein and splenic vein thrombosis, or variants in the anatomy of the venous pattern have been found in most of the cases. Rarer causes are compression from pancreatic fibrosis or tumor or from an aneurysm of the splenic artery.

The hematologic changes observed in the Banti syndrome are attributable to the unequal distribution of the cells of the blood in the splenic vascular bed and the remaining parts of the circulation resulting from stasis of the portal circulation. Following splenectomy the blood values usually return to normal.

Pathology The spleen weighs 600 to 1,200 g as a rule, but may weigh as much as 5,000 g. At first one finds an increase in the reticulum, cellular hyperplastic pulp, degenerative changes in the follicular arterioles, and congestion. Later the follicles become smaller, while fibrosis of the reticulum, trabeculae, and capsule increases. Periarterial hemorrhages and siderotic nodules deposited in the fibrous tissue around the arterioles are found in many instances.

Symptoms The symptoms are primarily those of the underlying conditions and include the various manifestations of hepatic failure when this is responsible for the congestive splenomegaly. However, in a few patients, the initial symptoms may direct attention to the spleen itself. In such patients, the symptoms of anemia may be prominent, or a large mass in the left upper quadrant of the abdomen may be noted. In other instances the disorder may be announced explosively by the occurrence of a gastric hemorrhage.

The anemia is normocytic and moderate in degree unless hemorrhage has occurred, when it may be microcytic and hypochromic. In cases with long-standing and severe liver disease the anemia may be macrocytic. Leukopenia is found consistently, and thrombocytopenia is observed frequently. The bone marrow may show no abnormality, or slight myeloid hyperplasia may be present.

Diagnosis Other conditions leading to pancytopenia (Chap. 61) must be excluded, as well as the various causes of splenomegaly (Chap. 60). Even when gastrointestinal hemorrhage has occurred, the diagnosis should be made only after other possibilities have been excluded. Thus, a "silent" peptic ulcer may produce hypochromic microcytic anemia with slight splenic enlargement. Hookworm infection may produce chronic hypochromic anemia with moderate splenomegaly. Liver function should be studied in suspected cases, and esophageal varices should be looked for. Liver biopsy, roentgenographic examination with barium, and endoscopic study of the esophagus may be required. If liver function is good and other conditions have been excluded, portal or splenic vein thrombosis should be suspected. If a block is suspected, its site should be determined, if possible, by portal venography. Congestive splenomegaly due to extrahepatic causes is more likely to be found in patients below the age of eighteen than in older patients.

Prognosis and treatment In general, the large spleen and the associated hematologic abnormalities pose less of a threat to these patients than does hepatic failure or bleeding from gastric or esophageal varices. Splenectomy often leads to improvement or correction of anemia, neutropenia, and thrombocytopenia but is of little value in relieving portal hypertension. Therefore splenectomy as the sole surgical measure should be limited to such rare causes of congestive splenomegaly as splenic vein thrombosis or aneurysm of the splenic artery. In other circumstances, splenectomy should rarely be considered except in conjunction with a shunting operation designed to relieve the increased portal pressure. Portacaval shunt is usually preferred because of the large size of the vessels involved. If a large-caliber splenic vein is available or when the portal vein is obliterated, splenectomy and splenorenal shunts are recommended.

The risks of surgery in these patients are substantial, and surgical intervention is advocated only (1) in cases in which there is severe bleeding from the upper part of the intestine and in which the portal hypertension is due to extrahepatic block; and (2) in cases of portal hypertension associated with cirrhosis of the liver where ascites and icterus are minimal or absent and there is a reasonable degree of hepatic reserve.

HYPERSPLENISM The concept that the spleen may produce disease as the result of an exaggeration of its normal functions is based on the observation that anemia, leukopenia, or thrombocytopenia, or combinations of these manifestations, may disappear following splenectomy. When the above-mentioned hematologic manifestations accompany recognizable disease entities the "hypersplenism" is "secondary"; otherwise it is "primary." According to this concept, the destructive potential of the spleen has increased or, in other cases, its hypothetic inhibitory effect on the bone marrow has become exaggerated. "Autoimmune" acquired hemolytic anemia and idiopathic thrombocytopenic purpura are examples of conditions which some investigators would classify as forms of hypersplenism. Although a helpful concept, use of the term has led to loose thinking and careless diagnosis. As outlined earlier (Chap. 60), the functions of the spleen still are not fully understood.

"Big spleen syndrome" Well-marked splenomegaly accompanying a variety of diseases, such as lupus erythematosus, sarcoidosis, malignant lymphoma, chronic lymphocytic leukemia, myelofibrosis, and Gaucher's disease may be associated with moderate or marked anemia, together with moderate reticulocytosis (5 to 10 percent) and erythroid hyperplasia of the bone marrow. Overt signs of exaggerated blood destruction are not necessarily present. Counts over the spleen following tagging of the patient's own red cells with radioactive chromium (^{51}Cr) may indicate increased radioactivity there. In such cases there also may be leukopenia (due mainly to granulocytopenia) and thrombocytopenia. In other cases the granulocytopenia is the most prominent manifestation, as in Felty's syndrome and in kala azar. Splenectomy has been observed in some of these cases to be associated with disappearance of the hematologic manifestations in whole or in part.

Thrombocytopenia in association with splenomegaly probably indicates that an increased proportion of the total body platelet pool is sequestered in the spleen, but the size of the total platelet pool may not be reduced in some cases. Anemia accompanying splenomegaly may also be explained in part by increased splenic sequestration of red cells, but also is due, in part, to an increase in plasma volume. An increased rate of destruction of normal red cells may contribute to the anemia. As noted in Chap. 60, most red cells move rapidly through a normal spleen. Studies employing red cells labeled with radioactive chromium indicate not only increased splenic sequestration, but also a very slow splenic transit time for a portion of the sequestered cells. These slowly circulating, closely packed, sequestered red cells may have insufficient glucose available for glycolytic energy production, and, as a consequence, suffer membrane damage and destruction.

MYELOFIBROSIS Definition This term refers to a disorder characterized by splenomegaly, often of great proportion, together with varying degrees of fibrosis or osteosclerosis of the marrow cavity. Extramedullary blood formation is found in the spleen. *Agnogenic myeloid metaplasia, myeloid megakaryocytic hepatosplenomegaly,* and *chronic nonleukemic myelosis* are among the other names which have been used for this syndrome.

Etiology and pathogenesis Most instances are idiopathic, and while the idiopathic form may occur at any age, most patients are more than fifty years of age. Both sexes are affected in approximately equal proportion. Occasionally myelofibrosis has developed following what has appeared to be typical chronic myelocytic leukemia, but sometimes the converse has been observed; namely, marked myeloid leukocytosis and other changes typical of chronic myelocytic leukemia have developed in patients whose findings previously had suggested myelofibrosis. A similar paradoxic relation to polycythemia vera has been observed. Such cases have led to elaboration of the concept of *myeloproliferative disorders.* By this term, it is implied that myeloid leukemia, acute and chronic, polycythemia vera, myelofibrosis, and even "essential thrombocythemia" and the di Guglielmo syndrome (Chap. 316) result from overgrowth of all or some of the types of cells which are normally formed in the bone marrow and can be produced in sites where extramedullary blood formation occurs, such as the spleen. It is argued that one or more of the marrow elements may be produced in excess and that the bone marrow, initially hyperplastic, ultimately becomes fibrotic. The overlapping of the clinical and hematologic manifestations of these diseases which is seen occasionally gives support to the concept, but in the great majority of cases the manifestations and course of the various disorders named above are sufficiently distinct to permit a more specific diagnosis. Since the nature of the fundamental disturbance in these conditions is unknown and may be similar or quite different, the value of the term *myeloproliferative disorder* may be questioned. However, it does give comfort to those who gain security from having a name.

Myelofibrosis may follow chronic exposure to benzene and carbon tetrachloride, phosphorus poisoning, or irradiation exposure, as observed in radium-dial painters and atomic bomb survivors. Patients with tuberculosis and with carcinoma have developed a myelofibrosis-like syndrome, seemingly as a complication of their primary disease.

The pathogenesis of the anemia in myelofibrosis was discussed earlier (Chap. 58). It must be presumed that blood formation in this disease is not confined to the spleen, as was once assumed, since splenectomy has been carried out in some cases without serious aggravation of the disease.

Pathology The fibrosis is irregular and may be interspersed with fatty areas or even with marrow hyperplasia. It tends to be greatest in the flat bones and in time may become more pronounced. In certain patients, marrow fibrosis may be difficult to demonstrate in the early stages of disease. In such patients marrow aspirates are usually quite cellular and often contain increased numbers of megakaryocytes. The spleen tends to increase in size and may become huge. Extramedullary hematopoiesis is prominent, especially in the pulp, but areas of fibrosis and infarction may be found as well. Myeloid metaplasia may also be present in the liver, lymph nodes, kidneys, perirenal fat, or other sites.

Clinical manifestations Weakness, fatigue, and ultimately, an awareness of a left-upper-quadrant mass are the usual complaints. Weight loss, sometimes anorexia, and episodes of abdominal pain, perhaps from splenic infarction and perisplenitis, as well as pallor and gradual enlargement of the liver, ensue. Less commonly there may be hemorrhage or thrombosis, arthralgia, bone pain, intolerance to heat, fever, dependent edema, and even ascites.

Normal and even high hemoglobin values early in the course of the disease are followed by the development of anemia, which may become severe. However, severe anemia may be present at diagnosis, marked poikilocytosis is a feature, and "teardrop" poikilocytes are characteristic. Polychromatophilia, occasional normoblasts, and reticulocytosis are additional features of the blood smear. Leukocytosis, with some shift to the left, is the rule, but the leukocyte count may be normal or low. In contrast to chronic myelocytic leukemia, the leukocytes stain heavily with the alkaline phosphatase stain in most, but not all, patients. Thrombocytosis and the presence of large and bizarre platelets are common, but ultimately, thrombocytopenia may occur. Serum uric acid usually is elevated.

Diagnosis The dry tap on marrow examination contrasts with the finding in chronic myelocytic leukemia, as does the usual finding of increased leukocyte alkaline phosphatase. Trephine biopsy confirms the inactive state of the marrow. With one exception, the Philadelphia chromosome abnormality which is common in chronic myelocytic leukemia has not been observed in marrow cells from patients with myelofibrosis. Roentgenographic evidence of myelofibrosis or osteosclerosis is found in only about 40 percent of the cases. Other causes of splenomegaly should be ruled out, as discussed elsewhere (Chap. 60).

Prognosis and treatment The course is slow but is likely to be progressive. The great majority of patients survive 3 to 5 years, a number even 10 years or longer. Transfusion may be needed if the anemia is severe but should be held to a minimum. Busulfan, 2 to 4 mg per day, may reduce the leukocyte count and size of the spleen but must be used cautiously to avoid serious depression of hematopoietic activity. There is little evidence to suggest that busulfan is of overall benefit. Large doses of androgenic hormone, oxymetholone, 4 mg per kg per day for men and 1 mg per kg per day for women, may relieve the anemia, but thrombocytopenia, if present, is less likely to be affected. Androgens are most often of benefit in relatively young women with myelofibrosis. If the transfusion requirement is very great, or if severe thrombocytopenia is present, evidence of excessive splenic destruction should be sought by external counting over the spleen and liver following ^{51}Cr tagging of the red cells or platelets. Irradiation over the spleen to reduce its size is of limited value. When increased blood destruction is very troublesome and not relieved by other measures, as described above, splenectomy may be found to reduce the transfusion needs and lead to improvement of the platelet count.

Death is usually due to infection, often pneumonia complicating congestive heart failure, hemorrhage, or thrombosis. A few patients die with a picture closely resembling acute myeloblastic leukemia.

GAUCHER'S DISEASE Definition This designation is applied to two or more hereditary disorders of glucosyl ceramide metabolism. These compounds, previously referred to as *cerebrosides*, accumulate in the reticuloendothelial cells. This accumulation is secondary to a deficiency of the enzyme beta-glucosidase, which catalyzes the cleavage of glucose from glycosyl ceramide. As a consequence, the latter compound accumulates. Two, and perhaps three, phenotypic expressions of the disease are recognized. The first, which is usually referred to as the *infantile* or *acute neuronopathic* type, is distinguished from the *adult* or *nonneuronopathic* type by the presence of severe neurologic disease and death in infancy. A third type, intermediate between the two, is referred to as the *juvenile* or *subacute neuronopathic* type. The accumulation of ceramide-loaded storage cells leads to marked splenomegaly in all varieties and also often to hepatomegaly, bone lesions, skin pigmentation, and pingueculae of the sclera.

Etiology, morbid anatomy, and pathogenesis The acute neuronal form begins in early infancy, and while the chronic nonneuronal form may be diagnosed in early childhood, the diagnosis may be made at any age. Family studies in all forms of the disease suggest inheritance as an autosomal recessive, although in occasional families a dominant form of inheritance is suggested. The failure to note more than one type of disease in any particular family suggests that these are distinct inheritance patterns. Caucasians, Negroes, and Orientals may be affected by any form, but in the acute neuronal type there is a marked preponderance of Ashkenazi Jewish ancestry. There also is some excess of Jewish ancestry in the chronic nonneuronal variety.

The characteristic finding is widespread reticulum cell hyperplasia, the cells being filled with large amounts of glucosyl ceramide. As noted above, there is evidence for deficiency of beta glucosidase which cleaves glucose from this compound. Glucosyl ceramide is a metabolic product of many cells, including blood leukocytes; the reticulum cell hyperplasia seems simply to have occurred in response to an excessive demand for storage of this compound.

The Gaucher cell is distinctive in its morphologic appearance, being 20 to 80 μm in diameter, round, oval, or spindle-shaped, and possessing one or more small eccentrically placed nuclei. The cytoplasm has the appearance of crinkled tissue paper showing numerous wavy fibrillae. These are visible in ordinary Wright's stain smears, but are best seen in supravital preparations or with electron microscopy. On electron microscopy these fibrillae are seen to be tubular structures with diameters of 120 to 750 A which are up to 5 μm in length. Each structure contains 10 to 12 fibrils twisted around the long axis of the tubule with a distance between fibrils of about 80 A. Tubules of similar appearance can be formed in vitro from pure glucosyl ceramide.

Gaucher cells are found throughout the body, but are present in greatest concentration in the spleen, liver, bone marrow, and lymph nodes of the paraaortic and thoracic chain. They are found in significant concentration in the alveolar capillaries of the lung.

In the acute neuronal form, ganglion cell destruction, glial proliferation, and demyelinization may be found in the brain. However, abnormal accumulation of glucosyl ceramide has not been demonstrated in all cases.

Clinical manifestations The typical patient with the acute neuronopathic form appears normal at birth, but by three months of age has developed problems with feeding, has a cough with frequent pulmonary infections, and is found to have an enlarged liver and spleen. Neurologic signs usually appear by six months and most commonly involve cranial nerves and extrapyramidal tracts. The usual patient dies from either pulmonary infection, progressive neurologic disease, or thrombocytopenic bleeding by age nine months; few survive beyond their second year.

The chronic nonneuronopathic form, which is the most common form of the disease, may begin in childhood; most patients have signs and symptoms by age 15 to 20 years, but the diagnosis has been made in old age. The disease varies markedly in its severity from patient to patient, and a normal life expectancy is possible. The most common life-threatening problem is bleeding secondary to thrombocytopenia. That this is due to increased sequestration and destruction of platelets in a markedly enlarged spleen is suggested by the observation that splenectomy leads to a marked decrease of thrombocytopenia. Repeated pulmonary infections may also be a problem, particularly when the disease begins in childhood. Although the liver is often enlarged and liver function tests may be abnormal, liver failure is not common, but portal hypertension may occur. Pain in the limbs associated with expanding bone lesions is common. The reason for the development of this type of lesion is not entirely clear, for while it is associated with accumulation of Gaucher's cells at the site of bony expansion with thinning of the cortex, the cells do not completely fill the expanding area, as one would anticipate if it were simple necrosis secondary to tumor growth. Pathologic fractures may occur. Of the roentgenographic abnormalities of bone, the development of a radiolucent area in the lower end of the femur in the contour of an Erlenmeyer flask is the typical lesion. Yellow-brown pingueculae may be seen on the conjunctiva on either side of the cornea, and similar pigmentation may be found on the exposed areas of the skin.

The subacute neuronopathic variety usually begins in childhood, but this is the most poorly characterized of the three conditions. Increased glucosyl ceramide has not been demonstrated in nonneuropathic tissue of certain cases, and it is possible that some of these patients have been confused with the newly described disease of *fucosidosis*, which is associated with accumulation of glycolipids and mucopolysaccharides containing fucose. Although splenomegaly may occur, their primary clinical problems relate to the neurologic involvement, and most have died before reaching adulthood.

In all types the plasma acid phosphatase activity is markedly increased when measured with phenyl phosphate as substrate. In contrast to the prostatic enzyme, the acid phosphatase is not inhibited by L-tartrate. In addition to the severe thrombocytopenia that may develop in many patients, moderate anemia and neutropenia may be observed. Plasma glucosyl ceramide levels usually are not elevated unless the spleen has been removed.

Diagnosis The typical cells may be seen by ordinary light microscopy in sternal marrow aspirates or in aspirates from the spleen. Phase microscopy and electron microscopy reveal these unique cells to best advantage. Confirmation by tissue lipid analysis showing accumulation of glucosyl ceramide should be carried out before a definitive diagnosis is made.

Treatment and prognosis There is no known form of useful therapy in this disease with the exception of splenectomy for correction of thrombocytopenia. The decision as to when to do splenectomy must be individualized. Most would not recommend splenectomy unless severe thrombocytopenia associated with significant hemorrhage has developed. Relief of bone pain has been reported following steroid therapy or irradiation, but this is not a consistent finding.

NIEMANN-PICK DISEASE Definition This is a rare group of familial disorders, first described in 1914, in which sphingomyelin, the phosphorylcholine ester of *N*-acylsphingosine, accumulates in reticuloendothelial cells throughout the body. Increased cholesterol is also present in some cases, and sphingomyelinase is decreased in some but not all forms. On the basis of differences in age of onset, presence or absence of neurologic disease, and the heterogeneity of chemical expression in ratios of sphingomyelin:sphingomyelinase:cholesterol, it has been suggested that at least four phenotypic expressions exist, based on an unknown number of mutants. Hepatomegaly and retarded nervous and physical development are usually observed within the first six months of life, and death from inanition or intercurrent infection usually occurs within one to three years. However, a smaller number of patients follow a much more chronic course, and some, usually without neurologic disease, live well into adulthood.

Etiology and pathogenesis The disease is apparently inherited as a simple mendelian recessive trait, both sexes being equally involved. It has not been observed in more than one generation in a single pedigree. Over half the reported cases have been in Jews, but many other ethnic groups have been involved. Inbreeding may be the cause of the high incidence among the groups involved.

The characteristic *foam cells* are reticuloendothelial cells, 20 to 90 μm in diameter, and are so filled with vacuoles that they have a mulberry appearance. The nucleus is small and is placed eccentrically but may be multiple. The vacuoles have a faint bluish hue with Wright's stain, are positive to the periodic acid–Schiff reaction, and stain with Sudan III and other fat stains. Sphingomyelin is contained in the vacuoles. These cells may be found everywhere but are essentially prominent in the spleen, liver, lymph nodes, and bone marrow. It is generally assumed that the increase in storage cells reflects the excessive sphingomyelin. In some but not all cases it is possible to demonstrate decreased sphingomyelinase, the enzyme which catalyzes the cleavage of phosphorylcholine from sphingomyelin.

Swelling, vacuolization, and degeneration of Nissl substance are found in the ganglion cells of the nervous system. There are also demyelination, scarring and fibrosis, and proliferation of glial cells which become converted to foam cells. In the retina, destruction of ganglion cells in the surrounding area may leave a grayish background, against which the macula stands out as a cherry-red spot. Although the anatomic changes in the nervous system resemble closely those in Tay-Sachs disease (Chap. 333), these two diseases are distinctly separate entities.

Clinical manifestations The earliest sign usually is a poor feeding pattern in infants. In addition to hepatosplenomegaly there may be generalized lymphadenopathy, infiltrative lesions in the lung visible by x-ray, xanthomatous or infiltrative lesions of the skin, and skin pigmentation. Nutrition is poor and physical development is retarded. A relentless and widely varied pattern of neurologic disturbances follows (Chap. 333) until a nearly vegetative state is reached before death, which occurs in 1 to 3 years. However, in a few instances the disease may develop more slowly, and changes may be present for years in the absence of neurologic signs.

Anemia and thrombocytopenia are usually moderate in degree, although with long-standing disease and marked splenomegaly severe thrombocytopenia may develop. The leukocyte count usually is normal but may be increased or low. The lymphocytes and monocytes may show some vacuolization, but adequate histochemical studies of their contents have not been made.

Roentgenography may reveal diffuse miliary pulmonary mottling. Trabecular coarseness is occasionally demonstrable in the long bones, but widening and prominence of the medullary cavities is unusual.

Diagnosis There are no characteristic laboratory tests. Slight hyperlipemia is common, but plasma sphingomyelin levels are normal. The appearance of the foam cells, usually obtained by marrow aspiration, affords a tentative diagnosis. Biopsy of rectal mucosa showing changes in the ganglion cells of the myenteric plexus may also be helpful. A positive Smith-Dietrich stain is usually obtained, but specific histochemical tests for sphingomyelin are not available. Similar clinical and morphologic findings have been obtained in one family in which the stored lipid was a lipid phosphatide other than sphingomyelin. Diagnosis is made by lipid analysis of involved tissues. Cells from bone marrow propagated in tissue culture also contain excessive sphingomyelin, and such cells may be examined for confirmation when sufficient biopsy material is not available otherwise.

Treatment There is no specific therapy, but x-ray therapy may be helpful in the control of infiltrative skin lesions. Splenectomy is of little value unless severe thrombocytopenia has developed.

HISTIOCYTOSIS X Pathologic lesions containing common features in various degrees have led to the grouping of Letterer-Siwe disease, Hand-Schüller-Christian disease, and eosinophilic granuloma under a single heading, histiocytosis X. The common denominator is a distinctive, inflammatory histiocytosis. Reticuloendothelial proliferation and hyperplasia, and granulomatous changes, featuring eosinophils and giant cells, are followed by the conversion of reticulum cells and histiocytes to foam cells or xanthomas containing cholesterol and its esters. Ultimately fibrosis may occur. The similarity in pathologic picture does not prove etiologic identity, however, and the relation of these disorders to one another must as yet be considered unproved. Indeed, it has even been suggested that these disorders do not represent an entity and are perhaps misdiagnosed infections and malignant lymphomas.

These three disorders differ in the sites of involvement and the predominating stage of tissue reaction. In these conditions, lipid accumulation is a secondary and inconsistent feature, and there is no clear-cut tendency for familial involvement. The nature of the underlying defect is unknown.

LETTERER-SIWE DISEASE This has been observed most often in infants and young children, is variable in duration (a few weeks to several years), and has usually proved fatal. There is evidence of a wasting disorder, with enlargement of the spleen and liver, generalized lymphadenopathy, a hemorrhagic diathesis, especially petechiae and purpura, skeletal lesions, progressive anemia, and cutaneous manifestations. The last consist of discrete, yellowish-brown maculopapular lesions, or papules with a red border and yellow center. They are scattered over the face and trunk particularly, but may be found in the scalp and elsewhere. Whitish macules over the palate and tongue and weeping erosions in the axillas and other moist areas may develop. There may be a low-grade, persistent spiking fever. Diffuse histiocytic proliferation may occur in the lungs. Localized bone destruction may occur, especially in the calvarium.

Diagnosis is made by biopsy of bone or lymph nodes. The course is relatively acute, and secondary precipitation of cholesterol esters in histiocytes to form foam cells usually does not occur. *Treatment* involves supportive care, irradiation of the skin lesions and other areas of involvement, and antimicrobial therapy for secondary infections, as they occur. The disease is usually fatal, termination often being similar to that of acute leukemia. Steroid therapy or vinblastine (Chap. 316) may be helpful. Rarely, recovery occurs or a more chronic picture develops, as seen in Hand-Schüller-Christian disease.

HAND-SCHÜLLER-CHRISTIAN DISEASE This may represent in chronic form the same disorder which, in acute or subacute form, presents the picture of Letterer-Siwe disease, or it may represent a multifocal form of solitary eosinophilic granuloma. Occurring predominantly in children, Hand-Schüller-Christian disease may also be found in adults, rarely in older persons. The pathologic feature is a histiocytic granuloma. The histiocytosis or granulomatosis may or may not be accompanied by intense eosinophilic reaction; the characteristic lipogranuloma is now thought to be the late phase in the evolution of the histiocytic lesion. The histiocytes contain so much cholesterol that they have the appearance of foam cells. The granulomas are found in bones, especially the skull, and in skin and viscera. Thereby the characteristic triad, rarely observed together in the same patient, of exophthalmos, diabetes insipidus, and defects in the membranous bones is produced. In the scalp soft-tissue nodules overlying the cranial defects may be palpated.

Xanthoma disseminatum is a cutaneous manifestation that may or may not be associated with bone and visceral lesions. The yellowish-brown maculopapular lesions are most frequently scattered over the face, especially the eyes and mouth, trunk and perineum, and in the axillas. They may occur in the mouth. Histologically they reveal foam cells and intensive histiocytic proliferation with or without eosinophils. The lesions are not painful but tend to recur when removed surgically. Fibrotic lesions associated with extracellular lipid deposits located under the tongue and in the pharynx and larynx, so-called *lipid proteinosis,* may represent an end stage of xanthoma disseminatum.

Visceral lesions may occur in the liver, spleen, kidneys, perirenal fat, walls of the larger blood vessels, brain, and lungs. There may be diffuse pulmonary infiltration, but more often it is perihilar or central. Hepatosplenomegaly and lymph node enlargement are usually modest and anemia is usually mild, but pancytopenia may occur. Although tissue cholesterol may be many times greater than normal, the plasma cholesterol level is normal.

Growth may be retarded and puberty delayed. Otitis media is a common complication. The course waxes and wanes irregularly, and spontaneous remissions occur. The skeletal lesions may respond to x-ray, but widespread radiation of chronic relapsing lesions usually produces more harmful side effects than benefit. Large doses of steroid may reverse all manifestations of the disease temporarily and can produce remissions of at least several years' duration. Vinblastine (Chap. 316) may have some value. From 15 to 30 percent of cases terminate fatally, but complete recovery may occur. Diabetes insipidus is likely to persist, however, and pulmonary lesions may produce alveolocapillary block, pulmonary insufficiency, or right-sided heart failure. Rarely the disease becomes more acute, then resembling Letterer-Siwe disease.

EOSINOPHILIC GRANULOMA This is the most benign of these conditions. It is characterized by single or multiple granulomas and osteolytic lesions with no discernible associated visceral involvement. Found in infants, children, and young adults, eosinophilic granuloma occasionally is seen at a later age. The condition is somewhat more common in males than in females and is rare in Negroes. The eosinophilic and histiocytic proliferation begins in the bone marrow but gradually erodes the cortex until the bone expands. Roentgenologically lytic lesions can be demonstrated within the medullary cavity, about 1 to 4 cm in diameter and with borders less distinct than those of bone cysts. In patients over the age of twenty years the lesions are found almost exclusively in the flat bones. At an earlier age they may also be present in long bones, especially the femur or humerus. The swellings may be silent, or there may be pain and swelling at the site of involvement. Rarely there is mild fever, but usually there are no constitutional symptoms. Pathologic fractures may occur. The blood is normal. Eosinophilia is unusual.

The granulomas may remain unchanged for years, but eventually, at least in some patients, fibrosis develops, eosinophils disappear, and the histiocytes become lipophages. Solitary granulomas are best treated by curettement or excision. Irradiation is reserved for lesions that are inaccessible to such therapy. The results are usually good, and the prognosis is excellent.

When multiple lesions occur, and especially when they are extraosseous, the distinction from milder forms of Schüller-Christian disease is unclear, and perhaps unimportant.

REFERENCES

Avioli LV et al: Histiocytosis X (Schüller-Christian disease): A clinicopathological survey, review of ten patients and the results of prednisone therapy. Medicine 42:119, 1963

Crocker AC, Farber S: Niemann-Pick disease. Medicine, 37:1, 1958; Am J Clin Nutr 9:63, 1961

Fredrickson DS, Sloan HR: Glucosyl ceramide lipidoses: Gaucher's disease, sphingomyelin lipidoses: Niemann-Pick disease, in *The Metabolic Basis of Inherited Disease,* 3d ed., eds JB Stanbury et al, New York: McGraw-Hill, 1972

Lichtenstein L: Histiocytosis X: Integration of eosinophilic granuloma of bone, "Letterer-Siwe disease," and "Schüller-Christian disease" as related manifestations of a single nosologic entity. AMA Arch Pathol 56:84, 1953

Lieberman PH et al: A reappraisal of eosinophilic granuloma of bone, Hand-Schüller-Christian syndrome and Letterer-Siwe syndrome. Medicine 48:375, 1969

MacPherson AIS: Assessment of the results of surgical treatment in portal hypertension. Gastroenterology 38:142, 1960

Motulsky AG et al: Anemia and the spleen. N Engl J Med, 259:1164 and 1215, 1958

Pitcock JA et al: A clinical and pathological study of seventy cases of myelofibrosis. Ann Intern Med 57:73, 1962

Ward HP, Block MH: The natural history of agnogenic myeloid metaplasia and a critical evaluation of its relationship with the myeloproliferative syndrome. Medicine 50:357, 1971

Wintrobe MM et al: *Clinical Hematology,* 7th ed., Philadelphia: Lea & Febiger, 1974

318
HODGKIN'S DISEASE AND OTHER LYMPHOMAS

M. M. WINTROBE
D. R. BOGGS

In an earlier chapter (Chap. 60) the causes of lymph node enlargement were discussed and their differential diagnosis was considered. In this section the clinical manifestations of Hodgkin's disease and of other conditions chiefly affecting lymph nodes ("lymphomas"), such as lymphosarcoma, are described. These disorders are considered under one heading because their clinical manifestions are very similar.

DEFINITION Hodgkin's disease, lymphosarcoma, "giant follicular" lymphoblastoma (lymphoma), and reticulum cell sarcoma are included in this group. They are characterized by painless, progressive enlargement of lymphoid tissue. Lymphadenopathy is a characteristic feature, and the spleen is frequently enlarged. Cachexia, anemia, and, in many instances, fever usually are late symptoms.

HISTORY A disorder affecting the "absorbent glands and spleen" was described by Hodgkin in 1832. *Lymphoblastoma, malignant lymphogranuloma,* and many other terms were used in referring to the disease in subsequent descriptions. The picture of lymphosarcoma was described by Kundrat in 1893; Brill, Baehr, and Rosenthal differentiated giant follicular lymphoblastoma in 1925. Roulet (1932) separated reticulum cell sarcoma from the general group of malignant diseases of lymphoid tissue. Some pathologists differentiate still other groups or call these groups by other names; others seek to avoid fine separations.

CLASSIFICATION Clinically these disorders vary considerably in severity. Hodgkin's disease usually is readily differentiated from the other forms of lymphoma, but among the latter there is as yet no general agreement regarding classification. Histologically they show marked differences, but these differences are not necessarily correlated with the clinical picture. Reticulum cell sarcoma and lymphosarcoma are fairly uniform in appearance, and the proliferating cells tend to encroach upon, obscure, and finally replace the architecture of the lymph node. The histologic pattern of Hodgkin's disease, on the other hand, is more complex. Lymphocytes, plasma cells, granulocytes (eosinophilic and neutrophilic), monocytes, fibroblasts, and giant cells make up the picture. The giant Reed-Sternberg cells, 10 to 40 μm in diameter, are possessed of abundant cytoplasm, a multilobed nucleus or multiple nuclei, and prominent nucleoli. A variable amount of fibrosis and/or sclerosis may be present, and the lymph node architecture is often lost. In giant follicular lymphoma the striking feature is the presence of multiple, follicle-like nodules of various sizes.

ETIOLOGY Hodgkin's disease forms about one-third to one-half of all cases of this group. It affects a younger age group than the other conditions, being most common in the second and third decades. However, no age is immune. Males are more frequently affected than females.

The cause of these disorders is unknown. There may not even be the common denominator of neoplastic growth to unite them, for many investigators have considered Hodgkin's disease to be an infectious granuloma. Efforts to transmit the disease to animals have failed, however, and attempts to incriminate various organisms, including the tubercle bacillus (human and avian), diphtheroid bacilli, and *Brucella* organisms, have not succeeded. There is much speculative interest in the possibility of a viral etiology of all the lymphomas and in the likelihood that an altered immune system is involved, particularly in Hodgkin's disease.

SYMPTOMS In most cases lymph node enlargement, usually cervical, is the first symptom to attract attention. This may be bilateral but is more often unilateral. More rarely the axillary or the inguinal nodes are the first to enlarge. The nodes are discrete and movable at first; only later do they become matted together and fixed. As a rule, they are painless and not tender, and the overlying skin is normal. However, when they have developed rapidly or when nerves are infiltrated as well, they may be painful. This is true in Hodgkin's disease especially. The size of the nodes ranges from that of a pea to that of a large orange. There is a resilient firmness in most instances, but the growth of connective tissue may make the nodes of Hodgkin's disease harder in the course of time. Occasionally the nodes in the axillary or inguinal regions may become secondarily inflamed and even break down.

After an interval varying from months to years, evidence appears of lymph node involvement elsewhere. In most patients, spread of disease from the original site appears first in the contiguous lymph node area. Superficial nodes which may be affected include the supraclavicular, axillary, inguinal, subpectoral, brachial, or femoral. A common site, also, is the mediastinum, to which such symptoms as cough, dyspnea, stridor, or dysphagia should attract attention. Splenomegaly develops in more than half the cases of Hodgkin's disease and of giant follicular lymphoma; it appears less frequently in the other forms. The liver is often palpable. Ultimately cachexia develops and weight loss occurs.

The mode of onset of these disorders may vary greatly, however. The manifestations may arise first in the mediastinum, the lungs, the digestive tract, the genitourinary tract, the bones, and rarely, the nervous system. Infiltration of the lungs, atelectasis, or pleural effusion may occur. With obstruction of lacteals, the effusion may become chylous. Extranodal primary sites include the tonsils, nasopharynx, stomach, rectum, and spleen. In the gastrointestinal tract the tumor may be far advanced before it is first discovered. Colicky pain, loss of weight, anemia, a palpable tumor, and obstruction are signs produced by lymphosarcoma of the small intestine. The lacteals may be involved so extensively that fat absorption is impaired and steatorrhea results. When the retroperitoneal nodes are the chief ones to enlarge, the diagnosis may be very difficult to make and the chief symptoms may be fever, pain, and loss of weight. Diffuse involvement of the liver and, in Hodgkin's disease, fibrosis of the portal triads, may produce jaundice; more rarely, the latter is due to obstruction of bile flow by nodes at the hilum. Hematuria, pyuria, or pain may be found when the genitourinary tract is involved. Localized pain and tenderness, spontaneous fractures, and neurologic changes due to extension into the spinal canal from vertebral lesions are the most common manifestations of bone involvement. Areas of rarefaction may be demonstrable in roentgenograms, although symptoms may be present long before roentgenographic signs become evident. Subperiosteal infiltration may occur, or the bone marrow involvement may be extensive. Of cutaneous manifestations, pruritus is the most frequent; it is encountered particularly in Hodgkin's disease. Brownish skin pigmentation, herpes zoster, and nodules produced by infiltration by the specific cells are among other skin manifestations which may be seen. Single or multiple nodules may be found in the breast. Symptoms and signs may also develop which are secondary to swellings producing pressure in various areas.

Constitutional symptoms may appear early in Hodgkin's disease, but they occur late in the other lymph node disorders. Hodgkin's disease, in particular, may produce a great variety of manifestations. Fever is common in Hodgkin's disease, although the well-known Pel-Ebstein type of fever is actually uncommon, appearing no oftener than in 16 percent of cases. This form of fever consists of febrile periods of several days' to several weeks' duration in which the temperature remains at levels of approximately 102 to 104°F, alternating with periods of weeks to even months during which there is no fever whatever.

Blood picture The greatest degree of variation is found in the blood picture associated with these disorders. There may be no changes whatever. On the other hand, there may be profound anemia as well as striking changes in the leukocytes and platelets. In Hodgkin's disease, changes in the blood occur relatively early. The anemia in Hodgkin's disease is usually only moderate in degree and normocytic in type; very occasionally, hemolytic anemia develops late in the disease. The total leukocyte count in Hodgkin's disease may be slightly or moderately increased, it may be normal, or there may be leukopenia. Sometimes the leukocyte count may exceed 25,000 per μl. The differential count may show neutrophilia, relative and absolute lymphocytopenia, monocytosis, or eosinophilia. All these changes may be present at the same time, or there may be none of them. Eosinophilia, which is mentioned frequently as characteristic of Hodgkin's disease and which may sometimes be very pronounced, is found only in about 10 percent of cases. An absolute increase in the number of lymphocytes suggests some disease other than Hodgkin's. Neutropenia suggests extensive bone marrow or splenic involvement.

The leukocyte picture in the other forms of disease chiefly affecting lymph nodes is more frequently normal than in Hodgkin's disease. Relative and even absolute lymphocytosis may be seen. The lymphocytes may be of normal types, but unusual forms and "tumor cells" (Chap. 316) have been described. Monocytes may be increased in number, and young forms may be seen, but a consistent and characteristic picture has not been described.

The platelet count may be increased in Hodgkin's disease, and large, bizarre forms may be seen. It is more common, however, to find the platelet count normal. In some instances thrombocytopenia is present; this usually occurs when leukopenia is found as well. The presence of thrombocytopenia suggests extensive bone marrow or splenic involvement and is usually, although not necessarily, a grave sign.

Bone marrow picture As would be expected from this description of the blood findings, changes in the bone marrow are not characteristic and are seldom helpful. Needle biopsy of bone marrow discloses Hodgkin's disease in approximately 5 percent of cases at the time of diagnosis. In other forms of lymphoma, increased lymphocytes, lymphoid nodules, or increased lymphoblasts or reticulum cells may be found in as many as 50 percent of the patients. Marrow examination may reveal identical degrees of lymphocytosis in lymphocytic lymphosarcoma and chronic lymphocytic leukemia.

Immune mechanism Response to antigenic challenge with production of circulating antibody is usually normal except in certain patients with lymphosarcoma. In these patients there may be reduced production of serum gamma-globulin and circulating antibodies similar to that seen in patients with chronic lymphocytic leukemia (Chap. 316).

Many patients with Hodgkin's disease have impaired delayed hypersensitivity, as evidenced by lack of reaction to injection of skin test antigens, such as tuberculin, and abnormally long survival of tissue homografts. Patients with impaired delayed hypersensitivity responses are more likely to be lymphopenic, to have a pathologic picture of "lymphocyte depletion" in involved lymph nodes, and to be in a more advanced clinical stage than are those with normal responses.

DIAGNOSIS The differential diagnosis of lymph node enlargement was discussed in Chap. 60. Cases in which there is little or no enlargement of the superficial lymph nodes present the most difficult problem in diagnosis, for then a variety of inflammatory and neoplastic disorders of the mediastinum, lungs, gastrointestinal tract, or liver must be considered, and the possible presence of chronic infections such as brucellosis must be ruled out. Hodgkin's disease, in particular, may produce such varied manifestations that this disorder must be kept in mind almost whenever diagnosis is obscure. This disease is particularly suggested by such symptoms as relapsing fever, loss of weight, and splenic or hepatic enlargement, together with anemia, neutrophilia, and lymphopenia.

COURSE AND PROGNOSIS The most important factor which seems to determine the course of these disorders is their inherent character. Cases of Hodgkin's disease and of lymphosarcoma are known to have run a chronic course for many years. In other instances the course is rapid and progression occurs in spite of therapy. The average survival time from the onset of symptoms in lymphosarcoma and reticulum cell sarcoma is approximately 2 years, but variations range from a few months to 10 years or longer. About 25 percent of patients have survived 5 years or longer. The median survival of the writers' cases of Hodgkin's disease was 43 months, but 35 percent survived for 5 years after the onset of symptoms. Pregnancy is not unusual in young women with Hodgkin's disease and seems to exert no deleterious effect. Now that cure is a possibility in a significant proportion of patients with Hodgkin's disease, median survival has less meaning. However, even in the absence of cure, 5- and 10-year survivals are not unusual. In giant follicular lymphoma a median survival of 72 months has been reported, with more than 50 percent surviving longer than 5 years.

In general, cases with the most favorable outlook are those in which only one accessible lymph node group is affected and where evidence of systemic involvement such as fever, loss of weight, increased sedimentation rate, and changes in the blood are lacking.

Clinical staging is of value in determining the prognosis and the type of treatment which should be employed in Hodgkin's disease. The value of such staging in other forms of lymphoma remains to be determined. In addition to a careful medical history, physical examination, examination of the blood, and chest x-ray, proper staging requires a roentgenologic survey of the bones, liver function tests, bone marrow biopsy, and a lymphangiogram of abdominal lymph nodes (Chap. 60) as part of the initial examination of most patients. Exploratory laparotomy with splenectomy may be of value in patients in whom an attempt at curative radiotherapy is being considered.

The prognostic importance and therapeutic implications of the extent of Hodgkin's disease at the time of diagnosis have been recognized. This has caused clinical staging to be refined. According to the classification adopted at a 1971 symposium in Ann Arbor, Michigan, the following stages are now differentiated:

Stage I: Involvement of a single anatomic lymph node region (I) or of a single extralymphatic organ or site (I_E).

Stage II: Disease in two or more lymph node regions on the same side of the diaphragm (II) or localized involvement of extralymphatic organ or site and of one or more lymph node regions on the same side of the diaphragm (II_E).

Stage III: Disease in lymph node regions both above and below the diaphragm. This may be accompanied by localized involvement of extralymphatic organ or site (III_E), by involvement of the spleen (III_S), or both (III_{SE}).

Stage IV: Diffuse or disseminated involvement of one or more extralymphatic organs or tissues with or without associated lymph node enlargement. Lymphatic structures are defined as lymph nodes, spleen, thymus, Waldeyer's ring, appendix, and Peyer's patches. The most commonly involved nonlymphoid tissues are liver, lung, bone, bone marrow, kidneys, gastrointestinal tract, and skin.

A and B Designations: All stages are classed as *A* or *B* (II*A*, III*B*, etc.) on the basis of the absence (*A*) or presence (*B*) of one or more of the following three: fever, night sweats, and loss of 10 percent or more of body weight in the preceding 6 months for which no explanation other than Hodgkin's disease is apparent.

In addition, it is recommended that a clinical stage (*C*), based on physical and roentgenographic examination be recorded, and that a final pathologic (*P*) stage, based on organ biopsies, be recorded. Each biopsy is recorded as positive or negative with annotation of *N* for additional nodes, *H* for hepar (liver), *M* for bone marrow, and *S* for spleen. Thus, a patient in whom the diagnosis was made from a solitary cervical node and in whom lymphangiogram, liver biopsy, exploratory laparotomy, and splenectomy failed to disclose additional disease would have a final stage of *C*-I-*A*, $P\text{-I-}A_{N-,H-,S-,M-}$.

A febrile patient in whom a needle biopsy of bone marrow disclosed Hodgkin's disease would require no further work-up and would be staged *C*-III*B*, $P\text{-IV}B_{M+}$.

The *histologic type* of Hodgkin's disease, in addition to clinical staging, is of some prognostic value. Lukes and Butler, improving on an earlier classification by Jackson and Parker, were able to classify most cases on a continuum of pathologic appearance ranging from those with lymphocyte predominance to those with lymphocyte depletion. The extreme range of "lymphocyte predominance" corresponds to the morphologic classification of "paragranuloma" and that of extreme "lymphocyte depletion" to "sarcoma" in the classification of Jackson and Parker. In the presence of lymphocyte depletion the cellular pattern is dominated by reticulum cells and Reed-Sternberg cells or by diffuse fibrosis. Cases falling between lymphocyte predominance and depletion are spoken of as having "mixed cellularity." In addition, certain cases did not fit into this continuum, but rather were classed as "nodular sclerosis." This group was characterized by prominent trabecular bands of dense collagenous tissue and by Reed-Sternberg cells with relatively small nuclei and prominent, pale cytoplasm. Lymphocyte predominance and nodular sclerosis were found to have favorable prognostic implication, lymphocyte depletion unfavorable, and mixed cellularity intermediate.

The best survival rates can be expected for patients in stages I and II*A* and the poorest in stages III and IV. With intensive irradiation therapy, more than 70 percent of patients with all stages of Hodgkin's disease treated by Kaplan have survived for 5 years. Actuarial survival figures for patients in stages I and II have exceeded 80 percent at 5 years, the majority surviving without recurrence of disease and have possibly been cured. Survival in the III*A* and IV*A* stages has exceeded 70 percent at 5 years, but a lesser percent have survived free of disease than those in stages I and II. Survival has been less than 50 percent in stages II*B* and IV*B*. In Hodgkin's disease, fever, weight loss, leukopenia or marked leukocytosis, anemia before therapy has begun, and skin infiltration are bad prognostic signs, but pruritus may be associated with relatively good survival. In the last analysis, a therapeutic trial should be attempted, for a prolonged remission may sometimes be encountered even in cases in which the general examination suggests a hopeless prognosis.

Terminally, patients with these diseases are plagued with severe anemia and great susceptibility to infection.

Antibody production is impaired, and dormant tuberculosis may become active. This is especially true in patients who are receiving adrenocorticosteroids. Fungal and antibiotic-resistant infections may also present very serious therapeutic problems. Secondary amyloidosis is a rare complication of Hodgkin's disease.

TREATMENT Surgical excision, irradiation, and chemotherapy all have their place in the treatment of these disorders. In general, it may be stated that irradiation is useful in localized disease, chemotherapy is useful in widespread disease, and surgery's usefulness is limited to diagnostic biopsy and a few special situations. In certain circumstances combined radiation and chemotherapy is of benefit.

The goal of therapy in Hodgkin's disease should be to cure, although this cannot be accomplished in all cases. In the other lymphomas, at the present time cure is an unrealistic goal except when the disease is limited to a single, extranodal site.

The hope that Hodgkin's disease can be cured was spurred by the experience of Peters in employing intensive irradiation in patients with localized disease. *Cure* as used in Hodgkin's disease is difficult to define. In patients treated for localized disease the incidence of recurrence is reduced with each succeeding disease-free year, most relapses having occurred in the first 3 years following initial therapy. Analysis of series of such patients has suggested that if no recurrence develops by 10 to 15 years, life expectancy is the same as that of the normal population. Recurrences after 10 years are unusual, but their existence makes it difficult to denote a finite disease-free period of time which constitutes a cure.

Surgical excision of localized, apparently solitary lymphomas should be limited to situations in which such surgery represents excisional biopsy. Radiotherapy of localized masses is reported to produce a higher "cure" rate than is surgical excision, even when widespread radical excision is employed. Surgical excision is also useful in treating localized masses whose quick removal is necessary to relieve organ dysfunction, as in a patient with paraparesis from a tumor compressing the spinal cord.

Radiation therapy is the treatment of choice for patients presenting with stage I or II Hodgkin's disease. The recommended tumor dose is 4,000 rad, delivered in about 1 month's time. With this dosage fewer than 5 percent of patients have developed a recurrence at the irradiated site, while with decreasing doses such recurrences become increasingly frequent. This dose of irradiation cannot be delivered safely unless equipment with energy in the millions of electron volts range is employed (linear accelerator, betatron, or telecobalt-therapy apparatus).

As stated earlier, the most common pattern of spread of Hodgkin's disease from clinically involved areas appears to be from one to another contiguous group of lymph nodes. Because of the likelihood that undetectable spread of disease has already occurred in areas adjacent to obviously involved nodes, "prophylactic" irradiation of areas adjacent to the proven tumor is commonly administered. If the involved area is cervical or supraclavicular (the most common site for localized involvement), irradiation is given to axillary and mediastinal areas, and some advise treatment of the paraaortic lymph nodes as well, particularly when left supraclavicular lymph nodes are enlarged or when constitutional symptoms are present. Similarly, if inguinal nodes are the primary site of disease, the entire pelvis and paraaortic abdominal area is treated.

With proper supravoltage equipment, skin damage is minimal with this type of irradiation therapy. However, this dose of irradiation can produce irreparable damage to such organs as the bone marrow, lungs, heart, and liver. Thus, meticulously constructed, individually designed shields must be employed to protect as much of each vital organ as is possible.

A number of radiotherapy research centers are presently attempting "curative" therapy in stage III*A* and a few are even studying the results of such therapy in stages III*B* and IV. Thus, whether chemotherapy or radiotherapy, or combinations thereof, is the treatment of choice in stage III is unsettled. However, there is little disagreement that chemotherapy, or chemotherapy combined with radiotherapy, is the treatment of choice in stage IV, and most would consider chemotherapy the treatment of choice in stage III*B*.

Chemotherapy was initiated with the discovery in 1946 of the effects of nitrogen mustard (HN2), which often were dramatic. Since that time, a number of agents of proved benefit in the lymphomas have been introduced: chlorambucil, cyclophosphamide, vinblastine, vincristine, procarbazine, bis-chloronitrosourea (BCNU), and bleomycin, as well as the adrenal glucocorticosteroids. Dosage, route, and method of administration, as well as toxicity, are discussed in Chap. 320.

Combination chemotherapy appears to be superior to chemotherapy with a single agent, at least in *Hodgkin's disease*. Thus, MOPP [nitrogen mustard, Oncovin (vincristine), procarbazine, and prednisone] given in the schedule shown in Table 318-1 produces an 80 percent complete remission rate in previously untreated patients with widespread disease (stages III*B* and IV). A number of patients have remained disease-free without receiving further therapy for 4 and 5 years following MOPP therapy, raising the possibility that some may have been cured. Comparable results have been observed in patients relapsing following attempts at curative radiotherapy, but

TABLE 318-1
A combination chemotherapy regimen for patients with Hodgkin's disease

Total of six courses, each course beginning every 28 days.*

Each course:
- M: Nitrogen mustard, 6 mg/m²†, on day 1 and day 7, i.v.
- O: Vincristine (Oncovin), 1.4 mg/m², on day 1 and day 7 (should not exceed 2 mg/dose), i.v.
- P: Procarbazine, 100 mg/m², on day 1 through day 10, by mouth
- P: Prednisone, 40 mg/m², on day 1 through day 14, in 1st and 4th courses only, by mouth

* *Frequency and intensity of each course is modified if toxicity develops.*
† *Square meter of body surface area.*

when extensive prior radiotherapy and chemotherapy have been employed, results have been less encouraging. The favorable results of radiotherapy and of combination chemotherapy have led to trials of their sequential use in patients with relatively advanced disease. The results of such trials, while encouraging from the standpoint that toxicity has been less than anticipated, are too preliminary to indicate whether these combined modalities will prove to be superior to either used alone.

Combination chemotherapy of *non-Hodgkin's lymphomas* also produces a high remission rate, but most patients have relapsed within a year following MOPP therapy or similar combinations. Combined prednisone and cyclophosphamide, or these two drugs together with vincristine (COP), may yield as high a remission rate as combinations of still more drugs.

In general, it may be said that Hodgkin's disease should always be treated with radiotherapy or with combination chemotherapy, depending upon the clinical extent of disease. Patients relapsing after an attempt at curative radiotherapy should be given a trial of combination chemotherapy. In the case of non-Hodgkin's lymphomas, therapy is palliative, except in instances of localized disease, as mentioned above. Consequently, observation may be the wiser course in asymptomatic patients, and in others the aggressiveness of therapy may be tailored to the observed aggressiveness of the disease. Similarly, the patient with Hodgkin's disease who is no longer responsive to MOPP may be watched, if relatively asymptomatic, or given therapy directed toward relief of symptoms, rather than cure, with single agents or combination of agents. It must be kept in mind that resistance to one of a class of chemotherapeutic agents usually signals resistance to another of the same class; the patient who is no longer responsive to HN2 is unlikely to respond to other alkylating agents such as chlorambucil or cyclophosphamide. However, cross resistance of BCNU and bleomycin is not observed with drugs used in the MOPP regimen, and responses to vinblastine may be observed in patients no longer responsive to MOPP.

The effect of irradiation may be dramatic, with large masses melting away in the course of a week. Pressure symptoms may disappear; fever and pruritus, if present, may be relieved; and pain caused by bone involvement may be alleviated. Pulmonary lesions may decrease in size, and pleural effusions may clear up. Anemia may disappear, and the leukocyte count, if elevated, may drop to normal. Primary reticulum cell sarcoma of bone is especially radiosensitive. In other cases, irradiation is less effective, in some instances being of scarcely any benefit. Prediction in advance as to the likelihood of benefit from therapy is often difficult. In general, the more chronic and slowly growing forms respond best to therapy. Remission following treatment may last but a few weeks or may persist for years. In some cases such improvement can be achieved many times by additional therapy.

The results of chemotherapy also may be dramatic. Fever often disappears promptly, enlarged nodes or other masses decrease in size, and anemia, if present, also is alleviated. Abnormalities in the leukocytes may revert toward normal, although the immediate effect may be leukopenia and an increase of anemia.

The use of radiotherapy with intent to cure for lymphomas other than Hodgkin's disease rarely is a practical goal. Disease usually is widespread and rarely is localized to a single lymph node area. Even when such localization seems to be present, relapse following radiotherapy is the rule. However, when disease is limited to extranodal tissue, apparent cures can be obtained with some frequency. The most common localized extranodal disease is lymphosarcoma of the small intestine, although localized disease in skin, lung, and many other organs may be observed. In such cases cure has followed simple excision, excision plus radiotherapy, or radiotherapy alone.

In addition to these measures, general supportive and symptomatic therapy will be required in individual cases, as discussed in Chap. 316.

REFERENCES

Aisenberg AC: Hodgkin's disease—Prognosis, treatment and etiologic and immunologic considerations. N Engl J Med 270:508, 565, and 617, 1964

Carbone PP et al: Report of the committee on Hodgkin's disease staging classification. Cancer Res 31:1860, 1971 (symposium)

Kaplan HS: *Hodgkin's Disease*, Cambridge, Mass.: Harvard, 1972

Lukes RJ et al: Natural history of Hodgkin's disease as related to its pathologic picture. Cancer, 19:317, 1966

Peters MV et al: Natural history of Hodgkin's disease as related to staging. Cancer 19:308, 1966

Rosenberg SA et al: Lymphosarcoma: A review of 1269 cases. Medicine 40:31, 1961

——: Report of the committee on the staging of Hodgkin's disease. Cancer Res 26:pt. 1, 1310, 1965

Wintrobe MM et al: *Clinical Hematology*, 7th ed., Philadelphia: Lea & Febiger, 1974

319
PRINCIPLES OF NEOPLASIA

EMIL FREI III
GERALD P. BODEY

INTRODUCTION A general understanding of the newer knowledge concerning the etiology and pathogenesis of cancer will aid the internist in individual patient care and counseling and also in public health problems. Improvements in the methodology of detection and diagnosis may be applied directly by the internist, and, if not, it is essential that he have definitive knowledge concerning the contribution of modern techniques in this area. He often plays a major integrating role in the multidisciplinary approach to the diagnosis and particularly in the management of neoplastic disease. While this has always been true in regard to the hematologic malignancies, it is becoming increasingly true for the so-called "solid tumors." It is here that the internist's expertise in playing an integrative role, his knowledge of clinical pharmacology and chemotherapy, of supportive and symptomatic care, and of the management of the medical complications that occur is essential.

In the following discussion, no attempt is made to be comprehensive, but rather to deal with the principles of neoplasia.

ETIOLOGY OF CANCER While at a molecular level there may be "a final common pathway" in the etiology of cancer, the interplay of a number of factors is responsible for the development of malignant disease. These include genetic, viral, chemical, and physical factors, as well as the response of the host.

Genetic factors Certain familial and genetic disorders significantly increase the risk of cancer, e.g., multiple polyposis of the colon. In virtually all cases this disorder leads to carcinoma as the patient's age advances, so that a prophylactic colectomy is indicated. In addition, family members who may be asymptomatic should be examined. In a number of other, relatively rare, hereditary neoplasms such as retinoblastoma and multiple endocrine adenomatosis the hereditary pattern is well defined and the frequency in family members is high. The physician should be aware of the hereditary patterns for these diseases and provide genetic counseling where appropriate.

Genetic factors also play a role in some of the more common types of tumors such as breast cancer. Thus, the risk of developing breast cancer in the first degree relatives of a patient is fivefold that of the general population. Routine detection techniques such as physical examination and mammography should be advised in such patients. Finally, there are the relatively rare, usually familial, diseases associated with cytogenetic abnormalities (Down's syndrome, Bloom's syndrome, Fanconi's syndrome) and the immunologic deficiency states (agammaglobulinemia, ataxia telangiectasia, etc.) which are associated with an increased risk of neoplasia. Strong direct support for genetic susceptibility to cancer in Bloom's and Fanconi's syndromes derives from the fact that cultured fibroblasts from such patients have an increased "sensitivity" to transformation by oncogenic viruses.

Viruses Viruses have been demonstrated to cause leukemia in a number of mammalian and other species. Most of these are the so-called C-type RNA viruses. Induction of neoplasia by these viruses results in persisting changes which consist of morphologic and biologic features of neoplasia in the progeny of the transformed cell. The fact that an RNA virus could produce cellular transformation, that is a change in the genome or DNA, at first was not comprehensible since the transfer of information was formerly thought to be exclusively unidirectional, i.e., from DNA to RNA (transcription). The discovery of the RNA-dependent DNA polymerase (reverse transcriptase), by revealing that information can flow from RNA to DNA, supplied the link necessary to explain the change in genome (DNA) that these RNA leukemogenic viruses are capable of imparting. Most of these viruses have a relatively narrow host range. However, the cat RNA leukemia virus is capable of infecting a number of mammalian species including human embryonic cells in culture. Virus leukemia in rodents is not contagious and in nature is transmitted vertically through the ovum or through the mother's milk.

Intensive investigation is currently under way concerning the virus etiology of human neoplasia. The fact that viruses cause leukemia in so many different mammalian species strongly suggests that this may be the case in man. C-type particles have occasionally been observed in human neoplastic tissues by electron microscopy, particularly in leukemia and lymphoma. Also, reverse transcriptase, while clearly present in normal and embryonic tissues, is also present, probably in greater quantity, in human leukemias. As in experimental systems, there is little or no evidence that leukemia is spread laterally, that is, by contagion, in man. B-type RNA viruses cause breast cancer in animals, and DNA viruses such as the polyoma virus may cause a variety of types of neoplasia in experimental systems. The development of leukemia in donor cells (as evidenced by cytogenetic studies) in two leukemic girls treated with total body irradiation and infused with bone marrow from HLA-compatible normal male siblings provides circumstantial evidence for viral induction of human leukemia.

The practical implication of virus research in relation to neoplasia would be the development of a vaccine and possibly other preventive measures. The ubiquity of the C-type virus in some rodent systems and some of the current hypotheses concerning virus etiology suggest that oncogenic viral infection is common, and that the phenotypic expression of neoplasia is determined by control mechanisms within the cell. Modulation of these mechanisms may be critical in the expression of neoplastic behavior on the part of the cell. Thus the study of these mechanisms may lead to means of prevention and treatment.

Chemical factors The role of chemicals as a cause of cancer in man was first demonstrated in the nineteenth century, when Sir Percival Pott described scrotal cancer in chimney sweeps in London. In subsequent studies by Kennaway and Yoshida, the coal-tar carcinogens which are capable of producing a variety of tumors in experimental systems were described. Since then other classes of chemical compounds which are potent carcinogens in experimental systems have been studied. The number of chemicals already present in our environment is substantial, and the rate of introduction of new agents is increasing very rapidly. These include such substances as food additives, animal growth-stimulating hormones, air pollutants, and cosmetics, among others. The most important established carcinogen in man's environment at the moment is cigarette smoke. The etiologic relation of cigarette smoking to lung cancer, upper respiratory cancer, and, interestingly, bladder cancer has been clearly established. Similarly, the relation of aniline dyes to bladder cancer and asbestos to lung cancer and mesotheliomas has been demonstrated. Benzene has been implicated as a possible cause of myelogenous leukemia. The observation of a number of cases of carcinoma of the vagina occurring in women under the age of 20 whose mothers received estrogens during pregnancy has important implications.

In experimental systems and in man, the evidence strongly suggests that, as with viruses, there is a long latent period between exposure to chemical carcinogens and neoplasia. For cigarettes, for example, this period is a minimum of 15 to 20 years. Thus, one of the most important problems in chemical carcinogenesis research is to develop methods of determining whether a current chemical or new chemicals introduced into the environment are likely to be carcinogenic. Chronic toxicity studies of all such agents conducted over a number of years in experimental in vivo systems would be enormously expensive. Moreover chemical carcinogenesis may be relatively species-specific so that the significance of experimental studies for man is uncertain. The demonstration of a "final common pathway" for molecular events in chemical carcinogenesis would allow for the identification of chemicals which may be carcinogenic. In vitro systems such as the cytogenetic effects of chemicals on cells in culture provide an important approach, though false positives are common, and such systems do not take into account the metabolism of the compound by the host.

Perhaps the most difficult problem is the statistical one. A compound such as a food additive or a cosmetic which produces a 1 or 2 percent increase in risk of cancer in man over a 10-year period would be unacceptable. The development of techniques for the preclinical identification of such quantitatively slight but important neoplastic potential poses enormous problems.

Chemical carcinogens produce tumors probably as a result of mutation. It has been demonstrated that an increase in the mutation rate in a given population will result in an increase in abortion, and an increase in the ratio of female to male births. This is because mutations on the X chromosome of the male are lethal since the male does not have the complementary X chromosome, as does the female. Thus, monitoring the rate of spontaneous abortion and the female-to-male-birth ratio has been proposed as a method for determining the cumulative mutation rate and thus the risk of cancer in a given population. This, plus careful monitoring of the incidence of various types of cancer in different populations over a specified time period, may provide leads regarding the presence of carcinogenic elements in the environment.

Radiation Exposure to x-rays may cause leukemia and other forms of cancer in experimental systems. Clinical studies, particularly those relating to the Hiroshima-Nagasaki experience and studies of patients receiving radiotherapy for rheumatoid spondylitis, clearly indicate a relation between radiation exposure and risk of neoplasia. It is now clear that (1) there is a long latent period (minimum of 5 years from time of exposure to development of neoplasia); (2) there is a dose-response relation, that is, the higher the dose, the greater the risk of neoplasia; and (3) myelogenous leukemia is the most common resulting neoplasm, though others may occur. The relation of bone-seeking radioactive material such as radium in radium dial workers to bone and mesenchymal tumors is well established.

All the above observations relate to major doses of radiation. There is considerable question, however, whether the relation of dose to incidence of neoplasia is linear down through small doses of radiation. There is controversy also concerning the duration of increased risk of neoplasia following exposure to radiation. It is possible that a subgroup of the population exists with an increased "sensitivity" to induction of neoplasia by radiation. These uncertainties have focused attention on the difficult and extraordinarily important problem as to how much radiation should be tolerated in our environment. With development and application of nuclear energy and the increasing use of external sources of radiation for diagnostic purposes and of radioisotopes in nuclear medicine and research, many radioactive materials have been introduced into our environment, and these must be monitored. Such procedures, particularly fluoroscopy, may deliver significant amounts of radiation and should be ordered with discretion. The risk of neoplasia from radiation is an inverse function of age. Thus, infants, children, and pregnant women are particularly susceptible. In the near future, technologic improvements such as more sensitive x-ray film will reduce radiation exposure incident to diagnostic procedures. The importance of ultraviolet light is indicated by the fact that skin cancer has a positive correlation with solar radiation and a negative correlation with the degree of natural pigmentation of the skin.

Immunologic surveillance It has been demonstrated in experimental systems and for a number of tumors in man that the surface and interior of certain tumors contain new antigens, some of which act as weak tumor-specific transplantation antigens. These observations, plus the fact that tumors occur with increased frequency in patients with congenital deficiencies and also in patients with acquired or induced immunologic deficits, have resulted in the "immunologic surveillance" hypothesis. This postulates that neoplastic transformation of cells is a frequent occurrence, but, in the vast majority of instances, these cells are destroyed immunologically by the host. If the host response is depressed acutely or chronically, such cells may multiply and develop into overt neoplasms. An example of the failure of such immunologic surveillance is the observed increase in the incidence of cancer in renal allograft recipients. This has been attributed to the use of immunosuppressive agents and, in particular, antilymphocytic serum.

EPIDEMIOLOGY Epidemiologic studies of cancer provide important information regarding hereditary and environmental causal factors. Thus, epidemiologic studies have defined the relations between certain congenital disorders and neoplasia and showed the relation of cigarette smoking and x-ray exposure to cancer. The continuous monitoring of the frequency of various types of cancer in population groups should provide other important etiologic leads. For instance, gastric cancer in Japan is very frequent, while colon cancer is infrequent. In contrast, in inbred migrant Japanese populations in Hawaii and the United States, the incidence of these cancers has changed significantly, suggesting that environmental factors are important, and perhaps food and other ingestants. On the other hand, the incidence of breast cancer is relatively low in Japanese populations and does not change in migrant populations. This would suggest that genetic factors are operative.

Epidemiologic studies of Burkitt's lymphoma in Africa indicate that a high incidence of this tumor is associated with certain climatic and geographic features and with holoendemic malaria. This has strongly suggested an infectious etiology transmitted by an insect vector.

CANCER DETECTION In general, the probability of curing cancer is directly related to early detection. Because of this, increasing emphasis is being given to the education of physicians, public health groups, and the lay population concerning cancer detection. Research efforts to devise better methods of early detection of cancer also are under way. In general, cancer detection clinics form an integral part of overall disease detection facilities. These often involve self-questionnaires, a battery of laboratory and, in some instances, radiographic tests, and review of such data by paramedical personnel, often aided by computer techniques. The physician's role is to monitor such studies and to follow up leads that suggest cancer. Such early signs as weight loss, change in bowel habits, bleeding, and persistent ulceration should bring the patient to the physician. The significance of precancerous lesions must be recognized. Thus, leukoplakia, senile keratosis, and cystic mastitis, to mention but a few, must be removed or observed carefully. The routine application on an annual or biannual basis of mammography and other techniques such as thermography and xerography is partially effective in the detection of early cancer, but their application to the population as a whole on a routine basis is not yet practicable. The Papanicolaou stain has proved highly effective in the detection of early cervical cancer, but the application of this and other techniques to the population as a whole has proved extraordinarily difficult.

It is particularly important to identify populations at increased risk and to apply the appropriate detection techniques to those populations, e.g., the first-degree female relatives of a woman with breast cancer, heavy smokers, and populations among whom sexual activity begins at an early age, since the risk of cervical cancer among these is substantially greater.

Advances in tumor immunology offer hope concerning the early detection of cancer. Thus, it has been demonstrated that human tumor cells from the gastrointestinal tract have carcinoembryonic antigens on their surface which may be released into the blood. These can be detected by the highly sensitive radioimmunoassay technique. While methodologic problems exist, particularly with respect to the purification of the antigen, the principle has been demonstrated. In addition to cancer detection, the evaluation of circulating carcinoembryonic antigens may prove useful in following the results of treatment. Carcinoembryonic antigens apply to tumors other than bowel cancer, and it may be anticipated that such detection techniques will be developed for other tumors.

CANCER PREVENTION Much of cancer prevention is implicit in the above discussion of etiology and epidemiology. However, identifying the approximate cause of a major type of cancer such as cigarettes in relation to lung cancer does not automatically lead to effective prevention. Education regarding risks obviously is important. The population in which smoking has been greatly reduced includes physicians, probably because the adverse effects of smoking are continuously brought home to them. Needless to say, the physician who smokes will be ineffective in persuading patients not to smoke.

PATHOLOGY OF CANCER While cytogenetic, biochemical, and other techniques eventually may provide a more quantitative and fundamental definition of, as well as diagnostic criteria for, cancer, the diagnosis still rests with morphology and the pathologist. Neoplastic cells were once thought to have lost the functional capacity of the cell of origin and to have become autonomous. While this is partially true, the majority of neoplasias continue to exhibit morphologic and often functional characteristics of the tissue of origin. Indeed, they may assume functions such as the production of ectopic hormones (see below) which are not associated with the tissue of origin.

In essence, the neoplastic cell is one in which the mechanisms within the cell and in its microenvironment which are responsible for restraint of growth are defective. Cancer cells tend to converge to a "primitive" or embryonic pattern. Thus, the nucleus of cancer cells often is large and irregular, and its DNA is coarsely distributed and tends to aggregate near the nuclear membrane; the nucleoli are large and usually are increased in number. Polyploidy is common. Mitoses are increased in more rapidly growing tumors, and abnormal multipolar mitoses and multinucleated cells may occur. In contrast to the nucleus, the cytoplasm is comparatively scanty and stains with basophilic dyes more deeply than does normal cytoplasm, indicating relatively greater RNA concentration.

In addition to the characteristics of the individual cells, the organization of the tumor as observed microscopically is helpful in distinguishing neoplasia. The stroma of certain tumors may be markedly desmoplastic, and the vasculature is quantitatively deficient. Destruction or invasion of normal architecture such as the lymph node, nodal capsule, and blood vessel wall is characteristic.

Electron microscopy has been of limited help in distinguishing neoplasia. The presence of intracellular organelles such as premelanosomes may aid in determining that a given neoplasm is of melanoblast origin. There is frequently a decrease in intercellular substance, and desmosomes are not normally maintained. Endocrine tumors, glandular carcinomas, and carcinoid tumors may reveal their identity by the presence of a particular type of secretory granule. Immature tumor cells of the reticuloendothelial system can be recognized with greater accuracy by their fine structural characteristics. Abnormal vacuoles or ingested material are frequently seen within cancer cells, since they are often phagocytic and can absorb fluids by the process of pinocytosis. Histochemistry may also distinguish the type of tumor, but it is less useful in distinguishing benign from malignant neoplasms. Thus, the presence of mucin may distinguish certain types of adenocarcinomas. Also melanin can be distinguished from phagocytized hemosiderin and aid in the diagnosis of melanoma.

PATHOGENESIS OF CANCER

Preneoplastic changes Definitive studies, particularly of lung and cervical cancer, indicate that neoplasia develops insidiously and perhaps in a stepwise fashion, as illustrated by studies of the respiratory tract of smokers. The bronchial mucosa shows progressive changes in both the nucleus and cytoplasm, in the form of cellular atypia and proliferative changes. Up to a point, these may be reversible, if the inciting agent is removed. The bronchial tree in patients with squamous-cell carcinoma of the lung almost always shows atypical preneoplastic changes in areas not directly involved by tumor, and, in fact, carcinoma *in situ* at other sites in the bronchial mucosa is not uncommon. Similar changes occur in skin malignancies and in the uterine cervix. Such preneoplastic changes almost certainly occur in other organs, but have not been as well studied because of lack of accessibility.

Preneoplastic lesions such as senile keratosis and leukoplakia represent stages in the process of development of neoplasia that may or may not proceed to cancer. Cytogenetic studies of carcinoma of the cervix suggest that in dysplasia and in carcinoma *in situ*, chromosomal abnormalities are infrequent, but they almost invariably occur with the development of an invasive lesion. Hyperplastic and dysplastic changes are found in the ducts of some patients with cystic mastitis and probably represent preneoplastic changes. Indeed, the distinction between late preneoplastic change and cancer may be extremely difficult.

Tumor invasion The basic mechanism of tumor invasion is not fully understood. Certain tissues such as cartilage, fascial planes, and ligaments are resistant to invasion and, in part, determine patterns of spread. On the other hand, soft tissues are invaded with relative ease. Certain experimental tumors produce proteolytic enzymes or collagenase which may destroy or modify adjacent normal tissue and facilitate tumor invasion. While tissue pressure created by cellular multiplication may lead to expansion and pressure atrophy of surrounding tissue and cause the formation of a capsule, it probably does not contribute significantly to invasion per se. Thus, malignant tumors invade even when they grow very slowly.

Locomotion is characteristic of most mammalian cells in vitro. Thus, normal cells on a solid surface spread as a monolayer until the area is covered and growth and spread cease. This self-limiting process has been termed *contact inhibition*. Malignant tumor cells, on the other hand, will continue to grow and extend over each other in a somewhat chaotic fashion. Assuming that loss of contact inhibition also applies to tumor growth in vivo, this behavioral feature would constitute an essential factor in the invasive process. In vivo cinematographic studies have demonstrated that cancer cells move in a random, nondirectional, and complex fashion, invade adjacent normal tissue, and metastasize. This contrasts to normal cells such as leukocytes which are subject to homeostatic mechanisms such as chemotaxis and contact inhibition. In addition, tumor cells have decreased cohesiveness as compared with normal cells and, thus, may more readily detach themselves from the main mass and exfoliate.

Metastases Metastases may be vascular or lymphatic. Venous invasion is much more common than arterial invasion, presumably because of the elastic wall of the artery. Thus, venous invasion can be demonstrated microscopically in 40 to 80 percent of the more common primary tumors. This presumably explains the relatively common finding of tumor cells in the blood, but the prognostic significance of this finding is debatable since many patients with venous invasion and circulating tumor cells survive for many years after surgical excision of the primary growth. In experimental studies large numbers of tumor cells may have to be injected intravenously to produce a single metastasis. In fact, small detached clumps of tumor cells are much more likely to produce metastatic foci than single cells. Such cells adhere to the vascular endothelium of a small postcapillary venule, initiate fibrin formation, multiply, and invade through endothelial defects. Experimental approaches to the prevention of metastases, such as the administration of substances that reduce endothelial stickiness and the use of anticoagulants, are based on these observations. Following lymphatic invasion, tumor may spread to regional lymph nodes. Such nodes may serve as immunologic and perhaps mechanical barriers to further spread of disease but, in some instances, may provide fertile soil for growth and spread. In experimental studies and also in man, the development of hyperplastic reactions within lymph nodes surrounding metastatic tumor tissue suggests an immunologic reaction.

BIOLOGY OF NEOPLASIA Tumor growth (cytokinetics) Advances in cytokinetic techniques have provided considerable insight into the biology of tumors. Experimentally small tumor nodules tend to increase exponentially for a limited period of time, after which the growth rate decreases with increasing tumor size and finally levels off. This is known as the *Gompertzian growth curve*. The biologic basis for this is as follows: the tumor will increase to 2 to 3 mm in diameter without vascular supply. Further growth requires vascularization from the surrounding stroma. This is very likely stimulated by a tumor product known as *tumor angiogenesis factor*. Such vascularization will allow for continued exponential growth for a while. However, for most tumors the replication of tumor cells exceeds the replication capacity of normal endothelium. Thus, tumors in fact "outgrow their blood supply." Angiographic studies have indicated decreasing arterial supply as the tumor increases in size, irregularity of the surface of blood vessels within tumors, and the "tumor blush." Experimentally, the replicative capacity of tumor cells that are removed by three to four layers of cells from the capillary is markedly reduced, and they eventually die because of both lack of vascular supply and injury by the products of dying or necrotic cells.

By the use of tritiated thymidine, which labels only cells during DNA synthesis, it has been possible to determine precisely the cytokinetics of experimental tumors and to some extent those of man. It has been found that the proportion of cells in DNA synthesis may be as high as 50 to 60 percent in patients with Burkitt's lymphoma and less than 5 percent in many of the relatively slow-growing solid tumors such as myeloma and breast cancer. There is evidence that the DNA synthesis period of the cell cycle is relatively constant and that variation in the intermitotic time is largely the result of variation in the G_1 period. The difference between very rapidly growing tumors as compared with slow-growing ones is due primarily to the low growth fraction and high cell loss in the latter tumors; the DNA synthesis period and the intermitotic times tend to be only slightly longer in the slow-growing tumors.

In experimental studies, it has been demonstrated that cells which are not in cycle are not necessarily nonviable, end-stage maturing cells. Some of these cells are resting stem cells (clonogenic cells) which are capable of reentering cycle, particularly when the size of the tumor is reduced by chemotherapy or radiotherapy. Most chemotherapeutic agents affect cells which are in cycle (such as inhibitors of DNA biosynthesis or mitotic arrestors). These observations have major implications for chemotherapy. Cytokinetic perturbation of tumors by various forms of treatment is under study. In addition to fundamental information with respect to regulatory mechanisms as compared with normal tissues, such as the bone marrow and gastrointestinal tract, such studies should provide important leads as to the tactics of chemotherapy. In addition, in experimental systems considerable emphasis is being given to the identification of agents which will affect noncycling cells.

Cytogenetics Advances in the methodology of cytogenetics have resulted in important observations in tumor biology. The observation that chromosomes have specific banding patterns when exposed to certain fluorescent or Romanovsky stains is a major advance in chromosome technology. The increased incidence of neoplasias, particularly leukemias and lymphomas, in persons with congenital or acquired (e.g., following radiation exposure) cytogenetic defects was mentioned earlier.

Approximately 50 percent of patients with acute leukemia have cytogenetic abnormalities in their leukemic cells. These are not common for the disease as a class, but with any given patient tend to remain stable. The abnormalities are usually relatively minor, consisting of slight hyperdiploidy, pseudodiploidy, or hypodiploidy. Chronic myelogenous leukemia is the only neoplastic disease in man which is associated with a specific and characteristic cytogenetic abnormality. This consists of loss of the arms of chromosome 22 resulting in the Ph^1 chromosome. As patients with chronic myelogenous leukemia enter the acute or blast phase of their disease, additional chromosome abnormalities develop.

A limited number of studies have been performed on metaplastic and preneoplastic lesions. In patients with carcinoma *in situ* of the cervix, cytogenetic abnormalities are unusual. On the other hand, in primary lesions, particularly when there is evidence of invasion, cytogenetic abnormalities are frequent. Thus, in difficult cases, cytogenetic studies may aid in distinguishing neoplastic from nonneoplastic and preneoplastic lesions. In the limited number of studies of metastatic solid tumors such as in patients with melanoma and lung cancer, cytogenetic abnormalities are frequent and major. In addition, there is substantial variation from cell to cell; this is evidence for multiple stem lines, cytogenetic instability, and rapid clonal evolution. The changes are almost invariably hyperdiploid, including triploid, tetraploid, and hypertetraploid cell lines, in marked contrast to the relatively slight and stable cytogenetic abnormalities which occur in the leukemias. Multiple stem-cell lines and rapid clonal evolution represent an ideal circumstance for the selection and/or development of drug-resistant lines. This may in part explain the relatively poor response to chemotherapy of the majority of solid tumors as compared with the leukemias.

Biochemistry It has long been known that undifferentiated tumors have defective aerobic glycolysis and increasing dependence on anaerobic glycolysis (the Warburg theory), but important insights into tumor biochemistry and etiology have not derived from this observation; it almost certainly represents a secondary biochemical manifestation associated with rapid tumor growth and perhaps rapid growth of many normal cells.

Experimental models which have been of considerable value in identifying fundamental biochemical abnormalities in tumor cells have been the so-called "minimum deviation tumors." These are carcinogen-induced hepatomas in rodents which vary in differentiation from rapidly growing anaplastic tumors to very slowly growing morphologically mature but biologically neoplastic (minimum deviation) hepatomas. Biochemical studies of these systems as compared with those of normal liver have indicated that many of the abnormalities are quantitatively related to the rapidity of growth. Subtle changes in regulatory mechanisms and in cell membranes have been demonstrated in some of the minimum deviation tumors.

While isoenzyme patterns differ in tumor tissue as compared with the normal tissue of origin, these changes are similar to those in the embryonic counterpart. In this regard they are similar to the carcinoembryonic antigens. RNA-dependent DNA polymerase was mentioned above. Consistent with the protovirus hypothesis of Temin, this enzyme has also been demonstrated in certain normal tissues, though in considerably lesser quantities.

Endocrine factors The endocrine system influences the growth of certain tumors. In some instances tumor growth may be dependent upon certain hormones, usually those which are essential for the growth and function of the corresponding normal tissue. Examples include estrogens and androgens for premenopausal breast and prostatic carcinoma, respectively. In contrast, in the elderly patient with breast cancer, estrogens may cause tumor regression instead of tumor stimulation. Carcinoma of the endometrium may resemble morphologically the type of endometrium which has been stimulated by estrogen in the absence of adequate progesterone. Endocrine studies support this interpretation. Substantial regression may occur in such tumors with the administration of progesterone.

Advances in the mechanism of action of steroid hormones may have practical implications in the near future. Thus, for estrogens, androgens, and corticosteroids, specific binding proteins have been demonstrated in the cytoplasm of tissues, including tumors, responsive to the hormone. These binding proteins transport, either directly or through mediators, the hormone into the nucleus where it apparently interacts with DNA. In experimental systems, and provisionally in man, there is good correlation between the quantity of specific binding protein in the cytoplasm and the responsiveness of that tissue to the specific hormone. Thus, it may be possible to predict the effects of a given endocrinologic manipulation.

Immunologic factors The spontaneous regression which may occasionally occur in human tumors and the positive correlation between prognosis and mononuclear-cell infiltrate surrounding tumors long has suggested that the host exerts some immunologic restraint on tumors. The rapid development of immunologic techniques and the use of inbred strains of animals have conclusively demonstrated that new antigens, some of which function as tumor-specific transplantation antigens, may appear within and on the surface of tumor cells. This has been demonstrated not only in viral and chemical carcinogen-induced tumors but in spontaneous experimental tumors as well. By use of a variety of approaches including indirect membrane immunofluorescence, the various sandwich techniques, colony inhibition, and others, it has been conclusively demonstrated that some human tumors contain antigens not shared by normal tissues. Some of these, as indicated above, represent carcinoembryonic antigens, but some apparently are not shared even by the corresponding embryonic tissue. The weight of evidence indicates that tumor restraint by the immunologic apparatus is similar to allogeneic transplant immunity and results primarily from cellular immune mechanisms. While in some systems humoral cytotoxic antibodies may occur, in others humoral "enhancing" or "blocking" substances have been described, which in experimental systems accelerate or "enhance" tumor growth. These substances can interfere with the ability of lymphocytes to kill tumor cells in tissue culture and presumably can interfere with the cellular immune response to the tumor in in vivo systems. The blocking substances may consist of antigens, antibodies, or immune complexes.

The adoptive transfer of cellular immunity and immunostimulation by substances such as bacillus Calmette-Guérin (BCG) which stimulate primarily cellular immunity may result in tumor regression in experimental systems. Also the important clinical observation that the induction of cellular immunity within and adjacent to superficial tumors by dinitrochlorobenzene (DNCB) or BCG results in tumor regression provides strong evidence for the importance of such immunity to tumor restraint. Studies concerning the mechanisms of cellular immunity are moving at an extraordinarily rapid rate (Chap. 63).

HOST EFFECT OF CANCER The neoplastic process may produce secondary host effects which often present the primary challenge to the physician. The *psychologic effects* of cancer and the production of *pain* require major attention. *Weight loss* and cachexia result primarily from anorexia, the mechanism of which is not understood. It has been demonstrated in experimental systems that tumors may have priority for various metabolites and divert them from appropriate host tissues (the nitrogen trap).

While it has been demonstrated that subjects with defective *immune mechanisms* generally have an increased risk of cancer (see above), immune response is normal in the majority of patients, at least early in their course. However, in many neoplastic diseases, particularly Hodgkin's disease, immune mechanisms, particularly cellular immune mechanisms, progressively fail as the disease progresses. This may result in accelerated growth and spread of the tumor. It has been demonstrated for some neoplastic disease categories that the degree of cellular immunity correlates positively with response to treatment (surgery or chemotherapy) and survival.

Improvement in supportive care and improved treatment, particularly chemotherapy and radiotherapy, have resulted in prolongation of effective survival but also have increased and prolonged chemotherapeutically induced myelo- and immunosuppression. As a result of this, and as a result of improving antibiotic programs for the more common bacterial *infections*, an increasing incidence of opportunistic infections with gram-negative rods, mycotic organisms, viruses, and protozoa (such as *Pneumocystis carinii*) is being reported. In addition, the natural history of infections may be substantially modified by the presence and degree of immunosuppression and myelosuppression.

The tumor may produce substances such as *ectopic hormones* which affect the host. It is possible that certain unexplained manifestations such as anorexia result from, as yet unidentified, tumor products. Ectopic hormone production usually consists of the polypeptide hormones (ACTH, parahormone, antidiuretic hormone, etc.) and has been associated most frequently with oat-cell carcinoma of the lung, though a variety of other tumors may infrequently or rarely produce ectopic hormones. The glycoprotein hormone erythropoietin is produced in some patients with hypernephroma. The mechanism of ectopic hormone production is incompletely understood. The dedifferentiation associated with neoplasia and other evidence of reversion to the embryonic state, as well as biochemical studies relating to histones, have suggested that repressor mechanisms for DNA transcription, which progressively increase with the process of differentiation, decrease as a result of neoplastic change (unmasking of DNA).

Other effects of tumor upon the host include *neuromuscular syndromes* which clinically and pathologically usually resemble degenerative changes (Chap. 333), *dermatologic effects* such as acanthosis nigricans (Chap. 367), and *skeletal effects* such as clubbing and osteoarthropathy (Chap. 353). The mechanisms leading to these changes are not understood.

Those tumors associated with marrow invasion such as the leukemias are associated with *anemia, granulocytopenia, and thrombocytopenia*, as discussed elsewhere (Chap. 316). In fact the management of the acute leukemias depends in considerable part on the prevention and treatment of the hemorrhagic and infectious complications associated with granulocytopenia and thrombocytopenia. Anemia also occurs with nonhematologic malignancies, and its mechanism is similar to that of other chronic diseases (Chap. 308).

Some of the most common host effects of cancer are *iatrogenic*. The effects of radiotherapy and chemotherapy may mimic and exacerbate the host effects of cancer. Since patients with cancer almost invariably require substantial symptomatic and supportive care, they very frequently receive tranquilizers, hypnotics, analgesics (including narcotics), and antibiotics, which may mimic host effects produced by cancer per se. It is essential that this be kept in mind in evaluating the clinical status of such patients.

REFERENCES

M.D. Anderson Hospital and Tumor Institute: *Carcinogenesis: A Broad Critique*, Baltimore: Williams & Wilkins, 1967

M.D. Anderson Hospital and Tumor Institute: *The Proliferation and Spread of Neoplastic Cells*, Baltimore: Williams & Wilkins, 1968

Folkman J et al: Isolation of a tumor factor responsible for angiogenesis, J Exp Med 133:275, 1971

Holland JF, Frei E III (eds): *Cancer Medicine*, Philadelphia: Lea & Febiger, 1973

Sandberg AA, Hossfeld DK: Chromosomal abnormalities in human neoplasia. Ann Rev Med 21:379, 1970

Shirakawa S et al: Cell proliferation in human melanoma. J Clin Invest 49:1188, 1970

320
MEDICAL THERAPY OF CANCER

GERALD P. BODEY
EMIL FREI III

The management of the patient with cancer has become increasingly important as our abilities to cure more of the patients improve through the use of new surgical, radiation, and chemotherapeutic procedures. At the present, the possibility of curing most malignant diseases lies in early detection. Usually the family physician or general internist has the first contact with the patient, and his judgments regarding the significance of the patient's complaints and his skills in physical examination often are a major factor influencing the patient's survival. Failure to investigate the etiology of newly discovered anemia or recent changes in a patient's bowel habits may eliminate the possibility of curative surgery for carcinoma of the colon. Inclusion of digital examination of the rectum and prostate in the routine physical examination may lead to the early diagnosis of unsuspected carcinoma of these organs. About 50 percent of the malignancies originating in the large bowel can be detected by digital examination.

New diagnostic techniques have been introduced in recent years which facilitate earlier detection of malignant disease. The diagnosis of cervical carcinoma can be made by cytologic examination or Papanicolaou smears while the disease is still localized and can be cured by surgery. Mammography is a useful technique for the early detection of breast carcinoma. Abnormal constituents can be detected in the blood of patients with certain malignancies. Carcinoembryonic antigen can be detected in patients with gastrointestinal malignancies, and α-fetoglobulin has been found in patients with hepatomas. The routine application of these and other new diagnostic procedures should lead to a reduction in the number of patients with incurable disease at the time of diagnosis.

The treatment of cancer is complex and requires the knowledge and skills of multiple disciplines. Physicians skilled in surgery, radiotherapy, and chemotherapy should be involved in planning the management of most patients with either curable or incurable cancer. As an increasing number of effective antitumor agents become available, the medical oncologist will assume a central role in the management of the cancer patient. The patient requires the sympathetic support of many persons, including physicians, nurses, and associated personnel. The nursing staff maintains close contact with the patient and is a major source of support. The socioeconomic impact of this disease is formidable, and most patients require the professional assistance of social workers. As the patient faces the prospects of suffering and death, the clergyman can offer comfort, strength, and meaning to life. Some patients are unable to cope with their problems and require psychiatric assistance. The medical oncologist is usually responsible for the long-term care of the patient with incurable cancer and should coordinate the interdisciplinary approach to his management.

SURGICAL THERAPY Although surgery is the only modality capable of curing certain neoplastic diseases, many patients are no longer amenable to surgical cure at the time of diagnosis. For example, over 10 percent of carcinomas of the colon are unresectable at the time of operation, and an additional 25 percent have visible metastases which cannot be resected. Even the results obtained with surgical procedures presumed to be curative based on the appearance of the tumor at operation are discouraging for some types of malignant diseases. Autopsy examination of patients dying within 1 month after presumed curative surgery for bronchogenic carcinoma revealed that 25 percent had either residual local disease or distant metastases. The 5-year survival following what was assumed to be curative surgery in this disease is only 25 percent. In addition to the extent of disease, factors which limit surgical approaches include the general condition of the patient, interference with vital organ function by the surgical procedure, and disfigurement resulting from extensive surgical dissection.

The surgeon nevertheless often plays an important role in the treatment of patients where curative surgery is not possible. Removal of large tumor masses may increase the effectiveness of subsequent chemotherapy or radiotherapy. Surgical procedures may be necessary to relieve obstruction of the gastrointestinal or genitourinary tracts or to remove tumor masses impairing the function of other vital organs. Palliative procedures are sometimes necessary to relieve intractable pain, and when this is not possible, chordotomy may be indicated. The surgical removal of single metastases in certain malignancies such as thyroid and renal carcinoma occasionally results in long-term survival. This is especially important when a single metastasis involves the brain or spinal cord. Local perfusion of chemotherapeutic agents is currently under investigation by surgeons as a means of delivering high doses of drug to the tumor without causing serious systemic toxicity.

RADIOTHERAPY Radiation has a role in curative, adjuvant, and palliative therapy of malignant diseases. Radiation is the treatment of choice for most head and neck tumors, cancer of the uterine cervix, and some tumors of the urinary bladder. Seminomas are quite radiosensitive, and although they usually disseminate widely, they can be effectively controlled and cured with radiotherapy. For many years radiation was used as palliative therapy for lymphomas, but recently curative therapy has been attempted, especially in stages I to III of Hodgkin's disease. The use of doses of 3,500 to 4,000 rads (rd) and treatment of lymph node areas contiguous to tumor sites have produced 5-year survival rates of over 70 percent. Although radiotherapy is also efficacious against other types of localized lymphoma, most of these patients have widespread disease at diagnosis. Radiation has been used as adjuvant therapy with surgery or chemotherapy. Preoperative radiation may reduce the size of certain tumors, thus facilitating the surgical removal and providing a greater opportunity for cure. Postoperative radiation to areas where tumor involvement is likely, such as regional lymph nodes, improves results in some malignancies.

Palliative radiotherapy has many applications. Immediate radiation is often required for the treatment of tumor-induced superior mediastinal syndrome, increased intracranial pressure, or spinal cord compression. It can provide relief of obstruction of the gastrointestinal or genitourinary tracts in patients with extensive disease. Radiotherapy is useful for the control of severe bone pain and prevention of imminent fractures due to metastatic disease. Radiation should be administered promptly for metastases in large weight-bearing bones in an effort to prevent pathologic fracture. Palliative localized radiotherapy is often combined with systemic chemotherapy.

OBJECTIVES OF CHEMOTHERAPY The ultimate objective of chemotherapy is to cure the patient of his malignant disease. This has been achieved in patients with Burkitt's lymphoma and Wilm's tumor and in women with trophoblastic tumors. The initial objective of chemotherapy is to produce complete remission, which means to eliminate all clinical evidence of disease. It is estimated that remission induction therapy produces about a 90 to 99 percent reduction in malignant cells. This objective can be accomplished in 90 percent of children with acute lymphoblastic leukemia, 70 percent of patients with Hodgkin's disease, and 50 percent of patients with testicular tumors.

A major obstacle to curative therapy of malignant disease is the inability to measure the amount of residual cancer during complete remission. Clinical, laboratory, and radiologic examinations may be entirely normal, and yet the patient eventually relapses, presumably because of persisting neoplastic disease. Leukemic infiltrates have been demonstrated at autopsy examination of patients with acute leukemia who died of other causes while in complete remission. Trophoblastic tumors in the woman are an exception to this problem since the tumor cells secrete chorionic gonadotropin. Measurement of this hormone in the urine of patients can detect the presence of as few as 1,000 persistent tumor cells.

Once a patient has achieved complete remission, the main objective is to maintain the remission as long as possible. Since a large number of tumor cells probably still remain when the patient achieves remission, maintenance therapy should be designed to cause the maximum reduction of this tumor burden. Most studies of remission maintenance therapy have been conducted in children with acute lymphoblastic leukemia. Following successful remission induction with adrenal corticosteroids, the median duration of remission was 6 months for patients receiving maintenance therapy with 6-mercaptopurine compared with only 2 months for patients receiving placebo. Chemotherapeutic agents differ with respect to their effectiveness during remission induction and remission maintenance. Vincristine induces complete remission in about 50 percent of patients with acute lymphoblastic leukemia, and the median duration of these remissions is only 6 weeks. Methotrexate, on the contrary, induces complete remission in about 21 percent of patients, but the median duration is 6 months. Intermittent intensive therapy has been more effective than low-dose daily therapy for remission maintenance (Table 320-1). The duration of remission is probably affected by many factors, including host defense mechanisms, proportion of cells undergoing mitosis, and emergence of drug-resistant tumor cells.

A major difficulty in the evaluation of the effect of antitumor agents is the lack of uniform criteria for responses less than complete remission. In general, a partial response is defined as a 50 percent reduction in two diameters of a tumor mass. However, the problem of defining partial response is more complex. Patients with multiple metastases may have some tumor masses which regress while others progress. Chemotherapy may only stabilize tumor masses which were previously proliferating rapidly, yet cause extended patient survival. Furthermore, major reduction in tumor size may have little effect on survival. Busulfan reduces the white blood cell count and spleen size of over 90 percent of patients with chronic myelogenous leukemia. Although this drug definitely improves the quality of life, whether it increases duration of survival is debatable.

The only judicious approach to chemotherapy is that which promises the greatest chance of producing complete remission. The concept of administering a little chemotherapy to delay the progress of tumor growth is untenable. However, the more intensive chemotherapy required to produce complete remission increases the risk of serious complications. Nevertheless, the duration of survival is directly related to the degree of response to chemotherapy. For example, among patients with advanced Hodgkin's disease who achieve complete remission, over 90 percent are still alive at 3 years. The median duration of survival is about 18 months for patients achieving a partial remission and only 4 months for patients failing to respond to therapy.

Chemotherapeutic research has focused primarily on the goal of achieving maximal destruction of neoplastic cells. Recently it has been recognized that acute myelogenous leukemia stem cells are capable of maturation in vitro and that there are macromolecular regulators of stem-cell proliferation and differentiation. These observations suggest that a different approach to therapy may be possible in which the objective is modification of the behavior of the neoplastic cell rather than its destruction.

LIMITATIONS OF CHEMOTHERAPEUTIC AGENTS

In general, antitumor agents are relatively nonspecific, that is, their activity is directed against both normal cells and tumor cells. The major difference in effect is quantitative rather than qualitative, resulting in greater destruction of tumor cells. In general, rapidly dividing cells are the most sensitive to the majority of antitumor agents. In addition to tumor cells, certain normal cells such as those of the bone marrow and gastrointestinal tract proliferate rapidly and, hence, are most susceptible to the destructive effects of antitumor agents. Normal cells, generally, can regenerate more rapidly and thus have an advantage over tumor cells.

In experimental tumors, small increases in the dosage of antitumor agents result in substantial increases in tumor-cell destruction. A twofold increase in dose may result in a tenfold increase in tumor-cell destruction. However, the therapeutic range is often quite narrow, and small increments in dosage may cause a substantial and intolerable increase in toxicity.

The antitumor effects of a drug depend on many factors. Parenteral administration is usually preferable to oral administration since absorption from the gastrointestinal tract is variable and is influenced by nausea, diarrhea, presence of food, pH of the contents, gastrointestinal ulcerations, and lipid solubility. Once in the bloodstream, the plasma half-life varies greatly, depending upon the agent, which may affect both the antitumor activity and toxicity. For example, the half-life in the blood varies from a few minutes for mechlorethamine to several days for daunorubicin and L-asparaginase. Tissue distribution can favorably or adversely influence effectiveness. Many agents are not lipid soluble and do not cross the bloodbrain barrier, thus having no effect on meningeal disease. Meningeal leukemia frequently develops during systemic chemotherapy and requires intrathecal medication. The nitrosoureas cross the blood-brain barrier and are effective against brain tumors. Inadequate concentrations may be present at tumor sites because the drug is firmly bound to serum proteins. Other drugs

TABLE 320-1
Effect of schedule of drug administration on therapeutic response

		Optimum schedule		*Suboptimum schedule*	
Drug	*Disease*	*Regimen*	*Response*	*Regimen*	*Response*
Methotrexate*	Acute lymphocytic leukemia	10–30 mg/m² semiweekly	52 weeks† median duration	3 mg/m²/day	12–20 weeks† median duration
Cyclophosphamide	Burkitt's lymphoma	40 mg/kg every 3–4 weeks	70% remissions, 15% long-term survivors	Daily therapy	30% remissions
Melphalan*	Myeloma	0.25 mg/kg/day, 4-day courses	40% responses	0.025 mg/kg/day daily	20% responses
Cytosine arabinoside*	Acute leukemia	200 mg/m²/day, 5-day course	39% remissions	500 mg/m²/day, 2-day courses	24% remissions

* *Randomized comparative studies.*
† *Used as remission maintenance therapy.*

accumulate intracellularly. For example, methotrexate is actively transported across cell membranes, whereas arabinosyl cytosine accumulates intracellularly because of enzymatic conversion to the nucleotide. Drugs may be catabolized quickly, affording only a brief exposure to tumor cells. Arabinosyl cytosine is rapidly converted to inactive uracil arabinoside by deaminases in the serum, resulting in a very short serum half-life, whereas methotrexate is not catabolized but is excreted unchanged in the urine. The effect of other drugs on the metabolism of antitumor agents has not been studied adequately. One known example is the inhibition of xanthine oxidase by allopurinol, thus preventing the catabolism of 6-mercaptopurine to inactive 6-thiouric acid.

The schedule of administration may influence the activity of antitumor agents (Table 320-1). This was first demonstrated with methotrexate in animal studies. Later it was shown that when methotrexate was used for remission maintenance therapy of acute lymphocytic leukemia, intermittent high dosage produced substantially longer remissions than daily lower dose therapy. For multiple myeloma, 4-day courses of melphalan probably are superior to daily treatment. Arabinosyl cytosine is an agent which is active only during the period of the cell cycle when DNA is being synthesized. The proportion of tumor cells surviving exposure to this drug in tissue culture is related more to the duration of exposure than to the concentration of the drug. The surviving cells retain their sensitivity to arabinosyl cytosine. This importance of schedule has been demonstrated in acute leukemia of animals and humans (Table 320-1). The degree of myelosuppressive toxicity is also related to the duration of therapy. No myelosuppression was observed when the drug was given to cancer patients by a single intravenous injection, even at very high doses. Mild myelosuppression was observed following a 24-hr continuous infusion, but dose-limiting myelosuppressive toxicity was observed when the drug was given in 48- or 96-hr infusions.

Drug resistance is a major problem in cancer chemotherapy. Some tumors are inherently resistant to certain drugs, whereas others are not affected because of pharmacologic considerations. However, most tumors originally sensitive to an antitumor agent eventually develop resistance. Some tumors have variable populations of cells with different genetic constitutions, and a few cells may be inherently resistant. As the sensitive cells are destroyed, these resistant cells gain the ascendency. Other cells acquire resistance by mutation. Although the mechanisms for resistance have been demonstrated infrequently in human tumors, they have been characterized in some animal tumors. Alterations in membrane transport prevent deliverance of active drugs intracellularly. Deletion of an enzyme results in failure of conversion of the drug to its active metabolite. For example, deletion of inosinic pyrophosphorylase prevents conversion of 6-mercaptopurine to the active nucleotide. Alternate pathways may circumvent the damage inflicted by the agent. Tumors resistant to L-asparaginase have increased amounts of asparagine synthetase which is required for the synthesis of L-asparagine. Understanding of these mechanisms may lead to methods of eliminating drug resistance.

SINGLE-AGENT CHEMOTHERAPY Five major types of antitumor agents are available: alkylating agents, antimetabolites, plant alkaloids, antibiotics, and endocrine agents. The important antitumor agents with their major toxicity and mechanism of action are described in Table 320-2. Most of the neoplastic diseases for which significant chemotherapy is currently available are shown in Table 320-3 with the appropriate agents or combinations.

Alkylating agents Mechlorethamine (nitrogen mustard) was the first chemical agent used in the treatment of cancer. It was originally investigated as a potential agent for chemical warfare. The observation that it caused marrow aplasia and lympholysis led to the administration of mechlorethamine in hematologic malignancies, where it was found to have major activity against lymphomas. The activity of alkylating agents results from internal ionization of the compound forming highly reactive intermediates which combine with molecules such as proteins, nucleic acids, and amino acids, all of which have replaceable protons. Mechlorethamine contains two β-chloroethyl groups which transfer into ethylenimonium derivatives that are positively charged and combine with negatively charged guanine moieties of complementary DNA strands. This results in cross-linking of the DNA strands. Mechlorethamine also causes linking of DNA to protein and protein to protein. Mechlorethamine causes nausea and vomiting during the day of infusion and myelosuppression. It is a vesicant on the skin, and care must be used in its administration.

Three major types of modification have altered the properties of mechlorethamine. The substitution of electrophilic groups on the nitrogen atom, as in chlorambucil, reduces the reactivity, producing a more stable drug with a longer half-life in the serum. An amino acid or nucleic acid precursor added to the nitrogen atom as a carrier enhances delivery to sites of greatest tumor activity. Melphalan is an L-phenylalanine congenor which would be expected to be most active at sites of protein synthesis. It has major activity against multiple myeloma, a tumor which synthesizes gamma-globulins. Cyclophosphamide is a derivative in which the reactivity of the chloroethyl groups is eliminated by reducing the basicity through the substitution of groups on the nitrogen atom. This drug is totally inactive until converted to intermediate derivatives by microsomal enzymes of the liver.

Although the alkylating agents are similar in their mechanism of action and spectrum of activity, there are differences among them. Busulfan has a greater effect on granulopoiesis, whereas chlorambucil has a greater effect on lymphopoiesis. Nausea and vomiting are prominent side effects of mechlorethamine, cyclophosphamide, and melphalan, but are infrequent with busulfan and chlorambucil. Cyclophosphamide causes alopecia and cystitis, whereas busulfan causes skin hyperpigmentation and occasionally pulmonary fibrosis. Also, while there is overlapping of the therapeutic effects of the alkylating agents, there are important differences. Thus, melphalan and cyclophosphamide are the most effective agents for patients with myeloma. Cyclophosphamide is the only alkylating agent which can produce and maintain complete remissions in acute lymphocytic leukemia. Busulfan is more effective in chronic myelogenous leukemia, whereas chlorambucil is more effective in chronic lymphocytic leukemia, a reflection of their selective greater activity against a single cell type. The toxicity of the various alkylating agents is shown in Table 320-2.

Antimetabolites An antimetabolite is a substance which resembles a normal metabolite so closely that it enters the same metabolic system, but differs sufficiently so that it interferes with the metabolic pathway. Antimetabolites currently in use are methotrexate, 6-mercaptopurine, 6-thioguanine, 5-fluorouracil, and arabinosyl cytosine (Tables 320-2 and 320-3).

Folic acid antagonists Methotrexate was the first important antimetabolite to undergo clinical investigation. Folic acid, an essential dietary factor in humans, is reduced by the enzyme dihydrofolate reductase to dihydrofolic acid and tetrahydrofolic acid. The latter substance accepts single carbon fragments to form the coenzyme citrovorum factor. Several coenzymes exist which differ depending upon the oxidation of the carbon fragment. One of these enzymes, N^{10}-formyltetrahydrofolic acid, donates a single carbon fragment to form deoxythymidine monophosphate, an immediate precursor of DNA. This inhibition of thymidine synthesis and, consequently, DNA synthesis is largely responsible for the biologic effect of methotrexate. Some of the folic acid antagonists have an affinity for dihydrofolate reductase which is 10,000 times greater than folic acid and, thus cannot be readily displaced. However, when citrovorum factor, the product of the enzymatic reactions, is given concurrently, it will prevent the effect of the antagonist.

TABLE 320-2
Important antitumor agents

Agent	*Mechanism of action*	*Myelo-suppression*	*Toxicity, gastro-intestinal*	*Other*
Alkylating agents				
Mechlorethamine	Cross-linking of DNA	4+	2+	Local vesicant to skin
Cyclophosphamide	Cross-linking of DNA	3+	1+	Alopecia, cystitis
Melphalan	Cross-linking of DNA	3+	1+	
Busulfan	Cross-linking of DNA	3+	0	Pigmentation, pulmonary fibrosis
Chlorambucil	Cross-linking of DNA	3+	0	
Hexamethylmelamine	Cross-linking of DNA	3+	3+	Peripheral neuropathy
Antimetabolites				
Methotrexate	Inhibits dihydrofolate reductase	4+	4+	Hepatotoxicity, alopecia
6-Mercaptopurine	Inhibits purine metabolism	3+	2+	Hepatotoxicity
5-Fluorouracil	Inhibits thymidylate synthetase	3+	4+	
Arabinosyl cytosine	Inhibits DNA polymerase	4+	3+	Alopecia
Plant alkaloids				
Vinblastine	Metaphase arrest	3+	1+	Paresthesias
Vincristine	Metaphase arrest	1+	2+	Paresthesias, motor weakness, alopecia
Antibiotics				
Actinomycin D	Inhibits DNA-dependent RNA synthesis	3+	4+	Alopecia, skin changes
Mithramycin	Inhibits RNA synthesis	3+	3+	Hemorrhage
Daunorubicin	Alters DNA and inhibits RNA synthesis	4+	3+	Alopecia, myocardopathy
Adriamycin	Alters DNA and inhibits RNA synthesis	4+	3+	Alopecia, myocardopathy
Bleomycin	Alters DNA and inhibits DNA synthesis	0	1+	Alopecia, skin changes, pulmonary fibrosis
Miscellaneous agents				
Hydroxyurea	Inhibits ribonucleoside reductase	4+	1+	
Procarbazine	Monoamine oxidase inhibitor	2+	3+	Paresthesias
Nitrosourea	Alkylating agent	4+	2+	Hepatotoxicity, pulmonary toxicity
L-Asparaginase	Depletion of asparagine	0	1+	Fatty liver, hyperglycemia, pancreatitis, hypofibrinogenemia, CNS toxicity
Adrenal corticosteroids (prednisone)	Lympholysis	0	0	Cushingoid features, hyperglycemia, muscle weakness, bone necrosis, salt retention
Imidazole carboxamide	Unknown	3+	4+	

Citrovorum factor is of little benefit for reversing the effects of the antagonist once they are initiated.

Methotrexate exemplifies the relation between the mechanism of action of an antitumor agent and its toxicity. Since the primary action of this drug is to inhibit DNA synthesis, it affects only proliferating cells. Consequently, toxicity is primarily limited to the bone marrow, gastrointestinal tract, and skin. Marrow toxicity is manifested by marked decrease in erythropoiesis, with reticulocytopenia appearing within several days after drug administration. Megaloblastosis may occur due to greater impairment in DNA synthesis than in RNA and protein synthesis. Methotrexate causes an immediate decrease in mitoses of granulocyte precursors of the bone marrow,

TABLE 320-3
Malignant diseases responsive to chemotherapy

Neoplastic disease	*Current status with chemotherapy*	*Active chemotherapeutic agents*	*Response, %*	*Effective combinations*	*Response, %*
Hematologic malignancies					
Hodgkin's disease	Complete remission in 80% of patients; median survival of about 4 years in advanced disease.	Prednisone	30	Mechlorethamine + vincristine + prednisone + procarbazine (MOPP)	83
		Mechlorethamine	60		
		Cyclophosphamide	60		
		Procarbazine	60		
		Vincristine	60		
		Vinblastine	65		
		BCNU	47		
		Adriamycin	46		
Lymphosarcoma	Complete remission in 50% of patients.	Cyclophosphamide	60	Cyclophosphamide + vincristine + prednisone (COP)	88
		Prednisone	40		
		Vincristine	50		
		Vinblastine	30		
		Mechlorethamine	50		
		Adriamycin	40		
Reticulum-cell sarcoma	Complete remission in 40% of patients.	Cyclophosphamide	55	Cyclophosphamide + vincristine + prednisone (COP)	78
		Prednisone			
		Vincristine	60		
		Vinblastine	30		
		Mechlorethamine	20		
		Adriamycin	70		
Acute lymphoblastic leukemia	Complete remission in 90% of children; median duration of over 2 years.	Vincristine	47	Vincristine + prednisone	90
		Prednisone	57	Prednisone + 6-mercaptopurine	82
		6-Mercaptopurine	35	Prednisone + vincristine + methotrexate + 6-mercaptopurine (POMP)	80
		Methotrexate	30		
		Daunorubicin	40		
		Adriamycin	40		
		Cyclophosphamide	20		
		L-Asparaginase	30		
		Arabinosyl cytosine	20		
Acute myelogenous leukemia	Complete remission in about 50% of adults; median duration of 14 months.	Arabinosyl cytosine	32	Cyclophosphamide + vincristine + arabinosyl cytosine + prednisone (COAP)	59
		Daunorubicin	35		
		Adriamycin	35		
		6-Mercaptopurine	12	Arabinosyl cytosine + 6-thioguanine	53
		Cyclophosphamide	10	L-Asparaginase + daunorubicin + arabinosyl cytosine	65
		Methotrexate	18		
Chronic myelogenous leukemia	Symptomatic control of disease.	Bulsulfan	90		
		Hydroxyurea	90		
		6-Mercaptopurine	10*		
		Dibromomanital			
Chronic lymphocytic leukemia	Symptomatic control of disease.	Chlorambucil	60		
		Cyclophosphamide	40		
		Prednisone	70		
Multiple myeloma	Response in 70% of patients; median survival of 2 years.	Melphalan	40	Melphalan + prednisone	70
		Cyclophosphamide	30		
		Prednisone			
Sarcoma					
Wilms's tumor	Over 50% long-term survivors.	Dactinomycin	30		
		Vincristine	50		
		Cyclophosphamide	25		
Neuroblastoma	Median survival 1 year; cure achieved in some patients.	Cyclophosphamide	67	Vincristine + cyclophosphamide	
		Vincristine	50		
		Dactinomycin	30		
		Prednisone			
		Adriamycin	40		
		Daunorubicin	40		

resulting in granulocytopenia beginning 3 to 6 days later and reaching a maximum at 7 to 10 days. Four hours after large doses of methotrexate the mitotic index of jejunal crypts markedly decreases and remains low for about 48 hr. Inhibition of proliferation of these cells leads to ulceration and invasion by microorganisms. Buccal ulceration is a frequent side effect of methotrexate therapy. Cells in the papillae of hair follicles have a very high turnover; hence hair loss is common during methotrexate therapy. Resting hair, such as axillary and pubic hair, eyebrows, and eyelashes, is spared. Tumors sensitive to methotrexate are shown in Table 320-3.

Purine analogues 6-Mercaptopurine is a structural analogue of hypoxanthine which is converted to the active nucleotide, 6-mercaptopurine-9-ribose phosphate, by the enzyme, inosinic pyrophosphorylase. The nucleotide interferes with several steps in purine biosynthesis. It decreases the synthesis of 5-phosphoribosylamine, the first step in purine biosynthesis, by pseudofeedback inhibition. It also interferes with the conversion of inosinic monophosphate to xanthine monophosphate and the conversion of inosinic monophosphate to adenosine monophosphate. 6-Mercaptopurine is metabolized to 6-thiouric acid by xanthine oxidase. Allopurinol, which is used to prevent uric acid synthesis, blocks the activity of this enzyme; hence, when they are used together, the dose of 6-mercaptopurine should be reduced to about 30

TABLE 320-3 *continued*

Neoplastic disease	*Current status with chemotherapy*	*Active chemotherapeutic agents*	*Response, %*	*Effective combinations*	*Response, %*
Rhabdomyosarcoma	Response in 50% of patients with embryonal rhabdomyosarcoma.	Dactinomycin	30		
		Cyclophosphamide	50		
		Vincristine	50		
		Adriamycin	30		
Soft-tissue sarcomas	Infrequent complete remission.	Dactinomycin	20	Adriamycin + imidazole carboxamide	40
		Cyclophosphamide	20		
		Adriamycin	23		
		Imidazole carboxamide	20		
Carcinoma					
Trophoblastic	About 75% of patients are cured.	Methotrexate	60		
		Dactinomycin	50		
Testis	Complete remission in about 15% of patients.	Methotrexate	40	Methotrexate + chlorambucil + dactinomycin	50
		Dactinomycin	30		
		Chlorambucil			
		Vincristine			
		Mithramycin	30		
		Bleomycin	30		
Breast	Partial response in most patients.	Androgens	25	Vincristine + cyclophosphamide + prednisone + 5-fluorouracil + methotrexate	55–80
		Estrogens	30		
		5-Fluorouracil	28		
		Cyclophosphamide	30		
		Chlorambucil	30		
		Methotrexate	40		
		Prednisone	10		
		Vincristine	20		
		Adriamycin	43		
		Melphalan	30		
Ovary	Complete remissions in 20% of patients; median survival of over 2 years.	Melphalan	47	Dactinomycin + 5-fluorouracil + cyclophosphamide	40
		Chlorambucil			
		Cyclophosphamide	70		
		5-Fluorouracil	25		
		Thio-TEPA	22		
Uterine corpus	Partial response only.	Progestins	30		
Melanoma		Imidazole carboxamide	20		
		Vincristine	20		
		BCNU	20		
		Hydroxyurea	20		
Head and neck		Methotrexate	45		
		Bleomycin	30		
		Vinblastine	20		
		Cyclophosphamide	35		
Colon		5-Fluorouracil	25		
Lung		Mechlorethamine			
		Cyclophosphamide	30		
		Methotrexate	25		
		Procarbazine	20		

* *Results in blastic transformation of chronic myelogenous leukemia.*

percent. The major usefulness of this drug is in the treatment of acute leukemia (Table 320-3). 6-Thioguanine has similar activity and toxicity as 6-mercaptopurine but is not metabolized by xanthine oxidase and is not affected by allopurinol administration.

Pyrimidine analogues The introduction of 5-flouro-uracil was an important advance in cancer chemotherapy because it is active against many carcinomas. 5-Fluorouracil must be converted to the active agent, fluorodeoxyuridine monophosphate, which inhibits DNA synthesis by blocking the enzyme thymidylate synthetase. This prevents the methylation of deoxyuridine monophosphate to deoxythymidine monophosphate. The nucleotide is incorporated into RNA, and prevents the incorporation of uracil and orotic acid, thus inhibiting RNA synthesis. The activity and toxicity of 5-fluorouracil are shown in Tables 320-2 and 320-3. It is most useful against carcinomas of the gastrointestinal tract and breast.

Arabinósyl cytosine is a pyrimidine nucleoside analogue which interferes with DNA synthesis by inhibiting DNA polymerase. It is structurally related to deoxycytidine and is converted to the active nucleotide by the enzyme deoxycytidine kinase. The drug is active only against proliferating cells which are synthesizing DNA. Arabinosyl cytosine is metabolized by a deaminase to uracil arabinoside which is excreted in the urine. There is some evidence to suggest that the ratio between tumor kinase and deaminase activity relates to the effectiveness of arabinosyl cytosine. Studies in both animals and humans indicate that the schedule of administration influences the antitumor effect and toxicity of this drug (Table 320-1). A major advantage of arabinosyl cytosine is that serious toxicity is virtually limited to myelosuppression. The major activity of this drug is against acute leukemia.

Plant alkaloids The plant alkaloids, vincristine and vinblastine, are derived from the periwinkle plants. Medical folklore attributed to periwinkle effectiveness in diabetes mellitus. When subjected to experimental studies in animals, the extracts were found to cause granulocytopenia and, subsequently, were demonstrated to be active against transplanted rodent lymphocytic neoplasms. The periwinkle alkaloids produce metaphase arrest in dividing cells, presumably by a direct adverse effect on spindle proteins. Although these drugs do not interfere with total RNA synthesis, a marked diminution in transfer RNA biosynthesis occurs which can be reversed by glutamic acid. It may be that interference with transfer RNA synthesis is the primary effect, and the effect on spindle protein is only of secondary importance.

Vincristine differs structurally from vinblastine only by replacement of a methyl group with a formyl group. Although they have similar activity, there are some important differences. Vincristine is capable of producing complete remissions in about 50 percent of patients with acute lymphoblastic leukemia, an accomplishment not observed with vinblastine. The major toxicity of vinblastine is myelosuppression, whereas the major toxicity of vincristine is paresthesias, peripheral muscle weakness, and constipation. Most of these differences in toxicity are only quantitative and can be observed with both drugs, depending upon the dose administered. The periwinkle alkaloids have a wide spectrum of activity, as indicated in Table 320-3.

Antibiotics Antibiotics are substances produced by organisms which interfere with the growth of other living cells. As new antibiotics are isolated, they are tested not only for antimicrobial activity but also for antitumor activity. Some of these substances, such as puromycin, are potent antitumor agents, but their formidable toxicity precludes clinical usefulness. The important antitumor antibiotics in clinical use are dactinomycin, mithramycin, daunorubicin, adriamycin, and bleomycin.

Dactinomycin was the first antibiotic used extensively in cancer chemotherapy. The drug forms a complex with DNA which inhibits DNA-dependent RNA synthesis. It has proved to be especially useful in the treatment of childhood malignancies, such as Wilms' tumor, neuroblastoma, and rhabdomyosarcoma, and trophoblastic tumors of women.

The antitumor activity of mithramycin is limited to testicular tumors. The drug can also rapidly reduce serum calcium levels in patients with hypercalcemia secondary to various malignant diseases. This effect appears to be due to inhibition of bone resorption by the drug. Mithramycin inhibits DNA-dependent RNA synthesis, presumably by binding with DNA. The drug causes myelosuppression which results in thrombocytopenia, but additionally produces an acute hemorrhagic diathesis of uncertain etiology which causes death in about 5 percent of patients receiving the drug.

Daunorubicin and adriamycin are anthracycline antibiotics with activity against a broad spectrum of animal and human tumors (Table 320-3). Adriamycin differs from daunorubicin only by the addition of a hydroxyl group. However, in animal tumor systems it has twice the therapeutic index of daunorubicin. The anthracycline antibiotics inhibit DNA synthesis and DNA-dependent RNA synthesis by binding with DNA in a fashion different from dactinomycin. Daunorubicin has a very long serum half-life and binds to tissues for as long as 1 month. A poorly understood side effect of these drugs is cardiotoxicity which consists of tachycardia, hypotension, and heart failure that usually results in death. Cardiotoxicity is dose-related and is more likely to occur in elderly patients. It seldom occurs in patients receiving a total dose of less than 750 mg per m^2 daunorubicin or 600 mg per m^2 adriamycin.

Bleomycin is an antibiotic complex consisting of seven polypeptides of similar structure. At low concentrations bleomycin inhibits cell division, and at high concentrations it inhibits DNA synthesis. It is most active against malignancies of the head and neck, larynx and skin, lymphomas, and testicular tumors (Table 320-3). Its activity against tumors of epithelioid organs is due to its preferential localization in these tissues. Responses generally are of short duration, lasting a median of only 6 to 12 weeks, largely because of the fact that its toxicity precludes long-term maintenance therapy. An unusual toxic manifestation of bleomycin is pulmonary fibrosis which has been observed in 10 percent of patients and is usually fatal. This toxicity is dose-related and occurs more commonly in older patients. It usually can be avoided by restricting the total dose to less than 300 mg.

Miscellaneous agents *Hydroxyurea* is an agent which may be used as an alternative to busulfan in the treatment of chronic myelogenous leukemia (Table 320-3). Hydroxyurea may potentiate the antitumor effects of radiotherapy in head and neck tumors. It also is useful for quickly reducing very high white blood counts in patients with acute myelogenous leukemia who have rapidly proliferating disease. Hydroxyurea is a simple derivative of urea which is rapidly absorbed from the gastrointestinal tract. It inhibits ribonucleoside diphosphate reductase and is active only against cells synthesizing DNA. The only major side effect of this drug is myelosuppression.

In the search for new monoamine oxidase inhibitors, 1-methyl-2-benzylhydrazine was synthesized and was found coincidentally to have antitumor activity. A number of related compounds were prepared, and *N*-isopropyl-α-(2-methylhydrazine)-*p*-toluamide hydrochloride (*procarbazine*) was found to be the best. Its major usefulness is for the treatment of patients with Hodgkin's disease. Procarbazine is not cross-resistant with other antitumor agents in animal tumor systems and is active in patients with Hodgkin's disease resistant to other therapeutic modalities. Hence, its mechanism of action is qualitatively different from other antitumor agents. It apparently acts like an alkylating agent, but its precise mechanism of action is unknown. Besides inhibiting monoamine oxidases, it may undergo autooxidation with formation of hydrogen peroxide and damage to DNA. In experimental systems procarbazine causes decreased mitotic activity and chromatin breaks.

The *nitrosoureas* are drugs which are quite active against a variety of animal tumors. One of these compounds, 1,3-bis-(2-chloroethyl)-1-nitrosourea (BCNU), has been evaluated clinically and is beneficial in the treatment of brain tumors and advanced Hodgkin's disease refractory to other agents. These drugs appear to act as alkylating agents but have the unique property of crossing the blood-brain barrier. An unusual feature of these agents is the delayed myelosuppressive toxicity which develops 3 to 4 weeks after drug administration.

Imidazole carboxamide (dimethyl-triazeno-imidazole carboxamide) produces responses in patients with malignant melanoma and soft-tissue sarcomas. The drug is an analogue of 5-amino-imidazole-4-carboxamide, a precursor in purine synthesis, but its exact mechanism of action has not been identified. Side effects are nausea, vomiting, myelosuppression, and a flu-like syndrome.

Guinea pig serum used as a source of complement for immunologic experiments was found to have activity against experimental lymphomas. The active constituent was found to be *L-asparaginase*. This drug is an enzyme which converts L-asparaginase to L-aspartic acid, thus depleting body stores of L-asparagine. Many experimental leukemias and lymphomas require exogenous L-asparagine, whereas normal tissues are able to synthesize this amino acid. L-Asparagine is synthesized from L-aspartic acid by the enzyme L-asparagine synthetase. Fairly good correlation exists in experimental systems between the absence of L-asparagine synthetase and requirement for exogenous L-asparagine. Furthermore, tumors which do not respond to L-asparaginase tend to undergo a marked increase in L-asparagine synthetase after exposure to L-asparaginase. L-Asparaginase was initially hailed as being a unique antitumor agent with specific activity limited to tumors. Unfortunately, this has been found to be incorrect, and the drug interferes with protein synthesis, thereby causing a wide variety of toxic effects. Important toxicity includes hypofibrinogenemia and hyperglycemia due to impaired synthesis of insulin (Table 320-2).

ADJUVANT CHEMOTHERAPY Chemotherapy as an adjunct to definitive surgery or radiotherapy would be anticipated to improve results for several reasons. Systemic chemotherapy could eradicate small recognized or unrecognized metastases without eradicating a large primary tumor. Chemotherapy is known to be less effective against large tumor masses, probably owing to inadequate diffusion or differences in proliferative activity of tumor cells. Adjuvant chemotherapy may destroy residual tumor cells at the operative site or released into the circulation or into a body cavity during surgery. Malignant cells have been demonstrated in the blood and wound washings during primary surgery for breast carcinoma. However, in most studies of adjuvants, chemotherapy has been given only during the immediate postoperative period, often with negative results. It may be that these residual tumor cells are susceptible to chemotherapy only at a later period when they are proliferating. However, since most antitumor agents are immunosuppressive, their administration may facilitate establishment of metastases by inhibiting the host's immune mechanisms which would destroy these tumor cells rather than by improving results.

Chemotherapy with dactinomycin as an adjuvant to surgery and radiation has been successful in Wilms' tumor. The addition of dactinomycin increased the 2-year survival from 43 to 92 percent. Long-term dactinomycin therapy was superior to a single course at the time of surgery, reducing the recurrence rate from 86 to 46 percent. Sixty percent of recurrences took place 6 months after surgery, emphasizing the necessity of prolonged treatment. Recently, it has been demonstrated that use of the four-drug combination of mechlorethamine, vincristine, procarbazine, and prednisone (MOPP) following radiotherapy of advanced Hodgkin's disease prolongs the duration of remission and decreases the relapse rate.

COMBINATION CHEMOTHERAPY In vitro studies with microorganisms have shown that several results may be obtained when two drugs are used in combination. (1) The result may be additive; that is, the activity of the combination is equal to the sum of the activity of each drug separately. (2) The result may be synergistic, wherein the activity obtained is greater than that from the sum of each agent alone. An example of synergism in cancer chemotherapy is the combination of vincristine and prednisone in acute lymphocytic leukemia. The expected remission rate if the drugs were additive would be about 75 percent, whereas the observed remission rate exceeds

90 percent. Two drugs may be antagonistic or nonadditive because of the interference or inactivity of one drug in the presence of the other.

It is reasonable to assume that combination chemotherapy decreases the potential for the emergence of resistant cells. The likelihood of a mutation occurring which confers multiple drug resistance is considerably less than one which confers resistance to a single agent. Since there may be differing sensitivities to a single agent among a population of tumor cells, only a combination may be capable of destroying all the cells. An established example of the prevention of resistance is the combination of isoniazid and para-aminosalicylic acid in the treatment of tuberculosis.

Combination chemotherapy is of greatest advantage when it is designed to exploit the different toxicities of antitumor agents. Myelosuppression is the dose-limiting toxicity for most agents, and the effects of two myelosuppressive agents are additive. Consequently, when used in combination, the dose of each drug must be substantially reduced. However, drugs with different toxicities can each be given in combination at full dose. The three-drug combination of cyclophosphamide, vincristine, and prednisone (COP) in lymphomas is an example of such a combination.

Substantial benefits have resulted from clinical studies of combination chemotherapy (Table 320-4). The four-drug combination prednisone, vincristine, methotrexate, and 6-mercaptopurine (POMP) for acute lymphocytic leukemia produces complete remission in 80 percent of patients and a median survival of 3 years, which is far superior to any single-agent therapy. Over 80 percent of patients with advanced Hodgkin's disease achieve complete remission with the combination of mechlorethamine, vincristine, prednisone, and procarbazine (MOPP), and the median duration of survival exceeds 5 years, suggesting that some of these patients have been cured. The superiority of combination over single-agent chemotherapy has also been demonstrated for acute myelogenous leukemia, other lymphomas, breast carcinoma, and childhood tumors.

ENDOCRINE THERAPY Tumors derived from organs which are normally responsive to or are dependent upon hormones often behave similarly, and this responsiveness or dependency can be exploited as therapy. Endocrine therapy consists of ablation of hormone-producing organs or specific hormonal therapy (Table 320-5). The major diseases responsive to hormonal therapy are carcinomas of the breast, prostate, uterine endometrium, and thyroid. Adrenal corticosteroids are unique because they are also active against nonendocrine-related tumors such as lymphomas and leukemias.

Ablative procedures Ablative surgery has been used extensively in women with breast carcinoma (see Chap. 93). About 35 percent of premenopausal women respond to oophorectomy, but it is seldom effective in postmeno-

TABLE 320-4
Comparison between single-agent and combination chemotherapy

Disease	*Single agent*	*Complete response, %*	*Combination*	*Complete response, %*
Acute lymphocytic leukemia	Vincristine	47	Vincristine + prednisone + methotrexate + 6-mercaptopurine	80
	Prednisone	57		
	6-Mercaptopurine	27		
	Methotrexate	21		
Acute myelogenous leukemia*	Arabinosyl cytosine	32	Vincristine + prednisone + arabinosyl cytosine + cyclophosphamide	48
Hodgkin's disease	Mechlorethamine	10	Vincristine + mechlorethamine + procarbazine + prednisone	83
	Vincristine	10		
	Procarbazine	30		
Multiple myeloma*†	Melphalan	32	Melphalan + prednisone	70
Breast carcinoma†	Vincristine	20	Vincristine + cyclophosphamide + prednisone + 5-fluorouracil + methotrexate	88
	Cyclophosphamide	30		
	5-Fluorouracil	28		
	Methotrexate	40		
	Prednisone	10		
Testicular tumors	Actinomycin D	30	Chlorambucil + methotrexate + actinomycin D	50

* *Randomized comparative studies.*
† *These figures represent partial responses which are not comparable to what is achieved in acute leukemia and Hodgkin's disease.*

TABLE 320-5
Endocrine therapy for metastatic carcinoma

Agent or approach	Tumor	Response, %	Comments
Ablative type of therapy			
Oophorectomy	Breast, female	35	Minimally effective in postmenopausal female.
Adrenalectomy	Breast, female	30	Most effective in patients who
	Breast, male	50	respond to castration.
Hypophysectomy	Breast, female	30	Benefit similar to that achieved with
	Breast, male	50	adrenalectomy.
Orchiectomy	Prostate	90	These diseases are usually hormone-
	Breast, male	70	dependent and quite responsive to castration.
Radioactive iodine (^{131}I)	Thyroid	15	Effective only in iodine-concentrating tumors.
Hormonal type of therapy			
Androgens:			
methyltestosterone, fluoxymesterone, methandrosteneolone, testosterone propionate, nandrolone phenpropionate, dromostanolone, testolactone	Breast, female	25	Most beneficial in postmenopausal females. Less effective than estrogens.
Estrogens:			
stilbesterol, chlorotrianisene, diethylstilbesterol diphosphate,	Breast, female	30	Most effective in postmenopausal females.
polyestradiol phosphate, ethinyl estradiol	Prostate		Most beneficial when used following recurrences after orchiectomy.
Progestins:			
hydroxyprogesterone caproate, medroxyprogesterone acetate	Endometrium	30	Most effective in older women with well-differentiated tumors.
Thyroid:			
thyroxine or triiodothyronine	Thyroid		
Adrenal corticoids:			
prednisone, prednisolone, hydrocortisone, cortisone, methylprednisolone, dexameth-	Acute lymphocytic leukemia	57	Of little value as maintenance therapy.
asone, triamcinolone, betamethasone, paramethasone	Chronic lymphocytic leukemia	70	Most useful in combination with other agents.
	Hodgkin's disease	30	
	Lymphosarcoma	40	
	Multiple myeloma		
	Breast	10	

pausal women. Castration is most beneficial to premenopausal women in whom there has been a long interval between mastectomy and recurrence and who have mainly osseous and soft-tissue metastases. Patients who do not respond to this procedure are unlikely to respond to additional endocrine manipulations and should be given chemotherapy. Nearly 50 percent of patients who relapse after responding to castration respond to adrenalectomy or hypophysectomy. These procedures may also benefit postmenopausal women who have responded to estrogen therapy. The procedures are equally effective, and selection should be made on an individual basis depending upon the patient's general condition, other illnesses and sites of metastases.

Castration is an especially useful procedure in men with breast carcinoma, producing a response rate of nearly 70 percent. Following recurrence, about 50 percent of these patients will respond to adrenalectomy or hypophysectomy. Nearly all patients with prostatic carcinoma will benefit for 2 to 3 years from orchiectomy.

Estrogens Estrogens have been used successfully in breast carcinoma in women and in prostatic carcinoma. Responses occur in about 35 percent of women with breast carcinoma, and they are most effective in postmenopausal women. Estrogens have been used in men with recurrent prostatic carcinoma following orchiectomy; however, they are of no benefit when given simultaneously with castration. Although estrogens clearly have an antitumor effect, this is somewhat negated by an increase in mortality from cardiovascular disease. Several estrogens have been used with equal success.

Their mechanism of action is unknown, but in breast carcinoma responsiveness has been related to the presence of an estrogen receptor protein in the tumors. Undesirable effects of these drugs include nausea, vomiting, vaginal bleeding, sodium retention, stress incontinence, hypertension, and increased capillary fragility.

Androgens Androgen therapy produces responses in about 20 percent of women with breast carcinoma. This therapy is most effective in postmenopausal women. The effects of therapy are not seen for several weeks, but 90 percent of those responding will have begun to show a response within 8 weeks. A variety of androgens have been used with equal success. However, in comparative studies, androgens have not been as effective as estrogens. The mechanism of action of these hormones is unknown, but the histologic changes resemble those observed during radiation therapy. Side-effects from androgens include hirsutism, deepening of the voice, and increased libido.

Progestins Progestins are related to progesterone, which is produced by the corpus luteum and placenta. They produce responses in 30 percent of women with endometrial carcinoma. Remissions usually last for several years. Best results are seen in older women with well-differentiated tumors who have had a long interval between the appearance of the primary and recurrent disease. Their mechanism of action is unknown. The only side effects from these drugs are mild fluid retention and rarely hypercalcemia.

Adrenal corticosteroids Prednisone is the adrenal corticosteroid most commonly used for antitumor therapy. It produces complete remission in about 60 percent of patients with acute lymphoblastic leukemia and partial responses in 70 percent of patients with chronic lymphocytic leukemia. It is also active against lymphomas and myeloma and in about 10 percent of breast carcinoma. The usual dose of prednisone is 40 mg per m^2 per day. Adrenal corticosteroids suppress mitosis and cause lysis of normal and abnormal lymphocytic elements, presumably by inhibiting cellular protein synthesis. Their activity in breast carcinoma is presumed to be due to suppression of estrogen production by the adrenal cortex. Major toxicity includes sodium retention, hyperglycemia, Cushingoid features, muscle weakness, and bone necrosis.

Thyroxine About 15 percent of thyroid carcinomas accumulate iodine for the synthesis of thyroxine. Radioactive iodine can destroy these thyroid tumors and their metastases. Most responsive tumors are follicular adenocarcinomas. Recent evidence indicates that some thyroid malignancies can be suppressed with thyroid hormone. These hormones inhibit the secretion of thyroid-stimulating hormone by the pituitary, and apparently some thyroid tumors.

IMMUNOTHERAPY Since the host's immunologic system may be involved in the control of the malignant process, immunologic approaches to cancer therapy are under investigation (see Chap. 319). Animal tumors have been treated successfully with both active and passive immunotherapy. Certain principles have been established from these animal experiments which are probably applicable to human studies. Maximum tumor reduction must be accomplished by surgery, radiation, or chemotherapy before attempting immunotherapy. The host must be immunocompetent, and there may be an optimum time following other treatment for the administration of immunotherapy. Most antitumor agents are immunosuppressive, but as the patient recovers from these effects, his immunologic reactivity may be temporarily enhanced, and this could be an optimum time for immunotherapy.

Passive immunotherapy involves the transfer of immune serums from syngeneic, allogeneic, or xenogeneic animals into tumor-bearing hosts. Specific antiserum has prevented the development of chemical and viral-induced tumors and has caused established tumors to regress or disappear. Passive immunotherapy has been attempted in patients with chronic lymphocytic leukemia. The administration of animal antihuman lymphocyte serum or high-titer isoantibody serum from multiparous or multiple-transfused subjects reduced the white blood count and the size of lymph nodes in these patients but had no effect on bone marrow infiltration.

Active nonspecific immunotherapy has been attempted with substances such as bacillus Calmette-Guérin (BCG), pertussis vaccine, and *Corynebacterium parvum.* These substances augment both cellular and humoral immunity. This approach is under investigation as maintenance therapy following chemotherapy-induced remission in acute leukemia, as therapy of cutaneous tumors by direct injection, and as therapy following resection of various solid tumors.

Active specific immunotherapy consists of immunization of the host with tumor cells or cellular extracts. Greatest success has been achieved with live cells. Preimmunization prevents subsequent tumor transplantation in animals. Since most tumor antigens are weak, attempts have been made to enhance their antigenicity by coupling the antigens with other substances. Patients with various malignancies have been injected with their own tumor cells or cell extracts, plus Freund's adjuvant; this resulted in some responses and increased survival. It has been possible to demonstrate cytotoxic antitumor antibodies in patients immunized in this fashion.

The infusion of immune lymphocytes or their extracts to tumor-bearing hosts is known as *adoptive immunotherapy.* This approach has been used successfully in some animal tumors. Allogeneic lymphocytes which have not been sensitized to the host's tumor also may be effective, providing the host is immunosuppressed so that transplantation of these lymphocytes becomes possible. Adoptive immunotherapy also has been attempted in human beings; e.g., pairs of patients with the same malignancy were immunized with each other's tumor cells. When rejection occurred, they were given leukocyte transfusions from each other over a period of several weeks. This therapy produced some response in 20 percent of patients with malignant melanoma, breast carcinoma, and sarcomas, but very few remissions.

Local immunotherapy utilizes delayed hypersensitivity reactions at the site of skin tumors. Local injection of BCG or concanavalin A has eliminated skin tumors in a majority of animals. Delayed sensitivity has been produced in patients by cutaneous application of dinitrochlorobenzene. Subsequent application of this substance to superficial squamous epitheliomas and basal-cell carcinomas has cured the majority of these tumors. Other substances used successfully include vaccinia virus, and autologous lymphocytes activated with phytohemagglutinin.

The application of immunotherapy to the control of human malignancies appears promising. However, at present the approach has not produced responses comparable with other therapeutic modalities. Considerable additional investigation is necessary before the role of immunotherapy in the management of cancer patients can be defined. Its major usefulness probably will be as an adjuvant to surgery, radiation, or chemotherapy.

SUPPORTIVE CARE Metastatic carcinoma often interferes with many body functions. Patients with hematologic malignancies or bone marrow invasion often have anemia, leukopenia, or thrombocytopenia. Deficiencies in these blood elements may lead to serious infections or hemorrhagic complications. Immunologic deficiencies occur in patients with hematologic malignancies and advanced carcinoma. Malnutrition is usually a serious complication in patients with advanced carcinoma. Metabolic complications such as hypercalcemia or hyperuricemia can lead to serious renal impairment. Endocrine and anaplastic tumors may produce excessive amounts of hormones resulting in problems such as Cushing's syndrome or hypoglycemia. Furthermore, the recognition of an incurable disease has a profound psychologic and socioeconomic impact on the patient. All these aspects must be appreciated and corrected for successful management of the cancer patient.

Cancer chemotherapy also has substantial side effects. Many agents cause myelosuppression with consequent anemia, neutropenia, and thrombocytopenia, making them susceptible to hemorrhage and infectious complications. Antitumor agents are also immunosuppressive and inhibit both antibody production and delayed hypersensitivity reactions. Other adverse effects of these drugs include nausea and vomiting which may prevent adequate nutrition. Gastrointestinal ulceration may interfere with nutrition and may also serve as a portal of entry for infectious agents.

Anemia As discussed in Chaps. 308, 316, and 318, anemia may be the first manifestation of malignant disease and is present in 60 percent of patients with disseminated cancer. The major causes of anemia are blood loss, hemolysis, myelophthisis, and inadequate erythropoiesis due to the tumor or its treatment. Occasional patients have megaloblastic anemia due to malabsorption of folic acid or vitamin B_{12} (Chap. 305), microangiopathic hemolytic anemia (Chap. 306), or sideroblastic anemia (Chap. 304). The most characteristic anemia is due to both increased destruction of red blood cells and inadequate compensatory erythropoiesis. The half-life of red blood cells in these patients is usually less than 35 days, and normal cells transfused into these patients have a similar short half-life. Over 90 percent of these patients have no overt clinical evidence of hemolysis. Autoimmune hemolytic anemia of both "warm" and "cold" types occurs in patients with lymphomas and chronic lymphocytic leukemia, and less frequently in other cancers. Adrenal corticosteroids usually control autoimmune hemolytic anemia, especially of the "warm" type. Splenectomy or splenic irradiation is beneficial in selected cases. Hemolytic anemia is best ameliorated by controlling the underlying malignancy. Except in cases of blood loss, autoimmune hemolytic anemia, and vitamin deficiencies, there is no specific therapy. Most patients will remain asymptomatic if their hemoglobin is maintained above 8 g per 100 ml with transfusions.

Hemorrhage Tumor invasion of blood vessels, thrombocytopenia, and disseminated intravascular hemolysis are the major causes of hemorrhage in cancer patients. Occasional patients with normal or excessive numbers of platelets bleed because of defects in platelet function (Chap. 313). Major bleeding due to vascular invasion by tumor requires immediate surgical intervention, if that is possible.

Thrombocytopenia occurs in 90 percent of patients with acute leukemia and is a common manifestation of drug toxicity. Life-threatening hemorrhage is unusual unless the platelet count falls below 20,000 per μl blood, unless additional coagulation defects are present. Nearly 90 percent of these hemorrhagic episodes can be controlled by the administration of platelet transfusions, and the routine use of platelet transfusions in severely thrombopenic patients has reduced fatal hemorrhage by over 50 percent. Platelets may be obtained by plasmapheresis of normal donors or as a by-product of whole blood.

Disseminated intravascular coagulation (Chap. 315) has been described in patients with acute leukemia, carcinoma of the lung, prostate, cervix, colon, pancreas, and stomach. The process is probably initiated by the release of thromboplastic substances from cancer cells. Characteristics of this disorder are a prolonged clotting time with poor clot formation, prolonged prothrombin time, thrombocytopenia, hypofibrinogenemia, and clotting-factor deficiencies, especially of factors V and VIII. The diagnosis can be established by demonstrating increased levels of fibrin split products in the blood. The process can be interrupted by the administration of heparin. Fibrinogen should not be administered while the process is active, since it may aggravate thrombosis. Permanent reversal of disseminated intravascular coagulation in cancer patients can be accomplished only by successful treatment of the underlying malignancy.

Infection Fever occurs in 70 percent of hospitalized cancer patients and is usually due to infection. Local factors such as obstruction to normal drainage or recent surgery play a prominent role in infections occurring in patients with metastatic carcinoma. Patients undergoing cancer chemotherapy are especially susceptible to infectious complications because they develop neutropenia and impaired host defense mechanisms. Patients with chronic lymphocytic leukemia and multiple myeloma have decreased levels of normal immunoglobulins and respond inadequately to antigenic stimuli. Patients with generalized Hodgkin's disease characteristically have impaired cellular host defense mechanisms and are particularly susceptible to infections caused by obligate intracellular parasites such as the tubercle bacillus, *Brucella*, and *Listeria*.

Cancer patients are susceptible to a wide variety of infectious complications (Table 320-6). The majority of infections occurring in cancer patients are caused by gram-negative bacilli, especially *Escherichia coli*, *Klebsiella* sp., and *Pseudomonas aeruginosa*. However, organisms of low pathogenicity, such as *Bacillus* sp., *Staphylococcus epidermidis*, and *Flavobacterium* sp., may cause fatal infections in neutropenic patients. Hence, all organisms cultured from the blood or sites of infections should be considered as the possible etiologic agent in these patients until proved otherwise. Fungal infections are also a major problem in patients with hematologic malignancies and are increasing in frequency. Candidiasis and aspergillosis are the most common fungal infections. Histoplasmosis and coccidioidomycosis are no more common in cancer patients than in the general population, but when infection occurs, it usually disseminates widely. The group of DNA viruses, especially cytomegalovirus and varicella-zoster, may cause serious infections in cancer patients. *Pneumocystis carinii* pneumonia has been recognized increasingly in patients with a wide variety of malignant diseases. Like cytomegalic inclusion disease, it is more prevalent in children and may occur in epidemics.

TABLE 320-6
Organisms responsible for infections in cancer patients

Infection	*Organism*	*Predisposing malignant disease*
Bacterial	Gram-negative bacilli	All types, especially leukemia
	Salmonella sp.	Intraabdominal tumors, hepatic metastases
	Listeria monocytogenes	Lymphoma
	Clostridium sp.	Gastrointestinal and genitourinary malignancies, acute leukemia
	Mycobacterium tuberculosis	Lymphoma, ? bronchogenic carcinoma
	Nocardia asteroides	Lymphoma
Fungal	*Candida* sp.	Acute leukemia, lymphoma
	Aspergillus sp.	Acute leukemia
	Cryptococcus neoformans	Lymphoma
	Phycomycetes	Acute leukemia
Viral	Cytomegalovirus	Acute leukemia
	Herpes zoster, varicella	Lymphoma, chronic lymphocytic leukemia, acute leukemia
	Herpes simplex	All types, especially lymphoma
	Vaccinia	Chronic lymphocytic leukemia, lymphoma
Protozoal	*Pneumocystis carinii*	All types, mainly leukemia and lymphoma
	Toxoplasma gondii	Lymphoma

Many patients are neutropenic when they develop infection. Infection in these patients may disseminate widely if not treated promptly. Often, the classic signs and symptoms of infection are absent. Gram-negative bacilli and, especially, *Pseudomonas* infections are common in this population. The best initial antibiotic regimen is probably carbenicillin and cephalothin. The effectiveness of aminoglycoside antibiotics is greatly reduced in neutropenic patients. Patients who fail to respond to antibiotic therapy should be carefully evaluated for fungal, viral, or protozoal infections. Granulocyte transfusions are beneficial for the treatment of infections in neutropenic patients. They may be obtained by plasmapheresis of patients with chronic myelogenous leukemia or from normal donors using the white blood cell separator. Gamma-globulin is of little benefit in the prophylaxis or treatment of cancer patients with hypogammaglobulinemia.

Malnutrition Patients with advanced malignant disease are usually malnourished owing to poor caloric intake. They often have vitamin deficiencies because of an imbalanced diet. Anorexia is almost universal in advanced cancer, for a variety of reasons. Many patients are depressed, and some have ulcerative or obstructive lesions of the gastrointestinal tract, making eating difficult. In some cancer patients intestinal structure and function are abnormal, resulting in malabsorption. Many cancer chemotherapeutic agents cause nausea, vomiting, and gastrointestinal ulcerations. Patients with rapidly growing tumors may have an elevated basal metabolic rate and hypermetabolism. Body tissue wasting is often out of proportion to weight loss because of fluid retention which may be present even without clinically apparent edema. Moderate to marked hypoalbuminemia is usual in patients with advanced carcinoma because of decreased production and increased utilization.

The maintenance of good nutritional status in patients with extensive cancer is difficult. Short-term tube feeding may lead to temporary symptomatic improvement but eventually proves ineffective. Vitamin supplements and correction of electrolyte imbalance help some patients. The intravenous administration of protein hydrolysates, glucose, vitamins, and minerals in hypertonic solutions via subclavian vein catheters will benefit some patients. Those patients whose tumors respond to therapy quickly return to normal nutritional status.

Hypercalcemia Extensive bone involvement is characteristic of some tumors such as multiple myeloma, breast carcinoma, and prostatic carcinoma and may result in hypercalcemia. Some tumors, such as bronchogenic carcinoma, may produce parathyroid hormone–like substances which also cause hypercalcemia. In some patients symptoms of hypercalcemia such as nausea, polyuria, constipation, and mental confusion may first lead to the diagnosis of malignancy. This complication requires prompt attention since it may rapidly worsen. Chronic hypercalcemia may lead to nephrocalcinosis and irreversible impairment of renal function. The mainstay of therapy consists of adequate hydration which should approximate 4 liters fluid daily. Adrenal corticosteroids reduce the serum calcium level to normal in 60 percent of patients. Electrolytes such as sodium sulfate and sodium phosphates facilitate excretion of calcium in the kidney. Phosphates must be used cautiously since they may cause extraosseous calcification. Mithramycin has been used successfully to reduce the serum calcium level acutely. Long-term management of hypercalcemia requires control of the underlying malignancy.

Hyperuricemia Hyperuricemia is most common in patients with acute leukemia, but occasionally occurs in other malignancies. The high serum uric acid levels are due to the increased formation and destruction of tumor cells and accompanying breakdown of nucleoproteins. Chemotherapy may cause further elevations of serum uric acid and urinary urate excretion. Uric acid is actively secreted by the kidney, and its solubility is highest in alkaline urine. When the concentration exceeds the solubility, uric acid precipitates in the tubules, causing obstruction and decreased glomerular filtration which eventually leads to anuria. Urate nephropathy can be prevented by inducing water diuresis. Administration of sodium bicarbonate is sometimes necessary to maintain the urine pH above 7.0. Allopurinol, a structural isomer of hypoxanthine, is a xanthine oxidase inhibitor which prevents the formation of uric acid from xanthine and hypoxanthine. This drug should be administered to prevent the formation of additional uric acid. Occasionally these measures are unsuccessful, and the patient becomes anuric. Mannitol will initiate urine flow in some patients. When mannitol infusion fails to increase urine output, peritoneal dialysis or hemodialysis may be necessary. Ultimately, control of urate nephropathy requires control of the underlying disease process.

Psychologic aspects Realization by the patient that he has an incurable malignant disease has profound psychologic and socioeconomic impact, particularly if the disease strikes him in youth or middle age. Unlike many other diseases, the patient has little personal influence on the course of cancer. An important aspect of cancer therapy is the hope of improvement that it offers the patient. Even experimental chemotherapy which fails to alter the disease may be beneficial because it gives some meaning to an otherwise dismal existence. The patient feels he is contributing to the welfare of others with the same ailment even if the drug fails to help him. As the disease progresses, the patient may pass through a variety of mental processes, including rejection, hostility, despair, and finally acceptance of the inevitable. Feelings of deprivation are a major component of the psychologic impact of this disease. The cancer patient is deprived of many of the pleasures of life. The physician should provide hope, encouragement, understanding, sympathy, and support. When therapy is no longer effective, the patient needs attention rather than abandonment. During this difficult period the physician should rely upon the nursing staff, clergyman, and social workers for assistance in the care of the patient. Occasional patients become incapacitated from severe depression and require psychiatric consultation even though their disease is responding to therapy (see Chap. 338).

REFERENCES

Holland JF, Frei E III (eds): *Cancer Medicine*, Philadelphia, Lea & Febiger 1973

Frei E III, Freireich EJ: Progress and perspectives in the chemotherapy of acute leukemia, in *Advances in Chemotherapy*, New York: Academic, 1965, vol. 2, p. 269

——, Gamble Jr: Progress in the chemotherapy of Hodgkin's disease. Cancer 19:378, 1966

Skipper HE et al: Experimental evaluation of potential anticancer agents: XXI. On the criteria and kinetics associated with "curability" of experimental leukemia. Cancer Chemother Rep 39:1, 1964

Rall DP, Zubrod GC: Mechanisms of drug absorption and excretion. Annu Rev Pharmacol 7:109, 1962

Livingston RB, Carter SK: *Single Agent Chemotherapy of Cancer*, New York: Plenum, 1970

321 APPROACH TO THE PATIENT WITH NEUROLOGIC AND PSYCHIATRIC DISEASE

RAYMOND D. ADAMS

Neurology is often regarded as one of the most difficult and exacting specialties of medicine. The student coming to the neurology clinic for the first time tends to be easily discouraged by what he sees. Already he is somewhat intimidated by the complexity of the nervous system through his brief contact with neuroanatomy, neurophysiology, and neuropathology and often has a defeatist attitude. The ritual he then witnesses, of putting the patient through a series of maneuvers designed to evoke certain mysterious signs named after famous neurologists or called by unpronounceable terms, does not reassure him. In fact it often appears to conceal the very intellectual processes by which neurologic diagnosis is attained. Moreover, the student has had no training in the many special tests which are used, such as the lumbar puncture and cerebrospinal fluid examination and the electroencephalographic, pneumoencephalographic, and arteriographic examinations, and he does not know how to interpret the results of such tests when they are given him. Neurologic textbooks only confirm his fears as he reads the details of the countless rare diseases of the nervous system.

THE CLINICAL METHOD

The author believes that many of the student's difficulties with neurology may be overcome by proper instruction in the basic principles of clinical medicine. First and foremost he must know and acquire facility in use of the *clinical method.* Without a clear comprehension of this method he is virtually as helpless with a new problem as would be the botanist or chemist who attempted to do research without having an understanding of the steps in the scientific method.

The importance of the clinical method stands out more clearly in the study of neurologic diseases than in certain other fields of medicine, but the following remarks nevertheless have universal application. The solution of any clinical problem is reached by a series of inferences and deductions, each an attempt to explain an item in the history of an illness or a physical finding. Diagnosis is the mental act of selecting the one explanation most compatible with all the facts of clinical observation. An analysis of the clinical method used will show that it generally consists of an orderly series of steps, as follows:

1 The essential clinical data are secured by history and physical examination.
2 Those clinical data which are considered relevant to the current problem are interpreted and translated in terms of anatomy and physiology. Certain complexes of symptoms and signs are recognized as having a meaningful relationship. This may be called *syndrome diagnosis.*
3 From these data the physician is able to determine the anatomic localization that best explains these findings. This may be called the *anatomic diagnosis.*
4 The course of the illness, the associated medical findings, and the accessory laboratory data are then ascertained.
5 Finally the *etiologic diagnosis* is deduced from these data and from the location of the disease process.

The elicitation of accurate and reliable data concerning the disordered functioning of the nervous system is the first step in diagnosis. If these data are incorrect, the diagnosis will surely be erroneous. The taking of the history and the performance of the physical examination, then, are the primary and fundamental steps in diagnosis. Where there is disagreement as to the diagnosis it will often be discovered that the source of the difficulty is an uncertainty as to the significant items in the history or physical examination. Repeated examination may be necessary in order to establish them beyond doubt. This is why it is said that the second examination is the most helpful diagnostic test in a difficult neurologic case.

Different disease processes may cause identical symptoms, which is understandable from the fact that several diseases may involve the same parts of the nervous system. For example, a spastic paraplegia may result from spinal cord tumor, syphilitic meningomyelitis, or multiple sclerosis. Conversely, one disease may cause several different symptoms. Despite the almost infinite number of possible combinations of symptoms and signs, a few occur with greater frequency than others in a given disease, and indeed some do not occur at all; and these can be recognized as the characteristic symptom complexes or syndromes. The experienced clinical worker acquires the habit of attempting to categorize every clinical case by placing it under one or another syndrome. In doing so he more or less determines the anatomic basis of the illness in question and at the same time narrows the range of possible etiologic factors.

The final diagnosis must state the locality of the disease as well as its nature and, to be complete, should express the degree of functional impairment as well. Anatomic diagnosis has precedence over etiologic diagnosis. To seek the cause of a disease without first ascertaining the part or parts of the nervous system affected would be analogous in internal medicine to an attempt at etiologic diagnosis without knowledge of whether the disease involved the lungs, stomach, or kidneys.

The student must learn the identity and differential diagnosis of the common syndromes before the details of individual diseases. It should be kept clearly in mind, however, that syndromes are not diseases but rather abstractions set up by clinical workers in order to facilitate the diagnosis of disease. The inherent danger in the method is that it may inculcate a rigidity of thinking and keep one from conceiving of diseases in new relationships.

TAKING THE HISTORY

The following three points about history taking in neurology deserve comment.

1 Special care must be exercised to avoid suggesting to the patient the symptoms that one seeks. The clinical interview is a bipersonal engagement, and the conduct of the examiner has a great influence on the patient. Psychiatrists have talked and written about this so much that the repetition may seem tedious, but it is evident that many of the conflicting histories presented on ward rounds can be traced to leading questions that have suggested to the patient the symptoms that the examiner expects to find or to an unconscious distortion of the patient's story. Errors and inconsistency in recording the history are as often the fault of the physician as of the patient. Here the practice of making bedside notes is particularly to be recommended. The suggestible and highly circumstantial patient can be kept on the subject of his illness by discreet questions which draw out essential points.

2 The mode of onset and the course of the illness are of paramount importance. Often the nature of the disease process can be decided by these facts alone. One must know how each symptom began and progressed from the onset of the illness to the present. If the patient cannot supply this information, it may be necessary to judge the course of the symptoms by what he was able to do at different times, i.e., how far he could walk, whether he could carry on his work, etc., or by changes in the clinical findings between successive examinations. Following a case and allowing time for a disease to evolve, a method relied upon by all astute physicians, takes advantage of the latter procedure.

3 Since neurologic diseases often derange the patient's mind, it is necessary in every case to decide by assessment of the mental status and the circumstances under which symptoms occurred whether or not he is competent to give the story of his own illness. If not, the history must be obtained from an outside source such as a relative, friend, or employer. The nature of certain illnesses, such as a convulsion, obviously precludes the patient's knowledge of all the details of that part of his illness. In general, students and some physicians, as well, tend to be careless in the estimation of the mental capacities of their patients. An attempt is sometimes made to take a history from a patient who is feeble-minded or so confused that he has no idea why he is in a doctor's office or a hospital, or from one who could not possibly have been aware of the details of the illness.

THE NEUROLOGIC EXAMINATION

The neurologic examination begins always with the history. The manner in which the patient tells the story of his illness may betray lack of coherence or confusion in thinking, defection of memory, faultiness of judgment, or difficulty in comprehending or in expressing ideas. Observation of such matters is an essential part of the examination of every medical case and provides information as to the adequacy of cerebral function. Usually this type of information can be obtained without embarrassment to the patient. The physician should maintain the same objective attitude toward the verbal responses of his patient and the thoughts expressed as he does in auscultation of the chest. A common error is to pass over inconsistencies in history and inaccuracies about dates and symptoms as being unimportant, only to discover later that these are the major symptoms of the illness.

The remainder of the neurologic examination should be performed as a part of the general physical examination, not as a special procedure, to be done later if indicated. It should always be carried out in an orderly, systematic manner, proceeding from the examination of the cranial nerves, to the upper extremities, trunk, and lower extremities, in order to avoid omissions. The cranial nerves can be tested along with the examination of the eyes, ears, nose, and throat. The arms should be examined after the cervical structures and before the heart and lungs, and the legs before the pelvic and rectal examination. Gait and station should be observed at some time during the procedure, usually before or after the rest of the examination.

The thoroughness of the examination of the nervous system must of necessity depend on the type of clinical problem presented by the patient. To spend a half-hour testing motor and sensory function in a patient seeking treatment for a sprained ankle is pointless and uneconomical. Furthermore, the procedure must be varied according to the condition of the patient. If he is comatose, obviously many tests cannot be done; infants and small children and psychotic patients must be examined in special ways. The following comments about the examination procedure apply to these particular clinical circumstances.

THE AVERAGE MEDICAL OR SURGICAL PATIENT WITHOUT NEUROLOGIC SYMPTOMS Brevity is desirable in the neurologic examination, but any test that is undertaken should be done well and recorded accurately on the patient's chart. In the examination of the cranial nerves, the pupil size, reaction to light, ocular movements, visual acuity and auditory acuity (by question), movements of face, jaw, palate, and tongue should be scrutinized. Observing the bare, outstretched arms for atrophy, weakness, tremor, or abnormal movements, inquiring about strength and subjective sensory disturbances, and tapping the supinator, biceps, and triceps tendons to evoke reflexes are usually sufficient for the upper extremities. Inspection of the legs as the feet, toes, and knees are actively flexed and extended, elicitation of the knee and ankle jerks, and stroking the lateral border of the foot for the plantar reflexes complete the essential part of the neurologic examination. The only sensory tests that should be attempted are vibration and position in the fingers, ankles, and feet. Coordination may be tested by watching the patient place his finger on the tip of his nose and run the heel up and down the front of his leg. This entire procedure does not add more than 3 or 4 min to the physical examination. The routine performance of these few simple tests may offer clues as to the presence of diseases of which the patient is not aware. For example, by finding Argyll Robertson pupils, absent tendon reflexes, and diminished vibratory and position sense in the legs the physician is alerted to the possibility of the gastric crises of tabes when there are no other symptoms of neurosyphilis.

Accurate recording of negative data may be useful in relation to some future illness.

PATIENTS WHO PRESENT SYMPTOMS OF A DISEASE OF THE NERVOUS SYSTEM Several monographs have been written on the neurologic examination of such patients. For a full account of the methods the interested reader is referred to the books of Denny-Brown, Monrad-Krohn, and DeJong, each of whom approaches the subject from a special point of view. A large number of tests have been devised, and it is not proposed to review them. Many are of doubtful value and should not be taught to students of neurology. Merely to perform all these tests on any one patient would require several hours, and probably in many instances would not make the examiner any the wiser. The danger with all clinical tests is that the student and physician may regard them as the inscrutable symbols of disease rather than as ways of uncovering disordered functioning of the nervous system. In general the following tests, which provide the most useful information, are few in number and relatively simple.

Testing of cerebral function Cerebral function is tested in detail only if there is a reason to suspect some defect from the patient's behavior during the general examination. Questions should then be directed toward determining orientation in time and place and insight into the current medical problem. Attention, speed of response, ability to give relevant answers to simple questions, and in general the capacity for sustained mental effort, all lend themselves to straightforward observation. Useful bedside tests of attention, memory, and clarity of thought are the repetition of a series of digits in forward or reverse order, serial subtraction of 7's from 100, the recall of the names of three objects after an interval of 3 min, and of the last six presidents. Day-to-day recollection of the medical procedures and incidents in the hospital is an excellent test of memory. Other tests can be devised for the same purpose. Often the examiner can obtain a better idea of the clearness of the patient's sensorium and the soundness of his intellect by giving him a few tests and noting the manner in which he deals with them than by relying on a crude score of a formal intelligence or achievement test (see Chap. 27).

If there is any suggestion of aphasia, a record of the patient's spontaneous speech should be made. In addition, accuracy in the naming of objects, in the execution of spoken commands, and the ability to read and write should also be noted (see Chap. 25).

Testing the cranial nerves The function of the cranial nerves must be investigated more fully than in the previous examination procedure. Tests of smell are carried out only if one suspects a lesion in the anterior fossa, and then it usually suffices to determine whether odors are perceived in each nostril. The visual fields should be outlined by the confrontation test; if any abnormality is suspected it should be checked on a perimeter and scotomas sought on the Bjerrum screen. Pupil size and reactivity to light and accommodation and range of ocular movements should next be observed.

Sensation over the face should be tested with a pin and wisp of cotton, and the corneal reflexes should be tried. Facial movements should be observed as the patient speaks and smiles, for a slight weakness may be more evident then than during voluntary movement. Audiograms and special tests of auditory recruitment and labyrinthine tests are needed if there is any suspicion of disease of the eighth nerve. The vocal cords should be inspected in cases of medullary disease, especially when there is hoarseness. Corneal and pharyngeal reflexes are usually of value only if there is a difference on the two sides; bilateral absence of gag and corneal reflexes is seldom significant. Inspection of the protruded tongue is helpful; atrophy, fibrillation, weakness, and instability of posture may be seen. Slight deviation of the protruded tongue to one or the other side as a solitary finding may usually be disregarded. Articulation and the pronunciation of words should be noted. The jaw jerk, tapping of orbicularis oculi or globella, buccal and sucking reflexes should be elicited, particularly if there is suspicion of dysphagia or dysarthria (see Chap. 25).

Tests of motor function In the assessment of motor function the student must remind himself that observations of the speed and strength of movements, of muscle bulk, and of tone and coordination are usually more informative than the tendon reflexes. It is essential to have the limbs fully exposed and to watch the patient maintain the arms in the outstretched position; to perform simple tasks, such as touching first the examiner's finger and then his own nose; to make rapid alternating movements that necessitate sudden acceleration and deceleration and changes in direction; and to do simple tasks such as buttoning clothes, opening a safety pin, or handling common tools. Estimates of the strength of leg muscles with the patient in bed are often unreliable; there may seem to be no weakness even though the patient cannot step up on a chair or arise from a squatting position. Running the heel down the front of the other shin, and alternately touching the examiner's finger with the toe, then the opposite knee with the heel is the only test of coordination that can be carried out in bed. The maintenance of both arms or both legs against gravity is a useful test; the weak one, tiring first, soon begins to sag. Also, abnormalities of movement and posture and tremors may appear (see Chap. 18).

Tests of reflex function The biceps, triceps, and supinator or radial-periosteal reflexes, the knee and ankle reflexes, and the cutaneous abdominal and plantar reflexes permit an adequate sampling of reflex activity of the spinal cord. The plantar response offers special difficulty because there are several different reflex patterns that can be evoked by stimulating the sole of the foot along its outer border from heels to toes. These are the high-level, quick-avoidance response, the spinal flexor nocifensor (extension of toes and foot and flexion of knee and hip) reflex, or Babinski's sign, and grasp and support reactions.

Testing of sensory function The testing of sensory function is undoubtedly the most difficult part of the neurologic examination. If the findings are to be reliable, it should be reserved for the end of the examination procedure and not prolonged for more than a few minutes. Usually an explanation of the purpose of the test should be given; yet too much discussion of it with a meticulous, introspective patient may encourage the reporting of useless minor variations of stimulus intensity. It is well to ask whether or not stimuli on opposite sides of the body feel the same, not whether they feel different. If the patient is highly suggestible, in which case sensory tests are unreliable, differences that demand further investigation will not then be reported.

The skin surface of the body is large, and it is not necessary to examine all areas. A quick survey of the face, neck, arms, trunk, and legs with a pin takes only a few seconds. One is of course usually seeking differences between the two sides of the body, a level below which sensation is lost, or a zone of relative or absolute anesthesia. Regions of sensory deficit can then be tested more carefully and mapped out. Hyperesthetic zones are usually not much help in diagnosis (more often than not an area appears to be hyperesthetic because of faulty technique); nevertheless they may call attention in some patients to areas of peripheral sensory disturbance. Variations in the sensory findings from one examination to another reflect differences in technique of examination as well as inconsistency in the responses of the patient.

The details of sensory testing methods are described in Chap. 21.

Testing of gait and stance No examination is complete without seeing the patient on his feet and walking. An ataxia of gait may be the only neurologic abnormality, as in certain cases of cerebellar tumor. Stance, posture, and lack of certain highly automatic adaptive movements may provide the most definite clues in an early case of paralysis agitans (see Chap. 17).

THE COMATOSE PATIENT Although subject to obvious limitations, examination of the stuporous or comatose patient may yield considerable information concerning the function of the nervous system. The special techniques involved have been presented in Chap. 22.

The demonstration of signs of focal cerebral or brain stem disease or of meningeal irritation is of aid in the differential diagnosis of the diseases which cause coma and which are the basis of the three syndromes outlined in Chap. 22.

THE PSYCHIATRIC PATIENT One is compelled in the examination of psychiatric patients to rely less on the cooperation of the patient and to be unusually critical of his statements and opinions. The depressed patient, for example, may declare that his limbs are weak or useless when actually there is little or no diminution in muscular power; or the psychopathic patient may feign paralysis. The opposite is sometimes true—that the most psychotic patient may make accurate observations of his own symptoms, only to have them ignored because the attending physician has been in the habit of disregarding his complaints.

If the patient will speak and cooperate to the slightest degree, much may be learned as to the functional integrity of different parts of the nervous system. Aphasia can, in nearly every instance, be diagnosed by the manner in which the patient uses words in phrases and sentences, or responds to spoken or written commands. Often it is possible to determine whether there are hallucinations, defective memory, or other symptoms of recognizable brain disease merely by watching and listening to the patient. The visual fields can often be tested with fair accuracy by observing the patient's response to a moving stimulus or threat in all four quadrants of the fields. The tests of cranial nerve, motor, and reflex function in the legs, already outlined for the examination of the stuporous and comatose patient, can be carried out even better if minimal cooperation is obtained from the patient. It must be remembered, however, that the neurologic examination is never complete unless the patient will speak and carry out the usual tests. On numerous occasions mute and resistive patients judged to be schizophrenic have had some widespread cerebral disease such as hypoxic or hypoglycemic encephalopathy, a brain tumor, a vascular lesion, or extensive demyelinative lesions.

INFANTS AND SMALL CHILDREN The reader is referred to the methods of examination outlined in the monographs of Gesell, André-Thomas, and Paine.

IMPORTANCE OF A WORKING KNOWLEDGE OF NEUROANATOMY AND NEUROPHYSIOLOGY

Once the technique of obtaining reliable clinical data is mastered, the student may find himself handicapped in the interpretation of the findings by a lack of facility in neuroanatomy and neurophysiology. These are highly complex subjects, and to acquire a practical working knowledge of them is time-consuming. Fortunately these subjects are taught well in most schools, and those principles which are immediately applicable to the clinical neurologic problem are to be found in most textbooks.

DIFFERENTIAL DIAGNOSIS

The differential diagnosis of the cause of a clinical syndrome requires knowledge of an entirely different order. One must be conversant with the clinical details and the course and natural history of the more common disease entities. Many of these facts are simple and well known and will be presented in later chapters of this textbook.

The findings in the general medical examination are of importance. To illustrate: low-grade fever, anemia, heart murmur, and splenomegaly indicate that in a case of unexplained apoplexy subacute bacterial endocarditis with embolic occlusion of a brain artery is the most likely cause. Pleocytosis in the cerebrospinal fluid with elevated protein level, abnormal gold sol, and a positive Wassermann test reaction establish a syphilitic etiology in a patient with symptoms of apoplexy, a progressive dementia, or blindness.

The anatomic diagnosis may suggest the cause of a disease. Thus when a unilateral Horner's syndrome, cerebellar ataxia, paralysis of a vocal cord, and analgesia of the face are combined with loss of pain and temperature sensation in the opposite arm, trunk, and leg, an occlusion of the posterior inferior cerebellar artery is suggested, because all the involved structures lie within the territory of this artery. In a sense the anatomic diagnosis determines and limits the disease possibilities. If the signs point to disease of the peripheral nerves, it is not necessary usually to consider the causes of disease of the spinal cord. Some signs themselves are almost specific, e.g., Argyll Robertson pupils for neurosyphilis or oculogyric crises for postencephalitic parkinsonism.

If one adheres faithfully to the clinical method outlined here, neurologic diagnosis becomes relatively simple. In most patients one can reach an anatomic diagnosis. The cause of the disease may prove more elusive. Even the most experienced neurologist is unable to ascertain the cause of many neurologic syndromes.

THE PURPOSE OF THE CLINICAL METHOD OF NEUROLOGY

Finally, a word about the main purposes of the clinical method of neurology. Actually, diagnosis accomplishes two purposes: (1) it enables the physician to decide on the proper method of treating the ailing patient; (2) it serves as an essential method in the scientific study of the disease by permitting the identification and segregation of clinical phenomena. The medical profession is primarily concerned with the prevention and cure of illness, and all our knowledge is applied to this well-defined end. The practical physician attempts to diagnose diseases for which he has an effective treatment. Each of the treatable causes of a given syndrome must be carefully considered and excluded by clinical and laboratory methods. For example, in the study of a case of disease of the spinal cord one must take special care to diagnose a tumor, subacute combined degeneration, spinal syphilis, epidural abscess, ruptured disk, and cervical spondylosis, for these are treatable spinal cord diseases. Failure to recognize amyotrophic lateral sclerosis is a less serious error as far as the patient is concerned.

One cannot agree with those who hold that neurologic diagnosis is merely an intellectual pastime. It is true that means are available for treating only a few of the many diseases known to affect the nervous system. But there is no doubt that the first step in the scientific study of a disease process is the identification of it in the living patient. Until this is achieved it is impossible to apply adequately the "master method of controlled experiment." The clinical method of neurology thus serves both the physician, in the practical diagnosis and treatment of a patient's condition, and the clinical scientist, who seeks the ultimate cause of the disease.

Finally, accurate diagnosis permits prognosis, which is advantageous to both the physician and the patient.

CLINICAL CLASSIFICATION OF DISEASES OF THE NERVOUS SYSTEM

The logical classification of the several hundred diseases to which the human nervous system is subject should be based on cause, mechanism, and established pathologic change. Unfortunately, this is not possible because of lack of data. But even if this could be done such a classification in this book, even if the data were available, would have certain disadvantages, for it would presuppose on the part of the student or physician a sufficient knowledge of each of these diseases so that they could be recognized at the bedside. Given such knowledge, it would be a relatively simple matter to find an account of methods of therapy under the appropriate heading in a medical encyclopedia. But seldom does the physician start from such a vantage point. Instead he proceeds in his study of a given patient from cardinal symptoms to the diagnostic syndrome and finally to the group of diseases most likely to underlie that syndrome. Syndromic diagnosis is an intermediary step which must precede the recognition of a disease, and it is the one most easily attained by clinical study alone. Hence we have grouped the major diseases of the nervous system around the following common syndromes.

1 Stroke (Chap. 326)
2 Convulsion or faint (Chap. 337, see also Chaps. 16 and 24)
3 Cranial or spinal injury (Chaps. 325 and 327)
4 Fever, headache, and stiff neck (Chap. 329)
5 Major disorders of consciousness (Chaps. 327, 332, and 337; see also Chap. 22)
6 Sensory and motor paralysis of a pattern indicative of *peripheral nerve disease* (Chaps. 323, 325; see also Chaps. 17 and 21—*spinal root or spinal tract disease*)
7 Major impairment of intellectual functions (Chap. 333); dementia (see also Chaps. 18 and 27)
8 Special cerebral deficits—speech, calculation, thinking, visual function (Chaps. 326, 328 and 333; see also Chaps. 26 and 27)
9 Special disorder of cranial nerves, vision, hearing, facial movement, swallowing, voice, etc. (Chap. 324; see also Chaps. 19 and 20)
10 Disorder of gait and motility beginning in childhood (Chap. 334; see also Chap. 19)
11 Headache, vomiting, and signs of increased intracranial pressure (Chap. 328)
12 Chronic disorder of coordination, movement, or posture and the presence of tremor (Chap. 333; see also Chap. 328)
13 Failure in mental development (Chap. 334)
14 Abnormalities of cranial and spinal formation (Chap. 334)
15 Recurrent headache (Chaps. 6 and 336; see also Chap. 328)
16 Recurrent vertigo (Chap. 324; see also Chap. 19)

17 Uncontrollable drowsiness (Chap. 335; see also Chap. 23)
18 Nervousness, anxiety, depression (Chaps. 338, 339, and 341; see also Chap. 14)
19 Chronic fatigue (Chaps. 338, 339, and 341; see also Chap. 15)
20 Queer behavior (Chaps. 340 and 342)

REFERENCES

André-Thomas et al: *The Neurological Examination of the Infant*, London: National Spastics Society, 1960

DeJong Russell N: *Neurologic Examination: Including the Fundamentals of Neuroanatomy and Neurophysiology*, New York: Hoeber, 1950

Denny-Brown D: *Handbook of Neurology and Case Recording*, Cambridge, Mass.: Harvard, 1942

Gesell A, Amatruda CS: *Developmental Diagnosis*, New York: Hoeber, 1941

Monrad-Krohn GH, Refsum S: *The Clinical Examination of the Nervous System*, 12th ed., New York: Hoeber, 1964

Paine RS, Opfré TE: *Neurologic Examination of Children*, The Spastics Society of Medical Education and Information, London: Heinemann, 1966

322 DIAGNOSTIC METHODS IN NEUROLOGY

RAYMOND D. ADAMS
ROBERT R. YOUNG

The strict analysis and interpretation of the data elicited by a careful history and examination may prove to be adequate for diagnosis; special laboratory tests can then do no more than corroborate the initial impression. But it more often happens that the final conclusion as to the nature of the disease is not reached by simple case study. The possibilities may be reduced to two or three, but the correct one cannot be determined. Under these circumstances, one resorts to some one or several of the laboratory tests outlined below.

It must be stressed that laboratory procedures should follow rather than precede clinical case study, except in emergencies when the disease threatens life and time does not allow detailed clinical observation. Laboratory procedures are but a part of the clinical method outlined in Chap. 321. They should be undertaken only for the specific purpose of obtaining certain otherwise unavailable data which should shed light on the clinical problem. The procedures are costly, time consuming, occasionally dangerous or painful (unless done with skill), may require hospitalization, and are misleading if the data are not gathered or interpreted competently. During every young neurologic physician's clinical training, he should master each of these special procedures and learn to recognize their limitations and to interpret the results correctly. Some of these tests are regularly performed by the general physician or internist.

LUMBAR PUNCTURE AND EXAMINATION OF CEREBROSPINAL FLUID

The information yielded by the examination of the cerebrospinal fluid (CSF) is often of crucial importance.

INDICATIONS FOR LUMBAR PUNCTURE

1 To obtain pressure measurements and to secure a sample of CSF for cellular, chemical, and bacteriologic examination.
2 To aid in therapy by the administration of spinal anesthetics and occasionally antibiotics or antitumor agents.
3 To inject air, as in pneumoencephalography, a radiopaque substance (Pantopaque) as in myelography, or a radioactive substance [e.g., radioactive iodinated serum albumin (RISA)] for diagnosis of hydrocephalus.

Lumbar puncture is risky if the CSF pressure is high (evidenced by headache and papilledema) for it increases the possibility of a fatal cerebellar or tentorial pressure cone. However, if it seems important, in a given case of suspected increased intracranial pressure, to have the information yielded by CSF examination, the lumbar puncture may be performed with a fine-bore (No. 22 or 24) needle as the last part of the clinical study.

Cisternal puncture, although safe in the hands of the expert, is too hazardous a procedure to entrust to those without experience. The lumbar puncture is to be preferred except in obvious instances of spinal block requiring a sample of cisternal fluid or myelography above the lesion.

Experience teaches the importance of meticulous technique. Lumbar puncture should always be done under sterile conditions. If procaine is injected in and beneath the skin, the procedure should be painless. Failure to enter the lumbar subarachnoid space after two or three trials can usually be corrected by doing the puncture with the patient in the sitting position and then assisting him to lie on his side for pressure measurements and fluid removal. The "dry tap" is more often due to an improperly placed needle than to a pathologic obliteration of subarachnoid space by compressive lesion of the spinal cord or chronic adhesive arachnoiditis. A bloody tap, due to transfixion of a meningeal vessel, may result in hopeless confusion, as regards diagnosis, if it is falsely interpreted as indicating subarachnoid hemorrhage.

EXAMINATION PROCEDURES Once the lumbar puncture is successful, some of or all the following aspects of the CSF should be studied: (1) pressure and "dynamics," (2) Queckenstedt test, if indicated by a lesion of the spinal cord, (3) gross appearance of CSF, (4) number and type of cells and presence of microorganisms, (5) protein, sugar, colloidal gold reaction, and, in special instances, analysis of pigments, (6) exfoliative cytology using millipore filters, (7) Wassermann reaction and appropriate serologic precipitation reactions, (8) protein immunoelectrophoresis for determination of gamma-globulin levels, and other special biochemical tests (for NH_3, pH, CO_2, enzymes, etc.), and (9) bacteriologic cultures and virus isolation. See the Appendix for normal values of CSF.

RADIOLOGIC EXAMINATION OF SKULL AND SPINE

Plain x-rays of the skull or spinal column, according to the nature of the symptoms, constitute an indispensable part of the thorough study of traumatic and neoplastic diseases and less often of infectious or metabolic ones. The procedure is relatively simple, and the findings are interpretable by most general radiologists. Space does not permit an illustration of such common findings as fractures, bone erosion, intracerebral calcifications, premature closure or separation of sutures, or alterations of skull configuration. These have been presented in a companion volume to the present book (E. J. Potchen et al: *Principles of Diagnostic Radiology*, McGraw-Hill, 1971).

More specifically of value in neurology and neurosurgery are four special radiologic procedures which now permit the visualization of most parts of the brain and spinal cord and their vessels.

1 *Angiography* has been developed over the last 30 years to the point where it is a relatively safe and extremely valuable method in the diagnosis of tumors, abscesses, intracranial hemorrhages, and occluded arteries. Following local anesthesia, a needle or cannula can be placed percutaneously into the lumen of any of the larger arteries of the neck; or a catheter can also be used to cannulate any of the major cervical vessels in a retrograde fashion after being introduced into the brachial or femoral artery. In these ways radiopaque contrast media can be injected to visualize the arch of the aorta, the origins of carotid and vertebral systems, and their extent through the neck into the cranial cavity. There, cerebral arteries down to about 0.1 mm lumen diameter under optimal conditions, as well as small veins of comparable size, vascular abnormalities (angiomas, aneurysms), occluded arteries, delayed circulation from increased intracranial pressure as with masses or occlusion of dural sinuses and veins, displacement of vessels by mass lesions, or complete failure of intracranial vascular filling with cerebral death can often be shown with clarity.
2 *Pneumoencephalography* and *ventriculography*. In recent years, the injection of air or oxygen into the lumbar subarachnoid space with the patient in the sitting position has largely replaced the direct injection of air into the ventricles (ventriculography). Pneumoencephalography permits visualization in considerable detail of the size and position of the ventricles, the subarachnoid space (upper spinal and cerebral), and, indirectly, the structures which lie between the ventricles and the meninges. Hydrocephalus, mass lesions which displace or deform the ventricles, and atrophic states of the cerebrum are revealed by this technique.
3 *Pantopaque myelography* (and ventriculography). By injecting 5 to 15 ml Pantopaque through a lumbar puncture needle and then tipping the patient on a tilt table, the entire spinal subarachnoid space may be visualized. The procedure is almost as harmless as the lumbar puncture, provided that the Pantopaque is afterward removed through the needle. Ruptured lumbar and cervical disks and spinal cord tumors can be diagnosed accurately. Intraventricular injection of Pantopaque is occasionally done to visualize the third and fourth ventricles and the aqueduct of Sylvius in tumors of the posterior fossa, for instance, when air does not enter from below. In some clinics air has been used instead of Pantopaque to visualize masses within the spinal canal but is less accurate and more painful.
4 *Radioactive isotopes*. Radioactive isotopes of mercury, technetium, and arsenic are in regular use for the visualization of tumors, inflammatory masses, and some vascular lesions. Since this is a simple, noninvasive procedure, the only limitation in its use is the expense. The more vascular the lesion, the more consistent its demonstration by these methods. Ultrasound can also be used to show displacement of central structures of the brain by a mass lesion.

ELECTROMYOGRAPHY (EMG)

This examination supplements the clinical study of patients with neurologic diseases which affect the neuromuscular apparatus or with primary or secondary diseases of the skeletal musculature. It is described in relation to muscle diseases (see Chap. 344).

ELECTROENCEPHALOGRAPHY

The electroencephalographic examination is part of the clinical study of the neurologic patient suspected of having a cerebral disease; it is also used in the evaluation of the CNS effects of many medical diseases.

The modern console model electroencephalograph has 8 to 16 or more separate amplifying units capable of recording from many areas of the scalp at the same time. The amplified brain rhythms are strong enough to move an ink-writing pen, which produces the waveform of the brain activity of frequency range 0.5 to 30 Hz on paper moving at a standard speed of 3 cm per sec (cf. standard ECG paper speed of 2.5 cm per sec). The resulting electroencephalogram (EEG) or *voltage-versus-time graph* appears as a number of parallel, wavy lines as many as there are units, or "channels." Electrodes, which usually are solder or silver-silver chloride disks 0.5 cm in diameter, are placed on the head by means of adhesive material such as bentonite or collodion, using ordinary ECG paste under the electrode to make contact with the scalp. Patients are usually examined with their eyes closed and while relaxed in a comfortable chair or bed. The procedure is entirely painless and takes $^3/_4$ to $1^1/_4$ hr. The ordinary EEG, therefore, represents the electrocerebral activity recorded under restricted circumstances usually during the waking state, from several parts of the cerebral convexities during an almost infinitesimal segment of the person's life.

In addition to the resting record, a number of so-called "activating" procedures are usually carried out.

1 The patient is requested to breathe deeply 20 times a minute for 3 min. The resulting alkalosis and cerebral vasoconstriction may activate characteristic seizure patterns or other abnormalities (Fig. 322-1*H*).

2 A very powerful light (a stroboscope) is placed over the patient's face and flashed at frequencies from 1 to 20 per sec with his eyes opened and closed. The EEG leads may then show abnormal discharges (Fig. 322-1*D*).

3 The EEG is recorded after the patient is allowed to fall asleep naturally or following sedative drugs by mouth or by vein. Procedures 1 and 2 are more commonly employed, but sleep is extremely helpful in bringing out abnormalities, especially where temporal lobe epilepsy and certain other seizures are concerned (Fig. 322-1*G*), and all too often is omitted from study.

4 Special activating procedures, such as the parenteral administration of pentylenetetrazol (Metrazol) or insulin, can usually be worked out in advance with the electroencephalographer. Though they are hazardous and rarely used now, their purpose is to produce diagnostically useful abnormalities without actually inducing convulsions.

Through the medium of all-night EEG recordings, sleep has been shown to consist of two very different states, as was described in Chap. 23. One type, associated with rapid eye movement (REM) and a relatively desynchronized EEG, is that during which most dreams occur. The other variety (non-REM) occupies most of sleep time, consists of slow waves and recurring sharp complexes, and has been subdivided, according to depth, into four electroencephalographic *stages*.

Normal subjects sleep for more than an hour before passing into the REM state, whereas patients with narcolepsy enter REM sleep immediately. This abnormality of the physiology underlying sleep, demonstrable by EEG, is one example of many fascinating observations being made by use of such techniques. Some of these promise to be important clinically, and the same may be said of EEGs recorded by telemetry from freely moving, active ambulatory patients.

The EEG consists of 150 to 300 or more pages, each representing 10 sec in time. These are obtained by a technician who is primarily responsible for the entire procedure, including notation of movements or other events responsible for artifacts and successive modifications of technique based upon what the record shows. The technician provides the electroencephalographer with the record which he attempts to interpret in the absence of the patient. These records are studied in the same careful manner as x-rays or electrocardiograms, though because of the continuously changing nature of the EEG, their interpretation usually takes longer. Competent EEG analysis requires considerable experience with normal and abnormal recordings as well as with the limitations of the technique and all the numerous artifacts produced by the recording system or other events involving the patient.

Certain preparations are necessary if electroencephalography is to be most useful. The patient should not be sedated and should not have been for a long time without food, for both sedative drugs and relative hypoglycemia modify the normal EEG pattern. The same may be said of mental concentration, extreme nervousness or drowsiness, all of which tend to suppress the normal alpha rhythm and increase muscle and other artifacts. When dealing with patients suspected of having epilepsy who are already being treated for it, most physicians prefer to record the first EEG while the patient continues to receive drugs. If it is normal, and if the referring physician and the electroencephalographer agree, the test can be repeated 24 hr after withdrawal of anticonvulsants; it is well known that they reduce the incidence of abnormal interictal records in patients with proved epilepsy. Though it is unusual for seizures to begin during this short interval, it may happen; longer periods without therapy are hazardous. It is helpful to indicate on the request form the suspected site of lesion or question to be answered.

TYPES OF NORMAL RECORDINGS The normal electroencephalographic record in adults is usually easy to identify. The pattern frequently shows somewhat asymmetric 8 to 12 per sec, 50 μV sinusoidal *alpha* waves in both occipital and parietal regions. These waves wax and wane spontaneously and disappear promptly when the patient opens his eyes or fixes his attention on something (Fig. 322-1*A*). Faster waves than 13 per sec of lower amplitude (10 to 20 μV), called *beta* waves, are also seen symmetrically in the frontal regions. Very slow waves (*delta* waves), spikes, or other unusual patterns are absent in a normal record. When the normal subject falls asleep, the rhythm slows symmetrically, and characteristic wave forms (vertex sharp waves and sleep spindles) appear; if the sleep is induced by barbiturates, an increase in the fast frequencies is seen and is considered to be normal (Fig. 322-1*B*).

An occipital response to each flash may be seen in the normal EEG during stroboscopic stimulation and is called the *evoked response*, or, at faster repetition rates, photic "driving." The arrival of the visual response in the calcarine part of the occipital lobe occurs 20 to 30 msec after the flash of light. In animals it has been shown that this produces an extremely brief spike discharge, only a few milliseconds long and only 50 μV in amplitude when recorded from the surface of the cortex. Since the scalp electrodes are 2 cm away from the brain and with the ink-writing oscillograph one cannot follow or record discharges of such brief duration, this primary evoked response is not seen in the EEG. The primary response, however, secondarily activates a great many more neurons, which communicate with cells in the thalamus, with other areas in the cortex, and with the reticular formation in the brainstem, this discharge in turn reverberating back to the occipital and adjacent cortices. This latter discharge is some 60 to 80 msec long and 200 μV in amplitude. It appears some 50 or 60 msec after the primary response, the total latency between the flash and the secondary evoked response (Fig. 322-1*C*) being 70 to 90 msec. It is called the secondary *evoked response* and can be seen in the EEG of 75 percent or more of all subjects, even in the presence of the background brain

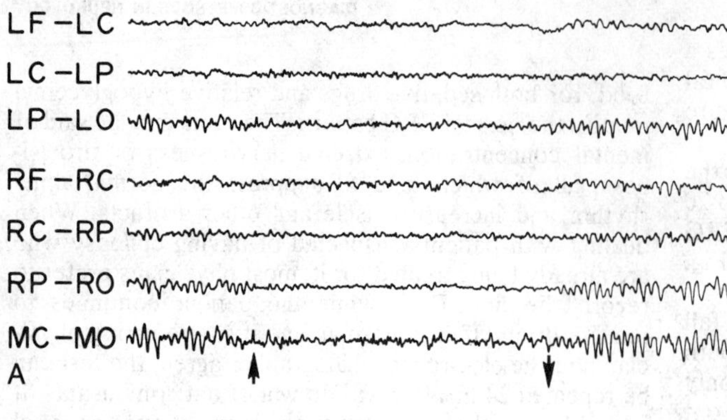

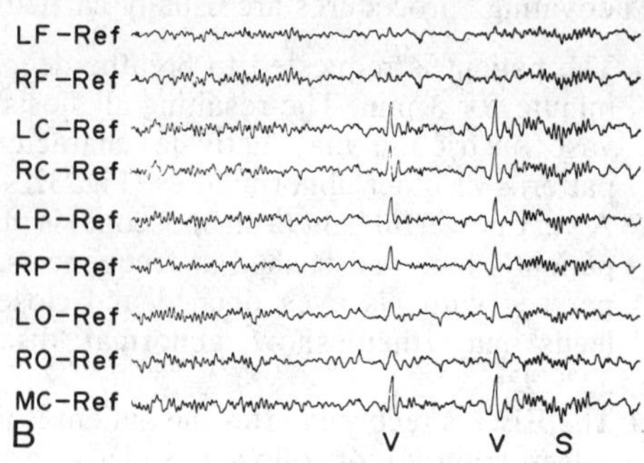

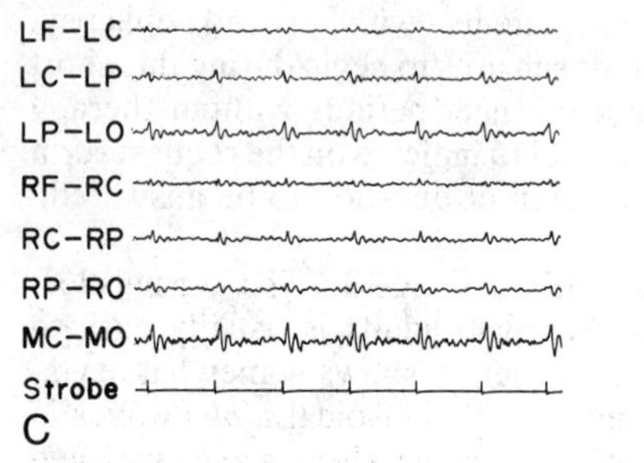

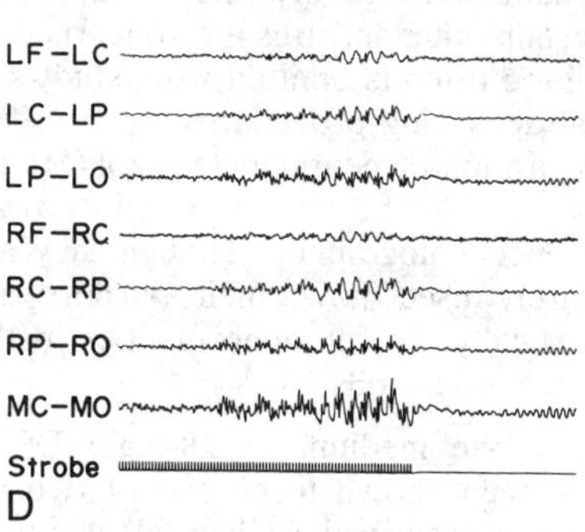

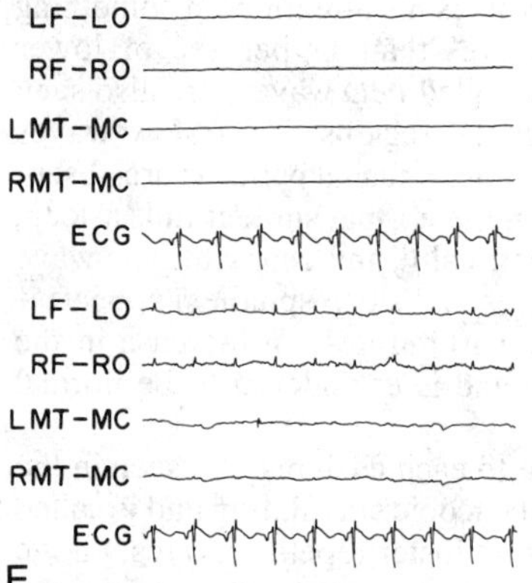

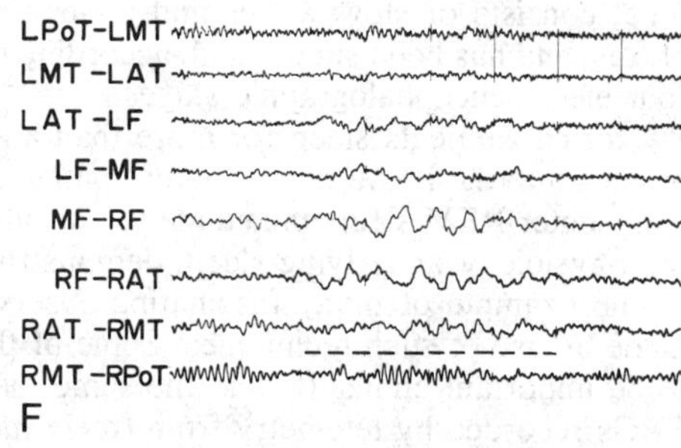

FIGURE 322-1

Abbreviations used in illustrations: R, right; L, left; A, anterior; M, mid; Po, posterior; F, frontal; C, central (sensorimotor area); T, temporal; P, parietal; O, occipital; V, vertex; Ref, reference or inactive lead (such as to neck and chest or both ears); strobe, stroboscopic stimulation. Calibrations are 1 sec and 100 μV except for the bottom half of E *where it is 10 μV.*

A *Normal* alpha *activity is present posteriorly over both hemispheres at 9 to 10 per sec. The arrows signify eye opening and closure. Note the striking reduction in alpha activity while the eyes are open.*

B *This recording is with the subject asleep (stage II of slow wave or non-REM sleep). The* vertex sharp waves *(V) and* sleep spindles *(S) are normal accompaniments of this stage of sleep. Note that the background consists of slow waves and that alpha activity is not present.*

C *During stroboscopic stimulation of a normal subject a visual-*evoked response *is seen posteriorly in both hemispheres and in the midline shortly after each flash of light (signaled on the bottom channel).*

D *Stroboscopic stimulation at 20 flashes per sec (bottom channel) has produced a* photoconvulsive *response in this epileptic patient. Note the abnormal spike and slow-wave activity toward the end of stimulation which is replaced then by normal alpha activity.*

E *This record, from a patient in deep coma following barbiturate overdose, shows* electrocerebral silence. *With the highest amplification (bottom half), ECG and other artifacts may be seen so that, while no cerebral rhythms are visible, the record does not consist of a series of truly flat or isoelectric lines. This patient recovered completely, but the record is identical with those recorded from patients with irreversible coma or brain death.*

F *Large, slow, irregular* delta waves *may be seen in the right frontal region (above the dotted line). A metastatic tumor was found in the underlying brain, but the EEG picture does not differ basically from that produced by a stroke, abscess, contusion, or other comparable cerebral lesion.*

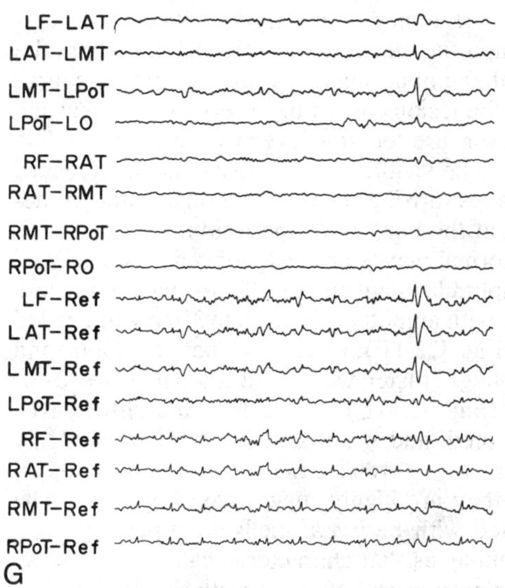

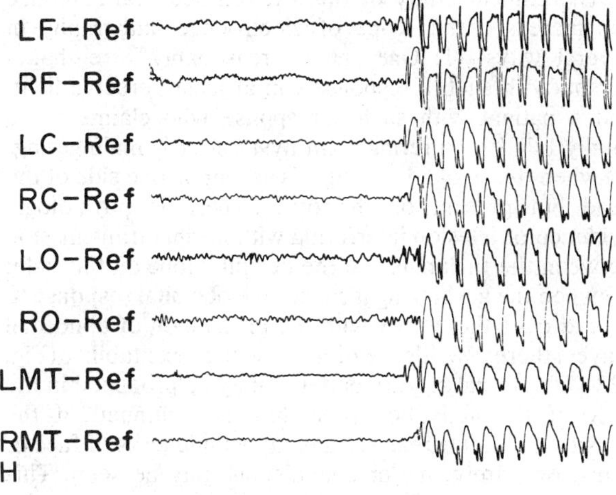

FIGURE 322-1 (*continued*)

G *A left frontotemporal focal* spike *discharge is seen to occur during light sleep in this patient with temporal-lobe epilepsy.*

H *Hyperventilation activates a generalized 3-per-sec* spike and wave *discharge in this patient with petit mal epilepsy. Note the abrupt onset of the abnormal activity which arises from a normal background.*

I *Bifrontal slow, occasionally* triphasic waves *(arrows) are present during hepatic coma in the upper half of the figure. They disappear after the administration of* L*-dopa and are replaced by normal activity (lower half). Note the artifacts produced by eye blink (above the dotted line) in the normal record.*

J *The grossly disorganized background activity (ranging from brief isoelectric periods to irregular slowing) interrupted by repetitive discharges consisting of large, sharp waves from all leads about once per second is characteristic of* Jakob-Creutzfeldt disease. *Note the ECG on channel 8 which serves to differentiate the sharp waves from ECG artifacts.*

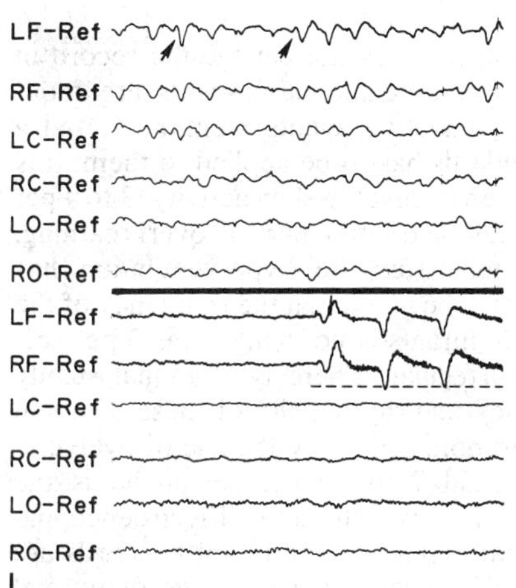

Calibrations:

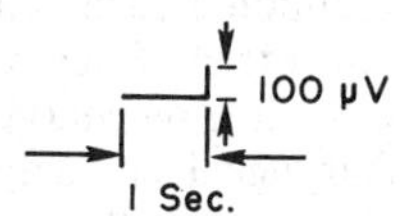

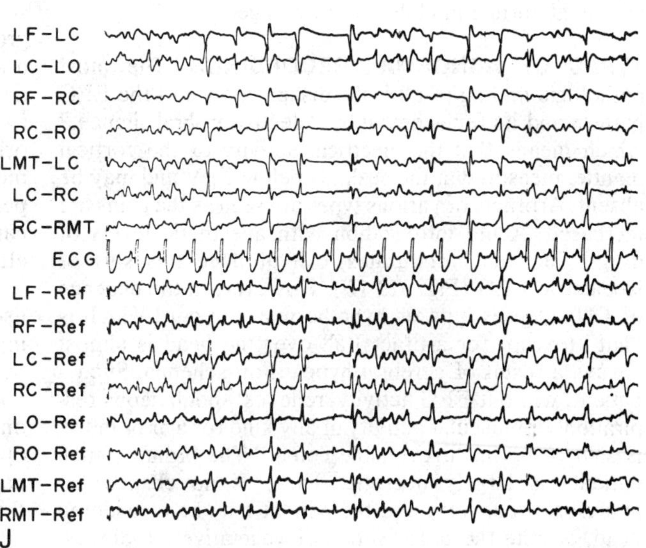

waves. In the remaining 25 percent, averaging techniques are necessary for its demonstration.

The clinical utility of this evoked occipital response has increased the scope of electroencephalography in several ways: (1) One can be reasonably sure that a person with such a response can at least perceive light, and a patient with such a response who claims to be totally blind is suffering from hysteria or is malingering; (2) when this evoked response is absent on one side of the head but present on the other, there is physiologic evidence of a lesion interfering with normal transmission between the thalamus and the occipital lobe on this side; (3) when the flashing light causes the occipital response to spread over the cortex with the production of abnormal waves, there is evidence of an abnormal excitability (Fig. 322-1*D*). Actual seizure patterns may be produced in the EEG if the activation procedure is continued; if the sensitivity is still greater, frank myoclonic jerks of face or arms, or, rarely, major convulsions may be seen. This finding is to be differentiated from the purely muscular response, also myoclonic, produced normally in contracting scalp muscles and often visible in routine EEGs (*photomyoclonus*).

Overbreathing usually does not change the record in the normal adult. Children and adolescents are more sensitive to all the activating agents mentioned, and a different set of standards has to be applied to them. It is customary for children to develop slow activity (3 to 4 per sec) during the middle and latter part of overbreathing. This disappears soon after the hyperventilation has stopped. Here it should be noted that the frequency of the dominant rhythms in infants is normally about 3 per sec, and they are very irregular. There is a gradual steady increase in frequency and rhythmicity of these occipital rhythms with maturation, and so by the age of twelve to fourteen years, normal 9 to 10 per sec alpha is the dominant pattern in most children. Electroencephalographers agree that children's and infant's records are difficult to interpret because the wide range of normal values at each age makes rigid classification, using frequency criteria for instance, impossible. Nevertheless, asymmetric records, or records with seizure patterns, are clearly abnormal in children of any age.

TYPES OF ABNORMAL RECORDINGS The most pathologic finding of all is the disappearance of the EEG pattern and its replacement by "electrocerebral silence," which means that the electrical activity of the cortical mantle, measured at the scalp, is below 2 μV and may be absent. Artifacts of various types are seen as the gains are increased. Acute intoxication with anesthetic levels of drugs, such as barbiturates, can produce this sort of isoelectric EEG (Fig. 322-1*E*). However, in the absence of CNS depressants or hypothermia, a record which is "flat" (except for artifacts) all over the head is almost always a result of cerebral hypoxia or ischemia. Such a patient, without EEG activity, reflexes, spontaneous respiration, or muscular activity of any kind for 6 hr or more, is said to be in "irreversible coma." The brain of such patients is largely necrotic. There is no chance for neurologic recovery, and the patient may be considered dead, despite the preservation of vegetative (cardiovascular) functions supported by mechanical means, such as respirators.

Localized regions of such absence of EEG may rarely be seen when there is a large area of softening or an extensive surface tumor or clot lying between the cerebral cortex and the electrodes. With such a finding, the localization of the abnormality is precise, but of course the nature of the lesion cannot be ascertained. Most such lesions, however, are too small, relative to the recording arrangement, to be visible, and the EEG may then record abnormal waves arising from functional, though deranged, brain at the borders of the lesion.

These abnormal waves are best defined as slower and of higher amplitude than normal. Those which are less than 4 per sec with amplitude from 50 to 350 μV are called *delta* waves (Fig. 322-1*F*); from 4 to 7 per sec, *theta*; and the higher-voltage, faster waves are known as *spikes* or *sharp waves* (Fig. 322-1*G*). These fast and slow waves may be combined, and when a series of them suddenly interrupts relatively normal EEG patterns in a paroxysmal fashion, they are highly suggestive of epilepsy. The ones associated with *petit mal* spells are 3 per sec spike and wave complexes that characteristically appear in all leads of the electroencephalogram at the same time and disappear almost as suddenly at the end of the seizure (Fig. 322-1*H*). This had led to the theoretic localization of a pacemaker for petit mal discharge in the thalamus or other deep gray structures ("centrencephalon"), but such clinical and experimental evidence as exists tends to refute this hypothesis.

NEUROLOGIC CONDITIONS WITH ABNORMAL EEG In the following groups of neurologic disorders, the EEG may be of considerable help in reaching the correct diagnosis. In others, as will be mentioned, it is of less value.

Epilepsy All types of generalized epileptic seizures (grand mal and petit mal) are associated with some abnormality in the EEG, provided it is being recorded at the time. The EEG is also usually abnormal during the more restricted types of seizure activity (psychomotor, myoclonic, Jacksonian). One exception is certain deep temporal lobe foci where the discharge fails to reach the scalp in sufficient amplitude to be seen against the background activity of the normal EEG, particularly if there is a strong alpha rhythm. If in these exceptional cases an anterior temporal electrode, which is most free of occipital alpha frequencies, does not show such a discharge originating deep and medially, a nasopharyngeal lead may pick it up, especially during sleep. In perhaps 2 to 5 percent of cases, the only way in which this deep activity can be sampled is by opening the skull and inserting an electrode into the substance of the brain. Some electroencephalographers are enthusiastic about the possible uses of depth electrodes and feel that a great deal of information about temporal lobe epilepsy can be obtained by this technique. Certainly most neurologists would be unwilling to allow depth electrode recordings to be made on any of their patients except the few who are having an operation on the brain. Although it is true that a rare patient with temporal lobe epilepsy and a normal EEG at the time of the seizure may be erroneously labeled as hysteric from the EEG alone, the clinical state itself is of help. Other exceptions in which, on occasion, no EEG abnormality may be recorded during a seizure include other focal seizures (sensory, Jacksonian, myoclonic, and *epilepsia partialis continua*). This fact presumably means that the neuronal discharge is too deep, discrete, fast, or asynchronous to be transmitted by volume conduction through the skull and recorded via the EEG electrode, which is some 2 cm from the cortex. Some of the different types of seizure patterns are shown in Fig. 322-1*D*, *G*, and *H*. The petit mal, myoclonic jerk, and grand mal patterns correlate closely with the clinical seizure type and may be present in the interictal EEG.

A fact of importance is that between seizures as many as 20 percent of patients with petit mal and 40 percent with grand mal epilepsy show a normal pattern. Anticonvulsant therapy also tends to diminish the EEG abnormalities. The records of another 30 to 40 percent of epileptics, though abnormal between seizures, are nonspecifically so, and therefore the diagnosis of epilepsy can be made only by the correct interpretation of the EEG abnormality in relation to the clinical data.

Brain tumor, abscess, and subdural hematoma Clinically significant intracranial space-occupying lesions are characteristically associated with abnormalities in the EEG, depending on their type and location, in some 90 percent of patients. In addition to diffuse changes, to be described below, the classic abnormalities are focal or localized slow wave (usually delta, as in Fig. 322-1*F*) or, occasionally, seizure activity and decreased amplitude and synchronization of normal rhythms. As a rule, those with the more rapidly expanding lesions (abscess, some metastases, glioblastoma) especially situated supratentorially, have the greatest frequency of EEG abnormalities (90 to 95 percent of the latter two and virtually 100 percent of abscesses). More slowly growing tumors (astrocytomas) and particularly those outside the cerebral hemispheres (meningiomas, pituitary tumors) often produce no change in the EEG, though they may be very evident clinically. The EEG abnormality has the correct lateralization in as many as 75 to 90 percent of patients with subdural hematomas and supratentorial tumors or abscesses. Therefore, when a patient in whom one of these conditions is suspected has a normal EEG, there are nine chances to one or more against its presence. Thus both the positive and negative values of the EEG in such situations may be helpful, particularly when integrated with the other laboratory and clinical findings. A normal EEG and brain scan together almost exclude the presence of a supratentorial brain tumor. The EEG may be normal, however, in 20 to 25 percent of patients with infratentorial tumors.

Cerebrovascular disease Both the diffuse and localized EEG changes produced by vascular lesions such as cerebral infarcts and intracranial hemorrhages depend on their location and size rather than their type. The EEG has been shown to be useful in the differential diagnosis of vascular hemiplegia. If the lesion responsible is in the internal carotid or major cerebral artery, an area of decreased normal activity and excessive slowing is practically always seen acutely in the appropriate region. If the hemiplegia is due to small-vessel disease and a lacunar infarction deep in the cerebrum (cf. Chap. 326), the EEG is usually normal. Large hemispheral lesions associated acutely with depressed levels of consciousness, also produce widespread, diffuse, slow wave activity of a nonspecific type as is seen with stupor or coma from any cause. Though a few very large infarctions betray themselves by ipsilaterally depressed EEG activity, most are not associated with asymmetric abnormalities acutely. Resolution begins after a few days, cerebral edema subsides, and focal activity may then be seen (slow-wave activity or suppression of normal background rhythms). Smaller infarctions are associated with focal abnormalities acutely which lateralize the lesion well but do not localize it precisely. In contrast with tumors, further resolution occurs, and after 3 to 6 months roughly 50 percent of patients with cerebrovascular accidents have a normal EEG despite the persistence of clinical abnormalities. Once this occurs, the prognosis for further recovery is poor. Perhaps half of these patients will have normal EEGs even when recorded in the week or two following the ictus. This is often true with discrete lesions, especially small, deep ones, which have the best prognosis. The same may be said for patients with any type of mild and short-lived EEG abnormalities. Large lesions of diencephalon or midbrain produce bilaterally synchronous slow waves, but, interestingly, those of pons and medulla may be associated with normal or near-normal EEGs despite profound and catastrophic clinical changes. The EEG may be of lateralizing value in acute subarachnoid hemorrhage depending upon the extent to which the adjacent cerebrum is affected.

Brain injury Cerebral concussion in animals is accompanied by a transitory disturbance in brain waves, but in man this is usually over before a recording can be made. Cerebral contusion or laceration produces EEG changes similar to those described for cerebrovascular disease. Diffuse changes often give way to focal ones, especially if the lesions are on the lateral or superior surface of the brain, and these in turn usually disappear over a period of weeks or months. Sharp waves or spikes sometimes emerge as the focal slow-wave abnormality resolves and may precede the occurrence of posttraumatic epilepsy. Following head injury, therefore, serial EEGs may be of prognostic value as regards the prospect of epilepsy. They may also aid, as mentioned above, in evaluating patients for subdural hematoma.

Diseases which cause coma and states of impaired consciousness The EEG is abnormal in almost all conditions in which there is some impairment of consciousness (cf. brainstem infarctions above). With hypothyroidism the rhythms are normal in configuration but are usually slow. In general, the more profound the change in consciousness, the more abnormal the EEG recording. In these latter situations the slow waves (delta) are bilateral, of high amplitude, and tend to be more conspicuous over the frontal regions (see Fig. 322-1*F*). This pertains to such differing conditions as acute meningitis or encephalitis, severe disorders of blood gases, glucose, electrolyte and water balance, uremia, diabetic coma, liver coma, or impairment of consciousness accompanying the large cerebral lesions discussed above. In hepatic coma, the degree of abnormality in the EEG corresponds with the degree of confusion, stupor, or coma. Moreover, paroxysms of bilaterally synchronous large, sharp "triphasic waves" are characteristic (Fig. 322-1*I*), though they may also be seen with other metabolic encephalopathies associated with renal or pulmonary failure. Diffuse degenerative diseases (e.g., Alzheimer's disease and senile dementia) affecting the cerebral cortex are accompanied by relatively slight degrees of diffuse, slow-wave abnormality in the theta (4 to 7 Hz) range. Certainly more rapidly progressive ones, such as subacute sclerosing panencephalitis (SSPE), Jakob-Creutzfeldt disease, and to a lesser extent the cerebral lipidoses have, in addition, very characteristic, almost pathognomonic, EEG changes consisting of recurring bursts of sharp, spiky, and slow activity (Fig. 322-1*J*). Even in situations where the EEG abnormality is not specific or diagnostic, it is useful in emphasizing the presence of physiologic, biochemical, and, sometimes, structural abnormalities of the brain. A normal EEG in a patient who is apathetic, slow, depressed, or forgetful is a point in favor of the diagnosis of an affective disorder or schizophrenia.

An EEG may also assist the physician in caring for a comatose patient when the pertinent history is unavailable. It may point to such otherwise unexpected causes as hepatic encephalopathy (bilaterally synchronous triphasic waves), intoxication with barbiturates or tranquilizers (excess fast activity), clinically inapparent continuous epileptic discharges, a large space-occupying lesion, or diffuse anoxia-ischemia.

Other diseases of the cerebrum There are many disorders of nervous function that cause little or no alteration in the EEG. Multiple sclerosis and other demyelinating diseases are examples, though as many as 50 percent of *advanced* cases will have an abnormal record. Delirium tremens and Wernicke-Korsakoff disease, despite the dramatic nature of the clinical picture, cause little or no change in the EEG. Some degree of slowing usually accompanies confusional states which have been designated eslewhere as hypokinetic delirium (see Chap. 26). Interestingly, neuroses and psychoses, such as manic-depressive disorders or schizophrenia, hallucinogenic drugs such as LSD, and the majority of cases of mental retardation are associated with no important modification of the normal record or with minor nonspecific abnormalities. The EEG has not assisted us in the understanding of these conditions.

SPECIAL APPLICATIONS OF THE EEG Because the EEG provides information about the status and function of the cerebrum, it is useful as a monitor in the operating room to ensure the presence of a viable brain during the increasingly extensive procedures of modern cardiovascular surgery. EEG apparatus has long been available for indicating the level of anesthesia, and such simple equipment should eventually be used by the anesthetist to monitor both the cardiac and cerebral status of *all* patients during surgical anesthesia.

In the neurosurgical operating room the EEG can be recorded from the exposed brain (*electrocorticogram*), and seizure patterns can be localized more precisely than from the scalp so that resection of such physiologically abnormal tissue may be undertaken.

The routine EEG can be of value in the diagnosis of hysterical blindness, as stated above. Similarly, a response evoked by noise during light sleep can be of help in confirming the presence of hearing in a patient who feigns total deafness. These responses may also be helpful in evaluating hearing and vision in infants.

In many subjects, however, the visual and auditory evoked responses are too small to be visible in the mélange of base-line noise and background activity of the routine EEG. Averaging techniques (computerized) may then be used to record them. This interesting new field of electroencephalography so far has proved to be useful clinically only in the evaluation of hearing in children and, to a lesser extent, in the study of vision.

CLINICAL VALUE OF MINOR EEG ABNORMALITIES

The gross EEG abnormalities discussed above are, by themselves, clearly and definitely abnormal and of obvious clinical significance. Any formulation of the patient's clinical status should consider and attempt to account for them. They include seizure discharge, generalized and extreme slowing, definite slow waves with a clear-cut asymmetry or a focus, and absence of normal rhythms. Certain other findings are of more doubtful significance and represent lesser degrees of abnormality which form a continuum between the undoubtedly abnormal and the completely normal. These records, which comprise such activity as 14- and 6-per-sec positive spikes, small, sharp spikes, scattered 5- to 6-per-sec slowing, voltage asymmetries, and moderate "breakdown" with hyperventilation, are termed *borderline* and are the most difficult to interpret. Ideally, the patient's physician should interpret the EEG himself just as he does the tests for cerebellar function or tendon reflexes. The EEG findings placed thus in the clinical context would be weighted appropriately, but, unfortunately, this is not always technically possible. The physician then depends upon the report he receives in which the EEG is usually described as "normal" or "abnormal." Such categorization in borderline records is difficult, arbitrary, and often meaningless. It is important, therefore, for the physician to realize the clinical value of minor EEG abnormalities which may be meaningful only if correlated with certain clinical phenomena. Whereas borderline deviations in an otherwise entirely normal person have no clinical significance, the same EEG findings, when associated with certain clinical signs and symptoms, even if they, too, are of minimal severity, become important. For example, a patient with tension headaches for 20 years is under neurologic study because of insomnia, weight loss, and an increase in the frequency of her headaches. The neurologic examination, spinal fluid, and x-rays of skull are all within normal limits. The EEG shows a clear-cut reduction of voltage in the left occipitoparietal area and less alpha than the same area on the right side. The finding of such an asymmetry in the brain wave has no clinical significance in this case and may be disregarded. On the other hand, this same finding in someone who was rendered unconscious in an accident 9 days before and who shows slight awkwardness in his right hand and a continuous dull headache with a lack of usual alertness now carries considerable diagnostic meaning. It points to the left hemisphere, which might show contusion or the presence of a subdural hematoma. The value of a normal or "negative" EEG in certain patients suspected of having a cerebral lesion has been discussed above.

In conclusion, the results of the EEG, like those of the EMG and ECG, are part of the clinical findings and are meaningful only in relation to the clinical status of the patient at the time they were recorded.

PSYCHOMETRY, PERIMETRY, AUDIOMETRY, AND TESTS OF LABYRINTHINE FUNCTION

These methods, drawn largely from the field of physiologic psychology, are of utility in quantitating and defining the nature of the psychic or sensory deficits produced by disease of the nervous system. Limitations of space do not permit a description of them here. The precise indications for doing these tests are (1) to obtain confirmation of a functional disorder in particular parts of the nervous system and to ascertain its nature; (2) to quantitate the disorder in order to determine, by subsequent examinations, the natural course of the underlying illness.

CONCLUDING REMARKS

Many of the procedures outlined here are highly technical and require special apparatus and carefully trained technicians. If the referring physician has never worked with these techniques, he must depend on the results of the technicians and also on their interpretations. Frequently he overestimates the power and objectivity of the special laboratory procedures and abdicates his role as the responsible physician by placing undue reliance upon them. This practice is to be discouraged. No one is better able to judge the significance of an abnormal laboratory datum in an abstruse clinical problem than a well-trained, experienced clinician. Therefore, it behooves every physician, using these several laboratory procedures, to find out enough about them so that he will know their limitations and the reliability of the data which they provide.

REFERENCES

Berger H: über das Elektrenkephalogramm des Menschen. Arch Psychiatr Nervenkr 87:527, 1929

Dement W, Kleitman N: Cyclic variations in EEG during sleep and their relation to eye movements, body motility, and dreaming. Electroencephalogr Clin Neurophysiol 9:673, 1957

Gibbs FA, Gibbs EL: *Atlas of Electroencephalography*, 2d ed., vols. 1–3, Reading, Mass.: Addison-Wesley, 1950–1964

Hill D, Parr G (eds): *Electroencephalography: A Symposium on Its Various Aspects*, 2d ed., New York: Macmillan, 1963

Kiloh LG, Osselton JW: *Clinical Electroencephalography*, 2d ed., London: Butterworth, 1966

Kooi KA: *Fundamentals of Electroencephalography*, New York: Harper & Row, 1971

Magnus O et al (eds): *Electroencephalography and Cerebral Tumors*, Amsterdam: Elsevier, 1961

Newton TH, Potts DG (eds): *Radiology of the Skull and Brain*, vols. 1–3, St. Louis: Mosby, 1971–72

Peterson HO, Kieffer SA: *Introduction to Neuroradiology*, New York: Harper & Row, 1972

323 DISEASES OF THE PERIPHERAL NERVOUS SYSTEM

RAYMOND D. ADAMS
ARTHUR K. ASBURY

Disease of the peripheral nervous system stands as one of the most difficult subjects in neurology. Since the structure and function of this system are relatively simple, one might suppose that knowledge of its diseases would be complete. Such is not the case. At present a suitable explanation cannot be offered in as many as half the patients who enter a general hospital with a disease of the peripheral nervous system; nor have the pathologic changes been fully determined in any one of them. Moreover, the physiologic basis of many of the symptoms of peripheral nerve disease continues to elude experts in the field.

With these rather discouraging remarks behind us, we shall attempt to present a distillate of our personal experience that may be of value to the reader.

GENERAL CONSIDERATIONS

It is well to have clearly in mind the extent of the peripheral nervous system and the scope of the possible pathogenetic mechanisms whereby it can be affected.

The peripheral nervous system (PNS) includes all nervous structures lying outside the piarachnoid membrane of the spinal cord and brainstem, with the exception of the optic nerves and olfactory bulbs, which are special extensions of the brain. The parts of it within the spinal canal and cranial cavity and attached to the ventral and dorsal surfaces of the cord and ventrolateral surface of the brainstem are the *spinal* and *cranial nerve roots*, respectively. The dorsal roots (sensory) containing afferent fibers (the central axonal processes of the dorsal root ganglion cells) extend for a variable distance into the posterior columns (funiculi) of the spinal cord. The efferent ventral roots, composed of the emerging axons of anterior and lateral horn cells, finally terminate on muscle fibers or in sympathetic or parasympathetic ganglions. Traversing, as they do, the subarachnoid space, and lacking an epineural and in part a perineural sheath, the cranial and spinal roots are bathed by cerebrospinal fluid (CSF), the lumbosacral roots presenting the longest exposure. The vast extent of the peripheral ramification of cranial and spinal nerves is noteworthy, as are their thick protective sheaths of perineurium and epineurium and their unique vascular supply through longitudinal arrays of richly anastomosing nutrient arterial branches. Sensory endings, freely branching or corpuscular, are the site of termination of the peripheral axons of dorsal root ganglion cells. Sympathetic afferent fibers, arising on blood vessels and in viscera, and the sympathetic and parasympathetic ganglions, with their rami communicantes and peripheral extent, complete this system. Segments of myelin, special extensions of Schwann cell plasma membrane, cover the axon but always maintain a morphologically independent though symbiotic relation to it.

These many anatomic features reveal the possible pathways and mechanisms of peripheral nerve disease. Pathologic processes directed at the anterior or lateral horn cells of the spinal cord, the nerve cells of dorsal root ganglions, or the nerve cells of sympathetic or parasympathetic ganglions may reflect themselves secondarily in degeneration of axons and myelin sheaths of the peripheral nerve fibers of these cells. Disease processes involving the oligodendrocytes or astrocytes in the ventral or dorsal columns (funiculi) of the spinal cord, wherein lie the axons of anterior horn cells or dorsal root ganglion cells, may also affect the function and structure of the peripheral nervous system. A pathologic process in the leptomeninges and CSF may damage the latter differently from the former because of their intimate relation to groups of specialized arachnoidal cells (villi) where CSF is absorbed. Pathogenic processes confined to various components of connective tissue may affect the peripheral nerves which lie enveloped within their sheaths. Diffuse or localized arterial diseases injure nerves by narrowing or obliterating the nutrient arteries, thus curtailing their blood supply. Noxious agents which selectively damage the Schwann cells or their membranes composing the myelin sheaths cause demyelination of peripheral nerves, but leave axons intact. Finally one might suppose that axoplasm of either motor or sensory nerve fibers or their peripheral endings and end organs might each have their particular liabilities to disease.

All this is theoretical and somewhat speculative. At present we can cite examples of diseases which are based on only a few of these potential disease pathways, e.g., diphtheria toxin, which acts directly on the membranes of the Schwann cells near the dorsal root ganglions and adjacent nerves; polyarteritis nodosa, which causes widespread occlusion of vasa nervorum; tabes dorsalis, in which there is a treponemal meningoradiculitis of lumbosacral segments. But analogous anatomic possibilities doubtless are implicated in other diseases whose mechanisms remain to be divulged.

Pathologically several distinct processes are recognized, although they are not disease-specific and may be present in varying combinations in any given patient. The major processes are Wallerian degeneration, sequential demyelination, and axonal degeneration. The myelin sheaths themselves are the most susceptible element of nerve, for they may break down as part of a primary process involving the Schwann cells (or some component thereof or secondarily to axonal or nerve cell destruction). When the myelin sheath itself degenerates, the highly structured lipoprotein disintegrates into fine particles, which are then converted through the action of macrophages into cholesterol esters and removed via the bloodstream. Focal myelin sheath degeneration is called *segmental demyelination.* Breakdown of axons causes fragmentation of myelin into blocks or ovoids in which lie fragments of axons. This is a feature typical of Wallerian degeneration. Degeneration of both axon and myelin sheath may occur either distal to axonal interruption (Wallerian degeneration) or as a "dying back" phenomenon in more generalized, metabolically determined polyneuropathies (axonal degeneration). In segmental demyelination, recovery may be rapid, because the intact axon need only become remyelinated over denuded segments to become functional once more. In contrast, with Wallerian or axonal degeneration, recovery is slower, often requiring months to a year or more, because the axon must regenerate and reconnect to its peripheral ending before function returns.

Aside from difference in pathologic pathway and the effects of disease on parenchymal elements of nerve, the various forms of polyneuropathy are distinguished by other characteristics of the lesions and by the topography of the nerve fiber changes. In fact these are the only available criteria for "differential diagnosis." In acute idiopathic polyneuritis and infectious mononucleosis, infiltrations of lymphocytes, plasma cells, and other mononuclear cells in the spinal roots, sensory and sympathetic ganglions, and nerves and a frequent perivenous location of myelin destruction characterize the disease. In polyarteritis nodosa with polyneuropathy, "necrotizing panarteritis" with occlusion and focal infarction of nerve and, less often, rupture and hemorrhage are the dominant findings. In amyloid polyneuropathy, it is the deposits of this foreign material in endoneurial connective tissue and the walls of vessels secondarily affecting the nerve fibers either by compression or ischemia that are the basis of diagnosis. In diphtheritic polyneuropathy, the aforementioned location in and around the roots and sensory ganglions, the purely demyelinative character of the nerve fiber change, and the lack of inflammatory reaction permit its identification under the microscope. Other polyneuropathies (carcinomatous, nutritional, porphyric, arsenical, uremic) are topographically symmetric but are not presently distinguishable from one another by histopathologic means. They await more definitive study. The least is known about the familial types of polyneuropathy. Although genetic factors can be envisaged, the biochemical mechanisms are just beginning to be recognized.

Concerning the causes of pathogenetic mechanisms and pathology of the mononeuropathies, even less is known. Compression, producing local or segmental ischemia, violent stretch, laceration from penetrating injuries are understandable, and the pathologic changes they cause have been reproduced in animals. Of localized infections of single nerves only leprosy, sarcoid, and zoster represent identifiable disease states. For the larger number of acute lesions the pathology has yet to be defined, since they are benign, reversible states usually, which allow no opportunity for postmortem examination.

The clinician is usually faced with two problems: (1) To establish the existence of disease of the peripheral nervous system; (2) to ascertain its nature and the possibilities of treatment. When muscular weakness, areflexia, atrophy, and sensory loss are demonstrable and conform to the region of distribution of one or many nerves, this is not difficult. The tendency for these diseases to affect the feet and lower legs more than the proximal parts, and the legs more than the arms, the frequent sparing of the trunk, the escape of vesical and anal sphincters, phenomena which probably reflect involvement of the largest and longest nerves, already com-

TABLE 323-1
Principal causes of peripheral neuropathy

I Poisons
- *A* Metals: arsenic, lead, mercury, antimony, bismuth, copper, phosphorus, thallium
- *B* Drugs: Nitrofurantoin and related nitrofurazones, isoniazid, thalidomide, vincristine, diphenylhydantoin, stilbamidine, tetraethylthiuram disulfide
- *C* Organic substances; carbon monoxide, carbon disulfide, trichoroethylene, methyl alcohol, triorthocresylphosphate, immune serums, benzene and derivatives, acrylamide, organophosphorus compounds

II Deficiency states and metabolic disorders
- *A* Chronic alcoholism, beriberi, pellagra, subacute combined degeneration, pregnancy, chronic gastrointestinal disease
- *B* Carcinoma of lung, diabetes mellitus, porphyria, amyloidosis, multiple myeloma, macroglobulinemia, uremia, hypoglycemia, lupus erythematosus

III Specific inflammatory states and infections
- *A* Acute idiopathic polyneuritis (Landry-Guillain-Barré syndrome)
- *B* Polyneuropathy, complicating acute or chronic infection: diphtheria, Boeck's sarcoid, infectious mononucleosis
- *C* Local infection of nerves: leprosy

IV Vascular disease: polyarteritis nodosa, arteriosclerosis, diabetes mellitus, rheumatoid arthritis

V Genetically determined disorders: progressive hypertrophic polyneuropathy, peroneal muscular atrophy, and others

VI Polyneuropathy of obscure origin: chronic progressive or recurrent polyneuropathy

mented upon in Chaps. 17 and 21, are relatively certain clues to diagnosis. But at times pain or dysesthesias may be the major symptoms, and the other subjective and objective neurologic findings are more difficult to put in evidence. Or the disorder may be purely motor, raising a question of myopathy, of motor end plate disorder or anterior horn cell disease; again, only paresthesias, ataxia, and sensory loss may be found, suggesting as alternative possibilities a disease of the posterior roots or the posterior columns of the spinal cord, such as tabes dorsalis. Under these circumstances one must resort to a number of laboratory procedures, such as (1) biochemical tests to rule in or out those metabolic or toxic states which will produce neuropathy; (2) measurement of nerve conduction velocity (lowered in chronic nerve disease but not in spinal cord or muscle diseases); (3) electromyography, which distinguishes disorders of muscle due to primary disease (myopathy) denervation, and neuromuscular block; (4) CSF examination (increase in protein and sometimes in cells with radicular and meningeal diseases); and (5) nerve (sural) and muscle biopsy.

Taking advantage of all available clinical and laboratory techniques and knowledge of the natural course of illnesses, the physician will find it helpful to be familiar with the following peripheral nerve syndromes. Stated another way, whenever one of the following syndromes can be identified, one is justified in considering any one of the several diseases of the peripheral nerve system listed in the following classification.

Only minor semiological differences separate (1) acute idiopathic polyneuritis of Landry-Guillain-Barré, (2) acute infectious mononucleosis, (3) porphyria, (4) diphtheritic polyneuropathy, (5) acute idiopathic hepatitis with polyneuritis, and (6) other toxic polyneuropathies, the diseases which induce this syndrome.

ACUTE IDIOPATHIC POLYNEURITIS Landry-Guillain-Barre syndrome This disease seems to occur at all seasons, as if it is an endemic process, and it affects children and adults of all ages and both sexes. Its cause is unknown; all attempts to isolate a virus or microbial agent have failed. A mild respiratory or gastrointestinal infection has preceded the neuritic symptoms by 1 to 3 weeks in approximately half the patients. Other preceding events include surgical procedures, viral exanthems, and antirabies inoculations.

The principal symptoms of peripheral nerve involvement conform to the general description given above. The weakness, which advances over a period of days, involves proximal as well as distal limb and also trunk muscles. Pain is exceptional; paresthesias (tingling and numbness) are frequent but are occasionally absent throughout the illness. The enfeeblement of muscle is so acute that it is not attended by atrophy, though hypotonia and areflexia are obvious. There is usually tenderness on deep pressure or squeezing of muscles. At an early stage the arms may be spared or their muscles may be less weakened than the leg muscles. Facial diplegia, occurring in half of all cases, usually comes later, after the arms are affected. However, other cranial nerves (ocular, bulbar) are often affected. When retention of urine occurs, it seldom requires catheterization for more than a few days.

The temperature is usually normal, and lymphadenopathy and splenomegaly do not occur. Electrocardiogram alterations of minor degree have often been reported. The CSF is under normal pressure and is acellular; elevations of protein level are found in most cases, but the values on the first lumbar puncture in the first few days of the disease are usually normal or only slightly raised. In about 10 percent of patients a pleocytosis of 10 to 50 cells per ml (rarely to 200 cells per ml, predominantly lymphocytes and mononuclear cells) is found. The white cell count and differential count tend soon to fall within normal limits. The pathologic changes in fatal cases have had a consistent pattern and form. When the disease was fatal within a few days, perivascular, lymphocytic infiltrates have been found. Later the diagnostic inflammatory cell infiltrates and perivenous demyelination are combined with segmental demyelination and some Wallerian degeneration. Inflammation of roots accounts, evidently, for the CSF changes. Infiltrates in liver, spleen, lymph nodes, heart, and other organs are occasionally found and reflect the systemic nature of the disease. From a pathogenetic standpoint, most of the evidence suggests that the clinical manifestations of this disorder are the result of a cell-mediated immunologic reaction directed at peripheral nerve.

The differential diagnosis includes poliomyelitis (distinguished usually by epidemic occurrence, meningeal symptoms, fever, and pure areflexic paralysis) and acute myelitis (marked by sensorimotor paralysis below a given spinal level and sphincteric paralysis). The forms of acute polyneuropathy described below must also be differentiated from this syndrome.

A therapeutic trial of prednisone (45 to 60 mg per day) with low salt diet and precautions against peptic ulceration of stomach and duodenum is warranted, but should be omitted in a few days if a definite response is not observed. Respiratory assistance is given when the vital capacity falls below 800 to 1,000 ml, and tracheostomy is usually performed at this time, especially if the patient has difficulty in removing secretions from the pharynx and tracheobronchial tree. Careful tracheal toilet, treatment of bronchial and pulmonary infections by the use of an appropriate antibiotic, and support of the blood pressure in the face of hypotension by vasopressor agents complete the therapeutic regimen. The best results are obtained by an efficient respiratory unit skilled in maintaining adequacy of ventilation and of cerebral circulation. Under the most ideal conditions the mortality is reduced to less than 5 percent.

Physiotherapy (passive-movement positioning of limbs and later mild resistance exercises) should be given, particularly to avoid pseudocontractures. Decision to discontinue respiratory aid and to close the tracheostomy are based on the degree of recovery of the patient's respiratory mechanism.

Prognosis for complete recovery is good. More than 85 percent of patients are restored to normal function; the remaining usually have only mild residual deficit. Speed of recovery varies. Usually it takes place within a few weeks or months, but if nerves have degenerated, their regeneration may require 6 to 18 months.

Infectious mononucleosis with polyneuritis Three neurologic syndromes have been described with this disease: (1) Ascending sensorimotor paralysis, identical with that of the Landry-Guillain-Barré syndrome, (2) aseptic meningitis, and (3) meningoencephalitis. All three appear during the midphase of the infection. The polyneuritis varies in severity and has rarely been fatal. The few autopsied cases have shown heavy infiltrations of lymphocytes, monocytes, and plasma cells in the nerves, roots, and meninges. The CSF contains as many as several hundred mononuclear cells, and the protein level is raised. The diagnosis is suggested by the other typical physical and laboratory findings in this disease (see Chap. 224).

Infectious hepatitis with polyneuritis Jaundice accompanied or followed by signs of disease of the peripheral nerves occurs most frequently as a complication of alcoholism and nutritional deficiency but has also been observed in familial amyloidosis. In our experience with this syndrome, the polyneuritis has followed the jaundice by several days or a few weeks and has the same relation to it as to respiratory or intestinal infections. Usually the diagnosis of the type of hepatitis has remained unclear. Antibodies to Epstein-Barr virus are found in some cases. There is no basis for believing it homologous serum hepatitis or infectious mononucleosis. It may be that the mild interstitial hepatitis found in many fatal cases of acute idiopathic polyneuritis is more marked than usual. Recovery from the hepatitis has been the rule.

TABLE 323-2
Principal neuropathic syndromes

I Syndrome of acute ascending motor paralysis with variable disturbance of sensory function
- *A* Acute idiopathic polyneuritis (Landry-Guillain-Barré syndrome)
  - *1* Infectious mononucleosis and polyneuritis
  - *2* Hepatitis and polyneuritis
  - *3* Diphtheritic polyneuropathy
  - *4* Porphyric polyneuropathy
  - *5* Toxic polyneuropathies (triorthocresyl phosphate poisoning, Jamaica ginger)

II Syndrome of subacute sensorimotor paralysis
- *A* Symmetric polyneuropathies
  - *1* Alcoholic polyneuropathy and beriberi
  - *2* Arsenic polyneuropathy
  - *3* Lead polyneuropathy
  - *4* Nitrofurantoin and other intoxications
- *B* Asymmetric polyneuropathies
  - *1* Diabetic
  - *2* Polyarteritis nodosa
  - *3* Subacute idiopathic polyneuritis
  - *4* Sarcoidosis

III Syndrome of chronic sensorimotor polyneuropathy
- *A* Acquired
  - *1* Carcinoma, myeloma, and other malignancy
  - *2* Paraproteinemias
  - *3* Uremia
  - *4* Beriberi
  - *5* Diabetes
  - *6* Connective tissue diseases
  - *7* Amyloidosis
  - *8* Leprosy
- *B* Genetically determined disorders
  - *1* Peroneal muscular atrophy (Charcot-Marie-Tooth disease)
  - *2* Hypertrophic polyneuropathy (Dejerine-Sottas disease)
  - *3* Portuguese amyloidosis (Andrade's disease) and other types
  - *4* Heredopathia atactica polyneuritiformis (Refsum's disease)
  - *5* Abetalipoproteinemia
  - *6* Tangier disease
  - *7* Metachromatic leukodystrophy

IV Syndrome of chronic relapsing polyneuropathy
- *A* Idiopathic polyneuritis
- *B* Porphyria
- *C* Beriberi or intoxications

V Syndrome of mono- or multiple neuropathy
- *A* Pressure palsies
- *B* Traumatic neuropathies
- *C* Idiopathic brachial and sciatic neuritis
- *D* Serum neuritis
- *E* Zoster
- *F* Tumor invasion with neuropathy
- *G* Leprosy
- *H* Paratubercular (polyneuritis cranialis multiplex)

Diphtheritic polyneuropathy Typical diphtheria (see Chap. 151) follows pharyngeal and laryngeal infections. Local action of the exotoxin may paralyze pharyngeal and laryngeal muscles within a few days and may also cause blurring of vision due to loss of accommodation. But these and other cranial nerve symptoms may be overlooked. The first signs of the neuropathy, coming 4 to 8 weeks later, are then an acute to subacute weakness of limbs with paresthesias and distal loss of vibratory and position sense. The weakness characteristically involves all four extremities at the same time or may descend from arms to legs. After a few days to a week or more the patient may be unable to stand or walk, and occasionally the paralysis is so severe and extensive as to impair respiration. The CSF protein level is usually elevated (50 to 200 mg per 100 ml). After the pharyngeal infection is controlled, death in diphtheria is due usually to myocardiopathy or to polyneuropathy with respiratory paralysis.

Postmortem examination discloses a demyelination without inflammatory reaction of spinal roots, sensory ganglions, and adjacent spinal nerves. Axons anterior horn cells, peripheral nerves distally, and muscle fibers remain normal.

The disease should be considered in all cases of acute polyneuropathy. Throat culture may demonstrate the *Corynebacterium* many weeks after the throat infection has subsided. Usually the history of nasal voice, dysphagia, blurred vision, and numb lips with a throat infection several weeks before provides the clue to the diagnosis. The ECG may be abnormal at the time of the polyneuritis. Occasionally the polyneuropathy has followed a local wound infection with *Corynebacterium.* Titers of antitoxin in the blood and a positive Schick test reaction have usually not been helpful (for treatment see Chap. 151).

The prognosis for full recovery is excellent, once respiratory paralysis is circumvented.

Porphyric polyneuropathy As was stated in Chap. 102, a severe, rapidly advancing, more or less symmetric polyneuropathy with or without psychosis (delirium confusion) and convulsions may occur in the course of acute intermittent porphyria. The neuropathy may affect principally the motor or both the sensory and motor nerves; it may begin in the feet and legs and ascend, or it may begin in the arms and later spread to the trunk and legs. Often it is predominantly proximal in distribution. The CSF protein level is usually normal.

The course of the polyneuropathy is variable. If the disease is mild, it may be quite transitory, with regression of symptoms in a few weeks. If severe, it may rapidly progress to a fatal issue in a few days, the advance occurring without warning; or it may progress in a saltatory fashion over a period of weeks, finally resulting in a severe sensorimotor paralysis that may regress only over a period of months. Disorder of the central nervous system is more likely to precede the acute severe forms of neuropathy, but it may not appear at all.

The pathologic changes in the peripheral nervous system vary according to the stage of the illness at which death occurs. If the patient dies in the first few days, the myelinated fibers may appear entirely normal, despite an almost complete paralysis. If symptoms had been present for weeks, a severe degeneration of both the axons and myelin sheaths often is found in most of the peripheral nerves. No inflammatory reaction, vascular lesion, or other change distinguishes this form of neuropathy. The relation between the metabolic abnormality centering about porphyrin biosynthetic pathway in the liver and nervous dysfunction has never been satisfactorily explained.

See Chap. 102 for a discussion of treatment.

The prognosis for ultimate recovery is excellent, though relapse of the porphyria may result in further involvement of the peripheral nervous system (see Relapsing Polyneuropathy, below).

Polyarteritis nodosa with polyneuropathy Occasionally this form of neuropathy develops as rapidly as acute idiopathic polyneuritis. Most of the cases evolve more slowly, however, and the syndrome has been either symmetric or asymmetric in its distribution. For this reason the description will be given in the next section. At times a muscle biopsy may be needed to distinguish this acute form from acute idiopathic polyneuritis.

Other toxic polyneuropathies that may cause paralysis in a few days An example is triorthocresyl phosphate intoxication, in which the purely motor paralysis ultimately proves to be due to involvement of upper and lower motor neurons (see Chap. 110 for discussion of other chemical agents). The acute stages are accompanied by an encephalopathy with delirium and coma. Stilbamidine, used in the treatment of kalaazar, produces a purely sensory neuropathy predominating in the trigeminal nerves.

SUBACUTE SENSORIMOTOR PARALYSIS

SYMMETRIC DISTRIBUTION Reference is made here to a neurologic disorder that develops over a period of a few weeks and pursues a variable course. Pain, hypersensitivity of skin, tenderness of muscles, and a mixture of dysesthesias and paresthesias are often prominent features of this clinical state. A purely symmetric syndrome of this type usually proves to be due to alcoholism, vitamin B deficiency (beriberi), arsenic, lead, nitrofurantoin, or isoniazid therapy.

Alcoholic polyneuropathy and beriberi All data point to a common nutritional factor for both these diseases, though it remains unclear whether the deficiency is one of thiamine, pyridoxine, pantothenic acid, or of several of the B vitamins. We have not been able to define a form of polyneuropathy due solely to the direct effect of alcohol.

In North America and Western Europe this form of polyneuropathy is rarely observed in the nonalcoholic person. Pure starvation does not produce it, the ideal conditions being a vitamin B deficiency in the face of a relatively high carbohydrate consumption. Of course, eccentricity of diet, gastrointestinal disorders, sprue, rice diet for hypertension with neglect of vitamin supplements, all may create the circumstances for such a neuropathy.

After several months (approximately three) of dietary inadequacy, numbness, tingling, and tenderness of the feet appear and are accompanied by weakness of the more distal muscles of the lower extremities, spreading within a few days to the calves and later the thighs. The leg muscles are always affected before the thighs, and foot drop, accompanied by weakness of the plantar flexors, is the first stage of the motor paresis. Involvement of the thighs is indicated by difficulty in arising from a squatting position. The tendon reflexes (ankle and knee jerks) are abolished, the skin and muscles are tender and vibratory, and position and touch senses are diminished to a variable degree, increasing as one proceeds distally. The nerves supplying the muscles and skin of the trunk are usually spared, and as the disease progresses, numbness and sensitivity of the fingers, hands, and forearms, weakness of hand grip, and wrist drop are next to appear. Cranial structures are always spared unless Wernicke's disease is conjoined, in which instance there will be bilateral abducens and lateral gaze palsy and nystagmus, as well as cerebellar ataxia of gait, confusion, and memory defect (Korsakoff's psychosis). If pellagra or nutritional myelopathy also occur, signs of retrobulbar neuropathy, deafness, and pyramidal tract signs may be found resembling subacute combined degeneration.

This form of neuropathy produces a manifest sensorimotor disorder, which demands medical attention in only about half the patients in whom the diagnosis can be made. Once started, the syndrome often progresses over a period of days and weeks until the patient becomes confined to bed. But many alcoholics come to the physician with only a subclinical neuropathy (thin leg muscles, questionable sensory disorder over the shins and feet, and reduced or absent tendon reflexes). They give no history of having had a subacute symptomatic polyneuropathy. If untreated, the symptomatic form may progress over weeks and months to a severe atrophy of leg muscles, the polyneuropathy then becoming chronic. Edema is not infrequent (wet beriberi) and is due to dependency of limbs and stasis, more than to coincidental myocardial involvement.

Alcoholic Laennec's cirrhosis and a nutritional anemia as well as autonomic dysfunction, weight loss, myocardiopathy, hypoglycemia, and electrolyte disturbance may coexist. The CSF is normal in nearly all the cases (rarely is the protein elevated).

The pathologic changes of the neuropathy have not been fully described. The primary change encountered is axonal degeneration with destruction of both axon and myelin sheath, but variable amounts of segmental demyelination may also occur. Cursory studies show the most pronounced lesions to be in the distal parts of the longest and largest myelinated fibers in the crural and, to a lesser extent, the brachial nerves. Vagi, phrenic, and trunk nerves are implicated only in the more advanced and fatal cases. Anterior horn cells and sensory ganglion cells undergo chromatolysis indicating axonal damage. Exceptionally, spinal roots and posterior columns of the spinal cord have shown degenerative changes. Recovery awaits remyelination and regeneration.

The disease process is invariably arrested by adequate diet, and the amount of B vitamins in the average food ration of the American public will be curative, though there is no harm in supplementing the diet with B vitamins (see Chap. 78). Positioning and splinting paralyzed limbs to prevent undue stretching and passive motion to prevent contracture are important. Occasionally pain and tenderness are so severe as to require analgesic medication. The pain may be of a burning type (causalgic) with excessive perspiration and only slight weakness and reflex changes. This latter, called the *burning foot syndrome*, has been ascribed to pantothenic acid deficiency, but we have not been able to prove its relation to this vitamin or to separate it clearly from the usual alcoholic neuropathy. Cooling lotions, Darvon, aspirin, and codeine are needed. Sometimes sympathetic blocking agents are helpful. The pain subsides after some few weeks.

The prognosis for full functional recovery is good, but if the paralysis is complete, one may anticipate a period of invalidism for 6 months or more. Vitamins do not hasten recovery. The tendon reflexes may remain absent or diminished. Fatalities have usually been the result of coincidental beriberi, heart disease, or cirrhosis rather than of the polyneuropathy. Vitamin supplements will prevent the polyneuropathy.

Arsenic polyneuropathy Nerve involvement from chronic arsenic poisoning is relatively infrequent. The symptoms develop rather slowly over a period of weeks and have the same sensory and motor distribution as was described in beriberi. A single acute ingestion of arsenic may be followed in 14 to 21 days by a more rapidly advancing polyneuropathy. The condition may be preceded by mental disturbances, convulsions, confusion, and coma, i.e., arsenic encephalopathy. Diagnosis is based on the subacute course of the polyneuropathy coupled with symptoms of gastrointestinal disorder, anemia, jaundice, brownish cutaneous pigmentation, hyperkeratosis of palms and soles, and white transverse banding of nails (Mees' lines).

See Chap. 110 for diagnostic tests and treatment.

Poisoning due to mercury, thallium, antimony, and nitrofurantoin may produce a similar picture; the first three of these intoxications respond to British antilewisite (BAL).

Lead neuropathy Lead neuropathy occurs following chronic exposure to lead, and its most characteristic feature is the predominantly motor affection involving mainly the upper extremities. The radial nerves are most frequently involved, producing wrist and finger drop with few or no sensory manifestations. Less commonly, weakness of the proximal shoulder-girdle muscle occurs, and in the lower extremities foot drop may appear. Lead neuropathy is seldom combined with encephalopathy. Important associated findings are anemia, basophilic stippling of red blood cells, lead line along the gingival margins, colicky abdominal pain, and constipation. Neuropathy occurs usually in adults and is infrequent in children. In contrast, lead encephalopathy, manifested by increased intracranial pressure, convulsions, blindness, and coma, occurs almost exclusively in children. The diagnosis of lead neuropathy is established by the history of lead exposure, the characteristic motor involvement, the associated medical findings, and increased urinary excretion of lead and coproporphyrins. Treatment consists of withdrawal from exposure to lead and measures to eliminate lead from the bloodstream (see Chap. 110). Recovery may be slow.

Nitrofurantoin neuropathy The earliest symptoms of nitrofurantoin neurotoxicity are tingling dysesthesias of the toes and feet, followed shortly by similar sensations in the fingers. If the offending agent is not discontinued, this may progress to a severe, sensorimotor, distal, symmetric polyneuropathy. Usually neuropathic symptoms appear only after the drug has been administered in high dosage for several weeks or months, but rare patients have experienced dysesthesias after brief periods. Patients with chronic renal failure and azotemia are particularly prone to neurotoxicity with nitrofurantoin, presumably because of diminished excretion in the urine and consequent high tissue levels of the drug. To make matters more difficult, the uremic state itself may be responsible for a clinically similar polyneuropathy, so that the distinction between uremic polyneuropathy and nitrofurantoin neuropathy in the presence of chronic renal failure may be impossible.

SUBACUTE ASYMMETRIC POLYNEUROPATHIES

The most notable examples of this syndrome are diabetes mellitus, polyarteritis nodosa and other vasculitides, and a more or less obscure form of idiopathic polyneuritis. Rarely, sarcoidosis presents in this fashion.

Diabetic neuropathy Only about 15 percent of patients with diabetes mellitus have both symptoms and signs of neuropathy, but nearly 50 percent either complain of neuropathic symptoms or exhibit slowing of nerve conduction velocity. Neuropathy is most common in older diabetics over fifty years of age, is uncommon under thirty years of age, and is rare in childhood diabetes.

A number of clinical syndromes have been delineated as follows: (1) Diabetic ophthalmoplegia (described in Chaps. 20 and 324); (2) acute mononeuropathy; (3) painful, asymmetric mononeuropathy multiplex, which may pursue an acute, subacute, or chronic course and which usually recovers; (4) distal, symmetric, primarily sensory polyneuropathy, affecting feet and legs more than hands in a chronic, slowly progressive manner; and (5) an autonomic neuropathy involving bowel, bladder, and circulatory reflexes. Combinations of these neuropathies often coexist, particularly the autonomic disturbance in conjunction with other types.

The acute mononeuropathy involves most commonly the femoral or sciatic nerves and is presumably due to occlusion of vessels within or supplying the nerve. The outlook for recovery is good.

Painful, asymmetric mononeuropathy multiplex tends to occur in older patients with mild or unrecognized diabetes. Pain often begins in the low back or hip and spreads to thigh and knee on one side. It usually has a deep, burning character with superimposed, tearing, lancinating jabs and a propensity to become most severe at night. Muscle weakness and atrophy are usually most evident in pelvic girdle and thigh, although the distal muscles may not be spared. The upper extremities are usually unaffected. Sensory loss for position, vibration, touch, and pain is not generally severe and may conform to either a multiple nerve or root distribution, or to both. The vesical and anal sphincters may be involved, and the knee jerk is often lost on the affected side. Recovery from this type of neuropathy is the rule, although months and even years are often required. There is a tendency for the same syndrome to recur after a lapse of months or years in the opposite lower extremity.

When the clinical picture is dominated by lancinating pain and sensory ataxia, with only slight weakness and bowel and bladder derangements, it resembles that of tabes dorsalis so closely that the condition goes by the name of *diabetic tabes*. The syndrome known as *diabetic amyotrophy*, in which one finds proximal pelvic girdle weakness, wasting, weight loss, absent knee jerks, and often sphincteric symptoms and sexual impotence, probably represents a chronic form of the mononeuropathy multiplex.

The distal, symmetric, primarily sensory form is the most common type of diabetic neuropathy. Numbness and tingling with relatively little pain are the main symptoms and are usually confined to the feet and lower legs. The ankle jerks are rarely preserved. Trophic changes in the form of deep ulcerations and neuropathic joints are occasionally encountered, presumably due to severe denervation of skin and joints. Muscle weakness is usually mild, but in some cases a crural weakness with only minor sensory disturbance may predominate.

Pathologically, severe nerve fiber loss is a prominent finding in this form of neuropathy. In addition, evidence of segmental demyelination and remyelination of remaining axons is apparent in teased nerve fiber preparations. Since myelin is formed from the cell membranes of Schwann cells, one may infer that the Schwann cell is a primary target of the pathologic process in the distal, symmetric type of diabetic neuropathy. Whether the nerve fiber loss is explained by this same process remains uncertain. The blood vessels in these nerves do not appear abnormal.

Symptoms of autonomic involvement include impairment of sweating and vascular reflexes, nocturnal diarrhea, atonic bladder, sexual impotence, and occasionally postural hypotension. The basis for this type of nerve damage is unknown.

In all forms of diabetic neuropathy, the CSF protein may be elevated (50 to 200 mg per 100 ml), and similar increases may be seen in diabetics with no clinical evidence of neuropathy. An explanation for this phenomenon has not been discovered.

Many uncertainties persist about the pathogenesis of the diabetic neuropathies. Both the cranial mononeuropathies (diabetic ophthalmoplegia) and the proximal asymmetric mononeuropathy multiplex are thought to be ischemic in origin secondary to disease of the vasa nervorum. The other forms are rather vaguely ascribed to an undefined metabolic defect.

The only known treatment is meticulous regulation of the diabetes mellitus along the lines described in Chap.

88. Maintenance of the blood sugar level in a relatively normal range is desirable, for there is some evidence that uncontrolled hyperglycemia is harmful. Vitamin supplements may have some merits, but no clear results have been obtained. Improvement and eventual recovery may be expected over a period of months, but during that time the management of the painful forms of neuropathy may be trying, because analgesic medication is required and one is faced with the possibility of drug addiction.

Polyarteritis nodosa with polyneuropathy Involvement of the intraneural vessels happens in perhaps as many as 90 percent of cases (autopsy figures), but a symptomatic form of neuropathy develops in only 10 to 20 percent. Yet such involvement may be the principal clue to the diagnosis of the underlying disease when, up to that time, the main components of the clinical picture—abdominal pain, hematuria, fever, eosinophilia, hypertension, vague limb pains, and possibly asthma—have not fully declared themselves.

As was stated above, the polyneuropathy may develop acutely and be diffuse and more or less symmetric in distribution, but more often it is subacute, multiple, and asymmetric, i.e., a mononeuropathy multiplex. Both spinal and cranial nerves may be affected. No two cases are identical. The CSF protein level is usually normal. Muscle biopsy, taken near the motor point so as to include nerve, is useful in corroborating the clinical impression in the majority of cases.

Fatal issue is the rule. Corticosteroid therapy has not been successful in most cases. Spontaneous remission and therapeutic arrest are known, however, and a healed or healing form has been observed at autopsy, death having been due to other causes.

Subacute asymmetric idiopathic polyneuritis A few patients who consult the physician with an illness which at first glance has all the appearance of acute idiopathic polyneuritis will continue to become worse over a period of weeks or months. Some have an extremely high CSF protein level (600 to 1,500 mg per 100 ml), with a virtual Froin CSF syndrome (xanthochromia and spontaneous clotting). The higher concentration of protein fluids may induce headache, papilledema, and high CSF pressure, possibly because of the osmotic effect of the protein in increasing CSF volume. As the months pass, some symptoms improve as others appear. Ultimately most patients recover, though late fatality is known to occur; corticosteroids in full doses have proved to be beneficial in the majority of cases but may have to be continued over a period of months.

The pathology of these subacute forms has not been defined, nor is their relation to the acute varieties of idiopathic polyneuritis settled.

Sarcoidosis Another cause of subacute or chronic polyneuropathy, sarcoidosis, is discussed in Chap. 223. It may be associated with signs of central nervous system involvement (stalk of the pituitary with diabetes insipidus and the cerebellum with ataxia) or with lesions in muscles (polymyositis). Facial nerve weakness is the single commonest manifestation of peripheral nerve involvement (Chap. 324).

CHRONIC PROGRESSIVE ATROPHIC MUSCLE WITH SENSORY LOSS

In this syndrome weakness and muscular atrophy tend to progress over a period of months or years. The time of onset is often uncertain. In infants the condition is often mistaken for muscular dystrophy or infantile muscular atrophy until sensory tests become possible. In the developing child whose musculature naturally increases in power and volume, it may be difficult to decide whether the disease is progressive. Ataxia of limbs may be pronounced at a stage when sensory loss exceeds paresis. The atrophy of muscle and trophic changes in the skin are more marked than in the acute and subacute forms of polyneuropathy, which is why the syndrome must be differentiated from the other forms of severe muscular atrophy, i.e., motor system disease, muscular dystrophy (distal type), and syringomyelia. In some cases the distribution is quite asymmetric, e.g., in leprosy, or only in a few of the nerves of the legs may be involved, e.g., in familial perforating ulcer. The feet and hands may be extremely wasted and subject to painless injuries, loss of digits, and Charcot's joints (Morvan's syndrome), while proximal structures are sound. In the majority of cases symmetry of pattern is the rule. The CSF protein level may remain elevated over a period of years.

Two main categories of disease are known to present with this syndrome, one acquired, the other familial. The familial analgesic varieties such as the perforating ulcer syndrome, Tangier disease, and amyloidosis cause little weakness or loss of reflexes and leave all forms of sensation except pain and temperature relatively intact. Diffuse anhydrosis, impotence, or orthostatic hypotension, fixity of pupils, and lack of saliva and tears due to involvement of sympathetic nerves are often added. Most of the acquired forms are of obscure cause and mechanism.

ACQUIRED FORMS Carcinomatous and myelomatous polyneuropathy A slowly developing symmetric sensory or sensorimotor polyneuropathy may accompany the development of a carcinoma or multiple myeloma. Severe weakness, atrophy, ataxia, and sensory loss of the limbs may advance to the point where the patient is confined to a wheelchair or bed; and all this happens months or even a year or more before a small malignant tumor is found. The CSF protein level is often moderately elevated. This form of polyneuropathy has occurred most frequently with carcinoma of the lung but actually has been joined to every tumor. It may accompany either a solitary plasmocytoma of bone or multiple myeloma and in a few instances has been seen in macroglobulinemia without tumor formation. Thus polyneuropathy must be added to polymyositis or dermatomyositis, with which it is frequently conjoined as a neurologic complication of malignant tumor growths. A peculiar type of myasthenia, spinocerebellar degeneration (particularly with carcinoma of the ovary), and multifocal leukoencephalopathy, the other neurologic complications of neoplasia, may coexist. The pathology of the neuropathy has been incompletely defined. The only known therapy consists of removing or controlling the tumor growth, which has resulted at times in improvement. Corticosteroid therapy has helped some patients.

Paraproteinemia (see Chap. 63) More than a dozen patients with mild chronic, sensorimotor neuropathies have been seen on our wards in recent years in whom no associated metabolic disturbance other than an abnormality of the immunoglobulins was found. In general, three protein abnormalities have occurred: (1) Isolated macroglobulinemia (IgM); (2) diffuse increase in all three immunoglobulins (IgM, IgG, and IgA), and (3) a specific disorder of (IgA) immunoglobulin in ataxia-telangiectasis (see Chap. 334). In the latter disease, peripheral nerve dysfunction is evidenced by hyporeflexia, decreased nerve conduction velocities, and severe nerve fiber loss on sural nerve biopsy. In macroglobulinemia and diffuse immunoglobulinemia (not to be confused with multiple myeloma), the neuropathies have been chronic, some exquisitely so, relatively mild, and occasionally asymmetric and distributed in a multiple nerve trunk pattern. Either prednisone or chlorambucil have at times led to reversal of neuropathy, although recovery has usually been incomplete.

Uremic polyneuropathy Some uremic patients whose renal impairment is chronic will develop a slowly progressive sensorimotor paralysis of the legs and then of the arms. Almost as frequently, the polyneuropathy has developed subacutely. Muscle atrophy, areflexia, and distal distribution in the limbs of neurologic defect leave little doubt of the peripheral nerve character of the disorder. Improvement has been observed after treatment on the artificial kidney, and recovery is the rule after successful renal transplantation. The CSF protein level may be moderately elevated (50 to 150 mg per 100 ml).

The pathology is that of a nonspecific degeneration of large myelinated fibers in nerves and spinal roots. Axons degenerate with the expected chromatolysis of their cell bodies. Amyloid deposit in the nerve has not been found; there is no evidence of vitamin deficiency or of diabetes during life and no sign of polyarteritis nodosa at autopsy. The neuropathy has been observed with all types of chronic kidney disease.

Beriberi In all the regions of the world where nutrition is borderline and treatment for an evolving beriberi may of necessity be delayed or even impossible to obtain, the motor paralysis and atrophy of the legs and, to a lesser extent, thighs and arms may reach an extreme degree. Thus this disease, though subacute in its evolution, becomes a frequent cause of chronic polyneuropathy. Uncontrolled diabetes may behave similarly.

Chronic polyneuropathy with connective tissue diseases In a clinic where many patients with connective tissue disease are being studied, occasional examples of either subacute or chronic polyneuropathy or a mononeuropathy have appeared. The latter are usually related to rheumatoid arthritis and are difficult to distinguish from pressure palsies clinically. The polyneuropathy is diffuse, often symmetric, and variably painful. Little is known of its cause, mechanism, or pathology. Some of the most extremely painful polyneuropathies we have seen, extending over long periods of time, have had only minimal sensory loss, weakness, or reflex change in some part of the body, and the diagnosis has been difficult. An unexpected rise in CSF protein level or electromyographic evidence of denervation may sometimes prove to be important leads. Occasionally a chronic symmetric polyneuropathy may accompany lupus erythematosus. It may be due to a small-vessel arteritis. Perhaps more of the obscure polyneuropathies fall into this group of connective tissue diseases than is presently realized.

Amyloidosis with chronic polyneuropathy As was pointed out in Chap. 107, primary amyloidosis may occur as a sporadic or a familial disease, the latter being particularly common in Portugal and Brazil. The polyneuropathy usually begins in middle adult life, is often severe, and is usually preceded by gastrointestinal symptoms (anorexia, indigestion, diarrhea). Sensory and motor nerve fibers are affected; in the familial varieties autonomic disturbance may predominate. Symmetry of involvement is the rule. The tongue may be enlarged and weak, and ocular muscles may be paretic. Cerebrospinal fluid protein level is elevated. The diagnosis is suggested by the clinical picture, the polyneuropathy being combined with hepatomegaly (often jaundice), anemia, cardiac enlargement, and EEG change. The nerves are probably enlarged in some patients. Restricted syndromes (eye muscles, tongue, etc.) are known.

Leprous polyneuritis This is the classic example of an infectious neuritis, for the inflammatory reaction in the nerve is evoked by the leprous bacillus. In the early stages of the disease, the neuropathic process is restricted. The nerves most involved are ulnar, greater auricular, tibial, supraorbital, and peroneal. As a rule the condition is painless. The symptoms are principally those of sensory loss or paresis. Anesthesia permits unrecognized injury, infections, trophic changes, and loss of digits. The nerves may be palpably enlarged and beaded.

Diagnosis depends on the character of the clinical picture, skin and nerve changes often being associated.

See Chap. 157 for diagnostic tests and therapy.

GENETICALLY DETERMINED NEUROPATHIES

Two chronic familial polyneuropathies (peroneal muscular atrophy and progressive hypertrophic polyneuropathy) have been recognized for many years, but in neither has an associated metabolic disturbance been discovered. Several other genetically determined neuropathies have been described (Refsum's disease, abetalipoproteinemia, metachromatic leukodystrophy, and Tangier disease) with which a known metabolic disorder is associated. Familial amyloidosis with neuropathy also belongs to the group and is discussed above.

Peroneal muscular atrophy (Charcot-Marie-Tooth disease) This is a dominant hereditary disease with onset during adolescence or adult years. There is chronic degeneration of peripheral nerves and roots, resulting in distal muscle atrophy, beginning in the feet and legs and later involving the hands. Early symptoms are muscular wasting and weakness affecting the extensor and abductor muscles of the feet and producing an equinovarus deformity. Later, all muscles below the middle third of the thigh may atrophy, resulting in a "stork leg" appearance of the legs. After a period of years, atrophy of hand and forearm muscles develops. The wasting seldom extends above the elbows or above the middle third of the thighs. The feet are short and arched, sometimes with perforating ulcers. Pain, paresthesias, and cramps are common. The objective sensory disorder is usually rather slight. There is impairment of position and vibratory sensation in the feet, and touch and pain sensation are lost in the feet. Reflexes are absent in the involved limbs. The progression of the illness is very slow, and it may arrest at any stage (see Chap. 333 for more complete descriptions).

Progressive hypertrophic polyneuropathy (Dejerine-Sottas disease) This type of neuropathy is uncommon and is frequently familial, with a recessive type of inheritance pattern. It begins usually in childhood and is slowly progressive. Pain and paresthesias in the feet are early symptoms, followed by development of symmetric weakness and wasting of the distal portion of the limbs. Sensation is impaired in a distal distribution, and the tendon reflexes are absent. Miotic pupils, nystagmus, and kyphoscoliosis have been observed in some cases. Patients are usually confined to a wheelchair at an early age. Other patients present with a recurrent polyneuropathy and enlargement of peripheral nerves because of hypertrophy and proliferation of the cells of Schwann and fibroblasts. Hypertrophic changes in nerve are not specific for this condition, but may also occur diffusely in Refsum's disease (see below), certain forms of peroneal muscular atrophy, relapsing polyneuropathy, or in a single nerve or multifocal distribution, and possibly in diabetes mellitus. Palpable thickening of the ulnar and peroneal nerves may be conspicuous. In the absence of palpable enlargement of nerves, the diagnosis can be established by biopsy of a cutaneous nerve. The treatment is symptomatic.

Chronic polyneuropathy with ichthyosis, deafness, and retinitis pigmentosa (Refsum's disease) This rare, genetically determined disorder begins in childhood or early adolescence, and the polyneuropathy is sensorimotor, distal, and symmetric in distribution, affecting legs more than arms. Although the nerves may not be enlarged clinically, hypertrophic changes with "onion-bulb" formation are an unfailing pathologic feature. The metabolic defect has been shown to be tissue accumulation of phytanic acid, a tetramethylated 16-carbon fatty acid. The relation between this biochemical lesion and the polyneuropathy remains uncertain. Diets low in phytanic acid may be beneficial.

Abetalipoproteinemia (Bassen-Kornzweig syndrome; acanthocytosis) (see also Chap. 106) The clinical manifestations of this unusual syndrome include (1) near absence of beta-lipoprotein in the serum; (2) retinitis pigmentosa; (3) acanthocytosis of the red blood cells; and (4) a chronic, progressive neurologic deficit, usually beginning in childhood. Extreme proprioceptive sensory loss, ataxia, and areflexia are the most constant features, although muscular weakness and atrophy, kyphoscoliosis, and corticospinal signs may also be encountered. The main burden of the neurologic disorder falls upon the peripheral nervous system, but the relation between the neuropathy and the deficiency of beta-lipoprotein remains unknown.

Tangier disease (see also Chap. 106) In this rare familial disorder, which is marked by alpha-1-lipoprotein deficiency, some cases have had neuropathic symptoms and signs of a relapsing nature and denervation atrophy of muscle.

Metachromatic leukodystrophy (see also Chap. 333) Massive sulfatide accumulation throughout the central and peripheral nervous systems, and to a lesser extent in other organs, occurs in this disorder, apparently because of congenital absence of the degradative enzyme, sulfatase. The abnormality is transmitted as an autosomal recessive trait. Progressive cerebral deterioration is the most obvious clinical aspect, but hyporeflexia, muscular atrophy, and diminished nerve conduction velocity indicate a neuropathic element. Metachromatically staining granules accumulate in the cytoplasm of Schwann cells in all peripheral nerves, as well as in central white matter. Sural biopsy may be used to establish the diagnosis, even early in the course of the illness.

RELAPSING POLYNEUROPATHY

Two diseases most regularly take this form: porphyria, in which the attacks recur because of the administration of barbiturates or spontaneous relapses, and idiopathic polyneuritis. The latter has no proved cause. Enlargement of nerves may occur in the latter disorder so that it is probable that some patients with hypertrophic polyneuropathy may fall into this category. Amyloidosis may also cause palpable enlargement of nerves, but by an obviously different mechanism.

MONONEUROPATHY OR MULTIPLE NEUROPATHY

This group of diseases differs in that one or a few of the nerves are involved in the disease process. The diagnosis rests on the finding of motor, reflex, or sensory changes confined to the territory of the nerve and the presence of other data pointing to its causation. A part of a plexus may also be involved. One variety, mononeuropathy multiplex, which has already been discussed, is due to leprosy, sarcoid, diabetes, and polyarteritis nodosa.

Common brachial and crural mononeuropathies

BRACHIAL PALSIES The fifth to eighth cervical and first thoracic spinal nerves innervate the muscles of the shoulder girdles and upper extremities. The brachial plexus is formed by components of these nerves, and lesions of the nerves or their branches result in characteristic palsies. The following are the brachial palsies most likely to be observed on the medical wards of a hospital.

Long thoracic nerve This nerve is derived from the fifth, sixth, and seventh cervical nerves and supplies the serratus magnus muscle. Paralysis of the serratus magnus muscle results in inability to raise the arm over the head from a forward position, and there is winging of the medial border of the scapula on pushing forward against resistance. It is injured most commonly by pressure on the shoulder, from either a sudden blow or prolonged pressure from carrying heavy weights. It is also involved at times in diabetic patients and as a manifestation of brachial and serum neuritides and in other idiopathic forms of neuritis (pleurodynia, Coxsackie disease).

Suprascapular nerve This nerve is derived from the fifth and sixth cervical nerves and supplies the supra- and infraspinatus muscles. Lesions may be diagnosed by the presence of weakness of abduction and external rotation of the arm and atrophy of the supra- and infraspinatus muscles. The nerve may be injured by blows on top of the head shoulder joint.

Upper brachial plexus paralysis This is due to injury to the fifth and sixth cervical nerves and roots caused most commonly by forceful separation of the head and shoulder during difficult delivery or by pressure in the supraclavicular region during anesthesia. The muscles affected are the biceps, deltoid, brachialis anticus, supinator longus, supra- and infraspinatus, and rhomboids. The arm hangs at the side, internally rotated, with the elbow extended. The forearm is pronated. Hand motion is unaffected. The prognosis for spontaneous recovery is generally good, especially in cases of birth injury. This condition as a result of birth injury (Erb-Duchenne brachial plexus palsy), which may persist throughout life, is discussed in Chaps. 17 and 334.

Lower brachial plexus paralysis This is due to injury to the eighth cervical and first thoracic roots as a result of traction on the abducted arm in falls, during operation, and with tumors of the apex of the lung (superior sulcus or Pancoast's syndrome). Injury may occur during birth (Dejerine-Klumpke brachial plexus injury). There is paralysis and wasting of the small muscles of the hand and a characteristic claw-hand deformity. Sensory loss is limited to the ulnar border of the hand and inner side of forearm, and there may be an associated paralysis of the cervical sympathetic nerve with a Horner's syndrome if the T_1 motor root is involved.

Lesions of the cords of the brachial plexus The outer and inner cords are most commonly affected. Dislocation of the head of the humerus, pressure of the cervical ribs, and stab wounds are the most frequent causes. Injury to the outer cord results in paralysis of the biceps and coracobrachialis muscles and all muscles supplied by the median nerve except the intrinsic hand muscles. There is some loss of sensation over the radial

aspects of the forearm. Involvement of the inner cord, as may occur in compression by the cervical rib, results in paralysis of the muscles supplied by the ulnar nerve together with the median-innervated intrinsic muscles of the hand and sensory loss over the ulnar aspect of the hand and forearm.

Axillary nerve This nerve arises from the posterior cord of the brachial plexus and supplies the teres minor and deltoid muscles. It may be involved in injuries resulting from fractures of the neck of the humerus, serum neuritis, brachial neuritis, or as a part of a disease of unknown cause. The anatomic localization depends on the recognition of a paralysis of abduction of the arm, wasting of the deltoid muscle, and slight impairment of sensation over the outer aspect of the shoulder.

Musculocutaneous nerve This nerve is derived from the fifth and sixth cervical nerves and is a branch of the outer cord of the brachial plexus. It innervates the biceps and brachialis anticus muscles. Lesions of the nerve result in weakness of elbow flexion. Rarely is it injured alone.

Radial nerve This nerve is derived from the fifth to eighth cervical nerves and is the termination of the posterior cord of the brachial plexus. It innervates the triceps muscle and the supinator and extensor muscles of the forehand and hand. Complete radial paralysis results in inability to extend the elbow, paralysis of supination of the forearm, and complete wrist and finger drop. Sensation is impaired over the posterior aspect of the forearm and a small area over the radial aspect of the dorsum of the hand. The nerve may be injured in the axilla, for example in "crutch" palsy, but most commonly traumatism occurs in the lower arm where the nerve winds around the humerus. Common types of injury at this site are fractures and pressure palsies incurred during sleep.

Median nerve This nerve is derived from the sixth cervical to the first thoracic root and is formed by the union of two heads from the inner and outer cords of the brachial plexus. It innervates the pronators of the forearm, long finger flexors, and abductor and opponens muscles of the thumb and is a sensory nerve to the palmar aspect of the hand. Complete median nerve paralysis results in wasting of the affected muscles and inability to pronate the forearm or deviate the hand in an ulnar direction, paralysis of flexion of the index finger and terminal phalanx of the thumb, weakness of flexion of the remaining fingers, weakness of abduction and opposition of the thumb, and sensory impairment over the radial two-thirds of the palmar aspect of the hand and over the distal phalanges of the dorsum of the index and third fingers. The nerve may be injured in the axilla by shoulder dislocation and in any part of its course by laceration, stab, or gunshot wounds. The wrist is the most common site of external injury. Compression of the nerve at the wrist (carpal tunnel syndrome) may occur secondary to prolonged occupational pressure or local infiltration, for example, by a thickening of connective tissue and deposit of amyloid with multiple myeloma. Other systemic diseases associated with carpal tunnel syndrome are acromegaly and hypothyroidism. Incomplete lesions of the median nerve between the axilla and wrist may result in *causalgia* (see Chap. 5).

Ulnar nerve This nerve is derived from the eighth cervical and first thoracic roots. It innervates the ulnar flexor of the wrist, the inner half of the deep finger flexors, the adductors and abductors of the fingers, the adductor of the thumb, the two medial lumbricals, and muscles of the hypothenar eminence. It is the sensory nerve to the fifth and ulnar half of the fourth fingers and the ulnar border of the hand. Complete ulnar paralysis results in a characteristic claw-hand deformity owing to wasting of the small hand muscle and hyperextension of the fingers at the metacarpophalangeal joints and flexion at the interphalangeal joints. The flexion deformity is most pronounced in the fourth and fifth fingers. Sensory loss occurs over the fifth finger, the ulnar aspect of the fourth finger, and the ulnar border of the palm. The ulnar nerve is most commonly injured at the elbow because of fracture or dislocation involving the joint. *Delayed ulnar palsy* may occur many years after an injury to the elbow joint which has resulted in a cubitus valgus deformity of the joint. Because of the deformity, the nerve is stretched in its course over the ulnar condyle. The superficial location of the nerve at the elbow makes it a common site of pressure palsy. Prolonged pressure on the outer part of the palm may result in damage to the deep palmar branch of the ulnar nerve, causing weakness of small hand muscles but no sensory loss.

CRURAL PALSIES The twelfth thoracic, first to fifth lumbar, and first, second, and third sacral spinal nerve roots compose the lumbosacral plexuses and innervate the muscles of the lower extremities and "saddle" region. The following are the common crural palsies.

Lateral femoral cutaneous nerve This nerve is derived from the second and third lumbar roots. It is a sensory nerve supplying the lateral aspect of the thigh. The nerve enters the thigh beneath the lateral end of the inguinal ligament and then enters the fascia lata, where it may become constricted. Compression of the nerve results in uncomfortable paresthesias along its cutaneous distribution and in sensory impairment. The condition is called *meralgia paresthetica* (mentioned below).

Obturator nerve This nerve is derived from the second, third, and fourth lumbar roots. It supplies the adductor muscles of the thigh, and injury to the nerve results in almost complete paralysis of adduction of the thigh. The nerve is most frequently injured during the course of a difficult labor and also as a result of dislocation of the hip or an obturator hernia. It may be affected in diabetes, polyarteritis nodosa, osteitis pubis, retroperitoneal carcinoma of the cervix of the uterus, and other tumors, etc.

Femoral nerve This nerve is derived from the second, third, and fourth lumbar roots. It supplies the iliacus, pectineus, sartorius, and quadriceps muscles and carries sensory impulses from the anteromedial aspect of the thigh and medial side of the lower leg. Following injury to the nerve, there is paralysis of extension of the knee, with wasting of the quadriceps muscle and also some weakness of hip flexion. The knee jerk is abolished. The nerve may be involved in fractures and dislocation of the hip and in fractured pelvis. It may be affected in diabetes, polyarteritis nodosa, and in retroperitoneal, pelvic, or abdominal lesions such as psoas abscess or tumor. Because of the femoral triangle, wounds in this region may be fatal.

Sciatic nerve This nerve is derived from the fourth and fifth lumbar and first, and second sacral roots. It provides the motor innervation of the hamstring muscles and all those below the knee; it carries sensory impulses from the posterior aspect of the thigh and posterior and lateral aspects of the leg and entire sole. In complete sciatic paralysis, the knee cannot be flexed and all muscles below the knee are paralyzed. The sciatic nerve is commonly injured in fractures of the pelvis or femur, in gunshot wounds of the buttock and thigh, and by the inadvertent injection of toxic substances such as paraldehyde. It may also be involved by pelvic tumors and in both diabetes mellitus and polyarteritis nodosa. Cryptogenic forms also occur and are actually more frequent than those with an identifiable cause. A ruptured lumbar disk often simulates sciatic neuropathy. Incomplete lesions of the sciatic nerve occasionally result in causalgia.

Common peroneal nerve This nerve is one of the terminal divisions of the sciatic nerve in the popliteal fossa. It supplies the dorsiflexors of the foot and toes and everters of the foot and sensation to the dorsum of the foot and lateral aspect of the lower half of the leg. These functions are lost with lesions which completely interrupt the nerve. Pressure or sleep palsy is one of the most frequent types of injury, the compression being of that part of the nerve which passes over the head of the fibula. It is also commonly involved by fractures involving the upper end of the fibula and in diabetic neuropathy.

Tibial nerve This nerve is the other of the two terminal divisions of the sciatic nerve in the popliteal fossa. It supplies all the calf muscles and the flexors of the foot. Complete paralysis of the nerve results in a calcaneovalgus deformity of the foot, which no longer can be plantar-flexed. There is loss of sensation over the plantar aspect of the foot.

SOME DISEASES WHICH INVOLVE SINGLE NERVES OR PLEXUSES

INFECTIONS In faucial diphtheria, selective involvement of the vagi and nerves to the ciliary muscles of the eye results in palatal paralysis and paralysis of accommodation. The palatal palsy occurs in the first 2 weeks of infection and the loss of accommodation about a week later. Both tend to improve rapidly. In cutaneous diphtheria, involvement of nerves locally results in paralysis of the muscles supplied by the spinal segment from which the infected region is innervated. In leprosy, granulomatous involvement of skin and cutaneous nerves, particularly in the cooler parts of the body, dominates the clinical picture. Several nerves become involved at sites where they lie superficially, for instance, the median nerve at the wrist, the ulnar nerve at the elbow, and the peroneal nerve on the dorsum of the foot. Herpes zoster is a sensory neuritis of viral etiology, characterized by acute inflammation of one or more posterior root ganglions, spinal nerves, and roots and gray matter of the spinal cord. Lancinating pain and hyperalgesia over the skin surface supplied by affected roots occur for 3 or 4 days, followed by the appearance of a segmental herpetic eruption. If the inflammatory process spreads to involve adjacent motor roots of anterior horns of the cord, segmental motor weakness and wasting disappear. Paralysis of the oculomotor nerves may occur in conjunction with involvement of the gasserian ganglion (opthalmoplegic zoster). Facial paralysis may occur with involvement of the geniculate ganglion (Ramsay Hunt syndrome). Sarcoidosis may involve single or multiple peripheral nerves, producing asymmetric mononeuritis or polyneuritis. Unilateral or bilateral facial paralysis is common in association with parotitis and uveitis in sarcoidosis.

TRAUMA External trauma may result in complete transection of a peripheral nerve or may impair conduction without interrupting the anatomic continuity of the involved nerve. Complete division of a mixed peripheral nerve results in paralysis and sensory loss corresponding to the region supplied by the damaged nerve. Recovery of function after complete division can take place only when the divided ends lie in apposition or have been sutured. Growth of nerve fibers from the center proceeds at a rate of 1 to 2 mm a day, and the recovery time can be estimated by the distance between the site of injury and the destination of the nerve. An early indication of regeneration is the presence of tingling sensation below the lesion (Tinel's sign due to sensitivity of thinly myelinated fibers) on tapping the nerve. Sensory recovery precedes the return of motor power. All forms of cutaneous sensation begin to return together. Appreciation of pain and temperature improves, but the stimuli are poorly localized for some time. Eventually there is recovery of the discriminative aspects of sensation, including localization of sensory stimuli, postural sense, recognition of slight differences in temperature, and appreciation of very light touch.

PRESSURE PALSIES AND ENTRAPMENT NEUROPATHIES A period of prolonged compression of a nerve against an underlying bone results in temporary paralysis owning to local ischemia. Mild degrees of compression are followed by fairly rapid recovery. Severe compression, such as may occur during a bout of alcoholic intoxication, deep sleep, or anesthesia, may result in focal disintegration of myelin, damage to axis cylinders, and Wallerian degeneration of distal segments. Recovery may be rapid by reversal of functional disorder or slow awaiting regeneration. Common varieties of pressure palsy are radial nerve paralysis with wrist drop due to prolonged pressure against the back of the arm (Saturday night palsy), ulnar palsy due to repeated trauma to the nerve at the elbow, especially after an old fracture that changes the relation of the nerve to the bicipital groove, and peroneal nerve palsy with foot drop caused by compression of the nerve against the fibula, as in sitting with legs crossed or during obstetric procedures with legs in stirrups.

The entrapment neuropathies result from repeated compression of a nerve against bone or a point where it passes through a narrow space. Slowly the perineurium and epineurium thicken and strangulate the nerve with injury to some of its larger, more peripheral, fibers. Several unique syndromes are known: (1) median nerve entrapment in carpal tunnel (see above); (2) *meralgia paresthetica.* This is a sensory neuropathy characterized by pain and paresthesia over the lateral aspect of the thigh because of compression of the lateral femoral cutaneous nerve in the fascia lata; (3) Morton's toe from pressure of plantar nerves giving rise to pain and paresthesia of third and fourth toes on walking. Pressure on nerve roots in the cervical and lumbar regions by *herniated intervertebral disks* results in pain, sensory impairment, and variable motor weakness corresponding to the area supplied by the involved root (see Chap. 9). Compression of the inner cord of the brachial plexus by a *cervical rib or by some other malformation of the thoracic outlet* (thoracic outlet syndrome) results in atrophy of small hand muscles and sensory loss in the ulnar nerve distribution. Usually the subclavian artery is compressed. When the median nerve is compressed at the wrist beneath the transverse carpal ligament (carpal tunnel syndrome), there are pain and paresthesias in the palmar surface of the hand and first three fingers, the naratrophy, weakness in flexor of thumb and opponens muscle, and sensory impairment over the median nerve distribution.

TUMOR Peripheral nerves may be compressed or invaded by primary or metastatic tumors arising in other tissues. Solitary tumors of nerve sheaths, or neuromas, commonly occur along the roots of spinal nerves, chiefly in the thoracic and lumbar regions. Compression of the nerve root and adjacent spinal cord may occur. Root compression causes pain referred to the distribution of the involved nerve, and there may be associated sensory impairment and motor weakness. Lymphomatosis and carcinomatosis of the cranial and spinal meninges may implicate single or multiple nerve roots. Tumor cells may be found in the cerebrospinal fluid. Solitary neuromas may involve any of the peripheral nerves, producing local pain and tenderness to palpation. Multiple neuromas occur in von Recklinghausen's disease and are associated with multiple congenital anomalies, as well as kyphoscoliosis, cutaneous pigmentation, and cutaneous fibromas. The treatment of solitary expanding nerve tumors of the limbs is wide excision with nerve graft or suture, if that is possible.

IDIOPATHIC NEUROPATHY *Bell's palsy* is due to inflammation of the facial nerve in the facial canal as a result of an obscure, possibly infective process. Edema may play a part leading to compression of nerve fibers, with resulting acute unilateral paralysis of facial muscles (see Chap. 324).

Brachial neuritis is an acute affection of the brachial plexus, characterized by the acute or subacute onset of severe pain in the neck, arm, and hand, followed by moderate muscle weakness, slight impairment of sensation in the fingers and hand, numbness or hyperesthesia, and depressed reflexes in the involved arm. The pain is usually severe and constant and is aggravated by moving the arm or stretching the brachial plexus. Muscle wasting is rarely severe, but some cases of brachial neuritis, especially those described by the term *neuralgic amyotrophy*, may be followed by localized paralysis and atrophy of the shoulder girdle and arm muscles. Some of these have a familial incidence. Recovery slowly occurs over a period of several weeks to months. Symptomatic treatment, including complete rest of the involved arm and analgesics in the acute phase, followed by mild massage and exercise, usually suffices.

Sciatic neuritis causes pain in the lumbar region and behind the leg from buttock to ankle. The pain is aching or burning in quality and is aggravated by movement or straining. The sciatic nerve is tender to palpation or stretching. There may be slight weakness of the hamstrings and muscles below the knee. The ankle jerk is absent. Sensory impairment is usually slight. It is necessary to distinguish the symptoms of sciatic neuritis from those of sciatic compression. In compression (e.g., by tumor) the onset is more gradual, symptoms are progressive, muscle wasting is more conspicuous, the nerve is less tender to palpation, and sensory loss is greater. The course of sciatic neuritis is stationary at first, followed by slow improvement.

Serum neuritis develops several days after the onset of serum sickness. The fifth cervical nerve root is most commonly involved, with pain, paralysis, and atrophy corresponding to the distribution of the nerve. Occasionally the entire brachial plexus may be involved, and there is sometimes, but rarely, a generalized polyneuritis. The cause is not known, but the condition is attributed to perineural edema, comparable to the urticaria of serum sickness, with compression of affected roots or nerves. Recovery is usually complete but may take weeks or months.

REFERENCES

Asbury AK et al: Uremic polyneuropathy. Arch Neurol 8:413, 1963

——et al: Acute idiopathic polyneuritis. Medicine 48:173-215, 1969

Dyck PJ: Peripheral neuropathy. Postgrad Med 41:279, 1967

Raff MC et al: Ischemic mononeuropathy multiplex in association with diabetes mellitus. Arch Neurol 18:487, 1968

Thomas PK, Lascelles RG: The pathology of diabetic neuropathy. J Med 35:489, 1966

324 DISEASES OF CRANIAL NERVES

MAURICE VICTOR
RAYMOND D. ADAMS

The cranial nerves are susceptible to many diseases that rarely if ever affect the spinal peripheral nerves, and for that reason alone they deserve to be considered separately. Reference has already been made to some of these diseases in Chaps. 19 and 20. But there the emphasis was on cardinal manifestations and the ways of demonstrating the disordered function. Here we are concerned with the principal syndromes in which the disordered functions of these nerves are expressed and the diseases which cause them.

SYNDROME OF ANOSMIA AND AGEUSIA AND RELATED DISORDERS OF OLFACTION The delicate filaments of the olfactory nerve, as they pass from the nasal mucous membrane through the cribriform plate of the ethmoid bone to the olfactory bulbs, are easily damaged by diseases of the nasal mucosa, skull fractures, and meningeal lesions. If unilateral, *hyposmia* or *anosmia*, as the defect is called, will not be recognized by the patient. Bilateral anosmia, on the other hand, is a frequent complaint, and the patient is usually convinced that he has lost sense of taste as well. This calls attention to the fact that much of taste is olfactory, and often it can be shown that such patients are able to distinguish perfectly the elementary taste sensations (sweet, sour, bitter, and salty). The olfactory defect can be verified readily enough by presenting the patient with a series of nonirritating olfactory stimuli (vanilla, lemon, cigarette, coffee, etc.), first in one nostril, then in the other, and asking him to distinguish between them. Ammonia and similar pungent substances should not be used because they stimulate the trigeminal nerve.

The sudden development of anosmia and impaired taste is related most often to a nasal infection. Little is known of its cause and nothing of its pathology. It may be transitory or permanent, and nothing can be done about it. In time the patient adjusts to the fact that the world no longer presents an interesting array of olfactory stimuli and that he no longer savors his food. Sometimes swelling of the mucous membranes by allergic rhinitis may intermittently interfere with olfaction. These nerve filaments may be ruptured by head injury, especially if it is severe enough to cause fracture; the damage may be unilateral or bilateral and is usually permanent. Cranial surgery (especially if much cerebrospinal fluid escapes while the patient is on his back so that the olfactory bulbs retract from the ethmoid bones), subarachnoid hemorrhage, and chronic meningeal inflammation may have a similar effect.

The gradual development of anosmia should prompt an investigation of the anterior base of the skull. Meningiomas of the olfactory region may not only implicate the olfactory nerves but may extend posteriorly to involve the optic nerves. Upward extension into the frontal lobes causes a lack of initiative (abulia), personality change (apathy, silliness, or witzelsucht), and forgetfulness. Large aneurysms of the anterior cerebral and anterior communicating arteries may produce a similar syndrome. Children with anterior meningoencephaloceles are usually anosmic and, in addition, may exhibit cerebrospinal fluid (CSF) rhinorrhea when the head is held in certain positions (demonstrated by examination of the fluid and by watching, under ultraviolet light, fluorescein issue from the nostrils after it has been instilled in the spinal subarachnoid space). Head injury, nasal injury, and hydrocephalus are other more frequent causes of CSF rhinorrhea.

Parosmia, or perversion of the sense of smell, may occur with local nasal conditions such as empyema of the nasal sinuses and ozena. It may also be a troublesome symptom in middle-aged and elderly persons who have depressive symptoms. Every article of food may have a horrid odor. Nothing is known of the basis of this state; there is no loss of discriminative sensation. Minor degrees of parosmia are not necessarily abnormal, for unpleasant odors have a way of lingering for several hours and of being reawakened by other olfactory stimuli, as every pathologist knows.

Olfactory hallucinations are always of central origin. As described in Chap. 24, a disagreeable odor may be the aura of a seizure. The evocative lesion is usually on the inferior and medial surface of one temporal lobe, in or near the uncus, and the seizure it produces is therefore called *uncinate*. Schizophrenic patients sometimes complain of smelling disagreeable odors about themselves, which they believe cause other persons to shun them. These olfactory sensations rarely have the objectivity of a hallucination but are rather in the nature of a delusion. The sense of smell is demonstrably intact.

SYNDROME OF RETROBULBAR NEUROPATHY The acute development of impaired vision in one eye or both eyes (in the latter case the eyes may be affected either simultaneously or successively) gives rise to a number of interesting and troublesome problems. The most frequent clinical setting is one in which a child, adolescent, or young adult notes a rapid diminution of vision in one eye (as though a veil or haze covered every object seen). The condition may progress to complete blindness. The optic disk and retina appear normal, but in some cases the optic disk is elevated or choked, and the disk margins are obscure and surrounded by hemorrhages (papilledema). Papillitis is distinguished from the papilledema of increased intracranial pressure by the effect on visual acuity. In retrobulbar neuropathy, after some few days or weeks the other eye may become similarly involved, the blindness then being complete except for slight peripheral vision. The pupillary light reflex is impaired. In a high percentage of patients, no cause can be found and after several more weeks there is spontaneous recovery. Vision may return to normal in more than two-thirds of all instances; occasionally a scotoma is left, or even blindness. The optic disk later becomes slightly pale in many of the patients. The CSF may be normal or may contain from 10 to 200 lymphocytes, and the protein level may be elevated.

Nearly half of such patients will develop other symptoms and signs consistent with multiple sclerosis within 10 to 15 years, and even more will do so if the patients are observed for longer periods. Less is known about children with retrobulbar neuropathy, but the prognosis for them is probably similar to that for adults. Formerly the syndrome was blamed on sinusitis and treated as such, but Cushing long ago proved the error of the assumption. Sinus disease rarely affects vision except for an occasional mucocele which presses on an ocular or optic nerve. Demyelination is the only common cause of a unilateral retrobulbar neuritis (see Chap. 331). Regression of symptoms has been observed to accompany the administration of ACTH (45 units per day for 3 weeks) or Meticorten (45 mg per day for 3 weeks).

Simultaneous impairment of vision in the two eyes, with central or centrocecal scotomas, usually is due not to a demyelinative process but rather to a toxic or nutritional disorder. The former condition (so-called "tobacco-alcohol amblyopia") is observed most commonly in the chronic alcoholic patient. Impairment of visual acuity evolves over several days or weeks, and examination discloses bilateral, roughly symmetric central or centrocecal scotomas, the peripheral fields being intact. With appropriate treatment (nutritious diet and B vitamins), partial or complete recovery is possible, although some patients are left with a permanent defect in central vision and pallor of the temporal portions of the optic disks. The same disorder may be seen in nonalcoholic patients, under conditions of severe nutritional deprivation and in pernicious anemia. Impairment of vision due to methyl alcohol intoxication is more abrupt in onset and is characterized by large symmetric central scotomas, as well as by symptoms of systemic disease and acidosis (see Chap. 111). Treatment is directed mainly to correction of the acidosis.

Rarely amblyopia is due to cranial arteritis, some other vascular disease, or diabetes. Congenital and hereditary forms of optic atrophy are known. In the adult syphilitic meningitis may lead to optic neuritis and atrophy (see Chaps. 159 and 333).

SYNDROME OF BITEMPORAL HEMIANOPIA This type of visual disorder is usually related to a pituitary adenoma (ballooned sella shown in x-rays of the skull) but may also be due to craniopharyngiomas, saccular aneurysms of the circle of Willis, meningiomas of the tuberculum sellae (normal sella or thickened tuberculum by radiography), and rarely sarcoidosis, metastatic carcinoma, and Hand-Schüller-Christian disease. The lesion is always in the chiasm, involving the decussating nasal fibers from each retina.

SYNDROMES OF HOMONYMOUS HEMIANOPIA See Chap. 20.

SYNDROME OF VISUAL AGNOSIA See Chap. 27.

SYNDROME OF OPHTHALMOPLEGIA Rarely, children or adults may have one or more attacks of ocular palsy in conjunction with an otherwise typical migraine (*migrainous ophthalmoplegia*). The muscles innervated by the oculomotor or, less often, the abducens nerve are affected. Presumably, intense vascular spasm in branches of the ophthalmic artery causes a transitory ischemia of nerve. Arteriograms, done after the onset of the palsy, usually reveal no abnormality. Recovery is the rule.

The acute development of a sixth or third nerve palsy on one side is a relatively common occurrence in the adult. The pupil is usually spared. In more than half the patients so affected no cause can be assigned; fortunately, most of them recover in a few weeks to months. Other patients prove to have diabetes mellitus or, rarely, cranial arteritis; in these instances the disorder may be ascribed to vascular occlusion. Exophthalmic ophthalmoplegia and myasthenia gravis must always be ruled out.

The slow development of a complete ophthalmoplegia is most often due to an aneurysm, tumor, or inflammatory process in the cavernous sinus or at the superior orbital foramen (syndrome of Foix) (see Table 324-1).

Gaze palsies or mixed ophthalmoplegia and gaze palsies, due usually to vascular, demyelinative, or neoplastic processes in the brainstem, have already been discussed in Chap. 20.

SYNDROME OF FACIAL PAIN (TRIGEMINAL NEURALGIA, TIC DOULOUREUX) The most striking disorder of the trigeminal nerve is tic douloureux. This occurs in middle-aged and elderly persons and consists of excruciating paroxysms of pain in the lips, gums, or chin, and, very rarely, in the distribution of the ophthalmic division of the fifth nerve. The pain seldom lasts more than a few seconds or a minute or two but may be so intense that the patient winces, hence the term *tic*. The paroxysm recurs frequently, both day and night, for several weeks at a time. Another characteristic feature is the initiation of pain by obvious stimuli applied to certain areas on the face, lips, or tongue, or by movement of these parts, the so-called "trigger zones." Sensory loss cannot be demonstrated in these cases. In studying the relationship between stimuli applied to the trigger zone and the pain paroxysm, it is found that the adequate stimulus for precipitating an attack is touch and possibly tickle, rather than pain or temperature. Usually a spatial and temporal summation of impulses is necessary to trigger an attack, which is followed by a refractory period of up to 2 or 3 min. This suggests that the mechanism for the paroxysmal pain involves the nucleus of the spinal tract of the fifth nerve.

The diagnosis of this disorder must rest upon these strict clinical criteria, and the condition must be distinguished from other forms of facial and cephalic neuralgia and pain arising from diseases of the jaw, teeth, or sinuses. Tic douloureux is usually without assignable cause, although occasionally it is a manifestation of multiple sclerosis (may be bilateral) or of herpes zoster. Very rarely a tumor in the posterior fossa which has caused only an early irritative lesion in the nerve or its root may produce pain clinically indistinguishable from that of tic douloureux. Usually, however, space-occupying lesions, such as aneurysms, neurofibromas, or meningiomas, produce a loss of sensation.

The conventional treatment for tic douloureux is alcohol or phenol injection of the affected nerve at the foramen ovale and rotundum or section of the root of the trigeminal nerve between the ganglion and the brainstem. Stereotaxic electrolyte lesions have also been made. Antiepileptic drugs such as diphenylhydantoin (Dilantin) and 5-carbamoyl-5*H*-dibenz(*b, f*) azepine (Tegretol) have been found to suppress or shorten the duration of the attacks. Temporizing and using these drugs may permit a spontaneous remission to occur. Most of the patients with severe pain come to surgery.

Anesthesia and analgesia of the face may be induced by stilbamadine (in the treatment of kala-azar and multiple myeloma) and trichloracetic acid intoxication. Pain and itching may occur during recovery. An idiopathic form of bitrigeminal anesthesia has also been observed, and leprosy may involve these nerves.

Tonic spasm of the masticatory muscles, known as *trismus*, is symptomatic of tetanus, although it may occur in patients treated with phenothiazine drugs; lesser degrees may be associated with disease of the pharynx and temporomaxillary joint, the teeth, and gums or may be a manifestation of encephalitis.

SYNDROME OF FACIAL PALSY (BELL'S PALSY) AND FACIAL SPASM The seventh cranial nerve is mainly a motor nerve supplying all the muscles concerned with facial expression on one side. The sensory component is small (the nervus intermedius of Wrisberg); it

TABLE 324-1
Cranial nerve syndromes

Site	*Cranial nerves involved*	*Eponym*	*Usual cause*
Sphenoidal fissure	III, IV, ophthalmic V, VI, sometimes II		Invasive tumors of sphenoid bone, aneurysms
Lateral wall of cavernous sinus	III, IV, ophthalmic V, VI, often with proptosis	Foix's syndrome	Aneurysms of cavernous sinus, cavernous sinus thrombosis, invasive tumors from sinuses and sella turcica
Petrosphenoidal space	II, III, IV, V, VI	Jacob's syndrome	Large tumors of middle cranial fossa
Apex of petrous bone	V, VI	Gradenigo's syndrome	Petrositis, tumors of petrous bone
Internal auditory meatus	VII, VIII		Tumors of petrous bone (dermoids, etc.), infectious processes
Pontocerebellar angle	V, VII, VIII, and sometimes IX		Acoustic neuromas, meningiomas
Jugular foramen	IX, X, XI	Vernet's syndrome	Tumors and aneurysms
Posterior laterocondylar space	IX, X, XI, XII	Collet-Sicard syndrome	Tumors of parotid gland, carotid body, and secondary tumor
Posterior retroparotid space	IX, X, XI, XII, and Bernard-Horner syndrome	Villaret's syndrome	Tumors of parotid gland, carotid body, secondary tumor, lymph node tumors, tuberculous adenitis

conveys taste sensation from the anterior two-thirds of the tongue and probably cutaneous sensation from the anterior wall of the external auditory canal. The taste fibers originally traverse the lingual nerve (a branch of the mandibular) but then leave this nerve to join the chorda tympani. Secretomotor fibers innervate the lacrimal gland through the greater superficial petrosal nerve, and others travel to the sublingual and submaxillary glands via the chorda tympani.

Several other anatomic facts are worth remembering. The motor nucleus of the seventh nerve is anterior and lateral to the abducens nucleus, and in their intrapontine course the facial nerve fibers hook around the abducens nucleus before they emerge from the pons at a point just lateral to the corticospinal tract. After leaving the pons they enter the internal auditory meatus with the acoustic nerve. The facial nerve then bends sharply forward and downward around the anterior boundary of the vestibule of the inner ear. At this angle lies the sensory ganglion (named *geniculate* because of its close proximity to the genu). The nerve continues its course in its own bony channel, the facial canal, and makes its exit from the skull at the stylomastoid foramen. It then passes through the parotid gland and subdivides to supply the facial muscles, the stylomastoid, and the posterior belly of the digastric muscle. Within the facial canal, just distal to the geniculate ganglion, it gives off the branch to the sphenopalatine ganglion, i.e., the greater superficial petrosal nerve, and somewhat more distally it gives off a small branch to the stapedius and is joined by the chorda tympani.

A complete interruption of the facial nerve at the stylomastoid foramen paralyzes all muscles of facial expression. The corner of the mouth droops, the creases and skin folds are effaced, the forehead is unfurrowed, the palpebral fissure is widened, and the eyelids will not close. Upon attempted closure of the lids, the eye on the paralyzed side is seen to roll upward (Bell's phenomenon). The lower lid sags also, and the punctum falls away from the conjunctiva, permitting tears to spill over the cheek. Food collects between the teeth and lips, and saliva may dribble from the corner of the mouth. The patient complains of a heaviness or numbness in the face, but no sensory loss is demonstrable and taste is intact.

If the lesion is in the facial canal above the junction with the chorda tympani but below the geniculate ganglion, all the above symptoms occur and, in addition, taste is lost over the anterior two-thirds of the tongue on the same side. If the nerve to the stapedius is paralyzed, there is hyperacusis (painful sensitivity to loud sounds), and the sound produced by moving the jaw and facial muscles is no longer present in the ear on the affected side. If the geniculate ganglion or the motor root proximal to it is involved, lacrimation may be reduced. Lesions at this point may also affect the adjacent auditory nerve, causing deafness, tinnitus, or dizziness. Intrapontine lesions that paralyze the face usually affect the abducens nucleus and often the corticospinal and sensory tracts.

If the peripheral facial paralysis has existed for some time and return of motor function has begun but is incomplete, a kind of contracture may appear. The palpebral fissure becomes narrowed and the nasolabial fold deepens. Attempts to move one group of facial muscles result in contraction of all of them (associated movements or synkinesis). Facial spasms develop and persist indefinitely, being initiated by every facial movement. This condition, called *facial spasms*, may also appear in adults who have never had a Bell's palsy. Presumably it is due to a benign constrictive lesion of the seventh nerve, which results in volleys of motor impulses spreading to all the muscles of facial expression. Anomalous regeneration of the seventh nerve fibers may result in other curious disorders. If fibers originally connected with the orbicularis oculi become connected with the orbicularis oris, closure of the lids may cause a retraction of the mouth; or if fibers originally connected with muscles of the face later come to innervate the lacrimal gland, anomalous tearing (crocodile tears) may occur with any activity of the facial muscles, such as eating (Bogorad's syndrome). With the passage of time, the face and even the tip of the nose become pulled to the unaffected side.

The most common disease affecting the facial nerve is Bell's palsy, presumably due to an inflammatory reaction in or around the nerve near the stylomastoid foramen. The onset is acute, and the paralysis may evolve over a few hours, although pain behind the ear may have been present for a day or two. Occasionally taste sensation is lost, and more rarely hyperacusis is present. In some cases there is mild pleocytosis in the cerebrospinal fluid. Fully 80 percent of patients recover within a few weeks. Electromyographic evidence of denervation after 10 days indicates a long delay until regeneration occurs, and sometimes it is incomplete. Thus electromyography may be of value in distinguishing temporary conduction defects from a pathologic interruption in continuity of nerve fibers. Protection of the eye during sleep, massage of the weakened muscles, and a splint to prevent drooping of the lower part of the face are the measures generally employed in the management of such cases. The use of ACTH and the unroofing of the facial nerve in the facial canal have been tried in isolated cases, but the results are impossible to evaluate.

Tumors which invade the temporal bone (carotid body, cholesteatoma, dermoid) may produce a facial palsy, but the onset is insidious and the course progressive. The Ramsay Hunt syndrome, due to herpes zoster of the geniculate ganglion, gives a severe facial palsy associated with a vesicular eruption in the external auditory canal and other parts of the cranial integument; often the eighth cranial nerve is affected as well. Acoustic neuromas frequently involve the facial nerve. Vascular lesions or tumors are the common forms of pontine disease which may cause facial palsy. Bilateral facial paralysis (facial diplegia) occurs in acute idiopathic polyneuritis and in a variety of sarcoidosis known as *uveoparotid fever* (*Heerfordt's syndrome*). *Melkersson's syndrome* consists of a rarely encountered triad of recurrent facial paralysis, recurrent—and eventually permanent—facial (particularly labial) edema, and less constantly, plication of the tongue. The cause is unknown. In the Far East leprosy may be the cause.

All these forms of nuclear or peripheral facial palsy must be distinguished from the supranuclear type. In the latter the frontalis and orbicularis oculi muscles are involved less than those of the lower part of the face, since the upper facial muscles, unlike the lower ones, receive upper motor neuron innervation from both hemispheres. In supranuclear lesions there may be a dissociation of emotional and voluntary facial movements, and often some degree of paralysis of the arm and leg or an aphasia (in dominant hemisphere lesions) is conjoined.

A curious disorder is the *facial hemiatrophy of Romberg.* It occurs mainly in females and is characterized by a disappearance of fat in the dermal and subcutaneous tissues on one side of the face. It usually begins in adolescence or early adult years and is slowly progressive. In its advanced form the face is gaunt and the skin is thin, wrinkled, and rather dark. The hair may turn white and fall out, and the sebaceous glands become atrophic. The muscles and bones are as a rule not involved. The condition is probably a form of lipodystrophy, and the localization with a dermatome indicates the operation of some neural factor of unknown nature.

The facial muscles on one side may be affected by irregular clonic contractions of varying degree (*facial hemispasm*). This condition may be due to an irritative lesion of the facial nerve (e.g., an acoustic neuroma) or may represent a transient or permanent sequela to a Bell's palsy. It may be caused by a plaque of multiple sclerosis. In the most common form, however, the cause and pathology are unknown. An involuntary recurrent spasm of both eyelids (blepharospasm) may occur in elderly persons as an isolated phenomenon or with varying degrees of spasm of the facial muscles. Relaxant and tranquilizing drugs are of little help, although in many cases this disorder may subside spontaneously. In very severe and persistent instances, the only effective treatment has been crushing of the facial nerve innervation of the orbicularis oculi muscles.

SYNDROME OF AURAL VERTIGO AND MÉNIÈRE'S DISEASE *Ménière's disease,* or *Ménière's syndrome,* is the name applied to recurrent aural vertigo, accompanied by tinnitus and deafness. The latter symptoms may be absent during the initial attacks of vertigo, but they invariably assert themselves as the disease progresses and are increased in severity during an acute attack. With milder forms of the syndrome the patient may complain more of head discomfort and of difficulty in concentration than of vertigo and may be considered neurotic. Provided that deafness is not complete, the recruitment phenomenon can be demonstrated (see Chap. 20). Ménière's syndrome has its onset most frequently in the fifth decade of life, though young adults and the elderly are not spared. The pathologic changes in Ménière's syndrome are said to consist of a dilatation of the endolymphatic system which leads to a degeneration of the delicate vestibular and cochlear hair cells. The relation of these changes to paroxysmal disorder of labyrinthine function is unknown. During an acute attack, rest in bed is the most effective treatment, since the patient can usually find a position in which vertigo is minimal. Dimenhydrinate (Dramamine) or cyclizine (Marezine) in doses of 25 to 50 mg t.i.d. is useful in the more protracted cases. A low salt diet is still used in treatment, but its value is difficult to judge. Mild sedative and hypnotic drugs may help the anxious patient between attacks. Usually the deafness is progressive, and when it is complete, the vertiginous attacks cease. However, the course is variable, and if the attacks persist in a severe manner, permanent relief can be obtained by the administration of 10 to 12 g streptomycin in doses of 2 g per day or by surgical destruction of the labyrinth or section of the vestibular portion of the eighth nerve intracranially. Of course, the streptomycin effect is bilateral; hence it should not be used unless both sides are affected.

Another disorder of labyrinthine function is characterized by the occurrence of paroxysmal vertigo and nystagmus with the assumption of certain critical positions of the head. This is the *positional vertigo of Bárany,* of the so-called "benign paroxysmal type" (see Chap. 19).

There are many other causes of aural vertigo, such as purulent labyrinthitis complicating meningitis, serous labyrinthitis due to infection of the middle ear, "toxic labyrinthitis" due to drug intoxication (e.g., from alcohol, quinine, streptomycin, and salicylates), motion sickness, trauma, and hemorrhage into the internal ear. In these instances the attacks of vertigo tend to last longer than in the recurrent form, but in other respects the symptoms are similar. Streptomycin may damage the fine hair cells of the vestibular end organs and cause a permanent disorder of equilibrium.

There has been described a dramatic clinical syndrome, characterized by the abrupt onset of severe vertigo, nausea, and vomiting, without tinnitus or hearing loss. The vertigo persists for several days or weeks, and labyrinthine function is permanently ablated on one side. Occlusion of the labyrinthine division of the internal auditory artery would logically explain this syndrome, but so far postmortem confirmation of this idea has not been obtained.

Vertigo of vestibular nerve origin may occur with diseases that involve the nerve in the petrous bone or the cerebellopontine angle. Except that it is less severe and is less frequently paroxysmal, it has many of the characteristics of labyrinthine vertigo. The adjacent auditory division of the eighth cranial nerve may also be affected, which explains the frequent coincidence of tinnitus and deafness. The function of the eighth cranial nerve may be disturbed by tumors of the lateral recess (especially acoustic neuroma), as well as by meningeal inflammation in this region or, very rarely, by compression from an abnormal vessel.

Vestibular neuronitis and epidemic vertigo are the names that have been applied to a clinical syndrome which occurs mainly in young adults and is characterized by the abrupt onset of vertigo, nausea, and vomiting, without impairment of hearing.

A particular variety of paroxysmal vertigo of childhood has been described by Basser. The attacks of vertigo occur in a setting of good health and are of sudden onset and brief duration. Pallor, sweating, and immobility are prominent manifestations, and occasionally vomiting and nystagmus occur. No relation to head posture or movement has been observed. The attacks are recurrent but tend to cease spontaneously after a period of several months or years. The outstanding abnormal finding is demonstrated by caloric testing, which shows impairment or loss of vestibular function, bilateral or unilateral, frequently persisting after the attacks have ceased. Cochlear function is unimpaired. The pathologic basis of this disorder has not been determined.

Cogan has described a peculiar syndrome in young adults, in which a nonsyphilitic interstitial keratitis is associated with vertigo, tinnitus, nystagmus, and rapidly progressive deafness. The prognosis for life and vision is good, but the deafness is usually permanent. The causation of Cogan's disease is not understood, although several patients later developed periarteritis nodosa.

The question of *viral infections of cranial nerves* is always raised by these acute palsies of the facial, trigeminal, and auditory nerves, especially when the affection is bilateral, involves several nerves in combination, or is associated with pleocytosis of CSF. Actually, the only proved virus etiology in this group of cases is that of herpes zoster, and search for this virus from cases of Bell's palsy or of vestibular neuronitis has not been rewarding . Since perceptive deafness, vertigo, and other cranial nerve palsies have been observed in conjunction with the parainfectious encephalomyelitis of varicella, measles, rubella, mumps, and scarlet fever and also with Landry-Guillain-Barré syndrome, an allergic etiology must be considered. Nothing is known of the pathology of the peripheral lesion or of the localization of a virus in the nervous system in these diseases. We have studied a number of cases of acute bilateral facial palsy, or facial palsy, numbness, and deafness or vertigo on one side and pleocytosis of CSF without succeeding in isolating the causative agent. There is no treatment other than symptomatic; fortunately the prognosis for complete recovery is excellent.

SYNDROME OF DEAFNESS See Chap. 20.

SYNDROME OF GLOSSOPHARYNGEAL NEURALGIA Glossopharyngeal neuralgia is a syndrome which resembles trigeminal neuralgia in many respects. The pain is intense and paroxysmal; it originates in the throat, approximately in the tonsillar fossa. In some cases the pain is localized in the ear or may radiate from the throat to the ear, because of implication of the tympanic branch (Jacobson's nerve). Spasms of pain may be initiated by swallowing. There is no demonstrable sensory or motor deficit. A trial of Dilantin or Tegretol is the recommended therapy, but if this is unsuccessful, division of the nerve near the medulla is the treatment of choice.

Very rarely, herpes zoster may involve the glossopharyngeal nerve. One may occasionally observe a glossopharyngeal palsy in conjunction with vagus and accessory nerve involvement due to a tumor or aneurysm in the posterior fossa. Hoarseness due to vocal cord paralysis, some difficulty in swallowing, deviation of the soft palate to the sound side, anesthesia of the posterior wall of the pharynx, and weakness of the upper part of the trapezius and sternomastoid muscles comprise the syndrome (see Table 324-1, jugular foramen syndrome).

SYNDROME OF DYSPHAGIA AND DYSPHONIA Complete interruption of the intracranial portion of one vagus nerve results in a characteristic paralysis. The soft palate droops and does not rise in phonation. There is loss of the gag reflex on the affected side, as well as of the "curtain movement" of the lateral wall of the pharynx, whereby the faucial pillars move medially as the palate rises in saying "ah." The voice is hoarse, often nasal, and the vocal cord lies immobile in an abducted or cadaveric position. There may also be loss of sensibility at the external auditory meatus and back of the pinna. Usually no change in visceral function can be demonstrated.

Complete bilateral paralysis is said to be imcompatible with life, and this is probably true if the nuclei are involved in the medulla by poliomyelitis or some other disease. However, in the cervical region, both vagi have been blocked with procaine (Novocaine) for the treatment of intractable asthma, without mishap. The pharyngeal branches of both vagi may be affected in diphtheria; the voice has a nasal quality, and regurgitation of liquids through the nose occurs during the act of swallowing.

The vagus nerves, especially the left, are most often damaged as a result of thoracic disease. Aneurysm of the aortic arch, an enlarged left atrium, and tumors of the mediastinum and bronchi are much more frequent causes of an isolated vagus palsy than are intracranial disorders. The nerve may be implicated at the meningeal level by tumors and infectious processes and within the medulla by tumors and vascular lesions, e.g., the lateral medullary syndrome of Wallenberg, and by motor system disease. Herpes zoster may attack this nerve. Polymyositis and dermatomyositis, which cause hoarseness and dysphagia owing to direct involvement of laryngeal and pharyngeal muscles, may be confused with disease of the vagus nerves.

When confronted with a case of laryngeal palsy, the physician must attempt to determine the site of the lesion. If it is intramedullary, there are usually other signs, such as ipsilateral cerebellar signs, loss of pain and temperature sensation over the ipsilateral part of the face and contralateral arm and leg, and ipsilateral Bernard-Horner syndrome. If the lesion is extramedullary, the glossopharyngeal and spinal accessory nerves are frequently involved (jugular foramen syndrome). If it is extracranial in the posterior laterocondylar or retroparotid space, there may be a combination of ninth, tenth, eleventh, and twelfth cranial nerve palsies and Bernard-Horner syndrome. Combinations of these lower cranial nerve palsies are sometimes called the *syndrome of Collet-Sicard* and the *syndrome of Villaret,* respectively. If there is no sensory loss in the palate and pharynx, or no palatal weakness, the lesion is below the origin of the pharyngeal branches, which leave the vagus nerve high in the cervical region. The usual site of disease is then the mediastinum.

SYNDROME OF BULBAR PALSY This syndrome is the result of weakness or paralysis of those muscles which are supplied by the bulb or medulla oblongata, namely the tongue, pharynx, larynx, sternomastoid, and upper trapezius. If development is rapid, as may happen in diphtheria or poliomyelitis, there is no time for muscle atrophy. The more chronic disease, progressive bulbar palsy (a form of motor system disease), or tumors or aneurysms of the posterior fossa result in marked wasting and fasciculation of the tongue, sternomastoid, and trapezius muscles. The condition must be distinguished from progressive muscular dystrophy and a restricted form of

TABLE 324-2
Brainstem syndromes which involve cranial nerves

Eponym	*Site*	*Cranial nerves involved*	*Tracts and nuclei involved*	*Signs*	*Usual cause*
Weber's syndrome	Base of midbrain	III	Corticospinal tract	Oculomotor palsy with crossed hemiplegia	Vascular occlusion; tumor; aneurysm
Claude's syndrome	Tegmentum of midbrain	III	Red nucleus	Oculomotor palsy with contralateral cerebellar ataxia and tremor	Vascular occlusion; tumor; aneurysm
Benedikt's syndrome	Tegmentum of midbrain	III	Red nucleus and corticospinal tract	Oculomotor palsy with contralateral cerebellar ataxia, tremor, and corticospinal signs	Softening; hemorrhage; tuberculoma; tumor
Nothnagel's syndrome	Tectum of midbrain	Unilateral or bilateral III	Superior cerebellar peduncles	Ocular palsies, paralysis of gaze, and cerebellar ataxia	Tumor
Parinaud's syndrome	Tectum of midbrain	Supranuclear coordinating mechanism for upward gaze	Superior colliculi	Paralysis of upward and sometimes downward gaze; fixed pupils; divergence of eyes	Pinealoma
Millard-Gubler syndrome and Raymond-Foville syndrome	Base of pons	VII and often VI	Corticospinal tract	Facial and abducens palsy and contralateral hemiplegia; sometimes palsy of gaze to side of lesion	Softening or tumor
Avellis's syndrome	Tegmentum of medulla	X	Corticospinal tract Sometimes descending pupillary fibers, with Bernard-Horner syndrome	Paralysis of soft palate and vocal cord and contralateral hemiplegia	Softening or tumor
Jackson's syndrome	Tegmentum of medulla	X, XIII	Corticospinal tract	Avellis's syndrome plus ipsilateral tongue paralysis	Softening or tumor
Wallenberg's syndrome	Tegmentum of medulla	Spinal V, IX, X, XI	Lateral spinothalamic tract Descending pupillodilator fibers Spinocerebellar and olivocerebellar tracts	Ipsilateral V, IX, X, XI palsy, Bernard-Horner syndrome, and cerebellar ataxia Contralateral loss of pain and temperature sense	Occlusion of posteroinferior cerebellar artery

polymyositis which may be limited to neck muscles; these latter disorders seldom affect the tongue, however. It must also be differentiated from pseudobulbar palsy (see Chap. 17).

MULTIPLE CRANIAL NERVE PALSIES As will be readily understood, several cranial nerves may be affected by the same disease process. One of the clinical problems that arises is whether the disease lies within or outside the brainstem. Lesions lying on the surface of the brainstem usually are featured by an adjacent cranial nerve palsy (or a succession of them) and late and rather slight involvement of the long sensory and motor pathways and segmental structures lying within the brainstem. The opposite is true of intramedullary, intrapontine, and intramesencephalic lesions. The extramedullary lesion is more likely to cause bone erosion or enlargement of the foramens of exit (seen radiographically). The intramedullary lesion involving cranial nerves often produces a crossed sensory or motor paralysis (cranial nerve on one side, evidence of tract involvement on the other). In this way a number of distinctive syndromes to which eponyms have been attached are produced. These are listed in Table 324-1.

Involvement of multiple cranial nerves outside the brainstem is frequently the result of trauma (sudden onset), localized infections such as zoster (acute onset), granulomatous disease (subacute onset), or tumors and saccular aneurysms (chronic development). Of the tumors, neurofibromas, meningiomas, cholesteatomas, carcinomas, and sarcomas have all been reported. The chordoma (see Chap. 328) may implicate a succession of lower cranial nerves. Owing to their anatomic relationships, the multiple cranial nerve palsies form a number of distinctive syndromes, listed in Table 324-2.

From time to time one observes a benign form of multiple cranial nerve involvement on one or both sides of the face. The disease may recur over a period of years with variable degrees of recovery between attacks. Sarcoidosis is found to be the cause of some, and chronic glandular tuberculosis (scrofula), the cause of others. The condition is called *polyneuritis cranialis multiplex.* The malignant granuloma of the nasopharynx may also affect multiple cranial nerves, as do also nasopharyngeal tumors, platybasia, and adult Arnold-Chiari malformation. A purely motor disorder without atrophy raises the question always of myasthenia gravis (see Chap. 347).

REFERENCES

BRODAL A: *The Cranial Nerves,* Springfield, Ill.: Charles C Thomas, 1959

COGAN DG: *Neurology of the Ocular Muscles,* 2d ed., Springfield, Ill.: Charles C Thomas, 1956

——: *Neurology of the Visual System,* Springfield, Ill.: Charles C Thomas, 1966

MAYO CLINIC, STAFF: *Clinical Examinations in Neurology,* 2d ed., Philadelphia: Saunders, 1963

WOLFSON RJ (ed): *The Vestibular System and Its Diseases,* Philadelphia: University of Pennsylvania Press, 1966

325 DISEASES OF THE SPINAL CORD

FUAD SABRA
RAYMOND D. ADAMS

Diseases of the nervous system may at times limit themselves to the spinal cord and also produce a number of distinctive syndromes. This relates to special anatomic features such as great length in proportion to width, peripheral location of medullated fibers next to pia, tight envelopment by meninges, arrangement of blood vessels, and vertebras. Because of the frequency and gravity of these diseases, and the special difficulties attendant upon diagnosis, we have grouped them in a special chapter under a series of relatively common syndromes, the basis of which will be understood after reading Chaps. 17 and 21.

GLOBAL PARALYSIS OF LEGS OR ALL EXTREMITIES DUE TO MASSIVE TRANSVERSE LESION OF THE SPINAL CORD

This condition may best be considered in relation to trauma, one of the most frequent causes of it, but it also occurs with certain types of myelitis, infarction and hemorrhage in the spinal cord, and rapidly advancing compressive myelopathy.

INJURIES TO THE SPINE AND SPINAL CORD

Although injuries to the spinal cord may be the sole manifestation of a traumatic disease, it is seldom that the vertebral column is not harmed at the same time. Often there is an associated head injury, as is pointed out in Chap. 327.

A useful classification of spinal injuries is one which divides them into fracture-dislocations, pure fractures, and pure dislocations. The relative frequency of these types is about 3:1:1. Direct violence to the spine is an uncommon cause of vertebral disruption; except for stab and bullet wounds, most spine injuries are the result of force *applied at a distance.* All three types of injury are produced by a similar mechanism, usually a vertical compression of the spinal column to which flexion is almost immediately added. Or, in the neck the mechanism may be one of extension. The two important variables in the mechanics of vertebral injury are the nature of the bones and the strength, direction, and point of impact of the force.

Strength, direction, and point of impact of the force If the injuring body striking the cranium is hard and the velocity is high, a skull fracture occurs, the elastic quality of the skull absorbing the force of the injury. If the injuring body is soft yet heavy, the spine and particularly its cervical portion will be the part injured. If the neck happens to be rigid and straight and the force is quickly applied to the head, the atlas and the odontoid process of the axis may break. If the force is less quickly applied and removed, an element of flexion occurs. Flexion movement plus a vertical force constitute the essential factors in fracture-dislocation or pure dislocation.

The other common mechanism of cord injury, sudden extension of the neck, is called the *whiplash injury.* It is especially frequent in civilian motor accidents and in forward falls, and more often it affects supporting structures of the head than spinal nerves or cord. Cervical spondylosis adds to the hazard of spinal cord damage.

A special type of spine injury, occurring most often in military life, is that in which missiles of high velocity pass through the vertebral canal and destroy the spinal cord. In some cases they may strike the vertebral column without entering the spinal canal and agitate it so violently that the cord suffers injury. The term given to temporary spinal paralysis is *spinal concussion.* This condition may also be produced by violent falls flat on the back.

A study of 2,006 cases collected from the literature by Jefferson shows that most vertebral injuries occur at the first to second cervical, fourth to sixth cervical, and eleventh thoracic to second lumbar vertebras. Industrial accidents most often involve the dorsolumbar vertebras. Accidents caused by falling or with head down as in diving accidents, affect the cervical region. In the author's neuropathologic material, which contains 26 cases, the usual circumstances of spinal injury were a state of alcoholic intoxication and a fall down a flight of stairs, automobile accidents, crushing industrial accidents, gunshot or stab wounds, and birth injury, in that order of frequency. The majority of these fatal cases had fracture-dislocations or dislocations of the cervical spine.

Mechanism of spinal cord injury The spinal cord may escape injury even though there is vertebral dislocation, especially in regions where the spinal canal is large, i.e., in the cervical and lumbar regions. Rarely the spinal cord may be damaged without radiologic evidence of fracture or dislocation. One cannot easily determine the full extent of spinal injury by radiology or even at autopsy because of the difficulty in examining the vertebras. By far the most satisfactory technique for demonstrating the degree of spine injury and the presence of a tearing of ligaments with dislocation is the x-ray, taken laterally, but one must be careful to avoid flexion or extension of the neck which may inflict further injury to the spinal cord. The most frequently established mechanism is a vertebral dislocation with or without fracture. The upper vertebras are displaced anteriorly, and there is a break in the posterior longitudinal ligament and intervertebral disk. The spinal cord is most often subjected to a shearing force between the pedicles of the vertebra above and the body and laminae of the vertebra below the dislocation.

When the cervical spine is sharply extended, especially in the presence of cervical spondylosis, the damage to the spinal cord is due to the sudden narrowing of the spinal canal. The spinal cord is caught between the laminas of the lower vertebra and body of the higher one. Also, the ligamentum flavum may buckle and compress the cord. There may be no x-ray evidence of the spinal lesion.

In direct trauma of the spine, as when it is struck in some part by a bullet, the means of spinal concussion is said to be *agitation.* Little is known of the underlying pathology. This term has led to much confusion because it is not employed here in the usual sense of cerebral concussion, i.e., a transient interruption of neural function by trauma without perceptible structural change.

Pathology of spinal cord injury As a result of squeezing or shearing of the cord, there is destruction of gray matter and a variable amount of hemorrhage, chiefly in the more vascular parts. These changes are maximum at the level of injury and one or two segments above and below it. Rarely is the cord cut in two, and seldom is the piarachnoid lacerated. The condition is best designated as *traumatic necrosis of the spinal cord.* As the lesion heals, it results in cavitation or a gliotic focus. Separation of such pathologic entities as hematomyelia, concussion, contusion, and hematorrhachis is of little value either clinically or pathologically.

As with most lesions, the total disease picture is compounded of an irreversible structural lesion and a disorder of function, each of which may vary in degree. The extent and permanence of the clinical manifestations are determined by the relative proportions of these two. An exception to this statement might be made for gunshot wounds of the vertebras. Here the explosive force of the missile may shatter myelinated fibers with maximal functional disturbance.

CLINICAL EFFECTS OF SPINAL CORD INJURY The "classic" description of traumatic paraplegia by Riddock cannot be excelled. He divides the clinical picture into two stages: spinal shock and reflex activity.

Spinal shock or muscular flaccidity The loss of function which is inflicted at the time of injury (fourth to fifth cervical vertebras—quadriplegia, thoracic vertebras—paraplegia, both with paralysis of bladder and bowel sphincters and loss of sensibility below the level corresponding to the spinal lesion) is accompanied by a complete or almost complete suppression of reflex activity of all spinal segments below the lesion. This is the condition known as *spinal shock.* The plantar reflexes are first variable and may be absent, flexor, or extensor. The lower extremities lose heat if left uncovered and swell if dependent. Sweating is abolished. Cutaneous ulcerations may develop over bony prominences. Urine and feces are retained to the point where overflow or involuntary leakage results. Occasionally there is priapism because of venous congestion. A paralytic ileus may occur.

Reflex activity If the lumbosacral segments are undamaged, spinal shock wears off in 2 to 3 weeks. The first sign of this is contraction of the hamstrings and flexion or extension of the toes on plantar stimulation. Then gentle and later strong involuntary flexor spasms make their appearance. Ankle jerks and then knee jerks return. Retention of urine and feces becomes less complete, and at irregular intervals urine is expelled by active contraction of the detrusor muscle. Reflex defecation and sweating also return. At times flexor spasms and later extensor spasms, often accompanied by profuse sweating and micturition, all occur after stimulation of the skin, viz., the *mass reflex.* This stage of reflex activity may last for years unless sepsis intervenes, in which case the state of spinal shock may return.

Less complete lesions of the spinal cord may result in little or no spinal shock or extensor spasm. Incomplete voluntary motor paralysis, a flaccid atrophic paralysis, variable sensory impairment in the arms, a spastic weakness of the legs, and a partial or complete Brown-Séquard syndrome are some of the resulting clinical pictures.

The final result may be permanent and complete disability, rarely consistent with survival for more than a short time (days, weeks, months); or a gradual improvement and complete or almost complete recovery may occur. Any residual symptoms after 6 months are likely to be permanent.

The level of the cord lesion can be determined by the clinical picture. A complete paralysis of arms and legs usually indicates a dislocation at the fourth to fifth cervical vertebras. If the legs are paralyzed and the arms can still be abducted and flexed, the dislocation is likely to be at the fifth to sixth cervical. Paralysis only of hands and of legs indicates the level of vertebral disorder to be the sixth to seventh cervical. When the motor paralysis involves muscles above the knees and sensory loss includes the twelfth thoracic dermatome, the site is the eleventh to twelfth thoracic. If the paralysis is below the knees and the first lumbar escapes, the lesion is at the twelfth thoracic, first lumbar vertebras. Prognosis for the latter group of patients, with preponderantly cauda equina lesions, is better than for those with injury to the eleventh to twelfth thoracic vertebras. In all cases of spinal cord injury any elicitable movement or preserved sensation during the first 48 to 72 hr gives a favorable prognosis for recovery.

Treatment In general, the treatment for spinal cord injuries is conservative and symptomatic. The degree of injury can be lessened by assuring that no movement of cervical spine (especially flexion) is made from the moment of the accident. Corticosteroid therapy, as for brain swelling (Chap. 327), may reduce the swelling of spinal cord tissue. If the spinal cord injury is associated with dislocation of the vertebras, traction on the neck is necessary to secure proper alignment. This is accomplished by a head halter attached through the head of the bed over a pulley to a weight of 10 to 15 lb or, even better, the use of tongs which fasten onto the skull (Crutchfield). In thoracic crush injuries, hyperextension can be maintained by placing a narrow pillow under the affected area. Traction should be continued for 4 to 6 weeks, and then a brace may be substituted. In some centers for the treatment of spinal cord injury early fixation and traction of spine have almost completely replaced decompression by laminectomy. The aftercare of patients with paraplegia and disturbance of vesical or rectal function is similar to that of patients with like symptoms from other causes. Decubitus ulceration can be prevented by special skin care. Tidal drainage is a valuable adjunct in preventing infection, stone formation, and contracture and in securing return of function. Daily enemas are usually the most effective means of controlling fecal incontinence. Physiotherapy, muscle reeducation, and the application of proper braces are all important in the rehabilatation of the patient. All this is best carried out in centers for rehabilitation of spine injuries.

MYELITIS The spinal cord appears to be vulnerable to three types of inflammatory processes, all of which have been called *myelitic*. First there are the specific viral infections which tend to involve principally the gray matter (hence called *poliomyelitic*). Zoster and the three viruses of poliomyelitis are the most frequent examples. Secondly, all the subacute and chronic primary meningeal infections may induce damage of the spinal roots and outer surfaces of the spinal cord, i.e., to the white matter of posterior, lateral, and anterior funiculi (meningoradiculitis and meningomyelitis), or there may be occlusion of meningeal vessels. Syphilis offers the best known and most numerous examples of this category of inflammatory diseases, viz., tabes dorsalis (which is essentially a treponemal lumbosacral meningoradiculitis), syphilitic meningomyelitis, and arteritis with myelomalacia. Tuberculous meningitis and fungous meningitis provide other examples. Thirdly, there is a group of primary inflammations of white matter, the leukomyelitides. Although the white (and gray) matter may be the site of an infective inflammatory process as in abscess, tuberculoma, gumma and parasitic inflammations, such conditions are rare. Most of the leukomyelitides are of unknown cause. Three varieties of the latter have been delineated: (1) Postinfectious and postvaccinial myelitis, (2) demyelinative myelitis (acute or chronic relapsing multiple sclerosis), and (3) acute or subacute necrotizing myelitis.

Whereas any one of the above forms of chronic meningitis or leukomyelitis may induce the clinical picture of a tranverse cord lesion, this lesion is usually due to one of the demyelinative or necrotizing forms of myelitis. A painless (rarely painful) paraplegia, beginning simultaneously in both legs, or more often first in one leg and then the other, or in sacral segments, ascends to the abdomen and thorax. Either sensory or motor symptoms may initiate the disease, but both are present as it progresses. Like all cord lesions with involvement of tracts, the loss of sensory and motor function affects all parts of the body below a certain level, and sphincters as well and, if acute, overflow incontinence and obstipation are included. In only a few patients will vaccination against smallpox, or rabies inoculation, or a frank chickenpox or measles be found to have preceded the neurologic symptoms by days to 1 to 2 weeks; in all the rest, the illness develops without explanation. The conjunction of retrobulbar neuritis with the cord lesion is called *neuromyelitis optica* or *Devic's disease*. This is not a disease but a syndrome occurring in necrotizing myelitis (usual cause), multiple sclerosis, and postinfectious myelitis. If the spinal cord lesion is severe and paralysis is complete, spinal shock supervenes, with the same flaccidity and areflexia of legs mentioned under spinal cord trauma. The CSF may be normal or may contain lymphocytes and mononuclears (numbering from 20 to 1,000 or more per ml), and the protein is sometimes raised. If the cord lesion swells, as it rarely does, there may be a dynamic block (positive Queckenstedt test). When the latter is found, it always suggests the possibility of an *epidural spinal abscess*, another important and treatable cause of the rapid development of a transverse cord lesion with spine ache and fever.

Treatment of the demyelinative and necrotizing myelitides consists of ACTH (40 units twice a day for a week, then once a day for 2 to 3 weeks) or prednisone (60 mg per day for 3 weeks). Improvement usually occurs, but the relation to therapy is uncertain. Except for patients with the postinfectious form of myelitis there is always danger of later progression or relapse. Prevention of decubitus ulceration, early catheterization and bladder care, and rehabilitation measures, the usual procedures in the management of the paraplegia patients, must also be employed.

SPINAL EPIDURAL ABSCESS Children or adults may be affected. An injury to the back, often trivial, at the time of a furunculosis or other skin infection or a bacteremia may permit seeding of the spinal epidural space or of vertebral body. The latter gives rise to osteomyelitis with extension to the epidural space. The suppurative process is accompanied at first only by fever and aching in the region of the spine and later by radicular pain. After several days or a few weeks there is a rapid onset and progression of paraplegia, sensory loss in the lower parts of the body, urinary and fecal retention, and sphincteric incontinence. Percussion of the spine elicits tenderness over the site of the infection. Examination reveals all the signs of transverse cord lesion with spinal shock. The CSF contains small numbers of cells (neutrophilic leukocytes and lymphocytes), and the protein is relatively high (100 to 400 mg per ml). More importantly there is a dynamic block (positive Queckenstedt test). If not treated surgically by laminectomy and drainage at the earliest possible moment, the spinal cord lesion, which is due in part to ischemia (compression mainly of veins), becomes irreversible. Emergency myelography must be used to determine the level of block and the operative site. Antibiotic therapy must also be given.

Another circumstance in which an acute spinal epidural abscess may develop is in a patient with some combination of chronic medical diseases in which a septicemia occurs. Here the symptoms of spine disease may be minimal until the onset of the spinal cord lesion some weeks later. Staphylococci or some other organism may reach the epidural or subdural spinal space via a lumbar puncture needle or during epidural anesthesia. The localization is then over lumbar and sacral roots. Pain may be severe and neurologic symptomatology minimal.

Subacute pyogenic infections and granulomatous infections (tubercular, fungal) may also arise in the spinal epidural space causing symptoms and signs of disorder of spinal tracts at the level of the lesion. The clinical picture is less dramatic, and the diagnosis depends on the demonstration, in a patient with weakness and/or sensory loss or ataxia of the legs, of a partial or complete block by contrast myelography. The treatment depends on the nature of the underlying disease and the general condition of the patient (see Chap. 125).

INFARCTION OF SPINAL CORD (MYELOMALACIA) AND HEMORRHAGE (HEMATOMYELIA) Unlike the brain, the spinal cord is rarely the site of vascular disease. The spinal arteries are not susceptible to atherosclerosis, and emboli rarely lodge there. As was stated in relation to chronic meningeal infections, an endarteritis of surface arteries may lead to thrombosis with devastating ischemic necrosis of the spinal cord. Polyarteritis nodosa may have a similar effect though the localization in the nervous system in this disease is usually peripheral. Atherosclerotic thrombosis of the aorta or dissecting aortic aneurysms may cause myelomalacia by occluding nutrient arteries at cervical, thoracic, or lumbar levels. Paralysis during cardiac surgery requiring clamping of the aorta for more than 30 min and aortic arteriography may result in the syndrome. Sudden development of symptoms referable to lesions of spinal tracts (sensory or motor or both) always bespeaks an infarctive or hemorrhagic vascular lesion of the spinal cord. The onset of symptoms in such cases is more rapid than in the myelitides.

Hemorrhage into the spinal cord is rare. Aside from the aforementioned traumatic variety of hematomyelia, it is usually traceable to a vascular malformation or a hematologic disease.

SUBACUTE OR CHRONIC SPINAL SYNDROMES

These take several forms for the reason that the responsible diseases have a variety of different localizations in the tracts and gray matter. Most of the remaining diseases of the spinal cord may be grouped around the following syndromes.

SPASTIC ATAXIC PARAPARESIS The gradual development of ataxia and weakness of the legs is the common manifestation of several diseases. In late childhood or adolescence a syndrome of this type which begins insidiously and progresses steadily over a period of years usually indicates the existence of Friedreich's ataxia or one of its variants. In early adult life multiple sclerosis, syphilitic meningomyelitis, and chronic adhesive spinal arachnoiditis are the more frequent causes of it. And in middle and late years of life subacute combined degeneration, nutritional combined system disease, and cervical spondylosis reach their highest incidence.

FRIEDREICH'S ATAXIA This classic form of hereditary ataxia, first clearly depicted by Nikolaus Friedreich of Heidelberg in 1863, forms a relatively distinct symptom complex which generally runs true to form, although it overlaps other heredodegenerative syndromes, particularly the chronic familial polyneuropathies and progressive optic atrophy (discussed in Chaps. 323 and 333). In some families, the disorder occurs with dominant inheritance; more often it is a recessive trait.

Clinical aspects As with other progressive ataxias, the disorder first appears in the legs. Thus, the patient, previously healthy, begins to stagger and lurch in walking and is unsteady on standing, often in a tremulous fashion. Clumsiness and intention tremor of the hands and arms appear later along with faulty articulation and abnormal rhythm (scanning) of speech. These symptoms usually result from changes in the cerebellum. The limbs, in addition to being ataxic, generally show considerable weakness. Examination usually discloses nystagmus and skeletal deformities: kyphoscoliosis, the basis of which is not certain, and a peculiar foreshortening and high arching of the feet (pes cavus) with cocking of the toes (sometimes called the "Friedreich foot" and best ascribed to atrophy and contractures of the musculature of the feet at a time when the bones of the feet are malleable). Typically, there is the unusual combination of total absence of tendon reflexes with extensor plantar reflexes (Babinski sign). This results from the presence of degeneration of pyramidal tracts together with a mild affection of peripheral sensory neurons. The presence of the latter is further indicated by impairment of position and vibration sense in the extremities and, in some patients, of the sensations of pain, temperature, and light touch in a distal and roughly symmetric distribution. The optic disks may be pale, indicating optic atrophy, although actual blindness is relatively rare. Rarely patients are of low intelligence or may become demented late in the course of the disease. Survival beyond early adult life is rare, with death frequently the result of associated myocardial disease.

Occasionally very mild or fragmentary forms of the disorder (such as pes cavus and absent or hyperactive tendon reflexes) may be encountered with little if any disability or progression. Such abnormalities are most likely to be seen in other members of the family of a patient afflicted with the fully developed form of the disease.

Pathology The principal changes are in the spinal cord and peripheral nerves; they are typical of a chronic degenerative process. In the cord the disease affects chiefly the sensory fibers of the posterior columns, the spinocerebeller tracts, and the corticospinal (pyramidal) tracts. Additional lesions of varying extent may be found in the brainstem and in the cerebellum itself, although the latter structure occasionally is intact. Involvement of other parts of the central nervous system at higher levels occasionally occurs. In the peripheral nerves the lesions vary likewise in severity and extent. They consist of degeneration of dorsal root ganglion cells and their central and peripheral fibers. In addition to the neuropathologic changes there is in some cases a peculiar form of myocardial degeneration resulting in thickening and fibrosis. There are no other associated visceral lesions.

Differential diagnosis The classic form of Friedreich's ataxia is readily recognizable and cannot easily be confused with other conditions. It is to be expected, however, that variations in the clinical manifestations may occur because of the variable pathologic changes. Chronic familial polyneuropathies are particularly difficult to distinguish since they also give rise to sensory ataxia, but signs of pyramidal tract disease are absent (see Chap. 323). Familial spastic paraplegia with or without optic atrophy (Behr's syndrome) is another closely related disease. In the absence of a family history, and with atypical clinical findings, further diagnostic studies to exclude tumor, chronic basal meningitis, intoxication, or congenital malformation will be necessary.

No treatment is known. Physical medicine and rehabilitation measures are of little value in cerebellar ataxia.

MULTIPLE SCLEROSIS Probably an ataxic paraparesis ranks as the most common manifestation of an established form of multiple sclerosis. Asymmetric involvement of limbs and signs of cerebral, optic nerve, brainstem, and cerebellum manifestations provide important information for the diagnosis of this disease. Nevertheless, purely spinal involvement may occur, no lesions being found outside the spinal cord even at autopsy. See Chap. 331 for further details.

SYPHILITIC MENINGOMYELITIS Here as in multiple sclerosis the degree of alteration of vibratory and position sense and ataxia is variable. Some patients with primary lateral sclerosis, such as Erb described, have almost pure pyramidal spasticity and weakness of the legs requiring differentiation from motor system disease and familial spastic paraplegia. In others sensory ataxia and posterior column signs predominate. The confirmation of diagnosis depends on the finding of a positive Wassermann reaction in the CSF, but a late and advancing form of the disease may appear with a negative CSF in a known syphilitic patient. See Chap. 159 for a discussion of pathology and treatment.

SUBACUTE COMBINED DEGENERATION OF SPINAL CORD AND BRAIN DUE TO B_{12} DEFICIENCY AND SYNDROME OF NUTRITIONAL COMBINED SYSTEM DISEASE (STRACHAN SYNDROME) These two forms of the more treatable diseases of the spinal cord are fully described in Chap. 332.

Progressive spastic or spastic-ataxic paraparesis may also develop in conjunction with hepatic decompensation.

CERVICAL SPONDYLOSIS Osteophytic overgrowth in the cervical spinal canal during the late years of life encroaches upon the spinal cord, narrowing it, and compressing it or possibly impairing its circulation by occlusion of nutrient radicular arteries. Stiff neck, cervical pain, numbness, and weakness or atrophy of hands are combined with ataxia, spastic weakness of legs, or an ataxic paraparesis. X-rays disclose the bony overgrowth, which can be confirmed by myelography. The CSF protein may be elevated and the Queckenstedt test may be positive. Immobilization of the head with a cervical collar has resulted in relief of symptoms in some cases. Decompressive laminectomy has halted the disease in the majority of instances and has often permitted some degree of recession of symptoms. An anterior approach, permitting removal of osteophytes, promises to give even better results.

SPASTIC PARAPARESIS WITH OR WITHOUT CERVICOBRACHIAL AMYOTROPHY

Although a few such cases are traced to multiple sclerosis, syringomyelia, cervical pachymeningitis, or cervical meningomyelitis, the purely motor syndrome is nearly always traceable to amyotrophic lateral sclerosis. Paralysis, atrophy, and fascicular twitching of hands and arms are joined with spastic weakness and hyperreflexia in legs with Babinski signs (see Chap. 333). Cervical spondylosis and high cervical tumors must also be considered in the differential diagnosis. Pure spastic paraparesis may occur in multiple sclerosis, spondylosis, liver failure, and hereditary spastic paraplegia with or without dementia.

SEGMENTAL SENSORY DISSOCIATION WITH BRACHIAL MUSCULAR ATROPHY (SYRINGOMYELIC SYNDROME)

This syndrome is most often ascribable to a syringomyelia, but examples have been found in patients with intramedullary cord tumors, traumatic myelopathy, postradiation myelopathy, syphilitic cervical pachymeningitis, cervical spondylosis, extramedullary tumors, or high cervical canal and necrotizing myelitis. For a description of syringomyelia, see Chap. 334.

OTHER SYNDROMES CAUSING ASYMMETRIC WEAKNESS OF LEGS, SENSORY LOSS (ATAXIA), AND SPHINCTERIC DISTURBANCES

Here a miscellany of diseases (vascular malformations, chronic adhesive arachnoiditis following spinal anasthesia, and infections and metabolic and nutritional diseases, etc.) would have to be considered, but only spinal cord tumor will be discussed.

Spinal cord tumors

Growths and other space-occupying lesions within the spinal canal can be conveniently divided into two groups: (1) those which arise within the substance of the spinal cord and invade and destroy tracts and central gray structures (intramedullary) and those which arise outside the spinal cord (extramedullary) arising in the vertebral bodies and epidural tissues (extradural), and in the meninges, or roots (intradural). The relative frequency of spinal tumors in these different locations in a general hospital is about 5 percent intramedullary, 40 percent intradural-extramedullary, and 55 percent extradural. The percentages of extradural lesions in a general hospital population is usually higher than in most neurosurgical services (e.g., Elsberg's figures of 10, 67, and 16 percent respectively), which often do not include many of the lymphomas, metastatic carcinomas, etc., most of which are extradural.

The cellular origin of the intramedullary gliomas has been mentioned in the section on intracerebral tumors. The proportions of the different cell types differ, however. Ependymoma makes up 40 percent of the cases, and the remainder are more or less evenly distributed among astrocytomas, glioblastomas, oligodendrogliomas, ganglioneuromas, medulloblastomas, hemangiomas, and hemangioblastomas. The hemangioma is the common source of spontaneous hematomyelia, and the hemangioblastoma may give rise to a syringomyelia.

SYMPTOMATOLOGY Patients with spinal cord tumor are likely to manifest one of two clinical pictures: either a purely sensorimotor spinal tract and rarely a syringomyelic syndrome or a radicular-spinal syndrome, nearly always painful.

COMPRESSION OF SENSORIMOTOR SPINAL TRACTS The predominant clinical syndrome relates to spinal cord compression. With intraspinal tumors, the onset of the compressive symptoms is usually gradual over a period of weeks and months, and the course is progressive. The initial disturbance is likely to be motor, and often the distribution is asymmetric. With cervical lesions the order of motor impairment is first the arm, then the ipsilateral and contralateral leg, and finally the opposite arm. With thoracic lesions one leg usually becomes weak and stiff before the other one. Subjective sensory symptoms (tingling paresthesias) of the spinal tract type take the same pattern. Pain and temperature are more likely to be affected than touch, vibration, and position senses and are contralateral to the maximum motor weakness (Brown-Séquard syndrome). Nevertheless the posterior columns are also frequently involved. The bladder and bowel usually become paralyzed coincident with motor paralysis of the legs. If the compression is relieved, there is recovery from these sensory-motor symptoms in the reverse order of their affection. The first part affected is the last to recover, and sensory symptoms disappear before motor.

COMPRESSIVE-IRRITATIVE RADICULAR SYMPTOMS This syndrome of spinal cord compression is often combined with radicular pain, i.e., pain in the distribution of a spinal root. It is described as knifelike or as merely a dull ache with superimposed sharp pains which are intensified by cough, sneeze, or strain and radiation in a distal direction, i.e., away from the spine. Segmental sensory changes (paresthesias, hyperalgesia, impairment of pain and touch) or motor disturbances (spasm, cramp, twitching, atrophy, fascicular twitching, and loss of tendon reflex) and an ache in the spine are the usual manifestations of a compressive-irritative lesion of roots. Tenderness of spinous processes over the growth is found in half the patients. These segmental changes, particularly the sensory ones, often precede the signs of spinal cord compression by months or years if the lesion is benign. Sphincter disturbances usually appear late.

The clinical findings are (1) spastic weakness of the legs, in one leg more than in the other, with thoracolumbar lesions, and of the arms and legs with cervical lesions, (2) a sensory level for pain on the trunk below which pain sense is reduced or lost, (3) posterior column signs, and (4) a spastic bladder under weak voluntary control.

The diagnosis is established by x-rays of the spine (erosion of vertebras, widened spinal canal), lumbar puncture, and electromyography to demonstrate the fasciculations and denervation resulting from involvement of motor roots. The most important diagnostic test of all is contrast myelography for the direct visualization of the compressive lesion. Occasionally lumbar puncture may exacerbate the symptoms and signs.

SPECIAL SPINAL SYNDROMES Unusual clinical syndromes may be found in patients with tumors near the foramen magnum. They may produce a quadriparesis with pains in the back of the head and stiff neck, a weakness and atrophy of the hands and dorsal neck muscles, and either bizarre sensory changes or no sensory loss whatsoever. Lesions of the tenth, eleventh, and twelfth thoracic and the first lumbar vertebras may result in a curious syndrome of mixed cauda equina and spinal cord symptoms. *Lesions of the cauda equina* alone, always difficult to separate from those of the plexus and multiple nerves, are usually attended in the early stages with pain which is variously combined with an asymmetric, atrophic, areflexic paralysis, radicular sensory loss, and later sphincteric disorder. This must be distinguished from *tumors of the conus medullaris* (lower sacral segments of spinal cord) in which there are early disturbances of sphincters of the bladder and bowel, back pain, hypesthesia, and anesthesia over the sacral dermatomes, a lax anal sphincter with loss of anal and bulbocavernosus reflexes, and sometimes weakness of lower leg muscles. A Babinski sign means that the spinal cord is involved above the fifth lumbar segment. Pain and stiffness of the back may precede signs of spinal cord disease or dominate the clinical picture in some extramedullary tumors.

PATHOLOGY, ANATOMY, AND PHYSIOLOGY Peculiarities of anatomic structure are decisive factors in determining the symptomatology of tumor growths. The structure of the spine was described in Chap. 9, Pain in the Back and Neck. Epidural growths arise from hematogenous deposits or tumors which extend from the vertebral bodies or from extraspinal spaces through intervertebral foramena.

Intramedullary growths both invade as well as compress and distort fasciculi in the adjacent white matter. As the cord enlarges from the tumor growing within it or is compressed from a tumor growing without, the free space around the cord is consumed and the cerebrospinal fluid below the lesion becomes isolated or loculated from the rest of the so-called "circulating cerebrospinal fluid" above. This can be demonstrated by a positive Queckenstedt test, Froin's syndrome of xanthochromia and clotting of CSF, and interruption of the flow of a contrast medium in the subarachnoid space (myelogram).

DIFFERENTIAL DIAGNOSIS Several problems may arise in the diagnosis of patients with spinal cord tumors. In the early stages spinal tumor must be distinguished from other diseases which cause pain over certain segments of the body, i.e., those affecting the gallbladder, kidney, stomach and intestinal tract, pleura, etc. Here the localization of the pain to a dermatome, its intensification by effort, segmental sensory changes, and minor alterations of motor, reflex, or sensory function in the legs will usually provide the clues to the compressive-irritative radicular lesion. Examination of the cerebrospinal fluid, x-ray of the spine, and myelography will settle the diagnosis in most instances.

If symptoms and signs of disorder of sensory and motor tracts of the spinal cord are present, there is still the problem of locating the segmental level of the lesion.

At first the sensory and motor deficiencies may be more pronounced in those parts of the body farthest removed from the lesion, i.e., in feet or lumbosacral segments. Later these sensory and motor levels may ascend, but at any time they may continue to be far below the lesion. Of greatest help in determining the level of the lesion are the locality of the root pains and atrophic paralysis and lastly the upper level of hypalgesia.

Once vertebral and segmental levels are settled, there is still the necessity of determining whether the lesion is neoplastic and extradural, intradural-extramedullary, or intramedullary. This is important from the standpoint of etiologic diagnosis. If there is a visible or palpable spinal deformity or x-ray evidence of vertebral destruction, one may confidently assume an extradural localization. Without x-ray changes one still suspects extradural lesion if root pain developed early and is bilateral, spine ache is prominent, and percussion tenderness is marked, if motor symptoms below the lesions precede sensory changes, and sphincter disturbances are late. To distinguish between intradural-extramedullary and intramedullary lesions is almost impossible. Radicular pain, asymmetry of signs of motor and sensory tract involvement, and early cerebrospinal fluid blockage (positive Queckenstedt test and high protein) favor the extramedullary localization. With extradural lesions one must differentiate between ruptures of disk, spondylosis (hypertrophic spurring and osteophyte formation in cervical spinal canal), tuberculous caries, other pyogenic, fungous, or syphilitic granulomatous lesions, secondary carcinoma, or lymphoma. With intradural-extramedullary lesions, meningioma, neurofibroma, meningeal carcinomatosis, cholesteatoma, teratomatous cyst, or meningomyelitic process is most likely. Intramedullary lesions are usually gliomas or vascular malformations. A negative Queckenstedt test, normal or relatively low protein in cerebrospinal fluid, and a negative myelogram will serve to rule out intraspinal tumors or granulomatous lesions in most instances.

TREATMENT This varies with the nature of the lesion and the clinical condition of the patient. Intradural-extramedullary tumor should be removed. Laminectomy, decompression, marsupialization of cysts, and x-ray therapy are the treatment of intramedullary gliomas. Extradural malignant growths are best managed by the use of opiates for pain, x-ray therapy, endocrine therapy (for carcinoma of breast and prostate), or nitrogen mustard treatment (for certain lymphomas). Sometimes laminectomy and decompression are necessary for diagnosis and prevention of irreversible compressive effects and infarction of the spinal cord. With tuberculous caries, immobilization of the spine in hyperextension and streptomycin therapy are indicated, and laminectomy should be reserved for exceptional cases with complete and irreversible spinal block. For spondylosis surgery (extradural decompression) is advised if these are serious neurologic deficits. Syndromes of lesser severity or patients with other important diseases may best be treated with a Thomas collar to immobilize the spine.

In conclusion it is always well to remind oneself that of the more than 30 diseases of the spinal cord, there are available effective means of treating only a few—spondylosis, extramedullary spinal cord tumors, syphilis (meningomyelitis and tabes), epidural granulomas (pyogenic, tuberculous, fungous), subacute combined degeneration, and nutritional myelopathy. The physician's major responsibility is to determine whether his patient has one of the treatable diseases.

INJURIES TO SPINAL ROOTS, PLEXUSES, AND PERIPHERAL NERVES See Chaps. 9 and 322.

REFERENCES

Brock S (ed): *Injuries of the Brain and Spinal Cord and Their Coverings*, 3d ed., Baltimore: Williams & Wilkins, 1949, p. 71

Elsberg CA: *Tumors of the Spinal Cord*, London: Paul B. Hoeber, 1925

Kernohan JW et al: Intramedullary tumors of the spinal cord. Arch Neurol 25:679, 1931

Kuhn WG Jr.: Care and rehabilitation of patients with injuries to the spinal cord and cauda equina: Preliminary report on 113 cases. J Neurosurg 4:40, 1947

Prather GC, Mayfield FH: *Injuries of the Spinal Cord*, Springfield, Ill: Charles C Thomas, 1953

Seddon HJ: Pott's paraplegia: Prognosis and treatment. Br. J Surg 22:769, 1934-35

Wyburn-Mason, R: *Vascular Abnormalities and Tumors of the Spinal Cord*, London: Kimpton, 1943

326 CEREBROVASCULAR DISEASES

C. MILLER FISHER
JAY P. MOHR
RAYMOND D. ADAMS

Vascular diseases of the nervous system rank first in frequency amongst all the neurologic diseases. Furthermore, it is evident to all who work in this field of medicine that the cerebrovascular diseases provide one of the best approaches to the study of neurology since they compose about 50 percent of all neurologic hospital admissions to adult wards. Both in the past and in the present, the neurologist has depended heavily on the focal ischemic lesion in his attempts to learn the secrets of the function of the human brain.

The term *cerebrovascular disease* refers to any disease implicating one or more of the blood vessels of the brain in a pathologic process. By *pathologic process* is meant any abnormality of the vessel wall, an occlusion by thrombus or embolus, rupture of a vessel, a failure of cerebral blood flow due to a fall in blood pressure, a change in the caliber of the lumen, altered permeability of the vascular wall, or increased viscosity or other quality of the blood. The pathologic process within the vessel may be described not only according to its grosser aspects — thrombosis, embolism, rupture of a vessel, etc. — but also in terms of the more basic vascular disorder, i.e., atherosclerosis, hypertensive arteriosclerosis, arteritis, trauma, aneurysm, developmental malformation. Furthermore, in classifying cerebrovascular diseases it is not sufficient to consider only the primary vascular lesion; equal weight must be given the resulting parenchymal changes in the brain. These latter are of two types, ischemia with or without infarction, and hemorrhage. Aside from these the vascular lesion is silent, the only exceptions being the local pressure effects of an aneurysm, vascular headache (migraine, hypertension, arteritis), and occasionally increased intracranial pressure as in hypertensive encephalopathy and venous thrombosis.

Brain tissue is dependent for its existence on the moment-to-moment supply of oxygenated blood. In Stokes-Adams attacks unconsciousness occurs within 10 sec of cardiac arrest. In animal experiments the stoppage of blood flow for longer than 3 min produces irreversible damage. When brain tissue is deprived of blood and oxygen, it undergoes ischemic necrosis (infarction) and is destroyed. Obstruction of the nutrient artery by thrombus or embolus is the usual cause, but failure of the systemic circulation and hypotension, if severe and prolonged enough, can also produce infarction. Cerebral infarcts vary greatly in the amount of congestion and hemorrhage found within the softened tissue. Some infarcts are strikingly pallid (pale infarction); others show mild congestion (dilatation of vessels and some extravasation of red blood cells); still others show an extensive scattering of petechial hemorrhages throughout the damaged gray matter (red infarction). Thrombotic infarcts are usually pale, while embolic infarcts are sometimes pale, sometimes red; red infarction is usually a sign of embolism. The reason for the simultaneous occurrence of pale and red infarctions in cases of embolic infarction is not known, although the hypothesis which we favor attributes it to the fragmentation and the migration of embolic material from its original site of arrest, the movement distally allowing blood to enter the part of the infarct lying more proximally.

In hemorrhage an extravasation of blood occurs into the parenchyma, the subarachnoid space, or both. Once the leakage stops, the blood is slowly resorbed over a period of weeks and months. Damage to the brain results from the pressure of the mass of blood on the surrounding tissue combined with physical disruption of the region directly involved.

In classification of cerebrovascular disease it is most practical from the clinical viewpoint to preserve the three classic divisions, thrombosis, embolism, and hemorrhage, and our descriptions will follow this scheme, listing the causes of each in the corresponding section. These three make up the majority of strokes. The plan has some disadvantages in not providing a precise niche for disorders such as reversible ischemia, hypertensive encephalopathy, and venous thrombosis, but these will be discussed.

THE STROKE SYNDROME

The clinical picture resulting from vascular disease is in most instances so distinctive that the diagnosis is more readily made than any other in the realm of neurology. The cardinal feature is the *stroke*, a term which connotes the sudden and dramatic development of a focal neurologic deficit. In its severest form, the patient falls hemiplegic and even unconscious—an event so striking as to deserve its own separate designation, namely, apoplexy, stroke, shock, or cerebrovascular accident. In its mildest form, it may consist of only a trivial neurologic disorder insufficient to disturb the customary activities of the patient or to demand medical attention.

Undoubtedly, the most characteristic feature is the sequence of events which may be called the *temporal profile* of the stroke. It is the suddenness with which the neurologic deficit develops that especially stamps the disorder as vascular. The speed of evolution, though variable, depending on the cause, is comparatively rapid, and the deficit appears in a matter of seconds, minutes, hours, or at most a few days. Embolic stroke characteristically begins suddenly, with the deficit reaching its maximum almost immediately. Thrombotic strokes frequently begin in a similar fashion. When a thrombotic stroke develops over a period of several days, it usually progresses in a stepwise fashion, i.e., in a series of sudden changes, rather than smoothly. In hemorrhage related to hypertension, the deficit evolves smoothly over minutes or hours. By contrast, a slow, gradual, downhill course over a period of several days to a few weeks or more indicates that the process is probably not vascular in nature. Later in the course of a stroke illness, if the attack is not fatal, stabilization occurs, and is followed by some degree of improvement, especially in cases with deficits in language function. Not infrequently an extensive deficit reverses itself dramatically within a few hours or a day. More often, however, the improvement is gradual, taking place over weeks and months.

It must not be supposed that every neurologic abnormality in patients with cerebrovascular disease can be related by the patient or his family to a stroke. Often the exact date of onset of a given symptom cannot be remembered. Vascular incidents, especially in the hypertensive patient, may be so mild that they do not attract notice until their cumulative effects become manifest. Furthermore, patients with lesions in the right (nondominant) parietal region often have anosognosia (unawareness of motor deficit) and cannot be depended upon to give any of the important details of their illness. In dominant hemispheral lesions, aphasia hampers history taking.

The neurologic deficit in a stroke depends, of course, on the location of the infarct or hemorrhage in the brain and the size of the lesion. Hemiplegia is the classic sign of vascular disease and occurs chiefly with lesions of either cerebral hemisphere or of the brainstem. A stroke, however, may give rise to many manifestations other than a hemiplegia, e.g., numbness, sensory deficit, dysphasia, blindness, diplopia, dizziness, and dysarthria. In the following paragraphs these manifestations will be emphasized equally with hemiplegia.

CEREBRAL THROMBOSIS

Of the many causes listed in Table 326-1, thrombosis with atherosclerosis accounts for the overwhelming majority of cases seen clinically. Several others (hypotension, cerebral herniation, with ruptured aneurysm) are conveniently included here although they are really examples of infarction without actual thrombosis.

Thrombosis with atherosclerosis

Atherosclerosis in the arteries of the brain is similar to that elsewhere in the body. The atheromatous plaques tend to form at branchings and curves. The severity of the process runs parallel to but is somewhat less severe than that of other arteries—aorta, lower limbs, and heart. Thrombosis is most likely to occur where the plaque narrows the lumen to the greatest degree. The most common sites of thrombosis are the internal carotid artery at the carotid sinus in the neck, at the main bifurcation of the middle cerebral artery, in the vertebral and basilar arteries in the region of their junction, in the posterior cerebral artery as it winds round the cerebral peduncle, and in the anterior cerebral artery as it curves upward over the corpus callosum. The abundant collateral arterial pathways make it uncommon that occlusion of the common carotid, brachiocephalic, or subclavian arteries in the upper thorax is responsible for cerebral ischemia. The vertebral arteries may be narrowed at their origins from the subclavian, resulting in cerebral ischemia. Hypertension aggravates the atherosclerotic process and in addition is associated with a special segmental arterial disorganization, which then results in involvement of smaller vessels (1 mm and less). Thrombosis in the small, penetrating branches of the middle cerebral, posterior cerebral, and basilar arteries may produce small infarcts called *lacunes* in the internal capsule, central white matter, deeper parts of the basal ganglions, and brainstem. In hypertension the cerebellar and ophthalmic arteries also are liable to involvement. However, ordinarily it is extremely rare for the cerebral arteries to be significantly affected beyond their first major branching; i.e., thrombotic occlusion over the convexities seldom occurs. Occlusion of arteries in these regions is almost always of embolic origin.

The details of the process by which thrombosis becomes superimposed on atherosclerosis are poorly understood, and according to the encrustation theory, the two processes are closely related.

The effects of both thrombotic and embolic arterial occlusion are subject to ischemic modifying factors, not always predictable in the individual case. If the obstruction lies proximal to the circle of Willis, collateral flow via the circle may be and often is adequate to prevent infarction. In occlusion of the internal carotid artery in the neck, anastomotic flow may pass along the external carotid artery and retrograde in the ophthalmic artery or other smaller external-internal connections. In vertebral artery blockage low in the neck, blood may reach the upper part of the vertebral artery via the deep cervical, thyrocervical, or occipital artery. If the occlusion is distal to the circle of Willis, i.e., in the stem of one of the cerebral or cerebellar arteries, a series of subarachnoid interarterial anastomoses that join many of the branches of the major cerebral arteries end-to-end may carry sufficient blood into the compromised territory to prevent or lessen the ischemic damage (Fig. 326-4). However, this capillary anastomotic system between adjacent brain arteries, although always appearing to be the source of some collateral supply, is probably inconsequential. In occasional cases, however, the collateral flow is so great that a major arterial trunk can be entirely occluded without visible damage to the parenchyma. In other cases, occlusion may lead to softening throughout a vast area which extends to the outermost boundaries of the territory nourished by the affected vessel. Between these two extremes are countless variations in the size, shape, and completeness of an infarct, depending on factors

TABLE 326-1
Causes of cerebral thrombosis

I Atherosclerosis
II Ruptured saccular aneurysm
III Cerebral thrombophlebitis: secondary to infection of ear, paranasal sinus, face, etc.; with meningitis and subdural empyema; debilitating states, post-partum, postoperative, cardiac failure, hematologic disease (polycythemia, sickle-cell disease), and of undetermined cause
IV Arteritis
  A Meningovascular syphilis, arteritis secondary to pyogenic and tuberculous meningitis, rare types [typhus, schistosomiasis mansoni, malaria (?), trichinosis (?), mucormycosis, etc.]
  B Connective tissue diseases: polyarteritis (necrotizing, granulomatous, allergic, Wegner's), temporal arteritis, Takayasu's disease, granulomatous arteritis of aorta, lupus erythematosus
V Hematologic disorders: polycythemia, sickle-cell disease, thrombotic thrombocytopenic purpura, thrombocytosis, etc.
VI Trauma to carotid
VII Dissecting aortic aneurysm
VIII Systemic hypotension: "simple faint," acute blood loss, myocardial infarction, Stokes-Adams syndrome, traumatic and surgical shock, sensitive carotid sinus, severe postural hypotension
IX Complications of arteriography
X Migrainous aura with persistent deficit
XI With tentorial-foramen magnum and subfalcial herniation
XII Hypoxia
XIII Miscellaneous types: radioactive or x-ray radiation, lateral pressure of intracerebral hematoma, unexplained middle cerebral infarction in closed head injury, pressure of unruptured saccular aneurysm, mural thrombus in fusiform aneurysm, local dissection of carotid or middle cerebral artery, complication of contraceptive medication
XIV Undetermined cause as in children and young adults

such as the availability of collateral flow, the speed of occlusion (time for compensation), and the level of the systemic blood pressure. These factors and possibly others such as hypoxia and altered physical state of the blood may also at times operate adversely to produce ischemia in the territory of partially occluded vessels.

The actual state of the arterial lumen during the period when the stroke is evolving varies from case to case. Judging from arteriographic and surgical findings in the carotid and vertebral arteries in the neck, it is likely that when prodromal transient ischemic attacks are occurring, atherosclerosis and superimposed thrombus only incompletely occlude the affected artery; yet blood flow for reasons not yet understood is intermittent in the territory distal to the stenosis. Or, the main vessel is totally occluded while a compensating collateral channel is stenotic. By the time the neurologic deficit persists and is advancing, the superimposed thrombus will in the majority of cases have progressed to block completely the main vessel of supply. When the stroke becomes fully established, complete occlusion is the rule. It is common to find more than one vessel affected by stenosis or occlusion, and then it is especially difficult to decipher the interplay of hemodynamic factors leading to symptoms, transitory or persistent. On the other hand stenosis or occlusion of the carotid and vertebral arteries may remain "silent" or nearly so.

CLINICAL PICTURE In general, the evolution of the total clinical picture in cerebral thrombosis is much more variable than in embolism and hemorrhage. In approximately 80 percent of cases, the main part of the stroke (paralysis or other deficit) is preceded by minor signs or by one or more transient, warning ischemic attacks, which in a sense herald the oncoming vascular catastrophe. *A history of such prodromal episodes is of paramount importance in establishing the diagnosis of cerebral thrombosis.* Such episodes rarely precede embolism and intracerebral hemorrhage. Transient warning attacks in carotid-middle cerebral disease consist of mono- or hemiplegia, mono- or hemiparesthesia, blindness in one eye, speech disturbance, confusion, etc. In the vertebral-basilar system, they consist of dizziness, diplopia, numbness, impaired vision in one or both visual fields, dark vision, dysarthria, headache, etc. (described more fully below under Vertebral-Basilar Posterior Cerebral System). The attacks last from a few seconds up to 8 hr or so, and the final stroke may be preceded by hundreds of attacks or by only a single one. The stroke may come within a day of the first one or may be delayed for weeks or even months, and sometimes the attacks die away without leading to a stroke. When these minor ischemic attacks are not part of the picture, one must depend on other factors in identifying the cerebrovascular process as one of cerebral thrombosis.

The main part of the thrombotic stroke, whether or not it is preceded by warning attacks, develops in one of several ways. There may be but a single attack, the whole illness developing in a few hours. Another pattern is for the stroke, once it commences, to have a stuttering intermittent progression in the next several hours or days. Or a partial stroke may develop, and after the patient has improved for several hours, there is progression to a full paralysis. Again, after one or more fleeting episodes, there may be a longer-lasting attack, succeeded in a day or two by the occurrence of a complete and permanent paralysis. The affection may involve several parts of the body simultaneously or, only one part, such as a limb or one side of the face, and the other parts become involved serially in steplike fashion until the stroke is fully developed. This may take several days or weeks, during which time there may be improvement and superimposed transient episodes of worsening. All these various modes of development bespeak cerebral thrombosis, and the whole process may be referred to as *thrombosis in evolution.* It might be commented that the transitory attacks and the abrupt episodes of progression reflect the temporal profile of the stroke syndrome in miniature. The principle of *intermittency* seems to characterize the thrombotic process from the beginning to the end. In thrombotic strokes either the onset or progression of the stroke is particularly common during sleep or shortly after arising (60 percent of cases). Occasionally a thrombotic stroke comes on in what appears to be a slow, gradual fashion, but in most of these cases careful inquiry will reveal an uneven or saltatory progression, and actually there are only a few cases—these are usually pure motor hemiplegia—in which it can be said that the evolution of the thrombotic stroke was truly gradual over a period of several days. Table 326-2 shows the way in which the clinical picture developed in 125 cases of cerebral thrombosis diagnosed clinically, for the most part.

Headache, although absent in the majority of cases, is not uncommon in cerebral thrombosis. It is not so violent as in cases of intracranial hemorrhage, generally being on one side in the front part of the head in occlusion of the carotid system and at the back of the head or simultaneously in the forehead in basilar disease. Its cause is unknown. Presumably it is related in some way to the disease process within the vessel, since it may antedate the other symptoms of the stroke. Stiffness of the neck rarely occurs with cerebral infarction.

Hypertension, an important aggravating factor in atherosclerosis, is more often present than not. Diabetes is not infrequent. Often there is evidence of vascular disease elsewhere, e.g., angina pectoris, electrocardi-

TABLE 326-2
Development of the clinical picture in 125 cases of cerebral thrombosis

Clinical development	*No. of cases*	*Percentage*
Transient ischemic attacks progressing to a persistent neurologic deficit, major or minor	53	42
Stepwise development of a stroke, with or without transient ischemic attacks	23	18
Stroke developing as a single event	21	17
Abrupt (hours), with or without fluctuations	*14*	
Slow, gradual (a few days), with or without minor fluctuations	*7*	
Transient ischemic attacks only	17	14
Development of a limited stroke followed by transient ischemic attacks	11	9

ographic abnormality, myocardial infarction, absence of one or several peripheral pulses in the lower limbs, or intermittent claudication. The retinal arteries may show uniform or focal narrowing, increase and irregularity of the light reflex, or displacement of the veins, but these alterations cannot be correlated with cerebral atherosclerosis. The patient is usually elderly but may be in the fourth decade or even younger when stricken.

The *specific neurologic abnormality* depends on the location and size of the infarct or the focus of ischemia. The territory of any vessel, large or small, deep or superficial, may be involved. The carotid and basilar systems are approximately equally affected. In involvement of the carotid system, *unilateral* signs predominate: hemiplegia, hemihypesthesia, hemianopia, aphasia, and agnosia. In basilar disease, one more commonly finds *bilateral* signs, motor and/or sensory, in combination with a disturbance of cranial nerves, cerebellum, or other structures localized in or related to the brainstem. In order that carotid occlusion cause bilateral signs, the vessels to both hemispheres would have to be affected at the same time (bilateral carotid occlusion) or one carotid have been occluded silently in the past, neither a common event. It is important therefore to determine if the signs and symptoms indicate unilateral or bilateral lesions.

Neurovascular syndromes

In order to understand the particular groupings of neurologic symptoms and signs, the student must be familiar with certain points of neurovascular anatomy which will now be presented. The clinical syndrome associated with occlusion of each of the cerebral and cerebellar arteries will then become clear. It has already been pointed out that, because of differences in collateral blood flow, speed of occlusion, etc., the ischemic effect of occlusion at any one site is somewhat variable. Therefore the clinical picture resulting from the occlusion of any particular artery differs in minor ways from one patient to another; partial syndromes are in the majority. The following descriptions apply particularly to infarction and ischemia due to thrombosis or embolism. Although hemorrhage within these vascular territories may give rise to many of the same effects, the total clinical picture is apt to differ, because in its deep extension the hemorrhage may involve the territory of more than one vessel. Also it displaces tissues and causes an increase in intracranial pressure.

MIDDLE CEREBRAL ARTERY The middle cerebral artery through its cortical branches supplies the lateral surface of the hemisphere except for the frontal pole, a strip along the superomedial border irrigated by the anterior cerebral, and the lowest temporal convolutions, which are in the territory of the posterior cerebral artery.

Its area includes the cortex and white matter of the lateral and inferior aspects of the frontal lobe, the motor cortex (areas 4 and 6, the centers for contraversive eye movements, and in the dominant hemisphere the motor speech area of Broca), the cortex and white matter of the

FIGURE 326-1
Diagram of a cerebral hemisphere, coronal section, showing the territories of the major cerebral vessels.

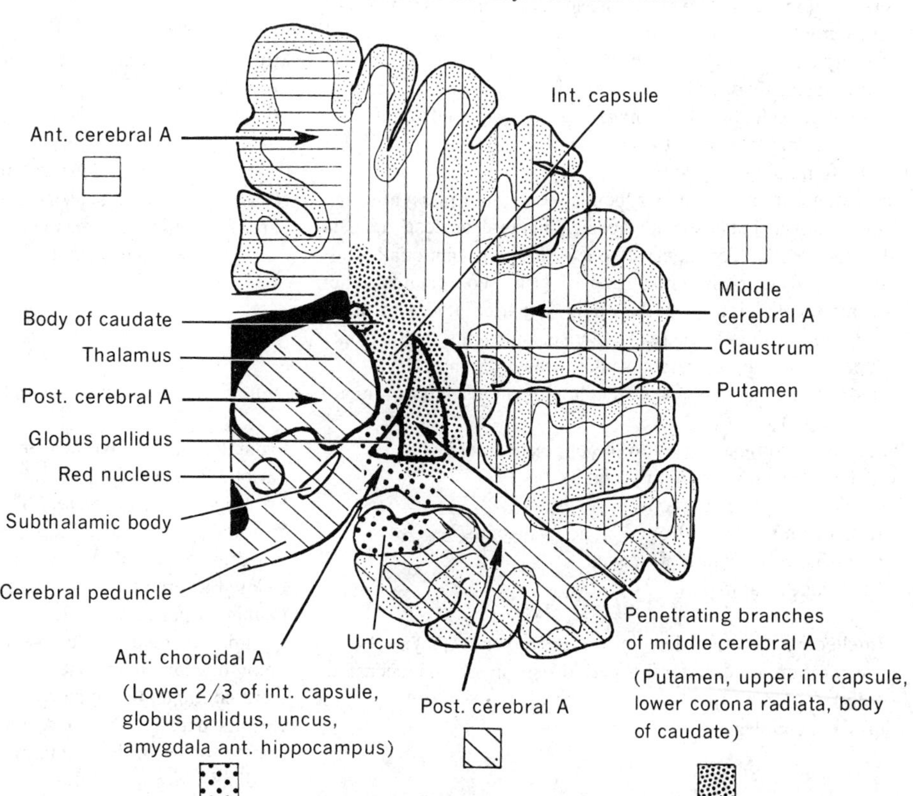

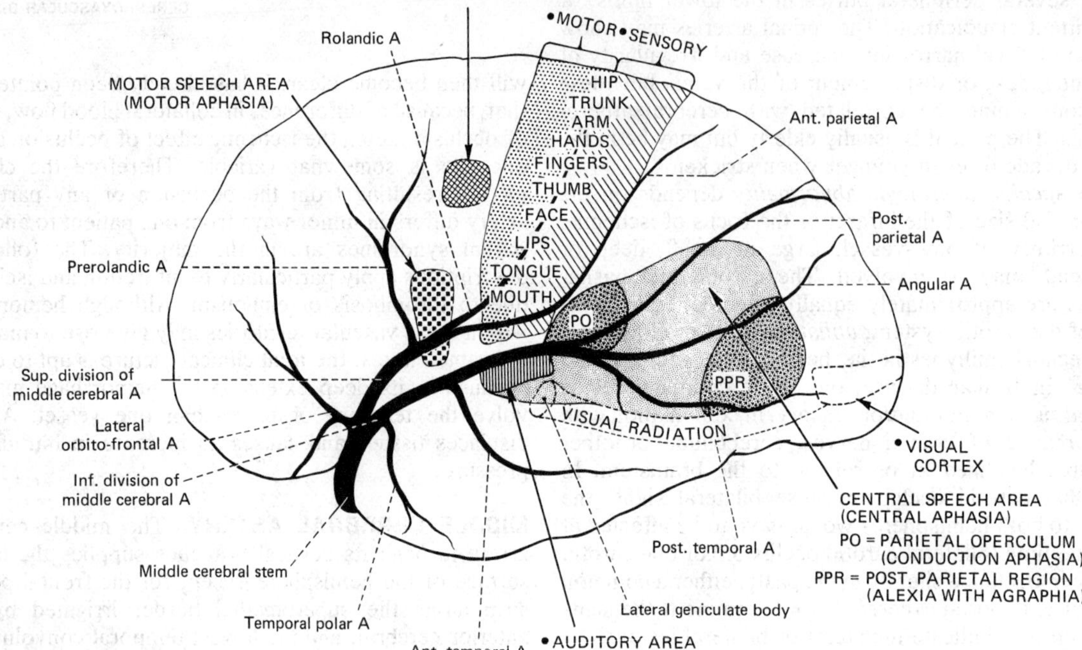

FIGURE 326-2

Diagram of a cerebral hemisphere, lateral aspect, showing the branches and distribution of the middle cerebral artery and the principal regions of cerebral localization. Below is a list of the clinical manifestations of infarction in the territory of this artery and the corresponding regions of cerebral damage.

Signs and symptoms	*Structures involved*
Paralysis of the contralateral face, arm, and leg	Somatic motor area for face and arm and the fibers descending from the leg area to enter the corona radiata
Sensory impairment over the contralateral face, arm, and leg (pinprick, cotton touch, vibration, position, two-point discrimination, stereognosis, tactile localization, barognosis, cutaneographia)	Somatic sensory system corresponding to motor involvement described above
Motor aphasia	Motor speech area of the dominant hemisphere
Central aphasia word deafness, anomia, jargon speech, sensory agraphia, acalculia, alexia, finger agnosia, right-left confusion (the last four comprise the Gerstmann syndrome)	Central, supramodal speech area and parietooccipital cortex of the dominant hemisphere
Conduction aphasia	Central speech area (parietal portion)
Apractognosia of the minor hemisphere (amorphosynthesis), anosognosia, hemiasomatognosia, unilateral neglect, agnosia for the left half of external space, dressing "apraxia," constructional "apraxia," distortion of visual coordinates, inaccurate localization in the half field, imparied ability to judge distance, upside-down reading, visual illusions (e.g., it may appear that another person walks through a table)	Nondominant supersensory zone (area corresponding to speech area in dominant hemisphere). Loss of topographic memory is usually due to a nondominant lesion, occasionally to a dominant one.
Homonymous hemianopia (often homonymous inferior quadrantanopia)	Optic radiation deep to second temporal convolution
Paralysis of conjugate gaze to the opposite side	Frontal contraversive field or fibers projecting therefrom
Avoidance reaction of opposite limbs	Parietal lobe lesion
Miscellaneous: frontal ataxia	Frontopontine tract lesion(?)
Loss or impairment of optokinetic nystagmus	Supramarginal or angular gyrus lesion
Disturbance of caloric nystagmus	Posterior temporal lobe lesion
Limb-kinetic apraxia (?)	Related to premotor cortical damage
Asymbolia for pain	Dominant parietal lobe lesion
Intellectual deterioration, mirror movement, Cheyne-Stokes respiration, contralateral hyperhidrosis, mydriasis (occasionally)	Location of responsible lesions not known. Acute lesions of the nondominant hemisphere may cause some degree of amnesia and confabulation mimicking Korsakoff's syndrome
Capsular hemiplegia	Results usually from a softening of the upper portion of the posterior limb of the internal capsule and the adjacent corona radiata. Motor paralysis is the chief sign, and dysphasia, homonymous hemianopia, and significant sensory loss seldom

lateral parietal lobe (sensory cortex, angular and supramarginal convolutions), the lateral and superior parts of the temporal lobe, and the insula. The penetrating branches of the middle cerebral artery supply the putamen, outer globus pallidus, the posterior limb of the internal capsule above the plane of the upper border of the globus pallidus, the adjacent part of the corona radiata, the body of the caudate nucleus, and the superior and lateral portion of the head of the caudate nucleus (Fig. 326-1).

The middle cerebral territory is the region most frequently affected in embolic and thrombotic cerebrovascular disease. The artery may be occluded in its stem,[1] blocking the mouths of the penetrating vessels as well as the flow to the superficial (cortical) vessels, or its major branches can be involved individually. The classic picture of total superficial and deep middle cerebral infarction is a contralateral hemiplegia, hemianesthesia, and homonymous hemianopia (Fig. 326-2). If the dominant hemisphere is involved, global or total sensorimotor aphasia also is present. If the nondominant hemisphere is affected, speech is spared but apractognosia is added to the clinical syndrome (see below). When collateral circulation limits the ischemia to a part of the territory, only some of the symptoms and signs listed in Fig. 326-2 will occur.

Thrombotic occlusion of the stem of the middle cerebral artery is relatively uncommon compared with embolic. When the circulation falters, ischemic threat first appears in the distal reaches of the middle cerebral territory, but collateral flow from the anterior cerebral artery through the meningeal interarterial anastomoses will compensate. Depending on the effectiveness of this influx, the area of infarction is more or less limited, with the production of partial middle cerebral syndromes of varied severity. Infarcts from embolic occlusion tend to be more extensive.

Branch occlusion is usually embolic, the embolus entering any of the middle cerebral branches and producing a corresponding partial deficit. It may block predominantly either the superior or inferior division of the middle cerebral (Fig. 326-2) with involvement, on the one hand, of the anterior or motor part of the hemisphere (superior division) or, on the other hand, the posterior or sensory part of the hemisphere (inferior division). Selective involvement of the posterior part of the hemisphere, e.g., receptive aphasia without paralysis, is a reliable sign of embolic occlusion of the inferior division of the middle cerebral artery. A similar rule applies to involvement of the superior division, i.e., a motor-sensory deficit in the limbs and a speech disorder without receptive aphasia, is almost as reliable in indicating embolism, but occlusion of the anterior cerebral or internal carotid artery occasionally produces this picture.

Lacunar state in middle cerebral territory and other vascular fields Hypertension combined with atherosclerosis results in thrombotic occlusion of individual penetrating branches running to the internal capsule and putamen, resulting in lacunes 2 to 15 mm in extent. When they involve the internal capsule, a pure motor hemiplegia results, recovery from which is often nearly complete. In the thalamus or above such lacunes are manifested by a pure hemisensory defect; in the midbrain the common syndrome is hemiparesis with cerebellar ataxia on the same side as the weakness; in the pons the most frequent syndrome is dysarthria with a clumsy hand or a pure hemiplegia. Other syndromes such as pure hemiballismus will be defined. In all, the neurologic syndrome develops abruptly without change in state of consciousness. Multiple lacunes involving the corticospinal and corticobulbar motor tracts cause the clinical picture of "pseudobulbar palsy" (more appropriately called *bipyramidal palsy*), featuring bilateral upper motor neuron signs, viz., spasticity, increased tendon reflexes, Babinski sign, dysarthria, and dysphagia. Spasms of excessive crying or laughing, short-step gait, and mental impairment are also part of the picture. Lacunes are sometimes said to be the basis of so-called "arteriosclerotic parkinsonism," but proof that such an entity exists is wanting.

ANTERIOR CEREBRAL ARTERY The anterior cerebral artery, through its cortical branches, supplies the anterior four-fifths of the medial surface of the cerebral hemisphere, the medial part of the orbital surface of the cerebral hemisphere, the medial part of the orbital surface of the frontal lobe, the frontal pole, a strip of the lateral surface along the superomedial border, and the anterior seven-eighths of the corpus callosum. The deep branches, which arise near the circle of Willis, run chiefly to the anterior limb of the internal capsule and inferior part of the head of the caudate nucleus (see Fig. 326-3).

Well-studied cases of infarction of the territory of the anterior cerebral artery are not numerous, and the syndrome of this artery has not been clearly determined as yet. Again the clinical picture will depend on the size and location of the infarct, which in turn depend on the site of the occlusion, the pattern of the circle of Willis, and the other ischemia-modifying factors. Occlusion of the stem of the anterior cerebral artery proximal to the anterior communicating artery is usually well tolerated, since collateral flow will come from its mate of the opposite side. The maximal disturbance occurs when both anterior cerebral arteries happen to arise from one anterior cerebral stem, occlusion of which then results in a devastating infarction of the anterior cerebral territory of both hemispheres. This may include bilateral pyramidal signs with paraplegia and profound mental symptoms. The components of the typical syndrome resulting from occlusion of one anterior cerebral artery distal to the circle of Willis are indicated in the legend of Fig. 326-3.

ANTERIOR CHOROIDAL ARTERY A few incomplete clinicopathologic studies have been the basis of present knowledge of the syndrome of the anterior choroidal artery. It is said to consist of contralateral hemiplegia, hemianesthesia (hypesthesia), and homonymous hemi-

[1] *The term stem refers to the section of artery lying between the origin of the middle cerebral and the first major branching. The stem of the anterior cerebral artery lies between its origin and the junction with the anterior communicating artery. The stem of the posterior cerebral stretches from its origin to the posterior communicating artery. The stem of the internal carotid artery extends from the region of the clinoid process to the bifurcation into the middle and anterior cerebral arteries.*

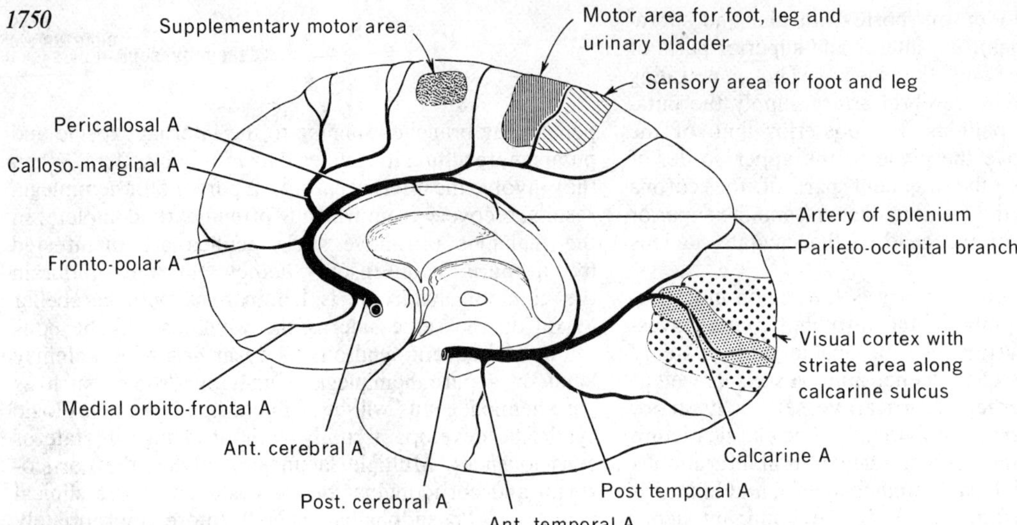

FIGURE 326-3
Diagram of a cerebral hemisphere, medial aspect, showing the branches and distribution of the anterior cerebral artery and the principal regions of cerebral localization. Below is a list of the clinical manifestations of infarction in the territory of this artery and the corresponding regions of cerebral damage.

Signs and symptoms	*Structures involved*
Paralysis of opposite foot and leg	Motor leg area
A lesser degree of paresis of opposite arm	Involvement of arm area of cortex or fibers descending to corona radiata therefrom
Cortical sensory loss over toes, foot, and leg	Sensory area for foot and leg
Unwitting urinary incontinence	Sensorimotor area in paracentral lobule
Contralateral grasp reflex, sucking reflex, gegenhalten (paratonic rigidity), "frontal tremor"	Medial surface of the posterior frontal lobe (?) supplementary motor area
Abulia (akinetic mutism) slowness, delay, intermittent interruption, lack of spontaneity, whispering, motor inaction, reflex distraction to sights and sounds	Uncertain localization—probably interomedial lesion near subcallosum
Impairment of gait and stance (gait apraxia)	Frontal cortex near leg motor area
Mental impairment (perseveration) and dysmemory	Localization unknown
Miscellaneous: dyspraxia of left limbs	Corpus callosum
Tactile aphasia in left limbs	Corpus callosum
Frontal ataxia (that this disorder may mimic cerebellar ataxia is disputed)	Not reported with vascular lesions
Cerebral paraplegia	May be due to bilateral occlusion of anterior cerebral artery

Note: aphasia and hemianopia do not occur, although the occasionally observed abulia and echolalia may at first appear to be aphasia

anopia, all due to involvement of the posterior limb of the internal capsule and the white matter posterolateral to it, through which the first part of the geniculocalcarine fibers passes. In the reported cases, however, the clinical syndrome usually fell far short of what was expected on anatomic grounds. Surgical occlusion of the vessel also produced little or no deficit. It has yet to be demonstrated that such a syndrome exists.

INTERNAL CAROTID ARTERY The clinical picture of occlusion of the internal carotid artery is variable. Not infrequently occlusion is completely asymptomatic, while in other cases it produces a devastating, massive infarction which leads to death in a few days. Between these two extremes lies every shade of variation. As a rule, the infarct involves some part of the middle cerebral territory, but when the anterior communicating artery is very small, the ipsilateral anterior cerebral territory may be affected too, in which case the anterior part of the hemisphere (the frontal lobe) bears the brunt of the insult, while the region posterior to the rolandic fissure tends to be spared. When both anterior cerebral arteries arise from a common stem on one side, infarction may involve the anterior cerebral territory bilaterally. The posterior cerebral artery also may be supplied from the internal carotid rather than from the basilar artery, in which case its territory, too, may be softened, and thus the entire hemisphere and even part of the other may be involved. Not infrequently the tissue in the territory of the anterior choroidal artery is also infarcted. When one carotid has been asymptomatically occluded at a previous time, occlusion of the other can result in bilateral hemispheric infarction. In such cases, coma with quadriparesis and continuous horizontal conjugate roving eye movements may be seen.

In symptomatic occlusion of the internal carotid artery, when the deficit is advanced, the picture usually resembles that of middle cerebral occlusion with a contralateral hemiplegia, and hemihypesthesia and aphasia, (with involvement of the dominant hemisphere). When the anterior cerebral territory is also infarcted, the clinical picture will include some of or all the features already mentioned under Anterior Cerebral Artery. Patients with infarction in the combined territories of the middle and anterior cerebral arteries are much less responsive than those with lesions in only one territory, and often they are in a coma. Headache may also occur with both cerebral thrombosis or embolism in the carotid artery; the pain is situated just above the eyebrow. That associated with occlusion of the middle cerebral artery is usually more lateral, at the temple with occlusion of the posterior cerebral artery, in the eyebrow.

When the circulation in one carotid is compromised and collateral flow is restricted, the most distal or terminal parts of the middle and anterior and at times the posterior cerebral territories suffer first and most. This gives rise to an irregular and asymmetric *border-zone* configuration of infarction in which the contiguous distal fields of each vessel are disproportionately affected, the heaviest involvement usually falling on the middle cerebral artery territory. When well developed the zone of damage forms an elongated strip of variable width extending from the frontal pole to the occipital. Therefore carotid infarcts of less than maximal extent tend to be located distally rather than proximally in the Sylvian region. Likewise it is in this most vulnerable region that transient ischemic attack symptoms are liable to arise in carotid stenosis, taking the form of weakness or paresthesias in the upper extremity and, only if more extensive, in the face and tongue. The relative sparing of the posterior part of the hemisphere is reflected in a low incidence of homonymous hemianopia and central aphasia.

In addition to nourishing the brain, the internal carotid artery supplies the optic nerve and retina via the ophthalmic artery (Fig. 326-4). Transient monocular blindness occurs intermittently as a warning symptom prior to the onset of the stroke in almost 25 percent of cases of symptomatic carotid occlusion. Surprising, however, is the fact that the picture of central retinal artery occlusion rarely appears under such circumstances.

Whereas most cerebral vessels are inaccessible within the skull and topical diagnosis is made only by inference, in carotid occlusion more direct diagnostic tests are available. Pressure in the central retinal artery is usually reduced on the side of carotid occlusion or severe stenosis, and a pressure difference in the two eyes on careful ophthalmodynamometry will point strongly to carotid occlusion. Dilated collateral channels coursing over the forehead may also suggest carotid occlusion. Retinal embolism, either of shining white or plain type, may point to carotid disease. Severe stenosis within the carotid sinus due to an atherosclerotic plaque—with or without superimposed thrombus—may give rise to a local bruit, which can be an important finding in disease of the carotid artery. Occasionally the murmur results from stenosis at the mouth of the external carotid artery and can then be misleading. The murmur may be on the side of the stenosed artery. The narrowing may be unilateral or bilateral. If the murmur is heard at the angle of the jaw, the stenosis is in the carotid sinus; if lower in the neck, the stenosis is in the common carotid artery, or subclavian. (Distal propagation of an aortic valvular murmur must be distinguished from carotid bruits.) An additional sign of carotid occlusion is the presence of an intracranial murmur over the *opposite* carotid artery. This is heard best by placing the bell of the stethoscope over the eyeball. The murmur is presumably due to augmented blood flow through the remaining patent vessel. Pulsation may be reduced or absent in the internal or common carotid arteries in the neck, in the external carotid branch in front of the ear, or in the internal carotid artery when palpated in the pharynx. *Because of the possibility* of precipitous onset of unconsciousness, seizures, or an electroencephalographic change, compressing the patent contralateral carotid artery in the neck is a test not to be recommended.

The common carotid arteries may be occluded at their origin, as in "pulseless disease" or *aortic arch syndrome.* The neurologic symptoms and signs of carotid occlusion, just discussed, may or may not be present, depending on the adequacy of the circle of Willis and of the vertebral-basilar system. The following manifestations, for the most part nonneurologic, have been reported in the aortic arch syndrome: absence of pulsation in carotid and radial arteries, faintness on arising from the horizontal position, recurrent loss of consciousness, headache, neck pain, paresthesias of various parts of the body, transient blindness (unilateral or bilateral), dimness of vision with exercise, premature cataracts, retinal atrophy and pigmentation, atrophy of the iris, leukomas, peripapillary arteriovenous anastomoses, optic atrophy, claudication of the jaw muscles, perforation of the nasal septum, saddle nose deformity, trophic ulceration of the face, facial atrophy (unilateral or bilateral), indolent infections of the face, abnormal facial pigmentation, and loss of hair. This condition was originally described in Japan, particularly in young women who were found to be suffering from a granulomatous arteritis involving all three major trunks arising from the aortic arch (Takayasu's disease, see Chap. 246). An incomplete aortic arch syndrome consisting of various combinations of carotid, subclavian, or innominate occlusion or stenosis is not uncommon. The majority of the cases of pulseless disease in the United States and Europe, both the partial and the complete syndrome, have been due to severe atherosclerosis, which has often been mistakenly called *Buerger's disease.* Occlusion of the cervical arteries proximal to the internal carotid is frequently asymptomatic, because of the abundant collateral circulation.

VERTEBRAL-BASILAR POSTERIOR CEREBRAL SYSTEM **Posterior cerebral artery** In 71 percent of cases both posterior cerebral arteries arise from the basilar artery; in 22 percent one comes from the basilar and one from the internal carotid artery; and in 7 percent both come from the internal carotid. The terminal or cortical branches of this vessel supply the undersurface of the temporal and occipital lobes, as well as the entire medial surface of the occipital lobe including the visual area (areas 17, 18, and 19). From the more proximal part of the artery between its origin at the bifurcation of the

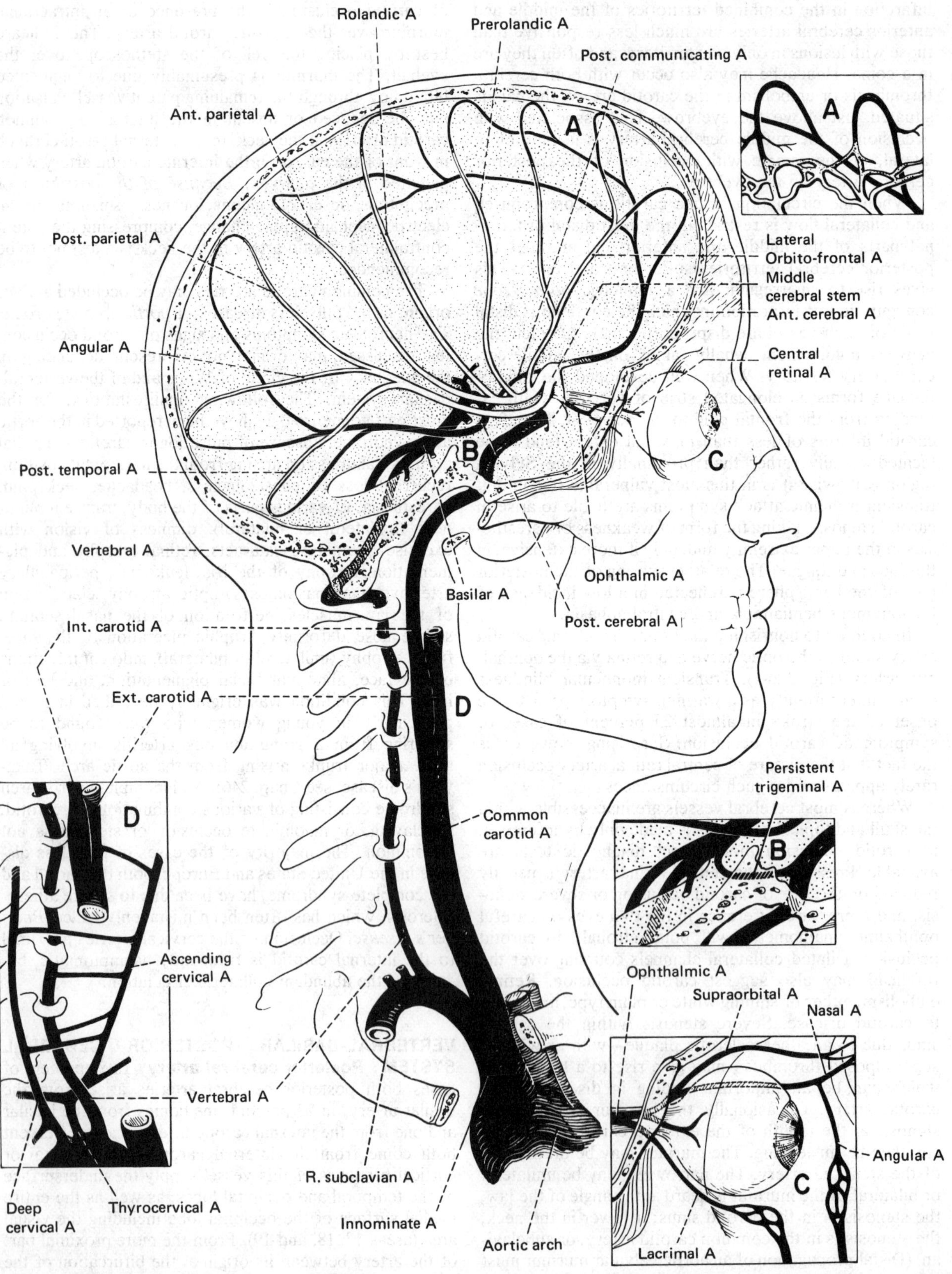
Rolandic A
Prerolandic A
Post. communicating A
Ant. parietal A
A
A
Post. parietal A
Lateral
Orbito-frontal A
Middle
cerebral stem
Ant. cerebral A
Angular A
Central
retinal A
B
C
Post. temporal A
Vertebral A
Ophthalmic A
Basilar A
Post. cerebral A
Int. carotid A
Ext. carotid A
D
Persistent
trigeminal A
D
Common
carotid A
B
Ascending
cervical A
Ophthalmic A
Supraorbital A
Nasal A
Vertebral A
Angular A
C
R. subclavian A
Deep
cervical A
Thyrocervical A
Innominate A
Aortic arch
Lacrimal A

basilar artery and the cortical distribution many important branches arise.

The interpeduncular branches arising near its origin penetrate the brainstem to supply the red nucleus, subthalamic nucleus of Luys, substantia nigra, the most medial part of the cerebral peduncle, the oculomotor nucleus, the reticular substance of the midbrain, the decussation of the superior cerebellar peduncles, rubrothalamic tract, medial longitudinal fasciculus, and the medial lemniscus. The thalamoperforating branches also arise here and pass to the inferior medial and anterior parts of the thalamus. Branches arising serially along the parent vessel as it encircles the midbrain supply the cerebral peduncle, lateral part of the medial lemniscus, corpora quadrigemina, pineal gland, lateral geniculate bodies, choroid plexus, and hippocampus. The thalamogeniculate branches supply the pulvinar and the lateral nuclei of the thalamus (Fig. 326-5).

Again the clinical picture resulting from occlusion will depend on the site of the obstruction, the ischemia-modifying factors, and the site and size of the resultant infarct. Occlusion proximal to the posterior communicating artery may be tolerated if collateral flow via that vessel is adequate (point A in Fig. 326-5); however, the penetrating branches arising from the stem of the posterior cerebral artery may be occluded at their mouths. Even distal to the posterior communicating artery, occlusion may cause no damage if collateral flow via the meningeal interarterial border zone anastomoses is sufficient.

Classically, occlusion of the cortical or superficial branches of the posterior cerebral artery gives rise to a contralateral homonymous hemianopia because of involvement of the primary visual area in the calcarine region. This syndrome and the effects of branch occlusions are indicated at C in Fig. 326-5.

Bilateral lesions of the occipital lobes, if extensive, cause total blindness of the cortical type, because of a bilateral homonymous hemianopia. The pupillary reflexes are retained, and funduscopically the optic nerves are not atrophic (unlike the situation in disease of the optic nerves). Often the patient is unaware of the blindness and may in fact deny it when questioned specifically. More frequently the bilateral lesions are incomplete and a sector of the visual field is left intact. When the remnant is very restricted, vision may fluctuate greatly from moment to moment, suggesting hysteria. In small calcarine lesions there may be loss of central vision only (bilateral homonymous central scotomas); on the other hand, in larger calcarine lesions, only central vision may be spared, and vision is likened to looking through a narrow pipe (gun-barrel vision). With bilateral lesions, there is usually a loss of memory, the severity of which varies from case to case. There may or may not be the various cortical disturbances described under unilateral lesions.

FIGURE 326-4

Arrangement of the major arteries on the right side carrying blood from the heart to the brain. Also shown are vessels of collateral circulation that may modify the effects of cerebral ischemia. For example, the posterior communicating artery connects the internal carotid and the posterior cerebral arteries, and may provide anastomosis between the carotid and basilar systems. Over the convexity, the subarachnoid interarterial anastomoses linking the middle, anterior, and posterior cerebral arteries are shown, with insert A *illustrating that these anastomoses are a continuous network of tiny arteries forming a border zone between the major cerebral arterial territories. Occasionally a persistent trigeminal artery connects the internal carotid and basilar arteries proximal to the circle of Willis, as shown in insert* B. *Anastomoses between the internal and external carotid arteries via the orbit are illustrated in insert* C. *Wholly extracranial anastomoses from muscular branches of the cervical arteries to vertebral and external carotid arteries are indicated by insert* D.

When occlusion of the *posterior cerebral artery* occurs more proximally, as at A in Fig. 326-5 (one might speak of anterior syndromes), the clinical picture will comprise signs of damage to thalamus, cerebral peduncle, midbrain, and subthalamus, and possibly, in addition, the manifestations just described (hemianopia, etc.), depending on the collateral inflow of blood. Best known is the *thalamic syndrome of Dejerine and Roussy*, which results from infarction of the region of the sensory nucleus in the posterolateral part of the thalamus (supplied by the thalamogeniculate vessel at B in Fig. 326-5). The lesion may be so small as to be overlooked on pathologic examination. The central feature is a sensory loss on the opposite side of the body, usually affecting deep and superficial sensation (pain, temperature, touch, proprioception); or rarely, it may be of the dissociated type, either pain and temperature or vibratory and position sense being affected while the other sensory modalities are relatively spared. It may take a monoplegic pattern. Sometimes there develops later an associated intractable agonizing pain in the affected parts of the body (thalamic pain), occurring spontaneously and augmented by all types of stimulation of the affected parts. However, this spontaneous pain is often entirely missing, whereas hyperpathia is common. Distortion of taste is not infrequent. In the motor sphere there may be a mild evanescent hemiparesis, and in some patients the affected limbs show hemiballismus, choreoathetosis, incoordination, intention tremor, asynergy, cramplike spasms, and a postural abnormality of the hand (see Chap. 18). The mind is usually spared.

Occlusion of the stem of the posterior cerebral artery may lead to a hemiplegia owing to infarction of the cerebral peduncle, but this is uncommon. Occlusion of the thalamoperforate branches which originate from the most medial part of the posterior cerebral stem gives rise to several different syndromes, depending on the branches involved: (1) a superior syndrome in which the upper part of the red nucleus or dentatothalamic tract is involved, producing on the opposite side of the body a gross ataxia (see Chap. 19); (2) an inferior syndrome (Claude's syndrome), in which a third-nerve palsy and contralateral cerebellar sings are combined; (3) Weber's syndrome, i.e., a third-nerve palsy combined with a contralateral hemiplegia (see Chap. 324); (4) *hemiballismus*, which probably arises also from an occlusion of the branch of the posterior cerebral artery running to the

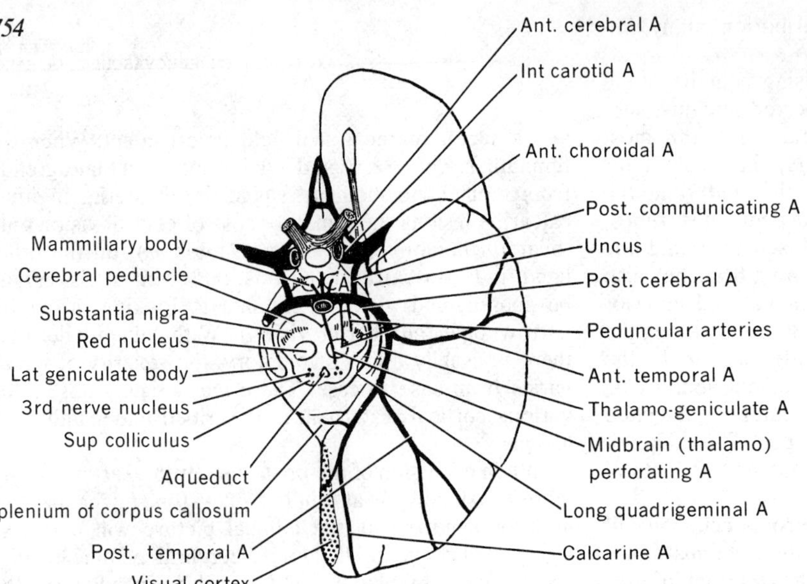

FIGURE 326-5
Inferior aspect of the brain with the branches and distribution of the posterior cerebral artery and the principal anatomic structures shown. Below is a list of the clinical manifestations producted by infarction in its territory and the corresponding regions of damage.

Signs and symptoms	*Structures involved*
Peripheral territory	
Homonymous hemianopia (often upper quadrantic)	Calcarine cortex or optic radiation nearby; hemoachromatopsia may be present. Macular or central vision tends to be preserved because occipital polar striate is spared
Bilateral homonymous hemianopia, cortical blindness, unawareness or denial of blindness; tactile naming, achromatopsia, failure to see to-and-fro movements, inability to perceive objects not centrally located, apraxia of ocular movements, inability to count or enumerate objects, tendency to run into things which the patient sees and tries to avoid	Bilateral occipital lobe with possibly the parietal lobe also involved
Verbal dyslexia without agraphia, color anomia	Dominant calcarine lesion of posterior part of corpus callosum
Memory defect	Hippocampal lesion bilaterally or on the dominant side only; or involvement of hippocampal system at another level (mammillary bodies, psalterium)
Topographic disorientation and prosopagnosia	Usually with lesions of nondominant, calcarine, and lingual gyri
Simultanagnosia, perseveration	Dominant visual cortex
Unformed visual hallucinations, peduncular hallucinosis, metamorphopsia, teleopsia, illusory visual spread, irreminiscence, paliopsia, distortion of outlines, central photophobia	Calcarine cortex. Complex hallucinations, usually nondominant
Central territory	
Thalamic syndrome: sensory loss (all modalities), spontaneous pain and dysesthesias, choreoathetosis, intention tremor, spasms of hand, mild hemiparesis	Posteroventral nucleus of thalamus in territory of thalamogeniculate artery. Involvement of the adjacent subthalamic body or its afferent tracts results in hemiballismus and choreoathetosis
Thalamoperforate syndrome: (a) superior, crossed cerebellar ataxia; (b) inferior, crossed cerebellar ataxia with ipsilateral third nerve palsy (Claude's syndrome)	Dentatothalamic tract and issuing third nerve
Weber's syndrome—third nerve palsy and contralateral hemiplegia	Third nerve and cerebral peduncle
Contralateral hemiplegia	Cerebral peduncle
Paralysis or paresis of vertical eye movement, skew deviation, sluggish pupillary responses to light, slight miosis and ptosis (retraction nystagmus and "tucking" of the eyelids may be associated)	Supranuclear fibers to third nerve, interstitial nucleus of Cajal, nucleus of Darkschewitsch, and posterior commissure
Contralateral rhythmic, ataxic action tremor; rhythmic postural or "holding" tremor (rubral tremor)	Dentatothalamic tract (?) after decussation. Site of the lesion actually unknown

subthalamic nucleus of Luys; (5) Parinaud's syndrome, paralysis of conjugate vertical gaze which results from damage to the region of the posterior commissure; (6) peduncular hallucinosis (visual hallucinations of brightly colored scenes and objects) has been observed in occlusion of the posterior cerebral artery, but the site of the lesion has not been determined. More often an intracerebral hemorrhage is responsible. Finally, (7) extensive infarction of the upper part of the midbrain results in deep coma, bipyramidal signs, and "decerebrate rigidity" (reflex extensor posture).

Lacunar infarction in the posterolateral thalamus causes a pure sensory or paresthetic stroke consisting of numbness and sensory loss in the face, arm, and leg on one side.

Vertebral artery The vertebral arteries are the chief arteries of the medulla, and each supplies the lower three-fourths of the pyramid, the medial lemniscus, all or nearly all the retroolivary region (the lateral medullary region), the restiform body, and the posteroinferior part of the cerebellar hemisphere (see Fig. 326-6). The relative size of the vertebral arteries varies a good deal, and in approximately 10 percent of cases, one vessel is so small that the other can be considered the only artery of supply to the brainstem. In this case, if collateral inflow from the carotid system via the circle of Willis is unavailable, occlusion would be equivalent to occlusion of the basilar artery or bilateral occlusion of the vertebral arteries. The posterior inferior cerebellar artery is usually a branch of the vertebral artery, but not infrequently it has a common origin with the anterior inferior cerebellar artery from the basilar artery. It is necessary to keep these anatomic variations in mind when visualizing the effects of vertebral artery occlusion.

The results of vertebral occlusion are quite variable. When there are two good-sized vertebral arteries, occlusion on one side occurs not infrequently without any recognizable symptoms and signs or pathologic changes. If the subclavian artery is blocked proximal to the origin of the vertebral artery, exercise of the arm on that side may draw blood from the vertebral-basilar system into the arm, sometimes resulting in the symptoms of basilar insufficiency. Fisher has called this the "subclavian steal" syndrome. If the occlusion of the vertebral artery is so situated as to block the mouth of one or more arteries supplying the lateral medulla, the lateral medullary syndrome may be precipitated, and this is probably the most common picture in vertebral occlusion (see below). When the branch to the anterior spinal artery is blocked, collateral influx from the spinal artery branch of the opposite side is usually sufficient to prevent infarction. If the branch to the pyramid is occluded, that part of the corticospinal tract may be infarcted unless collateral flow is adequate. Also, any of these branches may become occluded in its course after leaving the vertebral artery and may produce similar effects. Rarely, occlusion of the vertebral artery or one of its medial branches produces an infarct which involves the medullary pyramid, the medial lemniscus, and the emergent hypoglossal fibers [contralateral paralysis of arm and leg (face spared), contralateral loss of position and vibration sense, and ipsilateral paralysis and atrophy of the tongue]. This is the medial medullary syndrome (see Fig. 326-6D). Vertebral occlusion can also lead to symptoms by blocking the posterior inferior cerebellar artery. Occlusion of the vertebral arteries low in the neck is usually compensated for by anastomotic flow to the upper part of the vertebral arteries via the thyrocervical, deep cervical, and occipital arteries, or an influx from the anterior part of the circle of Willis may occur.

The *posterior inferior cerebellar artery* supplies the inferior portion of the lateral medullary region, the restiform body, and the inferior surface of the cerebellar hemisphere. It may be occluded at its mouth, i.e., by thrombosis of the vertebral artery, or anywhere along its course. Some patients tolerate obstruction of the vessel with little or no ill effect; in others an extensive infarct results in the cerebellum and/or the posterolateral medulla. It should be pointed out that the various cerebellar arteries are connected to their neighbors by subarachnoid interarterial anastomoses, in the same way as the main arteries of the cerebrum, and the potential for collateral flow to a compromised territory is excellent.

The clinical picture resulting from occlusion of the posterior inferior cerebellar artery is variable. Often no serious damage results. Occasionally the *lateral medullary syndrome* may be evoked through blockage of flow along the inferior artery of the lateral medulla. Although occlusion of the posterior inferior cerebellar artery is usually stated to be the cause of the lateral medullary syndrome, this appears to be true in only a very small minority of patients; more careful studies show that in 8 out of 10 cases the vertebral artery is occluded, and in the other 2 cases either the posterior inferior cerebellar artery is occluded or no arterial occlusion is found. Infarction in the posterior medullary region causes ipsilateral cerebellar ataxia and rarely hiccup. The symptoms associated with infarction of the inferior part of the cerebellum have not been clearly determined, but they also probably include ataxia.

The *lateral medullary syndrome* is produced by infarction of a small wedge of lateral medulla lying posteriorly to the inferior olivary nucleus (see Fig. 326-6D). The classic syndrome consists of the symptoms and signs listed below the figure. This syndrome,

---

Decerebrate attacks	Damage to motor tracts of upper brainstem

Resting tremor or tremor not easily abolished by relaxation has been omitted because of the uncertainty of its occurrence in the posterior cerebral artery syndrome

Peduncular hallucinosis may occur in thalamic-subthalamic ischemic lesions, but the exact location of the lesion is unknown

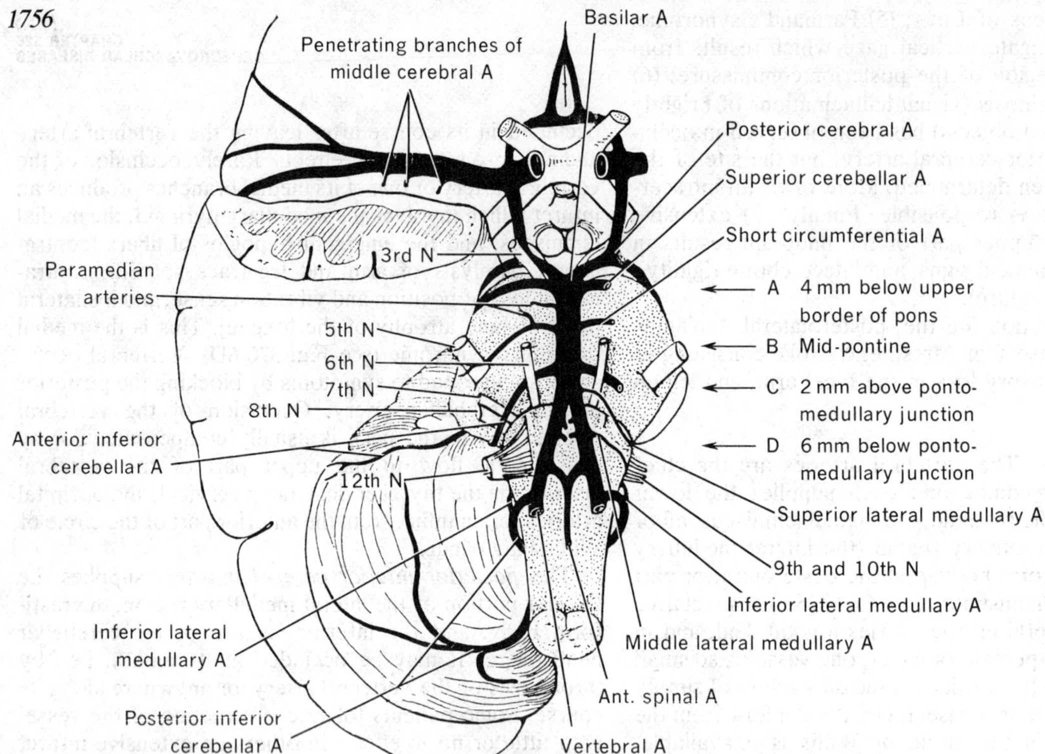

FIGURE 326-6
Diagram of the brainstem showing the principal vessels of the vertebral-basilar system. The letters and arrows on the right indicate the levels of the four cross sections A, B, C, and D which follow. Although typical vascular syndromes of the pons and medulla have been designated by sharply outlined shaded areas, the student must appreciate that since satisfactory clinicopathologic studies are far from numerous, the diagrams are not necessarily accurate, nor do they always represent established fact. The great frequency with which infarcts fail to produce a well-recognized syndrome and the special tendency for syndromes to merge with one another must be emphasized.

one of the most striking in neurology, is almost always due to infarction.

Basilar artery The basilar artery supplies not only the pons and upper part of the cerebellum but also in most cases the tissue in both posterior cerebral territories. Occlusion may occur in the trunk of the basilar artery or in any one of its branches.

The branches of the basilar artery may be conveniently grouped as follows: (1) paramedian, seven to ten in number, supplying a wedge of pons on either side of the midline; (2) the short circumferential branches, five to seven in number, supplying the lateral two-thirds of the pons and the middle and superior cerebellar peduncles; and (3) the long circumferential, two in number on each side, running laterally across the pons to reach the cerebellar hemispheres (the superior cerebellar artery and the anterior inferior cerebellar artery).

Occlusion of the basilar artery evokes a vast array of clinical manifestations reflecting involvement of a large number of structures [corticospinal and corticobulbar tracts, cerebellum, middle and superior cerebellar peduncles, medial and lateral lemnisci, spinothalamic tracts, medial longitudinal fasciculi, pontine nuclei, vestibular and cochlear nuclei, descending hypothalamospinal sympathetic fibers, the upper medulla, and the third, fourth, fifth, sixth, seventh, and eighth cranial nerves (including the nuclei, the segment within the brainstem, and the peripheral nerve itself)] (see Fig. 326-6).

The picture of basilar occlusion due to thrombosis may arise in several ways: (1) occlusion in the basilar artery itself, usually in the lower third at the site of an atherosclerotic plaque; (2) occlusion of both vertebral arteries, with closure of the second amounting to basilar obstruction; (3) occlusion of a single vertebral artery, when there is only one of good size. It must be emphasized that thrombosis may involve only a branch of the basilar artery rather than the trunk, and this is the most common cause of basilar symptoms. When the obstruction is embolic, the embolus usually lodges at the upper bifurcation of the basilar or in one of the posterior cerebral arteries, since if it is small enough to pass through the vertebral artery, it should easily traverse the length of the basilar artery, which is usually of greater diameter than either vertebral artery.

The composition of the complete basilar syndrome is given in Fig. 326-6D. In the presence of the full syndrome, it is usually not difficult to make the correct diagnosis. The aim should be, however, to recognize basilar insufficiency long before the stage of total deficit has been reached. The early manifestations occur in many combinations, and it would be difficult to list all the possibilities.

In regard to occlusion of individual basilar branches, the main signs of thrombosis of the *superior cerebellar artery* are severe ipsilateral cerebellar ataxia (middle and/or superior cerebellar peduncles), nausea and vomiting, slurred speech, and loss of pain and temperature over

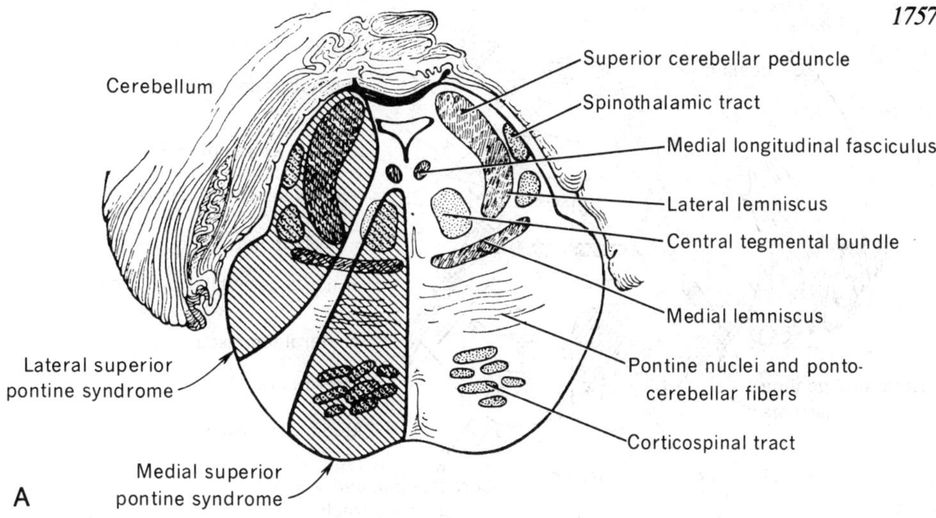

FIGURE 326-6A

1. Medial superior pontine syndrome (paramedian branches of upper basilar artery)

Signs and symptoms	*Structures involved*
On side of lesion	
Cerebellar ataxia (probably)	Superior and/or middle cerebellar peduncle
Internuclear ophthalmoplegia	Medial longitudinal fasciculus
Myoclonic syndrome, palate, pharynx, vocal cords, respiratory apparatus, face, oculomotor apparatus, etc.	Localization uncertain—central tegmental bundle (?), dentate projection (?), inferior olivary nucleus (?)
On side opposite lesion	
Paralysis of face, arm, and leg	Corticobulbar and corticospinal tract
Rarely touch, vibration, and position are affected	Medial lemniscus

2. Lateral superior pontine syndrome (syndrome of superior cerebellar artery)

On side of lesion		
Ataxia of limbs and gait, falling to side of lesion	Middle and superior cerebellar peduncles, superior surface of cerebellum, dentate nucleus	
Dizziness, nausea, vomiting	Vestibular nucleus	Territory of descending branch to middle cerebellar peduncle from superior cerebellar artery
Horizontal nystagmus	Vestibular nucleus	
Paresis of conjugate gaze (ipsilateral)	Uncertain	
Loss of optokinetic nystagmus	Uncertain	
Skew deviation	Uncertain	
Miosis, ptosis, decreased sweating over face (Horner's syndrome)	Descending sympathetic fibers	
Static tremor reported in one case	Dentate nucleus (?), superior cerebellar peduncle (?)	
On side opposite lesion		
Impaired pain and thermal sense on face, limbs, and trunk	Spinothalamic tract	
Impaired touch, vibration, and position sense, more in leg than arm (There is a tendency to incongruity of pain and touch deficits.)	Medial lemniscus (lateral portion)	

the extremities, body, and face of the opposite side (spinothalamic tract). Partial deafness, a static tremor of the ipsilateral upper extremity, Horner's syndrome, and bulbar myoclonus have also been reported. In occlusion of the *anterior inferior cerebellar artery* the extent of the infarct is extremely variable. The size of this artery and the territory it supplies vary inversely with that of the posterior inferior cerebellar artery. The principal findings are ipsilateral cerebellar ataxia (middle cerebellar peduncle), Horner's syndrome, ipsilateral deafness, whirling dizziness, nystagmus, tinnitus, nausea, vomiting, and paresis of conjugate lateral gaze. Pain and temperature sensation may be lost on the opposite side of the body. If the occlusion is close to the origin of the artery, the corticospinal fibers may also be involved, producing a hemiplegia. Occlusion of the *artery to the retroolivary space* will produce the lateral medullary syndrome. Occlusion of a *paramedian branch* will result in infarction of the corticospinal fibers, the adjacent pontine nuclei, and the pontocerebellar fibers on one side of the pons. If the infarct extends deep to reach the tegmentum, as it occasionally does, paralysis of conjugate lateral gaze and a contralateral sensory deficit will result. Occlusion of smaller branches in patients with hypertension and atherosclerosis results in small infarcts (lacunes), which cause a pure motor hemiparesis and dysarthria, and

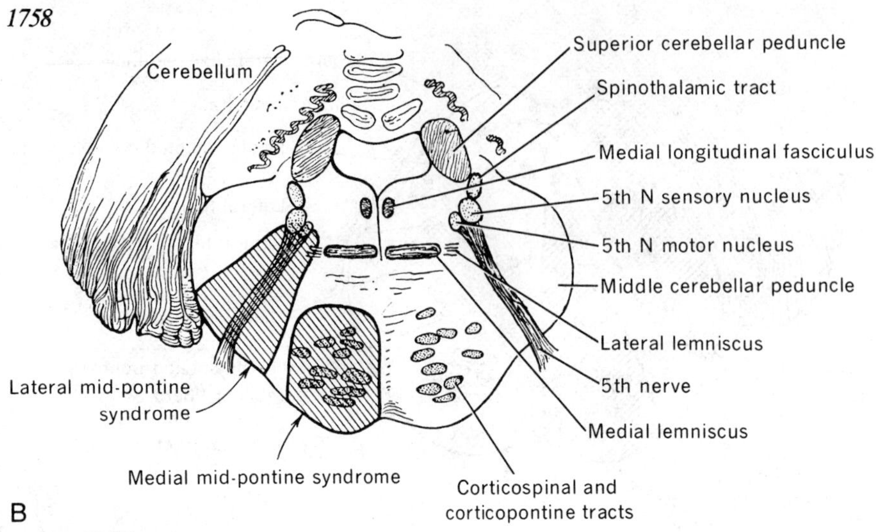

FIGURE 326-6B

1. Medial midpontine syndrome (paramedian branch of midbasilar artery)

Signs and symptoms	*Structures involved*
On side of lesion	
Ataxia of limbs and gait (more prominent in bilateral involvement)	Middle cerebellar peduncle
On side opposite lesion	
Paralysis of face, arm, and leg	Corticobulbar and corticospinal tract
Deviation of eyes	
Variable impaired touch and proprioception when lesion extends posteriorly. Usually the syndrome is purely motor	Medial lemniscus

2. Lateral midpontine syndrome (short circumferential artery)

On side of lesion	
Ataxia of limbs	Middle cerebellar peduncle
Paralysis of muscles of mastication	Motor fibers or nucleus of fifth nerve
Impaired sensation over side of face	Sensory fibers or nucleus of fifth nerve

which in the long run contribute to the lacunar state and the syndrome of pseudobulbar palsy.

One of the hallmarks of a brainstem lesion is *bilateral* motor and sensory signs. Within the brainstem, tracts descending to and ascending from each side of the body either cross each other or run in close proximity, in contrast to the cerebral hemispheres, where tracts serving the two sides of the body are widely separated.

Other cardinal brainstem signs are a "crossed" cranial nerve and long tract deficit or peripheral involvement of the cranial nerves III to XII. Although it is correct to emphasize that bilaterality of a lesion strongly suggests brainstem involvement, it must be pointed out with equal force that in many instances of infarction within the basilar territory the lesion is limited to one side, bespeaking occlusion of a basilar branch, not of the main trunk.

In the diagnosis of disease of the brainstem it is impossible from motor signs alone to distinguish a hemiplegia of pontine origin from one of cerebral origin, and we are dependent on coexisting phenomena. In a lower brainstem hemiplegia the eyes may move more easily to the side of the paralysis just opposite to the supratentorial lesions. In brainstem lesions, as in cerebral, a flaccid paralysis gives way to spasticity in the following days, weeks, or months, and there is no satisfactory explanation for the variability in this period of delay. The pattern of sensory disturbance may be helpful in localization. A dissociated sensory deficit over the face or one-half the body usually indicates a lesion within the brainstem, while a sensory loss over one side of the body involving all modalities with no suggestion of dissociation in any region indicates a lesion at the thalamic level or higher. When position sense, two-point discrimination, and tactile localization are affected relatively more than pain, temperature, and tactile sense, a cortical lesion is suggested; the converse suggests a brainstem location. When both motor and sensory manifestations are bilateral, it is almost unequivocal evidence that the lesion lies infratentorially. When hemiplegia or hemiparesis and sensory loss are coextensive, the lesion lies supratentorially. Additional manifestations which point unequivocally to a brainstem site are whirling dizziness, diplopia, cerebellar ataxia, Horner's syndrome, and deafness. The several brainstem syndromes illustrate the important point that the cerebellar system, spinothalamic tract, trigeminal nucleus, and sympathetic fibers can be involved at differ-

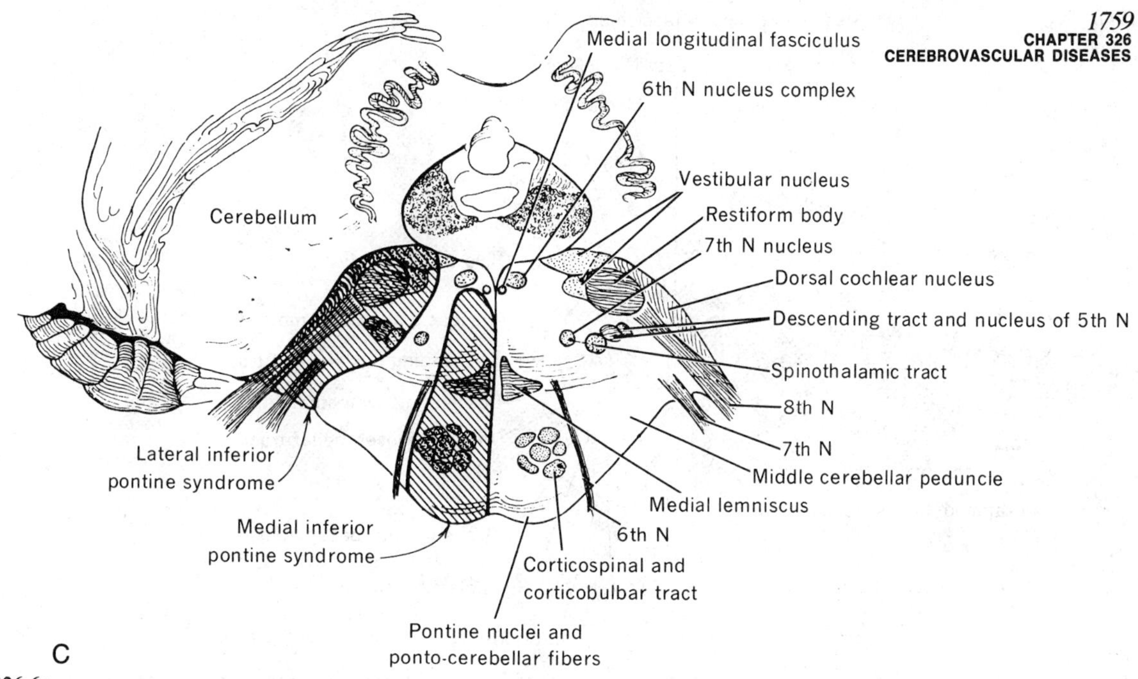

FIGURE 326-6C

1. Medial inferior pontine syndrome (occlusion of paramedian branch of basilar artery)

Signs and symptoms	*Structures involved*
On side of lesion	
Paralysis of conjugate gaze to side of lesion (preservation of convergence)	"Center" for conjugate lateral gaze
Nystagmus	Vestibular nucleus
Ataxia of limbs and gait	Middle cerebellar peduncle (?)
Diplopia on lateral gaze	Abducens nerve
On side opposite lesion	
Paralysis of face, arm, and leg	Corticobulbar and corticospinal tract in lower pons
Impaired tactile and proprioceptive sense over half of the body	Medial lemniscus

2. Lateral inferior pontine syndrome (occlusion of anterior inferior cerebellar artery)

Signs and symptoms	*Structures involved*
On side of lesion	
Horizontal and vertical nystagmus, vertigo, nausea, vomiting, oscillopsia	Vestibular nerve or nucleus
Facial paralysis	Seventh nerve
Paralysis of conjugate gaze to side of lesion	"Center" for conjugate lateral gaze
Deafness, tinnitus	Auditory nerve or cochlear nucleus
Crossed diplopia	Uncertain
Ataxia	Middle cerebellar peduncle and cerebellar hemisphere
Impaired sensation over face	Descending tract and nucleus fifth nerve
On side opposite lesion	
Impaired pain and thermal sense over half the body (may include face)	Spinothalamic tract

3. Total unilateral inferior pontine syndrome (occlusion of anterior inferior cerebellar artery). Lateral and medial syndromes combined

ent levels, and neighborhood phenomena must be used in order to identify the exact site.

Lacunar infarction in the pons may cause a pure motor hemiparesis or the dysarthria-clumsy-hand syndrome (dysarthria, facial weakness, slight impairment of the hand). Pontine lacunes are particularly associated with pseudobulbar emotional lability.

A myriad of eponymic brainstem syndromes, e.g., Weber, Claude, Benedict, Foville, Raymond-Cestan, Millard-Gubler, already mentioned in Chap. 324, have been described in relation to brainstem lesions. In their classic descriptions most of these syndromes relate to tumors and other nonvascular diseases, and only occasionally is one of them encountered in association with vascular disease. The diagnosis of vascular disorders in this region of the brain is not greatly facilitated by a knowledge of

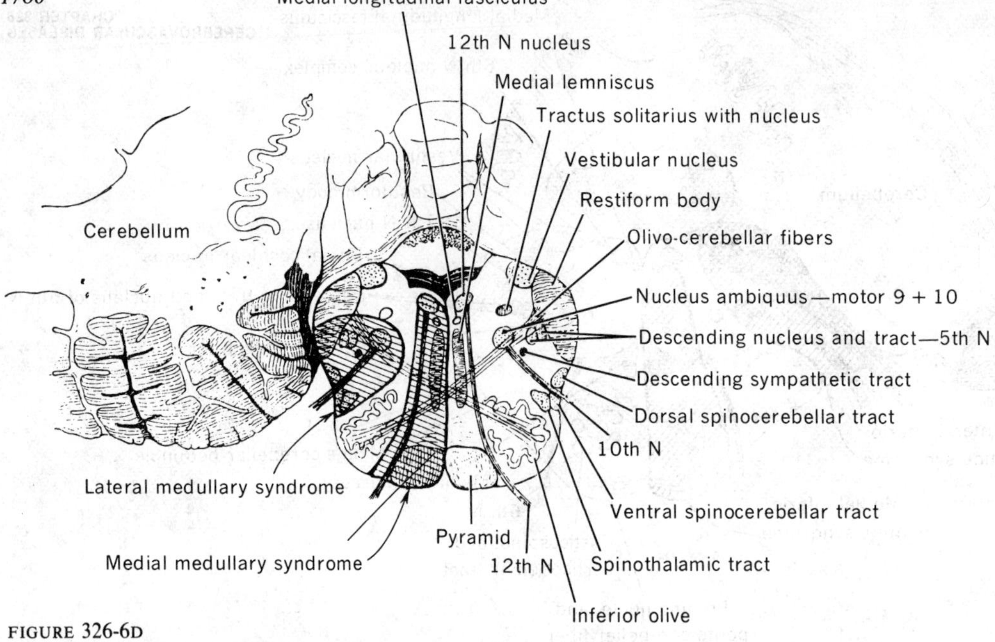

FIGURE 326-6D

1. Medial medullary syndrome (occlusion of vertebral artery or of branch of vertebral or lower basilar artery)

Signs and symptoms	*Structures involved*
On side of lesion	
Paralysis with atrophy of half the tongue	Issuing twelfth nerve
On side opposite lesion	
Paralysis of arm and leg sparing face	Pyramidal tract
Impaired tactile and proprioceptive sense over half the body	Medial lemniscus

2. Lateral medullary syndrome (occlusion of any of five vessels may be responsible—vertebral, posterior inferior cerebellar, or superior, middle, or inferior lateral medullary arteries)

On side of lesion	
Pain, numbness, impaired sensation over half the face	Descending tract and nucleus fifth nerve
Ataxia of limbs, falling to side of lesion	Uncertain—restiform body, cerebellar hemisphere, olivocerebellar fibers, spinocerebellar tract (?)
Vertigo, nausea, vomiting	Vestibular nucleus
Nystagmus, diplopia, oscillopsia	Vestibular nucleus
Horner's syndrome (miosis, ptosis, decreased sweating)	Descending sympathetic tract
Dysphagia, hoarseness, paralysis of palate, paralysis of vocal cord, diminished gag reflex	Issuing fibers ninth and tenth nerves
Loss of taste	Nucleus and tractus solitarius
Numbness of ipsilateral arm, trunk, or leg	Cuneate and gracile nuclei
Hiccup	Uncertain
On side opposite lesion	
Impaired pain and thermal sense over half the body, sometimes face	Spinothalamic tract

3. Total unilateral medullary syndrome (occlusion of vertebral artery). Combination of medial and lateral syndromes

4. Lateral pontomedullary syndrome (occlusion of vertebral artery). Combination of lateral medullary and lateral inferior pontine syndromes

5. Basilar artery syndrome (the syndrome of the lone vertebral artery is equivalent). A combination of the various brainstem syndromes plus those arising in the posterior cerebral artery distribution. The clinical picture comprises bilateral long-tract signs (sensory and motor) with cerebellar and peripheral cranial nerve abnormalities

Paralysis or weakness of all extremities, plus all bulbar musculature	Corticobulbar and corticospinal tracts bilaterally

these syndromes, and it is preferable to memorize the neuroanatomy of the brainstem.

The great desirability of being able to categorize brainstem vascular cases with accuracy need hardly be mentioned. An analysis of the authors' experience with a large number of these cases shows that too often it has been impossible to either designate the vessel involved or fit the clinical picture to an eponym. It seems more practical, therefore, to classify the cases according to the topography of the lesions within the brainstem, and for this purpose the classification shown in Fig. 326-6 was drawn up. There are some twelve syndromes in all, eight being medial and lateral lesions at four different levels of the brainstem—upper pons, midpons, lower pons, and midmedulla. Three are combinations of two or more of these eight syndromes, and the final one represents a full brainstem infarction. The principal syndromes are full basilar, lateral medullary, anterior inferior cerebellar artery, superior cerebellar, medial pontine, ponto-medullary, and medial medullary, in that order. Possibly division of the pons into three levels is excessive, and two would have sufficed. The medial superior pontine syndrome is very rare. However, a list has been useful in cataloging day-to-day clinical cases.

LABORATORY The cerebrospinal fluid pressure is normal in patients with cerebral thrombosis, unless the infarct is large and associated with severe swelling of the damaged tissue. Cerebral thrombosis never causes blood in the spinal fluid, which is "crystal clear" unless the infarct is especially congested, when a very faint xanthochromia (1 to 2 on a scale of 10) may occur. A slight increase in the leukocytes of the spinal fluid (3 to 8 polymorphonuclears) is common in the first few days of the illness. Rarely, and for unexplained reasons, a brisk, transient pleocytosis (400 to 2,000 polymorphonuclears per mm^3) occurs on about the third day. A persistent increase in the number of white blood cells of the cerebrospinal fluid suggests the presence of chronic meningitis (syphilis, tuberculosis, torula), granulomatous arteritis, septic embolism, cerebral thrombophlebitis, or a nonvascular process. The total amount of protein may be normal, but frequently it is raised to 50 to 80 mg per 100 ml. Rarely is it over 100, in which case some other diagnosis should be seriously considered. A Wassermann or some other specific test for syphilis is still routinely made in many clinics but can be dispensed with unless the rest of the clinical and laboratory picture points toward neurosyphilis. A positive test in a bloody fluid is not valid, since syphilitic reagin may have been carried into the fluid by the contaminating blood. Skull x-rays are not remarkable, and the pineal gland will not be shifted unless severe cerebral swelling has occurred, in which case the patient will usually be stuporous or comatose. Reference has already been made to the use of ophthalmodynamometry in the diagnosis of carotid obstruction.

The electroencephalogram is still of limited value in indicating infarction or distinguishing it from hemorrhage and from nonvascular conditions. In cerebral infarction the electrical activity may be found to be of a slightly slower frequency and lower voltage than normal. High-voltage slow waves (3 to 5 per sec) are evidence in favor of hemorrhage or tumor. The pneumoencephalogram may be normal or show local swelling in the acute stages of arterial occlusion, but in the healed stages local ventricular dilatation (or diverticulation) may occur at the site of tissue loss due to infarction. This procedure is not recommended as a diagnostic laboratory test in patients with occlusive cerebrovascular disease because of the danger of precipitating progression of the neurologic syndrome, due to the hypotensive state which so often attends the introduction of air. Carotid arteriography will demonstrate the blocked artery if it is in the carotid or in the proximal parts of the middle cerebral or anterior cerebral stems. To detect occlusion in the proximal parts of the common carotid or vertebral arteries or the innominate and subclavian trunks, injection via a catheter from femoral or brachial artery into the subclavian or the arch of the aorta is necessary. Arteriography provides essential information about cerebral hemodynamics. It is not without risk, and in patients with vessels narrowed by atherosclerosis the infarction may be extended. It should be used when the diagnosis of vascular disease is uncertain, when vascular surgery may be possible, or when anticoagulant therapy is contemplated in an indefinite case. Radioactive concentration studies (e.g., technesium, arsenic or mercury scan) used for the detection of tumor, abscess, etc., often show a mildly positive picture over infarcts, especially in the second or third week. Scintillation counting over the two sides of the skull after the intravenous injection of radioactive material may provide a comparative index of circulation in the two carotid systems.

COURSE AND PROGNOSIS When the patient is seen early in the course of cerebral thrombosis, it is extremely difficult to give an *immediate prognosis*. Where does the patient stand in the stroke process when first examined?

Signs and symptoms	*Structures involved*
Diplopia, paralysis of conjugate lateral and/or vertical gaze, internuclear ophthalmoplegia, horizontal and/or vertical nystagmus	Ocular motor nerves, apparatus for conjugate gaze, medial longitudinal fasciculus, vestibular apparatus
Blindness, impaired vision, various visual field defects	Visual cortex
Bilateral cerebellar ataxia	Cerebellar peduncles and the cerebellar hemispheres
Coma	Tegmentum of midbrain, thalami
Sensation may be strikingly intact in the presence of almost total paralysis. Sensory loss may be syringomyelic or the reverse or involve all modalities	Medial lemniscus, spinothalamic tracts or thalamic nuclei

Is worsening to be anticipated or not? No rules have yet been laid down which allow one to predict the course. A mild paralysis today may become a disastrous hemiplegia tomorrow, or the patient's condition may only worsen temporarily for a day or two. In basilar artery occlusion, dizziness and dysphagia may progress in a few days to total paralysis and deep coma. The course of the deficit is so often progressive that a pessimistic attitude on the part of the physician is justified in what appears to be a mild case.

Progression of the stroke is probably due to increasing stenosis of the involved artery by mural thrombus or to extension of the thrombus along the artery to block side branches and hinder anastomotic flow. In the basilar artery, thrombus may gradually build up along its entire length. In the carotid system, thrombus at times propagates distally from the site of origin in the neck to the intracranial supraclinoid portion, and possibly into the anterior cerebral artery, preventing collateral flow from the opposite side. In middle cerebral occlusion, retrograde thrombosis may occur back to the mouth of the anterior cerebral, perhaps secondarily infarcting the territory of that vessel. Some of the ischemia-modifying factors already referred to probably also play a part in the progression.

Several other circumstances influence the *immediate prognosis* in cerebral thrombosis. In the case of large infarcts, swelling of the infarcted tissue may occur, tentorial herniation follow, and the patient dies in 2 to 4 days. Milder degrees of swelling and increased intracranial pressure, though causing an apparent progression for 2 to 3 days, may not prove fatal. In extensive basilar infarction associated with deep coma, the patient seldom lives for more than a few days. If coma or stupor is present in a case from the beginning, survival may be largely determined by the success in keeping the airway clear and maintaining fluid and electrolyte balance (see Chap. 22). Respiratory and urinary infections are constant dangers, and once they begin, there is usually a rapid decline in the patient's condition as his temperature rises.

As for the *eventual, or long-term, prognosis* of the neurologic deficit, there are too many possibilities to recount them in detail. In the introduction it was pointed out that improvement is the rule if the patient survives. Lacunar infarcts with a pure motor hemiparesis fare very well. In the case of small infarcts, recovery may start within hours or a day or two, and restoration may be complete. In cases of severe deficit there may be no significant recovery whatsoever, and after months of assiduous efforts at rehabilitation, the patient may remain bereft of speech, with the upper extremity still totally useless and the lower extremity serving only as an uncertain prop in attempting to walk. Between these two extremes there is every degree of recovery. It is safe to say that the longer the delay before movement begins, the poorer the prognosis becomes. If recovery is not started in 1 or 2 weeks, the outlook is gloomy both for motor activity and speech, and in general it may be said that whatever motor paralysis remains after 5 to 6 months will probably be permanent. Aphasia, dysarthria, and cerebellar ataxia may improve for a year or longer, and sensory improvement has been detected for up to 2 years. A hemianopia which has not cleared in a few weeks will usually remain permanently, although reading and color discrimination may continue to improve. In lateral medullary infarction difficulty in swallowing may be protracted (4 to 7 weeks), and yet relatively normal function may be restored finally.

Characteristically, the paralyzed muscles are flaccid in the first days or weeks following a stroke, and the tendon reflexes may be unchanged, slightly increased, or decreased. Gradually spasticity develops, and the tendon reflexes become brisker. The arm tends to assume a flexed adducted posture, whereas the leg is usually extended and adducted. Function is rarely if ever restored after the slow evolution of spasticity. Conversely, the early development of spasticity in the hand, or the appearance of a grasp reflex, and other postural reactions may presage a favorable outcome. Bowel and bladder control usually returns and sphincteric disorders persist only in patients with the most severe hemiplegia or bilateral motor deficit. Not infrequently the hemiplegic limbs are at first tender and ache on manipulation, interfering with the physical therapy program. Nevertheless, physiotherapy should be initiated early in order to prevent contracture of muscles at shoulder, elbow, wrist, knuckles, knee, and ankle, a frequent complication and often the source of pain and added disability, particularly in relation to the shoulder. A typical Sudeck type of pain and bone atrophy of the hand may accompany the shoulder pain (shoulder-hand syndrome) as described in Chap. 10. An annoying, unsteady, "dizzy" feeling in the head often persists after damage to the vestibular system in brainstem infarcts.

Recurrent cerebral (epileptic) seizures are a complication in some 20 percent of cases of infarction in which the cerebral cortex has been involved. They are infrequent during the evolution of a thrombotic stroke and usually appear within a few weeks or months. The occurrence of a seizure followed by postictal (Todd's) paralysis must not be construed as extension of an infarct.

Many patients complain of fatigability and are depressed. The explanation of these symptoms is uncertain; some are expressions of a reactive depression (see Chap. 341). Only a few patients become serious *behavior problems* or are psychotic after a stroke, but paranoid trends, ill temper, stubbornness, and peevishness are common.

Finally, in regard to prognosis, it must be mentioned that having had one thrombotic stroke, the patient is in danger in the ensuing months and years of suffering delayed progression of his deficit or having a stroke at another site. The latter is especially true if there is hypertension.

TREATMENT OF CEREBRAL THROMBOSIS The treatment of cerebrovascular disease and strokes may be divided into four parts: (1) general medical management in the acute phase, (2) measures to restore the circulation and arrest the pathologic process, (3) physical therapy and rehabilitation, (4) preventive measures against strokes and vascular disease.

General medical management in the acute phase In essence, this is the care of the comatose or helpless patient (see Chap. 22).

Measures to restore the circulation and arrest the pathologic process Once a thrombotic stroke has developed fully, no therapy so far devised is of any value in restoring the cerebral tissue or its function. *To be effective, therapy must be preventive.* The diagnosis of thrombosis must be made at the earliest possible stage and the full catastrophe circumvented by every means. It will be appreciated, therefore, that all the measures used in combating a stroke in so far as they are designed to alleviate, check, or prevent the cerebral ischemic process are really preventive in nature. They will be instituted at various stages of the process—when only transient ischemic attacks are occurring or at any point in the progression of a thrombosis-in-evolution or when almost the full neurologic deficit has appeared. Even when persistent signs and symptoms have appeared, it is conceivable that some of the tissues affected, particularly at the edges of the infarct or islands within, have not been irreversibly damaged and will survive if blood flow can be increased.

The following therapeutic methods are being tried at present or have been tried in the recent past:

MEDICAL MEASURES TO IMPROVE THE BLOOD SUPPLY TO THE BRAIN Clinical observation indicates that strokes and ischemic attacks in many cases develop when the patient gets up from his bed, particularly in the morning or postoperatively. On the assumption that decrease in the cerebral circulation resulting from the upright position can aggravate cerebral ischemia, it is recommended that patients with a stroke as the result of ischemic infarction should remain horizontal in bed for 7 to 10 days initially and that, when ambulation starts, special attention should be given to preservation of the systemic circulation (avoid standing quietly for prolonged periods, sit with the feet up, etc.). Elevating the foot of the bed 14 in. or more in the acute stage may be beneficial. It is of great importance that the systemic blood pressure be maintained (correction of blood loss, use of Levophed in myocardial infarction with vascular collapse, avoidance of autonomic blocking agents, etc.). Injections of epinephrine have been recommended as a means of raising the systemic blood pressure above the usual levels. Although this enhances cerebral blood flow and might be beneficial, a systematic trial in thrombotic cases has not been undertaken. Anemia must be corrected. Polycythemia, if severe, may slow the circulation locally and must be treated.

ANTICOAGULATION According to present reports, anticoagulant therapy prevents transient ischemic attacks and postpones the arrival of an impending stroke whether the carotid or vertebral system is involved. Anticoagulants also halt the advance of a progressive thrombotic stroke, but not in all cases. In assessing anticoagulant therapy, one faces the question of where in the course of the stroke the patient stands when he is first examined. Will his course be benign or disastrous? There are no reliable rules for prediction at the present time. Anticoagulants are not of value in the fully developed stroke. Whether when given for a prolonged period of time they prevent the recurrence of a thrombotic stroke is still under study, but the incidence of severe hemorrhagic complications appears to limit their value in these cases.

When *anticoagulant therapy* is instituted in thrombotic cases, heparin is used intravenously in a dose of approximately 50 mg every 4 hr in cases with a progressing stroke or with transient ischemic attacks occurring more than once in 2 days. Heparin therapy is maintained for 1 to 3 weeks, when Coumadin therapy is instituted and continued well-regulated for 1 year or more. Coumadin therapy can be used alone from the beginning when transient ischemic attacks are infrequent. Anticoagulant therapy is not recommended in lacunar strokes unless they are at the stage of frequent transient ischemic attacks.

The use of anticoagulant drugs makes an accurate clinical diagnosis imperative. Intracranial hemorrhage must be ruled out by relying primarily on examination of the cerebrospinal fluid; it is to be remembered, however, that a clear fluid does not necessarily exclude hemorrhage (see Laboratory Findings below). A control prothrombin concentration and coagulation time are desirable before therapy is started, but if this is not feasible, the initial doses of anticoagulant drugs can usually be given safely if there is no evidence of active bleeding anywhere in the body. The question whether severe hypertension is a contraindication to anticoagulant therapy has not been accurately answered. There is no reliable evidence that complications are more frequent in the presence of hypertension if the prothrombin activity is maintained at 25 percent or higher, and therefore the authors have not withheld anticoagulant therapy in these patients; however, when the diastolic blood pressure is in the range of 130 mm Hg or more, an attempt is made at the same time to lower the pressure gradually with hypotensive agents, exercising care not to prejudice further the circulation in the region of the infarct by too great a reduction in the systemic pressure. It is preferable to avoid reduction of the blood pressure in the 2-week period immediately following a thrombotic stroke.

Anticoagulant therapy is relatively safe provided the prothrombin concentration is determined regularly (once a day, for the first 10 days, thence thrice a week, and finally once every week or 10 days) at a laboratory using reliable methods. Therapy can be prolonged for months and years, and only occasionally is it necessary to interrupt treatment because of unexplained disturbances of coagulation. Coumadin overdosage will cause hemorrhage from the kidney, nose, bowel, skin, or into muscle, as well as subdurally and into brain. Although most of these accidents are not serious, vitamin K_1 should be administered immediately.

SURGERY In recent years surgical management of the arterial obstruction in the neck and thorax has been used with increasing frequency, employing thromboendarterectomy or bypass grafts. The region of the carotid sinus is most frequently amenable to such therapy, but operation must be carried out at the stage of carotid stenosis rather than during total occlusion; otherwise secondary clot will have formed in the distal reaches of the artery, whence removal is impossible. Other sites suitable for surgical management include the common carotid, innominate, and subclavian arteries. Operation on the vertebral artery at its origin has not proved beneficial. Before operation the existence of the lesion and its extent must be determined by arteriography. Surgery is undertaken at the stage of transient ischemic attacks or early in the course of thrombosis-in-evolution. When total infarction has occurred, surgery will be ineffective even though patency of the vessel is restored. Surgery is not without risk, and its place in the treatment of cerebrovascular diseases has not been fully determined. In only a small minority of the total number of thrombotic strokes are the lesions so situated that surgery becomes feasible.

THERAPY FOR CEREBRAL EDEMA In the initial days following major cerebral infarction, cerebral edema may threaten life. In such instances, dexamethasone in intramuscular doses of 4 mg every 4 to 6 hr may prove helpful. Oral therapy with glycerin in doses of 30 ml every 4 to 6 hr or glycerol in doses of 50 g dissolved in 500 ml of 25% saline solution given intravenously daily are other forms of therapy available. The value of these agents in improvement of the neurologic deficit apart from therapy for edema alone remains a subject of dispute.

CEREBRAL VASODILATORS Despite experimental evidence that these agents increase the cerebral blood flow, as measured by the nitrous oxide method, they have not proved beneficial in careful studies in human stroke cases at the stage of transient ischemic attacks, thrombosis-in-evolution, or in the established stroke. This is true of nicotinic acid, Priscoline, alcohol, papaverine, and inhalation of 5% carbon dioxide. A few clinical trials have indicated that histamine, aminophylline, acetazolamide, and intraarterial papaverine have some merit. In opposition to the use of these methods is the suggestion that vasodilators are harmful rather than beneficial, since by lowering the systemic blood pressure they reduce the intracranial anastomotic flow.

THROMBOLYTIC AGENTS Fibrinolysin and profibrinolysin activator have not proved helpful in cases of transient ischemia, thrombosis-in-evolution, and the established stroke.

Physical therapy and rehabilitation Beginning within a few days, the joints of the paralyzed limbs should be passively carried through a full range of movement fifty times a day. Contracture (and periarthritis) must be avoided, especially at the shoulder, elbow, and ankle. Pain, soreness, and aching in the paralyzed limbs may temporarily interfere with exercises. The patient can be placed in a chair after 1 week or so, depending on the severity of his illness. Nearly all hemiplegics can learn to walk again to some extent, usually within a 3- to 6-month period, and this should be a primary aim in rehabilitation. A short or long leg brace is often required. Speech therapy is of questionable value but should be tried. At least it is of value in improving the morale of the patient. Physical therapy seems not to benefit patients with cerebellar ataxia. As the hemiplegic patient improves, and if mentality is preserved, instruction in the activities of daily living, using various special devices, can assist him in becoming at least partially independent in the home.

General preventive measures against strokes and vascular disease AVOIDING SITUATIONS IN WHICH STROKES ARE LIKELY TO OCCUR (1) Particular care should be taken to maintain the systemic blood pressure, oxygenation, and intracranial blood flow during surgical procedures, especially in elderly patients; (2) hypotensive agents, whether given therapeutically or for diagnostic procedures, should be administered with care; (3) in the elderly patient in whom deep sleep might help to precipitate cerebral ischemia, oversedation should be avoided; (4) systemic hypotension, severe anemia, and polycythemia should be treated promptly; (5) rapid diuresis may be contraindicated.

FACTORS WHICH DETERMINE ULTIMATE OUTCOME The ultimate solution of the problem of cerebrovascular disease lies in more fundamental fields. Atherosclerosis and hypertension must be prevented or alleviated (see Chap. 244 for prophylaxis of atherosclerosis and Chap. 245 for the treatment of hypertension).

Transient ischemic attacks of cerebral origin

It has already been pointed out that when transient ischemic attacks precede a stroke, they almost always stamp the process as thrombotic. Furthermore, neuropathologic studies indicate that these attacks are linked almost exclusively to atherosclerotic thrombosis. They belong, therefore, under the heading of cerebral thrombosis, but they are discussed separately here because of their importance clinically and therapeutically. Occasionally the development of cerebral embolism is associated with a few transient ischemic attacks and, rarely, cerebral hemorrhage.

In recent years increasing attention has been directed to these attacks, with the purpose of averting the threatening stroke by administering anticoagulant drugs or performing surgical endarterectomy at the stage of prodromal symptoms. There would seem to be little doubt that they are due to transient focal ischemia, and they might be referred to as temporary strokes which fortunately reverse themselves. Corresponding to the higher incidence of atherosclerosis in hypertension and in the male population, about two-thirds of all patients with transient ischemic attacks are men and/or hypertensive.

CLINICAL PICTURE Thrombosis of virtually any cerebral or cerebellar artery, deep or superficial, can be associated with transient ischemic attacks, e.g., common carotid, internal carotid, middle cerebral, anterior cerebral, ophthalmic, vertebral, basilar, posterior cerebral, the cerebellar arteries, and the penetrating branches to the deep structures of the basal ganglions and brainstem. If the posterior cerebral arteries are included in the vertebral-basilar system, ischemic episodes are slightly more common in that system than in the carotid. Transient ischemic attacks can occur by themselves, or they may precede, accompany, or follow the development of a stroke. So far, it has not been possible to distinguish the early cases destined to do well from those in which a full-blown stroke will develop.

Transient ischemic attacks last a few seconds up to 12

hr, the most common duration being a few seconds up to 5 to 10 min. It is uncommon for recurrent discrete attacks to last more than 30 min. There may be only a few attacks or several hundred. Between attacks, the neurologic examination may disclose no abnormalities. A stroke may ensue after the second episode or may be postponed until hundreds of attacks have occurred over a period of weeks or months. Not infrequently the attacks gradually cease and no important paralysis occurs, a fact which makes any form of therapy difficult to evaluate.

The neurologic features of the transient episode indicate the territory or artery involved and are fragments borrowed from the stroke which often is approaching. In the carotid system ischemia occurs foremost in the distal middle cerebral territory and adjacent border zone region, producing weakness or numbness of the opposite hand and arm. However, many different combinations may be seen: face and lips, or lips and fingers, fingers alone, hand and foot, etc. Other manifestations include transient monocular blindness or blurring of vision, aphasia, difficulty in calculation and other temporo-parieto-occipital disturbances (when the dominant hemisphere is involved), confusion, veering to one side, headache, and occasionally jerking or twitching, mimicking a focal epileptic seizure. Lack of pulsation in the carotid artery in the neck or pharynx, reduced pressure in the appropriate central retinal artery, and a carotid bruit in the neck indicate carotid disease.

The clinical picture in the vertebral-basilar system is exceedingly diverse, since so much motor and sensory traffic is sustained by the blood carried in these vessels. Occurring in the most varied combinations, the following manifestations in their approximate order of frequency may be recognized: dizziness, diplopia (vertical or horizontal); dysarthria; weakness of a part or all of one side of the body, or both sides; headaches; staggering gait; veering to one side; numbness of a part or all of one side, or both sides, or crossed numbness (one side of face and opposite limbs); a feeling of cross-eyedness; dark vision, blurred vision; tunnel vision; partial or complete blindness; scintillating scotomas; pupillary change; ptosis; paralysis of gaze; speechlessness; and dysphagia. Less common symptoms include noise or pounding in the ear or in the head, head or face pain, peculiar head sensations, vomiting, hiccups, memory lapse, confused behavior, drowsiness, unconsciousness (rare), impaired hearing, deafness, a feeling of movement of a part, hemiballismus, peduncular hallucinosis, forced deviation of the eyes, sweating, and facial redness.

It is not always easy to identify the territory affected. However, the occurrence of monocular blindness with or without contralateral weakness or numbness always points to the carotid system, as does receptive or sensory aphasia. The hallmarks of vertebral-basilar involvement are bilateral weakness and/or numbness, i.e., a disturbance of the long motor or sensory tracts bilaterally.

The attacks may all take approximately the same pattern or they may vary considerably in detail, although maintaining the same basic pattern. For example, weakness or numbness may involve fingers and face in some episodes and fingers only in others; or dizziness alone may occur in some attacks, while in others diplopia is added to the picture. In basilar artery disease each side of the body may be affected alternately. All the involved parts may be affected simultaneously, or a definite march or spread from one region to another can occur in a period of 10 to 60 sec, or even a few minutes; e.g., numbness may spread from the hand to the face, or the reverse. The individual attack may cease abruptly or fade gradually.

MECHANISM The onset of attacks in some patients is clearly related to standing up after lying or sitting. In general, attacks are likely to occur when the patient is up and around rather than lying down, but in many cases the episodes bear no relation to position or activity. They have been encountered in relation to exercise, exertion, emotional outbursts of anger or joy, and during bouts of coughing. Transient symptoms present on awakening from sleep usually indicate that a stroke is in the offing.

Ophthalmoscopic observations of the retinal vessels made during episodes of transient monocular blindness show either arrest of the blood flow in the retinal arteries and breaking up of the venous column to form "boxcar" pattern or white material temporarily blocking the retinal arteries. This indicates that in ischemic attacks a temporary, complete or relatively complete cessation of blood flow occurs locally, possibly with associated microembolism. Currently, recurrent ischemia is widely held to be the result of platelet emboli from sites of atherothrombosis, but proof is lacking. In the past, transient ischemic attacks have been attributed to cerebral vasospasm or to transient episodes of systemic arterial hypotension with resulting compromise of the intracranial circulation. Neither of these factors has been established. Although dropping the blood pressure to 90 or even 80 mm Hg by tilting the patient upright on a tilt table may cause electroencephalographic changes, it has not in the authors' experience reproduced the attacks. Vasodilator drugs have been without effect. There is good evidence that the attacks are abolished by anticoagulant drugs, but the mechanism of this is not known. Whatever their exact cause, they are closely related to vascular stenosis due to atherosclerosis and thrombosis. A proper recognition of the transient ischemic episode is of importance, since the use of anticoagulant drugs may prove of value in warding off an oncoming stroke.

DIFFERENTIAL DIAGNOSIS The following conditions must be differentiated: cerebral seizures (epileptic seizures), Ménière's syndrome, migraine accompaniments, Stokes-Adams attacks, hypersensitive carotid sinus reflex, transient global amnesia, insulin reactions, attacks of anxiety and depression, akinetic falling spells of the aged, and recurrent cerebral embolism.

Frank motor *convulsions* rarely if ever occur in ischemic attacks. The patient may report a feeling of movement, distortion, drawing, jumping, or jerking, but an isolated frank focal seizure has not been encountered. On the other hand, a cerebral seizure rarely displays as its own manifestation a temporary paralysis of a limb or of one side of the body. Unconsciousness is rare in ischemic attacks, and its occurrence even in only a few attacks indicates another diagnosis (seizure, Stokes-Adams attack, etc.). Incontinence of bowel and bladder, tongue biting, cyanosis, and residual sleepiness or muscle soreness are indicative of a seizure rather than an ischemic episode. In the sensory sphere, the distinction between ischemic episodes and seizures is less clear, for numbness or scintillating visual phenomena are seen in both conditions, and therefore in making a differentiation one must rely on the presence of associated phenomena (dizziness, diplopia, etc.). When numbness appears simultaneously in face, hand, and leg, i.e., when there is no "march," ischemia rather than a seizure is probably responsible. When a sensory march occurs, the pace of it may serve to distinguish the two in exceptional cases, for the numbness spreads from one part to another in a few seconds in a seizure and often over a period of many minutes in one of the ischemic episodes.

Dizziness associated with brainstem ischemia is less likely to have a clear rotatory component than that seen in *Ménière's syndrome or labyrinthitis.* In making a diagnosis, however, one depends on the presence of associated symptoms and signs. It is a simple matter to decide that the dizziness is of central origin when there are other evidences of brainstem involvement, by history or by neurologic examination: diplopia, dysarthria, cerebellar ataxia, vertical nystagmus, persistent horizontal nystagmus, numbness, weakness, dysphagia, etc. On the other hand, the isolated presence of the triad—recurrent dizziness, tinnitus, and chronic deafness (i.e., signs of both auditory and vestibular involvement)—is almost certain evidence of Ménière's syndrome. In the early stages the pictures at times resemble each other closely, however, and only an especially thorough search will reveal signs indicating that the disorder is due to ischemia of the brainstem. Tinnitus of a constant hissing or ringing type is a rare complaint in brainstem vascular disease. When dizziness is the sole symptom in an elderly person, it is often impossible to make an accurate diagnosis, and only after observing the patient for a period of time will the nature of the underlying disease be disclosed. Finally, it must be remembered that since both basilar artery disease and Ménière's syndrome are common conditions, the two may coexist.

The visual, sensory, and motor phenomena which precede the headache (or occur in its absence) in some cases of *migraine* bear a close resemblance to ischemic manifestations, but since migraine originates in early life, its differentiation from ischemic attacks does not ordinarily pose a problem. An important point is that migrainous accompaniments in 75 percent of cases develop gradually over a period of 5 to 10 min, marching across the affected region, whereas transient ischemic phenomena rarely do this. When vascular disease has its onset in the twenties or thirties, the two may be confused until the history is carefully taken. A migrainous accompaniment may return after a headache-free interval of 10 to 20 years. It is not rare for migrainous accompaniments to appear for the first time in the forties or fifties. Still more important, periodic headaches may not be obvious, leading to a denial of migraine. Headache, at times of great intensity, can accompany cerebral thrombosis, and in an elderly person the occurrence for the first time of periodic headache associated with numbness or weakness should suggest atherothrombosis rather than migraine. *Stokes-Adams attacks* and *hypersensitivity* of the *carotid sinus reflex* cause "collapsing spells" with unconsciousness, confusion, pallor, sweating and jerking, but almost never do they produce focal neurologic manifestations such as numbness, weakness, diplopia, etc. Difficulty in differentiation of these conditions will arise only when the clinical details of the episode are not available, and usually a careful minute-by-minute description of the attack will enable the physician to make the correct diagnosis. Only in an occasional case of basilar artery insufficiency will an ischemic episode result in unconsciousness, usually accompanied by other symptoms such as weakness, numbness, blindness, or dysarthria. In *akinetic falling spells of the aged,* the patient falls unconscious without convulsive movements, color change, or alteration in pulse, blood pressure, or respiration. Within a few seconds or a minute or two consciousness is restored.

Occasionally ischemic attacks may be confused with tussive syncope, multiple sclerosis, ulnar neuropathy, carpal tunnel syndrome, overhydration (hyponatremia), cataplexy with narcolepsy, brachial discomfort with hiatus hernia, cervical disk disease, severe postural hypotension, unusual symptoms in angina pectoris, recurrent pulmonary embolism, etc.

Cerebral embolism is frequently suggested as an explanation for recurrent cerebrovascular episodes. However, this seems unlikely if all the attacks are of approximately identical pattern, for successive emboli coming from a distance could not be expected to enter the same arterial branch. Moreover, one would expect the involved cerebral tissue to be at least partially damaged, leaving some residual signs. When only a single transient episode has occurred, the factor of recurrence does not assist in the diagnosis, and cerebral embolism must then be strongly considered. Single transitory episodes and multiple episodes of different pattern, suggesting embolism, must be clearly distinguished from recurrent attacks *of the same pattern,* which suggest thrombosis.

TREATMENT The therapy of transient ischemic attacks has already been discussed under Treatment of Cerebral Thrombosis, where it was pointed out that anticoagulants or surgical endarterectomy usually stop the attacks and prevent indefinitely the onset of a threatening stroke. Surgery must be seriously considered in carotid and subclavian cases. In many patients the attacks cease spontaneously, and anticoagulant therapy can be withheld if the episodes are few and spaced at long intervals. In nonsurgical cases, however, anticoagulants are indicated if the attacks are becoming more frequent, more severe, or of longer duration, or if each attack no longer clears away completely, and a persistent neurologic deficit is accumulating.

Other measures that have been recommended include administration of phenobarbital, papaverine, or nicotinic acid, inhalation of 5% carbon dioxide, breathing into a paper bag, and stellate block or cervical sympathectomy, but none of these has proved effective under careful clinical testing. On several occasions the authors have been impressed with the salutary effect of having the patient stop smoking cigarettes. For the more general therapeutic measures applicable in these cases, see the entire section, Treatment of Cerebral Thrombosis, above.

Other causes of cerebral thrombosis (infarction)

It will be seen from the list at the beginning of this chapter that there are a few causes of cerebral thrombosis other than atherosclerosis. There are fewer still that are important in the stroke picture. In some of those included, the mechanism is ischemia without actual thrombosis.

Venous thrombosis is a rather uncommon condition and rarely mimics a cerebrovascular stroke. Arising in relation to extracranial and intracranial sepsis, surgical operations, parturition, and chronic wasting illnesses, particularly in children, it can cause a relatively mild neurologic illness with raised intracranial pressure, headache, visual obscurations, and focal seizures, or on the other hand, it can lead to extensive cerebral infarction and hemorrhage, with grave neurologic manifestations and death.

Systemic hypotension usually results in unconsciousness (syncope) without focal motor and sensory signs. But if the state of vascular collapse persists for a sufficient length of time, ischemia distal to the point of stenosis may result. Infarction will occur in the border zone and adjacent distal regions of major arterial territories of the cerebrum and cerebellum. It has already been mentioned that transient ischemic attacks and persistent strokes often develop under circumstances which suggest that a fall of the systemic blood pressure was the precipitating factor. Hypotension occurs in "simple faint," acute blood loss, myocardial infarction, Stokes-Adams syndrome, traumatic and surgical shock, cardiac arrest or anesthetic accident during surgery, hypersensitivity of the carotid sinus reflex, and in the several types of postural hypotension [idiopathic, postsympathectomy, tabetic, diabetic, with autonomic blocking agents, with reserpine (Serpasil), and on getting up and around after surgical operations].

Arteriography occasionally causes cerebral infarction. In some cases this is the result of cerebral thrombosis, but the pathogenesis of other cases requires further study. *Arteritis* is no longer a common cause of cerebral thrombosis, at least in North America, owing to the present satisfactory treatment of syphilis. Necrotizing or granulomatous arteritis, whether limited to the cerebral vessels or occurring as part of a polyarteritis, usually produces a series of small ischemic deficits in brain, optic nerve, or spinal cord, and only rarely mimics a stroke. Idiopathic giant-cell arteritis involving the large arteries arising from the aortic arch is a rare cause of unilateral or bilateral carotid occlusion but must be kept in mind. It appears to be much more common in young women in Japan, the aforementioned Takayasu's syndrome or "pulseless disease." Cranial arteritis or temporal arteritis is usually limited to the extracranial arteries except for the small vessels supplying the optic and oculomotor nerves. Unfortunately, in over 50 percent of cases permanent blindness or a severe impairment of vision results. The process usually involves the internal or common carotid arteries, but rarely causes a stroke (Chap. 363). Occasionally vertebral-basilar ischemia is reported.

Polycythemia is stated to be a cause of cerebral thrombosis, but further study of the matter is required. *Thrombotic thrombocytopenic purpura* usually leads to multiple small infarcts and fluctuating, changing neurologic symptoms, but it is capable of causing infarcts several centimeters in diameter.

Idiopathic thrombocytosis with platelet counts of more than 10^6 per ml due to megakaryocytosis may result in multiple episodes of focal cerebral ischemia. Antimitotic drugs have suppressed the attacks. Hyperproteinemia (greater than 9 to 10 g per 100 ml) may produce impairment of circulation through small cerebral and retinal vessels (Bing-Neal syndrome). As in polycythemia the increased viscosity of blood, correctable by bleeding or plasmapheresis, tends to cause more general cerebral symptoms (confusion, coma, blurred vision) rather than strokes. Sickle-cell disease is associated with obstruction of small arteries, including the cerebral. A *dissecting aortic aneurysm* may involve the large vessels arising from the arch and result in carotid occlusion and hemiplegia, a concomitant fall in systemic blood pressure probably contributing to the picture. *Carotid occlusion* may be the result of direct *trauma* to the neck, or it may be precipitated by a "closed head injury," sometimes of a seemingly trivial nature. *Hypoxia* usually produces a diffuse destruction of neurons rather than frank infarction, but bilateral softening of the globus pallidus is a classic feature. *Tentorial and subfalcial herniation* and sometimes a cerebellar pressure cone can cause infarction by a compression of the posterior cerebral, anterior cerebral, and inferior cerebellar arteries, respectively. Under the rare types of infarction, it should be mentioned that carotid occlusion has been described following tonsillectomy, in association with *cavernous sinus thrombophlebitis*, and the trigeminal ganglionitis of herpes zoster. Also, a previously transient and harmless migrainous aura can be transformed into a persistent deficit, presumably because of infarction as the result of excessive ischemia. This complication most frequently takes the form of a homonymous hemianopia. Contraceptive therapy with progestin-estrogen combinations can cause cerebral infarction with or without vascular occlusion. Finally, a category for *cerebral infarction of undetermined cause* is included, for it must be admitted that in some cases even at neuropathologic examination it is impossible to determine the exact cause of an infarct.

Omitted here is *Binswanger's chronic progressive subcortical encephalitis*, a rare disease of cerebral white matter tentatively attributed by Binswanger to atherosclerosis. In some instances extensive softening of white matter is a form of border-zone ischemia, between the penetrating cortical arteries and periventricular ones.

CEREBRAL EMBOLISM

In most cases of cerebral embolism, the embolic material consists of a fragment which has broken away from a thrombus within the heart. Embolism due to fat, tumor cells, or air is a rare occurrence and seldom enters into the differential diagnosis of strokes. The embolus usually becomes arrested at a bifurcation or other site of narrowing of the lumen. Ischemic infarction usually follows and is pale, red, or mixed; red infarction, as pointed out earlier, nearly always indicates embolism. Any region of the brain may be affected, but the territory of the middle cerebral artery is most frequently involved. The two hemispheres are approximately equally affected. Large embolic masses will block larger vessels (sometimes the carotids in the neck), while tiny fragments may reach vessels as small as 0.2 mm, in which case the resultant infarct might be so small as almost to escape detection at autopsy. The exact behavior of embolic material is not fully understood. Often, it remains arrested and plugs the lumen solidly, but in many cases it breaks up into fragments which enter smaller vessels and disappear completely, so that careful pathologic examination fails to reveal their final location. The anatomic diagnosis must then be made by inference, e.g., the absence of a vascular occlusion at the proper site to explain the infarct, the absence of atherosclerosis or other cause for thrombosis in the cerebral vessel, a ready source of embolus, infarcts in other organs such as kidney and spleen, the occurrence of hemorrhagic infarction, and last, but not least, the clinical history.

Because of the rapidity with which occlusion develops in embolism, there is not much time for collateral influx to become established. Thus sparing of territory distal to the site of occlusion is not so common as in thrombosis. However, all the ischemia-modifying factors mentioned under thrombosis are still operative and will influence the size, shape, and severity of the infarct.

Brain embolism is essentially a manifestation of heart disease. Many kinds of heart disease can be associated with embolism. The commonest direct cause is *chronic atrial fibrillation* due to atherosclerotic or rheumatic heart disease, the source of the embolus being mural thrombus deposited within the atrial appendage. Atrial fibrillation due to other types of heart disease can, of course, also lead to embolism, e.g., hypertensive, congenital, thyrotoxic, or syphilitic. Embolism probably occurs also during paroxysmal atrial fibrillation or flutter, but there is need for further exact documentation of such cases. *Mural thrombus* deposited on the damaged endocardium overlying a myocardial infarct is the second most frequent source of cerebral emboli. Emboli can also arise from arterial thrombus associated with severe mitral stenosis without atrial fibrillation. *Cardiac surgery*, especially valvoplasty, may disseminate fragments of thrombus or particles of a calcified valve leaflet. Mitral and aortic valve prostheses are presently associated with embolism in 70 percent of cases. Paradoxic embolism can occur when an abnormal communication exists between the right and left sides of the heart, or when both ventricles communicate with the aorta. Thus embolic material arising in the veins of the lower extremity or, indeed, anywhere in the systemic venous tree may, particularly in conditions of pulmonary hypertension (often from previous pulmonary embolism), bypass the pulmonary circulation and reach the cerebral vessels. Subendocardial fibroelastosis, idiopathic myocardial hypertrophy, cardiac tumors, and cardiac lesions in trichinosis are rare causes of embolism.

TABLE 326-3
Causes of cerebral embolism

I Cardiac origin
- *A* Atrial fibrillation and other arrhythmias (with rheumatic, atherosclerotic, hypertensive, or congenital heart disease)
- *B* Myocardial infarction with mural thrombus
- *C* Acute and subacute bacterial endocarditis
- *D* Heart disease without arrhythmia or mural thrombus (mitral stenosis, etc.)
- *E* Complications of cardiac surgery
- *F* Valve prostheses
- *G* Nonbacterial thrombotic (marantic) endocardial vegetations
- *H* Paradoxical embolism with congenital heart disease
- *I* Trichinosis

II Noncardiac origin
- *A* Atherosclerosis of aorta and carotid arteries (mural thrombus, atheromatous material)
- *B* From sites of cerebral artery thrombosis (basilar, vertebral, middle cerebral)
- *C* Thrombus in pulmonary veins
- *D* Fat
- *E* Tumor
- *F* Air
- *G* Complications of neck and thoracic surgery

III Undetermined origin

The *vegetations of acute and subacute bacterial endocarditis*, being infected, give rise to septic embolism, which results in several different pathologic pictures in the brain. In some cases the infarcts (they are usually multiple) do not differ from those due to bland emboli; in others, tiny septic infarcts develop, or as in acute bacterial endocarditis, there may be miliary abscess into which a small amount of hemorrhage may occur (focal embolic encephalitis) and even meningitis. Mycotic aneurysm, now seen infrequently, is another complication of septic embolism and may be a source of intracerebral or subarachnoid hemorrhage. *Marantic or nonbacterial endocarditis* occasionally causes cerebral embolism and can produce a most baffling clinical picture, especially when associated, as it often is, with carcinomatosis.

The following sources of embolic material are less frequent or more difficult to prove: (1) Mural thrombus, deposited upon ulcerated atheroma in the arch of the aorta or in the carotid arteries, may break loose and find its way into brain arteries. Massage of the carotid sinus, a favorite site for atherosclerosis, may dislodge mural thrombus, with the production of a hemiplegia. This is one of the reasons why carotid massage should always be carried out gently. (2) Atheromatous material may be washed out of a large plaque in the aorta or carotid arteries and carried distally into the branches of the cerebral tree. (3) The pulmonary veins are a source of cerebral emboli, as indicated by the occurrence of cerebral abscesses in association with pulmonary suppurative processes and by the high incidence of cerebral deposits secondary to pulmonary carcinoma. (4) Surgery of the neck and thorax can be complicated by cerebral embolism. A rare type is that which follows thyroidectomy, in which thrombosis in the stump of the superior thyroid artery extends proximally until a section of it, protruding into the lumen of the carotid, is carried away into the cerebral arteries.

Cerebral embolism must always have occurred when secondary tumor is deposited in the brain, and cerebral embolism regularly accompanies septicemia. However, a mass of tumor cells or bacteria seldom is large enough to occlude a cerebral artery and produce the picture of a stroke. Nevertheless tumor embolism has been reported secondary to cardiac myomyxomas and occasionally with other tumors. It must be distinguished from the marantic endocarditis and embolism which occasionally complicate carcinomatosis. Embolism in the course of septicemia usually means that a vegetative endocarditis is present with thrombus formation. Cerebral fat embolism is usually related to trauma. As a rule, the emboli are minute and widely dispersed, giving rise to multiple petechial hemorrhages; accordingly the clinical picture is usually not focal, as in a stroke. Cerebral air embolism is a rare complication of criminal abortion or of cervical and thoracic operations and was formerly encountered as a complication of pneumothorax therapy. This condition is usually difficult to separate on clinical grounds from the deficits following hypotension or hypoxia, which frequently coexist.

Not infrequently at autopsy the diagnosis of cerebral embolism is made with full justification without finding a source. The same is true of embolism elsewhere in the body. Possibly the routine search for a thrombotic nidus is not sufficiently thorough, and small thrombi in the atrial appendage, the pulmonary veins, or the endocardium between the papillary muscles of the heart may be overlooked. Nevertheless, in some cases studied most carefully, no source of embolic material has been discovered.

CLINICAL PICTURE Of all strokes, those due to cerebral embolism develop most rapidly. "Like a bolt out of the blue," the full-blown picture evolves within several seconds or a minute, exemplifying most strikingly the temporal profile of a stroke. The neurologic deficit nearly always comes in a single sudden attack, only rarely in stuttering fashion. As a rule, there are no warning episodes whatsoever. This statement is possibly too stringent, for in occasional cases a transient episode may precede the final arrival of the stroke. However, any emphasis on these exceptions is misleading. The embolus strikes at any time of the day or night. Getting up to go to the bathroom is a time of danger. When the stroke occurs during sleep, its exact mode of development will not be known.

The neurologic picture will depend on the artery involved and where the obstruction lies. The syndromes related to each cerebrovascular territory are the same as those outlined under Cerebral Thrombosis above. A large embolus may plug the internal carotid artery or the stem of the middle cerebral artery, producing a severe hemiplegia. More often the embolus is smaller and passes into one of the branches of the middle cerebral artery, producing a strikingly focal disorder: motor aphasia, a monoplegia (or part thereof), a central type of aphasia with little or no motor paralysis, or a sensorimotor paralysis with little or no involvement of the supersensory zone. In fact, most patients diagnosed as having middle cerebral artery thrombosis prove to have emboli in the middle cerebral artery (or an atherosclerotic thrombosis of the carotid artery). It is important to realize that an embolus in its passage along an artery may produce a severe neurologic deficit which is only temporary and which clears up almost as quickly as it came, as the embolus finally passes into a small branch supplying a relatively silent part of the hemisphere. In other words, embolism is one of the causes of a single evanescent stroke, and a common one. Also it can give rise to multiple transient attacks of differing pattern. It has already been pointed out that recurrent transient ischemic attacks of the same pattern are not likely to be embolic, since successive emboli would hardly lodge at identical sites. Embolic material entering the vertebral-basilar system occasionally lodges in the vertebral artery just below its union with the basilar, but more often it traverses the vertebral and also the basilar, which is larger, and is not held up until it reaches the upper bifurcation. If arrested here, it abruptly produces deep coma and total paralysis. More often the embolus enters one, or both, of the posterior cerebral arteries and, by infarcting the visual cortex, causes a unilateral or bilateral homonymous hemianopia. Embolic infarction of the undersurface of the cerebellum is common, whereas embolic material rarely enters the penetrating branches of the pons.

The general neurologic disturbance associated with embolic strokes is not significantly different from that seen in thrombotic cases, and the reader is referred to the description of the changes in consciousness, respiration, etc., under Course and Prognosis, above. Again the patient may have a most devastating hemiplegia and yet be alert. Headache is not uncommon.

Although the abruptness with which the stroke develops and the lack of prodromal symptoms point strongly to embolism, it is the total clinical picture upon which the diagnosis is based. If hemorrhage is ruled out, there remains only thrombosis to be excluded. The presence of atrial fibrillation, a history of myocardial infarction (recent or in the preceding months), or the occurrence of embolism to other regions of the body all support the diagnosis of embolism. Embolism merits the most careful consideration in young persons in whom atherosclerosis is rather unlikely. Not infrequently the first sign of myocardial infarction is the occurrence of embolism; therefore, it is advisable that *an electrocardiogram be made in all patients with cerebrovascular stroke of uncertain origin.*

Acute and subacute bacterial endocarditis do not usually present as a stroke due to infarction, although this happens occasionally. The signs of endocarditis, anemia, splenomegaly, and often a pleocytosis in the cerebrospinal fluid should point to the correct diagnosis.

The diagnosis of the other causes of cerebral embolism—cardiac surgery, neck surgery, pulmonary vein thrombosis, marantic endocarditis, paradoxic embolism, tumor, fat, and air—need not be enlarged upon here.

LABORATORY FINDINGS The description under Cerebral Thrombosis above applies for the most part to embolism except insofar as hemorrhagic infarction and septic embolism (focal embolic encephalitis) are concerned. Cerebral embolism in some 30 percent of cases produces a hemorrhagic infarct, which in most instances does not cause the cerebrospinal fluid to be bloody. However, in some excessively hemorrhagic infarcts, the fluid may be grossly bloody and contain as high as 10,000 or more red cells per mm^3. In the milder cases of hemorrhagic infarction, a slight xanthochromia (grade 1 to 3 on the scale of 1 to 10) may appear after a few days. The possibility that an embolic infarct is unusually bloody underlines the danger of administering anticoagulants routinely without a careful examination of the cerebrospinal fluid in cases of cerebral embolism. Also, it is the single exception to the rule that blood in the spinal fluid is unequivocal evidence that the stroke is due primarily to a hemorrhage.

In septic embolism resulting from subacute bacterial endocarditis the white blood cells in the cerebrospinal fluid may be increased, usually numbering up to 200 per mm^3 and occasionally reaching several hundred; the proportion of lymphocytes and polymorphonuclears varies with the acuteness of the septic process. There may also be several hundred or more red blood cells, and a faint xanthochromia is often present. The protein values are elevated, and the sugar content is within normal limits. No bacteria are seen or obtained by culture. In acute bacterial endocarditis there may be either the cerebrospinal fluid formula of subacute endocarditis or a frank purulent meningitis.

COURSE AND PROGNOSIS The remarks made concerning the *immediate prognosis* in cerebral thrombosis apply as well here. As a rule, all but the most aggravated cases survive the initial insult. Massive brainstem infarction as a result of basilar embolism is almost always fatal. The *eventual prognosis* as to survival is determined by the occurrence of further emboli and the gravity of the underlying illness—cardiac failure, rheumatic heart disease, myocardial infarction, bacterial endocarditis, malignant growth, etc. The threat of an early recurrence of embolism is very real, and it is not uncommon to have the second embolus strike within a few days or weeks of the first. The urgency of anticoagulant therapy is thereby emphasized. The *eventual prognosis* regarding the neurologic deficit is not different from that given for cerebral thrombosis (see Course and Prognosis above). The fact that an embolic episode may last only minutes or hours before clearing up should be stressed, especially in estimating the effect of any therapeutic measure.

Treatment The first three phases of therapy—(1) general medical management in the acute phase, (2) measures directed to restoring the circulation, and (3) rehabilitation—are much the same as described under Treatment of Cerebral Thrombosis above. Attempted embolectomy at the bifurcation of the common carotid artery has usually failed but should be considered. If pulsation in the temporal artery in front of the ear is present, it means the embolus is not at that bifurcation but has passed up into the internal carotid system, and embolectomy will probably be unsuccessful. The same is true of embolectomy of the middle cerebral artery. Fibrinolysin therapy has not been effective. In the field of prophylaxis there is strong evidence that the use of long-term anticoagulant therapy is effective in the prevention of embolism in cases of atrial fibrillation, myocardial infarction, and valve prosthesis. After cerebral embolism has occurred, the question arises as to the necessity of delaying anticoagulant therapy for several days to avoid precipitating bleeding into a hemorrhagic infarct. It is the authors' practice always to perform a lumbar puncture first in order to rule out gross hemorrhage from the infarct. If the cerebrospinal fluid is clear, the authors proceed with anticoagulant therapy, since there is the constant danger of another embolus breaking away from the heart. We have not encountered a case in which the use of anticoagulant drugs has seemed to increase the degree of hemorrhage within a hemorrhagic infarct, and indications are that such therapy is relatively safe. Rare exceptions to this statement may be expected. The use of anticoagulant therapy in patients with acute myocardial infarction, including those judged to be in the "good risk" category, is advisable. In cerebral embolism associated with subacute bacterial endocarditis, anticoagulant therapy is usually held to be contraindicated because of the danger of intracranial bleeding, but this viewpoint is not well founded. Nevertheless caution is advisable in this matter, and it is preferable to rely on a rapid sterilization of the bloodstream.

Valvoplasty and amputation of the atrial appendage have substantially reduced the incidence of embolism in rheumatic heart disease. The need for special care in preventing emboli from entering the carotid arteries during the performance of cardiac valvoplasty is appreciated by all thoracic surgeons.

INTRACRANIAL HEMORRHAGE

Although more than a dozen causes of intracranial hemorrhage have been listed (Table 326-4), hypertensive intracerebral hemorrhage and ruptured saccular aneurysm account for most of the hemorrhages which give rise to the clinical picture of a stroke. Duret hemorrhages, hypertensive encephalopathy, and idiopathic brain purpura will not simulate a stroke and are included only for the sake of completeness.

Hypertensive intracerebral hemorrhage

Hypertensive intracerebral hemorrhage is the ordinary, well-recognized brain hemorrhage. Although sometimes the levels of blood pressure are only in the range of 160 to 170/90, in most cases they are much higher. Hypertensive hemorrhage occurs within brain tissue, and rupture of the arteries lying in the subarachnoid space is practically unknown, apart from aneurysm. It is a mistake to think of hypertensive hemorrhage as arising from the large arteries at the base of the brain. The extravasation which results from rupture of an artery forms a roughly circular or oval mass, which disrupts the tissue as the bleeding continues and it grows in volume. Adjacent brain tissue is displaced and compressed. If the hemorrhage is large, midline structures are displaced to the opposite side and vital centers are compromised, leading to coma and

TABLE 326-4
Causes of intracranial hemorrhage (including intracerebral, subarachnoid, ventricular, and rarely subdural)

1. Hypertensive and intracerebral hemorrhage
2. Ruptured saccular aneurysm
3. Ruptured angioma
4. Trauma including posttraumatic delayed apoplexy
5. Hemorrhagic disorders: leukemia, aplastic anemia, thrombopenic purpura, liver disease, complication of anticoagulant therapy, hyperfibrinolysis, hypofibrinogenemia, hemophilia, Christmas disease
6. Undetermined cause (normal blood pressure and no angioma)
7. Hemorrhage into primary and secondary brain tumors
8. Septic embolism, mycotic aneurysm
9. With hemorrhagic infarction, arterial or venous
10. Hypertensive encephalopathy
11. Idiopathic brain purpura
12. Secondary brainstem hemorrhage
13. With inflammatory disease of the arteries and veins
14. Miscellaneous rare types: after vasopressor drugs, upon exertion, during arteriography, during painful urologic examination, as a late complication of early-life carotid occlusion, complication of carotid-cavernous arteriovenous fistula, with anoxemia, migraine, teratomatous malformations. (Acute inclusion body encephalitis produces xanthochromia and up to 2,000 red blood cells or more per ml of cerebrospinal fluid; acute necrotizing hemorrhagic encephalopathy may be associated with up to 100 red blood cells per ml of cerebrospinal fluid; tularemia and snake venom poisoning may cause bloody cerebrospinal fluid.)

death. Rupture or seepage into the ventricular system usually occurs, and the spinal fluid becomes bloody in more than 90 percent of cases. A hemorrhage of this type almost never ruptures directly into the subarachnoid space through the cerebral cortex, and the blood reaches the subarachnoid spinal fluid via the ventricular system. When the hemorrhage is small and placed at a distance from the ventricles, the cerebrospinal fluid may remain clear even on repeated examinations.

Extravasated blood undergoes a series of changes beginning with phagocytosis at the outer rim producing a brown-orange zone of hemosiderin-filled macrophages. The mass gradually decreases in size, and after a period of some 2 to 6 months, only an orange-stained cleft is left at the site of the hemorrhage.

Hemorrhages might be classified as massive, small, slit, and petechial. *Massive* refers to huge hemorrhages several centimeters in diameter; *small* to those 1 to 2 cm in diameter; *slit* applies to a special type of hypertensive hemorrhage which lies subcortically at the junction of white and gray matter and which in the healing stage becomes narrowed to a long, thin, orange cavity.

In order of frequency, the most common sites for hypertensive hemorrhage are (1) the putamen and adjacent internal capsule (50 percent of cases), (2) thalamus, (3) cerebellar hemisphere, (4) pons, and (5) various parts of the central white matter (frontal lobe, corona radiata, etc., probably extensions from the putamen). The vessel involved is usually a penetrating artery. The nature of the vascular lesion which leads to arterial rupture is not known, and indeed, the site of the rupture has not been reliably identified. Atherosclerosis is held by many to be a factor, but there is no proof for this view, and hemorrhages are encountered in the absence of grossly visible atherosclerosis. Small aneurysmal dilatations were reported by Charcot and Bouchard to be the basis for the rupture. Hyalinosis and necrotizing change in the small arteries due to hypertension have also been described as the precursor of hemorrhage; this cannot at the moment be affirmed or denied. Another hypothesis attributes the hemorrhage to a confluence of myriads of smaller diapedetic hemorrhages rather than a single extravasation, but this is entirely without grounds and represents a confusion of hemorrhagic infarction and massive hemorrhage.

CLINICAL PICTURE The clinical picture conforms accurately to the temporal profile of a cerebrovascular stroke; namely, it has an abrupt onset and rather rapid evolution. The stroke usually evolves gradually and steadily over an appreciable length of time, taking minutes, hours, or occasionally days (average of 1 to 24 hr) to reach its peak, depending on the speed of bleeding. Usually there are no recognizable warning or prodromal symptoms. Often the patient has been well, and headache, dizziness, and epistaxis have not occurred with any consistency as prodromal symptoms. There is no sex or age predilection except that the younger are usually spared. However, average age of occurrence is less than in thrombotic infarction. In the great majority of cases, the hemorrhage comes on while the patient is up and active, and onset during sleep is a rarity. Hypertension is maintained early in the course of the stroke or may even rise higher, so that the existence of hypertension will be easily established when the patient is first examined. Hypertension is usually of the "essential" type, but other causes must always be considered—renal disease, toxemia of pregnancy, pheochromocytoma, ACTH overdosage, injection of excessive amounts of epinephrine, and rarely, violent exertion or an intense emotional experience. Cardiomegaly is usually present.

There is ordinarily only one episode of hemorrhage, and recurrence of bleeding from the same site, as occurs in cases of saccular aneurysm, is not encountered. Once bleeding has become arrested, rebleeding in the near future, i.e., after the first few days, is not to be anticipated. When blood is spilled into the tissues, it is removed slowly, over a period of weeks and months, during which time symptoms and signs persist. Hence the neurologic deficit is never transitory in intracerebral hemorrhage, as it so often is in thrombosis and embolism, and, for the same reason, rapid fluctuations in the neurologic deficit from one examination to another are not to be expected.

The neurologic signs and symptoms vary with the site and size of the extravasation. The most common picture is that associated with a *putaminal hemorrhage,* in which the adjacent internal capsule is implicated. The patient complains of something going awry within the head. In a few minutes the face sags on one side, speech becomes slurred or aphasic, the arm and leg gradually weaken, and the eyes tend to deviate away from the side of the paretic limbs. A carefully taken history often reveals that these events occurred gradually over a period of 5 to 30 min.

This type of evolution is virtually diagnostic of intracerebral bleeding. Gradually the paralysis worsens, the affected limbs become flaccid, pinprick is not appreciated, a Babinski sign appears, speaking becomes impossible, and confusion gives way to stupor. In the worst cases, signs of upper brainstem compression appear—coma, Babinski sign bilaterally, deep, irregular, or intermittent respiration, dilated fixed pupils, and occasionally decerebrate rigidity.

Thalamic hemorrhage of moderate size also produces a hemiplegia or hemiparesis via pressure on the adjacent internal capsule. The sensory deficit equals or outstrips the motor weakness. Aphasia may be present with lesions of the dominant side and apractagnosia of the nondominant. A homonymous field defect if present usually clears in a few days. Thalamic hemorrhage by virtue of its extension medially and into the subthalamus causes a series of ocular disturbances, including paralysis of vertical gaze, forced deviation of the eyes downward, inequality of pupils, with absence of light reaction, skew deviation with the eye opposite the hemorrhage being displaced downward and medially, ipsilateral ptosis and miosis, absence of convergence, an assortment of lateral gaze abnormalities (paresis or pseudoparesis of the sixth nerve), retraction nystagmus, and tucking of the eyelids. Another unusual sign is so-called "peduncular hallucinosis." Neck retraction may be prominent. Hemorrhage into the nondominant thalamus is liable to produce mutism.

In *pontine hemorrhage,* deep coma ensues in a few minutes, and the clinical picture includes total paralysis, prominent decerebrate rigidity, and small (1 mm) pupils that react to light. Lateral eye movements, evoked by head turning or irrigation of the ears with ice water, are impaired. The cerebrospinal fluid will be sanguineous. Death usually occurs within a few hours, but there are rare exceptions where consciousness is retained and the clinical manifestations indicate a lesion in the tegmentum of the pons, e.g., disturbances of lateral ocular movements, crossed sensory or motor disturbances, small pupils, cranial nerve palsies, and bilateral signs of pyramidal tract involvement.

Cerebellar hemorrhage usually develops over a period of several hours, and loss of consciousness at the onset is almost unknown. Repeated vomiting is a hallmark of cerebellar hemorrhage, along with inability to walk or stand, occipital headache, and vertigo. There is a paresis of conjugate lateral gaze of the eyes to the side of the hemorrhage, forced deviation of the eyes to the opposite side, or an ipsilateral sixth nerve weakness. In the most acute phase of the illness there may be little or no evidence of cerebellar disease, and only a minority of cases show nystagmus or cerebellar ataxia of the limbs, although these signs must always be sought. Other ocular signs include "ocular bobbing," blepharospasm, involuntary closure of one eye, skew deviation, and maintenance of vertical eye movements including small pupils which continue to react until very late in the illness and exhibit slight inequality. A mild ipsilateral facial weakness and a diminished corneal reflex are common. Dysarthria and dysphagia may be prominent. Contralateral hemiplegia and facial weakness do not occur. Occasionally at the onset there is a quadriplegia with preservation of consciousness or a spastic paraparesis. The plantar reflexes are flexor early, extensor late. As the hours pass, the patient becomes stuporous, then comatose as a result of brainstem compression.

It will be noted that in the localization of intracerebral hemorrhages, ocular signs are important. In putaminal hemorrhage the eyes are deviated to the side opposite the paralysis; in thalamic hemorrhage the eyes are deviated downward and the pupils may be unreactive; in pontine hemorrhage the eyeballs are fixed and the pupils tiny and reactive; and in cerebellar hemorrhage the eyes are deviated laterally in the absence of paralysis.

At each of the above sites the hemorrhage is usually massive, and the patient survives only a few hours or a few days, succumbing as a result of secondary brainstem insult. Rarely does a patient survive once deep stupor supervenes, although in some cases he may linger in an unresponsive state for a week or two. In some 30 percent of cases, however, the hemorrhage is less extensive and survival is possible, hemorrhage into the thalamus especially tending to be somewhat smaller than putaminal or cerebellar hemorrhage.

A *severe headache* is often considered to be a constant accompaniment of intracerebral hemorrhage, and in many cases it is a prominent and helpful diagnostic point. Nonetheless in almost 50 percent of our cases headache has been absent or insignificant. *Nuchal rigidity* is frequently found, but again it is so often absent that failure to find it must by no means detract from the diagnosis. If the neck becomes stiff, it will become supple again as coma deepens. *Vomiting* occurs once or twice at the onset of intracerebral hemorrhage, and it is more frequent in hemorrhage than in infarction, but of equal importance is the fact that the patient often is far from comatose and may even be alert and responding accurately when first seen. This is true with grossly bloody spinal fluid, and thus the adage that hemorrhage into the ventricular system always precipitates coma is quite incorrect. Only if bleeding into the ventricles is massive will coma result. *Cerebral seizures,* usually focal, occur in some 10 percent of cases of supratentorial hemorrhage in the first few days, especially as the result of a subcortical "slit" hemorrhage. The fundi often show hypertensive changes in the arteries, and rarely fresh preretinal (subhyaloid) hemorrhages occur, the latter being much more common in ruptured aneurysm or angioma. Severe hypertension accompanied by papilledema need by no means be present for cerebral hemorrhage to occur.

Many of the less precisely localized neurologic manifestations described under cerebral thrombosis are also encountered in intracerebral hemorrhage, including coma, stupor, drowsiness, confusion, Cheyne-Stokes respiration, grasping and sucking reflexes, incontinence of bowel and bladder, and unilateral and bilateral extensor rigidity.

Although the proper interpretation of this array of clinical data allows the correct diagnosis to be established in most cases, the examination of the cerebrospinal fluid for blood is the single most important step in the detection of intracranial bleeding.

LABORATORY FINDINGS Any urinary abnormalities will for the most part reflect coexisting renal disease, although transient glucosuria has been reported to result specifically from intracranial hemorrhage. The white blood cell count often rises to 15,000 to 20,000 per mm^3, a higher figure than in thrombosis. The sedimentation rate is elevated. In cases of massive hemorrhage, the cerebrospinal fluid is often under increased pressure, but in almost half of our cases readings under 200 mm were obtained. The fluid is usually grossly bloody, although not so bloody as in ruptured saccular aneurysm (the count ranging from a few thousand cells up to 1 million). In smaller hemorrhages into central structures the cerebrospinal fluid contains a lesser amount of blood, and in occasional cases of intracerebral hemorrhage, particularly in those of the "slit" type, between cortex and white matter, it remains free of blood and clear of xanthochromia in repeated taps. In these latter cases, slight xanthochromia may appear after a few days to a week. At times the spinal fluid may be clear grossly but contain some 200 to 400 red cells, and it is then difficult to decide if this represents intracranial bleeding or a traumatic tap. These details are mentioned because they are of great importance in the essential task of making an accurate diagnosis of the type of stroke prior to the use of therapeutic measures such as anticoagulant drugs, surgical exploration, hypothermia, etc.

A *traumatic bloody spinal tap* greatly complicates the diagnostic problem. In a bloody tap the pressure tends to be low, the fluid that first flows from the needle is more bloody than that which comes later (third tube less bloody than the first), the fluid often clots in the test tube, and xanthochromia is either absent or at most present only in proportion to the amount of serum bilirubin admixed with the fluid. Bloody fluid due to cerebral hemorrhage is often under increased pressure, there is an even admixture of blood in all samples, the cerebrospinal fluid will not clot, and if more than 8 to 12 hr has elapsed since the hemorrhage, a definite xanthochromia will be present in the supernatant fluid after centrifugation, which should always be carried out if there is any question of the reliability of the tap. However, the presence of xanthochromia after centrifugation may be due to the bilirubin contained in the blood spilled by a traumatic tap and therefore is not an infallible index of subarachnoid or brain hemorrhage. The white blood cells of the cerebrospinal fluid are accounted for by the amount of hemorrhage, and their ratio to red cells is usually the same as in the circulating blood. After hemolysis of red blood cells, the white cell count may be disproportionately increased. Sometimes after a questionably traumatic tap it is worthwhile to perform immediately another puncture at a higher level.

Lumbar puncture is not completely innocuous, since temporal lobe or cerebellar herniation may be aggravated in cases of massive supratentorial hemorrhage or softening and in cerebellar hemorrhage. Despite this danger, the procedure is necessary if specific therapeutic measures are contemplated or if any doubt exists as to the diagnosis of cerebrovascular disease. X-ray of the skull early in the stroke sometimes shows a shift of the calcified pineal gland to the side of the cranium opposite the lesion, a change not seen in infarction. The electroencephalogram does not show a typical or diagnostic pattern, but high-voltage, slow waves are the most common finding with hemorrhage into the cerebral hemisphere. X-ray of the chest will often show cardiomegaly.

COURSE AND PROGNOSIS The immediate prognosis is grave, some 70 to 75 percent of patients dying in 1 to 30 days. Either the hemorrhage extends into the ventricular system, or temporal lobe herniation and midbrain compression occur. Sometimes the hemorrhage appears to seep gradually into vital centers. Gastric erosion and gastrointestinal hemorrhage of neurogenic origin may occur at any time within the first week or two. When the hemorrhage is smaller, survival is possible, and the restitution of motor function, speech, etc., can be excellent, since, in contrast to infarction, the hemorrhage has to some extent pushed brain tissue aside instead of destroying it. Function may be slow to return, because extravasated blood is slow to be resorbed or removed from the tissues. Since rebleeding from the same site is unlikely, the patient may live for many years. In some instances of medium-sized cerebral and cerebellar hemorrhages, the patient survives and his condition gradually stabilizes, but definite papilledema appears after several days of increased intracranial pressure. This does not mean that the hemorrhage is increasing in size or swelling, only that papilledema is slow to develop. Healed scars impinging on the cortex are liable to be epileptogenic.

TREATMENT *The general medical mangement of the comatose, apoplectic patient is the same as that outlined under Cerebral Thrombosis* above and in Chap. 22. Measures to stem the hemorrhage and restore the integrity of damaged tissue have been relatively ineffective.

Surgical removal of the clot in the acute stage, either by evacuation or aspiration, has seldom proved beneficial except in patients with a hemorrhage lying near the surface and who are not comatose. Acute cerebellar hemorrhage may be amenable to surgical therapy. In the smaller hemorrhages that reach a subacute stage, when papilledema appears, in many instances it has dictated unnecessary surgical evacuation of the hemorrhage when the patient's condition stabilized. Although the prognosis in hemorrhage into the cerebral hemisphere is probably little altered by surgery, the outlook for cerebellar cases seems to be improved.

Attempts to halt the hemorrhage by lowering the systemic blood pressure through the use of autonomic blocking agents have not been effective, and in many instances the inadvertent occurrence of disastrously low levels of blood pressure has complicated the illness. Artificial hypothermia has been used sporadically, but there are insufficient data to permit appraisal of this procedure. Intermittent compression of the ipsilateral carotid in the neck may be beneficial in acute putaminal cases.

The *only preventive measure* is lowering the blood pressure in cases of essential hypertension by every possible means. If ACTH or one of the adrenal steroids is being given, toxicity must be watched for. When hypotension threatens during surgical procedures, injections of excessive amounts of epinephrine or ephedrine must be avoided. Toxemia of pregnancy must be detected early.

Ruptured saccular aneurysm

This is the fourth most frequent of the cerebrovascular disorders following atherosclerosis, embolism, and hypertensive intracerebral hemorrhage. Saccular aneurysms take the form of small, thin-walled blisters protruding from the arteries of the circle of Willis or the major branches arising therefrom. These saccules or *berries*, as they have been called, are located for the most part at bifurcations and branchings (Fig. 326-7) and are presumed to be the result of developmental defects in the media and elastica. A small number of aneurysms have been attributed to incomplete involution of embryonic vessels. Owing to the local weakness, the intima bulges outward, covered only by adventitia; the sac gradually enlarges, until finally dissolution of the wall and rupture occur. Saccular aneurysms vary in size from tiny nubbins 2 mm in diameter up to spheric masses 2 or 3 cm in diameter, averaging 8 to 10 mm. They vary greatly in form; some are round and connected to the parent artery by a narrower stalk; others are broad-based without a stalk; still others are narrow cylinders. The site of rupture is always the dome of the aneurysm which may present one or more secondary sacculations. Enlargement is the result of dilatation of the lumen and the accretion of clot to the external surface.

In routine autopsies the incidence of ruptured aneurysms is 1.8 percent, of unruptured ones, 2.0 percent. Saccular aneurysms are rare in childhood, even at routine postmortem examination, and increase in frequency to reach their highest plateau of incidence in persons between thirty-five and sixty-five years of age. Therefore, they are not congenitally formed anomalies but develop over the years on the basis of the developmental arterial defect. There is an increased incidence of congenital polycystic disease of the kidney and coarctation of the aorta in association with saccular aneurysm. Hypertension is more frequently present than in the average population, but aneurysms occur in persons with normal blood pressure. Atherosclerosis, although present in the walls of about 50 percent of aneurysms, probably plays no part in their formation or enlargement.

From 85 to 90 percent of saccular aneurysms lie on the anterior part of the circle of Willis. The four most common sites are (1) in relation to the anterior communicating artery, (2) at the origin of the posterior communicating artery from the stem of the internal carotid, (3) at the first major bifurcation of the middle cerebral artery, and (4) at the bifurcation of the internal carotid into middle and anterior cerebral arteries (see Fig. 326-7). Other sites include the internal carotid in the cavernous sinus, at the origin of the ophthalmic artery, at the junction of the posterior communicating artery with the posterior cerebral, at the bifurcation of the basilar artery, and at the origins of the three cerebellar arteries. In 8 percent of cases there is more than one aneurysm, and they may be situated unilaterally or bilaterally.

Several types of aneurysm other than saccular occur, e.g., mycotic, fusiform, diffuse, and globular. The last three are named for their predominant morphologic aspects and consist of enlargement or dilatation of the entire circumference of the involved vessels, usually the internal carotid, vertebral, or basilar arteries. Frequently showing atherosclerotic deposition in their walls, they are often referred to as arteriosclerotic, but most likely they are at least partly developmental in nature. They press on neighboring structures or become occluded by thrombosis and rupture only infrequently.

FIGURE 326-7
Diagram of the circle of Willis to show the principal sites of saccular aneurysm. Approximately 90 percent of aneurysms are on the anterior half of the circle.

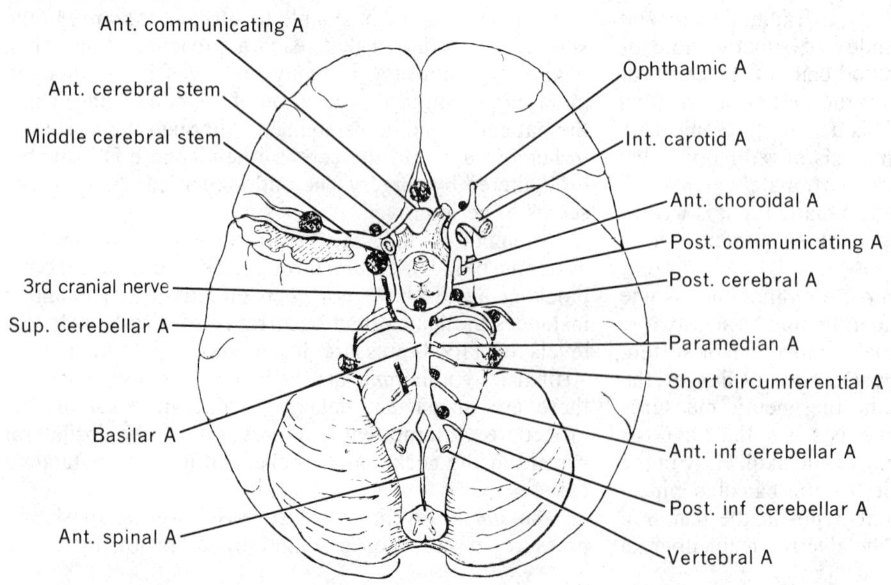

CLINICAL PICTURE Prior to rupture, saccular aneurysms are usually asymptomatic and rarely cause even headache. Occasionally, large aneurysms immediately distal to the cavernous sinus may compress the optic nerves or chiasm, third nerve, hypothalamus, or pituitary gland. In the posterior fossa, one or more of the cranial nerves may be compressed adjacent to the brainstem.

When rupture occurs, blood under high pressure is discharged into the subarachnoid space (the circle of Willis lies in the subarachnoid space), and the resulting clinical events fall into one of three patterns: (1) the patient may be stricken with an excruciating generalized headache and fall unconscious almost immediately; (2) headache may develop as in (1), but the patient remains relatively lucid; (3) consciousness may be lost quickly without any preceding complaint. Focal convulsive seizures or decerebrate rigidity occur at the onset of hemorrhage in about 10 percent of patients. If the hemorrhage is massive, a fatal issue may ensue in a matter of minutes, hours, or a day or two, deep coma persisting in association with irregular respiration, attacks of extensor rigidity, and finally respiratory arrest and circulatory collapse. In these rapidly fatal cases, the blood has usually dissected intracerebrally and entered the ventricular system. Death occasionally occurs within 5 min, and ruptured aneurysm must be considered in the differential diagnosis of sudden death.

In mild cases, consciousness, if lost, may be regained within a few minutes as the blood diffuses through the subarachnoid space, but a residuum of confusion and amnesia accompanied by severe headache and stiff neck persists for a day or two. It is not uncommon for drowsiness and confusion to last 10 days or longer. In major hemorrhages, headache may persist over a week, and remain severe during this time. If the hemorrhage is confined to the subarachnoid space, there are few or no lateralizing neurologic signs.

In most patients there are no warning symptoms; in some, however, minor leakage from the aneurysm sometimes precedes devastating rupture by a few days or weeks, headache and a transitory weakness of one side or speech disturbance being the chief signs of such an event. Aneurysmal rupture usually occurs while the patient is active rather than during sleep, and in many instances sexual intercourse or other exertion precipitates the ictus.

Gross lateralizing signs in the form of hemiplegia, hemiparesis, or aphasia are absent in the majority of cases, but can occur and are due to an intracerebral clot or infarction in the territory of the involved artery. The aneurysm may rupture partly into the subarachnoid space and partly into brain tissue (subarachnoid-cerebral hemorrhage) and even reach the ventricular system (subarachnoid-ventricular hemorrhage), rendering the patient stuporous or comatose. The initial neurologic deficit may clear in a matter of days, indicating that hemorrhage into tissues was not responsible for the focal signs. The pathogenesis of such manifestations is not fully understood, but a transitory fall in pressure in the circulation distal to the aneurysm is postulated. Transient deficits, still more evanescent, are not uncommon; paresis or aphasia, for example, may be present for only a few minutes or so after the onset of bleeding, constituting a reliable telltale of the site of the ruptured aneurysm. A delayed hemiplegia or other deficit may occur a few days after rupture. This is attributable to focal narrowing of a large artery at the base, usually interpreted as vasospasm resulting from the presence of extravasated blood. Areas of ischemic necrosis of tissue in the territory of the vessel bearing the aneurysm, usually without thrombosis of the vessel, may be found postmortem.

Although in most patients the neurologic manifestations do not point to the exact site of the aneurysm, in many instances there are clues to the localization. For example: (1) Third nerve palsy (ptosis, diplopia, mydriasis, and oculomotor paralysis) usually indicates an aneurysm at the junction of the posterior communicating artery and the internal carotid stem. The third nerve passes immediately lateral to this point. (2) Transient paresis of one or both of the lower limbs at the onset of the hemorrhage is suggestive of an anterior communicating aneurysm which has interfered with the circulation in the anterior cerebral arteries, causing ischemia of the motor areas for the lower extremities. (3) Hemiparesis or aphasia often points to an aneurysm at the bifurcation of the middle cerebral artery which has critically reduced the circulation in the middle cerebral system. (4) Unilateral blindness or amblyopia indicates an aneurysm which lies anteromedially in the circle of Willis (at the origin of the ophthalmic artery, at the bifurcation of the internal carotid artery, or in the anterior communicating region). (5) A stage of retained consciousness with akinetic mutism or abulia favors an aneurysm of the anterior communicating artery which has caused ischemia of or hemorrhage into one or both of the frontal lobes, hypothalamus, or corpus callosum. (6) The side on which the aneurysm lies may be indicated by a unilateral preponderance of headache or preretinal hemorrhages, by the occurrence of monocular pain, or by the lateralization of an intracranial sound heard at the time of rupture of the aneurysm. Sixth nerve palsy, unilateral or bilateral, results from the presence of subarachnoid blood and raised intracranial pressure and is seldom of localizing value. Other neurologic signs which have relatively little localizing value include sucking and grasping reflexes, choreoathetosis, and extensor rigidity.

In summary, the clinical sequence of sudden violent headache, collapse, brief unconsciousness and confusion, combined with an absence of prodromal symptoms and a paucity of lateralizing signs, is diagnostic of a ruptured saccular aneurysm.

Other clinical data may be of assistance in reaching a correct diagnosis. Nuchal rigidity is usually present. Examination of the fundi not infrequently reveals smooth-surfaced, sharply outlined collections of blood which cover the retinal vessels—the so-called "preretinal" or "subhyaloid" hemorrhages. These are usually a sign of ruptured aneurysm or angioma but can occur in hypertensive hemorrhage and cranial trauma. Bilateral Babinski signs are found in the early days following rupture. The patient may appear to be normally alert, when impairment of memory and confabulation are found on more careful testing. A fever with the temperature rising to 102°F is common in the first week. The escaping blood occasionally enters the subdural space and produces a subdural hematoma, evacuation of which may be lifesaving. Aneurysmal rupture may complicate pregnancy, but pregnancy is not associated with an increased incidence of aneurysmal rupture. Spontaneous intracranial bleeding with normal blood pressure should always suggest ruptured aneurysm, ruptured angioma, or hemorrhage into a cerebral tumor.

LABORATORY FINDINGS Any urinary abnormality is usually due to concomitant renal disease. Rarely diabetes insipidus occurs. A leukocytosis of 15,000 to 18,000 cells per mm^3 is common. The cerebrospinal fluid is usually extremely bloody, with red cell counts reaching to 1 million per mm^3 or higher. When the hemorrhage is very slight, there may be only a few thousand cells. It is unlikely that an aneurysm can rupture entirely into brain tissue without some leakage of blood into the subarachnoid fluid, and therefore the diagnosis of ruptured saccular aneurysm must never be made unless blood is present in the spinal fluid. Only expanding saccular aneurysms which either compress the optic nerves, chiasm, cranial nerves, or brainstem or lie within the cavernous sinus produce symptoms without hemorrhage. Usually deep xanthochromia is found after centrifugation. The cerebrospinal fluid is under greatly increased pressure, as high as 1,000 mm (see Laboratory Findings, above, regarding traumatic tap). The white blood cells in the spinal fluid are usually present in the same proportion to red blood cells as in the circulating blood, but in some patients within 48 hr a brisk leukocytosis appears, reaching 2,000 to 3,000 cells per mm^3.

X-rays of the skull are usually negative, though in a few patients one or both of the anterior clinoid processes show erosion by the pressure of an adjacent aneurysm, or calcification has occurred in the region of a previous hemorrhage. A calcified pineal gland may be displaced by an intracerebral or subdural clot.

Carotid and vertebral angiography, using Hypaque, will demonstrate the aneurysm in some 85 percent of patients in whom aneurysm appears to be the correct diagnosis on clinical grounds, i.e., in cases of so-called "spontaneous subarachnoid hemorrhage."

Acute subarachnoid hemorrhage may be associated with electrocardiographic abnormalities suggestive of myocardial ischemia. The electroencephalogram is of little help in localizing the lesion unless a gross neurologic deficit is present, in which case the lateralization is probably already evident clinically. The abnormality usually consists of slow waves.

COURSE AND PROGNOSIS The outstanding characteristic of this condition is the tendency for the hemorrhage to recur. This threat colors all prognostications, and unfortunately there appears to be no way of determining reliably which cases will rebleed. The cause of the intermittency of bleeding is not understood.

Patients with the typical clinical picture of spontaneous subarachnoid hemorrhage but in whom the angiogram shows no aneurysm or angioma have a better prognosis than those in whom the lesion is demonstrated.

McKissock et al. found that the patient's state of consciousness at the time of arteriography was the best single criterion of prognosis. By use of their data as representative of any large medical center, it can be shown that of every 100 patients coming to arteriography, 17 will be stuporous or comatose, and 83 will appear to be recovering from the ictus. At the end of the next 6 months, of the first 17, 7 will have died from the original hemorrhage and 7 more will have had a fatal recurrence, making a total of 14 deaths and 3 survivors. Of the other 83, one will have died of the original hemorrhage and 52 will have had a recurrence, of which 33 will have died, making a total of 34 deaths and 49 survivors. Thus, of the total of 100, at the end of 6 months, 8 will have died of the original hemorrhage, 59 more will have had a recurrence, with 40 deaths, making a total of 48 deaths and 52 survivors. The gravity of the illness is immediately apparent. In regard to the recurrence of bleeding, it was found that of every 50 patients seen on the first day of the illness, 5 will rebleed in the first week (all fatal), 8 in the second week (5 fatal), 6 in the third and fourth weeks (4 fatal), and 2 in the next 4 weeks (2 fatal), making a total of 21 recurrences in 8 weeks (16 fatal). Rerupture did not occur in the first 2 days; thereafter it occurred at a steady rate for the next 19 days and tapered off abruptly.

Of the survivors in the first group, all but one returned to work, and in the second group, 36 went back to full work, 12 were partly disabled, and 4 were totally disabled. The disability was due to paralysis, mental deterioration, or epilepsy.

TREATMENT General medical management in the acute stage is similar to that described under Cerebral Thrombosis above. The earlier the case comes under medical purview and the more severe the impairment of consciousness, the less certain are any known therapeutic measures to be beneficial. Those surviving in good condition for several days have the best outlook, and with the passage of time the risk of recurrent bleeding diminishes. Rational medical measures are based on the assumption that decreasing the arterial blood pressure is the most reasonable way of arresting the hemorrhage and preventing recurrence. Absolute bed rest for 4 to 8 weeks is prescribed, with the head of the bed raised some 15 to 20°. Straining during bowel movement is forbidden, and laxatives or gentle enemas are administered. Coughing and all forms of exertion are avoided. The patient is fed. The duration of the period of bed rest is empiric and not founded on any reliable clinical observations or the formation of scar tissue around aneurysms. Sedatives (barbiturates) and analgesics (opiates, acetylsalicylic acid) are important in aiding relaxation. Hypotensive agents (reserpine, aldomet) are used to bring hypertensive blood pressures to normal. In the presence of severe hypertension, blocking agents may be cautiously used to lower the blood pressure to 160/100, great care being exercised not to precipitate excessive hypotension and cerebral infarction. Drug therapy is usually not very effective in lowering the blood pressure of normotensive patients confined to bed. Promazine intramuscularly is used to control nausea and vomiting. Dilantin or phenobarbital may be prescribed to prevent cerebral seizures.

The place of repeated drainage of the cerebrospinal fluid by lumbar puncture is still uncertain, although several workers have concluded that it does not affect the outcome of the illness. At present, one lumbar puncture is usually carried out for diagnostic purposes, and thereafter it is performed only for the relief of intractable headache, to detect recurrence of bleeding, or to measure the intracranial pressure prior to surgery.

In maintaining fluid balance, intravenous fluids should be used sparingly and in the proper electrolyte combination (a mixture of equal parts of 5% glucose in water and normal saline solution or balanced electrolytes) in order to minimize the danger of aggravating brain swelling. Any abnormality of concentration of electrolytes in the blood must be corrected. If diabetes insipidus has occurred, it should be treated with Pitressin. Vitamins C and K have been recommended routinely, but there is no evidence that they are beneficial. Disorders of blood coagulation should be amended. Body hypothermia for 2 to 5 days in the stage of acute hemorrhage has been used with uncertain efficacy. Intravenous hypertonic urea of mannitol may be effective in temporarily reducing the intracranial pressure.

After resting in bed for 6 weeks, the patient is gradually allowed to resume activity and may return to work in 4 months. It seems logical to advise that heavy labor not be resumed.

SURGICAL THERAPY Apart from occasionally evacuating an associated intracerebral clot, surgical treatment is for the most part directed to the prevention of recurrence of the hemorrhage. The procedures are either *extracranial* (ligation of the common carotid in the neck) or *intracranial* (resection of the aneurysm; ligation of the neck of the aneurysm; wrapping or tamponade of the aneurysmal sac by muscle, fascia, plastic coating, or arterial graft; trapping the aneurysm; ligation of the main vessel proximal to the aneurysm). Occasionally extracranial and intracranial procedures are combined. Because of the high operative mortality if surgery is undertaken early, operation has usually been delayed until the patient's condition has stabilized following the first hemorrhage. During the waiting period, however, the patient is likely to suffer a further hemorrhage, and in an effort to intervene before this happens neurosurgeons are now attempting to operate much earlier than formerly, sometimes using hypothermia and hypotension during surgery. Before treatment is undertaken, the site, size, and form of the aneurysm must be determined by angiography. At the same time the pattern of the anterior half of the circle of Willis is noted, as it may influence the choice of operative procedure. It has been demonstrated that surgical treatment improves upon the natural outlook for aneurysms at the posterior communicating artery and the bifurcation of the middle cerebral artery. The mortality for anterior communicating aneurysms remains unchanged.

After aneurysmal rupture a chronic obstructive or communicating hydrocephalus may develop, causing persistent stupor, which is relieved by ventriculoatrial shunting.

Other causes of intracranial hemorrhage

An *angioma,* or hemangioma, consists of a tangle of abnormal vessels forming an abnormal communication between the arterial and venous systems, really an arteriovenous fistula. It is a developmental abnormality, not a neoplasm, but the constituent vessels enlarge with growth and the passage of time. Angiomas vary in size from a small blemish a few millimeters in diameter lying in the cortex to a huge mass of tortuous channels comprising an arteriovenous shunt of sufficient magnitude to raise the cardiac output. Hypertrophic dilated arterial "feeders" approach the main lesion, disappear below the cortex, and break up into a network of thin-walled blood vessels which connect directly with draining veins. The latter often form huge, dilated, pulsating channels, carrying away arterial blood. The blood vessels forming the tangle interposed between arteries and veins are usually abnormally thin and do not have the normal structure of arteries or veins. Angiomas occur in all parts of the brain, brainstem, and spinal cord, but the larger ones are more frequently found in the posterior half of the hemispheres, commonly forming a wedge-shaped lesion extending from the cortex to the ventricular lining.

Angiomas predominate in males over females about 2:1. They may occur in more than one member of a family in the same or successive generations. Although the lesion is present from birth, the onset of complaints is most common between the ages of ten and thirty, but occasionally it is delayed as late as the fifties. The chief clinical features are epileptic seizures and cerebral or cerebral-subarachnoid hemorrhage occurring in a child or young adult. In 50 percent the first manifestation is a seizure, in 20 percent an intracerebral hemorrhage with hemiplegia, and in 20 percent a typical subarachnoid hemorrhage. The seizure pattern depends on the site of the lesion; when focal motor in type the seizure may be followed by a temporary postictal paralysis. When hemorrhage occurs, blood may enter the subarachnoid space almost exclusively, producing a picture identical with that of ruptured saccular aneurysm, but since the angioma lies within the cerebral tissue, the bleeding is more likely to be partly intracerebral, causing hemiparesis, hemiplegia, or death. Before rupture, chronic nondescript headache is a frequent complaint. Occasionally typical migraine with accompaniments is associated, but this is probably a coincidence. Huge angiomas may produce a slowly progressive neurologic deficit because of depletion of blood from adjacent brain tissue. Proptosis has been encountered. When the vein of Galen is involved, hydrocephalus may result. Not infrequently one or both carotid arteries pulsate unusually forcefully in the neck. A systolic bruit heard over the carotid in the neck, the mastoid process, or the eyeballs in young adults is almost pathognomonic of angioma. The patient should be exercised in order to bring out a bruit if none is present at rest. A bruit may be heard over a spinal angioma of large size. The blood pressure may be raised or normal, and it is axiomatic that the occurrence of intracranial bleeding with normal blood pressure should lead to the suspicion of an angioma, ruptured saccular aneurysm, or hemorrhage into a tumor. The eye grounds may reveal a retinal vascular abnormality. Preretinal hemorrhages may be found after hemorrhage has occurred. X-ray of the skull occasionally shows crescentic linear calcification in the vicinity of larger angiomas. Pneumoencephalography may show the picture of an expanding lesion combined with cerebral atrophy, a combination typical of angioma. Arteriography is necessary to establish the diagnosis with certainty and will demonstrate angiomas larger than 5 mm in diameter. Small angiomas may be obscured by the resulting hemorrhage, and even at autopsy a careful microscopic search may be necessary to find them.

Most angiomas bleed sooner or later. The first hemorrhage may be fatal, but in more than 90 percent of cases bleeding stops, and the patient survives. Recurrence of hemorrhage with a fatal outcome is a constant danger. In recent years it has been the practice of neurosurgeons to perform a block dissection of angiomas of suitable size and location.

Although *intracranial bleeding due to head trauma* does not rightfully fall within the scope of the stroke problem, it must be mentioned here because of the great frequency with which it enters into the differential diagnosis, especially in cases in which the history is inadequate or the patient falls and injures himself at the onset of the stroke. *Acute extradural* and *acute subdural hemorrhage* must always be considered in the patient who under unknown circumstances has rather abruptly developed a neurologic deficit such as hemiparesis or confusion, whether the spinal fluid is bloody or not. In *chronic subdural hemorrhage,* which can occur without known trauma, the indefinite picture of drowsiness, confusion, and mild hemiparesis may be erroneously attributed to a stroke, especially in elderly persons. These conditions must be constantly kept in mind, since failure to make the correct diagnosis deprives the patient of lifesaving surgical intervention. There should be no hesitation in carrying out arteriography or placing diagnostic burr holes in all patients in whom subdural hemorrhage cannot be excluded on clinical grounds. *Cerebral contusion and laceration* may be a cause of subarachnoid hemorrhage, and if the patient has fallen and struck his head at the time of the onset of the stroke, it may be difficult or impossible to decide if the red blood cells in the cerebrospinal fluid are due to a cerebrovascular stroke or to cerebral contusion. Trauma may also cause *acute* or *delayed intracerebral hemorrhage, acute intracerebellar hemorrhage, acute infratentorial subdural hemorrhage, acute brain swelling,* and on rare occasions, extensive *focal infarction* of undetermined pathogenesis (see Chap. 327).

Several *hemorrhagic hematologic disorders* are not infrequently complicated by hemorrhage into the brain. The most frequent of these are leukemia, aplastic anemia, and thrombocytopenic purpura. As a rule this complication signals a fatal issue. Any part of the brain may be involved, and not infrequently the lesions are multiple. Usually there is already evidence of abnormal bleeding elsewhere (skin, mucous membranes, kidney) by the time cerebral hemorrhage occurs. Intracranial bleeding is a complication of anticoagulant therapy.

Hemorrhages of undetermined origin are of importance, since both clinically and pathologically hemorrhages are found in which the blood pressure is normal and neither an aneurysm nor angioma can be demonstrated. In some postmortem cases a careful microscopic search discloses a small angioma in the cerebral tissue at one side of the hemorrhage, and on this basis it is suspected that in other cases, too, an overlooked angioma may have been the cause of the extravasation of blood. Primary intraventricular hemorrhage, a rare event, is at times due to angioma or neoplasm of the choroid plexus, which may not have been seen by the prosector.

Hemorrhage into primary and secondary brain tumors is not rare, and when it is the first manifestation of the neoplasm, the correct diagnosis may be extremely obscure. Choriocarcinoma, melanotic carcinoma, renal cell carcinoma, bronchogenic carcinoma, pituitary adenoma, glioblastoma multiforme, and medulloblastoma may present in this way. Careful inquiry will usually disclose the fact that signs of a neurologic disorder compatible with intracranial tumor growth have preceded the onset of hemorrhage. Examination clinically and by x-ray may reveal evidence of intracranial tumor or of secondary tumor deposits in other organs. A chest film will frequently show metastatic or primary neoplasm and should be performed in all cases of obscure intracerebral hemorrhage.

Septic embolism may lead to massive fatal intracranial bleeding via a *mycotic aneurysm.* Any part of the circulatory tree may be involved, but usually the aneurysm lies at a branching or forking of a small vessel (about 0.5 mm in diameter) within the subarachnoid space.

On infrequent occasions bleeding within an area of *hemorrhagic infarction* as a result of cerebral embolism or venous thrombosis reaches major proportions, forming an intracerebral hematoma, and the cerebrospinal fluid becomes bloody.

Hypertensive encephalopathy may in its most advanced stage result in intracerebral hemorrhages, which can vary in size from petechial to massive.

Idiopathic brain purpura, or hemorrhagic encephalitis, consists of multiple petechial hemorrhages scattered throughout the white matter of the brain. The picture is that of a diffuse cerebral disease. There is never blood in the spinal fluid, and the condition should never be confused with a typical stroke.

Brainstem hemorrhages secondary to temporal lobe herniation are extremely common but never present as a cerebrovascular stroke.

Inflammatory disease of arteries and veins, especially polyarteritis nodosa and lupus erythematosus, occasionally cause hemorrhage into the nervous system. In polyarteritis rupture of a vessel may occur on the basis of a concomitant hypertension or local vascular disease. In lupus erythematosus—if it can be included in the arteritides—hemorrhage is attributable to hypertension or disease of the vascular wall of undetermined nature. Bleeding nearly always occurs into the parenchyma rather than the subarachnoid space.

The rarer types of hemorrhage listed in the classification in Table 326-4 are self-explanatory.

Hemorrhages of *intraspinal* origin may be the result of angiomas, hematomyelia, bleeding into tumors, subdural extravasation (trauma, anticoagulants, spontaneous) and circulatory changes around benign tumors.

HYPERTENSIVE ENCEPHALOPATHY

This term refers to an acute syndrome in which severe hypertension is associated with headache, nausea, vomiting, convulsions, confusion, stupor, and coma. Focal or lateralizing neurologic signs, either transitory or lasting, are rare and always suggest some other form of vascular disease (hemorrhage, embolism, or atherosclerotic thrombosis). By the time the neurologic manifestations appear, the hypertension has usually reached the malignant stage, with retinal hemorrhages, exudates, papilledema (*hypertensive retinopathy* grade IV), and evidence of renal and cardiac disease. In many of but not all the cases, the cerebrospinal fluid pressure and the protein values are both elevated, the latter sometimes to over 100 mg per 100 ml. The hypertension may be essential or due to chronic renal disease, acute glomerulonephritis, acute toxemia of pregnancy, pheochromocytoma, Cushing's syndrome, or ACTH toxicity. Lowering of the blood pressure with hypotensive drugs may reverse the picture in a day or two. If the hypertension cannot be controlled, the outcome is fatal. Neuropathologic examination may reveal a rather normal-looking brain, but usually cerebral swelling and/or hemorrhages of various sizes from massive to petechial will be found. A cerebellar pressure cone may cause fatality, and in some instances the event was seemingly encouraged by a lumbar puncture. Microscopically there are in addition to small hemorrhages clusters of glial cells, necrosis of arterioles, and minute cerebral infarcts.

The term *hypertensive encephalopathy* should be reserved for the above syndrome and not used to refer to chronic recurrent headaches, dizziness, epileptic seizures, recurrent transient ischemic attacks, or small strokes which often occur in association with high blood pressure. For further discussion, see Chap. 245.

INFLAMMATORY DISEASES OF BRAIN ARTERIES

Inflammatory diseases of the vessels of the brain have been mentioned on several occasions in the preceding paragraphs, and here they are reviewed and discussed briefly.

Meningovascular syphilis, formerly one of the most frequent causes of occlusive vascular disease in patients of all ages, has become a rarity since the introduction of penicillin therapy (see Chap. 159).

Tuberculous meningitis, fungous meningitis, and the subacute forms of bacterial meningitis (influenzal bacillus, staphylococcus, pneumococcus) may also be accompanied by vascular disorders of the occlusive type, in either the cerebral arteries or veins. Occasionally in tuberculous meningitis a stroke may be the first clinical sign of meningitis; more often it develops after the meningeal symptoms are established.

Typhus, schistosomiasis mansoni, mucormycosis, malaria, and *trichinosis* are rare types of infective inflammatory diseases of the arteries and, unlike the above, are not secondary to meningeal inflammation. In typhus and other rickettsial diseases, capillary and arteriolar changes and perivascular inflammatory cells are found in the brain, and presumably they underlie the convulsions, acute psychoses, and coma which reflect the central nervous system involvement. The internal carotid artery may be occluded in diabetic patients during orbital and cavernous sinus infections with mucormycosis. In trichinosis the sudden onset of convulsions, aphasia, hemiplegia, and coma may either accompany or, as happens more often, follow the systemic and muscular symptoms. The cause of the cerebral symptoms has not been established. Parasites have been found in the brain; in one of our cases the cerebral lesions were produced by bland emboli arising in the heart and related to a severe myocarditis. Malaria of the malignant or falciparum variety is frequently attended by a clinical state known as *cerebral malaria* in which convulsions, coma, and sometimes focal symptoms appear to be due to blockage of capillaries and precapillaries by masses of parasitized red blood corpuscles.

The *arteritides of obscure origin* include polyarteritis nodosa, disseminated lupus erythematosus, granulomatous arteritis, giant-cell arteritis, temporal (cranial) arteritis, and rheumatic arteritis (see Chap. 363).

Lupus erythematosus causes cerebral symptoms in over 50 percent of cases. Seizures and psychoses are common. Small cerebral infarcts lead to widespread focal deficits. Accompanying hypertension may precipitate hemorrhage or hypertensive encephalopathy, or endocarditis may cause cerebral embolism.

Temporal arteritis (cranial arteritis) is an uncommon affliction of elderly persons in which the external carotid system, particularly the temporal branches, is the seat of a subacute granulomatous inflammation with an exudate of lymphocytes, monocytes, neutrophilic leukocytes, and giant cells. Usually the most severely affected parts of the artery become thrombosed. Headache or head pain is the chief complaint. Systemic manifestations include anorexia, loss of weight, malaise, and polymyalgia rheumatica. The inflammatory nature of the illness is indicated by some one or several of the following: fever, slight leukocytosis, increased sedimentation rate, and anemia. Occlusion of branches of the ophthalmic artery results in blindness in one or both eyes in over 25 percent of patients, and occasionally an ophthalmoplegia due to involvement of ocular nerves occurs. An arteritis of the aorta and its major branches, including carotid, subclavian, coronary, and femoral arteries, is found at postmortem examination. Significant inflammatory involvement of intracranial arteries is rare, but strokes occur occasionally, on the basis of internal carotid, middle cerebral, or vertebral occlusion. The diagnosis depends on the finding of a tender thrombosed or thickened cranial artery and the demonstration of the lesion in a biopsy. Meticorten and ACTH bring striking subjective relief and prevent blindness. See Chap. 363 for further discussion.

Another type of *giant-cell arteritis,* which occurs in younger people, is described in Chap. 363.

Thromboangiitis obliterans of cerebral vessels (Winiwarter-Buerger disease) has not been included in the foregoing list. Despite the large amount of literature on the subject, the pathology is so dubious that it does not merit further exposition. All the patients that the authors have studied proved to have had either atherosclerosis of the carotid or cerebral arteries with "stasis thrombosis" of more distant cerebral branches. Buerger's disease of the legs has an equally uncertain status.

DIFFERENTIATION OF CEREBROVASCULAR DISEASE FROM OTHER NEUROLOGIC ILLNESSES

It has already been stated that the diagnosis of a vascular lesion rests solely on recognition of the stroke syndrome and that without evidence of this the diagnosis must always be in doubt. Three useful criteria in the identification of the stroke have already been emphasized: (1) the tempo of the clinical syndrome, (2) evidence of focal brain disease, and (3) the clinical setting. The temporal profile can usually be defined by means of a clear history of premonitory phenomena, the mode of the onset, and the evolution of the neurologic disturbance taken in relation to the medical status at the time of examination. If these data are lacking, the course may still be determined by extending the period of observation for a few more days or weeks. An inadequate history is probably the most frequent cause of diagnostic errors.

Few other neurologic illnesses mimic cerebrovascular disease. When the details of the history are missing, however, subdural hematoma, brain tumor, brain abscess, and senile dementia may lead to diagnostic difficulties. The reader should refer to Chaps. 322, 328, 329, and 333 for further discussion of differential diagnosis.

REFERENCES

FIELDS WS: *Pathogenesis and Treatment of Cerebrovascular Disease,* Springfield, Ill.: Charles C Thomas, 1961

FISHER CM: Cerebral ischemia—less familiar types. Clin Neurosurg 18:267, 1971

WALTON J: *Subarachnoid Hemorrhage,* Edinburgh: E. and S. Livingstone, Ltd., 1956

327 TRAUMATIC DISEASES OF THE BRAIN

KARL-ERIK ASTRÖM
HENRI VANDER EECKEN

Head injury, which is the basis of some of the most frequent and serious neurologic disorders in these times of high-velocity transport and mechanization in industry, poses many problems to the practicing physician. To deal effectively with this condition demands a knowledge of the clinical manifestations as well as a sound grasp of fundamental physiologic mechanisms. The physician must stand prepared at all times, for he may at any moment be summoned to render aid or to assess the clinical status of a person who has suffered an injury of the head or spine. The present chapter undertakes to review the salient facts concerning these injuries of the nervous system and to outline an approach to these problems that has been useful to the authors.

PHYSIOLOGIC AND PATHOLOGIC CONSIDERATIONS

The very language with which certain types of head injury are discussed divulges a number of misconceptions that have been inherited from previous generations of physicians. Words have crept into medical vocabulary and have often been retained long after the ideas for which they stood have been refuted—clear evidence of the disadvantage of prematurely adopting explanatory rather than descriptive terms. The word *concussion,* for example, implies the violent shaking and agitation of an organ or the functional impairment which results therefrom. Yet despite numerous experiments to demonstrate these physical changes within the nerve cells (vibration effects, formation of intracellular vacuoles, etc.), no confirmation of their existence has been possible. Similarly the word *contusion,* meaning a bruising or crushing without interruption of physical continuity, is applied rather indiscriminately to a variety of clinical states, some of which could not depend on a pathologic change of this type, e.g., "minor contusion state or syndrome"—an expression introduced by Wilfred Trotter, who was himself most critical of words that "embalm a fallacious theory."

In all attempts to analyze the mechanism of brain damage in head injury one fact stands preeminent—that there must be the sudden application of a physical force of considerable magnitude to the head. Unless the head is struck, the brain suffers no injury—except in the rare and somewhat controversial cases of crush injury to the chest or explosive injury with raised intrapulmonary pressure. A second fact, also susceptible of easy verification, is that the size of the area on the skull over which the force is exerted is of importance. High-velocity missiles destroy a small part of the skull and penetrate the cranial cavity without significant displacement of the head or brain; and heavy, crushing injuries which result from the skull being compressed between two converging objects may crush the brain. In these two circumstances it is interesting to note that the patient may suffer severe and often fatal injury without immediate loss of consciousness. Hemorrhage, destruction of brain tissue, and, if the patient survives for a time, meningitis or abscess, are the principal pathologic changes created by injuries of this type. They offer little difficulty to understanding.

The common civilian injury is one in which a rapidly moving blunt object strikes the head or the head is flung against a hard surface. Injuries of this type, often termed *blunt head injuries,* are remarkable in two respects: (1) they almost always induce at least a temporary loss of consciousness; (2) even though the skull is not penetrated and fragments of bone are not driven into its cavity, the brain may suffer gross damage, i.e., contusion, laceration, hemorrhage, swelling, herniation, etc. Clinicians as well as experimental physiologists have sought a theory which would bring into plausible form all gross neuropathologic changes, the skull fracture and the transient paralysis of nervous function (concussion) or prolonged coma, so often observed in fatal cases. It may be said that a comprehensive theory, acceptable to all workers in this field, has not been developed as yet.

The relation of skull fracture to injury of the cerebral tissues has been viewed in changing perspective through the entire history of this subject. In earliest times fractures dominated the thinking of the medical profession, and cerebral lesions were regarded as secondary. Later it became known that the skull, although rigid, is still flexible enough to yield to a blow severe enough to injure the brain without fracture. Therefore, the presence of a fracture, although a rough measure of the violence to which the brain has been exposed, is not an infallible index. Even in fatal head injury autopsy may reveal an intact skull in some 20 to 30 percent of cases. Also many patients suffer skull fractures without serious or prolonged disorder of cerebral function.

The modern trend is to be interested more in the presence or absence of brain injury than in the fracture of the skull itself. Nevertheless fractures cannot be dismissed without a few comments, for they assume importance in indicating the site and possible severity of brain damage, in providing an explanation for cranial nerve palsies, and in affording potential pathways for the ingress of bacteria and air or the egress of cerebrospinal fluid (CSF).

CRANIAL NERVE INJURY The existence of a basal skull fracture may be indicated by signs of cranial nerve damage. Cranial nerves which are particularly liable to injury are the olfactory, optic, oculomotor, first and second branches of the trigeminal, the facial, and the auditory. Anosmia and an apparent loss of taste (actually a loss of perception of aromatic flavors, elementary tastes—salt, sweet, bitter, sour—being retained) are frequent sequelae of head injury, especially of falls on the back of the head. In the majority of cases the anosmia is permanent. If unilateral it will not be noticed by the patient. The mechanism of these disturbances is believed to be displacement of the brain and tearing of the olfactory nerve filaments. A fracture in or near the sella may tear the stalk of the pituitary gland, with resulting diabetes insipidus amenorrheas. A fracture of sphenoid bone may lacerate the optic nerve, with complete blindness from the beginning. The pupil is dilated and unreactive to a direct light stimulus but still takes part in the consensual reflex. The optic disk becomes pale, i.e., atrophic, after an interval of several weeks. Partial injuries may result in a troublesome blurring of vision. Injury to the eighth cranial nerve with petrosal fractures causes loss of hearing and/or dizziness, immediately after injury. The deafness due to nerve injury must be distinguished from that caused by rupture of the eardrum or the presence of blood in the middle ear, and the vertigo, from posttraumatic nervous giddiness. In oculomotor nerve injury there is a divergent squint, with loss of internal and vertical movement of the eye and a fixed, dilated pupil. Diplopia only on looking down suggests trochlear nerve affection. Direct injury of the facial nerve by a basal fracture may be present immediately after the injury or may be delayed, coming on after several days. This delayed form is usually transitory, and its mechanism is not known. It may be misinterpreted as an important progression of the traumatic intracranial lesion. Injury to the ophthalmic or maxillary divisions of the trigeminal nerve may be the result either of a basal fracture across the middle cranial fossa or of a direct extracranial injury to the branches of the nerves. Numbness and paresthesias over the area of skin supplied by the nerve or a troublesome neuralgia are the sequelae of these injuries.

If the skin is lacerated over the skull fracture and the underlying meninges are torn, or if the fracture passes through the posterior wall of a nasal sinus, bacteria or air may enter the cranial cavity with resulting meningitis, abscess, and aerocele (air in the ventricles). Cerebrospinal fluid may also leak into the sinus and present as a watery discharge from the nose (cerebrospinal fluid rhinorrhea). Persistence of the rhinorrhea or the occurrence of episodes of recurrent meningitis (headache, convulsions, fever, and stiff neck with pleocytosis and sometimes bacteria) is often an indication for a repair of the torn dura mater over the fissure. Depressed fractures are of significance only if the underlying dura is lacerated by spicules of bone or the brain is compressed.

CONCUSSIVE INJURY Much has been written about the mechanism of coma in closed or blunt head injury. Two facts concerning this condition stand out clearly: (1) it bears only an indefinite relationship to skull fracture; (2) the optimal conditions for its production are those in which there is some change in the momentum of the head; i.e., movement is suddenly imparted to it by a blow, or its movement is suddenly arrested. Striking the stationary head of an experimental animal will cause a loss of brainstem reflexes only if the head was free to move, not if it is clamped in one position (Denny-Brown and Russell). This finding alone would stand in refutation of such theories of concussion as a wave of high intracranial pressure due to the indentation of the skull or a subsequent wave of negative pressure (Kahn, Ward, and Clark), cerebral anemia (Trotter), shattering of the myelinated fibers of cerebral white matter (Strich and Symonds), or a general vibration or agitation transmitted via the skull. The speed of acceleration or deceleration of the head necessary for this concussive effect must exceed 7 m per sec. The initial action of the blunt injury of this type is to excite the nervous system (the "stars" that one sees with a minor injury, the gasp of the animal); and this is followed by transient paralysis of cerebral function, i.e., abolition of consciousness, suppression of reflexes, arrest of respiration, etc. The means whereby the latter effects are produced is not known. Equally obscure is the site of injury, whether diffuse in the cerebral cortex (Denny-Brown and Meyer) or in the diencephalon and midbrain.

In fatal cases of severe head injury, where this concussive injury must also have existed, the brain is almost invariably bruised or lacerated, and often there is hemorrhage, either meningeal or intracerebral. The observation of these gross pathologic findings has led to the widely prevalent view that head injuries are largely matters of bruises and hemorrhages and of urgent operations. That this can hardly be the case is suggested by the fact that some patients survive head injuries almost as severe as the fatal ones and yet make an excellent recovery. At autopsy years later old contusions (*plaques jaunes*) and hemorrhages of approximately the same distribution and extent as those observed in some of the immediately fatal cases are found. One can only conclude, therefore, that most of the immediate symptoms of severe head injury, both general and localized, depend on invisible and highly reversible changes in the brain, probably of the same nature as those which underlie concussion. Nevertheless these bruises, lacerations, hemorrhages, and localized swellings of tissues cannot be disregarded, because they are probably responsible for many of the fatalities that occur 12 to 72 hr or more after the injury. Of these lesions the most important are the surface bruising of the brain beneath the point of impact (*coup* injury) and the more extensive lacerations and contusions on the opposite side of the brain (*contrecoup* injuries). The inertia of the malleable brain, which causes it to be flung against the side of the skull that was struck and to be pulled away from the contralateral side, has been invoked to explain these coup-contrecoup contusions. This theory has been further elaborated by Holburn, who points out that the brain is roughly spherical and that all movements of the head describe an arc with its axis centered where skull is attached to spine. Sudden changes in the momentum of the head, therefore, induce a swirling motion to the brain, which may then suffer injury against all rough, bony prominences (wings of sphenoid bones, petrous parts of temporal bones, rough surfaces of orbital and frontal bones).

CLINICAL MANIFESTATIONS OF HEAD INJURY

The physician upon being called to see a patient who has had a head injury will generally find him in one of three clinical conditions; each must be dealt with differently. It is usually possible to place the patient in one of these three categories by assessing his mental and general neurologic status when he is first seen and at intervals of time after the accident.

PATIENTS WHO ARE CONSCIOUS OR ARE RAPIDLY REGAINING MENTAL CLARITY WHEN FIRST SEEN (MINOR HEAD INJURY) The typical example is a patient who was rendered unconscious by a knock on the head and then regains his senses within seconds, minutes, or hours. Roughly two degrees of disturbance of consciousness may have occurred. First, there is the patient who was never unconscious at all. He was observed to have struck his head and was stunned or "saw stars." By all criteria his head injury was insignificant when judged in terms of life and death and severe brain damage, though in exceptional cases there is always the possibility of skull fracture or epidural or subdural hematoma. Nevertheless, a troublesome group of symptoms may have developed at once or within a few days. These are described below.

If consciousness was temporarily abolished, the patient is said to have suffered a *concussion*, defined by Trotter as "an essentially transient state due to head injury which is instantaneous in onset, manifests widespread symptoms of a purely paralytic kind, does not as such comprise any evidence of structural cerebral injury and is nearly always followed by amnesia for the actual moment of the impact." The patient, if observed immediately after the injury, shows a complete paralysis of nervous function. In a few instances death has occurred at this time, from respiratory arrest or cardiac arrhythmia, and no lesion was found at postmortem examination. However, the usual sequel is for the pulse and respiration (if they were depressed or arrested) to return at once and for muscle tone, reflexes, voluntary movement, and mental clarity to be regained within a few minutes. Only an amnesia for the accident and the events that immediately preceded (retrograde amnesia) and followed it (anterograde amnesia) will remain. Thereafter the patient may suffer the same headaches, giddiness, and nervousness described above.

These relatively trivial head injuries may rarely be followed by a number of other puzzling features, all of which indicate the occurrence of some process in addition to concussion: (1) *Delayed traumatic collapse:* following an accident a few patients, after walking about and seeming to be mentally normal, will turn pale and fall unconscious for a few minutes. This is a vasomotor syncopal attack and is probably related to injury, pain, and emotional upset. Rarely does the patient exhibit any focal or lateralizing neurologic signs. The suggestion that this represents medullary edema is hardly tenable. (2) *Immediate traumatic paraplegia* or *blindness:* with falls on top of the head, which may injure the motor areas for the lower extremities, both legs may become temporarily weak and numb, sometimes with bilateral Babinski signs and sphincteric incontinence. Concussion of the cervical section of the spinal cord is another possible mechanism of the paraplegia. Temporary blindness may have a similar base in occipital injuries. (3) *Immediate hemiplegia or monoplegia:* these conditions may develop immediately after a minor injury, with or without blood in the cerebrospinal fluid, and are commonly attributed to a relatively circumscript injury with minimal concussion or a direct contusion or laceration of the underlying brain (cerebrospinal fluid is then sanguineous). (4) *Immediate traumatic epilepsy:* a series of focal seizures may occur with a minor bruise of the cortex and may be followed by a postepileptic paralysis of short duration. (5) *Delayed hemiplegia* or *monoplegia:* an "interval" paralysis in cases of minor or major injury usually signifies an epidural hemorrhage, a subdural hemorrhage or hygroma, arterial thrombosis, spreading venous thrombosis, or intracerebral hemorrhage. (6) *Acute drowsiness, confusion,* and *headache* or *coma,* due presumably to localized and generalized traumatic brain edema; children who have concussions are especially liable to headache, drowsiness, and vomiting, which may have its onset some hours after the injury. In these children infusions and clyses of water and 5 percent glucose are particularly dangerous; such treatment may prove fatal, owing to a water intoxication and severe brain swelling. Apparently an excessive output of antidiuretic hormone and water retention occur under these circumstances. (7) *Posttraumatic nervous instability* (see below).

PATIENTS WHO ARE AND HAVE BEEN UNCONSCIOUS SINCE THE TIME OF THE ACCIDENT (MAJOR HEAD INJURY) The clinical state In this group, which includes the patients with the more severe head injuries, the outlook is obviously less favorable and one is concerned at first for their life. However, within this group there is still a wide variation in the severity of the traumatic brain disease. A certain number of patients die at once or within a few minutes, and it may be assumed that the direct injury to the brain or some other organ was incompatible with life. Other patients in this group recover consciousness rapidly after several hours, but a few remain deeply comatose for days or even weeks. If the pupils dilate and become fixed and all brainstem reflex mechanisms, including the maintenance of respiration, are paralyzed and remain so over a period of hours (EEG usually isoelectric as described on page 1714), the outlook is hopeless. The mortality rate in those who reach a hospital in coma has been approximately 20 percent, and most of them die within the first 12 to 24 hr. Of those alive after 24 hr, the mortality is 7 to 8 percent, and after 48 hr the figure falls to 1 percent.

In the patient whose prognosis is favorable, the coma is less deep; i.e., he is confused, stuporous, or semicomatose (see Chap. 22). For a time he may be restless and difficult to control. The reflexes are normal, as are pulse, blood pressure, and respiration. He is able to swallow and may or may not speak. There are no obvious neurologic signs. In contrast, those patients whose illness will end fatally may be moribund from the beginning. Their coma is profound. The limbs may be flaccid and without reflexes. The corneal and pharyngeal (gag) reflexes are absent. The pupils are small and unreactive to light, or dilated and fixed, or unequal. The ocular axes are divergent or askew. The jaw sags, the tongue falls back in the throat, saliva drools from the mouth, and swallowing is obviously lost. There may be surgical shock at first for a brief period, with the usual findings of pale and moist skin, weak and rapid pulse, subnormal temperature, and a blood pressure that is difficult to obtain. Within a few hours, however, the temperature usually rises, and this may continue until death. The breathing may be stertorous and later feeble and irregular. The state of consciousness and the temperature chart provide information of great value in appraising the status of the patient. An ascending pulse rate, possibly interspersed by short periods in which there is a bounding, slow pulse, and rising temperature or a combination of fast pulse and subnormal temperature, is a sign of grave prognosis.

In the group of patients whose outlook is less bleak, deep coma soon gives way to semicoma. The blood pressure stabilizes, and the temperature and pulse, having risen to 101 to 102°F and 100 to 110 per min, respectively, remain at these levels. Muscular tone is regained in the limbs, and the tendon reflexes are present. This is a critical period, for a sudden rise in temperature, cyanosis, and increasing respiratory difficulty may result in a fatal outcome. Once the patient regains consciousness sufficiently to respond to a spoken command, the physician no longer needs to be concerned about survival and may begin to think about the possibility of focal brain damage and prospects for recovery. There is still a substantial risk in the first 2 or 3 weeks, however, from pneumonia, meningitis, or epidural and subdural hemorrhage, which may intervene and impair the chances of survival. It is often said that death during the first 12 hr is the result of the direct injury of the brain; that which occurs later is usually the result of some complication of cranial trauma (intracerebral or subarachnoid hemorrhage, herniation of the temporal lobe, localized or generalized edema, epidural or subdural hemorrhage, meningitis, pneumonia).

There is another group of patients to which some reference must be made for they represent difficult problems in diagnosis and therapy. Here a known or evident head injury is not followed by deep or lasting coma, but instead the patient is awake and able to respond upon arrival at the hospital. Yet as the hours pass it is apparent that his condition is deteriorating, and within a day or two he lapses into coma. A sanguineous cerebrospinal fluid under slightly elevated pressure attests to the existence of contusion. The progressive nature of the illness suggests intracerebral, epidural, or subdural hemorrhage; yet at postmortem examination only contusion, localized edema (sometimes generalized), and temporal lobe pressure cone are found to be the basis of the clinical syndrome. The point to remember is that consciousness may return early, i.e., within minutes or hours, after a head injury severe enough seriously to contuse the brain and to lead to death, after some few days.

The course of clinical events in those who survive the first 24 to 48 hr is much like that in patients with brief concussion, except that it is likely to be more prolonged, so that one may witness all the varying stages of recovery in slow motion. As coma lessens, the patient opens his eyes; he may pause in his restless activity and seem to listen to what is said. He reacts briskly to painful stimuli applied to the face, passive manipulations of the head, and pinching the inner surface of the arms and legs. Moaning and groaning are the first vocal activities to return; their absence in patients who are beginning to respond always suggests aphasia. Restlessness, irritability, and hyperactivity may assume such proportions that the patient must be restrained. For example, he may resist all attempts to help him, struggle against restraints, yell, talk incessantly and without sense, strike at everyone near the bed, etc. This state, sometimes loosely called *traumatic delirium*, may last hours or days but eventually is replaced by a more quiet confusional state. Then the patient will begin to speak, unless the injury has caused a lack of impulse to act (abulia) or incapacity for speech (aphasia); and he is variably able to engage in conversation. But his thinking processes are slow and inefficient, and his thoughts are likely to be incoherent. Often he cannot understand the purposes of his splints, bandages, catheters, etc., and will remove them even when asked repeatedly not to do so. Movements and reactions to stimuli are more or less automatic. Memory is obviously faulty. As confusion lessens, there may be a brief period when mental function is nearly normal; yet later there will be little or no memory of what transpired. From a close study of this clinical sequence it is obvious that the capacity to form, retain, and reproduce new experiences is one of the best tests of the mental status. Not until the patient reaches the stage of continuous anterograde memory will he regard himself as fully normal. In looking back upon this period he can recall only a few events and has the impression that he was unconscious all this time. Retrograde amnesia for the accident and for the events which preceded it, which often extends over a period of minutes, hours, or even days, is another invariable accompaniment of severe head injury. This period of retrograde memory defect shortens as convalescence proceeds.

Focal and lateralizing neurologic symptoms and signs, as would be anticipated, will be observed with notable frequency in this group of patients. These abnormalities are presumably related to hemorrhage and contusion; and inasmuch as they are usually engrafted on a severe concussive injury, they become manifest as consciousness is regained. Local injury to the brain without a disturbance of consciousness occurs exceptionally, and then more often with the penetration of the skull with missiles or a direct glancing blow by a relatively small object (golf ball, stone), and sometimes with depressed fractures. Of the focal symptoms, hemiparesis is probably the most frequent. The weakness in the arm and leg may be evidenced even during coma by the hypotonia, the less frequent movement of the limbs, inequality of tendon reflexes, and a more persistent Babinski sign on one side. Complete hemiplegia is rarely observed. Hemihypesthesia, although occasionally found, is less common, possibly because sensory tests are difficult to interpret until mental clarity is regained. Homonymous hemianopia is not at all infrequent and may present early as an inattentiveness of visual stimuli on one side. Aphasia, usually of mixed type, may be noted in a number of cases. A series of focal seizures may occur within a few days of the time of injury and, as said before, is probably due to cortical contusion. Such seizures usually cease after a few days and do not necessarily signify that epilepsy is to be a sequel to the trauma. Diabetes insipidus, disturbances of sleep (reversal of rhythm, somnolence, later narcolepsy), diplopia, heteronymous visual field defects, gastrointestinal hemorrhage, amenorrhea, and impotence in the male indicate damage to the hypothalamus and walls of the third ventricle. Midbrain or diffuse cerebral lesions are evidenced by ocular palsies, protracted coma (weeks, months, or years), decerebrate rigidity, crossed ocular-limb paralyses, bilateral Babinski's signs, and, later, dysarthria, ataxia of limbs on one side, and sensory disturbances.

Laboratory findings In this group of patients with severe head injury there is a high incidence of skull fracture. The cerebrospinal fluid is usually sanguineous (red blood cells usually 100,000 per mm^3 or less) and under elevated pressure (between 200 and 300 mm) in the majority of patients. The prognosis is distinctly less good in those with more than 100,000 red cells per cubic millimeter and pressures in excess of 300 mm. Nevertheless death may occur in patients who have no skull fracture, a subnormal intracranial pressure, and relatively clear cerebrospinal fluid. The electroencephalogram regularly shows focal and diffuse abnormalities.

Neuropathologic findings In patients who die during the first few hours or days after a severe head injury, hemorrhage and necrosis of tissue will frequently be observed. In 50 consecutive autopsies summarized in Rowbotham's excellent monograph, only 2 showed no macroscopic change. Lacerations of cerebral cortex (28 percent), surface contusions (48 percent), subarachnoid hemorrhage (72 percent), acute subdural hemorrhage (16 percent), and extradural hemorrhage (20 percent) were the usual findings. As a rule, several of these pathologic changes were found in the same case. Skull fractures were discovered in 72 percent.

PATIENTS WHO ARE UNCONSCIOUS WHEN FIRST SEEN BUT WHO ARE SAID TO HAVE BEEN CONSCIOUS AFTER THE ACCIDENT (PRESENCE OF LUCID INTERVAL)

This group of patients is smaller than the other two but is of great importance because it includes many who are in urgent need of surgical treatment. The initial coma may have been brief or there may have been none at all, in which instance one might conclude that there was neither concussion nor contusion. The following conditions must be considered in every case of this type.

Acute epidural hemorrhage This condition is due as a rule to a temporal or parietal fracture with laceration of the middle meningeal artery and vein. Less often there is a tear in a dural venous sinus. The injury, even when it fractures the skull, may not have produced coma. A typical example is seen in a child who has fallen from a bicycle or a swing or has suffered a hard blow to the head in a fight and was only momentarily unconscious. A few hours or a day or two later (exceptionally the interval may be as long as several days or a week, especially with venous bleeding), he develops headache of increasing severity, vomiting, drowsiness, confusion, seizures (which may be one-sided), hemiparesis, with slightly increased tendon reflexes and Babinski's sign. As coma develops, the hemiparesis with Babinski's sign may give way to spastic limbs, and Babinski's sign bilaterally. There may be aphasia. Respirations become deeper and stertorous, then shallow and irregular, and finally stop. The pulse is often slow (below 60) and bounding, with a concomitant rise in systolic blood pressure. The pupil may dilate on the side of hematoma. The cerebrospinal fluid is usually under increased pressure, though normal and subnormal pressures do not exclude the possibility of an epidural hematoma. The fluid may be clear or sanguineous, depending on whether or not there is an associated contusion, laceration, or subarachnoid hemorrhage. Death, which is almost invariable if the clot is not removed surgically, comes at the end of a comatose period, rarely if ever in a conscious patient, and is due to respiratory arrest. The visualization of a fracture line across the groove of the middle meningeal artery and a knowledge of the side of the head struck (the clot is usually on that side) are of aid in diagnosis and of lateralization of the lesion. The surgical procedure consists of placement of several burr holes (a single one may miss the clot), drainage, identification of the bleeding vessel, and ligation. The operative results are excellent, except in the cases with extended fractures and laceration of the dural venous sinuses, in which instance the epidural hematoma may be bilateral rather than unilateral, as it ordinarily is. If coma, bilateral Babinski's signs, spasticity, or decerebrate rigidity supervenes before operation, the prognosis for life becomes poor. This usually means that a temporal lobe herniation and crushing of the midbrain have already occurred.

Acute and chronic subdural hematoma The problems created by the acute and chronic subdural hematoma are so different that they must be discussed separately. In *acute subdural hematomas*, which may be unilateral or bilateral, the latent interval is usually longer than in epidural hemorrhage—many days or 1 to 2 weeks. Headaches, drowsiness, sometimes agitation, slowness in thinking, and confusion, all of which progressively worsen, are the most frequent symptoms. Focal or lateralizing signs (hemiplegia) are late and tend to be less prominent than the disturbance of consciousness. Frequently the acute subdural hematoma is combined with cerebral contusion and laceration, so that the clinical effects of these several lesions are difficult to distinguish; and there are some patients in whom it is impossible before operation to state whether the surface clot is epidural or subdural in location. Arteriography, which shows inward displacement of cerebral arteries from the skull, provides quick, accurate diagnosis. The treatment is to place bilateral temporal burr holes and to evacuate the clot; placing of the burr holes is also one of the most certain diagnostic procedures. The surgical results are less certain than in chronic subdural hematoma. If the clot that is found is too small to explain the symptoms, the surgeon usually proceeds to do a right subtemporal decompression. Exceptionally the subdural hematoma forms in the posterior fossa and gives rise to headache, vomiting, pupillary inequality, dysphagia, cranial nerve palsies, ataxia of trunk and gait, and stiff neck, in some combination.

In *chronic hematoma*, the traumatic etiology is less clear. The head injury, especially in the elderly person, may be trivial (striking the head against the branch of a tree, or on the mantel of a fireplace during a faint, etc.), and it may have been forgotten completely. A period of weeks then follows when headaches (not invariable), giddiness, slowness in thinking, confusion, exaggeration of certain personality traits, and rarely a seizure or two are the main symptoms. The initial impression may be that the patient has a vascular lesion, a brain tumor, a drug intoxication, or a depressive, senile, or other type of psychosis. As with acute subdural hematoma, the disturbance of consciousness (drowsiness, inattentiveness, incoherence of thought, stupor, or coma) is more prominent than focal or lateralizing signs. The latter usually consist of hemiparesis and rarely of an aphasic disturbance. Hemianesthesia and homonymous hemianopia are seldom observed, probably because the anatomic structures subserving these functions are deep and not easily compressed (in the case of the geniculocalcarine pathway) and sensory changes are likely to be overlooked in a stuporous, confused patient. Hemiplegia, i.e., complete paralysis of one arm and leg, is usually indicative of an intracerebral lesion rather than of a compressive surface lesion. Another important feature of the hemiparesis is that it may be contralateral or ipsilateral, depending on whether or not herniation of the temporal lobe through the notch of the tentorium into the posterior fossa and compression of the contralateral cerebral peduncle are present; if they are present, corticospinal signs are then ipsilateral to the clot or bilateral. As the condition progresses, the patient becomes comatose but often with striking fluctuations of awareness. The ipsilateral pupil dilates (Hutchinson's pupillary sign), owing, it is believed, to direct pressure of the herniating temporal lobe upon the oculomotor nerve. The dilated pupil and ptotic eyelid are more reliable indications of the side of the hematoma than the hemiparesis, though they, too, may be misleading in certain cases. Convulsions are usually seen only in alcoholics or patients with a contusion and cannot be regarded as a cardinal sign of subdural hematoma, even though they are not infrequent. Roentgenograms of the skull are usually negative except for a shift of a calcified pineal to one side or an occasional unexpected fracture line. The electroencephalogram is usually bilaterally abnormal, sometimes with reduced voltage or electrical silence over the subdural hematoma and high-voltage slow waves over the opposite sides because of the damping effects of the clot and displacement of the brain respectively. The branches of the middle cerebral artery are separated from the skull and displaced contralaterally in an arteriogram. The cerebrospinal fluid may be clear, bloody, or xanthochromic, depending on the presence or absence of recent or old contusion and subarachnoid hemorrhage, and the pressure may be elevated, normal, or subnormal. Of all these diagnostic procedures, arteriography and direct burr hole exploration are the most reliable.

The acute, rapidly evolving subdural hematomas are due to tearing or bridging veins and direct compression of the brain by an expanding clot of fresh blood. Unlike the epidural arterial hemorrhage, which is progressive, the bleeding is usually arrested by the rising intracranial pressure. The chronic subdural hematoma is believed to cause symptoms by becoming encysted by fibrous membranes (pseudomembranes) which grow from the dura. In its encysted state, as red corpuscles hemolyze and blood proteins disintegrate, the osmotic pressure rises and fluid enters the hematoma, with the result that the hematoma enlarges and the compressive effects increase. Severe cerebral compression and displacement with temporal lobe–tentorial herniation are the usual causes of death. Treatment consists of placing burr holes and evacuating the clot before deep coma has developed.

Subdural hygromas (collections of blood and cerebrospinal fluid in the subdural space) may also form after an injury, as well as meningitis (in an infant) and pneumoencephalography (see Chap. 329). It is said that a tear of the arachnoid permits bacteria to enter and excite a serous reaction in the subdural space. Drowsiness, confusion, irritability, and fever are relieved when the subdural fluid is aspirated or drained.

Cerebral hemorrhage (immediate and delayed) Acute, massive brain hemorrhages are more frequent in elderly than in young patients and are usually fatal within a few hours. The clinical picture is similar to that of hypertensive brain hemorrhage (deepening coma with hemiplegia, a dilating pupil, bilateral Babinski's signs, stertorous and irregular respirations). Indeed the problem that cannot be solved even at postmortem examination is whether the patient had a hemorrhagic type of stroke and then fell, or a fall that caused the head injury and hemorrhage. If the bleeding is slow, there may be an interval of 2 to 3 days between injury and the symptoms of the oncoming hemorrhage. Coma or confusion, if present from the time of the injury, may obscure the signs of the intracerebral hemorrhage. Craniotomy with evacuation of the clot has given a successful result in a few cases.

TRAUMATIC OCCLUSION OF CAROTID ARTERY In this relatively rare and most dramatic form of cranial trauma, the patient is usually young and athletic, and the mechanism of the injury is usually unclear. An accident on the playing field of seemingly trivial type is followed after an interval of hours or days by a massive hemiplegia, hemianesthesia, homonymous hemianopia, and, if left-sided, aphasia. Occlusion is demonstrable by arteriography. Hemorrhage into the wall of the common or internal carotid artery has been found in a few patients (see Chap. 326).

REPEATED CONCUSSION (PUNCH DRUNK) The cumulative effects of repeated injuries, observed almost exclusively in professional boxers, constitute a type of head injury difficult to classify for it has never been well studied pathologically. It is a common observation that after a number of years in the ring, pugilists often become forgetful, slow in thinking, and slightly dysarthric. Their movements are stiff and uncertain, especially those involving the legs, there is an unsteadiness of gait, and occasionally there are involuntary movements. The plantar reflexes may be extensor on one or both sides. The electroencephalogram shows slow waves of theta and sometimes of delta type. The anatomic basis of this disease is unknown. The postulation of showers of petechial hemorrhages from repeated blows on the jaw should not be given credence until demonstrated pathologically. The brain is atrophied, and a pneumoencephalogram will reveal dilated lateral ventricles. The findings of diffuse degeneration of the cerebral white matter have been demonstrated in rabbits and monkeys which have been subjected to repeated concussions (Jakob) and offer a more acceptable possibility. Low-pressure hydrocephalus is another possibility.

SEQUELAE OF SEVERE HEAD INJURY

The signs of focal brain disease, whether due to open and penetrating or closed head injuries, tend always to ameliorate as the months pass. A hemiplegia is often reduced to a minimal hemiparesis or ineptitude of voluntary motor function with exaggerated reflexes and an equivocal Babinski's sign on that side, and aphasia improves to become a stuttering or hesitant paraphasia which is not disabling except in a professional worker, speaker, or writer. Many of the signs of brainstem disease improve, often to an astonishing degree.

PROTRACTED TRAUMATIC COMA AND PSEUDO-COMA Of particular interest is the outcome of those rare conditions in which the patient remains comatose for weeks or months or even years. The authors have examined the brains of nearly a dozen cases of this type, and nearly all have shown numerous foci of hemorrhage and ischemic necrosis in the midbrain and subthalamus, especially in the tegmentum and tectum. They were probably due in most instances to temporal lobe herniation and midbrain compression, for one could see where one side of the base and tegmentum had been indented by the free edge of the tentorium. In others there may have been direct injury to the midbrain and pons, with numerous small hemorrhages. Presumably these pathologic changes are not constant, for scattered lesions in the cerebral cortex (contusions of the summits of convolutions, ischemia with necrosis in the depths of sulci) and a remarkable diffuse degeneration of cerebral white matter have also been observed in cases of this type (Strich). These patients, while comatose (i.e., unreceptive to stimuli and unresponsive) or in a state of pseudocoma (receptive and capable of signaling by blinking their eyes but otherwise unresponsive), usually exhibit a variety of neurologic abnormalities: unequal pupils; dilated, fixed pupil and oculomotor palsy on one side and hemiplegia on the other; disturbances of gaze; bilateral corticospinal paralysis with Babinski's sign; extensor postures of arm and leg on one side and flexed arm and extended leg on the other; brainstem attacks (extension of limbs, increased respiration, blood pressure, and sweating on stimulation of any kind); and involuntary movements (tremor, chorea, athetosis). Some remain in this reduced mental state until death (after nearly 10 years in one of the author's cases, but usually after a few months or a year or two). The majority, however, may regain enough function to leave the hospital; not a few, surprising as it may seem, are restored to full alertness and adequate mental function. Residual weakness of limbs, slurred speech, ocular palsies, ataxia of an arm or leg, or involuntary movements are frequent. During convalescence, language mechanisms may be found disturbed in various ways, i.e., mutism, akinesia or adynamia (lack of volition or impulse to speak or move), dysarthria, and, if there are contusions of the cortex of the dominant hemisphere, an aphasia as well. Any one or a combination of these abnormalities may be present.

EPILEPSY Posttraumatic epilepsy, which occurs in 20 to 40 percent of patients, is one of the most dreaded complications of head injury. Its basis is nearly always a contusion or laceration of the cortex. The likelihood of epilepsy is said to be greater in parietal and posterior frontal lesions, but it may arise from lesions in any area of the cerebral cortex. The incidence of epilepsy is much greater in "open" than in "closed" head injuries. Indeed, in cases of pure concussion without contusion or laceration, seizures are not much more frequent than in the general population. The interval between head injury and the first seizure averages about 9 months, but it may be much longer, i.e., many years, particularly in children. The longer the interval, the less certain one is of its relationship to the traumatic incident. There is a slightly greater tendency for those patients who had seizures at the time of head injury to become subject to recurrent seizures later. The seizures are always of focal character, or grand mal; petit mal is rarely if ever due to trauma. The significance of the different patterns of focal seizures, which vary according to the location of the lesion, has been worked out in detail by Penfield and his associates (see Chap. 24) and by Russell et al. The frequency of seizures in any given patient varies widely; some patients have only a few, others many, with episodes of status epilepticus. The electroencephalogram is of value in diagnosis; a focus of spike or sharp waves is the characteristic finding. Usually the seizures can be controlled by anticonvulsant medications, and only the recalcitrant cases are likely to require excision of the epileptic focus. The surgical results vary according to the methods of selection and technique of operation. Seizures are abolished in approximately 50 percent of cases by excision of the focus. They tend to decrease in frequency as the years pass, and some patients (an estimated 10 to 30 percent) stop having them.

IMPAIRMENT OF MENTAL FUNCTION Fortunately this is a rare sequela to head trauma. Although mental function may be disturbed by focal lesions which produce dysphasia, agnosia, apraxia, etc., intellectual functions and memory are usually preserved. The exceptions are usually elderly persons in whom the injury may have uncovered an early senile dementia or the development at any age of a hydrocephalus secondary to subarachnoid hemorrhage.

POSTTRAUMATIC NERVOUS INSTABILITY Undoubtedly the most troublesome sequela of head injury is that alluded to above in the discussion of the first group of cases under Clinical Manifestations—*headache, giddiness*, and *nervous instability*. This has been called the *postconcussional syndrome* or the *minor contusion syndrome* (Trotter), or *posttraumatic vasomotor neurosis* (Friedmann). All these terms are objectionable on the grounds that they suggest an explanatory hypothesis, as yet unproved. Headache is the central symptom, usually, at times localized to the part struck. It is variously described as an aching, throbbing, pounding, stabbing, pressing pain and is remarkable for its variability. The intensification of symptoms by mental and physical effort, straining, stooping, and emotional excitement has already been mentioned. Rest and quiet may relieve them. Thus the headache becomes a major obstacle to convalescence, which demands always a resumption of normal activities. The dizziness is usually not a true vertigo but a giddiness. The patient feels suddenly unsteady, dazed, weak, or faint. However, a certain number of patients report symptoms which suggest a labyrinthine disorder. For example, objects in the environment are said to move momentarily, and looking upward or to the side may cause a sense of unbalance. Labyrinthine tests may show either hypo- or hyperreactivity, or the results may prove to be normal. The data are usually so indefinite that it is impossible to state whether or not the labyrinth and vestibular mechanisms have been injured. Exceptionally, vertigo is accompanied by diminished excitability of both the labyrinth and the cochlea, and one may assume the existence of direct injury to the nerve or end organ. The giddy patient usually is intolerant of noise, emotional excitement, and crowds. Tenseness, restlessness, inability to concentrate, a feeling of nervousness, fatigue, worry, apprehension, and an inability to tolerate the usual amount of alcohol complete the clinical picture. In contrast to the multiple subjective symptoms, detailed tests of intellectual functions and memory show little or no impairment. This syndrome, once established, may persist for months or even years, but usually the symptoms lessen as time passes. Strangely, it is almost unknown in children. Its intensity and duration are augmented by compensation problems and litigation, suggesting a psychopathologic process.

EXTRAPYRAMIDAL AND CEREBELLAR DISORDERS The question of *posttraumatic Parkinson's syndrome* has been discussed many times, usually with the general conclusion that a true traumatic parkinsonism does not exist. Most patients have merely had paralysis agitans or postencephalitic Parkinson's disease brought to light by head injury. Cerebellar ataxia is a rare consequence of cranial trauma. When present, it is frequently unilateral and due to injury of the superior cerebellar peduncle. An ataxia of gait may reflect a communicating hydrocephalus.

POSTTRAUMATIC HYDROCEPHALUS The not infrequent examples of posttraumatic hydrocephalus exhibit intermittent headaches, vomiting, confusion, and drowsiness, and autopsy has demonstrated an adhesive basilar meningitis, attributed to subarachnoid or ventricular hemorrhage. Later, mental dullness, apathy, and psychomotor retardation are the principal manifestations. The CSF pressure may then have fallen to a normal level (low-pressure hydrocephalus). Since symptoms like these have been observed occasionally after the rupture of a saccular aneurysm with massive subarachnoid hemorrhage, due presumably to blocking of the aqueduct and fourth ventricle by blood clot, this mechanism has also been suggested as a possible explanation of traumatic hydrocephalus in patients with cerebral confusion. Response to ventriculoatrial shunt may be dramatic.

POSTTRAUMATIC PSYCHIATRIC DISORDERS In contrast to nervousness and nervous instability, which are common sequelae of injuries of all types, posttraumatic psychoses are relatively infrequent. The most distressing psychiatric syndromes have been suspiciousness and paranoid delusions, unaccountable outbursts of violent temper, sometimes with homicidal or suicidal tendencies, progressive hyperactivity, delirium, and mania, and episodes of bizarre behavior with subsequent amnesia, reminiscent of temporal lobe seizures. Alcoholism may provoke some of these behavioral abnormalities. Some of these illnesses are undoubtedly due to residual brain damage in individuals of peculiar personality makeup. However, attempts to account for psychoses of this type by reference to constitutional peculiarities and predisposition, laid bare, so to speak, by head injury, have not been convincing.

TREATMENT

The physician who undertakes to treat the "head injury case" must at all times bear in mind that assiduous attention to detail may prove to be lifesaving, and that accurate documentation of all diagnostic findings and therapy is desirable if the medical data are later to be used in the arbitration of insurance claims, worker's unemployment compensation, etc. The suggestions which follow can do no more than serve as guides, for every patient presents a combination of problems that the physician has not encountered before and may not observe again in identical form.

Exact data concerning the patient's medical status before the accident (previous illnesses, work and social record, emotional stability), the nature and precise circumstances of the accident, the duration of retrograde and anterograde amnesia, and all that transpired afterward should be obtained and recorded. Verbatim statements should be written down whenever possible.

The treatment problems presented by each of the three groups of clinical cases discussed above are as follows.

MINOR HEAD INJURY In this group are included patients who (1) were never unconscious at any time, (2) were briefly unconscious at the time of the first examination, (3) are rapidly regaining consciousness.

Circumstances dictate how each case is managed. If the injury was trivial and the scalp was not lacerated, and if the patient is entirely clear mentally, little or nothing need be done. When the patient is unable to give an accurate account of what has happened and appears still to be somewhat confused or incoherent, he should be compelled to lie down or at least remain in one place. It often happens that the confusion is not detected and the patient is permitted to resume activity while still acting in an irrational manner. He may get into his car and attempt to drive, only to have another accident; or if he is an athlete he may continue to play a game and make a series of errors.

When a conscious or nearly conscious patient is admitted to a general hospital, it is tempting to let him go his way. Experience teaches caution, however. A complete examination, with the patient fully undressed, should be carried out. It is well, if there is any likelihood of litigation, to obtain x-rays of the skull and an electroencephalogram. Whether to perform a lumbar puncture will usually depend on how serious the injury was, on the prominence of posttraumatic headache, etc. A simple fracture without involvement of paranasal sinuses requires no special treatment but is believed to contraindicate vigorous athletic activities for several months or a year.

Posttraumatic headache, dizziness, and nervousness are the most difficult symptoms; an optimistic prognosis and the institution of a program of graded mental and physical activities to the point of tolerance stand the best chance of restoring the patient to a useful life. The patient should be told that he must expect a certain amount of headache and should carry on in spite of it. Meprobamate, 200 mg t.i.d., is useful for anxiety, and a non-habit-forming analgesic medication should be given for the more severe headaches (Empirin or aspirin). Insomnia may require a barbiturate medication or chloral hydrate at first, but these drugs should be discontinued as soon as possible. Any litigation that may be involved should be settled within 6 to 9 months. To delay settlement usually works against the best interests of the patient. The severity of his injury can be ascertained within this period of time, and a longer period of observation only enhances his worries and fears and reduces his motivation to return to work.

PATIENTS WHO ARE UNCONSCIOUS WHEN FIRST SEEN If the physician arrives on the scene of the accident, a hurried examination should be made before the patient is moved in order to determine whether there is dangerous hemorrhage from a laceration of the scalp or other parts of the body and whether there is a likelihood of a fracture-dislocation of the cervical part of the spine, which is occasionally associated with head injury. If the patient is in shock, with cold clammy skin and feeble pulse, he should be covered with warm blankets. In moving an individual with a potential cervical spine injury, the spine should be kept straight at all times and flexion of the neck should be avoided. This can best be done by placing sandbags or firm pillows on either side of the head and warning everyone against neck flexion. An even safer method is to place the patient on a stretcher face down and arrange pillows to assure a clear airway. Bleeding from the scalp can usually be controlled with a firm pad unless an artery is divided, and then a suture becomes necessary.

In the hospital, where all such patients should be taken, the first steps should be to control shock. This can usually be done by the application of warmth, keeping the head low, and leaving the patient alone for a few minutes. The shock will usually come under control in a few minutes with or without vasopressor drugs or transfusions. Persistent shock is rare in head injury and always raises the suspicion of a ruptured viscera with internal bleeding, extensive fractures, or traumatism of the cervical part of the spinal cord. A quick survey will enable one to estimate the depth of coma, size of pupils, and presence of obvious fractures; and if shock is not present, or after the blood pressure has stabilized, a more detailed examination can be performed. The skull should be carefully inspected and palpated. The hair should be cut off around the scalp wound. A bogginess of the temporal or postauricular region (Battle's sign), bleeding from the nose or ear, extensive conjunctival edema, and hemorrhage are useful signs of underlying skull fracture. However, it should be remembered that rupture of the eardrum or a blow on the nose may also cause bleeding from the ear and nose, respectively. Fractures of the orbital bones may cause displacement of the eye, with resulting diplopia, and fracture of the jaws, disalignment of the teeth, and great discomfort on attempting to open the mouth. Careful notes should be made regarding temperature, pulse, blood pressure, state of consciousness, pupil size, ocular movements, corneal reflexes, facial movements during grimace, swallowing, tone of limb muscles, movements of limbs, predominant postures, and reflexes. Vital signs and consciousness should be checked and recorded by the nurse or physician every 2 hr. A proper airway must be maintained. The best position for the patient is semisupine, with the head on a pillow and turned to one side. If urine is retained and the bladder is distended, a catheter should be inserted and kept there. If coma persists for more than 48 to 72 hr, a nasal tube should be passed and fluids and nourishment given by that route. Intravenous fluids should be administered slowly and not in excessive amounts; even hypertonic glucose may increase oncoming pulmonary and cerebral edema, the danger of the latter being especially great in children. Lumbar puncture should be done as soon as practicable for diagnostic purposes (immediately if bacterial meningitis is suspected), and if the pressure is elevated it should be lowered to 100 to 150 mm. The practice of daily lumbar punctures has its advocates and its opponents. The authors have tended to use them only if the pressure is elevated and the patient's condition is not improving. Hypertonic solutions intravenously are of therapeutic value. One hundred milliliters of hypertonic urea, or if not available, 50 to 100 ml of 25 percent mannitol may be injected intravenously in an attempt to lower CSF pressure. Recently corticosteroids, dexamethasone, e.g., (16 to 48 mg per day), have been strikingly effective in reducing brain swelling and permitting vital signs to stabilize. X-rays of skull and other parts should be taken after the first day or two, unless there is a suspicion of an epidural hemorrhage, in which case they should be made at once, to visualize a crack across the course of the middle meningeal artery. Restlessness is controlled by sodium phenobarbital or paraldehyde, but only if careful nursing does not quiet the patient and permit him to sleep for a few hours at a time.

Once the patient has regained consciousness, the danger of suffocation, aspiration pneumonia, thrombophlebitis, and pulmonary embolism has usually passed, and therapy can proceed along the lines indicated for the first group.

Death from head injury in the first 12 hr is the direct effect of primary brain injury and probably cannot be prevented. The advisability of any surgical procedure during the period is much debated. If the patient survives for one, two, or more days and remains in coma, the control of brain swelling and hemorrhage by surgical means must be considered. Should the condition of the patient then begin to deteriorate (pulse rising, temperature subnormal or rising, state of consciousness worsening, hemiplegia more obvious, plantar reflexes more clearly extensor), a decision must be made concerning an epidural or subdural hemorrhage and of increasing brain edema with temporal lobe herniation. Rowbotham, who has had a large experience with cases of this type, recommends a right-sided temporal decompression and two inspection burr holes in the left, one at the Sylvian point and one at the parietal eminence, for some of these patients. In his opinion the indications for surgery are (1) retrogression following a period of improvement, which cannot be controlled by lumbar puncture and oral and rectal hypertonic solutions or intravenous dehydration measures; (2) decerebrate rigidity which has its onset after an interval of 24 hr (early decerebrate rigidity implies primary brainstem injury), if meningitis is ruled out; (3) a dilated fixed pupil on one side, with no improvement after 12 hr; (4) prolonged unconsciousness associated with persistently high cerebrospinal fluid pressure. Not all neurologists and neurosurgeons are agreed on the value of this plan and would insist on diagnostic arteriography as a guide. But, certainly the removal of a large epidural or subdural hemorrhage, which cannot be diagnosed easily in the comatose patient, may be a lifesaving procedure.

In recent years a striking reduction in the mortality rate from these acute head injuries has been obtained by the application of intensive care together with the free use of tracheostomy. Many of the comatose patients who would otherwise have succumbed to respiratory obstruction, pulmonary infections, or dehydration are thereby saved. Also, greater efforts to evacuate intracranial hematomas as soon as possible seem to have helped. The mortality rate of a group of patients in a state of decerebrate rigidity is reduced by 50 percent, and the total mortality rate of all hospitalized patients has fallen from about 10 to 3.5 percent. Survivors may be left permanently disabled, but a surprising number, the percentage increasing up to 7 years, return to productive work.

The treatment of the patient with protracted coma has been outlined in Chap. 22. Every patient presents special problems which must be dealt with individually.

PATIENTS WHO TEMPORARILY RECOVERED CONSCIOUSNESS (LUCID INTERVAL) AND THEN BECAME STUPOROUS OR COMATOSE The treatment is that of epidural, subdural, and delayed cerebral hemorrhage. This has already been discussed.

GENERAL CONVALESCENCE

A head injury carries dire import to most lay persons, who often fear for their mind and are concerned about their capacity to resume their place in society. In former times, therapeutic measures often involved long discussions of the seriousness of the injury, protracted bed rest, and inactivity, all of which served only to engender greater anxiety. Even worse, these measures were not of proved value. It is now widely acknowledged that the patient does better if his physician tends to minimize the seriousness of his head injury and to reassure him that he will recover. Early rehabilitation should be encouraged. It may safely begin as soon as the cerebrospinal fluid becomes clear, usually within a few weeks at the most, except of course in the rare cases of protracted coma.

The prognosis of head injury, in good hands, is influenced by several variables. Elderly patients often remain disabled, especially when compensation is involved. Young and middle-aged adults do better if they are not entitled to compensation (Russell's figures: 70 percent of patients with compensation benefits back at work in 18 months; 83 percent of those without compensation working at the end of this period). Russell also pointed out that the severity of the injury as measured by the duration of traumatic amnesia was a factor. If the period of amnesia was less than 1 hr, 95 percent of patients were back at work within 2 months; if longer than 24 hr, only 80 percent had returned to work within 6 months. About 60 percent, however, still had symptoms at the end of 2 months, and 40 percent at the end of 18 months. Of the most severely injured (those comatose for several days), many will remain permanently disabled. However, recovery is always better than one expects, and the motor impairment, aphasia, and dementia tend to clear. Improvement may continue over a period of five or more years. Children seem to recover more completely than adults. Rehabilitation centers are of great help in restoring morale and reeducating the patient.

(For discussion of traumatism of spinal cord, nerve roots, and peripheral nerves, see Chaps. 325 and 323.)

REFERENCES

Brock S (ed): *Injuries of the Brain and Spinal Cord and Their Coverings*, 3d ed., Baltimore: Williams & Wilkins, 1949, p. 71

Merritt HH: Diagnostic considerations in patients with head injury. Res Publ Assoc Res Nerv Ment Dis 24:379, 1943

Munro D: *The Treatment of Injuries to the Nervous System*, Philadelphia: Saunders, 1952

Rowbotham GF: *Acute Injuries of the Head*, 4th ed., Baltimore: Williams & Wilkins, 1964

328 NEOPLASTIC DISEASE OF THE BRAIN

HENRY deF. WEBSTER
RAYMOND D. ADAMS

Tumors of the central nervous system play a very important part in neurologic medicine and occupy a distinct field by themselves. It may be said of them generally that they occur in great variety; produce neurologic symptoms because of size, location, and invasive qualities; usually destroy the tissues in which they are situated and displace those around them; are a frequent cause of increased intracranial pressure; and are often lethal.

For the student of medicine the most important facts to know are that (1) many types of tumor occur in the cranial cavity and spinal canal and that certain ones are much more frequent than others (see Table 328-1); (2) some of these tumors, such as the craniopharyngioma, meningioma, and schwannoma, have a disposition to grow in certain parts of the cranial cavity, thereby evincing certain syndromes; (3) their growth rates vary, some like the glioblastoma being highly malignant and invasive, others like the meningioma being benign and compressive. These pathologic peculiarities are important for they have valuable clinical correlations, providing the explanation of slowly or rapidly progressive clinical states, excellent or poor prognosis after surgical excision, etc.

The one place where these pathologic-clinical correlations tend to fail is in the glioma group of tumors, i.e., astrocytoma-glioblastoma series, and this is regrettable because tumors of this type are so common. Often these gliomas are of mixed cell type. For example, one part of the tumor may be a typical astrocytoma and another an oligodendrocytoma. Also the degree of differentiation or its opposite, the degree of anaplasia, varies from one part of the tumor to another. Therefore a biopsy sample is often misleading with reference to the expected clinical behavior of the tumor. For example, the clinician may be led to believe that a tumor which in a biopsy is composed of astrocytes is benign, whereas actually the main mass of it still in the brain is a glioblastoma.

TYPES OF BRAIN TUMORS AND THEIR INCIDENCE

Most of the available statistics on the different types of tumors of the central nervous system have been collected in special neurosurgical clinics and are somewhat misleading, for they fail to reveal their natural incidence in an unselected population. The figures in Table 328-1, compiled by Peer, are thus rather exceptional, for they avoid this error of selection and represent the natural incidence of these tumors in postmortem material during the period 1900–1930, at a time when very little neurosurgery was being performed in the hospital from which they were taken (Boston City Hospital).

These data reveal that the central nervous system and its enveloping tissues are fruitful soil for tumor growth and, further, that the bulk of these tumors are gliomas, metastatic tumors, and meningiomas. The increasing rarity of gummas and tuberculomas is noted in all pathologic material from the United States. Of the gliomas, approximately half are glioblastoma multiforme, and the remainder are divided between astrocytoma, oligodendroglioma, ependymoma, medulloblastoma, and undiagnosed gliomas. Tumors composed of neurons (postmitotic cells) are extremely rare. All statistics show the peak age incidence to be the fifth decade of life, with a fairly symmetric curve which reflects the lessening incidence at the extremes of age—infancy and senescence. In children, tumors of the posterior fossa (medulloblastomas, ependymomas, and gliomas) predominate; in adults, supratentorial tumors (glioblastomas, meningiomas, and metastatic carcinomas) are more frequent. Males appear to be more susceptible to intrinsic tumors of the brain (gliomas) than females, the ratio being 2:1. In contrast the meningioma occurs more frequently in elderly women.

TABLE 328-1
Incidence of intracranial and intraspinal tumors at Boston City Hospital, 1900–1930

Total no. of autopsies	10,592
Total no. of tumors	1,458
Tumors of other organs	1,270
Intracranial and intraspinal tumors	188 (12.7%)
Gliomas	81 (43.1%)
Pituitary adenomas	6 (3.2%)
Sheath tumors	22 (11.7%)
Meningioma	18
Acoustic neuroma	4
Metastatic tumors	29 (15.4%)
Blood vessel tumors	6 (3.0%)
Congenital tumors	8 (4.3%)
Granulomas	19 (10.1%)
Spinal cord tumors	4 (2.1%)
Unclassified	13 (7.1%)

INTRACRANIAL TUMORS

PATHOPHYSIOLOGY The cranium, according to the Monro-Kellie law, contains three elements—nervous tissue, blood, and cerebrospinal fluid—the total bulk of which must always be constant. Any increase in the volume of the brain, for example, can take place only at the expense of one of the other elements; and a diminished volume of brain (as in cerebral atrophy) is compensated by an increase in the amount of cerebrospinal fluid. Another noteworthy fact is that the cerebrospinal fluid pressure, while reflecting the volume of the intracranial mass, is largely maintained by the pressure under which the blood is delivered to the skull. In profound shock the raised cerebrospinal fluid pressure with tumors falls, and at death it is zero.

When a tumor or other space-occupying mass forms in the cranial cavity, the volume of cerebrospinal fluid within the subarachnoid and ventricular spaces is reduced and the cerebrospinal fluid is displaced into the spinal and perioptic subarachnoid spaces. Soon, however, the limits of these adjustments are surpassed, and the pressure throughout the ventricles and in all parts of the subarachnoid space rises. Presumably the veins in the cerebral tissues adjacent to the tumor are compressed, with resulting increase in venous pressure locally—the conditions necessary for *regional swelling*, or *edema*. Inasmuch as any general increase in venous pressure results in retarded absorption of cerebrospinal fluid and an increase in its volume, the pressure in the subarachnoid space must exceed that in the veins at all times. If the rise in cerebrospinal fluid pressure is slow, the stasis of blood resulting from this elevated venous pressure can be compensated for by vasodilatation of arteries and arterioles; if the rise is rapid, the blood pressure must rise, usually the systolic more than the diastolic. As a rule this is accompanied by a slowing of cerebral blood flow and bradycardia. Presumably these circulatory reflexes, which result in the rise of blood pressure and bradycardia, are initiated by venous stasis and accumulation of carbon dioxide in the vasomotor center in the medulla oblongata. The respiratory centers also become affected, for increases in intracranial pressure usually cause an irregularity and finally a cessation of respiration.

These changes in blood pressure, pulse, and respiration are of importance in the clinic, for they may afford valuable clues as to the existence of increased intracranial pressure. Not less valuable is the papilledema, or "choked disk," that can be seen with an ophthalmoscope in the optic fundi of most patients who have elevated intracranial pressure of more than a few days' standing. The papilledema is best accounted for by the high pressure in the subarachnoid space surrounding the optic nerves.

Raised intracranial pressure due to a mass or enlargement of the ventricles (blockage of cerebrospinal fluid circulation), when severe, causes obtundation of cerebral function. This is manifested clinically by a number of characteristic symptoms such as reduced mental activity, apathy, and drowsiness and electroencephalographically by diffuse slowing of the electrical activity of the cortex. The rate of cerebral blood flow is slowed.

Another extremely important anatomic fact is that the closed cranial "box" is subdivided into fairly rigid compartments by two infoldings of dura mater, one the falx, which lies between the two cerebral hemispheres, and the other the tentorium, which separates the cerebellum from the occipital lobes. These anatomic arrangements and the opening at the base of the skull through which the spinal cord and medulla are joined leave three important apertures, the foramen magnum, the tentorial opening or "notch," and the subfalcial or supracallosal space. A tumor growth in one compartment, say the right middle cranial fossa, raises the pressure in that compartment more than in the others, and either brain or tumor tissue tends to be displaced along lines of least resistance, i.e., through the subfalcial space to the left half of the cranial cavity and through the tentorial opening into the posterior fossa on the right side. These brain displacements are exceedingly dangerous and contribute to the death of the patient in most cases of intracranial tumor, abscess, trauma, and subdural and epidural hemorrhage. The temporal lobe—tentorial hernia is said to stretch the ipsilateral oculomotor nerve (Hutchinson's pupil—a dilated pupil on the side of a lesion, and also a drooping eyelid); to displace and compress the midbrain with resulting stupor or coma, bilateral pyramidal signs (often greater on the side of the hernia), decerebrate postures of extension of all four extremities, and periodicity (of Cheyne-Stokes type), then irregularity and finally arrest of respiration; and to distort and partially block the aqueduct of Sylvius and to narrow the perimesencephalic subarachnoid space with communicating hydrocephalus and rising intracranial pressure. Also, the posterior cerebral arteries may be occluded on one side or both sides, with infarction of the occipital lobes. The cerebellar-foramen magnum pressure cone (herniation of cerebellar tonsils), in which the cerebellar tissue or tumor mass is displaced into the cervical spinal canal with compression of the medulla oblongata, results in tilting or altered posture of the head, dilated pupils, impairment of consciousness, and death due to respiratory arrest. The physiologic and clinical effects of subfalcial herniation are not known.

A knowledge of these effects of elevated intracranial pressure and of the herniations and displacements of tissue is necessary if one is to understand the clinical behavior of intracranial growths.

CLINICAL AND PATHOLOGIC CHARACTERISTICS

It may be said at the very outset that tumors of the brain may exist with hardly any symptoms. Often only a slight deficiency in mental power, a slowness in comprehension, or a loss of capacity in sustaining continuous mental activity suggests any deviation from normal health. Specific signs that would lead to a suspicion of any real cerebral disease may be wholly wanting. In some patients, on the other hand, there is evidence of cerebral disease in the form of a seizure or some other dramatic symptom, but the evidence is not clear enough to warrant the diagnosis of a cerebral tumor. In a third group, the existence of a new growth in the brain may be determined with much probability by the presence of signs of elevated intracranial pressure, but without symptoms which disclose localization of the growth. Lastly, the symptoms may be so clear and definite as to make it probable not only that there is a new growth within the cranium but that it is located in one particular region. In fact, these localized growths may create certain unique syndromes seldom evinced by any other disease.

In the further exposition of this subject, all intracranial tumors are considered in relation to the common clinical circumstances in which they are likely to be encountered, as follows:

1 The patient whose presenting symptom is either a decline in general mental ability or a seizure.
2 The patient with unmistakable evidence of raised intracranial pressure.
3 Specific intracranial tumor syndromes.

PATIENTS WITH GENERAL SYMPTOMS OF CEREBRAL DISEASE OR A SEIZURE AS THE MAIN COMPLAINT These are the patients who give the most trouble in diagnosis and about whom decisions are often made with a great degree of uncertainty. Their initial symptoms are vague, and not until some time has elapsed will signs of focal brain disease appear; when they do, they are not always of accurate localizing value. Altered psychic function, headache, giddiness, and seizures are the usual symptoms in this group of patients.

Some *change in mental function* may be found in nearly every patient of this type, but it may be necessary to obtain the observations of a person who knows the patient intimately to learn of it. A lack of persistent application to the tasks of the day, an undue irritability, emotional lability, a "peculiar inertia," faulty insight, forgetfulness, reduced range of mental activity, indifference to common social practices, lack of initiative and spontaneity, all of which may be falsely attributed to worry, anxiety, or depression, are the usual symptoms. Much of this behavior is accepted by the patient with forbearance, and if he has any complaint it is of being weak, tired, dizzy (nonrotational), or "queer in the head." Inordinate drowsiness, a remarkable equanimity or apathy, and stoicism may be primary findings. Usually within a few weeks or months the drowsiness and mental dullness increase. When questioned, a long pause precedes each reply, and at times he may not bother to respond at all. Or at the very moment when the examiner has decided that the patient has not heard the question and prepares to repeat it, an appropriate, sensible answer is given, usually in relatively few words. The responses are often much more intelligent than would be expected from the torpid mental state. There are, in addition, patients who are confused or demented (see Chap. 27). The dullness and somnolence may gradually increase, and finally, as increased intracranial pressure supervenes, they end in stupor or coma.

Mental symptoms of this type cannot be ascribed to disease in any particular part of the brain. Tumors are most likely to be accompanied by intellectual disturbance when they interfere with large association fiber systems of the cerebral white matter; growths limited to the cortex and subcortical white matter are less likely to affect the mind. Much of the drowsiness, torpor, inertia, lack of spontaneity, and general restriction of mental horizon is related to increased intracranial pressure and is unrelated to the site and nature of the lesion.

The *headaches* in the "tumor patient" are variable. In some the pain is slight, temporary, and dull in character; in others it may be severe and unendurable, being either dull or sharp, but as a rule transitory or intermittent. If there are any characteristics of the headache, it would be its nocturnal occurrence, its presence on first awakening, and its deep nonpulsatile quality. However, these are not specific attributes, since migraine, hypertensive vascular headaches, etc., may also begin early in the morning on first awakening. The patient does not always complain of the pain even when it is present, and often he betrays its existence by placing his hand on his forehead and looking distressed.

The mechanism of the headache is not known. In the majority of instances, the intracranial pressure is normal during the first weeks when the headache is present, and one can attribute it only to distortion or alteration of blood vessels in or around the tumor. Later the headache appears to be related to rises in intracranial pressure. Tumors above the tentorium cause headache on the side of and in the vicinity of the tumor, usually in the orbital, frontal, temporal, or parietal regions. Tumors in the posterior fossa usually cause ipsilateral retroauricular or occipital headache. With elevated intracranial pressure, bifrontal and bioccipital headache is the rule, regardless of the location of the tumor.

Vomiting appears in about one-third of the patients with tumor syndromes of this type and usually accompanies the headache. It is more frequent with tumors of the posterior fossa. Some patients may vomit unexpectedly and forcibly, without preceding nausea (projectile vomiting), but others suffer both nausea and great pain. Usually the vomiting is not related to the ingestion of food, often occurring before breakfast.

No less frequent is the complaint of *giddiness* or *dizziness*. As a rule it is not described with accuracy and consists of a more or less confused sensation in the head, coupled with feelings of strangeness and insecurity when the position of the head is altered.

One or more generalized *convulsions* are the other major symptom calling attention to the existence of cerebral tumor. Their frequency in various statistical analyses is 20 to 50 percent of all patients with cerebral tumors. The onset of a seizure during adult years and the existence of a localizing aura are always suggestive of tumor. The localizing significance of seizure patterns has already been discussed (see Chap. 24). The seizures may occur once or many times and may precede other symptoms for as long as 10 years or more in cases of astrocytoma or meningioma.

The management of patients who present any one of the aforementioned symptoms requires brief discussion. Any clinical problem of this type, especially if accompanied by recurrent headache of a type which the patient recognizes as different from his customary headaches, or a seizure, appearing for the first time, justifies a careful review of the patient's general behavior. In obtaining further data, one must rely heavily on the observations of other members of the family. A thorough neurologic examination with careful inspection of optic fundi, a test of visual fields, motor, reflex, and sensory functions in the limbs, alertness, memory, facility in language (speaking, reading, writing, and understanding the spoken word), calculation, and tests of visuospatial orientation must follow. Sooner or later other regional or localizing symptoms and signs will be discovered, and it is only by repeated examinations that one will note earliest stages of a hemiparesis, aphasia, visual field defect, hemianesthesia, etc. Unmistakable signs of increased intracranial pressure may become manifest and establish the diagnosis of tumor with reasonable certainty (see Astrocytoma, below).

The decision as to the appropriate time for doing confirmatory diagnostic tests requires balanced clinical judgment. Since many of the symptoms described above could be due to any number of diseases, for a time it is wise to follow the patient by repeated examinations and not proceed too quickly to expensive and difficult diagnostic tests. As more of the clinical picture unfolds, there comes a time when x-rays of the skull and chest (always done to help rule out metastatic carcinoma), lumbar puncture (for pressure, cells, protein, and Wassermann reaction), localizing electroencephalogram, and radionuclide scan should be made, preferably by admitting the patient to a hospital. Perimetry, audiograms, vestibular tests, and psychometric tests are also helpful in the study of many of these patients. Pneumoencephalography and carotid arteriography are reserved in most medical neurologic clinics for those in whom the total clinical syndrome is already strongly suggestive of tumor. These procedures are too costly and hazardous to be used routinely in every "tumor suspect."

TUMORS WHICH TEND TO PRODUCE GENERAL CEREBRAL SYMPTOMS OR SEIZURES The following tumors are most likely to produce initial convulsions or a vague syndrome of headache, giddiness, vomiting, dull or stuporous state, and psychic changes: glioblastoma multiforme, astrocytoma, oligodendroglioma, metastatic carcinoma, meningioma, and primary reticulum cell sarcoma of the cerebrum.

Glioblastoma multiforme In all statistic analyses of surgical and postmortem material, glioblastoma multiforme is responsible for more than 25 percent of intracranial gliomas and for more than 90 percent of gliomas of the cerebral hemispheres in adults. Approximately 20 to 30 percent of the cerebral tumors are bilateral, occupy more than one lobe of a hemisphere, or show multicentric foci of growth. Although predominantly cerebral in location, similar tumors may be observed in the brainstem, cerebellum, or spinal cord. The peak incidence is in middle adult life, but no age group is spared.

The glioblastoma is a highly malignant tumor which infiltrates the brain extensively and may attain enormous size before attracting medical attention. It may extend to the meningeal surface or the ventricular wall, which probably accounts for the elevation of protein level (more than 100 mg per 100 ml in many cases), as well as an occasional pleocytosis of 10 to 100 cells or more, mostly lymphocytes. The tumor has a variegated appearance, being a mottled gray, red, orange, or brown, depending on the degree of necrosis and whether hemorrhage is recent or old. It is highly vascular, and in an arteriogram one can often see a network of abnormal vessels, mistaken at times for a hemangioma, and the displacement of normal vessels which may result from any "mass lesion." Some part of one lateral ventricle is often distorted, and both lateral and third ventricles are displaced contralaterally, which may be demonstrated by pneumoencephalography or ventriculography. The vessels in the tumor are excessively permeable to radioactive phosphorus (^{32}P), radioactive arsenic, mercury and technetium, which is the basis for radioactive scanning techniques. The characteristic microscopic pathologic findings are great cellularity with pleomorphism of cells and hyperchromatism of nuclei; identifiable astrocytes with fibrils in combination with astroblasts, tumor giant cells, and cells in mitosis; a curious neoplastic proliferation of the cells of small vessels (adventitial and endothelial); necrosis, pseudopalisading of viable cells, hemorrhage, and thrombosis of vessels. Temporal lobe–tentorial herniation, midbrain compression, midbrain and pontine hemorrhages, and increased intracranial pressure are usually the immediate causes of death.

Clinically the diffuse cerebral symptoms and seizures (present in 30 to 40 percent of cases) usually give way to a more definite frontal, temporal, parietooccipital, or callosal syndrome in a few weeks or months. Seldom, however, do the symptoms and signs point to one lobe, and often one is satisfied to be able to specify the region of the hemisphere which is involved.

Astrocytoma The astrocytoma may occur anywhere in the brain or spinal cord. Favored sites are cerebrum, cerebellum, thalamus, optic chiasm, and pons. It is a slowly growing tumor of infiltrative character with a tendency to form large cavities or pseudocysts. Others of these tumors are noncavitating, grayish-white, firm, and relatively avascular, almost indistinguishable from normal white matter, with which they may merge imperceptibly. Calcium deposits may occur in parts of the tumor and may be seen in a plain x-ray of the skull. The cerebrospinal fluid is acellular, the only abnormality being the increased pressure and elevated protein level in some cases. The tumor by its mass may distort the lateral and third ventricles (seen in pneumoencephalogram or ventriculogram) and may be seen to displace the anterior and middle cerebral arteries in a carotid arteriogram. Microscopically the tumor tissue is composed of well-differentiated astrocytes of fibrillary, protoplasmic, or transitional type.

The majority of cerebral astrocytomas undergo malignant degeneration and present as mixed astrocytomas and glioblastomas.

The astrocytoma may cause trivial symptoms for a long period of time. Seizures, headaches, and bizarre mental symptoms may be present for several years, in a few instances more than 10, before the diagnosis is made. The average survival period after the first symptom is 67 months in cerebral growths and 89 months in cerebellar ones. The cystic astrocytoma of the cerebellum is particularly benign, and some patients are alive and well as long as 30 years after part of the cyst was excised. In such cases, of course, accuracy of the original diagnosis of neoplasm is always open to question. The astrocytoma of the pons, optic nerves, and chiasm are discussed in more detail later on in this chapter (see Glioma of the Brainstem).

Oligodendrocytoma The oligodendrocytoma is a relatively rare cerebral tumor (5 to 10 percent of gliomas) and is usually slow in its rate of growth (average span of evolution is 66 months). It is generally a soft solid tumor, rarely cystic, and through its tendency to calcify (spherules and particles of calcium in microscopic sections) often casts a shadow in the roentgenogram of the skull. Microscopically it is composed of small round cells with spheric nuclei and cytoplasm that stains poorly, forming a halo around the nucleus. The usual location is cerebral. Seizures are uncommon, and generalized or focal symptoms may be present for a long time before the mass of the tumor declares its presence by increased intracranial pressure.

Ependymoma and ependymoblastoma Although occasionally this tumor presents as a solitary mass in a cerebral hemisphere in adults, presumably arising from the ependymal wall of the lateral ventricle, its most distinctive form is a papillary growth filling the fourth ventricle of children. It is discussed further below.

The treatment of all forms of glioma of the cerebral hemispheres is partial excision, if feasible, after surgical biopsy. Opinion is divided as to whether x-ray treatment is beneficial; probably it is. In many cases the diagnosis of glioblastoma multiforme can now be made from clinical, arteriographic, radioactive isotope, and EEG, and one is justified, at least in some cases, in withholding surgery and giving radiation therapy. The control of intracranial pressure is maintained by the use of dexamethasone, 6 to 8 mg every 6 hr, while radiation therapy is being given and in lesser dose thereafter. The value of antitumor drugs is unproven.

Meningioma (arachnoidal fibroblastoma or endothelioma) This is a benign tumor composed of specialized arachnoidal lining cells, arising usually in places where there are arachnoidal villi. Since these clusters of arachnoidal cells penetrate the dura in the vicinity of the venous sinuses, they often appear to originate from the dura itself, hence the old term *dural endothelioma.* Grossly the tumors are firm, gray-white, lobulated, bulbous, or plaquelike masses which indent or compress but do not invade brain tissue. Many of them are highly vascular. In size they are variable; those which have produced symptoms have attained a size of 3 to 4 cm or more. The cellular composition permits easy identification. The cells are of uniform type and have the peculiar disposition to encircle one another and to form characteristic whorls and psammoma bodies. The common sites of these tumors are the olfactory groove, tuberculum sellae, parasagittal region, Sylvian fissure, cerebellopontine angle, and spinal canal. Inasmuch as they lie on the surface of the brain in or next to the dura, changes in the skull are frequent. The skull may be eroded over the tumor, and the diploic vessels, which provide part of the blood supply of the tumor, dilate and are usually prominent in an x-ray. Or the tumor cells may invade the bone and stimulate osteoblastic activity, as a consequence of which a bony bulge may be seen and felt, or an endostosis is visualized on the inner table of the skull in an x-ray. The meningioma must be listed with bone-metastasizing carcinoma and the true cholesteatoma of the skull as the three tumors most likely to cause a visible cranial boss in relation to cerebral symptoms (*benign, exotoses are neurologically asymptomatic*). Offering a broad vascular meningeal surface as they do, these tumors often elevate the protein level of the cerebrospinal fluid. Their striking vascularity accounts for a characteristic "blush" seen in arteriograms; the excessive permeability of the vessels, as well as the superficial location of the tumors, makes them ideal subjects for localization with radioactive isotopes. The displacement without invasion of cerebral tissue probably explains the interruption locally of normal alpha frequencies in the electroencephalogram with sharp waves or theta waves, in contrast to the delta waves so often found in infiltrative gliomas. Multiple meningiomas may occur, particularly in cases of neurofibromatosis.

These tumors may be found at any age but are more frequent in advanced years, especially in women.

Reticulum cell sarcoma This tumor may be primary in the brain (microglioblastoma) and present a clinical picture nearly identical to that of glioblastoma multiforme. It is highly radiosensitive.

Metastatic carcinoma Of the secondary tumors of the brain only metastatic carcinoma will be discussed here because the other tumors that metastasize to the brain are decidedly rare. Carcinomas reach the brain by hematogenous spread. Probably 35 to 40 percent of them come from the lung, and approximately 15 percent each from the breast, gastrointestinal tract (usually colon or rectum), and kidney. Melanotic carcinoma of the skin, carcinoma of the stomach, gallbladder, liver, thyroid, testicle, uterus, ovary, etc., account for the remainder, no one of them usually being responsible for more than 3 or 4 percent of secondary tumors of the brain. Carcinoma of the prostate, esophagus, oropharynx, or skin (except for melanocarcinoma) rarely if ever is disseminated in the brain. In more than 75 percent of cases the metastases are multiple and are scattered through both the cerebrum and cerebellum, often near the surface and involving white matter, cortex, and meninges. The hypernephroma and thyroid carcinoma have a greater tendency to form solitary metastases than other tumors, and as with the chorioepithelioma and some lung tumors, the metastases are likely to be hemorrhagic. The tumor tissue generally has all the gross and microscopic features of any carcinomatous implant and excites rather little glial reaction but much edema.

The usual clinical picture in metastatic carcinoma of the brain does not differ from that of glioblastoma multiforme. However, a number of other rather striking clinical neurologic syndromes also occur. One that is particularly difficult to diagnose is a widespread *carcinomatous meningoencephalopathy* with headache, nervousness, depressed mood, trembling, mental confusion, and forgetfulness, the whole picture looking very much like that of general paresis. Carcinomatosis of the cerebellum with headache, dizziness, and ataxia, the ataxia being brought out only by having the patient walk, is another difficult condition to diagnose during life. Symptoms and signs referable to one or several cranial and spinal nerve roots may be combined with headache and confusion in widespread *carcinomatosis of the craniospinal meninges* (carcinomatous meningitis). Usually the cerebrospinal fluid contains a few white blood cells (lymphocytes) and an elevated protein level. Tumor cells can often be identified in Papanicolaou stains of cerebrospinal fluid sediment, and if many are present in the meninges, the sugar values may be subnormal, even as low as zero.

When the syndromes due to these several varieties of metastatic tumor are fully developed, diagnosis is relatively easy. If only headache and vomiting are present, a common error is to explain these symptoms on a psychologic basis. One should make a psychiatric diagnosis only if the patient has the standard symptoms of some mental illness. A lumbar puncture, a chest x-ray, sedimentation rate (increased in metastatic carcinoma but not glioblastoma), and other x-rays (gastrointestinal series, barium enema, and pyelograms if symptoms point to these organs) are advisable. The inflammatory neurologic syndromes which accompany carcinoma but which are not due to tumor invasion of the central nervous system, such as polyneuritis (especially with carcinoma of the lung), polymyositis, and spinocerebellar degeneration (ovarian and other carcinomas) may be the initial illness.

TUMORS OF INFECTIVE ORIGIN (GRANULOMAS AND PARASITIC CYSTS) Tuberculoma is much less frequent in the United States than it was 20 years ago, and gumma has become almost nonexistent. In fact a patient with serologic syphilis and a positive Wassermann reaction of the cerebrospinal fluid has a greater chance of having two diseases, a cerebral tumor and asymptomatic neurosyphilis, than a gumma. The tuberculoma may occur in any part of the brain, but in children it is more likely to develop in the posterior fossa, i.e., in the cerebellum or brainstem, than in the cerebrum. Often there are a small number of cells and an increased protein content in the cerebrospinal fluid because the lesion frequently lies contiguous to the meninges; it may at any time give rise to a tuberculous meningitis with typical cerebrospinal fluid formula (50 to 300 cells, increased amount of protein, decreased sugar content, and decreased chloride content).

In South America tuberculoma and gumma are much more frequent, and one can usually obtain clues as to their nature from similar disease in other parts of the body, especially the lungs, and characteristic changes in the cerebrospinal fluid (see Chap. 322). In addition, cysticercus cellulosae and hydatid cysts are common lesions and should always be suspected when seizures, increased intracranial pressure, or diffuse cerebral symptoms develop in the adult. X-rays of the skull and skeletal muscles (e.g., thigh) may reveal characteristic calcific deposits in cysticercosis. Torula and other fungous granulomas and *Schistosoma japonicum* infection may also present as space-occupying cerebral lesions.

PATIENTS WITH UNMISTAKABLE SIGNS OF INCREASED INTRACRANIAL PRESSURE WHEN FIRST SEEN A certain number of patients show all the characteristic symptoms and signs of increased intracranial pressure (periodic bifrontal and bioccipital headaches which awaken the patient during the night or are present upon awakening, vomiting that may or may not be expected and may or may not be projectile, mental torpor, unsteady gait, sphincteric incontinence, and papilledema) when first seen. The physician confronted with this clinical problem is forced to take immediate action, for the condition is potentially dangerous. A critical rise in intracranial hypertension may occur at any time and result in coma, respiratory arrest, and death. Admission to a hospital with a neurosurgical service is therefore usually urgent. Nevertheless all the medical aspects of the patient's problem should first be worked out.

Three questions demand immediate answers: (1) Does the patient have a space-occupying intracranial lesion? (2) Where in the cranial cavity is it situated? (3) What is its nature? With respect to the first question it is well to keep in mind that a number of medical conditions may simulate an intracranial growth that causes only the general symptoms of increased intracranial pressure. These are (1) "pseudotumor cerebri," (2) hypertensive encephalopathy, (3) chronic pulmonary disease with hypercapnia and hypoxia, (4) chronic meningitis or adhesive arachnoiditis and/or aqueductal stenosis, (5) thrombosis of cerebral veins and dural sinuses, (6) Addison's disease, hypoparathyroidism, (7) excessive vitamin A and chloromycetin therapy in children, and (8) withdrawal from corticosteroid therapy in children. Several of these conditions are discussed elsewhere in this book, and it is sufficient to mention them briefly; others have not been considered before and will be discussed in detail.

PSEUDOTUMOR SYNDROMES In the condition of *pseudotumor cerebri* (meningeal hydrops) the patient, more often than not a child or young woman, complains of headaches of some weeks' standing and when first examined is found to have papilledema or choked disk, with slightly constricted visual fields and enlarged blind spots. Except for a vague dizziness, diplopia due to a slight abducens weakness, or paresthesias of some part of the body, neurologic signs are conspicuously absent, and the patient appears remarkably "bright" and well. The cerebrospinal fluid is acellular with normal protein content, a ventriculogram shows small or normal-sized ventricles, and an arteriogram shows patency and normal position of arteries and veins, including the superior sagittal and lateral sinuses. With the use of corticosteroid drugs (dexamethasone, 6 to 12 mg every 6 hr) and daily, then biweekly, then weekly lumbar punctures to lower the cerebrospinal fluid pressure, most of the patients gradually recover over a period of weeks to months. Extremely high cerebrospinal fluid pressure with episodes of cloudy vision (obscurations) may herald the onset of blindness and require a right subtemporal decompression as an emergency measure. The cause of the condition is unknown.

Extreme hypertension (diastolic pressures of 120 mm or over), retinal arteriolar changes with hemorrhages and exudates in the periphery of the optic fundi, signs of renal disease, and headache, convulsions, confusion, stupor, or coma (due to multifocal ischemia and brain swelling) are the basis of the diagnosis of *hypertensive encephalopathy* (see Chap. 326). *Chronic emphysema or other lung disease*, with cyanosis, dyspnea, cough, signs of cor pulmonale with right-sided congestive heart failure, and secondary polycythemia, may be attended by bilateral papilledema, elevated cerebrospinal fluid pressure (small ventricles), high venous pressure, severe headache, drowsiness, stupor, or coma and a peculiar lapse in the posture of the outstretched limbs and other contracted skeletal muscles (flapping movements or asterixis similar to the flap in impending liver coma). The finding of an elevated P_{CO_2} and diminished arterial oxygen concentration substantiate the diagnosis (see Chap. 248). *Chronic meningitis or adhesive arachnoiditis* due to chronic fibrosing meningeal diseases such as syphilis, postspinal anesthesia arachnoiditis, and cryptogenic meningeal diseases may be attended by headache, papilledema, seizures, blindness, paraplegia, or quadriplegia. Other benign causes of adult hydrocephalus are aqueductal stenosis and the Arnold-Chiari malformation. The cerebrospinal fluid protein level may be normal or elevated, with or without a "dynamic block"; the lateral, third, and fourth ventricles are enlarged in the ventriculogram. Syphilis and the other chronic meningitides may also cause *aqueductal stenosis* owing to a proliferative gliotic ependymitis, with enlargement of the lateral and third ventricles (see Chap. 159). *Thrombosis of the jugular veins and of the lateral and posterior parts of the superior sagittal sinus* may result in increased intracranial pressure, with otherwise normal cerebrospinal fluid and usually small ventricles (see Chap. 329). No explanation can be given for the papilledema with headache, drowsiness, and confusion and elevated cerebrospinal fluid pressure observed in conjunction with *Addison's disease*, corticosteroid withdrawal, vitamin A overdosage, and also, in rare cases, hypoparathyroidism. The mechanism is not known; usually the ventricles are of normal size.

"TRUE" AND "FALSE" LOCALIZING SIGNS If the clinical findings permit the exclusion of the aforementioned conditions, there is reasonable certainty that the patient has an intracranial growth. The problem then is to search for signs that will localize the lesion. In doing this, several pitfalls must be avoided. One common source of error is to place undue reliance on a sign which proves to have no localizing value whatsoever. One should distrust any symptom or sign which develops late, after headache and increased intracranial pressure have been established, for it often turns out to be a false localizing sign. Under these circumstances drowsiness, slowness in response, inattentiveness, and emotional blunting can be found as often with cerebellar as with cerebral growths. Ataxia of gait, urinary incontinence, and psychomotor retardation may occur as part of a communicating hydrocephalus from any cause. Unilateral or bilateral abducens palsy is another common false localizing sign, and reference has already been made to the drooping eyelid, dilated pupil, ipsilateral hemiparesis and bilateral Babinski signs, and coma in temporal lobe herniation. Jacksonian and generalized seizures and ipsilateral or bilateral pyramidal signs may be observed in the advanced stages of a cerebellar tumor. Early and sometimes relatively slight focal signs that may be easily overlooked are sometimes the most reliable guides to the localization of the tumor. Examples are a mild weakness or stiffness and hyperreflexia of an arm and leg in a frontal tumor; ataxia of gait (but not of limbs) and head tilt in cerebellar tumors; paralysis of upward gaze with the Argyll Robertson pupillary phenomenon in pinealomas; pale optic disks and chiasmal field defects in craniopharyngiomas; and homonymous visual inattentiveness and sensory extinction (see Chaps. 20 and 21) in posterior cerebral tumors.

TUMORS WHICH TEND TO PRODUCE ELEVATED INTRACRANIAL PRESSURE WITHOUT CONSPICUOUS LOCALIZING SIGNS The tumors most likely to cause increased intracranial pressure with few or no focal or lateralizing signs are medulloblastoma, ependymoma of the fourth ventricle, hemangioblastoma, pinealoma, colloid cysts of the third ventricle, gliomas of tegmentum of the midbrain with blocking of the aqueduct, and craniopharyngioma. In addition, in some of the cerebral gliomas discussed above, particularly those of the corpus callosum and frontal lobes, increased intracranial pressure may precede focal cerebral signs.

Medulloblastoma This is a rapidly growing tumor which arises in the posterior part of the vermis of children and rarely in the cerebrum of adults. The tonsils of the cerebellum are forced down into the cervical spinal canal (cerebellar pressure cone) in fatal cases. Seedings of the tumor may be seen on the walls of the third and lateral ventricles, on the meningeal surfaces of the brain, and around the spinal cord. The tumor is solid, reddish gray in color, and poorly demarcated from the adjacent brain tissue. It is very cellular, and the cells are small, closely packed with little cytoplasm, many mitoses, and scant stroma, and have a tendency to form clusters or pseudorosettes. Bailey and Cushing introduced the name *medulloblastoma* in 1925. Although medulloblasts as such have not been described in the fetal or adult human brain and the cell type is not known for certain, the term is retained if for no other reason than its familiarity.

The clinical picture is distinctive. Typically, the patient becomes listless, vomits repeatedly, and has a morning headache. The first diagnosis which suggests itself may be gastrointestinal disease or abdominal migraine. Soon, however, a stumbling gait, frequent falls, and a squint lead to a neurologic examination and the discovery of papilledema. Ataxia of the limbs may be absent at all times. Decerebrate attacks (tonic cerebellar fits) may occur in the late stages of the disease. The tumor is highly radiosensitive, and surgery with x-ray treatment may prolong life for several years. Recent trials of intrathecal methotrexate and vincristine have yielded promising results in some cases.

Ependymoma and papilloma of the fourth ventricle This tumor also arises from the walls of the fourth ventricle, more often in children, and from lateral ventricles in adults. It is a soft, whitish-gray, lobulated growth composed of small cells arranged in the form of small rosettes around vessels or central clear areas and containing blepharoplasts in their cytoplasm. The clinical syndrome of the fourth ventricle tumor is much like that of the medulloblastoma except for the absence of ataxia of gait. The tumor is not very sensitive to x-ray, and surgical removal offers the only hope of survival. Prolongation of life is sometimes attained through ventriculoatrial shunting of cerebrospinal fluid (CSF). The papilloma or papillary adenocarcinoma of the choroid plexus of the fourth ventricle gives rise to a similar syndrome but tends to occur later in life.

Hemangioblastoma of the cerebellum The disease of Lindau is described in Chap. 334. Dizziness, ataxia of gait or of the limbs on one side, symptoms and signs of increased intracranial pressure, and in some instances a retinal angioma (von Hippel's disease) and polycythemia constitute the neurologic syndrome. Familial incidence is well known. Craniotomy with opening of the cerebellar cyst and excision of the mural hemangioblastomatous nodule may be curative.

Pinealoma This may be either a teratoma or a glioma of the pineal gland. The teratoma is a firm, discrete, noninvasive mass which usually reaches 3 to 4 cm in greatest diameter. It compresses the superior colliculi and sometimes the superior surface of the cerebellum, with narrowing of the aqueduct of Sylvius. Often it extends anteriorly into the third ventricle and may then compress the hypothalamus. Microscopically it is composed of large, spheric epithelial cells (much like those of a seminoma), separated by a network of reticular connective tissue which contains many lymphocytes. The gliomas have the usual morphologic characteristics of an astrocytoma of varying degrees of malignancy. Children, adolescents, and young adults, either male or female, may be affected. In some cases the clinical syndrome consists solely of symptoms and signs of increased intracranial pressure, and the diagnosis can be made only by a ventriculogram which reveals the tumor. The most characteristic localizing sign, an inability to look upward (Parinaud's syndrome) and slightly dilated pupils which react on accommodation but not to light is related to hydrocephalus and not to the local pressure effects of the tumor. Sometimes an ataxia of the limbs, choreic movements, or spastic weakness appears in the later stages of the illness. A Torkildsen ventriculocisterna magna shunt of cerebrospinal fluid and x-ray therapy have been remarkably successful in controlling the symptoms. Attempts at surgical removal of the tumor have seldom been successful (see also Chap. 94).

Colloid (paraphyseal) cyst of the third ventricle This is a papillomatous structure always situated in the anterior extremity of the third ventricle between the interventricular foramens and attached to the roof of the ventricle. Usually it is about a centimeter in diameter, is oval or round with a smooth external surface, and is filled with a glairy colloid material. The wall is composed of a layer of epithelial cells surrounded by a capsule of fibrous connective tissue. These benign cysts may exist for long periods of time; they produce neurologic symptoms by blocking the third ventricle and causing an obstructive hydrocephalus. This tumor should be suspected when the following clinical syndromes are found: dementia with or without headache, intermittent severe bifrontal-bioccipital headaches, sometimes modified by posture (ball valve obstruction of the third ventricle), crises of headache with obtundation, "frontal lobe" incontinence, unsteadiness of gait, bilateral paresthesias, dim vision, and weakness of legs with sudden falls. The treatment is surgical excision, but recently, satisfactory results have been obtained by ventriculoatrial shunt of CSF, leaving the benign growth untouched.

Craniopharyngioma (suprasellar or Rathke's pouch cyst, hypophyseal duct tumors, adamantinomas, ameloblastomas) This is a benign congenital or "rest cell" tumor. By the time it has grown to a diameter of 3 to 4 cm, it is almost always cystic. Usually it lies above the sella turcica, depressing the optic chiasma and extending up into the third ventricle. Less often it is subdiaphragmatic, i.e., within the sella, where it compresses the pituitary body, erodes one part of the wall of the sella or a clinoid process, but seldom balloons the sella like a pituitary adenoma. The tumor is oval, round, or lobulated and has a smooth surface. The wall of the cyst and the solid parts of the tumor consist of cords and whorls of epithelial cells (often with intercellular bridges and keratohyalin), separated by a loose network of stellate cells. The cyst contains dark albuminous fluid and cholesterol crystals. Calcium deposits are found in nearly all of them and can be seen in plain x-rays of the suprasellar region in about 40 percent of cases. The sella beneath the tumor tends to be flattened and enlarged. In children, adiposity, delayed or infantile physical and sexual development (Froehlich's or Lorain syndrome—see Chaps. 83 and 84), headaches, vomiting, dim vision with chiasmal field defects (see Chap. 20), optic atrophy, or papilledema comprise the clinical picture. In adults, waning libido, amenorrhea, slight spastic weakness of the legs, headache without papilledema, and mental dullness and confusion are often found. Later drowsiness, diabetes insipidus, and disturbances of temperature regulation may occur, indicating hypothalamic involvement.

In the differential diagnosis of these several tumor syndromes a careful clinical analysis is often more important than laboratory procedures. Arteriography and electroencephalography are not as helpful as in cerebral tumors. The tests which, though somewhat hazardous, are likely to give the most useful information are the air ventriculogram or a combined ventriculogram-pneumoencephalogram and the Pantopaque ventriculogram (injection of radiopaque fluid). Modern neurosurgical techniques reinforced by corticosteroid therapy before and after surgery and careful control of temperature and water balance postoperatively permit complete excision of the tumor in the majority of cases.

In certain marginal states of hydrocephalus benefit may accrue from the administration of acetazolamide (Diamox) in doses of 250 mg three or four times a day but surgical shunting of CSF has given the best results.

PATIENTS WITH SYMPTOMS AND SIGNS OF A SLOWLY PROGRESSIVE LESION IN A PARTICULAR REGION OF THE CRANIAL CAVITY In this group of conditions general cerebral symptoms and the signs of increased intracranial pressure occur late or not at all. The physician arrives at the correct diagnosis by being able to make an anatomic or regional diagnosis from a set of neurologic findings and by reasoning that the etiology must be neoplastic because of the slowly progressive nature of the illness. Special x-rays of the skull, cerebrospinal fluid examination, and, depending on the location of the disease, either pneumoencephalography or arteriography will usually confirm the clinical impression.

The following tumors produce unique syndromes usually diagnostic of a special type of tumor.

Acoustic neurofibroma or neurinoma This slowly growing benign tumor may occur as a solitary lesion or as a part of the syndrome of neurofibromatosis. By the time of operation the tumor has usually attained a size of 4 to 6 cm in diameter. It arises from the extramedullary part of the eighth cranial nerve, usually within the internal auditory meatus, where the intracranial part of the nerve first acquires the histologic character of a peripheral nerve, i.e., has Schwann cells and fibroblasts. The space in which it lies is the cerebellopontine angle, i.e., between the cerebellum, pons, and medulla posteriorly, the petrous pyramid anteriorly, and the tentorium above. The internal auditory meatus is usually enlarged (visible in x-rays), the middle cerebellar peduncle and the anterolateral part of the cerebellum are depressed, and the trigeminal, facial, glossopharyngeal, and vagus nerves are displaced and stretched over the surface of the growth. The fourth ventricle is deformed, displaced, and narrowed (visible in a pneumoencephalogram), and there is hydrocephalic enlargement of the aqueduct and of the third and lateral ventricle in the late stages. The tumor is vascular, and the surrounding cerebrospinal fluid has a high protein content (cerebrospinal fluid protein of 300 mg per 100 ml or over is not infrequent). The microscopic picture is that of a typical neurofibroma (axis cylinders mixed with masses of fibrous connective tissue in interlacing strands, palisaded nuclei, and mononuclear giant cells without mitoses).

The typical clinical syndrome, which usually occurs in adult men or women, consists of tinnitus, deafness, and rotational vertigo (seldom in discrete attacks as in Ménière's syndrome, Chap. 324) of several years' standing, followed by postauricular or suboccipital pain, disturbance in balance, spasms and twitching or slight weakness of the face, paresthesias in the face or facial weakness, dysophonia and dysphagia, and homolateral cerebellar ataxia of the arm and leg. Headache, vomiting, and choked disk are late findings. Variations of this syndrome are numerous. Early in its development only progressive deafness, tinnitus, and vague vertigo may be present, and the abnormal audiogram, impaired vestibular function, elevated cerebrospinal fluid protein level, widened internal auditory meatus, and obliteration of the lateral recess of the fourth ventricle in a pneumoencephalogram must be depended upon for diagnosis. Tomography and positive contrast encephalography improve diagnostic accuracy. Dementia may later be the presenting syndrome, and the deaf ear may be attributed to some other disease. Unilateral cerebellar ataxia and dizziness may predominate, and definite signs of involvement of the fifth, seventh, and eighth cranial nerves may not be found. The only treatment is surgical excision. Combined translabyrinthine and intracranial approach permits total removal in more than two-thirds of all cases.

The *neurinoma* of the *trigeminal* or *gasserian ganglion* and *meningioma* of the *cerebellopontine angle* may be indistinguishable from an acoustic neurinoma. They should always be considered if early tinnitus, deafness, and an unresponsive labyrinth ("dead labyrinth") are not the initial symptoms of the cerebellopontine angle syndrome. A true *cholesteatoma* of *the temporal bone* may simulate this clinical picture, but usually the facial weakness is early and severe, the ear is deaf, and labyrinthine function is absent, whereas the other cranial nerve signs, cerebellar ataxia, and increased intracranial pressure are absent. The *tumor* of *the glomus jugulare* (a flat ovoid body, found in the adventitia of the jugular bulb, immediately below the floor of the middle ear and near the ramus tympanicus of the ninth cranial nerve) may, like the acoustic neurofibroma, basal meningioma, metastatic cancer, syphilitic meningitis, neurofibroma of other cranial nerves, and vascular malformation, cause unilateral lower cranial nerve palsies (see Chap. 324). It is a purplish-red, highly vascular tumor composed of large epithelioid cells in an alveolar pattern and an abundant capillary network. Partial deafness, facial palsy, dysphagia, and unilateral atrophy of the tongue, combined with a vascular polyp in the auditory meatus and a palpable mass below and anterior to the mastoid eminence, often with a bruit, compose the syndrome. The jugular foramen is eroded (visible by x-ray), and the level of cerebrospinal fluid protein may be elevated. Women are affected more than men, and the peak incidence is during middle adult life. The tumor grows slowly over a period of many years, sometimes 10 or more. The treatment is x-ray radiation. Surgical excision has usually been unsuccessful.

Pituitary adenomas These tumors, which are so common, particularly in late adult life, often are discovered when a patient begins to complain of a visual disturbance. A partial or complete bitemporal hemianopsia progressing to blindness, with optic atrophy, is the usual finding and with x-ray evidence of an expanded sella turcica and endocrine disorder leads to a diagnosis of pituitary adenoma. As the growth enlarges and extends laterally, an oculomotor palsy is occasionally seen, and large suprasellar extensions may involve the hypothalamus or temporal lobe. If there are signs of acromegaly, one may assume that an eosinophilic adenoma is present; if not, and signs of pituitary insufficiency are present (amenorrhea without "hot flashes," sexual impotence, etc.—see Chap. 83), the tumor is usually a chromophobe adenoma. Basophilic adenomas, one of the causes of Cushing's syndrome, rarely produce enlargement of the sella or visual symptoms. The diagnosis is made from the endocrine picture (see Chap. 83). The cerebrospinal fluid is usually under normal pressure, and protein level is elevated only in exceptional cases.

Other conditions may rarely expand the sella (craniopharyngioma, carotid aneurysm, cysts of pituitary, and "the hollow sella syndrome"), and there are also rather wide normal variations in its size. The empty or hollow sella results from a defect in the dural diaphragm of the sella and nontumorous enlargement. Raised intracranial pressure may cause the floor of the third ventricle to protrude into the sella. Downward herniation of the optic chiasma may cause visual disturbances simulating a pituitary adenoma. This syndrome may follow surgical excision of a pituitary adenoma or pituitary apoplexy. Hence the diagnosis of pituitary adenoma should not be made because of minor enlargements of the sella in the absence of endocrine and neighborhood neurologic signs. A pneumoencephalogram permits visualization of the suprasellar extension of the tumor or an empty sella. Treatment of the adenoma is x-ray radiation; if vision is threatened despite x-ray therapy, ablation by the proton beam or either transnasal or transfrontal surgical excision is indicated. Replacement endocrine therapy is also needed.

Meningioma of the sphenoid ridge This tumor is situated over the lesser wing of the sphenoidal bone. As it increases in size, it may expand medially to encroach on structures in the wall of the cavernous sinus, anteriorly to invade the orbit, or laterally to erode or invade the temporal bone. Most prominent among the symptoms are a slowly developing unilateral exophthalmos, slight bulging of the bone in the temporal region, and roentgenologic evidence of thickening or erosion of the lesser wing of the sphenoid bone. Variants of the clinical syndrome include oculomotor palsy or syndrome of Foix (see Chap. 324), blindness in one eye with optic atrophy, anosmia (and sometimes the Kennedy syndrome—see below), mental changes, uncinate fits, and increased intracranial pressure. Sarcomas arising from the skull bones, metastatic carcinoma, orbitoethmoidal osteoma, tumors of the optic nerve, and angiomas of the orbit must be considered in the differential diagnosis. Auscultation of the skull, x-ray of the skull, and carotid arteriography are helpful in differentiating these lesions.

Meningioma of the olfactory groove This tumor is a growth derived from arachnoidal cells along the cribriform plate. The diagnosis depends on the finding of ipsilateral or bilateral anosmia, ipsilateral or bilateral blindness, often with optic atrophy on one side and papilledema without atrophy on the other (Kennedy syndrome), and mental changes. The tumors may reach enormous size before coming to the attention of the physician. The anosmia, if unilateral, is rarely if ever reported by the patient. The unilateral visual disturbance may consist of a slowly developing unilateral central scotoma. Confusion, forgetfulness, inappropriate jocularity (witzelsucht) are the usual psychic disturbances, cf. Chap. 29. The patient is indifferent to or jokes about blindness. Usually there are x-ray changes along the cribriform plate and an extremely high cerebrospinal fluid protein level (200 to 400 mg per 100 ml).

Glioma of the brainstem Astrocytomas of the brainstem (formerly called *bipolar spongioblastomas*) are slow-growing, firm, white infiltrating growths which insinuate themselves between tracts and nuclei. They produce a variable clinical picture, depending on their exact location in the medulla, pons, and midbrain (see Chaps. 19 and 20 for syndromes). The characteristic features, in the early stages, are signs of crossed motor or sensory disturbances, which always indicate brainstem disease. Headache, vomiting, and papilledema occur late. The course is slowly progressive over years unless some part of the tumor becomes more malignant (glioblastoma multiforme), in which instance the illness may terminate fatally within months. The main clinical problem is to differentiate between this disease, multiple sclerosis, and vascular malformations of the pons. Pneumoencephalography to visualize the fourth ventricle and aqueduct and occasionally vertebral arteriography are helpful in diagnosis. The treatment is x-ray radiation and, if intracranial pressure is increased, a Torkildsen ventriculocisterna magna shunt.

Glioma of the optic nerves and chiasma This tumor is often found in patients with von Recklinghausen's disease and, like the glioma of the brainstem, arises most frequently during the period of childhood and adolescence. The initial symptoms are dimness of vision with constricted fields, bizarre bilateral field defects of homonymous, heteronymous, sometimes bitemporal type, blindness, and optic atrophy with or without papilledema. Hypothalamic signs (infantilism, adiposity, polyuria, somnolence, and genital atrophy) are common. X-rays reveal an enlargement of the optic foramen. With this finding and the lack of ballooning of the sella or suprasellar calcification, pituitary adenoma, Hand-Schüller-Christian disease, and craniopharyngioma can be excluded. The treatment is surgical excision or x-ray, depending on the exact location. Nontumorous gliotic lesions of optic nerves may occur in von Recklinghausen's disease and be difficult to distinguish from tumors.

Chordoma This is a soft, jellylike gray-pink growth composed of cords or masses of large cells with granules of glycogen in their cytoplasm and often multiple nuclei and intercellular mucoid material. They are locally invasive but do not metastasize. Any part of the vertebral column or the base of the cranium are the most common sites, especially the base of the skull (from physaliphora ecchondrosis) or the lumbosacral region (giving rise to a cauda equina syndrome). Those in the base of the skull create a remarkable clinical picture in which all or any combination of cranial nerve palsies from the second to twelfth on one side or both sides are combined with a retropharyngeal mass and erosion of the clivus of sphenoid bone and the occiput. It is one of the lesions that may present both as an intracranial and as an extracranial mass. The others are the meningioma, neurofibroma, glomus jugulare tumor, carcinoma of sinuses or pharynx, and midline granuloma. The treatment is x-ray therapy.

Nasopharyngeal growths which erode the base of the skull These are rather common in a general hospital and arise from the mucous membrane of the paranasal sinuses or the nasopharynx near the eustachian tube, i.e, the fossa of Rosenmueller (*transitional cell carcinoma*, *Schmincke tumor*). In addition to symptoms of nasopharyngeal or sinus disease, which may not be prominent, facial pain and numbness (trigeminal), abducens palsy (sixth cranial nerve), and other cranial nerve palsies may occur. Diagnosis depends on inspection and biopsy of a nasopharyngeal mass, biopsy of an involved cervical gland, and x-ray evidence of erosion of the base of the skull. The treatment is x-ray therapy. Carcinoma of ethmoid or sphenoid sinuses may produce a similar clinical picture.

Prognosis The prognosis of intracranial tumor is influenced by the nature of the growth, its location, and other factors. As a general rule, unless an operation is performed, almost all intracranial tumors end fatally. Death in most instances is preceded by a critical rise in intracranial pressure and tentorial or foramen magnum herniation. The more malignant tumors, such as the glioblastoma multiforme, medulloblastoma, and metastatic carcinoma, end fatally within a year, as a rule, whereas the slowly growing meningiomas and astrocytomas often permit survival for many years.

The prospects for recovery after surgery depend largely on the type of tumor. With meningiomas and acoustic neurofibromas, if completely excised, there may be a complete cure. In gliomas the outlook is more bleak. Cure is rare, for seldom can complete excision be accomplished. Nevertheless with the slow-growing gliomas, partial excision, the marsupialization of a cyst, and the relief of increased intracranial pressure by long-term corticosteroid therapy may lead to improvement and resumption of a useful life for many years. With metastatic growth the outlook is dismal, though if there are no metastases in other organs and the cerebral deposit appears to be solitary, operation has occasionally resulted in temporary recovery for a few months or a year or two.

Conclusions The physician's responsibilities in this field of intracranial tumors are (1) diagnosis—he must separate the tumor cases from all the others which pass through his hands; (2) exclusion of the possibility that the intracranial mass is part of a general disease which would contraindicate surgery, i.e., metastatic carcinoma, syphilis, tuberculosis, parasitic infection, etc.; (3) exclusion of the several pseudotumor syndromes; (4) maintenance of the patient in the best possible condition, until surgery can be undertaken (fluids, electrolytes, corticosteroid therapy, etc.); (5) assisting the surgeon in the postoperative medical management.

(For tumors of spinal cord and nerves, see Chaps. 323 to 325.)

REFERENCES

Bailey P: *Intracranial Tumors*, 2d ed., Springfield, Ill.: Charles C Thomas, 1948

Lumsden CE: Study of tumors by tissue culture, in *Pathology of Tumors of the Nervous System*, 3d ed., eds DS Russell, LJ Rubenstein, Baltimore: Williams & Wilkins, 1971

Milhorat TH: *Hydrocephalus and the Cerebrospinal Fluid*, Baltimore: Williams & Wilkins, 1972

Ojemann RG, Montgomery WW: Evaluation and surgical treament of acoustic neuroma. N Engl J Med 287:895, 1972

329 PYOGENIC INFECTIONS OF THE CENTRAL NERVOUS SYSTEM

RAYMOND D. ADAMS
ROBERT G. PETERSDORF

All pyogenic infections of the cranial contents originate in one of two ways, by hematogenous spread (emboli of bacteria or infected thrombi) or by extension from surface structures (ears, paranasal sinuses, osteomyelitic foci in the skull, penetrating cranial injuries, or congenital sinus tracts).

Concerning the hematogenesis pathway surprisingly little is known, for human autopsy material seldom divulges information on this point and animal experiments involving the injection of virulent bacteria into the bloodstream have yielded somewhat contradictory results. In most instances of bacteremia or septicemia the nervous system seems not to be infected, yet in certain cases of pneumonia bacteremia is the only apparent forerunner of meningitis. In chronic pulmonary diseases septic emboli have been seen in veins in the lung and as emboli in the brain, and in acute and subacute bacterial endocarditis bacterial emboli are found in cerebral and meningeal arteries. The ideal sites of lodgment of these emboli for the production of meningitis, whether in choroid plexuses or in meningeal or superficial cerebral vessels, have not been ascertained.

With respect to the formation of brain abscess, the experimental data inform us that the cerebral tissues are resistant to infection. Direct injection of virulent bacteria into the brain of an animal seldom results in abscess formation. In fact, this condition has been successfully produced only by injecting the culture medium with the bacteria or by first causing necrosis of the tissue and then inoculating it with bacteria. In human beings infarction of brain tissue by arterial occlusion (embolism) or venous occlusion (thrombophlebitis) appears to be the common and perhaps necessary antecedent.

The cranial epidural and subdural spaces evidently are noticeably inaccessible to bloodborne infective agents in contrast to the spinal epidural space, where this happens not infrequently. Furthermore, the cranial bones and the dura mater, which serves essentially as the inner periosteum of the skull, protect the cranial cavity against the ingress of bacteria. This protective mechanism may fail if suppuration occurs in the middle ear, mastoid cells or frontal ethmoid, and sphenoid sinuses. Two pathways have been demonstrated in postmortem material.

1 Infected thrombi may form in diploic veins and spread along these vessels into the dural sinuses (into which they flow) and from there in retrograde fashion along the meningeal veins in the brain.

2 An osteomyelitic focus may form, with erosion of the inner table of bone and invasion of the dura, subdural space, piarachnoid, and even the brain substance. Each of these pathways may be visualized in some fatal cases of epidural abscess, subdural empyema, leptomeningitis, cranial venous sinusitis and meningeal thrombophlebitis, and brain abscess. However, in many cases coming to autopsy one cannot determine the pathway.

Hematogenous infections during bacteremias usually permit a single type of virulent organism to gain entry to the cranial cavity (meningococcus, pneumococcus, influenza bacillus, staphylococcus, or streptococcus). In contrast, septic cerebral emboli from chronic lung infections, in congenital heart disease and thrombotic or direct extensions from ear or sinus infections the whole bacterial flora common to these organs may be transmitted. In such infections multiple types of organisms, e.g., staphylococcus, fusiform bacillus, oral spirochetal organisms, resulting in "mixed infections," offer rather more complex problems in therapy. Not infrequently, in these latter conditions when active suppuration has occurred, the demonstration of the causative organism, even from the pus of an abscess, may be unsuccessful.

BACTERIAL MENINGITIS (LEPTOMENINGITIS)

This condition consists essentially of an inflammation of the piarachnoid and the fluid residing in the space which it encloses and also that in the ventricles of the brain. Since the subarachnoid space is continuous around the brain and spinal cord and the optic nerves, an infective agent (or tumor cells or blood) gaining entry to any one part of it may extend immediately to all of it, even its most remote recesses; viz., meningitis is always *cerebrospinal.* It also reaches the ventricles, either directly or by reflux through the basal foramens of Magendie and Luschka.

The effect of bacteria or other organisms in the subarachnoid space is to cause an inflammatory reaction in the pia and arachnoid and in the cerebrospinal fluid (CSF); in the pyogenic forms, pus accumulates in this space. The infective agent or its toxin, if allowed sufficient time to act, injures those structures which lie within the subarachnoid space (cranial and spinal roots) or ventricles (choroid plexuses) and adjacent to it (pial arteries and veins, underlying cerebral and cerebellar cortices, subpial white matter of the spinal cord, peripheral fibers of optic nerves, ependymal and subependymal tissues). In addition purulent material may interfere with the flow of CSF from the ventricles or along the subarachnoid space over the brainstem, with resulting obstructive or communicating hydrocephalus, respectively. Although the outer arachnoidal membrane proves to be a remarkably effective barrier to the extension of infection, nevertheless some reaction in the cranial subdural space and even the inner surface of the dura and spinal epidural space may occur. This happens more often in infants (subdural effusions) than in adults.

The most immediate clinical effects of acute subarachnoid suppuration, distinguishing it from infections in other parts of the body, are severe headache, generalized convulsions, and a disorder of consciousness (i.e., drowsiness, stupor, or coma). The one clinical sign of importance is stiffness of the neck (resistance to passive movement) on forward bending. The Kernig and Brudzinski's signs are of the same nature but less reliable. The basis of these symptoms and signs is explained below. Any circumstance which prolongs the meningitis should increase the risk of injury to all the enumerated structures; this fact accounts for many features of the clinical picture in the subacute and chronic varieties of meningeal infection. The potential pathologic-clinical relations of acute, subacute, and chronic meningitis are summarized in Table 329-1.

TYPES OF BACTERIAL MENINGITIS Eighty to ninety percent of cases of bacterial meningitis are caused by *Hemophilus* influenza (Chap. 137), *Neisseria* meningitis (Chap. 131), and *Diplococcus pneumoniae* (Chap. 128). The remaining 15 to 20 percent are composed of *Staphylococcus aureus* and group A streptococci, usually in association with brain abscess, epidural abscess, head trauma, neurosurgical procedures, or cranial thrombophlebitis; *Escherichia coli* (in newborns) and the other *Enterobacteriaceae* such as *Klebsiella enterobacter, Proteus,* and citrobacter; and *Pseudomonas* which is usually a consequence of lumbar puncture, spinal anesthesia, or shunting procedures to relieve hydrocephalus. Rare meningeal pathogens include *Salmonella, Shigella, Clostridium perfrigens,* and *N. gonorrhea.* Two unusual ones are *Listeria monocystogenes,* which is easily confused with diptheroids, and *Mima-polymorphia,* which may be difficult to distinguish from *Hemophilus* and *Neisseria.*

EPIDEMIOLOGY Pneumococcal, *H. influenza,* and meningococcal meningitis have a worldwide distribution tending to occur primarily in males during the fall, winter, and spring. Each has a relatively constant seasonal incidence, although epidemics of meningococcal meningitis appear to follow roughly a 10-year cycle. *Hemophilus* influenza meningitis is encountered almost exclusively in children between two months and seven years of age. Meningococcal meningitis occurs most often in children and adolescents, but is also encountered throughout much of adult life with a sharp decline in incidence after the age of fifty. Pneumococcal meningitis predominates in the very young and in adults over forty years of age.

PATHOGENESIS The three common meningeal pathogens are invasive and depend upon antiphagocytic capsular or surface antigens for survival in the tissues of the infected host; all express their pathogenicity largely in the form of extracellular proliferation. All three are inhabitants of the nasopharynx in a significant part of the population. It is evident from the frequency with which the carrier state is detected that nasal colonization is not a sufficient explanation of infection of the meninges. The factors which predispose the colonized patient to bloodstream invasion, which is the usual route by which bacteria reach the meninges, are obscure but include antecedent viral infections of the upper respiratory passages or, as in the case of the pneumococcus, infections in the lung. Once bloodborne, the factors which lead to meningeal localization of bacteria are unknown, but it has been postulated that pneumococci, *H. influenzae,* and meningococci possess a unique predilection for the meninges. Other hypothetic possibilities are that the entry of bacteria into the subarachnoid space is facilitated by disruption of the blood-CSF barrier by trauma, circulating endotoxin, or an initial viral infection of the meninges.

Avenues other than the bloodstream by which bacteria can gain access to the meninges include congenital neuroectodermal defects, craniotomy sites, diseases of the middle ear and paranasal sinuses, and severe cranial trauma, notably skull fractures. Occasionally brain abscesses may rupture into the subarachnoid space or ventricles, thus infecting the meninges. The isolation of anaerobic streptococci, *Bacteroides* sp. or *Actinomyces*, or a mixture of microorganisms in the CSF should suggest the possibility of a brain abscess occurring in conjunction with meningitis.

In most patients the precise route by which bacteria infect the meninges cannot be determined.

SYMPTOMATOLOGY The aforementioned symptoms of fever, headache, seizures, impairment of consciousness, and stiff neck and back, which compose the meningitic syndrome, are common to each of the three main types of bacterial meningitis. Diagnosis may offer difficulty only when the initial symptoms are pain in the neck or abdomen, or a confusional psychosis or delirious reaction.

There are certain special clinical features that correlate with particular types of meningitis. Meningococcus meningitis should always be suspected in epidemics of meningitis, when the evolution is extremely rapid, when the onset is attended by a morbiliform, petechial, or purpuric skin eruption and larger echymoses and lividity of skin of lower parts of the body, and if circulatory collapse has occurred. Since a rash accompanies approximately 50 percent of meningococcus infections, its presence should dictate immediate institution of therapy for a Neisserian infection, even though similar rashes may be observed with echo 9 meningitis, *Mima-polymorphia*, and rarely staphyloccus, *H. influenzae*, and streptococcal meningitis. Pneumococcus meningitis is usually preceded by an infection in the lungs, ears, and sinuses, and the heart valves may be affected. In addition a pneumococcus etiology should be suspected in patients suffering from alcoholism, sickle-cell disease, and basal skull fracture, and following splenectomy. *Hemophilus influenzae* meningitis usually follows upper respiratory and ear infections in the small child.

TABLE 329-1

Pathologic-clinical relations of acute, subacute, and chronic meningitis

I In acute meningitis

A Pure piarachnoiditis; headache, stiff neck, and Kernig and Brudzinski's signs. These signs depend on activation of protective, flexor reflexes which shorten the spine and immobilize it (extension of neck and flexion of hips and knees reduce stretch on inflamed spinal structures; all the clinical signs of meningitis, it will be noted, involve maneuvers which oppose these postural reflexes).

B Subpial toxic encephalopathy—the tissue beneath the pia is not penetrated by bacteria; hence the change must be toxic: confusion, stupor, coma, and convulsions are related to this lesion, though cerebral infarction due to cortical vein thrombosis may underlie this syndrome in some cases.

C Inflammatory or vascular involvement of cranial nerve roots: ocular palsies, facial weakness (exception is direct involvement of eighth nerve and cochlea with ear infections, or antimicrobial agents). Note: Deafness may be due either to middle ear infection or to extension of meningeal infection to the inner ear.

D Thrombosis of meningeal veins: focal convulsions, focal cerebral defects such as hemiparesis, aphasia (rarely prominent), etc., which may appear during the first days but more often after the first week or two of meningeal infection.

E Ependymitis, choroidal plexitis; it is doubtful if there are any recognizable clinical effects aside from those of the associated hydrocephalus.

II In more subacute and chronic forms of meningitis

A Obstructive or communicating hydrocephalus, due at first to purulent exudate around the base of the brain, later to meningeal fibrosis and rarely to aqueductal stenosis: variable degrees of impairment of consciousness, decorticate postures (arms flexed, legs extended), grasp and sucking reflexes, and sphincteric incontinence. Later, enlarging head, inability to look upward (eyes turn down and lids retract on effort to look up: sunset sign) in a child. In the mildest form only psychomotor retardation, unsteadiness of gait, and incontinence occur. Cerebrospinal fluid pressure in adults may at first be elevated; as the ventricles enlarge and the plexuses are compressed, it may fall within limits of normal (low-pressure hydrocephalus).

B Subdural effusion and empyema with sterile and infected effusions; impaired alertness, refusal to eat and vomiting, immobility, bulging fontanels, and persistence of fever despite clearing of CSF. In infants the effusion causes an exaggerated transillumination. With subdural empyema: fever is more pronounced, CSF is under increased pressure, and there are one-sided convulsions, hemiplegia, etc. (If fever is present but CSF pressure is normal and one-sided cerebral signs are clearly in evidence, thrombophlebitis is the leading possibility.)

C Extensive venous or arterial infarction: unilateral or bilateral hemiplegia, decorticate or decerebrate rigidity, cortical blindness, stupor or coma with or without seizures.

III Late effects or sequelae

A Meningeal fibrosis around optic nerves, or spinal cord and roots: blindness and optic atrophy, spastic paraparesis with sensory loss in the lower segments of the body, respectively (spinal arachnoiditis and meningomyelitis).

B Severe cerebral damage: dementia, stupor or coma, and paralysis, chronic meningoencephalitis with hydrocephalus (general paresis of the insane). If lumbosacral posterior roots are chronically damaged, tabes dorsalis.

C Persistent hydrocephalus in the child: with blindness, arrest of all mental activity, bilateral spastic hemiplegia.

Other specific bacterial etiologies are suggested by certain unusual clinical settings. Furunculosis or the occurrence of a recent neurosurgical procedure should raise the possibility of coagulase-positive staphylococcal meningitis. Ventriculovenous shunts inserted for control of hydrocephalus are particularly prone to infection with coagulase-negative staphylococci. Brain abscess, myelo- or lymphoproliferative disorders, defects in cranial bones (tumor, osteomyelitis), collagen diseases, metastatic cancer, and therapy with immunosuppressive agents are clinical conditions which favor the invasion of the craniospinal cavities by such pathogens as *Enterobacteriaceae*, *Listeria*, *Mima-Herellea*, and *Pseudomonas*.

SPECIAL PHYSICAL FINDINGS IN TYPES OF BACTERIAL MENINGITIS The signs of meningeal irritation—stiff neck or positive Kernig and Brudzinski's signs—may be absent in the very young, the very old, or the severely obtunded. Signs of focal cerebral disease, as mentioned above, although seldom prominent, are more frequent in pneumococcal and influenzal meningitis. Seizures are encountered most often in infants with *H. influenzae* meningitis, but it is difficult to ascertain their significance since persons of this age may convulse with fevers of any cause. Some of the more transitory focal cerebral signs may represent postictal phenomena (Todd's paralysis), whereas stable, local, cerebral lesions are consequent to vasculitis, occlusion of cerebral veins, and infarction of cerebral tissue. Cranial nerve abnormalities are particularly frequent with pneumococcal meningitis, being due to invasion of the nerve by the infective agent as it traverses the subarachnoid space.

LABORATORY FINDINGS Pleocytosis of the *cerebrospinal fluid* is diagnostic. The number of leukocytes in the CSF ranges between 1 and 100,000 per μl but averages 5 to 20,000. Cell counts above 50,000 raise suspicion of the possibility of a brain abscess having ruptured into the ventricle (ventricular empyema). Neutrophilic leukocytes generally predominate, but an increasing proportion of mononuclear cells are found in the exudate as the infection continues, especially in partially treated meningitis. In the early stages careful cytologic examination may disclose that some of the mononuclear cells are myelocytes or young neutrophils. Later as treatment takes effect, the proportions of lymphocytes, plasma cells, and histiocytes steadily increase.

The pressure of the *cerebrospinal fluid* is so consistently elevated (above 180 mm water) that a normal or low pressure on the initial lumbar puncture in a case of suspected bacterial meningitis should raise the possibility that the needle was partially occluded or the spinal arachnoid space was blocked.

The *protein levels* of CSF are higher than 45 mg per 100 ml in 90 percent of cases, and most determinations fall in the range of 100 to 500 mg per 100 ml.

The sugar concentration of CSF is depressed, usually to a level lower than 40 mg per 100 ml, or less than 40 percent of the blood sugar concentration (measured concomitantly), provided the latter is less than 250 mg per 100 ml. However in atypical or "culture-negative cases," other conditions associated with a depressed CSF glucose should be considered. These include hypoglycemia from any cause, sarcoidosis of the central nervous system, meningeal carcinomatosis or gliomatosis, fungal or tuberculous meningitis, and subarachnoid hemorrhage.

Gram stain of sedimented CSF permits identification of the causative agent in most cases of bacterial meningitis; pneumococci and *H. influenzae* are identified more readily than meningococci. Small numbers of gram-negative diplococci present within leukocytes may be indistinguishable from nuclear material which may also be gram-negative and of the same shape. In such cases a thin film of uncentrifuged CSF may lend itself more readily to morphologic interpretation than a smear of sedimented CSF. The commonest error in reading gram-stained smears of CSF is misinterpretation of precipitated dye or debris as gram-positive cocci, or a confusion of pneumococci with *H. influenzae*. *Hemophilus* organisms may stain heavily at the poles so that they resemble gram-positive diplococci, and older pneumococci often lose their capacity to take a gram-positive stain.

Cerebrospinal fluid cultures are positive in 70 to 90 percent of cases.

Measurements of lactic dehydrogenase (LDH) *isoenzyme* appear to yield data of prognostic and diagnostic value in bacterial meningitis. A rise in total LDH activity is consistently observed in patients with bacterial meningitis; most of this is due to fractions 4 and 5 which are derived from granulocytes. Lactic dehydrogenase fractions 1 and 2, which are presumed to come from brain tissue, are only slightly elevated in bacterial meningitis but rise sharply in patients who die or who develop neurologic sequelae. Thus the test may be helpful in singling out the patient who is most at risk. Cerebrospinal fluid lysozyme, derived from leukocytes, meningeal cells, or plasma, may also be increased in meningitis, but the clinical significance of this observation is unknown.

In addition to CSF cultures, *blood cultures* should always be obtained because they are positive in 40 to 60 percent of patients with *H. influenzae*, meningococcal, and pneumococcal meningitis and may provide the only definitive clue as to the causative agent (if CSF cultures are negative). Routine cultures of the pharynx or external ear are as often misleading as helpful because pneumococci, *H. influenzae*, and meningococci are such common inhabitants of healthy persons. The *leukocyte count* in the blood is generally elevated, and usually there is a shift to the left. Most meningitic patients are sufficiently ill to require determination of blood urea nitrogen and serum electrolytes. These may be abnormal because of severe dehydration. In addition, inappropriate secretion of antidiuretic hormone (ADH) with resultant severe hyponatremia may occur.

ROENTGENOGRAPHIC STUDIES Patients with bacterial meningitis should have x-rays of the chest, skull, and sinuses as soon as possible after admission. Chest x-rays are particularly important because they may reveal a silent area of pneumonitis or abscess. Sinus and skull films may provide clues to the presence of cranial osteomyelitis, paranasal sinusitis, and mastoiditis.

RECURRENT MENINGITIS

Recurrent attacks of bacterial meningitis usually follow in the wake of trauma. The interval between the traumatic episode and the initial bout of posttraumatic meningitis may be as long as several years. *Diplococcus pneumoniae* is the usual bacterial pathogen. Often it proves to be one of the higher serologic types, reflecting the predominance of such strains in nasal carriers. *Cerebrospinal fluid rhinorrhea* is present in most of these patients but may be transient. The patient with recurrent meningitis of inapparent origin should always be suspected of having fistulous connection between the nasal sinuses and the subarachnoid space. The fistula is usually traumatic (basal skull fracture), and the site is the frontal or ethmoid sinuses or the cribriform plate. The rhinorrhea may be difficult to demonstrate except by injection of a dye, such as carmine red, or radioactive albumin into the spinal fluid and watching for its appearance in nasal secretions. Cerebrospinal fluid rhinorrhea may also be detected by measuring the glucose concentration of nasal secretions. The usual mucous secretions contain little glucose, but in CSF rhinorrhea the amount approximates that in CSF. The prognosis in recurrent meningitis is remarkably benign, and the mortality is much lower than in ordinary pneumococcal meningitis. Treatment of recurrent meningitis is outlined below. Attempts to demonstrate CSF rhinorrhea should be made after the acute infection has subsided; if evidence of a fistula is found, surgical repair should be considered.

PROGNOSIS The mortality rate of *H. influenzae* or meningococcal meningitis has remained fixed at 5 to 15 percent for many years. Also in meningococcal infection, because of the fulminating nature of the disease and often a complicating adrenocortical necrosis (Waterhouse-Friderichsen syndrome), there is still a significant mortality rate. Old age, infancy, abrupt onset, bacteremia, coma, seizures, and a variety of concomitant diseases including alcoholism, diabetes mellitus, multiple myeloma, and head trauma all worsen the prognosis. In some series, very low CSF glucose concentrations (less than 10 mg per 100 ml) and very high CSF protein concentrations were noted to be favorable signs. The triad of pneumococcal meningitis, pneumonia, and endocarditis has a particularly high fatality rate.

It is often impossible to explain the death of the patient or at least to trace it to a single specific mechanism. Bacteremia with hypotension or brain swelling and cerebellar herniation are clearly implicated in the deaths of some patients during the initial 48 hr. These events may occur in bacterial meningitis of any etiology; however, some observations suggest that they are more important in meningococcal infection. Deaths occurring later during the course of illness may be attributable to cerebral necrosis and respiratory failure, often consequent to aspiration pneumonia.

Residual defects are encountered in relatively few cases of meningococcal meningitis, whereas at least 10 percent of children with *H. influenzae* meningitis and up to 30 percent of patients with pneumococcal meningitis exhibit sequelae. The abnormalities include dementia, epilepsy, deafness, hemiplegia and hydrocephalus.

DIFFERENTIAL DIAGNOSIS The diagnosis of bacterial meningitis is not difficult, providing a high index of suspicion is maintained. All febrile patients with lethargy, headache, or confusion of sudden onset, even if only low-grade fever is present, should be subjected to lumbar puncture. It is particularly important to consider meningitis in febrile, confused alcoholic patients. Too often one incorrectly ascribes the symptoms to inebriation, delirium tremens, or hepatic encephalopathy until the CSF reveals a meningitis.

Bacterial meningitis can be diagnosed definitively only by examination of the CSF. Viral meningoencephalitis, tuberculous, leptospiral meningitis, and fungal meningitides often enter into the differential diagnosis. Also to be considered are Behçet's syndrome, a disease characterized by recurrent oral and genital ulcers along with meningitis, and Mollaret's meningitis, which consists of recurrent episodes of fever, headache, and meningeal irritation accompanied by a leukocytosis in the CSF.

The diagnosis of other intracranial suppurative diseases is detailed below.

ANTIBIOTIC TREATMENT Bacterial meningitis is a medical emergency; the rapid destruction of bacteria in the meninges and in the CSF is essential to survival. For this reason, bactericidal drugs should be used where possible. The following therapeutic regimens are recommended:

1 For adults with pneumococcal or meningococcal meningitis, penicillin G, 12 to 15 million units intravenously each day in four to six divided doses, is recommended; for children the dose of penicillin G should be 200,000 to 300,000 units per kg. For children over two months of age with *H. influenzae* or uncomplicated meningitis of unknown etiology, ampicillin, 150 to 250 mg per kg body weight intravenously in divided doses, is the treatment of choice; adults with this type of meningitis should receive 12 g per day. An alternate plan of therapy for children with influenzal B meningitis is chloramphenicol 100 mg per kg per day intravenously in a continuous infusion or in divided doses for two to three days, then 50 mg per kg by the same route.

In adult patients with any of these types of bacterial meningitis who may be allergic to the penicillins, chloramphenicol in a dosage of 6 g per day intravenously may be used. Cephalothin or cephaloridine is a questionable alternate for pneumococcal meningitis, and there have been some failures also in *H. influenzae* and meningococcal meningitis; hence, chloramphenicol is preferred in infections due to these organisms. Another plan favored in some clinics for the patient who is allergic to penicillin is chloramphenicol in divided doses of 4 g per day in combination with erythromycin, 4 g per day.

2 For meningitis due to *Enterobacteriaceae*, the drug of choice is gentamicin in dosage of 5 mg per kg per day administered in divided dosages at 6-hr intervals. This drug can be given intravenously, but many prefer the intramuscular route to avoid high blood levels which may lead to respiratory paralysis and permanent damage to inner ears. *Pseudomonas* meningitis should also be treated with gentamicin; polymyxin B in dosage of 2.5 to 5 mg may be given intrathecally at the onset of therapy.

3 Meningitis due to *Staph. aureus* should be treated with a penicillinase-resistant penicillin (oxycillin is much the most preferred) in a dosage of 12 g a day.

Foci of infection in the paranasal sinuses, mastoids, in an infected shunt, or in cranial osteomyelitis should be identified so that appropriate drainage may be carried out when the acute episode of meningitis has subsided.

Duration of therapy In most patients bacterial meningitis need not be treated for longer than 10 days except when there is a persistent parameningeal focus of infection. Antibiotics should be administered in full doses parenterally (preferably intravenously) throughout the period of treatment. Treatment failures with several drugs, notably ampicillin, are attributable to oral or intramuscular administration, resulting in inadequate concentration in the CSF. Repeated lumbar punctures are not necessary to follow the course of therapy as long as the patient is doing well. The CSF sugar may remain low for many days after suppression of the infection and should occasion concern only if bacteria are present.

Prolongation of fever due usually to subdural effusion, sinus thrombosis, mastoiditis, intercurrent infection, phlebitis, or rarely abscess of brain requires continuation of therapy for a longer period. Bacteriologic relapse after treatment is discontinued requires immediate reinstitution of therapy.

Adrenocortical steroids The few controlled studies available have demonstrated that steroids exert no beneficial effects in pyogenic meningitis. These drugs should not be used except possibly in overwhelming meningococcal sepsis.

Other forms of therapy Intrathecal administration of enzymes to lyse excessive subarachnoid cellular exudate which may be associated with spinal block or hydrocephalus in the subacute stages of bacterial meningitis is not of proved value. There is also no evidence to support the therapeutic efficacy of repeated drainage of CSF. In fact, increased CSF pressure in the acute phases of bacterial meningitis is largely a consequence of cerebral edema, and the lumbar puncture may predispose to cerebellar herniation and death. Mannitol or urea have been employed apparently successfully in some cases of severe brain swelling with unusually high initial CSF pressures (> 400 mm). Acting as osmotic diuretics, these agents enter cerebral tissue slowly, and their net effect is to decrease brain water and sodium. The administration of both of these agents may be associated to some extent with the occurrence of a late rebound phenomenon. Neither agent has been studied in controlled fashion. An adequate but not excessive amount of parenteral fluids should be given, and anticonvulsants should be prescribed when seizures are present. In children care should be taken to avoid hyponatremia and water intoxication—a cause of brain swelling. Subdural effusions should be drained repeatedly by subdural taps; if persistent after infection has subsided, surgical removal may become necessary.

SUBDURAL EMPYEMA

DEFINITION Subdural empyema is a suppurative process in the cranial subdural space, usually on one side, between the inner surface of the dura and the outer of the arachnoid. The proper term for this condition is not *abscess* but *empyema*, indicating suppuration in a preformed space.

ETIOLOGY The infection usually gains entry to the subdural space from the frontal or ethmoid sinuses, or, less often, from the mastoid cells. Occasionally the subdural space becomes infected by extension of bacteria from the CSF or from a brain abscess. Rarely has it been observed with bloodstream infections. The microorganisms are usually anaerobic, nonhemolytic streptococci (*Strep. fecalis* and *Bacteroides*), and less often *Staph. aureus*, *E. coli*, *Proteus*, and *Pseudomonas*.

PATHOLOGY A collection of subdural pus in quantities of a few milliliters to 100 to 200 ml lies over the cerebral hemisphere. It is often mistaken for meningitis. The arachnoid, when cleared of exudate, is cloudy, and thrombosis of meningeal veins may be seen. The underlying cerebral hemisphere is depressed, and in fatal cases there is often an ipsilateral temporal lobe pressure cone. Microscopic studies demonstrate various degrees of organization of the exudate on the inner surface of the dura, and infiltration of the underlying pia with small numbers of neutrophilic leukocytes, lymphocytes, and mononuclear cells. The thrombi in cerebral veins appear to begin on the outer side (toward the empyema). The superficial layers of the cerebral cortex undergo ischemic necrosis, which probably accounts for the unilateral seizures and signs of disordered cerebral function.

SYMPTOMATOLOGY AND LABORATORY FINDINGS The usual history includes reference to chronic sinusitis and mastoiditis with a recent flare-up and evidence of local pain and increase in purulent nasal and aural discharge. Generalized headache and fever are the first indications of intracranial spread. They are followed within a few days by unilateral motor seizures, hemiplegia, hemianesthesia, and aphasia. Stupor or coma develops rapidly as the cerebral symptoms progress. Fever is always present and the neck is stiff. When CSF is examined, increased pressure, raised white cell count in the range of 50 to 1,000 per μl including both neutrophils and lymphocytes, elevated protein concentration (75 to 300 mg per 100 ml), and normal sugar values are the usual findings. The CSF is sterile. If the patient is stuporous or comatose, there is risk in performing a lumbar puncture because it may aggravate a threatening pressure cone of the temporal lobe. Instead, one should proceed with other diagnostic procedures.

DIAGNOSIS Skull films usually show involvement of the sinus or mastoid. The single most useful diagnostic procedure is carotid arteriography which discloses inward displacement of meningeal vessels and contralateral shift of the anterior cerebral arteries. A temporal burr hole with exposure of the dura demonstrates pus under increased pressure. Four conditions need to be distinguished clinically from subdural empyema: cerebral thrombophlebitis, brain abscess, acute hemorrhagic leukoencephalitis, and acute hemorrhagic viral (inclusion body) encephalitis (Chap. 330).

TREATMENT Single or multiple burr holes should be made to drain pus; appropriate antibiotic therapy consists of 20 million units penicillin per day plus chloramphenicol, 2 to 4 g per day, or tetracycline, 2 g per day, aimed particularly at *Bacteroides*, administered intravenously. Without such massive antimicrobial therapy and surgery, most patients will die, usually within 7 to 14 days, often while the unsuspecting physician and surgeon are waiting for better localization of an assumed cerebral abscess, the most commonly mistaken diagnosis. On the other hand, successfully treated patients may make a surprisingly good recovery, including full or partial resolution of their focal neurologic deficits, within a few months.

EXTRADURAL ABSCESS

This condition is almost invariably associated with osteomyelitis in a cranial bone which originates from an infection in the ear or paranasal sinuses. Pus and granulation tissue accumulate on the outer surface of the dura, separating it from the cranial bone. Symptomatically, the effects are those of a local inflammatory process: frontal or auricular pain, purulent discharge from sinuses or ear, and fever and local tenderness. Sometimes the neck is slightly stiff. Localizing neurologic signs are usually absent. Rarely a fifth and sixth cranial nerve palsy appears with infections of the petrous part of the temporal bone (petrositis with Gradenigo's syndrome), or a focal seizure may occur. The CSF is usually clear and under normal pressure but may contain a few lymphocytes and neutrophils (20 to 100 per ml) and slightly raised protein concentration. Treatment consists of antibiotics aimed at the appropriate pathogen which is often *Staph. aureus*. Later the primary sinusitis or mastoiditis, from which the extradural infection has arisen, may require a surgical procedure.

SPINAL EPIDURAL ABSCESS

This type of abscess possesses unique clinical features and constitutes an important neurologic and neurosurgical emergency. It is discussed in Chap. 325.

INTRACRANIAL THROMBOPHLEBITIS

The lateral, cavernous, and superior longitudinal sinuses are the common sites of infection. Usually there is evidence that the intracranial process has extended from the middle ear and mastoid cells, the paranasal sinuses, and skin around the upper lip, nose, and eyes. Fever tends to be high and intermittent.

LATERAL SINUS THROMBOPHLEBITIS In lateral sinus thrombophlebitis, which usually follows chronic mastoiditis, the earache and mastoid tenderness are succeeded, after a period of days to a few weeks, by generalized headache and papilledema. As a rule there are no other neurologic signs. Pulmonary embolism may occur but is usually asymptomatic. As a diagnostic aid, compression of the jugular veins separately, during the Queckenstedt maneuver, will demonstrate failure of the CSF pressure to rise when the ipsilateral one is compressed (Tobey-Ayer test). When the intracranial pressure is greatly elevated, the suspicion of cerebellar abscess is raised, but this process is usually characterized by other neurologic signs, especially nystagmus to the side of the lesion and ataxia of the arm and leg.

CAVERNOUS SINUS THROMBOPHLEBITIS In this condition, which is usually secondary to oculonasal infections, the clinical syndrome is one of orbital edema, chemosis, venous congestion, and evidence of palsy of the third, fourth, ophthalmic fifth, and sixth cranial nerves. Later spread through the circular sinus to the opposite cavernous sinus results in bilateral symptoms. The posterior part of the cavernous sinus may be infected via the superior and inferior petrosal veins without the occurrence of orbital edema or ophthalmoplegia. The CSF is usually normal unless there is an associated meningitis or subdural empyema. The only effective therapy in the fulminant variety, associated with thrombosis of the anterior portion of the sinus, has been antimicrobial therapy usually aimed at coagulase-positive staphylococci (Chap. 129), and occasionally gram-negative pathogens as well. Anticoagulants have been used occasionally, but their value has not been proved. Cavernous sinus thrombosis must be differentiated from mucormycosis which may cause a similar clinical picture in uncontrolled diabetics (Chap. 172).

THROMBOPHLEBITIS OF THE SUPERIOR LONGITUDINAL SINUS Although occasionally this may be asymptomatic, the typical clinical syndrome is one of unilateral convulsions and hemiplegia, first on one side of the body, then on the other, because of extension into the superior cerebral veins. The paralysis may be predominantly monoplegic and involve mainly the legs. Headache, papilledema, and increased intracranial pressure may accompany these signs. The diagnosis can be corroborated by demonstrating a sluggish circulation and failure of the superior sagittal sinus to fill during the late stage of the carotid arteriogram. Treatment consists of large doses of antibiotics and temporization until the thrombus recanalizes.

All types of thrombophlebitis, especially those related to ear and paranasal sinus infection, may be complicated by other forms of intracranial suppuration including bacterial meningitis, subdural empyema, or brain abscess. Therapy in these patients must be individualized. The initiating focus should be brought under control even by surgery if necessary, once the patient's condition permits such a procedure. To operate on the primary focus before medical treatment is instituted is to court disaster. The better plan is to treat the intracranial disease and to decide, after it has been brought under control, whether surgery on the offending ear or sinus is necessary. In complicated cases, the treatment of bacterial meningitis usually has to take precedence over the surgically treatable diseases like brain abscess and subdural empyema.

ASEPTIC THROMBOSIS OF INTRACRANIAL VENOUS SINUSES This may develop after sinus and ear infections, and may lead to an obscure increase in intracranial pressure because of the occlusion of one lateral or superior sagittal sinus. The more common conditions which may be accompanied by aseptic thrombosis are postpartum and postoperative states, which are often characterized by thrombocytosis and hyperfibrinogenemia; congenital heart disease, marasmus in infants; sickle cell disease; and primary or secondary polycythemia.

BRAIN ABSCESS

PATHOGENESIS Most of the focal suppurative intracranial processes of this type are linked to chronic ear and sinus or pulmonary infections. Approximately 40 percent of all brain abscesses are secondary to disease of the middle ear and mastoid cells, and of these about one-third arise in the anterolateral part of the cerebellar hemisphere and the remainder (lying above the tegmen tympani) in the middle and inferior part of the temporal lobe. Frontal sinusitis accounts for roughly 10 percent of the cases, the abscess being almost invariably situated in the anterior and inferior part of the frontal lobe. Of the remaining 50 percent of cases, a small portion are due to penetrating wounds and the rest are metastatic. Of these latter, about half are traceable to a primary septic focus in the lung, usually bronchiectasis, empyema, lung abscess, or bronchopleural fistual, and in the rest, the source of infection may be the skin, bone, i.e., a focus of osteomyelitis, or the heart. In 5 to 10 percent of cases, the source cannot be ascertained. Brain abscess is almost never a consequence of bacterial meningitis.

Brain abscesses are particularly frequent with congenital heart disease with right-to-left shunts (e.g., tetralogy of Fallot), and they may also complicate arteriovenous vascular abnormalities of the lung, as in cases of familial telangiectasia. With cranial trauma the location of the abscess will depend on the site of the penetrating wound. Metastatic abscesses are most likely to occur in the distal territory of the middle cerebral arteries. In contrast to the otogenic and rhinogenic abscesses they may be multiple.

Bacterial endocarditis rarely gives rise to brain abscess. Instead, the picture is one of the focal embolic encephalitis with or without signs of embolic vascular disease elsewhere (Chap. 127). In subacute endocarditis the emboli are sterile and cause only infarction, miliary foci of tissue necrosis, focal meningeal inflammation, and rarely mycotic aneurysms. The CSF may contain a mixture of neutrophilic leukocytes, lymphocytes, and red cells; the protein level may be elevated, but cultures are sterile and sugar values remain normal. In acute bacterial endocarditis, miliary abscesses and purulent meningitis may develop, or there may be infarcts, and meningeal or cerebral hemorrhages, secondary to mycotic aneurysms. Rarely do the miliary abscesses progress to large ones. Rapidly evolving cerebral signs in endocarditis are nearly always caused by embolic infarction or hemorrhage.

ETIOLOGY The most common organisms causing brain abscess are streptococci, many of which are anaerobic or microaerophilic. These organisms are often found in combinations with other anaerobes, notably *Bacteroides*, and may also be combined with *Bacteriaceae*, such as *E. coli* and *Proteus*. Staphylococci also may cause brain abscess, but pneumococci, meningococci, and *H. influenza* rarely do so. In addition to *Bacteroides* and anaerobic streptococci, anaerobic actinomyces and veillonellae have been isolated. The bacterial species vary with the site of the abcess; staphylococcal abscesses are usually a consequence of penetrating head trauma or of bacteremia; enteric organisms are almost always associated with otitic infections, while anaerobic streptococci are commonly metastatic from the lung.

PATHOLOGY Localized inflammatory necrosis and edema, septic thrombosis of vessels, and aggregates of degenerating leukocytes (suppurative encephalitis), represent the early reaction to bacterial invasion of the brain. This is followed within a few weeks by encapsulation of the liquefied brain and of accumulated pus. The lesion becomes encapsulated by fibroblasts and newly formed vessels, and the capsule thickens over a period of weeks. The meninges adjacent to the abscess, especially near the point of entry of infection, are infiltrated by neutrophils, lymphocytes, and plasma cells.

CLINICAL MANIFESTATIONS In patients who harbor chronic ear, sinus, or pulmonary infections, a recent reactivation of the infection usually precedes the onset of cerebral symptoms. In a number of patients evidence of central nervous system invasion is acute with fever, headache, vomiting, increasing obtundation, seizures, and a variety of localizing neurologic signs appearing within a few days. In other patients, bacterial invasion of the brain substance may be asymptomatic or may be attended only by a transitory focal neurologic disorder, as may happen when a septic embolus lodges in a brain artery. Sometimes stiff neck accompanies generalized headache, suggesting the diagnosis of meningitis (especially a partially treated one). However, the CSF shows only a few cells, normal or increased protein concentration, and normal sugar concentration. These early symptoms may subside or may appear to respond to antimicrobials, but within a few weeks, recurrent headache, slowness in mentation, focal or generalized convulsions, and obvious signs of increased intracranial pressure provide evidence of an inflammatory mass in the brain. At this stage, the symptoms of infection are not conspicuous. While fever is characteristic of the invasive phase characterized by suppurative encephalitis, as the abscess becomes encapsulated, the temperature returns to normal. Indeed, if the invasive stage of cerebral infection is inconspicuous, the entire clinical picture does not differ from that of brain tumor. In the later stages of the abscess formation, the CSF pressure is usually elevated and there is nearly always pleocytosis between 25 and 300 cells per ml consisting both of neutrophils and lymphocytes and an elevation of protein between 75 and 300 mg per 100 ml with CSF glucose remaining normal.

The focal neurologic signs depend on the location of the abscess as follows.

Temporal lobe abscess Headache is usually on the side of the abscess and is localized to the frontotemporal region. If the abscess lies in the dominant hemisphere, there is a dysphasia of of the amnestic type (inability to name objects—see Chap. 25). A homonymous upper quadrantic field may also be demonstrable—the inferior portion of the optic radiation is interrupted, and thus may be the only sign in abscess of the right temporal lobe. Contralateral motor or sensory defects in the limbs tend to be minimal, though weakness of the lower face is often observed.

Cerebellar abscess Headache in the postauricular or suboccipital region is usually the first symptom and may at first be ascribed to the infection in the mastoid cells. Coarse nystagmus and gaze weakness to the side of the lesion and a cerebellar ataxia of the ipsilateral arm and leg are present in most of the patients, though the ataxia may be difficult to demonstrate if the patient is very ill. As a rule, the signs of increased intracranial pressure are more prominent than those of cerebral disease. Mild contralateral or bilateral pyramidal signs are evidence of ipsilateral brainstem compression; in the late stages as consciousness becomes impaired they are ominous signs.

Frontal lobe abscess Headache, drowsiness, inattention, and general impairment of the mental function are prominent. Hemiparesis with unilateral motor seizures and motor or expressive dysphasia are the most frequent neurologic signs.

DIAGNOSIS The diagnosis of a brain abscess depends on (1) a demonstrated source of infection in the ears, sinuses, or lungs; or the presence of a right-to-left cardiac shunt; (2) evidence of increased intracranial pressure; and (3) focal cerebral or cerebellar signs. Although the CSF shows a characteristic inflammatory reaction, some neurosurgeons feel that lumbar puncture in brain abscess is dangerous, particularly when intracranial pressure is obviously elevated. Several other diagnostic maneuvers are useful.

1 The EEG demonstrates a focal slow wave (delta) abnormality over the cerebral abscess and may be used to follow its development or regression after therapy.

2 Radioactive technetium scanning is strongly positive and has become one of the most reliable methods for localizing brain abscesses. There is little likelihood of cerebral abscess if both the radioactive isotope scan and EEG are negative. These procedures have supplanted arteriography in many instances.

3 Arteriography may provide evidence of a cerebral mass by showing displacement of the anterior, middle, or posterior cerebral arteries. This technique is accurate in localizing only about 60 percent of abscesses and may be unreliable early in the course of disease before liquefaction and encapsulation has occurred.

4 Ventriculography may disclose deformities of the ventricles. Not infrequently the placement of the ventricular needle has resulted in penetration of a parieto-occipital metastatic abscess.

When the classic clinical picture is present and EEG, x-rays, and scan corroborate the presence of a mass lesion, the diagnosis is easy. If there is no source of infection and there are only signs and symptoms of a mass lesion, the diagnosis includes differentiation of abscess from glioma, subdural hematoma, and hemorrhage. Sometimes only surgical exploration will settle the issue. Once the inflammatory nature of the intracranial mass has been established, brain abscess must then be distinguished from subdural empyema, intracranial thrombophlebitis with hemorrhage and infarction of brain, necrotizing viral encephalitis, and acute hemorrhagic leukoencephalitis (Chap. 331).

TREATMENT During the stage of acute suppurative encephalitis, intracranial operation accomplishes little and probably causes only additional traumatization and swelling of the brain tissue and a wider dissemination of the infection. There is good evidence that many brain abscesses can be cured at this stage by the administration of adequate doses of antimicrobials. Since the bacteriologic diagnosis must be presumptive, the best regimen consists of 20 million units penicillin G intravenously in divided doses and 4 to 6 g chloramphenicol or 2 g tetracycline, both drugs being given intravenously in divided doses. This choice of antimicrobial agents is based on the preponderance of anaerobic streptococci and *Bacteroides* that are usually isolated from the abscess in such patients. If there is evidence of staphylococcal infection, adequate amounts of a penicillinase-resistant penicillin or a cephalosporin drug should be added. Treatment should be continued for 6 weeks, and if there is clinical improvement and recovery during the course of therapy, surgical intervention can be withheld. The initial elevation of intracranial pressure and threatening temporal lobe or cerebellar pressure cone should be managed by intravenous injection of urea or mannitol followed by dexamethasone, 6 to 12 mg every 6 hr. Persistence of progression of high intracranial pressure manifested by deepening coma and threat of herniation often forces one to operate, regardless of the stage of the abscess. Likewise, clear-cut evidence of a mass lesion which is not improving with antimicrobial therapy is an indication for surgery. The usual methods of treatment are unroofing of the abscess and drainage, or aspiration. If superficial and encapsulated, total excision should be attempted; if deep, aspiration and the injection of antimicrobial agents into the abscess are the only treatment, which may have to be repeated. The combination of antimicrobial therapy and surgery has reduced the mortality in brain abscess from more than 50 to 10 percent. The least satisfactory results are obtained in multiple metastatic abscesses. Neurologic residua occur in about 30 percent of surviving patients. Of these, focal epilepsy is one of the most troublesome.

Following successful treatment of a cerebral abscess in patients with congenital heart disease, correction of the cardiac anomaly is indicated to prevent recurrence.

PROGNOSIS With appropriate therapy, the prognosis is reasonably good. However, if brain abscess is not recognized and treated, it terminates either by development of a tentorial or foramen magnum pressure cone or by rupture of the abscess into the ventricles (ventricular empyema). Rarely the abscess becomes thickly encapsulated and chronic; in this form it may be only mildly symptomatic over a period of months or years.

REFERENCES

BHANDARI YS et al: Subdural empyema: A review of 37 cases. J Neurosurg 32:35, 1970

CARPENTER RR, PETERSDORF RG: The clinic spectrum of bacterial meningitis. Am J Med 23:262, 1962

GARFIELD J: Management of supratentorial intracranial abscess: A review of 200 cases. Br Med J 2:7, 1968

HAND LW, SANFORD JP: Post-traumatic bacterial meningitis. Ann Intern Med 72:869, 1970

HEINEMAN HS et al: Intracranial suppurative disease. JAMA 218:1542, 1971

MATHIES AW: Penicillins in the treatment of bacterial meningitis. J R Coll Physicians Lond 6:139, 1972

SWARTZ MN, DODGE PR: Bacterial meningitis—A review of selected aspects. N Engl J Med 272:725, 779, 842, 898, 954, 1003, 1965

——: Anaerobic bacteria in central nervous system infections. J Fla Med Assoc 57:19, 1970

WEISS W et al: Prognostic factors in pneumococcal meningitis. Arch Intern Med 120:517, 1967

330
VIRAL INFECTIONS OF THE NERVOUS SYSTEM:
ASEPTIC MENINGITIS AND ENCEPHALITIS

BYRON KAKULAS
RAYMOND D. ADAMS

More than 40 viruses are known to be capable of causing infection and symptomatic injury to the nervous system. In many instances the neurologic manifestations are only a part of a generalized disease with its own peculiarities and easy means of identification, such as mumps, chickenpox, or pleurodynia. But it may happen that overt evidences of the infection are limited to the nervous system, and the resulting syndrome can be either relatively stereotyped or highly varied. If the latter condition prevails, clinical diagnosis may be difficult and one must, perforce, turn to laborious and complicated laboratory procedures for the identification of the causative agent. But these diagnostic methods are not always successful, and even the most experienced laboratories have failed to establish the nature of the disease in as many as 30 to 50 percent of cases.

Those viruses which affect the nervous system primarily are said to be *neurotropic*. There are a considerable number of them, and their clinical manifestations are diverse, as might be expected. However, five clinical syndromes recur with regularity, and should be familiar to all students of medicine. These are the syndromes of (1) poliomyelitis, almost invariably a result of infection by one of the polioviruses; (2) zoster ganglionitis; (3) acute aseptic, nonsuppurative, or ("lymphocytic") meningitis; (4) acute and subacute encephalitis or meningoencephalitis; and (5) slow virus infections simulating degenerative diseases. The first and second of these (poliomyelitis and herpes zoster) are discussed in Chaps. 192 and 200, respectively; the third, fourth, and fifth are described below.

THE SYNDROME OF ASEPTIC MENINGITIS

The term *aseptic meningitis* was first introduced to designate what was thought to be a specific disease, but it is now applied to a symptom complex that can be produced by any one of several dozen infective agents, the majority of which are viral. In bold outline the syndrome consists of fever, signs of meningeal irritation, and mononuclear and lymphocytic pleocytosis of the cerebrospinal fluid (CSF).

Headache, out of proportion to that often associated with febrile states, ranks as the most frequent symptom in this group of diseases. A variable degree of drowsiness, confusion, stupor, or rarely coma, may occur, but as a rule the derangement of consciousness tends to be relatively mild. Stiffness of the neck and spine on forward bending attest to the presence of meningeal irritation, but at first it may be so slight as to pass unnoticed. Here the Kernig and Brudzinski's signs help very little, for they are often absent in the presence of a manifest viral meningitis. Frank neurologic signs of other types are infrequent; included are isolated strabismus and diplopia, vague weakness, pain or paresthesias in an extremity, a slight inequality of reflexes, or a wavering Babinski sign. The meningitis may be asymptomatic.

The CSF findings consist of pleocytosis (mainly mononuclear, except in the initial stage when a proportion of the cells are neutrophilic leukocytes), small and variable increase in protein, and no demonstrable microorganisms by smear and culture. The concentration of glucose in the CSF is normal; this is important because a low sugar value in an infection which evokes a lymphocytic or mononuclear pleocytosis usually signifies tuberculous (Chap. 156), mycotic (Chaps. 166 to 168) meningitis, or rarely metastatic carcinoma, lymphoma, or sarcoid of the meninges. Since the CSF glucose level may be normal in the early stages of tuberculosis or cryptococcosis, this determination should be repeated at intervals until the diagnosis is established or the patient is definitely convalescent.

VIRAL INFECTIONS THAT ARE PREDOMINANTLY MENINGEAL The majority of cases of aseptic meningitis are accounted for by nonparalytic poliomyelitis (Chap 192), Coxsackie viruses (Chap. 186), echo viruses

(Chaps.186), mumps (Chap. 205), and lymphocytic choriomeningitis (LCM) (Chap. 191). Indeed, these viral infections together with leptospirosis comprise about 95 percent of all cases of aseptic meningitis of established etiology. But in every series of cases published from virus isolation centers as many as one-fourth or more have an indeterminate cause.

Of the rarer types of aseptic meningitis one should mention the milder forms of postvaccinal meningoencephalitis or the meningoencephalitis which follows measles (Chap. 195), rubella (Chap. 196), chickenpox (Chap. 199), and prophylactic treatment of rabies (Chap. 193). Here the diagnosis is made on the history of the recent infection (usually within a few days or a week) or inoculation (usually within a few weeks).

Herpes simplex (Chap. 200) and the arthropod-borne (arbo-) encephalitis viruses (Chap. 207) are responsible for a small proportion of cases of aseptic meningitis. Infections by arboviruses are likely to be encountered in epidemics along with cases of frank encephalitis and tend to occur in certain geographic areas, points which facilitate early clinical recognition, though specific identification of the virus may still be difficult.

Neurologic manifestations, including the syndrome of aseptic meningitis, may appear in the course of syphilis (Chap. 159), influenza (Chap. 188), infectious mononucleosis (Chap. 224), psittacosis (Chap. 189), lymphogranuloma (Chap. 203), Rift Valley fever and encephalomyocarditis, Q fever, Behçet's disease, Vogt-Koyanagi disease, Harada's disease, Mollaret's recurrent meningitis, and other of the viral agents mentioned in Chap. 209.

The icteric stage of infectious hepatitis (Chap. 294) rarely is preceded by mild meningitis, the nature of which is evident when the jaundice appears. Among diseases of possible or probable viral causation, infectious mononucleosis (Chap. 224) sometimes produces what appears to be a primary meningitis; rarely a primary atypical pneumonia (Chap. 187) is complicated by aseptic meningitis or other neurologic disorder.

DIFFERENTIAL DIAGNOSIS OF INFECTIVE AND NONINFECTIVE FORMS OF LYMPHOCYTIC MENINGITIS Clinical distinctions between the many forms of aseptic meningitis cannot be made with a high degree of reliability, but useful leads can be obtained by careful attention to certain details of history and physical examination. The *season* during which the illnesses occur may be helpful. Enteroviral infections (poliomyelitis, Coxsackie, and echo) are diseases of midsummer and early fall, August and September usually being the peak months. The arthropod-borne diseases also occur in summer and fall (coinciding with the population of insect vectors), and though leptospirosis may appear at any season, its incidence in the United States shows a striking peak in August. Mumps and infectious mononucleosis are diseases of late winter and spring. Lymphocytic meningitis is particularly common in late fall and winter, presumably because field mice enter dwellings at this time. A definite past history of mumps aids in excluding the disease, second attacks being unusual. A preceding upper respiratory infection of a week's duration suggests LCM. Sore throat, lymphadenopathy, and rash point to infectious mononucleosis or echo infection. Severe back and leg pain occur in poliomyelitis, leptospirosis, and trichinosis. Aseptic meningitis during pregnancy is likely to be poliomyelitis. Exposure to such animals as mice (LCM), dogs, rats, or swine (leptospirosis) may suggest a diagnosis. A skin rash favors the presence of infectious mononucleosis, echo viral infections, and leptospirosis (often a transient, blotchy erythema). Icterus suggests infectious mononucleosis or viral hepatitis; it is not present in pure meningeal leptospirosis. Conjunctival suffusion is common in leptospirosis and may be seen in trichinosis. Slight tenderness and swelling of salivary glands and testes may be the only signs of mumps. Pulmonary infiltrates suggest LCM, infectious mononucleosis, psittacosis, or leptospirosis.

Aside from viral isolation, few laboratory tests are helpful. The peripheral leukocyte count is often normal, but leukopenia may be present. However it accompanies so many of the diseases responsible for aseptic meningitis (infectious mononucleosis, Colorado tick fever, LCM, lupus erythematosis, etc.) that rarely is it a useful finding. Eosinophilia should suggest a parasitic infection, and in most cases infectious mononucleosis may be identified by the blood smear. Lymphocytic choriomeningitis produces the most intense pleocytosis in the CSF (counts above 1,000 cells per ml are almost always due to this disease), and mumps gives an almost pure lymphocytic pleocytosis. Serologic tests on the CSF should be interpreted with caution because inflammation of many types can produce a false positive reaction; infectious mononucleosis and lupus erythematosus often evoke biologic false positive serum tests for syphilis. Liver function tests are abnormal in many patients with infectious mononucleosis and in anicteric hepatitis; hepatic abnormalities are not regularly present in the other entities under consideration.

Three other categories of disease may cause an apparently sterile, predominantly lymphocytic or mononuclear reaction in the leptomeninges: bacterial infections lying adjacent to the meninges; specific infections or parainfectious diseases in which the organism is difficult to isolate; and neoplastic invasion (usually lymphoma or carcinoma). The recognition of these is of great importance, since they require vigorous antibiotic therapy or some other form of treatment, as in syphilis, tuberculosis, cryptococcosis.

With respect to pyogenic infections in which the CSF does not show a purulent meningitis and is sterile, it must be remembered that antibiotic therapy given in inadequate dosage during a systemic or pulmonary infection may suppress a coexistent meningitis to the point where mononuclear cells predominate, glucose level is normal, and organisms are not detected in the CSF. A mistaken diagnosis of aseptic meningitis may then be made when the CSF is examined. The true state of affairs becomes evident only when the patient worsens and bacteria again appear. Careful attention to the history of recent antimicrobial therapy sometimes permits recognition of these cases before symptoms recur. A smouldering paranasal sinusitis or mastoiditis may produce a similar CSF change because of intracranial extension (epidural or subdural infection). Or a brain abscess, the localizing signs of which are obscure, may deceive the clinician into making a diagnosis of aseptic meningitis (see Chap. 329).

In the second group of diseases, acute syphilitic meningitis is of importance and may be symptomatic or asymptomatic. In former times it was likely to develop as a neurorecurrence after inadequate arsenic therapy, but now it may be merely the first manifestation of a florid syphilitic infection (see Chap. 159). Tuberculous meningitis often masquerades as an innocent aseptic meningitis; the diagnosis may at first be difficult because the tubercle bacillus is hard to see in stained smears, and cultures and guinea pig inoculations require considerable time. Similarly the cryptococcus may not be diagnosed for the reason that the organisms may exceptionally be present in such low number as to be overlooked in smears.

Children with scarlet fever or streptococcus pharyngitis rarely have been noted to develop meningeal signs and pleocytosis, the result of a sterile "serous" inflammation that does not involve invasion of the meninges by visible organisms. The same is true of subacute bacterial endocarditis.

In the third group, leukemias and lymphomas are the most conspicuous source of neoplastic meningeal reactions. In children with myelogenous leukemia, a leukemic meningitis with cell counts numbering into the thousands occurs not infrequently in the late stages of the illness. In adults a pleocytosis with lymphocyte or lymphoblast counts reaching as high as 4,000 per ml fluid may complicate lymphocytic and lymphoblastic lymphomas with or without leukemia. The sugar values may fall to 0, and the protein level is elevated.

In carcinomatous "meningitis" (from breast, stomach, lung, melanoma, or other organ) great numbers of cells may extend through the leptomeninges, involving cranial and spinal nerve roots, and produce a picture of meningoradiculitis with low sugar values. Gliomatous infiltration of ependyma and meninges also may have the same effect. Millipore filter preparations usually permit identification of the tumor cells.

Finally, in a number of other subacute or chronic infections of obscure origin, probably viral, the CSF formula corresponds to that of aseptic meningitis. These are (1) Behçet's disease, distinguished clinically by the triad of genital ulceration, uveitis, and involvement of central nervous system (cranial nerve palsies, seizures, mental disturbance, aphasia, hemiparesis, cerebellar ataxia); (2) Vogt-Koyanagi and Harada's diseases with various combinations of uveitis, depigmentation of hair and skin around the eyes, loss of eyelashes, dysacousis, and deafness; (3) Mollaret's recurrent meningitis (Chap. 329); and allergic or hypersensitivity meningitis, occurring in the course of serum sickness and diseases of connective tissue such as lupus erythematosus.

In summary, though clinical findings, season occurrence, and laboratory tests can sometimes enable the physician to direct further diagnostic efforts along specific lines, they may not be conclusive. Most important is to keep in mind always the possibility of tuberculosis, cryptococcosis, syphilis, inadequately treated pyogenic meningitis, and brain abscess, all of which may simulate aseptic meningitis. These diseases offer more pressing diagnostic problems, for they may take the life of the patient if they are not diagnosed and treated. In contrast, the various forms of aseptic viral meningitis are usually self-limiting and benign.

THE SYNDROME OF ENCEPHALITIS

From the above discussion it is evident that the separation of the clinical syndrome of aseptic meningitis and encephalitis is not always easy, because in some patients with the former condition a nonspecific drowsiness or confusion may be present when in fact there is no evidence of an inflammatory reaction in the substance of the brain. Conversely, in some patients with encephalitis the cerebral involvement may be so mild as to escape notice, and only the meningeal symptoms and CSF abnormality may be manifest. These facts make it difficult to place complete reliance on statistical data about the relative incidence of encephalitis collected in surveys from various virus laboratories. It is our impression that many cases of mumps and LCM are little more than examples of intense meningitis. They rarely have caused death with postmortem demonstration of cerebral lesions, and surviving patients seldom have residual signs.

The core of the encephalitis syndrome is an acute febrile illness with evidence of meningeal involvement, added to which are various combinations of the following symptoms and signs: convulsions, confusion, stupor, or coma; aphasia or mutism; hemiparesis with asymmetry of tendon reflexes and Babinski signs; involuntary movements, ataxia, and myoclonic jerks; nystagmus, ocular palsies, and facial weakness. Some one or other of these groups of findings predominate in certain types of encephalitis, as will be pointed out below, but always the clinical diagnosis in the setting of a febrile aseptic meningitis rests on the demonstration of focal derangement of the function of the cerebrum, brainstem, or cerebellum. The illnesses produced by these viral agents vary in duration but are usually measured in terms of weeks or, exceptionally, months. Death occurs in 5 to 20 percent of patients with viral encephalitis. Residual signs such as mental deterioration, amnestic defect, personality change, and hemiparesis are seen in about 20 percent of patients. This overall figure fails to reflect, however, the wide variation in the incidence of late changes that follow infection by different viruses. For example, neurologic sequelae have been observed in 80 to 90 percent of patients with Eastern equine encephalitis and in only 5 to 10 percent of those with Western equine infections.

ETIOLOGY Whereas numerous virus, bacterial, fungus, and parasitic agents are listed as causes of the encephalitis syndrome, only the viral ones are being considered here, for reference is usually being made to them when the term *encephalitis* is used. The number of viral infections or postviral allergic reactions is large, and one might suppose that clinical problems would be infinitely complex. However, those forms of viral encephalitis that occur with sufficient frequency to be of diagnostic importance are relatively few, and they tend to have geographic and seasonal incidence. In the United States, Eastern and Western equine encephalitis have been observed mainly in California; there have been only two recognized outbreaks of Eastern equine encephalitis in New England, each in the early autumn. St. Louis encephalitis, another arthropod-borne late-summer encephalitis, has rarely been encountered in Eastern United States. Japanese B encephalitis, Russian spring-summer, and Murray Valley encephalitis (Australian X disease) are virtually unknown in the United States. Definite cases of epidemic (lethargic) encephalitis have not been observed in the acute form in the United States or Western Europe since 1930, though patients with residual symptoms (Parkinson's syndrome) are still to be seen in neurology clinics.

In addition to the viruses that primarily exert their effects on the central nervous system, there is another large group in which cerebral involvement is an unusual complication in the course of a well-defined clinical illness. Infectious mononucleosis is the most frequent cause of encephalitis in adolescents and young adults. These diseases are fully described elsewhere in this text.

ACUTE ARTHROPOD FORMS OF ENCEPHALITIS

The clinical picture of this group of viruses, which attack principally the cerebral hemispheres, is described in Chap. 207.

Rabies stands apart because of its relatively long latency after the bite of a rabid animal and by the predominance of dysphagia (hence salivation), throat spasms induced by attempts to swallow water (hence hydrophobia), dysarthria, numbness of face, and facial spasms, to which are added a confusional psychosis. The localization indicates the intensive involvement of the tegmental medullary nuclei in the rabid form of the disease (paralytic form is due to spinal cord affection) (see Chap. 193).

ENCEPHALITIS LETHARGICA (VON ECONOMO'S DISEASE, SLEEPING SICKNESS)

This disease first occurred in the wake of the pandemic of influenza during and for about 10 years after World War I. No disease like it can be found in medical annals before 1914. Although the viral agent was never identified, the clinical and pathologic features were typical of viral infection. The unique symptoms were pronounced somnolence, from which the disease takes its name, and ophthalmoplegia. A small proportion of the patients were overly active rather than somnolent and manifested a disorder of movement in the form either of chorea or myoclonus. Headache, insomnia, dizziness, fatigability, or frank confusional psychosis were not infrequent. In contrast, paralysis (hemiplegia), cortical sensory loss, aphasia, disorders of hearing or vision, and convulsions were virtually unknown. The onset was acute or subacute, and the symptoms persisted for several weeks. Lymphocytic pleocytosis was found in half the patients, together with variable elevation of protein level. More than 20 percent of the victims died within a few weeks. A high proportion of the survivors developed within months or years (sometimes after an interval as long as 25 years) the syndrome of parkinsonism (see Chaps. 18 and 333). In fact, this is the only form of encephalitis known to cause an immediate or delayed extrapyramidal syndrome of this type. Myoclonus, dystonia, bulimia, obesity, reversal of sleep pattern, and in children a psychopathic personality with compulsive behavior were other distressing sequelae.

The pathology was typical of a neurotropic viral infection (nerve cell destruction and neuronophagia, perivascular cuffing with lymphocytes and mononuclear cells, and meningeal infiltrations of similar cells), localized principally to the region of the midbrain, subthalamus, and hypothalamus. In the patients who die years later of Parkinson's syndrome, fibrillary changes in the nerve cells of substantia nigra, oculomotor, and adjacent nuclei; destruction of nerve cells; and gliosis are the only findings.

Few if any new cases have been seen in the United States and Western Europe since 1930. The only treatment available for the survivors consists of antiparkinsonism drugs and surgery, as outlined in Chap 333.

ACUTE AND SUBACUTE INCLUSION BODY ENCEPHALITIS

First described by Dawson in 1939 and extensively studied by van Bogaert, in both subacute and chronic forms, this rather remarkable group of diseases is the only one which occurs sporadically throughout the year and in patients of all ages and in all parts of the world. Whereas herpes simplex has been isolated from many of the acute cases and rubeola virus from subacute sclerosing ones, no causative agent has been found in others. Identity of etiology has been claimed on the basis of the pathology, particularly the large intranuclear (Cowdry type B) inclusion bodies in the astrocytes, oligodendrocytes, and nerve cells, but the evidence now is clearly against a unitary concept.

Nothing is known of the incubation period of these diseases. In acute encephalitis rarely have there been herpetic lesions of the skin or mucous membranes. A febrile onset and convulsions, confusion, hallucinations, and stupor or coma have been the usual initial symptoms. Swelling and herniation of one or both temporal lobes through the tentorium may occur, leading to deep coma and respiratory arrest during the first 24 to 76 hr. The later clinical picture, which is relatively unique, evolves over a period of days or weeks, and the confusional psychosis shows elements of delirium or Korsakoff's amnestic state, the latter being more evident as the weeks pass. Age at onset has varied from childhood to the most advanced years (greater than sixty to seventy years in several of our patients). The CSF has shown a pleocytosis and increased protein content in most of the patients. The herpes simplex virus has been isolated from the brain (biopsy, autopsy) and CSF in only a few patients, and a rising titer of neutralizing antibodies has been demonstrated in others. The mortality rate is high (30 percent), and many of the survivors have been left with the most severe mental sequelae in the form of a complete Korsakoff's psychosis or global dementia. Prognosis is not hopeless, however, for a few patients have recovered to the point where they can resume an independent life.

The subacute and chronically progressive forms of

inclusion-body encephalitis have affected children and adolescents for the most part. Widespread myelin destruction in the cerebral hemispheres with gliosis (sclerosing encephalitis) is combined with focal lesions of the brainstem. The clinical picture is that of a slowly evolving mental deterioration (dementia) associated with myoclonic jerks, falling spells, and cerebellar ataxia. The CSF may contain no cells, but the protein level may be elevated, particularly the γ-globulin fraction (first zone gold sol curve). High levels of neutralizing antibody to measles virus have been found in serum and CSF, but this infective agent has been isolated from the brain tissue in only a few instances. It is still uncertain as to whether this virus has been seen in electron microscopic sections of the brain. The course of the disease is progressive, death usually occurring within a few months or years.

The pathology of the acute inclusion-body encephalitis is marked by an intense hemorrhagic necrosis of the medial and inferior parts of the temporal lobes, and the orbital parts of the frontal ones. This distribution of lesion is so characteristic that the diagnosis can be made by simple inspection. The subacute sclerosing form involves the cerebral cortex and white matter of both hemispheres as well as brainstem and cerebellum. Destruction of nerve cells, neuronophagia, and perivenous cuffing by lymphocytes and mononuclear cells indicate the viral nature of the infection. Degeneration of medullated fibers (myelin and axis cylinders) occurs in the white matter and is accompanied by perivascular cuffing and fibrous gliosis. The inclusion bodies in nerve and glial cells may be difficult to find. Treatment with some of the new antiviral agents is being tried.

The diagnosis may be difficult. The acute inclusion body encephalitis must be distinguished from acute hemorrhagic leukoencephalitis (see Chap. 331), acute subdural empyema, acute cerebral abscess, thrombophlebitis, and septic embolism (see Chap. 329). The subacute to chronic variety simulates the childhood and adolescent dementing diseases such as lipid storage disease (see Chap. 333) and Schilder's disease (see Chap. 331).

CHRONIC "SLOW" VIRAL ENCEPHALITIS

The idea that viral infections may lead to chronic disease, especially of the nervous system, has been entertained for half a century but only recently has received firm support from the following observations: (1) The demonstration of a slowly progressive noninflammatory degeneration of nigral neurons long after an attack of encephalitis lethargica; (2) the discovery in Iceland and England of a chronic viral degenerative disease of white matter in sheep (visna and scrapie); (3) the finding of inclusion bodies in the most chronic cases of sclerosing encephalitis and the demonstration by electron microscopy of viral particles in multifocal leukoencephalopathy; (4) the transmission of kuru and Creutzfeldt-Jakob disease to chimpanzees by Gajdusek and Gibbs; and (5) late onset of motor system disease after poliomyelitis. Claims have also been made for a viral causation of multiple sclerosis by Schubladze, of amyotrophic lateral sclerosis by Zilber, of epilepsia partialis continua and Vilynisk encephalomyelitis by Chumakov, but the evidence is questionable. From these observations has emerged the concept of the "slow viruses," the common features of which are long period of latency (months or years); protracted progression of illness after onset of symptoms; limitation of infections to a single host species; and localization of noninflammatory degenerative lesions in a particular part of the nervous system.

These slow viruses so perfectly simulate a purely degenerative disease that views of all the major degenerative diseases of white and gray matter of the brain are being altered. One of the most exciting prospects in medical neurology is thus unfolding before us. This concept of slow virus effects is discussed at greater length in Chap. 194.

There is presently no known treatment for any of these diseases.

CREUTZFELDT-JAKOB DISEASE (SUBACUTE SPONGIFORM ENCEPHALOPATHY) Creutzfeldt-Jakob disease is the most dramatic representative of a degenerative disease of purely noninflammatory type caused by what is presumed to be a virus.

H. G. Creutzfeldt (1920) and A. M. Jakob (1921, 1923) described a diffuse disorder of the central nervous system of adults that was characterized clinically by progressive dementia, spasticity or rigidity, and ataxia and pathologically by neuronal degeneration in the cerebral cortex, basal ganglia, and spinal cord. These reports have subsequently given rise to the concept that there is a clinicopathologic entity combining dementia with prominent motor impairment (including progressive weakness with muscular atrophy in some instances) and very widespread neuropathological changes to which the name *Creutzfeldt-Jakob* (or *Jakob-Creutzfeldt*) *disease* is applicable. This term is now firmly established in the nomenclature of neurologic diseases; its precise definition and limitations, however, remain uncertain.

Meanwhile, there has been increasing awareness of the existence of another distinctive cerebral disease of rapid evolution, in which profound dementia is associated with ataxia and diffuse myoclonic jerks. The major neuropathologic changes in this disorder are in the cerebral and cerebellar cortex; the outstanding features of the lesions are widespread neuronal loss and gliosis accompanied by a striking vacuolation or spongy state of the affected regions. These changes, both clinical and pathologic, occur so regularly and with such remarkable uniformity from case to case that there can be no doubt that they form a distinct nosologic entity. This disease state has come in recent years to be designated as subacute spongiform encephalopathy. At the same time, because of some features in common with what Creutzfeldt and Jakob had earlier described, it has frequently been referred to as Creutzfeldt-Jakob disease. It seems to us hardly likely, however, that subacute spongiform encephalopathy and the somewhat ill-defined syndrome of Creutzfeldt and Jakob, previously referred to, can truly be the same disease. Pending further knowledge, at any rate, we believe that they should be kept distinct from one another, or at least whenever Creutzfeldt-Jakob disease is spoken of, it should be clearly stated whether subacute spongiform encephalopathy is meant, or the slower progressive dementia with signs of pyramidal and extrapyramidal dysfunction. Preciseness in definition of these states is of greater importance now than before, because recent evidence obtained by Gibbs et al. suggests that subacute spongiform encephalopathy may be due to a transmissible agent.

Pathology In subacute spongiform encephalopathy, as already indicated, the disease affects principally the cerebral and cerebellar cortex, generally in a diffuse fashion, although in some cases the occipitoparietal regions are almost exclusively involved, as in those described by Heidenhain (1929). The degeneration and disappearance of nerve cells is associated with extensive astroglial proliferation; ultrastructural studies have shown that the microscopic vacuoles which give the tissue its typically spongy appearance are located within the cytoplasmic processes of glial cells. Despite the possibility referred to above that the disease may be the result of an infection, the lesions show no evidence of an inflammatory reaction.

In the cases that conform to what Creutzfeldt and Jakob described, the disease process in the cerebral cortex is more focal than in spongiform encephalopathy, the rolandic regions being chiefly affected, and there is more extensive involvement of the basal ganglia. Furthermore, the spinal cord typically shows some loss of anterior horn cells and degeneration of the corticospinal tracts in a manner reminiscent of amyotrophic lateral sclerosis, a condition that is discussed in a later section of this chapter.

Clinical aspects Subacute spongiform encephalopathy is in most cases a disease of late middle age, although it can occur in young adults and very possibly in children as well.

In early stages, a great variety of clinical manifestations may be seen, but those most frequently observed are changes in behavior, emotional responses, memory, and reasoning, together with abnormalities of vision such as peculiar distortions of the appearance of objects or actual impairment of visual acuity. Hallucinations, confusion, delusional ideas, and other evidences of delirium are frequently seen in the early phases of the disease. The disease characteristically progresses with great rapidity, so that obvious deterioration may be seen from week to week. Sooner or later, in all cases, sudden myoclonic contractions of various muscle groups appear, perhaps unilaterally at first, but later becoming generalized. These generally are brought on by sudden sensory stimuli of all sorts, but they occur spontaneously as well, particularly in the late stages. Twitches of individual fingers are typical. Ataxia and dysarthria are likewise prominent. These changes gradually give way to stupor and coma, but the myoclonic contractions may continue to the end. In all cases, the electroencephalogram shows distinctive abnormalities, especially when the disease is fully developed. The total course of the illness is generally less than a year from onset; it may last only a few weeks or months. The outcome is invariably fatal, with death from intercurrent infection. Investigations of blood and cerebrospinal fluid consistently show no significant findings.

When the cases of subacute spongiform encephalopathy are set apart as a distinct group, the remaining cases that have been classified as Creutzfeldt-Jakob disease have as their outstanding features progressive dementia and spastic weakness of the limbs coming on in late middle age and progressing to death within a year or two. Other neurologic abnormalities that have been described include generalized rigidity, inexpressiveness ("masking") of the face, ataxia, convulsions, and muscular atrophy. Cases of this kind are the ones to which *Creutzfeldt-Jakob disease* is most applicable, if this name is to be used at all. On the whole, though, it would be preferable if complex or unclassifiable cases of diffuse degenerative disease of the nervous system were given descriptive names, rather than being grouped under what gives the impression of being a specific diagnostic term. At any rate, if the eponym is to be retained, those using it should make entirely clear what syndrome they are applying it to.

Differential diagnosis In the earliest stages, the mental changes may be misinterpreted as an atypical or unusually intense emotional reaction to environmental factors or as one of the major psychoses. Intoxication, as with bromides or other central nervous system depressants, or infection, such as neurosyphilis, may have to be considered, but none of these is likely to produce so dramatic a clinical picture. In its fully developed form, the only other disease process that resembles it is subacute sclerosing panencephalitis (SSPE) (see above), but this is chiefly a disease of children or young adults, rather than middle age or the presenile period. The cerebrospinal fluid regularly shows elevation of gamma-globulin (IgG) in SSPE, however, whereas it is normal in subacute spongiform encephalopathy. Cerebral lipidosis in children or young adults can result in a similar combination of myoclonus and dementia, but in such cases there are retinal changes that do not occur in any of the varieties of Creutzfeldt-Jakob disease.

No treatment is known. Antiviral agents have been ineffective. See Chap. 194 for further discussion of virologic aspects of these diseases.

OTHER CAUSES OF ENCEPHALITIS

The most important nonviral diagnostic possibilities to be considered in a patient with the syndrome of encephalitis are syphilis, pertussis, leptospirosis, relapsing fever, epidemic typhus, scrub typhus, Rocky Mountain spotted fever, trypanosomiasis, toxoplasmosis, cerebral malaria, trichinosis, schistosomiasis, and cysticercosis.

REFERENCES

Brody JA et al: *Chronic Infectious Neuropathic Agents (CHINA) and Other Slow Virus Infections,* vol. 40 in *Current Topics in Microbiology and Immunology,* New York: Springer-Verlag, 1967

Gagdusek DC et al: Slow, latent and temperate virus infections. Public Health Service Pub. no. 1378, 1965

Van Bogart L et al (eds.): *Encephalitides: Proceedings,* Amsterdam: Elsevier, 1961

Von Economo C: *Encephalitis Lethargica,* New York: Oxford, 1931

331 MULTIPLE SCLEROSIS AND OTHER DEMYELINATING DISEASES

DAVID C. POSKANZER
RAYMOND D. ADAMS

A large and important group of neurologic disorders are termed the *demyelinating diseases* because they share the common pathologic feature of foci of degeneration, involving the myelin sheath of nerve fibers. These foci vary in size, shape, distribution, and rate of development in the different illnesses. The axon often suffers damage as well, but the destruction of myelin is considered the primary change.

Because no clear cause has been ascertained for this group of diseases and a wide variety of etiologic theories have been proposed, including infective, metabolic, allergic, and vascular ones, a classification must be based on a combination of clinical and pathologic factors. It is, of course, possible that the process of demyelination may have several different causes and may be a common manifestation of different diseases. Although intermediate and transitional cases exist among the various demyelinating diseases, four syndromes can be clearly distinguished on the basis of history, clinical examination, and pathologic findings.

1 Acute disseminated encephalomyelitis (including postinfectious and postvaccinial encephalomyelitis)
2 Acute necrotizing hemorrhagic leukoencephalitis
3 Multiple sclerosis
4 Diffuse cerebral sclerosis

ACUTE DISSEMINATED ENCEPHALOMYELITIS

Acute disseminated encephalomyelitis may be defined as an acute encephalitic or myelitic process of variable course and severity, characterized by symptoms indicating damage chiefly to the white matter of the brain or spinal cord and pathologically by perivascular cellular infiltration and perivenous demyelination.

An acute encephalitis, myelitis, or encephalomyelitis of this type may occur concurrently or follow shortly upon the exanthem of measles, smallpox, chickenpox, and rubella. A similar demyelinating illness with multiple perivascular foci of demyelination occurs following vaccination against rabies and against smallpox. Some cases, clinically and pathologically indistinguishable from these two categories of acute disseminated encephalomyelitis, appear to develop without any clearly defined preceding illness or vaccination. The disease has grave significance because of the substantial death rate and the frequency of persistent neurologic defects in patients who recover. The cause of the process is unclear, but it is generally thought to represent a form of hypersensitivity. A laboratory model for the disease, the experimental allergic encephalomyelitis of animals, can be produced by inoculating the animals with a combination of sterile brain tissue and adjuvants.

PATHOLOGY No distinctive changes are seen on naked-eye examination of the brain. Microscopically, the white matter shows innumerable small zones of demyelination from 0.1 to 1 mm in diameter, which invariably surround small and medium-sized veins. The axons are more or less intact. There is a perivascular infiltration with lymphocytes, histiocytes, and plasma cells. Multifocal meningeal infiltration is another invariable feature but is rarely marked.

POSTVACCINIAL ENCEPHALOMYELITIS A severe demyelinating illness may occur following vaccination against rabies, with an incidence reported between 1 in 1,000 and 1 in 4,000 persons vaccinated. The lesion is presumably due to sensitization of brain tissue contained in the vaccine. The use of killed duck embryo vaccine which is free of nerve tissue has substantially reduced the incidence of the encephalomyelitic complications of rabies vaccination. More than 90 percent of the 30,000 rabies vaccinations performed in the Central states each year now employ the safer duck embryo vaccine.

Encephalomyelitis following vaccination against smallpox has been known since 1860 but appears to have occurred only in isolated instances until 1922, when a real epidemic of postvaccinial encephalomyelitis was first recognized. The disease usually begins in the tenth to twelfth day after vaccination, though it may appear at any time between the second and twenty-fifth days. The mortality rate is high, between 30 and 50 percent, but varies among epidemics. If recovery occurs, it is usually complete. A typical estimate of incidence is 1 in 5,000 vaccinated. The disease occurs much more frequently, perhaps as much as twenty times more often, after primary vaccination than after revaccination. Smallpox vaccination is no longer recommended as part of routine pediatric immunization schedules in the United States. The occurrence of the disease, as might be expected, parallels an increase in the number of persons vaccinated when smallpox threatens, but there is good evidence that the incidence of postvaccinial encephalomyelitis varies considerably from time to time and from one place to another. The source of material used for the vaccination seems to have no bearing on its occurrence.

The onset of the illness is generally abrupt, with headache, drowsiness, fever, and vomiting. There may be stiffness of the neck and other signs of meningeal irritation. Convulsions are occasionally seen. Soon afterward, signs of spinal cord involvement usually appear, with flaccid paralysis generally involving all four limbs, though hemiplegia may occur. Tendon reflexes disappear, and the plantar responses become extensor. Sphincter control is generally lost, and sensory loss, though variable, may be extensive and severe. Nystagmus, ocular palsies, and pupillary changes give evidence of brainstem involvement, and stupor and deepening coma indicate diencephalic or cerebral lesions. The onset of coma and evidence of brainstem involvement signify a rapid worsening of prognosis. Despite the general features of the typical case, variations are common. One patient may suffer a predominantly encephalitic illness with convulsions and coma and little evidence of cord damage, another may have a hemiplegia, or a pure transverse myelitis may occur without headache, neck stiffness, or clouding of consciousness. The site of vaccination has no influence on the neurologic syndrome, and the florid skin lesions in the form of a generalized vaccinia or erythematous rash do not increase the likelihood of neuroparalytic accident. Spinal fluid almost invariably shows an increase in protein and lymphocytes, but in rare cases it is normal.

The association of the neurologic disorder with vaccination or inoculation usually leaves the diagnosis in little doubt, and the characteristic combination of encephalitic and myelitic features will help to distinguish the condition from meningitis, virus encephalitis, and poliomyelitis. Rarely, an atypical case may mimic any one of these disorders. On occasion, the disease may suggest involvement of nerve roots and peripheral nerves and resemble idiopathic polyneuritis (Landry-Guillain-Barré syndrome).

Improvement involving recovery of consciousness and regression of neurologic signs may be surprisingly complete. A significant proportion of patients may show residual neurologic signs, intellectual impairment, and psychoneurotic sequelae many years after the illness, however.

POSTINFECTIOUS ENCEPHALOMYELITIS This syndrome is often referred to as parainfectious encephalomyelitis because of its onset prior to, in association with, or after the rash of measles or other exanthem.

Clinically evident neurologic complications occur in 1 in 800 to 1 in 1,000 cases of measles. Prior to widespread measles vaccination, a measles epidemic in a large city might have included 100,000 cases and therefore resulted in a substantial number of neurologic complications. The mortality rate among patients with such complications ranges from 10 to 20 percent, and about 50 percent of the victims are left with persistent neurologic damage. The rate of neurologic complications may, in fact, be considerably higher than is apparent clinically. A high rate of abnormalities in the spinal fluid and in the electroencephalogram is observed in the studies of children with measles. Patients without clinically apparent neurologic residua may undergo significant and sometimes permanent changes in behavior. The neurologic complications of measles alone provide adequate justification for the prevention of the disease through the use of vaccine.

Following smallpox the incidence of neurologic complications is approximately 2.5 cases out of 1,000. The occurrence of encephalomyelitis complicating chickenpox is less common, and that complicating rubella is quite rare. An acute demyelinating process probably occurs in association with mumps, but the clinical picture is complicated by the presence of a true viral encephalomyelitis in mumps and often cannot be differentiated from a postinfectious process in the living patient.

The syndrome generally begins 2 to 4 days after the rash. The most common clinical picture is one dominated by convulsions and deepening coma. Less commonly, the patient may develop hemiplegia, show evidence of cerebellar disease, or occasionally develop a transverse myelitis or polyradiculitis. Chorea and athetoid movements are also seen infrequently. In many cases the disease is much less severe and the patient suffers transient encephalitic illness with headaches, confusion, and signs of meningeal irritation. It is not entirely clear that all the neurologic complications described are truly encephalomyelitic; in some cases cerebrovascular disease, particularly thrombophlebitis, acute toxic encephalopathy (Reye's syndrome, Chap. 299), or hypoxic encephalopathy may be responsible.

The cerebrospinal fluid, as in postvaccinial encephalomyelitis, contains lymphocytes and an elevated protein level.

PREVENTION AND TREATMENT Selective use of smallpox vaccination in travelers and high-risk populations will considerably reduce the risk of encephalomyelitis.

The use of killed duck embryo vaccine may well have largely eliminated the occurrence of post-rabies-vaccination encephalomyelitis. Measles vaccine has eliminated the largest group of the postinfectious encephalomyelitides in the United States.

The use of ACTH or high-potency steroids appears to be the treatment of choice, though controlled trials of this treatment have not been carried out. The steroids, if given early, appear to be effective in controlling the manifestations of experimental allergic encephalomyelitis in animals.

ACUTE NECROTIZING HEMORRHAGIC ENCEPHALOMYELITIS

In a small number of patients dying from a fulminating encephalopathic illness, certain distinctive pathologic features may be found. On section of the brain, the white matter of one or both hemispheres is seen to be destroyed almost to the point of liquefaction. The involved tissue is pink or yellowish gray and flecked with multiple small hemorrhages. Sometimes similar changes are localized to the brainstem or spinal cord. On histologic examination one finds widespread necrosis of small blood vessels, necrosis of brain tissue around the vessels with intense cellular infiltration, multiple small hemorrhages, and a violent inflammatory reaction in the meninges. The pathologic picture resembles that of disseminated encephalomyelitis in its perivascular distribution, with the added feature of more widespread necrosis leading to diffuse sclerosis and a tendency to congregate into large foci in the cerebral hemispheres.

The clinical course of the illness resembles that of acute disseminated encephalomyelitis save for its apoplectiform onset and rapidity of progress, sometimes leading to death within 48 hr; it is also true that neurologic signs are frequently unilateral or purely bulbar in type, reflecting the localized nature of the pathologic process. It is probable that certain patients showing an explosive myelitic illness are suffering from a necrotizing myelitis of similar type, but pathologic evidence in support of this view has been difficult to obtain. The cerebrospinal fluid examination discloses a more intense reaction than in other demyelinating diseases. Often a polymorphonuclear pleocytosis of up to several thousand cells and a considerable increase in amount of protein are detected.

The etiology of this condition remains obscure, but the resemblance to the other demyelinating diseases should be noted, a resemblance which is strengthened by the fact that certain patients showing the typically fulminating clinical picture have recovered, some completely, others with neurologic sequelae of variable severity. Later, a few may develop typical multiple sclerosis. Acute encephalitis due to herpes simplex or other viruses also figures in the differential diagnosis. The points of similarity to other demyelinative diseases are sufficient to suggest that steroid drugs should be used in such cases; in several personally observed patients, we have had the impression that they produced a favorable result.

MULTIPLE SCLEROSIS

Multiple sclerosis, referred to in the British Commonwealth as *disseminated sclerosis* and among French-speaking physicians as *sclérose en plaque*, is one of the most common chronic neurologic diseases. It is characterized clinically by episodes of focal disorders of the central nervous system (spinal cord and brain) which remit and recur over a period of 20 to 30 or more years. Though it is pleomorphic in its clinical presentation, the picture it presents is determined by the location of foci of demyelination, which tend to have a predilection for certain portions of the nervous system. The result is a group of symptom complexes which can often be readily diagnosed.

Classical features include impaired vision, nystagmus, dysarthria, intention tremor, ataxia, impaired perception of position and impaired vibratory senses, bladder dysfunction, paraplegia, and alteration in emotional responses. For purposes of diagnosis, it is generally required that both evidence of more than one discrete lesion and a history of exacerbation and remission be present.

Diagnosis may be uncertain in the early years of the disease. Long latent periods between a minor initial symptom, which may not even come to medical attention, and the subsequent development of more characteristic ones may delay the final diagnosis. In most cases, relapses are interspersed with periods of remission, but in other cases (as many as half the total number) the disease presents as an intermittently or steadily progressive illness.

PATHOLOGY Macroscopically, the brain before being sectioned generally shows no evidence of disease, but the surface of the spinal cord may feel uneven. On section, numerous scattered lesions are seen which are slightly depressed and which, by virtue of their pinkish gray appearance (due to loss of myelin) stand out in contrast to the surrounding white matter. The lesions may vary in diameter from less than 1 mm to several centimers; they affect principally the white matter of brain and spinal cord and do not extend beyond the root entry zone of brainstem and spinal cord. They also encroach frequently on cerebral gray matter but do not destroy nerve cells. The lesions appear to have a predilection for elongate structures where myelin abuts pial veins, hence the frequent involvement of spinal cord and the optic nerves

and chiasm. They are frequently seen in the paraventricular areas of the brain in relation to the veins in the walls of the lateral ventricles.

The histologic appearance depends on the age of the lesion. Relatively recent lesions show a predominantly perivenous distribution of the demyelination with sparing of axis cylinders, degeneration of oligodendroglia, neuroglial reaction, and perivascular infiltration with mononuclear cells. Later large numbers of microglial phagocytes infiltrate the lesion, and astrocytes in and around it increase in number and size. A long-standing lesion, on the other hand, will show thickly matted, relatively acellular fibroglial tissue, with only occasional perivascular macrophages; in such a lesion intact axis cylinders may still be discovered, but many are destroyed, and this in turn leads to descending and ascending degeneration of long-fiber tracts. All gradations of pathologic change between these two extremes may be found in lesions of variegated size and shape.

ETIOLOGY The cause or causes of multiple sclerosis remain undetermined. A number of epidemiologic facts have been clearly established, however, which must eventually be incorporated in any etiologic hypothesis. The disease has been shown to be rare between the equator and latitudes 30 and 35° north and south. It becomes more common with increasing latitude thereafter. For example, the prevalence of multiple sclerosis is six times as great in Winnipeg, Mannitoba, as in New Orleans, Louisiana. An exception to the geographic pattern appears to exist in Japan, where the prevalence rates are uniform and extremely low. Several studies indicate that a person who migrates from a high risk to a low risk zone carries the high risk of multiple sclerosis with him, even though the disease may not become apparent until 20 years after migration. This pattern has been demonstrated both in South Africa and in Israel. However, if emigration occurs prior to age fifteen the risk of acquiring multiple sclerosis is that of the country into which the person has migrated.

An increase in familial occurrence of multiple sclerosis has long been recognized. The disease is about eight times more common in immediate relatives (parents and sibs) than in patients in the general population. Twin studies have failed, however, to corroborate a genetic predisposition, and within families with more than one affected member, no consistent genetic pattern is evident. There is a tendency to consider all diseases with an increased familial incidence, such as multiple sclerosis, as hereditary. Instances of the same condition in several members of the family may actually reflect common exposure to a similar environmental factor, however. For example, paralytic poliomyelitis is also eight times more common in immediate family members than in the general population.

The age distribution of the disease follows a normal distribution, with a mean between thirty and thirty-five. Women have a higher prevalence and incidence than men.

Several studies have now demonstrated a shift toward

higher socioeconomic groups in the general pattern of distribution of the disease in the population.

All these data favor an infection, presumably viral, contracted early in life and capable of evoking disease over the entire span of adolescence and adulthood. Its mechanism may be that of an autoimmune reaction, attacking myelin, but in its most intense form destroying all tissue elements, including axis cylinders. At the present time there has been no confirmation of this theory. The data favoring an infectious etiology with a long incubation period are epidemiologic.

PRECIPITATING FACTORS A variety of events occurring immediately before the onset of illness have been regarded as precipitating factors in relation to multiple sclerosis. These include various types of infection, emotional trauma, injury, and pregnancy. Though there is a definite increase in the number of exacerbations during the pregnancy year, other traumatic factors during the course of the illness, including lumbar puncture and surgical procedures, have not been shown to be of statistical significance.

CLINICAL MANIFESTATIONS About 40 percent of patients with multiple sclerosis have an episode of optic neuritis as their initial symptom. The syndrome is one of rapid onset over a period of several days of partial or total loss of vision in one eye, often associated with pain on movement of the eye. Characteristically, a scotoma will be present involving macular vision, but a wide variety of field defects may occur. Some patients will develop bilateral optic neuritis simultaneously or within a few days to weeks. In about half the patients, if serial examination is carried out some evidence of inflammation or elevation of the optic nerve, termed *optic papillitis,* will be seen. The occurrence of papillitis depends on the proximity of the demyelinating lesion to the nerve head. It should be recalled that the optic nerve is in fact a tract of the brain, because demyelinating lesions in multiple sclerosis are known not to occur outside the central nervous system. Of patients with optic neuritis about one-third recover completely, one-third will show considerable improvement, one-third will show no evidence of improvement whatever. As in most acute exacerbations of demyelinating disease, improvement in the majority of cases will have begun within 2 weeks of the onset of neurologic damage. Much longer periods of up to months may elapse, however, during which improvement in neurologic function may occur. It should be noted that a maximum of 40 percent of patients who develop optic neuritis will go on to have other lesions of multiple sclerosis. It is unclear at this time whether optic neuritis when it occurs alone and is not followed by other evidence of demyelinating disease is a subclass of multiple sclerosis with only a single lesion or a manifestation of other disease processes. No other etiology for optic neuritis has been established at this time.

The remaining 60 percent of patients with multiple sclerosis will present with some evidence of a lesion of the spinal cord or brainstem. The frequency of involvement of the posterior columns of the cord is responsible for the commonly related symptoms of tingling of the extremities and the tight bandlike sensations around trunk or limbs.

Numbness or weakness of a limb or one side of the body (arm and leg) or in an asymmetric distribution in all four extremities follows retrobulbar neuritis in frequency. The resulting clinical syndromes vary from mere dragging or poor control of one or both legs, to an ataxic paraparesis or spastic paraparesis. The tendon reflexes are hyperactive; the abdominal reflexes are absent, and plantar responses are extensor.

Diplopia, as a result of brainstem lesions, is another common presenting complaint. These lesions may cause an internuclear opthalmoplegia that is due to involvement of the medial longitudinal fasciculus and is characterized by inability to adduct one or the other eye on lateral gaze in either direction or by nystagmus present to a greater degree in the abducting than the adducting eye. An internuclear opthalmoplegia, when present bilaterally in a young adult, is virtually diagnostic of multiple sclerosis. Other ocular palsies also occur but less frequently. Other manifestations of brainstem involvement include transient facial anesthesia and vertigo and vomiting because of affection of the vestibular connections. The occurrence of tic douloureux in a young person should immediately bring to mind the diagnosis of multiple sclerosis due to involvement of the fifth cranial nerve.

Nystagmus and cerebellar ataxia, with or without weakness and spasticity of the limbs, represent another common syndrome and reflect involvement of the cerebellar and corticospinal tracts and their connections. The ataxia of cerebellar type can be recognized by scanning speech, tremors and titubation of the head, intention tremors of arms and legs, and incoordination of voluntary movements. It may be mixed with sensory ataxia from involvement of the posterior columns of the spinal cord. Ultimately spinal cord involvement becomes predominant in most advanced cases. It is a common aphorism that the patient with multiple sclerosis presents with symptoms in one leg and signs in both. The patient will complain of weakness, ataxia, or sensory loss in one lower extremity and have evidence of bilateral corticospinal tract disease manifested by Babinski's sign in both lower extremities.

Symptoms of bladder dysfunction, including hesitancy, urgency, frequency, and incontinence, occur commonly with spinal cord involvement. In males, these symptoms are often associated with impotence, a symptom which the patient will not often report unless specifically questioned in this regard. About 5 percent of patients with multiple sclerosis, over the course of their disease, will have a seizure, presumably as the result of involvement of subcortical connections.

It has often been pointed out that patients with multiple sclerosis develop euphoria, a pathologic cheerfulness or lack of concern which seems inappropriate in relation to their obvious neurologic deficit. This syndrome, the result of lesions of the white matter, probably of the frontal lobes, is often associated with other signs of cerebral impairment. There are, however, a large number of patients who are depressed, irritable, and short-tempered, as a reaction to the disabling features of the disease. They may also have other psychologic deficits, such as loss of memory, because of lesions in other locations.

CLINICAL COURSE The symptoms described above may occur individually or in combination during exacerbations. Some patients will have a series of exacerbations of the disease, each with complete remission. Often such exacerbations may be severe enough to cause total quadriplegia or even coma. Most patients will have a series of exacerbations, each followed by a remission or stabilization and leaving in its wake some evidence of permanent neurologic deficit upon which succeeding acute manifestations are superimposed. After a period of years some patients who have had a series of acute exacerbations tend to develop an inexorably progressing downhill course. When the initial course of the disease is steadily progressive and the lesion is limited to the spinal cord, diagnosis is particularly difficult. Such cases tend to occur among the older group of patients. It has been suggested that this syndrome be considered a special subclass of multiple sclerosis, but it probably represents only a late phase of the disease. Diagnosis can be made only by exclusion or may be confirmed by abnormality of spinal fluid.

CEREBROSPINAL FLUID In a small number of cases, particularly the acute ones, there may be a slight mononuclear pleocytosis in the spinal fluid. This pleocytosis is in fact the only way in which activity of the disease may be measured. None of the other laboratory tests aid in measuring the activity or inactivity of the disease.

The proportion of gamma-globulin in the spinal fluid appears to be altered in multiple sclerosis, while the protein content is usually normal. The alteration in distribution of globulins may be demonstrated by an abnormality of the colloidal gold curve, usually a first-zone abnormality, but occasionally midzone in type, in the presence of a negative Wassermann reaction. When gamma-globulin content is measured directly, it is abnormal in about 60 percent of the patients with multiple sclerosis. The gamma-globulin abnormality, however, tends to reflect the duration of the disease, and therefore is usually abnormal in the established case rather than in an initial exacerbation when an abnormal laboratory test would be helpful in establishing the diagnosis.

Some patients with demyelinating disease will have elevations of spinal fluid protein, but a spinal fluid protein in excess of 100 mg per 100 ml is so uncommon in multiple sclerosis that another diagnosis should be entertained.

Acute multiple sclerosis Occasionally, multiple sclerosis runs an acute or subacute course leading to death in weeks or months. Alternatively, an acute course may develop rapidly, then remit partially or completely, to be followed by characteristic relapses. In some of these cases, the onset is marked by headache, vomiting, delirium, and by a succession of symptoms indicating severe involvement of the brainstem or the brain, optic nerves, and spinal cord. In the so-called "cerebral" cases, there may be mental changes, convulsions, aphasia, hemianopia, and variable long-tract signs; the spinal type may show the picture of transverse myelitis. These forms of the disease are uncommon and are difficult to distinguish from disseminated encephalomyelitis, with which we tend to group them. They differ pathologically in the larger size of lesions, being more like those of multiple sclerosis.

Neuromyelitis optica syndrome This disorder, referred to as *Devic's disease*, is said to represent a combination of bilateral optic neuritis and transverse myelitis. Attempts at clinical description of patients with this combination of symptoms have failed to provide any data of prognostic value. Perhaps it is best to consider neuromyelitis optica as a particular form of multiple sclerosis. Pathologic studies of fatal cases, particularly those in which cavitation of white matter is found, have revealed a more acute and uniformly destructive process than is often seen in multiple sclerosis, however. Recurrence of this necrotizing form gives rise to a clinicopathologic state known as subacute necrotizing myelitis (see Chap. 325).

DIAGNOSIS In the characteristic case with evidence of wide dissemination of the lesions throughout the nervous system, the diagnosis of multiple sclerosis is in little doubt. It is an excellent clinical rule that the disease should not be diagnosed when all the patient's symptoms and signs can be explained by a single lesion. Disseminated encephalomyelitis is a self-limited, monophasic disease, and stupor and coma occur only rarely in multiple sclerosis. The other acute manifestations may mimic labyrinthitis, meningovascular syphilis, and encephalitis.

Confusion may occasionally arise with the hereditary ataxias, which are generally distinguished by their familial incidence and other associated genetic traits and by their stereotyped clinical pattern. Amyotrophic lateral sclerosis and subacute combined degeneration may occasionally be mimicked by demyelinating disease, but muscle wasting, fasciculations, and the total absence of sensory involvement will identify the former, and the latter can be confirmed by a low level of vitamin B_{12} in the serum, the presence of megaloblasts in the bone marrow, anemia present in many cases, and the absence of acid in the gastric secretions.

Patients with a progressive spastic paraplegia should be carefully evaluated for the presence of intrathecal neoplasm or cervical spondylosis. Radicular pain at some point in the illness is a frequent manifestation of neoplasm and is rare in multiple sclerosis, and severe muscle wasting due to anterior horn or spinal root involvement, as is sometimes seen in spondylosis, is almost unknown in multiple sclerosis except in the rare cases of necrotizing myelitis. The occurrence of nystagmus in association with other neurologic symptoms should be carefully evaluated. A common cause of nystagmus is the ingestion of barbiturates or diphenylhydantoin. The possibility that an anxious patient with another neurologic lesion has taken a barbiturate to aid him in sleep should never be disregarded when nystagmus in association with evidence of a lesion elsewhere might establish a diagnosis of multiple sclerosis.

Basilar impression of the skull, or platybasia, should also be considered in the differential diagnosis, but patients with these conditions have a characteristic shortening of the neck, and careful radiographs of the base of the skull will be diagnostic. Occasional tumors of the posterior fossa have been misdiagnosed as multiple sclerosis because of the affection of a wide variety of neurologic systems in the brainstem.

Careful clinical appraisal will usually lead to accurate diagnosis, but the label "multiple sclerosis" should not be placed upon a patient until the evidence is unequivocal. Such a diagnosis will explain almost any subsequent neurologic event, and attention may be directed away from the possibility of another, perhaps treatable, disease.

PROGNOSIS The duration of the disease is exceedingly variable. Though some patients die within a few months, the average duration of the disease is in excess of 20 years. At the end of 25 years one-third of patients are still actively carrying out their work and two-thirds of those surviving are still ambulatory. Patients with milder and quiescent disease are, of course, less likely to come to the attention of the hospital-oriented physician. In a recent epidemiologic study, 74 percent of patients with multiple sclerosis survived 25 years, as compared with 86 percent of the comparable general population.

The final state of the bedridden, incontinent patient, racked by painful flexor spasms of the lower limbs and febrile episodes of intercurrent infection from bedsores is one of the most distressing in medicine.

TREATMENT A large number of remedies have been tried in the treatment of multiple sclerosis, and many have been thought to be successful because of its remitting nature. Only the use of adrenocorticotrophic hormone (ACTH) has withstood evaluation in reasonably controlled trials of exacerbations of both optic neuritis and multiple sclerosis. A substantial group of patients, however, fail to respond to this treatment in the acute exacerbation.

ACTH has been generally preferred over the corticosteroids in the treatment of multiple sclerosis because the initial trials and control studies have been carried out with it. A variety of dosage regimens have been employed. It seems important that a high dose be used initially to be effective. We give ACTH intravenously in a dose of 80 units in 500 ml dextrose and water for 3 days, followed by 40 units of gel intramuscularly every 12 hr for 7 days. The dose is then reduced by 10 units every 3 days. Many patients who show improvement on this therapy continue to improve or maintain their previous improvement even though the medication is gradually reduced and discontinued. Other patients begin to have a recurrence of symptoms as the dose is gradually reduced and are often maintained on small doses of ACTH (20 to 40 units) every other day for a period of several months. Because of the risk of potassium depletion, the patients are given potassium supplement in a dose of 60 mEq a day. Euphoria and depression may be severe enough to terminate medication, and a tranquilizer may be necessary because of the complaints of difficulty in sleeping and nervousness. The occurrence of peripheral edema due to sodium retention can be treated with mild diuretics and salt restriction. Gastrointestinal bleeding and the activation of tuberculosis should be considered as possible complications of the treatment. Hirsutism and acne cannot be prevented but disappear when the medication is stopped.

The importance of an understanding and sympathetic physician cannot be overemphasized in the care of patients with a chronic debilitating neurologic disease of this kind. Some patients consider the uncertainty of prognosis worse than true disability. General support can be rendered by providing bedrest in acute exacerbations, prevention of excessive fatigue, and meticulous attention to the prevention of bedsores in the disabled patient by the use of alternating pressure mattresses, silicone gel pads, and other special devices. The use of belladonna alkaloids and bethanechol chloride in the treatment of bladder dysfunction can be helpful. Antibiotics and acidifying drugs to treat and suppress urinary tract infections should also be employed. In patients with disorders of bowel function a program of bowel training can often be successfully undertaken. Injections of dilute solutions of phenol either into peripheral nerves or intrathecally for relief of spasticity and flexor spasms have been of value.

DIFFUSE CEREBRAL SCLEROSIS

In 1912 Schilder first called attention to a disease causing progressive massive demyelination of the white matter often beginning in one or both occipital or temporal lobes. It has been referred to as *Schilder's disease* or *encephalitis periaxialis diffusa.* Since that time, many other cases have been described, some resembling Schilder's original description, others differing with respect to familial occurrence and widespread symmetric destruction and gliosis of the white matter, often with metachromatic bodies and globoid bodies representing catabolic products of myelin.

The diffuse types of cerebral sclerosis constitute a group of entities, including the globoid body leukodystrophy of Krabbe, sudanophilic leukodystrophy, and the metachromatic leukodystrophy of Greenfield which may involve peripheral nerves as well as central nervous system tissue. For the moment, they are a group of diseases with unknown etiology, occurring sporadically, though occasionally running in families, characterized clinically by progressive visual failure, mental deterioration, and spastic paralysis and pathologically by massive demyelination of the white matter of the cerebral hemispheres. Each entity is unquestionably a specific inherited biochemical defect in the metabolism of myelin proteolipids. The causes of these diseases for the moment are unknown, and there is no treatment. For further discussion see appropriate heading under degenerative nervous diseases (Chap. 333).

REFERENCES

ADAMS RD, KUBIK CS: The morbid anatomy of the demyelinative disease. Am J Med 12:510, 1952

MCALPINE D et al: *Multiple Sclerosis, a Reappraisal,* Edinburgh and London: Livingston, 1965

MILLAR JHD: *Multiple Sclerosis. A Disease Acquired in Childhood,* Springfield, Ill.: Charles C Thomas, 1971

PERCY AK et al: Multiple sclerosis in Rochester, Minnesota. A 60-year appraisal. Arch Neurol 25:105, 1971

POSKANZER DC: Epidemiological evidence for a viral etiology for multiple sclerosis, in *Slow, Latent, and Temperate Virus Infections*, U.S. Department of Health, Education and Welfare, NINDB Monograph no. 2, 1965, p. 55

332 METABOLIC AND NUTRITIONAL DISEASES OF THE NERVOUS SYSTEM

HUGO MOSER
MAURICE VICTOR
RAYMOND D. ADAMS

Each of these categories of diseases is based on intricate and often unique biochemical changes within the nervous system, and for this reason they are described here in one chapter, even though their causes and pathogeneses are widely divergent.

METABOLIC DISEASES OF THE NERVOUS SYSTEM

One large group of metabolic diseases of the nervous system is related to a demonstrable fault in general metabolism, traceable to a disease of the heart and circulation, lungs, liver, kidneys, and endocrine glands. Acute hypoxia, hypercapnia, acute hepatic stupor or coma, uremia, hypoglycemia, hyperglycemia with hyperosmolarity, hyponatremia, hypo- and hyperkalemia, acidosis (diabetic, uremic, and other), Addison's disease, Cushing's syndrome, hyper- and hypothyroidism, and hypoparathyroidism are the most typical examples. A second group comprises disorders of the nervous system and other organ systems in which a metabolic abnormality affects both the brain and other organs. Here reference is made to such conditions as mucopolysaccharidoses, the lipidoses, leukodystrophies, hepatolenticular degeneration, porphyria, galactosemia, glycogen storage disease, several of the syndromes of aminoaciduria with mental defect, and the serum lipoprotein abnormalities. Many of these diseases are familial, as are others of still a third group which encompasses cerebral disorders of assumed metabolic origin in which no evidence of disease in other viscera or in blood can presently be evoked. Representative of this third class of disease are some of the leukodystrophies and lipid storage diseases, Friedreich's ataxia, dystonia musculorum deformans, Jakob-Creutzfeldt-Heidenhain's disease, and many others discussed in the chapter on degenerative diseases. It requires no imagination to see that only a thin veil of ignorance separates the disease of this third category from those called *degenerative* (see Chap. 333).

A classification of the above type provides a conceptual locus for all the known varieties of metabolic nervous disease and ultimately will bring them into orderly relation to the chemistry of the nervous system. However, it leaves the clinician without a practical approach to the subject until he has been able to reach a diagnosis. Only then is it possible to turn to the relevant published literature for detailed information concerning his patient. More helpful, it would seem, would be a classification in which diseases with similar clinical manifestations are grouped together. Final diagnosis would depend then on the differentiation by a combination of clinical and laboratory methods of the several diseases subsumed in a single syndrome. Such is the scheme which follows.

Only a few of these many diseases will be considered in detail here, and the reader is referred to other sections of the book for the definitive discussion of the metabolic aberration and its main clinical expression, if generalized. Also, in attempting to classify any given patient, reference should be made to the syndromes listed in Chaps. 333 and 334.

Syndrome of impaired consciousness

The general character of these types of derangement has been described in detail in Chap. 22, and it was there stated that a metabolic disorder of the brain should be considered when there was an acute disturbance of consciousness without localizing or lateralizing signs and without change in the cerebrospinal fluid. Intoxication with alcohol or other drugs enters prominently in the differential diagnosis, as do nutritional disorders due to lack of B vitamins.

ACUTE HYPOXIC ENCEPHALOPATHY The mechanism of cerebral damage from hypoxia has already been described in Chap. 22. But it is important for the clinician to realize that a hypoxic or ischemic accident (the two are virtually indistinguishable neurologically) encountered in the emergency room or on the wards of a general hospital is one of the more frequent complications of many diseases, causing death or, even worse, permanent coma or mental enfeeblement. The medical situations which most often have led to this have been strangulation (vomitus or blood in bronchi, surgical pack, sponge, or foreign body in trachea); respiratory-cardiac arrest during inhalation, spinal, or intravenous anesthesia; cardiac disease with arrest; infective and traumatic shock; any disease which causes paralysis of respiratory muscles, such as poliomyelitis or acute idiopathic polyneuritis; and central nervous system disease (cerebrovascular lesions, encephalopathies in children, epilepsy, or respiratory arrest). Carbon monoxide intoxication has similar effects.

Mild hypoxia induces only inattentiveness, poor judgment, and motor incoordination and has no lasting effects if corrected. Severe hypoxia causes coma within less than a minute, but again recovery will be complete if breathing, oxygenation of blood, and cardiac action are restored within 3 to 5 min. Periods of hypoxia with coma that exceed 5 to 6 min usually result in serious and permanent injury to the brain, particularly in those parts most susceptible to injury because of the marginal efficiency of their circulation (globus pallidus, cerebral cortex, especially that of the hippocampus and parieto-occipital regions, "border-zone regions," and cerebellar cortex). However, it is difficult to judge clinically the degree of hypoxia since slight heart action or an imperceptible blood pressure may serve to maintain some degree of circulation. Hence some individuals have made an excellent recovery after alleged cerebral hypoxia of 8 to 10 min or longer. *An important clinical rule is that degrees of hypoxia which do not at any time abolish consciousness rarely if ever cause permanent damage to the nervous system.*

The patient who has suffered a serious hypoxic episode may be breathing normally and have good color and normal heart action when first seen. The hypoxic crisis has already terminated. Yet he may be profoundly comatose with dilated, fixed pupils, eyes slightly divergent and motionless, the limbs inert, and tendon reflexes diminished or absent. Within a few minutes after cardiac action and breathing have been restored, generalized convulsions and also isolated or grouped twitches of muscles (myoclonus) supervene. If the damage is severe, coma persists and decerebrate postures may be present or occur upon pinching the limbs, and bilateral Babinski signs can also be evoked. In the first 24 to 48 hr death may terminate this state in a setting of rising temperature, deepening coma, and circulatory collapse. If the patient survives this period, he usually begins to respond in varying degrees. A period of restlessness and chaotic movement, sometimes clearly revealing ataxia, and myoclonic jerks or choreoathetosis may then appear and endure for variable periods of time.

The most severe degree of hypoxia, often complicated by circulatory collapse (ischemia), is manifested by complete unreceptiveness and unresponsiveness with abolition of all brainstem reflexes. Natural respiration cannot be sustained. *Only the cardiac action and blood pressure are maintained.* No electrical activity is seen in the patient's electroencephalogram (it is isoelectric). This is called the *brain death syndrome.* At autopsy nearly all the cerebral, cerebellar, and brainstem structures are found to have been destroyed.

When this syndrome of cerebral death occurs, the outlook for recovery is hopeless, and one must consider the advisability of discontinuing all supportive measures (respiratory aid, vasopressor agents, etc.). Such victims often become donors of vital organs. However, one must exercise caution in reaching the conclusion of irreversible brain damage unless the evidence of hypoxia and ischemia is definite, for anesthesia, drug intoxication, and hypothermia may also cause deep coma and an isoelectric electroencephalogram but permit recovery.

When improvement takes place, as it usually does in the less damaged patients, consciousness may be regained and then confusion, visual agnosia, or any one of several types of abnormal movement (action or intention myoclonus, extrapyramidal rigidity, choreoathetosis) becomes manifest. Some of these patients quickly pass

TABLE 332-1
Classification of metabolic diseases of the nervous system

I Metabolic diseases presenting as a syndrome of episodic confusion, stupor, or coma
- *A* Hypoxia
- *B* Hypercapnia
- *C* Hypoglycemia
- *D* Hyperglycemia
- *E* Acidosis (including ketotic hyperglycinemia and isovaleric and methylmalonic aciduria)
- *F* Uremia
- *G* Hypo- and hypernatremia and hypo- and hyperkalemia
- *H* Hepatic failure and Eck fistula
- *I* Addison's disease
- *J* Maple syrup urine disease (in infants)
- *K* Argininosuccinic aminoaciduria, hyperglycinemia, citrullinemia, hyperammonemia, isovaleric acidemia (in children), and methylmalonic aciduria

II Metabolic diseases presenting as progressive extrapyramidal syndrome
- *A* Acquired and familial hepatocerebral degeneration
- *B* Kernicterus
- *C* Fahr's disease
- *D* Lesch-Nyhan hyperuricemia

III Metabolic diseases presenting as progressive cerebellar ataxia
- *A* Lipid storage diseases
- *B* Bassen-Kornzweig disease
- *C* Argininosuccinic aciduria and Hartnup disease
- *D* Cerebrotendinous xanthomatosis
  (Friedreich's ataxia and the familial cerebellar ataxias, the degenerative diseases from which the above must be differentiated, will ultimately by brought into this category.)
- *E* Ataxia telangiectasia

IV Metabolic diseases presenting as polyneuropathy
- *A* Refsum's disease
- *B* Porphyria
- *C* Tangier disease
- *D* Macro- and cryoglobulinemias
- *E* Some cases of Bassen-Kornzweig syndrome and ataxia telangiectasia
  (Probably Charcot-Marie-Tooth peroneal muscular atrophy, Dejerine-Sottas hypertrophic polyneuropathy, and other of the chronic familial degenerative diseases of the peripheral nervous system will eventually fall into this group.)

V Metabolic diseases presenting as mental retardation
- *A* Phenylketonuria
- *B* Milder forms of maple syrup urine disease
- *C* Homocystinuria
- *D* Galactosemia
- *E* Histidinemia, cystathioninuria, argininosuccinic aciduria, hyperlysinemia, citrullinemia, hyperammonemia, isovaleric acidemia, carnosinemia, hyperalininemia, methylmalonic aciduria, sulfituria, hyperglycinemia, hypervalinemia, hydroxyprolinemia, Lowe's syndrome or oculocerebrorenal syndrome (see Table 96-1).

VI Metabolic disorders associated with dementia
- *A* Hypothyroidism
- *B* Cushing's disease
- *C* Hypoparathyroidism and Fahr's syndrome
  (Lipid storage diseases and leukodystrophies will eventually fall into this category.)
- *D* Chronic hepatic encephalopathy

through this acute hypoxic phase and proceed to make a full recovery; others are left with a permanently disabling syndrome. Seizures may or may not continue to be a problem. One unexplained phenomenon is an initial improvement for 1 to 2 days followed by a relapse, further progression of the neurologic syndrome, and death after 1 to 2 weeks. In some instances of carbon monoxide poisoning this hypoxic relapse, delayed for 1 to 2 weeks, has been found associated with a widespread cerebral demyelination.

The permanent neurologic sequelae, which may be classed as the *posthypoxic syndromes*, are *dementia* with or without extrapyramidal signs, *visual agnosia, parkinsonian syndrome, choreoathetosis, cerebellar ataxia*, and *intention or action myoclonus*.

The essential mechanism in hypoxic encephalopathy is a lack of oxygen and an arrest of all aerobic metabolic processes necessary for the Krebs tricarboxylic cycle and the electron transport system. Neurons are injured to such a degree they cannot survive. The phenomenon of delayed progression is not understood but may be due to the blockage or exhaustion of some enzymatic process during the period when brain metabolism is restored or even increased (as in hyperthermia).

Diagnosis depends on (1) the history of the hypoxic event and evidence of reduced oxygenation of arterial blood or CO intoxication (the latter is indicated by its cherry red color or spectroscopic band only for a few minutes to hours after the episode), blood pressures below 70 systolic, or cardiac arrest; (2) the typical sequences of events outlined above after a possible hypoxic episode has terminated. Renal damage (anuria) and injury to the myocardium may also have occurred, and provide corroborative evidence of hypoxia (see Chap. 33).

Treatment is mainly the prevention of a critical degree of hypoxic injury. After the physician quickly secures a clear airway, artificial respiration, external thoracic cardiac massage and open-chest surgery, and the use of a cardiac defibrillator or pacemaker all have their place, and every second counts in their prompt utilization. Once cardiac and pulmonary function are restored, there is some evidence from the work of Blalock and his associates that reducing cerebral metabolic requirements by continuous hypothermia for 48 to 72 hr may prevent the delayed worsening referred to above. Oxygen may be of value during the first hours and days, but it is probably of little use after the blood becomes well oxygenated. Dexamethasone intravenously in doses of 8 to 12 mg every 6 hr helps combat brain swelling. Seizures should be controlled by intramuscular sodium hydantoin (Dilantin), 100 mg every 6 hr, or sodium phenobarbital, 120 mg every 4 hr by mouth or stomach tube or four times a day parenterally. If the seizures are severe, continuous, and unresponsive to drugs, controlled respiration and curare may be helpful. Often the seizures cease after a few days. If they persist, they are often myoclonic, and Mebaral, in divided doses up to 500 mg per day, or phenobarbital, 300 mg per day, may be useful in their control.

HYPERCAPNIA (AND HYPOXIA) IN PULMONARY DISEASE Chronic emphysema, chronic fibrosing lung disease, and in some instances a seeming inadequacy of the respiratory center (Chap. 249) lead to chronic respiratory acidosis, with an elevation of P_{CO_2} and a reduction in arterial P_{O_2}. Secondary polycythemia, cor pulmonale, and heart failure often accompany these diseases of the lungs, and pulmonary infection may be superimposed. The clinical syndrome comprises an action tremor and a coarse twitching of all muscles sustained in a state of contraction (termed *asterixis*), *headache, papilledema, mental dullness, drowsiness, confusion*, and *coma*.

The cerebrospinal fluid is under increased pressure. P_{CO_2} may exceed 75 mm Hg, and the oxygen content of arterial blood ranges from 85 percent to as low as 40 percent. The mechanism of cerebral damage is said to be CO_2 narcosis, but the biochemical details are not known. The danger of administering morphine, which depresses the respiratory center, or the inhalation of oxygen, which removes the sole stimulus to the respiratory center, is now widely recognized; many patients so treated in the past have lapsed into coma (CO_2 narcosis) and have died.

Forced ventilation with an intermittent positive-pressure device, inhalation of oxygen if hypoxia is severe, the treatment of heart failure with digitalis and diuretic measures, venesection to reduce the viscosity of the blood, and antibiotics to combat pulmonary infection have been the most effective program of therapy and have often resulted in a surprising degree of improvement that may be maintained for months or years. If coma should persist, the arterial O_2 level should be rechecked; it may be critically reduced. Or the pH of cerebrospinal fluid (CSF) may be very low, in the range of 7.15 to 7.25. In CO_2 narcosis the correction of the acidosis of blood is easier than CSF, which tends to lag.

Unlike pure hypoxic encephalopathy, prolonged coma due to hypercapnia is exceptional. The papilledema and the jerky, intermittent postures or asterixis (the latter characteristic only of liver failure, hypercapnia, uremia, and, rarely, other metabolic disorders) are features of diagnostic import. The syndrome is apt to be mistaken for brain tumor, a confusional psychosis of nondescript type, or a disease causing chorea or myoclonus. In the latter instance it must be distinguished from a chronic extrapyramidal syndrome, as outlined below.

HYPOGLYCEMIC ENCEPHALOPATHY This condition is discussed in Chaps. 22 and 90. It is a rather frequent cause of profound coma, episodic confusion, and convulsions and merits separate consideration as a metabolic disorder of brain function. The essential biochemical datum is a blood sugar level of less than 25 to 30 mg per 100 ml, lasting 1 to 2 hr, and leading to exhaustion of the store of cerebral glucose and glycogen. Within this brief span of time, as cerebral oxidation proceeds without exogenous glucose, the structural components of neurons i.e., lipid and protein substances, are metabolized, and irreversible damage occurs.

Clinically the most common situations in which severe hypoglycemia develops are (1) accidental or deliberate overdose of insulin or of one of the oral antidiabetic agents, (2) insulin therapy in schizophrenia, (3) an islet cell insulin-secreting tumor of the pancreas, (4) rarely, following an alcoholic debauch or some form of acute liver disease such as acute nonicteric hepatoencephalopathy of childhood (Reye's syndrome), (5) glycogen storage disease in infancy, (6) an idiopathic state in the neonatal period. In functional hyperinsulinism the hypoglycemia is rarely of sufficient severity or duration to damage the central nervous system.

The clinical picture has already been sketched. The initial symptoms, as the level of blood glucose descends, are nervousness, hunger, and cold, and these gradually give way to confusion, drowsiness, and occasionally excitement or overactivity. In the next stage forced sucking, grasping, motor restlessness, muscular spasms, and finally decerebrate rigidity occur, in that sequence. Myoclonic twitching and convulsions may develop in some patients but are by no means the rule. Deepening coma is attended by dilatation of pupils, pale skin, shallow respiration, slow heart, and hypotonicity of limb musculature—the so-called "medullary phase" of hypoglycemia. If glucose is administered before this medullary phase appears, the patient is restored to normalcy, retracing the aforementioned steps in reverse order. However, once this medullary phase is reached, and particularly if it persists for a time before the hypoglycemia is corrected by intravenous glucose or spontaneously by the so-called "gluconeogenic activities" of the adrenal glands and liver, recovery is delayed for a period of days or weeks and may be incomplete. Although the lowering of blood sugar is equally severe in both instances, a huge dose of insulin with intense hypoglycemia, even of relatively brief duration (30 to 60 min), is more dangerous than smaller ones, possibly because it impairs or exhausts essential enzymes. This condition cannot then be overcome by large quantities of glucose intravenously. The cerebral cortex suffers major damage; cortical nerve cells degenerate and are replaced by microgliacytes and astrocytes. The distribution of lesions is not quite the same as in hypoxic encephalopathy.

The major difference, clinically, between hypoglycemia and hypoxia lies in the clinical setting of the illness and the mode of evolution of the neurologic disorder. Hypoglycemia usually unfolds more slowly over a period of 30 to 60 min rather than suddenly within seconds or a few minutes. The recovery phase and sequelae of the two conditions bear close resemblance and may not be easily differentiated. Recurrent hypoglycemia, as with an islet cell tumor, may masquerade for some time as an episodic confusional psychosis or convulsive illness, and diagnosis awaits a period of demonstrably low blood sugar or hyperinsulinism (see Chap. 90).

The correction of the hypoglycemia at the earliest moment is the obvious therapy. It is not known whether hypothermia or other measures will increase the tolerance of safety period in hypoglycemia or alter the outcome.

HEPATIC STUPOR AND COMA Chronic hepatic insufficiency with portacaval shunting of blood is often punctuated by epidoses of mental dullness, drowsiness, confusion, stupor or coma, "flapping tremor" of outstretched limbs, or intermittency of sustained postures (asterixis). This condition is described fully in Chap. 296. Less widely known is the fact that a pure portal-systemic shunt (Eck fistula) may be attended by a similar clinical picture. Also, there are a number of hereditary diseases of childhood which may lead to episodic coma with or without seizures. A special type of acute nonicteric hepatoencephalopathy, first described by Reye and his associates, occurs in children, presenting a picture of an acute toxic encephalopathy (acute brain swelling).

In many patients the syndrome does not advance beyond the stage of "flapping" (asterixis) and confusion with mild electroencephalographic changes. In this mild form it must be differentiated from other acute confusional psychoses and delirium. A disorder of posture and movement may be prominent (grimacing, tremor, ataxia of gait, choreoathetosis), and the condition must then be distinguished from the other extrapyramidal syndromes.

Reducing the protein intake, ridding the intestinal tract of blood, suppressing the bacterial action on protein in the intestinal tract with neomycin or kanamycin, and administering sodium glutamate intravenously, which sometimes lowers the NH_3 levels of the blood, have been found to restore many of these patients to a relatively normal state. Should these therapeutic measures not control the protein intolerance, surgical exclusion of the bowel may be undertaken, but even this measure has proved of limited value in preventing a fatal outcome. L-Dopa may be beneficial.

Although the biochemical mechanism is not fully understood, the most plausible hypothesis is that the levels of blood NH_3 are elevated because the diseased or bypassed liver fails to convert it into urea; glucose metabolism of the brain at the Krebs cycle stage is disturbed by withdrawal of alpha-ketoglutarate from the metabolic pool as the cerebral tissues attempt to remove the NH_3 formed *in situ*.

In acute hepatitis, delirious, confusional, and comatose states also occur, but their mechanisms are still obscure. NH_3 may be elevated but usually not to a degree that would be expected to affect central nervous system function.

OTHER METABOLIC ENCEPHALOPATHIES Limitations of space permit only brief reference to other important metabolic disturbances of the brain. *Metabolic acidosis*, such as that due to diabetes mellitus or renal failure, produces the typical drowsiness, stupor, and coma with dry skin and Kussmaul breathing described in Chap. 88. Acidosis in infancy and childhood may occur in the course of hyperammonemia, isovaleric acidemia, maple syrup urine disease, hyperglycinemia, etc. There is no recognizable neuropathologic change. High-voltage, slow electrical activity predominates in the electroencephalogram, and correction of the acidosis restores nervous function to a normal level, provided coma has not persisted for too long a time and become complicated by hypoxia or hypotension, in which instance death supervenes. Extreme degrees of hyperosmolarity of the blood may develop in the course of diabetes mellitus (blood glucose greater than 400 mg) and in childhood in hypernatremic dehydration, resulting in both instances in convulsions, tremulous movements, and coma. Hyponatremia, usually with water intoxication, is another cause of infantile episodic coma. *Uremic encephalopathy* is poorly understood because of the existence of two neuro-

TABLE 332-2
Inborn errors of metabolism which cause neurologic symptoms in adults or older children

Disease	*Mental subnormality*	*Extra-pyramidal syndrome*	*Inter-mittent coma*	*Convul-sions*	*Cere-bellar syn-drome*	*Periph-eral neurop-athy*	*Spastic paralysis*	*Somatic abnormalities*	*Laboratory tests*	
									Blood	*Urine*
Phenylketonuria	90%			25%				Eczema—20% diminished rejuvenation	Phenylalanine <15 mg per 100 ml	Phenylpyruvic acid present Ferric chloride test positive
Maple syrup urine disease (intermittent form)	Present except in intermittent form		+	50%			Except in intermittent form	Maple syrup odor	Elevated leucine, valine, isoleucine	Branched chain keto acids present Ferric chloride test positive
Homocystinuria	60%			10–30%			Due to infarcts	Dislocated lenses, malar flush, long, thin extremities, genu valgum	Methionine increases	Cyanide nitroprusside test positive Homocystine increases
Hyperglycinemia	+		+ (In ketotic form)	+			+		Glycine increases	Glycine increases
Argininosuccinic aciduria	95%		20%	70%	30%			Short, stubby hair (trichorhexis nodosa), 60%	Ammonia (postprandial) increases	Argininosuccinic acid present
Histidinemia	About 50%								Histidine increases	Imidazolepyruvic acid present Ferric chloride test positive
Hartnup disease	20%				45%			Pellagralike rash (75%)		Monoamino monocarboxylic amino acids and indoles in excess
Hurler's syndrome	+							Cloudy cornea, small stature, lumbar gibbus, large liver and spleen, gargoyle facies, hydrocephalus	Alder-Reilly granules in leukocytes and α-L-iduronides deficiency	Polysaccharides increase (Chondroitin sulfate B, heparan sulfate)
Hunter's syndrome	Variable							Resemble Hurler's but less severe. No corneal clouding or lumbar gibbus	Alder-Reilly granules	Same as Hurler's
Sanfilippo syndrome	+							"Coarse" features, moderately small stature, moderate joint stiffness	α-Glucosaminidase or heparan sulfatase deficiency	Polysaccharides increase (heparan sulfate)
Wilson's disease	+	+		+	+			Kayser-Fleischer ring, cirrhosis of the liver	Ceruloplasmin decreases	Aminoaciduria
Hallervorden-Spatz syndrome	+	+								
Lesch-Nyhan syndrome	+	+					+	Self-mutilation, kidney stones, tophi	Uric acid increases Hypoxanthine-guanine and phosphoribosyl-transferase deficiency	Uric acid increases
Metachromatic leukodystrophy	+ (late)	Rarely		Up to 50%	+	+	+	Mild "cherry red spot" in macula	Arylsulfatase A decreases	Sulfatides increases Arylsulfatase A decreases
Refsum's disease					+	+		Retinitis pigmentosa ichthyosis	Phytenic acid increases	
Bassen-Kornzweig syndrome		Rarely			+	+		Retinitis pigmentosa	Acanthocytes absent, low density lipoproteins absent	
Tangier disease						+		Large tonsils with yellow or orange discoloration, occasionally large spleen	High density lipoprotein decrease Low cholesterol	
Cerebrotendinous xanthomatosis	+				+		+	Tendon xanthomata cataracts	Occasionally high cholesterol	
Lipidoses Juvenile (Speilmeyer-Vogt) Adult (Kuf's)	+			+	+		+	Pigmentary degeneration of retina		
Acute intermittent porphyria				+		+				Porphobilinogen increases
Ataxia telangiectasia		Rarely			+	+		Telangiectasia on conjunctiva and other characteristic areas	IgA immuno-globulin decrease (80%)	

logic syndromes, one of hypertensive encephalopathy, the other a somnolent twitching-convulsive syndrome (uremic twitching) which is highly characteristic of renal failure but still of obscure cause (see Chap. 268). Encephalopathy due to *Addison's disease* (adrenal insufficiency) may be attended by episodic confusion, stupor, or coma without special identifying features. Its basis remains unclear. Hypotension and diminished cerebral circulation and hypoglycemia are the principal mechanisms presently being proposed, and measures which correct these conditions appear to have been beneficial in some instances. Brain atrophy from whatever cause, if complicated by a febrile state, may result in coma.

A point not previously emphasized is that an episode of stupor or coma with or without convulsions in infancy and childhood may be the first medical datum to suggest a hereditary metabolic disease. In the case of maple syrup urine disease the first episode within the first week or two of life may prove fatal, and the physician's only role would be to watch for biochemical evidence of the disease in the next fetus or child; but milder forms also occur and induce a stupor or coma periodically or in conjunction with each infection which the child has. If the disease passes unrecognized, he becomes more and more retarded. Isovaleric acidosis, methylmalonic aciduria, and the ketotic form of hyperglycinemia may result in a comatose state due to acidosis.

Syndrome of extrapyramidal tremor, rigidity, dystonia, and choreoathetosis (See also Chap. 18)

Unlike the group of diseases that cause episodic coma, only a few of which are genetic in origin, the diseases that cause progressive extrapyramidal syndrome (and the other syndromes which follow—cerebellar ataxia, polyneuropathy, and mental retardation) are frequently hereditary. As is pointed out in Chap. 18, the patient is usually normal at birth, and the neurologic disorder becomes manifest in childhood and adolescence after its biochemical basis has existed for months or years. This fact tells us that the injury of the nervous system is a secondary phenomenon. The complexity of structure and organization and slow development of the nervous system account for the delayed onset and wide diversity of syndromes. But other organs do not escape altogether, and they may show manifest dysfunction early. These facts are important from the diagnostic point of view, for prevention of the neurologic syndrome looms as a possibility, providing the biochemical abnormality can be detected early and controlled. This required screening programs for the study of blood and urine. Thus a novel concept is introduced—that a patient comes to the attention of the physician not because of a complaint or clinical sign but a laboratory datum. The latter now stands as a cardinal manifestation of disease, a theme which is elaborated in the introduction to Chap. 2. Physicians and pediatricians must join forces in case finding and application at a community level of biochemical screening techniques and cytologic studies of the blood and other tissues (including amniotic fluid during the first and second trimesters of pregnancy). These diagnostic tests, new ones of which are being introduced every few months, are described in connection with special diseases.

The outstanding examples are the von Woerkom nonhereditary and the Wilson-Westphal-Strumpell hereditary types of hepatocerebral degeneration. In the *acquired hepatocerebral degeneration*, any type of chronic liver cirrhosis or portosystemic shunt (usually both factors are operative) including hemochromatosis may give rise to the *episodic stupor* and *coma*, mentioned above, and to a *slowly evolving predominantly faciocervical choreoathetosis* and *cerebellar ataxia of limbs*. Rarely a progressive spinal spastic paraplegia is added to the clinical picture (primary hepatic degeneration of pyramidal tracts of spinal cord; see Chap. 325). Neuronal loss and hyperplasia of protoplasmic astrocytes are found in the basal ganglia and cerebral and cerebellar cortices. Ceruloplasmin levels in blood and copper excretion in urine are normal. Control of the hyperammonemia, which usually attends this disease, is beneficial. In the *familial hepatocerebral degeneration* the syndrome is predominantly extrapyramidal. During adolescence and in early adult life a tremor of one or both arms or a slowly developing extrapyramidal rigidity of face, trunk, and limbs, resembling Parkinson's disease, introduces the disease, and evidence of liver disorder is difficult to discern. However, a cirrhosis of subacute hypertrophic type invariably precedes the onset of the neurologic abnormality, and, more importantly, there is a stage when a deficiency of ceruloplasmin and an abnormality of copper transport exist without evidence of malfunction of either liver or brain, as is pointed out in Chap. 103. In the late and relatively irreversible neurologic stages of the disease the clinical picture assumes a more striking form, consisting of rigidity, flexion dystonia, tremors, dysarthria and dysphagia, cerebellar ataxia, and occasionally choreoathetosis. Personality change and intellectual impairment appear at some point in the course of the illness and teminate in dementia or even as akinetic mutism. But, unlike the acquired hepatocerebral degeneration, episodic coma is rare. Easy substantiation of the diagnosis of the hereditary form of the disease is secured by the finding of the corneal (Kayser-Fleischer) rings of golden-brown copper pigment. The differential diagnosis includes consideration of the acquired forms of liver disease and degenerative diseases such as juvenile Parkinson's syndrome, Hallervorden-Spatz disease, or a late variety of lipid storage disease.

At an earlier period of life (late childhood) the gradual development of progressive rigidity, dystonia, and choreoathetosis, progressing over a period of 5 to 15 years, should suggest *Hallervorden-Spatz disease* (Chap. 333). Surely it, too, represents an inborn error of metabolism, affecting only the cerebrum, where degenerative changes in basal ganglia are accompanied by deposit of organic ferruginous compounds. However, there is no systemic disturbance of iron metabolism.

In hypoparthyroidism or pseudohypoparathyroidism, seizures and tetany tend to occur at some interval of time after the level of ionized calcium in the blood is lowered. In exceptional cases athetosis of an arm or leg may appear later (announcing the onset of a slowly progressive extrapyramidal syndrome which may in its complete form simulate Parkinson's disease), a cerebellar ataxia, or athetosis. Radiographs of the skull reveal deposits of calcium within the lenticular nuclei and dentate regions of the cerebellum. Postmortem examination discloses calcium salt in the walls of small vessels and as isolated rods or spherules, not unlike those seen in lesser degree in some normal elderly individuals. Measures which elevate serum calcium may halt the progress of the extrapyramidal syndrome and at the same time suppress the seizures and tetany. A similar picture of calcium deposits, severe enough to cause a mild progressive choreoathetosis, may be observed without any change in levels of serum Ca, in which instance it is called *Fahr's syndrome.* Some of our patients have also been mentally retarded.

Choreoathetosis, becoming manifest within the first year of life and persisting into adulthood, stands as a well-known sequela to hypoxia at birth and also to kernicterus. The latter is a complication of a neonatal Rh or ABO blood incompatibility (erythroblastosis fetalis) which usually develops in the first 3 to 5 days of postnatal life and is due to serum bilirubin levels in excess of 25 mg per 100 ml. The acute rise of bilirubin, occasioned by hemolysis and immaturity of the glucuronide pathway of the liver, destroys neurons in the subthalamic nuclei of Luys, the globus pallidi, and certain other brainstem nuclei. Lesions in the latter structures account for deafness and ocular gaze disorder. Exchange transfusions of female blood or other measures to lower serum bilirubin or to bind it have greatly reduced the incidence of this frequently fatal or permanently disabling neurologic condition (see Chap. 293).

There are obviously other conditions in childhood which give rise to rigidity and athetosis, but the cause of most of them cannot presently be ascertained. One new entity has recently been isolated—*Lesch-Nyhan syndrome* of hyperuricemia and hyperuricosuria due to a deficiency of hypoxanthine-guanine phosphoribosyl transferase. Feeblemindedness and a compulsive self-mutilation are other characteristics of this syndrome.

Syndrome of cerebellar ataxia (See also Chaps. 18 and 19)

As was stated above, signs of cerebellar disease, slowly becoming apparent during adult life, may be the first manifestation of acquired hepatocerebral degeneration. The speech becomes slurred (more than scanning or explosive), the gait mildly ataxic, and the limbs slow and clumsy or tremulous. Clues as to the nature of the difficulty are usually provided by the episodic coma and cirrhosis or portal hypertension. Later a faciocervicotrunkal choreoathetosis and dementia are added.

Young children who develop a cerebellar ataxia with or without a choreoathetosis, apraxia of ocular movements, delayed mental development, and recurrent sinopulmonary infections may later be found to have telangiectasia of ears and conjunctivas. Familial incidence and deficiency of a gamma-globulin (IgA) are other features that help to identify the disease before the telangiectasia appears; the relation of the latter to the pathogenesis remains unclear.

Cerebellar ataxia may also present as a hereditary, dominant neurologic syndrome in the more slowly evolving lipid storage diseases. It also constitutes one of the features of Bassen-Kornzweig's disease, cerebrotendinous xanthomatosis, and, rarely, Refsum's disease (see Chaps. 106 and 323).

Episodic cerebellar ataxia with or without seizures demarcates a special clinical state peculiar to childhood when it is traceable to Hartnup disease, argininosuccinic aminoaciduria, hyperalanimemia, and several other hereditary metabolic diseases of infancy. In the former condition there are skin lesions not unlike those of pellagra. The ataxia may appear after a seizure and last several days. Mental retardation may be added (see Chap. 96).

Syndrome of subacute or chronic polyneuropathy (See also Chap. 323)

An acute or slowly progressive sensorimotor polyneuropathy of varying severity, afflicting several members of a family, has come to be recognized as another of the common clinical denominators of a number of diseases. In recent years several metabolic aberrations have been discovered. The best-known member of the group is porphyric polyneuropathy. Attacks of the disease are related in some obscure manner to increased urinary excretion of porphobilinogen and of coproporphyrin I and III. The importance of barbiturates in provoking an outbreak of the disease has been amply verified (see Chap. 102 for details of the metabolic abnormality). The other chronic metabolic polyneuropathies are discussed in Chap. 323.

Syndrome of mental subnormality in child or adult

Among the patients in an institution for the mentally retarded who are most severely affected but yet retain normal facial and somatic features and relatively intact motility and sensation, one finds a small percentage (estimated at 1 to 5 percent) who suffer from some one of the inborn errors of metabolism listed in Table 332-2. The largest number of these are disorders of amino acids. A few of the more common types are described in Chap. 96. The internist should know something of these diseases for they are found also in the adult.

The clinical picture is relatively monotonous. Apart from the delay in psychosensorimotor development, beginning in infancy, these patients show few other distinctive abnormalities. A mild spasticity or chorea may be observed, but this is exceptional. Unlike the cases of congenital malformation of the brain and chromosome anomalies, gross deformities of face, eyes, ears, jaw, etc., are also lacking. The details of the syndrome are described further in Chaps. 27 and 332. The laboratory tests used in the detection of these diseases are very simple, require only a small quantity of the patient's urine, and can be performed in the physician's office. These include the ferric chloride test (positive in phenylketonuria, maple syrup urine disease, and histidinemia), the dinitrophenylhydrazine test for ketones (positive in phenylketonuria, maple syrup urine disease, and tyrosinosis), tests for reducing sugar but not the enzymatic assay for glucose (galactosemia, pentosuria, fructose intolerance), the nitroprusside test (homocystinuria, cystinuria), and the Berry spot test (for disorders of polysaccharide metabolism). In the adult or older child these simple tests will almost always permit detection of the disorders mentioned. In newborn infants, however, more refined techniques are frequently needed. Other recommended tests include examination of blood and urinary amino acids by paper chromatography and/or high voltage electrophoresis and measurement of blood ammonia concentration 2 to 4 hr after eating a meal containing 1 g protein per kg body weight (normally, this should be less than 70 μg per 100 ml). Special tests to be considered under certain circumstances (see Table 332-2) include measurement of serum uric acid, calcium, cholesterol, and ceruloplasmin.

Very recently a variety of enzymatic assays have been developed which measure the ability of extracts of serum, white blood cells, or cultured fibroblasts to cleave radioactively labeled compounds which are identical to or resemble the substrates which accumulate in the lipidoses or mucopolysaccharidases. These assays, which are beginning to be generally available, permit the early and precise diagnosis of most of these disorders.

These methods of "metabolic screening" are being refined in a number of centers; semiautomated techniques should make it possible to perform a large number of pertinent tests on small samples of blood or urine at reasonable cost.

Syndrome of progressive dementia with or without spastic paralysis (See also Chap. 27)

In many of the inborn errors of metabolism, such as phenylketonuria, damage to the nervous system occurs during the first few years of life, but after that no further deterioration occurs, and in fact to a limited degree, maturation and development may proceed, but at a retarded rate. In certain other disorders, however, the function of the nervous system may be relatively normal during the first few years and then become progressively impaired. The clearest example of this is metachromatic leukodystrophy (sulfatide lipidosis), which allows normal development for the first 2 to 3 years and then a progressive gait disturbance, due to a mild involvement of peripheral nerves and more severe affection of pyramidal and cerebellar systems, all in conjunction with a deterioration of intellect. The course may be so slow that if the history is not evaluated carefully, this disease is mistaken for "cerebral palsy" or some static defect in the nervous system resulting from birth injury. The onset is usually early childhood, but in a small number of patients symptoms do not begin until adolescence or adult years, and in this "late onset" type, the initial symptoms are apt to be in the mental or emotional sphere. Diagnosis depends upon demonstration of a deficiency or complete absence of arylsulfatase A activity and excessive sulfatide excretion in the urine. The juvenile (Batten-Spielmeyer-Vogt) and adult (Kufs') form of lipid storage disease may also give rise to a clinical syndrome, characterized by seizures, dementia, ataxia, visual loss, and progressive paralysis. The biochemical basis of these disorders is described in Chap. 106, and the diagnosis may be corroborated in most instances by enzymatic assays of serum or white blood cells.

NUTRITIONAL DISEASES OF THE NERVOUS SYSTEM

The general principles of deficiency disease have been presented in Chap. 74, and the reader should review them as an introduction to this discussion of deficiency disease of the nervous system. The term *deficiency* is used here in its strictest sense, to designate those diseases or syndromes which result from the lack of an essential nutrient in the diet or from a conditioning factor which increases the need for that nutrient. The neurologic diseases which comprise this category are the following:

1 Pellagra
2 Wernicke's disease and Korsakoff's psychosis (also "alcoholic" cerebellar degeneration)
3 Nutritional polyneuropathy
4 Strachan's syndrome
5 Subacute combined degeneration of the spinal cord due to B_{12} deficiency
6 Nutritional retrobulbar neuropathy or amblyopia

Before discussing each of these disorders, some general remarks, applicable to all of them, may suitably be made. Of the known vitamin deficiencies, only those of the B group are of importance in neurologic disease. A lack of them affects the brain, spinal cord, peripheral nerves, and muscles of man. Thiamine chloride, nicotinic acid, pyridoxine, pantothenic acid, and riboflavin all play a role in carbohydrate metabolism, upon which the central nervous system depends for its principal source of energy. These vitamins are essentially coenzymes in the Krebs citric acid cycle, and, in addition, thiamine is involved in the hexose-monophosphate shunt. Vitamin B_{12} is known to be required for the conversion of methylmalonyl to succinyl–coenzyme A, and for the conversion of homocystine to methionine (see Chap. 72).

Except for subacute combined degeneration of the spinal cord (vitamin B_{12} deficiency) and certain components of Wernicke's disease (vitamin B_1 deficiency), it is not possible to relate the clinical deficiency syndromes in man to a lack of single vitamins. For example, polyneuropathy may result from one of several vitamin deficiencies [thiamine chloride, pyridoxine (vitamin B_6), pantothenic acid, and probably vitamin B_{12}]. Moreover, such syndromes as pellagra and beriberi are often the result of a simultaneous deficiency of multiple vitamins.

In patients with nutritional disease, it is usual for both the central and peripheral nervous systems to be involved, a combination found in few other circumstances. Also, the examination of these patients frequently discloses nonneurologic signs of malnutrition such as general wasting, lesions of the skin and mucous membranes, and circulatory abnormalities. In general, however, one should think of the possibility of a nutritional disease if a patient presents himself with a neurologic illness that conforms to one of the following syndromes:

1 A subacute confusional, delirious or amnesic state
2 A symmetric subacute sensorimotor polyneuropathy
3 A symmetric subacute posterolateral degeneration of the spinal cord
4 Subacute bilateral degeneration of optic nerves

Throughout the world the nutritional disorders of the nervous system are most often observed in the alcoholic population of the large urban centers. The role of alcohol is mainly to displace food in the diet, but it also increases the demand for B vitamins, which are necessary to metabolize the carbohydrate furnished by alcohol itself. There is also some evidence to indicate that alcoholism impairs the gastrointestinal absorption of vitamins.

Subacute confusional, delirious or amnesic syndrome (See Chaps. 26 and 27)

PELLAGRA This disease has already been described in Chap. 77. The discussion here is concerned only with the neurologic manifestations, which in themselves are extremely diverse. Pellagra is essentially an encephalopathy, although minor involvement of other parts of the nervous system may occur. The early mental symptoms, insomnia, fatigue, nervousness, irritability, and feelings of depression, may be mistaken for those of a psychoneurosis. However, careful examination as the disease advances will reveal slowing and inefficiency of mental processes and impairment of memory. Sometimes the patient passes rather rapidly (over a few days) into an acute confusional psychosis combined with changing rigidity of the limbs, grasping and sucking reflexes, and Babinski signs. The manifestations of involvement of the spinal cord have not been clearly delineated, perhaps because the mental state of the patients has precluded accurate testing. In general, they are referable to both the posterior and the lateral columns, predominantly the former. Neuropathic signs are frequent and are often difficult to distinguish from affection of the posterior columns. Other manifestations such as tremors, extrapyramidal rigidity, sucking and grasping reflexes, and coma have been included in the pellagrous syndrome, as have various disorders of the special senses. Thus, pellagra may be the cause of insanity or occasionally result from it, because certain illnesses are accompanied by anorexia and unbalanced diet, including alcoholism.

Pathologic changes The distinctive neuropathologic changes in pellagra are most readily discerned in the large cells of the motor cortex, the cells of Betz, which appear swollen and rounded with eccentric nuclei and loss of the Nissl particles. This central neuritis of pellagra, as it is called, is probably not dependent on injury to the axons of the Betz cells, but it appears to represent a primary affection of the whole motor cell. The spinal cord lesions take the form of a symmetric degeneration of the dorsal columns, especially of Goll, and to a lesser extent of the pyramidal tracts. The posterior column degeneration affects a specific system of fibers and is secondary to the degeneration of the posterior roots. The nature of the pyramidal tract lesion in pellagra is not known; one can only speculate that this change is secondary to the pyramidal cell degeneration.

A *spastic paretic syndrome,* apart from the other symptoms and signs of pellagra, may be a rare manifestation of deficiency disease. The chief clinical signs are spastic weakness of the legs with absent abdominal and increased tendon reflexes, clonus, and extensor plantar responses. These signs are usually accompanied by other signs of nutritional deficiency, such as Wernicke's disease and retrobulbar and peripheral neuropathy. Spastic weakness of the legs has also been observed in conjunction with chronic liver disease.

WERNICKE'S DISEASE In 1881, Carl Wernicke described an illness of sudden onset, characterized by mental disturbance, paralysis of eye movements, and ataxic gait. Swelling of the optic disks with retinal hemorrhages was also said to be present, and in all three of his patients there was a progressive depression of the state of consciousness and death, so that a fatal outcome was at one time thought to be a universal feature of this disease. Wernicke described focal vascular lesions, primarily affecting the gray matter around the third and fourth ventricles and aqueduct of Sylvius. He regarded the disease as inflammatory in nature and suggested the name *acute superior hemorrhagic polioencephalitis.*

Since Wernicke's time, views regarding this disease have undergone considerable modification, clinically, pathologically, and etiologically.

Symptoms and signs The crux of the clinical picture is the ocular disturbance (the clinical diagnosis of Wernicke's disease can hardly be made without it) which consists of weakness or paralysis of the external recti, nystagmus, both horizontal and vertical, and various palsies of conjugate gaze. These signs show a considerable diversity. The paralysis of conjugate movement varies from merely a nystagmus on extreme gaze in one direction to a complete loss of ocular movement in that direction. Vertical movements may be affected. Paralysis of downward gaze and internuclear ophthalmoplegia are less usual manifestations. The sixth nerve palsy is always bilateral, though not always symmetric, and is accompanied by diplopia and internal strabismus. With complete ocular paralysis nystagmus is absent, but it becomes evident as the weakness improves. In advanced stages of the disease there may be a complete loss of ocular movement, and the pupils, which ordinarily are spared, may become miotic and nonreacting.

The ataxia affects stance and gait predominantly. It may be so severe initially that the patient is unable to stand or walk without support. Caloric responses are usually absent in these patients. With specific treatment the gross disorder of equilibrium improves and the patient is left with a wide-based, uncertain gait. The mildest degree of ataxia may be brought out only by special tests, such as heel-to-toe walking. In contrast to the gross disorder of locomotion is the relative infrequency of a clear-cut intention tremor. When present, it affects the legs more than the arms. Scanning speech is present only in isolated instances. The ataxia of gait is vestibular and cerebellar in origin, but it is often mistakenly attributed to a polyneuropathy.

Symptoms of deranged mental function are found in over 80 percent of patients and take one of several forms. (1) A small proportion of patients show alcoholic withdrawal symptoms of delirium tremens or its variants (see Chap. 111). (2) The majority of patients are apathetic, listless, and severely confused. Unconsciousness as part of the initial episode is distinctly rare, but mild drowsiness is common. The patient's mental state is best described as one of disinterest or indifference. His spontaneous speech is minimal, and he is inattentive and cannot concentrate on the simplest tasks. Many questions directed to him go unanswered, or he may suspend conversation in the middle of a sentence to turn over and sleep. He is readily roused from this state, however. Whatever questions the patient answers betray disorientation in time and place, misidentification of those around him, and an inability to grasp the meaning of his illness or immediate situation. Many of his remarks are irrational and show no consistency from one moment to another. Under these circumstances a more extensive evaluation of intellectual function is seldom possible. (3) Some patients, from the time they are first seen, show a disorder of retentive memory and other cognitive functions characteristic of *Korsakoff's psychosis* (see Chap. 27).

The outcome of Korsakoff's psychosis varies. In approximately 20 percent of patients complete or almost complete recovery occurs. More commonly there is slow and incomplete recovery over a year or longer. Depending on the severity of the residual symptoms, the patient may or may not be able to lead a supervised existence out of a hospital. The residual mental state is usually one in which the patient shows large gaps in memory and the inability to sort out events in their proper temporal sequence. If the patient is seen for the first time during this stage, the diagnosis of "alcoholic deteriorated state" or "organic brain syndrome due to alcohol" is commonly made.

The symptoms of Wernicke's disease may all appear simultaneously and rather acutely, but more frequently the ophthalmoplegia and ataxia precede the mental signs by a few days or 1 to 2 weeks. The patient may also show other stigmata of malnutrition, the most frequent of which is polyneuropathy. The signs of neuropathy are usually slight and could not account for the disordered gait. Nevertheless, in a small proportion the neuropathy is so severe that stance and gait cannot be tested. Occasionally, amblyopia or spinal spastic ataxia may be added to the clinical picture. The advanced stages of beriberi heart disease are rarely observed in Wernicke's disease, although indications of disordered cardiovascular function, such as tachycardia, exertional dyspnea, postural hypotension, and minor electrocardiographic abnormalities, are common. Occasionally the patient may die suddenly, the mode of death suggesting *cardiovascular collapse.* It has been shown that Wernicke's disease is characterized by a state of high cardiac output which is out of proportion to the oxygen consumption. This is probably due to an abnormal state of vasodilatation, which in turn may be related specifically to thiamine deficiency. Death occurs in about 15 percent of hospitalized patients and is usually due to the complications of cirrhosis of the liver or to infection.

Pathologic changes Postmortem examination reveals symmetrically located lesions in the paraventricular regions of the thalamus and hypothalamus, the mammillary bodies, the periaqueductal region of the midbrain, the floor of the fourth ventricle, and the anterior lobe of the cerebellum, particularly the vermis. The lesions are invariably found in the mammillary bodies and less consistently in the other areas. Microscopically the principal change consists of varying degress of necrosis of parenchymal structures. Many nerve cells and fibers are destroyed; others remain intact and are seen against a background of reactive glial elements, both astrocytes and microgliacytes. The blood vessels are prominent, owing to adventitial and endothelial proliferation. Hemorrhagic lesions, as the original name suggests, are present in only a small proportion of cases. When present, they give the appearance of being of recent origin. The oculomotor and vestibular nuclei are involved only to a mild degree, as a rule. Correlation of the clinical manifestations with anatomic localization of lesions indicates that the ocular muscle and gaze palsies are attributable to lesions of the sixth and third nerve nuclei. The latter lesions are probably responsible as well for the loss of caloric responses and to some extent for the gross abnormalities of equilibrium that characterize the initial stages of the disease. The lack of significant destruction of nerve cells in these lesions accounts for the rapid improvement in oculomotor and vestibular function.

The persistent ataxia of stance and gait is attributable to the loss of cortical neurons in the superior vermis; ataxia of individual movements of the legs is attributable to an extension of the lesion into the anterior parts of the anterior lobes. The latter lesions are indistinguishable from those of *alcoholic cerebellar degeneration* (see Chap. 111). The latter designation is used when the cerebellar abnormalities occur without the characteristic ocular and mental disorder.

The amnesic defect is related to lesions in the diencephalon, more specifically in the medial dorsal nuclei and perhaps the medial pulvinar. Lesions in the mammillary bodies are probably not critical in respect to memory function since they are found in patients who have shown no disorder of memory during life.

Etiology Wernicke's disease is no longer regarded as inflammatory in nature or the result of the neurotoxic effects of alcohol. Nutritional deficiency is now established as the causal factor. Outbreaks have been encountered in prisoner-of-war camps, and occasional cases have been reported in wasting diseases of varied origin where alcohol played no part. The specific nutritional factor in most, if not all, of the symptomatology of Wernicke's disease is thiamine. The experimental evidence for this statement, both in animals and in man, is quite convincing. The marked sensitivity of the ophthalmoplegia to the administration of thiamine accounts for the rapid disappearance of this sign following the ingestion of one or two meals. The quality of prompt reversibility suggests that these symptoms are due to a biochemical abnormality and not to structural change. On the other hand, the memory loss responds slowly or not at all, suggesting that this symptom is the result of structural changes, presumably in the medial dorsal nuclei of the thalamus.

On the basis of clinical observation, nutritional studies, and the neuropathologic findings, the details of which cannot all be given here, one may say that Wernicke's disease, Korsakoff's psychosis, alcoholic cerebellar ataxia, and polyneuropathy are but different facets of one disease process.

Treatment of the Wernicke-Korsakoff syndrome

Wernicke's disease represents a medical emergency, and its recognition demands the immediate administration of thiamine. A delay of a few hours may be crucial in determining whether the patient who presents only ocular and ataxic signs will be prevented from developing mental signs and whether the patient with early Korsakoff's changes will be restored to a state of mental competency. Although 2 to 3 mg thiamine is sufficient to modify the ocular signs, much larger doses are usually employed—50 mg intravenously and 50 mg intramuscularly, the latter dose being repeated each day until the patient resumes a normal diet. The other B vitamins may be given by mouth in the dosages outlined in Chap. 173. If the patient cannot or will not eat, parenteral feeding and administration of B vitamins become necessary.

A particular danger attends the treatment of the severely depleted alcoholic patient with intravenous glucose solution. This solution may exhaust the patient's last reserve of B vitamins and either precipitate Wernicke's disease, where it was not present before, or cause a rapid worsening of the athiaminotic state with circulatory collapse and death. For this reason, B vitamins must be added in all cases requiring parenteral glucose. If there are signs of cardiac weakness as shown by pulmonary edema, feeble heart sounds, tachycardia, and low blood pressure, rapid digitalization should be undertaken. Since these patients are confused and forgetful, they must be supervised continually, preferably on a medical ward.

A special problem in management arises when the patient recovers from the acute phase of the illness and the amnesic psychosis becomes prominent. The disposition of the patient to family, nursing home, or mental institution should be undertaken on the basis of the severity of the mental illness as well as the existing family and social circumstances.

Syndrome of subacute and chronic symmetric sensorimotor polyneuropathy (See also Chap. 323)

Polyneuropathy of alcoholism, a deficiency state equivalent to alcoholic beriberi, is variably combined with Wernicke-Korsakoff disease. When the B vitamin deficiency is acute, death may occur without neurologic symptoms; when subacute, Wernicke-Korsakoff disease dominates the clinical picture and peripheral neuropathy is mild; when chronic, the peripheral neuropathy is prominent and there are no signs of central nervous system involvement. The clinical features of alcoholic beriberi are described in Chap. 323, and the nutritional disorder is explained in greater detail in Chap. 78.

Syndrome of subacute posterolateral degeneration of spinal cord (See also Chap. 325)

STRACHAN'S SYNDROME Beginning with the report of Strachan in 1888 and culminating in the recent observations among prisoners of war and civilian internees, there has appeared a large number of reports concerning a nutritional disorder of the nervous system which cannot be forced into the boundaries of the classic syndromes described above. Strachan was the first to describe this syndrome, although he did not recognize its nutritional etiology.

Strachan's syndrome is essentially a disorder of the peripheral and optic nerves. Clinically, sensory symptoms and signs dominate the picture; in this respect the syndrome differs from beriberi. Paresthesias of the extremities, face, and trunk, painful "hyperesthesia" of the feet, loss of superficial and deep sensation, and ataxia are the common manifestations. On the other hand, foot drop and muscle weakness occur very rarely. A frequently associated disorder is failing vision, which may go on to complete blindness and pallor of the optic disks. In general, deafness and vertigo are rare complications, but in some outbreaks these symptoms were so common as to earn the epithet "camp dizziness." Along with the neurologic signs there may be varying degrees of stomatoglossitis, corneal degeneration, and genital dermatitis. These mucocutaneous lesions are often spoken of together as the *orogenital syndrome* and are quite distinct from those of pellagra.

There have been only a few pathologic studies of this syndrome. Aside from the damage to the papillomacular bundle in the optic nerve, the most consistent abnormality has been a loss of medullated fibers in each column of Goll adjacent to the midline. This indicates a systematized degeneration of the central process of the bipolar sensory neuron of the lumbosacral spinal ganglions. The fact that the primary sensory neuron is the chief site of disease is consistent with the predominant sensory symptomatology.

Patients with this syndrome are occasionally found amongst the alcoholic population of the United States. It may also accompany chronic liver disease and non-tropical sprue or occur as an inexplicable illness in late adult life.

SUBACUTE COMBINED DEGENERATION OF THE SPINAL CORD AND BRAIN DUE TO B_{12} DEFICIENCY (see also Chaps. 305 and 325) Subacute combined degeneration of the spinal cord, the neurologic component of pernicious anemia, is due to vitamin B_{12} deficiency but is clearly different from the other nutritional disorders. The disease results not from the lack of vitamin B_{12} in the food but from the inability to transfer minute amounts of this nutrient across the intestinal mucosa. Such "starvation in the midst of plenty" has been called *conditioned deficiency disease* because it depends on the lack of an intrinsic factor in the gastric secretion.

Clinical manifestations Symptoms of nervous system disease are present in the large majority of patients with pernicious anemia. The patient first notices general weakness and paresthesias consisting of tingling, "pins and needles" feelings, or other vaguely described sensations. The paresthesias tend to be constant, to progress steadily, and to be the source of much distress. They are localized in the distal parts of all four limbs in a symmetric distribution, the lower extremities usually being involved before the upper ones. As the illness progresses, stiffness and weakness of the limbs, especially the legs, develop, which combined with a defect in postural sensation produce a weak, unsteady gait and awkwardness of the limbs.

Early in the course of the illness, when only paresthesias are present, there may be no objective signs. Later, the neurologic examination discloses a disorder of the posterior and lateral columns of the spinal cord, predominantly of the former. Loss of vibration sense is by far the most consistent sign; it is more pronounced in the legs than in the arms, and frequently it extends over the trunk. Position sense is involved somewhat less frequently. The motor signs include loss of power, spasticity, changes in the tendon reflexes, clonus, and extensor plantar responses. These signs are usually limited to the legs. At first the patellar and Achilles reflexes are found to be diminished as frequently as they are increased, and they may even be absent. With treatment the reflexes may return to normal or become hyperactive. The gait at first is predominantly ataxic, later ataxic and spastic.

Isolated instances of loss of superficial sensation below a segmental level on the trunk do occur, implicating the spinothalamic tracts, but such a finding should always suggest the possibility of some other disease of the spinal cord. The defect of cutaneous sensation may take the form of a mild blunting of touch, pain, and temperature sensation over the limbs in a distal distribution, but such a finding is also uncommon.

The nervous system involvement in subacute combined degeneration is characteristically, though not always, symmetric. A definite asymmetry of motor or sensory findings, maintained over a period of weeks or months should always cast doubt on the diagnosis.

Mental signs are frequent, ranging from irritability, apathy, somnolence, suspiciousness, emotional instability to a marked confusional or depressive psychosis, or intellectual deterioration. Signs of visual impairment are distinctly rare; when present, they take the form of centrocecal scotomata. If involvement of the optic nerve is severe, optic atrophy may occur. Although dementia and amblyopia are relatively uncommon, they may be the initial manifestations of the disease.

Neuropathologic changes The pathologic process takes the form of diffuse, although uneven, degeneration of the white matter. There are multiple foci of spongy degeneration, often in relation to small blood vessels. The myelin sheaths and the axis cylinders are both affected, the former perhaps earlier and to a greater extent than the latter. There is relatively little fibrous gliosis in the early lesions, but in the older treated cases gliosis is pronounced. The changes begin in the posterior columns of the thoracic cord and spread from this region up and down the cord, as well as forward into the lateral columns. The lesions are not limited to specific systems of fibers within the posterior and lateral funiculi but are scattered irregularly through the latter. The CNS lesions have now been traced to a metabolic disorder which allows methylmalonic acid to appear in the urine. They are not related to interference with the synthesis of DNA which underlies the anemia.

Treatment The treatment of subacute combined degeneration of the cord differs in no way from the treatment of the other manifestations of pernicious anemia. Theoretically, 1 μg of parenterally administered vitamin B_{12} is adequate, but in practice much larger doses are used.

The most important factor influencing *response* to treatment is the duration of the disease. Recovery may be complete if therapy is instituted within a few weeks of the onset of symptoms. For this reason subacute combined degeneration represents a medical emergency. If symptoms have been present for longer than a month or two, only partial recovery can be expected, and in long-standing cases the best that can be expected is arrest of progression.

The chief obstacle to *early diagnosis* is the lack of parallelism between the hematologic and neurologic signs. This is particularly the case in patients who have received folic acid, which serves to maintain a hematologic remission for an indefinite period while the neurologic signs worsen, often to an irreversible stage. Under these circumstances the most reliable diagnostic procedure is the Schilling test (Chap. 305).

Syndrome of bilateral retrobulbar neuropathy (nutritional amblyopia) (See also Chaps. 20 and 324)

This term refers to the visual failure which occurs in nutritional disease and which is not due to a lesion of the cornea or other parts of the eye concerned with refraction. The optic nerve lesion consists of a degeneration of myelinated fibers more or less confined to the zone of the papillomacular bundle.

Deficiency amblyopia was particularly prevalent during World War II in the prisoner-of-war and civilian internment camps of the Far East. Although it had previously been described in association with beriberi and pellagra, the peak incidence did not coincide with that of either of these syndromes but with the syndrome of mucocutaneous lesions in the orogenital regions and "burning feet." In the United States many, if not all, of the cases of retrobulbar neuropathy attributed to the toxic effects of alcohol or tobacco are probably of nutritional origin. Retrobulbar neuropathy may occur as the only manifestation of deficiency, but far more frequently it is combined with other nutritional syndromes, such as peripheral neuropathy and the Wernicke-Korsakoff syndrome.

Although the nutritional origin of this type of amblyopia seems established, the specific nutrient responsible is uncertain. Isolated reports have implicated riboflavin, thiamine, and vitamin B_{12}, but the evidence provided is inconclusive. Methylmalonic aciduria has also been demonstrated in this disease. Since a specific nutritional deficiency can rarely be determined in this disorder, treatment consists of the administration of a balanced diet and supplementary B vitamins and interdiction of alcohol, where this is a factor.

REFERENCES

Courville CB: *Cerebral Anoxia*, Los Angeles: San Lucas Press, 1953

Holmes LB et al: *Mental Retardation: An Atlas of Disorders with Associated Physical Abnormalities,* New York: Macmillan, 1972

Silber R, Moldon DF: The biochemistry of B_{12} mediated reactions in man. Am J Med 48:549, 1970

Spillane JD: *Nutritional Disorders of the Nervous System,* Baltimore: Williams & Wilkins, 1947

Stanbury JB et al (eds): *The Metabolic Basis of Inherited Disease,* 3d ed., New York: McGraw-Hill, 1972

Victor M: Diseases of the nervous system due to nutritional deficiency, in *Practice of Medicine*, vol. X, chap 24, Hagerstown, Md.: Harper & Row, 1971

—— et al: *The Wernicke-Korsakoff Syndrome*, Philadelphia: Davis, 1971

333 DEGENERATIVE DISEASES OF THE NERVOUS SYSTEM

EDWARD P. RICHARDSON, JR.
RAYMOND D. ADAMS

The term *degenerative* as applied to diseases of the nervous system is used to designate a group of disorders in which there is gradual, generally symmetric, relentlessly progressive wasting away of structural elements of the nervous system, for reasons still unknown. Many of the conditions so designated depend on genetic factors and thus appear in more than one member of the same family; this general group of diseases is, therefore, frequently referred to as *heredodegenerative.* A number of other conditions, not apparently differing in any fundamental way from the hereditary disorders, occur only sporadically, i.e., as isolated instances in a given family. For all diseases of this class Sir William Gowers in 1902 suggested the now-familiar term *abiotrophy*, by which he meant "defective vital endurance" of the structures affected, leading to their premature death. This term, of course, tells nothing of the true nature of the defects. It is to be assumed that their basis must be some disorder of the metabolism of the parts involved.

Within relatively recent times there has been some elucidation of the nature of a number of metabolic nervous disorders which, in their symmetric distribution and gradually progressive course, resemble the degenerative diseases under discussion. It is to be expected that with advances in knowledge others of the latter group will eventually find their place in the metabolic category. Others may turn out to be the result of atypical virus infections, as has been demonstrated in one disease previously classified with the degenerative group, Jakob-Creutzfeldt disease—subacute spongiform encephalopathy (see Chap. 330).

The degenerative diseases of the nervous system manifest themselves by a number of common syndromes easily distinguished by their clinical attributes, the recognition of which can assist the clinician in arriving at the diagnosis of a disorder of this class. Some of these syndromes and the particular diseases which give rise to them are summarized in the following paragraphs.

GENERAL CONSIDERATIONS It is a characteristic of the degenerative diseases that they begin insidiously and run a gradually progressive course which may extend over many years. The earliest changes may be so slight that it is frequently impossible to assign any precise time of onset. However, as with other gradually developing conditions, the patient or his family may give a history implying an abrupt appearance of disability. This is particularly likely to occur if there has been an injury, or if some other dramatic event has taken place in the patient's life, to which illness might conceivably be related. In such a case, skillful taking of the history may bring out that the patient or family has suddenly become aware of a condition which had, in fact, already been present for some time but had passed unnoticed. Whether trauma or other stress may bring on or aggravate one of the degenerative diseases is still a question that cannot be answered with certainty. From all that is known it would seem highly improbable that this could happen. In any event, it must be kept in mind that the disease processes under discussion by their very nature develop spontaneously without relation to external factors.

The family history is of great importance, but one cannot always be immediately satisfied with that obtained on first contact with the patient. One reason for this is that patients or their relatives may be ashamed to disclose a neurologic disease that has occurred in the family. Another is that it may not be realized that an illness is hereditary when other members of the family have a much less severe form of the disorder such that the patient and family may have been unaware of the abnormality—as not infrequently occurs in the hereditary ataxias and related conditions. Moreover, in modern Western families the small sibships may prevent even well-established hereditary diseases from expressing themselves. It must, of course, be remembered that familial occurrence of a disease does not always mean that it is hereditary; it may indicate instead that more than one member of a family has been exposed to the same infectious or toxic agent.

Another significant feature of the degenerative nervous diseases is that in general their ceaselessly progressive course is uninfluenced by all medical or surgical measures. Dealing with a patient with this type of illness is often, therefore, an anguishing experience for all concerned. Yet symptoms can often be alleviated by wise and skillful management, and the physician's kindly interest may be of great help even when curative measures cannot be offered.

The bilaterally symmetric distribution of the changes brought about by these diseases has already been mentioned. This feature alone may serve to distinguish conditions in this group from many other diseases of the nervous system. At the same time, it should be pointed out that, in the earliest stages, greater involvement on one side or in one limb is not uncommon. Sooner or later, however, despite the asymmetric beginning, the inherently generalized nature of the process asserts itself.

A striking feature of a number of disorders of this class is the almost selective involvement of anatomically or physiologically related systems of neurons. This is clearly exemplified in amyotrophic lateral sclerosis, in which the process is almost entirely limited to cortical and spinal motor neurons, and in the cases of progressive ataxia, in which the Purkinje cells of the cerebellum are alone affected. Many other examples could be cited (e.g., Friedreich's ataxia) in which certain neuronal systems disintegrate, leaving others perfectly intact. An important group of the degenerative diseases has therefore been called "system diseases" ("progressive cerebrospinal system atrophies"—Spatz), and many of these are strongly hereditary. It must be realized, however, that selective involvement of neuronal systems is not exclusively a property of the degenerative group, since several disease processes of known cause have similarly circumscribed effects on the nervous system. Diphtheria toxin, for instance, selectively attacks the myelin of the peripheral nerves, and triorthocresyl phosphate affects particularly the corticospinal tracts in the spinal cord as well as the peripheral nerves. Another example is the special vulnerability of the Purkinje cells of the cerebellum to hyperthermia. On the other hand, several of the conditions included among the degenerative diseases are characterized by pathologic changes that are diffuse and unselective. These exceptions nevertheless do not detract from the importance of affection of particular neuronal systems as a distinguishing feature of many of the diseases under discussion.

Typically, the pathologic process in the nervous system is one of slow involution of nerve cell bodies or their prolongations as nerve fibers, unaccompanied by any intense tissue reaction or cellular response. The cerebrospinal fluid, therefore, shows little if any change—at most a slight elevation of protein, without abnormalities in pressure, cell count, or in other constituents. Moreover, since these diseases invariably result in tissue loss, rather than in new tissue formation (as with neoplasms or inflammation), x-ray visualization of the ventricular system or subarachnoid space shows either no change or an enlargement of these compartments. These negative laboratory findings thus help to distinguish the degenerative disorders from the other large classes of progressive disease of the nervous system—tumors and infections.

CLASSIFICATION Since etiologic classification is impossible, subdivision of the degenerative diseases into individual syndromes rests on descriptive criteria, based

TABLE 333-1

Clinical classification of the degenerative diseases of the nervous system

I Syndrome in which progressive dementia is an outstanding feature, in the absence of other prominent neurologic signs
- *A* Diffuse cerebral atrophy
  - *1* Senile dementia
  - *2* Alzheimer's disease
- *B* Circumscribed cerebral atrophy (Pick's disease)

II Syndrome in which progressive dementia is combined with other neurologic signs
- *A* Principally in adults
  - *1* Huntington's chorea
  - *2* Cerebrocerebellar degeneration
- *B* In children and adults
  - *1* Amaurotic family idiocy (neuronal lipidoses)
  - *2* Leukodystrophy
  - *3* Familial myoclonus epilepsy
  - *4* Hallervorden-Spatz disease
  - *5* Wilson's disease (hepatolenticular degeneration; Westphal-Strümpell pseudosclerosis)

III Syndrome chiefly manifested by gradual development of abnormalities of posture or involuntary movements
- *A* Paralysis agitans (Parkinson's disease)
- *B* Dystonia musculorum deformans (torsion dystonia)
- *C* Hallervorden-Spatz disease and other restricted dyskinesias
- *D* Familial tremor
- *E* Spasmodic torticollis

IV Syndrome chiefly manifested by slowly developing ataxia
- *A* Cerebellar degenerations
- *B* Spinocerebellar degenerations (Friedreich's ataxia; Marie's hereditary ataxia)

V Syndrome with slowly developing muscular weakness and wasting
- *A* Without sensory changes; motor system disease
  - *1* In adults
    - *a* Amyotrophic lateral sclerosis
    - *b* Progressive muscular atrophy
    - *c* Progressive bulbar palsy
    - *d* Primary lateral sclerosis
  - *2* In children or young adults
    - *a* Infantile muscular atrophy (Werdnig-Hoffman disease)
    - *b* Other forms of familial progressive muscular atrophy (including Wohlfart-Kugelberg-Welander syndrome)
    - *c* Hereditary spastic paraplegia
- *B* With sensory changes
  - *1* Progressive neural muscular atrophy
    - *a* Peroneal muscular atrophy (Charcot-Marie-Tooth)
    - *b* Hypertrophic interstitial neuropathy (Dejerine-Sottas)
  - *2* Miscellaneous forms of chronic progressive neuropathy

VI Syndrome chiefly manifested by progressive visual loss
- *A* Hereditary optic atrophy (Leber's disease)
- *B* Pigmentary degeneration of the retina (retinitis pigmentosa)

largely on pathologic anatomy but to some extent on clinical aspects as well. In the terms used to designate many of these syndromes, the names of a number of distinguished neurologists and neuropathologists are commemorated. A useful way of keeping in mind the various disease states is to group them according to the outstanding clinical features that may be found in an actual case. The following classification, intended to be of practical help to the physician, is based on such a plan.

SYNDROMES IN WHICH PROGRESSIVE DEMENTIA PREDOMINATES

In the disease entities about to be discussed, the clinical picture is dominated by gradual loss of intellectual capacities, i.e., by dementia. Other neurologic abnormalities, except in the terminal stages, are absent or relatively insignificant. (For further discussion of dementia, including its clinical evaluation, Chap. 27 should be consulted.)

Diffuse cerebral atrophy: senile dementia; Alzheimer's disease

Some degree of shrinkage in size and weight of the brain, i.e., "atrophy," has been shown to be the inevitable accompaniment of advancing age. In many instances, this is of no clinical significance, and there are many very old people who remain alert and perceptive, with keen intellect, to the end. Nevertheless, severe degrees of diffuse cerebral atrophy are as a general rule associated with some evidence of dementia. When these changes occur in old age (and the definition of when old age begins is largely subjective), it is usual to speak of *senile dementia*. That this is a fairly frequent condition is common experience. Much more infrequent is a pathologically identical progressive dementia with diffuse brain atrophy coming on well before the senile period—a presenile dementia. This condition, classically described in 1906 by Alois Alzheimer, has since become generally known as *Alzheimer's disease*. The distinction between the two conditions is purely clinical; pathologically, they differ only in that the characteristic abnormalities tend to be more severe and widespread in cases beginning at an earlier age than at the senile period.

PATHOLOGY The brain presents a generally shrunken appearance, with atrophy of the convolutions and symmetric enlargement of the lateral and third ventricles. Frequently, these changes are especially pronounced in the frontal and temporal lobes. Microscopically, there is widespread loss of nerve cells, most apparent in the cerebral cortex, but often present likewise in the basal ganglions, with secondary glial proliferation. In addition, two types of lesion give this disease process its distinctive character: (1) Microscopic deposits of amorphous material, scattered throughout the cerebral cortex and most easily seen with silver staining methods—the so-called "senile plaques"; (2) the Alzheimer fibrillary change in nerve cells. This striking abnormality consists of the presence within the cytoplasm of thick fiberlike strands of silver staining material, often in the form of loops, coils, or tangled masses. Recent investigations have greatly advanced knowledge as to the structural aspects of these lesions, in that the senile plaques are now known to contain amyloid, and the fibrillary change is characterized by masses of twisted microtubules. Their pathogenesis is still unknown, however.

CLINICAL ASPECTS Although Alzheimer's disease has been described as occurring during every age period, it is most frequently a disease of the later decades of life. A number of well-documented familial cases have been recorded, but there is not sufficient evidence to indicate that this is truly a hereditary disorder. Most of the cases actually seen in practice are sporadic. The onset is insidious and subtle, with changes most noticeable first in memory for recent happenings and in range of mental activity. Emotional disturbances such as depression or anxiety states, or odd, unpredictable quirks of behavior, may be salient features in the early stages. Progression is very slow and gradual, and unless the condition is earlier brought to a close by the effects of advanced age, it may smolder on for some 10 to 15 years.

In the milder cases, including those of the senile period, the noteworthy features are those of simple dementia, as described in Chap. 27. More unusual disorders of thought and intellect, including aphasia, apraxic disturbances, and abnormalities of space perception, may be seen, such as occur in the presenile group. Exceptionally, in the advanced stages of the disease extrapyramidal signs appear; the patient walks in a shuffling manner with short steps, and there is a generalized stiffness of the musculature with slowness and awkwardness of all movements. These abnormalities have been attributed to involvement of the basal ganglions. Terminally the patient may become nearly decorticate, losing all ability to think, perceive, speak, or move. This is unusual, and the neurologic examination more characteristically discloses no other significant findings. Additional investigative procedures, including the usual blood and cerebrospinal fluid determinations, do not yield any conclusive or pertinent data. There *is* a diffuse slowing in the electroencephalogram in the more advanced stages of the disease. The enlargement of the ventricular system and subarachnoid space resulting from the diffuse brain atrophy can be demonstrated by pneumoencephalography; otherwise, no characteristic roentgenographic findings are seen. During the course of the illness, occasional convulsive seizures may occur, but they are relatively rare and should raise suspicion of other diseases. Terminally, in a state of total helplessness the patient dies from intercurrent disease. Usually, long before the end, institutional care is necessary.

DIFFERENTIAL DIAGNOSIS Several disease states for which effective treatment is available may give rise to progressive intellectual deterioration closely resembling what may be seen with the diffuse cerebral atrophy above described. It is imperative that these be looked for. Specific examples include chronic subdural hematoma, chronic "normal pressure" hydrocephalus, frontal meningioma, bromide intoxication, myxedema, pernicious anemia (vitamin B_{12} deficiency), and neurosyphilis. Various other forms of intoxication, infection, metabolic disorder, or neoplasm may have to be considered. Thus, in addition to careful clinical assessment, and whatever laboratory investigations may be indicated to exclude the various possibilities listed above, special procedures such as pneumoencephalography or carotid angiography may be necessary. Vascular disease of the brain is often included in the differential diagnosis, but dementia on the basis of cerebrovascular disorders characteristically progresses in a halting or stepwise fashion with conspicuous focal cerebral signs, whereas progression in senile dementia or Alzheimer's disease is gradual and steady and focal signs are absent.

No specific therapy is known. The management should be along the lines of that described in Chaps. 26 and 27 for the delirious and demented patient.

Pick's disease (circumscribed cerebral atrophy)

This remarkable form of cerebral disease, which is characterized by the circumscription of the atrophy (lobar sclerosis), was first described in a series of publications by Arnold Pick in Prague, around the turn of the century. In the differential diagnosis of dementia in the presenile period, it is often mentioned in the same breath with Alzheimer's disease. It is, however, an extremely rare condition as compared with diffuse cerebral atrophy of the Alzheimer type.

PATHOLOGY So striking are the gross pathologic changes in the brain that in typical cases the diagnosis can be made at a glance. One sees severe atrophy of the anterior portions of the frontal and temporal lobes, and there is a curiously sharp line of demarcation between the atrophied portions and the remainder of the brain, which appears normal or nearly so. In some cases, the frontal atrophy is more prominent; in others, the temporal lobes are more severely involved; in general, both regions are affected. Characteristically, there likewise are atrophic changes in a number of subcortical structures: caudate nucleus, putamen, thalamus, and substantia nigra, and in the descending frontopontine fiber system. In the diseased regions, the local destruction of central and convolutional white matter is out of proportion to the degree of loss of nerve cell bodies in corresponding areas of the cortex. A noteworthy histologic feature of this condition is the occurrence of numerous swollen "ballooned" nerve cells in the atrophic regions, a finding which has been interpreted as an axonal reaction or retrograde cell change secondary to the degenerative process in the periphery. Another frequent cell nerve change is the presence of spheric intracytoplasmic inclusions that stain deeply with silver impregnation methods; the significance of these is unknown.

CLINICAL ASPECTS There is no satisfactory way of differentiating between Alzheimer's and Pick's disease during life, nor is this of any practical importance. Familial occurrence is on record in a number of instances. Progression is slow and relentless, the average duration of Pick's disease being about 7 years.

DIFFERENTIAL DIAGNOSIS The considerations noted above with respect to Alzheimer's disease apply to Pick's disease as well.

SYNDROME COMBINING DEMENTIA WITH OTHER NEUROLOGIC SIGNS

Huntington's chorea (chronic progressive hereditary chorea)

This condition, which genetically follows the pattern of a mendelian dominant trait, was classically described in 1872 by George Huntington, who, with his father and grandfather, both physicians, observed cases in members of a family living near their home on Long Island, New York. Unmistakable in its typical form, the affliction combines progressive dementia with bizarre involuntary movements (chorea) and odd postures. Atypical cases have also been recognized (see below), but in general the disorder runs true to form.

PATHOLOGY The brain has a generally atrophic appearance, especially noticeable in the frontal lobes. Particularly characteristic is severe bilateral atrophy of the caudate nucleus, which becomes flattened and concave instead of projecting as a convex rounded eminence into the anterior horn of the lateral ventricle. The putamen, likewise, is shrunken, although not to the same extent as the caudate nucleus. The globus pallidus is generally involved to some degree, but less severely than the caudate nucleus and putamen. Microscopically, the affected regions show severe nerve cell loss with reactive glial changes.

CLINICAL ASPECTS This distressing condition generally makes its appearance in early to middle adult years. Its typical hereditary nature (mendelian dominant) has been emphasized, but it is not at all rare for sporadic cases to occur. The involuntary movements (bizarre grimacing, respiratory irregularity, faulty articulation of speech, and irregular, arrhythmic, unpatterned movements of the limbs, imparting to the gait a peculiar dancing quality) tend to be less quick and more athetoid than in Sydenham's chorea (see Chap. 18). A few reported cases which on genealogic and pathologic grounds must be classified with Huntington's chorea have shown progressive rigidity, rather than choreiform movements. As a general rule, dementia runs parallel with the motor disorder. Occasionally it may appear before or after chorea; very rarely it may be slight or lacking altogether. The advance of the disease is slow. There is increasing disability because of both involuntary movements and mental changes, terminated after many years by death from intercurrent infection or, not rarely, by suicide.

DIFFERENTIAL DIAGNOSIS There is no difficulty in the recognition of typical cases. The relatively late onset, the slowly progressive course, the prominent dementia, and lack of association with rheumatic fever help to exclude Sydenham's chorea. Hepatolenticular degeneration (Wilson's disease) and nonfamilial forms of hepatocerebral degeneration may display clinical abnormalities resembling those of Huntington's chorea, but the specific changes characteristic of these disorders, including liver disease, corneal Kayser-Fleischer rings (in Wilson's disease), and the typical biochemical abnormalities, are absent in Huntington's chorea. Choreoathetosis appearing during the second postnatal year and lasting throughout life is due to hypoxic birth injury or kernicterus. Sporadic cases of choreiform movements beginning in middle or late life may present a difficult problem in exact diagnosis. The occasional cases of violent choreiform movements produced by vascular lesions, classically in the subthalamic region, are characterized by sudden onset, unilateral distribution (hemiballismus), and a tendency to improve after a period of initial severity. Virus encephalitis may occasionally be associated with choreiform movements; acute development, fever, and pleocytosis in the cerebrospinal fluid help in recognition of such cases. Phenothiazine drugs may induce generalized chorea, unassociated with dementia. Finally, there is a form of self-limited chorea that may appear in older persons without identifiable cause.

TREATMENT It is impossible to halt the progress of this disease by any of the suggested forms of treatment. Chlorpromazine in doses of 25 to 50 mg thrice daily and haloperidol, 2 to 4 mg thrice daily, help to control the chorea.

Cerebrocerebellar degeneration

The progressive cerebellar degenerations of late life, and some cases of spinocerebellar degeneration, may be accompanied by significant dementia, the pathologic basis for which is not always easily demonstrated. These disorders are dealt with more fully below in the section devoted to conditions manifested by ataxia.

Lipidoses of the nervous system

The conditions to be considered here differ from other degenerative disorders in that the underlying biochemical abnormality is better defined. They are characterized by a more or less widespread derangement of lipid metabolism, which results in abnormal accumulations of lipids in the cytoplasm of cells of the nervous system and often of other organs as well. (For information relating to the problem of the lipidoses in general, Chaps. 106 and 334 should be consulted.) This process leads to abnormal function and, eventually, to death of the affected nerve cells. There is ample evidence for hereditary transmission of these disorders, the basis for which must consist of genetically determined abnormalities of enzyme systems concerned with intracellular lipid metabolism. This group of diseases is currently the subject of much intensive biochemical and ultrastructural investigation, such that for several of them it has been possible to identify the enzymes that are deficient.

SPECIAL CLINICAL TYPES The forms of lipidoses which affect the nervous system exclusively are often classified together as *amaurotic family idiocy*. This term emphasizes the important hereditary aspect, but it is not entirely satisfactory, since it can be correctly applied only to cases occurring in infancy. In the older child and adult, blindness (amaurosis) may never develop, and "idiocy," strictly speaking, implies defective intelligence existing from earliest infancy. Another name frequently given to this group of lipidoses is *cerebromacular degeneration*, but it is accurate only for infantile cases and for patients with the combination of cerebral lesions and degeneration of the macular part of the retina.

Within the group of diseases designated as amaurotic family idiocy, the following varieties are generally distinguished.

Tay-Sachs disease This is the classic form of amaurotic family idiocy occurring in infants, almost exclusively in Jewish families. It is characterized by extremely widespread neuronal involvement (see Chap. 106 for further details).

Late infantile form (Janský-Bielschowsky) This variety, which is rare, begins at a somewhat later age than Tay-Sachs disease (age three to four years) and has a more chronic course. It is biochemically and pathologically (by electron microscopy) distinguishable from both Tay-Sachs disease and juvenile amaurotic idiocy, but has features in common with both. However, vision and the appearance of the retina may be normal.

Juvenile form (Batten-Spielmeyer-Vogt) This form of lipidosis is not confined to patients of Jewish parentage. Clinically, the onset is between the ages of five to ten years, and the course is relatively prolonged, with death at the time of adolescence or early adulthood. The retinal lesions take the form of pigmentary degeneration (atypical retinitis pigmentosa). The intraneuronal accumulations differ considerably from those encountered in lipidoses of the Tay-Sachs and Janský-Bielschowsky types both under light and electron microscopy, although, in common with these disorders, they have the histochemical properties of a glycolipid. Their chemical composition has not as yet been fully determined, but can be classed with the lipofuscins.

Adult form (Kufs') This is an extremely rare disorder with ataxia, athetosis, or other extrapyramidal signs and dementia, pursuing a very prolonged course. In all essential respects, it is identical to the juvenile form, except that retinal lesions may be completely absent.

GENERALIZED LIPIDOSES WITH CNS INVOLVEMENT In addition to the group of lipidoses exclusively affecting the nervous system, there are a number of more generalized disorders of lipid metabolism in which the nervous system participates.

Generalized gangliosidosis Two rare forms of generalized lipidosis in infants have lately been recognized, both of them characterized by abnormal accumulations of gangliosides in many organs in addition to the nervous system. One of them closely resembles Tay-Sachs disease in that the substance that accumulates abnormally is the same monoganglioside (G_{M2} in the Svennerholm classification) that is present in excess in the neurons in Tay-Sachs disease. This is generally referred to as *Tay-Sachs disease with visceral involvement.* The other, termed *generalized gangliosidosis*, is characterized by excessive amounts of G_{M1} ganglioside.

Niemann-Pick disease This disease has already been discussed in Chap. 106. The typical accumulation of large amounts of lipid in macrophages (reticuloendothelial cells) in many organs, including particularly the liver and spleen, is accompanied by lipidosis of the nervous system, similar to that occurring in the various forms of amaurotic family idiocy. The lipid involved here is mainly sphingomyelin.

Hunter-Hurler syndrome This disorder belongs to the group of mucopolysaccharidoses, in which there are abnormalities of connective tissue in many organs. In the Hunter-Hurler variety, mental retardation is a prominent clinical feature, and there are striking intraneuronal accumulations of lipid (ganglioside) resembling those found in amaurotic family idiocy. The peculiar facial appearance of patients affected with the disease has led to its being referred to in the older literature as gargoylism (mucopolysaccharidoses).

Gaucher's disease This generalized metabolic disorder of childhood, already described in Chap. 106, resembles Niemann-Pick disease in many respects, inasmuch as it likewise is characterized by extensive lipid accumulations in various organs, especially the spleen, liver, and bone marrow. The nervous system, however, is much less regularly affected; it may be entirely normal in cases occurring in late childhood or adult life, although it usually is involved in infants.

CLINICAL ASPECTS The majority of cases of lipidosis occur in infancy and childhood, after a period of normal development. Motor regression, disinterest, and loss of visual capacity are the leading features and are well covered by the term *amaurotic family idiocy.* At later stages the limbs become enfeebled and the reflexes exaggerated. The fundamental change—"cherry-red spots" at maculae, surrounded by a gray halo—gives the diagnosis. Its absence suggests the possibility of another infantile cerebral disease, i.e., spongy degeneration of the white matter, in which progressive blindness is combined with psychomotor regression (see below). Excessive startle to sound (auditory myoclonus) is another characteristic finding of cerebral lipidosis. Later the child becomes decerebrate and dies in 2 to 3 years. In patients with onset later in life cerebellar ataxia, epilepsy, and myoclonic dementia suggest the diagnosis, especially when associated with atypical retinitis pigmentosa. In the adult form choreoathetosis and dementia may be conjoined and retinas are normal. (See Chap. 334 for differential diagnosis.)

Leukodystrophy (degenerative diffuse cerebral sclerosis)

The disorders to be considered here, which typically show an autosomal recessive pattern of inheritance, are characterized by a widespread disintegration of white matter in association with a remarkable sparing of the nerve cell bodies in the gray matter. There is thus a superficial resemblance to Schilder's disease (encephalitis periaxialis diffusa), which is best considered as an unusual variant of multiple sclerosis; in fact, the leukodystrophies have frequently been grouped together as *familial Schilder's disease.* It is now apparent, however, that the leukodystrophies represent disorders of metabolism involving components of the myelin sheath. Some of them are related to the neuronal lipidoses previously discussed.

PATHOLOGY The distinguishing feature is diffuse disintegration of myelin at all levels of the central nervous system and often of the peripheral nerves as well. As a rule, axons suffer damage to approximately the same degree as the myelin sheaths. The two major varieties of leukodystrophy (see below) are characterized by the presence, within the devastated regions, of lipid breakdown products of myelin which show distinct histochemical differences from the familiar lipid products encountered in all the other disease processes destroying myelin, such as infarction, traumatic necrosis, secondary fiber tract degeneration, demyelinative lesions in multiple sclerosis or Schilder's disease, and so on. The relative intactness of the nerve cell bodies forms a striking contrast to the extensive white matter lesions.

VARIETIES OF LEUKODYSTROPHY Metachromatic leukodystrophy This is now known to be a genetically determined metabolic disorder of sphingolipid metabolism in which cerebroside sulfate (sulfatide) accumulates excessively in many organs, especially brain and kidneys, because of deficient activity of the enzyme cerebroside sulfatase. Since neutral cerebrosides and sulfatides are among the chief lipid components of myelin, all myelin-containing parts of the nervous system, both central and peripheral, are affected in this disease. The metabolic abnormality is well tolerated by other organs, as far as their functional integrity is concerned, but in the nervous system the excessive accumulation of sulfatides leads to breakdown of myelin at all levels. Sulfatides have the property of altering the absorption spectrum of dyes such as toluidine blue and cresyl violet, so that in their presence the color obtained is purple or red or even brown instead of the expected blue or violet—a phenomenon known as *metachromasia.* The name *metachromatic leukodystrophy* comes from the fact that the diseased cerebral white matter stains intensely metachromatically because of the large amounts of phagocytosed sulfatide that accompany the breakdown of the myelin. Metachromatic material indicative of sulfatide can also be readily demonstrated postmortem in kidney tubule cells, Kupffer cells of the liver, and in other organs, unaccompanied by any evidence of tissue damage. In the gallbladder the sulfatide deposits apparently do lead to destructive tissue changes, with the result that nonfunctioning of the gallbladder on radiographic examination is one of the manifestations of the disease.

The disease is mostly seen in infants and young children, but it occasionally occurs in adults, including a few of fairly advanced age.

Krabbe's form of leukodystrophy In this variety, first described by Krabbe in 1916 as a familial disorder of infants, the lipid breakdown products also are atypical as compared with those occurring in most pathologic processes which destroy myelin. They differ histochemically from the metachromatic material just described in several ways, including absence of metachromasia. Typical of this disorder is the presence of unusual multinucleated phagocytic cells (globoid cells) which contain galactocerebrosides. In this disease, the biochemical abnormality is apparently the result of a deficiency of galactocerebroside-β-galactosidase.

Spongy degeneration of the nervous system (Van Boegaert-Bertrand; Canavan) This rare inherited disease of infants is generally classified with the leukodystrophies because the cerebral white matter is the chief site of pathologic changes. Characteristic of the disease is a fine-meshed spongy degeneration of the tissue associated with breakdown of myelin in some regions and, probably, failure of myelination in others. This spongy state is apparently the result of a large increase of water, some of which is within the myelin sheaths, resulting in their disruption. The pathologic findings suggest failure of regulation of intracellular fluid balance, perhaps mainly affecting glial cells, but the biochemical and enzymatic defects that underlie this disease have not yet been identified.

Late-life leukodystrophy In recent years, a few cases have been described of a very chronic form of white matter degeneration occurring in the presenile period, in which the atypical lipid products most closely resemble the lipofuscins, the "wear and tear" lipid pigment of advancing age. This is an extremely rare condition, about which very little so far is known.

Pelizaeus-Merzbacher disease In this condition, which is characterized clinically by a pronounced familial tendency and a very chronic course, the white matter lesions are patchy and irregular, rather than evenly distributed as in the other forms of leukodystrophy. Furthermore, there is relative sparing of axons. Another distinguishing feature of this disorder is that the breakdown products of the myelin, although very sparse (as would be expected from the prolonged course), are of the usual sort regularly seen with myelin destruction, rather than being atypical as in metachromatic leukodystrophy. What has been called *sudanophilic leukodystrophy* may well be identical with Pelizaeus-Merzbacher disease. The underlying basis for the lesions is still wholly unknown.

CLINICAL ASPECTS The symptoms and signs in all the forms of leukodystrophy are mainly those indicative of involvement of tracts of sensory and motor fibers (corticospinal, thalamocortical, geniculocalcarine, pontocerebellar, and cerebellomesencephalic) in combination with a progressive dementia. In the early stages there is weakness and unsteadiness of gait. Likewise prominent are spasticity and exaggeration of tendon reflexes, referable to the destructive lesions in the corticospinal motor system. In contrast to the neuronal lipidoses and other gray matter diseases, seizures are rare. In metachromatic leukodystrophy there is at first spastic weakness of limbs, but because of later involvement of the peripheral nervous system, muscle-stretch reflexes are lost.

On the whole, though, clinical differentiation of leukodystrophy from other forms of diffuse progressive cerebral disease is difficult. The metachromatic and globoid cell varieties can now be accurately identified by demonstrating the enzymatic deficiency in tissue cultures of leukocytes or fibroblasts, and metachromatic leukodystrophy can be recognized by the presence of sulfatides in the urine. In the other varieties of leukodystrophy, there are as yet no reliable biochemical tests whereby the diagnosis can be made during life. The disease can generally be identified in a brain biopsy, but this is a procedure which is justifiable only under very rare circumstances—such as direction of therapy, genetic counseling, or a carefully thought out research project in which a specimen of fresh tissue might lead to some new insight into an otherwise hopeless disease.

DIFFERENTIAL DIAGNOSIS Familial occurrence, signs referable to a disorder of long projection and associative fiber systems, and relative lack of convulsive manifestations may suggest the diagnosis during life. Final verification, however, requires, except in those conditions where a biochemical abnormality can be detected, pathologic examination by appropriate biochemical tests.

Progressive familial myoclonic epilepsy (Unverricht-Lundborg-Lafora disease)

This rare disorder forms a distinct clinicopathologic syndrome characterized by recessive heredity. Typically, it appears in adolescence or early adult life, beginning with generalized convulsive seizures, which are followed after an interval of years by myoclonic jerks of increasing frequency and severity and progressive dementia. Death follows, usually within 5 to 10 years. The pathologic features suggest a disorder of nerve cell metabolism, the nature of which is under current investigation.

PATHOLOGY In many of the cases on record, distinctive intracytoplasmic inclusion bodies within nerve cells may be found at all levels in the central nervous system, although they are most frequent in the cerebral cortex, dentate nucleus of the cerebellum, substantia nigra, and thalamus. These bodies were initially described by Gonzalo Lafora (1911) and are generally known as Lafora bodies. Material with similar staining properties has also been found in heart-muscle fibers and in liver cells in several cases. They have been found to be composed of polymers of glucose (polyglucosans), but the reasons for the accumulation of these polysaccharides are still unknown.

CLINICAL ASPECTS The onset in most cases is at about the time of puberty. The convulsive seizures, with which the disorder usually begins, are in no way distinctive. The myoclonic jerks are sudden, asymmetric or symmetric brief contractions of muscle groups of the limbs, face, and trunk, occurring arrhythmically and unpredictably, usually with sufficient force to displace the parts affected. They characteristically are provoked by all sorts of stimuli, but occur spontaneously as well. The sudden contractions may interfere seriously with willed movements, or may cause the patient to fall abruptly. The disorder progresses gradually, running a course over several years, with terminal stages characterized by profound dementia and total helplessness. Treatment with anticonvulsant medication may relieve the generalized convulsive seizures and reduce the frequency of the myoclonic jerks, but has no effect on the dementia.

DIFFERENTIAL DIAGNOSIS Other forms of progressive familial dementia with myoclonus may have to be considered. These are discussed elsewhere in the descriptions of Jakob-Creutzfeldt disease (Chap. 330) and the lipidoses. There is in addition a more benign form of myoclonic epilepsy which begins in childhood or adolescence and permits survival to middle age or longer. In cases of this kind, some degree of ataxia is frequently observed, and, whereas there are no distinctive pathologic changes, degeneration of fiber systems related to the cerebellum have been found. In Unverricht-Lafora myoclonic epilepsy, convulsive seizures are more prominent than in the other disorders mentioned. The diagnosis of these different forms of myoclonus is based on clinical picture and course of illness. All forms of treatment have hitherto been ineffective.

Hallervorden-Spatz disease

This unusual disorder, often familial, is associated with a rather variable clinical picture in which abnormalities of posture and muscle tone, involuntary movements, and progressive dementia predominate. Pathologically, there are characteristic abnormalities in the basal ganglions, suggesting a localized disorder of metabolism. The features of the condition were classically described in an affected family by Hallervorden and Spatz (1922).

PATHOLOGY Distinctive for this condition is the accumulation of large amounts of pigmented material in the globus pallidus and zona reticulata of the substantia nigra, resulting in grossly visible brownish discoloration of these regions. Microscopically, there are irregular pigmented, ferruginous concretions and granules of varying brownish or greenish hues, depending on the stains used. Although much of this pigment contains iron, serum iron and transferrin are normal, and there is no systemic disorder of iron metabolism in these regions. There also is loss of nerve cells and fibers. Another feature of the disease is the presence of focal swelling of axons, most probably in their terminal portions; this is especially pronounced in the regions affected by the pigmentary disorder, but typically can be found at all levels of the central nervous system, including the cerebral cortex.

CLINICAL ASPECTS The disorder typically makes its appearance in childhood or adolescence, with abnormalities in muscle tone and movements such as rigidity and choreoathetosis. Abnormal postures of the trunk characteristic of torsion spasm (dystonia) may be seen. Cerebellar ataxia and myoclonus are also present in some instances, or the clinical picture may be reminiscent of parkinsonism. Speech becomes indistinct, and there is progressive intellectual impairment. Eventually, the involuntary movements give way to increasing generalized rigidity, and death comes as a rule about 10 years after onset.

DIFFERENTIAL DIAGNOSIS No feature of the clinical picture serves to distinguish this particular disorder from other conditions showing dementia with extrapyramidal motor abnormalities. Wilson's disease must be excluded by appropriate laboratory tests. The clearly progressive course sets this condition apart from clinically similar abnormalities resulting from accidents or illnesses at birth or in the neonatal period. There is at present no effective treatment for the disease. A recent (unpublished) attempt at using a chelating agent (deferoxamine mesylate) in one case led to no definite benefit, and L-dopa and other antiparkinsonian medication, tryptophan, and megavitamin therapy have been of only temporary and questionable help.

Familial hepatolenticular degeneration (Wilson's disease)

This condition is discussed in Chap. 103.

Acquired hepatocerebral degeneration

This condition is discussed in Chap. 332.

EXTRAPYRAMIDAL SYNDROMES OF ABNORMAL POSTURE OR INVOLUNTARY MOVEMENT

Paralysis agitans (Parkinson's disease)

This by no means rare condition was named and classically described by James Parkinson in 1817. His remarkably complete account gives this definition:

> *Involuntary tremulous motion, with lessened muscular power, in parts not in action and even when supported; with a propensity to bend the trunk forward, and to pass from a walking to a running pace, the senses and intellects being uninjured.*

Typically, paralysis agitans is a disorder of middle or late life, with very gradual progression and a prolonged course. Although it has been seen to occur in families (the estimated familial incidence is 5 percent), it usually is sporadic. It is well recognized, however, that the epidemic encephalitis of von Economo, which occurred in a worldwide distribution in the years following World War I, was followed by a syndrome clinically indistinguishable from paralysis agitans. It is usual in such instances to speak of postencephalitic parkinsonism, whereas the term Parkinson's disease should be reserved for true paralysis agitans of unknown cause. Paralysis agitans bears no consistent relation to any known disease process such as arteriosclerosis, trauma, or intoxication, although such conditions have often been invoked as etiologically significant and may at times produce somewhat similar clinical manifestations.

PATHOLOGY Despite the general medical familiarity with the condition and an extensive literature on the subject, it cannot be said that the pathologic changes of paralysis agitans are yet fully understood. The only regularly observed changes have been in the aggregates of melanin-containing nerve cells in the brainstem (substantia nigra, locus caeruleus), where there are varying degrees of nerve cell loss with reactive gliosis (most pronounced in the substantia nigra) along with distinctive eosinophilic intracytoplasmic inclusions (Lewy bodies, after their description by F. H. Lewy in 1913). Changes have also been described in other structures of the basal ganglions, but they are not clearly different in nature or degree from what may be encountered in other patients of similar age without extrapyramidal motor disorders. The histopathologic evidence therefore suggests that paralysis agitans can be considered as belonging with the system diseases, the affected system being that of the pigmented nuclei of the brainstem. Significantly, extensive lesions in these same pigmented nuclei characterize the pathologic findings in postencephalitic parkinsonism in which Lewy bodies typically are absent. Recent biochemical studies, which show a decrease of dopamine in the caudate nucleus and putamen—an alteration consistently found on experimental ablation of the substantia nigra—lend further support to the idea that Parkinson's disease is indeed a disorder of a particular neuronal system (see Chap. 18).

CLINICAL ASPECTS In its fully developed form, this disorder cannot be mistaken for any other. The stooped posture, the stiffness and slowness of movement, the fixity of facial expression, and the rhythmic tremor of the limbs which subsides on active willed movement or complete relaxation are familiar to every clinician. Although symmetric in the later stages, the disorder typically begins asymmetrically, e.g., as a slight tremor of the fingers of one hand or in one leg. Also typical are more or less general hypokinesia and stiffness of the musculature so that even where tremor is inapparent, the disease may betray itself by a somewhat staring and immobile facial expression, a monotonous voice, a general slowness and diminution of all motor activity, and a curious lack of the little spontaneous movements of postural change that are so characteristic of the normal individual. When tremor is minimal, patients often are able to alleviate it by resting their hands on a table or the arms of a chair or by keeping them in their pockets. The tremor, although fluctuating from moment to moment in amplitude, characterizes the later course. The tremor is generally most pronounced in the hands but may involve also the legs (and thus secondarily the trunk), lips, tongue, and neck muscles, and is easily seen in the eyelids when they are lightly closed. Its frequency is 4 to 5 per sec but another faster tremor (7 to 8 per sec) predominates in some patients. There is no total paralysis, although general enfeeblement of voluntary movement is characteristic of the fully developed disorder. Together with the stooped attitude, there is the typical festinating gait, whereby the patient, prevented by the abnormality of postural tone from making the appropriate reflex adjustments required for effective walking, progresses with quick shuffling steps at an accelerating pace as if to catch up with his center of gravity. Clinical examination of the tendon and plantar reflexes discloses no abnormalities. There are no sensory changes, although deep aching in joints and muscles is common. Eventually, the patient may become so incapacitated by rigidity and tremor as to be helpless in caring for himself. It has often been observed, however, that even severely disabled patients may under great emotional stress perform complex motor acts quickly and efficiently. Although the temporary alleviation under extreme provocation can never be long maintained, it is nevertheless true that the severity of the symptoms is considerably influenced by emotional factors, being aggravated by anxiety, tension, and unhappiness, and minimal when the patient is in a contented frame of mind. Despite the inherently progressive nature of the condition, much can be achieved with good medical management, and patients may continue for years to live effective, happy lives in spite of this affliction. Intellectual deterioration is not a consistent feature of paralysis agitans, but it must be conceded that in very advanced stages of the condition dementia may be encountered.

DIFFERENTIAL DIAGNOSIS In typical cases, this is not difficult. The extrapyramidal syndromes associated with most diseases of known cause or established nature such as cerebral vascular disease, cerebral hypoxia (including carbon monoxide asphyxia), or metallic poisoning differ from paralysis agitans in a number of respects, such as atypical behavior or tremor, presence of signs of pyramidal tract deficit, or early onset of dementia. The differentiation from postencephalitic parkinsonism may be impossible; a clear history of an attack of epidemic encephalitis (prolonged somnolence, disturbance of consciousness, diplopia) and relatively early age of onset of the disorder and the presence of tics, localized spasms, and oculogyric crises may be the only clues to this diagnosis. In recent years, a neurologic disorder strikingly similar to Parkinson's disease has been seen following the prolonged administration of large amounts of reserpine and phenothiazine drugs, which subsides on withdrawal of the offending drug—a matter of considerable theoretic and practical importance. Parkinsonism is rarely, if ever, produced by cerebral neoplasms.

TREATMENT Although there is no treatment that is known to halt or reverse the neuronal degeneration that presumably underlies Parkinson's disease, methods are now available which can bring about a considerable degree of relief from symptoms in many patients. An important part of any therapeutic program is the maintenance of optimum general health and neuromuscular efficiency by planned programs of exercise, activity, and rest; expert physical therapy may be of great help in achieving these ends. In addition, the patient often needs much emotional support in meeting the stress of the illness, in comprehending its nature, and in carrying on courageously in spite of it. Along with these general supportive measures, which are applicable to many chronic illnesses, patients generally require a carefully thought out program of treatment specifically aimed at counteracting the pathophysiologic disorder that produces their disabilities. This treatment can be medical (with drugs) or surgical, or a combination of both. Experience over many years has shown that the drugs that are most beneficial in the symptomatic treatment of Parkinson's disease are anticholinergic agents related to atropine. Several synthetic preparations of this kind are now available, including trihexyphenidyl (Artane), cycrimine (Pagitane), procyclidine (Kemadrin), biperiden (Akineton), and benztropine methanesulfonate (Cogentin), among others. Whereas these drugs differ little from one another in their overall effectiveness in large groups of patients, an individual patient may respond better to one of them than to another, and occasionally after a patient has received one of these medications for a prolonged period, change to another one may be attended by some additional improvement—perhaps only from the psychologic effect of a change in regimen. In order to obtain maximum benefit from the use of these drugs, they should be given in gradually increasing dosage to the point where toxic side effects begin to appear. The side effects are those expected from anticholinergic agents: dryness of the mouth (which can be beneficial when drooling of saliva is a problem), blurring of vision from pupillary mydriasis (for which corrective spectacle lenses may be indicated), constipation, and sometimes urinary retention (especially with prostatism). Mental slowing, confusional states, hallucinations, and impairment of memory, especially in patients with already impaired mental functioning, can occur as troublesome toxic effects of these drugs and may sharply limit their usefulness under these circumstances. The optimum dosage level for a patient is when the greatest relief from tremor and rigidity is achieved within the limits of tolerable side effects. This may occur with trihexyphenidyl, for example, within a range of 6 to 20 mg daily in divided doses, or in a sustained-release capsule. With any of these drugs, a dosage level is reached when a further increase serves only to precipitate severe toxic effects with no further alleviation of the symptoms of the disease. The dose must then, of course, be reduced. It is possible, nevertheless, once maximum benefit from one of the anticholinergic agents has been achieved, to then add one of the antihistaminic drugs such as diphenhydramine (Benadryl) or phenindamine (Thephorin). These drugs have some ameliorating effect on the motor derangement, but it is insufficient for them to be used as the primary therapeutic agent. However, an antihistamine in combination with an anticholinergic drug can give better results in many patients than either one alone. Drowsiness is the chief side effect of the antihistamines, and this in turn can be combated with one of the analeptics such as dextroamphetamine (Dexedrine). From what has been said, it is clear that the drugs to be used, and how much, vary from patient to patient: what is inadequate for one is too much for another. The patients who can be expected to benefit the most from treatment with classic anti-Parkinson drugs are those with relatively mild disease in whom relief from the symptoms is sufficient to warrant tolerance of some side effects. In those more severely affected, the relief is partial at best, and as the disease advances, eventually a degree of incapacity is reached which is not significantly responsive to even the most carefully planned regimen of medications. Even so, there is no doubt that for a significant period the patient's effectiveness and well-being can be considerably enhanced by the wise use of these drugs. An important note of warning must be provided at this point: Under no circumstances should a medication program with anticholinergic agents be stopped suddenly. If this happens, the patient is likely to become totally immobilized and incapacitated by an abrupt and severe increase of tremor and rigidity.

To the list of anti-Parkinson drugs must now be added L-dihydroxyphenylalanine (L-dopa). The theoretic basis for the use of this compound is the decrease of catecholamines in extrapyramidal motor centers, to which reference has already been made. At the present, L-dopa is unquestionably the most effective method available, and the results even in those with far-advanced stages of the disease are far better than have ever been obtained by other drugs. This new agent should be given in doses starting at 250 mg t.i.d. and increasing every few days until doses of 4.0 to 5.0 g per day are reached. The drug is not without serious toxic effects, so that it is not universally applicable. Many patients are at first troubled by nausea, especially if the medication is not taken with meals, and a few have hypotensive episodes. Above a certain daily dose which varies from patient to patient (usually 4 to 6 g), choreic movements of head and neck may appear, forcing a reduction in dosage. Nausea can be allayed by antiemetic medication, but usually it disappears with continued usage of the drug. At present the most efficacious program of medical therapy consists of 3 to 6 g of L-dopa in six divided doses plus 2 to 4 mg Artane and 10 to 20 mg ethopropazine (Parsidol) thrice daily. Amantadine (Symmetrel) in doses of 50 to 100 mg thrice daily is also an excellent anti-Parkinson drug and may be given with L-dopa.

Another important advance in the attempt to relieve the symptoms of Parkinson's disease has been the recent development of stereotaxic surgery. This involves the placement of precisely localized focal lesions in the central nuclei of the brain, either in the globus pallidus or ventrolateral thalamus, contralateral to the side of the body chiefly affected. The best results occur in patients who are relatively young and in good general health with sound mentality, in whom unilateral tremor or rigidity, rather than akinesia, are the predominant symptoms. Opinions among neurosurgeons still differ as to the best way of making the lesion, and studies are still in progress as to what its ideal location should be. Success with L-dopa has greatly diminished the call for surgical therapy.

Dystonia musculorum deformans (torsion spasm)

This is a clinical term denoting a state characterized by slow, nonrhythmic, involuntary movements which produce abnormal, at times bizarre, postures of the trunk and limbs. With passage of time, these postures tend to become more or less fixed. Underlying the clinical disorder may be any of several pathologic conditions, such as the residual lesions of epidemic encephalitis, the pigmented deposits of Hallervorden-Spatz disease (described above), hepatolenticular degeneration (Wilson's disease), or the scars of cerebral birth injury in the broad sense, or kernicterus. More frequent and puzzling, however, is a hereditary form of relatively early onset and progressive course without a definitive lesion.

PATHOLOGY Until lately, very few cases of dystonia musculorum deformans not due to one of the definable disease processes indicated above had been adequately studied neuropathologically. Reported results from the few that had been examined led to uncertainty as to what the pathologic-anatomic basis of the clinical state might be, although it was generally assumed that the basal ganglia were diseased. A careful study by Zeman and Dyken in 1967, which included comparison of the findings in patients with the disease with control material, demonstrated that there is, in fact, no definable neuronal or other histologically demonstrable disease process to which the clinical abnormalities can reasonably be attributed. These negative findings, which are perhaps surprising, must not be interpreted as indicating that there is "no disease" in the brain, but rather that the pathologic state is not one that can be disclosed by the usual histopathologic techniques.

CLINICAL ASPECTS The motor abnormalities are described in Chap. 18. In the early stages, the involuntary muscular contractions are intermittent and variable in location and severity, but typically interfere with motor performance by superimposing an unwanted posture upon parts in use. One leg may briefly be pulled into a flexed or extended position or one shoulder elevated. Later the lingual, pharyngeal, neck, and thoracic muscles participate, and grimacing may occur. These latter may also be the first and only signs of disease for several years. Progression may be relatively rapid in cases with onset during early childhood, but is slow in those beginning in late childhood or adult life. The end result is extreme disability, with grossly distorted postures of the trunk and contractures of the limbs. Affection of face and tongue muscles results in faulty articulation of speech, which eventually becomes incomprehensible. The tendon and plantar reflexes, which can be assessed only during moments of relaxation of the affected parts, are characteristically normal.

Dementia is not a necessary accompaniment of the condition, except perhaps in the terminal stages; but with severe derangement of all available methods of communication, an adequate evaluation of mental capacity may be impossible.

Spasmodic torticollis (see below) may well be a form of dystonia, but it typically does not progress to involve the musculature generally. However, torticollis may be an early symptom in cases which later show the typical generalized motor abnormalities.

DIFFERENTIAL DIAGNOSIS Hepatolenticular degeneration should be seriously considered in any case presenting these motor symptoms, and appropriate measures should be undertaken for its investigation (see Chap. 103). The progressive course, and possibly the family history, differentiate the degenerative group from the "symptomatic" dystonias resulting from infections or metabolic disorders occurring at birth or later. Hallervorden-Spatz disease, however, cannot be distinguished on clinical grounds alone.

TREATMENT This is most unsatisfactory. Dystonia is notoriously unresponsive to drug therapy, although antispasmodic drugs such as those used for parkinsonism should be tried. Neurosurgical treatment of the sort used for Parkinson's disease has been sufficiently promising to be worth serious consideration in every case, especially if the patient is young.

Spasmodic torticollis and other restricted dyskinesias

With advancing age a large variety of degenerative "movement disorders" come to light. Supposedly there is loss of neurons in certain parts of the motor system. Groups of muscles begin to manifest arrhythmic involuntary spasms. The patient's lack of success in suppressing them and his recognition that they are beyond voluntary control distinguish them from the common tics, habit spasms, and mannerisms described in Chap. 18. If the muscle contraction is frequent and prolonged, an aching pain accompanies it and may be mistakenly blamed for the spasm. Worsening under stress and improvement during quiet and relaxation are typical of this group of disorders.

Surely the most frequent and familiar type is torticollis, wherein an adult, more often a woman, becomes aware of turning of the head to one side as she walks. It gradually worsens to a point where it may be more or less continuous, not even relieved when lying down. On the assumption of a psychogenic factor in the illness many patients receive psychotherapy, but always without benefit. When followed over the years, the condition is observed to remain limited to the same muscles (scalene, sternocleidomastoid, and upper trapezius). There is little if any response to various drugs. Section of upper cervical roots bilaterally (anterior and posterior roots) is the only form of treatment that has given satisfactory results.

Other restricted dyskinesias involve the neck in combination with facial muscles, the orbicularis oculi (blepharospasm and blepharoclonus), the throat, and respiratory muscles ("spastic dysarthria," respiratory, and phonatory spasms). All these conditions, once started, are persistent, unpleasant, and relatively unresponsive to all modes of therapy other than denervative surgical procedures. Presumably, the abnormality lies in the basal ganglions, but its pathologic substratum has never been divulged.

Familial tremor

One of the commonest hereditary disorders of man's nervous system is that which gives rise to a fast-frequency (6 to 7 or 8 to 9 per sec) action tremor. This may appear at any age but more often during adolescence and adult years; once started, it lasts throughout life. The heredity is dominant. Probably all cases are not the same, for some have tremors of slower frequency, looking more like those of Parkinson's disease but lacking the slowness of movement, rigidity, and flexed postures. In patients of advanced age it is called *senile tremor.* Imbibition of alcohol suppresses the fast-frequency forms, as does a beta-adrenergic blocking agent (propranolol) in doses of 20 to 40 mg thrice daily. Usually the tremor is the only abnormality, but in a few patients a cerebellar ataxia may appear years later. The pathologic basis is unknown.

SYNDROMES OF SLOWLY DEVELOPING ATAXIA

The conditions about to be considered are distinguished clinically by progressive unsteadiness in standing and walking, along with more or less impaired coordination of other motor acts. Pathologically, they are characterized by degeneration of the cerebellum and/or its related fiber systems, and thus constitute classic examples of the system diseases. Although sporadic instances occur, hereditary transmission is an outstanding feature in many cases; thus, this group of disorders is often referred to as the *hereditary ataxias.* Their subdivision into more or less separate entities is largely arbitrary, with pathologic changes of varying distribution underlying clinically indistinguishable symptom complexes. Furthermore, there is considerable overlapping with other forms of hereditary nervous disease, so that in a given case a remarkable combination of defects may be encountered. These facts have led to the idea that in the ataxias there is a group of closely related genetically determined abnormalities which may occur together in an almost infinite series of combinations, so that it is not possible to separate well-defined disease pictures. Nevertheless, certain constellations of symptoms and pathologic findings occur with sufficient regularity to warrant their separation for purposes of discussion. The classification about to be given is not entirely satisfactory but is designed to be of practical help to the physician confronted with a case.

Cerebellar degenerations

To be discussed are the forms of progressive ataxia which are associated with pathologic changes predominantly in the cerebellum. These include both hereditary and sporadic cases and, in addition, the rather rare subacute spinocerebellar degeneration associated with the presence of carcinoma of various types elsewhere in the body. The hereditary and sporadic forms of cerebellar degeneration resemble one another so closely that, for the purposes of the present discussion, they will all be referred to as *hereditary cerebellar degeneration.* Most cases are seen in adults, with the onset occurring in middle life.

PATHOLOGY In hereditary cerebellar degeneration the cerebellum is obviously atrophied. In one group of cases, these changes are chiefly localized to the superior vermis and adjacent parts of the cerebellar cortex, whereas in an even larger group, the entire cerebellar cortex is affected. Microscopically there is loss of nerve cells principally affecting the Purkinje cells, although the granule cells are often involved as well. In most cases, there is an associated atrophy of nerve cells in the inferior olivary nuclei in a distribution dependent on the location and extent of the changes in the cerebellar cortex. It no longer seems justifiable to separate the cases with associated olivary degeneration from the rest and to designate them as "cerebello-olivary degeneration," as has been done in the past. In *olivopontocerebellar degeneration*, there are extensive degenerative changes in the pontine nuclei, middle cerebellar peduncles, and olivary nuclei. In addition changes in the cerebellar cortex such as have been noted above may or may not be present. In all varieties of cerebellar degeneration, affection of other neuronal systems—as, for instance, the cerebral cortex and basal ganglions—may be encountered. In some cases, there are changes in the dentate and roof nuclei of the cerebellum and their projections in the superior cerebellar peduncles (*dentatorubral atrophy*), but these are always found in association with more diffuse cerebellar or spinocerebellar degeneration. *Carcinomatous cerebellar* (*spinocerebellar*) *degeneration* is characterized by extensive cell loss in all parts of the cerebellar cortex, often associated with inflammatory (lymphocytic) infiltrations in the perivascular and subarachnoid spaces. In addition there are degenerative changes in the long-fiber tracts of the spinal cord. These lesions do not depend on the presence of tumor implants anywhere in the nervous system or its coverings, but rather are thought to be due to an obscure infectious (? metabolic) process somehow resulting from the presence of carcinoma.

CLINICAL ASPECTS In the hereditary form of cerebellar degeneration the abnormality appears first in the legs, resulting in unsteadiness of stance and gait of the peculiar wavering, lurching character so typical of cerebellar ataxia (see Chap. 18). This has been correlated with the localization of changes in the superior vermis of the cerebellum and adjacent parts of the cerebellar cortex. With more extensive cerebellar involvement, a disturbance in articulation and rhythm of speech occurs that may progress to total incomprehensibility, and the arms likewise become ataxic. There may be nystagmus, but it is often absent. Where there is affection of other neuronal systems, additional neurologic abnormalities, such as exaggerated tendon reflexes, extensor plantar responses, rigidity, tremor, and dementia, may be encountered (*cerebrocerebellar degeneration*). Progression is gradual and slow, being measured in years and sometimes decades, and may not necessarily shorten life.

No specific treatment is available for any of the progressive ataxias, although encouragement to remain active and gait training may enable a patient to overcome his disability to some extent.

We have not been able to clinically differentiate a cortical parenchymatous from the olivopontocerebellar degeneration with any degree of consistency, though the latter tends to be sporadic, speech is affected early, and extrapyramidal signs of other type appear late. In dentatonigral degeneration, gaze palsy and spasticity are combined with cerebellar ataxia.

In the cases associated with carcinoma, the tempo of evolution of the process is relatively rapid, with severe disability coming on within a period of months. Vertigo, diplopia, and nausea may be prominent. In an occasional patient, the neurologic symptoms have appeared before there was any obvious evidence of carcinoma. In contrast to the consistently normal cerebrospinal fluid findings in the forms of cerebellar degeneration noted above, the cerebrospinal fluid may show increased lymphocytes and protein.

DIFFERENTIAL DIAGNOSIS The slow but relentless progression in the absence of abnormalities in the cerebrospinal fluid distinguishes the hereditary group from other forms of cerebellar ataxia such as may occur with neoplastic, infectious, or demyelinative disease, with drug intoxications (e.g., barbiturates), or with hyperpyrexia. The degenerative disorders under discussion tend to occur in a setting of otherwise good general health; this, together with the other clinical differences, distinguishes them from alcoholic cerebellar ataxia or deficiency disease, with or without Wernicke-Korsakoff syndrome. Alcoholic cerebellar degeneration usually develops rapidly, and then may remain more or less stationary for the remainder of the patient's life (Chap. 332). The form of spinocerebellar degeneration associated with carcinoma may be distinguished from direct carcinomatous involvement of the nervous system by the symmetry of the findings and the absence of increased intracranial pressure.

Hereditary ataxia of Pierre Marie

This designation has been applied to cases of hereditary progressive ataxia with onset in early adulthood. Considerable doubt has been raised as to the validity of retaining the concept of Marie's hereditary ataxia, because pathologically this is by no means a uniform group. When Pierre Marie wrote about the subject in 1893, Friedreich's ataxia (see Chap. 325) had relatively recently become recognized as a distinct entity. Marie pointed out, on the basis of case reports in the literature, that there were other cases of hereditary ataxia, of later onset, which could not be fitted into Friedreich's description. He offered the suggestion that the cerebellum itself was the major site of disease in these cases. Subsequent pathologic examination of the cases he reviewed have shown that he was partly in error in this supposition; nevertheless, following his report, the concept of Marie's ataxia has appeared repeatedly in the writings on hereditary ataxia. Cases that might be classified with this group either are indistinguishable from those discussed above under the cerebellar degenerations or are variants of Friedreich's ataxia.

SYNDROME OF MUSCULAR WEAKNESS AND WASTING, WITHOUT SENSORY CHANGES

Motor system disease

This general term is used to designate a progressive disorder of motor neurons in the cerebral cortex, brainstem, and spinal cord, manifested clinically by muscular weakness, with muscle atrophy and spasticity with exaggeration of tendon reflexes in varying combinations. It is a disease of middle life, generally appearing in the fifth or sixth decade. Customarily a subdivision is made on the basis of the particular grouping of symptoms and signs observed. Thus, the most frequent form, in which muscular atrophy and hyperreflexia are combined, is called *amyotrophic lateral sclerosis*. Rather more rare are the cases in which weakness and atrophy exist alone without clinical evidence of corticospinal tract dysfunction; for these, the term *progressive muscular atrophy* is used. Where the disorder affects predominantly the musculature innervated by the cranial nerves, it is usual to speak of *progressive bulbar palsy*. Very rarely, the clinical state is dominated by spasticity and hyperreflexia without obvious muscular wasting; such cases are classed as *primary lateral sclerosis*. There is no reason to believe that these subgroupings are anything other than clinical variants of the same disease process, which is another classic example of a system disease. Most cases are sporadic, but occasionally this disorder occurs in families in a manner suggesting genetic transmission.

PATHOLOGY There are widespread selective atrophy and loss of motor nerve cells at all levels of the central nervous system, including the Betz cells in the motor areas of the cerebral cortex. Some evidence of disease in the corticospinal motor system is usually found pathologically, even when physical signs referable to such changes were not observed during life. The atrophy of fibers in skeletal muscles is typically that due to loss of motor innervation.

CLINICAL ASPECTS The disease begins insidiously and may be well advanced before the patient is aware of it. Although often asymmetric initially, the weakness and muscular wasting gradually become symmetric and widespread. Classically, the disorder becomes first evident in the small muscles of the hands, but it may begin in one or both of the legs, or in muscles supplied by cranial nerves. Vague feelings of discomfort in the muscles, tightness, numbness (without objective sensory changes), and recurrent cramps may be early symptoms. The progressive enfeeblement and atrophy of the musculature are accompanied by widespread visible fascicular twitchings of groups of muscle fibers, a classic feature that can be related to degeneration of the motor nerve cells supplying the involved muscles. Despite extensive involvement of skeletal muscles generally, sphincter control remains intact. Sooner or later the disease affects muscles supplied by the brainstem, resulting in weakness, atrophy, and fasciculations in the tongue and facial musculature associated with dysarthria and impairment of chewing or swallowing. The ocular nuclei, oddly enough, are invariably spared. In most cases, the weakness and muscular wasting are accompanied by exaggeration of tendon reflexes, extensor plantar reflexes and spasticity, to a degree dependent on the severity of degeneration in the corticospinal (pyramidal) motor system. Affection of corticobulbar fibers results in manifestations of pseudobulbar palsy such as involuntary weeping or laughter, exaggerated reflex movements of the facial msucles or expression, and sucking reflexes. These latter may be the first manifestations of the disease. Progression is unhalting and relatively rapid, leading to extensive paralysis, with death from respiratory weakness or aspiration pneumonia, generally within about 2 to 5 years or more from onset. Intelligence and awareness are typically preserved to the end.

DIFFERENTIAL DIAGNOSIS Spinal cord compression from tumors in the cervical region or from cervical spondylosis with osteophytes projecting into the vertebral canal can at times give rise to weakness, wasting, and fasciculations in the upper limbs and spasticity in the legs, thus closely resembling amyotrophic lateral sclerosis. The absence of cranial nerve involvement may be helpful in differentiation, although some compressive lesions at the foramen magnum may implicate the twelfth cranial (hypoglossal) nerve, with resulting affection of the tongue. Absence of pain or of sensory changes, normal function of bowels and bladder, normal roentgenographic studies of the spine, and absence of changes in the composition of dynamics of the cerebrospinal fluid are all points in favor of motor system disease and against spinal cord compression. Where doubt exists, contrast myelography should be performed and the cervical region should be visualized.

Chronic inflammatory disorders of the meninges and spinal cord, exemplified by syphilitic meningomyelitis or some cases of adhesive arachnoiditis, may have to be considered. These conditions can readily be recognized by cerebrospinal fluid changes and, if necessary, by abnormal myelographic findings. Nutritional myelopathy can be excluded by history and on other clinical grounds.

Although fasciculations are a prominent feature of motor system disease, they are not, in the absence of weakness, muscle atrophy, or loss of tendon reflexes, valid signs of it, for they may occur in a variety of metabolic or toxic disorders (e.g., thyrotoxicosis, salt depletion) as well as in otherwise healthy individuals. Careful clinical evaluation suffices in such instances to exclude serious neurologic disease.

Progressive weakness from intrinsic disease of muscle (myopathy, polymyositis) may occasionally be difficult to distinguish from progressive muscular atrophy of the type under discussion; yet the differentiation is important from the standpoint of prognosis or treatment. Under such circumstances, the diagnosis can be made by muscle biopsy and electromyography.

There is no known treatment for any form of motor system disease.

Infantile muscular atrophy (Werdnig and Hoffmann), amyotonia congenita (Oppenheim)

The form of progressive muscular atrophy described by Werdnig and Hoffman is a disease of infants and young children, typically afflicting several members of a family. Pathologically, it closely resembles the adult disease described above. Amyotonia congenita is a purely clinical term, used to designate abnormal laxness of somatic musculature observed at birth or in early infancy; it may occur in a number of different pathologic processes, including Werdnig-Hoffmann disease. For further details of these conditions, Chap. 334 should be consulted.

OTHER FORMS OF FAMILIAL PROGRESSIVE MUSCULAR ATROPHY In addition to the infantile form there are several other familial syndromes of progressive muscular atrophy. They begin later in childhood, adolescence, and adult life and, though progressive, are extremely chronic. One form affects predominantly the proximal limb muscles (Wohlfart-Kugelberg-Welander syndrome) and must be distinguished from limb girdle dystrophy. In any given family the disease tends to have the same pattern and time course in all affected members.

Hereditary spastic paraplegia

This very rare disorder is characterized by weakness and spasticity of the legs, with early onset (childhood or adolescence) and slow progression. Later the arms may be affected, but usually to a lesser degree. The pathologic changes closely resemble those of Friedreich's ataxia, and there is reason now to believe that this condition is in fact an incomplete form of Friedreich's disease in which spastic weakness overshadows minimal or absent ataxia and sensory changes. The diagnosis is made by the family history and by excluding other possible causes of bilateral spastic weakness of the limbs. The relation to Friedreich's ataxia is further confirmed by the occurrence of pes cavus and optic atrophy in some cases. One group of patients also has progressive dementia. The combination of optic atrophy and spastic paraparesis beginning in childhood is called Behr's syndrome.

SYNDROMES COMBINING WEAKNESS AND WASTING WITH SENSORY CHANGES

Progressive neural muscular atrophy

The degenerative disorders characterized by progressive weakness and wasting of skeletal muscles combined with sensory changes are chronic diseases of peripheral nerves, often occurring as hereditary conditions. Although clinical and pathologic subvarieties exist, there is no sharp dividing line between them, and they are best considered together under the designation given above, in which the term *neural* emphasizes the peripheral nerve affection. Chronic peripheral neuropathy is an associated disorder in some of the hereditary ataxias and is regularly encountered in the classic form of Friedreich's ataxia. An additional connecting link with other genetically determined nervous diseases is the occurrence of progressive optic atrophy or pigmentary degeneration of the retina in some cases. Common to all is for the peripheral neuropathy to begin distally and to progress in a centripetal fashion and for the feet and legs to become first affected, with involvement of the hands and more proximal parts only after a considerable interval.

The variety most usually seen is that generally called *peroneal muscular atrophy* (*Charcot-Marie-Tooth disease*), a name which draws attention to the changes in the lower legs, although the disorder affects far more than the peroneal group of nerves. This condition was first clearly differentiated from other forms of muscular atrophy by Charcot and Marie in France, and independently by H. H. Tooth in England, in 1886. In rare cases which are otherwise similar, there is a remarkable palpable thickening of peripheral nerve trunks. Such cases are generally designated as *hypertrophic interstitial neuropathy* (*of Dejerine and Sottas*, the French neurologists who, in 1893, first described the condition clinically and pathologically). In a few cases, there are pronounced trophic and vasomotor abnormalities of the affected parts, chiefly the feet, which may lead to chronic, poorly healing, perforating ulcers on the ball of the foot, among other abnormalities (*familial neurovascular dystrophy*, Wadulla, 1949, Krücke, 1955; *hereditary sensory neuropathy*, Denny-Brown, 1951).

The rare condition described by Refsum (1946) and called by him *heredopathia atactica polyneuritiformis* (now generally referred to as *Refsum's disease*) is characterized by a hypertrophic neuropathy in association with ataxia, progressive nerve deafness, retinitis pigmentosa, and a high cerebrospinal fluid protein. This disorder is now known to be the result of a metabolic disorder in which an exogenous fatty acid (phytanic acid) accumulates in the tissues in abnormal amounts. Some success has been reported in treating patients with a diet low in phytanic acid. (For further details, see Chap. 323.)

PATHOLOGY The lesions are typical of a chronic multiple peripheral neuropathy with secondary atrophic changes in muscles. The degenerative process in the nerve fibers is associated with abortive regenerative phenomena and with proliferation of connective tissue and Schwann cells which, in the hypertrophic variety, may reach extreme degrees. In the central nervous system, there are varying degrees of overlap with the lesions found in the various forms of hereditary ataxia already discussed.

CLINICAL ASPECTS The disorder usually begins in childhood and progresses very slowly. In the classic cases of peroneal muscular atrophy, the combination of pes cavus with extreme atrophy of the anterior tibial and calf muscles ("stork legs") and wasting of the lower thigh musculature (giving an appearance like an "inverted champagne bottle") presents a striking picture. There is total absence of deep reflexes, and sensation is altered as described in Chap. 325. The possibility of combinations with other hereditary neurologic syndromes has already been pointed out. Although death in a state of extreme debility in early adult life is common, progression in some cases may be extremely slow and may lead to very little disability. Measurements of phytanic acid, alpha- and beta-lipoproteins, cholesterol, and gamma-globulins in the serum serve to distinguish some of the recently discovered metabolic neuropathies.

DIFFERENTIAL DIAGNOSIS It may be necessary to consider various other forms of chronic polyneuropathy (toxic, metabolic, nutritional), described in Chap. 323. The familial incidence, early onset, very slow progression, and absence (usually) of significant blood and cerebrospinal fluid changes, except for increased amount of protein in some patients, are generally sufficient for the accurate recognition of the hereditary neuropathies under discussion. In occasional sporadic or atypical cases, biopsy of muscle and of a small cutaneous nerve twig (most conveniently the sural cutaneous nerve) will be necessary.

TREATMENT Although no specific treatment is available (except possibly in Refsum's disease, as indicated above), patients whose disease is of slow progression and in whom conditions are otherwise favorable may be greatly helped by measures to ensure a stable walking surface, such as corrective shoes, braces to prevent foot drop, and even orthopedic procedures to stabilize the joints.

SYNDROME OF PROGRESSIVE VISUAL LOSS

As already stated in previous sections, progressive impairment or loss of vision, due to degenerative changes in the visual system (retinas and optic nerves), may be an accompaniment of morbid processes affecting the nervous system diffusely—in particular, the nervous system lipidoses and the hereditary ataxias. Occasionally, however, the peripheral visual system is the major, or only, site of disease. In such cases, the disorders are strongly hereditary. For detailed discussion of these conditions, standard reference works on ophthalmology should be consulted. Nevertheless, two entities, because of their close relationship with other degenerative diseases of the nervous system, warrant some discussion here.

Hereditary optic atrophy (Leber)

This rare condition is characterized by the relatively rapid development of bilateral blindness with optic atrophy, coming on in early adult life. It was first thoroughly described by Leber in 1871. Typically, it occurs as a sex-linked recessive trait, chiefly affecting men, but it may be seen in women.

PATHOLOGY In the only recorded case with autopsy, the changes occurred primarily in the ganglion cells of the retina, with secondary degeneration in optic nerve fibers. Because of the limited examination in this case, it is not known whether there were lesions in other parts of the nervous system.

CLINICAL ASPECTS The condition often begins asymmetrically, with blurring of vision in one eye followed in days or weeks by similar affection of the other eye. Vision then deteriorates rapidly over ensuing weeks or months, generally with eventual total blindness as a result, although arrest before this stage has been seen, or even a little improvement after initial steady progression. In the early stages, examination of the visual fields shows large central scotomas. The optic disks may be normal at first, or may be swollen (optic neuritis); later the appearance is typically that of optic atrophy, with pale, clearly outlined disks.

DIFFERENTIAL DIAGNOSIS Multiple sclerosis may at times act in a manner identical to that just described, but without a definite hereditary background and with a much better outlook for improvement of vision. Toxic or nutritional amblyopia can generally be excluded by history and associated clinical findings. In some cases it may be necessary to eliminate the possibility of a tumor compressing the chiasmal region and optic nerves, although some evidence of bitemporal defects would be then expected, rather than bilateral central scotomas alone. In addition to careful roentgenograms of the skull and cerebrospinal fluid examination, pneumoencephalographic visualization of the chiasmal region may be indicated in cases of serious doubt. Early onset of optic atrophy with spastic paralysis of legs (Behr's syndrome) should also be distinguishable on clinical grounds.

Pigmentary degeneration of the retina (retinitis pigmentosa)

This may at times occur as a relatively independent disorder, although it is often associated with other abnormalities, of which cataracts, deafness, and mental deficiency are outstanding. It is strongly hereditary, chiefly as a recessive trait, although dominant inheritance has been seen. Pigmentary degeneration of the retina is one of the features of the Laurence-Moon-Biedl syndrome. Special varieties of the condition also accompany some cases of neuronal lipidosis or hereditary neuropathy as already noted.

PATHOLOGY The principal lesion is a degeneration of the rods and cones, associated with displacement of melanin-containing cells from the pigment epithelium into more superficial parts of the retina. Other retinal structures are relatively intact.

CLINICAL ASPECTS The disorder typically begins in childhood, first as night blindness. The visual fields become concentrically narrowed from the periphery to the center, until eventually (by adolescence, or perhaps not until middle age) very little useful vision remains. Ophthalmoscopic examination may be normal at first, but generally discloses irregular patches of dark pigment in the periphery of the retina. When cataracts are likewise present, as sometimes is the case, visual acuity may be significantly improved by their removal. The frequent association of the retinal lesions with other neurologic abnormalities has been mentioned in previous paragraphs.

DIFFERENTIAL DIAGNOSIS Chorioretinitis from other causes (e.g., syphilis) may present a similar ophthalmoscopic appearance and should be excluded. The hereditary background and the progressive course, with night blindness and peripheral constriction of the visual fields, may lead to the diagnosis even in the rare cases where pigmentary deposits in the retina are absent. The slowly progressive or relatively stationary tapetoretinal degenerations of childhood can be distinguished clinically and by electroretinogram. In most instances, the opinion of a qualified ophthalmologist must be obtained.

REFERENCES

BLACKWOOD W. et al: *Greenfield's Neuropathology,* Baltimore: Williams & Wilkins, 1963

GAMBETTI P et al: Myoclonic epilepsy with Lafora bodies: Some ultrastructural, histochemical and biochemical aspects. Arch Neurol 25:483, 1971

PRATT RTC: *The Genetics of Neurological Disorders,* London: Oxford, 1967

VOLK BW, ARONSON SM (eds): *Sphingolipids, Asphingolipidoses and Allied Disorders,* New York: Plenum, 1972

WANGER SL: The management of Parkinson's syndrome. Med Clin N Am 56:693, 1972

WIGBOLDUS JM, BRUYN GW: Hallervorden-Spatz disease, in *Handbook of Clinical Neurology,* eds PJ Vinken, GW Bruyn, Amsterdam: North-Holland Publishing Co., 1968, p. 604

WOSTENHOLME GEW, O'CONNOR M (eds): *Alzheimer's Disease and Related Conditions,* London: J & A Churchill, 1970

ZEMAN W, DYKEN P: Dystonia musculorum deformans: Clinical, genetic and pathoanatomical studies. Psychiat Neurol Neurochir 70:77, 1967

DEVELOPMENTAL AND OTHER CONGENITAL ABNORMALITIES OF THE NERVOUS SYSTEM

RAYMOND D. ADAMS
G. ROBERT DeLONG

The human nervous system is subject to a variety of developmental abnormalities which may be traced to genetic faults or diseases acquired *in utero*, at birth, or during the early years of life. These conditions may be manifest at birth or may be recognized only in late infancy and childhood, after some degree of maturation of the nervous system has occurred. Together they comprise the principal problems of pediatric neurology, and to discuss them fully would be pointless in a textbook of medicine. But many individuals so afflicted reach adolescent and adult age and come under the care of internists and general physicians; hence some understanding of the basic problems in this field is requisite.

Adult disorders of the nervous system that originate in early life may be classified under the following headings:

1 Congenital malformations of head, spine, and other structures, including dwarfism
2 Diseases which retard motor, speech, and intellectual development
3 Hereditary diseases which begin during childhood and persist throughout lifetime
4 Epilepsy

Unlike many of the common neurologic problems that begin in adult years, those of infancy and childhood bring to light a number of pathogenic mechanisms unique to the early period of life. A genetic fault or exogenous agent may destroy the embryonal germ plasm in the first three postconceptional months, thereby blighting the formation and subsequent development of the nervous system as well as other somatic structures. Again, more subtle hereditary factors may alter the complex program of cerebral maturation so that it will not unfold in an even and harmonious way, leaving the person deficient in certain skills such as dexterity, speaking, reading, mathematic ability, music appreciation, etc. Or a disease may strike the rapidly maturing nervous system at birth (a unique event with its own possibilities of pathogenesis) or in the first years of life, leaving the victim with fixed and persistent deficits, such as retarded intellect, cerebral palsy, and epilepsy, for the entire span of life. For example, the myelination of the brain, which is one of the main developmental processes in infancy, is thought by some investigators to be permanently impaired by protein malnutrition. Finally, an unusually large proportion of special hereditary diseases declare themselves during childhood and continue into adult years, such as von Recklinghausen's neurofibromatosis and tuberous sclerosis.

MALFORMATIONS OF CRANIUM, SPINE, AND LIMBS The intimate relationship between craniovertebral structures and the growth and development of the brain and spinal cord deserves comment. In embryonic life the most rapidly growing parts of the neural tube induce special changes in and at the same time are influenced by the overlying mesoderm (a process known as induction which is important in the formation of skull, orbits, nose, and spine). During early fetal life the cranium and vertebral arches enclose and protect the developing brain and spinal cord. And all during the rapid phases of brain growth the skull accommodates to the increasing size of the brain as the latter exerts pressure on its inner surface. In addition, statural growth is controlled by the nervous system, as shown by the fact that the majority of severe mental retardates are dwarfed. Thus, the craniovertebral growth disorders assume importance not merely because of their unsightly appearance but also because of their frequent association with abnormalities of the brain and spinal cord.

Certain alterations in the size and shape of head observed in the adult can nearly always be assumed to be connected with a neurologic disease that began during intrauterine life or childhood. Beyond the first 4 to 5 years the skull has so nearly attained adult size and the sutures are so firmly closed that later acquired disease will have relatively little effect on the skull. Tumor invasion and trauma are the only exceptions. Enlargement of the head (macrocephaly) is as a rule due to childhood hydrocephalus or to macroencephaly; smallness of the head (microcephaly) may be the result of a lack of brain growth and development. Craniostenosis is the consequence of premature closure of the sutures. If the sagittal suture fuses, the head is long and narrow with prominent brow and occiput; if the coronal suture closes prematurely, the head is wider than long (brachycephaly). Closure of all sutures produces a characteristic high skull (turricephaly) and shallow orbits with bulging eyes. If this condition is not recognized during early life and treated surgically, the volume of the skull may be so limited as to prevent brain growth and to raise the intracranial pressure. Apert's syndrome (craniostenosis with syndactyly or "mitten hands") is often associated with mental retardation. Achondroplasia results in a normal-sized skull which looks disproportionately large because of the patient's short limbs. Flatness of one occiput and the opposite side of the forehead (plagiocephaly) is usually due to a condition that caused prolonged recumbency in infancy with the head turned to one side. Any disease that destroys brain tissue in early life leaves the head abnormally small (<50 cm in circumference), but there is also a hereditary form of cerebral maldevelopment in which the skull never grows. The small cranium contrasts with the normal size of facial structures. One can usually recognize such individuals at a glance because of their resemblance to primitive man or anthropoids. Many of the diseases that impair the development of the brain also deform the bridge of the nose, the distance between the eyes (hyper- and hypotelorism), the shape of the ears, and the growth of the maxillae. Such somatic stigmata may be used as indications that impaired brain function is a maldevelopment.

ABNORMALITIES OF THE SPINE A remarkable variety of lifelong neurologic syndromes is associated with abnormality of the vertebral column. Some of these, such as hemivertebra, platybasia, fusion of the atlas and occiput or of vertebras (Klippel-Feil syndrome), or congenital dislocation of the atlas, are the consequence of a malformation of the spine itself, and the enclosed spinal cord may or may not be involved. Others, such as spina bifida occulta, spinal meningocele or myelomeningocele or dysraphism, involve the whole neural tube, including spinal cord, investing meninges, vertebral bodies, and even the overlying skin and subcutaneous tissues.

In many of these patients the neurologic defect which appears in infancy does not shorten life and will be seen in the adult. In a few it may not appear until adult life.

PRIMARY MALFORMATIONS OF VERTEBRAE These are most frequent in the upper cervical region. *The Klippel-Feil deformity* consists of maldevelopment and fusion of two or more cervical vertebras, resulting in a short neck of limited mobility. The hairline is low, often at the level of the first thoracic vertebra. There may or may not be associated neurologic symptoms or signs. The importance of the spinal deformity lies in its frequent association with other abnormalities, especially platybasia and syringomyelia, the symptoms of which may not become manifest until adolescence or adult life.

Platybasia and basilar impression In this rare maldevelopment either the base of the skull is flattened or the occiput and upper cervical spine are invaginated in the posterior fossa. Often the foramen magnum itself is imperfectly developed, or the atlas and occiput are fused. The exact teratogenesis of these anomalies is uncertain. The conditions may be asymptomatic, but frequently there is "crowding," distortion, or compression of the spinal cord, medulla, and cranial and spinal nerves.

The resulting clinical picture is variable. Symptoms may be present from early life or may begin in late childhood, adolescence, or even adult years. Early symptoms consist of "dizzy" or "weak" spells and downward nystagmus on tilting the head; evidences of increased intracranial pressure such as headache; occipital neuralgia; vomiting; transient paresthesias in the occipital region, neck, or arm; facial paresthesias, deafness, nasal voice, and dysphagia; cerebellar ataxia; and spastic weakness of the legs. The symptoms may first be intermittent and at any time in the course of the illness may be aggravated by straining, moving the head, or placing the head and neck in certain positions. Inspection alone provides a clue to diagnosis. The whole configuration of the head and neck is abnormal. The neck is short; the ears and hairline are low; the neck movements are obviously restricted; and the normal cervical lordosis is lost or greatly exaggerated, sometimes to the extent that the occiput lies almost on the upper dorsal spine and shoulders.

Instability of the junction of axis on atlas (atlantoaxial dislocation) may cause compression of the spinal cord. This may also occur as a consequence of rheumatoid arthritis, other debilitating diseases, and trauma (tear of ligaments which bind the odontoid process to the body of the first cervical vertebra). The treatment is surgical.

Platybasia and these related anomalies of the spine should be suspected in all cases presenting progressive cerebellar, brainstem, and cervical cord syndromes. Many of these cases have been misdiagnosed as multiple sclerosis. Others present a typical syringomyelic syndrome and have been so labeled. The clinical suspicion of platybasia and other spine anomalies can be confirmed by a true lateral roentgenogram of the skull. In such a projection the extension of a line drawn from the hard palate and posterior border of the foramen magnum (Chamberlain's line) and another through the spine and body of the first cervical vertebra (Bull's line) when extended, instead of being more or less parallel as they normally are, intersect. The relation of cervical vertebras is also seen. An acquired form of *basilar impression* occurs with rickets and Paget's disease. It is usually asymptomatic but sometimes involves the lower cranial nerves.

The Arnold-Chiari malformation This condition, in which medulla and inferior-posterior portions of the cerebellar hemispheres project caudally through the foramen magnum, often to the level of the second cervical vertebra, is a common cause of hydrocephalus. It is usually associated with a spinal meningocele or myelomeningocele, and often there are deformities of the cervical spine and cervicooccipital junction. The symptoms of hydrocephalus dominate the clinical picture in infants; but in milder cases, there may develop during adolescence or adult years any one of the several syndromes already described under Platybasia and Basilar Impression. When platybasia and the Arnold-Chiari malformation coexist, it is generally impossible to decide which of the two is responsible for the clinical findings.

The treatment of platybasia and the Arnold-Chiari malformation has not been entirely satisfactory. If clinical progression is slight or uncertain, it is probably advisable to do nothing. If progression is certain and disability is increasing, upper cervical laminectomy and enlargement of the foramen magnum are indicated. Often this procedure halts the course of the illness or results in improvement. The surgical procedure must be done cautiously, however, for extensive manipulation of these structures may aggravate the symptoms or even cause death.

Malformations associated with a defect in closure of the neural arch Many deformities along the posterior surface of the body are accompanied by an abnormality in the formation of the posterior aspect of the neural arch and closure of the primitive neural tube. The entire neural canal, including the cranium, may fail to close (*craniorhachischisis totalis*), or there may be only a minute defect in one or more of the vertebral arches, demonstrable by roentgenograms (*spina bifida occulta*). The latter is said to occur in one-quarter of the population. It has been estimated that in approximately 1 of every 900 births there is a serious closure defect in the spine or, more rarely, in the cranium. Heredity cannot usually be established, but the defect is several times more frequent in siblings than in the general population.

Defects of this type may be found at any point along the neuraxis. They are most frequent in the lumbosacral and cranial regions, less so in the cervical, and rare in the thoracic. The character of the abnormality varies. There may be an outpouching of neural elements (nerve root and cord) through a defect in mesenchymal tissue and skin (myelomeningocele); less often, actually in less than one-fifth of all cases, only a thin-walled cyst composed of meninges and containing no neural tissue can be found. The cranial defect similarly may consist of an encephalocele with evagination of cerebral tissue and meninges through a midline defect in the membranous bones of the skull. These are most often occipital in location (and are accompanied by visual defects, mental retardation, and ataxia of gait), though a few may be frontal, presenting either anteriorly or inferiorly into the nasal cavity. The latter may be asymptomatic except for an occasional cerebrospinal rhinorrhea.

Meningocele and myelomeningocele Meningocele may exist alone, unaccompanied by any symptoms or signs. Myelomeningocele (much the more frequent), in contrast, is associated with some dysfunction of those nervous structures that lie within the wall of the sac. The signs may be minimal, limited to sensorimotor dysfunction of a few segments, or pronounced, with total paraplegia and incontinence of urine and feces.

Sinus tracts and congenital cysts These are often indicated by a small dimple in the skin or by a tuft of hair along the posterior surface of the body in the midline. These signs occur most often in the lumbosacral and occipital regions and are thought to represent failure of closure of the anterior or posterior neuropores. (The pilonidal sinus, in the opinion of the authors, should not be included in this group.) Small *sinus tracts* may exist at these points and are of clinical importance because they frequently connect with the central nervous system or its coverings and are not uncommonly associated with dermoid cysts at the central part of the tract. These cysts most often occur in the cerebellum or in the lumbosacral regions, and the sinus tracts which connect them to the skin provide free access for bacteria and are often a source of *abscess* and *recurrent meningitis*. Evidence of such tracts should be sought in every instance of meningitis, especially when infection has recurred.

There are, in addition, other *congenital cysts* and *tumors* which may produce progressive symptoms and signs by compressing the spinal cord or by implicating nerve roots.

Diastematomyelia is another unusual abnormality of the spinal cord. Here a bony spicule or ridge protrudes into the spinal canal from the body of one of the thoracic or upper lumbar vertebras. If the bony abnormality is in the thoracic region, there will be no duplication of, or splitting of, the spinal cord (diplomyelia); with growth, this leads to a "traction myelopathy."

All these spinal abnormalities are of particular interest to internists when they begin to produce symptoms for the first time in an adolescent or adult. Several clinical syndromes have been delineated: (1) Progressive spastic weakness in some of the weak muscles of the legs during late childhood or adolescence in a patient known to have had a meningocele or myelomeningocele. Presumably the spinal cord, which is securely attached to the lumbar vertebras, is stretched during the period of rapid lengthening of the vertebral column. (2) An acute cauda equina syndrome following some unusual activity or incident, e.g., rowing or a fall in a sitting position, in patients who have had an asymptomatic or symptomatic spina bifida or meningocele. The implicated sensory and motor roots are believed to be injured by sudden or repeated stretching. Weakness of bladder control, impotence (in the male), and numbness of feet and legs or footdrop comprise the clinical syndrome. (3) Progressive cauda equina syndrome in the lumbosacral region. (4) Syringomyelia.

SYRINGOMYELIA This is a term that refers to a cavity (from the Greek *syrinx*, meaning "pipe" or "tube"). The cavity occupies the central parts of the spinal cord in the cervical region but may extend upward into the medulla oblongata (syringobulbia) or downward into the thoracic or even lumbar segments. In approximately 15 percent of cases studied post mortem, an intramedullary tumor (hemangioblastoma or glioma) has been found in or near some part of the syrinx. The syrinx is independent of, but connected with, the central canal and replaces the gray matter of the posterior or anterior horns of the spinal cord and also interrupts the crossing pain and temperature fibers in the anterior commissure in several successive cord segments. The cavity is lined with astrocytic glia and a few thick-walled blood vessels. It may enlarge the spinal cord and even widen the interpedicular spaces. The cerebrospinal fluid in the cavity always has a relatively low protein level. The cause is unknown, but it is clearly linked to malformations at the craniocervical junction. Familial incidence is rare. A blastomatous formation akin to tuberous sclerosis or central von Recklinghausen's disease but with tendency for the abnormal tissue to cavitate is one explanation. A hydromyelia, sometimes associated with hydrocephalus in early life and diverticulation, appears more plausible. Elevated pressure of cerebrospinal fluid within the spinal canal may not only widen it, but dissect into zones of pressure necrosis of the spinal cord, leading to the formation of central cavities.

The clinical triad upon which the diagnosis is based consists of (1) segmental sensory loss or dissociation (loss of pain and temperature sense and preservation of sense of touch) over neck, shoulders, and arms; (2) amyotrophy, and (3) thoracic scoliosis. Symptoms may begin in late childhood and adolescence, but more often in adult life, and progress irregularly, often being arrested for long periods of time. The segmental sensory loss or dissociation and amyotrophy are caused by cavitation, destruction, and stretching of the ventral commissural fibers and the anterior and posterior horns, respectively. Analgesia and thermoanesthesia account for severe painless ulcers, injuries, and burns; Charcot joints, also common in this disease, result from injury of the denervated joint tissue. Areflexia without atrophy may be due to involvement of the afferent limb of the reflex arc; but destruction of anterior horn cells is a frequent cause, particularly if accompanied by muscle atrophy. A useful clinical rule is that a neurologic disease which leaves all deep tendon reflexes in the arms intact is probably not syringomyelia. A Horner's syndrome on the affected side may result from involvement of cells of the intermediolateral cell column of the eighth cervical to first thoracic segments of the spinal cord. Pyramidal tract signs in the legs tend to appear late in the course of the disease and are attributable to extension of the syrinx into the lateral columns of the cord or into the decussation of corticospinal tracts at the first cervical segment, or to compression of these tracts by a distended syrinx. If the cavity enlarges the spinal cord, a spinal subarachnoid block may result, and prolonged pressure may cause widening of the spinal canal and erosion of pedicles. The kyphoscoliosis, which may antedate other evidence of disease by several years, is thought to result from asymmetric weakness of paravertebral muscles.

A syrinx in the brainstem (syringobulbia) usually extends into the lateral tegmentum of the medulla, being so placed as to result in nystagmus and sensory impairment over one or both sides of the face. Unilateral palatal and vocal cord paralysis, as well as weakness and atrophy of one side of the tongue, are other clinical signs which call attention to lesions at this level of the neuraxis. Syringobulbia never occurs without syringomyelia.

The association of cavitation of the spinal cord with myelomeningocele (so-called "myelodysplasia"), Arnold-Chiari malformation, platybasia, and other congenital defects about the cervicocranial junction has been commented on in previous sections.

The treatment of syringomyelia is unsatisfactory. The fact that the disease process may remain stationary for some months or years before progressing makes evaluation of any mode of therapy difficult. Decompression of a distended syrinx up to the foramen magnum may alleviate temporarily those symptoms and signs resulting from local compression of ascending and descending spinal tracts, but relief is seldom lasting. Reducing the pressure within the cavity by occluding the upper end of the central canal, opening it, or making a ventriculosubarachnoid shunt has given unpredictable results. X-ray treatment, based on the belief that symptoms result from a gliomatous malformation of the cord which subsequently cavitates, is probably worthless, unless there is an underlying tumor.

MALFORMATIONS OF THE EXTREMITIES A variety of primary skeletal defects, such as absence of or increase in number of digits or extremities, fusion or webbing of digits (*syndactylism*), and deformity of digits or limbs or abnormalities of size may have neurologic import, for they tend to be associated with malformations of the central nervous system. For example, *syndactylism* is frequently combined with oxycephaly (Apert's syndrome). In *mongolism* (Down's syndrome) the middle phalanx of the fifth digit is usually short and the finger curved (clinodactyly), the hands are broad and simian-like, and there is usually only a single transverse crease in the palm. Gigantism of a limb may occur with neurofibromas and hemangiomas of that part of the body.

In some cases the deformity of the extremities is the direct consequence of a congenital neuromuscular defect. In fact, this happens so often that whenever smallness and deformities of the limbs are known to have begun early in life, one should at once evaluate the status of the nervous system. In most cases of *clubfoot* (talipes equinovarus), no abnormality of the nervous system can be ascertained. In a few, however, the deformity results from paralysis of the anterior tibial and peroneal muscles because of a primary defect in the anterior horn cells of the lumbrosacral segments of the spinal cord. The contracture of calf muscles is secondary to their unopposed activity. Widespread weakness and contractures of many limb muscles may cause extensive deformities (*arthrogryposis multiplex* or *amyoplasia congenita*). This syndrome may also be the result of any one of several other primary neural or muscular diseases such as congenital absence of muscles (muscular dystrophy) and rarely may result from congenital absences of anterior horn cells and *Werdnig-Hoffmann infantile muscular atrophy*. Reconstructive surgery and the techniques of physical medicine may permit a certain measure of rehabilitation in those patients with nonprogressive diseases and otherwise normal development.

DWARFISM IN RELATION TO NEUROLOGIC DISEASE Dwarfs (in contrast to midgets, who are more or less normally proportioned) suffer usually from a disorder of cartilaginous growth. Their head and trunk are large and out of proportion to their limbs. Achondroplasia would be an example. But it is noteworthy, as remarked above, that the majority of mentally retarded individuals fall below average in statural growth, and in a few dwarfism is part of any one of many special syndromes. The mongoloid and persons with most of the other chromosomal abnormalities are examples, and there are others in which an inherited or acquired metabolic defect of definable type blights brain and skeletal growth (e.g., cretinism and mucopolysaccharidoses). Microcephaly characterizes many of the dwarfs with cerebral diseases.

The 30 or 40 neurologic syndromes with statural underdevelopment and neurologic diseases are described and illustrated in the *Atlas of Mental Retardation* by Holmes, Moser, et al.

THE PHAKOMATOSES

A number of neurologic abnormalities are combined with congenital defects of skin or retina, explained usually by their common ectodermal origin. The terms *congenital ectodermal dysplasias*, *congenital neurocutaneous syndromes*, or *phakomatoses* (Greek *phakos*, lentil, mole, or freckle) are used frequently to designate this general class of disorders. The major syndromes include *neurofibromatosis*, *tuberous sclerosis*, *encephalotrigeminal syndrome*, and rarely the *cerebelloretinal hemangioblastomatosis*. Another variant of the latter is the *myelocutaneous* (Klippel-Trelauney) *syndrome*, in which a vascular malformation of spinal cord and meninges is associated with a vascular nevus within the area of skin innervated by the involved spinal segments. Recently it has been suggested that *ataxia telangiectasia* be included with this group of conditions.

NEUROFIBROMATOSIS (VON RECKLINGHAUSEN'S DISEASE) This is an inherited disease (mendelian dominant) in which spots of increased skin pigmentation are combined with multiple neurofibromas. The pigmented spots are irregular in shape with relatively even borders, vary in size from a few millimeters to several centimeters, and are of brownish coffee color (café au lait). They are most prominent over the trunk, in the axilla (axillary freckles), and about the pelvis. Similar lesions occur in individuals without neurofibromatosis but in such instances are generally smaller than 3 cm in diameter and fewer than five in number. The tumors arise from the neurilemmal sheath (Schwann cells) and fibroblasts of the peripheral nerve. They are usually multiple and vary in size from minute lesions to large tumors several centimeters in diameter. The majority are smoothly rounded or lobulated, soft or firm, and can sometimes be seen or felt along the course of a peripheral nerve. Often they sink into the subcutaneous fat on gentle pressure. Like the pigmented lesions, the tumors are more frequent over the trunk than on the extremities. The pigmented areas, because of giant melanosomes in pigment epithelial cells, become increasingly apparent with age; also the tumors of nerve sheaths are often not demonstrable early in life. Most of the tumors are asymptomatic; but occasionally, if they attain a large size or occupy an unusual position, they may produce pressure upon contiguous structures. Tumors of the spinal nerve roots may compress the spinal cord and at the same time extend through the intervertebral foramens to form a large mass in the posterior mediastinum (dumbbell tumors). Acoustic neurinomas, usually bilateral in patients with neurofibromatosis, may produce deafness and symptoms and signs of a cerebellopontine angle lesion (see Chap. 328). Other histopathologic types of tumor (meningioma, glioma) are encountered more frequently in neurofibromatosis than in the general population. Diffuse overgrowth of Schwann cells and fibroblasts may also occur, giving rise to plexiform neuromas. They may cause hideous deformities, often with overgrowth of underlying bone. Bone cysts may also form. Most of these associated tumors are rare in infancy and childhood, though pontine glioma and glioma of the optic nerve are exceptions to the clinical rule. The latter condition should always be considered in the differential diagnosis of unilateral (rarely bilateral) blindness, proptosis, and extraocular muscle paralysis in childhood, especially if there are signs of von Recklinghausen's disease. Enlargement of the optic foramens, demonstrable by roentgenogram, is a valuable aid in diagnosis. *Pulsating exophthalmos* (usually due to an orbital hemangioma) may result from congenital absence of part of the sphenoid bone. *Pheochromocytoma* is an infrequent accompaniment of the disease. In about 5 to 10 percent of cases of neurofibromatosis one of the tumors will become sarcomatous.

Fibrous dysplasia, congenital vertebral anomalies, local gigantism of an extremity, subperiosteal bone cysts, and pseudoarthrosis of the tibia may be associated with neurofibromatosis. Any of these can lead to scoliosis, a common skeletal deformity in children with this disease, so that neurofibromatosis must be added to the list of neurogenic kyphoscolioses (the others are syringomyelia, Friedreich's ataxia, and poliomyelitis). Stenosis of the aqueduct of Sylvius with obstructive hydrocephalus is at times observed in neurofibromatosis. Also there may be a mild degree of mental retardation, related presumably to developmental abnormalities of the cerebral cortex. Spina bifida, hypospadias, glaucoma, and elephantiasis are occasionally seen.

About one-third of cases of neurofibromatosis are discovered accidentally on routine examination, there being no complaints. Another third of these patients come seeking advice about the cosmetic aspects of the disease, and the remainder have neurologic syndromes. There is no treatment for the disease other than excision of symptomatic tumors.

TUBEROUS SCLEROSIS (BOURNEVILLE'S DISEASE) This curious disease, of dominant inheritance, is manifested by the clinical triad of convulsive seizures, progressive mental deficiency, and adenoma sebaceum. The latter are fine, wartlike lesions predominantly in a butterfly distribution over the cheeks and forehead. The individual adenomas vary in size from 0.1 to 1.0 cm and are elevated and pinkish or pinkish yellow in color. In addition, the skin over the lower part of the back may be thick, rough, and of yellowish color like sharkskin or pigskin (shagreen patch). Actually the earliest lesions are foliate light spots ("white spots") over the trunk, which are seen most clearly under ultraviolet light (Wood's lamp). They are distinguishable on the basis of size, shape, and character from avascular nevi and vitiligo, and are highly diagnostic, often providing the earliest clue to mental retardation or infantile epilepsy. The mental deficiency may be relatively stationary or progressive. The seizures are usually generalized but may be focal. Retinal tumors, optic atrophy and cataracts, syndactylism, spina bifida, and other visible malformations may be conjoined.

The most advanced examples of tuberous sclerosis usually are to be found in institutions for the mentally retarded, but it would be a mistake to assume that all are so severely disabled. In general hospital clinics it is not at all unusual to see patients with average intelligence and only seizures and a few skin lesions. Occasionally a focal cerebral syndrome will prove at biopsy to have a typical "tuber" or an associated glioma as its basis in a patient not known to have this disease. Family history is frequently unhelpful because the disease arose as a mutation.

The lesions of the skin are pathologically fibromas and not true adenomas. Some are rather vascular and suggest telangiectasia. The brain lesions consist of areas of malformed cortex with extensive astrogliosis and a peculiar mixture of glioblasts and monster nerve cells. Calcification may or may not be present. Masses of subependymal glial tissue account for nodules which project into and form "candle gutterings" on the walls of the ventricles that are often seen in pneumograms. In Bourneville's original case, death was due to rhabdomyoma of the heart, and most cases of this benign tumor of heart muscle are associated with tuberous sclerosis. This disease is also combined with vascular malformations of kidney, liver, adrenal glands, and pancreas.

The diagnosis is aided by roentgenograms of the skull. Calcified nodules occur particularly in the temporal lobes. The center of the nodule tends to be more densely radiopaque than the periphery. The electroencephalogram is usually abnormal but without specific pattern. The cerebrospinal fluid may be normal; rarely the total protein level is elevated.

The only treatment is symptomatic. The prognosis for life beyond the third decade is poor, especially for patients with advanced cases. Death may be due to seizures, associated tumors, or intercurrent diseases.

CEREBELLORETINAL HEMANGIOBLASTOMATOSIS (HIPPEL-LINDAU SYNDROME) This condition is discussed here though the skin is seldom involved. As the name implies, the syndrome consists of a vascular malformation of the retina and cerebellum. The retinal lesion usually has the characteristics of a malformation; the cerebellar lesion consists of a slowly growing cystic tumor. The clinical symptoms and signs consist of progressive cerebellar ataxia, headache, and papilledema. Seldom is a vascular bruit audible over the head. Polycythemia, possibly related to the production of erythropoietin, has been observed in many cases and has in a few instances disappeared after excision of the tumor. Rarely do these tumors appear before adolescence. Some cases are familial. The cerebellar lesions may be multiple and associated with one or more spinal hemangioblastomas. One should consider this diagnosis in all patients with a cerebellar tumor syndrome (see Chap. 328). Not all have a retinal lesion—the von Hippel part of the disease. The hemangioblastoma of the cerebellum is usually but one part of a constellation of abnormalities including angiomas of the liver, cysts of the pancreas and kidneys, and tumors of the epididymis and kidney, the latter being the cause of death in some cases. Pheochromocytomas have been described in this and in other of the phakomatoses. Syringomyelia has been observed in a few cases, and if a careful search is made, a hemangioblastoma can often be found in relation to the syrinx at some level.

The cerebellar hemangioblastoma demands surgical treatment, and if the nodule of the tumor is found in the wall of the cyst and is excised, the results can be excellent; if the tumor cannot be operated on because of size or multiplicity, radiation should be tried.

ENCEPHALOTRIGEMINAL SYNDROME (STURGE-WEBER DISEASE) This disease consists of capillary or cavernous hemangiomas, within the cutaneous distribution of the trigeminal nerve and of a predominantly venous hemangioma of the leptomeninges. If the skin lesion is within the area of supply of the ophthalmic division of the trigeminal nerve, the occipital lobes are more commonly involved, whereas a facial nevus is more often associated with involvement of the parietal and frontal lobes. The intracranial or cutaneous lesion may occur separately.

Pathologically, in addition to the large number of abnormal blood vessels in the meninges, the cortex is destroyed, and in some cases a band of calcium develops within the lesion. This band, following the convolutional pattern as it does, is responsible for the characteristic "railroad track" roentgenographic picture.

The first neurologic symptom is usually a focal seizure on the side opposite the skin lesion. Transient postictal (Todd's) paralysis or permanent paralysis may follow the seizure. Sensorimotor paralysis or permanent visual field defect, the most frequent findings, may be either of insidious onset with slow progression or apoplectic. Hemorrhage into the meninges has been reported, but this must be a rare event. Possibly occlusion of cortical vessels is, in certain instances, responsible for neurologic deficits. Blindness in the eye on the side of the nevus is frequent and is nearly always due to glaucoma. Most patients with this malformation survive for many years, often with residual mental defects and hemiparesis.

The lesions are usually too extensive to be treated surgically, though hemispherectomy has been advised by some surgeons for intractable epilepsy. Anticonvulsant medication is indicated, but the seizures may be difficult to control.

Hemangioma of the trunk or upper or lower extremity may be associated with a spinal cord vascular malformation (Weber-Trelawney syndrome). The extremity may be hypertrophied. The cord lesion may bleed into or cause infarction in the nervous tissue, producing a spinal sensorimotor paralysis. Surgical exploration and decompression are seldom beneficial to the patient.

ATAXIA TELANGIECTASIA (LOUIS-BAR DISEASE) This condition has attracted considerable interest because of theoretical implications of its apparent cause and pathogenesis. Inherited as a recessive trait, the disease is characterized neurologically by a progressive cerebellar ataxia, apraxia of ocular movement, and choreoathetosis beginning during the early years of life. Telangiectases of bulbar conjunctivas and skin, especially about the ears, neck, and in flexor creases at the elbows and knees, appear somewhat later in childhood or adolescence. Recurring pulmonary and sinus infections have been prominent in many cases, and a deficiency in the IgA globulins and a defect of delayed hypersensitivity are found. The associated pathologic changes consist of an extensive loss of Purkinje cells of the cerebellum and degeneration of the neurons in other parts of the basal ganglions. Inclusion bodies are seen in some of the Purkinje cells of the cerebellum, suggesting a slow viral infection. The changes in the latter and in the spinal nerves have not been adequately characterized. Dysplasia of the thymus has been well documented, and death usually occurs by the second or third decade of life from infection or a reticuloendothelial tumor.

FAMILIAL DYSAUTONOMIA (RILEY-DAY SYNDROME)

This disease is characterized by autonomic instability (abnormal sweating, loss of vasomotor control, labile hypertension), impaired taste with absence of fungiform papillae, diminished pain and temperature sensation, hyporeflexia, episodic fever, vomiting attacks, and lack of lacrimation (alacrima), with corneal ulceration. Studies by Brunt and McKusick of 172 families show the disease to be inherited in a pattern consistent with an autosomal recessive trait and to be limited for the most part to Ashkenazi Jews.

The clinical manifestations become apparent in the first months of life and are increasingly evident in childhood. A few patients reach adult years, but the mortality rate is high because of recurrent pulmonary infections with inappropriate autonomic responses. Emotional instability presents a problem in most patients, but it has not been decided whether it is primary or secondary to prolonged illness. Nevertheless, there is a consistent electroencephalographic abnormality in most of the patients; and, although intelligence has been within normal limits in some patients, in others it has been slightly subnormal. Special studies reveal evidence of a small-fiber peripheral neuropathy, hypersensitivity of the pupil to 2.5% solutions of methylcholine (like Adie's myotonic or denervated pupils), and disturbed esophageal motility which accounts for aspiration pneumonia. Growth seems to be delayed for unclear reasons, and the natural tendency is to undernutrition and scoliosis. Neuropathic (Charcot) joints due to lack of pain and related injury have been reported.

Proof of the disturbance of the autonomic nervous system comes from special tests such as absence of skin flare after histamine and skin stroking (axonal reflex blockage), hypersensitivity to both cholinergic and adrenergic agents, altered pattern of nerve conduction, and abnormalities of catecholamine metabolism (change in urinary vanillomandelic and homovanillic acid ratios). Critical quantitative pathologic studies of peripheral and autonomic nervous systems have not been performed. A paucity of neurons in the lateral horns of the spinal cord would be consistent with a peripheral autonomic defect.

By inference it is suggested that the disease is due to a unitary biochemical defect, probably a deficiency of a single enzyme and perhaps related to the "nerve growth factor." Recently a deficiency of serum dopamine beta-hydroxylase has been found which might explain the disturbances in brain function.

In the differential diagnosis one must consider other forms of small-fiber polyneuropathy with analgesia and dysautonomia (including congenital indifference to pain and amyloidosis) (see Chap. 323), as well as the Shy-Drager syndrome (a degenerative disease of lateral horn cells and basal ganglions (see Chap. 333).

Picrotoxin is said to increase tearing of eyes, and the Heller-type myotomy has been successful in some few instances in improving esophageal function. Orthopedic measures are needed to stabilize neuropathic joints. Injury must be avoided and wounds treated carefully.

ABNORMALITIES OF MOTOR FUNCTION (CEREBRAL PALSY)

In this category of neurologic defect a major disturbance of motor function, usually nonprogressive, has been present since infancy or childhood. The popular term for these conditions is *cerebral palsy*. The name is not altogether appropriate, nor is such a crude classification of nervous disorders particularly useful from the viewpoint of the physician, because it results in a collocation of diseases of widely differing etiologic and anatomic types. The hereditary and acquired, the intrauterine, natal, and postnatal diseases lose their identity. Nevertheless, the term has been adopted as a slogan for fund-raising societies and for a major rehabilitation movement throughout the United States, and it will not soon disappear from medical terminology.

CLINICAL ASPECTS OF MOTOR DISTURBANCES WHICH HAVE BEEN PRESENT SINCE INFANCY OR CHILDHOOD Motor abnormalities which have had their onset early in life are so numerous and diverse in their manifestations that it is necessary to refer to the discussion of the motor system (Chaps. 17 and 18) in order to interpret them. In order to ascertain etiologic factors it is helpful to attempt to categorize a given case according to the extent and nature of the abnormality. Many patients with these motor abnormalities of infancy and childhood, which are relatively frequent, reach adult years.

SPECIAL TYPES Infantile spastic and rigid paralyses The pattern of paralysis or rigidity is important, for it provides information as to the etiology and possible pathogenic mechanism.

Cerebral spastic diplegia (Little's disease) In 1862 Little called attention to the concurrence of "Abnormal parturition, difficult labours, premature birth, and asphyxia neonatorum" and of a spastic weakness that affected legs more than arms. He emphasized the prenatal or natal origin, the diplegic distribution of the paralysis (legs more than arms), and the nonprogressive course. Little was of the opinion that asphyxia caused the cerebral damage; the present view attributes most cases to this factor and to cerebral circulatory insufficiency of posterior frontal and parietal lobes (border zone infarcts). Other factors such as prematurity are contributory in many cases.

Actually, the pattern of paralysis is more variable than the title implies. Three types may be distinguished, the paraplegic, diplegic, and the generalized and pseudobulbar. These differ from one another only with respect to the severity of affection of the arms and bulbar musculature. Pure paraplegias and pure pseudobulbar cases are relatively rare. Usually all four extremities are involved but the legs much more than the arms, which is the real meaning of diplegia. As a rule the damage to the nervous system is recognized at birth or soon thereafter by some abnormality of breathing, sucking and swallowing, color of mucous membranes, or responsiveness. These latter signs may indicate either a congenital defect of the nervous system or birth injury of the brainstem. However, the stiff, awkward movements of the legs, maintained in an extended, adducted posture, do not usually attract attention until several weeks or months have passed. Seizures occur in some cases, and it is not uncommon to observe a delay in all normal developmental sequences, especially those which depend on the motor system. Once walking is attempted, usually much later than in the normal child, the characteristic stance and gait become manifest. The legs are advanced stiffly in short steps, each describing part of the arc of a circle; adduction is often so strong as to lead to actual crossing (scissors gait), with lower legs slightly splayed out and the feet flexed and turned in, the heels not touching the ground. In the adolescent and adult, the legs tend to be short and small, but the muscles are not markedly atrophic, as in infantile muscular atrophy and dystrophy. Passive manipulation of the limbs reveals marked spasticity in the extensors and adductors and also slight shortening of the calf muscles. The hands and arms may be affected only slightly, if at all; there may be awkwardness and stiffness of the fingers; and in a few, pronounced weakness and spasticity. Speech may be well articulated or noticeably slurred, and in some instances the face is set in a spastic smile. The deep-tendon reflexes are exaggerated, those in the legs more than in the arms, and the plantar reflexes are extensor. Usually there is no disturbance of sphincteric function, though delay in acquiring voluntary control is usual. Athetotic postures and movements of the face, tongue, and hands are present in some patients and may actually conceal the pyramidal weakness. Ataxic and hypotonic forms also exist. The mentality in the pure form of diplegia tends to be relatively normal.

Surprisingly little exact information has been obtained concerning the cause, mechanism, and morbid anatomy of this syndrome. A higher incidence of spastic diplegia is known to be associated with prematurity. Only exceptionally are the Apgar scores of vital function in the first minutes and hours after birth reduced. The claim that physical birth injury is responsible has been challenged, and the existence of an antenatal lesion in some cases can no longer be doubted. Clinical study is handicapped by the fact that some of the infarcts of the cerebral cortex and white matter may occur *in utero* when the fetus cannot be tested, and the possibility of silent injuries to the nonfunctioning cerebrum can never be excluded. The condition must be distinguished from familial types of spastic paraparesis.

Infantile hemiplegia, double hemiplegia, and quadriplegia Hemiplegia is a not uncommon condition of infancy and childhood, and the functional difference between the two sides may be noticed soon after birth or during the first 6 to 12 months of life. The condition results usually as a consequence of a predominantly unilateral infection or thrombosis of cerebral arteries that may have happened before or after birth or during childhood. The parents may be the first to notice that movements of prehension and exploration are carried out with only one arm. The affection of the leg is usually recognized later, i.e., during the first attempt to stand and walk.

Mental defect may be associated with infantile hemiplegia but is even less common than with cerebral diplegia and much less than in bilateral hemiplegia. Convulsions occur in 35 to 50 percent of children with congenital hemiplegia, and these may persist throughout life. If the hemiplegia was acquired during childhood, seizures often accompany the onset. They may be generalized but are frequently unilateral and limited to the hemiplegic side. Often, after a series of seizures, the affected side will be weak for several hours or longer (Todd's paralysis).

In double hemiplegia, a much less frequent condition, the bilateral weakness of face, arms, and legs arises under conditions of more severe acquired cerebral disease and at any age. The arms are severely affected, in contrast to their minimal involvement in cerebral diplegia.

The quadriplegic state differs from bilateral hemiplegias in that the bulbar musculature is not involved. The condition is relatively rare but may result from a bilateral cerebral lesion. However, one should also be alerted to the possibility of a high cervical cord lesion. Although this may occasionally result from cysts, tumors, and other malformations, it is usually produced in the infant by a fracture-dislocation of the cervical spine, incurred during a difficult breech delivery. Similarly, in *paraplegia*, with weakness or paralysis limited to the legs, the lesion may be either a cerebral form of diplegia or a spinal one. Sphincteric disturbances and a definite loss of somatic sensation below a certain level on the trunk always favor a spinal localization. Congenital cysts, tumors, and diastematomyelia are more frequently the cause of paraplegia than of quadriplegia.

Encephaloclastic disorders underlie all these conditions. The pathologic change is essentially that of ischemic necrosis. In many cases, the lesions must have been incurred *in utero* and thus are not dependent on perinatal events. For the most part, the lesions reflect not pure asphyxia (anoxia) but circulatory insufficiency (ischemia) resulting from hypotension or circulatory collapse. The ischemia of circulatory failure tends to affect the tissues lying in arterial border zones, and there may also be venous stasis with congestion and hemorrhage (occurring particularly in the deep central structures such as the basal ganglions and periventricular matrix zones).

CONGENITAL EXTRAPYRAMIDAL SYNDROMES IN INFANCY AND CHILDHOOD

The spastic and rigid cerebral diplegias discussed above shade almost imperceptibly into the congenital extrapyramidal syndromes. Many such patients are found in every cerebral palsy clinic, and they ultimately may reach adult medical clinics. Pyramidal tract signs may be completely absent, and the inexperienced student, familiar only with the pure cerebral spastic diplegia syndrome, is always puzzled as to their classification. Some extrapyramidal cases of this type undoubtedly are attributable to severe perinatal hypoxia; others represent separate diseases such as erythroblastosis fetalis with kernicterus. In the interest of being able to state accurately the probable pathologic basis and future course of these illnesses, it is desirable to separate the extrapyramidal syndromes due to prenatal and natal diseases, which usually become manifest during the first year of life, from the acquired or hereditary postnatal syndromes such as familial athetosis, dystonia musculorum deformans, and cerebellar ataxia. The latter have been discussed in Chap. 333.

CONGENITAL CHOREOATHETOSIS (DOUBLE ATHETOSIS) Probably the most frequent representative of this group, this condition is like the spastic states in that it may not be recognized at birth but only after several months or a year have elapsed. The nature of the chorea and athetosis has been discussed in Chap. 18. Syndromes may be mixed, however. All combinations of chorea, athetosis, hemiballismus, myoclonus, and even dystonia may be found in a single case, or one or another type of movement disorder may predominate. However, in all instances there is in addition a primary defect in voluntary movement.

Choreoathetosis in infants and children varies in severity. In some the disorder is so mild that the abnormal movements are misinterpreted as restlessness or "the fidgets"; in others, every voluntary act is marred by intense involuntary movements, leaving the patient nearly helpless. In the latter the tongue may extrude itself from the mouth with unsightly drooling, and the face is contorted in a never-ending series of grimaces. Speech is slurred or inarticulate and punctuated by grunts and unpleasant throat sounds. The hands and arms are engaged in a constant play of writhing, twisting movements, and all attempts to use the limbs result in a slow, spreading spasm of the entire limb or all the musculature (intention spasm). Bizarre postures may assert themselves. The arms may be carried in a flexed or extended position in front of or behind the body, and the legs may be extended. The feet may be deformed; walking on the heels or side of the foot is more common than the "toe walking" of the cerebral diplegic. The neck may be extended or twisted. Movements may also be ataxic, and tremors are not uncommon. A retardation of motor development is the rule in these cases. Upright posture and walking may be delayed until the age of three to five years, and in some, may never be attained. Tonic neck reflexes or fragments thereof are commonly noted. The tendon reflexes are not consistently abnormal; plantar reflexes are characteristically flexor, though they may be difficult to interpret because of the continuous flexion and extension of the toes. The various sensory pathways usually function normally.

It is because of the motor and speech impairment that patients are many times erroneously classified as mentally defective. No doubt, in some patients this conclusion is correct, but others retain adequate intellectual function and can be educated. With growth and development new postures and new motor capacities are acquired. The less severely affected patients can even make successful occupational adjustments. However, the severely handicapped patients, even with the help of rehabilitation clinics and corrective orthopedic operations, rarely achieve a degree of motor control that will permit them to lead an independent life, and they continually need supportive treatment and help as adults. One sees some of these unfortunate persons bobbing and twisting as they walk in public places.

The most frequently observed pathologic change in the brain has been a curious whitish, marble-like appearance of the shrunken putamen, thalamus, and the border zones of the cerebral cortex. These whitish strands represent foci of nerve-cell loss and gliosis with peculiar condensations of myelinated fibers and even myelination of astroglial fibers (hypermyelination), the so-called *status marmoratus*. They do not arise beyond infancy, after the "myelination glia" have finished their developmental cycle.

Kernicterus is of importance in this context for it may also be a cause of generalized athetosis in children and adults. It is true that the majority of infants who suffer this disease die within the first week or two of life, and those who survive are often mentally retarded, deaf, and totally unable to sit, stand, or walk, so that the tendency is always to put them in homes for the feebleminded. But there are exceptional patients, obviously less damaged, who are mentally normal or at most only slightly backward. These are the ones who develop a variety of other neurologic sequelae that persist throughout life. Either athetosis or ataxia may be present, and a few have also shown rigid limbs and a picture not too different from that of cerebral spastic diplegia with involuntary movements. Kernicterus should always be suspected if an extrapyramidal syndrome is accompanied by bilateral deafness and ocular palsies. The neuropathologic changes in these surviving patients with milder cases consist of symmetrically distributed nerve-cell loss and gliosis in the subthalamic nucleus of Luys, the globus pallidus, thalamus, and oculomotor and cochlear nuclei. These lesions are the result of the hyperbilirubinemia. In the newborn, unconjugated bilirubin can pass through the poorly developed blood brain barrier into these central and brainstem nuclei, where it is directly toxic. Acidosis and hypoxia exacerbate the effect.

CONGENITAL AND ACQUIRED ATAXIAS The combination of cerebral diplegia with cerebellar ataxia has already been mentioned. In these patients difficulty in standing and walking cannot be attributed to spasticity or paralysis. Incoordination, similar to that seen in cerebellar disease, and hypotonia are the principal findings. The motor defect may be so great that the individual is never able to sit or stand; the muscles are of normal size, and voluntary movements, though weak, are possible in all the limbs. In less severe cases sitting, standing, and walking are merely delayed, and with advancing years cerebellar ataxia and tremor become manifest. Relative improvement may occur in later years. The tendon reflexes are present, and the plantar reflexes are either flexor or extensor. Many of these patients suffer a degree of amentia and retardation of speech development that results in their placement in homes for the feebleminded. In relatively few of the recorded cases have the pathologic changes of this condition been studied. Aplasia or hypoplasia of the cerebellum has been reported only a few times.

As to causes of this condition, radiation of the abdomen of a parturient woman during the first trimester of pregnancy is said to have resulted in cerebellar hypoplasia. A cerebral and cerebellar lesion may coexist with congenital ataxia, which is the reason for its classification as cerebrocerebellar diplegia.

Aside from the congenital ataxias, some of which are cerebellar and others probably of cerebral type, there are other forms of childhood ataxia which have an acute onset and which persist during adolescence and adult life. Batten has written informatively on this subject. Some are sequelae of an infection (a postinfectious encephalitis, especially postvaricella), and a few may be due to virus infections which affect the cerebellum more than other parts of the nervous system. Hyperthermia, with temperatures over 106°F, may result in extensive destruction of Purkinje cells and ataxia. Some of these patients with cerebellar ataxia have other more prominent neurologic disturbances such as opsoclonus (lightning-like jerks of eyes) and truncal myoclonus (see Chap. 18). This syndrome may occur as an infectious "encephalitis," or in association with neuroblastomatous occult carcinoma without explanation. In the latter instance the motor disorder may be permanent. ACTH surprisingly may suppress the myoclonic jerks and has been given in doses of 40 units on alternate days for months or longer. Cerebellar tumors and demyelinative and lipid storage diseases also occur at this age and may at times give rise to a more slowly evolving cerebellar ataxia. Labyrinthine injury resulting from streptomycin therapy or mumps and polyneuritis are the common causes of noncerebellar ataxia, which must be differentiated from the above condition.

The hereditary ataxias are likely to begin at a later age and are progressive. They are discussed in Chap. 333.

THE FLACCID PARALYSES The cerebral form, first described by Foerster and called *cerebral atonic diplegia*, has already been mentioned. It can usually be distinguished from spinal and peripheral nerve paralysis and muscular dystrophy by the retention of postural reflexes (flexion of the legs at the knee and hip when the patient is lifted from the axillas), the preservation of tendon reflexes, and the failure of mental development.

The syndrome of infantile muscular atrophy (Werdnig-Hoffmann disease) is the leading example of the category of infantile spinal muscular atrophies, and, since it terminates life in the first year or two, is not of importance in "adult medicine." But in recent years, several other types of familial progressive muscular atrophy have been described in which the onset is in late childhood, adolescence, or early adult life. Weakness, atrophy, reflex loss without sensory change are the diagnostic features and are discussed in further detail in Chap. 333. Unlike "motor system disease," these conditions are inherited, usually in an autosomal recessive pattern and less often in dominant patterns. A few patients suspected of having infantile or childhood muscular atrophy prove, with the passage of time, to be merely rather inactive, "slack" children, whose motor development has proceeded at a slower rate. A few may remain rather weak throughout life, with thin musculature. Such cases fall into the group called *benign congenital hypotonia* (Walton) or *benign congenital myopathy* (Turner). These and several other myopathologic entities, i.e., "central core disease," "rod-body myopathy," pleoconial, megaconial, and myotubular myopathies, are described in Chap. 346. Probably other types of myopathy will also be discovered as causes of this syndrome of congenital hypotonia and lifelong weakness. Muscle biopsy reveals a definite abnormality in only a few cases, and the electromyogram is often normal. Polymyositis and acute idiopathic polyneuritis may rarely manifest themselves as a syndrome of congenital hypotonia.

Infantile muscular dystophy and lipid and glycogen storage diseases may also produce a clinical picture of progressive atrophy and enfeeblement of muscles. The diagnosis of *glycogen storage* disease (the Pompé form) should be entertained when the syndrome of progressive muscular atrophy is associated with clinical enlargement of heart, liver, or spleen. The motor disturbance in this condition may be related in some way to the abnormal deposits of glycogen found in skeletal muscle, though it is more likely due to the degeneration of the anterior horn cells of the spinal cord, which are distended with glycogen and other substances.

Brachial plexus palsies, well-known complications of dystocia, usually result from forcible extraction of the fetus by downward traction on the shoulder in a breech presentation, or from traction and tipping of the head in a shoulder presentation. The effects of such injuries are sometimes lifelong, and in adults, their early onset is betrayed by the small size and inadequate osseous development of the affected limb. The upper brachial plexus and roots of the fifth cervical or the lower plexus and roots of the seventh and eighth cervical and first thoracic nerves suffer the brunt of the injury. Sometimes the entire plexus is involved. The upper plexus injuries (*Erb's upper plexus syndrome*) are estimated to be twenty times more frequent than the lower (*Klumpke's lower plexus syndrome*) (see Chap. 323).

Facial paralysis, due to injury of the facial nerve immediately distal to its exit from the stylomastoid foramen by the application of forceps, is another common peripheral nerve affection in the newborn. The failure of one eye to close and the difficulty in suckling make this condition easy to recognize. It must be distinguished from congenital facial paralysis or facial diplegia usually with weakness of muscles innervated by the facial and abducens nerves (*Moebius's syndrome*). In most cases of facial paralysis function is recovered after a few weeks; in some the paralysis is permanent and may account for an asymmetry observed in later life (see Chap. 324).

MENTAL RETARDATION

The mentally retarded (feebleminded) individual poses special problems not only in childhood but also in the adult. They become the concern of the internist for several reasons. Firstly, failure to recognize the mentally subnormal patient means that one depends on a history that is inadequate, instead of turning to the guardian; also one must rely more on objective signs of disease than on subjective complaint. Then, too, the reactions of such patients to drugs and fever may be more devastating and less predictable. Recognition of the type of disease underlying impaired mentality also becomes important in genetic counseling for the prevention of similar disease in other members of the family.

The more severely retarded individuals nearly always are forced to reside in institutions, and the brain is so extensively damaged that many do not survive beyond childhood. There are special severe types of mental retardation, such as mongolism (Down's syndrome), that are less lethal and many persons with such conditions live with their families until adulthood. Their condition raises a number of interesting problems for the internist (i.e., tendency to develop leukemia and premature senile dementia). Other milder forms of mental subnormality are much more numerous, however, amounting to 3 percent of the general population, and they are more often familial and peculiar to the lower economic stratum of society. Their anatomic basis is uncertain. In many instances they probably represent examples of persons who fall within the lower distribution of normal human intelligence.

The clinical manifestations of mental retardation are relatively easy to perceive. Silly behavior and inability to give a sensible account of the medical problem constitute one useful datum. Slowness in motor development, inability to learn, lack of a concept of time or space, ineducability, poor school progress (individuals unable to pass beyond the sixth grade usually have an IQ of 60 to 70), inability to secure and hold a job or to perform more than menial tasks of society are other useful indices. Such persons are prey to the effects of a poor social environment and may easily be led into criminal practices, prostitution, etc. The differentiation of the various classes of mental backwardness by clinical criteria is facilitated if the framework of reference in Table 334-1 is used.

In spite of the wide spectrum of specific disease entities causing mental retardation, perhaps half of all mentally retarded persons cannot presently be classified in terms of specific etiology by clinical criteria. Many of these cases are familial, the patients coming from families in which other members are retarded or have important mental disorders, and the heritable factors are probably polygenic. There also appears to be another group of disorders, due to single gene defects affecting only the brain, which have been poorly defined clinically and pathologically; included are several types of maldevelopment of the cerebral cortex. Finally, malnutrition as a cause of impaired brain growth and consequent poor mental development has received much attention; its role in mental retardation has not yet been fully determined.

CLINICAL CHARACTERISTICS As an aid to the general physician who must undertake the diagnosis and management of backward children, the following comments may be of some value. Mental retardation manifests itself most obviously in the spheres of motor, language, social, and intellectual development. The severely retarded child at idiot level with an IQ of less than 20 and unable to look after himself often does not sit up, walk, or stand, and if any one of these motor activities is

TABLE 334-1
Types of mental retardation

I Mental defect with associated developmental abnormalities in nonnervous structures
- *A* Those affecting cranioskeletal structures
  - *1* Microcephaly
  - *2* Macrocephaly
  - *3* Hydrocephalus (including myelomeningocele with Arnold-Chiari malformation and associated cerebral anomalies)
  - *4* Down's syndrome (mongolism)
  - *5* Cretinism (congenital hypothyroidism)
  - *6* Mucopolysaccharidoses (Hurler, Hunter, and Sanfilippo types)
  - *7* Acrocephalosyndactyly (craniostenosis)
  - *8* Arthrogryposis multiplex congenita (some cases)
  - *9* Rare specific syndromes: Rubinstein-Taybi
  - *10* Dwarfism, short stature: Russell-Silver dwarf, Seckel's bird-headed dwarf, Cockayne-Neel dwarf, etc.
  - *11* Hypertelorism; median-cleft-face syndromes; agenesis of corpus callosum
- *B* Those affecting nonskeletal structures
  - *1* Neurocutaneous syndromes: tuberous sclerosis, Sturge-Weber, neurofibromatosis (uncommonly)
  - *2* Congenital rubella syndrome (deafness, blindness, congenital heart disease, small stature)
  - *3* Chromosomal disorders: Down's syndrome; some cases of Klinefelter's syndrome (XXY); XYY; Turner's (XO) syndrome (occasionally); others
  - *4* Laurence-Moon-Biedl syndrome (retinitis pigmentosa; obesity; polydactyly)
  - *5* Eye disorders: toxoplasmosis (chorioretinitis); galactosemia (cataract); congenital rubella

II Mental defect without developmental anomalies in nonnervous structures, but with focal cerebral and other neurologic abnormalities
- *A* Cerebral spastic diplegia
- *B* Cerebral hemiplegia, unilateral or bilateral
- *C* Congenital choreoathetosis or ataxia
  - *1* Kernicterus
  - *2* Status marmoratus
- *D* Congenital atonic diplegia
- *E* Posthypoglycemic, posttraumatic, postmeningitic, and postencephalitic states
- *F* Those associated with other neuromuscular abnormalities (muscular dystrophy, Friedreich's ataxia, etc.)
- *G* Cerebral degenerative diseases (lipidoses)
- *H* Lesch-Nyhan syndrome

III Mental defect without signs of other developmental abnormality or neurologic disorder (epilepsy may or may not be present)
- *A* Simple mental retardation; familial mental retardation
- *B* Some cases of encephaloclastic disease (hypoxia, hypoglycemia)
- *C* Infantile autism
- *D* Associated with inborn errors of metabolism (phenylketonuria, other aminoacidurias, organic acidurias)
- *E* Congenital infections (some cases of congenital syphilis; cytomegalic inclusion disease)

acquired, it appears late and is imperfectly performed. Language is not mastered, or at most a few words are understood and uttered. The patient is continuously idle and can only vocalize in meaningless way. He does not interact with people and objects around him, nor does he make known his needs for water, food, excretion, etc. He does nothing for himself and exhibits only primitive emotional reactions. Physical growth is usually retarded, nutrition may be poor, and susceptibility to respiratory infections is common. Sphincteric control may never be accomplished. A variety of physical deformities, particularly microcephaly, is common in this group, and they always suggest that the brain disease originated in the antenatal period because of either a genetic disorder or a disease (during the first 12 weeks of pregnancy). Such persons are to be found among the adult populations of state hospitals. Affections of the nervous system which have their onset later in life are usually not attended by bodily disfigurement.

If the mental defect is less pronounced, with an IQ of 20 to 50 (i.e., imbecile), or 50 to 70 (i.e., moron), and if specific motor defects do not coexist, then sitting, walking, and speech are acquired, but after a delay in many cases. The existence of a cerebral defect may be noted for the first time when the child fails to speak normally during the second and third years of life and seems not to be able to learn the usual household tasks and play activities as well as other children. However, delay in language development must not by itself be taken as a mark of mental retardation, for many bright children who are obviously intelligent and who show remarkable talent in communicating by gesture are slow in talking. Also the deaf child may be singled out by his indifference to noise and reduced vocalization but otherwise normal development. Toilet training also may be difficult to accomplish in the retarded child, but again it may be delayed in an otherwise normal child.

Within the spectrum of types of mental retardation, even within a group of persons of similar IQs, there are vast differences and contrasts in overall behavioral functioning. Some mentally retarded persons are pleasant and amiable, and achieve a rather satisfactory social adjustment; this is especially true of simple mental retardates. At the opposite extreme is the ill-understood syndrome of autism, associated with varying degrees of retardation, in which the child or older person fails to manifest any kind of interpersonal, social contact—including communicative language—and demonstrates a limited and bizarre interest primarily in inanimate objects. It is impossible to list all variations of mental retardation here, but the point should be made that all aspects of intellectual life and personality are touched in differing degrees. Many retarded individuals are dull, apathetic, and underactive. Others display an incessant hyperactivity, characterized by a very short attention span, a restless inquisitive searching of the environment, and low frustration tolerance; they may be destructive or recklessly fearless, and may seem strangely impervious to injury. Some display a peculiar "anhedonia" and are indifferent to either punishment or reward. Strangely, as with the mentally normal but hyperactive, inattentive child, improvement in these children can often be achieved by using amphetamines. Other types of behavior, such as violent aggressiveness and even self-mutilation, are not uncommon. Rhythmic rocking, rolling, head banging, and bouncing movements feature the motor activities of retarded persons, and may be performed hour after hour without fatigue, often to the accompaniment of bleating sounds, squeals, and other ejaculations. Here the abnormality is not the appearance of rhythmic movements of the body, which are to be observed at one period in the development of many normal children, but their persistence. Music may encourage rhythmic movement and gives pleasure to many retarded children and adults.

It is apparent that the clinical and behavioral characteristics of individuals with retarded development cannot be adequately described by a single parameter, the IQ. There are many other factors which determine the social success of the retarded child and should give direction to his education and training. These include recognition of specific sensory or motor handicaps, such as blindness and deafness as well as athetosis or hemiplegia, specific language or speech deficits, behavioral disturbances, such as autism or hyperactivity, and the presence of seizures. Measures can be taken which help the handicapped person to compensate for these deficiencies. This becomes a primary consideration in functional diagnosis and in guiding the parents or guardians.

The least severely retarded individual (IQ of 50 to 70) grows and develops in many ways not different from normal ones, and he can be taught useful occupational skills. A few of these persons can work under careful supervision. All scholastic pursuits are relatively unsuccessful, and vocational training is of more value than other types of education.

SPECIAL VARIETIES OF MENTAL RETARDATION

Several of the special types of mental retardation are discussed in other chapters (see Lipidoses and Cerebral Sclerosis, in Chap. 333). In the following pages are presented only those with special features likely to be seen in adults.

Mongolism (Down's syndrome) This is a unique condition, and, although accounting for only about 1 percent of all mental defectives, it is the reason for nearly one-third of the admissions to state schools. The degree of mental retardation varies from mild to severe and is associated with a curious facial configuration and a dwarfed physical stature. A number of stigmas of mongolism can be recognized in the neonatal period. The head tends to be small and oval, with sloping forehead. The ears are set low and are oval, with small lobules. The eyes slant slightly upward and outward owing to the presence of a medial epicanthal fold, which partly covers the angle of the palpebral fissure. The bridge of the nose is generally absent or poorly developed. The mouth tends to hang open, and the tongue is usually enlarged, heavily fissured, and protruding. Gray-white specks of depigmentation are seen in the iris (Brushfield's spots). The little fingers are often short and curved, owing to a hypoplastic middle phalanx. The hands are broad and simian-like, with a single transverse palmar crease. A number of other characteristic dermal markings are noted in fingers and toes. Lenticular opacities and congenital heart lesions (septal defects) are found in some cases. At birth the mongoloid child is of average size, but at later periods of life he is characteristically small. The average adult person with mongolism never exceeds the stature of a ten-year-old child. The resemblance to the Oriental is at most superficial; in fact the differences are so striking that it is quite easy to recognize the condition in those of Oriental heritage.

Aside from having a rather rounded shape, which conforms to that of the skull, a subnormal weight, and a relatively simple convolutional pattern, with particular smallness of the frontal lobes and superior temporal convolutions, the brain of the mongoloid shows no abnormalities.

The mortality rate is high in the first years of life, death usually being due to respiratory infections, interventricular cardiac lesion with failure, or leukemia. Of the mongoloid patients who survive to puberty, many live to middle adult life only to suffer then a premature form of Alzheimer's cerebral degeneration (onset in the majority by the age of forty).

Older mothers are more apt to have mongoloid babies than are young mothers. The mean age of the mother at the time of birth of the mongoloid child is thirty-seven. Trisomy of chromosome 21 or translocation of parts of this chromosome has been found consistently in patients with Down's syndrome and is responsible for the disorder.

Cretinism This is due to congenital deficiency of thyroid secretion and is distinguished from myxedema, a form of hypothyroidism acquired later in life (see Chap. 85).

Gargoylism (Hunter-Hurler disease) This condition is discussed in Chap. 333.

Phenylketonuria (phenylpyruvic oligophrenia) This condition is discussed in Chap. 96.

Galactosemia Another congenital metabolic disease, galactosemia is transmitted by a single, autosomal recessive gene. It is characterized clinically by mental defect, cataract, nausea, vomiting, hepatomegaly, jaundice, and the excretion of large quantities of galactose in the urine (Chap. 105).

Autism Autism is a mysterious and provocative condition identified in young children. Long considered primarily psychiatric, it is now generally thought to represent an organic defect in brain development. It is characterized by failure of children to develop communicative language or any form of social communication. By contrast, they often show motor and other skills far beyond what is to be expected of a mentally retarded person. Often they are obsessively preoccupied with inanimate objects, such as lights, running water, or spinning objects. Many of the youngsters prove later to be retarded, and the ultimate prognosis depends largely on the child's IQ. Some few gradually acquire language and may then exhibit certain exceptional talents, such as mathematic ability. Upon reaching adult life they are found to retain all the above characteristics. Not more than 1 in 30 will seem to have made any progress. Imprecision of diagnosis allows the inclusion of other brain diseases under the rubric of autism. The patients at a later age do not resemble schizophrenics, despite claims that autism is an unusually precocious form of schizophrenia. No biochemical abnormality has been discovered. Brain volume appears to be normal by contrast studies and gross examination, but few detailed histopathologic studies have been made. There is no therapy for this condition.

Simple mental retardation Although presented last, this category includes the great number of cases of defective mentality of indeterminate etiology in which neither somatic nor neurologic abnormality is exhibited. The degree of mental impairment tends to be mild (moron, educable) or moderate (imbecile, trainable). Penrose found that this group of retardates constituted 25 percent of 1,280 institutionalized individuals, and of course those who are in institutions represent only the more severely damaged individuals in our society. Their physical appearance is usually not strikingly abnormal; yet many of the aforementioned characteristics of the mentally retarded individual are to be observed. Seizures occur in a significant number, being several times more frequent than in a normal population. Within the limits of their intelligence, the success of these individuals in learning to look after themselves is often determined by how effectively their parents and teachers have inculcated or reinforced good work habits and stable personality traits. The brighter ones can profit to some extent from formal education. Those less well endowed may be trained to care for their personal wants and needs and may profit from a limited amount of manual training. Special schools and classes are of great help. Later in life supervised work situations are possible solutions to their occupational needs.

Society, in the final analysis, determines the eventual disposition of these unfortunates. Many of them, being not unattractive and giving less trouble than many other defective persons, are able to adjust to foster families and live in a community. They need protection, for they are easily led astray and may commit infractions of the law, usually of a minor sort. Institutionalization is required when family and society cannot or do not wish to look after them. Reproductivity is frequently impaired in those with severe mental defects but may be distressingly undisturbed in many of the less defective individuals.

The problem of eugenics assumes great importance. This type of mental defect is often seen in families in which one or both of the parents are dull or retarded. The term *familial* may be applied to this group. However, the majority of cases are sporadic. Probably multiple etiologic factors may lead to simple mental retardation. The pathologic change is variable, ranging from "no demonstrable lesion" to several different gross and microscopic abnormalities.

EPILEPSY

The majority of adult patients with recurrent seizures acquire the tendency toward seizures during childhood. They represent the sequelae of disease processes which may have begun and ended in the distant past. In early life the pattern of the seizures varies widely, depending in part on the level of maturation of the nervous system. Certain types such as fragmented neonatal seizures, infantile spasms, photic epilepsy, febrile seizures, etc., are peculiar to the earlier periods of life. Others, such as petit mal, grand mal, and psychomotor, are identical in child and adult. The latter types are discussed in Chaps. 24 and 337.

ABNORMALITIES OF BEHAVIOR AND SPECIAL DEFECTS IN CEREBRAL DEVELOPMENT

Aggressiveness, undisciplined and impulsive behavior, delays in speaking and reading, and peculiarities of personality come as often to the attention of the pediatric neurologist as to that of the psychiatrist. Such abnormalities extend into adult life and require that every physician have some knowledge of the normal cycles of maturation of instinctive life, intelligence, and personality of the patient. He must be familiar with the results of current investigations of the malevolent effects of undernutrition, chronic illness, sense deprivation and insufficiency of stimulation, emotional deprivation, lack of parental discipline, and impoverished social environment. These neurologic and psychopathologic factors were discussed at length in the sixth edition of the *Principles of Internal Medicine* but are omitted in this edition to conserve space. The interested reader may refer to the references below, and will find mention of these factors in Chaps. 338 and 339.

REFERENCES

ADAMS RD, REED WB: Neurocutaneous disease, in *Dermatology in General Medicine*, eds TB Fitzpatrick et al, New York: McGraw-Hill, 1971, p. 1379

COOPER IS: *Involuntary Movement Disorders*, New York: Hoeber-Harper, 1969

HOLMES LB et al: Mental retardation, in *An Atlas of Diseases with Associated Physical Abnormalities*, New York: Macmillan, 1972

335 NARCOLEPSY AND CATAPLEXY

RAYMOND D. ADAMS

This clinical entity has long been known to the medical profession. Westphal described attacks of uncontrollable natural sleep in 1877, and Gélineau gave it the name *narcolepsy* in 1880. But it was not until 1916 that Henneberg called attention to the common association of temporary paralysis of cranial muscles and limbs during laughter or other emotional states (cataplexy). Paralysis during the period of falling asleep (hypnopompic) and paralysis at the time of awakening (hypnogogic), the so-called "sleep paralyses," were added to the syndrome by Wilson in 1916; episodic diplopia was included by Levin in 1943.

CLINICAL STAGE The above tetrad of symptoms appears to be not infrequent, as shown by the fact that several hundred cases were observed in the Mayo Clinic over a period of years. Males are affected more often than females. As a rule the condition begins in late childhood, adolescence, or early adult life, and narcolepsy is the presenting symptom. The essential disorder is one of uncontrollable sleepiness. Several times a day, usually while sitting in class, the subject is assailed by an uncontrollable desire to sleep. His eyes close, his muscles relax, his breathing deepens slightly, and he has all the appearances of a person who is dozing. A noise, a touch, or even the cessation of the lecturer's voice are enough to awaken him, and he may feel momentarily refreshed. Often the impulse to sleep is so frequent and insistent that a student so afflicted will never remain awake for a single period in class. Somnolence may occur in unusual situations, as while standing or carrying on a conversation.

Approximately 70 percent of these patients, if questioned carefully, will admit to having cataplexy. Reference is made here to the curious circumstance that hearty laughter, more rarely excitement, sadness, or anger, will cause the patient's head to fall forward, his jaw to drop, his knees to buckle, even with falling to the ground, all with perfect preservation of consciousness. The attack lasts only a minute or two. Much less frequent are the sleep paralyses and episodic diplopia. The narcolepsy does not alter the nocturnal sleep pattern.

Once the condition begins, it usually continues over most of adult life, perhaps becoming less frequent with age. No other neurologic abnormality is associated with it, nor does one later develop. All investigative procedures usually yield negative results, and one has only the patient's description or the observed phenomena on which to make a diagnosis.

The Kleine-Levin syndrome is a closely related condition. It consists of periodic hypersomnolence lasting for periods of 2 to 3 weeks and hyperphagia. The attacks occur two to three times a year. Onset is usually during adolescence with a striking male predominance. The cause and pathogenesis of this mesodiencephalic disturbance are unknown.

CAUSE AND PATHOGENESIS The cause of true narcolepsy is unknown. Attempts to impute it to encephalitis lethargica carry little conviction, since the disease long antedated the outbreak of this infection. It bears no relation to epilepsy or migraine. A psychogenesis has been offered, but the relevance of the psychologic observations remains open to question. No autopsies in which the brain was thoroughly examined have been reported. Rarely, a narcoleptic state may accompany multiple sclerosis, idiopathic epilepsy, cerebral trauma, or a craniopharyngioma.

In recent years much interest has centered on the nature of the sleep and its EEG pattern. In many patients the normal sequence of slow wave and rapid eye movement (REM) sleep is altered, and in an attack the REM is predominant. It is associated sometimes with peculiar dreamlike or hallucinatory experiences.

The greatest difficulty in diagnosis relates to the problem of separating narcolepsy from the normal sleep pattern. Many sedentary, obese adults doze readily after breakfast, if unoccupied, or after dinner, during a game of bridge, or in the theater. But characteristic of narcolepsy is the irresistible urge to sleep under unusual circumstances (such as standing up) and the tendency of the sleep to recur many times a day. When cataplexy is conjoined, diagnosis becomes virtually certain. Excessive somnolence, easily mistaken for idiopathic narcolepsy, may attend obesity and hypercapnia, heart failure, hypothyroidism, excessive use of barbiturates and alcohol, etc.

TREATMENT There is no therapy which will control all the symptoms. The narcolepsy responds best to (1) strategically placed naps (during lunch hour, before or after dinner, etc.) and (2) the use of analeptic drugs, such as amphetamine sulfate (Benzedrine), methylphenidate (Ritalin), or pipradrol (Meratran). The time of medication should be adjusted to the study or work habits of the patient. The usual dose of amphetamine varies from 5 to 10 mg given three to five times a day. This is ordinarily well tolerated and does not cause wakefulness at night. The dose of Ritalin is 10 to 20 mg thrice daily, and of Meratran, 2.5 to 5.0 mg twice or thrice daily. These have rather little effect on cataplexy but are partially effective in the Kleine-Levin syndrome. Fortunately the latter is less frequent and is said to be controlled by avoidance of emotional situations.

The newest addition to the pharmacology of narcolepsy and cataplexy is imipramine (Tofranil) which, in doses of 25 mg three to four times a day, markedly reduces attacks, presumably by abolishing REM sleep (see Chap. 23).

REFERENCES

Brock S, Wiesel B: The narcoleptic-cataplectic syndrome. J Nerv Ment Dis 94:700, 1941

Goggi Auto (ed): *The Abnormalities of Sleep in Man*, Proc XVth European Meeting Electroencephalography, p. 147, Bologna, 1967

Levin M: The pathogenesis of narcolepsy. J Neurol Psychopathol 14:1, 1933

Wilson SAK: The narcolepsies. Brain, 51:63, 1928

336 MIGRAINE

RAYMOND D. ADAMS
JOHN F. GRIFFITH

The term *migraine* refers to periodic, hemicranial, throbbing headaches which begin in childhood, adolescence, or early adult life and continue to recur with diminishing frequency during advancing years.

Two closely related clinical syndromes have been identified. The first is called "classic" or "typical" migraine, the second "common" or "atypical." The typical syndrome is ushered in by a disturbance of neurologic function (hemianopsia or central blindness, hemiparesthetic disturbance, slight speech abnormality or aphasia, or hemiparesis) followed in a few minutes by hemicranial headache, nausea, and vomiting, all of which last for hours or as long as a day or two. The other syndrome is characterized by an unheralded onset of hemicranial or generalized headache with or without nausea and vomiting but following the same temporal pattern. Both headache syndromes respond to ergot preparations, if administered early in the attack. Their genetic nature is evidenced by concurrence in several members of the family of the same and successive generations in 60 to 80 percent of cases; but inheritance is somewhat less clear in the atypical than the typical variety, perhaps because diagnosis is less certain.

Classic migraine presents such a dramatic and at times confusing sequence of events that it merits further description. On awakening in the morning, or at any time of day, the patient may have a kind of vague premonition of an attack. Then abruptly there is a disturbance of vision consisting usually of bright spots or dazzling zigzag lines which give way within minutes to scotomatous defects; usually they are bilateral and often of homonymous and congruent pattern (corresponding parts of the field of vision of each eye). Soon thereafter, numbness and tingling of lips, face, hand (on one or both sides), slight confusion of thinking, weakness of an arm or leg, mild aphasia, dizziness and uncertainty of gait, drowsiness, or confusion (rarely coma) are added to the clinical picture. Only one or a few of these neurologic phenomena are present in any given patient and they tend to occur in the same combination in each attack. They last 5 to 15 min, and if the weakness or numbness spreads from one part of the body to another or one symptom follows another, it does so slowly in a period of minutes (not in seconds as in a convulsion). Just as inexplicably as they come, they soon begin to recede, and within minutes they are followed by a unilateral throbbing headache, usually on the side of the cerebral disturbance, which slowly increases in intensity. At its peak, in an hour or so, nausea and vomiting may occur. The headache lasts hours or a day or two and is always the most unpleasant feature of the illness.

Much variation occurs. When this "sick headache," as it is called, is most severe, the patient is forced to lie down and to shun light and noise. Milder forms, especially if partially controlled by medication, do not force withdrawal from accustomed activities. Any one of the three principal components—neurologic derangement, headache, or vomiting—may be absent. Particularly with advancing age there is a tendency for the headache and vomiting to become less severe, finally leaving only the neurologic abnormality. The neurologic symptomatology is also subject to variation. Although visual disturbances are far and away the most common manifestation, they differ in detail from patient to patient; numbness and tingling of the lips and fingers of one hand are probably next in frequency, with transient aphasia or a thickness of speech following in that order. A relatively rare syndrome of vertigo, staggering drowsiness, and stupor has been delineated by Bickerstaff and called *basilar artery migraine*. Also, he has reported the loss of consciousness at the onset, especially in migrainous young women. Recurrent unilateral headaches associated with extraocular muscle palsies have been called *ophthalmoplegic migraine*. A transient third nerve palsy with associated ptosis of one eyelid is the usual picture; rarely, the abducens nerve is affected and lateral movement is impaired. Disturbances of the mind may appear—a strange excitement, an unaccountable irritability or depression, or a slight mental confusion, which is the more common. The headache, though typically hemicranial (the word *migraine* is said to be derived from *megrim*, meaning hemicrania), may be frontal, temporal, or generalized. In children abdominal pain and vomiting may accompany the headache (abdominal migraine). The attacks, instead of beginning in childhood and recurring in the usual fashion every few weeks or months with diminishing frequency in middle and late adult years, may begin in adult life or even middle age or suddenly increase in frequency during menopause or when hypertension and vascular disease develop. The neurologic symptoms, instead of being transitory, may leave a permanent deficit (e.g., a homonymous visual field defect) reminiscent of an ischemic stroke. The use of hormones to prevent pregnancy has increased the frequency and severity of migraine and in several reported instances has resulted in a permanent neurologic deficit.

Between attacks the migrainous patient is essentially normal. For a time, when psychosomatic medicine was much in vogue, there was insistence on a migrainous personality characterized by tenseness, rigidity in thinking, meticulousness, and perfectionism. The migrainous attack was said to occur often during the let-down period, after many days of hard work or stress. But further personality analyses have not borne out these ideas, and the temporal relations between headache and the day's activities have not been consistent. Moreover, the fact that the headaches may begin in early childhood, when the personality is relatively amorphous, would argue against this idea.

During an attack, the electroencephalogram reveals a nonspecific slowing of wave frequencies in one-third to one-half of all patients. Carotid arteriograms show arterial constriction at the onset of the headache, and the cerebral circulation is found by blood flow studies to be slowed early in the attack and speeded up once headache begins. Migraine is frequent, found in an estimated 5 percent of general population; females are slightly more susceptible than males, and there is a tendency for the headaches to occur during the period of premenstrual tension and fluid retention. The migrainous attacks usually cease during pregnancy. Reserpine treatment and estrogens and progesterone may increase their frequency. A few patients have linked their attacks to certain articles of diet, such as chocolate. There is no clear relationship, despite many statements to the contrary, between migraine and vascular malformations of the brain and psychoneurosis. The relationship to epilepsy is less clear; convulsions are slightly increased in frequency in the migrainous patient and his relatives.

Vasodilatation and excessive pulsation of branches of the external carotid artery have been observed during the headache. Further, as the pulsation decreases, either spontaneously or after the administration of ergotamine, the headache disappears. Vasoconstriction was early postulated as the basis of the neurologic symptoms; it has been confirmed in at least one chance carotid arteriogram and has been inferred from prompt abolition of the visual or neurologic disorder upon administration of nitrites. Thus the vascular theory of migraine has come to be accepted, supported further by surgical observations, that the extracranial arteries can be a source of pain. However, it is quite apparent that the theory does not explain why the intracranial and extracranial arteries should periodically undergo spasm and dilatation in the migrainous individual, nor does it account for the nausea and vomiting (infrequent in all other headaches except those due to tumor) or the tenderness and swelling of the temporal vessels and surrounding tissues.

A new hypothesis has been put forth—that the observed vasospasm and later hyperemic pulsations are induced by a release of amines such as norepinephrine and epinephrine and serotonin in individuals whose vessels are peculiarly sensitive. These substances are known to be powerful vasoconstrictors. It was found that some migraine patients during their attack excrete increased amounts of the terminal metabolites of the catecholamines, particularly 5-hydroxyindoleacetic acid (5-HIAA) derived from serotonin, and of vanillylmandelic acid (VMA), a product of norepinephrine and epinephrine. A corresponding reduction in serotonin levels in the blood has also been detected. Other observations in line with this are that (1) reserpine, which reduces the level of serotonin in platelets, brain, and other tissues, may provoke migraine; (2) the injection of serotonin gives partial or complete relief of headache, and (3) a serotonin antagonist, methysergide, wholly prevents attacks. However, it is still difficult to reconcile these data with the finding that a heat-stable polypeptide with some of the properties of bradykinin (one of the plasma kinins) not only can be aspirated from the edematous subcutaneous tissue but, if reinjected at another site, will cause increased capillary permeability, pain, and lowered skin threshold in the overlying skin. Its algogenic action is potentiated by serotonin. Whether this substance, called *neurokinin,* escapes secondarily during the phase of vasodilatation or initiates the vasodilatation is not known. While this humoral amine theory is incomplete and several of the findings need verification, nonetheless it does promise clarification of the migraine syndrome and possibly other forms of vascular headache.

DIAGNOSIS Typical migraine should occasion no difficulty in diagnosis if the above facts are kept in mind and if a good history is obtained. That is possible, as a rule, for migraine patients tend to be intelligent.

The real difficulties come from three sources: (1) ignorance of the fact that a progressively unfolding neurologic syndrome may be migrainous in origin; (2) lack of appreciation that the neurologic disorder may occur without headache; (3) lack of awareness that recurrent headaches, which may be an isolated phenomenon, may take many forms, some of which may prove difficult to distinguish from the other common types of headache described in Chap. 6.

Some of these problems merit further elaboration because of their practical importance, as follows:

The neurologic part of the migraine syndrome may resemble focal epilepsy, the clinical picture of a vascular malformation such as an angioma or aneurysm, or some other vascular disease such as a thrombotic or embolic stroke. Here it is the pace of the neurologic symptoms of migraine more than their character that reliably distinguishes the condition from epilepsy. The clinical profile of the aura of epilepsy is measured in seconds, for it depends on spreading neural excitation, in contrast to the slow progression of migraine, which is based on spreading vascular spasm.

Ophthalmoplegic migraine will always suggest a carotid aneurysm, but in relatively few cases has carotid arteriography revealed such an abnormality. Despite many claims that hemicranial painful attacks invariably on the same side of the head (unlike migraine) should raise the question of a vascular malformation, in a large series of cases this has not been confirmed by arteriography. Of course, focal epilepsy, protracted headache, stiff neck and bloody cerebrospinal fluid, a persistent neurologic deficit, and cranial bruit would be indicative of a vascular type of headache associated with angioma or aneurysm. Only in the earlier stages, when periodic throbbing headache is the sole symptom, might it be confused with true migraine.

Attacks indistinguishable from epilepsy may also appear in association with hypertensive and the cerebral arteriosclerotic vascular diseases of late life. Here one is aided by late age of onset, more persistent and frequent headaches, and the evidence of vascular disease of heart, lower extremities, and brain.

A special problem relates to paroxysms of throbbing headache, not hemicranial in distribution, not preceded by a neurologic aura, and not accounted for by other known cause. Are they examples of atypical, or common, migraine? Unfortunately, since diagnosis depends on the interpretation of the patient's description of symptoms and since there is as yet no biologically valid confirmatory laboratory test, the controversy as to where migraine begins and ends is of the armchair type. Favoring the diagnosis of migraine are lifelong history, childhood onset, positive family history, and response of the headache to ergot derivatives.

A variety of episodic attacks have been described as migraine equivalents: attacks of abdominal pain with nausea, vomiting, and diarrhea; pain localized in the thorax, pelvis, and extremities; bouts of fever; transient disturbances in mood (psychic equivalents); recurrent nocturnal orbital (cluster) headache, or migrainous neuralgia (see Chap. 6). The only advantage of considering such attacks as migrainous is that this view protects some patients from unnecessary diagnostic procedures and surgical intervention—but it may also prevent necessary surgery.

From all this discussion the reader should be left with the idea that the migraine syndromes are rather larger and more protean than the rigid stereotyped descriptions we have given would suggest. In these days of complicated diagnostic procedures it is tempting to take x-rays of the skull and perform arteriography and electroencephalography on every patient. A conservative approach would lead to temporization, reserving a single lateral skull film or EEG for the exceptional case.

TREATMENT Migraine may require no treatment at all, other than an explanation of its nature to the patient and a reassurance that it will do him no harm. Some patients know, or allege to know, that certain acts induce attacks, and it is obvious enough that they should be urged to avoid these acts, if possible. In certain persons it has been claimed that the correction of a refractive error, an elimination diet, or psychotherapy for some personality disorder has relieved their migraine. However, this is so exceptional that a cause and effect relationship must be doubted, in view of the variability of the disease itself.

Treatment of the neurologic aura is rarely required because of its brevity. If the deficit is lasting, inhalation of an ampul of amyl nitrate should be tried; used at the first premonition of the attack, the drug might prevent it. The time to initiate treatment of the oncoming headache is during the neurologic disorder. If many of the headaches are mild, the patient may already have learned that 0.6 g acetylsalicylic acid and possibly 5 mg Dexedrine will suffice to control the pain so that he can carry on. More severe attacks respond only to ergot preparations (ergotamine and dihydroergotamine). In such patients the attack can be cut short by the intravenous injection of 1 mg dihydroergotamine methane sulfate or 0.5 mg ergotamine tartrate, the former being less likely to induce vomiting. The injection should be repeated in 30 min, if necessary. When these drugs are administered early (within 30 to 60 min of onset), some 90 percent of patients will be relieved of the headache. Oral medication in the form of three 1-mg tablets, to be held under the tongue until dissolved, and repeated in 2-mg doses every half hour until the headache is relieved or until a total of 9 mg is taken, is almost as effective. Caffeine, 100 mg with 1 mg of ergotamine (Cafergot), is a useful combination when taken in the form of a tablet (two at onset of headache and a third in half an hour) or as a rectal suppository (2 mg ergotamine and 100 mg caffeine) if vomiting prevents oral administration.

Because of the danger of prolonged vascular spasm in patients who have vascular disease or are pregnant, ergot preparations must be used cautiously, if at all. Even in healthy individuals more than 10 to 15 mg ergotamine per week is risky. For the frequent atypical migraine headaches, some of which respond poorly to ergot, one should prescribe a preparation containing 150 mg acetylsalicylic acid, 160 mg acetophenetidin, and Dexedrine, 5 mg, with phenobarbital, 30 mg. This can be repeated once or twice in a severe attack. Once the headache has become intense, ergot is of little help, and one must resort to codeine sulphate, 30 mg, or meperidine (Demerol), 50 mg, as the only means of terminating the pain.

In individuals with frequent migrainous attacks (one to three times a week) efforts at prevention are worthwhile. Some success has been obtained with preparations of ergot, 0.5 mg, atropine, 0.3 mg, and phenobarbital, 15 mg (Bellergol) twice or three times a day for a few weeks. ACTH (40 units per day) or prednisone (45 mg per day for 3 to 4 weeks) have also been helpful in some difficult refractory patients. Recently methysergide (Sansert) in a dose of 6 to 8 mg per day given for several weeks or months has proved to be most promising in reducing the frequency of or abolishing attacks. The main contraindication has been retroperitoneal fibrosis; this complication has been reported in several dozen cases, when the patient has been treated continuously for more than six months. Discontinuing treatment for 1 month out of every 6 has greatly reduced the incidence of this complication.

All experienced physicians appreciate the importance of helping the patient rearrange his schedule so as to control his tensions and hard-driving ways of living, so often a feature of many migrainous patients. There is no one way of accomplishing this, but in general, long and costly psychotherapy has not been helpful, or at least one can say there is no substantial data as to its value.

REFERENCES

CHAPMAN LF: A humoral agent implicated in vascular headache of the migraine type. Arch Neurol 3:223, 1960

GRAHAM JR, WOLFF HG: The mechanism of the migraine headache and the action or ergotamine tartrate. Arch Neurol Psychiat 39:737, 1938

LANCE JW, HINTZENBERGER H: The control of cranial arteries by humoral mechanisms and its relation to the migraine syndrome. Headache 7:93, 1967

PARRY CH: *Collections from the Unpublished Medical Writing of the Late Caleb Hillier Parry,* vol. 1, London: Underwood, 1825

SICUTERI F: Vasoneuroactive substances and their implication in vascular pain, chap. 2 in *Research and Clinical Studies of Headache*, ed A Friedman, Baltimore: Williams & Wilkins, 1967

SMITH R: *Background of Migraine*, New York: Springer, 1967

337 IDIOPATHIC EPILEPSY

RAYMOND D. ADAMS

In Chap. 24 the general problem of convulsive disorders and their medical implications were presented. The common seizure patterns, their underlying cerebral anatomy and physiologic mechanism, and the relevant biochemical changes, not too well known, to be sure, were described. With respect to the possible causes of seizures it was pointed out that they differ according to the age of the patient at the time of their onset. In the adult who begins to have a convulsive disorder, the cause is likely to be discovered sooner or later; but in the infant or child, or the adult who has had seizures since childhood, our success is limited and the greater number of cases fall into the category of idiopathic epilepsy. It is about this latter group, which makes up the majority of patients seen by the medical profession, especially during the first three decades of life, that the following remarks are made.

Many physicians will find it curious, indeed almost comic, that neurology should be concerned with the treatment of an important entity when it has little or no idea of its cause. The plain fact is that the very nature of the human nervous system and this particular manifestation of the nervous disease have defied analysis. In the development of such a complex structure as the brain a minor disturbance may occur and be expressed by a seizure tendency. During the long intrauterine period a noxious factor might injure the brain without betraying itself by other symptom or sign. And we know that in infancy and childhood, diseases of the brain may masquerade as a relatively trivial infection, etc. To make the problem more difficult, seizures have a way of occurring not at the time of a cerebral insult but months or years later when the disease has become inactive. Thus, it is possible for the cerebrum of man to harbor one or more potentially epileptic lesions of indeterminate type, and they are usually nonprogressive. Since epilepsy is rarely fatal, the only chance at pathologic study may come years after the onset of the responsible disease, when all distinguishing marks have vanished; and if the lesions are small and unobtrusive, only special cytologic methods, i.e., serial sections of the whole cerebrum, might reveal their residual effects.

The fact that a group of idiopathic epileptic disorders is set apart from all convulsive states of known cause should not discourage one from attempting a complete diagnosis in every patient: (1) to obtain knowledge of the existence of the convulsive state, (2) to ascertain the cause of the cortical lesion, and (3) to determine its localization. But in the younger subject, whose brain is more disposed to seizure activity than that of an older person, and in whom stationary lesions are more frequent, the pursuit of causation tends to be less vigorous.

THE CLINICAL STATE

Idiopathic epilepsy tends to express itself with maximal frequency at two periods in life, between the ages of two and five years and around puberty. More often than not the first seizure is generalized, though a series of petit mal, "staring spells," may precede its appearance. Up to this moment development may have been normal, and a neurologic examination is likely to disclose no other abnormality. Although the seizures may be either of generalized motor type (51 percent of cases) or petit mal (8 percent) in the beginning, as the years pass and the seizures continue, approximately 40 percent of patients will have both these types or psychomotor seizures in addition. The latter are also frequent in pure form. See Chap. 24 for further description of seizures.

The severity of the convulsive state varies from a single attack every several years to many per day. If the generalized seizures are at all frequent, they pose a constant threat of injury or social embarrassment, often preventing the further education of the child or the gainful occupation of the adult. Of the milder form of disorder, however, sufficient medical control may be achieved so that there is no interference with the normal life activities. In enlightened communities no longer is an intelligent epileptic stigmatized by teachers or employers, and virtually all patients without other neurologic abnormalities can find their place in society. If there is evidence of mental retardation, character changes, hemiparesis, etc., as not infrequently happens, the other problems may be more important than the idiopathic epilepsy.

The common diagnostic procedures performed in the interval between seizures are usually uninformative, i.e., the cerebrospinal fluid is normal, x-rays of skull are normal, pneumoencephalogram and arteriograms, where they have been done, are negative. Only the electroencephalogram will demonstrate an abnormality in 60 to 75 percent of cases, either a generalized paroxysmal 3-per-sec spike–slow wave complex (dart-dome), sharp waves, or some other alterations (see Ch. 322).

PROGNOSIS

Without doubt the appearance of a convulsion poses a serious problem for the patient, his family, and his physician. There is first of all the possibility of its being the initial manifestation of a neurologic disease which will take the life of the patient (e.g., infiltrating glioma). But even if the convulsion is due to a stationary, healed lesion, life expectancy is slightly reduced owing to the danger of injury or, rarely, unexplained death. If seizures are frequent or difficult to control, mentation may be altered; the patient is dull, vague, querulous, and illogically argumentative. If seizures are infrequent and the EEG relatively normal between attacks, prognoses for successful schooling, occupational adjustment, and marriage are excellent. Mental deterioration, fortunately, occurs rarely, contrary to lay opinion, and when it becomes evident over a few weeks, one must suspect (1) wrong initial diagnosis (not idiopathic epilepsy but seizures due to some definable cerebral disease), (2) drug intoxication from anticonvulsant medication, (3) recurrent subclinical seizures, (4) subdural hematoma resulting from head injury.

TREATMENT

The treatment of epilepsy of all types can be divided into three parts: the removal of causative and precipitating factors, the regulation of physical and mental hygiene, and the use of anticonvulsant drugs.

REMOVAL OF CAUSATIVE AND PRECIPITATING FACTORS Infections of the central nervous system, such as the meningitides and syphilis, that may give rise to convulsive seizures should be treated by appropriate measures. The same may be said of hyponatremia, hypocalcemia, or other conditions. Disturbances of the endocrine system resulting from adenomas of the pancreas or hypoparathyroidism require surgery and appropriate replacement therapy, respectively. Of course, these remarks do not apply to idiopathic epilepsy.

Whenever convulsive seizures are associated with a surgically removable lesion of the brain, such as tumor or abscess, removal of such a lesion is usually indicated. It must be remembered, however, that convulsive seizures will be relieved in only about 50 percent of cases of meningioma of the brain and in a much smaller percentage of cases of glioma or abscess of the brain. In such cases, further treatment with drugs is necessary.

Surgery has also been advocated for the removal of cortical scars secondary to cerebral trauma, of vascular lesions, and birth injuries on the assumption that such scars are surrounded by irritable foci which act as a trigger mechanism for the seizures. Reduction in the frequency of seizures has been reported as a sequel to these operations by a number of neurosurgeons. This treatment should be limited to the group of patients with focal attacks which do not respond to medical therapy. In addition, such lesions should be excised only by neurosurgeons who have facilities for the adequate localization of the lesion. Medical treatment will still be required for most of these patients after operation.

The anterior tip of the temporal lobe and the amygdaloid nuclei have been removed or destroyed by stereotaxis in patients with psychomotor seizures who have failed to respond to medical therapy and in whom it was possible to demonstrate a temporal lobe focus by electroencephalography. Favorable results have been reported for this procedure by some neurosurgeons, but experience is too limited to evaluate its efficacy.

PHYSICAL AND MENTAL HYGIENE The epileptic patient should have a wholesome, regular diet consisting of simple foods with an abundance of vegetables and fresh fruits. Excessive quantities of alcoholic beverages of any sort are ill-advised. Constipation can be a troublesome symptom and should be avoided by the establishment of regular bowel habits. This can be developed by training and the use of mild laxatives when necessary.

The patient should be encouraged to maintain regular hours of sleep. Physical activity is desirable, and a moderate amount of physical exercise should be recommended. With proper safeguards, even the more dangerous sports, such as swimming, may be permitted. The uncontrolled epileptic patient, however, should not be allowed to drive an automobile or operate unguarded machinery.

Simple, superficial psychotherapy will frequently prevent or help overcome feelings of inferiority and self-consciousness of many epileptic patients. Both the patient and his family will benefit from such therapy, and a proper family attitude should be established. Oversolicitude and overprotection should be discouraged. It is important to emphasize that the patient should be allowed to live as normal a life as possible.

Every effort should be made to keep children in school, and adults should be encouraged to work. Many communities have vocational rehabilitation centers, and advantage should be taken of such facilities. Patients should be encouraged to participate in available recreational activities, such as movies, dancing, and parties.

THE USE OF ANTICONVULSANT DRUGS Success in the management of patients with epilepsy depends on the ability of the physician to prevent the occurrence of seizures. Approximately 75 percent of patients with convulsive seizures can have their attacks controlled or reduced in frequency by the use of anticonvulsant drugs. Although these drugs are not a cure for epilepsy, their use is the most important step in the treatment of patients with convulsive disorders.

The drugs commonly used at present in the treatment of patients with convulsive seizures (see Table 337-1) are the barbiturates, hydantoins, oxazolidinediones, and, to a lesser extent, the acetylureas and bromides. The available products which have been given a thorough clinical trial and their daily dosages are given below:

General principles Certain drugs are more effective in one type of seizure than in another, and it is necessary to use the proper drugs in the optimum dosages for the different types of seizures. If satisfactory results are not obtained with one of the drugs, the others should be tried, but frequent shifting of drugs is not advisable, and each should be given an adequate trial before another is substituted. In some patients a combination of two or more drugs will produce better results than one alone.

Intelligent management of drugs depends on having the patients chart daily their medication and the number, time, and circumstances of their seizures. Ideally such a base line should be established before medication is begun, since each patient tends to have his own pattern of seizures, but often this is impractical. Changes in medication should be made only when a given program is shown to be inadequate. Frequent measurements of blood levels of diphenylhydantoin and barbiturate are useful. For Dilantin, the therapeutic level is 10 to 15 μg per ml, and one-half of patients have side effects at 30 or more μg per ml. These consist of ataxia, slurred speech, staggering, nystagmus, diplopia, mental dullness, forgetfulness, and confusion. Coma occurs when the level exceeds 50 μg. Clinical and electroencephalographic improvement are not obtained if the level is below 10 μg per ml. The therapeutic level for phenobarbital is probably about 10 to 15 μg per ml, though the range has not yet been exactly determined. Side effects appear in patients on long-term treatment at 25 μg per ml.

When changing medication, the dosage of the new drug should be gradually increased to an optimum level at the same time as the dosage of the old drug is gradually decreased. The sudden withdrawal of a drug may lead to status epilepticus, even though a new drug is substituted. Once an anticonvulsant or a combination of anticonvulsants is found to be effective, its use should be maintained for a period of years.

The therapeutic dose for any patient must be determined to some extent by trial and error. Not uncommonly a drug is discarded as being ineffective, whereas in reality a slightly increased dosage would have led to a complete disappearance of all the attacks. It is, however, inadvisable to administer a drug to the point where the patient is so dull and stupid that he is more incapacitated by the toxic effects than by the seizures. It is highly doubtful whether the prolonged administration of anticonvulsant medication is a factor in the development of the mental deterioration that occurs in a small percentage of the patients with convulsive seizures. However, there is some evidence, albeit contradictory, that chronic Dilantin intoxication can lead to cerebellar degeneration (loss of Purkinje cells) and to polyneuropathy. It is not uncommon to note an improvement in the mental faculties of some patients following control of the seizures by the use of anticonvulsant drugs. The recent claim of pulmonary fibrosis after prolonged Dilantin therapy seems to be unfounded. An antifolate effect on blood serum and a reduction of protein-bound iodine (without lowering of the BMR) have been reported.

Indications for use of specific drugs GRAND MAL SEIZURES For those patients with infrequent grand mal seizures (from one to four per year), phenobarbital can be tried first because of its high therapeutic index and its relatively low toxicity. When the seizures are more frequent, Dilantin is the drug of choice. A combination of Dilantin (0.3 to 0.4 g) and phenobarbital (0.1 to 0.2 g) is more often effective than either of the drugs used alone. When these drugs are used in combination, a full therapeutic dose of each drug must be given. Occasionally, Mesantoin or a combination of this drug with the Dilantin or Mysoline will succeed where Dilantin alone has failed. Only rarely will bromides or a combination of bromides and phenobarbital or Dilantin prove to be more effective.

The toxic effects of phenobarbital, which are drowsiness and mental dullness, nystagmus, and staggering, should be used as indications of excess dosage. Only skin eruption is a contraindication to its further use; otherwise these symptoms can be controlled by reducing the dose. Dilantin almost always leads to hirsutism, hypertrophy of gums, and, as was stated above, ataxia, stupor, or coma. If skin rashes and other hypersensitivity phenomena (polyarteritis) occur, discontinuation of the medication is necessary. Reduction of dose controls the other symptoms.

PSYCHOMOTOR ATTACKS Drugs effective in the treatment of grand mal seizures are effective in the treatment of patients with psychomotor attacks. Dilantin, 300 to 400 mg per day, and Mysoline, 750 to 1,000 mg per day, have given the best results. The results on the whole are not as good as in grand mal epilepsy.

PETIT MAL ATTACKS As a rule, drugs effective in the treatment of grand mal and psychomotor seizures are relatively ineffective in the treatment of patients with petit mal attacks. Zarontin, 750 to 1,500 mg per day, has been most successful and has the advantage over trimethadione (Tridione), paramethadione (Paradione), and phenisuxamide (Milontin) in producing less side effects. It is wise to begin with a single dose of 250 mg per day and increase it every week until therapeutic effect is achieved. Toxic symptoms to Tridione and Paradione are skin eruptions and photophobia. Aplastic anemia has been reported; hence monthly blood counts during the first year are indicated. Methylphenylsuccinamide (Celontin), (adult dose 0.3 g three or four times a day) and acetazolamide (Diamox) (adult dose 0.25 to 0.75 g per day) have been useful in controlling difficult cases of petit mal and massive myoclonus in children.

MINOR SEIZURES AND FOCAL ATTACKS The same drugs effective in the treatment of grand mal and psychomotor seizures are effective against minor seizures and focal attacks. Minor seizures, which appear in patients whose grand mal attacks have been controlled, can occasionally be checked by simply increasing the dose of the drug or drugs that the patient is already taking. If the minor attacks are very infrequent and nonincapacitating, no great effort need be made to treat them.

PETIT MAL PLUS OTHER TYPES When patients are subject to petit mal seizures as well as grand mal or psychomotor seizures, they should receive Zarontin plus diphenylhydantoin sodium, phenobarbital, or Mesantoin. The treatment of the special types of convulsions in infancy and childhood is discussed in Chap. 334.

MYOCLONIC EPILEPSY Mebaral (0.2 to 0.5 g) and phenobarbital (0.1 to 0.2 g) have been the most effective agents in this type of seizure. In the treatment of massive myoclonus in infants, ACTH or a combination of Mogadon and Diamox have been most effective.

STATUS EPILEPTICUS Recurrent convulsions at a frequency which does not allow consciousness to be regained in the interval between seizures (status epilepticus) probably constitute the most serious therapeutic problem. Most patients who die of epilepsy do so because of uncontrolled recurrent seizures or an injury sustained as a result of seizure. Rising temperature, circulatory collapse, and lower nephron nephrosis is a sequence of events which may be encountered in fatal cases.

TABLE 337-1
Anticonvulsant medications*

Generic name	*Trade name*	*Total daily dose per kg body wt; and usual adult dose*	*Principal therapeutic purposes*
Phenobarbital	Luminal	1–5 mg; 60–200 mg	Major seizures; partial seizures; psychomotor seizures; and petit mal
Diphenylhydantoin	Dilantin	4–7 mg; 200–500 mg	Major seizures; psychomotor seizures; partial epilepsy
Primidone	Mysoline	10–25 mg; 750–1,500 mg	Major seizures; psychomotor seizures; partial epilepsy
Ethosuximide	Zarontin	20–30 mg; 1,000–1,500 mg	Petit mal
Trimethadione	Tridione	10–25 mg; 500–1,250 mg	Petit mal
Paramethadione	Paradione	10–25 mg; 500–1,250 mg	Petit mal
Mephenytoin	Mesantoin	7–12 mg; 300–600 mg	Major seizures; psychomotor seizures; focal epilepsy
Mephobarbital	Mebaral	2.5–10 mg; 200–500 mg	Same as phenobarbital; myoclonic epilepsy
Methsuximide	Celontin	10–20 mg; 500–1,000 mg	Petit mal
Phenisuxamide	Milontin	10–20 mg; 500–1250 mg	Petit mal
Acetazolamide	Diamox	5–15 mg; 250–750 mg	Petit mal; infantile spasms; major seizures
Diazepam	Valium	0.15–2 mg; 15–30 mg	Petit mal; major seizures; status epilepticus
Nitrazepam	Mogadon	0.15–2 mg; 10–100 mg	Infantile spasms; myoclonic epilepsy
Ethotoin	Peganone	10–20 mg; 500–1,000 mg	Major seizures; focal seizures
ACTH		40–60 units per day	Infantile spasms

* *Children usually need larger doses than adults, if dose is calculated according to body weight. Excessive drowsiness can often be diminished by dextroamphetamine (Dexedrine), methamphetamine (Desoxyn), or methylphenidate (Ritalin).*

It must be conceded that at present no known drug will safely control all recurrent convulsions. This is not surprising, for there are many causes of convulsions and not all cases are alike. Clinical experience teaches that in some patients the convulsive tendency is so overwhelming that no amount of anticonvulsant medication, even deep ether anesthesia, will prevent recurrence of seizures. In others the liability to recurrent convulsions lasts only a few hours or at most a few days, regardless of whether anticonvulsant medication is given. The real hazard in treating resistant recurrent convulsions is that consciousness and vital functions may be suppressed to a degree incompatible with life. The risk of deep coma without convulsions is greater than semicoma or stupor with an occasional convulsion.

The following medications have been recommended for recurrent convulsions with brain disease and for status epilepticus:

1 Sodium phenobarbital in doses of 0.3 to 0.4 g intramuscularly, and a repeated dose of 0.1 to 0.2 g every 2 hr until a maximum of 0.8 to 1.0 g/24 hr is reached.
2 Thiopental (Pentothal Sodium) in doses of 0.3 to 0.6 g intravenously or intramuscularly.
3 Diazepam (Valium) in intravenous doses of 5 to 10 mg repeated every few hours (to a maximum of 50 mg per 24 hr) has proved to be one of the most effective means of controlling status epilepticus.
4 Diphenylhydantoin sodium (Dilantin) in doses of 0.4 to 0.5 g per day orally (through stomach tube) or intravenously. This is usually given morning, noon, late afternoon, and evening.
5 Tribromoethanol (Avertin) by rectum in doses of 25 mg per kg body weight and followed by 10 to 15 mg per kg body weight at 15- to 30-min intervals as indicated by the response of the patient.
6 Ether by inhalation.
7 Paraldehyde intravenously in doses of 1.0 to 4.0 ml given slowly (over 2 min), or 4 to 8 ml intramuscularly (avoiding injection near nerves, which may be destroyed by it), is a rapidly acting anticonvulsant.

These many treatments attest that no one of them is altogether satisfactory. The author has had the most success with the following program: When the patient is first seen, an intramuscular injection of 0.3 g sodium phenobarbital is given. Diphenylhydantoin sodium, 0.1 to 0.2 g, is then administered intravenously or through a stomach tube, and additional amounts are added later to a total of 0.5 g per day. If seizures continue for the next 2 hr, 0.2 g sodium phenobarbital is again injected. If the seizures continue for the next 1 to 2 hr, 0.2 g sodium phenobarbital is again injected. If the seizures cease for an hour or two and then recur, this amount of barbiturate may be given in repeated doses up to a total amount of 1.0 g per 24 hr. If the seizures are not controlled by the first two injections of phenobarbital and diphenylhydantoin, 10 mg Valium may be injected intravenously. If seizures continue, all medication except diphenylhydantoin sodium should be discontinued, and either a light ether anesthesia or a light Pentothal anesthesia, up to 0.5 g intravenously, should be tried. Should the seizures continue despite all these medications, one is justified in the assumption that the convulsive tendency is so strong that it cannot be checked by reasonable quantities of anticonvulsants. One then depends entirely on diphenylhydantoin sodium, 0.5 g, and sodium phenobarbital, 0.4 g per day. For infants and children, correspondingly smaller doses should be administered. For special types of recurrent seizures such as those associated with brain abscess, subdural empyema, or thrombophlebitis, paraldehyde is highly effective. The dose is 4.0 to 8.0 ml injected intramuscularly, taking care to avoid nerves, and it may be repeated every 3 to 4 hr.

Hyperthermia, which occurs in most cases of severe status epilepticus, must be controlled by the measures outlined in Chap. 11.

REFERENCES

Lennox W, Lennox M: *Epilepsy and Related Disorders*, Boston: Little, Brown, 1960

Penfield W, Jasper H: *Epilepsy and Functional Anatomy of the Human Brain*, Boston: Little, Brown, 1954

Schmidt RP, Wilder BJ: *Epilepsy*, vol. 5 in *Contemporary Neurology Series*, eds F Plum, FH McDowell, Philadelphia: Davis, 1968

Yahr MD: *Anticonvulsants—Clinical Considerations*, ARNMD, vol. 37, Baltimore: Williams & Wilkins, 1959, pp. 57–71

338 INTRODUCTION TO MENTAL DISORDERS

PETER REICH
MARTIN J. KELLY

When first compared with other medical entities the *mental disorders* may seem intangible and confusing. The wide variations in human behavior and personality make it difficult for the physician to determine where the normal ends and the abnormal begins. He may recognize some of the features of mental disorders in his friends, colleagues, or even in himself. The methods used in the study of the mind may seem subjective, relying mainly on the perceptions of the observer and on the memories and descriptive powers of the patient. Diagnoses cannot be corroborated by laboratory findings or confirmed at the autopsy table. However, clinical observations have shown that the mental disorders fall into distinct diagnostic clusters which have implications for the management of the patient. These clinical entities can be identified through the application of basic medical principles. A thorough history and the examination of the patient are fundamental to psychiatric diagnosis. However, the physician needs to understand the nature of mental disorders in order to apply these familiar techniques.

The mind as the composite of the higher activities of the nervous system provides the basis of the life style of each individual, his ways of satisfying his inner needs, of conforming to a society, and of dealing with reality. The accomplishment of these tasks requires the continuing function of adaptive and regulatory mechanisms. The mental disorders may be characterized as disorders of these mechanisms. In some disorders these mechanisms are chronically inadequate or maladaptive, apparently as the result of disturbed development or of hereditary factors. In others, a breakdown or decompensation of previously adequate adaptive mechanisms occurs. Mental disorders cannot be separated from the general state of the body. The mind reflects disturbances in physiologic homeostasis and in turn may influence other organs and bodily systems through nervous and endocrine pathways.

When a patient is assessed for a mental disorder, he serves as his own base line. There is no relevant concept of an average or normal person. Has the patient's own way of adapting to life enabled him to accomplish the basic tasks? To what extent is his present state of adaptation a change from his usual state? The style of function among people is so variable that differences in customs and modes of adaptation may be confused with pathologic processes and may distract the observer from his view of the underlying functions themselves. The life style of a patient may seem eccentric or even offensive to certain moral or ethical considerations, but this does not necessarily indicate the presence of a psychiatric disorder.

It follows that one of the major goals in the treatment of mental disorders is the restoration of the patient's own adaptive mechanisms. Reduction of stress, resolution of conflict, support of psychologic mechanisms, and, at times, the learning of new and more flexible means of adaptation are all useful approaches.

CLASSIFICATION OF MENTAL DISORDERS

The present system of classification of mental disorders was adopted by the World Health Organization in 1966, to answer the need for a unified international system of nomenclature in psychiatry. Table 338-1 lists only the mental disorders with no known organic basis, entities to be discussed in this section. The other part of this classification system includes diseases of the nervous system that cause an impairment of intellect or other derangements of mental function. This system provides a basis for improved communication regarding psychiatric disorders throughout the medical world. Of necessity the diagnoses are descriptive and functional, not implying any special theory of etiology. Some of the entities may be true diseases, in the sense of being outward manifestations of an as yet unrecognized lesion of the nervous system, others may be the expressions of hereditary tendencies, still others the outcome of disturbances of learning or adverse environmental or nutritional factors, and some may be due to combinations of factors. Present understanding of the nervous system does not allow an explanation of these mental disorders on a physiologic, morphologic, or biochemical basis. Until such correlates are elucidated, physicians must be satisfied with a classification system based on the behavior of the patient. However, this classification has clinical validity and provides a rational basis for the understanding and treatment of mental disorders.

The *neuroses* are relatively benign episodes of disordered mental function, usually involving anxiety and the maladaptive exaggeration of elements of the patient's personality. There is usually a lifelong susceptibility to neurosis, with recurrences of overt symptoms at times of stress. Patients will often have mild subclinical symptoms between episodes. For example, during the 3 months following an elective herniorrhaphy, a meticulous and anxious young history professor was unable to concentrate on work, experienced an old stage fright at his lectures, and suffered from fatigue, insomnia, and diarrhea. He also had waves of diffuse anxiety, especially on weekends, and, in open competition with his young children, he made excessive demands for his wife's attentions. Such patients suffer inwardly, often from depression as well as anxiety, but seldom lose their grip on reality. They usually have achieved an adequate adjustment to life with the exception of their neurotic episodes.

In contrast, the *psychoses* involve major disturbances of thinking, mood, or behavior which grossly interfere with the patient's capacities to meet the ordinary demands of life. For example, an isolated, overconscientious college freshman, away from home for the first time, kept to his room for several weeks, reading books on mystical religions, before appearing at the health services tense and disheveled, complaining that his heart was stopping. He later said that he was struggling with the devil, who spoke to him through his father's voice. Unlike the symptoms of neuroses, the symptoms of psychoses represent a more complete derangement of nervous functioning in which both primary and secondary phenomena probably occur; and in the psychotic state itself there is an indefinable alteration in the state of consciousness. Whatever the cause of the psychosis, there appears to be a reduction to a lower level of nervous functioning or, in psychodynamic terms, a breakthrough of primitive areas of the mind. Thus psychosis represents a specific disruption of the integrative mechanisms of the brain. The approach to a psychotic patient, therefore, should emphasize the search for the source of the disruption and its correction as a means of restoring neurologic and psychologic integration.

A *personality disorder* involves deeply ingrained, chronic maladaptive patterns of behavior, suggesting an arrest or distortion in the development of the personality. For example, during her eighth admission to a hospital for leg pain, muscle weakness, and fever, a 33-year-old x-ray technician was found to be hiding thermometers in her bedside stand. Prior to this she had provoked an argument between the intern and the attending neurologist regarding her pain medications and had alienated the nurses through her childlike temper tantrums and frequent demands. The history revealed two suicide attempts by drug overdose, an erratic work record, frequent medical consultations, and chronic abuse of medications. She complained that her physicians were incompetent and insensitive to her problem. Such patients have few periods in their lives when their maladaptive patterns are not in evidence. They tend to blame others for their distress and have little capacity for insight.

Transient situational disturbances are the direct result of the impact of stress and generally resolve themselves when the stress is over. For example, during his third day on a coronary unit, a 64-year-old businessman became agitated, pulled off his chest electrodes, and demanded to leave the hospital. He refused to talk to the doctors, claiming they were murderers. The man in the next bed had died the night before after an unsuccessful attempt at resuscitation. The patient calmed down after being moved to a private room near the unit and showed no signs of mental disorder during the remainder of his stay. Most of the acute mental disturbances seen in response to sickness and hospitalization are in this category. They may take the form of neuroses or psychoses, but there is usually no history of a previous mental disorder. At times such acute reactions can be adaptive, sparing the patient from the full effects of reality.

The *psychophysiologic disorders* are disturbances in the homeostatic relationship between the mind and the body. The classical "psychosomatic disorders" are included in this category, e.g., peptic ulcer, bronchial asthma, migraine, and essential hypertension. However, in recent years, the concept has been broadened to include all those instances in which a vulnerable organ is affected adversely by emotional factors, generally mediated by the autonomic nervous system. The earlier view of relating specific psychologic conflicts to specific disorders is invalid and no longer widely held. The use of this diagnosis reflects the emotional *component* of the disorder. As pointed out in Chap. 13, it does not imply that the emotional element is the cause of the disease. The relationships between emotional tension and the disorders of specific organs are covered elsewhere.

CLINICAL APPROACH TO THE MENTAL DISORDERS

Evaluation of the patient

Without a thorough history and physical evaluation, the mental examination does not enable the physician to make the distinction between the primary mental disorders and those which are secondary to other conditions. The mind has only a limited range of reactions. A depressive episode might be related to an occult carcinoma, to a stressful aspect of illness or hospitalization, to the effects of a medication, or to a long-standing mental disorder. Often such factors are interwoven. Sometimes the symptoms of a mental disorder will distract the

TABLE 338-1
Mental disorders

I Neuroses
- *A* Anxiety neurosis
- *B* Hysterical neurosis
  - *1* Conversion type
  - *2* Dissociative type
- *C* Phobic neurosis
- *D* Obsessive compulsive neurosis
- *E* Depressive neurosis
- *F* Neurasthenic neurosis
- *G* Depersonalization neurosis
- *H* Hypochondriacal neurosis
- *I* Other neurosis

II Psychophysiologic disorders

III Personality disorders and other nonpsychotic disorders
- *A* Personality disorders
  - *1* Paranoid personality
  - *2* Cyclothymic personality
  - *3* Schizoid personality
  - *4* Explosive personality
  - *5* Obsessive compulsive personality
  - *6* Hysterical personality
  - *7* Asthenic personality
  - *8* Antisocial personality
  - *9* Passive aggressive personality
- *B* Sexual deviations
- *C* Alcoholism
- *D* Drug dependence

IV Psychoses (nonorganic)
- *A* Schizophrenia
- *B* Major affective disorders
- *C* Paranoid states
- *D* Other psychoses

V Transient situational disturbances

SOURCE: *From the International Classification of Diseases (ICD-8).*

physician from his pursuit of the physical complaints. If a patient tends to develop hysterical symptoms, he will probably respond to a physical illness with hysterical mechanisms. However, physical and mental disorders can also be concomitant and unrelated. The discovery of a mental disorder should no more deter the physician from completing a medical examination than should the discovery of a physical disorder deter him from the appropriate evaluation of the personality of his patient.

The first clues of the presence of a mental disorder may be the physician's own inner responses to his patient, for example, a sense of uneasiness or a feeling that something has changed that cannot be explained by physical or laboratory findings. Prior experience with the patient gives the physician a base line for the evaluation of mood, behavior, and thought processes. The patient may openly complain about mental symptoms, or he may describe changes in his habits or way of life, or he may only refer to tension states, such as insomnia, restlessness, or fatigue.

THE INTERVIEW Given a relaxed and private setting, the physician's natural manner and genuine interest in his patient's feelings and experiences will lead to a useful interview. Patients usually enjoy the chance to talk to a sympathetic listener. Those who refuse or are evasive are probably displaying some aspect of their mental life, such as depression, paranoid fears, or a deep-seated problem in the forming of relationships. Others may be concealing suicidal thoughts or other sources of guilt. Patients are seldom if ever hurt by talking freely, even though they may cry or confess hidden fears or impulses. In fact, sharing feelings often brings relief. In a hospital, the presence of neighboring patients may be a serious impediment to an honest exchange, and it may be necessary to move the patient or his neighbors. A special challenge is presented by the problem of assessing the psychologic functioning of a patient from an unfamiliar ethnic, socioeconomic, or national background.

The technique of interviewing is best learned by experience. It is an inquiry into the patient's background, his manner of coping with problems, especially those relating to social relationships, and his immediate situation. An interrogatory attitude should be avoided, but beyond that the natural style of the interviewer is the preferred approach. A concept of the important areas to investigate, based on the principles of psychiatric diagnosis, can provide a road map, but the patient should be allowed to choose his own way. Occasional questions or expressions of interest are usually sufficient to bring him to another subject. The art is in watching the game while playing it.

The psychiatric evaluation consists of the history and the mental status examination, but in practice both these elements are combined in the interview. The physician observes the patient's thought processes, emotions, and behavior, and at the same time helps him to tell his story.

The history The *present illness* can be characterized in terms of its duration, extent, symptoms, and relationship to stress. An acute disorder precipitated by stress generally has a better prognosis than one with an insidious onset and no apparent precipitant. The feelings, personal experiences, and private interpretations of the patient are as important as the realistic sequence of events. Related symptoms, often involving bodily functions, may be overlooked. Insomnia, anorexia, constipation, sexual disturbances, difficulty in concentrating, and irritability are useful diagnostic signs. The strengths of the patient are often as important to evaluate as his disorders of function. His islands of adequate function, his satisfying relationships, and his capacities for work or enjoyment may play significant roles during treatment. Sometimes a patient who complains loudly about emotional distress will prove to have adequate function in every significant area, while another patient who makes only a vague allusion to an emotional problem may reveal major disorders of function when he is interviewed. In many instances it is important to inquire about the use of drugs. Amphetamines, LSD, and the heavy use of marijuana, as well as certain prescribed medications to control blood pressure or sleep, are significant factors. Which drugs were taken, when, and how much, are basic questions. Delusions or other distortions of reality can usually be identified in the patient's story and in his manner of presentation.

An understanding of the premorbid personality and of the previous levels of function of the patient can be obtained through the *past history.* The nature of the present illness is best evaluated against this base line. Chronic maladjustments or impairments will influence the prognosis. The patient's previous reactions to stressful events or significant transitions in life are useful landmarks. Severe emotional or physical trauma, especially in early life, may have a lasting effect on later adaptation. The *family history* can help in understanding the influence of innate or familial patterns of behavior.

Mental status examination The interaction in the interview is a microcosm of the patient's current level of function. His ability to organize his thoughts, conceptualize causal relationships, communicate ideas and emotions, and exercise judgment can all be observed. At times examples of delusions or bizarre affect occur during an interview. Body language is an important dimension, and tension states that are not verbalized are sometimes communicated through posture, voice tone, and body movements. Depression may first be detected through such clues. Hesitations, changes in tone, and avoidance of subjects may indicate painful areas. Characteristic mental mechanisms, such as obsessive attention to detail, hypochondriacal preoccupations, or denial of affect may appear in the interview, much as they appear in the patient's other relationships. His manner of telling his story, whether freely or only in response to pressure, may also indicate his state of mind. The various mental disorders often appear in characteristic form during the interview, especially if the interaction is relatively unstructured and if it focuses mainly on the patient's emotional distress.

An underemphasized source of information is the *physician's response* to the patient. An intuitive empathy for the deeper distress of the patient may occur in the absence of corresponding mental content. Too often this information is discarded because it does not seem to be objective and is difficult to communicate to colleagues. The extent of a patient's inner sense of helplessness may be measured by the physician's impulse to protect or rescue the patient. Other nonverbalized emotions in the patient may be reflected in the physician's responses of anger or frustration. At times the earliest perception of a psychosis is a feeling of not being able to make real contact with the patient or of not being able to fathom the real meaning of a patient's complaints. Such intuition is also sensitive to underlying tensions, bizarre qualities, and an inner sense of despair.

SUICIDE RISK Though the evaluation of suicide risk is part of the approach to patients with mental disorders, many suicides occur in patients with no prior history of significant mental disturbances. Suicide correlates with aging, physical disorders, alcoholism, loneliness, and personal losses, as well as with depression and psychosis. The suicides that occur in general hospitals are often associated with delirium. At best it is difficult to predict suicidal behavior. An acute mental decompensation may occur without warning. Suicidal patients may be reluctant to confess their plans or impulses because of guilt or shame. However, desperate people often come to their physicians for help, because suicidal impulses are usually accompanied by the wish to live. Any hint of suicide risk, including a sudden change in the patient's mental status or an ill-defined sense of alarm on the part of the physician, is an indication for active investigation. Raising the issue of suicide with the patient often provides welcome relief. Relatives or other responsible people should be involved promptly.

OTHER SOURCES OF INFORMATION When psychosis or personality disorder is being considered, it may be useful to get information from other sources that seem more reliable than the patient. However, the patient's privacy should be protected whenever possible. Relatives, friends, and other observers will have their own biases and may also provide information of questionable reliability. The records of past hospitalizations and of other medical contacts are especially useful in documenting a diagnosis. The past history of a psychosis, of drug abuse, or of manifestations of personality disorder can often clarify a confusing clinical picture.

PSYCHOLOGIC TESTING When administered and interpreted by a skilled psychologist, psychologic tests are useful diagnostic adjuncts. They are especially important in the differentiation of organic brain syndromes from functional disorders and are also helpful in revealing latent psychoses and in examining guarded or overcontrolled patients. These tests also have a wide use in general medicine and neurology. They include (1) intelligence tests (Wechsler Adult Intelligence Scale), which assess intellectual functions and performance against standardized criteria, (2) tests of perceptual and motor functions (Bender Gestalt), (3) personality inventories (Minnesota Multiphasic Personality Inventory), which give profiles of character and personality and which can be self-administered, and (4) projective tests (Rorschach, Thematic Apperception Test), which elicit responses to unstructured but standardized stimuli.

TREATMENT

During an episode of decompensation, the therapeutic approach focuses on *protection of the patient, reduction of stress and internal tension*, and *reconstitution of adaptive mechanisms.* The treatment of chronic disorders is more likely to involve support, insight, and reeducation. Many disorders can be managed effectively by the physician during his medical relationship with the patient. When referral to a psychiatrist is necessary, the preparation of the patient by the physician is often the crucial element in the process. Psychiatric treatments take various forms—psychologic, somatic, and environmental. Whatever the treatment or combination of treatments, the relationship with the physician is the most sustaining feature.

Psychotherapy can provide both support and the opportunity to learn new modes of adaptation. During an acute decompensation the active process of investigating psychologic factors is often a very effective way to restore equilibrium. Long-term psychotherapy may be helpful in the prevention of exacerbations of mental disorders and in the treatment of chronic disabilities. Often a medical relationship provides extended support for patients who might otherwise be more disabled by mental symptoms. Newer approaches involving families, couples, or groups focus on problems in interpersonal relationships. Intensive group experience, such as "marathon sessions" or encounter groups, is being used in the treatment of personality disorders, notably the addictions. The occasional adverse effects of these intense experiences on patients with psychoses underscore the importance of the diagnosis in treatment selection. *Behavior modification* using conditioning techniques has been applied to specific symptoms and behavior problems.

Pharmacologic agents will have increasingly important influence on the treatment of mental disorders as biochemical approaches to emotional states are elucidated. At present, effective agents are available for the management of the psychoses, anxiety states, and certain forms of depression. The treatment of psychophysiologic reactions often involves the pharmacologic management of an anxiety state. The potential for addiction or suicide should be considered carefully when prescribing drugs for the treatment of mental disorders. In practice, the psychopharmacologic approach is best combined with other treatment modalities, and frequent contact with the patient, often in the form of psychotherapy, is advisable in order to monitor dosage and to evaluate therapeutic effectiveness. *Electroconvulsive therapy* continues to have an important role in the treatment of patients with severe depression and with suicidal tensions. When modified by succinylcholine and when performed under anesthesia with adequate respiratory exchange, electrically induced seizures have very few complications even with elderly patients or with patients suffering from heart disease. *Neurosurgical approaches* to severe mental disorders using stereotactic techniques are being reinvestigated.

Hospitalization may be needed in order to reduce

stress and to protect the patient from the consequences of his impulses and his disturbances of judgment. The milieu available in a hospital setting in itself constitutes an important treatment modality. With the development of community-based mental hospitals and psychiatric units in general hospitals, there is a movement toward active treatment and short-term hospitalization rather than custodial care. This trend also facilitates partial hospitalization, such as day care, night care, and the halfway house. Even with these developments, some patients will continue to require long-term hospitalization.

The implementation of the Community Mental Health Act in the United States, passed in 1963, has shifted the emphasis from large poorly supported hospitals located at some distance from centers of population to smaller units serving individual communities. The aim of the community mental health movement is to mobilize available community resources, including lay and professional members of the community, to deal with mental problems of the locale.

There has also been an increased emphasis on *social approaches* to mental disorders through the study of families, work situations, communities, and treatment facilities. This interest extends to larger issues, such as poverty, racism, and war. Attempts are being made at the *primary prevention* of mental disorders through work with social systems and with those families or groups of children thought to be in the high-risk category. The results of these efforts are being evaluated.

The specific mental disorders will be discussed in more detail in the next four chapters. Depression, a symptom occurring in all mental disorders, will be discussed in a separate chapter because of its importance in medical practice.

REFERENCES

American Psychiatric Association, Committee on Nomenclature and Statistics: *Diagnostic and Statistical Manual of Mental Disorders,* 2d ed., Washington: American Psychiatric Association, 1968

Freedman AM, Kaplan HI: *Comprehensive Textbook of Psychiatry,* Baltimore: Williams & Wilkins, 1967

Havens LL: Clinical methods in psychiatry. Int J Psychiatry 10:7, 1972

MacKinnon RA, Michels R: *The Psychiatric Interview in Clinical Practice,* Philadelphia: Saunders, 1971

Mayer-Gross W et al: *Clinical Psychiatry,* 3d ed., London: Baillière, 1967

Whitehorn J: Guide to interviewing and clinical personality study. Arch Neurol Psychiatry 52:197, 1944

339 THE NEUROSES

PETER REICH
MARTIN J. KELLY

Although neuroses are among the more common disorders seen in medical practice, probably no other entities are more widely misunderstood. To some extent the confusion arises from misuse of the term. Literally meaning "full of nerves," it was used during the nineteenth century as a general term for nervous disorders. When Freud made his observations on the psychogenic basis of hysteria and obsessional states, he designated a subgroup of the mental disorders as *psycho*neuroses. The term *neurosis* is now used for this subgroup alone, and its more general meanings have been eliminated. However, for lack of a better word, it is still commonly used to designate all those minor mental aberrations that defy classification and characterize troublesome, eccentric, or maladjusted patients, giving a somewhat pejorative connotation and depriving it of its specific meaning.

With the occurrence of a neurosis the patient may find himself as puzzled as his physician. For no apparent explanation he may experience waves of diffuse anxiety or feelings of guilt, pessimism, and despondency. He may lose his self-confidence and be plagued with doubts, become preoccupied with minor signs of illness, or feel compelled to perform senseless rituals. Physical symptoms may develop that cannot be explained by his physician, and he may be troubled by persistent insomnia and fatigue. Although in all likelihood he will identify his symptoms as originating in his own mind, he will be unable to overcome them through force of will and may be left with a sense of shame and inadequacy.

The understanding of such a syndrome can come as a great relief both to the physician and to his patient. Characteristically the patient retains his grasp of reality and will benefit from a rational explanation of his difficulties. Although neurotic episodes may be self-limiting, the application of appropriate treatment can reduce the morbidity and duration of the symptoms.

DEFINITION The neuroses are episodes of psychologic decompensation that occur in people who have already achieved relatively adequate mental function. The symptoms often include anxiety and the exaggeration or overactivity of mechanisms usually employed by the patient to cope with anxiety and stress. Thus, specific neuroses take their form from the personality type of the patient. For example, an intellectual lawyer may become obsessed with doubts or a shy girl fearful of crowds. Neuroses are usually recurrent, taking the same form throughout a patient's lifetime. An elderly patient who develops an anxiety neurosis may find himself experiencing the same feelings and symptoms that he can remember from his adolescence. Although neuroses seem to be reactions to stress, often no apparent source of stress can be found, and even when a precipitant is identified it seldom seems to be sufficient to account for the extent of the reaction.

Neuroses may vary in severity from mild episodes to severe incapacitating illnesses that may even require hospitalization. Rarely if ever does a neurosis develop into a psychosis. The personality is not disrupted and impulsive, antisocial, or bizarre actions are not seen. Instead, patients generally become more inhibited and more limited in their activities, losing their capacities to enjoy habitual pleasures. They may become preoccupied, unable to relax; they may lose their interest in work. Often physical symptoms occur reflecting the physiologic components of anxiety, such as tachycardia, urinary frequency, and tremulousness, and these may then become the foci of hypochondriacal concerns. Childhood fears of loneliness and separation reappear, and patterns of petulance, demanding irritability, or clinging dependency occur in patients who may ordinarily be mature and independent. Many of these behavioral aspects are tendencies that the patient recognizes in himself during his healthier periods of adjustment. Feelings of guilt and depression are usually prominent, partly because the patient experiences his illness as a sign of weakness and partly because deeper and forbidden feelings arise during the course of neurotic episodes.

DIAGNOSIS Neuroses are always decompensations in the individual's level of adaptation, and the patient serves as his own base line in making this assessment. Almost everyone has habits, minor symptoms, or inhibitions that resemble features of the neuroses. These are aspects of the character of the patient and usually are not associated with suffering or disability. The patient's attitude toward these manifestations helps to distinguish them from neurotic symptoms. He usually feels they are part of himself and are not matters of concern.

Neuroses can usually be distinguished from the psychoses by the absence of delusions, hallucinations, and bizarre affect. Psychoses are generally more global in their effects on function and involve more disorganization of the personality. The history of the onset of an episode usually makes this point clear. Premorbidly or between episodes the patient with neurosis usually functions more effectively than the patient with psychosis, especially in the area of interpersonal relationships. There are, however, instances when a severe neurosis may be difficult to differentiate from a psychosis because of the incapacitating nature of the illness. Persistent hypochondriacal neurosis, severe obsessive-compulsive neurosis, and phobic neurosis are in this category. During the onset of psychosis, patients may go through a phase of neurotic symptoms. Usually these manifestations are more chaotic and polymorphous than those of a true neurosis, do not necessarily follow the character type of the patient, and often are accompanied by intense agitation and anxiety.

Whenever chronic maladaptive patterns resembling neuroses are seen, the possibility of a personality disorder should be considered. Careful attention to the question of chronicity is advisable when patients come to the physician with hysterical, hypochondriacal, obsessive-compulsive, or depersonalization symptoms. In dealing with personality disorders, a detailed history of previous medical contacts will often reveal disturbed relationships with physicians and occasionally malingering.

A neurosis may be confused with a transient situational reaction if the acute stress is not apparent during the initial evaluation. The identification of the stress and the rapid return of function after the termination of stress will make the differentiation clear. If the situation is not too pressing, the various mental disorders can often be differentiated by observing the patient over a period of time.

Many physical and emotional disorders resemble a neurosis at some point in their presentation or course. Multiple sclerosis may be confused with conversion symptoms. Temporal lobe epilepsy often resembles hysterical dissociative neurosis or depersonalization neurosis. Endocrine problems, especially thyrotoxicosis, frequently present some of the symptoms of anxiety states. The neurasthenic and depressive neuroses should be differentiated from physical and emotional states associated with undiagnosed tumors. Anxiety states are also commonly seen with chronic amphetamine abuse and after the heavy use of marijuana.

In the diagnostic approach to the neuroses, the mental-status examination, personal history, medical evaluation, and ongoing observations of the clinical course each provide an important facet. In addition, psychologic testing, especially with the Rorschach test, is very useful in identifying neuroses and in differentiating them from psychoses and organic conditions.

INCIDENCE Studies on the incidence of neuroses are difficult to interpret because of variations in definition and in case finding. However, it is clear from population studies of midtown New York and of Stirling County, Canada, a rural community, that neuroses are not specifically associated with urbanization or with racial, cultural, or socioeconomic factors. Furthermore, there is no evidence to support the popular belief that neuroses are related to the stresses of modern society. Neuroses occur throughout the life cycle, and there is no significant sex difference in their incidence.

PATHOGENESIS Symptomatically the neuroses appear to be heterogeneous, but the central and unifying position of anxiety in their genesis becomes apparent when patients with various entities are examined closely. Even in hysterical neurosis, when a patient may be blandly indifferent to a physical disability, a deep underlying anxiety can be seen and often the history will reveal episodes of anxiety preceding the onset of physical symptoms. In fact, each neurotic pattern represents a mechanism for coping with anxiety, although these mechanisms are only partially successful. The intensity of the panic experienced when neurotic patterns are thwarted or impaired is a measure of the full force of the anxiety involved in neurotic decompensations. The origins of this anxiety and the reasons for its persistence in the absence of overt danger are puzzling features.

An adequate theory of the etiology of neuroses not only must explain the anxiety but also should take into account the other general features. These include the regressive, childlike aspects of the illness, the lifelong patterns of susceptibility, the presence of irrational guilt, and the specificity of precipitants. This last feature is illustrated by the patient with obsessive-compulsive neurosis who faced the bombing of his city with relative equanimity but was thrown into a panic by the need to decide between two makes of automobiles.

The various hypotheses that have been advanced stress the importance of constitutional predispositions, of parental attitudes, of early experiences and life events, of socioeconomic and cultural conflicts, and of biochemical factors. At one level the neuroses undoubtedly represent disorders of nervous system function. Nevertheless, within the limits of our knowledge, the psychodynamic hypothesis is the one most widely accepted at this time. It provides a clinically useful basis for psychotherapy, although biochemical, environmental, social, and behavioral approaches may also be needed.

In brief, the psychodynamic hypothesis holds that neuroses arise from unresolved intrapsychic conflicts concerning the expression of sexual or aggressive drives. During development, primitive drives are normally transformed into socially acceptable ambitions and activities. This process can be arrested if some aspect of the expression of a drive becomes a threat to the basic security of the child. This segment of the drive is then suppressed in its immature form, and the child becomes inhibited in the corresponding area of behavior. The inhibitions become part of the conscience of the child, and the conflict is internalized in the personality. Later in life, if the drive is stimulated, the old fears that led to its original suppression are reactivated. Thus an intense fear not appropriate to the adult situation develops. Old mechanisms associated with the control of the drive also reappear. Insofar as the conflict also involves the conscience, guilt is experienced.

A simple example of this formulation of a neurosis would be the following. A mother is intolerant of her child's aggression and he learns to inhibit the expression of his anger at her through fear of losing her sustaining love. Her prohibitions become internalized as part of his conscience. His aggressive drives, especially toward women, then fail to undergo transformation through experience and, instead, are held in an immature form removed from his consciousness. Later in life, if events lead to the development of anger toward a woman he depends upon, perhaps his wife or another representation of his mother, he will reexperience his early fears of loss of support and fall back on the childhood mechanism he originally employed when controlling his anger at his mother because he has failed to learn any other mechanisms. These early mechanisms and the unchanged childhood form of his aggression give an immature cast to his thoughts and behavior. The old conflict between his anger and his conscience then leads to an inappropriate sense of guilt. He may be quite capable of functioning aggressively at work or in competitive activities with men. The specificity of the precipitant is accounted for by the underlying conflict.

CLINICAL TYPES The International Classification of Diseases recognizes eight specific types of neuroses, differentiated by their principal psychologic mechanisms. These types and their major characteristics are listed in Table 339-1. Clinically they are rarely seen in pure form. Usually a neurosis involves more than one mechanism.

TABLE 339-1
The neuroses

Type of neurosis	*Characteristics*
1 Anxiety neurosis	Episodic diffuse anxiety in attacks or waves; somatic complaints such as palpitations, paresthesias, weakness, dizziness; pessimism and irritability
2 Hysterical neurosis:	
a Conversion type	Physical symptoms involving voluntary musculature and sensory system, such as paradoxic paralyses, seizures, sensory deficits, and pain; attitude of indifference
b Dissociative type	Alterations in consciousness and sense of identity, such as fugue states, amnesias, somnambulism; anxiety not evident
3 Phobic neurosis	Intense irrational fears of objects or situations; anxiety attacks may occur with corresponding physical symptoms
4 Obsessive-compulsive neurosis	Persistent or intrusive thoughts, often distressing in content, and uncontrollable minor acts, often to expiate, cleanse, or counteract evil; depression and guilt are prominent; preoccupations with disease may occur
5 Depressive neurosis	Episodic excessive self-criticism, low self-esteem, and lowered vitality, often accompanied by physical complaints
6 Neurasthenic neurosis	Weakness, fatigability, exhaustion, with low self-esteem but little self-criticism
7 Depersonalization neurosis	Feelings of unreality and estrangement from self, body, and surroundings; panic may occur
8 Hypochondriacal neurosis	Morbid preoccupations with bodily processes and diseases, accompanied by multiple physical complaints; anxiety and agitation may occur; depression is common

Anxiety, depression, and the occurrence of physical symptoms are seen throughout the spectrum of neuroses. The various clinical types reflect major character traits and mental mechanisms. Neuroses are also grouped according to characteristic mental manifestations, including anxiety, depression, conversion, and hypochondriasis. These manifestations are general phenomena and are seen throughout the range of mental disorders as well as among patients without disorder.

Anxiety neurosis and depressive neurosis, by far the most common of these syndromes seen in medical practice, should be distinguished from depressive psychosis, especially in middle-aged or elderly patients. Hysterical, hypochondriacal, and obsessive-compulsive neuroses are also important entities in medicine. The range of depressive disorders will be covered in Chap. 341. Neurasthenia and hypochondriasis have been discussed in Chaps. 14 and 15.

Anxiety neurosis This common syndrome, also described in Chap. 14, varies in severity from self-limited periods of mild agitation to major incapacitating states of tension. Unlike the other neuroses, where the symptoms serve to protect the patient from the direct impact of anxiety, here the anxiety itself in acute attacks or wave-like episodes dominates the clinical picture. Obsessions, phobias, hypochondriacal concerns, and other neurotic manifestations may appear in transitory form. The physiologic manifestations—palpitations, hyperventilation, excessive sweating, tremulousness, insomnia, anorexia—are common complaints and may form the basis of hypochondriacal concerns. An episode of anxiety may be painful and debilitating, and patients often suffer from fatigue, weakness, and irritability between episodes.

Patients with this disorder often give a history of a lifelong tendency toward excessive anxiety, beginning with phobias, nightmares, and inhibitions in childhood, and continuing in their adolescence and adult life as chronic insecurity, nervousness, and low self-esteem. A family tendency toward excessive anxiety is a common finding. The episodes of neurosis usually occur during times of insecurity, and such patients are especially sensitive to loneliness and loss. After experiencing recurrent episodes, patients may recognize and dread the early manifestations of anxiety and lose their capacity to use anxiety as a cue for adaptive behavior. Instead, they develop rigid patterns of avoidance and feelings of pessimism and vulnerability. When an anxiety syndrome occurs in an adult patient with no past history of similar episodes, other diagnoses should be entertained. Almost any physical disorder that disturbs the homeostasis of an individual may include anxiety as one of its manifestations.

Acute anxiety attacks may be confused with medical catastrophes. The onset of terror, hyperventilation, suffocation, dizziness, paresthesias, and other ominous sensations will often lead a patient to seek emergency care. Hyperventilation may lead to tetany. Again, the history of similar attacks will favor the diagnosis of neurosis. Other causes to consider include cardiovascular episodes, hypoglycemia, perforated viscus, internal hemorrhage, or other major disorders of sudden onset. Anxiety attacks are also seen during incipient schizophrenia, LSD "bad trips," amphetamine and cannabis intoxication, withdrawal states from addicting agents, and in alcoholic hallucinosis. Most of these states include fragmented paranoid delusions or other psychotic manifestations and may be associated with desperate efforts to escape or with impulsive suicide attempts.

Anxiety neurosis can complicate the management of medical illnesses, especially during hospitalization. The fears associated with illness may be exaggerated, and patients may become too agitated to listen to reassurance or accept medical advice. At times anxiety takes the form of anger and patients will attempt to leave the hospital against advice. Hospitalization itself has stressful features, including forced passivity, immobilization, infantilizing routines, intimate examinations, injections, and other intrusive procedures that may activate inner psychologic conflicts and touch off anxiety states.

The management of an anxiety state in a patient recovering from a myocardial infarction may be a critical factor. Such patients may fight sleep and resist tranquilizers because of fear of death. Here the importance of interpersonal contact cannot be overemphasized. In general, anxiety states are very responsive to the presence of a calm person, but reassurances alone will rarely work. The patient should be encouraged to express his fears. Dramatic therapeutic effects can be obtained by sitting at the patient's bedside and listening to him talk.

In the management of anxiety states it is important to help the patient regain his confidence in his ability to control his symptoms. Helping him understand that anxiety is self-limited and has no ominous significance in itself will enable him to endure his uncomfortable feelings with more courage. Physical activity often brings relief, especially if it involves contact with other people. Sometimes the reassuring feel of a bottle of tranquilizers in the pocket will enable the patient to resume his usual activities.

Hysterical neurosis Hysterical neurosis is a much more limited disorder than the common usage of the word hysteria would suggest. Most of the patients with symptoms of physical disorder in the absence of objective findings are showing *conversion* phenomena, the representation of psychologic conflicts through motor or sensory manifestations. Conversion is a general phenomenon of the mind-body relationship; it occurs throughout the range of mental disorders and also serves as an adaptive mechanism. In hysterical neurosis, conversion occurs within the framework of a neurotic disorder.

Two types of hysterical neuroses are distinguished, the *conversion type*, in which symptoms involve the neuromuscular and sensory systems, and the *dissociative type*, in which disorders of consciousness occur. At times the patient with hysterical neurosis appears to be gaining some satisfaction or advantages from his disabled state, leading to the confusion of this neurosis with malingering. However, in neurosis the symptoms are not under conscious control. True malingering is usually a manifestation of a serious personality disorder and is generally accompanied by features such as immaturity, chronically disturbed interpersonal relations, or antisocial tendencies (sociopathy). Patients who feign illness may be protecting themselves from a major emotional crisis and should be handled tactfully and cautiously.

Whether or not hallucinations can occur as hysterical manifestations is a matter of controversy. Isolated visual hallucinations not accompanied by delusional thinking are sometimes reported by patients with other features of hysterical neurosis. However, many of the more dramatic examples of hysterical phenomena occur among patients with hysterical personality disorders. For example, the patients who have undergone numerous abdominal operations for unexplained pain or those who display grossly inappropriate histrionic or sexualized behavior during hospitalization are usually in this category. Hysterical neuroses are discrete episodes, often having their onset after emotionally significant events. An initial anxiety phase is replaced by the physical symptoms, and the patient is left apparently calm and strangely indifferent to his illness. These episodes often terminate as suddenly as they begin. At times simple suggestion will lead to relief of symptoms. However, recurrences are common. The conversion type is more prevalent among women than men; there is no sex difference in the incidence of the dissociative type. The relative lack of anxiety differentiates these disorders from the psychophysiologic disorders.

A wide variety of confusing symptoms may occur in the conversion type, including the classical manifestations of "grand hysteria," such as motor paralyses or blindness, now relatively rare, and a myriad of symptoms simulating disorders of the nervous system, including gait disturbances, tremors, localized paralyses, anesthesias, paresthesias, and bizarre seizure-like states. These symptoms can usually be distinguished from true physical disorders by history and physical examination. For example, hysterical sensory deficits or paralyses usually do not follow the anatomic distribution of the nervous system, and hysterical seizures do not often include the characteristic cry, loss of consciousness, free fall, and incontinence seen in true seizure episodes. Conversion neuroses often occur after industrial accidents or automobile injuries. When secondary gain involves compensation, the recovery process may be prolonged, again on an unconscious basis. Abdominal pain, chest pain, head pain, and dizziness may also be manifestations. Conversion symptoms sometimes arise during the course of an organic illness, making the differential diagnosis between the physical symptoms and the conversion symptoms extremely difficult. Hospitalization may then be prolonged by the persistence of these psychogenic symptoms, especially when the patient has fears associated with leaving the hospital. Often patients with hysterical neurosis are dependent and immature and will need the support of the physician during the recovery process.

The symptoms of the dissociative type include amnesias, fugue states, multiple personality states, and somnambulism. The amnesias may be brief, covering only specific incidents, or they may be global and prolonged. The familiar story of the man who finds himself in a strange city with no memory of his journey is characteristic of this syndrome. Complex acts can be performed during fugue states, and the patient may appear to be normal to the casual observer. Often such states have their onset in traumatic situations associated with real dangers, such as bomb explosions, train wrecks, or physical assaults. Events associated with guilt, shame, or anxiety may also be precipitants. Dissociative states may be brought on by the sudden emergence into consciousness of primitive destructive impulses. Such states sometimes occur after patients have committed violent acts and may present difficulties during the legal assessment of responsibility.

In the diagnosis of hysterical neurosis, a history of previous episodes is helpful. The patient with hysterical pain often will not show the characteristic facial expressions and bodily tensions of patients with organic pain. Response to placebo is of little use diagnostically, since most patients with organic pain will experience some relief following the injection of normal saline solution.

Hypochondriacal neurosis Hypochondriasis, the morbid preoccupation with bodily processes or physical symptoms, is a common expression of emotional distress. It appears in various forms throughout the range of psychiatric disorders. In neurosis, hypochondriasis does not have the bizarre, fixed delusional aspects that it may show in psychotic depressions and schizophrenia. Unlike the hypochondriacal personality, in which concern for health and relationships with physicians are involved in chronic patterns of adaptation, the hypochondriacal neurosis is a decompensation from a healthier, more mature level of adjustment. Unlike hysterical neuroses and psychophysiologic disorders, in which there also may be morbid preoccupations with physical processes, this neurosis entails no disorder of bodily function.

The patient usually has a preexisting tendency to focus his worries on his body. Often there is a family atmosphere of overconcern about health. As a child he may have received special care when he was sick. The common misconception that bad behavior leads to sickness may have made illness an expression of his guilt. His symptoms express both his anxiety and an element of self-punishment and may lead to a retreat to a less mature state in which protection and care are available. The doctors and nurses become involved in his struggle with anxiety. This may be a replay of earlier scenes with his parents, when he tried to excite their fears in order to relieve his own tensions. The insatiable need for reassurance is often an expression of hostility toward the people who are unable to quiet his real inner fears.

The physician and nurse may be drawn into this old pattern, making the management of hypochondriasis very difficult in a medical situation. The anxieties of the hypochondriacal patient may drive the physician to carry out unnecessary procedures. The minor elements of doubt that realistically accompany all medical findings will only inflame the patient's anxieties. Once the physician is satisfied that no physical disorder is present, the patient should be told that his problem is a neurosis, a real and painful entity that requires further medical assistance. Through this approach, the patient will be spared the termination of his relationship with physicians, an important element of support for him during his neurotic episode. The simple announcement that he is in perfect health will only stimulate his anxiety and will lead him into new hypochondriacal preoccupations. Hypochondriasis in adults often represents an aspect of depression (see Chap. 341) and responds to appropriate treatment.

Obsessive-compulsive neurosis Minor variations of this neurosis are extremely common, and the full-blown picture described here is relatively rare, but when it occurs, it constitutes one of the most painful and incapacitating of the neurotic syndromes. Predisposed individuals are often meticulous, perfectionistic, rigid, insecure people who lack spontaneity and who are intolerant of their own anger. Uncontrollable thoughts (obsessions) and acts (compulsions) that seem irrational to the patient are characteristic. The patient may feel forced to knock on wood, wash his hands, check the electric outlets or gas jets. He may have to whisper nonsense phrases or magic formulas. Words that are repugnant to him may pop into his mind. Sequences of ideas, scenarios of perverse behavior or violent acts, or ruminations of revenge may dominate his thoughts. Prayers, promises, resolutions, and denials may also be present. These acts may seem childish or unnecessary and the thoughts repulsive, irrelevant or out of character, but they are driven by a sense of urgency, and if they are inhibited there will be increasing anxiety approaching panic. These symptoms are often accompanied by doubting, vacillation, and indecision. The doubts may reach a frenzy when the deadline for an important decision approaches. Depression is frequently present, and the patient often feels a pervasive sense of guilt or shame. Insomnia, restlessness, and fatigue result from the tension state that invariably accompanies this disorder. These patients present special management problems during illness. If possible, one physician should provide all the medical information and instructions, keeping them clear and unambiguous. Patients with this disorder are very sensitive to ambiguities of meaning. When a medical regimen that can be turned into a ritual needs to be instituted, patients should be told when to stop as well as when to begin. A patient who was once advised to drink plenty of water was found years later to be drinking 16 glasses of water every morning. These patients may ask innumerable questions and may insist on repeated reassurances. This state of mind is best handled by a firm statement that the doctor is in charge of the situation and that everything is under control. Guilt is especially prominent in this neurosis, and patients may conceal their symptoms and maintain an image of health even while they are suffering severely.

Phobic neurosis The patient with a phobic neurosis has an intense, irrational fear or aversion for an object or situation. He can recognize that he has little realistic basis for his feelings but cannot master his reactions. His fear mounts as he approaches the focus of his phobia and reaches panic proportions if he is confronted directly by the object or situation. Mild phobias, such as fears of animals or of darkness, are often seen in childhood and many minor phobias may be part of everyday life, some of them accepted culturally, such as fears of mice or snakes. In phobic neurosis the patient may be severely incapacitated and may have feelings of helplessness, pessimism, despondency, and low self-esteem. Often the neurosis has obsessive-compulsive symptoms as well. Hypochondriasis may occur and in itself has many of the features of a phobia.

The most widely accepted explanation of phobias is that anxiety has been displaced from an internal source to the external focus of the phobia. The anxiety can then be controlled by avoidance mechanisms and by inhibitions. The focus of the phobia itself often symbolizes the inner fear or has been associated historically with it. The functional disturbance resulting from a phobia may be so severe that the patient appears to be in a withdrawn, psychotic state, although reality testing has been preserved. A patient may be unable to leave the house, unable to eat a variety of foods, engage in sexual relations, ride in elevators or streetcars, eat in public, enter a crowd, or ride in an automobile. At times the patient is able to face the phobia with a companion when he cannot face it alone. For example, the patient may be unable to travel to work or even leave the house without being accompanied by a relative. Often confronting the phobic object or situation is the equivalent of facing a forbidden thought or impulse. A fear of being trapped is common. This often is tied to the fear of loss of control.

Phobias also develop in anxiety neurosis, hysterical neurosis, and obsessive-compulsive neurosis, and at times phobic states occur in schizophrenia. Severe phobic neurosis generally occurs in immature and inhibited people who have long histories of minor phobias and come from anxious families. These patients are often disabled and require long-term treatment. Milder phobias, especially those that are long-standing and not attached to major fears, may respond to deconditioning techniques or suggestion. Tranquilizers can help the patient to face phobic situations and learn that his fears are not justified.

Depressive neurosis Here there is excessive reaction of depression when conflict occurs, especially loss, with a ready-made attitude of self-criticism, self-depreciation, brooding, and helplessness. This is often based on a character tendency. The reactions are characterized by loss of self-esteem, inhibition of aggressive impulses, distancing from others. Instead of feeling forbidden impulses, especially aggressive impulses, a depressive reaction arises, a defense which immobilizes and punishes. Guilt over forbidden impulses is also expressed. Hence the guilt appears to be far out of proportion to the minor self-depreciating content. Often hostility itself is expressed in the depressed state because subtly it makes the other person feel helpless, unable to please, and rejected. The range of depressive disorders will be dealt with in Chap. 341. The concept of depressive neurosis shows not only that depression may be a neurotic disorder in terms of a continuum but that depression is a defense against or an alternative to anxiety.

Neurasthenic neurosis Weakness, fatigability, exhaustion without secondary gain characterize this disorder. There are often depression and feelings of low self-esteem. The disturbance often has a chronic character. It was previously called psychophysiologic nervous system reaction. It is often seen in late adolescence and may be a persistent syndrome, more approaching a character type than a neurotic reaction. The state itself may also be seen following an acute psychotic episode and has certain mild equivalents in patients who have successful adaptive mechanisms but who at times may avoid conflict by this bland, weakened, apparently helpless state. Physicians may be called upon to do diagnostic evaluations on patients with neurasthenic states. Often the family is the motivating force in such an evaluation. Retreat from hostile impulses may be a factor in the syndrome.

Depersonalization neurosis In this neurosis, feelings of unreality, with estrangement from self, body, and surroundings, are the dominant symptoms. It is relatively rare as a circumscribed entity. Such feelings may arise in a minor form in everyday life. They also may occur as an aspect of a psychotic state and often are associated with the early stages of a schizophrenic reaction. This neurosis is similar to the dissociated states seen, in hysterical neurosis and should be distinguished from acute situational reactions, which are brief and have less serious implications. Symptoms resemble some neurologic states involving temporal and parietal lobes.

TREATMENT Compared with other mental disorders, the overall prognosis in the neuroses is good because the population involved is relatively healthy and neuroses are characteristically self-limited. The presence of stable interpersonal relationships, satisfying work, capacities for introspection and for the expression of emotions, and a motivation to return to health are all highly favorable signs. Insidious onset, compelling secondary gain, and the paucity of interpersonal relationships are unfavorable signs. The influence of age on prognosis has been overemphasized. Elderly patients with neuroses are often as responsive to treatment as their younger counterparts. Because they are self-limited, most neuroses can be managed by the physician without psychiatric referral. In the rare instances of severe disability or suicide risk, hospitalization may be indicated.

Psychotherapy is an effective approach. During acute episodes the active investigation of the source of anxiety often leads to relief of symptoms. An understanding of the influence of unsettled issues from the past may give the patient the opportunity to develop more flexible and mature solutions to his conflicts. Long-term insight-oriented psychotherapy may be helpful in preventing recurrences.

The reduction of anxiety by pharmacologic agents is effective in the treatment of anxiety neurosis, phobic neurosis, neurasthenic neurosis, and some instances of hypochondriacal neurosis. These agents have not been as useful with obsessive-compulsive, hysterical, depressive, or depersonalization neuroses, or in the treatment of chronic anxiety states. Depressive and hysterical neuroses are often quite responsive to the placebo effect. The benzodiazepines are usually sufficient for the management of neurotic anxiety. In severe cases, the phenothiazines are helpful. It is wise to prescribe medications for a few days and then discontinue them if they are ineffective. If they achieve the reduction of anxiety, the patient may be instructed to take them as needed within dosage limits. In contrast to patients with personality disorders, most patients with neuroses are not likely to become habituated to medications and, given the option, will discontinue them when the target symptoms remit. However, if they are put on a medical regimen, they may continue to take medications long after the remission of symptoms, and habituation may develop. Chronic maintenance on benzodiazepines should be avoided. Withdrawal symptoms, including seizures, may occur after prolonged use.

Behavior modification has been effective in the treatment of monosymptomatic neuroses, especially the phobias. Group therapy has no special application in the neuroses, except in helping patients develop more skills in socialization.

THE PERSONALITY DISORDERS The patient with a personality disorder shows immaturity on a chronic basis, not as a retreat from a healthier adjustment. Intrapsychic

TABLE 339-2
Personality disorders

Type of personality disorder	Characteristics
1 Paranoid	Chronic wariness, suspiciousness, litigiousness; lack of insight or humor; tendency to blame others; sense of self-importance and entitlement
2 Cyclothymic	Recurring periods of depression and elation not readily explained by circumstances; severe moodiness
3 Schizoid	Isolation, seclusiveness, secretiveness; discomfort in relationships; often eccentric and lacking in energy; few friends
4 Explosive	Outbursts of rage and aggression not in keeping with usual personality, often in response to minor provocation; sense of loss of control followed by regret
5 Obsessive-compulsive	Chronic worries about standards; excessive concern about self-image; tension in relationships, leading to isolation; inability to relax and excessive inhibitions; predisposition to depression
6 Hysterical	Immaturity, histrionic behavior, sexualization of relationships, low frustration tolerance, and shallow interpersonal ties; dependency
7 Asthenic	Chronic weakness, easy fatigability, sense of vulnerability, poor response to stress, little ambition or aggression
8 Passive, aggressive	Obstructive behavior, stubbornness, intentional errors or omissions; intolerance of authority with struggles over control often creating difficulties in medical settings; externalization of conflicts and blaming others for untoward events
9 Inadequate	Chronic inability to meet ordinary life demands in the absence of mental retardation; severe dependency on others; tendency to become institutionalized or to become dependent on institutions
10 Antisocial	Unsocialized or antisocial behavior in conflict with society; selfishness, callousness, impulsiveness, lack of loyalty, and little guilt; frustration tolerance is low; tendency to blame others and have a long history of interpersonal and social difficulties and arrests

conflict is not a significant factor. The patient feels his distress in terms of his relationship with the world around him. The history will show chronic lifelong patterns of maladaptation with episodes of more serious disturbance, usually during periods of stress. The distinction between personality disorders and the neuroses is important because of the marked differences in prognosis and response to treatment. A list of these disorders and their major characteristics is given in Table 339-2.

Patients with these disorders often are distressed in the manner of a fretful child when frustrated, angry, and dissatisfied. They often have a deep sense of longing and loneliness, although they lack the skills to satisfy their dependency needs in socially acceptable ways. They may use physicians and medical institutions in an effort to make up for the emptiness in their lives. However, their low tolerance for discomfort, lack of objectivity, and inability to accept limits create many difficulties in the doctor-patient relationship. In every arena in their lives they tend to re-create their childlike versions of human relationships.

The etiology of these disorders is not well understood. A failure or distortion in the process of growth of the personality has taken place, perhaps related to constitutional factors and perhaps to emotional deprivation in early childhood. The evidence from studies of emotionally deprived children suggests that severe trauma and deprivation may lead to premature self-sufficiency with closure of development at an immature level. The concept of developmental arrest can be applied to the various personality disorders. For example, the inadequate personality shows global defects in its capacities to meet the day-to-day demands of life, the explosive personality has a defect in the control of anger, and the hysterical personality has generalized immaturity with poor impulse control.

The treatment of the personality disorders requires patience and flexibility. Often the actual relationship with a physician over many years may be a stabilizing influence and may gradually lead to growth. The use of tranquilizers should be avoided because of the problem of abuse of medications. Unless the patient seeks treatment for himself because of inner distress he is not likely to benefit from psychotherapy. Often patients with personality disorders are coerced into psychiatric consultation. This seldom leads to effective therapy. At times such patients may seek medical assistance to give them relief from the pressures of the world, especially from their families or from law-enforcement agencies.

By understanding these disorders, the physician can do a lot to help prevent the patient from sabotaging needed medical care. During hospitalization, firm limits often bring relief to the patient and to the staff. The physician's skill as the leader of the therapeutic team and as a student of human nature will help him in the care of these difficult and sometimes exasperating patients.

REFERENCES

English OS, Pearson G: *Emotional Problems of Living*, New York: Norton, 1945

Fenichel O: *The Psychoanalytic Theory of Neurosis*, New York: Norton, 1945

Freedman AM, Kaplan HI: *Comprehensive Textbook of Psychiatry*, Baltimore: Williams & Wilkins, 1967

Kolb LC: *Noyes' Modern Clinical Psychiatry*, 7th ed., Philadelphia: Saunders, 1968

Mayer-Gross W et al: *Clinical Psychiatry*, 3d ed., London: Baillière, 1967

Zinberg NE (ed): *Psychiatry and Medical Practice in a General Hospital*, New York: International Universities Press, Inc., 1964

340 ANTISOCIAL PERSONALITY (SOCIOPATHY)

ELI ROBINS

Antisocial personality was formerly called psychopathy or constitutional psychopathy or sociopathy (see Table 339-2). The sociopathic state comes to medical attention under three sets of circumstances: (1) when signs and symptoms develop that are suggestive of medical or some other psychiatric illness; (2) when the patient, usually an adult, is referred by social agencies, various "counselors," or the police for medical or psychiatric opinion; and (3) when an adolescent is referred by police or social agencies or is brought by a parent because of incorrigible behavior. Generally, referral to physicians is from an institutional setting—school, military service, jail—since such patients tend to do poorly and stand out strikingly in situations where they are required to adjust to other individuals.

Clinical description Sociopathy begins early in life, virtually always before age fifteen; in more than one-half the patients the onset is before age ten, and sometimes by age five or six. Diagnosis before the age of twenty-one is difficult because there has been too little time for the full pattern of antisocial behavior to emerge. The occasional turmoils and antisocial outbreaks of childhood and adolescence may represent only transient behavioral disorders in youths who turn out to be stable, productive adults.

There is no pathognomonic or specifically diagnostic symptom or sign of sociopathy in adolescents and adults. Instead, it is the total pattern of social adjustment that provides clues to the nature of the illness. This is revealed by the following troubles in life activities: poor work history, unstable family relationships, disturbed marital history, prolonged financial dependency, difficulties with the law, excessive use of alcohol, school problems, impulsive behavior, aberrant sexual behavior, wild adolescence, vagrancy, belligerency, social isolation, difficulties with the military, use of aliases, pathologic lying, use of drugs, and suicide attempts. If there are abnormalities in at least five of the above areas of adjustment the diagnosis of sociopathy is reasonably secure. Actually the frequencies of such abnormalities in a large group of sociopaths varies from 85 percent with a poor work history to 11 percent who have attempted suicide before age forty-five. There are difficulties in the majority of the above life areas in over 50 percent of patients.

These antisocial symptoms are not merely the expression of a neurosis (Chap. 339). Nevertheless, somatic complaints do occur, and many of the symptoms (e.g., nervousness, back pain, headache, death wishes, nausea, dizzy spells, dyspnea, palpitation, insomnia, excessive sensitivity, fatigue, anxiety attacks, vomiting, weight loss, chronic unhappiness, weakness, sexual diffidence, blurred vision, anxiety in crowds, fainting spells, anorexia, lump in throat, inability to work, paranoid ideas, obsessions and blindness, paralysis, astasia-abasia, trances, amnesia, and obsessive thoughts) are the same as those of the neuroses. Furthermore, all are more frequent than in the general population (47 to 7 percent of the patients), according to one statistical analysis.

This mixture of antisocial and neurotic symptoms brings these patients to the physician with a wide variety of clinical problems. Clues to the nature of the patient's difficulty are obtained by learning during the elicitation of the history that the patient is unstable and has exhibited impulsive job quitting, abandoned his family, engaged in thievery, has taken excess alcohol, engaged in serious fights, and has amnesia for parts of his own history. The medical problem may be quite dramatic, such as difficulty in walking, apparent but unexplained bleeding from different body orifices, unexplained fever that disappears when the patient is closely supervised while his temperature is being taken, uncontrollable temper outbursts, and suicidal attempts.

At the time of examination the patient may be cheerful, charming, and lively, or morose, sullen, and irritable. Historically, large segments of his life appear to have been forgotten or are ignored. He seems to lack the ability to judge the implications of his behavior, to profit from past mistakes, and to adhere to any moral or ethical standard. There is no sense of guilt. Some psychiatrists have referred to this state as "moral imbecility." When caught in the act of putting blood from his finger into his urine or rubbing the thermometer against the bed sheet to cause an apparent fever, the patient may be ostensibly bewildered or uninterested and leaves the hospital saying he is sorry the doctors did not believe him.

Childhood manifestations The child who will become an adult sociopath already betrays the trends that will characterize his entire life. Usually he manifests antisocial symptoms in many areas of his life before the age of fifteen. By then he has indulged in theft, is an incorrigible truant, runs away from home overnight, has "bad" associates, fights, is impulsive, reckless, and irresponsible, appears slovenly, lies pathologically, indulges in indiscriminate premarital sexual relations as well as (generally brief) homosexual activities, and is frequently held back in school. The study of a group of sociopaths has shown that on an average they have exhibited at least seven such antisocial symptoms and four nonantisocial (nervous) symptoms during childhood.

Cause and pathogenesis The cause or causes of antisocial personality are unknown, but there are interesting leads. In a study conducted by the author it was found that when the number of antisocial symptoms in childhood is zero, the number of such children developing adult sociopathy is zero; when the number of childhood antisocial symptoms is 1 or 2, the proportion developing adult sociopathy is 4 percent, if the number is 3 to 5, adult sociopathy is 15 percent, etc. In the most disturbed childhood group, with 10 or more antisocial symptoms, 43 percent of the adults will exhibit sociopathy. This suggests that the stronger the trend to abnormal behavior, from either habit or other cause, the more likely it is to continue. Of course, the fact that the child who shows many of the antisocial symptoms is more apt to turn out badly in adult years may only be another way of saying that the worst illnesses are manifest at a younger age. It is noteworthy that even of the most disturbed children less than half will develop adult sociopathy. Sociopathy tends to run in families, but the reason for this is not known. A specific type of inheritance has not been established. Male predominance stands as an unassailable fact. Having an antisocial or alcoholic father only raises the liability to adult sociopathy from 43 to 50 percent. An antisocial or alcoholic father appeared actually to have a more deleterious effect on the less disturbed child. A total lack of parental discipline favors slightly the development of sociopathy. Social standing of the family seems not to matter; hence one cannot explain sociopathy simply on the basis of an unstable home environment, lack of discipline, etc. Left open is the possibility, however, that during early life when each person develops a moral code the environment offered insufficient sources of love, security, and guidance.

From time to time over the years it has been claimed that the psychopath or sociopath has an abnormal brain. Sociopathy occurred in a considerable number of children who had had encephalitis lethargica after World War I. The incidence of abnormal electroencephalograms is said to be increased in this group of patients. Close study of the available data, making allowance for imprecision of diagnosis, does not support these statements, but the matter is still far from settled.

Antisocial behavior that expresses itself in violence, sometimes resulting even in homicide, is one of the most extreme forms of sociopathy. Although in exceptional instances episodic violence may be a manifestation of psychomotor epilepsy, the majority of habitual culprits are psychopaths. Two-thirds of patients who stand apart because of violent temper, overt aggressiveness, and repeated criminal actions are found to have electroencephalographic abnormalities. The abnormality in the encephalogram is usually bilateral and predominantly in the anterior temporal regions. There are approximately 15 to 20 reported examples of episodic violence in which tumors or other lesions in these parts of the brain were found at autopsy. Such data lend credence to the proposition that subnormal development or disease of the amygdaloid nuclei and related parts of the limbic system interfere with the control of impulse and emotionality, and that some forms of sociopathy might have a neuropathologic basis.

Diagnosis The key to diagnosis is a fully documented history of frequent, repetitive, multiple antisocial acts going back to childhood. The outstanding diagnostic characteristics are (1) the invariability of early age of onset, before age fifteen; (2) the frequency, variety, and intensity of antisocial behavior; (3) the repetitiveness and chronicity of the antisocial acts without even temporary periods of remission; (4) the large number of life areas deranged by the illness; (5) the display by the patient of callousness, egocentricity, lack of deep attachments, lack of loyalty, poor judgment, impulsivity, and seeming inability to profit by experience. The frequency of the latter qualities, which are the marks of the antisocial personality, has never been ascertained. That sociopathy is five to ten times more frequent among men than women is of some help in differential diagnosis.

Sociopathy may be distinguished from chronic alcoholism. It is true that nonsociopathic alcoholics behave in many ways like sociopaths, once they become addicted, but they lack the other elements of sociopathic behavior. A special problem arises when sociopathy and alcoholism are combined (75 percent of sociopaths drink excessively). A careful history will show that in the sociopath, in contrast to the alcoholic, the antisocial behavior was manifest long before the person turned to drink or drugs. Other illnesses that must be separated from sociopathy are hysteria, mania, and schizophrenia, but this can usually be done by a detailed history and examination. Behavioral disorders in an epileptic with psychomotor seizures may at times be confused with sociopathy. Indeed, a rather impressive number of sociopaths have electroencephalographic abnormalities, and there is said to be a higher incidence of seizures among them than in the normal population. Nevertheless, frank convulsions are rarely observed, which is helpful in differential diagnosis. Chromosomal abnormalities are found in only a few of all sexual offenders (XYY karyotype).

Treatment There is no known way of modifying the personality defect that underlies sociopathy. Unsupported claims have been made to the contrary, but at best they show only that an occasional juvenile delinquent (not a true sociopath) has responded to psychologic guidance, psychotherapy, or a pharmacologic agent. It is important to try to help the family and to aid the patient in attaining more limited goals. If the electroencephalogram is abnormal, a trial on Dilantin Sodium is sometimes helpful in stabilizing the patient's behavior, even when frank seizures have not been observed. Early recognition of the syndrome may enable the family to avoid embarrassment and the spending of large sums of money on useless psychiatric therapy.

Prognosis There appears to be some amelioration of the condition with age. Antisocial behavior tends to diminish between the ages of twenty-five and fifty, although less than half the patients are able to achieve a more or less stable adjustment afterwards. It is the grosser elements that subside; those patients whose disorder is in remission tend to remain irascible and relatively asocial, and to show less flagrant aberrations. Those who improve or seem to recover seldom attribute their improvement to physicians, counselors, or other professionals. Marriage, children, fear of further incarceration, maturity, or "I don't know why" are the reasons usually given for remission.

Public health considerations Sociopathy tends to be ignored by psychiatrists and other physicians, perhaps because of the mistaken belief that it is not "really" an illness at all but a gross social maladjustment induced by a miserable environment, such as is often found in the lowest socioeconomic stratum of urban society. A large segment of offenders arraigned in civil courts is made up of sociopaths. Of the 600,000 felons in state and federal prisons or on parole, 80 percent suffer from sociopathy. The costs of incarceration and parole supervision of these 480,000 sociopaths is incalculable. Although the number of patients in hospitals with other psychiatric illnesses is greater, the expense of the sociopath in terms of costs and crimes and human misery may be far more important. The necessity for preventing and rectifying this condition is apparent.

Malingering The question of malingering comes up frequently in relation to the actions of persons diagnosed as antisocial personalities. Such patients feign illness, lie, claim compensation for unreal illness, etc. Malingering is difficult to prove, and, even worse, the allegation of it requires the adoption of an unprofessional attitude toward a patient. Certainly malingering is more common in sociopathy than in any other single illness and is particularly frequent when such a patient stands to gain money or avoid military service or legal prosecution. The symptoms of hysteria may also lead to a suspicion of malingering, which is sometimes verified. The distinction that in hysteria the motivation is not conscious is also an assumption difficult to prove, especially in compensation neurosis. When pushed to extremes by adversity, most persons may prevaricate. Drug addicts who desire to obtain opiates may be expected to falsify their symptoms, especially when abstinence begins to bring on painful symptoms.

The sociopathic malingerer tends to avoid exhaustive examination and does not give a clear-cut history. These two characteristics help in at least suspecting malingering. It is well to remember that whatever its basis, malingering signifies mental illness. Once evidence of malingering has been observed, the physician does well to confront the patient with the facts in a simple direct fashion without sign of contempt or loss of temper, and to indicate a willingness to help him, if he so desires.

SEXUAL DEVIATION Of the seven forms of sexual deviations listed in the Official Classification of Psychiatric Disorder *only three will be discussed*: homosexuality, pedophilia, and exhibitionism. The others (fetishism, transvestitism, voyeurism, sadism, and masochism) are rare, and little reliable information has been obtained about them. Since the physician's counsel is often sought on matters of abnormal sexual behavior, he should know something of the normal development of sexuality. The work of Kinsey et al. is a most valuable reference.

Homosexuality This condition is defined as a state in which a person admits to being a homosexual or in which there is repetitive homosexual behavior (leading to orgasm) after age eighteen. Its frequency is difficult to ascertain. Kinsey suggests that in the United States approximately 4 percent of men and 1 to 2 percent of women are homosexuals. These data refer to overt homosexuality, not to the so-called latent form, which is more frequent but diagnosed often only by inference. Female homosexual behavior and fantasies have a somewhat later onset than those of the male. Whereas 86 percent of the males had already indulged in homosexual practices before age fifteen, only about one-fourth of the females have done so. Males tend to have their first sexual experience with an adult of the same sex prior to the age of sixteen, and the female at a later time. Members of neither sex attribute their sexual aberration to such experiences in early life.

The predominant homosexual practices among men and women naturally differ; in the younger male it is usually mutual masturbation, or manual-genital contact, and later (after age twenty) oral-genital contact (fellatio) and anal intercourse. In both younger and older women manual-genital stimulation (masturbation) is more frequent than oral-genital contact. The homosexual partnership is less stable for men than for women; more than 80 percent of women remain faithful to one partner, while only 20 percent of men do so.

At present it cannot be decided whether homosexuality is an illness, "a way of life," or an elaborate habit pattern. Surprisingly, other sexual deviations among homosexuals are rare to nonexistent. Initially mental illness proves to be no more common than in heterosexuals. But homosexuality does lead to psychologic problems, and these occur more frequently in women than in men. By the age of thirty to thirty-five, 7 percent of the homosexual men have made a nonserious suicide attempt, whereas 12 percent of the women have done so.

Alcoholism or alcohol abuse is as common among the women as among the men, which is unusual, since ordinarily there is a male predominance for this condition.

Medical studies, such as measurements of gonadotropins, ketosteroids, and other hormones, have revealed no consistent abnormalities. The chromosomal karyotype and results of nuclear typing for Barr bodies are normal. Early-life patterning of the nervous system is a currently favored hypothesis.

More homosexual women seek medical aid than men (37 percent versus 26 percent), usually in order to change sexual orientation or because of a reactive mood disorder or excessive alcohol intake. However, only 5 percent obtained sufficient help to continue therapy for a prolonged period, and their goal then was not to change their sexual orientation but to rid themselves of some other problem. There is no known specific treatment for homosexuality. Psychotherapy usually fails, and hormonal treatment and pharmacologic agents are of value only for reactive psychologic symptoms.

Pedophilia Pedophilia (literal meaning, "love of children") is among the three or four most common sexual deviations. The term refers to sexual advances made by adults and adolescents to prepubertal children. In heterosexual pedophilia the child is almost always between six and twelve years of age, whereas in homosexual pedophilia the limits of the definition are somewhat less clear, since the number of victims increases into puberty, resulting in some overlap with adult homosexuality. Whether homosexual pedophilia is a consistent entity is uncertain. Heterosexual acts rarely involve intercourse, but consist instead of fondling, sex play, looking, or showing. Homosexual acts are similar to those that occur between adult homosexuals, except that anal and intercrural intercourse are even less frequent than between adults. The offenders fall into three age groups: puberty, mid-to-late thirties, and mid-to-late fifties. Studies show that almost all girl "victims" age fourteen and over indulge in mutual-consent coitus, and the act can hardly be classified as pedophilic. The victim, contrary to widely held beliefs, is seldom a stranger to the offender. The most common relationships are family members, friends, neighbors, and youth club associates. Heterosexual acts ordinarily take place in the home of the offender or victim. Orgasm is rarely sought in heterosexual acts but is achieved in about one-half of homosexual acts.

Violence and force are fortunately infrequent in pedophilic acts. Murder is rare, usually unplanned, and results from panic or violent passion. The main effects on the victim are usually minimal, and only in one-sixth (or less) of the cases is there said to be any long-term psychologic ill effect. The offenders usually have a normal intelligence, but a few are mentally defective.

These findings and the data indicating that violence is rare, should lay to rest a number of myths about pedophilia. Pedophiles come from all occupational and social groups. More often than not their home was broken during childhood, but not more so than in patients with other psychiatric illnesses. Repetition of pedophilic acts approximates 10 percent for first offenders but rapidly rises in those offenders with records of previous sexual offenses. Pedophilia manifests itself as a pathologic impulse but is not part of an ordinary obsessive-compulsive neurosis. Psychoses are almost nonexistent.

Treatment of pedophilia is still a subject for debate. Individual therapy, psychoanalytic therapy, group therapy, castration, have each given results that show no striking superiority. In fact it is questionable whether they have any effect at all.

Exhibitionism This deviation is common. It is a relatively innocuous practice, and the offenders are only fined or arrested for a misdemeanor. Coitus and sexual assault are not part of the act. Essentially it consists of a showing of male genitalia to females, usually to strangers and often to more than one female simultaneously. The impulsive nature of the act has been noted by most investigators. The apparent responses desired by the offender are fright, laughter and amusement, and indignation. Two-thirds of exhibitionists are in their twenties, some are in their teens, and a few somewhat older than thirty. Little is known of the genesis of the personality disorder that leads to this sexual deviation. About one-third of all sexual offenses reaching public notice are for exhibitionism. About 3 percent to 15 percent of exhibitionists suffer from a psychosis; the exhibitionism may then be considered symptomatic, not a primary diagnosis. Sociopathy is rarely a concomitant diagnosis.

Psychiatric treatment of exhibitionism has involved individual or group therapy. The results are uncertain. Treatment appears not to have affected the rate of recidivism. Voyeurism (compulsive looking at the genitals of the opposite sex or at individuals copulating) is assumed to be the one deviation most closely related to exhibitionism, but the evidence even on this point is anything but convincing.

ALCOHOLISM This condition may be said to occur when a patient drinks sufficiently to impair his health or his social or personal functioning, or when alcohol becomes a prerequisite for apparently normal functioning. The illness begins in the late teens or early twenties in over 90 percent of patients, and the risk of alcoholism is over by the age of forty. The condition tends to be familial, especially in the males of the family. One form of it (episodic drinking) bears a relationship to manic-depressive illness, and both the chronic and episodic forms bear some relation to sociopathy, but the details have not been fully explored. Studies of half-siblings suggest a genetic element in its causation.

A diagnosis of "definite" alcoholism may be made in the event of (1) any manifestation of alcohol withdrawal, such as tremulousness, convulsions, hallucinations, or delirium; (2) a history of medical complications, e.g., cirrhosis, gastritis, myopathy, pancreatitis, polyneuropathy, Wernicke-Korsakoff's syndrome; (3) alcoholic blackouts, i.e., amnesic episodes during heavy drinking not accounted for by head trauma; (4) alcoholic binges or benders lasting 48 hr or more and associated with default of ordinary obligations. Less certain evidence is provided by the circumstance of a patient not being able to stop drinking when he wants to do so or being forced to curtail drinking, being arrested for drinking, having traffic difficulties, fights, or trouble at work because of drinking.

The sex ratio of alcoholism in several studies varies from 2:1 to 6:1 (men to women). Women show the more blatant symptoms about 10 years later than men. Complications of alcoholism, excluding the strictly medical complications, include death by accident, suicide, homicide, divorce, severe friction in the family, belligerence, and wife beating. These various complications, even apart from the medical ones, reduce the life span.

There is no certainty that any one mode of therapy has proved beneficial. Certainly an understanding physician can help a compliant patient, but few are willing to accept help. Unfortunately, there are no long-term studies documenting the value of any one method of therapy, such as the use of drugs (Disulfiram), psychotherapy, deconditioning techniques, Alcoholics Anonymous, and industrial programs (see Chap. 111).

OPIATE ADDICTION The statement "once an addict, always an addict" is relatively true. The relapse rate once opium (heroin or morphine) addiction is established is high, and there is no doubt that it constitutes a serious chronic illness. About 90 percent of addicts who have once reached the Federal Addiction Center in Lexington resume usage of the drug once they are discharged; only 10 percent seem to remain drug-free for the period of a decade. Though addiction is more frequent among individuals from the lower socioeconomic class and "ghettos," nonetheless it occurs among the middle class and also among medical and paramedical personnel. Long-term studies of opiate addiction show that about 30 percent are functioning effectively 5 to 10 years later, despite relapses and imprisonments.

The factors that are conducive to narcotic addiction are difficult to define. The majority of present-day addicts come from depressed districts in metropolitan slum areas. Economic privation and availability of illicit drugs, laxity of social controls, unstable family relationships, and prevalence of psychopathic attitudes are characteristics of this segment of society. The use of drugs often represents a retreat from a hopeless environment. On the Minnesota Multiphasic Personality Inventory (MMPI) the opiate addicts show psychopathic deviation and hypomanic reactions. Contrary to popular belief, overtreatment of painful illness is an infrequent cause of addiction.

The most effective treatment appears to be confinement in an addiction center for more than 9 months, followed by supervised parole in the community. Attempts to break the drug habit in a general hospital nearly always fail. Currently the use of methadone is being widely advocated. It consists of replacing the usual opiate with this longer-acting, less disturbing, addicting drug. Striking social benefits have been reported, but methadone treatment is only a way station until a better method is found. Apart from its own addicting properties, the methadone treatment requires careful supervision, for there is the possibility of complications and misuse of the drug. It is still probably best handled by specialized clinics or physicians who have had much experience with it.

The link between drug addiction and criminality is difficult to assess. Unquestionably addiction promotes crime, but one cannot estimate the number and types of crime this same group might have committed had they not become addicted.

The synthetic analgesics with morphine-like properties generally possess the same addicting properties and lead to the same tolerance and withdrawal phenomena as heroin. The leading example is Demerol.

It should be noted that the effects of dependence on short-acting barbiturates and other sedatives and hypnotics differ from those of opium dependence. After barbiturates are taken daily in a dose large enough to cause direct physiologic effects, withdrawal results in hallucinations, delirium, disorientation, hyperpyrexia, convulsions, and rarely death. To avoid these effects, withdrawal should be slow, beginning with reduction of the habitual dosage by not more than 10 percent per day. Fortunately, there is enough cross reaction among the barbiturates so that either secobarbital or pentobarbital may be given to prevent withdrawal symptoms.

Dependence on marijuana is not a true physical dependence. Psychologic dependence and habituation may occur to the extent that numbers of "reefers" are smoked daily. When a large amount of marijuana is used instead of single exposures for simple pleasure and sedation, hallucinations, overactivity, and certain other unpleasant psychic experiences may occur. At high dosages over a period of a year or more marijuana is said to cause intellectual deterioration and finally atrophy of the cerebrum, but this has not been reliably documented.

There are a number of other drugs loosely called hallucinogens (LSD, dimethyltryptamine, DOM, and mescaline), each of which is capable of inducing visual distortions, hallucinations, "feeling of being at one with the world," and in general of giving a "good trip." But "bad trips" also occur, even among persons who previously have had good ones. The patient has frightening hallucinations and distortions of his thought processes and becomes panicky. Ordinarily he can be "talked down" or "out" of a "bad trip," but sometimes medications such as chlorpromazine, Valium, or secobarbital become necessary to control him. Persons having a "bad trip" should not be left alone even if treated with medication, at least until the medication has had time to take effect.

The stimulants (e.g., amphetamines, metamphetamine, phenmetrazine, methylphenidate) are potentially much more serious in their effects than was once thought. In low dosages they reduce fatigue and impart a sense of euphoria, but by the time the dose reaches about 50 mg, especially if given intravenously, depression and irascibility are seen. With doses of from 120 to 700 mg, many patients become paranoid, have persecutory delusions and ideas of reference while retaining a relatively clear state of consciousness; they also show a lack of concentration, changes in motor activity, anxiety, fear, belligerence, and rarely disorientation, or thought disorganization. It is not certain whether some of these patients may have had a psychosis prior to taking the drug; however, a number of studies have shown that most of them recover when use of the drug is discontinued.

REFERENCES

JAFFE JH: Drug addiction and drug abuse, in *Pharmacological Basis of Therapeutics*, eds LS Goodman, A Gilman, New York: Macmillan, 1970, p. 276

ROBINS LN: *Deviant Children Grown Up*: A Sociological and Psychiatric Study of Sociopathic Personality. Baltimore: Williams & Wilkins, 1966

SAGHIR MT, ROBINS E: Homosexuality. I. Sexual behavior of the female homosexual. Arch Gen Psychiatry 20:192, 1969

—— et al: Homosexuality. II. Psychiatric disorders and disability in the male homosexual. Am J Psychiatry 126:1079, 1970

SCHNEIDER K: *Psychopathic Personalities*, Springfield, Ill.: Charles C Thomas, 1958

341 GRIEF, REACTIVE DEPRESSION, MANIC-DEPRESSIVE PSYCHOSIS, INVOLUTIONAL MELANCHOLIA, AND HYPOCHONDRIASIS

THOMAS P. HACKETT
RAYMOND D. ADAMS

Each term in the title of this chapter stands for a highly distinctive clinical state which will receive separate description in the following pages. Nevertheless, they bear close relationship to one another, which is the justification for considering them as a related group of diseases. Depression is the most important member of the group and, as pointed out in Chap. 14, is the most frequent of all major psychiatric illnesses, accounting for an estimated 50 percent of all psychiatric illnesses and 12 percent of all medical admissions to a hospital for diagnosis. Each year from 4 to 8 million Americans are treated for depression, of whom about 250,000 require hospitalization. A conservative calculation places the cost of depressive illness in this nation between $1.3 and $4 billion per annum.

Aside from the prevalence of depression, mania, and hypochondriasis, physicians should be well acquainted with these symptom complexes for several reasons. One of the paramount dangers is suicide, which may be attempted and successfully executed, often before the depressive symptoms have been recognized, i.e., while the patient is being treated for "low blood pressure," "nerves," "emotional problems," and "chronic infection," or even before he has sought medical care. Prompt diagnosis may therefore prevent a tragedy. Furthermore, the majority of depressive reactions can be successfully treated.

Because of their frequent occurrence in medical practice, the symptoms common to this entire group of illnesses were presented as constituting one of the cardinal manifestations of disease (see Chap. 14). The point was made in the introduction to the section on psychiatric diseases that the physician must assume the responsibility for recognizing the depressed state and distinguishing it from a number of other medical and psychiatric conditions.

Depression is a state of mind characterized by sadness. Normally it comes in response to a loss, but pathologic depressions may occur for a variety of reasons, the majority of which are not known. Depression is always accompanied by a variety of physical complaints, the most common of which are anorexia, insomnia, decreased energy, and diminished libido. At one extreme are depressions of psychotic proportions, such as manic-depressive reactions, which chaotically disrupt the individual's life and the lives of those who are close to him. At the other extreme are the normal disappointments of living, such as the failure to gain recognition, or the loss of a friend. No one can go through life without experiencing depression in some form. Feelings of sadness and discouragement are very much a part of living. The precise point at which the normal experience of depression becomes abnormal or pathologic can rarely be pinpointed. There are, however, diagnostic guidelines which should enable the practitioner to recognize these important medical conditions. The issue of recognition is significant; it is estimated that the nonpsychiatric physician overlooks or wrongly diagnoses 50 percent of the depressions he encounters in his patients. Next to recognition, the most critical consideration in this discussion is the separation of patients who can be treated successfully by the nonpsychiatric physician from those who require careful psychiatric handling.

CLASSIFICATION

There is no satisfactory classification of the depressive disorders. In this country the most commonly used nomenclature has been prepared by the American Psychiatric Association and can be found in the third edition of their *Diagnostic and Statistical Manual of Mental Disorders.* Because the nosology is both confusing and unnecessary for the nonpsychiatrist, it has been entirely omitted in this section. There are three main types of depression with which the physician should be acquainted, and he can become familiar with them without adverting to an elaborate classification. The first is the reactive depression. It is by far the most common and is typified by the grief reaction. Manic-depressive psychosis is the second type. It is included because it represents the standard model for a psychotic depression and because it is often used incorrectly as a diagnosis by nonpsychiatric physicians. The third, involutional melancholia, deserves recognition since it is frequently encountered in general practice and carries an excellent prognosis if given proper treatment.

REACTIVE DEPRESSION

GRIEF An important contemporary view of depression uses the grief reaction as a prototype. Grieving occurs in response to a loss. The loss may be real, as in the death of a spouse, or imagined, or even symbolic. The typical acute grief reaction comprises five characteristics:

1 An intense subjective sensation of mental pain accompanied by a feeling of exhaustion
2 Preoccupation with the image of the deceased
3 A sense of guilt concerning the relationship to the deceased
4 An inexplicable and unwarranted hostility toward friends and relatives
5 A loss of the usual pattern of conduct; bereaved individuals are unable either to initiate or to organize their daily affairs and tend to perform routine tasks in an automatic and uninterested fashion

The natural course of the normal grief reaction occupies a period of 4 to 12 weeks, by which time most of these five characteristics begin to abate, and within a few more months normal activities are resumed. Grieving thus defined is a natural human reaction to loss or to a personal tragedy, and its absence in circumstances where it is called for seldom bodes well.

There are many distortions of the normal reaction to distress or personal loss; they are referred to by psychiatrists as *pathologic grief.* The most frequent one is undue prolongation of the reaction, i.e., there is no sign of resolution by the end of a 3-month period. Under certain circumstances this may occur in the absence of psychopathology. For example, it is known that mothers who have lost young children tend to suffer for a long period of time, and the elderly who have lost a spouse of many years may never recover completely. Patients with a history of previous depressive episodes may also remain in mourning for longer periods. In general, when the bereaved or depressed patient has shown no improvement within 3 to 4 months of his loss, it would be wise to consider psychiatric consultation. Prolonged grief is a not unusual setting for suicide.

The second variation of the grief reaction is *delayed* or *postponed grief.* Often, in an attempt to sustain the morale of others or to avoid the unpleasant spectacle of mourning, the patient may show little or no reaction to the loss for weeks or months. This type of "stiff upper lip" control is frequently admired and consequently reinforced. The result is that grief remains unexpressed for long periods of time. The difficulty is that grief may eventually find expression, often unexpectedly and embarrassingly. Thus, an individual may go into a major depression following the death of someone he scarcely knew. Upon close examination it will be found that the more recent death excited a depression that should have transpired years before in response to the loss of a significant figure, but which for various reasons had been postponed.

In an effort to avoid distress and sadness, the bereaved person may become hyperactive and apparently imbued with a sense of well-being. This is a situation in which elation appears to be a defense against depression. It usually ends in a sudden reversal of mood, whereupon the individual plummets into a depressed state. In another variation of unacknowledged grief, the individual acts out a series of social or economic misadventures that are invariably detrimental. He may invest or gamble recklessly, turn away from old friends, or take up high-risk activities such as car racing or sky diving. Rarely does the person recognize the self-punitive nature of his activity or sense the guilt that lies behind it. Sometimes simply pointing this out helps such a patient.

Occasionally a patient will acquire the same symptoms as the deceased. He may believe he has developed a disease identical with that of the lost person. This may be the origin of the hypochondriasis which accompanies so many depressive reactions. As a means of identifying this variant in the grieving process, it is important in examining patients who have sustained a recent loss to inquire into the illness that took the life of the deceased.

The management of reactive depression in its normal form is sympathy, helping the bereaved person to acknowledge his loss and to face the changes required as a result of it. Stoicism should not be encouraged or reinforced. To express sadness through tears, anguish, and even hostility is advantageous in the end. The sooner the patient comes to grips with the loss, the more swiftly the painful process will reach closure. Undue restlessness and anxiety can be assuaged by minor tranquilizers, and insomnia by carefully prescribed hypnotics. Diazepam (Valium), 5 mg t.i.d., or the equivalent dose of chlordiazepoxide (Librium) or oxazepam (Serax) is suitable for daytime sedation and can be used at bedtime for sleep if the dose is doubled. None of the three drugs alone has been successfully used as a means of committing suicide, despite extremely high doses, for each has a wide margin of safety. The possibility of suicide must be entertained in handling all depressed patients, including mourners, and careful attention must be given to ensure that a lethal dose of hypnotics is not inadvertently supplied.

Pathologic grief reactions often require specialized psychiatric help. The wise general practitioner should turn to a psychiatric colleague to see if his plan of treatment is sound. The practice of some physicians of treating grief-stricken patients with antidepressants is seldom effective and attempts to suppress what is a natural and necessary human reaction.

OTHER FORMS OF REACTIVE DEPRESSION Depressed patients seldom, if ever, express feelings of sadness or despair without mentioning physical concomitants, such as the ease with which they tire, their loss of appetite, reduced interest in life and love, and trouble in falling asleep or in premature awakening; therefore, whenever these symptoms become manifest in the course of medical disease they should arouse suspicion of a depressive reaction. Chronic pain is a particularly frequent somatic complaint in depression. The pain may be vague in nature and will remain recalcitrant to most straightforward medical and surgical approaches. One should question such individuals about recent losses or changes in status, disappointments, or dissatisfactions. All patients with chronic pain syndromes should be evaluated psychiatrically, as pointed out in Chap. 5.

In a number of major medical illnesses depressive symptoms occur with such frequency as to constitute important diagnostic and therapeutic problems; and in certain chronic, occult diseases, symptoms such as lassitude and fatigue resemble those of a depressive reaction. For example, infectious mononucleosis, infectious hepatitis, carcinoma of the head of the pancreas, malnutrition, and frontal lobe tumors deplete energy and often simulate depression for several weeks or months before the diagnosis becomes evident. Drugs such as reserpine, or any of the *Rauwolfia* derivatives, and phenothiazines may also evoke a depressive reaction; and the steroids can induce a peculiar psychiatric state in which confusion, insomnia, and depression or elevation of mood are combined. Depression may emerge during the tapering-off period of steroid medication.

Of far more significance, however, are the depressions which occur in the wake of medical diseases. Often each emotional reaction, which the medical profession has tended to ignore, may dominate the symptoms of devastating diseases that threaten the life pattern and independence of the patient. Medical catastrophes such as heart disease, cancer, multiple sclerosis, Parkinson's disease, and cerebrovascular accidents are almost always followed by a reactive depression.

An example is the depression that comes after myocardial infarction. It begins usually toward the end of the patient's stay in the critical care ward and continues through the rest of the hospitalization period. Usually, too, it is a covert or silent depression and attracts little attention. The clinical manifestations are at first obscured by bedrest, sedation, and hypnotic medication. Discouragement and a gloomy preoccupation about the future are the principal indications of the state. The patient seldom mentions these concerns to his doctor, assuming them to be trivial or likely to be misinterpreted as signs of fear or weakness of character. Once home, the depression becomes much more apparent both to the patient and to his family. Fatigability which approaches exhaustion is the primary complaint and interferes with accustomed activities. It may be falsely attributed to a failing heart. Irritability, anxiety, and despondency occur next in order of frequency, followed by insomnia and a feeling of aimlessness and boredom. When the time comes to return to work, fearful anticipation mounts and often results in long, unwarranted delays in ending the convalescent period. These are more apt to intrude themselves when the patient's occupation is physically or mentally stressful.

Though it is true that most of these patients do ultimately recover without medical assistance (the disorder is, in this sense, self-limited), the toll that depression exacts in suffering and anguish is enormous. Depression is probably the main cause of extended convalescence and retarded rehabilitation following myocardial infarction. Much of it could be prevented by proper intervention.

The first step in the management of such patients is recognition. This can be greatly simplified if one assumes that all patients after a coronary are liable to depression and if a plan to deal with this is started during the acute stage of the illness. Such a program would carry no risk for those unusual individuals who may not be depressed, and would offer considerable benefit to those who are. One begins by assuring the patient that a sense of sadness and discouragement are normal and to be expected. Next, he should be advised that his activities may not need to be curtailed as much as he dreads. This can be supplemented by giving examples of public figures, such as former Presidents Eisenhower and Johnson, who returned to active life following an infarction. The patient should then be given a program of graduated activity consistent with his cardiac condition. Physical conditioning is the best antidote for depression in the coronary patient. It can raise self-esteem and reinstate a feeling of independence even when he is on bed rest. Once established, this schedule of activity should be carried through convalescence and kept up long after the patient has returned to work.

Another point in treating post-coronary depression is giving instructions about the disease. Patients have their own ideas about illness, which often do not conform to the facts. Misconceptions must be actively uncovered and corrected. The most prevalent misbeliefs surrounding cardiovascular disease include the following: (1) Exertion, even when mild, can kill you. (2) Sexual intercourse should never again be attempted. (3) Cardiac infarctions tend to recur at orgasm. (4) Recurrence is apt to take place on the anniversary of the first infarction. (5) One is likely to die at the same age as did a parent from heart disease. (6) Recurrent infarctions are more likely to take place in sleep. After these misunderstandings have been corrected, the patient may be informed as to what he can and cannot do. The spouse and children should be included in the discussions. Warning a patient what to expect almost always reduces the actual stress of an event and spares him much torment. If the patient is told it is normal to feel weak when he returns home from the hospital and that this is not a sign of a failing heart, he is not alarmed when it occurs. The family should be cautioned against being overprotective or becoming upset if the patient is irritable and rebellious.

These measures are simple and require little time. The tricyclic antidepressants and MAO inhibitors are generally considered unsafe for use with coronary patients unless great care is taken in their administration. Electric shock therapy has been successfully and safely employed in post–myocardial infarction patients with depressions severe enough to warrant it.

Victims of milder stroke exhibit almost identical symptoms, which should be managed in the same way.

Cancer is another medical illness which is almost invariably attended by a depressive reaction. Aside from the prognosis, an important determinant of the severity of this depressive response is the attitude of the physician. In the nineteenth century, physicians tended to be quite open with their patients and gave an honest diagnosis and a straightforward prognosis. A midtwentieth century survey of physicians' attitudes toward the truthful disclosure of these vital factors in cancer revealed a disinclination toward candor. There seemed to be a direct relationship between the seriousness of the prognosis and the degree to which truth was espoused or rejected. Thus, over 90 percent of dermatologists treating skin cancer favored openness, while less than 20 percent of gynecologists chose to be frank. This disparity relates to the control the specialist can exert over the malignancy. Basal-cell carcinoma can usually be removed entirely and survival ensured. The outlook in carcinoma of the breast or cervix is far less hopeful. Thus the type of tumor, rather than the patient's personality, decides what is said. It is assumed that when intervention offered but negligible success, the patient, upon hearing this would fall into a hopeless depression and that hence it would be wiser to withhold information that could serve no useful purpose.

In the last 15 years there has been a gratifying change in the psychologic management of the cancer patient. It is agreed that patients should learn the truth in most instances and that withholding or distorting information seriously undermines the doctor-patient relationship. Furthermore, the facts of the illness, no matter how grim, can be coped with more readily than a tangle of half truths, hollow reassurances, and furtive falsifications. The notion that a patient can be kept blissfully unaware of his jeopardy while his closest relatives are fully informed is absurd. This situation, which has aptly been called "the conspiracy of silence," not only fails to accomplish its purpose but cruelly isolates the patient at a time when he needs all the human support available. In being truthful the physician need not thrust the harsh realities on each patient the moment the biopsy report returns, but he must make available whatever information is requested and maintain open communication with his patient throughout the course of the illness. Though it is true that some individuals cannot bear to hear the truth and ask not to be told, most patients want to know and should be told. It is important to remember that the cancer patient often phrases crucial questions indirectly, especially when he is fearful of the answer. He might talk of buying a new house in an effort to get his doctor's opinion as to whether he will be around long enough to justify the expense. Such questions ought not to pass unnoticed. The doctor should ask the patient what he means or rephrase the question to bring out the hidden query.

A worry common to the patient with cancer, yet seldom mentioned openly, is that the doctor will give up on him. This is particularly so in this era of the specialist, in which so often no one doctor is in overall charge. A firm, supportive doctor-patient relationship with mutual trust and respect is the best insurance against the fear of abandonment. Once this has been established, the patient is usually able to cope with his depression without specific help from the doctor. However, the latter should be ready to supply minor tranquilizers such as diazepam, 2 to 10 mg q. i. d., if necessary. The dose may be doubled or tripled for use as a hypnotic at bedtime. If depression persists, it is justifiable to try a tricyclic antidepressant or a monoamine oxidase inhibitor.

Neurologic diseases, such as paralysis agitans (Parkinson's disease), are complicated by a depressive reaction in more than half the cases. Weakness and fatigability, the principal psychologic manifestations, are added to the akinesia of this disease, and the resulting therapeutic problem becomes formidable.

Since grief in one of the forms described is, without doubt, the most common form of reactive depression that the general practitioner is likely to encounter, we have taken it as our model. However, some psychiatrists question whether depression and grief are the same process. There are two schools of thought. Adolf Meyer and his followers regard depression as a continuum, with sadness and disappointment at one end and psychotic depressions at the other. The school associated with Emil Kraepelin considers depression as a disease process quite distinct from grief and other everyday mood swings. They distinguish two types of depression: exogenous and endogenous. Exogenous, or reactive depressions, have a known external cause, such as a loss of a loved one, loss of one's fortune or position, or a life-threatening illness. The grief reaction would exemplify a typical reactive or exogenous depression. In contrast, the endogenous depressions have no apparent external cause; they seem to occur in susceptible individuals as a response to some unknown biologic stimulus. Manic-depressive psychosis and involutional melancholia are typical endogenous depressions. To date there has been no definitive study to support either point of view.

MANIC-DEPRESSIVE PSYCHOSIS

DEFINITIONS AND EPIDEMIOLOGY Manic-depressive psychosis is a disorder of affect (mood) which may consist of episodes of mania and/or depression. Although it has been traditionally regarded as a periodic or circular condition in which one major mood swing is followed by an equal but opposite excursion, this is seldon in fact the case. Depression is far more prevalent than mania, and the mixed or bipolar variety containing both extremes is uncommon. As a consequence, manic-depressive psychosis is divided into three subtypes: manic, depressed, and circular.

The disease was given its name by Kraepelin in 1896, and it is with him that our current clinical concept of this disorder originates. He viewed the manic and depressive attacks as opposite poles of the same underlying process and pointed out that unlike schizophrenia, manic-depressive psychosis entails no intellectual deterioration with recurrent episodes.

Differing criteria for diagnosis account for disparity in statistics. British psychiatrists diagnose the disease more frequently than their American colleagues. Moreover, in the United States either the disease is being diagnosed by different standards today than at the turn of the century or its incidence has changed. In 1900, for example, 17 percent of all patients admitted to the Boston State Hospital and 37 percent of those admitted to the McLean Hospital were diagnosed as having manic-depressive disease, whereas in 1950 the figures were 8 percent and 16 percent, respectively. The prevalence at present is 3 to 4 cases per 100,000 population.

Manic-depressive psychosis is an illness largely confined to the middle and later adult years. Not many patients develop their first attack prior to their fiftieth year, and the peak age of onset is between fifty-five and sixty-five for both sexes. The disease is two or three times more frequent among females. It is more common in individuals of Jewish and Irish heritage and occurs more frequently among those of upper socioeconomic strata. The manic form tends to occur at an earlier age than the depressive, but at any age, episodes of depression are far more frequent than are episodes of mania.

CLINICAL PICTURE The depressive phase may develop into a full-blown picture within a surprisingly few days. The symptoms and signs of depression were described in Chap. 14. It need only be stressed that the patient is apathetic and despondent, with reduced energy for mental and physical activity. There is a lack of interest in all pleasurable activity. Overwhelmed by feelings of helplessness and indecisiveness, the patient becomes increasingly dependent and incapable of acting in his own behalf. In despair, he expresses the desire for death and may become suicidal with very little warning. As pointed out in Chap. 15 any combination of weakness, easy fatigue, anorexia, insomnia, and loss of libido may dominate the clinical picture and may therefore simulate several medical diseases. At its worst the illness takes the form of a depressive stupor; the patient becomes mute and indifferent to nutritional needs and neglectful even of bowel and bladder functions. His condition at this time resembles catatonia. He must be fed and his vital functions tended to until therapy (usually electroconvulsive therapy) brings about an improvement.

The manic phase is, in most ways, the mirror opposite of the depressed phase. Patients are hyperactive, with increased appetite and sex urge. With a minimum of sleep they awake in the morning filled with joy and expectation. They appear to possess great drive and confidence, yet lack the ability to carry out their plans. Setbacks do not perturb them, but rather act as goads for new activities. Euphoria and expansiveness sometimes bubble over into delusions of power and grandeur, which in turn may make them offensively aggressive. Their mirth and good spirits are contagious, and they make others laugh with them; however, if thwarted, their warmth can suddenly change to anger. Their threshold for paranoid thinking is low, which makes them sensitive and suspicious. They tend to neglect themselves to the point of dishevelment and poor personal hygiene. In its most advanced form, a condition described as *delirious mania* develops, in which the patient becomes totally incoherent and his behavior altogether disorganized. At this stage visual and auditory hallucinations and paranoid delusions may be rampant. Furthermore, as the term implies, the patient in a delirious mania may be disoriented in time, place, and person, and his sensorium may be clouded as well. Fortunately, this extreme is rarely encountered.

Hypomania represents a milder degree of the disorder, but this term has also been used to depict normal behavior which is unusually animated or colorful. In such form it need not arouse concern unless it is totally out of character for the individual. In this sense hypomania is a personality trait found in many talented people.

First attacks of either depression or mania last an average of 6 months if untreated. Modern therapy can reduce this by more than half. Over 93 percent of manic-depressive patients recover from their first attack. For those who do not recover, there is often some pertinent reason in terms of their family or environment which serves to retard improvement. Attacks tend to be longer in older age groups.

ETIOLOGY The following are some of the theories that have been put forth to explain the origin of depression:

Genetic theories The capacity to experience sadness and depression is common to all mankind. There is no question that depression can be caused by adverse circumstances; however, in response to the same degree of loss, some individuals are more liable to depression than others. In general, there seems to be a familial diathesis for most depressive illness, but especially for manic-depressive psychosis and involutional melancholia. Much work has been done on the inheritance of depression, most of which has dealt with these two affective psychoses. If one parent has a severe depression bordering on psychosis, there is a 10 to 15 percent chance that his child will be severely depressed as well. If both parents have severe depression, their offspring stand a 50 percent chance of being depressed. Although it is not known how the genetic components are transmitted, it is known that depression is not produced by either a simple dominant or a simple recessive gene. It is the opinion of Aaron Beck that the available research data from pedigree studies in identical twins do not establish conclusively whether affective disorders are genetic, environmental, both, or neither.

Biochemical The biogenic amines (norepinephrine, serotonin, and dopamine) are the key elements in this theory. Following the observations that antidepressant drugs, such as the tricyclic antidepressants and the monoamine oxidase (MAO) inhibitors, exert their effect by increasing one or another of the biogenic amines at the central adrenergic receptor sites (limbic system and hypothalamus) and that drugs which often cause depression, such as reserpine, deplete biogenic amines, the theory logically followed that naturally occurring depressions might be associated with a deficiency of these substances. Research on the amphetamines, cocaine, electroconvulsive shock treatment and lithium salts has produced data that agree with the biogenic amine hypothesis. Although this possibility has received much attention and is generally well accepted, it leaves many questions unanswered. How is a genetic abnormality transcribed into a disorder of biogenic amines? Why are the therapeutic results so inconsistent with either the tricyclic antidepressants or the MAO inhibitors, both of which should favorably influence the balance of biogenic amines at the proper receptor site? How can one explain the observation that steroids play a part in the etiology of affective disorders? Further knowledge of the metabolism and physiology of the transmitter function of the biogenic amines is needed before a complete theory can be developed.

Psychoanalytic Karl Abraham was the first psychoanalyst to study manic-depressive patients. He pointed out their tendency to have obsessive-compulsive personalities and claimed that they possessed unusually strong oral needs. The mother-child relationship was marked by strong ambivalent feelings, which resulted in the infant's constant sense of unfulfillment. This, in turn, set the stage for the deep depressions in adult life. Abraham viewed depression in manic-depressive patients as a regression to an earlier period of development, the oral stage of hostile dependency. He looked upon the manic phase as an acting out of the infant's unbridled freedom.

Freud used mourning as a model for depression. He pointed out that the melancholic behaved like someone who was in mourning—i.e., someone who has sustained a loss. In the case of the melancholic, however, the loss is symbolic. Edward Bibring believed that the predisposition to depression occurred in response to a series of early childhood and adolescent traumatic events. Central to Bibring's concept of depression is the loss of self-esteem and a sense of helplessness. There are many other psychoanalytic explanations of depression, but none is universally accepted.

INVOLUTIONAL MELANCHOLIA

DEFINITIONS AND EPIDEMIOLOGY This is a severe depression of psychotic proportions which occurs in the involutional phase of life. It is characterized by agitation, insomnia, and a profound sense of worthlessness. Multiple physical complaints, some of which may be delusional in nature, generally accompany the condition. Typically, there is no history of previous episodes.

There appears to have been a steady increase in the prevalence of this disorder over the last 50 years. This probably reflects the growing awareness of the condition by the lay population and the appreciation that such an entity as "middle-life depression" exists and can be treated, rather than an actual increase. As in manic-depressive psychosis, there is a sex difference. Three times as many females as males fall victim to it. There is no known cause for this sexual distribution, but some have speculated that just as many men are depressed only they deny it or turn to alcohol. Women are more apt to develop signs of involutional melancholia between the ages of fifty-one and sixty, whereas men usually fall prey to it some 5 to 10 years later. Unlike manic-depressive psychosis, this depression is more common in lower socioeconomic categories.

CLINICAL PICTURE The onset is most apt to be insidious, characterized by increased irritability, insomnia, psychomotor restlessness, easy fatigue, loss of interest in sexual and gustatory pleasures, and an ever-mounting worry about health. These manifestations accrue over one or more years before the clinical picture is complete. As time passes, the individual's life narrows to a single-minded concern about his physical deterioration, his mental decline, or both. Before long, every conversation comes to balance on the fulcrum of symptoms, no matter how hard the patient may try to avoid that topic. In dialogue his rejoinders become so stereotyped that the listener can soon predict exactly what is going to be said. There is a poverty of ideation and a notable absence of insight. Consciousness is clear, and though there is usually no evidence of a schizophrenic type of thought disorder, paranoia is not infrequently part of the picture. The suspicions and delusions are generally not as fixed or bizarre as in schizophrenia. However, if hallucinations are present, the possibility of an associated early organic brain syndrome must be considered.

In contrast to the physical inactivity and mental slowness of the depressed manic-depressive patient, the principal behavioral manifestation of involutional melancholia is agitation, the source of which is an underlying anxiety state. As a consequence, these patients usually pace restlessly about the room and have great difficulty sitting still. Furthermore, they tend to be overtalkative and vexed in their manner of expression, so that the examiner is acutely aware of their mental distress. Attempts at reassurance may meet with initial success, only to be unseated in the next rush of doubts. Involutional melancholics remain inaccessible to reason and logic as these apply to their symptoms, even though they retain the capacity to exercise these functions in other areas of their life.

ETIOLOGY One of the consistent observations made by the many psychiatrists who have studied this illness pertains to the patient's premorbid character structure. The person most apt to develop an involutional depression is compulsive, rigid, and overconscientious, with a great capacity for work and an obsessive concern about conforming to the customs of his community. The specific relationship between these personality traits and the depression is unknown. However, it is reasonable to assume that the man who sets high goals for himself, making no allowance for aging, will surely suffer disappointment and dissatisfaction, which are the forerunners of depression. Since this disorder occurs in conjunction with either menopause or the male climacteric, endocrine depletion has been thought to play a role in its genesis. However, since there is no specific accompanying endocrinologic abnormality and its course has never been influenced by hormone replacement, such does not seem to be the case.

The most important concern in this particular illness is that the responsible physician be aware of the risk of suicide. Since so many of these individuals have reputations for being sound, dependable, and stable, one's psychologic set toward them is to reject the possibility of self-destructiveness. Furthermore, consumed as they often are in hypochondriac ruminations, they may deny being depressed. This is in marked contrast to manic-depressive illness, in which the depression is so evident that suicidal precautions are thought of as a matter of course. Despite the absence of obvious suicidal intent, involutional melancholia carries with it a high suicide risk. As a consequence, one should seek the advice of a psychiatrist as soon as the diagnosis is suspected.

TREATMENT

For the depressed phase of manic-depressive psychosis and of other serious depressions as well, the plan of therapy revolves around five points:

1 *Enlisting the help of a psychiatrist.* The untrained physician would be rash to attempt the management of these patients without psychiatric assistance.
2 *The prevention of suicide.* This involves the question of hospitalization. If there is any doubt about the patient's intention of suicide it is better to hospitalize him than to take a chance. In manic-depressive illness, attacks of depression or elation are remarkably similar in the same individual. Thus one can predict the course and content of the present spell on the basis of the last. If suicide attempts were made then, the chance is they will be made again.
3 *Antidepressant medication.* There are two categories of antidepressants, the tricyclic compounds and the monoamine oxidase (MAO) inhibitors. Representing the former are imipramine (Tofranil) and amitriptyline (Elavil), and the latter, phenelzine (Nardil), tranylcypromine (Parnate). In the treatment of depression, most psychiatrists start with the tricyclic antidepressants because they are far safer. With imipramine and amitriptyline, doses range from 100 to 200 mg each day. The starting dose is usually 100 mg per day, which is then raised in stepwise fashion as is needed. The therapeutic effect of tricyclic medication is often not evident for 2 or 3 weeks after treatment has been initiated. As a consequence it would be premature to stop the drug before that time. Common side effects are orthostatic hypotension, dry mouth, constipation, tachycardia, and urinary retention. Because of their effect on the cardiovascular system, the tricyclic compounds should not be given to patients who have coronary heart disease. If these are not effective, they are discontinued for 2 weeks and administration of an MAO inhibitor is started. Phenelzine is regarded as the least likely of the MAO inhibitors to produce serious side effects. As a consequence, it is usually the first one prescribed. The usual starting dose is 15 mg t.i.d., which is gradually increased as needed to a maximum of 45 mg t.i.d. The most serious side effect of this class of antidepressants is hypertensive crisis. As a consequence, all MAO inhibitors should be dispensed with extreme caution in patients with a history of cardio- or cerebrovascular disease. Patients taking MAO inhibitors should avoid foods with high tyramine content. The latter is a pressor amine that is normally inactivated by MAO, and ingestion under such circumstances may result in a hypertensive crisis. Proscribed foods (aged cheese, pickled herring, chicken liver, etc.) are always listed on the manufacturer's information insert.

   Since patients are usually responsive to one or the other but not to both, it is important to find out whether tricyclics or MAO inhibitors have been more helpful in the past. This will guide one in current management. Interestingly enough, it has been found that members of the same family are apt to have a similar response to the same antidepressant. Thus, if a patient's mother was helped by an MAO inhibitor, then her children would probably react well to drugs in this category.
4 *Lithium carbonate.* Lithium carbonate has been used since 1949. It is the drug of choice in treating the manic phase of manic-depressive illness. Because it takes a few days to weeks to act effectively against mania, the patient should be hospitalized and sedated with chlorpromazine or haloperidol until the lithium has taken effect. Lithium carbonate has been found to be an effective prophylactic against further attacks of both mania and depression. Since it is not a specific antidepressant, the depression must be controlled by either an antidepressant or electroconvulsive therapy before lithium can be started. The blood level of lithium must be followed closely, both to ensure that a therapeutic dose is being given and to guard against toxicity.
5 *Electroconvulsive therapy (ECT).* Electroconvulsive therapy is an effective treatment for the depressed phase of manic-depressive psychosis and involutional melancholia and can also be used to interrupt manic excitements. The latter often require only two or three treatments. The technique is quite simple. The patient is premedicated with a muscle relaxant (Anectine) and then anesthetized by an intravenous injection of a short-acting barbiturate (Brevital). An electrode is then placed over each temple and an alternating current of about 400 mamp and 70 to 120 V is passed between them for $^{1}/_{10}$ to $^{1}/_{2}$ sec. The Anectine prevents strong and sometimes injurious muscle spasm. The patient is awake within 5 to 10 min and is up and about in $^{1}/_{2}$ hr. Convulsions can also be induced chemically by injecting Metrazol or by inhaling the gas Indoklon. The mechanism by which convulsive therapy works is not known. In treating depression, ECT is usually given every other day for 14 to 20 treatments. The only absolute contraindication is the presence of an intracranial mass such as a neoplasm or hematoma. Its one major drawback is a transient impairment of recent memory for the period of treatment and the days which follow, the degree of impairment being related to the

number of treatments given. Placing both electrodes on the nondominant side (unilateral ECT) produces less memory disturbance but is thought to be less effective against the depression.

In manic-depressive illness the best program of management relies on a physician who is willing to follow the patient's course over a long period of time and who is known to the family. Although the prognosis for any individual attack is relatively good, it is wise to arrange for a plan of action which is set in operation as soon as the first symptoms of a recurrence become manifest. A physician who works in conjunction with the family and who has ready access to a psychiatrist would be helpful in arranging for the early treatment of each recurrence.

The manic phase of manic-depressive psychosis also usually requires hospitalization to prevent the patient from impulsive and often aggressive behavior which might jeopardize his career or standing in the community. Judgment is so poor in mania that patients may gamble away fortunes or make reckless investments. Chlorpromazine (Thorazine) or haloperidol (Haldol) can be used to control the mania while lithium carbonate is started. If tranquilizers are ineffective in slowing hyperactivity, ECT can be used.

Until the advent of the antidepressant drugs, electroconvulsive therapy was the treatment of choice for involutional melancholia. Of all the conditions for which ECT is used, it is the one that is most predictably benefited. Close to 90 percent of patients with involutional melancholia recover within less than 2 months following a course of 6 to 14 ECTs. Prior to electroconvulsive therapy this depression could be expected to last 2 to 7 years before remission occurred. Although there are some who prefer to use drugs, most psychiatrists still favor ECT. It has the advantage of speed and safety, but carries the tariff of amnesia.

The tricyclic antidepressants and the MAO inhibitors have both been used successfully in the treatment of involutional melancholia. They have the disadvantage of acting more slowly and in some instances in producing unpleasant and even dangerous side effects. Since they cause no memory impairment, patients with jobs requiring an intact memory should first be given a trial of both types of antidepressants on the chance that their success would preclude the use of ECT. These trials, of course, must be conducted in a setting where behavior can be monitored in such a way as to greatly reduce the chance of suicide.

SUICIDE

There are approximately 225,000 suicide attempts in the United States each year, of which 25,000 end fatally. All psychiatrists agree that this is a conservative figure. Suicide ranks thirteenth of the 36 leading causes of death in America, a figure which should call every physician's attention to the importance of recognizing those depressions with a high potential for self-destruction. Furthermore, every doctor should be familiar with the few clues we possess to identify the patient who intends to end his life.

The depressions which take the highest toll of lives are manic-depressive psychosis, involutional melancholia, depression resulting from a debilitating disease, pathologic grief, and depression in an alcoholic or schizophrenic. Despite an extraordinary amount of work on the subject, only a few general guidelines have been found that can serve as clues, and these offer but limited help in the individual case. We have learned that most suicides are not impulsive but planned. Furthermore, the intention of suicide is more often than not communicated by the patient to a person who is significant in his life. This may be a direct verbal statement of intent or an indirect message, such as giving away a treasured possession or revising a will. It is known that successful suicide is three times more common in men than in women and more common among older people, especially those who have lost a mate through death, separation, or divorce. Those with a history of suicide in the family (i.e., suicide by either mother or father) carry a higher risk for self-destruction than those who do not. A previous attempt at suicide by the patient adds to the risk. Most successful suicides give as their motive, "a concern about ill health." Chronic illnesses such as alcoholism, cancer, heart disease, and progressive incurable neurologic conditions all contribute their toll of suicides. Thus, a portrait of a likely prospect for suicide might read as follows: an elderly man in poor health through heavy drinking who has recently lost his beloved wife, who attempted suicide a year ago, and whose father took his own life. There is no single trait that stands out as highly significant in terms of predicting suicide. As a consequence, we are left with our clinical judgment and our index of suspicion as our main guides. The only rule of thumb is that all suicidal threats are to be taken seriously and all patients who threaten to kill themselves should be evaluated by a psychiatrist.

There are physicians who claim a reluctance to question the presence of suicidal thoughts with depressed patients on the grounds that this might upset them. It is more probable that the doctor is himself upset, for surely mention of suicide will not alarm the person who is determined to end his life, nor offend the patient who has no such intention. Rather, a query of this type by the doctor is more apt to be appreciated by both types of depressed patients because it expresses his genuine concern. Furthermore, it forces the patient to realize that his behavior is being taken seriously. This in itself sometimes brings to awareness unrecognized suicidal urges. Should a patient's manner or conversation raise the doctor's suspicion, he should quickly voice it. If there is no immediate danger the doctor can make an appointment for his patient to see a psychiatrist in the next few days. If the danger is immediate, a bed should be obtained in a general hospital (preferably on the psychiatric ward) and a psychiatrist consulted. The point is to get the patient under cover until a psychiatrist arrives, and since a general hospital is far less threatening than an asylum, the patient is more apt to agree to enter. Once he has been admitted to the hospital, suicidal precautions should be initiated, including special nurses "around the clock." When the psychiatrist arrives he can determine the need for more or less security. If the patient refuses hospitalization, the family should be assembled, along with intimate friends and the clergy, if appropriate, to urge the patient's cooperation. Should all efforts fail, the only recourse is a commitment to a mental hospital. Though commitment procedures and laws vary from state to state, all provide temporary confinement of individuals who are thought to be self-destructive. Although an action of this sort is bound to be stressful for all concerned, the most useful dictum to remember in cases of doubt is that prudence and caution are more important than the patient's plea for freedom. Hard feelings over a short period of enforced confinement vanish in time. Those who mourn the loss of a loved one through a suicide which could have been prevented are apt to be unforgiving.

Patients who arrive at the hospital having attempted suicide should be under constant surveillance, once consciousness is regained, and a psychiatrist should be called in for consultation. Until he arrives the patient should have a nurse or attendant assigned to keep watch. It is unwise to allow the family to provide this service unless their competence is unquestioned. The psychiatrist should assume the responsibility for setting up a program of therapy and arrange for transfer to a psychiatric ward, if this is necessary, or for out-patient treatment.

HYPOCHONDRIASIS

Finally, a few remarks concerning the status of hypochondriasis as a psychiatric illness are in order. It is a condition which may be defined as the constant preoccupation with matters of health and an exaggerated concern about real or imagined signs and symptoms of illness. A hallmark of hypochondriasis is the failure of reassurance to affect either the symptoms or the patient's conviction of being sick. The most common complaint is pain, often vague and variable, most of which is referable to the head, chest, and lower part of the abdomen. It is a curious fact that over 70 percent of hypochondriacal complaints are on the left side of the body.

Hypochondriasis is considered to be not a specific psychiatric disorder but rather the somatic equivalent of depression or anxiety. As such, it is found in a number of psychiatric conditions such as depression (as described earlier in this chapter), schizophrenia, and the psychoneuroses. It is not uncommon to encounter hypochondriacal reactions in otherwise normal individuals during periods of stress. For example, medical students traditionally develop the symptoms of a variety of lethal diseases during the stress of their first exposure to clinical medicine. When adolescents or young adults present hypochondriacal symptoms that are not related to transient episodes of stress, one should suspect a more serious underlying disorder such as schizophrenia.

Though it is estimated that 85 percent of hypochondriasis is secondary to other mental disorders, chiefly depression, in about 15 percent of cases there appears to be no associated emotional illness. The term *primary hypochondriasis* is used to describe the disorder in this small group. The etiology is unknown. In this category are the habitués of medical outpatient clinics, who are passed from specialist to specialist, perplexing and angering doctors along the way because their symptoms defy both proper diagnosis and satisfactory cure. Often referred to as "crocks," these patients seldom benefit from conventional therapy. The first principle in the management of hypochondriasis is to determine what should be treated. Is the hypochondriasis part of another psychiatric syndrome such as depression, psychoneurosis, or schizophrenia? As a rule this question can best be answered by a psychiatrist, and it is advisable to have each case so evaluated in order to institute a suitable program of management. Should depression play an important part in the etiology, the patient could be given a trial of antidepressant medication, in the form of either a tricyclic compound or a monoamine oxidase inhibitor. Psychoneurotics and schizophrenics should be treated by a psychiatrist.

The treatment of primary hypochondriasis is difficult, if not impossible, unless the physician alters his goal of therapy. Since, for a variety of reasons, the patient needs to retain his symptoms, the concept of "curing" is inapplicable. The presence of symptoms is thought by some to provide the context for a relationship with a physician. It is the continuation of this relationship, which is often the only dependable human contact in the patient's life, that motivates some hypochondriacs. In this setting it is understandable why being reassured that vigor and health will be restored seldom moves the patient to improve. Physicians are so oriented toward the relief of suffering and the cure of disease that anger and frustration inevitably occur when they meet a patient who coexists with his symptoms in an immutable symbiosis. In this situation it is usually the doctor who is the most discomfited. Such patients are best managed by physicians who realize that these patients do not necessarily want or expect a cure, who are content with the small gains of avoiding unnecessary surgery, and who have an interest in the way symptoms persist rather than improve. Since this type of doctor is difficult to come by, some hospitals have found it economical to utilize the time of those on their staff who are able to provide such care by establishing special clinics under their leadership where all hypochondriacs are evaluated and treated and their course is followed. This is probably the most effective method for managing these cases from the standpoint of the physician as well as the patient.

REFERENCES

BECK AT: *Depression: Clinical, Experimental and Theoretical Aspects*, Hoeber-Harper, New York: 1967

DAVIS JM et al: Drugs used in the treatment of depression, in *Psychopharmacology: A Review of Progress, 1957–1967*, ed DH Efron, Washington: U.S. Government Printing Office, 1968, p. 719

KENYON FE: Hypochondriasis: A clinical study. Br J Psychiatry 110:478, 1964

LINDEMANN E: Symptomatology management of acute grief. Am J Psychiatry 101:141, 1944

SCHILDKRAUT JJ: Neuropsychopharmacology and the affective disorders. N Engl J Med 281:197, 302, 1969

SHNEIDMAN ES, FARBEROW NL: *Clues to Suicide*, New York: McGraw-Hill, 1957

WEISMAN AD: *On Dying and Denying*, New York: Behavioral Publications, 1972

342
THE SCHIZOPHRENIC SYNDROME AND RELATED PSYCHOSES

ROSS J. BALDESSARINI

DEFINITIONS The diagnostic classification of psychotic illnesses is still evolving. Current American and most international classifications accept as principal categories the organic brain syndromes due to degenerative, toxic, infectious, or metabolic conditions and the so-called "functional" psychoses of unknown etiology. Under the second subdivision are (1) the affective disorders (manic-depressive reaction, involutional melancholia, and psychotic depressive reaction), (2) the paranoid states, and (3) schizophrenia.

Currently, "schizophrenia" is believed to comprise a large and common group of mental disorders bearing some similarity to one another. From one point of view, schizophrenia is that which is left over of the psychoses when organic brain syndromes and purely affective disorders are excluded. As such, schizophrenia is clearly *not a single disease.*

The schizophrenias present characteristic disturbances of thinking, mood, and behavior. The presence of thought disorder in the face of a relatively clear sensorium is essential for the diagnosis, which is reached by recognition of specific psychologic symptoms. Other features include altered concept formation, misinterpretation of reality, and sometimes frank delusions and hallucinations. Mood is usually described as flat, withdrawn, or inappropriate to the situation. Behavior and appearance are often odd or even bizarre. Currently, most authorities would include a paranoid form as one of the schizophrenias, but also recognize other less common forms of paranoia in which a single fixed idea or delusion is the major feature.

A debate still rages as to whether the usual medical model of "disease" is really appropriate to schizophrenia. It is likely that future research will show it to be a syndrome subsuming several diseases which will come to have firmer biologic and psychologic identities. Extreme views are that the illness of schizophrenia exists only in the imagination of certain central European psychiatrists or that the schizophrenias are merely forms of idiosyncracy or aberrant life style.

HISTORICAL HIGHLIGHTS Emil Kraepelin's contribution was to bring diagnostic order out of the chaotic mass of chronic asylum inmates by lumping together most of the psychoses which were not clearly organic dementias or deliriums or simply affective disorders. He adopted the term dementia praecox, introduced by Morel in the 1860s. The original conception included a pattern of onset early in life and a chronic downhill course.

Eugen Bleuler in the early 1900s coined the somewhat unfortunate, but generally accepted, term *schizophrenia,* which implies a splitting or fragmentation of psychic functions, and which has led to the popular but incorrect notion of "split or multiple personality." Another lasting contribution was Bleuler's distinction between more primary or fundamental symptoms (especially disturbances of the association process or logical continuity in the stream of conscious thought), usually summarized in the mnemonic of the "four As" (loose *a*ssociations, flat *a*ffect, *a*mbivalence, and *a*utism); and secondary or reactive symptoms, including delusions and hallucinations, passivity phenomena, and other peculiarities of thought, speech, and behavior.

Adolf Meyer, the late dean of American psychiatry, contributed the basic concept of the psychobiologic approach, which suggests that to understand any major psychiatric illness requires an understanding of the patient's life history and his habitual reactions to life situations. Sigmund Freud sought explanations for psychotic behavior in problems surrounding early developmental crises and, in contrast to Kraepelin, thought of schizophrenia not as deterioration into dementia, but as regression to very early or infantile levels of function.

INCIDENCE Schizophrenia appears in all societies studied so far, although local cultural patterns may modify the clinical picture. One problem in estimating incidence rates is that local definitions of schizophrenia vary widely. American psychiatrists have relatively loose diagnostic criteria for it and tend to include cases that might elsewhere be called severe neuroses, character disorders, or acute reactive psychoses.

Worldwide prevalence rates (number of existing cases per 100 persons) are on the order of 0.3 percent, and life-expectancy rates (chance of becoming schizophrenic at some time) are about 1 percent. Incidence figures (new cases) in the world vary from about 0.05 to 0.2 percent per year, depending on real local differences and upon the methods of data gathering. Since most studies are from Europe, the English-speaking countries, and Japan, they may not be truly representative of the rest of the world. Nevertheless, it is estimated that there are about 4 or 5 million new cases of schizophrenia a year in the world and a prevalence of some 9 million cases!

Although patterns of hospital care are changing rapidly, schizophrenics still account for about 25 to 30 percent of new admissions to public mental hospitals in the United States; they occupy more than half of all the beds in most mental hospitals, and approximately a quarter of all the hospital beds in the country. There are about a quarter of a million new cases a year in the United States (0.1 to 0.2 percent yearly incidence), more than 300,000 hospitalized schizophrenics, and at least an equal number outside hospitals (0.2 to 0.3 percent prevalence). The incidence based on admission rates appears to have been relatively stable in this country for the past century, or as long as accurate hospital statistics have been recorded.

The incidence of schizophrenia is about equal for males and females. The rates seem to be higher in areas of high mobility and social disorganization, in crowded urban areas, and in the lowest social classes. These observations have led to the "drift versus origin" debate, which is still unsettled: i.e., do schizophrenics drift into poor, crowded, mobile, and disorganized areas and social strata as a result of their disabilities, or do these aspects of society "cause" increased risks? The formerly much lower reproductivity rates for schizophrenics are now approaching 90 percent of those of the general population. These increased birth rates should eventually cause incidence rates for schizophrenia to increase. Ironically, this appears to be an "ecologic" side effect of improved treatment or rehabilitation.

ETIOLOGY Simply stated, the etiology of schizophrenia is unknown. Research in this area is beset with great fundamental difficulties, including the lack of clear and objective definitions of "schizophrenia," the limitations and distortions produced by the traditional "medical-disease" model, the difficulty in separating genetic and environmental factors, and the illogical assumption that measurable descriptive differences imply something about causes.

GENETICS Early in the last century, clinical investigators were impressed not only that a family history of psychosis was common, but also that the clinical type usually ran true to form. A crude summary of the present status of the genetic approach is that the greater the degree of relatedness of a family member to a schizophrenic and the more severe his illness, the greater is the risk of schizophrenia. Thus, family studies have found that up to the first degree of kinship, risk is little if at all greater than in the general population, while the risks for a full sibling, a fraternal twin, or a child of a schizophrenic are about equal and several times that of less closely related persons. If both parents are schizophrenic, the risk is greater still (probably more than 50 percent), and exceeded only for an identical twin of a schizophrenic, for whom the illness is almost inevitable, according to the classic studies of Kallmann. More recent studies conclude that a monozygote has a three- to fourfold greater risk than a dizygotic twin of a known schizophrenic. There is no evidence that the experience of being a twin itself contributes to increased risk of schizophrenia.

Another approach to this problem has been to study the incidence of psychopathology among natural and adoptive families of schizophrenic patients adopted and separated from their parents early in life; again, schizophrenia is much more common among the biologic relatives. Several studies have shown a general increase of psychopathologic change among close relatives of schizophrenics, including a variety of characterologic and psychotic disorders (exclusive of manic-depressive psychosis).

Genetic hypotheses offering nearly every conceivable mendelian model have been suggested and attest to the fact that the data do not permit the construction of an unambiguous single-gene hypothesis. Currently popular are polygenic theories which draw analogies to the inheritance aspects of other complex functions such as intelligence.

BIOLOGIC FACTORS Among the earliest attempts to find biologically unique features of schizophrenics were descriptions of their general body types. It had been said that schizophrenics are often slender or odd-looking and rarely short and plump. This idea is of very doubtful validity or usefulness and is not supported by several modern studies.

There are many documented differences between schizophrenics and other subjects, including physiologic responses to drugs or to a variety of stresses. Unfortunately, they probably reflect the general clinical effects of inactivity and social withdrawal, especially in chronic hospitalized schizophrenics, and tell us nothing about etiology.

Pathologic changes in the brain had been reported from time to time in many poorly conceived and uncontrolled studies. By the 1950s the conclusion became unavoidable that the histopathologic changes described were no more than coincidences, artifacts, or misjudgments of normal histologic variation. More recently, some rather subtle morphologic distinctions about schizophrenics have been suggested, and while there is no evidence of specific chromosomal abnormalities in schizophrenia, there are some preliminary hints that these persons may have unique fingerprint patterns and unique finger-web and nailbed capillary patterns.

In recent decades, the prevailing theme has been the search for metabolic or biochemical abnormalities. So far all investigations have been unsuccessful or inconclusive. Several suggestions have been made that a circulating serum factor may be abnormal in schizophrenia. Levels of histamine, serotonin, or the catecholamines are said to be altered, and methodologically poor experiments with blood or urine purport to reveal differences in amino acid metabolism. Serum of patients has been claimed variously to alter tadpole development, to cause rats to behave strangely, to lead to irregularities of spider web spinning, and to drive normal volunteers mad. None of these findings has been corroborated in well-controlled and objectively evaluated experiments. Macroglobulins are found to be abnormal, but not specifically so in relation to schizophrenia. There are claims that a copper-containing globulin fraction ("taraxein"), said to be directly or indirectly psychotomimetic, and a mysterious lysing factor that leads to changes in glucose metabolism in chicken erythrocytes have been isolated from the blood of schizophrenic patients. These findings either have not been confirmed or have been found to be nonspecific.

The fact that mescaline and several other methylated aromatic amines are hallucinogenic has led to speculation that altered methylation of biogenic amines might produce an endogenous psychotogen. In support of this idea, there are several independent observations that large doses of methionine, an important source of methyl groups, can lead to psychotic exacerbations in some schizophrenics, although the significance of this possibly toxic effect is not clear. Findings of increased amounts of methylated amines in the urine of schizophrenics (including dimethoxyphenethylamine and N-methylated indoleamines) have not been confirmed consistently or demonstrated by unambiguous methods.

The initial enthusiasm for the study of hallucinogens such as mescaline or lysergic acid diethylamide (LSD) has also waned as it has become apparent that the interesting toxic effects of these substances have little in common with schizophrenia. More recently, attention has been drawn to the toxic psychotic effects of large doses of stimulant drugs, including the amphetamines, since they and the antipsychotic phenothiazine and related drugs appear to exert specific and opposite effects on the limbic system and other important subcortical centers. These stimulant intoxications appear uniquely to produce thought disorders, particularly paranoid thinking, in a relatively clear sensorium, as well as stereotyped peculiarities of movement. However, even paranoid thinking is not specific to schizophrenia.

The many observations that severely disturbed metabolism of endogenous hormones (e.g., in hyperthyroidism, myxedema, or Cushing's disease) or the administration of exogenous hormones (particularly steroids) can produce serious organic-toxic psychotic effects have also led to searches for endocrine dysfunction in schizophrenics, but, again, without demonstration of consistent or unique abnormalities that cannot be interpreted as nonspecific responses to stress. No consistent abnormality has been observed in the electroencephalogram of schizophrenic patients.

PSYCHOSOCIAL FACTORS In general, psychosocial studies have greatly enriched the *description* of schizophrenia, but have contributed little that is certain about etiology. Much of modern psychoanalytic and psychologic thought has emphasized defects in ego function in schizophrenia, i.e., in modulation of drives, formation of human relationships, formal thought processes and cognitive functions, psychologic defense mechanisms, and the organization of experience. It is generally believed that such deficits are the primary core of schizophrenic psychopathology and that many other symptoms follow from them secondarily. One difficulty in studying the many abnormalities of thought processes is that present psychologic techniques do not permit distinctions among those that are due to intrinsic organic deficit, to faulty learning, or to abnormal motivation.

Pathologic relationships within the family might also contribute to the development of schizophrenia. For example, the picture of a cold, rejecting, but controlling and perhaps overprotective "schizophrenogenic" mother has emerged. Another popular concept has been the "double bind," or the giving of conflicting double messages to a child, which makes it impossible for a "correct" or satisfying response to be given. However, these phenomena are not unique to families of schizophrenics. Other behavior patterns in families include elements of coercion, threats of separation, rigidity and recrimination, lack of mutual support, and the phenomenon of "pseudomutuality" in which individuals are forced to conform to family expectations in order to satisfy the need to stay together. The essential theme of these observations is that such interactions would make it difficult for a child to mature and to become an individual.

Though interesting, these observations are always made after the fact and might as easily be consequences of severe mental illness as causes. Furthermore, though psychoanalysts have suggested that problems around maternal-child relationships may have occurred early in the life history of schizophrenics, the data to support this idea are gathered retrospectively by observers deeply committed to a point of view. It may very well be impossible to study the problem prospectively. Other problems for psychosocial theories include the facts that many different forms of mental illness arise after similar early life experiences, and that among children exposed to very stressful and disorganized early lives, very few later become schizophrenic.

CLINICAL FEATURES Since the early descriptions of the syndrome, there has been a tendency to divide the symptoms of schizophrenia into the more central, important, or primary ones versus the lesser, associated, nonspecific, variable, or secondary ones. Bleuler suggested four important areas: (1) the loosening of associations leading to confusing, illogical, and peculiar use of language in communication of thought, (2) autism or withdrawal into subjective preoccupations and fantasy, (3) abnormal affect, with exaggeration, inconsistency, or inappropriateness, or, most often, flatness, blunting, or shallowness, and (4) ambivalence, or mixed (love-hate) simultaneous feelings. Schneider also emphasized the importance of immediate and sudden peculiar feelings or ideas ("primary delusions"), sometimes including frank auditory hallucinations, but more often odd and indefinable sensations, suspiciousness, and the experience of passivity feelings or of external control or influence.

Other general characteristics of schizophrenics include an overwhelming *lack of will, drive, enthusiasm,* and *assertiveness.* Also typical are oddness, incommunicativeness, vagueness, social withdrawal, extreme sensitivity, great preoccupation with thoughts, feelings, meanings, and symbols, and severe hypochondriasis. These phenomena are expressions of the psychoanalytic concept of *narcissism,*

Closely related is the so-called indefiniteness of ego boundaries, or the ability to be comfortable and secure in knowing "self" from "not-self," often reflected in the following subjective phenomena: *depersonalization,* the loss of certainty about what is real and not real, uncertainty of gender identity, ideas of reference (being talked about), passivity of feelings (being powerless and externally influenced or controlled), and feeling remote, isolated, or "numb." Psychoanalysts consider such phenomena to represent very early, primitive or infantile experiences and suggest that schizophrenics attain such mental states by "regression" to a lower or earlier level of function.

The *cognitive disorder* in schizophrenia, often designated as "primary-process" thinking, is quite different from that of dementias and deliriums. Thus schizophrenics, depending on their ability to cooperate with the examiner, have relatively intact formal intelligence which may even be quite high, although during acute states of disorganization the inability to attend and concentrate may lead to marked variability in performing psychologic tests. Orientation and memory are also not usually impaired. *Primary-process,* or primitive, thought of schizophrenia includes a general disregard for the logical limits of time and space, the confusion of parts for wholes, lumping and condensation of separate items, acceptance of identity of opposites, reversal and substitution of parts of a thought in an illogical way, and a variety of other distortions of conceptual relationships. These phenomena are exaggerations of mystical and magical thinking and may occur normally in dreams.

Schizophrenics are often very concrete and literal and lose the ability to think abstractly, to generalize, or to "get the point" of figurative statements, proverbs, and the like, and there is much difficulty in separating the relevant from the irrelevant. In conversation with a schizophrenic, an observer may only after some time be struck with the marked circumstantiality, tangentiality, and lack of communicability. Often, there is a tendency to be overinclusive, rather than to miss features of a stimulus, as might occur with a retarded, demented, or delirious patient. It is as if there were an inability to filter out or to select and sort incoming stimuli, or as if higher central nervous system centers were flooded with input. In this setting, it is quite common for blocking or abrupt interruption of the stream of conscious thought to occur, sometimes leading to overt perplexity and apparent "confusion," or in the extreme, mutism.

Schizophrenic thought disorder is manifest in speech, writing, and art, in all of which there are certain common characteristics. Again, combinations of excessive concreteness and symbolic, esoteric interpretations come to the foreground. The patient seems to have his own elaborate and consistent but autistic and idiosyncratic rules of logic and language. Language is often stiff, stilted, inflexible, repetitious, and even stereotyped. It becomes a means of self-expression rather than of communication. There is a cryptic, inscrutable, and strangely intriguing quality. Other features of schizophrenic language include neologisms and incoherent "word salad" in the most extreme form.

Usually *hallucinations* and more clearly formulated *delusions* are considered secondary symptoms. They are less specific to schizophrenia and vary greatly among patients. Auditory hallucinations are the most common, and they may include voices which are accusatory, obscene, or controlling. Other odd illusions or perceptual distortions may also occur, and occasionally, very bizarre and delusional notions about internal bodily states or functions are reported. Delusions and hallucinations are often considered to have a reactive quality and may represent attempts to cope with the distressing and peculiar states of feeling that precede them. Schizophrenic patients usually realize that such phenomena are "crazy" and may be reluctant to reveal them on casual examination.

Characteristic *behavioral changes* may include gross catatonic stupor, as well as mannerisms, automatisms and repetitious stereotypes, negativism, uncooperativeness, and sometimes impulsivity. In appearance, over a period of time, severe chronic schizophrenics tend to become deteriorated, thin, neglectful of their personal care and appearance and of social amenities, and may even become incontinent of urine and feces and may smear feces or openly masturbate. The extremities may be mottled and cyanotic, and the fingers may be densely stained from heavy smoking. Nevertheless, many of the characteristics of chronic patients are modifiable artifacts of prolonged institutionalization, isolation, boredom, and neglect.

SUBTYPES OF SCHIZOPHRENIA Among the classical types are the following:

Simple schizophrenia In contrast to a mere schizoid personality style, this diagnosis requires some evidence of a gradual downward course of social maladjustment, blandness, and apathy. The psychotic manifestations are rarely dramatic; such persons are often seen among hoboes and prostitutes and may not come to medical attention.

Hebephrenic schizophrenia One of the earliest described of the schizophrenic syndromes, it is perhaps the most malignant form, and usually leads to marked deterioration. Thinking is grossly disorganized and affect is shallow, inappropriate, unpredictable, silly, or fatuous. Mannerisms are frequent, and hypochondriasis is common. Florid symptoms are not usual, and delusions are usually fragmented and rather simple. Such patients are extremely inaccessible and often eventually require chronic institutional care.

Catatonic schizophrenia This is historically another very old syndrome and one of the most florid. In addition to thought disorder, there are striking anomalies of behavior. Excited and withdrawn forms are recognized. Thus, there may be either extreme excitement, restlessness, or even dangerous rages, or the more typical muteness, posturing, negativism, "waxy flexibility," or frank stupor, occurring despite a good deal of awareness of the surroundings. There may be echolalia, echopraxia, peculiar stereotyped mannerisms, grimacing, posturing, and frank catalepsy, although there is no evidence of organic disorder of the central nervous system. Such patients may be unpredictable, impulsive, and dangerous. Their management may constitute a medical emergency; they require careful attention during periods of anorexia and insomnia and may become dehydrated and exhausted. The occurrence of catatonia in the current American culture is relatively unusual. The course of the illness is variable, though tending toward chronicity or recurrence. Periodically recurrent forms (Gjessing's syndrome) occur rarely.

Paranoid schizophrenia This is the most common form of the illness at the present time in the United States. The personality often remains relatively intact, and premorbid adjustment is often quite good as well, partly since the illness tends to occur relatively later in life. Delusions and auditory hallucinations are the rule, in addition to more ordinary features of thought disorder. Typical characteristics are mistrust, hostility, suspiciousness, "touchiness," projection, coldness, aloofness, resentfulness, litigiousness, and ideas of reference. Delusions are usually persecutory, sometimes grandiose or religious, or, rarely, amorous; they are usually quite well organized, consistent, and pseudological, although in severely psychotic cases they may be more primitive and disorganized. Such patients may initially come to medical attention because of hypochondriasis.

There has always been a problem in classifying paranoid disorders. They are clearly very different from catatonic and hebephrenic cases; some of these patients manage to adjust quite well and can learn to conceal their delusions. The current practice is to separate certain paranoid disorders from the schizophrenias. Paranoid personalities and relatively transient reactive paranoid states are recognized. There is also a rare but venerable diagnosis of "paranoia," a form of psychosis with a single isolated delusional system and little else in the way of thought disorder, and there is the fairly common involutional paranoid psychosis of later life. Another exotic form of paranoid illness is *folie à deux*, or a shared delusion between two persons, usually intensely interdependent and relatively isolated, and sometimes with sadomasochistic behavior.

Acute schizophrenia These relatively time-limited episodes may occur as reactions to situational stresses; they have also been referred to as "acute undifferentiated," "atypical," "benign," or "psychogenic" schizophrenia. The diagnosis is relatively well accepted in this country, but abroad some psychiatrists question whether illnesses lacking a positive family history, apparent "endogenicity," and a relatively chronic and progressive course should be associated with the more classical forms of schizophrenia. On the other hand, the phenomenon of acute exacerbation in relatively stable schizophrenic patients is generally accepted, although in such cases it would be preferable to use one of the more classical diagnoses.

Latent schizophrenia This category, too, is difficult diagnostically and includes a somewhat vague group of syndromes peculiar to contemporary American psychiatry, with its tacit assumption that severe ego dysfunction is tantamount to actual psychotic illness or a strong potential for it. Included are the "ambulatory" or functionally compensated cases of schizophrenia, as well as "borderline" or "incipient" cases and the recently fashionable syndrome of polyneurosis and extreme anxiety called "pseudoneurotic" schizophrenia.

Residual schizophrenia This term refers to the condition of patients who have had more acute episodes of psychosis but who are not currently actively psychotic.

Chronic undifferentiated schizophrenia This widely accepted category is for those cases that do not readily fit into a more specific classification. In this or the "residual" category is included the condition of those patients who no longer seem to be actively struggling with psychotic turmoil and are said colloquially to be "burned out."

Schizoaffective schizophrenia This is another recently defined category and is probably overused. In principle, this syndrome should include cases with clear evidence of schizophrenic thought disorder but with strong affective elements of elation or depression. The diagnostic problem is to exclude cases of agitated or withdrawn schizophrenics of other types on the one hand, and manic-depressives or cases of psychotic depressive reaction on the other.

Childhood schizophrenia This concept is also very controversial outside the United States, but is commonly diagnosed here and includes a broad range of severe developmental and adjustment problems of children. Whether such disturbed children bear even superficial resemblance to adult schizophrenics or whether they become adult schizophrenics later are difficult questions to resolve since the term is used very loosely. Though psychotic illnesses certainly occur in children, great care is required to rule out organic brain syndromes, primary sensory disturbances (especially deafness), aphasia, mental retardation, and infantile autism (Kanner's syndrome).

CLINICAL COURSE Occasionally a chronic schizophrenic illness will apparently originate with an acute psychotic decompensation in a relatively intact and well-functioning personality, but often close examination will reveal a long history of maladjustment. Typically, the diagnosis of schizophrenia is first made in adolescence or early adulthood; a number of cases of "adolescent turmoil" are the start of a schizophrenic illness. Many psychiatrists are reluctant to make the diagnosis in younger patients. Though it is very unusual to find typical adult schizophrenics with a history of childhood psychosis, not infrequently such patients retrospectively were known to have been odd, difficult, distant, or neurotic as children, and for families to be perceived retrospectively as disorganized or as a source of stress. No single personality pattern is unique to schizophrenics, but the schizoid personality is common, and the patients may be described as having been cold, withdrawn, eccentric, sensitive, socially isolated, and solitary. Another pattern is the so-called "stormy" personality, with a history of instability, alternating aggression and submissiveness, and with many defiant, dyssocial characteristics. Paranoid schizophrenia is often preceded by a paranoid personality style, and such patients may have been suspicious, mistrustful, envious, disdainful, and irritable, though inwardly insecure and fearful. Marked obsessive-compulsive features are also common in most paranoid illnesses.

The prodrome of schizophrenia usually includes a series of neurotic complaints, especially hypochondriacal symptoms and increasing preoccupation with the self, followed by vague feelings that all is not well and that strange changes are taking place. Fear and anxiety may then escalate, leading to a sense of impending disaster or frank depersonalization. Thinking may be filled with grossly exaggerated adolescent themes, including meanings, principles, and abstract religious or philosophic preoccupations. Changes in basic drives are usual, with insomnia, anorexia, and loss of interest in sex and work. Most often these changes are seen without obvious precipitating stresses, although the general situation is usually that of increasing pressure to assume independent adult responsibility, and occasionally a loss, separation, disappointment, or physical illness may set off an acute break with reality. At this point features of thought disorder are usually present. It is important to realize that in early or acute phases of psychosis, patients are often extremely anxious and terrified, and have some insight into the fact that something is happening to them. Both homicide and suicide are very real problems, and the risk of suicide is often not adequately appreciated. Even though suicide *rates* may be higher among the psychotically depressed, there are probably more schizophrenic suicides than any other kind! Such suicides are often not predicted, and frequently occur among young adults, including college students, living in relative isolation or apart from their families. During such crises, there is often a pathologic sensitivity to rejection, and such "fragile egos" may respond to relatively slight and unintentional hurts from a friend, lover, teacher, nurse, or physician with profound dejection. Suicide may also represent a confused psychotic response to terror, to delusions, or to commanding hallucinated voices.

DIFFERENTIAL DIAGNOSIS The most typical cases will present little difficulty, particularly if one looks for the thought disorder, oddness, and narcissistic withdrawal in contrast to the dominant mood of sadness, hopelessness, or angry agitation in depressives, or the restless, pressured, hyperactive, intrusive, dysphoric elation in manics. Onset in youth, a preceding schizoid personality, and a positive family history also help to make the diagnosis of schizophrenia. In older patients, depressions, involutional psychoses, presenile dementias, and organic psychoses are the more common psychotic illnesses. Paranoid conditions may be difficult to diagnose accurately until the previous history and the outcome of the case are clearer. Paranoid symptoms per se are remarkably common and nonspecific; they occur in organic and toxic syndromes; they are very frequent in involutional psychoses; and they may even color depressive and manic illnesses. Toxic and metabolic psychoses may occasionally cause some diagnostic confusion (e.g., alcoholic auditory hallucinosis, Chap. 112). Also, some cases of porphyria may resemble schizophrenia, at least superficially. A useful generalization is that the majority of psychotic reactions for which psychiatric consultation is requested on general medical wards are organic, toxic confusional brain syndromes, including many iatrogenic drug reactions, which should readily be differentiated from schizophrenia by the clouded sensorium (see Chap. 26). Another current problem is posed by reactions to psychotomimetic drugs such as LSD and the methylated aromatic amines; furthermore, high doses of amphetamines, cocaine, other stimulants, and the marijuana alkaloids can produce some puzzling psychotic reactions resembling acute schizophrenia (see Chap. 114). Certain interictal epileptic states (including temporal lobe seizures) may also be troublesome unless a complete history is available (Chap. 24). In an earlier era, paretics and pellagrins caused some diagnostic problems. Another serious problem for physicians is that schizophrenics may present serious medical illnesses in very confusing and atypical ways.

OUTCOME The typical picture for classical schizophrenic psychoses is for a more or less acute illness, or possibly an insidious onset to evolve over months or years into a more chronic pattern, occasionally accentuated by more acute exacerbations. The chronic state is usually dominated by marked passivity and by poverty of ideation and motivation. There is a gradual cooling of fear, anger, and resentment, as well as a dulling or encapsulation of delusional thinking. The older term, *dementia praecox*, is somewhat misleading, as the mental defect is not so much in the sphere of formal intelligence or memory, but is rather a defect in the personality, with loss of feeling, motivation, volition, and the ability to take responsibility and to relate to others. Generally, life expectancy is somewhat reduced for chronic schizophrenics, even though the older picture of severe deterioration, malnutrition, neglect, and infection in public institutions is becoming uncommon. The current practices of maintaining chronic schizophrenics on neuroleptic medications and of early return to the community have produced increasing rates and durations of functional remissions. Spontaneous remissions also occur, particularly in the first year or two after an initial breakdown.

Since the mid-1950s, coincident with the introduction of the phenothiazines and newer methods of hospital care, the total population of schizophrenic patients in American public mental hospitals has been dropping steadily, at a rate of 1 to 2 percent (but up to 10 percent) per year, despite an even faster *rise* in the national population. Unfortunately, new admission and readmission rates have been increasing (the "revolving door" phenomenon), and the total numbers of very young and very old hospitalized schizophrenics have actually increased, partly because of problems of placement upon discharge. Furthermore, the rates of decline in numbers of hospitalized schizophrenics as a group have been slower than for other diagnostic categories.

Perhaps the most common picture today for chronic schizophrenics is one of recurring brief breakdowns and periods of more or less sustained adequate-to-marginal functional compensation. Complete "cures" are exceptional, although the current very loose use of the term "acute schizophrenic reaction" will include many patients with excellent prognoses whom traditionalists might not call schizophrenic at all. Many psychiatrists divide schizophrenia roughly into "process" and "reactive" types. Process schizophrenia corresponds to the classical Kraepelinian syndromes, with an insidious onset and a persistent chronic course in which social or functional recovery is rare; reactive types would include cases with a better prognosis. Better prognostic features include the lack of a family history, origin in a high social class, high intelligence, a good premorbid adjustment with some degree of social, educational, and occupational success, marriage, an ability to relate effectively and affectively with others, an athletic or plump physique, breakdown later in adult life, a relatively brief and acute illness, important situational stress as a precipitant to breakdown, a strong affective component to the psychosis, lack of bizarre delusions and hallucinations, lack of hebephrenic features, and lack of complicating problems such as secondary alcoholism or preexisting brain damage or epilepsy. That is to say, briefly, the "healthier" schizophrenics (or other psychotics) tend to have a more favorable outcome.

TREATMENT AND MANAGEMENT Although some physicians may find schizophrenic patients difficult to understand and to manage, it is often possible for a family physician or internist to manage selected patients quite efficiently, with or without assistance of a consulting psychiatrist. Indeed, a family physician may be in a unique position to support such patients and their families during periods of remission and rehabilitation. At times, because of severe psychotic decompensation, imminent risk of injury or suicide, or severe management problems in the community, hospitalization is necessary. Modern psychiatric in-patient management can often be handled very well in a general community hospital. Public psychiatric hospitals have changed greatly since the 1950s by adopting the principles and practices of milieu therapy. Very infrequently are locked doors, physical restraints, and the untoward consequences of chronic institutionalization necessary. The basic principles now accepted for most psychotic patients are to offer a flexible program of planned activities, physical treatments, vocational rehabilitation, and the involvement of the patient in the clinical unit as an important contributing member of it, along with the staff. The aim of hospitalization should be to foster self-esteem and to provide a structure that supports and clarifies reality and counteracts seclusiveness and institutionalization. Hospitalization can usually be quite brief, with a goal of early return to the community, family, or a protected after-care facility.

The essential feature of treatment has become neuroleptic medication in adequate dosage. These drugs have helped to revolutionize the modern management of schizophrenia. The original antipsychotic drugs were the *Rauwolfia* alkaloids and the phenothiazines, of which chlorpromazine (Thorazine) is still the most commonly prescribed. There are now several modifications of the original phenothiazines, including the piperazine derivatives, which are higher in milligram potency [e.g., trifluoperazine (Stelazine) and perphenazine (Trilafon)], as well as new types of molecules, including the thioxanthenes [e.g., chlorprothixene (Taractan)] and the butyrophenones [e.g., haloperidol (Haldol)]. These compounds are sometimes called "tranquilizers," but this is a misnomer, as it implies that they merely reduce anxiety, in the way that barbiturates or the benzodiazepines (e.g., Librium, Valium) do. The neuroleptic drugs are in fact relatively ineffective for neurotic anxiety and should not be used for that purpose. They appear to be uniquely antipsychotic medications and produce a variety of rather specific neurologic ("neuroleptic") effects as well. Thus, side effects include pseudo-Parkinsonism, acute and chronic ("tardive") dyskinesias, and motor restlessness (akathisia), as well as annoying atropine-like anticholinergic effects (e.g., dry mouth, blurred vision, decreased intestinal and bladder motility). Acute dystonias can be managed with parenteral antihistaminic drugs [e.g., diphenhydramine (Benadryl), 25 mg] or one of the anticholinergic drugs used in Parkinson's disease [e.g., benztropine (Cogentin), 2 mg]. The sustained use of anti-Parkinson drugs to avoid the extrapyramidal effects of the neuroleptic drugs is a very questionable practice, and in high doses they themselves can produce toxic psychoses. The tardive dyskinesias are quite common among chronically medicated schizophrenics, and neuroleptic drugs may suppress the symptoms so that these very difficult and persistent reactions may be overlooked. Other side effects include postural hypotension and, less commonly, transient cholestatic jaundice and skin rashes, as well as blood dyscrasias, which, while unpredictable and catastrophic, are rare. Addiction and tolerance do not occur with these drugs, and they can be used safely for several years. Their turnover rates are slow, so that most or all of a day's dose of the less potent phenothiazines may be given at bedtime to help deal with insomnia and to avoid excessive daytime sedation. The barbiturates, other sedatives, and so-called "minor tranquilizers" really have no place in the treatment of schizophrenia; they are impotent and many are potentially toxic and addicting. Doses of neuroleptic drugs should be individualized, but usually the required daily oral antipsychotic doses range from 300 or 400 mg, up to 1,000 mg or more of chlorpromazine, or an equivalent dose of another drug of this type. These drugs are also effective in managing affective and even organic psychoses, and are of value for various types of paranoid patients as well.

Reserpine in high doses (up to 5 or 10 mg a day) is still occasionally used when other medications are ineffective or toxic. Electroconvulsive treatment (ECT) is sometimes used, although its general efficacy is somewhat questionable; it may have a place in dealing with very stuporous or agitated catatonics or in patients with a serious affective disturbance, in whom it might be lifesaving; it may also have some legitimate use in severe cases responding poorly to medications.

Other physical treatments are largely of historical interest. Insulin coma therapy is difficult, dangerous, and no longer generally employed in this country. Prefrontal lobotomy has little to offer except in very rare cases. Even in its more modern selective leukoablation variants, which are still in the experimental stage, psychosurgery should be reserved for the most extremely unmanageable cases and should be used then only as a last resort. Other treatments, including prolonged sleep, narcosis, or delirium induced by drugs or frequent ECT, are measures of desperation and are currently rarely employed.

From time to time, the chronic and poorly understood nature of schizophrenia has led to unfortunate therapeutic fads and misleading claims, and sometimes to extreme measures taken to assist desperate and uncritical families of chronic schizophrenic patients. There have been recent claims that massive doses of vitamins C or B, and particularly of nicotinic acid, may be of some benefit. There is no compelling scientifically acceptable evidence that such treatments are effective, and their long-term safety is not established. At the present time, the only generally recognized means of physical treatment with scientifically demonstrated efficacy and relative safety are the neuroleptic drugs.

The contributions of dynamic and psychoanalytic psychiatry to the *understanding* of the schizophrenic condition have been important, and a few highly motivated psychotherapists have devoted their lives to the psychologic management of such patients, with some success. Nevertheless, as a general rule, psychotherapy has relatively little to offer as a primary mode of *treatment* for severe schizophrenics and may be contraindicated if analytic or "uncovering" techniques are used. On the other hand, active supportive psychotherapy has much to offer. The general strategy is to attempt to assist the patient in maintaining a grasp on reality and to strengthen psychologic defenses. Special problems with such severely disabled, dependent, and sometimes too fascinating patients include their exploitation for selfish reasons, overinvolvement, the risk of becoming callously domineering or of being put off by their strangeness or fearing their openness and often terrifying honesty. The goal is to be understanding and accepting but also firm and professional, without being either rejecting or too quick to gratify unreasonable demands.

In summary, while much is unknown about the nature and etiology of the schizophrenias, some cautious optimism is justified in that modern pharmacotherapy and rehabilitation methods can help to improve the level of function and to hasten and support remissions.

REFERENCES

ARIETI S: *Interpretation of Schizophrenia*, New York: R. Brunner, 1955

ARTISS KL: *Milieu Therapy in Schizophrenia*, New York: Grune & Stratton, 1962

BELLAK L, LOEB L (eds): *The Schizophrenic Syndrome*, New York: Grune & Stratton, 1969

BLEULER E: *Dementia Praecox or the Group of Schizophrenias*, New York: International Universities Press, Inc., 1950

FREEDMAN AM, KAPLAN H (eds): *Comprehensive Textbook of Psychiatry*, Baltimore: Williams & Wilkins, 1967

GRUENBERG, EM (ed): *Diagnostic and Statistical Manual of Mental Disorders* (DSM-II), Washington: American Psychiatric Association, 1968

HILL LB: *Psychotherapeutic Intervention in Schizophrenia*, Chicago: The University of Chicago Press, 1955

KRAEPELIN E: *Dementia Praecox*, London: E and S Livingstone, 1918

ROSENTHAL D, KETY SS (eds): *The Transmission of Schizophrenia*, Oxford: Pergamon, 1968

SEARLES HJ: *Collected Papers on Schizophrenia*, New York: International Universities Press, Inc., 1965

SLATER E, ROTH M: Mayer Gross' *Clinical Psychiatry*, Baltimore: Williams & Wilkins, 1969

SOLOMON P, PATCH VD: *Handbook of Psychiatry*, Los Altos, Calif.: Lange Medical Publications, 1971

SULLIVAN HS: *Schizophrenia as a Human Process*, New York: Norton, 1962

WYATT R et al: Biochemical and sleep studies in schizophrenia: A review of the literature—1960–1970. Schizophrenia Bull 4:10, 1972

section 12 | Diseases of striated muscle

343 CLINICAL MYOLOGY AND CLASSIFICATION OF MUSCLE DISEASES

JEAN REBEIZ
MARIA Z. SALAM
RAYMOND D. ADAMS

The muscle fiber has been more thoroughly studied than any other cell of the human or animal body, but until comparatively recent times little had been learned of the diseases to which it is subject. However, clinicians, pathologists, and biochemists are now beginning to concentrate on the conditions which impair its function and imperil its survival, and even in the period of time which has elapsed since the last edition of this book, several monographs devoted exclusively to diseases of muscle have appeared.

GENERAL CONSIDERATIONS The striated muscle tissue constitutes the principal organ of locomotion as well as a vast metabolic reservoir. Disposed in more than 600 separate muscles, this tissue comprises as much as 40 percent of the weight of adult man. Intricacy of structure undoubtedly accounts for its diverse susceptibilities to disease, and for this reason reference to the following anatomic characteristics provides an appropriate introduction to this chapter.

A single muscle is composed of thousands of fibers which course for variable distances along its longitudinal axis. Some fibers extend the entire length of the muscle; others are joined end to end by connective tissue. Each fiber is a relatively large and complex multinucleated cell varying in length from a few millimeters to several centimeters (34 cm in the human sartorius muscle) and in diameter from 10 to 100 μm. Although the fiber represents an indivisible anatomic and physiologic unit, disease may affect only one part of it, leaving the remainder to atrophy, degenerate, or regenerate depending on the nature and severity of the disease. The nuclei of each cell, which are oriented parallel to the longitudinal axis of the fiber and number into the thousands, lie beneath the cytoplasmic membrane (true sarcolemma) and hence are called "sarcolemmal." The cytoplasm (sarcoplasm) of the cell is abundant and contains myofibrils and various other organelles such as mitochondria, microsomes, and endoplasmic reticulum. The myofibrils in turn are composed of longitudinally oriented interdigitating filaments (myofilaments) of contractile proteins (actin and myosin). Droplets of stored fat, glycogen, various proteins, many enzymes, and myoglobin, the latter imparting the red color to muscle, have been identified within the sarcoplasm or its organelles.

The individual muscle fibers are enveloped by delicate strands of connective tissue (endomysium) which provide for their support and permit unity of action. The blood vessels, of which there may be several for each fiber, and nerve filaments lie within the endomysium. Similar reticular tissue and sheets of collagen (perimysium) bind together groups or fascicles of fibers and surround the entire muscle (epimysium). These latter connective tissue tunics are also richly and variably vascularized, different types of muscle having different arrangements of arteries and veins; and fat cells (lipocytes) are embedded within the interstices. The muscle fibers are attached at their ends to tendon fibers, which in turn connect with the skeleton. By this means contraction maintains posture and effects movement.

Other notable characteristics of muscle are its natural mode of activation, i.e., innervation, by nerve and the necessity of intact nerve supply for the maintenance of its nutrition. Each muscle fiber receives a nerve twig from a motor nerve cell in the anterior horn of the spinal cord or nucleus of a cranial nerve, which joins it at a point called the neuromuscular junction (also called motor end-plate). And, as was pointed out in Chap. 17, groups of muscle fibers with a common innervation from one anterior horn cell constitute the "motor unit" which is the basic physiologic unit in all reflex, postural, and voluntary activity. Acetylcholine and cholinesterase, which play a special role in neuromuscular transmission, are concentrated at this junction zone. In addition to the motor nerves there are two types of sensory receptors (proprioceptors), the muscle spindles and Golgi tendon organs, which participate in reflexes; and finally there are free nerve endings which subserve pain sensation.

It would be a mistake to predicate that apparent similarity of structure renders all muscles equally susceptible to disease. In point of fact, no disease affects all muscles in the body and each disease has as one of its features a unique topography within the musculature. These topographic differences between diseases provide incontrovertible evidence of unique structural qualities, not presently disclosed by the light microscope. One factor may relate simply to fiber size. Consider, for example, the large diameter and length of the fibers of the glutei and paravertebral muscles in comparison with the ocular muscles. Again, the number of fibers composing a motor unit may be of significance in explaining selective vulnerability; e.g., in the ocular muscles they contain only 6 to 10 muscle fibers, whereas in the gastrocnemius, as many as 1,800 fibers. Allusion has already been made to individual differences in vascular patterns of supply, permitting some muscles to withstand the effects of hypoxia or vascular occlusion better than others. Subtle metabolic differences between fibers within any one muscle have been revealed by enzyme studies, certain fibers being richer in glycolytic and poorer in oxidative enzymes than others. Doubtless other differences will be discovered.

These anatomic and biochemical qualities inform us of some of the possibilities of pathogenesis of myopathic disease. Thus, one may envisage causative agents which affect each of the different components of sarcoplasm, namely, an enzyme, an essential substrate, the filamentous proteins, the endoplasmic reticulum, or the sarcolemma itself. Again, the endomysial connective tissue could be the primary pathway in disease, since it so closely invests the muscle. Inadequacy of blood supply in relation to the metabolic requirement of oxygen by active muscle, or frank ischemia from vascular occlusion could be postulated as another mechanism of disease. Finally, the nerve or its cell of origin in the spinal cord is known to bear the brunt of certain pathologic processes paralyzing all the fibers of the respective muscle and causing it to reflect the unique trophic influence of nerve on muscle.

Normal muscle possesses a limited capacity to regenerate, a point often forgotten. Acute destructive processes of the muscle fiber, e.g., inflammatory, metabolic, and certain other diseases, are usually followed by fairly complete restoration of the muscle cells, providing some part of each fiber has survived and the endomysial sheaths of connective tissue have not been disturbed. Unfortunately many pathologic processes of muscle are chronic and unrelenting and destroy completely the muscle fibers. Under such conditions any regenerative activity fails to keep pace with the disease, and the loss of muscle fibers is permanent.

PRINCIPLES OF MYOPATHOLOGY OF MUSCLE CONTRACTION

Several basic disorders (see below) may be distinguished in biopsy material from patients with neuromuscular diseases, and the procedure of muscle biopsy is in common usage in most medical centers.

1 Degeneration atrophy: reduction in size of fibers in motor units, with enlargement of intact units (collateral regeneration of nerves) and delayed degenerative changes in some fibers. This typical change in all peripheral nerve and spinal cord diseases is particularly well shown in histochemical stains for ATPase, phosphorylase, and oxidases, where the pattern of fiber types is altered.

2 Segmental necrosis of muscle fibers with myophagia, regeneration, and forking or branching. This is the typical change in idiopathic polymyositis (in combination with infiltrates of inflammatory cells), in infective polymyositis (in the presence of trichina, toxoplasma, etc.), in Zenker's degeneration, in Meyer-Betz paroxysmal myoglobinuria, in Duchenne's and other dystrophies, and in alcoholic polymyopathy.

3 Disfigurative changes of muscle fibers: sarcoplasmic masses and ringbinden in myotonic dystrophy, glycogen masses in glycogen storage diseases, rod (nemeline) and other cytoplasmic bodies in the congenital myopathies, aggregation and other abnormalities of mitochondria. Here histochemical stains for fiber typing and electron microscopy have been useful adjuncts.

4 Disturbances in number and size of fibers as a reflection of abnormalities of growth, maturation, and aging. Many states of dwarfism, congenital myopathies of a myotubular type, show principally as numerical or volumetric changes, which must be distinguished from denervation, disuse effects, cachexia, and work hypertrophy.

5 Disorders of conduction apparatus (neuromuscular junctions, sarcolemma, and sarcoplasmic reticulum), in which nerve fibers and muscle fibers appear to be intact and the abnormality can be revealed only by special techniques such as the methylene blue staining of nerve twigs (Cöers and Wolff), Kolle stain of cholinesterase, and electron microscopy of neuromuscular junctions. Myasthenia gravis, botulism, the periodic paralyses, states of spasm, and contracture fall into this category.

Further details of pathology will be presented with the descriptions of specific muscle diseases.

BIOCHEMISTRY OF MUSCLE CONTRACTIONS

(See Chap. 344)

CLINICAL MANIFESTATIONS OF MUSCLE DISEASE (CLINICAL MYOLOGY)

It would appear that the large number and diversity of diseases of striated muscle exceed the number of symptoms and signs by which they express themselves clinically. Different diseases thus must share certain common symptoms and even syndromes. To avoid excessive repetition in the description of individual diseases there is some advantage to discussing in one place all the clinical manifestations, a subject which we propose to call *clinical myology*.

WEAKNESS AND PARALYSIS Reduced strength of contraction, reflected in diminished power of single contractions [peak or power factor (*PF*) in performance] or of repeated contractions [endurance factor (*EF*)], stands as the indubitable sign of muscle disease. Fatigability per se less reliably denotes muscle affection, since it is most often due to some psychic aberration linked to anxiety and depression or to systemic illness (see Chap. 15). It is noteworthy that slight weakness of muscle may be present, even though tests of *PF*, because of crudeness of clinical measurement, lack of quantitation, and the uncertainty of gaining the patient's full cooperation, may seem to reveal no definite diminution in power. Theoretically, with milder degrees of weakness, a diminution in *EF* elicited in a series of timed contractions against a fixed resistance (ergogram) may more reliably demonstrate the disorder than does *PF*. Furthermore, sustained or repeated maximal muscle contraction over a given period of time evinces optimally the myasthenic reaction, i.e., a rapid failure of contraction, with the power being restored within minutes by rest. This, in fact, in combination with a restoration of power, i.e., disappearance of the myasthenic state, by neostigmine and edrophonium (Tensilon) and a worsening of it by small doses of curare (see Chap. 347), stands as the most valid diagnostic criterion of the various forms of myasthenia gravis.

Qualitative changes in the contractile process In addition, there are other qualities of muscular contraction and relaxation that may be discovered by observing, during one or a series of maximal actions of a group of muscles, the speed and efficiency of contraction and relaxation. Slow waves of contraction in a muscle such as the quadriceps may be seen on change in posture (contraction myoedema) in hypothyroidism. Here it is often associated with percussion myoedema and slowness of tendon reflex. Slowness in relaxation is another indication of a thyroid deficiency state, accounting for the complaints of uncomfortable tightness and firmness of proximal limb muscles.

A prolonged failure of relaxation with after-discharge is a characteristic of myotonia, as in the diseases congenital myotonia (of Thomsen) and dystrophic myotonia (of Steinert). But a true myotonia, with its long electrical discharges of action potentials, unlike the electrically silent myoedema and contracture (see below), requires strong contraction for its elicitation, is more evident after a period of relaxation, and tends to disappear with repeated contractions (see Chap. 344). This persistence of contraction is demonstrable upon tapping a muscle (percussion myotonia), a phenomenon easily distinguished from the electrically silent local bulge (myoedema) induced by a sharp tap of a muscle in the myxedematous or cachectic patient.

Increase in power in a series of several voluntary contractions in the absence of myotonia is a feature of the inverse myasthenic syndrome of small-cell carcinoma of the lung. It, too, has its electromyographic equivalent—a rapid increase in the voltage of a series of action potentials (see Chap. 344).

The effect of cold on muscle contraction may also prove informative; either paresis or myotonia, lasting for a few minutes, may be evoked or enhanced by cold as in the paramyotonia of von Eulenberg.

Myotonia and myoedema must be distinguished from the recruitment and spread of involuntary spasm induced by strong and repeated contractions of limb muscles in patients with mild or *localized tetanus*, which is not a phenomenon of muscle but is due to an abolition of inhibitory spinal mechanisms.

The repeated contraction of forearm and leg muscles after the application of a tourniquet (above arterial pressure) to the proximal part of a limb will often elicit latent tetany. The latter state must be separated from ordinary cramp by its special mode of development, duration, its enhancement by hyperventilation, the presence of accompanying tingling, prickling paresthesias, and also from true contracture.

In *true contracture* a group of muscles, after a series of strong contractions, may remain shortened for many minutes, unable to relax because of failure of the metabolic mechanism necessary for relaxation; and the muscle in this shortened state remains electrically silent in the electromyogram, in contrast to the tremendous high-voltage, rapid discharges observed with cramp, tetanus, and tetany. Such contracture occurs in McArdle's phosphorylase deficiency, where it is aggravated by arterial occlusion, but it has been seen in phosphofructokinase deficiency and possibly in another disease, as yet undefined, where the tourniquet has no effect and phosphorylase seems to be present in adequate amounts, at least as judged by histochemical stains (see Chap. 104).

Pseudocontracture (myostatic contracture) which inevitably follows all conditions which occasion prolonged fixation and complete inactivity of the normally innervated muscle, is another common disorder. But here the shortened state of the muscle, which may persist for days or weeks, has no established anatomic, physiologic, or chemical basis. It is distinguished from *ankylosis* by the springy nature of the resistance coincident with increased tautness of muscle and tendon during passive motion, and from *Volkmann's contracture*, where there is evident fibrosis of muscle and the surrounding tissues due to ischemic injury, usually after a fracture of the forearm.

Topography of paralysis: patterns of paralysis As we stated above, in the majority of the diseases under consideration, some of the muscles are affected and others are spared. Each disease exhibits its own pattern. Moreover, the topography or distribution of involvement tends to follow the same pattern in all patients with the same disease. Thus, determination of the topography of muscular involvement becomes another of the most valid diagnostic attributes of a disease, ranking next in importance after altered quantity and quality of contraction.

To ascertain the extent and severity of muscle weakness requires a systematic examination of all the main groups of muscles from forehead to feet. The patient is asked to contract each group quickly with as much force as he can muster, while the examiner opposes the movement and offers a graded resistance in accordance with the degree of residual power. If the weakness is unilateral one has the advantage of being able to compare it with the action of muscles on the normal side. If it is bilateral, the physician must refer to his idea of what constitutes normalcy, based on experience in muscle testing. Ocular, facial, lingual, pharyngeal, laryngeal, cervical, shoulder, upper arm, lower arm and hand, truncal, pelvic, thigh, and lower leg-foot muscles are examined quickly in this order. To facilitate description and comparison a rating scale must be used. Five graded steps, from normal power to paralysis, are readily distinguishable: 5 = normal power; 4 = barely detectable weakness; 3 = moderate weakness; 2 = severe weakness with ability to overcome gravity and slight resistance; 1 = trace of movement if gravity and opposition are removed; 0 = no movement. With practice one can distinguish pseudoparalysis from pain, unwillingness to cooperate, and feigned weakness (see Chap. 17).

The following topographic patterns are so well known that they constitute a core of essential clinical knowledge in this field.

1 *Ocular palsies presenting more or less exclusively as diplopia, ptosis,* or *strabismus*, sometimes in association with exophthalmos, enophthalmos, and pupillary change.

As a rule muscle diseases do not affect the pupil, and in most instances their effects are bilateral. In single-nerve lesions the neural origin is revealed by the combination of paralyses of eye muscles or sympathetic paralysis of the pupil. When weakness of the orbicularis oculi muscle (muscle of eye closure) is added to ocular palsies and ptosis, it nearly always signifies myopathic disease.

Myasthenia gravis, progressive ocular dystrophy of Kiloh and Nevin, exophthalmic ophthalmoplegia of thyroid disease, curare-sensitive nonmyasthenic ophthalmoplegias, myotonic dystrophy of Steinert, ocular dystrophy (with retinitis pigmentosa, heart block, dwarfism and ovarian dysgenesis, myotubular myopathy) and botulism are the principal conditions to be considered. When ptosis or weakness of eye closure occurs alone or in combination with weakness of other skeletal muscles, one should think of Landouzy-Dejerine facioscapulohumeral dystrophy and oculopharyngeal dystrophy and the nemeline form of congenital myopathy.

2 *Bifacial palsy presenting as an inability to smile and expose teeth and to close eyes.* Mild bifacial weakness is observed in myasthenia gravis, and ptosis and ocular palsies are usually conjoined (90 percent of cases) in this disease. The same is true of myotonic dystrophy. More severe or complete facial palsy occurs in facioscapulohumeral dystrophy, in Landry-Guillain-Barré syndrome (nearly always with other weaknesses), and in combination with abducens palsies in the Moebius syndrome. Sometimes polyneuritis cranialis multiplex causes bilateral facial paralysis.

3 *Bulbar palsy presenting as dysphonia, dysarthria, and dysphagia with or without a hanging jaw or facial weakness.* Myasthenia gravis is the most frequent cause of this syndrome and must also be considered whenever there is the solitary finding of a hanging jaw or fatigue of jaws while eating or talking; but usually ptosis and ocular palsies are conjoined (>90 percent of cases). The same is true of myotonic dystrophy and botulism. Progressive bulbar palsy of upper or lower neuron type (or both) may be the basis of this syndrome, and the diagnosis is most obvious when the tongue is withered and twitching. The neurologic condition known as pseudobulbar palsy is readily distinguished by the lack of atrophy of muscle, the mode of onset (usually sudden), and the associated clinical findings. Platybasia and the Arnold-Chiari malformation may also reproduce some of these findings by involving the lower cranial nerves and their nuclei. Diphtheria and bulbar poliomyelitis are often diseases that may present in this way. Pure dysphonia and dysphagia may be early manifestations of polymyositis.

4 *Cervical palsy presenting often as the hanging-head syndrome, or inability to lift the head from the pillow.* The patient may be unable to hold up his head owing to weakness of the posterior neck muscles, or to lift it from a pillow because of weakness of the anterior neck muscles. If this condition is severe, the head may loll unless it is held up by the patient's hands.

This condition occurs most often in idiopathic polymyositis or dermatomyositis. It tends to be combined with slight dysphagia and dysphonia. The major types of progressive muscular dystrophy, when advanced, usually weaken neck flexors and extensors, but seldom to the point where the head must be held in the hands. Rarely syringomyelia, syphilitic meningoradiculitis, subacute poliomyelitis (in conjunction with carcinomatosis), and motor system disease (Kugelberg-Welander syndrome) may differentially paralyze the neck muscles.

5 *Bibrachial palsy presenting sometimes as the dangling-arm syndrome.* Weakness, atrophy, and fasciculations of hands and arms and sometimes of the shoulders characterize the commonest syndrome of motor system disease, namely, amyotrophic lateral sclerosis. Primary muscle disease hardly ever selects these parts or weakens them disproportionately to other muscles. Rarely, a diffuse arm weakness may

also occur early in acute idiopathic polyneuritis and porphyric polyneuropathy, but it soon becomes part of a more generalized paralysis.

6 *Bicrural palsy presenting as lower leg weakness with floppy feet and inability to walk on the heels and toes, or as paralysis of all leg and thigh muscles.* In lower leg weakness, polyneuropathy is the usual explanation, although peroneal and anterior tibial muscles are often weakened in dystrophy. Diabetic polyneuropathy may weaken thigh and pelvic muscles asymmetrically with little sensory change. In total leg and thigh weakness, one first thinks of a disease of the spinal cord, and then there is often loss of control of the bladder and bowel sphincters, as well as loss of sensory function below a certain level. Motor system disease may also begin in these parts and affect them out of proportion to others. Thus the differential diagnosis of patterns of leg weakness involves more diseases than do the restricted paralyses of other parts of the body.

7 *Limb-girdle palsies presenting as inability to raise the arms or to arise from a squatting, kneeling, or sitting position.* Two groups of diseases most often manifest themselves in this fashion—poly- and dermatomyositis and the progressive muscular dystrophies. The Duchenne type and Leyden-Moebius variant tend first to affect the muscles of the pelvic girdle and lumbar region, resulting in a waddling gait, difficulty in arising from the floor, in climbing stairs without the assistance of the arms, lumbar lordosis, and protuberant abdomen. The Landouzy-Dejerine type affects muscles of face and shoulder girdles foremost, and is manifested by incomplete eye closure, pouting lips, inability to raise the arms above the head, winging of the scapulae, and thinness of the upper arms (Popeye appearance). The lower parts of the deltoid and at times the biceps and brachioradialis may be relatively spared. In polymyositis, weakness may be limited to either neck muscles or those of the shoulder or pelvic girdles, but sometimes it involves all muscles, including distal ones as well, whereas the muscles of the face and eyes are spared (except in rare instances where there is an associated myasthenia gravis). It is the milder form of polymyositis that causes weakness of either shoulder and neck or of the pelvic girdle alone, and, similarly, it is the early or mild forms of dystrophy that may selectively involve only the peroneal and scapular muscles (scapuloperoneal dystrophy). A metabolic myopathy, such as the adult form of acid-maltase deficiency or late hypokalemic dystrophy, may affect only the pelvic and thigh muscles. Unfortunately, proximal muscles are occasionally implicated in progressive spinal muscular atrophy, as in the syndrome first described by Kugelberg and Welander, which adds to confusion in diagnosis.

8 *Distal limb palsies presenting usually as foot drop, with steppage gain (and pes cavus), weakness of all lower leg muscles, and later wrist drop and weakness of hand grips (claw hand).* The principal cause of this neuromuscular syndrome is a familial polyneuropathy, such as the peroneal muscular atrophy of Charcot-Marie-Tooth, hypertrophic polyneuropathy of Dejerine and Sottas, and the hereditary polyneuropathy of Refsum. Chronic nonfamilial polyneuropathies may also present in this fashion. But once more, there are exceptions, such as some forms of familial progressive muscular atrophy and distal types of progressive muscular dystrophy (Gowers, Welander). Steinert's myotonic dystrophy also weakens peroneal and posterior tibial muscles as well as those of the forearm, sternomastoid, face, and eyes. Despite these exceptions, the principle that girdle weakness means myopathy and distal weakness neuropathy holds firm.

9 *Generalized or universal paralyses: limb and cranial muscles—involved either in attacks or in persistent, progressive deterioration.* When acute in onset and episodic, this syndrome is usually traceable to an electrolyte imbalance, as in familial hypokalemic or normokalemic periodic paralysis. One variety of the former type is associated with hyperthyroidism. A paresis, rather than paralysis of acute onset that lasts many weeks, is a feature of a peculiar disease called paroxysmal myoglobinuria of Meyer-Betz, and at times of a severe form of idiopathic or parasitic polymyositis (trichinosis) as well. Polymyositis of the idiopathic type may involve all limb and trunk muscles but usually spares the facial and ocular muscles, and trichinosis causes only mild ocular and lingual weakness. In children a chronic and persistent generalized weakness of all muscles except those of the eyes always raises the question of the Werdnig-Hoffmann infantile muscular atrophy or, if it is in lesser degree, of one of the relatively nonprogressive congenital myopathies or polyneuropathy. In all these diseases, paucity of movement, hypotonia, and retardation of motor development may be more obvious in the infant than weakness.

Universal ascending paralysis, developing over a few days, with involvement of cranial (including ocular) muscles, is usually due to the idiopathic polyneuritis of Landry-Guillain-Barré. Slow onset and progression of paralysis, atrophy, and fasciculation of limb and trunk muscles, without sensory loss, over months to years characterizes motor system disease. Mild degrees of generalized weakness are features of a number of metabolic myopathies, such as thyrotoxic myopathy, glycogen storage disease, vitamin D deficiency, rickets, etc.

10 *Paralysis of single muscles or a group of muscles.* This is almost always neuropathic, or rarely spinal. Muscle disease does not need to be considered except possibly in its earliest stages, and then the weakness is always mild.

From this exposition of the topographic aspects of weakness one can appreciate that each neuromuscular disease exhibits a certain predilection for particular groups of muscles. As a corollary of this—a given pattern of weakness always suggests certain possibilities of disease and excludes others.

Diagnosis depends also on features of the paralysis other than its topography, such as mode of onset and duration, the coexistence of medical disorders, and certain laboratory findings (serum enzymes, creatine-creatinine excretion, electromyogram, and biopsy findings). Consideration should also be given to other of the differentiating features, such as the natural course of the diseases in question, age of onset, and its genetic determinations.

VOLUMETRIC CHANGES IN MUSCLE Altered volume of muscular mass stands as another feature of disease which may be evidenced in all except the most obese patient. There are, of course, innate differences in muscle development, a greater salience of muscle in the male than in the female, and differences due to use and disuse. Greatly increased size and strength of muscles (hypertrophia musculorum vera) may be observed in *congenital myotonia* (circus freaks with phenomenal muscular development often have this disease), in rare instances of a pathologic cramp syndrome, in some patients destined to develop muscular dystrophy, and in deLange's syndrome of congenital athetosis with feeblemindedness. Muscle enlargement in progressive muscular dystrophy more often takes the form of pseudohypertrophy, where increased size is accompanied by weakness. Here large and small fibers are mixed with fat cells which have replaced many of the degenerated muscle fibers. Other muscles are atrophied in the same patient. Cachexia, malnutrition, and lipodystrophy tend to reduce muscle bulk without significantly reducing power of contraction (pseudoatrophy). Denervation due to lesions of the peripheral nerve or spinal cord, which if complete leads to a loss of bulk up to 75 percent of the original volume within 3 months, is invariably attended by paralysis. The most severe degrees of atrophy usually signify denervation or dystrophy.

TWITCHES, SPASMS, CRAMPS, AND CONTRACTURE Fascicular twitches during rest, if pronounced and combined with muscular weakness and atrophy, usually signify motor neuron disease (amyotrophic lateral sclerosis, progressive muscular atrophy, or progressive bulbar palsy); but they may be seen in lesser degree in other diseases of gray matter of the spinal cord (e.g., syringomyelia or tumor), in lesions of anterior roots (e.g., ruptured intervertebral disk), and in peripheral neuropathies. Widespread fascicular twitches spreading in a wavelike pattern along the entire length of a muscle with associated weakness progressing to complete flaccid paralysis within minutes form the striking clinical picture of organic phosphate insecticide poisoning. The same sequence evolving at a slightly slower pace may occur in poliomyelitis. Fasciculations during contraction indicate, instead, a state in which the muscle is excessively irritable, often for reasons that are not known, or in a condition which leaves muscle with some paralyzed motor units, so that during contraction small and large units are not enlisted smoothly. One may observe this latter phenomenon years after a poliomyelitis has left a muscle weakened. *Benign fasciculations*, a common finding in otherwise normal individuals, can usually be distinguished by the lack of muscular weakness and atrophy; and *myokymia* is a rare form of the condition in which innumerable twitchings impart a rippling appearance to the muscle.

Cramps at rest or with movement (action cramps) are frequently reported in motor system disease, tetany, and dehydration after excessive sweating and salt loss and other metabolic diseases (uremia, hypocalcemia, and hypomagnesemia), but there is a benign form (idiopathic cramp syndrome), in which no other neuromuscular disturbance can be found. One form of it is known as *myokemia with persistent spasm.* A particularly malignant and progressive form of painful spasm is known as the *stiff man syndrome;* this appears to be an obscure disease of the central nervous system. Continuous spasm, with no demonstrable disorder of a neuromuscular level, intensified by the action of muscles, is a common manifestation of tetanus and also follows the bite of the black widow spider.

PALPABLE ABNORMALITIES OF MUSCLE Altered structure and function of muscle are not accurately revealed by palpation. Of course, the difference between the firm hypertrophied muscle of a well-conditioned athlete and the slack muscle of a sedentary person is as apparent to the palpating finger as to the eye. And the persistent contraction in myxedema, contracture, tetanus, cramp, etc., is easily felt. In muscular dystrophy the muscles are said to have a "doughy" or "elastic" feel, but this is difficult to judge. In the Pompé type of glycogen storage disease attention may be attracted to the musculature by an unnatural firmness and increase in bulk. The swollen, edematous weak muscles in acute paroxysmal myoglobinuria or severe polymyositis may feel taut and firm but are usually not tender. Areas of tenseness in muscles which otherwise function normally, a state called *myogelosis*, may be found in patients with fibrositis or fibromyositis, and their nature has not been divulged by biopsy.

A mass developing in one part of a muscle, or throughout a muscle, poses a special clinical problem. It may, if chronic, be a tumor (rhabdomyosarcoma, angioma, metastatic carcinoma, or desmoid) or a granulomatous inflammation (sarcoid, tuberculoma, or mycosis). Hard masses are usually calcium (myocalcinosis) or bone deposit (myositis ossificans). If a muscle mass develops rapidly, hemorrhage, either spontaneous or traumatic, must be considered. A ruptured tendon may take this form but always causes a bulge which, for obvious reasons, becomes manifest on contraction, and the muscle exhibits a diminished power of contraction.

TENDON (STRETCH) REFLEXES The tendon reflexes are altered in the majority of muscle diseases, particularly those which involve peripheral nerves. In muscular dystrophy and polymyositis they tend to be reduced in proportion to the reduction in muscular power. In the myopathy of hypothyroidism, in which the contractile process is slowed, there is a characteristic prolongation of the tendon reflex, and the opposite condition of quickening and brevity of the tendon reflex is less reliably demonstrated in hyperthyroidism.

MUSCLE PAIN Pain localized to a group of muscles is extremely severe in wry neck, fibrositis and fibromyositis, acute brachial neuritis, radiculitis, Bornholm's disease, or pleurodynia, but little is known of its cause in any of these diseases. In contrast, the established forms of muscle disease, even the most serious ones such as polymyositis, are usually painless. In the latter condition, if pain is present, it usually indicates coincident involvement of connective tissues and joint structures. Tenderness of muscle is a variable state normally, and it tends to be more definite in polyneuritis, poliomyelitis, and polyarteritis nodosa than in polymyositis and in the various forms of dystrophy and other myopathies in which there is usually no increase in the sensitivity of muscle tissue.

TABLE 343-1
Syndromic classification of muscle diseases

- *I* Acute (days) or subacute (weeks) paralytic disorders of muscle (may cause weakness or paralysis)
  - *A* Primary diseases of muscle
    - *1* Rarely fulminant myasthenia gravis
    - *2* Polymyositis and dermatomyositis
    - *3* Alcoholic polymyopathy
    - *4* Acute paroxysmal myoglobinuria (*Note*: first attack of episodic weakness may enter into differential diagnosis; see below)
    - *5* Botulism
    - *6* Organophosphate poisoning

      See also acute spinal or peripheral nerve diseases (denervation paralysis where paralysis is often severe and widespread and atrophy may or may not be present)
      - *a* Poliomyelitis
      - *b* Acute idiopathic polyneuritis, or other forms of polyneuropathy (porphyria, beriberi, etc.)
      - *c* Rarely polyarteritis nodosa with polyneuropathy and other neuropathy
- *II* Chronic (i.e., months to years) paralytic disorders of muscle (weakness usually with severe atrophy)
  - *A* Progressive muscular dystrophy
    - *1* Duchenne type
    - *2* Facioscapulohumeral type (Landouzy-Dejerine)
    - *3* Limb girdle type (Erb's)
    - *4* Distal type (Gowers', Welander's)
    - *5* Myotonic dystrophy (Steinert's disease)
    - *6* Progressive ophthalmoplegic or oculopharyngeal types
  - *B* Chronic polymyositis

    See also the progressive muscular atrophies and other forms of motor system disease (amyotrophic lateral sclerosis, progressive bulbar palsy) and infantile muscular atrophy (Werdnig-Hoffman disease), as well as chronic neural muscular atrophies such as peroneal muscular atrophy (Charcot-Marie-Tooth), hypertrophic polyneuritis (Dejerine-Sottas), amyloid polyneuropathy, chronic nutritional, arsenical, leprous, and other polyneuropathy
  - *C* Chronic thyrotoxic and other myopathies
  - *D* Chronic slowly progressive or relatively stationary polymyopathies
    - *1* Central core disease
    - *2* Rod body and related polymyopathies
    - *3* Pleoconial, megaconial and myotubular polymyopathies
    - *4* Glycogen storage disease
    - *5* Congenital benign hypotonia and congenital universal hypoplasia of muscle
- *III* Episodic weakness of muscle
  - *A* Myasthenia gravis
  - *B* Symptomatic myasthenia of other types
    - *1* With lupus erythematosus disseminatus
    - *2* With polymyositis
    - *3* With rheumatoid arthritis
    - *4* With nonthymic carcinoma
  - *C* Familial periodic paralysis
  - *D* Hereditary adynamia [normokalemic periodic paralysis (Gamstorp's)]
  - *E* Paramyotonia congenita (von Eulenberg's)
  - *F* Hyper- and hypokalemia (including primary hyperaldosteronism)
  - *G* Acute thyrotoxic myopathy (also thyrotoxic periodic paralysis)
- *IV* Stiffness, soreness, involuntary spasm, and cramp
  - *A* Congenital myotonia (Thomsen's disease), paramyotonia congenita, and myotonic dystrophy
  - *B* Tetanus
  - *C* Tetany
  - *D* Black widow spider bite
  - *E* Hypothyroidism with pseudomyotonia (Debré-Semelaigne and Hoffman syndromes)
  - *F* Myopathy resulting from myophosphorylase deficiency (McArdle's syndrome) and other forms of contracture
  - *G* Contracture with Addison's disease
  - *H* Idiopathic cramp syndrome
- *V* Myalgic states
  - *A* Connective tissue diseases (rheumatoid arthritis, menopausal arthritis, lupus erythematosus, polyarteritis nodosa, scleroderma, polymyositis)
  - *B* Localized fibrositis or fibromyositis
  - *C* Many forms of polyneuritis
  - *D* Trichinosis
  - *E* Myopathy of myoglobinuria and McArdle's syndrome
  - *F* Myopathy with hypoglycemia
  - *G* Bornholm's disease
  - *H* Anterior tibial syndrome
- *VI* Localized muscle mass(es)
  - *A* Rupture of a muscle
  - *B* Muscle hemorrhage
  - *C* Muscle tumor
    - *1* Rhabdomyosarcoma
    - *2* Desmoid
    - *3* Angioma
    - *4* Metastatic nodules
  - *D* Localized idiopathic myopathy
  - *E* Localized and generalized myositis ossificans
  - *F* Fibrositis (myogelosis)
  - *G* Granulomatous infections
    - *1* Sarcoidosis
    - *2* Tuberculosis
  - *H* Pyogenic abscess

DIAGNOSIS OF MUSCLE DISEASE

These various clinical phenomena, along with certain laboratory data including muscle biopsy, when integrated with information concerning the natural course of the pathologic process, enable one to diagnose relatively easily most of the diseases of muscle.

The clinical recognition of myopathic diseases is facilitated, as a rule, by a prior knowledge of a few syndromes. The following ones recur with regularity, and their identification and proper analysis in terms of common underlying diseases are indicated. Diagnostic accuracy will be aided by an intelligent use of the laboratory methods described in Chap. 344.

We have grouped in Table 343-1 all the common diseases around their manifest syndromes.

REFERENCE

ADAMS RD: Principles of myology and myopathology (Thayer Lectures). Johns Hopkins Med J 131:24, 1972

344 LABORATORY AIDS IN DIAGNOSIS OF NEUROMUSCULAR DISEASE

ROBERT R. YOUNG
LEONARD W. JARCHO
JACK H. PETAJAN

Clinical suspicion of neuromuscular disease now finds ready confirmation in the laboratory. Absolute proof of diagnosis, however, is rarely forthcoming from this source. All laboratory data must be evaluated in the light of clinical findings based on broad knowledge of muscle disease.

BIOPHYSICS AND BIOCHEMISTRY OF NEUROMUSCULAR DISEASE

The biochemical tests presently in use fall into two categories: measurement of serum electrolytes and enzymes and detection of myoglobin and abnormal amounts of creatine and creatinine in the urine. Current research on sarcoplasm promises even more valuable microchemical analysis of bits of muscle taken at biopsy.

ELECTROLYTES AND THEIR EFFECTS ON NEUROMUSCULAR EXCITABILITY The concentration of electrolytes and their fluxes in relation to neuromuscular activity are now known to be the basis of the electrical events of impulse conduction along nerve and muscle fiber.

In the resting state all nerve and muscle fibers are *polarized* with the interior of the cell negative to the outside surface by a potential difference of 70 to 90 mV. This *resting membrane potential* is closely related to the electrochemical equilibrium for potassium ions, the interior of the cell being some thirty times richer in this ion than the extracellular fluid on the other side of the nerve or muscle membrane. At equilibrium, the chemical forces tending to promote diffusion of K ions outward (down their concentration gradient) are counterbalanced by electrical forces, since the relative external positivity opposes the movement of further K ions to the outside. At the resting potential, the situation for Na ions is quite the opposite. Since their external concentration is ten to twelve times that within the cell, they tend to be driven inward because of both their concentration gradient and the electrical attraction of the relative negativity inside the cell. Under resting conditions, however, these forces are ineffective by virtue of the very low permeability of the sarcolemma to Na ions. Any leakage of Na into the cell is overcome, initially by the diffusion of an equal amount of K outward, and subsequently by the metabolically active expulsion of Na ions (*sodium pump*).

The membrane permeability to Na is controlled by the membrane potential—depolarization producing increased permeability to Na. With slight electrically or chemically mediated depolarization there is a brief influx of Na, but the subsequent diffusion of K outward repolarizes the membrane and, therefore, reduces its permeability to Na. This is "passive decay" of change in resting potential. If, when the depolarization is greater and a *threshold* is reached at which the outward K current is unable to stabilize the situation, the membrane is further depolarized, it becomes progressively more permeable to Na, and an explosive *regenerative Na current* develops (positive feedback). Na rushes down its chemical and electrical gradients into the cell, eventually reaching the equilibrium potential for Na with the interior of the cell now 40 mV or so positive. This *action potential* lasts a millisecond or less because the membrane now becomes almost impermeable to Na and much more permeable to K. The resulting efflux of K repolarizes it to the resting level.

The regenerative Na current cannot be activated by another depolarizing stimulus during the *refractory period* until the membrane has been repolarized. If this process of recovery is delayed, *depolarization inactivation* prevents the development of further action potentials until the resting membrane potential has been restored. These various membrane phenomena responsible for the resting and action potentials do not themselves depend directly upon energy-rich substrates, though such metabolically active processes are essential for the sodium pump and the long-term maintenance of resting ionic concentrations.

When, at the site of the action potential, one region of membrane becomes polarized oppositely to the remainder, *action currents* flow into the former from the surrounding regions and depolarize the latter. The depolarization may reach the threshold for development of an action potential there, and the new zone of increased Na permeability then spreads in this way in an all-or-none fashion down the length of the nerve or muscle membrane as a *conducted action potential.*

Clearly, these events, the hallmarks of all excitable tissues, are modified by the concentration of K ions in extracellular fluids. Other ions, particularly Ca, Mg, and Cl, are also influential.

The *neuromuscular junction* (motor end plate) has

properties of special importance. Here a terminal motor nerve twig indents the surface of the muscle fiber which it innervates. The membranes of the two cells, the neurilemma and the sarcolemma, remain separated by a narrow space, the *synaptic cleft.* Across this space acetylcholine diffuses, liberated from presynaptic vesicles in the terminal nerve filaments by the arrival of the *nerve action potential.* Ca ions facilitate the release of packets (*quanta*) of acetylcholine from the vesicles, whereas botulinus toxin or a very high concentration of Mg ions interferes with this release. The specialized, chemically excitable area of muscle membrane which forms the postsynaptic portion of the end plate reacts to the presence of acetylcholine by local increase in conductance of Na, K, and other small cations, producing a depolarization which can be recorded as the *end plate potential.* If this shunt across the membrane is large enough, current flowing into it from the neighboring electrically excitable areas of muscle membrane depolarize them. If the threshold is reached, an independent, all-or-nothing *muscle action potential* arises and, in the same manner as the nerve action potential is conducted, propagates over the surface of the sarcolemma toward both ends of the fiber. The electrical change appears to be distributed from the surface of the muscle fiber inward to all the myofibrils via the transverse tubular sarcoplasmic reticulum (T system) to activate the contractile mechanism. Calcium is released from the depolarized membrane of this endoplasmic reticulum into the sarcoplasm, activates myosin adenosine triphosphatase (ATPase), energy is released by the dephosphorylation of adenosine triphosphate (ATP), cross-bridges form between the actin and myosin filaments, and they slide past one another producing tension. In resting muscle, actin exists as filaments to which tropomyosin is attached at regular intervals. Interaction between troponin and Ca somehow releases myosin to interact with actin. The resultant shortening occurs in each sarcomere and constitutes the ultrastructural equivalent of contraction (*excitation-contraction coupling*). This mechanical change or *twitch* lasts a great deal longer than the action potential. A second electrical wave can, therefore, arrive before the muscle fiber has relaxed, prolonging the contraction, and if the anterior horn cell fires (or the motor axon is stimulated) at frequencies of 10 to 20 per sec, the twitches fuse into a prolonged contraction (tetanus). The mechanical event can thus be smoothed into a continuous process, but the electrical potentials remain a series of peaks of external negativity, separated by plateaus during part of which the membrane is in its resting polarized state. This *repolarization* after passage of an action potential is necessary if the membrane is to be capable of transmitting a second impulse. At the end plate, repolarization is possible only if acetylcholine is removed, a process achieved by the enzyme cholinesterase. If this fails, the end plate remains depolarized and cannot respond to further nerve impulses. *Anticholinesterases* such as neostigmine (Prostigmin), pyridostigmine (Mestinon), edrophonium (Tensilon), physostigmine (Eserine), diisopropyl fluorophosphate (DFP), tetraethylpyrophosphate (TEPP), and several of the "nerve gases" and pyrophosphate insecticides act in this way to paralyze muscle. These substances and the so-called *depolarizing blocking agents* (succinylcholine and decamethonium) paralyze by maintaining the end plate region in a depolarized state (depolarization inactivation) refractory to the arrival of further nerve impulses. Curare-like substances including most of the quaternary ammonium ions, the so-called "competitive blocking agents," paralyze muscle in a different way by occupying receptor sites for acetylcholine at the end plate, thereby preventing it from depolarizing the muscle fiber.

Biochemical disturbances may account not only for impairment of neuromuscular activity, resulting in weakness or paralysis, but also for its enhancement, reflected in excessive irritability. In the latter case, "spontaneous" discharges may occur, or a single nerve impulse may set off a train of action potentials in nerve or muscle. Hypocalcemic (and hypomagnesemic) *tetany* ensues in this way when the membrane of the nerve fiber becomes unstable. Ca and Mg both tend to stabilize the membrane, and changes in their concentrations within the range seen clinically affect conduction in peripheral nerve rather than function at the neuromuscular junction where their actions are opposite or competitive but require changes in concentrations usually incompatible with life. Ischemic paresthesias also arise on the basis of neurolemmal irritability. The common cramps of calf and foot muscles (painful, sustained, involuntary contractions with motor unit discharges at frequencies up to 200 per sec) may in part be due to increased excitability of the peripheral parts of the motor nerve. Hyponatremia or Na loss predisposes to cramps, as does the unaccustomed use of a muscle. Quinine, procainamide, diphenhydramine (Benadryl), and warmth tend to prevent them.

The manner in which the muscle action potential may initiate the contractile process has been discussed. The energy for this process is derived from the interaction of ATP with the special muscle proteins, actin and myosin. The change in shape of these protein molecules results in shortening with increased tension within the myofilaments and hence the myofibrils and whole fiber. The pyrophosphate bonds of ATP supply the energy for this process, and they must be replenished constantly, a reaction which involves interchanges with the muscle phosphogen, creatine diphosphate, where high-energy phosphate bonds are stored. These interchanges in both directions require the action of creatine phosphokinase (CPK). Myoglobin, another important muscle protein, plays a part in the transfer of oxygen, and a series of oxidative enzymes is involved in this exchange. The intracellular calcium which, as noted above, is released by the muscle action potential must be reaccumulated within the sarcoplasmic reticulum before actin and myosin filaments can slide back past one another with relaxation. This re-uptake of calcium (*relaxing factor*) requires the expenditure of considerable energy. When ATP is lacking, the muscle remains contracted as in *rigor mortis* or the electrically silent *contracture* of phosphorylase deficiency (McArdle's syndrome). The same sort of contracture occurs under normal conditions in the "catch muscles" of certain mollusks.

Many glycolytic and other enzymes (transaminases, aldolase, creatine phosphokinase) are also implicated in the metabolic activity of muscle, particularly under relatively anaerobic circumstances. Muscle fibers differ in their content of oxidative versus glycolytic enzymes; the latter determine their ability to sustain anaerobic metabolism during periods of contraction when blood flow is compromised. Muscle cells with primarily aerobic metabolism have high concentrations of oxidative enzymes, are rich in mitochondria, contain greater concentrations of myoglobin (appear red), have slower rates of contraction and relaxation, fire more tonically, and are less fatigable than muscle cells poor in oxidative enzymes and myoglobin ("white") but rich in glycolytic enzymes, which fire phasically in short bursts. The speed of contraction, a function of the amount of myosin ATPase activity (number of myofibrils), is low in the former and high in the latter type of muscle cell. The calcium-activated myosin ATPase at pH 9.4 has been used to classify muscle fibers into two major types: type I possesses low and type II high activity. All the muscle fibers within one motor unit are of the same metabolic type.

To summarize, the muscle fiber, which is totally dependent on nerve for its stimulus to normal contraction, may be paralyzed in a number of ways. There may be failure of nerve to conduct an impulse, insufficiency of acetylcholine to depolarize the muscle cell, inaccessibility of the motor end plate to normally released acetylcholine because of the presence of a competing substance, or excess of a depolarizing substance, preventing repolarization of the end plate. Finally, the sarcolemmal membrane itself may fail to distribute the muscle impulse throughout the fiber, or the metabolic or contractile elements of the muscle may be temporarily or permanently deficient. Similarly, fascicular twitching, cramps, and muscle spasms may be due to excessive activity at a number of points in the neuromuscular apparatus. There may be unstable polarization of the nerve fiber, as in tetany, or unexplained hyperirritability of the motor neuron, as in amyotrophic lateral sclerosis. The threshold level for mechanical activation or electrical reactivation of the sarcolemmal membrane may be reduced, as with myotonia, or a change may occur within the muscle fiber itself, which, once shortened, may have insufficient energy for restoration to a relaxed state (contracture).

When the musculature is acutely and diffusely weakened, or when twitchings, spasms, and cramps occur, serum electrolytes should be studied. They reflect extracellular levels, and the ECG (see Chap. 229) may betray alterations in intracellular content in cardiac muscle, which tend to parallel those in skeletal muscle. If the plasma level of *potassium falls below 2.5 mEq or rises above 7 mEq per liter*, weakness of extremity and trunk muscles results. When the concentration reaches 2 mEq or 9 mEq per liter, there is almost invariably flaccid paralysis of these muscles and later of the respiratory ones as well, only those of cranium, e.g., extraocular, tending to be spared. In addition, the tendon reflexes are diminished or absent. The reaction of muscle to percussion is also reduced or abolished, suggesting impairment of transmission along the sarcolemmal membranes themselves. *Hypocalcemia* of 7 mg per 100 ml or less (as in rickets or hypoparathyroidism) or relative reduction in the proportion of ionized calcium (as in hyperventilation) causes increased irritability and spontaneous discharge of sensory and motor nerve fibers, i.e., *tetany* (see Chap. 348) and sometimes convulsions. Frequent repetitive and finally prolonged spontaneous discharges appear in the electromyogram (EMG). *Hypercalcemia* above 12 mg per 100 ml (as in vitamin D intoxication, hyperparathyroidism, and carcinomatosis) causes lethargy and weakness, perhaps on a central basis. *Reduction in the plasma concentration of magnesium* results in tetanic muscle spasms and convulsions; a considerable *increase in magnesium levels* leads to muscle weakness and depression of central nervous function (confusion). The weakness of muscle may be due, in part at least, to reduced release of acetylcholine at the motor end plate.

CHANGES IN THE SERUM LEVELS OF ENZYMES ORIGINATING IN THE MUSCLE CELLS In all diseases which cause extensive damage to striated muscle fibers, intracellular enzymes leak out of the fiber and enter the blood. Those which are now being measured in most hospital laboratories are the transaminases, lactic acid dehydrogenase, aldolase, and creatine phosphokinase. But, as is noted in Chap. 292, high concentrations of these enzymes are found in heart muscle and/or liver cells; hence raised serum values may be due to myocardial infarction or hepatitis, as well as to the necrobiotic diseases of striated muscle (polymyositis, muscle trauma, muscle infarction, Meyer-Betz paroxysmal myoglobinuria, and the more rapidly advancing muscular dystrophies). For the serum levels to be interpretable, one must have evidence of the integrity of heart and liver. Creatine phosphokinase (CPK), though present in heart and brain, is found in highest concentration in striated muscle. If the normal level is 0 to 65 IU per liter of serum, it may exceed 1,000 IU in patients with destructive lesions of striated muscle. Even more interesting is its rise in some patients with progressive muscular dystrophy before there is enough destruction of fibers for the disease to be clinically manifest, at least as judged by random biopsies. Moreover, the unaffected female carriers of Duchenne's pseudohypertrophic form may now be identified because they often show slight elevations of serum CPK level. All workers are agreed that alterations of serum enzyme levels are nonspecific for dystrophy since they occur in all types of disease which destroy the muscle fiber. Moreover, in the more slowly evolving types of dystrophy, such as that of Landouzy-Déjerine, the serum levels of CPK may be normal. It would be expected that the values would always be normal in denervation paralysis and muscular atrophy, but unfortunately they may be slightly elevated in some patients with progressive muscular atrophy and amyotrophic lateral sclerosis.

ENDOCRINOPATHIES In a number of disorders of endocrine glands, muscle weakness may be a prominent feature, and occasionally it becomes even a chief complaint. While these diseases are discussed in detail elsewhere (Chaps. 347 and 348), it should be noted that such weakness, local or generalized, acute or chronic, may occur in the absence of changes in serum electrolytes or enzymes. Specific hormone assays are then necessary for diagnosis. This is particularly true of thyrotoxicosis, where severe muscle paresis may appear without the classic signs of Graves' disease.

MYOGLOBINURIA The red pigment, myoglobin, responsible for much of the color of muscle, is an iron-protein compound present in the sarcoplasm of striated skeletal and cardiac fibers. Of the total body hematin compounds, about 25 percent is in muscle, the remainder in red corpuscles and other cells. Destruction of striated muscle, regardless of the process, liberates myoglobin, and because of its relatively small size, the molecule filters through the glomerulus and appears in the urine, imparting to it a burgundy-red color. The serum is effectively cleared and retains its normal color. In contrast, hemolysis of red corpuscles frees hemoglobin, coloring both serum and urine because of the high renal threshold. Myoglobinuria should thus be suspected when the urine is deep red and the serum normal in color. As in hemoglobinuria, the guaiac and benzidine tests are positive, and the final demonstration depends on spectroscopic analysis, which shows an absorption band at 581 nm. The urine does not fluoresce, as it does in porphyria. Myoglobin appears in the urine in the following conditions: spontaneous myoglobinuria of unknown cause, e.g., Meyer-Betz paroxysmal myoglobinuria; as a result of crushing or infarction of muscles; in rare cases of polymyositis and alcoholic and other myopathies such as McArdle's disease; following extreme muscular activity; and after the ingestion of certain toxic substances (from fish poisoned by waste products, as in Haff disease).

CREATINURIA Creatine, an amino acid, is a prominent constituent of striated muscle tissue. It may be ingested (exogenous creatine) but is also synthesized in the liver from glycine, arginine, and methionine and then delivered to the skeletal muscles, which contain the largest amount of this compound of any organ (150 mg per 100 g fresh weight muscle tissue). Creatinine, the anhydride of creatine, is a degradation product which is excreted in the urine. The creatinine content of muscles is low (about 5 mg per 100 ml), since it diffuses readily through the sarcolemma. Normal male serum contains 0.2 to 0.6 mg per 100 ml creatine; female serum 0.4 to 0.9 mg. Creatinine serum levels range from 0.8 to 1.4 mg and are increased only in serious renal disease. Adult 24-hr urine excretion of creatine averages from 60 to 150 mg in normal men and 100 to 300 mg in women. Creatinine excretion is remarkably constant at 1.0 to 1.6 g per day. In diseases such as progressive muscular dystrophy, the creatine content of the muscle fiber is diminished, and there is a decrease in creatinine excretion, increase in creatine excretion, and hypercreatinemia. The same alterations occur in neurogenic atrophy and with reduction in muscle mass in polymyositis, hyperthyroidism, Addison's disease, and male eunuchoidism. Ingestion of 1 to 3 g creatine will not significantly raise its level in blood or urine in a normal person, for his muscles are not saturated, but in an individual with a reduced muscle mass, creatinemia and creatinuria result. This type of creatine tolerance test thus merely indicates reduction in functional muscle mass.

PHYSIOLOGY OF NEUROMUSCULAR ACTIVITY

Electromyography

It was discovered long ago that muscle responds to pulses of current, especially if applied to the motor point where the nerve enters. Normally, a twitch can be produced by a brief pulse, less than 1 msec long (faradic) which stimulates motor nerve fibers within the muscle. After denervation, contraction can be produced only by much longer pulses (galvanic) which are necessary to stimulate the muscle fibers directly. This difference (Erb's reaction of degeneration) led to the plotting of strength-duration curves, a technique which is rarely necessary now.

Functional organization of movement was clarified by Sherrington, who introduced the most important concept of the *motor unit*: a motor neuron, its axon, and all the muscle fibers which it innervates. All movement, posture, and reflex activity are now interpreted in terms of the organization and integration of large numbers of these motor units by spinal and supraspinal mechanisms. Strength of muscle contraction can be reduced to the number of motor units enlisted at a given time and the frequency of their discharge, and the speed of contraction to the rate of recruitment of phasic versus tonic units. A tendon reflex is caused by a volley of sensory impulses from receptors within muscle spindles which briefly activate a group of the large (alpha) spinal motoneurons. Effectiveness of movement is related to the manner in which motor units of different muscles are activated and inhibited in reciprocal relations. Coordination of movements, posture, and automatic movements such as walking and running are understandable in terms of more complex spinal integrations of muscles. Paralysis represents the reverse, an inactivation of motor units or whole muscles, complete only upon severance of the peripheral motor innervation and followed then by extreme atrophy of muscle fibers with fibrillation and unusual sensitivity to acetylcholine.

Unlike the heart, which can be sampled effectively from a relatively limited number of fixed electrode positions, the striated muscles, on the other hand, are numerous, scattered, and, in some instances, of large size. As a result, no small series of leads will give an average picture of their electrical activity. They must be tested laboriously, one at a time, because disease may be spread irregularly through many of them, so that normal findings in one area do not exclude the possibility of pathologic phenomena close by. External plate or surface electrodes, such as those used in electrocardiography and electroencephalography, will pick up potentials representing the chance summation of many motor units, giving only an average picture. A more detailed physiologic analysis requires needle electrodes, which register the activity of only a small number of motor units or muscle fibers.

Concentric needle electrodes, 0.3 to 0.8 mm in diameter, in which recordings are made between the tip of a thin wire in the lumen and the shaft of the hypodermic needle, are to be recommended for ease of comparison and reproducibility. The needles are positioned within the muscle so that maximal recordings are made of the potentials under observation. This implies that one or more active muscle fibers lie near the central or "active" recording electrode, whereas the shaft of the needle is in contact over most of its length with a pool of tissue fluid and a great many muscle fibers, forming an "indifferent" or reference electrode.

As an impulse travels down the active muscle fiber, current begins to flow outward through the normally polarized region under the recording electrode toward the depolarized zone. Therefore, as in Fig. 344-1, the recording electrode becomes positive relative to the reference electrode, and the beam of the cathode ray oscilloscope (CRO) is deflected, by convention, downward (at *A*). When the depolarized region moves under the recording electrode, the latter rapidly becomes quite negative (upward deflection at *B*). As the active region moves further down the sarcolemma, away from the electrode, the membrane under the latter slowly becomes repolarized. Current again begins to flow outward through the membrane toward the distant depolarized region, and the electrode, therefore, becomes relatively positive once again, as at *C*, before becoming isopotential to the

FIGURE 344–1

The shaded area represents the zone of the action potential which is negative to all other points on the fiber surface. It is shown at three points in its course (from left to right) along the fiber. At each point, the correspondingly lettered portion of the triphasic muscle action potential displayed on the cathode ray oscilloscope (CRO) reflects the potential difference between the active (vertical arrow) and reference (Ref.) electrodes. Polarity in this and subsequent figures is negative upward as depicted. The time calibration is on the CRO screen; for further details see the text.

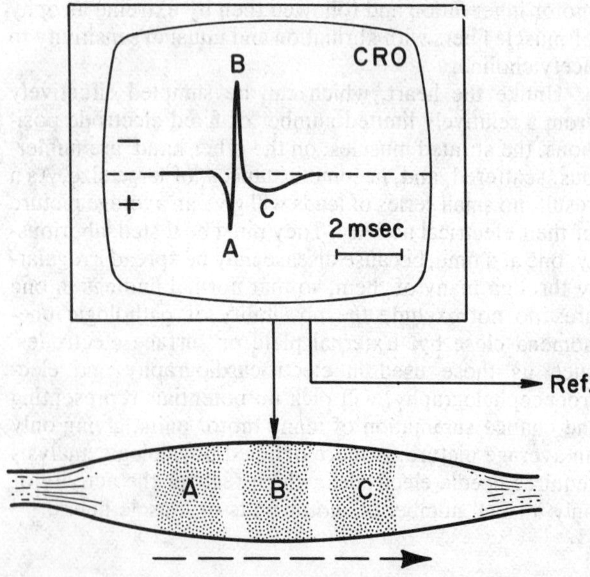

reference electrode at rest. The net result is a triphasic action potential recorded on the CRO as in Fig. 344-1, with a very rapid negative-going phase, a configuration typical of fibrillations recorded from denervated and spontaneously active single muscle fibers. Because these potential changes are completed in less than 5 msec, the inertia-free CRO must be used to record them (ink writers do not have the necessary frequency response).

RECORDING OF MOTOR UNIT ACTIVITY The simple triphasic potentials discussed above result from the activity of single muscle fibers, but in healthy muscle, single fibers do not act alone. Normally, excitation arrives via the motor nerves so that all the fibers of one motor unit are activated by any one impulse from a motoneuron (as indicated in Chap. 17). The size of the normal motor unit varies from several muscle fibers per motor axon in extraocular or laryngeal muscles to several thousand muscle fibers per axon in some of the large limb-girdle muscles. In these motor units, which are the smallest fraction of the muscle under central nervous system control, the fibers are not of uniform diameter, length, or shape, and their spatial orientation with regard to the electrode will vary. In normal muscle, the fibers of one motor unit are not packed tightly together in groups but are spread out in one general region of the muscle interspersed with the fibers of adjacent motor units. Such muscle activated by its nerve, therefore, produces rather complex motor unit potentials, presumably the result of summation of potentials of varying characteristics from each fiber of that motor unit within recording range of the electrode.

THE NORMAL ELECTROMYOGRAM Normal muscle is electrically silent when it is at rest. Once *insertion activity*, produced by the trauma of placing the needle, has died down, the electrodes record no propagated action potentials. When a muscle is voluntarily contracted, action potentials appear on the CRO screen. Slowly graded contraction allows one to observe the manner in which force normally builds up (Fig. 344-2*A*). As contraction begins, potentials of one motor unit appear at rates of 4 to 5 per sec and increase to 8 or 10 per sec; with increasing power of contraction, a second, or even third, unit will be *recruited*, slightly larger in size than the first. In still stronger contractions more and larger motor units enter the picture, and their potentials begin to overlie each other until there results a disorderly crowd of action potentials of many sizes and shapes, firing at rates of 20 to 30 per sec. Since individual motor unit potentials can no longer be distinguished, this is referred to as a complete *interference pattern*. The maximal amplitude is many millivolts. Obviously, a muscle contracting weakly because of less than full effort or disease of central or peripheral nervous or muscular systems will have fewer than normal active fibers and will produce a smaller total potential than normal. However, unless reduction in output is sufficient either to break up the interference pattern just described so that individual motor unit potentials become identifiable or to reduce its amplitude strikingly, one obtains no certain electrical evidence of abnormality. As long as a normal muscle is held actively contracted, the interference pattern continues. Gradual relaxation will show a progressive dropping out of motor units until only a few are left firing, then one, then none.

Skeletal muscle may also be artificially stimulated by the application of brief electric pulses to the skin overlying its motor nerve. With proper stimulating conditions, there will be one maximal muscle response for each shock, the form of which will depend upon the number of motor units activated and the number sampled by the recording electrodes. If repeated shocks are given, each response will have the same form and amplitude, until fatigue supervenes. Normal muscle will follow rates of stimulation greater than 25 per sec for periods of at least 60 sec before decrement of the action potential indicates the failure of some fibers to respond, probably because of failure of nerve impulse transmission at branching points of the terminal axon. This ability of muscle to follow repetitive stimulation is altered in certain diseases.

THE ABNORMAL ELECTROMYOGRAM Deviations from normal are detected in (1) the appearance of excessive irritability upon insertion of the recording needle; (2) the occurrence of "spontaneous" activity during relaxation (fibrillation, positive sharp wave, and fasciculation); (3) abnormalities in the amplitude, duration, and shape of single-motor-unit potentials; (4) a decrease in the number of motor units which can be recruited; (5) alteration in size and duration of action potentials recorded during graded single or successive voluntary or electrically induced muscular contractions; and (6) the demonstration of special phenomena, such as myotonia, coupling (tetany), bizarre high-frequency potentials, or electrical silence during obvious shortening of the muscle (contracture).

"Spontaneous activity" during complete relaxation At the moment the needle is placed in the muscle, there is usually a brief burst of action potentials which cease once the needle is stable, providing it is not in a position to irritate an intramuscular nerve fiber. Myotonic muscle is extremely irritable; long runs of high-frequency discharges, waxing and waning in frequency with a "dive-bomber" sound, may be produced and recur at the slightest movement of the needle. Irritability is also found with conditions which dispose to muscle cramp and in certain denervated muscles. Spontaneous activity of motor units and of single muscle fibers, known respectively as fasciculation and fibrillation, is abnormal.

FIBRILLATION The two phenomena of fibrillation and fasciculation are often confused with each other. Fasciculation, discussed below, consists of synchronous contraction of *groups of muscle fibers* integrated by a single axon into a motor unit. Fibrillation is the contraction of *single muscle fibers* and appears only when destruction of a motor axon has disintegrated its motor unit.

When a motor neuron is destroyed by disease, or when its axon is severed, the distal part of the axon degenerates, a process which takes several days. The muscle fibers formerly innervated by the branches of the dead axon, viz., the motor unit, are disconnected from the nervous system. For reasons which are still obscure, the chemosensitive region of the sarcolemma at the motor end plate "spreads" after denervation to involve the entire surface of the muscle fiber. Then, 10 to 25 days after death of the axon, the denervated fibers develop spontaneous activity, similar perhaps to that found in the sinoatrial (SA) node of the heart; i.e., even while no effort is being made by the patient to contract the muscle, each fiber contracts at its own rate and without relation to the activity of its fellows. There results a totally random conglomeration of brief, triphasic potentials (Fig. 344-3*A*). Fibrillation potentials have a duration of 1 to 5 msec, are di- or triphasic, the initial phase being positive, and rarely exceed 300 μV in amplitude, but with much smaller ones recorded from fibers relatively distant from the electrodes. When brief, spontaneous potentials of this sort are observed at two or three different locations outside

FIGURE 344–2
Patterns of motor unit recruitment. A *Normal. Note that with each successive increment of voluntary effort, more and larger units are brought into play until, with full effort at the extreme right, a complete "interference pattern" is seen in which single units are no longer recognizable.* B *After denervation, only a single motor unit is recorded despite maximal effort. It is seen to fire repetitively.* C *With myopathic diseases, a normal number of units is recruited, though the amplitude of the pattern is reduced from normal, and the maximum tension produced is quite deficient. Calibrations: 50 msec (horizontal) and 1 mV in* A *and* B, *200 μV in* C.

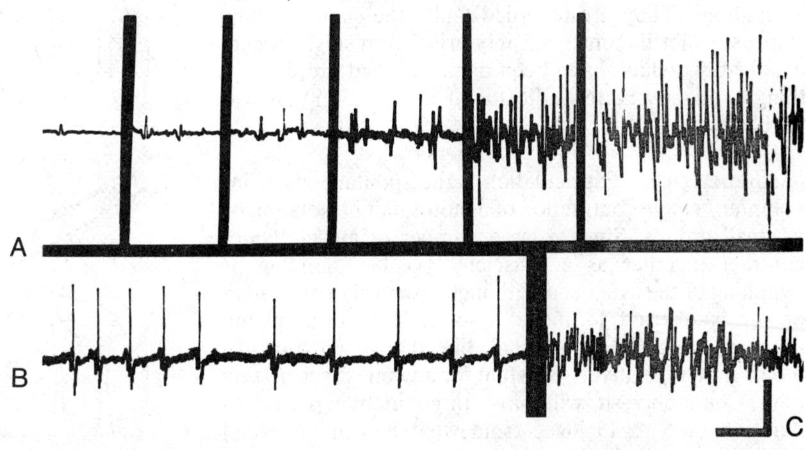

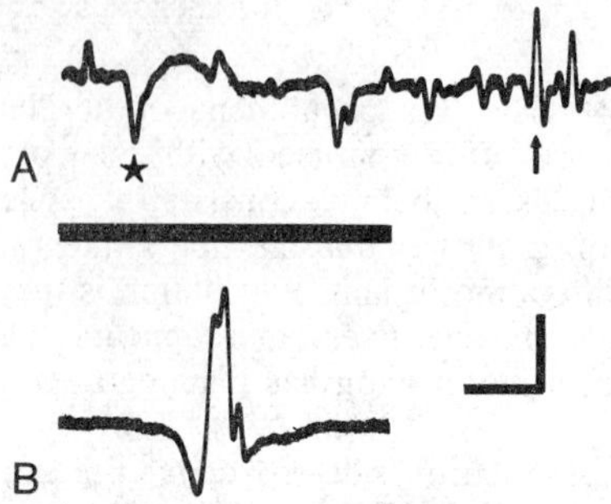

FIGURE 344–3
A *Fibrillations and positive sharp waves. This spontaneous activity was recorded from a totally denervated muscle—no motor unit potentials were produced by attempts at voluntary contraction. The fibrillations (such as above the arrow) are 1 to 2 msec in duration, 100 to 300 μV in amplitude, and largely negative in polarity (upward) following an initial positive deflection. A typical positive sharp wave is seen above the star.* B *Fasciculation. This spontaneous motor unit potential was recorded from a patient with amyotrophic lateral sclerosis. Its dimensions and configuration are normal; it fired once every second or two. Calibrations denote 5 msec (horizontal) and 200 μV in* A *and 1 mV in* B *(vertical).*

the end plate zone of a resting muscle, the conclusion can be reached that some of the fibers are denervated. While found to a slight degree in certain primary diseases of muscle, such as polymyositis, or occasionally in dystrophy, nevertheless, if at all prominent, they may be taken as a mark of denervation hypersensitivity. Diseases such as poliomyelitis which cause degeneration of motor axons, or injuries of peripheral nerves or anterior spinal roots, frequently produce only partial denervation of the involved muscles. In such muscles, one electrode placement may pick up fibrillation at rest in denervated fibers and normal potentials during activity from nearby healthy fibers. Fibrillation continues until the muscle fiber is reinnervated by the outgrowth of new axons, either from nearby healthy nerve fibers or from the central nervous system, or until the fiber is replaced by connective tissue, a process which may not take place for many years. In addition one often observes *positive sharp waves*, i.e., spontaneous diphasic potentials, as their name suggests, of longer duration and slightly greater amplitude than fibrillations. They are recorded under the same circumstances as fibrillations, probably arise from single denervated fibers which have been damaged, and are, if anything, a slightly better indicator of denervation than are fibrillations.

FASCICULATION Fasciculation is the spontaneous or involuntary single contraction of a motor unit in isolation or in small groups. Since a large number of muscle fibers contract together as a "fascicle," visible dimpling or twitching of the skin occurs, though ordinarily not enough power is exerted to move a joint. The form of the accompanying EMG potential, like that of an ordinary motor unit, is relatively constant for any one fasciculating unit. Commonly, it will have three to five phases, a duration of 5 to 15 msec (somewhat less in the facial muscles), and an amplitude of several millivolts (Fig. 344-3*B*). With "benign fasciculations" seen in normal subjects, the same unit tends to repeat at a fairly regular rate of one per second, or even faster, indicating a rhythmic activation of the fibers by the responsible axons. With the "malignant fasciculations" described below, the rate is considerably slower at one per 3 or 4 sec and slightly less regular.

Traditionally, fasciculation occurs in chronic, slowly advancing, destructive disease of the anterior horn cells, such as amyotrophic lateral sclerosis and progressive

FIGURE 344–4
The shaded muscle fibers are functional members of one motor unit, the axon, which enters from the upper left and branches terminally to innervate the appropriate muscle fibers. The motor unit action potential produced by each motor unit is seen in the upper right; its duration is measured between the two vertical lines. The normal-appearing but unshaded fibers belong to other motor units. A *The normal situation is schematized with five muscle fibers in the active unit.* B *In this myopathic unit, only two fibers remain active, the other three (shrunken) have been affected by one of the primary muscle diseases.* C *Four fibers which belonged to other motor units and had been denervated have now been reinnervated by the terminal axon sprouting from the healthy active motor unit. Both the motor unit and its action potential are now larger than normal. Note that only under these abnormal circumstances do fibers in the same unit lie next to one another.*

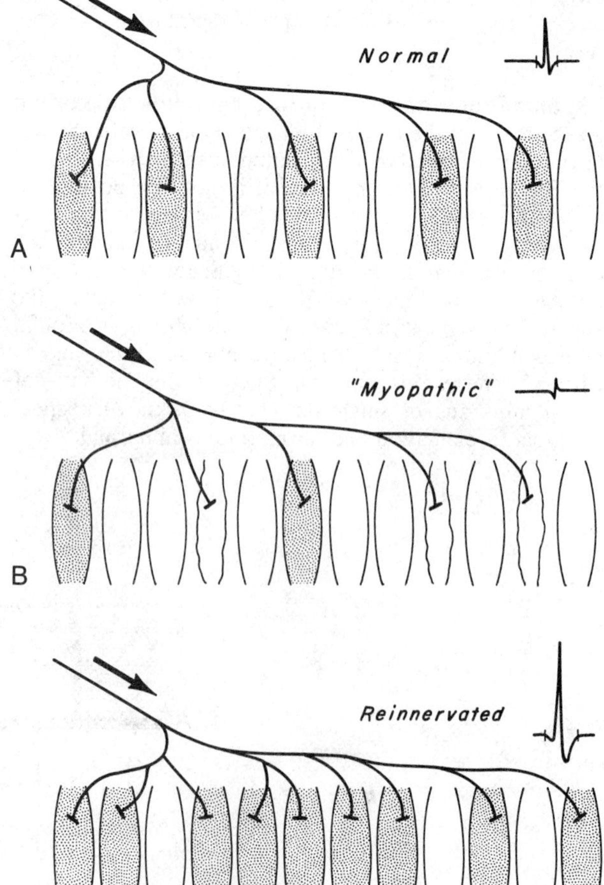

spinal muscular atrophy. In these diseases, fasciculation potentials are numerous and may exceed 15 msec in duration. They are often seen in the early stages of poliomyelitis but are recorded less commonly than in the chronic diseases mentioned, perhaps because the affected cells die too rapidly. They are also seen with compressive root lesions and early in the course of some patients with acute idiopathic polyneuritis. With peripheral lesions such as those caused by herniated nucleus pulposus (ruptured disk), large numbers of axons may be affected with the result that the fasciculations (or even cramps) may be more obvious to the patient than the twitching with disease of anterior horn cells. In all these cases, the damaged neuron seems to be "irritated" by the disease process, fires repetitively, and, in so doing, produces activity in all the muscle fibers that it innervates. It has been shown that fasciculation may also follow peripheral nerve lesions, giving way to fibrillation upon death of the axon. More important is the fact that fasciculation, particularly in the calves and hands, occurs occasionally in many normal persons and constantly in some, and so it need not be evidence of disease at all. Shivering induced by low temperature and the twitchings associated with depressed serum calcium levels are also forms of fasciculation.

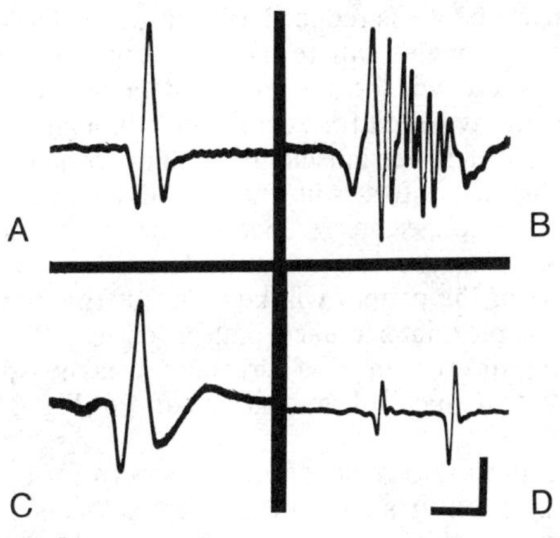

FIGURE 344–5
Single voluntary motor unit potentials. A *Normal.* B *Prolonged polyphasic potential seen with reinnervation.* C *"Giant unit"—normally shaped but of much greater amplitude than normal.* D *Brief, low-amplitude "myopathic" units. Calibrations: 5 msec (horizontal) and 1 mV in* A *and in* B, *5 mV in* C, *and 100 μV in* D *(vertical).*

Abnormalities in amplitude, duration, and shape of motor units potentials ENLARGED MOTOR UNIT POTENTIALS IN PARTIALLY DENERVATED AND REINNERVATED MUSCLE Figure 344-4 depicts, schematically, ways in which disease processes affect the motor unit and, therefore, the motor unit potential recorded by EMG. Early in the course of denervation, any motor units with functional connections to the spinal cord are unaffected, and though the number of motor unit potentials appearing during contraction is reduced, the configurations of the remaining ones are quite normal. In time, those remaining often increase in amplitude, perhaps to two to three times normal, and become longer in duration and *polyphasic* (more than four phases). Such large and, sometimes, *giant potentials* (Fig. 344-5*C*) are believed to arise from motor units, as in Fig. 344-4*C*, containing more than the usual number of muscle fibers spread out over a greatly enlarged territory within the muscle. Presumably, new nerve twigs have *sprouted* from these undamaged axons, reinnervated previously denervated fibers, and added them to their own motor units. Some of these reinnervated units may become extremely polyphasic and prolonged, a finding pathognomic of reinnervation (Fig. 344-5*B*). These units are to be differentiated from (1) those with lesser degrees of polyphasicity which are of normal duration and make up 10 to 20 percent of the activity recorded from normal muscles, particularly at the end plate zone, and (2) the polyphasic but brief units seen with primary muscle disease.

REDUCED AMPLITUDE AND DURATION OF ACTION POTENTIALS Diseases such as polymyositis, the muscular dystrophies, and myopathies which destroy scattered fibers within a motor unit or render them nonfunctional, as in Fig. 344-4*B*, obviously reduce the population of fibers per motor unit. When such a unit is activated, its potential is, therefore, of lower voltage and shorter duration than normal (Fig. 344-5*D*), and it may also appear polyphasic as the compound motor unit potential is fragmented into its constituent single-fiber potentials. When most of the muscle fibers are affected, the motor unit potentials from these very small units may be difficult to differentiate from fibrillation potentials, and when destruction of all fibers is completed, electrical activity ceases. These small, brief, voluntary motor unit potentials, with their characteristic high-pitched crackling sound from the audio monitor, occur in all forms of progressive muscular dystrophy and, unfortunately, are indistinguishable from those of polymyositis, dermatomyositis, and other chronic myopathies. In the myositides, however, fibrillation potentials may often be seen, perhaps because of the destruction of terminal nerve twigs by the inflammatory process. In myasthenia gravis, where transmission of impulse fails progressively at one neuromuscular junction after another in any one motor unit, the EMG potential of that unit may be normal at first and become more *myopathic* as fatigue progresses. Potentials from muscles which are chronically weak in myasthenics are then proportionately myopathic. It can be seen, therefore, from Fig. 344-4*B*, that the motor unit potentials will appear equally myopathic whether the disease process directly affects single muscle fibers within the unit as in dystrophy, disturbs neuromuscular transmission at single junctions as in myasthenia gravis, or blocks transmission of the nerve impulse in single axon terminals.

DECREASE IN THE NUMBER OF MOTOR UNITS AVAILABLE Diseases which reduce the population of functional lower motor neurons or motor axons within the peripheral nerve obviously decrease the number of motor units which can be recruited in the affected muscles (see Fig. 344-2*B*). The number of motor units available for activation vary then in proportion to the strength of a maximal voluntary contraction, showing no longer as an interference pattern but only as a *single unit pattern* (Fig. 344-2*B*) or a *mixed pattern*.

If muscle power is reduced in diseases such as myopathies or dystrophies, where individual muscle fibers are affected, there will be no reduction in the number of motor units available for recruitment, though each unit will consist of fewer muscle fibers than normal. A maximal voluntary effort will then be associated with a normally complete interference pattern despite marked weakness. Because fewer muscle fibers are active, the amplitude of the pattern will be reduced from normal. A highly complex interference pattern of less than usual amplitude, in the face of dramatic weakness, is the hallmark of a so-called *myopathic pattern* (Fig. 344-2*C*).

PROGRESSIVE REDUCTION OR AUGMENTATION OF ACTION POTENTIALS WITH SUCCESSIVE CONTRACTIONS In certain disorders, the initial motor unit potentials are normal with voluntary contraction, as is the compound muscle action potential produced by electric stimuli applied to the nerve. After a few shocks at rates as low as 1 to 10 per sec, the amplitude of the potentials falls off, though not to zero, and then increases again after the fourth or fifth stimulus (Fig. 344-6*A*), while normal muscles respond to the electrical stimuli with little decrement or facilitation over a minute or two at rates as high as 30 to 40 per sec. This phenomenon is characteristic of *myasthenia gravis*. It is superficially similar to the partial block at the neuromuscular junction produced by curare and, like it, may be relieved by neostigmine, though the pathophysiology is largely prejunctional in myasthenia gravis and postjunctional with curare. Similar but less definite decline of the action potentials with repetitive stimulation may occur in poliomyelitis or certain other diseases of the motor unit, but the pattern described for myasthenia gravis is not present.

FIGURE 344–6
Compound action potentials evoked in hypothenar muscles by electrical stimulation of the ulnar nerve at the wrist. A *Patient with myasthenia gravis—typical pattern of decrement in first four responses followed by slight increment. At this rate of stimulation (4 per sec) the responses do* not *continue to decrement toward zero.* B *Patient with Eaton-Lambert syndrome and "oat-cell" carcinoma—typical marked increase toward normal amplitude with rapid repetitive stimulation (20 per sec). Horizontal calibration, 250 msec.*

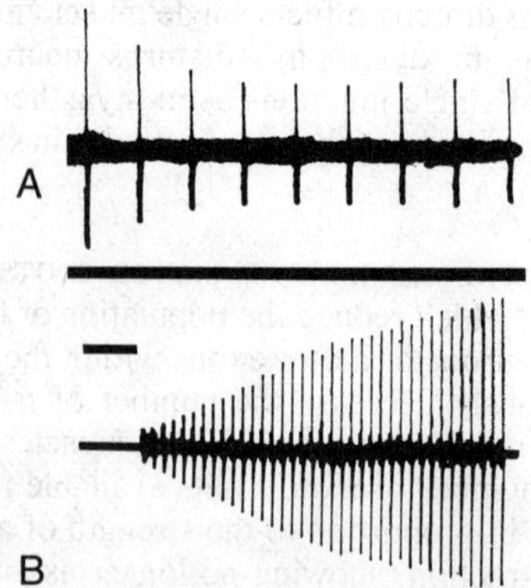

In some cases of "oat-cell" carcinoma of the lung and sarcoidosis with muscular weakness, the *Eaton-Lambert syndrome*, a condition with somewhat opposite findings, may be observed. If electrical stimulation through nerve is rapid (20 to 30 per sec) or following a brief voluntary contraction, muscle action potentials which were small or practically absent with the first stimulus now increase in voltage with each successive one until a more nearly normal amplitude is attained (Fig. 344-6*B*). Neostigmine has no effect on this phenomenon, but it may be reversible with guanidine (20 to 35 mg per kg per day in divided doses). The pathophysiology of this *myasthenic syndrome* is similar to that produced by botulinus toxin or neomycin and certain other antibiotics (see Chap. 347).

SPECIAL ABNORMALITIES IN THE EMG In *myotonia*, muscle contraction persists despite voluntary attempts at relaxation. The symptom occurs in several hereditary diseases, myotonia congenita (Thomsen's disease), dystrophia myotonica (Steinert's disease), and hyperkalemic periodic paralysis (Eulenburg's paramyotonia). Minor forms occur sporadically under other circumstances. Myotonia consists of high-frequency repetitive discharges which wax and wane in amplitude and frequency, producing a "dive-bomber" sound on the audio monitor. It is produced mechanically by percussion or movement of the needle electrode. The characteristic electrical picture is also seen following voluntary contraction or electrical stimulation of the muscle via its motor nerve. The motor unit potentials appear normal, but they are not followed by the silence which normally occurs on relaxation. Instead there is a burst of rapid activity which may take as long as several minutes to subside (Fig. 344-7*A*). Some of the potentials of this prolonged discharge have the duration, amplitude, and form of single-fiber activity, while others appear to have the characteristics of motor unit potentials. If the muscle is activated repeatedly at short intervals, the late discharge becomes briefer and briefer and eventually disappears (Fig. 344-7*B*) as the patient becomes able to relax the exercised muscle at will.

Pseudomyotonia, or bizarre high-frequency discharges without waxing and waning, is seen in hypothyroidism or with certain types of denervation. High-frequency *coupling* of action potentials into doublets, triplets, or higher multiples of single units, indicating instability in repolarization of the nerve fiber, occurs in tetany.

Contracture, as with cramping in McArdle's disease, percussion and contraction myoedema, and percussion fasciculation have no electrical counterpart (the EMG is silent). This aspect of these phenomena is important in their definition.

STATISTICAL ANALYSIS

In electrocardiography, it is frequently possible to decide that a single complex is abnormal because its configuration lies outside well-established limits for the lead under consideration. For reasons discussed above, it is often difficult to make this decision in the case of an individual motor unit potential in skeletal muscle. As a result, Buchthal and others have established tables of the frequency distribution of potential durations in normal muscles using their techniques, and similar ranges of normal

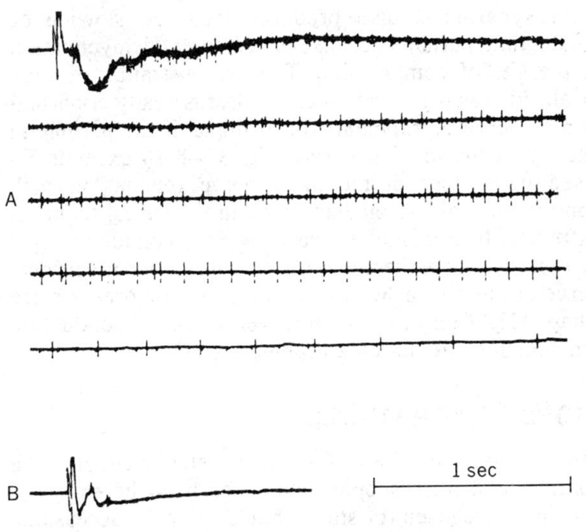

FIGURE 344–7
A *Myotonia congenita (Thomsen's disease). The five lines are a continuous record of activity in the biceps brachii following a tap on the tendon. The initial response is within normal limits, but it is followed by a prolonged burst of rapid activity, gradually subsiding over a period of many seconds or minutes.* B *Same electrode placement as in* A. *Response to the fifth of a series of tendon taps. "Warm-up" has occurred, and the characteristic prolonged myotonic activity is no longer evident.*

values must be established for each laboratory using its own recording system. Such durations, it has been found, vary from one to another normal muscle and tend to increase with age.

ELECTRONEUROGRAPHY

Disease of peripheral nerve may produce the electromyographic evidences of denervation discussed above, but more quantitative observations of neural function can be made by studies of the electrical activity of nerves themselves. Hagbarth and colleagues have, by means of fine needle electrodes within peripheral nerves *in situ*, pioneered in the recording of single-fiber activity from muscle afferents and from autonomic and other subgroups within peripheral nerves. This promises to be of critical importance in the understanding of many aspects of human physiology but is not yet available in every adequately equipped EMG laboratory, as are measurements of conduction velocity.

CONDUCTION VELOCITY OF NERVE

Painless and harmless techniques are now available for both percutaneous stimulation of the larger peripheral motor and sensory nerve fibers and recording of their conducted action potentials. These routine techniques provide numeric data which are of considerable clinical interest. The results of these *motor and sensory nerve conduction studies*, expressed simply as conduction velocity or peripheral latency, are more objective than the results of electromyography and afford certain information unavailable from EMG studies.

An accessible nerve is stimulated through the skin by surface electrodes, and the resulting compound action potential is recorded by electrodes on the skin (1) over the nerve more proximally in the case of orthodromic activity in large sensory fibers stimulated in the digital nerves or (2) over the muscle more distally in the case of motor fibers in a mixed nerve (Fig. 344-8). The conduction time from the most distal stimulating electrode, measured in milliseconds from the stimulus artifact to the onset of the response, is also termed the *distal* or *peripheral latency*. If a second stimulus can be applied to a mixed nerve more proximally (or if recording electrodes can be placed more proximally in the case of activity in sensory fibers), a new and longer conduction time can be measured. When the distance (in millimeters) between the two sites of stimulation of motor fibers or recording of sensory fibers is divided by the difference in conduction times (in milliseconds), a *maximal conduction velocity* (in meters per second) is obtained which describes the velocity of propagation of the action potentials in the largest and fastest nerve fibers. These velocities in normal subjects vary roughly from a minimum of 40 or 45 m per sec, depending upon which nerve is studied, to a maximum of 75 or 80 m per sec. Values are lower in infants, reaching the adult range by the age of two to four years. Normal values also exist for peripheral latencies from the distalmost site on various mixed nerves to the appropriate muscles; when one stimulates the median nerve at the wrist, for example, the latency (Fig. 344-8*A'*) for conduction through the carpal tunnel to the abductor pollicis brevis muscle in the thenar eminence is always less than 4.5 msec in normal adults. Similar tables of normal values have been compiled for orthodromic sensory conduction velocities and distal latencies.

When motor fibers in a mixed nerve are stimulated and even one is in functional continuity with its many muscle fibers, the compound action potential of many hundreds of microvolts can easily be recorded from electrodes on the skin over the muscle. However, when one is dealing with sensory potentials, activity is recorded from nerve fibers themselves; one lacks the "amplification" provided by all the muscle fibers in one motor unit, as noted above, and much greater electronic amplification is required. In the clinic, therefore, abnormal sensory potentials tend to be very small or absent even when powerful computer averaging techniques are used, and sensory conduction measurements are more often impossible to record than abnormally slow. In contrast, a reliable motor conduction velocity is possible if one functional nerve fiber remains. These conduction velocities reflect the status of surviving fibers and, if the latter are unaffected by the disease process, may be normal despite widespread denervation: following incomplete transection of a nerve by a sharp object, the maximal motor conduction velocity may be normal in the few remaining fibers, although the muscle involved is almost paralyzed.

Disease processes which preferentially affect larger fibers in peripheral nerve should reduce the maximal conduction velocity slightly because the remaining fibers with smaller diameters conduct more slowly. Such a reduction in velocity is often not great enough to place it outside normal limits, and nerve conduction studies can then be used to document the presence of neuropathy in the disease under question only by comparison of values recorded from the patient population with those from a control group of the same age and sex.

In most neuropathies the axon itself is affected (either by the "dying-back" phenomenon or Wallerian degeneration), and nerve conduction studies are then relatively uninformative. This is true for typical alcoholic, nutritional, paracarcinomatous, uremic, other metabolic, and most diabetic neuropathies where conduction velocities range from low in the normal range to 35 or 40 m per sec. On the other hand, diseases such as acute idiopathic polyneuritis (Landry-Guillain-Barré syndrome), diphtheria, infantile metachromatic leukodystrophy, Krabbe's disease, and Charcot-Marie-Tooth disease (as it is seen in most kinships) affect Schwann cells primarily and produce segmental demyelination with conduction velocities as low as 10 to 15 m per sec.

Focal compression of nerve, as in the various entrapment syndromes, also produces localized slowing of conduction, perhaps because of segmental demyelination at the site of compression. The demonstration of such localized slowing of conduction affords ready confirmation of nerve entrapment; for example, if the peripheral latency in the median nerve (Fig. 344-8*A'*) exceeds 5.0 msec while that in the ulnar nerve remains normal, compression of the median nerve in the carpal tunnel is extremely likely. Similar focal slowing of conduction may be recorded from the ulnar nerve at the elbow or peroneal nerve at the fibular head when they are compressed (see Chap. 323). Contrariwise, however, a normal conduction time cannot rule out an entrapment syndrome.

FIGURE 344–8

The median nerve may be stimulated through the skin at the wrist (1) or in the antecubital fossa (2) and the resultant compound muscle action potential may be recorded as the potential difference between a surface electrode over the thenar eminence (arrow) and a reference electrode (Ref.) more distally. Sweep 1' on the CRO depicts the stimulus artifact (moment of stimulation at 1) followed by the muscle potential. The distal latency *is the time* A' *on the CRO sweep (3.0 msec, for example) which corresponds to conduction over distance* A *in the hand. The same is true for sweep 2' where stimulation is at point 2 and the time from artifact to response is* A' + B'. *The maximal motor conduction velocity from points 2 to 1 is obtained by dividing distance* B *by time* B'.

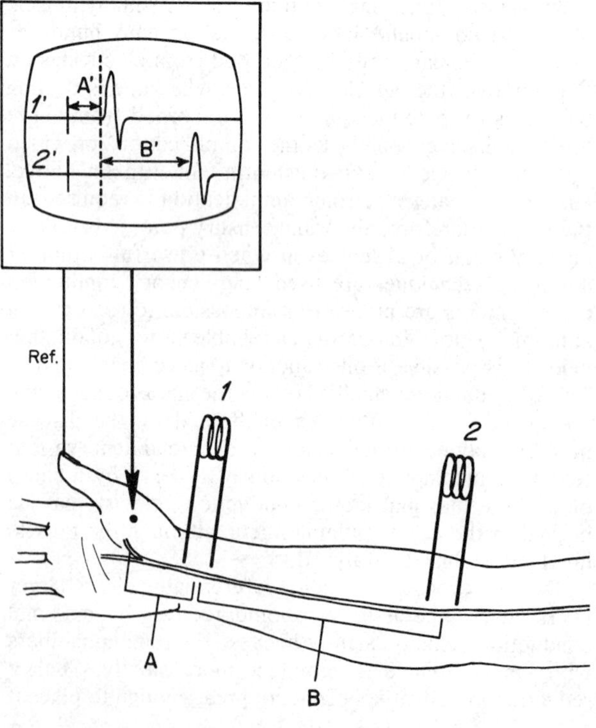

BIOPSY MYOPATHOLOGY

Muscle biopsy can be of great diagnostic value, but both surgical and microscopic techniques must be exacting. The muscle chosen for study should be easily accessible; there should be evidence that it has been affected but not totally destroyed by the disease in question, and it should not recently have been studied electromyographically since the trauma of the needle electrodes produces focal inflammatory lesions. Muscle biopsy is indicated (1) to attempt to differentiate among neuropathic atrophy, dystrophy, metabolic myopathy, and polymyositis; (2) to support the diagnosis of diffuse diseases of connective tissue and blood vessels (e.g., polyarteritis nodosa, lupus), or special infections (e.g., trichinosis, toxoplasmosis); (3) for diagnosis of metabolic diseases involving muscle (e.g., glycogen storage disease) and the special myopathies (rod body and central core myopathies); (4) in the scientific study of disorders of neuromuscular transmission (e.g., myasthenia gravis, periodic paralysis), usually by a combination of histochemical technqiues and methylene blue staining of nerve endings. In most instances, it is possible to distinguish histologically the effects of denervation, the dystrophies and other necrotizing myopathies, special disfigurative myopathies, and polymyositis.

As a rule, the biopsy procedure requires no more than a cleanly excised block of muscle 1.0 by 1.0 by 2.0 cm which is then fixed in 10% neutral Formalin, embedded in paraffin, sectioned in a cross and longitudinal fashion, and stained by hematoxylin and eosin, phosphotungstic acid hematoxylin, or Mallory trichrome methods. Special techniques may be applied, if it is desirable to visualize special qualities of a disease, such as the methylene blue–cholinesterase technique for nerve endings and myoneural junctions (method of Cöers and Woolf) or various histochemical stains for enzyme content of muscle fibers (phosphorylase in McArdle's disease, etc). The latter require rapid freezing rather than Formalin fixation. Electron microscopy can also be performed on carefully selected blocks of fixed muscle and nerve, fixed in glutaraldehyde. Sural nerve biopsies, processed by the fixation, staining, and embedding techniques of electron microscopy, can, when studied by ordinary microscopy, provide very useful histopathologic data. These biopsies can also be studied physiologically in vitro where fibers of all sizes can be stimulated and their activity recorded—in contrast with routine nerve conduction studies where only the largest fibers can be sampled. All these latter are of interest to research workers and are available in centers where nerve and muscle diseases are under investigation.

USE OF LABORATORY TESTS IN THE STUDY OF MUSCLE DISEASE

The results of none of the diagnostic laboratory procedures described above may be taken as infallible indexes of specific diseases of muscle. Each procedure is subject to technical error and the findings to misinterpretation. A biopsy specimen may be excised from an unaffected muscle or portion of a muscle and be negative in the face of clinical evidence of obvious disease; rough excision and improper fixation and staining may produce artifacts which the unwary may misinterpret as marks of disease when, in fact, the muscle is microscopically normal. Similarly, EMG study may fail to record fibrillations in obviously denervated muscle, or a few fibrillations may be seen in an otherwise typical dystrophic process. As in the study of all disease, laboratory data have important significance only if viewed against the background of the clinical findings.

REFERENCES

Adams RD et al: *Diseases of Muscle: A Study in Pathology*, 2d ed., New York: Hoeber-Harper, 1962

Buchthal F, Rosenfalck A: Evoked action potentials and conduction velocity in human sensory nerves. Brain Res 3:1, 1966

Cöers C, Woolf AL: *The Innervation of Muscle: A Biopsy Study*, Springfield, Ill.: Charles C Thomas, 1959

Elmqvist D, Lambert EH; Detailed analysis of neuromuscular transmission in a patient with the myasthenic syndrome associated with bronchogenic carcinoma. Mayo Clin Proc 43:689, 1968

Goodgold J, Eberstein A: *Electrodiagnosis of Neuromuscular Diseases*, Baltimore: Williams & Wilkins, 1972

Hagbarth KE, Wohlfart G: The number of muscle-spindles in certain muscles in cat in relation to the composition of the muscle nerves. Acta Anat (Basel) 15:85, 1952

Hubbard JI et al: *Electrophysiological Analysis of Synaptic Transmission*, Baltimore: Williams & Wilkins, 1969

Katz B: *Nerve, Muscle and Synapse*, New York: McGraw-Hill, 1966

Sherrington CS: On the anatomical constitution of nerves of skeletal muscles: With remarks on recurrent fibres in the ventral spinal nerve-root. J Physiol 17:211, 1894

Walton JN: *Disorders of Voluntary Muscle*, 2d ed., Baltimore: Williams & Wilkins, 1970

345 ACUTE AND SUBACUTE MYOPATHIC PARALYSIS

FRANK H. TYLER
RAYMOND D. ADAMS

As remarked in Chap. 17, sudden paralysis of skeletal muscles in a limb or sector of the body, developing over a period of minutes or hours, can usually be traced to a vascular disorder of spinal cord or brain, and rarely to a myelitis or encephalitis. Acute paralysis developing in the course of days (1 to 14) is usually due to poliomyelitis or acute idiopathic polyneuritis (Landry-Guillain-Barré syndrome) and rarely another form of polyneuropathy (porphyria, polyarteritis). The primary diseases of muscle, by contrast, rarely cause a rapidly developing widespread paralysis. Instead, their course is usually subacute (2 to several weeks) or chronic. The only exceptions that we have observed are rare cases of myasthenia gravis in which the evolution of the disease to a severe and incapacitating paresis has been over 2 or 3 days, rare cases of polymyositis, and some of the cases of acute thyrotoxic myopathy which we have suspected of being a combination of myasthenia gravis and hyperthyroidism. In some of the cases of paroxysmal myoglobinuria, a moderately severe weakness of the limbs has appeared within a few hours of physical exertion, but usually the clinical picture has been at once complicated by renal damage and anuria. Occasionally an attack of myoglobinuria has followed an infection and has led to severe paralysis of trunk and limb muscles within a few days to 2 or 3 weeks. A pronounced, rapidly developing paralysis of the limbs and respiratory and cranial musculature may occur after the bite of certain species of ticks (tick-bite paralysis); and botulism causes a fulminant paralysis beginning in ocular and other cranial muscles, extending to trunk and limb muscles, and leading to respiratory failure and death in a few hours or days (see Chap. 153). The initial attack of periodic paralysis or of hyper- or hypopotassemia must also enter the differential diagnosis of the acute muscle paralysis. The clinical analysis of these acute syndromes is aided by certain laboratory data such as the electrocardiogram, serum potassium level, sodium and chloride values, serum enzymes such as creatine phosphokinase, and protein-bound iodine measurement; and the cerebrospinal fluid may be of great help. The response to neostigmine or edrophonium (Tensilon) (Chap. 347) aids in the diagnosis of acute myasthenia gravis.

The two principal categories of subacute myopathy are dermatomyositis (polymyositis if there is no skin involvement) and polymyopathy due to metabolic diseases.

DERMATOMYOSITIS AND POLYMYOSITIS

DEFINITION These are relatively common diseases which affect primarily the striated muscle, skin, and other connective tissues of the body. The term used varies according to the distribution of the pathologic process. If restricted clinically to the striated muscles, the disease is called polymyositis; if the skin is involved, it is designated as dermatomyositis; and if other connective tissues are implicated, the term of choice is dermatomyositis with rheumatoid arthritis, rheumatic fever, lupus erythematosus, or scleroderma.

HISTORY Polymyositis has been known since the original descriptions by Wagner in 1863 and 1887, and the dermatomyositic form was first reported by Unverricht in 1887. The literature since that time and a general statement of present knowledge are found in the monographs of Walton and Adams and of Walton in 1969.

ETIOLOGY The cause of the disease is unknown. All attempts to isolate an infective agent have been unsuccessful. Several electron microscopists have observed virus particles of two types in muscle fibers, but their causative role has not been proved. Rising titers of antibodies have not been demonstrated, nor has a polymyositic illness been induced in animals by injections of infected muscle. A disease which resembles polymyositis has been provoked in laboratory animals by injections of sterile muscle extracts with Freund's adjuvants, suggesting an autoimmune mechanism. Its close association with diseases of connective tissue favors the notion of common etiology or pathogenesis, also in keeping with an autoallergic inflammation. It must be conceded, however, that the category of disease called polymyositis is not precise and probably has been used to include other diseases of noninflammatory type, namely, metabolic myopathies.

CLINICAL MANIFESTATIONS This type of muscle disease tends to assume several clinical forms, as follows.

Polymyositis *A subacute symmetric weakness of proximal limb and trunk muscles without dermatitis or with minimal skin lesions.* The onset is usually insidious and the course slowly progressive over a period of several weeks or months. The disease may develop at almost any age (from one to eighty years) and in either sex. However the majority of patients range from thirty to sixty years of age, and females outnumber males 2:1. A respiratory or obscure systemic infection may precede the muscle weakness, but in many patients the first symptoms develop during excellent health.

The patient first becomes aware of a painless weakness of the proximal limb muscles, especially of the hips and thighs, and acts such as arising from a squatting or kneeling position, climbing or descending stairs, walking, putting an object on a high shelf, or combing the hair become increasingly difficult. In restricted forms of the disease only the neck muscles or quadriceps may be involved. Pain of an aching variety, in buttocks, joints, and calves, is experienced in only a small percentage of cases (15 percent) and often indicates a combination of polymyositis and arthritis or other connective tissue disease. The weakness progresses over a period of weeks and months.

When the patient is first seen, the facial, anterior, and posterior neck muscles (the head may loll), the pharyngeal and laryngeal muscles (dysphagia and dysphonia), all the trunk, the girdle muscles of shoulders and hips, upper arms, and the thighs are usually involved. Ocular muscles are almost never affected; the forearm, hand, leg, and foot muscles are spared in all but about 25 percent of cases. The muscles are usually not tender, and atrophy and reduction in tendon reflexes, though present, are not so pronounced as in denervation diseases. When reflexes are disproportionately reduced, one must think of carcinomatosis with polymyositis and neuritis. The skin and mucous membranes and joints are unchanged.

In a review of our cases of polymyositis and dermatomyositis a surprising number of cardiac abnormalities were observed. Most of these were relatively minor ECG changes, but several patients had arrythmias of significance. Among the fatal cases about half showed clinical evidence of severe cardiac disease and had necrosis of myocardial fibers at autopsy, usually with only modest inflammation. As a rule, evidence of systemic infection is absent. Exceptionally there is low-grade fever, especially if joint pain coexists, and a spot or a few spots of dermatitis may be present at one stage of the illness.

Dermatomyositis The skin changes may precede, accompany, or follow the muscle syndrome and take the form of a localized or diffuse erythema, maculopapular eruption, scaling eczematoid dermatitis, or even an exfoliative dermatitis. Of particular importance is the occurrence of a lilac-colored (heliotrope) change in the skin over the bridge of the nose, cheeks, forehead, and around the fingernails. Itching may be troublesome in some cases. The skin lesions are restricted and unimportant in some cases, consisting, as mentioned, of only a patch or more of dermatitis. Periorbital and perioral edema is frequent, particularly in more fulminating episodes. Also skin lesions are frequent over the joints, particularly in childhood. In the healing stage they become depressed, with a flat, scaly base. Periarticular and subcutaneous calcification may occur. Signs of other connective tissue disease are more frequent (in one-third to one-half of all patients) than in examples of pure polymyositis. The limb weakness is usually proximal but may be diffuse, i.e., distal and proximal, just as in polymyositis. Raynaud's phenomenon is reported in nearly a third of the patients. Others will develop a mild form of scleroderma. Esophageal weakness may be demonstrated by fluoroscopy in approximately 30 percent of all patients. The superior constrictors are involved almost universally, but careful analysis by cinefluorography may be required to demonstrate the abnormality.

Connective tissue diseases with polymyositis or dermatomyositis This combination involves rheumatic fever, rheumatoid arthritis, scleroderma, or lupus erythematosus when there is greater muscular weakness and atrophy than can be accounted for by the original disease. Inasmuch as pain in arthritis may limit motion, result in atrophy, and impair the power of voluntary movement, the diagnosis is not easy, and sometimes reliance must be put on muscle biopsy, urinary excretion of creatine and creatinine, and measurements of muscle enzymes in the serum. Malaise, aches, and pains may be the only symptoms in the early stages of the disease. Sjögren's syndrome of keratitis desiccans, swelling and diminished secretion of salivary glands, and xerostomia and rheumatoid arthritis may accompany polymyositis (see Chap. 356).

Carcinoma with polymyositis or dermatomyositis This syndrome is placed in a separate category, although the muscle and skin changes are indistinguishable from those in the above forms of the disease. Approximately 10 percent of all adults, especially the elderly, who have polymyositis or dermatomyositis are found to have a carcinoma or some other tumor. Some cases of thymoma are accompanied by polymyositis. The incidence of this neoplastic syndrome is slightly higher in men than in women. Over 1,000 examples have been reported in the literature, being linked most often with bronchogenic carcinoma. The tumors, however, have occurred in every organ of the body. The muscle and skin tissues show no evidence of tumor cells. The polymyositis may antedate the clinical manifestations of the malignancy by 1 to 2 years. The relationship is not understood but the most likely possibility is an altered immune stage which fosters occult infection.

LABORATORY FINDINGS Regardless of the clinical associations, in all forms of polymyositis the creatine excretion in the urine is moderately elevated in most cases and creatinine excretion is low. The serum levels of the several types of transaminase and other tissue enzymes such as creatine phosphokinase and aldolase are elevated. Serum α_2- and γ-globulin values may be raised. Tests for circulating rheumatoid factor (latex fixation and sensitized sheep cell procedure) are positive in less than half the cases. Myoglobin is occasionally found in the urine when the muscle affection is acute and severe. The sedimentation rate may be normal or elevated. Lupus erythematosus preparations of blood smears are negative, as a rule. The electromyogram reveals a typical "myopathic pattern," i.e., many abnormally brief action potentials of low voltage and, in addition, numerous fibrillation potentials and salvos of pseudomyotonic activity (see Chap. 344). As stated, the electrocardiogram has been abnormal in a few of our cases. The muscle biopsy, if taken from an affected muscle, usually demonstrates the typical pathologic changes of the disease. Poor sampling may result in a negative biopsy.

PATHOLOGY The principal changes in muscle tissue consist of widespread destruction of muscle fibers, with all the expected cellular reaction thereto (myophages), and infiltrates of inflammatory cells (lymphocytes, mononuclear leukocytes, plasma cells, and rare neutrophilic leukocytes). Evidences of regenerative activity in the form of proliferating sarcolemmal nuclei, basophilic (ribonucleic acid–rich) sarcoplasm, and new myofibrils are almost invariable. Many of the residual muscle fibers are small, with increased numbers of sarcolemmal nuclei. Either the degeneration of muscle fibers or the infiltrations of inflammatory cells may predominate in any given biopsy specimen, though at autopsy both types of change are in evidence. There are also inflammatory changes in the skin and other organs.

DIAGNOSIS Patients with a pure polymyositis are often suspected of having progressive muscular dystrophy because of the similar distribution of weakness (in the proximal and trunk muscles). Polymyositis is unlike dystrophy, however, in that the development is much more rapid, individuals may be affected at all ages (one rarely sees a dystrophy begin after thiry years of age), and the laryngeal, pharyngeal, and neck muscles and the esophagus are usually involved. It must be conceded, however, that in some patients, especially children, it is virtually impossible, even with biopsy, to distinguish a chronic polymyositis from a rapidly advancing dystrophy.

A few patients with poly- or dermatomyositis and malignancy will exhibit signs of one of the other paraneoplastic syndromes (polyneuritis, subacute cerebellar degeneration, combined system disease, or multifocal leukoencephalopathy). A peculiar type of inverse myasthenia has also been reported, especially with small-cell carcinomas of the lung (oat cell, squamous cell). A sense of stiffness and pain on motion in these latter patients may be mistaken for rheumatoid arthritis.

The painful varieties of the polymyositis must be separated from early connective tissue disease. If the latter is not established, it may be impossible to reach a correct diagnosis even after all the laboratory data have been obtained. Such patients may be classified as hysteric, neurotic, or depressed or may be suspected of having some metabolic disease.

Trichinosis may be confused with idiopathic polymyositis, especially if the history of pork ingestion is not obtained. The high eosinophil counts in the blood, the relatively slight weakness of limbs, the conjunctival edema, the ocular and lingual weakness, the symptoms of cerebral involvement (hemiplegia, aphasia, coma, etc.), the positive skin reaction to trichinae antigen, and the muscle biopsy establish the diagnosis in most cases.

TREATMENT The various measures which have been suggested are of uncertain value. Our most gratifying results have been obtained by a program which consists of (1) prednisone, 40 to 60 mg per day for a month, gradual reduction in steps of 5 mg, and finally 1 mg every week over a period of a year; the therapy should be monitored by careful tests of strength and serum enzyme levels [once the dosage is reduced to 20 mg per day, it is best to give double this amount on alternate days (i.e., 40 mg)]; (2) acetylsalicylic acid, 0.6 g every 4 hr except during the night (blood levels of 20 to 30 mg per 100 ml); and (3) physiotherapy—gentle massage, passive movement, and then "resistance exercises" as the evidences of activity (elevated sedimentation rate and high serum enzyme values) subside. Vitamin E or alpha-tocopherol has been used with doubtful benefit.

Elderly patients in particular should be reexamined every few weeks for malignancy. If a malignant lesion is found, it should be excised, if possible, or treated by x-ray or chemical agents. The muscle weakness may disappear if the tumor is eradicated. Response to corticosteroids may occur in patients with polymyositis associated with tumor.

PROGNOSIS Only a few of the patients will die, usually with some pulmonary, renal, or cardiac complication. The majority improve upon therapy, and in fact, the muscle weakness may lessen even in those patients with an advancing malignancy. A few patients recover completely, but more often some weakness of the shoulders and hips, usually not disabling, remains at the conclusion of treatment. Relapse may occur at any time up to 1 to 15 years or more. Corticosteroids should not be discontinued too soon, for the relapse which may follow is often more difficult to treat than the original symptoms of the disease. Acetylsalicylic acid may possibly reduce the likelihood of the relapse.

SARCOID POLYMYOPATHY In the medical literature there are some 25 or so cases of a subacutely progressive polymyositis involving proximal limb and trunk muscles, in which biopsy has demonstrated a noncaseating granulomatous involvement of muscle. In all other respects the patients are indistinguishable from those with the idiopathic polymyositis described above. Most of them have not shown many of the other characteristic manifestations of sarcoid and it is only proper to inquire as to whether the finding of a few Langhans-type giant cells in the muscle is a sufficient basis for the diagnosis of sarcoid. We are skeptical of this entity, but the problem is presently unresolved. Response to corticosteroid therapy is not different from that of idiopathic polymyositis.

POLYMYOPATHY WITH HYPOKALEMIC PERIODIC PARALYSIS A rare complication of *familial periodic paralysis* (see Chap. 347) takes the form of a subacute or chronic persistent weakness of thigh and pelvic musculature. Onset may be in the middle adult years, long after a troublesome adolescent periodic paralysis has ameliorated or ceased altogether. Biopsy reveals the extreme degrees of vacuolization and hydropia so characteristic of this form of periodic paralysis, and muscle fiber degeneration may be consequent to it. Slight increase in muscle enzymes in serum and a myopathic electromyogram substantiate the diagnosis already indicated by the sequence of clinical events. Administration of potassium (4 to 5 g orally per day), which alleviates or suppresses the periodic paralysis, may be beneficial.

METABOLIC DISEASES OF MUSCLE

The boundaries of this category of disease cannot be sharply drawn at this time. With advance in knowledge it is probable that many diseases presently classified as degenerative, and possibly some labeled as polymyositic, will be linked to specific defects in enzymes within the muscle cells. Limitations in space permit the description of only a few representative forms of the better known metabolic myopathies.

THYROID MYOPATHIES During the past three decades several myopathic diseases related to alterations in thyroid function have been recognized. These are (1) chronic thyrotoxic myopathy, (2) exophthalmic ophthalmoplegia (infiltrative ophthalmopathy), (3) myasthenia gravis associated with toxic diffuse goiter or with hypothyroidism, (4) periodic paralysis associated with toxic diffuse goiter, and (5) muscle hypertrophy and slow muscle contraction and relaxation associated with myxedema and cretinism. Although not frequent, several examples of each of these diseases may be seen in a single year in any large general hospital.

Chronic thyrotoxic myopathy is a disease characterized by progressive weakness and atrophy of skeletal musculature, occurring in conjunction with overt or covert (masked) hyperthyroidism. The latter is usually chronic, and the goiter is of the nodular rather than the diffuse type seen in Graves' disease. The muscular disorder may reach proportions such as to suggest progressive muscular atrophy (motor system disease). It is estimated that the middle-aged patient is most likely to suffer from this complication of hyperthyroidism and that men are more susceptible than women. The onset is insidious, the weakness progresses over weeks and months, and exophthalmos need not be present. The pelvic girdle and thigh muscles are weakened more than others (Basedow's paraplegia), though all are affected to some extent, even bulbar and rarely ocular muscles. However, the shoulder and hand muscles are the ones which show the most conspicuous atrophy. Tremor and coarse twitching during contraction may occur, but we have not seen fasciculations at rest or true fibrillations (in the electromyogram). The tendon reflexes are normal or lively. Creatine excretion in the urine is increased, and tolerance to ingested creatine diminished, but the degree of this impairment has not correlated with the degree of weakness. Serum enzyme levels are not elevated. Electromyograms have disclosed no definite abnormality, and biopsies of muscle, except for slight volumetric reduction in fibers, have been normal. Injections of neostigmine have no effect. Muscle power and bulk are gradually restored when thyroid function is reduced to normal levels.

Exophthalmic ophthalmoplegia is a weakness of external ocular muscles (pupillary and ciliary muscles are always spared) which is conjoined with the exophthalmos of Graves' disease. The exophthalmos varies in degree, being sometimes absent at an early age of the disease, and is not in itself responsible for the muscle weakness. Both the ocular weakness and exophthalmos may precede the hyperthyroidism or follow the effective treatment of it. The ocular palsy may occasionally be unilateral, especially in the beginning. Many of the fibers of the eye muscles in biopsies and in autopsy material are seen to have degenerated, and infiltrations of lymphocytes, mononuclear leukocytes, and lipocytes are present; hence the term *infiltrative ophthalmopathy*. All external eye muscles may be affected, often one more than others, accounting for strabismus and diplopia; upward movements are usually limited to the greatest degree. Neostigmine has no effect. The condition often runs a self-limited course as does the exophthalmos itself, and therapy is difficult to evaluate. Certainly the maintenance of a euthyroid state is desirable (see Chap. 85 for treatment of hyperthyroidism). If the exophthalmos reaches a degree which threatens injury of the cornea, tarsorrhaphy, or orbital decompression by removal of the roof of the bony orbit, may save the eyesight.

In patients with marked periorbital and conjunctival edema high dosage of corticosteroids (about 80 mg prednisone per day) may give partial control of the ophthalmic problem, including the extraocular muscle weakness. Because of the toxicity of the corticoid, it should be reserved for patients who would otherwise require surgical intervention. However, in a number of patients it has been possible to carry them over the crisis and avoid the trauma and risks of surgery.

Thyrotoxic periodic paralysis resembles familial periodic paralysis (Chap. 347) and consists of attacks of mild to severe weakness of limb and trunk muscles, usually with sparing of those of the cranium, which develops in a few minutes or hours and lasts part of a day or longer. In some series as many as half the cases of periodic paralysis have been in patients who suffered from hyperthyroidism. Unlike what has been found in typical hypokalemic periodic paralysis, a family history is not obtained. In most cases the serum potassium levels have been low during the attacks and the administration of several grams of KCl has terminated the attack. Treatment of the hyperthyroidism abolishes the symptomatic manifestations of the muscular disorder.

Myasthenia gravis in typical neostigmine-responsive form may accompany hyper or hypothyroidism. In hyperthyroidism the typical weakness and poorly sustained contraction of the aforementioned chronic thyrotoxic myopathy are added to the myasthenia, without appearing to affect the response to or requirement for neostigmine. In constrast, hypothyroidism, even of mild degrees, seems to aggravate the myasthenia gravis, greatly increasing the need for neostigmine and at times inducing a myasthenic crisis. Thyroxine is beneficial and, with respect to myasthenia, restores the patient to his status before the onset of the thyroid insufficiency. However, the myasthenia gravis (described in Chap. 347) is independent of thyroid disease. Each disease must be treated separately.

Hypothyroidism, whether in the form of myxedema or of cretinism, is often accompanied by a series of changes in skeletal muscle consisting of increased volume, stiffness, and slowness of contraction. Action myospasm and percussion myoedema, along with the slowness of tendon reflexes, assist the examiner in making a bedside diagnosis (see Chap. 85). These changes probably account for the large tongue and typical dysarthria seen in this disease. The clinical syndrome simulates hypertrophia musculorum vera and myotonia congenita. Cretinism manifesting these muscle symptoms is known as *Debré-Semelaigne syndrome,* and myxedema with a similar muscle picture is called *Hoffmann's syndrome.* In neither of these two syndromes is there real evidence of myotonia by either clinical test or electromyogram, and muscle biopsies have revealed only large fibers. In the rare condition where myotonia and hypothyroidism coexist, the myotonia appears to be accentuated by the hypothyroidism. Creatinine excretion is reduced, and creatine tolerance is increased. Transaminase values in the serum are normal, but the creatine phosphokinase (CPK) level is usually slightly elevated. The administration of thyroxine, corrects the abnormality of muscle.

The effect of thyroid secretion on the muscle fiber in all these myopathies is still a matter of conjecture. Clinical data indicate that this hormone influences in some manner the contractile process without interfering in any way with the transmission of impulses in the peripheral nerves or across the myoneural junctions. In hyperthyroidism this functional disorder enhances the speed of the contractile process and reduces its duration, the net effect being a weakening, an excess fatigability, and a loss of endurance in muscle action. In hypothyroidism the converse of these changes occurs.

The thyroid hormone also acts on the central nervous system, and in some syndromes, such as myxedema and the acute toxic encephalopathy and myopathy of hyperthyroidism, it is possible to observe the effects of both a neurologic and a muscular disorder.

ALCOHOLIC POLYMYOPATHY WITH CARDIOPATHY Occasionally in alcoholics during a severe drinking bout one observes the rapid development of universal muscle weakness over a period of a few days. At the onset muscle pain and cramps are common. The condition may reach such proportions as to render the patient bedfast, and biopsy reveals extensive segmental necrosis of sarcoplasm. All the limb and trunk muscles may be affected; there is no record of its extending to ocular and other cranial muscles. Myonecrosis is reflected by high levels of muscle enzymes (CPK and aldolase). Myoglobin may appear in the urine, leading to renal failure. Signs of cardiac enlargement and decompensation accompany the polymyopathy in some instances. Most patients recover within a few weeks, but relapse in another spree of drinking has been noted. Restoration of motor power is attendant upon regeneration but may be complicated by polyneuropathy in other syndromes of neuromuscular disability associated with alcoholism.

First observed in Swedish alcoholics, this condition has appeared in American clinics. Perkoff and his associates find some evidence that it is due to a transient suppression of myophosphorylase during bouts of alcoholism. It is too frequent (in milder degrees) to represent an inborn error of metabolism. Some cases formerly described as beriberi cardiopathy may fall in this group.

MYOPATHY The widespread use of adrenal corticosteroids in recent years has brought to light a new muscle disease, probably not dissimilar to that which has been noted in rabbits receiving cortisone. The proximal limb and girdle musculature becomes extremely weak, to the point where it is difficult to elevate the arms and to arise from a sitting, squatting, or kneeling position, and walking itself may be hampered. The electromyogram shows the myopathic pattern of small but abundant action potentials and also fibrillations; in biopsies there is evidence of scattered atrophic and a few degenerating and regenerating muscle fibers without infiltrates of inflammatory cells. The serum creatine kinase and aldolase levels are raised, and there is a creatinuria. Discontinuation of corticosteroid administration leads to recovery within a few weeks. The dose levels of corticosteroid have frequently been high and sustained over a period of months, and fluorinated preparations are more culpable, though all corticosteroids may produce the disorder. There is only a poor correlation between total dose and severity of myopathy. Improvement upon lowering the dose has been reported. A similar myopathy occurs regularly in patients who suffer from Cushing's syndrome. The mechanism of the muscle disease is unknown.

MYOPATHY AND MYOGLOBINURIA In any disease that results in rapid destruction of striated muscle fibers, myoglobin and other muscle proteins may enter the bloodstream and appear in the urine. The latter is dark red or burgundy-colored, much like the urine in hemoglobinuria. However, in hemoglobinuria the serum initially is pink because hemoglobin but not myoglobin is bound to haptoglobin. This complex is not excreted in the urine. The complex of hemoglobin-haptoglobin is removed from the blood plasma over a period of hours, and if hemolysis continues, the haptoglobin may be depleted so that hemoglobinuria is present without grossly evident hemoglobinemia. Differentiation of the two pigments in urine is difficult. Very small differences are seen on spectroscopic examination, but both pigments are rapidly degraded to other compounds, such as hematin, with differing spectrums. Thus great care must be taken with such procedures.

When myoglobinuria is severe, renal damage may ensue and lead to anuria. The mechanism of the renal damage is not clear; probably it is not simply a mechanical obstruction of tubules by precipitated myoglobin. Alkalinization of the urine by the ingestion of sodium bicarbonate is said to protect the kidney by preventing the formation of myoglobin casts, but in severe cases it is of doubtful value, and the sodium may actually be harmful if anuria has already developed. Therapy is the same as in the anuria which follows surgical shock (see Chap. 269).

The following conditions may give rise to myoglobinuria:

1 Crush injury to a limb.
2 Strain or excessive use of muscles, especially the pretibial muscles, which are confined in the tight pretibial compartment (pretibial syndrome).
3 Extensive infarction, as in occlusion of the main artery of a limb or a subcutaneous infusion into the lower leg (with resultant swelling and probable ischemia).
4 Polymyositis.
5 Haff disease, which results from eating fish poisoned by toxic resinous acids derived from cellulose. This was first reported in the bay (Haff) of Königsberg, Germany.
6 Alcoholic polymyopathy and McArdle's disease (see Chap. 343).
7 Familial myoglobinuria (Meyer-Betz disease) occurs in families with or without a diffuse chronic myopathy or dystrophy. The attack of myoglobinuria may be precipitated by strenuous exertion or possibly by an infection. Weakness, stiffness, and tenderness or swelling of muscles are the principal symptoms, and they vary in intensity. The muscle fibers are later found in various stages of degeneration and regeneration. The degree of renal injury usually determines the outcome. No therapy is known except that of complete inactivity and measures which assist return of renal function. Some patients will be shown to have a lifelong disposition to attacks of myoglobinuria; hence strenuous physical activity must be curtailed. In others there may be but a single attack with complete or nearly complete recovery. Nothing is known of the precise mechanism by which the muscle fibers are damaged, but presumably an enzymatic defect of the muscle fibers reduces the tolerance of the muscle to maximal activity (a fault in anaerobic metabolism?). It is probable that more than one disease is presently included in this category.
8 Extreme hyperthermia, especially with convulsions.

OTHER METABOLIC MYOPATHIES A progressive areflexic muscular atrophy giving rise to a syndrome of infantile muscular atrophy, or slack child, has been recorded in two of the five established forms of glycogen storage disease (see Chap. 346).

A syndrome of painful muscles and generalized weakness has been reported in hypoglycemia (see Chap. 90).

In hyperparathyroidism and osteomalacia resulting from renal tubular acidosis (a form of Milkman's syndrome), muscular weakness, fatigability, atrophy, and discomfort after exercise have been noted. The tendon reflexes are normal or hyperactive. In hypophosphatemic rickets the skeletal muscles may be markedly weakened. In several reported cases a bone tumor (an ossifying angioma) was found and its removal restored muscle power to normal.

A contracture of hamstring muscles which prevents upright stance has been found several times in patients with Addison's disease. Biopsy has revealed normal muscle tissue; the electromyogram is normal; and the tendon reflexes are retained.

A primary defect of phosphorylase has been established as the cause of another condition known as McArdle's syndrome. This is a chronic familial myopathy with weakness, stiffness, and discomfort in the muscles following exercise. Therefore it is more logically considered in connection with the myalgic and muscle stiffness syndromes (Chap. 348).

Central core disease, described by Shy and McGee in 1956, is a familial, nonprogressive polymyopathy which manifests itself by hypotonia and delay in locomotion in childhood and by thinness and slight weakness of proximal muscles. The tendon reflexes are preserved. Muscle biopsy has shown large fibers with a conglomerate core of central fibrils which are devoid of both oxidative and phosphorylase enzymes. *Nemeline* or *rod body, pleoconial, megaconial,* and *myotubular polymyopathies,* presenting somewhat similar clinical pictures, have been described. Details are to be found in the monograph by Adams and Pearson.

REFERENCES

Adams RD, Pearson C: *Diseases of Muscle: A Study in Pathology,* 3d ed., New York: Hoeber, 1973

WALTON JN: *Disorders of Voluntary Muscle,* 3d ed., Baltimore: Williams & Wilkins, 1973

——, ADAMS RD: *Polymyositis,* Edinburgh and London: Livingstone, 1955

346 PROGRESSIVE MUSCULAR ATROPHY AND PARALYSIS

RAYMOND D. ADAMS
FRANK H. TYLER

As intimated in the clinical classification in Chap. 343 (see Table 343-1), one of the major causes of the syndrome of progressive weakness and wasting of the musculature of the limbs and trunk is muscular dystrophy. This category of disease can usually be differentiated from the familial or nonfamilial varieties of neuropathy by the pattern of the muscle involvement (usually proximal in the dystrophies and distal in most of the neuropathies), by the absence of sensory disturbances, the less severe reduction of tendon reflexes, the normal cerebrospinal fluid, the characteristic electromyogram, and the findings in a muscle biopsy. It can usually be distinguished from spinal muscular atrophy, exemplified in the adult by motor system disease and in the infant by Werdnig-Hoffmann muscular atrophy, by the proximal and symmetric pattern of muscle involvement (total lack of pattern in motor system disease and asymmetry of involvement in the muscles of forearms and hands or feet and legs), lack of coarse fasciculations, and the characteristic electromyogram and biopsy changes. These two forms of chronic muscular atrophy due to diseases of the nervous system are described in Chaps. 17 and 333 and will not be discussed further in this section.

THE MUSCULAR DYSTROPHIES

HISTORY AND TERMINOLOGY Progressive muscular dystrophy *(dystrophia musculorum progressiva)* was described by several prominent physicians in the middle and latter half of the nineteenth century. The many names used since that time to designate types of this condition have been a source of confusion. Duchenne reported a group of young patients, mostly males, with muscular enlargement as well as atrophy; this disease has since been referred to as *pseudohypertrophic muscular dystrophy.* Leyden and Möbius called attention to a clinically similar group in which, however, muscular enlargement was lacking. Thus arose the name *simple atrophic* type. Landouzy and Dejerine described muscular dystrophy of the facial, pectoral, and shoulder girdle muscles, which they called the *facioscapulohumeral* type; and Erb reported a condition of limb-girdle dystrophy with little or no facial involvement, which he termed *juvenile dystrophy.* Recently, Walton and others have insisted on the distinction between "limb-girdle dystrophy" and facioscapulohumeral dystrophy because the former has earlier onset and lack of typical dominant inheritance as well as the lack of facial involvement. However, reexamination of many of these cases revealed a proximal form of hereditary progressive muscular atrophy secondary to disease of motor neurons (Wolfahrt-Kingellberg-Welander syndrome). Hence its nosologic position remains in doubt. Many cases do not fit into this classification, and a number of other syndromes have been described. It is now generally agreed that all these groups represent the end stage of more than one disease process. Clinical and genetic evidence permits the separation of at least six syndromes; Duchenne's pseudohypertrophic, facioscapulohumeral, limb-girdle, distal, ocular, and myotonic dystrophy. The criteria for each group are mode of inheritance, age of onset, rate of progression, localization of initial involvement, morphologic changes, and associated dystrophy of other organs (eye, testicles, skin, brain). It should be emphasized that other much rarer types do exist, but description of their characteristics is beyond the scope of this discussion.

CAUSES AND PATHOGENESIS The cause of muscular dystrophy is an abnormality of genes. Although in many instances a family history cannot be obtained by direct questioning, in approximately 40 to 50 percent of cases other affected individuals are found on careful examination of the members of the pedigree. Other considerations lead to the conclusion that the disease may be caused either by a previously latent recessive trait or by the occurrence of a mutation (see Chap. 62). Although it is quite possible that the same clinical manifestations may occur occasionally as the result of a nongenetic mechanism, the occurrence of the genetic pattern in the majority of instances must be considered in forming any concept of the mechanism of these disorders.

By analogy with the other known genetic disorders, it must be presumed that some abnormality in the intracellular metabolism of the muscle fibers is caused by the genetic abnormality. This could be a modified or absent enzyme system within the muscle cell or some defect in the muscle metabolism resulting from inability to absorb or to metabolize normally a substance vital to muscle function.

The occurrence of creatinuria in patients with muscular dystrophy has led to extensive study of creatine synthesis as the basis of the metabolic anomaly. Although there is some evidence of both increased synthesis and imperfect control of normal synthesis, the significance of this to the fundamental anomaly is as yet unknown. Many other metabolic systems in the muscle are under investigation or have been investigated in the past. As yet no clear-cut mechanism by which the observed chemical changes could lead to the muscular damage has been proposed.

The pattern of development of muscular atrophy is remarkably similar from one patient to another with the same type of dystrophy. It has been suggested, concerning diseases that affect a local group of muscles, that the affection bears a relationship to their order of development in the embryo; those muscles which appear earliest manifest the first and most severe weakness and atrophy. Even when one part of the muscle develops earlier than another, the atrophy follows this order. Thus, the lower fibers of the trapezius muscle form very early, in contrast to the upper fibers, which are dependent on late innervation by the spinal accessory cranial nerves. The lower fibers of the pectoral muscle are among the earliest of girdle muscles to develop; and the disease always involves the lower part of this muscle most severely. On the other hand, the variation in severity of the disease in different patients and variation in area of initial involvement in the various types make this embryologic explanation not completely apposite. Other subtle differences (probably biochemical) between muscles are most likely being revealed by these diseases.

As in other genetically determined metabolic disorders, it is probable that a single enzymatic abnormality underlies the entire disease process and accounts for all its manifestations, even in such a disease as myotonic dystrophy, in which many systems are involved. Only continued search at the basic level of metabolic processes will lead to an understanding of the pathogenesis of these disorders.

CHILDHOOD TYPE OF DUCHENNE'S PSEUDOHYPERTROPHIC PELVIFEMORAL MUSCULAR DYSTROPHY Although several of the different varieties of muscular dystrophy begin in infancy and childhood (e.g., myotonic dystrophy facioscapulohumeral dystrophy), the most frequent and dreaded form in this age period is that first described by Duchenne.

The Duchenne type has been subdivided into three distinct categories as follows: (1) severe, sex-linked recessive form; (2) mild, sex-linked recessive form; (3) mild autosomal recessive form. These occur, according to Walton, Milhorat, and others, in a ratio of 27:3:5 respectively.

The severe sex-linked variety, which has been the most thoroughly studied, may begin in fetal life and is not infrequently (in nearly half the cases) manifest during the second and third years of life, thus interfering with the beginning of locomotion. More often such children are normal at birth and their early muscular and other development is normal. Onset after ten years of age would place the case in the second category of milder disease.

Females may transmit the disease but do not suffer from it, as a rule. The carrier female may be identified (with about 80 percent accuracy) by the creatine kinase test on serum (which is slightly elevated), muscle biopsy (slight dystrophic changes), and a slightly myopathic electromyogram.

The most frequent initial complaints relate to the early involvement of pelvifemoral muscles, resulting in frequent falls, difficulty in rising from the floor or climbing stairs, awkward, peculiar gait, and inability to run properly. Muscle weakness often is not recognized initially by the family. The onset is insidious, and the course is slowly progressive over months and years. Later, shoulder, girdle, and trunk muscles become affected, and usually the child becomes confined to chair or bed before the age of twelve years. Fatality is frequent during the second decade of life owing to obesity and kyphoscoliosis, sudden cardiac failure, and pulmonary insufficiency or infection.

When the patient is examined, the findings naturally vary with the stage of the disease, but early the calves and sometimes the quadriceps and deltoid muscles are unusually large and firm even though weak, i.e., pseudohypertrophy. The weakness is evidenced by a typical waddling gait (weak glutei), a curious manner of "climbing up one's legs" (weak extensors of hip and spine), the so-called Gower's sign, and winging of scapulae on elevation of arms. The abdomen is protuberant because of weak abdominal muscles, and an exaggerated lordosis is required to maintain balance. Facial muscles are entirely spared or affected late in the course of the illness. More specifically one may find weakness of the iliopsoas, quadriceps, gluteus, and anterior tibial muscles in the lower extremities and later of the serrati, pectorals, latissimi, biceps, and brachioradialis muscles in the upper extremities. The forearm and hand muscles and the gastrocnemius and foot muscles retain good power until late in the illness. Early in the disease the tendon reflexes in the arms are preserved, and even at a late stage it is usually possible to obtain ankle reflexes. The neurologic findings are otherwise within normal limits.

Cardiac involvement is commonly observed in the late stages of the disease, manifest as tachycardia and also by signs of decompensation. Prolongation of the P-R interval, slurring of the QRS complex, bundle branch block, and elevation or depression of the S-T segments are seen in the ECG. The shafts of long bones are thin (disuse atrophy). Intelligence seems to be normal, though when large groups of patients are examined it is often found to be mildly reduced, i.e., about 10 percent below that of the general population. Mental retardation, when present, tends to be proportional to the severity of the muscular dystrophy. It is nonprogressive.

The mild sex-linked variety and the less definite autosomal recessive form differ from the above only in later age of onset, slower progression (permitting survival into adult years), less frequent fatality, and in that they affect females.

The Leyden-Möbius pelvicrural, atrophic dystrophy is probably a variety of either Duchenne's or Erb's juvenile, limb-girdle dystrophy.

FACIOSCAPULOHUMERAL TYPE OF LANDOUZY-DEJERINE This disease is inherited as an autosomal dominant disorder with complete penetrance. This, plus the fact that affected persons are often not incapacitated during the childbearing period, accounts for the high familial incidence and also for the high prevalence in a community. Males and females are equally affected.

Facioscapulohumeral dystrophy often begins later than the Duchenne type, though we have seen mild facial weakness at two to three years of age. The average age of onset is thirteen years, with a range between nine and twenty years. A few patients even beyond fifty years of age are found on close examination to have the disorder, although they have not recognized their disability. As this implies, the degree of involvement may be extremely slight. Other patients, however, are significantly incapacitated before the age of twenty.

The pattern of muscular involvement differs from that of other dystrophies, as is indicated by the name. Weakness of facial muscles is nearly always present. All the facial muscles are involved in the process, but the orbicularis oris may show a weakness which results in abnormal movements and inability to pucker the mouth or whistle normally. There are weaknesses of the orbicularis oculi and diffuse flattening of the face; and asymmetric movements, particularly about the mouth, are extremely characteristic. The diagnosis may be suspected after watching the patient's face while he gives his history. The facial weakness may be the earliest change.

Usually, however, it is weakness of the muscles of the pectoral girdle and winging of the scapulae which bring the patient to the physician. In contrast, the pelvifemoral muscles are strong and there is no pseudohypertrophy. These patients cannot raise their arms above their heads, but they frequently maintain normal strength in the forearms and hands until an advanced age.

The axial and pelvic musculature becomes involved later in the disease, and the tibial and peroneal groups may also become weak and atrophic.

The same complications and associated abnormalities as were described in childhood dystrophy will eventually occur, but there are fewer associated congenital anomalies; and heart disease due to dystrophy and severe scoliosis is extremely rare. The average patient lives out a normal life span, becoming completely incapacitated only very late in life. This disease, like the limb-girdle dystrophy, must be distinguished from the proximal forms of hereditary motor system disease, chronic polymyositis, and syringomyelia (see Chaps. 333, 334, and 343).

Laboratory data Laboratory examinations yield no abnormalities except creatinuria, which is usually not so marked as in childhood dystrophy, and creatinine excretion is not as much reduced as in childhood dystrophy. Some patients, particularly those with minimal involvement, may have relatively insignificant creatinuria. The serum enzyme levels are raised only slightly.

LIMB-GIRDLE DYSTROPHY OF ERB This form of muscular dystrophy is characterized by occurrence in either sex; onset during the second and third decades of life; transmission as an autosomal recessive trait and, in rare instances, as a dominant one; primary involvement of the muscles of either the shoulder girdle or the pelvic girdle, usually with spread to the other after a variable period of time; pseudohypertrophy in the calves and other muscles in only a small proportion of cases. The course of the illness is variable, but usually the rate of progression is slow, and severe disability does not occur until the disease has been present for 20 years or more. Facial muscles are spared. *Formes frustes* are known, one type being limited to the quadriceps muscles.

The purity of this entity, as stated above, has been much debated. It evidently overlaps clinically with the third subvariety of Duchenne's dystrophy and with Landouzy-Dejerine dystrophy. The muscles involved are essentially the same as in Duchenne's dystrophy. Cardiac impairment is rare, and the range of intelligence, like that of the Landouzy-Dejerine groups, is normal.

Laboratory findings These are the same as in Landouzy-Dejerine dystrophy.

DISTAL TYPE OF DYSTROPHY Gowers and Spiller many years ago and Welander more recently have called attention to patients with slowly progressive atrophy of the muscles of the hands and feet. In these patients muscle biopsy has shown the characteristic lesions of muscular dystrophy. The disorder apparently begins in middle adult life (average age, forty-seven years) and is slowly progressive but produces only moderate disability. Welander was able to show the existence of an autosomal dominant transmission of the trait in some of the families which she studied. The disorder must be unusual, for we have observed only a few such patients in Boston and Salt Lake City over a period of years. It should be noted that the cardinal manifestation of this disorder, i.e., atrophy and weakness of the lower leg and hand muscles, is characteristic of peroneal muscular atrophy and the hereditary types of progressive muscular atrophy (motor system disease). The former disease is also a genetically determined disorder of autosomal dominant inheritance in which the patients usually develop more severe atrophy and weakness with minimal sensory loss in the lower leg, the forearm, and hand, in contrast to the distal type of dystrophy. This and other features of neuropathy, such as delayed conduction velocity of peripheral nerves, prove to be useful in differential diagnosis.

MYOTONIC DYSTROPHY Definition Myotonic dystrophy (myotonia dystrophica, myotonia atrophica, Steinert's disease) is a hereditary disease characterized by myotonia, muscular wasting of a characteristic pattern, cataracts, testicular atrophy, and frontal baldness.

Clinical pattern The myotonia in the early years may be more prominent than the other manifestations. Although the disease usually begins in early adult life, it may be observed in infancy and childhood. Myotonia, as was stated in Chap. 343, consists of an inability to relax a muscle normally after its contraction and is the result of repetitive discharge of the contractile mechanism of the fiber. It is a symptom which may be seen in an occasional patient with any of several other neuromuscular disorders. Most characteristically it is demonstrable in the adductors of the thumb, forearm muscles, and tongue. The patient's inability to let go after shaking hands may give the clue to the proper diagnosis. This difficulty tends to disappear after repeated contractions and to return after inactivity. Idiomuscular contractions elicited by direct percussion of the muscle are also delayed in relaxation. This latter sign (percussion myotonia) may be present when the grasp response and other clinical evidence of myotonia are not found. The muscular atrophy which develops is in some respects similar to that in the diseases described above. A different type of facial involvement occurs, however. In general the patient exhibits a rather dull, expressionless facies, with ptosis of the eyelids due to weakness of levator muscles. The forehead is furrowed as a compensatory effort on the part of the frontalis muscle to overcome the ptosis. The latter may become so severe that the patient must tip his head back to see straight ahead. Closure of the eyes (orbicularis oculi) is also weak, which in combination with ptosis is invariably myopathic. The "dystrophic" facial movements of the facioscapulohumeral dystrophy do not occur. The voice becomes nasal and expressionless. Atrophy of the temporalis muscles is usually severe. Atrophy of the sternocleidomastoids is disproportionately marked; the other muscles of the anterior part of the neck may be so atrophic that the trachea is seen immediately beneath the skin. Extreme difficulty in flexing the neck, with moderately strong extension, is explained by the preservation of the spinalis group of muscles. The long flexors and extensors of the fingers are involved. In the lower extremities the weakness begins in the anterior tibial group but soon spreads to the peronei and gastrocnemii and later to the quadriceps and hamstrings. The tendon reflexes are reduced, and contractures may occur late in the illness.

These patients, whether male or female, also develop progressive *alopecia*, usually frontal, at an early age. Testicular atrophy with androgenic deficiency usually develops in males. The latter are frequently sterile and sometimes impotent. In some patients, gynecomastia and elevated gonadotropin excretion are found. Testicular biopsy may show peritubular fibrosis. Thus, all the clinical characteristics of Klinefelter's syndrome may be present. However, the nuclei of skin or bone marrow cells only rarely have been shown to have "sex chromatin mass"; the majority of patients are of the usual sex chromosome constitution. Ovarian deficiency occasionally develops in females. This is seldom severe enough to interfere with the menstrual pattern or fertility. The lens opacities of myotonic dystrophy are of two types. The first consists of fine dustlike subcapsular deposits which frequently appear scintillating and colored under the slit lamp but often cannot be seen with the ordinary ophthalmoscope. This type of opacity is virtually always present in patients with other signs of the disorder. Its appearance is so characteristic as to be virtually diagnostic. The second type of cataract is like the usual senile cataract and seldom appears except in elderly patients, being of little diagnostic usefulness. *Blepharoconjunctivitis* is an extremely common finding, even in patients with little weakness of facial muscles, and is universal in advanced cases. The disease affects the gastrointestinal tract, causing in particular weakness and dilatation of the esophagus.

Neurologic examination reveals no sensory or other motor abnormalities. Mental retardation is a common finding in these patients or in their siblings. The brain weight in such cases is reduced below normal levels by more than 200 g, and there is an abnormality of cortical lamination. *Dystrophic heart disease* is also a frequent finding, as it is in childhood dystrophy (contrasting with the facioscapulohumeral type), but because it usually occurs at an advanced age and presents no specific features, it is difficult to differentiate from other types of heart disease common in elderly persons. Atrial arrhythmias are notably frequent.

Among all the dystrophies the myotonic variety is the most variable. Rarely a patient may exhibit only one of the features, such as myotonia or the characteristic cataracts; and in many of the more complete cases one or more of the dystrophic features may be missing. Nonetheless diagnosis is seldom difficult on physical examination alone, if care is taken to look for the features described. The diagnosis is obvious in patients who suffer significant disability from their myotonic dystrophy.

Two rare but distinct diseases are closely related to myotonic dystrophica and need mention in order that they may not be confused with it: *myotonia congenita* (*Thomsen's disease*), a familial disorder of dominant inheritance in which there is lifelong myotonia, which is most severe following rest, excitement, or anxiety, but lacks the other manifestations of myotonia dystrophica; and *paramyotonia congenita*, an even rarer disorder, in which myotonia along with episodic weakness occurs only following exposure to cold. The latter is also familial, of dominant inheritance, of lifelong duration, and benign in character. It is clinically and genetically separable from the other myotonias. All forms of myotonia respond to quinine and procainamide, as described below.

Myotonia dystrophica is inherited as a typical mendelian dominant trait, but certain members of a given line may manifest only one or two of the usual group of findings. Myotonia is the most common finding on physical examination, while cataracts are often mentioned in family histories. Care must be used, however, in evaluating this latter datum, because cataracts of other causation may occur in the nondystrophic line and lead to confusion. Search by history and examination for other features of the syndrome in persons with cataracts will usually prevent such errors.

Routine laboratory data are of no aid in making the diagnosis. Creatinuria is irregular and frequently absent. The characteristic afterpotentials of myotonia can be demonstrated electromyographically and may be useful, especially where clinical demonstration of myotonia is difficult. In addition, the electromyogram shows the usual myopathic pattern of many low-voltage, brief action potentials of myopathy.

Hyperostosis frontalis interna has been reported in relation to myotonic dystrophy. The sella turcica is often small. The 17-ketosteroid levels in urine are low.

PROGRESSIVE OPHTHALMOPLEGIA AND OCULOPHARYNGEAL DYSTROPHY Isolated dystrophic involvement of the extraocular muscles is another relatively rare form of muscle dystrophy. These disorders must be differentiated from other causes of ophthalmoplegia. Two separate syndromes have been identified. One consists of a progressive external ophthalmoplegia (sparing of pupils and muscles of accommodation), ptosis, and sometimes weakness of orbicularis oculi. It begins in childhood, adolescence, or early adult life and slowly progresses over many years. Isolated involvement of other cranial or spinal muscles may later be conjoined. Affection of eye muscles is a relatively uncommon feature of the other forms of muscular dystrophy. Similarity of the histologic findings on biopsy to those in other varieties of dystrophy has been the means by which Kiloh and Nevin were able to establish the myopathic character of this disorder. The second form, demonstrated to be a myopathy by Hayes, Adams, and Victor, consists of a progressive ptosis and dysphagia developing in late life (beyond fifty years of age). The disease appears to be inherited as a mendelian dominant trait. Each patient complains of increasing difficulty in swallowing and eventually suffers inanition. Biopsy of temporal muscles and electromyograms were compatible with muscular dystrophy, not with denervation, as E. W. Taylor had previously supposed.

LABORATORY DATA Apart from the ECG abnormalities already mentioned, the electrical reactions of skeletal muscle are reduced and the electromyogram exhibits the characteristic pattern of low voltage and brief action potentials. Excretion of creatine in the urine is increased, and that of creatinine is decreased. Levels of transaminases, aldolase, and creatine kinase, the most sensitive and specific of these tests, may be raised (>4, or, by the new standard, 50 units) even before the disease is recognized clinically, and they are also slightly elevated in the normal female carriers of this trait.

PATHOLOGY OF THE MUSCULAR DYSTROPHIES

The atrophic muscles appear white or fatty, coming to resemble fish flesh, and the diagnosis may be suspected from the gross appearance. Microscopically, probably the most important change is necrosis of single fibers. Some of the remaining fibers are enlarged, and many others are atrophic; the sarcolemmal nuclei are increased in number, forming chains and appearing centrally in the fibers. Other fibers within a microscopic field look entirely normal. The distribution of involved muscle fibers in any muscle is entirely random, quite unlike the pattern of "group atrophy" of spinal and neural atrophic diseases. The damaged and atrophic fibers ultimately disappear and are progressively replaced by fibrous tissue and fat cells.

The lesions are more or less similar in all types of dystrophy. Myotonic dystrophy differs in that there are spiral annulets of myofibrils, zones of sarcoplasm free of organized myofibrils, and unusually prominent "rowing" of nuclei, in addition to the usual dystrophic changes. In the very advanced cases, in which all muscle fibers have disappeared, it may be difficult to recognize the tissue as muscle. The peripheral nervous system and spinal cord are unchanged, and even in late stages of the disease nerve cells and fibers are preserved.

Under the electron microscope the earliest changes are fragmentation and dissolution of myofilaments, together with abnormalities in the structure and organization of endoplasmic reticulum and mitochondria. In myotonic dystrophy myofilamentous loss tends to be subsarcolemmal, with nuclear increase.

Despite the many biochemical studies that have been undertaken, no important insights have been forthcoming. In sum, one finds a lowering in the level of the intramuscular enzymes involved in the glycolytic systems (with the exception of hexokinase and lactic dehydrogenase); normal oxidative enzymes and metabolism (cytochrome oxidases, succinoxidase, and succinic dehydrogenase remain proportional to residual muscle substance); diminished total body potassium, but always in proportion to residual muscle mass; increased excretion of all amino acids in urine; and change of myoglobin pattern, especially in Duchenne's dystrophy, to a fetal type (probably a regenerative phenomenon). None of these changes seems to be specifically related to the dystrophic process.

TREATMENT OF THE MUSCULAR DYSTROPHIES

There is no treatment for any of the dystrophies of muscle, and the physician is forced to stand by helplessly and witness the spectacle of unrelenting progressive paralysis. The various preparations recommended in the past, such as vitamin E, inositol, anabolic steroids, amino acid and protein supplements to diet, and Levadosin and digitalis preparations, have not been shown to have a beneficial effect.

Quinine has a mild curare-like action at the motor end-plate and thus relieves the myotonia. Although symptomatic relief of the myotonia is usually achieved, the drug has no effect on the progress of the muscle atrophy or other degenerative aspects of the disease. The usual dose is 0.3 to 0.6 g orally, repeated as needed about every 6 hr. Mild toxic symptoms such as tinnitus may develop before enough quinine has been given to obtain satisfactory relief of the myotonia. Some patients find the side effects more distressing than the myotonia and prefer not to take quinine except on special occasions when the myotonia is troublesome in a particular activity. Procainamide and diphenylhydantoin also have some effect but are only occasionally useful.

Surgical management of the cataracts when they are mature is indicated.

Androgens may be administered in cases of myotonic dystrophy and provide symptomatic benefit when deficiency is apparent, but a relation of the hormone to the pathogenesis of the disease is not established.

Two factors are of importance in the management of these patients—avoidance of prolonged bed rest and inactivity, and encouragement of the patient to maintain as full and normal a life as possible. These measures help to prevent the rapid worsening associated with inactivity and to conserve a healthy attitude of mind. Obesity should be avoided; this may require careful attention to diet. Contractures and skeletal deformities in Duchenne's dystrophy can be prevented or delayed by passive and active stretching exercises. Fasciotomy or tendon-lengthening operations and long leg braces may aid in preserving ambulation for several additional years.

CHRONIC, SLOWLY PROGRESSIVE, OR RELATIVELY STATIONARY MYOPATHIES (OTHER THAN MUSCULAR DYSTROPHY)

Central-core myopathy (Shy and Magee); nemeline myopathy (Engel and Shy); pleoconial, megaconial, and myotubular polymyopathies; McArdle's phosphorylase deficiency; some cases of familial periodic paralysis; and familial paroxysmal myoglobinuria are examples of diseases in which a congenital thinning and weakness of muscles progresses slowly over a long period of time. Many of the children with this type of condition have been described as "floppy" or hypotonic. In each instance the basic pathologic process induces a distinctive alteration (disfiguration) of the muscle fibers, and the increasing weakness is due to a mild necrobiosis of individual muscle fibers, leading ultimately to a numerical reduction. Diagnosis, as a rule, depends on some other attribute, either clinical or pathologic, or an associated episodic disorder of function. In the latter case, the disease must be considered in another context, as indicated in the clinical classification in Chap. 343.

Central-core disease and nemeline myopathy are rare familial affections of muscle beginning in childhood. In the former, each striated muscle fiber is marked by a core of hyaline appearance; in the latter, myriads of rodlike structures resembling bacilli collect in aggregates beneath the sarcolemma. In both diseases thinness of proximal limb and trunk muscles imparts a myopathic aspect to the patient's bodily configuration. Progression of the disease is so slow that in childhood it is more than counterbalanced by the natural growth and development of the musculature. In pleoconial, megaconial, and special inclusion body myopathies, these fibers are observed to contain unusually large or otherwise altered mitochondria or central tubes. Diagnosis depends on biopsy.

Paroxysmal (familial) myoglobinuria, McArdle's disease, and familial periodic paralysis are described in Chaps. 345 and 348. In most patients, muscular power and bulk are preserved between attacks of myoglobinuria, contracture, or weakness; however, if the attacks are frequent and severe, necrosis of muscle fibers will occur and result in a gradual loss of fibers (numerical reduction).

REFERENCES

TYLER FH, STEPHENS FE: Studies in disorders of muscle. II. Clinical manifestations and inheritance in facioscapulohumeral dystrophy in a large family. Ann Intern Med 32:640, 1950

WALTON JN: *Disorders of Voluntary Muscle*, 3d ed., Baltimore: Williams & Wilkins, 1973

——, NATTRASS FJ: On the classification, natural history, and treatment of the myopathies. Brain 77:169, 1954

347 EPISODIC MUSCULAR WEAKNESS

RAYMOND D. ADAMS

Characteristic of most of the muscular diseases included in this chapter is the episodic nature of the weakness, the patient being normal or only slightly weak between attacks, and the evident disorder of neuromuscular transmission or of muscle membrane excitability (see Chap. 344).

The diseases listed under Episodic Weakness in the classification in Chap. 343 should be considered when a patient with an apparently intact nervous system and relatively normal-appearing muscles complains of episodic or fluctuating weakness or paralysis.

In myasthenia gravis and thyrotoxic myopathy with myasthenia or periodic paralysis, some degree of weakness is persistent at all times but is made worse by activity. Exhaustion and fatigability with drug intoxication (organophosphates, neostigmine, certain antibiotics, phenothiazine drugs, barbiturates, and bromides), neurasthenia, depression, and other states of excessive fatigability can be separated as a rule on clinical grounds (see Chap. 16).

MYASTHENIA GRAVIS

DEFINITION The disease, first described in 1672 by Thomas Willis and later by Goldflam and Jolly, is characterized by weakness and easy fatigability; it most frequently affects the facial, oculomotor, laryngeal, pharyngeal, and respiratory muscles. Partial recovery with rest and after the administration of anticholinesterase drugs is another important attribute.

CLINICAL PATTERN Myasthenia gravis occurs at all ages and in both sexes, but females are affected twice as often as males. The period of highest incidence is in the third decade of life. No significant familial occurrence has been noted, though the disease has rarely been observed in siblings or parent and child.

The onset may be insidious but is often subacute and rarely acute, being precipitated by infection or emotional upset. Weakness of ocular muscles with drooping of the eyelids, which may be unilateral at first, occurs in 90 percent of cases. Diplopia due to unequal weakness of the ocular muscles is usually the first symptom; it is often transient and intermittent, but may persist and at times progresses to complete paresis of ocular movement. The pupils are never affected. Facial and pharyngeal muscles are weakened in 70 percent of cases. The facial involvement gives rise to a smooth, relatively immobile facies. The smile has an unnatural appearance in that the lips elevate but do not retract; it resembles a snarl. The tongue may be weak and is bilaterally furrowed, the so-called "trident tongue."

Weakness of the laryngeal and pharyngeal muscles may be the initial symptom in a smaller number of patients. Choking and aspiration of food are then common and obvious symptoms. As a result of paresis of palatal muscles, fluids may be regurgitated through the nose when swallowing is attempted. The involvement of tongue, laryngeal, and facial muscles results in abnormal speech of a rather feeble, "mushy" type, and the voice has a nasal quality; if the patient continues to talk for a short time, the abnormality becomes more severe, to the point where speech becomes unintelligible. This is in striking contrast to the psychoneurotic patient, who also complains of weakness but can talk interminably without change in voice or enunciation. Affection of masseter muscles may prevent closure of the mouth ("hanging-jaw sign"), and the patient habitually holds his hand under his jaw.

A generalized weakness of skeletal muscles is also present in advanced cases of myasthenia gravis but seldom occurs in the absence of involvement of muscles innervated by cranial nerves. As in other myopathies, the proximal or girdle muscles, especially those of the shoulder girdle, are most severely affected. In the most advanced or severe stages, weakness may be universal.

Easy fatigability and relatively prompt, partial recovery after rest, revealed by history or clinical examination, can be elicited in most cases. The best test is to have the patient perform a repetitive long-sustained motion with an involved muscle or group of muscles. As the disease process becomes more severe and of longer duration, the weakness also tends to be more extensive. There are no other neurologic abnormalities in the average patient.

The disease may be aggravated to a variable extent by a number of factors. The most frequent of these are infections of the upper part of the respiratory tract, excitement, general fatigue, loss of sleep, menstruation, high-carbohydrate meals, and the intake of alcohol. Medications which increase the neural and muscular block, such as curare, quinine, and quaternary ammonium compounds, and sometimes hypothyroidism may add to the myasthenia, resulting in more severe paralysis, and should be avoided or treated.

Muscular atrophy is not seen in the great majority of patients but may be present, particularly if the process has been of long duration. It is most frequently seen in a few muscles, such as the temporal masseter, cervical, and proximal shoulder-girdle muscles. Exceptionally a denervative process in one or a few muscles may occur and account for weakness. The tendon reflexes are preserved even with severe myasthenia. Stiffness and paresthesias of face or hands are frequent complaints, but usually there is no evidence of sensory impairment. The external vesical and anal sphincters may be weakened, with stress incontinence.

Approximately 8 to 10 percent of myasthenic patients have a small-celled tumor of the thymus gland. Macrocytic anemia has been reported in a few such patients. Thyrotoxicosis, polymyositis, rheumatoid arthritis, and lupus erythematosus may occur in conjunction with myasthenia gravis, and there is a special variety (Eaton-Lambert inverse myasthenia) which accompanies malignant tumors.

Having developed over a few days or weeks, the disease may advance irregularly or remain at the same level of severity for a long time. Remissions, partial or complete, occur in about half the patients, usually in the first few years. There may also be relapses, completely unpredictable as to time of occurrence or severity, and they usually reproduce the initial syndrome. Certainly the most distressing state is that in which the myasthenic patient, unable to breathe independently, must pass long periods of time in a respiratory unit, intubated, exposed to repeated respiratory infections, and needing a gastrectomy for tube feeding. Certain muscles (eye, tongue, cervical) may almost cease to function and are unresponsive to anticholinergic drugs and thymectomy.

The life of the patient with severe myasthenia is endangered by progression of paralysis. Fatality most frequently occurs in the first year of the disease and in the period between the fourth and seventh years. If the disease has been present for 10 years or more, it usually remains benign. Respiratory infections are a threat and should be treated by appropriate sulfonamides and antibiotics. Some female patients have a reduced fertility, but pregnancy does occur and may be followed by a normal delivery. Remissions and occasionally relapses have accompanied pregnancy. The offspring may exhibit a mild or severe *myasthenia* at birth which may threaten their lives. This type of neonatal myasthenia lasts only a few weeks, and spontaneous recovery is the rule. Later in childhood the usual variety of myasthenia may develop.

Respiratory insufficiency may come on quite abruptly or may be insidiously progressive. This is the complication that still terminates life in some 5 to 10 percent of patients. Fatal accessions of profound weakness may be evoked by an overdose of neostigmine.

PATHOLOGY Collections of small round cells, presumably lymphocytes, are seen among the muscle fibers and around the small blood vessels in a majority of cases. Other organs may also show similar cellular infiltrations. Single muscle fibers or groups of fibers in a state of degeneration have been found in a few muscles in about half the fatal cases. Chronically paralyzed muscles may show atrophy of single fibers and rarely motor unit atrophy though anterior horn cells and nerves are of normal appearance. Replacement of muscle fibers by fat and fibrous tissue accounts for the permanent paralysis seen sometimes in eye and tongue muscles. There is no lack of acetylcholine or cholinesterase at myoneural junctions in histochemical stains, but two groups of investigators have noted that the motor end-plates are abnormally thin and unbranched. The latter have been examined under the electron microscope, and a patchy decrease in electron density of the muscle membrane within the end-plate zone and a diminution in the number of nerve filaments and infoldings of the sarcolemma have been observed. The thymic tumors have been of both lymphoblastic and epithelial types. They are more frequent in elderly patients. The tumor, whether called benign or malignant, remains confined to the mediastinum. In the nontumor cases, the thymus shows hyperplasia of lymph follicles.

PATHOGENESIS The disease is believed to be the result of a specific functional abnormality at the *neuromyal junction.* Normally, acetylcholine, released at this junction, facilitates the passage of impulses across from nerve terminals to the muscle fiber. Cholinesterase is normally present and hydrolyzes the acetylcholine; physostigmine and neostigmine antagonize cholinesterase. The block in neuromuscular transmission is evidenced in the electromyogram (Chap. 344) as a progressive decline in the voltage of action potentials. The exact nature of the block has eluded all investigators. It is not.corrected by acetylcholine given intraarterially. Curare, quinine, or the quaternary ammonium compounds, which normally impair transmission across the neuromyal junction or over the surface of the muscle fiber, act in unusually small dosages to enhance the weakness in myasthenic patients. A circulating curare-like factor has never been demonstrated in the blood, and exchange transfusions of blood from normal patients have been of no value. A faulty catabolism of acetylcholine has also been postulated.

Antinuclear, anti-end-plate, and antimuscle antibodies have been demonstrated in a considerable proportion of cases, and the possibility has been suggested that one of these antibodies inhibits the action of either acetylcholine or cholinesterase, more likely the latter, at receptor sites on the muscle fibers.

DIAGNOSIS The diagnosis usually is made without difficulty if one carefully evaluates the history and thinks of the disease. The characteristic pattern of *myasthenic fatigability* is easy to demonstrate by having the patient make some repetitive or sustained movement, such as looking up toward the ceiling for 2 to 3 min. The eyelids progressively droop until they cover the iris. Strength returns to the levator palpebrae muscles after a few minutes of rest. Intramuscular injection of 0.5 to 2.0 mg neostigmine usually results in prompt relief of the muscular weakness, which is evident both to the patient and to the physician. When the larger doses of neostigmine are used, it is important to administer about 1 mg atropine prior to the neostigmine in order to minimize the parasympathomimetic effects of the neostigmine. Many times a patient who is unable to sit up, speak, or swallow will in the course of 5 to 15 min after neostigmine administration regain strength in a dramatic fashion. Occasionally patients with localized ocular palsies do not respond promptly to neostigmine, but then the effect is nearly always obvious in other groups of muscles. Edrophonium chloride (Tensilon) is very similar in its action to neostigmine. For diagnostic testing it has the advantage that the response to an intravenous injection is always instantaneous and the action is dissipated within a few minutes. The usual dose is 10 mg. Also, severe side reactions are uncommon, making it unnecessary to administer atropine except in patients with asthma or cardiac disease. Although the short duration of action of this drug makes it unsatisfactory for maintenance therapy, in a myasthenic crisis it may be given by continuous intravenous drip. Another use is to determine if the weakness which develops in a myasthenic patient on neostigmine or similar therapy is the result of an exacerbation of the myasthenia gravis or of overtreatment with neostigmine or related compounds, which of themselves may cause weakness. If the weakness is due to the latter, 5 or 10 mg edrophonium administered intravenously, briefly worsens the patient's condition. If, on the other hand, improvement ensues, higher doses of neostigmine or other long-acting agent can be given safely. The weakness of thyrotoxic myopathy and motor system disease and the tiredness of neurasthenia which are sometimes confused with myasthenia gravis do not show the fluctuations of myasthenia gravis or respond to neostigmine. Such patients develop large numbers of fasciculations after neostigmine, as do many normal persons. In thyrotoxicosis, however, a typical myasthenia may occur and be added to the thyroid myopathy, and, as was stated above, hypothyroidism, if present, may actually enhance myasthenic weakness (see Chap. 85).

TREATMENT The management of these patients is divided into two parts: the treatment of acute episodes of severe paralysis and the long-term management. Neostigmine is by far the most useful drug during acute attacks and should be given parenterally in doses of 1 mg and in multiples of this amount until the desired degree of improvement has been attained. The side reactions are gastrointestinal and uterine cramps, which may be partially controlled by the simultaneous administration of atropine.

Other problems which must be taken care of during the acute episode include the protection of the patient from hypostatic pneumonia and other infections and the prevention of impaired respiratory exchange with resulting cyanosis and respiratory acidosis due to failure of respiratory excretion of normal amounts of carbon dioxide. At times a respirator for maintaining respiratory exchange may be lifesaving. If these complications are prevented, most patients will experience a remission after a few weeks or months. Some recover completely. Others, as time goes on, relapse, and a slow general trend toward increasing severity of the disease may become apparent.

Mild cases may require no special medical attention except during relapse. In the slightly more severe case, neostigmine in oral doses of 15 mg every 2 or 3 hr, or multiples of this dose, as needed, is the most useful medication and may be quite effective. Over a period of months or years, the dosage may have to be increased progressively, and the cost becomes nearly prohibitive for some families. The maximal effect of neostigmine given orally appears in half an hour and decreases rapidly after that time. If the patient becomes resistant to this medication, Mestinon bromide (60 mg is equivalent to 15 mg neostigmine) may be substituted, tablet for tablet. Mytelase chloride (5 to 7.5 mg is equivalent to 15 mg neostigmine) may also be tried, beginning always with a small dose of 5 mg every 2 hr and increasing to tolerance and to maximum therapeutic effect. All three of these drugs are available in syrup form (for tube feeding and for small children) and in delayed time-spaced tablets which have an effect for 3 to 12 hr.

Supplementing neostigmine with ephedrine (25 mg three times daily) and potassium salts (KCl, 25% aqueous solution in doses of 4 to 6 ml t.i.d.) may be of slight therapeutic value in certain cases, particularly in relieving the weakness which occurs between doses of neostigmine. The possible usefulness of these agents must be investigated for each patient. Many anticholinesterase agents other than neostigmine have been investigated in an attempt to find an agent with more prolonged action and fewer side effects. Of these pyridostigmine (Mestinon) is probably the best and does have a more prolonged period of activity. Ambenonium (Mysuran) is also said to be effective in some patients. The most severe and chronic forms of myasthenia gravis do not respond to any of these drugs, and the patient is forced to live a miserable existence in and out of a respirator. As a rule thymectomy is performed on patients in whom severe weakness prevents independent activity. The repeatedly hospitalized patient with recalcitrant myasthenia gravis often needs tracheostomy and gastrectomy, for he can neither breathe nor eat without the help of neostigmine. Brief periods of 1 to 2 weeks in which all anticholinesterase drugs are withheld while respirations are maintained by machine may restore responsivity to neostigmine. Also 100 units of ACTH per day for 10 days, or 60 mg prednisone, though temporarily worsening the myasthenia, may be followed by a respite. Rarely a low-maintenance dose of corticosteroid medication benefits a patient with chronic myasthenia.

Variation in the intensity of the disease at different times makes evaluation of any type of management extremely difficult. This statement is nowhere better demonstrated than in the attempt to assess the results of thymectomy and radiation of the thymus. Dramatic and apparently permanent cures have been effected by these measures, particularly by excision of the thymus, in as many as 30 to 40 percent of cases; the majority of patients continue to have symptoms of myasthenia after thymectomy. Some proponents of the procedure believe that only patients with early, chronically active, but not too severe cases should be selected for operation. One authority has noted particularly beneficial effects of thymectomy in young women. However, it should be noted that these are the patients in whom spontaneous remissions are most frequent. The postoperative management of these patients is difficult (see books by Osserman and by Viets and Schwab if it is to be undertaken); it requires oxygen, a respirator, an aspirator, and excellent nursing. Preferably the patients should spend the postoperative period in a special-care unit with a trained team of nurses and physicians. With proper respiratory aid, antimyasthenic medication can be omitted during the postoperative period and then later begun, as the patient recovers from surgery. Parenterally administered neostigmine should at first be used in place of oral medication. Intravenous prostigmine (1 mg being equivalent to 15 mg of the oral dose) in 1 liter of 5% glucose and water or normal saline solution may be administered over a 4-hr period. The adequacy of treatment may be checked by the response to Tensilon. Because of the unpredictability of remissions, the relatively few examples of striking improvement, and the great danger to the patient, thymectomy cannot be recommended as a routine procedure.

Thymomas usually respond to x-ray therapy, and the associated myasthenia improves.

SYMPTOMATIC MYASTHENIA GRAVIS Typical myasthenia gravis has been reported most frequently in conjunction with thyroid disease. It has been shown that hyperthyroidism adds its typical muscle weakness to the myasthenia without increasing the requirement of anticholinesterase drugs. Hypothyroidism if present may make the myasthenia worse, and the latter improves as the thyroid deficiency is treated. A few of our patients with lupus erythematosus and polymyositis have had myasthenia gravis. Perhaps the most interesting form is that special one which accompanies the small-cell carcinoma of the lung (Eaton-Lambert syndrome). Weakness in these patients is usually in the pelvic, thigh, and shoulder-arm muscles and is accompanied by aching and stiffness. Contrary to what happens in true myasthenia gravis, ocular and bulbar muscles are usually spared. Initial movements are weak, and strength improves with each of the first several contractions. The reason for this is seen in the electromyogram, where low-voltage action potentials increase in amplitude with rapid frequencies of neuromuscular stimulation (20 to 30 per sec) and diminish in amplitude with low frequencies (1 to 2 per sec). Neostigmine has little effect on the weakness; tubocurarine and decamethonium make it worse, even when very small doses, easily tolerated by the normal person, are given. Guanidine HCl in oral doses of 250 mg three to four times a day has dramatically improved strength in most patients. Muscle biopsies have shown degeneration of end-plates, according to McDermott. The condition may precede the appearance of the malignant tumor by as long as 2 years, but not all patients develop a tumor. The same peculiar muscle disorder has been observed in sarcoidosis.

EPISODIC PARALYSIS OF OTHER TYPES

At least four different syndromes of recurrent muscle weakness have now been identified: (1) familial periodic paralysis, (2) hyperthyroidism with periodic paralysis; (3) congenital paramyotonia (von Eulenberg's); and (4) hereditary periodic adynamia (Gamstorp's). In each of these conditions the patient may develop over a period of a few hours a disorder of skeletal muscles which may vary from weakness of trunk and limb muscles to total paralysis, and which subsides and disappears completely after a few hours or days. Differences among them are small, but von Eulenberg's disease appears to exhibit, in some instances at least, a mild degree of restricted myotonia. The syndrome must be differentiated from cataplexy (always of seconds' or a few minutes' duration, precipitated by strong emotion and conjoined with narcolepsy), from syncope (the physical weakness is always combined with impairment of consciousness), from hydrocephalic attacks with limb weakness (headache and signs of increased intracranial pressure), and from "drop seizures," one of the varieties of epilepsy (see petit mal triad and myoclonus).

FAMILIAL PERIODIC PARALYSIS Clinical pattern Familial periodic paralysis is a very rare disorder which occurs in certain families, usually being inherited as a mendelian dominant trait. The clinical story is striking. The patients are normal except for well-demarcated episodes in which intense weakness or complete paralysis of limb and trunk muscles develops. The attacks begin in early life and may come at varying intervals throughout life, being more frequent in adolescence or early adult life.

A single attack may last from a few minutes to several days, the average duration being 12 to 48 hr. The attacks in many patients have a periodicity and duration characteristic for that individual or family. During the episode there are marked hypotonia of the affected muscles and hyperextensibility of the joints. The tendon reflexes are absent or greatly reduced but return to normal as strength and tone return. The muscles are refractory to electric stimulation. The facial, pharyngeal, thoracic, and diaphragmatic muscles are affected only in very severe cases, but respiratory embarrassment and death have been reported.

The attacks are precipitated by several factors, such as violent exercise or a large high-carbohydrate meal. Attacks often begin during sleep or are present on awakening. Profuse diaphoresis may precede the attack. Usually no definite precipitating cause can be discovered.

In the average patient there is no evidence of progressive muscular disease, and physical examination of a patient between attacks frequently demonstrates no abnormality. Exceptionally some degree of weakness, usually mild, persists after the termination of the attack and is cumulative in successive attacks. Creatine phosphokinase values in serum rise. More common, however, is a slowly progressive myopathic weakness of pelvifemoral muscles during middle and late adult life, long after the attacks of periodic paralysis have ceased.

Pathology The principal change is a striking vacuolization of muscle fibers. The vacuoles are filled with clear fluid, but in glycogen stains a few positive-reacting granules may be seen. Under the electron microscope the endoplasmic reticulum is also dilated. In the degenerative stage one may see the same vacuolization but also segmental necrosis and abortive regeneration, but leading eventually to a loss of muscle fibers.

Pathogenesis During the attack the *serum potassium level* drops sharply. This apparently results from the sudden passage of potassium into the cells of the body, because the urinary excretion of potassium falls at the same time. The intracellular potassium of muscle has been demonstrated to rise during attacks. The relation to excess carbohydrate intake has frequently been noticed; there are a fall in serum potassium level and a rise in intracellular muscle and liver potassium levels during rapid glycogen storage. However, the timing of the two events is frequently not similar. The initial potassium changes are observed in all individuals during the first few hours after carbohydrate ingestion, while the paralysis in periodic paralysis is frequently delayed by 8 to 12 hr and is associated with a second series of changes in potassium levels. Thus the mechanism of the metabolic anomaly is not entirely clear. Biopsies of muscle taken during the attacks of paralysis reveal sarcoplasmic vacuolization, but this is seen also in patients who have had no attacks of paralysis for years.

HYPERTHYROIDISM WITH PERIODIC PARALYSIS See Chaps. 85 and 345.

CONGENITAL PARAMYOTONIA (VON EULENBERG'S DISEASE) The principal feature of this disease is stiffness (myotonia), weakness, or paralysis which follows exposure to cold. It is inherited as a mendelian dominant trait. At first only the myotonic features of this disease were described, and it was always regarded as a variant of congenital myotonia (Thomsen's syndrome). It has been known for a long time, however, that in some cases there are attacks of weakness similar to those of periodic paralysis. The latter may or may not be related to cold. It is of interest that the serum potassium level is not reduced in attacks, and in fact the administration of potassium may induce an attack, in which respect this condition differs from the usual variety of familial periodic paralysis. In this way it is similar to if not identical with Gamstorp's *adynamia episodica hereditaria* (see below). The resting potential of muscle fibers during attacks is diminished. The myotonia of von Eulenberg's syndrome may be limited to the eyelids or tongue. Muscle biopsy reveals no abnormality. Vacuolization is seldom seen in this variety of periodic paralysis.

The relationships among myotonia congenita, myotonia dystrophica, paramyotonia congenita, adynamia episodica hereditaria, and familial periodic paralysis are close and remain somewhat controversial.

ADYNAMIA EPISODICA HEREDITARIA (GAMSTORP'S DISEASE) This is also a hereditary disease (mendelian dominant) characterized by periods of weakness or paralysis of skeletal muscle not unlike that described in familial periodic paralysis. The onset is between the ages of five and ten years. The attacks, which are frequent and may last for one to many hours, tend to occur during rest after physical exertion, particularly if the patient is wet, cold, or hungry. Tingling of lips, fingers, and toes may occur at the onset of attacks. Weakness varies in degree. Respiratory embarrassment has not been noted. Between attacks the patient is symptom-free, though in a few cases mild weakness persists for days at a time.

Serum potassium level rises transiently during the attack but not necessarily to high levels (paralysis may be present with serum K concentration of 5.5 mEq), and in the electrocardiogram the T waves are high and peaked. The amount of urinary potassium does not increase before or during attacks. Administration of 2 to 5 g KCl induces an attack. Glucose tends to prevent this phenomenon. Reducing the serum K below a certain level, which varies from patient to patient, has been effective in preventing attacks.

This condition is worse during puberty; after this period the prognosis is good both for survival (no fatal cases) and for effective work.

HYPERALDOSTERONISM AND OTHER ALTERATIONS OF POTASSIUM METABOLISM Another syndrome of potassium depletion recognized recently has been called *primary hyperaldosteronism, Conn's syndrome*, or potassium-losing nephritis. This disorder results in marked hypopotassemia, with episodes of paralysis similar to those of periodic paralysis. Tetany, polyuria, hypertension, and other manifestations, not found in the hereditary cases, are commonly present. Most of the patients have adrenal tumors which secrete aldosterone and possibly other steroids (see Chap. 86). Care should be taken to distinguish this disease from familial periodic paralysis.

The same clinical picture may be observed in patients with other disorders when serum potassium is depleted, as in severe diarrhea or in overtreatment of a patient with Addison's disease with deoxycorticosterone; the plasma potassium levels observed are usually lower than those found during attacks of familial periodic paralysis.

Extreme hypokalemia is also accompanied by muscular weakness or paralysis.

TREATMENT OF PERIODIC PARALYSIS Episodes of familial periodic paralysis with hypokalemia are treated by the oral administration of potassium salts in doses of 2 to 8 g until the attack is relieved. In the rare instance when acute respiratory or pharyngeal paralysis appears, it may be necessary to give potassium intravenously. Great care should be observed in its use, for it may be toxic if administered too rapidly. Normal renal function, sufficient fluids to maintain a good urine volume, and slow administration (50 mEq over several hours) are the most important precautions which should be taken in giving potassium salts intravenously. In patients with periodic paralysis who have frequent episodes, attacks may be prevented by giving 4 to 8 g potassium chloride in divided doses per day by mouth.

In the flaccid paralysis which results from von Eulenberg's paramyotonia and adynamia episodica hereditaria with hyperkalemia, potassium is of course contraindicated. Diuril, on the other hand, will prevent attacks by keeping the potassium levels below a critical point.

REFERENCES

Grob D: Course and management of myasthenia gravis. JAMA 153:529, 1953

Osserman KE ed: *Myasthenia Gravis*, New York: Grune & Stratton, 1958

Simpson, JA: Myasthenia gravis and myasthenic syndromes, in *Disorders of Voluntary Muscles*, 2d ed., ed JN Walton, London: Churchill, 1969, p. 541

Viets HR, Schwab RS: in *Myasthenia Gravis*, ed KE Osserman, Grune & Stratton, 1958

348 OTHER MAJOR MUSCLE SYNDROMES

RAYMOND D. ADAMS

This chapter considers the syndromes not covered in preceding chapters by which diseases of muscles declare themselves clinically.

THE SPASM AND STIFFNESS SYNDROMES

Quite apart from spasticity and rigidity, which are forms of excessive motility due to a disinhibition of spinal motor mechanisms (see Chaps. 17 and 18), there are forms of muscular spasm that can be traced to abnormalities of motor neurons themselves or of their terminal axons to the sarcolemma of muscle fibers and their intrinsic conducting apparatus. Examples of each type of abnormality have been discovered. Thus, muscles may go into spasm because of an unstable depolarization of their axons, in myokymia, hypokalemic tetany, pseudohypoparathyroidism, and motor system disease. The contraction of muscle may be normal but persists despite attempts at relaxation, in myotonia; after one or a series of contractions the muscle may be slow in decontracting, in hypothyroidism, or may lack the energy to relax, in the contracture of McArdle's phosphorylase deficiency and phosphofructosekinase deficiency.

Each of these conditions evokes complaint, termed by the patient as cramp or spasm, which is variably painful and interferes with free and effective voluntary activity. Each condition has its own identifying clinical characteristics, registered also in the electromyogram, and a gratifying response to therapy may be obtained. Premium attaches, therefore, to the clinical differentiation of cramp, spasm, tetany, tetanus, and contracture, of which the following descriptions are presented.

MUSCLE CRAMP As mentioned in Chap. 343, everyone at some time or other has had the experience of muscle cramp. Usually it happens during the night after a day of unusually strenuous activity. As the feet become cold, a random restless movement will induce a hard contraction of a muscle of foot and leg which cannot be voluntarily relaxed. The muscle is visibly and palpably taut and painful, and the condition is readily distinguished from an illusory sensory experience of painful cramp where little or no contraction occurs, as in intermittent claudication and in certain diseases of peripheral nerve. Only by massage and by vigorous stretch of the cramped muscle will the spasm suddenly yield, though for a time the muscle remains excitable and subject to recurrent cramp. Visible fasciculation may precede and follow cramp, disclosing an excessive excitability of the motor nerve fibers supplying the muscle. In the electromyogram the cramp is attended by high-frequency action potentials and, in precramp phases, by runs of activity in motor units. Why cramp should be painful is not known; probably the demands of the overactive muscle exceed metabolic supply, causing a relative ischemia and accumulation of metabolites. Overwork of muscle with or without impairment of circulation is also painful.

Cramps are known to increase in frequency under certain conditions and with certain diseases. They are frequent during pregnancy for reasons not fully understood. Dehydration and sweating favor cramp, and athletes try to prevent this by the ingestion of sodium chloride. Exertional cramps are frequent in motor system disease. Diphenhydramine HCl (Benadryl) 50 mg at bedtime, quinine sulfate, and procainamide are useful medications.

TETANY As pointed out in Chap. 344 hypocalcemia and hypomagnesemia induce cramplike involuntary spasms which in their mildest form tend to be distal (carpopedal spasm) but may spread to all except eye muscles. Stimulation of the nerve leading to a muscle at fast frequencies (15 to 20 times per second) characteristically reproduces the cramp, and hyperventilation and ischemia increase the tendency. Indeed the Trousseau sign takes advantage of this phenomenon—carpal spasms accompany occlusion of the blood supply to the arm. That hypocalcemic tetany is due to an unstable depolarization of the distal segments of the motor nerves is shown by the following facts: (1) the sensitivity of nerve to percussion (tapping over facial nerve near its foramen of exit induces facial twitch (Chvostek's sign); (2) fast-frequency doublets and triplets of motor unit potentials are seen in the EMG; (3) cramp is evoked by tourniquet applied to proximal parts of limb (causing ischemia of segments of nerve beneath tourniquet); (4) there is a regular association of tingling, prickling paresthesias from excitation of sensory nerve fibers. Hypocalcemia also causes a change of lesser importance in the muscle fibers themselves; hence nerve block does not completely eradicate tetany.

A condition resembling tetany without measurable hypocalcemia occasionally presents itself as a *pathological cramp syndrome.* Here all skeletal muscles may be continuously or intermittently locked in spasm, and every strong movement leads to cramp. The muscles often hypertrophy. One can demonstrate the same effects of nerve tapping, nerve ischemia, hyperventilation, and fast-frequency nerve stimulation. In this way it differs from the myokymic syndrome described below, and response to quinine and procainamide is variable.

MYOKYMIA WITH CONTINUOUS MUSCLE ACTIVITY (NEUROMYOTONIA) Numerous patients have been observed whose muscles are continuously active. All attempts at relaxation fail. The twitching and spasm are involuntary. In the mildest degree there is persistent activity of hand and foot muscles resulting in clawlike postures, but when the condition is severe, it spreads to axial, facial, and bulbar muscles as well, sparing only the eyes. At rest there are almost continuous fasciculations which combine to impart a rippling motion to the muscle, the term for which is *myokymia.* Typically the muscles are well developed, the tendon reflexes difficult to elicit, and excessive sweating and elevated basal metabolism rate are almost constant features. The spasms continue at rest, unlike the spasms of myotonia, and during sleep, unlike the muscles of the "stiff-man syndrome." Spinal anesthesia does not abolish the spasms. No changes in blood chemistry have been found. Ischemia has no effect on the cramps. There is evidence in some cases of a mild peripheral neuropathy, hence the term "neuromyotonia." The EMG shows closely grouped, fast-frequency action potentials unlike that of tetany. That the condition is due to instability of terminal parts of motor axons is revealed by the effects of curare and succinylcholine, which by acting on neuromuscular junctions abolish the spasms. Diphenylhydantoin (100 mg every 6 hr) has effectively controlled the condition in most instances. Carbamazepine (Tegretol) and potassium chloride have also helped.

A condition resembling myokymia has been observed in aberrant regeneration of nerve after injury of any type to spinal root or nerve, which may result in a pseudomyotonia, where voluntary contraction is slow and prolonged. Unlike true myotonia it does not "wear off" after repeated contractions but actually worsens, and the electromyogram also differs. A similar condition is seen also in intoxication by the herbicide dichlorophenoxyacetic acid (2,4-D), and Parathion and other anticholinesterase drugs may evoke widespread fasciculations but not cramp.

CONTRACTURE (PSEUDOMYOTONIA) McArdle's phosphorylase deficiency and phosphofructosekinase deficiency provide another example of a type of painful shortening and hardness of muscle of entirely different type. Here muscle contraction and relaxation is normal when the patient is rested, but strenous activity, especially under conditions of ischemia, cause the muscles to shorten, unable to relax. Unlike muscles in cramp and other involuntary spasms the contracted muscles no longer use energy, and they are more or less electrically silent. Moreover lactic acid is not produced. The condition complies with the definition of true *contracture.* The affected muscles cannot then be used in voluntary contraction. Thus there is limitation of full activity which is also hampered by mild pain. See Chap. 343 for further description. In ischemia circulatory glucose is not available, and the muscle cannot function adequately on fatty acid and nonglucose substrates.

A kind of pseudomyotonia also accompanies hypothyroidism, where the muscle fiber, once contracted, is slow in relaxation. The muscles are large and slow in response, and reflex relaxation is delayed (see Chap. 85). The muscles when used may show waves of slow contraction and are subject to myoedema and are enlarged. The basis of this disorder appears to be a slowness in the reaccumulation of calcium ions in the endoplasmic reticulum and in the disengagement of thin actin and thick myosin filaments. The electromyogram does not reflect the abnormality.

TETANUS AND THE STIFF-MAN SYNDROME In tetanus the skeletal muscles are persistently contracted, owing to the effect of the tetanus toxin on spinal neurons whose natural function is to inhibit the motor neurons. As the condition develops, activities that normally excite the neurons, i.e., repeated voluntary contraction, startle, visual and auditory stimulation, evoke involuntary spasms. Sleep tends to quiet them, and they are suppressed by spinal anesthesia and curare. The EMG shows the expected interference patterns of action potentials. Once the muscle is involved in spasm, it is said that the shortened state may persist after procaine block of nerve or severance of nerve (in animal), but this so-called *myostatic contracture* has not been demonstrated in man.

The *stiff-man syndrome* originally described by Woltman and Moersch bears many resemblances to tetanus but is obviously different. It has been observed in isolated instances all over the world. The usual clinical picture is that of an adult man or woman who begins to complain of intermittent, then more of less continuous, spasms of limb and trunk muscles. Once started, the condition continues for years. Pharmacologic study and electromyography have led to the postulation of a disinhibition of spinal motor neurons, akin to that of tetanus; curare, tubocurarine, and spinal anesthesia abolish the spasms, and they cease during sleep. No abnormality of muscle has been detected.

The spasms of abdominal and trunk muscles consequent to the bite of the black-widow spider (effect of the Latrodectus toxin) have been little studied because of their transient nature. Presumably a hyperexcitability of motor neurons occurs here as well. Our uncertainty as to their nature is reflected in the wide variety of drugs used in treatment (magnesium sulfate, methocarbonal, atropine, epinephrine, and chlorpromazine).

The other conditions that give rise to involuntary spasms such as myotonia and phenothiazine or piperazine dyskinesias are discussed below under Thomsen's disease, and in Chap. 18, respectively.

CONGENITAL MYOTONIA (THOMSEN'S DISEASE)

Definition This is a hereditary disease in which a difficulty in initiating movement is combined with slowness of relaxation. Originally described by Julius Thomsen, who suffered from the disease himself, later descriptions by Strumpell, Erb, and Westphal served to establish its nosologic position as a lifelong, familial disease. Erb provided the first description of its pathology and called attention to two additional unique features, muscular hyperexcitability and hypertrophy.

Clinical manifestations The disease begins in the first years of life (usually by the age of six to eight years) and persists throughout its span. The disorder appears to be transmitted in two forms: one as an autosomal dominant, the other as an autosomal recessive trait. However, the patient frequently fails to give a family history, and myotonia may be difficult to demonstrate clinically in some individuals who nonetheless have typical electrical myotonia. It may be present in a milder subclinical degree early in life and interfere with learning to stand and walk. However, its chief feature, myotonia, is seldom demonstrable before the end of the first months or even the first 1 to 2 years of life unless unusually severe, and it becomes more intense at adolescence (in myotonia dystrophica, myotonia usually is milder and has a later onset). Muscular hypertrophy may also be noted during the early years of life.

The typical slowness of contraction and persistence of contraction upon attempted relaxation is best provoked by strong voluntary movements after a period of inactivity, but it may be induced by electrical stimulation or by percussion. It is most prominent in the legs, where the first movements of walking or running after a period of rest are slow and stiff. It is also present in the hands and arms and even the face and eye muscles. Characteristically a certain intensity of voluntary contraction is required to elicit the symptom pattern. It is not present in gentle contractions such as blinking. With repetition of the contraction, the movement characteristically becomes more facile and rapid and relaxation more prompt (warm-up effect), until both are normal. Clinically the slowness of relaxation is most easily demonstrated in the forearm and hand muscles and in the orbicularis oculi during voluntary effort. Percussion myotonia, which may be evoked in any of these muscles and in the tongue, consists of a persistent contraction, for half a minute or more, of a segment of a muscle which has been tapped. Myotonia does not accompany the tendon reflex, but it may alter the abdominal and cremasteric reflexes. The muscles being repeatedly involved in these strong contractions are hypertrophied, though Patterson and Maas call attention to the development of a mild dystrophic change in some cases. Cataract, temporal baldness, testicular atrophy, and muscle weakness and wasting do not occur in Thomsen's disease. When present, they always signify myotonic dystrophy.

Laboratory data The only metabolic abnormality is a mild creatine intolerance and increased urinary excretion in some patients. The electromyogram is characteristic (see Chap. 344) in that voluntary attempts to arrest muscle contraction are followed by a persistence of action potentials for several seconds. The biopsy of muscle reveals little or nothing of interest except large fibers with occasional rows of central sarcolemmal nuclei.

Treatment Quinine sulfate 0.3 to 0.6 g three times daily reduces or relieves the myotonia, but often patients dislike it because of side effects (tinnitus, etc.). Procainamide in doses of 250 to 500 mg orally three times daily is said to be superior to quinine.

Prognosis The disease remains unchanged throughout the patient's life. The later development of dystrophy must be exceptional.

PARAMYOTONIA CONGENITA (VON EULENBERG'S)

This rare disease, already discussed, is one in which slowness and stiffness of movement are most clearly evoked by cold. The myotonia tends to be rather mild and is often restricted to the hands and tongue or facial muscles (eyelids). The aforementioned episodes of weakness may also be induced by cold but may occur spontaneously. The myotonia is seldom of sufficient intensity to require treatment (see Chap. 347).

MYOTONIA DYSTROPHICA This third disease which features myotonia has already been discussed in Chap.

346 for the reason that muscle weakness and atrophy are the principal manifestations.

MYALGIC STATES

Diffuse muscle pain, which merges with malaise, is a frequent expression of a large variety of systemic infections, e.g., influenza, brucellosis, dengue, Colorado tick fever, glanders, measles, malaria, relapsing fever, rheumatic fever (cf. growing pains), salmonellosis, toxoplasmosis, trichinosis, tularemia, and Weil's disease. When this pain is remarkably intense, and especially if it is localized to one group of muscles, the most likely diagnostic possibility is epidemic myalgia (also designated as pleurodynia, devil's grip, painful neck, and Bornholm's disease). Poliomyelitis also may be accompanied by intense pain at the onset of neurologic involvements, and later the paralyzed muscles may ache. Herpes zoster is another well-known cause of segmental pain. Nothing is known of the pathologic basis for the pains of either pleurodynia or poliomyelitis. Inflammation in spinal nerves and dorsal root ganglia, which may precede the vesicular skin eruption by as long as 72 to 96 hr, is the cause of the segmental pain in herpes zoster. The muscle tissue has been little studied by pathologists, and random biopsies have proved to be relatively uninformative in all these diseases.

Fibromyositis and *myogelosis* (see Chap. 363) would appear by definition to represent an inflammation of the fibrous tissues of the muscles, fascia, aponeuroses, and probably nerves as well. Unfortunately, the pathologic changes remain obscure. Only the clinical facts are at hand: a muscle or group of muscles becomes painful and tender after exposure to cold, dampness, or minor trauma, or for no reason that can be discerned. The neck and shoulders are the common sites. Firm, tender zones, sometimes several centimeters in diameter, are found within the muscles, and palpation and active contraction or passive stretching of them increases the pain—points of diagnostic value. In Europe, following the descriptions by Lange and Schadé in 1921, the term *myogelosis* was applied to this condition, but it has never gained popularity in the United States. Usually the condition clears up in a few days, and local heat and massage are found to give comfort while symptoms are present. The condition is a "favorite" with physiotherapists and osteopaths, who believe their maneuvers and adjustments to be helpful, as indeed they may. Rarely a similar syndrome is but the forerunner of what proves after some days, with the onset of neurologic signs, to be a radiculitis, brachial neuritis, or an outbreak of herpes zoster.

Diffuse muscular soreness and aching may at times be the initial symptoms in rheumatoid arthritis, preceding the signs of joint involvement by a period of weeks or months. The muscles are tender, but since this may be found in otherwise normal individuals, particularly women, it is difficult to interpret. Often the patient observes that aching pain occurs not at the time of activity but some hours or even a day or two later, resembling the discomfort following the excessive use of unconditioned muscles. However, a program of conditioning exercises does not alleviate the pain. An increased sedimentation rate, a positive latex-fixation test, or other of the laboratory aids listed in Chap. 356 may clarify the diagnosis. Muscle biopsy may reveal a nonspecific interstitial nodular myositis. Occasionally a localized weakness of muscle, a slightly reduced tendon reflex, or a zone of impaired cutaneous sensation within the territory of a nerve will indicate the existence of a disease of the peripheral nervous system—an interstitial mononeuritis simplex or multiplex (see Chap. 323)—which can sometimes be confirmed by the finding of infiltrates of lymphocytes, mononuclear leukocytes, and plasma cells in a nerve or muscle biopsy.

In thin, asthenic adults who exhibit this rather ambiguous symptomatology without other abnormalities, the authors have found it difficult to exclude hysteria or other psychoneurosis or depression. In every such individual it is well to search for evidence of rheumatic state and brucellosis as well as the metabolic myopathy which accompanies hyperparathyroidism and renal tubular acidosis, hypoglycemia, the intrinsic phosphorylase defect (McArdle's syndrome), phosphofructokinase defect, and myoglobinuria before calling for a psychiatric consultant. Patients with these latter diseases often complain of soreness, stiffness, and lameness after any strenuous muscular effort.

The treatment for each of these conditions will be found in the appropriate section of the book.

LOCALIZED MUSCLE MASSES

Masses may be found in one or many muscles in a variety of clinical settings, and the clinical findings in each one have a different significance.

Muscle rupture giving rise to a large bulge upon contraction is usually caused by a violent strain attended by an audible snap and then a bulge which appears when the muscle contracts. A weakening in contractile power and mild discomfort are usually noted by the patient. The biceps muscle is the one most often affected. Treatment is immediate surgical repair; if delayed, little can be done for the condition.

Hemorrhage into muscle may occur as a consequence of trauma, as a complication of the use of anticoagulants, in hematologic diseases, or after a minor trauma in a patient with Zenker's degeneration who is convalescing from typhoid fever or other infection.

Tumors include *desmoid tumor* (a benign massive growth of fibrous tissue in parturient women and after surgery), *rhabdomyosarcoma* (a highly malignant tumor with strong liability to local recurrence and metastasis), and *angioma.*

Thrombosis of arteries or, more often, *of veins* causes congestion and infarction of muscle.

Myositis ossificans refers to the deposit of bone within the substance of a muscle. Two types are recognized. One is a localized form which appears in a single muscle or group of muscles after trauma, and the other is a progressive, widespread ossifying process in many muscles of the body and entirely unrelated to trauma. In the localized traumatic form, after a single traumatic blow or the tear of a muscle or repeated minor trauma, a painful area develops in the muscles. It is gradually replaced by masses of solid cartilaginous consistency, and within 4 to 7 weeks' time a solid mass of bone can be felt and becomes visible in the x-ray. As would be expected, this most frequently happens in vigorous adult men, and the pectoralis major, biceps, brachii, or thigh muscles of militiamen, cavalrymen, and athletes are the usual sites of the abnormality. Symptoms tend to subside if the patient desists from the activity which produced the mass.

GENERALIZED MYOSITIS OSSIFICANS This is a disease of unknown origin and consists of bone formation within muscles of children, adolescents, or young adults. Only this disease need be discussed in any further detail here.

Pathology The first stage is believed to be as an interstitial myositis or fibrositis. Biopsies of early indurated swellings have revealed extensive proliferation of interstitial connective tissue in which little inflammatory cell reaction is found. The adjacent muscle fibers become compressed by the connective tissue, which retracts and calcifies. Osteoid and cartilage formation occur at a later stage, developing in the connective tissue and enclosing intact muscle fibers.

Clinical manifestations Nearly 75 percent of all reported cases have had congenital anomalies, the most frequent of which is a failure of development of the great toes or thumbs and less often other digits. The first symptom is often a firm swelling in a vertebral or cervical muscle. There is, in addition, a mild tenderness and a discomfort during muscle contraction, and the overlying skin may be reddened and slightly swollen. A trauma may have been recalled as the initiating factor, but as the months pass, other muscles not injured in any recognizable way become similarly involved. At first x-rays reveal no important changes, but within 6 to 12 months calcium deposits are observed and one can feel stony-hard masses within the muscle. As the disease advances, limitation of movement, contractures, and deformities become increasingly evident, and occasionally the patient is converted into a virtual "stone man." Scoliosis, rigidity of spine, abnormal postures, and limited expansion of the thorax may ultimately occur.

Diagnosis The principal problem in diagnosis is to differentiate this condition from calcinosis universalis, which usually occurs in relationship to scleroderma or polymyositis. It is not clear whether a sharp dividing line can be drawn between the two conditions. In calcinosis universalis there is said to be calcinosis (calcium deposit) in the skin, subcutaneous tissues, and connective tissue sheaths around the muscles, whereas in myositis ossificans there is actual bone formation within the muscles. Probably the pathologic data are too meager to justify this distinction at present. Vitamin D calcinosis, resulting from the prolonged ingestion of large doses of vitamin D, may also produce widespread deposition of masses of calcium around muscles, joints, and subcutaneous tissue.

Prognosis The disease may undergo spontaneous remissions and exacerbations and may halt at a point where the patient is capable of adequate function, remaining in this state for years. If death is to occur, it is related to the enfeebled, debilitated, malnourished condition of the patient, the final illness often being a terminal pneumonia or other intercurrent infection.

Treatment No medical treatment is of proved value. Excision of bony deposits may be undertaken if it is certain that they are causing particular trouble. Some of the calcium deposits in calcinosis universalis have disappeared under prednisone therapy, and because of the unclear relationship of this disease to generalized myositis ossificans, it is probably advisable to try this form of therapy, using the same plan as that described in the chapter on diseases of connective tissue (Chap. 356).

REFERENCES

Adams RD et al: *Diseases of Muscle*, 2d ed., New York: Hoeber-Harper, 1962

—— et al: *Neuromuscular Disorders*, Baltimore: Williams & Wilkins, 1961

Layzer RB, Rowland LP: Cramps. N Engl J Med 285:31, 1971

Walton JN: *Disorders of Voluntary Muscle*, 2d ed., Baltimore: Williams & Wilkins, 1970

section 13 | Disorders of bone and bone mineral metabolism

349
SKELETAL REMODELING AND FACTORS INFLUENCING BONE AND BONE MINERAL METABOLISM

STEPHEN M. KRANE
JOHN T. POTTS, JR.

BONE STRUCTURE AND METABOLISM (see also Chap. 352) Bone is a dynamic tissue, constantly remodeling itself throughout life. The skeleton is highly vascular and receives about 10 percent of the cardiac output. The skeleton has extraordinary mechanical functions that are suited to the requirements for mobility that all vertebrates possess. The particular arrangement of compact cancellous bone provides a combination of strength and density ideal for these mechanical functions. In addition, bone provides a store of calcium, magnesium, phosphorus, sodium, and other ions necessary for the support of a variety of homeostatic functions.

In the following chapters a number of disorders will be discussed in which the metabolism of cartilage, bone, and mineral ions are affected. A brief review of skeletal remodeling, the metabolism of mineral ions, and the major factors which influence mineral metabolism is therefore pertinent.

The properties of bone as a tissue are a function of the particular organization of its extracellular components: a solid mineral phase in close association with an organic matrix, consisting of 90 to 95 percent collagen, small amounts of protein polysaccharides, and a variety of glycoproteins. The mineral phase is composed of hydroxyapatite [empiric formula $Ca_{10}(PO_4)_6(OH)_2$] of small crystal size and poor crystallinity and so-called "amorphous" calcium phosphate with a lower molar calcium/phosphorus ratio than that of hydroxyapatite. In addition, other ions are present predominantly in the surface layers. The mineral phase of bone is deposited in intimate relation to the collagen fibrils and is located largely in specific locations within the "holes" of the collagen fibrils which result from the particular manner in which the collagen molecules are packed. This architectural organization of mineral and matrix results in a two-phase material uniquely suited to withstand mechanical stresses. The formation as well as the localization of the inorganic phase is probably determined at least in part by the organic matrix, particularly the collagen.

Bone is formed by cells of mesenchymal origin which synthesize and secrete the organic matrix. Mineralization of the matrix, particularly in osteons, begins soon after secretion (primary mineralization) but is not completed until after several weeks (secondary mineralization). As an osteoblast secretes matrix which is then mineralized, this cell becomes surrounded by matrix and becomes an osteocyte, still connected with its blood supply through a series of canaliculi. Resorption of bone is carried out by cells which include the mononuclear cells as well as multinucleated osteoclasts, characterized by their elaborately infolded border adjacent to the bone and their location in scalloped resorption spaces (Howship's lacunas). Some resorption of bone may also take place around the osteocytes. The cells of bone are thought to be derived from more primitive, mesenchymal osteoprogenitor cells; there is evidence that transformation or modulation of one type of cell to another can occur, for example, in the response of bone to injury.

In the embryo and in the growing child, bone develops either by remodeling and replacing previously calcified cartilage (endochondral bone formation) or it is formed without a cartilage matrix (intramembranous bone formation). The young new bone, especially in embryos and infants and that newly formed in adults during repair, has a relatively high ratio of cells to matrix and is characterized by coarse fiber bundles of collagen which are interlaced and randomly dispersed (woven bone). In adults, the more mature bone is organized with fiber bundles regularly arranged in parallel or concentric sheets (lamellar bone). In long bones, the lamellar bone is deposited in a highly ordered concentric arrangement around blood vessels along their length, and forms the haversian systems, or osteons. Growth in length of bones is dependent upon proliferation of cartilage cells and the endochondral sequence at the growth plate. Growth in width and thickness is accomplished by formation of bone at the periosteal surface and resorption at the endosteal surface with the rate of formation exceeding that of resorption. In adults, after the epiphyses close, growth in length and endochondral bone formation cease, except for some activity in the cartilage cells beneath the articular surface. However, even in adults, remodeling of bone (remodeling of haversian systems as well as trabecular bone) is a continuous process through life, as can be shown by microradiographic studies utilizing radioisotopes or fluorescence of tetracyclines fixed in bone in regions of new mineralization. Newly forming surfaces are characterized by smooth character, uptake of tetracycline, and relatively low mineral density. The osteoid seam which results from the relative lag in mineralization of the newly formed organic matrix is normally no greater than about 12 μm. Resorption areas are characterized by their irregular configurations and the presence of osteoclasts. In adult man, approximately 10 percent of the surface of bone such as iliac crest is involved in active formation and resorption. Kinetic studies using isotopes such as radioactive calcium (^{47}Ca) provide estimates that as much as 18 per cent of the total skeletal calcium may be deposited and removed each year. Thus bone is an active metabolizing tissue, with its cells dependent upon an intact blood supply. Throughout life bone is constantly being remodeled, in a manner which is somehow related to the continuous mechanical stresses to which it is subjected. Bone also serves as an important reservoir of mineral ions, particularly calcium, which are critical for a variety of processes in other tissues.

The response of bone to injuries such as fractures, infection, interruption of blood supply, or the presence of expanding lesions is relatively limited. Dead bone must be resorbed and new bone formed, a process which normally is carried out in association with new blood vessels growing into the involved area. In injuries that are severely disruptive to the organization of the tissue such as a fracture in which apposition of fragments is poor and much motion occurs at the fracture site, the osteoprogenitor cells differentiate into cells with functional capacities other than those of osteoblasts, and the repair is accompanied by varying amounts of fibrous tissue and cartilage. In instances in which there is good apposition and fixation and little motion at the fracture site, there is repair predominately by bone without other scar tissue. Remodeling of this bone is subsequently accomplished along lines of force determined by mechanical stresses, somehow translated into biologic response.

Expanding lesions in bone, such as tumors, tend to induce resorption at the surface in contact with the tumor and increased formation at the outer circumference. A bowing deformity tends to result in increased new bone formation at the concave surface and resorption at the convex surface, all seemingly designed to produce the strongest mechanical structure. Even in a disorder architecturally disruptive as Paget's disease of bone, remodeling appears to be dictated by mechanical forces. Thus the biologic plasticity of bone is due to the response of cells interacting with each other and the environment.

Mechanisms of bone formation and resorption Bone formation is an orderly process in which inorganic mineral is deposited in relation to an organic matrix. The mineral phase is composed of calcium and phosphorus, and therefore the concentration of these ions in the plasma and extracellular fluid influences the rate at which the mineral phase is formed. In vitro, mineralization can proceed and crystals of hydroxyapatite grow at concentrations of calcium and phosphorus similar to those in an ultrafiltrate of plasma. However, it is not known what the concentration of these ions is at the sites of mineralization, and it is possible that the cells involved (osteoblasts, osteocytes) somehow regulate the local concentration of calcium, phosphorus, and other ions. Collagens from a variety of sources can catalyze the nucleation of a mineral phase of calcium and phosphorus from solutions of these ions, and the initial mineral phase is deposited in specific location in the holes produced by the particular packing arrangement of the collagen molecules. It is likely that the particular organization of collagen influences the amount and type of mineral phase that is formed. The collagen of bone is similar in its primary structure to that of skin [contains two α_1 (I) chains and one α_2 chain] but differs by virtue of modification of that structure in hydroxylation, glycosylation, and the type, number, and distribution of intermolecular cross-links. In addition, there is evidence that the "holes" in the packing structure of the collagen are larger in normally mineralized collagen of bone and dentin than those of a normally unmineralized collagen such as tendon. Other noncollagenous organic components such as glycoproteins may also play a role in the formation and localization of the mineral phase of bone. In order to explain how collagens from tissues normally not mineralized can catalyze nucleation of an inorganic phase from solutions of concentration similar to that of normal extracellular fluid, regulation of mineralization by inhibitory substances has been suggested. Inorganic pyrophosphate is a potent inhibitor of mineralization at concentrations several orders of magnitude below those necessary to bind calcium ions. Since alkaline phosphatase, present in osteoblasts and other cells, can catalyze the hydrolysis of inorganic pyrophosphate at neutral pH, this enzyme could play a role in the regulation of mineralization by controlling the concentrations of pyrophosphate. In addition, macromolecular inhibitors such as the protein polysaccharides may also influence the rate and extent of mineralization. In cartilage undergoing calcification, membrane-bound vesicles containing mineral have been identified outside of the cells, and it has been suggested that this is the initial mineral phase.

In bone, the initial mineral phase is probably the "amorphous" solid with relatively low molar calcium/phosphorus ratio of about 1.5. With maturation, part of the "amorphous" phase is converted to a poorly crystalline hydroxyapatite. However, even mature bone from old animals still contains considerable amounts of the amorphous calcium phosphate. Fluoride ions, when incorporated into the mineral phase, tend to decrease the proportion of amorphous calcium phosphate and increase crystallinity.

There is a limit for the concentration of calcium and phosphorus ions in the extracellular fluid below which the mineral phase will not be formed. A "solubility product" for bone mineral is difficult to calculate since the mineral phase itself is of variable composition and the true nature of species in solution governing this solubility product is not known. Nevertheless when the concentrations of calcium and phosphorus, particularly the latter, in extracellular fluid are excessive, a mineral phase may be formed in areas that are not normally mineralized.

When bone is resorbed, calcium and phosphorus ions from the solid phase are released into solution in the extracellular fluid, and subsequently the organic matrix is also resorbed. It is not entirely clear how these processes occur. A decrease in pH, the presence of a chelating substance, and the operation of a cellular pump mechanism to shift the equilibrium between solids and solution are possibilities to explain mineral release. Resorption occurs at specific sites either adjacent to osteoclasts or surrounding osteocytes and requires normal metabolism of these cells. The matrix is resorbed presumably through the action of collagenases released from the resorbing cells; these enzymes attack collagen in a specific manner but are incapable of degrading the protein before the mineral phase is removed. The rate at which resorption occurs is influenced by several hormones, particularly parathyroid hormone and calcitonin, and is accelerated by the action of other substances such as heparin. The effect of the hormones is discussed in more detail later.

CALCIUM METABOLISM Before considering the effects of hormones and vitamin D, a brief summary of calcium and phosphorus homeostasis in man is indicated.

There is about 1 to 2 kg calcium in the average adult human body of which over 98 percent is found in the skeleton. The calcium of the mineral phase at the surface of the crystals is in equilibrium with ions of the extracellular fluid, but only a minor proportion of the total calcium (about 0.5 percent) is exchangeable as determined by isotope dilution techniques. Although the calcium in the extracellular fluid is only a small fraction of the total, its concentration is critical for a variety of functions, and it is kept remarkably constant. In plasma, in normal adults, the range of concentration is 8.8 to 10.4 mg per 100 ml (2.2 to 2.6 mM). The calcium in the plasma is present in three forms: as free ions, bound to plasma proteins, and, to a small extent, as diffusible complexes. It is the concentration of free calcium ions that is of critical importance in regulating the level of neuromuscular irritability and that is subjected to exquisite hormonal control, especially through parathyroid hormone, as is described below. The concentration of serum proteins is an important factor in prediction of the concentration of calcium ions; most of the protein binding is to albumin. One formula that approximates the amount of calcium bound to proteins is:

$$\% \text{ protein bound Ca} = 8 \text{ albumin} + 2 \text{ globulin} + 3$$

where albumin and globulin are measured in grams per 100 ml. Thus the concentration of ultrafiltrable calcium is usually about 50 percent of the total calcium. In most clinical laboratories only total calcium is determined, and therefore knowledge of the concentration of proteins is essential to estimate concentration of calcium ions. The introduction of calcium-specific electrodes may eventually make it possible to measure free ions directly as a practical routine procedure.

Decrease in the concentration of free calcium ions in plasma results in increased neuromuscular irritability and the syndrome of tetany. This syndrome is characterized, when fully expressed, by peripheral and perioral paresthesias, carpal spasm, pedal spasm, anxiety, seizures, bronchospasm, laryngospasm, Chvostek's, Trousseau's, and Erb's signs, and lengthening of the Q-T interval of the electrocardiogram. In infants tetany may be manifested only by irritability and lethargy. The level of calcium ions that determines which features of tetany will be manifested is highly variable in different individuals.

Increases in total serum calcium are as a rule accompanied by increases in calcium ions and may be associated with a variety of symptoms and signs including anorexia, nausea, vomiting, constipation, some degree of hypotonia, and depression, occasionally leading to lethargy and coma. Persistent hypercalcemia, especially when accompanied by normal or elevated levels of serum phosphate, may eventually result in deposition of a solid mineral phase of calcium and phosphate in abnormal sites such as walls of blood vessels, connective tissue about the joints, gastric mucosa, cornea, and renal parenchyma. Hypercalcemia per se alters renal function in addition to the pathologic effects of deposition of calcium-phosphate deposits in the lumen of renal tubules and in the interstitial areas of the kidney.

The concentration of calcium ions in the extracellular fluid is kept constant by the interaction of a number of processes which are constantly feeding calcium into and withdrawing calcium from the extracellular fluid. Calcium enters the plasma via absorption from the intestinal tract and by resorption of ions from the bone mineral. Calcium leaves the extracellular fluid via secretion into the gastrointestinal tract, urinary excretion, deposition in bone mineral, and, to a minor extent, via losses in sweat. It is probable that movement of ions into and out of the skeleton are the processes of greatest magnitude influencing concentration of calcium ions. Resorption and formation are usually tightly coupled, estimates having been made of approximately 500 mg calcium entering and leaving the skeletal sources daily.

The average diet in the United States provides about 600 to 1,000 mg calcium daily, mostly in the form of dairy products. However considerably less than half of the calcium in the diet is absorbed in adults. The percentage of calcium absorbed increases during periods of rapid growth in children, in pregnancy, and in lactation, and decreases with advancing age. If adequate vitamin D is available, a greater percentage of dietary calcium is absorbed (adaptation). Most of the calcium is absorbed in the proximal small intestine, and the efficiency of absorption decreases in the more distal intestinal segments. Adequate calcium absorption requires the availability of a functioning surface and is critically dependent upon the presence of vitamin D and the formation of its active metabolites.

Calcium is also secreted into the lumen of the gastrointestinal tract in all the secretions, estimated on the basis of calcium content to average 760 mg per day in normal man. When isotopes of radiocalcium are administered intravenously, radioactivity appears in the feces, leading to the calculations of *endogenous fecal calcium* of about 60 to 130 mg per day. Why such discrepancy exists in these two estimations is not clear, although it is generally agreed that no control of calcium balance is exerted by regulation of intestinal calcium secretion. It is possible that all forms of calcium in the diet are not equally absorbed; even with defined salts, calcium as the chloride is probably absorbed more efficiently than that in other preparations.

The urinary calcium of normal adults on average calcium intakes ranges between 100 and 300 mg per day. When the dietary calcium is reduced to below 200 mg daily, urinary calcium excretion is usually less than 200 mg per day. However, the level of dietary intake over a wide range has relatively little effect on the urinary excretion of calcium. Estimations of calcium clearance have been reported based on a calculation of calcium concentration obtained by ultrafiltration methods. Ratios of calcium to creatinine clearance are thus calculated to be less than 0.05. However, the amount of calcium excreted in the urine is minute compared with that estimated to be filtered through the glomerulus (about 12 g per day), and it is not certain whether some non-protein bound, nonionic forms of calcium (e.g., calcium citrate) are cleared at rates considerably greater than others. The excretion of other electrolytes also affects the urinary excretion of calcium. For example, calciuresis is usually proportional to natriuresis, and other ions, such as sulfate, also increase calcium excretion.

PHOSPHORUS METABOLISM Phosphorus is not only a major component of the mineral phase of bone but is among the most abundant constituents of all tissues and in some form is involved in almost all metabolic processes. The total amount of phosphorus in the normal adult is about 1,000 g, of which about 85 percent is located in the skeleton.

In normal human plasma most of the phosphorus is present as inorganic orthophosphate in concentrations which range in the fasting state from 2.8 to 4.0 mg (P) per 100 ml. In contrast to calcium where about 50 percent is bound, only about 12 percent of the phosphorus in plasma is bound to proteins. Free HPO_4^{--} and $NaHPO_4^-$ normally are about 75 percent of the total plasma phosphorus and free $H_2PO_4^-$ is 10 percent. Since so many species are present, depending upon pH and other factors, it has been the convention to express concentrations in terms of mass of elemental phosphorus, i.e., milligrams phosphorus per 100 ml. Total phosphorus levels are higher in children and tend to rise in women after the menopause. In addition, phosphorus levels fluctuate considerably throughout the day by as much as 1 mg per 100 ml or more. Ingestion of carbohydrate depresses serum phosphorus, presumably by cellular uptake and formation of phosphate esters. Ingestion of phosphorus per se increases serum levels. Therefore, it is essential for the interpretation of serum levels and urinary clearances that samples be obtained in the postabsorptive state. Decreases in plasma phosphorus also occur during induction of alkalosis.

No definite symptoms result from hyperphosphatemia. However, when high levels are maintained for long periods, the driving force for mineralization is increased, and calcium phosphate deposits may occur in abnormal sites as discussed earlier. Severe hypophosphatemia, when acute, may be unaccompanied by symptoms. However, persistent hypophosphatemia may be associated with a syndrome consisting of varying degrees of anorexia, dizziness, bone pain, proximal muscular weakness, and waddling gait. The bone pain and waddling gait are attributed to the osteomalacia which develops as a result of phosphate depletion. Defective growth in children may also be due to phosphate depletion. It has been shown that hypophosphatemia results in decreased levels of 2,3-diphosphoglyceric acid and adenosine triphosphate (ATP) in erythrocytes which in turn alter the dissociation of oxyhemoglobin so that less oxygen is delivered in the periphery. Hemolytic anemia may also be produced by the effects of decreased ATP on the ability of erythrocytes to deform in small peripheral vessels.

Whereas only a small proportion of dietary calcium is absorbed from the intestine, phosphorus absorption is remarkably efficient. At low levels of dietary intake (less than 2 mg per kg per day) 80 to 90 percent of ingested phosphorus is absorbed. Even at higher levels of intake (greater than 10 mg per kg per day) usually encountered in average diets in the form of dairy products, cereals, eggs, and meat, absorption is about 70 percent.

The major control of phosphorus economy is exerted at the level of the kidney. Phosphorus filtered through the glomerulus is largely reabsorbed in the proximal tubule so that normally only about 10 percent of that filtered reaches the distal tubule. When filtered loads of phosphorus decrease, the proximal tubular reabsorption increases. Conversely when phosphorus loads are increased, tubular reabsorption decreases and clearance rises. Thus the urinary excretion of phosphorus normally reflects dietary intake, and conservation or elimination of excessive amounts of the ion depend upon adequate renal handling. There is no good evidence for renal tubular phosphate secretion. Proximal reabsorption of phosphorus is dependent upon parallel sodium reabsorption, but whereas the sodium rejected by the proximal tubule may be reabsorbed distally, the rejected phosphorus is not. Therefore the effects of volume expansion and decreased sodium reabsorption are to increase phosphorus clearance; similarly diuretics such as acetazolamide, which act proximally, are phosphaturic parallel to the degree to which they are natriuretic.

PARATHYROID HORMONE (see also Chap. 350) The physiologic function of parathyroid hormone in man as well as in other mammalian species is to maintain extracellular fluid calcium concentration. The hormone acts on bone, kidney, and intestine to increase serum calcium; in turn, parathyroid hormone production is closely regulated by serum calcium concentration. This feedback system involving the parathyroids is one of the most important homeostatic mechanisms for the close regulation of extracellular fluid calcium concentration. Any tendency toward hypocalcemia, such as might be induced by prolonged starvation, is counteracted by an increased rate of secretion of parathyroid hormone. This in turn (1) acts to increase the rate of dissolution of bone mineral, thereby providing an increased flow of calcium from bone into blood, (2) reduces the renal clearance of calcium, returning more of the calcium filtered at the glomerulus into extracellular fluid, and (3) increases, perhaps by an indirect mechanism, the efficiency of calcium absorption in the intestine. The relative physiologic importance of these three actions of parathyroid hormone, stimulation of calcium transport in bone, kidney, and intestine, is not definitely resolved.

Most workers have believed that the effect of the hormone on bone is the most important in maintaining extracellular fluid calcium homeostasis. Evidence from calcium kinetic studies indicates a transfer between extracellular fluid and bone of as much as 500 mg calcium daily (an amount large in relation to the total extracellular fluid calcium pool), and parathyroid hormone is known to influence this movement of calcium from bone into blood. However, the action of parathyroid hormone on kidney to preserve calcium by increasing the percentage reabsorption of filtered calcium may also be important in rapid regulation of blood calcium concentration.

There is evidence for a dual action of parathyroid hormone on bone. These two effects have been termed the *calcium replacement* and the *bone remodeling* effects of parathyroid hormone. It can be shown in vitro that there is an increased rate of release of calcium from bone into blood within minutes of the administration of parathyroid hormone; in vivo, a rapid efflux of calcium out of blood, presumably into bone cells, can be shown to precede the release of calcium. On the other hand, the more chronic effects of parathyroid hormone, mainly an increase in the number and activity of osteoclasts and a general increase in the remodeling of bone, appear only hours after the hormone is given. These actions, which involve increased protein synthesis, persist for hours after parathyroid hormone has been given. It is the latter effect, bone remodeling, which seems to be most closely related to the radiologic and histologic picture of the bone disease that results from long-standing excessive parathyroid action, osteitis fibrosa cystica. It is not clear whether the two effects of parathyroid action on bone represent a continuous spectrum with a common initiating biochemical event.

The often discussed possibility that different forms of the hormone are active on bone and kidney separately is not supported by analyses of the relation between parathyroid hormone structure and physiologic actions. Although the role of the parathyroid glands in the prevention of tetany and maintenance of normal plasma calcium levels has been appreciated since the late nineteenth century, a reliable method for extraction of an active principle from parathyroid tissue was not accomplished for many years afterward. However, there has been rapid progress in our knowledge of the chemical properties of parathyroid hormone and of the structural requirements for biologic activity. The complete amino acid sequences of the major form of the bovine and the porcine hormones have been defined. The peptides consist of a single-chain structure composed of 84 amino acids. The molecules lack cysteine or cystine; the sequence of the bovine and porcine hormones differs in 7 of the 84 residues. Studies of the human hormone, although still less complete, show that the structure of the human hormone is similar but not identical to that of the bovine and porcine hormones.

The structural requirements for biologic activity of parathyroid hormone have been defined by synthesis of peptides based on the structures deduced. Numerous sequences of the bovine and porcine hormones consisting of portions of the amino terminal 34 residues and various analogues have been synthesized.

It can now be concluded on the basis of these studies that any fragment of parathyroid hormone, in order to be biologically active, must consist of a continuous peptide sequence beginning with residue 2, valine, and extending as far as residue 27, lysine.

These observations are of particular interest because the biosynthesis and peripheral metabolism of parathyroid hormone have been found to be more complex than initially thought. Furthermore, parathyroid hormone which is extracted from glands differs both from the hormone which is initially synthesized and from the hormone found in the peripheral circulation. It has been shown that parathyroid hormone in human plasma is immunologically different from the hormone extracted from human adenomas.

The hormone secreted in vivo from normal bovine and human parathyroid glands and from parathyroid adenomas is indistinguishable by immunologic criteria and by molecular size from the 84-amino-acid peptide (molecular weight: 9,500) extracted from glands. However, much of the immunoreactive hormone found in the peripheral circulation of man and animals (cow, dog) is smaller than the extracted or secreted hormone. One fragment of immunoreactive hormone (approximate molecular weight: 7,000) lacks a portion of the critical amino terminal sequence required for biologic activity and, hence, must constitute a biologically inactive hormonal fragment(s).

Since cleavage of the native peptide by an endopeptidase would be expected to result in formation of at least two fragments, one might have expected to find a second fragment with a molecular weight of approximately 2,500. Such a small fragment with an approximate molecular weight of 2,500, and the large fragment of approximately 7,000 molecular weight, have been detected in animals.

A report also states that such a smaller fragment can be found in human blood concentrates. Biosynthesis of a precursor (proparathyroid hormone) to human and bovine parathyroid hormone has been demonstrated. Studies suggest that the prohormone sequence is added as a short sequence of residues to the amino terminus of the parathyroid hormone sequence.

Thus we now know that human and bovine parathyroid hormone undergo at least two specific cleavages from the point of initial cellular biosynthesis to ultimate disappearance from the circulation. The first of these cleavages occurs in the parathyroid cell; proparathyroid hormone (approximate molecular weight: 10,500) is converted to parathyroid hormone (molecular weight: 9,500), the latter being the predominant species of the hormone that is secreted into the circulation. After secretion, the hormone rapidly undergoes a second cleavage in yet undefined peripheral site(s). The latter, peripheral cleavage results in at least two fragments, one with an approximate molecular weight of 7,000 (which appears to be biologically inactive) and a smaller fragment with an approximate molecular weight of 2,500 (the biologic activity of the smaller fragment is at present uncertain).

Many issues remain to be clarified about the biosynthesis and peripheral metabolism of parathyroid hormone. If peripheral cleavage occurs carboxyl terminal to position 27, the resulting, smaller, amino terminal fragment might be biologically active. In addition, these specific cleavage steps may serve as points of metabolic control to regulate both the amount of biologically active hormone available for secretion and the concentration of hormonally active polypeptides in the circulation. The peripheral metabolism, in turn, may also be affected by pathologic processes.

It is not known whether prohormone is secreted into the circulation. It seems possible that in the syndrome of hypercalcemia due to ectopic production of a parathyroid-like hormone by malignant tumors, the malignant tissue may lack the cleavage enzyme found in the parathyroid cells. If this were true, secretory products from these tissues might be largely or exclusively proparathyroid hormone. A radioimmunoassay, specific for prohormone, would be of special diagnostic value in detecting ectopic hyperparathyroidism.

Classic in vivo and in vitro experiments have shown that blood calcium concentration controls the secretion of parathyroid hormone, and that the ionized fraction of blood calcium is the important determinant of hormone secretion. These studies were performed prior to the appreciation of the complex nature of immunoreactive parathyroid hormone in blood resulting from peripheral cleavage. It is now appreciated that the true concentration of intact or biologically active hormone in blood is unknown and that measurements of hormone concentration reflect intact hormone plus metabolic products. There are probably different rates of clearance for each form of immunoreactive parathyroid hormone (PTH). Nonetheless, good correlations, as would be expected, are found from one day to the next or from one patient to another between secretory activity and concentration of immunoreactive hormone.

Earlier studies indicated that there was a linear inverse correlation between parathyroid hormone concentration and plasma calcium as calcium varied between 4 and 12 mg per 100 ml. These observations are probably still valid but require reexamination with more specific assays. It seems likely that the fundamental mechanism of control of hormone secretion rate with calcium is proportional rather than differential or integral. However, derivative control may also occur; that is, hormone production under certain conditions may be sensitive to rate of change as well as absolute magnitude of blood calcium.

There is suggestive evidence that magnesium may also influence hormone secretion in the same direction as calcium. It has not been determined whether physiologic variations in magnesium concentration affect parathyroid secretion, however.

The mode of action of parathyroid hormone at the biochemical level involves effects of parathyroid hormone on adenyl cyclase in the cells of the target tissue. The initial effect of parathyroid hormone on kidney cells both in vivo and in vitro and on bone cells in vitro is a stimulation of adenyl cyclase. Stimulation of enzyme activity during specific hormone–target cell membrane interaction leads to an increase in intracellular 3′,5′ cyclic AMP. It seems likely that this rapid rise in intracellular 3′,5′ cyclic AMP is the initial biochemical step in all the physiologic effects of parathyroid hormone. It has been shown that following the administration of parathyroid hormone there is, within minutes, a rise in urinary cyclic AMP that precedes in time any observable increase in phosphate excretion in the kidney. Likewise, the effects on bone cell adenyl cyclase activity can be detected within 1 min of the addition of parathyroid hormone to a suspension of bone cells. In addition, administration of dibutyryl cyclic AMP, which, as a more soluble analogue of 3′,5′ cyclic AMP, penetrates cells more effectively, simulates the actions of parathyroid hormone in parathyroidectomized animals. Dibutyryl cyclic AMP leads to a rise in serum calcium, a lowering of serum phosphate, and an increased excretion of calcium, phosphate, and hydroxyproline in urine.

Data have been provided concerning the cellular mechanism whereby an increased intracellular concentration of cyclic AMP may lead to changes in calcium and phosphate ion translocation. In a number of tissues responsive to hormones through a cyclic AMP mechanism there is evidence for stimulation of protein kinases causing, in turn, phosphorylation of critical proteins that initiate the hormonal effect. The postulated sequence of events in parathyroid hormone–driven, cyclic AMP–mediated calcium (and phosphate) transport can be summarized as follows. Cyclic AMP binds to a specific binding protein causing it to dissociate from and thereby activate a protein kinase. The protein which, in turn, is phosphorylated by the kinase is at present unknown, but certain evidence suggests that microtubular proteins are the site of phosphorylation.

Whatever the cellular sites affected by the increased concentration of intracellular cyclic AMP, the mediating role of cyclic AMP in hormone action seems rather firmly established. The initial effect, within minutes of parathyroid hormone administration, is a hypocalcemia due to flow of calcium out of blood into cells, apparently skeletal cells. Thus, both cyclic AMP and calcium may serve as "second messengers" for mediating parathyroid hormone effects in receptor cells.

CALCITONIN (see also Chap. 351) Calcitonin is the potent hypocalcemic, hypophosphatemic peptide hormone which, in many ways, acts as the physiologic antagonist to parathyroid hormone. Calcitonin reduces bone resorption and has opposing effects to parathyroid hormone on the kidney in that calcitonin increases renal calcium clearance. This hormone, whose existence in nature was unsuspected only about 10 years ago, has already been the subject of intensive physiologic studies, and the hormone has been extensively evaluated as a therapeutic agent of potential value in skeletal disease characterized by excessive demineralization. Although it is appreciated that calcitonin exerts its hypocalcemic, hypophosphatemic action principally by an overall inhibition of bone resorption, the initial step in hormone action or the exact sequence of effects on target cells influenced by the hormone is not known.

The thyroid gland is the major source of the hormone in many mammalian species. In submammalian vertebrates calcitonin is found in a separate organ, the ultimobranchial body, which contains cells of a similar embryologic origin to the C cells of the thyroid. Extensive embryologic and histologic studies have established that the cells involved in calcitonin synthesis arise originally from neural crest tissue. These cells during embryogenesis migrate into the ultimobranchial body. The latter body or gland arises from the last branchial pouch, hence the name *ultimobranchial body*. In submammalian vertebrates the ultimobranchial body remains as a discrete organ, anatomically separate from the thyroid gland. In mammals the ultimobranchial gland fuses with the thyroid gland, and the calcitonin-secreting cells become part of the thyroid gland in adult life. Calcitonin is found in all vertebrate classes that have been examined.

The amino acid sequences of seven calcitonins from five species, including man, have been determined. The naturally occurring calcitonins consist of a peptide chain composed of 32 amino acids. Although there are certain common structural features, there is a considerable amount of variability in sequence. The entire chain of 32 amino acids appears to be required for biologic activity. Details of the factors that regulate the synthesis of calcitonin in the parafollicular or C cells are not known.

In animals, the concentration of the hormone rises within minutes of induced hypercalcemia. The secretion of the hormone is under the directly proportional control of blood calcium: an increase in calcium concentration causes an increase in the concentration of calcitonin, and a decrease in calcium concentration causes a decrease in the concentration of calcitonin. Calcitonin disappears rapidly from the circulation once secreted, with a half-life of 2 to 15 min. However, the concentration of calcitonin in the peripheral blood of human beings is unknown; in fact, there is no convincing evidence that calcitonin has been detected in the peripheral circulation of normal man. Development of more sensitive assays will be required to decide whether calcitonin does circulate in man, but at very low concentrations, or whether the hormone is not secreted under normal physiologic conditions.

Studies of the metabolism of calcitonin have been stimulated by the observation that calcitonin from salmon, when tested in various animal species, is 25 to 200 times more potent by weight in lowering serum calcium than are other forms of calcitonin. In fact, the salmon hormone has proved to be at least ten times more potent in man than human calcitonin. Greater resistance to metabolic destruction may explain in part the greater biologic potency of salmon calcitonin.

The physiologic role of calcitonin is still, in many ways, quite unclear. It is clear that in mammals calcitonin acts to lower both blood calcium and blood phosphate; the principal action of calcitonin is blockade of bone resorption. The importance of calcitonin in increasing urinary calcium and phosphate clearance is synergistic with its effects on bone resorption. The actions of calcitonin on kidney and bone are in turn modulated by the regulation of calcitonin production by serum calcium; hypercalcemia stimulates and hypocalcemia suppresses calcitonin release. The view that calcitonin serves physiologically to protect against hypercalcemia is thus explained by the hypocalcemic effects of calcitonin triggered in response to hypercalcemia.

However, there are numerous paradoxes and uncertainties about the role of calcitonin in vertebrates and in man. Calcitonin is present in high concentration in certain fish that have an entirely cartilagenous skeleton. The role of calcitonin, if any, in normal human physiology is unknown. It is not certain that calcitonin is normally secreted in human beings, nor are there any definite effects in man of calcitonin deficiency (totally thyroidectomized patients replaced only with thyroxine) or excess (patients with the calcitonin-secreting tumor, medullary carcinoma of the thyroid).

Present gaps in understanding of the physiologic role of calcitonin and the effects of the peptide at physiologic concentrations on organs other than the bone in turn complicate efforts to understand the biochemical mode of action of the hormone. However, evidence has been obtained that calcitonin may exert its effects through stimulation of membrane-bound adenyl cyclase in receptor cells in kidney and bone. Calcitonin has been shown to bind to renal cells and to stimulate membrane-bound adenyl cyclase. The cells responsive to calcitonin are located in different regions of the kidney than are cells affected by parathyroid hormone or vasopressin. Although it is not clear which ion translocation is primary in the overall action of calcitonin, data have pointed to mediation of calcitonin effects on calcium transport and bone metabolism through initial effects on phosphate transport. In this view, calcitonin acts by causing an initial influx of phosphate into cells; this in turn results in effects on calcium transport.

Calcitonin has shown promise as a therapeutic agent. The effectiveness of calcitonin in osteoporosis and in Paget's disease of bone is being evaluated. Preliminary results are encouraging; toxicity in chronic use has not proved to be a problem, and beneficial effects have been reported in long-term control of excessive bone turnover in Paget's disease.

VITAMIN D (see also Chap. 352) It is now clear that an understanding of the normal physiologic role of vitamin D in calcium homeostasis, as well as the effective use of vitamin D–like compounds in therapy of calcium-deficient states, requires a knowledge of the metabolic fate of vitamin D in the body.

Analysis of the patterns of endogenous biosynthesis and metabolism of an essential vitamin seems a contradiction in terms. The classic definition of a vitamin implies a trace substance which must be obtained by dietary means (because of a lack of capacity to synthesize the compound); in the classic view, the vitamin then acts as a critical metabolic cofactor. However, in certain respects vitamin D is a hormone. 7-Dehydrocholesterol, the precursor, is stored in large abundance in skin and can be converted by sunlight into vitamin D. Hence, vitamin D is not, in conditions of adequate sunlight, a dietary requirement at all.

Vitamin D is also obtainable from dietary sources. Preformed vitamin D is absorbed after ingestion of fish-liver oils or irradiated yeast. Most other foods, plant or animal, contain only inactive vitamin D precursors, 7-dehydrocholesterol or ergosterol. In order to prevent rickets when exposure to sunlight is inadequate, vitamin D is added to a variety of foodstuffs such as milk, milk products, and cereals.

It is now clear that, whether ingested or formed by ultraviolet irradiation in skin, vitamin D by itself is metabolically inert and must undergo endogenous transformation into active metabolites. The first step in metabolism involves conversion of vitamin D_3 into 25-hydroxycholecalciferol (25-HCC). The responsible enzyme system is located in the liver, and has been shown in in vitro studies to be under feedback suppression by the product 25-HCC. The details of this hepatic control have yet to be worked out in vivo, however. A second step in vitamin D metabolism occurs in the kidney. Two compounds, 1,25-dihydroxycholecalciferol (1,25-DHCC) and 24,25-dihydroxycholecalciferol (24,25-DHCC), are formed via further specific hydroxylation in the kidney from 25-HCC.

The nature of the metabolic control of kidney hydroxylation is not well defined at present. Calcium and phosphate ions and parathyroid hormone and calcitonin have all been reported to affect the efficiency of conversion of 25-HCC to 1,25-DHCC. However, observations from different groups appear contradictory. There is general agreement that low calcium concentration stimulates, and high calcium suppresses, 1,25-dihydroxy D formation. However, an important role for phosphate has been stressed (low phosphate, stimulation; high phosphate, suppression of 1,25-dihydroxy D formation). It is clear that further work will be required to clarify this important aspect of vitamin D metabolism.

These findings support the concept that in the presence of adequate ultraviolet exposure, vitamin D is actually a hormone. There are (1) large supplies of precursors, (2) specific syntheses occur in two sites, the liver and kidney, (3) the active products are secreted into the general circulation to be taken up by the target tissues, bone, and gut, and (4) biosynthesis is under metabolic control.

The role of these newly discovered metabolites and metabolic control points is consistent with earlier physiologic and clinical observations that indicated physiologic regulation of vitamin D action. It is known that the body adapts to increased calcium requirements (growth, pregnancy, lactation) or a low-calcium diet by increasing the efficiency of calcium absorption. This facultative increase in absorptive efficiency is absolutely dependent on the presence of vitamin D. It has been suggested that regulation of production of 1,25-DHCC by the kidney plays the important role in this adaptation. Further indirect evidence supporting regulation of vitamin D activation in man is the rarity of hypervitaminosis D despite wide variations in ultraviolet light exposure and dietary vitamin D intake. In fact, induction of hypervitaminosis D (as in the treatment of hypoparathyroidism) requires 50 to 100 times the minimum daily dose of the vitamin needed to prevent rickets.

Vitamin D, 25-OH vitamin D, and 1,25-dihydroxy D do not circulate free in the circulation, but are bound to specific high-affinity vitamin D transport proteins. The transport protein(s) appear to play an important role in the metabolism and transport of vitamin D. The vitamin must be transported to liver and hydroxylated. Product (25-OH D) must be removed and transported to kidney for a second hydroxylation to 1,25-dihydroxy D. Then the dihydroxylated compound must again be transported from kidney to the sites of action in intestine and bone. In each transport sequence, the vitamin and metabolites are tightly bound to the carrier proteins. Other dihydroxy metabolites, including the 25,26-; 21,25-; and 24,25-dihydroxy metabolites, are formed in the liver, kidney, and possibly other sites.

It has been suggested that 1,25-dihydroxycholecalciferol is the principal form of the vitamin acting to stimulate calcium transport by the intestine. 1,25-dihydroxycholecalciferol can also act to mobilize bone calcium, with a time course somewhat faster than, but a total effect no greater than, 25-hydroxycholecalciferol. 1,25-dihydroxycholecalciferol is more active than 25-hydroxycholecalciferol in mobilizing calcium from fetal rat calvaria (vitamin D is inactive in this system), and the dihydroxy metabolite alone is effective in mobilizing bone calcium in anephric rats. 21,25-Dihydroxy D also facilitates the mobilization of skeletal calcium in the vitamin D–deficient animals but has only limited potency on intestinal calcium transport. The physiologic significance of this metabolite and that of 24,25- or 25,26-dihydroxy D_3, if any, has yet to be established.

Even more subtle evidence of the importance of small structural changes in the vitamin D molecule is indicated by the finding that the 5,6-trans analogues of vitamin D_3, 5,6-trans-D_3, and 5,6-trans-25-hydroxy D_3, are active on intestinal transport without hydroxylation at the 1 position. The biologic activity of the 5,6-trans compounds seems explained by steric factors; trans configuration of the A ring results in placing of the original 3-hydroxy group in the steric position occupied normally by the 1-hydroxy. Activity requirements are satisfied even though the 1 position is lacking a hydroxy group.

There are striking differences in the relative potency and spectrum of biologic activity of dihydrotachysterol and vitamin D_2 or D_3 in man. Dihydrotachysterol is much less effective in calcium regulation than vitamin D_2 or D_3 in normal man or animals. However, on a weight basis dihydrotachysterol is three to ten times as effective as vitamin D_2 or D_3 in hypoparathyroid subjects or in patients with chronic renal failure. Two recent findings may, in part, explain the unique properties of dihydrotachysterol (DHT) in states of relative vitamin D resistance. It has been suggested that DHT, because of its trans-diene configuration, may act directly without 1-hydroxylation on intestinal transport, as has been confirmed with the 5,6-trans derivatives of vitamin D_3. It has also been demonstrated that DHT is more efficiently converted to the monohydroxyl form than is vitamin D_2 or D_3. These overall observations have led to widespread interest in DHT in therapeutic applications such as for chronic renal failure and hypoparathyroidism. The cost is greater for DHT, but easily justified in complex treatment problems.

The ultimate physiologic and pharmacologic significance of these vitamin D analogues is not yet fully evaluated, but the overall results suggest that important new advances, particularly in therapy of disorders of calcium and skeletal metabolism, may be forthcoming in the next several years.

The principal action of vitamin D (active metabolites) is to increase the efficiency of intestinal calcium absorption and thereby to prevent calcium deficiency. In higher doses the vitamin also appears to act directly on bone to increase bone mineral release. There has been considerable speculation that the vitamin may also affect directly (rather than through effects on intestinal calcium absorption) deposition of bone mineral. In addition, effects of vitamin D on renal calcium and/or phosphate transport have been suspected. However, there is no convincing proof, at present, in support of either of the latter two effects, bone formation or renal calcium and/or phosphate clearance by any direct action of vitamin D metabolites.

Effects of vitamin D on intestinal calcium transport and on bone resorption may be mediated through vitamin D–directed synthesis of a specific calcium-binding protein. Inhibitors of protein synthesis block vitamin D action on bone and intestine (the latter effect being only partial). The exact role of a calcium-binding protein or a second protein, a calcium-dependent adenosine triphosphatase believed to be synthesized under vitamin D control, in intestinal calcium transport has not been clarified, however. There is also evidence that vitamin D may increase calcium absorption, in part by direct membrane or extranuclear actions leading to facilitation of calcium diffusion across the intestinal cell mucosal border.

It is difficult to adequately assess the cellular events important in expression of vitamin D action at the present time in view of the large number of vitamin D metabolites which have been identified. However, it is clear that vitamin D and the active metabolites of the vitamin play a central role in maintaining positive calcium balance. In the absence of vitamin D, severe calcium deficiency results in man; this calcium deficiency, in combination with associated disturbances in phosphate metabolism, leads to blockade of normal bone mineralization—rickets or osteomalacia (Chap. 352).

HORMONAL AND IONIC INTERACTIONS IN CALCIUM HOMEOSTASIS The metabolic actions of parathyroid hormone, thyrocalcitonin, and vitamin D are closely interrelated. Investigations into the control of calcium homeostasis and the transport of calcium and phosphate by renal, intestinal, and bone cells have suggested not only a complex interaction between parathyroid hormone, thyrocalcitonin, and vitamin D but also critical effects due to the extracellular and intracellular concentration of the calcium and phosphate ions themselves. These complex interactions must be appreciated in efforts to ultimately understand the nature of the pathophysiologic changes in diseases such as primary hyperparathyroidism or lack of vitamin D.

Vitamin D promotes the increased intestinal transport of calcium and, secondarily, of phosphate even in the absence of the parathyroids and of thyrocalcitonin. In addition, the vitamin in high doses sustains increased levels of bone resorption and thereby provides skeletal calcium and phosphate to maintain extracellular fluid calcium and phosphorus concentrations near normal levels. This has been amply evident clinically since high concentrations of vitamin D have been shown to be therapeutically useful in the management of patients with postsurgical or idiopathic hypoparathyroidism. However, even in the case of vitamin D, expression of biologic action is influenced by the presence of the parathyroids. Patients with hypoparathyroidism require much greater doses of vitamin D than the normal nutritional requirement.

In experimental severe vitamin D deficiency, serum calcium levels are very low. Parathyroid hyperplasia may be evident, yet parathyroidectomy produced little further decline in blood calcium. This suggests a state of parathyroid hormone resistance in the face of vitamin D deficiency. Most investigators have found that large doses of PTH are needed to raise the serum calcium in vitamin D–deficient animals and patients or else have found that parathyroid hormone is completely ineffective. The mechanism whereby vitamin D deficiency results in PTH resistance is still unresolved. Some have suggested it is the calcium deficiency and hypocalcemia of vitamin D deficiency, rather than vitamin D lack per se, which causes PTH resistance. Other workers emphasize that vitamin D is an absolutely essential cofactor for PTH effects on the skeleton. According to this view, the integrity of certain cellular transport systems on which parathyroid hormone acts are dependent on vitamin D action. By contrast, it seems likely that the phosphaturic effect of parathyroid hormone is not impaired in vitamin D deficiency. The severe hypophosphatemia associated with certain osteomalacic states may be, at least in part, a consequence of this disparity between the relative effectiveness of parathyroid hormone on calcium versus phosphate transport in vitamin D deficiency. Due to hypocalcemia, parathyroid hypersecretion develops as an adaptation. The increased secretion of parathyroid hormone with normal sensitivity of the renal tubule to parathyroid-induced effects on phosphate reabsorption results in excessive renal phosphate wasting.

Extracellular fluid and renal cell concentrations of calcium and phosphate may directly affect renal tubular phosphate transport. Increased phosphate clearance can be induced in hypoparathyroid subjects whose serum calcium concentration is normal by the administration of oral phosphate loads under conditions in which blood phosphate concentration has apparently not changed. In other words, increased phosphate loads lead directly to enhanced phosphate clearance by the kidney. The concentration of serum calcium appears to have a biphasic effect on tubular absorption of phosphate. Raising the level of serum calcium from low to normal or to slightly elevated levels leads to increased phosphate clearance, whereas marked elevations of serum calcium (as, for example, by infusion of calcium) lead to a reduction in renal phosphate clearance, even in parathyroidectomized subjects.

The varied observations made on the closely related interaction of parathyroid hormone, vitamin D, and the concentrations of calcium and phosphate in blood and cells on responses to any given metabolic challenge undoubtedly reflect the great evolutionary pressure to preserve calcium and phosphate homeostasis in mammals. Knowledge of the various hormonal and ionic interactions involved in mineral ion homeostasis is only fragmentary at present. The practical importance of these concepts is in the interpretation of diagnostic studies and in the planning of medical management of patients with mineral ion deficits or hormonal deficiency. For example, the demonstration that a patient with hypophosphatemia exhibits a sharp reduction in renal phosphate clearance after calcium infusion need not imply an overproduction of parathyroid hormone since similar effects are noted after calcium infusion in hypoparathyroid subjects. The appropriate amount of supplemental vitamin D and oral calcium given to control temporary hypoparathyroidism after extensive parathyroid surgery may suddenly change if parathyroid function returns. Hence, frequent reexamination of blood and urine calcium concentration is necessary in such patients. Further examples of the implications of these complex interactions in calcium homeostasis are discussed in connection with specific disease entities in subsequent chapters.

REFERENCES

Aurbach GD et al: Structure, synthesis and mechanism of action of parathyroid hormone. Rec Prog Horm Res 28:353, 1972

Bourne GH (ed): *The Biochemistry and Physiology of Bone*, vol. 3, New York: Academic, 1971

Canterbury JM, Reiss E: Multiple immunoreactive molecular

forms of PTH in human serum. Proc Soc Exp Biol Med 146:1393, 1972

DeLuca HF: 1,25-Dihydroxycholecalciferol: Isolation, identification, regulation and mechanism of action. Proc 3d Int Symposium Endocrinol, ed S Taylor, London: Heinemann, 1972, p. 452

Foster GV et al: Calcitonin, in *Clinics in Endocrinology and Metabolism*, vol. 1, ed I MacIntyre, London: Saunders, 1972, p. 93

Glimcher MJ, Krane SM: The organization and structure of bone and the mechanism of calcification, in *A Treatise on Collagen*, vol. 2, part B, eds GN Ramachandran, BS Gould, London: Academic, 1968, p. 67

Holick MF et al: Isolation and identification on 1,25-dihydroxycholecalciferol: A metabolite of vitamin D active in intestine, Biochemistry 10:2799, 1971

Kemper B et al: Proparathyroid hormone: Identification of a biosynthetic precursor to parathyroid hormone. Proc Natl Acad Sci USA 69:643, 1972

Kodicek E: Recent advances in vitamin D metabolism, in *Clinics in Endocrinology and Metabolism*, vol. 1, ed I MacIntyre, London: Saunders, 1972, p. 305

Krane SM: Calcium, phosphate and magnesium, in *The International Encyclopedia of Pharmacology and Therapeutics*, ed H Rasmussen, New York: Pergamon, 1970, p. 19

Potts JT Jr et al: The chemistry of parathyroid hormone and the calcitonins, in *Vitamins and the Hormones*, vol. 29, eds RS Harris et al, New York: Academic, 1971, p. 41

Segre GV et al: Parathyroid hormone in human plasma: Immunochemical characterization and biological implications. J Clin Invest 51:3163, 1973

Singer FR et al: Pharmacological effects of salmon calcitonin in man, in *Calcium, Parathyroid Hormone and the Calcitonins*, eds RV Talmage, PL Munson, Amsterdam: Excerpta Medica, 1972, p. 89

Talmage RV et al: Effect of calcitonin and calcium infusion on plasma phosphate. Endocrinology 92:146, 1973

350 DISORDERS OF PARATHYROID GLANDS

JOHN T. POTTS, JR.

PRIMARY HYPERPARATHYROIDISM

NATURAL HISTORY AND INCIDENCE Primary hyperparathyroidism is a generalized disorder of calcium, phosphate, and bone metabolism that results from an increased secretion of parathyroid hormone. The excessive concentration of circulating hormone usually leads to hypercalcemia and hypophosphatemia; there may be recurrent nephrolithiasis, peptic ulcers, mental changes, and less frequently, excessive bone resorption. However, with improved recognition of the disease and wider use of diagnostic techniques, particularly multiphasic screening of blood calcium, the diagnosis is being made with increasing frequency and earlier in the course of the illness. Because of this it has become evident that the clinical manifestations and laboratory evidence of hyperparathyroidism may be quite subtle. There are many patients in whom an incidental blood calcium determination establishes hypercalcemia, without any apparent symptoms. These patients, in turn, raise obvious questions about the natural history of the disease and the indications for surgery.

The disease most commonly occurs in adults, with peak incidence between the third and fifth decades. However, primary hyperparathyroidism has been detected in young children, and the initial diagnosis has been made in the very elderly. Patients may go for years with undetected hyperparathyroidism because of the minimal symptoms. Occasionally, the disease seems to appear abruptly, and patients may exhibit severe complications, such as marked dehydration and coma associated with severe hypercalcemic parathyroid crisis. If the incidence of the disease is at all accurately reflected by the apparent frequency in referral centers, it would appear that hyperparathyroidism is more common than previously appreciated; one projection has been made that the incidence of primary hyperparathyroidism is 1 case per 1,000 persons per year.

ETIOLOGY AND PATHOLOGY In greater than 80 percent of patients, primary hyperparathyroidism results from neoplastic transformation of one parathyroid gland; all but a few percent of the neoplasms are benign adenomas. "Double adenomas," by which was meant neoplastic transformation of two parathyroids with the remaining glands entirely normal, is now felt to be extremely rare. Most cases of supposed double adenoma represented unrecognized hyperplasia involving all parathyroids. The two most likely possibilities to be considered by the surgeon and pathologist in their analysis of the pathology present in a given patient are (1) disease in a single gland with an incidence of approximately 85 percent (81 percent adenoma, 4 percent histologically carcinoma) or (2) hyperplasia of all glands in approximately 15 percent of cases. These considerations are of practical importance in the surgical management of hyperparathyroidism, as discussed below.

An adenoma is the most common cause of hyperparathyroidism; often the tumor is in the inferior parathyroid glands. However, the tumor is found in an unusual location in 6 to 10 percent of patients; such ectopic parathyroid adenomas may be located in the thymus, the thyroid, or even the pericardium. Retroesophageal adenomas have also been reported. Adenomas vary in size from 0.5 to 5 g; in some instances, however, tumors as large as 10 to 20 g are found. Histologic examination usually reveals that the adenoma is composed primarily of chief cells; the nodule can be surrounded by a rim of normal tissue. This latter feature can sometimes be useful in distinguishing adenomas from primary chief-cell hyperplasia. Rarely adenomas are composed of oxyphil cells or a mixed population of cells.

For many years, occasional patients with hyperparathyroidism had been recognized to have clear cell (Wasserhelle) hyperplasia of all four glands. Chief-cell hyperplasia of the parathyroid glands, on the other hand, had usually been seen in secondary hyperparathyroidism. However, it was recognized that chief-cell hyperplasia could also be found in primary hyperparathyroidism. This diagnosis is now being made with increasing frequency. Chief-cell hyperplasia is especially common in those instances of hyperparathyroidism which are familial or which are part of the syndrome of multiple endocrine adenomatosis.

Some hyperplastic glands may exhibit compression of tissue around an area of hyperplasia, giving the appearance of a capsule (pseudoencapsulation) and, hence, may be mistaken for an adenoma. It can be difficult to distinguish adenoma from hyperplasia by histologic criteria. Findings at surgery must be combined with microscopic examination of biopsy specimens of several glands. When an adenoma is present, examination of other glands indicates that they are of normal size, approximately 25 mg average weight, and histologically there is a normal distribution of all cell types, rather than only chief cells, and normal areas of fat. With hyperplasia all glands may be enlarged; even if certain glands are not clearly increased in size, histologic examination reveals a uniform pattern of chief cells and *disappearance of fat.*

Carcinoma of the parathyroid glands is rare; fewer than 50 cases have been reported. The tumor usually secretes excessive amounts of parathyroid hormone, although nonfunctioning tumors have been reported. Parathyroid carcinoma is usually slow growing but eventually metastasizes, often to the lungs and the liver. It is often difficult initially to decide if the primary tumor is carcinoma; even benign adenomas may show histologic changes that suggest malignant disease. Hyperparathyroidism resulting from a parathyroid carcinoma may be clinically indistinguishable from other forms of primary hyperparathyroidism.

A variety of nonparathyroid tumors have been associated with a clinical syndrome resembling primary hyperparathyroidism. This syndrome has been termed *pseudohyperparathyroidism* or *ectopic hyperparathyroidism.* The clinical evidence that some nonparathyroid tumors produce a parathyroid hormone–like peptide has been confirmed by immunologic studies, which indicate that parathyroid-like activity is present in extracts of such tumors and in the blood of affected patients. The true incidence of ectopic hyperparathyroidism is difficult to assess. The entity must be suspected particularly in older patients. Lung tumors, particularly squamous-cell carcinoma, and renal tumors are the most common type of nonparathyroid tumors associated with ectopic hyperparathyroidism. However, tumors of many types and origin have been described in association with this form of hyperparathyroidism.

The occurrence of hyperparathyroidism in a familial pattern is well documented and may occur without other endocrinologic abnormality. More often, however, hereditary hyperparathyroidism is found as part of a multiglandular endocrinopathy. It is now appreciated that there are probably two genetically distinct syndromes with multiple endocrine disorders. The syndrome originally described (Wermer's syndrome) consisted of hyperparathyroidism and tumors of the pituitary and pancreatic islet cells. This multiglandular disorder is often associated with peptic ulcer and gastric hypersecretion (the Zollinger-Ellison syndrome). Another distinct constellation of endocrinologic abnormalities which consists of hyperparathyroidism associated with pheochromocytoma and medullary carcinoma of the thyroid has also been described (see Chap. 351).

In both of these syndromes the hyperparathyroidism can be due to adenomas or hyperplasia, the latter usually of the chief-cell variety. There is a very high familial incidence of both syndromes that fits inheritance pattern as an autosomal dominant. Tumors of the thyroid and adrenal medulla are not found in Wermer's syndrome, and pancreatic and pituitary tumors are not found in the kindreds with a high incidence of medullary carcinoma of the thyroid and pheochromocytoma. In this revised classification Wermer's syndrome is termed *multiple endocrine adenomatosis* type I (MEA type 1), and the more recently described syndrome involving thyroid tumors MEA type 2. Since the different endocrine tumors can occur at widely separated intervals, hyperparathyroidism and the related endocrine disorders should be carefully and repeatedly searched for in all members of kindreds afflicted with the multiple endocrine adenomatosis syndromes.

SIGNS AND SYMPTOMS Most of the signs and symptoms of hyperparathyroidism reflect known pathophysiologic consequences of hypercalcemia. Many organ systems can be affected by hyperparathyroidism. However, characteristically, involvement of the kidneys and skeletal system is most prominent. *Kidney involvement,* due either to deposition of calcium in the renal parenchyma or to recurrent nephrolithiasis, is found in 60 to 70 percent of patients. Renal stones are usually composed of either calcium oxalate or calcium phosphate. Repeated episodes of nephrolithiasis or the formation of large calculi may lead to urinary tract obstruction and repeated episodes of infection. These complications may also contribute to progressive loss of renal function. Nephrolithiasis and nephrocalcinosis rarely occur in the same patient. Nephrocalcinosis may be accompanied by decreased renal function and phosphate retention.

Bone disease sufficiently severe to produce symptoms is reported in 10 to 25 percent of patients; this incidence is much lower than was characteristic of the clinical picture of hyperparathyroidism several decades ago. This changing pattern of frequency of involvement of the skeleton has not been adequately explained. The classic pattern of bone involvement in hyperparathyroidism is osteitis fibrosa cystica. In the United States, x-ray evidence of osteitis fibrosa cystica is not commonly found in patients at the time that the diagnosis of hyperparathyroidism is made, even though there may be a long history of renal and other complications of the disease. However, bone biopsy studies reveal almost invariably microscopic evidence of abnormality in bone turnover such as osteocytic osteolysis, even in the absence of osteitis fibrosa. Thus, although nearly all patients give evidence of excessive effects of parathyroid hormone on bone, only a few develop severe skeletal involvement.

Clinically, a number of features of the bone disease are of importance, when present, in evaluating the symptoms of the patient, in providing diagnostic clues to the presence of the disease, or in helping to assess the response of the patient following surgical correction of the hyperparathyroidism. Histologic examination of bone specimens from patients with severe osteitis fibrosa reveals a number of changes that collectively define the presence of parathyroid overactivity. There is a reduction in the number of trabeculae, an increase in giant multinucleated osteoclasts seen in scalloped areas on the surface of the bone (Howship's lacunas), and a marked replacement of normal cellular and marrow elements by fibrous tissue. In milder forms of skeletal involvement early changes can sometimes be detected by x-rays of the hands and skull. *The phalangeal tufts* may be resorbed, and an irregular outline replaces the normally sharp cortical outline of the bone in the digits. This change is termed *subperiosteal resorption.* Detection of loss of the *lamina dura* of the teeth is also helpful diagnostically, but is found less frequently than subperiosteal resorption. Tiny, "punched-out" lesions in the skull, so-called "salt-and-pepper" appearance, are very characteristic.

In addition, it has been appreciated that hyperparathyroidism may be associated with symptoms or signs referable to *neuromuscular function, the gastrointestinal tract, the skin, and the joints.* Sometimes, quite vague or minor complaints from a patient, particularly neuromuscular or gastrointestinal symptoms, are the only clue to the diagnosis; awareness of the subtle manifestations of the disease may prompt a request for blood calcium determination as part of a diagnostic evaluation.

Central nervous system manifestations of hyperparathyroidism are multiple and varied. Reported symptoms range from mild personality disturbances to severe psychiatric disorders; mental obtundation or coma is seen with severe hypercalcemia. In some instances, the patient experiences multiple and vague complaints which can often be mistaken for psychoneurosis.

Frequently, there are varied and sometimes subtle manifestations of hyperparathyroidism in the *gastrointestinal tract.* In addition to a variety of vague abdominal complaints, diseases of the stomach and pancreas are frequent. *Duodenal ulcers* have been reported in as many as 25 percent of the patients with proved hyperparathyroidism. In addition, in patients with hyperparathyroidism resulting from multiple endocrine adenomatosis syndrome (type 1), there is a very high incidence of ulcer as a result of the associated pancreatic tumors that secrete excessive quantities of gastrin, the Zollinger-Ellison syndrome. Cases of pancreatitis have been reported in association with hyperparathyroidism, but the absolute incidence is not firmly established. Various mechanisms have been proposed to explain the apparent increased incidence of pancreatitis, but there is no convincing explanation.

Calcification in the cornea of the eye (*band keratopathy*) may be clinically recognizable, usually when renal insufficiency and phosphate retention are present; slit lamp examination may, however, be necessary to detect the calcification.

It has also been noted that chondrocalcinosis and pseudogout are seen in association with hyperparathyroidism. Occasionally pseudogout is the initial clinical manifestation of the hyperparathyroidism.

DIAGNOSIS Except in those situations in which the parathyroid immunoassay is applied, the diagnosis of hyperparathyroidism in a patient with proved hypercalcemia usually proceeds by exclusion.

The disease is most often sought for in patients with recurrent kidney stones or, in rarer instances, with symptoms and/or signs of osteitis fibrosa. With the increased recognition of the disease, blood calcium measurements may lead to detection of hypercalcemia in a patient with vague constitutional complaints, ulcer, or atypical arthritis. Finally, hypercalcemia may be detected as a result of multiphasic routine blood testing in asymptomatic subjects. Repeated measurements of plasma calcium should be made in patients with suspected hypercalcemia. One may detect either a sustained hypercalcemia or a pattern of high normal blood calciums alternating with occasional definitely elevated values. If errors due to altered concentration of blood protein or variation in laboratory range of normal can be eliminated, such findings establish the presence of hypercalcemia.

Obviously, the efforts to establish the diagnosis are most exhaustive in patients with clear-cut symptoms referable to hyperparathyroidism, particularly with recurrent kidney stones. The philosophy of approach is different at the other extreme, a totally asymptomatic patient in whom hypercalcemia is detected coincidentally. However, since hypercalcemia can be the presenting evidence for malignancy or other serious disease, a thorough evaluation of possible etiologies including hyperparathyroidism by application of at least standard screening procedures is indicated even in asymptomatic subjects. If the diagnosis of hyperparathyroidism is suspected after such an evaluation, a decision can still be made to follow the patient for a time rather than recommend surgery.

Hypercalcemia is the most invariant manifestation of hyperparathyroidism. In fact, without definite hypercalcemia there is almost never a justification for surgical exploration. There continue to be reports of so-called "normocalcemic hyperparathyroidism," that is, patients with surgically proved hyperparathyroidism with normal calcium. However, careful scrutiny of the reports reveals that in those with adenomas, the patients were, in fact, hypercalcemic at some time in their course; they could more correctly be described, therefore, as having intermittent hypercalcemia, perhaps an early feature of hyperparathyroidism. If normocalcemic hyperparathyroidism does occur, it is extremely rare. Reports of removal of all four glands, found to be normal grossly and by light microscopy in normocalcemic patients with kidney stones, cannot be accepted as valid examples of hyperparathyroidism.

Hypercalcuria is also commonly seen in hyperparathyroidism. However, it should be kept in mind that parathyroid hormone actually reduces calcium clearance. In fact, the 24-hr urine excretion of calcium is lower in patients with hyperparathyroidism than in patients with equivalent degrees of hypercalcemia from nonparathyroid causes.

Serum phosphate is usually low but may be normal, especially if renal failure has developed. Detection of hypophosphatemia can be useful but is less specific than hypercalcemia. In addition, samples must be obtained in the morning, under fasting conditions, to be useful.

Other electrolyte abnormalities have also been described; however, these abnormalities are not sufficiently specific to be of diagnostic value. Serum magnesium levels have been reported to be low. Serum chloride and citrate are often elevated.

Blood alkaline phosphatase and urinary hydroxyproline concentrations are usually elevated when there is significant bone involvement. Renal involvement can be reflected by a decreased concentrating ability, by specific tubular defects such as tubular acidosis, and finally by frank renal failure with the chemical findings of azotemia.

Special tests *Glucocorticoid administration* has been useful in differentiating the hypercalcemia of hyperparathyroidism from that associated with sarcoidosis, multiple myeloma, vitamin D intoxication, and some malignant diseases with osseous metastases. In the latter disease, doses of hydrocortisone of 100 mg per day (or an equivalent dose of another steroid such as prednisone) given for 10 days often result in a lowering of the serum calcium, whereas calcium does not fall in hyperparathyroidism, except that if osteitis is present in the hyperparathyroidism, the calcium has been reported to drop. Occasional false positive and false negative results have been reported. The mechanism of the effect is not explained.

A variety of tests of parathyroid function are based on the known effects of the hormone on the *renal handling of phosphate*. These tests are designed to take advantage of the decrease in tubular resorption of phosphate caused by parathyroid hormone. To perform the test, any of several convenient indexes of phosphate handling by the kidneys is determined. Because of the diurnal variation in plasma phosphate concentration and the marked fluctuations in phosphate that occur with eating, long periods of urine collection are not useful in determinations of phosphate clearance.

Phosphate clearance is determined by standard clearance techniques involving simultaneous measurement of urinary and blood phosphate concentrations; usually urine samples are collected over a 1- to 2-hr period. Normal subjects have a phosphate clearance of 10.8 $\pm$2.7 ml per min. Values 50 or more percent above this figure have been detected in hyperparathyroidism. The tubular resorption of phosphate can be derived from the estimation of the phosphate clearance and the additional measurement of the glomerular filtration made by measuring creatinine clearance. The ratio of phosphate clearance over creatinine clearance indicates the percent of filtered phosphate that was excreted. In normal subjects the tubular resorption of phosphate exceeds 85 percent; in hyperparathyroidism tubular resorption of phosphate may be as low as 50 to 60 percent. Unfortunately, these tests are all influenced by the many other factors that affect the renal handling of phosphate, and their value seems limited.

Thiazide diuretics in the usual doses can produce sustained, frank hypercalcemia in patients with hyperparathyroidism and borderline calcium values. Since such a response is not seen in normal subjects (there may be some elevation in blood calcium in normal subjects, but any effect seen is lost in a few days despite continued administration of thiazides), thiazide administration has been suggested as a provocative test for the presence of hyperparathyroidism.

The development of a *specific radioimmunoassay* sufficiently sensitive to detect the circulating human parathyroid hormone has provided, for the first time, a specific test for parathyroid function. Independent assay procedures have now been developed in several centers in this country, elsewhere in England, and Europe as well. There have been and continue to be, however, numerous problems with the application and interpretation of the assay. It is necessary to use a nonhomologous assay system-labeled bovine parathyroid hormone and antiserum to bovine parathyroid hormone to measure human parathyroid hormone. There occur in plasma several immunologically (and biologically) distinct species of parathyroid hormone (see Chap. 349). Despite these problems, when appropriate precautions are observed, the immunoassay for parathyroid hormone can be uniquely useful in the diagnostic evaluation of patients with primary hyperparathyroidism and/or with hypercalcemia.

Most workers find that the concentration of hormone in some subjects with proved hyperparathyroidism is no higher than that found in some normal subjects. However, many of the patients with hyperparathyroidism have concentrations of hormone clearly elevated above the normal range. In these latter patients, the assay result strongly confirms the diagnosis. It has been recently appreciated that hormone concentration in blood in patients with hyperparathyroidism changes in response to induced changes in blood calcium. This, in part, explains the overlap found between hormone concentrations in patients with hyperparathyroidism and increased blood calcium level versus normal subjects with normal calcium concentrations. The assay is helpful in the differential diagnosis of hypercalcemia; a clear distinction exists in values found in hypercalcemia of parathyroid origin and nonparathyroid origin. Patients with hypercalcemia not due to parathyroid disease have undetectable concentrations of parathyroid hormone; in these patients, since parathyroid gland function is normal, secretion is suppressed because of the hypercalcemia. Patients with hypercalcemia due to hyperparathyroidism have detectable, if not elevated, concentrations of hormone despite hypercalcemia.

In addition to its usefulness in diagnostic studies, the immunoassay for parathyroid hormone has been applied to the study of the control of secretion of the peptide by abnormal parathyroid tissue. In patients with primary hyperparathyroidism, it has been observed that hormone secretion is not autonomous as was previously believed, but that the concentration of hormone is responsive to induced changes in blood calcium concentration. These findings emphasize that the disorder of parathyroid function in primary hyperparathyroidism cannot be explained simply on the basis of a fixed rate of hormone secretion; the defect in control of secretion, responsible for excessive hormone production, must be more subtle than simple autonomy. The nature of the defect has not yet been defined.

Because of the small size of the parathyroids, even when hyperplastic or neoplastic, the variable position of the glands, and the complex anatomy of the neck, localization of abnormal parathyroid tissue at surgery is often difficult. For this reason several methods have been devised to attempt preoperative localization of abnormal parathyroid tissue. *Roentgenographic examination of the esophagus* during barium swallow can reveal an indentation on the esophagus due to pressure from a large parathyroid. Because it is a simple procedure and occasionally rewarding, it should probably be performed routinely prior to surgery. Some success has been reported with *selenomethionine scans* and *arteriography*. These procedures are not routinely applied in most centers, and there is little systematic experience.

The technique of *percutaneous venous catheter sampling* of the veins of the neck and thorax, and parathyroid hormone radioimmunoassay of the samples so obtained, has been introduced as a method for preoperative localization of parathyroid tissue. In patients in whom a single adenoma is subsequently found at surgery, a marked unilateral gradient in hormone concentration is seen in the small thyroid veins on the side of the neoplasm. In patients who have abnormal parathyroid tissue on both sides of the neck (hyperplasia), on the other hand, gradients in hormone concentration are found on both sides of the thyroid plexus. The technique has permitted preoperative localization to be made in most patients tested, even in patients who had had prior unsuccessful neck surgery. It has been possible to distinguish preoperatively a single adenoma from hyperplasia of all four glands. However, since the radiologic expertise necessary to catheterize thyroid veins is not available in many centers and overall experience is still limited, the technique is recommended only for patients who present special diagnostic problems, or in whom previous neck surgery has failed to locate hyperfunctioning parathyroid tissue.

DIFFERENTIAL DIAGNOSIS The differential diagnosis of hyperparathyroidism is best considered under three general headings: (1) hypercalcemia, (2) nephrolithiasis, and (3) bone disease.

It must be emphasized that hyperparathyroidism is a chronic disorder. It is important to obtain historical features or clinical evidence of the chronicity of a disorder in calcium metabolism such as recurrent renal calculi, documented hypercalcemia many months earlier, or evidence of occult renal stones. Such evidence of chronicity usually favors the diagnosis of hyperparathyroidism rather than malignancy. On the other hand, if hypercalcemia has been detected only recently without other historical features of chronicity, the search for other causes of hypercalcemia must be particularly thorough. The pattern of high calcium with low phosphate is believed typical of hyperparathyroidism in contrast to many other causes of hypercalcemia where phosphate levels are normal or increased. However, it has been shown that severe hypercalcemia per se lowers phosphate.

Malignancy Hypercalcemia is a frequent complication of malignant disease. The elimination of malignancy as the underlying cause of hypercalcemia can be one of the most difficult problems in differential diagnosis, particularly when one considers the possibility of ectopic hyperparathyroidism. The patient's medical history, as well as physical and laboratory findings, are helpful in the differentiation. If a patient with hypercalcemia has a history of vague complaints and recurrent symptoms extending over several years prior to evaluation, it is much less likely that occult malignant disease is responsible; if malignancy were the cause of the hypercalcemia, there should be definite evidence of the primary tumor or metastatic lesions.

Hypercalcemia complicating malignancy results from one of three processes: (1) Osteolytic metastases, such as occur in carcinoma of the breast, (2) pseudohyperparathyroidism with ectopic production of parathyroid hormone, and (3) pseudohyperparathyroidism secondary to production of humoral substances chemically distinct from parathyroid hormone. The syndrome of pseudohyperparathyroidism is usually suspected, rather than hypercalcemia caused by osteolytic metastases, if hypophosphatemia in addition to hypercalcemia is detected, and skeletal x-ray survey or bone scan fail to reveal osteolytic lesions. Mild alkalosis rather than acidosis is often seen in pseudohyperparathyroidism. Hypercalcemia in malignant disease not involving ectopic humoral production usually occurs as a result of a direct invasion of bone by the tumor. A metastatic series or skeletal x-ray survey may point to osteolytic lesions.

Sarcoidosis The hypercalcemia of sarcoidosis can also present a difficult problem in differential diagnosis, especially since sarcoidosis may have existed for several years but with many typical features of the disease lacking. In sarcoidosis the hypercalcemia presumably results from increased absorption of calcium from the gastrointestinal tract secondary to exaggerated sensitivity to vitamin D (this phenomenon may explain the hypocalcemic effect of steroids—inhibition of formation of the active forms of vitamin D). Hypercalcemia, when present in sarcoidosis, is usually a manifestation of severe involvement and disseminated disease. Hence evidence of pulmonary involvement is usually seen; chest x-ray may reveal a diffuse fibronodular infiltrate and/or prominent hilar adenopathy. An elevated blood gamma-globulin may also be detected. In severe cases there may also be direct involvement of bone by the granulomatous process. The most definitive procedure is to demonstrate noncaseating granulomas by liver biopsy or lymph node biopsy, the latter usually of a scalene node.

Multiple myeloma Hypercalcemia is seen in approximately 40 percent of patients with multiple myeloma. It is presumably due to direct erosion of bone by the neoplastic cells. Typical "punched-out" lesions in bone may be detected on x-ray, particularly of the skull. Glucocorticoids lead to a reduction in the increased bone turnover; a lowering of blood calcium occurs within several days to a week following institution of therapy (a typical regimen is 40 mg prednisone per day). Steroids act by direct tumor suppression; improvement in marrow morphology, rise in hemoglobin, and reduction in abnormal urinary and plasma protein are found.

Vitamin D intoxication The chronic ingestion of large doses of vitamin D can produce hypercalcemia. Usually the ingestion of doses in excess of 100,000 units vitamin D_2 or D_3 for many months is necessary for this complication to occur. The diagnosis in self-induced cases is usually established by uncovering the history of excessive vitamin D intake. In considering vitamin D intoxication, it should be noted that the hypercalcemia may persist for weeks to months after vitamin D ingestion is stopped. Excessive quantities of the vitamin are stored in the body and released slowly. Hence, in addition to the use of steroids to confirm the diagnosis through an acute suppression of hypercalcemia (cortisone suppression test), treatment with glucocorticoids may be necessary to control hypercalcemia and to prevent irreversible renal damage due to persistent hypercalcemia.

Milk-alkali syndrome (Burnett's syndrome) In this unusual syndrome hypercalcemia and renal failure occur as a complication of long-term ingestion of large amounts of milk or calcium and absorbable antacids. This syndrome seems much less prevalent since the nonabsorbable antacids have been used in ulcer therapy. It seems possible that some of these patients have a pattern of excessive gastrointestinal absorption similar to that predicated to be present in idiopathic hypercalcuria. Alkalosis contributes to deposition of calcium phosphate in abnormal locations including the kidney. Because of the increased incidence of ulcer disease in primary hyperparathyroidism, the possibility that the milk-alkali syndrome may coexist with hyperparathyroidism should always be considered.

Thyrotoxicosis Significant hypercalcemia is a rare complication of thyrotoxicosis. However, minimal elevations of calcium have been reported in as many as 25 percent of patients with hyperthyroidism. Hypercalcemia in hyperthyroidism is presumably related to increased bone resorption. The diagnosis usually offers no difficulties since, in most cases, it is the thyrotoxicosis rather than the hypercalcemia that brings the patient to the physician. However, particularly in the elderly, the signs of thyrotoxicosis may be minimal. During treatment of a patient with thyrotoxicosis and hypercalcemia, repeated determinations of serum calcium should be made. If the serum calcium does not return toward normal as the thyrotoxicosis is brought under control, another cause for the hypercalcemia should be suspected.

Adrenal insufficiency Hypercalcemia has been reported to occur in adrenal insufficiency, especially acute adrenal failure. The cause of the hypercalcemia has not been determined. There is evidence that glucocorticoids and vitamin D have opposing actions on blood calcium. High doses of steroids lower blood calcium when given as replacement in adrenal crisis; it is assumed by some that the elevation in calcium in the state of adrenal insufficiency reflects in some way the result of glucocorticoid deficiency. Others, however, have suggested that the hypercalcemia is due merely to hemoconcentration and that the ionized calcium is normal. In any event, in acute adrenal failure hypercalcemia is only a transient phenomenon; blood calcium returns to normal with adrenal replacement therapy.

Idiopathic hypercalcemia of infancy This is a rare syndrome characterized by hypercalcemia, often in association with multiple congenital cardiovascular lesions. Hypersensitivity to vitamin D has been postulated. The distinctive clinical features and age distribution of the syndrome make it unlikely to be a problem in the differential diagnosis of most cases of hypercalcemia.

Other causes of hypercalcemia Prolonged immobilization of a patient may lead to hypercalcemia, especially in patients with high rates of bone turnover, such as those with Paget's disease. Immobilization may also cause hypercalcemia in young patients who are undergoing rapid growth and, therefore, have higher bone turnover rates. The hypercalcemia and associated hypercalcuria resolve when the patient becomes ambulatory. Hypercalcemia may occur in renal disease as a complication of secondary hyperparathyroidism, particularly in subjects undergoing chronic hemodialysis or renal transplantation.

Nephrolithiasis Nephrolithiasis must be considered in any discussion of the differential diagnosis of hyperparathyroidism. Recurrent episodes of formation of calcium-containing kidney stones are most often associated with metabolic or renal abnormalities unconnected with hyperparathyroidism. Nonetheless, a detailed search for hyperparathyroidism is indicated in patients who form calcium-containing kidney stones, even if hypercalcemia is not present at the time when nephrolithiasis first occurs.

A difficulty frequently encountered in the differential diagnosis of nephrolithiasis is to distinguish idiopathic hypercalcuria from hyperparathyroidism. In idiopathic hypercalcuria, there is a strong familial incidence, a preponderance in males, an increased urinary excretion of calcium, and a tendency to hypophosphatemia. In most patients the disorder reflects excessive dietary absorption of calcium with high calcium intake leading secondarily to increased urinary calcium (and thereby can be diagnosed).

Hypercalcuria and the formation of calcium-containing stones have been recognized in a number of disorders in addition to hyperparathyroidism and idiopathic hypercalcuria. These include metastatic cancer, multiple myeloma, senile osteoporosis, Cushing's syndrome, phosphate diabetes, milk-alkali syndrome (in the initial phases), vitamin D intoxication, sarcoid, gout, and idiopathic hypercalcemia of infancy. In some instances hypercalcemia is present; in others blood calcium is normal. The differential diagnosis involves a careful examination for the cause of the hypercalcemia when present (as discussed in the preceding section). Hypercalcuria without hypercalcemia is noted with renal tubular disorders such as renal tubular acidosis, in which systemic acidosis may be responsible for increased bone resorption.

Bone disease Discussion of the differential diagnosis of the common types of metabolic bone disease occurs in subsequent chapters. A few points should be stressed in considering the differentiation of hyperparathyroidism from other skeletal disorders. The only commonly occurring disorder in which hypercalcemia is found as well as demineralization and localized areas of bone resorption is malignant disease with osteolytic metastases; patients with severe Paget's disease may develop hypercalcemia during periods of enforced immobilization.

The possibility of underlying hyperparathyroidism should always be considered when solitary bone rarefactions are detected; such a lesion could represent a bone cyst or brown tumor of the bone.

MEDICAL TREATMENT Once the presumptive diagnosis of primary hyperparathyroidism has been made, surgery is the treatment of choice. However, a decision may be made to defer surgery. This is particularly true when mild asymptomatic hypercalcemia is discovered in an elderly patient or when other factors such as cardiovascular or pulmonary disease make the patient a poor operative risk. Too little is known about the natural history of hyperparathyroidism to automatically recommend surgery initially, particularly in older patients, if no signs or symptoms are present that are attributable to hyperparathyroidism. One may elect to follow the patient carefully if hypercalcemia is not severe, e.g., less than 11.5 to 12.0 mg per 100 ml. Alternatively, if the relation of vague constitutional symptoms to hypercalcemia is raised, it may be useful to evaluate the symptomatic response following the lowering of blood calcium. Since blood phosphate is low, administering sodium or potassium phosphate in doses of 1 to 2 g phosphate phosphorus daily may be useful. Phosphate promotes the deposition of calcium into the skeleton. However, complications such as metabolic calcification may develop during phosphate therapy. The occurrence of metastatic calcification appears related to the concentration of serum phosphate; therefore, phosphate should not be used in patients who have impaired renal function.

The alternate, and rather dramatic, indication for medical therapy develops when a patient without previous medical history of disorders related to calcium metabolism presents with severe hypercalcemia. When the etiology is unknown, a curable disease such as primary hyperparathyroidism must be considered. Under the circumstances, it may be lifesaving to rapidly lower blood calcium to safe levels so that diagnostic studies can be performed.

After rehydration has been accomplished, it is now agreed that the most effective mode of therapy is intravenous infusion of sodium chloride, 4 to 5 liters daily, plus administration of potent natriuretic agents such as furosemide. This mode of therapy can be undertaken only if renal function is adequate; strict records of intake and output and avoidance of fluid overload must be observed. Several grams of calcium may be excreted daily, resulting in rapid lowering of blood calcium. The beneficial effects result from the linkage of sodium and calcium transport in the kidney tubule.

Intravenous phosphate is effective in lowering calcium but increases the hazard of widespread metastatic calcification. Mithramycin given as a single intravenous dose of 25 to 50 μg per kg body weight may lower calcium to normal within several days; this approach serves as an alternate therapy if the saline/furosemide regimen cannot be applied.

SURGICAL TREATMENT Parathyroid exploration should be undertaken only by an experienced surgeon with the help of an equally astute pathologist. There are many critical decisions regarding management that can be best made only during the operation. The examination of tissue removed at surgery by frozen section should direct the subsequent course of the operation. The usual procedure, if an abnormal gland is identified and removed, is to search for at least one additional gland. If the second gland is normal in size and normal histologically (frozen section), a single adenoma is most likely. Some surgeons recommend identification of all four glands; others advocate stopping exploration when an enlarged gland and a normal gland are identified.

Hyperplasia involves more difficult diagnostic criteria and questions of surgical management. Once a diagnosis of hyperplasia has been established, it is necessary to identify all the glands. It usually is recommended that three glands be totally removed and that the fourth gland be partially excised; care should be taken to leave a good blood supply for the remaining glands. There are documented cases of five or six glands, as well as unusual locations for adenoma. If no glandular abnormalities are found in the neck, further exploration must be undertaken. When parathyroid carcinoma is encountered, it is important that the tissue be widely excised; great care should be taken to avoid rupture of the capsule to prevent local seeding of the tumor.

Decline in serum calcium invariably occurs within 24 hr after successful surgery; usually blood calcium falls to low normal values for 4 to 5 days until the remaining parathyroid tissue resumes hormone secretion. Severe postoperative hypocalcemia is likely to occur if there has been significant osteitis fibrosa or if there has been injury to the normal parathyroid glands during surgery.

For mild symptomatic hypocalcemia, oral calcium supplementation may suffice; if hypocalcemia is severe, intravenous calcium is necessary. It is usually convenient to prepare a solution of calcium (gluconate or chloride) at a concentration of 1 mg per ml in 5% dextrose/water. The rate and total duration of intravenous calcium therapy are determined by severity of symptoms and the response detected by frequently monitoring blood calcium levels. A rate of infusion of 0.5 to 2 mg per kg per hr or 30 to 100 cc per hr of the 1 mg per ml solution will usually suffice to relieve symptoms. Generally, parenteral therapy in most instances will be required for only a few days. If symptoms and/or need for parenteral calcium continues for more than 4 to 5 days, replacement therapy with vitamin D and/or calcium should be started (as outlined below under Treatment). A sudden rise in blood calcium after several months on vitamin D replacement therapy may indicate restoration of parathyroid function to normal.

Magnesium deficiency may also complicate the postoperative course of parathyroid surgery and represents an additional cause of tetany. A normal concentration of magnesium may be necessary for the biologic effects of parathyroid hormone, and resistance to the action of parathyroid hormone has been demonstrated in magnesium deficiency.

Magnesium deficiency, indicated by hypomagnesemia, should therefore be corrected whenever detected. $MgCl_2$ is sufficiently soluble to be effective by mouth, but preparations of this compound are not widely available. Accordingly, repletion must usually be parenteral. Only a small fraction of total body magnesium is present in extracellular fluid, but total body Mg deficiency is reflected by hypomagnesemia. Since the depressant effect of magnesium on central and peripheral nerve functions is not seen below 4 mEq per liter (normal range 1.5 to 2 mEq per liter), parenteral replacement can be given at a vigorous rate. A dose as great as 2 mEq per kg can be given if severe hypomagnesemia is detected. The magnesium is given either as an intravenous infusion over 8 to 12 hr or in divided doses intramuscularly (magnesium sulfate, USP, is the preparation normally used, available as a 20% solution, 1 g or 8 mEq per ml, or as a more concentrated solution, 50%).

SECONDARY HYPERPARATHYROIDISM

Secondary hyperparathyroidism is a metabolic disorder characterized by excessive production of parathyroid hormone; this disorder is encountered in various disease states in which there is resistance to the metabolic actions of parathyroid hormone. Because of the resistance to the action of the hormone, these disease states are usually characterized by a mild degree of hypocalcemia, at least in the ionized fraction of blood calcium, despite the excessive secretion of parathyroid hormone.

Secondary hyperparathyroidism occurs in patients with some forms of osteomalacia, pseudohypoparathyroidism and chronic renal disease. Correction of the osteomalacia with adequate vitamin D therapy or reversal of renal failure (as with successful renal transplant) should lead to regression of the hyperparathyroidism. This has been documented in patients with a successful renal transplant. In turn, these considerations lead to an important distinction between the character of abnormal growth in secondary hyperparathyroidism (reversible) and primary hyperparathyroidism (presumably irreversible). A variable picture of bone disease may develop in association with hyperparathyroidism in chronic renal failure. (This is discussed in Chap. 352.) Occasionally, in chronic renal failure, severe bone pain, widespread ectopic calcification, and severe pruritis may develop, and the question of subtotal parathyroidectomy may be raised. While this may be necessary, appreciation of the reversibility of the parathyroid hyperplasia has led to a more conservative attitude toward surgical intervention. Subtotal parathyroidectomy may lead to severe postoperative hypoparathyroidism. Medical treatment such as reduction of excessive blood phosphate by dietary phosphate restriction and use of nonabsorbable antacids, and better management of renal failure, may reverse ectopic calcification and eliminate the need for surgery of the parathyroids in favor of eventual renal transplant.

The stimulus responsible for hyperplasia of the parathyroids has not been identified. It seems possible that in all the conditions in which secondary hyperparathyroidism is found, resistance to hormone action accounts for persistent hypocalcemia in spite of increased hormone secretion. Chronic, even though partly compensated, hypocalcemia may be the stimulus that directly causes parathyroid hyperplasia. Specific aspects of the clinical features and approaches encountered in states of secondary hyperparathyroidism in pseudohypoparathyroidism, chronic renal failure, and osteomalacia are reviewed below.

In summary, present knowledge concerning the complex pattern of biosynthesis, secretion, and metabolism of parathyroid hormone, even in normal subjects, must be taken into account in attempting to understand the origins or predict the course of secondary hyperparathyroidism. Attempts to manage hyperparathyroidism by correction of underlying defects seems the most reasonable approach whenever feasible in view of the potential reversibility of this adaptive disorder of the parathyroids.

HYPOPARATHYROIDISM

Hypoparathyroidism is a metabolic abnormality characterized by hypocalcemia and consequent neuromuscular symptoms; the disease results from a deficiency of parathyroid hormone production or end organ resistance to the action of the hormone.

ETIOLOGY Postoperative hypoparathyroidism

The most common cause of hypoparathyroidism is excision of the parathyroids or damage to the glands or their vascular supply during surgery for thyroid disorders, hyperparathyroidism and radical neck dissections for cancer. Postoperative hypoparathyroidism is now much less frequent, not only because of improved awareness of the potential problem during thyroid surgery, but also because of the increased use of medical therapy for treatment of thyrotoxicosis. Although the symptoms of hypoparathyroidism usually develop several days after the operation, there can be a delay of months to years after neck surgery before the diagnosis is made. Although it has been speculated that in these patients the glands may slowly atrophy because of progressive ischemic damage to the glands following surgery, it is possible that signs and symptoms of hypocalcemia were overlooked. A different situation can also take place: transient hypoparathyroidism may occur immediately following thyroid surgery. In this situation it seems likely that the glands are initially injured, but gradually recover, or that a small remnant of remaining parathyroid tissue gradually hypertrophies.

Idiopathic hypoparathyroidism Idiopathic hypoparathyroidism is a relatively rare disease. A total lack of parathyroid function can be detected as (1) an isolated entity, idiopathic hypoparathyroidism; (2) in association with agenesis of the thymus (the Di George syndrome); or (3) in association with a familial disorder in which there may be a deficiency of thyroid, adrenal, and ovarian function, pernicious anemia, and other defects. The Di George syndrome is a rare disorder in which there is congenital absence of the thymus and the parathyroids, organs embryologically derived from the third and fourth branchial pouches. Patients with this syndrome usually die at one to two years of age of severe hypocalcemia, persistent infection, or both. The immune deficiency is of the cellular type. Delayed hypersensitivity reactions are deficient, and allograft rejections are absent. Humoral and circulating antibody mechanisms are intact. These striking features that result from the absence of the thymus make this syndrome quite distinctive.

The familial syndrome of hypoparathyroidism is unusual in several respects. An autoimmune basis for this disease has been suspected. These patients frequently have moniliasis, particularly in the fingernails. Recognition of the associated features is important because of the clinical problems encountered when adrenal failure or anemia develops. Careful periodic evaluation of a given patient or family members with respect to hematopoietic, adrenal, ovarian, and thyroid status is important. Antibodies have been detected to parietal cells, the parathyroids, adrenal cortex, thyroid, and ovary. However, there are poor correlations between the occurrence of the given endocrine deficiency and detection of endocrine organ-specific antibodies. The frequency of expression of the disease or of antibodies does not fit any simple pattern of inheritance. Nonetheless, it is clear that the several endocrine deficiency states may all appear eventually in a given individual or in family members.

Other causes of true hypoparathyroidism Hypoparathyroidism secondary to radiation therapy is very rare but has been reported. The gland presumably atrophies secondary to radiation damage after radioactive iodine (^{131}I) therapy for thyrotoxicosis. An unusual form of hypoparathyroidism is its occurrence in an infant born of a mother with hyperparathyroidism. The high level of the circulating calcium in the mother's blood apparently inhibits the activity or development of the parathyroid glands in the infant. This form of hypoparathyroidism is usually transient.

Pseudohypoparathyroidism Pseudohypoparathyroidism is a rare hereditary disorder characterized by symptoms and signs of hypoparathyroidism in association with distinctive skeletal and developmental defects. The hypoparathyroidism is due to *deficient end organ response* to the endogenous hormone. Pseudohypoparathyroidism is characterized by excessive secretion of parathyroid hormone and hyperplasia of the parathyroids, a response to the resistance to hormone action at the target tissues—kidney and bone.

Many aspects of pseudohypoparathyroidism remain unclarified, including the relation between the skeletal and developmental defects and the hypoparathyroidism. Relatives of patients with pseudohypoparathyroidism often exhibit skeletal and developmental defects without any symptoms or chemical evidence of hypoparathyroidism, so-called "pseudopseudohypoparathyroidism." Details of the pathophysiology of pseudohypoparathyroidism remain uncertain, although studies have suggested that defective stimulation of membrane-bound adenyl cyclase is the biochemical defect responsible for end organ resistance to the hormone. It has been shown that (1) there is an increased concentration of circulating parathyroid hormone in all subjects with pseudohypoparathyroidism (at least, if studied when they are hypocalcemic prior to the institution of vitamin D therapy), (2) there is no evidence for circulating antiparathyroid antibodies in any of these patients, and (3) there is evidence that the hormone made by these patients is biologically active.

Since, by definition, all patients with the complete syndrome are hypocalcemic and hyperphosphatemic, it has generally been believed that both bone and kidney are unresponsive, but certain observations are not consistent with a unitary view concerning pathophysiology. Some patients show an essentially normal phosphaturia following the injection of parathyroid hormone. Some patients show a detectable, even though subnormal, increase in 3′,5′-adenosine monophosphate (cyclic AMP) after administration of parathyroid extract. In one patient with pseudohypoparathyroidism previously treated with vitamin D, the removal of all four parathyroid glands was accomplished by a striking fall in serum calcium, requiring a massive increase in vitamin D to restore serum calcium toward normal. This may mean that at least in some patients, on long-term vitamin D treatment, there is a significant contribution to extracellular fluid calcium from parathyroid hormone-driven bone resorption when sufficient parathyroid hypersecretion has developed, despite osseous resistance to parathyroid action.

Reports have accumulated concerning approximately a dozen patients with hypocalcemia and hyperphosphatemia in whom evidence of osteitis fibrosa has been found by both x-ray and biopsy. This has led to the speculation that the renal end organ defect may be the most severe if not the sole abnormality in some patients. A report has also appeared which carefully documents the restoration of a normal sensitivity to parathyroid hormone after vitamin D therapy in a patient with typical pseudohypoparathyroidism. Subjects with pseudohypoparathyroidism, unlike patients with true hypoparathyroidism, usually do not excrete excessive quantities of calcium in urine when their blood calcium is made normal after vitamin D treatment. This suggests that there is a normal renal end organ response with regard to the action of the hormone to reduce renal calcium clearance.

These varied observations suggest that end organ resistance may be less severe in some patients than in others or that vitamin D treatment alters end organ sensitivity. In addition, it may be true that bone is more responsive to hormone than kidney in certain patients with pseudohypoparathyroidism.

Little can be said at the present time about the pathophysiology of the multiple skeletal and developmental effects in these patients. The genetic transmission of the disorder is compatible with an abnormality in the X chromosome. Since identical short stature, abnormal metacarpals and metatarsals, and other physical features of the disease are found without hypocalcemia or hyperphosphatemia in patients with pseudopseudohypoparathyroidism (who have an apparently normal renal cell adenyl cyclase system), it seems likely that the skeletal and developmental defects are an independently inherited aspect of the illness reflecting X-chromosome deficits rather than a consequence of hypoparathyroidism per se.

In any event, the hereditary aspects of pseudohypoparathyroidism have been well established. Pseudohypoparathyroidism is usually found within kindreds in which some other family members also have pseudohypoparathyroidism or the metabolically normal variant of the disorder, pseudopseudohypoparathyroidism. However, the exact mode of genetic inheritance is still uncertain, and the variable expression of metabolic abnormalities in affected individuals is not understood. Some analyses have suggested that the two linked disorders, pseudopseudohypoparathyroidism and pseudohypoparathyroidism, are transmitted as a sex-linked dominant. The sex incidence is 2:1 affected females versus males. However, the disease is extremely rare, and so the total numbers of patients or of involved sibships is small for purposes of suitable statistical analysis. Furthermore, acceptance of cases as authentic examples of the syndrome on the basis of literature reports is difficult, particularly with respect to the metabolically normal individuals, those with pseudopseudohypoparathyroidism. Certain of the developmental defects such as short stature, short metacarpal or metatarsal bones, and/or even basal ganglion calcification are found in Turner's syndrome, Gardner's syndrome, basal-cell nevus syndrome, and other hereditary disorders that are believed to be genetically distinct.

SIGNS AND SYMPTOMS Most of the symptoms of hypoparathyroidism reflect altered neuromuscular irritability due to the decreased concentration of ionized calcium. The age of onset of symptoms is earlier in pseudohypoparathyroidism than in idiopathic hypoparathyroidism.

Tetany and convulsions represent the most serious complications in hypoparathyroidism. Latent tetany can be elicited by tapping the facial nerve and producing a contraction of the facial muscles (Chvostek's sign), or by application of a tourniquet or blood pressure cuff leading to carpopedal spasm (Trousseau's sign). Increased bone density may occasionally be shown in hypoparathyroidism. However, there may be no detectable skeletal abnormalities; in pseudohypoparathyroidism, as mentioned above, there are reports of osteitis fibrosa.

A complication, perhaps related to the hyperphosphatemia, is the frequent occurrence of *soft-tissue calcification.* In pseudohypoparathyroidism the mineral deposits in ectopic sites may include the development of true bone. True bone formation in ectopic sites is never seen in idiopathic hypoparathyroidism. Amorphous deposits of calcium and phosphate are also found in the basal ganglions. Calcification of the basal ganglions is noted in as many as 50 percent of the patients. Most patients with pseudopseudohypoparathyroidism do not have ectopic calcium deposits.

The multiple skeletal and developmental abnormalities that are found in both pseudohypoparathyroidism and pseudopseudohypoparathyroidism include short stature, round face, short neck, thick, stocky body build, and multiple discrete abnormalities in individual bones of the skeleton. Abnormally short metacarpal and metatarsal bones and sometimes phalanges have been reported. These defects seem to be due to premature closure of the epiphyses. The most classic finding is an *abnormally short fourth and fifth metacarpal and metatarsal.* This defect may be unilateral. Exostoses are frequently reported. Usually only one or two are detected, but occasionally multiple exostoses are found. Radius curvus may be present in some patients.

Multiple abnormalities are detected in tooth formation. The nails may be fragile and skin-dry; moniliasis is commonly found in true hypoparathyroidism but not in pseudohypoparathyroidism. Mental deficiency is rather common in patients with pseudohypoparathyroidism. It seems most probable that this is part of the inherited syndrome. In any event, there is little improvement in mental status even with adequate therapy with calcium and vitamin D. Distinctive impairment in olfaction and taste has also been reported in the majority of patients examined, and in addition, unusual dermatoglyphic abnormalities have been noted.

In pseudohypoparathyroidism there is a much-increased incidence of either frank diabetes or an abnormal glucose tolerance curve and hypothyroidism. Recent studies have indicated that hypothyroidism, at least in some patients, is due to isolated thyrotropin deficiency.

DIAGNOSIS AND DIFFERENTIAL DIAGNOSIS Typically, the diagnosis of hypoparathyroidism is considered in a patient who has symptoms of hypocalcemia and is found to have both hypocalcemia and hyperphosphatemia in the presence of normal renal function. Clinically, the patient's history of physical features may be helpful in suggesting the probable diagnosis. A history of neck surgery with difficulties dating from that time points to postsurgical hypoparathyroidism. Pseudohypoparathyroidism is more likely than true hypoparathyroidism if unusual skeletal and developmental defects are detected or if there is a family history of other sibs with short stature and skeletal abnormalities. However, a definitive diagnosis, particularly for pseudohypoparathyroidism, must be established through application of specific laboratory tests. Two specific tests should be used, namely, the *parathyroid hormone radioimmunoassay* and *measurement of urinary cyclic AMP excretion* following the administration of parathyroid hormone.

Patients with *symptomatic hypocalcemia,* particularly if the history and physical examination suggest chronicity of the hypocalcemia (such as gradual onset of symptoms and evidence of ectopic calcification), would be expected to have secondary hyperparathyroidism if the parathyroid glands are functional. If no parathyroid hormone is detected by radioimmunoassay, notwithstanding the stimulus of marked hypocalcemia, then true hypoparathyroidism is the most likely diagnosis; if elevated concentrations of parathyroid hormone are found, pseudohypoparathyroidism on the basis of end organ resistance is more likely. If high circulating concentrations of hormone are found, the renal end organ resistance to the parathyroid hormone can be demonstrated by measuring the urinary excretion of cyclic AMP in response to the injection of a standard dose of parathyroid hormone. Normal subjects, patients with idiopathic or postsurgical hypoparathyroidism and pseudopseudohypoparathyroidism, exhibit a ten- to twentyfold increase in urinary cyclic AMP secretion. In those with pseudohypoparathyroidism, very little, if any, response is noted.

Hypocalcemia may be encountered not only in hypoparathyroidism but also in malabsorption, osteomalacia secondary to true vitamin D lack or vitamin D resistance, renal failure, hypoproteinemia, pancreatitis, and acute, nutritional deficiency with associated hypomagnesemia. In patients with *malabsorption*, true vitamin D lack, vitamin D resistance, or renal failure, the parathyroid radioimmunoassay has invariably shown an increased concentration of hormone in the plasma. Secondary hyperparathyroidism apparently results from the chronic hypocalcemia that accompanies these diseases. The manifestations of *renal failure*, including phosphate retention, are usually obvious when hypocalcemia is found. Patients with *osteomalacia* usually show a low serum phosphorus, an apparent reflection of the persistence of the action of parathyroid hormone on renal phosphate excretion in spite of the deficiency of the vitamin D that interferes with the effective action of the hormone on bone.

Hypoproteinemia causes a reduction in total serum calcium because of reduced binding protein. Subjects with this abnormality have a normal ionized serum calcium concentration and lack symptoms of hypocalcemia. Correction for the total calcium concentration in patients with hypoproteinemia is based on the known binding of calcium by albumin and globulin. Episodes of *acute pancreatitis* are associated with hypocalcemia, but this is present only during the acute phase of the illness. The explanation for the hypocalcemia in pancreatitis, although much discussed, remains unknown.

There is an increasingly frequent recognition of the syndrome of hypocalcemia in patients with a recent history of a poor nutritional intake and *hypomagnesemia*. In some alcoholics with severe hypomagnesemia, hypocalcemia and refractoriness to exogenous parathyroid hormone are found, including a lack of the normal urinary cyclic AMP response. Parenteral correction of the hypomagnesemia over several days completely restores normal parathyroid responsiveness, including urinary cyclic AMP response. It has also been observed in similar patients that, with an improved dietary intake, serum magnesium rises and the hypocalcemia disappears within a week without specific treatment. Recognition of this syndrome is important in order to avoid unnecessary and expensive diagnostic evaluation for some unusual cause of parathyroid failure in patients with hypomagnesemia.

TREATMENT The principal aim of treatment is to restore calcium toward normal by use of supplementary dietary calcium and vitamin D and thereby relieve symptoms of increased neuromuscular irritability. However, it is not clear whether the other complications of hypoparathyroidism can be as readily controlled despite therapy which appears to be adequate for regulation of blood calcium. It has been noted that lenticular opacities may progress despite therapy.

There are numerous problems in achieving proper regulation of calcium metabolism in patients with hypoparathyroidism. Continued treatment with adequate doses of vitamin D presents several difficulties. Urinary calcium excretion is often excessive in hypoparathyroidism owing to the lack of the normal parathyroid effect to lower urine calcium clearance. This leads to the anomalous result that patients with hypoparathyroidism may develop nephrolithiasis during therapy which maintains blood calcium only at low normal concentration. Excessive urinary calcium excretion is typically not seen in pseudohypoparathyroidism. Vitamin D intoxication may develop without any apparent change in a dosage of vitamin D and calcium that has been optimal for several years. If hypercalcemia occurs, the long duration of action of vitamin D may result in persistence of hypercalcemia for weeks after the vitamin D has been discontinued. Despite these potential complications, most patients with hypoparathyroidism can be adequately regulated; complications can be avoided if the effects of therapy are continually monitored by frequent determinations of urinary as well as blood calcium concentration.

A practical approach to the chronic treatment of hypoparathyroidism at present involves initial use of less expensive agents with careful attention to complications and the use of newer, more expensive analogues of vitamin D only if more conventional measures prove inadequate for various reasons. Vitamin D is given, usually as ergocalciferol (vitamin D_2), in a dose of 50,000 to 100,000 units per day; several grams of additional elemental calcium as citrate, lactate, or gluconate are usually provided (calcium lactate contains 13 percent calcium). Appropriate adjustments in dosage are made to achieve a blood calcium of 8.5 to 9.0 mg per 100 ml; it is important to appreciate that often weeks are required before the full effects of an increased dose of vitamin D are manifest. Patients should be seen at frequent intervals, particularly when dose schedules are initially established or readjusted; blood and urine calcium estimations provide the early clues to excessive or inadequate dosage of vitamin D.

Crystalline dihydrotachysterol (DHT) is theoretically preferable in view of preferential rates of formation of the 25-hydroxyl intermediate or the possibility that DHT, because of the steric configuration of the A ring, acts directly on intestinal transport (as discussed in the preceding section on vitamin D). However, the greater cost of DHT at the present time makes routine use more expensive. If a patient is unusually resistant to vitamin D and therefore difficult to maintain symptom-free, if the therapeutic margin between hypocalcemia and hypercalcuria in a given patient is excessively narrow, or if one or more episodes of vitamin D intoxication have occurred, dihydrotachysterol in doses of 1.0 to 1.5 mg per day may be substituted for vitamin D.

Interesting effects of magnesium administration have been noted during evaluation and management of patients with hypoparathyroidism. It has been reported that in several patients in whom vitamin D resistance of unusual degree was observed, hypomagnesemia was discovered. Supplemental magnesium therapy led to much greater responsiveness to a given dose of vitamin D, and such patients maintained a more normal blood calcium concentration. The explanation for the beneficial effect of magnesium is not understood, but hypomagnesemia should be searched for in patients who are difficult to control.

In general, it can be concluded that satisfactory maintenance of mineral ion deficits can be achieved in hypoparathyroid subjects with supplemental calcium plus vitamin D or vitamin D analogues. However, vitamin D is not a perfect substitute for parathyroid hormone, particularly in view of different effects on renal calcium conservation and the much higher requirement for vitamin D in parathyroid deficiency. Hence all patients with hypoparathyroidism, particularly idiopathic or postsurgical hypoparathyroidism, must be reexamined at appropriate intervals of 6 months to 1 year to ensure adequate treatment schedules and particularly to detect complications, hypercalcuria, or onset of more severe vitamin D intoxication.

REFERENCES

BLIZZARD RM et al: The incidence of parathyroid and other antibodies in the area of patients with idiopathic hypoparathyroidism. Clin Exp Immunol 1:119, 1966

BURNETT CH et al: Hypercalcemia without hypercalcuria or hypophosphatemia. Calcinosis and renal insufficiency: A syndrome following prolonged ingestion of milk and alkali. N Engl J Med 240:787, 1949

CHASE LR et al: Metabolic abnormality in pseudohypoparathyroidism: Defective renal excretion of cyclic 3′5′-AMP in response to parathyroid hormone. J Clin Invest 47:18a, 1968

HARRISON HE et al: Comparison between crystalline dihydrotachysterol and calciferol in patients requiring pharmacologic vitamin D therapy. N Engl J Med 276:894, 1967

Keating Memorial Symposium—Hyperparathyroidism, 1970, eds SF Haines, CD Arnaud. Am J Med 50:557, 1971

KRANE SM: Selected features of the clinical course of hypoparathyroidism. JAMA 178:472, 1961

——— et al: The effect of thyroid disease on calcium metabolism in man. J Clin Invest 35:874, 1956

PARSONS JA, POTTS JT JR: Physiology and chemistry of parathyroid hormone, in *Clinics in Endocrinology and Metabolism*, ed I MacIntyre, London: Saunders, 1:33, 1972

POTTS JT JR: Pseudohypoparathyroidism, in *The Metabolic Basis of Inherited Disease*, 3d ed., eds J Stanbury et al, New York: McGraw-Hill, 1972, p. 1305

———, DEFTOS LJ: Parathyroid hormone, thyrocalcitonin, vitamin D, and bone and bone mineral metabolism, in *Duncan's Diseases of Metabolism*, 7th ed., eds PK Bondy, LE Rosenberg, Philadelphia: Saunders (in press)

POWELL D et al: Non-parathyroid humoral hypercalcemia in patients with neoplastic disease. N Engl J Med 289:176, 1973

PRIEN EL et al: Secondary hyperparathyroidism, in *The Handbook of Physiology* Sect. 7: Endocrinology (in press)

STEINER AC et al: Study of a kindred with pheochromocytoma, medullary thyroid carcinoma, hypoparathyroidism and Cushing's disease: Multiple endocrine neoplasma, type 2. Medicine 47:371, 1968

WERMER P: Endocrine adenomatosis and peptide ulcer in a large kindred: Inherited multiple tumors and mosaic pleiopropism in man. Am J Pathol 35:205, 1963

ZOLLINGER RM, ELLISON EH: Primary peptide ulcerations of the jejunum associated with islet cell tumors of the pancreas. Ann Surg 142:709, 1955

351 MEDULLARY CARCINOMA OF THE THYROID

JOHN T. POTTS, JR.

Medullary carcinoma, an unusual thyroid malignancy composing 5 to 10 percent of all thyroid tumors, is recognized as a distinct type of tumor involving neoplasia of the parafollicular cells normally concerned with calcitonin synthesis. Medullary carcinoma is, in fact, the first disease state in which an abnormality of calcitonin secretion has been described. Medullary carcinoma has received much attention because of appreciation of its role in calcitonin overproduction, the association of the tumor with other endocrine tumors, and the familial as well as the sporadic incidence of the disease. Since medullary carcinoma does not involve the follicular cells of the thyroid which synthesize thyroxine, medical management such as suppressive therapy with exogenous thyroid hormone or radioiodine is of no avail. In addition, the parafollicular cells present in this form of thyroid tumor have also been shown to secrete a variety of other bioactive substances which may contribute additional metabolic features to the disease.

EMBRYOLOGY AND HISTOLOGY The parafollicular cells, the stem cells of medullary thyroid carcinoma, are of different embryologic origin than the other thyroid elements (see Chap. 349). In medullary thyroid carcinoma, these parafollicular, calcitonin-secreting cells undergo malignant transformation and produce an excess of calcitonin. Parafollicular cells are very difficult to identify in the normal human thyroid. The cells are epithelial in appearance and are located in the stroma between the thyroid follicles. Secretory granules, presumably containing calcitonin, have been identified.

The typical medullary carcinoma of the thyroid is a firm, rounded tumor up to 8 cm in diameter, lying within the substance of the thyroid gland. It is usually well demarcated from adjacent normal thyroid tissue. On microscopic examination, the tumor is seen to be made up of sheets and nests of granular cells with eosinophilic-staining properties, and a second type of cell, more spindle-shaped. One of the most characteristic features of medullary thyroid carcinoma is the dense amyloid stroma that separates the cells.

The amyloid is usually, but not invariably, a conspicuous feature of the tumor; when detected, however, the presence of amyloid in a thyroid tumor is of value to the pathologist in establishing the diagnosis.

CLINICAL FEATURES The growth of medullary thyroid carcinoma is usually slow and indolent. The manifestations of the tumor itself are therefore usually local, although distant metastases occur and the disease can be rapidly fatal. This tumor can occur either sporadically or with a familial incidence (it has been estimated that as many as 20 percent of reported cases are familial). In the sporadic form, the tumor usually presents in middle or late life and is often unilateral in its location. In the familial form, the tumor usually becomes manifest within the first three decades of life and is usually multicentric. The familial form of the disease is thought to be inherited as a dominant autosomal trait (19 cases were reported in one kindred alone), and it is now well documented that this familial form of medullary thyroid carcinoma is part of a discrete multiple endocrine adenomatosis syndrome (MEA 2). The two most common associated findings are pheochromocytomas, usually bilateral in distribution, and hyperparathyroidism, usually due to parathyroid hyperplasia. The association between a peculiar type of thyroid carcinoma, now recognized as medullary carcinoma, and bilateral pheochromocytomas was described earlier and became known as *Sipple's syndrome.*

In the *familial form of the disease*, in addition to the bilateral pheochromocytomas, there are other neuroectodermal features leading to a striking and distinctive facial appearance. These features include small polypoid neuromas of the eyelids, lips, and tongue, usually with profuse thickening of the lips. The proliferation of nerves, which causes these neuromas, can also occur throughout the intestine and sometimes may involve the bronchial tree and the bladder. Often a Marfanoid habitus is seen. Hypocalcemia is not found in the majority of patients, even with widespread disease, nor are definite skeletal abnormalities reported.

The high incidence of *hyperparathyroidism* in patients or in family members with the familial form of medullary thyroid carcinoma probably represents an independent expression of the underlying genetic mechanism that is responsible for the syndrome. Although both adenomas and hyperplasia have been reported, parathyroid hyperplasia of the chief-cell type seems more common. It had been speculated that the hyperparathyroidism seen in these patients is a compensatory response to the high levels of calcitonin. However, in many patients parathyroid hormone levels were found to be normal despite high levels of calcitonin. Support for an independent genetic mechanism for the hyperparathyroidism rather than a reactive disorder of the parathyroids also comes from the observation that some relatives of patients with medullary thyroid carcinoma have high circulating levels of parathyroid hormone prior to development of medullary carcinoma or increased secretion of calcitonin.

Another associated endocrinologic disturbance in patients with medullary carcinoma of the thyroid is the occurrence of *Cushing's disease*; 17 cases were reported by 1971. In such patients, the Cushing's disease has been shown to be due to the ectopic production by the medullary thyroid carcinoma of adrenocorticotrophic hormone. When the thyroid carcinoma can be completely removed, the Cushing's syndrome remits.

Diarrhea is a common clinical manifestation of medullary thyroid carcinoma. It has been stated that the diarrhea is due, in part, to excessive amounts of prostaglandin secreted by these tumors. However, evidence for increased prostaglandin production could not be found in some patients with diarrhea. Another contributing mechanism to the diarrhea may be the high incidence of ganglioneuromatosis and diverticulosis of the intestinal tract which is seen in these patients.

DIAGNOSIS The presence of medullary thyroid carcinoma, even in occult form, should be carefully searched for in the relatives of patients who have the disease, particularly in view of the importance of early diagnosis. Medullary carcinoma should also be suspected in patients who have a thyroid tumor with histology that is atypical. The possibility of ACTH-producing medullary thyroid carcinoma should be considered in patients with otherwise unexplained Cushing's syndrome where ectopic ACTH production is suspected. Since most patients with medullary thyroid carcinoma do not have hypocalcemia, the finding of a normal blood calcium does not argue against the diagnosis.

It is now established that the most reliable method for establishing the diagnosis of medullary thyroid carcinoma is the immunoassay for calcitonin. Most patients with medullary thyroid carcinoma have increased fasting, basal concentrations of plasma calcitonin. In fact, plasma calcitonin concentration may be increased before there is any clinical evidence of the presence of the tumor. Therefore, especially in familial cases, the presence of high levels of calcitonin may be a very early clue to the presence of this malignancy. In one extensively studied kindred, 11 patients without clinical evidence of disease were detected by prospective essays. However, some patients with this tumor may have levels of plasma calcitonin that are not clearly diagnostic. In every such patient tested, stimulation of calcitonin secretion by provocative testing, principally calcium infusion, led to clearly abnormal hormone concentrations, to confirm the presence of the disease. The secretion of calcitonin by these malignant parafollicular cells seems to be responsive to the same stimuli that influence secretion of calcitonin by normal parafollicular cells. Not only does hypercalcemia induced by calcium infusion cause a stimulation of calcitonin secretion by these tumors, but hypocalcemia induced by infusions of ethylenediaminetetraacetic acid, which suppresses the secretion of calcitonin by normal parafollicular cells, leads to suppression of secretion of calcitonin by the tumors as well. Provocative tests with agents such as glucagon and pentagastrin, known to stimulate calcitonin release in other species are less reliable than a test with calcium infusion. All family members from suspected kindreds should be examined and given appropriate urine and blood tests for the presence of pheochromocytoma, adrenal cortical overactivity, and hyperparathyroidism.

Although several other bioactive substances have been identified (prostaglandins, serotonin, and histaminase) as secretory products of medullary carcinoma of the thyroid, the detection of these substances has not been reported with sufficient consistency to recommend their measurement in searching for disease in family members, although histaminase measurements may help to identify the presence of metastatic disease.

TREATMENT The only effective treatment for patients with medullary thyroid carcinoma is surgical removal of the tumor. In advanced cases, surgery can be only palliative and directed at the symptoms, because of local obstruction by the tumor of large veins or of the trachea. However, with growing awareness of the familial nature of the disease and with the introduction of the immunoassay for calcitonin, the disease can be detected very early in some individuals from affected kindreds; consequently, surgery in these cases may be curative.

Because of the multifocal distribution of the disease, total thyroidectomy should be undertaken. Wide excision of lymph nodes is recommended, but radical neck dissection does not seem to be indicated. If lymph nodes are positive, mediastinal lymph node exploration is also recommended. Surgical management is influenced by the presence of other associated endocrinopathies. For example, when pheochromocytomas are present, it may be expeditious to first perform adrenalectomy, which should be bilateral. There is no substantial experience with radiotherapy or chemotherapy in the treatment of this disease.

PROGNOSIS It is difficult to assess prognosis, particularly in light of the changing pattern of recognition leading to earlier diagnosis. Earlier reports suggested, despite the slow growth of tumor, a poor 5- and 10-year overall survival (less than 50 percent), but many of these patients had known lymph node metastases at the first exploration.

REFERENCES

DEFTOS LJ et al: Immunoassay for human calcitonin: II. Clinical studies. Metabolism 20:1129, 1971

—— et al: Suppression and stimulation of calcitonin secretion in medullary thyroid carcinoma. Metabolism 20:428, 1971

MELVIN KEW et al: Studies in familial (medullary) thyroid carcinoma. Recent Prog Horm Res 28:399, 1972

SIZEMORE GW et al: Relations of calcitonin and gastrin in the Zollinger-Ellison syndrome and medullary carcinoma of the thyroid. New Engl J Med 288:641, 1973

TASHJIAN AH et al: Immunoassay of human calcitonin in normal and diseased states. N Engl J Med 283:890, 1970

WILLIAMS ED: Histogenesis of medullary carcinoma of the thyroid. J Clin Pathol 19:114, 1966

352
METABOLIC BONE DISEASE

STEPHEN M. KRANE

OSTEOPOROSIS

GENERAL CONSIDERATIONS Osteoporosis is the term used to describe a group of diseases of diverse etiology which are characterized by a reduction in the mass of bone per unit volume to a level below that required for adequate mechanical support function. The reduction in mass is not accompanied by a significant reduction in the ratio of the mineral to the organic phase, nor by any reproducible abnormality in the structure of either the mineral or the organic matrix. Histologically, osteoporosis is characterized by a decrease in the number and size of the trabeculae of cancellous bone with normal width of the osteoid seams. Osteoporosis is the commonest of the metabolic bone diseases, disorders in which all the skeleton is involved, presumably as a result of systemic factors acting on the skeleton, and is an important cause of morbidity in elderly subjects.

The remodeling of bone (its formation and resorption) is a continuous process throughout life. Any combination of changes in the rates of formation and resorption which results in bone resorption exceeding bone formation could therefore cause a decrease in bone mass. In osteoporosis the bone mass *is* decreased, indicating that the rate of bone resorption must exceed that of bone formation. In most studies formation rate is normal in osteoporosis, although low rates are sometimes found. Current evidence suggests that in normal individuals for many years after closure of the epiphyses and after longitudinal growth has ceased, skeletal mass remains constant and the rates of bone formation and resorption are relatively low and approximately equal. After the age of forty to fifty skeletal mass begins to decline, at a faster rate in women than in men, and at a different rate in different parts of the skeleton. For example, the rate of loss is greater in the metacarpals, in the femoral neck, and in the vertebral bodies than in the midshaft of the femur, the tibia, and the skull. Over the next three or four decades the total loss in skeletal mass may be 30 to 50 percent of that at age thirty or forty. Evidence obtained from kinetic studies, using radioactive isotopes of calcium and strontium and from quantitative microradiography indicates that in most older subjects the resorption rate is high, whereas the bone formation rate remains at a level similar to that of younger adults. As discussed earlier, radiocalcium kinetics indicate that as much as 400 to 500 mg calcium may enter and leave the normal adult skeleton daily. At some critical point if the difference between formation and resorption rates is maintained, loss of bone substance may become so marked that the bone can no longer resist the mechanical forces to which it is subjected, and fracture results. Osteoporosis would now be evident as a clinical problem, although the level of reduction in bone mass sufficient to result in fractures after minimal trauma is variable. The strength of the vertebral body may depend upon additional factors such as adequacy of ligamentous support and the age-related changes in the intervertebral disks.

In the process of remodeling of lamellar bone in adults, most of the net resorption occurs at the corticoendosteal surface. The abnormal remodeling in osteoporosis follows the same pattern; most of the bone loss occurs at the endosteal surface, resulting in enlargement of the medullary cavity and thinning of the cortex. Since bone formation at the periosteum continues at a very slow rate, the diameter of the bone does not decrease, and the periosteal surface retains its smooth configuration. In addition, the cancellous bone also undergoes progressive resorption, with some trabeculae being resorbed at rates faster than others, particularly those vertebral trabeculae with horizontal orientation.

It is not clear what is the cause of this age-associated decrease in bone mass and increase in bone resorption or the accelerated loss in that form of osteoporosis occurring particularly in older women after the menopause. The decrease in mass is similar in a number of different populations throughout the world. Although blacks in the

United States have a lower incidence of clinically significant osteoporosis than do whites, they also have a larger initial skeletal mass, and adequate bone could remain even in the presence of age-associated losses. Estrogens often used to treat osteoporosis tend to inhibit bone resorption and decrease the hypercalcemia of hyperparathyroidism. However, there is no direct evidence of increased parathyroid hormone secretion with increasing age. Epidemiologic surveys have shown that there is no relation between the degree of bone loss and age of onset or type of menopause. There is also no difference in the calcium intake of osteoporotic compared with control subjects of similar age and sex. Osteoporotic subjects tend to have lower body weight and muscle mass than do controls, but the significance of these findings is uncertain. No consistent changes in adrenocortical function have been documented in osteoporotics, although there are suggestions that subtle alterations in pituitary, adrenal, and gonadal functions may play a role in the production of osteoporosis. In patients with primary hypogonadism due to gonadal dysgenesis or pituitary failure, osteoporosis is frequently noted radiologically. This has been attributed to the failure to attain full adult skeletal mass rather than to an increased rate of bone loss associated with age.

Another factor which some have implicated in bone loss is the possibility that excessive acid intake, particularly in the form of high-protein diets, results in "dissolution" of bone in an attempt to buffer the extra acid. It has also been observed that prolonged use of heparin as an anticoagulant is associated with osteoporosis and that heparin potentiates bone resorption in vitro. Patients with osteoporosis have increased numbers of mast cells, presumably capable of producing heparin, in their bone marrow. Circumscribed and diffuse areas of osteoporosis are also seen in patients with systemic mastocytosis.

As mentioned earlier, the remodeling of bone is physiologically responsive to mechanical forces of many types. The early response to immobilization in the normal skeleton is an increase in bone resorption while bone formation remains normal or is decreased; later there is a compensatory increase in bone formation. In osteoporosis, immobilization tends to aggravate the defect by further increasing the gap between formation and resorption. It is therefore possible that a sedentary life in an individual with poor musculature would tend to reduce mechanical forces exerted on the skeleton and to increase the tendency to bone loss.

CLASSIFICATION OF OSTEOPOROSIS In only a few forms of osteoporosis is the cause certain, such as in that associated with Cushing's syndrome, both endogenous and exogenous. In other cases, the occurrence of osteoporosis together with other disorders is a frequent association, although it is not clear how these other disorders are related to the pathogenesis of the osteoporosis. In the majority of cases of osteoporosis the etiology is not apparent. While most of these occur in older women past the menopause, it is not certain how the osteoporosis is related to the postmenopausal state, although the terms *senile* or *postmenopausal osteoporosis* are frequently used. When osteoporosis occurs in younger individuals, it is usually termed *idiopathic osteoporosis*. However, most of these disorders should be considered idiopathic since details of their pathogenesis are not known. A suggested classification is provided in Table 352-1.

GENERAL CLINICAL FEATURES OF OSTEOPOROSIS Although osteoporosis is a generalized disorder of the skeleton, its major clinical manifestations involve the axial skeleton. Fractures of long bones are also somewhat more frequent in osteoporotic subjects than in others of similar age without osteoporosis and are most common in the hip, humerus, and wrists. The most frequent symptoms are pain in the back and deformity of the spine. Pain usually results from collapse of the vertebral bodies, especially in the lower dorsal and upper lumbar regions, and typically is acute in onset after radiating anteriorly around the flank into various portions of the abdomen, depending upon the location of the fracture. Such episodes frequently occur after sudden bending, lifting, or jumping movements which may seem to have been trivial; on some occasions they cannot be related to trauma. The pain may be increased even with slight movements such as turning in bed or by the Valsalva maneuver. Rest in bed in one position may relieve the pain temporarily, but it then may recur in spasms of variable length. Radiation of pain down one leg is uncommon, and symptoms or signs of spinal cord compression are very rare. The acute episodes of pain

TABLE 352-1
Classification of osteoporosis

I Common forms of osteoporosis of unknown cause unassociated with other disease
- *A* Idiopathic osteoporosis (juvenile and adult)
- *B* Postmenopausal osteoporosis
- *C* Senile osteoporosis

II Disorders or conditions in which osteoporosis is a common feature or pathogenesis partially understood
- *A* Hypogonadism
- *B* Hyperadrenocorticism
- *C* Thyrotoxicosis
- *D* Malabsorption
- *E* Scurvy
- *F* Calcium deficiency
- *G* Immobilization
- *H* Chronic heparin administration
- *I* Systemic mastocytosis
- *J* Adult hypophosphatasia
- *K* Associated with other metabolic bone diseases

III Osteoporosis as a feature of heritable disorders of connective tissue
- *A* Osteogenesis imperfecta
- *B* Homocystinuria due to cystathionine synthase deficiency

IV Disorders in which osteoporosis is associated but pathogenesis not understood
- *A* Rheumatoid arthritis
- *B* Malnutrition
- *C* Alcoholism
- *D* Epilepsy
- *E* Diabetes
- *F* Chronic obstructive pulmonary disease

may also be accompanied by abdominal distention and ileus, thought to be due to retroperitoneal hemorrhage, but the use of narcotics at this stage also contributes to the ileus. Loss of appetite and apparent muscular weakness probably due to fear of reproducing pain may also be present. Episodes of pain usually subside after several days to a week, and by 4 to 6 weeks patients may be fully ambulatory and able to resume their normal activities. Although the acute pain may be minimal, many patients continue to have nagging, deep, dull, uncomfortable sensations localized to the area of fracture brought about by straining or sudden changes in position. They may be unable to sit up in bed and have to arise by rolling over on their sides and then propping themselves up. Most patients have disappearance or marked diminution of pain between episodes of vertebral body collapse. Others never have acute episodes but complain of varying degrees of backache often made worse by standing or moving suddenly. Tenderness over involved areas of the spinous processes or rib cage is commonly noted. The collapse fractures of the vertebral bodies are usually anterior, producing a wedge-shaped deformity and contributing to loss in height. This is particularly common in the upper dorsal region where collapse may be unassociated with pain but result in a dorsal kyphosis and exaggerated cervical lordosis described as a "dowager's" or "widow's" hump. Postural slumping with increase of existing curves also contributes to the loss of height. Generalized skeletal pain is uncommon, and between fractures most patients are free even of pain localized to the spine. Although recurrent episodes of collapse-fractures of vertebral bodies, increasing spine deformity, and loss of height are common in osteoporosis, the course of the disorder in any one subject is not predictable, and there may be intervals of several years between fractures.

RADIOLOGIC FEATURES OF OSTEOPOROSIS Prior to fracture and collapse the osteoporotic vertebral body shows a decrease in mineral density, an increase in prominence of vertical striations due to a relatively greater loss of the horizontally oriented trabeculae, and prominence of the endplates. The bodies may become increasingly biconcave because of weakening of the subchondral plates and expansion of the intervertebral disks, resulting in the so-called "codfish" vertebras. When collapse occurs, most frequently in lower dorsal and upper lumbar spine, it usually produces a decrease in the anterior height of the vertebral body and irregularity in the anterior cortex. Older compression fractures may show reactive changes and osteophytes about the anterior margins. Although the cortices of long bones may be thin because of excessive endosteal resorption, the outer margins are sharp in contrast to the typical effects of the subperiosteal resorption of hyperparathyroidism. Pseudofractures or Looser's zones are not present in osteoporosis without osteomalacia.

LABORATORY FINDINGS The concentrations of calcium and inorganic phosphorus in the blood are usually normal in patients with osteoporosis; slight hyperphosphatemia is present in women who are past the menopause. The alkaline phosphatase in uncomplicated instances is normal, although slight increases may be seen after fractures. Only about 20 percent of postmenopausal women with osteoporosis have significant hypercalcuria. Urinary excretion of peptides containing hydroxyproline, an index of bone resorption, is usually normal or slightly increased.

DIFFERENTIAL DIAGNOSIS Since decrease in skeletal mass is an age-associated finding, it is particularly difficult to evaluate asymptomatic decreased bone density observed radiologically in older women, especially when unaccompanied by marked increase in biconcavity of vertebral bodies or fractures. In the presence of bone pain with or without fracture or deformity, it is important to establish the presence or absence of known causes of osteoporosis as listed in Table 352-1 and to be certain that osteoporosis in the broad sense is the correct diagnosis. Malignancies of various types, particularly *multiple myeloma*, *lymphoma*, *leukemia*, and *carcinomatosis*, may result in diffuse loss of bone, especially the trabecular bone of the vertebral column, even in the absence of hypercalcemia. The absence of anemia, elevated erythrocyte sedimentation rate, abnormal electrophoretic patterns of serum proteins, and Bence Jones proteinuria is helpful in eliminating the possibility of multiple myeloma. However, bone marrow aspiration is an important procedure in cases of severe osteoporosis.

Radiologic osteoporosis is commonly present in patients with *hyperparathyroidism* who may not have specific evidence of osteitis fibrosa (discrete lytic lesions of varying size and subperiosteal resorption) or elevation of serum alkaline phosphatase. Although hyperparathyroidism could accelerate bone loss in the pattern of osteoporosis and contribute to it, it is not clear that excessive secretion of parathyroid hormone is the sole cause of the bone disease, even in these cases, rather than an associated finding. Repeated determinations of serum calcium and phosphorus are therefore necessary.

Osteomalacia may mimic osteoporosis or be associated with it, yet specific radiologic signs of osteomalacia may not always be present. Although the presence of abnormalities such as hypophosphatemia would suggest the possibility of osteomalacia, these too may be absent in some cases of osteomalacia, and bone biopsy may be essential for diagnosis, as discussed below. Since osteomalacia of various causes is more responsive to specific therapy than the usual case of osteoporosis, such diagnostic procedures are often warranted and provide, in addition, adequate specimens for examination for the presence of malignant cells.

In an occasional patient with *Paget's disease* the radiologic features may be almost purely lytic and be confused with osteoporosis. However, high alkaline phosphatase levels and moderately or markedly increased urinary excretion of hydroxyproline-containing peptides would be clues to the presence of Paget's disease. Scanning procedures with bone-seeking isotopes would not be helpful in differential diagnosis if fractures are present, because in any disease fractures demonstrate preferential uptake of isotope. However, in the absence of fracture, "hot spots" would suggest presence of tumor or early Paget's disease.

IDIOPATHIC OSTEOPOROSIS Most of the comments about osteoporosis in the preceding sections are particularly pertinent to elderly patients, especially women with bone loss sufficient to produce significant symptoms. Although its ultimate cause is unknown, this type of osteoporosis is often termed *senile* or *postmenopausal. Idiopathic osteoporosis* is the term used to describe the disorder in younger men or in premenopausal women in whom no other etiologic factor is detected. It is likely that these patients will eventually be shown to have a number of different disorders with superficial resemblances. In some women the onset and deterioration of their bone disease appear to be related to pregnancy, whereas in others no adverse effect of pregnancy is observed. Some patients tend to have low levels of serum alkaline phosphatase but not low enough to fit into the group of patients with so-called hypophosphatasia. Estrogens are ineffective in therapy. Losses of calcium and phosphorus are probably excessive, and it is unwise to permit women to breast-feed their infants since additional calcium losses via lactation are appreciable. It is possible that some patients have a disorder similar to the late-onset forms of osteogenesis imperfecta, although such features as family history, blue scleras, and deafness are lacking. The course of this disorder is variable, and although recurrent episodes of fractures are characteristic, progressive deterioration does not occur in all patients, and in some the clinical problem is rather benign.

GLUCOCORTICOID EXCESS The presence of glucocorticoid excess has not been established in osteoporosis of the idiopathic, senile, or postmenopausal variety. However, osteoporosis commonly accompanies Cushing's syndrome, both endogenous and exogenous, and in some instances is rapidly progressive. This is probably accounted for by the low rate of bone formation in glucocorticoid excess while the rate of bone resorption is increased. Glucocorticoids depress collagen synthesis in organs other than bone, as evidenced by delayed wound healing, thinning of the dermis, characteristic striae, and tendency to blue scleras. In some disorders in which glucocorticoids in pharmacologic doses are administered, such as rheumatoid arthritis, a tendency to thin skin and osteoporosis is initially present, and the skeletal effects of the glucocorticoids may become particularly apparent. Once osteoporosis develops in Cushing's syndrome in adults, the abnormal appearance of the vertebras may persist indefinitely following alleviation of the glucocorticoid excess. In children, however, cure of the Cushing's syndrome may result in striking improvement in the appearance of the spine due to new endochondral bone formation which can surround the less dense, older osteoporotic bone. This does not occur in adults since endochondral bone formation has ceased. Usually withdrawal of glucocorticoids is the only way to halt progression of the osteoporosis. Anabolic steroids have not been proved to be effective in this regard. In Cushing's syndrome, spontaneous, symptomless fractures may occur in bones such as ribs and pubic and ischial rami even in the absence of marked osteoporosis of the spine. These fractures often heal partially with an exuberant calcified callus surrounding a radiolucent zone of nonunion, which superficially resembles the pseudofractures of osteomalacia. If they appear in the thorax superimposed upon the lungs, they may be confused with nodules suggesting primary or metastatic tumor.

GONADAL DEFICIENCY Estrogen lack is present in the postmenopausal woman with osteoporosis, and the administration of estrogen to such an individual reduces the negative calcium balance and decreases urinary hydroxyproline excretion as is consistent with a decrease in bone resorption. However it does not necessarily follow that estrogen deficiency per se is the cause of the osteoporosis. In patients of either sex castrated at an early age, the adult skeleton is smaller to begin with, and therefore age-related losses are more significant.

THYROTOXICOSIS In many patients with hyperthyroidism, there is excessive bone resorption, occasionally marked in degree and far exceeding that in the usual patient with osteoporosis, associated with increased excretion of calcium and phosphorus in urine and feces. The excessive bone resorption is usually accompanied by a compensatory increase in bone formation. If the hyperthyroidism is of short duration, skeletal losses are inconsequential. However in patients with chronic hyperthyroidism, especially in women after the menopause, this accelerated bone loss becomes clinically significant, and it is important to eliminate hyperthyroidism as a contributing cause of osteoporosis. Although typical osteitis fibrosa (resorption lacunas containing osteoclasts and a fibrous stroma) may be seen on biopsy, even in these cases the skeletal lesions have the appearance of osteoporosis when examined radiologically.

ACROMEGALY Hypercalcuria and overall net negative calcium balance occur in acromegaly, and occasionally osteoporosis is an associated finding. The panhypopituitarism secondary to a pituitary adenoma and gonadal insufficiency may be factors in production of the osteoporosis. In adult animals growth hormone decreases endosteal resorption and stimulates bone formation, and it is therefore unlikely that excessive secretion of growth hormone would in itself produce osteoporosis.

CALCIUM DEFICIENCY AND MALABSORPTION Although calcium deficiency may be a factor in some instances of osteoporosis, it cannot be the sole or major cause in idiopathic, senile, or postmenopausal osteoporosis. Osteoporosis is an associated finding in a significant number of cases of steatorrhea, prolonged obstructive jaundice, and lactose intolerance, and in patients following gastrectomy. In other patients there are suggestions of a specific defect in calcium absorption or a failure to adapt adequately to a low-calcium diet either by increasing the percentage of dietary calcium absorbed or by decreasing urinary calcium excretion. Presumably adequate vitamin D is available in these instances to prevent osteomalacia.

HERITABLE DISORDERS OF CONNECTIVE TISSUE In the strict sense, the bone disease of osteogenesis imperfecta is osteoporosis. *Osteogenesis imperfecta* is a disorder(s) of unknown mechanism, of variable degree of severity, transmitted as an autosomal dominant, and associated with blue scleras and, later, deafness. Although the disease may be apparent *in utero* and in infancy, other cases are not detected until childhood; it is possible that some cases of idiopathic osteoporosis represent forms of osteogenesis imperfecta. Osteoporosis is also seen in all patients with *homocystinuria* due to cystathionine synthase deficiency, transmitted as an autosomal recessive. Other characteristics of this disorder should suggest its presence, such as ectopia lentis, various deformities of the extremities, mental retardation, decreased pigmentation of hair and skin, and thromboembolism. The diagnosis is established by the finding of homocystine in urinary chromatograms. The defect may be due to the effect of homocysteine or other metabolites in interfering with the cross-linking of collagen.

THERAPY Before considering the use and efficacy of various modes of treatment advocated for osteoporosis, it should be emphasized that one is dealing with a group of disorders rather than a single entity. Even in patients considered to fall within the same category, e.g., those with idiopathic osteoporosis, the etiologies may be different. In addition, it is difficult to predict the course and the rate of progression of the disease in any one patient, especially when seen initially because of pain and collapse-fracture. Many patients in the idiopathic, senile, and postmenopausal groups have a few episodes of vertebral body collapse with symptom-free intervals of months or years, lose some height consistent with the extent of collapse, but then go for many years without symptoms or further loss in height. Furthermore the acute pain associated with vertebral body fracture tends to subside in a matter of weeks, and *any* treatment administered at that time might be considered efficacious. Even the use of high doses of glucocorticoids has not been shown to produce osteoporosis consistently in patients with normal skeletons, and even after fractures with glucocorticoid-induced osteoporosis, there is no proof that the osteoporosis will steadily worsen. It is also evident in view of the number of different therapeutic programs available for all forms of osteoporosis that therapy is far from ideal, despite claims to the contrary.

General measures Patients who present with acute pain secondary to fracture of vertebral bodies will frequently require hospitalization with rest in bed in any position of maximum comfort, local heat, adequate analgesics, and avoidance of constipation. Use of traction or plaster jacket splints is not indicated. As soon as pain permits, it is prudent to have the patient attempt to move out of bed, slowly at first, perhaps with support of a walker or crutches. It is best not to have the patient become too fatigued when starting ambulation. Braces of various types are commonly employed, but most patients tolerate them poorly, and it has not been proved that they are efficacious in preventing progression of spinal deformity. If a well-made corset provides sensation of support and comfort, wearing it is worthwhile. Supervised exercises to correct postural deformity and increase muscle tone are useful. It is also important to instruct patients to avoid sudden painful movements such as jumping and how to lift and carry objects with minimal back strain.

Estrogens and androgens The use of estrogens in postmenopausal women with osteoporosis was first advocated by Dr. Fuller Albright and his colleagues. Decrease in urinary calcium and hydroxyproline excretion results from such therapy, especially during the first few months of treatment. Estrogens act by decreasing the rate of bone resorption, but bone formation does not increase, and eventually usually decreases. Thus estrogens produce significant, although modest, calcium retention, decrease the difference between formation and resorption, and therefore tend to retard the progress of osteoporosis, but they are not capable of restoring skeletal mass. The magnitude of calcium retention also tends to decrease with continuous therapy. Therefore it is not surprising that no change in radiologic features of the osteoporosis can be appreciated with such therapy. It is likely that estrogens have their role in preventing osteoporosis in menopausal women rather than treating clinical disease already developed, although they are probably the best preparations to use in the postmenopausal woman with mild or moderate disease. Testosterone preparations are useful in treatment of men with gonadal deficiency, but there are no convincing reports of their efficacy in men with normal gonadal function. So-called anabolic steroids are weak androgens, and there is no advantage to their use in women in view of their masculinizing properties. There is also no proved advantage to combinations of estrogens and androgens. The chronic use of estrogens does restore menses in postmenopausal women and does induce breast swelling and hyperpigmentation. The incidence of mammary and uterine cancer is not increased as compared with that in women of similar age not receiving estrogens.

A typical program would be oral administration of 0.625 to 1.25 mg conjugated estrogens per day or 1 to 3 mg diethylstilbestrol per day for 4 weeks, followed by abstinence for 1 week to allow for withdrawal bleeding. Subsequently dosage may be increased to as much as 2.5 to 5.0 mg daily. Occasionally it is advisable to add a progestational agent for the last 5 days on estrogens. Pelvic examination and vaginal smear for cytology is indicated at annual intervals.

Calcium preparations Use of oral calcium preparations in doses greater than 1.0 g elemental calcium per day (e.g., calcium glycerophosphate 2 g three times daily) has been shown to increase calcium retention in some osteoporotic subjects and decrease indexes of bone resorption. However, as with the use of estrogens, this eventually results in decrease in bone formation and tends to arrest rather than "cure" the osteoporosis. In patients with malabsorption, calcium may be effective in addition to vitamin D given orally in doses of 25,000 to 50,000 IU once or twice weekly. Both serum and urinary calcium should be monitored at intervals of several months to be certain that hypercalcemia does not result, although this would be very unusual with such a dose. Calcium preparations might be of greater use in patients with normal gonadal function and relatively mild disease. Intermittent intravenous infusions of calcium have also been advocated, but the efficacy of this form of therapy has yet to be established.

Fluoride Fluoride ions are promptly deposited in the skeleton where they become incorporated into the crystal lattice of hydroxyapatite, substituting for hydroxyl ions. This process results in a mineral phase of greater crystallinity. Fluoride ions in chronic high doses also increase new bone formation and in excess produce a form of hyperostosis with dense bones, exostoses, neurologic complications due to bony overgrowth, and ligamentous calcification. The use of fluoride in treating osteoporosis has therefore been reported without uniformly satisfactory results, possibly because of variations in dosage of fluoride ion, retention of absorbed ion, and calcium intake while on fluoride. The stimulation of new bone formation, a desirable effect not seen with the other agents mentioned previously, is unfortunately associated with the production of bone which is poorly mineralized and also, presumably, structurally unsound. It has recently been suggested that if the dose of fluoride ion is moderate (25 mg per day) and calcium supplements are given in doses of at least 1 g daily plus vitamin D, 50,000 IU twice weekly, considerable new bone is produced. Significant toxicity is absent, although weight-bearing pain, especially in ankles and knees, is noted by some patients and disappears when fluoride is discontinued. Such therapeutic programs are still in the process of evaluation.

Other measures The efficacy of calcitonin in inhibiting bone formation in osteoporosis is still under evaluation, although it appears unlikely that it will prove to be of great benefit. Oral phosphates (greater than 1 g elemental phosphorus per day in divided doses) may decrease urinary calcium excretion in patients with marked hypercalcuria and thereby improve calcium tolerance. However, phosphate has not been shown to be of value in the treatment of patients with postmenopausal osteoporosis who have normal levels of serum phosphorus. Growth hormone may eventually be shown to be of therapeutic value in osteoporosis, in view of its effects in stimulating new bone formation in animals.

RICKETS AND OSTEOMALACIA

The terms *rickets* and *osteomalacia* are used to describe a group of disorders in which there is defective mineralization of the newly formed organic matrix of the skeleton. In *rickets* the growing skeleton is involved, and defective mineralization occurs not only in bone but also in the cartilage matrix of the growth plate; the term *osteomalacia* is usually reserved for the disorder of mineralization of the adult skeleton where the epiphyseal growth plates are closed. There are a number of conditions that result in rickets and/or osteomalacia: inadequate dietary intake of vitamin D, inadequate exposure to ultraviolet radiation to form endogenous vitamin D, intestinal malabsorption of vitamin D, chronic acidosis, and renal tubular defects which produce hypophosphatemia or acidosis as well as chronic administration of diphenylhydantoin and other anticonvulsants. In the renal tubular disorders rickets and osteomalacia develop in the presence of normal intestinal function and are not cured by treatment with doses of vitamin D adequate to cure deficiency rickets. Thus the term *vitamin D–resistant* (or *refractory*) has been applied in these instances. Renal insufficiency, especially in children, is also associated with rickets or osteomalacia. A classification of rickets and osteomalacia is given in Table 352-2.

PATHOGENESIS AND HISTOPATHOLOGY In order for mineralization of matrices of skeletal tissues to take place, a particular concentration of calcium and phosphate is required at the mineralization sites. Although it is not known what the optimal concentration is at these sites, mineralization does not proceed normally when the concentrations of calcium and inorganic phosphate in the plasma (and extracellular fluid) are too low. Other conditions required for normal mineralization include intact metabolic and transport functions of osteoblasts and chondrocytes, adequate collagen matrix, possibly phosphorylation of matrix components, and low concentrations of inhibitory substances such as specific protein polysaccharide fractions and inorganic pyrophosphate. If the osteoblast continues to produce matrix components which cannot be adequately mineralized, the typical features of rickets and osteomalacia result. If calcification continues to be inadequate, the production of organic matrix (osteoid) must also gradually decrease. In bone there will be an increase in the forming surface covered by incompletely mineralized osteoid seams (usually less than 12 μm) and a decrease in the staining intensity of the so-called calcification front. A variety of methods are available to measure the thickness of the osteoid seam

TABLE 352-2
Classification of rickets and osteomalacia

I Vitamin D lack (insufficient dietary intake plus insufficient endogenous production)
II Vitamin D loss (various forms of malabsorption syndrome)
III Vitamin D "resistance"
- *A* Renal tubular disorders
- *B* Chronic renal insufficiency
- *C* Systemic acidosis
- *D* Excessive metabolism of vitamin D (e.g., anticonvulsant therapy)
- *E* "Pseudovitamin D deficiency"

IV Renal phosphate leak
- *A* "Primary" (includes phosphate diabetes, particularly adult onset, and other renal tubular disorders in which high phosphate clearance is not due to secondary hyperparathyroidism alone)
- *B* "Secondary" (e.g., giant-cell tumors, granulomas, and hemangiomas associated with osteomalacia)

V Rapid bone formation in excess of resorption
- *A* Postparathyroidectomy in the osteitis fibrosa of hyperparathyroidism
- *B* Osteopetrosis in children

VI Hypophosphatasia

and the presence of a calcification front. In routine histologic sections stained with hematoxylin and eosin, if the specimens are not overdecalcified in preparation, the more heavily mineralized areas tend to appear violet or blue, whereas the osteoid seams appear pink. Subtle degrees of osteomalacia may not be appreciated with routine preparations, and undecalcified sections are necessary to establish its presence. In addition to these features, rickets is also characterized by inadequate mineralization of the cartilage matrix of the growing epiphyseal plate. Calcification in the interstitial regions of the hypertrophic zone is defective, the growth plate increases in thickness, the arrangement of the columns of cartilage cells (usually highly ordered) is disorganized, and there is a variable degree of cupping of the epiphyses. The rachitic bones are often incapable of withstanding usual mechanical stresses and in the process of growth tend to undergo bowing deformities. If rickets is untreated, growth at the epiphyseal plates is slowed and the eventual length of the long bones is diminished.

Vitamin D does not have a major effect directly on mineralization. Its primary role after conversion to its more active polar metabolites (25-hydroxycholecalciferol and 1,25-dihydroxycholecalciferol) is to permit the regulation and enhance absorption of calcium ions from the intestinal lumen. The pathogenesis of inadequate skeletal mineralization when there is insufficient vitamin D present, from whatever cause, is probably as follows. Lack of vitamin D causes plasma calcium concentration to fall, there is increased secretion of parathyroid hormone (PTH), and, later, there is increased synthesis of PTH and hyperplasia of the parathyroid glands. The increased circulating concentration of PTH tends to raise plasma calcium concentrations but also stimulates increased renal phosphate clearance, which, in turn, produces hypophosphatemia. When the concentration of phosphorus in the extracellular fluid falls below a critical level, mineralization cannot proceed normally. In severe degrees of vitamin D lack, normocalcemia cannot be maintained, and the driving force for mineralization is further decreased.

Phosphate depletion alone can produce osteomalacia such as is seen in patients consuming large amounts of nonabsorbable antacids. Excessive renal loss of phosphate due to decreased tubular reabsorption may also result in the hypophosphatemia responsible for the osteomalacia in some of the renal tubular disorders. Secondary hyperparathyroidism is probably not present in many of these patients. Hypophosphatemia cannot account for the osteomalacia in all the disorders listed in Table 352-2. In chronic renal failure, for example, plasma phosphorus levels are not decreased and usually are increased. Similarly plasma phosphorus levels are not depressed in infants and children with osteomalacia secondary to hypophosphatasia, a hereditary deficiency in alkaline phosphatase.

CLINICAL FINDINGS The clinical problems of rickets are the result of skeletal deformities, susceptibility to fractures, weakness and hypotonia, and disturbances in growth. In extreme instances of vitamin D–deficiency rickets, hypocalcemia may be sufficient to produce tetany which, when severe, may be accompanied by laryngeal spasm and convulsive seizures.

In infants and young children features include listlessness, irritability, and often profound hypotonia and muscular weakness. As the disorder progresses, children become unable to walk without support. In the skull abnormal parietal flattening appears, as well as frontal bossing. The calvaria is softened (craniotabes), and widening of sutures may be evident. Prominence of the costochondral junctions is called the "rachitic rosary," and the indentation of the lower ribs at the site of attachment of the diaphragm is known as *Harrison's groove*. If the rickets is untreated, progressive deformities of the pelvis and extremities result with bowing particularly common in the tibia, femur, radius, and ulna. Because of inadequate structure of the bones, fractures are frequent. Dental eruption is often delayed, and enamel defects are common.

The presentation of osteomalacia in adults usually is not as dramatic as that of rickets in infants and children. The skeletal deformities may be overlooked, and the features of the underlying disorder may dominate, as, for example, in the vitamin D loss associated with nontropical sprue. Major symptoms, when they occur, include varying degrees of diffuse skeletal pain and bony tenderness. Pain may be especially prominent about the hips and may result in an antalgic gait. Muscular weakness is also common in adults with osteomalacia, although it may be difficult to distinguish muscular weakness from hesitancy to move because of skeletal pain. Weakness, usually proximal in distribution, may be prominent, however, and may be severe enough to mimic that of primary muscle disorders and may contribute to the waddling gait. In some patients pain and muscular weakness may be sufficient for them to be confined to bed and chair. Fractures of involved bones may occur with minimal trauma. When the ribs are involved, severe deformities may result in the thoracic cage, and collapse of vertebral bodies may produce loss of height.

RADIOLOGIC FEATURES Radiologic changes in the skeleton in rickets and osteomalacia reflect the pathologic changes. In rickets the alterations are most evident at the epiphyseal growth plate which is increased in thickness, cupped, and reveals a haziness at the diaphyseal border due to decreased calcification of the hypertrophic zone and inadequate mineralization of the primary spongiosa. The trabecular pattern of the metaphyses is abnormal, the cortices of the diaphyses may be thinned, and bowing of the shafts may be present.

In osteomalacia there is usually some decrease in bone density associated with loss of trabeculae and variable degrees of thinning of the cortices. In some patients the radiologic changes are indistinguishable from those seen in osteoporosis. The finding that suggests osteomalacia more specifically is the presence of radiolucent bands ranging from a few millimeters to several centimeters in length, usually perpendicular to the surface of the bones. They are particularly common at the inner aspects of the femur, especially near the femoral neck, in the pelvis, in the outer edge of the scapula, in the upper fibula, and in the metatarsals. These usually symmetric radiolucent bands, called *pseudofractures* or *Looser's zones*, occur most often at sites where major arteries cross the bones, and are thought to be due to the mechanical stress of the pulsation of these vessels. Arteriography has confirmed that the origins of the pseudofractures correspond to the location of major vessels in some instances. Subperiosteal erosions along the diaphyseal cortices are sometimes seen in patients in whom secondary hyperparathyroidism is present.

In some patients with osteomalacia increased rather than decreased density of bones may be observed. This is seen in patients with renal tubular disorders, rather than with vitamin D deficiency, and may produce a striking degree of thickening of the cortices and trabeculae of spongy bone. Despite the increase in mass of bone per unit volume, microscopically the trabeculae are covered with abnormally thickened osteoid seams typical of osteomalacia. Similar findings may be noted in patients with chronic renal failure. The reason for the hyperostosis is unknown; the bone is still architecturally abnormal and subject to fracture with relatively minimal trauma.

LABORATORY FINDINGS Changes in plasma concentrations of calcium and inorganic phosphorus vary with the different disorders. In states of vitamin D deficiency, whether due to dietary lack, inadequate sunlight exposure, or intestinal malabsorption, serum calcium levels are normal or low, whereas phosphorus levels are characteristically low. In adults phosphorus concentrations less than 2.8 mg per ml are abnormal; in children the lower limit of normal is closer to 4.0 to 4.5 mg per 100 ml. In *severe* states of vitamin D depletion, hypocalcemia may also be seen, occasionally sufficient to produce tetany. Mild acidosis and generalized aminoaciduria may also be found, as a result of secondary hyperparathyroidism. As a rule, patients with renal tubular disorders maintain normal serum calcium levels while hypophosphatemia is characteristic. Other laboratory findings such as glucosuria, aminoaciduria, acidosis, and hypouricemia reflect variable degrees of disturbance of proximal tubular function or features of the underlying disease (e.g., low plasma ceruloplasmin in Wilson's disease or abnormalities of immunoglobulins in multiple myeloma). In chronic renal failure hyperphosphatemia and some degree of hypocalcemia are usually seen. Serum phosphorus levels are also normal or elevated in hypophosphatasia. Increased excretion of hydroxyproline peptides is a component of those conditions in which secondary hyperparathyroidism and excessive bone resorption are associated with the defect in mineralization. Levels of alkaline phosphatase in plasma are usually elevated in rickets or osteomalacia, but typical and even severe osteomalacia, especially that due to renal tubular disorders, may be accompanied by normal or only borderline elevations. Levels may increase during the early phases of therapy.

DIETARY VITAMIN D DEFICIENCY AND INADEQUATE ENDOGENOUS SYNTHESIS Rickets was first described in England in about 1650 where it affected largely the poor people in sunless urban areas. Most foods unfortified with vitamin D contain insufficient amounts of the vitamin to prevent rickets in growing children or osteomalacia in adults living in temperate-zone cities. As discussed in Chap. 349, in the absence of supplements, vitamin D must be formed endogenously through the ultraviolet irradiation of precursor 7-dehydrocholesterol in the skin. Many factors decrease the formation of cholecalciferol (vitamin D_3) from its precursor: increased melanin pigmentation, hyperkeratosis, limited exposure of the body, short days of sunlight, oblique angle of ultraviolet irradiation, and factors in the atmosphere, such as smog, which prevent adequate penetration of the required radiation. Since fortification of dairy products and routine use of vitamin D supplements for infants have been in effect, deficiency rickets is very unusual in the United States. Poor, dark-skinned infants living in crowded Northern cities are most susceptible. However, osteomalacia due to vitamin D deficiency still is observed in adults, especially in elderly individuals who tend to remain indoors and whose dietary intake of vitamin D is inadequate (probably less than 70 to 100 IU per day).

VITAMIN D LOSS AND INTESTINAL MALABSORPTION Osteomalacia may be seen in patients with intestinal malabsorption such as in adult celiac disease and regional enteritis. Prior to the discovery of gluten sensitivity in some of these cases, celiac disease was among the more common disorders underlying osteomalacia. Vitamin D absorption, which normally occurs via chylomicrons, is impaired in diseases causing steatorrhea such as chronic biliary obstruction where emulsification of fat is disturbed. Osteomalacia is less frequent in chronic pancreatic deficiency. Patients who have had gastric surgery may also develop osteomalacia, possibly due to malfunction of the proximal small bowel. Factors other than failure to absorb vitamin D may contribute to the osteomalacia in patients with small-bowel disease, such as inadequate absorbing surface and failure of intestinal cells to respond to the active metabolites of vitamin D. Secondary hyperparathyroidism is usually present in intestinal malabsorption, as it is in dietary lack of vitamin D.

ABNORMAL METABOLISM OF VITAMIN D It is probable that some instances of familial so-called vitamin D–resistant rickets (see below) will be shown to be due to specific defects in the metabolism of vitamin D. In some cases, modest doses of 25-hydroxycholecalciferol have been found to induce healing whereas in other cases, relatively large doses have been ineffective. It is likely that what is called vitamin D–resistant rickets represents a group of similar but not identical defects. Insufficient formation of the essential metabolite of vitamin D, 1,25-dihydroxycholecalciferol may be responsible for vitamin D resistance in some cases although this has yet to be demonstrated conclusively. There is evidence that individuals consuming anticonvulsants such as diphenylhydantoin and phenobarbital develop osteomalacia (or rickets) due to the effects of the drugs on normal vitamin D metabolism. For example, it has been suggested that there is induction of hepatic microsomal enzyme activity capable of increasing the formation of more polar, inactive metabolites of vitamin D. Intake of anticonvulsants may be especially important in this regard in individuals whose intake of vitamin D is barely optimal, whose exposure to sunlight is minimal, or in whom mild intestinal malfunction exists such as in the post-gastrectomy state.

A disorder superficially resembling vitamin D–resistant osteomalacia has been termed pseudovitamin D deficiency. These patients have rickets or osteomalacia, a tendency to hypocalcemia but normal or only slightly depressed serum phosphorus levels, a response to a variable but moderate dose of vitamin D which is usually excellent and complete, and an autosomal recessive inheritance. No other renal tubular abnormalities are found. Some defect in the metabolism of vitamin D has been suspected but not proven.

RENAL TUBULAR DISORDERS Rickets and osteomalacia develop in association with a variety of disorders of proximal renal tubular function. These disorders have in common increased renal clearance of inorganic phosphorus and hypophosphatemia with normal, or near normal, glomerular filtration rate. Most frequently, increased phosphate clearance with resultant hypophosphatemia is an isolated defect with no other abnormalities present except for some increase in urinary glycine excretion (hyperglycinuria). Primary hypophosphatemia (phosphate diabetes and vitamin D–resistant rickets are terms applied to these cases especially when the disorder presents in early childhood) is characterized by increasingly severe skeletal deformities, dwarfism, and sex-linked dominant inheritance. In some of these patients there may be spontaneous remissions followed by recurrences in adult life associated, for example, with pregnancy and lactation. Early reports suggested that there was a defect in the conversion of cholecalciferol to 25-hydroxycholecalciferol in members of some of the pedigrees, but replacement doses of this metabolite have usually been unsuccessful in curing the skeletal disorder, whereas pharmacologic doses have been of benefit. It is likely that the biochemical defect is not the same in all these kindreds and that other defects in metabolism of vitamin D will be defined in some. Sporadic cases of hypophosphatemia have also been described in adults in whom family histories have been negative and where proximal muscle weakness has been a prominent feature. In sex-linked hypophosphatemic rickets, muscle weakness is not characteristic. As mentioned above, in most of the untreated cases of renal tubular disorders with rickets and osteomalacia, secondary hyperparathyroidism is not present.

In other patients the disorder in tubular function may be more widespread involving (besides phosphorus) glucose, potassium, amino acids, and uric acid; the various combinations are termed the de Toni-Debre-Fanconi syndrome. The more complete renal tubular defects may also occur sporadically or in families. In some instances the lesion is simply part of a more widespread disorder such as in Wilson's disease and cystinosis. The acidosis of proximal tubular defects also plays a role in development of osteomalacia, possibly by altering metabolism of vitamin D or altering renal handling of calcium and phosphorus. In this regard osteomalacia has accompanied the hyperchloremic acidosis of ureterocolic anastomosis.

A number of cases have been reported in which hypophosphatemic osteomalacia and high renal phosphate clearance have been associated with a variety of tumors, such as giant-cell tumors (benign and malignant) or reparative granulomas, but hemangiomas of soft tissues have also been implicated. In some instances removal of the tumor has resulted in normalization of renal phosphate clearance, rise in serum phosphorus, and remission of the rickets or osteomalacia. The mechanism of this response has not been elucidated.

CHRONIC RENAL FAILURE Histologically osteomalacia is common in patients with chronic renal failure; it often tends to be the predominant phase of renal osteodystrophy in younger patients and statistically is more frequent in those with the lower plasma levels of calcium and phosphorus. There is almost always a component of secondary hyperparathyroidism and osteitis fibrosa accompanying the defect in mineralization. The defect itself probably involves a decreased conversion of 25-hydroxycholecalciferol to 1,25-dihydroxycholecalciferol which is somehow associated with the renal disease, probably in addition to a primary defect in intestinal calcium absorption. In the presence of near-normal plasma concentration of calcium and hyperphosphatemia, it is not clear why mineralization of the organic matrix should be incomplete. Although it has been postulated that inhibitors of mineralization are present to account for this anomaly, the osteomalacic component usually does respond to large doses of calciferol or dihydrotachysterol. In some patients with renal osteodystrophy the total bone mass may be increased (osteosclerosis), resulting in increased density of bone seen radiologically. This is particularly evident in the spine where a characteristic appearance is that of dense bone at the superior and inferior margins of the vertebral bodies with more radiolucent central portions ("rugger jersey sign"). Histologically, although there is more bone per unit area, each trabecula is covered by an abnormally wide osteoid seam.

HYPOPHOSPHATASIA Rickets is a feature of this heritable deficiency of alkaline phosphatase in infants and children, although osteomalacia has been an inconstant finding in adults with hypophosphatasia. Serum phosphorus levels are not reduced. Phosphorylethanolamine is excreted in excessive amounts in the urine, but it is not clear how this is related to the inadequate skeletal mineralization. There is a direct correlation between plasma alkaline phosphatase and inorganic pyrophosphatase. Since patients with hypophosphatasia are also deficient in pyrophosphatase, it is possible that concentrations of inorganic pyrophosphate, a potent inhibitor of mineralization, are too high at the sites where mineralization occurs to allow it to proceed normally.

OTHER DISORDERS ASSOCIATED WITH DEFECTIVE MINERALIZATION Some decrease in mineralization of newly forming matrix, increase in surface covered by osteoid, and increase in the width of the osteoid seams are seen in several conditions that are not usually considered as osteomalacia except by these criteria. Biopsies in some of these conditions would show a normal calcification front. Examples include patients with the osteitis fibrosa of hyperparathyroidism in the weeks to months following surgical cure, and some patients with extensive Paget's disease. In these circumstances there is a temporary imbalance between the rate at which mineral is supplied to bone and the rate at which bone matrix is formed. Wide osteoid seams as well as hypophosphatemia are also seen in the bones of children with osteopetrosis in whom there is inadequate resorption of bone and calcified cartilage but active bone formation.

A condition which resembles osteomalacia and is associated with a coarsened, mottled bony trabecular pattern, pseudofractures, and bone pain, but normal plasma levels of calcium and phosphorus is fibrogenesis imperfecta ossium. Histologically the bone has a distinctive appearance, with wide osteoid seams and a distortion of the birefringent pattern of normal bone suggesting an abnormality in the collagen recently deposited. The nature of the abnormality is not known.

TREATMENT OF RICKETS AND OSTEOMALACIA

The therapeutic approach to each of the disorders associated with rickets and osteomalacia is somewhat different. In rickets and osteomalacia due to dietary absence of vitamin D or inadequate exposure to sunlight, vitamin D (as calciferol) is given orally in doses of 2,000 to 4,000 IU (0.05 to 0.1 mg) daily for 6 to 12 weeks, followed by daily supplements of 200 to 400 IU, which are adequate to prevent the development of the disorder in otherwise normal subjects. In infants and children with such treatment improvement in muscle tone and strength and rise in serum calcium and phosphorus are noted within several weeks, and alkaline phosphatase levels fall. Radiologic evidence of healing is first noted within weeks and may be complete by a few months. Calcium supplements and larger initial doses of vitamin D may be necessary in infants and children with tetany. In adults with nutritional osteomalacia healing of pseudofractures may be evident within 3 to 4 weeks after therapy with as little as 2,000 IU (0.05 mg) calciferol daily. Healing is complete usually by 6 months.

Patients with osteomalacia due to intestinal malabsorption do not respond to the relatively small doses of vitamin D that can cure deficiency-nutritional osteomalacia. In the presence of active steatorrhea, oral doses of vitamin D of 40,000 to 100,000 IU (1.0 to 2.5 mg) daily may be required in addition to large doses of calcium (e.g., 15 to 20 g calcium lactate per os daily). In some instances oral calciferol is ineffective, and the parenteral route is required (e.g., 10,000 IU intramuscularly per day). Another approach is the use of ultraviolet irradiation, e.g., total body erythema doses daily for several weeks, in addition to supplemental calcium. Inorganic phosphate therapy is not indicated in either deficiency osteomalacia or in intestinal malabsorption, since hypocalcemia will develop and intestinal and calcium absorption remain inadequate. In all patients in whom large doses of vitamin D are used, monitoring of plasma calcium levels at intervals is essential. Semiqualitative urinary calcium measurements alone are inadequate.

In patients who have been using anticonvulsants, it is often necessary to continue the drugs while adding supplemental vitamin D and monitoring levels of serum calcium at biweekly intervals until a therapeutic response (evidence of radiologic healing, improvement in symptoms) is obtained. Doses varying from 4,000 to 40,000 IU daily have been recommended.

Treatment of rickets and osteomalacia in the presence of renal tubular disorders is more difficult, and there is not uniform agreement as to the exact regimen to be followed. The X-linked form of hypophosphatemic osteomalacia has usually been treated with large doses of calciferol from 40,000 IU to several hundred thousand IU or more daily. With vitamin D therapy alone, there is radiologic evidence of healing in many patients, but this is usually incomplete, some hypophosphatemia persists, linear skeletal growth remains abnormally slow, and bony deformities continue to develop. In addition, the potential hazard of hypercalcemia and its consequences exists. The addition of oral supplements of inorganic phosphate in divided doses of 1.0 to 3.6 g P daily have improved the clinical and radiologic response, allowed the use of smaller doses of vitamin D, and improved the rate of linear growth in many younger subjects. In some adults, therapy with inorganic phosphate alone has been successful in abolishing muscle weakness and bone pain and in producing radiologic and histologic healing. However, the addition of vitamin D improves calcium balance and maintains a higher level of serum phosphorus to permit complete healing. In some patients there may be a temporary increase in bone pain and rise in serum alkaline phosphatase level during the early phases of treatment.

In the osteomalacia associated with the chronic acidosis of renal tubular disorders, the use of alkali may be of value in supplementing therapy with phosphate and vitamin D. In patients with ureterosigmoidostomy, oral sodium bicarbonate has reversed acidosis, improved serum phosphate level, and healed the bone disease; with maintenance use of alkali, recurrence of symptoms has been prevented.

In chronic renal failure high doses of calciferol, similar to those needed to treat osteomalacia of renal tubular disorders, are used. Dihydrotachysterol, which may not require hydroxylation past the initial 25-hydroxylation, has been reported to be particularly effective in therapy of renal osteodystrophy. Phosphate supplements are, of course, contraindicated.

In patients who have had rickets in childhood, the abnormal mechanical stress of severe deformities may contribute to the development of degenerative joint disease, particularly in hips and knees. Osteotomies at the proper time after healing has occurred may help to prevent this complication and avoid more extensive arthroplasties later in life.

REFERENCES

Osteoporosis

Barzel UA (ed): *Osteoporosis,* New York: Grune & Stratton, 1970

Dent CE, Watson L: Osteoporosis. Postgrad Med J 42:581, 1966

Jowsey J: Quantitative microradiography: A new approach in

the evaluation of metabolic bone disease. Am J Med 40:485, 1966

Nicholas JA, Wilson PD: Osteoporosis of the aged spine. Clin Orthop 26:19:1963

Smith RW Jr: Dietary and hormonal factors in bone loss. Fed Proc 26: 1737, 1967

Wallach S (ed): Drug treatment of bone. Semin Drug Treatment 2:1, 1972

Rickets and osteomalacia

Arnstein AR et al: Recent progress in rickets and osteomalacia. Ann Intern Med 67:1296, 1967

Dent CE: Rickets (and osteomalacia), nutritional and metabolic. Proc R Soc Med 63:401, 1970

——, Smith R: Nutritional osteomalacia. Q J Med 38:195, 1969

Hahn TJ et al: Effect of chronic anticonvulsant therapy on serum 25-hydroxycholecalciferol levels in adults. N Engl J Med 287:900, 1972

Nagant deDeuxchaisnes C, Krane SM: The treatment of adult phosphate diabetes and Fanconi syndrome with neutral sodium phosphate. Am J Med 43:508, 1967

Salassa RM et al: Hypophosphatemic osteomalacia associated with "nonendocrine" tumors. N Engl J Med 283:65, 1970

Steinbach HL, Noetzli M: Roentgen appearance of the skeleton in osteomalacia and rickets. Am J Roentgenol Radiotherapy 91:955, 1964

Winters RW et al: A genetic study of familial hypophosphatemia with vitamin D resistant rickets with a review of the literature. Medicine 37:97, 1958

353
PAGET'S DISEASE OF BONE

STEPHEN M. KRANE

Paget's disease of bone (osteitis deformans) is among the most common of the chronic skeletal diseases. In the strict sense it is a focal disease, although occasionally it may be widespread. Histologically the inital event is excessive resorption of bone mediated by cells such as osteoclasts, followed by the replacement of normal marrow by vascular, fibrous connective tissue. At some stage in the disease, and to a variable degree, the resorbed bone is replaced by coarse-fibered, dense trabecular bone organized in haphazard fashion. The irregular and often rapid deposition of this new bone causes an increase in the number of prominent, irregular cement lines which gives the bone its characteristic "mosaic" pattern. Some areas of bone may show evidence of both excessive resorption and the chaotic new bone formation.

INCIDENCE The prevalence of Paget's disease is difficult to determine since it is most often asymptomatic and is detected usually when roentgenograms are obtained for other reasons. On the basis of autopsy examination, the incidence of Paget's disease has been estimated to be about 3 percent in individuals over the age of forty; there is increased likelihood of occurrence with increasing age. Figures based on radiologic surveys indicate less than 1 percent in the adult population in the United States, Great Britain, and Australia. However, the incidence varies markedly in different parts of the world; in some areas, including India, Japan, the Middle East, and Scandinavia, the disease is exceedingly rare.

ETIOLOGY Almost a century after the original description of the disorder, and despite intensive study and widespread interest, the etiology of Paget's disease is unknown. No convincing evidence of endocrine abnormality has been produced. Although pagetic bone can be exceedingly vascular, out of proportion to any other disorder, it has not been established that the vascular abnormality is primary. The observations that some of the manifestations of the disease can be suppressed with the use of adrenal corticosteroids, salicylates, and cytotoxic drugs are of interest, although there is not sufficient information to support earlier hypotheses that an inflammatory process is the fundamental lesion.

PATHOPHYSIOLOGY The characteristic feature of Paget's disease is the increased resorption of bone accompanied by an increase in bone formation, which is usually adequate to compensate. In the early phase of Paget's disease, bone resorption predominates (for example, in the variant, *osteoporosis circumscripta*), and the bones are exceedingly vascular. This has been termed the *osteoporotic, osteolytic,* or *destructive phase* of the disease in which the external calcium balance may be negative. Commonly the excessive resorption is followed closely by formation of new pagetic bone. In this so-called "mixed" phase of the disease, the rate of bone formation is so geared to that of bone resorption that the magnitude of the increase in bone turnover is not reflected in the overall calcium balance.

As the activity of the disease decreases, a progressive decrease in resorptive rate may occur, eventually leading to the occurrence of hard, dense, less vascular bone (the so-called *osteoplastic* or *sclerotic* phase) and a positive external calcium balance. Techniques measuring disappearance rates of injected radioisotopes of calcium or strontium have shown that the rates of bone turnover may be increased enormously in patients with active Paget's disease, occasionally more than twenty times normal. The magnitude of the increase in turnover varies with the extent as well as the activity of the disease. The increase correlates well with the increased levels of plasma alkaline phosphatase, which are higher in Paget's disease than in any other condition with the exception of hereditary hyperphosphatasia. Although increased bone resorption enhances release of calcium and phosphate ions from the inorganic mineral phase of bone, utilization of these ions for new bone formation and, presumably, feedback control of parathyroid hormone secretion usually maintain the concentration of calcium ions in the plasma at normal levels. The concentration of phosphate in the plasma is normal or slightly elevated. When marked imbalance between bone formation and resorption occurs in favor of resorption, such as after prolonged immobilization or fractures, urinary calcium excretion may be increased, and rarely hypercalcemia may be encountered. Resorption involves the organic phase of bone as well as the mineral phase. Although the inorganic ions of the mineral phase are reutilized for bone formation, amino acids such as hydroxyproline and hydroxylysine released during resorption of the collagen matrix of bone are not reutilized for collagen biosynthesis. The urinary excretion of small peptides containing hydroxyproline is increased in Paget's disease, reflecting the increased bone resorption. Peptides of higher molecular weight (about 5,000), also containing hydroxyproline and other amino acids in proportions characteristic of collagen, are also excreted in increased amounts in the urine, and are correlated with increased bone formation.

RADIOLOGIC CHANGES The radiologic findings in Paget's disease reflect the underlying pathology and the phase of the disease which predominates at the time of the examination. The pelvic bones are most commonly involved, followed by the femur, skull, tibia, lumbosacral spine, dorsal spine, clavicles, and ribs in that order; small bones are not as frequently diseased. The lytic phase of the disease may be overlooked except when it occurs in the skull as *osteoporosis circumscripta*, with areas of sharply demarcated radiolucency in the frontal, parietal, and occipital bones. In the long bones the lytic areas are usually first seen at one end from which they progress toward the other end with a V-shaped advancing edge. The lesion may produce expansion of the cortex and exhibit other features which suggest malignancy. Usually the lytic area is followed by a zone of increased density, representing the new bone formation of the mixed phase of the disease. In general, the bone shows enlargement with irregularly widened cortex in a coarse, striated pattern and increased density, occasionally focal in distribution. Perpendicular lines of radiolucency (cortical infractions) are frequent and occur on the convex side of bowed long bones, particularly the femur and tibia. Transverse fractures may also occur, some initiated at the sites of these cortical infractions. The remodeling of the pagetic bone usually follows the lines of stress produced by muscle pull or gravity, accounting for the characteristic lateral bowing of the femur or anterior bowing of the tibia and the tendency for most of the dense bone to be deposited on the concave side of the bowed bone. In the skull, in the mixed stage, there is enlargement and thickening, especially of the outer table with irregular areas of increased density, often spotty. Basilar invagination is common with involvement of the base of the skull. The changes in the pelvis also consist of the combination of bone resorption and new bone formation and are frequently accompanied by a thickening of the pelvic rim, a characteristic of Paget's disease. In the sclerotic phase of the disease, the bone may show uniform increase in density often in the absence of striations. This is common in the facial bones, but is occasionally seen as well in the vertebras where a homogeneous, dense pattern gives an "ivory" appearance similar to that produced typically by Hodgkin's disease, although the involved vertebras are not enlarged in Hodgkin's disease.

CLINICAL PICTURE The clinical presentation of patients with Paget's disease is extremely variable and is a function of the extent of the disease, the particular bones involved, and the presence of associated complications. Many patients are asymptomatic. In these individuals the disorder is discovered because of radiologic findings during the course of examination of the pelvis or spine for an unrelated disease or complaint, or because of the finding of an elevated level of plasma alkaline phosphatase. Other individuals may gradually become aware of a swelling or deformity of a long bone or develop a disturbance in gait due to unequal length of and change in the distribution of mechanical forces in the lower extremities. Enlargement of the skull is often not noticed by the patient; individuals may be aware of increasing hat size. Pain in the face and headache are initial complaints in some patients; backache and pain in the lower extremities are common. The pain is usually dull, but occasionally shooting or knifelike pains are described. Pain in the lower extremities may be associated with the transverse cortical infractions which occur along the convex lateral surface of the femur or the anterior surface of the tibia. Pain may also be due to involvement of the hip joint resembling degenerative joint disease and characterized by narrowing of the joint space, bony lipping at the margin of the acetabulum, and deepening of the acetabulum. Angioid streaks of the retina have been observed in patients with Paget's disease. Hearing loss, usually of the nerve deafness type, is also common and is believed to be related to involvement of the temporal bone. More serious neurologic complications can result from overgrowth of pagetic bone at the base of the skull (platybasia) due to compression of the brainstem. Compression of the spinal cord with paraplegia has been observed, particularly with involvement of the middorsal spine. Pathologic fractures of vertebras have also produced spinal cord lesions.

COMPLICATIONS The increased vascularity of the bones involved with Paget's disease in the active, destructive phase is responsible for the increased warmth noted through the skin over such bones. When the disease is widespread, involving over one-third of the skeleton, the increased blood flow through the involved skeleton may be associated with *high cardiac output*. In the rare patient with Paget's disease at this stage so-called "high-output heart failure" may result. However, heart disease in pagetic individuals is usually accounted for by the same conditions that occur in other patients of similar age. *Pathologic fracture* is a frequent complication in patients with Paget's disease, usually occurring in bones involved in the destructive phase of the disease. In the weight-bearing bones fractures are often incomplete, multiple, and on the convex side of the bone. They may occur spontaneously or follow only slight trauma and result in pain but heal spontaneously with no major disability. More serious fractures may also occur. Under these circumstances the fracture itself or immobilization accompanying the fracture may upset the delicate balance between bone formation and resorption in favor of resorption. At this stage the imbalance may be reflected by increased urinary calcium excretion, and in rare instances the serum calcium level may rise to dangerous levels.

There is no characteristic level of urinary calcium excretion in Paget's disease, although there is a tendency for calcium excretion to be higher at any point in the disease when the resorptive phase predominates. This may be a factor which accounts for the somewhat higher incidence of *urinary stone* in these patients, although many of the urinary calculi reported may be unrelated to the pagetic process.

Sarcoma is the most dreaded complication of Paget's disease. Fortunately, the incidence is low, probably no greater than 1 to 2 percent, although higher incidence has been noted in some series which include many patients with polyostotic involvement. The sarcomas most frequently arise in the femur, humerus, skull, face,.and pelvis, and rarely in the vertebra. In about 20 percent the tumors are multicentric. Histologically, they are usually osteosarcomas, although fibrosarcomas and chondrosarcomas have also been found. Increase in pain and swelling are the most common complaints which lead to recognition of the sarcomas. The level of alkaline phosphatase in the serum of patients with sarcomas reflects the activity and extent of the Paget's disease, although in occasional patients an "explosive rise" of the phosphatase level may accompany the growth of the sarcoma. However, in some patients with limited involvement, phosphatase levels may be only slightly elevated and give no clue to the development of the malignant lesion. The prognosis is extremely poor following the development of sarcomas, and ablative operative therapy is rarely successful. Giant-cell tumors also occur with an increased frequency in Paget's disease and are usually benign. Pagetic bone is rarely the site of metastases despite its great vascularity.

THERAPY Most patients with Paget's disease require no treatment, since the disease is usually localized in its distribution and does not cause symptoms. Possible indications for therapy include persistent pain in involved bones, neural compression, rapidly progressive deformity resulting in disabling disturbance of posture and/or gait, high-output congestive heart failure, hypercalcemia, and severe hypercalcuria with or without formation of renal stones. *Acetylsalicylic acid* is an effective analgesic, and if it can be tolerated in large enough doses (3.6 to 4.0 g per day) for periods of months or years, there may be some suppression of the disease activity, as shown by decreases in the level of plasma alkaline phosphatase and urinary hydroxyproline excretion. *Indomethacin*, 25 mg three or four times daily, may also relieve pain, especially in the presence of hip involvement. *Corticosteroids* will suppress the disease but only in large doses (greater than 60 mg per day prednisone) which are usually not tolerated and, therefore, are not recommended. It is of interest, however, that the high cardiac output of some patients with Paget's disease may be reduced significantly after only a few days of steroid treatment. Although the use of *sodium fluoride* (80 to 120 mg sodium fluoride per day) for more than a year has produced amelioration of symptoms and decrease in the indexes of activity of the disease, this high dose may lead to poorly mineralized bone. Orthopedic procedures also have a role in the management of selected cases. Total hip replacement may be indicated in the patient with severe hip involvement, and osteotomy is useful to correct marked bowing deformities. In patients with fractures or orthopedic procedures or in patients immobilized for any reason, determinations of urinary and serum calcium levels should be performed at intervals to anticipate the development of hypercalcuria and hypercalcemia. Early ambulation and adequate fluid intake are essential. Preparations of sodium phytate or inorganic phosphate to reduce hypercalcuria may be useful under these circumstances (5 to 6 g neutral sodium phosphate daily in divided doses).

Several agents have been introduced which are effective in reducing the excessive bone resorption of Paget's disease and are of possible therapeutic value. Porcine, salmon, and human *calcitonin* have been administered subcutaneously for prolonged periods to pagetic patients, accompanied by decrease in plasma alkaline phosphatase levels and urinary hydroxyproline excretion. Treatment with calcitonin has produced variable decrease in bone pain, improvement in neurologic symptoms, and decrease in elevated cardiac output. Some patients have not continued to respond to porcine and salmon calcitonins because of the development of neutralizing antibodies. In others in whom diminution in response was not associated with development of antibodies, the development of secondary hyperparathyroidism has been postulated, although this cannot account for resistance in all cases. The calcitonins will probably be found to have a limited usefulness in the treatment of Paget's disease.

Cytotoxic drugs such as mithramycin and actinomycin D are potent agents in pagetic patients. Parenteral administration of mithramycin, 10 to 25 μg per kg for 10 to 14 days, has produced striking decrease in urinary hydroxyproline excretion with subsequent decreases in plasma alkaline phosphatase level and clinical improvement. Potential toxicity has limited use of these drugs.

Disodium etidronate, a diphosphonate compound, given orally in doses up to 20 mg per kg per day has also been effective in reducing indexes of bone resorption and producing clinical improvement in some cases. This drug may produce poorly mineralized bone, and its ultimate usefulness will require more information.

REFERENCES

AVIOLI L, BERMAN M: Role of magnesium metabolism and the effects of fluoride therapy in Paget's disease of bone. J Clin Endocrinol 28:700, 1968

BARRY HC: *Paget's Disease of Bone*, Edinburgh: E and S Livingstone, 1969

MCKENNA RJ et al: Osteogenic sarcoma arising in Paget's disease. Lancet 17:42, 1964

NAGANT DEDEUXCHAISNES C, KRANE SM: Paget's disease of bone: Clinical and metabolic observations. Medicine 43:233, 1964

RYAN WB et al: Experiences in the treatment of Paget's disease of bone with mithramycin. JAMA 231:1153, 1970

SINGER FR et al: An evaluation of antibodies and clinical resistance to salmon calcitonin. J Clin Invest 51:2331, 1972

SMITH R et al: Diphosphonates and Paget's disease of bone. Lancet 1:945, 1971

STEINBACH HL: Some roentgen features of Paget's disease. Am J Roentgenol 86:950, 1961

WOODHOUSE NJY et al: Radiological regression in Paget's disease treated by human calcitonin. Lancet 2:992, 1972

354 HYPEROSTOSIS, NEOPLASMS, AND OTHER DISORDERS OF BONE AND CARTILAGE

STEPHEN M. KRANE

HYPEROSTOSIS

A number of disease states have in common an increase in the mass of bone per unit volume (hyperostosis). Such increase in bone mass is detected radiologically as increased density of the bone, often associated with a variable degree of disturbance in the architecture of the tissue. In most of these disorders, it is not possible to distinguish between an increase in bone mass due to excessive formation of new bone or decreased resorption of bone already formed. When bone deposition is rapid, the new bone may be of the woven type, but if the process is more chronic, true lamellar bone is formed. The additional bone may be located at the periosteum, within the compact bone of the cortex, or in the trabeculae of the cancellous regions. In the medullary area, the new bone is deposited on and between the trabeculae and encroaches upon the medullary spaces. Typical examples of such responses are seen in areas adjacent to tumors or in association with infection. In some diseases the increase in bone mass may be spotty, as in osteopoikilosis, whereas in others most of the skeleton may be involved, as in the malignant form of osteopetrosis in children. The mechanism of the increase in mass is usually not due to an abnormal increase in the ratio of mineral to matrix, except in some disorders such as osteopetrosis where islands of calcified cartilage may persist. (The mineral density of calcified cartilage is greater than that of bone.) In some diseases such as in the osteosclerosis of renal insufficiency, the bone mass and radiodensity may be increased, even though the new bone formed is poorly mineralized and contains widened osteoid seams. A classification of the causes of hyperostosis is presented in Table 354-1.

Several of these conditions will be discussed in more detail in other chapters, although some general comments are pertinent. Bone that is denser than normal may be seen occasionally in the osteitis fibrosa associated with active hyperparathyroidism. When the hyperparathyroidism is successfully treated, the rate of bone resorption is decreased abruptly out of proportion to the rate of bone formation; this imbalance may lead to the production of areas of bone of density greater than in the surrounding skeleton, especially in the healing of brown tumors. In hypothyroidism, the rates of both bone formation and resorption may be decreased, but the balance may be in favor of formation, resulting in bones that are of increased density but normal architecture. The occurrence of increased bone density in renal tubular abnormalities associated with osteomalacia has been appreciated only recently. The increased mass of bone occurs together with widened osteoid seams, as in chronic renal glomerular insufficiency. In the vertebral bodies the bone appears denser in transverse bands at the upper and lower margins, with a relatively radiolucent center. This "sandwich" appearance is similar to that seen in some patients with osteopetrosis and has been termed by the British the "rugger jersey sign."

OSTEOPETROSIS Osteopetrosis (marble bone disease of Albers-Schönberg) is a rare disorder which varies in severity and age of clinical presentation. The most severe form occurs in infants and children and is inherited as an autosomal recessive, while a clinically more benign form is transmitted as an autosomal dominant. The so-called "malignant" variant starts *in utero* and progresses rapidly with marked anemia, hepatosplenomegaly, hydrocephalus, cranial nerve involvement, and death, often due to infection. In the less fulminant form, the anemia is not as severe, neurologic abnormalities are not as frequent, and recurrent pathologic fractures are the main feature. Although the majority of cases are in infants and children, many are discovered first in adult life when roentgenograms are obtained because of fractures or unrelated diseases. There is no particular predilection for either sex.

TABLE 354-1
Causes of hyperostosis

I Endocrine disorders
- *A* Healing phase of osteitis fibrosa cystica
- *B* Hypothyroidism
- *C* Acromegaly

II Radiation osteitis

III Chemical poisoning
- *A* Fluoride
- *B* Elemental phosphorus
- *C* Beryllium
- *D* Arsenic
- *E* Vitamin A intoxication
- *F* Lead
- *G* Bismuth

IV Osteomalacic disorders
- *A* Renal tubular osteomalacia (vitamin D resistance or phosphate diabetes)
- *B* Chronic renal glomerular failure

V Osteosclerosis (localized) associated with chronic infection

VI Osteosclerotic phase of Paget's disease

VII Osteosclerosis associated with carcinomatous metastases and with malignant lymphoma

VIII Osteosclerosis of erythroblastosis fetalis

IX Unclassified diseases
- *A* Osteopetrosis (marble bone disease of Albers-Schönberg)
- *B* Pyknodysostosis
- *C* Osteomyelosclerosis
- *D* Hyperostosis corticalis generalisata
- *E* Hyperostosis generalisata with pachydermia
- *F* Hereditary hyperphosphatasia
- *G* Progressive diaphyseal dysplasia (osteopathia hyperostotica multiplex infantilis; Camurati-Engelmann disease)
- *H* Melorheostosis
- *I* Osteopoikilosis
- *J* Hyperostosis frontalis interna

The increased bone mass is generally thought to be due to a defect in the normal remodeling of bone. Both bone formation and resorption are depressed, particularly resorption. Islands of unresorbed calcified cartilage encased in bone are frequently seen. The defect in remodeling results in marked disorganization of bone structure with thickened cortices and lack of funnelization of metaphyses. Despite its increased density, the bone is abnormal mechanically and fractures readily. Osteomalacia or rickets is sometimes a component of the osteopetrosis in children.

The histologic changes are reflected in the roentgenograms, which reveal uniformly dense, sclerotic bone often without distinction between the cortical and cancellous regions. The long bones are usually involved, with increased density along the entire shaft. Foci of increased density may be seen in the epiphyses corresponding to regions of unresorbed calcified cartilage. The metaphyses have a characteristic clubbed or splayed appearance. Horizontal bandings of increased density alternating with zones of decreased density are seen in the long bones and vertebras and suggest that the defect may be intermittent during periods of growth. The skull, pelvis, ribs, and other bones may also be involved. The phalanges and the distal humerus may appear normal when the disease is not severe.

Encroachment of bone upon the marrow cavity is associated with anemia of the myelophthisic type with foci of extramedullary hematopoiesis in liver, spleen, and lymph nodes and enlargement of these organs. Neurologic abnormalities are associated with encroachment on cranial nerves, which may result in optic atrophy, nystagmus, papilledema, exophthalmos, and impairment of extraocular motility. Facial paralysis and deafness are frequent; trigeminal lesions and anosmia have also been described. In infants with severe disease, macrocephaly, hydrocephalus, and convulsions may occur. Infections such as osteomyelitis are frequent in these children.

In the milder dominant osteopetrosis, about half of the patients have no symptoms, and the disorder is discovered incidentally on roentgenograms. Other such patients present because of fractures, bone pain, osteomyelitis, and cranial nerve palsies.

Fractures are a common complication even with trivial trauma. Healing of such fractures is usually satisfactory, although delayed union may occur. When the disease is manifested first in adult life, fractures may be the only clinical problem. Levels of calcium and alkaline phosphatase in the plasma are usually normal in adults, although in children hypophosphatemia and, occasionally, moderate hypocalcemia have been noted. Serum acid phosphatase levels are usually increased. The mechanism of the skeletal abnormality in osteopetrosis is not known. However, a disorder resembling osteopetrosis has been described in the so-called "gray-lethal" strain of mice. These animals have an increased number of parafollicular cells in their thyroid glands, hypocalcemia, and high circulating levels of a hypocalcemic factor thought likely to be calcitonin. It has therefore been postulated, but not established, that excessive secretion of calcitonin is the cause of the osteopetrosis in these mice and may play some part in the disease in human beings.

Attempts to affect the altered remodeling of bone in patients with osteopetrosis have been unsuccessful. Despite the extramedullary hematopoiesis that has been found in the spleen, splenectomy can occasionally decrease erythrocyte destruction in this organ and increase the life span of the erythrocytes.

PYKNODYSOSTOSIS *Pyknodysostosis* is a disorder which resembles osteopetrosis but is a more benign condition not associated with hepatosplenomegaly, anemia, or cranial nerve involvement. In addition to a generalized increase in bone density, features of the disease include short stature, separated cranial sutures, hypoplasia of the mandible, persistence of deciduous teeth, and partial aplasia of the terminal phalanges. Longevity is not decreased, and the patient usually presents to the physician because of frequent fractures. Pyknodysostosis is inherited as a mendelian recessive trait. It has been suggested from karyotope analysis that the gene which determines this disorder is located on the short arm of a small accrocentric chromosome.

OSTEOMYELOSCLEROSIS *Osteomyelosclerosis* is a disorder in which the marrow cells are replaced by diffuse fibroplasia, occasionally accompanied by osseous metaplasia. When the latter is prominent, increased skeletal density is seen on roentgenograms. Osteomyelosclerosis is probably a phase in the course of the myeloproliferative disorders and is characteristically accompanied by extramedullary hematopoiesis.

A disease distinct from those described above has been termed *hyperostosis corticalis generalisata* (van Buchem's disease). It is characterized by osteosclerosis of the skull (base and calvaria), lower jaw, clavicles, and ribs, and thickening of the diaphyseal cortices of the long and short bones. Alkaline phosphatase levels in the serum are elevated, and histologic observations suggest that the disorder is due to increased formation of bone of normal structure. The major clinical manifestations are due to neural compression and consist of optic atrophy, facial paralysis, and perception deafness. In *hyperostosis generalisata with pachydermia* (Uehlinger), the sclerosis is due to increased formation of subperiosteal spongy bone and involves the epiphyses, metaphyses, and diaphyses. Pain and swelling of joints and thickening of the skin of the lower arms are common.

HEREDITARY HYPERPHOSPHATASIA This disorder is characterized by severe structural deformities of the skeleton with increase in thickness of the calvaria, large homogeneous areas of increased density at the base of the skull, and widening and loss of normal architecture of the shafts and the epiphyses of the long and short bones. There is a failure to deposit normal bone, with haphazard orientation of lamellae suggesting active remodeling. Plasma alkaline phosphatase level and urinary excretion of hydroxyproline peptides and other collagen degradation products are markedly increased. The disorder is apparently inherited as an autosomal recessive.

PROGRESSIVE DIAPHYSEAL DYSPLASIA A disorder in which a symmetric osteosclerosis occurs, usually limited to the diaphyses of the long bones, especially the femur and tibia, has been termed *progressive diaphyseal* *dysplasia* (Camurati-Engelmann disease). The alkaline phosphatase levels are normal. Pain in the legs, fatigue, abnormal gait, and muscle wasting are the major manifestations.

MELORHEOSTOSIS This is a rare condition which begins usually in childhood, characterized by areas of sclerosis that appear in the bones of one limb. All segments of the bone may be involved, with the dense structures appearing as sclerotic areas which have a "flowing" distribution. The involved limb is often extremely painful.

OSTEOPOIKILOSIS This is a benign disorder usually discovered by chance and is not associated with symptoms. It is characterized by dense spots of trabecular bone less than a centimeter in diameter, usually of uniform density, that are located in the epiphyses and adjacent parts of the metaphyses. All bones may be involved except the skull, ribs, and vertebras.

HYPEROSTOSIS FRONTALIS INTERNA *Hyperostosis frontalis interna* is an abnormality of the inner table of the frontal bones of the skull first described by Morgagni and consisting of smooth, rounded enostoses covered by dura and projecting into the cranial cavity. These enostoses are usually less than 1 cm at their greatest diameter and usually do not extend posteriorly beyond the coronal suture. The abnormality is found almost exclusively in women, who are frequently obese, hirsute, and who have a variety of neuropsychiatric complaints (Morgagni-Stewart-Morel syndrome). However, hyperostosis frontalis interna has also been seen in women with no obvious illness or particular associated disease. There is no good evidence that the finding in the skull is a manifestation of a generalized metabolic disorder.

NEOPLASMS OF BONE

Primary neoplasms of the skeletal system reflect in their histology the cellular and extracellular components of the skeleton. However, it is not always possible to prove that a tumor arises from the same type of tissue that it produces. The precursor cell of bone tissue is the osteoprogenitor cell which may be transformed by modulation into the specialized cells of bone tissue: the osteoblast, osteocyte, and osteoclast. It is likely that these cells can modulate back to the osteoprogenitor cell. Under certain conditions osteoprogenitor cells may also be transformed into nonosteogenic cells such as chondroblasts and fibroblasts. Each of these cells can produce its characteristic extracellular matrix, and neoplasms arising from them may thus be recognized. Primary neoplasms of bone can arise also from hematopoietic, vascular, and neural elements.

PATHOPHYSIOLOGY Tumors in bone produce resorption of normal skeletal tissue by (1) production of substance(s) that can lyse bone, (2) inducing modulation of cells of the osteogenic series into cells involved in the process of resorption, such as osteoclasts, and (3) interfering with blood supply. Tumors will also produce some reaction in surrounding bone and alter the normal contour. The epiphyseal plate, articular cartilage, cortex, and periosteum of bone often offer a barrier to the spread of neoplastic tissue. Alteration of the contour of the cortex is not due to "expansion" but to remodeling of the bone in the area and formation of new bone with the new contour. Some tumors induce primarily an osteoplastic or sclerotic reaction in surrounding bone, which results in increased radiodensity. Primary neoplasms may appear as less radiopaque than surrounding bone or more radiopaque, depending upon the degree of calcification or ossification of the matrix and the density of the tissue. Bone tumors may be recognized because of (1) the presence of a mass in the soft tissues, (2) deformity of a bone, (3) pain and tenderness, and (4) pathologic fractures. Tumors of bone may also be detected incidentally on roentgenograms obtained for other clinical reasons.

There are numerous pitfalls in the clinical diagnosis and interpretation of histologic features of tumors of bone. Bone scans can detect the presence of bone tumors but would not distinguish this from benign tumors or fractures. Management of the patient therefore requires cooperation of experts in several disciplines.

BENIGN TUMORS The most common benign tumors are *osteochondromas* (exostoses) and *chondromas* (which may be multiple in Ollier's disease), *benign giant-cell tumors*, *aneurysmal bone cysts*, and *fibromas*. As a rule benign tumors are not painful except for osteoid osteomas, benign chondroblastomas, and benign chondromyxoidfibroma. The usual clinical problem is that of slowly progressing mass and deformity. Treatment is usually accomplished by removal of the tumor and/or curettage and bone grafting.

MALIGNANT TUMORS The most common malignant tumor of bone is multiple myeloma (see Chap. 65), which arises from hematopoietic cells. Reticulum cell sarcoma also may be a primary bone tumor. Malignant tumors of nonhematopoietic origin include chondrosarcomas, osteosarcomas, fibrosarcomas, Ewing's tumor, malignant giant-cell tumor, and chondromas. *Osteogenic sarcoma* arises presumably from the osteoprogenitor cell and shows a wide variation in its histopathology. These tumors usually contain some osteoid tissue, at least in small foci, and may contain in addition cartilaginous and fibrous elements. They are most common in the second and third decades and are less common under the age of ten and over the age of forty years. When they do occur in older individuals, some predisposing cause is usually present such as Paget's disease or prior radiation therapy. In primary osteogenic sarcomas the lesions usually arise in the metaphyseal region of long bones, especially in the distal femur and the proximal tibia. The most common symptoms are pain and swelling which may be present for weeks or months. The roentgenographic features of osteosarcomas depend upon the degree of bone destruction, the extent to which bone is formed by and within the tumor, and the type of reaction in the surrounding bone. Thus the lesions may vary from ones purely lytic in character to those with dense areas containing radiopaque lumps, clouds, or spicules of tumor bone in varying patterns of organization. Discontinuities in the cortex surrounding the lesion are common. In other cases, there may be hyperostotic periosteal reactions of laminated bone. When the tumor growth is very rapid, it penetrates and destroys the cortex, growing directly into the soft tissue surrounding the bone, and it leaves only a cuff of periosteal new bone at the peripheral margin of the tumor, just at the point of penetration (Codman's triangle). High plasma alkaline phosphatase levels are often present in those sarcomas that are predominantly osteogenic, and the level of this activity parallels the course of the tumor. When lesions are adequately treated by amputation or radiation, the level of alkaline phosphatase falls, and when metastases appear, the level rises again, often reaching values higher than those present initially. When values are initially very high, the course is often rapidly fatal. Metastases occur primarily by the hematogenous route especially to the lung. Osteogenic sarcomas are relatively radio-resistant, and although some use radiotherapy as an adjuvant to primary ablative treatment, i.e., amputation, the mortality is extremely high even when treatment is promptly instituted.

Chondrosarcomas are clinically distinguishable from osteogenic sarcomas. In contrast to the latter, chondrosarcomas arise usually in adulthood and old age, with the peak incidence in the fourth, fifth, and sixth decades. Most are located in the pelvic girdle, ribs, and upper ends of the femur and humerus and are rare in the distal portions of the extremities. Chondrosarcomas may also arise by malignant transformation of osteochondromas. As a rule chondrosarcomas are slow growing and slow to recur. Radiographically the lesions appear destructive, with mottled increases in radiodensity which reflect the variable degree of calcification of cartilage matrix and ossification. Radical excision is the treatment of choice.

Ewing's tumor This is a malignant sarcoma composed of small, round cells which occurs most frequently in the first three decades of life. Most are located in some portion of the long bones, although any bone may be involved. Ewing's sarcoma is a highly malignant lesion with an extremely low incidence of cure whether by ablative surgery or irradiation.

TUMORS METASTATIC TO BONE The skeleton is one of the most common sites of metastases from carcinomas and sarcomas. Skeletal metastases may be relatively silent or may produce symptoms by the same mechanism that primary tumors do, i.e., pain, swelling, deformity of a bone, encroachment on hematopoietic tissue in the marrow, compression of spinal cord or nerve roots, and pathologic fractures. In addition, rapidly lytic skeletal metastases can result in hypercalcemia and in some instances renal insufficiency secondary to the hypercalcemia. The bones involved most commonly are the vertebras, proximal femur, pelvis, ribs, sternum, and proximal humerus, in that order of frequency. The carcinomas that most frequently metastasize to bone arise in prostate, breast, lung, thyroid, kidney, and bladder.

Malignant cells reach the skeleton via the bloodstream. Those that survive may proliferate and distort the normal architecture, probably by production of substances which cause dissolution of the mineral phase and the organic matrix.

Osteolysis most often results from stimulated modulation of osteoprogenitor cells to osteoclasts in the surrounding bone. Parathyroid hormone–like polypeptides, prostaglandins, and other as yet unidentified substances capable of stimulating bone resorption may be formed by malignant cells. Examples of carcinomatous metastases which are usually predominantly osteolytic are those arising from thyroid, kidney, and lower bowel. Other tumors induce an *osteoblastic* response in which the new bone arises from skeletal cells and not the tumor itself. The resulting lesion may appear more dense than the surrounding tissue. Occasionally the increase in radiodensity is uniform, simulating osteosclerosis. Carcinoma of the prostate characteristically produces osteoblastic metastases. Carcinoma of the breast produces both osteolytic and osteoblastic metastases. Malignant carcinoid tumors arising from the embryonic foregut and hindgut metastasize to bone with high frequency, producing an osteoblastic reaction. Hodgkin's disease in bone also produces an osteoblastic response both focal and diffuse. More malignant lymphomas in bone produce predominantly destructive lesions. As a rule, osteolytic metastases are the ones which produce hypercalcemia, hypercalcuria, and increased hydroxyprolinuria (reflecting matrix destruction) and are associated usually with normal or slightly increased levels of serum alkaline phosphatase. Osteoblastic metastases, on the other hand, are often accompanied by hyperphosphatasia and may even be associated with hypocalcemia. With some metastases, (such as in carcinoma of the breast) there may be phases in which osteolysis predominates (with hypercalcuria, hypercalcemia, and normal alkaline phosphatase levels) alternating with phases in which alkaline phosphatase levels rise and the skeletal lesions become more sclerotic.

Treatment of skeletal metastases is usually palliative. In the case of slowly growing localized lesions such as in some instances of carcinoma of the thyroid or occasionally in carcinoma of the kidney, local radiation is useful to relieve pain or reduce compression of surrounding structures. Many patients with carcinomas of breast or prostate will survive for years even after extensive skeletal metastases are recognized. Castration and estrogen therapy will slow the progress of the lesions in patients with metastatic prostatic carcinoma (see Chap. 91). When patients with mammary cancer are treated with estrogens or androgens, the character of the reaction to the metastases may temporarily shift from a predominantly osteoplastic to a lytic phase with resultant hypercalcemia (see Chap. 93). It is also important to recognize that hypercalcemia in patients with malignant tumors is not due solely to skeletal metastases, although this is the most common situation. Production of parathyroid hormone–like polypeptides and other osteolytic substances by extraskeletal neoplasms may also result in elevation of serum calcium levels. In the latter, hypophosphatemia is often encountered, whereas in the hypercalcemia associated with skeletal metastases serum phosphorus levels are usually normal or elevated. Hypercalcemia per se, whether spontaneous or induced by therapy, may produce symptoms such as anorexia, polyuria, polydipsia, depression, and eventually coma. In addition, nephrocalcinosis can result from hypercalcemia, and death may result from renal insufficiency. Treatment of hypercalcemia of any cause is discussed in Chap. 350.

OTHER DISORDERS OF BONE AND CARTILAGE

FIBROUS DYSPLASIA (ALBRIGHT'S SYNDROME)

Albright and his associates, in 1937, described a syndrome characterized by "osteitis fibrosa disseminata, areas of pigmentation and endocrine dysfunction, with precocious puberty in females." It was subsequently recognized that the bony lesions, called *fibrous dysplasia*, may occur in the absence of the other features of Albright's syndrome. The fundamental nature of the osseous disorder is unknown; the disease does not appear to be heritable. The frequency of the disease is approximately the same in both sexes.

Incidence The lesions of fibrous dysplasia may be confined to one bone or be polyostotic in distribution. In patients with monostotic involvement, the majority of the lesions are in craniofacial bones and ribs; other features of the syndrome are usually absent in these subjects. In contrast, the polyostotic lesions occur in almost every bone, occasionally including over 50 percent of the skeleton. They may be confined to one side and be striking in extent. Involvement of the lower extremities is especially frequent. Approximately one-half of the females (girls) with the polyostotic form have abnormal pigmentation and sexual precocity. Abnormal pigmentation is also seen in about one-half of the males (boys).

Pathology The lesions of polyostotic fibrous dysplasia are of uniform reddish-gray color and are finely gritty in texture. Microscopically they are composed of fibrous tissue having the appearance typical of fibromata embedded in which are areas of coarse fiber bone with wide osteoid seams. Cement lines are prominent. Mature lamellar bone does not form. Occasionally multiple islands of cartilage and fluid-filled cysts are present. The lesions of monostotic fibrous dysplasia are similar to those in the polyostotic form except that cartilage and fluid-filled cysts are not found.

Radiologic changes The roentenographic appearance of the lesions is that of a radiolucent area with a smooth border, typically associated with focal thinning of the cortex of the bone. These lesions are not usually cysts in the strict sense, since they are not fluid-filled cavities. They occasionally appear multiloculate. The so-called *ground-glass appearance* reflects the content of thin, calcified trabeculae of fiber bone. Frequently deformities are present such as coxa vara, shepherd's-crook deformity of the femur, bowing of the tibia, Harrison's grooves, and protusio acetabuli. Involvement of facial bones usually with lesions of increased radiodensity may create a leonine appearance (leontiasis ossea) superficially resembling that seen in some patients with leprosy. Advanced skeletal age may be noted, which in females is correlated with sexual precocity but may also be seen in males without sexual precocity. Although the lesions tend to spare the epiphyseal regions before puberty, in older individuals fibrous dysplasia may develop in the epiphyses.

Clinical picture The clinical course is highly variable. Skeletal lesions are usually detected because of deformity or fractures. In some females sexual precocity is the presenting complaint, occasionally present years before the appearance of skeletal symptoms. Serum calcium and phosphorus values are usually normal. In approximately one-third of patients with polyostotic fibrous dysplasia, levels of serum alkaline phosphatase may be elevated in some instances to very high values, and urinary hydroxyproline excretion is often increased. In some subjects, high cardiac output similar to that seen in extensive Paget's disease may be found. In general, patients with extensive involvement have widespread disease when symptoms first appear, whereas with mild disease at the onset extensive disease does not usually develop.

The abnormal cutaneous pigmentation that is seen in most patients with Albright's syndrome consists of isolated dark-brown to light-brown macules which tend to remain on one side of the midline. The border is usually, although not always, irregular or jagged ("coast of Maine") in contrast to the smooth borders of the pigmented macules of neurofibromatosis ("coast of California"). As a rule there are fewer than six of the lesions, which range in size from 1 cm to those covering very large areas. When the lesions are present in the scalp, the overlying hair may be more deeply pigmented than that over the remainder of the scalp. There is a strong tendency for the pigmentation to be on the same side as the skeletal lesions and actually overlie them.

The sexual precocity of unknown cause previously mentioned is usually restricted to females, although it has been described rarely in males. Premature vaginal bleeding and development of axillary and pubic hair and of breasts are the main features. In the few ovaries that have been examined, no corpora lutea have been seen. Precocious sexuality is not limited to patients with cranial involvement, and although the characteristic pigmented macules are usually found, this association is not invariable. Another endocrine abnormality present with increased frequency is hyperthyroidism. Rarer associations include Cushing's syndrome and acromegaly.

Although the lytic lesions of fibrous dysplasia resemble superficially the brown tumors of hyperparathyroidism, the age of the patient, normocalcemia, increased density of bone in the skull, and areas of cutaneous pigmentation identify the former condition. However, fibrous dysplasia and hyperparathyroidism may coexist. Neurofibroma may involve bone and produce cutaneous pigmentation as well as nodules in the skin. The pigmented macules of neurofibromatosis are more numerous and more widely distributed than in fibrous dysplasia, usually have smooth borders, and tend to involve areas such as the axillary folds. Other lesions which may have a roentgenographic appearance similar to that of isolated fibrous dysplasia are unicameral bone cysts, aneurysmal bone cysts, and nonossifying fibromata. Leontiasis ossea is most often due to fibrous dysplasia, although other disorders may also produce this appearance such as craniometaphyseal dysplasia, hyperphosphatasia, and, in adults, Paget's disease.

Treatment Fibrous dysplasia, when symptomatic, can be managed by a variety of orthopedic operative procedures such as osteotomy, curettage, and bone grafting. Indications for such procedures include progressive deformity, nonunion of fractures, and persistent pain unresponsive to conservative treatment.

DYSPLASIAS AND CHONDRODYSTROPHIES A variety of diseases of bone and cartilage have been called dystrophies or dysplasias. Classification has been difficult, since the underlying defect is not usually known. It is possible that a biochemical lesion, such as that in the metabolism of the mucopolysaccharides demonstrated in the Hunter and Hurler syndromes, will also be found in a number of these disorders and permit more than a descriptive classification. However, a useful scheme has been proposed by Rubin based on the consideration of errors in modeling of bone and cartilage as departures from normal development (Table 354-2). Pathologic processes in the skeletal dysplasias may be expressed as a deficiency (hypoplasia) or excess (hyperplasia) in relation to normal development. Several of the more common of these will be described.

Spondyloepiphyseal dysplasia The spondyloepiphyseal dysplasias are disorders in which abnormalities of growth occur in various bones including the vertebras, pelvis, carpal and tarsal bones, and the epiphyses of tubular bones. On the basis of roentgenographic findings, this group can be divided into: (1) those with generalized platyspondyly, (2) those with multiple epiphyseal dysplasias, and (3) those with epiphysometaphyseal dysplasias. *Morquio's syndrome*, a mucopolysaccharidosis inherited as an autosomal recessive character and associated with corneal opacities, dental defects, and variable disturbances in intellect and characterized by increased urinary excretion of keratosulfate, belongs in the first group. Other forms of spondyloepiphyseal dysplasias show no abnormality in mucopolysaccharide metabolism and are sometimes not recognized until late in childhood. Flat vertebral bodies are associated with other abnormalities in shape and alignment. The disordered development of the capital femoral epiphyses leads to irregularities in shape and flattening of the femoral heads and early onset of osteoarthritis of the hips.

Achondroplasia *Achondroplasia* is an example of a physeal dysplasia in which dwarfism results from decrease in the proliferation of cartilage in the growth plate. This disorder of unknown cause is among the more common types of dwarfism and is inherited as an autosomal dominant trait. Histologic sections through the growth plate show a thin zone of cartilage cells with absence of the normal columnar arrangement and zone of provisional calcification. Formation of the primary spongiosa is defective. However, formation and maturation of the secondary ossification centers and articular cartilage are not disturbed. Appositional growth at the metaphysis continues, with resulting flare in this region of the bone; intramembranous bone formation at the periosteum is normal. The result of abnormal proliferation at the growth plate, leaving other areas relatively unaffected in the tubular bones, is the production of short bones which are proportionately thick. However, the length of the spine is almost always normal. The appearance of short limbs with a normal trunk is characteristically accompanied by a large head, saddlenose, and an exaggerated lumbar lordosis. The disease is usually recognized at birth. Those who survive the period of infancy usually have normal mental and sexual development, and longevity may be unimpaired. However, spinal deformity may lead to neurologic signs of cord compression and nerve root encroachment in a significant number of affected individuals, especially those with kyphoscoliosis.

Enchondromatosis (dyschondroplasia, Ollier's disease) This is also a disorder affecting the growth plate in which the hypertrophic cartilage is not resorbed and ossified in a normal fashion. It results in masses of cartilage with disorderly arrangement of the chondrocytes showing variable proliferative and hypertrophic changes. These masses are located in the metaphyses in

TABLE 354-2
Proposed classification of bone dysplasias

- *I* Epiphyseal dysplasias
  - *A* Epiphyseal hypoplasias
    - *1* Failure of articular cartilage; spondyloepiphyseal dysplasia, congenita and tarda
    - *2* Failure of ossification of center: multiple epiphyseal dysplasia, congenita and tarda
  - *B* Epiphyseal hyperplasia
    - *1* Excess of articular cartilage: dysplasia epiphysalis hemimelica
- *II* Physeal (growth plate) dysplasias
  - *A* Cartilage hypoplasias
    - *1* Failure of proliferating cartilage: achondroplasia, congenita and tarda
    - *2* Failure of hypertrophic cartilage: metaphyseal dysostosis, congenita and tarda
  - *B* Cartilage hyperplasias
    - *1* Excess of proliferating cartilage: hyperchondroplasia
    - *2* Excess of hypertrophic cartilage: enchondromatosis
- *III* Metaphyseal dysplasias
  - *A* Metaphyseal hypoplasias
    - *1* Failure to form primary spongiosa: hypophosphatasia, congenita and tarda
    - *2* Failure to absorb primary spongiosa: osteopetrosis, congenita and tarda
    - *3* Failure to absorb secondary spongiosa: craniometaphyseal dysplasia, congenita and tarda
  - *B* Metaphyseal hyperplasia
    - *1* Excessive spongiosa: familial exostosis
- *IV* Diaphyseal dysplasias
  - *A* Diaphyseal hypoplasias
    - *1* Failure of periosteal bone formation: osteogenesis imperfecta, congenita and tarda
    - *2* Failure of endosteal bone formation: idiopathic osteoporosis
  - *B* Diaphyseal hyperplasias
    - *1* Excessive periosteal bone formation: Engelmann's disease
    - *2* Excessive periosteal bone formation: hyperphosphatasia

close association with the growth plate. The disorder is usually recognized in childhood by the appearance of deformities or retardation in growth. The most common sites of involvement are the ends of long bones, usually in that region where rate of growth is most marked. The pelvis is often involved, but bone such as ribs, sternum, and skull are seldom affected. There is also a tendency toward unilateral involvement. Chondrosarcoma develops rarely in the enchondromata. The association of enchondromatosis and cavernous hemangiomata in the soft tissues is known as Maffucci's syndrome.

Multiple exostoses (diaphyseal aclasis) This is a disorder of the metaphysis, inherited as an autosomal dominant character, in which areas of the growth plate become displaced and are followed by formation of spongiosa in an abnormal position in relation to the shaft. Usually the growth of these exostoses ceases when growth of the adjacent plate ceases. The lesions may be solitary or multiple and are usually located in the metaphyseal areas of long bones with the apex of the exostosis directed toward the diaphysis. Often the lesions produce no symptoms, but occasionally interference with the function of a joint or tendon or compression of nerves may result. Dwarfing is seen occasionally. The metacarpals may be shortened, resembling those seen in Albright's hereditary osteodystrophy. Indeed, multiple exostoses are sometimes seen in patients with the pseudohypoparathyroid syndrome.

An exostosis may suddenly begin to enlarge long after growth should have ceased, and occasionally, chondrosarcomas develop at the site of an exostosis. Although the exact incidence of this complication is not known, estimates as high as 7 to 11 percent have been made.

RELAPSING POLYCHONDRITIS Relapsing polychondritis is an inflammatory disease of cartilaginous structures. The cause is unknown, and although it may occur as a separate entity, it is often associated with other disorders of connective tissue such as rheumatoid arthritis and systemic lupus erythematosus. It may occur at any age, and both sexes are equally affected. The course is commonly a relapsing one with attacks which last from a few days to several months occurring from several times a month to once in several years. The external ear and the cartilage of the nose are the common sites, but other cartilages may also be involved, including those of joints, trachea, larynx, bronchi, costal cartilage, and epiglottis. During an acute attack in a cartilaginous structure such as the ear, there is swelling, redness, pain, and tenderness. Fever and malaise are prominent systemic manifestations; subsequently the ear may become softened and atrophic. Saddlenose deformity may result from involvement of the nose. The joint disease resembles rheumatoid arthritis in some patients, whereas in others, articular symptoms are ascribable to a tendonitis. Cardiac involvement with aortic insufficiency and mitral regurgitation has also been described. Ocular involvement with episcleritis, iritis, and conjunctivitis is also seen. During acute attacks the erythrocyte sedimentation rate is usually elevated, and urinary excretion of acid mucopolysaccharides is increased. In the patients with involvement of the trachcobronchial tree respiratory obstruction may result in death if not treated promptly with tracheostomy.

Histologic sections from biopsy or necropsy material have shown diffuse destruction and alteration in the staining properties of the cartilage matrix, focal calcification, metaplastic bone formation, replacement of cartilage with fibrous tissue, and a variable, chronic inflammatory reaction. Salicylates may be helpful in the mild cases, although corticosteroids are indicated in patients with severe involvement. Initial dose of prednisone or its equivalent usually is 30 mg daily with gradual tapering as the clinical signs permit.

TIETZE'S SYNDROME (COSTOCHONDRAL SYNDROME) Tietze's syndrome is a disorder of unknown cause which is characterized by painful tender swellings of the costochondral junctions. Individuals in the third and fourth decades are most commonly affected, and the disorder is rare before puberty and after the age of sixty. There is no predilection for either sex. Most patients have single episodes involving a single area, with the gradual or sudden onset of pain followed by swelling in the same area. The second costal cartilage on either side is the most common area but almost all the costochondral articulations have been involved. In some individuals multiple areas are tender in an individual attack. On examination a firm, tender swelling is palpable without warmth or fluctuation. Fever and systemic symptoms are absent, and all laboratory examinations, including the erythrocyte sedimentation rate, are normal. Pain lasts from weeks to months, and swelling lasts for a longer period. When biopsies have been performed, the cartilage appears normal. The disorder is self-limited, and no treatment is indicated except for nerve block and local infiltration with corticosteroids only in those instances where pain is unbearable. The major interest in Tietze's syndrome is that the pain in the anterior chest region may mimic that of myocardial infarction or angina pectoris. Neoplasms and suppurative, rheumatoid, and gouty arthritis may all have to be considered in the differential diagnosis.

REFERENCES

Bone and cartilage

ALBRIGHT FA et al: Syndrome characterized by osteitis fibrosa, disseminate areas of pigmentation and endocrine dysfunction, with precocious puberty in females: Report of five cases. N Engl J Med 216:727, 1937

ALTERMAN SL, LIEBER AL: Albright's hereditary osteodystrophy: The effect of treatment during adolescence. Ann Intern Med 63:140, 1965

BAILEY JA: Orthopaedic aspects of achondroplasia. J Bone Joint Surg [Br] 52A:1285, 1970

BENEDICT PH: Endocrine features in Albright's syndrome (fibrous dysplasia of bone). Metabolism 11:30, 1962

—— et al: Melanotic macules in Albright's syndrome and in neurofibromatosis. JAMA 209:72, 1968

BURCH GE, DEPASQUALE NP: Tietze's disease. Geriatrics 19:61, 1964

DANES BS, GROSSMAN H: Bone dysplasias, including Morquio's

syndrome, studied in skin fibroblast cultures. Am J Med 47:708, 1969

Hall R, Warrick C: Hypersecretion of hypothalamic releasing hormones: A possible explanation of the endocrine manifestations of polyostotic fibrous dysplasia (Albright's syndrome). Lancet 1:1313, 1972

Harris WH et al: The natural history of fibrous dysplasia: An orthopaedic, pathological and roentgenographic study. J Bone Joint Surg 44A:207, 1962

Hemry DA et al: Relapsing polychondritis, a "floppy" mitral valve, and polytendonitis. Ann Intern Med 77:576, 1972

Kaye RL, Sones DA: Relapsing polychondritis: Clinical and pathologic features in fourteen cases. Ann Intern Med 60:653, 1964

Langer LO Jr, Carey LS: The roentgenographic features of the KS mucopolysaccharidosis of Morquio (Morquio-Brailsford's disease). Am J Roentgenol 97:1, 1966

Levey GS, Calabro JJ: Tietze's syndrome: Report of two cases and review of the literature. Arthritis Rheum 5:261, 1962

Rubin P: *Dynamic Classification of Bone Dysplasias*, Chicago: Year Book, 1964

Hyperostosis

Collins DH, Dodge OG: *Pathology of Bone*, London: Butterworth, 1966

Dent CE et al: Studies in osteopetrosis. Arch Dis Child 40:7, 1965

Elmore SM et al: Pyknodysostosis, with a familial chromosome anomaly. Am J Med 40:273, 1966

Follis RH Jr: A survey of bone disease. Am J Med 22:469, 1957

Johnston CC et al: Osteopetrosis: A clinical, genetic, metabolic and morphologic study of the dominantly inherited benign form. Medicine 47:149, 1968

Murphy HM: Calcitonin-like activity in the circulation of osteopetrotic grey-lethal mice. J Endocrinol 53:139, 1972

Thompson RC Jr et al: Hereditary hyperphosphatasia. Am J Med 47:209, 1969

Van Buchem FSP et al: Hyperostosis corticalis generalisata. Am J Med 33:387, 1962

Neoplasms

Jaffe HL: *Tumors and Tumorous Conditions of the Bones and Joints*, Philadelphia: Lea & Febiger, 1958

Lodwick GS: *The Bones and Joints*, Chicago: Year Book, 1971

Moseley JE: *Bone Changes in Hematologic Disorders*, New York: Grune & Stratton, 1963

Muggia FM, Heinemann HO: Hypercalcemia associated with neoplastic disease. Ann Intern Med 73:281, 1970

section 14 | Disorders of the joints and connective tissues

355 APPROACH TO DISORDERS OF THE JOINTS

BRUCE C. GILLILAND
MART MANNIK

The causes of joint disorders are numerous and include traumatic, infectious, metabolic, immunologic, and neoplastic processes. However, often the cause remains unknown, and at times the disease mechanisms have been partially elucidated. Many classifications of joint disorders have been proposed, but they seldom serve as a useful guideline in arriving at a logical diagnosis. The purpose of this chapter is to present an approach to the patient with joint disease, without giving detailed discussion of the differential diagnoses. Table 355-1 should serve as a guide to a group of disorders with common manifestations that may be divided further by means of historical, physical, or laboratory information. Because specific tests are frequently not available for each branching point in the flow sheet, clinical judgment and bedside information become highly important for achieving the correct diagnosis. The detailed differential diagnoses are discussed in the appropriate chapters.

Disorders of joints can produce pain, stiffness, swelling, redness, increased warmth, or limitation of motion. Involvement of a single joint or of several joints may be a manifestation of a systemic illness or may be due to a disorder confined to the joints. Therefore, a complete history and physical examination are mandatory to seek extraarticular features of specific diseases. The number of joints involved, the location of involved joints (peripheral small joints, proximal large joints, spine), and the pattern of involved joints (symmetric or asymmetric) provide useful diagnostic clues. The course of joint involvement is important because some disorders are self-limited and leave no residua, whereas other disorders are chronic and may lead to progressive joint destruction. Specific radiographs and laboratory tests can provide useful diagnostic information. Synovial fluid examination and synovial tissue biopsy also can yield specific diagnostic information.

The initial step is to determine whether the symptoms attributed to joint(s) are articular or periarticular. Periarticular disease may produce symptoms related to the joint. Bursitis, tendonitis, and cellulitis can be differentiated from articular disease by a negative joint examination and positive evidence of periarticular disorders. The depressed or anxious patient may have joint symptoms; patients with psychogenic rheumatism have no musculoskeletal abnormalities. However, patients with early rheumatoid arthritis or other joint diseases may have no

TABLE 355-1
Approach to joint disorders*

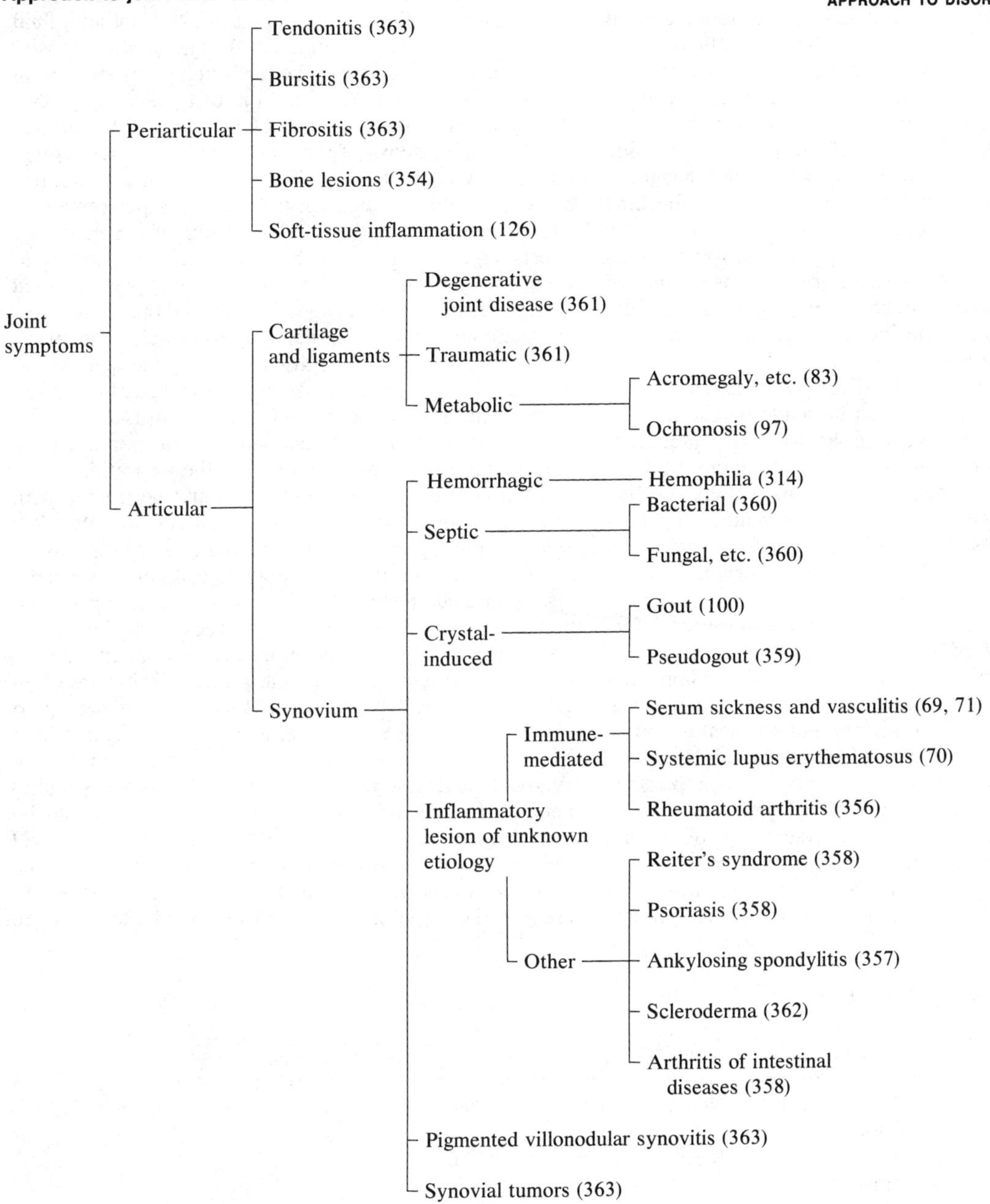

* *Numbers in parentheses indicate chapters containing detailed discussions.*

objective evidence of disease, and therefore reevaluation with the passage of time is necessary. Articular involvement is manifested by joint tenderness, increased warmth, erythema, synovial effusion, synovial hypertrophy, and restriction of joint motion or crepitation. A synovial effusion in the knee and other joints is best detected by a fluid wave (bulge sign) or by transmission of pressure by the fluid that distends the joint. In the knee a patellar click or ballotement can help in identifying a large amount of fluid, but the bulge sign permits detection of as little as 5 ml of synovial fluid. Synovial fluid may be present in knee joints in edematous states even in the absence of an underlying joint disorder. Fluid in other joints may be more difficult to demonstrate, especially in the hip joint. Synovial hypertrophy is palpable as boggy tissue around the joint margins. Joint involvement is also suggested by the finding of pain on firm compression of the joint and by decrease in muscle strength adjacent to the involved joint (e.g., quadriceps atrophy and weakness with knee disease, or decreased grip strength with involvement of the wrists and small joints of the hand). The joint examination should include assessment of all joints even though symptoms are localized to one joint or a few joints.

Joint symptoms may originate primarily from diseased cartilage and supporting structure involvement or from synovial tissue disease. The inflammatory arthritides are characterized by synovitis and accumulation of inflammatory cells in the synovial fluid. Degenerative joint disease, ochronosis, and some of the metabolic diseases such as acromegaly and hyperparathyroidism involve primary cartilage and supporting structures; synovial inflammation tends to be chronic and low grade.

Inspection and examination of the joint may provide information about the underlying pathologic change. A history of antecedent trauma is important in establishing traumatic arthritis. In inflammatory joint disease, the joint is swollen and often warm. Synovial hypertrophy may be present. In degenerative joint disease, synovial effusion may be found but the overlying tissues usually do not show inflammation; bony overgrowth at the joint margins may be present.

Among the disorders that affect primarily the synovium, further discrimination can be made by the history, such as bleeding episodes in hemophilia, antecedent infections in septic arthritis, recurrent attacks of gout, multisystem involvement in systemic lupus erythematosus, associated intestinal diseases in ulcerative colitis, etc., and physical examination such as lesions in psoriasis, butterfly rash in systemic lupus erythematosus, etc. However, the examination of synovial fluid becomes mandatory to establish the specific diagnosis of infections, crystal-induced arthritides, pigmented villonodular synovitis, and neoplasms involving the joint. Inflammatory joint diseases of unknown cause often can be diagnosed on the basis of the history and physical examination without the examination of synovial fluid. However, the synovial fluid should be examined when possible because it may provide a precise diagnosis or further clues to an accurate diagnosis. Aspiration of a joint should be performed under aseptic conditions.

Table 355-2 lists the characteristics of joint fluid for the major types of arthritis. Normal joint fluid is clear and straw-colored. Turbidity is produced by inflammatory cells and occasionally by a chylous effusion. Fragments of cartilage and fibrin may be present. Normal joint fluid is quite viscous, because of hyaluronic acid. The viscosity is reduced in inflammatory arthritides, especially in chronic rheumatoid arthritis. Viscosity can be grossly evaluated by forcing a drop of fluid from the syringe. Fluid of high viscosity forms a string several inches long; fluid of low viscosity drops like water. The mucin clot test correlates with the viscosity. This test is performed by adding acetic acid to joint fluid from which cells and debris have been removed by centrifugation. The formation of a tight, ropy clot that remains intact is interpreted as indicating qualitatively good mucin and the presence of adequate molecules of intact hyaluronic acid. The mucin clot in degenerative joint disease is of good quality and quantity. Fluid from an inflammatory effusion often forms a fibrin clot and should not be confused with the mucin clot. Normal joint fluid will not clot spontaneously unless blood enters the joint during the aspiration.

Synovial fluid for cell counts should be treated with anticoagulants. Normal joint fluid contains less than 200 cells per mm^3, predominantly mononuclear white cells. In degenerative joint disease the white cell count is usually less than 2,000 per mm^3 and the cells are also predominantly mononuclear. Variable degrees of leukocytosis, consisting mainly of neutrophils, are seen in inflammatory joint diseases; cell counts in septic arthritis are often greater than 50,000 per mm^3. White cell counts up to 50,000 per mm^3 or even higher may occasionally be found in nonseptic joints. For proper interpretation of the synovial fluid glucose, blood should be drawn simultaneously for glucose analysis; both samples should be obtained 6 hr after a meal. The synovial fluid glucose level falls with increasing inflammation, and the difference between levels of serum and synovial fluid glucose increases. The level in septic arthritis may be less than 50

TABLE 355-2
Synovial fluid characteristics in major joint diseases

Diagnosis	*Appearance*	*Fibrin clot*	*Mucin* clot*	*WBC/ mm³*	*PMN†, %*	*Sugar, % of blood level*
Normal	Straw-colored, clear	None	Good	<200	<25	~100
Degenerative joint disease	Slightly turbid	Small	Good	<2,000	<25	~100
Traumatic arthritis	Straw-colored, bloody or xanthochromic	Small	Good	2,000	<25	~100
Rheumatoid arthritis	Turbid	Large	Fair to poor	5,000–50,000	>65	75‡
Other types of inflammatory arthritis§	Turbid	Large	Fair to poor	5,000–50,000	>50	75
Acute gout or pseudogout	Turbid	Large	Fair to poor	5,000–50,000	>75	90
Septic arthritis	Very turbid or purulent	Large	Poor	50,000–200,000	>80	<50
Tuberculous arthritis	Turbid	Large	Poor	~25,000	Variable	<50

* *Correlates with viscosity.*
† *PMN, polymorphonuclear cells.*
‡ *May be less than 50 percent.*
§ *Includes Reiter's syndrome, psoriatic arthritis, ankylosing spondylitis (peripheral joints), arthritis associated with intestinal diseases.*

percent of the serum glucose. A low synovial glucose level also can be seen in rheumatoid arthritis.

Synovial fluid should be examined under polarized light for the presence of crystals. The crystals of gout and pseudogout are differentiated by their size, shape, and properties under compensated polarized light. The fluid to be used for examination of crystals should be anticoagulated with heparin, since crystalline anticoagulants may be mistaken for crystals in synovial fluid.

A gram stain and stains for tubercle bacilli should be performed on the sediment of synovial fluid. Bacterial, fungal, and viral cultures should be obtained when these infections are suspected.

Determination of the joint fluid complement is useful, but specific diagnostic information is not obtained from this measurement. Synovial fluid complement level is low in comparison to serum complement, in normal subjects as well as in patients with degenerative joint disease, because these macromolecules do not readily enter the uninflamed synovial cavity. The inflamed synovium is more permeable to large molecules, and therefore the synovial fluid complement approaches serum levels in inflammatory joint disease. However, the complement level in inflammatory conditions may be quite low because of consumption by antigen-antibody complexes; thus, the joint fluid complement in rheumatoid arthritis may be low when compared with the serum complement level. In rheumatoid arthritis the low joint fluid complement is found in patients with a high titer of rheumatoid factor. In some patients with Reiter's syndrome, the level of joint fluid complement is higher than that found in other inflammatory arthritides.

Needle biopsy of the synovium can provide precise diagnostic information. With currently available needles, a biopsy can be performed on most large joints with relatively little discomfort. If bedside observations and synovial fluid studies have not yielded a diagnosis, a biopsy should be considered. In systemic diseases with joint involvement (tuberculosis, hemochromatosis, etc.), synovial biopsy is necessary to ascertain whether the articular disease is due to the underlying systemic disorder. Synovial biopsy may lead to a diagnosis of tuberculosis, coccidioidomycosis, hemochromatosis, sarcoidosis, amyloidosis, pigmented villonodular synovitis, or synovial tumors. A biopsy may support the diagnosis of rheumatoid arthritis, systemic lupus erythematosus, or Reiter's syndrome, but the biopsy alone will not suffice for a diagnosis in these diseases.

REFERENCES

HOLLANDER JL: Introduction to arthritis and the rheumatic diseases, chap. 1, and Intrasynovial corticosteroid therapy, chap. 32, in *Arthritis and Allied Conditions*, 8th ed., ed JL Hollander, Philadelphia: Lea & Febiger, 1972

JESSAR RA: The study of synovial fluid, chap. 6 in *Arthritis and Allied Conditions*, 8th ed., ed JL Hollander, Philadelphia: Lea & Febiger, 1972

LOCKIE LM: Examination of the arthritic patient, chap. 2 in *Arthritis and Allied Conditions*, 8th ed., ed JL Hollander, Philadelphia: Lea & Febiger, 1972

MCCARTY DJ JR: A basic guide to arthrocentesis. Hosp Med p. 77, Nov. 1968

PEKIN TJ, ZVAIFLER NJ: Hemolytic complement in synovial fluid. J Clin Invest 43:1372, 1964

RUDDY S, AUSTEN KF: The complement system in rheumatoid synovitis. Arthritis Rheum 13:713, 1970

SCHUMACHER HR, KULKA JP: Needle biopsy of the synovial membrane—experience with the Parker-Pearson technique. N Engl J Med 286:416, 1972

356
RHEUMATOID ARTHRITIS

BRUCE C. GILLILAND
MART MANNIK

INTRODUCTION Rheumatoid arthritis (subsequently abbreviated RA) is a chronic systemic disease of unknown etiology, manifested primarily by inflammatory arthritis of peripheral joints, usually in a symmetric distribution. Systemic manifestations include hematologic, pulmonary, neurologic, and cardiovascular abnormalities.

PATHOGENESIS The serum and joint fluid of the majority of patients with RA contain antibodies specific for IgG (rheumatoid factor). These antibodies are heterogeneous and consist of IgM, IgG, and IgA. The stimulus for rheumatoid factor synthesis appears to be chronic antigenic challenge. Studies have shown that animals immunized with altered autologous IgG form antibodies to IgG. In addition, similar antibodies appear in the serum of animals repeatedly immunized with *Escherichia coli.* Patients with subacute bacterial endocarditis or with other forms of chronic infection develop rheumatoid factors which disappear from the serum after successful treatment of the infection. These observations suggest that IgG, altered as a result of combining with an antigen, can serve as the immunogenic stimulus for the synthesis of rheumatoid factors (antibodies to IgG). Chronic arthritis does not appear in the above-mentioned patients or in the immunized animals, indicating that the presence of rheumatoid factors alone does not contribute to the pathogenesis of rheumatoid arthritis. In RA, the reasons for the appearance and continued production of rheumatoid factors remain unknown.

Though the presence of rheumatoid factor in the serum apparently does not lead to the development of rheumatoid arthritis, increasing evidence shows that immunologic mechanisms play an important role in the pathogenesis of synovitis in RA. Lymphocytes and plasma cells in the synovium synthesize immunoglobulins, including some with antibody specificity to IgG. Immunoglobulin (IgG, IgA, IgM) deposits, together with complement components, are found in articular cartilage, in synovium, and in phagocytic cells of the synovial membrane. Immunoglobulins, including some with antibody specificity to IgG, and complement occur in vacuoles of polymorphonuclear cells in the synovial fluid. Immune complexes composed of IgG and antibodies to IgG exist in synovial fluid. In addition, antinuclear antibodies and deoxyribonucleic acid (DNA) appear in the synovial fluid of some patients. The activation of complement by these immune complexes apparently leads to the generation of chemotactic and vasoactive factors, resulting in the influx of neutrophils into the joint. The finding of decreased complement components and total hemolytic complement and the presence of breakdown products of complement in synovial fluid support this notion. Phagocytosis of immune complexes by polymorphonuclear cells results in the release of lysosomal enzymes capable of producing tissue injury. Among other enzymatic effects, collagenase activity exists in the synovial fluid. The role of cellular immunity in RA has not yet been clearly defined. However, the abundance of lymphocytes in the inflamed synovium suggests that these cells are important in the inflammation of RA.

The pathogenic mechanisms of extraarticular manifestations of RA have not been identified with certainty. However, mounting evidence indicates that humoral immune mechanisms participate in this process. The acute vasculitic lesions of RA contain immunoglobulins and complement components. Patients with such lesions tend to have minimally depressed serum complement level, and these patients frequently have circulating immune complexes consisting of IgG and rheumatoid factors (IgM-rheumatoid factor or IgG-rheumatoid factor).

The etiologic factor or factors that set into motion the above immunologic events are not known. An infectious agent, viral or bacterial, may well initiate the inflammatory process in rheumatoid arthritis, but there is no unequivocal evidence for an infectious etiology.

EPIDEMIOLOGY The onset of RA may occur anytime in life. Approximately 70 percent of RA occurs between the third and seventh decades; the peak onset is in the fourth decade. The prevalence in North America ranges from 0.5 to 3.8 percent in women and from 0.15 to 1.3 percent in men, depending on which diagnostic criteria are applied in population studies. Women are affected approximately three times more often than men; however, this difference disappears in older age. Unknown environmental factors may play a role in the observed family aggregation of RA. Race and occupation appear to have no significance; climate may modify symptoms, but not the disease.

PATHOLOGY The synovium in rheumatoid arthritis shows edema, hypercellularity, and hyperemia. The synovium develops numerous folds consisting of large villi; it spreads to cover the articular cartilage with what is referred to as a *pannus.* The synovium invades the subchondral bone at the margin of the joint where the articular cartilage ends and the synovium is reflected from the periosteum, the so-called bare area. The earliest bony erosions are observed in this location. The pannus produces dissolution of the underlying articular cartilage. Later the opposing joint surfaces may form fibrous adhesions and subsequently bony ankylosis. The invasion of the subchondral bone and cartilaginous destruction are mediated by hydrolytic enzymes emanating from phagocytic cells in the synovial membrane and fluid. The inflammatory process weakens the joint capsule and supporting ligaments. The combination of joint destruction, loss of supporting structures, muscle atrophy, and imbalance of opposing muscle groups results in joint instability and subluxation. Persistent inflammation in the tendon sheaths may cause weakening and even rupture of the tendons.

Hypercellularity of the synovium results from the influx of lymphocytes, plasma cells, and mononuclear cells. The synovial lining cells proliferate and lose their organization. In more chronic disease, lymphocytes form follicles in the synovium.

The so-called rheumatoid nodules are fairly characteristic of RA. The center of the nodule consists of an area of fibrinoid necrosis and cellular debris, surrounded by several layers of pallisading large monocytic cells. The periphery is infiltrated with lymphocytes and monocytes. Small-vessel vasculitis is considered to be the initiating event in the formation of the nodule. Nodules are most often found in subcutaneous tissue over pressure points such as the elbows. They may be bound to the underlying periosteum. Nodules may appear on the dorsum of the fingers and may be attached to tendons. Solitary or multiple nodules may appear in the lung parenchyma. Nodules may be found in the pleura, in heart valves, in myocardium, and rarely in vocal cords.

Vasculitis involving small to medium-sized vessels occurs in RA. The histologic picture ranges from focal perivascular accumulation of lymphocytes to necrotizing lesions showing fibrinoid necrosis, disruption of the intima, and infiltration of polymorphonuclear cells. Immunoglobulins and complement deposits can be demonstrated by immunofluorescence in the vessel of acute lesions. Vasculitis of vasa nervorum may lead to peripheral neuropathy. Nail-fold thrombi, digital gangrene, and leg ulcers may occur. Necrotizing vasculitis involving intestinal wall, coronary, and cerebral arteries has also been described.

Atrophy of skeletal muscles with interstitial accumulation of lymphocytes is present. Rarely, myositis occurs that is indistinguishable histologically and clinically from polymyositis.

Lymphadenopathy next to the inflamed joint, as well as generalized lymphadenopathy, may be present. Histologically, the nodes show hyperplasia and in some instances may resemble those of giant follicular lymphoma.

CLINICAL MANIFESTATIONS The onset of RA in the majority of patients is insidious. A prodrome of fatigue, weakness, joint stiffness, and vague arthralgias and myalgias may precede by several weeks the appearance of joint swelling. Several joints are usually involved at the onset, especially those of the hands and feet. Disease, however, may initially be confined to a single joint, often the knee, before spreading to other joints in a symmetric pattern. Unlike the migratory polyarthritis of rheumatic fever, RA usually continues in the initially involved joints as other joints become affected. Some patients may have an acute onset, with fever and multiple swollen, painful joints. Raynaud's phenomenon occurs in some patients.

The course of RA is highly variable, making prognosis very difficult in the individual patient. Spontaneous remissions and exacerbations are characteristic; remissions are more apt to occur early in the disease. The majority of patients will experience progressive joint damage of varying degrees over the years. Fortunately, many patients will be able to function at home or at work, though often in limited capacity. Another group of patients, approximately 10 percent, will have relentless, destructive, crippling disease, leading ultimately to confinement in a wheelchair or bed. There is yet another group with mild, intermittent disease who seldom, if ever, seek medical attention.

Examination of involved joints reveals increased warmth, tenderness, and swelling, which early in the disease may be subtle. The synovium becomes palpable as boggy tissue around the joint margin. The skin over small joints often has a ruddy cyanotic hue; marked erythema is unusual. Muscle weakness and atrophy adjacent to the affected joint often parallel the severity of joint disease. Range of joint motion, especially extension, becomes limited. Flexion contractures and in some instances fibrous or bony ankylosis develop. Terms such as "swan neck," "boutonnière," and "cock-up toes" are used to describe joint deformities in the hands and feet. Another frequently observed deformity consists of volar subluxation and ulnar deviation of the fingers at the metacarpal-phalangeal joints. Flexion contractures of the knees and hips greatly hinder ambulation.

The duration of morning stiffness may be useful in assessing disease activity. During periods of active joint disease, the patient may complain of morning stiffness lasting an hour or more. With improvement, the duration of morning stiffness will decrease. Disease activity in the hands and wrist can be followed by measurement of grip strength, which is performed by having the patient compress a rolled-up, partially inflated sphygmomanometer cuff. Disease activity in lower extremities is assessed by recording the time required to walk a standard distance (e.g., 50 ft).

Though the disease may occur in any diarthrodial joint, the joints most commonly affected are the proximal interphalangeal, metacarpal-phalangeal, metatarsal-phalangeal, wrist, knees, elbows, and ankles. Cervical spine disease is common; however, the lower part of the spine is relatively spared. Unilateral sacroiliitis occurs but is of little clinical significance. A serious complication is *subluxation of the atlantoaxial joint*, which may lead to compression of the spinal cord by the odontoid process. Symptoms and signs of cord compression, such as bladder dysfunction, anal sphincter laxity, circumanal hypesthesia, and long-tract signs, should be sought. Sudden death has resulted from laceration of the cord by the odontoid process. *Temporomandibular disease* may interfere with mastication, and pain from this joint may be referred to the middle ear and throat. *Arthritis in the cricoarytenoid* joints can cause hoarseness or even life-threatening upper-airway obstruction if the joints are fixed in adduction. Tenosynovitis in the wrist may compress the medial nerve, causing a carpal tunnel syndrome.

Popliteal cyst may develop in patients with synovitis of the knee. The cyst forms either from herniation or rupture of the synovium posteriorly through the joint capsule or from communication of the joint with the semimembranosus bursa. The cyst enlarges because synovial fluid is forced into it by motion of the joint. The pressure of fluid is always greater in the knee than in the cyst. Hence, the communication between the knee joint and the cyst can be demonstrated only by injecting radiopaque dye into the knee joint. A popliteal cyst may extend down into the calf or up into the posterior thigh. A clinical picture resembling thrombophlebitis is produced by rupture of the popliteal cyst or by rupture of synovium of the knee even in the absence of a cyst. This diagnosis may be confirmed by performing an arthrogram.

Rheumatoid nodules are found in 20 percent of patients and are most commonly located over the extensor surface of the elbows. They may also be present over the extensor surface of the fingers and in other areas exposed to excessive pressure, such as the back of the head and over the sacrum in bedridden patients. The nodules may be freely movable or attached to tendons or the periosteum. They are usually firm and nontender but may be cystic. The overlying skin may break down and lead to chronic drainage. Nodules are usually associated with active disease and a positive test for rheumatoid factor.

The hands of a rheumatoid patient are often cool and damp, reflecting autonomic nervous system dysfunction. Palmar erythema is also seen. In advanced disease, the skin over the fingers may become shiny and atrophic.

Nail-fold thrombi, small infarcts on the volar surface of the hands, digital gangrene, and ulcers of the lower part of the leg and the ankle are manifestations of rheumatoid vasculitis. Both sensory and motor types of neuropathy result from vasculitis of the vasa nervorum. Vasculitis of the cranial, coronary, and mesenteric vessels has been observed. Steroid therapy has been implicated in the development of vasculitis; however, vasculitis is seen in patients who have never received steroids.

The most common ocular manifestation is keratoconjunctivitis sicca (Sjögren's syndrome), which occurs in 15 percent of patients. Uveitis is encountered occasionally. Episcleritis may occur; this may evolve into a rheumatoid nodule that eventually perforates the sclera (scleromalacia perforans).

Pulmonary involvement may take the form of diffuse interstitial fibrosis, single or multiple nodules in the lung parenchyma, or a pleural effusion with or without antecedent symptoms of pleurisy. A distinguishing characteristic of some pleural fluids is their low glucose concentration. The pleural fluid may show a distinctive cytologic picture, consisting of a background of amorphous necrotic material, large elongated cells, and giant multinucleated cells. These cells are thought to be shed from rheumatoid nodules in the pleura. Parenchymal rheumatoid nodules may lead to cavitation, which is easily seen on x-ray films. Caplan's syndrome, described originally in Welch coal miners, is the combination of RA and multiple pulmonary nodules (rheumatoid granulomas) developing in patients with underlying pneumoconiosis.

Clinical heart disease is unusual, even though evidence of previous pericarditis is often found at necropsy. Rarely, pericarditis with cardiac tamponade occurs. Aortic regurgitation and conduction abnormalities are occasionally seen. These problems result from rheumatoid granulomas in the aortic valve leaflets and conduction system respectively.

Splenomegaly is present in 10 percent of patients. Lymphadenopathy of the nodes proximal to the involved peripheral joints or generalized lymphadenopathy may be present. The extreme degree of lymphadenopathy in some patients may suggest a malignant lymphoproliferative disease. Amyloidosis may occasionally develop and produce renal failure in patients with long-standing disease.

Felty's syndrome is the combination of rheumatoid arthritis, splenomegaly, and neutropenia. Anemia and thrombocytopenia may occur in these patients. The syndrome usually appears in patients with long-standing disease. Vasculitis manifested by leg ulcers and peripheral neuropathy may be present. Infection may be a serious complication in patients with marked neutropenia. In such patients, splenectomy may improve the neutropenia and decrease infections. Neutropenia, however, may recur after splenectomy. The course of the arthritis is not affected by splenectomy.

LABORATORY FINDINGS Normocytic, hypochromic (hypoproliferative) anemia is often present in active disease. The serum iron level is low, but the total iron-binding capacity remains normal. The ineffective erythropoiesis, also seen with other chronic inflammatory disorders, is due in part to a block in the release of iron from the reticuloendothelial system. Iron therapy is of no value except in those cases where superimposed blood loss has occurred and when no stainable iron can be demonstrated on bone marrow. Rarely, a Coombs-positive hemolytic anemia is present.

A mild leukocytosis may be present. A few patients may have neutropenia and a mild thrombocytopenia. Eosinophilia of 5 percent or greater has been observed, especially in patients with extraarticular manifestations of vasculitis, pleuropericarditis, pulmonary fibrosis, and subcutaneous nodules.

The erythrocyte sedimentation rate (ESR) is commonly elevated and can be used as a parameter for following disease activity. However, the ESR may not always reflect the activity of the disease.

Protein electrophoresis often shows a reduced albumin, moderately elevated gamma-globulin, and elevated alpha-2-globulins. Measurements of immunoglobulins may show increased levels of IgG, IgM, and IgA. These findings, however, are not diagnostic.

Rheumatoid factor as indicated by the latex agglutination test is positive in approximately 80 percent of patients with "classical" or "definite" RA as defined by the criteria of the American Rheumatism Association. Rheumatoid factors are immunoglobulins (IgG, IgM, and IgA) with antibody activity specific for IgG globulin. Only IgM rheumatoid factor is readily measured by the currently available methods, which include latex agglutination, bentonite flocculation, and sensitized sheep or human red cell and the tanned red cell tests. The basic principle of all these tests is the same because the antigen, human or rabbit IgG, is coated onto a carrier particle (red cell, latex, bentonite), allowing agglutination to be visible when rheumatoid factor (antibody to IgG) reacts with IgG. Methods for detecting IgG and IgA rheumatoid factors are at present technically too difficult to be of practical use.

Patients with a variety of nonrheumatoid diseases, characterized usually by chronic inflammation with persistent antigenic challenge, will have positive test results for rheumatoid factor. These include other connective tissue diseases (systemic lupus erythematosus, Sjögren's syndrome, polymyositis, scleroderma) and infectious diseases (tuberculosis, leprosy, syphilis, subacute bacterial endocarditis, bronchitis due to bacteria, parasitic infections, viral hepatitis, infectious mononucleosis, influenza). Positive results are also found in patients with idiopathic pulmonary fibrosis, pneumoconiosis, sarcoidosis, hypergammaglobulinemic purpura, mixed cryoglobulinemia, chronic active hepatitis and cirrhosis, lymphomas, renal homografts, and repeated blood transfusions. An occasional Waldenström's macroglobulin will show rheumatoid factor activity. Rheumatoid factor has been reported to appear transiently in the serum of army recruits after extensive prophylactic immunizations. Population studies of apparently healthy persons show an increasing prevalence of rheumatoid factor with age. The overall prevalence in persons below the age of sixty is less than 4 percent. However, in persons over the age of sixty, positive results have been encountered in 40 percent of subjects in some surveys. The titer of rheumatoid factor is usually low in the elderly apparently normal persons.

Rheumatoid factor will usually be present either when the patient is first seen or within the first year of disease. The titer of rheumatoid factor correlates poorly with disease activity. However, those patients with high titers tend to have more severe disease and thus a poorer prognosis than seronegative patients. Positive tests are almost always found in patients with nodules or with clinical evidence of vasculitis. A positive test does not make the diagnosis of RA but must be interpreted in the light of other clinical features.

Antinuclear antibodies are found in 20 to 60 percent of patients. Antibodies with specificity for native DNA are usually not detected. The lupus erythematosus (LE) cell test is positive in 10 to 20 percent of patients. Serum complement level is usually normal or elevated. Slightly reduced levels have been reported in patients with rheumatoid vasculitis.

Synovial fluid has a turbid appearance because of increased numbers of white cells. The cells are predominantly neutrophils and range from 10,000 to 50,000 per mm^3. The fluid may clot spontaneously because of the presence of fibrinogen. This fibrin clot should not be confused with the mucin clot formed by adding 1 percent acetic acid to the fluid. In rheumatoid synovial fluid the viscosity is decreased and the mucin clot is poor because of smaller than normal polymers of hyaluronic acid. Cytoplasmic inclusions in polymorphonuclear cells, containing ingested immune complexes, are not specific for RA. In contrast to normal levels of serum complement, the synovial fluid complement or complement components tend to be low in patients who have positive tests for rheumatoid factors. The synovial fluid glucose level may be low in some patients, possibly because of decreased transport across the membrane or increased utilization by inflammatory cells.

Radiographs of the joints in early disease show only soft-tissue swelling and mild juxtaarticular osteoporosis. Later, bony erosions, initially quite subtle, appear at the joint margins; these are most readily seen in the small joints of the hands and along the ulnar and radial styloid processes. Joint space narrowing is seen as cartilage is destroyed. In advanced disease destruction of subchondral bone and diffuse osteoporosis develop. When the cervical part of the spine is involved, flexion and extension films should be obtained to check for atlantoaxial subluxation.

DIAGNOSIS The diagnosis of RA is readily made in the patient with symmetric inflammatory arthritis of small joints, rheumatoid nodules, characteristic radiographic abnormalities, and a positive test result for rheumatoid factor. The patient who presents a history of fatigue and vague arthralgias without definite evidence of arthritis frequently poses a diagnostic problem. Such a patient may be in the prodromal phase of RA; however, these symptoms are often found in depressed middle-aged patients, especially women. The patient's course should be followed, to see if objective evidence of arthritis develops, before the case is labeled with the diagnosis of RA. Other types of inflammatory arthritis deserve consideration, especially in the patient who has only a few joints involved in an asymmetric distribution. Reiter's syndrome (Chap. 358), psoriatic arthritis (Chap. 358), systemic lupus erythematosus (Chap. 70), and arthritis associated with gastrointestinal diseases (Chap. 358) should be considered in the differential diagnosis. Some patients with ankylosing spondylitis (Chap. 357) may have peripheral arthritis. Arthritis of rheumatic fever and that of viral infections, especially rubella and hepatitis associated with Australia antigen, may mimic RA early in their course. Degenerative joint disease is easily distinguished from RA, but erosive osteoarthritis (Chap. 361) may be confused with RA. The finding of a positive test result for rheumatoid factor in an elderly person should not by itself lead to the diagnosis of RA.

The definite diagnosis of RA depends primarily on the presence of characteristic clinical features and the exclusion of other inflammatory arthritides.

TREATMENT The patient and his family should be given a clear understanding of the chronic nature of RA and the value of careful and continuous medical supervision. Since many patients associate RA with severe disability, the patient should be appraised of the variable course of RA, and should be encouraged to continue working within reasonable limits. This may necessitate retraining in work that is physically less demanding. Adequate rest is important. Depression and passive behavior, not surprisingly, are common in RA, and require careful attention. The question of moving to a warm climate is often raised, but the patient should be advised that a warm climate does not cure RA even though it may cause him to feel better.

The goal of therapy is to maintain the patient's ability to function. To accomplish this, every effort should be made to reduce joint inflammation and pain, prevent joint deformities, maintain motion and strength, and correct deformities. The proper utilization of anti-inflammatory drugs, splints, physical therapy, and orthopedic surgery is directed to this end.

Drug therapy *Salicylates* remain the mainstay of drug therapy and should be given an adequate trial in the initial treatment of RA. They have been shown to be superior to placebo and to exert both an anti-inflammatory and an analgesic action. A dosage of 3 to 6 g per day should be administered in divided amounts four times a day, preferably after meals. Periodic checks of the blood salicylate level are useful to determine whether adequate blood levels are being achieved. The blood sample should be obtained 2 to 3 hr after a regular dose. A level between 15 to 30 mg per 100 ml is in the therapeutic range.

An increase in fecal blood is commonly observed with salicylate usage regardless of the route of administration, and is not necessarily due to bleeding from a peptic ulcer. However, salicylates may aggravate peptic ulcer disease. The gastrointestinal upset, a common complaint, can be alleviated by giving the drug with meals and by the use of antacids. Salicylates have been reported to cause urticaria or asthma. Signs of toxicity such as tinnitus, deafness, hyperventilation, or confusion should be carefully monitored, especially in older patients.

Acetylsalicylic acid (aspirin) is the most effective preparation on a weight basis. Choline salicylate or salicylsalicylic acid may be better tolerated in patients with gastrointestinal upset or with peptic ulcer disease. Enteric coated preparations have the disadvantage of delayed and unpredictable absorption.

Phenylbutazone is not recommended for long-term therapy in RA. It may be useful for short periods during an acute exacerbation. The dose should not exceed 400 mg per day. Complications include fluid retention, peptic ulcer disease, and bone marrow toxicity, primarily leukopenia.

The response to *indomethacin* has been variable, but the drug may be effective in some patients. It probably has little if any advantage over salicylates. The usual dosage is between 75 and 150 mg per day in divided doses, and the drug is best tolerated if the dosage is gradually increased to these amounts. Side effects of lightheadedness, headaches, an "unreal" feeling, depression, dyspepsia, or peptic ulcer disease may curb its use.

When salicylates prove ineffective in controlling the disease, gold salts or chloroquin are the next order of drugs to be used. In controlled studies both *chloroquin* and *hydroxychloroquin* have been shown to be effective. The recommended daily dose of chloroquin is 250 mg, and of hydroxychloroquin, 200 to 400 mg. A response is not usually seen until 4 to 6 weeks of therapy. Once improvement is noted, the dosage should be reduced. Long-term use of these drugs is curtailed by the risk of blindness from irreversible retinal degeneration, which may progress even after therapy when the drug has been discontinued. The drug should not be given unless an initial and regular eye examination every 4 to 6 months is performed by an ophthalmologist. Other complications include neuromyopathy, gastrointestinal distress, band keratopathy, and bleaching of hair.

Gold salts are beneficial in suppressing disease activity in some patients. In a controlled study patients treated with a total of 1 g gold sodium thiomalate over a 20-week period experienced greater clinical improvement than those given placebo. The clinical improvement was not lasting, since no differences between the two groups were found approximately 2 years after the last gold injection. In general, patients with recent onset of RA are more likely to respond than those with long-standing disease. Also, patients who previously failed to respond to an adequate course of gold are not likely to respond to another course.

The two gold salts most commonly used are gold sodium thiomalate (Myochrysine) and gold thioglucose (Solganol); they are administered intramuscularly, usually on a weekly basis. The initial dose is 10 mg, followed by 25 mg the next week. If no adverse effects are noted, 50 mg is given weekly until definite improvement is observed or a total dose of 1 g is reached. When no improvement results, the drug is discontinued. With a favorable response, the interval between injections is gradually increased until the patient is receiving 50 mg monthly. The value of maintenance therapy is not proved. The beneficial effects of gold therapy usually do not become apparent until at least 400 to 500 mg has been given.

Dermatitis and stomatitis are the most common toxic manifestations of gold therapy. The rash is often pruritic and accompanied by development of eosinophilia. The mucocutaneous lesions are reversible when gold therapy is discontinued. Early detection of a rash is important, since continuation of gold may lead to a generalized exfoliative dermatitis. A mild rash may be treated with local steroid preparations; however, systemic steroids may be necessary for severe extensive dermatitis.

Gold toxicity can cause renal damage, the earliest manifestations being proteinuria and/or hematuria. These signs may be followed by the nephrotic syndrome. Bone marrow toxicity may present as an aplastic anemia, agranulocytosis, and/or thrombocytopenia with severe marrow depression. The use of a chelating agent may be necessary for treatment of severe gold toxicity.

In view of the potential serious toxicity of gold, the decision to use gold carries with it the obligation of careful medical supervision. Each week the patient should be asked about and examined for evidence of skin and/or mouth lesions. White blood counts and analysis of the urine for protein should be performed on alternate weeks. If rash, proteinuria, or leukopenia appears, gold should be discontinued.

The use of corticosteroids should be reserved for patients whose disease is not adequately controlled by the previously mentioned drugs. When corticosteroids are initially given, the patient may experience dramatic symptomatic relief; however, their continued use does not appear to alter the natural course of the disease or to prevent joint destruction. Low dose therapy, however, may provide sufficient symptomatic relief to permit a patient to continue functioning. The dose of prednisone or its equivalent should be the smallest amount providing symptomatic relief and should not exceed 10 to 15 mg per day. Continued use of larger doses provides no added advantage and increases the well-known side effects of these drugs. Larger doses, however, may be necessary in patients with severe extraarticular complications of RA, especially in patients with vasculitis. Supplemental steroids should be given to patients receiving steroids or to patients who have recently received steroids when these patients undergo surgery or develop severe intercurrent stressful illnesses.

Intraarticular steroid injections are useful in temporarily suppressing joint inflammation, especially when only a few joints show active disease. In patients with multiple joint involvement, injection of a few of the most symptomatic joints may serve to supplement other forms of therapy. Following injection of small finger joints, inflammation may be suppressed for as long as 1 year. Numerous and frequent injections of a joint have the potential danger of predisposing the joint to damage from overuse because of the suppression of pain, which serves to protect an already injured joint. A possible deleterious effect of intraarticular steroid on cartilage has not been demonstrated with therapeutic doses. Some patients experience a transient exacerbation of joint inflammation a few hours after injection which is due to a "crystal-induced synovitis" from corticosteroid crystals. Sterile technique should be used to prevent possible introduction of infection.

Immunosuppressive (*cytotoxic*) *drugs* are being evaluated for the treatment of rheumatoid arthritis. The rationale for their use is based on evidence that immunologic mechanisms mediate synovitis and other manifestations of RA. These drugs are effective in suppressing the primary humoral and cellular responses, provided that the drug is given in the proper dose and time in relation to the introduction of antigen. They diminish ongoing cellular immune responses but have little, if any, effect on ongoing humoral immune responses. These drugs are anti-inflammatory, as shown in experimental animals and in human beings. Their action in RA has not been clarified but may be related in large part to their anti-inflammatory properties.

The immunosuppressive drugs that have been used in RA include cyclophosphamide, azathioprine, 6-mercaptopurine, chlorambucil, and methotrexate. Favorable responses have been reported with all these drugs; however, few carefully controlled studies have been performed. A controlled study of cyclophosphamide, over an 8-month period, showed that patients receiving high doses (up to 150 mg per day) had greater improvement than those on a nontherapeutic dose (up to 15 mg per day). Patients treated with the high-dose regimen had improved grip strength, a decrease in the duration of morning stiffness, a decrease in the number of painful swollen joints, and a decrease in the number of new articular erosions. Sedimentation rates did not correlate well with improvement. Controlled studies carried out with azathioprine have also shown favorable results. The beneficial effect of these drugs on a long-term basis is not known, nor has the beneficial effect of their intraarticular injection been proved.

The toxicity and side effects of cytotoxic drugs limit their use. These agents can cause bone marrow depression with severe leukopenia, infection (especially with opportunistic microorganisms), sterility, and an increased risk of neoplasia. Because of their mutagenic potential, contraception should be recommended when they are being used. In addition, there are specific adverse manifestations of the individual drugs. Methotrexate is hepatotoxic and causes cirrhosis. Cyclosphosphamide causes cystitis, resulting in hemorrhage and bladder wall fibrosis. Alepecia occurs frequently. At present immunosuppressive therapy is experimental and, if used at all, should be restricted to patients who have not responded to more conventional forms of therapy. The use of these drugs requires constant and close supervision. White blood cell counts should be carefully monitored.

Physical therapy This form of treatment plays an important role in the treatment of RA. Heat helps to relieve muscle spasm and reduce stiffness. Paraffin baths and heat lamps can be used at home. Passive range-of-motion exercises can help to prevent or minimize loss of joint motion. Isometric exercises increase muscle strength and thereby help to maintain joint stability. Splinting of an actively involved joint for short periods of time is useful in reducing pain and possibly inflammation. The use of night splints is helpful in preventing flexion contractures, especially of the knees and wrists. The wise use of physical therapy along with occupational therapy will enhance the patient's ability to continue functioning at an independent level.

Orthopedic surgery This modality plays an important role in the treatment of RA. Function may be improved by surgical correction of joint deformities and stabilization of certain joints. Resection of the metatarsal heads is often beneficial in relieving forefoot pain. The carpal tunnel syndrome necessitates surgical release and synovectomy. Ruptured tendons should be repaired. Removal of rheumatoid synovium involving the extensor hood over the dorsum of the wrist and hands may prevent tendon rupture. Resection of the distal ulna, together with synovectomy of the wrist, helps to relieve pain and improve function. Synovectomy of the knee may be needed when a symptomatic popliteal cyst is present. Removal of the cyst is not necessary, since the "pumping" of fluid from the knee by motion is responsible for the expansion of the cyst. Atlantoaxial subluxation with symptoms of cord compression requires surgical stabilization. Patients with atlantoaxial subluxation but without evidence of cord compression should protect themselves by wearing a collar, especially when riding in an automobile. Prophylactic synovectomy may diminish joint pain and temporarily retard the disease in the joint that is operated on. A prospective study by the American Rheumatism Association is presently being conducted to evaluate this procedure. Development of a total hip prosthesis has given new hope to patients with severely damaged hip joints. Preliminary results of a total knee prosthesis are encouraging. Rehabilitation of many patients is now possible through orthopedic procedures that improve function and reduce pain.

JUVENILE RHEUMATOID ARTHRITIS

Rheumatoid arthritis in children has a peak onset between the ages of one to three years and is more common in girls. Approximately 5 percent of all patients with rheumatoid arthritis are children under sixteen. Juvenile rheumatoid arthritis (JRA) differs from the disease in adults by the more frequent occurrence of systemic manifestations, by monoarticular and oligoarticular joint involvement, by iridocyclitis, and by infrequent occurrence of typical rheumatoid factor and rheumatoid nodules.

In about 25 percent of the patients, especially in those less than seven years old, JRA is characterized by prominent systemic manifestations. These patients may have high fever (103°F and over). The fever has wide diurnal fluctuations and is highest in the afternoon and evening. The child may appear ill or may be remarkably little affected by the fever. Fever may be present for weeks or months before the appearance of arthritis. An evanescent, salmon-colored, nonpruritic macular to maculopapular rash may appear, especially during the fever. The lesions are usually discrete, show central clearing, and are more common on the trunk than on the extremities. Generalized lymphadenopathy, splenomegaly, and hepatomegaly are often present. Cardiac involvement includes pericarditis and rarely myocarditis; pneumonitis and pleuritis also occur. The arthritis in these patients is polyarticular and may affect any joint. The name "Still's disease" is sometimes used for this form of disease, but this eponym is also used for all forms of JRA.

One-third of the patients have monoarticular or pauciarticular arthritis; a knee or an ankle is most often involved. Iridocyclitis occurs frequently in monoarticular JRA and may lead to band keratopathy, cataracts, and loss of vision. Since eye symptoms may be minimal, patients should regularly have slit-lamp examinations by an ophthalmologist. Polyarticular arthritis, similar to that in adults, occurs in another one-third of the patients, particularly in older children. The onset is usually insidious; the initial joint involvement is in the small joints of the hands and feet. The remaining patients with JRA have a mixture of these forms of the disease.

Joint manifestations are rare but when present resemble those in adults. In children, arthritis may first be suspected because of a limp or guarding of joints. The cervical part of the spine is involved in 50 percent of patients; the apophyseal joints are affected, especially at the second to third cervical vertebras. Atlantoaxial subluxation or fusion between cervical vertebras may be present. Sacroiliitis is also common, but the dorsolumbar part of the spine is spared. Involvement of the temporomandibular joints may produce micrognathia because of impaired mandibular growth. Inflammation of the Achilles tendon may cause heel tenderness; calcaneal erosions and spurs are observed radiographically. Rheumatoid nodules occur much less frequently than in adult disease and histologically tend to resemble more closely those found in rheumatic fever.

Impairment of general growth is common, especially during active disease. Joint inflammation may cause early closure of epiphysis and overgrowth of epiphyseal plates.

The course in all forms of JRA is highly variable. Patients with pauciarticular disease have a favorable prognosis and rarely have persistent active disease. Patients with acute-onset systemic disease are more likely to develop crippling joint deformities. About 20 percent of patients with the adult type of onset of JRA continue with active disease into adulthood; however, many retain relatively good joint function.

Laboratory findings show a peripheral blood neutrophilic leukocytosis; the counts sometimes reach 50,000 per mm^3. Rheumatoid factor as measured by standard tests is positive in 10 to 20 percent of patients, usually in the older children with adult-type onset. IgG and IgA rheumatoid factors have been found by a new technique in over half the patients seronegative by standard methods. Antinuclear antibodies have been reported in as high as 30 percent of the patients. Synovial fluid findings are the same as in adult disease.

The diagnosis of JRA presenting with fever and generalized lymphadenopathy but without arthritis requires the exclusion of infections and neoplasms, especially leukemia (Chap. 12). Rheumatic fever may present a diagnostic problem initially but can usually be distinguished by the evidence of carditis and by the nature of the arthritis, which is migratory, does not involve small joints in a symmetric fashion or affect the cervical part of the spine, and does not persist. In systemic lupus erythematosus, the arthritis is usually milder and nephritis is more common. Juvenile ankylosing spondylitis with peripheral joint involvement may be mistaken for JRA. Clinical features in the early stages that suggest ankylosing spondylitis are the late onset in childhood (especially in a male), the relative sparing of the hands and wrists, the infrequent involvement of the cervical part of the spine, and the radiographic finding of sacroiliitis with sclerosis.

Chronic polyarthritis may be seen in congenital X-linked agammaglobulinemia and is considered a distinct entity, separate from JRA (Chap. 64). With monoarticular or pauciarticular disease, tuberculosis and other infections as well as sarcoidosis should be excluded by skin test, needle biopsy of synovium, and synovial fluid culture.

The principles of therapy in JRA are the same as in adult disease. Adequate rest, exercise, prevention of deformities by the judicious use of splints, the use of anti-inflammatory drugs are important. Iridocyclitis is treated with local or intraocular steroids and mydriatics.

SJÖGREN'S SYNDROME

This consists of dry eyes (keratoconjunctivitis sicca, xerophthalmia), dry mouth (xerostomia), and a chronic arthritis. The syndrome can be diagnosed when any two of the three clinical features (dry eyes, dry mouth, arthritis) are present. The lack of secretions may also involve the entire respiratory tract, vagina, and skin. The syndrome occurs most commonly in middle-aged women; fewer than 10 percent of patients are men. The histologic and immunologic findings suggest that abnormalities of both humoral- and cellular-mediated immunity are involved in the pathogenesis of Sjögren's syndrome.

The decrease in tears and saliva (sicca syndrome) results from lymphocytic infiltration of the lacrimal and salivary glands. The earliest histologic finding is periductal lymphocytic infiltration, which progresses to produce atrophy of the acini. The cells are predominantly small lymphocytes, but large lymphocytes, plasma cells, and reticulum cells may be present. Lymph follicles with germinal centers form in the gland. Hyperplasia of the ductal lining cells narrows and obstructs the duct and leads to cystic dilatation of the distal duct. Focal hyperplasia of ductal cells produces epimyoepithelial islands surrounded by lymphocytes. Hyalinization of these islands may occur. Later in the course of the disease, the atrophied parenchymal tissue is replaced by adipose tissue. Lip biopsy specimens show infiltrates of plasma cells and lymphocytes in the minor (accessory) salivary glands. Features that are helpful in distinguishing this syndrome from malignant lymphoma are the benign appearance of the small lymphocytes, the preservation of the lobular architecture of the gland, and the presence of epimyoepithelial cells.

Rheumatoid arthritis is present in approximately one-half the patients with Sjögren's syndrome; the arthritis usually appears first. Rheumatoid nodules, splenomegaly, leukopenia, and vasculitis may be present in these patients. Rarely Sjögren's syndrome is associated with systemic lupus erythematosus, polymyositis, scleroderma, and periarteritis nodosa. The syndrome has also been found in some patients with autoimmune liver disease (chronic active hepatitis, primary biliary cirrhosis, and cryptogenic cirrhosis).

Keratoconjunctivitis sicca produces symptoms of burning, itching, and blurring of vision. The patient may complain of a sensation of sand in the eye. Thick secretions accumulate in the conjunctival sac, and the conjunctiva may be reddened. The diagnosis is made by demonstrating decreased lacrimation (Schirmer's test), corneal or conjunctival erosions (rose bengal or fluorescein dye staining), and filamentary keratitis (slit-lamp examination).

Patients with xerostomia may have difficulty in swallowing solid foods, a decrease in taste acuity, and a rapid progression of dental caries. Cracks and fissures may appear at the corners of the mouth. The buccal mucosa has a parchment-like appearance, and the tongue is red and smooth. Bilateral parotid gland enlargement is observed in one-half the patients. Other salivary glands also may enlarge. The glands are usually smooth, firm, and only slightly tender but may be nodular and hard. Fluctuation in size is common. The diagnosis of xerostomia may be confirmed by measurement of salivary flow, by sialography, and by sequential salivary scintigraphy with pertechnetate.

Dryness of the nasal mucosa may cause epistaxis and decreased acuity of smell. Hoarseness may occur with laryngeal dryness. Patients also may have recurrent bronchitis and pneumonitis because of the decrease of protective mucous secretions.

The development of lymphadenopathy and extrasalivary lymphoid abnormalities in patients with Sjögren's syndrome may suggest malignant lymphoma. These patients are considered to have a disorder falling between neoplasia and hyperplasia, which is diagnosed as *pseudolymphoma*. Serum IgM levels are usually elevated.

Lymphadenopathy, splenomegaly, leukopenia, purpura, neuropathy, vasculitis, and Raynaud's phenomena are more frequently observed in patients with extrasalivary gland lymphoid abnormalities than in those with abnormalities confined to the salivary glands. In some patients, malignant reticulum-cell sarcoma has been reported at sites other than the salivary glands.

Other features sometimes associated with Sjögren's syndrome are hypergammaglobulinemic purpura, thrombotic thrombocytopenic purpura, and renal tubular acidosis. Gastric achlorhydria and acute pancreatitis may also occur.

Mild anemia, leukopenia, and eosinophilia may be present. Approximately one-half the patients have hypergammaglobulinemia. Positive rheumatoid factor test results are found in almost all the patients, and approximately 70 percent have antinuclear antibodies. Antithyroglobulin antibodies may also be present. Complement fixing antibodies to tissue homogenates, not specific for salivary tissue, may also be demonstrated. These antibodies and antinuclear antibodies are much more common in patients with the sicca syndrome alone than in those with Sjögren's syndrome and rheumatoid arthritis. Antibodies specific for the cytoplasm of salivary ducts have been demonstrated in Sjögren's syndrome but can also be found in systemic lupus erythematosus without the sicca syndrome. Impairment of delayed hypersensitivity can be demonstrated in some patients by the failure to become sensitized with dinitrochlorobenzene.

In the differential diagnosis, parotid gland tumors should be considered when enlargement is unilateral and other features of the syndrome are absent. Features favoring Sjögren's syndrome are the absence of pain, fluctuation in gland size, and the chronicity of the swelling without extension into the adjacent tissues. The differentiation between a benign and malignant lymphoproliferative disease may be difficult and confusing. Enlargement of the lacrimal and salivary glands (Mikulicz's syndrome) may occur in lymphoma, lymphocytic leukemia, and sarcoidosis. The sicca syndrome is usually not present in malignant lymphoproliferative involvement of the salivary and lacrimal glands, but occurs in sarcoidosis. The diagnosis of sarcoidosis is established by the finding of noncaseating granulomas in the involved gland.

The treatment of RA in patients with Sjögren's syndrome is the same as for RA alone. Dry eyes can be temporarily relieved by the use of 0.5% methylcellulose drops or other types of artificial tears. Methylcellulose (1 or 2%) may be used as a mouthwash in patients with dry mouth. Gelatin and glycerine lozenges may be helpful. Systemic steroids are not recommended for treatment of the enlarged glands. Though they may reduce the size of the glands, dryness is not helped. Steroids may be indicated in patients with extrasalivary lymphoid infiltrates and with clinical manifestations of vasculitis. Improvement of the sicca syndrome by treatment with cyclosphamide has been observed; however, further controlled observations are necessary before immunosuppressive drugs can be recommended for this use. Irradiation of the enlarged parotids is contraindicated because reticulum-cell sarcoma may develop in patients who have received this form of therapy during the early phases of their Sjögren's syndrome.

REFERENCES

American Medical Association: *Primer on the Rheumatic Diseases,* reprinted from JAMA 190:127, 425, 509, 741, 1964

American Rheumatism Association, Cooperating Clinics Committee: A controlled trial of cyclophosphamide in rheumatoid arthritis. N Engl J Med 283:883, 1970

Anderson LG et al: Salivary gland immunoglobulin and rheumatoid factor synthesis in Sjögren's syndrome. Am J Med 53:456, 1972

Bianco NE et al: Immunologic studies of juvenile rheumatoid arthritis. Arthritis Rheum 14:685, 1971

Block KJ et al: Sjögren's syndrome: A clinical, pathological and serological study of sixty-two cases. Medicine 44:187, 1965

Calabro JJ, Marchesano MD: The early natural history of juvenile rheumatoid arthritis. Med Clin North Am 52:567, 1968

Empire Rheumatism Council, Research Sub-committee: Gold therapy in rheumatoid arthritis—final report of a multicentre controlled trial. Ann Rheum Dis 20:315, 1961

Jeremy R et al: Juvenile rheumatoid arthritis persisting into adulthood. Am J Med 45:419, 1968

Ruddy S, Austen KF: The complement system in rheumatoid synovitis. Arthritis Rheum 13:713, 1970

Winchester RJ et al: Occurrence of γ-globulin complexes in serum and joint fluid of rheumatoid arthritis patients: Use of monoclonal rheumatoid factors as reagents for their administration. J Exp Med 134:286s, 1971

357
ANKYLOSING SPONDYLITIS

BRUCE C. GILLILAND
MART MANNIK

INTRODUCTION Ankylosing (rheumatoid) spondylitis (Strümpell-Marie disease) is a chronic and usually progressive inflammatory disease involving the articulations of the spine and adjacent soft tissues. The sacroiliac joints are always affected. Involvement of the hip and shoulder joints commonly occurs; peripheral joints are affected infrequently. The disease predominantly affects young men and begins most often in the third decade. The clinical features of this disease are distinctly different from those of rheumatoid arthritis. The etiology is not known.

EPIDEMIOLOGY Ankylosing spondylitis is found throughout the world. The frequency of disease in the general population is approximately 1 per 2,000; however, in blacks, the prevalence is one-fourth that observed in the white population.

Precipitating factors have not been identified. A small number of patients attribute their disease to prior back trauma, but most likely trauma served to focus attention on the underlying disease. Hereditary factors appear to play a role in the development of disease, since spondylitis is twenty to thirty times more frequent in relatives of spondylitic patients than in appropriate controls. The disease is thought to be transmitted by a single autosomal dominant gene with 70 percent penetrance in males and 10 percent in females.

PATHOLOGY The earliest histopathologic changes usually occur in the sacroiliac joints but may start anywhere in the spine. The disease usually progresses up the spine, and occasionally segments will be skipped.

Synovitis of the involved diarthrodial joints of the spine (apophyseal and costovertebral joints) and of the sacroiliac, hip, shoulder, and peripheral joints resembles that of rheumatoid arthritis. Synovial hyperplasia and focal accumulation of lymphoid and plasma cells are seen histologically. Bony erosions and cartilage destruction ensue, followed later by fibrosis and bony ankylosis. In cartilagenous joints (intervertebral disks, manubriosternal, and symphysis pubis), granulation tissue invades the fibrocartilage and adjacent bone is replaced later by fibrosis and ossification.

Occasionally, fibrous tissue invades the vertebral body to produce a radiolucent cyst which may be confused with an infectious process. Erosions at the anterior corners of the vertebral bodies destroy their normal anterior concavity and give the vertebra a square appearance on lateral radiographs. Ossification of the outer layers of the annulus fibrosus at its lateral margins produces the syndesmophytes and "bamboo spine" observed radiographically. Ossification also involves the anterior portion of the annulus fibrosus and occasionally the inner aspect of the anterior longitudinal ligament. The radiographic appearance of the ossification at the anterior disk margins has led to the misconception that only the anterior longitudinal ligament is involved. Bony erosions and new bone formation also occur at the insertion of tendons, most notably at the spinous processes, greater trochanters, pelvic bones, and heels.

Focal medial necrosis at the root of the aorta causes dilatation of the aortic ring. The aortic cusps may be shortened and thickened but are not fused. These processes lead to aortic valve incompetence. Fibrous tissue may enter the membranous septum and invade the AV bundle, resulting in conduction defects.

MANIFESTATIONS The disease occurs most commonly between the ages of fifteen and forty years and rarely after age fifty. The initial symptoms are low back pain and stiffness, often worse in the early morning. Pain in the hips, buttocks and shoulders is often present. Nocturnal back pain may force the patient to walk around in an attempt to gain relief.

In approximately 10 percent of patients, early symptoms resemble sciatica, with pain in the buttocks and in back of the thighs. The pain may alternate from side to side and seldom radiates below the knee. Neurologic manifestations are rare.

Patients may have the simultaneous onset of peripheral arthritis and back pain; however, peripheral arthritis uncommonly precedes back symptoms. Approximately one-fourth of patients will have peripheral arthritis during the course of their disease, but residual joint damage occurs in less than half of them.

Hip disease may be a major cause of disability. Severe involvement early in the disease may result in ankylosis. Other patients may come to the physician several years later with hip disease indistinguishable from degenerative joint disease. It is not known whether this is due to the previous inflammation in the joint or the abnormal stresses exerted on the joint because of the spine disease.

Occasionally, patients may experience radicular chest pain from involvement of the costovertebral joints, which at times may mimic angina pectoris. Pain on deep breathing also may occur. Other causes of chest pain are involvement of the manubriosternal and sternoclavicular joints. Radicular pain from the lumbar part of the spine may radiate to the abdomen, suggesting visceral disease.

Atlantoaxial subluxation occurs less commonly than in rheumatoid arthritis. Patients with fused cervical spines are especially susceptible to fractures of the neck on falling.

Aortic valve incompetence is present in 3 percent of patients and may result in severe aortic regurgitation, requiring surgical repair. Conduction abnormalities include varying degrees of heart block and left bundle branch block. The conduction defects are more apt to appear in patients with aortic valve incompetence, but they may exist alone. Some patients require implantation of a pacemaker.

Iritis is observed in twenty to thirty percent of patients and may be recurrent. Occasionally, iritis may be the presenting symptom, calling attention to the diagnosis of ankylosing spondylitis. Amyloidosis is found in a small number of patients at autopsy and is a cause of uremia in this disease.

The constitutional symptoms are usually mild at the onset and throughout the disease, but in a few patients with severe disease, fatigue, anemia, fever, and weight loss may be present.

Symptoms may be persistent or intermittent for months or years. In some patients ankylosis of the spine may progress with little or no pain. The degree of spinal involvement varies among patients, ranging from only sacroiliac joint involvement to complete ankylosis of the spine. Once ankylosis of joints occurs, pain usually disappears.

Physical findings early in the disease may be minimal. Tenderness over the sacroiliac joints can be elicited by direct palpation or percussion, or by maneuvers that stress the joint. The lumbar part of the spine will show loss of the normal lordosis, and paraspinal muscle spasm. An objective method for assessing anterior flexion of the lumbar part of the spine is available. Costovertebral involvement is best measured by chest expansion. The more advanced changes of spondylitis are easily recognized by the rigid spine, often fused in varying degrees of flexion, which may be quite pronounced in the thoracic part of the spine.

LABORATORY FINDINGS The erythrocyte sedimentation rate (ESR) is elevated in the majority of cases, but its level reflects fluctuations of disease activity poorly, and the ESR is normal in 20 percent of patients with mild disease. A mild hypoproliferative anemia may be present during severe active disease. Sheep cell agglutination and latex fixation tests for rheumatoid factor are negative even when peripheral joint disease is present. Mild to moderate elevations of the spinal fluid protein level may be present in active spondylitis. Synovial fluid from peripheral joints usually shows a moderate neutrophilic leukocytosis.

Radiographs of the sacroiliac joints in early disease show blurring of the margins, irregular subchondral erosions, and patchy sclerosis. These changes are initially more pronounced in the lower third of the joint. Both sacroiliac joints are characteristically involved, but findings may first appear on one side. With progression, sclerosis becomes more marked, the joint space is lost, and later osteoporosis appears. Similar changes are observed in other articulations of the axial skeleton, including the symphysis pubis and apophyseal joints. At points of tendon insertions (e.g., pelvis, os calcis) the adjacent bone shows erosions, sclerosis, and fluffy new bone formation. Lateral films of the os calcis may show bony spurs at the site of attachment for the Achilles tendon and for the plantar fascia.

Radiographs of the spine in early phases of the disease may show straightening of the lumbar part of the spine and squaring of the lumbar and lower thoracic vertebras. With progression, syndesmophytes appear along the lateral and anterior surfaces of the intervertebral disks and bridge adjacent vertebras. They are characteristically present on both lateral sides of the intervertebral disk at any given level and usually arise from the margin of the vertebral body. The widespread distribution of syndesmophytes in advanced disease produces the picture of the "bamboo spine." Syndesmophytes must be differentiated from the osteophytes observed in degenerative joint disease. The syndesmophyte extends vertically from the adjacent vertebral margins along the outer aspect of the intervertebral disk, while osteophytes project horizontally before curving to form an intervertebral bridge. The radiographic changes in involved peripheral joints are similar to those of rheumatoid arthritis.

DIAGNOSIS A patient with ankylosing spondylitis in the advanced stage is easily recognized by the characteristic bent-over posture, rigid spine, exaggerated dorsal kyphosis, and waddling gait. When peripheral arthritis is present in the early stages of ankylosing spondylitis, confusion with rheumatoid arthritis may occur. Ankylosing spondylitis is predominantly a disease of young men, rheumatoid factor tests are negative, and rheumatoid nodules are not present. Radiographs of the spine show bilateral sacroiliitis and syndesmophytes, which are features not seen in adult rheumatoid arthritis. Back symptoms and hip involvement are not infrequent in juvenile rheumatoid arthritis. Fusion of the upper cervical vertebras and of both sacroiliac joints may occur; however, the lumbar and thoracic sections of the spine do not show the characteristic changes of ankylosing spondylitis. Differentiation from other diseases with spondylitis early in the course may be difficult. Since the spondylitis is indistinguishable from that associated with ulcerative colitis and regional enteritis, symptoms and signs of intestinal disease should always be sought, especially in female patients. The spondylitis with Reiter's syndrome and psoriatic arthritis have common radiographic features, but differ from ankylosing spondylitis in having a greater tendency for syndesmophytes to appear at only one lateral margin of the intervertebral disk at any given level and to arise beyond the margin of the vertebral body. The distribution of syndesmophytes is more random, and the degree of spinal involvement is usually less than in ankylosing spondylitis. Other clinical features of Reiter's syndrome and psoriatic arthritis allow for easy separation of these diseases from ankylosing spondylitis. Features that distinguish ankylosing hyperostosis are the lack of involvement of sacroiliac and apophyseal joints and its more frequent occurrence in older men. Spondylitis of hypoparathyroidism rarely involves the sacroiliac joints. Sciatica of ankylosing spondylitis can be differentiated from that of disk disease, since it may alternate from side to side, the pain seldom radiates below the knee, and neurologic signs are usually absent. Malignant disease should be considered in both youngsters and older patients with symptoms of back pain.

TREATMENT The goal of therapy is to prevent or minimize the deformities of the spine inherent in this disease. With minimal deformity, patients may be able to continue working and living in a reasonably normal fashion if hip disease is not severe. The patient should be instructed to maintain an erect posture whether walking, standing, or sitting. He should be encouraged to sleep in a prone position or, if this is not possible, in a supine position on a flat firm mattress using a small pillow or none at all. Breathing exercises should be encouraged.

Drugs will not halt the progression of the disease, but they provide adequate relief to permit maintenance of posture. Phenylbutazone or indomethacin is effective in this respect. The maintenance dose of phenylbutazone is 200 to 300 mg per day, and of indomethacin, 75 to 150 mg per day. Therapy should be discontinued when symptoms abate. Salicylates are not as effective but may be useful in mild disease. Gold and chloroquine have not been beneficial. Any benefit from corticosteroids is outweighed by their side effects. Iritis can usually be treated with intraocular steroids.

X-ray therapy localized to the sacroiliac joints and involved regions of the spine may give symptomatic relief; however, the natural course of the disease probably is not favorably influenced.

Surgical correction of extreme flexion deformities of

the spine by wedge resection and refusion in an improved position may be helpful in selected patients. The potential danger of spinal cord damage and the long convalescent period should be carefully considered before advising surgery. Patients with crippling hip disease may benefit from a total hip replacement.

REFERENCES

BERENS DL: Roentgen features of ankylosing spondylitis. Clin Orthop 74:20, 1971

CALABRO J, MALTZ BA: Ankylosing spondylitis. N Engl J Med 282:606, 1970

CRUICKSHANK B: Pathology of ankylosing spondylitis. Clin Orthop 74:43, 1971

MCEWEN C et al: Ankylosing spondylitis and spondylitis accompanying ulcerative colitis, regional enteritis, psoriasis, and Reiter's disease. Arthritis Rheum 14:291, 1971

MACRAE IF, WRIGHT V: Measurements of back movement. Ann Rheum Dis 28:584, 1969

WEED CL et al: Heart block in ankylosing spondylitis. Arch Intern Med 117:800, 1966

358 REITER'S SYNDROME, PSORIATIC ARTHRITIS, AND ARTHRITIS ASSOCIATED WITH GASTROINTESTINAL DISEASES

BRUCE C. GILLILAND
MART MANNIK

REITER'S SYNDROME Reiter's syndrome is the clinical triad of arthritis, urethritis, and conjunctivitis, but characteristic mucocutaneous lesions occur frequently enough to be included in the syndrome. The complete syndrome may not be present at any given time. The diagnosis should be entertained when arthritis is associated with any of the other manifestations.

Epidemiology, pathogenesis, and pathology Reiter's syndrome occurs most frequently in young men between the ages of twenty and forty and is uncommon in women or children. In North America, many cases are closely related to sexual exposure. Reiter's syndrome may also follow bacillary dysentery. The cause is unknown, and the pathogenesis of the syndrome has not been clarified. Reports that mycoplasma have been isolated from synovium have not been confirmed. More recently, chlamydia (formerly termed *Bedsonia agents*) have been implicated, but their role remains uncertain. Both T-strain mycoplasma and trachoma-inclusion conjunctivitis (Tric) agents have been recovered from the urethra of patients with nongonococcal urethritis, in which they are considered to be of possible etiologic significance. However, most patients with nongonococcal urethritis do not develop Reiter's syndrome. No evidence exists for an etiologic role of *Shigella*. It is possible that these different types of infection expose the patient to other yet-unknown factors responsible for Reiter's syndrome. A primary immunologic abnormality has not been demonstrated. The mechanisms for the inflammatory lesions in eyes and skin have not been elucidated.

Histologically, the cutaneous and mucosal lesions are very similar, even though their gross appearances are different. In the cutaneous lesions, the epidermis shows hyperkeratosis, parakeratosis, and acanthosis. Spongiform pustules or microabscesses are present in the epidermis and are formed by focal infiltration of neutrophils, with degeneration of epithelial cells. The dermis shows edema, infiltration of lymphocytes, plasma cells, and neutrophils. The skin lesions are termed *keratodermia blenorrhagica* and are indistinguishable microscopically from those of pustular psoriasis. In the mucosal lesions, the inflammatory changes are similar, but keratinized cells do not accumulate. The synovium in the superficial vascular region shows edema, erythrocyte extravasation, and infiltration of neutrophils and lymphocytes. In synovitis of several months' duration, the synovium resembles that of rheumatoid arthritis, with villous hypertrophy, pannus formation over the articular cartilage, and infiltration of lymphocytes and plasma cells.

Clinical manifestations Reiter's syndrome often begins with urethritis after sexual exposure, followed in a few days to 4 weeks by conjunctivitis, mucocutaneous lesions, and arthritis. The onset of the arthritis is usually acute, affecting two or more joints. The joints are usually warm, erythematous, and painful. There is a predilection for joints of the lower extremities; ankles, knees, and metatarsophalangeal and proximal interphalangeal joints of the toes are commonly affected. Arthritis also occurs in the wrist, interphalangeal joints of the hand, costosternal joints, sacroiliac joints, and low part of the back, but is relatively uncommon in the hips and shoulders. Tenderness under the heel may be prominent because of periostitis at the insertion of the plantar fascia. Achilles tendonitis may also be present. The distribution of the arthritis tends to be asymmetric and is extremely variable; multiple or single joints may be affected. The arthritis usually reaches a maximum within 2 weeks and begins to subside after 2 to 6 weeks. The duration is usually from 2 to 4 months, with a spontaneous remission occurring within the first year in the majority of patients. Some patients, however, may continue to have recurrent attacks of arthritis for several years; these flare-ups may be accompanied by one or more of the other clinical features of the syndrome. Recurrent attacks, similar to the first, may be precipitated by sexual exposure followed by urethritis. In patients with a self-limited course, little joint damage occurs, but with persistent or recurrent arthritis, flexion contractures and permanent joint damage may result.

Urethritis is characterized by a mucopurulent discharge and dysuria, but may be asymptomatic and may be overlooked unless the urethra is milked. The urethral meatus may be edematous and reddened, and urethral strictures may develop. Prostatitis and seminal vesiculitis occasionally occur, but epididymitis and orchitis are rare. Cystitis, which may be hemorrhagic, can occur and lead to urinary frequency, suprapubic pain, hematuria, and rarely to obstruction of the ureters. Since gonococcal urethritis may usher in the nonspecific urethritis of Reiter's syndrome, urethral smear and culture should be performed in all patients. When gonococcal urethritis is present, the purulent discharge will usually clear when penicillin is given, but will be replaced by the less purulent mucosal discharge of nonspecific urethritis.

Conjunctivitis is usually bilateral, mild, and evanescent, lasting only a few days. It may be present only at the lateral aspect of the tarsal conjunctiva. Conjunctivitis at times may be quite severe and produce burning, itching, and a profuse mucopurulent discharge, which may last several weeks. A nongranulomatous anterior uveitis which appears in some patients may lead to photophobia, glaucoma, cataracts, and even blindness. Subsequent attacks of anterior uveitis may appear in the absence of other clinical features of Reiter's syndrome. Painful superficial keratitis occurs occasionally.

Mucocutaneous lesions occur in over half the patients and appear most commonly on the glans penis, on the palms and soles, and in the mouth. They are typically painless and transient, and may go unnoticed unless the patient is examined carefully. On the glans penis, the lesion begins as a small vesicle, which evolves to a superficial reddened erosion with well-demarcated borders. In the circumcised male, the lesions may be covered with scales. Only a few lesions may be present on the glans penis, usually around the meatus, or lesions may completely circumscribe the glans (circinate balanitis). Lesions are occasionally found on the shaft and prepuce of the penis and on the scrotum. They also have been observed by endoscopy on the mucosa of the urethra and bladder. In the mouth, the lesions begin as small vesicles, papules, or plaques and later become superficial erosions with a surrounding area of erythema. The erosions may be covered by a thin grayish membrane. The mouth lesions are found on the soft palate, buccal mucosa, and the dorsum of the tongue. Keratodermia blenorrhagica describes the cutaneous lesions, which are found most commonly on the soles but are also occasionally observed on the palms, the extremities, and the trunk. These lesions begin as brownish-red macules, which develop into crusted scaling papules. Such lesions may coalesce to cover the sole with a thick layer of crusted scales, which peel off in the ensuing weeks. The nails may become thickened, opaque, and brittle; keratotic debris accumulates under the nail. None of the mucocutaneous lesions leaves residual scarring.

Cardiac conduction abnormalities and aortic regurgitation have been reported. The pathogenesis of the aortic valve incompetence is similar to that of ankylosing spondylitis, resulting from medial necrosis of the aortic root and dilatation of the aortic ring. Neurologic abnormalities, including optic neuritis, peripheral neuropathy, and transient hemiplegia, are exceedingly rare.

Laboratory findings A mild leukocytosis and an elevated erythrocyte sedimentation rate are often present. Tests for rheumatoid factor are negative. Synovial fluid examination shows an increase in white cells, predominantly neutrophils, ranging usually from 5,000 to 20,000 cells per mm^3. Large mononuclear cells, some containing ingested polymorphonuclear cells, are observed frequently but are not specific for Reiter's syndrome. The viscosity of the fluid may be reduced, and the mucin clot is fair to poor. The synovial fluid complement tends to be high, especially when compared to levels found in some patients with rheumatoid arthritis.

Radiographs of the involved joint may show only soft-tissue swelling. With recurrent disease, bony erosions and joint narrowing may appear. A suggestive, but not diagnostic, finding is periosteal new bone formation along the shaft adjacent to the involved joint and on the posterior and inferior aspects of the os calcis. Calcaneal spurs appear later. One or both sacroiliac joints may show irregularity, sclerosis, and fusion. With involvement of the spine, syndesmophytes may be observed and tend to be randomly distributed in the thoracic and lumbar parts of the spine. These syndesmophytes often arise at the upper or lower third of the vertebral body.

Diagnosis The most important immediate differential diagnosis is gonococcal arthritis, because gonococcal urethritis may be present simultaneously. Gonococcal arthritis is confirmed by a positive synovial fluid culture but is not excluded by a negative one. The presence of conjunctivitis or characteristic mucocutaneous lesions is helpful, since these are not associated with gonococcal arthritis. When in doubt, the arthritis associated with gonococcal urethritis should be treated as gonococcal arthritis, with adequate doses of penicillin (Chap. 132). If Reiter's syndrome is present, the arthritis will persist and other features of the syndrome may appear subsequently.

There is usually no problem differentiating Reiter's syndrome from rheumatoid arthritis. The sudden onset preceded by urethritis, the absence of nodules, negative rheumatoid factor, and the asymmetric joint involvement contrast sharply with the insidious, symmetric joint disease of rheumatoid arthritis.

Psoriatic arthritis and ankylosing spondylitis share several features of Reiter's syndrome. The pustular form of psoriasis is similar in appearance to keratodermia blenorrhagica but tends not to involve mucous membranes, soles, or palms. Psoriatic arthritis may be differentiated from Reiter's syndrome by the more gradual onset of arthritis, the chronic nature of the skin lesions, the absence of urethritis and conjunctivitis, and the rarity of mucous membrane lesions. At times, however, differentiation of these two diseases may not be possible. Compared to ankylosing spondylitis, the spondylitis associated with Reiter's syndrome is usually less severe and progressive. Radiographically, spondylitis of both Reiter's syndrome and psoriatic arthritis shows syndesmophytes which are randomly distributed and which often arise at the lower or upper third of the vertebral body. In addition, ligamentous ossification is less common. In ankylosing spondylitis, the syndesmophytes more often completely bridge adjacent vertebras, arise at the margins of the vertebras, and appear on all sides of an intervertebral disk. Dilatation of the aortic ring, conduction abnormalities, calcaneal periostitis and spurs, and iritis occur both in Reiter's syndrome and in ankylosing spondylitis. The sudden onset of the peripheral arthritis associated with urethritis and conjunctivitis and typical mucocutaneous lesions help to distinguish Reiter's syndrome. Hip involvement is rare in Reiter's syndrome and common in ankylosing spondylitis.

Treatment The treatment of the nongonococcal urethritis with 2 g tetracycline per day for 10 to 14 days may affect the urethritis but probably has no effect on the arthritis. No treatment is necessary for conjunctivitis and other mucocutaneous lesions; however, iritis may require corticosteroid therapy. The arthritis is usually responsive to phenylbutazone or indomethacin. With phenylbutazone, a loading dose of 600 to 800 mg is given initially to obtain a rapid therapeutic blood level, followed by a daily maintenance dose of 200 to 300 mg. The dose of indomethacin is 100 to 150 mg per day. Salicylates may be effective in some patients. Corticosteroids are rarely indicated. The same is true of immunosuppressive drugs.

PSORIATIC ARTHRITIS The prevalence of arthritis in patients with psoriasis is higher than that found in the general population, even when degenerative joint disease and rheumatoid arthritis are excluded.

The *etiology* and *pathogenesis* are not known; however, studies showing aggregation of psoriatic arthritis in first-degree relatives of psoriatic patients suggest that hereditary factors may play a role.

The age of onset is similar to that of rheumatoid arthritis, and the sex distribution slightly favors women. Psoriasis usually precedes the onset of arthritis by months or years; however, the onset of both may coincide or, very uncommonly, arthritis may precede psoriasis. In general, the prognosis of chronic psoriatic arthritis is more favorable than that of rheumatoid arthritis, except in patients with severe destructive arthritis (arthritis mutilans).

On the basis of the pattern of joint involvement three clinical groups may be distinguished. The first is characterized by having predominantly distal interphalangeal joint involvement affecting one or several joints and usually lacking symmetry. The adjacent nail may have changes of psoriasis. A second group has arthritis of several peripheral joints and may be confused with rheumatoid arthritis. The asymmetry of the arthritis, the negative tests for rheumatoid factor, and the absence of nodules are features uncommon to rheumatoid arthritis. Patients with a positive rheumatoid factor test are considered to have both rheumatoid arthritis and psoriasis, although this point is controversial. The third group, termed arthritis mutilans, has a severe destructive polyarthritis, often with associated spondylitis.

Spondylitis, manifested most commonly by sacroiliitis, is found in approximately 20 percent of patients, with varying degrees of peripheral joint involvement. Spondylitis is rarely, if ever, the sole manifestation of psoriatic arthritis. These patients have less back pain, stiffness, and restriction of chest expansion than those with ankylosing spondylitis; however, the disease may result in severe ankylosis of the spine. The peripheral joints are warm, swollen, and tender, and show synovial proliferation. Flexion contractures and ankylosis of joints may occur, with long periods of joint inflammation.

No definite correlation exists between the degree of skin involvement and joint disease, but in some patients the activity of both tends to be parallel. A closer temporal relationship has been found between psoriatic nail lesions and arthritis than between the skin lesions and arthritis.

Laboratory abnormalities include hypoproliferative anemia and an elevated erythrocyte sedimentation rate, which are nonspecific findings. Tests for rheumatoid factor are negative. Hyperuricemia is observed in 10 to 20 percent of patients, the same incidence as in uncomplicated psoriasis. Synovial fluid and biopsy findings are those of nonspecific inflammation.

Several *radiographic* features are characteristic of psoriatic arthritis. These include severe destruction of isolated joints, osteolysis, bony ankylosis, whittling of bone at the distal end of terminal phalanges, and the "pencil-in-cup" deformity, which is most commonly observed in the joints of the fingers and toes. Resorption of the distal end of the bone produces the "pencil," which projects into a widened, cuplike erosion in the adjacent joint surface. The radiographic findings in spondylitis associated with psoriatic arthritis are similar to those found in spondylitis with Reiter's syndrome.

The *diagnosis* of psoriatic arthritis is suggested by the presence of an inflammatory arthritis in a patient with typical skin or nail lesions of psoriasis. The asymmetry of joint involvement, negative test for rheumatoid factor, and the absence of rheumatoid nodules help to distinguish psoriatic arthritis from rheumatoid arthritis. The differentiation of psoriatic arthritis from Reiter's syndrome and ankylosing spondylitis has been discussed under Reiter's syndrome. Psoriatic arthritis presenting as an acute arthritis, especially in a toe or finger, may be mistaken for gouty arthritis. In addition, hyperuricemia, which may occur in association with psoriasis, may also be present. The appearance of the joint also may suggest septic arthritis. These diagnostic considerations are easily excluded by examining synovial fluid for sodium urate crystals and for microorganisms with appropriate cultures.

The *treatment* of the arthritis is similar to that outlined for rheumatoid arthritis except for use of antimalarials. These drugs are contraindicated because they may produce an exfoliative dermatitis in patients with psoriasis. The value of gold has not been established. The use of immunosuppressive agents may be beneficial; methotrexate has been used most extensively. However, in view of their toxicity, these drugs should be restricted to patients with severe psoriasis and destructive polyarthritis. Adequate control of skin disease may lead to improvement of the joint disease in an occasional patient.

ARTHRITIS ASSOCIATED WITH GASTROINTESTINAL DISEASES **Ulcerative colitis** Arthritis is the most common nonintestinal manifestation of ulcerative colitis; it occurs in approximately 20 percent of patients. Two patterns of joint involvement may be distinguished in patients with arthritis of ulcerative colitis: arthritis of peripheral joints (colitic arthritis), which occurs in 75 percent of patients; and spondylitis, which occurs in 25 percent of patients.

The peripheral arthritis of ulcerative colitis most commonly begins between the ages of twenty-five and forty-five years and affects both sexes equally. Arthritis usually

An Atlas of common lesions encountered during the physical examination of the skin

The skin and mucous membrane may frequently contain a variety of lesions that are rarely a major complaint (Fig. 52-1). They are, therefore, incidental findings in the general physical examination. The recognition of the "bumps and blemishes" is a necessary first step for the physician, inasmuch as he will be required to distinguish the trivial from the serious and important skin changes. For example, such a serious lesion as a malignant melanoma may be incidentally discovered during a routine physical examination (see color Figs. 6-1, 6-2, 6-3 and the discussion in Chap. 366).

The common disorders of the skin that every physician should be able to recognize are presented in this series of color photographs (Plates 1 to 4).

A

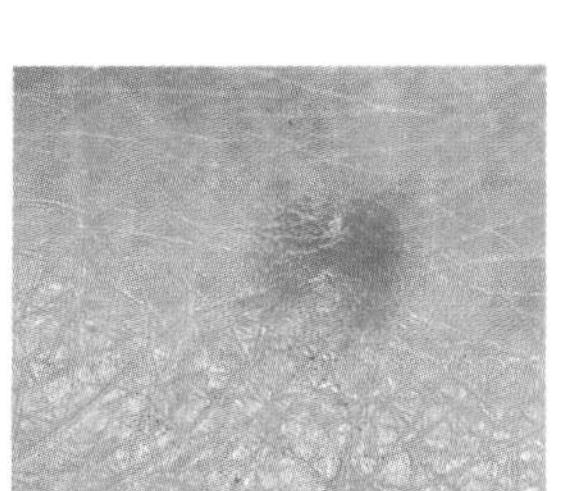

B

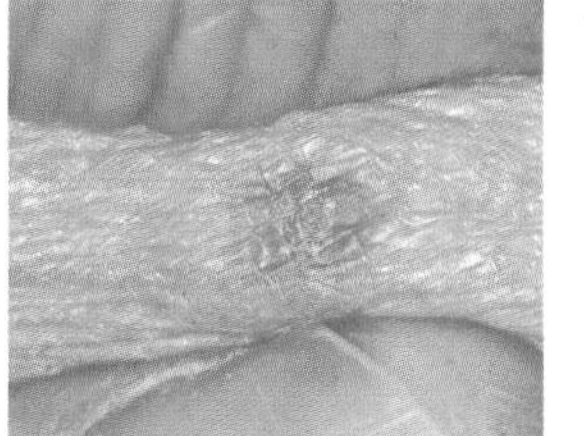

1-1 **Dermatofibroma** is especially common in middle life and in females. The lesions, when pigmented, are occasionally confused with malignant melanoma. They appear as isolated, slightly elevated, hard, button-like nodules *(A)*. In fair-skinned persons, the lesions are not usually skin color, but are pink or dark red, yellowish brown, or gray-black. They are usually less than 1 cm in diameter. A diagnostic sign is that a dermatofibroma dimples or becomes depressed *(B)* when it is laterally compressed; melanocytic nevus and melanoma, however, with which dermatofibroma may be easily confused, become elevated with lateral compression.

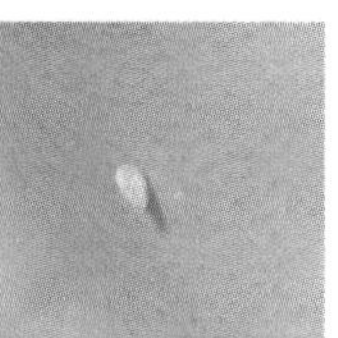

1-2 **Acrochordon** (skin tag) is very common after middle life and appears on the neck, especially in females, in the axillae, and on the upper part of the trunk. The lesions are small (1 to 5 mm), soft, pedunculated papules, usually of normal skin color.

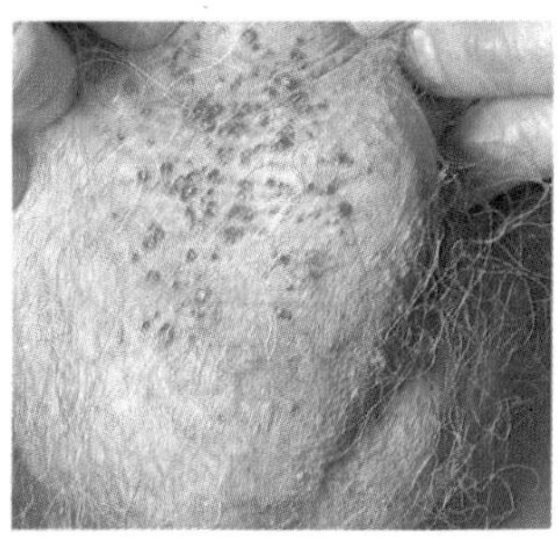

1-3 **Angiokeratomas** are bizarre vascular dilatations that occur under the tongue and on the scrotum and consist of myriads of 2- to 3-mm purplish red papules. They are of no known significance. When they occur on the trunk and extremities, a biopsy is indicated to rule out glycolipid lipidosis, or Fabry's disease.

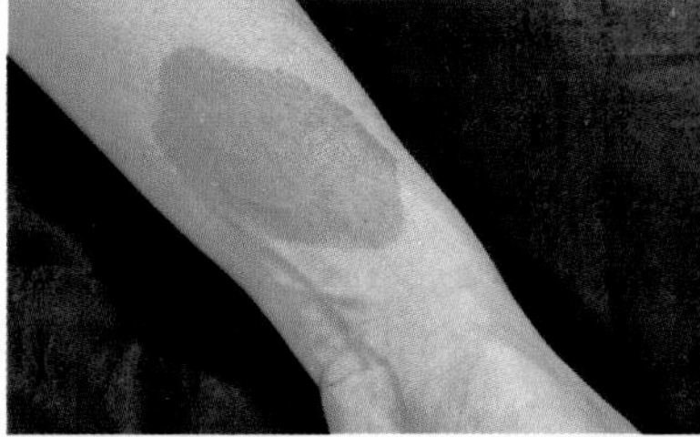

1-4 **Café au lait macules** are found in about 10 percent of the normal population and, in fair-skinned persons, are light-yellowish brown macules, which may also be markers of neurofibromatosis and polyostotic fibrous dysplasia (Albright's syndrome). The presence of six or more café au lait macules with a diameter of 1.5 cm or greater is diagnostic of neurofibromatosis.

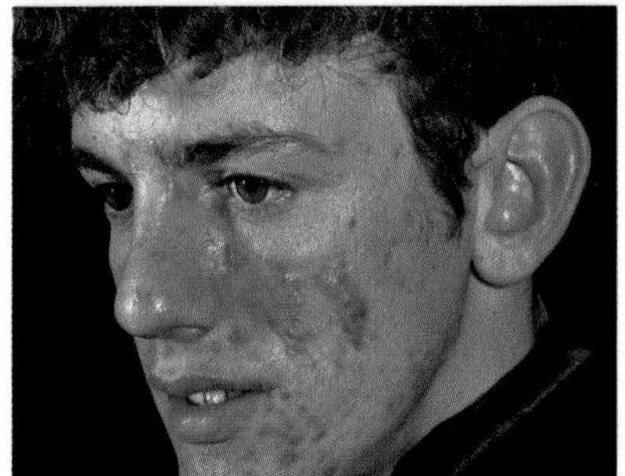

1-5 **Acne** is a condition in which the most characteristic lesion is the comedo, or "blackhead," that later becomes a conical erythematous papule or pustule. A third type of lesion is the "blind boil," which is a dermal cyst without an orifice. This lesion is often associated with atrophic or hypertrophic scarring. Cystic acne may appear with only a very few comedones; also, comedo-like acne may occur with few cysts, or erythematous papules.

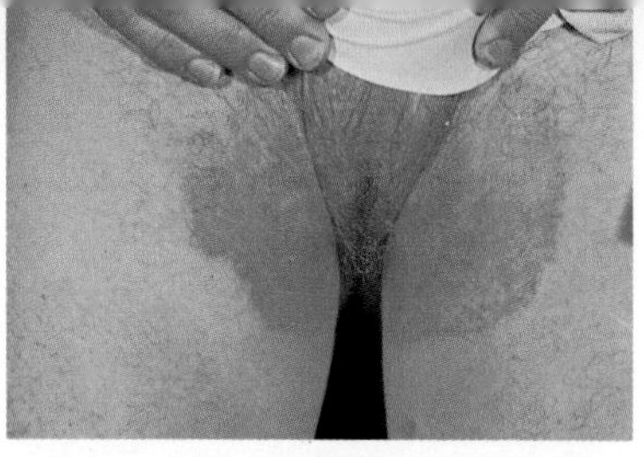

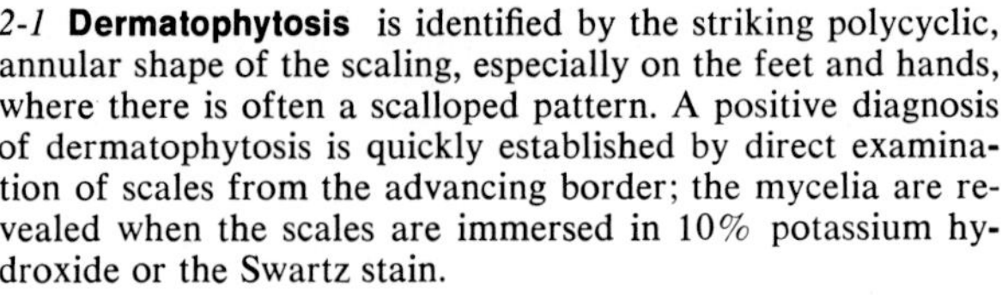

2-1 **Dermatophytosis** is identified by the striking polycyclic, annular shape of the scaling, especially on the feet and hands, where there is often a scalloped pattern. A positive diagnosis of dermatophytosis is quickly established by direct examination of scales from the advancing border; the mycelia are revealed when the scales are immersed in 10% potassium hydroxide or the Swartz stain.

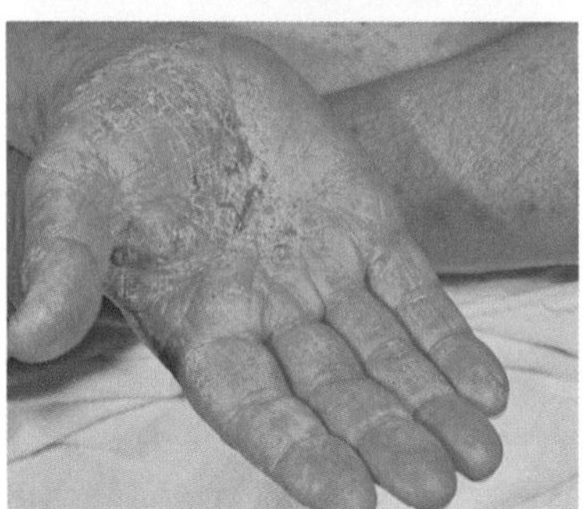

2-2 **Eczematous dermatitis** is a very common cutaneous reaction that is localized to the hands of housewives, to the legs in patients with chronic venous insufficiency, and behind the ears in patients with seborrheic dermatitis. In subacute eczematous dermatitis, there are mild erythema, dry scales, and often small red papules, many of which are excoriated. In chronic eczematous dermatitis, lichenification is the most prominent feature.

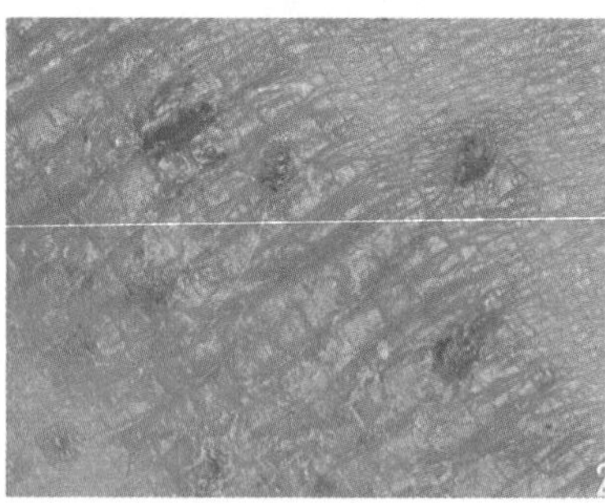

2-3 **Localized lichenification** results from repeated rubbing of the skin and consists of isolated, circumscribed plaques. These single lesions vary in size from 2 to 10 cm and occur most often on the extensor aspect of the forearm and in the scrotal, nuchal, inguinal, and anogenital areas. The perianal and vulvar areas may become diffusely lichenified. Lichenification is thought to be more frequent in persons with an atopic background.

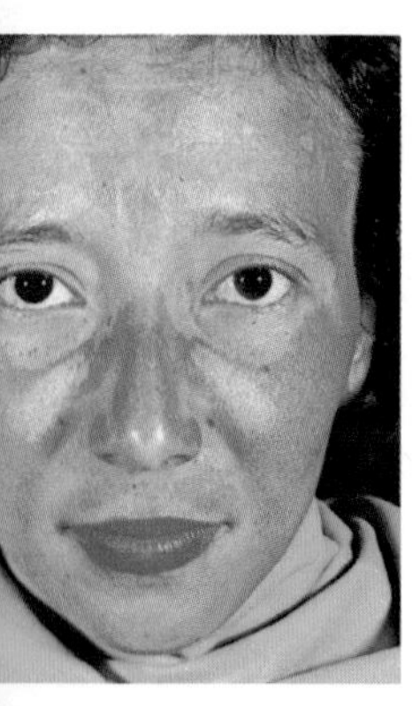

2-4 **Melasma (chloasma)** is the so-called "mask" of pregnancy, but it also occurs in men and in women taking progestational agents. The pigmentation is uniform and is limited to the exposed areas of the face. There is no scaling or epidermal change. In fair-skinned persons, the pigment may be any shade from light tan to a very dark brown. It is most often seen on the cheeks and upper lip, as here, and on the forehead.

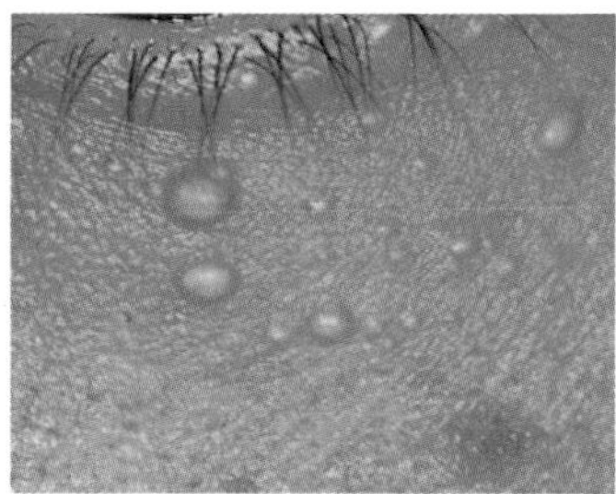

2-5 **Milia** are a collection of lesions occurring most commonly on the face, and consist of tiny (1- to 2-mm) white, hard, rounded, superficial papules. There is no orifice, and the keratinous contents are easily expressed by lateral compression after the making of a tiny incision in the dome of the lesion.

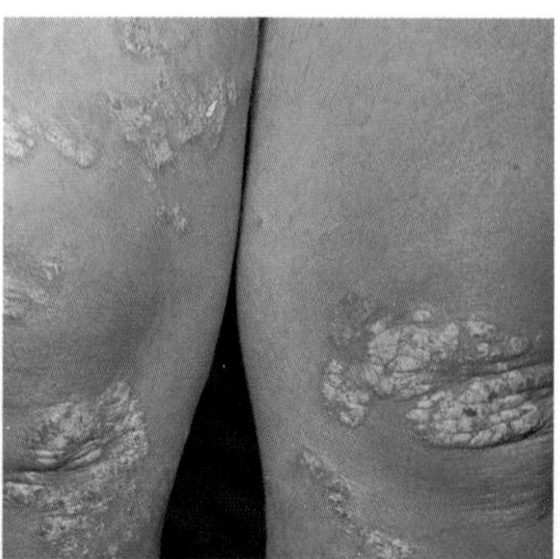

2-6 **Psoriasis,** affecting more than 2 percent of the population, consist of isolating scaling papules or plaques and is quite commonly observed in the routine physical examination. The lesions occur most frequently on the scalp, elbows, and knees. The color and type of scales are the identifying features of the lesions. The scales are either dense and lamellated with peripherally detached edges or loose and branny. The plaques are pink to deep red, and the borders are distinct.

3-1 **Perlèche** consists of painful small fissures at the angles of the mouth, often covered with yellow crusts. Perlèche most often occurs with poorly fitting dentures and in moniliasis and secondary syphilis.

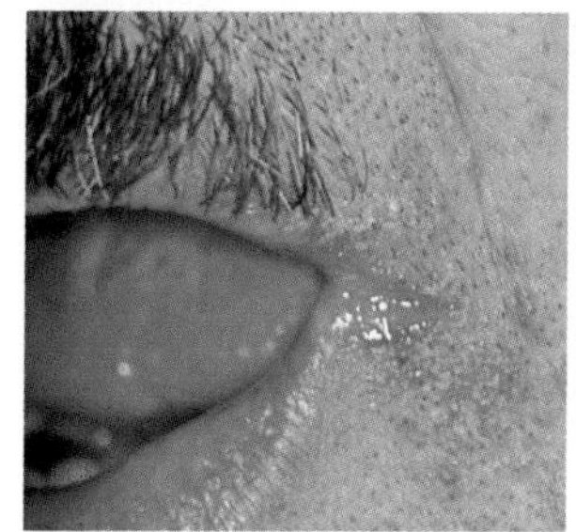

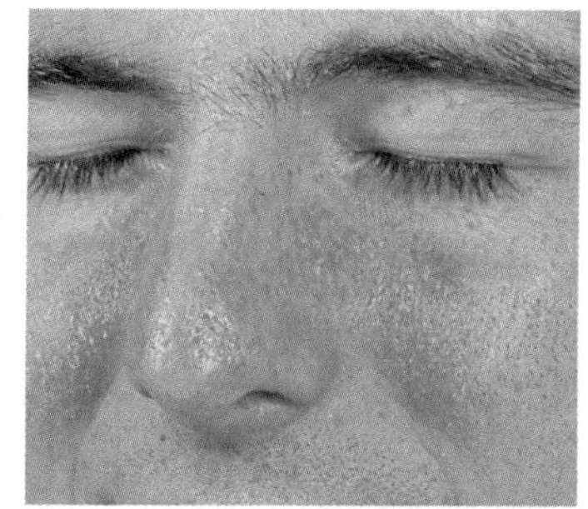

3-2 **Rosacea,** usually limited to the face, consists of tiny, erythematous papules and pustules 1 to 5 mm in size. The pustules, often tiny and sometimes hardly visible, sit on the dome of the papules. The diffuse redness of the face is due to a vasodilatation, as well as to myriads of telangiectases. In males, rhinophyma, a disfiguring enlargement of the nose, may occur.

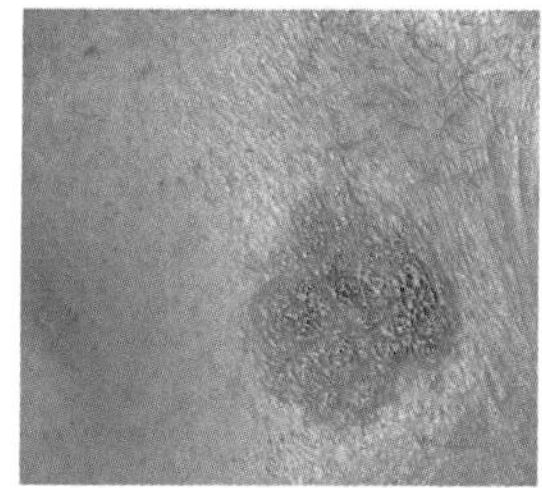

3-3 **Seborrheic dermatitis,** a common disorder found in all age groups, occurs most frequently on the scalp, eyebrows, and nasolabial folds, and behind the ears. Scaling is the prominent feature and is loose and branny; it may be yellow and oily or dry and white. The lesion may become exudative and crusted or eczematous.

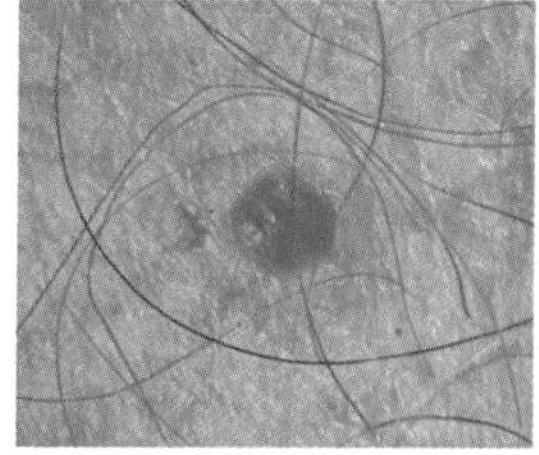

3-4 **Seborrheic keratosis** appears in middle life and may be on the exposed or unexposed areas but is especially common on the trunk. The lesions are irregularly round or oval flat-topped papules or plaques that seem "stuck" on the skin. The margins are distinct, and the surface is often warty or consists of multiple tiny projections (vegetation). In fair-skinned persons, the lesions are light brown at first but, enlarging, become more heavily pigmented and may be confused with malignant melanoma.

3-5 **Senile angioma ("cherry-red spot")** appears in the third decade. On the lip, the lesion is usually singular and consists of a bluish-red round nodule. On the trunk, the lesions are small (2- to 3-mm), bright red, globular papules.

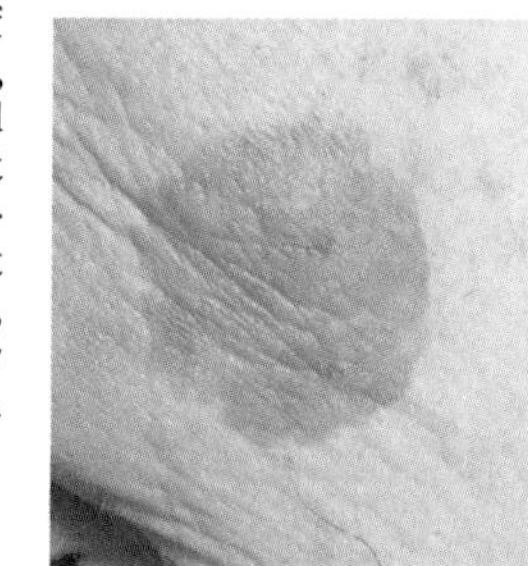

3-6 **Senile lentigo** occurs as a single macule or as a group of isolated, sharply circumscribed macules on the exposed areas, especially on the dorsal surfaces of the hands and arms and on the forehead and cheeks. The macules are usually light yellowish brown, but may be dark brown; the color is somewhat variegated, rather than uniform as it is in a café au lait macule. Rarely, dark brown *papules* develop in these lesions, and then the condition is called *lentigo maligna,* which may slowly develop, over a period of years, into a melanoma (lentigo maligna melanoma).

PLATE 4

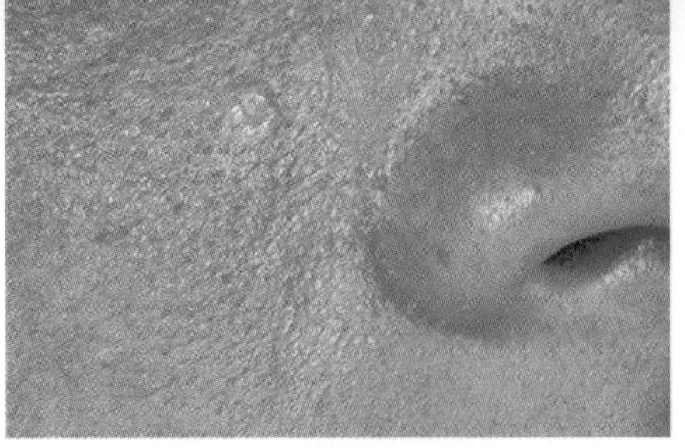

4-1 **Senile sebaceous adenoma** occurs on the face in patients over forty and is often diagnosed as basal-cell carcinoma. The lesions are soft, small, flat-topped papules, varying in size from 1 to 8 mm, and are characterized by a minute central depression from which sebaceous material can be exuded by lateral compression.

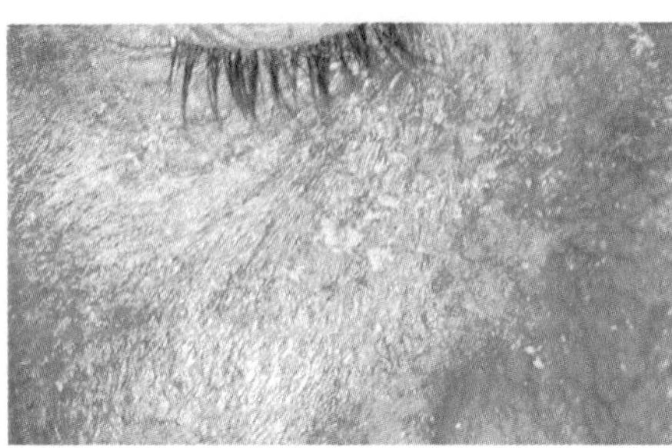

4-2 **Solar keratosis** (1) occurs usually in persons with light skin prone to sunburn or with darker skin after chronic excessive exposure; (2) is strictly limited to exposed skin, especially on the face and dorsal surfaces of the hands; (3) is more easily felt than seen (gritty and sandpaperish); (4) in fair-skinned persons, consists of skin-colored or light brown macules or slightly raised papules with superficial adherent scales not easily removed; (5) is associated with marked wrinkling, telangiectasia, and often diffuse, tiny pale yellow papules indicating solar degeneration of connective tissue ("turkey skin").

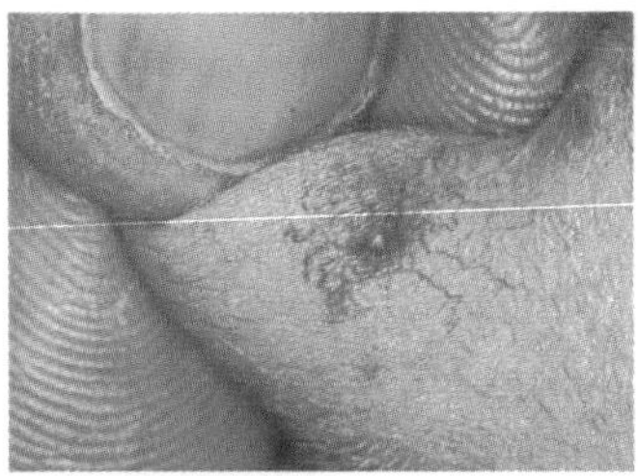

4-3 **Spider nevus** consists of a central, punctate, bright red macule or papule (the body) from which fine red lines radiate like spider legs. There is often a red flare between the radiating vessels. On diascopy, the central body pulsates.

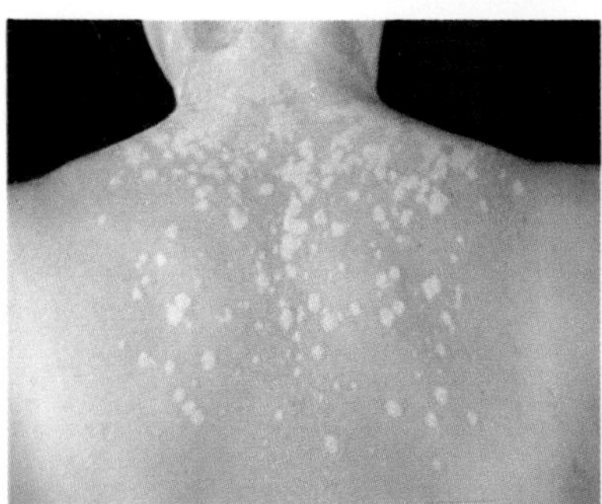

4-4 **Tinea versicolor** is a relatively common disorder occurring primarily on the trunk and appearing in two forms: as scattered, 3- to 5-mm, very slightly scaling brown macules; or as whitish macules that may be confused with vitiligo. The fungal spores and hyphae can be easily demonstrated on direct examination of the scales using the Swartz stain.

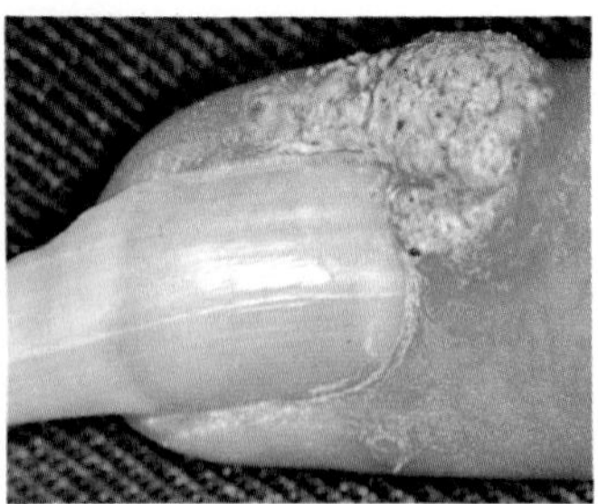

4-5 **Verruca vulgaris** may occur at any age, but it is most common in children. The lesions may be from 0.5 to 2.0 cm, and they are round or oval, firm, skin-colored papules with multiple tiny keratotic, rounded or filiform, projections covering the surface (vegetation). They occur most frequently on the hands and soles.

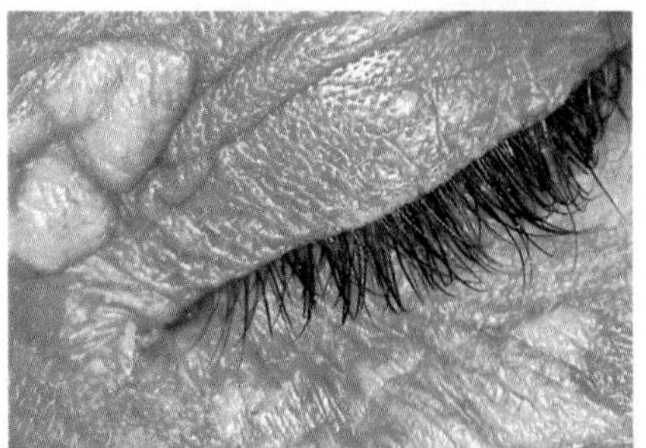

4-6 **Xanthelasma** consists of one or more bright yellow, sharply marginated plaques with no epidermal change, usually occurring on the eyelids. All patients with xanthelasma should be investigated for evidence of plasma lipid abnormalities.

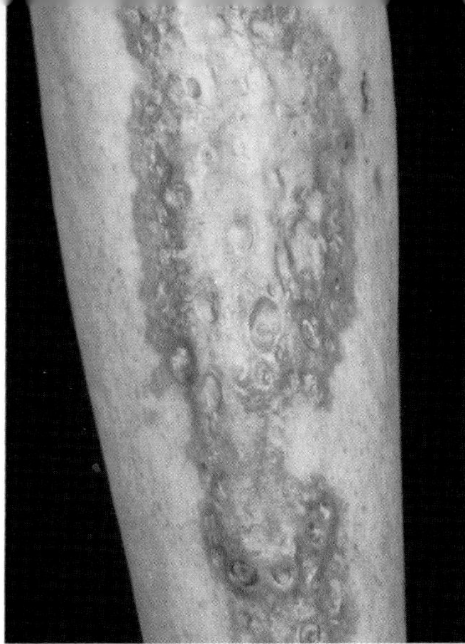

5-1 Necrobiosis lipoidica diabeticorum. Note vivid colors (brown and yellow) and fine, arborizing blood vessels traversing atrophic skin.

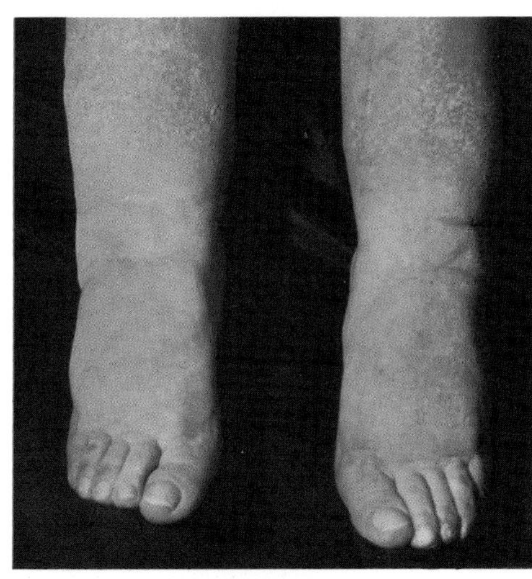

5-2 Pretibial myxedema.

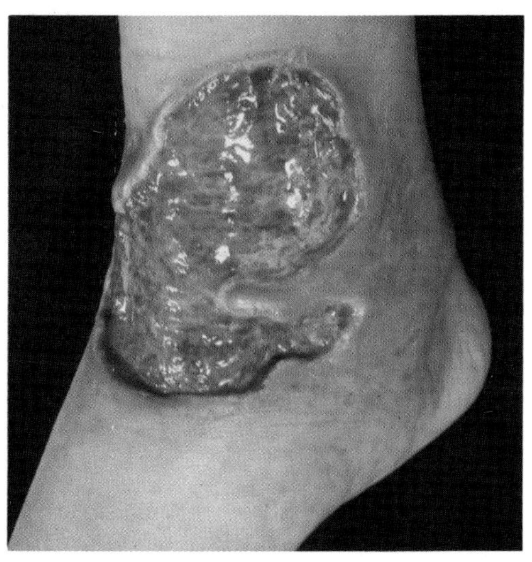

5-3 Pyoderma gangrenosum in a patient with ulcerative colitis.

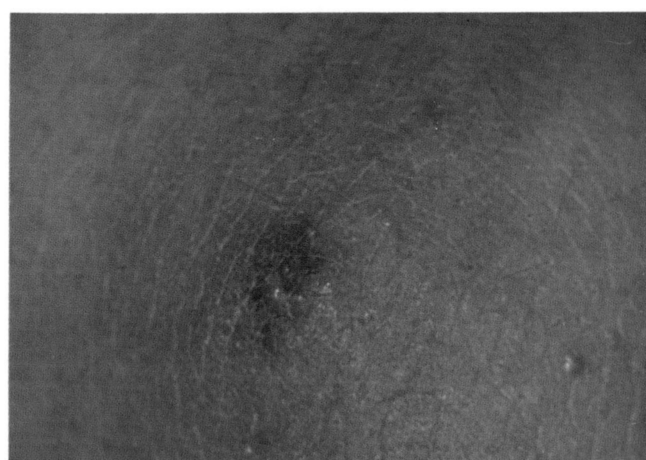

5-4 "Palpable" purpura with inflammation occurring in gonococcemia. An identical lesion may be seen in meningococcemia. staphylococcemia, and systemic vasculitis.

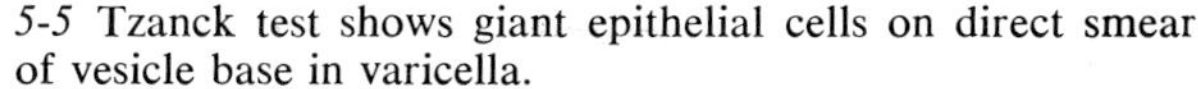

5-5 Tzanck test shows giant epithelial cells on direct smear of vesicle base in varicella.

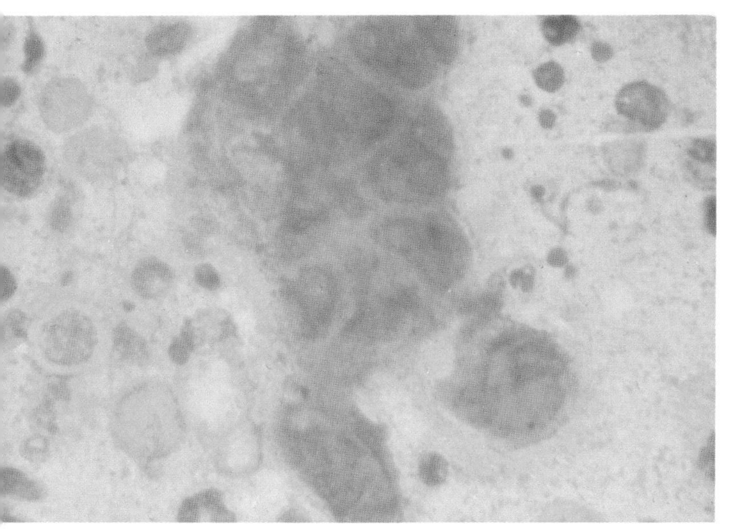

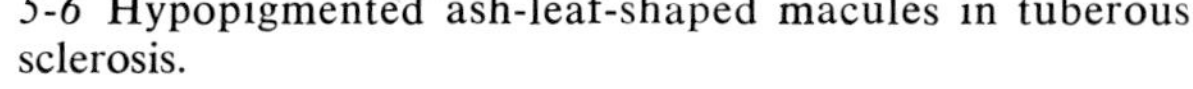

5-6 Hypopigmented ash-leaf-shaped macules in tuberous sclerosis.

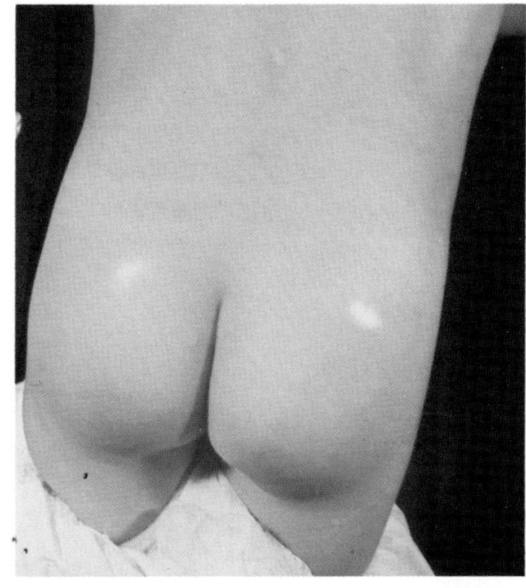

PLATE 6

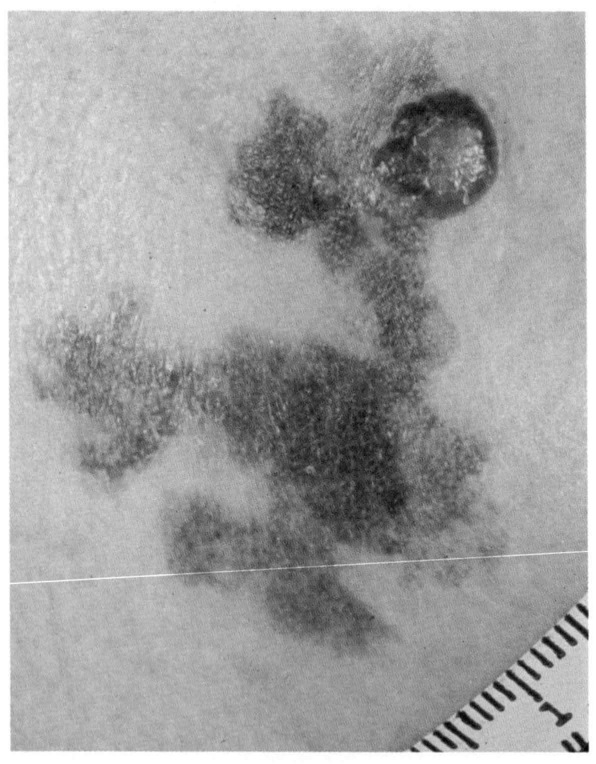

6-1 In Type I malignant melanoma, the lesion is predominantly flat, but there may be a few nodules or papules. The color consists mainly of shades of brown and black, admixed with whitish gray and, occasionally, with reddish brown, bluish gray, and bluish black.

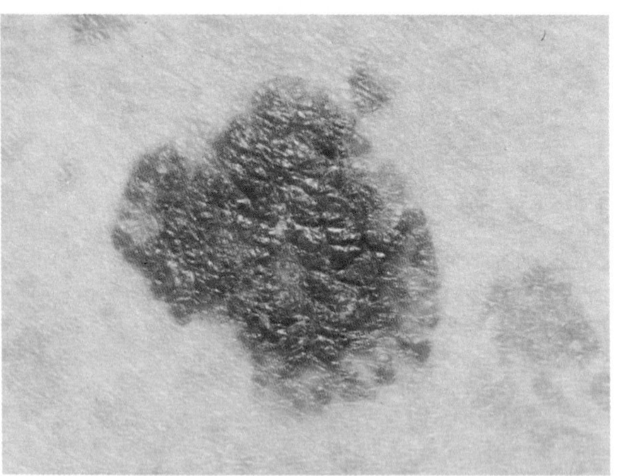

6-2 In Type II malignant melanoma, the lesion is usually just slightly raised in its entirety and is punctuated with papules and, sometimes, nodules. The color consists mainly of brown and black, admixed with bluish red (violaceous), bluish gray, bluish black, reddish brown, and often whitish pink.

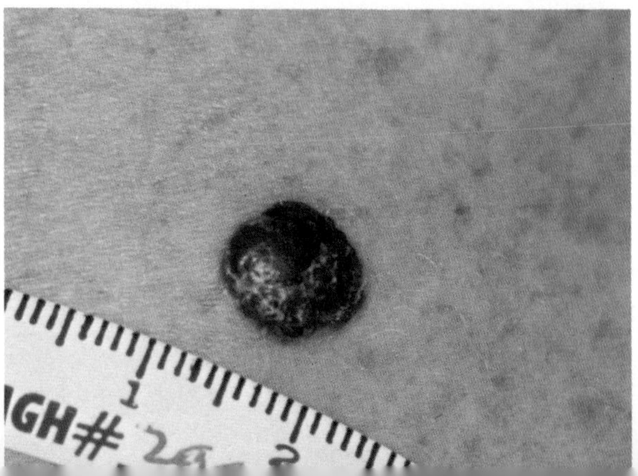

6-3 In Type III malignant melanoma, the lesion is always raised and may be dome-shaped or polypoid. The color is usually uniform bluish black, but there may rarely be shades of reddish blue (purple) or an admixture of bluish black with brown or black.

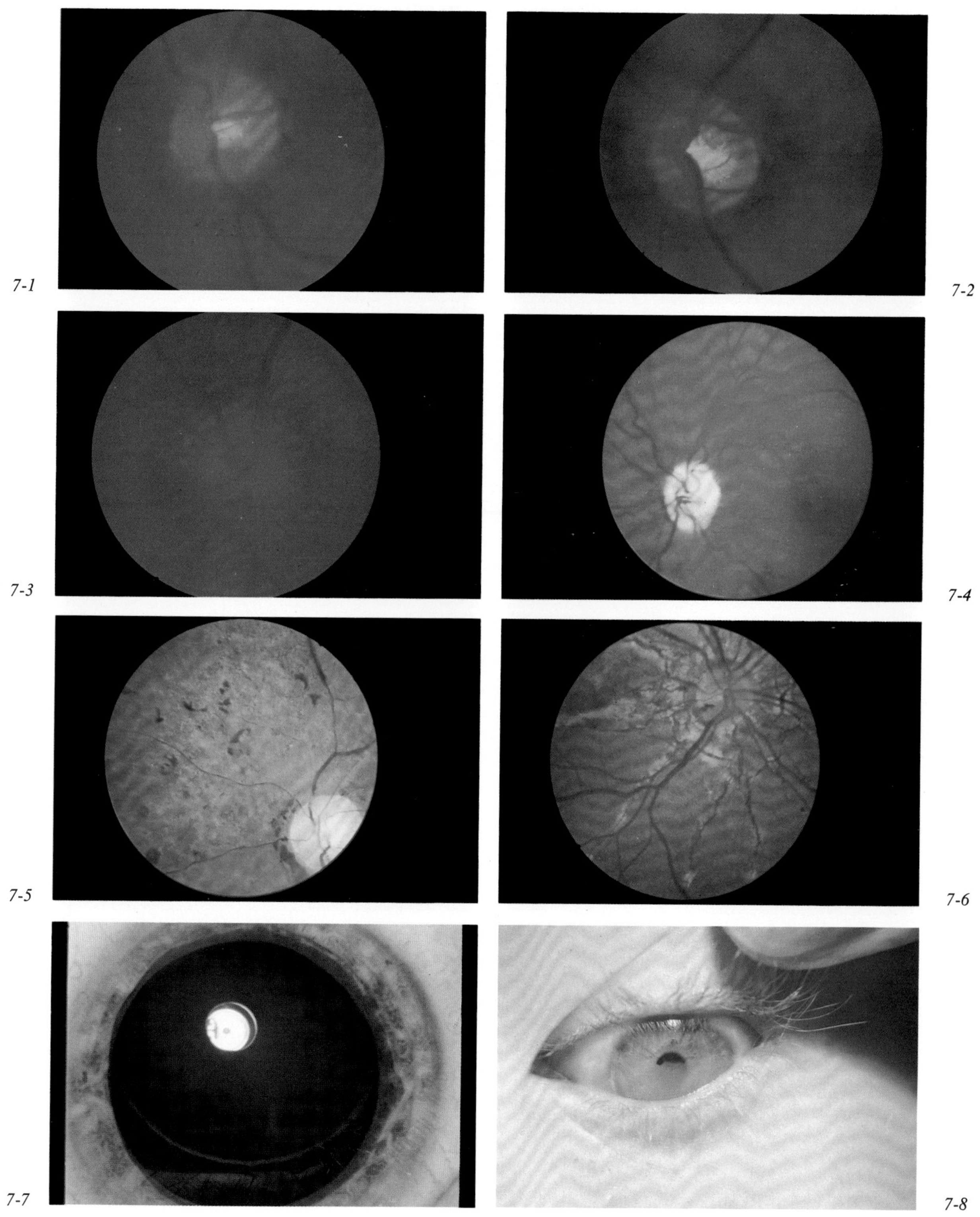

7-1 Normal optic nervehead, right eye *7-2* Temporal pallor, optic nervehead, left eye. Compare with normal right optic nerve figure 1.
7-3 Papilledema *7-4* Optic atrophy
7-5 Retinitis pigmentosa *7-6* Angioid streaks
7-7 Dislocation of crystalline lens *7-8* Band keratopathy

PLATE 8

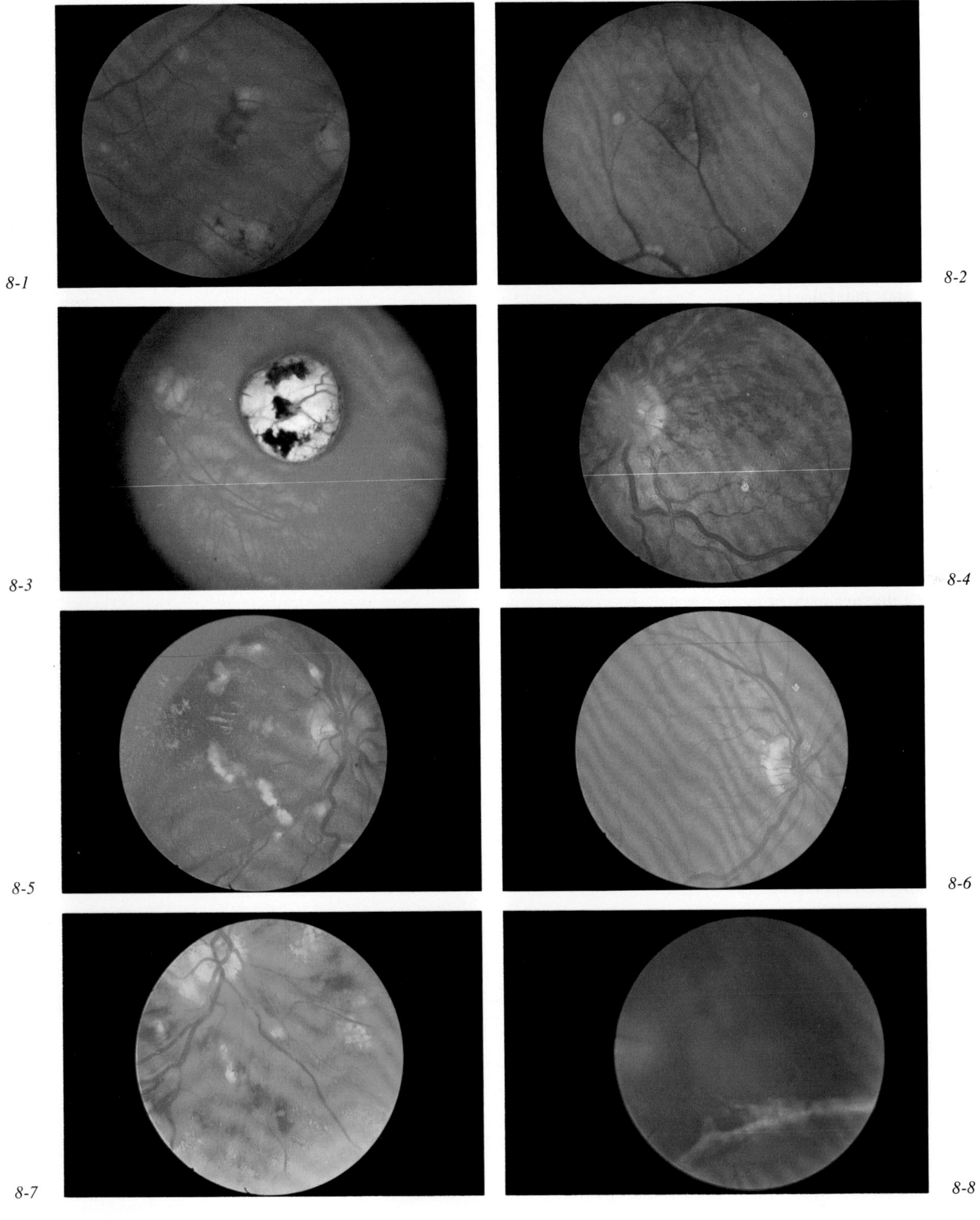

8-1 Histoplasmosis *8-2* Sarcoid *8-3* Toxoplasmosis
8-4 Occlusion of superior temporal vein with edema of macula
8-5 Hypertensive retinopathy *8-6* Early intraretinal diabetic retinopathy
8-7 Advanced intraretinal diabetic retinopathy
8-8 Advanced extraretinal (proliferative) diabetic retinopathy

follows the onset of colitis by 6 months to several years, but rarely the onset of both may coincide or the arthritis may precede colitis. Arthritis tends to be more common in patients with diffuse intestinal involvement, with continuous or intermittent chronic intestinal disease, or with intestinal disease complicated by perianal disease or pseudopolyposis. Patients with recurrent mouth ulcers, uveitis, pyoderma gangrenosum and erythema nodosum are also more likely to have arthritis. When erythema nodosum is present, it is not clear whether to attribute the arthritis to that often associated with idiopathic erythema nodosum or to that associated with colitis.

The typical attack of arthritis presents acutely, often affecting a single joint in the lower extemity. Involvement of other joints, without definite symmetry, may follow over the next few days. The involved joint is usually red, swollen, and painful. The knee and ankle are most frequently affected, followed by the proximal interphalangeal, elbow, shoulder, and wrist joints. The arthritis usually subsides within several weeks, but occasionally lasts for months. Complete resolution without residual damage is the general rule. Recurrent attacks of arthritis tend to occur with flare-ups of colitis and occasionally may herald an impending exacerbation of colitis. Peripheral arthritis usually subsides following colectomy.

Spondylitis with ulcerative colitis is indistinguishable from ankylosing spondylitis. However, the usual male preponderance observed in ankylosing spondylitis is not seen in patients with ulcerative colitis and spondylitis. In addition, uveitis and erythema nodosum are rare with the spondylitis that accompanies ulcerative colitis. The onset of spondylitis more often precedes the colitis than does peripheral arthritis, and spondylitis tends to progress regardless of colectomy or remission of intestinal disease. The disease may progress to complete ankylosis of the spine.

The peripheral blood white cell count, anemia, and elevated erythrocyte sedimentation rate usually reflect the intestinal disease. Tests for rheumatoid factor are negative. Synovial fluid shows a moderate leukocytosis, in the range of 10,000 cells per mm^3, consisting predominantly of polymorphonuclear leukocytes.

Radiographs of involved peripheral joints usually are normal except for soft-tissue swelling. An occasional patient with recurrent or persistent disease will show small bony erosions at the joint space narrowing. Films of the spine show changes indistinguishable from those of ankylosing spondylitis.

Treatment with salicylates or phenylbutazone is of benefit in reducing symptoms. Physical therapy is directed toward maintenance of posture in spondylitis and prevention of contractures in the peripheral form of arthritis. Colectomy or systemic steroids are not indicated for treatment of the arthritis alone.

Regional enteritis Peripheral arthritis or spondylitis similar to that of ulcerative colitis is found in approximately 5 percent of patients with regional enteritis. Nonspecific musculoskeletal complaints without objective arthritis are common. Arthritis is more common in patients with ileocolitis, and the peripheral arthritis tends to follow the activity of the intestinal disease. The arthritis comes on acutely, tends to be migratory, and most commonly affects the knees. With involvement of numerous small joints of the hand, especially the proximal interphalangeal joints, it may be confused initially with rheumatoid arthritis. The peripheral joint disease is mild, subsiding in a few weeks without residual joint damage. The spondylitis is identical to that of ulcerative colitis. The management of the arthritis is the same as in ulcerative colitis.

Whipple's disease Whipple's disease (intestinal lipodystrophy) is a rare disorder affecting predominantly middle-aged males and is characterized by arthritis, serositis, diarrhea, malabsorption, weight loss, and lymphadenopathy. The diagnosis is confirmed by the identification of PAS (periodic acid–Schiff)-positive bacilliform structures intercellularly or as inclusions in foamy macrophages. These bacilli can be seen in the mucosa and lamina propria of the small intestine, in abdominal and peripheral lymph nodes, and in other tissues (Chap. 285).

Arthritis occurs in approximately two-thirds of the patients and usually precedes the appearance of intestinal symptoms by months or years, making the diagnosis of the arthritis difficult. With the onset of intestinal symptoms, the arthritis may subside. The joint disease involves predominantly peripheral joints, affecting knees and ankles most commonly, followed by fingers, hips, shoulders, elbows, and wrists. It is typically acute, migratory, and transient, lasts only a few days, and causes no permanent joint damage. Long irregular periods of remission are common. Some patients with peripheral joint involvement have radiographic changes in the sacroiliac joints similar to those of ankylosing spondylitis. Synovial fluid shows only a mild monocytosis without characteristic foamy macrophages. A report of PAS-positive inclusion bodies in synovial lining cells has not been confirmed. This disease responds well to therapy with tetracycline, chloramphenicol, or ampicillin. Corticosteroids may be necessary in addition to antimicrobials in severely ill patients but are not indicated for the treatment of arthritis alone. Salicylates or phenylbutazone may be helpful in controlling joint symptoms.

REFERENCES

Ford DK: Reiter's syndrome. Bull Rheum Dis 20:588, 1970

——: Reiter's syndrome, in *Arthritis and Allied Conditions*, 8th ed., ed JL Hollander, Lea & Febiger: Philadelphia, 1972

Kulka JP: The lesions of Reiter's syndrome. Arthritis Rheum 5:195, 1962

McEwen C et al: Ankylosing spondylitis and spondylitis accompanying ulcerative colitis, regional enteritis, psoriasis and Reiter's disease. Arthritis Rheum 14:291, 1971

Maizel H et al: Whipple's disease—a review of 19 patients from one hospital and a review of the literature since 1950. Medicine 49:175, 1970

Wright VW, Moll JMH: Psoriatic arthritis. Bull Rheum Dis 21:627, 1971

——, Watkinson G: The arthritis of ulcerative colitis. Brit Med J 2:670, 1965

359 CRYSTAL-INDUCED ARTHRITIS

BRUCE C. GILLILAND
MART MANNIK

GOUT See Chap. 100.

PSEUDOGOUT Pseudogout is an acute and sometimes chronic inflammatory arthritis of older individuals, caused by the presence of calcium pyrophosphate dihydrate crystals in the joint. Pseudogout is characteristically accompanied by the radiographic finding of calcification of articular cartilages. The knee and other large joints are the most frequent sites of involvement. The mechanism for the deposition of crystals in the articular cartilage (chondrocalcinosis) is unknown.

The disease most commonly occurs in persons over age fifty, and its prevalence increases with age. Both sexes are affected. In some instances, chondrocalcinosis is considered to be genetically determined, since several family members and young adults develop the disease.

Elevated levels of inorganic pyrophosphate are found in the synovial fluid of many patients. Plasma levels are normal. The interpretation of these observations, together with reports of low synovial fluid pyrophosphatase activity, requires further study.

Chondrocalcinosis has been found in association with metabolic diseases and other disorders, including diabetes mellitus, gout, hyperparathyroidism, pernicious anemia, and hemochromatosis. The relationship of these disorders to the pathogenesis of chondrocalcinosis is presently unknown.

The *pathologic change* in the joint involves deposits of calcium pyrophosphate dihydrate crystals in the joint capsule, in the midzonal area of articular hyaline cartilage, and diffusely in fibrocartilage. The menisci of the knee are a common site of crystal deposition. Crystals can be seen at the margin of degenerating cartilage and surrounding the lacunae of chondrocytes; this site is considered the earliest detectable lesion. The deposition of crystals varies from microcrystalline aggregates to large masses intermixed with fibrous tissue. Crystals may also be observed in normal-appearing cartilage.

The synovium in acute arthritis is edematous, with numerous polymorphonuclear leukocytes. Crystals are seen in the superficial portion of the synovium. In chronic arthritis, mononuclear cell infiltration and fibroblastic proliferation are present; crystals are rarely observed.

Acute arthritis can be experimentally induced by the injection of calcium pyrophosphate dihydrate crystals into the normal joint. In chondrocalcinosis, the arthritis is thought to be initiated by the rupture of crystals from cartilage into the joint cavity, resulting in the activation of vasoactive and chemotactic factors. Polymorphonuclear leukocytes are attracted into the joint and phagocytize the crystals, leading to the release of lysosomal hydrolytic enzymes into the joint fluid.

The onset of the acute attack of pseudogout is rapid and reaches a peak usually in 12 to 36 hr. The involved joint is erythematous, swollen, very warm, and extremely painful. The acute attack is usually confined to a single joint, but in some patients, involvement of other joints may follow in rapid progression. The knee is by far the most frequent site of acute arthritis, but attacks occur in the ankles, wrists, elbows, hips, and cervical and lumbar parts of the spine. As in gout, the first metatarsal joint of the great toe may also be a site of involvement. The acute arthritis is most commonly intermittent, and the same joint is often involved in subsequent attacks. The acute episode usually subsides in 1 to 2 weeks. Between attacks the previously involved joint appears relatively normal. Some patients have almost continuous acute attacks, often affecting several joints at one time. Other patients may have a chronic form of arthritis, predominantly affecting larger joints. Symptoms may be indistinguishable from those of degenerative joint disease; however, in some of these patients, superimposed episodes of acute arthritis occur. Finally, some patients may show typical articular calcification radiographically but are free of symptoms.

The microscopic examination of *synovial fluid* in an acute attack shows large numbers of polymorphonuclear leukocytes. Calcium pyrophosphate dihydrate crystals are invariably found extracellularly and in polymorphonuclear leukocytes. In chronic arthritis, the crystals are observed less frequently and are most often extracellular. With polarized light, the crystals appear as short blunt rods, rhomboids, and cuboids. They show weakly positive birefringence under compensated polarized light, in contrast to the strongly negative birefringence of sodium urate crystals. X-ray diffraction studies are necessary to identify them definitely as calcium pyrophosphate dihydrate crystals. However, the diagnosis can be made with the finding of weakly positive birefringent crystals under compensated polarized light in combination with radiographic evidence of typical articular calcifications.

Radiographically, calcifications in articular hyaline cartilage appear as fine linear densities parallel to the subchondral bone surface. In the knee, this line is best observed on a lateral film. Calcifications in fibrocartilage, ligaments, and joint capsule usually appear as more diffuse punctate and linear densities. Common sites of fibrocartilage involvement include the menisci of the knee, articular disk of the distal radioulnar joint, symphysis pubis, and the annulus fibrosus of the intervertebral disk. Evidence for chondrocalcinosis can usually be obtained with radiographs of the knees, wrists, and pelvis. Radiographic findings of osteoarthritis are also present, particularly in patients with chronic arthritis of pseudogout.

Gout and septic arthritis are the main considerations in the *differential diagnosis* of the acute arthritis. Gout and pseudogout are frequently indistinguishable clinically, and the diagnosis depends on the identification of their characteristic crystals under compensated polarized light. Both crystals occasionally have been found together in the synovial fluid of patients with typical radiographic articular calcifications of chondrocalcinosis. Bacterial smears and cultures should be performed on synovial fluid in all patients with an acute monarticular arthritis. The symptoms of osteoarthritis and chronic pseudogout are very similar, and radiographic evidence for both is often present. The role played by each is difficult to determine. Pseudogout should be considered in these patients when intermittent attacks of acute arthritis occur. Also, the finding of a large chronic effusion in patients with symptoms of osteoarthritis suggests the possibility of pseudogout. The diagnosis of pseudogout should not be made only on the radiographic findings of intraarticular calcific deposits, but depends also on the identification of the characteristic crystals, since other forms of inflammatory arthritis may affect the same joints. Radiographic evidence of calcific deposits is found not infrequently in knees of elderly patients who have no joint symptoms.

For the *treatment* of acute pseudogout, phenylbutazone is usually effective. A loading dose of 600 mg is given, followed by 200 to 300 mg per day until symptoms subside. Indomethacin 75 to 150 mg per day may also be used. Remarkable relief is sometimes achieved with aspiration of the synovial fluid. Colchicine is not as effective as in acute gout. In chronic arthritis, salicylates may give symptomatic relief. The deposition of calcium pyrophosphate crystals in articular tissues cannot be prevented or reversed.

REFERENCES

McCarty DJ: On the crystal deposition diseases. Disease-a-Month, March, 1970

—— et al: Inorganic pyrophosphate concentrations in the synovial fluid of arthritic patients. J Lab Clin Med 78:216, 1971

360
INFECTIOUS ARTHRITIDES

BRUCE C. GILLILAND
MART MANNIK

ACUTE BACTERIAL ARTHRITIS Septic arthritis is a medical emergency which must be recognized promptly and treated appropriately to avoid permanent joint damage. Microorganisms usually reach the joint by hematogenous spread from a primary infection elsewhere, but occasionally no source can be found. Joint sepsis may also occur by direct extension of infection from adjacent bone or soft tissue.

The purpose of this discussion on infectious arthritides is to provide a general approach to the diagnosis and management of articular infections. The bacteriology and specific antimicrobial therapy are considered in the chapters on the respective infections.

Acute *bacterial arthritis* is caused by many different types of bacteria; the ones most commonly encountered are *Neisseria gonorrhoeae, Staphylococcus aureus, Diplococcus pneumoniae, Streptococcus pyogenes, Hemophilus influenzae,* and gram-negative bacilli (*Escherichia coli, Salomonella* sp., *Pseudomonas,* etc.). Septic arthritis due to *H. influenzae* occurs mostly in children; gonococcal arthritis is a disease of young adults. Joint sepsis with gram-negative bacilli tends to occur in patients with underlying infection of the urinary tract or intestine, and in patients with impaired resistance to infection. Patients with salmonella arthritis often have evidence of underlying osteomyelitis. Infectious arthritis of the spine is seen in brucellosis and salmonella infections.

An increased susceptibility to joint infection occurs in patients with diabetes, in those with lymphomas, and in those receiving corticosteroids or immunosuppressive drugs. In addition, joints previously damaged by arthritis, such as rheumatoid arthritis or trauma, are more liable to infections.

The onset of bacterial arthritis is usually abrupt and accompanied be fever and chills. One or a few joints may be involved. The affected joint is warm, erythematous, swollen, and painful; however, these signs may be masked in patients receiving corticosteroids. Marked guarding of the joint and muscle spasms are common. The larger joints, such as the hips, knees, and shoulders, are more commonly affected, and the wrists, ankles, elbows, and sternoclavicular and sacroiliac joints less often. The articulations of the spine or any peripheral joint may be a site of infection. In the spine, infection involves the vertebral body and adjacent intervertebral disk space, and may extend to the adjacent apophyseal joint. Localized tenderness and spasm of the paraspinal or psoas muscles are often present. The diagnosis of septic arthritis of the hip is often delayed, since the swelling of this joint is not readily detected and aspiration is difficult. Pain from the hip is frequently referred to the knee. Initially, patients hold the thigh in adduction and internal rotation; subsequently it is held in abduction, flexion, and external rotation. In some instances, the thigh becomes edematous and swelling appears in the anterior groin.

The synovium in the early stages of infection is edematous and infiltrated by neutrophils. An effusion with many neutrophils forms rapidly. Lysosomal proteolytic enzymes are released from neutrophils and destroy articular cartilage, subchondral bone, and joint capsule. Small abscesses appear in the synovium and subchondral bone, and necrotic debris collects in the joint space. During healing, proliferation of fibroblasts may lead to ankylosis.

Joint aspiration should be performed in any patient suspected of having a septic joint. The synovial fluid is initially cloudy and later may be grossly purulent. The white blood cell count usually ranges from 50,000 to 100,000 per mm^3 or higher, and more than 90 percent of the cells are neutrophils. The concentration of glucose in the joint cavity is often less than 50 percent of a simultaneous blood sugar reading when obtained at least 6 hr after a meal. Gram stain frequently reveals microorganisms. Cultures of the synovial fluid and blood should be performed even if the gram stain is negative. Radiographs of the joint early in infection show only distention of the joint capsule, but later x-rays reveal juxtaarticular osteoporosis, joint space narrowing due to cartilage destruction, and bony erosion on the articular surface. In the spine, radiographic changes may not be seen for several months. The first changes consist of narrowing of the involved disk space or vertebra and proliferation of bone at the vertebral margins. Subsequently, lytic lesions appear in the vertebra and may extend to the disk space.

During healing adjacent vertebras may become fused.

The diagnosis of septic arthritis is confirmed by a positive culture from synovial fluid or tissue. With spinal involvement, needle biopsy or open surgical biopsy is usually required to obtain tissue for culture. The acute arthritis of gout or pseudogout may be mistaken for septic arthritis because of the monarticular involvement and manifestations of acute joint inflammation. They are easily distinguished by the finding of the respective characteristic crystals in synovial fluid. Other types of inflammatory arthritis, such as psoriatic arthritis, Reiter's syndrome, rheumatoid arthritis, or rheumatic fever, may also be confused with a septic arthritis, especially when only one or a few joints are involved. In a patient with generalized arthritis (such as rheumatoid disease) who develops fever and chills and has one joint disproportionately more inflamed than other joints, the possibility of septic arthritis should be carefully ruled out by examination of the synovial fluid cells and by culture of synovial fluid. The possibility of infectious arthritis should also be entertained in patients with unilateral sacroiliitis and fever.

Septic arthritis requires prompt treatment with the appropriate antibiotic. Table 360-1 shows the preferred antibiotic regimen for the more common types of septic arthritis. Bactericidal levels of antibiotics are achieved with systemic administration. Direct administration of an antibiotic into the joint is not recommended and may in itself produce a chemical synovitis. During treatment, bactericidal assays of synovial fluid may be performed to assure that therapeutic levels of antibiotic have been achieved. Aspiration of the joint once or several times a day should be done to reduce the pressure and to remove pus that generates proteolytic enzymes. Open surgical drainage is usually not indicated except in septic arthritis of the hip or in a joint with chronic suppuration. Splinting of the affected joint will make the patient more comfortable and reduce the degree of flexion deformity. Prolonged splinting, however, should be avoided, since it may lead to a permanent joint stiffness. When the inflammation has subsided, physical therapy will aid the return of joint function. When a weight-bearing joint has been severely damaged, bony fusion may be necessary.

TABLE 360-1
Recommended therapy for the major types of acute bacterial arthritis

Organism	*Drug and dose*
Neisseria gonorrhoeae	Penicillin G, 1–2 million units q.6h. for 10–14 days
Hemophilus influenzae	Ampicillin, 1 g q.6h. IM for 10–14 days
Staphylococcus aureus	
Penicillin G–sensitive	Penicillin G, 4 million units q.6h. IV for 2 weeks,* then oral therapy for 4–6 weeks
Penicillin G–resistant	Methicillin, 2 g q.6h. IV for 2 weeks,* then dicloxacillin, 1 g q.6h. orally for 4 weeks
Diplococcus pneumoniae	Penicillin G, 2 million units q.6h. IV for 10–14 days
β-Hemolytic streptococcus, group A	Same as for *Diplococcus* pneumoniae

* *Intravenous therapy should be continued until infection is controlled.*

TUBERCULOUS ARTHRITIS Tuberculous arthritis is a chronic destructive form of septic arthritis caused by *Mycobacterium* tuberculosis. Most patients have a focus of tuberculosis elsewhere in the body; however, in some patients no primary lesion can be detected. The bacilli infect the synovium either through the circulation or by extension from a tuberculous lesion in the adjacent bone. Tuberculous arthritis is more common in children but occurs at any age.

The tuberculous process in the joint produces synovitis, with the formation of a pannus of granulation tissue over the articular cartilage. The subchondral bone is involved, and areas of necrosis occur. Destruction of articular cartilage occurs later in the course, followed by fibrous ankylosis.

In the spine, the infection begins in the vertebral body; the thoracic spine is affected most frequently. Destruction of bone leads to vertebral collapse and angulation of the spine. Extension of the infection into the adjacent soft tissues produces a cold abscess, which may spread down the anterior aspect of the spine to form a psoas abscess. The abscess may eventually point in the anterior groin.

Tuberculous arthritis has an insidious onset, is usually monarticular, and usually affects the spine, hips, and knees. The affected peripheral joint is swollen, warm, and tender and has a decreased range of motion. Erythema is minimal, and pain is usually a later manifestation. The hypertrophied synovium gives the joint a boggy, doughy feeling. Muscle atrophy and spasm of the affected extremity occur. Tenosynovitis of the flexor tendon sheaths of the wrist may compress the median nerve and produce a carpal tunnel syndrome. Regional lymphadenopathy is usually present.

With spine involvement (Pott's disease), tenderness and muscle spasm over the affected area are found. Subsequent vertebral collapse in the dorsal part of the spine leads to kyphosis. Paralysis and tuberculous meningitis are serious complications.

The patient may have only slight fever. Weight loss is common. The course of untreated disease is one of progressive joint destruction, but spontaneous remission sometimes occurs.

Examination of synovial fluid shows usually more than 10,000 leukocytes per mm^3. Differential counts are not helpful. The tubercle bacilli may be seen on smears of synovial fluid but are more likely to be found on biopsy of synovial tissue or of regional lymph nodes.

Radiographs of peripheral joints in early disease show joint capsule distention and juxtaarticular osteoporosis. Bony erosions at the joint margin, subchondral bone destruction, and joint space narrowing are observed later in the disease. Films of the spine show destruction of the vertebral body, vertebral collapse, and loss of intervertebral disk space.

The diagnosis of tuberculous arthritis is made on the

demonstration of the tubercule bacilli in synovial fluid or tissue by smear, histology, or culture. The tuberculin skin test is almost always positive.

Antimicrobial therapy is described in Chap. 156. Surgical treatment may be necessary and includes debridement, synovectomy, and joint fusion.

MYCOTIC, SYPHILITIC, AND VIRAL ARTHRITIDES

The systemic mycoses (coccidioidomycosis, histoplasmosis, blastomycosis, cryptococcosis, actinomycosis, and sporotrichosis) may involve bone and joints. In the primary phase of coccidioidomycosis, a transient polyarthritis, lasting up to 1 month, may occur in association with erythema nodosum (desert arthritis), but no residual joint damage ensues. However, with disseminated disease, bone and joint involvement leads to joint destruction. Joint involvement by actinomycosis results from extension of infection from adjacent bone. Sporotrichosis, however, may produce synovial infection. In the other mycotic diseases, joint involvement is infrequent.

The diagnosis of fungal arthritis is established by the identification of the organisms in synovial fluid or in a biopsy specimen. Treatment with amphotericin B is usually successful; however, surgical debridement may be necessary.

Syphilitic arthritis occurs in congenital, secondary, or tertiary syphilis. During the first year of life, congenital syphilis may produce an osteochondritis in the juxtaepiphyseal region which results in the breakdown of bone and articular cartilage (Parrot's pseudoparalysis). At puberty, congenital disease may cause a synovitis which most commonly involves the knees and elbows (Clutton's joints). The joint is often red, swollen, and tender, but pain may be minimal. Synovial fluid shows a leukocytosis, predominantly lymphocytes.

In secondary syphilis, transient polyarthritis and polyarthralgia occur. Gummatous involvement of the synovium may occur in tertiary syphilis and most often involves the larger joints.

In addition to direct involvement of the joint, syphilis also produces a neuropathic joint (Chap. 159).

The proper diagnosis of the joint disease can be established only after the correct diagnosis of syphilis. A positive serologic test for syphilis is not diagnostic, since biologic false positive tests may occur in rheumatic diseases such as systemic lupus erythematosus. Treatment of syphilis is considered in Chap. 159.

A self-limited *polyarthritis* may be a manifestation of several *viral diseases* (e.g., mumps, arboviral infection, rubella, hepatitis, infectious mononucleosis), especially in the prodromal stages of the illness.

Rubella infection may manifest a polyarthritis, usually involving the small joints of the extremities. The arthritis is seen most often in young adults, especially women. Arthritis has also been observed in children and young adults after vaccination with rubella vaccine. The onset of arthritis coincides with or shortly follows the appearance of the rash. The arthritis lasts up to 2 weeks and leaves no residual joint damage. Synovial fluid has been reported to show an increased numbers of lymphocytes. Rheumatoid factor tests are usually negative.

Arthritis is a relatively common manifestation of viral hepatitis, especially when hepatitis is associated with Australia antigen (serum hepatitis, type B hepatitis, hepatitis-associated antigen). Arthritis, sometimes accompanied by a rash, usually precedes the onset of clinical jaundice by a few days to 2 weeks, but disappears with the appearance of jaundice. The arthritis may be migratory, involves both small and large joints, and leaves no residual joint damage. Symmetric joint involvement of the hands may be confused with rheumatoid arthritis. Synovial fluid shows a mild leukocytosis with predominantly lymphocytes. Rheumatoid factor tests usually are negative.

Serum and joint fluid complement levels are usually low during arthritis. Serum complement level returns to normal with the appearance of overt liver disease. Australia antigen can be detected in both serum and joint fluid during the prodromal period of hepatitis. The synovitis is thought to be induced not by the virus itself, but by immune complexes consisting of antibodies and viral antigens.

REFERENCES

ALPERT E et al: Pathogenesis of arthritis associated with viral hepatitis: Complement component studies. N Engl J Med 285:185, 1971

HOLLANDER JL: *Arthritis and Allied Conditions* 7th ed., Philadelphia: Lea & Febiger, 1966

KELLY PJ, KARLSON AG: Musculoskeletal tuberculosis. Proc Mayo Clin 44:73, 1969

PARKER RH, SCHMID FR: Antibacterial activity of synovial fluid during therapy of septic arthritis. Arthritis Rheum 14:96, 1971

WILLERSON JT et al: Septic arthritis, the unexpected complication. Postgrad Med 45:127, 1969

361 DEGENERATIVE JOINT DISEASE

MART MANNIK
BRUCE C. GILLILAND

INTRODUCTION Degenerative joint disease (subsequently abbreviated DJD) is characterized by loss of joint cartilage and by hypertrophy of bone. Synonyms for degenerative joint disease include osteoarthritis and hypertrophic arthritis. DJD occurs in a very high percentage of elderly persons, as determined by radiologic or pathologic examinations. However, many persons with such abnormalities have no musculoskeletal complaints. In young persons changes identical to the degenerative changes in advanced age are encountered when cartilage has been damaged by injury, infection, or congenital deformities. The exact mechanisms for cartilage loss in

DJD have not been defined, but abnormal stress and subchondral bone changes contribute to the damage. Treatment of DJD is directed to amelioration of symptoms, decrease in excessive stress, and corrective procedures in properly selected subjects.

PATHOGENESIS AND ETIOLOGY Two schools of thought have evolved in the study of pathogenesis of primary DJD. One suggests that DJD is primarily a disease of cartilage. Degeneration of cartilage then leads to secondary changes of bone, such as subchondral sclerosis and osteophyte formation (overgrowth of bone at the joint margins). The other thesis is that the first alterations are due to microfractures of subchondral bone. Remodeling then leads to loss of deformability of bone, with a concomitant decrease in energy dissipation by bone. These primary changes in bone increase stress on cartilage, which then breaks down, with further distortion of weight-bearing surfaces. Thus a "vicious cycle" of bone and cartilage damage evolves. In this theory, no predisposing biochemical defects are postulated; the repetitive application of stress on joints is thought to be the important initiating factor. For example, in the distal interphalangeal joints the stress on the joint is applied only in a longitudinal direction over a small area of the joint, while in the ankle the load is distributed over a relatively large area with less shearing stress on motion; hence the digit is a frequent site of DJD, and the ankle an infrequent one. Work patterns can change the usual stresses of joints, for example, air hammer operators develop DJD of the elbows and shoulders. In contrast, the development of DJD is slow in paralyzed limbs. These concepts emphasize the universality of DJD and the role of recurrent and excessive force on the joints as the most important cause of initial injury to cartilage or bone. Other forms of injury to cartilage, including sequelae of inflammatory joint disease and probably biochemical and metabolic changes in articular cartilage, may lead to a degenerative change indistinguishable from the usual form of DJD. In the damaged joint cartilage, chondrocytes are thought to release lysosomal proteases that in turn degrade proteoglycans of the cartilage matrix and thereby decrease the biophysical performance of the cartilage.

PATHOLOGY Early pathologic changes of DJD occur in the joint cartilage. Subsequently new bone formation develops in subchondral bone and at the margins of the articular cartilage. Progressive loss of metachromasia (histologic evidence of proteoglycan loss) occurs in the cartilage, beginning at the surface. Chondrocytes increase in number and form clusters. This has been interpreted as a reparative attempt in response to cartilage loss. With progression of the process the surface of cartilage begins to loosen and flake along superficial collagen fibers that parallel the joint surface; upon reaching the deeper radial layer the damage is reflected in fissuring of cartilage. Abrasion of damaged cartilage may ultimately lead to total loss of the cartilage. This progressive loss of cartilage is apparent radiologically as "joint space" narrowing.

The bone at joint margins responds to cartilage damage with osteophyte formation. These lesions usually extend from the margin of the joint along the contour of the joint surface. Alternatively, osteophytes may develop within and extend along ligamentous and capsular attachments of the joint margin. The denuded subchondral bone becomes dense, smooth, and glistening, and looks like ivory (eburnation). In addition, cystic areas may develop below the joint surface and become filled with fibrous tissue. These "pseudocysts" are thought to result from transmission of intraarticular pressure through cartilaginous defects into underlying cancellous bone. Minimal inflammatory changes are present in the synovium and joint capsule, but the capsule is subject to thickening with fibrosis.

CLINICAL MANIFESTATIONS Clinically degenerative joint disease is divided into *primary* and *secondary* forms. In primary DJD no predisposing abnormality or cause can be found, and the usual symptoms of the illness begin after the fifth and sixth decades of life. In secondary DJD an underlying abnormality or injury can be found, and the clinical symptoms may begin several decades earlier. The clinical findings in primary and secondary DJD are similar, except that in secondary DJD unusual or single joints are more likely to be involved.

The cardinal complaint in DJD is pain confined to joints, especially on motion and weight bearing. The pain is frequently described as aching and only seldom is intense. Patients complain of definite joint stiffness; this occurs after resting and subsides in a few minutes upon resuming motion. In the morning the stiffness lasts only a short time (usually reported in minutes), whereas the morning stiffness of rheumatoid arthritis lasts an hour or more. On examination the joints may show a restricted range of motion, local tenderness, bony enlargement, small effusions, and crepitus. Erythema and increased heat are unusual in DJD.

DJD of the distal interphalangeal joints of fingers leads to bony enlargement of the joint. These dorsolaterally located nodules at the base of the terminal phalanx are called *Heberden's nodes.* A quarter of the patients who have nodes of the distal interphalangeal joints also have similar deformities at the proximal interphalangeal joints, called *Bouchard's nodes.* The primary Heberden's nodes usually evolve insidiously and without pain. However, some patients develop redness, swelling, and tenderness that lasts a few weeks. Subsequently the initial relatively soft and painful swelling is replaced by a hard, bony, painless enlargement and complaints are on cosmetic grounds only. Heberden's nodes are more common in females than males, and in females heredity seems to play a role. The mother and sisters of a woman with Heberden's nodes are more likely to have the nodes than controls of the same age and sex. Heberden's nodes may involve single joints as a result of trauma (e.g., "baseball fingers," "karate fingers"). Metacarpophalangeal joints are virtually never involved. The carpometacarpal joint of the thumb is frequently involved (Fig. 361-1).

DJD of the wrists, elbows, and shoulders is relatively uncommon. However, occupational trauma may enhance DJD in elbows and shoulders, as in air hammer workers.

With mild osteoarthritis of the spine, patients complain of stiffness, pain, and decreased motion of the involved area. Encroachment of osteophytes on spinal foramens may lead to cervical and lumbar nerve root compression. Radicular pain, muscle spasms, muscle atrophy, and neurologic abnormalities help to localize the problem. X-rays of the spine show characteristic lipping and spur formation. Most elderly persons have these changes, but in relatively few do the changes evolve to symptomatic DJD of the spine.

DJD of the hip is perhaps the most disabling form of the illness, with considerable loss of function in the advanced stages. Groin pain, at times referred to the knee, and loss of range of motion are the important findings. Radiologic examination is important in evaluation of the extent of the involvement. *Secondary DJD* of the hip occurs earlier and is often unilateral. The causes of secondary DJD of the hip and other joints include trauma, fractures, infection, and damage by inflammatory joint diseases such as rheumatoid arthritis. Developmental abnormalities are also important, including congenital dislocation of the hip, dysplasia of the acetabulum, anomalies of the upper femur, adolescent slipped epiphyses, and avascular necrosis (aseptic necrosis). Avascular necrosis occurs in divers, alcoholics, patients receiving corticosteroids, and those with sickle-cell disease. Severe pain follows collapse of the subchondral bone; a characteristic wedge-shaped defect is seen on radiographs. The destruction of cartilage and subchondral bone then hastens the development of DJD.

Occupational or sport injuries are frequent causes of degenerative changes in the knees. Torn menisci and ligamentous instability contribute to early changes. Tenderness, limitation of motion by pain, crepitation, and joint effusions may be present. *Chondromalacia patellae* produces softening and loss of cartilage from the articular surface of the patella. This is usually an early development of DJD, but at times is seen in young persons. Pain and crepitus are frequently present on patellar motion.

Extensive DJD is found late in the course of acromegaly. The early articular changes in acromegaly include thickened synovial tissues and considerable overgrowth of the joint cartilage, presumably resulting from excessive secretion of growth hormone.

Erosive osteoarthritis Occasionally middle-aged or older females are encountered who have an acute and transient inflammatory joint disease, particularly in the joints of the hands, in association with typical changes of DJD. These patients have tender and red distal and proximal interphalangeal joints. Subsequently Heberden's nodes evolve. Single or several joints may be involved at any one time. On radiographs these patients are seen to have developed osteophytes and subchondral sclerosis but may also have erosions of the joint surface. Periarticular osteoporosis is not a feature of this condition. On histologic examination, mild to moderate inflammation is present during the acute phase, with lymphocyte and plasma cell infiltration and even mild pannus formation—quite similar to that in mild rheumatoid arthritis. However, patients with erosive osteoarthritis can be distinguished from patients with rheumatoid arthritis by the characteristic presentation and pattern of joint involvement, the absence of prolonged morning stiffness, absence of typical rheumatoid deformities, lack of palpable synovial hypertrophy, radiologic presence of degenerative changes, normal erythrocyte sedimentation rate, and negative tests for rheumatoid factor. A weakly positive test for rheumatoid factor does not exclude erosive osteoarthritis, since normal elderly persons may have a positive test.

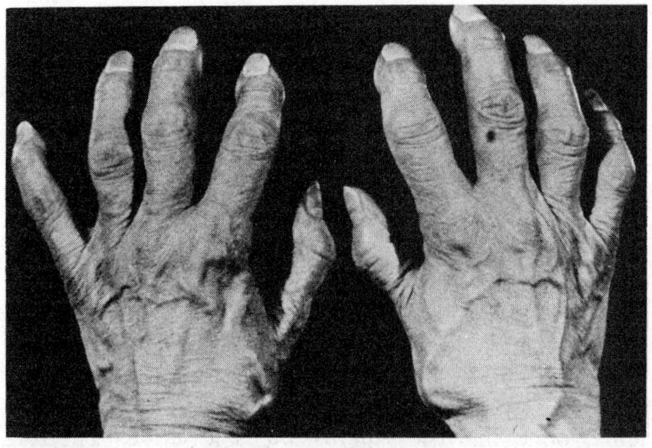

A

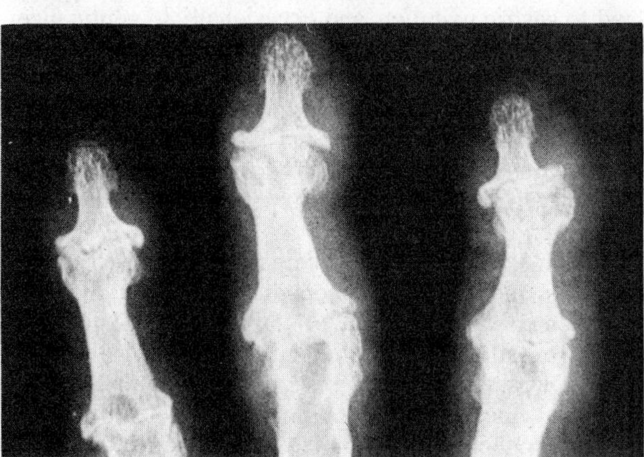

B

FIGURE 361–1

Degenerative joint disease. A *Heberden's nodes of the distal interphalangeal joints and Bouchard's nodes of the proximal interphalangeal joints of the fingers. The carpometacarpal joints of both thumbs are swollen.* B *X-rays of the middle three fingers of the left hand from the same patient. Note the marked joint space narrowing, osteophyte formation in the distal and proximal interphalangeal joints, cystic changes in subchondral bone, and absence of osteoporosis.*

DIAGNOSIS The usual laboratory tests show no abnormalities in DJD. The erythrocyte sedimentation rate is normal for the age of the patient. The characteristics of joint fluid have been discussed (Chap. 355). Radiological changes are most helpful for diagnosis. Joint pain in elderly persons without other abnormalities usually means DJD. However, caution should be exercised in ascribing joint complaints to DJD on the basis of radiographic changes alone because spurs, lipping, and joint space narrowing occur along with infections, rheumatoid arthritis, pseudogout, and gout in this age group.

TREATMENT Following evaluation of a patient with DJD, realistic goals for treatment should be established.

Reassurance is important, because patients frequently equate any joint disease with total disability. Steps should be taken to eliminate excessive and recurrent trauma. A weight-reduction program should be initiated for overweight individuals. Moderate exercise is recommended, but prolonged pain and discomfort after motion lead to decreased activity.

Acetylsalicylic acid in an adequate dose (2 to 4 g per day) is the drug of choice for relief of pain. Other salicylate preparations may be equally useful (sodium salicylate, choline salicylate, salicyl salicylate). Indomethacin (25 mg t.i.d. to q.i.d.) provides relief in some patients who do not benefit from salicylates. Phenylbutazone (100 mg b.i.d. to q.i.d.) should be employed only for short periods, and care must be exercised to detect toxicity. Dermatitis and salt retention are common problems; bone marrow suppression is a serious but fortunately uncommon complication. All these drugs may lead to gastric irritation, and occasionally to peptic ulcer.

Local heat is useful in many patients with mild DJD. In severe joint involvement, physical therapy with infrared heat, ultrasound, or hot packs may help to relieve pain. Isometric exercises may be useful, especially to strengthen the quadriceps muscle when knees are involved. Cervical traction may be helpful in relieving compression of the nerve roots.

Patients with intractable pain and advanced DJD can benefit significantly by orthopedic procedures, including debridement and removal of loose bodies, osteotomy, partial prosthetic replacement, and total joint replacement. Outstanding results have been achieved with total hip replacement in patients who were disabled by DJD of the hips. Other artifical joints are being developed. The potential benefits should be carefully weighed against the risks in each patient who is being considered for these procedures.

REFERENCES

BOLLET AJ: An essay on the biology of osteoarthritis. Arthritis Rheum 12:152, 1969

HOWELL DS et al: A comprehensive regimen for osteoarthritis. Med Clin North Am 55:457, 1971

PETER JB et al: Erosive osteoarthritis of the hands. Arthritis Rheum 9:365, 1966

RADIN EL et al: Role of mechanical factors in pathogenesis of primary osteoarthritis. Lancet I:519, 1972

362 PROGRESSIVE SYSTEMIC SCLEROSIS (DIFFUSE SCLERODERMA)

BRUCE C. GILLILAND
MART MANNIK

Progressive systemic sclerosis (subsequently abbreviated PSS) is a disorder of connective tissue leading to fibrosis that involves the skin (scleroderma) and a variety of internal organs, most notably, the gastrointestinal tract, lungs, heart, and kidney. The clinical hallmark of PSS is the tight, firm skin, which may be present several years before visceral involvement becomes apparent. However, in some patients visceral disease occurs in the absence of skin involvement.

ETIOLOGY AND PATHOGENESIS This uncommon disease has a worldwide distribution but is apparently exceedingly rare in Asia, especially among the Chinese, Indians, and Malaysians. The onset of disease is usually in the third to fifth decades, and women are affected twice as often as men. The etiology and pathogenesis of PSS are not known; hereditary factors are not involved. The increased fibrosis in the various organ systems is considered to be due to the overproduction of collagen. Tissue cultures of skin fibroblasts from scleroderma patients showed these cells to synthesize increased amounts of collagen and glycoprotein as compared with appropriate controls. Qualitative abnormalities of collagen have not been found in PSS.

Vascular injury at the level of the small arteries and capillaries has been proposed as the primary event in the pathogenesis of PSS. Evidence in support of the concept is the finding of vascular abnormalities in the absence of sclerosis in the adjacent tissue. Decreased vascularization has been documented in the skin, skeletal muscles, and lungs, which may lead to fibrosis in these tissues as a secondary event. However, it is not clear whether vascular sclerosis is only another manifestation of a generalized fibrotic process or is the result of primary vascular injury.

The role of immunologic abnormalities in the pathogenesis of PSS has not been established. Autoantibodies occur in this disorder, and PSS is associated with other rheumatic diseases in which immunologic mechanisms are of pathogenic importance. In particular, patients with combined features of scleroderma, systemic lupus erythematosus, and myositis have been described. In addition PSS is sometimes associated with Sjögren's syndrome.

PATHOLOGY In the skin, a thin epidermis overlies compact bundles of collagen which lie parallel to the epidermis. Fingerlike projectures of collagen extend from the dermis into the subcutaneous tissue and bind the skin to the underlying tissue. Dermal appendages are atrophied, and rete pegs are lost.

In the lower two-thirds of the esophagus, the histologic findings consist of a thin mucosa and increased collagen in the lamina propria, submucosa, and serosa.

The degree of fibrosis is less than that seen in the skin. Atrophy of the muscularis in the esophagus and throughout the involved portions of the gastrointestinal tract is more prominent than the amount of fibrotic replacement of muscle. The muscle atrophy is probably secondary to a neurogenic cause, not a result of a primary muscle abnormality or fibrosis. Ulceration of the mucosa is often present and may be due to either PSS or superimposed peptic esophagitis. Striated muscles in the upper one-third of the esophagus are relatively spared. Similar changes may be found throughout the gastrointestinal tract, especially in the second and third portions of the duodenum, jejunum, and large intestine. Atrophy of the muscularis of the large intestine may lead to the development of large-mouth diverticula. In later stages of the disease, the involved portions of the gastrointestinal tract become dilated. Infiltration of lymphocytes and plasma cells in the lamina propria are also present.

With pulmonary involvement, diffuse interstitial fibrosis, thickening of the alveolar membrane, and peribronchial fibrosis are observed. Bronchiolar epithelial proliferation accompanies the pulmonary fibrosis. Rupture of septums produces small cysts and areas of bulbous emphysema. Small pulmonary arteries and arterioles show intimal thickening, fragmentation of the elastica, and muscular hypertrophy; however, bronchial vessels and pulmonary veins are usually spared.

The synovium in patients with PSS and arthritis is similar to that seen in early rheumatoid arthritis and shows edema with infiltration of lymphocytes and plasma cells. Later in the disease the synovium may become fibrotic. Fibrinous deposits appear on the surfaces of tendon sheaths and in the overlying fascia, and may lead to audible creaking over moving tendons.

Histologic features of muscle involvement consist of interstitial and perivascular lymphocytic infiltrations, degeneration of muscle fibers, and interstitial fibrosis. Arterioles may be thickened, and capillaries may be decreased in number.

In the heart, myocardial interstitial fibrosis replaces myocardial fibers. Fibrosis also involves the conduction system, leading to AV conduction defects and arrhythmias. The wall of smaller coronary arteries may be thickened, and lymphocytic infiltration is seen. Fibrinous pericarditis and pericardial effusions are found in some patients.

Renal involvement is found in over half the patients and consists of intimal hyperplasia of the interlobular arteries, fibrinoid necrosis of the afferent arterioles, including the glomerular tuft, and thickening of the glomerular basement membrane. These lesions result in cortical infarctions and glomerulosclerosis. The renal pathologic change is often indistinguishable from that observed in malignant hypertension. Renal vascular lesions, however, may be present in the absence of hypertension. Electron-microscopic examinations of the kidney have revealed endothelial cytoplasmic inclusions resembling myxovirus particles, similar to those reported in systemic lupus erythematosus and polymyositis.

Primary liver involvement is not common, but diffuse cirrhosis, intrahepatic cholestasis, and chronic passive congestion occur occasionally. Fibrosis of the thyroid may occur. Thickening of the periodontal membrane with replacement of the lamina dura is demonstrated radiographically as widening of the periodontal space and rarely causes loosening of the teeth.

Small arterial and arteriolar lesions are found in many tissues; they consist of concentric acellular thickening of the intima with narrowing or occlusion of the lumen. These lesions are found in digital arteries and arterioles in patients with PSS and Raynaud's phenomenon. Vascular abnormalities have been described in the lung, skin, kidney, muscle, gastrointestinal tract, pancreas, synovium, vasa vasorum, and the central nervous system. Arteritis with fibrinoid necrosis and round-cell invasion of all three layers is occasionally observed.

CLINICAL MANIFESTATIONS PSS usually begins insidiously; the first symptoms are often Raynaud's phenomenon or symmetric swelling or stiffness of the fingers. Raynaud's phenomenon may precede the skin changes by months or even years. In some patients, the first manifestation is pitting edema of the extremities and face.

The fingers and hands in the early stages are tightly swollen. Subsequently the skin becomes very firm, tight, waxy in appearance, and bound to the underlying subcutaneous tissue. The skin changes spread to involve the arms, face, upper part of the chest, abdomen, and back. The lower extremities are relatively spared. The taut skin over the fingers gradually limits full extension, and fixed flexion contractures may develop. Ulcers may appear on the fingertips and over bony prominences and may become infected; they are refractory to treatment. The soft tissue of the fingertips is lost, and in some instances the bone of terminal phalanges is resorbed. The skin may become darkly pigmented in the absence of exposure to the sun; areas of depigmentation and numerous telangiectases may appear on the skin. In some patients, calcific deposits develop in the subcutaneous and periarticular tissue. The overlying skin may break down, with draining of calcific material. Involvement of the face results in the loss of normal skin wrinkles, loss of facial expression, and limitation in opening of the mouth.

The coexistence of calcinosis, Raynaud's phenomenon, sclerodactyly, and telangiectasia has been termed the CRST syndrome and initially was considered a benign form of PSS. However, some of these patients have subsequently developed visceral and more extensive cutaneous lesions of PSS.

More than half the patients with PSS complain of pain, swelling, and stiffness of fingers and knee joints. A symmetric polyarthritis, resembling rheumatoid arthritis, may be seen. In more advanced stages of the disease, leathery crepitation can be palpated over moving joints, especially the knee. Extensive fibrotic thickening of the tendon sheaths in the wrist can produce a carpal tunnel syndrome.

Generalized muscle atrophy is a common manifestation. Myositis with proximal muscle weakness and elevated level of muscle enzymes is seen in some patients and is indistinguishable from polymyositis.

Symptoms attributable to esophageal involvement, which are present in more than 50 percent of patients, include epigastric fullness, burning pain in the epigastric or retrosternal regions, and regurgitation of gastric contents. These symptoms, most noticeable when the patient is lying flat or bending over, are due to the reduced tone of the gastroesophageal sphincter and to dilatation of the distal esophagus. Peptic esophagitis frequently occurs and may lead to strictures and narrowing of the lower part of the esophagus. However, it seldom results in bleeding. Dysphagia, particularly of solid foods, may occur independent of other esophageal symptoms and is caused by the loss of esophageal motility. Gastric involvement, which is not common in PSS, produces symptoms that are difficult to distinguish from esophageal symptoms. Balloon pressure studies and cineradiography reveal decreased amplitude or disappearance of peristaltic waves in the lower two-thirds of the esophagus. A closer correlation exists between this finding and Raynaud's phenomenon than with cutaneous manifestations of PSS. Later in the course of the illness, dilatation and atony of the lower portion of the esophagus as well as reflux are seen. With gastric involvement, barium studies show dilatation, atony, and delayed gastric emptying.

Symptoms referrable to involvement of the small intestine by PSS include bloating and abdominal pain and may suggest intestinal obstruction or paralytic ileus. Malabsorption syndrome with weight loss, steatorrhea, and anemia also occur and may be due in some patients to bacterial overgrowth in the atonic intestine. Involvement of the large intestine may cause chronic constipation and fecal impaction with episodes of bowel obstruction. Roentgenographic features of the second and third portions of the duodenum and of the jejunum include dilatation, loss of the usual feathery pattern, and delayed disappearance of barium. Pneumatosis intestinalis, which occasionally occurs in PSS, is seen as radiolucent cysts or linear streaks within the wall of the small intestine. Benign pneumoperitoneum may result from the rupture of these cysts. Barium studies of the large intestine may show dilatation, atony, and large-mouth diverticula.

Patients with pulmonary fibrosis often complain of a dry cough and exertional dyspnea; however, shortness of breath as a presenting complaint is unusual. Bilateral basilar rales may be present. Though pleural involvement is not infrequent at postmortem, pleurisy is unusual. Restriction of chest movement may rarely occur with extensive skin involvement of the thorax. Additional pulmonary problems result from aspiration pneumonia secondary to esophageal malfunction. Superimposed bacterial or viral pneumonia may be a serious complication in patients with pulmonary fibrosis. Malignant alveolar or bronchiolar cell neoplasms have been reported in some patients with PSS and pulmonary fibrosis. However, no other association of PSS with malignancy has been shown. Pulmonary function test results are abnormal even in early disease and show most frequently a low diffusion capacity and a low P_{O_2} on exercise. Roentgenograms of the chest may show a pattern of linear densities, mottling and honeycombing. These changes are more evident in the lower two-thirds of the lungs.

Cardiac involvement by PSS often goes clinically unrecognized; however, varying degrees of heart block and arrhythmias may be seen. Cardiomyopathy attributable to diffuse myocardial fibrosis may also occur. Other cardiac manifestations may be secondary to pulmonary disease and hypertension. Left ventricular failure develops more frequently than cor pulmonale, even with the presence of pulmonary fibrosis. In some patients, pulmonary hypertension appears without pulmonary fibrosis, presumably secondary to pulmonary arterial and arteriolar narrowing. Pericarditis and pericardial effusions are occasionally seen.

Renal involvement may give rise to abrupt onset of malignant hypertension, with rapid development of azotemia and oliguria leading to death. Rapidly progressive renal failure has been attributed to corticosteroid administration, but the same rapidly progressive course may be seen in patients who have not received steroids.

PROGNOSIS The disease in the majority of patients is characterized by a prolonged, relentless course of progressive skin and/or visceral involvement. Weight loss is a prominent manifestation. In some patients remissions occur, including partial improvement of the skin, and the disease progresses slowly; 80 percent of one group of patients were alive 2 years after onset of symptoms, and 20 percent were alive 10 years after onset. Patients with CRST syndrome or only restricted skin involvement have a more gradual and favorable course than those with extensive skin and/or visceral disease, especially of the heart, kidney, and lung. Among Caucasians the prognosis is worse in males than in females, and it is worse in patients whose onset of disease occurs at an older age. The disease tends to be more severe in blacks, especially black females. Death stems from cardiac, renal, and pulmonary involvement.

LABORATORY FINDINGS The erythrocyte sedimentation rate may be elevated. Hypergammaglobulinemia, with elevated level mainly of IgG, is found in approximately half the patients. Rheumatoid factor, in low titer, is present in 25 percent of patients. Antinuclear antibodies are reported in 40 to 80 percent of patients and include antinucleolar antibodies, antideoxyribonucleoprotein, and antibodies to extractable nuclear antigens. The latter give a speckled pattern on immunofluorescent tests and are most frequently found in the so-called mixed connective tissue syndrome (see below).

DIAGNOSIS The diagnosis of PSS presents no difficulty in the presence of Raynaud's phenomena, with typical skin lesions and visceral involvement. PSS should always be included in the differential diagnosis of patients with Raynaud's phenomenon. Linear scleroderma and morphea are localized forms of PSS and may be associated with Raynaud's phenomenon and hypergammaglobulinemia. PSS may be confused with rheumatoid arthritis, systemic lupus erythematosus, or polymyositis when articular or muscle involvement is prominent early in the disease. PSS without cutaneous involvement should be considered in patients with unexplained pulmonary fibrosis, cardiomyopathies, heart block, dysphagia, or malabsorption syndrome.

Mixed connective tissue disease A distinct rheumatic syndrome occurs with clinical features of scleroderma, systemic lupus erythematosus, and polymyositis. The serums of all these patients have hemagglutinating antibody specific for an extractable nuclear antigen which is composed largely of protein and ribonucleic acid. The serums of these patients also have high titers of antinuclear antibodies, which give a speckled pattern on immunofluorescent tests. These antibodies are probably identical to the hemagglutinating antibodies.

Arthralgia or arthritis is present in most of the patients, but deformities are infrequent. The clinical appearance of skin over the hands and the skin biopsies are consistent with scleroderma. Raynaud's phenomenon and esophageal hypomotility occur frequently. Some patients show heliotropic discoloration of the upper eyelids and erythematous patches over the dorsum of the fingers similar to that observed in dermatomyositis; myalgias, proximal muscle weakness, elevated levels of muscle enzymes, and electromyographic changes of myositis are found in the majority of patients. Other features are pleuritis, pericarditis, generalized lymphadenopathy, and splenomegaly. Renal involvement is exceedingly rare in these patients. Anemia, leukopenia, and diffuse hypergammaglobulinemia are present frequently. In contrast to patients with typical PSS, these patients usually show a favorable response to corticosteroids.

TREATMENT Many drugs have been used in the treatment of PSS without any consistent or prolonged benefit. Systemic corticosteroids may produce improvement in the early edematous phase of the disease. They have no effect on visceral lesions. Since patients with mixed connective tissue disease respond favorably to steroids, it is important to distinguish these patients from those with PSS. Para-aminobenzoic acid was claimed to improve the skin in PSS, especially in patients with morphea; however, its therapeutic value remains unproved. This drug frequently causes nausea and skin eruptions. In addition, hypoglycemia may occur in patients who have decreased food intake. D-penicillamine has been tried with variable results. Toxic reactions, fever, rash, nephrotic syndrome, and leukopenia occur with this drug. Chlorambucil has recently been reported to be beneficial in PSS; however, further documentation is needed.

Intraarterial reserpine may temporarily improve Raynaud's phenomenon when vasospasm is the major component, but is of little benefit in patients who already have anatomic narrowing of the arterioles. Likewise, oral vasodilators are usually of little value in these patients. Sodium versenate has been shown to be of no value in reducing subcutaneous calcinosis. Patients with severe Raynaud's phenomenon should be advised to wear warm mittens and to use hand warmers when out in the cold. Infected skin ulcers are treated with local antibiotics. Physiotherapy may help to reduce flexion deformities.

Patients with reflux esophagitis are treated with small frequent meals, antacids, and elevation of the head of the bed. Malabsorption syndrome may improve with tetracycline therapy. Patients with cardiac failure usually respond poorly to digitalization and have a tendency to develop digitalis toxicity. Pulmonary infections in patients with pulmonary fibrosis require prompt treatment with antibiotics and other supportive measures.

REFERENCES

COHEN S et al: The pathogenesis of esophageal dysfunction in scleroderma and Raynaud's disease. J Clin Invest 51:2663, 1972

D'ANGELO WA et al: Pathologic observations in systemic sclerosis (scleroderma). Am J Med 46:428, 1969

LEROY EC: Connective tissue synthesis by scleroderma skin fibroblasts in cell culture. J Exp Med 135:1351, 1972

MEDSGER TA et al: Survival with systemic sclerosis (scleroderma). Ann Intern Med 75:369, 1971

NORTON WL, NARDO JM: Vascular disease in progressive systemic sclerosis (scleroderma). Ann Intern Med 73:317, 1970

RODNAN GP: Progressive systemic sclerosis, chap. 64 in *Immunological Diseases*, vol 2, ed M Samter, Boston: Little, Brown, p. 1052

SHARP GC et al: Mixed connective tissue disease—an apparently distinct rheumatic disease syndrome associated with a specific antibody to an extractable nuclear antigen (ENA). Am J Med 52:148, 1972

363 MISCELLANEOUS ARTHRITIDES AND EXTRAARTICULAR RHEUMATISM

MART MANNIK
BRUCE C. GILLILAND

HYPERTROPHIC OSTEOARTHROPATHY Hypertrophic osteoarthropathy is characterized by the presence of periosteal inflammation and new bone formation, arthritis, and clubbing of digits. This syndrome frequently results from disorders in the lungs and hence is frequently called *hypertrophic pulmonary osteoarthropathy* or *secondary hypertrophic osteoarthritis.* It also occurs because of disorders of other organs, as well as in familial and idiopathic forms.

In hypertrophic osteoarthropathy round-cell infiltration and edema develop in the periosteum, synovial membrane, and joint capsule. The periosteum is lifted, and new bone matrix is put down and calcified. At the same time endosteal bone is resorbed. These changes occur at the distal ends of long bones at the wrists and ankles, as well as in the distal ends of metacarpal and metatarsal bones. With progression of the disease, these changes may affect ribs, clavicles, and scapulae. At the same time soft-tissue edema, fibroblast proliferation, and minimal mononuclear infiltration lead to enlargement of the distal ends of digits, a process termed *clubbing.*

The mechanisms that cause hypertrophic osteoarthropathy are not known, but arteriovenous shunts and humoral and neurogenic factors are suspected because the process may be reversed upon correction of cardiac shunts, removal of pulmonary tumors, and vagotomy.

Hypertrophic osteoarthropathy occurs in 5 to 10 percent of patients with primary intrathoracic malignancies, notably bronchogenic carcinomas and pleural tumors, but is very rare with metastatic tumors of the lung. Chronic suppurative lung lesions, such as lung abscesses, bronchiectasis, and empyema, are frequent causes of hypertrophic osteoarthropathy. However, with decline of these problems, due to antibiotics, tumors are now the most frequent cause. This disorder also may accompany cyanotic cardiac malformations, biliary cirrhosis, and, rarely, intestinal disorders such as ulcerative colitis or regional enteritis. When no associated disorders have been identified, the disorder is called *idiopathic hypertrophic osteoarthropathy*. Hereditary hypertrophic osteoarthropathy (pachydermoperiostitis) is a disorder characterized by marked thickening of skin of the limbs and face, in addition to the typical features of hypertrophic osteoarthropathy.

Hypertrophic osteoarthropathy frequently occurs with digital clubbing, but may precede clubbing or develop without it. Similarly, clubbing of digits occurs without any evidence of hypertrophic osteoarthropathy. Hypertrophic osteoarthropathy may cause mild arthralgias. Other patients develop severe or burning pain in the hands and feet. Erythema and effusions may be present in wrists, ankles, and metacarpophalangeal or metatarsophalangeal joints. Tenderness is likely to be present in joints of these patients as well as over the adjacent bones. Dependency may aggravate these symptoms. At times the periosteal changes evolve without symptoms.

Radiographs show increased thickness of the periosteum with new bone formation over the distal ends of bones. However, this may not be evident if the symptoms and signs have been present for only a short time. Presence of lung lesions and other associated diseases must be sought. No specific laboratory tests are available for hypertrophic osteoarthropathy, and its treatment must be directed toward search for and treatment of the underlying disorder. The symptoms may be controlled with analgesics.

NEUROPATHIC JOINT DISEASE (CHARCOT JOINTS) Neuropathic joint disease develops in a variety of neurologic disorders in which proprioception and/or deep pain sensation are disrupted. Increased trauma and stress are thought to occur during normal joint motion because of relaxation of the supporting structures of the joint. This leads to cartilage degeneration, recurrent fractures of subchondral bone, and marked proliferation of bone. The most frequently involved neuropathic joints in *tabes dorsalis* are knee, hip, ankle, and lumbar vertebras; in *diabetic neuropathy*, tarsal, tarsometatarsal, and metatarsophalangeal joints; and in *syringomyelia*, shoulder, elbow, and cervical vertebras. Neuropathic joints also occur in meningomyelocele, congenital insensitivity to pain, leprous neuropathy, and peripheral nerve injuries.

On pathologic examination, cartilage degeneration, formation of loose bodies, and marginal osteophytes are seen. The osteophytes are larger and more disorganized than in degenerative joint disease. Fractures occur in the articular facets, osteophytes, epicondyles, or condyles, with callus formation and further osteophyte formation. This process ultimately results in disorganization of the joints, which is characteristic of this disease. These alterations of the bone and joint space are easily recognized radiologically. The synovium shows fibrosis, fragments of calcified cartilage, and hemosiderin deposits.

Neuropathic joint disease, regardless of the underlying disorder, begins insidiously in a single joint and then progresses to involve other joints. The distribution of involved joints is influenced by the underlying neurologic disorder. The involved joint enlarges because of effusion and overgrowth of bone; instability develops later. The discomfort is strikingly mild in relation to the structural abnormalities. Intraarticular fractures may cause sudden onset of pain. The examination may show increased mobility and instability. Effusions are common. Crepitus is frequent and marked in the late stages of the disease. Presence of many loose bodies may give the joint a feeling of a "bag of bones" on examination. The synovial fluid is bloody and similar to that in traumatic effusions.

To diagnose a neuropathic joint, the underlying neurologic disorder must be identified, but the treatment of the underlying neuropathologic condition seldom influences the progression of the joint disease. Therefore, the treatment should be directed to providing stability and relief of pain. External supports are useful, but the braces have to be carefully adjusted and checked, since patients with neurologic disorders are not sensitive to maladjustments. Arthrodesis may provide stability but sacrifices motion. Joint replacement should be considered in selected patients.

ARTICULAR PROBLEMS IN RENAL HOMOTRANSPLANTATION One to several months after renal homotransplantation about a third of the recipients develop musculoskeletal complaints. *Avascular necrosis* of bone may occur in these patients. The hips are most frequently involved, but other joints may be affected as well. Corticosteroid therapy is thought to contribute to this problem. Some patients have only transient musculoskeletal pain; in others acute or chronic synovitis and joint effusions may occur. The cause of these abnormalities has not been elucidated. The joint symptoms may last for months and tend to appear first after reduction of steroid dosage. In one study elevated blood lipid levels were associated with these clinical symptoms, and intracellular lipoid inclusions were noted in synovial fluid leukocytes. These patients, as well as about 90 percent of all transplant recipients, develop positive tests for rheumatoid factor, but the significance of this remains unknown.

SARCOID ARTHRITIS See Chap. 223.

ARTHROPATHY OF HEMOCHROMATOSIS See Chap. 101.

ARTHRITIS OF FAMILIAL MEDITERRANEAN FEVER See Chap. 225.

HEMOPHILIC ARTHRITIS See Chap. 314.

PIGMENTED VILLONODULAR SYNOVITIS Pigmented villonodular synovitis usually affects a single joint, most commonly the knee. However, hip, ankle, tarsus, carpus, and elbow may be involved. The cause of this disorder is unknown. The synovium is brownish in color and covered with elongated and enlarged villi; fusion of villi leads to formation of pedunculated nodules. Histologically the synovial lining cells appear normal, but the stroma of the villi contains large numbers of round and polyhedral cells. Hemosiderin granules and cholesterol crystals are abundant in cytoplasm of synovial cells and in interstitial spaces. Multinucleated giant cells may be present. Invasion of other tissues does not occur.

The clinical picture of pigmented villonodular synovitis is characterized by insidious onset of monarticular swelling in young adults, accompanied by pain. These symptoms tend to be continuous, but exacerbations occur from time to time. The synovial fluid frequently contains blood, and it is dark brown, indicative of previous episodes of bleeding from the synovium.

Complete removal of the affected synovium is recommended. With incomplete synovectomy, recurrences are common. Irradiation has been used successfully in some patients.

TRAUMATIC ARTHRITIS Joints are subject to many forms of trauma. The immediate damage may include capsular tears, detachment of menisci and joint cartilage, laceration of cartilage, and articular fractures. As a result of such damage hemorrhagic effusions are frequent. The product of such effusions changes to a serous, amber-colored fluid within 2 to 3 weeks. Bleeding may occur from injury of the synovial membrane alone, without bone or cartilage damage.

The symptoms of joint trauma are obviously confined to the damaged joint. Swelling, ecchymoses, muscular spasms, and tenderness tend to be present. Pain is present, particularly on motion. Radiologic examination is essential to exclude fractures. Obvious rupture of ligaments must be excluded on examination, but internal derangement of the joint may become apparent only later. Air-contrast arthrograms are helpful in defining internal derangements, particularly meniscal tears.

Treatment should include rest and removal of large hemorrhagic effusions. Physical therapy is necessary during convalescence. Orthopedic evaluation and surgery are frequently indicated. Severe damage to a joint hastens the onset of degenerative joint disease.

Patients frequently attribute the onset of a generalized joint disease to trauma. The diagnosis of *traumatic arthritis* should be reserved for patients in whom: (1) a specified traumatic insult was severe enough to produce acute pain, swelling, effusion, and dysfunction of the affected joint, (2) the affected joint(s) alone shows the abnormalities mentioned, (3) these abnormalities did not exist prior to trauma.

RELAPSING POLYCHONDRITIS Relapsing polychondritis is a disease of unknown cause that leads to inflammation and destruction of cartilage. The cartilage loses its characteristic basophilic staining with hematoxylin and eosin. The chondrocytes degenerate, and the cartilage is fragmented and replaced with fibrous connective tissue. Lymphocytes and plasma cells are present at the interface of cartilage and new connective tissue.

This disorder occurs predominantly in middle age. Involvement of the ears and nose is most common (in 80 to 90 percent of patients). Disease activity fluctuates and involves different sites. The affected ears or nose becomes swollen and tender, and destruction of cartilage leads to floppy ears and a collapsed nose. Hearing loss may ensue from collapse of the external auditory meatus. Fever and arthralgias are frequent. Involvement of the larynx, trachea, and bronchi leads to hoarseness, recurrent pulmonary infections, stenosis, and even acute suffocation from collapse of the cartilagenous structures. Episcleritis is seen in about 60 percent of patients. Aortic insufficiency occurs occasionally.

No specific laboratory tests are available, but the erythrocyte sedimentation rate is usually elevated, and mild anemia occurs. Biopsy of cartilage is helpful in establishing the diagnosis. Corticosteroids in moderate doses suppress the disease's activity.

TIETZE'S SYNDROME Tietze's syndrome consists of swelling, pain, and tenderness in the upper costochondral cartilages. The cause of this disorder is unknown. This syndrome tends to evolve gradually but may be acute. Patients often associate the onset with trauma. The involved costochondral joints are swollen and tender but not warm, and the disorder must be differentiated from bacterial infections and rheumatoid arthritis. Single joints are frequently involved, and multiple joint involvement tends to be unilateral. The location and character of pain may mimic the symptoms of myocardial infarction. Injection with procaine and corticosteroids tends to provide relief. Excision has been tried. Analgesics and physical therapy have been helpful sporadically.

BURSITIS AND TENOSYNOVITIS Bursitis is inflammation of unknown cause of any of the many bursae between tendons, muscles, and bony prominences. The most common type of bursitis occurs in the shoulder. Other common types of bursitis are *trochanteric bursitis* (bursae around the gluteus medius insertion to the trochanter of the femur), which causes pain on external rotation of the hip and is recognized by tenderness over the trochanteric area; *olecranon bursitis*, recognized by tenderness and inflammation at the point of the elbow; *ischiatic bursitis* (also called "weaver's bottom"), in which tenderness is present over the ischial tuberosities and is caused by prolonged sitting on hard surfaces; *prepatellar bursitis* (also called "housemaid's knee"), or swelling and tenderness over the kneecap, produced by frequent or prolonged kneeling; *anserine bursitis*, an inflammation of the sartorius bursa, in which tenderness is present at the insertion of the conjoined tendon of the sartorius, semitendinosus, and gracilis muscles on the inner aspect of the tibia, and in which characteristically pain occurs on ascending or descending stairs.

In the shoulder, *subacromial bursitis* and *bicipital tenosynovitis* are the most common problems. In the former the supraspinatus tendon or other rotator cuff tendons become inflamed as they pass just below the subacromial or subdeltoid bursa. Calcifications are frequently seen adjacent to the tendon, but the presence of calcium does not necessarily relate to the symptoms. With acute subacromial bursitis or supraspinatus tendinitis, the onset of symptoms is sudden and the pain may be severe. Any abduction or external rotation causes agony. Marked tenderness is present over the lateral humeral head below the acromion. In chronic forms, a nagging, intermittent pain may be present, particularly during any motion that includes abduction and rotation of the shoulder.

Bicipital tenosynovitis consists of inflammation of the synovial sheath of the tendon of the long head of the biceps as it passes through the bicipital groove of the humeral head. In the acute form of this illness, pain develops along the biceps area and may radiate to the forearm. Abduction and forceful supination cause increase in pain. Marked tenderness is present over the bicipital groove. In chronic bicipital tenosynovitis the symptoms are milder but tenderness is present. Muscle atrophy and adhesive capsulitis of the shoulder may develop because of decreased usage.

The treatment of any type of bursitis should include rest, use of analgesics, and physical therapy upon recovery from the acute phase, to prevent loss of function. Phenylbutazone (100 mg. t.i.d.) may be helpful. Injection of corticosteroids and local anesthetics hastens recovery and provides marked relief from acute symptoms.

Tenosynovitis (inflammation of the synovial lining of tendons) occurs with other types of rheumatic disease (rheumatoid arthritis, systemic lupus erythematosus, gout), in bacterial infections (gonococcal, tuberculous), secondary to trauma, and without known causes (idiopathic).

SHOULDER-HAND SYNDROME The shoulder-hand syndrome is the most common form of *reflex neurovascular dystrophy*. An external injury or an internal disorder initiates the reflex neurovascular dystrophy, that includes pain, reflex vasomotor reactions, disability, swelling, tenderness, and osteoporosis. Both upper or lower extremities may be involved. The shoulder-hand syndrome is due to a number of disorders: in about one-fifth of patients the underlying cause is myocardial infarction; in one-fifth the symptoms develop secondary to cervical disk disease or cervical degenerative joint disease; in two-fifths an underlying disorder cannot be found or identified with certainty; trauma and hemiplegia each are the contributing cause in one-tenth of patients. The pathogenic mechanisms have not been identified. The most widely accepted hypothesis suggests that pain fibers carry impulses to the spinal cord where they initiate a cycle of reflexes through the interconnecting pool of neurons stimulating efferent autonomic and motor neurons, which in turn are responsible for the symptoms and signs.

The onset of the shoulder-hand syndrome may be insidious or acute, with stiffness and weakness in the upper extremity or only in the shoulder or hand, weeks or months after the causative insult. These symptoms are followed by swelling, vasomotor changes, hyperesthesia, and disability after a variable period of time. This stage lasts 3 to 6 months. Thereafter, the vasomotor signs diminish and atrophy and contractures develop. Finally the atrophy and contractures remain but improve gradually. The syndrome may run its course in one to several years. Radiographs will show varying degrees of osteoporosis in the head of the humerus, wrist, and phalanges. Other laboratory tests provide no useful information. The early diagnosis of a shoulder-hand syndrome may be difficult, because it may resemble the early phases of rheumatoid arthritis.

Exercises and reassurance are the cornerstones of therapy. Salicylates provide some symptomatic relief. Corticosteroids in small doses or stellate ganglion blocks have been recommended, but there have been no controlled studies on the efficacy of this type of therapy. The most encouraging results are achieved when exercises are initiated early in the course of the shoulder-hand syndrome. Reflex neurovascular dystrophy of the lower extremities is treated according to similar principles.

FIBROSITIS Fibrositis is a term used for an ill-defined, poorly understood set of symptoms, consisting of aching pain and stiffness in one or several parts of the body. These symptoms occur deep in tissues, including muscles, tendon insertions, and bony prominences. The lower back, gluteal regions, neck, shoulders, and thighs are the areas most frequently involved. These patients tend to be middle-aged and depressed. Illnesses like rheumatoid arthritis, systemic lupus erythematosus, myositis, neuropathy, and giant-cell arteritis must be considered and excluded. Reassurance, exercises, massage, and salicylates tend to provide relief.

PSYCHOGENIC RHEUMATISM Psychogenic rheumatism is a term applied to rheumatic symptoms that are manifestations of psychoneurosis. Common complaints are stiffness and limitation of motion and painful joints, tendons, or muscles. These patients are in good general health and have no objective abnormalities of joints. Radiologic and laboratory study results are normal. The complaints tend to vacillate and do not improve with analgesics.

CARPAL TUNNEL SYNDROME (ENTRAPMENT NEUROPATHY) Carpal tunnel syndrome may be due to trauma, edema, fibrosis, tuberculosis and other granulomatous diseases, rheumatoid arthritis, acromegaly, amyloidosis, edema of pregnancy, and premenstrual edema. It is caused by pressure on the median nerve as it passes through the space formed by the bones of the wrist and the transverse carpal ligament. Any space-occupying process may cause compression and malfunction of the median nerve or other nerves similarly confined, such as the ulnar nerve or posterior tibial nerve.

Patients with the carpal tunnel syndrome complain of burning pain on the palmar surface of the first three digits of the hand. This pain may be referred proximally up the arm. Characteristically the pain is more severe at night, and numbness may develop. Adduction of the thumb is weakened, and atrophy of the thenar eminence develops. Pain and tingling may be elicited by sustained flexion of the wrist or by tapping the area of the median nerve. Nerve conduction studies across the wrist will confirm the diagnosis.

Surgical decompression of the carpal tunnel with

release of the transverse ligament and debridement is the definitive treatment. Analgesics, splinting, and injection of corticosteroids may provide temporary relief.

TUMORS OF THE JOINTS Primary tumors of the joints are relatively uncommon but should be considered a rare cause of monarticular symptoms. In addition, primary bone tumors and metastases to bone may produce articular symptoms when adjacent to joints.

In *synovial chondromatosis* multiple metaplastic growths of cartilage occur in the synovium or tendon sheaths. Later these may calcify and become evident on radiographs. Single joints are involved and include the knee, hip, elbow, and shoulder. The involved joint may enlarge because of effusions. Pain and limitation of motion occur because of loose bodies. Synovectomy is the definitive treatment.

Hemangiomas may occur in the synovial or tenosynovial membranes. Symptoms usually develop in childhood. Bloody effusions occur. The hemangioma should be excised. *Lipomas* may occur in subsynovial fat and extend into the joint space, particularly into the knees.

Synoviomas or synovial sarcomas develop in the immediate periarticular tissues, not in the synovial cavity. These highly malignant tumors develop in adolescents or young adults. They present as a slowly growing mass adjacent to a joint. Biopsy is required for diagnosis, and radical resection is recommended for treatment.

Synovial chondrosarcoma may occur in joints or tendon sheaths.

Metastatic tumors to bone rarely extend to the synovial cavity. Destruction of adjacent bone and bloody effusions are characteristic.

REFERENCES

BRAVO JF et al: Musculoskeletal disorders after renal homotransplantation. A clinical and laboratory analysis of 60 cases. Ann Intern Med 66:87, 1967

DOLAN DL et al: Relapsing polychondritis: Analytical literature review and studies on pathogenesis. Am J Med 41:285, 1966

HOLLANDER JL (ed): *Arthritis and Allied Conditions*, 8th ed., Philadelphia: Lea & Febiger, 1972

section 15 | Genetic disorders of supporting tissues

364 INHERITED DISORDERS OF CONNECTIVE TISSUE

VICTOR A. McKUSICK

These are generalized, or at least widespread, disorders of connective tissue due to the effects of a single mutant gene, as demonstrated by their occurrence in families in mendelian pedigree patterns. The disorders may be divided into those of the fibrous elements (collagen, elastin) and those of mucopolysaccharides. They may be further classified as either primary (if the mutation concerns one of the steps by which collagen, elastin, or mucopolysaccharide is synthesized or degraded) or secondary (if the mutation results in a block in intermediary metabolism with damage to connective tissue by accumulated metabolites, as in homocystinuria and alkaptonuria). Table 364-1 gives a partial listing of heritable disorders of connective tissue according to this classification.

EHLERS-DANLOS SYNDROME AND ITS FORMS

The Ehlers-Danlos syndrome (synonyms: cutis hyperelastica, "India rubber men," dermatorrhexis with dermatochalasis and arthrochalasis) is a heritable and generalized disorder of connective tissue, manifested by fragility, hyperelasticity, and bruisability of the skin, and by loose-jointedness. Several distinct forms may be identified.

Characteristically, the skin can be stretched through an unusually great range, but returns promptly to its normal position on release. Later on, the skin may lose its elasticity, become truly cutis laxa, and hang in flabby folds or wrinkles. The skin is fragile, so that minor traumas are likely to produce gaping, "fish-mouth" wounds which bleed little and hold sutures poorly. There is easy bruisability. Firm spherules, up to about 1 cm in diameter, develop subcutaneously, can be moved about through a considerable range, and can be demonstrated radiographically because of calcification. "Cigarette pa-

TABLE 364-1
Heritable disorders of connective tissue (a partial list)

I Disorders of fibrous elements
- *A* Primary
  - *1* The Ehlers-Danlos syndrome
  - *2* Cutis laxa
  - *3* Osteogenesis imperfecta
  - *4* The Marfan syndrome
- *B* Secondary
  - *1* Homocystinuria
  - *2* Alkaptonuria
  - *3* Pseudoxanthoma elasticum (?)
  - *4* Menkes "kinky hair" syndrome

II The genetic mycopolysaccharidoses

per" scars develop over the knees, shins, etc. So-called "molluscoid pseudotumors" develop on the knees, ankles, and elbows as soft, poorly outlined swellings that may be several centimeters in diameter.

The loose-jointedness results in genu recurvatum, habitual dislocation of various joints, or flatfoot. Recurrent hydrarthrosis may result from the repeated trauma due to poor stabilization, especially in the knees (Fig. 364-1).

Internal ramifications include diaphragmatic hernia or eventration of the diaphragm, ectasia or diverticula of portions of the gastrointestinal and respiratory tracts, and spontaneous pneumothorax. Spontaneous rupture of the intestine and of large arteries is a rare complication of one form of the disorder, and dissecting aneurysm of the aorta has been observed in some patients.

Six forms of the Ehlers-Danlos syndrome may be distinguished:

Ehlers-Danlos syndrome I, or gravis type Skin hyperextensibility, fragility, and bruisability are marked, and joint hyperextensibility is generalized and severe. Friable tissues create difficulties at operation. Prematurity as a result of early rupture of fetal membranes is frequent. The inheritance pattern is autosomal dominant.

Ehlers-Danlos syndrome II, or mitis type The cutaneous and joint manifestations are mild. Joint hyperextensibility is limited mainly to the hands and feet. Tissue friability and prematurity are not problems. This and type I might be allelic. Each "breeds true" within families and is autosomal dominant.

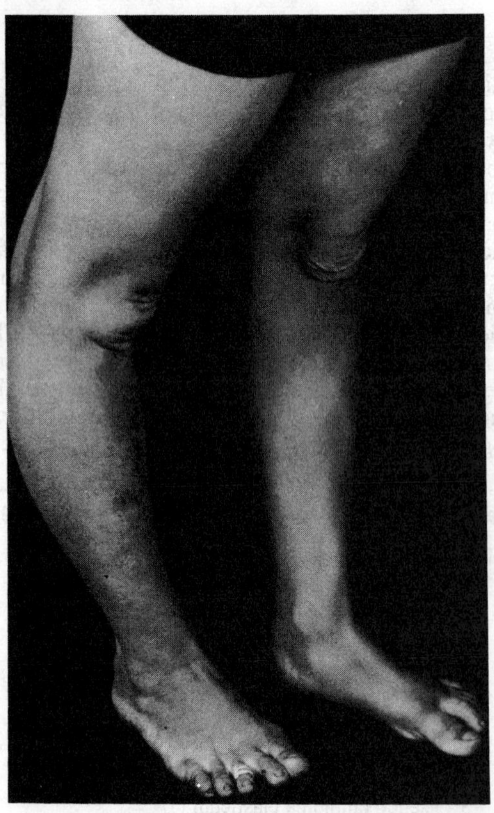

FIGURE 364–1
The loose-jointedness and the "cigarette paper" scarring of the Ehler-Danlos syndrome.

Ehlers-Danlos syndrome III, or benign hypermobile type Joint hypermobility is generalized and severe, and although skeletal deformity, such as severe scoliosis, is usually not present, other complications such as effusions and dislocations are troublesome. Skin manifestations are mild. This appears to be an autosomal dominant disorder.

Ehlers-Danlos syndrome IV, ecchymotic, arterial, or Sack's type Joint hypermobility is limited largely to the digits, and skin hyperextensibility is minimal. However, the skin is characteristically thin and pale, with a prominently evident venous network. Bruisability is severe. Minor trauma or muscle strain leads to extensive ecchymoses. Rupture of the intestine and large vessels occurs predominantly in this form of the disease. It is thought to be an autosomal dominant disorder.

Ehlers-Danlos syndrome V, or X-linked form Skin stretchability is more striking than joint hypermobility. The main distinguishing feature of this form is its mode of inheritance: X-linked recessive.

Ehlers-Danlos syndrome VI, hydroxylysine-deficient collagen, or ocular type Although this form also has striking skeletal and cutaneous features, ocular abnormalities are out of proportion to those in the other forms and include microcornea, glaucoma, and retinal detachment or corneal rupture on mild trauma. The inheritance mode is autosomal recessive. Deficiency has been found in the enzyme which catalyzes the hydroxylation of lysine in collagen. Since hydroxylysine is important to the cross-linking of collagen, the manifestations observed are well explained.

The basic defect in the other forms appears likewise to be abnormality in the way the collagen "wickerwork" is arranged, such that excessive extensibility of collagenous structures is possible. Various defects in cross-linking of collagen will probably be found.

OSTEOGENESIS IMPERFECTA

Osteogenesis imperfecta (synonyms: OI, fragilitas ossium, osteopsathyrosis idiopathica, disease of Eddowes, Lobstein, van der Hoeve, Vrolik) is a heritable, generalized disorder of connective tissue with clinical manifestations in the eye (blue scleras), ear (progressive deafness), skeleton (especially multiple fractures), joints (loose-jointedness), and skin. The nosology of this syndrome has been much confused because of wide variability in its clinical expression. Osteogenesis imperfecta congenita and tarda have been separated. A further separation of the tarda type into levis and gravis forms has been suggested. A hereditary disease characterized by fragility of bones without blue scleras has been claimed as a separate entity and called specifically osteopsathyrosis idiopathica. Although the evidence for autosomal dominant and autosomal recessive forms is convincing and indicates the existence of at least two distinct forms, further separation into subtypes does not appear to be warranted.

CLINICAL MANIFESTATIONS **Skeleton** Multiple fractures with trivial trauma are a main feature. Intrauterine fractures may permit antenatal diagnosis. Usually after puberty, the victims become less subject to fractures; susceptibility may return in later life, especially after the menopause in the female. Bowing of bones, porotic appearance on the roentgenogram without fracture, "codfish" or "hourglass" vertebras, platybasia (basilar impression of the skull) are all features. Dwarfism, with short legs and relatively large head, may be confused with achondroplasia. The calvarium tends to bulge laterally, and the head and face have a triangular configuration which often permits diagnosis from photographs alone.

Eye The change in the sclera, which may be various shades of blue, is the only important ocular feature.

Ear The deafness has the clinical features of conventional otosclerosis: variable age of onset, steady progression, and tendency to begin during pregnancy. The tympanic membrane may be blue like the sclera.

Joints Loose-jointedness is one of the four cardinal features of the disease. It is responsible, at least in part, for the flatfoot, kyphoscoliosis, and habitual dislocation of joints. Weakness of ligaments and tendons responsible for the loose-jointedness sometimes results in rupture of tendons from relatively minor stress.

Others Hernia is frequent. The teeth are characteristically small, misshapen, and bluish yellow. Kyphoscoliosis may lead in later life to cardiorespiratory complications.

INHERITANCE Usually, osteogenesis imperfecta is clearly inherited as an autosomal dominant disorder. An autosomal recessive form, presenting usually as OI congenita, is much rarer.

PATHOLOGY AND BASIC DEFECT In the bones, peculiar basophilic-staining material is found in place of osteoid. In other tissues, there are a sparsity of collagen fibers and replacement by fibers with tinctorial and other characteristics of reticulin. There appears to be a generalized defect in the maturation of collagen.

MARFAN SYNDROME

The Marfan syndrome is a heritable, generalized disorder of connective tissue, clinically manifested by abnormalities of the eye (especially ectopia lentis), of the skeletal system (especially excessive length of the long bones), and of the cardiovascular system (especially diffuse and/or dissecting aneurysm of the ascending aorta). In individual cases, manifestations may not be present in all three systems.

CLINICAL MANIFESTATIONS **Skeleton** Characteristically, the tubular bones are excessively long, resulting in arachnodactyly and in anomalous proportions. Normally after puberty the ratio of the upper segment of the body (top of pubic symphysis to crown) to the lower segment (pubic symphysis to sole) is about 0.92 (SD = 0.04) in whites and 0.85 (SD = 0.03) in Negroes. Because of the excessively long lower segment, the ratio is usually lower in patients with the Marfan syndrome. The arm span exceeds the height. The patient with the Marfan syndrome is taller than the average for his age and family; however, the deviation from the normal skeletal proportion is of more specific diagnostic significance. Excessive longitudinal growth of ribs may result in outward displacement of the sternum (pigeon breast, pectus carinatum) or inward displacement (pectus excavatum, *Trichterbrust*). Redundant ligaments, tendons, and joint capsules result in loose-jointedness, hyperextensibility of joints, genu recurvatum (backward curvature of the legs at the knees), flatfoot, kyphoscoliosis, and habitual dislocation of the hips, patella, clavicles, mandible, and other joints. Hernia occurs with increased frequency. In general, patients with the Marfan syndrome display a sparsity of subcutaneous fat (Fig. 364-2).

FIGURE 364–2
Typical features of the Marfan syndrome in an eleven-year-old boy.

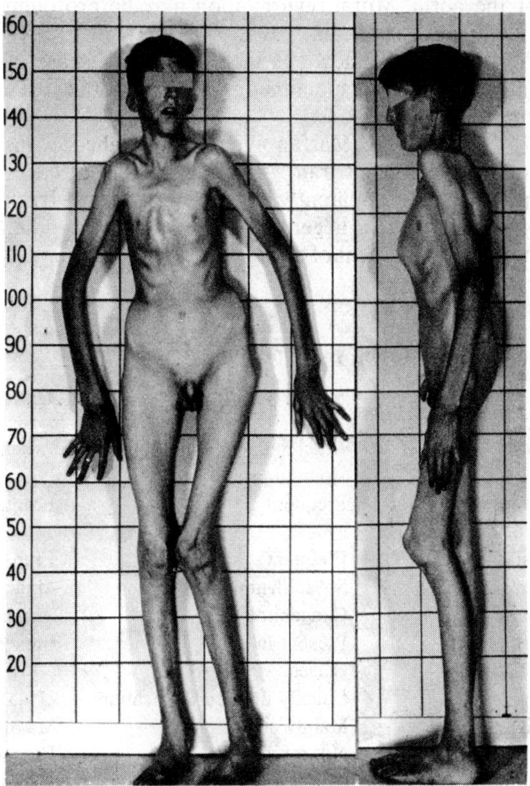

Eye Ectopia lentis (subluxation of the lens, dislocated lens) is the ocular hallmark of Marfan's syndrome. Iridodonesis (tremor of the iris) is often a clue to the presence of dislocated lenses. Occasionally the margin of a dislocated lens is visible through the undilated pupil, and rarely the lens may be totally dislocated into the anterior chamber. To exclude minor subluxation, it is necessary to dilate the pupil maximally and perform a careful slit-lamp examination. Under these circumstances one sees in the severely affected person that the suspensory ligaments are redundant, attenuated, and fragmented.

Myopia, often of high grade, is usually present; a long globe generally occurs as in integral part of the syndrome. Spontaneous detachment of the retina is frequent.

Cardiovascular system The principal cardiovascular manifestation of the Marfan syndrome is a weakness of the aortic media such that the portion subject to greatest hemodynamic stress of certain types—the ascending aorta—tends to undergo progressive dilatation or acute dissection. The dilatation, beginning as early as the first year or as late as the fifth decade, occurs first in the coronary sinuses. Profound aortic regurgitation may precede evidence of dilatation of the aorta on ordinary radiographic study. The clinical features of acute dissection are discussed in Chap. 246.

Less common cardiovascular complications are bacterial endocarditis superimposed on minor changes of heart valves, "partial" mitral regurgitation due to redundant cusps and chordae tendineae producing systolic clicks and late systolic murmurs, and incomplete coarctation of the aorta. Mitral regurgitation may be profound and functionally significant.

Other internal ramifications include cystic disease of the lung and recurrent spontaneous pneumothorax.

INHERITANCE The Marfan syndrome is inherited as an autosomal dominant trait. About 15 percent of cases are sporadic and apparently are the result of fresh mutation occurring in a germ cell of one or the other parent; about 85 percent of patients have one parent also affected. Paternal age effect is demonstrable in the sporadic cases; the average age of fathers of such patients is about 7 years higher than that of patients with inherited cases.

PATHOLOGY AND BASIC DEFECT The main histologic abnormality is that of the aortic media. Probably in most cases normal at birth if examined by the usual techniques, it undergoes changes which in the mildest form are identical with Erdheim's cystic medial necrosis seen in other settings (Chap. 246). In its advanced form, there are loss of elastic fibers, scarring, hyperplasia of smooth muscle in large whorls, and dilatation of the vasa vasorum. Which element of connective tissue is fundamentally defective is unknown.

DIFFERENTIAL DIAGNOSIS Given cardiovascular and skeletal manifestations consistent with the Marfan syndrome but not pathognomonic for it, one cannot be certain of the diagnosis unless ectopia lentis, the most specific of the components of the syndrome, can be demonstrated, or unless close relatives display unmistakable evidence of the disease. Some patients without ectopia lentis or definitely affected relatives have the Marfan syndrome, but a specific test is lacking. Confusion results from the fact that there is wide variability in the clinical severity of this syndrome, and its individual components display some independence in their severity ("expressivity") or even in whether they are present at all ("penetrance"). When the mutant gene for this syndrome occurs in pyknic stock, the affected person is likely to display less impressive skeletal abnormalities. The patient must be judged against the background of his family.

The main condition to be distinguished from the Marfan syndrome is *homocystinuria* (Table 364-2), which is identified by specific tests on the urine. Homocystinuria qualifies as a heritable disorder of connective tissue because of the ocular, skeletal, and cardiovascular features which simulate those of the Marfan syndrome. The features (Fig. 364-3) are ectopia lentis, chest deformity, scoliosis, generalized osteoporosis, recurrent thromboses in arteries and veins, and mental retardation. The patients tend to be tall and have chest deformity and scoliosis as in

TABLE 364-2
Comparison of Marfan syndrome and homocystinuria

	Marfan syndrome	*Homocystinuria*
Skeleton	Arachnodactyly and loose-jointedness	Arachnodactyly less striking; reduced joint mobility
Deformity of anterior part of chest	Frequent	Frequent
Scoliosis	Frequent	Frequent
Skin	Striae distensae frequent	Malar flush and livedo reticularis frequent
Ectopia lentis	Congenital	Acquired and progressive
	Present in about 75% of cases	Present in almost 100% of untreated cases by their 20s
	Usually upward dislocation	Usually downward dislocation
Vascular disease	Mainly aortic	Mainly thrombotic
Mental retardation	Not a feature	Frequent (about two-thirds of cases)
Inheritance	Autosomal dominant	Autosomal recessive

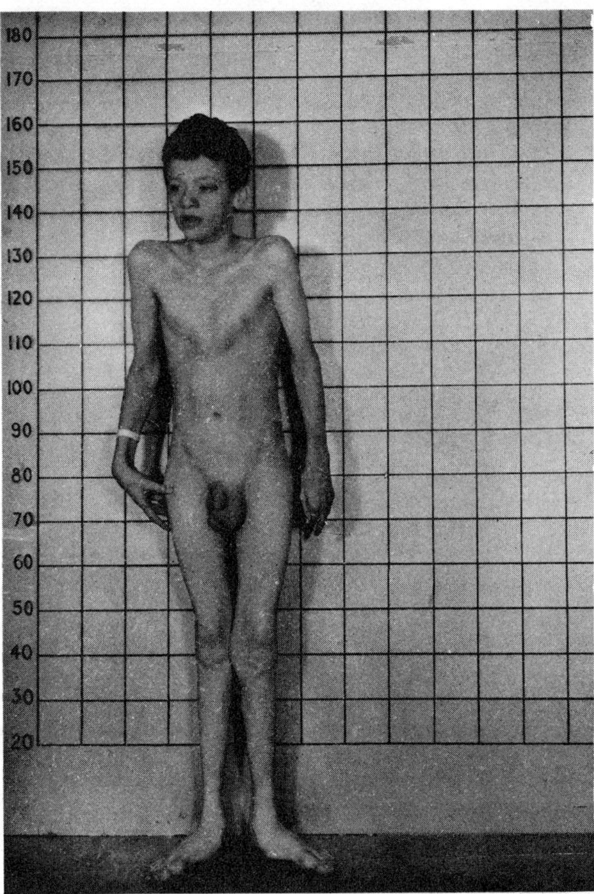

FIGURE 364–3
An eleven-year-old boy with homocystinuria manifested by severe mental retardation, bilateral dislocated lenses, pectus carinatum, "rocker-bottom feet," genu valgum, spinal curvature, and generalized osteoporosis.

the Marfan syndrome, although usually none of these features is as extreme. Loose-jointedness is not impressive, and the fingers usually show reduced joint mobility. Ectopia lentis is progressive and is demonstrable in the great majority of patients by the age of ten years. Generalized osteoporosis, with "codfish vertebras" and proneness to fracture in severe cases, is present in some degree in all patients. Thrombosis in arteries and veins may occur at any age and at any site. Coronary artery occlusion, bilateral thrombosis of the internal carotid artery, and thrombosis of the inferior vena cava have been observed in children and teenagers with homocystinuria. Mental retardation in some degree occurs in about two-thirds of cases.

The diagnosis of homocystinuria rests on demonstration of homocystine in the urine. The cyanide nitroprusside test is positive for both cystine and homocystine. Further tests, such as high-voltage paper electrophoresis, permit the differentiation. Enzymatic confirmation is provided by demonstrating very low activity of cystathionine synthetase in liver biopsy material or in fibroblasts grown in culture from skin.

Like other Garrodian inborn errors of metabolism, homocystinuria is inherited as an autosomal recessive trait. The fundamental defect in homocystinuria is deficient activity of cystathionine synthetase, the enzyme which normally catalyzes the condensation of homocysteine and serine to form cystathionine. Ectopia lentis, osteoporosis, and skeletal deformity may result from interference of accumulated sulfhydryl groups with cross-linking in collagen. The mechanism of vascular thrombosis is obscure. Both damage to the vessel wall by homocysteine and abnormality of the platelets have some evidence to support them. The cause of mental retardation is also not understood, although intracranial thromboses undoubtedly contribute in many cases. Furthermore, the normal presence of cystathionine and cystathionine synthetase in brain and their absence from the brain of the homocystinuric patient suggest that deficiency of a substance synthesized distal to the enzyme block is involved in the mental retardation.

The *Weil-Marchesani syndrome* is characterized by ectopia lentis, short stature, stiff joints, congenital pulmonic stenosis (in some cases), and autosomal recessive transmission.

TREATMENT In some girls who are already very tall by the age of nine or ten, precocious puberty has been induced with estrogen, with satisfactory results in terms of reducing the adult height. In markedly asthenic children and perhaps in adults with signs of aortic dilatation, anabolic steroids may have a place. In patients with early dilatation of the aorta (as signaled, for example, by the murmur of aortic regurgitation), reserpine or propanolol in subhypotensive doses may protect the aorta by reducing the abruptness of the ventricular ejection. The ascending aorta and aortic valve are being replaced surgically with increasing success in patients with the Marfan syndrome.

Homocystinuria should be treated along the lines of phenylketonuria and galactosemia, in which pathologic effects of metabolites accumulating proximal to an enzyme block are averted by specific dietary restrictions; patients with homocystinuria are being treated with low-methionine diet (supplemented by cystine, which in homocystinurics becomes an essential amino acid). The results are difficult to evaluate. Pyridoxine (vitamin B_6) is a coenzyme for cystathionine synthetase, and some patients show clearing of homocystinuria and probable benefit when vitamin B_6 is given in pharmacologic dosage (100 to 500 mg per day). Long-term anticoagulants of the coumadin type are of doubtful benefit. Because of the evidence that platelets are implicated in the thrombotic complications, agents which have a platelet suppressive effect, such as phenylbutazone and sulfinpyrazone, are under trial.

PSEUDOXANTHOMA ELASTICUM

Pseudoxanthoma elasticum (synonyms: PXE, Groenblad-Strandberg syndrome) is a hereditary, generalized

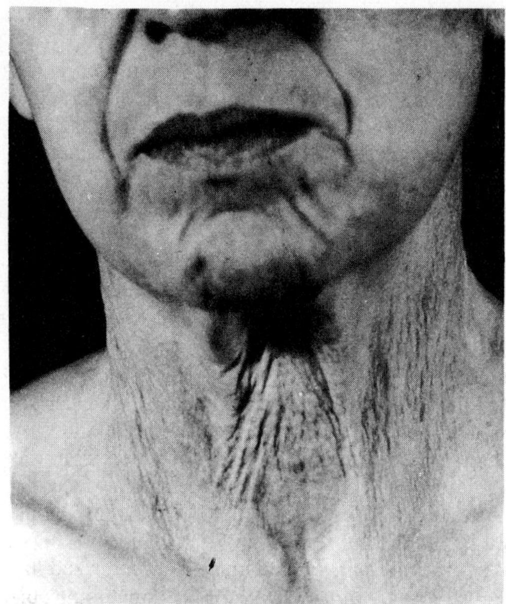

FIGURE 364-4
The skin in pseudoxanthoma elasticum.

disorder of one element of connective tissue, resulting in premature breakdown of the skin in certain areas, angioid streaks in the fundus oculi, and hemorrhage from arterial degeneration.

CLINICAL MANIFESTATIONS **Skin** In the second, third, or fourth decade of life, patients affected by PXE are likely to develop changes in the skin of the neck, axillas, inguinal areas, and periumbilical zone, consisting of thickening, grooving, and formation of yellowish, diamond-shaped, rectangular, or polygonal nodules (Fig. 364-4). The skin in involved areas becomes inelastic, lax, and redundant. In women, the changes in the neck may be cosmetically disturbing. The skin changes simulate those in actinic elastosis (senile elastosis, sun dermatosis), which differs from PXE, however, by lack of involvement in unexposed areas such as the axilla and groin and by the presence of changes on the hands.

Eye Angioid streaks develop at a variable time, often as early as the second decade. They are brownish or gray and four or five times wider than the veins but resemble vessels in the manner in which they course over the fundus. Proliferative changes occur in the retina, with angioid streaks as points of origin. Hemorrhage contributes further to the ocular damage, which may progress to near-blindness.

Arterial tree Pulses may be weak or absent in the extremities. Calcification of arteries is often demonstrable by radiography early in life. Brachial arteriograms show characteristic occlusion of the radial and/or ulnar arteries, with blood supply to the hands through dilated interosseous arteries. Intermittent claudication and easy fatigability of the arms and legs occur. Many of the affected persons suffer from angina pectoris and hypertension. Recurrent gastrointestinal hemorrhage is the problem which most often brings the patient to the attention of the internist. Occasionally, some lesion such as peptic ulcer or hiatus hernia is discovered and the vascular disease of PXE is considered only an aggravating factor. More often, no such lesion is found. Hemorrhage from other sites—uterine, urinary, nasal, or subarachnoid—may occur.

INHERITANCE Pseudoxanthoma elasticum behaves genetically as an autosomal recessive trait.

PATHOLOGY AND BASIC DEFECT The skin and media of arteries of intermediate and smaller size (and occasionally the endocardium and pericardium) become the site of markedly altered connective tissue fibers, which are basophilic, have an affinity for calcium, and display the tinctorial characteristics of elastic fibers. In some areas, material of this description is reduced to amorphous or granular accumulations. The basis for angioid streaks appears to be basophilic change and subsequent crazing (cracking) of Bruch's membrane behind the retina. The earliest histologic change detectable involves the elastic fibers. The exact biochemical defect is not known. Indeed, it is not known whether the defect is primarily in the elastic fiber or in some other biochemical process, e.g., intermediary metabolism or intestinal absorption, with secondary effects on elastic fibers.

THE GENETIC MUCOPOLYSACCHARIDOSES

Table 364-3 shows the classification of the mucopolysaccharidoses, as revised because of recent findings on the basic defects. The mucopolysaccharidoses are lysosomal diseases, i.e., each has a mutation-produced deficiency in the activity of a lysosomal enzyme important to the degradation of one or more mucopolysaccharide. As a result mucopolysaccharide accumulates in the lysosomes of the cells of various organs. Other characteristics of these and other lysosomal diseases include their progressive nature, heterogeneity of the accumulated material (because of lack of substrate specificity of the deficient enzyme), and the potential for treatment by enzyme replacement.

MUCOPOLYSACCHARIDOSIS I, HURLER TYPE The Hurler syndrome (Fig. 364-5) is the prototype of the mucopolysaccharidoses. The cardinal features are gross facies, dwarfism, lumbar gibbus and radiologic changes from involvement of the osseous skeleton, stiff joints including claw hand, corneal clouding, hepatosplenomegaly, cardiac disorders, and mental retardation. Clinically this is the severest of the mucopolysaccharidoses (MPS), usually leading to death in the first decade. The child usually seems normal at birth. The several manifestations appear in the first year or two and are progressive. There may be dyspnea, precordial pain, and congestive heart failure, and murmurs referable to any of the valves of the heart may occur. Death is attributable to cardiac causes or intercurrent respiratory infection. MPS I H (see Table 364-3) is an autosomal recessive condition.

Pathology and basic defect As in all the mucopolysaccharidoses, metachromatically staining inclusions of mucopolysaccharide may be found in the circulating polymorphonuclear leukocytes (Reilly granulation) or lymphocytes, and are most consistently seen in the clasmatocytes of the bone marrow. Cells of an inflammatory exudate and fibroblasts cultured from skin also show the mucopolysaccharide.

Connective tissue from many sites shows characteristic "gargoyle cells," which are probably fibroblasts distended with mucopolysaccharide. Collagenosis is stimulated. Storage material "balloons" the neurons of the central nervous system, peripheral ganglions, and retina, the Kupffer and parenchymal cells of the liver, the reticulum cells of spleen and lymph nodes, and the epithelial cells of endocrine glands. The material stored in the nervous system is partly glycolipid in nature. That

TABLE 364-3
The genetic mucopolysaccharidoses

Designation		*Clinical features*	*Genetics*	*Excessive urinary MPS*	*Substance deficient*
MPS I H	Hurler syndrome	Early clouding of cornea, grave manifestations, death usually before age 10	Homozygous for MPS I H gene	Dermatan sulfate; heparan sulfate	α-L-Iduronidase (formerly called Hurler corrective factor)
MPS I S	Scheie syndrome	Stiff joints, cloudy cornea, aortic regurgitation, normal intelligence, normal life-span (?)	Homozygosity for MPS I S gene	Dermatan sulfate; heparan sulfate	α-L-Iduronidase
MPS I H/S	Hurler-Scheie compound	Phenotype intermediate between Hurler and Scheie	Genetic compound of MPS I H and I S genes	Dermatan sulfate; heparan sulfate	α-L-Iduronidase
MPS II A	Hunter syndrome, severe	No clouding of cornea, milder course than in MPS I H, but death usually before age 15	Hemizygous for X-linked gene	Dermatan sulfate; heparan sulfate	Hunter corrective factor
MPS II B	Hunter syndrome, mild	Survival to 30s to 50s, fair intelligence	Hemizygous for X-linked allele for mild form	Dermatan sulfate; heparan sulfate	Hunter corrective factor
MPS III A	Sanfilippo syndrome A	A and B have an identical phenotype:	Homozygous for Sanfilippo A gene	Heparan sulfate	Heparan sulfate sulfatase
MPS III B	Sanfilippo syndrome B	mild somatic, severe central nervous system effects	Homozygous for Sanfilippo B gene (at different locus)	Heparan sulfate	N-Acetyl-α-D-galactosaminidase
MPS IV	Morquio syndrome	Severe bone changes of distinctive type, cloudy cornea, aortic regurgitation	Homozygous for Morquio gene	Keratan sulfate	Unknown
MPS V	Vacant				
MPS VI A	Maroteaux-Lamy syndrome, classic form	Severe osseous and corneal change, normal intellect	Homozygous for M-L gene	Dermatan sulfate	Maroteaux-Lamy corrective factor
MPS VI B	Maroteaux-Lamy syndrome, mild form	Severe osseous and corneal change, normal intellect	Homozygous for allele at M-L gene	Dermatan sulfate	Maroteaux-Lamy corrective factor
MPS VII	β-Glucuronidase deficiency	Hepatosplenomegaly, dysostosis multiplex, white cell inclusions, late mental retardation	Homozygous for mutant gene at beta-glucuronidase locus	Dermatan sulfate	β-Glucuronidase

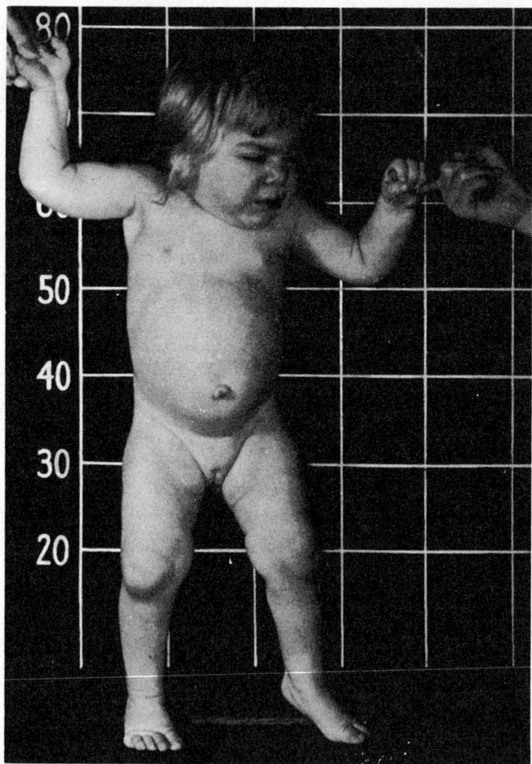

FIGURE 364-5
Mucopolysaccharidosis I H (the Hurler syndrome).

deposited elsewhere is largely mucopolysaccharide. Extensive intimal deposits of mucopolysaccharide are found in the aorta and all other arteries, large and small, resulting in "pseudoatherosclerosis." The heart valves become scarred and deformed. Involvement of the meninges results in internal hydrocephalus.

Two mucopolysaccharides are excreted in the urine and are identified in various organs: dermatan sulfate and heparan sulfate (formerly called chondroitin sulfate B and heparitin sulfate). The lysosomal enzyme deficient in MPS I H is α-L-iduronidase. The enzyme is present in normal plasma and urine. The use of plasma or plasma fractions in the treatment of this and the other mucopolysaccharidoses is under active investigation.

MUCOPOLYSACCHARIDOSIS I, SCHEIE TYPE This disorder is characterized particularly by stiff joints and clouding of the cornea, with long survival and little impairment of intellect. By about ten years of age, stiff joints, especially in the hands and feet, are noted. The mouth is broad. Hypertrichosis is generalized. Corneal clouding is first detected in the teens and is progressive, with greatest density in the peripheral portions (Fig. 364-6). Disability from stiffness of the fingers is aggravated by the carpal tunnel syndrome, manifested by atrophy of the thenar muscles and numbness in the distribution of the median nerve to the fingers. Intellect is impaired little if at all, but psychosis occurs in some cases. Aortic regurgitation is present in most of these patients by the third decade. Survival to age fifty-five years has been observed.

The Scheie syndrome is an autosomal recessive disorder.

As in MPS I H, (the Hurler syndrome) both dermatan sulfate and heparan sulfate are excreted in the urine in excess. Collagenosis, e.g., in the fingers and carpal tunnel, appears to be induced by the primary disturbance in mucopolysaccharide metabolism.

MUCOPOLYSACCHARIDOSIS II (THE HUNTER SYNDROME) The Hunter syndrome (Fig. 364-7) differs from the Hurler syndrome in its milder course, lack of corneal clouding, and mode of inheritance. Two forms may be recognized.

Clinical manifestations Grotesque facies, stiff joints, hepatosplenomegaly, and cardiac involvement occur as in MPS I H (the Hurler syndrome). Lumbar gibbus and corneal clouding do not occur, and mental retardation is less severe and more slowly progressive. Progressive deafness is a consistent feature. In one form of the disease the patients are so mildly affected that they may survive to age sixty years and children have been produced. In the more severe form, death usually occurs before age fifteen years.

The Hunter syndrome is an X-linked recessive condition. In about a third of cases the disorder in the patient is the result of fresh mutation.

Qualitatively the histologic changes are similar to those of MPS I H. The same two mucopolysaccharides are excreted in excess in the urine.

A Hunter corrective factor, missing in patients with MPS II, has been identified in normal urine by its ability to correct the degradative defect in cultured fibroblasts. The factor has been characterized in terms of molecular weight and certain other properties, but its enzymatic nature is not yet known. The two clinical forms of MPS II, the mild and the severe, lack the same corrective factor and are presumably allelic, i.e., produced by a different type of mutation in the same X-linked gene.

FIGURE 364–6
Corneal clouding, greatest at periphery in mucopolysaccharidosis I S (Scheie type).

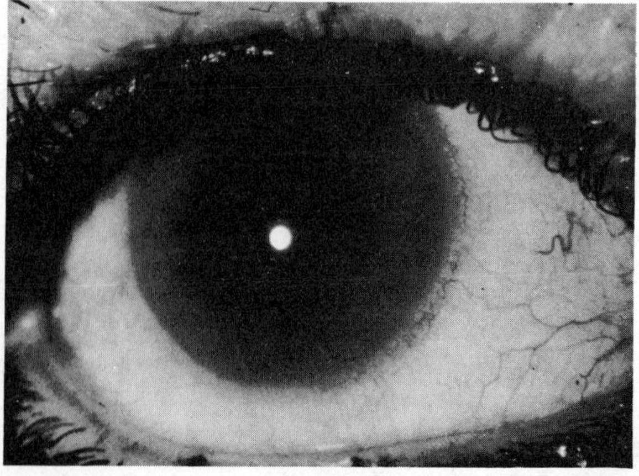

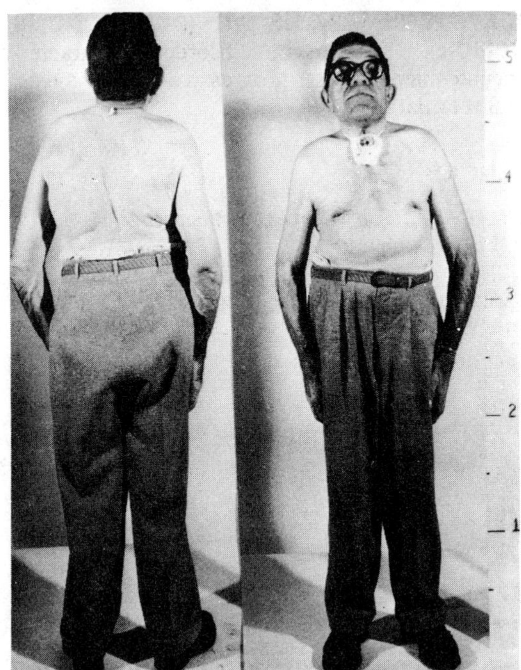

FIGURE 364-7
Mucopolysaccharidosis II (the Hunter syndrome), in a forty-six year-old man. (Courtesy of Dr. John F. Murray and the New England Journal of Medicine)

MUCOPOLYSACCHARIDOSIS III (THE SANFILIPPO SYNDROME) This syndrome is characterized by severe mental retardation with relatively mild somatic changes and by excretion of heparan sulfate in the urine.

Agitation and mental retardation first become evident between three and six years of age and rapidly progress, with loss of speech and deterioration to imbecility by age ten or twelve. Gross facies, generalized hypertrichosis, hepatosplenomegaly, and stiff joints are less striking than in the other mucopolysaccharidoses. Corneal clouding does not occur. Skeletal changes, in the spine for example, are minimal. The calvarium is markedly thickened, however.

The Sanfilippo syndrome is an autosomal recessive condition.

Only heparan sulfate is excreted in the urine in large amounts. Two clinically indistinguishable forms of Sanfilippo syndrome have been demonstrated by studies of corrective factors in fibroblast cultures supplemented by enzymatic studies. The Sanfilippo syndrome A has deficiency of heparan sulfate sulfatase, whereas the Sanfilippo syndrome B has deficiency of N-acetyl-α-D-galactosaminidase.

MUCOPOLYSACCHARIDOSIS IV (THE MORQUIO SYNDROME) The Morquio syndrome (Fig. 364-8) is characterized by typical skeletal changes, corneal clouding, aortic regurgitation, and excretion of excessive keratan sulfate in the urine.

Flat vertebras, drastic hip changes, generalized osteoporosis, and thoracic deformity, including sternal abnormality, are typical of the skeletal changes. The wrists are loose-jointed rather than stiff. Hepatosplenomegaly is only moderate. The skeletal features are evident early and bring the patients to medical attention. By their teens most patients have "steamy" corneas and aortic regurgitation. Evidence of spinal cord compression and cardiorespiratory symptoms are usually present by this stage. Hypoplasia of the odontoid process of the second cervical vertebra and subluxation of the first on the second cervical vertebra may lead to quadriplegia. Death occurs between fifteen and thirty years of age in most patients, although one of Morquio's patients is alive in his fifties.

The Morquio syndrome is an autosomal recessive disorder.

Keratan sulfate is excreted in the urine in excessive amounts and is deposited in macrophages and various parenchymal cells. A nonkeratan sulfate-excreting type of the Morquio syndrome is closely similar in many of its clinical manifestations (which are milder, however) and is a mucopolysaccharidosis, as indicated by accumulations in fibroblasts. The basic defect is presumed to concern the degradation of keratan sulfate because of deficiency of a specific lysosomal enzyme. The exact nature of the defect has not been defined, however.

MUCOPOLYSACCHARIDOSIS V The Scheie syndrome, previously designated MPS V, is now known to be a variant of (and presumably allelic to) the Hurler syndrome. It is therefore classed as MPS I S.

FIGURE 364-8
Mucopolysaccharidosis IV (the Morquio syndrome) in brothers of ages fifteen and six.

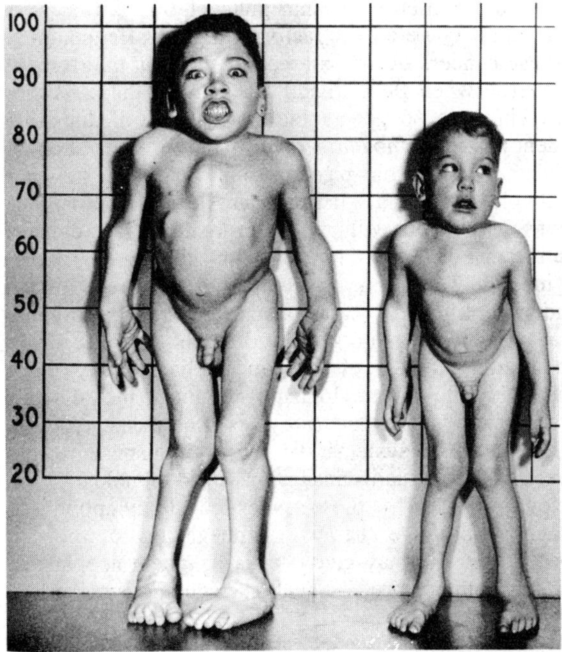

MUCOPOLYSACCHARIDOSIS VI (MAROTEAUX-LAMY SYNDROME) The classic form of this disorder is characterized by severe somatic features, e.g., corneal clouding and skeletal deformity, with good retention of intelligence until late. There is, however, a mild form which has clouding of the cornea, stiff joints, and somewhat short stature as features and resembles the Scheie syndrome. There are presumably allelic disorders, i.e., the patients are homozygous for different genes at the same locus.

MUCOPOLYSACCHARIDOSIS VII (β-GLUCURONIDASE DEFICIENCY) This rare disorder is characterized by hepatosplenomegaly, progressive bone changes, and mental retardation.

REFERENCES

McKusick VA: *Heritable Disorders of Connective Tissue*, 4th ed., St. Louis: Mosby, 1972

Pinnell SR et al: A new heritable disorder of connective tissue with hydroxylysine-deficient collagen. N Engl J Med 286:1013, 1972

section 16 Skin cancer and cutaneous manifestations of malignancy

365 PRIMARY CANCER OF THE SKIN

HARLEY A. HAYNES

Carcinoma of the skin is the most common carcinoma occurring in Caucasoid individuals. Inasmuch as the lesions can be seen with the naked eye when they are in an early stage, the potential for cure is well over 90 percent. Although not responsible for all carcinomas of the skin, chronic exposure to ultraviolet light of the sunburn wavelengths (290 to 320 nm) in individuals not protected by intense melanin pigmentation is the most important single etiologic factor (Chap. 56). Hence, most of these cancers occur on areas of the skin that remain uncovered when the individual is fully clothed. As discussed in Chap. 56, genetic factors markedly mediate this tendency for carcinogenesis. Heritable diseases such as albinism, xeroderma pigmentosum, and the nevoid-basal-cell carcinoma syndrome are less common conditions associated with a greater risk of skin cancer. The routine local use of effective sun-screen preparations by individuals at risk can undoubtedly reduce tumor incidence. Chemical carcinogens, especially inorganic arsenicals and certain organic hydrocarbons, are separate and additional causes of skin cancers, particularly of the squamous-cell variety. Ionizing radiation, including x-rays, grenz rays, and gamma rays, is also carcinogenic. As with other organ systems, the skin is predisposed to the development of malignant lesions in immunologic deficiency states, such as those associated with lymphoma or immunosuppressive therapy. Although any of the cell types in the skin may give rise to malignant neoplasms, the most common are basal-cell and squamous-cell carcinoma.

BASAL-CELL CARCINOMA Basal-cell carcinoma accounts for over 75 percent of all skin cancers. These carcinomas arise from the epidermis, cytologically resemble the normal basal cells, and show little tendency to undergo the usual differentiation into squamous cells which produce keratin. Although these tumors very rarely metastasize, they are locally invasive and, if neglected, may invade widely and deeply into underlying structures, including nerves, bone, and brain. Like most cancers, these tumors are remarkably painless in their course. This lack of symptoms often leads to prolonged neglect of a lesion. The typical basal-cell carcinoma is a noninflamed, smooth, waxy nodule that appears translucent, usually has numerous telangiectatic vessels visible near the surface, and may have variable amounts of melanin pigment in the form of small dots. Such nodules often ulcerate and form a crust. This ulceration may reepithelialize, causing the patient to assume that the nodule is resolving. Basal-cell carcinomas may take many other forms, including subtle infiltrating lesions that do not produce elevated nodules. Biopsy for confirmation of the diagnosis should be routine. The patient with one basal-cell carcinoma is likely to have others, either at the same time or in following years. Some patients come to the physician with a dozen or more concurrent primary basal-cell carcinomas. Although there is no visible premalignant lesion that precedes a basal-cell carcinoma, the lesion is usually seen in patients who manifest the stigmata of skin damage from sunlight (or x-radiation). Treatment is selected according to the size, depth, type, and location of the lesion, as well as the particular abilities of the physician. If a simple excision will suffice, there is no other procedure that can equal the cosmetic result. Curettage and electrodesiccation for small lesions give a cure rate of more than 95 percent in experienced hands, as does x-radiation. Cryosurgery is beginning to be used and seems to give excellent results. Local chemotherapy with 5-fluorouracil is not recommended as routine treatment of basal-cell carcinomas, but may have a role in the treatment of multiple superficial lesions.

SQUAMOUS-CELL CARCINOMA Squamous-cell carcinoma also arises from the epidermis but shows significant squamous differentiation and usually keratin production. These tumors have a variable tendency to metastasize, depending upon their size, extent of invasion, location, and whether or not they arise from a premalignant lesion, a burn scar, a chronic inflammatory condition, or from apparently normal skin. The typical squamous-cell carcinoma is a painless, firm, red nodule or plaque with visible scales on the surface. Ulceration and crusting may occur. Relatively undifferentiated lesions that do not produce much keratin may fail to show noticeable scaling on the surface. In contrast to the basal-cell variety, squamous-cell carcinomas most commonly arise from preexisting *actinic* or *solar keratoses.* These premalignant keratoses are scaly, rough, red plaques that occur in chronically sun-damaged skin. Although very few of these keratoses progress to carcinoma, most squamous-cell carcinomas on exposed skin do arise from such keratoses. This type of squamous-cell carcinoma has the lowest frequency of metastasis (under 2 percent). However, because of the potential of malignant change in solar keratoses, which though small is real, it seems prudent to remove them, especially in younger patients. At present, the local application of 5-fluorouracil (1 to 5%) in cream or lotion seems to be the most effective method and one that generally produces no scarring. Squamous-cell carcinomas arising from mucous membranes, mucocutaneous junctions, burn scars, chronic ulcers, or sinus tracts or from apparently normal skin have a much higher tendency to metastasize. An *in situ* stage of cutaneous squamous-cell carcinoma is known as Bowen's disease. Although some of these *in situ* lesions are the result of chronic sun damage, a significant proportion occurs in patients who had received inorganic arsenic preparations either accidentally or for medicinal purposes a decade or more before. In these patients there is also an increased risk of carcinomas of the respiratory, genitourinary, and gastrointestinal systems.

Patients with squamous-cell carcinoma must be examined carefully for the presence of metastases so that therapy may be appropriate. In the absence of metastases, therapy of the local lesion may generally be as indicated for basal-cell carcinoma, with preference for surgical excision or x-irradiation in view of the potential for metastasis. Extensive local or metastatic lesions may benefit from systemic chemotherapy, sometimes via local perfusion.

MYCOSIS FUNGOIDES LYMPHOMA *Lymphoma of the skin* may be a primary or secondary manifestation of various types of lymphoma. Reticulum-cell sarcoma and lymphoblastic lymphoma may occasionally begin with only skin lesions, but Hodgkin's disease rarely does so. The most common lymphoma of the skin is *mycosis fungoides*, which always begins with cutaneous lesions, usually with no evidence of visceral infiltration for several years. The initial lesions may be clinically confused with eczema, contact dermatitis, or psoriasis, and the biopsy may not be diagnostic. Later, more typical patches of infiltrated skin develop, often with a tendency for central clearing or in an arciform or polycyclic arrangement. At this point, the biopsy may be diagnostic. In some patients, diffuse exfoliative erythroderma develops, and there may be circulating mycosis fungoides cells in the blood, at times causing diagnostic confusion with chronic lymphocytic leukemia. The skin biopsy may resolve the confusion if it is sufficiently characteristic, as may electron microscopy of the atypical cells, which are quite distinct in mycosis fungoides. The atypical cells found in the skin appear to be the same cells found in the blood or in visceral infiltrates. In blood smears these cells resemble large lymphocytes with scant cytoplasm and folded nuclei. In routine tissue sections these cells sometimes look like lymphocytes and sometimes like reticulum cells with the characteristic infolded nucleus. Electron-microscopic examination shows the nucleus of this cell to be highly irregular, convoluted, lobulated, and drawn into narrow threads and ribbons. At some point in time, most patients develop larger tumors as well. Although any of the viscera may be affected, disability from internal involvement usually does not occur until quite late in the course of the disease. For a patient with the early stage of the disease, the prognosis is for survival for several decades. After ulcerated tumors or lymphatic involvement have occurred the prognosis is usually for less than 5 years' survival.

Treatment is best planned so as to not restrict unnecessarily the future options of therapy. Topical applications of dilute, nonvesicant concentrations of mechlorethamine are often very effective for months or even years. Selected lesions can be treated with grenz rays. Several courses of whole-skin electron-beam treatment may be given without fear of hematologic suppression, since the voltage is regulated to control the depth of penetration of electrons. The use of orthovoltage x-irradiation of multiple sites should be carefully restricted, so as not to compromise the marrow or complicate future therapy with electron beam. Systemic chemotherapy with agents such as methotrexate, cyclophosphamide, vinca alkaloids, procarbazine, and steroids often can cause dramatic objective regression of disease, but has not yet been proved to prolong life expectancy. Even though most patients at necropsy are found to have infiltrates in various viscera, early systemic chemotherapy has not been found advantageous, as a rule, perhaps because of the adverse effect of such therapy on the clinically very apparent resistance of the host with this lymphoma. In fact, this lymphoma was the first human malignancy to regularly show regression of lesions that were challenged locally with delayed hypersensitivity reactions.

REFERENCES

EPSTEIN EH et al: Mycosis fungoides: Survival, prognostic features, response to therapy, and autopsy findings. Medicine, 15:61, 1972

FITZPATRICK TB et al (eds): Neoplasms of skin: Neoplasms of epithelium, chap. 10 in *Dermatology in General Medicine*, New York: McGraw-Hill, 1971

LEVER WF: Tumors of the surface epidermis, chap. 24, and Tumors of the epidermal appendages, chap. 25, in *Histopathology of the skin*, 4th ed., New York: Lippincott, 1967

VAN SCOTT EJ, WINTERS PL: Responses of mycosis fungoides to intensive external treatment with nitrogen mustard. Arch Dermatol 102:507, 1970

ZACARIAN SA: *Cryosurgery of Skin Cancer and Cryogenic Techniques in Dermatology*, Springfield, Ill.: Charles C Thomas, 1969

366 MALIGNANT MELANOMA

THOMAS B. FITZPATRICK

Inasmuch as primary malignant melanoma of the skin is the most serious disease involving skin, the detection of early lesions must be the task for every physician, regardless of specialty. At every occasion when all the skin can be viewed, a careful search for suggestive pigmented lesions should be made.

Pigmented moles are among the most common growths on the skin of man, and yet cancer involving pigment cells (i.e., malignant melanoma) is relatively uncommon, constituting about 1.5 percent of all cancers. Cutaneous malignant melanoma, however, is virtually untreatable by chemotherapy or x-ray, and, so far, hope for survival has been based on surgical excision during the very early primary stages before deep invasion occurs. The problem for the physician, therefore, is to recognize, among the large number of pigmented lesions that occur on the skin, early primary malignant melanoma and also those precancerous lesions that will develop into malignant melanoma.

Primary malignant melanoma of the skin, even in the early stages, is now considered relatively easy to detect just by clinical examination. In the past, the clinical description of primary cutaneous malignant melanoma was presented incompletely, inasmuch as physicians and patients were told to have concern only for those pigmented lesions that show changes in growth pattern or color or are bleeding or ulcerated—criteria indicating deep invasion in the skin and, usually, a poor prognosis.

Follow-up study of more than 300 patients with primary melanoma has provided evidence indicating that a primary cutaneous melanoma may exist in a "silent," intraepidermal, preinvasive form for several years. These early "silent" primary malignant melanomas, even when 3 to 4 mm in size, can be recognized by certain simple criteria, which will be delineated in the following paragraphs.

Variegation of color and, to a lesser extent, irregularities in surface pattern and configuration are so characteristic of primary cutaneous malignant melanoma that histologic examination is mandatory when they are present. The important color changes that are signs of primary malignant melanoma are listed below:

Red	*White*	*Blue*
Reddish blue (purple)	Whitish gray	Blue
Reddish brown	Whitish pink	Bluish red (violaceous)
		Bluish gray
		Bluish black

(These colors may all be admixed with brown or black, or a lesion may be uniformly colored—e.g., bluish black or bluish red, etc.)

The diagnostic significance of various shades of brown or black, or both, in pigmented primary cutaneous malignant melanoma has been stressed in the past. It is, however, the diagnostic significance of the various shades of red or white or blue, or all three admixed with brown or black, that needs to be stressed. Of the colors present in pigmented primary cutaneous malignant melanomas, shades of blue (bluish red, bluish gray, and bluish black) are the most significant in the diagnosis.

Before 1967, malignant melanoma was considered to be a single morphologic type with a uniformly grave prognosis. Later investigations, especially by Clark of the United States and McGovern of Australia, have permitted a new approach to the classification of pigmented primary cutaneous melanomas, based on the correlation of the clinical and histologic features with prognosis. Three types of primary malignant melanoma have been delineated:

Type I — Malignant melanoma with an adjacent intraepidermal component (malignant Hutchinson's melanotic freckle) (Plate 6-1)

Type II — Malignant melanoma with an adjacent intraepidermal component (superficial spreading melanoma) (Plate 6-2)

Type III — Malignant melanoma *without* an adjacent intraepidermal component (nodular melanoma) (Plate 6-3)

Some of the features of these types are listed in Table 366-1.

It should be emphasized that these three types of malignant melanoma may exist for several years in the preinvasive stage. Hence, early diagnosis of malignant melanoma of the skin makes excision of the identified lesions possible before deep invasion has occurred. The survival rate of malignant melanoma differs in the three different types, and in each different type the prognosis is related to the level of invasion of the tumor. These levels of invasion have been arbitrarily classified as follows:

Level 1 — Tumor confined to the epidermis

Level 2 — Tumor invading the papillary layer but not extending to the reticular layer

TABLE 366-1
Clinical features of malignant melanoma

Type	*Site*	*Average age at diagnosis, yr*	*Duration of known existence*	*Color*
Type I	Exposed surfaces usually, and particularly malar region of cheek and temple; on unexposed surfaces sometimes	70	5–20 yr* or longer	In flat portions, shades of brown and black predominant, but whitish gray occasionally present; in nodules, shades of reddish brown, bluish gray, bluish black only
Type II	Any site (possibly, more common on exposed surfaces)	40–50	1–7 yr	Shades of brown and black admixed with bluish red (violaceous), bluish black, reddish brown, and often whitish pink
Type III	Any site	40–50	Months to less than 5 yr	Reddish blue (purple) or bluish black, either uniform in color or admixed with brown or black

* *During much of this time, type I has a precursor stage, lentigo maligna; malignant melanoma supervenes in this preinvasive lesion.*
SOURCE: *Adapted from Mihm et al (1971)*

Level 3 Tumor filling and expanding the papillary layer but not invading the reticular layer
Level 4 Tumor penetrating into the reticular layer of the dermis
Level 5 Tumor invading the subcutaneous fat

For example, type I and type II malignant melanomas that have not extended beyond level 2 usually cause death in 5 years in fewer than 5 percent of the patients. Type III melanoma, however, has usually extended to level 3 when it is first recognized and is responsible for death in 5 years in approximately 45 percent of the patients. In type II and type III, the survival rate decreases progressively according to the depth of invasion at the time of excision, thus making the earliest possible identification obligatory.

Treatment of malignant melanoma at the present time is primarily by surgical excision of the primary lesions; there is no agreement as to whether prophylactic lymph node dissection affects the course of the disease. Early stages of types I and II, i.e., invasion to levels 1 and 2, can be treated successfully by simple excision and, if necessary, skin grafting. The advanced stages of type II (i.e., invasion to levels 3, 4, and 5) and type III melanomas at any level of invasion should be treated by wide local excision down to the deep fascia, followed by skin grafting; radical lymph node dissection when the tumor drains to only one lymph node group also is advocated by most surgeons.

In the past few years, considerable interest has been directed toward the factors that influence both the development of primary malignant melanomas of the skin and also the rate and degree of dissemination of the tumor. The possibility that there is a population with a high risk for the development of primary malignant melanoma of the skin is being studied. It is suspected that persons, both male and female, who have poor tolerance to sunlight and develop sunburn on short exposures have a higher incidence of malignant melanoma. It is certainly true that the incidence of primary malignant melanoma of the skin is higher in the sunniest parts of Australia than in any other place in the world. Thus in northeastern Australia, the incidence of primary malignant melanoma of the skin is 17 per 100,000 population, whereas in Boston the incidence is less than 2 per 100,000 population. Only a few factors are presently known that influence the dissemination of melanoma. There is a higher incidence of melanoma in females, although the survival rate seems to be correlated with hormonal factors. Premenopause females have a better survival rate once metastases have occurred, whereas postmenopause females have a survival rate that is equal to or shorter than that of males. The immune status of the patient is another factor under investigation. The possibility that immunologic factors are involved in the course of malignant melanoma is suggested by the high rate of spontaneous regressions of melanoma, by the long periods of freedom from the time of excision of the primary lesion to the development of metatases, and by the histologic changes seen in early lesions but not seen in more invasive advanced lesions—a lymphocytoid response, which occurs in the early, but not in the later, lesions.

The general physician examining a patient with many pigmented lesions should recognize the features that are highly suggestive of primary malignant melanoma of the skin and necessarily indicate that the lesion must be removed, or, if it is very large, at least biopsied. If these early lesions can be detected and excised, the 5-year survival rate of patients with malignant melanoma will be markedly improved. The most important criteria in the detection of primary malignant melanoma are the areas of bluish gray, bluish red, bluish black, and whitish gray. Certain pigmented lesions, however, such as all congenital hairy nevi, and pigmented lesions of the scalp and soles, do not have these telltale color changes but should be prophylactically removed anyway.

REFERENCES

CLARK WH JR: A classification of malignant melanoma in man correlated with histogenesis and biological behavior, in *The Pigmentary System*, eds W Montagna, F Hu, vol. 8 of *Advances in Biology of Skin*, New York: Pergamon, 1967

MIHM MC JR et al: The clinical diagnosis, classification and histogenetic concepts of the early stages of cutaneous malignant melanomas. N Engl J Med 284:1078, 1971

367 CUTANEOUS MANIFESTATIONS OF INTERNAL MALIGNANCY

HARLEY A. HAYNES
THOMAS B. FITZPATRICK

One of the most satisfying aspects of dermatologic diagnosis is the detection of previously unknown malignant disease in a treatable stage by recognizing an apparently irrelevant alteration of the skin as a clue to the presence of the neoplasm. Although less satisfying, the recognition of the probability of a neoplastic disease may be of great assistance in clarifying a difficult diagnostic problem, even if the neoplasm should be untreatable when discovered. Sometimes these skin changes are induced directly by infiltration of the neoplasm into the skin, but more often they are induced indirectly by a variety of mechanisms.

This chapter is an attempt to classify the wide range of skin signs of internal malignancy in a logical fashion (Table 367-1). Since the types of skin alterations and the number of neoplasms are extremely large, grouping of the alterations by pathogenetic mechanisms was selected. There remains a substantial idiopathic category; the entities therein will be grouped by pathogenesis when this becomes understood. The skin alterations induced by neoplasms of the endocrine organs are not included here as they generally are the alterations one would expect from excess or deficiency of the hormone in question and are mentioned in the appropriate chapters.

SKIN INFILTRATION BY AN INTERNAL MALIGNANCY

METASTASES FROM CARCINOMA Cutaneous metastases of malignant lesions occur in 3 to 5 percent of patients with metastatic disease. These lesions may provide the first indication of recurrence in a patient with a known primary tumor or may be the presenting lesions of a hitherto unsuspected tumor. Typical skin metastases are dermal nodules, varying from skin color to purple, which are more easily felt than seen, and are very firm to the touch; they ulcerate rarely. Metastases from renal and thyroid carcinomas may be pulsatile and have a bruit. Breast carcinomas may produce an erysipelas-like appearance on the chest. The location of skin metastases may give a clue to the origin of the primary tumor. The abdominal wall is the most common site in both sexes for lesions initially presenting as metastases. In this situation, the primary sites are usually the lung, stomach, or kidney in men, and the ovary in women. In women with metastases on the chest wall, the most likely primary site is the breast. Other skin areas that tend to be involved by metastases are the scalp, from lung, kidney, or breast; the chest, in men, from lung; the back, from lung or breast; the extremities, from malignant melanomas; and the face, from oropharyngeal carcinomas. Histologic examination of a skin metastasis may reveal the identity of the primary tumor.

METASTASIS FROM LEUKEMIA Leukemic deposits in skin are more common in myelomonocytic leukemia than in lymphocytic or granulocytic leukemias (Chap. 316). Firm papules or nodules ranging in color from pink to purple are the usual lesions, although ulcerations may develop. If thrombocytopenia is present, purpura often occurs in the nodules. Leukemic infiltrates may develop in recent scars, in traumatized areas, and in lesions of herpes zoster and herpes simplex. Cytologic examination of "touch" preparations from the cut surface of a nodule more readily identifies the cell type than examination of histologic sections. The only clinically pathognomonic lesion of any of the leukemias is chloroma, named for its green color, which is due to myeloperoxidase in the cells of acute granulocytic leukemia. In addition to specific leukemic cell infiltrates, a variety of lesions occur that are nonspecific on biopsy.

INTRAEPIDERMAL METASTASES: PAGET'S DISEASE *Paget's disease of the nipple* and areola is an uncommon but well-known skin sign of underlying intraductal carcinoma of the breast. The primary ductal carcinoma extends upward within the epithelium of the mammary ducts and into the epidermis, where it causes the skin lesion. The clinical appearance is that of an eczematous, weeping, crusted, or scaly lesion resembling atopic eczema or contact dermatitis. Paget's disease is unaffected by topical corticosteroids, in contrast to the responsiveness of eczema. Therefore, any such "eczematous" lesions that fail to respond to treatment must be biopsied. The histopathologic appearance of Paget's disease is diagnostic; the presence in the epidermis of clear cells containing mucopolysaccharides is apparent.

Extramammary Paget's disease is a similar eczematous-appearing lesion occurring on the pubis, perineum, thighs, or genitalia, related usually to underlying apocrine or eccrine sweat gland carcinoma, but occasionally to rectal or urethral adenocarcinoma. Occasionally, a primary malignant origin cannot be found. The histopathologic appearance of extramammary Paget's disease of apocrine gland origin is identical to that of Paget's disease of the breast, which is an apocrine gland. Special staining of the mucopolysaccharides will permit differentiation between Paget's disease of cloacagenic or apocrine gland origin.

LYMPHOMA Lymphomatous deposits in the skin secondary to an internal lymphoma are seen most often in reticulum-cell sarcoma and lymphoblastic lymphoma. Such cutaneous deposits are rare in Hodgkin's disease. Mycosis fungoides, the most frequent lymphomatous

TABLE 367-1
Classification of skin signs of internal malignancy

I Skin infiltration by an internal malignancy
- *A* Metastatic, lymphatic, hematogenous, or by surgical implantation
  - *1* Carcinoma
  - *2* Leukemia
- *B* Metastatic, intraepidermal
  - *1* Paget's disease of the breast
  - *2* Extramammary Paget's disease
- *C* Autochthonous or metastatic (?)
  - *1* Lymphoma
  - *2* Malignant histiocytosis

II Skin changes due to exposure to a carcinogen that also induces internal malignancy
- *A* Arsenical keratoses
- *B* Bowen's disease

III Skin malignancies associated with increased risk of separate primary internal malignancy
- *A* Bowen's disease
- *B* Kaposi's sarcoma
- *C* Any skin malignancy (??)

IV Skin changes due to metabolic products of nonendocrine malignancies
- *A* Malignant carcinoid syndrome (Chap. 99)
- *B* Addisonian hyperpigmentation with Cushing's syndrome, from carcinomas producing MSH- and ACTH-like peptides
- *C* Generalized dermal melanosis (slate gray), from malignant melanoma
- *D* Nodular fat necrosis, due to lipases from pancreatic carcinoma
- *E* Raynaud's syndrome with cryoproteinemia, from multiple myeloma
- *F* Amyloidosis, from multiple myeloma

V Skin changes due to functional disturbances in other systems induced by nonendocrine malignancies
- *A* Jaundice, obstructive (Chap. 42)
- *B* Addisonian hyperpigmentation from adrenal infiltration by a tumor (Chap. 86)
- *C* Purpura, thrombocytopenic (Chap. 313)
- *D* Pallor, from anemia (Chap. 58)
- *E* Herpes zoster (Chap. 199)
- *F* Herpes simplex, severe, protracted, recurrent (Chap. 200)
- *G* Pyoderma, recurrent
- *H* Delayed hypersensitivity, exaggerated to mosquito bites

VI Skin changes, idiopathic
- *A* Changes frequently related to internal malignancy
  - *1* Dermatomyositis, adult-onset (Chap. 343)
  - *2* Acanthosis nigricans
  - *3* Thrombophlebitis, migratory
  - *4* Ichthyosis, adult-onset
  - *5* Alopecia mucinosa, adult
  - *6* Pachydermoperiostosis, acquired
  - *7* Hypertrichosis lanugosa, acquired ("malignant down")
- *B* Changes occasionally related to internal malignancy
  - *1* Pruritus, without causative skin lesions
  - *2* Clubbing, with and without hypertrophic osteoarthropathy
  - *3* Erythroderma
  - *4* Normolipemic xanthomatosis
  - *5* Erythema multiforme
  - *6* Urticaria and erythema perstans
  - *7* Bullous disease (bullous pemphigoid and dermatitis herpetiformis)
  - *8* Dermatoses, bizarre

VII Heritable diseases with skin manifestations and the propensity to develop internal malignancy (see Table 367-2)

skin disorder, is discussed in Chap. 365. Lymphoma lesions in the skin are dermal or subcutaneous nodules that typically have a purple or red-brown color. The lesions usually are covered by relatively normal intact epidermis. Skin infiltrates may be the initial manifestations or may appear at any time in the course of the disease. Biopsy of these lesions is necessary to establish the correct diagnosis. The nonspecific skin changes in lymphoma are discussed below.

MALIGNANT HISTIOCYTOSIS In the Letterer-Siwe, Schüller-Christian disease complex a variety of skin lesions may occur: (1) scaly papules or vesicles with or without purpura on trunk or scalp, (2) pruritic seborrheic or eczematous lesions in intertriginous areas that do not respond to local treatment for the benign conditions, (3) petechiae due to perivascular infiltrates, thrombocytopenia, or both, (4) scaly or exudative eruptions of the scalp, and (5) xanthomas, usually late in the course. When there is lack of response to local therapy, directed at presumptive diaper dermatitis, seborrheic dermatitis, moniliasis, or intertrigo, early biopsy of these various lesions should be done and is usually diagnostic if histiocytosis is present. Skin lesions may be the presenting sign and may lead to the correct diagnosis, or they may appear late in the course of the disease if it is not controlled (Chap. 317).

SKIN CHANGES DUE TO EXPOSURE TO A CARCINOGEN THAT ALSO INDUCES INTERNAL MALIGNANCY

ARSENICAL KERATOSES Inorganic arsenicals are the only well-recognized carcinogens which cause both skin and visceral malignancies. These salts were widely used in medicine a few decades ago for the treatment of a large variety of disorders, such as arthritis, asthma, and psoriasis, and were also used as herbicides in agriculture. Arsenic contamination of drinking water occurs in many parts of the world. Exposure may therefore be intentional and known or accidental and wholly unsuspected. Multiple, discrete, hard hyperkeratotic wartlike lesions, termed arsenical keratoses, on the palms and soles occur characteristically in patients a decade or more after exposure to arsenic. These lesions are similar to actinic or solar keratoses in that they are premalignant lesions, but they have a very low incidence of malignancy. The histopathologic changes produced by these two types of keratoses also are similar.

BOWEN'S DISEASE Squamous-cell carcinoma of the skin *in situ* is known as Bowen's disease. The lesions are single or multiple, sharply defined plaques that are slightly thickened and brownish red, and have a varying amount of scale. At times the lesions of Bowen's disease resemble eczema or psoriasis but fail to respond to local therapy. Such lesions must be biopsied. Arsenical exposure is definitely the cause of many cases of Bowen's disease and may be the cause of nearly all. The lesions are easily treated by surgical excision or by various methods of local destruction. Although about 5 percent become invasive, less than 2 percent metastasize. More important is the recognition of the fact that the patient is at significant risk of developing carcinomas of the respiratory, genitourinary, and gastrointestinal systems. This risk is especially high in patients in whom Bowen's disease develops on skin that is not usually exposed to sunlight. Thorough examinations to detect visceral neoplasia must be performed at intervals, as the average latent period between the onset of Bowen's disease and the development of visceral neoplasia is more than 8 years. Even without a history or stigmata of arsenical exposure, there is an increased risk of visceral neoplasms in patients with this condition.

SKIN MALIGNANCIES ASSOCIATED WITH INCREASED RISK OF SEPARATE PRIMARY INTERNAL MALIGNANCY

BOWEN'S DISEASE See preceding section.

KAPOSI'S SARCOMA Initially Kaposi's sarcoma may be a multiple, autochthonous, reactive, lymphoreticular and endothelial cell proliferation rather than a neoplasm.

TABLE 367-2
Heritable diseases with skin manifestations and propensity to develop internal malignancy

Disorder	*Skin signs*	*Alterations of other systems*	*Predominant malignancy*
Dominant inheritance			
Gardner's syndrome	Epidermal cysts Sebaceous cysts Dermoid tumors Lipomas Fibromas	Polyposis of colon Osteomas	Colonic adenocarcinomas (very high incidence, unless colectomy done)
Multiple mucosal neuromas	Neuromas on eyelids, lips, tongue, nasal or laryngeal mucosae	Parathyroid adenomas Hypertension	Pheochromocytoma Medullary carcinoma of thyroid (high incidence)
Neurofibromatosis (Recklinghausen's)	Neurofibromas Café au lait spots Axillary "freckles" Giant nevi	Acoustic and spinal neuromas Meningiomas Osseous fibrous dysplasia	Malignant neurilemmoma (5% incidence) Pheochromocytoma (uncommon) Astrocytoma, glioma (uncommon)
Nevoid basal-cell carcinoma syndrome	Multiple basal-cell carcinomas Epidermoid cysts "Pits" on palms and soles	Jaw cysts Rib and vertebral abnormalities Short metacarpals Ovarian fibromas Hypertelorism	Medulloblastoma Fibrosarcoma of jaw (low incidence)
Palmar-plantar hyperkeratosis (tylosis)	Hyperkeratosis of palms and soles (usually onset after age 10)	None	Esophageal carcinoma (95% incidence)
Peutz-Jeghers syndrome	Pigmented macules on lips, oral mucosa, digits	Intestinal polyposis (predominantly small intestine)	Gastric, duodenal, and colonic adenocarcinomas (low incidence)
Tuberous sclerosis	Hypopigmented macules Shagreen patches Adenoma sebaceum Subungual fibromas	Epilepsy Mental retardation Hamartomas in brain, kidneys, heart	Astrocytomas Glioblastomas (low incidence)

It usually behaves in an indolent fashion, although frank, aggressive sarcomatous change develops in a small percentage of patients. The lesions begin on the feet or ankles, then may progress proximally and also occur on the hands and arms. Extracutaneous lesions are most frequently seen in the gastrointestinal tract, where bleeding is the major complication. The respiratory tract is the second most frequently involved extracutaneous site. Generally these extracutaneous lesions are not clinically significant, unless frankly sarcomatous. There is a marked genetic predisposition to the disease among Jews, Italians, and the Bantus in the Congo. A pronounced male predominance of 9:1 has been noted. The skin lesions of Kaposi's sarcoma are rather distinctive, dark blue or purple-brown nodules or plaques, primarily located on the distal extremities. The color is due to the vascular nature of the lesions and the chronic extravasation of erythrocytes, resulting in hemosiderin deposition. Almost invariably, chronic lymphedema is associated with, and at times precedes, the lesions. Lymphoma and leukemia are associated in about 10 percent of cases in the Western Hemisphere, but not in the Eastern. The histopathologic picture is sufficiently characteristic for confirmation of the clinical diagnosis. For the average case, very conservative therapy, such as elastic support hose to reduce edema and low-dose x-irradiation of symptomatic skin lesions, is all that is required. Chemotherapy should be considered only in the presence of clinically significant visceral lesions or aggressive sarcomatous behavior.

ANY SKIN MALIGNANCY Neoplasia of the skin of any type may be an indication of increased risk of

TABLE 367-2 (*Continued*)
Heritable diseases with skin manifestations and propensity to develop internal malignancy

Disorder	*Skin signs*	*Alterations of other systems*	*Predominant malignancy*
Autosomal recessive			
Ataxia telangiectasia	Telangiectasia: Neck, Malar, Antecubital fossae, Popliteal fossae, Ears	Cerebellar ataxia Sinopulmonary infections IgA deficiency ± IgE deficiency	Lymphoma, leukemia (10% incidence)
Bloom's syndrome	Telangiectasia of sun-exposed skin Photosensitivity	Short stature Fine features Dolichocephaly	Leukemia (high incidence)
Chediak-Higashi	Dilution of skin and hair color Recurrent pyoderma Giant melanosomes	Recurrent infections Azurophilic leukocytic inclusions Nystagmus Iris translucence Photophobia Pancytopenia	Lymphoma (high incidence)
Fanconi's anemia	Patchy hyperpigmentation	Bone anomalies Chromosomal aberrations	Leukemia (high incidence)
Werner's syndrome (adult progeria)	Premature aging Scleroderma-like changes Graying hair and baldness Leg ulcers	Arteriosclerosis Cataracts	Sarcoma Meningiomas
Sex-linked recessive			
Bruton's sex-linked agammaglobulinemia	Recurrent infections	Recurrent infections Agammaglobulinemia	Leukemia, lymphoma (5% incidence)
Dyskeratosis congenita	Reticulate hyperpigmentation Leukoplakia of mucosae Loss of nails Hyperkeratosis of palms and soles Atrophy of skin of extensor surfaces	Pancytopenia	Carcinomas (high incidence) Leukemia (occasional)
Wiscott-Aldrich syndrome	Eczematous dermatitis Petechiae—purpura Recurrent pyoderma	Decreased IgM Thrombocytopenia	Leukemia, lymphoma (10% incidence)

visceral neoplasia, but the exact relationship is difficult to ascertain because of the high incidence of skin malignancies.

SKIN CHANGES DUE TO METABOLIC PRODUCTS OF NONENDOCRINE MALIGNANCIES

MALIGNANT CARCINOID SYNDROME The hallmark of the syndrome (Chap. 99) is the sudden onset of bright-red flushing of the skin, especially of the face, neck, and upper part of the chest.

ADDISONIAN HYPERPIGMENTATION WITH CUSHING'S SYNDROME (see Chap. 86) Some nonendocrine tumors, particularly oat-cell carcinoma of the lung, secrete polypeptide hormones. The most commonly observed syndrome is Addisonian hyperpigmentation with Cushing's syndrome. Intense hyperpigmentation combined with proximal muscle weakness, hypertension, diabetes mellitus, edema, and confusion are typical features. Hypokalemic alkalosis and elevated serum cortisol levels are more frequent findings than are the usual physical signs of Cushing's disease. The syndrome is caused by the production of ACTH and β-MSH (melanocyte-stimulating hormone) by the tumor.

GENERALIZED DERMAL MELANOSIS (SLATE GRAY) In some patients with widespread metastases from malignant melanoma, metabolic precursors of melanin enter the circulation and are deposited in all tissues, where they become oxidized to melanin. Excretion of these intermediates results in urine that turns black upon exposure to air. Inasmuch as most of the visible melanin in this type of melanosis is in the dermis, the Tyndall effect causes the skin to look gray or blue-black rather than brown.

NODULAR FAT NECROSIS The syndrome of tender subcutaneous nodules, fever, eosinophilia, and polyarthritis of the small joints is produced by pancreatic adenocarcinoma as well as by pancreatitis. In this syndrome, the subcutaneous nodules are various shades of red, and may undergo central necrosis with discharge of oil material. The increased circulating levels of lipase and other pancreatic enzymes are probably responsible for the syndrome. The histopathologic picture of the nodules usually permits the diagnosis of pancreatic fat necrosis, but does not permit differentiation of benign from malignant etiology.

RAYNAUD'S PHENOMENON (see Chap. 247) The production of cryoglobulins in patients with myeloma may cause Raynaud's phenomena. Such an etiology should be especially suspected when the syndrome is atypical in males, or begins in individuals over fifty years of age.

SYSTEMIC AMYLOIDOSIS From 10 to 20 percent of patients with multiple myeloma develop amyloidosis (Chap. 107). The characteristic presentation resembles "primary" amyloidosis and includes macroglossia, extraordinarily easy bruising, and, occasionally, yellowish papules or plaques or plaques visible in the skin. All organs may be affected. The purpura appears to result from vascular fragility as a consequence of deposition of amyloid. Purpura may often be induced by gentle stroking or pinching of apparently normal skin, particularly the eyelids and body folds. When the skin lesions of amyloidosis are isolated rather than scattered diffusely, the etiology is unlikely to be systemic. Such local skin amyloidosis is not rare and must be differentiated from systemic amyloidosis.

SKIN CHANGES DUE TO FUNCTIONAL DISTURBANCES IN OTHER SYSTEMS INDUCED BY NONENDOCRINE MALIGNANCIES (See Table 367-1)

IDIOPATHIC SKIN SIGNS OF INTERNAL MALIGNANCY

Signs frequently related to internal malignancy

DERMATOMYOSITIS (see Chap. 345) Adults with dermatomyositis have an associated malignancy in at least 15 percent of cases, the association being slightly higher in men than in women. The skin changes may be either subtle and transient initially or widespread, persistent, and rapid in onset. Transient, blotchy, red or violaceous areas, with or without fine scaling, may be incorrectly diagnosed as contact dermatitis, eczema, or seborrheic dermatitis. When the initial lesions are sudden in onset and marked on the face, neck, and other sun-exposed areas, a photosensitivity dermatitis or contact dermatitis may be simulated. Indeed, photosensitivity is frequently noted in dermatomyositis. Later, telangiectasia develops in the lesions, and often edema and telangiectasia of the malar area or the eyelids may result in the violaceous (heliotrope) color. Linear telangiectasia adjacent to the cuticles on the nail folds within areas of periungual erythema are usually seen, as in systemic lupus erythematosus. Accentuation of cutaneous lesions over the joints on the dorsum of the hands, as well as over large joints, is often noted.

ACANTHOSIS NIGRICANS This skin sign is a highly significant marker of probable malignant disease when it develops in adults. The clinical problem is to differentiate between the different types of acanthosis nigricans, all of which look the same clinically and histopathologically. The lesions typically involve the axillas, groin, umbilicus, and nipples, but more extensive lesions may occur. The epidermis shows brown-to-black hyperpigmentation in areas of multiple confluent papillomas, resulting in a velvety elevation of the surface of the epidermis. Pruritus is sometimes present. The histopathologic appearance of the lesions confirms the diagnosis of acanthosis nigricans but does not permit differentiation between the various types. It is the history, the family history, and the physical examination which provide the most helpful data in classifying the type of acanthosis nigricans. Lesions present at birth or developing in childhood or at puberty are genetically determined and not related to malignancy. Obese individuals may develop intertriginous acanthosis nigricans without underlying disease. Various endocrinopathies, particularly Cushing's syndrome, acromegaly, and Stein-Leventhal syndrome, may be associated with acanthosis nigricans. When these conditions are absent and acanthosis nigricans develops in an adult, an underlying malignancy will be associated in most of the cases. Adenocarcinomas are the usual type of malignancy, and 60 percent of these are gastric (Chap. 283). Occasionally an undifferentiated or squamous-cell carcinoma or a lymphoma is the associated neoplasm. Though the course of the acanthosis nigricans in two-thirds of cases tends to parallel the course of the neoplasm, including remission with cure, intervals as long as 6 years between the skin lesion and the onset of the malignancy have been observed. If no benign explanation can be found for acanthosis nigricans in an adult, periodic efforts to locate a neoplasm are mandatory.

MIGRATORY THROMBOPHLEBITIS Superficial and multiple deep venous thromboses, not readily explained by the usual causes, are likely to be associated with a malignancy, usually pancreatic carcinoma (Chap. 302). Involvement of atypical sites, such as upper extremities, should also alert the physician to this possible association. An involved area may resolve in a few days. Pulmonary embolism is not a frequent complication. The migratory thrombophlebitis may precede detection of the neoplasm by several months. Unfortunately, the neoplasms associated with recurrent phlebitis tend to be inoperable.

ICHTHYOSIS The development of ichthyosis in adults having no personal or family history of the disorder is very likely to be associated with lymphoma (usually Hodgkin's disease), although occasionally other types of malignancy have been reported. The skin appears dry, and the stratum corneum cracks to produce rhomboidal scales with flaky edges. Hyperkeratosis of the palms and soles may occur as well. The histopathologic changes are epidermal atrophy and hyperkeratosis, but they do not distinguish ichthyosis as a manifestation of malignancy from certain hereditary types. Although the association of this ichthyosiform alteration with lymphoma is strong, only a small number of cases have been reported.

ALOPECIA MUCINOSA Dermal papules, often with follicular accentuation and usually with hair loss in affected areas, are the typical findings. Usually this disorder is benign and self-limited, especially in patients under forty and with a small number of lesions. In patients over forty and when there are multiple infiltrated plaques with alopecia, the lesions are likely to represent a lymphoma with associated follicular mucinosis. However, alopecia mucinosa may develop before the lymphoma can be diagnosed in a certain number of patients.

PACHYDERMOPERIOSTOSIS This term describes hypertrophic osteoarthropathy combined with acromegaloid features (Chap. 83). Thickening of the skin of the hands, forearms, and legs, as well as marked accentuation of facial folds, is typical. When the scalp is involved, the skin is reduplicated and furrowed (cutis verticis gyrata). A familial form of the disorder occurs and is unrelated to malignant disease. The acquired form usually occurs in men over forty years of age who have bronchogenic carcinoma. Some acquired cases are associated with pulmonary infections, congenital heart disease, and hepatic disease.

HYPERTRICHOSIS LANUGOSA This sign is quite rare but so striking in its appearance and in its association with internal malignancy that it deserves discussion. A congenital form, often familiarly known as "dog face" or "monkey face," is inherited as an autosomal dominant trait and has no association with malignancy. Acquired hypertrichosis of lanugo hair type in adults has been associated with malignant disease. The associated neoplasms have been carcinomas of the breast, urinary bladder, lung, gallbladder, colon, and rectum. The hypertrichosis in this condition is composed of extremely fine, silky, and lightly pigmented hairs of the lanugo type. This hair growth is most apparent on the face and ears, but may occur on the trunk and extremities. Care must be taken to differentiate this lanugo hair growth from adult-type hair growth in women with disorders of androgen excess and in either sex with porphyria cutanea tarda, erythropoietic porphyria (Chap. 56), and diphenylhydantoin administration.

Signs occasionally related to internal malignancy

PRURITUS Since pruritus is one of the major symptoms expressed in the skin (Chap. 54), it is obvious that most causes of pruritus are not related to malignant disease. Yet pruritus may be a significant symptom in up to 30 percent of patients with Hodgkin's disease. Other lymphomas are less frequently associated with pruritus, excepting mycosis fungoides, in which pruritus is almost universal. Occasionally carcinomas of the lung, stomach, colon, breast, or prostate are associated with pruritus. In such patients the pruritus usually is not limited to a small discrete area. An association with malignancy should be considered in any patient in whom pruritus cannot be explained by the finding of a metabolic cause (Chap. 54) or a local skin disease, aside from excoriations, which could explain it. Hodgkin's disease is the most likely malignancy in patients in their teens through the thirties. In the elderly, xerosis (dry skin) is common and presents a tempting explanation for pruritus. However, if decreased frequency of bathing and the use of emollients do not eliminate the pruritus, then a malignant disease must be considered. The pruritus of malignant disease will cease upon successful therapy of the malignancy.

CLUBBING This alteration of the fingers and toes may sometimes be a manifestation of tumors either arising intrathoracically or metastatic to the thorax (Chap. 260).

ERYTHRODERMA This dramatic reaction of the skin is a response to a variety of stimuli (Chap. 53). Approximately 8 percent of persons with generalized erythroderma are patients with lymphoma, particularly mycosis fungoides, or leukemia. Only occasionally is erthyroderma a manifestation of a carcinoma. In patients with erythroderma due to mycosis fungoides, atypical cells are present in the skin, and a skin biopsy will often be diagnostic. In erythroderma related to other types of lymphoma, leukemia, or carcinoma, there is not usually a definable infiltration of the skin by the atypical cells, and the diagnosis must be made from the blood smear, the bone marrow, involved lymph nodes, or other such tissue. In such cases, this erythroderma syndrome may represent an expression of a hypersensitivity reaction to tumor products. The course of the erythroderma parallels the response of the malignant disease to therapy, but it may precede the detection of the malignancy by a year or more, making repeated diagnostic investigations necessary.

NORMOLIPEMIC XANTHOMATOSIS Malignant diseases of the reticuloendothelial system have been reported in approximately one-half the reported cases of normolipemic plane xanthomatosis. Multiple myeloma is the most frequent type of associated malignant process, but several cases of lymphoma and malignant histocytosis have been reported. Lesions are yellow to yellow-brown, flat or slightly elevated plaques. There is marked variation in size, and the lesions may be sharply demarcated or may have indistinct borders. The eyelids, sides of the neck, and upper trunk are favored sites, but lesions may appear on any portion of the body. The histopathologic appearance of these xanthomas does not differ from that of clinically similar lesions not associated with malignant disease.

ERYTHEMA MULTIFORME (see Chap. 53) This skin reaction occasionally occurs days to weeks after deep radiation therapy of internal malignant disease, perhaps representing a hypersensitivity reaction to components of the tumor tissue. Erythema multiforme is also occasionally reported as an apparent manifestation of a lymphoma, leukemia, or carcinoma, in the absence of radiation therapy. The number of cases which are related to malignant disease is a very small fraction of the total number. This skin reaction tends to resolve spontaneously even in the presence of persistent malignant disease.

URTICARIA (see Chap. 53) This frequent skin reaction is an uncommon manifestation of malignant disease. A cause-effect relationship is difficult to establish unless a clear effect on the urticaria results from therapy of the associated condition. In a few patients with chronic urticaria in whom investigation disclosed a malignant disease, removal of the malignant process was associated with remission of the urticaria. Variants of urticaria present with wheal-like lesions that persist for days to months in the same site, possibly slowly changing position to form annular, arcuate, polycyclic, concentric, or other patterns. This reaction pattern is often classified under the heading of *erythema perstans.* One clinically spectacular but rare syndrome is known as *erythema gyratum repens,* in which concentric, arcuate lesions look like the grain of a soft wood. Only a few cases have been reported, but all were associated with a malignant disease, and in several the skin reaction cleared after successful treatment of the malignancy. These urticarial cutaneous vascular reactions are presumed to represent a hypersensitivity reaction to some component of the malignant disease.

BULLOUS DISEASE Blistering disorders of various types may occur as a manifestation of malignant disease. The most common type is the subepidermal bullous disease known as *bullous pemphigoid* (Chap. 53). This disorder usually occurs in the elderly and may affect any or all of the skin and mucosal surfaces. There may be an increased incidence of malignant disease in such patients, but this point is not proved. In a few cases, removal of a neoplasm was associated with remission of the dermatosis. Another bullous reaction which should cause the physician to think of the possibility of a malignant disease is *dermatitis herpetiformis.* The disease is characterized by intensely pruritic, grouped vesicles which tend to be symmetrically distributed on the extensor surfaces of the limbs and over the scalp, buttocks, and back. It is the patient over forty or fifty years of age who has a dermatitis herpetiformis–like disorder which is atypical and which does not respond well to sulfone or sulfapyridine therapy, who should be suspected of having an occult malignant process. This situation is distinctly uncommon.

DERMATOSES, BIZARRE From time to time patients present very strange skin reactions, difficult to identify, and are discovered to have a malignant process. Some of these patients appear to have a cutaneous vasculitis, but this eventually is recognized to be a lymphoma. The variety of such skin reactions is great and cannot be clearly defined. The major importance of including this category is to alert the physician to the possibility of occult malignancy in a patient who presents an unusual, atypical, or bizarre skin reaction.

HERITABLE DISORDERS WITH SKIN MANIFESTATIONS AND THE PROPENSITY TO DEVELOP INTERNAL MALIGNANCY

The role of heredity in neoplasia is interesting and complex. At times congenital immunologic deficiency states predispose to malignancy, as does acquired immune deficiency. In other cases the relationship between the hereditary condition and neoplasia is unclear. Both types are listed here to increase the awareness of the association. The list is not complete but has been selected to include the most significant syndromes. The manifestations in the skin and other organ systems, as well as the predominant type of malignancy, are presented in Table 367-2. The reader should refer to specific discussions of these entities for more complete information.

REFERENCES

BRAVERMAN IM: *Skin Signs of Systemic Disease,* Philadelphia: Saunders, 1970

BROWNSTEIN MH, HELWIG EB: Metastatic tumors of the skin. Cancer 29:1298, 1972

CROCKER AC: The histiocytosis syndromes, p. 1328, and HO Curth: Cutaneous manifestations associated with malignant internal diseases, p. 1561, in *Dermatology in General Medicine*, eds TB Fitzpatrick et al, New York: McGraw-Hill, 1971

LYNCH HT: *Skin, Hereditary, and Malignant Neoplasms*, Flushing, New York: Medical Examination Publishing Company, 1972

MULLER SA et al: Herpes simplex infections in hematologic malignancies. Am J Med 52:102, 1972

NEWBOLD PCH: Skin markers of malignancy. Arch Dermatol 102:680, 1970

APPENDIX | LABORATORY VALUES OF CLINICAL IMPORTANCE

ASCITIC FLUID
(See Table 43-1, p. 229)

BODY FLUIDS AND OTHER MASS DATA

Body fluid, total volume: 56% (in obese) to 70% (lean) of body weight
 Intracellular: 30 to 40% of body weight
 Extracellular: 23 to 25% of body weight
Blood:
 Total volume:
  Male: 69 ml/kg body weight
  Female: 65 ml/kg body weight
 Plasma volume
  Male: 39 ml/kg body weight
  Female: 40 ml/kg body weight
 Red cell volume:
  Male: 30 ml/kg body weight (1.15-1.21 L per m^2 body surface area)
  Female: 25 ml/kg body weight

$$\text{mEq/L} = \frac{\text{mg/100 ml} \times 10 \times \text{valence}}{\text{atomic weight}}$$

$$\text{mg/100 ml} = \frac{\text{mEq/L} \times \text{atomic weight}}{10 \times \text{valence}}$$

TABLE A-1
Atomic weights of elements commonly encountered in clinical medicine

Calcium	40.08	Magnesium	24.32
Carbon	12.01	Nitrogen	14.008
Chlorine	35.46	Oxygen	16.00
Copper	63.54	Phosphorus	30.98
Hydrogen	1.008	Potassium	39.100
Iodine	126.91	Sodium	22.997
Iron	55.85	Sulfur	32.07

CEREBROSPINAL FLUID

Cells: 5 per mm^3, all lymphocytes
Pressure, initial (horizontal position): 70-200 mm water
Colloidal gold test: Not more than one to two in first few tubes
Creatinine: 0.4-1.5 mg/100 ml
Glucose*: 44-100 mg/100 ml
pH*: 7.35-7.70
Protein:
 Lumbar: 14-45 mg/100 ml; gamma globulin, < 10% of total
 Cisternal: 10-20 mg/100 ml
 Ventricular: 1-15 mg/100 ml

CHEMICAL CONSTITUENTS OF BLOOD†
(See also under Function Tests, especially Metabolic and Endocrine)

Acetone, serum: 0.3-2.0 mg/100 ml
Albumin, serum: 3.5-5.5 g/100 ml
Aldolase: 0-8 IU/L
Alpha amino nitrogen, plasma: 3.0-5.5 mg/100 ml
Ammonia, whole blood, venous: 30-70 μg/100 ml
Amylase, serum (Somogyi): 60-180 units/100 ml; 0.8-3.2 IU/L
Arterial blood gases:
 HCO_3^-: 21-18 mEq/L
 P_{CO_2}: 35-45 mm Hg
 pH: 7.38-7.44
 P_{O_2}: 80-100 mm Hg
Ascorbic acid, serum: 0.4-1.0 mg/100 ml
 Leukocytes: 25-40 mg/100 ml
Barbiturates, serum: 0
 "Potentially fatal" level (Schreiner) phenobarbital: approx. 8 mg/100 ml
 Most short-acting barbiturates: 3.5 mg/100 ml
Base, total, serum: 145-155 mEq/L
Bilirubin, total, serum (Mallory-Evelyn): 0.3-1.0 mg/100 ml
 Direct, serum: 0.1-0.3 mg/100 ml
 Indirect, serum: 0.2-0.7 mg/100 ml
Bromides, serum: 0
 Toxic levels: above 17 mEq/L; 150 mg/100 ml
Bromosulphalein, BSP (5 mg/kg body weight, i.v.): 5% or less retention after 45 min
Calcium, ionized: 2.3-2.8 mEq/L; 4.5-5.6 mg/100 ml
Calcium, serum: 4.5-5.5 mEq/L; 9-11 mg/100 ml
Carbon dioxide-combining power, serum (sea level): 21-28 mEq/L; 50-65 vol%
Carbon dioxide content, plasma (at sea level): 21-30 mEq/L; 50-70 vol%
Carbon dioxide tension, arterial blood (sea level): 35-45 mm Hg
Carbon monoxide content, blood: Symptoms with over 20% saturation of hemoglobin
Carotenoids, serum: 50-300 μg/100 ml
Ceruloplasmin, serum: 27-37 mg/100 ml
Chlorides, serum (as Cl): 98-106 mEq/L
Cholesterol:
 Total, serum (Man-Peters method): 180-240 mg/100 ml
 Esters, serum: 100-180 mg/100 ml
Cholesterol ester fraction of total cholesterol, serum: 68-72%
Complement, serum, total hemolytic (CH_{50}): 200 ± 50 units/ml
Copper, serum (mean ± 1 SD): 114 ± 14 μg/100 ml
Corticosteroids, plasma (Porter-Silber) (mean ± 1 SD): 13 ± 6 μg/100 ml at 8:00 A.M.
Cortisol (competitive protein binding): 5-20 μg/100 ml at 8:00 A.M.
Creatine phosphokinase, serum:
 Female 5-25 U/ml
 Male 5-35 U/ml
Creatinine, serum: 1-1.5 mg/100 ml
Dilantin, plasma:
 Therapeutic level, 10-20 μg/ml
 Toxic level, >30 μg/ml
Ethanol, blood:
 Mild to moderate intoxication: 80-200 mg/100 ml
 Marked intoxication: 250-400 mg/100 ml
 Severe intoxication: above 400 mg/100 ml
Fatty acids, serum: 380-465 mg/100 ml
Fibrinogen, plasma: 160-415 mg/100 ml
Folic acid, serum: 6-15 ng/ml
Gastrin, serum: 40-150 pg/ml
Globulins, serum: 2.0-3.0 g/100 ml
Glucose (fasting);
 Blood (Nelson-Somogyi): 60-90 mg/100 ml
 Plasma: 75-105 mg

Since cerebrospinal fluid concentrations are equilibrium values, measurement of blood plasma obtained at the same time is recommended.
†IU = International units.

Hemoglobin, blood (sea level):
  Males: 14–18 g/100 ml
  Females: 12–16 g/100 ml
Immunoglobulins, serum:
  IgA: 90–325 mg/100 ml
  IgG: 800–1500 mg/100 ml
  IgM: 45–150 mg/100 ml
Iron, serum;
  Males and females (mean ± 1 SD): 107 ± 31 μg/100 ml
Iron-binding capacity, serum (mean ± 1SD): 305 ± 32 μg/100 ml
  Saturation: 20–45%
Ketones, total: 0.5–1.5 mg/100 ml
Lactic acid, blood: 0.6–1.8 mEq/L
Lactic dehydrogenase, serum:
  200–450 units/ml (Wrobleski)
  60–100 units/ml (Wacker)
  25–100 IU/L
Lead, serum: <20 μg/100 ml
Lipase, serum (Cherry-Crandall): 1.5 ml *N*/20 NaOH (upper limit of normal). (However, values above 1.0 should be regarded with suspicion.)
Lipids, total, serum: 500–600 mg/100 ml
Lipids, triglyceride, serum: 50–150 mg/100 ml
Magnesium, serum: 1.5–2.5 mEq/L; 2–3 mg/100 ml
Nitrogen, nonprotein, serum: 15–35 mg/100 ml
5′-Nucleotidase, serum: 0.3–2.6 Bodansky units/100 ml
Nutrients, various: See Table 75-3
Osmolality, serum: 280–300 mOsm/L
Oxygen content:
  Arterial blood (sea level): 17–21 vol %
  Venous blood, arm (sea level): 10–16 vol %
Oxygen percent saturation (sea level):
  Arterial blood: 97 vol %
  Venous blood, arm: 60–85 vol %
Oxygen tension, blood: 80–100 mm Hg
pH blood: 7.38–7.44
Phosphatase, acid, serum:
  Bessey-Lowry method: 0.10–0.63 units
  Bodansky method: 0.5–2.0 units
  Fishman-Lerner (tartrate sensitive): <0.6 unit/100 ml (up to 0.15/100 ml)
  Gutman method: 0.5–2.0 units
  International units: 0.2–1.8
  King-Armstrong method: 1.0–5.0 units
  Shinowara method: 0.0–1.1 units
Phosphatase, alkaline, serum:
  Bessey-Lowry method: 0.8–2.3 units (3.4–9)*
  Bodansky method: 2.0–4.5 units (3.0–13.0)*
  Gutman method: 3.0–10.0 units
  International units: 21–91 U/L at 37°C incubation
  King-Armstrong method: 5.0–13.0 units (10.0–20.0)*
  Shinowara method: 2.2–8.6 units
Phospholipids, serum: 150–250 mg/100 ml
Phosphorus, inorganic, serum: 1–1.5 mEq/L; 3–4.5 mg/100 ml
Potassium, serum: 3.5–5.0 mEq/L
Proteins, total, serum: 5.5–8.0 g/100 ml
Protein fractions, serum:
  Albumin 3.5–5.5 g/100 ml (50–60%)
  Globulin 2.0–3.5 g/100 ml (40–50%)
    α_1 0.2–0.4 g/100 ml (4.2–7.2%)
    α_2 0.5–0.9 g/100 ml (6.8–12%)
    β 0.6–1.1 g/100 ml (9.3–15%)
    γ 0.7–1.7 g/100 ml (13–23%)
Pyruvic acid, serum: 0–0.11 mEq/L
Salicylate, plasma: 0
  Therapeutic range: 20–25 mg/100 ml
  Toxic range: over 30 mg/100 ml
Sodium, serum: 136–145 mEq/L
Steroids: See under Function Tests: Metabolic and Endocrine
Transaminase, serum glutamic oxalacetic (SGOT): 10–40 Karmen units/ml; 6–18 IU/L
Transaminase, serum glutamic pyruvic (SGPT):
  10–40 Karmen units/ml; 3–26 IU/L
Urea nitrogen, whole blood: 10–20 mg/100 ml
Uric acid, serum: 3–7 mg/100 ml
Vitamin A, serum: 50–100 μg/100 ml
Vitamin B_{12}, serum: 200–600 pg/ml
Zinc, serum: 120 ± 20 μg/100 ml

** Values in parenthesis are those found in children.*

FUNCTION TESTS

Circulation

Cardiac output (Fick): 2.6–3.6 L/m²/min
Circulation time: Arm to lung, ether: 4–8 sec
  Arm to tongue:
    Calcium gluconate: 12–18 sec
    Decholin: 10–16 sec
    Saccharin: 9–16 sec
Ejection fraction:
  Stroke volume/end-diastolic volume (SV/EDV), normal range: 0.55–0.78; A_1: 0.67
Pressures, intracardiac and intraarterial:
  Aorta: Systole: 120 mm Hg
    Diastole: 80 mm Hg
  Atrium: Left (mean): 2–12 mm Hg
    Right (mean): 0–5 mm Hg
  Pulmonary artery: Systole: 12–28 mm Hg
    Diastole: 3–13 mm Hg
    Wedge (mean): 3–11 mm Hg
  Ventricle, left: Systole: 120 mm Hg
    Diastole: 2–12 mm Hg
  Ventricle, right: Systole: 25 mm Hg
    Diastole: 0–5 mm Hg
Venous (antecubital): 70–140 mm H_2O
Systolic time intervals (see Table A-2)

TABLE A-2
Systolic time intervals in normal individuals (in msec)

Regression equation	SD *of index*
QS_2 (M) = −2.1 HR + 546	14
QS_2 (F) = −2.0 HR + 549	14
PEP (M) = −0.4 HR + 131	13
PEP (F) = −0.4 HR + 133	11
LVET (M) = −1.7 HR + 413	10
LVET (F) = −1.6 HR + 418	10

QS_2 = total electromechanical systole, PEP = preejection phase, LVET = left ventricular ejection time. HR = heart rate, M = male, F = female, SD = standard deviation of the systolic time interval index. (From A. M. Weissler, and C. L. Garrard: Mod Concepts Cardiovasc Dis 40:1, 1971)

Gastrointestinal (See also Stool)

Absorption tests:

d-Xylose absorption test: After an overnight fast, 25 g xylose is given in aqueous solution by mouth. Urine collected for the following 5 hr should contain 5–8 g (or > 20% of ingested dose). Serum xylose should be 25–40 mg/100 ml 1 hr after the oral dose.

Vitamin A absorption test: A fasting blood specimen is obtained and 200,000 units vitamin A in oil given by mouth. Serum vitamin A levels should rise to twice fasting level in 3 to 5 hr.

Gastric juice:

Volume: 24 hr, 2–3 L; nocturnal, 600–700 ml; basal, fasting 30–70 ml/hr

Reaction: as pH, 1.6–1.8; titratable acidity of fasting juice, 15–35 mEq/hr

Acid output:

Basal: females 2.0 ± 1.8 mEq/hr
males 3.0 ± 2.0 mEq/hr

Maximal (after subcutaneous histamine acid phosphate 0.04 mg/kg, preceded by 50 mg Phenergan; or Histalog 1.7 mg/kg):
females 16 ± 5 mEq/hr
males 23 ± 5 mEq/hr

Basal acid output/maximal acid output ratio: 0.6 or less

Tubeless gastric analysis with azure A dye: acid present if more than 0.6 mg dye is excreted in urine over a 2-hr period. (CAUTION: A negative test is meaningless and requires performance of the ordinary test with a gastric tube.)

Metabolic and endocrine

Adrenal-pituitary function tests (see Chap 86)

Adrenocortical inhibition test (Liddle) (see p. 497)

Aldosterone, secretion rate: 50–250 μg/24 hr on 100 mEq sodium diet (see Table 86–1)

Corticotropin (ACTH) response tests (see p. 496–497)

Cortisol, secretion rate: 5–25 mg/24 hr

Insulin tolerance test: Blood glucose usually falls to 50% of fasting level in 20–30 min and returns to normal levels in 90–120 min after i.v. administration of 0.1 unit crystalline insulin per kg body weight

Metyrapone test (see p. 498)

Basal metabolic rate: −15% to +15% of mean standard

Catecholamines, urinary excretion (24 hr):

Free catecholamines, epinephrine and norepinephrine: 100 μg

Metanephrine, normetanephrine: 1.3 mg

VMA: 0.7–6.8 mg

Estrogens, urinary (Brown method):

Females (postpubertal, premenopausal):
Estrone: 5–20; estradiol: 2–10; estriol: 5–30 μg/24 hr

Females (postmenopausal):
Estrone: 0.3–2.4; estradiol: 0–14; estriol: 2.2–7.5 μg/24 hr

Males and prepubertal females:
Estrone: 0–5; estradiol: 0–5; estriol: 0–10 μg/24 hr

Glucose tolerance test, oral: 100 g glucose or 1.75 g glucose/kg body weight. Blood sugar not more than 160 mg/100 ml "true glucose" (Somogyi-Nelson) after $\frac{1}{2}$ hr; return to normal by 2 hr; sugar not present in any urine specimen.

Hyperparathyroidism, tests for (see p. 538–539)

Iodine, butanol extractable: 3.2–6.5 μg/100 ml

Iodine, protein bound: 4.0–8.0 μg/100 ml

Iodine, radioactive (^{131}I), uptake: Range 15–45% in 24 hr; mean 35%

Iodine, thyroxine (column method) (T_4I): 3.2–6.4 μg/100 ml

Resin T3 (Triosorb sponge): 25–35% (expressed as a ratio: 0.82–1.17)

Thyroxine (binding displacement): 4–11 μg/100 ml

TSH test (see p. 470)

Renin test (see p. 498)

Tolbutamide test, and other tests for hypoglycemia (see p. 555–557)

Plasma and urine steroids

	Plasma	Urine
17-hydroxy-corticoids	7–25 μg/100 ml (8 A.M.)	2–10 mg/24 hr (Porter-Silber) 5–23 mg/24 hr (ketogenic)
17-ketosteroids		7–25 mg/24 hr (male) 4–15 mg/24 hr (female)
Testosterone	0.37–1.0 μg/100 ml (male) 0–0.1 μg/100 ml (female)	47–156 μg/24 hr (male) 0–15 μg/24 hr (female)
Aldosterone	0.015 μg/100 ml	2–10 μg/24 hr

T_3 suppression test (Werner): Measure ^{131}I neck uptake before and after 1 week of T_3 75 units/day p.o. ^{131}I uptake should go below 20% in 24 hr.

Triiodothyronine uptake, erythrocyte (RBC-T_3): 11.0–17.0% (female); 11.8–19.0% (male)

T_3 concentration (radioimmunoassay): 96–172 ng/100 ml

Pancreatic islet cell function tests (see pp. 559–560)

Water loading test (Soffer): More than 50% excretion of a 1,500-ml water load in 5 hr

Metanephrine urinary excretion: Up to 1 mg/24 hr volume

Pulmonary

TABLE A-3
Specific airway conductance and resistance, normal values in adults

	SGAW (sec^{-1} cm H_2O^{-1})	*SRAW* (sec cm H_2O)
Male		
NS	0.24	4.1
S	0.23	4.3
Female		
NS	0.22	4.5
S	0.16	5.0

SGAW = specific airway conductance = airway conductance per unit lung volume
SRAW = specific airway resistance = 1/SGAW
NS = nonsmoker
S = smoker

TABLE A-4
Lung volumes for seated subjects of average size, range of normal values

Age	Men	Women
Vital capacity, in liters		
20-39	3.35-5.90	2.45-4.38
40-59	2.72-5.30	2.09-4.02
60	2.42-4.70	1.91-3.66
Residual volume, in liters		
20-39	1.13-2.32	1.00-2.00
40-59	1.45-2.62	1.16-2.20
60	1.77-2.77	1.32-2.40
Total lung capacity, in liters		
20-39	4.80-7.92	3.61-6.18
40-59	4.50-7.62	3.41-6.02
60	4.35-7.32	3.31-5.86
Residual volume/total lung capacity × 100		
20-39	20-30	26-33
40-59	30-39	32-39
60	35-44	38-42

Note: First value in each column is for shorter individual. Height: men, 62-72 in. (157-183 cm); women, 56-70 in. (142-178 cm).

TABLE A-5
Normal spirometric values for seated subjects

Age	Men	Women
Forced expiratory volume in 1 sec (FEV_1), L		
20-39	3.11-4.64	2.16-3.65
40-59	2.45-3.98	1.60-3.09
60-70	2.09-3.32	1.30-2.53
FEV_1/vital capacity (FEV%)		
20-39	77	82
40-59	70	77
60-70	66	74
Maximal midexpiratory flow ($MMEF_{25-75\%}$) L/sec		
20-39	3.8	3.4
40-59	2.8	2.2
60-70	2.2	1.6

Arterial blood gas measurements in normal subjects:
P_{CO_2} in mm Hg: 38 (± 2.9 SD) seated; no change with age
P_{O_2} in mm Hg: seated, 104.2 − 0.27 × age in years; supine, 103.5 − 0.42 × age in years

TABLE A-6
Prediction formulas* for lung volumes and spirometric tests in seated subjects

	Age, to nearest year (A)	Height, m (H)	Weight, kg (W)	Constant (G)	Residual standard deviation (RSD)
Men					
TLC, L		+6.92	−0.017	−4.30	0.67
VC, L	−0.020	+4.81		−2.81	0.50
FRC, L	+0.015	+5.30	−0.037	−3.89	0.56
FRC/TLC, %	+0.18		−0.12	+52.3	6.8
FEV_1, L	−0.033	+3.44		−1.00	0.50
FEV%	−0.37			+91.8	7.2
$MMEF_{25-75\%}$	−0.0523			+5.85	1.00
Women					
TLC, L	−0.015	+6.71		−5.77	0.48
VC, L	−0.022	+4.04		−2.35	0.40
FRC, L		+5.13	−.028	−4.50	0.41
FRC/TLC, %	+0.16		−0.08	+45.2	4.7
FEV_1, L	−0.028	+2.67		−0.54	0.36
FEV%,	−0.26			+92.1	5.4
$MMEF_{25-75\%}$	−0.0579			+5.63	0.71

**Answer* = (*A* × *age*) + (*H* × *height*) + (*W* × *weight*) + *C* ± 2 *RSD Example: The normal value and lower limit for the* FEV_1 *are sought in a man, age forty years, height 1.77 m, and weight 76 kg. The following equation gives the normal value:*
$FEV_1 = (-0.033 \times 40) + (3.44 \times 1.77) + (-1.00) = 3.77$ *liters*
The lower limit of normal: 3.77 − 2 × 0.50 = 2.77 liters
Only 2.5% of a normal population will fall below this value (2 SD below the mean).
Key: FRC, functional residual capacity; FEV_1, *forced expiratory volume in 1 sec; FEV%,* FEV_1 *expressed as percent of nonforced expiratory VC;* $MMEF_{25-75\%}$ *mean flow rate during the middle half of the forced expiratory vital capacity.*
SOURCE: *Birath et al, Acta Med Scand 173:193, 1963; Grimby and Soderholm, Acta Med Scand 173:199, 1963*

Renal

Clearances (corrected to 1.73 m² body surface area):
- Measures of glomerular filtration rate:
  - Inulin clearance (C_I):
    - Males: 124 ± 25.8 ml/min
    - Females: 119 ± 12.8 ml/min
  - Endogenous creatinine: 91-130 ml/min
  - Urea: 60-100 ml/min
- Measures of effective renal plasma flow and tubular function:
  - Para-aminohippuric acid (C_{PAH}):
    - Males: 654 ± 163 ml/min
    - Females: 594 ± 102 ml/min
  - Tubular maximum for *PAH*, males and females: 77.2 mg/min
  - Diodrast: 600-800 ml/min; 20-30% excretion in 15 min

Concentration and dilution test:
- Specific gravity of urine:
  - After 12 hr fluid restriction: 1.025 or more
  - After 12 hr deliberate water intake: 1.003 or less

Phenolsulfonphthalein:
- After intravenous injection:
  - Excretion in urine in 15 min: 25% or more
  - Excretion in urine in 2 hr: 55-75%
- After intramuscular injection:
  - Excretion in urine in 2 hr: 55-75%

Protein excretion, urine
Males, 0–60 mg/24 hr
Females, 0–90 mg/24 hr
Specific gravity, maximal: 1.002–1.028
Tubular reabsorption phosphorus:
79–94% of filtered load

HEMATOLOGIC EXAMINATIONS
(See also Chemical Constituents of Blood)

Bone marrow
(See Table 58–5, p. 299)

Erythrocytes and hemoglobin
(See also Table A–7)

Carboxyhemoglobin:
Nonsmoker: 0–23%
Smoker: 2.1–4.2%
Fragility, osmotic:
Slight hemolysis: 0.45–0.39%
Complete hemolysis: 0.33–0.30%
Haptoglobin, serum: 128 ± 25 mg/100 ml
Hemochromogens plasma: 3–5 mg/100 ml
Hemoglobin, fetal: <2% of fetal
"Life span":
Normal survival: 120 days
Chromium, half-life ($T\frac{1}{2}$): 28 days
Methemoglobin: Up to 1.7% of total
Plasma iron turnover rate: 20–42 mg/24 hr (0.47 mg/kg)
Protoporphyrin, free erythrocyte (E.P.):
16–36 μg/100 ml RBCs
Reticulocytes: 0.5–2.0% of red cells
Sedimentation rate:
Westergren: <15 mm/1 hr
Wintrobe: Male: 0–9 mm/1 hr
Female: 0–20 mm/1 hr

Leukocytes

TABLE A–8
Normal values

	Percent	*Average*	*Minimum*	*Maximum*
Total number, per mm³		7,000	4,300	10,000
Neutrophils:				
Juvenile and band	0–21	520	100	2,100
Segmented	25–62	3,000	1,100	6,050
Eosinophils	3–8	150	0	700
Basophils	0.6–1.8	30	0	150
Lymphocytes	20–53	2,500	1,500	4,000
Monocytes	2.4–11.8	430	200	950

Platelets and coagulation

Bleeding time (Ivy method, 5-mm wound) 1–9 min; Duke method, 1–4 min
Clot retraction:
Qualitative: Apparent in 60 min, complete in <24 hr, usually <6 hr
Coagulation time (Lee-White):
Majority and range (glass tubes): 9–15 min, 2–19 min
Majority and range (siliconized tubes): both 20–60 min
Whole clot lysis: >24 hr
Prothrombin time (Quick one stage): Comparable to normal control (with most thromboplastins, 11–16 sec)
Partial thromboplastin time (P.T.T.) (Nye-Brinkhous method): Comparable to normal control. With standard technique, 68–82 sec; activated, 32–46 sec
Plasma thrombin time: 13–17 sec
Platelets, per mm³, Brecher-Cronkite method: 290,000 (140,000–440,000)

TABLE A–7
Normal values at various ages

Age	*Red cell count, millions/mm³*	*Hemoglobin, g/100 ml*	*Vol. packed RBC, ml/100 ml*	*Corpuscular values** *MCV, fl*	*MCH, pg*	*MCHC, g/100 ml*	*MCD, μm*
Days 1–13	5.1 ± 1.0†	19.5 ± 5.0†	54.0 ± 10.0†	106–98	38–33	36–34	8.6
Days 14–60	4.7 ± 0.9	14.0 ± 3.3	42.0 ± 7.0	90	30	33	8.1
3 mon–10 yr	4.5 ± 0.7	12.2 ± 2.3	36.0 ± 5.0	80	27	34	7.7
11–15 yr	4.8	13.4	39.0	82	28	34	
Adults:							
Females	4.8 ± 0.6	14.0 ± 2.0	42.0 ± 5.0	90 ± 7	29 ± 2	34 ± 2	7.5 ± 0.3
Males	5.4 ± 0.9	16.0 ± 2.0	47.0 ± 5.0	90 ± 7	29 ± 2	34 ± 2	7.5 ± 0.3

Note: MCV = mean corpuscular volume. MCH = mean corpuscular hemoglobin. MCHC = mean corpuscular hemoglobin concentration. MCD = mean corpuscular diameter.
(Wintrobe et al: Clinical Hematology, *7th ed., Philadelphia, Lea & Febiger, 1974)*
**fl = cu μ; pg = μμg*
†The range of values represents almost the extremes of observed variations (93 percent or more) at sea level. The blood values of healthy persons should fall well within these figures.

Schilling test

Excretion in urine of orally administered radioactive vitamin B_{12} following "flushing" parenteral injection of B_{12}: 7–40%

STOOL

Bulk:
- Wet weight: <197.5 g/day (mean 115 ± 41)
- Dry weight: <66.4 g/day (mean 34 ± 16)

Fat, on diet containing at least 50 g fat: <7.0 g/day when measured on a 3-day (or longer) collection (mean 4.0 ± 1.5)
- As percent of dry weight: <30.4 (mean 13.3 ± 8.07)
- Coefficient of fat absorption: >93%

Fatty acid:
- Free: 1–10% of dry matter
- Combined as soap: 0.5–12% of dry matter

Nitrogen: <1.7 g/day (mean 1.4 ± 0.2)
Protein content: Minimal
Water: Approximately 65%
Urobilinogen: 40–280 mg/24 hr
Coproporphyrin: 400–1,000 μg/24 hr

URINE
(See also Function Tests: Metabolic and Endocrine)

Acidity, titratable: 125–150 mEq/24 hr
α-Amino nitrogen: 0.4–1.0 g/24 hr
Ammonia: 30–50 mEq/24 hr
Amylase (Somogyi): 35–260 units/hr
Calcium, 10 mEq or 200 mg calcium diet:
<7.5 mEq/24 hr or <150 mg/24 hr
Catecholamines: Less than 100 μg/24 hr
Copper: 0–25 μg/24 hr
Coproporphyrins (types I and III): 100–300 μg/24 hr
Creatine, as creatinine:
- Adult males: <50 mg/24 hr
- Adult females: <100 mg/24 hr

Creatinine: 1.0–1.6 g/24 hr
D-Xylose excretion: 5–8 g/5 hr after oral dose of 25 g
Glucose, true (oxidase method): 50–300 mg/24 hr
5-Hydroxyindoleacetic acid (5HIAA) 2–9 mg/24 hr
Ketones, total (mean ± 1 SD): 50.5 ± 30.7 mg/24 hr
Lactic dehydrogenase: 560–2,050 units/8 hr urine
Lead: <0.08 μg/ml or mercury < 120 μg/24 hr
Protein: <50 mg/24 hr
Porphobilinogen: 0 μg/24 hr
Potassium: 25–100 mEq/24 hr (varies with intake)
Sodium: 100–260 mEq/24 hr (varies with sodium intake)
Urobilinogen: 1–3.5 mg/24 hr
Vanillylmandelic acid (VMA): 0.7–6.8 mg/24 hr

Index

Boldface page numbers refer to the principal discussion of a subject. Under a general category the subentries for specific conditions may refer to the principal discussion only, and more information will be found under the name of the condition. See muscle diseases and muscular dystrophy.